Fifteenth Edition

CECIL

Textbook of Medicine

Edited by

PAUL B. BEESON, M.D.

Distinguished Physician, United States Veterans Administration,
Professor of Medicine, University of Washington School of Medicine

WALSH McDERMOTT, M.D.

Emeritus Professor of Public Health and Medicine, Cornell University
Medical College; Special Advisor to the President, Robert Wood Johnson Foundation

JAMES B. WYNGAARDEN, M.D.

Frederic M. Hanes Professor and Chairman,
Department of Medicine, Duke University Medical Center

W. B. SAUNDERS COMPANY · Philadelphia · London · Toronto

W. B. Saunders Company: West Washington Square
                           Philadelphia, PA   19105

                           1 St. Anne's Road
                           Eastbourne, East Sussex BN21 3UN, England

                           1 Goldthorne Avenue
                           Toronto, Ontario M8Z 5T9, Canada

Listed here are the latest translated editions of this book, together
with the language of the translation and the publisher.

Portuguese (14th Edition)—Editora Interamericana Ltda., Rio de Janeiro, Brazil

Serbo-Croat (11th Edition)—Medicinska Knjiga, Belgrade, Yugoslavia

Spanish (14th Edition)—Nueva Editorial Interamericana S.A. de C.V., Mexico

                                          Single Vol: ISBN 0-7216-1663-1
                                              Vol I: ISBN 0-7216-1664-X
                                             Vol II: ISBN 0-7216-1666-6
Textbook of Medicine   Set: ISBN 0-7216-1667-4

Last digit is the print number: 9   8   7   6   5   4   3

What is a textbook? It is a putting-together of discrete pieces of information into a cohesive, meaningful pattern. In the weaving of the pattern, the editors of this Fifteenth Edition of the *Textbook of Medicine* have been mindful, as in the previous editions, of the original purposes of Russell Cecil and Robert Loeb to provide authoritative clinical guidance and a reasoned, scientific basis for the pursuit of medicine. The two ideas are complementary, for an understanding of the mechanisms of disease and its manifestations enables the physician to select appropriate diagnostic procedures and therapy. This guiding principle is underscored by introducing each major section with an overview of pathophysiology and the principles of approach to the clinical problem.

The period of time covered by the editions of this textbook extends from 1927, soon after the epochal discoveries of insulin for diabetes and the liver treatment of pernicious anemia, through an era of unprecedented productivity in biomedical research and clinical investigation; hence each succeeding edition has required substantial revision to keep pace with emerging knowledge and technology. The first edition came to about 800,000 words and had 130 contributors. The present edition runs well over 2,000,000 words and has 237 contributors. The number of individual clinical entities and syndromes has grown from about 550 in the first edition to an almost uncountable number in the current edition. For example, the subject of intestinal malabsorption, of which 41 forms are now described, was dealt with only under the term "tropical sprue" in 1927. Sickle cell anemia was given a nine-line paragraph in the first edition; there are now five chapters dealing with disorders associated with 180 different hemoglobins. The diagnostic procedures available in 1927 were relatively simple and crude (blood sugar, blood urea nitrogen, x-ray, and the use of rigid endoscopes). Modern diagnostic capabilities are, by comparison, immensely refined, including such precise aids as angiography, ultrasound, and computerized tomography, together with many new chemical determinations, some so delicate that they can measure hormone concentrations in picogram quantities.

Our therapeutic capabilities have similarly expanded. In 1927 two favorite drugs, arsenic (Fowler's solution) and potassium iodide, were each recommended for 30 to 40 different diseases. The current edition discusses the use of scores of effective and well-tested compounds, along with such high technologies as renal dialysis, parenteral nutrition, platelet transfusion, assisted respiration, and cardiac pacemakers. Surgery of the heart has revolutionized the practice of cardiology, and the replacement of joints has gained an established place in the field of rheumatology.

The flow of new ideas and new procedures continues, as reflected in this new edition. Several major Parts have been completely revised and rewritten: Respiratory Disease, Cardiovascular Diseases, Renal Diseases, Diseases of Bone, and Certain Cutaneous Diseases with Significant Systemic Manifestations. Indeed, all continuing chapters have been revised to a greater or lesser extent to fit today's situation.

Several new Parts have been added. First is one on Human Growth and Development. The remarkable lengthening in average life span that is taking place in this century calls for greater textbook emphasis on the changes that occur over time in the structure and function of the human body. Inasmuch as older patients make disproportionate demands on health services, it can be predicted that when our present medical students and house officers reach mid-career, about half their work will be in the care of people over the age of 65 years.

Another new Part—Critical Care Medicine—has been made necessary by advances both in the understanding and in the technology of supportive measures for failing respiratory, cardiac, or renal function. Coronary care units and medical intensive care units are now commonplace in general hospitals, and the specialty of critical care medicine has emerged. Inevitably, some of the matters discussed in this Part must also be mentioned in other chapters; nevertheless, it seemed desirable to bring together a general discussion of the principles of this kind of treatment in a separate Part.

Oncology is now a formal subspecialty of internal medicine, with a rapidly expanding body of knowledge from research and from clinical experience. The editors felt it appropriate, therefore, to consolidate chapters on cancer into a new Part, to give the user easier access to information, and to underscore the importance of the subject in clinical practice.

Ocular manifestations accompany many systemic diseases, and it was decided that this edition should include a Part dealing with those aspects of ophthalmology that should be part of the working knowledge of the internist or primary care physician. Special emphasis is laid on the funduscopic changes that may provide clues to the existence or progress of such conditions as lupus erythematosus, leukemia, hypertension, and hereditary disorders.

Another new Part deals with the subject of Drug-Drug Interactions. Although the detail of this subject is immense, the editors believe that certain principles which underlie such interactions can be illustrated in examples and that they would be helpful to users of the book.

Diagnostic techniques have undergone remarkable changes since the last edition; consequently much more emphasis is given to use of such procedures as fiberscopic endoscopy, ultrasound, computerized tomography, Doppler studies, nuclear imaging, and selective angiography.

This body of information is now so vast that the place

of importance of each individual piece cannot be finally judged solely by the editors; they must have expert help. For Disorders of the Nervous System and Behavior there is a separate editor, Fred Plum. In addition, nine physicians widely recognized as expert authorities in particular branches of medicine have served as Consulting Editors: Alexander Bearn (Medical Genetics), Nicholas Christy (Diseases of the Endocrine System), Philip Marsden (Protozoan and Helminthic Diseases), John Murray (Respiratory Disease), Ralph Nachman (Hematologic and Hematopoietic Diseases), Roscoe Robinson (Renal Diseases), Marvin Sleisenger (Diseases of the Digestive System), Andrew Wallace (Cardiovascular Diseases), and Sheldon Wolff (Microbial Diseases). A book is ideas made visible. This process could not have been accomplished without these consulting editors and the contributors. We are greatly indebted to them all for their selfless help.

In order to assist our users to cope with the increasing need for continuing medical education and recertification, a companion book is in preparation, to be used in self-assessment study. Its questions and answers are being devised by members of the Departments of Medicine at Duke University and the University of California, San Francisco.

To have attempted to put the essence of contemporary medicine within the covers of this textbook is an exciting and demanding adventure in which the three of us have joined as Co-Editors. For Beeson and McDermott this edition will be the last, and Wyngaarden will be joined by Lloyd H. Smith, Jr., as Co-Editor of the next edition. This change is in keeping with the book's history of orderly transition.

We cannot close without expressing our pleasure in the friendship and invaluable advice of Jack Hanley, Vice President and General Manager for Health Sciences of the W. B. Saunders Company. We wish also to thank the many other able and devoted people in the Company from whom we have learned so much. It is a special pleasure to acknowledge with gratitude the skill and untiring efforts of Dave Kilmer, Special Projects Editor at Saunders, who has so ably helped us to bring together this large assemblage of writings. Finally, we must acknowledge special indebtedness to Helen Miller, who has now been with the book for five editions, and to Patsey Sutphin, for whom this edition has been the first. Together these editorial assistants have done a splendid job not only in faultlessly handling hundreds of manuscripts and proofs, but in providing the linkage that binds contributors, publisher, consulting editors, and ourselves to the facts and ideals of medicine. Their help deserves, and has, our deepest thanks.

PAUL B. BEESON
WALSH McDERMOTT
JAMES B. WYNGAARDEN

DOSAGE NOTICE

Extraordinary efforts have been made by the authors, the editors, and the publisher of this book to ensure that dosage recommendations are precise and in agreement with the highest standards of practice.

It does happen, however, that dosage schedules are changed from time to time in the light of accumulating clinical experience and continuing laboratory studies. This is most likely to occur in the case of recently introduced products.

It is urged, therefore, that you check the package information data for the manufacturer's recommended dosage. In addition, there are some quite serious situations, each encountered only rarely, in which drug therapy must be individualized and expert judgment advises the use of a higher dosage or administration by a different route than is included in the manufacturer's recommendations. Throughout the text many such instances are indicated by a footnote.

THE EDITORS

CONTRIBUTORS

FRANCOIS M. ABBOUD, M.D.

Shock

Professor of Medicine and Physiology; Head, Department of Medicine; and Director, Cardiovascular Center, College of Medicine, University of Iowa. Chief of Medicine, University Hospitals, Iowa City, Iowa.

ALBERT J. AGUAYO, M.D., F.R.C.P.(C.)

Mechanical Lesions of the Nerve Roots and Spinal Cord

Professor of Neurology and Neurosurgery, McGill University. Senior Physician, The Montreal General Hospital, Montreal, Quebec, Canada.

CURTIS P. ARTZ, M.D.

Electric Shock and Electric Injury

Late Distinguished University Professor and Chairman, Department of Surgery, Medical University of South Carolina. Late Chief of Surgery, Medical University Hospital, Charleston, South Carolina.

G. D. AURBACH, M.D.

Parathyroid

Chief, Metabolic Diseases Branch, National Institute of Arthritis, Metabolism, and Digestive Diseases, National Institutes of Health, Bethesda, Maryland.

K. FRANK AUSTEN, M.D.

Connective Tissue Diseases ("Collagen Diseases") Other Than Rheumatoid Arthritis: Introduction; Periarteritis Nodosa

Theodore B. Bayles Professor of Medicine, Harvard Medical School. Physician-in-Chief, Robert B. Brigham Hospital, Boston, Massachusetts.

LOUIS V. AVIOLI, M.D.

Diseases of Bone

Shoenberg Professor of Medicine, Washington University School of Medicine. Chief of Endocrinology, The Jewish Hospital of St. Louis; Attending Physician, Barnes Hospital, Jewish Hospital, and St. Louis Children's Hospital; Director, Division of Bone and Mineral Metabolism, and Director, Metabolic Bone Unit, Shriner's Hospital, St. Louis, Missouri.

ROBERT W. BALOH, M.D.

Hearing Loss

Associate Professor of Neurology, Reed Neurologic Research Center, UCLA School of Medicine. Director, Neurotology Clinic, UCLA Center for the Health Sciences, Los Angeles, California.

J. RICHARD BARINGER, M.D.

Herpes Simplex Encephalitis

Professor of Neurology and Pathology, Vice-Chairman, Department of Neurology, University of California, San Francisco. Chief, Neurology Service, Veterans Administration Hospital, San Francisco, California.

ALEXANDER G. BEARN, M.D.

Heredity; Genetic Principles: Introduction; Pedigree Analysis in Inherited Disease; Inborn Errors of Metabolism and Molecular Disease; Polygenic and Multifactorial Inheritance; Pharmacogenetics; Population Genetics; Congenital Malformations; Prevention and Management of Genetic Disease; Albinism; Wilson's Disease; The Mucopolysaccharidoses; Marfan's Syndrome; Acatalasia; Familial Dysautonomia; Laurence-Moon Syndrome; Lipoatrophic Diabetes; Lipoid Proteinosis; Werner's Syndrome

Stanton Griffis Distinguished Medical Professor and Professor of Medicine, Cornell University Medical College. Attending Physician, The New York Hospital, New York, New York.

MARGARET R. BECKLAKE, M.D., F.R.C.P.

Physical and Chemical Irritants

Professor, Department of Medicine and Department of Epidemiology and Health, McGill University. Associate of the Medical Research Council of Canada. Senior Physician, Royal Victoria Hospital, Montreal, Quebec, Canada.

PAUL B. BEESON, M.D.

On Becoming a Clinician; Granulomatous Diseases of Unproved Etiology: Introduction; Polymyalgia Rheumatica and Cranial Arteritis; Relapsing Polychondritis; Weber-Christian Disease; Fibrosing Syndromes; Eosinophilic Syndromes; Epidemic Neuromyasthenia

Distinguished Physician, United States Veterans Administration; Professor of Medicine, University of Washington, Seattle, Washington.

VICTOR S. BEHAR, M.D.

Diseases of the Myocardium: Introduction; Asymmetric Septal Hypertrophy; Familial Cardiomyopathy; Inflammatory or Infective Cardiomyopathy; Nutritional Cardiomyopathy; Cardiac Amyloidosis; Other Cardiomyopathies

Associate Professor of Medicine and Associate Director, Cardiovascular Laboratory, Duke University Medical Center, Durham, North Carolina.

JOHN E. BENNETT, M.D.

Nocardiosis; Cryptococcosis; Mucormycosis; Aspergillosis; Candidiasis

Head, Clinical Mycology Section, Laboratory of Clinical Investigation, National Institute of Allergy and Infectious Disease, Bethesda, Maryland.

ROBERT N. BERK, M.D.

Diagnostic Imaging Procedures in Gastroenterology

Professor and Chairman, Department of Radiology, University of California, San Diego School of Medicine, La Jolla. Director, Department of Radiology, University Hospital, San Diego, California.

ERNEST BEUTLER, M.D.

Galactosemia

Chairman, Department of Clinical Research, and Member, Scripps Clinic and Research Foundation, La Jolla, California.

EDWIN L. BIERMAN, M.D.

Obesity

Professor of Medicine and Head, Division of Metabolism and Endocrinology, University of Washington School of Medicine. Attending Physician, University of Washington Affiliated Hospitals, Seattle, Washington.

IRA B. BLACK, M.D.

Idiopathic Autonomic Insufficiency

Associate Professor of Neurology, Cornell University Medical College. Associate Attending Neurologist, New York Hospital, New York, New York.

LEO F. BLACK, M.D.

Cysts and Neoplasms of the Lung

Associate Professor of Medicine, Mayo Medical School. Consultant, Division of Thoracic Diseases and Internal Medicine, Mayo Clinic, Rochester, Minnesota.

DANE R. BOGGS, M.D.

The Leukopenic State

Professor of Medicine, and Chief, Division of Hematology-Oncology, University of Pittsburgh School of Medicine, Pittsburgh, Pennsylvania.

PHILIP K. BONDY, M.D.

Medical Treatment of Hormone-Dependent Cancers

Professor of Medicine, Yale University School of Medicine. Associate Chief of Staff for Research, West Haven Veterans Administration Hospital; Attending, Yale–New Haven Hospital, New Haven, Connecticut.

THOMAS H. BOTHWELL, M.D., D.Sc., F.R.C.P., F.A.C.P.(Hon.)

Hemochromatosis

Professor of Medicine, University of the Witwatersrand Medical School. Chief Physician, Johannesburg Hospital, Johannesburg, South Africa.

M. C. BRAIN, D.M., F.R.C.P., F.R.C.P.(C.)

The Anemias: Introduction; Aplastic Anemia; Sideroblastic Anemia; Myelophthisic Anemia

Professor of Medicine, McMaster University. Physician, McMaster University Medical Centre and Hamilton Civic Hospitals, Hamilton, Ontario, Canada.

LLOYD L. BRANDBORG, M.D.

Neoplastic Diseases of the Alimentary Tract: Introduction; Neoplasms of the Esophagus; Malignant Neoplasms of the Stomach; Benign Neoplasms of the Stomach

Clinical Professor of Medicine, University of California, San Francisco. Chief, Gastroenterology Section, Veterans Administration Hospital, San Francisco; Consultant, Letterman Army Medical Center, U.S. Public Health Service Hospital, San Francisco, Oakland Naval Hospital, Oakland, and David Grant Air Force Medical Center, Travis Air Force Base, California.

BARRY M. BRENNER, M.D.

Structure and Function of the Kidneys

Samuel A. Levine Professor of Medicine, Harvard Medical School. Director, Renal Division, and Physician, Peter Bent Brigham Hospital, Boston; Consultant, Veterans Administration Hospital, West Roxbury, Massachusetts.

RUBIN BRESSLER, M.D.

Drug-Drug Interactions

Professor and Head, Internal Medicine, Professor of Pharmacology, and Chief, Clinical Pharmacology, Department of Internal Medicine, University of Arizona Medical Center, Tucson, Arizona.

NEAL S. BRICKER, M.D.

The Pathophysiology of Chronic Renal Disease; Acute Renal Failure

Professor of Medicine, School of Medicine, University of California, Los Angeles. Attending Nephrologist, UCLA Hospital and Clinics, Los Angeles, California.

FRANK P. BROOKS, M.D., Sc.D.(Med.)

Diseases of the Pancreas

Professor of Medicine and Physiology, School of Medicine, University of Pennsylvania. Member, Gastrointestinal Section, Hospital of the University of Pennsylvania, Philadelphia, Pennsylvania.

ELMER B. BROWN, M.D.

Acute Hemorrhagic Anemia; Anemia Associated with Infection and Chronic Systemic Diseases; Hypochromic Anemias

Professor of Medicine and Associate Dean for Continuing Medical Education, Washington University School of Medicine. Associate Physician, Barnes Hospital, St. Louis, Missouri.

ANTHONY D. M. BRYCESON, M.D., F.R.C.P.E., D.T.M. & H.

Relapsing Fever; Tropical Phagedenic Ulcer; Leishmaniasis

Senior Lecturer, London School of Hygiene and Tropical Medicine. Consultant Physician, Hospital for Tropical Diseases, London, England.

THOMAS M. BUCHANAN, M.D.

Brucellosis

Associate Professor of Medicine, University of Washington. Head, Immunology Research Laboratory, U.S. Public Health Service Hospital, Seattle; Attending Physician in Medicine and Infectious Diseases, U.S. Public Health Service Hospital, Harborview Medical Center, and Fred Hutchison Cancer Research Center, Seattle, Washington.

BENJAMIN BURROWS, M.D.

Diseases Associated with Airways Obstruction; Abnormalities of Lung Aeration

Professor of Internal Medicine, University of Arizona College of Medicine. Director, Division of Respiratory Sciences, and Staff Physician, Arizona Health Sciences Center, Tucson, Arizona.

GEORGE F. CAHILL, Jr., M.D.

Diabetes Mellitus

Director of Research, Howard Hughes Medical Institute; Professor of Medicine, Harvard Medical School. Physician, Peter Bent Brigham Hospital, Boston, Massachusetts.

PAUL CALABRESI, M.D.

Principles of Oncologic Treatment: Irradiation, Cytotoxic Drugs, and Immunostimulatory Procedures

Professor of Internal Medicine, Brown University. Chief of Medicine, Roger Williams General Hospital, Providence, Rhode Island.

PAUL P. CARBONE, M.D.

Lymphoreticular Neoplasms: Introduction; Burkitt's Lymphoma

Professor and Chairman, Department of Human Oncology, Professor of Medicine, University of Wisconsin. Attending, University Hospitals and Middleton Veterans Administration Hospital, Madison, Wisconsin.

CHARLES C. J. CARPENTER, M.D.

Shigellosis; Cholera

Professor and Chairman, Department of Medicine, Case Western Reserve University. Physician-in-Chief, University Hospitals of Cleveland, Ohio.

HUGH CHAPLIN, Jr., M.D.

Hemoglobinuria; Transfusion Reactions

Professor of Medicine and Preventive Medicine, Washington University School of Medicine. Associate Physician, Barnes Hospital, St. Louis, Missouri.

CHARLES L. CHRISTIAN, M.D.

Diseases of the Joints

Professor of Medicine, Cornell University Medical College. Physician-in-Chief, Hospital for Special Surgery; Attending Physician, The New York Hospital, New York, New York.

NICHOLAS P. CHRISTY, M.D.

Endocrine Syndromes Associated with Cancer; Diseases of the Endocrine System: Introduction; The Anterior Pituitary

Professor of Medicine, College of Physicians and Surgeons, Columbia University. Director of Medical Service, Roosevelt Hospital; Attending Physician, Presbyterian Hospital, New York, New York.

LEIGHTON E. CLUFF, M.D.

Diseases Caused by Malleomyces; Anthrax; Listeriosis; Erysipeloid of Rosenbach

Adjunct Professor of Medicine, University of Pennsylvania School of Medicine, Philadelphia. Vice-President, Robert Wood Johnson Foundation, Princeton, New Jersey.

JAY D. COFFMAN, M.D.

Diseases of the Peripheral Vessels

Professor of Medicine, Boston University School of Medicine. Section Head, Peripheral Vascular Section, and Visiting Physician, University Hospital, Boston, Massachusetts.

C. LOCKARD CONLEY, M.D.

Hemoglobin, the Hemoglobinopathies, and the Thalassemias

Distinguished Service Professor of Medicine, Head of the Hematology Division, Department of Medicine, The Johns Hopkins University School of Medicine. Physician, The Johns Hopkins Hospital, Baltimore, Maryland.

ROBERT B. COUCH, M.D.

Mycoplasmal Diseases

Professor of Microbiology and Immunology and Medicine, Baylor College of Medicine. Attending Physician, Baylor Affiliated Hospitals: Ben Taub General Hospital, Veterans Administration Hospital, and The Methodist Hospital, Houston, Texas.

ANTHONY N. DAMATO, M.D.

Cardiac Arrhythmia

Chief, Medical Department, U.S. Public Health Service Hospital, Staten Island, New York.

JEFFERSON C. DAVIS, M.D., M.P.H.

Alterations in Atmospheric Pressure

Chief, Hyperbaric Medicine, U.S. Air Force School of Aerospace Medicine; Clinical Assistant Professor, Anesthesiology, University of Texas Health Science Center, at San Antonio; Visiting Scientist, Department of Biology, Texas A & M University.

THOMAS E. DAVIS, M.D.

Non-Hodgkin's Lymphomas

Assistant Professor of Human Oncology and Medicine, University of Wisconsin School of Medicine. Attending Physician, University Hospitals, Madison, Wisconsin.

LESLIE J. DeGROOT, M.D.

The Thyroid

Professor of Medicine, University of Chicago, Pritzker School of Medicine. Head of Endocrine Section, Billings Hospital, University of Chicago, Chicago, Illinois.

ROGER M. DES PREZ, M.D.

Tuberculosis; Extrapulmonary Tuberculosis

Professor of Medicine, Vanderbilt University Medical School. Chief, Medical Service, Veterans Administration Hospital, Nashville, Tennessee.

BERTRAM D. DINMAN, M.D., Sc.D.

Carbon Monoxide Poisoning

Adjunct Professor, Occupational Health, Graduate School of Public Health, University of Pittsburgh. Vice President, Health and Safety, Aluminum Company of America, Pittsburgh, Pennsylvania.

PHILIP R. DODGE, M.D.

Infections and Inflammatory Diseases of the Central Nervous System and Its Coverings: Introduction; Aids to Diagnosis in Intracranial and Intraspinal Inflammatory Disease; Spinal Epidural Infections; Transverse Myelitis or Myelopathy; Syphilitic Infections of the Nervous System

Professor of Pediatrics and of Neurology, Head of the Edward Mallinckrodt Department of Pediatrics, Washington University School of Medicine. Medical Director, St. Louis Children's Hospital; Pediatrician-in-Chief and Neurologist, Barnes and Affiliated Hospitals, St. Louis, Missouri.

RAPHAEL DOLIN, M.D.

Viral Gastroenteritis Caused by Norwalk-Like Agents and Rotaviruses

Head, Medical Virology Section, National Institute of Allergy and Infectious Diseases, National Institutes of Health, Bethesda, Maryland. Associate Professor of Medicine, Uniformed University of the Health Sciences.

C. T. DOLLERY, M.B., F.R.C.P.

Arterial Hypertension

Professor of Clinical Pharmacology, Royal Postgraduate Medical School. Consultant Physician, Hammersmith Hospital, London, England.

DAVID A. DRACHMAN, M.D.

Dizziness and Vertigo

Professor and Chairman, Department of Neurology, University of Massachusetts Medical Center. Attending Physician, University of Massachusetts, Worcester City Hospital, and St. Vincent Hospital, Worcester, Massachusetts.

PIERRE M. DREYFUS, M.D.

Nutritional Disorders of the Nervous System

Professor and Chairman, Department of Neurology, School of Medicine, University of California, Davis. Chief, Neurology Service, Sacramento Medical Center of the University of California, Davis, Sacramento; Consultant, U.S. Air Force Base Hospital, Travis, and Veterans Administration Hospital, Martinez, California.

PETER JAMES DYCK, M.D.

Diseases of the Peripheral Nervous System

Professor of Neurology, Mayo Medical School, Rochester, Minnesota.

DAVID L. EARNEST, M.D.

Other Diseases of the Colon, Rectum, and Anus

Associate Professor of Medicine, University of Arizona College of Medicine. Chief of Gastroenterology, University of Arizona Health Sciences Center, Tucson; Consultant, Veterans Administration Hospitals, Tucson and Phoenix, Arizona.

THEODORE C. EICKHOFF, M.D.

Colorado Tick Fever

Professor of Medicine and Head, Division of Infectious Disease, University of Colorado Medical Center, Denver, Colorado.

BRYAN T. EMMERSON, M.D., Ph.D.

Toxic Nephropathy

Professor of Medicine, University of Queensland Medical School. Physician in Charge, University Medical Unit, Princess Alexandra Hospital, Brisbane, Australia.

KARL ENGELMAN, M.D.

The Adrenal Medulla and Sympathetic Nervous System; The Carcinoid Syndrome

Associate Professor of Medicine and Pharmacology, University of Pennsylvania School of Medicine. Attending Physician, Hospital of the University of Pennsylvania, Philadelphia Veterans Administration Hospital, and Childrens Hospital of Philadelphia; Director, Clinical Research Center, Hospital of the University of Pennsylvania, Philadelphia, Pennsylvania.

ALLAN J. ERSLEV, M.D.

Polycythemia

Cardeza Research Professor of Medicine and Director, Cardeza Foundation for Hematologic Research, Thomas Jefferson University. Attending Physician, Thomas Jefferson University Hospital, Philadelphia, Pennsylvania.

ANTHONY S. FAUCI, M.D.

Wegener's Granulomatosis; Midline Granuloma; Familial Mediterranean Fever

Head, Clinical Physiology Section, Laboratory of Clinical Investigation, Deputy Clinical Director, National Institute of Allergy and Infectious Diseases, National Institutes of Health, Bethesda, Maryland.

ALVAN R. FEINSTEIN, M.D.

Science, Clinical Medicine, and the Spectrum of Disease

Professor of Medicine and Epidemiology, and Director, Robert Wood Johnson Clinical Scholar Program, Yale University School of Medicine. Attending Physician, Yale–New Haven Hospital, New Haven; Senior Biostatistician, Cooperative Studies Program Coordinating Center, West Haven Veterans Administration Hospital, West Haven, Connecticut.

F. ROBERT FEKETY, Jr., M.D.

Staphylococcal Infections

Professor of Internal Medicine, University of Michigan School of Medicine. Attending Physician and Chief, Infectious Disease Service, University Hospital, Ann Arbor, Michigan.

HARRY A. FELDMAN, M.D.

Meningococcal Disease

Professor and Chairman, Department of Preventive Medicine, State University of New York, Upstate Medical Center, Syracuse, New York.

PHILIP FELIG, M.D.

Nutritional Maintenance and Diet Therapy in Acute and Chronic Disease

C. N. H. Long Professor and Vice Chairman, Department of Medicine, and Chief, Section of Endocrinology, Yale School of Medicine. Vice Chairman, Department of Medicine and Chief of Endocrinology, Yale–New Haven Hospital, New Haven, Connecticut.

THOMAS F. FERRIS, M.D.

Renal Disease in Pregnancy

Professor and Chairman, Department of Medicine, University of Minnesota. Consultant, Veterans Administration Hospital, Minneapolis, Minnesota.

SYDNEY M. FINEGOLD, M.D.

Disease Due to Nonsporeforming Anaerobic Bacteria; Lung Abscess and Bronchiectasis

Professor of Medicine, UCLA School of Medicine. Chief, Infectious Disease Section, Wadsworth Hospital Center, Veterans Administration, Los Angeles, California.

ALFRED P. FISHMAN, M.D.

Heart Failure

William Maul Measey Professor of Medicine, University of Pennsylvania School of Medicine. Director, Cardiovascular-Pulmonary Division, Hospital of the University of Pennsylvania, Philadelphia, Pennsylvania.

ROBERT A. FISHMAN, M.D.

Intracranial Tumors and States Causing Increased Intracranial Pressure

Professor and Chairman, Department of Neurology, University of California, San Francisco. Chief, Neurology Service, University of California Hospitals, San Francisco; Attending Neurologist, San Francisco General Hospital; Consultant in Neurology, Veterans Administration Hospital, San Francisco, California.

EDMUND B. FLINK, M.D., Ph.D.

Heavy Metal Poisoning

Professor of Internal Medicine, West Virginia University Medical Center, Morgantown, West Virginia.

KATHLEEN M. FOLEY, M.D.

Neurologic Diagnostic Procedures

Assistant Professor of Neurology, Cornell University Medical College. Assistant Attending Neurologist, Memorial Sloan-Kettering Cancer Center, New York, New York.

NOBLE O. FOWLER, M.D.

Diseases of the Aorta

Professor of Medicine, University of Cincinnati College of Medicine. Director, Division of Cardiology, University of Cincinnati Medical Center; Chief Clinician, Cardiac Clinic, Cincinnati General Hospital, Cincinnati, Ohio.

DONALD S. FREDRICKSON, M.D.

Gaucher's Disease; Niemann-Pick Disease

Director, National Institutes of Health, Bethesda, Maryland.

NORBERT FREINKEL, M.D.

Hypoglycemic Disorders

Kettering Professor of Medicine; Director, Center for Endocrinology, Metabolism and Nutrition; and Chief, Section of Endocrinology, Metabolism and Nutrition; Northwestern University Medical School. Attending Physician, Northwestern Memorial Hospital; Consultant in Endocrinology and Metabolism, Veterans Administration Lakeside Hospital, Chicago, Illinois.

JOHN I. GALLIN, M.D.

The Compromised Host

Head, Bacterial Disease Section, Laboratory of Clinical Investigation, National Institute of Allergy and Infectious Disease, National Institutes of Health, Bethesda, Maryland.

KENNETH D. GARDNER, Jr., M.D.

Cystic Diseases of the Kidney

Professor of Medicine, University of New Mexico School of Medicine. Chief, Division of Renal Diseases, Bernalillo County Medical Center; Attending Nephrologist, Albuquerque Veterans Administration Hospital; Consulting Nephrologist, Presbyterian Medical Center, Albuquerque, New Mexico.

JEFFREY A. GELFAND, M.D.

Complement

Assistant Professor of Medicine, Tufts University School of Medicine. Assistant Physician, Department of Medicine, Tufts–New England Medical Center, Boston, Massachusetts.

PARK S. GERALD, M.D.

Chromosomes and Their Disorders

Professor of Pediatrics, Harvard Medical School. Chief, Clinical Genetics Division, Children's Hospital Medical Center, Boston, Massachusetts.

NORMAN GESCHWIND, M.D.

Focal Disturbances of Higher Nervous Function

James Jackson Putnam Professor of Neurology, Harvard Medical School. Neurologist-in-Chief, Beth Israel Hospital, Boston, Massachusetts.

GILBERT H. GLASER, M.D., Med.Sc.D.

The Epilepsies

Professor of Neurology and Chairman, Department of Neurology, Yale University School of Medicine. Chief of Neurology, Yale–New Haven Hospital, New Haven; Consultant in Neurology, Veterans Administration Hospital, West Haven, Connecticut.

RICHARD J. GLASSOCK, M.D.

Mechanisms of Renal Injury

Professor of Medicine, UCLA School of Medicine. Chief, Division of Nephrology and Hypertension, Los Angeles County Harbor–UCLA Medical Center, Torrance, California.

JAMES F. GLENN, M.D.

Anomalies of the Urinary Tract; Tumors of the Kidney

Professor of Urology, Duke University School of Medicine. Chief of Urology, Duke University Medical Center, Durham, North Carolina.

MARTIN GOLDBERG, M.D.

Interstitial Nephritis and Interstitial Nephropathy

Professor of Medicine, University of Pennsylvania School of Medicine. Chief, Renal-Electrolyte Section, Hospital of the University of Pennsylvania, Philadelphia, Pennsylvania.

RALPH GOLDMAN, M.D.

Aging and Geriatric Medicine

Formerly Professor of Medicine, UCLA School of Medicine. Assistant Chief Medical Director for Extended Care, Veterans Administration Central Office, Washington, D.C.

ROBERT A. GOOD, Ph.D., M.D.

The Primary Immunodeficiency Diseases

President and Director, Sloan-Kettering Institute for Cancer Research; Professor of Medicine and Pediatrics, Cornell University Medical College; Adjunct Professor, Rockefeller University, New York, New York. Attending Physician, Departments of Medicine and Pediatrics, Memorial Hospital for Cancer and Allied Diseases, New York, New York.

ROBERT A. GOODWIN, Jr., M.D.

Pulmonary Tuberculosis; Diseases Due to Mycobacteria Other Than M. tuberculosis and M. leprae

Professor of Medicine, Vanderbilt University School of Medicine. Chief, Pulmonary Disease Section, Veterans Administration Hospital, Nashville; Visiting Staff, Vanderbilt University Hospital; Consultant, St. Thomas Hospital, Nashville, Tennessee.

SHERWOOD L. GORBACH, M.D.

Typhoid Fever

Professor of Medicine and Microbiology, Tufts University

School of Medicine. Chief, Infectious Disease Service, Tufts–New England Medical Center Hospital, Boston, Massachusetts.

GARETH M. GREEN, M.D.

Infiltrative Diseases of the Lung

Professor of Environmental Health Sciences, Johns Hopkins School of Hygiene and Public Health, Baltimore, Maryland.

B. M. GREENWOOD, M.D., F.R.C.P.

African Trypanosomiasis

Senior Lecturer in Medicine, Ahmadu Bello University, Zaria, Nigeria.

MORTON I. GROSSMAN, M.D., Ph.D.

Peptic Ulcer: Pathogenesis and Pathophysiology

Professor of Medicine and Physiology, UCLA School of Medicine. Senior Medical Investigator, Veterans Administration Wadsworth Hospital Center, Los Angeles, California.

J. CAULIE GUNNELLS, Jr., M.D.

Vascular Disorders of the Kidney

Professor of Medicine, Duke University School of Medicine, Durham, North Carolina.

THORSTEIN GUTHE, M.D., M.P.H.

Nonsyphilitic Treponematoses

Former Chief Medical Officer, Venereal Diseases and Treponematoses, World Health Organization, Geneva, Switzerland. Director, Institute of Medicine, Alkem-Spigerverket, Oslo, Norway.

ROBERT J. HAGGERTY, M.D.

Common Accidental Poisoning

Roger I. Lee Professor of Health Services and Pediatrics, Harvard School of Public Health, Harvard Medical School. Senior Physician, Children's Hospital Medical Center, Boston, Massachusetts.

JAMES B. HANSHAW, M.D.

Cytomegalovirus Infections

Professor and Chairman, Department of Pediatrics, University of Massachusetts Medical School. Chief of Pediatrics, University of Massachusetts Medical Center and St. Vincent Hospital, Worcester, Massachusetts.

EDWARD D. HARRIS, Jr., M.D.

Systemic Sclerosis

Professor of Medicine, Dartmouth-Hitchcock Medical Center; Director, Arthritis Center, and Chief, Connective Tissue Disease Section. Staff Physician, Mary Hitchcock Memorial Hospital, Hanover, New Hampshire; Veterans Administration Hospital, White River Junction, Vermont.

RICHARD J. HAVEL, M.D.

Disorders of Lipid Metabolism

Professor of Medicine, University of California School of Medicine, San Francisco, California.

LEE W. HENDERSON, M.D.

Hemodialysis

Professor of Medicine in Residence, University of California, San Diego. Associate Chief of Staff for Research, Veterans Administration Hospital, San Diego; Staff Physician, University Hospital, San Diego, California.

VICTOR HERBERT, M.D., J.D.

Megaloblastic Anemias

Professor of Medicine, State University of New York, Downstate Medical Center, Brooklyn. Chief, Hematology and Nutrition Laboratory, Veterans Administration Hospital, Bronx, New York.

ALBERT HEYMAN, M.D.

Syncope; Hyperventilation

Professor of Medicine (Neurology), Duke University Medical Center, Durham, North Carolina.

HOWARD H. HIATT, M.D.

Environment

Dean, Harvard School of Public Health; Professor of Medicine, Harvard Medical School. Consultant in Medicine, Beth Israel, Peter Bent Brigham, and Children's Hospitals, Boston, Massachusetts.

JAMES F. HOLLAND, M.D.

The Acute Leukemias

Professor and Chairman, Department of Neoplastic Diseases, Mt. Sinai School of Medicine of the City University of New York. Director, Cancer Center, Mt. Sinai Hospital, New York, New York.

EDWARD W. HOOK, M.D.

Pneumococcal Pneumonia; Salmonella Infections Other Than Typhoid Fever

Henry B. Mulholland Professor of Medicine and Chairman, Department of Medicine, University of Virginia School of Medicine. Physician-in-Chief, University of Virginia Hospital, Charlottesville, Virginia.

DOROTHY M. HORSTMANN, M.D.

Mumps

Professor of Epidemiology and Pediatrics, Yale University School of Medicine. Attending, Pediatrics, Yale–New Haven Hospital, New Haven, Connecticut.

CHARLES M. HUGULEY, Jr., M.D.

The Chronic Leukemias

Professor of Medicine and Director of Cancer Center, Emory University School of Medicine. Attending Staff, Emory University Hospital and Grady Memorial Hospital, Atlanta, Georgia.

JON I. ISENBERG, M.D.

Peptic Ulcer: Diagnosis; Peptic Ulcer: Medical Therapy

Professor of Medicine, UCLA School of Medicine. Chief, Gastroenterology Section, Wadsworth Veterans Administration Hospital, Los Angeles, California.

GEORGE GEE JACKSON, M.D.

The Common Cold; Rhinoviral Respiratory Disease; Viral Pharyngitis, Laryngitis, Croup, and Bronchitis; Adenoviral Infections; Respiratory Syncytial Viral Disease; Parainfluenza Viral Diseases

Professor of Medicine, Abraham Lincoln School of Medicine; Chief, Section of Infectious Diseases. Attending Physician, University of Illinois Hospital and Veterans Administration West Side Hospital; Consultant in Infectious Diseases, Veterans Administration West Side Hospital, Chicago, Illinois.

HARRY S. JACOB, M.D.

Hemolysis Due to Intracorpuscular Abnormalities

Professor of Medicine and Chief, Section of Hematology, University of Minnesota Medical School. Attending Physician, University of Minnesota Hospitals, Minneapolis Veterans Administration Hospital, Hennepin County General Hospital, Minneapolis, and St. Paul–Ramsey General Hospital, St. Paul, Minnesota.

ERNST R. JAFFÉ, M.D.

Methemoglobinemia and Sulfhemoglobinemia

Professor of Medicine, Albert Einstein College of Medicine; Head, Division of Hematology; Senior Associate Dean; Associate Dean for Faculty. Attending Physician, Bronx Municipal Hospital Center and Hospital of the Albert Einstein College of Medicine, Bronx, New York.

D. GERAINT JAMES, M.A., M.D.(Cambridge), F.R.C.P.

Sarcoidosis

Dean and Physician, Royal Northern Hospital, London, England; Consultant Ophthalmic Physician, St. Thomas' Hospital, London. Adjunct Professor of Medicine, University of Miami, Florida. Consulting Physician, Royal Navy.

HENRY D. JANOWITZ, M.D.

Chronic Inflammatory Diseases of the Intestine

Clinical Professor of Medicine, Mount Sinai School of Medicine. Head, Division of Gastroenterology, Mount Sinai Hospital, New York, New York.

ERNEST JAWETZ, M.D., Ph.D.

Trachoma and Inclusion Conjunctivitis; Lymphogranuloma Venereum

Professor of Microbiology and Medicine, University of California Medical Center, San Francisco, California.

GRAHAM H. JEFFRIES, M.B., Ch.B. (N.Z.), D.Phil.(Oxon.)

Diseases of the Liver

Professor and Chairman, Department of Medicine, Pennsylvania State University College of Medicine. Chief, Medical Service, The Milton S. Hershey Medical Center Hospital, Hershey, Pennsylvania.

KARL M. JOHNSON, M.D.

Arthropod-Borne Viral Fevers, Viral Encephalitides and Viral Hemorrhagic Fevers: Introduction; Dengue; West Nile Fever; Fevers Caused by Group A Arboviruses; Rift Valley Fever; Sandfly Fever; Arthropod-Borne Viral Encephalitides; Viral Hemorrhagic Fevers: Introduction; Hemorrhagic Fever Caused by Dengue Viruses; Crimean Hemorrhagic Fever; Hemorrhagic Diseases Caused by Arenaviruses; African Hemorrhagic Fever; Epidemic Hemorrhagic Fever

Chief, Special Pathogens Branch, Virology Division, Bureau of Laboratories Center for Disease Control, Atlanta, Georgia.

MARIE-LOUISE JOHNSON, M.D., Ph.D.

Certain Cutaneous Diseases with Significant Systemic Manifestations

Professor of Dermatology, New York University School of Medicine. Attending, New York University Medical Center; Chief, Dermatology Service, Bellevue Hospital Center, New York, New York.

RICHARD T. JOHNSON, M.D.

Viral Infections of the Nervous System: Introduction; Viral Meningitis and Encephalitis; Herpes Zoster; Slow Infections of the Nervous System

Eisenhower Professor of Neurology and Professor of Microbiology, The Johns Hopkins University School of Medicine. Neurologist, The Johns Hopkins Hospital, Baltimore, Maryland.

THOMAS C. JONES, M.D.

Malaria; Toxoplasmosis; Pneumocystosis; Babesiosis; Trichomoniasis

Associate Professor of Medicine and Associate Professor of Public Health, Cornell University Medical College. Associate Attending Physician, The New York Hospital, New York, New York.

DESMOND G. JULIAN, M.D., F.R.C.P.

Disorders of the Coronary Arteries: Introduction; Angina Pectoris; Myocardial Infarction; Sudden Death

Professor of Cardiology, University of Newcastle-upon-Tyne. Cardiologist, Freeman Hospital, Newcastle-upon-Tyne, England.

FRED S. KANTOR, M.D.

Serum Sickness; Drug Allergy; Allergic Rhinitis; Vasomotor Rhinitis; Urticaria; Angioedema; Insect Stings

Professor of Medicine, Yale University School of Medicine; Chief, Allergy and Clinical Immunology Section, Department of Medicine. Attending Physician, Yale–New Haven Hospital, New Haven, Connecticut.

NATHAN KASE, M.D.

The Ovaries

Professor of Obstetrics and Gynecology, Yale University School of Medicine. Attending Physician, Yale–New Haven Hospital, New Haven; Consultant, Greenwich Hospital, Greenwich, Griffin Hospital, Derby, New Britain General Hospital, New Britain, St. Raphael Hospital, New Haven, Stamford Hospital, Stamford, Norwalk Hospital, Norwalk, and William W. Backus Hospital, Norwich, Connecticut. National Consultant, Department of the Air Force.

HERANT A. KATCHADOURIAN, M.D.

The Life-Cycle Perspective in Medicine; Development to Adulthood; Adulthood

Professor of Psychiatry and the Behavioral Sciences, Stanford University School of Medicine; Vice Provost and Dean of Office of Undergraduate Studies, Stanford University, Stanford, California.

DONALD KAYE, M.D.

Infective Endocarditis; Gonococcal Disease

Professor and Chairman, Department of Medicine, The Medical College of Pennsylvania. Chief of Medicine, Hospital of the Medical College of Pennsylvania; Consultant in Medicine, Veterans Administration Hospital, Philadelphia, Pennsylvania.

HUGH L. KEEGAN, Ph.D.

Arthropods as Environmental Agents of Disease; Pentastomiasis; Leeches as Agents of Disease; Snakebite; Venomous Marine Animals

Professor of Preventive Medicine, University of Mississippi School of Medicine, Jackson, Mississippi.

C. HENRY KEMPE, M.D.

Variola and Vaccinia

Professor of Pediatrics and Microbiology, University of Colorado School of Medicine. Consultant, Colorado General Hospital, Fitzsimons Army Hospital, Children's Hospital, and Veterans Administration Hospital, Denver, Colorado.

D. N. S. KERR, M.S., F.R.C.P., F.R.C.P.E.

Investigation of Renal Function; Investigation of Renal Structure and Regional Function; Chronic Renal Failure

Professor of Medicine, University of Newcastle-upon-Tyne. Consultant Physician, Royal Victoria Infirmary, Newcastle-upon-Tyne, England.

JOHN H. KERR, D.M., F.F.A., R.C.S.

Tetanus

Clinical Lecturer in Anaesthetics, University of Oxford. Consultant Anaesthetist, Oxford Area Health Authority (Teaching), Nuffield Department of Anaesthetics, Radcliffe Infirmary, Oxford, England.

SIDNEY KIBRICK, M.D., Ph.D.

Varicella

Professor of Pediatrics and Microbiology, Boston University School of Medicine. Visiting Physician for Pediatrics, Boston City Hospital, Boston, Massachusetts.

EDWIN D. KILBOURNE, M.D.

Introduction to Viral Diseases; Influenza; Measles; Rubella

Professor and Chairman, Department of Microbiology, Mount Sinai School of Medicine of the City University of New York.

PRISCILLA KINCAID-SMITH, M.D., F.R.C.P., F.R.A.C.P., D.C.P., F.R.C.P.A.

Treatment of Irreversible Renal Failure by Transplantation and Dialysis: Introduction; Renal Transplantation

Professor of Medicine, University of Melbourne. Physician-in-Charge, Department of Nephrology, Royal Melbourne Hospital, Melbourne, Australia.

S. J. KLEBANOFF, M.D., Ph.D.

Neutrophil Function; Neutrophil Dysfunction Syndromes

Professor of Medicine, University of Washington School of Medicine, Seattle, Washington.

RICHARD KNIGHT, M.B., B.Chir., M.R.C.P., Ph.D., D.T.M. and H.

Amebiasis

Senior Lecturer, Department of Tropical Medicine, Liverpool School of Tropical Medicine. Honorary Consultant Physician, (Tropical Medicine), Liverpool Area Health Authority, Liverpool, England.

HILARY KOPROWSKI, M.D.

Rabies

Wistar Professor of Research Medicine, University of Pennsylvania School of Medicine, Philadelphia, Pennsylvania.

RICHARD M. KRAUSE, M.D.

Rheumatic Fever

Director, National Institute of Allergy and Infectious Diseases, National Institutes of Health, Bethesda, Maryland.

CALVIN M. KUNIN, M.D.

Enteric Bacterial Infections; Urinary Tract Infections and Pyelonephritis

Professor of Medicine and Chairman of the Department of Medicine, Ohio State University School of Medicine, Columbus, Ohio.

HENRY G. KUNKEL, M.D.

Immune Disease: Introduction

Professor of Immunology and Medicine, Rockefeller University; Adjunct Professor of Medicine, Cornell University Medical School, New York, New York.

HAROLD P. LAMBERT, M.D., F.R.C.P.

Food Poisoning

Professor of Microbial Diseases, St. George's Hospital Medical School, London. Consultant Physician, St. George's Hospital, London, England.

MAURICE B. LANDERS, III, M.D.

Diseases of the Eye

Professor of Ophthalmology, Duke University Medical Center. Attending Ophthalmologist, Veterans Administration Hospital, Durham; Chief of Ophthalmology, Veterans Administration Hospital, Asheville, North Carolina.

DAVID H. LAW, M.D.

Gastrointestinal Bleeding

Professor of Internal Medicine (Vice Chairman), University of New Mexico School of Medicine. Chief, Medical Service, Veterans Administration Hospital, Albuquerque, New Mexico.

ALEXANDER LEAF, M.D.

Posterior Pituitary

Jackson Professor of Clinical Medicine, Harvard Medical School. Chief, Medical Services, Massachusetts General Hospital, Boston, Massachusetts.

ROBERT I. LEVY, M.D.

Prevalence and Epidemiology of Cardiovascular Disease

Director, National Heart, Lung, and Blood Institute, National Institutes of Health, Bethesda, Maryland.

HERBERT L. LEY, Jr., M.D., M.P.H.

Trench Fever; Q Fever; Bartonellosis

Medical Consultant in foods and drugs, Rockville, Maryland.

GRANT W. LIDDLE, M.D.

Adrenal Cortex

Professor and Chairman, Department of Medicine, Vanderbilt

University School of Medicine. Physician-in-Chief, Vanderbilt University Hospital, Nashville, Tennessee.

PHILIP H. LIEBERMAN, M.D.

Eosinophilic Granuloma and Related Syndromes

Associate Professor of Pathology, Cornell University School of Medicine. Attending Pathologist and Chief, Surgical Pathology Service, Memorial Hospital for Cancer and Allied Diseases, New York, New York.

HAROLD I. LIEF, M.D.

Medical Aspects of Sexuality

Professor of Psychiatry, University of Pennsylvania School of Medicine. Director, Marriage Council of Philadelphia, Inc., Philadelphia, Pennsylvania.

MORTIMER B. LIPSETT, M.D.

The Testis

Director, The Clinical Center, National Institutes of Health, Bethesda, Maryland.

JOHN N. LOEB, M.D.

Mode of Action of Hormones

Associate Professor of Medicine, College of Physicians and Surgeons, Columbia University; Adjunct Associate Professor, Rockefeller University. Associate Attending Physician, Presbyterian Hospital, New York, New York.

DANIEL S. LUKAS, M.D.

Pulmonary Hypertension

Associate Professor of Medicine, Cornell University Medical College. Associate Attending Physician, The New York Hospital; Consultant, Cardiopulmonary Service, Memorial Hospital, New York, New York; Vice President of Medical Affairs, Elliot Hospital, Manchester, New Hampshire.

VANIZE MACEDO, M.D.

Chagas' Disease

Professor of Tropical Medicine, University of Brasilia. Physician, Sobradinho Hospital, Brasilia, Brazil.

ANDREW M. MARGILETH, M.D.

Cat Scratch Disease

Professor and Associate Chairman, Department of Child Health and Development, George Washington University School of Medicine; Associate Professor of Pediatrics, Howard University School of Medicine. Director, Outpatient Department, Senior Attending Staff Physician, Children's Hospital National Medical Center, Washington, D.C.

PAUL A. MARKS, M.D.

Human Carcinogenesis

Frode Jensen Professor of Medicine and of Human Genetics

and Development Director, Cancer Center, Columbia University. Attending Physician, Presbyterian Hospital, New York, New York.

PHILIP D. MARSDEN, M.D.

Protozoan and Helminthic Diseases: Introduction; Protozoan Diseases: Introduction; Trypanosomiases: Introduction; Other Protozoan Diseases: Introduction; Giardiasis; Balantidiasis; Primary Amebic Meningoencephalitis; Isosporiasis; Sarcosporidiosis; Helminthic Diseases: Introduction; The Cestodes; Hermaphroditic Flukes; The Nematodes; Disorders with Some Relation to Helminths

Professor of Tropical Medicine, University of Brasilia. Physician, Sobradinho Hospital, Brasilia, Brazil.

JOHN H. McCLEMENT, M.D.

Diseases of the Pleura, Mediastinum, Diaphragm, and Chest Wall

Professor of Medicine, New York University School of Medicine. Director, Chest Service, Bellevue Hospital, New York; Attending Physician, University Hospital, New York, New York.

WALSH McDERMOTT, M.D.

Medicine in Modern Society; Chemical Contamination of Water and Air; The Nature of Microbial Diseases; Foot-and-Mouth Disease; Bacterial Diseases: Introduction; Granuloma Inguinale; Drugs and Microbes

Emeritus Professor of Public Health and Medicine, Cornell University Medical College; Special Advisor to the President, Robert Wood Johnson Foundation, Princeton, New Jersey.

FLETCHER H. McDOWELL, M.D.

Cerebrovascular Diseases

Professor of Neurology, Cornell University Medical College. Attending Neurologist, The New York Hospital; Medical Director, Burke Rehabilitation Hospital; Consulting Neurologist, Memorial Hospital, New York, New York.

PAUL R. McHUGH, M.D.

Dementia; Psychologic Illness in Medical Practice; Psychologic Testing in Clinical Medicine

Henry Phipps Professor of Psychiatry, Department of Psychiatry, and Behavioral Science, The Johns Hopkins School of Medicine. Psychiatrist-in-Chief, The Johns Hopkins Hospital, Baltimore, Maryland.

PATRICK A. McKEE, M.D.

Thrombosis

Professor of Medicine and Assistant Professor of Biochemistry, Duke University Medical Center, Durham, North Carolina.

BYRON D. McLEES, M.D., Ph.D.

Critical Care Medicine

Chief, Department of Critical Care Medicine, Clinical Center, National Institutes of Health, Bethesda, Maryland.

JACK H. MENDELSON, M.D.

Alcohol Abuse and Alcohol-Related Illness

Professor of Psychiatry, Harvard Medical School. Director, Alcohol and Drug Abuse Research Center, McLean Hospital, Belmont, Massachusetts.

JAMES H. MEYER, M.D.

Peptic Ulcer: Complications and Surgical Treatment

Associate Professor of Medicine, University of California, Los Angeles. Chief, Division of Gastroenterology, Veterans Administration Hospital, Sepulveda, California, and UCLA/San Fernando Valley Medical Program.

ROBERT B. MILLMAN, M.D.

Drug Abuse, Dependence, and Intoxication: Introduction; The Opiates; Central Nervous System Depressants; Central Nervous System Stimulants; Cannabis; Psychedelics; Miscellaneous Inhalants

Clinical Associate Professor of Public Health, Assistant Professor of Psychiatry, Cornell University Medical College. Director, Alcohol and Drug Abuse Programs, The New York Hospital–Cornell Medical Center, New York, New York.

STANLEY R. MOHLER, M.D.

Motion Sickness and Problems of Air Travel

Professor and Vice-Chairman, Department of Community Medicine, Director of Aerospace Medicine, Wright State University School of Medicine, Dayton, Ohio.

THOMAS P. MONATH, M.D.

Yellow Fever

Director, Vector-Borne Diseases Division, Bureau of Laboratories, Center for Disease Control, Public Health Service, U.S. Department of Health, Education, and Welfare, Fort Collins, Colorado.

STEPHEN I. MORSE, M.D.

Whooping Cough

Professor and Chairman, Microbiology and Immunology, State University of New York, Downstate Medical Center, Brooklyn, New York.

ARNO G. MOTULSKY, M.D.

Genetic Counseling

Professor of Medicine and Genetics, Director, Center for Inherited Diseases, University of Washington School of Medicine. Attending Physician, University Hospital, University of Washington, Seattle, Washington.

FRANCIS P. MULDOWNEY, M.D., F.R.C.P.

Obstructive Nephropathy

Research Professor of Medicine, University College, Dublin. Physician in Charge, Metabolic and Renal Unit, St. Vincent's Hospital; Consultant Physician, Metabolic Diseases, National

Maternity Hospital; Visiting Consultant, Meath Hospital; Visiting Consultant, St. Luke's Hospital, Dublin, Ireland.

JOHN F. MURRAY, M.D.

Respiratory Disease: Introduction; Respiratory Structure and Function; Respiratory Failure

Professor of Medicine, University of California, San Francisco. Chief of the Chest Service, San Francisco General Hospital, San Francisco, California.

W. P. L. MYERS, M.D.

Cancer and Internal Medicine: An Internist's Approach to Cancer and Its Medical Manifestations; The Care of the Patient with Terminal Illness

Professor of Internal Medicine and Associate Dean, Cornell University Medical College. Vice President for Educational Affairs, Memorial Sloan-Kettering Cancer Center; Attending Physician, Memorial Hospital for Cancer and Allied Diseases and The New York Hospital; Member, Sloan-Kettering Institute for Cancer Research; Formerly Chairman, Department of Medicine, Memorial Hospital for Cancer and Allied Diseases, New York, New York.

RALPH L. NACHMAN, M.D.

Hematologic and Hematopoietic Diseases: Introduction; Hemorrhagic Disorders: Disorders of Primary Hemostasis

Professor of Medicine, Cornell University Medical College. Chief, Division of Hematology, Cornell University Medical College; Attending Physician, The New York Hospital, New York, New York.

JAMES C. NIEDERMAN, M.D.

Infectious Mononucleosis

Clinical Professor of Epidemiology and Medicine, Yale University School of Medicine. Medical Staff Member, Yale–New Haven Medical Center, New Haven, Connecticut.

THOMAS F. O'BRIEN, Jr., M.D.

Neoplasms of the Small Intestine; Neoplasms of the Large Intestine

Professor of Medicine, East Carolina School of Medicine. Chief, Gastroenterology Section, East Carolina School of Medicine; Attending Physician, Pitt County Memorial Hospital, Greenville, North Carolina.

ROBERT K. OCKNER, M.D.

Vascular Diseases of the Intestine; Diseases of the Peritoneum, Mesentery, and Omentum

Professor of Medicine, University of California School of Medicine, San Francisco. Attending Physician, University of California–Moffitt, Veterans Administration, and San Francisco General Hospitals, San Francisco, California.

ELLIOTT F. OSSERMAN, M.D.

Plasma Cell Dyscrasias

American Cancer Society Professor of Medicine, Associate

Director, Institute of Cancer Research, Columbia University College of Physicians and Surgeons. Attending Physician, Presbyterian Hospital, New York, New York.

DEMOSTHENES PAPPAGIANIS, M.D., Ph.D.

Coccidioidomycosis

Professor and Chairman, Department of Medical Microbiology, School of Medicine, University of California, Davis, California.

WILLIAM W. PARMLEY, M.D.

Circulatory Function and Control

Professor of Medicine, University of California, San Francisco, School of Medicine. Chief of Cardiology, H. C. Moffitt Hospital, San Francisco, California.

RUSSEL H. PATTERSON, Jr., M.D.

Injuries of the Head and Spine

Professor of Surgery (Neurosurgery), Cornell University Medical College. Attending Surgeon-in-Charge (Neurosurgery), The New York Hospital, New York, New York.

JOSEPH K. PERLOFF, M.D.

Congenital Heart Disease

Professor of Medicine and Pediatrics, Center for the Health Sciences, School of Medicine, University of California, Los Angeles, California.

SHELDON R. PINNELL, M.D.

Ehlers-Danlos Syndrome

Investigator, Howard Hughes Medical Institute, and Professor of Medicine (Dermatology), Duke University Medical Center, Durham, North Carolina.

FRED PLUM, M.D.

Disorders of the Nervous System and Behavior: Introduction; Consciousness and Its Disturbances: Introduction; The Pathogenesis of Stupor and Coma; Acute Drug Poisoning; The Hypothalamus and Neurologic Disorders; Headache; Acute Anterior Poliomyelitis

Professor of Neurology, Cornell University Medical College. Neurologist-in-Chief, New York Hospital, New York, New York.

JEROME B. POSNER, M.D.

Delirium and Exogenous Metabolic Brain Disease; Pain; Nonmetastatic Effects of Cancer on the Nervous System

Professor of Neurology, Cornell University Medical College. Chairman, Department of Neurology, Memorial Sloan-Kettering Cancer Center, New York, New York.

OSCAR D. RATNOFF, M.D.

Hemorrhagic Disorders: Coagulation Defects

Professor of Medicine, Case Western Reserve School of Medicine. Career Investigator of the American Heart Association; Physician, University Hospitals of Cleveland, Cleveland, Ohio.

SEYMOUR REICHLIN, M.D., Ph.D.

The Control of Anterior Pituitary Secretion; The Pineal

Professor of Medicine, Tufts University School of Medicine. Chief, Endocrine Division, and Senior Physician, New England Medical Center Hospital, Boston, Massachusetts.

HERBERT Y. REYNOLDS, M.D.

Introduction to Pneumonia; Pneumonia Due to Klebsiella pneumoniae; Legionnaires' Disease; Pneumonia and Nosocomial Respiratory Infections Caused by Aerobic Gram-Negative Bacilli

Associate Professor of Internal Medicine and Head, Pulmonary Section, Department of Internal Medicine, Yale University School of Medicine. Attending Physician, Yale–New Haven Hospital, New Haven; Pulmonary Consultant, West Haven Veterans Administration Hospital, West Haven, Connecticut.

RICHARD A. RIFKIND, M.D.

Diseases of the Spleen

Professor of Medicine and of Human Genetics and Development, Columbia University College of Physicians and Surgeons. Attending Physician and Director, Division of Hematology, Presbyterian Hospital, New York, New York.

JOHN B. ROBBINS, M.D.

Hemophilus Infections with Special Emphasis on Hemophilus influenzae Type b

Director, Division of Bacterial Products, Bureau of Biologics, Food and Drug Administration, Department of Health, Education, and Welfare, Bethesda, Maryland.

RICHARD B. ROBERTS, M.D.

Antimicrobial Therapy

Professor of Medicine and Head, Division of Infectious Diseases, Cornell University Medical College. Attending Physician, The New York Hospital, New York, New York.

ROSCOE R. ROBINSON, M.D.

The Major Renal Syndromes

Florence McAlister Professor of Medicine, Duke University School of Medicine. Director, Division of Nephrology, Duke University Medical Center, Durham, North Carolina.

HEONIR ROCHA, M.D.

Diphtheria

Professor of Medicine, Faculty of Medicine, Federal University of Bahia, Salvador-Bahia, Brazil.

ROGER N. ROSENBERG, M.D.

Inherited Degenerative Diseases

Professor of Neurology and Physiology, Chairman, Department of Neurology, The University of Texas Health Science Center, Southwestern Medical School, Dallas. Chief, Neurology Service, Parkland Memorial Hospital; Attending Neurologist, Parkland Memorial Hospital and Children's Medical Center, Dallas, Texas.

SAUL A. ROSENBERG, M.D.

Hodgkin's Disease

Professor of Medicine and Radiology, Stanford University School of Medicine. Chief, Division of Oncology, Stanford University School of Medicine, Stanford, California.

JOHN ROSS, Jr., M.D.

Acquired Valvular Heart Disease

Professor of Medicine and Head, Division of Cardiology, University of California, San Diego, School of Medicine. Attending Physician, University of California Medical Center, San Diego, California.

WENDELL F. ROSSE, M.D.

Hemolytic Disorders: Introduction; Hemolysis Due to Acquired Abnormalities

Investigator, Howard Hughes Medical Institute, and Professor of Medicine and Immunology, Duke University Medical Center. Chief, Division of Hematology–Medical Oncology, Duke University Medical Center, Durham, North Carolina.

LEWIS P. ROWLAND, M.D.

Diseases of Muscle and Neuromuscular Junction

Henry and Lucy Moses Professor and Chairman, Department of Neurology, College of Physicians and Surgeons, Columbia University. Director, Neurological Service, Neurological Institute, Presbyterian Hospital, New York, New York.

GERALD F. M. RUSSELL, M.D., F.R.C.P., F.R.C.P.Ed., F.R.C.Psych.

Anorexia Nervosa

Professor of Psychiatry, Royal Free Hospital School of Medicine, University of London. Consultant Psychiatrist, Royal Free Hospital and Friern Hospital, London, England.

DAVID C. SABISTON, Jr., M.D.

Surgical Treatment of Coronary Artery Disease

James B. Duke Professor of Surgery and Chairman of the Department of Surgery, Duke University Medical Center, Durham, North Carolina.

HERBERT A. SALTZMAN, M.D.

Therapeutic Hyperbaric Oxygen

Professor of Medicine, Duke University Medical Center, Durham, North Carolina.

JAY P. SANFORD, M.D.

Plague; Rat-Bite Fever; Leptospirosis

Professor of Medicine and Dean, Uniformed Services University School of Medicine. Attending Physician, Walter

Reed Army Medical Center, Washington, D.C., and National Naval Medical Center, Bethesda; Consultant, Clinical Center, National Institutes of Health, Bethesda, Maryland.

WILLIAM SCHAFFNER, M.D.

Psittacosis

Associate Professor of Medicine and Preventive Medicine, Vanderbilt University School of Medicine. Hospital Epidemiologist, Vanderbilt University Hospital, Nashville, Tennessee.

PHILIP S. SCHEIN, M.D.

Tumor Markers

Professor of Medicine and Pharmacology, Georgetown University School of Medicine. Assistant Director, Vincent T. Lombardi Cancer Research Center, Georgetown University Medical Center, Washington, D.C.

LABE C. SCHEINBERG, M.D.

The Demyelinating Diseases

Professor of Neurology, Albert Einstein College of Medicine of Yeshiva University. Director of Neurology and Psychiatry, St. Barnabas Hospital, Bronx, New York.

RUDI SCHMID, M.D., Ph.D.

Porphyria

Professor of Medicine, University of California, San Francisco, School of Medicine. Attending Physician and Consultant, Moffitt-University Hospital, Veterans Administration Hospital, and U.S. Army Letterman General Hospital, San Francisco, California.

ROBERT W. SCHRIER, M.D.

Other Specific Renal Diseases

Professor and Chairman, Department of Medicine, University of Colorado Medical Center, Denver, Colorado.

PETER H. SCHUR, M.D.

Systemic Lupus Erythematosus

Associate Professor of Medicine, Harvard Medical School. Physician, Robert B. Brigham Hospital, Boston, Massachusetts.

MARVIN M. SCHUSTER, M.D.

Disorders of Motility

Professor of Medicine and Assistant Professor of Psychiatry, The Johns Hopkins School of Medicine. Chief, Division of Digestive Diseases, Baltimore City Hospitals, Baltimore, Maryland.

WILLIAM B. SCHWARTZ, M.D.

Disorders of Fluid, Electrolyte, and Acid-Base Balance

Professor of Medicine, Tufts University School of Medicine. Professor of Medicine, Tufts–New England Medical Center Hospital, Boston, Massachusetts.

NEVIN S. SCRIMSHAW, Ph.D., M.D., M.P.H.

Nutrient Requirements; Assessment of Nutritional Status; Nutrition and Infection; Kwashiorkor, Marasmus, and Intermediate Forms of Protein-Calorie Malnutrition; Undernutrition, Starvation, and Hunger Edema; Deficiencies of Individual Nutrients: Vitamin Diseases

Head, Department of Nutrition and Food Science, Massachusetts Institute of Technology. Director, Clinical Research Center, Massachusetts Institute of Technology, Cambridge, Massachusetts.

CHARLES R. SCRIVER, M.D., F.R.S.C.

Hyperaminoaciduria; Branched-Chain Aminoaciduria; Hyperhistidinemia; The Hyperprolinemias and Hydroxyprolinemia; Diseases of the Urea Cycle; β-Aminoisobutyricaciduria; The Hyperglycinurias; Renal Hyperaminoacidurias; Fanconi's Syndrome; The Hyperphenylalaninemias

Professor of Biology and Pediatrics, McGill University. Director, De Belle Laboratory for Biochemical Genetics, McGill University–Montreal Children's Hospital Research Institute, Montreal, Quebec, Canada.

WILLIAM R. SHAPIRO, M.D.

Sleep and Its Disorders

Professor of Neurology, Cornell University Medical College. Attending Neurologist, Memorial Sloan-Kettering Cancer Center and The New York Hospital, New York, New York.

SOL SHERRY, M.D.

Thrombophlebitis and Phlebothrombosis; Pulmonary Embolism and Infarction

Professor and Chairman, Department of Medicine, Temple University School of Medicine. Physician-in-Chief, Temple University Hospital, Philadelphia, Pennsylvania.

J. B. SIDBURY, Jr., M.D.

Glycogen Storage Disease; Pentosuria; Fructosuria and Hereditary Fructose Intolerance

Professor, Pediatrics, Duke University Medical School; Lecturer, Pediatrics, Johns Hopkins Medical School; Professor, Child Health and Development, George Washington University School of Medicine and Health Sciences. Scientific Director, National Institute of Child Health and Human Development, National Institutes of Health, Bethesda, Maryland.

DONALD H. SILBERBERG, M.D.

Encephalitic Complications of Viral Infections and Vaccines

Professor and Vice Chairman, Department of Neurology, University of Pennsylvania School of Medicine. Neurologist, Hospital of the University of Pennsylvania, Philadelphia, Pennsylvania.

RICHARD T. SILVER, M.D.

Leukemoid Reactions; Myeloproliferative Disorders

Clinical Professor of Medicine, Cornell University Medical College. Chief, Oncology Service, Division of Hematology-Oncology, and Attending Physician, The New York Hospital, New York, New York.

MARVIN H. SLEISENGER, M.D.

Diseases of the Digestive System: Introduction; Malabsorption; Other Inflammatory Diseases of the Intestine

Professor of Medicine and Vice-Chairman, Department of Medicine, University of California, San Francisco. Chief, Medical Service, Veterans Administration Medical Center, San Francisco, California.

LLOYD H. SMITH, Jr., M.D.

Primary Hyperoxaluria; Gout; Xanthinuria; Disorders of Pyrimidine Metabolism

Professor of Medicine and Chairman, Department of Medicine, University of California, San Francisco. Chief of Medicine, Moffitt Hospital, San Francisco, California.

GORDON L. SNIDER, M.D.

Special Diagnostic Procedures in Pulmonary Disease

Professor of Medicine and Head, Pulmonary Medicine Section, Boston University School of Medicine; Lecturer, Tufts University School of Medicine. Chief, Pulmonary Medicine Section, Veterans Administration Hospital, Boston; Attending Physician, University Hospital and Boston City Hospital; Consultant Pulmonary Physician, U.S. Public Health Service Hospital, Boston, Massachusetts.

P. FREDERICK SPARLING, M.D.

Syphilis

Professor of Medicine and Bacteriology, University of North Carolina School of Medicine. Chief, Division of Infectious Diseases, Department of Internal Medicine, Memorial Hospital, Chapel Hill, North Carolina.

CHARLES J. STAHL, M.D.

Drowning

Captain, Medical Corps, United States Navy. Professor of Pathology, School of Medicine, Uniformed Services University of the Health Sciences; Professor of Pathology, School of Medicine, Georgetown University. Chairman, Department of Laboratory Medicine, National Naval Medical Center, Bethesda, Maryland; Consultant in Laboratory Medicine, Bureau of Medicine and Surgery, Washington, D.C.

GENE H. STOLLERMAN, M.D.

Streptococcal Diseases: Introduction; Group A Streptococcal Infection; Clinical Syndromes of Group A Streptococcal Infection; Treatment of Group A Streptococcal Infection and Chemoprophylaxis of Nonsuppurative Complications; Prophylaxis of Streptococcal Infection

Goodman Professor and Chairman, Department of Medicine, University of Tennessee College of Medicine. Physician-in-Chief, City of Memphis Hospital, Memphis, Tennessee.

MORTON N. SWARTZ, M.D.

Bacterial Meningitis; Parameningeal Infections

Professor of Medicine, Harvard Medical School. Physician and Chief, Infectious Disease Unit, Massachusetts General Hospital, Boston, Massachusetts.

WILLIAM C. THOMAS, Jr., M.D.

Renal Calculi

Professor, Department of Medicine, College of Medicine, University of Florida. Associate Chief of Staff for Research, Veterans Administration Hospital, Gainesville, Florida.

C. CRAIG TISHER, M.D.

Renal Changes in Other Systemic Diseases

Professor of Medicine, Associate Professor of Pathology, Duke University Medical Center, Durham, North Carolina.

H. RICHARD TYLER, M.D.

Polymyositis and Dermatomyositis

Professor of Neurology, Harvard Medical School. Head, Section of Neurology, Peter Bent Brigham Hospital; Consultant in Neurology, Children's Hospital Medical Center, Beth Israel Hospital, Robert Breck Brigham Hospital, West Roxbury Veterans Administration Hospital, and Boston Lying-In Hospital, Boston, Massachusetts.

JOHN P. UTZ, M.D.

Actinomycosis; The Mycoses: Introduction; Histoplasmosis; Blastomycosis; Paracoccidioidomycosis; Maduromycosis; Chromomycosis; Sporotrichosis

Professor of Medicine, School of Medicine, Georgetown University, Washington, D.C.

NIEL WALD, M.D.

Radiation Injury

Professor and Chairman, Department of Radiation Health, Graduate School of Public Health, and Professor of Radiology, School of Medicine, University of Pittsburgh. Active Medical Staff (Radiology) and Director, Radiation Medicine Department, Presbyterian-University Hospital, Pittsburgh; Consultant Staff, University Health Center of Pittsburgh Hospitals, Pittsburgh, and Aliquippa Hospital, Aliquippa, Pennsylvania.

ANDREW G. WALLACE, M.D.

Approach to the Patient with Cardiovascular Disease

Professor of Medicine, Duke University Medical Center. Chief, Division of Cardiology, Duke University Medical Center, Durham, North Carolina.

JOHN H. WALSH, M.D.

Peptic Ulcer: Clinical and Endocrine Aspects

Professor of Medicine, UCLA School of Medicine. Deputy Director, Center for Ulcer Research and Education, Veterans Administration Wadsworth Hospital Center, Los Angeles, California.

KENNETH S. WARREN, M.D.

Schistosomiasis

Adjunct Professor, Rockefeller University; Professor of Medicine, New York University, New York, New York.

M. F. R. WATERS, M.A., M.B., F.R.C.P., F.R.C.Path.

Leprosy

Senior Lecturer, London School of Hygiene and Tropical Medicine. Consultant Leprologist, Hospital for Tropical Diseases, London, England. Member of the Senior Scientific Staff, British Medical Research Council.

LAWRENCE W. WAY, M.D.

Diseases of the Gallbladder and Bile Ducts

Professor of Surgery, University of California School of Medicine, San Francisco. Chief of Surgery, Ft. Miley Veterans Administration Hospital, San Francisco, California.

PAUL WEBB, M.D.

Disorders Due to Heat and Cold

Principal Associate, Webb Associates, Yellow Springs, Ohio.

ROBERT E. WHALEN, M.D.

Disorders of the Pericardium; Tumors of the Heart

Professor of Medicine, Duke University Medical Center. Director, Cardiovascular Disease Service, Duke University Medical Center, Durham, North Carolina.

CHARLES L. WISSEMAN, Jr., M.S., M.D.

Rickettsial Diseases: Introduction; The Typhus Group; Rocky Mountain Spotted Fever; Tick-Borne Rickettsioses of the Eastern Hemisphere; Rickettsialpox; Scrub Typhus

Professor and Chairman, Department of Microbiology, University of Maryland School of Medicine, Baltimore, Maryland.

SHELDON M. WOLFF, M.D.

Introduction to Microbial Diseases

Endicott Professor and Chairman, Department of Medicine, Tufts University School of Medicine. Physician-in-Chief, New England Medical Center Hospital; Adjunct Professor of International Health, Fletcher School of Law and Diplomacy, Tufts University, Boston, Massachusetts.

EMANUEL WOLINSKY, M.D.

Clostridial Diseases: Introduction; Clostridial Myonecrosis; Other Clostridial Diseases; Clostridial Gastroenteritis

Professor of Medicine, Case Western Reserve University School of Medicine. Director of Microbiology and Chief of Division of Infectious Diseases, Department of Medicine, Cleveland Metropolitan General Hospital, Cleveland, Ohio.

HARVEY WOLINSKY, M.D., Ph.D.

Atherosclerosis

Professor of Medicine and Pathology, The Albert Einstein College of Medicine. Attending Physician, Bronx Municipal Hospital Center, Bronx, New York.

THEODORE E. WOODWARD, M.D.

Tularemia

Professor of Medicine and Chairman of Department of Medicine, Physician-in-Chief, University of Maryland School of Medicine and Hospital, Baltimore, Maryland.

O. M. WRONG, D.M., F.R.C.P.

Glomerular Disease: Introduction; Nephrotic Syndrome; Glomerulonephritis; Renal Involvement in Connective Tissue Diseases; Hereditary Nephritis

Professor of Medicine, University College Hospital Medical School, University of London. Consulting Physician, University College Hospital, London, England.

JAMES B. WYNGAARDEN, M.D.

Biological Science and Medical Practice; Diseases of Metabolism: Introduction; Fabry's Disease; Alcaptonuria; Cystinuria; Homocystinuria; The Lesch-Nyhan Syndrome; 2,8-Dihydroxyadenine Renal Stones; Miscellaneous Diseases of Purine Metabolism; Normal Laboratory Values of Clinical Importance

Frederic M. Hanes Professor and Chairman, Department of Medicine, Duke University Medical Center, Durham, North Carolina.

MELVIN D. YAHR, M.D.

The Extrapyramidal Disorders: Introduction; The Parkinsonian Syndrome; Essential Tremor; Senile Tremor; The Choreas; Tics; Athetosis; Dystonia Musculorum Deformans; Spasmodic Torticollis; Hemiballism

Henry P. and Georgette Goldschmidt Professor of Neurology, Chairman, Department of Neurology, Mt. Sinai School of Medicine, City University of New York. Neurologist and Chief, Mt. Sinai Hospital; Director, Neurological Service, Mt. Sinai Medical Center, New York, New York.

NATHANIEL A. YOUNG, M.D.

Enteroviral Diseases

Head, Section of Viral Oncology and Molecular Pathology, Laboratory of Pathology, National Cancer Institute; Senior Attending Physician in Infectious Diseases, Clinical Center, National Institutes of Health and National Naval Medical Center, Bethesda, Maryland.

CONTENTS

PART I   The Nature of Medicine 1
PART II   Human Growth and Development 11
PART III   Genetic Principles 31
PART IV   Environmental Factors in Disease 60
PART V   Immune Disease 126
PART VI   Connective Tissue Diseases ("Collagen Diseases")
              Other Than Rheumatoid Arthritis 164
PART VII   Diseases of the Joints 184
PART VIII   Granulomatous Diseases of Unproved Etiology 209
PART IX   Microbial Diseases 227
PART X   Protozoan and Helminthic Diseases 565
PART XI   Disorders of the Nervous System and Behavior 639
PART XII   Respiratory Disease 931
PART XIII   Critical Care Medicine 1031
PART XIV   Cardiovascular Diseases 1059
PART XV   Renal Diseases 1316
PART XVI   Diseases of the Digestive System 1463
PART XVII   Diseases of Nutrition 1670
PART XVIII   Hematologic and Hematopoietic Diseases 1713
PART XIX   Medical Oncology 1898
PART XX   Diseases of Metabolism 1949
PART XXI   Diseases of the Endocrine System 2060
PART XXII   Diseases of Bone 2225
PART XXIII   Certain Cutaneous Diseases with Significant Systemic
              Manifestations 2266
PART XXIV   Diseases of the Eye 2313
PART XXV   Drug-Drug Interactions 2336
PART XXVI   Normal Laboratory Values of Clinical Importance 2342

              Index i

*(Detailed Table of Contents begins on the
following page)*

xxiii

VOLUME 1

Part I.   The Nature of Medicine

1.   On Becoming a Clinician, *Paul B. Beeson* 1
2.   Science, Clinical Medicine, and the Spectrum of Disease,
      Alvan R. Feinstein 3
3.   Biological Science and Medical Practice, *James B. Wyngaarden* 6
4.   Medicine in Modern Society, *Walsh McDermott* 8

Part II.   Human Growth and Development

5.   Heredity, *Alexander G. Bearn* 11
6.   Environment, *Howard H. Hiatt* 12
7.   The Life-Cycle Perspective in Medicine, *Herant A. Katchadourian* 16
8.   Development to Adulthood, *Herant A. Katchadourian* 17
      8.1.   Biologic Processes in Puberty 17
      8.2.   Psychosocial Development 20
9.   Adulthood, *Herant A. Katchadourian* 22
      9.1.   Introduction 22
      9.2.   Issues, Changes, and Stages 22
      9.3.   Crises of Adult Life 23
10.   Aging and Geriatric Medicine, *Ralph Goldman* 25
      10.1.   Introduction 25
      10.2.   Structural and Functional Changes with Age 25
      10.3.   The Gompertz Concept 27
      10.4.   Theories of Aging 28
      10.5.   Psychosocial Problems of the Aged 29
      10.6.   Special Problems of Management 29
      10.7.   The Physician's Responsibility 30

Part III.   Genetic Principles

11.   Introduction, *Alexander G. Bearn* 31
12.   Pedigree Analysis in Inherited Disease, *Alexander G. Bearn* 34
13.   Inborn Errors of Metabolism and Molecular Disease,
      Alexander G. Bearn 40
14.   Polygenic and Multifactorial Inheritance, *Alexander G. Bearn* 44
15.   Pharmacogenetics, *Alexander G. Bearn* 45
16.   Population Genetics, *Alexander G. Bearn* 46
17.   Congenital Malformations, *Alexander G. Bearn* 48
18.   Chromosomes and Their Disorders, *Park Gerald* 49
      18.1.   Introduction 49
      18.2.   Meiotic and Mitotic Nondisjunction 51
      18.3.   Changes in Chromosome Number 53
      18.4.   Changes in Chromosomal Structure 53
19.   Prevention and Management of Genetic Disease,
      Alexander G. Bearn 54
20.   Genetic Counseling, *Arno G. Motulsky* 56

Part IV.   Environmental Factors in Disease

21.   Chemical Contamination of Water and Air,
      Walsh McDermott 60
22.   Food Poisoning, *Harold P. Lambert* 64
      22.1.   Introduction 64
      22.2.   Bacterial Food Poisoning 64
      22.3.   Botulism 67
      22.4.   Poisonous Plants and Animals 68
      22.5.   Chemical Food Poisoning 70
23.   Common Accidental Poisoning, *Robert J. Haggerty* 71

24. Heavy Metal Poisoning, *Edmund B. Flink* 76
    24.1. Introduction 76
    24.2. Arsenic Poisoning.. 76
    24.3. Lead Poisoning 77
    24.4. Mercury Poisoning 80
    24.5. Antimony Poisoning.. 81
    24.6. Cadmium Poisoning 81
    24.7. Thallium Poisoning.. 82
25. Carbon Monoxide Poisoning, *Bertram D. Dinman*............................ 82
26. Disorders Due to Heat and Cold, *Paul Webb* 84
    26.1. Introduction 84
    26.2. Heat Stroke.. 84
    26.3. Heat Syncope 85
    26.4. Heat Exhaustion 85
    26.5. Hypothermia 85
27. Radiation Injury, *Niel Wald* 86
28. Electric Shock and Electric Injury, *Curtis P. Artz* 92
29. Motion Sickness and Problems of Air Travel, *Stanley R. Mohler*............ 94
    29.1. Motion Sickness... 94
    29.2. Problems of Air Travel... 95
30. Alterations in Atmospheric Pressure, *Jefferson C. Davis* 97
    30.1. Introduction 97
    30.2. Direct Effects of Changes in Atmospheric Pressure................. 98
    30.3. Indirect Effects of Changes in Atmospheric Pressure............... 99
31. Therapeutic Hyperbaric Oxygen, *Herbert A. Saltzman*...................... 103
32. Drowning, *Charles J. Stahl* 105
33. Arthropods as Environmental Agents of Disease, *Hugh L. Keegan*......... 108
    33.1. Introduction 108
    33.2. Pediculosis.. 108
    33.3. Flea-Bite.. 110
    33.4. Scabies 110
    33.5. Myiasis... 111
    33.6. Allergy to Arthropod Products 112
    33.7. Stings by Bees, Wasps, Hornets, and Ants...................... 113
    33.8. Blister Beetles... 114
    33.9. Spider Bite.. 114
    33.10. Scorpion Sting 116
    33.11. Centipedes and Millipedes 117
    33.12. Tick Paralysis 117
    33.13. Allergy to House-Dust Mites 118
    33.14. Dermatitis Caused by Caterpillars and Moths 118
34. Pentastomiasis (Porocephaliasis, Linguatuliasis),
    Hugh L. Keegan.. 119
35. Leeches as Agents of Disease (Hirudiniasis), *Hugh L. Keegan*............... 120
36. Snakebite, *Hugh L. Keegan*.. 121
37. Venomous Marine Animals, *Hugh L. Keegan* 123

Part V. Immune Disease

38. Introduction, *Henry G. Kunkel* 126
39. Complement, *Jeffrey A. Gelfand*.. 135
40. The Primary Immunodeficiency Diseases, *Robert A. Good*.................. 138
    40.1. Introduction 138
    40.2. X-Linked Infantile Agammaglobulinemia 139
    40.3. DiGeorge's Syndrome.. 140
    40.4. Severe Combined Immunodeficiencies (SCID, Swiss
           Type Immunodeficiency) 141
    40.5. Severe Combined Immunodeficiencies with
           Adenosine Deaminase Deficiency 141
    40.6. Thymoma with Immunodeficiency 142

40.7.   Common Variable Immunodeficiency..................................... 142
40.8.   Isolated Absence of Immunoglobulins—Selective
        Deficiency of IgA... 143
40.9.   Immunodeficiency Diseases with Ataxia
        Telangiectasia and Wiskott-Aldrich Syndrome........................ 143
40.10. Other Primary Immunodeficiencies 144
41. The Compromised Host, *John I. Gallin*................................. 145
42. Serum Sickness, *Fred S. Kantor*...................................... 153
43. Drug Allergy, *Fred S. Kantor*.. 154
44. Allergic Rhinitis (Hay Fever), *Fred S. Kantor*...................... 157
45. Vasomotor Rhinitis, *Fred S. Kantor* 160
46. Urticaria, *Fred S. Kantor*... 160
47. Angioedema (Angioneurotic Edema), *Fred S. Kantor*................... 162
48. Insect Stings, *Fred S. Kantor* 163

Part VI.   Connective Tissue Diseases ("Collagen Diseases") Other Than Rheumatoid Arthritis

49. Introduction, *K. Frank Austen* 164
50. Systemic Sclerosis (Scleroderma), *Edward D. Harris, Jr.*........... 168
51. Polymyositis and Dermatomyositis, *H. Richard Tyler* 171
52. Systemic Lupus Erythematosus, *Peter H. Schur* 174
53. Periarteritis Nodosa (Polyarteritis Nodosa), *K. Frank Austen*...... 180

Part VII.   Diseases of the Joints, *Charles L. Christian*

54. Introduction... 184
55. Arthritis Associated with Known Infectious Agents................... 185
    55.1.   Bacterial Arthritis... 185
    55.2.   Viral Arthritis... 186
    55.3.   Other Forms of Infectious Arthritis 186
56. Rheumatoid Arthritis 186
57. Variants of Rheumatoid Disease 193
    57.1.   Felty's Syndrome 193
    57.2.   Sjögren's Syndrome 193
58. Other Forms of Polyarthritis of Unknown Etiology 194
    58.1.   Ankylosing Spondylitis (Marie-Strümpell Spondylitis,
            von Bechterew's Syndrome, Rheumatoid Spondylitis)............. 194
    58.2.   Juvenile Rheumatoid Arthritis 195
    58.3.   Psoriatic Arthritis 196
    58.4.   Reiter's Syndrome 197
    58.5.   Palindromic Rheumatism 198
    58.6.   Intermittent Hydrarthrosis 198
59. Diseases with Which Arthritis Is Frequently Associated 198
60. Miscellaneous Forms of Arthritis 200
61. Degenerative Joint Disease (Osteoarthritis) 202
62. The Painful Shoulder.. 205
63. Nonarticular Rheumatism... 207

Part VIII.   Granulomatous Diseases of Unproved Etiology

64. Introduction, *Paul B. Beeson* 209
65. Sarcoidosis, *D. Geraint James* 209
66. Polymyalgia Rheumatica and Cranial Arteritis (Temporal
    Arteritis, Giant Cell Arteritis, Polymyalgia Arteritica),
    Paul B. Beeson.. 216
    66.1.   Introduction 216

66.2. Polymyalgia Rheumatica.................................... 217
66.3. Cranial Arteritis 217
67. Relapsing Polychondritis, *Paul B. Beeson* 218
68. Wegener's Granulomatosis, *Anthony S. Fauci*...................... 218
69. Midline Granuloma, *Anthony S. Fauci* 220
70. Weber-Christian Disease (Relapsing Febrile Nodular
Nonsuppurative Panniculitis, Panniculitis), *Paul B. Beeson*................. 221
71. Fibrosing Syndromes (Multifocal Fibrosclerosis), *Paul B. Beeson* 222
71.1. Introduction 222
71.2. Retroperitoneal Fibrosis (Periureteral Fibrosis) 223
71.3. Mediastinal Fibrosis..................................... 224
71.4. Sclerosing Cholangitis 224
71.5. Fibrosclerosis in Other Organs 224
71.6. Practolol Peritonitis 224
72. Eosinophilic Syndromes, *Paul B. Beeson* 225
72.1. Introduction 225
72.2. Eosinophilic Pulmonary Syndromes 225
72.3. Eosinophilic Syndromes Affecting Other Organ Systems........... 225
72.4. Diseases in Which Eosinophilia Occurs Occasionally 226

Part IX. Microbial Diseases

73. The Nature of Microbial Diseases, *Walsh McDermott*...................... 227
74. Introduction to Microbial Diseases, *Sheldon M. Wolff* 227

SECTION ONE. VIRAL DISEASES, 229

75. Introduction to Viral Diseases, *Edwin D. Kilbourne* 229

Viral Infections of the Respiratory Tract, 230

76. The Common Cold (Acute Coryza), *George Gee Jackson*.................... 230
77. Rhinoviral Respiratory Disease, *George Gee Jackson* 234
78. Viral Pharyngitis, Laryngitis, Croup, and Bronchitis,
George Gee Jackson.. 235
79. Adenoviral Infections, *George Gee Jackson*........................... 236
80. Respiratory Syncytial Viral Disease, *George Gee Jackson* 238
81. Parainfluenza Viral Diseases (Croup), *George Gee Jackson*................. 239
82. Influenza, *Edwin D. Kilbourne* 240

Viral Diseases Characterized by Cutaneous Lesions, 246

83. Measles (Morbilli, Rubeola), *Edwin D. Kilbourne*..................... 246
84. Rubella (German Measles), *Edwin D. Kilbourne* 250
85. Varicella (Chickenpox), *Sidney Kibrick* 253
86. Variola and Vaccinia, *C. Henry Kempe* 255
86.1. Introduction and History 255
86.2. Variola (Smallpox)..................................... 255
86.3. Vaccinia (Vaccination) 259
87. Foot-and-Mouth Disease (Aphthous Fever), *Walsh McDermott* 261
88. Mumps, *Dorothy M. Horstmann* 261

Viral Disease of Lymphoid Tissue, 264

89. Infectious Mononucleosis, *James C. Niederman*................................ 264

Enteroviral Diseases, *Nathaniel A. Young*, 268

90. Introduction... 268
91. Paralysis and Other Neurologic Complications of Nonpolio
Enteroviral Infections 270
92. Herpangina 270
93. Epidemic Pleurodynia (Bornholm Disease, Epidemic
Myalgia, Devil's Grip, Sylvest's Disease) 271

94. Pericarditis and Myocarditis Caused by Enteroviruses 272
95. Exanthems Caused by Enteroviruses... 274
96. Acute Hemorrhagic Conjunctivitis... 274
97. Diarrhea Associated with Coxsackie- and Echoviruses........................ 275
98. Respiratory Illness Due to Enteroviruses.. 275

Arthropod-Borne Viral Fevers, Viral Encephalitides, and Viral Hemorrhagic Fevers (Arboviruses and Arenaviruses), 276

 99. Introduction, *Karl M. Johnson*... 276
100. Undifferentiated Fevers 277
      100.1. Dengue, *Karl M. Johnson*... 277
      100.2. West Nile Fever, *Karl M. Johnson*..................................... 278
      100.3. Fevers Caused by Group A Arboviruses:
              Chikungunya, O'nyong-nyong, Mayaro, and
              Ross River, *Karl M. Johnson* 279
      100.4. Colorado Tick Fever, *Theodore C. Eickhoff* 280
      100.5. Rift Valley Fever, *Karl M. Johnson* 281
      100.6. Sandfly Fever, *Karl M. Johnson* 282
101. Arthropod-Borne Viral Encephalitides, *Karl M. Johnson*...................... 283
      101.1. Introduction 283
      101.2. Western Equine Encephalitis 284
      101.3. Eastern Equine Encephalitis 285
      101.4. Venezuelan Equine Encephalitis 286
      101.5. California Encephalitis 288
      101.6. St. Louis Encephalitis 288
      101.7. Japanese B Encephalitis... 289
      101.8. Murray Valley Encephalitis 290
      101.9. Tick-Borne Group B Arbovirus Diseases: Russian
              Spring-Summer Encephalitis, Louping Ill, Kyasanur
              Forest Disease, Omsk Hemorrhagic Fever 290
102. Viral Hemorrhagic Fevers... 292
      102.1. Introduction, *Karl M. Johnson* 292
      102.2. Yellow Fever, *Thomas P. Monath* 292
      102.3. Hemorrhagic Fever Caused by Dengue Viruses,
              Karl M. Johnson 296
      102.4. Crimean Hemorrhagic Fever, *Karl M. Johnson* 298
      102.5. Hemorrhagic Diseases Caused by Arenaviruses:
              Argentine and Bolivian Hemorrhagic Fevers and
              Lassa Fever, *Karl M. Johnson* 298
      102.6. African Hemorrhagic Fever (Marburg Disease),
              Karl M. Johnson 300
      102.7. Epidemic Hemorrhagic Fever: Hemorrhagic
              Nephrosonephritis, *Karl M. Johnson* 301

Viral Diseases (Presumptive), 302

103. Cat Scratch Disease (Benign Nonbacterial Regional
      Lymphadenitis, Inoculation Lymphoreticulosis),
      Andrew M. Margileth 302
104. Viral Gastroenteritis Caused by Norwalk-Like Agents and
      Rotaviruses (Acute Infectious Nonbacterial Gastroenteritis,
      Epidemic Diarrhea, Winter Vomiting Disease), *Raphael Dolin* 305
105. Epidemic Neuromyasthenia (Iceland Disease, Benign
      Myalgic Encephalomyelitis), *Paul B. Beeson* 307

SECTION TWO. BACTERIAL DISEASES, 307

106. Introduction, *Walsh McDermott*.. 307

Rickettsial Diseases, 309

107. Introduction, *Charles L. Wisseman, Jr.* 309

108. The Typhus Group, *Charles L. Wisseman, Jr.*.. 318
    108.1. Epidemic Louse-Borne Typhus Fever (Classic, Historic, European Typhus; Jail, War, Camp, Ship Fever; Fleckfieber; Typhus Exanthématique; Tifus Exantemático, Tabardillo; Dermotypho)............................... 318
    108.2. Brill-Zinsser Disease (Recrudescent Typhus)........................ 320
    108.3. Murine or Flea-Borne Typhus Fever 320
109. Rocky Mountain Spotted Fever (Spotted Fever, Tick Typhus, Fiebre Manchada, Fiebre Petequial, Febre Maculosa, São Paulo Typhus), *Charles L. Wisseman, Jr.* 322
110. Tick-Borne Rickettsioses of the Eastern Hemisphere, *Charles L. Wisseman, Jr.* 324
111. Rickettsialpox, *Charles L. Wisseman, Jr.*... 326
112. Scrub Typhus (Chigger-Borne Rickettsiosis, Tsutsugamushi Disease, Japanese River or Flood Fever, Mite-Borne Typhus, Tropical Typhus, Rural Typhus, Mossman Fever), *Charles L. Wisseman, Jr.* 327
113. Trench Fever (Five-Day or Quintana Fever, Shin Bone Fever, Volhynian Fever), *Herbert L. Ley, Jr.* 329
114. Q Fever, *Herbert L. Ley, Jr.* 329
115. Bartonellosis (Carrión's Disease, Oroya Fever, Verruga Peruana), *Herbert L. Ley, Jr.*... 331

Diseases Caused by Chlamydiae, 332
116. Trachoma and Inclusion Conjunctivitis, *Ernest Jawetz*........................ 332
117. Lymphogranuloma Venereum, *Ernest Jawetz* 335
118. Psittacosis (Ornithosis, Parrot Fever), *William Schaffner*..................... 336

Pneumonia, 338
119. Introduction to Pneumonia, *Herbert Y. Reynolds* 338
120. Mycoplasmal Diseases, *Robert B. Couch*.. 343
    120.1. Introduction 343
    120.2. Pneumonia and Other Respiratory Diseases Caused by *M. pneumoniae*....................................... 343
    120.3. Mycoplasmas in Genitourinary Disease............................... 346
121. Pneumococcal Pneumonia, *Edward W. Hook* 347
122. Pneumonia Due to *Klebsiella pneumoniae* (Friedländer's Pneumonia), *Herbert Y. Reynolds*.............................. 357
123. Legionnaires' Disease, *Herbert Y. Reynolds*.................................... 359
124. Pneumonia and Nosocomial Respiratory Infections Caused by Aerobic Gram-Negative Bacilli (*Pseudomonas, Escherichia coli,* and *Serratia*), *Herbert Y. Reynolds* 361

Streptococcal Diseases, 366
125. Introduction, *Gene H. Stollerman* 366
126. Group A Streptococcal Infection, *Gene H. Stollerman* 367
127. Clinical Syndromes of Group A Streptococcal Infection, *Gene H. Stollerman* 371
    127.1. Streptococcal Sore Throat.. 371
    127.2. Streptococcal Skin Infections 374
    127.3. Hemolytic Streptococcal Pneumonia.................................. 375
128. Treatment of Group A Streptococcal Infection and Chemoprophylaxis of Nonsuppurative Complications, *Gene H. Stollerman* 375
129. Prophylaxis of Streptococcal Infection, *Gene H. Stollerman* 376
130. Rheumatic Fever, *Richard M. Krause*... 377

Endocarditis, 386
131. Infective Endocarditis, *Donald Kaye*.. 386

Staphylococcal Infections, F. Robert Fekety, Jr., 396

  132. Introduction 396
  133. Cutaneous Staphylococcal Infections 399
       133.1. Furuncles 399
       133.2. Carbuncles 400
       133.3. Impetigo 400
       133.4. The Scalded Skin Syndrome 400
       133.5. Treatment of Cutaneous Infections 400
       133.6. Prevention of Cutaneous Infections 401
  134. Staphylococcal Pneumonia 401
  135. Staphylococcal Osteomyelitis 402
  136. Staphylococcal Bacteremia and Endocarditis 403
  137. Miscellaneous Infections 404
  138. Staphylococcal Gastroenteritis and Enterocolitis 404

Diseases Caused by Neisseria, 405

  139. Gonococcal Disease, *Donald Kaye* 405

Bacterial Meningitis, 411

  140. Bacterial Meningitis, *Morton N. Swartz* 411
  141. Meningococcal Disease, *Harry A. Feldman* 417
  142. *Hemophilus* Infections with Special Emphasis on
        Hemophilus influenzae Type b, *John B. Robbins* 423

Whooping Cough, 426

  143. Whooping Cough (Pertussis), *Stephen I. Morse* 426

Granuloma Inguinale, 429

  144. Granuloma Inguinale, *Walsh McDermott* 429

Diphtheria, 429

  145. Diphtheria, *Heonir Rocha* 429

Clostridial Diseases, 433

  146. Introduction, *Emanuel Wolinsky* 433
  147. Clostridial Myonecrosis (Gas Gangrene), *Emanuel Wolinsky* 433
  148. Other Clostridial Diseases, *Emanuel Wolinsky* 436
  149. Clostridial Gastroenteritis, *Emanuel Wolinsky* 436
  150. Tetanus, *John H. Kerr* 436

Anaerobic Bacteria, 441

  151. Disease Due to Nonsporeforming Anaerobic Bacteria,
        Sydney M. Finegold 441

Typhoid Fever and Salmonellosis, 446

  152. Typhoid Fever, *Sherwood L. Gorbach* 446
  153. *Salmonella* Infections Other Than Typhoid Fever,
        Edward W. Hook 449

Other Bacterial Infections, 453

  154. Enteric Bacterial Infections, *Calvin M. Kunin* 453
  155. Shigellosis, *Charles C. J. Carpenter* 457
  156. Cholera (Asiatic Cholera), *Charles C. J. Carpenter* 460
  157. Plague, *Jay P. Sanford* 463
  158. Tularemia, *Theodore E. Woodward* 465
  159. Diseases Caused by *Malleomyces, Leighton E. Cluff* 468
       159.1. Glanders (Farcy) 468
       159.2. Melioidosis 469

160. Anthrax, *Leighton E. Cluff* 470
161. Listeriosis, *Leighton E. Cluff* 471
162. Erysipeloid of Rosenbach, *Leighton E. Cluff* 473
163. Actinomycosis, *John P. Utz* 473
164. Nocardiosis, *John E. Bennett* 474
165. Brucellosis, *Thomas M. Buchanan* 475

Diseases Due to Mycobacteria, 479

166. Tuberculosis, *Roger Des Prez* 479
167. Pulmonary Tuberculosis, *Robert A. Goodwin, Jr.* 484
168. Extrapulmonary Tuberculosis, *Roger Des Prez* 491
    168.1. Introduction 491
    168.2. Principles of Drug Therapy 491
    168.3. Tuberculosis of the Pleura 491
    168.4. Endobronchial Tuberculosis 491
    168.5. Tuberculosis of the Larynx 491
    168.6. Gastrointestinal Tuberculosis 492
    168.7. Miliary Tuberculosis 492
    168.8. Tuberculous Meningitis 493
    168.9. Tuberculomas 494
    168.10. Tuberculous Pericarditis 494
    168.11. Tuberculous Peritonitis 495
    168.12. Tuberculous Lymphadenitis 495
    168.13. Genitourinary Tuberculosis 496
    168.14. Tuberculosis of Bones and Joints 496
    168.15. Rare Forms of Tuberculosis 498
169. Diseases Due to Mycobacteria Other Than
    M. tuberculosis and *M. leprae, Robert A. Goodwin, Jr.* ... 498
170. Leprosy (Hansen's Disease), *M. F. R. Waters* 501

Treponemal Diseases, 505

171. Syphilis, *P. Frederick Sparling* 505
172. Nonsyphilitic Treponematoses, *Thorstein Guthe* 518
    172.1. Yaws (Frambesia Tropica, Pian, Bouba, Parangi, Patek) 518
    172.2. Bejel (Endemic Syphilis, Nonvenereal Childhood
        Syphilis, Belesh, Dichuchwa, Njovera, Skerljevo) 522
    172.3. Pinta (Mal del Pinto, Carate) 524

Spirillary and Leptospiral Diseases, 526

173. Relapsing Fever, *Anthony D. M. Bryceson* 526
    173.1. Introduction 526
    173.2. Louse-Borne Relapsing Fever (Yellow Plague,
        Yellow Famine Fever, Vagabond Fever, Bilious
        Typhoid, Recurrent Fever) 526
    173.3. Tick-Borne Relapsing Fever (Tick Fever) 529
174. Tropical Phagedenic Ulcer, *Anthony D. M. Bryceson* 530
175. Rat-Bite Fever, *Jay P. Sanford* 531
176. Leptospirosis, *Jay P. Sanford* 532

SECTION THREE. THE MYCOSES, 535

177. Introduction, *John P. Utz* 535
178. Histoplasmosis, *John P. Utz* 536
179. Coccidioidomycosis (Valley Fever), *Demosthenes Pappagianis* 537
180. Blastomycosis (North American), *John P. Utz* 540
181. Paracoccidioidomycosis (South American Blastomycosis),
    John P. Utz 541
182. Maduromycosis (Mycetoma, Madura Foot), *John P. Utz* 542
183. Chromomycosis, *John P. Utz* 542
184. Cryptococcosis (European Blastomycosis, Torulosis),
    John E. Bennett 543

185. Sporotrichosis, *John P. Utz* 544
186. Mucormycosis, *John E. Bennett* 545
187. Aspergillosis, *John E. Bennett* 546
188. Candidiasis (Candidosis, Moniliasis, Thrush), *John E. Bennett* 547

SECTION FOUR. CHEMOTHERAPY OF MICROBIAL DISEASE, 549

189. Drugs and Microbes, *Walsh McDermott* 549
190. Antimicrobial Therapy, *Richard B. Roberts* 553

Part X. Protozoan and Helminthic Diseases

191. Introduction, *Philip D. Marsden* 565

SECTION ONE. PROTOZOAN DISEASES, 566

192. Introduction, *Philip D. Marsden* 566
193. Malaria, *Thomas C. Jones* 566
194. Trypanosomiases 575
      194.1. Introduction, *Philip D. Marsden* 575
      194.2. African Trypanosomiasis (Sleeping Sickness),
              B. M. Greenwood 576
      194.3. Chagas' Disease (American Trypanosomiasis),
              Vanize Macedo 579
195. Leishmaniasis, *Anthony D. M. Bryceson* 583
      195.1. Introduction 583
      195.2. Visceral Leishmaniasis (Kala-Azar, Ponos) 584
      195.3. Cutaneous Leishmaniasis of the Old World
              (Oriental Sore) 587
      195.4. Cutaneous Leishmaniasis of the New World (Including
              American Mucocutaneous Leishmaniasis or Espundia) 589
196. Amebiasis, *Richard Knight* 589
197. Toxoplasmosis, *Thomas C. Jones* 594
198. Pneumocystosis, *Thomas C. Jones* 598
199. Babesiosis (Babesiasis, Piroplasmosis), *Thomas C. Jones* 600
200. Other Protozoan Diseases 602
      200.1. Introduction, *Philip D. Marsden* 602
      200.2. Giardiasis, *Philip D. Marsden* 602
      200.3. Trichomoniasis, *Thomas C. Jones* 602
      200.4. Balantidiasis, *Philip D. Marsden* 603
      200.5. Primary Amebic Meningoencephalitis, *Philip D. Marsden* 603
      200.6. Isosporiasis (Coccidiosis), *Philip D. Marsden* 604
      200.7. Sarcosporidiosis, *Philip D. Marsden* 604

SECTION TWO. HELMINTHIC DISEASES, 605

201. Introduction, *Philip D. Marsden* 605

The Cestodes (Tapeworms), Philip D. Marsden, 606

202. Introduction 606
203. *Diphyllobothrium latum* (The Fish Tapeworm) 607
204. *Taenia saginata* (The Beef Tapeworm) 607
205. *Taenia solium* (The Pork Tapeworm Causing Human
      Cysticercosis Due to *Cysticercus cellulosae*) 608
206. Treatment of Infections with Adults of the Fish, Beef,
      and Pork Tapeworm 608
207. *Hymenolepis nana* (Dwarf Tapeworm) 609
208. Echinococcosis (Hydatid Disease) 609
209. Other Tapeworms 610

Diseases Caused by Trematodes (Flukes), 611

210. Schistosomiasis (Bilharziasis), *Kenneth S. Warren* 611
211. Hermaphroditic Flukes, *Philip D. Marsden* 617
    211.1. Introduction 617
    211.2. Hepatic Hermaphroditic Flukes 617
    211.3. Lung Hermaphroditic Flukes (Paragonimiasis) 619
    211.4. Intestinal Hermaphroditic Flukes 620

The Nematodes (Roundworms), Philip D. Marsden, 621

212. Introduction 621
213. Intestinal Nematodes 622
    213.1. Strongyloidiasis (Cochin-China Diarrhea) 622
    213.2. Capillariasis 623
    213.3. Hookworm Disease (Ancylostomiasis, Miner's Anemia) 624
    213.4. Cutaneous Larva Migrans (Creeping Eruption) 625
    213.5. Trichostrongyliasis 626
    213.6. Gnathostomiasis 626
    213.7. Oesophagostomiasis 626
    213.8. Ascariasis 626
    213.9. Toxocariasis (Visceral Larva Migrans) 627
    213.10. Anisakiasis 628
    213.11. Trichuriasis (Whipworm Infection, Trichocephaliasis) 628
    213.12. Enterobiasis (Oxyuriasis, Pinworm or Seatworm
        Infection) 629
214. Tissue Nematodes 630
    214.1. Trichinosis (Trichiniasis, Trichinellosis) 630
    214.2. Angiostrongyliasis 631
    214.3. Filariasis 632

Disorders with Some Relation to Helminths, Philip D. Marsden, 638

215. Eosinophilia in Relation to Helminthic Infections 638
216. Tropical Pyomyositis 638

Part XI. Disorders of the Nervous System and Behavior

217. Introduction, *Fred Plum* 639

SECTION ONE. CONSCIOUSNESS AND ITS DISTURBANCES, 640

218. Introduction, *Fred Plum* 640
219. The Pathogenesis of Stupor and Coma, *Fred Plum* 640
220. Delirium and Exogenous Metabolic Brain Disease,
    Jerome B. Posner 644
221. Sleep and Its Disorders, *William R. Shapiro* 651

SECTION TWO. FOCAL DISTURBANCES OF HIGHER NERVOUS
                FUNCTION, *Norman Geschwind*, 656

222. Language, Aphasia, and Related Disorders 656
223. Aphasia 656
224. Other Disorders of the Higher Functions 658
225. Memory 658

SECTION THREE. DEMENTIA, *Paul R. McHugh*, 660

226. Introduction 660
227. Alzheimer's Disease 661
228. Pick's Disease 662
229. Creutzfeldt-Jakob Disease 663

230. Huntington's Chorea 663
231. Treatment of the Demented Patient 663

SECTION FOUR. PSYCHOLOGIC ILLNESS IN MEDICAL
                        PRACTICE, *Paul R. McHugh*, 664

232. The Concept of Disease in Psychiatry... 664
233. Functional Psychoses 665
    233.1. Introduction 665
    233.2. Schizophrenia 665
    233.3. Manic-Depressive Psychosis 669
234. Personality Disorders and Neurotic Symptoms 672
    234.1. Introduction 672
    234.2. Anxiety 673
    234.3. Depression 675
    234.4. Hysteria... 678

SECTION FIVE. PSYCHOLOGIC TESTING IN CLINICAL
                        MEDICINE, *Paul R. McHugh*, 681

235. Introduction.. 681
236. Intelligence 681
237. Personality 682

SECTION SIX. MEDICAL ASPECTS OF SEXUALITY, *Harold I. Lief*, 684

238. The Physician's Role... 684
239. Sexuality... 686
240. Classification of Sexual Dysfunctions.. 687
241. Additional Problem Areas 689
242. Homosexuality 691

SECTION SEVEN. DRUG ABUSE, DEPENDENCE, AND INTOXICATION, 692

243. Introduction, *Robert B. Millman* 692
244. The Opiates, *Robert B. Millman* 694
245. Central Nervous System Depressants, *Robert B. Millman*.................. 698
246. Central Nervous System Stimulants, *Robert B. Millman* 701
247. Cannabis (Marijuana and Hashish), *Robert B. Millman* 702
248. Psychedelics, *Robert B. Millman*.. 703
249. Miscellaneous Inhalants, *Robert B. Millman* 705
250. Alcohol Abuse and Alcohol-Related Illness, *Jack H. Mendelson* 705
251. Acute Drug Poisoning, *Fred Plum*... 711

SECTION EIGHT. THE HYPOTHALAMUS AND NEUROLOGIC
                        DISORDERS, *Fred Plum*, 715

252. Introduction.. 715
253. Functional Anatomy.. 715
254. Sleep and Arousal.. 715
255. Memory and Emotion.. 716
256. Heat Regulation 716
257. Sympathetic and Parasympathetic Functions 717
258. Feeding Behavior and Caloric Balance 717
259. Water Balance.. 718

SECTION NINE. PROMINENT NEUROLOGIC SYMPTOMS AND
                        THEIR MANAGEMENT, 720

260. Pain, *Jerome B. Posner*... 720
261. Headache, *Fred Plum*... 728
262. Hearing Loss, *Robert W. Baloh* 734
263. Dizziness and Vertigo, *David A. Drachman* 737

264. Syncope, *Albert Heyman* 742
265. Hyperventilation, *Albert Heyman* 745

SECTION TEN.   NEUROLOGIC DIAGNOSTIC PROCEDURES,
            Kathleen M. Foley, 746

266. Introduction 746
267. Computerized Transaxial Tomography (CT Scan, CAT) 747
268. Lumbar Puncture 747
269. Conventional Roentgenography 748
270. The Radionuclide Brain Scan 748
271. Electroencephalography 749
272. Selected Neurodiagnostic Procedures 749

SECTION ELEVEN.   THE EXTRAPYRAMIDAL DISORDERS, 750

273. Introduction, *Melvin D. Yahr* 750
274. The Parkinsonian Syndrome (Paralysis Agitans, Shaking
     Palsy), *Melvin D. Yahr* 752
     274.1.   Introduction 752
     274.2.   Paralysis Agitans (Parkinson's Disease) 752
     274.3.   Secondary or Symptomatic Parkinsonism 753
     274.4.   Management of the Parkinsonian Syndrome 754
275. Essential Tremor (Familial Tremor), *Melvin D. Yahr* 756
276. Senile Tremor, *Melvin D. Yahr* 757
277. The Choreas, *Melvin D. Yahr* 757
     277.1.   Introduction 757
     277.2.   Acute Chorea (Sydenham's or Infectious Chorea,
            St. Vitus' Dance) 757
     277.3.   Hereditary Chorea (Chronic Progressive Chorea,
            Huntington's Disease) 758
     277.4.   Senile Chorea 759
278. Other Extrapyramidal Disorders 759
     278.1.   Tics (Habit Spasms), *Melvin D. Yahr* 759
     278.2.   Athetosis (Mobile Spasms), *Melvin D. Yahr* 760
     278.3.   Dystonia Musculorum Deformans (Torsion Dystonia),
            Melvin D. Yahr 760
     278.4.   Spasmodic Torticollis, *Melvin D. Yahr* 761
     278.5.   Hemiballism, *Melvin D. Yahr* 762
     278.6.   Idiopathic Autonomic Insufficiency (Idiopathic
            Orthostatic Hypotension, Shy-Drager Syndrome),
            Ira B. Black 762

SECTION TWELVE.   INHERITED DEGENERATIVE DISEASES OF
                THE NERVOUS SYSTEM, *Roger N. Rosenberg*, 764

279. Introduction 764
280. Striatonigral Degeneration 764
281. Motor Neuron Diseases 765
     281.1.   Introduction 765
     281.2.   Amyotrophic Lateral Sclerosis 765
     281.3.   Werdnig-Hoffmann Disease 766
     281.4.   Wohlfart-Kugelberg-Welander Disease 766
282. Spinocerebellar Degenerations 766
     282.1.   Introduction 766
     282.2.   Friedreich's Ataxia 767
     282.3.   Olivopontocerebellar Degenerations 768
283. Syringomyelia 768
284. The Phakomatoses or Neurocutaneous Syndromes 769
     284.1.   Neurofibromatosis (Von Recklinghausen's Disease) 769
     284.2.   Tuberous Sclerosis (Bourneville's Disease) 770

284.3.   Sturge-Weber Disease 771
284.4.   Hippel-Lindau Disease 771
284.5.   Ataxia Telangiectasia 771

SECTION THIRTEEN.   NUTRITIONAL DISORDERS OF THE
                    NERVOUS SYSTEM, *Pierre M. Dreyfus*, 772

285.   Introduction 772
286.   Nutritional Polyneuropathy (Dry Beriberi, Alcoholic Neuropathy) 772
287.   Wernicke-Korsakoff Syndrome 773
288.   Nutritional Amblyopia (Tobacco-Alcohol Amblyopia,
       Nutritional Retrobulbar Neuropathy) 774
289.   Cerebellar Cortical Degeneration 775
290.   Central Pontine Myelinolysis 775
291.   Marchiafava-Bignami Disease 776
292.   Vitamin B_{12} Deficiency 776

SECTION FOURTEEN.   CEREBROVASCULAR DISEASES,
                    Fletcher H. McDowell, 777

293.   Introduction 777
294.   Cerebral Ischemia and Infarction 778
295.   Intracranial Hemorrhage 794

SECTION FIFTEEN.   INFECTIONS AND INFLAMMATORY DISEASES
                   OF THE CENTRAL NERVOUS SYSTEM AND
                   ITS COVERINGS, 802

296.   Introduction, *Philip R. Dodge* 802
297.   Aids to Diagnosis in Intracranial and Intraspinal Inflammatory
       Disease, *Philip R. Dodge* 802
298.   Parameningeal Infections, *Morton N. Swartz* 804
299.   Spinal Epidural Infections, *Philip R. Dodge* 810
309.   Transverse Myelitis or Myelopathy, *Philip R. Dodge* 811
301.   Syphilitic Infections of the Central Nervous System, *Philip R. Dodge* 812

SECTION SIXTEEN.   VIRAL INFECTIONS OF THE NERVOUS SYSTEM, 816

302.   Introduction, *Richard T. Johnson* 816
303.   Viral Meningitis and Encephalitis, *Richard T. Johnson* 817
304.   Herpes Simplex Encephalitis, *J. Richard Baringer* 821
305.   Herpes Zoster, *Richard T. Johnson* 824
306.   Cytomegalovirus Infections, *James B. Hanshaw* 827
307.   Acute Anterior Poliomyelitis, *Fred Plum* 829
308.   Rabies (Hydrophobia, Lyssa), *Hilary Koprowski* 833
309.   Encephalitic Complications of Viral Infections and
       Vaccines, *Donald Silberberg* 836
       309.1.   Introduction 836
       309.2.   Acute Disseminated Encephalomyelitis 836
       309.3.   Neuroparalytic Accidents Following Antirabies Vaccination 838
       309.4.   Reye's Syndrome 839
310.   Slow Infections of the Nervous System, *Richard T. Johnson* 839
       310.1.   Introduction 839
       310.2.   Kuru 840
       310.3.   Creutzfeldt-Jakob Disease 840
       310.4.   Subacute Sclerosing Panencephalitis (Dawson's
                Encephalitis, Subacute Inclusion Body Encephalitis) 841
       310.5.   Progressive Multifocal Leukoencephalopathy 841
       310.6.   Other Neurologic Diseases 842

SECTION SEVENTEEN.   THE DEMYELINATING DISEASES,
                     Labe C. Scheinberg, 843

311.   Introduction 843

312. Multiple Sclerosis 845
313. Possible Multiple Sclerosis Variants.................................... 848
314. Leukodystrophies 850

SECTION EIGHTEEN. THE EPILEPSIES, 851

315. The Epilepsies, *Gilbert H. Glaser* 851

SECTION NINETEEN. INTRACRANIAL TUMORS AND STATES
CAUSING INCREASED INTRACRANIAL
PRESSURE, *Robert A. Fishman*, 863

316. Intracranial Tumors 863
317. Radiation Injury of the Nervous System............................. 869
318. Benign Intracranial Hypertension (Pseudotumor Cerebri) 870
319. Intracranial Hypotension.. 873
320. Hydrocephalus.. 873
321. Anomalies of the Craniovertebral Junction, Spine, and Meninges 874

SECTION TWENTY. NONMETASTATIC EFFECTS OF CANCER ON
THE NERVOUS SYSTEM, *Jerome B. Posner*, 876

322. Introduction.. 876
323. Brain and Cranial Nerves 876
324. Spinal Cord 878
325. Peripheral Nerves.. 878
326. Neuromuscular Junction and Muscles 879
327. Muscle Weakness 879

SECTION TWENTY-ONE. INJURIES OF THE HEAD AND SPINE,
Russel H. Patterson, Jr., 879

328. Injuries of the Head... 879
329. Injuries of the Spine.. 885
330. Severe Spinal Cord Dysfunction and Paraplegia.................. 886

SECTION TWENTY-TWO. MECHANICAL LESIONS OF THE NERVE
ROOTS AND SPINAL CORD, *Albert J. Aguayo*, 889

331. Symptoms of Nerve Root and Spinal Cord Compression...... 889
332. Laboratory Aids to Investigation....................................... 892
333. Management of Patients with Suspected Nerve Root or
Spinal Cord Compression.. 893
334. Specific Disorders That Cause Nerve Root or Spinal Cord
Compression.. 893
   334.1. Intervertebral Disc Protrusion 893
   334.2. Myelopathy and Nerve Root Compression Due
   to Spondylosis,... 894
   334.3. Spinal Cord Tumors... 896
   334.4. Spinal Arachnoiditis... 897
   334.5. Arteriovenous Malformations and Other Vascular
   Lesions of the Spinal Cord.................................... 897
   334.6. Spinal Epidural Hematoma.................................... 898

SECTION TWENTY-THREE. DISEASES OF THE PERIPHERAL
NERVOUS SYSTEM, *Peter James Dyck*, 899

335. Definition of Peripheral Neuropathy 899
336. Mononeuropathies and Plexus Neuropathies 899
   336.1. Cranial Nerves.. 899
   336.2. Mononeuropathy 900
   336.3. Multiple Mononeuropathy..................................... 902
   336.4. Plexus Neuropathies 902
337. Polyneuropathy 903

337.1. Differential Diagnosis of Peripheral Neuropathy 903
337.2. Neuropathy Associated with Infection 905
337.3. Neuropathy Associated with Inflammation and
        Presumed Altered Immunity... 906
337.4. Acute Inflammatory Polyradiculoneuropathies.......................... 906
337.5. Chronic Inflammatory Polyradiculoneuropathy
        (Including Recurrent Polyradiculoneuropathy)......................... 908
337.6. Sarcoid Neuropathy... 908
337.7. Neuropathy Associated with Mesenchymal Disease
        and Necrotizing Angiopathy... 908
337.8. Neuropathy Associated with Diabetes Mellitus 908
337.9. Neuropathy Associated with Uremia 909
337.10. Neuropathy Associated with Hepatic Disease 909
337.11. Neuropathy Associated with Endocrine Diseases.................... 909
337.12. Amyloidosis 910
337.13. Neuropathy Associated with Carcinoma and Other
        Malignancy.. 910
337.14. Neuropathy Associated with the Use of Drugs....................... 910
337.15. Neuropathy Associated with Household and
        Industrial Poisons... 910
337.16. Inherited Disorders of Peripheral Neurons 911
337.17. Disorders of Peripheral Sensory Neurons............................ 911
337.18. Inherited Disorders of Peripheral Motor, Sensory,
        and Autonomic Neurons.. 912

SECTION TWENTY-FOUR.   DISEASES OF MUSCLE AND
                       NEUROMUSCULAR JUNCTION, *Lewis P. Rowland,* 914

338.   Introduction.. 914
339.   Inherited Diseases 915
       339.1.   Muscular Dystrophies 915
       339.2.   Other Inherited Biochemical Disorders 919
       339.3.   Congenital Myopathies... 919
       339.4.   Myotonia Congenita (Thomsen's Disease) 920
       339.5.   Familial Myoglobinuria... 920
       339.6.   Familial Periodic Paralysis....................................... 921
       339.7.   Myositis Ossificans 922
340.   Sporadic Disorders 923
       340.1.   The Problem Presented by Dermatomyositis and
                Polymyositis.. 923
       340.2.   Other Acquired Myopathies....................................... 923
       340.3.   Sporadic Myoglobinuria... 924
       340.4.   Myasthenia Gravis 925
       340.5.   Eaton-Lambert Syndrome (Myasthenic Syndrome)................... 929
       340.6.   Unusual Causes of Neuromuscular Block.......................... 929
       340.7.   Syndromes of Muscular Overactivity: Cramps and
                Related Disorders... 930

Part XII.   Respiratory Disease

341.   Introduction, *John F. Murray* 931
342.   Respiratory Structure and Function, *John F. Murray*.................... 931
       342.1.   Introduction 931
       342.2.   Ventilation 932
       342.3.   Diffusion... 936
       342.4.   Perfusion 938
       342.5.   Control of Breathing 938
       342.6.   Gas Exchange... 939
343.   Special Diagnostic Procedures in Pulmonary Disease,
       Gordon L. Snider.. 941

343.1. The Chest Roentgenogram.. 941
343.2. Radionuclide Imaging.. 944
343.3. Ultrasonography... 945
343.4. Skin and Serologic Tests.. 945
343.5. Examination of the Sputum.. 947
343.6. Examination of Pleural Fluid... 948
343.7. Bronchoscopy... 949
343.8. Biopsy Techniques.. 949
343.9. Miscellaneous Procedures... 950
344. Diseases Associated with Airways Obstruction, *Benjamin Burrows*......... 951
344.1. Generalized Airway Diseases.. 951
344.2. Localized Airway Obstruction... 964
345. Abnormalities of Lung Aeration, *Benjamin Burrows*....................... 965
346. Infiltrative Diseases of the Lung, *Gareth M. Green*...................... 966
346.1. Introduction 966
346.2. Pulmonary Infiltrate with Eosinophilia (PIE).......................... 968
346.3. Hypersensitivity Pneumonitis (Extrinsic
       Allergic Alveolitis).. 970
346.4. Pulmonary Vasculitis and Granulomatous
       Vasculitis (Including Wegener's Granulomatosis)....................... 972
346.5. The Connective Tissue Disorders 973
346.6. Drug-Induced Reactions.. 974
346.7. Infiltrative Diseases Associated with
       Capillary Bleeding 976
346.8. Sarcoidosis... 977
346.9. Miscellaneous Infiltrative Diseases................................... 978
347. Lung Abscess and Bronchiectasis, *Sydney M. Finegold*.................... 979
347.1. Lung Abscess.. 979
347.2. Bronchiectasis.. 982
348. Physical and Chemical Irritants, *Margaret R. Becklake*................. 983
348.1. Introduction 983
348.2. Inorganic Dusts: Dosage, Clearance, and
       Cellular Reaction... 985
348.3. Inorganic Dust Pneumoconioses: Diagnosis, Lung
       Function, and Disability 986
348.4. Noncollagenous Pneumoconioses.. 987
348.5. Collagenous Pneumoconioses (Nodular)................................. 988
348.6. Collagenous Pneumoconioses (Diffuse) 990
348.7. Complicated Pneumoconiosis 992
348.8. Inorganic Dust Pneumoconioses: Treatment and Prevention............. 993
348.9. Neoplasia Associated with Dust Exposure............................. 994
348.10. Occupational Bronchitis.. 995
348.11. Acute Airway Reactions to Organic Particles......................... 996
348.12. Airway Obstruction (Eventually Chronic) Due
       to Organic Particles 997
348.13. Interstitial (Lipoid) Pneumonia 998
348.14. Asthma-Like Reactions to Chemical Agents 999
348.15. Acute Chemical Bronchitis and/or Pneumonitis 1000
348.16. Chemical Pulmonary Edema.. 1001
348.17. Radiation 1001
349. Cysts and Neoplasms of the Lung, *Leo F. Black*........................ 1002
349.1. Cystic Lesions of the Lung, Bullous Disease of
       the Lung, and Unilateral Hyperlucent Lung........................... 1002
349.2. Neoplasms of the Lung 1005
350. Diseases of the Pleura, Mediastinum, Diaphragm,
     and Chest Wall, *John H. McClement*................................... 1013
350.1. The Pleura 1013
350.2. The Mediastinum 1018
350.3. The Diaphragm... 1019
350.4. The Chest Wall.. 1019
351. Respiratory Failure, *John F. Murray*................................. 1021

351.1.   Introduction 1021
351.2.   Pathophysiology of Respiratory Failure........................... 1021
351.3.   Causes of Respiratory Failure 1022
351.4.   Clinical Manifestations... 1024
351.5.   Treatment of Acute Respiratory Failure........................... 1025
351.6.   Treatment of Chronic Respiratory Failure 1028

Part XIII.   Critical Care Medicine, *Byron D. McLees*

352.   The Medical Intensive Care Unit 1031
    352.1.   Introduction 1031
    352.2.   Instrumentation for the Intensive Care Unit................. 1032
    352.3.   Acute Respiratory Failure................................... 1033
    352.4.   Shock... 1045
    352.5.   Renal Function in the Critically Ill Patient................ 1050
    352.6.   Massive Blood Transfusions.................................. 1051
    352.7.   Coagulation Disorders in the Critically Ill Patient 1052
353.   Cardiopulmonary Resuscitation.. 1053

Part XIV.   Cardiovascular Diseases

354.   Introduction... 1059
    354.1.   Prevalence and Epidemiology of Cardiovascular
        Disease, *Robert I. Levy*.................................... 1059
    354.2.   Circulatory Function and Control, *William W. Parmley* 1063
    354.3.   Approach to the Patient with Cardiovascular
        Disease, *Andrew G. Wallace*................................ 1072
355.   Heart Failure, *Alfred P. Fishman* 1080
356.   Shock, *Francois M. Abboud* 1107
357.   Thromboembolic Diseases... 1122
    357.1.   Thrombosis, *Patrick A. McKee*............................. 1122
    357.2.   Thrombophlebitis and Phlebothrombosis, *Sol Sherry* 1124
    357.3.   Pulmonary Embolism and Infarction, *Sol Sherry*........... 1129
358.   Pulmonary Hypertension, *Daniel S. Lukas*........................... 1135
    358.1.   Introduction 1135
    358.2.   Primary Pulmonary Hypertension 1137
    358.3.   Other Causes of Pulmonary Vascular Disease................. 1141
    358.4.   Left Atrial and Pulmonary Venous Hypertension.............. 1144
    358.5.   Pulmonary Diseases and Disorders of Respiration 1146
359.   Congenital Heart Disease, *Joseph K. Perloff*....................... 1149
    359.1.   Introduction 1149
    359.2.   Common Congenital Cardiac Defects in Which
        Postpediatric Survival Is Expected 1155
    359.3.   Uncommon Congenital Cardiac Defects in Which
        Postpediatric Survival Is Expected 1166
    359.4.   Common Congenital Cardiac Defects in Which
        Postpediatric Survival Is Exceptional...................... 1170
    359.5.   Uncommon Congenital Cardiac Defects in Which
        Postpediatric Survival Is Exceptional...................... 1172
360.   Acquired Valvular Heart Disease, *John Ross, Jr.*................... 1174
    360.1.   Introduction 1174
    360.2.   Mitral Stenosis.. 1179
    360.3.   Mitral Regurgitation....................................... 1185
    360.4.   The Mitral Valve Prolapse Syndrome 1188
    360.5.   Aortic Stenosis 1190
    360.6.   Aortic Regurgitation 1194
    360.7.   Tricuspid Valve Disease.................................... 1197
    360.8.   Pulmonic Valve Disease 1199
361.   Arterial Hypertension, *C. T. Dollery*.............................. 1199

362. Atherosclerosis, *Harvey Wolinsky* 1218
363. Disorders of the Coronary Arteries... 1223
    363.1. Introduction, *Desmond G. Julian* 1223
    363.2. Angina Pectoris, *Desmond G. Julian* 1223
    363.3. Myocardial Infarction, *Desmond G. Julian* 1229
    363.4. Sudden Death, *Desmond G. Julian*................................. 1237
    363.5. Surgical Treatment of Coronary Artery Disease,
        David C. Sabiston, Jr. 1238
364. Cardiac Arrhythmia, *Anthony N. Damato*............................... 1242
    364.1. Introduction 1242
    364.2. Arrhythmias 1243
    364.3. Antiarrhythmic Drugs 1264
    363.4. Cardioversion of Arrhythmias by DC Electroshock................... 1266
    364.5. Pacemakers 1267
365. Disorders of the Pericardium, *Robert E. Whalen*...................... 1268
    365.1. Introduction 1268
    365.2. Acute Pericarditis... 1269
    365.3. Pericardial Effusion.. 1273
    365.4. Pericardial Constriction 1274
    365.5. Neoplastic Diseases... 1276
    365.6. Congenital Lesions of the Pericardium 1276
    365.7. Diseases of Diverse Unknown Cause 1276
366. Diseases of the Myocardium.. 1276
    366.1. Introduction, *Victor S. Behar* 1276
    366.2. Asymmetric Septal Hypertrophy, *Victor S. Behar*............ 1278
    366.3. Familial Cardiomyopathy, *Victor S. Behar*..................... 1280
    366.4. Inflammatory or Infective Cardiomyopathy
        (Myocarditis), *Victor S. Behar* 1281
    366.5. Nutritional Cardiomyopathy, *Victor S. Behar*................. 1283
    366.6. Cardiac Amyloidosis, *Victor S. Behar*........................... 1285
    366.7. Other Cardiomyopathies, *Victor S. Behar* 1286
    366.8. Tumors of the Heart, *Robert E. Whalen* 1288
367. Diseases of the Aorta, *Noble O. Fowler* 1288
    367.1. Introduction 1288
    367.2. Congenital Diseases of the Aorta 1289
    367.3. Heredofamilial Diseases of the Aorta.............................. 1291
    367.4. Effects of Aging upon the Aorta..................................... 1292
    367.5. Increased Aortic Dimensions 1292
    367.6. Traumatic Aortic Disease 1293
    367.7. Syphilitic Aortitis and Syphilitic Heart Disease 1294
    367.8. Dissecting Aneurysm of the Aorta 1295
    367.9. Miscellaneous Forms of Aortitis and the Aortic
        Arch Syndrome.. 1297
    367.10. Aortic Occlusion Syndromes.. 1298
368. Diseases of the Peripheral Vessels, *Jay D. Coffman* 1299
    368.1. Peripheral Vascular Diseases Due to Organic Arterial
        Obstruction 1299
    368.2. Peripheral Vascular Disease Due to Abnormal
        Vasoconstriction or Vasodilatation 1305
    368.3. Peripheral Vascular Diseases Due to Exposure to Cold 1309
    368.4. Peripheral Vascular Diseases Due to Abnormal
        Communications Between Arteries and Veins 1312
    368.5. Diseases of the Peripheral Veins..................................... 1313
    368.6. Diseases of the Peripheral Lymphatic Vessels................... 1314

VOLUME 2

Part XV.   Renal Diseases

369. Introduction.. 1316
    369.1. Structure and Function of the Kidneys, *Barry M. Brenner*......... 1316
    369.2. Mechanisms of Renal Injury, *Richard J. Glassock* 1323

369.3. The Major Renal Syndromes, *Roscoe R. Robinson* 1331
369.4. Investigation of Renal Function, *D. N. S. Kerr* 1336
369.5. Investigation of Renal Structure and Regional
Function, *D. N. S. Kerr* 1341
370. The Pathophysiology of Chronic Renal Disease, *Neal S. Bricker* 1346
371. Chronic Renal Failure, *D. N. S. Kerr* 1351
372. Acute Renal Failure, *Neal S. Bricker* 1367
373. Treatment of Irreversible Renal Failure by Transplantation
and Dialysis 1375
373.1. Introduction, *Priscilla Kincaid-Smith* 1375
373.2. Hemodialysis, *Lee W. Henderson* 1376
373.3. Renal Transplantation, *Priscilla Kincaid-Smith* 1382
374. Glomerular Disease 1386
374.1. Introduction, *O. M. Wrong* 1386
374.2. Nephrotic Syndrome, *O. M. Wrong* 1387
374.3. Glomerulonephritis, *O. M. Wrong* 1390
374.4. Renal Involvement in Connective Tissue Diseases,
O. M. Wrong 1400
374.5. Hereditary Nephritis (Alport's Syndrome), *O. M. Wrong* 1402
374.6. Renal Changes in Other Systemic Diseases,
C. Craig Tisher 1402
375. Vascular Disorders of the Kidney, *J. Caulie Gunnells, Jr.* 1407
375.1. Renal Infarction from Arterial Thrombi and Emboli 1407
375.2. Renal Vein Thrombosis 1408
376. Urinary Tract Infections and Pyelonephritis, *Calvin M. Kunin* 1409
377. Renal Disease in Pregnancy, *Thomas F. Ferris* 1414
378. Interstitial Nephritis and Interstitial Nephropathy,
Martin Goldberg 1416
379. Toxic Nephropathy, *Bryan T. Emmerson* 1422
380. Other Specific Renal Diseases, *Robert W. Schrier* 1435
380.1. Nephrogenic Diabetes Insipidus 1435
380.2. Hypokalemic Nephropathy 1437
380.3. Hypercalcemic Nephropathy 1438
380.4. Uric Acid Nephropathy 1440
380.5. Renal Tubular Acidosis 1441
380.6. Miscellaneous Disorders 1442
381. Renal Calculi, *William C. Thomas, Jr.* 1443
382. Obstructive Nephropathy, *Francis P. Muldowney* 1447
383. Cystic Diseases of the Kidney, *Kenneth D. Gardner, Jr.* 1450
384. Anomalies of the Urinary Tract, *James F. Glenn* 1456
385. Tumors of the Kidney, *James F. Glenn* 1458

Part XVI.   Diseases of the Digestive System

386. Introduction, *Marvin H. Sleisenger* 1463

SECTION ONE.   DIAGNOSTIC IMAGING PROCEDURES IN
GASTROENTEROLOGY, *Robert N. Berk*, 1464

387. Abdominal Ultrasonography 1465
388. Computerized Tomography 1466
389. Radionuclide Imaging 1468
390. Visceral Angiography 1470
391. Endoscopic Retrograde Cholangiopancreatography 1472
392. Percutaneous Transhepatic Cholangiography 1473

SECTION TWO.   DISORDERS OF MOTILITY, *Marvin M. Schuster*, 1475

393. Normal Physiology of Motor Activity 1475
394. Relation of Symptoms to Disordered Motor Activity 1476
395. Pathophysiology and Cardinal Symptoms of Disordered Motility 1476

395.1.	Pain	1476
395.2.	Vomiting	1477
395.3.	Disorders of Swallowing	1478
395.4.	Diarrhea	1479
395.5.	Constipation	1480
395.6.	Incontinence	1482
396.	Disorders of Esophageal Motility	1483
397.	Disorders of Gastroduodenal Motility	1488
398.	Intestinal Obstruction (Ileus)	1490
399.	Disorders of Colonic Motility	1492
400.	Gastrointestinal Allergy and Food Intolerance	1498
401.	Diverticula of the Intestinal Tract	1499

SECTION THREE. PEPTIC ULCER, 1502

402.	Peptic Ulcer: Pathogenesis and Pathophysiology, *Morton I. Grossman*	1502
403.	Peptic Ulcer: Clinical and Endocrine Aspects, *John H. Walsh*	1507
404.	Peptic Ulcer: Diagnosis, *Jon I. Isenberg*	1509
405.	Peptic Ulcer: Medical Therapy, *Jon I. Isenberg*	1513
406.	Peptic Ulcer: Complications and Surgical Treatment, *James H. Meyer*	1516

SECTION FOUR. GASTROINTESTINAL BLEEDING, 1520

| 407. | Gastrointestinal Bleeding, *David H. Law* | 1520 |

SECTION FIVE. MALABSORPTION, 1523

| 408. | Malabsorption, *Marvin H. Sleisenger* | 1523 |

SECTION SIX. DISEASES OF THE PANCREAS, *Frank P. Brooks*, 1550

409.	Introduction	1550
410.	Pancreatitis	1550
410.1.	Introduction	1550
410.2.	Acute Pancreatitis	1550
410.3.	Chronic Pancreatitis	1554
411.	Carcinoma of the Pancreas	1557
412.	Cystic Fibrosis of the Pancreas (Mucoviscidosis)	1559

SECTION SEVEN. INFLAMMATORY DISEASES OF THE INTESTINE, 1560

413.	Chronic Inflammatory Diseases of the Intestine, *Henry D. Janowitz*	1560
413.1.	Introduction	1560
413.2.	Regional Enteritis (Crohn's Disease of Small Bowel)	1560
413.3.	Ulcerative Colitis	1568
413.4.	Crohn's Disease of the Colon (Granulomatous Colitis)	1576
414.	Other Inflammatory Diseases of the Intestine, *Marvin H. Sleisenger*	1578
414.1.	Acute Appendicitis (Including the Acute Abdomen)	1578
414.2.	Diverticulitis	1582
414.3.	Radiation Enterocolitis	1584
414.4.	Pseudomembranous Enterocolitis	1585
414.5.	Primary Nonspecific Ulceration of the Small Intestine	1585

SECTION EIGHT. VASCULAR DISEASES OF THE INTESTINE, *Robert K. Ockner*, 1586

| 415. | Anatomy, Physiology, and Pathophysiology of the Mesenteric Circulation | 1586 |

416. Chronic Intestinal Ischemic Syndromes 1587
417. Acute Intestinal Ischemic Syndromes.. 1588
418. Miscellaneous Disorders... 1590

SECTION NINE. DISEASES OF THE PERITONEUM, MESENTERY, AND OMENTUM, *Robert K. Ockner*, 1591

419. Diseases of the Peritoneum 1591
420. Diseases of the Mesentery and Omentum 1595

SECTION TEN. NEOPLASTIC DISEASES OF THE ALIMENTARY TRACT, 1596

421. Introduction, *Lloyd L. Brandborg*.. 1596
422. Neoplasms of the Esophagus, *Lloyd L. Brandborg* 1597
423. Malignant Neoplasms of the Stomach, *Lloyd L. Brandborg*................. 1599
424. Benign Neoplasms of the Stomach, *Lloyd L. Brandborg*...................... 1604
425. Neoplasms of the Small Intestine, *Thomas F. O'Brien, Jr.*................... 1604
426. Neoplasms of the Large Intestine, *Thomas F. O'Brien, Jr.* 1606

SECTION ELEVEN. OTHER DISEASES OF THE COLON, RECTUM, AND ANUS, *David L. Earnest*, 1611

427. Introduction... 1611
428. Colitis Cystica Superficialis and Profunda.. 1611
429. Pneumatosis Cystoides Intestinalis 1611
430. Endometriosis 1612
431. Malakoplakia 1613
432. Melanosis Coli, Cathartic Colon, and Soap Colitis.............................. 1613
433. Fecal Impaction and Stercoral Ulcer.. 1615
434. Nonspecific or Solitary Ulcer of the Colon.. 1615
435. Nonspecific Ulcerative Proctitis 1616
436. Diseases of the Anus.. 1616

SECTION TWELVE. DISEASES OF THE GALLBLADDER AND BILE DUCTS, *Lawrence W. Way*, 1618

437. Introduction... 1618
438. Clinical Evaluation of Jaundice 1621
439. Roentgenologic Examination.. 1622
440. Asymptomatic Gallstones... 1623
441. Chronic Cholecystitis and Biliary Colic 1624
442. Acute Cholecystitis.. 1625
443. Gallstone Ileus.. 1628
444. Choledocholithiasis and Cholangitis 1629
445. Biliary Stricture.. 1631
446. Uncommon Causes of Bile Duct Obstruction 1632
447. Carcinoma of the Gallbladder 1633
448. Benign Tumors and Pseudotumors of the Gallbladder......................... 1634
449. Malignant Bile Duct Tumors 1634
450. Benign Tumors of the Bile Ducts 1635
451. Postcholecystectomy Syndrome 1635

SECTION THIRTEEN. DISEASES OF THE LIVER, *Graham H. Jeffries*, 1637

452. Mechanisms of Hepatic Disease... 1637
453. Diagnostic Procedures... 1645
454. Metabolic Disorders.. 1648
455. Acute Viral Hepatitis 1650

456. Fulminant Hepatitis 1655
457. Hepatitis Due to Other Viruses.. 1656
458. Liver Disease Associated with Bacterial Infections 1656
459. Acute Liver Abscess.. 1656
460. Protozoan or Helminthic Disease of the Liver................................ 1657
461. Toxic and Drug-Induced Liver Disease.. 1657
    461.1. Toxic Hepatitis.. 1657
    461.2. Liver Disease Due to Hypersensitivity Drug
        Reactions.. 1659
462. Fatty Liver.. 1660
463. The Liver in Acute Heart Failure and Shock................................... 1661
464. Hepatic Vein Occlusion (Budd-Chiari Syndrome)............................... 1661
465. Chronic Liver Disease.. 1661
    465.1. Chronic Active Hepatitis... 1661
    465.2. Cirrhosis of the Liver... 1663
466. Congenital Hepatic Fibrosis 1667
467. Infiltrative Disease of the Liver.. 1667

Part XVII. Diseases of Nutrition

468. Nutrient Requirements, *Nevin S. Scrimshaw*.................................. 1670
469. Assessment of Nutritional Status, *Nevin S. Scrimshaw* 1675
470. Nutrition and Infection, *Nevin S. Scrimshaw*............................... 1678
471. Kwashiorkor, Marasmus, and Intermediate Forms of
    Protein-Calorie Malnutrition, *Nevin S. Scrimshaw*.......................... 1680
472. Undernutrition, Starvation, and Hunger Edema, *Nevin S. Scrimshaw* 1684
473. Deficiencies of Individual Nutrients: Vitamin Diseases,
    Nevin S. Scrimshaw 1684
    473.1. Hypovitaminosis A (Including Xerophthalmia and
        Keratomalacia)... 1684
    473.2. Ariboflavinosis... 1686
    473.3. Pellagra 1687
    473.4. Beriberi 1688
    473.5. Scurvy... 1689
    473.6. Hypervitaminosis A and D 1691
474. Obesity, *Edwin L. Bierman* 1692
475. Anorexia Nervosa, *Gerald F. M. Russell*.................................... 1699
476. Nutritional Maintenance and Diet Therapy in Acute and
    Chronic Disease, *Philip Felig* 1703
    476.1. Introduction 1703
    476.2. Fuel Homeostasis in Health and Disease................................ 1703
    476.3. Parenteral Nutrition.. 1705
    476.4. Diet Therapy.. 1708

Part XVIII. Hematologic and Hematopoietic Diseases

477. Introduction, *Ralph L. Nachman*.. 1713

SECTION ONE. THE ANEMIAS, 1714

478. Introduction, *M. C. Brain* 1714
479. Megaloblastic Anemias, *Victor Herbert* 1719
480. Normochromic Normocytic Anemias 1729
    480.1. Acute Hemorrhagic Anemia, *Elmer B. Brown*............................ 1729
    480.2. Anemia Associated with Infection and Chronic
        Systemic Diseases (Simple Chronic Anemia, Anemia
        of Chronic Disorders), *Elmer B. Brown*............................... 1731
    480.3. Aplastic Anemia, *M. C. Brain* 1733
    480.4. Sideroblastic Anemia, *M. C. Brain*.................................. 1740

480.5.   Myelophthisic Anemia, *M. C. Brain* 1742
481.   Hypochromic Anemias, *Elmer B. Brown* 1743
    481.1.   Iron Deficiency Anemia 1743
    481.2.   Hypochromic Anemias Not Caused by Iron Deficiency............. 1751

SECTION TWO.   HEMOLYTIC DISORDERS, 1751

482.   Introduction, *Wendell F. Rosse*...................................... 1751
483.   Hemolysis Due to Intracorpuscular Abnormalities, *Harry S. Jacob*......... 1755
    483.1.   Introduction 1755
    483.2.   Membrane Abnormalities... 1756
    483.3.   Enzyme Deficiencies.. 1758
    483.4.   Other Intracorpuscular Abnormalities 1761
484.   Hemolysis Due to Acquired Abnormalities, *Wendell F. Rosse* 1762
    484.1.   Introduction 1762
    484.2.   Immunologic Alteration of the Membrane........................... 1762
    484.3.   Hemolysis Due to Traumatic Alteration of the Membrane.......... 1766
    484.4.   Hemolysis Due to Acquired Dysplastic Alteration
        of the Membrane.. 1768
    484.5.   Hemolysis Due to Chemical Alteration of the Membrane.......... 1769
    484.6.   Hemolysis Due to Overactivity of the Reticuloendothelial
        System 1770
485.   Hemoglobin, the Hemoglobinopathies, and the
    Thalassemias, *C. Lockard Conley*.. 1771
    485.1.   Introduction 1771
    485.2.   Oxygen Affinity of the Red Cells 1771
    485.3.   Abnormalities of Hemoglobin 1771
    485.4.   Clinical Syndromes Associated with Hemoglobinopathies........... 1773
    485.5.   Hemolytic Anemias Caused by Unstable Hemoglobins.............. 1776
    485.6.   Disorders Caused by Hemoglobins with Abnormal
        Oxygen Affinity.. 1777
    485.7.   The Thalassemia Syndromes 1778
486.   Methemoglobinemia and Sulfhemoglobinemia, *Ernst R. Jaffé* 1780
487.   Hemoglobinuria, *Hugh Chaplin, Jr.* 1782

SECTION THREE.   TRANSFUSION REACTIONS, 1785

488.   Transfusion Reactions, *Hugh Chaplin, Jr.*.............................. 1785

SECTION FOUR.   HEMOCHROMATOSIS, 1790

489.   Hemochromatosis (Iron Storage Disease), *Thomas H. Bothwell* 1790

SECTION FIVE.   POLYCYTHEMIA, *Allan J. Erslev*, 1792

490.   Introduction.. 1792
491.   Relative Polycythemia.. 1793
492.   Absolute Polycythemia.. 1793
    492.1.   Primary Polycythemia (Polycythemia Vera)......................... 1794
    492.2.   Secondary Polycythemia.. 1798

SECTION SIX.   DISEASES OF THE WHITE BLOOD CELLS, 1800

493.   Neutrophil Function, *S. J. Klebanoff*.................................... 1800
494.   Neutrophil Dysfunction Syndromes, *S. J. Klebanoff*....................... 1803
495.   The Leukopenic State, *Dane R. Boggs*.................................... 1807
496.   Leukemoid Reactions, *Richard T. Silver*................................. 1812
497.   The Acute Leukemias, *James F. Holland*.................................. 1813
498.   The Chronic Leukemias, *Charles M. Huguley, Jr.*......................... 1821

498.1. Chronic Granulocytic Leukemia (Chronic Myelocytic Leukemia [CML], Chronic Myeloid Leukemia, Chronic Myelogenous Leukemia) 1821
498.2. Chronic Lymphocytic Leukemia (Chronic Lymphatic Leukemia) 1824
499. Myeloproliferative Disorders, *Richard T. Silver* 1826
499.1. Introduction 1826
499.2. Agnogenic Myeloid Metaplasia 1827

SECTION SEVEN. LYMPHORETICULAR NEOPLASMS, 1829

500. Introduction, *Paul P. Carbone* 1829
501. Non-Hodgkin's Lymphomas, *Thomas E. Davis* 1830
502. Burkitt's Lymphoma, *Paul P. Carbone* 1838
503. Hodgkin's Disease, *Saul A. Rosenberg* 1839

SECTION EIGHT. EOSINOPHILIC GRANULOMA AND RELATED SYNDROMES, *Philip H. Lieberman*, 1848

504. Introduction 1848
505. Eosinophilic Granuloma 1848
506. Letterer-Siwe Syndrome 1850
507. Further Notes on Terminology 1850
508. Treatment 1850

SECTION NINE. PLASMA CELL DYSCRASIAS, *Elliott F. Osserman*, 1852

509. Introduction 1852
510. Clinical Patterns of the Plasma Cell Dyscrasias 1858
510.1. Multiple Myeloma (Plasma Cell Myeloma, Myelomatosis) 1858
510.2. Macroglobulinemia (Primary or Waldenström's Macroglobulinemia) 1862
510.3. Amyloidosis 1863
510.4. Lichen Myxedematosus 1865
510.5. γ Heavy Chain Disease 1865
510.6. IgA Heavy Chain (α-Chain) Disease 1866
510.7. IgM Heavy Chain (μ-Chain) Disease 1866
510.8. Plasma Cell Dyscrasia of Unknown Significance and Plasma Cell Dyscrasia Associated with Chronic Infections, Biliary Disease, and Nonreticular Neoplasms 1866
510.9. Association Between Plasmacytic and Monocytic Dyscrasias 1867

SECTION TEN. DISEASES OF THE SPLEEN, *Richard A. Rifkind*, 1867

511. Introduction 1867
512. Hyposplenism 1869
513. Splenomegaly and Hypersplenism 1869

SECTION ELEVEN. HEMORRHAGIC DISORDERS: DISORDERS OF PRIMARY HEMOSTASIS, *Ralph L. Nachman*, 1871

514. Introduction 1871
515. Quantitative Platelet Abnormalities 1872
515.1. Thrombocytopenia 1872
515.2. Thrombocytosis 1877
516. Qualitative Platelet Abnormalities 1878
517. Vascular Purpura 1879
518. Hereditary Hemorrhagic Telangiectasia (Osler-Weber-Rendu Disease) 1880

SECTION TWELVE.   HEMORRHAGIC DISORDERS: COAGULATION
                  DEFECTS, *Oscar D. Ratnoff*, 1881

   519.   Introduction.. 1881
   520.   Heritable Disorders of Blood Coagulation.............................. 1883
      520.1.   Introduction 1883
      520.2.   Classic Hemophilia 1883
      520.3.   Other Heritable Disorders of Blood Coagulation....... 1886
   521.   Acquired Disorders of Blood Coagulation.............................. 1889
      521.1.   Vitamin K Deficiency 1889
      521.2.   Liver Disease 1890
      521.3.   Renal Disease... 1891
      521.4.   Acquired Deficiency of Stuart Factor 1891
      521.5.   Acquired Hypofibrinogenemia and Syndromes of
            Intravascular Coagulation and Fibrinolysis 1891
      521.6.   Fibrinolytic States 1896
      521.7.   Anticoagulants... 1896

Part XIX.   Medical Oncology

   522.   Cancer and Internal Medicine: An Internist's Approach to
       Cancer and Its Medical Manifestations, *W. P. L. Myers*....................... 1898
      522.1.   Internist's Approach to the Cancer Patient 1898
      522.2.   Medical Manifestations of Cancer 1901
   523.   Human Carcinogenesis, *Paul A. Marks*.................................... 1907
   524.   Tumor Markers, *Philip S. Schein*... 1911
      524.1.   Introduction 1911
      524.2.   Oncofetal Antigens 1911
      524.3.   Placental Proteins... 1912
      524.4.   Ectopic Polypeptides..................................... 1913
      524.5.   Miscellaneous 1913
   525.   Endocrine Syndromes Associated with Cancer, *Nicholas P. Christy*........ 1914
   526.   Medical Treatment of Hormone-Dependent Cancers,
       Philip K. Bondy.. 1918
   527.   Principles of Oncologic Treatment: Irradiation, Cytotoxic
       Drugs, and Immunostimulatory Procedures, *Paul Calabresi*.................... 1922
      527.1.   General Principles of Antineoplastic Therapy.............. 1922
      527.2.   Therapy by Irradiation 1927
      527.3.   Therapy with Cytotoxic Drugs 1930
      527.4.   Therapy with Immunostimulatory Procedures 1938
      527.5.   Supportive Care.. 1941
   528.   The Care of the Patient with Terminal Illness, *W. P. L. Myers*............ 1941

Part XX.   Diseases of Metabolism

   529.   Introduction, *James B. Wyngaarden* 1949
   530.   Disorders of Fluid, Electrolyte, and Acid-Base
       Balance, *William B. Schwartz* 1950
   531.   Disorders of Carbohydrate Metabolism 1969
      531.1.   Diabetes Mellitus, *George F. Cahill, Jr.*.................... 1969
      531.2.   Hypoglycemic Disorders, *Norbert Freinkel*.................. 1989
      531.3.   Galactosemia, *Ernest Beutler* 1997
      531.4.   Glycogen Storage Disease, *J. B. Sidbury, Jr.*............ 1999
      531.5.   Pentosuria (Essential Pentosuria), *J. B. Sidbury, Jr.*.... 2000
      531.6.   Fructosuria and Hereditary Fructose Intolerance,
            J. B. Sidbury, Jr. 2000
      531.7.   Primary Hyperoxaluria, *Lloyd H. Smith, Jr.*............... 2001
   532.   Disorders of Lipid Metabolism, *Richard J. Havel* 2002
      532.1.   Introduction 2002
      532.2.   Transport of Lipids in the Blood......................... 2002

532.3. Classification of Disorders of Lipid Transport 2003
532.4. Normal Regulation of Plasma Lipoprotein Concentration 2003
532.5. Inborn Errors of Lipoprotein Metabolism 2004
532.6. Acquired Disorders of Lipoprotein Metabolism 2009
532.7. Hyperlipoproteinemia in Atherosclerotic Vascular Disease 2010
533. Lipid Storage Diseases 2011
    533.1. Fabry's Disease (Glycosphingolipidosis),
        James B. Wyngaarden 2011
    533.2. Gaucher's Disease (Glucosyl Ceramide Lipidosis),
        Donald S. Fredrickson 2012
    533.3. Niemann-Pick Disease (Sphingomyelin Lipidosis),
        Donald S. Fredrickson 2014
534. Inborn Errors of Amino Acid Metabolism 2015
    534.1. Hyperaminoaciduria, *Charles R. Scriver* 2015
    534.2. Branched-Chain Aminoaciduria, *Charles R. Scriver* 2021
    534.3. Hyperhistidinemia, *Charles R. Scriver* 2022
    534.4. The Hyperprolinemias and Hydroxyprolinemia
        (Iminoacidopathies), *Charles R. Scriver* 2022
    534.5. Diseases of the Urea Cycle, *Charles R. Scriver* 2022
    534.6. β-Aminoisobutyricaciduria, *Charles R. Scriver* 2022
    534.7. The Hyperglycinurias, *Charles R. Scriver* 2023
    534.8. Renal Hyperaminoacidurias, *Charles R. Scriver* 2023
    534.9. Fanconi's Syndrome, *Charles R. Scriver* 2023
    534.10. The Hyperphenylalaninemias, *Charles R. Scriver* 2024
    534.11. Alcaptonuria, *James B. Wyngaarden* 2026
    534.12. Cystinuria, *James B. Wyngaarden* 2027
    534.13. Homocystinuria, *James B. Wyngaarden* 2028
    534.14. Albinism (Oculocutaneous Albinism), *Alexander G. Bearn* 2029
535. Disorders of Purine and Pyrimidine Metabolism 2029
    535.1. Gout, *Lloyd H. Smith, Jr.* 2029
    535.2. Xanthinuria, *Lloyd H. Smith, Jr.* 2041
    535.3. The Lesch-Nyhan Syndrome (HGPRT Syndrome),
        James B. Wyngaarden 2042
    535.4. 2,8-Dihydroxyadenine Renal Stones (APRT Deficiency),
        James B. Wyngaarden 2043
    535.5. Miscellaneous Diseases of Purine Metabolism,
        James B. Wyngaarden 2043
    535.6. Disorders of Pyrimidine Metabolism, *Lloyd H. Smith, Jr.* 2043
536. Porphyria, *Rudi Schmid* 2044
    536.1. Introduction 2044
    536.2. Congenital Erythropoietic Porphyria (Congenital
        Photosensitive Porphyria, Günther's Disease) 2045
    536.3. Hepatic Porphyrias 2045
    536.4. Protoporphyria (Erythropoietic Protoporphyria) 2049
537. Wilson's Disease (Hepatolenticular Degeneration),
    Alexander G. Bearn 2049
538. Inherited Disorders of Connective Tissue 2051
    538.1. The Mucopolysaccharidoses, *Alexander G. Bearn* 2051
    538.2. Marfan's Syndrome (Arachnodactyly, Dolichostenomelia),
        Alexander G. Bearn 2053
    538.3. Ehlers-Danlos Syndrome, *Sheldon R. Pinnell* 2054
539. Miscellaneous Disorders 2055
    539.1. Familial Mediterranean Fever (Paroxysmal Polyserositis,
        Familial Recurrent Polyserositis, Periodic Fever),
        Anthony S. Fauci 2055
    539.2. Acatalasia (Acatalasemia, Takahara's Disease),
        Alexander G. Bearn 2057
    539.3. Familial Dysautonomia (Riley-Day Syndrome),
        Alexander G. Bearn 2057
    539.4. Laurence-Moon Syndrome (Laurence-Moon-Biedl
        Syndrome), *Alexander G. Bearn* 2058

539.5.   Lipoatrophic Diabetes, *Alexander G. Bearn* 2058
539.6.   Lipoid Proteinosis (Cutaneous-Mucosal Hyalinosis),
         Alexander G. Bearn 2058
539.7.   Werner's Syndrome, *Alexander G. Bearn* 2058

Part XXI.   Diseases of the Endocrine System

540.   Introduction, *Nicholas P. Christy* 2060
541.   Mode of Action of Hormones, *John N. Loeb* 2070
542.   The Control of Anterior Pituitary Secretion, *Seymour Reichlin* 2074
543.   The Anterior Pituitary (Adenohypophysis), *Nicholas P. Christy* 2083
       543.1.   Introduction 2083
       543.2.   Anterior Pituitary Function in Normal Subjects and
                in Patients with Systemic Diseases 2084
       543.3.   The Hormones of the Anterior Pituitary 2085
       543.4.   Assessment of Anterior Pituitary Function 2091
       543.5.   Diagnosis and Treatment of Pituitary Tumors 2094
       543.6.   Hypopituitarism 2100
       543.7.   Hyperpituitarism 2105
544.   Posterior Pituitary, *Alexander Leaf* 2109
       544.1.   Antidiuretic Hormone 2109
       544.2.   Diabetes Insipidus 2110
545.   The Pineal, *Seymour Reichlin* 2111
546.   The Thyroid, *Leslie J. DeGroot* 2114
       546.1.   Introduction 2114
       546.2.   Graves' Disease and Hyperthyroidism 2120
       546.3.   Thyroiditis 2128
       546.4.   Hypothyroidism and Myxedema 2132
       546.5.   Multinodular Goiter 2135
       546.6.   Endemic Goiter 2137
       546.7.   Metabolic Defects in Thyroid Hormone Formation,
                Transport, and Action 2138
       546.8.   Thyroid Neoplasms 2141
547.   Adrenal Cortex, *Grant W. Liddle* 2144
       547.1.   The Adrenal Steroids and Their Functions 2144
       547.2.   Regulation of Adrenal Steroid Secretion 2146
       547.3.   Addison's Disease (Primary Adrenal Cortical
                Insufficiency) 2147
       547.4.   Adrenal Apoplexy 2150
       547.5.   Adrenal Insufficiency Secondary to Hypopituitarism 2150
       547.6.   Adrenal Insufficiency Secondary to Pituitary-
                Adrenal Suppression by Corticosteroids 2151
       547.7.   Cushing's Syndrome 2152
       547.8.   Primary Aldosteronism 2157
       547.9.   Secondary Aldosteronism 2158
       547.10. Congenital Adrenal Hyperplasia 2158
       547.11. Virilizing Tumors 2161
       547.12. Feminizing Adrenal Tumors 2162
548.   The Testis, *Mortimer B. Lipsett* 2162
       548.1.   Introduction 2162
       548.2.   Pubertal Development in the Male 2166
       548.3.   Sexual Precocity 2166
       548.4.   Hypogonadism 2167
       548.5.   Male Pseudohermaphroditism 2172
       548.6.   Cryptorchidism 2173
       548.7.   Impotence 2174
       548.8.   "Male Climacteric" 2174
       548.9.   Orchitis 2174
       548.10. Tumors of the Testis 2174
549.   The Ovaries, *Nathan Kase* 2175

549.1. Ovarian Structure and Function.. 2175
549.2. Ovarian Disorders Pertinent to General Medicine.................... 2179
550. The Adrenal Medulla and Sympathetic Nervous System,
      Karl Engelman.. 2199
551. The Carcinoid Syndrome, *Karl Engelman*...................................... 2207
552. Parathyroid, *G. D. Aurbach*.. 2213
      552.1. Parathyroid Hormone and Calcitonin.............................. 2213
      552.2. Hyperparathyroidism 2214
      552.3. Hypoparathyroidism 2220
      552.4. Pseudohypoparathyroidism and Pseudopseudo-
              hypoparathyroidism 2221
      552.5. Tetany... 2223
      552.6. Calcitonin and Medullary Carcinoma of the Thyroid 2223

Part XXII.   Diseases of Bone, *Louis V. Avioli*

553. Calcium, Phosphorus, and Bone Metabolism 2225
      553.1. Calcium 2225
      553.2. Phosphorus 2228
      553.3. The Structure of Bone and Its Relation to Calcium
              Homeostasis 2230
554. Vitamin D 2232
555. Hypercalcemia 2233
556. Hypocalcemia 2241
557. The Osteoporotic Syndromes.. 2242
558. Osteomalacia and Rickets 2247
559. Renal Osteodystrophy 2254
560. Paget's Disease (Osteitis Deformans)... 2257
561. Osteonecrosis... 2259
562. Osteomyelitis 2260
563. Radionuclide Bone Toxicity.. 2261
564. Fluorosis... 2262
565. Fibrous Dysplasia... 2262
566. Hypertrophic Osteoarthropathy... 2263
567. Other Congenital and/or Hereditary Disorders Involving Bone.............. 2263

Part XXIII.   Certain Cutaneous Diseases with Significant Systemic Manifestations, *Marie-Louise Johnson*

568. Introduction... 2266
569. Pathophysiology 2267
570. The Examination of the Skin 2272
571. Principles of Therapy 2275
572. The Differential Diagnosis.. 2277
      572.1. The Head and Neck 2278
      572.2. The Thorax 2279
      572.3. Dermatitis of the Hands and Feet 2283
573. Significant Dermatologic Signs of Disease..................................... 2284
      573.1. Introduction 2284
      573.2. Acanthosis Nigricans 2285
      573.3. Ichthyosis.. 2285
      573.4. Acquired Erythrodermas.. 2286
      573.5. Pigmentary Disturbances 2289
      573.6. Neurofibromas 2293
      573.7. Pseudoxanthoma Elasticum.. 2294
      573.8. Nodose Lesions of the Leg 2295
      573.9. Cutaneous Manifestations of Internal Malignancy.................. 2295
      573.10. Cutaneous Correlations with Specific Organ Systems 2300
574. Selected Significant Dermatologic Diagnoses.................................. 2301

574.1.   The Blistering Diseases.. 2301
574.2.   Mucocutaneous Lymph Node Syndrome............................... 2306
574.3.   Behçet's Disease... 2306
574.4.   Mast Cell Disease... 2307
574.5.   Malignancy... 2308

Part XXIV.   Diseases of the Eye, *Maurice B. Landers, III*

575.   Introduction... 2313
576.   The Differential Diagnoses of the Acute Red Eye.................... 2313
577.   Arthritic Diseases.. 2314
578.   Connective Tissue Diseases 2316
579.   Diabetes Mellitus... 2320
580.   Glaucoma.. 2322
581.   Ocular Histoplasmosis... 2323
582.   Systemic Hypertension and Arteriolosclerosis 2325
583.   The Optic Nerve 2327
584.   Ocular Sarcoidosis... 2329
585.   Sickle Cell Diseases... 2330
586.   Thyroid Eye Disease... 2332
587.   Ocular Toxoplasmosis 2334

Part XXV.   Drug-Drug Interactions, *Rubin Bressler*

588.   Introduction... 2336
589.   Physical-Chemical Processes 2336
590.   Drug Disposition 2338
591.   Adverse Drug Reactions... 2341

Part XXVI.   Normal Laboratory Values of Clinical Importance, *James B. Wyngaarden*

592.   The Use and Interpretation of Laboratory-Derived Data............ 2342
593.   Common Laboratory Values of Clinical Importance 2346

Index... i

PART I
THE NATURE
OF MEDICINE

1. ON BECOMING A CLINICIAN

Paul B. Beeson

This essay is addressed to the student entering upon the study of clinical medicine. To leaf through a modern medical textbook for the first time must be a daunting experience for you. How can anyone hope to master so much scientific and technical information? The task *is* difficult, indeed impossible. Nevertheless, some encouragement should come from observing that senior medical students and young doctors on the hospital staff appear to have made a satisfactory adjustment to the challenge. Furthermore, as your acquaintance with clinical teachers grows, you will observe that although each of them has special knowledge and experience in some area of clinical medicine, they make no pretense of knowing it all. You will also find that clinicians frequently disagree, and that each of them comes to wrong conclusions from time to time. Clinical teachers must in fact appear to be very different from those under whom your preclinical work was done. Biochemists and pharmacologists have "hard" facts to propound. We, on the other hand, deal with such commodities as pain and nausea. We must accept any kind of problem. We cannot insist on working with inbred strains of people, we cannot control the environment from which they come, we know that their recollection of past events is faulty, and we cannot reduce them to subcellular fractions in order to determine what is going on. We must even question the opinions of our colleagues. We live, therefore, in an atmosphere of doubt and uncertainty, and make our decisions and take our actions on the basis of probabilities. You will have the same handicaps, and you too will make mistakes. Simply try to ensure that each mistake constitutes a learning experience which leaves you a better doctor.

Students as a rule accommodate to clinical medicine with astonishing speed. They learn by their own study and practice, by attending lectures and conferences, by observing senior people at work, and by informal discussions with fellow students and residents in ward offices, corridors, and dining rooms. Good-natured arguments facilitate the process, because debate tends to fix the information that emerges. In that connection you will find it helpful to adopt a habit of offering your point of view tentatively rather than in the form of a positive assertion.

But how should you *begin* the study of clinical medicine? I have not found it helpful (except as an editor!) to read a book like this in systematic cover-to-cover fashion. Instead, you should use it the way the mature clinician does, as a place in which information can be obtained about problems being dealt with at the time.

Inasmuch as common disorders occur commonly, this practice will in good time ensure that you will have read and thought about such frequently encountered disorders as peptic ulcer, angina pectoris, and urinary tract infection. Furthermore, although at first glance a medical text seems to be a sort of dictionary describing hundreds of unrelated entities, you will find that knowledge of one helps the study of another, because there often are dovetailing aspects or useful contrasts. I suggest that you always examine the references which accompany the discussions, and make it a practice to consult some of them. That is the kind of study doctors must carry on for themselves throughout life. Reading in connection with specific clinical problems is likely to provide knowledge that sticks.

What about the many uncommon maladies described in textbooks? The student of any age really needs only to know how to find out about them. One test of a good doctor is ability to achieve a correct diagnosis without having met the disease before.

Medical knowledge and practice are continually changing. In order to incorporate the steady flow of new information, a textbook must be extensively rewritten every few years. Let me illustrate this by citing a few examples of changes that have taken place during my own clinical career.

The third edition of this Textbook appeared in 1933, the year I graduated from medical school. It contained no mention of effective treatments for bacterial, mycobacterial, or fungal diseases; consequently, such entities as bacterial endocarditis, miliary tuberculosis, and cryptococcal meningitis were described as fatal infections with hopeless outlook. Adrenal steroids and steroid-like compounds had not been discovered. Diuretics were not available for treatment of heart failure; nor were there any drugs for control of hypertension. Anticoagulant drugs had not been introduced. The brief section entitled "Diseases of Allergy" contained nothing about lymphocytes, immune complexes, complement, or the structure of immunoglobulins. Sprue was described as an infectious disease, probably caused by *Monilia albicans*. Sydenham's chorea was thought to be due to toxins produced by an unidentified nonhemolytic streptococcus. The section on treatment of rheumatoid arthritis stated: "The most important single factor is the removal of foci of infection." The only deficiency diseases described were pellagra, beriberi, scurvy, and rickets; there was virtually no information about the nature of the responsible vitamins or of the metabolic consequences of such deficiencies. Discussions of "acidosis" and "alkalosis" were based on only one clinical chemical test — i.e., measurement of the carbon dioxide combining power of the blood. Removal of tonsils and adenoids was enthusiastically recommended: "The beneficial results of this operation are so great and so prompt that unless there is a distinct reason for its omission, it is folly to wait for spontaneous shrinking. . . ." For "falling of the stomach," recommended treatments included cacodylate of iron, strychnine in tonic doses, retention enemas of olive oil, or such surgical measures as pyloroplasty. For treatment of peptic ulcer it was mentioned that injections of nonspecific protein such as dead bacteria or milk may be followed by some success. The management of bleeding peptic ulcer called for application of an ice bag to the epigastrium; complete starvation; morphine hypodermically; and water, glucose, and soda given by rectal drip. Blood banks were unknown, and transfusion of a single unit of blood was a formidable procedure; consequently: "If the symptoms increase, transfusion of blood is advisable; in certain cases this may have to be repeated several times. When properly grouped blood cannot be quickly obtained, 10 cc of horse serum may be injected. . . ." Ulcerative colitis was covered in two brief descriptive paragraphs, which offered no suggestions as to medical or surgical treatment. Systemic lupus erythematosus, regional enteritis, and mycoplasmal pneumonia were not mentioned at all! The pathologic lesion of catarrhal jaundice (now viral hepatitis) was said to be an inflammatory swelling of the mucosa of the common bile duct. Diagnostic procedures in clinical biochemistry, endocrinology, and immunology, which now seem commonplace, had not come into use. Diagnosis by angiography, sonography, nuclear medicine, computerized tomography, and fiberscopic endoscopy were still unknown.

Nothing would be gained by a continuation of such examples; they are sufficient to illustrate the point that the conventional wisdom called clinical medicine changes rapidly. Without question, in a few decades another reader will be able to characterize much material in this edition of the Textbook as equally quaint.

The medical student should be aware, however, that exciting advances in medicine sometimes create serious new problems. Our therapy makes use of powerful drugs, all of which can do harm. Few hospital patients receive less than half a dozen different medications. In addition to intrinsic toxicity, these can interact with each other to produce unwanted effects. Part of hospital medicine today is in fact devoted to overcoming untoward effects of therapy. Knowing when to stop a certain treatment is as important as knowing when to bring it into use. There are risks, too, in many of our present invasive diagnostic procedures. In a manner of speaking, the recent scientific and technologic explosion in clinical medicine has created its own kind of pollution. One of the most important qualities needed by today's physician is ability to restrain curiosity. We should adhere to the rule that a potentially injurious diagnostic procedure should be carried out only when its possible benefit to that patient justifies the risk. A test should never be done just for the sake of "thoroughness," that is to say, before someone else suggests that it be done, or because a specialist feels it must be done to protect his or her reputation, "just in case. . . ."

Advancement in knowledge of clinical medicine is now mainly accomplished by full-time clinical scientists in medical schools and research institutes throughout the world. They concentrate on specific problems and nearly always make use of new findings and techniques developed in other biologic and physical sciences. This kind of investigation-in-depth is essential, but requires concentration on a limited field. We have, for all time, departed from the era of clinical "giants" who were re-

garded as authorities on many aspects of internal medicine. That is why a modern textbook must be compiled from the writings of scores of contributors.

Having recognized the essential role of the specialist investigator in bringing about what are really immense advances in clinical medicine, we should give some consideration to the impact of this on trends in the practice of medicine as well as the training of future doctors. Does it follow, because we owe our advances in medical sciences to specialists, that the best medical care can only be given by specialists? Shall we say to young people now entering the profession that the age of specialization is here, and advise each of them to select a narrow field for his or her medical practice? I believe that much medical care can, and should, be the work of generalists. Diseases do not always present themselves in pure culture, and indeed the perspective of the clinical scientist can sometimes be skewed. It seems fair to say, for example, that a good general physician (now, alas, in short supply in America) can deal effectively with the great majority of episodes for which patients seek a doctor's help. When we focus on the field with which this book is concerned, it can be said with assurance that the well-trained internist is capable of dealing with most medical illnesses, including those for which hospital care is required. To do that in exemplary fashion is, however, a full-time job, which does not permit allocation of substantial portions of time and effort to research. The medical student and the house officer in a teaching hospital may need to be reminded that outside the medical school orbit much excellent medical care is provided by generalist physicians. The funds available for salaries in medical school departments go mainly to doctors who are active investigators, inasmuch as acquisition of new knowledge is a major responsibility of a university. In the setting of a teaching hospital, the clinical investigator can be a superb teacher of undergraduate and graduate medical students, and can, by combining forces with many other subspecialists in the institution, provide sophisticated medical service for patients there. This, however, is an expensive and somewhat inefficient way of offering medical care, which, although well suited to the diverse functions of a teaching institution, does not offer a realistic pattern for professional care in the outside community. In other words, specialized skill, although essential to any good system of medical care, is not needed in the proportion found among the members of medical school faculties.

Now finally, you must not only study the factual basis of clinical diagnosis and treatment, but at the same time work toward an equally difficult goal: cultivation of a proper relationship with each of your patients. This is the art of clinical practice. As Peabody described so vividly half a century ago, a hospital setting, in which you will spend the next few years, tends to be impersonal. It is easy for all of us to blend into that ambience of impersonality. More and more, people "get the bad news" during the course of a hospital stay. More and more, people must die in hospitals instead of at home. Our patients, therefore, are anxious, uncomfortable, often embarrassed, and confused by the unfamiliar surroundings. We must constantly remind ourselves of this, because successful medical care may be directly dependent on establishing an understanding and trusting relationship between ourselves and our patients. Often a good doctor scores where others have failed simply by listening to the patient and asking the right questions. Here is the way Wilfred Trotter, a great English neurosurgeon, put it:

". . . As long as medicine is an art, its chief and characteristic instrument must be human faculty. We come therefore to the very practical question of what aspects of human faculty it is necessary for the good doctor to cultivate. . . . The first to be named must always be the power of attention, of giving one's whole mind to the patient without the interposition of oneself. It sounds simple but only the very greatest doctors ever fully attain it. It is an active process and not either mere resigned listening or even politely waiting until you can interrupt. Disease often tells its secrets in a casual parenthesis. . . ."

Pickering has recently recalled an observation of Trotter at work:

". . . I asked Trotter to see a notoriously difficult patient, and marvelled how the anxious angular woman became clay in Trotter's hands. He had made it clear to her that he had listened, and that he had not only listened but had understood. I suspect that that had never happened to her before and it was for this reason that she had been, up to then, a difficult patient; that was the first time that her message had been heard. Hearing the patient's message is the *sine qua non* of a great physician. To hear that message requires first the physician's interest, second his understanding of the meaning of language, and third his sympathy and his knowledge and understanding of the circumstances of that patient's life; these again he learns best by listening to the patient."

So these are some precepts you might consider: Give each patient enough of your time. Sit down; listen; ask thoughtful questions; examine carefully; go back and do it again. Learn how to study clinical medicine, and be appropriately critical of what you read or hear. Train yourself to concentrate on each patient's problem to the exclusion of all else. Follow the example set by William Osler: "Do the kind thing and do it first."

Emerson, C. P.: Reminiscences of Sir William Osler. Internat. Assoc. Med. Museums Bull., 1926, p. 294.

Peabody, F. W.: The care of the patient. JAMA, 88:877, 1927.

Pickering, G. W.: Medicine at the crossroads: Learned profession or technological trades union? Proc. Roy. Soc. Med., 70:16, 1977.

Trotter, W.: Collected Papers. London, Oxford University Press, 1941, pp. 97–98.

2. SCIENCE, CLINICAL MEDICINE, AND THE SPECTRUM OF DISEASE

Alvan R. Feinstein

A textbook of medicine contains concepts and data for at least two distinctly different types of clinical decisions. With *explicatory** decisions, doctors choose names, causes, and mechanisms that provide intellectual explanations for the ailments observed in patients. With *interventional* decisions, doctors choose therapeutic strategies intended to prevent or to remedy the ailments. Thus, for a patient who describes his ailment as

---

*The word *explicatory* is used here to refer to diagnostic citations or pathogenetic explanations or both.

a substernal pressure provoked by exertion and relieved by rest, the doctor may make the explicatory decisions contained in such phrases as *angina pectoris, coronary artery disease,* and *myocardial ischemia.* The doctor's interventional decisions may then be expressed in recommendations about permissible physical activities, use of pharmaceutical substances, and the possible value of surgical therapy.

The explicatory decisions of clinical medicine are often regarded as its main scientific challenge. For diagnostic selections, modern technology has allowed diseases to be identified more precisely than ever before. The morphologic abnormalities that formerly could be demonstrated only at necropsy are now often revealed during life with the aid of roentgenography (including CAT scanners), biopsy, cytology, or surgical exploration; and many other ailments that cannot be depicted morphologically are identified with the aid of chemical, microbial, electrophysiologic, or other laboratory procedures. For ideas about causes and mechanisms of disease, doctors have received scientific confirmation both from the diagnostic tests performed in individual patients and from the many experimental models that have been tested during clinical investigation. The explicatory decisions thus enable doctors to apply at the bedside the major advances that laboratory research has brought to diagnostic medical science.

A doctor's interventional decisions, on the other hand, are often regarded mainly as art. The pharmaceutical, surgical, and other agents used for therapeutic intervention are highly developed from the scientific standpoint, but the decisions made about them are still often made as acts of judgment, generally unsupported by the type of scientific evidence that sustains the explicatory activities. The available evidence to prove the value of a treatment may be quantitatively defective, consisting mainly of anecdotal reports of clinical experiences that have not been thoroughly enumerated; or the evidence may seem qualitatively unappealing, depending on such "soft" data as a patient's pain, a family's anxiety, or an employer's forbearance. Even when treatments have been tested in controlled clinical trials, the results may be inconclusive because the patients under study, the investigated therapeutic regimens, or the methods of observation may differ substantially from those of customary clinical practice.

With medical activities demarcated into explicatory science and interventional art, a medical student (or a practicing clinician) often develops the belief that the purely clinical work of patient care does not present any scientific challenges. According to this belief, a clinician's principal science is contained in the "workup" that reveals diagnostic names and pathogenetic mechanisms. Once this challenge is completed, no further scientific thinking may seem necessary. After choosing a therapeutic agent according to the established diagnosis, the clinician would need only the arts of human perception and communication for telling the patient what is wrong and what is planned.

Despite popular acceptance, this demarcation of art and science in clinical work has at least three major inaccuracies. The demarcation is based on the idea that science consists only of explication, but science contains another major component: prediction. In dealing with a sick patient, a clinician is scientifically challenged not merely to explain what is wrong and how it went wrong, but also to predict what may happen and how its occurrence can be altered. To perform these predictions, a clinician must make the same type of interventional decisions with which prognosis is estimated, therapy chosen, and results evaluated. A second conceptual error arises from the belief that the choice of treatment depends almost entirely on the diagnostic citation. Although diagnosis is usually an important first step, the scientific selection and appraisal of therapy require analysis of data much more intricate than the mere identification of a disease. The most cogent information often includes symptoms, signs, and other clinical phenomena rather than a diagnostic title alone. A third misconception is the idea that important clinical phenomena cannot be expressed in "hard" scientific terms because the descriptions usually contain verbal categories rather than measured dimensions. The fallacy here is that "hard" information must be precise and reproducible, but it need not be dimensional. Some of the outstanding accomplishments of biologic science — including the work of Darwin, Virchow, and modern geneticists and electron microscopists — have been based on precise, reproducible, but nondimensional descriptions. With better standards of observation and classification, the verbal categories of "soft" clinical data could readily be improved into "hard" scientific quality.

Even when these attributes of clinical work are recognized, they may be regarded as scientifically unimportant because ordinary medical practice does not provide the experimental challenges offered by laboratory research. This belief is also inappropriate, however, because every act of clinical therapy is constructed in the same architectural sequence used for an experiment: a prepared entity is exposed to a planned maneuver and undergoes an observed response. This basic construction of an experiment can be used to outline all of a doctor's interventional decisions in clinical practice.

Despite similar challenges in the applicability of scientific methods, the "experiments" of the laboratory and bedside contain major differences in goals, reasoning, and procedures. In motive, the laboratory investigator seeks to understand how nature works and what it does; the clinician wants to change what nature has done or to thwart what it might do. In hypothesis, the laboratory investigator is innovative, wanting to test a new idea; the clinician is repetitive, wanting to reproduce the successful result achieved with the therapy used in a similar situation of the past. In cause-effect comparisons, the laboratory investigator can contrast the results of a concurrent "control group"; the clinician often relies on the "historical controls" of previous experience. In choice of data, the laboratory investigator can confine his observations only to the immediate events that seem most pertinent; the clinician must note all phenomena that can indicate a change in the patient's medical condition and way of life. These major differences in orientation require different strategies for the scientific methods used in the experiments of laboratory explication or clinical intervention, but both sets of activities offer the intellectual challenges of planning and evaluating an experiment.

In contemporary medicine, however, the methods used for acquiring and analyzing clinical data are not yet as scientifically well developed as the techniques that have been employed in laboratory research. Consequently, a doctor's explicatory decisions are often supported by excellent scientific evidence, but the interventional decisions are not. The purely clinical activities of contemporary medicine may thus seem more like art than science. The scientific improvement of this clinical art offers a prime target for future research, but in the meantime the reader of any compendium of clinical knowledge must deal with the state of the art in its existing form. The remainder of this essay will be concerned with certain caveats to help warn about some of the imperfections, and with a few suggestions to help resolve some of the difficulties.

One of the principal problems arises from the complex clinical spectrum associated with a disease. With increasing frequency in modern medicine, diseases are diagnostically identified as abnormalities not in a patient's clinical state (such as fever, jaundice, or chest pain), but in a paraclinical entity. The paraclinical abnormalities of disease can be diagnostically cited in such terms as morphologic structure (*coronary artery disease, carcinoma*), biochemical function (*diabetes mellitus, hyperthyroidism*), physiologic function (*atrial fibrillation, malabsorption*) or microbial invasion (*viral infection, meningococcemia*). Although the aid of modern diagnostic technology allows these paraclinical abnormalities to be diagnosed with unprecedented specificity and consistency, the principal "lesion" of each such paraclinical disease has an associated spectrum of diverse clinical manifestations that may not always occur specifically or consistently.

Some of the clinical manifestations represent the primary effects of the disease's principal abnormality, whereas other manifestations can be regarded as secondary effects or complications. In coronary artery disease, for example, angina pectoris is a primary effect and congestive heart failure is secondary. In peptic ulcer, pain is a primary effect and pyloric obstruction is secondary. Since different primary and secondary manifestations can appear alone or in various overlapping combinations, the disease in a particular patient may occur with some, all, or none of the possible clinical manifestations. For example, among patients with lung cancer, some may be wholly asymptomatic; others can have primary features, such as hemoptysis; others can have the secondary features of systemic or metastatic manifestations; and yet others may have various combinations of these primary and secondary elements. The complexity of a disease's spectrum will thus produce subsets of patients who have the same diagnosis but different clinical manifestations, and who may also differ in prognosis and therapy.

The existence of these different subsets creates important defects in any "textbook picture of disease." Since the author can seldom describe all the diverse possibilities, the "classic" textbook description is usually based on the most common or pathognomonic manifestations. The reader who expects that the disease will always occur in this classic manner may then be surprised, perplexed, or dismayed by the many occasions in which a patient appears from a less common subset. For example, in 1032 patients with lung cancer, the most common single subset consisted of 340 patients with the concurrence of pulmonic and systemic manifestations; 271 patients had pulmonic features only, and 196 had pulmonic, systemic, and metastatic manifestations; but 70 patients were wholly asymptomatic, and 34 had metastatic features only. Similarly, coronary artery disease can occur without angina pectoris in certain patients who have no symptoms or in others with manifestations only of congestive heart failure; hepatitis may first be found as advanced cirrhosis in a patient who never had jaundice.

The occurrence of an asymptomatic subset in a disease's spectrum is responsible for the frequent practice of "screening" in modern medicine. The purpose of the screening tests is to find the disease in circumstances in which it has produced no overt manifestations to arouse diagnostic suspicion. The occurrence of the many diverse subsets in a disease's spectrum is also responsible for some of the major current difficulties in evaluating prognosis and therapy. Despite similarity in diagnosis, the patients in the different subsets may have striking differences in prognosis. Thus, among a total of 1032 patients with lung cancer, the six-month survival rate was 44 per cent, but the rate ranged from 84 per cent in the localized asymptomatic subset to 14 per cent in patients who had both anatomic and symptomatic evidence of metastasis. In acute myocardial infarction, a patient with only chest pain has a much better prognosis than a patient with shock and pulmonary edema.

These natural prognostic distinctions will substantially affect the selection and appraisal of therapy. Since the "experiments" of routine clinical treatment are based on a repetitive hypothesis, a doctor chooses treatment for an individual patient by reviewing previous clinical experience, recalling the patients with similar manifestations, noting the outcomes of the therapy given to the "resemblance group," ascertaining which treatment gave the best result, and trying to reproduce that success in the current patient. To select the appropriate resemblance group, the doctor must have data for suitably demarcated subsets of patients.

Such data may not always be available. The results of previous treatment are often reported for all patients with the same disease, regardless of subsets; or the subsets distinguished in the reported results may be different from the particular one in which a subsequent patient is encountered. The absence of these details often creates difficulty in choice of treatment for an individual patient and arouses controversy in comparative evaluations of treated groups. One physician, treating diabetes mellitus with Regimen X, may have had a group of patients whose prognostic expectations were substantially different from those of another physician's patients treated with Regimen Y. One surgeon's Stage I cancer patients may be predominantly asymptomatic, whereas another surgeon's Stage I patients may have a high proportion of weight loss and fatigue. During arguments about the merits of the compared therapy, the clinicians may not realize that some of the crucial post-therapeutic differences arose not from different methods of treatment, but from prognostic differences in the subsets who constituted the treated groups.

To this complexity of clinical subsets for a single disease is added the further complexity introduced by comorbidity and demography. Since an individual patient may have more than one disease, the presence of associated ailments will create extra subsets in the spectrum of the "principal" disease, and may produce pathologic effects that alter prognosis and treatment in those subsets. The number of potential subsets for a disease becomes even larger when the cited clinical and comorbid demarcations are augmented by such demographic features as age, race, sex, and occupation.

This enormous variability of individual patients and diseases would pose insurmountable problems in clinical decisions if each decision depended on determining a unique subset for that patient and on having adequate background information for previous experience with that subset. Fortunately, many small subsets can be combined into larger "determinant" groups for which therapeutic decisions can be based on satisfactory amounts of previous data or experience. For example, a patient with acute rheumatic fever is usually treated with salicylate if there is no clinical evidence of carditis, and with steroids if severe carditis is present. In this decision, the *no carditis* and *severe carditis* groups act as therapeutically determinant subsets, regardless of the many smaller subgroups into which the patients could be classified by virtue of demography or other clinical phenomena.

The selection of therapeutically determinant "super" subsets has traditionally been a fundamental decision in clinical judgment. The formation of the judgment may be substantially aided in the future by the availability of electronic data processing and computers for storing, augmenting, and analyzing the data of previous experience. The use of a computerized "data bank" for this type of quantification in estimating prognosis and choosing therapy offers an intriguing clinical addition to some of the other activities in which computers now receive useful medical applications. Among such activities are the calculation of complex mathematical formulas in diagnostic and therapeutic technology, the storage and display of inventories of laboratory results, the maintenance of selected components of patients' medical records, and the construction of "protocols," depicted in the flow-chart patterns of an algorithmic computer program, that provide instructions for making diagnostic or therapeutic decisions in a standard manner.

A different type of therapeutic intervention is aimed not at a disease or a determinant subset, but at a specific clinical manifestation, such as pain, constipation, or insomnia. Thus a patient may receive an antimicrobial drug for the disease pneumococcal pneumonia, but codeine for the associated symptom of pleuritic pain. Radiation or chemotherapy may be given for Hodgkin's disease, and blood transfusions for the associated weakness and anemia. For patients with acute myocardial infarction, the only treatment directed at the disease itself is bed rest. All other treatments are chosen according to the associated clinical manifestations: e.g., narcotics or analgesics for pain, diuretics or digitalis for congestive heart failure, and appropriate agents for arrhythmia.

For the many minor ailments encountered in primary medical care or family practice, a specific disease may not be diagnosed and treatment may be intended only to relieve symptoms. Encountering such ailments as an upper respiratory infection, a sprained muscle, or a gastrointestinal upset, the practitioner may decide prognostically that the ailment is self-limited and does not require more extensive diagnostic or therapeutic efforts. Another common event in general medical practice is a temporary, acute exacerbation of a chronic major ailment that has been relatively stable. In these events, which may occur in such conditions as chronic alcoholism, irritable colon syndrome, or neurotic anxiety, patients are also often treated for symptoms only.

In all the circumstances just described, the clinician's scientific challenges in interventional decisions were to determine the target(s) to be treated and to choose the best mode(s) of therapy. A different set of challenges consists of evaluating the patient's condition afterward to decide what the treatment accomplished and whether it has been successful. For this purpose, the clinician again often uses individual manifestations, rather than a disease diagnosis, as an index of accomplishment. Furthermore, the evaluation of a particular response may depend on graded subsets composed of changes in clinical manifestations. Thus the effect of treatment on congestive heart failure may be called *excellent* if both dyspnea and edema disappear; *fair* if one disappears while the other remains; and *poor* if both remain.

The data used to identify transitions in clinical state often require additional details that may not have been necessary for decisions about diagnosis, prognosis, and therapy. For example, a description of substernal chest pain provoked by exertion and relieved by rest will often suffice for a clinical diagnosis of coronary artery disease, but the evaluation of response of the angina to treatment will usually depend on further information about the angina's frequency and the associated amounts of exertion or rest. Similarly, the amount of jaundice may not be crucial for a diagnosis of hepatitis, but may be a valuable index of therapeutic response. Other examples of clinical details that are sometimes diagnostically unimportant but therapeutically valuable are the patient's weight (in treatment of edematous congestive heart failure), the size of a massive spleen (in treatment of chronic monocytic leukemia), the frequency of bowel movements (in treatment of various gastrointestinal disorders), and the frequency of urination (in treatment of cystitis or prostatitis).

The challenges of directly communicating with patients are often regarded as a nonscientific form of clinical art, mainly because the contents of the communications, which are much more complex than any of the complexities already cited, create diverse data and subsets that are even more difficult to specify. Nevertheless, many of the decisions made during these communications require the intellectual discipline used by a scientist to select suitable information, organize data, recapitulate previous experience, and evaluate responses. The discipline of scientific reasoning may not contribute to a clinician's creative insight and artful perception in dealing with the personal attributes of people, but without such reasoning the insight and perception will often be used ineffectually.

Whether a practicing doctor is involved in decisions of communication, explication, or intervention, clinical medicine will always contain and unite elements of both art and science. The complexity of people and human ailments will demand many artful judgments that cannot be expressed in scientific terms, but a scientific discipline is required for the optimal use of modern technology in identifying, explaining, preventing, or treating the ailments. To be properly adapted to its human recipients, this scientific discipline must contain suitable provision for the important personal and clinical information that is not perceived with "scientific" equipment or expressed in "scientific" dimensions. The art and science of clinical medicine are intermingled, symbiotic, and inseparable. Without the art, there can be no data for the science. Without the science, there can be no reason for the art.

3. BIOLOGICAL SCIENCE AND MEDICAL PRACTICE

James B. Wyngaarden

Every medical student and practitioner knows that the advances of clinical medicine depend in large part upon discoveries in the basic biological sciences. Much of scientific medicine derives from basic research conducted by fundamental scientists in the pursuit of truth for its own sake and eventually applied by others to medical problems. Another part stems from basic research conducted by physician-scientists with a specified clinical goal in mind—for example, the elucidation of a disease mechanism. Still other parts involve direct observations by clinical investigators or astute practitioners upon individual patients, or by epidemiologists upon populations of people. This essay is restricted to considerations of the interdependence of clinical medicine and biological science.

Most of us accept as an article of faith that applied research in the absence of basic research would sooner or later founder for the lack of a continually expanding bank of fundamental knowledge. It follows that some fraction of research in every field must always be at a basic level, conducted for its own intrinsic merit as a contribution to human understanding. Yet it is difficult to know what fraction of research should be basic and what proportion of resources should be allocated to pure science; even informed planners and policy makers are not agreed. Furthermore, it is often difficult to draw a sharp distinction betweeen pure and programmed basic science. Hypotheses, methods, and technical complexities are not qualitatively different. The same scientist may engage in both types of research, responding to different motives at one time or another.

It has been useful as an argument for support of basic science to analyze the significant antecedent discoveries that have made possible a particular practical advance. In a recent study, Comroe and Dripps chose ten major clinical innovations in cardiovascular and pulmonary medicine and traced their roots. With the help of panels of experts they concluded that over 60 per cent of the enabling discoveries were in the category of basic science, and that over 40 per cent were the result of research conducted without a particular clinical advance in mind at the time. The lags between discovery and application showed a wide range and averaged over 20 years. Often substantial development, refinement, and testing were required before the introduction of a potential new procedure or drug into clinical medicine was shown to be useful, appropriate, and safe. They concluded that some lag was essential and protective of patient and public interest.

It would not be correct, of course, to imply that all new clinical knowledge represents the final stage of a univectorial trail of development of which the seminal observations are always based in pure science. There are many positive and negative feedback loops in the process. A substantial amount of basic scientific discovery has been stimulated by clinical observations. Most of the coenzyme vitamins were recognized on the basis of human deficiency states. Most of the blood clotting factors were identified as substances present in normal blood capable of correcting a clotting defect in a patient with a hereditary bleeding condition. Many of the complex mucopolysaccharides were first identified and characterized from storage material in patients with hereditary mucopolysaccharidoses. The structure of antibodies was worked out in large part from urinary proteins of patients with multiple myeloma. Many clues to functions of the nervous system came from patients with neurologic lesions or behavioral aberrations.

However, the present bioscientific character of medical practice is a relatively recent development. Throughout most of recorded history medicine was anything but scientific, being dominated by empiricism and shackled by dogma. Diagnoses were inexact, causes of diseases poorly understood, and therapies frivolous and haphazard. Interventions by physicians consisted of bleeding, purging, cupping, administration of infusions of every known plant and of solutions of every known metal, and prescription of every possible diet — based entirely on experience, with no scientific foundation for these practices. Nor could there be such a foundation in the absence of a body of scientific biomedical knowledge.

Harbingers of change emerged slowly in the early nineteenth century, as new principles of physics and chemistry were applied to medicine. Physiologists stressed functions of organs and tissues. Its exemplars, especially Claude Bernard (1813–1878), emphasized the experimental method in establishing biological knowledge and the necessity of basing medical practice in such knowledge. Pathologists, led by Virchow (1821–1902), stressed the critical study of normal and abnormal tissues and the correlation of features of disease with precise anatomical observations. Bacteriologists, with Pasteur (1822–1895) and Koch (1843–1910) in the vanguard, began to identify the microorganisms and to implicate specific organisms in specific diseases—the anthrax bacillus in anthrax, the tubercle bacillus in consumption, the pneumococcus in lobar pneumonia, the streptococcus in puerperal fever. The groundwork for future therapies was being laid by these great Western European scientists, but there was relatively little the physician could do about most illnesses at the time. His major contributions were diagnostic, prognostic, and supportive. By correct diagnosis he could advise concerning outcome. By common-sense supportive measures he could provide comfort and maximize opportunities for recovery. But interventions were as likely as not to make things worse. The first edition of Osler's *Textbook of Medicine* in 1892 was influential for its skepticism and its therapeutic nihilism, as this outstanding physician condemned the majority of nostrums and remedies as useless, even harmful.

Slowly, specific therapies — insulin for diabetes, liver extract for pernicious anemia — or specific immunizations — diphtheria antitoxin, pneumococcic antisera — appeared. But it was not until the decade 1935–1945 that the entry of sulfonamides and penicillin into clinical medicine made a large number of previously lethal and untreatable diseases curable. It is customary to date the beginnings of modern medicine from these relatively recent events.

The language of contemporary biological science has become increasingly biochemical. The compositions of organs, tissues, cells, organelles, and membranes have been defined. The biosynthesis and catabolism of hundreds of compounds have been elucidated. The regulation of body processes has been described at progressively finer levels, and in chemical language. Pharmacologic agents are progressively understood in terms of specific loci and mechanisms of action. The expansion of new knowledge continues at a pace that is bewildering to all but experts in a given field. Current advances are particularly rapid in immunology, molecular biology, and peptide research. A beginning has been made in explaining human behavior in mechanistic terms, as more and more chemical mediators and pharmacologic modifiers are discovered.

We have entered a molecular age of basic biological science, and molecular biology is now a recognized discipline. The molecular influence pervades all the traditional disciplines underlying clinical medicine. Approximately 200 inborn errors are now understood in terms of specific missing or abnormal enzymes or other proteins. There are more than 240 known abnormal human hemoglobins, and for each of these the precise structural defect in the DNA of the mutant gene can be defined. Membrane, cytoplasmic, and nuclear receptors for hormones and drugs are exploding upon us, and old as well as new diseases are being defined in terms of receptor abnormalities — for example, type II hypercholesterolemia and nephrogenic diabetes insipidus. Recognition of opiate receptors has led to the discovery of endogenous peptides (endorphins) with analgesic activity. Their localization gives promise of further understanding of the limbic system, affective states, and addictions. Revolutionary techniques such as cell hybridization and fast-reaction measurement are reducing the gene, the cell, and even the brain to molecular terms.

Much of the recent fundamental information in science has been obtained by the process of reductionism — the exploring of details, and then details of details, until all the smallest bits of the structure, or the smallest parts of the mechanism, are exposed to scrutiny. Many of the most exciting observations of molecular biology have been made in microorganisms, which can be grown by the billions and selected for specific characteristics. Some scientists interested in mechanisms of DNA replication have even found that organisms such as *Escherichia coli* are too complex, and have switched to tiny bacterial DNA viruses whose chromosomes are about a thousandth the size of those of *E. coli*. These studies throw new light on biological mechanisms that could not at present be studied directly in eukaryotic cells.

In the biochemistry laboratory, proteins are isolated, purified, sequenced, and synthesized, their three-dimensional structure elucidated, and their active sites defined. Some of the best work has involved human proteins and has led to new understanding of clinical disorders. Islet cell tumors secrete insulin and proinsulin derived from pre-proinsulin. Lung tumors produce immunologically active parathormone-like material, resembling the C-terminal piece, or the N-terminal piece; only the latter is associated with biological activity.

The scientists responsible for our evolving understanding of biological systems know that the reductionist approach must often precede reconstitutive endeavors. Scientific progress rests on myriads of small observations, tedious measurements, and the findings of investigators asking humble, answerable questions. Instead of reaching for the whole truth, the scientist examines small, defined, and clearly separable phenomena. The pattern of science is a stepwise extension of what came before.

Critics of the bioscientific strategy of medicine have pointed out that the great advances that have dramatically reduced mortality rates consist in the improvement of the environment, the correction of malnutrition, and the control of infectious diseases through immunizations and antimicrobial agents, and that the relevant medical breakthroughs largely occurred before the prodigious expansion of federal support of biomedical science began in the early 1950's. They contend that the enormous expenditures that have made the United States pre-eminent in biomedical research have produced too little in the way of medical advance to justify their continuation, and have instead fostered the development of an extremely costly technology which has had only a minimal effect upon mortality statistics. They propose that the bioscientific strategy of medicine should be replaced by an ecological strategy for health.

These critics ignore several important realities. (1) Strategies for medicine and strategies for health are neither the same nor mutually exclusive. (2) Major advances have occurred since 1950 that have revolutionized the outlook in individual diseases or disease groups — for example, in Hodgkin's disease, acute lymphocytic leukemia of children, Parkinson's disease, and Wilson's disease. (3) Such advances have rested in most instances on a deeper and clearer understanding of underlying disease mechanisms. (4) The elucidation of a disease mechanism and the devising of rational therapy usually depend upon the application of basic scientific knowledge to a clinical problem in the laboratory or ward — for instance, the definition of pathways and rates of uric acid synthesis in gout, and the development of a xanthine oxidase inhibitor (allopurinol) for the control of hyperuricemia and hyperuricaciduria. (5) The expansion of the knowledge bank of the past quarter century justifies great optimism for the eventual control and cure of major diseases and the possible elimination of premature death from illness.

The list of human diseases for which there are as yet no definitive measures for prevention or cure is still formidable. Fresh insights into the nature of these diseases are needed. These insights can come only from continued basic research. Those who believe that there is an abundance of scientific information locked in the laboratory merely awaiting a new emphasis on human application are mistaken. Those who believe that a series of crash programs will lead to ready cures of cancer and heart, vascular, arthritic, emotional, and mental disease are misled. The essential pieces of background information are not merely awaiting assembly; most have yet to be discovered.

It is the record of recent decades that each time a major disease has come under control, through either prevention or cure, the solution has been much simpler and less costly than the half-way technologies devised during earlier stages of incomplete knowledge. Two of today's conspicuous examples of the high cost of half-way technologies are the use of the artificial kidney and renal transplantation for the treatment of chronic renal failure, and of bypass grafts for the treatment of coronary artery disease. Our lack of adequate information concerning the basic mechanisms of chronic nephritis and of atherosclerosis delays more rapid progress in prevention or cure of these conditions.

The practice of medicine is both a science and an art.

A skilled physician must have extensive medical knowledge, which is the bedrock of technical competence. In addition, he or she must have judgment, tact, decisiveness, restraint, compassion, interest, time, and other personal qualities of caring and dedication. This essay does not contend that technical competence is enough. It does contend that compassion without knowledge is insufficient. The science and the art of medicine must always be intimately linked. The student studies the science of medicine first, masters it early, and returns to it frequently. The student acquires the art of medicine — the skillful application of medical knowledge in the optimal care of the patient — more gradually and with experience.

Keeping abreast of the bioscientific, technological, and therapeutic advances of medicine has become an almost insuperable challenge for the physician. Review articles, postgraduate courses, and recertification examinations all help. But the surest way, given the realities of professional demands, is to look upon each patient as a learning experience, and to use each experience as a stimulus to self-renewal and to excellence. Internal drive will cause the student or physician to read about the condition in question and to inquire into the advances in scientific knowledge and application that have occurred since the topic was last reviewed. In this way the highest standards of personal care will be maintained. Given the pace of advance, review must occur at frequent and regular intervals. A wide range of experts must be consulted. Each edition of the *Textbook of Medicine* is a compendium of pertinent information selected and presented by experts, designed to maximize the opportunities for learning and to minimize the lag between discovery and application.

Comroe, J. H., and Dripps, R. D.: The top ten clinical advances in cardiovascular-pulmonary medicine and surgery between 1945 and 1975: How they came about. Bethesda, Md., 1977. Public Inquiries and Reports Branch, National Heart, Lung, and Blood Institute, National Institutes of Health, 1977.

Kornberg, A.: Research, the lifeline of medicine. N. Engl. J. Med., 294:1212, 1976.

Thomas, L.: Biomedical science and human health: The long-range prospect. Daedalus, 106:163, 1977.

4. MEDICINE IN MODERN SOCIETY

Walsh McDermott

Medicine is not a science but a learned profession deeply rooted in a number of sciences and charged with the obligation to apply them for man's benefit. So complex a process could hardly be reduced to a neat symmetrical design and fitted within the covers of a book. Yet this subject, the beneficial uses of medical science, is not without any design at all — it has a conceptual base on which all medical teaching and all medical books should rest. To consider this base, or certain aspects of it, seems proper at the start of a textbook of medicine. Although the book itself is addressed to medical students and graduate physicians of all ages, this essay is presented mainly for those now entering the profession.

One part of the conceptual base is set forth above in the opening sentence that ends ". . . to apply them for man's benefit." Traditionally this applying is made with compassion and in accord with a widely recognized moral and ethical code. The responsibilities of medicine are thus threefold: to generate scientific knowledge and to teach it to others; to use the knowledge for the health of an individual or a whole community; and to judge the moral and ethical propriety of each medical act that directly affects another human being. These three areas of responsibility command the efforts of individuals from a wide range of scientific disciplines and professions. The physicians who actually apply the knowledge, however, are of two sorts: those who deal through a personal encounter with one patient at a time and those who deal with people as groups.

The activities of both sorts of physicians are based on the concept that each disease entity has its own pathogenic chain — the whole series of events that determine its causation and maintenance — and that understanding this chain for a particular disease not only permits clearer recognition of its clinical manifestations, but reveals any weak links that might be exploited for prevention or therapy.

Approach to the body of knowledge organized in this way (both in books and elsewhere) is made from one of two viewpoints. The physician in public health or community medicine is constantly reaching for ways in which pathogenic chains can be broken by some continuing intervention that affects a number of people at once, e.g., to reduce the incidence of goiter by putting iodine in table salt. By contrast, physicians acting through the personal encounter system will search the same knowledge sectors and with educated discrimination will extract those elements appropriate for the solution of a problem in an individual. The viewpoints from which the knowledge is scrutinized are different, but the body of knowledge about each disease is the same. Textbooks about diseases and their pathogenic chains serve both these viewpoints and form important instruments for this process of the beneficial uses of science.

The physician who treats one patient at a time and the physician who deals with a community as a whole both exert compassion, but it is of two quite different sorts. The compassion exercised by the physician who treats individuals takes the form of a cultivated instinct to lend support and comfort to a particular fellow human being. By contrast, the "group" compassion of the public health or community physician necessarily takes the form of what the writer has previously termed "statistical compassion." By this is meant an imaginative compassion for people whom one never gets to see as individuals and, indeed, can know only as data on a graph. This compassion — the deep-seated instinct to try to help those whom one never gets to see — is a characteristic form of motivation for political leaders and other social activists, and "statistical" successes bring them major satisfactions. Such is really not the case with most physicians, who usually do not derive as much satisfaction from seeing improvement on a graph as they do from seeing improvement in an individual. *Indeed, part of the self-selection in choosing medicine as a career seems to be a self-image of a person whose professional activities are to relate directly with individuals rather than with groups.* Thus the system of public health or community medicine — based on physicians *not* seeing patients as individuals — runs contrary to most medical instincts. Yet until we have significant numbers of physicians for whom "statistical compas-

sion" is as rewarding as it is to the leaders in certain other walks of life, we will fail as a society to derive the full measure of the benefits of our medical science.

The scientific basis of medicine had been building up throughout the whole nineteenth century, but the *uses* of that science in the sense of decisively altering or preventing disease were largely accomplished through the public health or "community" physicians who dealt with people as groups. Chlorination of water supplies and the pasteurization of milk are cases in point. It was not until the discovery of insulin in 1921, and not really until the advent of the modern antimicrobial era more than 40 years ago, that the clinical physicians had much in the way of decisive therapies or preventives derived from science. Since that time most of the practical uses of biomedical science and technology have been of a nature fitted to the clinical or personal system, and, despite recent efforts, the other system has been allowed to languish. Indeed, the evolution of the highly complex and extraordinarily effective instrument that is today's university-based medical center has been almost exclusively devoted to the one system — the personal encounter system of one patient at a time.

We could tolerate this so long as what medicine had to offer was technologically simple and physicians were spread out across the whole of society much more evenly than they are now. But the coincidence of massive scientific innovation and wide social change has created a situation in which the application of medical science for man's benefit can no longer be managed by just one of the two systems — we desperately need both.

For there are two critically different populations involved, each of which is the primary responsibility of one of the systems. These two populations are the *constituency* and the *community*. The members of the constituency represent a progressively selected group, in part self-selected, and the selection is based on the presence of a medical problem, frequently one that is quite complex. Each member, in effect, has *voted* to obtain the services of a physician (or center or medical group) and has cast this vote as an individual without reference to others. The constituency is thus a collection of individuals who share in common only the fact that each has perceived a self-problem of illness or disease. It is the group known familiarly as the physician's "practice." The community, by contrast, is made up of people distinguished by the possession in common of some factor not directly related to disease. Usually, but not invariably, this common factor is a domicile located within some geographically defined boundary. In health terms, therefore, the community is a wholly unselected group, and at any one point in time many more of its members are well than are sick. *The community and the constituency thus differ strikingly in the prevalence of significant illness and disease. Because of this difference, an institutional form appropriate to meet the needs of one group would be markedly different from the form appropriate for the other.* Our challenge today is to develop such a two-type institutional form so that the needs of both groups may be equally served.

What the community needs is recognition of weakness in pathogenic chains that may be exploited in the prevention of disease. For nonpreventable disease the community needs straightforward medical care close to home, safeguarded by continuous mechanisms for identifying those who need care in the first place and mechanisms for sifting the few who need complex care from the many who do not. These few needing complex care join with a similar few from the constituency — that group of people self-selected from a much larger population base than could be satisfactorily served by a single personal encounter physician. What these properly sifted members of the constituency need is an institution that can offer a complete array of talents appropriate for the solution of any currently solvable medical problem, no matter how rarely occurring or complicated it might be. Whether for the community or for the constituency, the actual provision of the care is the responsibility of the personal encounter physician. Community medicine (or the larger public health system of which it is a part) is thus responsible *not* for the delivery of personal health services to the members of a community, but for ensuring that the community receives the proper health services of all sorts. And prominent among these are the invention of better mechanisms than we have now for both the continuous community scan of who needs care at any moment and appropriate entry points for the care of those identified. Neither of these two systems is inherently of greater social value than the other, but in the course of developing the personal encounter system to its present high point of technologic effectiveness for the individual, we have failed to mount a comparable effort for the nourishment of the other system responsible for the medical welfare of every member of the group. Without such a healthy watchdog we have allowed the personal encounter system to become unevenly distributed throughout our population. The correction of this imbalance is the critical challenge facing medicine today, and how well we meet it will determine the role of the physician in our society. For the imbalance of the two systems affects our efforts for the beneficial uses of science not only at the level of medical care for the community and the constituency, but in those even larger health matters that have to do with how the developing individual can be aided in his or her continuous interaction with the environment.

Health, like happiness, is an abstraction; it cannot be defined in exact measurable terms because its presence is so much a matter of subjective judgment. Health is a relative condition that represents the degree to which an individual can operate with effectiveness within the particular circumstances of his or her heredity and physical and cultural environment. Disease *can* be measured, and it occurs in patterns that closely reflect the major features of a particular society. The term "level of health" of a society designates which of some four or five possible patterns is present. Serious misunderstanding has arisen in recent years about the respective impacts of the two delivery systems on a society's health. Economists and other health planners have failed to recognize that there are virtually no established indicators by which to measure the impact of the personal encounter system on our nation's health. What gets measured, using the customary health indices, is the impact of the other two forces — the public health system and the life style afforded by the material culture. Each of us is under the constant influence of all three forces, and in that setting the disease pattern of the United States, including certain chronic conditions with a significant cultural linkage, has shown a steady trend toward a better level of health in recent years.

It is not possible to do justice to all these issues in this book, although some are indeed considered. For others, certain key references to the literature that has been developing in recent years are set forth below. There remain a few, however, that are so vital to the conceptual base forming the theme of this chapter that they deserve special mention.

Moral judgments must be made by the physician engaged in individual patient care, but they are to be made on his own professional acts and those of his colleagues, not on the actions of those who sought his care. Any moral judgments he might make on his patients' behavior are private matters to be kept within himself; he must not permit them to influence his own professional acts. This has long been the medical tradition, and it is important that it not be forgotten in the tumult of today's world of clashing value systems. The prospect of moral and ethical problems of an essentially new type is also now emerging before us. There is general awareness that advances in medical science are leading to various ethical conflicts that have to be faced by the personal encounter physician. What is less well recognized, however, is that this situation will also become socially serious for the nonclinical system, whether it be called public health or community medicine. Critical phenomena in human development formerly thought to represent the hand of fate are now found to be, at least in part, environmentally determined, and hence manipulable — such matters as the full expansion of an individual's intelligence or perhaps his or her degree of educability. If we develop the power to significantly influence such critical matters — and scientifically we are getting closer to it every day — we may find ourselves faced with seeking to protect the "interests" of an unborn or newborn child in the receipt of a particular intervention against the "rights" of its parents to be free from outside interference. And this question of how to ensure the best opportunity for the individual without destroying family structure in the process will not be an ethical problem to be faced by medicine in rare instances, but one that will involve whole societies. Yet we cannot run away from such questions, for it is the wise application of our science and technology, made with either form of compassion, that allows us to approach one of our major goals — that of ensuring that every child born into the world has the maximal chance to make the run through life's most productive years.

Finally, we must heed a concept of medicine that is ageless. In the life of an individual there ultimately may come a time when all the knowledge so carefully presented by the contributors to this book no longer has usefulness, yet life must go on, at least for a time. Whenever this happens, and it happens every day, it is up to each of us to follow to the fullest measure the charge laid down long ago for "the physician to become himself the treatment."

Beeson, P. B.: Some good features of the British National Health Service. Arch. Intern. Med., 133:708, 1974.
Dubos, R.: So Human an Animal. New York, Charles Scribner's Sons, 1969.
McDermott, W.: Demography, culture, and economics and the evolutionary stages of medicine. *In* Kilbourne, E. D., and Smillie, W. G. (eds.): Human Ecology and Public Health. 4th ed. New York, The Macmillan Company, 1969.
McDermott, W.: The public good and one's own. Perspect. Biol. Med., 21:167, 1978.
Morison, R. S.: Where is biology taking us? Science, 155:429, 1967.
Rogers, D. E.: The Changing Face of American Medicine. Cambridge, Mass., Ballinger Publishing Company, 1978.

PART II
HUMAN GROWTH AND DEVELOPMENT

5. HEREDITY

Alexander G. Bearn

Man is a singular creature exhibiting much genetic diversity, and able to adapt with extraordinary versatility to a wide range of environmental circumstances, some of them extreme. His genetic constitution has evolved over the last 10 to 20 million years—the period that has elapsed since we began to diverge from our nearest relative, the chimpanzee (presently vying with the gorilla for this dubious honor), who unlike man has 48 chromosomes in each diploid cell. The cranial capacity of man's immediate ancestors increased rapidly, trebling in 10 million years, although there is scant evidence that it has undergone further enlargement during the last 100,000 years. However, domestication of plants and animals as sources of food some 10,000 years ago accelerated man's cultural evolution and increased his independence from nature.

During evolution, a number of irreversible biologic steps have been taken. From the time that mammals began to evolve from amphibia and gill structures were lost, perhaps 200 million years ago, future man was condemned to a terrestrial existence. Dependence on oxygen for metabolism and life was set even earlier in the long evolutionary process.

Although man has been able to adjust to a variety of hostile environments, including ocean depths and outer space where he survives at 0 g, he has been able to do so only because his intellectual ingenuity has allowed him to equip himself with the necessary life support systems. Thus, man's present genetic constitution has established the boundary conditions for his biologic future and the cultural structures which he is able to fashion.

The revolution in biology over the past 25 years has established, in minute particulars, the sequential events that determine the structure of proteins as a result of information encoded in DNA. But the inevitability and fidelity of this information transfer have sometimes been obscured by environmental factors that influence the ultimate expression of the genetic message. In the final analysis, it is not possible to separate genes from the environment in which they act. The nature-nurture polemic is a Victorian abstraction, of no concern to modern biologists.

Despite this, it remains conventional to regard all diseases of man as due principally to either hereditary or environmental influences. The limitation of such a classification is exposed when we realize that many diseases classified as genetic can be managed by manipulating the environment rather than the abnormal gene. Restricting phenylalanine in the diet of infants with phenylketonuria is one example. Conversely, the disease scurvy, usually regarded as due to an environmental deficiency of vitamin C, could just as well be

thought of as an inborn error of metabolism in which the hepatic enzyme that converts L-gluconalactone to L-ascorbic acid (present in all mammals except man, monkey, and the guinea pig) is genetically deficient.

In some diseases, such as achondroplastic dwarfism, genetic influences appear decisive and environmental factors undetectable, whereas in microbial disease and other disorders caused by exogenous environmental agents, the genetic component is considered trivial. Yet even here genetic susceptibility or resistance may play an important role. For example, human red cells which have on their surface the Duffy blood group antigen are susceptible to infection by *Plasmodium vivax* malaria. In contrast, cells which lack the Duffy factor are not subject to this infection. Many West Africans lack the Duffy marker on their cells; the parasites rarely gain entry to the red cell, and *Plasmodium vivax* malaria is rare. The uniqueness of the molecular specificity that determines the infection is evident not only from the regional absence of vivax malaria, but from the prevalence of falciparum malaria: the falciparum parasite is totally indifferent to the molecular architecture of the Duffy factor, and infection proceeds unhindered.

Thus, although in many infections the environmental agent is crucial, the importance of the genotype of the host, as in vivax malaria, should not be discounted. It seems likely that, in the past, infectious diseases were powerful selective agents, and that the ability to survive epidemic disasters was dependent at least in part on the individual's genotype (see Ch. 12).

For more than half a century, comparative studies of identical and nonidentical twins have been used to draw distinctions between hereditary and environmental influences. However, even when identical twins are reared apart, they have a shared common environment before birth, and dogmatic conclusions are treacherous.

Indeed, quantifying the balance of genetic and environmental influences in disease has been overemphasized by geneticists who have substituted algebra for biology and abstraction for reality. The greatest difficulty in sorting out the relative importance of genetic and environmental influence is encountered with common diseases. In disorders such as cancer, essential hypertension, and coronary artery disease, genetic influences are important but hard to identify in specific biochemical terms. It is occasionally possible to identify single genes that have a specific metabolic effect, such as those responsible for hypercholesterolemia and hypertriglyceridemia, but more often genetic factors are elusive.

Recently, the nature-nurture polemic, so frequently revived in sterile discussions of educability and intelligence, has been refreshingly illuminated by many fundamental studies on gene regulation. One only will be noted; evidence has now accumulated which suggests that, at any given time, as much as 80 per cent of the genetic material in the cells of higher organisms is inactive. This inactivity can be reversed by certain environmental influences. Certain steroid hormones, for example, possess the capacity to influence gene activity, and a number of these have now been shown to influence directly the synthesis of mRNA and tRNA. Indeed, the administration of estrogen to a rooster can activate genes in the rooster's liver cells so that they synthesize egg yolk proteins — proteins of more interest to the molecular biologist than to the rooster.

We can summarize by re-emphasizing that genetics is concerned with the study of hereditary variations. Most of these variations are not harmful; indeed, they confer a distinct biologic advantage by enabling the species to adapt to an ever-changing environment. When they are extreme they may be associated with clinical disease and come directly to the attention of the physician. Only by understanding the complexity of the interaction between genes and environment will the old concept of genetic diathesis be clothed in scientific reality. In the future, environmental and social change will assuredly create new diseases. Man will continue to learn more and more about his genetic constitution and, as he does, he must try to make the most of its virtues and outwit its defects.

Although the fabric of human diversity is brilliantly close-woven, it is not man's individuality that sets him apart but his awareness of it. For those who would truly understand human disease, the individuality of man's response to an ever-changing and often hostile environment is the ultimate basis of medical practice. Upon this foundation the precious and humane responsibility for the care of our patients must be built.

Bodmer, W. F., and Cavalli-Sforza, L. L.: Genetics, Evolution and Man. San Francisco, W. H. Freeman and Company, 1976.

6. ENVIRONMENT

Howard H. Hiatt

All disturbances in health reflect the interplay of environmental and genetically determined host factors. In that sense a textbook of medicine is concerned in its entirety with a consideration of man and his environment. However, the complexity of environmental factors affecting health makes it appropriate to offer a few introductory generalizations about them. Further, attention to how alteration of environmental factors can prevent or ameliorate disease is particularly urgent at this time of justifiable concern with the limitations and economic costs of therapeutic medicine.

The dimensions of man's environment are suggested when we consider that it encompasses everything that impinges on man other than the genes of the germ cell. Indeed, studies in other forms indicate that the genetic apparatus itself often includes material that was once "environment." For example, a bacterial cell may become resistant to an antimicrobial drug as a result of infection with a virus containing the information necessary for the synthesis of enzymes that inactivate the drug. Not only is the bacterium thus able to make the enzymes in question, but because viral nucleic acid may become a part of the genetic apparatus of the cell, the cell can pass on to its progeny the capacity to inactivate the drug. A related phenomenon may explain the presence of tumor viral nucleic acid in certain animal

cells. The expression of the nucleic acid in terms of tumor production may require one or more further environmental exposures — for example, to x-rays or to a chemical. This multifactorial etiology is characteristic of all diseases, and the complex interaction of causes has been likened by MacMahon and Pugh to a "web" of causation. Fortunately, effective action does not require complete unraveling of such webs — the disruption of any one thread may be sufficient to induce a favorable change in health status.

DETERMINANTS OF RESPONSE TO ENVIRONMENTAL FACTORS

It has long been recognized that many environmental substances are harmful only to individuals of a specific genetic constitution. Individuals with genetic defects in metabolic pathways may be poisoned by substances that are readily tolerated by most people. An example is the damage done by the muscle relaxant drug suxamethonium to people with abnormal forms of the enzyme pseudocholinesterase. A diet containing "normal" amounts of phenylalanine will be profoundly damaging to persons homozygous for a particular gene. People unable to convert certain dietary constituents to biologically active forms, such as those with vitamin D resistant rickets, will manifest deficiency states even when receiving the substance in amounts adequate for "normal" individuals. Such conditions are worthy of special emphasis, for although they are infrequent, they are but recognized manifestations of individual variations that are ubiquitous. Responses to drugs, chemicals, microorganisms, stress, and other environmental factors, particularly at low doses, reflect in part the genetically determined constitution of the person exposed. Differences from the "normal" in lipoprotein metabolism have already been well documented in the families of patients with complications of atherosclerosis; thus genetic predisposition probably makes the cardiovascular system of certain people more susceptible to the ravages of such known potentially harmful factors as hypertension, obesity, and too little exercise. Similarly, individual susceptibility likely explains in part why many but not all cigarette smokers develop lung cancer. Critical to preventive medicine is the development of methods for identifying people for whom specific environmental factors are hazardous, so that appropriate measures can be directed at those at risk.

Response to environmental factors is greatly affected by other environmental conditions prevailing at the time of exposure. One example is a drug the administration of which leads to altered metabolism of, and thereby to altered action of, a second drug or other chemical. Another is the effect of nutritional status on the response to infectious agents; malnutrition may explain in large part why the fatality rate from measles is so much greater in rural Guatemala than in the United States. An individual with compromised function as a result of earlier exposure to one environmental factor may be particularly prone to the effects of another; for example, people with pneumoconiosis are sensitive to carbon monoxide and those with coronary artery disease to carbon monoxide and carbon disulfide.

Timing of exposure may also be important, particularly during prenatal life. A few of the known congenital malformations and spontaneous abortions have thus far been traced to identified environmental insults, but over 80 per cent are of unknown cause. Drugs, other chemicals, viruses, bacteria, carbon monoxide, and ionizing radiation are among factors known to cause congenital malformations, but only if exposure occurs during the first trimester of pregnancy. Thalidomide, for example, given to pregnant women caused serious anomalies in their offspring. Exposure of the pregnant woman early in the sensitive period led to ear anomaly in the offspring, later to arm deformity, and later yet to leg deformity. Exposures after the first trimester produced no deformity.

Environmental factors may affect the incidence or the course of a disease, or both; the condition of the host at the time of exposure helps determine which. For example, in mice, x-rays may activate a pre-existing tumor virus, thereby producing cancer. However, even in the absence of latent oncogenic viral DNA, x-rays may themselves lead to cancer by inducing a mutation of cellular DNA. Finally, by their lethal effects on cells, x-rays may be used to destroy cancer, and thus are used therapeutically. Similarly, diethylstilbestrol will produce temporary remissions of breast cancer in some patients; however, it is also known to lead to the appearance of cancer, and some young women have developed cancer of the vagina after exposure to diethylstilbestrol during intrauterine life many years earlier. Since many environmental factors cause disease only after latent periods measured in decades, alertness and continued monitoring of potential hazards are required.

CLASSIFICATION OF ENVIRONMENTAL FACTORS

In considering the variety of environmental factors known to be harmful to health, it must be emphasized that the field is in a state of flux, and there are few broadly accepted organizing principles. Some environmental influences of major importance, particularly in developing countries, are naturally occurring. Increasingly, however, attention is focused throughout the world on the health hazards of environmental conditions created by man. Some factors are detrimental to health when present in excess, and others when deficient; many lead to problems under either circumstance. Many, and probably most, environmental factors injurious to health have yet to be identified, and new ones are constantly appearing as a result of increased population, increased affluence, and technologic advances.

A prevailing classification breaks down the principal environmental factors into chemical, physical, biologic, and social. A few examples of each follow.

CHEMICAL FACTORS. The role of chemicals in inducing human disease is variable and complicated. No chemical can be considered completely nontoxic, even though many are required in small amounts for physiologic processes. For example, the benefits of small amounts of fluoride on tooth development are now accepted. Studies of disease patterns in areas of hard and soft water supply suggest that as yet unidentified factors in water may offer some protection against atherosclerosis. Lead, arsenic, mercury, cadmium, cobalt, selenium, tin, manganese, and other metals can produce acute poisoning and may be introduced by contaminated food or water. Polychlorinated biphenyls, organochlorine, and organophosphorus insecticides may gain access via the same routes. A variety of chemicals, including silica, asbestos, lead, vinyl chloride, and many solvents, may be present in toxic amounts in the air, particularly in and near industrial plants. The exposure of workers to harmful chemicals is often reflected in higher mortality and morbidity rates in areas where certain industries are concentrated.

Over 15,000 chemicals are now in commercial production in amounts between 500 and 1 million kilograms per year, and an additional 500 are introduced annually. Some are carcinogenic, some mutagenic, some teratogenic, and some toxic in other ways. Because the long-term effects of a substance cannot be known with certainty for decades, testing for chronic as well as acute effects should be carried out before widespread human exposure is permitted. However, since it is impossible to test comprehensively all new compounds, it is particularly important to pay attention to those structurally related to other substances known to be toxic. Of crucial importance has been the recent development of short-term in vitro tests for measuring the mutagenic effects of chemicals on cultured bacterial and mammalian cells. Increasing evidence points to a close (but not perfect) correspondence between mutagenicity in cultured cells and carcinogenicity in animals. Thus the in vitro tests are now widely used as an early warning system. They have already obviated the introduction into the environment of many potentially harmful substances and have led to the withdrawal of others. In many instances in which relation between cancer and environmental exposure is well established, the specific chemicals responsible remain to be identified, as for example the carcinogenic constituents of cigarette smoke.

PHYSICAL FACTORS. Home accidents accounted for 1.3 per cent of all deaths and 4 million injuries in the United States in 1975, and automobile accidents caused 44,570 deaths and 1,800,000 injuries. Modern transportation has had detrimental effects on health in addition to the loss of life and limb caused by automobile accidents; there is evidence that one factor contributing to coronary artery disease is lack of exercise.

Excessive heat, cold, and noise are harmful, as are both nonionizing and ionizing radiation. Less than 2 per cent of our total exposure to ionizing radiation comes from occupational sources and fallout consequent to nuclear weapons testing and nuclear power development. Almost one third of our exposure is from medical diagnostic procedures, and two thirds from natural sources. However, with increasing dependence on nuclear power likely in the years ahead, this could change significantly. The effect of ionizing radiation on the gene pool is cumulative. The most important known somatic effect is carcinogenesis. Whether radiation effects contribute to mortality from causes other than cancer is uncertain.

BIOLOGIC FACTORS. Man may be exposed to pathogenic bacteria, viruses, and parasites through inspired air, ingested food and water, and skin contact. The soil is a common source of pathogenic microorganisms and parasites, and many occupations have special biologic hazards, such as anthrax and brucellosis. Many infectious agents produce both acute and chronic disease. Some virus-induced conditions, such as kuru, become manifest only after a latent period of years. Although there have been many claims and much speculation, no unequivocal evidence yet exists for a microbiologic agent as a cause of cancer in man. However, it is likely that some forms of human cancer are viral in origin. At present, the herpes viruses seem to be the best candidates.

SOCIAL FACTORS.   Social factors, including economic, psychologic, and cultural factors, all affect health. Brenner has found that there is a significant statistical relationship between unemployment and the incidence of cardiovascular disease, cirrhosis of the liver, suicide, mental illness, homicides, and the rate of imprisonment. In addition, there is evidence that schizophrenia, crime, suicide, alcoholism, and drug abuse have higher rates in impoverished and crowded areas. Infant mortality is as much as three times higher in the poverty sectors than in more affluent parts of the same cities. Knobloch and Pasamanick have shown that although black and white infants manifest no differences in developmental tests at 40 weeks of age, by three years the performance of black children is significantly behind

that of the white. Whether poverty itself, poor housing, inadequate diet, less education, a combination of these, or other factors are responsible is yet to be established. However urgent the need for more knowledge in this area, existing information is sufficient to provide strong incentive for improving conditions.

Examination of mortality data for the eighteenth, nineteenth, and early twentieth centuries reveals that some major improvements in health have resulted to a much greater extent from changes in a variety of environmental factors than from medical measures. This is particularly apparent in studies of deaths from infectious diseases in the preantimicrobial era (see accompanying figure). There is reason to believe that the improvements resulted from better nutrition, removal of hazards from the physical environment by improved water supply and sewage disposal, and a decrease in the birth rate. Other factors may also have contributed, including changes in the virulence of some of the microorganisms, notably the streptococci.

A, Respiratory tuberculosis: mean annual death rate, England and Wales. *B*, Scarlet fever: mean annual death rate of children under 15, England and Wales. (From McKeown, T., and Lowe, C. R.: An Introduction to Social Medicine. Oxford, Blackwell, 1974.)

BEHAVIORAL CHANGE

It was earlier pointed out that in order to prevent or alter an illness we do not always require an understanding of the mechanism whereby an environmental factor contributes to it, and often not even a precise identification of the specific offending factor. On the other hand, however difficult it may be to establish a cause-and-effect relationship between environmental factor and disease, it may be far more difficult to exploit such knowledge. Consider, for example, the difficulties in inducing the attitudinal and behavioral changes required to take greater advantage of the knowledge that gonorrhea is transmitted sexually and that a variety of pulmonary, cardiac, and other diseases are aggravated by cigarette smoking. One important step is, of course, behavioral change in the physician. It is unlikely that even the most enlightened patients will be appropriately moved by statistics relating cigarettes, obesity, or lack of exercise to disease if those statistics are offered by physicians who pay them no heed. Further, just as physicians who have diagnosed a condition that requires penicillin must ensure that the drug is received, so they must do everything possible to achieve the environmental and behavioral changes that they feel are dictated by their patients' health.

Much of the health benefit resulting from a recognition of responsible environmental factors and their alteration can be achieved only through action directed at population groups. Here the responsibilities of the physician include participation with other members of society in those socially acceptable actions necessary to achieve the desired ends.

CONCLUSIONS

An examination of the present state of knowledge of the relationships of environmental factors and health leads to certain conclusions. First, there is great need for careful and extensive data collection and analysis. The paucity and unreliability of available data and the complexity of the problems that confront us have led too often in this chapter and in this book to the use of such expressions as "is believed to," "may," "conflicting reports exist," and so on, and undoubtedly even more often to our overlooking associations. Better patient records and information systems are required to help correlate data concerning illness, drugs, chemicals, and physical, nutritional, social, and other environmental factors that affect health in order to alert society to dangers as early as possible. However, even these will never replace the contribution of the astute physician who regards every patient not only as a human being in need of attention and devotion, but also as one presenting a problem in need of a solution. It is relevant to recall that rubella and thalidomide were recognized as teratogens not in a research laboratory or by a computerized medical record system, but by astute clinicians in the course of their practice. (It is true, of course, that had better record systems been available at the time, the teratogenic effects might have been recognized earlier.)

The most sophisticated techniques of modern science will help demonstrate mutagenic, carcinogenic, teratogenic, and other effects of environmental factors on human cells and test organisms. Modern technology can contribute greatly needed quantification to environmental health studies. We require methods for assessing the effects of a variety of factors on human behavior and emotions and on other mental functions, although precise methodology in this area is likely to be a long way in the future. Cost-benefit studies, both medical and economic, are necessary for the physician to make enlightened decisions concerning the risks to which diagnosis and treatment inevitably expose his patient. The risk of anaphylaxis to penicillin is surely worth taking in the individual with pneumococcal pneumonia who has never had the drug previously. The risk of side effects such as thromboembolic disease from oral contraceptives now seems reasonable in the young woman seeking birth control. (Whether this will continue to be the case when all their health effects are uncovered remains uncertain.) Many other more difficult choices exist, and with the growing medical armamentarium and increasing information concerning the effects of drugs, chemicals, and procedures, many more difficult decisions are placed daily before the physician in his practice.

In recent decades there has been no improvement in over-all mortality rate from cancer.* More than 80 per cent of cases of cancer in the United States are thought to be the result, at least in part, of environmental factors. Similarly, a variety of environmental factors are known to aggravate cardiovascular disease. These and related facts make mandatory increased attention to preventive measures. The exciting implications of the application of our rapidly growing understanding of biology and chemistry to medical problems are widely recognized, and fundamental and clinical research has been and must continue to be encouraged. However, it is at least equally important that we address the present neglect of the benefits that can be achieved from available knowledge. Social and individual action could surely lead to the prevention or amelioration of many diseases, including several that are occupationally related. In this area the physician is often in a unique position to help identify problems and contribute to campaigns to alter responsible conditions.

---

*However, some changes, including a marked increase in survival of children with acute leukemia, are not reflected in the over-all data.

Brenner, H.: Estimating the Social Costs of National Economic Policy: Implications for Mental and Physical Health, and Criminal Aggression. Study prepared for the Joint Economic Committee, Congress of the U.S., October 26. Washington, D.C., U.S. Government Printing Office, 1976.

Gregg, N. M.: Congenital cataract following German measles in mother. Trans. Ophthalmol. Soc. Australia, 3:35, 1942.

Health Hazards of the Human Environment. Geneva, World Health Organization, 1972.

Knobloch, H., and Pasamanick, B.: Environmental factors affecting human development, before and after birth. Pediatrics, 26:210, 1960.

MacMahon, B., and Pugh, T. P.: Epidemiology: Principles and Methods. Boston, Little, Brown & Company, 1970.

McBride, W. G.: Thalidomide and congenital abnormalities. Lancet, 2:1358, 1961.

McKeown, T., and Lowe, C. R.: An Introduction to Social Medicine, 2nd ed. Oxford, Blackwell, 1974.

7. THE LIFE-CYCLE PERSPECTIVE IN MEDICINE

Herant A. Katchadourian

The perception of the individual in the context of the life cycle is essential for understanding patients and for dealing efficiently with their ailments and infirmities. In the seventeenth century Sir Thomas Browne wrote:

"Confound not the distinctions of thy Life which Nature hath divided, that is, Youth, Adolescence, Manhood, and old Age; nor in these divided Periods, wherein thou art in a manner Four, conceive thyself but One. Let every division be happy in its proper Virtues, nor one Vice run through all. Let each distinction have its salutary transition, and critically deliver thee from the imperfections of the former; so ordering the whole, that Prudence and Virtue may have the largest Section."

It is not merely convention that requires case histories to begin with a statement of the patient's age. Considerations related to chronologic age enter into the interpretation of the history of illness and the findings of physical examinations and laboratory tests. Since the prevalence and manifestations of illness are often age related, the fact that one is dealing with a child or an adult, an adolescent or an elderly person, significantly influences probabilistic judgments in differential diagnosis. At an even more fundamental level, the developmental phase itself determines the fact and nature of illness. Bedwetting or the presence of immature blood cells in the circulation does not carry the pathologic connotations in an infant that it would in an adult. Treatment, too, is age dependent, because the choice of procedure and dosage and even the expected outcome are significantly linked to age.

Even though a person's age is an unequivocal chronologic fact, to declare that someone is a child or an adult implies that the life span is divisible into phases and that childhood and adulthood are definable periods within it. But despite their pervasive use, terms like *child, adolescent,* or *adult* have no precise medical definition. Even more ambiguous are terms that refer to various subphases of these periods, such as *late adolescence* or *middle age.*

We take it for granted that such life phases are universal because they are biologically determined. Yet our notions about life phases are culturally defined. In spite of obvious physical differences between young and old, social differentiation is comparatively recent. Until the seventeenth century, there was no special emphasis on childhood as a separate phase of life in Western societies. In the Middle Ages, after the age of seven or so, when children could presumably look after themselves, they simply joined the world of adults, dressed like adults, and shared adult work and play. Although some went to school, there was no age grading in classrooms, and the ten- and twenty-year-olds could be taught together.

The shift away from viewing children as miniature adults began with the Reformation and the Counter Reformation in the seventeenth century. The philosophies of John Locke (1632–1704) and Jean Jacques Rousseau (1712–1778) were important early influences in shaping modern views of childhood. It was only after children had been recognized by society as a class of individuals different from adults that physicians began to make the same distinction systematically. Thus, although references to diseases of children can be found even in the most ancient of medical texts (such as the Ebers Papyrus of 1550 B.C.), medical specialization based on the age of the patient dates back only to the middle of the nineteenth century, when pediatrics began to emerge as a distinct field.

Since the turn of the century, both social and medical perspectives of the life span have tended toward further differentiation. Our modern concept of adolescence was greatly influenced by Granville Stanley Hall (1844–1924), a leading figure in American psychology and education. During the last several decades, adolescent medicine and geriatrics have become fairly well established subspecialties, even though neither of them yet qualifies for board certification. Currently there is growing interest in the specific processes and problems of adulthood itself.

Although most of the research on the life span has been done by social scientists (Goulet and Baltes; Nesselroade and Reese; Baltes and Schaie), there are now some good books by physicians in this field (Engel; Lidz). The concept of the life-cycle and life-span developmental psychology hold considerable promise for contributing to our understanding of people and how to take care of them.

The advantages to the physicians of adopting a life-cycle or life-span view can be subsumed under three general areas. First, this view extends the developmental focus beyond childhood and adolescence, so that adulthood and old age also can be seen as dynamic and changing phases of life, rather than static plateaus punctuated by periods of illness. This approach allows not only a more coherent longitudinal view of life but also a better understanding of its components over time and in a broader context. For example, sexual physiology and behavior make better sense if understood in terms of their varied manifestations at different phases of life and in relation to other significant biologic and psychosocial events occurring concurrently.

The second advantage of a life-cycle perspective is that it facilitates a multidisciplinary, integrative approach to human development and behavior. It furnishes a conceptual umbrella broad enough to incorporate a variety of views and approaches toward making cumulative sense out of the diversity of human life.

Finally, when the field of life-span developmental psychology has reached sufficient maturity, it may provide useful indices of the normative tasks and critical events that characterize the various nodal points and transitional periods of the life cycle. Such indices will help the physician assess the patient in a set of normative contexts and will facilitate more intelligent judgments in pathology. Furthermore, to the extent that such normative crises are predictable, there is allowance for anticipation and preparation to cope with them. The physician stands to gain from such knowledge not only in dealing with patients but also in the conduct of his or her own life. Although we share our patients' experiences only infrequently, in living out our own lives we are basically no different from those we set out to help.

On the other hand, the concept of the life cycle, like any other model or theory, is not a panacea. When theory becomes dogma, it entraps us into expectations that become self-fulfilling prophecies. By accepting the notion of "growing pains," we may be inclined to take lightly serious pain in a growing person. If adolescence is considered a turbulent period, then adolescents will oblige us by becoming turbulent. If middle age is expected to be a time for finding new directions, then middle-aged people may be inclined to throw away the worthwhile with the worthless in their vocational and personal lives.

Concepts like the cycle are useful at best as modest aids to our understanding the awesome complexity of human beings. Such concepts are not meant to be devices with which to wrap up life and put it in our pockets.

Aries, P.: Centuries of Childhood. New York, Knopf, 1962.

Baltes, P. B., and Schaie, K. W. (eds.): Life-Span Developmental Psychology: Personality and Socialization. New York, Academic Press, 1973.

Browne, T.: Part III, Sect. 8 of Christian Morals. In Religio Medici, Letter to a Friend, Urn-burial and Other Papers. Boston, 1878.

Engel, G. L.: Psychological Development in Health and Disease. Philadelphia, W. B. Saunders Company, 1962.

Goulet, L. R., and Baltes, P. B. (eds.): Life-Span Developmental Psychology: Research and Theory. New York, Academic Press, 1970.

Lidz, T.: The Person: His and Her Development Throughout the Life Cycle. New York, Basic Books, 1976.

Muuss, R. E.: Theories of Adolescence. New York, Random House, 1968.

Nesselroade, J. R., and Reese, H. W. (eds.): Life-Span Developmental Psychology: Methodological Issues. New York, Academic Press, 1973.

Simons, R. C., and Pardes, H.: Understanding Human Behavior in Health and Illness. Baltimore, Williams & Wilkins Company, 1977.

8. DEVELOPMENT TO ADULTHOOD

Herant A. Katchadourian

The terms "adolescent" and "adult" are both derived from the Latin "to grow" (*adolescere*): an adolescent is someone who is growing up, and an adult is someone who has grown up. Although this designation is overly simple to encompass the complex changes entailed in attaining adulthood, bodily growth and reproductive maturation are in fact among the cardinal events in this process. The period of life during which these biologic changes occur is properly referred to as "puberty," to differentiate it from the psychosocial developmental phase of "adolescence" with which it overlaps but does not coincide.

8.1. BIOLOGIC PROCESSES IN PUBERTY

The changes that constitute puberty have been classified by Marshall and Tanner as follows: (1) Acceleration and then deceleration of skeletal growth (the adolescent growth spurt). (2) Altered body composition as a result of skeletal and muscular growth, together with changes of the quantity and distribution of fat. (3) Development of the circulatory and respiratory systems, leading, particularly in boys, to increased strength and endurance. (4) The development of the gonads, reproductive organs, and secondary sex characters. (5) A combination of factors, not yet fully understood, which

modulates the activity of those nervous and endocrine elements which initiate and coordinate all these changes.

These changes result in two major biologic outcomes that have profound psychosocial repercussions. First, the child attains the physique and physiologic characteristics of the adult, including reproductive capacity. Second, most of the major adult physical sex differences become established through this process, greatly enhancing sexual dimorphism in adulthood.

These changes are virtually universal but with important differences between normal individuals in the onset, order, and rate of growth at puberty. We shall be mainly concerned here with the general patterns.

SOMATIC CHANGES. One usually becomes aware of the onset of puberty through its somatic manifestations. But these are preceded by hormonal changes, which in turn are triggered by activities in hypothalamic and other brain centers. The precise mechanisms that determine the onset of puberty are as yet unknown.

Among contemporary Western youth, the first signs of puberty become apparent at about age 10 to 11 among girls and 11 to 12 among boys (see accompanying figure). There is, however, a wide range of normal variability extending from 8½ to 13 years for girls and 9½ to 15 for boys. Most children do enter puberty within these ages (95 per cent of girls show at least one sign of puberty by age 13½); yet even at that, perfectly normal exceptions are possible at both extremes.

Puberty entails a whole host of changes, some of which are shown in the accompanying figure. Each of these events has its own schedule and range of variability. The general sequence of these events is more predictable than the ages at which they are likely to unfold. Girls enter puberty consistently earlier than boys by about two years, but here again the magnitude of discrepancy depends on what is being compared; girls grow pubic hair a year and a half earlier, but breast budding antedates testicular enlargement by six months.

It is essential to appreciate the normality of this wide range of variability during puberty. The physician must be prepared to confront adolescents of precisely the same chronologic age with dramatic differences in physical appearance, depending on whether they have entered puberty, are part way through it, or have completed the process.

Height and Weight. The pubescent growth spurt is among the more dramatic events encountered during development. Growth in stature is in progress throughout childhood. Actually, by age 10, boys have already attained 78 per cent and girls 84 per cent of their adult height. What makes the growth spurt at puberty noteworthy is mainly its rate rather than its magnitude. The height spurt typically starts at about 10½ years among girls, reaches peak velocity at 12, and ends by 14. But it may start as early as 9½ or end as late as 15 years. Among boys, the onset is usually at about 12 to 13 (or as early as 10½ and as late as 16), the peak at 14, and the end at 16 (or between 13½ and 17½). During the year of peak height velocity, a boy grows on an average of 3 to 5 inches and a girl somewhat less. This means an actual doubling in velocity of growth and approximates the rapid growth rate of the two-year-old child. Following the growth spurt, the rate of growth decelerates rapidly. Most girls at 14 years and most boys at 16 years reach 98 per cent of their ultimate adult height.

Sequence of events of puberty in girls (above) and boys (below). (From Tanner, J. M.: Sci. Am., 229:40, 1973. Copyright © 1973 by Scientific American, Inc. All rights reserved.)

Further noticeable growth in stature ceases at about 18 years in women and at 20 years in men.

Stature is determined by a host of genetic and environmental factors. It varies among children as it does among adults. During puberty further differences emerge which are transient artifacts of discrepant rates of growth. Thus an early maturing adolescent may move ahead of his peers but eventually end up no taller.

How tall a youngster will be as an adult is generally of considerable consequence to the individual and the family. Boys are usually worried about not being tall enough and girls about growing to be too tall. Physicians dealing with adolescents need to know the various normal patterns of maturation and the methods of predicting final stature by reference to skeletal age rather than chronologic age.

The gain in weight during puberty follows a similar pattern to height, but it is a more labile index of development than height. The nonskeletal growth increments are more marked than those for skeletal growth; by age 10, boys have gained only 55 per cent and girls 59 per cent of their adult weight. The factors which contribute to gain in weight are the increased size of the skeleton, muscles, and internal organs, and the amount of fat.

There is a marked sex difference between the amount and distribution of subcutaneous fat which contributes to shaping bodily contours. Infants accumulate subcutaneous fat (more in the case of females), but children gradually lose their chubbiness until shortly before puberty when they regain some of it. With the growth spurt a negative fat balance is established among boys, but not among girls, who usually enter adulthood with more body fat than males, particularly in the region of the pelvis and breasts.

Musculature and Strength. There is a marked increase in the size and strength of the musculature at puberty in both sexes but more so for males. This is the result of muscle cells becoming more numerous and larger. Among boys, the increase in number of cells is fourteen-fold; among girls, ten-fold. In females, maximum muscle cell size is reached by age 10½, whereas in males muscle cells continue to enlarge until the end of the third decade.

Body Proportions. The difference between the physique of the child and the adult is determined by variation in body proportions as well as size. During puberty body proportions undergo marked changes, and when these are in progress they may become sources of concern and distress to the adolescent who feels that he looks neither like his former childhood self nor quite like an adult. For example, legs accelerate in growth a year before the trunk, contributing to the stereotype of the gangling adolescent. Leg growth itself is not uniform; the foot accelerates first (though it stops growing soon), followed by the calf and the thigh. Similarly, hand and forearm grow ahead of the upper arm.

The adult face becomes distinctive through changes undergone during puberty. The neural pattern of growth, which also characterizes the growth of the cranium, places it ahead of other systems in the developmental schedule. Thus, throughout the growth period the size of the head becomes progressively smaller relative to the rest of the body. With the growth spurt at puberty, which affects the size of the cranium much less than the other parts of the skeleton, this trend is further exaggerated.

Other changes affect the head itself. The bones of the face grow faster than those of the cranial vault, so that at puberty the face is said to "emerge from under the skull." The profile of the adult becomes straighter, the nose and the jaw more prominent, and the lips fuller. Facial appearance is further altered by the recession of the hairline and in males by the growth of facial hair. All these changes are more marked among males.

Some sex differences in physical features are present at birth and become further exaggerated at puberty. For example, the male forearm is larger relative to height and contributes to his stronger hand grip. Other differences that emerge at puberty include the male's broader shoulders, narrower hips, and longer legs relative to trunk length.

Internal Changes. Numerous internal changes accompany the more evident manifestations of puberty. The heart, like other muscles of the body, participates in the growth spurt and its weight nearly doubles. The steady rise of systolic blood pressure throughout childhood accelerates and soon attains adult values. The concurrent decline in pulse rate is checked, and there may even be a slight increase in the resting heart rate. Blood volume, hemoglobin, and the number of red blood cells are all increased. All these changes are more marked among males.

The respiratory system undergoes similar changes. Lung size and respiratory capacity increase during puberty, whereas respiratory rate continues to decrease. These changes once again favor the male, including a greater efficiency in oxygen exchange.

The net effect of these and related physiologic alterations in puberty greatly increases the capacity for physical exertion and allows quicker recovery from its effects. Greater exercise tolerance combined with superior strength permits individuals of both sexes to vastly outperform their prepubescent selves in physical effort.

Not all changes at puberty are in the direction of growth and better performance. The lymphoid system regresses markedly. Myopic children become more so, and many new cases of myopia appear during this time.

Reproductive Maturation. The maturation of the reproductive system is the quintessential mark of puberty. It involves the accelerated growth of the internal sex organs and the external genitalia (figure). This is accompanied by the development of the so-called secondary sexual characteristics, which include the development of the female breast, the sprouting of pubic and axillary hair, the lowering pitch of the voice, and the appearance of facial hair in the male. In physiologic terms, the key events are the activation of ovulation and the menstrual cycle in females and the production of sperm and the ability to ejaculate in males. At least some prepubescent children have orgasmic capability but do not ejaculate semen prior to the development at puberty of the prostate gland, which produces most of the seminal fluid.

FEMALE REPRODUCTIVE MATURATION. Breast development is usually the first visible sign of female puberty; it starts between the ages of 8 and 13 and is completed between 13 and 18. Transient asymmetry is not unusual. Pubic hair ordinarily appears next, starting at age 11 to 12 and developing into the adult pattern by about 14; it precedes the growth of axillary hair by about a year. Breast and pubic hair growth follow predictable patterns which have been standardized and are used as indices of pubertal development.

The external genitalia become enlarged and their erotic sensitivity heightened. The internal sex organs rapidly increase in weight. Uterine musculature develops more fully, and the endometrium undergoes its elaborate cyclical changes following menarche. The vagina enlarges, with thickening of its epithelium.

Menarche does not commonly herald puberty as is sometimes erroneously assumed, but it is one of the late events. In the United States, the average age at menarche currently ranges from about 9 to 18 years (mean, 12.83). Contrary to earlier assumptions that a secular trend of decreasing ages at menarche was in progress, current data show that the age at menarche has not changed for the past three decades at least among American middle class girls.

MALE REPRODUCTIVE MATURATION. The onset of puberty in males is signaled by enlargement of the testes, which usually starts between 10 and 13½ and remains in progress until ages 14½ to 18. Pubic hair growth occurs between 12 and 16. The growth of the facial and axillary hair lags behind by two years. The first ejaculation usually occurs at 11 or 12, but mature sperm take a few more years to appear. This relative pubescent sterility in girls and boys who have otherwise matured sexually does not amount to reliable contraceptive security.

The penis begins to grow markedly about a year after testicular and pubic hair development. Deepening of the voice results from enlargement of the larynx. It is a late event in puberty and much less marked among females. Some breast enlargement may be observed in males, which eventually regresses as a rule.

NEUROENDOCRINE CONTROL OF PUBERTY. A complex set of neuroendocrine mechanisms underlies the initiation and control of puberty. They involve the interaction of hypothalamic hormones, anterior pituitary hormones (somatotropin, gonadotropins — FSH, LH) and steroid hormones from the gonads and adrenal cortex (estrogens, progestins, androgens). Other substances such as thyroid hormones and insulin also take part in these regulating mechanisms.

The nature and actions of these hormones are discussed elsewhere (see Ch. 548.2 and 549.2). The precise mechanism that initiates puberty is not known. The hypothalamus, pituitary, gonads, and body tissues have the capacity to be stimulated into adult function long before the normal ages of puberty. This means that puberty is due to the further activation of an already functional system.

The current postulate is that as the child matures, the hypothalamic receptor sites become less sensitive to inhibition by circulating low levels of steroid hormones. Consequently, under hypothalamic prompting, larger amounts of gonadotropins are produced by the pituitary, which in turn increases gonadal hormonal output. Through continuing readjustment of the equilibrium between pituitary and gonadal activities, gonadal steroids required to suppress the hypothalamus reach a level which exceeds the threshold of sensitivity of peripheral tissues to these hormones, and the physical changes of puberty are set into motion.

FACTORS AFFECTING PUBERTY. A wide range of genetic and environmental factors influence the onset and course of events in puberty. Some of these factors are well established; others are conjectural. The human pattern of puberty is the culmination of an evolutionary process starting with primates and successively carried further by monkeys, apes, and man. The current pattern of puberty in humans probably evolved with early man and has basically not changed except for relatively minor aspects such as its time of onset.

The presence of racial differences in pubertal patterns remains unsettled. The force of genetic factors is discernible in familial tendencies. Randomly chosen girls reach menarche differing on the average by 19 months; for sisters who are not twins, the difference is 13 months; for nonidentical twins, it is 10 months; for identical twins, 2.8 months.

The influence of climate is dubious; that of seasons more certain: height increases twice as fast in the spring, and growth in weight is four or five times as fast in the autumn; during spring there is a significant reduction in the incidence of menarche.

Malnutrition stunts growth and will interfere with the pubertal process. The effects are selective, as growth of sexual organs is relatively less retarded than that of other tissues. Boys are more vulnerable than girls. Differences in menarchal age in various countries and between social classes are due at least in part to nutritional factors. The effects of illness are highly variable. Most acute conditions have no lasting effect; disorders specific to the endocrine systems in question will have profound influence (see Ch. 548.2 and 548.3 and Ch. 549.2). Finally, emotional factors have considerable bearing on the developmental process, but in ways that are as yet poorly understood.

8.2. PSYCHOSOCIAL DEVELOPMENT

A comprehensive account of psychosocial aspects of normal adolescence would include psychologic reactions to the changes of puberty; emotional maturation; sexual behavior; cognitive and ideologic development; identity formation; restructuring of parental, sibling, and peer relationships; school experiences and vocational choice; participation in the youth subculture; socialization into the adult world; and so on. These events include so many complex variables and uncertainties that no concise and generally acceptable account of adolescent development is currently feasible.

We shall selectively focus here on those aspects of adolescent development that are likely to be of significance to the clinician who encounters adolescents in two contexts: first, when the issue is directly related to the process of adolescence itself and may be manifested in somatic or psychologic symptoms; and second, when some other illness, such as diabetes, occurs in an adolescent. In both cases some understanding of the normative developmental processes at work is helpful.

A central problem in adolescent psychology is whether normal adolescence is characterized by psychic turmoil. The concept that adolescence constitutes a stormy stage of life has been dominant in psychiatric thinking of the last half century (usually referred to as *Sturm und Drang*, or storm and stress). A contending view that "coming of age" need not necessarily entail turmoil has recently gained more credence through research involving adolescent populations at large rather than relying on extrapolations from clinical experience. A sensible compromise is to view adolescence as a labile period when emotional turmoil may commonly occur, without either expecting that it necessarily do so or viewing youngsters who show no such distress as pathologic.

Adolescent development is often assessed in terms of "tasks" the person must accomplish in order to successfully emerge from this stage. Beyond obvious requirements, such as the need to move toward economic self-sufficiency, the tasks that are set forth usually reflect a particular theoretical view or social value system. Some of these schemes are nevertheless quite useful for the clinician, because they provide him with a convenient framework in which to assess the young individual.

STAGES OF ADOLESCENT DEVELOPMENT. Tasks of adolescence are often subdivided as characterizing one of three subphases of adolescence. Thus, in early adolescence there is the task of psychologically integrating the ongoing somatic changes of puberty. Changes in body proportions and body image, menstruation, and enhancement of the sexual drive are among the developments that require psychologic adaptation and adjustment.

There is some reshuffling of peer groups at this time, but these remain largely monosexual. Likewise, intense outside relationships begin to form as exemplified by strong attachments and "crushes." But the home still remains the center of the youngster's life.

The adolescent makes important strides in cognitive development at this time, constituting Piaget's stage of "formal operations." Starting with age 11 to 12 and going on to 14 or 15, this process endows the adolescent with the capacity to use propositional and deductive logic. The youth can now reason abstractly, formulate hypotheses, and manipulate ideas in sophisticated adult fashion.

Similarly, Kohlberg has categorized stages of moral development that begin with "premoral" concern with avoiding punishment which is a carryover from childhood. The teenager then moves on to conventional role conformity to remain in the good graces of the family and to win approval. Only by about 16 or 17 are right and wrong understood as self-accepted moral principles.

Mid-adolescence raises the issues of dealing with family attachments and controls, revolt and conformity, participation in youth subcultures, further differentiation of gender identity, sexual experiences, and falling in love. Late adolescence is preoccupied by the task of self-definition and the identity crisis which, according to Erikson, is the phase-specific task of adolescence. The capacity for intimacy and more mature forms of love and sexual relationships characterizes adolescents approaching the threshold of adulthood.

RESTRUCTURING RELATIONSHIPS. Common social expectations require that the adolescent increasingly relate to others as an adult. This implies being less dependent and more dependable, along with a host of other expectations that are by no means consistently fulfilled by the majority of adults themselves.

The most crucial set of relationships to be redefined involves parents or other adults on whom the adolescent is economically and psychologically dependent.

Anna Freud has proposed that this detachment or emancipation from childhood ties is managed through a number of psychologic mechanisms in which the person engages without himself being quite conscious of them.

One mechanism for the adolescent to detach himself from the parents is to displace his intense feelings of attachment for them onto other people and interests. If this occurs slowly, the youngster experiences periods of moodiness and other reactions akin to those seen in mourning over a serious loss. The need to become separate may make him act seclusive or be "like a stranger" in the home. These feelings need not entirely dominate his life and may well be hidden under the continuing cordiality he maintains with his parents as well as the new and rewarding experiences he begins to develop in relating to them more like an adult.

A more abrupt expression of detachment is to run away from home. Some homes are so intolerable that this move is no less than an act of self-preservation. There are also many socially approved forms of leaving home, such as going away to boarding school or college, joining the armed forces, and so on, which may be at least in part motivated by the need to break away.

The attachment to others may take the form of friendships with peers, teachers, employers, or more distant figures such as rock stars or sports or movie figures to whom the adolescent becomes uncritically and helplessly attached as he was earlier to his parents.

A second mechanism is to reverse the feelings held toward the parents whereby love, dependence, and respect turn into various intensities of hate, revolt, and contempt. More often, positive feelings simply become tinged with ambivalence. This process is in part the result of seeing parents for who they really are and in part a means of facilitating giving them up by dwelling on their shortcomings. Since it is safer and less painful for the conflict to be shifted from the private to the public arena, the fault finding may become focused on parental substitutes, public institutions, society, and the world at large. But youth can also be critical of society on justifiable grounds quite apart from personal considerations.

Another mechanism involves the adolescent turning inward as it were and investing his own self with the intense feelings formerly reserved for parents. This would account for the narcissism and selfishness of young people, their preoccupation with their bodies, and their inflated ideas of beauty, strength, and competence. An adolescent may only indulge these thoughts in fantasies or may impose them on the world. In contrast, he may so totally lose himself in others that he thinks and acts as if he were someone else. This, too, may be indulged only in daydreams without his losing touch with reality, or it may take on pathologic expressions.

DEALING WITH DRIVES. Sexuality long antedates adolescence, yet there is a distinct upsurge in sexual interest and activity with the maturation of the reproductive system in puberty. Most societies attempt to regulate sexual behavior to widely divergent extents. So the task confronting the adolescent in this regard is socially dependent. When sexual expression in youth is frowned upon, there may be an attempt to give up the sexual impulse. When this repression is extended to all feelings of pleasure, it leads to various degrees of asceticism. The flight from sexuality may take the form of preoccupation with abstract intellectual issues or rigid and uncompromising stands toward all forms of seeming or real moral laxity.

Currently, rather than resort to such repression, many adolescents engage in various forms of sexual expression, including sexual intercourse. This confronts the physician with difficult dilemmas over such issues as contraception and abortion when he has to deal with individuals who are biologically adult but socially considered not to be so.

The expression of aggression in adolescence is a very serious social and medical problem. Violent deaths such as those resulting from accidents represent by far the leading cause of death in the second decade of life, accounting for over half of all deaths from all causes between the ages of 10 and 19. Homicide is the fifth most common cause of death among 10- to 14-year-olds. In 15- to 19-year-olds, homicide ranks second and suicide fourth.

IDENTITY FORMATION. Mainly as a result of Erikson's work, the concept of identity as the central task of adolescence has gained wide currency. Erikson's theory of psychosocial development postulates a sequence of eight phases or "ages of man." These phases derive from Freud's stages of psychosexual development, but they also go beyond them and encompass the entire life span. Each stage is defined by a phase-specific task and follows a general chronology without being linked to specific age limits.

These assignments hold true only in the sense that the phase-specific tasks reach their critical point of resolution during their respective phases. Otherwise, their solutions are prepared in previous stages and elaborated in subsequent ones.

The psychosocial transition to adulthood is accomplished during adolescence (Stage V) through the achievement of a sense of ego identity. In everyday terms, identity refers to a person's individuality, the response to the question of "Who am I?" But what Erikson means by identity is more complex. It includes a conscious sense of individual identity, an unconscious striving for a continuity of personal character, certain aspects of "ego synthesis," and the maintenance of an inner solidarity with a group's ideals and identity. The issue of identity is not settled once and for all during adolescence. What occurs at best is a clarification and reworking of earlier solutions and enough of a consolidation to provide the person with a self-sameness, even though many aspects of his personality continue to be reworked and refined in successive phases of the life cycle.

In more global terms, the criterion of attaining adulthood may be phrased in terms of achieving competence in a variety of spheres. Biologically, this means completing growth and becoming endowed with reproductive capacity. Psychologically, it requires a sufficient differentiation of the self whereby one can perceive the uniqueness of oneself in the context of other relationships. It implies the ability to recognize people for who they are and to relate to them effectively. As a minimum, it entails being able to look after oneself as well as being able to look after others in one or another context of one's choosing. It involves the capacity to help run society and be run by it.

In the final analysis, the task of becoming adult and what it means to be adult resolve into philosophical quests about the meaning and purpose of life. These are not ordinarily medical issues; yet since the physician at some level must deal with the patient as a person within a given social context, these considerations become relevant to medical practice.

Berenberg, S. R. (ed.): Puberty: Biologic and Psychosocial Components. Leider, H. E., Stenfert Kroese, B.V., 1975.

Erikson, E.: Childhood and Society. New York, Norton, 1963.

Freud, A.: Adolescence. In The Psychoanalytic Study of the Child, New York, International Universities Press, 13:255, 1958.

Grumbach, M. M., Grave, G. D., and Mayer, F. E.: Control of the Onset of Puberty. New York, John Wiley & Sons, 1974.

Heald, F. P., and Hung, W. (eds.): Adolescent Endocrinology. New York, Appleton-Century-Crofts, 1970.

Inhelder, B., and Piaget, J.: The Growth of Logical Thinking from Childhood to Adolescence. New York, Basic Books, 1958.

Kohlberg, L.: Development of moral character and ideology. In Hoffman, M. L., and Hoffman, L. W. (eds.): Review of Child Development Research, Vol. 1. New York, Russell Sage Foundation, 1964, pp. 383–433.

Marshall, W. A., and Tanner, J. M.: Puberty. In Davis, J. A., and Dobbing, J. (eds.): Scientific Foundations of Pediatrics. London, William Heinemann Medical Books, 1974.

Root, A. W.: Endocrinology of puberty: I. Normal sexual maturation. J. Pediat., 83:1, 1973.

Tanner, J. M.: Physical growth. In Mussen, P. (ed.): Carmichael's Manual of Child Psychology, Vol. I. 3rd ed. New York, John Wiley & Sons, 1970.

Zacharias, L., Rand, W. M., and Wurtman, R. J.: A prospective study of the sexual development and growth in American girls: The statistics of menarche. Obstet. Gynecol. Survey, 3:325, (Suppl.), 1976.

9. ADULTHOOD

Herant A. Katchadourian

9.1. INTRODUCTION

Unlike the pediatrician, who can turn to a vast literature on child development, physicians who deal with adults can find no comparable source of information on normative adult development. Until recently the prevailing view was that after childhood and adolescence, nothing of major consequence happened in developmental terms until toward the latter part of the normal life span, when the individual began to age. Currently gaining credence is an alternative viewpoint, whereby adulthood is seen not as a simple plateau interposed between the ascending steps of childhood and the descending steps of old age, but rather as a phase of life with its own discernible normative tasks and predictable transitions and stages. Although there is as yet no generally accepted developmental sequence for the adult years, and considerable disagreement over whether a stage theory for adulthood has any validity, knowledge accumulated in this field is of potential usefulness to the physician in understanding and treating adults.

Just as there is a great deal of normal variability in the ages at which biologic adulthood is attained, there is even more variance in the ways various cultures de-

fine an adult in psychosocial terms. Some investigators of the life cycle find it convenient nevertheless to divide the adult life span tentatively into several chronologic periods. Thus the transition to adulthood is expected to take place during the second decade of life (Katchadourian, 1977). Adulthood itself is subdivided by Levinson et al. into early adulthood, which corresponds to the age period of 20 to 40 years; middle adulthood (ages 40 to 60); and late adulthood (age 60 and older). Gerontologists divide old age into periods, such as early old age (ages 65 to 70) and advanced old age (75 years and older) (Butler).

Formidable difficulties confront investigators in this field. In order to obtain a proper time frame, for example, they must consider the interweaving of "historical time," which defines the period and hence the nature of the culture; "life time," or chronologic age of the individual; and "socially defined time," representing the age-graded expectations of appropriate behavior (Neugarten). The expectation is that during each adult developmental period a variety of biologic, psychodynamic, cultural, and social structural developmental timetables are in operation in variable degrees of synchronization. There are currently serious differences pertaining to fundamental aspects of adult developmental processes, in addition to disagreements over details, but some of the insights that are generally agreed upon will benefit the physician in his or her work.

9.2. ISSUES, CHANGES, AND STAGES

In attempting to understand the unfolding of adult life, the simplest approach is to identify those issues pertinent to adult life that are readily observable among a wide sector of the adult population. More ambitious is the attempt to delineate stages of adult development through which most individuals pass and which therefore constitute significant nodal points and predictable landmarks of adult life.

Factors within the first category are easier to identify, but because of their ubiquity and high variability they are also more difficult to systematize. Certain biologic changes become manifest more or less universally among people who live long enough. We refer to this process as "aging," but until the confounding effects of disease are eliminated, it is impossible to say whether changes in mental and physical abilities with age are due to the pathologic effects of disease or the manifestations of a normative developmental process of progressive biologic decline characteristic of all organisms. Furthermore, we have no systematic knowledge as yet as to whether these changes over time follow a discernible sequence that could conceivably be subsumed under chronologic phases or stages. Although a few physiologic events such as the menopause would seem to be notable exceptions, precisely what it is that transpires during the menopause is still far from clear.

Similarly, innumerable variables can be identified in the social realm in terms of the various adult roles individuals take on, maintain, change, or abandon. For example, a large segment of the adult population goes through divorce in addition to the sequence of courtship, marriage, parenthood, and separation from grown-up children. Similar sequences exist in vocations and other social realms. Yet the voluminous social science literature that elucidates these issues does not always help us understand how these events fit into a life-cycle perspective.

In addition to very wide cross-cultural variability in these institutions, one encounters within a given culture changes that occur over relatively short periods of time and redefine the ages at which most individuals experience these roles and what the roles signify for them. For example, Americans are getting married later and becoming parents later; from 1960 to 1976 the estimated median age at first marriage increased from 22.8 to 23.8 years for men and from 20.3 to 21.3 years for women. In 1960 there were 35 divorced persons per every 1000 people who were partners in intact marriages; by 1976 the ratio had risen to 75 per 1000. Meanwhile, women are going to work in increasingly higher proportions. The number of married women in the labor force rose from 30.5 per cent of women with husbands present in 1960 to 44.4 per cent in 1976.

Investigators have identified certain trends that are characteristic of some phases of adult life. Neugarten, for example, has described an increased tendency during middle age toward "interiority," which consists of increased emphasis upon introspection and stocktaking and conscious reappraisal of the self. Another characteristic of middle age is a change in one's perception of time. Whereas in earlier years the individual reckons time in terms of "time lived," with middle age the focus shifts to "time left to live." Although younger individuals are quite aware of their mortality, it is experienced in more personal terms during middle age and later, when a shift occurs from more abstract concern about death to a more personalized perception of its certainty and significance to one's everyday life. Additional discriminations between age groups center on attitudes toward the self and others. For instance, age-related responses have been obtained to questions such as whether marriage has been a good thing, whether parents are a cause of problems, and the possibility of changing careers (Gould).

Of various stage theories, the most widely known is Erikson's eight phases of the life cycle. In Erikson's view, the psychosocial transition to adulthood is accomplished during adolescence (Stage V) through the achievement of a sense of Identity, which in turn makes possible the establishment of a sense of Intimacy, the first phase-specific task of adulthood proper (Stage VI). Erikson defines these phase-specific tasks in terms of polar opposites of successful outcome or failure. Thus the counterpart to Intimacy is Isolation. Stage VII revolves around the issue of Generativity versus Stagnation. Using a heterosexual paradigm, Erikson sees as the central task at this phase the establishment of the next generation through the production and care of offspring, or, alternatively, through other altruistic and creative acts. The final phase of adult life confronts the task of Integrity versus Despair and Disgust. Integrity is the outcome of having taken care of things and people, originated others and generated things and ideas, and adapted to triumphs and disappointments. Because adulthood has received less attention in Erikson's work than adolescence, a great deal of Erikson's thinking about the derivatives and precursors of these adult stages of development has yet to be enunciated.

A more recent attempt to delineate stages in development comes from the work of Levinson and his associates. So far, this investigation has reported on male subjects between the ages of 18 and 45 only. Developmental phases in the lives of these men have been discerned to consist of the following: First is a transitional phase ("leaving the family") that usually stretches from the end of high school into the early twenties. During this period the young man may go through a phase of institutional living outside the home, such as in college or the military. Or, should he join the labor force, he may continue living at home but substantially outside parental control. Next is the phase of "getting into the adult world," which extends from the early twenties to the end of the twenties. During this period an initial definition of oneself as an adult is attained, and the individual fashions an initial life structure providing a link between the self and the adult world. This is a time of exploration and choice, when provisional commitments are made to an occupation. Those who resist making even tentative choices tend to develop a desperate need to settle down later on, or forfeit the chances of ever forming a reasonably satisfying life structure. Next is the "age 30 transition," a phase one passes through between the ages of 28 and 32. Like all transitional periods, this phase may be characterized by considerable turmoil, confusion, and struggle within oneself and with others, or it may simply entail a quiet reassessment of one's state and moving on.

The next period, "settling down," extends to the end of the thirties. The person now makes deeper commitments, investing more of himself in work, family, and other interests. There is a strong tendency toward maintaining order, stability, and security, while simultaneously striving to move ahead in order to "make it." In conflict with both these tendencies is the residual need to be free and unfettered. An important component of the settling-down period is "becoming one's own man," which typically is accomplished between the ages of 35 and 39 and represents the high point of early adulthood. During this phase a man has a profound need to be affirmed by society in the roles that he values most. In most instances this need involves some key event in the person's vocational career.

The "mid-life transition" ushers in another turning point, in which, irrespective of past accomplishments, the person confronts the issue of disparity between what has been gained and what one wants for himself. Major issues include the sense of bodily decline and recognition of one's mortality. There is a more acute sense of aging and further reorganization of the person's sense of gender identity. The crucial issue at mid-life is the changing relationship to the self. The mid-life transition occurs around the age of 40 and usually encompasses several years. By the mid-forties there is a period of restabilization that ushers the individual into middle adulthood.

9.3. CRISES OF ADULT LIFE

Just as a major problem in adolescent psychology is whether normal adolescence is characterized by psychic turmoil, a similar controversy involves whether certain phases of adult life have a higher potential for psychologic turbulence. Most often it is the period of mid-life that is singled out as hazardous.

Traditionally the menopause has served as an example of mid-life crisis. It represents a fairly discrete biologic event, and its psychologic repercussions have been taken to constitute a coherent entity. Physicians who treat middle-aged women could testify to having seen countless such cases. Yet what has been generally lacking is empirical research with women who go through the menopause without being seen by physicians. When examined within a broader population base, the menopause emerges as a very different entity. For instance, in one nonmedical sample studied by Neugarten, only a few of the women viewed the menopause as a major source of worry. (The women were much more concerned about getting older, developing cancer, or losing their husbands.) Although many women presumably experience the symptoms of vasomotor instability ("hot flashes") and other physiologic signs of hormonal withdrawal, the majority seem to take these events in stride without major loss of feminine identity or sexual function. Furthermore, women who have difficulty during the menopause turn out to be the same women who had difficulty with menarche, menstrual periods, and pregnancy, which would indicate that the problem is idiosyncratic, rather than related to a normative developmental crisis.

Another so-called crisis commonly assumed to affect predominantly women is related to the "empty nest" created when grown-up children leave home. A more systematic investigation reveals that the postparental stage of life is associated with a higher, rather than lower, level of life satisfaction for women. Some studies show that marital adjustment improves for both sexes during middle age, possibly because of increased companionship after the children have left home (Burr; Rollins and Feldman).

The question has been raised repeatedly whether men undergo a counterpart of the female menopause. In a literal sense, of course, they do not; but the question is more difficult to answer in the broader sense of a climacterium encompassing bodily and psychic involutional changes during the transition from middle age to old age. Unlike ovarian function, which generally ceases between the ages of 48 and 50, testicular function declines gradually in adulthood, so that the production of sperm and testosterone declines gradually over decades. Yet many of the psychologic symptoms associated with the female menopause, such as irritability and depression, seem to characterize significant numbers of middle-aged males also.

Sexual function in middle life is another common source of concern. It has long been observed that potency generally suffers with age, but age is only one factor that has a bearing on this issue, and it is by no means clear that declining potency is predominantly due to aging as such rather than illness. Without denying the possibility that a fundamental biologic process related to aging affects sexual function, one can also assume that in a large number of cases failing potency with increasing age is an artifact of psychologic factors and social expectations. It is also important to recognize the changing nature of sexual response without equating such altered responses with sexual failure. The middle-aged or older male generally requires more physical stimulation to attain erection, for example, although in his younger years psychologic arousal would often be sufficient. But once having attained an erection, an older man is likely to maintain it longer or

delay ejaculation at will, thus enhancing his lasting capacity during sexual intercourse. Other changes of sexual function at the physiologic level for aging men and women have been described (Masters and Johnson). None of these alterations in sexual function can yet be linked to a particular stage or phase of adult life.

Numerous other issues critical to mid-life have been proposed in the realms of economic life, social roles, and intrapsychic processes (Butler). On reviewing the more current literature, Brim derives the following six statements that sum up theories of the male mid-life crisis and may possibly be extrapolated to women crossing the threshold of middle life:

First, the mid-life male is likely to be undergoing profound personality changes.

Second, these changes will have more than one cause.

Third, a "male mid-life crisis" will occur for some men if there are multiple, simultaneous demands for personality change; if, for instance, during the same month or year the man throws off his last illusions about great success; accepts his children for what they are; buries his father and his mother and yields to the truth of his mortality; recognizes that his sexual vigor and, indeed, interest, are declining, and even finds relief in the fact.

Fourth, these challenges may be stretched out over ten or twenty years. Some men are obsessed about their achievements, but not yet confronting the fact of death; other men are sharply disappointed in their children's personalities but not yet concerned about sexual potency. The events come sooner for some men, much later for others. There is no evidence that they are related to chronologic age in any but the most general sense — e.g., "sometime during the forties."

Fifth, there is as yet no evidence for either developmental periods or "stages" in the mid-life period, in which one event must come after another or one personality change brings another in its wake. The existence of "stages," if proved true, would be a powerful concept in studying mid-life; meanwhile, there is a danger of our using this facile scheme as a cover for loose thinking about human development, without carrying forward the necessary hard-headed analyses of the evidence.

Sixth, the "growing pains" of mid-life, like those of youth and of old age, are transitions from one comparatively steady state to another, and these changes, even when they occur in crisis dimensions, bring for many men more happiness than they found in younger days.

Brim, O. G., Jr.: Theories of the male mid-life crisis. Counseling Psychologist, 6:2, 1976.
Burr, W. R.: Satisfaction with various aspects of marriage over the life cycle: A random middle class sample, J. Marriage Family, 32:29, 1970.
Butler, R. N.: Psychiatry and psychology of the middle-aged. In Freedman, A. M., Kaplan, H. I., and Sadock, B. J. (eds.): Comprehensive Textbook of Psychiatry, Vol. 2. 2nd ed. Baltimore, Williams & Wilkins Company, 1975, pp. 2390–2404.
Erikson, E. H.: Growth and crises of the healthy personality. In Identity and the Life Cycle: Selected papers by Erik H. Erikson. Psychological Issues, 1:18, 1959.
Gould, R. L.: The phases of adult life: A study in developmental psychology. Am. J. Psychiatry, 129:521, 1972.
Katchadourian, H. A.: Biology of Adolescence. San Francisco, W. H. Freeman and Company, 1977.
Katchadourian, H. A.: Medical perspectives on adulthood. Daedalus, 105:29, 1976.
Levinson, D. J., Darrow, C. M., Klein, E. B., Levinson, M. H., and McKee, B.: Periods in the adult development of men: Ages 18 to 45. Counseling Psychologist, 6:21, 1976.

Masters, W. H., and Johnson, V. E.: Human Sexual Response. Boston, Little, Brown & Company, 1966.

Neugarten, B. L.: Adaptation and the life cycle. Counseling Psychologist, 6:16, 1976.

Rollins, B. C., and Feldman, R.: Marital satisfaction over the life cycle. J. Marriage Family, 32:20, 1970.

U. S. Bureau of Census: A statistical portrait of women in the United States. Current Population Reports, Special Studies, Series P-23, No. 50, April 1976, p. 31.

U. S. Bureau of Census: Population characteristics. Current Population Reports, Series P-20, No. 306, January 1977, pp. 1–5.

10. AGING AND GERIATRIC MEDICINE

Ralph Goldman

10.1. INTRODUCTION

Few individuals live to maturity in a world of great environmental danger. The persistence of a species requires that enough members survive and reproduce so that a balance can be established. Once this is assured, individual survival is no longer essential. In fact, postreproductive or inefficiently reproducing individuals compete for the resources of an ecologic niche and may threaten species survival. In humans the control of infections and malnutrition, improved management of trauma, and the reduction in death associated with reproduction have produced a profound social as well as scientific revolution. Figure 1 shows changes in survival over a prolonged historical period. The magnitude of this change is exemplified by the following data: During the sixteenth century, in the city of York, England, only 45 per cent of girls survived their first year, 18 per cent reached age 20, 11 per cent reached age 40, and 3 per cent reached age 65. These data are worse than what must have been the norm for that period, but cities with similar statistics existed well into the current century. In the United States and most developed countries, more than 96 per cent of white women will now reach age 40, 82 per cent will reach age 65, and 62 per cent will reach age 75. The outlook for men is less favorable, yet 93 per cent will reach age 40 and 67 per cent will reach age 65.

The very existence of a large older population means that serious disease and injury at younger ages have decreased. Thus, although medical researchers and practitioners have been chiefly concerned with acute injuries and illnesses of younger patients, the focus of their activities must now be shifted to chronic conditions, including their acute episodes, and to a consideration of the nature and implications of the aging process itself. Since human survival no longer depends upon adequate reproduction, we have both practical and moral imperatives for the study of gerontology and the practice of geriatrics.

The word *gerontology* derives from the Greek *gerontos*, old man, and *logos*, discourse upon, and refers to the study of the aging process. The word *geriatrics* is derived from *gerontos*, and *iatros*, physician, or *iatreia*, cure, literally physician or treatment of old men. The age at which a patient becomes eligible for geriatric care is artificial and arbitrary and usually relates to a statutory criterion, such as eligibility for Social Security or the age of mandatory retirement. Geriatrics uses the knowledge of gerontology, but the latter must study the aging process, which starts much earlier in life. Aging can be said to start at conception, but for practical purposes growth and development are associated with incremental processes, whereas during maturity and senescence decremental processes predominate.

Life span refers to the longest survival for a member of a species and serves as an index of maximum potential under ideal natural conditions. *Life expectation* refers to the average length of survival from a specific age, most commonly from birth, for a given cohort. Scientific and social improvements have increased life expectancy, but have not altered life span.

Geriatrics is not limited to management of decremental disease, dementia, and death. A large portion of the practice of medicine must, by the very fact of general survival to advanced age, be with older patients not thought of as a geriatric clientele. It is necessary for the concept of geriatric care to include both ambulatory and acute, as well as chronic, disease. The role of geriatrics is to integrate the information developed by gerontology with traditional medical knowledge to increase the well-being of aging patients.

10.2. STRUCTURAL AND FUNCTIONAL CHANGES WITH AGE

A primary problem of gerontology is to identify changes which are due to age alone and to differentiate these changes, if they exist, from pathologic processes.

Figure 1. Cohort survival of women in different eras. A, Townswomen of York, England, sixteenth century. B, Aristocrats, England, sixteenth century. C, White women, United States, 1900. D, White women, United States, 1972.

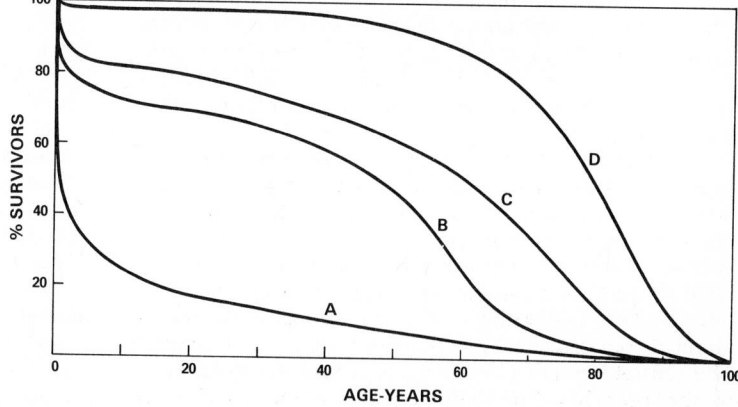

Growth and development are universal and proceed according to an intrinsically determined pattern which can be modified by the environment within limits compatible with survival. Changes which are due to aging must also be universal. They should be unidirectional, and experience indicates that they are decremental. Although there is no a priori reason that age change should be either extrinsic or intrinsic in origin, the evidence now supports an intrinsic mechanism. The following are some of the major structural and functional changes with age which have been observed in humans and most mammals.

CELLS. Postmitotic cells, primarily muscle and nerve cells, are incapable of multiplication; they are not replaced when lost, and their number decreases with age. Mitotic cells have a limited capacity for replacement and are not immortal, as was once thought. Some cells, particularly the postmitotic cells, accumulate pigment within storage granules, and all cells show degeneration of intracellular organelles.

TISSUES. The regularity of tissue structure is lost, the individual cells enlarge, but the total number of cells decreases approximately 30 per cent. Fat deposition increases and conceals much of the loss of active cell mass. Intercellular collagen and elastin increase. The proportion of soluble collagen decreases, and there may be increased cross-linking between the long-chain collagen macromolecules. Elastin loses its discrete structure and elasticity and has an increased calcium content.

HEART. There is myocardial hypertrophy and fibrosis, and the valves become stiffer with age. The maximum cardiac rate and stroke volume, and thus the cardiac output, are progressively decreased, and the return to resting rate is prolonged. The isometric contraction and relaxation times are prolonged. Although there is a statistically valid increase in ECG intervals, there is no visually discernible abnormality in the normal pattern.

BLOOD VESSELS. The increased collagen, altered elastin, and increased calcium result in arterial rigidity with elevation of the systolic pressure, accelerated pulse wave velocity, and a loss of 10 per cent in cardiac systolic efficiency. The peripheral resistance is increased, whether due to arteriolar atrophy or spasm is not established, and the diastolic pressure is slightly elevated. The capillary basement membrane thickness increases from 700 to 1100 Angstroms between youth and old age.

EXCRETORY SYSTEM. The number of nephrons decreases 30 to 40 per cent between 25 and 85 years. The filtration rate, renal blood flow, and tubular functions are proportionately reduced, although the serum creatinine level is maintained because of reduced release from the decreasing muscle mass. The capacity for compensatory hypertrophy diminishes with age and increasingly depends upon cellular hypertrophy rather than hyperplasia.

RESPIRATORY SYSTEM. Upper respiratory infections become less frequent because of immunologic experience. The anteroposterior diameter of the chest increases and the compliance of the chest wall is decreased. The total lung capacity is unchanged, but the residual volume is doubled and the vital capacity is reduced. The maximum breathing capacity decreases about 50 per cent between the third and ninth decades. The reduced cough efficiency, decreased ciliary activity of the bronchial epithelium, and the increased dead space enhance the potential for mechanical and infectious respiratory complications of surgery and enforced bed rest in the aged individual.

GASTROINTESTINAL SYSTEM. Hiatus hernia, atrophic gastritis, appendiceal involution, and colonic diverticulosis are increasingly common. Motility may be disorganized, and fecal incontinence is frequent in the mentally impaired. Salivary, gastric, and fasting pancreatic secretion are decreased, but after stimulation pancreatic secretion is normal. Digestion and absorption are generally adequate, although iron and calcium may be less well absorbed. The liver shows characteristic change and atrophy. There is a decreased albumin production, with a 20 per cent fall in the serum concentration. Bromsulphalein storage in hepatic cells is linearly decreased, but the secretory transport maximum is unchanged. The frequency of cholelithiasis approaches 40 per cent by the eighth decade.

ENDOCRINE SYSTEM. Blood levels of GH may be decreased and those of TSH, ACTH, and ADH are maintained. Blood levels of FSH are increased fifteen-fold and LH three-fold in postmenopausal women, whereas in men these changes are marginal. Large doses of estrogen fail to suppress FSH, and the feedback control mechanism in women is probably impaired. The serum T_4 remains normal, although the rate of turnover is decreased; T_3 is reduced 25 to 40 per cent. Responses to stress and to TSH are normal. The status of PTH is not certain, but the postmenopausal decrease in estrogen may allow an unopposed PTH effect and predispose to osteoporosis. The glucose tolerance decreases with age, and if the usual standards are used, 50 per cent of all individuals aged 70 or older would have diabetes. An adjustment in diagnostic criteria is obviously necessary. This reduced tolerance may be due to a delay in insulin release by the beta cells. Glucagon levels are unchanged. The plasma cortisol level and the circadian cycle persist, but a decreased secretion rate is matched by reduced disposal and excretion rates. The response of cortisol secretion to stress still needs clarification. The blood level and urinary excretion of aldosterone decrease 50 per cent between youth and old age, and the response to sodium depletion is reduced two thirds. The secretion of renin has a similar age-related decrease. Adrenal androgen also decreases progressively to less than one half of young adult values. Recent studies show a decrease in norepinephrine and an increase in monamine oxidase and serotonin in the brain with age. Stimulation results in a delayed but quantitatively normal increase in the excretion of epinephrine. After the menopause all female estrogen is adrenal in origin and thus decreases markedly; in males there is little age-related change. Since progesterone is a precursor of cortisol, adrenal production is probably sustained in both sexes. The production and clearance of testosterone decline, but there is no agreement that blood levels are reduced.

BLOOD. There is no decrease in the blood volume before age 80, red cell survival time is normal, and anemia is usually secondary to iron depletion. The number and distribution of leukocytes is unchanged, except for T lymphocytes, which are probably decreased. The leukocytosis of inflammation and immunoglobulin production after antigenic challenge are both decreased. Immune surveillance is markedly decreased despite an increase in total gamma globulin. Platelets may have increased adhesiveness and fibrinogen may be increased, but there is no conclusive evidence of hyper-coagulability. The erythrocyte sedimentation rate may be markedly accelerated without evidence of disease.

MUSCULOSKELETAL SYSTEM. Muscle cell loss and disorganization cause a progressive reduction in muscle strength. The poor reparative characteristics of cartilage lead to deterioration as early as the third decade, with progressive loss of joint surfaces and resultant degenerative arthritis. Throughout life there is a continuous remodeling of bone by reabsorption of interior surfaces and formation on exterior surfaces. By age 40 the reabsorption exceeds bone formation. Both the protein matrix and the bone mineral are involved, and clinical osteoporosis may result. In women 25 per cent of the bone is lost. Fractures of the vertebral body and femoral neck may result. The cumulative risk of hip fracture by age 90 approaches 25 per cent for women and 10 per cent for men.

THE INTEGUMENT. Wrinkling and sagging of the skin and graying of the hair are hallmarks of aging. The epidermis thins and contains less melanin, and cell replacement slows, resulting in delayed healing. The epidermal glands are reduced in number and function, and the skin is dry. A significant reduction in subcutaneous fat, increased collagen, and fragmented, inelastic elastin cause the observed wrinkling. The blood supply is reduced, but capillary fragility results in the common subcutaneous senile purpura. The loss of subcutaneous fat, reduction of vascularity, and slowed cell replacement contribute to the frequency and severity of decubitus ulceration. Hair distribution is subject to genetic and racial variation, but in each individual is determined by the number of active and resting hair follicles in local areas more than by follicular atrophy. Luxuriant scalp hair in youth decreases with age; facial hair appears at puberty and may persist in males, but it may appear after the menopause in Caucasian women; axillary and pubic hair appear at puberty and, in women, decrease after the menopause. Graying is due to decreased melanin production by the hair follicle. The rate of nail growth decreases 40 per cent.

NERVOUS SYSTEM. Nerve cells are postmitotic, and when lost are not replaced. The weight of the brain is essentially constant, but careful studies have shown not only a significant loss of cells, as many as 45 per cent in some cortical areas, but, more important, a loss of cellular integrity and of cellular interconnections. A consensus of several studies shows that from age 17 to age 80 years the cerebral blood flow declines from 79 to 46 ml per minute per 100 grams of brain tissue and the cerebral oxygen consumption rate decreases from 3.6 to 2.7 ml per minute per 100 grams of brain. The mean arterial pressure is constant at 90 to 100 mm Hg, but the derived cerebrovascular resistance increases from 1.3 to 2.1 mm Hg per ml blood per minute per 100 grams of brain. Patients with senile dementia cluster at the lowest levels of blood flow and oxygen utilization, but there is overlap with subjects lacking overt intellectual deterioration. Motor nerve conduction velocity decreases about 15 per cent, and sensory nerve conduction velocity may decrease 30 per cent between 20 and 95 years. Sleep levels 3 and 4 become less prominent and brief arousals more frequent with age, but total sleep time may be little affected. A reciprocal increase of monamine oxidase and decrease of norepinephrine in brain tissue may be causal to the depression and apathy so often associated with aging.

SENSORY ORGANS. Visual acuity decreases with age, primarily due to reduction in transparency of the optical portions of the system. There is also loss in the extent of the visual fields, decrease in the speed of dark adaptation, elevation in the minimal threshold of light perception, and reduction in the critical speed of flicker fusion. There is a continuous, but decelerating, formation of cells on the lens surface, which gradually lose their nuclei and become transparent. Thus the lens thickens with age and there is progressive loss of the elasticity needed to adaptively deform the lens. Between ages 42 and 45 years, previously normal individuals will need corrective glasses for near vision. Hearing decreases, particularly for high tones after age 60, especially in men. There is a decrease in the senses of taste, smell, and touch. Pain fibers appear to be intact, but clinical experience suggests that pain threshold may also be reduced.

10.3. THE GOMPERTZ CONCEPT

Benjamin Gompertz, a British actuary, proposed a concept in 1825 which did not fully arouse the interest of biologists until more than a century later. Based on data then available from Northhampton, England, he noted that at advanced ages the age-specific risk of death increased geometrically, and could be computed by the formula:

$$q_x = q_0 e^{ax}$$

where q_x is the death rate at age x, q_0 is the death rate at age o, and a is a constant. When age is plotted against the log of the age-specific death rate, the portion of the curve which corresponds to Gompertz's formula is essentially a straight line (Fig. 2). Thus at these ages the risk of death is determined by age, indepen-

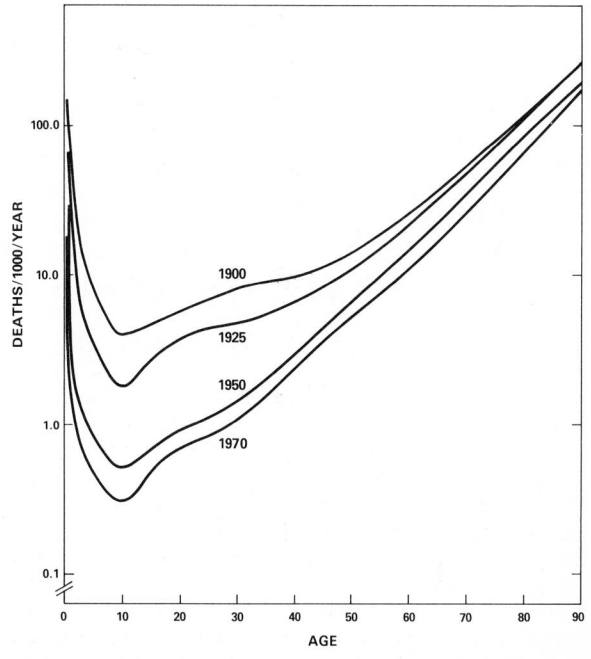

Figure 2. Mortality rates for white women, United States, 1900, 1925, 1950, and 1970.

dent of cause. The Gompertz concept has been found to be valid for all mammals.

Figure 2 shows the changes in age-specific mortality during the present century for American white women and demonstrates features which would be magnified by a longer time frame. The biggest gains have resulted from the reduction of infections and infant and maternal mortality, and in the better management of trauma. First exposures to infections occur most frequently early in life prior to the development of specific immunity. Immunization, sanitation, and antibiotics reduce the hazards of infection. The risks of childbirth are early for the infant, and in young adulthood for mothers in a society in which massive reproduction is no longer necessary. Accidents are most common as a result of the inexperience and recklessness of youth. As a result, a number of changes can be seen in the mortality risk curves. First, there is a large decrease in early mortality risk where the deviation from the Gompertz prediction is greatest. Second, the linear portion of the curve starts at an earlier age and at a lower risk level. Third, the slope of the curve is steeper. This slope defines the time required for the risk of death to double. At present the doubling time is seven years, and, if the slope remains constant, any maneuver which would eliminate 50 per cent of the causes of death (such as heart disease) would reduce the age-specific mortality by seven years. However, since the slope accelerates as the risk is reduced at lower ages, the benefits at advanced age are less prominent, and there may be a limit to the amount of reduction that can be achieved without modification of the aging process itself.

As the risk of death after maturity more closely follows the Gompertz projection, two phenomena become apparent. First, the lethality of an episode of acute disease or injury tends to parallel the Gompertz curve, suggesting that the total capability of the organism to cope with stress is decreasing with age at an accelerating rate. Second, a large number of chronic conditions, including arteriosclerosis and its manifestations, cancer, senile dementia, arthritis, diabetes, and osteoporosis, become apparent at frequencies which are less than but also parallel to the Gompertz curve. Although these conditions may manifest themselves acutely, it is clear that they are the result of progressive changes over long periods of time. These changes could result from constitutional factors, single traumas which set in motion a slow but progressive response, or multiple and continuing stimuli acting over a long period of time.

10.4. THEORIES OF AGING

The search for perpetual youth and immortality has given rise to many theories of aging, most now only of historical interest. Genetic factors are undoubtedly important, because each species has a characteristic life span, and within species there are strain differences in survival distribution. Genetic theories raise the possibility of programmed senescence or of program exhaustion. Recent knowledge of genetic mechanisms has resulted in the development of a number of error theories based on the concept that defects in protein synthesis can accumulate over time. Postmitotic cells, because of their long life, should be vulnerable particularly at the levels of transcription and translation, whereas mitotic cells should be vulnerable to somatic mutation during replication. Chromosome studies show an increase in gross abnormalities visible by light microscopy.

Another group of theories has arisen from developments in immunology. Both humoral and cellular immunocompetence decline, but autoimmune manifestations increase with age and amyloid deposits become common, particularly in the walls of blood vessels. The constant occurrence of somatic mutations could result in an ongoing immunologic response, possibly to a cell product from within a cell otherwise not distinguishable on its surface as alien, and thus free to continue producing its aberrant product. Mutation of immunocompetent cells which no longer recognize "self" would produce a graft-versus-host reaction.

In addition to the theories already noted, several others, not necessarily mutually exclusive, have attained some support. The progressive loss or impairment of postmitotic cells is a self-evident mechanism of aging. The finite limit of the reproductive capacity of mitotic cells, now very conclusively established, indicates that some limits to mortality exist on a cellular level. With age there is an accumulation of storage granules within the cellular cytoplasm, particularly lipofuscin, which may interfere with cellular functions. Quantitative increases in the amount and cross-linkage of collagen and related macromolecules have been shown for the connective tissue matrices. A similar cross-linkage of intracellular macromolecules, particularly DNA and RNA, could impair cell function. The existence of free radicals and exposure to natural radiation could produce irreversible changes in genetic and protein structures.

The accumulating evidence makes it unlikely that aging is a unitary phenomenon for which a specific therapy may be found. For the present it may be more practical to reconcile the observations of aging with certain clinical phenomena. Since aging is conceived as universal, any process which affects only a segment of the population has been considered to be a disease. However, if every individual has a potential for cancer which is held in check by immunosurveillance, the development of cancer would depend upon the level of the defense and the strength of the carcinogenetic mechanisms. Since immune competence decreases with age, cancer should occur when the defense is no longer adequate to cope with the stress. The rate of development of atherosclerosis has been linked to risk factors, particularly blood pressure, glucose tolerance, and blood lipid levels. Each increment in arterial pressure is linked with a statistical increase in mortality. Whether an individual dies of a vascular complication, cancer, or some other cause depends upon the individual vulnerability of a particular system. The risk for each potential cause of aging death and the likelihood that more than one will be present increases geometrically with age, as does the risk of death. The phenomenon of the one-horse shay, in which all parts wear out at the same moment, is just as improbable in biology as in mechanics.

The same concept could be applicable to other, non-lethal phenomena. For example, there is clear evidence that both the protein matrix and mineral content of bone decrease after the fourth decade. If this decrease were proportional in all individuals, those with the least dense bone at early maturity would be the most probable candidates for osteoporosis. There are few convincing data that therapy is effective once osteoporosis is present; it may be possible to increase maximum bone density, but this would require increased bone formation during growth. Similarly, treatment of vascular degeneration and cancer may be less effective than long-term control of appropriate risk factors. Changes in dietary patterns and effective control of blood pressure may provide future information, but the length of the human life span makes the accumulation of reliable data a prolonged process.

10.5. PSYCHOSOCIAL PROBLEMS OF THE AGED

Very few members of migratory, hunting societies lived to old age, and those few must have had unique qualities. Despite the obvious value of their wisdom, they probably were not spared if their incapacity endangered the group. The development of fixed, agricultural communities increased the security of the aged, especially after the development of property rights and rules of inheritance. Science and technology further increased the number of survivors to old age. However, the industrial revolution also broke up the family as a social and economic unit, increased social and geographic mobility, and so altered the social position of the aged that new social models have become necessary.

The popular image of the aged is negative. They are thought of as reduced in intelligence, limited in memory, rigid in concept, and uncongenial in personality. In fact, intellectual competence usually persists until quite late in life, and for a long period established knowledge and experience compensate for any slowness of learning. Even flexibility of thought is greater than was once believed. The increasing level of general education is improving the ability of the aged to adapt and to maintain interests.

Nevertheless, aging is associated with losses. There is the loss of occupation, as a source both of income and of meaningful activity. The loss of income may be more important because of reduced social leverage than lowered standard of living. Yet, with adequate income noneconomic activities can often become significant and satisfying. The loss of friends and family and separation from children become increasingly painful. The loss of vigor and attractiveness and, ultimately, the loss of health are the final reminders that the cycle is closing. Women now live eight years longer than men and are several years younger at the time of marriage. Geriatrics as a specialty must deal primarily with older women who will be widowed for an average of ten years with reduced economic resources and social contacts.

Under these conditions it is not surprising that depression is common and is often manifest as insomnia or dementia. In the latter the apparent intellectual decline is really a loss of attention created by the depression, and effective therapy can be gratifying.

In caring for aging patients, the physician must be aware of a range of problems which are less important in other age groups. First, the life experience of the patient encompasses a time period which the younger physician knows only indirectly, and the patient may be conditioned by lifetime social and ethnic considerations which also may be quite alien to him. Second, the patient may not have the economic or social resources to adhere to a prescribed regimen. Third, the patient has an increased probability of multiple problems which may be self-treated or lie in the area of another specialist. Multiple medications may be utilized with potential incompatibilities. Fourth, the patient may often be incompetent, and both the history and the therapy may suffer as a result. Fifth, the longer the survival, the more likely the loss or absence of a spouse or companion. Sixth, the need for social welfare, visiting nurse, homemaker, and related services is extensive, and when properly used can often help maintain an older patient at home as the preferred medical, social, and economic solution.

Despite the enumerated decrements associated with aging, most older individuals live remarkably active and satisfying lives. Social Security, pensions, Medicare and health insurance, and a long period of relative economic prosperity have greatly improved the economic aspects. If the individual survives, the general enfeeblement of aging is infrequently incapacitating before age 75 or 80. It is becoming usual to speak of early and late old age, since the two periods may be quite different.

It is during advanced old age that the stereotypes may be more typical. Significant senile dementia may be present in 20 per cent. Losses of hearing and vision reduce sensory input and with reduced physical mobility may aggravate the other problems of social isolation. These patients are often best managed in a home for the aged or in a skilled nursing facility if they are unable to perform the activities of daily living. It is revealing that the average age of residents in these homes is often more than 80 years.

10.6. SPECIAL PROBLEMS OF MANAGEMENT

DIET. There is little evidence that age alters the need for specific nutrients, but the total calories should be reduced to compensate for decreased metabolic activity and cell mass. Because a reduced total diet may result in an inadequate intake of vitamins and iron, a single appropriate supplement may be prescribed. No specific diet to promote longevity has yet been confirmed. The older patient will have an increased probability of need for a specific therapeutic diet, and the ability to conform to the dietary prescription must be determined.

MEDICATION. The age-related concerns of clinical pharmacology are those of drug level, receptor and effector competence, and drug toxicity. Drug levels are determined by absorption, volume of distribution, biodegradation, and excretion. Quantitatively, the 40 to 50 per cent decrease in renal function is the most important age-related factor for substances which are excreted in active form in the urine. The decrease in renal function may produce a significant increase in blood levels if dose is not adjusted. An important factor in dose level is patient compliance. Reliable information requires frequent review of all drugs taken, including over-the-counter drugs, and their amounts. Each patient should be instructed periodically to bring in all actively used drugs in their containers to determine the exact drugs taken and their amounts. This is a most instructive exercise for both patient and physician.

Recent studies have shown quantitative and qualitative changes in the receptor sites, particularly of the nervous system, heart, and muscle. The reduced number and integrity of effectors are the natural result of the changes previously described. Further information should do much to rationalize geriatric pharmacology.

Drug misadventures increase in frequency with age. The patient has had more opportunity for prior sensitization. In addition, the multiple medical problems increase the number of drugs to be administered. The frequency of pharmacologic incompatibilities and of drug-drug interactions increases geometrically with the number taken. Safe and effective drug therapy requires knowledge of the drugs used, their probable pharmacologic changes with age, tests for blood level or effect (e.g., suppression of FSH by estrogen) when possible, and close titration for effect if not. In addition, drug prescription should be selective and minimal, and the patients closely observed for untoward responses.

DECUBITUS ULCERS AND CONTRACTURES. Every attempt should be made to prevent both these complications. Frequent movement, aggressive skin care, smooth sheets, and appropriate padding are essential. Pulling, rather than lifting, a patient into the upright position may damage fragile skin by a shearing effect. Every attempt must be made to get the patient out of bed daily. When ulcers develop, care must be intensified if they are to heal. Careful enzymatic and surgical debridement, antibiotics, and occasional skin grafting are utilized when needed. Large, infected ulcers have a high mortality.

SENILE DEMENTIA. The frequency of senile dementia increases with age. The physician must rule out and treat all medical, psychologic, and social causes of decreased intellectual function and minimize their effects whenever possible. Nevertheless, true senility is a frequent reality which the family and society must be helped to accept and to manage in a positive and humane manner. In the early stages the awareness of intellectual losses may be magnified by an understandable depression which often can be minimized by social support and the proper use of mood-elevating drugs. Paranoid manifestations may also appear and also can often be controlled. The appropriate social setting may be difficult to obtain, and cooperation with a variety of social agencies is usually necessary. As with mental disease at earlier ages, the family usually has intense feelings of shame and guilt. Much support and counseling are required. Since the costs of care may be large, the family must often be reassured that there is no currently effective therapy, and that expensive searches are unnecessary and usually unwise. The development of computerized brain scanning, although rarely positive, provides a noninvasive and probably decreasingly expensive method for ruling out many potentially treatable lesions such as subdural hematomas and brain tumors.

DYING AND DEATH. Dying and death are periods of stress for the patient, family, friends, and attendants. Every attempt must be made to keep the patient comfortable. There is no excuse for a dying patient to be in pain. Analgesia, if clearly needed, as for cancer, should be prescribed on a regular schedule, and in adequate amounts. Less medicine is required to prevent than to relieve pain. The obviously dying patient should be spared unnecessary tests and procedures. Visits should be encouraged and facilitated, but governed primarily by the sense of the patient's need and desire. One of the great tragedies of modern institutional medicine is the tendency to isolate the dying patient. The family is kept at a distance, and the staff reduces interaction out of frustration and discomfort. If necessary, psychiatric consultation should be obtained, but this must be arranged with caution and sensitivity. The patient should be allowed to be dependent or hostile if it makes adjustment easier. Ideally, he should be helped to work through his own mourning reaction with its sequence of denial, anger, bargaining, depression, and final acceptance. The family and friends should also be helped through this period. The physician should always be available to his patient when needed.

10.7.   THE PHYSICIAN'S RESPONSIBILITY

Humans are mortal. Not all diseases will be cured or deaths prevented. It is only within this century that the physician's intervention has been decisive in more than occasional situations. We must not allow our newfound technical competence to separate us from our larger role as physicians. Now that our patients live out their life spans, we will more frequently be unable to cure and to prevent death. Yet, as with physicians in millenia past, we are not freed of our responsibilities to comfort, to console, to reassure, to be available. This is a responsibility which cannot be delegated; it is the essence of medical practice.

The inevitability of death and the presence of incurable disease should not lull the physician into nihilism or neglect. Most individuals are socially competent and lead active and enjoyable lives until their terminal illness. Many conditions, as with younger patients, are either self-limited or curable. Chronic disease is often subject to control, and symptoms can usually be reduced if not eliminated. Much can be done to assist the patient in maintaining independence and dignity. Most older individuals do not expect to have the capabilities of youth; nor are they afraid of death. They demand of us only that we keep them as comfortable and functional as possible, so that they can make what remains of their lives meaningful and enjoyable.

Binstock, R. H., and Shanas, E. (eds.): Handbook of Aging and the Social Sciences. New York, Van Nostrand Reinhold Company, 1976.

Birren, J. E., and Schaie, K. W. (eds.): Handbook of the Psychology of Aging. New York, Van Nostrand Reinhold Company, 1977.

Brocklehurst, J. C. (ed.): Textbook of Geriatric Medicine and Gerontology. Edinburgh and London, Churchill Livingstone, 1973.

Finch, C. E. and Hayflick, L. (eds.): Handbook of the Biology of Aging. New York, Van Nostrand Reinhold Company, 1977.

Reichel, W. (ed.): Clinical Aspects of Aging. Baltimore, Williams & Wilkins Company, 1978.

Rossman, I. (ed.): Clinical Geriatrics. Philadelphia, J. B. Lippincott Company, 1971.

PART III
GENETIC PRINCIPLES

11. INTRODUCTION

Alexander G. Bearn

After Gregor Mendel established the principle of genetic transmission, Johannsen, in 1909, introduced the word *gene* to denote a unit of heredity. A structural gene is now defined, operationally, as a functional unit of inheritance situated on a chromosome and responsible for the synthesis of a specific polypeptide. It has been estimated that there are probably at least 10,000 genes in man. Since the number of well documented examples of genetic variability is of the order of 1000, it is apparent that despite the acceleration in discovery of new genetic entities 90 per cent of the human genome remains to be discovered.

MODERN GENETICS AND ITS RELATION TO INTERNAL MEDICINE. The chemical nature of the gene was unrecognized until 1944, when a soluble extract derived from pneumococci of one genotype was found to effect a stable heritable change when added to a growing culture of pneumococci of another genotype. The recognition that the transforming substance in the extract was deoxyribonucleic acid (DNA) launched the present era of molecular biology.

THE GENE AND PROTEIN SYNTHESIS. The genetic information encoded in the double-stranded DNA that determines polypeptide structure is brought to the ribosome, where the polypeptides are synthesized by a unique type of single-stranded RNA, known as messenger RNA, or mRNA. This mRNA is complementary to one of the strands of DNA, and the linear sequences in the polypeptide are precisely determined by the linear sequences of the coding units ("codons" — triplets of nucleotides coding for different amino acids) in the mRNA. These relationships are often referred to as the central dogma of molecular biology, and can be depicted schematically as shown at the bottom of this page.

The universality of this biologic truth was abruptly shaken by the discovery in 1970 that several RNA animal tumor viruses contain polymerase activity (reverse transcriptase), which used RNA as a template for the synthesis of double-stranded DNA and thus reversed the familiar direction of genetic transcription. This discovery raised the possibility that an RNA-dependent DNA polymerase might indicate the presence of an oncogenic virus which can transform normal cells into genetically stable cancer cells. Although this enzyme has now been detected in certain nononcogenic viruses as well, the function of viral reverse transcriptase remains a question of central biologic importance in the problem of neoplasia.

DEOXYRIBONUCLEIC ACID (DNA). Deoxyribonucleic acid is constructed from three essential components: the five carbon sugar 2-deoxy-*D*-ribose; phosphoric acid, which confers on DNA its acidic properties; and nitrogenous bases. Two of the bases are purines, aden-ine (A) and guanine (G), and two are pyrimidines, thymine (T) and cytosine (C). In 1953 Watson and Crick assembled the available physical and chemical data on DNA into a molecular model for the structure of DNA. Two polynucleotide chains are twisted together to form a double helix. The two chains are held together by hydrogen bonds between the bases which face inward forming the core, and the phosphate-sugar groups form an external helical backbone. Adenine must always pair with thymine (A-T), and guanine with cytosine (G-C). The result of this pairing leads to a precise complementary relationship between the bases on the two chains. Thus, if part of the base sequence were TTGCC, the corresponding portion of the complementary strand would read AACGG.

REPLICATION OF DNA. One of the chief attractions of the Watson-Crick model for DNA is that it contains a built-in system for self-replication. As the double helix of a parent molecule unwinds, the sequence of bases in each strand acts as a template for the synthesis of a new strand of DNA in two daughter molecules. The replication is catalyzed by the enzyme DNA polymerase and has been termed *semiconservative*, because both parental strands are conserved in the next generation, each now paired with a newly synthesized complementary partner. Recent evidence suggests that normal replication occurs in short fragments which start with an RNA primer and are then joined by a specific ligase. It is also evident that there are at least three distinct DNA polymerases, α, β, and γ. Only DNA polymerase α can initiate new DNA synthesis with an RNA primer provided by RNA polymerase. All three can function in DNA repair.

RIBONUCLEIC ACID (RNA). Ribonucleic acid differs from deoxyribonucleic acid in three important ways. (1) The sugar D-ribose replaces the 2-deoxy-*D*-ribose of DNA. (2) The pyrimidine base uracil (U) replaces the thymine of DNA. (3) RNA is a single-stranded polymer in contrast to double-stranded DNA.

MESSENGER RIBONUCLEIC ACID (mRNA). The genetic information encoded in the DNA of the chromosomes must be conveyed from the nucleus to the cytoplasm where the proteins are synthesized. Messenger RNA is formed by the transcription of one of the strands of DNA and is catalyzed by RNA polymerase II. The sequence of bases in mRNA is complementary to that in the corresponding uncopied strand of DNA except that uracil replaces thymine. In this way single-stranded RNA carries into the cytoplasm the genetic information originally encoded in nuclear DNA. In bacteria, mRNA has a half-life of about two minutes, and it has been calculated that during this time about 10 to 20 molecules of protein can be synthesized. In cells of higher organisms mRNAs vary in their stability over a range from minutes to many hours. For example, the half-life of globin mRNA is about 14 hours.

TRANSFER RNA (tRNA). Before amino acids are as-

DNA (double-stranded) $\xleftarrow{\text{transcription}}$ RNA (single-stranded) $\xrightarrow{\text{translation}}$ polypeptide

Figure 1. A schematic diagram of the genetic control of protein synthesis. A=adenine, T=thymine, G=guanine, C=cytosine, U=uracil. The codons indicated represent code words for the amino acids indicated. The messenger RNA (mRNA) moves across the ribosomes in the direction of the arrow. tRNA=transfer RNA; rRNA=ribosomal RNA. AA= amino acids.

sembled into polypeptide chains, they must first be "activated." This activation is accomplished by the enzymes known as aminoacyl-tRNA synthetases, each of which is specific for one amino acid. Such an enzyme combines ATP and an amino acid to form aminoacyl-adenylate, with the release of pyrophosphate. The activated amino acid is now joined to another type of RNA called transfer RNA, with the release of adenylic acid. Mammalian cells contain more than 20 different transfer RNA's, which are transcribed from DNA by RNA polymerase III. At least one transfer RNA is specific for each of the amino acids. Each transfer RNA molecule is folded into a cloverleaf pattern and has two recognition sites. One site recognizes the "activated" amino acid, whereas the second, often called the anticodon, recognizes the codon in the mRNA. Thus the fidelity of translation is assured by the specific binding of the amino acid to the appropriate tRNA catalyzed by the specific activating enzyme, and by complementary pairing of the anticodon of tRNA with the codon of the mRNA.

RIBOSOMAL RNA (RRNA).   More than 80 per cent of the RNA of most cells is found in cytoplasmic particles called ribosomes. These ribosome particles represent the protein synthetic machinery of the cell and are com-

posed of about half protein and half RNA. Ribosomes from *Escherichia coli* consist of a 30 S subunit, consisting of 21 proteins and 16 S RNA, and a 50 S subunit with some 34 proteins, 5 S, and 23 S RNA. Mammalian ribosomes are somewhat larger; they have a diameter of about 200 Å and a sedimentation coefficient of 80 S and dissociate into 40 S and 60 S subunits in low concentrations of magnesium. Messenger RNA, bearing the instructions for protein synthesis, forms a complex with the smaller subunit and the initiator tRNA. The larger subunit then attaches to this complex from the functional ribosome, and the sequential assembly of amino acids into protein can now begin.

PROTEIN SYNTHESIS.   Protein synthesis on the ribosome occurs in three main steps: initiation, elongation, and termination. These steps are complex and require the involvement of many protein components of the ribosome as well as rRNA.

Initiation, in bacteria, can be said to begin when the codon AUG binds N • formylmethionyl-tRNA to the 30 S ribosome subunit and mRNA becomes bound to the ribosomes. Thus most bacterial proteins have, as their first amino acid, N-formylmethionine. Since there are no formylated end groups in bacterial proteins, this means that the formyl group must be cleaved soon after the beginning of protein synthesis. The second codon, recognizing its specific tRNA, brings the second amino acid in sequence into alignment. A peptide bond is now formed and the messenger RNA moves along the ribosome so that the third amino acid comes into position, with further elongation of the peptide chain (Fig. 1). The messenger RNA has a distinct polarity as it moves along the ribosome, always reading from the 5' to the 3' end. The information that a polypeptide chain is completed and that its synthesis must be terminated is specified by a special chain-terminating codon. A ribosome takes about ten seconds to read an entire mRNA molecule of average length, and a single mRNA molecule may move over the surfaces of several ribosomes simultaneously. This explains why a cell needs relatively little mRNA to synthesize a great deal of protein. A cluster of several ribosomes all translating the same mRNA is called a polyribosome; polyribosomes synthesizing hemoglobin (a protein of molecular weight 64,500), consist, on the average, of four to six ribosomes.

CODONS. Because most proteins are composed of 20 different amino acids and because DNA has only four different nucleotide bases, it is evident that more than one base is required to prescribe for a particular amino acid. A sequence of three bases (a codon) is needed to code for each amino acid. Thus a gene with 1500 nucleotide pairs would determine the sequence of a polypeptide chain consisting of 500 amino acids. Since the four-letter code is triplet in nature, there are 64 (4 × 4 × 4) possible codons, of which 61 have been shown to code for one of the 20 amino acids. Three remaining codons, UAA, UAG, and UGA, represent signals that the polypeptide chain is completed and are called chain-terminating codons and do not code for any amino acid. Two codons serve to initiate polypeptide synthesis as well as to insert amino acids and are sometimes designated chain-initiating codons. One of the unresolved problems in eukaryotic organisms, such as man, is that they appear to possess more DNA in their genome than can be accounted for by the estimated number of unique genes. However, some genes occur

in multiple copies, and there are also stretches of noncoding DNA. The genetic code is said to be *universal* in the sense that all plant and animal species have thus far been found to use the same genetic code, and *degenerate* because certain amino acids can be specified by more than one triplet.

Certain acridine dyes, e.g., proflavine, induce mutations in bacteriophage by leading to the insertion of an extra nucleotide into the pre-existing (normal) sequence. Because of this extra nucleotide, the reading frame becomes altered distal to the point of insertion and results in a disruption of normal protein synthesis. The correct reading frame of the code can be restored by deletion of a nucleotide (or by the insertion of two extra nucleotides) distal to the insertion. This model makes the prediction that a double mutant, consisting of an insertion followed by a deletion, will result in a polypeptide chain with an altered amino acid sequence between the two mutations. If the segment of DNA between the two mutations is short, and does not code for amino acids vital for functional specificity, a protein with a normal function may still be produced. A mutation in the codon which terminates the reading of the code is referred to as a terminator mutation.

Three hemoglobin variants have been found affecting the terminating codons UAG or UAA. In each variant, the alpha chain of hemoglobin has 171 residues instead of 141. Each of these hemoglobins has an identical amino acid sequence, the alteration being at residue 141 (glutamine in Hb Constant Spring, serine in Hb Koya Dora, and lysine in Hb Icaria). The codons for each of these amino acids can be derived from UA (G or A) by a point mutation. The predicted mutation in which an amino acid–specifying codon is changed to a terminator codon has also been found. Hb McKees-Rock is a 144 residue beta chain variant which lacks the two C-terminal amino acids tyrosine and histidine, and is the result of the single step conversion of UA (C or U) tyrosine specifying codon to a terminator codon (Fig. 2).

Crossing-over between synapsing chromatids can also yield structurally abnormal proteins. In Hb Tak, for instance, misalignment and crossing-over between two

Figure 2. Hemoglobin mutants affecting terminator codons. *Key:* UCU=Serine. UCA=Serine. CAA= Glutamine. AAA=Phenylalanine. UAA=Asparagine. CAC=Histidine. UAA=Terminator. UAU=Tyrosine. AAG=Phenylalanine.

beta chains results in the insertion of two nucleotides. As a consequence, the terminating codon is not read in phase and the mRNA continues to add another 11 amino acids until the next termination codon is read at residue 157. Similar molecular rearrangements account for Hb Cranston and Hb Wayne. Hb Wayne can be derived from Hb Constant Spring by a frameshift mutation (deletion) involving the alpha 138 serine.

GENETIC REGULATORY MECHANISMS. Genetic mechanisms for the control of protein synthesis are much better understood in microorganisms than in man. The original hypothesis of Jacob and Monod postulated two classes of genes: structural genes which controlled the amino acid structure of the protein, and regulatory genes which influenced the rate of protein synthesis. Structural genes were linked together as a single functional unit, termed an operon. Thus this genetic model suggested a simple transcriptional control of protein synthesis; the amount of protein synthesis was determined by the amount of mRNA.

Direct application of this model to mammalian systems cannot be made, although the report of Ingram, in 1956, that sickle cell hemoglobin differed from normal hemoglobin in a single amino acid substitution appeared to be a neat example of a structural mutation. Since Ingram's initial observation, many structural mutants in man have been described, but whether there are regulatory mutations in man, corresponding to those seen in microorganisms, is quite unclear. Many structural mutations affect the rate of synthesis of the abnormal protein. From such observations the concept that genes controlling the structure of a protein also influence the amount of protein synthesized has gained ground, and has been termed the structure-rate hypothesis. In most instances, the mutational event leads to decreased synthesis; however, an increased enzymatic activity has been observed in G6PD Hektoen, a structural mutant in the glucose-6-phosphate dehydrogenase system, and in a pseudocholinesterase mutant, designated Cynthiana.

The molecular basis of the various forms of thalassemia (see Ch. 485.7) has become increasingly understood in recent years. Alpha thalassemia is the result of a deletion of the whole or part of the alpha-chain genes. The beta thalassemias exhibit a variety of molecular defects. Patients with classic Cooley's anemia (beta$^+$ thal) have a reduced beta-chain mRNA synthesis; those with the less common Cooley's anemia (beta^0 thal) have absent beta-chain mRNA, although the beta-chain genes are present (see Ch. 485.7).

In contrast to microorganisms, in which protein synthesis is controlled predominantly by genetic regulatory mechanisms, hormonal influences have a profound effect in man and other eukaryotic organisms. In certain cells, thyroxine and adrenocortical hormones influence the rate of RNA synthesis and the activity of DNA-dependent RNA polymerase. Another regulatory mechanism of protein synthesis in man involves the histones, which are closely associated with mammalian DNA. It seems likely that histones play an important role in controlling the transcription of DNA; temporary removal, or modification, of the DNA-associated histone results in an increased transcription of the DNA. When this histone modification is reversible, it provides a molecular mechanism which can adjust protein synthesis to physiologic need. Histone modification is also thought to play a key role in differentiation and development. Recent techniques for hybridizing animal cells will enable genetic regulatory mechanisms in man to be examined at the cellular level.

Watson, J. D.: Molecular Biology of the Gene. 3rd ed. New York, Benjamin, 1976.

12. PEDIGREE ANALYSIS IN INHERITED DISEASE

Alexander G. Bearn

Inspection and analysis of human pedigrees form the basis for an understanding of the application of the laws of Mendel to human disease. Analysis of a pedigree begins with the affected individual, who is referred to as the propositus, proband, or index case. Using the propositus as the point of departure, a pedigree is constructed, and the pattern of the pedigree is analyzed. It is worth emphasizing, however, that the construction of human pedigrees beyond first- and second-degree relatives is an occupation more likely to please the physician than to provide a deeper genetic understanding of the patient's disease. Human memories are notoriously untrustworthy, and great care must be exercised when very large pedigrees are compiled and recorded.

AUTOSOMAL INHERITANCE. When there are two alleles, A and a, at a locus, three possible genotypes exist, which can be represented AA, Aa, and aa. The genotypes AA and aa are called *homozygotes;* Aa is a *heterozygote.* A gene can be recognized only by the effect it produces; thus in the strictest sense it is incorrect to speak of dominant or recessive genes, but only of dominant or recessive effects. If the phenotype Aa cannot be easily distinguished from the phenotype AA, but is clearly different from aa, the effect of gene A is said to be dominant over the effect of gene a. In this circumstance there are only two phenotypes corresponding to the three genotypes AA, Aa, aa. However, the failure to detect a phenotypic difference between the genotypes AA and Aa is usually testimony to the insensitivity of the methods employed. If the gene products of A and a can both be detected in the heterozygote Aa, the genes are said to exert an effect which is *co-dominant.* It would be preferable to discard the terms "dominant" and "recessive" and instead to state whether the genes concerned are phenotypically expressed in a single or double dose; for the sake of convenience, however, the terms are often retained. Although logically indefensible, it is pragmatically useful practice to designate a trait as dominant even though the homozygote has never been observed and in fact might have quite a different phenotype.

Autosomal Dominant Traits. Autosomal genes are those genes situated on chromosomes other than the X and Y. Dominant traits are defined as those traits that are fully manifested by the presence of a gene in the heterozygous state. Thus far, approximately 750 well established autosomal dominant traits have been identified in man. (Satisfactory examples of dominant traits are those responsible for the formation of certain blood group antigens. In the ABO system, the genes controlling the formation of A and B substances are dominant over O. Thus it is not ordinarily possible to distinguish serologically AA from AO individuals, or BB from BO individuals. However, heterozygous individuals of type

Autosomal Dominant

Autosomal Dominant (mutation)

Figure 3. Pedigrees of autosomal dominant traits. In the lower pedigree the normal parents of the affected individual suggest the possibility of a new mutation. Solid symbols indicate those affected. (For details see text.)

AB can be recognized because the product of genes A and B can be detected.)

An autosomal dominant trait can be recognized in human pedigrees by its transmission from one generation to the next. Except for sporadic cases in which a fresh mutation in the germ line has arisen in either the father or the mother, and provided illegitimacy can be excluded, every affected individual has at least one affected parent and may have affected offspring and sibs (Fig. 3). The more severe the condition, the larger is the proportion of sporadic cases caused by fresh mutation. According to mendelian laws, a heterozygous affected individual married to a normal homozygote will, on the average, transmit the trait to half his offspring, both sexes being equally affected.

In contrast to recessive disorders, most dominant traits in man frequently exert only mild effects, and marked variation in the expression of the trait is the rule. In many instances the disease is not manifest until adult life. Occasionally the expression of the abnormal gene may be so weak that a generation appears to be skipped because the carrier of the abnormal gene is clinically normal. When a gene that can be clinically expressed in the heterozygous condition occurs in the homozygous state, the effect is usually more severe and may be lethal. Although examples are common in species in which experimental matings can be constructed, such examples are exceptional in man, because marriage of two clinically affected heterozygotes is rare. Possible examples include achondroplasia and the Osler-Weber-Rendu syndrome. An increased paternal age effect has been demonstrated among parents of sporadic cases of achondroplastic dwarfism, Marfan's syndrome (see Ch. 538.1), and certain other dominantly inherited disorders.

The molecular basis for the more than 750 genetically dominant diseases now known is quite obscure. It is of interest that in contrast to recessively inherited diseases in which an impairment of enzyme function is the rule, defective enzymes are only rarely found in dominant diseases. A deficiency of the inhibitor of the first component of complement, *C1-esterase inhibitor,* in hereditary angioedema and a deficiency of *uroporphyrinogen-1-synthetase* in acute intermittent porphyria are exceptions to this general rule (see Ch. 47 and 536.3). It appears that in most dominantly inherited disorders the abnormal

gene determines a protein with a nonenzymatic function. In familial hypercholesterolemia the defect lies in an abnormality in the cell surface receptor that binds low density lipoprotein. Several hemolytic disorders are due to the presence of a single unstable mutant hemoglobin (see Ch. 485). The presence of one of these abnormal hemoglobin genes is sufficient to shorten the life of the red cells.

Autosomal Recessive Traits. In an autosomal recessive trait, the father and the mother of the affected individual are usually normal, as are more distant ancestors. On the average, one fourth of the brothers and sisters of the index case will be affected. If the trait is rare, an increased consanguinity will often be observed among the parents of those affected. According to mendelian laws, two normal parents, both heterozygous for a recessive trait, will produce offspring of whom, on the average, one quarter will be homozygous for the normal allele, one quarter homozygous for the abnormal allele and thus affected, and one half heterozygous for the abnormal allele, like the parents. Affected individuals usually have phenotypically normal offspring who are all carriers of the abnormal gene. If an affected individual marries an individual heterozygous for the same gene, one half of the offspring will be affected and one half will be heterozygous carriers (Fig. 4). Approximately 800 well established recessive traits have been identified in man.

Certain aspects of the segregation ratio in autosomal recessive conditions must be emphasized. Because of the small size of families and because ascertainment of the family is usually through an affected member, the mean observed proportion of affected individuals will be greater than expected. Only when the size of the sibships is large will the expected ratio of one affected to three unaffected be realized in pooled data. Thus the analysis of the expected ratio in families of various sizes requires a correction factor whose magnitude depends on the number of children in the sibship. The simplest correction is to subtract in each family the index case from the total number of affected individuals and then determine the proportion of affected children among the remaining sibs.

The disadvantage of the term "recessive" is emphasized by the increasing number of instances in which refined biochemical observations enable the recognition of the trait in the clinically normal heterozygote. Indeed, because of its importance in genetic counseling, the detection of healthy heterozygous carriers of genes that in the homozygous condition cause overt disease is

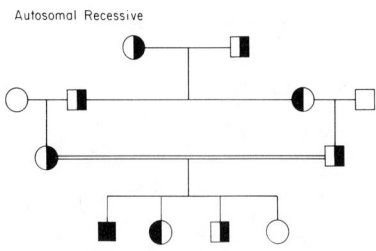

Autosomal Recessive

Figure 4. Pedigree of autosomal recessive trait. Note: both parents are heterozygous. One sib is affected, two are carriers, and one is normal. Double line (══) indicates that parents are related by descent (first cousins).

Figure 5. Pedigree of dominant X-linked trait. The X chromosome bearing the abnormal gene is designated by a small white dot.

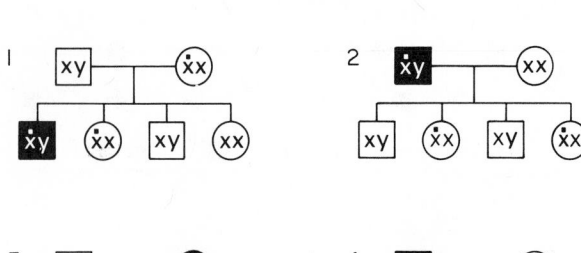

Figure 6. Pedigrees of recessive X-linked trait. The X chromosome bearing the abnormal gene is designated by a small dot. Affected individuals are indicated by solid squares (males) and circles (females). Pedigree 1 is commonly observed; pedigree 4 is rare.

becoming one of the most significant aspects of medical genetics. Detection of the sickle cell gene in black populations and the Tay-Sachs gene among Ashkenazic Jews are classic examples of the usefulness of heterozygote detection. In recent years, the biochemical detection of heterozygotes for autosomal recessive diseases has been greatly facilitated by the development of techniques to culture skin fibroblasts. Although the culturing of human fibroblasts has been relatively uninformative in dominant disorders, in approximately 25 per cent of all autosomal recessive diseases the precise biochemical defect can be detected in cultured fibroblasts derived from a simple skin biopsy.

Genetic Compounds. Heteroallelic compounds represent those conditions which are due to the inheritance of two different mutant genes derived from the same locus. Thus individuals with Hb SC disease have inherited an Hb S gene from one parent and an Hb C gene from the other. Certain unusual mucopolysaccharidoses may also represent genetic compounds (see Ch. 538.1).

X-LINKED INHERITANCE.   Dominant X-Linked Traits. This mode of inheritance is uncommon. Heterozygous affected females will transmit the trait to both sexes with a frequency of 50 per cent. Affected males will transmit the trait to all their daughters, but to none of their sons (Fig. 5). This rule of X-linked dominant inheritance enables critical distinction from traits inherited in an autosomal dominant fashion, in which an affected male transmits the trait to both sons and daughters. The variability of expression of an X-linked dominant trait is less in males than in females. If the trait is uncommon, the incidence in females is roughly twice that in males. The erythrocyte antigen Xg[a] and vitamin D resistant rickets (hypophosphatemic rickets) are inherited as X-linked dominant traits. Approximately 100 loci have been identified on the human X chromosome.

Recessive X-Linked Traits. Recessive X-linked traits

are relatively common. On the average, half the sons of normal heterozygous females will be normal, and half will be affected. If the trait is rare, parents and relatives will be normal except for male relatives in the female line; for instance, on the average, one half of the maternal uncles will be affected. An affected male married to a normal female will have normal offspring. All their daughters will be carriers, and they, in turn, can transmit the trait to the next generation. The rare event of an affected male married to a carrier female will result in equal proportions of affected male and female offspring. The unaffected males will be genotypically normal; the unaffected females, however, will be heterozygous carriers (Fig. 6). The common red-green color blindness is inherited as an X-linked recessive trait. In the general population the frequency of affected females will be roughly the square of the frequency of affected males.

Some common mendelian disorders that are inherited in a dominant autosomal and X-linked fashion are illustrated in Table 1.

THE LYON HYPOTHESIS. Since the female bears two X chromosomes, it might have been expected that the concentration of proteins determined by genes on the X chromosome would be twice that observed in males who have only one X chromosome. Thus it might have been expected that the concentration of factor VIII (antihemophilic factor) in females would be twice that found in males. This is not the case, and the explanation is provided by a hypothesis first advanced by Mary Lyon.

TABLE 1.   Some Relatively Common Mendelian Disorders

Autosomal Dominant	Autosomal Recessive	X-Linked
Familial monogenic hypercholesterolemia	Cystic fibrosis	Hemophilia A
Marfan's syndrome	Deaf mutism	Classic agammaglobulinemia (Bruton)
Adult polycystic disease	Phenylketonuria and other hereditary aminoacidurias	Pseudohypertrophic muscular dystrophy
Huntington's chorea	Wilson's disease	Glucose-6-phosphate dehydrogenase deficiency
Acute intermittent porphyria	Homocystinuria	Fabry's disease
Hereditary hemorrhagic telangiectasia	Albinism	Testicular feminization
Neurofibromatosis	Emphysema (due to alpha-1-antitrypsin deficiency)	Chronic granulomatous disease
Osteogenesis imperfecta	Friedreich's ataxia	Vitamin D resistant rickets
von Willebrand's disease		
Achondroplastic dwarfism		

In all adult female cells only one of the two X chromosomes is genetically active. Early in differentiation one of the X chromosomes becomes inactive and forms the Barr body. Inactivation is random; but once one of the two X chromosomes in any cell is inactivated, the same X chromosome remains inactive during all its subsequent cell divisions. For example, only half the X chromosomes are genetically active and synthesizing antihemophilic globulin, and thus the amount of antihemophilic globulin synthesis is approximately the same in males and females. Greater variability in expression of an X-linked trait is a natural consequence of the Lyon hypothesis. The number of cells determining a specific function at the time of inactivation is small, and thus chance alone could influence the number of such cells inactivated.

Y-LINKED INHERITANCE. If a trait is determined by a gene in the Y chromosome, it will be transmitted through the father to all his sons and none of his daughters. Thus far, the only genes that have been shown to be located in the Y chromosome are those that determine "maleness" and an antigen that influences graft rejection. (See also XYY Syndrome in Ch. 548.4.)

SEX LIMITATION. Autosomal genes that are expressed only in males may mimic sex-linkage but can be formally distinguished if affected individuals reproduce. If a gene is on an autosome, affected males can transmit the trait to their sons; if the gene is on the X chromosome, they cannot. Linkage analysis may also serve to distinguish between autosomal and X-linked genes.

MODIFICATION OF GENE EXPRESSION. The manifestation of an abnormal gene is influenced not only by its normal allele, but also by alleles at other loci, and by environment. The terms expressivity and penetrance have been employed to describe the variable manifestation of a gene. These vague words are usually best avoided unless they can be used with precision; e.g., it would be precise but cumbersome to say that the gene for Huntington's chorea is 0 per cent penetrant at the age of 10 and 95 per cent penetrant at 65. Some genetically determined traits such as those determining the blood antigens are present at birth, whereas others such as Huntington's chorea appear only in adult life. A negative correlation between the age of onset of a trait in parents and sibs suggests that the expression of a gene may be influenced by the type of normal allele present. The effect can be seen in certain dominant diseases such as the nail-patella syndrome and in the dominant form of muscular dystrophy. The concept of anticipation, which asserts that hereditary diseases tend to have a progressively earlier age of onset with successive generations, is a statistical artifact which is based on a bias of ascertainment.

CONSANGUINITY. The most common error in taking a family history is to fail to inquire about consanguinity. When confronted with a patient, particularly a child, whose disorder does not fit any clear-cut diagnosis, a history of consanguinity in the parents is often the first clue that the patient is suffering from a rare, recessively inherited disorder. In all autosomal recessive disorders the affected individual has inherited one abnormal gene from each parent. It is thus evident that an individual will be more likely to inherit the same allele from each parent if the two parents have genes inherited from a common ancestor. First cousins share, on the average, one eighth of their genes, which were derived from a common ancestor. When two first cousins marry, an offspring has, on the average, one sixteenth of the loci homozygous for a gene derived from a common ancestor. It is frequently of interest to calculate the expected frequency of first-cousin marriages among parents of those with rare autosomal recessive disorders. Providing that the frequency of the disease in the population can be estimated and the frequency of first-cousin marriages in the general population is known, the calculation can be made according to the following formula. If k is the frequency of first-cousin marriages in a rare recessive disease, then as a first approximation $k = c/16q$, where c is the frequency of first-cousin marriages in the general population and q is the frequency of the abnormal gene. The frequency of cousin marriages is variable. In some isolated populations a frequency of as high as 30 per cent has been recorded, whereas in the United States in an urban population the frequency may be as low as 0.05 per cent. Let us suppose a recessively inherited disease has a frequency in the population of 1 in 10,000 (q^2); then the frequency of the gene, which in double dose causes the disease, is 1 in 100 (q). If the frequency of consanguinity in the general population is 0.5 per cent, then k, the parental consanguinity, is 3 per cent, a six-fold increase over normal. If the disease is much rarer, 1 in 100,000, then 10 per cent of the individuals affected by the disease will have parents who are first cousins. As the frequency of c increases, the expected frequency of parents who are first cousins will also increase. In some geographically isolated populations c may reach as high as 2 per cent. If a recessively inherited disease in such an isolate has a frequency of 1 in 100,000, 40 per cent of the parents of the affected individuals will be first cousins.

It is important to realize that an increased frequency of consanguinity will not be observed if the recessive disease is common. Thus in cystic fibrosis of the pancreas, which has a frequency of approximately 1 in 2500, no increase in parental consanguinity can be detected. Although the frequency of albinism in the general population is approximately 1 per 20,000, the unexpectedly high consanguinity in the parents (k = 20 per cent) of some patients is due to the existence of more than one gene for this condition. No increase in consanguinity would be expected in dominant or X-linked traits or genetic compounds.

Although in most populations the consanguinity rate is less than 1 per cent, certain geographic and cultural isolates remain in which there is a high coefficient of inbreeding. These isolates may shelter rare genes which because of the high consanguinity rate are likely to become manifest. More than 90 per cent of patients described with the Ellis–van Creveld syndrome have been found in the Old Order Amish living in Pennsylvania, Ohio, Indiana, and Ontario. Other rare recessive diseases found within this genetic isolate include pyruvate kinase deficiency, a form of dwarfism associated with hypoplasia of the cartilage and hair, and a form of limb-girdle muscular dystrophy. It is worth remembering that, in general, the offspring of first-cousin marriages are slightly more likely to have congenital malformations, as well as mental and physical defects, than are children born to unrelated parents.

ASSOCIATION. The occurrence of two traits in the same person more often than would be expected by chance is called association. A consistent positive association between blood group A and carcinoma of the stomach, and between duodenal ulceration and blood group O, has long been recognized. Such an association may be due to many causes, and does not indicate that the genes controlling blood group antigens are on the same chromosome as those associated with the development of duodenal ulceration. If an association is found between two characters in the general population, it is important to determine whether the association persists when the two characters are examined in sibships. If geographic or social stratification is the cause of the association, the correlation will disappear. If, for example, a mixed population of Africans and Europeans is examined, a positive association between cDe Rhesus blood group (common in African populations) and dark skin color would be found. This association disappears within a sibship, but the small size of human sibships and the statistical problems associated with pooling data from different sibships make it difficult to provide a simple test.

PLEIOTROPISM. Sometimes two characters are associated because they are due to the action of a single gene. Thus clouding of the cornea and mental retardation are two traits that are associated in Hurler's syndrome. The two traits are not caused by two genes, but are due to a single gene with a so-called pleiotropic effect. When a gene causes a pleiotropic effect, the association found in the general population persists when sibships are examined. Pleiotropic effects of genes are common, and may be of clinical importance. Familial intestinal polyposis (see Ch. 426) is an early consequence of the effect of a gene that later commonly leads to carcinoma of the colon.

AUTOSOMAL LINKAGE. The site of a gene on a chromosome is termed a *locus*. Alternative forms of genes which occupy corresponding sites on homologous chromosomes are called alleles. Applied to human genetics, Mendel's law of independent assortment states that traits controlled by two or more pairs of allelic genes will be transmitted to the children of the next generation, either together or separately, by chance alone. The law holds only for genes situated on different chromosomes or at widely separated loci on the same chromosome. However, if two genes occupy closely adjacent sites on the same chromosome, they tend to segregate together and are then said to be linked. The frequency of crossing over gives an estimate of closeness of the linkage. It is important to remember that even if two genes are present on the same chromosome, they will appear unlinked if they are so widely separated that free (50 per cent) recombination between two loci can take place.

The application of somatic cell genetics as well as the development of more discriminating methods for chromosome identification has enabled the assignment of specific loci to individual autosomes. Structural loci can be assigned to all 22 autosomes. In many instances more than one genetic locus can be assigned to a particular chromosome. Chromosome 1 has 22 loci assigned, including the Rh locus.

Linkage of two genes does not cause association of the two characters in the general population unless the population is heterogeneous, as it would be in an American city, recently derived from several parts of the world. In any one sibship the two characters may be associated, in which case the genes are on the same chromosome and are said to be linked in coupling (cis configuration). If the characters are dissociated, the genes responsible are distributed on each of the two homologous chromosomes and are described as being linked in repulsion (trans configuration). A common error is to suppose that the association of two characters in the single sibship implies genetic linkage. If true linkage exists, sufficient pedigrees are collected, and the genes concerned are in equilibrium, an equal number of sibships will be found in which the two characters are not associated. If, however, the genes concerned are not in equilibrium (genetic disequilibrium), as in the case with HLA-B27 and ankylosing spondylitis, then the specific allele B27 at the HLA locus will be much more frequent in patients with the disease (see below). There are many instances of autosomal linkage in man, including the ABO blood group locus and the locus for the nail-patella syndrome; the Rh blood groups and one form of elliptocytosis; and Lutheran blood group and the secretor locus (which determines whether soluble ABO blood substances are present in saliva and other body fluids). The loci determining the β and δ chains of hemoglobin are also very closely linked (see Ch. 485.1). The development of somatic cell genetics has enabled the human chromosome map of the autosomes to be rapidly filled. One hundred fifteen genes are now assigned to the autosomes and 96 to the X chromosome. The increased information now available on the linkage of genes to specific chromosomes has been greatly enhanced by these techniques.

The linkage relationships of human genes have one important practical consequence for clinical medicine. If a mutant causing a serious inherited disease is closely linked to one causing a common trait, healthy carriers of the disease may be detected in unaffected members of the family by the presence or absence of the common trait. It would, of course, be important to know whether the two linked genes in the family under investigation were in the coupling or repulsion phase. Accurate information regarding the phase can be obtained by studying the distribution of the two traits in three generations.

THE HISTOCOMPATIBILITY LOCUS (HLA). The HLA system comprises four closely linked highly polymorphic loci on chromosome 6 (Fig. 7). These loci as ordered on the chromosome are HLA-A, HLA-C, HLA-B, and HLA-D. The A, B, and C loci are defined serologically; the D locus controls lymphocyte (LD) antigens detectable by the mixed lymphocyte test (MLD). Multiple alleles are found at each locus; HLA-A and HLA-B have more than 20 alleles, whereas at the HLA-C locus only five alleles have been identified thus far. Closely adjacent to the HLA locus are loci controlling some of the complement components. These include the genes that determine C2 and C4 deficiency and the Chido (Ch) and Rodgers (Rg) loci coding for red cell antigens. The C2 deficiency locus is particularly closely associated with DW2. Many diseases with strong associations with the HLA-B region frequently have an even stronger association with HLA-D. Since linkage of the HLA antigen to many diseases is particularly marked at the D locus, further definition of this complex area is likely to lead to information of extreme clinical importance. The immune response genes, which may serve as the T cell receptor in the mouse, have not yet been identified in man.

The association of the HLA system and disease has an unusual feature; in most disease associations such as the gene for sickle cell trait and resistance to infection with *Plasmodium falciparum*, or the Duffy blood group

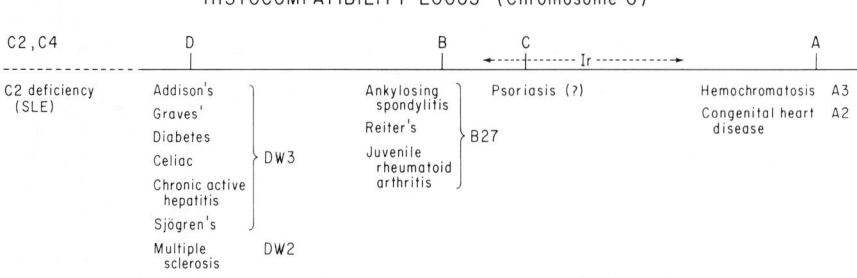

Figure 7.

and *Plasmodium vivax*, the association is with a specific disease entity. The association of specific HLA genes and disease is far ranging, and a specific HLA allele may have a significant association with several diseases.

Ankylosing Spondylitis. The frequency of the HLA-B27 allele in the white population is approximately 8 per cent. In patients with ankylosing spondylitis the frequency of B27 is over 90 per cent. In Australian aboriginals and black Africans the B27 antigen is virtually absent, and the frequency of ankylosing spondylitis in these populations is sharply reduced. In contrast, B27 occurs in 50 per cent of the adult Haida Indians of the United States, and sacroiliitis is present in 10 per cent of the adult male population. A Caucasian with the B27 antigen is approximately 100 times more likely to develop ankylosing spondylitis than one who does not possess this antigen; the increased liability in Japanese populations of B27 individuals is 300. Between 5 and 20 per cent of all individuals of both sexes, above the age of 30, with the B27 antigen have some clinical or radiologic evidence of sacroiliac joint disease.

Rheumatoid Arthritis, Sjögren's Syndrome, Reiter's Syndrome, and Multiple Sclerosis. The frequency of HLA-DW4 in patients with rheumatoid arthritis is 42 per cent compared to 16 per cent in controls, irrespective of whether the individual is positive for the rheumatoid factor. HLA-B8 is more common in patients with Sjögren's syndrome (53 per cent) than in a control population (17 per cent). Reiter's syndrome usually follows an infection of the urinary tract or bowel with *Shigella, Salmonella,* or the *Yersinia* organism. No less than 20 per cent of B27 positive individuals with *Shigella* infections will develop Reiter's syndrome. Although multiple sclerosis is strongly associated with HLA-DW2, at least 40 per cent of patients are DW2 negative.

Graves' Disease, Juvenile Diabetes, and Addison's Disease. These diseases, all of which are associated with disturbances in the immune response, are associated with an increased frequency of HLA-DW3.

Gluten Enteropathy and Chronic Active Hepatitis. The highest known disease association with the HLA system occurs in gluten enteropathy, in which 98 per cent of patients have HLA-DW3 antigen.

An association between HLA-B8 and DW3 and chronic active hepatitis has been reported, and is particularly correlated with the presence of the hepatitis associated antigen (HAA); as many as 80 per cent of the HAA positive individuals possess the B8 antigen. Recent evidence, from renal dialysis units, suggests that HLA-B8 is associated with rapid elimination of the hepatitis virus,

even though the risk of developing chronic disease is enhanced.

Mechanisms of Disease Associations. Almost all the associations of the HLA locus relate to susceptibility to disease rather than resistance. Although well over 90 per cent of patients with ankylosing spondylitis are B27 positive, no more than 20 per cent of B27 positive individuals develop the disease. Several mechanisms have been proposed to explain the association between HLA specificity and susceptibility to disease.

The immune response gene hypothesis is based on the reasonable assumption that the immune response genes (Ir gene) will map within the HLA locus in man close to the D locus, as it does in the mouse. Ir genes are dominant, as is disease susceptibility, and might cause an effect by the formation of antigen-antibody complexes or by influencing cell-mediated immunity. An alternative hypothesis suggests that the HLA gene product interacts directly with the pathogen. Certain allelic products would fail to interact with the HLA receptor on the surface of the cell, and cell-based immunity toward the virus would be affected. A third mechanism suggests that if the HLA product is molecularly similar to that of the pathogen, tolerance will obtain and the host will be unable to mount an immunologic defense.

LINKAGE DISEQUILIBRIUM. The frequency of the HLA-A1 antigen in European populations is about 0.31, and the frequency of the antigen HLA-B8, 0.21. Thus the expected frequency of individuals who possess the A1 and B8 antigens would be $(0.31 \times 0.21) = 0.065$. The observed frequency of A1+ B8+ individuals is approximately 0.17 — three times higher than expected if there were no association. The frequency of the A1 allele is 0.17 and that of B8 is 0.11. Thus the expected haplotype (a shorthand word for "haplogenotype") frequency A1, B8, if there were no association, would be $(0.17 \times 0.11) = 0.019$. In fact, the observed frequency of the A1, B8 haplotype is 0.088 — four times the expected frequency. The difference between the observed and expected frequencies is called the linkage disequilibrium $(0.088 - 0.019) = 0.069$. Thus the association between traits and linked genes, such as A1 and B, depends on the disequilibrium. Linkage disequilibrium is common among alleles on the HLA locus and accounts for the disease associations; the biologic reasons remain obscure. An interesting reason for the existence of linkage disequilibrium has been postulated. Strong selection for certain alleles at the HLA locus could have arisen in the past if catastrophic epidemic infectious disease favored the survival of individuals of a specific HLA type. Thus the HLA linkage disequilibrium we see today may represent an important relic of our evolutionary past.

Fraser, F. C., and Nora, J. J.: Genetics of Man. Philadelphia, Lea & Febiger, 1975.

McKusick, V. A.: Human Genetics. 2nd ed. Englewood Cliffs, N. J., Prentice-Hall, 1969.

Nora, J. J., and Fraser, F. C.: Medical Genetics: Principles and Practice. Philadelphia, Lea & Febiger, 1974.

Stern, C.: Principles of Human Genetics. 3rd ed. San Francisco, W. H. Freeman, 1973.

13.   INBORN ERRORS OF METABOLISM AND MOLECULAR DISEASE

Alexander G. Bearn

Development of the concept of an inborn error of metabolism by Archibald Garrod in the first decade of this century was one of the most brilliant insights in the history of genetics, for it introduced the far-reaching hypothesis that the primary action of a gene is to control the synthesis of a specific enzyme. Subsequent work has fully substantiated Garrod's belief that the block in a metabolic pathway arises from an inherited deficiency of a specific enzyme. More recently the term inborn error of metabolism has been extended to include hereditary alterations in proteins that have no enzymatic functions.

The development of precise chemical methods that enable a comparison to be made between normal and genetically altered proteins led to the introduction of the term *molecular disease*, to emphasize that the difference between a normal and an affected individual might rest in the substitution of a single amino acid residue in the primary sequence of a protein molecule. Although the metabolic block may affect protein, carbohydrate, lipid, nucleic acid, porphyrin, or pigment metabolism, the *primary* defect invariably lies in the genetic specification of the synthesis of a protein.

In some inborn errors of metabolism the mutational event occurs at the active site of the enzyme. In these instances, although the enzyme will be functionally altered, the presence of cross-reacting material can be detected by immunologic methods. In other instances the mutation results in a protein which is functionally inert, and no cross-reacting material can be detected immunologically. Using the terminology of microbial genetics, the former class of mutants is frequently termed CRM (cross-reacting material) (+) and the latter CRM (−). At the pseudocholinesterase locus, for instance, 17 CRM (+) mutants and 18 CRM (−) mutants have been recognized. In the Lesch-Nyhan syndrome there is only one CRM (+) mutant; by contrast, 13 CRM (−) have been described. Even when there is no cross-reacting material detectable by immunologic methods, the protein, although no longer recognizable by antisera developed against the normal protein, may be present.

Some of the clinical conditions for which a demonstrated abnormality in a specific protein has been observed are listed in Table 2. In most of these a deficiency in a specific enzymatic activity is demonstrable, whereas in others a normal quantity of a structurally abnormal nonenzymic protein is synthesized. The classic example of a "molecular disease" affecting a nonen-

zyme is sickle cell anemia, in which the only difference between normal and sickle cell hemoglobin is the substitution of a valine for a glutamic acid in the β chain of hemoglobin.

It is increasingly being recognized that many of the inborn variations in metabolism are unassociated with clinical disease (Table 3). These biochemical variations represent the more conspicuous examples of the importance of human biochemical diversity. In some instances they provide a critical genetic background for the expression of an environmentally controlled disorder; in others the physiologic effect of the genetic variation is not apparent.

GENETIC HETEROGENEITY. It is becoming increasingly evident that identical or closely similar clinical syndromes may be determined by different mutant genes. In some instances, the mutations may be at different loci (nonallelic genes) (Table 4), whereas in others they occur at the same locus (allelic genes). In an individual cistron, genes may be allelic at the same codon (eualleles) or at a different codon (heteroalleles). In hemoglobins S and C the mutations occur at the same codon and are thus examples of eualleles. Hurler's and Scheie's syndromes are examples of heteroalleles, for in these instances the mutations occur at different codons but in the same cistron (see Ch. 538.1).

Even before the syndromes of recessive albinism yielded to biochemical probes, it was evident that the two clinical syndromes must be caused by genes at different loci, because it was well known that two albinos may marry and produce normally pigmented offspring. Indeed, it is a safe generalization to assume that the majority of inherited diseases presently regarded as homogeneous entities represent the clinical effects of different mutant genes.

Genetic heterogeneity can be detected at several different levels of biologic organization. Although Hurler's and Hunter's syndromes appear clinically similar, genetic heterogeneity is evident, because family studies indicate that Hurler's syndrome is controlled by a gene on an autosome, whereas in Hunter's syndrome the disease is X-linked. Similar variations exist among the spastic paraplegias: some pedigrees indicate autosomal inheritance, whereas others are clearly X-linked. Genetic heterogeneity can be demonstrated in recessive deaf mutism. Moreover, nonallelism can be definitely inferred, because marriage between deaf mutes, as with marriage between albinos, can result in normal offspring. Sometimes genetic heterogeneity can be strongly suspected from the clinical spectrum of a disease, as is the case in the various inherited mucopolysaccharidoses. When the syndromes associated with nonspherocytic anemias are examined biochemically, it is also evident that a number of different genes are involved. Heterogeneity among the X-linked hemophilias is strongly suggested as a result of functional and immunologic studies of factor VIII in different families. Heterogeneity is also evident in families exhibiting C'3 esterase deficiency. In some instances "genetic compounds" result in additional phenotypic variation. These genetic compounds arise when the individual carries two different mutant alleles. Hemoglobins S and C are controlled by euallelic genes, and individuals who have hemoglobin SC disease can thus be said to illustrate the phenotypic consequences of a genetic compound (euallelic homozygotes).

TABLE 2. Selected Inborn Errors of Metabolism

Disorder	Primary Defect	Carrier Detection	Prenatal Diagnosis
Amino acid metabolism:			
Phenylketonuria	Phenylalanine hydroxylase	+	
Albinism I	Tyrosinase		
II	?		
Tyrosinemia	p-Hydroxyphenylpyruvate oxidase (?)		
Tyrosinosis	Tyrosine transaminase		
Homocystinuria	Cystathionine synthetase	+	(+)
(a) Pyridoxine responsive			
(b) Pyridoxine unresponsive			
Cystathioninuria	γ-Cystathionase	+	(+)
Alcaptonuria	Homogentisic acid oxidase		
Maple syrup urine disease	Oxidative decarboxylase of branched chain ketoacids	+	+
Intermittent branched-chain ketoaciduria	Oxidative decarboxylase of branched chain ketoacids		(+)
Hypervalinemia	Valine transaminase		
Isovaleric acidemia	Isovaleryl-CoA-dehydrogenase		(+)
Beta-hydroxyisovaleric aciduria	Beta-methylcrotonyl-CoA-carboxylase	+	
Methylmalonic aciduria			+
(a) Vitamin B_{12} responsive	Deoxyadenosyl transferase		(+)
(b) Vitamin B_{12} unresponsive	Methylmalonyl-CoA-mutase		(+)
Hyperammonemia I	Carbamyl phosphate synthetase		
II	Ornithine transcarbamylase	+	
Citrullinemia	Argininosuccinic acid synthetase	+	(+)
Argininosuccinicaciduria	Argininosuccinase	+	(+)
Hyperargininemia	Arginase	+	
Hyperlysinemia	Lysine-ketoglutarate reductase		
Saccharopinuria	Aminoadipic semialdehyde–glutamate reductase		
Histidinemia	Histidase		
Hyperprolinemia I	Proline oxidase	+	
II	Δ'-pyrroline-5-carboxylate dehydrogenase	+	
Hydroxyprolinemia	Hydroxyproline oxidase (?)		
Ketotic hyperglycinemia	Propionyl-CoA-carboxylase	+	+
Nonketotic hyperglycinemia	Glycine decarboxylase (?)		
Hyper-beta-alaninemia	Beta-alanine-alpha-ketoglutarate amino transferase		
Carnosinemia	Carnosinase	+	
Hypersarcosinemia	Sarcosine dehydrogenase	+	
Cystinosis	?	+	+
Hartnup disease	Tubular reabsorption of monoamino-monocarboxylic acids		+
Cystinuria (three types)	Transepithelial transport of cystine and dibasic amino acids	+	
Iminoglycinuria	Transport of imino acids and glycine	+	
α-Methyl-β-hydroxybutyric acidemia	?	+	(+)
Hyperdibasic aminoaciduria	?	+	
Carbohydrate metabolism:			
Pentosuria	Xylitol dehydrogenase	+	
Fructosuria	Liver fructokinase		
Fructose intolerance	Fructose-1-phosphate aldolase		
Fructose-1,6-diphosphatase deficiency	Fructose-1,6-diphosphatase	+	
Glycogenosis I	Glucose-6-phosphatase	+	
II	Alpha-1,4-glucosidase	+	+
III	Amylo-1,6-glucosidase	+	(+)
IV	Amylo(1-4 to 1-6)-transglucosidase		(+)
V	Muscle phosphorylase		
VI	Liver phosphorylase		
VII	Muscle phosphofructokinase		
VIII	Liver phosphorylasekinase	+	
Galactosemia	Galactose-1-phosphate uridyl transferase	+	+
Galactokinase deficiency	Galactokinase	+	
Hyperoxaluria I	Alpha-ketoglutarate:glyoxalate carboligase		
II	D-Glyceric dehydrogenase		
Renal glycosuria	?		
Pyruvate decarboxylase deficiency	Pyruvate decarboxylase	+	(+)
Lactase deficiency	Lactase		
Sucrase-isomaltase deficiency	Sucrase, isomaltase		
Glucose-galactose malabsorption	?	+	
Hurler's syndrome	Alpha-L-iduronidase	+	+
Hunter's syndrome	Sulfoiduronate sulfatase	+	+
Sanfilippo's syndrome A	Heparan sulfate sulfatase	+	+
B	N-acetyl-alpha-glucosaminidase	+	(+)
Morquio's syndrome	N-acetylhexosamine-6-sulfate sulfatase	+	(+)
Scheie's syndrome	Alpha-L-iduronidase		
Maroteaux-Lamy syndrome	N-acetyl galactosamine-4-sulfatase	+	+
β-Glucuronidase deficiency	β-Glucuronidase	+	+
I-cell disease	?	+	+
Mannosidosis	Alpha-mannosidase		(+)
Fucosidosis	Alpha-1-fucosidase	+	(+)
Gaucher's disease (three types)	Glucocerebrosidase	+	+
Globoid cell leukodystrophy	Galactocerebroside beta-galactosidase	+	+
Pyruvate carboxylase deficiency	Pyruvate carboxylase		

Table continues on following page

TABLE 2.   Selected Inborn Errors of Metabolism (Continued)

Disorder	Primary Defect	Carrier Detection	Prenatal Diagnosis
Lipid metabolism:			
Lipoprotein lipase deficiency	Low density lipoprotein receptor	+	+
Hypercholesterolemia	?		
Hypertriglyceridemia	?		
Combined hyperlipidemia	?		
Abetalipoproteinemia	Betalipoproteins		
Hypobetalipoproteinemia	Low density lipoproteins	(+)	
Tangier disease	?	+	
Norum disease	Lecithin:cholesterol acetyl transferase		
Gangliosidosis GM$_1$ (types I and II)	Beta galactosidase	+	+
Gangliosidosis GM$_2$ (Tay-Sachs)	Hexosaminidase A	+	+
Gangliosidosis GM$_2$ (Sandhoff)	Hexosaminidase A and B	+	+
Gangliosidosis GM$_2$ (juvenile, Type 3)	Hexosaminidase A	+	+
GM$_6$ (hematoside) sphingolipodystrophy	?		(+)
Fabry's disease	α-Galactosidase A	+	+
Metachromatic leukodystrophy I	Arylsulfatase A	+	+
II	Arylsulfatase A, B, C, and steroid sulfatase	+	
Lactosylceramidosis	Lactosylceramidase		
Niemann-Pick disease	Sphingomyelinase	+	+
Wolman's disease	Acid lipase	+	(+)
Cholesterylester storage disease	Acid lipase	+	(+)
Cerebrotendinous xanthomatosis	?		
Refsum's disease	Phytanic acid alpha hydroxylase	+	(+)
Ceramide lactoside lipidosis	?		(+)
Nucleic acid metabolism:			
Gout	?		
Lesch-Nyhan syndrome	Hypoxanthine-guanine phosphoribosyl transferase	+	+
Xanthinuria	Xanthine oxidase		
Xanthurenic aciduria	Kynureninase		
Orotic aciduria I	Orotidylic pyrophosphorylase and decarboxylase	+	(+)
II	Orotidylic decarboxylase		
Xeroderma pigmentosum	UV-specific endonuclease		
Porphyrin and heme metabolism:			
Erythropoietic porphyria	Uroporphyrinogen-III cosynthetase and uroporphyrinogen-I synthetase	+	(+)
Acute intermittent porphyria	Uroporphyrinogen-I synthetase	+	+
Porphyria variegata	?		
Coproporphyria	Coproporphyrin oxidase	+	
Porphyria cutanea tarda	Uroporphyrinogen decarboxylase	+	
Protoporphyria	Ferrochelatase	+	
Crigler-Najjar syndrome (two types)	Glucuronyltransferase		
Gilbert's syndrome	Bilirubin uptake		
Dubin-Johnson syndrome	Bilirubin excretion		
Erythrocyte metabolism:			
Hemolytic anemia	Pyruvate kinase	+	
	Hexokinase	+	
	Glucosephosphate isomerase	+	
	Triosephosphate isomerase	+	
	2,3-Diphosphoglyceromutase	+	
	Phosphoglycerate kinase	+	
	Glucose-6-phosphate dehydrogenase	+	(+)
	6-Phosphogluconate dehydrogenase		
	Glutathione reductase		
	Glutathione peroxidase		
	Glutathione synthetase		
Methemoglobinemia	NADH-methemoglobin reductase	+	

Table continues on opposite page.

TABLE 2. Selected Inborn Errors of Metabolism *(Continued)*

Disorder	Primary Defect	Carrier Detection	Prenatal Diagnosis
Leukocyte metabolism:			
Myeloperoxidase deficiency	Myeloperoxidase	+	
Chronic granulomatous disease	?	+	
Chédiak-Higashi syndrome	?	+	
Abnormalities of plasma proteins:			
Analbuminemia	Albumin		
Atransferrinemia	Transferrin		
Afibrinogenemia	Fibrinogen		
Alpha₁-antitrypsin deficiency	Alpha₁-antitrypsin	+	
Acatalasemia	Catalase	+	(+)
Suxamethonium sensitivity	Pseudocholinesterase		
Hereditary angioedema	C1-inhibitor		
C1q deficiency	C1q		
C1r deficiency	C1r		
C2 deficiency	C2		
C3 deficiency	C3		
X-linked agammaglobulinemia	?		
Severe combined immunodeficiency	Adenosine deaminase (?)	+	+
Selective IgA deficiency	?		
X-linked immunodeficiency with increased IgM	?		
Hemophilia A	Factor VIII	+	
Hemophilia B	Factor IX	+	
von Willebrand's disease	?	+	
Hageman trait	Factor XII	+	
PTA deficiency	Factor XI	+	
Parahemophilia	Factor V	+	
Hypoprothrombinemia	Factor II	+	
Factor VII deficiency	Factor VII	+	
Factor X deficiency	Factor X	+	
Fibrin-stabilizing factor deficiency	Factor XIII	+	
Hormone and vitamin metabolism:			
Adrenogenital syndrome	21-Hydroxylase		+
	11-Hydroxylase		
	3-Beta-hydroxysteroiddehydrogenase		
	17-Hydroxylase		
	Desmolase		
Aldosterone deficiency	18-Hydroxylase		
Familial goiter	Iodide transport		
	Peroxidase		
	Iodotyrosine coupling		
	Iodotyrosine deiodinase		
	Thyroglobulin synthesis		
Renal diabetes insipidus	?	+	
Vitamin D dependent rickets	25-Hydroxycholecalciferol-1-hydroxylase		
Formiminotransferase deficiency	Formiminotransferase		
Miscellaneous:			
Cystic fibrosis	?		
Wilson's disease	?	+	
Hemochromatosis	?		
Menkes' kinky hair syndrome	Intestinal copper absorption		
Sulfite oxidase deficiency	Sulfite oxidase		
Hypophosphatasia	Alkaline phosphatase (?)	+	
Lysosomal acid phosphatase deficiency	Acid phosphatase	+	+
Renal tubular acidosis I	Gradient defect		
II	Bicarbonate wastage		
Aspartylglucosaminuria	N-aspartyl-β-glucosaminidase	+	+

(+) = Prenatal diagnosis is likely to be possible, because the enzyme defect can be detected in cell culture.

TABLE 3. A Selection of Common Inherited Polymorphisms

Blood groups, e.g., ABO, MNS, Rh
Leukocyte groups
Platelet groups
Histocompatibility antigens (HLA)
Hemoglobin (α, β, γ, δ chains)
Myoglobin
Serum proteins:
  Albumin
  Alpha$_1$-antitrypsin
  Group-specific component (Gc)
  Haptoglobin (α, β chains)
  Ceruloplasmin
  Alpha$_2$-macroglobulin (Xm)
  Complement (C3, C4)
  Beta-lipoprotein (Ag-, Ld-, Lp-types)
  Transferrin
  Fibrinogen
  Immunoglobulins (Am, Gm, InV)
Enzymes:
  Glucose-6-phosphate dehydrogenase
  Phosphoglucomutase (PGM 1, 2, 3)
  Phosphohexoseisomerase
  Lactate dehydrogenase
  Adenine phosphoribosyl transferase
  Hypoxanthine-guanine phosphoribosyl transferase
  Peptidases (A, B, C, D, E)
  Pseudocholinesterase (E1, E2)
  Amylase
Phenylthiocarbamide testing
Beta-aminoisobutyric aciduria
Color blindness

Now that it is firmly established that genes control the specificity of particular proteins, genetic heterogeneity can also be detected by immunologic and biochemical techniques that discriminate between closely similar protein molecules. The application of these techniques to serum protein and red cell enzymes has disclosed a surprising degree of heterogeneity in normal persons. However, any estimate of genetic heterogeneity based on the application of electrophoretic techniques will be too low, because it seems that less than half the mutational events leading to a specific amino acid substitution will result in an altered net charge of the protein.

SCREENING FOR INBORN ERRORS OF METABOLISM. The central purpose of any screening program is the detection of individuals in whom it is likely that a specific hereditary disease will develop and against which preventive or therapeutic measures are potentially available. It is important to emphasize this latter point, because screening large populations for a disease such as Duchenne muscular dystrophy, for which there is presently no treatment, is neither useful nor humane. Screening for genetic diseases can be performed at three principal phenotypic levels. In many instances the recognition of overt clinical disease represents the only phenotypic level at which the inborn error can be recognized. Thus in Huntington's chorea no biochemical abnormality has been found to be characteristic of the

TABLE 4. Some Illustrative Examples of Genetic Diseases Showing Nonallelic Heterogeneity

Albinism
Deafness
Diabetes insipidus, neurohypophyseal type
Osteogenesis imperfecta
Pituitary dwarfism
Retinitis pigmentosa
Sanfilippo's syndrome A and B

disease, and early recognition of signs and symptoms represents the only sure means to arrive at a diagnosis. Early diagnosis of polyposis of the colon is important because of the frequency of malignant transformation. The recognition of genital abnormalities at birth in females may aid in early detection of the adrenogenital syndrome. Inborn errors can also be recognized by the presence of an abnormal metabolite in physiologic fluids. The enzymatic deficiency may lead to accumulation of the substrate for the reaction catalyzed by the normal enzyme and to a deficiency of the product. An increased level of blood galactose in galactosemia and of phenylalanine in phenylketonuria are examples in which the disturbance of the normal metabolic relationships leads to detection of disease.

Since genes control the synthesis of proteins, the most direct way of identifying an inborn error is to utilize a screening program which detects a qualitative change in the structure of the protein, e.g., electrophoretically, or by its altered enzymatic or immunologic activity. Mass screening for rare inborn errors of metabolism in the general population is expensive and time consuming, and a careful estimate of the cost of such a program must be balanced against the potential gains. For most countries the cost of extensive screening programs for genetically determined disease is prohibitive. For the moment it seems wiser to focus, with the exception of phenylketonuria, on families and populations who are particularly at risk and for whom effective therapy for the inborn errors of metabolism is available. More than 90 per cent of babies born in the United States are tested for phenylketonuria. Although the incidence of false negative tests (5 to 10 per cent) can be minimized by performing a second test after the third day of life, the practical problem of guaranteeing a second screening is insurmountable. Despite these and other difficulties, such as the devastating effect of maternal phenylketonuria on the fetus, the PKU testing program has been effective in preventing one form of mental retardation. Screening for Tay-Sachs disease among Ashkenazic Jews and sickle cell hemoglobin among black populations are examples of screening programs which, when carefully carried out, can be of undoubted benefit. Amniocentesis and the use of cultured fibroblasts to identify certain inborn errors of metabolism before birth can be expected to increase sharply in the years ahead and will increase the usefulness of screening programs.

Harris, H.: The Principles of Human Biochemical Genetics. *In* Neuberger, A., and Tatum, E. L. (eds.): Frontiers of Biology. Vol. 19. New York, American Elsevier Publishing Company, 1970.
McKusick, V. A.: Mendelian Inheritance in Man: Catalogs of Autosomal Dominant, Autosomal Recessive, and X-linked Phenotypes. 4th ed. Baltimore, The Johns Hopkins Press, 1975.

14. POLYGENIC AND MULTIFACTORIAL INHERITANCE

Alexander G. Bearn

Traits determined by the collaboration of many genes at different loci are called polygenic, in contrast to those traits which are determined by a single gene (monogenic). Most of the differences among normal people are determined by the interaction of many ge-

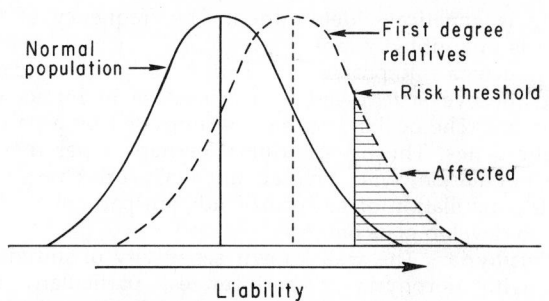

Figure 8. Diseases which conform to a polygenic multifactorial model of inheritance lead to an increased incidence of disease among the relatives of affected individuals. This increased incidence is most evident among first degree relatives.

netic and environmental factors (multifactorial inheritance).

Polygenic inheritance, in which many genes each contribute a minor effect, is best established for those traits which show continuous variation in the form of a "normal" distribution curve. Height is an example of a polygenic (and multifactorial) trait in which the extremes of the normal distribution are not considered abnormal. The degree of resemblance among relatives can be deduced from the number of genes they have in common. Dizygotic twins, however, will have 50 per cent of their genes in common, as will all sibs. Parents and children also have 50 per cent of their genes in common. Thus it would be expected that if one parent is 72 inches tall and the other 66 inches tall, all the children, on the average, would be 69 inches tall. For a variety of reasons (dominance, environment, and epistasis), the offspring are usually closer to the population average than to the average of their parents. Polygenic models have been advanced for inheritance of high blood pressure, diabetes mellitus, and rheumatoid arthritis, as well as a variety of congenital defects.

In clinical medicine polygenic and multifactorial inheritance should be suspected when the disease under consideration is "known to run in families," and when, in addition, examination of the affected and unaffected sibs in any sibship does not support inheritance in a simple dominant or recessive fashion. When this occurs, it is reasonable to suspect that within such families a large number of "risk genes" are present. "Risk genes" are of course present in the normal population, but in low frequency. If in any one individual there is a particularly large number of high "risk genes," the latent disorder becomes overt. This phenomenon is known as the "threshold effect" (Fig. 8). When examining a pedigree for a possible polygenic inheritance pattern, it is worth remembering that (1) the frequency of affected individuals is very roughly the square root of the frequency in the population, and (2) the frequency of the disease in first degree relatives will fall off in a nonlinear fashion as the relationship to the affected individual decreases; thus the frequency of cleft lip is 40 per 1000 for first degree relatives, 7 for second degree relatives, and 3 for third degree relatives. This latter fact is particularly important in genetic counseling. Thus, in distinction to monogenic traits, in which the recurrence risk in a sibship is one fourth or one half, the recurrence risk in sibs of those affected with threshold traits depends on the incidence of the trait. The elegance and complexity of the mathematical models advanced for

polygenic-multifactorial disease should not obscure the fact that each of the "risk genes" has, like any other gene, a specific biochemical consequence. Eventually, the vague concept of genetic susceptibility of polygenic inheritance must yield to the central dogma that genes control the synthesis of specific proteins each of which has a specific function.

Carter, C. O.: Genetics of common disorders. Br. Med. Bull., 25:52, 1969.

15. PHARMACOGENETICS
Alexander G. Bearn

It has long been recognized that certain people respond unusually to the administration of specific drugs. In some instances the altered reaction has an immunologic basis; in others it appears to be idiosyncratic without obvious cause; and in some the difference appears to be contingent on the genetic constitution of the host. Pharmacogenetics is concerned with those deviant responses to specific drugs that are genetically determined. The breakdown and disposal of drugs in the body are usually dependent on a series of specific gene-controlled enzymatic reactions. Mutant genes in the population that alter these reactions can result in serious clinical consequences.

INHERITED DISEASES DISCOVERED OR PRECIPITATED BY THE USE OF DRUGS. Several diseases have been disclosed or precipitated as a direct result of the administration of drugs which for their proper metabolic disposal require an intact enzyme system. In the absence of pharmacologic overload, the defective enzyme system is not stressed enough to cause clinical manifestations.

Glucose-6-Phosphate Dehydrogenase Deficiency. A severe hemolytic anemia (favism) may be produced by the ingestion of the broad bean *Vicia fava*. The anemia is due to deficiency of the X-linked enzyme glucose-6-phosphate dehydrogenase in the erythrocytes of susceptible subjects (see Glucose-6-Phosphate Dehydrogenase in Ch. 483.3). A deficiency of the enzyme is a necessary but not sufficient cause for the anemia that follows ingestion of fava beans. Additional genetic factors, presently poorly identified, are also required if the disease is to be manifest. Severe neonatal jaundice in the Mediterranean basin and Far East may occasionally be associated with glucose-6-phosphate dehydrogenase deficiency.

Persons with glucose-6-phosphate dehydrogenase deficiency are particularly susceptible to hemolytic reactions after administration of the antimalarial drug primaquine and certain other drugs, including aspirin and phenacetin. A severe hemolytic anemia may also occur during the course of acute viral hepatitis and infectious mononucleosis in individuals with deficiency of glucose-6-phosphate dehydrogenase. The mutation in the black population is characterized by a mean enzyme activity of 10 to 20 per cent of normal, and the increased susceptibility to hemolysis is restricted to the older red cells. The risk of hemolysis is significantly less than in the Mediterranean type of glucose-6-phosphate dehydrogenase deficiency in which the residual enzymatic activity is less than 5 per cent of normal and increased susceptibility to hemolysis occurs in young as well as old cells. The trait is present in about 10 per cent of blacks in the United States and may reach as high as 35 per cent in certain African and Mediterranean populations. The deficiency provides some protection against falciparum malaria and accounts for the persistence of the gene at a very high level in these populations. The relationship of glucose-6-phosphate dehydrogenase deficiency and resistance to falciparum malaria affords one of the better examples of a balanced polymorphism in which a heterozygous advantage can be clearly demonstrated.

Isoniazid. When a group of individuals is given a standard dose of the antituberculosis drug isoniazid (INH), two subpopulations can be identified. In one group the blood level of isoniazid is high and very little acetylated INH is excreted in the urine (slow inactivators), whereas in the second group the blood isoniazid is considerably lower and acetylated INH appears in the urine in large quantities (rapid inactivators). Twin studies show a similar metabolic response in monozygotic twins, whereas notable differences are apparent in dizygotic twins. Pedigree analysis indicates that the capacity to acetylate isoniazid is inherited as a simple recessive trait. The "slow inactivators" lack the liver enzyme N-acetyltransferase present in "rapid inactivators." Although it is clinically reassuring that rapid acetylators show an impairment of the antituberculosis effect of the drug, slow acetylators are more likely to encounter undesirable side effects such as peripheral neuropathy, a mischance which can be avoided if pyridoxine is administered concomitantly. It is of some clinical importance that the absence of the acetylating enzyme also makes more likely the toxic effects of the antiepileptic drug phenelzine and the antihypertensive agent hydralazine, because both these agents are acetylated by N-acetyltransferase.

The gene determining N-acetyltransferase deficiency occurs in 60 per cent of the black and white populations, but in only 10 per cent of Eskimo and Japanese populations. This polymorphism is of particular interest, because the aberrant gene has no recognizable clinical effect unless drugs which require acetylation for their metabolism are administered.

Suxamethonium (Succinylcholine). Suxamethonium is a commonly employed short-acting muscle relaxant. Its short action is due to the rapidly inactivating influence of the serum enzyme cholinesterase. Genetic variants of the enzyme are known which fail to hydrolyze suxamethonium and as a consequence cause a prolonged, but fortunately rarely fatal, apnea. This increased sensitivity to suxamethonium occurs in about 1 in 3000 patients and can be caused by a large number of different alleles at the pseudocholinesterase locus.

Hemoglobin Zürich and Other Drug-Sensitive Hemoglobins. The red cells from patients with the unstable hemoglobins (Zürich, Shepherd's Bush, and Torino) exhibit an unusual tendency to hemolysis when exposed to certain drugs. The sulfonamides are particular offenders, but all drugs which cause hemolysis in patients with glucose-6-phosphate deficiency may be potentially harmful.

Anticoagulant Resistance. Two families have been reported in which some members are extremely resistant to warfarin and other coumarin congeners. Approximately ten times the usual dose of warfarin was needed to increase the prothrombin time to an expected level. This provides an example in which resistance to a drug is genetically determined. The frequency of the trait is undoubtedly rare.

Glaucoma. Repeated instillation of glucocorticoids into the eye is followed by an increase in intraocular pressure. The ocular response is controlled by a pair of allelic genes. Those individuals, perhaps 5 per cent of the population, who have an unusually brisk response to the instillation of glucocorticoids are particularly liable to develop glaucoma.

Porphyria. The well known sensitivity of individuals with porphyria to barbiturates, particularly the short-acting compound thiopental (thiopentone), is a classic example of a genetically determined altered response to a drug.

Malignant Hyperthermia. This is an autosomal dominantly inherited condition causing a frequently fatal hyperthermia associated with muscle rigidity that may follow the administration of anesthetic agents such as halothane, succinylcholine, or methoxyflurane. It is particularly important to inform affected individuals that half of their first-degree relatives are at a similar risk. This condition occurs in 1 out of 20,000 anesthetized patients.

Vesell, E. S.: Advances in pharmacogenetics. *In* Steinberg, A. G., and Bearn, A. G. (eds.): Progress in Medical Genetics. Vol. 9. New York, Grune & Stratton, 1973, p. 291.

16. POPULATION GENETICS

Alexander G. Bearn

GENE FREQUENCY. Although genes are expressed in individuals, it is often of interest to consider the distribution of mutant genes in the general population. The basis of population genetics is the Hardy-Weinberg law, which was formulated in a context of concern that a dominant trait would eventually displace a normal trait in the population. In particular, it arose in response to the startling assertion that because brachydactyly is a dominant trait, then "in the course of time, one would expect in the absence of counteracting factors to get three brachydactylous persons to one normal." This is quite fallacious, as the following argument will show.

If the frequency of a particular gene A is p, then its alternate allele is $(1-p)=q$; the population will consist of individuals of three genotypes: those who are homozygous AA, those who are heterozygous Aa, and those who are homozygous aa. The frequency of these genotypes in a randomly mating population will be in the proportion p^2 (AA), $2pq$ (Aa), and q^2 (aa). One important consequence of this formulation is that whatever the initial frequency of the genes A and a in the population, the proportion of the three genotypes will tend to remain constant during succeeding generations, providing that the three genotypes are equally fertile. If the mating in the population is not random or if there is unequal viability of three genotypes, the frequency calculations require considerable adjustment, and in small populations substantial changes in gene frequency may occur simply as a matter of chance.

The Hardy-Weinberg law has a very useful practical consequence. If the frequency of a recessive disease in a particular population is known, the frequency of heterozygous carriers as well as the frequency of the abnormal gene can be calculated. Thus for a recessively inherited disease aa (q^2) with a frequency of 1 per 10,000, the frequency of the gene a (q) will be the square root of 1/10,000 or 1/100. The frequency of heterozygous carriers will be $2 \times p \times q = 2 \times 99/100 \times 1/100$ or approximately 1/50. Thus for this particular inherited disease there will be 200 clinically unaffected carriers of the abnormal gene in the population for every affected individual. Cystic fibrosis of the pancreas, the most frequent recessively inherited disease in the white population, has a frequency of approximately 1 in 2500 (q^2); thus the frequency of heterozygous carriers is approximately 1 in 25 (2pq).

MUTATION AND SELECTION. A mutation is a stable heritable change in the genetic material. This change may affect a single locus, or it may consist of chromosome breakage with loss or rearrangement of the fragments. In molecular terms a point mutation can be regarded as an alteration, addition, or deletion of one of the bases of the DNA molecule. The simplest mutational event is the substitution of one nucleotide for another in the DNA sequence. Although this usually results in the substitution of one amino acid for another in the polypeptide chain (e.g., glutamic acid at position 6 of the beta polypeptide chain is replaced by valine in hemoglobin S), it is not invariable, because several different triplets can code for the same amino acid. Mutations which either insert or delete nucleotide into the genetic code usually cause more extensive substitutions in the polypeptide synthesis than single nucleotide substitutions. It will be recalled that the genetic code is read as successive triplets; an insertion or deletion will upset the regularity of the triplets, and the translation of the code into amino acids distal to the point of insertion or deletion will be altered. From what is known about the genetic code, about 75 per cent of mutations will result in a single base change, resulting in the substitution of one amino acid for another; about 20 per cent of the mutations will be synonymous, in which the base change in the codon does not change the amino acid specified; and in about 5 per cent the base triplet change will result in a nonsense triplet, leading to a chain termination and the synthesis of a polypeptide lacking a variable portion of its carboxyl terminal amino acid sequence. The effect of a mutation in a somatic cell is restricted to the life of an individual, whereas mutation in the germ line can be transmitted to future generations. The natural mutation rate can be greatly increased by x-rays, ultraviolet rays, increased temperature, and various chemical mutagens such as nitrogen mustard, ethylene sulfonate, and 5-bromouracil. Chemical mutagens are thought to achieve their effects by direct structural modification of a purine or pyrimidine base, by substitution of a base analogue for one of the normal bases, or by a frame-shift mutation.

The average spontaneous mutation rate is usually expressed as the number of mutations per locus per generation. The average spontaneous mutation rate for a number of autosomal, recessive, and X-linked traits is 3×10^{-5}. One common, often unavoidable, error in estimating mutation rates in man is the failure to recognize that indistinguishable clinical syndromes can be caused by different genes (see Genetic Heterogeneity in Ch. 13). Thus the frequencies deduced by the elegant studies of Haldane on mutation rate for hemophilia must be revised downward, because Christmas disease,

another bleeding disorder determined by a gene on the X chromosome, had not been discovered when the original calculations were made. Since heterogeneity appears to be the rule in inherited disease, all estimates of mutation rate are likely to be high. Nonhereditary conditions which mimic mutations are termed phenocopies and will also lead to overestimation of mutation rates. Spontaneous mutation rates tend to increase with advancing age. The occurrence of new mutations for chondrodystrophy is almost linearly related to paternal age. It is approximately three times more likely for a chondrodystrophic child to be born of unaffected parents if the father is 45 years of age or older than if he is 25 years old.

The frequency of most genes in the population is relatively stable. When a gene is rare and severely disadvantageous, the mutation rate is balanced by the elimination of the disadvantageous gene by natural selection. The frequency of a dominant lethal disease is twice the mutation rate; algebraically, the frequency of a dominant trait is twice the mutation rate divided by the selective disadvantage, S (S being one for a lethal). The frequency of the disadvantageous gene, however, can be stabilized at a high level if the heterozygotes are slightly favored and leave a greater number of progeny than either homozygote. The concept of *balanced polymorphism* has been defined as the existence of two or more discontinuous forms of a species in such proportion that the rarest of them cannot be maintained at its frequency in the population by recurrent mutation. As a general proposition, if the rarer of the two allelic forms occurs in a frequency that is greater than 1 per cent, the existence of balanced polymorphism should be entertained. An example of such a balanced polymorphism is the increased resistance of individuals heterozygous for sickle cell trait to falciparum malaria. Although patients with sickle cell disease (homozygotes) usually die before they can reproduce and thus cannot transmit the gene to the next generation, the incidence of the sickle cell trait may reach 40 per cent in certain West African populations. Theoretically, the high frequency of the sickle cell gene could be maintained if the heterozygote were 25 per cent more fit than the so-called normal homozygote. It has now been shown unequivocally that death from falciparum malaria is much less frequent in carriers of the sickle cell trait than in noncarriers, and thus the heterozygote does have an advantage. How much of the advantage is due to differential mortality and how much to differential fertility is uncertain, but this example serves to emphasize that the effect of genes can be assessed only in relation to a particular environment. It is, however, being slowly appreciated that the example of balanced polymorphism provided by the advantage to individuals heterozygous for the sickle cell trait may be atypical. In most instances a distinct advantage for the heterozygote cannot be demonstrated, and the possibility that certain polymorphic traits are genetically neutral is becoming increasingly discussed.

The term *genetic load* has been used to describe the total genetic disability of a population. It is composed of the *mutational load*, the load caused by recurrent mutations from a normal to a lethal or sublethal gene, and the *segregational load*, which is due to the segregation of harmful genes from favorable heterozygotes. The sickle cell gene is maintained in the population because of its heterozygous advantage, and thus contributes to the segregational load. It has been estimated that, on the average, each person has three to six genes which, if homozygous instead of heterozygous, would be lethal. The relative contribution of the segregational and mutational loads to the total load is unsettled.

Fraser, F. C., and Nora, J. J.: Genetics of Man. Philadelphia, Lea & Febiger, 1975.
Stern, C.: Principles of Human Genetics. 3rd ed. San Francisco, W. H. Freeman and Company, 1973.

17. CONGENITAL MALFORMATIONS

Alexander G. Bearn

The term congenital malformation is usually applied to important structural defects present at birth that are not caused by a birth injury. The relative importance of congenital malformation has increased as more effective control has been exercised over the environmental agents of disease. In 1900, in the United States, approximately 3.3 per cent of the total infant mortality could be ascribed to congenital malformations, whereas in 1964 congenital malformations accounted for 25 per cent of the total infant mortality. Congenital malformations are responsible for approximately 15 per cent of all deaths up to the age of 15. It has also been estimated that 7 per cent of children have a congenital malformation of consequence recognizable by the age of one year, yet only 43 per cent of such malformations are detectable at birth. In most malformations no major etiologic factor can be identified, and it must be presumed that their existence depends on complicated interactions of genetic and environmental influences or on particular genetic combinations. The frequency of many congenital malformations is compatible with a polygenic model with a threshold beyond which there is a risk of malformation. First-degree relatives (sibs and children) of an individual with a congenital malformation are at greater risk than members of the general population. This is because first-degree relatives will have a curve of distribution of high risk genes approximately halfway between the general population and those affected. The first-degree relatives of a patient with cleft lip and cleft palate are approximately 40 times more likely to develop the malformation than the population at large. The approximate frequency and sex ratio of the major malformations are shown in Table 5.

GENETIC FACTORS. With the exception of mongolism (trisomy 21) and Turner's syndrome, relatively few congenital malformations can be ascribed to specific genes or numerical chromosomal abnormalities. Congenital hydrocephalus is occasionally inherited in an X-linked fashion. Congenital pyloric stenosis is five times more frequent in males, and harelip and cleft palate twice as common. Congenital dislocation of the hip and spina bifida are more frequent in females. Twin studies and pedigree patterns seldom provide any useful genetic information in the common malformations. The offspring of consanguineous marriages show a slight increase in the frequency of congenital malformations.

ENVIRONMENTAL FACTORS. Contrary to popular belief, there is little direct evidence that environmental factors such as viral diseases, maternal ingestion of drugs, or maternal irradiation make a significant contribution to the *common* malformations, although each

TABLE 5. Approximate Frequency and Sex Ratio of Common Congenital Malformations

Malformation	Frequency/1000 Births	M:F
Congenital heart disease	2.5	1:1
Pyloric stenosis	3.0 (0.5–4.0)	4:1
Talipes equinovarus	2.0	2:1
Myelomeningocele	1.5 (0.5–4.4)	1:1
Anencephaly	2.0	1:2
Down's syndrome (mongolism)	1.6	1:1
Hydrocephalus*	1.2	1:1†
Congenital dislocated hip	1.0	1:6
Cleft lip ± cleft palate	1.0	2:1
Klinefelter's syndrome	1.0	1:0

*Without spina bifida.
†Excluding X-linked recessive hydrocephalus.

of these factors materially increases the frequency of certain *specific* malformations. Recent evidence suggests that approximately 70 per cent of mothers exposed to rubella during the first trimester give birth to children with severe congenital defects, including cataracts, deafness, heart disease, and neonatal thrombocytopenic purpura.

Some evidence indicates that first-born children are more likely to have a congenital defect than later children. This is particularly true of anencephaly, congenital dislocation of the hip, talipes equinovarus, and pyloric stenosis. Striking regional differences in the incidence of congenital defects have been recognized, and have been well documented for anencephaly and spina bifida. An increased frequency of congenital dislocation of the hip in Lapps and certain American Indians is well recognized. An inexplicable but marked seasonal variation in the incidence of certain malformations has also been reported. It has been estimated that nearly one third of the pregnancies complicated by hydramnios result in congenital malformations.

The risk that a congenital malformation will recur with subsequent pregnancies depends on the specific abnormality and its cause. For the three most common neurologic malformations, anencephaly, hydrocephalus, and spina bifida, the recurrence rate in subsequent children is approximately 4 per cent after the first malformation, but much higher after two malformations. If it is recalled that the recurrence rate for a simple recessively inherited disease is 25 per cent, the role of genetic factors in congenital malformation can be put in perspective.

DRUG-INDUCED EMBRYOPATHY. Fetal malformations may be regarded as the consequence of developmental asynchrony, and are likely to follow environmental insults during the first three months of fetal life. There is growing evidence that errors in embryonic development are particularly likely to arise between the sixth and eighth weeks. It is therefore clearly prudent to minimize frivolous medication during the first three months of pregnancy. The importance of the drugs as possible etiologic agents in congenital malformations has been emphasized, and perhaps overemphasized, by the thalidomide tragedy. Indeed, it is virtually impossible to specify a drug that will *not* result in an increased frequency of congenital malformations when administered to a sufficiently large panel of different laboratory animals. To assume that a drug that causes a congenital malformation in one species will necessarily cause one in man is as misguided as to assume that if a drug is harmless in animals, it will be harmless in man. It is certainly worth emphasizing that had thalidomide merely increased the frequency of a common malformation, such as cleft lip or cleft palate, rather than the strikingly tragic malformation of phocomelia ("seal extremities"), the causal association might still be unrecognized. During the two- to three-year period during which thalidomide (alpha-phthalimidoglutarimide) was freely available, approximately 7000 infants throughout the world were born with thalidomide-induced deformities.

Although convincing evidence of teratogenicity can be claimed only for thalidomide, steroid hormones, and folate antagonists, suspicion has fallen on alcohol, anticonvulsants, which may act by causing folate deficiency, warfarin, and an operating room environment (generally assumed to be related to anesthetic gases). Lysergic acid diethylamide (LSD) is mischievously and dangerously toxic, but whether it causes congenital malformations remains unproved.

Warkany, J.: Congenital Malformations. Chicago, Year Book Medical Publishers, 1971.

18. CHROMOSOMES AND THEIR DISORDERS

Park Gerald

18.1. INTRODUCTION

Modern human cytogenetics began in 1956, when Tjio and Levan employed techniques that had been created for use with other organisms to demonstrate the presence of 46 chromosomes (23 pairs) in cultured human fibroblasts. The field became of major medical importance with the observation in 1959 that an additional chromosome was present in patients with Down's syndrome (mongolism). It was soon thereafter brought to clinical maturity when simple means were discovered for obtaining chromosome preparations with cultured leukocytes from peripheral blood.

Modern cytogenetics entered its second and present period of growth with the introduction of a fluorescent stain which permitted identification of each of the 22 pairs of non-sex chromosomes (autosomes) as well as the 2 sex chromosomes (XX in the female and XY in the male). Additional staining procedures have since been developed which provide further evidence for the uniqueness of each chromosome pair and even of individual regions within chromosomes.

FREQUENCY OF CHROMOSOMAL ABNORMALITIES. Chromosomal abnormalities occur with greatly different frequencies at various times in life. The highest frequency and the greatest variety are found among spontaneous abortuses, 30 to 40 per cent of whom have a major chromosomal defect. Among liveborn infants, about 6 per 1000 have a chromosomal defect sufficiently severe to cause disability at some time in their lives. About half of these abnormalities involve the autosomes, whereas the remainder are sex chromosomal disorders. Among adults in the general population, the abnormalities are largely confined to the sex chromosomal disorders.

There are clinically definable subgroups within these population segments that have an increased risk for a chromosomal disorder. Infants with multiple congenital defects, for example, have a 5 to 10 per cent probability of possessing a major autosomal abnormality. The occurrence in a family of individuals with a similar group of congenital malformations is often the result of an inheritable chromosomal disorder. Such families may also have an increased number of spontaneous abortions. Sex chromosomal disorders occur with increased frequency among infertile males and among women with primary amenorrhea. They are also found to be unusually frequent among males incarcerated in penal institutions.

PREPARATION OF CELLS FOR CHROMOSOMAL ANALYSIS. The chromosomes in the nondividing (interphase) cell are so extended and intertwined that they cannot be individually distinguished. During cell division (mitosis), however, they become greatly condensed and are then visible as separate entities. Dividing cells can be arrested in that phase of mitosis (metaphase) at which the chromosomes are most contracted by treatment with colchicine. By the use of colchicine and by swelling the cells in hypotonic solution to increase the separation of the chromosomes, preparations can be produced in which each chromosome is clearly visible.

Dividing cells can be obtained directly from bone marrow or by culturing a small piece of skin. The procedure required for obtaining either of these specimens, however, is unpleasant for the patient. In addition, skin cells must be cultured for several weeks before a sufficient number of dividing cells is present. Fortunately, the normally nondividing leukocyte from peripheral blood can be stimulated to divide when exposed to phytohemagglutinin (PHA). PHA appears to act only on lymphocytes (specifically, the so-called T cell). Stimulated lymphocytes undergo a transient wave of mitoses that reaches a peak in three to four days. By a combination of PHA, colchicine, and hypotonic treatments, suitable chromosome preparations can be obtained from a few drops of capillary blood.

In view of the simplicity of the procedure, most chromosomal analyses are now carried out with peripheral blood specimens. Bone marrow cells may nonetheless be used in the study of diseases, such as myelogenous leukemia, which are confined to these cells. Skin cells may be examined when a difference between the skin cell and lymphocyte chromosome complement is suspected, or when blood samples cannot be obtained, as in abortuses.

AMNIOCENTESIS. The amniotic fluid comprises a special source of fetal cells which has attained great practical importance in recent years. Ten to 20 ml of fluid can be withdrawn with apparent safety as early as the fourteenth to fifteenth week of gestation. The amniotic cells may be examined directly for sex determination by staining for the Barr body (sex chromatin mass) or for the F body, as will be described later. More commonly, they are cultured and the dividing cells are treated to obtain metaphase preparations by the methods previously mentioned. Amniotic cells are unusual in that tetraploid cells (cells with two complete chromosomal complements) occur with significant frequency even when the fetus is cytologically normal. This may indicate that amniotic cells may arise in part from the fetal membranes and may not be totally representative of the fetus proper. Chromosomal examination of the fetus may alter in the future if procedures to obtain

Figure 1. Schematic representation of human metaphase chromosomes and the terms commonly used to describe their gross morphologic features.

fetal blood or skin biopsies through an amnioscope can be simplified.

Amniocentesis for chromosomal analysis can be con-

sidered for those pregnancies in which the risk of a chromosomally abnormal fetus is thought to be significantly greater than the risk of damage to the fetus from the amniocentesis procedure itself (see Ch. 20).

METHODS OF CHROMOSOME IDENTIFICATION. The chromosomes present in metaphase have replicated but have not yet longitudinally divided, as would have occurred if mitosis had proceeded further. The unseparated parts are known as *sister chromatids*, or *chromatids*, and remain attached together at the centromere (Fig. 1). This leads to an X-like or inverted V configuration. The portions of a chromatid extending above and below the centromere are the chromosome arms. Chromosomes are described as metacentric, submetacentric, or acrocentric, according to the position of the centromere (Fig. 1). The acrocentric chromosomes usually possess a small amount of chromosomal material, called a satel-

Figure 2. Karyotype of a normal male cell stained by the trypsin-Giemsa banding technique. Each chromosome pair can be identified and is given a specific number. The group designation (A, B, C, etc.), used before identification of individual chromosomes was possible, is also shown. The X chromosome in that system was classified in the C group, and the Y was frequently included in the G group. (Constructed from a karyotype kindly provided by Dr. K. Hirschhorn.)

lite, connected to the short arm by a constricted region (the secondary constriction). Secondary constrictions are also found near the centromere on the long arms of chromosomes 1, 9, and 16.

When conventional stains are used, the chromosomes display no longitudinal features other than the centromere and secondary constrictions (Fig. 1). When certain fluorescent stains, such as quinacrine mustard, are applied directly or when Giemsa stain is used after various pretreatments (e.g., trypsin, urea, heat), the chromosomes display a characteristic banded appearance (Fig. 2). The location and morphology of the individual bands in each chromosome are sufficiently constant that a system of nomenclature for each band has been devised (Fig. 3). This is becoming of great importance, because it is now possible to associate a particular gene with a particular band by such techniques as somatic cell hybridization.

The chromosomes from a single metaphase are customarily arranged in a standardized format, known as a *karyotype* (Fig. 2). Conventionally, the chromosomes are arranged in pairs and are ordered on the basis of decreasing length. Since the chromosome pairs could not be individually identified when the first karyotypes were prepared, chromosomes with similar morphology were originally classified into groups (A to G). Now that each pair can be recognized, the autosomes are numbered from 1 to 22, and the sex chromosomes are identified as X and Y (Fig. 2).

NOMENCLATURE FOR CHROMOSOMAL ABNORMALITIES. In the shorthand notation now generally used to describe the chromosome complement of an individual, the number of chromosomes is specified first, followed by the listing of the sex chromosomes. In this notation the normal female karyotype is 46,XX and the normal male is 46,XY. Any deviations from the normal karyotype are written after the sex chromosome listing. An individual autosome is referred to by number, its upper (shorter) arm by p and its lower arm by q. A plus or a minus sign written *after* the p or q indicates an increase (+) or decrease (−) in length of the arm. When written before a designated chromosome, the sign indicates that the chromosome is extra (+) or missing (−). (Examples: 46,XY, 18q− describes a male with 46 chromosomes, including one chromosome 18 whose long arm is diminished in length; 47,XX,+21 describes a female with 47 chromosomes, including an extra chromosome 21 in addition to the 46 chromosomes of the normal karyotype.)

THE BARR BODY AND THE F BODY. Despite the detail revealed by the various banding techniques, most are unable to distinguish between the two X chromosomes of the normal female. It is known that only one X chromosome is active in any cell; each X chromosome in excess of one condenses to form a sex chromatin mass (Barr body) visible at the periphery of the nucleus. The number of X chromosomes may be indirectly determined by examination of buccal mucosal cells for the number of Barr bodies.

Condensed, inactive X chromosomes are also delayed in the timing of their DNA synthesis, relative to the active X chromosome. The late-replicating X chromosome can be identified by autoradiography using tritiated thymidine, or by the incorporation into DNA of 5-bromodeoxyuridine (BUDR) in place of thymidine followed by staining with a dye that differentiates between BUDR and thymidine (the Hoechst-BUDR technique).

In over 99 per cent of males, the distal part of the long arm of the Y chromosome fluoresces brilliantly after staining with quinacrine. The intensity is sufficiently great that this region can be seen as a spot of fluorescence, the F body, in the interphase nucleus. Y-bearing cells can thereby be recognized in cells from blood, hair follicles, and tissue sections, and even in sperm.

POLYMORPHIC VARIATIONS IN THE HUMAN KARYOTYPE. In addition to those alterations in the karyotype which are directly or potentially associated with disease, some variations are known which are apparently without consequence to the individual who possesses them or to his progeny. These polymorphic variations, as they are called, may represent changes in the DNA sequence of the chromosomal region concerned. They are transmitted to progeny as part of the chromosome which contains them. The more commonly recognized variations of this type occur in the length of the short arms of the acrocentric chromosomes, the size of their satellites, the length of the fluorescent segment in the long arm of the Y, and the length of the secondary constrictions of 1, 9, and 16.

Figure 3. Schematic representation of human chromosomes 1 and X, showing their standardized banding patterns. A numbering system for the individual bands was adopted at the Paris conference (1971) on Standardization in Human Cytogenetics (Birth Defects Original Article Series, 8:1, 1972). The Rh blood group locus is in chromosome 1 near band 34 on the short arm. The loci for the following enzymes have been tentatively localized to the long arm of the X: phosphoglycerate kinase, hypoxanthine-guanine phosphoribosyl transferase, and glucose-6-phosphate dehydrogenase.

18.2. MEIOTIC AND MITOTIC NONDISJUNCTION

MEIOTIC NONDISJUNCTION. Since gametes (sperm or ova) contain only half as much genetic material as a somatic cell, the behavior of the chromosomes during their formation is obviously a unique process, to which the term meiosis is applied. Of the many steps involved in meiosis, those of concern here are only the steps that lead to a reduction in the chromosome number from 46 in the precursor cell to 23 in the ga-

Figure 4. Schematic representation of the behavior during meiosis of a single pair of acrocentric chromosomes, contrasted with their behavior during mitosis. The round bodies on the short arms represent the satellites which are characteristically present on acrocentric chromosomes.

GAMETES PRODUCED BY NONDISJUNCTION

Figure 5. Production of gametes with an altered number of chromosomes by the two types of meiotic nondisjunction. When polymorphic variation in the satellites of acrocentric chromosomes occurs, a distinction may be made between first and second meiotic nondisjunction of these chromosomes.

mete. Meiosis consists of two successive stages of divisions (Fig. 4). During first meiotic division, each replicated chromosome pairs with its identical partner. Next, each member of a pair enters one of the two new daughter cells formed. During second meiotic division, sister chromatids separate at the centromere, analogous to their behavior in mitosis, and the two new chromosomes enter the two daughter cells produced at this stage (Fig. 4). Of the four cells formed from a gonadal precursor cell, each contains one chromosome from every autosomal pair and one sex chromosome (either an X or Y). (In the formation of the female sex cell, only one of the four cells becomes a functional ovum. In the male, all four cells become spermatozoa.)

Maintenance of the normal chromosome number in the gametes requires the separation of the paired chromosomes at first meiotic division and the separation of sister chromatids at second meiotic division. The failure to disjoin properly (nondisjunction) at either first or second meiotic division will produce gametes with abnormal numbers of chromosomes (Fig. 5). This will result in formation of an individual with an abnormal number of chromosomes in each cell. By using marker genes or polymorphic variations (Fig. 5), it is sometimes possible to identify the parent in whom the nondisjunction occurred and even to distinguish between first and second meiotic division nondisjunction. It is now known that nondisjunction can occur during gametogenesis in either the male or the female and during either first or second meiotic division. Some types of meiotic errors, however, are more likely to be associated with certain kinds of chromosomal abnormalities than with others (see below).

MITOTIC NONDISJUNCTION. Mitosis resembles second meiotic division in that sister chromatids become separated, with one of the two newly formed chromosomes

Clinical and Cytogenetic Characteristics of Common Syndromes Associated with Change in Chromosome Number

Autosomal Abnormalities	Common Name	Approximate Frequency among Liveborn Infants	Mechanism of Origin	Major Clinical Findings
47, +21	Trisomy·21 or Down's syndrome	1:1000	Frequently maternal first meiotic division nondisjunction	Mental retardation, abnormal brain development (microgyria), characteristic facies, marked hypotonia
47, +18	Trisomy 18 or Edwards' syndrome	1:11,000	Meiotic nondisjunction	Mental retardation, severe failure to thrive, periarticular limitation of motion of distal interphalangeal joints
47, +13	Trisomy 13 or Patau's syndrome	1:15,000	Meiotic nondisjunction	Mental retardation, abnormal brain development (arrhinencephaly), cleft palate (and cleft lip), ocular colobomata, postaxial polydactyly
Sex Chromosomal Abnormalities				
45, X (45, XO)	Turner's syndrome	1:6000	Maternal (22%) or paternal (78%) meiotic nondisjunction	Short stature, failure of secondary sexual development, pterygium colli, neonatal edema of hands and feet
47, XXX	Triple X syndrome	1:2000	Possibly maternal meiotic nondisjunction	Usually clinically normal; may be mentally retarded and deficient in secondary sexual development
47, XXY	Klinefelter's syndrome	1:2000	Maternal (61%) or paternal (39%) meiotic nondisjunction	Mild increase in stature, micro-orchidism, infertility, gynecomastia, behavioral changes
47, XYY	XYY syndrome	1:2000	Paternal second meiotic division nondisjunction	Significantly increased stature, behavioral changes

going to each of the daughter cells. Failure of separation (mitotic nondisjunction) of the chromatids may occur and lead to creation of two cell lines, one with 47 chromosomes and one with 45 chromosomes. If mitotic nondisjunction occurs at the first cleavage division of the zygote (the cell formed by union of ovum and sperm), an individual with two cell lines (if both cell lines are viable), neither of which is normal in karyotype, will result. If mitotic nondisjunction occurs subsequent to the first cleavage division, a third and normal cell line will be present.

Individuals with two or more chromosomally distinct cell types are referred to as mosaics. Mosaicism usually results from mitotic nondisjunction or anaphase lag loss. In the latter, sister chromatids separate properly at mitosis, but one of the newly formed chromosomes fails to be incorporated in a daughter cell. This leads to creation of a new cell line with one chromosome less than the main cell line.

18.3. CHANGES IN CHROMOSOME NUMBER

Chromosomal abnormalities limited to a change in chromosome number are usually the consequence of nondisjunctional errors. This abnormality is much more common than the group of disorders which result from change in chromosomal structure. The presence of an additional autosome (trisomy) occurs with reasonable frequency, whereas the absence of an autosome is almost never found among liveborn individuals.

A change in the number of sex chromosomes is less deleterious than a change in the number of autosomes. Individuals with as many as three extra sex chromosomes are able to survive, although they are usually mentally defective and congenitally malformed. Individuals with a single sex chromosome (one X chromosome) are, surprisingly, only moderately affected. Individuals with only Y chromosomes, that is, without any X chromosome, have never been found.

The clinical features associated with the more frequently encountered changes in chromosome number are given in the accompanying table. Each type of chromosomal aberration is associated with a relatively characteristic group of clinical findings. It is therefore highly probable that the clinical findings associated with each chromosomal aberration are at least in part determined by the specific genes present on the chromosome involved.

18.4. CHANGES IN CHROMOSOMAL STRUCTURE

CHROMOSOMAL BREAKAGE. Changes in chromosomal structure are largely the consequence of chromosomal breakage. The constancy of the human karyotype from cell to cell and from individual to individual conceals the true frequency with which the continuity of the genetic material is interrupted. In most instances, a break in a chromosome is quickly repaired, with restoration of the normal chromosome structure and without harmful consequences. The exceptions to this are of two kinds and include, on the one hand, the produc-

A. Reciprocal Translocation   B. Reciprocal Translocation, Centric Fusion Type

C. Inversion (Pericentric)   D. Inversion (Paracentric)

Figure 6. Schematic representation of the mechanisms underlying some types of chromosomal rearrangements. The horizontal lines represent the points of chromosomal breakage and reunion. The chromosomes are depicted as having single chromatids (i.e., they are unreplicated). It is not known, however, whether rearrangements usually occur before or after replication.

tion of chromosomal rearrangements and, on the other hand, diseases characterized by the presence of unrepaired chromosomal breaks.

CHROMOSOMAL REARRANGEMENTS; RECIPROCAL TRANSLOCATIONS. If two or more chromosomal breaks occur simultaneously in the same cell, the repair process occasionally may unite the chromosomal fragments incorrectly, with production of a chromosomal rearrangement (Fig. 6). One of the most common rearrangements encountered is that which is produced by an exchange of terminal chromosomal segments between two different chromosomes, with formation of a reciprocal translocation (Fig. 6A). A reciprocal translocation occurring between two acrocentrics, with the chromosomal breakpoints in each being located very near to the centromere, is given the special name of *centric fusion translocation* (Fig. 6B). The two most common rearrangements observed in man are centric fusions between chromosomes 14 and 21 and between chromosomes 13 and 14. The minute chromosome produced during a centric fusion translocation (Fig. 6B) is usually lost so that a cell with only 45 chromosomes results. The minute chromosome appears to have little essential genetic material, because its loss has no effect on the cell or the individual.

The types of rearrangement illustrated in Figure 6 apparently produce no change in the amount of genetic material in the cells in which they occur. Such rearrangements are described as *balanced rearrangements,* and the individuals who possess them are carriers of the balanced rearrangement.

TRANSMISSION OF A RECIPROCAL TRANSLOCATION. When meiosis occurs in a reciprocal translocation carrier, the translocated chromosomes will pair with each other, as well as with their untranslocated partners. Separation of the individual members of this pairing group is often quite abnormal, with any one, two, three, or four chromosomes of the group being incorporated in a single gamete. Since gross amounts of genetic imbalance are poorly tolerated, only a few of the possible abnormal types of progeny will be liveborn. The remaining abnormal types may appear as abortuses or may not be detected at all (because the embryo expires before implantation).

The variety of liveborn progeny expected depends dramatically upon the specific reciprocal translocation. A carrier of a centric fusion translocation between chromosomes 14 and 21, for example, will produce equal numbers of children with the balanced rearrangement and children who are chromosomally normal. A smaller number will have the genetic equivalent of an extra chromosome 21 (and have Down's syndrome), the only type of abnormal progeny produced by this rearrangement able to survive until birth.

Individuals with balanced or unbalanced reciprocal translocation may also be born of chromosomally normal parents. In this case the reciprocal translocation is assumed to have originated during gametogenesis.

Occasionally, a somatic cell may develop a chromosomal rearrangement which may then be passed on to its cellular descendants. This has been observed particularly in some forms of leukemia and in some solid tumors. Chronic myelogenous leukemia, for example, is characterized by a rearrangement (probably a reciprocal translocation) occurring in the leukemic cell which involves chromosome 22 and another autosome, usually chromosome 9. One chromosome 22 in this case has the appearance of a 22q− and is referred to as the Philadelphia chromosome (Ph[1]) (see Ch. 498.1).

CHROMOSOMAL REARRANGEMENTS; DELETIONS. A chromosome may undergo breakage so that an interstitial or a terminal segment of one arm is lost. These abnormalities are known as *chromosomal deletions*. In general they are sporadic, because the abnormality is not present in the ancestors of the affected individual. The loss of genetic material leads to production of multiple congenital malformations if an autosome is involved or to abnormal sexual development if a sex chromosome is affected. The most commonly encountered autosomal chromosomal deletion syndromes have the karyotypes 46,XX or XY,5p− (the cri du chat syndrome) and 46,XX or XY, 18q−.

DISEASES ASSOCIATED WITH UNREPAIRED CHROMOSOMAL BREAKS. There are three diseases (Bloom's syndrome, Fanconi's anemia, and ataxia telangiectasia) now known in which unrepaired chromosomal breakage commonly occurs with several times the frequency observed in normal individuals. Each of these diseases is inherited as an autosomal recessive condition. In addition to the unrepaired breaks, other cytogenetic abnormalities are present with an abnormally high frequency. These include chromosomal rearrangements, deletions, *"fusion figures,"* and *endoreduplication* (in Fanconi's anemia). The fusion figures appear to result from a break in a single chromatid in each of two chromosomes, followed by union of the ends from nonsister chromatids. Endoreduplication is a different type of cytogenetic abnormality and results when two cycles of chromosomal replication occur without an intervening cell division — each metaphase chromosome possesses four juxtaposed sister chromatids instead of the normal two. Although chromosomal breaks and rearrangements as well as fusion figures are perhaps likely consequences of an abnormality in the DNA repair process, it is not yet possible to visualize a rational connection of this with endoreduplication.

Clinically, these three syndromes are also associated with congenital malformations and a predisposition to malignancy. This latter may also be the consequence of an alteration in a DNA repair process. By a modification of the Hoechst-BUDR technique, sister chromatids can be differentially stained. This permits the demonstration of the exchange of chromosomal segments between sister chromatids (sister chromatid exchanges). Sister chromatid exchanges (SCE) occur with considerable frequency in cells exposed to certain DNA-damaging agents, which suggests that they may be the result of repair of DNA. In Bloom's syndrome, SCE occur with *increased* frequency even without known exposure to DNA damaging agents, whereas in Fanconi's anemia SCE occur with unusually *low* frequency after such exposure.

de Grouchy, J., and Turleau, C.: Clinical Atlas of Human Chromosomes. New York, John Wiley & Sons, 1977.

Ford, E. H. R.: Human Chromosomes. New York, Academic Press, 1973.

Latt, S. A.: Optical studies of metaphase chromosome organization. Ann. Rev. Biophysics Bioengineering, 5:1, 1976.

Levine, H.: Clinical Cytogenetics. Boston, Little, Brown & Company, 1971.

Yunis, J. J.: New Chromosomal Syndromes. New York, Academic Press, 1977.

19. PREVENTION AND MANAGEMENT OF GENETIC DISEASE

Alexander G. Bearn

The cardinal principles underlying the prevention and management of disease are similar, whether the disease is determined primarily by environmental agents or by genetic influences; in both instances accurate diagnosis is a prerequisite. Treatment of the patient with inherited disease must not depend exclusively on alleviation of the metabolic defect; symptomatic treatment is often of the greatest value, and the need for sympathetic handling of a patient with a disease that is inherited, and which may be transmitted to subsequent generations, is paramount.

Although in this chapter considerable emphasis is placed on specific, individually rare, genetic syndromes, it must be realized that the magnitude of the genetic component in the causation of all disease must be assessed if control and treatment of the disease are to be optimal. Indeed, it has been a tragic misconception, too long held, that in contrast to disease caused by environmental agents, there is no effective prevention or treatment for inherited diseases. This misguided view is quickly drained of validity when it is remembered that the expression of a disease process requires the interaction of environmental and genetic influences. Realization that 20 per cent of the hyperlipidemic survivors of a myocardial infarct occurring under the age of 60 suffer from a monogenic inherited hyperlipidemic disorder suggests that it is prudent to investigate the first-degree relatives of such individuals to ascertain those particularly at risk. Moreover, an understanding of the genetic aspects of such common diseases as obesity, hypertension, and emphysema is necessary for a comprehensive approach to prevention and management. Furthermore, an awareness of genetic influences in the metabolism of many drugs will increase the effectiveness of a physician confronted with a variety of puzzling clinical syndromes.

In the balance of this chapter attention is drawn, in particular, to those specific modalities of treatment which can be applied to inherited disease, and which stem from an understanding of the nature of the primary molecular defect. Therapeutic manipulation of the cellular environment in which the gene must display its nature is an approach more tractable and less perilous than direct interference with the genetic material itself.

RESTRICTION OF SUBSTRATE. General dietary restriction is often an effective way to reduce the excessive substrate that accumulates behind an inherited metabolic block. A general reduction in protein intake will improve the clinical manifestations of a number of rare inherited diseases affecting the urea cycle, including argininosuccinicaciduria, citrullinemia, and hyperammonemia. In some rather more common diseases, such as phenylketonuria and galactosemia, specific dietary restrictions are needed. The elimination of phenylalanine from the diet of phenylketonuric infants, if instituted before two years of age, is increasingly recognized as effective therapy. Similarly, elimination of galactose in the neonatal period for patients with galactosemia has resulted in an increased mental alertness, as well as the prevention of cataracts in those individuals who have a recessively inherited galactokinase deficiency. Defective oxidation of phytanic acid is the specific inherited defect in Refsum's disease; dietary restriction of this lipid will significantly ameliorate the symptoms of this disorder.

REPLACEMENT OF THE BIOLOGICALLY ACTIVE END-PRODUCT. An inherited enzymatic defect will lead not only to an accumulation of the substrate on which the enzyme normally acts but also to a decrease in the end-product. When the end-product is of key biologic importance, simple replacement will overcome the consequences of the metabolic block. Many instances of familial goiter associated with a deficiency of a specific enzyme can be effectively prevented by the administration of thyroid hormone. Human growth hormone is effective treatment for the recessively inherited form of pituitary dwarfism, and the ill effects of X-linked diabetes insipidus can be prevented by supplying antidiuretic hormone. Oroticaciduria, in which there is an inherited deficiency of enzymes that transform orotic acid to uridine, can be circumvented by providing the uridine-starved cells with an increase in the uridine of the diet. Dietary phosphorus will overcome the excessive urinary loss of phosphate in X-linked hypophosphatemic rickets, and administration of dietary copper will effectively combat the inherited copper deficiency of Menkes' syndrome.

REMOVAL OF THE ACCUMULATION OF SUBSTRATE. In some hereditary diseases the accumulation of a "toxic product" may be responsible for the manifestations of the disease, and removal of the excess material may reverse the phenotypic consequences of the abnormal gene. Removal of the increased tissue copper in Wilson's disease by penicillamine is a particularly striking example of the effectiveness of this form of treatment. Similarly, removal of iron in hemochromatosis by phlebotomy is another example of therapy designed to remove accumulated toxic material.

AMPLIFICATION OF ENZYMATIC ACTIVITY. Active efforts are being directed toward increasing the residual enzymatic activity that is usually present in patients with autosomal recessively inherited diseases. The administration of barbiturates, for example, to patients with the Crigler-Najjar syndrome has been found to increase the activity of the enzyme glucuronyl transferase, and simultaneously to decrease the serum bilirubin level.

Many biologically important enzymes require essential cofactors for their activity. In some inborn errors of metabolism the mutational event affects the ability of the enzyme to combine with cofactor. Pyridoxine (vitamin B_6) is a cofactor for the enzyme cystathionine synthetase. In more than half the patients with homocystinuria, in whom there is a decrease in activity of this enzyme, the defect can be overcome by administration of large doses of pyridoxine (500 mg per day). Similarly, the metabolic ketoacidosis of some patients with methylmalonic aciduria can be overcome by the administration of pharmacologic doses of the cofactor vitamin B_{12}.

ENZYME REPLACEMENT. Direct replacement of the missing enzyme (or nonenzymatic protein) is an attractive and direct approach to the treatment of recessively inherited disease, and although there are a number of substantial obstacles to this simple concept, progress is being made. It should be emphasized, however, that to be effective the enzyme not only must retain its biologic activity when administered to the patient but must also gain access to the organs and cellular organelles in which excessive substrate has accumulated. Moreover, since the infused enzyme will have a finite half-life, continuous administration or gradual release from an implanted "depot store" must be achieved. Enzyme infusions have been attempted in the mucopolysaccharidoses, in which their therapeutic effect is still unproved, and in metachromatic leukodystrophy, in which the effect is rather more promising.

MODIFYING MUTANT PROTEIN. Although modification of hemoglobin by carbamylation of valine at position 6 in the beta polypeptide chain of hemoglobin S by cyanate has a profound antisickling effect in vitro, severe toxic reactions, such as peripheral neuropathy, sharply limit its clinical usefulness. This approach to the modification of mutant proteins, however, holds much promise for the future.

SURGICAL TREATMENT. Numerous examples of the application of surgery to the treatment of inherited disease could be cited. This is particularly likely to be effective in diseases transmitted in a mendelian dominant fashion. The prevention of neoplastic transformation in polyposis of the colon and the removal of the spleen in hereditary spherocytosis are examples of inherited diseases in which surgery can play an important therapeutic role. It should not be overlooked that surgery is a quick and permanent cure for polydactyly as well as for certain other dominantly inherited defects.

Allotransplantation of the organ in which the deficient enzyme is normally synthesized has been attempted in a variety of inherited diseases. Renal transplantation has been performed in patients with Fabry's disease and in cystinosis. In Fabry's disease renal transplantation appears to ameliorate the manifestations; in cystinosis allotransplantation is effective in overcoming uremic nephropathy but does not affect the disease itself. Although in general the results are encouraging, considerably more work will be needed before organ transplantation can be recommended as a routine therapeutic measure in any inborn error of metabolism. Bone marrow transplantation is presently the only effective therapy in patients with severe combined immunodeficiency disease.

20. GENETIC COUNSELING

Arno G. Motulsky

Genetic counseling includes a range of medical, genetic, and communication activities. Diagnosis of the underlying disease is followed by assessing the risks of genetic recurrence and providing information concerning these risks to the patient, to parents, or to other family members as may be required. Ideal genetic counseling should allow the individual or family to understand the full medical and genetic facts; the natural history of the disease, including its variability from patient to patient; the available modes of management; and the potential personal, economic, psychologic, and social burdens. All possible reproductive options and their advantages and disadvantages should be explained. The patient or the family should be helped to choose the most appropriate course of action considering the genetic risks, the family needs, and the ethical and religious standards of the family. Alleviation of guilt will frequently be required. Since genetic factors play an etiologic role in many different diseases, genetic counseling has become an important component of patient management. If there is a significant risk that a given disease will recur in future children, physicians should provide or arrange for genetic counseling even if the patient or parents do not specifically request such advice. Occasionally it may be appropriate to give firm and directive advice. More generally, genetic counseling should be nondirective and should provide the necessary information to allow a couple to make their own decision regarding future reproduction. The physician in his role of genetic counselor should not force his values on those who seek his advice.

DIAGNOSIS. Accurate diagnosis is a prerequisite for genetic counseling. Similar-appearing diseases may be inherited by different modes of transmission (heterogeneity) or may not be genetic at all. Apparently identical genetic diseases caused by different gene mutations may be of variable severity and carry a different burden ranging from trivial symptoms to extensive suffering. Accurate diagnosis requires a carefully obtained family history, which is best denoted by conventional pedigree symbols. Information about relatives regarding age, onset of a given disease, health status, and cause of death is obtained. Knowledge of the ethnic origin of the family may be helpful in considering certain genetic diseases; Tay-Sachs disease is common in Jews of European origin, and cystic fibrosis is rare in blacks. Advanced maternal age is a predisposing factor to chromosomal errors such as Down's and Klinefelter's syndromes. Advanced paternal age may be found when new mutations for autosomal dominant diseases such as Marfan's disease or achondroplasia are suspected. Historic data on the immediate family are more accurate than information regarding more remote relatives. Occasionally physicians' and hospital records have to be obtained for documentation of suspected diseases. Genetic diseases manifesting anomalies of stature or a characteristic physiognomy can sometimes be recognized in photographs of family members. If the parents are related, or if both the father's and mother's ancestors originated from a restricted rural area, autosomal recessive inheritance should be considered as the possible cause for an obscure disease. The mode of inheritance together with the clinical and laboratory findings of a given patient may be helpful in defining various subtypes of clinically similar-appearing genetic disorders such as Hurler's (autosomal recessive) and Hunter's (X-linked recessive) diseases, or Marfan's disease (autosomal dominant) and homocystinuria (autosomal recessive). Diagnosis and appropriate counseling for the majority of genetic diseases require knowledge of the clinical and genetic features of the disease rather than special "genetic tests." Suitable cytogenetic and enzymatic tests should be available in the investigation of some conditions. Some patients with complex birth defects or mental retardation and many patients with gonadal and other sexual abnormalities have various cytogenetic aberrations. Most of the patients owe their abnormal karyotype to isolated events, and their parents have normal chromosomes. Cytogenetic family investigations are therefore only rarely indicated. Four to 8 per cent of couples with repeated spontaneous abortions have chromosomal translocations carried in a balanced state by one of the parents. Chromosomal analysis using banding techniques is indicated in such situations.

RECURRENCE RISKS. If a disease is transmitted by a mendelian or monogenic pattern, recurrence risks can be well defined (Table 1). Lack of clinical manifestation (diminished penetrance), variable expression, or late onset is particularly frequent in autosomal dominant disorders. In addition to the information that a given gene will be transmitted with a certain probability, the actual recurrence risk of the clinical symptomatology and the risk for severe manifestations associated with that gene must be communicated to the patient. Thus, although the risk for coronary heart diseases among patients with familial hypercholesterolemia is high, about one half of men and women by the age of 50 years and 60 years, respectively, will not exhibit clinical manifestations of coronary heart disease. About 5 per cent of all men with myocardial infarction aged 60 or below carry the gene for familial hypercholesterolemia. Some genetic diseases transmitted by an autosomal dominant mechanism, such as polycystic kidneys and Huntington's chorea, usually only express themselves clinically in the middle aged. The risk for unaffected offspring of patients, which is 50 per cent at birth, becomes progressively less as a person remains unaffected beyond the age at which these diseases first manifest. Curves plotting the age of onset can be used to quantitate these risks more precisely. McKusick's catalogue of mendelian disorders gives helpful short descriptions and literature citations for the known mendelian genetic diseases. Many human genes have been assigned to their specific chromosomal location in recent years. It will be occasionally possible to detect the affected gene carriers for a disease by studying the segregation of closely linked marker genes in families in which variants for the marker gene exist (e.g., G6PD variants and hemophilia on the X chromosome; HLA genes,

TABLE 1. Risks for Rare Mendelian Disorders in Families

Mode of Inheritance	First Degree Relatives at Risk	Risk	Other Relatives at Risk	Risk
Autosomal dominant	Sibs, parents, children (both sexes)	50%	Uncles, aunts, nephews, nieces	25%
			First cousins	12.5%
Autosomal recessive	Sibs (both sexes)	25%	Uncles, aunts, nephews, nieces, cousins	Negligible
	Children	Negligible*		
X-linked recessive	Brothers	50%†	Maternal uncle	50%†
	Sisters (carriers)	25%†	Maternal aunt (carrier)	50%†
			Maternal male cousin	25%†
			Maternal female cousin (carrier)	25%†

*Risks for children of patients affected with common autosomal recessive diseases depend upon gene frequency (highest risk [2%] for sickle cell anemia [0.08×0.25]).

†Risks are negligible when the disease in an affected patient is caused by a new mutation. Recent work suggests that the proportion of new mutations may be much less than the expected 33 per cent in X-linked lethal diseases.

PGM_3, glyoxalase, and a type of spinocerebellar ataxia on chromosome 6; secretor gene and myotonic dystrophy on a yet unassigned chromosome).

Genetic counseling in the multifactorial conditions (birth defects, common diseases of middle life, major psychoses) lacks the precision possible with counseling involving mendelian genes, as the number of genes and their relative contributions are usually unknown. Empiric risk figures based on the frequency of recurrence of the disease in many affected families are utilized for such counseling. The recurrence risks for sibs and children of patients affected with birth defects and malformations usually range between 3 and 5 per cent. Recurrence risks in first degree relatives (sibs, parents, children) for the more common multifactorial diseases of middle life such as hypertension, schizophrenia, and the affective disorders are in the range of 10 to 15 per cent. These risks increase when several immediate relatives are affected.

Recurrence risks for diabetes mellitus are often requested by families. These figures have been particularly difficult to estimate because of the heterogeneity of the condition. Extensive current work on the genetics of juvenile and late onset diabetes should provide better data in the near future. The risk of juvenile diabetes if there is one affected child and normal parents ranges around 10 per cent. The risk becomes lower with late age onset of diabetes in the affected patients and higher when several relatives are affected.

Risk assessment requires recognition of the occasional monogenic variant in a given common disease by careful consideration of the family history and possible differentiating clinical and laboratory features. For instance, about 1 per cent of men with gout carry the X-linked gene for HGPRT deficiency. The transmission of chromosomal aberrations, such as translocations, does not usually follow mendelian principles, and counseling must be based on empirically derived risk figures.

Absolute recurrence risks are more meaningful to a family than relative risks. A 1000-fold increase in recurrence risk for a certain disease in a family as compared with the general population appears frightening. However, for a condition which occurs in 1 of 100,000 births, a 1000-fold increase means that the absolute or actual risk of recurrence is only 1 per cent — a rather low risk. In mendelian diseases the recurrence risk is fixed (e.g., 25 per cent for autosomal recessive disease), whether several or no affected children preceded. Chance has no memory! In multifactorial diseases, if two or more first degree relatives are affected in a given family, more disease-producing genes are operative in that sibship, and the risk for future offspring becomes higher.

COMMUNICATION. The meaning of genetic risks must be conveyed in terms understandable to patients. Qualitative terms such as "high" for 50 per cent risks, "substantial" for 25 per cent risks, and "low" for risks of 5 per cent or less may be helpful for optimal communication. The probability that approximately 3 per cent of all children of normal couples will develop serious birth defects, genetic disease, or mental retardation should be communicated as a measure against which the additional risks can be gauged. It is useful to discuss the concept of the total burden of the disease with the family. Some conditions may be very severe but invariably fatal in early life. The burden of such a disease would be less than one of somewhat later onset but associated with chronic crippling disease and prolonged suffering such as the Duchenne type of muscular dystrophy and others.

Once the significance of the recurrence risk and the contributions of heredity to the disorder have been considered, reproductive alternatives which are meaningful within the social, emotional, and religious framework of the particular family must be discussed. Since the issues under discussion may be complex and prove emotionally difficult for the patient and family or both, comprehension may not be optimal in a single interview. It has proved useful to have several sessions and to provide a written summary of the advice given, using lay language as much as possible. Since the full process of good communication can be time consuming, professionals known as "genetic associates" have been trained through programs in several colleges and universities in recent years. Such individuals have become useful for optimal communication with patients and families with genetic diseases in collaboration with medical geneticists who provide the medical and genetic expertise.

HETEROZYGOTE DETECTION. Heterozygote detection is particularly important in sisters of males affected with X-linked recessive diseases such as hemophilia and Duchenne type muscular dystrophy, because regardless of their husband's genetic constitution, there is a 50 per cent risk that the sons of female carriers will be affected. In contrast, autosomal recessive disease becomes evident only when *both* parents are carriers, and a heterozygote sib of an affected patient must mate with another heterozygote for the disease to occur. The chance that an unrelated mate will be a carrier is usually quite low. Specialized laboratory tests for carrier detection (such as creatine phosphokinase enzyme

TABLE 2.   Genetic Diseases—Carrier Detection* Advisable for Reproductive Decisions

Disorder	Mode of Inheritance	Method of Carrier Diagnosis	Preventive Measures in Carriers	Population Affected
Duchenne muscular dystrophy	X-linked	CPK level	Amniocentesis for male sex	All
Hemophilia	X-linked	AHG level and AHG cross-reactive material	Amniocentesis for male sex	All
Lesch-Nyhan syndrome	X-linked	HGPRT assay	Amniocentesis—HGPRT assay	All
Translocation Down's syndrome	Empirical recurrence risks apply	Chromosomal tests for balanced carrier	Amniocentesis—chromosomal study	All
Sickle cell anemia	Autosomal recessive	Hemoglobin electrophoresis	Genetic counseling	Blacks
β-Thalassemia major	Autosomal recessive	Red cell abnormalities, Hb A$_2$ increased	Genetic counseling	Mediterranean and tropical populations
Tay-Sachs disease	Autosomal recessive	Hexosaminidase A assay	Amniocentesis—hexosaminidase assay	Ashkenazic Jews

*Limited to translocation Down's syndrome, X-linked, and *frequent* autosomal recessive diseases. Detection of carriers for many rare inborn errors associated with enzyme deficiency is possible, but the risk for normal sibs of affected patients to have affected offspring is very small, because the frequency of the carrier state for such inborn errors is very low in the population.

assays in Duchenne muscular dystrophy and combined assay of antihemophilic globulin clotting and antigenic activity for hemophilia A) may be helpful but must be carefully standardized on normal subjects and known heterozygotes before applying them for individual carrier identification. Detection of carriers is relatively simple and accurate in the hemoglobinopathies, and an increasing number of heterozygote states for various enzyme deficiencies such as Tay-Sachs disease can be recognized. The significance of identical laboratory test results may differ, depending upon the a priori probability of the tested person being a carrier if there is overlap in laboratory values between "low" normals and "high" carriers. Tests which may be excellent for carrier detection in families may give too many "false positives" in screening studies of an extended kindred or particularly in the general population, in which the probability that the tested subject is a carrier is low. Heterozygote detection for cystic fibrosis — the most common recessive disease in the general American population — is not yet available. Some conditions for which carrier detection tests should be done are listed in Table 2.

REPRODUCTIVE OPTIONS. Various data suggest that couples who sought genetic counseling have had fewer children if the genetic risk was more than 10 per cent

and the burden of the disease is great. If a couple decides that the risks for further reproduction are too high, several options besides contraception should be discussed. Adoption is becoming less practicable because fewer babies are available. Sterilization of either husband or wife may be considered, but it must be emphasized that this is an irreversible procedure. Thus sterilization is undesirable for prevention of autosomal recessive conditions, because remarriage after possible divorce or death could eliminate the genetic risks almost entirely. Artificial insemination by a donor other than the husband may be acceptable to rare couples to prevent autosomal recessive disease or autosomal dominant disease contributed by the husband.

INTRAUTERINE DIAGNOSIS. Amniocentesis performed during the fourteenth to sixteenth week of pregnancy allows the diagnosis of genetic disease in fetuses. When performed by a trained gynecologist, the procedure has proved safe to mother and fetus. During amniocentesis amniotic fluid containing cells of fetal origin is aspirated transabdominally. After a 10- to 20-day period of cell culture, chromosomes can be visualized to ascertain fetal sex and to detect various chromosomal aberrations. Many enzyme deficiencies can be detected by suitable assays. An increased level of α-fetoprotein in amniotic fluid is frequently observed in spina bifida

TABLE 3.   Treatable and Preventable Adult Genetic Diseases with Autosomal Dominant Inheritance for Which Search in Family Members of Affected Patients Is Mandatory

Disorder	Method of Diagnosis	Treatment	Advantages of Early Diagnosis and Treatment
Hemochromatosis*	Liver biopsy most reliable	Venesection	Prevents liver, heart, and pancreatic disease
Hereditary spherocytosis	Incubated osmotic fragility test	Splenectomy	Prevents anemia and gallstones; protects against splenic rupture
Hereditary polyposis	Colonoscopy	Colectomy	Prevents colonic cancer
Gardner's syndrome	Colonoscopy—benign cysts, lipomas, fibromas on physical examination	Colectomy	Prevents colonic cancer
Familial hyperparathyroidism	Serum calcium, phosphorus, parathyroid hormone	Surgery	Prevents renal damage and other complications of hypercalcemia
Multiple endocrine adenomatosis	Serum calcium, phosphorus, blood sugar, gastrointestinal, skull x-ray, GI series	Surgery	Prevents complications of hyperparathyroidism, hypoglycemia, peptic ulcer, metastatic cancer
Medullary thyroid carcinoma–pheochromocytoma syndromes	Calcitonin, measurement of blood pressure	Surgery	Prevents thyroid carcinoma and complications of hypertension
Familial hypercholesterolemia	Serum cholesterol, LDL receptor	Diet, drugs?	Prevents premature coronary heart disease(?)

*Mode of genetic transmission may be autosomal recessive.

and other neural tube malformations. Amniocentesis is therefore indicated to rule out the following conditions: (1) chromosomal aberrations such as Down's syndrome, (2) detection of male fetuses who have a 50 per cent risk of being affected with serious X-linked diseases, (3) inborn errors of metabolism which can be detected by amniotic cell enzyme assay, and (4) spina bifida and anencephaly. Intrauterine diagnosis of the thalassemias and sickle cell anemia is possible in specialized laboratories following aspiration of fetal blood by placental puncture or fetoscopy and analysis of hemoglobin synthesis. Most amnioceses are performed in pregnant women over 35 years of age who have a significant chance of carrying babies with Down's syndrome or in women who had a previous child with that disorder. In both situations the recurrence risk for the defect is approximately 1 per cent; this risk becomes significantly higher if either parent is a D/G translocation carrier for Down's syndrome (5 per cent for male carriers and 20 per cent for female carriers).

Intrauterine diagnosis provides a definite diagnosis and replaces statistical likelihood with certainty. Parents may select abortion if the fetus is affected, and, with monitoring of future pregnancies by amniocentesis, may be assured of unaffected children.

DETECTION OF GENETIC DISEASE IN RELATIVES. Optimal genetic counseling in some diseases should include the testing of relatives at risk (Table 3). In some conditions the detection of latent disease in sibs and other relatives, if followed by suitable therapy, may be lifesaving. A sib of a patient with Wilson's disease (autosomal recessive) has a 25 per cent chance of being affected but may be too young to exhibit overt symptoms. Sibs of patients with hereditary polyposis of the colon or Gardner's syndrome (autosomal dominant) have a 50 per cent chance of being affected and therefore carry the certain risk of developing malignant transformation of one of the many polyps. In general, vigorous attempts should be made to examine relatives, using appropriate tests, when a genetic condition causes serious preventable or treatable disease. A case can also be made for early detection of diseases such as polycystic kidneys (autosomal dominant) in family members to allow those who are affected better reproductive decisions, choice of life style and appropriate occupations, and better preparation for ultimate renal transplantation or dialysis. Possible carriers for serious X-linked diseases (such as hemophilia and Duchenne muscular dystrophy) and for chromosomal carrier status (such as Down's syndrome associated with translocation) should be sought in families for prevention by intrauterine diagnosis.

GENETIC SCREENING. Genetic counseling has usually been retrospective and has followed the advent of a sick child or relative. In prospective counseling, advice is given before a sick person is born. Such an approach is possible for common autosomal recessive diseases such as sickle cell anemia, thalassemia major, and Tay-Sachs disease in populations with high frequencies of these genes. Eight per cent of the American black population are carriers of the sickling gene, and 4 per cent of the American Jewish population of European extraction are carriers of the Tay-Sachs gene. Mass screening for heterozygote detection followed by suitable genetic counseling has been frequently carried out.

Identification of the sickle cell trait before reproduction permits the prevention of sickle cell anemia if carriers refrain from mating with each other or if those already married have no children. Such programs raise many ethical and social problems, and it is doubtful whether mating and reproductive choices which are logical from the points of view of medicine, genetics, and public health would actually be made. Unfortunately, some sickling screening programs have been established without adequate counseling. Occasionally the mistaken notion has been promoted that the sickle cell trait represents a mild form of sickle cell disease. Needless anxiety and occupational discrimination against sickle cell trait carriers have resulted. Screening programs for Tay-Sachs disease have been more successful. Intrauterine detection of this condition is readily possible on amniotic fluid cells and does not require aspiration of fetal blood. Mass screening for the genetic hyperlipidemias remains a research procedure until better methods for identifying the genetic hyperlipidemias have been developed and effective means of preventing coronary heart disease by drugs and diet have been demonstrated.

With the present tendency for couples to have smaller families, there is greater concern that children should be healthy, and thus genetic counseling will become more important. The principles of genetic counseling are simple and should be mastered by every physician. Although referral to a medical genetics clinic in a medical center is necessary for complex genetic problems, increased education in the principles of human genetics will enable genetic counseling to be undertaken by primary care physicians in many instances.

Fuhrmann, W., and Vogel, F.: Genetic Counseling. 2d ed. New York, Springer-Verlag, 1976.

Lubs, H. A., and de la Cruz, F. (eds.): Genetic Counseling. New York, Raven Press, 1977.

McKusick, V. A.: Mendelian Inheritance in Man. 4th ed. Baltimore, The Johns Hopkins Press, 1975.

Milunsky, A.: The Prevention of Genetic Disease and Mental Retardation. Philadelphia, W. B. Saunders Company, 1975.

Nora, J. J., and Fraser, F. C.: Medical Genetics: Principles and Practice. Philadelphia, Lea & Febiger, 1974.

PART IV
ENVIRONMENTAL FACTORS IN DISEASE

21. CHEMICAL CONTAMINATION OF WATER AND AIR

Walsh McDermott

Chemical contamination may occur in one's own special environment, or it may occur in the environment we share with our community, that is to say, our environment at large. Both types of contamination stem in large measure from our skill in manipulating chemicals. Public attention is largely focused on the air and water "at large," but from the standpoint of health it is probably one's own special environment that is of the greater importance. There are two reasons for this: (1) The introduction of potentially harmful chemicals occurs more often in the workplace, in the home, or in an enclosed vehicle than in the environment at large. (2) In the enclosed environments much higher concentrations of toxic materials can occur and persist, and malfunctions may develop in apparatus designed for their control. More and more, all of us are spending most of our time in a controlled environment. Dr. Lawrence Hinkle conducted a Cornell diary-questionnaire type of survey of more than 1000 men employed in a wide range of occupations in the northeastern United States; it was revealed that from October to April for most of these men the amount of time spent outside buildings, homes, and vehicles during the average working day was *less than one hour*. Although such an umbrella of artificial environment has not yet covered all portions of our population, there is no reason to doubt that something closely approximating it will eventually happen. What it does is to provide an avenue through which essentially harmless amounts of chemicals in air or water can be greatly concentrated and, in effect, sharply focused on an individual or small group. Shortly after the conclusion of an Independence Day celebration in Philadelphia, 600 "running" automobiles were backed up at the pay-as-you-leave toll collectors in a three-level underground parking lot. An outside humidity of 70 per cent prevented the ventilators from exhausting the emissions adequately. As a consequence, a traffic jam that on an unroofed parkway would have been regarded as no more than one of life's daily urban annoyances made some 150 persons ill with vomiting and other symptoms, 61 of whom received outpatient hospital care. In this case the nature of the problem was clear. But one need not force the imagination far to think of how subtle could be the early effects of undetected breaks in environmental control such as the malfunctioning of pressurized cabins in commercial aircraft or of air-cooling systems. Today's physician, aware that for a large portion of the year the patient may be spending only one hour a day in an uncontrolled environment, must determine the significant environmental facts of the other 23 hours in considerable detail. To rail against the technology that makes this necessary is not logical, because much of it — properly functioning air-cooling systems, for example — is unquestionably a positive influence for health. A severe heat wave in the United States can temporarily double the death rate — a loss of life well exceeding that of the recorded air pollution disasters. At present we may conclude that some form of technologic control would appear here to stay, and by its very existence such a "special" environment forms a potential funnel for otherwise harmless contamination to become menacing.

Contamination of air or water at the workplace presents a somewhat different sort of problem. As our skill in manipulating chemicals continues, new chemical threats are inadvertently introduced into small clusters of people in the workplace environment. Once a particular chemical can be identified as a threat to health, its dangers can be neutralized in some way, or its use in the process or the product can be abandoned. It is the initial identification that may be quite difficult, for the health damage produced by a particular chemical may take the form of a well known disease entity — asthma or primary carcinoma of the liver, to mention two actual examples. Because the disease is well characterized and known to occur in many geographic areas, there seems little sense in suspecting that it might be related to some identifiable element in the environment. Thus to detect a correlation between one or only a few instances of a well known disease and some one of the many chemicals in a particular "occupational" environment is obviously difficult. Yet the feat must be accomplished early; otherwise, conceivably large numbers of people might be seriously harmed. By no means all of the threat to health comes from newly synthesized chemicals or the breakdown of sophisticated means for their control. When technology is at fault, it is not usually *because* it is modern and sophisticated, but rather because elementary provisions for heating and ventilating are either deficient or absent altogether, and dangerous makeshifts are substituted.

A constant vigilance and a keen epidemiologic sensitivity must be a prominent part of the skill of clinicians engaged in occupational medicine. In a sense these are the pioneers of the outermost frontier of the subject of environmental contamination. Likewise, the physician not engaged in occupational medicine should be quick to consult the medical staff of his patient's workplace when some disease arises in a setting that might be viewed as representing something of a surprise.

Some of the more common chemical offenders are discussed in the chapters that follow and in Ch. 348. But the chemical nature of occupational environments is ever changing. For comprehensive coverage the practitioner or student must consult the periodical literature or textbooks in occupational medicine.

For the physician one feature characterizes these two main forms of health threat from ambient chemicals. Although there may be a considerable delay in coming to suspect the environment as culprit, once this happens the actual proof of the environmental causation and the other medical decisions follow traditional medical logic. By contrast, in the third threat, that from the environment at large, both the nature of the threat and the decisions thus made necessary are highly abstract.

Like so many problems in medicine today, the one presented by chemical contamination of our air and water is only partly medical. The effects of contaminants on an individual would be medical; yet the forces that expose the individual to the contaminants would be technologic, economic, or cultural. As modulation of these forces requires social action on a broad scale, the physician's role has to be chiefly one of educator and counselor for those of his patients who are concerned citizen activists and for the public authorities. But the physician is frequently "a concerned citizen" too. It is imperative, therefore, that while serving as counselor or educator he be able to distinguish between his advice given as a physician based on scientific and professional evidence relating to *human health,* and his advice given as a concerned citizen — albeit one with a fairly broad background in biology.

The crux of the matter is that with a very few exceptions (see below) the risks to health posed by chemical contamination of our air and water are not tangible disease realities of the sort with which the physician is accustomed to deal. Instead the fact that there are health risks at all is an intellectual judgment based mainly on biologic analogies rather than on evidence established by direct medical observations. For example, it is believed that a considerable portion of human cancers are related to some factors in the environment (see Ch. 523). The evidence for this is that there are considerable variations in the incidence of particular cancers at the same time in various places in the world and in the same place at various times, and this can be observed in situations in which it is reasonable to discount an important genetic influence. So far only four substances (tobacco, alcohol, asbestos, and betel nuts) have been convincingly incriminated as environmental factors. Except for tobacco, the groups are associated with only a small portion of the total cancers discovered each year, and all more closely resemble the contaminations of "special" environments such as the workplace rather than the environment at large. Whether contamination of our air or water at large could facilitate development of cancer cannot yet be judged. The charge that fluoridation could do so has been convincingly disproved by Doll.

In traditional medical analyses and decisions, the physician is well schooled in weighing offsetting risks. Almost invariably, however, he is dealing with risks, all of which loom for the immediate future of his patient. In weighing chemical threats from the environment, however, he must frequently offset health gains that are clear and immediate against health risks that are far off and theoretical, and indeed might become a problem only for some future generation.

A splendid example of such offsetting threats may be seen in the chemical contamination of our streams and lakes, some of which serve as community water supplies. The availability of this water made it possible to build the United States as an urbanized society, but to do so required the development of a technology whereby the water could be decontaminated of its threats to health. These threats were all actual disease-producing agents. Because they were living organisms they had the property of death and dissolution, and a highly effective technology was based on these biologic properties. For the past 50 years or so, however, on an increasing scale, we have been contaminating the water not only with our microbes but with the direct or indirect products of our chemical industry. Whereas our microbes are biodegradable, many of these chemicals are not; indeed some are not simplified at all, either by biologic degradation or by any other process of decay. Technologic solutions for this part of the problem are to be expected in the form of substituting more readily degradable pesticides and detergents. The over-all problem, however, cannot be solved purely through technologic means. For the chemical contamination, like that by man's microbes, is part of his aura and is derived from his presence and way of life. To change the aura significantly would require major changes in the way of life; yet it is only the microbial part of his aura that can be clearly incriminated as producers of disease.

Microbes, however, can contribute to the process by more ways than one. The methylation of inorganic mercury in large bodies of water appears to take place through microbial action. This microbial process is of the greatest importance; it converts a form of mercury of rather low toxicity for man into one that is quite dangerous, because, unlike inorganic mercury, methyl mercury is readily absorbed and distributed throughout the tissues of man. Strictly speaking, the *demonstrable* dangerous contamination is in the food chain, i.e., the fish; but as fish cannot methylate inorganic mercury, it is clearly a contaminant of the water. Indeed two outbreaks in Japan (the Minamata Bay and River and the Agono River) of serious disease from methyl mercury acquired through this *microbe to water to fish to man* route represent one of the few solid examples of human disease from chemical contamination of a large body of water.

The many offsetting factors that must be weighed in a judgment on the health risks of chemical contamination of water in general are well illustrated by the story of chlorophenothane (DDT). Indeed the DDT situation may be regarded as a fine prototype of the whole problem. As a pesticide this chlorinated hydrocarbon has been marvelously effective in enhancing agricultural productivity; unfortunately it is relatively stable chemically over a wide range of conditions and thus persists for long periods in the environment. Here it produces a number of unsought ecologic effects. These include critically harmful disturbances of the calcium metabolism of predatory birds; interference with various forms of marine life; and persistence in the food chain whereby it can accumulate in the tissues of a number of organisms, including man. All these effects are reason enough for insisting on strict controls on the use of DDT and on an intensive effort to develop less stable but comparably effective substitutes. Moreover, the property of accumulation in human tissue is obviously disquieting from the standpoint of human health. Thus far, however, there is no evidence that this accumulation has led to recognizable disease in humans. The World Health Organization in a 20-year experiment involving more than 200,000 DDT spraymen has received no reports of toxic effect except from accidental swallowing, and even that caused no deaths. No adverse effects were observed in a clinical study of chronic low-grade exposure in which a group of volunteers received daily for 18 months a dosage 200 times the estimated usual exposure from food (Hayes, W. S., et al., 1956).

The physician must offset the theoretic risk that these accumulations might ultimately lead to human disease against the demonstrable health gains from controlling some of the world's major diseases such as malaria (or filariasis) and those caused by arboviruses and rickettsia. At the present time, despite the presence, particularly in Central America, of mosquitoes physiologically resistant to the insecticide, there is no wholly satisfactory substitute for DDT in disease control. Faced with this choice between the clear and present danger of vector-borne diseases and the theoretic risk that tissue accumulation of low concentrations of DDT might lead to disease a few decades hence, the physician has no choice but to opt for continued use of DDT under proper control. Yet in making this choice — and the DDT situation can be viewed as the prototype of many more — he must be keenly aware of the critical nature of the factors it was *not* possible to include in the decision.

For to say that low-grade continued exposure to DDT has produced no recognizable disease in man is not to say that it exerts no *physiologic effects*. On the contrary, it is a potent inducer of the microsomal enzyme system of the liver. As this system plays a critical role in the metabolism of drugs and other chemicals introduced to the body from the outside, it serves as a major protective mechanism against chemical threats from the environment, and hence consideration of its workings is appropriate.

The activity of the microsomal enzyme system is minimal at birth and in early life but increases steadily throughout adulthood. It is inducible; and the buildup of enzymatic capability as the individual grows older is thought to be a reflection of increasing experience with chemicals from the environment acting as inducers. Activity of the system induced by one chemical may also be effective on another. Consequently when more than one drug (or adventitious chemical) are being taken into the body simultaneously, the metabolic disposition of one of the drugs can be significantly altered by the presence and inducing capabilities of the other drug or adventitious chemical. Such "cross-over" effects have obvious implications for multiple drug therapies and conceivably might also attain significance when one of the chemical compounds was an environmental contaminant. The only endogenous materials metabolized via the hepatic microsomal system are the steroid hormones, and their hydroxylation can be considerably enhanced when the system is induced. In theory, therefore, it could be imagined that the presence of DDT with its known potency as an inducer of the hepatic microsomal system could lead to an increased demand for the synthesis of some hormone. There is no evidence that such a DDT phenomenon with steroid hormones actually occurs. But the postulated phenomenon can serve as an imaginary example of how an adventitious chemical in the environment could alter the course of bodily metabolic activities *through an adaptive hepatic system that is known to exist.*

The question arises whether the decades-long stimulation of such an adaptive mechanism in an individual carries with it a risk to the total organism or whether, on balance, such continued stimulation is a good thing. In general, the many bodily systems that work toward homeostasis are regarded as normal processes whose continued operation is not harmful in itself. But some of these systems require the synthesis of protein, and this requires an allocative process involving protein precursors. In effect, therefore, as emphasized by V. R. Potter, there is a "physiologic cost" involved in each of these adaptive enzymatic processes in the sense that one is accomplished at some cost to all possible others. When the "triggering" of the system comes chiefly from the external environment, as in the hepatic microsomal system, the long-continued engagement with a wealth of chemical stimuli conceivably might result in "physiologic costs" that would be harmful to the organism. This could be so; conversely, as our knowledge advances, the notion may prove to have been ridiculously naïve. Our current state of knowledge simply does not permit judgment of the question at this time. It is really the fact that we are dealing with so many "unknowns" that serves to temper any tendency to complacency based on the present absence of detectable disease resulting from chemical contamination of our water at large. For any situation in which a variety of chemicals pass through a series of living systems that at some stage may include the human body is bound to be not only complex but a situation that is continuously subject to change. It is this fact — that the door is wide open for trouble rather than that trouble has already occurred — that characterizes our present situation with respect to possible adverse effects on health from chemical contaminants of our water.

One expressed fear about pesticides in the water also concerns contamination of the air, specifically that the world's newly released oxygen content might be undergoing subtle reduction. Approximately 60 per cent of the world's newly released oxygen each year comes from the activity of oceanic plant life which it was feared might be harmed by the pesticide pollution of the oceans. However, careful studies of Machta and Hughes have revealed that there has been no change in the world atmosphere's content of oxygen in the 60-year period from 1910 to 1970. Their "negative" data can now serve as a baseline for monitoring this question throughout the future. Fears of reduction in the global oxygen supply from combustion on land can be set completely to rest by examining the quantitative aspects of the question.

With respect to chemical contamination of the air, the challenge to the physician is the same as with water — namely, he must learn to distinguish at any one point in time between what are presently demonstrable health hazards and what are *current stimuli* that conceivably might be generating health effects to be recognized only several decades later. In broad terms, two distinct types of widespread chemical contamination exist: a "London type," composed principally of sulfur compounds from burning coal or certain grades of oil; and a "Los Angeles type," composed mainly of petroleum products introduced into the atmosphere principally from automobiles, and consisting chiefly of carbon monoxide, carbon dioxide, oxides of nitrogen, lead, and unburned or partially oxidized hydrocarbons. None of these chemicals are present in concentrations sufficiently high in themselves to produce toxicity in man. In the Los Angeles type of contamination the visible and palpable "smog" is a result of *sunlight* acting on certain of these discharged chemicals to produce more reactive chemicals, whereas in London it frequently results from *fog* physically trapping the sulfur compounds from the coal. Both types exist in both countries, but in the United States it is the hydrocarbon type that is our basic problem. It is overlaid in certain localities by the sulfur type, for the use of coal varies considerably from region to region. It is highly probable that with both types, one of the important end-results — irritation of certain body and plant cells — is much the same.

In terms of presently demonstrable effects on health, the evidence is conflicting as to whether this irritation is definitely harmful to persons who have sustained damage to their cardiovascular or bronchopulmonary systems, notably that apparently enlarging number of patients with chronic obstructive pulmonary disease (see Ch. 344.1). One may presume that it is, but thus far it has not really been possible to demonstrate it in a convincing fashion. Nevertheless, although he must act mainly on a priori reasoning, the physician would seem to be on solid ground when he attempts to protect his patients with damaged lungs or bronchi from the aggravating effects of chemically polluted urban air. Sometimes this can be accomplished by emigration, sometimes by window fans with filters. Often, however, particularly among urban poverty groups, it cannot be accomplished at all. For these unfortunates, and indeed for the majority of those with chronic pulmonary disease in all socioeconomic groups, protection, if it is to come, will have to come from the community efforts now in progress in many localities to reduce chemical contamination of the air.

It must be appreciated that virtually the entire "health case" for the need to reduce the chemical contamination of the air rests on the protection of this population with damaged cardiopulmonary systems. For no convincing case has yet been assembled to the effect that chronic obstructive pulmonary disease with its frequent cardiac sequels can be *initiated* by continued exposure to the chemical contamination of urban air. This is not to say there is no medical case at all for continued efforts to minimize contamination of the air for the sake of the far larger population with undamaged bronchopulmonary structures. On the contrary, such a case does exist. The physician must recognize clearly, however, that the case for action to protect the population at large is of quite a different nature from that for action to protect those already damaged. For those damaged the evidence is of a conventional medical sort — i.e., it is based on systematic clinical, laboratory, and epidemiologic observations. For the population at large, however, the case is not derived from actual scientific observations. On the contrary, *as in the case of chemical contamination of the water*, the argument for decontaminating the air can be no more than an intellectual judgment based mainly on biologic analogies.

There is one difference between the problems with air and with water. As mentioned previously, at present there is no recognized disease of unknown pathogenesis that seems to have any relationship to widespread chemical contamination of water. By contrast, in the disease complex of bronchitis and emphysema (chronic obstructive pulmonary disease), there *is* a commonly occurring disease grouping of unknown pathogenesis that starts in early middle age; it appears to be aggravated by chemicals in the air, and hence might also be *initiated* by them. But to demonstrate convincingly that such a causative relationship exists is a difficult task that has not yet been accomplished despite careful and intensive studies of laboratory animals and man. The epidemiologic problems involved have to do with the great difficulties in separating for analysis the various factors of conceivable relevance such as cigarette smoking and degree of exposure to particular chemicals in the air. After the first five years of planned long-term studies in the Netherlands (Van Der Lende et al., Vlagtwedde/Vlaardingen), it was not possible to demonstrate that residence in areas of high air pollution was associated with abnormalities in pulmonary function. The factor of age seemed to produce a far greater decrease of pulmonary function than smoking or living in a polluted area. Conceivably the *impact* of the chemicals that lead ultimately to disease might be something that occurs relatively early in life. Studies in young children in the United Kingdom suggest that continued exposure to high levels of pollution increases the risk of serious respiratory disease in children (Colley and Reid, 1970).

But the major problem is how to study what are in effect "water dripping on stone" effects. The chemicals now contaminating the air, taken singly or collectively, are not present in quantities that produce detectable bronchopulmonary damage in the short run. Thus if the "current stimuli" represented by these chemicals play a significant role in the pathogenesis of such a major disease grouping as chronic obstructive pulmonary disease, the effects presumably would take the form of steady but individually minute episodes of damage that ultimately fail to heal completely and emerge to significance only when accumulated over decades. Questions of this type — i.e., 30- to 40-year effects in humans — are far more difficult to answer than questions of the role of environmental contaminants on plant life or other elements of the nonhuman ecology.

To be sure, the physician in his role of public educator and counselor should support well organized efforts to develop the new methods and the new institutional arrangements for the research needed for the productive study of these medical questions of this essentially new type. But he should also not fail to stress that because of the very nature of these questions as they apply to *human health*, it seems highly unlikely that answers concerning air pollution as an initiator of disease will be forthcoming in the near future. Whatever action is to be taken, therefore, must be based on the medical information that is available now.

From the standpoint of health, therefore, we are left with the following dilemma. On the one hand, most of the actions necessary to abolish air pollution as a potential danger to health are costly and likely to prove quite disruptive to the economy and the whole style of life. To campaign for these actions in the name of health without a convincing scientific case that the evils to be corrected represent a widespread danger to health might be unwise. On the other hand, if, a few decades hence, it were shown convincingly that long-continued chemical contamination of the air *of the present sort* did have the property of initiating chronic obstructive pulmonary disease, the proportion of the population of any industrialized country that would by then have been irreversibly affected would be large indeed.

There seems to be no obvious solution for this dilemma so long as the major case for minimizing air pollution is viewed as being primarily a "health matter" and health is considered principally in terms of detectable disease. But there are more subtle aspects to health than definable disease, including even definable mental disease. There is the whole spirit involved in one's response to one's environment. The intense love of their city shown by so many Leningraders when it was under siege in World War II is a case in point. These are not the kinds of phenomena that lend themselves readily to comparative weighing in the scale against the major economic factors that might be disrupted in "air reform." Nevertheless, they deserve attention too.

What it comes down to is that, except for those already afflicted with cardiopulmonary disease, the present chemical pollution of urban air is not really a health problem in the orthodox sense; it is a widespread *social evil* that is quite unacceptable on a number of counts, of which the possible health effects are only one (Dubos). Viewed in this way it becomes the physician's role to characterize continuously what is known or seems highly probable about the health aspects of the matter. Included should be encouragement of attempts to develop more sensitive methods for the essentially permanent monitoring of the possible effects of long-continued chemical stimuli. The physician presents this knowledge not as a determining reason in itself for air control, but as only one portion of a total argument for cleansing this part of our external environment. Once the medical contribution can be regarded as but one contribution to a much larger total effort, the physician can escape from the trap of seeming to be minimizing the significances of a particular form of contamination of the air on the grounds that it is not a *known* danger to health. For the physician to operate in such a cooperative professional-social role is not new; most of the impressive early twentieth century accomplishments of medicine in extending life expectancy from birth were made in exactly this way.

Bend, J. R., and Hook, G. E. R.: Hepatic and extrahepatic mixed-function oxidases. *In* Handbook of Physiology, Section 9: Reactions to Environmental Agents. Bethesda, Md., American Physiological Society, 1977.

Carter, L. J.: Asbestos: Trouble in the air from Maryland rock quarry. Science, 197:347, 1977.

Doll, R., and Kinlen, L.: Fluoridation of water and cancer mortality in the U.S.A. Lancet, 1:1300, 1977.

Dubos, R.: Reason Awake! Science for Man. New York, Columbia University Press, 1970.

Hack, J. T.: Letter to the editor. Science, 197:1232, 1977.

Hinkle, L. E.: Hudson Basin Project, Task Group Reports, No. 9, Human Health. New York, The Rockefeller Foundation, June 1974. (Library of Congress Catalog Card No. 76–6700 38.)

Machta, L., and Hughes, E.: Atmospheric oxygen in 1967 to 1970. Science, 168: 1582, 1970.

The New York Times, July 6, 1977.

Royal College of Physicians: Air Pollution and Health. London, Pitman Medical and Scientific Publishing Company, Ltd., 1970.

Summary Report: Drinking Water and Health. Safe Drinking Water Committee, Advisory Center on Toxicology; Assembly of Life Sciences, National Research Council (Safe Drinking Water Committee), 1977. 98 pp. (Available from the Office of Public Affairs, U.S. Environmental Protection Agency, Washington, D.C. 20460).

Van Der Lende, R., et al.: Epidemiological study of the correlation between air pollution and the prevalence of airway diseases. So. Ned. Tijdschr. Geneeskd. 119:577, 1975.

22. FOOD POISONING

Harold P. Lambert

22.1. INTRODUCTION

Food may cause illness in three ways. The most common varieties are produced by *contamination with microorganisms or their products*. Although the gastrointestinal tract is an important mode of entry for many viral, bacterial, and parasitic agents of disease, the term "food poisoning" is conventionally restricted to two main types of syndromes: various forms of acute gastroenteritis caused by bacteria or their products in food; and neurologic syndromes such as botulism or paralytic shellfish poisoning caused by the toxic products of microorganisms. Second, food may be *contaminated by poisonous chemicals*. Examples include heavy metal poisoning by mercury, antimony, cadmium, arsenic, or zinc; poisoning by simple salts such as sodium fluoride or potassium chlorate; and poisoning by organic compounds such as insecticides and orthotricresyl phosphate. Third, *poisonous plants or animals may be eaten in error*. The material may be inherently poisonous, as are some species of mushroom and many other plants; or it may have become secondarily poisonous by incorporating a substance toxic to man during its own food cycle, as in certain forms of shellfish and fish poisoning.

22.2. BACTERIAL FOOD POISONING

The infectious type of bacterial food poisoning requires the ingestion of living organisms, albeit often in very large numbers, and their subsequent multiplication in the gastrointestinal tract. The most important example of this type of illness is *Salmonella* gastroenteritis, which is dealt with in Ch. 153. *Shigella* species may give rise to very similar syndromes, but these are not conventionally classified as episodes of food poisoning, although water- or food-borne outbreaks of *Shigella* infection do sometimes occur. In the toxin type of bacterial food poisoning, such as that associated with staphylococci, the illness is caused by toxin formed in food before its ingestion, and does not depend on the ingestion of living organisms. Although a generally useful concept, the distinction between the "infection" and "toxin" types of food poisoning has become less rigid than formerly with the demonstration and partial identification of a number of enterotoxins produced by bacterial gut pathogens, including those which produce disease only when ingested as living organisms.

STAPHYLOCOCCAL FOOD POISONING

ETIOLOGY AND EPIDEMIOLOGY.   This common form of food poisoning is caused by the multiplication of an enterotoxin-forming strain of *Staphylococcus* in the food before ingestion. Contamination of food with staphylococci is extremely common, because the organism can be grown from the hands of about 50 per cent of people. Heavy growth may often be obtained from apparently noninfected minor cracks and cuts on the skin. Most outbreaks are caused by meat or confectionery contaminated by staphylococci of human origin, but about 10 per cent of them are milk borne, and the organism is then usually of bovine origin. The conditions needed to cause food poisoning of this type are contamination of a suitable food — most foods will support the growth of staphylococci — and a period of some hours after preparation during which the organisms are able to multiply. This may occur during a period of slow cooling after cooking or if food is held at ambient temperature in a warm climate after preparation. Later reheating or even boiling will not then prevent illness, because this is caused by preformed, heat-stable toxin and not by the ingestion of living staphylococci.

PATHOGENESIS. Detailed study of staphylococcal enterotoxin has been hindered by many technical difficulties. Strains which form enterotoxin are almost always coagulase positive, but enterotoxin production is otherwise not related to any easily measurable metabolic activities. Moreover, study of the toxin has hitherto been limited by lack of a satisfactory animal model; most workers use intraperitoneal injection of toxin in kittens as the test system. Some progress has been made in recent years, notably the differentiation of at least four and possibly five antigenic types. Enterotoxin B has been isolated in relatively pure form by Bergdoll and his colleagues. The types are antigenically specific and do not cross-react, but one staphylococcal strain may produce more than one type. The toxin, like the crude extracts, is relatively heat resistant and resistant to trypsin. Its precise mode of action is still in dispute, but experiments in monkeys suggest that this so-called enterotoxin probably has its primary site of action in the central nervous system, and that vomiting is a centrally induced response.

CLINICAL MANIFESTATIONS AND TREATMENT. The period between ingestion and illness is short, one to six hours, occasionally a little longer, and the illness is characterized by abdominal cramping pain with violent and often repeated retching and vomiting. Diarrhea is variable; it may be profuse, mild, or absent entirely. Although often violent, staphylococcal food poisoning is short lived, usually subsiding in six or eight hours and rarely lasting as long as 24 hours. It may occasionally threaten life in patients who are old or suffering from other serious disease. The patient is often recovering when first seen by a doctor, but may require an intramuscular injection of prochlorperazine, 12.5 mg, or metoclopramide, 10 mg, to control vomiting. Patients with evidence of serious depletion of extracellular fluid may require intravenous treatment using isotonic sodium chloride with added potassium.

PREVENTION. Careful training of food handlers in personal hygiene and immediate refrigeration of foods not due for immediate consumption are the most important preventive measures. Enterotoxin is not produced at ordinary domestic refrigerator temperatures. Foods should not be left to cool slowly, especially in large containers, and should be taken from the refrigerator and reheated, if this is required, immediately before serving.

Epidemiologic work on outbreaks of staphylococcal food poisoning involves standard methods of bacteriophage typing in identifying the source of the responsible strain. Since, however, terminal heating may kill the organisms in food without inactivating enterotoxin, staphylococci may not be grown from food under suspicion. Animal assays for the detection of enterotoxin are now being replaced by serologic methods. Precipitin techniques such as double gel diffusion and immunoelectrophoresis require preliminary extraction and concentration of the material, but more rapid and direct methods for detection of enterotoxin based on radioimmunoassay and reverse passive hemagglutination are being developed.

CLOSTRIDIAL FOOD POISONING

ETIOLOGY. *Clostridium perfringens* type A is responsible for about one third of the reported cases of food poisoning both in the United States and in Great Britain. It occurs in fairly large outbreaks, with an average of 35 affected people in each episode. The organism is ubiquitous. Strains can be isolated from the feces of man and of most domestic and farm animals, and samples of raw meat may often be contaminated with this organism. It has also been found in flies, soil, and dirt from kitchens. The conditions necessary for an outbreak are well defined. A meat or poultry dish, in the form of either a stew or a solid preparation such as a joint, pie, or mince, is cooked at a temperature not higher than 100° C, allowing the spores to survive. During a period of slow cooling the spores germinate, this process being provoked by "heat shock"; rapid multiplication of vegetative forms is encouraged by the rich medium and the low oxidation-reduction potential after cooking. These conditions are especially likely to apply with a large bulk of food, in which slow cooling and anaerobic conditions are likely to occur. Food eaten cold or merely warmed before serving may then cause an outbreak of food poisoning.

PATHOGENESIS. Human volunteer experiments indicate that ingestion of living organisms is necessary for the production of this form of food poisoning, and the responsible strain may often be found in large numbers in the feces of affected patients. Strains of *Cl. perfringens* type A which cause food poisoning do not differ from other strains in any way easily identifiable by routine methods, although outbreaks in Britain have most commonly been caused by strains with heat-resistant spores. The pathogenesis of the disease has yet to be defined in detail. It was believed for some time that phosphoryl choline, an end product of the action of alpha toxin (= lecithinase-phospholipase-C) was responsible for the outpouring of fluid into the bowel, but this substance has no effect in experimental systems and is probably inactive in the bowel. Recently, however, partial purification has been achieved of an antigenic heat-labile toxin, different from the other known toxins of *Cl. perfringens*, which causes accumulation of fluid in isolated loops of rabbit ileum. The toxin is a heat-labile, nondiffusible protein, antigenic and different from other known toxins produced by *Cl. perfringens*.

CLINICAL MANIFESTATIONS. The incubation period is 8 to 12 hours after ingestion of the infected food, occasionally as little as 6 or as long as 24 hours. The main features are diarrhea and griping abdominal pain. The feces are liquid but do not contain blood or mucus. A small proportion of patients suffer from nausea and vomiting. The illness is usually not severe, lasts less than 24 hours, and is unaccompanied by systemic disturbance or fever. A few deaths have been recorded in old or infirm patients.

Drug treatment is rarely necessary, but in longer attacks a kaolin mixture may be given, and patients with severe abdominal pain may need an analgesic.

PREVENTION. Preferably food should be served immediately after cooking. If it has to be kept, it should be rapidly cooled and held at a safe temperature. Cooked meat should always be kept either cold, below 5° C, or hot, over 60° C. Careful techniques of food hygiene are especially important in institutions in which large amounts of meat or poultry are cooked.

ENTERITIS NECROTICANS
(Pig-Bel)

Outbreaks of severe intestinal disease have been associated with ingestion of *Cl. perfringens* type C. A large outbreak was reported from Germany in 1948, and a similar syndrome known as pig-bel has more recently been described from parts of New Guinea in which pig feasts have an important economic and social function. The syndrome is characterized by severe abdominal pain, bloody diarrhea, and vomiting. Operation or autopsy reveals a severe hemorrhagic jejunitis and ileitis. Some patients die and some recover after resection of strangulated, perforated, and necrotic bowel. Others may pass through the acute phase to develop chronic small bowel obstruction and malabsorption, and some recover completely.

VIBRIO PARAHAEMOLYTICUS FOOD POISONING

V. parahaemolyticus is a halophilic marine vibrio long recognized as an inhabitant of coastal waters of Japan and as a cause of gastroenteritis associated with sea foods. More recently it has been found in American and British coastal sea waters. Techniques for its isolation and differentiation from nonpathogenic marine vibrios are now well established. In particular, pathogenic strains exhibit a specific in vitro hemolytic reaction.

In Japan gastroenteritis of this type is confined to the summer months. It is the most common cause of infective food poisoning in Japan, accounting for 59 per cent of 22,000 cases of identifiable cause in 1963. *V. parahaemolyticus* causes an infectious type of gastroenteritis and is associated with ingestion of raw fish or shellfish. Outbreaks in Japan have been associated with semidried young sardines, and especially with sushi, a food composed of cooked rice, raw fish, and shellfish. The organism, as well as episodes of food poisoning caused by its ingestion, has now been identified in many parts of the world, including the Atlantic, Pacific, and Gulf coasts of the United States, other parts of the Pacific, the United Kingdom, and Australia.

Incubation periods varying from a few hours to four days have been recorded, but the most frequent interval between ingestion and infection is 12 to 24 hours. The chief clinical features are severe diarrhea accompanied by cramping abdominal pain, nausea, and vomiting. Many patients also exhibit systemic symptoms of fever, chills, and headache. Less commonly the organism causes a dysenteric form of illness with fever and bloody diarrhea. The illness lasts for one to five days, and recovery appears to be complete. As with staphylococcal and clostridial food poisoning, the disease is rarely fatal, but old and debilitated patients may be at special risk. The role of antibiotics in treatment is uncertain, but tetracycline should be given to patients who are seriously ill.

BACILLUS CEREUS FOOD POISONING

Bacillus cereus is an aerobic, spore-bearing, gram-positive bacillus of wide natural distribution, and several outbreaks of food poisoning have been associated with high counts of the organism in the responsible food. Contamination has been traced to corn flour, rice, and other dried foods. In large outbreaks in Norway affecting as many as 600 people, the incubation period was 12 hours, and the main features were watery diarrhea, abdominal pain, and nausea lasting about 12 hours. More recently, fried or boiled rice in restaurants has been incriminated. Large quantities of rice are prepared and kept at warm kitchen temperatures for many hours, small portions being refried for a few minutes as orders are placed. In one such episode the rice contained 450×10^6 organisms per gram. The incubation period has been as short as 15 minutes to 3 hours when large inocula such as these are ingested. The pathogenesis of this form of food poisoning is not precisely established, but some strains of *B. cereus* cause accumulation of fluid in the rabbit ileal loop test, increased permeability in rabbit skin, and a necrotic reaction after intradermal injection in guinea pigs.

OTHER FORMS OF BACTERIAL FOOD POISONING

Many outbreaks cannot be assigned to one of the specific pathogens generally accepted as a cause of food poisoning, but many other bacteria have been implicated at one time or another as possible causes of acute gastrointestinal illness. The evidence is often inconclusive and is frequently based on high counts of the presumptive pathogen in samples of food which may have been kept at room temperature for long periods before reaching the laboratory, or on the isolation from patients' stools of organisms which form part of the normal fecal flora. Volunteer studies have often proved equivocal. With these reservations, it seems likely that diarrhea and vomiting may occasionally be caused by a considerable variety of bacteria, if circumstances have allowed their multiplication to high enough concentrations before ingestion. The genera most often implicated have been the enterococci (group D streptococci) and various members of the Enterobacteriaceae, notably *E. coli*, *Proteus*, *Providencia*, *Pseudomonas*, and *Citrobacter*. A remarkable and special example is the contamination of fermented coconut press cake (bongkrek), a common food in Central Java, by a species of *Pseudomonas*. The toxin produced causes hypoglycemia which is often fatal.

22.3. BOTULISM

ETIOLOGY. Botulism is a life-threatening illness characterized by muscle paralysis and variable gastrointestinal symptoms. It is caused by absorption from the gastrointestinal tract of ingested toxin produced by *Clostridium botulinum*. Botulism resulting from wound infection by this organism has also been recorded several times.

INCIDENCE. The unexpectedness of outbreaks of botulism, the dramatic and frightening nature of the illness, and its high mortality have attracted much attention from both laymen and doctors, but botulism is in fact an uncommon disease. From 1899 to 1969 there were 659 outbreaks in the United States, with 1696 cases and 959 deaths. The years 1970 to 1973 saw 30 outbreaks, in which 21 of the 91 patients died. Outbreaks have also been recorded in many other countries, especially in Canada, Japan, Western Europe, Scandinavia, and the U.S.S.R.

EPIDEMIOLOGY. The six strains of *Cl. botulinum* cause disease in man and in a variety of animals. Human disease is caused by types A, B, and E and occasionally by type F. Toxins produced by the different types are antigenically distinct. *Cl. botulinum,* a spore-bearing anaerobic bacillus, is widely distributed in nature. The organism has been identified in many parts of the world, in cultivated and virgin soils, in a variety of marine environments, and in many animals and animal products. The distribution of types varies in different areas, so that type A botulism is more common than type B in the United States, especially in the Western states, whereas in Europe this order is reversed. In recent years type E has superseded both types A and B in frequency. Type E organisms are especially but not exclusively associated with the aquatic environment in northern latitudes, being found in the sea bed of coastal and lake waters and in the intestinal tract of fish. However, types A and B may also be associated with a marine source.

PATHOGENESIS. Contamination of fresh food by spores of *Cl. botulinum* does not cause botulism. The spores must have germinated and toxin must have been produced by the vegetative organisms. Spores are destroyed at a temperature of 121° C or greater, as used in commercial canning processes, but can usually survive a temperature of 100° C. Type E spores are relatively heat sensitive, but smoking and light cooking may not kill them, so that food processed in these ways or preserved in the raw state may act as a vehicle of the disease. Another factor predisposing to type E botulism is the production of toxin by this organism at temperatures as low as 5° C. The cooking or preserving process is conducive to the germination of spores and, by reason of the lowered redox potential, to multiplication of the vegetative forms. Multiplication is inhibited in acid media, and botulism is rarely associated with food of pH below 4.5. All types of botulinum toxin are heat labile, and botulism could be entirely prevented by terminal heating for 20 minutes at 80° C or for 10 minutes at 90° C.

The types of food associated with botulism as a result of these contributory factors vary, with local food customs, from country to country. In the United States home-preserved vegetables constitute the most frequent source, followed by preserved fruit and fish products.

Meat and meat products are more commonly responsible in Europe. Preserved fish is the chief source of botulism in Japan, Scandinavia, and the U.S.S.R. Although most outbreaks are associated with domestic methods of preparing and preserving foods, outbreaks from commercially prepared foods also occur. Recent sources have included canned tuna fish, canned vichyssoise, and vacuum-packed smoked fish.

Ingested toxin is rapidly absorbed from the gastrointestinal tract. Toxemia may be demonstrated for periods of up to ten days or even three weeks, and it is possible that toxin continues to be formed in and absorbed from the bowel for some days after ingestion. Type E toxin is potentiated by proteolytic enzymes, including trypsin, and this phenomenon has been invoked as a mechanism which contributes to the pathogenicity of this type. Botulinum toxin is active in extremely low doses, nanogram quantities of pure toxin being lethal to mice. It prevents conduction in peripheral nerves by a presynaptic block, thus preventing release of acetylcholine without direct action on the acetylcholine release mechanism. Anticholinesterase drugs do not affect its action.

INFANT BOTULISM. This recently recognized syndrome is of special interest, since it is caused by production of toxin within the bowel lumen. Forty-two cases were described in the United States in 1977.

CLINICAL MANIFESTATIONS. Illness usually begins between 12 and 36 hours after ingesting the toxin-containing food. The first manifestations are often gastrointestinal, especially in type E disease, with nausea, vomiting, abdominal pain, and distention. Other common early symptoms are weakness, unsteadiness, and dryness of the mouth and throat. Neurologic symptoms may accompany the early gastrointestinal illness or may follow at an interval of 12 to 72 hours. Early features are blurring of vision, dysphagia, dysarthria, and weakness of a variety of muscles. Weakness spreads as the disease advances, affecting especially the respiratory system, the external ocular muscles, and muscles of the neck and proximal limb groups. Cherington, reviewing ten years' experience with botulism, found pupillary abnormalities uncommon, being present in only 2 of 14 patients. Retention of urine is common. Deep tendon reflexes are preserved. The patient remains mentally clear, and fever is not observed except as a terminal event. Paralysis may continue for many days or weeks. An occasional patient with mild disease shows myasthenic features with a response to injection of edrophonium chloride. Defects of cardiac conduction have occasionally been noted.

The chief causes of death are respiratory or bulbar paralysis or both, along with the infective complications resulting from these paralyses. Wound botulism usually follows severe injuries of the type associated with other anaerobic infections. The incubation period is 4 to 14 days, but the illness is otherwise identical with botulism caused by ingestion of toxin.

DIAGNOSIS. The illness is easily recognized if a group of patients, known to have eaten food of a type associated with botulism, present with characteristic symptoms. By contrast, diagnosis of the individual patient, in whom there may be no suspicion that the illness is a form of food poisoning, has often proved extremely difficult. The gastrointestinal features may be so severe as to stimulate intestinal obstruction, and the epigastric pain may be mistaken for that of myocardial infarction. The dry and sometimes painful throat may suggest various forms of acute pharyngitis, and the combination of sore throat and neurologic disease can cause confusion with diphtheria. The neurologic illness has been mistaken for acute polyneuritis (Guillain-Barré syndrome), encephalitis, a stroke, or myasthenia gravis. The dry mouth and fixed dilated pupils suggest atropine poisoning, as is produced by *Datura stramonium* (jimson weed). Paralytic poisoning caused by shellfish or by puffer fish (see below) is accompanied by prominent sensory symptoms not found in botulism. Electromyography is of some value, showing diminished response to a single stimulus but facilitation of action potentials with paired or repeated nerve stimulation. The changes thus resemble those found in the Eaton-Lambert syndrome.

Circulating toxin may sometimes be detected in the patient's blood or feces, even long after onset of the disease. It is detected by intraperitoneal injection in mice, controls simultaneously receiving antiserum of the different types. Suspected food is also tested for toxin in the same way, and the organism is sought by anaerobic culture.

TREATMENT. Since the greatest risk of botulism is respiratory failure, treatment is dominated by the prevention and management of this complication. Bulbar paralysis is treated by early tracheostomy, employing a cuffed endotracheal tube. Coincident or supervening respiratory muscle paralysis indicates the need for artificial ventilation applied through the tracheostomy. Specific antitoxin is probably effective in reducing the mortality of type E botulism. Although there is no such evidence in other forms of botulism, the high mortality of the disease and the difficulty of obtaining statistically valid data justify the use of antitoxin in all forms of the disease. Antitoxin should be given irrespective of the duration of illness when the diagnosis is made, because toxin may be present in the blood for many days. Unless the type of botulism is definitely known, multivalent antitoxin should be administered, because the type cannot be reliably inferred from the food source. After a preliminary test for hypersensitivity to horse serum, two vials of trivalent antitoxin (each containing 7500 IU type A, 5500 IU type B, and 8500 IU type E antitoxin) are administered by intravenous injection, and this is repeated in two to four hours. For botulism of known type, preparations containing A and B antitoxin or E antitoxin alone are available, as is a small stock of monovalent F antitoxin.

Guanidine, which enhances acetylcholine release, has been claimed as a useful adjunct in treatment. Both clinical and electromyographic improvement were observed in a number of patients who received guanidine by nasogastric tube in a dose of 15 to 50 mg per kilogram per day; unfortunately, it is less effective on respiratory than on ocular or limb weakness.

Since it is uncertain whether the long duration of toxemia in botulism is attributable to continued absorption from the bowel, gastric aspiration and colonic washouts are also used in treatment. A solution of sodium bicarbonate may be left in the stomach to promote breakdown of toxin.

PROGNOSIS. The over-all mortality of botulism is high, 60 to 70 per cent for type A, 10 to 30 per cent for type B, and 30 to 50 per cent for type E. Patients with type E botulism tend to die more quickly than those affected by other types, usually within three days of onset. Improved management of respiratory failure should lower the death rate, especially because patients who survive the stage of severe paralysis can recover completely.

SPECIAL NOTE. For assistance in suspected botulism, or for supplies of antiserum, in the United States, telephone the Center for Disease Control: 404-633-3311 (days) or 404-633-2176 (nights, weekends, and holidays).

22.4. POISONOUS PLANTS AND ANIMALS

PARALYTIC SHELLFISH POISONING

Shellfish may act as the vehicle of transmission of many pathogens, for example, infective hepatitis, *Vibrio parahaemolyticus* gastroenteritis, and diarrhea and vomiting of unknown cause. Ingestion may also give rise to an acute neurologic syndrome caused by the transmission to man of a neurotoxin acquired by shellfish from plankton on which they feed. Outbreaks are especially likely to follow a sudden increase in the population of dinoflagellate protozoa, the "red tide." The main responsible species in the Pacific Ocean is *Gonyaulax catanella*, which produces the paralytic poison *saxitoxin*, first isolated from the Alaskan butterclam *Saxidomus giganteus*. The toxin of *G. tamarensis*, responsible for outbreaks on Atlantic coasts, produces the same pharmacologic effects, although it may not be identical with saxitoxin. The toxins are water-soluble, heat-stable compounds, rapidly absorbed from the gastrointestinal tract and active in vitro at concentrations of 1 to 10 μg per milliliter. They act on vertebrate nerve fibers and on skeletal muscle fibers, abolishing action potentials by preventing depolarization. Their study has proved of great value in elucidating mechanisms of nerve conduction.

CLINICAL MANIFESTATIONS. Symptoms may begin as soon as 20 minutes after ingestion, with paresthesias of the hands and mouth, weakness of the limbs, and a floating feeling. Other common features are ataxia, headache, and vomiting, whereas in severe cases bulbar and respiratory paralysis supervene and may cause death. Mortality rates between 5 and 18 per cent have been reported in various outbreaks, but the illness is less likely to be severe if water used in cooking the shellfish has been discarded. Treatment is that of respiratory paralysis. No specific treatment is available, but patients are likely to recover if they survive the first 12 hours of the illness. The toxin of *Gymnodinium breve*, a flagellate producing red tides off the Florida coast, causes upper respiratory tract and ocular irritation in people living near the affected beaches.

A different form of paralytic shellfish poisoning is associated with ingestion of red whelk, *Neptunea antiqua*. This is caused by tetramine (tetramethylammonium hydroxide) which is produced in the salivary glands of this mollusk and causes curare-like effects on muscle.

FISH POISONING

A number of different mechanisms are involved in fish poisoning. Some species are inherently poisonous; the toxins of other species are acquired from organisms on which they feed; yet another form of fish poisoning is caused by breakdown products of bacterial action.

CIGUATERA POISONING. This can be acquired from a large number of species, about 300 in all, whose common characteristic is the narrow range of reef or coastal tropical waters which they inhabit. The toxin is thought to originate in blue-green algae consumed by herbivorous fish which are in turn the prey of carnivorous species. The toxin accumulates in the tissues and is excreted very slowly. Poisoning of this type is difficult to prevent, because the toxin is stable to heat, cold, and drying, and the taste and smell of the fish are unaffected. Symptoms commonly begin several hours after ingestion, but may be almost immediate. Nausea and vomiting are followed by paresthesias of the face, mouth, and limbs, dizziness, ataxia, muscular weakness, and severe muscle pain. The patient may die from respiratory paralysis during the first day, and in nonfatal cases the neuritic symptoms may persist for many weeks. No immunity is gained by an attack; indeed, a second episode of poisoning may be more severe.

TETRAODON POISONING. Many puffer fish found in the Pacific, Atlantic, and Indian Oceans are inherently toxic. The neurotoxin contained in their viscera (tetrodotoxin) is identical with that formerly known as tarichatoxin, found in the Californian newt *Taricha torosa* and some South American frogs. Its mode of action is similar to that of saxitoxin, and this is reflected in the syndrome of tetraodon poisoning which bears clear resemblances to paralytic shellfish poisoning (see above). Symptoms begin soon after ingestion and include paresthesias, dizziness, ataxia, and paralysis, often together with diarrhea, vomiting, and abdominal pain. The patient may die of respiratory paralysis.

SCOMBROID POISONING. Some species of the mackerel family, such as tuna and bonito, are susceptible to decomposition by *Proteus morganii*. Toxic products result from the breakdown of histidine normally contained in fish flesh. Within a few minutes of ingesting contaminated fish, the patient develops nausea, vomiting, headache, epigastric pain, dysphagia, dryness of the mouth, and severe urticaria. The illness usually lasts less than 24 hours.

OTHER FISH POISONS. Neurologic symptoms may follow ingestion of several other types of fish. Some of the toxins responsible are probably acquired from dinoflagellates, as in paralytic shellfish poisoning, but the source of other neurotoxins is still uncertain. In addition to these forms of fish poisoning, some species of the Gempylid group such as castor oil fish and snake mackerel contain a purgative oil, whereas the roe of some freshwater fish is toxic during the reproductive period, causing acute gastrointestinal symptoms with headache and fever.

MUSHROOM POISONING

In poisoning by muscarine-containing species such as *Amanita muscaria* (fly agaric) and *Amanita pantherina*, symptoms begin two or three hours after ingestion and consist of abdominal cramping, sweating, salivation, miosis, and bradycardia. Poisoning by these species is rarely fatal. By contrast, death-cup poisoning, by *Amanita phalloides* and *Amanita verna*, carries a mortality of 30 to 50 per cent or more. Two groups of toxins are contained in these mushrooms. Cyclic heptapeptides known as *phallotoxins* cause the violent symptoms of abdominal pain, vomiting, and diarrhea which begin 6 to 15 hours after ingestion. Symptoms then remit for about 48 hours. During this time tests of liver function become abnormal, and signs of hepatic and renal failure then develop, often accompanied by confusion, coma, and paralysis of the extremities. Small doses may lead to renal tubular necrosis without hepatic damage, but usually both organs are affected. This phase of the illness is probably caused by cyclic octapeptides known as *amatoxins*.

No specific treatment is available, but the stomach should be emptied by induced vomiting or gastric lavage, and atropine administered if muscarinic effects — that is, sweating, salivation, and colic — are observed. Otherwise, the general principles of management in acute hepatic and renal failure should be observed. For example, peritoneal dialysis or hemodialysis may be necessary in renal failure, and modern methods of managing acute hepatic failure may help to reduce the high mortality.

A number of pharmacologic agents have been shown to mitigate the effects of alpha-amanitin (the principal amatoxin of *A. phalloides*) in experimental systems, but their effect in human mushroom poisoning is not known.

TOXICANTS FOUND NATURALLY IN FOODS

Some substances found naturally in food cause forms of damage not usually thought of as food poisoning, partly because their effects are chronic rather than acute, and partly because the pathogenic role of many possible food toxicants is still uncertain. The mycotoxins have aroused special recent interest, but many other substances in food may be involved in the causation of chronic disease.

Antithyroid compounds in plants, mainly *Brassica* species, are thought to account for 4 per cent of the world incidence of goiter.

Cyanogenic glycosides, found especially in cassava or lima beans may be a causal agent of chronic cyanide poisoning. Tropical ataxic myelopathy and toxic amblyopia have been ascribed to this cause in several areas of high cassava consumption, but these syndromes are also found in other areas in which no such dietary factor can be invoked.

Lathyrism, a slowly progressive spastic paraplegia, is associated with the ingestion of pulse made from the seeds of *Lathyrus sativus* and other related species, which grow under adverse conditions and may become a staple diet in times of food shortage in Eritrea, parts of India, and Algeria. The toxic factor in the seeds is thought to be aminopropiononitrile.

MYCOTOXINS. Ergotism (see Ch. 368.2) is the most familiar of the illnesses caused by mold contamination of food. More recently, many other mycotoxins have been identified and their possible roles assessed in human and animal disease. Aflatoxins, products of *Aspergillus flavus* and allied species, were identified in the early 1960's after huge losses in turkey flocks, followed by outbreaks among ducks, pheasants, pigs, and calves, had been ascribed to contaminated peanut meal. In experimental animals, aflatoxin B1 causes liver necrosis, bile duct proliferation, and cirrhosis, whereas chronic or repeated administration leads to hepatocellular and cholangiocarcinoma. A probable role for this toxin in human disease is suggested by the association, established in Thailand and in several parts of Africa, between dietary intake of aflatoxin and the incidence of hepatic carcinoma.

Another group of mycotoxins, the trichothecenes, derived from *Fusarium* and other genera which cause spoilage of cereal grains, are now thought to have been responsible for alimentary toxic aleukia, widespread in the U.S.S.R. when conditions of war or famine compelled consumption of moldy grain. The main features were a hemorrhagic tendency, fever, leukopenia, agranulocytosis, and resulting sepsis.

Mycotoxins also have an indirect influence on human health by the depletion of livestock caused by moldy feed.

POISONING BY FLOWERING PLANTS

An immense number of plant species may contain constituents toxic to man, and only a few of the more common and important forms of plant poisoning can be considered here.

The first examples are all members of the family of *solanaceous plants,* in which toxic species are especially well represented.

Atropa belladonna (deadly nightshade) poisoning is caused by ingestion of the prominent black berries, which contain a number of alkaloids of the belladonna group. The symptoms and signs are those of atropine poisoning: dry mouth, dry skin, blurring of vision, dilated pupils, tachycardia and excitement, hallucinations, and delirium followed by coma — "hot as a hare, blind as a bat, dry as a bone, red as a beet, and mad as a hen."

Datura stramonium (thorn apple, jimson weed) also contains stramonium alkaloids, as do other species of this genus, and they may cause poisoning by ingestion of their seeds, of extracts of leaves, and even of nectar. Clinical manifestations are generally similar to those of atropine poisoning. Seeds may be ingested as a form of drug abuse, and the high dose thus received has led to alarming but fortunately transient syndromes characterized by hallucinations, hyperthermia, decerebrate posturing, hyperreflexia with extensor plantar responses, and electroencephalographic abnormalities.

Other familiar members of the Solanaceae are *Solanum americanum* and *S. nigrum* (common nightshade, black nightshade), *S. dulcamara* (woody nightshade, bittersweet), *Hyoscyamus niger* (henbane), and the potato plant, of which the green parts and tuber sprouts may be poisonous. Plants of this group contain a mixture of the stramonium alkaloids and of solanine, itself a mixture of alkaloids.

No specific treatment is available for these forms of poisoning. Peripheral effects caused by atropine can be antagonized by pilocarpine, but this does not affect its cerebral actions. Vomiting should be induced or the stomach emptied by gastric lavage.

The family Umbelliferae also includes many toxic species, in addition to familiar food species such as carrot, parsnip, and celery. *Conium maculatum* (hemlock), a common weed which looks somewhat like wild parsnip, contains several toxic alkaloids causing nausea and vomiting, progressive weakness, respiratory paralysis, and convulsions. Various species of *Cicuta*, the water hemlocks, are also toxic, the root containing cicutoxin, an unsaturated alcohol. Ingestion is followed by vomiting, salivation, delirium, convulsions, and paralysis. Effects similar to hemlock poisoning may result from ingestion of laburnum (family Papilionaceae), which contains the toxic alkaloid cytisine.

Some forms of poisoning are not confined to a particular plant family. Digitalis-like effects, for example, may be produced by oleander and lily-of-the-valley as well as by the foxglove.

The forms of plant poisoning discussed so far affect organs remote from the gastrointestinal tract. A number of plant products cause gastrointestinal symptoms, ranging from burning of the mouth and throat, through severe gastroenteritis (e.g., spurge laurel berries, roots and stems of pokeweed), to the hemorrhagic gastroenteritis which follows ingestion of seeds of the castor bean and certain other species.

22.5. CHEMICAL FOOD POISONING

Various forms of metallic poisoning are discussed in Ch. 24 and 379. Occasionally patients react idiosyncratically to a normal constituent of food, or to a food additive or preservative. The headache and hypertension induced by certain foods in patients receiving monoamine oxidase inhibitors are attributable to their natural tyramine content. The two examples which follow illustrate peculiar reactions to additives in food.

CHINESE RESTAURANT SYNDROME. A few people develop dramatic symptoms 10 to 20 minutes after eating some kind of Chinese food. These include tingling and burning in the back of the neck, radiating to the upper back, arms, and front of the chest. Some of them experience throbbing pain in the temples and infraorbital region. The symptoms fluctuate in severity and usually last for 45 minutes to 2 hours. The cause of this syndrome has been much disputed, but is probably the monosodium glutamate used in seasoning certain Chinese foods.

HOT DOG HEADACHE. A patient experienced several hours of bitemporal headache and facial flushing, starting within 30 minutes of eating certain kinds of cured meat. His symptoms were shown to be caused by sodium nitrite used in the curing process.

Arnon, S. S., Midura, T. F., Clay, S. A., Wood, R. M., and Chin J.: Infant botulism: Epidemiological, clinical and laboratory aspects. JAMA, 237:1946, 1977.

Barker, W. H., and Gangarosa, E. J.: Food poisoning due to *Vibrio parahaemolyticus.* Ann. Rev. Med., 25:75, 1974.

Blankenship, J. E.: Tetrodotoxin; from poison to powerful tool. Perspectives Biol. Med., 19:509, 1976.

Cherington, M.: Botulism, 10 years' experience. Arch. Neurol., 30:432, 1974.

Committee on Food Protection: Toxicants Occurring Naturally in Foods. 2nd ed. Washington, D.C., National Academy of Sciences Publication No. 73.8988, 1973, p. 346.

Crowther, J. S., and Holbrook, R.: Trends in methods for detecting food poisoning toxins produced by *Cl. botulinum* and *Staph. aureus.*

In Skinner, F. A., and Carr, J. G. (eds.): Microbiology in Agriculture Fisheries and Food. New York, Academic Press, 1976, p. 215.

Dadisman, T. A., Nelson, R., Molenda, J. R., and Garber, H. J.: *Vibrio parahaemolyticus* in Maryland. 1. Clinical and epidemiological aspects. Am. J. Epidemiol., 96:414, 1972.

Earampamoorthy, S., and Koff, R. S.: Health hazards of bivalve-mollusk ingestion. Ann. Intern. Med., 83:107, 1975.

Evans, M. H.: Mechanism of saxitoxin and tetrodotoxin poisoning. Br. Med. Bull., 25:263, 1969.

Hardin, J. W., and Arena, J. M.: Human Poisoning from Native and Cultivated Plants. 2nd ed. Durham, N. C., Duke University Press, 1973.

Hughes, J. M., Horwitz, M. A., Merson, M. H., Barker, W. H., Jr., and Gangarosa, E. J.: Foodborne disease outbreaks of chemical etiology in the U.S., 1970–74. Am. J. Epidemiol., 105:233, 1977.

Koenig, M. G., Drutz, D. J., Mushlin, A. I., Schaffner, W., and Rogers, D. E.: Type B botulism in man. Am. J. Med., 42:208, 1967.

Koenig, M. G., Spickard, A., Cardella, M. A., and Rogers, D. E.: Clinical and laboratory observations on type E botulism in man. Medicine, 43:517, 1962.

Lampe, K. F.: Systemic plant poisoning in children. Pediatrics, 54:347, 1974.

Loewenstein, M.: Epidemiology of *Cl. perfringens* food poisoning. N. Engl. J. Med., 286:1026, 1972.

Merson, M. H., and Dowell, V. R.: Epidemiologic clinical and laboratory aspects of wound botulism. N. Engl. J. Med., 289:1005, 1973.

Merson, M. H., Hughes, J. M., Dowell, V. R., Taylor, A., Barker, W. H., and Gangarosa, E. J.: Current trends in botulism in the United States. JAMA, 229:1305, 1974.

Mikolich, J. R., Paulson, G. W., and Cross, C. J.: Acute anticholinergic syndrome due to jimson seed ingestion. Ann. Intern. Med., 83:321, 1975.

Murrell, T. G. C., Roth, L., Egerton, J., Samels, J., and Walker, P. D.: Pig-bel; enteritis necroticans. Lancet, 1:217, 1966.

Nakamura, M., and Schulze, J. A.: *Clostridium perfringens* food poisoning. Ann. Rev. Microbiol., 23:359, 1970.

Portnoy, B. L., Goepfert, J. M., and Harmon, S. M.: An outbreak of *Bacillus cereus* food poisoning resulting from contaminated vegetable sprouts. Am. J. Epidemiol., 103:589, 1976.

Strong, F. M.: Toxicants occurring naturally in foods. Nutr. Rev., 32:225, 1974.

Symposium: Food, is it safe? Medlock, J. M. (ed.). Postgrad. Med. J., 50:593, 1974.

Wogan, G. N.: Mycotoxins. Ann. Rev. Pharmacol., 15:437, 1975.

Zen-Yoji, H., Sakai, S., Terayama, T., Kudo, Y., Ito, T., Benoki, M., and Nagasaki, M.: Epidemiology, enteropathogenicity and classification of *Vibrio parahaemolyticus*. J. Infect. Dis., 115:436, 1965.

23. COMMON ACCIDENTAL POISONING

Robert J. Haggerty

DEFINITION. The term "accidental poisoning" is usually limited to clinical illness that results from the introduction of exogenous chemicals into the body. These chemicals may be medications in excessive dose, other chemicals not intended for human metabolism, or biologic products, both plant and animal. The term, however, generally excludes disease produced by toxic products of microorganisms. An accident is (1) an observable tissue or biochemical injury that is (2) unplanned. This definition is too restrictive for accidental poisoning, for in many instances the physician is called upon to treat patients who have only ingested a poison but do not yet have any observable symptoms or signs of tissue or biochemical injury. Also, although most poisonings are unplanned in children, the same tissue or biochemical damage occurs when a chemical is introduced for homicidal or suicidal intent in adolescents and adults.

ETIOLOGY. Accidental poisoning is best understood

TABLE 1. Mortality: Agents Responsible for Accidental Poison Deaths in the United States, 1975*

	Less Than 5 Years of Age	Total All Ages
Medications: Total	65	3132
Salicylates and analgesics	24	1275
Sedatives and hypnotics	3	594
Psychotherapeutic drugs	11	178
Systemic and hematologic	6	61
Other	21	1024
Other substances:		
Total	49	1562
Alcohol	1	391
Petroleum and solvents	21	54
Pesticides	6	30
Heavy metals	2	13
Corrosives	4	16
Other	15	1058
Total poison deaths	114	4694

*From the National Center for Health Statistics, HRA, HEW; Reported in The National Clearinghouse for Poison Control Centers Bulletin, April, 1977.

as a problem of multiple causes — the interaction of an agent (the poison) with a host (the patient) in a particular environment. The major agents and the number of accidental poisoning deaths caused by each are listed in Table 1. In nonfatal accidental poisoning the agents responsible are quite different from those in fatal cases. The most common agents responsible for nonfatal accidental poisoning are listed in Table 2, together with the number of such accidents in different age groups. Strictly speaking, these are the etiologic agents, but to understand why a particular poisoning occurs requires knowledge of the interaction of the agent, environment, and host; this is discussed under Pathogenesis.

The route of entry of the poison (agent) is most often oral for solids and liquids, but may occasionally be by absorption through skin, rectum, or lung, or by parenteral injection.

INCIDENCE. Over 4500 accidental poison fatalities occur each year in the United States. Less than 5 per cent of these fatalities occur in children, but nearly two thirds of all accidental but nonfatal poisonings occur in preschool children. Not so evident from Table 2 is the second peak in the late teens and early twenties owing to suicide attempts. In children there are from 300 to 1000 nonfatal poison ingestions for each poison fatality. Some estimates place the total number of nonfatal poisonings as high as 300,000 to 500,000 per year in children in the United States. It is the most common medical, i.e., nonsurgical, emergency seen in preschool children. In one study, 12 per cent of all two-year-old children had experienced an accidental poisoning within the previous year. In addition to differences in the agents responsible for fatal as compared with nonfatal poisoning, the agents responsible for accidental poisoning vary considerably in their frequency between children and adults. Salicylates are the most common agent involved in children, whereas barbiturates are more common in adults. A multitude of household products (such as cleansers, solvents, and insecticides) are potentially poisonous and are available in the American home. They are more likely to be the cause of childhood than of adult poisonings.

TABLE 2.   Most Common Agents Responsible for Accidental Poisoning Reported to the National Clearinghouse
for Poison Information Centers, 1973

	Total All Ages	5 Years	5–14	15–24	25–44	45 and Over
Medicines	82,904	45,919	5144	15,662	12,001	4178
Internal*	73,086	37,428	4660	15,397	11,799	3802
Aspirin*	9182	6576	691	1347	453	115
Other*	63,904	30,852	3969	14,050	11,346	3687
External*	9818	8491	484	265	202	376
Cleaning and polishing agents	18,598	16,478	874	493	409	344
Petroleum products	5695	4381	505	508	243	58
Cosmetics	9167	8697	266	88	57	59
Pesticides	6414	5079	517	307	342	169
Gases and vapor	886	121	144	213	255	153
Plants	7719	6210	874	487	100	48
Turpentine, paints, etc.	6947	5937	446	300	182	82
Miscellaneous	11,290	8122	1650	718	496	304
Unknown	2140	732	206	618	405	179
Total	307,750	185,023	20,430	50,453	38,290	13,554

*These Totals are included in Medicines.

EPIDEMIOLOGY.   There are more epidemiologic data available on the role of the agent in causing accidental poisoning than on the host and environmental factors, and very few data on the complex interrelations of these three factors in causing accidental poisoning (Wehrle et al.). Most of the available information is of the retrospective epidemiologic type for accidental poisoning in children. It documents incidence by age (peak childhood age one to four years), sex (males more than females, except for the poison suicides of the late teens and early twenties), socioeconomic class (no difference), season (no overall significant variation, although there are some special variations such as medications that are more frequent in the winter and pesticides in the summer), hour of day (peak in midmorning), geographical area (lye and petroleum distillates more common in the South), and place where poisoning occurred (kitchen, bedroom, and bathroom are most common). Death *rate* for all age groups from accidental poisoning has remained steady for the past two decades at about 1 per 100,000 for all age groups. There has been a significant decrease in both the *actual number* of deaths in children under five years of age from accidental poisoning (from 422 in 1958 to 114 in 1975) and in the *rate* (from 2.5 per 100,000 in 1958 to under 1.0 in 1975). At the same time, poison fatalities in all ages rose from 3000 in 1969 to over 4500 in 1975. The most dramatic drop has occurred in aspirin poisoning. Over 20,000 total aspirin ingestions were reported to the National Clearinghouse in 1965 and only about 8000 in 1972, whereas the number of all ingestions reported actually increased. The reasons for the decline in children are probably multiple, but are likely to be from public and professional education, better therapy, safety enclosures for dispensing medicines (Schertz et al.), and limitation of the number of tablets in children's aspirin (1¼ grains) to 36 per bottle.

Since poisonous agents such as aspirin are available in nearly every home, the very real question is why more children are not poisoned when one considers the ubiquity of potentially poisonous agents.

Some children seem peculiarly susceptible to accidental poisoning (Sobel and Margolis). A child with a history of one poisoning episode is nine times as likely to have a second episode in the following year than is a child from a matched control group. Poisoned as compared to nonpoisoned control children appear to have different personalities. They are more impulsive and overactive and are likely to strike back when disciplined, to have more disturbed relationships with their parents, and to have other behavior problems. Their social environment is also different, for their parents are more likely to have marital problems, to be suffering acute illness at the time of the ingestion, or to show a more distant and tense family relationship. Whether this knowledge can lead to identification of the high-risk group before poisoning occurs and whether one can change the incidence of poisoning in this high-risk group are not known; prevention by alteration of social and environmental therapy has never been documented.

Among adults, suicide and homicide by poisoning obviously present a very different epidemiologic picture. Unlike immunization for infectious diseases, no one method of control can be expected to be effective for all types of poisoning.

PREVENTION.   Prevention of accidental poisoning, in spite of these negative statements about its effectiveness, should be attempted by many groups, including physicians. Better labeling of household products and prescriptions is of importance, but it should be remembered that children of the age most often poisoned cannot read. Parents should store such medications in safe places, but locked medicine cabinets are of little practical use because they are usually left unlocked when in use. Physicians treating adults should especially warn grandparents that the digitalis, quinidine, or other potent drugs they are receiving are toxic to small children and are often taken by the child from the grandmother's pocketbook. When prescribing analgesics, especially aspirin, for an acute illness in adults, the physician should warn that those are poisonous to children and should prescribe only the minimal amounts needed for an illness. All prescriptions should be dispensed in safety cap enclosures. New laws also require household cleansers to be dispensed in safety cap containers and should be effective. A common scenario of an accidental poisoning starts with a mother with an influenzal syndrome who may have aspirin prescribed; she falls asleep, and her two-year-old child ingests a fatal amount of aspirin left on the bedside table. Other acute family crises, social as well as medical, also seem to be factors in the pathogenesis of childhood poisoning (Meyer et al.). The physician who cares for such adult crises may be the most effective person to prevent childhood accidental poisonings by seeing that adequate supervision of children is arranged when parents are sick or upset.

Most poisonings in adults are the result of suicide attempts, and of course prevention is aimed at recognition of the person at risk.

Community aspects of poison prevention include public education concerning the hazards of poisons. The Consumer Product Act of 1970 and the Commission Coordinating Safety Packaging Regulations require special labeling of hazardous substances and the listing of toxic ingredients on the label. This important step is but one of many that have been taken by the community in an effort to reduce the frequency of accidental poisoning.

National Poison Prevention Week during the third week in March serves as a focal point for health education programs. But to have any chance of success, such measures should be carried out throughout the year. The rapid development of poison information centers since the first one was formed in Chicago in 1953 to the now more than 500 in the United States is another important community action. The National Clearinghouse for Poison Information Centers of the Public Health Service coordinates activities of the local centers and is a valuable repository of information, both for treatment of poisoned patients and for preventive programs. Several poison information centers now have on-line computer terminals to the National Center for rapid access to information on the ingredients of new products. In addition, many centers now have microfiche systems to facilitate retrieval and standardize treatment. These systems have as many as 200,000 trade-name items indexed and easily accessible. The Association of Poison Control Centers, a voluntary national group, has produced educational material designed to prevent poisonings, has established standards for operation of poison control centers, including an approved list of antidotes, their indications, and doses, and has promoted scientific study of poisonings. The American Academy of Clinical Toxicology and its Board in Clinical Toxicology serve as the academic organization for poison center personnel. These organizations have stimulated research in accidental poisoning. It seems clear that these multiple approaches to prevention of poisoning need to be continued, but there is a need to critically evaluate their effectiveness and to add imaginative new programs aimed at prevention.

DIAGNOSIS. Diagnosis of accidental poisoning is made from (1) the label on the poison container, (2) the characteristic signs and symptoms in the patient, and (3) chemical analyses, in that order of importance. In most cases of acute poisoning, especially in children, there is no problem in determining that ingestion of a poison has occurred. The patient is often observed to ingest the poison or is found with the empty container. Here the problem is only to determine the chemical ingredients of the compound ingested, how much was taken, and what toxicity is to be expected. On the other hand, unlabeled prescriptions or trade-name household products (of which there are estimated to be over 250,000 potentially poisonous ones available in American homes) may present a serious problem in identification of the precise chemical involved. Poison information centers are especially equipped to deal with this aspect of diagnosis, for they keep on file trade names of potentially poisonous products and their ingredients.

Most operate 24 hours a day and are listed in the telephone book. Information on management will also be provided by these centers. Of great use to the physician in diagnosis of poisoning, as well as in therapy, is a book (Gleason et al.) which contains a section with over 17,000 trade-name household products, their ingredients, toxicity, symptoms, and treatment.

When the label is missing, identification of the poison may be aided by knowing that certain ingredients are common to household products used for the same specific purpose; e.g., most solvent cleansers contain ketones or hydrocarbons. Federal labeling legislation, which requires most hazardous household chemicals to bear a label that plainly lists ingredients, has helped in diagnosis. *The label on the container is the single most useful diagnostic bit of information in accidental poisoning.*

When the patient has not been observed to ingest a poison, the problem of diagnosis may be great. Although some poisons produce pathognomonic signs or symptoms, most do not. Almost any acute disease may be simulated, and the range of symptoms and signs that may result is so vast that one can only advise that any symptoms or signs of unknown cause must be suspected of being due to poisoning until proved otherwise. Lists of such symptoms and signs with the various poisons that can produce them are available in standard toxicology texts.

Toxicologic analysis of body fluids or of the ingested substance itself plays a numerically small but important and increasing role in the diagnosis of accidental poisoning. In those instances in which analysis is useful, it is usually much easier to analyze the remains in the container from which the poison came than to analyze body fluids in which great dilution of the poison has occurred. Recent development of chemical analyses by mass spectrometry and gas-liquid chromatography now allows toxic screens for a wide variety of poisons from small amounts of blood. Commercial laboratories provide qualitative analyses for sedatives, narcotics, psychotropics, heavy metals and pesticides, which have made diagnoses much more specific in a period as short as a few hours.

Once the poison that was ingested has been identified, there remains the problem of determining its potential for harm to the patient. This depends on the amount ingested and the toxicity of the agent. The amount can sometimes be estimated by observers who may have seen the patient ingest the poison and by the amount remaining in the container. The toxicity of a particular poison can be assessed by reference to known data on LD_{50} and minimal lethal dose. A table has been prepared that is most useful in then estimating the degree of risk to the patient (Table 3).

TABLE 3. Toxicity Rating*

	Probable Lethal Dose	
Rating	mg/kg	For 70 kg Man
6 — Super toxic	<5	A taste <7 drops
5 — Extremely toxic	5–50	7 drops to 1 tsp
4 — Very toxic	50–500	1 tsp to 1 oz
3 — Moderately toxic	500 mg–5 grams	1 oz to 1 pint
2 — Slightly toxic	5–15 grams	1 pint to 1 quart
1 — Practically nontoxic	>15 grams	>1 quart

*From Gleason, M., Gosselin, R., Hodge, H., and Smith, R.: Clinical Toxicology of Commercial Products. 4th ed. Baltimore, Williams & Wilkins Company, 1973.

TREATMENT. A common mistake in the therapy of acute poisoning is to search for a specific antidote, of which there are very few, and to delay general therapy, which may be very effective and which is all that is available for the majority of poisonings.

General principles of therapy are (1) elimination of the poison from the body, (2) inactivation of the poison, and (3) supportive measures. **Elimination of the Poison.** INDUCED EMESIS. One of the most common poison problems brought to the physician is that of a child or adult who has just ingested a potential poison but is still asymptomatic. The most important part of therapy is removal of the poison from the stomach before significant absorption can occur. It is now clear that gastric lavage, the time-honored method for removal of gastric contents, is much *less* effective than induced vomiting because the stomach normally traps large quantities of material in several pouches inaccessible to the lavage tube. The most effective way to induce vomiting is to administer a large dose of syrup of ipecac (15 ml for a child one to four years old, 30 to 45 ml for adults), followed by a repeat dose if no vomiting occurs within 20 minutes (Robertson). This dose is considerably larger than is recommended in older texts, but it has been found safe and much more rapidly effective than smaller doses. Many physicians now prescribe a 1-ounce bottle of syrup of ipecac when children reach age one in order that parents will have it on hand in case of need. Vomiting is more complete if the patient drinks several ounces of fluid three to five minutes after administration of the syrup of ipecac. Mechanical induction of vomiting by gagging, although having the merit of speed, is so often not effective that it is not the first choice of methods. Parenteral administration of apomorphine has not proved to be useful. Vomiting should be induced even if several hours have elapsed after ingestion, for many poisons remain for long periods in the stomach when ingested in large quantities. Other methods of inducing vomiting such as use of a solution of powdered mustard or soap suds are not very effective.

CAUTIONS REGARDING INDUCED EMESIS. The only contraindications to induced emesis in the treatment of accidental poisoning are in patients who have ingested caustics (e.g., lyes, acids), strychnine, and hydrocarbons, and in the comatose patient. With any cause of altered consciousness, gag reflex may be altered sufficiently to increase the risk of aspiration. Ipecac does work even with ingestion of antiemetics and tranquilizers with antiemetic properties (Verhulst and Thoman). Whether one should remove hydrocarbons by careful gastric lavage is still a disputed point. A collaborative study suggests that it may be of slight advantage, and emesis is less safe and less effective than lavage. Saturated salt and sodium bicarbonate solutions should not be used as emetics.

GASTRIC LAVAGE. Even though less effective than emesis, gastric lavage is indicated for comatose poisoned patients to remove the poison from the stomach with less risk of aspiration than with emesis. A large-bore gastric lavage tube should usually be employed, and the stomach should be irrigated with copious amounts of water or physiologic saline. Aspiration can be prevented by having the patient lie on his side with the head slightly lower than the body. Sodium bicar-bonate should not be used because it increases absorption of many poisons (salicylates) and causes large amounts of carbon dioxide to be released in the stomach, increasing the risk of aspiration.

OTHER METHODS OF POISON REMOVAL. No data are available on the *effectiveness of catharsis* or *colonic irrigations*. Most do not use cathartics today unless activated charcoal is also used, for ipecac will cause catharsis and there is often diarrhea produced by the original poison.

Exchange transfusion has proved useful for removal of some poisons when plasma protein binding makes any form of dialysis less effective, i.e., with boric acid and some barbiturates.

Peritoneal dialysis and hemodialysis are effective means of removing many poisons. For preschool children, and even for many adults, peritoneal dialysis (Etteldorf et al.) is preferred because proper equipment and an experienced team for hemodialysis are less available. Use of commercially prepared solutions that contain properly balanced electrolytes and albumin, together with simple multiple-holed polyethylene tubing for insertion into the peritoneal cavity, provides a relatively convenient and simple technique. In certain adult patients in whom renal failure from the poisoning is the major problem, e.g., ethylene glycol poisoning, or for whom prolonged dialysis is needed, hemodialysis has proved very useful.

The kidney is the most effective organ for removal of many poisons. If renal function was normal prior to the poisoning, this route of excretion should be facilitated by adequate fluids, usually intravenously, and in some situations by the use of *osmotic diuretics*, such as mannitol (Cirksens et al.). In salicylate poisoning renal excretion is enhanced as much as twentyfold by making the pH of the urine alkaline with sodium bicarbonate. Acid diuresis with ammonium chloride for amphetamines and phencyclidine also increases excretion of these weak bases. For patients who are seriously ill, several of these routes of elimination of the poison should be used simultaneously, i.e., gastric lavage, enhancement of urinary excretion, and peritoneal dialysis.

Inactivation of the Poison. A time-honored agent designed to inactivate many poisons has been the "universal antidote" made of two parts charcoal, one part tannic acid, and one part magnesium oxide. This mixture is of no value, but there are new data to support the use of specially prepared activated charcoal to absorb poisons in the intestinal tract. Five to 6 teaspoonfuls of such charcoal (not burnt toast) mixed in a glass of water should be swallowed or administered by gastric tube and then, after absorption has occurred, within 30 minutes, removed from the stomach, followed by saline cathartics to remove the absorbed poisons (Corby and Decker). Neutralization of ingested acids or alkalis is probably of little value, because the tissue necrosis that results from such poisons occurs almost immediately upon contact. The use of demulcents, such as olive oil or milk, makes the patient who has ingested an irritant poison more comfortable but probably does little else and should be avoided if the poison is fat-soluble.

Supportive Measures. More lives are likely to be saved by careful, early, symptomatic treatment of complications such as peripheral vascular collapse, respiratory obstruction, urinary retention, fluid imbalance, and central nervous system excitement or depression than by frantic and usually unsuccessful search for specific antidotes. All these complications are treated by the standard methods that are used when they are due to other causes.

Poisonings for Which Specific Antidotes Exist. *Cyanide poisoning* produces death within minutes. Specific antidotes are available, but unless poisoning occurs in a laboratory there is rarely time to administer them. The antidotes are sodium nitrite injected intravenously (6 to 8 ml per square meter of body surface of a 3 per cent solution at a rate of 2.5 to 5 ml per minute), which produces methemoglobinemia, followed by sodium thiosulfate intravenously (50 ml of a 25 per cent solution). Amyl nitrite inhalation may be of value immediately while the sodium nitrite is being prepared.

Heavy metal poisoning can be successfully treated by various chelating agents — BAL, EDTA, or penicillamine (Ch. 24 and 379).

Iron salts produce acute gastroenteritis, shock, liver necrosis, and, frequently, death. As few as 10 tablets of the usual size (0.3 gram) may be fatal. The specific antidote, desferrioxamine, is useful intravenously to bind absorbed iron (2.0 grams in 5 per cent of levulose solution intravenously, dose 90 mg per kilogram); 140 mg of desferrioxamine can bind about 1 gram of ferrous sulfate — 200 mg of iron. It is contraindicated orally, for it probably enhances absorption. Fluid replacement, including blood plasma, should be used for shock.

Morphine and other opium derivatives can be successfully antagonized by naloxone HCl (adult dose 0.4 mg), repeated up to three times at three-minute intervals. If no improvement occurs, another cause of symptoms should be suspected. Since the action of the antagonist lasts only one to two hours and that of morphine for six or more hours, repeat doses may be needed after two hours (see Ch. 244).

Phosphate ester insecticides such as parathion are powerful anticholinesterases. In addition to peripheral parasympathetic stimulation they produce voluntary muscle paralysis, the most serious being to the muscles of respiration. Red cell cholinesterase is a valuable laboratory test to make the diagnosis and to follow therapy. Atropine in very large doses of 1 mg subcutaneously for a child, 2 to 3 mg for an adult, every 15 to 60 minutes until symptoms subside will antagonize these peripheral parasympathomimetic toxic effects. 2-Pyridine aldoxime methiodide (PAM), a cholinesterase regenerator, is dramatically effective in relieving skeletal muscle paralysis (1 gram intravenously over a five- to ten-minute period and repeated as a slow intravenous drip as needed for respiratory paralysis). Atropine is used first. PAM is not used alone. Airway obstruction must be treated by aspiration, positioning, and occasionally tracheostomy.

Treatment of Specific Common Poisons. A few words should be said about general management of the most common poisonings, but reference to standard texts is necessary for details of treatment of these as well as for the many poisonings that cannot be discussed here.

Amphetamine poisoning is common from an overdose of reducing pills or pep pills. After removal from the stomach, chlorpromazine should be administered in full dose to counteract mania and delirium. Barbiturates should not be used because the late-stage depression that occurs with amphetamines may be compounded.

Atropine poisoning may be produced by overdose or accidental ingestion of the drug or by accidental ingestion of one of several plants, such as the jimson weed. Symptoms include those of parasympathetic blocking, intense erythema, fever, and delirium. Antihistamines and many psychotropic drugs also have anticholinergic action plus central nervous system depression. Physostigmine is a very useful diagnostic agent (dose 0.5 mg for child under five, 1 to 2 mg for child over 10, given slowly intravenously over two to three minutes). It counters both central and peripheral actions.

DDT and other chlorinated hydrocarbon insecticides are relatively uncommon causes of acute poisoning, for fatal doses in man are in the range of 250 mg per kilogram, and this amount is difficult to ingest. Central nervous system stimulation and convulsions are the most serious symptoms. Treatment is entirely symptomatic.

Hydrocarbon ingestion, especially of gasoline and kerosene, produces a severe pneumonia due mainly to direct aspiration into the lung rather than to bloodstream transport to the lungs. Most of the aspiration probably occurs during the initial swallow, but some may also occur during subsequent vomiting. If large amounts have been ingested or the hydrocarbon is a vehicle for some other toxin (i.e., insecticide), removal by emesis is preferable to leaving in the stomach. Controversy still surrounds this recommendation. For the more volatile hydrocarbons, such as charcoal lighter fluid from which central nervous system depression can occur, most now agree it should be removed by emesis. For the low volatile waxes, there is no need to remove.

Probably the only effective therapy for the patient with severe pneumonia is oxygen. Although adrenocortical steroids and prophylactic antimicrobials have been used, there is little evidence that they are the crucial element in successful therapy of this poisoning. Again, lighter fluid is the exception, and adrenal steroids do seem useful for pneumonia caused by this agent.

Carbon tetrachloride produces prompt central nervous system depression and abdominal pain. Early death is due to depression of vasomotor and respiratory centers and convulsions. If the patient survives this, he may develop renal and hepatic necrosis. The management at this stage is the same as for other causes of failure of these organs.

Methyl alcohol can cause severe metabolic acidosis and blindness with a fatal dose from as little as 2 ounces. Treatment includes emesis, ethyl alcohol to inhibit the metabolic oxidation of methanol (whiskey, 30 ml every three to four hours for adults), and sodium bicarbonate intravenously for the metabolic acidosis.

Lye and other caustics produce severe, deep burns of the esophagus that may perforate or may later cause esophageal stenosis. Initial pain, airway obstruction, and shock are treated symptomatically. Early esophagoscopy, to determine whether burns have occurred, is followed by cortisone if burns are found. After several days for healing to progress, careful dilatation of the esophagus can be begun. Management should be a team effort with the esophagoscopist.

Salicylate poisoning is the single most common cause of poisoning in children. Emesis should always be carried out if the patient is awake, even though several hours have elapsed after ingestion. Salicylates produce an initial respiratory alkalosis that is transient in children but less so in adults, followed by severe metabolic acidosis, dehydration, and loss of body potassium. With severe poisoning several routes of elimination may have to be used, i.e., by increasing urinary excretion and by peritoneal dialysis. Initial hydration should be vigorous to initiate brisk diuresis, and the fluids should include sodium bicarbonate, 2 mEq per kilogram given over one hour. Once diuresis has begun, potassium salts, approximately 35 mEq per liter of fluid, should be added to the solution. Monitoring of serum pH and electrolytes and adjustment of fluid and electrolyte administration appropriately are important for optimal therapy. Milder degrees of poisoning can usually be treated with alkali and intravenous fluids alone. Other symptoms, such as respiratory depression or convulsions, are treated symptomatically.

Cirksens, W. J., Bastian, R. C., Malloy, J. P., and Barry, K. G.: Use of mannitol in exogenous and endogenous intoxications. N. Engl. J. Med., 270:161, 1964.

Corby, D. G., and Decker, W. J.: Management of acute poisoning with activated charcoal. Pediatrics, 54:324, 1974.

Etteldorf, J. N., Dobbins, W. T., Summitt, R. L., Rainwater, W. T., and Fischer, R. L.: Intermittent peritoneal dialysis using 5 per cent albumin in the treatment of salicylate intoxication in children. J. Pediat., 58:226, 1961.

Gleason, M., Gosselin, R., Hodge, H., and Smith, R.: Clinical Toxicology of Commercial Products. 4th ed. Baltimore, Williams & Wilkins Company, 1973.

Meyer, R. J., Roelofs, H. A., Bluestone, J., and Redmond, S.: Accidental injury to the preschool child. J. Pediat., 63:95, 1963.

Robertson, W. O.: Syrup of ipecac — a slow or fast emetic? Am. J. Dis. Child., 103:136, 1962.

Rumack, B.: Anticholinergic poisoning: Treatment with physostigmine. Pediatrics, 52:449, 1973.

Schertz, R. G., Latham, G. H., and Stracener, D. E.: Child-resistant containers can prevent poisonings. Pediatrics, 43:84, 1969.

Sobel, R., and Margolis, J. A.: Repetitive poisoning in children: A psychosocial study. Pediatrics, 35:641, 1965.

Verhulst, H. L., and Thoman, M. E.: Ipecac syrup in antiemetic ingestion. JAMA, 196:433, 1966.

Wehrle, P. F., DeFreest, L., Penhollow, J., and Harris, V. G.: The epidemiology of accidental poisoning in an urban population. III. Pediatrics, 27:614, 1961.

24. HEAVY METAL POISONING

Edmund B. Flink

24.1. INTRODUCTION

Many features of poisoning by the heavy metals are similar. The important metals from the standpoint of toxicology are arsenic, lead, mercury, antimony, cadmium, and thallium. The toxic and lethal doses of each metal are small. Antimony, arsenic, lead, mercury, and thallium all have effects on enzymes of the body. Antimony, arsenic, and mercury poison sulfhydryl groups. Mercuric ions even in fairly dilute solutions denature proteins and cause protein precipitation. Thallium and cadmium have recently assumed importance industrially.

Other metals may be toxic also. *Beryllium* intoxication is discussed in Ch. 348.6, and *bismuth, copper, gold, iron, silver, and uranium* intoxications are discussed in Ch. 379. *Barium* ions cause epigastric pain, nausea, vomiting, diarrhea, chills, cramps, muscle contractions, convulsions, hypertension, tachyarrhythmia, and cardiac arrest.

Sodium sulfate or magnesium sulfate should be given immediately to precipitate the barium as sulfate. *Cobalt* was added to beer from 1957 to 1967. Ingestion of large volumes of this beer caused serious and often fatal myocardiopathy. Cobalt has been eliminated as an additive. *Manganese* poisoning occurs in mining and smelting of manganese ores. Damage to the basal ganglia of the brain occurs with attendant Parkinson-like symptoms. When symptoms begin, removal from exposure is mandatory. Proper ventilation of mines and processing plants will prevent intoxication.

Browning, E.: Toxicity of Industrial Metals. New York, Appleton-Century-Crofts, 1969.

Goodman, L. S., and Gilman, A.: Pharmacological Basis of Therapeutics. 5th ed. New York, The Macmillan Company, 1975.

Lee, D. H. K.: Metallic Contaminants and Human Health. New York, Academic Press, 1972.

Vallee, B. L., and Ulmer, D. D.: Biochemical effects of mercury, cadmium, and lead. Ann. Rev. Biochem., 41:91, 1972.

24.2. ARSENIC POISONING

EXPOSURE. Many household and garden pesticides contain arsenous oxide, copper acetoarsenite (Paris green), or calcium or lead arsenate. Drugs that contain arsenic include sodium cacodylate, Fowler's solution, and the arsphenamines (now obsolete). Fowler's solution continues to be used in treatment of asthma in certain regions. Fruits sprayed with insecticides may contain enough arsenic to be toxic. Bootlegged whiskey has occasionally been contaminated with arsenicals. Arsenic trioxide (As_2O_3) or white arsenic has been a favorite for homicidal purposes. Accidental ingestion of arsenic-containing poison continues to be an important source of exposure, especially for children.

Although toxic exposure occurs in a variety of industries, only a few cases are reported. Poisoning does occur among agricultural workers using insecticide spray or dust. Arsine (AsH_3) is a very serious industrial hazard. It is produced accidentally by the exposure of nascent hydrogen to arsenic trioxide.

Arsenic is stored in liver, nervous system, nails, hair, and other viscera and can be detected in them after excretion in urine has ceased. A single dose requires 10 to 70 days for excretion, so accumulation is possible from small daily doses.

The minimal lethal dose of arsenic trioxide (As_2O_3) is 60 to 180 mg, but there is a great variability in susceptibility. The lethal dose of arsine is smaller than this.

MANIFESTATIONS. *Acute poisoning* may be overwhelming and may produce shock and death within 20 minutes to 48 hours. Ingestion of smaller doses causes vomiting, diarrhea, abdominal pain, and muscle cramps, but does not cause corrosion of mucous membranes. If the victim survives acute poisoning, he may recover without sequelae, or he may develop symptoms of chronic poisoning.

Intravascular hemolysis and renal damage are characteristic of arsenic poisoning, so hemoglobinuria, nausea, vomiting, and abdominal pain develop within six hours after exposure. This initial illness may be quickly fatal, or recovery may begin in a few days. Instances of chronic arsine poisoning have been reported.

Chronic poisoning results from repeated ingestion of small doses. This is the usual method for homicide.

Weight loss, diarrhea or constipation, nausea, anorexia, fatigue, drowsiness, peripheral neuropathy, headache, confusion, pigmentation and scaling of the skin, hyperkeratoses of palms and soles, and transverse white lines of all fingernails (Mee's lines) are the important symptoms and signs. Hyperkeratoses may go on to malignant changes in the form of multiple basal cell cancers (Bowen's disease). Perforation of the nasal septum is common. Myocardiopathy induced by arsenic may be fatal.

Hematologic findings of chronic arsenic poisoning include anemia, leukopenia, thrombocytopenia, basophilic stippling, and disturbed erythropoiesis, and myelopoiesis.

DIAGNOSIS. The diagnosis can be established by determining arsenic in the urine. Normal persons excrete an average of 0.015 mg per day, with a range of 0.005 to 0.04 mg. Most patients with manifestations of arsenic poisoning excrete more than 0.1 mg per day.

As in lead poisoning, urine coproporphyrin III excretion is increased markedly, but delta amino levulinic acid is not increased in experimental arsenic poisoning in rabbits and probably not in human intoxication.

Hair and nails store arsenic, so analysis of arsenic content may be of diagnostic value, particularly after removal of the patient from exposure. Hair and nail samples must be very carefully washed to exclude adhering dust and extraneous material. Normal values have ranged from 0.025 to 0.088 mg per 100 grams of hair. Over 0.1 mg per 100 grams is abnormal.

TREATMENT. When a poison has been ingested, immediate induction of emesis or gastric lavage is of prime importance. Dimercaprol or 2,3-dimercaptopropanol (BAL) should be given immediately. The initial intramuscular dose of BAL is 2.5 to 3.0 mg per kilogram of body weight, followed by the same dose every four hours for six doses. For very severe poisoning, the initial dose should be 5.0 mg per kilogram, followed by 2.5 mg per kilogram, as indicated above, with additional doses at 6- to 12-hour intervals for six doses, depending on the status of the patient. BAL has not proved to be effective in arsine poisoning or in chronic poisoning, probably because the damage has already occurred. Removal from exposure in chronic poisoning is mandatory and usually suffices.

Severe anemia must be treated by transfusion. Treatment of acute renal insufficiency requires the same considerations as that resulting from a variety of causes.

PREVENTION. Proper storage and labeling of poisons in general should prevent accidental poisoning of children. Avoiding direct contact with insect sprays and wearing appropriate masks when using dusting powders will control this industrial exposure.

Heyman, A., Pfeiffer, J. B., Jr., Willet, R. W., and Taylor, H. M.: Peripheral neuropathy caused by arsenical intoxication: A study of 41 cases with observation of the effects of BAL. N. Engl. J. Med., 254:401, 1956.

Kyle, R. A., and Pease, G. L.: Hematologic aspects of arsenic intoxication. N. Engl. J. Med., 273:18, 1965.

Vallee, B. L., Ulmer, D. D., and Wacker, W. E. C.: Arsenic toxicology and biochemistry. AMA Arch. Industr. Health 21:132, 1960.

24.3. LEAD POISONING

ETIOLOGY. Exposure to lead in the home is chiefly by ingestion of white lead paint scales by children (pica), from new water systems in which white lead has been used in joints of pipes, by ingestion of soluble lead salts in foods, wines, and distilled liquors, by use of pewter dishes and earthenware dishes with a glass glaze, and by use of tetraethyl lead gasoline for cleaning purposes. Drinking of "moonshine" whiskey distilled by use of an auto radiator as a condenser has resulted in epidemics of acute lead poisoning and constitutes an important cause of lead poisoning of adults.

Ingestion of lead paint scales by young children in areas of poor and old housing constitutes the greatest problem in the United States today. In New York City 4000 cases of lead poisoning were found in 1970 and 1971 because of increased interest and availability of appropriate tests. The incidence in children is greatest in summer months and reaches a peak at the age of one to three years. Black children are at greatest risk. Siblings of children with lead intoxication should be examined also, because about a third of them have been found to have serious exposure.

Lead is dissolved and absorbed from the gastrointestinal tract, deposited in the liver, and then released into the systemic circulation. About 10 per cent of ingested lead is absorbed. The respiratory tract epithelium absorbs lead fumes or may propel particles into the pharynx, where they are swallowed. Thirty to 50 per cent of lead in air is absorbed. Tetraethyl lead and related compounds may be absorbed through the skin. Soluble lead salts, such as lead acetate or lead carbonate, are readily absorbed and can cause acute poisoning when ingested.

There are many industrial uses of lead and, therefore, many opportunities for exposure. In recent years the industrial consumption of lead in the United States has averaged about 1,110,000 tons a year. The industries using or producing lead are petroleum, mining and smelting, storage battery manufacture, printing, paint and pigment, ceramic and glass, construction (mainly plumbing and insulation), ammunition, wrecking and salvage (acetylene torch and electric arc volatilizing lead paints and alloys), battery reclaiming, and brass polishing. Any procedure that produces lead vapor, mist, or dust exposes workers to inhalation and absorption of lead from respiratory tract epithelium. A new source is paint dust generated during restoring old houses with old lead paint.

The lead-using trades have set up standards and checking procedures that have controlled industrial hazards well. Smoking and eating are restricted to uncontaminated areas. Washing hands and changing clothes before eating and leaving work are the most important personal preventive measures. The gasoline industry has rigid standards for tetraethyl lead workers, but exposure to dangerous amounts still occurs when there is a break in procedure. Cleaning and repairing large storage tanks pose a particular hazard.

PATHOLOGY. In chronic poisoning no gross or microscopic lesions are pathognomonic of lead poisoning. Lead is stored in an inert form in bone and is not harmful except when mobilized. Most of the remaining lead is found in the bone marrow, blood, liver, and kidneys. An increased amount of lead in tissues indicates exposure but not necessarily toxicity. Absence of an increased concentration of lead in tissues practically excludes lead poisoning.

In the encephalopathic type, small perivascular hemorrhages, necrosis of cells, and serous exudate around blood vessels may be found anywhere in the brain. In children with acute poisoning, nuclear inclusions are found in liver cells and renal tubular cells. Occasionally inclusions are found in renal tubule cells of lead workers. In Australia chronic lead exposure from the dust of white lead paint has been incriminated as a common cause of chronic renal failure in young adults.

CLINICAL MANIFESTATIONS. Lead posioning is usually divided into acute and chronic forms. Although "chronic poisoning" correctly describes prolonged exposure, manifestations often are acute. It is convenient for descriptive purposes to divide symptomatology into an alimentary form, a neuromuscular form, and an encephalopathic form.

Anemia and attendant pallor and weakness are present in most patients with chronic exposure. *Insomnia, headache, dizziness,* and *irritability* are common symptoms without evidence of more serious encephalopathic disturbances. In a patient with poor oral hygiene, lead sulfide is deposited along the gingival margin of some or all teeth and produces a blue-black *"lead line."* *Stippling of the retina* adjacent to the optic disc has been described as an early sign in lead poisoning. Chronic renal failure results from chronic lead intoxication. *Saturnine gout* is particularly common in lead poisoning from "moonshine" whiskey. The renal clearance of uric acid decreases.

Alimentary Form. *Painter's* or *lead colic* is the most common feature and is the result of spasm of the bowel. Constipation is a natural consequence, and nausea, vomiting, and weight loss are common. Colic is intermittent and often severe enough to double the patient up. Between attacks there is merely a sense of pressure. Absence of tenderness differentiates the condition from appendicitis or other causes of peritoneal inflammation. Relief actually may be produced by pressure on the abdomen. Colic is not invariably present.

Neuromuscular Form. Extensor muscles of the upper extremities are more often paralyzed than flexors or lower extremity muscles. *Wrist drop* is a common and characteristic example. Muscle soreness and stiffness or hypertonus precede and accompany paralysis. The absence of sensory disturbance is important in differentiating this from other forms of peripheral neuropathy. Paralysis is confined to a functional muscle group and is not determined by the distribution of an entire motor nerve. Atrophy may occur after longstanding paralysis and may result in incomplete recovery of muscle function after termination of exposure (see Ch. 335 to 337).

Encephalopathic Form. At present this occurs primarily in children. The diagnosis is not suspected until a large amount of lead has been ingested. Because of the good safeguards in industry now, it rarely occurs in adults and then only after massive exposure to lead fumes or tetraethyl lead in a salvage operation, in cleaning large gasoline storage tanks, or in accidental breaks in techniques. Tetraethyl lead is lipid-soluble, so that exposure results almost exclusively in the encephalopathic form.

The presenting manifestations include *convulsions, aphasia, cortical blindness, mania, delirium,* or *coma.* There may be a history of antecedent behavioral changes such as irritability, insomnia, restlessness, loss of memory, hallucinations, and confusion. In fact, a toxic encephalopathy much like Korsakoff's psychosis may occur in adults.

Children may suddenly become very ill. Increased intracranial pressure may occur and is manifested by projectile vomiting, lethargy, convulsions, and coma. In very young children fontanelles bulge. The optic discs may not reflect increased pressure when the process is very acute in onset. Scattered neurologic findings indicate cerebral and cerebellar abnormalities. Blindness and deafness may occur and persist.

LABORATORY FINDINGS. The hematologic findings depend on the action of lead on hemoglobin synthesis. Lead interferes with enzymes ALA synthetase, ALA dehydrase, and heme synthetase. ALA dehydrase is uniformly low with increased burden of lead. A level of more than 600 IU per 100 ml excludes lead poisoning. ALA and coproporphyrin III accumulate and are excreted in the urine in excessive amounts, and protoporphyrin accumulates in erythrocytes as a result of the blocks in synthetic process. Normally 2 mg of ALA or less is excreted per 24 hours. Lead poisoning results in a 20- to 200-fold increase in excretion of ALA. ALA excretion is a sensitive indicator of lead intoxication. Normally 60 to 280 μg of coproporphyrin is excreted per 24 hours.

In lead poisoning free erythrocyte protoporphyrin (FEPP) ranges from 300 to 3000 μg per 100 ml (normal 15 to 60) and free erythrocyte coproporphyrin (FECP) ranges from 1 to 20 μg per 100 ml (normal 0 to 2). It is noteworthy that iron deficiency anemia and thalassemia result in FEPP values that overlap those of lead poisoning, but the range is not quite as great. If a fresh wet film of blood of a patient with lead poisoning is examined under ultraviolet light, 75 to 100 per cent of the erythrocytes have a red fluorescence. This fluorescence is the result of increased FEPP.

Lead poisoning and *hereditary acute intermittent porphyria* have manifestations that are similar. Both are characterized by colicky abdominal pain, mental symptoms, and paralysis. Acute intermittent porphyria regularly has a great increase in porphobilinogen excretion and uroporphyrin excretion, but lead poisoning usually does not result in excessive excretion of either substance.

Normochromic microcytic anemia, decreased red cell life span, decreased osmotic fragility, but increased mechanical fragility are found. Acute hemolytic anemia with hemoglobinemia, hemoglobinuria, and renal damage occur occasionally in acute poisoning. Death from shock may occur in two to three days. *Basophilic stippling* is nonspecific, is rarely found in tetraethyl lead intoxication, is seldom found in acute poisoning of children, and cannot be relied on for screening purposes. Nevertheless, it frequently furnishes the initial clue for clinical recognition of chronic lead poisoning.

Aminoaciduria, renal glycosuria, fructosuria, hyperphosphaturia, citraturia, and decreased uric acid clearance result from changes in the epithelium of the proximal convoluted tubules. These changes are like those in Fanconi's syndrome. Other toxins also cause these manifestations. The changes are usually reversible.

DIAGNOSIS. In children, particularly, the normal blood level is low. If the higher range is used with the upper limit of some 0.06 mg per 100 grams, children with serious acute poisoning will have normal levels (see accompanying table). In adults the upper limits of

Normal and Abnormal Values in Exposure to Lead

	Adults		
	Normal Industrial Exposure	"Safe" Industrial Exposure	Dangerous Industrial Exposure
Urine mg per liter	Range: 0.00 to 0.06 Mean: 0.03	0.01 to 0.15 0.08	0.08 to 0.4 0.2
Blood mg per 100 grams	Range: 0.01 to 0.05 Mean: 0.03	0.01 to 0.07 0.06	0.07 to 0.2 0.09
Feces mg per specimen	0.25	0.6 to 1.0	1.1+

	Children	
	Normal Range	Poisoning
Blood mg per 100 grams	British series	0 to 0.04	0.04 to 0.4
	American series	0.03 to 0.04	0.06+

normal coincide with the mean of "safe" exposure. Unfortunately, analytical precision is poor, often with poor agreement between laboratories.

A diagnosis of tetraethyl lead intoxication is made on the basis of history of exposure. Urine lead determination is the most valuable test. Blood values may be normal, but ALA dehydrase is low. ALA in urine is a poor indicator of tetraethyl lead poisoning.

Because of the medicolegal implications, it is important to be certain that there is evidence of increased lead excretion. Detection of an earlier exposure may be accomplished by the use of 25 mg per kilogram or a maximum of 1.0 gram of calcium disodium edetate (CaEDTA) in 5 per cent glucose solution intravenously. Striking augmentation of lead excretion to over 1.0 mg per day usually occurs. This proves previous exposure but not intoxication. There are three stages of lead poisoning: increased absorption, physiologic poisoning, and clinical poisoning.

Collection of samples for analysis must be done with great care to avoid contamination. Pyrex bottles or polyethylene flasks should be rinsed with nitric acid and distilled water. Urine and stool specimens should be passed directly into acid-cleaned containers. Tissues should be placed directly in acid-cleaned containers.

Blood now can be collected in special vacutainer 20 ml tubes (Becton, Dickinson Company) with pure gum rubber stoppers. These tubes have been chemically cleaned for lead analyses. The needle is a straight stainless steel tube. Duplicate samples are desirable.

Lead determinations on blood and urine can now be performed quickly and accurately, using an atomic absorption spectrophotometer. All state and many large city departments of health have such facilities available.

TREATMENT. Cessation of exposure is of prime importance. A saline cathartic should be given to rid the gut of any unabsorbed lead before chelation of lead is attempted, especially in the encephalopathic form in children.

Colic may be controlled temporarily by intravenous infusion of 1.0 gram of calcium gluconate. The infusion may be repeated as needed.

Fluid intake should be high unless there is increased intracranial pressure. Electrolyte concentrations should be determined and corrected if abnormal.

Chelation with CaEDTA is now the initial treatment of choice. For moderately severe intoxication of chil-

dren, 50 mg per kilogram is given per 24 hours by deep intramuscular injection in three divided doses for three to five days. For adults, 2 grams per day of CaEDTA is given in 5 per cent glucose solution continuously intravenously for five days. The minimal rest period between courses is two days but the rest period should preferably be 10 to 14 days. Urine should be collected, and an aliquot of the pooled sample should be analyzed for lead. For more severe intoxication, 2,3-dimercaptopropanol (BAL) should be given as the initial medication—4 mg per kilogram per dose intramuscularly in children and 2.5 mg per kilogram per dose intramuscularly in adults. Subsequently, BAL is given simultaneously intramuscularly, but in different sites, with 12.5 mg CaEDTA per kilogram per dose intramuscularly in children and 8.0 mg CaEDTA per kilogram per dose intramuscularly in adults every four hours for five days. In encephalopathy, the course may be extended to seven days if no improvement has occurred by the fourth day. Nephropathy has rarely been reported from therapy. When symptoms are severe, treatment should not be delayed for results of lead analysis but should be started immediately on the basis of clinical diagnosis. The use of oral CaEDTA or D-penicillamine in workers exposed to lead is not effective prophylactically and may be dangerous.

D-Penicillamine not only chelates lead but also supplies sulfhydryl groups. A dose of 30 mg per kilogram up to a total of 2.0 grams per day in four divided doses given orally is satisfactory. It is particularly useful to follow the initial CaEDTA therapy. It has the additional advantages that it can be given orally continuously, and that it is much less toxic than CaEDTA. For moderate lead intoxication, penicillamine is the agent of choice. Successful treatment with CaEDTA or penicillamine results in a return of ALA and coproporphyrin excretion to normal. Erythrocyte protoporphyrin declines very slowly after successful treatment.

The most serious manifestation is lead encephalopathy, which requires prompt and skillful treatment. Increased intracranial pressure may occur suddenly and must be treated vigorously. Infusion of urea solution in a dose of 100 mg per kilogram to 1000 mg per kilogram as 30 per cent urea in 10 per cent glucose solution or of mannitol solution (20 per cent) in a dose of 7 to 10 ml per kilogram can alleviate increased pressure effectively, but the benefit may last only a day or two, and repetition may be necessary. Dexamethasone sodium phosphate in a dose of 10 mg intravenously initially followed by 4 to 6 mg intramuscularly every four to six hours in adults is an effective alternative. Craniotomy may even be required for relief of pressure.

Physiotherapy is important for patients with neuropathy. Splinting to support the weak extremity prevents overstretching of muscles; otherwise, permanent disability can follow.

PROGNOSIS. In the gastrointestinal form the outlook is good for complete recovery after adequate treatment and prevention of re-exposure. Recovery from paralysis is usually complete even after many months of paralysis.

Encephalopathy is very serious. It causes a mortality rate of 25 per cent or more, and often leaves mental retardation and various permanent neurologic lesions in those who survive. In adults permanent blindness, extraocular muscle paralysis, or other lesions may result. The acute form caused by tetraethyl lead either is fatal or is followed by complete recovery. There is great urgency in treatment of this form. One cannot wait to get results of lead analysis before starting treatment.

Albahary, C.: Lead and hemopoiesis. Am. J. Med., 52:367, 1972.
Ball, G. V., and Sorensen, L. B.: Pathogenesis of hyperuricemia in saturnine gout. N. Engl. Med., 280:1199, 1969.
Beattie, A. D., Moore, M. R., and Goldberg, A.: Tetraethyl-lead poisoning, Lancet, 2:12, 1972.
Browder, A. A., Joselow, M. M., and Louria, D. B.: The problem of lead poisoning. Medicine, 52:121, 1972.
Chisholm, J. J.: Treatment of lead poisoning. Mod. Treatment, 8:593, 1971.
Feldman, F., Lichtman, H. C., Oransky, S., Ana, E. S., Reiser, L., and Malemud, C. J.: Serum delta aminolevulinic acid in plumbism. J. Pediat., 74:917, 1969.
Guinee, V. F.: Lead poisoning. Am. J. Med., 52:283, 1972.

24.4. MERCURY POISONING

ETIOLOGY. Acute mercury poisoning results from accidental or intentional ingestion of soluble mercuric salts such as mercuric chloride ($HgCl_2$, corrosive sublimate) and is characterized by very serious corrosive effects on the entire gastrointestinal tract and serious renal tubular cell damage.

Mercury is a liquid and is highly volatile at room temperature. In 1957 over 4 million pounds of mercury were used in the United States. It is used widely in medical research and clinical pathology laboratories, as well as in the manufacture of scientific instruments, electric meters, mercury vapor lamps, amalgams with copper, tin, silver or gold, in solders, and in the production of organic mercurial compounds. Mining cinnabar (HgS), refining mercury from it, and cleaning mercury distilling apparatus involve substantial hazards. Photoengraving, bronzing, and the production of certain paint colors such as vermilion and antifouling agents for hulls of ships all use mercury compounds.

As little as 0.1 gram of $HgCl_2$ may cause poisoning, but fatal doses are usually in excess of 1.0 gram. It is caustic and produces cell destruction by protein precipitation on direct contact. In more dilute solutions, such as concentrations effected by absorption from the intestinal tract after ingestion of a toxic dose, its effect is primarily due to selective affinity for sulfhydryl (-SH) groups of proteins, especially of enzymes. This property is counteracted by dimercaprol.

Chronic mercury poisoning results from inhalation of mercury vapor or ingestion of small amounts of mercuric nitrate or other salts, and is characterized by mental symptoms and stomatitis.

Alkyl mercury compounds (ethyl and methyl mercury) have become an important environmental problem. Alkyl mercury compounds are more readily absorbed than inorganic mercury or compounds. The compounds are soluble in organic solvents, and the covalent carbon-mercury bond is not degraded by biologic processes. Methyl mercury particularly is found in tuna and swordfish taken from waters heavily contaminated with mercury. Epidemics have occurred in Minamata and Niigata, Japan, and in several countries where seed grain treated with alkyl mercury compounds (as antifungal agents) has been diverted into food. Nearly complete intestinal absorption occurs; the liver excretes most of it into the intestine, resulting in continuous enterohepatic circulation. Methyl mercury passes the placental barrier very well and accumulates in the fetus with resultant cerebral palsy and mental retardation of the child.

ACUTE POISONING

See Ch. 379.

CHRONIC POISONING

CLINICAL MANIFESTATIONS. Stomatitis. Excessive salivation and a metallic taste are common. A blue line develops along the gingival margin. Gums become hypertrophied, bleed easily, and are sore. The teeth become loose.

Erethism. The term "erethism" is applied to the psychic disturbance characterized by irritability, shyness, and deterioration of family and social activities, suggesting hyperthyroidism. Since felt hat makers formerly used mercury salts in the manufacturing process and often became "mad," these symptoms gave rise to the phrase "mad as a hatter."

Tremors. Tremors of the eyelids, lips, tongue, fingers and extremities are characteristic of chronic poisoning. Coarse jerky movements and gross incoordination interfere with fine movements such as writing and eating. Atrophy of the cerebellar cortex and, to a lesser extent, of the cerebral cortex occurs. Microscopic changes occur in the granular layer of the cerebellum, ganglion cells, and posterior columns.

Nephrotic Syndrome. Contact with ammoniated mercury and other compounds has caused proteinuria and frank nephrotic syndrome. Removal from exposure is mandatory, so a careful history of medicinal or occupational exposure is needed.

Hypersensitivity. Hypersensitivity reactions to mercurial diuretic agents include asthma, urticaria, exfoliative dermatitis, and sudden death. Fatal accidents can be prevented by avoiding intravenous injections. Death is usually due to ventricular fibrillation.

Hypersensitivity to calomel (HgCl) results from long-term ingestion of HgCl. Hypersensitivity to ammoniated mercury or other compounds results from topical application. Fever, morbilliform rash, leukopenia, eosinophilia, and enlargement of the spleen and lymph nodes characterize this condition. Mercury fulminate used in percussion caps and detonators may cause dermatitis of exposed parts, with pruritus, papules, vesicles, and pustules.

Acrodynia or "Pink Disease." This disorder of infants and young children is characterized by irritability, insomnia, stomatitis, loss of teeth, hypertension, erythema of fingers, toes, nose, cheeks, and buttocks, and even acral gangrene. Fever, leukocytosis, and albuminuria occur. In 1948 Warkany and Hubbard suggested that sensitivity to mercury might be the cause, and that hypothesis is now fairly generally accepted. The diagnosis is established by finding excretion of more than 0.1 mg of mercury per day in the urine. An organic mercury compound, phenyl mercuric propionate, has been incorporated into house paint to prevent growth of mold. This paint has been incriminated as a'source of toxic exposure.

ORGANIC MERCURY INTOXICATION

Ethyl and methyl mercury compounds have an affinity for the central nervous system and produce fatigue, headache, loss of memory, apathy, emotional instability, paresthesia, generalized ataxia, deafness, dysarthria, progressive visual deterioration, dysphagia, and, occasionally, coma and death. Changes in the central nervous system similar to the lesions of chronic mercury poisoning are found.

DIAGNOSIS. Industrial exposure and characteristic symptoms usually make recognition of chronic mercury poisoning relatively straightforward, but, in the absence of known exposure, the diagnosis may be elusive. Patients with chronic mercury poisoning excrete in excess of 0.3 mg of Hg per liter of urine. Normal values range from 0.0001 to 0.001 mg per liter. An excretion of 0.1 mg per liter is considered evidence of toxic exposure. In instances of exposure to metallic mercury for more than five years, a brown reflex from the anterior lens capsule can be seen by slit lamp. Some observers consider it an early sign of mercury poisoning. Albuminuria and hematuria are common findings in chronic poisoning.

TREATMENT. Removal of the patient from all possible exposure is of paramount importance. The use of BAL in chronic poisoning has not been established as effective treatment. However, n-acetyl-DL-penicillamine, in a dose of 500 mg four times a day, increases mercury excretion and has been used successfully in therapy of chronic mercury poisoning and acrodynia. This treatment is ineffective in methyl mercury poisoning, but promising results have been obtained here, using ion-absorbing resin to interrupt the enterohepatic circulation of mercury.

PROGNOSIS. Recovery is slow even after removal from exposure. Patients with advanced intoxication fare poorly. Only 15 per cent of the more severely involved patients recovered completely in one series. Signs of cerebellar and cerebral damage persisted and prevented return to normal activities.

PREVENTION. Removal of $HgCl_2$, calomel, and mercury ointments from the market would eliminate acute poisoning and many instances of chronic poisoning. Good safe substitutes are available for each compound. Elimination of mercuric nitrate from the felt-processing industry has already occurred. Mercury salts for fingerprinting by police departments have been replaced by barium, zinc, or bismuth. Silver has replaced mercury in the manufacture of mirrors. Stopping discharge of all mercury-containing waste will eventually stop methyl mercury contamination of fish. This has been clearly demonstrated in Sweden.

Mercury-containing paints should have a warning label "For Outside Use Only." Mercury cannot be replaced in many electrical apparatuses and scientific instruments. Proper exhaust ventilation, scrupulous avoidance of any exposed metallic mercury, and good personal hygiene are necessary precautions. The maximal allowable concentration of Hg has been set at 0.1 mg per cubic meter of air. Medical supervision is necessary wherever potential exposure exists. Neurologic signs and especially visual field changes, tremor, ataxia, and dysarthria are serious danger signals.

Amin-Zaki, L., Majeed, M. A., Clarkson, T. W., and Greenwood, M. R.: Methyl mercury poisoning in Iraqui children: Clinical observations over two years. Br. Med. J., 1:613, 1978.

Battigelli, M. C.: Mercury toxicity from industrial exposure. A critical review of the literature. J. Occup. Med., 2:337, 1960.

Hirschman, S. Z., Feingold, M., and Boylen, G.: Mercury in house paint as a cause of acrodynia. N. Engl. J. Med., 269:889, 1963.

Joselow, M. M., Louria, D. B., and Browder, A.: Mercurialism. Environmental and occupational aspects. Ann. Intern. Med., 76:119, 1972.

24.5. ANTIMONY POISONING

Antimony and potassium tartrate (tartar emetic) is used for emetic purposes, and other organic antimony compounds are used in treatment of schistosomiasis, filariasis, and certain fungal infections. Antimony is encountered in metallurgic processes, mining and smelting, and in rubber manufacturing, but industrial poisoning is rare. Finely divided antimony is more toxic than compounds of antimony. Trivalent antimony combines with sulfhydryl groups of enzymes. The symptoms of acute poisoning are similar to those of acute arsenic poisoning. Vomiting is a prominent symptom. Dimercaprol (BAL) is an effective agent for treatment of antimony poisoning, and the regimen is like that for arsenic and mercury. Dermatitis and conjunctivitis occur from exposure to dust in the smelting process. Stibine (SbH_3) is more volatile than arsine and is very toxic also. It attacks the central nervous system and causes acute hemolysis. Death occurs when there is a 0.01 per cent concentration in the air. The chemical process of formation and the effects are like those of arsine.

24.6. CADMIUM POISONING

Cadmium sulfide is associated with zinc minerals and particularly with zinc sulfide. Cadmium exposure can occur in the manufacture of alloys, vapor lamps, and storage batteries, grinding and polishing alloys, cadmium plating, welding, zinc ore smelting, and glass blowing. Inhalation of cadmium fumes results in pulmonary edema, followed in two to three days by proliferative interstitial pneumonia. Various degrees of permanent lung damage and fibrosis occur. Cadmium can be inhaled in fatal concentrations without enough discomfort to warn the worker. The inhalation of fumes with cadmium produces dryness of throat, cough, headache, vomiting, sensation of constriction in the chest, severe dyspnea, and prostration. There is no effective treatment except symptomatic treatment of pulmonary edema. Pulmonary emphysema is the principal effect of industrial exposure. Cadmium is known to be carcinogenic. It has been implicated in the pathogenesis of hypertension, but this is not established.

Foods prepared and stored in cadmium-plated containers may be contaminated sufficiently to cause poisoning. Cadmium ingestion usually does not produce fatal poisoning, but causes rather violent gastrointestinal symptoms, with sudden onset 20 to 30 minutes after eating.

Chronic poisoning from food occurs particularly in Japan. There, a great deal of mining of cadmium, lead, and zinc sulfide, as well as zinc and cadmium smelters, contaminates the streams. Water is used for irrigation of rice fields, so rice is contaminated. Chronic cadmium poisoning is endemic in these areas. A disease called "itai-itai byo" or "ouch-ouch" disease is due to severe osteomalacia which causes pain. It primarily affects women 40 to 70 years old. A Fanconi-like renal dysfunction occurs with proteinuria (largely globulins), phosphaturia, and glucosuria. This leads to typical severe osteomalacia with kyphosis, pseudofractures, and waddling gait. Osteomalacia occurs only in Japan, but the renal lesion occurs in chronic cadmium poisoning in both men and women elsewhere. Vitamin D in large doses sometimes affords relief of pain. A number of deaths have occurred, primarily from severe osteomalacia.

Friberg, L., Piscator, M., Nordberg, G. F., and Kjellström, T.: Cadmium in the Environment. 2nd ed. Cleveland, C.R.C. Press, 1974.

24.7.   THALLIUM POISONING

Thallium sulfate (Tl_2SO_4) is an extremely toxic cumulative poison (lethal dose 0.2 to 1.0 gram). It has a mild metallic taste. Thallium is absorbed from the gut and from the intact skin. It has had wide use as a rodent, ant, and cockroach poison. Because of serious and frequent accidental and deliberate (homicidal) toxicity, the U.S. Department of Agriculture banned thallium formulations for household use in 1965. Unfortunately, some of it can still be found on shelves in homes and stores.

Alopecia is a very important and unique sign. *Accumulation in nervous tissue* accounts for critical symptoms which include ataxia, choreiform movements, vomiting, constipation, restlessness, delirium with hallucinations and delusions, and, finally, coma. Blindness, loss of other special senses, facial paralysis, paresthesias, and peripheral neuropathy occur. Central lobular necrosis of the liver and renal damage also occur. Liver radiopacity increases in some patients. Urinary excretion of 10 mg per day or more indicates serious poisoning.

Various therapeutic trials, including dithiocarb, dithizone, BAL, and KCl, have been used but either have failed to bring improvement or may even be dangerous because of mobilization of thallium and redistribution to the brain. Gastric lavage should be done immediately after diagnosis up to four hours after exposure. Prussian blue (potassium ferric hexacyanoferrate II) is an excellent chelator of thallium by exchange of potassium for thallium. Prussian blue is not absorbed from the gut and is nontoxic. The recommended dose of colloidal solution is 250 mg per kilogram per day in two to four divided doses. A vigorous laxative such as castor oil is necessary for the first day or two. After this an osmotic agent such as 50 ml of 15 per cent mannitol solution will suffice. Therapy should continue until thallium excretion is less than 0.5 mg per 24 hours.

Barbier, F.: Treatment of thallium poisoning. Lancet, 2:965, 1974.
Huff, J. E.: Special communication: Thallium poisoning. Clin. Toxicol., 5:89, 1972.
Kamerbeck, H. H., Rauws, A. G., TenHam, M., and VanHeijst, A. N. P.: Prussian blue therapy of thallotoxicosis. Acta Med. Scand., 189:321, 1971.

25.   CARBON MONOXIDE POISONING

Bertram D. Dinman

DEFINITION.   Carbon monoxide, a product of incomplete combustion of carbonaceous materials, is an odorless, colorless gas; its density is slightly less than air. The gas is commonly produced by the internal combustion engine, poorly vented heating devices, or gas refrigerators. Certain industrial operations such as those associated with blast furnaces and coke ovens, foundry cupolas, petroleum refineries, and underground mines also present risks of serious carbon monoxide intoxication. Less severe but potential exposures may exist in automobile repair shops, among traffic policemen, or in arc welding. Frank intoxication caused by vehicular exhausts is usually due to impaired integrity of exhaust systems and/or the automobile body. Poisoning associated with engine operation for in-car heating purposes occurs only with such defects or when the motor is run in confined spaces, e.g., deep snowdrifts, garages. Natural gas has replaced manufactured gas in the United States; since the former is free of carbon monoxide, illuminating gas per se no longer presents any risk of injury. However, carbon monoxide may be produced by the incomplete combustion of natural gas in faulty heating or other gas-burning apparatus. The most common human exposure to carbon monoxide is associated with smoking. Chronic cigarette smokers develop 3 to 8 per cent carboxyhemoglobin (COHb) concentrations. Although the foregoing exogenous sources of carbon monoxide have long been recognized, the phenomenon of endogenous carbon monoxide production is now well established; as a result of cleavage of the α-methylene bridge in the heme portion of hemoglobin, 0.3 to 1.0 ml per hour is normally produced. This leads to a normal blood COHb concentration of 0.5 to 0.8 per cent.

In contrast to the preceding anthropogenic sources of carbon monoxide, it has been estimated that approximately 3 to 25 times as much carbon monoxide is formed by natural processes. These sources of carbon monoxide are derived from atmospheric oxidation of biochemically produced methane, various free-floating components of the oceanic biomass, photo-oxidation of plant-produced terpenes, volcanic activity, and forest fires.

PATHOGENESIS.   Since carbon monoxide usually exists in a gaseous form, the only significant portal of entry is via the respiratory tract. The gas diffuses across the alveolar membrane in amounts proportional to the pressure gradient for carbon monoxide between alveolar air and blood. The rate of uptake is directly proportional to the respiratory rate, duration of exposure, and carbon monoxide concentration in air. The high affinity of carbon monoxide for hemoglobin (218 times greater than that of oxygen) is responsible for its primary pathologic effect, i.e., reduction of erythrocytic oxygen-carrying capacity. As a result, all signs, symptoms, and pathologic alterations are those of tissue hypoxia. In addition to reducing blood oxygen tension, carbon monoxide in association with hemoglobin (i.e., carboxyhemoglobin) impedes that pigment's discharge of oxygen at the capillary bed. Thus capillary oxygen tensions must be decreased lower than normal in order to dissociate oxygen from the erythrocyte to the tissues. This impairment of oxygen dissociation is expressed by a shift in the oxyhemoglobin curve to the left. Such effects are further complicated in that respiratory chemoreceptors respond only to decreased blood oxygen tension; since this is not decreased (i.e., there is simply a decrease in blood oxygen content), physiologic compensatory mechanisms are not brought into play.

Aside from the formation of carboxyhemoglobin and the resultant hypoxia, there is little evidence that carbon monoxide has any significant direct effect upon tissue except at high carboxyhemoglobin concentrations.

PATHOLOGY. Carboxyhemoglobin is characteristically cherry red in color. Accordingly, the tissues and skin of poisoned individuals always grossly present a characteristic pink color when blood levels of carboxyhemoglobin exceed 30 per cent concentration levels. (Rarely, severely poisoned individuals may not manifest this change at autopsy; this results from reduction of COHb below the 30 per cent level owing to therapeutically induced respiratory clearance prior to death.) The skin may present areas of vesiculation and ulceration at pressure points. Ischemic necrosis of the cardiac papillary muscles and renal tubular degeneration may be noted. Although animal experiments suggest that repeated carbon monoxide exposures may accelerate the development of coronary atherosclerosis, the design of these experiments makes extrapolation of the results to humans difficult. Although the brain of patients dying of acute intoxication (i.e., within the first 24 hours) is congested, pink, and edematous, under these conditions this organ does not usually demonstrate specific, localized degenerative lesions. However, those surviving this acute episode can later develop diffuse degenerative changes prominently involving the cerebral cortex, globus pallidus, cerebellum, and basal ganglia. It is frequently stated that carbon monoxide–induced lesions have a predilection for certain locations in the brain, e.g., basal ganglia, hippocampal region, but in fact a consistent pattern of brain localization is not evident.

CLINICAL MANIFESTATIONS. This disease is characteristically an acute poisoning. Although chronic forms of carbon monoxide intoxication have been claimed to exist, they are not adequately documented. Repeated episodes of mild acute poisoning can occur without cumulative effects.

The clinical picture of carbon monoxide poisoning is closely correlated with the blood concentration of carboxyhemoglobin. Although levels of less than 10 per cent COHb are said to produce no clinical effects, subtle changes of central nervous system function have been consistently demonstrated at the 5 to 20 per cent COHb level (e.g., increased visual threshold, impaired higher cognate function). In addition, precipitation of anginal episodes has been noted in patients with coronary artery disease during exercise with COHb levels of 3 to 5 per cent.

Although frontal, bandlike headaches may be experienced in the 10 to 20 per cent COHb range, more commonly these occur at the upper reaches of this range. In the 20 to 30 per cent COHb range the headaches become more severe. Dyspnea on exertion may be the only other manifestation. At the 30 to 40 per cent COHb levels, headaches become very severe, and are associated with nausea and vomiting, weakness, dizziness, dimness of vision, and possibly collapse. At the 40 to 50 per cent COHb level, ataxia, syncope, and collapse may be observed, in addition to tachycardia and tachypnea. As blood levels of 50 to 60 per cent COHb supervene, there may be coma associated with intermittent convulsions, and Cheyne-Stokes respiration may develop. In the 60 to 70 per cent COHb range, coma deepens, intermittent convulsions occur, and there is clinical shock. Death may terminate such exposures, although profound shock, respiratory and cardiovascular failure, and death have been reported to be delayed until 70 to 80 per cent COHb concentrations are attained. In severe cases, leukocytosis, proteinuria, glycosuria, hematuria, and cylindruria are usually demonstrated, in addition to temperature elevation of 39° C or more.

In contrast to the relatively high levels of carboxyhemoglobin required to produce the foregoing clinical symptoms in otherwise healthy individuals, special susceptibilities among other segments of the population are becoming more clearly defined. Individuals with symptomatic arteriosclerotic heart disease experience a more rapid onset of anginal symptoms when exercised at carboxyhemoglobin levels of 2.5 per cent. Likewise, fetal carboxyhemoglobin levels are 10 to 15 per cent greater than the maternal concentration at steady-state conditions. This enhanced exposure potential for the fetus is further aggravated by the relatively slower rate of elimination of carbon monoxide by the fetus than by the mother. Aside from a decreased birth weight similar to that seen in altitude-induced hypoxia, the clinical implications of these observations as regards carbon monoxide effects on the fetus are not clear.

DIAGNOSIS. Diagnosis is established by quantitative determination of blood carboxyhemoglobin concentration; analysis of alveolar air for carbon monoxide correlates well with blood COHb. The method of Coburn, utilizing a nondispersive infrared meter, is highly accurate; the hydrogen flame–ionization detector equipped gas chromatograph provides the highest level of sensitivity. Although spectrophotometry has long been used, its sensitivity and specificity are less than with more modern techniques.

The cherry-red skin and mucous membrane coloration are highly characteristic of carbon monoxide poisoning. However, it is not readily detected until a 30 to 35 per cent COHb concentration is attained.

TREATMENT. The patient must be immediately removed from the contaminated environment. In mild cases clearance of carbon monoxide from the blood is spontaneously accomplished if respiration is sustained. Fresh air and absolute rest are sufficient in such cases; attempts at exertion of any type within four to six hours can cause a rapid recrudescence of signs and symptoms. In the event of unconsciousness — no matter how transient — hospital management and emergency treatment are indicated. Respiration must be sustained by whatever method is available — i.e., artificial respiration, intermittent positive pressure breathing apparatus. Regardless of the level of COHb initially found, normal air breathing will result in 50 per cent clearance of blood carbon monoxide in about 250 to 300 minutes; 100 per cent oxygen inhalation will achieve a similar reduction of carbon monoxide loading in 35 to 80 minutes, and oxygen at three atmospheres of pressure results in the same clearance in about 25 minutes. The use of a 95 per cent oxygen–5 per cent carbon dioxide mixture hastens oxygenation, largely owing to the Bohr shift.

Persistence of coma and the presence of shock require the usual supportive treatments. Induction of hypothermia may help prevent irreversible brain damage.

PROGNOSIS. Patients who do not become comatose usually recover without permanent sequelae. Persistence of hyperthermia, shock, or acute hypoxia-induced clinical laboratory signs for two days after intoxication holds a grave prognosis. Among those who survive such severe intoxication, a small proportion will demonstrate residual changes — e.g., major seizures, dysphasia, parkinsonism or varying degrees of hyperkinesia, mental impairment. Such severely affected patients usually manifest such signs within one week of the acute episode. However, in approximately half of these severe cases there may be apparent recovery followed by relapse after a latent period of one to three weeks. In either case, if recovery is to supervene, it should be expected within two years of the acute episode.

Carbon Monoxide, Report of the Committee on Carbon Monoxide, Committee on Medical and Biological Effects of Environmental Pollutants. Washington, D.C., National Research Council–National Academy of Sciences, 1977.

Coburn, R. F. (ed.): Biological effects of carbon monoxide. Ann. N.Y. Acad. Sci., 174:430, 1970.

Haldane, J.: The action of carbonic oxide in man. J. Physiol., 18:430, 1895.

Meigs, J. W.: Acute carbon monoxide poisoning. An analysis of one hundred five cases. AMA Arch. Indust. Hyg. Occup. Med., 6:344, 1952.

Peterson, J. E., and Stewart, R. D.: The post-exposure relationship of carbon monoxide in blood and expired air. Arch. Environ. Health, 21:165, 1970.

Richardson, J. C., Chambers, R. A., and Heywood, P. M.: Encephalopathy of anoxia and hypoglycemia. Arch. Neurol., 1:178, 1959.

Shillito, F. H., Drinker, C. K., and Shaughnessey, T. J.: The problem of nervous and mental sequelae in carbon monoxide poisoning. JAMA, 106:669, 1936.

26. DISORDERS DUE TO HEAT AND COLD

Paul Webb

26.1. INTRODUCTION

When thermoregulation fails or is overwhelmed, life-threatening disorders develop from severe heat stress or cold stress. Profound hypothermia is the result of serious loss of body heat, whereas a major accumulation of body heat produces heat stroke. Both conditions require prompt and vigorous treatment. There are other, less serious disorders from heat exposure, in which heat is not stored in large quantity; these are the more common and more easily managed heat syncope and heat exhaustion. Cold and heat can cause local tissue injury, of course, as in frostbite, immersion foot (see Ch. 368.3), and burns, but this chapter deals only with the general disorders.

26.2. HEAT STROKE

A medical emergency, heat stroke is easily diagnosed when it is expected. Thus when military men begin

training in hot climates or when seamen work in the engine rooms and galleys of ships in tropical waters, heat casualties are common, and some of them may be heat stroke. In young, healthy men who have been working hard in heat, unconsciousness, high body temperature, strong rapid pulse, and hot flushed skin are presumptive evidence of heat stroke in the absence of another obvious diagnosis such as head injury or massive infection. But in older people who have not been exerting themselves in hot work places, the diagnosis of heat stroke is not so obvious. Deaths from "excessive heat and insolation" in the United States range from 1 to 12 per 100,000 in people over 65, and many cases are missed or not reported. Heat deaths in the elderly are presumably similar in mechanism to classic heat stroke.

Prodromal symptoms, which may not be notable, include faintness, dizziness, staggering, headache, and nausea. There is a clear history of heat exposure or of heavy exertion in heat. Classically the patient in heat stroke is unconscious, although any degree of impairment of the central nervous system may present initially, from lethargy, confusion, or irrational agitation, to coma and convulsions. The body temperature is high, 40° C or higher measured in the rectum; but if the patient is not seen immediately, and if even simple measures have been started to relieve heat stress and to start cooling, the body temperature may be lower. The pulse is strong, and its rate is usually 140 or higher. Blood pressure measurement will show a normal or elevated systolic pressure and a lowered diastolic pressure. However, in the late and severe stage of the disorder, blood pressure is low as the circulation fails. The skin is flushed, and sweating may be present, or — a bad sign — reduced or absent. Heat stroke is easily distinguishable from heat syncope or heat exhaustion, with their mildly elevated body temperatures, transient disturbances of consciousness, and mild circulatory signs. Heat stroke results from excessive heat storage, with high cardiac output, cutaneous vasodilation, and low peripheral resistance. Cessation of sweating and circulatory failure are late signs. There is evidence that the heart failure is right-sided, with low resistance in the systemic circulation and high resistance in the pulmonary circulation.

One should not always expect to see all the signs of heat stroke in an elderly person whose circulatory function is not what it used to be, and in whom there may be some pre-existing infectious disease. The diagnosis should be thought of if body temperature stays high and circulation is failing. Heat deaths during heat waves typically increase one or two days after the heat wave begins, and continue for one or two days after it is over. Predisposing factors are age, obesity, lack of acclimatization, and preceding infection or gastrointestinal upset.

The greater the heat storage and the longer it has been present, the worse the prognosis. Damage is done by general cellular degeneration and widespread hemorrhages, especially those in the central nervous system, kidneys, and liver. Laboratory findings in severe cases include reduced blood coagulation, low prothrombin, and low platelet count; low urine volume, high specific gravity, albumin, and renal casts; elevated blood urea; hemoconcentration; low serum potassium and normal to high serum chloride; changes in liver function; elevation of serum enzymes; and a hyperdynamic circulatory pattern unless circulatory failure has already developed.

Treatment of heat stroke should begin at once. Its aim is to lower body temperature and to support the circulation. Effective cooling methods, in ascending order of effectiveness, are wet towels and a strong fan in a cool dry room; icebags over much of the body; water-cooled sheets such as are used to induce hypothermia; and a tub bath of cold water. The higher the body temperature, the more aggressive the cooling technique should be. Sedation may be needed to control the patient, who may struggle or who may begin to convulse. A tranquilizing cocktail of pethidine, chlorpromazine, and phenergan may be used to prevent both convulsions and shivering, or simpler means of calming a person may suffice. Cooling should be continued until the rectal temperature goes below 38° C. After the initial lowering of body temperature, continued temperature monitoring is vital, for strong cooling may produce an after-drop of temperature, and somewhat later, patients will often start to store heat again despite being in a thermally comfortable environment.

Shock must be treated with fluid replacement and possibly isoproterenol. Fluid therapy should be started judiciously, with the amount and electrolyte content guided by laboratory findings. Other supportive measures are begun when problems are identified, e.g., platelet transfusions or renal dialysis.

Ellis, F. P.: Mortality from heat illness and heat-aggravated illness in the United States. Environ. Res., 5:1, 1972.
O'Donnell, T. F., Jr., and Clowes, George H. A., Jr.: The circulatory abnormalities of heat stroke. N. Engl. J. Med., 287:734, 1972.
Shibolet, S., Coll, R., Gilat, T., and Sohar, E.: Heatstroke: Its clinical picture and mechanism in 36 cases. Quart. J. Med., 36:525, 1967.

26.3. HEAT SYNCOPE

A person who becomes dizzy or suddenly tired after exercising in the heat may abruptly faint. As soon as he is recumbent, and especially if he is removed from direct exposure to heat, he recovers. In contrast to the patient with heat stroke, the person with heat syncope has a cool, sweaty, pale skin; his pulse is weak and either mildly elevated — 100 to 120 beats per minute — or slow, as in vasovagal syncope. His blood pressure falls just before fainting, and recovers quickly when he lies down or sits with head lowered.

Lack of acclimatization and lack of training for the exercise undertaken predispose to heat syncope. Cutaneous vasodilation and blood pooling in the erect position contribute to the hypotension. Treatment is a matter of allowing the person to rest, cool down a little, and drink some extra liquid.

26.4. HEAT EXHAUSTION

Taking much longer to develop than heat syncope (often several days), heat exhaustion results from loss of fluid or loss of fluid and salt. The symptoms of prolonged water depletion are thirst, fatigue, giddiness, elevated body temperature, oliguria, and finally delirium. The water depletion results from sweating and inadequate replacement by drinking, whether voluntary or involuntary. Voluntary dehydration in heat — the failure to replace water loss even though water is avail-

able — is common, but most people catch up at the end of the day when they get out of the heat. In the tropics it is sometimes not possible to cool off at night or keep up with water replenishment. This causes problems for the non-native dweller especially.

When both water and salt become depleted, muscle cramps are added to the picture of fatigue, nausea, and giddiness. The urine chloride will be low to absent, and serum chlorides reduced.

Heat exhaustion is treated by rest in bed away from heat, and restoration of body water, or water and electrolytes. Cool liquids should be given by mouth, up to 6 or 8 liters the first day. If body temperature does not return to normal spontaneously, alcohol sponging or wet towels and a fan may be used. If the patient cannot drink, intravenous therapy should be started. Continuation of fluid and electrolyte replacement should be guided by laboratory analyses.

Prevention of heat exhaustion is a matter of ensuring an adequate fluid intake, which means enough to replace losses from sweating. These losses can be as high as 6 to 8 liters per day in men working hard in hot dry conditions. People who are not yet acclimatized to heat need supplemental salt, because their sweat contains more electrolyte than that of the acclimatized. A daily intake of 15 to 25 grams of NaCl is recommended for newcomers to hot environments; about 10 grams of this can be consumed with a meat-containing diet. The additional 5 to 15 grams is best taken in the form of salted fruit drinks and enteric-coated salt tablets. But if water and fluids are in short supply, salt tablets should not be used. The routine use of salt tablets in hot situations is no longer encouraged except possibly for people who have little experience, and then only during the first days of becoming acclimatized.

Leithead, C. S., and Lind, A. R.: Heat Stress and Heat Disorders. Philadelphia, F. A. Davis Company, 1964.

26.5. HYPOTHERMIA

When the rectal temperature is below 35° C, hypothermia is said to be present. This major loss of body heat occurs in hikers and climbers exposed to cold, in elderly people who live alone in meagerly heated homes, in people who have been drinking heavily and have fallen asleep out of doors, in accident victims, and in people accidentally immersed in cold water. In profound hypothermia people are often assumed to be dead, for their vital signs are so depressed as to be missed even by trained observers. If only a clinical mercury thermometer is available, it will fail to register low enough to point to the diagnosis.

Estimates of the frequency of hypothermia vary widely, but the incidence is possibly higher than anyone suspects. In England it has been shown that elderly people are often forced to tolerate being chronically depleted of body heat, and the same may well be true in the United States for isolated old people. This would seem to be an ideal initial condition from which to develop hypothermia. Added hunger, fatigue, or minor injury could increase the heat depletion by rendering such people helpless. Drugs such as chlorpromazine may also contribute to it.

A person in profound hypothermia is in coma and cold to the touch. The skin is pale, usually grayish in color; the neck and extremities resist bending. No peripheral pulse can be found, breathing appears to be absent, and pupillary reflexes are absent. If a low-reading thermometer can be found, the rectal temperature will show 30° C or lower. Less profound hypothermia differs in degree; there will be some signs of consciousness, reaction to pain, a detectable if slow pulse, and flexible joints.

Additional findings are hypotension; cardiac irregularities on the EKG, typically atrial fibrillation and a J wave associated with the QRS complex; low pH in the blood from metabolic acidosis, especially in patients whose hypothermia was preceded by exhaustion and prolonged shivering; low blood CO_2 content; and high blood glucose.

Rewarming is the first order of business, and a decision must be made about passive or active rewarming and, if active, whether by external or core first means. A person who is still somewhat conscious, who has a reasonable heart rhythm, and whose rectal temperature is between 31 and 35° C is probably best handled by rewarming in a warm room or in a bed with blankets. If a person is acutely hypothermic from cold water immersion, the preferred approach is immersion in a warm tub bath the temperature of which is kept at 40 to 42° C. Inhalation rewarming is suitably employed by rescue personnel, since the equipment needed is a portable source of oxygen or air and a device for heating and humidifying the gas to be delivered at 45° C. It is a decided advantage to begin treatment at once, before the patient is transported to a building with a bathtub. A person with slowly developed hypothermia, in whom fatigue, injury, or old age has produced a poor condition beyond the hypothermia, should probably be warmed actively but less aggressively, e.g., with a heating blanket kept at 37° C. Rewarming the core first may be undertaken for profound hypothermia, for there is grave danger of ventricular fibrillation at heart temperatures from 27 to 30° C. The core-warming method avoids the early return of cold blood from the arms, legs, and skin, which commonly causes an unwanted after-drop in central temperature during external rewarming. But the methods of core-warming first are not simple ones; warm peritoneal dialysis and an extra-corporeal blood circuit with a heater are examples.

Other than a determined approach to restoring body heat, the management of hypothermia should be as conservative as circumstances warrant, i.e., trauma or infection must be heeded. Respiratory support, for example, should include intubation or tracheostomy only if absolutely necessary. These procedures affect an already irritable heart. Cardiac irregularities should be watched rather than treated; if arrest occurs, it should be treated by external cardiac massage, and use of a defibrillator for ventricular fibrillation. Fluid therapy should be guided by laboratory findings rather than by some predetermined rule; thus one should combat acidosis or hypokalemia specifically if present.

Anderson, S., Herbring, B. G., and Widman, B.: Accidental profound hypothermia. Br. J. Anaesth., 42:653, 1970.
Collis, M. L., Steinman, A. M., and Chaney, R. D.: Accidental hypothermia: An experimental study of practical rewarming methods. Aviat. Space Environ. Med. 48:625, 1977.
Fernandez, J. P., O'Rourke, R. A., and Ewy, G. A.: Rapid active external rewarming in accidental hypothermia. JAMA, 212:153, 1970.
Fox, R. H., Woodward, P. M., Exton-Smith, A. N., Green, M. F., Donnison, D. V., and Wicks, M. H.: Body temperatures in the elderly: A national study of physiological, social, and environmental conditions. Br. Med. J., 62:200, 1973.
Patton, J. F., and Doolittle, W. H.: Core rewarming by peritoneal dialysis following induced hypothermia in the dog. J. Appl. Physiol., 33:800, 1972.
Zingg, W.: The management of accidental hypothermia. Can. Med. Assoc. J., 96:214, 1967.

27. RADIATION INJURY
Niel Wald

DEFINITION. Radiation energy from sources of ionizing radiation which interacts with human cells, tissues, and organs produces a variety of clinical manifestations, depending on the magnitude and duration of radiation exposure and on the size and function(s) of the body area irradiated. The source of the radiation energy absorbed may be external, such as an x-ray machine, or it may be internal contamination from a radioactive isotope inhaled, ingested, injected, or absorbed through the skin or a wound.

Clinical manifestations of radiation energy absorption may be acute, with or without late sequelae, or they may be delayed and chronic. The acute manifestations include the acute radiation syndrome which typically follows whole body radiation exposure; local tissue or organ injury with little or no systemic manifestations after partial body exposure; and growth and developmental disturbances after exposure of the fetus. The clinical effects of intermittent or constant low level radiation exposure from external or internal sources may present as chronic progressive impairment of certain tissues or organs, or solely as the relatively late appearance of one or another of the long-term sequelae of radiation exposure, such as cancer and leukemia. In addition, any of these forms of exposure which impinge on the gonads may produce germ cell changes or mutations which can cause sequelae in subsequent progeny.

Tissue injury may be produced by cellular interactions with radiations of any part of the electromagnetic spectrum, including the output of the sun, lasers, or microwave equipment. Some of these, such as x-rays, gamma rays, and neutrons, are capable of penetration, and can produce internal tissue damage. Other radiations, such as alpha rays and low energy beta rays, have a very limited range in tissue and are only injurious when given off within the body by incorporated radioactive isotopes. The radiations *emitted* by ionizing radiation sources are quantitated in roentgens (r) of exposure, whereas the radiation energy *absorbed* by the tissues exposed is quantitated in rads. The same absorbed dose delivered at different rates will produce very different effects.

ETIOLOGY. Typical radiation injury is caused by exposure to *ionizing radiations*. Since the recognition of man-made radiation by Roentgen in 1895 and of natural radioactivity by Becquerel the following year, occupational and medical exposures have been the most usual sources of radiation injury, although the use of nuclear weapons in World War II produced a major addition in clinical cases. Injury from external sources occurred among the early x-ray workers, the employees of the nuclear weapons project, and the subsequent nuclear energy research and industrial organizations. In addition, unavoidable injury has been produced in some radiation therapy patients through exposure of normal tissues adjacent to the lesion under treatment.

Internal radionuclide exposure resulted in injury to employees of the radium watch dial painting industry in the 1920s. More recently, fallout from nuclear weapon tests has produced some internal radionuclide deposition in the general public. In the medical patient population, the uses of radium as a therapeutic agent and thorium as a diagnostic x-ray contrast medium have resulted in clinical sequelae decades after administration. Also, there have been instances of diagnostic and therapeutic radioisotope misadministration producing acute injury and occasionally causing death.

INCIDENCE AND PREVALENCE. The frequency with which radiation injury occurs is closely related to the availability of sources for radiation exposure and the understanding and care with which they are maintained and used. The largest potential source of radiation casualties is the military use of *nuclear weapons*. The Joint Commission for the Investigation of the Effects of the Atomic Bomb in Japan estimated the incidence of radiation injury in Hiroshima to be about 40 per cent and in Nagasaki about 50 per cent in the injured survivors. In Hiroshima about 30 per cent of the deaths in those who survived longer than one day were ascribed to radiation injury either alone or combined with blast and/or burn damage. In the survivor study population of 82,244, 141 cases of leukemia developed between 1950 and 1972. It is probable that the modern nuclear weapon effects would exceed these results. In nuclear weapon tests, some 300 people have inadvertently been exposed to local high levels of radioactive fallout, with resultant clinical manifestations in about 25 per cent.

Early peacetime uses of radioactivity led to an initial high incidence of injury. Within seven years of the demonstration of x-irradiation by Roentgen in 1895, some 200 cases of x-ray injury had been reported. After recognition of the hazard, radiation protection standards were developed internationally. There has been a marked reduction in this type of injury, although hand injuries still occur occasionally in industrial radiographers and the users of x-ray diffraction and other analytic equipment in research and development laboratories.

The discovery of natural radioactivity by Becquerel in 1896 led to the purification of radium by the Curies in 1911 and its use in medicine and industry. About 5000 watch dial painters, industrial chemists, and medical patients were involved. In 2500 of these, in whom medical information was compiled by A. M. Brues at Argonne National Laboratory through 1975, there were 408 malignant tumors, with the excess over the expected frequency involving bone and the air cavities of the head. The development of manmade radioactive material during and after World War II led to a nuclear industry population of several hundred thousand workers, but only 97 cases of clinical radiation injury had developed by 1969. Although data collection concerning medical misadministrations of radioactive isotopes designed for diagnostic and therapeutic purposes has not been systematic, several deaths and a number of injuries are known to have occurred in the very large American patient population, estimated at over 8 million annually, receiving these materials.

EPIDEMIOLOGY. The manifestations of acute or of late radiation injury are not produced solely by irradia-

tion. It is therefore essential to utilize epidemiologic methodology in order to establish the relationship of the etiologic agent to the clinical symptomatology. Two most helpful features have been the temporal relationship of the exposure to the development of clinical effects and the quantitative dose-response relationship.

The etiologic role of radiation in the clinical syndrome of *acute* radiation injury has been shown in epidemiologic studies of the Japanese atomic bomb survivors, the Marshall Islanders and Japanese fishermen exposed to fallout from a nuclear weapon test, several groups of radiation therapy patients, and the workers involved in various industrial radiation accidents. Epidemiologic studies relating *late* radiation effects such as neoplastic diseases and life-shortening to radiation exposure have dealt with radiologists and other physicians, the Japanese population under long-term follow-up by the Atomic Bomb Casualty Commission and its successor since 1975, the Radiation Effects Research Foundation, the radium watch dial painters, therapeutically x-irradiated patients (particularly those receiving thymic irradiation in infancy), patients receiving radioactive iodine therapy, and nuclear industry employees.

PATHOGENESIS. The basic pathology begins with the interaction of the radiation with tissue within the first second of exposure. The radiation energy in photons or particles penetrating the protoplasm may interact at the atomic level to produce ion pairs. These ions combine radiochemically with cell water, producing free radicals such as H and OH which further react to produce such forms as H_2O_2 and HO_2. These, in turn, may interact with critical molecules of the cell protoplasm such as nucleic acids or enzymes. If the dose is high and interactions are numerous, the cell may be killed directly by the radiation. At lower doses, the ability of the cell to divide may be impaired permanently or temporarily. If the DNA is involved, sublethal damage of this molecule may result in reproduction of the alteration (i.e., mutation) in daughter and descendant cells. Direct cell killing begins with exposures of one or more thousands of rads, in general, although some cells such as lymphocytes and spermatogonia are affected at much lower doses. Those cells which are rapidly dividing and differentiating are most vulnerable. Mitotic arrest occurs after several hundreds of rads and is characterized by continuing function of the existing cells but no new divisions. The continuing synthesis of proteins and enzymes, despite an irreversibly impaired mitotic apparatus, leads to "giant cells" which die after several weeks because their excessive size interferes with nutrition and metabolism. At doses of about 100 rads or more, mitotic delay results from temporary impairment of the mitotic mechanism. At still lower doses transient chromosomal "stickiness" is seen, presumably caused by denaturation of the DNA-histone molecules. Also, beginning at exposures as low as a few rads, are chromosome aberrations, i.e., breaks, deletions, gaps, and abnormal forms such as ring and dicentric chromosomes.

The effects of these cellular abnormalities on the various organs depend on the rate of proliferation of new cells required. In high turnover tissues such as the blood-forming tissue and the gastrointestinal tract, the relatively short life span of the predominant cells leads to rapid depletion before the onset of mitotic recovery and new cell production. In the period of mitotic inhibition of the blood-forming tissue, for example, the consequent depletion of mature cells results in increased probability of infection and hemorrhage. The resultant pathologic manifestations are nonspecific, although the inflammatory changes accompanying infection are deficient in polymorphonuclear cells.

In tissues which have little or no continuous proliferation, such as the liver or brain, this type of radiation injury is not apparent; however, functional impairment may be detected by appropriate means. In very slow turnover tissues, such as the lens of the eye or the thyroid gland, the manifestations of acute radiation effects may require months to years before becoming evident. Also, the small arterioles damaged by local radiation injury may show a compensatory increase in cell production, leading to endothelial thickening, obliterative endarteritis, and extensive fibrosis over a prolonged period of time.

Chromosomal abnormalities produced in injured cells may be reproduced and perpetuated for decades. A long-lived component of the lymphoid cells may even carry the original radiation damage for many years before dividing. Clones of cells with the same specific chromosome abnormality may develop over a period of years as well.

CLINICAL MANIFESTATIONS. Clinical manifestations of radiation injury can be subdivided into three major forms: the acute radiation syndrome, acute local radiation injury, and delayed effects. External penetrating irradiation, as well as external and internal radionuclide contamination and local traumatic injury with radionuclide contamination, may produce these manifestations.

Acute Radiation Syndrome. This syndrome is seen typically after exposure of most or all of the body to external sources of penetrating ionizing radiation, although high doses of ^{32}P, ^{131}I, and ^{198}Au have also evoked it. It appears in three major forms, in ascending severity of injury. These are the hematologic, the gastrointestinal, and the central nervous system–cardiovascular forms. Four discernible clinical stages can be recognized, particularly when the severity of injury allows for ultimate survival. These are the initial or prodromal stage which subsides into a latent stage, followed by a stage of manifest or overt illness, and a recovery stage. The duration of each stage is inversely related to the severity of injury.

Typical manifestations of the *hematologic form* are seen after an exposure in the midlethal range (about 300 rads without treatment). Prodromal anorexia, nausea, and possibly vomiting may commence within several hours and generally subside within 48 hours. Transient waves of skin erythema and conjunctivitis may be observed over the same period or longer. The patient may be asymptomatic after the prodromal stage for one to three weeks. Then the increasing inadequacy of the body's defenses against infection and hemorrhage becomes manifest, with development of fever, oropharyngeal lesions, abscesses, petechiae, purpura, and bleeding from body orifices. Other findings include scalp pain and epilation in the third postexposure week, and recurrent anorexia and nausea accompanied by weakness, fatigue, weight loss, and emaciation. Gradual recovery ensues, beginning about the fifth to sixth week after exposure and may require several months.

The earliest laboratory finding is lymphopenia, reaching absolute lymphocyte levels below 1000 per cubic millimeter within the first 48 postexposure hours. The reticulocytes may disappear in the same time period. A gradual fall in granulocyte counts begins during the first two weeks, reaches a plateau, or even shows an abortive rise, followed by a steep fall to a low point at about 30 days postexposure. The platelet count nadir occurs at the same time, after a more continuous fall. If the individual survives, an abrupt increase in all the cell lines mentioned, except the lymphocytes, will occur within the next week and they will rapidly reach normal levels. An initial increase in granulocyte count in the first 24 hours may occur on the basis of a nonspecific "alarm reaction," and should not mislead one to exclude radiation injury on this basis. Blood biochemical analyses may show nonspecific indicators of major cell and tissue damage such as creatinuria, increased excretion of DNA breakdown products such as beta-aminoisobutyric acid, deoxycytidine, and various other amino acids. Serum enzyme measurements such as LDH, SGOT, and SGPT may be elevated, and an early transient slight hyperbilirubinemia observed. Within 24 hours chromosome breakage and abnormal forms can be seen in peripheral blood cytogenetic preparations, with the frequency related to the magnitude of the radiation exposure.

The *gastrointestinal form* is associated with anorexia, nausea, vomiting, and diarrhea within the first few hours after exposure. These may be of sufficient severity to require active treatment but usually subside within 48 hours. A latent period follows which may last only a few days to a week before there is a major recurrence of all the gastrointestinal symptoms as well as those of infection and hemorrhage as described above. These patients generally die with a fulminating enterocolitis before the full appearance of epilation and other slower developing radiation sequelae.

Laboratory abnormalities in the gastrointestinal form of radiation injury are similar to those of the hematologic form but occur more promptly and with greater magnitude. In addition, the hematocrit may be increased as a result of hemoconcentration caused by fluid loss, which, with hypoglycemia and electrolyte imbalance, results from the loss of a functional intestinal mucosal lining.

In the *central nervous system and cardiovascular form*, immediate nausea, projectile vomiting, and explosive diarrhea are characteristic. These may be accompanied by disorientation, hyperesthesia, ataxia, sweating, prostration, and shock. There may be some improvement after several hours, but alternations develop between evidences of central nervous system hyperexcitability, including convulsions, and CNS depression, such as somnolence and coma. This is accompanied by hypotension which becomes irreversible, as does oliguria, leading to a fatal outcome in 24 to 48 hours.

Laboratory observations in the central nervous system and cardiovascular form of acute radiation injury show marked telescoping of the previously described injury syndromes with abnormalities occurring sooner and with greater severity. Complete lymphopenia and an initial granulocyte level of 30,- to 40,000 may be present within the next few hours. Prompt chromosome examination may show marked increase in aberrations, but as the circulating lymphocytes disappear, it may become difficult to find dividing cells. The biochemical evidences of tissue damage are much more striking in this form of the syndrome. In addition, biochemical evidences of azotemia secondary to hypotension become prominent.

Local Radiation Injury. Localized radiation injury may occur with acute and/or chronic clinical manifestations, depending on the total dose and dose rate at which the exposure takes place.

The early changes result in three major clinical findings: erythema, epilation, and transepidermal injury. *Erythema* comparable to a mild sunburn or a thermal burn of the first degree may appear on exposure to more than 200 to 300 rads. A transient first wave may be present within hours after exposure, associated with hyperesthesia, burning, or itching. The major redness appears two or three weeks later, the interval depending on the dose. In the lower dose range no further changes other than tanning may occur, and medical care is not necessary. A counterpart to this reaction has been described in the conjunctiva and in the anterior chamber of the eye, with inflammatory changes observed promptly after exposure.

Epilation, or loss of hair, may occur after exposure to any form of radiation, beginning with exposures to the skin of about 300 rads. It generally does not become apparent until the third week after exposure. Associated skin or scalp tenderness may occur one or two days preceding the actual hair loss. With doses greater than about 500 rads, epilation may be complete. If the exposure is much greater than 600 rads, hair may not regrow.

Transepidermal injury (dry or wet dermatitis) is comparable to a thermal second-degree burn with erythema, blistering, and pain. Confluent bullae may develop in about one and one-half to three weeks, depending on dose (usually exceeding 1000 rads). These may rupture, leaving open, weeping lesions vulnerable to infection.

With higher doses, probably on the order of 5000 rads, a more serious version of transepidermal injury occurs, in which the lesion resembles a third-degree burn. Pain occurs promptly and is intense. The raw areas may be very slow in healing, or may not heal until surgical resection and skin grafting are performed. Epilation is permanent.

Still higher doses may produce immediate tissue damage to structures below the skin. Such injuries, which have occurred in the abdominal wall, male genitalia, and extremities, are irreversible, requiring surgical excision and further reconstructive management.

Delayed Effects. Delayed effects of radiation exposure are of two varieties: those finally appearing in organs whose cells received the radiation exposure and are relatively slow in responding; and those late effects occurring in organs and tissues in which descendent cells ultimately express the initial radiation injury after a latent period which may be many years in duration. The first type of delayed effect can be seen in the male gonad, for example. Doses as low as 15 rads will produce *impairment in fertility* owing to moderate oligospermia beginning about 50 days after the exposure. Azoospermia will occur with doses of more than 200 to 300 rads for a period of roughly one to two years. Doses of 500 to 600 rads may produce permanent sterility in male or female survivors.

The lens of the eye is another late-responding tissue, with opacities appearing in the posterior subcapsular region in months to several years after exposures of about 200 rads or more. *Cataracts* of the posterior lens may develop in the majority of patients who receive more than 600 rads. The gradual development of *hypothyroidism* several years after exposure of several hundred rads is another example of delayed response. *Skin changes* constitute another late response to either acute injury or repeated low level radiation exposure. There may be loss of the detailed finger-ridge pattern and hair, abnormalities of the fingernails, and dryness of the skin. Localized hyperkeratosis may be seen, as well as breakdown of previously healed but atrophic skin, and, ultimately, neoplastic skin changes may develop in such areas.

In the *fetus* the clinical manifestations will depend largely on its age and the magnitude of exposure. If the exposure takes place in the first one to two weeks, resorption of the conceptus is probable. Between the second and sixth weeks, the effect will be on the particular organs under development at the time. Further along in gestation, there will be more subtle generalized effects ultimately expressed as deficits in growth and development, including microcephaly and mental retardation.

The most common *late effects* of radiation exposure are *neoplastic diseases*. The earliest to appear are the acute leukemias and chronic granulocytic leukemia, with a peak incidence of approximately four to seven years after the radiation exposure. Chronic lymphocytic leukemia is not increased by radiation exposure. Other neoplasms whose induction appears significantly increased by radiation exposure include cancer of the thyroid and salivary glands, lung, bone, and female breast tissues. Internally deposited radionuclides have been associated particularly with malignant neoplasms of bone and reticuloendothelial tissues such as liver, spleen, and lymph nodes. Radium deposition has involved the mastoid bones and those surrounding the paranasal sinuses in particular, whereas internally administered thorium dioxide has produced an increase of hemangiosarcomas of the liver. In addition, a generalized increase in incidence of all forms of cancer has been documented in the Japanese atomic bomb survivors. *Shortening of life expectancy* through somewhat earlier death from all causes has been demonstrated in the radiologist population but not yet in the Japanese A-bomb survivors.

DIAGNOSIS. Acute Radiation Syndrome. The manifestations of acute radiation injury are not unique to this causative agent. Therefore the diagnosis rests on the history and the evolving clinical pattern defined by time of onset and duration of the clinical signs, symptoms, and laboratory abnormalities, particularly the hematologic changes.

In the absence of an adequate history of radiation exposure, the diagnosis may be elusive. The various manifestations may suggest a wide range of conditions. Prodromes suggest psychoneurosis, food poisoning, or gastrointestinal viral infection; symptoms in the period of manifest illness may mimic aplastic anemia, leukemia, infectious gastroenteritis, typhoid fever, and even mumps (for radiation parotitis). When a radiation exposure history is elicited, hematologic and cytogenetic examinations may be used as well as physical dosimetry data obtained by personnel monitoring equipment, if any, and by reconstruction of the exposure situation, in order to obtain confirmatory and quantitative information concerning the potential severity of the injury.

However, it must be kept clearly in mind that the evolving clinical pattern is the final diagnostic criterion for the recognition and management of this form of injury.

Local Injury. Local radiation injury, particularly as it appears on the upper extremities, is often confused with thermal and chemical burns. Differentiating features are absence of waves of erythema in the latter as well as the more severe prolonged pain and slower healing associated with radiation. Recurrent tissue breakdown after healing is also suggestive of radiation injury as opposed to the other possibilities.

Delayed Effects. No clinical characteristics of the late effects of radiation exposure are unique to this etiologic agent.

Radionuclide Contamination. Radionuclides deposited on the surface of the skin may be absorbed, inhaled, or ingested into the body where they may act to produce delayed effects. In order to prevent such sequelae, the recognition of their presence is essential even though no immediate clinical manifestations are present. Such diagnostic procedures must involve close collaboration between the physician and the health physicist, the professional trained to recognize and quantitate radiation exposure in order to prevent deleterious effects of radiation. Radioactivity surveys of the suspected individual with appropriate radiation detection equipment should be carried out. It is most important to collect all urinary and fecal excretions in separate containers until sufficient data of the nature and magnitude of contamination are obtained. Some radionuclides such as radon may be sought in breath samples. An early postexposure blood sample should also be collected and preserved for radionuclide analysis. Finally, it may be necessary to carry out chest or whole body low-level radiation counting in an appropriate facility, i.e., a so-called "whole body counter."

If a traumatic wound is present, radionuclide contamination may be sought by measuring radioactivity of swabs used in cleaning the wound as well as by surveying over the surface with appropriate detectors. If the wound is the sole contaminated area, excreta samples will show whether the contaminant has been absorbed into the body and therefore is sufficiently soluble for circulation and translocation to sites remote from the wound.

TREATMENT. Acute Radiation Syndrome. The treatment of acute radiation syndrome is based on an understanding of its pathophysiology. The prodromal symptoms in the acute radiation syndrome are self-limited, but sedatives and antiemetics may be used if needed. Throughout the syndrome it is important to reduce anxiety by keeping the patient informed about the nature of his injury, the expected transient health impairment, and its anticipated duration and treatment. The prolonged weakness associated with this syndrome even during convalescence may be in some measure secondary to the prolonged anxiety and fear of the unknown often associated with radiation injury.

In the *hematologic form*, the inhibition of mitosis responsible for the overt illness is self-limited. Thus management is directed toward maintenance of the patient through the period in which his defenses against infection and hemorrhage are deficient. This is best achieved by conservative means. The threat of exogenous bacterial and viral infection is reduced by strict reverse isolation of the patient with maintenance of a clean environment by use of a laminar air flow or "life-island" methods. Attendant personnel must be screened for potential pathogens and treated prophylactically if necessary.

Prophylactic oral antimicrobial drugs to clear pathogenic bacterial and fungal organisms from the gastrointestinal tract have been used when the total granulocyte level falls below 1000 per cubic millimeter. Various blood elements may be given to replace deficiencies when needed. Donors should be limited in number and tissue typed to minimize systemic reactions to and inefficacy of transfused cells. Red cells are needed only if significant bleeding has occurred. Fresh platelets should be available for use if significant hemorrhage develops. Their use has been advocated even in the absence of bleeding when the platelet count falls below 10,000 per cubic millimeter. If available in concentrated form, normal granulocytes may be administered in the face of overt infection during the granulocytopenic phase. If not available, in the presence of a clearly life-threatening infection the use of the much greater numbers of granulocytes of patients with chronic granulocytic leukemia has been suggested, because they are capable of phagocytosis. On recovery, it is assumed that the patient's immune system will rid the body of such donor cells.

In the situation in which both biologic and dosimetric indicators suggest the high probability of a fatal outcome, bone marrow transplantation may be warranted. Because such marrow requires about two weeks to correct the deficit in circulating blood cells, such a decision should not be delayed much beyond the first postexposure week. The hazards of a graft reaction by the host if his radiation-induced immunosuppression is not sufficient, and of "graft versus host" reaction if it is too long lasting, define the narrow boundaries within which therapeutic benefit may be expected. The availability of an identical twin or a very close matching relative on tissue compatibility testing will also influence the decision. The transplantation procedures developed by Thomas et al. for managing leukemic patients after therapeutic whole body irradiation are helpful in accidental radiation injury patients also.

Management of the *gastrointestinal form* of acute radiation syndrome has not been successful thus far in the few human occurrences. Animal studies by Bond and Cronkite suggest that the vigorous and early utilization of adequate anti-infection agents, blood components, nutrients, electrolytes, and fluid may influence mortality favorably.

In the few human instances of the *central nervous system–cardiovascular form*, the progressive hypotension has not been improved by the administration of pressor agents, and the fluid administration involved has augmented the congestive heart failure which has ensued.

Local Radiation Injury. The treatment of local radiation injury is generally similar to that of thermal burns of the same severity. This includes the maintenance of asepsis, eventual removal of devitalized tissue to the degree necessary, and the use of skin grafting to cover nonhealing ulcerations. An additional feature in management is very careful and prolonged observation for possible early neoplastic changes of the skin.

Delayed Effects. Clinical management of the delayed effects of radiation exposure does not differ in any way from the management of similar pathologic conditions not caused by radiation.

Radionuclide Contamination. In the event of an accident in which radionuclide contamination is likely, only urgent first aid should be given and the patient evacuated from the site. Contaminated skin and wounds should be washed promptly, and all excreta collected.

Useful preparations for skin decontamination include soap and water, surgical and laundry detergents, and oxidizing agents. These should be accompanied by brushing and rinsing, with care taken not to abrade the skin.

Contamination of the eyes, nose, and mouth is treated initially with copious water washing as soon as possible. Isotonic irrigants may be substituted as soon as available.

For definitive wound care, the usual surgical principles apply, with modifications only in the aseptic procedures and debridement in order to avoid introduction of skin contamination into the wound. Prior to surgical treatment it may also be desirable to give intravenous diethylenetriaminepentaacetic acid (DTPA), a chelating agent available from the U.S. Department of Energy for investigational use, to minimize the retention of any contaminant which may get into circulation during surgery.

If radioactivity measurements of excreta and of the whole body suggest a residual body burden of a larger quantity than seems acceptable on the basis of medical and health physics judgment, various treatments may be used to minimize the absorption and enhance the excretion of the radionuclide.

To minimize respiratory absorption, the use of irritants, expectorants, and pulmonary lavage is under current investigation. Inhalation of DTPA aerosol mist is also currently being tested for transuranic isotope contamination.

To minimize gastrointestinal absorption, the simplest measure is to accelerate excretion with a mild laxative. For strontium-90, sodium alginate and aluminum hydroxide gel have been used orally to prevent uptake from the gut. For cesium-137, Prussian blue (ferric ferrocyanide) does the same. To promote excretion of nuclides already within the body and to reduce deposition in target organs, such as bone, a variety of agents are available. For plutonium, americium, yttrium, lanthanum, and fission products, intravenously administered chelating agents are useful, DTPA being the most effective. For strontium, the combination of high calcium intake and acidification of the blood with ammonium chloride has effectively reduced bone absorption.

PROGNOSIS. Acute Radiation Syndrome. The estimated short-term radiation exposure which would be lethal for 50 per cent of an untreated human population in 60 days ($LD_{50/60}$) is about 300 rads mean midline absorbed dose. This exposure would be expected to produce the hematologic form of the acute radiation syndrome, with half the exposed population dying within 60 days. However, an accidentally irradiated worker survived an estimated 600 rads absorbed whole body dose, with postexposure treatment, including isogeneic marrow transplantation, by Wald, Thomas, and coworkers, despite tissue damage severe enough to necessitate subsequent amputation of all four extremities. Also, Thomas et al. and others have used pre- and

postexposure treatment, including isogeneic marrow, in over 100 acutely ill leukemic patients receiving 1000 rads of whole body exposure with about 20 per cent early post-treatment fatalities.

Thus it appears that successful management of the hematologic form of acute radiation injury is possible under good therapeutic circumstances. It has therefore been suggested by Wald and Watson that active supportive treatment can raise the LD_{50} to over 500 rads and heroic therapy, such as bone marrow transplantation, to over 1000 rads in accidentally exposed individuals. Clearly, such prognostic optimism would not apply to the large-scale population exposure situation such as occurred in Hiroshima and Nagasaki. Furthermore, even the best clinical management has not yet succeeded in allowing the survival of those few individuals who accidentally have received exposures resulting in major gastrointestinal or central nervous system–cardiovascular damage.

Local Radiation Injury. The outlook for good recovery from local radiation injury depends in part on the adequacy of management of the acute changes, including the removal of devitalized tissue and the prevention of secondary infection. However, the main determinant of the ultimate outcome will be the severity of injury to the underlying blood vessels.

Delayed Effects. The likelihood of a radiation-exposed individual's developing a late effect of the exposure is increased in some relation to the magnitude of the exposure. Since most radiation exposure above the natural background is due to human activities and therefore presumably controllable, increasing recent effort has been given to quantitative risk assessment for radiation carcinogenesis to facilitate better benefit-risk judgments. In 1977, both the United Nations Scientific Committee on the Effects of Atomic Radiation (UNSCEAR) and the International Commission on Radiological Protection (ICRP) reviewed human epidemiologic data and published risk approximations for radiation-induced cancer in various tissues. Although the risk estimates cannot be determined with great accuracy, it is possible, in some instances in which mutually consistent epidemiologic data are obtainable from several different sources, to classify different tissues into groups with different degrees of sensitivity to induction of malignancies by radiation. It is important to note that most of the information is derived from exposures of 100 rads or more of x- or gamma radiation at high dose rates, and therefore may represent overestimates when extrapolated to exposures of a few rads or less delivered at very low dose rates, such as received by the occupationally exposed radiation worker population.

The approximate risk of induction of radiation cancer in various tissues estimated by UNSCEAR can be summarized in terms of the number of cases expected per million persons so exposed per rad of absorbed radiation exposure. In descending order of sensitivity, with the approximate number of cases per million per rad given in parentheses following each tissue, they include thyroid (100); female breast (100); lung (25 to 50); leukemia (20 to 50); stomach, liver, large intestine, brain, and salivary glands (10 to 15); and bone, esophagus, small intestine, urinary bladder, pancreas, rectum, lymphatic tissues, and mucosa of cranial sinuses (2 to 5). It must be recognized that these estimates are very broad generalizations and that for each tissue there are differing effects of such factors as sex and age at exposure, in addition to the kind of radiation, dose, and dose rate. For example, the pediatric population is more sensitive to thyroid cancer induction, female breast cancer is induced primarily by exposure during the early reproductive period, and lung cancer is highest in males exposed at over 35 years of age. Also, the induction of cancer in the fetus is distinctly elevated, estimated roughly as 200 to 250 cases per million per rad.

The duration of the period at risk also varies with different tissues. The mean interval between exposure and leukemia development is in the region of 10 years, for example, whereas the other malignancies typically appear in an exposed population with a mean of 25 years of latency. In a population exposure, the earlier appearing leukemia may serve as an indicator for the eventual total of all fatal malignancies, which ultimately may occur in four to six times as many individuals as developed leukemia alone.

The prognosis for the various delayed effects of radiation exposure is similar to that of the same pathology in the absence of such exposure. For this reason many of the radiation-induced cancers would be expected to respond to treatment. The ICRP therefore derived maximum risk rates for fatalities from radiation-induced cancers. In descending order of risk, with approximate numbers of fatal cases per million exposed per rad in parentheses, they are female breast (50), leukemia (20), lung (20), thyroid (5), bone (5), and all other organs together (50).

Prevention. Since the foregoing discussion has indicated that there are no specific methods of reversing the course of events initiated by radiation exposure, the best measure against radiation injury is prevention. The largest *potential* source of radiation exposure to the general population is the nuclear weapon. It is therefore essential that all measures be taken to minimize the possibility of any human population receiving such an exposure again. Another potential source of population exposure, the widespread and increasing utilization of nuclear energy as a source of electric power generation, has been controlled successfully thus far.

The largest *actual* source of population exposure consists of users of radiation in the healing arts. It is evident that such usage of ionizing radiation has produced untold benefit to the same population. Nevertheless, it is incumbent on the users of medical radiation sources to minimize the exposures needed to obtain the necessary diagnostic information. This requires not only optimal operation of existing equipment by current techniques but also a continuing research and development effort to improve the efficiency of such equipment to allow reduction of exposure while obtaining the necessary biomedical information. Adequate specialized education of all users of radiation sources in the philosophy and methods of radiation protection is another factor in the preventive approach to radiation injury.

Andrews, G. A., Balish, E., Edwards, C. L., Kniseley, R. M., and Lushbaugh, C. C.: Possibilities for Improved Treatment of Persons Exposed in Radiation Accidents. In Handling of Radiation Accidents. Vienna, International Atomic Energy Agency, 1969, p. 119.

Basic Radiation Protection Criteria. NCRP Report No. 39, Washington, D.C., National Council on Radiation Protection and Measurements, 1971.

Cleary, S. F. Biological effects of microwave and radiofrequency radiation. In Straub, C. P. (ed.): Critical Reviews in Environmental Control, Vol. 7, Issue 2. Cleveland, CRC Press, 1977, p. 121.

Dalrymple, G. V., et al.: Medical Radiation Biology. Philadelphia, W. B. Saunders Company, 1973.

Management of Persons Contaminated with Radionuclides. NCRP Report

in preparation. Washington, D.C., National Council on Radiation Protection and Measurements, 1979.

Medical Radiation Exposure of Pregnant and Potentially Pregnant Women. NCRP Report No. 54. Washington, D.C., National Council on Radiation Protection and Measurements, 1977.

Norwood, W. D.: Health Protection of Radiation Workers. Springfield, Ill., Charles C Thomas, 1975.

Radiation Protection. ICRP Publication 26, Recommendations of the International Commission on Radiological Protection. New York, Pergamon Press, 1977.

Robinson, D. W.: Surgical problems in the excision and repair of radiated tissue. Plastic Reconstruct. Surg., 55:41, 1975.

Rubin, P., and Casarett, G. W.: Clinical Radiation Pathology. Philadelphia, W. B. Saunders Company, 1968.

Sources and Effects of Ionizing Radiation. United Nations Scientific Committee on the Effects of Atomic Radiation. 1977 report to the General Assembly, with annexes. New York, United Nations, 1977.

Stannard, J. N.: Toxicology of radionuclides. Ann. Rev. Pharmacol., 13:325, 1973.

The Effects on Populations of Exposure to Low Levels of Ionizing Radiation. Report of the Advisory Committee on the Biological Effects of Ionizing Radiations. Washington, National Academy of Sciences — National Research Council, 1972.

Thomas, E. D., et al.: Bone marrow transplantation. N. Engl. J. Med., 292:832, 985, 1975.

Wald, N.: Radiation injury and its management. In Wang, Y. (ed.): Handbook of Radioactive Nuclides. Part IX. Cleveland, The Chemical Rubber Co., 1969, p. 837.

Wald, N., and Watson, J. A.: Medical modification of human acute radiation injury. In Proceedings, IVth Congress. Paris, International Radiation Protection Association, 1977, p. 1183.

28.   ELECTRIC SHOCK AND ELECTRIC INJURY

*Curtis P. Artz**

Electric shock and electric injury occur when the current of electricity passes through the body. Kouwenhoven pointed out six factors that determine the effects of electricity on the body. These are type of circuit, voltage, resistance offered by the body, value of the current, pathway of the current, and duration of the contact. Direct current does not produce the same contraction of muscles that is found with alternating current.

In high voltage injury there is greater cause for respiratory arrest, because of the very severe muscular contraction. High voltage currents also cause a greater amount of tissue damage. If the victim of an electric shock retains consciousness during and after the contact, there is often a ringing in the ears and partial deafness for a time. In addition there may be visual disorders such as flashes and brilliant luminous spots. If there is a prolonged period of apnea, the neurologic manifestations of anoxia may be present.

The resistance to electric current in tissue varies in order from the greatest to the least as follows: bone, fat, tendon, skin, muscle, blood, nerve. Thin skin is less resistant, of course, than thick skin. After an electric current has penetrated the skin, it passes rapidly through the body along the lines of least resistance — that is, through the tissue fluids and along blood vessels, where it may cause degeneration of vessel walls and formation of thrombi. If the resistance of the skin is low at the time it interrupts the electric current, the current passes readily into the body. It is generally be-

---

*Deceased.

lieved that the greater the skin resistance, the more severe the local burn; similarly, the less the resistance, the greater the systemic effect of the current.

The pathway of the current through the body is important. If it passes through vital organs such as the heart and the brain, the resulting injury is greater. It is always difficult, however, to tell from the cutaneous injury the exact pathway the current has taken. The difference in the susceptibility of the heart to electrical injury at different times in its contraction cycle also seems important. The longer the duration of contact, the greater the amount of damage.

INCIDENCE. There are about 1000 accidental deaths due to electric current in the United States each year. About 90 per cent of these occur in males. The highest fatality rate is experienced by men in the age range of 20 to 34. More than two fifths of the fatalities occur from June through August. Approximately two thirds of all fatal injuries from electric current occur on the job, and more than one fourth occur on home premises.

PATHOGENESIS. The wounds of electric injury are extremely variable because there are such differences in type and intensity of current, tissues through which the current passes, and degree of contact. Injuries associated with electricity may be divided into three types: true electric injury, arc burn, and flame burn.

True electric injury is caused by the passage of electric current through the skin. The entry wound is charred and depressed, whereas the exit wound is dry and gives the appearance that the electric current exploded as it made its exit. The extensive underlying tissue damage is evidenced by intense swelling. The cause of this damage is most likely due to the heat generated by the passage of the current through the tissues. The current follows blood vessels, and thrombosis even at some distance from the original injury is common. A limb that appears viable soon after an electric accident may in a few days become ischemic and finally gangrenous. Parts of the media of vessels may be weakened by cellular disintegration, and if thrombosis does not occur there may be serious hemorrhage. The death of muscle is usually very uneven. Sometimes there is a palpable pulse in the large arteries of an extremity but the nutrient artery to a muscle bundle is completely occluded.

This deeper destruction has led to the concept that electric injuries are more like crush injury than like a burn (see accompanying figure). Thermal burns usually destroy only the skin and subcutaneous tissue, whereas electric injury is deeper and frequently associated with muscle destruction.

Arc burns are produced by current coursing externally to the body from the contact point to the ground. Burns that follow the leaping of an electric arc from the conductor to the skin are mainly associated with high tension current. They are usually severe because an electric arc has a temperature of approximately 2500° C.

Flame burns result from ignition of clothing by electrical sparks or arcing.

CLINICAL MANIFESTATIONS. Tetanic contraction of muscles is common and sometimes causes fractures and dislocations. Delayed effect of electric injury includes the development of cataracts. However, the severe effects of electric injury are damage to the skin, subcutaneous tissue, and muscles. Most common is true electric injury accompanied by flame burns.

Electric injury is more like crush injury than like a burn. The damage is deep and frequently involves muscle.

Vascular Injuries. Delayed hemorrhage from large blood vessels is a threat when there is an area of extensive necrosis over the vessels. Rupture of major vessels distant from the areas of tissue necrosis may also occur. Progressive loss of blood supply to muscles may account for the fibrosis that is not uncommonly observed.

Spinal Cord Injury. Spinal cord injuries are more frequently encountered than is generally recognized, because many of these lesions are incomplete and are not associated with either vertebral fractures or the apparent path of the current. The clinical signs often are those of spastic paresis, and the patients may have little or no sensory deficit accompanying the motor changes. Such injury is difficult to diagnose, and the lesions are not suspected until ambulation provides evidence of neuromuscular imbalance.

Cardiopulmonary Injury. Anoxia and ventricular fibrillation are the principal causes of immediate death. Acute pulmonary complications are limited to pleural damage resulting in effusion and lobular pneumonitis directly adjacent to the contact point. Taylor reported electrocardiographic changes in patients who showed right bundle branch block, ectopic focus arrhythmias, or supraventricular tachycardia. There may be some longlasting cardiovascular effects, including disturbance of rhythm consisting essentially of disturbances in atrioventricular and intraventricular conduction, clinically and electrocardiographically established manifestations of acute coronary insufficiency, and subjective disturbances such as precordial pains and palpitations. Baxter reported that tachycardia and minor S-T segment alterations frequently persist for several weeks after electric injury.

Renal Effects. Renal damage is not uncommon. Most likely it is caused by a combination of the initial severe shock, direct electric current damage to the kidneys, and abnormal protein breakdown products from damaged muscles. Acute tubular necrosis is a recognized complication.

Abdominal Injury. Submucosal hemorrhages scattered throughout the gastrointestinal tract are not infrequently seen at autopsy after electric injury. This is probably because of the direct effect of the current. A most distressing diagnostic problem occurs in electric injuries to the abdomen. It is difficult to determine whether or not intra-abdominal injury is present. Too often abdominal symptoms are ascribed to nonspecific paralytic ileus. One must beware of making a diagnosis of paralytic ileus associated with electric injury and forgetting that intestinal damage as a result of the current may be present.

TREATMENT. An electric shock victim should be freed from contact with the current as quickly as possible. The rescuer must make sure that he is well insulated. If the victim is not breathing, artificial respiration must be started immediately. If the heart is not beating, there is probably ventricular fibrillation, and cardiac massage should be given until the patient can be moved to a facility where defibrillation is possible.

A most important aspect of initial resuscitation is replacement of isotonic fluid that has been rapidly lost into the area of injury. When there is true electric damage to muscle as well as to skin and subcutaneous tissue, large volumes of fluid are required. Since the injury is similar to crush injury, the principles associated with replacement therapy after crush injury are applicable. This means large quantities of lactated Ringer's solution, mannitol, and sodium bicarbonate. In extensive damage when the initial fluid therapy does not produce a clear urine, 25 grams of mannitol should be given intravenously. It should be followed by 12.5 grams per hour until the reddish brown urine clears or six doses are given. Sodium bicarbonate should be given to ensure alkalinization of the urine.

Wound Care. Management of the local wound is difficult because of the various types of injury. If the injury is small, such as is seen from low voltage current, the area should be treated with local antibacterial ointments and allowed to slough and heal.

High voltage injuries must be treated more aggressively. A surgeon should make sure that there is no underlying muscle damage. This can usually be ascertained by incising one or two areas and looking at the muscle. If there is dead muscle, the patient should be taken to the operating room as soon as his general physical condition permits, and all the dead skin, subcutaneous tissue, and muscle should be excised. Sometimes this requires amputation. In extensive injury to the extremities, fasciotomy and muscle debridement are usually accomplished at the first operation. Because of the progressive nature of the lesion, additional excision and debridement of muscle may be necessary. When there has been appreciable surface injury without deep destruction, the primary problem of management is the treatment of the entry and exit wound. Usually these are managed in the same way as a thermal burn. Associated thermal injury is treated by the application of a local antibacterial agent, and the wounds are closed by skin grafts after all the dead tissue has been removed.

Artz, C. P.: Changing concepts of electrical injury. Am. J. Surg., 128:699, 1974.

Baxter, C. R.: Present concepts in the management of major electrical injuries. Surg. Clin. North Am., 50:1401, 1970.

Kouwenhoven, W. B.: Effect of electricity on the human body. Elec. Engineering, 68:199, 1949.

Statistical Bulletin. New York, Metropolitan Life Insurance Company, May 1968.

Taylor, P. H., Pugsley, L. Q., and Vogel, E. H., Jr.: The intriguing electrical burn. J. Trauma, 2:309, 1962.

29. MOTION SICKNESS AND PROBLEMS OF AIR TRAVEL

Stanley R. Mohler

29.1. MOTION SICKNESS

DEFINITION. Motion sickness is the most likely reason for nausea experienced during travel on a pitching, rolling, and/or yawing conveyance, these three motions often interacting. The travel may be of any mode: air, land, sea, or space. Even riding a camel can cause motion sickness. The nausea that develops is often preceded by a feeling of fatigue, and may progress to retching and vomiting. Commonly, the skin becomes clammy and the victim prefers to withdraw from the presence of others. Vertigo (dizziness and disorientation) may be experienced, and nystagmus can often be observed (the slow motion opposite to the imposed angular acceleration, the quick return in the direction of the motion). When nystagmus occurs, some associated blurring of vision may be a major complaint.

ETIOLOGY. Repeated angular acceleration stimulations of the three semicircular canals in each ear, especially when visual contact with the actual outside horizon is lost, cause conflicting sensations of orientation. The afferent nerve signals sent to the brain centers from the body's entire motion- and position-detecting senses (semicircular canals for angular accelerations, saccule and utricle for linear accelerations, and the proprioceptive system for the gravity "downward" acceleration) are involved. The proprioceptive system contains the subcutaneous pressure and kinesthetic senses. It sends signals to the brain on the body responses to experiencing accelerations and segment position changes. When the brain can no longer resolve or ignore the aforementioned varieties of afferent signals, confusion and dismay often result. This may lead to fatigue, anxiety and adrenergic "fear" response, sweating, pallor, tachycardia, and, ultimately, nausea and vomiting.

The air traveler most often encounters motion sickness in the 0.1- to 0.7-Hz frequency range of linear acceleration. From one third to one half of airline passengers suffer motion sickness to various degrees when the linear acceleration levels (primarily in the vertical parameter) are in the range of 0.2 to 0.4 g root mean square. This is in the "moderately heavy" to "very heavy" turbulence range as described by pilots. About one in ten of the passengers of jet aircraft can be expected to experience an advanced degree of motion sickness in these frequency ranges.

In addition to the aforementioned linear acceleration aspect, the three semicircular canals in each ear detect angular accelerations at levels as low as 2.5 degrees per second^2 for a one-second period. At higher rotation rates, less time is required to detect motion. When one set of the three sets of canals (posterior, superior, lateral) is equilibrated to a constant angular velocity (for example, a constant rate turn) and the head is tilted, another set of canals receives stimulation. The canal endolymph must dissipate the angular momentum when moving to or from a given plane of rotation, producing canal sensor stimulations that the brain cannot resolve in regard to actual motion cues, giving the Coriolis effect (an uncomfortable disorientation feeling of movement different from the actual motion). At 0.6 degrees per second, the Coriolis effect can be detected. At 240 times this angular velocity, respiratory movements alone can cause the Coriolis symptoms.

It has been found that anxiety can lower the threshold for the onset of motion sickness. In addition, some persons are prone to experiencing motion sickness from childhood. No specific reason why these persons are susceptible has been found. In some cases, a labile emotional state has been implicated, as has a rigid, compulsive personality in others. However, more studies on these points are needed before positive statements can be made. The key role of the vestibular system in causing motion sickness is shown by the virtual absence of motion sickness in persons who have lost their left and right vestibular organs because of disease or surgery, or who suffered a congenital loss of these systems.

DIAGNOSIS. The progressive onset of sleepiness, fatigue, nausea, and/or vertigo, during air travel, is the prime symptom that aids in diagnosing motion sickness. This is especially so if the past history reveals prior occurrences in a given individual. The degree of the severity of the illness is usually associated directly with the degree of turbulence and maneuvering experienced. The progression of the symptoms to a state of frank vomiting is common. The signs include a clammy skin and, often, some degree of nystagmus.

The differential diagnosis must include (1) food poisoning (an occasional problem from meals served through airline caterers is staphylococcal food poisoning, often causing symptoms similar to severe motion sickness), (2) acute alcohol ingestion toxicity, (3) gastritis caused by intrinsic pathology (for example, peptic ulcer), and (4) shock. In repeated progressively severe instances of motion sickness involving a given individual, the possibility of increased intracranial pressure or some form of cranial tumor exists.

TREATMENT, PROGNOSIS, AND PREVENTION. The treatment of motion sickness is most effective when given one to two hours prior to exposure to accelerations. Reassurance is a useful aid for many travelers. Habituation of the vestibular system to accelerations usually occurs in the veteran traveler, markedly decreasing the times of motion sickness.

The following drugs have been found useful in treating motion sickness (*adult doses*):
1. Promethazine (Phenergan), 25 mg twice a day. (Note: When 25 mg ephedrine sulfate is also given simultaneously, a much more effective antimotion sickness effect results.)
2. Scopolamine (hyoscine), 1.2 mg.
3. Dimenhydrinate (Dramamine), 50 mg.
4. Cyclizine (Marezine), 50 mg.
5. Meclizine (Bonine), 50 mg.

In the 1960's, scopolamine and d-amphetamine were found to counteract motion sickness in an effective manner; but with the current trend away from prescribing amphetamines, this combination is not recommended in the routine practice of medicine.

It is quite possible that a strong placebo effect is operating in the case of drugs 4 and 5 above.

Since motion sickness is aggravated by the odors of vomitus, susceptible persons should move from its proximity. The motion-sick person should lie back and remain still, and may find that a cool damp cloth over the forehead provides comfort. The prognosis for the motion-sick person is excellent, because upon completion of the exposure to motions, recovery is usually rapid, taking place in a matter of minutes, and seldom exceeding a few hours. Prevention of motion sickness includes avoidance by susceptible persons of the types of accelerations that induce the syndrome. When this is not possible, the use of any one of the drugs given above should ameliorate or prevent motion sickness, especially if taken prior to the exposure to accelerations. It is emphasized that these drugs should not be taken by air crew members or others who must operate vehicles or machinery, because there are side effects that temporarily can impair higher mental functions and produce diminished alertness.

Gillingham, K. K.: A Primer on Vestibular Function, Spatial Disorientation, and Motion Sickness. USAF School of Aerospace Medicine, Brooks Air Force Base, Texas, Rev. 4-66, June 1966.

Graybiel, A., and Knepton, J.: Direction-specific adaptation effects acquired in a slow rotation room. Aerosp. Med., 43:1179, 1972.

Graybiel, A., Wood, C. O., Knepton, J., Hoche, J. P., and Perkins, G. F.: Human Bioassay of Antimotion Sickness Drugs. Naval Aerospace Medical Research Laboratory Report 1215, April 1975.

Lentz, J. M., and Collins, W. E.: Motion sickness susceptibility and related behavioral characteristics in men and women. Aviat. Space Environ. Med., 48:316, 1977.

von Gierke, H. E., and Clarke, N. P.: Effects of vibration and buffeting on man. *In* Randel, H. W. (ed.): Aerospace Medicine. Baltimore, Williams & Wilkins Company, 1971, p. 198.

Waite, R. E., and DeLucchi, M. R.: Labyrinthine and proprioceptive aspects of aerospace medicine. *In* Randel, H. W. (ed.): Aerospace Medicine. Baltimore, Williams & Wilkins Company, 1971, p. 254.

29.2. PROBLEMS OF AIR TRAVEL

GENERAL. U. S. airlines carried 232,100,000 passengers in 1977, many passengers characterized by extremes of age and physical status (Civil Aeronautics Board figure). Old age, infancy, and pregnancy do not alone preclude air travel. Complications accompanying these states may preclude safe travel, as may specific illnesses or conditions at any age. Persons in precarious health should be transported by air ambulance, although in individual instances safe travel may be possible if a trained health professional is along. Of course, serious contagions would preclude air travel in view of the risk to other passengers.

Passengers with specific chronic medical problems should have appropriate medications with them when traveling by air. It is very unlikely that a well provisioned medical kit will be available on a U. S. airline aircraft, as most U. S. airlines do not furnish this service at present (many non–U. S. airlines do). Therefore the diabetic, for example, should have extra insulin in his carry-on luggage, the cardiac patient should have appropriate medication along, and persons with other medical requirements should have available the appropriate drugs and equipment. Possible en route delays of several hours and even the possibility of diversions of the aircraft to another city should be considered in estimating the type and amount of medical items to carry. Possible delays in receipt of checked luggage make it wise to have all medicines in the carry-on luggage.

In addition to the above, a time factor should be included with reference to time zone changes and the relative time of taking medicine. When a diabetic travels west (lengthening the day by the number of time zones covered), a mild degree of hyperglycemia is preferable to risking hypoglycemia, and therefore the next *insulin injection* may be postponed until the local time of destination. However, when traveling several time zones to the east, resulting in a shortened day, the local destination time cannot be observed immediately for the next injection, as this would likely produce hypoglycemia. The injection may be postponed for the number of hours equivalent to the time zones crossed, or the dosage may be halved or otherwise diminished on the first day.

Persons with severe *emphysema* may arrange through the airline for airline-provided carry-on oxygen. This will assist the individual to have an adequate tracheal oxygen for the duration of the trip. Cabin altitudes may reach a maximum of about 8000 feet (2438.4 meters) equivalent altitude at the highest cruising flight altitude of the aircraft. Some advance planning to assure adequate oxygen availability in the departure and arrival terminals is also necessary. Certain other medical problems, including asthma and epilepsy, may require special medication, and this should be carried by the patient. Complicated pregnancies and advanced pregnancies are additional problems that can result in on-board flight emergencies. In all these instances, the advice of the patient's physician must be obtained, and the circumstances of the flight must be balanced against the medical condition and the purpose of the flight. In addition, the airline medical department (if the airline has one) can be consulted.

Handicapped persons with *paraplegia, blindness, deafness*, and other static problems may travel upon the advice of their physician and the airline. In some cases, an accompanying assistant will be required. Accommodation in the passenger cabin for the guide dog of a blind person can also be arranged. A major consideration in transport of the handicapped is the problem of using the toilet. If the passenger cannot tend to this alone, an accompanying attendant will be necessary, as the flight attendants do not undertake this type of care as part of their routine duties.

Persons who have upper respiratory infections with *sinusitis* or *otitis media* may experience severe discomfort as the passenger cabin repressurizes on the descent phase of flight. It is best to avoid air travel when these conditions exist, but if the problem is encountered, nasal inhalers can be of assistance in opening passageways. For aerotitis media, the Valsalva maneuver conducted with a closed mouth and nose will often open the eustachian tube and ventilate the middle ear. During the postflight period, an otolaryngologist should be consulted if symptoms persist.

Certain other potential problems preclude safe passenger flight. The few weeks following a myocardial infarction and the period of one or two weeks following abdominal or cranial surgery are generally not times for flight. In no case should flight be undertaken if there is any significant amount of trapped gas in any part of the body. A *pneumothorax* precludes safe flight.

A common bother to passengers with lower leg circulatory problems is that of *swelling of the feet and ankles* during the protracted time of sitting on long flights. This problem is due to venous stasis and can be serious from the standpoint of phlebothrombosis. Walking about the aisle during periods free from turbulence (and when the seat belt sign is off) helps diminish lower body venous stasis.

Prior to undertaking flight, crew members and passengers should allow 12 to 24 hours following *scuba diving*, depending on the depths to which the dive was carried. In the case of very deep dives, 36 hours should be allowed. If insufficient time elapses, the nitrogen stored in the fat tissue during the dive can evolve and cause the bends or chokes. Should these occur, rapid transport to a hyperbaric pressure facility is necessary for relief of symptoms and prevention of possible permanent injury (preferably by land if the distance is short; if by air, destination ground level cabin pressure should be maintained).

TIME ZONE EFFECTS, "JET LAG." A medical problem that is bothersome to air travelers undertaking lengthy flights that cover several time zones has been identified. The syndrome has been referred to by many terms, including circadian rhythm desynchronosis, transmeridian dysrhythmia, and "jet lag." The symptoms include a diminished degree of alertness, a feeling of considerable fatigue, and insomnia during nighttime hours, and may also include constipation and irritability. In addition, executives may find it difficult to solve complex problems, and athletes may find their performance markedly poorer, during the first day or two upon arrival at the destination.

The "jet lag" syndrome occurs most strongly during the two- to three-day period following east-west or west-east travel across time zones, at which time the individual is displaced geographically from the origin of the trip, although physiologically the individual is adapted to the time of the origin. If the displacement is in an easterly direction, the relative day-night cycle will be markedly shortened, and persons generally find displacement to the east to be the most fatiguing experience.

In the easterly direction, the individual is "driven" by the relatively shorter time for sleep in relation to associates. If the traveler has traversed five time zones to the east, the effective day at the destination is shortened by five hours. If he or she has flown all night, the low quality sleep acquired in the sitting position (good quality sleep necessitates a horizontal position in order that the pull of gravity along the long axis of the body be neutralized), leads to additional fatigue. It is noted that in order for refreshing stage four level sleep (the deepest sleep stage) to be achieved, the person must sleep in the horizontal position. Flights in the westerly direction lead to a stretched-out day and result in a prolonged wakeful period. This additional wakefulness is fatiguing, but is offset somewhat by the relatively longer time for sleep. Although flying to the west is not as fatiguing as flying to the east, the total time for readaptation is longer for westerly flights.

A rule of thumb for estimating readaptation following time zone dislocation is that the circadian rhythms of the body take approximately one day for each time zone (15 degrees of longitude) traversed. Serious psychophysiologic effects do not begin until three or more time zones are covered. There are wide differences in individual susceptibility to experiencing symptoms in this syndrome, and there are also wide variations in individual recovery. With increasing age, there is a general tendency for more difficulty in adapting to any time zone displacement. Recommendations for minimizing time zone displacement effects on circadian rhythms include recognizing the phenomenon, minimizing the amount of rich food and alcoholic beverages consumed during the transmeridian flights, and allowing one to two days of free rest period following arrival at the destination before engaging in complex or competitive activities. A short-acting barbiturate may be prescribed to assist sleep upon arrival at the destination should the wakeful portion of the circadian cycle be inhibiting the need for sleep.

SICKLE CELL ANEMIA. There are more than 100 identified inherited types of hemoglobinopathies that contain deletions or substitutions of certain amino acids in the alpha or beta chain of the heme moiety of hemoglobin A. Hemoglobin S is one of these hemoglobinopathies. The presence alone of the hemoglobin S genotype, sickle cell trait, does not result in any symptoms for the carrier. This genotype is detected only by laboratory tests.

The individual with hemoglobin S is most susceptible to sickling crises in the homozygous state. Crises may also occur in the heterozygous state if certain abnormal types of hemoglobin are associated with hemoglobin S. Examples are hemoglobins C, D (Los Angeles), and O (Arab). The individual with the homozygous hemoglobin S condition and the person with the combination of hemoglobin S and one or another of the various abnormal hemoglobins constitute phenotypes that experience sickle cell disease. The sickling crises of this disease occur in vivo when blood oxygen tension falls below 60 mm Hg. The total number of sickled cells depends in part upon the types of hemoglobin associated with the S type. The sickled cells can no longer pass through capillaries, and produce a cycle of vascular infarctions. It has been demonstrated that hemoglobins A and F confer resistance to sickling by the S hemoglobin. The combination of hemoglobin A and S hemoglobins does not sickle in vitro until the oxygen tension falls to about 10 mm Hg.

The hemoglobin AS genotype can be viewed as an incomplete dominance, in that although there are no sickling crises, hyposthenuria can usually be demonstrated, possibly the result of a slight tendency toward sickling in the kidneys. In World War II, 7 per cent of black pilots had the sickle cell trait. None showed any clinical manifestations of the genotype, in spite of arduous missions, including high altitude flight. There is evidence, however, that the AS genotype in some cases can have a fatal original crisis in extreme degrees of severe hypoxia. More study of this possibility must be done before definitive information is available.

In view of the aforementioned aspects concerning sickle cell anemia, the following conclusions can be made:

1. Persons with the sickle trait alone will experience no problems in air travel.
2. Persons with sickle hemoglobin in association with other abnormal hemoglobins may have sickling crises during air travel, especially if they have had a history of sickling.
3. Persons with homozygous sickle hemoglobin are very prone to hypoxic sickling crises and should avoid air travel unless absolutely necessary.

If air travel is unavoidable in categories 2 and 3 above, prophylactic oxygen should be considered, based on the past history of the individual. This must be available for the entire flight. To assure adequate kidney blood circulation with no stasis, good hydration during flight should be assured. If the cabin is to exceed an equivalent altitude of 8000 feet (2438.4 meters), the use of oxygen is essential.

Carruthers, M., Arguelles, A. E., and Mosovich, A.: Man in transit: Biochemical and physiological changes during intercontinental flights. Lancet, 1:977, 1976.

Klein, K. E., Wegmann, H. M., and Hunt, B. I.: Desynchronization of body temperature and performance circadian rhythm as a result of outgoing and homecoming transmeridian flights. Aerosp. Med., 43:119, 1972.

McKenzie, J. M.: The Aeromedical Significance of Sickle-Cell Trait: A Review. Office of Aviation Medicine Report, FAA-AM-76-15, Federal Aviation Administration, U.S.A., 1976.

Mohler, S. R.: Physiologic index as an aid in developing airline pilot scheduling patterns. Aviat. Space Environ. Med., 47:238, 1976.

Siegel, P. V., Gerathewohl, S. J., and Mohler, S. R.: Time zone effects. Science, 164:1249, 1969.

30. ALTERATIONS IN ATMOSPHERIC PRESSURE

Jefferson C. Davis

30.1. INTRODUCTION

Exposure to decreased barometric pressure in flight or to barometric pressure greater than sea level in diving presents unique pathophysiologic and therapeutic implications. In the past, medical care of workers in these environments was largely the province of flight surgeons and diving medical officers. In recent years, however, there has been rapid growth in air travel and in excursions to mountainous regions on vacation or business by the general public — often by ambulatory patients with significant medical problems. Participation in scuba (self contained underwater breathing apparatus) diving by people of all ages, in inland lakes as well as coastal waters, has expanded underwater medicine from the limited realm of the caisson worker and the commercial or military diver to include patients seen in any medical practice. Further, therapeutic use of intermittent high dose oxygen inhalation in hyperbaric or high pressure chambers (hyperbaric oxygen) has gained acceptance as an adjunct in clostridial myonecrosis and cellulitis and in carbon monoxide poisoning, as well as the promotion of healing in certain ischemic, hypoxic wounds. In order to understand the specific medical problems encountered, a brief review of the environments is necessary.

PHYSICS OF ENVIRONMENTAL PRESSURE. The weight of atmospheric air and water, at any point on or above the surface of the earth or beneath the surface of the water, can be expressed in various units of pressure. On ascent to altitude, we are passing through the blanket of air which extends from sea level to approximately 430 miles altitude, where the atmosphere is so thin that no molecular collisions occur. The atmosphere weighs 14.7 pounds per square inch, or 760 mm Hg (760 torr), at sea level. The pressure change for a given ascent is much greater at lower altitudes. For example, ascent from sea level to 3048 meters (10,000 feet) gives a pressure reduction of 237 mm Hg, from 760 mm Hg to 523 mm Hg; but the same 3048-meter altitude change, from 9146 meters (30,000 feet) to 12,192 meters (40,000 feet), gives a pressure reduction of only 85 mm Hg, from 226 mm Hg to 141 mm Hg. Contrast this pressure reduction to the linear pressure change at depth, in which each foot of sea water weighs 0.445 pound per square inch; thus, $14.7 \div 0.445 = 33$ feet of sea water, or 10 meters. The barometric pressure (P_B) at this depth can be stated in terms of gauge pressure (that in excess of sea-level pressure) or, more conveniently, as absolute pressure (the total of sea-level atmospheric pressure plus the water pressure). Pressure can be expressed in various units; most commonly used are mm Hg, feet of sea water (FSW), meters of sea water, or atmospheres absolute (ATA). Further descent to depth gives linear pressure changes, so that at 20 meters (66 FSW), the total pressure is 3 ATA or 2280 mm Hg. Barometric pressure at any altitude is available from standard altitude charts, and pressure at any depth can be easily derived; but for clarification and because certain pressures are key in the physiologic principles to follow, selected altitudes and depths are provided in Table 1.

The earth's atmosphere is composed of a mixture of gases — including nitrogen (78.98 per cent), oxygen (20.95 per cent), argon (0.93 per cent), and carbon dioxide (0.03 per cent) — with varying amounts of water vapor and other inert rare gases, totaling 760 mm Hg at sea level according to Dalton's law ($P_B = P_{N_2} + P_{O_2} + P_{others}$). For physiologic considerations, the atmospheric composition is usually considered to consist of 21 per cent oxygen and 79 per cent nitrogen, with the rare gases being included with the inert nitrogen. For practical purposes, these percentages remain constant through the range of pressure changes, so it is the partial pressures (P_{O_2}) of gases in the mixture which change. For example, at sea level, $P_{O_2} = 160$ mm Hg

(760×0.21), $P_{N_2} = 600$ mm Hg (760×0.79); at an altitude of 3048 meters (10,000 feet), $P_{O_2} = 110$ mm Hg (523×0.21), $P_{N_2} = 413$ mm Hg (523×0.79); and with air compressed to equal the water pressure at 20 meters (66 FSW), $P_{O_2} = 479$ mm Hg (2280×0.21), $P_{N_2} = 1801$ mm Hg (2280×0.79).

The medical problems created by changes in atmospheric pressure may be grouped into direct and indirect effects. The former result from mechanical forces created when pressure differentials develop across the walls of air-containing spaces within the body or upon its surface. Indirect effects result from alterations in partial pressures of the individual gases of the atmosphere.

Davis, J. C., and Hunt, T. K. (eds.): Hyperbaric Oxygen Therapy. Bethesda, Md., Undersea Medical Society, Inc., 1977.

Strughold, H.: The earth's atmosphere and aviation. In Randel, H. W. (ed.): Aerospace Medicine. Baltimore, Williams & Wilkins Company, 1971, pp. 22–34.

30.2. DIRECT EFFECTS OF CHANGES IN ATMOSPHERIC PRESSURE

Gases respond to pressure changes in accordance with Boyle's law ($P_1 V_1 = P_2 V_2$). Their volume varies inversely and their density, or molecular concentration, directly as the absolute pressure. The fluids and solids of the human body, being incompressible, transmit pressure freely and thus assume the pressure exerted upon the body's surface. Any alteration in pressure on the surface of the body is reflected almost instantly by an identical pressure change in body tissues and within air-containing spaces of the body. Gas pressures within the middle ears, paranasal sinuses, respiratory tract, and gastrointestinal tract can be maintained equal to external pressure only by appropriate adjustments either of the number of molecules of gas within the space or of the volume of the space. No medical difficulties arise as long as air can pass freely between such spaces and the environment. If additional air cannot enter such a space to increase its pressure during descent, a relative vacuum is created, the lining of the walls becomes hyperemic and swollen, and serum or blood may move in to eradicate the pressure differential. Conversely, during ascent with declining environmental pressure, expansion of gas volume in the fixed volume cavity produces increasing pressure. Unless air can be vented from the space, an increasing pressure gradient creates a distending force against the walls.

Pockets of air against various surfaces of the body may be produced by such factors as goggles, tight-fitting hoods, ear plugs, or wrinkles in diving suits.

CLINICAL MANIFESTATIONS. The most common direct or mechanical effect of descent from altitude, or from sea level to depth, is *barotitis media*. Because of the flutter valve effect produced by the nasopharyngeal end of the eustachian tube, equalization of middle ear pressure is usually automatic on ascent to altitude or to the surface from depth; but on descent — unless active measures (yawning, swallowing, or the modified Valsalva maneuver) are taken to open the tube — a relative vacuum is created in the middle ear. Surprisingly little pressure imbalance (60 to 100 mm Hg) produces pain as the tympanic membrane is retracted, followed by hy-

TABLE 1.   Representative Alterations in Barometric Pressure

Altitude/depth	Absolute Pressure (mm Hg)	Absolute Pressure Atmospheres (ATA)	Absolute Pressure (PSIA)
15,200 meters (50,000 feet)	87	0.11	1.7
13,106 meters (43,000 feet)	122	0.16	2.4
5486 meters (18,000 feet)	380	0.50	7.3
3048 meters (10,000 feet)	523	0.67	10.1
Sea level	760	1.0	14.7
10 meters (33 FSW)*	1520	2.0	29.4
20 meters (66 FSW)	2280	3.0	44.1
30 meters (99 FSW)	3040	4.0	58.8
40 meters (132 FSW)	3800	5.0	73.5
50 meters (165 FSW)	4560	6.0	88.2

*FSW = Feet of sea water; 32.8 FSW = 10 meters.

peremia and hemorrhage into the membrane; finally, the tympanic membrane perforates, or blood is drawn into the middle ear to equalize the pressure imbalance. Flying or diving with an upper respiratory infection may make equalization impossible and predisposes to this injury. *Barosinusitis* is less common, but the mechanisms are similar and pain can be quite intense. Barosinusitis can occur on ascent if edematous mucosa, a polyp, or mucus prevents escape of air from the sinus cavity to equalize pressure.

Prevention of these common problems is best achieved by teaching the diver not only to use techniques for pressure equalization but also to avoid pressure changes when acute coryza or allergic rhinitis restricts the eustachian tube or paranasal sinus orifices. During descent in diving, attempts to equalize middle ear pressure by a very forcible Valsalva maneuver result in elevated cerebrospinal fluid pressure. This hydrostatic pressure, transmitted by perilymph to the round window at the same time a relative vacuum exists in the middle ear, can result in *round window rupture.* The manifestations are sudden, severe vertigo, tinnitus, and persistent deafness in the affected ear. It is important to refer such a diver to an otolaryngologist immediately, so that evaluation and surgical repair can be performed.

The most serious direct effects of pressure, leading to important medical emergencies, involve the lungs. Reference to Table 1 clarifies important points. *First,* direct effects on the lungs are rare in altitude exposure, because breath-holding would have to be sustained over a long period of time during normal ascent or descent to realize sufficient pressure changes. An exception would be in the event of catastrophic aircraft cabin decompression; but here, also, breath-holding before and during the decompression would be required. The weight of water produces great pressure changes with small depth changes. *Second,* in diving, the greatest volume changes in gases trapped in body cavities occur at shallow depths. Ascent from 4 ATA (99 FSW) to 2 ATA (33 FSW) results in an attempt to double the volume of gas which, in a fixed volume cavity, means a doubling of pressure according to Boyle's law. At shallower depths, however, the same pressure-volume change occurs with ascent from only 2 ATA (33 FSW) to the surface. This very important concept has accounted for severe *pulmonary overpressure accidents* among scuba divers who breath-held from as little as 2.2 to 3.1 meters (7 to 10 feet) of water depth.

In order to understand the direct effects of pressure change on the lung, as well as some of the indirect changes (to be discussed in Ch. 30.3), a brief description of diving modes must be introduced. (The concept of pressurized aircraft cabins has already been presented in Ch. 29.2, and will not be repeated.) The breath-holding diver carries no supplemental breathing gas supply underwater, and his depth is limited by his breath-holding time, physical stamina, and lung volume. During descent, lung volume will decrease according to Boyle's law; and, when reduced to less than residual volume, a "lung squeeze" can result in pulmonary edema and hemorrhage. Compressed gas diving (e.g., air, nitrogen-oxygen, helium-oxygen) supplies breathing gas to the diver through regulators designed to match water pressure at any depth, either from the surface by means of hoses or by compressed air or mixed breathing gas carried in high-pressure cylinders by the diver (scuba). While the lung squeeze of the breath-holding diver is avoided, the major risks to the supplied diver are on decompression.

After breathing compressed gas at pressure equal to water pressure at depth, gas must be released from the lungs by normal breathing — or, in the event of loss of gas supply at depth, by slow exhalation during ascent. Failure to do so results in intrapulmonary gas expansion, increased intra-alveolar pressure, and introduction of extra-alveolar gas (pulmonary overpressure accidents). Lung tissue distal to a poorly communicating diseased bronchial passage may be similarly damaged, even if the diver vents his excess air during ascent. The air traveler with such bronchopulmonary disease, or one who happens to be holding his breath, may be similarly injured during a sudden loss of cabin pressure at high altitude. The result may be arterial gas (air) embolism, mediastinal and subcutaneous emphysema, and/or pneumothorax. The latter two manifestations are recognized by physical and radiographic examination, and can be managed by conventional measures. In diving, a gas embolism has been reported during ascents of as little as 2.2 meters (7 FSW), and is said to be exceeded in frequency only by drowning as a cause of accidental death among divers.

Knowledge of the character of the dive, including depth, duration, air supply, and patterns of descent and ascent in relation to symptoms, often simplifies the problem of diagnosing lung injury in divers. Frothy, bloody sputum may be produced in either thoracic squeeze or lung overpressure. The overriding clinical manifestations in arterial gas embolism result from arterial gas bubbles embolizing the brain. There is sudden onset of unconsciousness, focal or generalized seizure activity, visual field loss or blindness, weakness, paralysis, and hypesthesia or confusion. The diver with these manifestations must be presumed to have gas embolism or decompression sickness.

TREATMENT. Either gas embolism or decompression sickness requires treatment by recompression at the earliest possible moment. Transport to a recompression chamber should be by the fastest method available. An aircraft used for transportation must have cabin pressure kept at or near sea-level equivalent — or, if unpressurized, flown not more than a few hundred feet above sea level. Cardiopulmonary resuscitation and bicarbonate administration may be required, because many of these casualties are also near-drowning victims. Oxygen should be administered as well as intravenous solutions, such as dextran and normal saline. Positioning the suspected gas embolism patient in the Trendelenburg position, and on the left side, seems to be of benefit.

Bond, G. F.: Arterial gas embolism. *In* Davis, J. C., and Hunt, T. K. (eds.): Hyperbaric Oxygen Therapy. Bethesda, Md., Undersea Medical Society, Inc., 1977, pp. 141–152.

30.3. INDIRECT EFFECTS OF CHANGES IN ATMOSPHERIC PRESSURE

Gases in contact with liquids dissolve in direct proportion to their partial pressures and their solubility coefficients. Gases enter and leave the body in response to gradients of partial pressure between blood and alveolar gases. Gradients of partial pressure likewise determine the movement of gases within body fluids. Alterations in respiratory gas composition (caused by the reduced barometric pressure at altitude) and the high partial pressures of inspired gases (from compressed gas sources in diving) present a series of significant hazards.

HYPOXIA

Without supplemental oxygen, the physiologic effects of the reduced atmospheric partial pressure of oxygen (Po_2) at altitude are described as hypoxic hypoxia. Other factors which lead to tissue hypoxia can coexist and be additive. Thus a patient whose oxygen transport capacity is impaired by anemia or carbon monoxide bound hemoglobin ("hypemic hypoxia"), or whose tissue oxygen utilization is impaired by cyanide or ethanol ("histotoxic hypoxia"), will be more susceptible to hypoxia at altitude. A special potentiating factor in aviation is stagnant hypoxia in an aviator exposed to high head-to-foot acceleration forces, as in recovering from an aircraft dive. The increased weight of the column of blood reduces cerebral perfusion with resultant cerebral hypoxia. Although these factors can be important contributors to hypoxia in aviation, this discussion will center on hypoxia caused by reduction in Po_2 at the decreased barometric pressures at altitude.

Inspired air is humidified in the respiratory tract, rapidly equilibrating with the 47 mm Hg vapor pressure of water at body temperature. Alveolar Pco_2 of about 40 mm Hg and water vapor of 47 mm Hg are roughly constant at any altitude, so that alveolar partial pressure of oxygen (PA_{O_2}) can be approximated for any altitude by use of the simplified alveolar gas equation, assuming a respiratory quotient of 1:

$$PA_{O_2} = FI_{O_2} (P_B - PA_{H_2O}) - PA_{CO_2}$$
in which FI_{O_2} = fraction of inspired O_2
P_B = barometric pressure

For example, at 3048 meters (10,000 feet), breathing air:

$$PA_{O_2} = 0.21 (523 - 47) - 40$$
$$PA_{O_2} = 60 \text{ mm Hg}$$

Or, at 5846 meters (18,000 feet), breathing air:

$$PA_{O_2} = 0.21 (380 - 47) - 40$$
$$PA_{O_2} = 30 \text{ mm Hg}$$

Alveolar Po_2 rapidly equilibrates with arterial Po_2 at the alveolar-capillary interface in healthy people, and hemoglobin is saturated according to the alveolar Po_2. The shape of the oxygen-hemoglobin dissociation curve is of great importance at altitude, with the "knee" of the curve at Po_2 of 60 mm Hg, with a fairly flat slope above this point so that a drop from the normal 100 mm Hg PA_{O_2} at sea level to 60 mm Hg at 3048 meters (10,000 feet) causes a drop in arterial oxygen saturation of only 10 ml of oxygen per 100 ml of blood. Above this altitude, however, even small drops in PA_{O_2} result in large decreases in arterial saturation along the steep slope of

the curve. Thus, except for a decrement in night vision at about 1220 meters (4000 feet) to 1829 meters (6000 feet), there are no significant effects of hypoxia in healthy people below 3048 meters (10,000 feet). In general, pressurized aircraft cabins are maintained well below that equivalent air pressure, so no supplemental oxygen is required. Nevertheless, patients with reduced cardiac reserve may have difficulty tolerating even this small drop in arterial oxygen saturation, and require supplemental oxygen during flight.

MANIFESTATIONS. Table 2 summarizes the major manifestations of altitude hypoxia with corresponding PA_{O_2} breathing ambient air.

The time required for the onset of symptoms in Table 2 differs from person to person, depending on age, fitness, acclimatization, and individual variation. At higher altitudes, the progression of symptoms to the point of inability to perform useful functions (time of useful consciousness, or TUC) is quite rapid and within a narrower range of individual variation. For example, the TUC at 9146 meters (30,000 feet) is about 90 seconds, and at 13,106 meters (43,000 feet) is about 15 seconds.

PREVENTION. The use of pressurized cabins, which allows man to stay safely within the physiologically comfortable zone below 3048 meters (10,000 feet), is the main preventive factor in modern aviation. The percentage of supplemental oxygen required to maintain an alveolar Po_2 no less than the 3048 meters (10,000 feet) equivalent at an altitude can be derived by varying the FI_{O_2} in the simplified alveolar gas equation. For example, at 12,192 meters (40,000 feet), where the barometric pressure is 141 mm Hg and PA_{CO_2} is somewhat lower due to hyperventilation:

$$PA_{O_2} = 1.0 (141 - 47) - 35$$
$$PA_{O_2} = 59 \text{ mm Hg}$$

This example is equivalent to breathing air at 3048 meters (10,000 feet) and is the maximum altitude at which 100 per cent oxygen breathing is adequate to prevent hypoxia. At higher altitudes, positive pressure breathing and, finally, pressure suits are required.

TABLE 2.   Responses to Hypoxic Hypoxia

Altitude		Alveolar Po_2 (mm Hg)
3048 meters (10,000 feet)	Impairment of recent memory, judgment, and ability to perform complex calculations; increased heart rate and pulmonary ventilation	60
3658 meters (12,000 feet)	Dyspnea, impaired ability to perform complex tasks, headache, nausea, decreased visual acuity	52
4573 meters (15,000 feet)	Decrease in auditory acuity, constriction of visual fields, impaired judgment, irritability; exercise can lead to unconsciousness	46
5486 meters (18,000 feet)	Decrements in personality and intellect; threshold for loss of consciousness in resting unacclimatized individuals after several hours' exposure	40
6096 meters (20,000 feet)	Handwriting illegible in conscious subjects	33
6706 meters (22,000 feet) and above	Almost all individuals unconscious after sufficient exposure time	30

Holmstrom, F. M. G.: Hypoxia. *In* Randel, H. W. (ed.): Aerospace Medicine. Baltimore, Williams & Wilkins Company, 1971, pp. 56–85.

ACUTE MOUNTAIN SICKNESS

This is a clinical syndrome observed in unacclimatized persons, usually within a few hours after rapid exposure to high altitude. Individual tolerance varies widely. Some people experience symptoms at altitudes as low as 2134 to 2439 meters (7000 to 8000 feet), although others tolerate altitudes of 4267 meters (14,000 feet) with minimal symptoms. There appears to be no way to predict unusual susceptibility; but rapid ascent, physical exertion, and poor physical condition increase the likelihood. Initial symptoms are usually mild to incapacitating headache, exertional dyspnea, malaise, and weakness. Insomnia, anorexia, nausea, vomiting, diarrhea, and abdominal pain may occur. Mental capacity and judgment may be impaired. Inability to sleep is a common problem. Cyanosis of the lips and nail beds, Cheyne-Stokes breathing, and tachycardia are usually present. These manifestations usually subside gradually over a period of several days, but may recur at higher altitudes. In some instances, the symptoms are severe and unrelieved except by oxygen or descent to a lower altitude. Gradual ascent with periodic halts of several days to allow acclimatization will prevent or reduce the severity of symptoms. Acetazolamide, given in dosages of 250 mg every eight hours prior to and during exposure to altitude, has been reported to reduce the frequency and severity of symptoms. The mechanism of its effect is not clear; but increased ventilation and alveolar oxygen tension, decreased carbon dioxide tension and serum bicarbonate, and absence of alkalosis were observed in treated subjects. Furosemide, 80 mg every 12 hours, has produced relief of symptoms and signs usually within 48 hours, apparently in association with the induced diuresis.

Forward, S. A., Landowne, M., Follansbee, J. N., and Hansen, J. E.: Effect of acetazolamide on acute mountain sickness. N. Engl. J. Med., 279:839, 1968.
Singh, I., Khanna, P. K., Srivastava, M. C., Lal, M., Roy, S. B., and Subramanyam, C. S. V.: Acute mountain sickness. N. Engl. J. Med., 280:175, 1969.

HIGH ALTITUDE PULMONARY EDEMA

Acute pulmonary edema is an uncommon but serious and sometimes fatal complication of rapid exposure to altitudes above 2744 meters (9000 feet). Hypoxia is considered the primary etiologic agent. Many earlier fatal cases were erroneously diagnosed as pneumonia. Most susceptible appear to be young, unacclimatized persons and acclimatized residents who have sojourned at lower altitudes for a few days or weeks. Recurrences are common in those who have experienced an attack. Rapid ascent and heavy physical exertion increase susceptibility.

Autopsy findings have included wet lungs congested with serosanguineous edema fluid. Bronchiolar and alveolar edema with hyaline membranes, resembling those seen in hyaline membrane disease of the newborn, over the internal walls of alveoli, alveolar sacs, and alveolar ducts have been characteristic findings.

Dilatation of preterminal arterioles and thrombosis of septal capillaries and of small and medium-sized pulmonary arteries have also been observed. The exact pathogenic mechanism is conjectural. A comparative increase in capillary pressure is thought to be responsible for the alveolar edema. In a few cases, pulmonary artery pressure has been elevated, and electrocardiograms have suggested acute right ventricular overloading. The hyaline membrane formation, not a characteristic finding in death caused by simple hypoxia, has not been explained; but a deficient pulmonary fibrinolysis system has been postulated.

Symptoms usually appear 6 to 36 hours after exposure to altitude and may be preceded by acute mountain sickness. Exertional dyspnea, weakness, malaise, and a persistent, dry, irritating cough are the characteristic initial symptoms. Later, noisy respiration, rales, cyanosis, orthopnea, and hemoptysis develop. Unless continuous oxygen therapy is carried out or the patient descends to a lower altitude, these symptoms progress, and death occurs. Gradual acclimatization and avoidance of undue physical exertion during the early period of exposure to altitude are important preventive measures.

CHRONIC MOUNTAIN SICKNESS
(Monge's Disease)

Chronic mountain sickness is a clinical syndrome that occurs in residents at high altitudes, usually over 4267 meters (14,000 feet), characterized by loss of tolerance to hypoxia in a previously acclimatized person. The cause is not known, but associated are increased polycythemia, decreased pulmonary ventilation, increased Pco_2, lowered arterial saturation, and impaired sensitivity of the respiratory center as compared with asymptomatic residents at high altitude. Hemoglobin and hematocrit may be increased to as much as 25 grams per 100 ml and 80 per cent, as compared with 21 grams and 60 per cent in native residents. Hyperplasia and hyperactivity of marrow erythroid cells and pulmonary hypertension are greater than in the healthy residents.

The clinical manifestations are similar to those of polycythemia vera. They include marked cyanosis, dyspnea, cough, palpitations, headache, giddiness, muscular weakness, pain in the extremities, sensory and motor changes, and episodic stupor. The condition can be cured only by returning the patients to a lower altitude or to sea level.

Monge also described a less severe form of chronic mountain sickness in mountain residents that he called subacute mountain sickness. Many of the symptoms resemble those of acute mountain sickness, but they persist unless the patient descends to sea level or receives oxygen. The marked cyanosis and alveolar hypoventilation of chronic mountain sickness do not occur, and the laboratory findings are like those in asymptomatic natives.

Hultgren, H. N., and Grover, R. F.: Circulatory adaptation to high altitude. Ann. Rev. Med., 19:119, 1968.
Lenfant, C., and Sullivan, K.: Adaptation to high altitude. N. Engl. J. Med., 284:1298, 1971.
Weihe, W. H. (ed.): Physiological Effects of High Altitude. New York, The Macmillan Company, 1964.

DECOMPRESSION SICKNESS

Decompression sickness refers to the plethora of clinical manifestations first described in the middle 1800's among caisson workers who were decompressed to sea level after working in compressed air to keep water and mud out of tunnel construction (hence the previous term, "caisson disease"). Military, commercial, and, more recently, sport diving brought emphasis to studies of this complex disorder to determine safe decompression schedules and treatment of casualties. Since the 1930's, it has been recognized that decompression from sea level to altitude can produce the same disorder, and, since 1960, treatment of altitude decompression sickness persisting at ground level has been compression to greater than sea-level pressure in chambers, as has been the treatment of divers and caisson workers for decades.

PATHOPHYSIOLOGY. A brief description of diving techniques has already been given in Ch. 30.1. The compressed gas respired at increased atmospheric pressure must be a mixture of oxygen and an inert gas diluent to prevent oxygen toxicity. This inert gas is usually nitrogen for shallow depths and helium at greater depths to prevent the narcotic effects of nitrogen at high partial pressures. Here we will deal only with compressed air, which is the respiratory gas in question for cases encountered by most physicians, for deep helium oxygen diving represents a specialized area of commercial and military and scientific diving usually covered by fully trained diving medical officers.

When compressed air is breathed underwater, to balance the hydrostatic pressure of water on the thoracic wall, or from the environment of a compressed air pressurized chamber (hyperbaric chamber, compression chamber), the alveolar partial pressure of nitrogen (P_{N_2}) rises according to barometric pressure. For example, at 50 meters (165 FSW), the barometric pressure is 4560 mm Hg and the inspired P_{N_2} is $0.79 \times 4560 = 3602$ mm Hg. Allowing for water vapor, carbon dioxide, and oxygen ($P_{O_2} = 0.21 \times 4560 = 948$ mm Hg), the alveolar P_{N_2} approximates 3525 mm Hg. According to Henry's law (the amount of gas in solution varies directly with the partial pressure of gas in contact with the solution), there is rapid diffusion of the inert nitrogen across the alveolar-capillary membrane to physical solution in plasma. Upon reaching the tissues, the high P_{N_2} dissolved in arterial blood is diffused into tissues at a rate dependent on the perfusion rate of various tissues. The total nitrogen uptake by a given tissue is determined by its composition, with lipid-rich tissues taking on larger amounts of nitrogen. The body's uptake of nitrogen can thus be seen as a complex of uptake curves which results in variable loading of different tissues, increasing with time of exposure to the elevated pressure until full equilibration is achieved at approximately 24 hours (saturation). Upon decompression from the high pressure environment to lower pressures and finally to sea level, the reverse set of gradients is established for off-loading of inert gas from tissues, to venous blood, to the lung. Inert gas will stay in solution in tissues and blood within strictly defined pressure reductions; but if critical limits are exceeded, it comes out of solution into the gas phase as bubbles in blood and tissues. The limits of safe decompression are beyond the scope of this text, and represent the goal of

extensive research still ongoing after more than 70 years of work. Once formed, bubbles in tissues and blood cause a series of pathophysiologic events which can culminate in permanent paralysis or death. Local tissue distortion by bubbles may cause pain, and circulating venous gas emboli may produce congestive infarction of the spinal cord or gas pulmonary embolism. At the blood-bubble interface, platelet aggregation has been seen; and, with platelet damage, there is release of vasoactive substances — such as serotonin and epinephrine — complicating the picture with vasoconstriction, and alteration of the platelet membrane makes phospholipid (platelet factor 3) available and accelerates clotting. Further, untreated, bubble-induced tissue ischemia and hypoxia result in loss of capillary integrity with resultant edema and hemoconcentration. Therapy today is directed toward this entire spectrum of events.

The sea-level dweller is in equilibrium (saturated) with the nitrogen partial pressure in the atmosphere. Upon rapid exposure to decreased barometric pressure at altitude, a series of events comparable to those described above can occur with evolution of nitrogen bubbles. Because of the relatively higher proportion of CO_2 and water vapor at altitude, these gases diffuse into bubbles and play a larger role than in diving. The precise critical altitude for bubble formation has not been defined; but, of clinical importance, the lowest documented case of altitude decompression sickness occurred at 5640 meters (18,500 feet). The incidence rises sharply with increasing altitude and with time at altitude. Most patients recover upon recompression to sea level; but for those who do not, emergency treatment in a compression chamber is required to resolve bubbles which persist at sea level because of growth while at altitude. Exposure to altitude following diving can produce bubbles at much lower altitudes. Cases of decompression sickness have been seen at as little as 1220 meters (4000 feet) after safe decompression from diving.

CLINICAL MANIFESTATIONS. The onset of symptoms and signs of decompression sickness tends to be gradual and progressive, beginning minutes to hours after an inciting dive or exposure to altitude. With certain exceptions which will be noted, the manifestations resulting from both environments are the same and can be divided into Type I (minor manifestations) and Type II (serious manifestations), as summarized in Table 3. A late manifestation is the so-called dysbaric osteonecrosis of divers and caisson workers. The exact cause of this aseptic necrosis of bone in divers is still unclear, as is its relationship to untreated previous episodes of decompression sickness. The scope of this chapter does not allow a review of the monumental research in this area.

PREVENTION AND TREATMENT. All the varied manifestations of decompression sickness usually respond rapidly to early and adequate treatment by compression. Descent from altitude produces sufficient recompression to abolish the early manifestations, but merely retards the appearance of the more slowly developing serious forms of decompression sickness. In such cases, widespread bubble formation has presumably already occurred, and descent is entirely analogous to inadequate compression therapy during which symptoms subside only temporarily.

Divers can prevent decompression sickness by knowing and following established limits for depth and time

TABLE 3.   Clinical Manifestations of
Decompression Sickness

Diagnosis	Symptoms and Signs
Type I (minor)	
Bends	Mild to severe, deep, "boring" pain; single or multiple joints; aggravated by exercise; may be relieved by local pressure; local lymphedema may be present
Cutaneous	Pruritus, described by the diver as "the itches or creeps"; usually clears spontaneously in minutes; mottled or marbled skin lesion with a pale and cyanotic appearance; may accompany serious manifestations
Type II (serious)	
Pulmonary ("chokes")	Substernal pain, dyspnea, nonproductive cough, cyanosis
Neurologic	1. Spinal cord (diving chiefly): Any level may be affected, but most commonly lower thoracic and upper lumbar; low back and girdling abdominal pain, hypesthesia, weakness below that level; loss of anal sphincter tone and urinary bladder control; can result in permanent paraplegia 2. Brain (altitude chiefly): Diffuse, confusing, and poorly localized; range from blurred vision, visual field defects, spotty hypesthesia, weakness, paralysis, dysphasia, headache, vertigo, to focal or generalized seizures
Shock	Poorly responsive to fluid replacement without concurrent compression chamber treatment; may be accompanied by chokes, neurologic manifestations, and mottling of skin

at depth. Adequate denitrogenation, by breathing 100 per cent oxygen prior to and during ascent, is an effective preventive measure in fliers. Fliers who have experienced decompression symptoms during a flight should delay return to even relatively low altitudes for at least 72 hours, because the expansion of bubbles still present in tissues may cause a rapid recurrence of more serious symptoms. The hazard of exposure to altitudes as low as 1220 meters (4000 feet), even after safe depth-time dives, should be recognized.

Adequate compression performed at the earliest possible time is the specific therapy for decompression sickness. Every physician should be aware of the hyperbaric chamber closest to his city. All other measures are adjunctive. Those reported to be beneficial include 100 per cent oxygen by mask, dextran and standard replacement fluids to correct hypovolemia, and injectable steroids—such as dexamethasone, 10 mg intravenously initially, with diminishing doses every six hours.

Beckman, E. L., and Elliott, D. H. (eds.): Dysbarism — Related Osteonecrosis: Proceedings of a Symposium on Dysbaric Osteonecrosis. Superintendent of Documents, U. S. Government Printing Office, 1974.

Elliott, D. H., and Hallenbeck, J. M.: The pathophysiology of decompression sickness. *In* Bennett, P. B., and Elliott, D. H. (eds.): The Physiology and Medicine of Diving and Compressed Air Work. Baltimore, Williams & Wilkins Company, 1975, pp. 435–455.

Fryer, D. I.: Subatmospheric Decompression Sickness in Man. Slough, England, Technivision Services (Library of Congress Catalog Card No. 69–19960), 1969.

Kidd, D. J., and Elliott, D. H.: Decompression disorders in divers. *In* Bennett, P. B., and Elliott, D. H. (eds.): The Physiology and Medicine of Diving and Compressed Air Work. Baltimore, Williams & Wilkins Company, 1975, pp. 471–495.

OXYGEN TOXICITY

Aside from the well-known pulmonary oxygen toxicity which occurs with prolonged inhalation of elevated partial pressure of oxygen even at sea level, oxygen-enriched breathing media in diving introduce a unique problem. One hundred per cent oxygen breathing while under pressure, to speed nitrogen elimination and shorten decompression time, was introduced by the Royal Navy and the U. S. Navy during the early 1930's. It was quickly recognized that 100 per cent oxygen breathing at high barometric pressure produced a series of central nervous system events leading to a major seizure. There was a latent period before onset, markedly shortened at deeper than 20 meters (66 FSW). The onset was hastened by exercise while breathing oxygen at depth, and by breathing oxygen in the water. Systematic studies of safe oxygen time-pressure limits have been completed. Modern oxygen decompression, hyperbaric oxygen therapy (HBO) of decompression sickness, clostridial myonecrosis, carbon monoxide poisoning, and other accepted indications stay well within these limits.

Behnke, A. R., Johnson, F. S., Poppen, J. R., and Motley, E. P.: The effect of oxygen on man at pressures from 1 to 4 atmospheres. Am. J. Physiol., 110:565, 1934–35.

Clark, J. M., and Lambertsen, C. J.: Pulmonary oxygen toxicity: A review. Pharmacol. Rev., 23:37, 1971.

Donald, K. W.: Oxygen poisoning in man. Br. Med. J., 1:667, 1947.

NITROGEN NARCOSIS

It has long been recognized that breathing the high partial pressures of nitrogen in compressed air leads to behavioral and performance decrements. This effect, which is noticeable at 4 ATA or 30 meters (99 FSW) in most people, increases progressively at depth. The symptoms are euphoria, poor judgment, and impaired ability to concentrate. These symptoms can become quite serious when critical decisions need to be made during a dive. The symptoms do not occur if helium is used to replace nitrogen as the inert gas in a breathing mixture.

31.   THERAPEUTIC HYPERBARIC OXYGEN

Herbert A. Saltzman

Therapeutic application of hyperbaric oxygen is clearly beneficial in only a limited number of human illnesses. Although the full domain of clinical usefulness has yet to be determined, reasonable guidelines have been established. This review of basic principles, associated hazards, and clinical investigational experience is intended to help the reader distinguish between appropriate usage of hyperbaric oxygen, as currently understood, and costly exploitation in situations in which it is of no proved value.

DEFINITION, RATIONALE. The term hyperbaric oxygen is applied to the breathing of 100 per cent oxygen at greater than normal atmospheric pressures. This is achieved in special environmental chambers containing pressurized gas and at the same time providing technologic support for patient care. Hyperbaric oxygen provides a means for overcoming the barrier to increased oxygen transport imposed by the limited solubility of oxygen. Even though only 0.3 ml of oxygen dissolves in 100 ml of blood equilibrated at a P_{O_2} of 100 mm Hg, physically dissolved oxygen can be increased to almost 6 ml per 100 ml at an atmospheric pressure of 3 atmospheres absolute (ATA). Under these circumstances the Po_2 in blood will approach 2000 mm Hg. Increased oxygen concentrations have been thought to be clinically useful for the following reasons: (1) Function of hypoxic vital organs can be maintained or restored despite reduced perfusion of blood. This concept presumes satisfactory maintenance of other metabolic requirements. (2) There may be a specific desirable pharmacologic action of hyperbaric oxygen. The best example is the bactericidal effect, as employed in the treatment of clostridial myonecrosis. (3) In special circumstances wherein bubbles of gas form in tissues, removal can be expedited dramatically by treatment with hyperbaric oxygen. The increased pressure reduces bubble size, and the washout of dissolved inert gas from surrounding tissues yields a much larger and more favorable gradient for diffusion of inert gas molecules out of the bubble.

HAZARDS AND OTHER PROBLEMS. The major biologic limitations to therapeutic use of hyperbaric oxygen are (1) inability to deliver oxygen to a critical tissue if perfusion is interrupted or severely reduced by vascular disease, and (2) toxic consequences of excessive exposure. Severe and lethal pulmonary damage can be incurred in progressively shorter intervals as the inspired pressure of oxygen increases. Neurologic toxicity may occur, usually in the form of convulsions, at oxygen pressures greater than 2.5 ATA. These manifestations of toxicity are readily avoided by limiting the magnitude and duration of the exposure. Exposures of 90 minutes at an oxygen pressure of 3 ATA and longer treatments at 2 ATA have been widely employed and are very well tolerated. Intermittent exposures to hyperbaric oxygen profoundly constrain therapeutic expectations, however, as limited tissue reserves of oxygen are consumed within a few minutes. Thus sustained correction of hypoxia requires continuous treatment in the absence of other favorable biologic changes.

There are several technical problems associated with application of hyperbaric oxygen. Fire and explosive decompression are inherent risks. Exposed patients and personnel have been maimed or killed in hyperbaric chamber accidents. There are substantial costs incurred in maintaining a large hyperbaric facility. The substitution of small hyperbaric units capable of containing only a single patient, although more economical, compounds problems of adequate nursing support.

The decision to treat a patient with hyperbaric oxygen should be made after determining that alternative approaches fail to offer comparable dividends of efficacy, safety, and cost effectiveness. For example, although hyperbaric oxygen has been demonstrated to prevent or correct dangerous arrhythmias associated with myocardial ischemia, treatment with appropriate pharmacologic agents in a coronary care unit is clearly preferable.

CLINICAL EXPERIENCE. There are a small number of medical problems in which theoretical considerations, experimentation, and clinical experience justify confident employment of therapeutic hyperbaric oxygen.

Acute carbon monoxide poisoning causes profound hypoxia because hemoglobin combines with carbon monoxide preferentially, blocking oxygen transport to tissues. Concentrations of carboxyhemoglobin above 30 per cent adversely affect release of oxygen from oxyhemoglobin as well. The clinical consequences of cytochrome interactions with carbon monoxide are less well understood. Prompt treatment with hyperbaric oxygen at 2.5 ATA, for one hour, will greatly accelerate elimination of carbon monoxide from blood, while at the same time improving delivery of oxygen to the central nervous system. At the end of the treatment carboxyhemoglobin levels are generally below 10 per cent, and prompt recovery can be anticipated if irreversible brain damage has not already occurred.

Acute cyanide poisoning leads to profound tissue hypoxia because of blocked cytochrome function within cells. Ordinarily the process evolves so rapidly that death occurs before treatment can be implemented. Successful resuscitation with hyperbaric oxygen has been accomplished, however.

Smoke inhalation may lead to unconsciousness. Commonly carbon monoxide poisoning is the major underlying cause. Less commonly, cyanide poisoning is a significant factor. These presumptions merit prompt treatment with hyperbaric oxygen, if it is available.

In unusual circumstances of *exceptional blood loss* wherein the ensuing anemia cannot be corrected with sufficient rapidity, acute cardiorespiratory embarrassment may occur. An example is fulminant hemolytic anemia. Treatment with hyperbaric oxygen will improve oxygen transport sufficiently to avert cardiovascular decompensation, at least temporarily. The value of hyperbaric therapy in this setting is limited to unusual circumstances wherein direct blood replacement cannot be accomplished immediately.

Clostridial myonecrosis is a complex, rapidly progressive illness. Loss of limb and death are common. Adjunct therapy with hyperbaric oxygen has been shown to alter the clinical course favorably with a decrease in morbidity and increase in limb salvage. Most therapists administer five to seven treatments at 8- to 12-hour intervals. Each exposure lasts two hours, including 90 minutes at the maximum pressure of 3 ATA.

Decompression sickness is generally attributed to the formation of inert gas bubbles in tissues and blood. Brief exposures to hyperbaric oxygen have been dramatically effective in reversing the clinical manifestations of decompression sickness in most victims. There are well developed protocols of alternating exposures to oxygen and air at specified times and pressures. Experience has demonstrated these treatment schedules to be generally free of toxicity, and relief is prompt.

Air embolism, whether precipitated during ascent in the water or during open heart surgery or dialysis, generally causes a massive acute central nervous system deficit. Currently, the preferred treatment is immediate exposure to 6 ATA of air, facilitating reduction of the intravascular gas volume. Oxygen and air are breathed sequentially during decompression. Prompt improvement and recovery generally ensue if treatment is implemented within a few minutes. This requirement is readily achieved in specialized centers training personnel for rapid ascent in the ocean. In the usual hospital setting, practical considerations prevent immediate treatment and results are less satisfactory.

There are several additional illnesses in which the rationale, experimental evidence, and clinical experience are more limited but in which sufficiently promising results have been reported to justify employment of hyperbaric oxygen. *Osteoradionecrosis* is an uncommon affliction in which dissolution of bone, usually the mandible, occurs after radiation therapy. In many such patients intractable pain, sequestration of bone, and infection cause profound disability. Ultimately mandibulectomy may be necessary. Adjunct therapy with hyperbaric oxygen over an extended interval of 40 or more days, using two-hour treatments at 2 ATA, has been associated with dramatic relief of pain and healing in most patients so treated. Comparable observations have been reported for *refractory osteomyelitis*, a condition in which there are many similarities. *Meleney's ulcers* are uncommon, chronic debilitating skin lesions associated with a mixed bacterial infection. These seem to respond well to combined topical and inhalational treatment with hyperbaric oxygen. Although most *skin grafts* are accomplished successfully in modern practice, viability may be compromised by impairment of the blood supply and infection. In these circumstances some groups have reported enhanced survival of grafts after a series of intermittent two-hour treatments with hyperbaric oxygen. The need for this is rare, however. *Thermal burns* represent another acute and complex illness in which reduced complications of infection, more rapid healing, and shorter periods of hospitalization have been reported after use of hyperbaric oxygen as adjunct therapy. Benefit has been reported for the following conditions as well: actinomycosis, acute peripheral arterial insufficiency, *Bacteroides* infections, crush injuries, acute cerebral edema, acute traumatic head and spinal cord injury, intestinal obstruction, early osteomyelitis, radionecrosis of soft tissue, acute central renal artery insufficiency, retinopathy, as an adjunct to surgical restoration of continuity for a severed limb, chronic skin ulcers secondary to arterial insufficiency, and stasis ulcers. The role of hyperbaric oxygen in practical clinical management of these and other conditions is under continuing investigation.

The dramatic character of hyperbaric facilities has generated great interest among patients with unresolved chronic medical problems, and unfortunately this has led to exploitation. Hyperbaric oxygen has no proved merit in the treatment of "aging" or of such entities as wrinkles and impotence. These claims are properly rejected by responsible physicians.

Brown, I. W., Jr., and Cox, B. G.: Proceedings of the Third International Conference on Hyperbaric Medicine. Washington, D.C., National Academy of Sciences, 1966.

Davis, J. C., and Hunt, T. K.: Hyperbaric Oxygen Therapy. Bethesda, Md., Undersea Medical Society, Inc., 1978.

Hart, G.: Osteoradionecrosis. *In* Trapp, W. G., Bannister, E. W., Davison, A. J., and Trapp, P. A. (eds.): Fifth International Hyperbaric Congress Proceedings. Burnaby, Canada, Simon Fraser University, 1974, p. 845.

Holland, J. A., Hill, G. B., Wolfe, W. G., Osterhout, S., Saltzman, H. A., and Brown, I. W.: Experimental and clinical experience with hyperbaric oxygen in the treatment of clostridial myonecrosis. Surgery, 77:75, 1975.

Kindwall, E. P.: Carbon monoxide poisoning treated with hyperbaric oxygen. Resp. Ther., 5:29, 1975.

Slack, W. K., Thomas, D. A., and Perrins, D.: Hyperbaric oxygenation in chronic osteomyelitis. Lancet, 1:1093, 1965.

Wada, J., and Iwa, T.: Proceedings of the Fourth International Congress on Hyperbaric Medicine. Baltimore, Williams & Wilkins Company, 1970.

32. DROWNING

Charles J. Stahl

DEFINITION. Drowning is a pathologic condition, terminating in death, which may result from the complex biochemical, respiratory, and cardiovascular changes that follow the aspiration of fluid during immersion, or — less commonly — from asphyxia associated with obstruction of the airway. The term near-drowning implies survival after immersion, with or without aspiration of fluid, but delayed deaths of these survivors may occur several hours or several days later.

ETIOLOGY. Accidents account for most drownings. The victims are often children or other persons who have not learned to swim. Less frequently, it may result from suicide or homicide. The circumstances for accidental drowning may include the following: (1) disasters such as floods, tidal waves, shipwrecks, and vehicular accidents; (2) hazardous environmental conditions or careless acts while engaged in fishing, aquatic sport, or occupational activities; (3) impaired ability to swim because of pre-existing illness, intoxication, exhaustion, or exposure to cold water; and (4) unintentional falls into water.

INCIDENCE AND PREVALENCE. Over 8000 deaths by drowning and approximately the same number of near-drownings occur annually in the United States. This is the third most common type of accidental death. The majority of the victims are young men under 25 years of age. Several million Americans engage in the sport of underwater swimming, using either self-contained underwater breathing apparatus (scuba) or snorkel. When underwater accidents are considered alone, drowning is the most common cause of death. It occurs more frequently than deaths from barotrauma, including air embolism and decompression sickness, discussed in Ch. 30.2 and 30.3. A study by Goldhahn of fatalities among underwater swimmers using self-contained underwater breathing apparatus (scuba) indicates the need for more thorough investigation and evaluation of these cases.

PATHOGENESIS. Survivors of near-drowning have provided some knowledge of the sequence of events. The victim usually experiences panic at the time of immersion and struggles to reach the surface, unless previously incapacitated by alcohol, drugs, or injury. Breath-holding is common and persists until accumulation of carbon dioxide stimulates the respiratory center. When the victim can no longer restrain the urge to breathe, high pulmonary carbon dioxide and low pulmonary and arterial oxygen tensions are present. Gasping may result in aspiration of water or other liquid. In about 10 per cent of fatal cases, however, it is believed that the victims do not aspirate fluid, but die from asphyxia during reflex laryngospasm or breath-holding. Swallowing of water, vomiting, and coughing may occur. Convulsions precede death in some cases.

The pathophysiologic changes in drowning were poorly understood until the studies with experimental animals reported by Swann and Spafford (1951). They demonstrated that the hemodynamic and biochemical changes during drowning of dogs are affected by the type of fluid encountered. When drowning occurs in *fresh water*, rapid absorption of hypotonic water from the lungs into the circulation results in hypervolemia, hemodilution, and hemolysis. Serum electrolytes are decreased, except for potassium, which increases be-

The opinions and assertions contained herein are those of the author, and are not to be construed as official or as necessarily reflecting the views of the Department of the Navy or the Naval service at large.

cause of hemolysis. The altered ratio between sodium and potassium, as well as anoxia, may cause ventricular fibrillation in dogs. The mechanism for drowning in *sea water*, however, is probably different. As the result of the aspiration of sea water, salts pass into the circulation and fluids diffuse into alveoli. Serum electrolytes, particularly chloride and magnesium, increase markedly. Hypovolemia, hemoconcentration, and hypoproteinemia, as well as pulmonary edema, occur.

Studies of drowning and near-drowning in laboratory animals by Modell indicate that the biochemical and cardiovascular changes are dependent not only upon the tonicity of fluid but also upon the quantity of fluid aspirated. Sea water, volume for volume, is twice as lethal as fresh water, and causes more profound changes in serum electrolytes. The serum electrolytes of animals that survived aspiration of either fresh water or sea water quickly returned to normal concentrations. These studies confirm prior observations by Fuller (1963) that life-threatening changes in electrolytes may not occur in human victims of drowning. After near-drowning with aspiration of water by dogs, the most significant changes include hypoxemia, hypercarbia, and acidosis. Pulmonary edema and decreased pulmonary compliance are evident. Fresh water alters or destroys the normal surface-tension properties of *pulmonary surfactant*. Sea water only partially removes surfactant. The pathophysiologic effects are alveolar collapse, uneven ventilation, pulmonary edema, and hypoxemia. At least 20 ml of fresh water per pound of body weight must be aspirated by dogs to cause changes in electrolytes or ventricular fibrillation.

Although the pathophysiologic mechanisms seem less well understood and may differ from experimental findings, clinical evaluations of near-drowning victims indicate that fluid and electrolyte balance are restored rapidly. The majority of human drowning victims aspirate 10 ml of fluid or less per pound of body weight. Hemodilution has not been demonstrated, and hemolysis is uncommon. The changes in serum electrolytes and blood volume are often transient and depend upon the quantity and tonicity of fluid aspirated. Nonspecific electrocardiographic changes occur as the result of hypoxia. Ventricular fibrillation is uncommon in human victims. The initial effect of the aspirated fluid on the alveolar membranes and pulmonary surfactant results in collapse of alveoli, decreased compliance, and shunting of blood through nonventilated alveoli. Subsequently, hypoxia also occurs from the diffusion deficit resulting from pulmonary edema or pneumonia. The hypoxia caused by near-drowning with aspiration in human victims is manifested by arterial hypoxemia and metabolic acidosis. Retrospective clinical studies by Modell and his associates of patients who survived near-drowning show that the chance for survival is greater when the patient is alert upon admission, the initial chest roentgenograms and arterial oxygen tension are normal, and the ratio of arterial oxygen tension to the fractional concentration of oxygen in the inspired gas exceeds 150 mm Hg. Neither serum electrolyte, hematocrit, nor hemoglobin concentrations were useful predictive values of survival or threat to life. Vigorous resuscitative efforts are indicated for all near-drowning victims, as neurologic sequelae are less common than previously believed.

The pathologic findings of drowning are often nonspecific. White or bloody foam, usually seen in the mouth, nose, and tracheobronchial tree, may not be evident after attempts at resuscitation. The skin of the palms and soles is often wrinkled and pale. These changes are consistent with prolonged immersion, but are not pathognomonic of drowning. Lacerations or incised wounds of skin, without evidence of vital reaction, reflect the effects of tides, collision of the body with underwater obstacles, and postmortem injuries inflicted by sharp objects such as motorboat propellers. Mutilation of a body by aquatic animals is common, particularly about the soft tissues of the face.

The lungs are heavy and edematous. In children, however, the lungs are often pink and distended with entrapped air. Pressure on the cut surfaces of the lungs yields variable degrees of frothy fluid. Foreign material from the aquatic environment, as well as vomitus, is often seen in the mouth, upper airway, and tracheobronchial tree. Depending on the postmortem interval, the pleural cavities contain variable quantities of straw-colored to dark watery fluid, which is a transudate from the edematous lungs. A relatively dry appearance of the lungs, attributed in some cases to death by reflex laryngospasm and closure of the glottis, may also result from agonal absorption and elimination of water from the lungs after cessation of respiration. Water may be found in paranasal sinuses, and hemorrhagic fluid is frequently observed in the middle ear and mastoid air cells. The latter finding is not specific for drowning, as it is also seen in other asphyxial deaths. Diatoms are microscopic unicellular or colonial algae containing silica. The significance of diatoms in the diagnosis of drowning is controversial. They may offer evidence of the aspiration of water when the same types of diatoms are demonstrated not only in the lungs but also in the water in which the body was found. After prolonged immersion in water, the changes of decomposition and the effects of aquatic life obscure the usual anatomic findings, but the pleural spaces may contain unusual amounts of sanguineous, watery fluid. The microscopic findings in the lungs may include pulmonary edema, focal intra-alveolar hemorrhage, disruption of alveoli, and demonstration of diatoms.

In laboratory animals (rats), Reidbord and Spitz (1966) observed differences in the ultrastructural changes of lungs in drownings in fresh water from those in sea water. With sea water, cellular swelling and vacuolation, as well as discontinuity of alveolar lining cells, were noted. After drowning in fresh water, the lungs of rats showed endothelial destruction, mitochondrial swelling, and cellular disruption. Histochemical changes were also reported by Spitz (1969). An acute perivasculitis, consisting mainly of neutrophils, was seen in the lungs of rats after drowning in sea water. Similar changes, but to a lesser extent, were seen in fresh-water drowning. The distribution and amount of peroxidase-positive granules in the histologic sections parallel the density of the neutrophilic infiltration around vessels. These experimental studies may serve as the basis for a distinction between drowning in sea water and drowning in fresh water.

Numerous chemical and physical tests have been applied to the diagnosis of drowning. They include tests for concentrations of chloride or magnesium in whole blood, plasma, or serum; specific gravity of plasma; refractive index, electrical conductivity, and osmolarity of blood. None of them is entirely reliable, and all require considerable judgment in interpretation. There is yet no specific laboratory test for the diagnosis of drowning.

CLINICAL MANIFESTATIONS. The victim of drowning usually experiences breath-holding and a substernal burning sensation. Loss of consciousness and aspiration of fluid may occur. Most victims have a violent struggle prior to loss of consciousness, but a few people show passive behavior. After rescue, the patient is usually unconscious, flaccid, cold, and cyanotic. Respirations are absent, and the pulse is imperceptible. If the patient is conscious, tinnitus and visual abnormalities are often reported. Frothy fluid may be seen in the nose and mouth, and examination of the chest may disclose signs of pulmonary edema. If a significant amount of water has been swallowed, nausea and vomiting may occur and gastric distention may be evident. Nonspecific electrocardiographic changes are related to the effects of hypoxia. Cardiac arrhythmias such as ventricular fibrillation, as reported for animals, are uncommon in man. Evidence of arterial hypoxemia and metabolic acidosis is provided by studies of gas and pH in blood. Serum electrolyte changes are usually transient and depend on the quantity and tonicity of fluid aspirated. The postimmersion period is sometimes complicated by pneumonia, hemoglobinuria, acute tubular necrosis, or brain damage from prolonged cerebral anoxia.

DIAGNOSIS. When the patient is a victim of near-drowning, other physical causes for disability should be considered, including injury to the cervical cord from a dive into shallow water. In the differential diagnosis of near-drowning, other causes for aquatic accidents, especially air embolism and decompression sickness, must be considered. These untoward effects of barotrauma (see Ch. 30.2 and 30.3) are usually associated with underwater swimming, diving, or the use of self-contained underwater breathing apparatus (scuba). Recognition and differentiation from near-drowning are extremely important, as recompression, the appropriate method of treatment, may bring dramatic and lifesaving results.

The diagnosis of near-drowning is usually not difficult after the circumstances are known. Diagnostic studies include chest films, electrocardiograms, electroencephalogram, central venous pressure, serial determinations of arterial gas and pH, and appropriate laboratory tests, including hematocrit, hemoglobin, leukocyte count, serum electrolytes, and serum protein determinations. Respiratory complications, particularly pneumonia, are invariably present when fever, leukocytosis, pulmonary infiltrate on chest x-ray films, and decreased arterial oxygen tension are evident.

When the body of a dead person is found immersed in water, the diagnosis of drowning alone requires exclusion of other possible causes for death. A careful appraisal of the circumstances of death and of findings from pathologic and toxicologic studies and from postmortem chemical and physical tests is required. The role of a pre-existing illness, such as heart disease, as a precipitating factor in drowning depends on demonstration of pathologic features of the disease, as well as careful correlation with the circumstances and consideration of the hazards in the environment occupied by the victim immediately before the fatal incident. In some cases of suicide, particularly in bathtubs, if a concentration of a drug sufficient to cause coma is found in the blood, the investigator should suspect that the victim ingested a lethal dose of the drug, then went into coma, and drowned subsequently. Failure to find evidence of injury, intoxication, or pre-existing disease, as well as evidence that the person was alive during the period of immersion, favors the presumption that death was caused by drowning.

TREATMENT. Prompt rescue, first aid, and resuscitation offer the best chance for survival of drowning victims. The airway is cleared of any obstructions, and dentures are removed. Resuscitation by artificial ventilation is continued until oxygen is available, spontaneous breathing occurs, or signs of death are evident. If a heart beat or carotid pulse is not detectable, closed-chest cardiac massage, as well as artificial ventilation, is required. As soon as it is available, 100 per cent oxygen, with or without intermittent positive pressure, is administered continuously en route to a hospital. Survival depends not only upon the emergency care but also the prior health of the victim, the duration of immersion, and the amount of water aspirated.

Since there are both immediate and delayed effects of near-drowning, admission to a hospital for intensive pulmonary care is indicated. If the patient is alert, has normal chest roentgenograms and arterial oxygen tension upon admission, and survives the first 24 hours, he is likely to recover. Reoxygenation should be started, followed by aspiration of the airway and suction of the stomach. Tracheostomy is rarely necessary, but abnormalities of either blood gases or chest films may indicate the need for endotracheal intubation. After insertion of an endotracheal tube, 100 per cent oxygen is given with positive end-expiratory pressure and intermittent mechanical ventilation. Subsequently, the concentration of inspired oxygen is decreased to maintain the highest arterial oxygen tension without compromising the cardiac output. The administration of sodium bicarbonate solution intravenously in a dose of 0.3 to 0.4 mEq per pound of body weight is recommended upon admission to the hospital, for a significant number of near-drowning victims have metabolic acidosis associated with hypoxia. Based on serial determinations of gases and pH in the arterial blood, arterial hypoxemia and acid-base concentrations are corrected by effective ventilation, oxygenation, buffers, or bicarbonate. Respiratory stimulants are contraindicated. As indicated, bronchodilators, diuretics, digitalization, or transfusion of whole blood, plasma, or packed red cells are given. The need for antimicrobial drugs is determined by clinical signs and roentgenographic changes, as well as by culture of tracheal secretions. Although the role of steroids in the treatment of near-drowning is uncertain, the intravenous administration of methylprednisolone sodium succinate, 5 mg per kilogram per 24 hours divided into six equal doses, has been proposed. Intensive care is continued as long as necessary to correct hypoxemia and acidosis. As the patient improves, oxygen is given by catheter or mask and reduced in concentration to 40 per cent.

PREVENTION. Continuing education programs for the public, as well as for physicians, are required to prevent drowning. Instruction in swimming, water safety, rescue, lifesaving techniques, and cardiopulmonary resuscitation is indicated for persons of all ages. Physicians have a responsibility to their communities not only to assist in the training of paramedical personnel, such as emergency medical technicians, but also to carefully evaluate prospective swimmers and divers. Rescue units and hospitals with emergency facilities should be equipped for cardiopulmonary resuscitation and intensive pulmonary care, respectively. Fear of brain damage should not deter vigorous lifesaving efforts. Siebke (1975) has reported the survival of a patient, without neurologic deficit, who was immersed for 40 minutes. The retrospective study by Modell of 81 patients who survived near-drowning revealed that only two patients had neurologic sequelae. Among 54 children, apparently dead at the time of rescue who survived near-drowning, Pearn reported that over 95 per cent recovered without neurologic abnormalities.

Bradley, M. E. : Near-drowning: Pathophysiology and treatment. *In* Strauss, R. H. (ed.): Diving Medicine. New York, Grune & Stratton, 1976, pp. 317–327.

Bucklin, R.: Drowning: A review of the physiological, experimental, and pathological findings. *In* Wecht, C. H. (ed.): Legal Medicine Annual, 1972. New York, Appleton-Century-Crofts, 1972, pp. 93–104.

den Otter, G.: Low-pressure aspiration of fresh water and sea water in the non-anoxic dog. An experimental study on the pathophysiology of drowning. Forensic Sci., 2:305, 1973.

Edmonds, C., and Thomas, R. L.: Medical aspects of diving. Part 2. Med. J. Aust., 2:1256, 1972.

Goldhahn, R. T.: SCUBA diving deaths: A review and approach for the pathologist. *In* Wecht, C. H. (ed.): Legal Medicine Annual, 1976. New York, Appleton-Century-Crofts, 1977, pp. 109–132.

Modell, J. H.: The Pathophysiology and Treatment of Drowning and Near-Drowning. Springfield, Ill., Charles C Thomas, 1971.

Modell, J. H., Graves, S. A., and Ketover, A.: Clinical course of 91 consecutive near-drowning victims. Chest, 70:231, 1976.

Pearn, J.: Neurological and psychometric studies in children surviving freshwater immersion accidents. Lancet, 1:7, 1977.

Sladen, A., and Zauder, H. L.: Methylprednisolone therapy for pulmonary edema following near drowning. JAMA, 215: 1793, 1971.

The Committee on Allied Health: Water hazards. *In* Emergency Care and Transportation of the Sick and Injured. 2nd ed., revised. Chicago, American Academy of Orthopaedic Surgeons, 1977, pp. 330–332.

Wayne, K. S.: Positive end-expiratory pressure (PEEP) ventilation. A review of mechanisms and actions. JAMA, 236:1394, 1976.

33. ARTHROPODS AS ENVIRONMENTAL AGENTS OF DISEASE

Hugh L. Keegan

33.1. INTRODUCTION

The arthropods are invertebrates characterized as a group by bilateral symmetry, chitinous exoskeleton, jointed appendages, and a single body cavity — the hemocele — which contains the internal organs and a fluid, the hemolymph. Members of several of the classes of phylum Arthropoda are of medical importance. These include class Insecta (the insects — e.g., flies, lice, fleas); class Chilopoda (the centipedes); class Arachnida (spiders, scorpions, ticks, mites); and class Crustacea (crabs, lobsters, water fleas). The pentastomids or tongue worms were formerly considered as a class in phylum Arthropoda but the consensus at present is that these wormlike parasites represent a separate phylum.

From a medical viewpoint arthropods are of primary importance as vectors of disease. Transmission of pathogens is of two types: (1) *biological transmission,* in which the arthropod is essential for transmission of the disease; and (2) *mechanical transmission,* when a disease-producing agent, which may be acquired in a variety of ways, is transmitted to man by the bite of an arthropod or through contamination of food or water by the feces or bodies of the arthropods. The first of these, biologic transmission, is of far greater importance than the second. Examples are malaria, epidemic typhus, plague, and the various forms of leishmaniasis and trypanosomiasis. The true importance of mechanical transmission has yet to be evaluated. Although many types of disease-producing organisms may survive and multiply in insects and other arthropods in the laboratory and have been found in such arthropods in nature, it is difficult to assess the importance of the arthropod in transmission of an agent which also might be acquired in food or water or by personal contact. Some arthropods, particularly the crustaceans, indirectly affect man's health by serving as intermediate hosts for helminths which parasitize man. Examples of such organisms would be the lung fluke, *Paragonimus westermani,* and the broad fish tapeworm, *Diphyllobothrium latum.*

As the diseases transmitted to man by arthropods are discussed in detail elsewhere in this textbook, the present chapters will deal only with illness and death produced directly by arthropods. Although bites by many insects and other arthropods not usually regarded as venomous may produce painful reactions in some individuals, the discussion presented here will deal primarily with *entomophobia,* an abnormal or unreasonable fear of insects and other "bugs"; *dermatosis,* skin irritation caused by bites by flies, lice, fleas, ticks, mites, and bedbugs; *myiasis,* infestation by fly larvae (maggots); injury to sense organs, caused by entry of insects or other arthropods into the eyes or ears; *allergenic effects,* caused by contact with some arthropods, or by inhalation of scales or fragments of skins of insects or by sensitization to arthropod venoms, particularly those of wasps, bees, and ants; and finally, *envenomation,* injection of venom by bites, stings, or spines, or by deposition of blister-producing secretions on the skin. This latter group would include illness produced by the Hymenoptera (wasps, bees, and ants); the Arachnida (ticks, scorpions, and spiders); the Chilopoda and Myriapoda (centipedes and millipedes); and the blister beetles of order Coleoptera.

33.2. PEDICULOSIS

Species of lice which cause pediculosis in man are the body louse, *Pediculus humanus humanus;* the head louse, *Pediculus humanus capitis;* and the pubic or crab louse, *Phthirus pubis.* These obligatory, ectoparasitic, bloodsucking insects are of medical importance as irritating pests. The body louse may serve as a vector of epidemic typhus, trench fever, and louse-borne relapsing fever. Although the head louse can harbor disease agents in the laboratory, it is not thought to be a vector in nature. The pubic louse is not known to transmit disease.

Head and body lice are similar in appearance and in

life cycles. Adult female head lice are 3 to 4 mm in length; the males are slightly smaller. Both are larger than female and male body lice. These lice are dorsoventrally flattened, have a soft but tough skin, and are a dirty white to gray color. The legs are short and terminate in hook-like grasping organs which enable the parasite to cling firmly to hair and fibers of clothing.

After fertilization, a female body louse lays her eggs either on fibers of the clothing of the host (underclothing primarily) or on body hairs. In normal circumstances about 70 per cent of the eggs are fastened to clothing fibers. When an egg is deposited, it is "cemented" in place with a secretion which quickly hardens and renders the egg almost impossible to remove by bathing. The eggs, oval and grayish white, hatch in about a week. The nymphs which emerge are similar to the adults except in size. They molt three times before achieving maturity in eight to nine days. The total cycle from egg to egg under favorable conditions may require only 16 days.

Both immature and adult lice feed on blood. While feeding they may excrete dark red feces onto the skin. Lice are totally dependent upon the host and die in a week or less unless they can get a blood meal. They are also quite susceptible to either low or high temperatures. For this reason lice will often leave a patient and will also depart from a corpse as the body temperature lowers. This has been linked to the spread of louseborne diseases during epidemics.

The head louse is so called because it inhabits only the head hair, particularly on the nape of the neck and behind the ears. It is not known to occur on eyebrows or lashes. Head louse infestations rarely occur in black people.

The crab louse has the same general life cycle as the head and body lice but differs in appearance and habits. The body is almost circular instead of elongate, and the lice in all stages are much slower in movement than head and body lice. As the name implies, these lice usually infest the pubic and perianal regions but may also be found on eyelashes, hair of the face, the axillae, and body hair, but seldom on head hairs (on the scalp). Adults live about a month. During this period they produce about three nits a day. Of 200 adult crab lice removed from a host, only one survived as long as 24 hours. Because of the usual mode of transmission of crab lice, the physician should consider the possibility of venereal disease in the louse-infested patient.

Head and body louse infestation is generally transmitted under conditions of crowding and poor sanitation. Skin-to-skin contact, infested clothing and bedding, and even upholstered furniture are common sources. The use of common clothing, hair brushes, and towels in family situations and close contact among playmates in schools may be important factors. Crab louse infestation is usually acquired during coitus, but parasites may also be picked up from infested bedding, clothing, or even latrine seats.

Although a characteristic irritant roseate papular dermatitis and continuous scratching by the patient are good indications of louse infestation, diagnosis is easily achieved by direct examination for active forms and nits. In suspected head louse infestations a search for parasites should be made on the nape of the neck and behind the ears. In doing this the hair should be parted with applicator sticks. Usually the nits and active forms are visible to the naked eye, but a hand lens and flashlight may help. In active infestations the nits are found attached to hair shafts about 6 to 7 mm from the scalp. In "old" infestations the nits are found on hair shafts at greater distances from the scalp. The examiner should take care to avoid infestation. Surgical gloves and wooden applicator sticks should be used, and subsequently both should be discarded.

Physical effects of louse infestation are intense itching and consequent scratching, which result in secondary infections, particularly impetigo in children. Psychologic effects are common among persons who regard louse infestation as a sign of social inferiority. With the partial exception of crab louse infestations, in which coitus is a primary factor in transmission, most louse infestations are acquired under circumstances beyond control of the individual.

Control of louse infestations is accomplished through a combination of effective treatment of the individual; disinfestation of clothing, bed linen, towels, and other items which may be of common use; and administrative measures designed to keep infested persons and their clothing from contact with others. This is of particular importance in schools and other institutions where large numbers of persons are in close contact.

During World War II several effective louse powders were developed and used in many areas to prevent or control outbreaks of epidemic typhus and other louseborne diseases. In reaction to the developing of resistance to insecticides by lice, such powders, which at first contained DDT as the active ingredient, were later composed of formulations containing pyrethrins, lindane, dieldrin, and malathion. Because of governmental restrictions, only three of these compounds — pyrethrins, lindane, and malathion — are found in pediculicide formulations at present. Pediculicides, some of which may not be dispensed without prescription, which are currently registered with the Environmental Protection Agency, are in dust, shampoo, lotion, and cream foundations. Most contain lindane as the active ingredient. Others contain pyrethrins (in company with piperonyl butoxide), isobornyl thiocyanoacetate, carbaryl, tetrahydronaphthalene, malathion, and benzyl benzoate. Treatment should be conducted according to directions on the labels. It is probably desirable to repeat the treatment in ten days to kill newly hatched lice which may not have been affected by the original effort.

In addition to treatment of the individual, clothing, bed linen, and personal items such as hair brushes which might be in common use should be disinfested. Such items should be machine washed or dry cleaned if necessary. Combs and hair brushes should be soaked for an hour in 2 per cent Lysol solution or heated in water to a temperature of about 66° C for five to ten minutes. Freezing in a household refrigerator for about 30 minutes should also kill the parasites.

One of the most emotion-laden problems which can confront a school administrator or public health official is large-scale head louse infestation. Successful handling of such situations requires tact, knowledge, and effective organization. Control of head louse infestations depends upon prompt case finding, proper administrative handling of each case, effective treatment, and prevention of spread of the infestations. This should include examination of all students for head louse infestation as a part of routine physical examination at the beginning of each school year, administrative handling of each case to ensure that the parents understand need for treatment and will carry out such treatment, and prevention of transmission by proper assignment of lockers, wall hooks, or other methods to ensure that garments of students are not in contact. School officials should be trained in diagnosis of pediculosis, and cooperation of public officials is essential if programs are to succeed. Education of both parents and students as to the nature of the problem is of the utmost importance.

Ackerman, A. B.: Crabs — the resurgence of *Phthirus pubis*. N. Engl. J. Med., 278:950, 1968.

Buxton, P. A.: Louse: An Account of the Lice Which Infect Man, Their Medical Importance and Control. London, Edward Arnold, Ltd., 1939.

Controlling Head Lice. Atlanta, U.S. Department of Health, Education, and Welfare/Public Health Service, Center for Disease Control, 1975.

Gordon, R. M., and Lavoipierre, M. M. J.: Entomology for Students of Medicine. Oxford, Blackwell Scientific Publications, 1962.

33.3. FLEA-BITE

The fleas, members of the insect order Siphonaptera, are small, laterally compressed, wingless, blood-sucking ectoparasites which feed on a variety of avian and mammalian hosts, including man. They are of medical importance primarily because they may transmit plague and endemic (murine) typhus and cause irritating dermatitis by their bites. These insects vary in length from 1 to 8 mm. In order to deposit eggs a female must obtain a blood meal. The eggs, which are oval and pearly white or yellowish, are deposited in nests on the host or in crevices in floors, under rugs, or between cushions on overstuffed furniture upon which dogs and cats have been lying. During her lifetime a female will deposit as many as 300 to 500 eggs in small batches of up to a dozen at a time. The eggs hatch in from a few days to a few weeks. Temperature seems to be an important factor in this process. The legless, maggot-like larvae which emerge from the eggs are quite active and move about in the nest of the host, feeding on organic debris or on partially digested blood which has passed through the alimentary tract of the adults. Under optimal conditions the larvae reach maximum size in a few weeks, but this may be prolonged due to low temperature or humidity and when adequate food is not available. When conditions are favorable, the larvae spin cocoons in which the adults will develop. The duration of life in the cocoon is extremely variable. Adults may emerge in a week or so, or the process may be delayed for several months. Although temperature and humidity are undoubtedly important factors, it is believed that vibration is of particular importance; hence the sudden appearance of large numbers of fleas in a day or so after occupancy of homes which have been vacant for some time but in which dogs and cats had previously been kept.

Most fleas spend only a portion of their lives on the host, although a few embed themselves in the integument where they remain until death. The majority feed several times a day. In so doing much of the blood ingested passes through the gut and is excreted in a semidigested condition. Fleas are attracted to a host by body warmth, vibration of the substrate, CO_2 in the breath, and perhaps odor and movement of the host. Although some species are fairly host specific, when the usual host is not available almost any warm-blooded food source is acceptable. It is in these situations that man becomes a target. Fleas live as adults for several months. In general, feeding activity is increased by rise in temperature. A major factor in spread of plague is the tendency of fleas to abandon bodies of dead animals. This has led to the practice of directing control efforts first at the flea population, then at the rodent reservoirs of disease.

Aside from the plague vectors, the most important flea parasitic on man is *Tunga penetrans*, the "jigger flea" or "chigoe." This species, which is widely distributed in Central and South America and in tropical Africa is unique in habit in that the fertilized female burrows into the skin where her presence leads to intense itching, scratching, and often severe secondary infection. As with other fleas, both males and females are blood suckers. The male leaves the host after obtaining a blood meal, but the female burrows into the skin where it is soft, commonly between the toes or around the nail beds. When the posterior end of the body is almost level with the skin surface, the female ceases to burrow and stays in position as the ova develop. During this period the abdomen swells to a diameter of 6 mm or more in about a week. Egg laying then commences, and during the following week or ten days from 150 to 200 eggs are extruded and fall to the ground. The depleted female then shrivels and dies in situ. In severe infestations extensive secondary infections, including gangrene, often occur. It is recommended that the gravid female be extracted with a needle point and that suitable antibiotics be given for prevention or control of infection. A related species, *Echidnophaga gallinacea*, a parasite of chickens, other birds, and mammals, is occasionally a problem and may cause irritating dermatitis.

The most frequent complaints concerning fleas come from those moving into quarters formerly occupied by persons with dogs or cats as pets. When the normal blood source is available, fleas will usually not bother humans; but when the reverse is true, the first person entering a flea-infested room will quickly find the lower portions of the legs dotted with fleas which rapidly converge on the target. In such cases a residual insecticidal spray should be effective in reducing the nuisance. A repeat treatment may be necessary as additional fleas emerge from their cocoons.

Gordon, R. M., and Lavoipierre, M. M. J.: Entomology for Students of Medicine. Oxford, Blackwell Scientific Publications, 1962.

33.4. SCABIES

Scabies, also known as "the itch," "seven-year itch," and sarcoptic acariasis, is an infectious disease of the skin caused by the itch mite, *Sarcoptes scabiei*. The disease, which has been associated with wars, social upheaval, and poverty, seems to appear in epidemic cycles at 12- to 15-year intervals. Although it is most common in groups in which frequent bathing is not usual, scabies is no respecter of social or economic status. The sole requirement for infestation is contact. Close body contact, often through sexual intercourse and by sleeping with infested persons or even shaking hands, is the usual means of transmission of the parasite from one host to another. Clothing and bed linen may also be involved in the spread of the disease. Frequently, outbreaks occur in schools or other institutions where persons live in close proximity, and it is usual for all members of the family to develop infestations. *Sarcoptes scabiei* also causes sarcoptic mange in dogs, horses, and other domestic animals. Although mites found on such hosts are structurally identical with those parasitizing man, they differ physiologically and cause only transient, atypical dermatitis in humans.

As with other acarina (ticks and mites), adults of *S. scabiei* possess four pairs of legs, and immature stages have only three pairs. The adult female is usually about 350 μ long and 250 μ wide. The smaller male measures 250 by 170 μ. In the female the first two pairs of legs terminate in suckers and the last two end in long setae. The male possesses terminal suckers on the fourth pair of legs. The dorsum in both sexes bears backwardly directed spines.

There are four stages in the life cycle: egg, larva, nymph, and adult. The adult female remains in a molting pouch in the skin until she is fertilized by the male. She then extends the molting pouch into a tunnel and commences egg laying. The burrow is always superficial and never extends below the stratum corneum. Females usually extend the length of the burrow 2 or 3 mm in a 24-hour period, working chiefly at night. It has been shown that warmth provided by bed clothing or a hot shower or bath stimulates mite activity. As the female burrows, she deposits eggs. There is some difference of opinion as to whether this commences within hours after fertilization or after a four- to five-day delay. There is also some question as to the numbers of eggs produced and frequency of deposition. Some authorities believe that the female will deposit four to five eggs daily for about a month. Others are of the opinion that the eggs are deposited at two- to three-day intervals for about two months. It is agreed that the eggs, which measure about 150 by 100 μ, hatch in four to five days. The six-legged larvae which emerge from the eggs leave the tunnel, wander about the skin, and then burrow into the skin to construct almost invisible molting pouches. In these pouches males molt once and females molt twice to become nymphs, then adults. The adult male emerges from the molting pouch and wanders about over the skin surface in search of females. The adult female remains in the molting pouch until found and fertilized by the male. She then extends the molting pouch into a tunnel and commences egg laying. The cycle from egg to egg-laying female takes from 10 to 14 days. The female lives in the host for at least a month and has been known to survive off the host for ten days. It has been reported that less than 10 per cent of the eggs mature into adult mites.

Although in theory the only certain method of diagnosis of scabies is by demonstration of the parasite, the presence of papules, vesicles, and tiny serpentine burrows associated with a history of itching is adequate for diagnostic purposes. In fair-skinned persons the burrows, under magnification, may have a "peppered" appearance owing to accumulation of fecal pellets. At one end of the tunnel a tiny, pearl-shaped object, dark at one extremity, may be found. The pearl-shaped structure is the adult female, and the dark object is her mouth-parts. The parasite may be easily removed from the burrow with the point of a needle.

The burrows may vary in length from a few millimeters to several centimeters. They are usually located in areas where the skin is thin and wrinkled. Favorite spots seem to be skin between the fingers, the anterior surfaces of the wrists, the feet, the extensor surface of the elbows, the axillae, the belt line, the thighs and external genitalia in men, and under the breasts, the nipples, the abdomen, and lower portions of the buttocks in women. Itching is particularly intense at night when the mites are most active. Secondary infection by scratching is not uncommon and may also serve to reinoculate mites in new areas. Sensitization to the presence of *S. scabiei* may result in a follicular, papular eruption widely distributed over areas where mite burrows are absent. This rash seldom appears until about a month after a primary infestation, and until its appearance the patient may be unaware of his infestation. The severe itching which accompanies this rash may also lead to scratching and secondary infection. Occasionally, particularly in invalids or other persons not able to care for themselves, large numbers of mites may develop under serous crusts. This condition is commonly called "Norwegian scabies" or crusted itch.

In view of the discomfort produced by scabies infestation, it seems odd that the number of burrows and adult females parasitizing a person is usually about 10 to 15, although more than 100 may be occasionally present.

Control of scabies, particularly in schools and institutions, should be based on a program involving education, case-finding, proper treatment of individuals, and adequate laundering of underclothing and bedding. Treatment of scabies usually involves use of creams or lotions containing 1 per cent lindane, 10 per cent crotamiton, benzyl benzoate, or tetraethylthiuram monosulfide. It is generally agreed that these medications should be applied to the entire body below the chin. The medication is washed off the following day. An additional one or even two treatments may be required at seven- to ten-day intervals. One authority has urged caution to avoid overtreatment, as, even when all parasites have been killed, itching may sometimes persist for several days. Because of the long incubation period during which transmission may occur, treatment of all family members and others in close contact with the patient should be considered. Students found to be infested should be removed from school until properly treated.

Gordon, R. M., and Lavoipierre, M. M. J.: Entomology for Students of Medicine. Oxford, Blackwell Scientific Publications, 1962.
Herridge, C. F.: Norweigan scabies (crusted scabies). Br. Med. J., 1:223, 1963.
Mellanby, K.: Scabies. Middlesex, England, E. W. Classey, Ltd., 1972.
Thomsett, L. R.: Mite infestations of man contracted from dogs and cats. Br. Med. J., 2:93, 1968.

33.5. MYIASIS

Myiasis is the term for infestation of a living animal by fly larvae (maggots). Larvae of some species of flies are obligatory parasites; others are facultative in that they may develop in carrion, feces, or even vegetable debris as well as in living animals. Although some flies are fairly specific in host choice, man is not the sole host for any of the flies which cause myiasis. Several of the species which parasitize man are normally found in domestic or wild animals, and many others are accidental parasites.

Classification of myiasis is based on the portion of the body affected as well as on the symptoms produced; hence such terms as cutaneous myiasis, gastrointestinal myiasis, ophthalmomyiasis, furuncular myiasis, and creeping myiasis are encountered. The important medical problems involved are recognition of the infestation and prompt removal of maggots.

Gastrointestinal myiasis may be caused by flies of many species whose eggs or early stage larvae are accidentally ingested. One species often encountered is the rat-tailed maggot, the larva of *Eristalis tenax*. This type of myiasis may result in nausea, sharp pain, vomiting, diarrhea, and occasionally hemorrhage from the anus. *Genitourinary myiasis*, caused by several of the smaller diptera, may result from migration of maggots from the alimentary tract or from deposition of fly eggs near the genitals. Symptoms reported have been albuminuria, dysuria, hematuria, and pyuria. *Cutaneous myiasis*, including *furuncular myiasis* and *creeping myiasis*, is caused by several obligatory parasites. One of these, *Auchmeromyia luteola*, a species found only in tropical Africa, is unique in that the larva has a feeding habit similar to that of a bedbug. During the daytime it hides in crevices in the walls or floor, emerging only at night to feed on sleeping persons. *Dermatobia hominis*, the human botfly, a species widely distributed in neotropical portions of the Americas, does not directly approach the host animal but lays its eggs on mosquitoes and occasionally on ticks. When these blood-sucking arthropods contact a warm-blooded host, the eggs quickly hatch and the larvae penetrate the skin where they produce furuncular lesions as they grow. Although at first there is no pain at the invasion site, a serous exudate accompanied by swelling and severe pain may follow. The larvae may be removed by pressure, by application of petroleum jelly to the lesion (to block the spiracles through which the maggot breathes), or by surgical removal. The latter is preceded by local anesthetization to quiet the larvae as well as to relieve pain of the host.

Larvae of the botfly *Gasterophilus intestinalis*, normally a parasite of horses, may occasionally parasitize man, causing *creeping myiasis*. This is characterized by raised, reddish, serpentine lines on the skin. A larva may advance 1 to 2 cm daily, moving mainly at night. The larva is located just ahead of the inflammatory line, and because of its superficial location in the corneum it may be easily removed surgically. Another botfly, *Hypoderma lineatum*, the cattle grub, has frequently been reported as a parasite of man. As the larvae move through the subcutaneous tissues of this "unfamiliar" host, they may produce indefinite reddish lines on the skin or local painful swellings. During the infestation, which may last for months, the patient may experience severe discomfort and even temporary paralysis of limbs which have been invaded by the parasite. The most serious danger is that the maggots may enter an eye, where they have been found in both chambers. Conjunctival myiasis caused by larvae of *Oestrus ovis*, a parasite of sheep and goats, has been reported from many areas of the world. In the United States cases have frequently been reported in California.

Infestation of man by larvae of *Cochliomyia hominivorax*, the primary screw-worm, may result in serious illness. In nature these flies deposit their eggs adjacent to open wounds on cattle and other animals. The eggs quickly hatch, and, after entering the wound, the maggots burrow beneath the skin where they cause extensive tissue destruction. Infestations in man are usually nasal or aural. In such instances the flies are apparently attracted by purulent discharge. The growing larvae may cause severe local trauma and may also wander and eventually reach the brain. Removal of the larvae manually or by irrigation should be accomplished as quickly as possible, for, as the larvae mature and approach pupation, the tendency to migrate increases and so does the danger to the host.

A number of species of blue bottle, green bottle, and flesh flies which normally deposit their eggs on carrion will sometimes parasitize man if they are attracted to an open sore or to a discharge from the nose, eye, or ear. Eggs of some of these may also be swallowed along with food and give rise to gastrointestinal myiasis.

Baumhover, A. H.: Eradication of the screw worm fly: An agent of myiasis. JAMA, 196:240, 1966.
Gunther, S.: Furuncular Tambu fly myiasis of man in Gabon, Equatorial Africa. J. Trop. Med. Hyg., 70:169, 1967.
James, M. T.: The flies that cause myiasis in man. U.S. Department of Agriculture, Misc. Publ. No. 631, 1947.
Zumpt, F.: Myiasis in Man and Animals of the Old World. London, Butterworth and Company Ltd., 1965.

33.6.   ALLERGY TO ARTHROPOD PRODUCTS

Many arthropods which in most persons may cause only minor annoyance by their bites may stimulate severe allergic responses in some individuals. Others, which do not bite, may also cause similar effects by contact. Inhalant allergic response is of particular importance. Among the arthropods associated with this syndrome are spiders, ticks, mites, mayflies, caddis flies, lacewing flies, and aphids. In order for an arthropod to be of importance as an excitant of allergic symptoms, it must appear in large numbers and be widely distributed, particles from its body must be windborne at some stage in the life cycle, and the particles must be sufficiently buoyant to be carried considerable distances. Good examples are the mayflies and caddis flies. Both of these spend part of the life cycle in the water as larvae. They emerge from the water, molt, and become winged adults. The molted "skins" are light, fragile, and easily fragmented. These readily become airborne and are important causes of inhalant allergic response in areas surrounding lakes where these insects breed. In some persons, inhalation of scales and body fragments of houseflies, beetles, moths, and cockroaches may evoke allergic response.

Clinical effects may include rhinitis, expiratory wheezing, dyspnea, and a constricted feeling in the chest. Diagnosis is dependent not only on symptomatology but also on a consideration of the seasonal nature of attacks, and on a lack of response to treatment for other allergens such as pollens, molds, and housedust. Treatment consists of hyposensitization, oral bronchodilators and use of epinephrine for dyspnea and cyanosis.

TROMBICULID MITES

These mites, which include chiggers, red bugs, and harvest mites, have a wide geographic distribution; they parasitize man, other mammals, birds, amphibians, and reptiles. In most areas they are known primarily as causes of irritating dermatitis, but in Japan, portions of Central and Southeast Asia, and Australasia some are vectors of scrub typhus (tsutsugamushi disease). There is circumstantial evidence that they may be involved in the epidemiology of epidemic hemorrhagic fevers on the Asian mainland.

As with the other acarids, chiggers have four stages in the life cycle: egg, larva, nymph, and adult. Unlike the ticks, trombiculid mites are parasitic only in the larval stage. The tiny (150 by 300 μ), pale yellow or white larvae do *not* burrow into the skin but attach only while feeding. This process may require from a few hours to three or four days. The salivary secretions of the chigger dissolve the tissues adjacent to the inserted mouth-parts, so that a "feeding tube" or stylosome is formed. The actual food ingested is usually not blood but lymph and liquefied skin tissue.

Some persons develop intensely irritating dermatitis as a result of chigger attachment. Scratching may also lead to secondary infection. Although area control of chiggers in camping grounds has been achieved with DDT, dieldrin, and other insecticides (most of which are now banned by the Environmental Protection Agency), the only practical measure at present is prevention of chigger attachment by spraying clothing with insect repellent, especially with a product containing dimethylphthalate.

Baker, E. W., Evans, T. M., Gould, D. J., Hull, W. B., and Keegan, H. L.: A Manual of Parasitic Mites of Medical or Economic Importance, New York, National Pest Control Association, Inc., 1956.
Frazier, C. A.: Insect Allergy: Allergic and Toxic Reactions to Insects and Other Arthropods. St. Louis, Warren H. Green, 1969.

33.7. STINGS BY BEES, WASPS, HORNETS, AND ANTS

Except for vectors of disease agents, members of the order Hymenoptera are of far greater medical importance than all the other groups of phylum Arthropoda combined. In many regions they are also more frequent causes of illness and death than the venomous snakes, fishes, and marine invertebrates.

The stinging apparatus of the hymenopterans has been described as the "hypodermic syringe" of the arthropod world and as the most sophisticated of the invertebrate devices for envenomation. The stinging apparatus is located in the posterior part of the abdomen, between the rectum and ovaries in females, and shares a common orifice with these structures. In most species there is an "acid" and a "basic" gland associated with the stinging apparatus, but there is some disagreement as to whether the secretion of the latter is an active component of the venom. The length of the stinger varies according to species. The depth of insertion of the stinger of the honeybee is generally only 2 or 3 mm. The amount of venom injected varies from 0.2 to 0.5 mg. Although the stinger of the honeybee is lost in the act of stinging (remaining in the recipient), this is not true of other stinging hymenoptera, which may

sting repeatedly at intervals of only a few seconds. Some ants may bite and sting simultaneously; indeed, some cannot sting if they are unable to engage their mandibles.

Venom composition varies greatly among the hymenopterans. Because venoms of even closely related species may possess different allergens, generalizations which might be expected to lead to more effective treatment are not warranted. At least eight toxic fractions have been identified in bee venom. Although the effects of bee sting result from the combined action of these fractions, one component, melittin, is largely responsible for the local and general toxicity. Hyaluronidase, present in bee venom, is also found in venoms of other stinging hymenopterans. Bee venom also contains histamine and, in addition, causes release of histamine in tissues by the decarboxylation of histidine. The venom contains no cholinesterase, but may contain several basic protein components, several amino acids, and at least two enzymes.

Aside from the painful local reaction following stings by bees, wasps, hornets, or ants, more serious reactions, which may lead to the death of the victim, can occur in four circumstances: (1) *Massive envenomation by a large number of stings.* Although death has been reported after a person has received only 30 to 60 bee stings, it is the consensus that ordinarily at least 400 stings are necessary to cause death in an adult. Even single stings by some of the larger hymenopterans may produce grave illness. There have been reports of death of not only man but also water buffalo and even elephants following stings by the giant bee, *Apis dorsalis.* (2) *Particular localization of the sting.* Stings on the head have been known to cause central nervous system symptoms, and stings on the throat may produce edema of the glottis. (3) *Intravascular injection of venom.* Although this is extremely rare, it has been reported. (4) *Hypersensitivity.* In hypersensitive persons even a single sting may lead to death from anaphylactic shock or laryngeal edema.

In the majority of envenomations by a hymenopteran, the initial reaction is acute local pain followed within a few minutes by local swelling and itching. The area affected shows a small, clear, round central zone surrounded by a red halo. In the case of a honeybee sting, the stinger is found in the clear zone, often still moving spasmodically. This local reaction usually subsides after a few hours. More serious effects occur when the victim is hypersensitive to the venom. In such instances onset of symptoms is rapid, usually reaching a maximum within 30 minutes or less following the sting. Location of the sting in sensitized persons may affect the outcome. In a series of 53 persons who suffered anaphylactic shock following bee sting, 5 of 20 who were stung on the head died; 1 person stung on the arm died, but all others who were stung on the neck, trunk, and legs survived. In sensitized individuals the sting may be quickly followed by abnormal swelling, massive urticaria, and shock. There is often slight fever and sometimes diarrhea and polyuria. There may also be a hot flush over the entire body, severe dyspnea, wheezing and coughing, generalized trembling, and coma.

Effects of stings by fire ants vary somewhat from those caused by bees or wasps. Although the immediate reaction is an intense, burning sensation (hence the name "fire ant"), this sensation subsides within a short time and a wheal appears at the site of venom injection. A few hours later a superficial vesicle containing a clear fluid appears. After 24 hours, the fluid becomes purulent as a result of the necrotizing properties of the venom. The pustules are sterile and may persist as long as a week if they are not broken. During this time the fluid is absorbed, leaving a crust and, in many instances, scar tissue. Occasionally a person may have systemic reactions, including nausea and vomiting, dizziness, excessive perspiration, cyanosis, asthma, and other symptoms typical of severe allergic reaction.

It is recommended that all persons showing systemic reaction to hymenopteran stings undergo a hyposensitization program involving immunizing injections with whole-body, aqueous extracts of insects to whose venoms they are sensitive. In such a program a maintenance level is first achieved, and then for a three-year period the interval between injections is gradually increased — i.e., once a month during the first year, once every two months during the second year, and up to once every three months during the third year. Thereafter maintenance doses as tolerated, equal to the antigenicity of one or more average stings of the responsible insects, are given. It has been found that the RAST procedure (radioallergosorbent procedure) is an accurate method of documenting IgE-mediated allergic sensitivity to stinging insects. In one study involving 109 sera of persons who had immediate systemic allergic reactions following insect stings, it was found that the majority contained IgE antibodies to either yellow jacket or hornet venoms. Some sera had positive RAST reactions to two or three venoms, but others had only single venom-specific IgE antibodies. Of 24 patients who had large local reactions only, the sera of 13 contained venom IgE antibodies. Immune therapy for a three-year period seems to provide a high degree of protection for most patients. In one large series it was found that 5 per cent of the patients did not reach a complete protection level during treatment and that an additional 5 per cent had a decrease in protection after treatment was stopped.

For evident severe envenomation, epinephrine hydrochloride (0.5 ml or more of a 1:1000 solution intramuscularly or part of the dose intravenously) should be given. This should be followed by an injectable antihistamine. One hundred mg of hydrocortisone should then be injected intravenously. A sensitized person should carry several sublingual tablets of isoproterenol (15 mg for adults, 10 mg for children) and several uncoated antihistamine tablets on the person at all times. If a sting occurs, the patient should swallow the antihistamine tablet and place the isoproterenol tablet under the tongue. The parents or spouse of a sensitized person should know to inject epinephrine and should keep several ampules of 1:1000 epinephrine hydrochloride on hand at all times.

Beard, R. L.: Insect Toxins and Venoms. Ann. Rev. Entomol, Vol. 8. Palo Alto, Calif., Annual Reviews, Inc., 1963.

Brown, L. L.: Fire ant allergy. South. Med. J., 65:273, 1972.

Frazier, C. A.: Insect Allergy: Allergic and Toxic Reactions to Insects and Other Arthropods. St. Louis, Warren H. Green, 1969.

Frazier, C. A.: Biting insect survey: A statistical report. Ann. Allerg. 32:200, 1974.

Lello, E. D.: Bee venom: Glands, intoxication, accidents. Mem. Inst. Butantan Simp. Internac., 33:821, 1966.

Michener, C. D.: The Brazilian Bee Problem. Ann. Rev. Entomol., Vol. 20. Palo Alto, Calif., Annual Reviews, Inc., 1975.

Mueller, H. L., Schmid, W. H., and Rubinstein, R.: Stinging insect hypersensitivity: A 20 year study of immunologic treatment. Pediatrics, 55:530, 1975.

Reisman, R. E.: Stinging insect allergy treatment failures. J. Allerg. Clin. Immunol., 52:257, 1973.

Reisman, R. E., Wypych, J., and Arbesman, C. E.: Stinging insect allergy: Detection and clinical significance of venom IgE antibodies. J. Allerg. Clin. Immunol., 56:443, 1975.

33.8.   BLISTER BEETLES

Beetles of many species throughout the world qualify for the title "blister beetle." Effects of contact with these insects may vary from a vesicular dermatitis to frank blisters which may be 50 mm or more in length. Accidents occur when contact is made with beetles in vegetation or when beetles, attracted by light, enter unscreened buildings. When a beetle is brushed off the skin or crushed, a vesicant secretion deposited on the skin produces painful irritation within a few minutes. The blisters and surrounding areas are painful, but the most severe reactions occur when the secretions enter the eyes. In the tropics "whip-lash dermatitis," due to species of genus *Paederus,* is common. "Spanish fly," the supposed aphrodisiac, is actually cantharidin, secreted by beetles in the Mediterranean area. This substance, a powerful renal irritant, has frequently been misused with disastrous effects.

Treatment of dermatitis caused by blister beetles is symptomatic. As might be expected, in patients in whom large blisters are formed, prevention of secondary infection is important. In addition to antibiotics, topical and systemic administration of steroids has been reported as effective.

Armstrong, R. K., and Winfield, J. L.: *Paederus fuscipes* dermatitis. An epidemic on Okinawa. Am. J. Trop. Med. Hyg., 18:147, 1969.

Fain, A.: Toxic action of rove beetles (Coleoptera, Staphylinidae). Mem. Inst. Butantan Simp. Internac., 33:835, 1966.

33.9.   SPIDER BITE

Spiders are arachnids of the order Araneida, which is divided into two suborders, the mygalomorphs of suborder Orthognatha, and the true spiders of suborder Labidognatha. The former, commonly known as "tarantulas" or bird spiders, are distinguished from the true spiders in that their jaws or chelicerae are anterior in position on the cephalothorax, are parallel, and operate vertically in a stabbing motion. In the true spiders the jaws are ventrally located and operate from side to side as pincers. Spiders differ from the ticks and mites in that the body is distinctly divided into an anterior cephalothorax and a posterior abdomen, connected by a narrow pedicle. Spiders possess four pairs of legs in all stages of development.

With very few exceptions, spiders secrete venom which is used for killing prey. Although most spiders will bite under some circumstances, less than 100 of the approximately 30,000 species which have been described have been reported as causes of spider bite in man. Still fewer can be considered as of true medical importance. Although the large, hairy mygalomorphs inspire fear, bites by members of the group are rare. Only two species of genus *Atrax* in Australia and species of genus *Harpactirella* in South Africa have consistently been reported as causing envenomation in man.

Several of the mygalomorphs in Central and South America have been shown to possess venom potent against laboratory animals, but most apparently seldom bite man. Indeed, New World mygalomorphs seem to rely for protection more on urticating hairs on the dorsal surface of the abdomen than on their chelicerae. When disturbed, these spiders will vigorously rub their hind legs over the abdomen, releasing a cloud of tiny hairs. Upon contact with the eyes, nasal mucosa, or skin these may cause intense but transitory irritation. It is possible, of course, that some of the large mygalomorphs possess venom which could be lethal for man. Fortunately, lack of contact with forest-dwelling species and the mild temperament characteristic of many species leave the question open for speculation.

Although bites by many of the true spiders have been reported, the majority of cases of even moderately severe envenomation have been caused by the black widow spiders of genus *Latrodectus* in both the Old and New Worlds; the brown spiders of genus *Loxosceles* in North and South America; the "wandering spiders" of genus *Phoneutria* in South America; the wolf spiders of genus *Lycosa,* particularly in South America; and several species of genus *Chiracanthium* in both the Old and New Worlds.

Bites by the black widow spider *Latrodectus mactans* and other members of the genus, may at first go unnoticed, marked only by two tiny puncture marks and some slight local redness. However, in a matter of a few minutes to a few hours, severe muscular pains commence, usually accompanied by a feeling of pressure on the chest. Abdominal rigidity is also characteristic. Nausea, vomiting, profuse perspiration, intestinal spasms, shock, and visual difficulty may occur. Electrocardiographic changes have been reported, as has evidence of hepatic involvement. Treatment is both symptomatic and specific. Muscle relaxants of various types have been used. Although intravenous administration of 10 per cent calcium gluconate has been used for this purpose in the past, other muscle relaxants such as mephenesin (Tolserol) and orphenadrine citrate (Norflex) have been reported to be more effective. A specific antivenin produced by Merck Sharp & Dohme (Lyovac) is highly effective in neutralizing effects of envenomation. Apparently venoms of the various species of *Latrodectus* are antigenically similar to the extent that an antivenin produced with venom of one of the species will neutralize venoms of all other spiders of the genus.

Effects of bites by *Loxosceles reclusa,* the species of genus *Loxosceles* most widely distributed in the United States, and by other members of the genus are similar. First symptoms usually appear two to three hours after the bite as mild to severe pain. In many patients, a transient erythema at the site of envenomation is quickly followed by formation of a blister surrounded by concentric areas of ischemia and erythema. This combination, termed the "bull's eye" by some, has often been used as a criterion for separation of *Loxosceles* bites from those by other spiders. Unfortunately, however, the classic picture does not always appear. Usually, within 24 hours the color of the lesion changes from red to violaceous or black. Following collapse of the blister, local necrosis occurs, leaving a persistent, slowly growing ulcer which, showing a gravitational spread, may attain a diameter of up to 20 cm or more and cause extensive damage to skin and subcutaneous tissues. Healing may require weeks or even months. In addition to the local reaction, systemic involvement and secondary infection often follow the bite. Fever, chills, edema, nausea, vomiting, and joint pain, together with a generalized morbilliform and petechial eruption, may occur within 24 to 48 hours after envenomation. It has been suggested that the longlasting lesions following bites by *L. reclusa* may be due to stimulation of an autodestructive reaction in the host by a venom component. Rarely severe and sometimes fatal intravascular hemolysis may occur. In nearly all fatal cases, hemolytic anemia, thrombocytopenia, hemoglobinuria, and renal failure have been preterminal complications. Although this syndrome has occurred in adults, it is usually found in children 24 to 48 hours after envenomation.

An antivenin for treatment of loxoscelism in South America is produced at the Instituto Butantan in São Paulo, Brazil. Since no such product is available in the United States, management of envenomation by *L. reclusa* and related species which occur in the western states has been basically symptomatic. There have been recommendations for and against use of steroids, antihistamines, heparin, phentolamine methanesulfonate, and low molecular weight dextran. There seems to be consensus on the effectiveness of early excision of the cutaneous ulcerations. This, according to several reports, relieves pain, stops spread of the ulcer, helps control secondary infection, and prevents systemic manifestations. Antibiotics are routinely used for control of secondary infection.

In the event of intravascular hemolysis, blood replacement (particularly in the form of packed cells) may be needed. Peritoneal dialysis has been used with success in treatment of severe visceral arachnidism and renal shutdown. Hemodialysis and exchange transfusion are sometimes necessary.

House-infesting species of genus *Phoneutria* in Brazil and other areas in South America are both active and aggressive. Bites by these spiders are followed by intense pain, vertigo, visual difficulties, trembling, convulsions, hypothermia, tachycardia, urine retention, and profuse sweating. Wolf spiders of genus *Lycosa* found in the same geographic areas also enter houses and will usually bite upon contact. Effects of envenomation by these spiders may be painful, but are usually restricted to the area surrounding the bite. Treatment of envenomation by species of both these genera is based upon prompt administration of antivenin. A bivalent antivenin, effective against species of both genera and monovalent antivenins, one against species of *Phoneutria,* the other against venoms of the wolf spiders, are produced at the Instituto Butantan.

Arnold, R. E.: Brown recluse spider bites: Five cases with a review of the literature. JACEP, 5:262, 1976.

Berger, R. S.: A critical look at therapy for the brown recluse spider bite. Arch. Dermatol., 107:298, 1973.

Bücherl, W.: Spiders. *In* Bücherl, W., and Buckley, E. E. (eds.): Venomous Animals and Their Venoms, Vol. III. New York, Academic Press, 1971, p. 197.

Russell, F. E., Wainschel, J., and Gertsch, W. J.: Bites of spiders and other arthropods. *In* Conn, H. F. (ed.): Current Therapy 1973. Philadelphia, W. B. Saunders Company, 1973, p. 868.

Taylor, E. H., and Denny, W. F.: Hemolysis, renal failure and death presumed secondary to bite of brown recluse spider. South. Med. J., 59:1209, 1966.

33.10. SCORPION STING

In many areas of the world scorpion sting is a public health problem of some magnitude. Areas particularly affected are Africa, the Middle East, India, Mexico, the West Indies (particularly Trinidad), Central America, and South America (particularly Brazil and Argentina). One dangerously venomous species, *Centruroides sculpturatus*, is found in the southwestern United States. Although several hundred scorpion species have been described, published reports indicate that stings by only about 50 of these can cause serious illness and death in man.

Scorpions are arachnids with four pairs of legs and two main body divisions, the anterior cephalothorax and the posterior abdomen. The latter is further divided into a broad preabdomen and a narrow, tail-like postabdomen. This terminates in the telson, a structure which is vesicular in shape and possesses a sharp, hollow stinger. On either side of the stinger near its tip is a tiny pore which serves as an outlet for venom secreted by each of the two venom glands contained in the telson. At the anterior end of the scorpion are the conspicuous, pincer-like pedipalps which are used for seizing prey.

Scorpions produce living young and may require a year or more to reach maturity. Food consists of insects and arthropods of suitable size. These arachnids are nocturnal. During the daytime they remain hidden, and they emerge only at night to feed. Many scorpions hide under rocks, under loose tree bark, or in and around the habitations of man where they can be found in lumber piles, in crevices in walls, among clothing, behind furniture, and in any situation offering shelter and darkness. Every year thousands of accidents and many deaths are caused by contact with house-infesting species which will sting immediately if touched.

Immediate, sharp pain at the site of venom injection is a common feature of all scorpion stings; subsequent developments allow division of these accidents into two categories. In the first of these, symptoms are local and usually transitory, persisting for a few minutes or hours to a day or so. The second category includes those cases showing the systemic involvement characteristic of severe envenomation. There are no hard and fast guidelines for separation of scorpion species into "harmless" and "dangerous" groups. Some genera such as *Centruroides* and *Tityus* of the Western Hemisphere contain dangerously venomous species along with others whose stings produce relatively mild effects. Size and appearance alone are definitely *not* criteria for judgment of the medical importance of a scorpion.

Moderate local edema, which may be discolored, is frequently seen in cases of the milder type of scorpion envenomation. Regional lymph node enlargement, local itching and paresthesia, fever, nausea, and vomiting may occur. Swollen eyelids and "thick tongue," which are sometimes seen, may indicate an allergic response to the venom. In most cases of mild envenomation all signs and symptoms subside within 24 hours.

Because scorpion venoms vary greatly not only in chemical composition but also in their effects on man, it is impossible to give a simple clinical picture of scorpion sting. In various areas of the world where dangerous scorpions occur, a wide variety of characteristics of

severe scorpion envenomation have been described. Some of these are anxiety and/or agitation; excessive salivation and perspiration; hyper- or hypotension; cold clammy skin; irregular pulse; unstable temperature; involuntary micturition and/or defecation; pulmonary edema; respiratory difficulties, ranging from irregular movements to respiratory paralysis; muscle tone increases, ranging from twitching and contractures in abdomen, limbs, and pharynx to convulsions, syncope, delirium, mental cloudiness, hemiplegia, shock, blurred vision, blindness, oliguria, polyuria, and hematuria; hyperglycemia; glycosuria, myocarditis; VMA elevation; and SGOT elevation.

Some authorities have felt that death from scorpion sting is always due to respiratory failure; others are of the opinion that peripheral vascular failure and myocarditis are important causes of death. In such cases the view is that cardiovascular manifestations are related to the level of circulating catecholamines elicited by the direct effect of scorpion venom on the sympathetic nervous system. Although the convulsions so frequently seen in severe scorpion envenomation may be due to direct action of the toxin on the brain, in some instances they may be the result of ventricular tachycardia.

Onset of symptoms other than local pain vary from a few minutes to as long as 24 hours following the sting. The interval between the sting and death may vary from several minutes to 30 hours. The physician should be on the alert for the sudden reappearance of symptoms after the patient seems to be on the road to recovery. Respiratory difficulties are characteristic of such relapses. Mortality rate from scorpion sting is much higher among children than adults. In a series of cases in Trinidad, the mortality rate from scorpion sting was 25 per cent among children under five years of age but only 0.25 per cent in adults. Similar data are available for stings by *Tityus serrulatus* in Brazil.

It is generally agreed that administration of a potent antivenin is the most effective treatment for scorpion sting. Various measures have been advocated for use in instances when antivenin is not available and as adjuncts to serotherapy. In mild cases no medical treatment is required, although a cube of ice over the site of the sting will reduce pain. In serious envenomation both oxygen and positive pressure breathing assistance may be needed. Atropine has been recommended as a parasympatholytic drug, and sodium phenobarbital given by the intravenous route has been helpful when convulsions occur. In the treatment of scorpion sting in the United States, morphine and meperidine are contraindicated, as these drugs have a synergistic effect with venom of the only dangerous North American species, *Centruroides sculpturatus*. An authority on scorpion sting in the Old World has stated that barbiturates, too, are contraindicated, as they have an inhibitory effect on the bulbar respiratory centers. Intravenous injections of calcium gluconate have proved helpful in relief of muscle spasms. In some areas such as India, where dangerously venomous scorpions occur and no antivenins are available, treatment is purely symptomatic. Unfortunately, scorpion venoms differ greatly in antigenicity, and antivenins produced with them are usually not paraspecific in action. This means that in each area where severe envenomation by scorpions might occur, an antivenin produced with indigenous species must be used in treatment. At present there is no commercial production of scorpion antivenin in the United States. Although antivenins produced in Mexico for treatment of stings by Mexican species of *Centruroides* are effective in neutralization of effects of envenomation by *Centruroides sculpturatus* of the southwestern United States, importation and distribution of these products are, at present, illegal. An antivenin produced at the Antivenom Production Laboratory of Arizona State University against venom of *C. sculpturatus* is distributed free throughout the state of Arizona only. Although there are many published reports of studies to characterize scorpion venoms, none of these, at least to date, has resulted in increased effectiveness of treatment of envenomation.

Efforts to eliminate scorpion sting as a medical problem have included destruction of scorpions with pesticides, mechanical barriers to prevent entry of scorpions into buildings, general policing of yards around homes to remove litter which might harbor scorpions, and common sense measures to be followed by campers or others who might be living outdoors in areas where scorpions occur.

Bücherl, W.: Classification, biology, and venom extraction of scorpions. *In* Bücherl, W., and Buckley, E. E. (eds.): Venomous Animals and Their Venoms, Vol. III. New York, Academic Press, 1971, p. 317.

Ennik, F.: A short review of scorpion biology, management of stings, and control. Calif. Vector Views, 19:69, 1972.

Gueron, M., and Yaron, R.: Cardiovascular manifestations of severe scorpion sting. Chest, 57:156, 1970.

Reddy, C. R. R. M., Suvarkakum, G., Devi, C. C., and Reddy, C. N.: Pathology of scorpion venom poisoning. J. Trop. Med. Hyg., 75:98, 1972.

Stahnke, H. L.: Some aspects of scorpion behavior. Bull. South. Calif. Acad. Sci., 65:65, 1966.

Wainshel, J., Russell, F. E., and Gertsch, W. S.: Bites of spiders and other arthropods. *In* Conn., H. F. (ed.): Current Therapy 1974. Philadelphia, W. B. Saunders Company, 1974, p. 865.

Whittemore, F. W., Keegan, H. L., and Borowitz, J. L.: Studies of scorpion antivenins. 1. Paraspecificity. Bull. WHO, 25:185, 1961.

33.11. CENTIPEDES AND MILLIPEDES

The centipedes (order Chilopoda) and the millipedes (order Diplopoda) are superficially alike in that they are wormlike in form and possess several pairs of legs; however, the millipedes possess two pairs of legs on each body segment.

The body of a centipede is composed of a series of similar segments, each of which bears a pair of legs. The head bears one pair of long antennae and associated mouth-parts. The segment immediately behind the head possesses a pair of maxillipeds or "claws," which are used in capturing prey and for defense. At the tip of each of these claws is an orifice through which venom is extruded when the centipede bites. The number of leg pairs present varies from 15 to over 100. Although most centipedes are small, some, particularly in the tropics, may reach a length of over 25 cm. Many of the species of genus *Scolopendra* are striking in appearance, with black or blue-black bodies and orange legs.

All centipedes are carnivorous and move about at night in search of food. This habit brings them in contact with man with resulting accidents, as most centipedes will bite immediately if touched. Centipede bite may be intensely painful, and the bite of at least one

species, found in Malaysia, has been compared in severity to a bite by a pit viper. In experiments with a large centipede of genus *Scolopendra* found in Texas, a single bite killed a laboratory mouse in about 30 seconds. In spite of this and the severe local pain caused by centipede bite, effects are usually transitory and there seem to have been no verifiable human deaths from this cause. Treatment is entirely symptomatic.

Unlike the centipedes, the millipedes are vegetarians. They do not bite when touched, but may squirt an irritating secretion from pores on the sides of the body. This substance may cause transitory dermatitis, or severe irritation if it reaches the eyes. Again, treatment is symptomatic.

Bücherl, W.: Venomous chilopods or centipedes. *In* Bücherl, W., and Buckley, E. E. (eds.): Venomous Animals and Their Venoms, Vol. III. New York, Academic Press, 1971, p. 169.

Keegan, H. L.: Centipedes and millipedes as pests in tropical areas. *In* Venomous and Poisonous Animals and Noxious Plants of the Pacific Region. Oxford, Pergamon Press, 1963, p. 161.

33.12. TICK PARALYSIS

Tick paralysis is a progressive, ascending flaccid paralysis of man and domestic and wild animals, caused by a toxin secreted by attached adult female (usually) hard ticks during engorgement. Although several species of ticks have been incriminated in various regions of the world, cases in man in the United States have resulted from attachment by ticks of only two species: *Dermacentor andersoni*, the Rocky Mountain wood tick, and *D. variabilis*, the American dog tick. It is believed that the toxin responsible for this condition is secreted only after the tick has been attached and feeding for one or more days.

Onset of the condition may be marked by restlessness, irritability, and numbness or tingling of the extremities, lips, throat, and face. Difficulty in walking is soon followed by inability to stand. Swallowing may become difficult or impossible. Within a day or two paralysis of the limb and trunk muscles and bulbar involvement may lead to dysphagia, slurred speech, and impaired vision. Death may result from respiratory failure or aspiration pneumonia. During the illness leukocyte and erythrocyte counts and spinal fluid, hemoglobin, and urine levels are usually normal. The temperature is only slightly elevated.

In a recent typical case, a three-year-old girl awakened unable to walk, and fell. Her parents noted extreme weakness of the legs and lack of balance. The child was examined by a physician, but except for a bruise on the leg nothing unusual was noted. On the following day the child was still weak and unable to stand. On the third day of illness, there was still no sign of improvement. However, later the same day the child's mother noted a lump on the occipital area of the scalp and found a tick. A physician removed the blood-engorged tick, and the child recovered uneventfully within a day. The tick was a female specimen of *D. andersoni*. It was thought that the tick had been acquired three weeks previously when the family had been on a camping trip.

Unless paralysis is too far advanced, rapid and complete recovery occurs within a few hours or days after removal of the tick. In most cases ticks have been found concealed in the hair and, since their bite is painless, have not been noticed. In the past, tick paralysis was sometimes confused with poliomyelitis. In polyneuritis, myelitis, syringomyelia, and spinal cord tumor, sensory loss is usually present. Sensory signs are rare in tick paralysis.

Diagnosis of tick paralysis may be delayed because the condition is not often seen. From 1960 through 1974, only 13 cases were reported from Oregon, Washington, Oklahoma, Arkansas, Mississippi, North Carolina, and Virginia. During the same period cases were reported from ten other states. Most cases of tick paralysis have been among children and adolescents. Death rates in various series of cases have ranged from 10 to 12 per cent. Deaths have generally been due to respiratory paralysis.

In Australia a canine anti-tick serum has been produced which will protect dogs from paralysis caused by attachment of *Ixodes holocyclus*. In other areas prevention lies in the use of personal protective measures. Anyone going into woods or other areas which might be tick infested should wear protective clothing — i.e., trousers tucked into boots, shirts tucked into belts, and sleeves buttoned. In addition, and of greater importance, insect repellent should be sprayed or rubbed into clothing, particularly the lower portions of trouser legs. As frequently as possible, anyone in an area where ticks are numerous should search for attached ticks. In removing these the fingers should not come into direct contact with them. Using gloves, a leaf, paper, or forceps the ticks should be removed by a gentle and then a stronger pull. Insect repellent, mineral oil, and even a heated needle or knife blade have been used for this purpose.

Gregson, J.D.: Tick Paralysis — an Appraisal of Natural and Experimental Data. Ottawa, Canadian Department of Agriculture Monograph No. 9, 1973.

Kaire, G. H.: Isolation of tick paralysis toxin from *Ixodes holocyclus*. Toxicon, 4:91, 1966.

Nelson, B. C.: Tick paralysis in a dog caused by *Ixodes pacificus*. Calif. Vector Views, 20:80, 1973.

Stanbury, J. B., and Huyck, J. H.: Tick paralysis: A critical review. Medicine, 24:219, 1945.

33.13.   ALLERGY TO HOUSE-DUST MITES

Since 1964, when mites of genus *Dermatophagoides* were first shown to be important allergenic components of house dust, a veritable flood of papers by investigators throughout the world has appeared on the subject. Although 15 species of the genus have been described, much of the research concerning these arachnids has centered on two widely distributed species, *D. pteronyssinus* and *D. farinae*. It has been found in the laboratory that females of these species require an average of 30 days to develop from the egg to the adult stage. Various types of culture media have been used to rear these mites. These have included dog food, house dust, gelatin, dry hair, yeast, and skin scales. Even though mites may be present in large numbers in a home, they may not be noticed because of their small size (less than 500 μ in length) and pale color. In homes, species of the genus have been collected not only from house dust but also from overstuffed furniture, carpets, pillows, and bedding. Both temperature and humidity affect the abundance of mites. Low temperature and low humidity have adverse effects on mite development.

The allergic responses of man to house-dust mites do not differ from those evoked by contact with mite-free house dust. An examination of literature which has appeared in the past several years has revealed the same general symptoms reported from the many countries in which these mites occur. One problem has been the proper evaluation of epidemiologic data. It has been shown that there may be considerable variations in mite populations found in homes of dust-sensitive and non-dust-sensitive persons. In some localities mites are lacking from most dust samples. An additional difficulty is that house dust usually contains a variety of allergens. Recent development of commercially available pure extracts of house-dust mites has been of aid in diagnosis. Use of a vaccine prepared from cultures of *D. farinae* has shown promise in hyposensitization of asthmatic children. In addition to the techniques commonly used for protection of hypersensitive persons from contact with house dust, use of insecticides, vacuuming of infested rooms, and environmental measures involving manipulation of temperature and humidity have been suggested for mite control. However, none of these methods has been thoroughly evaluated in a field situation. In laboratory studies it has been found that cultures of *D. farinae* have been eliminated by predatory mites of two species.

Bernecker, C.: The antigenicity of house dust and mites. Acta Allerg., 25:392, 1970.

Kawai, T., March, E., Naey, S. M., and Norman, P. S.: The significance of *Dermatophagoides* allergens in house dust allergy in the Baltimore area: Assay by leukocyte histamine release. J. Allerg. 47:95, 1971.

Keh, B.: The common house dust mites of the genus *Dermatophagoides* (Acarina: Oyroglyphidae). Calif. Vector Views, 20:37, 1973.

Morita, Y., Miyamoto, T., Horiuchi, Y., Oshima, S., Katsuhata, A., and Kawai, S.: Further studies in allergenic identity between house dust and the house dust mites. Ann. Allerg., 35:362, 1975.

Wharton, G. W., and Brody, A. R.: Colloquium: The entomology of house-dust allergy. Proc. North Cent. Br. Ent. Soc. Am., 26:57, 1971.

33.14.   DERMATITIS CAUSED BY CATERPILLARS AND MOTHS

In many regions, moth caterpillars as well as adult moths are of seasonal medical interest because of the irritating dermatitis, pain, and systemic manifestations produced when they contact the skin of man. These effects are caused by venom contained in the sharp hairs and spines borne singly or in clusters on the body of the caterpillar. When adult moths are involved, it is because some of these hairs adhered to the insect when it emerged from the cocoon.

Structurally, the irritating hairs and spines range from those which act in a purely mechanical manner, analogous to glass wool fibers, to complicated types resembling the "hypodermic syringe" of the hymenopterans. In many species the urticating spines are hollow and lined with venom-secreting glandular epithelium. Upon slight contact the tip of the spine breaks off and its contents pour into the skin. It has been suggested that the toxic effects, in some cases, are a result of the chemical composition of the spine rather than the venomous secretions per se. Efforts to chemically characterize lepidopteran venoms have not, as yet, met with great success. Histamine has been found in venoms of several species. Irritating, water-soluble proteolytic enzyme components have been isolated from extracts of setae of others.

Species of several genera may produce dermatitis in man. Principal offenders in the United States are the puss-caterpillar, the larva of *Megalopyge opercularis;* and the saddle-back caterpillar, the larva of *Sibine stimulea.* In East and Southeast Asia dermatitis and other symptoms have been caused by a number of species. Both caterpillars and adult moths have been involved. It has been reported that on the Japanese island of Honshu about 250,000 cases of dermatitis result yearly from contact with adults and caterpillars of *Euproctis flava,* the Oriental tussock moth. Many other species cause both dermatitis and other symptoms in man.

Symptoms following contact with urticating species may be restricted to mere reddening of the skin, itching, and mild dermatitis, but may also include sudden burning pain, swelling, lymphangitis, numbness, papule-like eruptions, blistering, urticaria, and such systemic manifestations as nausea, vomiting, and shock. Persons who have contacted the puss-caterpillar often describe the sensation as one of "through-and-through" severe pain. Appearance of large numbers of caterpillars with resulting painful contacts has caused temporary closing of schools in some areas. In one instance a military maneuver had to be cancelled when about a third of the men in a battalion acquired painful dermatitis after a one-night bivouac in a pine grove. In this episode the cause of illness was contact with empty cocoons which littered the forest floor.

Treatment of caterpillar sting is symptomatic. No antisera or other products for direct action against the venom have been developed. Codeine, morphine sulfate, and meperidine have been used in treatment with varying results. Aspirin is usually not effective in relief of pain. It has been reported that 10 ml of a 10 per cent solution of calcium gluconate given intravenously provides quick relief from the intense pain caused by the puss-caterpillar. In event of severe urticaria, administration of epinephrine has proved effective. Ice packs are sometimes helpful. Antihistamines have not been of noticeable value in therapy.

Note: In addition to their role in urticarial dermatitis, adult moths in several countries in Southeast Asia have been reported to cause severe conjunctivitis when they feed on ocular secretions. These insects may be in a state of transition from a phytophagous to a hematophagous role.

Beard, R. L.: Insect toxins and venoms. Ann. Rev. Entomol., Vol. 8. Palo Alto, Calif., Annual Reviews, Inc., 1963.

Keegan, H. L.: Caterpillars and moths as public health problems. *In* Keegan, H. L., and Macfarlane, W. V. (eds): Venomous and Poisonous Animals and Noxious Plants of the Pacific Region. Oxford, Pergamon Press, 1963, p. 161.

McGovern, J. P., Barkin, G. B., McElhenney, T. R., and Wende, R.: *Megalopyge opercularis.* Observations on its life history, of its sting in man, and report of an epidemic. JAMA, 175:1155, 1961.

Pesce, H., and Delgado, A.: Poisoning from adult moths and caterpillars. *In* Bücherl, W., and Buckley, E. E. (eds.): Venomous Animals and Their Venoms, Vol. III. New York, Academic Press, 1971, p. 119.

Sakai, M., and Toshioka, S.: References of the irritating lepidoptera of Japan. Jap. J. San. Zool., 7:107, 1956.

Zaias, N., Ioannides, G., and Taplin, D.: Dermatitis from contact with moths (genus *Hylesia).* JAMA, 207:525, 1969.

34. PENTASTOMIASIS

(Porocephaliasis, Linguatuliasis)

Hugh L. Keegan

The pentastomids are endoparasitic invertebrates which, in spite of a worm-like appearance, are not helminths but probably constitute a separate phylum. As adults most pentastomids parasitize reptiles, especially snakes, although a few utilize birds and carnivorous mammals as definitive hosts. Immature stages have been found in all orders of vertebrates, including man. Of the approximately 70 species of pentastomids, only six have been shown to infest man. Over 90 per cent of reported infestations have been due to two species: *Armillifer armillatus,* a species which in the adult stage is found in pythons and some vipers in tropical Africa, and *Linguatula serrata,* a widely distributed parasite utilizing dogs, wolves, and other carnivores as definitive hosts, and herbivores such as goats and sheep as intermediate hosts. Human infestation occurs either by ingestion of eggs of the parasite or by eating tissues of the definitive host which contain infective stage larvae.

In the first type of infestation, usually caused by *Armillifer armillatus,* eggs of the parasite are ingested in food or water or when a definitive host is being handled or skinned. In such cases the primary larvae which emerge from the ingested eggs bore through the intestinal wall and migrate to various parts of the body where they may encyst and continue development. In addition to the inflammatory response elicited by these larvae, the increase in size during growth (probably over 1000-fold) can produce severe pressure effects, especially if cysts are adjacent to passages such as bile ducts and bronchi, or are within the central nervous system. In a series of 32 autopsied patients in Africa, cysts were found in the liver, intestinal wall, mesentery, mesenteric ganglia, parietal peritoneum (renal and splenic), greater omentum, and lung.

Encysted larvae are ordinarily well tolerated. The majority of infestations are found on autopsy or as a result of x-ray examination. However, in some instances, cysts have been so numerous as to cause intestinal obstruction or to compress bile ducts or bronchi. In a few cases they have been found in the conjunctiva or floating free in the anterior chamber of the eye.

Infestation with *Linguatula serrata* is particularly common in the Middle East and North Africa, where it results from eating raw or insufficiently cooked sheep or goat liver containing the infective third stage larvae. Ingested larvae migrate from the stomach to the throat and nasopharynx where they attach to the tonsils or nasopharyngeal membrane and produce symptoms in a matter of hours. These may include pain and itching in the throat, paroxysmal coughing and sneezing, lacrimal and nasal discharge, hoarseness, dysphagia, and vomiting. Occasionally hemoptysis and temporary loss of hearing occur. There may be enlargement of the submaxillary and cervical lymph nodes. Death caused by asphyxiation resulting from edematous swelling of the tonsillar region has been reported. Fortunately these parasites do not grow to maturity in man, and the infestations are self-limiting within a week or two. This type of illness is known in the Middle East as halzoun and in the Sudan as the marrara syndrome. Similar clinical effects may be produced by nasal leeches which occur in the same geographic region.

In asymptomatic infestations the encysted parasites are found at autopsy or during x-ray examinations. The crescent-shaped, calcified cysts may be confused with other encysted parasites such as tapeworm larvae (the sparganum stage) and arthropod parasites which may penetrate living tissue (the flea, *Tunga penetrans*, and fly larvae).

Burns Cox, C. M., Prathap, K., Clark, E., and Gillman, R.: Porocephaliasis in Western Malaysia. Trans. R. Soc. Trop. Med. Hyg., 63:409, 1969.

Fain, A.: Pentastomida of snakes — their parasitological role in man and animals. Mem. Inst. Butantan Simp. Internac., 33:167, 1966.

Hopps, H. C., Keegan, H. L., Price, D. L., and Self, J. T.: Pentastomiasis. *In* Marcial-Rojas, R. A. (ed.): Pathology of Protozoal and Helminthic Diseases. Baltimore, Williams & Wilkins Company, 1971, p. 970.

Lindner, R. R.: Retrospective x-ray survey for porocephalosis. J. Trop. Med. Hyg., 68:155, 1965.

Prathap, K., Lau, K. S., and Bolton, J. M.: Pentastomiasis: A common finding at autopsy among Malaysian aborigines. Am. J. Trop. Med. Hyg., 18:20, 1969.

Schacher, J. F., Saab, S., Germanos, R., and Boustany, N.: The aetiology of halzoun in Lebanon: Recovery of *Linguatula serrata* nymphs from two patients. Trans. R. Soc. Trop. Med. Hyg., 63:854, 1969.

35. LEECHES AS AGENTS OF DISEASE (Hirudiniasis)

Hugh L. Keegan

Leeches are classified as members of the class Hirudinea of the phylum Annelida. A leech is dorsoventrally flattened, possesses a ventral sucker at either end of the body, and is divided by transverse furrows into a series of annuli. The buccal cavity is located at the rear of the cavity of the oral sucker. Within the buccal cavity are three, rarely two, "jaws." These are muscular ridges, usually armed with a double or single row of tiny teeth. When a leech attaches to a host, the jaws are protruded and the teeth quickly cut through the skin as the jaws are moved in a rocking fashion. Feeding may require a half hour or more, and during this time ingested blood may increase the weight of the leech several-fold. Leeches feed infrequently and may live for months without a blood meal following a single engorgement. The shape of the leech may change considerably as the animal lengthens, contracts, or becomes distended with blood.

Blood-sucking leeches of importance to man include aquatic (freshwater) species of the genera *Hirudo*, the medicinal leeches; *Poicilobdella*, the buffalo leeches; the nasal leeches of genera *Dinobdella* and *Limnatis*; and several species of land leeches of genus *Haemadipsa*. With the exception of the nasopharyngeal leeches of genus *Limnatis*, which occur in Africa and the Middle East, the leeches of medical importance are widely distributed throughout the Pacific region, particularly on the mainland of Central and Southeast Asia and on the islands of Malaysia and Melanesia.

Initially at least, the feeding response of aquatic leeches is stimulated by disturbance of the water. After swimming toward and contacting a suitable host, the leech will attach with the anterior sucker and quickly (usually in less than one minute) cut through the skin and commence feeding. With the majority of species the bite is painless and the person bitten is unaware of the attachment unless the leech is seen.

Land leeches are found in shaded areas on damp ground or in vegetation. Some species may ascend bushes to a height of 1 or 2 meters. Species of *Haemadipsa* are often numerous along game or cattle trails. Even a shadow passing over a leech will evoke the feeding response. The leech will "stand up" on its posterior sucker and then unerringly move toward the host in inchworm fashion. Upon contact it will quickly attach to unprotected skin, or, if boots, socks, and trousers are worn, will quickly surmount these obstacles. Almost any opening, even eyelets of shoes, offers entrance to a hungry leech.

The nasal leeches usually enter the nares or mouth of the host when the animal or man is drinking, although infestations have been reported in man and guard dogs moving through wet vegetation. Although adult land leeches are rarely greater than 50 to 60 mm in length, extended specimens of several of the buffalo leeches and of the nasal leech *Dinobdella* may exceed 200 mm.

Although leeches are annoying pests in areas where they occur, they do not transmit disease agents to man. Their medical importance lies in the repugnance which many persons feel for them; the loss of blood ingested by the leeches during feeding and the often prolonged frank bleeding or oozing of blood from the bite; the two- or three-day period of intense itching at the site of each attachment; the possibility of infection; and, of greater importance, the entry of leeches into the eye, nose, anus, or urethra.

Attachment of leeches to buccal mucosa or to the pharynx or the larynx produces a variety of symptoms. These may include breaking through one or both nostrils, nosebleeds, and hemoptysis. Hoarseness and vomiting of blood are common in such infestations. In some areas, particularly among children, hemorrhage from leech infestation may be so severe as to cause anemia leading to death. Several techniques have been used for removal of leeches from the nasopharynx. In some cases a steady pull on the specimen with forceps has been successful. In others it may be necessary to narcotize the leech before it can be removed. In one case a 1:1000 solution of epinephrine hydrochloride sprayed into the nose was effective. A spray of 5 per cent cocaine hydrochloride has also been used successfully. In cases of urethral or vaginal involvement, a strong salt solution has caused the leeches to detach. The rather drastic technique of gripping the leech with a hemostat and pressing a burning cigarette end held against it in another hemostat has been used in the removal of leeches from the nostril, buccal wall, and tonsillar fossa.

Some protection against both aquatic and land leeches is afforded by clothing, particularly if full-length trousers and field or hunting boots are worn and trouser bottoms are tucked into sock tops. However, in areas heavily infested with land leeches, use of repellent on clothing and exposed skin is essential if leech bites are to be avoided. There are no commercially produced leech repellents. The ordinary insect repellents applied to the clothing and particularly to the boots and lower portions of trouser legs are fairly effective. However, since the active ingredients in most of these are water soluble, reapplications every three to four hours or more frequently during the period of exposure are necessary if the wearer is moving through wet vegetation, is caught in heavy rain, or wades through swamps.

Cameron, A.: Haematemesis from leeches. Br. Med. J., 2:679, 1950.
Chin, T. M.: A further note on leech infestation of man. J. Parasitol., 35:215, 1949.
Keegan, H. L., Radke, M. G., and Murphy, D. A.: Nasal leech infestation in man. Am. J. Trop. Med. Hyg., 19:1029, 1970.
Keegan, H. L., Toshioka, S., and Suzuki, H.: Blood sucking Asian leeches of families Hirudidae and Haemadipsidae. Special report, 406th Medical Laboratory, U.S. Army Medical Command, Japan, 1969.

36. SNAKEBITE

Hugh L. Keegan

Although snakebite, as a cause of morbidity and mortality, is of less public health importance than hypersensitivity to hymenopteran venoms on a worldwide basis, or to scorpion stings or spider bites in many areas, snakebite remains one of the most dramatic and feared accidents to affect man. As a result of a WHO survey conducted in 1954, it was estimated that between 30,000 and 40,000 persons die from snakebite each year. Since only a small percentage of snakebites result in fatalities, it seems likely that at least 500,000 persons are bitten yearly by venomous snakes. Most deaths occur in tropical Asia and Africa where venomous snakes are numerous and where adequate medical care is often unavailable.

The venomous snakes are classified in five families: (1) Elapidae (cobras, kraits, mambas, coral snakes, and all the venomous snakes of Australia and New Guinea); (2) Viperidae (Russell's viper and related species of the genera *Vipera, Bitis, Echis,* and *Cerastes* in the Old World); (3) Crotalidae (the pit vipers: rattlesnakes, copperheads, moccasins, the fer-de-lance, the bushmaster, many species of genus *Bothrops* in the New World, and related species in East and Southeast Asia); (4) Hydrophidae (the sea snake); and (5) Colubridae (most members of the family are nonvenomous, but some, such as *Dispholidus typus,* the boomslang of South Africa, the mangrove snakes of Southeast Asia, and several species in the New World, possess venom glands and fangs which are located in the rear of the upper jaws). Although references concerning snake morphology and classification are given at the end of this discussion, the precise identification of a snake species is seldom of practical importance to a clinician. Because usually less than five or six species occur in a single area and because bites by closely related species generally produce similar results and respond to polyvalent antivenins, the physician should be concerned primarily with accurate diagnosis and effective treatment.

The simplistic notion that snake venoms can handily be characterized as either neurotoxic or hemotoxic has long since been dispelled. It is now known that venoms previously thought to be solely hemorrhagic in action may contain neurotoxic fractions and that cobra venoms, once known only as neurotoxins, possess necrotizing elements. Nevertheless, the clinical picture presented by snakebite, at least in a given geographic area, is fairly consistent. Symptoms following snakebite and severity of the illness vary according to the size and species of the snake involved, the location of the bite, and the size and physical condition of the person bitten. However, it should be realized that a bite by a venomous snake does *not* always result in envenomation. Indeed, surveys in the United States and elsewhere have shown that in many instances a bite by even a large, dangerously venomous snake will result in no envenomation or only minimal effects.

Probably the most helpful early diagnostic sign of envenomation by a viper or pit viper is the appearance of local swelling which commences often within a few minutes of the bite. This swelling progresses rapidly in severe cases and is often accompanied by ecchymosis. Pain, which usually occurs immediately, varies in intensity even in severe cases and is not a reliable criterion for judgment of the degree of envenomation. Following the initial signs and symptoms, nausea, vomiting, bleeding from the fang punctures, bleb formation, visual difficulties, and shock may occur. Later in the course of the illness, severe necrosis is frequently seen. Other signs seen in envenomation by vipers are hemoptysis, bleeding from the gums, hematemesis, and hematuria. Renal shutdown and hepatic and cardiovascular changes may also occur, and convulsions are common, particularly in children. Although death may occur within less than an hour following the bite, most deaths from snakebite occur after a matter of hours or even days. In severely bitten patients there is likely to be massive extravasation of blood into the tissues so that an entire extremity may become deep purple or black. This, coupled with massive edema, results in oozing of blood and lymph through the skin and sometimes tearing of the skin. If the bite was on an upper extremity, this process may extend onto the chest wall.

Recovery is usually prolonged over a period of weeks or months. A 56-year-old man who was bitten on the dorsum of the hand by an Eastern diamondback rattlesnake continued to have swelling in the hand a year later, and the use of his index finger was markedly restricted.

Because of the great variation in severity of effects after viper bite, grading systems have been set up to categorize the degree of illness. One such system is as follows: *Grade I*: Minimal; puncture marks are present, but little or no local swelling or discoloration and no systemic effects. *Grades II, III, and IV*: Moderate, severe, and very severe, respectively; cases in which systemic effects are evident soon after the bite range from moderate to very severe in intensity.

Although in the past the venoms of cobras, coral snakes, kraits, and their allies were generally described as neurotoxins, it is now well documented that venoms of the snakes of family Elapidae vary greatly in their effects on man. Pain, lacking after bites by some species, may be prominent in other cases. Swelling and necrosis are important features of envenomation by some of the cobras, and venoms of some Australian elapids contain both neurotoxins and coagulant fractions, whereas others contain anticoagulants. Blurring of vision, ptosis, slurred speech, dysphagia, often severe abdominal pain, and excessive salivation and sweating early in the illness may be followed by respiratory failure requiring immediate tracheostomy and mechanical respiratory assistance.

Onset of symptoms after bites by elapids may commence less than an hour after the bite, or may be delayed for several hours. It is generally considered that the sooner the signs and symptoms commence, the more severe the case. In bites by the North American coral snake, euphoria, which may be delayed in onset until several hours after the bite, is one of the first symptoms of envenomation. This is quickly followed by drowsiness, ptosis, strabismus, double vision, excessive salivation, weakness, confusion, vomiting, and hematuria. In severe cases respiratory paralysis soon occurs. It has been reported that death from coral snake envenomation usually occurs within 24 hours of the bite.

The first symptom of envenomation after a bite by a sea snake is myalgia, which may appear as early as 30 minutes following the bite. This may cause only moderate discomfort at first, but within an hour or two discomfort may greatly increase in intensity, producing severe pain on passive movements of arm, thigh, leg, and trunk muscles. Appearance of myoglobinuria within an hour or two of a bite is evidence of severe envenomation. In such cases respiratory failure may follow in a few hours. Other evidences of severe envenomation are ptosis, weakness of external eye muscles, dilatation of pupils with sluggish light reaction, and leukocytosis exceeding 20,000.

There has always been a certain amount of disagreement over first aid for snakebite, particularly as to what recommendations should be given to persons with little or no medical training. It seems to be the consensus at present that an *untrained individual* can best help a snakebite victim in the following ways: (1) Within practical limits, immobilizing the bitten part in a position below the heart (most persons are bitten on the limbs). (2) Positioning of an improvised, lightly constricting tourniquet closer to the heart than the bite. If the bite is on the leg or arm, the tourniquet should be applied above the knee or elbow respectively, where a single bone is present. The tourniquet should be moved ahead of the swelling if it progresses up the limb. (3) Obtaining assistance from the nearest medical source, or, preferably, taking the patient to a treatment facility without delay. In addition to the measures listed above, *a person with some paramedical training* may wish to carry out incision and suction *if the patient is seen less than an hour after the bite has occurred* and unavoidable delay in obtaining specific care seems likely. If this is done, an incision about 12 mm in length, and just through the skin, should be made parallel to the long axis of the limb, and through each fang mark. Either oral suction or mechanical suction with a snakebite kit can then be instituted. Although some feel that this procedure is effective if properly carried out by a trained, cool-headed individual, it is generally agreed that it is virtually a waste of time if it is started more than an hour following the bite. In the absence of a physician, and when faced with probable delay in obtaining definitive medical help, a *trained* person can administer antivenin in the field if the patient appears to be seriously ill. This should be given intravenously only after tests for hypersensitivity to horse serum have been conducted. Materials and instructions for such tests are included in each package of antivenin. If the patient is sensitive to

horse serum, administration of antivenin in the field should be used only in a situation of extreme emergency.

Use of adequate amounts of specific antivenin is of basic importance in management of snakebite in the hospital. Symptomatic measures needed will vary according to the species of snake involved and the severity of illness but may include blood transfusion, maintenance of electrolyte balance, antibiotic therapy, and use of corticosteroids for treatment of allergic response to antivenin. Oxygen may be required for treatment of shock and respiratory failure, and, because of the latter, mechanical respiratory assistance should be at hand. Antitetanus prophylaxis is important. Those who have not been previously immunized should be given a prophylactic dose of tetanus immune globulin intramuscularly. The usual dose is 250 units. Previously immunized persons who have not had a booster injection within six months of the snakebite should be given 0.5 ml of fluid tetanus toxoid intramuscularly.

In pit viper and viper bites, it is highly important that a bitten limb be immobilized in the position of function during early hospitalization. Active and passive exercise to prevent contracture should be commenced as soon as the patient's condition permits. The necrotizing action of some venoms may increase swelling and tensions in the deep fascia to the extent that blood flow may be impaired and further tissue death likely. In such instances careful surgical intervention to allow drainage and reduce tensions may be necessary in order to save the function of a hand or foot.

Except for administration of antivenin, treatment of coral snake bite is symptomatic. Because of the delayed onset of symptoms in even severe cases, it is imperative that coral snake antivenin (produced by Wyeth Laboratories) be given intravenously immediately if it is certain that the patient was bitten by a coral snake. As respiratory failure is a prominent feature of severe envenomation by coral snakes, plans should be made for tracheostomy and availability of mechanical respiratory assistance.

Although antivenin remains the single most important factor in treatment of snakebite, none of the products available has reached the goal for potency recommended by WHO years ago — i.e., that 1 ampule of antivenin be sufficiently potent to neutralize the maximum amount of venom which could be injected in a bite by a snake of the species whose bites it was designed to treat. Up to 150 ml or more of antivenin may be required for treatment of seriously ill patients. Because of widespread sensitivity to horse serum and resulting anaphylaxis if antivenin is given in treatment, this problem can be of primary importance. Although use of animals other than equines for antivenin production has been suggested, latest information is that all antivenins now available either from governmental or commercial sources are prepared by immunizing horses. Although physicians have varied in their view toward administration of antivenin, many believe that it should be withheld in cases of obvious minimal envenomation or when it is known that the snake species involved is not dangerously venomous. Of course the size, age, and general physical condition of the patient must be taken into consideration in reaching a decision.

Although there has been much improvement in antivenin potency and in preparation of effective polyvalent antivenins in recent years, development in this field has not kept up with advances in knowledge of the biochemistry and pharmacology of venoms. It is to be hoped that much of this new knowledge can soon be translated into more effective treatment.

Bücherl, W., Buckley, E. E., and Deulofeu, V. (eds.): Venomous Animals and Their Venoms, Vol. I. New York, Academic Press, 1968.

Bücherl, W., and Buckley, E. E. (eds.): Venomous Animals and Their Venoms, Vol. II. New York, Academic Press, 1971.

Glass, T. G., Jr.: Early debridement in pit viper bites. JAMA, 235:2513, 1976.

Greenwood, B. M., Warrell, D. A., Davidson, N. McD., and Ormerod, L. D.: Immunodiagnosis of snake bite. Br. Med. J., 4:743, 1974.

Harris, A. R. C., Hurst, P. E., and Saker, B. M.: Renal failure after snake bite. Med. J. Aust., 2:409, 1976.

Minton, S. A. (ed.): Snake Venoms and Envenomation. New York, Marcel Dekker, Inc., 1971.

Ohsaka, A., Hayashi, K., and Sawai, Y.: Animal, Plant, and Microbial Toxins. New York, Plenum Press, 1976.

Reid, H. A.: Epidemiology of sea-snake bites. J. Trop. Med. Hyg., 78:106, 1975.

Reid, H. A.: Antivenom in sea-snake bite poisoning. Lancet, 1:622, 1975.

37. VENOMOUS MARINE ANIMALS

Hugh L. Keegan

Envenomation by marine animals of several phyla has been of increasing importance in recent years because of widespread interest in scuba diving, shell collecting, and water sports in general. Although accidents have been more numerous in warmer waters, venomous species are ubiquitous to the extent that a knowledge of locally occurring animals is of importance to both the hobbyist and the physician. As descriptions adequate for recognition of the many species of medical importance are beyond the scope of this work, references for that purpose are given at the end of this discussion.

COELENTERATES (JELLYFISH, CORALS, SEA ANEMONES). Skin contact with many of the coelenterates, particularly the jellyfish, may result in severe pain, allergic reactions, and even death. Most accounts of severe reactions have come from tropical regions, but dangerous species also occur in regions with temperate climates.

Phylum Coelenterata has been divided into three classes: *Class I*, Hydrozoa. The most important of the orders of this class, from a medical viewpoint, is the order Siphonophora, which consists of free-swimming or floating colonies composed of both feeding and reproductive individuals attached to a stem or disk. The upper end of the colony may be a balloon-like float. *Physalia*, the Portuguese man-of-war, is the most dangerous of the Siphonophora. The tentacles dangling from the float may exceed 30 meters in length. *Class II*, Scyphozoa, the "true" jellyfish, which are solitary, not colonial, individuals. These are free-swimming forms which vary considerably in size and in toxicity for man. The best known genera are *Carybdea*, *Dactylometra*, and *Chiropsalmus*. Because of the intensity of their stings, these are known in some areas as "sea wasps" or "fire medusae." *Class III*, Anthozoa. This class includes the sea anemones and corals.

Except for cuts from contact with coral, injury to man from coelenterates is caused by nematocysts, small intracellular structures present on the tentacles of all coelenterates. Each nematocyst consists of a capsule containing a hollow, coiled, intraverted thread. These are discharged to the exterior by eversion. Some types may penetrate the skin of man, injecting a toxic substance. The nature of the toxins found in the nematocysts of the many species of coelenterates is largely unknown. The cause of discharge of the nematocysts seems to be a selective reaction to mechanical and perhaps chemical stimuli.

Symptoms following contact with venomous coelenterates vary considerably. Contact is often followed immediately by intense, burning pain. If the species is one with long tentacles, lines of contact often appear as purplish, swollen wheals. These may disappear in a few hours or in some cases vesiculate. Systemic effects, sometimes absent, may appear a few minutes after contact, or may be delayed for as much as an hour. These effects frequently include muscle spasm, particularly in the abdomen, back, and diaphragm. The patient often has great difficulty in breathing and may be nauseated. Profuse lacrimation and nasal and bronchial secretion are usual. Cardiac weakness, generalized muscular weakness, anxiety, swelling, particularly of the extremities, profuse perspiration, erythema, elevated temperature, vertigo, rapid pulse, mental confusion, and moderate dilation of the pupils may occur. Some authorities believe that the chief danger from jellyfish sting is that the victim might drown because of cramps and respiratory muscle spasm. In one series of six cases from North Queensland which ended fatally, none of the victims survived more than ten minutes after being stung. The signs were those of anaphylactic shock. In these and similar cases there was no wheal at the point of contact, and in some cases there was a delay of a half hour or more before appearance of systemic effects.

For the most part, treatment of coelenterate sting has been symptomatic. Tentacles which have adhered to the skin should be removed as soon as possible, preferably after the nematocysts have been inactivated by application of alcohol. If this is not available, bath towels, clothing, or even sand may be used. Intravenous calcium gluconate has been found to be helpful in relieving muscle spasms. Codeine, morphine, sodium phenobarbital, epinephrine, diphenylhydramine, and atropine have been used in therapy with varying success. Artificial respiration and use of oxygen may be necessary if respiration is depressed. Norepinephrine has been used to combat cardiac failure. An antivenin for treatment of stings by the sea wasp *Chiropsalmus fleckeri*, a dangerous jellyfish found in Australian waters, is produced at the Commonwealth Serum Laboratories, Melbourne, Australia.

MOLLUSCS. The most important of the marine molluscs to affect man are the cone shells. These are large, attractively colored, carnivorous snails which are widely distributed, although the species which are dangerous to man are most often found in the western and southwestern Pacific from Japan to Australia. Though perhaps 200 species of these have been described, only about 15 have been reported as causing envenomation in man. The painful, sometimes fatal sting is inflicted with a hollow, needle-like tooth which is rapidly extruded through the opening in the shell. The venom injected in this way ordinarily serves to kill small fishes and marine invertebrates which are food for cone shells. The snails, of course, do not attack man. Almost without exception, persons stung by cone shells have been shell collectors or have been gathering snails for bait. In other words, only persons who have actually been handling shells have been stung.

The victim is always aware that he has been stung. The sting has been described as a very small puncture mark and, as might be expected, usually on the hand. The sequence of symptoms following the sting varies. In some cases sharp, burning pain commences immediately. In others, pain is absent and the initial symptom is a feeling of numbness, which extends rapidly up the arm. Rapidly developing flaccid paralysis, difficulty in speech, and blurred vision occur in severe cases. Dysphagia and a feeling of constriction of the chest are common. Death, when it occurs, is due to respiratory paralysis.

Treatment is entirely symptomatic. Support of respiration is essential in severe cases. In nonfatal cases on record, most symptoms had disappeared within 24 hours. In fatal cases, death occurred in less than 12 hours, usually in 6 or less.

ECHINODERMS (STARFISHES, SEA URCHINS, SEA CUCUMBERS, AND SEA LILIES). These animals are radially symmetrical and possess structures known as tube feet, which serve as tentacles or as organs of locomotion. The sea urchins are globular, cushion-shaped, or discoidal relatives of the starfish. Unlike the former, they do not possess arms but move by tube feet or with the aid of long, movable spines. Both starfishes and sea urchins possess pedicellariae, sets of two or three spines arranged to function as pincers. There are several types of pedicellariae, some of which bear venom glands in each "jaw."

Of all the echinoderms, the sea urchins are of greatest medical importance because of wounds and envenomation which may result from penetration of spines or attachment of venom-containing pedicellariae to the skin. Throughout the Far East sea urchins are numerous in shallow, coastal waters, and are often found among coral reefs or ledges or in the intertidal shore zone. Spines of some species may be over 30 cm in length. All are sharp, brittle, and easily fragmented so that particles may remain in punctures caused by them. Most accidents occur when persons wade in infested waters with bare feet. In addition to the problem of envenomation, infection may occur when deep penetration by the spines has taken place. Symptoms resulting from attachment to the finger of pedicellariae of sea urchins in Japanese waters have included instant severe pain, fainting, difficulty of respiration, paralysis of lips, tongue, and eyelids, and relaxation of muscles of the limbs. Generalized muscular paralysis and respiratory distress have led to death in some cases.

Treatment is symptomatic. Precautionary measures against injury from starfishes and sea urchins should include wearing of shoes while wading in infested areas and use of forceps if specimens with needle-like spines are collected.

VENOMOUS FISHES. Painful and sometimes fatal stings are caused by contact with venom-bearing spines of many species of fishes in both temperate and tropical waters. These spines, which are grooved, and may be serrated, are usually located in the dorsal, pectoral, or pelvic fins, but may be present in other areas, including the top of the head and the cheek. Venom-secreting tissue lines the grooves of the spines, and sac-like venom glands may be located at the base of each grooved spine. Often an integumentary sheath may enclose the spines, particularly those of the dorsal fin. Pressure on the spine by the hand or foot of a person forces back the sheath and venom flows along the groove into the wound. These sharp, sturdy spines can easily penetrate a glove or soft-soled shoe, and even slight penetration can result in agonizing pain.

Although many fishes possess venom-bearing spines, the groups of greatest medical importance are the stingrays, catfishes, weeverfishes, stargazers, scorpion fishes, and toadfishes. *Stingrays* are flat, disk- or kite-shaped animals which possess a long tail armed with one or more barbed spines. These fishes habitually lie partially buried on the bottom in shallow water and are a serious menace to waders. Several species of bottom-dwelling *catfishes* possess serrated, venom-bearing spines on dorsal and pectoral fins. The family Scorpaenidae includes several genera with extremely dangerous species. Among these are the *scorpion fishes* of genera *Scorpaenopsis,* *Scorpaena,* and *Dactylopterus;* members of genus *Pterois,* often known as zebra fishes, lion fishes, or butterfly cod; and the *stonefishes* of genus *Synanceja.*

Stingray injuries occur when the animals are stepped upon or grazed by persons wading or diving. When this happens the animal lashes out with its tail, producing deep punctures or lacerations. The injury plus effects of the venom causes immediate excruciating pain, which may be localized or radiating. The area surrounding the puncture is at first blanched, later hyperemic and edematous. Shock, muscular twitching, convulsions, irregular respiration, and cardiac arrhythmia indicates severe envenomation.

Stonefishes are grotesque in appearance and often bear a close resemblance to weed-covered rocks or pieces of bottom debris. They are extremely difficult to detect, as they lie half-buried in bottom mud or sand or among rocks. Unlike most fishes, they do not swim away when approached, but usually lie motionless unless touched. Some species possess as many as 13 venom-bearing spines in the dorsal fin. As with stings by the other venomous fishes, immediate pain is a first symptom following contact. This may be followed by edema, paralysis, and loss of sensation in the injured limb. General effects may include syncope, impairment of all sensations, and coma. Dyspnea and general weakness may last for several months following a sting. Deaths from stings by *Synanceja verrucosa* have been reported.

SCORPION FISHES AND LION FISHES (ALSO KNOWN AS ZEBRA FISHES AND BUTTERFLY FISHES). Like stonefishes, many of these animals greatly resemble their surroundings, and are bottom-dwelling, lethargic species. Perhaps the most dangerous of these is *Scorpaenopsis diabolus,* a species widely distributed from Japan southward through Indonesia and Oceania. When disturbed, this and related species turn to face the intruding object, then flip over the pectoral fins to display their brilliantly colored undersurfaces. If further molested, the fishes spread their operculae and "butt" the offending object. Lion fishes also do not show a tendency to flee but will rotate the body to bring the tips of venomous spines in the dorsal fin directly in the path of an approaching object. Symptoms produced are similar to those caused by stonefish envenomation.

Immediate, agonizing pain has been described as characteristic of stings by *marine catfishes*. Later, tissue necrosis may occur and may be so severe as to result in loss of a limb. Deaths from catfish stings have been reported.

Treatment of venomous stings by marine fishes should be directed toward achievement of three objectives: (1) alleviation of pain, (2) combating effects of the venom, and (3) prevention of secondary infection. In injuries of this type, the prompt cleansing of the wound by irrigation with cold salt water, followed by soaking of the injured limb in hot water for 30 minutes to an hour is recommended. Infiltration of the wound area with analgesics followed by debridement, and further cleansing may be necessary if tips of spines have broken off in the tissue. The wound should be protected with an antiseptic and a sterile dressing. Tetanus prophylaxis is advised. Treatment for shock may be necessary. This should be directed toward maintenance of cardiovascular tone and prevention of further complications.

The only specific remedy for fish sting is an antivenin produced at the Commonwealth Serum Laboratories, Melbourne, Australia, for treatment of envenomation by the stonefish, *Synanceja trachynis*. This product may be expected to have some effect in treatment of sting by related species. In the brochure containing the antivenin it is recommended that the severe pain which follows stonefish sting can usually be relieved by infiltration of the wound with emetine hydrochloride solution (65 mg per milliliter).

Cleland, J.B., and Southcott, R. V.: Injuries to Man from Marine Invertebrates in the Australian Region. National Health and Medical Research Council, Special Report Series No. 12, Commonwealth of Australia, Canberra A.C.T., 1965.

Halstead, B. W.: Poisonous and Venomous Marine Animals of the World (3 vols.). Washington, D.C., U. S. Government Printing Office, 1965–1970.

Halstead, B. W.: Venomous fishes. In Bücherl, W., and Buckley, E. E. (eds.): Venomous Animals and Their Venoms, Vol. II. New York, Academic Press, 1971, p. 587.

McMichael, D. F.: Molluscs — classification, distribution, venom apparatus and venoms, symptomatology of stings. *In* Bücherl, W., and Buckley, E. E. (eds.): Venomous Animals and Their Venoms, Vol. III. New York, Academic Press, 1971, p. 373.

Southcott, R. V.: Coelenterates of medical importance. *In* Keegan, H. L., and Macfarlane, W. V. (eds.): Venomous and Poisonous Animals and Noxious Plants of the Pacific Region. A symposium volume from Proceedings of the 10th Pacific Science Congress. Oxford, Pergamon Press, 1963, p. 41.

PART V
IMMUNE DISEASE

38. INTRODUCTION

Henry G. Kunkel

Immunology represents one of the most rapidly expanding areas of biology, and many new techniques for the study of alterations in disease have become available recently. This is particularly true at the cellular level, and much has been learned of the lymphocyte which is clearly the key cell involved in both cellular and humoral immunity. The concept of two major types of lymphocytes, T cells (thymus derived) and B cells (bone marrow derived), is firmly established. Alterations in level and defects in these cells are now recognizable.

Immunologic alterations, both at the cellular level and with respect to immunoglobulins (Igs) and antibodies, have been found in a wide variety of different diseases. However, in many instances it has proved uniquely difficult to pinpoint the abnormality as primary in the disease etiology. It is well recognized that similar changes can occur secondarily, particularly as a result of certain viral infections. In some diseases the significance of the immunologic alterations is clear, as for example in the allergic disorders, in thyroiditis, and in certain types of immune deficiency. In other diseases, such as systemic lupus erythematosus (SLE), Graves' disease, acquired hemolytic anemia, and pemphigus, immunologic alterations are present which appear to be involved in the disease process, but their origin and relative significance remain less clear. Finally, there are diseases such as rheumatoid arthritis, ulcerative colitis, and pernicious anemia in which the evidence for an immunologic disorder remains very tentative. Interest has centered in particular on the challenging question of autoimmunity and its possible pathogenic role in many of these disorders. One difficulty which has hampered investigators stems from the gradual realization that the occurrence of autoantibodies is by no means a rare phenomenon limited to specific diseases. Many normal persons appear to possess such antibodies. Some autoantibodies appear to be without harmful effects, and the possibility exists, at least in certain instances, that they may be of benefit.

Examples of widely prevalent autoantibodies that in most situations appear to be without harmful effects are immunoconglutinin or antibody to complement, the anti–gamma globulins frequently termed rheumatoid factors, and the antinuclear antibodies of many different types. All of these have been found in the serum of normal persons as well as in those with a wide variety of microbial diseases. Evidence has been obtained, however, that under certain conditions harmful effects can be produced by certain types of antinuclear and anti–gamma globulin antibodies. Characteristics such as concentration in serum, exact specificity (particularly toward antigens encountered in the serum), and physical properties such as solubility appear to govern this question.

One immunologic mechanism of tissue injury that is coming increasingly to the fore is the direct effect of antigen-antibody complexes from the circulation. This is particularly true of renal injury. Such a process appears to be involved in a number of diseases in which renal injury is manifest such as systemic lupus erythematosus and glomerulonephritis. The antigen reacting with antibody to form complexes may come from external sources such as streptococci and administered drugs, or it may come from autologous tissue breakdown products. The injury from such complexes is not limited to the kidney, a particularly sensitive target organ, but may also involve the blood vessels as a potential mechanism of vasculitis. Platelet damage represents a well documented example; complexes of drugs such as quinidine and its antibody in sensitive individuals adhere to platelets and bring about their destruction.

Considerable interest is currently centered on the important role of suppressor T cells and their special function in the regulation of immune responses. Increased suppressor cell activity appears to be involved in certain cases of immune deficiency in a situation in which B cell differentiation into antibody secreting plasma cells is inhibited. Decreased suppressor cell activity, on the other hand, may be important in the immunologic hyper-reactivity of patients with systemic lupus erythematosus and their proclivity to develop autoantibodies.

Another immunologic mechanism of disease that has come forward recently is the blockade of physiologically significant receptors by specific antibodies. Such a mechanism is well documented in myasthenia gravis and also appears involved in certain types of insulin resistance. Such a mechanism may well be more broadly significant in disease.

TYPES OF ANTIBODIES AND THEIR PROPERTIES

Five major classes of human antibodies have been characterized: IgG, IgM, IgA, IgD, and IgE. In addition, the IgG class has been divided into four subclasses which differ markedly in biologic properties: IgG1, IgG2, IgG3, and IgG4. The concentration in serum and some of the special properties of these classes and subclasses are shown in the accompanying table. All these proteins migrate in the gamma-beta area by electrophoresis, with IgG4, IgA, IgD, and IgE showing the most rapid mobility at pH 8.6. They have been determined quantitatively primarily through the use of specific antisera in radial immune diffusion assays. The five major classes are very distinct antigenically, and specific antisera are readily obtained. The four subclasses of IgG show marked cross-reactions, and it is primarily because of this distinction that they have been termed subclasses.

It is now apparent that all Igs and antibodies consist of two major polypeptide chains, the heavy or H chain and the light or L chain. Both the H and L chains have

Biologic Properties of Human Immunoglobulins

	IgG1	IgG2	IgG3	IgG4	IgA	IgM	IgD	IgE
Concentration mg/ml*	9.4	3.2	1.0	0.6	1.9	0.5	0.03	0.0003
Placental transfer	+	+	+	+	0	0	0	0
Complement fixation†	+	±	+	0	0	+	0	0
PCA‡ reactivity	+	0	+	+	0	0	0	0
P-K§ reactivity	0	0	0	0	0	0	0	+
Lymphocyte receptors¶	±	±	0	0	+	+	+	0
Macrophage binding	+	0	+	0	0	0	0	−

*Mean values in adult whites.
†Classic complement pathway.
‡Passive cutaneous anaphylaxis.
§Prausnitz-Küstner.
¶Ig receptors for antigen on the membranes of B lymphocytes.

a variable and a constant area. The variable portions are directly involved in the antibody combining site. The constant areas of the heavy chains differ among the classes and subclasses and are responsible for the different biologic properties shown in the table. Figure 1 illustrates the basic Ig chain structure, showing the variable and constant areas as they apply to IgG1 immunoglobulins. There are two L-H chain pairs which make up the two antigen combining sites of this type of molecule. Enzymatic splitting of the molecule has proved of great utility in the study of the various properties of antibodies. Papain produces an Fab and an Fc fragment, and each of these is readily isolated. Most of the properties of the different classes and subclasses shown in the table are based on structural differences in the Fc part of the molecule.

As shown in Figure 1, the common IgG globulin is made up of a single four-chain unit. In the case of IgM or 19S Ig as it is sometimes called, a similar four-chain monomeric unit is further polymerized into a macroglobulin consisting of five such units linked by disulfide bonds. The IgA globulin is more variable and sometimes consists of a simple four-chain 7S molecule and in other instances is polymerized to various larger sizes. Less is known about the IgD type, but this also appears to be a 7S protein made of two light and two heavy chains. The proteins of the IgE class also consist of two light and two heavy chains. However, longer heavy chains are present, making the four-chain molecule somewhat larger. These classes differ from each other in carbohydrate content, which plays an important role in solubility differences. They also differ in their ability to cross the placenta, an important property with regard to maternal-infant antibody relationships. The IgM and the IgA show little or no placental passage, in marked contrast to IgG globulin, which in cord blood reaches similar levels to those in maternal serum. A very significant special property of IgA antibodies is their occurrence as the dominant antibody in all external secretions. Saliva, tears, intestinal secretions, colostrum, and other body fluids contain primarily IgA antibodies.

Recently it has been demonstrated that IgD is of special significance on the membrane of B type lymphocytes. It appears that IgD and IgM act as the primary receptors for antigen on the lymphocyte surface.

The total amino acid sequence is now available for a number of Igs and it is clear that marked differences occur in the variable areas of the heavy and light chains, particularly in special regions which have been termed the hypervariable areas. These amino acid substitutions account for the specific combining properties of individual antibodies for antigen. The genetic mechanism by which the huge diversity of antibody molecules is produced with amino acid differences in the hypervariable areas remains unknown. The germ line theory proposes that there are sufficient DNA units in the genome to code for all the different antibodies. The somatic theory, on the other hand, considers a variety of different mechanisms arising during cell development and involving somatic mutations from a very limited number of DNA units.

Antibodies with autospecificity have been found that belong in each of the main classes of Igs, with the possible exception of IgE. Most of the diverse antibodies encountered in the sera of SLE patients are of the IgG type, which goes along with the usual marked elevation in the total serum IgG globulin. A few, however, have been described that fall into the IgM and IgA class, particularly among the antinuclear antibodies. The rheumatoid factors as well as the majority of other anti-

Structure of Immunoglobulins

Figure 1. Diagrammatic illustration of the basic structure of the Ig molecule. There are two L chains and two H chains linked by disulfide bonds; the amino terminal ends of the chains are on the left and the carboxy terminal ends at the right. The undulating lines represent the variable portions of both the H and L chains. The sites of cleavage by papain and pepsin to give Fab and Fc fragments are indicated. The Greek letters refer to the kappa and lambda light chains and the heavy chains of the various Ig classes. The position of a carbohydrate side chain (CHO) is shown.

gamma globulins are primarily IgM macroglobulins. Most of the cryoglobulins are macroglobulins; this is also true of the cold agglutinins. Decreased solubility in the cold is a general characteristic of the antibodies of high molecular weight. It is known that these antibodies are also very sensitive to sulfhydryl compounds such as cysteine and penicillamine, which act on the disulfide bonds responsible for their polymeric structure. Attempts have been made to utilize this effect for therapeutic purposes, particularly for the cold agglutinin disease, but with limited success thus far. The antibodies of high molecular weight usually fix complement very effectively and as a result produce severe cellular injury when cells are involved as antigens. Many such antibodies are involved in hemolytic reactions of erythrocytes. In other instances the specific properties of macroglobulin antibodies make them more benign. The IgG–anti-IgG complexes found in rheumatoid arthritis sera are readily soluble under most conditions, permitting them to circulate at high concentrations with surprisingly few harmful effects. However, some of the IgG–anti-IgG complexes have been shown to have very harmful effects. This is particularly true in the disorder known as mixed cryoglobulin disease in which severe kidney disease is frequently found.

The skin-sensitizing antibodies or reagins that appear to be responsible for most of the harmful effects in the allergic diseases have many unique properties. The most striking of these is the persistence in the skin for periods of weeks after transfer to normal persons. The demonstration that these properties are characteristics of antibodies of the IgE class has been a significant recent development in immunology. Quantitatively this is a very minor class, representing only approximately 0.05 per cent of the total immunoglobulins of the serum. However, it has become clear that it is specifically involved in histamine release from leukocytes and other cells. The finding of several myeloma proteins of the IgE type has aided greatly in our understanding of the specific characteristics of proteins of this class. Their molecular weight is somewhat higher than IgG proteins and their sedimentation rate is approximately 8S. They are rich in carbohydrate and do not fix complement. It is of particular interest that IgE forming cells are concentrated in the mucosal system of the nose and respiratory tract as well as the regional lymph nodes, raising the possibility that locally formed IgE may be involved in respiratory allergy. Other types of antibodies to allergens are also found in the sera of sensitive patients that do not have the unique skin-sensitizing properties and rapidly diffuse away from the site of the injection. These antibodies, which have been termed blocking antibodies, appear to be typical IgG globulins, in contrast to the reagins. They also combine with antigen and may prevent a reaction with the skin-sensitizing antibody.

LYMPHOCYTES AND OTHER IMMUNOLOGICALLY SIGNIFICANT CELLS

Two major classes of lymphocytes are now well documented which differ strikingly in their biologic properties. The B cell is distinguished by the presence of readily detected immunoglobulin receptors for antigen on its surface. Stimulation by antigen as well as certain mitogens cause it to differentiate into a plasma cell which is the primary antibody-producing cell. The T cell, on the other hand, plays a number of very different roles and appears to be much more heterogeneous. At least some of the T cells have specific receptors for antigen on the membrane surface; the nature of these receptors, which are not ordinary Ig, remains one of the challenging questions of immunology today. After stimulation by antigen and certain mitogens such as phytohemagglutinin and concanavallin A, individual members of T cell populations enlarge to blast cells that do not produce antibody but produce a wide variety of factors and mediators that are significant in many immunologic processes. One type, which has been termed helper factor or allogeneic factor, has a significant effect on B cells and their differentiation into antibody-producing cells. Another type, produced by suppressor T cells, has an opposing regulatory function with resulting suppression of B cell activity. Figure 2 illustrates diagrammatically some of the current concepts of these interrelationships, especially involving T cell regulation of B cell differentiation. Another important functional T cell product is the cytotoxic T cell, which specifically attaches to and destroys target cells such as tumor cells in certain instances. These cells, along with a variety of mediators produced by different T blasts, also are involved in other cellular immune reactions such as graft rejection.

A wide variety of other mediators have been described which are released by activated lymphocytes.

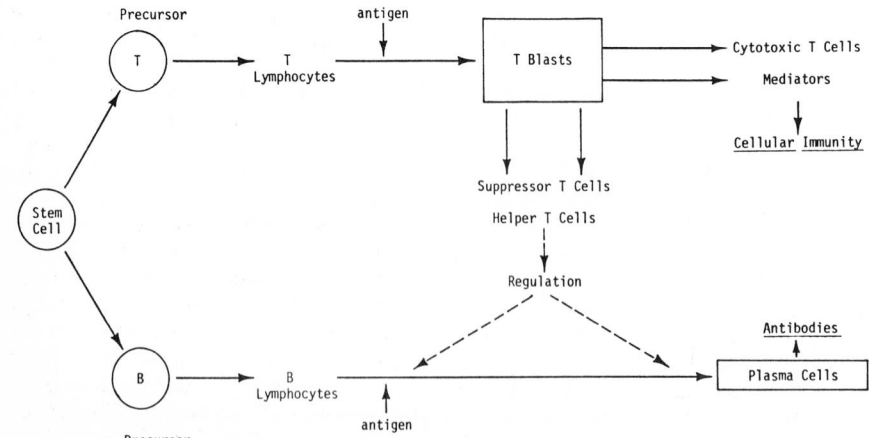

Figure 2. Diagrammatic representation of the development of immunologically active lymphoid cells of the T and B cell types from a common stem cell. Terminal differentiation of B cells to plasma cells producing antibodies and of T cells to T blasts responsible for different aspects of cellular immunity is shown. The regulating effects of T cells and their suppressor and helper functions on antibody production are also illustrated. The significant position of the macrophage in these processes is omitted.

None of these have been isolated, and it is not clear that they all represent different substances. The best known of these is "transfer factor," which is a low molecular weight dialyzable constituent that appears to transfer delayed hypersensitivity to specific antigens from a positive individual to a negative one; sensitivity to tuberculin, to diphtheria toxoid, and to coccidioidin represent three examples out of many that have been studied. Special interest has centered on "transfer factor" because of its potential value in therapy. Patients with various fungal infections, those with immune deficiency disorders, and even cancer patients have been injected with concentrated material prepared from donor lymphocytes in an attempt to produce a cellular immunity that may aid the immune response of these patients. Evidence has been obtained of therapeutic value for "transfer factor," but the final word on its usefulness is not in.

Migration inhibition factor (MIF) is another mediator released by T cells which has been widely studied. It is released in response to antigen and inhibits the migration of macrophages. This is usually measured by determining the diameter of the ring of macrophages moving out of the end of a capillary tube. It has become a widely used assay for the determination of cellular immunity to specific antigens. Other mediators include interferon, lymphotoxin, chemotactin, and skin reactive factor.

The macrophage clearly plays a key role in cellular immunologic reactions. Many aspects of this role remain poorly understood, but it is evident that a number of mediators described above affect the macrophage directly and increase its activity against bacterial or other targets. Evidence is available for the release of a variety of enzymes from macrophages after stimulation. In addition, the macrophage has been shown to play an important role in the interaction of antigen with T cells. Some workers view this as a presentation of antigen which otherwise would not activate the T cell.

Another cell type which appears to have broad significance is the K or killer cell. This cell appears to hold a high affinity for antibody and acts in conjunction with antibody to attack target cells, the so-called antibody mediated lympholysis. At present it is not known whether this is a special type of T cell or whether it represents a third type of lymphocyte. In the past it was confused with the classic cytotoxic T cell. However, it is very different and only acquires target specificity through the antibody with which it functions.

CHARACTERISTICS AND ESTIMATION OF B AND T LYMPHOCYTES

A number of different methods have been developed for differentiating B and T lymphocytes, and some of these provide quantitative results which are of use in assessing these immunologic parameters in diseased individuals. The most characteristic aspect of the B cell is the surface Ig which can be detected readily by a variety of techniques. The most widely used of these is the fluorescent antibody method in which anti-Ig antiserum that is fluorescent is used to stain the Ig on the living cell. Figure 3 illustrates the dot-like staining ob-

Figure 3. Surface Ig staining by the fluorescent antibody technique of a B type lymphocyte (lower frame). The upper frame shows two lymphocytes by phase contrast microscopy. One lymphocyte of the T type fails to show any Ig.

tained with such an antiserum on the surface of a B cell, whereas a T cell in the same field is entirely negative. This procedure reveals positive staining for Ig on approximately 10 per cent of normal peripheral blood lymphocytes. The Ig is primarily IgM and IgD and has been shown to be synthesized by the B cells. There are, however, numerous pitfalls in this method. The fluorescent antibodies may bind to other cells with Fc receptors, giving falsely high results. Antibodies to T cells may also interfere. These problems usually can be eliminated through the use of fluorescent antibodies in the $F(ab')_2$ form and through the use of short-term cultures.

Another method for determining B cells stems from the presence of a receptor for the third component of complement which is not found on T cells. Red cells that are coated with antibody and complement form rosettes around B cells, and the number of such rosettes is readily quantitated. A third procedure utilizes the B cell characteristic of reacting with the Fc portion of IgG immunoglobulins. This is a weak interaction, and stable binding occurs only when the Ig is aggregated or is in the form of an immune complex. Large aggregates of IgG are readily visualized by a variety of methods attached to B cells specifically. Other cells than B cells, however, carry the Fc receptor and to some degree the complement receptor, and falsely high values are obtained by these procedures unless these interfering cells are removed. Recently, a new antigen termed Ia has proved extremely useful for determining B cells; rabbit antisera to this component are widely available.

The T lymphocyte in the human can be detected by its selective binding of sheep red blood cells to give rosettes. This is a simple and accurate quantitative method that has come into wide use. The explanation for this useful binding procedure remains obscure. Both thymocytes and peripheral blood T cells give the rosettes. Approximately 85 per cent of blood lymphocytes are positive. Specific antisera that are T cell specific are also available and can be utilized in fluorescent antibody studies or cytotoxic assays to quantitate the T cell population. Results with the antisera usually give a lower percentage figure for blood lymphocytes than is obtained with the rosetting procedure. Specific mitogen stimulation of T cells is also used as an assay of T cell competence. Phytohemagglutinin and concanavalin A are the primary mitogens for this purpose, and the T cell response is measured by determination of the blast cells produced or through the incorporation of tritium labeled thymidine. The advantage of the mitogen procedures is that the functional competence of T cells is determined, rather than just an enumeration of T cells. The disadvantages lie in the difficulty in quantitation and the influence of other cells such as the macrophage in the response.

The *mixed lymphocyte culture* (MLC) reaction is also used as an assay of T cell function. This is usually carried out in a unidirectional system with a known stimulating lymphocyte population that is treated with mitomycin C. The latter reagent prevents these cells from responding but preserves their stimulating potential. The response is measured by the uptake of tritiated thymidine, and cells from different patients can be analyzed in terms of their response. The primary use of the MLC reaction, however, is in histocompatibility testing prior to grafting, in which compatibility is detected through an absence of any response, which is determined primarily by the MLC genes. These appear to differ from the classic HLA genes that are separate but closely linked. Because of the difficulties of the MLC test systems, the different phenotypes are only partially recognized. However, Ia antisera, obtained from pregnancy sera, are rapidly becoming available for a typing system that reflects MLC differences. One of the key developments in experimental immunology has been the delineation of immune response or *Ir* genes which are closely linked to the histocompatibility systems. The genes controlling the Ia (Ir associated) system and the MLC reactions relate closely to the Ir genes as defined in laboratory animals.

Alterations in the level and functional capacity of T and B lymphocytes have been found in a wide variety of diseases. The most striking findings are in the immune deficiency disorders (see Ch. 40.1 to 40.10), and analyses of the lymphocytes that are present are providing new insight into the basic defects. The delineation of a role of excess suppressor cells in certain individuals with immune deficiency represents one of the important developments. In Graves' disease and thyroiditis an increase in T cells and a fall in B cells have been demonstrated clearly. Alterations in Hodgkin's disease, leprosy, cancer, and connective tissue disease have been described. However, these studies are only beginning, and their significance remains to be determined. It is of special interest that the leukemic lymphocytes in the vast majority of cases of chronic lymphatic leukemia are of the B cell type. In acute lymphatic leukemia the picture is more complex. Approximately one third of the cases represent a proliferation of T cells. The remaining cases show a different and interesting new cell type that is not readily classifiable in the T or B category.

DELAYED TYPE OF HYPERSENSITIVITY

Delayed type of hypersensitivity is clearly a reaction of T cells which have been stimulated by antigen to react against targets such as infectious agents, grafts, and tumors. Antibody is not involved in this phenomenon, and disagreement exists among immunologists concerning the role of macrophages. The term "delayed type of hypersensitivity" arose from the delayed skin response of sensitive subjects to antigen; the reaction does not begin for several hours and reaches a maximum after two or three days. The term "cellular immunity" has also been used, although, as mentioned above, some types of cellular immunity also involve antibodies. Two major types of delayed hypersensitivity have been most widely studied: that induced by infection, and the other, termed contact sensitivity, resulting from exposure to a variety of substances ranging from oily resins of plants to simple chemicals employed for domestic, industrial, and medical purposes. Delayed hypersensitivity to autologous antigens has been difficult to demonstrate in humans, although it can be produced in laboratory animals by immunization with autologous antigens.

Delayed-type hypersensitivity is more strikingly evident in certain specific infections such as tuberculosis, brucellosis, lymphogranuloma venereum, mumps, vaccinia, and some fungal infections. Skin tests that depend on this type of cellular immunity have been utilized in these diseases. Tuberculin reactions have been extensively studied in humans and laboratory animals as a model for the delayed type of hypersensitivity. The skin reactivity to tuberculin can be transferred to normal recipients by means of cells from lymphoid tissue, peritoneal exudate, and peripheral blood. In laboratory animals viable cells are required, but in humans the supernatant fluid of disrupted leukocytes can transfer the reactivity. "Transfer factor," mentioned above in the discussion of mediators, represents the active principle involved.

GRAFT VERSUS HOST REACTION. Another probable manifestation of delayed-type hypersensitivity, or at least cellular immunity, is the graft versus host reaction. This has sometimes been termed "homologous disease." Initially it was largely a disorder of laboratory animals that are able to accept foreign bone marrow or lymphoid cells because they have been irradiated or otherwise treated so that these cells are not rejected. More recently it has been encountered frequently in humans who have received certain grafts, particularly bone marrow. The foreign cells react against various antigens in the host animal, resulting in a variety of clinical manifestations. The skin lesions are most characteristic: edema, erythema, and ulceration, followed by thickening, scaling, and loss of hair. Lesions of the joints and of the heart are also observed and these have aroused considerable interest because of certain similarities to those observed in some of the connective tissue disorders. Hemolytic anemia with a positive Coombs reaction has also been described. The possibility has been raised that in certain human diseases immunologically active cells react against the host in a fashion similar to that of the transferred cells in the laboratory animal experiments. The origin of such cells has been ascribed to some type of failure of tolerance mechanisms or to an alteration of host cells through somatic mutation.

SENSITIVITY TO FOREIGN ANTIGENS

Direct sensitivity to foreign antigens, the most common type of potentially injurious immunologic reaction in man, is usually a result of antigenic stimulation by foreign protein or polysaccharide antigens. These may gain entrance to the body through parenteral, oral, respiratory, or other routes. The classic example is serum sickness, usually resulting from the administration of horse or rabbit immune serum. An Arthus reaction is initiated through the direct union of antigen and antibody in the tissue spaces. Precipitates in and around small blood vessels cause secondary damage to cells, or, when antigen is in excess, soluble complexes are formed that may deposit in certain sensitive organs in the blood vessel walls and cause local inflammatory reactions.

In most of the human allergies such as hay fever and food allergy the exact mode of sensitization to external antigens is not directly apparent. Numerous factors such as heredity, intestinal absorption, respiratory secretion, and even emotional state appear involved. In such sensitive or atopic individuals the reaction to foreign antigens is more commonly of the anaphylactic type. Here the binding of antibody to tissue cells appears to play an important role. Local anaphylaxis results from the association or passive absorption of antibodies to local sites that come in contact with antigen. Not all antibodies have this property, and the IgE class is primarily involved. The antigen in turn reacts with the antibody and alters these cells, which then cause the release of histamine and other pharmacologic mediators into the tissue fluid and circulation. In the skin this gives rise to the wheal and erythema at the site of antigen introduction, as in ordinary prick and scratch diagnostic tests. Hay fever and allergic asthma are local manifestations of such reactions. Extensive urticaria may also represent an expression of local cutaneous anaphylaxis.

The antigens involved in these local allergic reactions are a very diversified group. A number have been isolated and partially characterized. The major allergen of *ragweed pollen* has been found to be a protein of approximately 37,000 molecular weight and represents a very small portion of the extractable solids of the pollen. The biologic activity of the isolated material is very high; as little as 10^{-12} grams causes a positive intracutaneous wheal and erythema reaction in sensitive individuals. A highly active protein has also been isolated from the *timothy hay pollen*. Low molecular weight nonprotein allergens have also been isolated. The best example of these is chlorogenic acid, which is the active material from castor beans. Just how this is effective is not clear, but the general hypothesis is that it acts as a hapten and combines with body proteins to become a complete antigen. Similar sensitivity to a wide variety of chemicals, particularly those belonging to the group of nitrogenous aromatic substances, has been observed.

The *drug reactions* represent an analogous type of sensitivity that may become manifest in an extremely variable manner. There is a growing awareness of the possibility that sensitivity to unknown foreign materials may play a role in a variety of diseases that at present remain obscure or have been classified as possibly autoimmune in nature. Particular insight into a variety of mechanisms of immunologic cell injury has been gained from the study of the sensitization caused by

drugs, particularly quinidine. In some persons thrombocytopenic purpura is the result of such sensitivity; in others it is a hemolytic anemia. It now appears that this effect is primarily the fortuitous result of the physical characteristics of the antibody produced. If the antibody is of low molecular weight, it forms a type of antigen-antibody complex with quinidine that has a particular predilection for platelets; if it is of high molecular weight, complexes are formed on union with the drug that affect primarily the erythrocytes. Complement is also intimately involved in the different effects. This system illustrates the vagaries involved in the selective action against individual target organs and may be of importance in consideration of disorders of unknown origin such as idiopathic thrombocytopenic purpura and "autoimmune" hemolytic anemia. The possibility of involvement of unknown foreign antigens, particularly haptens, is not excluded.

It has become increasingly evident that many antigens gain entrance into the body via the intestinal tract through the consumption of *food*. This has been demonstrated best for bovine milk proteins, and antibodies to a wide variety of these proteins have been found in the serum of many children and some adults. Clear precipitin reactions between bovine protein fractions and these human sera are readily observed. Usually, apparently, no ill effects result from these antibodies despite the fact that some bovine products that remain antigenic continue to gain entrance into the circulation. However, this is only one example of an antibody response to food products; many others must exist that may have important implications in, for example, certain of the intestinal disorders of unknown origin such as ulcerative colitis.

A somewhat different but very important type of reaction to foreign antigens is that produced by maternal-infant incompatibility in which the foreign antigen is introduced from the fetus. *Hemolytic disease of the newborn* is the outstanding example in which the mother produces antibodies that cause destruction of the erythrocytes in the fetus or newborn. The incompatibility leading to such effects may involve Rh antigens or those of the ABO system. Analogous phenomena have been described for leukocytes and platelets. Cytolytic or cytotoxic reactions occur in which complement is usually but not always necessary to effect the cellular damage. Many other antigens are probably involved in similar maternal-infant incompatibility, but the extent to which they lead to disease is not clear at present. One outstanding example that has become manifest recently is that for genetic types of gamma globulin. A high percentage of infants who lack the genetic gamma globulin character of the mother develop antibodies. These usually appear at approximately the sixth month after delivery and may remain throughout the life of the individual. Antibodies to IgA globulins appear to have special significance with regard to transfusion reactions. Most of these appear in individuals who lack all IgA in their serum and probably arise either through maternal immunization or through the administration of blood products.

Another indirect type of reaction to foreign antigens involves antigenic cross-reactions between such antigens and autologous tissues. In this situation an immune response is stimulated by a foreign antigen such as a bacterium, but since a constituent of the organism is antigenically similar to a constituent of the host the immune reaction damages the host tissue. Such cross-reactions have been identified, but the exact role of this mechanism in disease remains to be determined; the possibility exists that presumed autoimmune reactions may be initiated in certain instances by such foreign stimuli. Evidence has been obtained that material from the cell wall of hemolytic streptococci is related antigenically to human cardiac myofibers and the smooth muscle of blood vessel walls. This finding has led to the hypothesis that the cardiac damage of rheumatic fever thus results secondarily from the immune response to the streptococcal infection that preceded it.

SENSITIVITY TO AUTOLOGOUS ANTIGENS

It has become amply clear that many persons develop immunologic reactivity against autologous tissue antigens, but the mechanism by which this sensitivity arises remains obscure. In some instances it may be through the reaction to an unknown foreign organism that contains antigens, particularly polysaccharides, that cross-react with similar polysaccharides in the body tissues. In other instances it may arise through tissue breakdown with release of antigens into the circulation that are ordinarily buried and not subject to the usual tolerance mechanisms. Recent studies in laboratory animals indicate that autologous proteins such as gamma globulin readily become antigenic through slight alteration of the molecule. Antibodies are produced to new determinants not ordinarily exposed but, in addition, as immunization continues, additional antibodies may be produced that involve the native configuration of the protein and will react directly.

One of the best examples of autosensitization in human disease is that found in thyroiditis. There are many features that remain poorly understood, but the evidence is overwhelming that the various degrees of lymphadenoid change in the thyroid gland, particularly in Hashimoto's disease, involve some type of immune reaction against antigens in the thyroid gland. The fact that similar lesions can be produced in laboratory animals by immunization with autologous thyroid antigens lends strong support to such a view. Even in laboratory animals it remains unclear whether some type of cytotoxic antibody or a cellular autoimmunity plays the dominant role in the tissue injury.

In Goodpasture's disease antibodies reactive with autologous antigens of basement membranes have been demonstrated. These react primarily with renal and pulmonary tissues and have been eluted from these diseased organs obtained at autopsy. Clear evidence of a pathogenic role of the basement membrane antibodies in the renal disease of these patients has been obtained. The antibodies eluted from the human kidneys produce glomerulonephritis in monkeys after infusion. The evidence for a role in the pulmonary disease of these patients is more indirect. It has been demonstrated that antibodies eluted from the lung fix to renal glomerular basement membrane, and antibodies eluted from the kidney fix to pulmonary membranes. The origin of these antibodies remains obscure. Similar antibodies also appear to be involved in a few cases of idiopathic glomerulonephritis.

In many blood diseases antibodies occur in the serum that react with autologous cells and in some instances clearly produce disease. The cold agglutinin

syndrome is perhaps the clearest from the standpoint of the effect of the abnormal antibody in producing erythrocyte destruction. Anemia, jaundice, and hemoglobinuria can all be traced directly to the action of the cold agglutinin. An "idiopathic" type of the syndrome and one associated with histiocytic lymphoma and lymphocytic lymphoma frequently show IgM bands that represent the cold agglutinin. These relate closely to the bands in Waldenström's macroglobulinemia and probably do not arise as a result of antigenic stimulation. Another type of disease that is usually of shorter duration follows viral or mycoplasmal pneumonia. Paroxysmal cold hemoglobinuria of the Donath-Landsteiner type is closely related and usually is associated with prenatal syphilis, although many nonsyphilitic cases have been reported. The much more common idiopathic, acquired hemolytic anemia of the warm antibody type presents a more obscure picture. Here the relationship of the erythrocyte damage to a variety of red blood cell antibodies is much more tentative. Only in a minority of cases can the antibodies be shown to have a definite specificity. In these instances it is directed against an Rh antigen, usually anti-e. Few clues are available concerning the origin of these gamma globulins that react with autologous erythrocytes.

Idiopathic thrombocytopenic purpura is another disease in which circulating antibodies react with autologous cells — in this case platelets — and cause disease through the resulting cellular injury. These antibodies have proved surprisingly difficult to detect by conventional immunologic methods, but it is now clear that they are present. The role of leukocyte autoagglutinins as a cause of leukopenia has proved even more difficult to assess. Many of the antibodies reported by early workers have been shown to result from transfusions given to these patients, with the production of isoantibodies. However, recent work indicates that autoagglutinins do occur and are responsible for some cases of leukopenia.

Systemic lupus erythematosus (SLE) is probably associated with a greater variety of antibodies with autospecificity than any other condition. The best known of these are the antinuclear antibodies, certain of which are responsible for the LE cell phenomenon. Special interest has centered on the DNA antibodies because of evidence for an association with disease activity. Antibodies to native double-stranded DNA as well as antibodies specific for the single-stranded form are found in the sera of these patients. Recently antibodies to double-stranded RNA have been detected. It has become evident that antibodies to a wide spectrum of polynucleotides are uniquely present in this disease. Numerous additional antibodies to protein and carbohydrate antigens extracted from the cytoplasm as well as the nucleus of human cells have been described. Some of these appear to be responsible for various secondary manifestations of the disease as, for example, hemolytic anemia. This is associated with a positive Coombs test, suggesting the occurrence of antibodies to autologous erythrocytes. Idiopathic thrombocytopenic purpura, probably involving antiplatelet antibodies, also occurs in these patients. Abnormalities involving blood coagulation have been of special interest to investigators; antibodies to specific clotting factors appear to be involved. The origin of these many antibodies as well as others not discussed remains obscure. Some of them appear to represent a marked elevation of antibodies found at low levels in normal persons, which is compatible with the concept that in SLE a general hyperreactivity of the immune system exists. The new concept that this situation might result from a deficiency of suppressor T cells has received some experimental support. The high prevalence in females and the familial trend of the disease have not as yet been fitted into the immunologic concepts. Recent work with various strains of mice, particularly the New Zealand NZB strain, has shown that manifestations of a disease with many features resembling SLE occur in a high proportion of the animals. Most striking are the renal disease and the hemolytic anemia. This experimental model shows a marked similarity to the human disease, and the unique antibodies to double-stranded DNA and RNA are present. Studies in these mice have suggested a significant role for secondary viral infections in potentiating various disease manifestations. Whether this also applies to the human disease remains to be proved.

The possibility has been considered that a large number of other diseases in which the cause is unknown may have as their origin some type of autoimmune mechanism. This is particularly true of *rheumatoid arthritis*, primarily because it is associated with uniquely high incidence and levels of an unusual group of antibodies called rheumatoid factors. These have been clearly demonstrated to be antibodies to gamma globulin and are capable of reacting with autologous gamma globulin. No evidence is available to suggest that the rheumatoid factors play a direct role in the arthritis; however, many workers think they may be indicative of an as yet undefined immunologic reaction. The fact that they are produced at least in part in the synovial tissue of the joints from local accumulation of plasma cells adds some weight to this concept. On the other hand, it has also become clear that the rheumatoid factors could develop as a response to some type of foreign organism. Antibodies to the organism after reaction with the particulate antigen or fragment thereof would form secondary anti–gamma globulins to these antigen-antibody complexes. This possibility has been strengthened by the experimental production of anti–gamma globulins in rabbits after injection of coliform organisms, as well as their appearance in human sera after various types of infection. In bacterial endocarditis, for example, the rheumatoid factors disappear after elimination of the organism with antimicrobial therapy. Similar attempts with such therapy in rheumatoid arthritis patients is without effect on the rheumatoid factors. The accumulated evidence indicates that there must be some profound immunologic stimulus present in the rheumatoid arthritis patient to sustain the rheumatoid factors at the extreme levels often observed and for the prolonged periods in which they are present. The nature of this stimulus remains unknown.

Another disorder showing profound immunologic abnormalities associated with arthritis similar to that in rheumatoid arthritis is *Sjögren's syndrome*. It also has been considered a possible connecting link between rheumatoid arthritis and SLE. Extreme elevation of gamma globulin similar to that found in SLE patients is observed along with many similar antinuclear and anticytoplasmic antibodies. In addition, the vast majority of these patients have rheumatoid factors, often at extreme levels. Serologically they show the findings of both rheumatoid arthritis and SLE. The lesions observed in the lacrimal, salivary, and other glands of patients with Sjögren's syndrome are highly suggestive of a local immunologic reaction. They closely resemble those observed in the thyroid gland in chronic thyroiditis, in which an immunologic alteration has been more evident.

The immunologic aspects of *pernicious anemia* are of considerable interest. Antibodies to intrinsic factor have been demonstrated in a large number of cases, and antibodies to the parietal cells of the gastric mucosa are frequently found. These have been revealed by a variety of classic immunologic procedures. In addition, the intrinsic factor antibody inhibits labeled B_{12} absorption in tests in vivo. Many of the antibodies appear to be autoantibodies and are found in untreated cases; others appear to represent antibodies to hog intrinsic factor as a result of therapy. A direct role in the pathogenesis of the disease has not been established, but they at least are important in certain therapeutic considerations.

It has been known for a number of years that the serum of patients with *myasthenia gravis* contains a number of unusual antibodies directed to muscle constituents. The idea that this disease might be autoimmune in nature was widely held. Recently, however, definitive evidence on this score has come forward. The surprising finding was made that injection of the acetylcholine receptor of the electric eel into rats as well as other species produced specific antibodies to the receptor and a myasthenia syndrome. This also has now been done with acetylcholine receptor from mammals and the disease transferred by antibody. In addition a large amount of evidence has accumulated indicating that patients with myasthenia gravis have similar antibodies that relate to disease exacerbations. It thus appears that a specific antibody that reacts with the receptor and blocks its function causes the disease manifestations.

Antibodies with autospecificity of various types have been found in a variety of other diseases. In ulcerative colitis, antibodies to colon tissue and cellular immunity to colon cells have been described. Patients with liver disease show a wide variety of antibodies to autologous cell constituents. Antibodies reactive with mitochondria are of special interest because of their special occurrence in primary biliary cirrhosis. They are of diagnostic value, but a pathogenic role remains to be demonstrated. Pancreas antibodies have been described in patients with pancreatitis, and adrenal antibodies in patients with Addison's disease. In all these instances the major possibility that these represent antibodies secondary to tissue breakdown in the disease has not been excluded. As stressed earlier, autoantibodies are far more common than had previously been thought, and any assessment of an injurious role in a specific disease is extremely difficult.

IMMUNE COMPLEX DISEASE

When artificially made antigen-antibody complexes are injected into laboratory animals, they are deposited in a number of organs with resultant tissue injury. By far the most sensitive organ is the kidney, and acute and chronic renal disease has been produced in a number of species by this procedure. The complexes are trapped in the glomeruli and form lumpy deposits along the glomerular basement membrane. These have distinct histologic characteristics by electron microscopy and by fluorescent antibody staining techniques. In human glomerulonephritis similar deposits are frequently observed when these same procedures are utilized. In systemic lupus erythematosus such deposits in the glomeruli are particularly striking, and a large accumulation of additional evidence for antigen-antibody complex mediated renal injury is available.

Extensive studies in a number of different laboratories have demonstrated that DNA–anti-DNA complexes represent one type involved in SLE. Antibodies to DNA aroused considerable interest when they were first described in SLE approximately 17 years ago. However, they were relegated to the position of scientific curiosities, and it has only been recently that their harmful potential has been realized. Antibodies to double-stranded DNA have special significance because double-stranded DNA antigens can appear in the circulation as a result of tissue breakdown; antigen-antibody complexes are formed with fixation of complement and deposition in the most vulnerable organ, the kidney. Elution of antibody from isolated glomeruli of diseased kidneys has proved to be a very effective technique for the detection of antibodies deposited in the kidney. DNA antibody has been found in such eluates at specific concentrations as high as 1000 times those in the serum. DNA antigen has also been demonstrated in the granular deposits observed in the glomeruli. Other, more indirect evidence such as the close clinical relationship among the appearance of DNA antibodies, serum complement depression, and exacerbations of disease has also aided in establishing the significance of the DNA system. Other immune complex systems also have been demonstrated in certain of these patients, including IgG–anti-IgG, SDNA–anti-SDNA, and ribonucleoprotein–anti-ribonucleoprotein. Their exact role, as well as that of other undetermined complexes relative to the native DNA system, remains to be established. SLE, has clearly become the prototype of immune complex renal disease.

Another type of renal disease in which evidence for immune complexes is rapidly accumulating is that associated with various types of drugs. Some of these may present a picture very analogous to that of serum sickness; in others, chronic drug administration may lead to a slowly progressive glomerulonephritis. The latter situation is well illustrated in the case of penicillamine. Numerous instances of nephritis have been reported after long-term administration of this material for the treatment of cystinuria, Wilson's disease, or rheumatoid arthritis. Granular deposits of gamma globulin and complement, along the glomerular basement membrane are readily visualized in fluorescent antibody studies which closely resemble those produced in experimental animals by injection of complexes.

The presence of granular and ''lumpy'' deposits of gamma globulin and complement detected by fluorescent antibody techniques may be well visualized in renal biopsy specimens and have been found in a variety of different conditions such as malaria, bacterial endocarditis, and thyroiditis. Cases of chronic glomerulonephritis of unknown cause frequently show such a pattern. However, supporting evidence for specific antigen-antibody complexes is as yet unavailable for most of these. In poststreptococcal nephritis similar characteristics of complex-induced nephritis are present, and suggestive evidence for streptococcal antigens in the deposits has been obtained.

Eluates obtained from glomeruli isolated at autopsy from kidneys of patients who had subacute and chronic glomerulonephritis have in a number of instances shown high concentrations of gamma globulin. This appears to represent specific antibody, but its nature remains a mystery. The search is on in a number of laboratories for specific antigens that might react with such gamma globulin. Particular attention is being paid to various human viruses, because recent work in laboratory animals has demonstrated complexes of virus and antibody in the kidneys of mice. The task is a difficult one, however, and human tissue antigens, bacterial antigens, and even unknown drugs may be equally reasonable candidates. The possibility also seems likely that multiple antigen-antibody systems are involved in the different cases of idiopathic glomerulonephritis.

Another type of antigen-antibody complex that appears to be involved in some types of renal disease is that composed of IgG globulin and anti-IgG globulin. Such complexes are widely distributed in human sera and reach unusual levels in rheumatoid arthritis. Usually these are quite soluble, but in some patients they precipitate out in the cold as mixed cryoglobulins. Patients with such mixed cryoglobulins show a rather ill-defined clinical syndrome, but renal lesions are common. The components of such complexes along with complement have been identified in the glomeruli of these patients.

Evidence has been obtained that injury to circulating cells, particularly platelets, may be mediated by antigen-antibody complexes. A number of drug-induced thrombocytopenias fall into this category. Particular interest is currently centered on similar mechanisms in the joint inflammation of SLE and rheumatoid arthritis. Gamma globulin complexes are well known in the latter, and high concentrations have been observed in joint fluid, in which they appear to be involved in local complement depletion. Much work remains before a direct cause-and-effect relationship can be established. Lack of an adequate experimental model similar to those available for immunologic renal injury has hampered progress in this field. The recent introduction of a variety of sensitive methods for the detection of immune complexes in serum should facilitate progress in this area. One result that already is clearly of interest is the frequent detection of immune complexes in cancer patients, offering new approaches for the difficult area of human tumor immunology.

Benacerraf, B. (ed.): Immunogenetics and Immunodeficiency. London, MTP, 1975.

Dixon, F. J., and Kunkel, H. G. (eds.): Advances in Immunology, Vols. 23 and 24. New York, Academic Press, 1976.

Fudenberg, H. H., Stites, D. P., Caldwell, J. L., and Wells, J. V. (eds.): Basic and Clinical Immunology. California, Lange Medical Publications, 1976.

Möller, G. (ed.): Autoimmunity and Self-Nonself Discrimination. Transplantat. Rev. 31:1, 1976.

39. COMPLEMENT

Jeffrey A. Gelfand

GENERAL CONSIDERATIONS

The complement system is composed of a series of circulating inactive precursor proteins which, upon activation, mediate and amplify inflammatory and host defense reactions. Observations in the late 1800's led to the description by Pfeiffer and Bordet of a serum factor that would lyse cholera vibrios in combination with a specific heat-stable immune factor (antibody). This lytic factor was inactivated by heating to 56°C, and lytic activity was restored by the addition of nonimmune, fresh serum. Ehrlich and Morganroth hypothesized that antibody was necessary for the binding of the lytic factor, which they called *complement*. It is now known that this "factor," complement, is in reality a cascade of sequentially activated proteins following two major pathways of activation which merge to form a final common pathway that produces the majority of biologic effects. There have now been identified at least 15 major component proteins, as well as 5 inhibitor proteins which modulate complement reactions. Furthermore, one of these sequences, the alternative pathway, appears to function in the absence of specific antibody. This pathway contains its own primitive recognition system, being directly activated by such foreign, nonmammalian structures as repetitive polysaccharides and lipopolysaccharides. It appears to function as an "early warning system," being triggered to a variable degree by bacteria and fungi. Earlier work focused on the ability of complement to lyse antibody-sensitized erythrocytes. It is now apparent that cell lysis is not the only biologic function of complement. Opsonization, bloodstream clearance, the release of neutrophils from the bone marrow, chemotaxis of leukocytes, virus neutralization, antigen processing, histamine release, smooth muscle contraction, increased vascular permeability, and blood clotting may all be produced or enhanced by complement activation. These functions can serve to protect the host, or to produce host tissue damage. Human complement has even been identified as a necessary factor for the successful penetration and parasitization of human erythrocytes by a pathogenic protozoan, *Babesia rhodhaini*, which causes babesiosis (see Ch. 199). Finally, complement-mediated lysis of coronaviruses, virus-transformed cells, and other tumor cells may be important in immune surveillance against malignancy.

COMPLEMENT ACTIVATION. Complement activation is characterized by the conversion, in sequential fashion, of circulating precursor proteins into active ones. Some components undergo conformational changes, whereas others undergo limited proteolytic cleavage. Such changes in turn either render the component enzymatically active or complex it to a structure. A smaller fragment may be split off in the process, usually with phlogistic properties.

The classic complement pathway was the first elucidated. The components were numbered, in order of discovery, C1 to C9. Unfortunately, this did not turn out to completely correspond to the reaction sequence, hence some confusion. Components of the more recently described alternative pathway or properdin pathway are now, by convention, given capital letters (factor B

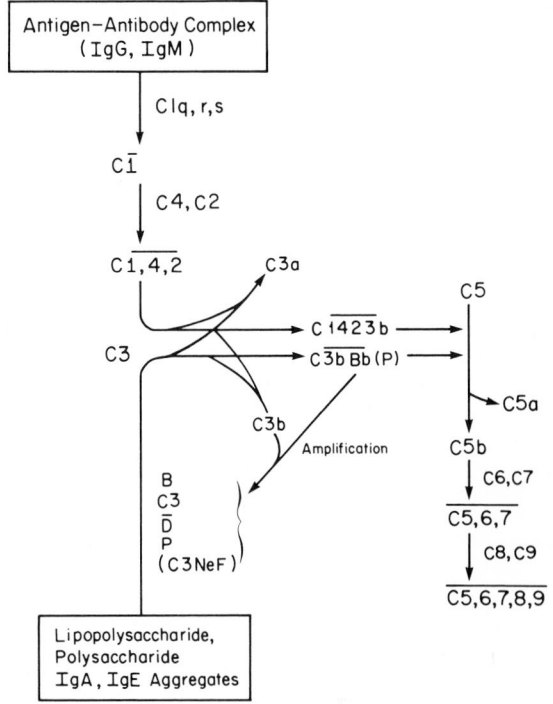

The pathways of complement activation.

or B, properdin or P). Activation of a component is indicated by a bar ($\bar{B}$ or $\overline{C1}$). Cleavage products are usually given the letter "a" for smaller, fluid phase products, whereas larger, complex-bound products are designated "b" (e.g., C5a, C5b, Bb). Further cleavage products may be termed "d," "e," and so on. An exception is C2, in which the complex-bound larger fragment is termed C2a. The pathways of activation are shown in the accompanying figure.

THE CLASSIC PATHWAY. Activation of the classic pathway occurs in the presence of antigen antibody complexes. IgG1, IgG2, IgG3, and IgM antibodies activate the classic pathway; IgA, IgD, and IgE do not.

**Biologic Functions of Complement
Components and Cleavage Products***

C1	Aggregates with antigen antibody complexes; combines directly with some viruses
C4b	Virus neutralization; binds to receptors on cells
C2 fragment	Kinin-like activity
C3b	Opsonic fragment; receptors for this fragment identified in neutrophils, monocytes, B lymphocytes, eosinophils, erythrocytes, renal glomeruli; cooperates in antigen processing, lymphocyte transformation
C3 fragment	Release of neutrophils from bone marrow
C3a	Anaphylatoxin (histamine release from mast cells, smooth muscle contraction, increased capillary permeability); chemotactic factor†
C5a	Anaphylatoxin (histamine release from mast cells, smooth muscle contraction, capillary permeability); chemotactic factor
C5b67	Chemotactic factor; may attach to unsensitized cells
C8	Incomplete membrane lesion, "slow leak"
C9	Complete membrane lesion, "fast leak"

*Adapted from Frank, M. M., and Atkinson, J. P.: Complement in clinical medicine. Disease-a-Month, January 1975.

†The role of C3a as a chemotactic factor is not certain.

Usually two IgG molecules fixed to antigen and in close proximity are required for C1 activation, whereas the pentameric IgM molecule does not require such a "doublet." This results in much more efficient complement activation by IgM. If one considers membrane-associated antigens on an erythrocyte, it would obviously take both spatially close antigenic sites and enough antibody to array two IgG molecules together in order to produce complement fixation with IgG.

Recent evidence suggests that C-reactive protein (CRP) can function analogously to immunoglobulin to activate the classic pathway. CRP is an acute phase serum reactant present in trace amounts in normal serum that can bind to the C-polysaccharide of the pneumococcus or other charged surfaces, and then bind and activate C1.

C1 circulates as a trimolecular complex of C1q, C1r, and C1s whose association is calcium dependent. C1q attaches to the Fc region of the antigen-bound antibody molecule, and undergoes a conformational change. This activates sequentially C1r and C1s. Activated C1 (C1̄) has enzymatic activity (as an esterase), and proteolytically cleaves its substrates, C4 and C2, thereby creating a new cell-membrane associated complex C1̄, 4, 2. The C42 moiety of this complex has proteolytic activity, and is termed the C3 convertase. C3 convertase splits C3 into C3a, with anaphylatoxin and possible chemotactic properties, and C3b which may be cell bound or released into the fluid phase. The bound C3b associated with the C3 convertase now becomes an enzyme that cleaves C5, termed C5 convertase. C5 is cleaved into C5b, which attaches to the cell membrane and begins the "membrane attack" sequence. C5a is released into the surrounding medium, where it effects potent chemotactic and anaphylatoxin activity. C5b binds C6 and C7, forming C5̄b67, which can dissociate from the cell membrane. It is a chemotactic factor itself, and can attach to unsensitized cells. Cell bound C5̄b67 will bind C8 and C9. The C5-9 complex produces holes in the cell membrane, presumably by disrupting the lipid bilayer. Exactly how this lesion is produced is not yet completely agreed upon, but it appears that C5̄-8 opens a small channel only intermittently, whereas C5̄-9 permanently opens a larger channel in the cell membrane, ultimately producing osmotic lysis of the target cell.

THE ALTERNATIVE PATHWAY. In 1954, a series of observations by Pillemer, Lepow, and associates led to the formulation of the existence of an antibody-independent system of complement activation. This was termed the properdin system, from the Latin *perdere* (to destroy). It represented a novel concept in theories of nonspecific host resistance to infection, as well as a radical departure from prevailing dogma about the requirement for specific antibody to activate complement. Although some of the details of what is now termed the alternative pathway are still unsettled, it is clear that the basic hypothesis of Pillemer is correct. Polysaccharides and lipopolysaccharides of bacteria and fungi, aggregated IgA, IgE, IgG, and even radiographic contrast media and renal dialyzer cellophane have been demonstrated to activate complement by this pathway. In the presence of these and possibly other initiating factor(s), factor D̄, factor B, and C3b can form an alternative pathway C3 convertase, C3̄bBb, which is stabilized by properdin (P). C3b produced by this convertase or the C42 convertase can continue to act as an

autocatalyst producing more C3 convertase with subsequent C3-C9 activation and its biologic effects. This is termed the "amplification loop." An IgG autoantibody with anti-C3bBb specificity, termed C3 nephritic factor (C3NeF), has been found in some patients with membranoproliferative glomerulonephritis and in patients with partial lipodystrophy. This factor stabilizes C3̄bB̄b in a manner analogous to P, thereby promoting complement consumption. It does not appear to be present in normal sera.

The interrelatedness of the two pathways can be appreciated when one considers that (1) C3b generated in the classic pathway can be "recruited" to enter the alternative pathway amplification loop; (2) C1 activation in animals congenitally deficient in C4 (and hence classic pathway activity) activates the alternative pathway; (3) antibody appears to increase the efficiency of alternative pathway activation; and (4) although the classic pathway is generally considered antibody dependent, recent reports indicate that viral nucleic acids can directly activate C1 and subsequent classic pathway components, in the absence of antibody. The activation of C1 by CRP bound to the C-polysaccharide of pneumococci is an additional example of antibody independent classic pathway activation.

MODULATION AND CONTROL OF COMPLEMENT ACTIVATION. Complement activation is regulated physiologically by the decay of unstable intermediates (i.e, C3̄bB̄b), the formation of unstable binding sites on the molecule (the binding of C3b to the cell surface), and the function of inhibitor proteins. There are currently at least five. C1 inhibitor (C1INH) inhibits the activated C1, an esterolytic enzyme. Deficiency in the amount of function of this inhibitor can be inherited or acquired, the former producing hereditary angioedema, the latter a similar acquired syndrome.

There is an inhibitor of C3b and the alternative pathway, C3b inactivator (C3bINA). This protein proteolytically degrades C3b into biologically less active subcomponents. It also inhibits the activity of C4b. Deficiency of C3bINA results in unchecked alternative pathway activation via the amplification loop, with resultant C3 consumption and the biologic consequences of C3 depletion. There is an additional inhibitory protein directed against C3b, the C3b inactivator accelerator (A-C3bINA, or β-1H globulin, for its electrophoretic mobility). This protein binds to C3b of the alternative pathway convertase, displacing properdin factor B. It does not affect immune adherence.

A C6 inactivator (C6 INA) has been demonstrated. Its physiologic significance is unknown. Finally, the anaphylatoxins C3a and C5a are inactivated by a carboxypeptidase, anaphylatoxin inhibitor (AI).

BIOLOGIC FUNCTION OF COMPLEMENT. Complement may be critical in facilitating or mediating host defense and inflammatory reactions. Complement activation by either the classic or alternative pathways results in the formation of C3a and C5a, which have potent anaphylatoxin and chemotactic factor activity (the latter activity of C3a is controversial). Chemotactic factor directs the migration of leukocytes into the site of infection or inflammation. The anaphylatoxin activity increases local capillary permeability, permitting egress of yet more antibody and complement into the site. The next contribution of complement is to phagocytosis. Complement was identified in the 1930's as an opsonin, a serum factor facilitating phagocytosis. Initial descriptions noted the requirement for antibody, but the properdin system of Pillemer suggested an antibody-independent opsonic system.

The dramatic discovery in the late 1960's of the existence of receptors on leukocytes for immunoglobulin and complement has enabled a more integrated view of humoral, phagocytic, and cell-mediated immune mechanisms. *Immune adherence*, the adherence of complement-sensitized particles to receptors on primate erythrocytes, had been described earlier, but its biologic function was unknown. It is now known that receptors for C3b, the major opsonic fragment, exist on neutrophils, monocytes and macrophages, eosinophils, B lymphocytes, and erythrocytes. Receptors for other complement fragments have been described; the significance of these is as yet unknown. It now appears that receptors provide a specific "latching" mechanism that enables the cell to contact and hold on to a specific opsonic particle. These receptors could help clear the bloodstream of complement (or immunoglobulin) sensitized microbes, immune complexes, or even host erythrocytes (as in autoimmune hemolytic anemia). Phagocytosis is facilitated, and antigen processing by macrophages is thus enhanced. An additional provocative discovery was provided by the demonstration of receptors for complement (C3b) in the human renal glomerulus. Pathologic studies revealed an inverse correlation between the degree of C3b deposition in specimens and the ability to demonstrate C3b receptors, suggesting that these receptors were "occupied" in the pathologic samples with C3 deposition. The possibility that these receptors are involved in the pathogenesis of some forms of glomerulonephritis is obvious, although highly speculative at present.

In addition to phagocytosis, complement may play a role in host defense by enhancing virus neutralization by antibody or, independently of antibody, by the alternative pathway. Complement-mediated bacterial lysis had been thought to be relatively unimportant until the recent discovery of gonococcal sepsis associated with deficiency of C6 or C8. This suggested at least some role for bacterial lysis in host defense.

As previously noted, complement may play a role in immune surveillance against malignancy. Alternative pathway lysis of lymphoma cells, and classic pathway lysis of tumor cells have been described.

The functions of complement may also produce host damage. The direct effects of opsonic, anaphylatoxin, and lytic activities, plus those produced by chemotactic factor–attracted leukocytes, may cause tissue inflammation and destruction.

The clearance of erythrocytes in autoimmune hemolytic anemia, lysis of paroxysmal nocturnal hemoglobinuria cells (PNH-cells), various forms of glomerulonephritis (e.g., systemic lupus erythematosus, poststreptococcal, membranoproliferative), joint disease (lupus, rheumatoid, gout) and perhaps septic shock involve complement-mediated damage. The reader is directed to the appropriate chapters of this text and several excellent reviews for details.

INTERACTIONS WITH OTHER SYSTEMS. The complement system interacts with the coagulation, fibrinolytic, and kinin systems. Plasmin can activate C1 and cleave C3b from C3, thereby enabling C3b to enter the amplification loop of the alternative pathway. C1 inhibitor (C1INH) blocks the effects of activated Hageman factor in initiating both coagulation and fibrinolysis, as well as directly inhibiting factor XI and plasmin. C1INH also blocks the effects of kallikrein kinin generation.

GENETICS AND METABOLISM. Recent evidence suggests that the genes controlling synthesis of C2, C4, C8, and properdin factor B are on chromosome 6, closely linked to the major histocompatibility complex (HLA) and to a region regulating lymphocyte responsiveness. The remaining complement loci are on other chromosomes or have not yet been identified.

The sites of synthesis of various components have been investigated. Current evidence suggests that C1 synthesis takes place primarily in intestinal epithelium, although even macrophages and fibroblasts have been reported to produce C1 in vitro. The liver appears to be the major synthetic site for C3, C6, C9, and C1 inhibitor. C2, C4, and C5 appear to be produced by macrophages.

The metabolism of complement has been studied, and those components investigated have a high turnover, in the range of 1 to 2.5 percent of the plasma pool per hour. C2 and C4 production by macrophages can be increased by exposing these cells to killed pneumococci, and C3 synthesis is increased by challenge with bacterial endotoxin. There is evidence to suggest that alternative pathway activation of C3 in membranoproliferative glomerulonephritis may result in decreased synthesis of C3. Finally, there may be hormonal modulation of the production of some complement components and their inhibitors. Evidence suggests that C4 levels in mice and C1INH levels in humans may be increased by androgens.

COMPLEMENT TESTS. The clinical assays for complement either involve a determination of the amount of antigenic (complement) protein present in serum or fluid or measure the ability of that fluid to support a complement-mediated function. An example of the latter is the total hemolytic complement titer, or CH_{50}, which measures the ability of a fluid to produce lysis of sensitized sheep erythrocytes. All nine components (C1 to C9) must be present to support lysis. Decreases in individual components affect the resultant titer to a variable degree — a 70 per cent fall in the C4 level may barely affect the CH_{50}, for example. The individual components may also be tested in lytic assays, as well as immunoprecipitation tests. Care must be taken in the handling of samples. Functional titers may fall, whereas C3 antigen levels may actually rise in "aged" serum. Finally, immunofluorescence may be used to detect the involvement of complement in reactions in tissue.

COMPLEMENT AND DISEASE

HEREDITARY COMPLEMENT DEFICIENCY DISEASES. Homozygous complement deficiencies are fortunately relatively rare. Homozygous C2 deficiency is the most common of these, and has an incidence of approximately 1:10,000. Several generalizations can be made regarding hereditary deficiency states. Deficiencies of C1, C4, and C2 may be associated with connective tissue disease syndromes, most notably an "SLE-related syndrome" described by Agnello and others. Components of this syndrome may include vasculitic rash, arthritis, and glomerulonephritis. Antibodies to single-stranded DNA, rheumatoid factor, and a positive C1q precipitin test may be present in these patients. C3 deficiency may result in recurrent severe pyogenic infections, whereas deficiency of terminal components C5-C8 may result in increased susceptibility to infection, particularly with *Neisseria gonorrhoeae* and *meningitidis*. This is presumably due to defective bacteriolysis.

Deficiency of C3b inactivator (C3bINA) has already been mentioned. In the absence of C3bINA activity, C3b autocatalytically continues to activate the alternative pathway "amplification loop," and C3 deficiency occurs, with attendant susceptibility to infection. Inherited $\overline{C1}$ inhibitor deficiency, caused by either decreased synthesis or synthesis of an inactive inhibitor protein, produces hereditary angioedema (HAE). HAE is manifested by recurrent episodes of swelling of the face, extremities, abdominal viscera, or airway, the last of which may produce asphyxiation (see Ch. 47). Uninhibited $\overline{C1}$ results in consumption of C4 and C2. C2 cleavage produces a fragment with kinin-like activity. Androgens have been used successfully to increase C1INH levels, with therapeutic success.

There are no known inherited deficiencies of alternative pathway components. C3bINA deficiency depletes this pathway. C3 nephritic factor (C3NeF), an IgG anti-C3bBb antibody, occurs in association with membranoproliferative glomerulonephritis and partial lipodystrophy. Alternative pathway activation and decreased C3 levels are seen. Finally, patients with sickle cell disease have been shown to have defective alternative pathway–mediated opsonization. Evidence suggests that these patients are deficient in factor B. The cause for this association with hemoglobin SS is unknown.

ACQUIRED ABNORMALITIES. The involvement of complement in many inflammatory and host defense reactions will predictably result in a variety of serum patterns of complement activation. Furthermore, complement levels have been determined in cerebrospinal, joint, pleural, pericardial, and even subcutaneous fluids. However, several generalizations can be made. In diseases involving circulating immune complexes, C1, C4, C3, and the CH_{50} may be lowered. These levels may fall before the actual clinical exacerbation which occurs, for example, in systemic lupus erythematosus (SLE) and serum sickness. Joint fluid may reflect the same pattern, and levels of C1, C4, C3 and the CH_{50} are diminished in SLE and rheumatoid arthritis (although serum levels are normal in the latter).

Alternative pathway activation has been noted in a variety of situations, notably gram-negative sepsis, in which it may participate in the shock syndrome, and membranoproliferative glomerulonephritis.

It is important to stress that the determination of complement levels either antigenically or functionally yields a result which represents the vectorial sum of the processes of synthesis and consumption. Either or both may be involved in a given pathologic state, and "complement levels," whether normal or abnormal, must be interpreted with caution.

Agnello, V.: Complement deficiency states. Medicine 57:1, 1978.

Alper, C. A., and Rosen, F. S.: Clinical applications of complement assays. Adv. Intern. Med., 20:61, 1975.

Cameron, J. S., Vick, R. M., Ogg, C. S., Seymour, W. M., Chantler, C., and Turner, D. R.: Plasma C3 and C4 concentrations in management of glomerulonephritis. Br. Med. J., 3:668, 1973.

Colten, H. R.: Biosynthesis of complement. Adv. Immunol., 22:67, 1976.

Frank, M. M., and Atkinson, J.P.: Complement in clinical medicine. Disease-a-Month, January, 1975.

Gelfand, M. C., Shin, M. L., Nagle, R. B., Green, I., and Frank, M. M.: The glomerular complement receptor in immunologically mediated renal glomerular injury. N. Engl. J. Med., 295:10, 1976.

Gigli, I.: Control mechanisms of the classical and alternate complement sequences. Transplant. Proc., 6:9, 1974.

Ruddy, S., Carpenter, C. B., Chin, K. W., Knostman, J. N., Soter, N. complement metabolism: An analysis of 144 studies. Medicine, 54:165, 1975.

40. THE PRIMARY IMMUNODEFICIENCY DISEASES

Robert A. Good

40.1. INTRODUCTION

Knowledge of the lymphoid cells, their functions, and their organization into two separate major immunity systems has advanced rapidly in recent years. Current views are summarized in Table 1. Understanding of the immunity functions has derived in considerable measure from study of the primary immunodeficiencies of man. In turn, new knowledge and understanding of the relation of structure to function in the lymphoid system have made possible better definition of the several primary immunodeficiencies. A continuing interplay between clinical analyses and advancing basic understanding of immunity and the immunologic apparatus represents a fine model of how progress in medicine can proceed most rapidly to the maximal benefit of humanity. Consequently, study of the primary immunodeficiencies has had importance to medicine in recent years far beyond the numerical frequency of patients who suffer from these relatively infrequent diseases.

In Table 2 is a listing of those diseases currently recognized by a WHO expert panel as the major primary

TABLE 1. The Cellular Basis of Immune Responses

T cell system:	$\xrightarrow{\text{+PHA or Con-A}\dagger}$	Blast cells	
Thymus-dependent T lymphocytes*	$\xrightarrow{\hspace{2cm}}$	Killer cells (e.g., graft rejection)	Cell-mediated immunity
	$\xrightarrow{\text{+antigen}}$	Soluble lymphocyte factors	
B cell system:			
Thymus-independent, "bursa-equivalent" B lymphocytes	$\xrightarrow{\text{+antigen}}$	Plasma cell line	Humoral antibody synthesis

*There is evidence that T cells plus antigen can cooperate with B cells to produce antibody.
†Phytohemagglutinin or concanavallin.

TABLE 2

Type	Suggested Cellular Defects			Inheritance		
	B Cells		T Cells	X-linked	Autosomal Recessive	Other§
	(a)*	(b)†				
X-linked agammaglobulinemia	X	(X)‡		X		
Thymic hypoplasia			X			X
Severe combined immunodeficiency	X	(X)	X	X	X	X
With dysostosis	X	?	X		X	
With adenosine deaminase deficiency	X		X		X	
With generalized hematopoietic hypoplasia	X		X		X	
Selective Ig deficiency						
IgA	?	X	(X)			X
Others		?				X
X-linked immunodeficiencies with increased IgM		X		X		
Immunodeficiency with ataxia telangiectasia		X	X		X?	
Immunodeficiency with thrombocytopenia and eczema (Wiskott-Aldrich syndrome)			X	X		
Immunodeficiency with thymoma	X*		X			X
Immunodeficiency with normo- or hypergammaglobulinemia	X	X	(X)			X
Transient hypogammaglobulinemia of infancy		X				X
Varied immunodeficiencies (largely unclassified and common)	X	X	(X)		(X)	X

*Absent or very low.
†Easily detectable or increased.
‡Some cases with circulation B-lymphocytes without detectable surface Ig have been found.
§Implies multifactorial or unknown genetic basis or no genetic basis.

immunodeficiencies of man. Included in Table 2, as well, is an effort to analyze each of the diseases in terms of its genetic basis and in terms of the types of cells primarily involved in the deficiency. Such an analysis must be recognized as ephemeral because of the rapidity of development of our knowledge and because rapid changes in understanding continue. Nevertheless, for the present these several diseases can be usefully viewed in light of this classification.

40.2. X-LINKED INFANTILE AGAMMAGLOBULINEMIA

Soon after Bruton initially described agammaglobulinemia in an eight-year-old boy, groups of patients, including multiple cases in several families, were studied in Boston, Minneapolis, and New York. From these studies, one form of agammaglobulinemia could be clearly established as being of sex-linked nature. This form has been called the Bruton type of agammaglobulinemia in recognition of the monumental contribution of the pediatrician who discovered the first of the primary immunodeficiencies and associated diseases with absence of gamma globulin in the blood. Bruton's discovery launched a period in which immunology has been maximally influenced by the "experiments of nature" represented by the several forms of primary immunodeficiency.

X-linked agammaglobulinemia is a disease in which fully developed B lymphocytes and plasma cells are absent from blood and bloodforming tissues. Production of immunoglobulins and synthesis and secretion of antibodies are grossly deficient or lacking altogether. Figure 1 represents a characteristic immunoelectrophoretic pattern comparing normal with agammaglobulinemic patients. Figure 2 compares an antigen-stimulated lymph node from a normal person (A) and a stimulated node from an eight-year-old aggammaglobulinemic child (B). Absence of germinal centers and absence of plasma cells characterize the node of the agammaglobulinemic patient. Plasma cells are not found anywhere in the body. Even the lamina propria of the intestinal tract and exudates of chronic inflammatory processes such as bronchiectasis are devoid of plasma cells in these patients.

Figure 1. Normal immunoelectrophoretic pattern (above) compared with immunoelectrophoretic pattern from a patient with X-linked infantile agammaglobulinemia. Note absence of demonstrable IgM, IgA, and IgG on the immunoelectrophoretic pattern.

Figure 2. Comparison of normal lymph node (*A*) and lymph node of patient with X-linked infantile agammaglobulinemia (*B*) after antigenic stimulation. Note abundant germinal center formation in the normal node and absence of germinal centers in the stimulated node from the agammaglobulinemic patient.

Clinically, children with X-linked agammaglobuline-mia are normal at birth, but during the second half of the first year of life they begin to have infections with the encapsulated, virulent pathogens such as pneumo-cocci, *Hemophilus influenzae,* and *Pseudomonas aerugino-sa.* Infections in these children usually respond well to appropriate drug therapy; but because of lack of hu-moral immunity, resistance to these infections is mini-mal. Untreated, the bacterial infections spread rapidly, and recurrent episodes of pneumonia, otitis, sinusitis, dermatitis, meningitis, and osteomyelitis are charac-teristic. By contrast, these patients seem able to resist well many other infections such as tuberculosis, histo-plasmosis, and fungal and viral infections. Herpes, vac-cinia, chickenpox, measles, paralytic poliomyelitis, and hepatitis, however, are unusually frequent in these children. Leukemia may also occur with inordinate fre-quency.

Even though immunoglobulins are virtually absent in serum and antibody synthesis is minimal or absent al-together, cell-mediated immunities, including delayed and contact allergies, are normal. Skin allograft rejec-tion occurs with nearly normal vigor. Specific delayed allergic reactions can be transferred from the agamma-globulinemic child to an immunologically normal per-son, using large numbers of peripheral blood lympho-cytes. Modern techniques for studying the peripheral blood lymphocytes reveal that X-linked agammaglobu-linemia may be heterogeneous. The majority of patients with this disease are completely lacking B lymphocytes, as defined by the presence of readily demonstrable im-munoglobulins at the cell surface. Recently, an early stage of B lymphocytes featured by cytoplasmic Ig but no surface Ig has been described in the bone marrow of patients with this disease. This interesting evidence that an early stage of B lymphocytes is present in the bone marrow needs confirmation because of its funda-mental significance. In these patients T cells are some-what increased in number, and one finds in the blood a third population of lymphocytes whose origin and exact nature are not absolutely clear. The latter may possess receptors for the third component of complement and also receptors for the Fc portion of the IgG molecule.

Diagnosis is established by analysis of the immuno-electrophoretic pattern of serum and by quantitation of each of the several immunoglobulins, using the Man-chini radioimmunodiffusion or other suitable immuno-chemical analyses. IgM, IgA, IgD, and IgE are regularly absent, and IgG is absent or present in extremely low concentrations, 100- to 1000-fold less than that of normal persons.

Treatment involves early detection and intensive and specific treatment of the bacterial infections, as well as prophylaxis using gamma globulin concentrates inject-ed intramuscularly at frequent intervals. Injections of 0.6 ml per kilogram of 16 per cent gamma globulin solu-tion given intramuscularly every two weeks is a good regimen with which to start prophylactic management. Exudative enteropathy is a common complication and is often due to infestation with *Giardia lamblia.* This infec-tion and the exudative enteropathy can be treated spe-cifically with metronidazole. The usual immunizations may be given, although no antibodies will be formed. Although vaccinia has been tolerated, it is recommend-ed that no live virus vaccines be used in any patient with primary or secondary immunodeficiency disease.

40.3. DiGEORGE'S SYNDROME

Counterpart to patients with X-linked agammaglo-bulinemia are those born without a thymus who as a consequent lack T lymphocytes in their blood and tis-sues. Such patients also frequently have no parathy-roids. Their ears are often of abnormal appearance, and they have a characteristic facies with prominent fore-head and bowed mouth. Frequently, they also have ab-normalities of the first portions of the great vessels and the outflow tract from the heart. Absence of thymus is not always complete. Absence of thymic shadow on chest roentgenograms and absence of T lymphocytes and T lymphocyte functions on immunologic analysis are characteristic. The stimulated lymph nodes show well developed far cortical areas, and in some cases ger-minal centers are present. In other cases, germinal centers have been deficient. In all instances, the thymic dependent lymphoid areas are very grossly depleted. Plasma cells are present and may be present in normal numbers in the lymphoid tissues. The number of B lymphocytes in the blood and lymphoid tissues is usually increased. Absence of thymus and T lymphocytes may be incomplete. Treatment of the endocrinopathy requires appropriate use of vitamin D and sterol therapy to raise serum calcium level. The immunodeficiency has now been repeatedly treated successfully, using transplantation of thymus obtained from allogeneic embryos. This form of treatment has in several instances seemed to correct completely the deficiency of T lymphocytes and the defects of immunologic functions. With the appearance and increase of T lymphocytes, B lymphocytes decrease in number. Failure of thymus and T cell development of nude mice represents an autosomal recessive defect that seems to be an experimental counterpart of DiGeorge's syndrome. The cause of the human disease is unclear, and a genetic basis has not yet been established for this rare disease in man. Selective deficiency of thymus and T lymphocyte development without the associated hypoparathyroidism or great vessel anomalies has been called Nezelof's syndrome. This disease has also apparently been treated successfully by allotransplantation of fetal thymus.

40.4. SEVERE COMBINED IMMUNODEFICIENCIES
(SCID, Swiss Type Immunodeficiency)

Several different genetically determined primary immunodeficiency diseases in which both T and B lymphocyte systems fail to develop normally have now been described. Each of these diseases is genetically determined. Forms with either autosomal recessive or X-linked inheritance have been defined. Infants with each of these distinct forms of severe combined immunodeficiency disease have very gross deficiencies of both T and B immunity systems. Lymphocyte numbers, generally under 1000 per cubic millimeter, are low, but these cells are usually not absent from blood. Both T and B lymphocytes are either missing or very much reduced. Levels of all classes of immunoglobulin are low.

The thymus, lymph nodes, and spleen are small and poorly developed. Indeed, these lymphoid organs are often almost completely devoid of lymphoid cells. Antibody production and development of cell-mediated immunities are extremely deficient or absent, and lymphocytes fail to respond to phytomitogens such as phytohemagglutinin, concanavalin A, and pokewood mitogen in vitro. In some of these children, responses of blood leukocytes to stimulation with allogeneic cells have been noted.

If these patients are not treated, they regularly succumb early in life to any of many different forms of infection, i.e. *Pneumocystis carinii*, cytomegalovirus, other viruses, fungi, or low- or high-grade bacterial pathogens. Live virus immunization often leads to lethal infections. Attempts to help these children, or children with DiGeorge's syndrome, by blood transfusion often leads to death from fulminating graft-versus-host disease, because these patients cannot defend themselves against the immunologically competent lymphocytes invariably present in whole blood. If blood or blood products must be given, they should be given only after irradiation of well oxygenated blood with 1500 to 3000 r or after freezing and centrifugation.

Since both B and T immunity systems are lacking in these children, attempts have been made to correct the immunodeficiency by transplantation of bone marrow. In more than 50 instances, marrow transplantation from an appropriately matched sibling donor has made possible apparently complete restoration of both T and B immunity systems in these children. Whenever definitive markers have been available, it has been possible to establish that the new immunity systems in such marrow-reconstituted children have been derived from the bone marrow cells of the donor. For successful marrow transplantation, a sibling donor selected by HLA tissue typing and mixed leukocyte culture matching has generally been necessary.

More recently, however, in absence of a matched sibling, a satisfactory matching of a kinship donor by mixed leukocyte reaction with an SCID child has permitted reconstitution of immunity function by bone marrow transplantation. Techniques have been developed which promise sufficient matching, even among unrelated persons, to permit reconstitution of the two missing immunity systems in such patients by marrow transplantation with a donor selected from the general population. In one such instance, correction of the immunodeficiency has been successful. Fetal liver transplantation, using livers from fetuses of less than 12 weeks' gestation, has also been used to correct the cellular deficiencies in this disease. Recently, treatment of a few patients with severe combined immunodeficiency by cultured human thymus transplantation has been reported. Definitive diagnosis and immunologic reconstitution of the rare children with this disease are highly technical undertakings that should be done only by those who specialize in this therapeutic approach.

40.5. SEVERE COMBINED IMMUNODEFICIENCIES WITH ADENOSINE DEAMINASE DEFICIENCY

An autosomal recessive, genetically determined disease similar to the severe combined immunodeficiency disorders described above has recently been found to be associated with absence of the enzyme adenosine deaminase (ADA) in red blood cells, lymphoid cells, and other cells of the body. Patients lacking nucleoside phosphorylase or inosine phosphorylase who have severe combined immunodeficiency (SCID) have also been described. Clinical manifestations, immunodeficiencies, cellular defects, and susceptibility to infection in this disease are all similar to those occurring in the X-linked and autosomal recessive forms of SCID in which ADA is normal, except that, quantitatively, the functional and cellular defects seem more variable.

Approximately 15 per cent of all patients with SCID lack the enzymes ADAse, nucleoside phosphorylase, or inosine phosphorylase. In the patients with SCID and adenosine deaminase deficiency, however, some lymphoid tissue development does occur, and the thymus contains Hassall's corpuscles and has characteristics of an involuted rather than an underdeveloped thymus. Patients with ADA deficiency and SCID have repeatedly been reconstituted by marrow transplantation.

The relationship between ADA deficiency and this form of SCID is not yet clear, but it is of great interest that three forms of SCID can now be associated with an inherited inability to produce an enzyme. Whether the immunodeficiencies are due to some toxic product consequent to the enzyme deficiency or whether the enzymes are essential for some crucial step in development of the lymphoid cells remains to be determined. When the immunodeficiency associated with ADA deficiency is corrected by marrow transplantation, the lymphoid cells possess normal amounts of adenosine deaminase, but the red cells continue to lack the enzyme completely. In one instance, administration of the normal enzyme in the form of red blood cells from a normal donor has led to remission of the disease. In this patient the disease and lymphoid abnormality reappeared when the ADA-carrying red blood cells were lost.

40.6. THYMOMA WITH IMMUNODEFICIENCY

More than 50 patients have been studied in which broadly based immunodeficiency, thymoma, and hypogammaglobulinemia have been associated. The first such case provoked the extensive laboratory inquiry which established the major role played by the thymus in developmental immunobiology. Both cellular and humoral immunity functions and both T and B cell numbers are deficient in such patients. They are susceptible to a broad range of bacterial, viral, and fungal infections. In one such infection encountered by Siegal et al., normal serum possessed a factor that permitted the patient's lymphoid cells to develop in vitro into B lymphocytes with readily demonstrable surface immunoglobulin. This factor was absent from the blood or serum of the patient with the thymoma-agammaglobulinemia syndrome. Red cell aplasia or hypoplasia may sometimes be associated. Some patients with the thymoma-agammaglobulinemia syndrome appear to lack both the marrow lymphoid cell precursor of the B cell line, B lymphocytes, and plasma cells. Removal of the thymus tumor, which is composed primarily of nonlymphoid, spindle-shaped stromal epithelial cells, does not correct the immunodeficiency. The bone marrow of several of these patients has been studied and found not to contain the B cell precursor lymphocyte that appears to be present in the bone marrow in Bruton's agammaglobulinemia.

40.7. COMMON VARIABLE IMMUNODEFICIENCY

Among the most frequent forms of primary immunodeficiency diseases is that presently called the common variable immunodeficiency. This rather cumbersome term is used as temporary nomenclature for what may indeed be several different diseases. However, in this form the immunodeficiency is variable from time to time in the same patient and from patient to patient in the same family. Inheritance may be autosomal recessive or autosomal dominant. In still other patients the disease is sporadic, and because of its onset later in life has been thought to be acquired. The initial agammaglobulinemic patient described by Bruton probably would now be classified with this group.

Immunodeficiency in these patients is associated with decreased concentration of all or several immunoglobulins. Antibody production is feeble, and even cell-mediated immunity responses may be decreased. Pneumonia, sinusitis, otitis media, gastrointestinal infection and malfunction, and *Giardia lamblia* infestation are common concomitants. A wide variety of autoimmune phenomena and autoimmune diseases have been frequently encountered. Pernicious anemia, histamine-fast achlorhydria, and gastric cancer occur with high frequency early in life in patients with this syndrome.

The occurrence in these patients of much autoimmunity, autoimmune disease, e.g., Coombs-positive hemolytic anemia, autoimmune thrombocytopenic purpura, pernicious anemia, and many collagen-vascular or mesenchymal diseases, including rheumatoid arthritis and vasculitis, has represented a set of fascinating but perplexing relationships. Sprue-like syndrome with or without giardiasis is frequent.

Diagnosis is made by history of frequent and persisting infections, immunoelectrophoretic pattern, and quantitation of each of the immunoglobulin classes by radial immunodiffusion. Enumeration of T and B lymphocytes is of interest because, in spite of deficiencies in producing immunoglobulins, most of these patients have normal or only slightly reduced numbers of B lymphocytes in the circulating blood. Plasma cells are deficient in the lymphoid tissue in direct proportion to the deficits of antibody production and immunoglobulin levels. In patients possessing normal or increased amounts of IgM who have low levels of IgG and IgA, lymph nodes, spleen, and intestinal lymphatic tissue may be grossly enlarged. Germinal centers may be extraordinarily hypertrophied, suggesting the erroneous diagnosis of follicular lymphoma. Waldmann discovered that some patients with the common variable immunodeficiency have lymphocytes which suppress differentiation of B lymphocytes to plasma cells that synthesize and secrete Ig. Whether these suppressor cells are responsible for the pathogenesis of hypogammaglobulinemia, as proposed, has not yet been established. At present writing the best indications are that in a few instances these suppressor cells are pathogenetically crucial, but in most instances they are not. It is of interest that such suppressor cells have also been seen in patients with Bruton-type agammaglobulinemia, in which it seems unlikely that they are responsible for the immunodeficiency.

Treatment, as in other forms of primary immunodeficiency, involves early recognition and specific antimicrobial therapy of the frequent bacterial infections. Careful diagnosis and specific treatment of *Giardia lamblia* and fungal infections are also important. Prophylactic administration of gamma globulin concentrates in very large doses, 0.6 ml per kilogram every three to four weeks, is helpful in reducing the frequency of infections in some patients. However, in these patients even more than in patients with Bruton's X-linked infantile agammaglobulinemia, prophylaxis with currently available preparations of gamma globulin is often inadequate. More satisfactory prophylaxis has sometimes been achieved using frequent infusions of plasma from carefully selected donors free of history of hepatitis and free of both Australia antigen and antibody to Au antigen. The latter precaution is extremely important, because chronic progressive hepatitis has been an especially difficult and sometimes lethal consequence of administration of blood products to these patients. What is needed are adequate preparations of gamma globulin concentrates that are suitable for intravenous administration.

In addition to the more specific forms of therapy, prophylactic regimens such as those introduced by Mathews for the ideal pulmonary toilet in patients with cystic fibrosis are helpful. Postural and positional pulmonic drainage, breathing exercises, and inhalation therapy have all been helpful in treating and apparently in preventing pulmonary disease in these patients. The autoimmune diseases should be treated as they are in persons of greater immunologic vigor, but with cognizance of the fact that the patients are immunologically compromised and that large doses of adrenal steroids, immunosuppressive agents, and splenectomy can further debilitate the bodily defense.

40.8. ISOLATED ABSENCE OF IMMUNOGLOBULINS — SELECTIVE DEFICIENCY OF IgA

Selected absence of any of the immunoglobulin classes or subclasses can occur, and such selective deficiencies have already been described for several, e.g., selective absence of IgG2. However, none of the other immunoglobulins are so frequently lacking from blood as is IgA. The frequency of selective absence of IgA ranges from 1:700 to 1:3000, according to studies of blood bank donors from several parts of the world. Many patients lacking IgA seem to be quite healthy, but a high proportion have severe atopy, autoimmune phenomena, and autoimmune diseases. Respiratory disease is frequent, especially in those patients who possess IgE. Gastrointestinal disease is also frequent, and severe progressive sprue has been reported. Soothill and his associates have observed that classic atopy caused by production of antibody of IgE class occurs with particular frequency when the IgA system is slow to develop. One possible basis for the increased frequency of autoimmune phenomena and disease with deficiency of IgA is that the dimeric form of IgA antibodies is transferred across the epithelial barrier onto the gut surface from the site of production in the lamina propria of the gastrointestinal tract. This local antibody system normally provides a barrier to absorption of foreign proteins and other antigens. Consequently, when the local immunity system is lacking or is deficient, antigens that are cross-reactive with host constituents can be absorbed and provide excessive stimulation of the remaining systemic immunity systems. This stimulation leads to production of antibodies and immune cells that in some instances cross-react with host constituents, producing autoimmune phenomena and autoimmune disease. In keeping with this view, patients lacking IgA frequently develop antibodies to IgA, serum proteins of the bovidae, and many other antigens in food and flora in amounts far in excess of those produced by normal persons. Most patients who fail to produce IgA antibody have in their circulation at least normal numbers of B lymphocytes that produce and have at their surface IgA molecules. For reasons currently poorly understood, these cells do not differentiate to IgA-secreting plasma cells. If these cells could be induced to develop to B cells capable of secreting IgA, these patients might be much improved. Wu et al., using pokeweed mitogen, and Waldmann et al., using blast forms of putative T lymphocytes obtained

from patients with Sézary's syndrome (presumably T-cell leukemia), have induced such differentiation of these IgA-producing B lymphocytes to IgA-secreting plasma cells. Some patients who fail to secrete IgA have circulating lymphocytes that inhibit differentiation of IgA secreting plasma cells. It has not been established whether these class-specific suppressor lymphocytes are of pathogenetic significance in IgA deficiency.

40.9. IMMUNODEFICIENCY DISEASES WITH ATAXIA TELANGIECTASIA AND WISKOTT-ALDRICH SYNDROME

Immunodeficiency diseases also accompany the Wiskott-Aldrich and ataxia telangiectasia syndromes. The former is a disorder of X-linked inheritance that is featured by a clinical triad, including eczema, thrombocytopenic purpura, and increased susceptibility to infection. The immunodeficiency in this syndrome is accompanied by low levels of IgM. These patients form antibody poorly to certain antigens, especially polysaccharide and small protein antigens, and show a progressive deficiency of T cell numbers and functions. The basic genetic fault is unknown, but the patients frequently succumb to infection with any of several viruses, bacteria, or fungi. Nearly 10 per cent of patients with the Wiskott-Aldrich syndrome die of cancer. Usually, but not always, the cancer takes the form of lymphoreticular sarcoma. Bleeding, especially accompanying infection, and intracranial bleeding are also frequent causes of death in these children. Treatment has generally been unsatisfactory, but platelet transfusions and plasma infusions from selected donors have been helpful in some instances. This disease has now been successfully treated by immunosuppression with alkylating agents and/or total body irradiation followed by bone marrow transplantation.

Patients with ataxia telangiectasia (see Ch. 284.5) reflect a familial and autosomal recessive, genetically determined clinical triad of progressive cerebellar ataxia, cutaneous telangiectases, and immunodeficiency. In this disease the thymus fails to develop normally and retains an embryonic appearance. T lymphocytes and T cell functions are regularly grossly deficient, and some 70 to 80 per cent of the patients lack IgA. IgE also is frequently absent from the circulation in both ataxia patients and healthy family members. These patients are troubled with frequent sinopulmonary infections, which seem to be related to the deficiency of IgA but not clearly to the deficiency of IgE.

More than 15 per cent of the patients with ataxia telangiectasia thus far studied have developed malignancies. The malignancies reported are predominantly reticulum cell sarcomas, lymphosarcomas, leukemias, and gastrointestinal cancers. Waldmann found that alphafetoprotein is present in inordinately high concentration in a majority of patients with ataxia telangiectasia. Chromosomal abnormalities, especially involving chromosome number 14, have been described, and this disease has been classified with the chromosomal instability syndromes along with Fanconi's anemia and Bloom's syndrome. How the immunodeficiency and chromosomal instability are related is not certain at present, but it seems likely that both the great susceptibility to certain forms of cancer in these patients and the immunodeficiency syndrome are in some way a function of the chromosomal dysmetabolism. Patients with Wiskott-Aldrich syndrome, who suffer from hematologic abnormality, profound immunodeficiency, and great susceptibility to certain malignancies, may also have a chromosomal instability at the base of all the disorders which make up the disease complex.

40.10. OTHER PRIMARY IMMUNODEFICIENCIES

Many other forms of immunodeficiency have been discovered in recent years, and the diseases and syndromes associated with them are only now being clarified. For example, selective deficiencies of the components of the complement system are associated with serious immunodeficiency in very high frequency. These deficiencies render the patients susceptible to infection, collagen-vascular diseases, overwhelming pneumonia, or skin and bowel infections, depending on which complement component is lacking. Ongoing studies will define these associations more clearly. Some of the complement components such as C2 and C4 and factor B of the alternative pathway are clearly linked in their inheritance to the major histocompatibility region (MHR) of chromosome 6. The immunodeficiencies associated with deficiencies of these components are thus linked as well to the MHR. Hereditary angioedema is a complement component deficiency inherited as an autosomal dominant trait that is associated with absence or abnormality of the inhibitor of the C1 esterase normally present in plasma. The sometimes life-threatening attacks of edema can be aborted by giving normal plasma. Recently, prevention has become possible by treating the patients with anabolic steroids related to testosterone. Such treatment appears to induce the production of normal C1 esterase inhibition by the liver. Untreated patients with C1 esterase deficiency may develop lupus erythematosus or chronic progressive renal disease.

Patients with genetically determined deficiency of C2, which is transmitted as an autosomal recessive trait, besides showing increased susceptibility to infection, frequently develop arthritis, anaphylactoid purpura, lupus erythematosus, or other mesenchymal vascular diseases. The basis for the association of the complement component immunodeficiencies to these as yet poorly understood mesenchymal diseases is not clear but may suggest that infection, probably with a virus, underlies all of them. Similarly, inherited deficiencies of the C1r, C1s, C4, and C5 components of complement predispose to both infection and mesenchymal vascular diseases. C1r deficiency has been corrected by renal transplantation, apparently because the kidney contains cells that produce C1r. Leiner's syndrome has been associated by Miller with an abnormality of C5, and patients with this disorder have been successfully treated by regular injection of normal plasma. Deficiencies of C3 have been associated with inordinate susceptibility to many different kinds of infection and deficiencies of C6 and C7 with increased susceptibility to infections with gram-negative pathogens.

It seems fair to predict that deficiencies of each of the specific proteins involved in the defenses of the body will occur and that diseases will be associated with these deficiencies. Such deficiencies will include deficiencies of each immunoglobulin class or subclass and deficiencies of the essential lymphokines produced by lymphocytes, complement components, and cellular or humoral components of the major effector processes. The latter already include diseases in which malfunction or deficiencies of development of granulocytes occur, as in congenital neutropenia or chronic granulomatous disease. Deficiencies or abnormal function of monocytes or other cells and molecular elements involved in bodily defense are being defined. Each disease will represent an experiment of nature capable of teaching us a new lesson about how the immunity system functions. Each will require treatment, which will be made possible by the advancing knowledge of immunity functions and their organization and development. It is thus to be anticipated that the constructive interplay between clinic and laboratory will continue to produce new knowledge and to test our advancing understanding of the immunologic systems in the bodily defense. Two good illustrations of this developing new knowledge are the chronic septic granulomatous disease of childhood (CGD) and Chédiak-Higashi anomaly. In the former, increased susceptibility to infection with catalase positive microorganisms may be associated with either complete absence of glucose phosphate dehydrogenase or absence of glutathione reductase. Both these disorders are inherited as autosomal recessive traits. The most frequent form of CGD is an X-linked recessive form in which failure to generate the oxidative burst culminating in production of H_2O_2 and bacterial singlet oxygen $'O_2$, superoxide O_2^-, and OH^- radicals has been demonstrated. This disease is associated with absence on leukocytes of the antigen Kx that is associated with production of red blood cell antigens of the Kell system. In still another form of chronic granulomatous disease of childhood, the disease is inherited as an autosomal recessive trait, but no enzyme defect has been identified to date. Any of these immunodeficiency diseases should be correctable by treatment with cyclophosphamide or total body irradiation plus bone marrow transplantation. Recently, a report of major improvement in a patient with CGD, using this approach to therapy, has been presented.

The Chédiak-Higashi anomaly is an abnormality of cellular development in which leukocytes as well as many other bodily cells possess gigantic single membrane-bound particles. The leukocytes in these patients perform poorly in chemotaxis and phagocytosis, probably accounting for the increased susceptibility to infection with which these patients are troubled. Persons with the Chédiak-Higashi abnormality develop malignancies of the lymphoid and lymphoreticular system in very high frequency. These malignancies have been classified as non-Hodgkin's lymphomas, Hodgkin's disease, and reticulum cell sarcomas. The leukocytes of patients with Chédiak-Higashi syndrome have been shown to lack microtubular structure, very likely accounting for their poor performance in chemotactic responses. In most exciting recent research, it has been shown that the microtubular abnormality and functional deficiencies can be corrected by treatment of the cells in vitro with ascorbic acid. In addition, treatment of patients with this disease with ascorbic acid corrects both the deficiency of microtubules in their leukocytes and monocytes and the functional defects of their leukocytes revealed in analyses of chemotaxis and phagocytosis. Further, this dramatic new therapy appears to improve their ability to defind themselves against infection. Whether this treatment will also improve their ability to defend themselves against cancer is still enigmatic, but it is a question that is most intriguing and the answer is urgently awaited.

Because of the multiplicity of cells, proteins, peptides, developmental processes, interactions of systems, biologic amplifications, and complex effector processes that are normally involved in the defense of the body against external and internal invaders, the primary immunodeficiency diseases, once thought to be infrequent or rare diseases, turn out to be quite frequent. Indeed, in the aggregate they are about as frequent as the combination of leukemias, lymphomas, and Hodgkin's disease. Study of these diseases has aided the analysis of deficiencies in immunologic function, which are often called secondary immunodeficiencies. This is important because the secondary immunodeficiencies, being associated with nutritional deprivation, aging, viral, bacterial, and fungal infection, myelomas, leukemias, lymphomas, Hodgkin's disease, sarcomas, carcinomas, infestations, and even endocrine disturbances, represent the most frequent serious diseases of man. Understanding of these defects and development of means to correct them promise to represent truly major therapeutic advances.

Alexander, J. W., and Good, R. A. (eds): Fundamentals of Clinical Immunology. Philadelphia, W. B. Saunders Company, 1977.

Bach, F. H., and Good, R. A. (eds.): Clinical Immunobiology, Vols. 1, 2, 3. New York, Academic Press, 1972, 1974, 1976.

Bergsma, D., Good, R. A., and Finstad, J. (eds.): Immunodeficiency in Man and Animals. Sunderland, Mass., Sinauer Associates, Inc., 1975. (Birth Defects: Original Article Series, Vol. XI, No. 1, 1975.)

Boder, E., and Sedgwick, R. P.: Ataxia-telangiectasia. In Goldensohn, E., and Appel, S. (eds.): Cellular and Molecular Bases of Neurological Disease. Philadelphia, Lea & Febiger, 1973.

Bruton, O. C.: Agammaglobulinemia. Pediatrics, 9:722, 1952.

Cooper, M. D., Faulk, W. P., Fundenberg, H. H., Good, R. A., Hitzig, W., Kunkel, H. G., Roitt, I. M., Rosen, F. S., Seligmann, M., Soothill, J. R., and Wedgwood, R. H.: Meeting Report, Primary Immunodeficiency in Man. Second International Workshop of the WHO Committee. Clin. Immunol. Immunopathol., 2:416, 1974.

Day, N. K., and Good, R. A. (eds.): Biological Amplification Systems in Immunology. New York, Plenum Press, 1977. (Comprehensive Immunology, Vol. 2.)

DiGeorge, A. M.: Congenital absence of the thymus and its immunological consequences. In Bergsma, D., and Good, R. A. (eds.): Immunologic Deficiency Diseases in Man. New York, The National Foundation Press, 1968, pp. 116-121. (Birth Defects: Original Article Series Vol. IV, No. 1, 1968.)

Dupont, B., Anderson, V., Ernst, P., Faber, V., Good, R. A., Hansen, G. S., Henriksen, K., Juhl, F., Killmann, S. A., Koch, C., Müller-Berat, N., Park, B. H., Svejgaard, A., Thomsen, M., and Wiik, A.: Immunological reconstruction in severe combined immunodeficiency with HL-A incompatible bone marrow graft. Donor selection by mixed lymphocyte culture. Transplant. Proc., 5:905, 1973.

Gelfand, J. A., Sherins, R. J., Alling, D. W., and Frank, M. M.: Treatment of hereditary angioedema with danazol. Reversal of clinical and biochemical abnormalities. N. Engl. J. Med., 295:1444, 1976.

Gell, P. G. H., Coombs, R. R. A., and Lachmann, F. J. (eds.): Clinical Aspects of Immunology. 3rd ed. Oxford, Blackwell Scientific Publications, Ltd., 1975.

Golub, E. S.: The Cellular Basis of the Immune Response. Sunderland, Mass., Sinauer Associates, 1977.

Good, R. A.: Studies on agammaglobulinemia. II. Failure of plasma cell formation in bone marrow and lymph nodes of patients with agammaglobulinemia. J. Lab. Clin. Med., 46:167, 1955.

Good, R. A.: Morphological basis of the immune response and hypersensitivity. In Felton, H., et al.: Host-Parasite Relationships in Living Cells. Springfield, Ill., Charles C Thomas, 1957, pp. 68-160.

Good, R. A.: Immunodeficiency in developmental perspective. Harvey Lect., 67:1, 1973.

Good, R. A., and Zak, S. J.: Disturbances in gamma globulin synthesis as experiments of nature. Pediatrics, 18:109, 1956.

Janeway, C. A., and Rosen, F. S.: The gamma globulins. IV. Therapeutic uses of gamma globulin. N. Engl. J. Med., 275:826, 1966.

Lawton, A. R., Wu, L. Y. F., and Cooper, M. D.: The cellular basis of IgA deficiency in humans. In Mestecky, J., and Lawton, A. R., III (eds.): International Symposium on the Immunoglobulin A System, Birmingham, Ala., 1973. New York, Plenum Press, 1974, pp. 373-380. (Advances in Experimental Medicine and Biology, Vol. 45.)

Siegal, F. P., and Good, R. A.: Human lymphocyte differentiation markers and their application to immune deficiency and lymphoproliferative diseases. Clin. Haematol., 6:355, 1977.

Soothill, J. F.: Interactions in immunodeficiency. In Bergsma, D., Good, R. A., and Finstad, J. (eds.): Immunodeficiency in Man and Animals. Sunderland, Mass., Sinauer Associates, Inc., 1975, pp. 50-52. (Birth Defects: Original Article Series, Vol. XI, No. 1, 1975.)

Waldmann, T. A., Broder, S., Durm, M., and Blackman, M.: Regulation of synthesis of immunoglobulins. In Bianchi, R., Mariani, G., and McFarlane, A. S. (eds.): Plasma Protein Turnover. Baltimore, University Park Press, 1976, pp. 265-275.

Waldmann, T. A., Durm, M., Broder, S., Blackman, M., Blaese, M., and Strober, W.: Role of suppressor T cells in pathogenesis of common variable hypogammaglobulinemia. Lancet, 2:609, 1974.

Waldmann, T. A., Broder, S., Krakauer, R., MacDermott, R. P., Durm, M., Goldman, C., and Meade, B.: The role of suppressor cells in the pathogenesis of common variable hypogammaglobulinemia and the immunodeficiency associated with multiple myeloma. Fed. Proc., 35:2067, 1976.

Walker, W. A., Isselbacher, K. J., and Bloch, K. G.: Intestinal uptake of macromolecules: Effect of oral immunization. Science, 177:608, 1972.

41. THE COMPROMISED HOST

John I. Gallin

COMPONENTS OF THE HOST DEFENSES. The host defenses comprise complex and interrelated systems which are outlined in Table 1. Familiarity with these systems provides a basis for the diagnosis and management of patients with compromised defenses.

Physical Barriers. Intact skin and mucous membranes prevent microbial invasion. The skin is a complex organ, consisting of several cell types which, in addition to providing a physical barrier, produce numerous antimicrobial agents such as lactic acid, ammonia, urea, and free fatty acids. These protect the host from superficial challenges. The mucous membrane secretions, which trap inhaled microorganisms, contain soluble factors such as immunoglobulin A, lactoferrin, lysozyme, and α_1-antitrypsin, which have antibacterial activity. Proper function of the nasal and respiratory passage cilia facilitates microbial clearance. In addition, host defenses require normal anatomy of the respiratory, genitourinary, and gastrointestinal symptoms.

Inflammatory Response. The circulating phagocytes (neutrophils, monocytes, eosinophils, and basophils) are the central components of the inflammatory response. The phagocytes are manufactured and undergo maturation in the bone marrow, and upon appropriate

TABLE 1. The Host Defenses

Physical barriers
    Skin
        Mucous membranes
Inflammatory response
    Circulating phagocytes
    Humoral mediators
Reticuloendothelial system
    Fixed phagocytes
Immune response
    T cells (cell-mediated immunity, delayed hypersensitivity)
    B cells (antibody responses)
    Other mediators (i.e., lymphotoxin)

stimulation are delivered to the bloodstream where they circulate and are distributed to local tissue sites. Recruitment of phagocytic leukocytes from the bloodstream involves a complex process called diapedesis or emigration. The initial step of this process is not completely understood but seems to require phagocyte aggregation and adherence to the endothelium. The phagocytic cells migrate between the endothelial cells as they migrate to tissue sites. The availability of the potential space between endothelial cells through which phagocytes migrate is modulated by local tissue products of the complement cascade (the anaphylatoxins, or small molecular weight cleavage products of the third and fifth complement components, C3a and C5a) and the potent vasodilator bradykinin produced by activation of the fibrinolytic and kinin generating systems. The complement cascade and the fibrinolytic and kinin generating systems are activated by microbial products such as endotoxin and a variety of substances secreted by leukocytes, platelets, and fibroblasts. Locomotion of phagocytes requires cell adherence to their substratum, deformability, machinery for random locomotion, and the ability to sense a gradient of a chemical signal (chemotactic factor) and convert random locomotion (kinesis) to directed locomotion (chemotaxis). The locomotory apparatus includes an intact actin and myosin system for movement and an intact microtubule system to stabilize the cell during locomotion and organize the intracellular granules, which are secreted extracellularly during locomotion and appear to be important modulators of the inflammatory process.

The chemotactic factors are humoral mediators and include products from activation of complement (C5a) and activation of the kinin generating system (kallikrein), from neutrophils, macrophages, lymphocytes (lymphokines), and fibroblasts (collagen), as well as oxidation products of certain fatty acids. Some chemotactic factors are highly preferential for particular cell types (i.e., histamine and other mast cell products are preferential for eosinophils, whereas an alveolar macrophage product is preferential for neutrophils). After recruitment, microorganisms that have been rendered palatable by proper opsonization by complement products and immunoglobulins adhere to the phagocyte membrane and then are ingested, killed, and digested. These events require complex biochemical and biophysical events with specific mechanisms for elimination of different classes of microorganisms (see Ch. 493).

Reticuloendothelial System. The reticuloendothelial system is the major system for the clearance of circulating microorganisms from the bloodstream. The main components of the system are the fixed phagocytes, consisting of splenic macrophages, alveolar macrophages, Kupffer cells, lymph node macrophages, and microglial cells in the brain. Many or perhaps all of these macrophages are derived from circulating monocytes which migrate from the bloodstream into tissues, where they differentiate into the fixed macrophages.

The Immune Response. The T and B lymphocytes are the main components of the immune response. T lymphocytes are the functional cells of cell-mediated immunity or delayed hypersensitivity. Mature B cells, or plasma cells, produce antibodies and are the cells of humoral immunity. The thymus gland controls the maturation of the T lymphocytes; factors controlling B cell maturation in humans are not known.

Upon appropriate signal, lymphocytes are released from the bone marrow into the circulation, where they are distributed throughout the body. The mechanism of mobilizing lymphocytes to tissue sites from the circulation is poorly understood but may involve chemotaxis and/or the process of emperipolesis. Emperipolesis is the transport of cells through, rather than between, endothelial cells. At tissue sites lymphocytes perform their specific tasks. The T lymphocytes are believed to be critical in eliminating such pathogens as *Mycobacterium tuberculosis, Histoplasma capsulatum, Candida albicans,* and certain viruses. The B cells respond to antigens (which may first have to be processed by macrophages) by synthesis of the immunoglobulins (antibodies), which have important roles in complement activation, virus neutralization, and opsonization. (For a detailed review of the various components of the immune response, see Ch. 38.)

ETIOLOGY. A host may be compromised as a consequence of extrinsic (environmental) factors or abnormalities of the intrinsic components of the host defense system. Extrinsic factors include conditions that increase the infectious challenges and factors which directly impair host defenses. Examples of the former are overcrowded living conditions, as in military recruit camps where outbreaks of infectious (meningococcal) meningitis are well known; exposure to pathogenic microorganisms from sexual activity; or occupational conditions or hospitalizations with exposure to contaminated equipment used in certain diagnostic or therapeutic procedures. Other extrinsic factors associated with compromised host defenses include protein-calorie malnutrition, thermal injury, alcoholism, irradiation, and depletion of or interference with function of cells involved in host defense by iatrogenic means. Host defense defects can also result from a number of inherited and congenital disorders, as well as from acquired defects associated with numerous diseases. The particular type of infection will depend on the nature of the fundamental defect.

PATHOGENESIS AND PATHOLOGY. Pathologic models in support of predicted abnormalities of host defenses are well described for certain components of the defense system. Other examples are emerging as we understand what parameters are important to assess. Examples related to infection from penetration of the skin are obvious and include penetrating trauma and severe burns.

Mucous membrane secretions are abnormally viscid in cystic fibrosis and mucous plug formation, and obstruction with subsequent pneumonia can result. Mucociliary movement is abnormal in Kartagener's syndrome (situs inversus, chronic sinusitis, and bronchiectasis), and there is evidence that this is related to absence of a particular cilial subunit (dynein arms). Mucous secretion and cilial integrity may also be damaged by decreases in temperature and humidity, exposure to inhalants such as cigarette smoke and atmospheric pollutants, supplemental oxygen, endotracheal tubes, and thermal injury. Infection by certain respiratory viruses (i.e., influenza) and *Mycoplasma pneumoniae* can damage the mucociliary system, resulting in increased susceptibility to bronchitis and pneumonia. Recurrent bacterial pneumonias result from anatomic derangement of bronchi by obstruction from neoplasm, foreign objects, mucous plugs, or local collapse secondary to bronchiectasis and from chronic aspiration.

Gastrointestinal "blind loops" following certain surgical procedures result in overgrowth with coliform bacteria which consume vitamin B$_{12}$ or folic acid and thereby contribute to neutropenic states. Genitourinary tract infections with gram-negative bacteria are associated with congenital and acquired abnormalities such as congenital ureteral abnormalities, urethral stricture, urethral changes following pregnancy, and urethral obstruction from stones, prostatic hypertrophy, and prostatic carcinoma.

Other anatomic defects increasing susceptibility to infection include damaged heart valves following endocarditis or rheumatic fever. Aortic aneurysms can be infected with salmonellae (particularly *Salmonella cholera-esuis*), staphylococci, and streptococci. Peripheral vascular disease of diabetes mellitus is associated with infection of the distal phalanges of the toes. Foreign objects, including prosthetic devices, sutures, gauze, and intravenous or Foley catheters, interfere with normal anatomic integrity and are subject to microbial colonization and subsequent microbial dissemination.

Patients who have had splenectomy are at increased risk for *Streptococcus pneumoniae* infection, especially infants and young children. The precise basis for this is not known, but decreased clearance of bacteria is thought to be important. Children with sickle cell hemoglobinopathies without autosplenectomy, as well as patients with hemoglobinopathies from a variety of causes, are susceptible to *Salmonella, Streptococcus pneumoniae*, and *Bartonella* infection. The host defect in the hemoglobinopathies may relate to splenic dysfunction, but abnormal alternative complement pathway function and impaired phagocytosis and killing of the indicated organisms by leukocytes have been described. Splenic dysfunction is also seen in splenomegaly from a variety of causes, including passive congestion, certain collagen-vascular diseases (systemic lupus erythematosus and Felty's syndrome), and lymphomas. These examples of splenic dysfunction are associated with neutropenia from neutrophil trapping and destruction in the spleen.

A number of other conditions predispose to compromised defenses. During viral influenza there is increased susceptibility to *Streptococcus pneumoniae* and staphylococcal pneumonia. The mechanism for this is poorly understood, but impaired mucociliary function, neutropenia, and adverse effects of the virus on phagocytic cell function have been implicated. Neoplasms, malnutrition, diabetes mellitus, and effects of a variety of pharmacologic agents, especially corticosteroids and myelosuppressive agents, compromise host defenses by affecting the production, distribution, and function of leukocytes. Prolonged use of antimicrobial drugs increases susceptibility to infection with microorganisms which colonize the host, particularly *Staphylococcus aureus*, resistant gram-negative bacilli such as *Pseudomonas, Serratia*, and the gram-negative coccobacillus *Mima-Herellea*, as well as fungi *(Candida)*.

Leukopenias. Perhaps the best evidence for a role of leukocytes in host defenses is the severe infections associated with leukopenias. Leukopenia exists when the peripheral white blood count is below 4000 per cubic millimeter. Although all leukocytes may be depressed, most commonly there are depressed granulocytes (neutrophils). In general, when the granulocyte count is below 500 to 1000 cells per cubic millimeter, patients are at increased risk of infection, and when there are fewer than 200 cells per cubic millimeter the inflammatory response is essentially absent and severe infection is the rule. Lymphopenia exists when the number of lymphocytes is below 1400 per cubic millimeter in children and 1000 per cubic millimeter in adults. The complete absence of leukocytes is not compatible with life in a normal environment. The particular type of infection associated with leukopenia depends upon which leukocyte population is depressed. Absence of thymus-dependent lymphocytes or T cells as in thymus aplasia (DiGeorge's syndrome) or thymus hypoplasia (Nezelof's syndrome) is associated with severe defects of cell-mediated immunity (see Ch. 40.3). Absent B lymphocytes (Bruton's X-linked agammaglobulinemia) is associated with a severe abnormality of humoral mediated immunity (see Ch. 40.2). Combined T and B cell lymphopenia (see Ch. 40.4) has a particularly poor prognosis.

The causes of leukopenias are multiple and are related to depressed marrow production (idiopathic, drug-induced, leukemias, tumor invasion of the bone marrow, and nutritional deficiencies), peripheral destruction (immune mechanisms, splenic trapping), or peripheral pooling with overwhelming bacterial infection. Leukopenia is seen following infection with bacteria (typhoid, paratyphoid fever, tuberculosis, brucellosis), viruses (influenza, measles, infectious mononucleosis, rubella), rickettsiae, and protozoa (malaria, kala-azar). (For a complete review of the leukopenias, see Ch. 495.)

Leukocyte Dysfunction. The leukocyte dysfunction syndromes also demonstrate the primary importance of leukocytes in host defenses. Patients with T cell dysfunction include those with mucocutaneous candidiasis and nucleoside phosphorylase deficiency. Combined T and B cell dysfunction are seen in adenosine deaminase deficiency and the Wiskott-Aldrich syndrome (see Ch. 40). Other patients with neutrophil dysfunctions attributable to abnormal adherence, chemotaxis, degranulation, and bactericidal activity are reviewed in Ch. 494. Defects of the humoral components of the inflammatory response include abnormalities of mediators. These include deficiencies of certain complement components (C3 and C5) with abnormal anaphylatoxin, opsonin, and chemotactic factor production. Inhibitors acting on the chemotactic factors have been described in patients with Hodgkin's disease, sarcoidosis, alcoholism, and cirrhosis. Patients deficient in the late complement components (C6 and C7) have increased susceptibility to *Neisseria* infections.

CLINICAL MANIFESTATIONS. The clinical history can be very important when evaluating a patient suspected of having a host defense defect. The type, frequency, duration, and location of infections, the intensity of the inflammatory reaction, and associated illnesses or clinical problems such as allergies or atopic dermatitis, as well as the family history, are important and are summarized in Table 2.

Leukopenias. The clinical manifestations of leukopenia without infection are minimal, or those of the underlying disease. With acute drug-induced leukopenia, chills, fever, and prostration may be the initial manifestations and may be attributed to invasion by bacteria. However, these symptoms may occur within an hour of administering a drug which results in a hapten-antibody type reaction, such as with aminopyrine, and may relate to release of endogenous pyrogens from immune lysis of leukocytes. The initial symptoms may transiently disappear, to be followed by recurrent fever,

TABLE 2. Infections in Patients with Host Defense Defects

Host Defect	Clinical Examples	Clinical Manifestation of Infections	Infectious Agents
Inflammatory response			
Neutropenia	Aplastic anemia Agranulocytosis Leukemias	Pneumonia; ulcers of skin, oral cavity, rectum, and vagina; fever; depressed inflammatory response	Gram-negative bacilli (especially *E. coli, Pseudomonas* sp., *Klebsiella, Staph. aureus*), fungi (*Candida, Aspergillus*), *Pneumocystis carinii*
Chemotaxis	Chédiak-Higashi syndrome Job's syndrome and variants	Subcutaneous abscesses "Cold" abscesses, bronchitis, otitis, pneumonia, bronchiectasis	*Staph. aureus, Strep. pyogenes* *Staph. aureus, Strep. pneumoniae, H. influenzae, E. coli, Klebsiella*
	Newborns Protein-calorie malnutrition; others (see text)	Bacteremia Bacteremia	Gram-negative bacilli Gram-negative bacilli
Phagocytosis			
Cellular defect	Systemic lupus erythematosus, megaloblastic anemia, chronic myelocytic leukemia	Otitis, bacteremia, pneumonias, meningitis	Encapsulated bacteria
Opsonin deficiency			
C3 deficiency	Inherited or acquired (i.e., systemic lupus erythematosus)	Otitis, bacteremia, pneumonia, meningitis	*Pseudomonas, Proteus, Staph. aureus, Strep. pneumoniae*
C5 dysfunction	Leiner's syndrome of newborn infants	Generalized seborrheic dermatitis, severe diarrhea, local and systemic infections	Gram-negative bacilli
Alternative complement pathway	Sickle cell disease	Pneumonia, osteomyelitis	*Salmonella, Strep. pneumoniae*
Bactericidal activity	Chronic granulomatous disease	Recurrent infection of lymph nodes, skin, lung, liver, bone, and other tissues	Catalase (+) microorganisms (*Staphylococcus, Klebsiella, E. coli, Serratia marcescens, Pseudomonas, Proteus, Salmonella, Candida, Aspergillus, Nocardia*)
Immune response			
T cells			
Deficiency	Thymic aplasia (DiGeorge's syndrome) and thymic hypoplasia (Nezelof's syndrome)	Otitis, pneumonia	Tuberculosis, *Listeria*, BCGosis, leprosy, *Candida*, cryptococci, aspergillosis, *Pneumocystis*, toxoplasmosis, *Strongyloides*, herpes simplex, herpes zoster, cytomegalovirus, measles
Dysfunction	Mucocutaneous candidasis	Candida of mucous membranes or oral cavity, esophagus, vagina, nailbeds	*Candida albicans*
	Purine nucleoside phosphorylase deficiency	Chronic pneumonias, diarrhea, candidiasis	Fungal and viral infections
B cells	Bruton's X-linked agammaglobulinemia	Sinusitis, otitis, dermatitis, pneumonia, meningitis, osteomyelitis	*Strep. pneumoniae, H. influenzae, Pseudomonas* sp.
	Dysgammaglobulinemias, agammaglobulinemia, multiple myeloma, chronic lymphocytic leukemias	Bacteremia, pneumonias, sinusitis	Fulminant hepatitis, poliomyelitis, measles, chickenpox
	IgA deficiency and nodular lymphoid hyperplasia of the intestine	Diarrhea, malabsorption	*Giardia lamblia*
Mixed T and B cells	Common variable hypogammaglobulinemia (may be due to excess T suppressor cells inhibiting B cells)	Sinusitis, bronchitis, pneumonia, bacteremia	High and low grade bacterial pathogens, *Pneumocystis*, cytomegalovirus
	Ataxia telangiectasia (decreased IgA and IgE)	Sinusitis, bronchitis, pneumonia	*Strep. pneumoniae, H. influenzae, rubella, Giardia lamblia*
	Wiskott-Aldrich syndrome (defective antibody response to polysaccharides, decreased IgE, IgM, abnormal monocyte chemotaxis)	Otitis, pneumonia	Infections seen in T and B cell dysfunction
	Severe combined immunodeficiency, adenosine deaminase deficiency	Severe infection involving multiple sites	Infections seen in T and B cell dysfunction
Mixed defects	Hodgkin's disease and lymphoma (lymphocytopenia, delayed hypersensitivity, abnormal monocyte chemotaxis)	Pneumonia, bacteremia, hepatitis	Tuberculosis, histoplasmosis, *Salmonella, Listeria, Pneumocystis*, cytomegalovirus, herpes zoster, herpes simplex, *Cryptococcus, Candida*, aspergillosis
	Diabetes mellitus (abnormal chemotaxis, phagocytosis, compromised neurovascular supply)	Cellulitis, urinary tract infections	*Staphylococcus aureus*, gram-negative *Candida*, mucormycosis
	Uremia (chemotactic defect, depressed, delayed hypersensitivity, lymphopenia)	Bacteremia, pneumonia, urinary tract infection	*Staph. aureus, E. coli, Klebsiella, Pseudomonas*

TABLE 2. Infections in Patients with Host Defense Defects *(Continued)*

Host Defect	Clinical Examples	Clinical Manifestation of Infections	Infectious Agents
Iatrogenic	Burns (chemotactic defect, necrosis)	Cellulitis, bacteremia, pneumonia	*Staphylococcus, Strep. pyogenes, Pseudomonas* sp., *Candida,* herpes simplex
	Cystic fibrosis (mucociliary dysfunction)	Bronchitis, pneumonia	*Staph. aureus, Pseudomonas*
	Splenectomy	Pneumonia and osteomyelitis	*Streptococcus pneumoniae, Salmonella*
	Foreign body (intravenous catheters, prosthetic devices)	Bacteremia, local abscesses	*Staph. aureus,* gram-negative bacilli, *Candida*
	Antibiotics	Bacteremia	*Staph. aureus,* gram-negative bacilli (*Serratia, Pseudomonas, Mima-Herellea*) *Candida*
	Corticosteroid therapy (depressed delayed hypersensitivity, neutrophil margination and adherence)	Bacteremia, pneumonia	*Candida, Pneumocystis, Staph. aureus,* gram-negative bacilli, others

chills, headaches, and frequently ulceration of the oropharynx and sometimes the rectum and vagina. These ulcerations are called aphthous ulcers and may be the initial clinical manifestation of neutropenia. The ulcers often have a gray membrane, but frank pus is absent. Patients receiving cytotoxic drug therapy get similar ulcers, independent of neutropenia, which may be difficult to distinguish from aphthous ulcers. Following or concomitant with this stage there are usually symptoms of local bacterial invasion. Frequently bacterial invasion is overwhelming without impressive clinical manifestations because of lack of an inflammatory reaction. Minimal skin lesions characterized by local erythema and tenderness or minimal roentgenographic findings often are the only indications of overwhelming infection with gram-negative bacilli. Careful and frequent inspection of the patient is thus required. With agranulocytosis, regional lymph nodes become enlarged. In the absence of aggressive therapy or spontaneous remission, death from overwhelming infection (usually gram-negative bacilli) ensues. If remission of the agranulocytosis occurs, immature granulocytes appear in the circulation before mature cells.

Patients with severe neutropenia also have an increased incidence of *Pneumocystis carinii* and cytomegalovirus infection as well as infection with the systemic mycoses, including candidiasis, invasive aspergillosis, and mucormycosis. Systemic candidiasis, defined as tissue invasion and not just colonization of superficial surfaces, is the most common mycosis in the neutropenic patient. Prolonged drug therapy for a bacterial infection predisposes to candidiasis and especially *C. albicans* because of normally occurring local colonization. The presence of thrush in the mouth, vagina, or skin indicates candidiasis in these patients, and indwelling catheters may serve as a portal of entry. In systemic candidiasis symptoms are usually confined to the distal esophagus or the bladder, with rare local symptoms in the lung, liver, spleen, or kidney. Symptomatic lesions in the distal esophagus in compromised hosts are usually indicative of candidiasis and are characterized by dysphagia, odynophagia, pyrosis, retrosternal pain, and gastrointestinal bleeding. On x-ray irregular scalloping of the esophageal lining is manifest. Aspergillosis (penetration of hyphae into tissues) is an infection seen in neutropenic patients who are also on corticosteroid therapy; mucormycosis is also seen in

this setting, especially in patients with diabetes mellitus. Invasion with aspergillosis almost invariably involves the lung, causing symptoms suggesting pneumonia or pulmonary emboli. Pulmonary mucormycosis is almost indistinguishable from aspergillosis.

Disorders of the Inflammatory Response. Patients with defective phagocyte chemotaxis present with minimal physical findings or findings characteristic of their underlying disease. The signs and symptoms of the infection are delayed because too few phagocytes arrive too late. Patients with defective leukocyte chemotaxis frequently have severe periodontal disease and dermatologic abnormalities, and these patients have frequent sinopulmonary infections with recurrent otitis media, bronchitis, and pneumonia. *Staphylococcus aureus* is the most frequent infectious agent, but *Streptococcus pneumoniae* and *Hemophilus influenzae* are also common. Perhaps the most common syndrome in which defective neutrophil and monocyte chemotaxis is the predominant host defect occurs in patients with eczematous and pustular dermatitis, markedly elevated IgE, recurrent "cold" staphylococcal skin infections, and recurrent bronchitis and pneumonias with subsequent bronchiectasis (Job's syndrome and its variants). The severity of the atopic dermatitis correlates with the severity of the chemotactic defect. These patients frequently have subcutaneous and lymph node abscesses requiring surgical drainage, and their facies have a characteristic broad nasal bridge. Many patients are in the teenage years at the time of evaluation for host defense defects, and few patients over 30 years of age have been noted. Usually these patients have had recurrent pneumonias since early childhood, and many have thoracotomy scars from lobectomy for the severe bronchiectasis. Some of these patients also have T cell dysfunction and mucocutaneous candidiasis. This syndrome appears to be familial in some cases. Similar clinical spectrums with high IgE and a chemotactic defect are seen in patients with incontinentia pigmenti and an unusual type of ichthyosis.

Defective neutrophil and monocyte chemotaxis and delayed degranulation of neutrophils are also noted in patients with the Chédiak-Higashi syndrome, a rare disease with autosomal recessive inheritance characterized by partial oculocutaneous albinism, nystagmus, neutropenia, recurrent cutaneous infections (particularly with *Staphylococcus aureus*), and giant lysosomes in all cells containing lysosomes. These patients usually have multiple subcutaneous scars from the recurrent infections.

An impressive list of diseases with chemotactic defects and recurrent infections has emerged in recent years and includes the following: diabetes mellitus, leukemias, malignancies (melanoma and breast carcinoma), rheumatoid arthritis, Felty's syndrome, systemic lupus erythematosus in some patients, thermal injury, bone marrow transplantation (associated with graft versus host disease and administration of antithymocyte globulin), congenital ichthyosis with *Trichophyton rubrum* infection, hypogammaglobulinemia, α-mannosidase deficiency, chronic renal failure (especially if the patient is on chronic hemodialysis), severe protein-calorie malnutrition, and severe bacterial infections and viral influenza. In most of these studies the mechanism for the chemotactic defect has not been delineated, and it is not clear whether the chemotactic defect is a cause or effect of the recurrent infections. However, a few well documented case reports of patients with severe pyogenic infections and defective leukocyte locomotion attributable to actin dysfunction or abnormal microtubule assembly clearly illustrate the importance of leukocyte chemotaxis in the host defense system.

Other phagocyte disorders include deficient phagocytosis related to abnormal opsonins as in sickle cell disease, dysfunction of the fifth complement component (Leiner's syndrome), and congenital deficiency of certain complement components (C3 and C5) or immunoglobulins. Clinical manifestations of these deficiencies are recurrent otitis media, bronchitis, pneumonia, and sepsis with encapsulated bacteria. These deficiencies, as well as those with abnormal killing of bacteria, as in chronic granulomatous disease in which there is defective hydrogen peroxide generation and recurrent severe infections of the skin, lymph nodes, lung, liver, and bone with catalase-positive microorganisms such as *Staphylococcus aureus*, enteric bacilli, *Candida*, *Aspergillus*, and *Nocardia*, are reviewed in Ch. 494.

Immune Dysfunctions. Patients with T cell abnormalities have recurrent infections from intracellular bacteria such as *M. tuberculosis*, leprosy, BCGosis, *Listeria*, and *Candida*. These patients also become infected with other fungi (cryptococcosis and aspergillosis), protozoa (*Pneumocystis carinii*, toxoplasmosis, and *Strongyloides*), and viruses (herpes simplex, herpes zoster, varicella, cytomegalovirus, and measles). The clinical presentation of these patients is discussed in Ch. 40.

In other patients the number of T cells is normal, but there is abnormal effector cell response to antigenic stimulation. Delayed skin responses to *Candida* and other naturally occurring antigens is absent, and lymphocytes from many of the patients do not respond to in vitro stimulation with antigens, especially *Candida*, by producing lymphokines or by replication. A well defined group of patients with T cell dysfunction have mucocutaneous candidiasis with *Candida albicans* infection restricted to the skin, nails, and mucous membranes. Another small group of patients deficient in purine nucleoside phosphorylase have T cell dysfunction with recurrent viral and fungal infections.

The prototype disease for B cell deficiency is Bruton's X-linked agammaglobulinemia with absent fully developed B cells and grossly deficient synthesis and secretion of antibody. These patients are subject to infection with encapsulated virulent pathogens such as *Strepto-*coccus pneumoniae, Hemophilus influenzae,* and *Pseudomonas aeruginosa*. Untreated, these infections spread rapidly, and patients have sinorespiratory infections with recurrent pneumonias and otitis media, as well as osteomyelitis, dermatitis, and meningitis. The patients usually respond to appropriate antimicrobial drugs, probably because of normal phagocyte and T cell function. Infections caused by intracellular microorganisms such as *M. tuberculosis*, *Histoplasma* and fungi are relatively infrequent.

Diseases with combined deficiencies of T and B cells are associated with severe infections. Such patients usually succumb early in life to many different forms of infection, including *Pneumocystis carinii*, cytomegalovirus, other viruses, and bacterial pathogens of high and low grade virulence.

DIAGNOSIS. Initial evaluation of patients with recurrent infections requires a thorough history. For example, a history of contact dermatitis (poison ivy) helps eliminate T cell dysfunction, whereas a history of mucocutaneous candidiasis suggests a T cell abnormality. Aphthous ulcers may be early signs of severe neutropenia. Staphylococcal skin infections and recurrent pneumonias suggest a chemotactic defect, and a history of recurrent infections with catalase positive microorganisms suggests chronic granulomatous disease.

Tests useful in the laboratory evaluation of compromised hosts are summarized in Table 3. Initial laboratory screening studies can be very informative. A white blood count and differential count will serve as a screen for the leukopenias. The morphology of the white cell can be particularly helpful. For example, multilobed nuclei are seen in polymorphonuclear leukocytes in vitamin B_{12} or folate deficiency, and when considering the Chédiak-Higashi syndrome the characteristic giant lysosomes can be seen. An excellent screening test used to diagnose chronic granulomatous disease is the ability of granulocytes to reduce nitroblue tetrazolium dye. This test, which is available in most medical centers, reflects leukocyte oxidative metabolism and is markedly abnormal in chronic granulomatous disease and a few related disorders of phagocyte function (see Ch. 494). Quantitative immunoglobulins assess B cell function, and in the presence of borderline hypogammaglobulinemia the capacity of patients to produce specific antibodies after immunization is important. Most hospital laboratories can measure typhoid H and O agglutinins before and after immunization with standard vaccines, and antibodies to common viruses are also usually available. T cell function can be screened by delayed hypersensitivity skin testing to common antigens (PPD, *Candida*, mumps, streptokinase, and streptodornase). A chest x-ray will help in evaluation of the thymus gland and may reveal evidence for recurrent pneumonias or bronchiectasis. Total hemolytic complement (CH_{50}) and C3 are available in many laboratories, although studies of individual complement components can be obtained only in a few research centers.

More specific studies are often necessary to define host defense defects. In addition to a bone marrow aspirate, marrow reserves can be evaluated with etiocholanolone. The inflammatory response can be estimated in vivo with a Rebuck skin window, which assesses the ability of leukocytes to accumulate at a superficial abrasion and to stick to a glass coverslip. More precise characterization of the cellular and humoral components of the inflammatory response re-

TABLE 3. Diagnostic Tests Used in the Evaluation of Host Defense Defects

Host Defense	Test
Bone marrow production	Peripheral white blood count*
	Marrow aspirate*
	Bone marrow reserve test†
Inflammatory response	Rebuck skin window*,†
	Leukocyte function
	Adherence*,†
	Chemotactic response*,†
	Phagocytosis‡
	Degranulation‡
	Bactericidal activity*,†
	Nitroblue tetrazolium dye reduction (NBT test)*,†
	Hexosemonophosphate shunt activity‡
	Leukocyte glucose-6-phosphate dehydrogenase and myeloperoxidase‡
	Chemotactic and opsonic activity of serum*,†
	Complement levels (CH$_{50}$,* C3*,†)
Immune response T cell system (cellular immunity)	Delayed hypersensitivity skin tests to common antigens*
	Sensitization to dinitrochlorobenzene‡
	Chest x-ray to assess thymus gland*
	Quantitation of T cells†
	T cell rosettes
	Specific membrane markers
	Lymphocyte transformation studies†
	Nonspecific mitogens (pokeweed, concanavallin A)
	Specific antigens (PPD, mumps, streptokinase-streptodornase, Candida albicans)
	Lymphokine production‡
	Chemotactic lymphokines
	Macrophage migration inhibitory factor
B cell system (humoral immunity)	Quantitative immunoglobulins*
	Immunoglobulin subclasses‡
	Kinetics of antibody synthesis following primary and secondary immunization‡
	Antibodies to common viruses†
	Specific antibody response after immunization* (typhoid H and O agglutinins)

*Screening tests.
†Generally available at major medical centers.
‡Available only in specialized laboratories.

quire in vitro studies. Leukocyte adherence is measured by the ability of cells to stick to nylon wool. Locomotion can be qualitatively evaluated by looking at cells moving on glass slides and can be quantitated by measuring cell migration into different kinds of filter paper. Chemotactic factors are assessed by their ability to attract normal leukocytes. These studies of the inflammatory response are generally available in medical centers, as are studies for the quantitation of leukocyte phagocytosis and killing of bacteria. Studies of leukocyte hexose monophosphate shunt activity, leukocyte actin and myosin, or microtubule function are presently restricted to a few clinical research laboratories.

In-depth studies of the immune system include quantitation of T and B cells (and their subpopulations), using specific membrane markers. B cell function can be evaluated by the kinetics of antibody synthesis following primary and secondary immunization. Measurement of immunoglobulin G subclasses is also available. T cell function can be further characterized in vivo by monitoring the delayed hypersensitivity response after contact sensitization with dinitrochlorobenzene. T cell functional correlates to delayed hypersensitivity can be assessed in vitro by measuring proliferative responses (tritium incorporation) to nonspecific stimuli such as mitogens (phytohemagglutinin, pokeweed mitogen, and concanavallin A) or specific stimuli such as antigens (PPD, mumps, streptokinase-streptodornase, or Candida albicans). Quantitation of the release of lymphokines (i.e., migration inhibitory factor or chemotactic lymphokines) are generally available in medical centers. Other specific tests of T cell function are available only in highly specialized laboratories.

Particularly puzzling patients with no demonstrable defect of host defenses should raise one's suspicion of the possibility of a psychologic disorder with self-inflicted lesions. Psychologic problems can be very serious, with patients inoculating fecal material subcutaneously or performing other manipulations that can manifest as severe abscesses or unexplained fevers; many of these patients are medical or paramedical professionals. Continual culture of fecal flora from wounds and localization of infections to conveniently reached areas (such as the left side of the body in right-handed individuals) should lead one to suspect psychologic problems.

MANAGEMENT. General Considerations. Management of the compromised host is based in part on the specific problems. Risk from environmental factors such as crowded living conditions, contaminated hospital respirators, or intravenous lines must be rigidly controlled. Intravenous lines should be used only when necessary; metal (scalp vein) devices should be used whenever possible, as microbial colonization with these is less than with plastic catheters. Similarly, all catheters, especially Foley catheters, should be used as little as possible, and they should be changed regularly. Antimicrobial agents should be carefully selected and used as briefly and with as much microbial specificity as possible.

Certain procedures are associated with bacteremia or local spread of infection, and compromised hosts undergoing these procedures may be at increased risk. In particular, dental manipulation, bronchoscopy, certain gastrointestinal studies (gastroscopy, jejunal biopsy, liver biopsy, sigmoidoscopy, barium enema, retrograde cholangiogams), urinary tract manipulations (catheterization, cystoscopy, retrograde pyelogram), angiograms (cardiac catheterization), orthopedic surgery, and, on rare occasions, bone marrow aspiration have been associated with bacteremia. In severely compromised hosts, administration of appropriate antimicrobials (depending on the expected bacteremia) prior to and for several hours after the procedure may prevent development of disseminated foci of infection.

Considerable controversy exists regarding the necessity for isolating patients with compromised defenses. Obviously judgment is required as to which patients require isolation. Patients with severely compromised defenses (such as patients with agranulocytosis plus corticosteroid therapy) may benefit by isolation from hospital personnel, as may those with draining staphylococcal wounds or herpes zoster. However, isolation is disruptive to hospital routine and should not be continued any longer than required. Hospital personnel with minor infections, including herpes simplex "cold sores," should not be restricted. Use of laminar flow isolation facilities may provide some benefit in selected situations; however, the availability of such units is limited to a few institutions.

Leukopenias. The compromised host with leukopenia, and in particular granulocytopenia, poses a particularly difficult management problem. This is especially true if immunosuppressive drugs such as corticosteroids are being used concurrently. If there is any possibility of an environmental or drug-induced leukopenia, the etiologic agent should be eliminated. When infections occur, inflammatory manifestations are markedly diminished or absent, and careful and frequent examination of the patient for subtle findings of infection is required. Surveillance cultures of the oral cavity, stool, and open wounds, as well as culture of withdrawn catheter tips, can be particularly helpful in the selection of initial antimicrobials when these patients become infected. Mycotic infections can be a particular problem in these patients. Heavy colonization with *Candida* (thrush of the mouth, esophagus, or vagina) should be treated with a topical antifungal agent such as mycostatin (Nystatin). Patients with urinary tract colonization with *Candida*, as judged by pseudohyphae in the urine, who have no fever or other evidence of infection, and in whom a Foley catheter is required, may benefit from bladder irrigation for several days with amphotericin B (50 μg per milliliter). If a bladder catheter is not in place, oral 5-fluorocytosine should be considered, especially if the clinical situation is not urgent and renal function is normal. With severe candidiasis, intravenous amphotericin B should be used. Patients with compromised defenses with transient candidemia that is thought to be related to contaminated intravenous lines may benefit from a short course of intravenous amphotericin B to try to prevent the establishment of disseminated foci. Fungemia in patients with malignancies and compromised defenses, especially lymphoreticular or hematopoietic malignancies, is frequently associated with disseminated fungal infection, and in these patients early use of amphotericin, sometimes prior to microbiologic confirmation, should be considered.

The use of bone marrow transplantation to reconstitute patients with agranulocytosis and other immunodeficiencies is attractive but still under investigation and at present is restricted to only a few medical centers. Use of leukocyte transfusions to transiently correct leukopenias may prove to be beneficial. Initial studies using leukocyte transfusions are encouraging, but methods for collection and storage of leukocytes and techniques for the prevention of antileukocyte antibody formation in recipients remain particular problems.

Disorders of the Inflammatory Response. Management of patients with neutrophil dysfunction syndromes requires aggressive therapy of particular infections with careful selection of antimicrobial drugs. Aggressive use of antimicrobials and early surgical drainage of abscesses in some patients (i.e., with chronic granulomatous disease) is appropriate. Long-term chemoprophylaxis has not been established as beneficial, although it may help in selected situations; chemoprophylaxis prior to procedures commonly associated with bacteremia is appropriate. Plasma transfusions may be particularly useful in infants with Leiner's syndrome (C5 dysfunction).

Manipulation of leukocyte function with pharmacologic agents may be an important future approach to management of patients with leukocyte dysfunction.

Ascorbic acid has improved granulocyte function in a few patients with the Chédiak-Higashi syndrome, although this has not been seen in every patient. Several patients with the syndrome of elevated IgE, recurrent bacterial infections, atopic dermatitis, and a leukocyte chemotactic defect showed improvement of the chemotactic defect after oral levamisole. Similarly, a monocyte chemotactic defect in patients with acute influenza was also corrected by levamisole. Clinical trials with these agents have not yet been completed. It is hoped that therapeutic manipulation of inflammatory components of the host defenses will emerge as important tools in the management of these patients.

Disorders of the Immune Response. Patients with IgG immunoglobulin deficiency with recurrent bacterial infections usually benefit from replacement therapy with human gamma globulin. Maintenance of plasma IgG around 200 mg per milliliter is reported to decrease severe infections, although sinusitis, bronchitis, and otitis may persist. Intramuscular injection of IgG (100 mg per kilogram) at monthly intervals is usually adequate. Globulin injection is beneficial only in patients deficient in immunoglobulin G. An alternative therapy is infusion of fresh plasma, 10 to 20 ml per kilogram, at intervals of three to four weeks. The advantage of this is that, in addition to replacing IgG, it replaces IgM and IgA, although the IgA never enters the secretory pools. The disadvantage is the risk of transmitting hepatitis. Despite gamma globulin, repeated infections and progression of pulmonary fibrosis and bronchiectasis may persist.

Treatment of patients with T cell deficiencies is largely a research procedure. Some patients have responded to fetal thymus graft with increased numbers of T cells and improved T cell function. Other patients have responded to immune reconstitution with transfer factor therapy. Transfer factor is prepared from dialysates of leukocyte extracts and was first shown by Lawrence in 1954 to have the potential for immune reconstitution. In some patients, when the candidiasis is first cleared with a short course of intravenous amphotericin, remissions have been sustained with transfer factor therapy. Transfer factor has also been used with variable success in the reconstitution of defective cell-mediated immune responses in the Wiskott-Aldrich syndrome, in severe combined immunodeficiency, and in patients who have coccidioidomycosis, tuberculosis, or leprosy. With the recent availability of highly purified preparations of the biologically active components in transfer factor, more defined benefits of this agent should emerge. At present, therapeutic use of transfer factor should be considered investigational and its use restricted to investigators actively evaluating its therapeutic potential.

Babior, B. M.: Oxygen-dependent microbial killing by phagocytes. N. Engl. J. Med., 298:659, 721, 1978.

Cooper, M. D., and Seligman, M.: B and T lymphocytes in immunodeficiency and lymphoproliferative disorders. *In* Loor, F., and Roelants, G. E. (eds.): B and T Cells in Immune Recognition. London, John Wiley & Sons, Ltd., 1977, pp. 377–406.

Fauci, A. S.: Mechanisms of host defense. *In* Current Concepts. The Upjohn Company, 1978.

Frank, M. M., and Atkinson, J. P.: Complement in clinical medicine. Disease-a-Month, January 1975.

Gallin, J. I., and Quie, P. G. (eds): Leukocyte Chemotaxis: Methods, Physiology and Clinical Implications. New York, Raven Press, 1978.

Kirkpatrick, C. H., and Gallin, J. I.: Treatment of infectious and neoplastic diseases with transfer factor. Oncology, 29:46, 1974.

Lichtman, M. A. (ed.): Granulocyte and monocyte abnormalities. Clin. Haematol., 4:483, 1975.

Quie, P. G.: Infections due to neutrophil malfunction. Medicine, 52:411, 1973.

Wanner, A.: Clinical aspects of mucociliary transport. Am. Rev. Respir. Dis., 116:73, 1977.

Young, R. C., Bennett, J. E., Geelhoed, G. W., and Levine, A. S.: Fungemia with compromised host resistance. Ann. Intern. Med., 80:605, 1974.

42. SERUM SICKNESS

Fred S. Kantor

DEFINITION. Serum sickness is a disease characterized by fever, arthralgia, skin eruptions, and edema which appears after injection of a foreign serum or serum proteins and is dependent upon an immune response of the patient to the injected serum. Hypersensitivity reactions to a variety of drugs may produce an identical illness.

ETIOLOGY. With the advent of antimicrobial therapy, the use of serum for the treatment of microbial diseases has declined markedly; the most common cause for "serum sickness" at present is not serum itself but exogenously administered drugs, particularly the antimicrobials. Serum therapy is still used primarily for the neutralization of bacterial toxins such as tetanus and botulinus toxins and also in the form of rabies antiserum.

The incidence and severity of the disease are clearly related to the type of serum preparation as well as to the amount administered. Of patients given prophylactic tetanus antitoxin prepared in horses, approximately 2 to 5 per cent will develop symptoms of serum sickness. The figure is considerably higher for those patients receiving equine rabies antiserum; approximately 16 per cent of these patients develop serum sickness. In general, there is an increasing incidence and severity through childhood, adolescence, and adulthood. Reactions in children are quite mild, lasting from one to four days, whereas in patients over the age of 15, the disease is more frequent and more severe.

Different methods of production of various equine antisera may have a profound effect upon the serum sickness liability of the product. Most tetanus antitoxin preparations involve a peptic digestion which does not impair antitoxic properties while hydrolyzing many of the proteins present in the serum. In contrast, antirabies antiserum is not subjected to peptic digestion because of the great loss of antibody encountered with the enzymatic treatment. The most important factor concerned with the development of serum sickness is the total amount of serum administered. Recommended doses of tetanus antitoxin and rabies antisera vary considerably from time to time; from 5 to 10 ml of tetanus antitoxin may produce serum sickness in 5 to 10 per cent of patients, whereas 80 ml will almost always result in illness. Age and dose relationships in serum sickness resulting from drugs are not as clear cut as with serum or serum proteins. In most cases the drug by itself is not capable of inducing the disease and must combine with a protein of the patient to form a complete antigen or immunogen. In such a situation the genetic potential of the patient of forming complete antigens and producing antibodies to them must be considered in addition to the patient's age and the dose and duration of the drug given.

MECHANISM. The essential basis of serum sickness is antigen-antibody interaction. A blood level of circulating foreign protein can be measured in patients shortly after beginning serum treatment. In the early stages the administered protein is catabolized in a manner similar to that seen in the animal from which it came. This is the latent period and usually lasts from four to ten days, during which time the patient develops an immune response that is evidenced by the appearance of antibody directed against the injected protein. As soon as antibody appears, it combines with circulating foreign protein antigen to form soluble complexes. These complexes have a varied fate, depending upon their nature and the ratio of antigen to antibody in the complex. Experimental studies, in the rabbit primarily, have shown a deposition of antigen-antibody complexes beneath the endothelium of blood vessels and within the basement membrane of these vessels. Complexes containing antibodies of the IgM or the IgG classes may initiate fixation and activation of the complement sequence. With localization of complement-containing complexes in the walls of blood vessels, polymorphonuclear leukocytes are attracted to the site and appear to injure the vessel by release of potent enzymes found in their lysosomal granules. The vascular injury mediated by complement and polymorphonuclear leukocytes may lead to thrombosis and hemorrhage, typified by the petechial or ecchymotic rash attendant on serum sickness.

Another manifestation of the interaction of antigen and antibody is the release of potent vasoactive materials such as histamine, serotonin, bradykinin, and slow-reacting substance (SRSA), all of which lead to vasodilatation and leakage of protein and fluid from the vascular space into the tissues, resulting in edema. The disease varies from species to species in laboratory animals. As most of the work has been done in the rabbit, it is pertinent to note that the renal disease, which is a frequent and important aspect of immune complex disease in the rabbit, is often nonexistent or a very mild component in the usual human patient.

Continuation of disease is dependent upon a continual supply of antigen. Removal by the reticuloendothelial system of the immune complexes is signified by a rise in serum antibody directed against the foreign proteins, and reduction of symptoms and signs of illness. Unless the foreign proteins are readministered, the disease is self-limited. During convalescence and for long periods thereafter, antibodies against the foreign proteins are readily demonstrable in the patient's serum. Readministration of foreign antigen promptly leads to formation of immune complexes and clinical manifestations of disease, which continue until antigen is entirely removed from the circulation.

CLINICAL MANIFESTATIONS. The onset of disease is often heralded by itching and discomfort, frequently at the site of serum injection. Fully developed serum sickness is a miserable disease. The unfortunate patient lies on his side in bed with a swollen, distorted face, often resulting in closure of both eyes so that he cannot see, with a skin itching all over and often covered with an urticarial or erythematous rash. He is reluctant to scratch his skin because of the pain in all his muscles and joints upon movement, and so he lies quietly in bed suffering from headache, itching, and joint pain. Especially frightening and discomforting is the appearance of neurologic manifestations which may result in weakness of an extremity or a sensory deficit, or occasionally an isolated facial palsy. Compounding the patient's difficulties may be abdominal pain, nausea, and vomiting. Upon examination a generalized lymphadenopathy may be palpated, especially prominent in the regions draining the site of injection of the serum. At that site there may be a local rash with erythema and either urticaria or tenderness, and this may provide a potent clue for the physician as to the nature of the illness. Occasionally, auscultation of the chest reveals a cardiac arrhythmia or a pericardial friction rub. The spleen is usually not palpable. A common manifestation is fever of 38.3 to 39°C, and, in addition to the subjective complaints of joint pain, the patient may manifest objective arthritis with swelling, redness, and accumulation of fluid in joints. The skin may show a petechial or purpuric rash in addition to the more common urticarial eruption.

LABORATORY STUDIES. Examination of the blood may reveal a mild leukocytosis, and circulating plasma cells have been observed. The sedimentation rate is usually normal or only slightly elevated. Eosinophilia occurs, but is relatively uncommon. The urine may show slight proteinuria, a few red cells, and occasionally a few casts; but there are rarely significant evidences of renal impairment. Examination of the patient's serum proteins reveals circulating horse gamma globulins and macroglobulins present early in the disease, and predominantly anti-horse IgA globulin antibodies late in the disease and during convalescence. The development of antibodies to horse alpha-2-macroglobulin in the sera of patients recovering from serum sickness suggests that this component of the equine serum which lacks any antibody value could be deleted in manufacture without impairing the antitoxic benefits of the serum. Serum complement levels are reduced for variable periods during the disease and then return to normal.

TREATMENT AND PROGNOSIS. Very mild symptoms of pruritus and skin rash may be controlled by an antihistamine, such as brompheniramine, 4 mg given every four hours. Epinephrine and sympathomimetic amines have been recommended in the past for the treatment of the urticaria of serum sickness, and salicylates for the treatment of joint pains. However, for all but the mildest symptoms, adrenocortical steroids in the form of prednisone can be given with great safety and efficacy, and the patient need not suffer with less effective medications. As this is a self-limited disease with a natural course of one to three weeks, the usual hazards of steroid therapy are not realized before treatment is stopped. A treatment course of 40 mg per day for four or five days may be sufficient, even for quite severe disease. Symptomatic improvement appears often within hours of the onset of steroid therapy and sometimes is remarkable within 24 hours.

PREVENTION. Tetanus antitoxin and rabies antiserum prepared from human sera are now commercially available in many parts of the world. If a human serum can be obtained, there is no reason to choose horse serum. When equine sera must be used in treatment, patients should be carefully questioned concerning prior exposure and for allergic symptoms to other horse products, such as horse dander or horsehair, as found in horse-hair mattresses. All patients, regardless of history, should be skin tested by production of a minimal wheal (0.01 to 0.02 ml) of a 1:10 dilution of the serum to be used. After 15 to 20 minutes the skin site is examined for an urticarial wheal, and in its absence treatment may be instituted. If the patient is allergic and the necessity for serum treatment is great, desensitization may be attempted by repeatedly injecting small amounts of serum beginning in dilutions of 1:100 and doubling the tolerated amount about every 15 or 20 minutes until the appropriate dose is achieved. Such treatment is hazardous because of possible anaphylaxis, and the indications for it should be scrutinized carefully.

In patients who have developed serum sickness after tetanus antitoxin, active immunization should be begun during the patient's convalescence from serum sickness. It is generally advisable to immunize against tetanus all individuals who are seen by the physician in connection with unrelated allergic disease and found to be sensitive to horse dander or horse products. The immunization can be accomplished by use of tetanus toxoid.

Occasionally, in the course of serum therapy *an acute anaphylactic reaction* occurs, consisting of sudden vascular collapse, severe pruritus of the face, hands, and feet, often accompanied by bronchospasm and incontinence of stool and urine. Such events must be treated promptly *with epinephrine and not adrenocortical steroids.* A tourniquet should be placed proximal to the injection site of the drug or serum, and 0.2 ml of epinephrine injected into the site of injection which will slow absorption from the site. An additional 0.3 to 0.5 ml of 1:1000 aqueous solution of epinephrine should be given subcutaneously above the tourniquet if the patient has an effective blood pressure. In the absence of adequate blood pressure, the epinephrine must be given intravenously notwithstanding the hazard of production of cardiac arrhythmia, because the drug will not be absorbed from the periphery. After epinephrine administration, diphenhydramine (Benadryl), 50 mg, should be given orally or intramuscularly. The outcome of anaphylactic reactions is usually decided in the first few minutes; rapid restoration of blood pressure with prompt treatment is an excellent prognostic sign. Fatalities are few but tend to occur when the possibility of anaphylaxis is not considered *prior* to the administration of serum or drugs so that effective measures are delayed.

Kunkel, H. G. (Chairman): Symposium on immune complex and disease. J. Exp. Med., 134:1s, 1971.
Moroz, L. A., Comerford, T. A., and Guttman, R. D.: Mixed IgG-IgA cryoglobulinemia in human serum sickness. Int. Arch. Allergy Appl. Immunol., 48:756, 1975.
Vaughan, J. H., Barnett, E. V., and Leadley, P. J.: Serum sickness: Evidence in man of antigen-antibody complexes and free light chains in the circulation during the acute reaction. Ann. Intern. Med., 67:596, 1967.
von Pirquet, C., and Schick, B.: Serum Sickness. Baltimore. Williams & Wilkins Company, 1951.

43.   DRUG ALLERGY

Fred S. Kantor

The value of therapeutic agents should constantly be weighed against their potential liability. Hypersensitivity reactions must be distinguished from two other untoward effects of drugs. The first is that of intolerance, in which the usual undesirable toxic effects occur at dosages of the drug well below that expected in a normal population. An example of this type of reaction includes visual disturbances and alterations in cardiac rhythm with very small doses of digitalis. The second form of drug reaction to be distinguished from hypersensitivity is that of idiosyncrasy. Whereas intolerance is a quantitative difference, idiosyncrasy is qualitative and is based upon a biochemical alteration in the way the patient handles the drug. Such a reaction does not depend on prior exposure to the drug, is not dose dependent, and does not resemble the other pharmacologic manifestations of the drug. An example of idiosyncrasy is the hemolytic anemia produced in patients with glucose-6-phosphate dehydrogenase deficiency when treated with primaquine. Altered reactivity (von Pirquet combined these two words to produce the word "allergy") on the part of the patient always follows prior exposure, even though this may not be apparent, and its mechanism is related to the hypersensitive state as reflected by delayed hypersensitivity or antibody production.

INCIDENCE. Any drug may produce a hypersensitivity reaction, but some drugs have a much higher liability in this regard than do others. Digitalis and tetracycline have a low liability in producing allergic drug reactions, even though reports of documented cases have appeared. On the other hand, several of the antimicrobials, notably novobiocin, and certain antiinflammatory agents, such as phenylbutazone, may have a high incidence of drug reaction. In addition to the variations produced by different drugs, equal liability is not shared by all patients for development of drug reactions to a single drug, such as penicillin. Patients with a history of allergic disease or previous drug reactions, as well as patients with certain inflammatory diseases such as lupus erythematosus, are generally thought to be more prone to the development of new drug allergies.

PATHOGENESIS. Certain therapeutic agents such as insulin are complex protein molecules which are known to be immunogenic. The majority of drugs represent classes of simple chemicals which require complexing with a tissue or serum protein of the patient in order to form an antigenic or immunogenic molecule. Drugs which are highly reactive chemicals usually are the most frequent sensitizers, and conversely the more inert members of the drug armamentarium are of less allergenic potential. Sensitization by means of a simple chemical involves the formation of covalent bonds with host protein which forms a hapten-carrier conjugate. Antibodies and hypersensitivity are directed against the hapten or the hapten and a closely adjacent portion of the carrier molecule, but never to the carrier protein itself. To form a hapten-protein conjugate, the administered drug may have to undergo considerable chemical rearrangement. This may occur during the metabolism of the drug, producing an antigenic determinant which is different from the administered drug. The necessity of chemical rearrangement of the drug to form the allergenic hapten-protein complex shows the difficulty of testing in vitro for drug allergy, because before testing it is necessary to know what the antigenic determinant is.

Drug allergy has been investigated with respect to the antigenic determinant in only a limited number of cases. One of the most recent and extensive investigations has been in the case of penicillin and a derivative, the penicilloyl determinant. This has been labeled the major determinant, and as many as three — and perhaps many more — as yet undescribed chemical rearrangements may account for minor determinants, all of which can produce sensitization in given individuals and produce allergic symptoms upon administration of the drug. It should be borne in mind that not all drug immunization implies drug allergy. A good example of this is that all patients recently treated with penicillin will have developed antibodies directed against the penicilloyl determinant.

Hypersensitive reactions have been divided into *delayed hypersensitivity* and two varieties of immediate hypersensitivity: *wheal-and-flare* and *Arthus reactivity*. Serum sickness, which is discussed in Ch. 42, is an excellent example of an immediate type of hypersensitivity involving complement-fixing antibody and producing reactions of the so-called "Arthus" type.

The other type of immediate hypersensitivity, i.e., wheal-and-flare, is manifested in two major, clinically recognizable situations, urticaria and anaphylaxis. In these cases, the interaction of the drug-protein conjugate with IgE antibodies leads to release of active mediators resulting in vasodilatation and smooth muscle contraction. In this form of reaction, the hapten-protein conjugate and its respective antibody do not enter into the pathogenesis of the reaction but merely cause the release of the vasoactive material which produces the clinical effects. The last type of well-recognized mechanism is that of cellular or delayed hypersensitivity. In this form of immunity, circulating antibody is not important, and the interaction of the drug-protein conjugate is with sensitized cells, causing a release of a variety of biologically active materials which lead to perivascular accumulation of mononuclear cells and the development of induration. The best example of delayed hypersensitivity induced by drugs is skin sensitization resulting from direct contact with a variety of medications. Paradoxically, antihistamines, which have been incorporated into a variety of topical preparations for treatment of itching, burning, or allergic skin conditions, are themselves skin-sensitizing, and by combining with skin proteins form potent sensitizing agents which lead to delayed hypersensitivity and the development of the typical skin lesions of contact sensitivity. A combination of reaction types is often present in typical drug allergy, but one or another of the reaction types usually predominates and treatment is most efficacious when directed against this reaction type.

CLINICAL MANIFESTATIONS. Fever may develop immediately after administration of a drug or, more commonly, may increase in a stepwise fashion after the seventh or eighth day of administration. The fever may show a sustained or remittent course and is usually low-grade in the range of 37.8 to 39°C, although hectic fevers are often observed, accompanied by constitutional symptoms. In general, the patient appears less ill than would be anticipated from the height of the fever. A drug reaction may mimic the septic picture entirely, but it usually pursues a more indolent course. Cessation of fever within a day or two of discontinuing the offending drug is to be expected. In some cases of fever alone, and if the drug reaction involves other organ systems, such as the skin and the joints, it may take several days, up to a week, for the symptoms to slowly subside. Penicillin, diphenylhydantoin (Dilantin), and barbiturates are frequent causes of drug fever.

Skin Rash. Skin rash as a manifestation of drug allergy may take several forms. A maculopapular, very fine rash appearing in the softer skin of the axillary line and on the extensor surfaces of the extremities and along the trunk may be unnoticed by the patient. Usually, *urticarial rashes* are reported because they are accompanied by pruritus. Persistent administration of an offending drug causing maculopapular eruptions may lead to confluent erythroderma and subsequent exfoliative dermatitis. Similarly, a rash may progress to an eczematous eruption with weeping papulovesicular lesions and ill-defined patches of erythema and edema, accompanied by intense pruritus. Erythema multiforme–like eruptions may be produced by a variety of drugs and are characterized by the formation of sharply circumscribed lesions that are usually symmetrical in distribution. The individual lesions seem to spread peripherally and clear centrally to form an annular pattern with secondary and tertiary rings evolving into a "target" or "iris" lesion.

Symmetrical lesions of the lower extremities closely resembling typical erythema nodosum may also be caused by drugs, including sulfones, penicillin, and iodides. The term "fixed eruption" is used to describe an erythematous and sharply defined lesion which recurs at the same site and in the same form upon re-exposure to the same drug. Withdrawal of the drug usually leads to healing, but hyperpigmentation of the area involved may remain. Photosensitivity reactions characterized by erythema, edema, and mild scaling are sharply limited to areas exposed to light, and a clue to the examiner may be provided by the V-shaped area at the neckline, usually at the site where the collar leaves the skin exposed to light and it becomes involved. Sulfonamides and thiazide derivatives are examples known to engender photoallergic reactions.

Other Organ Systems. Drug allergy is often manifested by reactions involving the hematopoietic system. Sedormid, a once popular sedative, resulted in thrombocytopenic purpura, which was shown to depend upon the presence of drug, a serum factor demonstrated to be antibody, and the presence of platelets. Several other drugs, such as quinine and quinidine, thiouracil, and the anticonvulsant hydantoin group, have been implicated as causes of thrombocytopenic purpura. Hemolytic anemia and agranulocytosis are also common adverse reactions ascribed to drugs. Sulfonamides and thiouracil have caused both types of reaction, but aminopyrine and phenylbutazone produced mainly agranulocytosis. Care should be taken in the interpretation of allergic causality of pathologic events leading to agranulocytosis or hemolytic anemia. One of the outstanding examples of a purported allergic hemolytic anemia was that induced by the fava bean. It was later shown that the presence of an enzyme defect in the red cells of these patients resulted in their shorter life span when exposed to drug and that sensitization in the immunologic sense was not required. Aplastic anemia, involving all the formed elements of the blood, is occasionally associated with drug administration; in particular it is described with chloramphenicol, gold, and the sulfonamides.

Gastrointestinal symptoms are common adverse reactions to the administration of therapeutic agents, but the mechanism of action is rarely allergic in nature. The kidney is involved in periarteritis nodosa caused by drugs. In this disease, antimicrobial drugs, notably the sulfonamides, have been frequently implicated. Interstitial nephritis has been described with the penicillinase-resistant penicillin preparation methicillin in association with hematuria, rash, and marked eosinophilia.

The lupus erythematosus syndrome has been described following ingestion of certain drugs, particularly hydralazine, procainamide, and the hydantoin derivatives. The severity of the syndrome induced by drug ingestion may vary from only a serologic manifestation, such as a positive lupus test, to the full-blown picture of fever, arthritis, polyserositis, and hematologic manifestations. Pulmonary infiltration and eosinophilia (PIE syndrome), peripheral neuritis, and hemorrhagic encephalitis have all been ascribed to allergic drug reactions, and probably represent varieties of allergic vascular injury resident in the particular organs involved. Liver damage has been attributed to treatment with heavy metals, thorazine, and sulfonamides; the evidence supporting the allergic basis of these reactions is meager. In recent times, the introduction of halothane, a potent, widely used anesthetic agent, has led to a series of symptoms, primarily involving liver dysfunction, which in some patients strongly suggest an allergic basis.

GENERALIZED ANAPHYLAXIS. Generalized anaphylaxis as a manifestation of drug allergy is a clinical catastrophe with which the physician must be prepared to deal promptly. The condition is usually initiated by an injected drug, although an orally administered tablet has been reported to produce a fatal reaction. Frequently the initial symptoms are generalized pruritus, particularly on the soles of the feet and the palms of the hands, and the general development of a hyperemia of the skin, particularly about the ears, so that the individual often looks as though he had acquired a recent sunburn. Angioedema may cause distortion of the face, swelling of the eyelids, and rapid loss of effective plasma volume, leading to vascular collapse and shock. The risk of developing an anaphylactic reaction, particularly to penicillin, is enhanced by the patient's having had a prior, less serious reaction, such as a maculopapular rash.

DIAGNOSIS. Discontinuance and challenge are still the best diagnostic means available to the physician, although challenge is often inadvisable because of the danger to the patient. Certainly in cases of anaphylactic reactions or urticarial eruptions, the challenge to the patient subsequent to the subsidence of the symptoms is not warranted and is extremely dangerous. However, in drug fever, when that condition appears alone, a fractional dose may be administered after the fever subsides to further identify the cause. Unfortunately, laboratory tests have been very disappointing. The basophil degranulation test, lymphocyte stimulation test, skin window technique, and others have been reported with some success from isolated laboratories, but in general they have been found to be difficult to reproduce and have not come into general use. The necessary information concerning the intermediary metabolites of each drug and the development of specific antigenic determinants is not available for the majority of drugs which cause allergic reactions. Until this information is known, laboratory tests are not likely to be useful. The leukocyte count may be high or low, and therefore not useful; eosinophilia is not a regular occurrence.

TREATMENT AND PROPHYLAXIS. Subsidence of allergic reactions to drugs usually occurs promptly after discontinuance of the drug, often within one or two days, but in many instances prolongation of symptoms for several days and, indeed, in some instances for several weeks and months, is well recognized. Many of our foodstuffs are contaminated with medications: Chickens are fattened with estrogenic hormones, hogs are fed antimicrobials, and cows, when suffering from mastitis, may be treated with large doses of penicillin which appears in the milk. When strongly suspecting a drug hypersensitivity which fails to subside after cessation of the drug, inadvertent environmental drug administration should be carefully investigated. In general, treatment of the drug reaction should be directed against the altered physiology. In the reactions involving vasoactive substances, the use of a direct vasoconstrictor such as epinephrine may be lifesaving and should be used first, instead of the more glamorous, but less effective, group of adrenocortical steroids. The latter group of agents are very useful in the treatment of the Arthus type of immediate hypersensitivity as manifested by serum sickness and polyarteritis, as well as in many forms of delayed hypersensitivity. Epinephrine should be given in dosages of 0.5 to 1 ml of 1:1000 dilution of aqueous epinephrine, given subcutaneously. Antihistaminics such as diphenhydramine (Benadryl, 50 mg) or brompheniramine (Dimetane, 4 mg) may be administered orally or parenterally, but the intravenous use of diphenhydramine is to be avoided because serious adverse reactions to this medication have occurred. Drug reactions are self-limited diseases, and the use of steroids in these diseases is most efficacious and generally does not impose the usual liabilities of steroid therapy. Accordingly, therapy may be instituted with full doses of prednisone, 40 to 60 mg a day, and 40 mg a day may be given for three or four days, dropped to 20 mg a day for an additional several days, and discontinued without a long tapering regimen.

Demis, D. J.: Allergy and drug sensitivity of skin. Ann. Rev. Pharmacol., 9:457, 1969.

Levine, B. B.: Immunochemical mechanisms of drug allergy. Ann. Rev. Med., 17:23, 1966.

Neely, C. L., and Kraus, A. P.: Mechanisms of drug induced hemolytic anemia. Adv. Intern. Med. 18:59, 1972.

Parker, C. W.: Drug allergy. N. Engl. J. Med., 292:511, 732, 957, 1975.

44. ALLERGIC RHINITIS

(Hay Fever)

Fred S. Kantor

DEFINITION. Hay fever is the common name applied to allergic rhinitis which recurs each year at a specific season — usually spring or fall. It is characterized by rhinorrhea, sneezing, itching of the eyes, nose, ears, and palate, and edema of the nasal mucous membranes. Nonseasonal allergens, such as feathers and animal danders, may produce year-round disease called perennial allergic rhinitis; vasomotor rhinitis is a "wastebasket" term which designates perennial rhinitis without an identifiable allergic basis.

ETIOLOGY AND EPIDEMIOLOGY. Susceptible persons exposed each year to airborne pollen of many varieties of plants, particularly trees, grasses, and weeds, develop a "wheal and flare" type of immediate hypersensitivity to protein components of the pollen grains called allergens. The exact heritable basis of hay fever is still unclear, but clustering of a variety of diseases which involve "wheal and flare" hypersensitivity in certain individuals, and in families, strongly supports the view that such a basis exists. The evidence suggests that sensitivity to a particular allergen, such as ragweed, may be dependent upon transmission of a specific immune response gene and therefore might be predictable in an individual before development of the disease.

Drab, colorless plants, unattractive to birds and bees, must depend upon the wind for pollination and release of huge amounts of airborne pollen. In contrast, colorful blossoms and odoriferous plants generally release smaller amounts of heavier, stickier pollen which is not widely disseminated. "Rose fever," a form of allergic rhinitis prevalent in early summer, is a misnomer; while roses are visually in full bloom, it is the pollen from grasses such as timothy, June, and orchard grass which produces the disease.

Ragweed and grass pollen are the most common causes of allergic rhinitis in the United States. Ragweed abounds in the midwestern states, and is prevalent in the eastern and southeastern part of the country. West of the Rocky Mountains and in the dry Southwest, very little ragweed appears. Each area has a distinctive potentially sensitizing flora, and sufferers fleeing from one part of the country to another are often disappointed when symptoms rapidly reappear in their new location. In the northern United States early spring hay fever (April and May) is usually due to tree pollen; the grasses pollinate and produce symptoms in early summer (June and early July) and the ragweed in late summer and early fall. Spores of ubiquitous molds are present throughout the year but increase in numbers at different times because of increased mold growth on decaying vegetation. Spores of *Hormodendrum* peak in number in July, whereas spores of *Alternaria* increase in the fall, overlapping the ragweed season, and may be the basis of an erroneous diagnosis of ragweed hay fever.

The trees are a varied and an important group; ash, beech, birch, cedar, hickory, maple, oak, sycamore, and poplar all produce important windborne pollen, whereas the less antigenic pollens of the firs and pines are not usual sources of disease. Each species of tree produces an antigenically distinct pollen with a relatively short period of pollination lasting two to four weeks. Hypersensitivity to multiple species of trees with overlapping pollinating periods, and to grasses, molds, and ragweed, may blur the seasonal aspects of the patient's problem and suggest a perennial allergic rhinitis. Unlike the trees, grasses such as timothy, fescue, orchard, redtop, and June (Kentucky bluegrass) share important antigenic determinants and in the extreme South and West may produce year-round symptoms. A careful account of seasonal variations in symptoms coupled with a knowledge of the flora of the patient's locality and the pollinating periods of the indigenous plants is vital to the specific diagnosis and management of this group of diseases. In the British Isles and the European continent, trees and grasses are important causes of pollinosis; allergic travelers would do well to check the season of their proposed trip. Europe has little or no ragweed, so American sufferers may doubly enjoy a late summer European vacation.

Pollen grains are about 20 to 40 μ in diameter, and each species has a distinctive appearance. By collecting grains on a glass slide with a simple timed exposure or with more sophisticated air-sampling devices, pollens may be identified and enumerated. The severity of symptoms of an allergic population will vary with the pollen numbers in an approximate way, but the use of daily radio broadcast pollen numbers as a diagnostic or predictive aid is of little value. The "counts" are derived from samples obtained the previous day, and at different locations and altitudes. Often the patient will ask why he doesn't feel better (or worse) because of the low (or high) pollen count!

Allergic rhinitis may be caused by any inhaled antigen; those often implicated, in addition to plant pollen, are house dust, feathers, fungus spores, and animal danders. Food allergy is often suggested as a basis for inhalant symptoms, but manifestations in the skin such as urticaria or angioedema (see Ch. 46 and 47) are the rule, and the respiratory tract is an unlikely target organ for this type of hypersensitivity.

PATHOGENESIS. Sensitization may occur at any time of life but usually occurs in childhood or adolescence. It is curious that an adult may become sensitized to a pollen to which he has been exposed each previous year of his life; this suggests that factors other than genetic proclivity and exposure are necessary. When pollens impinge upon the nasal mucous membrane, they release a variety of protein antigens called allergens which initiate the immune response. The major allergens of grasses and ragweed have been partially purified and are low molecular weight proteins of relatively low antigenicity. This means that for a given amount of antigen, the immune response in terms of amount and avidity of antibody produced is small. The important point is that this type of antigen in low doses tends to elicit an unusual response characterized by production of reaginic antibody, which is largely or completely of the IgE class. Such antibodies are present in nanogram quantities in serum, and "fix" to the surface of cells so that passive administration will sensitize a particular skin site for weeks. Because of this quality, reaginic antibodies are sometimes called homocytotropic. Contact with the specific allergen will cause "sensitized" cells to release potent vasoactive substances, largely histamine and slow reacting substance of anaphylaxis (SRS-A). These materials cause capillary vasodilatation with leakage of fluid and colloid into the tissues leading to the major symptoms of allergic disease.

Although the symptoms produced by inhalation of pollen are localized to the mucosa with which it comes in contact, the sensitization is systemic. When peripheral leukocytes of sensitive individuals are exposed to allergen in vitro, they release histamine. This reaction affords a rapid measurement of sensitivity, usually expressed in terms of amount of allergen necessary to produce release of 50 per cent of the cellular histamine. It also provides an objective measurement of the efficacy and mechanism of treatment. Production of IgE antibody is not limited to allergic individuals; normal

subjects or laboratory animals will develop this class of antibody response after subcutaneous injection of allergens. The presence of extracts of roundworms such as *Ascaris* facilitates production of IgE antibody in an unknown way. Similarly, the nasal route of allergen exposure in an allergic individual facilitates development of IgE antibody. Nonimmunologic factors also play a role in producing what may be called the "inertia" of allergic disease; patients who are well tend to remain well, whereas those who are sick tend to remain sick. Nonspecific irritants of all sorts can cause incapacitating sneezing and rhinorrhea in a patient suffering from allergic rhinitis; these might be tolerated without a sniffle at another time of year. Upper respiratory infections, particularly sinusitis, occur more frequently in the allergic patient owing to edema and obstruction of normal drainage. Similarly, the normal effects of emotional states upon the nasal mucosa are often exaggerated in the allergic patient.

CLINICAL MANIFESTATIONS. The abrupt onset of morning sneezing, usually in paroxysms of several sneezes in rapid succession, accompanied by rhinorrhea and itchiness of eyes, palate, and pharynx, is characteristic of allergic rhinitis. Symptoms recur each year at approximately the same time, corresponding to the appearance of the offending pollen in the air. Increased exposure will intensify symptoms: dry, windy days, riding in an open car, and working in a garden are frequently reported to worsen the symptoms. A hay fever sufferer notes that the morning and evening hours are the worst, with a relatively better period during the midday. Mucosal congestion and edema often lead to total blockage of the airway, necessitating mouth breathing. The conjunctivae are red and weepy, and the lids and periorbital tissues may be puffy.

Hay fever is not often accompanied by temperature elevations, and the name is therefore misleading. Fever should alert one to the common complications; sinusitis, otitis, or mastoiditis. Cough, wheezing and dyspnea are frequent companions of allergic rhinitis. Because pollen grains are too large to affect the terminal bronchioles, it was thought that the allergic reaction in the upper respiratory tract could trigger lower airway obstruction, but recent studies indicate that pollen fragments small enough to reach the bronchioles are present in the inspired air.

DIAGNOSIS. Early in the course, the differentiation of allergic rhinitis from that caused by irritants or infections is difficult, but in retrospect the patient will usually remember similar but milder symptoms at the same time in previous years. The seasonal history is the most important of all clues to correct diagnosis. Allergic rhinitis may be differentiated from viral upper respiratory infections by the presence of pruritus of eyes, nose, and pharynx and by the absence of fever, sore throat, and malaise. The nasal mucous membranes appear swollen, pale, and boggy in allergic rhinitis, and red and "angry" in viral infections; but inflammation secondary to sneezing and frequent blowing to clear the nose may blur these differences. Nasal secretions may be obtained by asking the patient to blow his nose into a piece of ordinary wax paper; smears stained with Wright's or Giemsa stains show an abundance of eosinophils in allergic rhinitis, whereas in infectious rhinitis smears reveal polymorphonuclear leukocytes.

Environmental allergens other than pollen are more

difficult to diagnose as the basis of allergic rhinitis, but a careful history will often elicit them. Inquiry should be made into the home: How old is it? What is the heating system? What are the floor, wall, and window coverings? What types of pillows, mattresses, quilts, and comforters are used by the patient and by his or her spouse? Frequently the nonallergic marriage partner will sleep on a feather pillow not five inches from the allergic one sleeping on a nonallergenic pillow. The question of what makes symptoms worse or better has a special significance in the allergic history. Often patients can specify a place or activity associated with symptoms which when avoided keeps them symptom-free.

Skin Tests. Since sensitization is systemic, the allergic individual reacts whenever contact with allergen occurs. Injection of minute quantities of allergens into the skin produces a wheal in 10 to 15 minutes in individuals with reaginic antibodies. Unfortunately, the presence of a positive skin test does not prove that the patient's symptoms are related to the allergen provoking the skin response. Often allergic individuals will have multiple positive skin reactions, such as to ragweed and grass allergen, but express symptoms in only one season and not the other. Skin tests are performed as either scratch tests or intradermal injections. Sets of skin test allergens are readily available and are often used indiscriminately. The patient may be tested with 200 to 300 skin tests with confusing results and erroneous diagnoses. A limited number of tests, 10 to 20, including house dust, common animal danders, feathers, common molds, and pollen, should suffice in all but the most difficult cases.

If skin tests are not diagnostic, why do them? They are often helpful in confirming a suspicion based on the history. The degree of skin reactivity in the untreated patient bears an approximate relationship to the degree of sensitivity and the amount of specific IgE antibody. Occasionally a positive skin test will point to a new direction of inquiry; e.g., a positive test to horse dander led to the finding that the patient was sleeping on a mattress with horse hair. Finally, when a decision is made to hyposensitize with allergen injections (see below), the degree of skin test reactivity provides guidance for a starting dosage.

Allergenic materials for testing and treatment are made by extraction of the solid allergen in a neutral buffer; usually a weight-to-volume ratio is employed, such as 1 gram of defatted ragweed pollen extracted with 100 ml of buffer producing 1:100 allergenic extract. In recent years, Kjehldahl analysis has led to standardization of extracts in protein nitrogen units (PNU) per milliliter. One PNU is equal to 10^{-8} gram N.

This "scientific"-sounding quantity may mislead the user, because only a small fraction of the extract contains the allergenic proteins and all the nitrogen is measured. Until the content of specific allergens is assayable, it is likely that the crude weight per volume or PNU per milliliter standard will be used. Extracts prepared in the same manner at different times may have wide variation in the amount of active allergen per milliliter. It is essential to be careful when using a new extract.

Intradermal tests are more sensitive than scratch tests but carry a greater likelihood of causing a constitutional reaction in a highly sensitive individual. Reactions are read after 10 to 15 minutes. A slight but definite wheal is considered 1+; a moderate reaction (wheal 6 to 10 mm) without pseudopods is read as 2+; a wheal of 10 to 15 mm with pseudopod formation is read as 3+; and wheals larger than 15 mm with a wide flare are read as 4+.

The initial intracutaneous tests with pollens should be made with solutions of antigen containing no more than 10 protein nitrogen units per milliliter, and not more than five to ten tests should be done at any one time. A minimal wheal (0.01 to 0.02 ml) is produced in the skin with a 27 needle attached to a tuberculin syringe. If little or no reaction is obtained, subsequent tests may be made with solutions containing 100 units and then 1000 units per milliliter. Reactions less than 2+ at 1000 PNU per milliliter are of doubtful significance in the untreated patient, whereas strongly positive reactions at 10 PNU per milliliter are almost always associated with symptomatic disease. The interpretation of positive reactions must be made in relation to the prevalence of the antigen in the area and the patient's history.

Circulating γE antibodies directed against a specific allergen can be evaluated by the radioallergosorbent (RAST) test. In this instance a *purified* allergen is adsorbed to an inert particle. The patient's serum is added, and the coated particles are washed. If the serum contained specific γE antibodies, they form complexes with the antigen on the particles and are measured by adding radiolabeled anti-γE antibodies. The promise of a simple in vitro test for diagnosis of allergic rhinitis is not yet fulfilled by the RAST test and, when applied, it is used in conjunction with, not instead of, skin tests.

TREATMENT. Treatment is directed toward avoiding the allergen, modifying the state of hypersensitivity, and ameliorating the symptoms. By far the most effective means is strict avoidance of the offending allergen. When this is due to an increased sensitivity to an animal dander such as that of horse or cat, merely identifying the cause will help greatly in avoidance. Often patients will "hide" their pets from the physician's inquiry because they have a strong suspicion of the offender but hope that something else will be found. Effective filtration of the air within the patient's house is now possible with a variety of electrostatic and barrier-type filters. Dust control and attention to bedding and furniture filling will be rewarding in selected cases.

Treatment with repeated injections of specific allergens has been in vogue for 70 years, and several studies have confirmed the efficacy of this mode of therapy and given insight to its mechanism. Preseasonal, coseasonal, and perennial administration of allergens all have their proponents, but perennial administration avoids the necessity of building up the dosage each year and results in the same number of patient visits. Increasing amounts of allergen are injected subcutaneously once or twice weekly, starting with a dose shown to be tolerated by skin tests. The goals of hyposensitization are two: production of a nonreaginic (blocking) antibody which can effectively compete with reaginic antibody for allergen, and reduction of the amount of reaginic antibody produced (tolerance induction), thereby decreasing cellular sensitivity to allergen. Addition of serum from a treated individual to sensitized leukocytes in vitro may increase by 100-fold the amounts of allergen necessary for 50 per cent histamine release from these leukocytes.

The increment of allergen injected at each visit is determined by the patient's skin reaction to the previous injection. If redness and swelling exceed the size of a 50-cent piece, the dose should be repeated or lowered until it is better tolerated. Often an increase in sensitivity occurs early in treatment; this may lead to a worsening in symptoms if it coincides with the patient's season. Usually patients are treated for two or more years after maximal benefit has been achieved, at which time hyposensitization is stopped. A proportion of patients will maintain their improvement, whereas, in many, a slow return of symptoms during the following year or 18 months is common. Patients should always be advised to remain in the office for 30 minutes after the injection, because the allergen may provoke a constitutional reaction. This is often heralded by reddening of the conjunctivae, nasal swelling, red ears and nose, and a feeling of faintness. Tourniquets should be applied above the injection sites and 0.2 to 0.5 ml of aqueous epinephrine 1:1000 injected above the tourniquet. Such reactions are uncommon. They are usually easily managed in the office or clinic; but if the patient leaves the office immediately after an allergen injection, the reaction at best will be very frightening and might possibly be fatal.

A variety of repository preparations, including alum-precipitated allergens, have generated interest because of a putative ability to administer more allergen in fewer injections with less likelihood of systemic reactions. The efficacy and safety of these preparations are still to be determined.

Symptomatic Treatment. Antihistamines are often helpful in ameliorating symptoms of allergic rhinitis. In general they are only partially effective, and patients complain of the soporific side effects. Brompheniramine (Dimetane) and chlorpheniramine (Chlor-Trimeton) are both available in 4 mg tablets and in long-acting preparations containing 8 or 12 mg. Both these preparations seem to have less soporific effects than Benadryl, which should be used only at bedtime. Response to these drugs is often quite variable in different patients, and several preparations should be tried if results are poor or side effects great. Dexamethasone (Decadron), administered locally by a special nasal spray inhaler, delivers 0.1 mg per spray, and it is often efficacious. Its use once on each side twice a day is often all that is necessary during a short pollen season. The local effect without systemic liability makes this therapy attractive. Systemic steroids are very effective but are used rarely because of their considerable side effects. A short course of four to five days of 30 mg per day of prednisone will help a new patient over the worst symptoms before other measures become effective or the peak of the season passes.

A variety of sympathomimetic drugs, such as Neo-Synephrine, 0.5 per cent, phenylephrine, 0.25 per cent, or Privine, 0.1 per cent, have been used intranasally to shrink the nasal mucosa, but the effects are short-lived and all cause a "rebound" swelling of the nasal mucosa which may be a self-propagating disease. These drugs are not recommended in allergic rhinitis. For relief of allergic conjunctivitis accompanying pollinosis, eye drops containing epinephrine (0.025 per cent), or dexamethasone (0.1 per cent drops) may be used for a brief period with excellent relief. Prolonged use of steroid eye drops is not recommended because of corneal thinning and cataract formation.

Ishizaka, T., and Ishizaka, K.: Biology of immunoglobulin E. Molecular basis of reaginic hypersensitivity. Prog. Allergy, 19:60, 1975.

Lichtenstein, L. M.: Allergic responses to airborne allergens and insect venoms. Fed. Proc., 36:1727, 1977.

Lieberman, P., and Patterson, R.: Immunotherapy for atopic diseases. Adv. Intern. Med. 19:391, 1974.

Norman, P.S.: Specific therapy in allergy: Pro (with reservations). Med. Clin. North Am., 58:111, 1974.

45. VASOMOTOR RHINITIS

Fred S. Kantor

Vasomotor rhinitis is a vague term describing chronic rhinitis without an allergic basis. It is indistinguishable from allergic rhinitis except for chronicity, absence of geographic or seasonal influences, and prevalence of coexistent nasal polyps. Frequently the patient has sought the use of sympathomimetic drugs administered as nose drops such as Neo-Synephrine or Privine. The problem is compounded by the recurrent rebound rhinitis produced by these agents. Often they are the sole propagating cause of rhinitis which was once allergic or viral in origin, but which has become chronic through the use of these drugs.

The causes of vasomotor rhinitis have been ascribed to bacterial and food allergies, but documentation of these agents is meager and the mechanism is really unknown. Occasionally, a patient with allergies to a variety of ubiquitous substances may present without a clear-cut seasonal environmental history because of the overlapping allergens. These patients may recall a time when their symptoms were seasonal, and skin tests may be helpful in sorting out the problem. In general, however, the bulk of patients with perennial rhinitis at home or away, in summer and winter, will not yield a definite etiologic agent.

Treatment is symptomatic. If nose drops or sprays have been abused, it is useful to discontinue these agents on one side only for a few days and then on the other side so that the patient can breathe through the treated side while the other is recovering from the rebound effects of the drug. Antihistaminics such as brompheniramine (Dimetane), 4 mg every four hours, are sometimes helpful but rarely very successful. Some patients are helped by a nasal dexamethasone spray (Turbinaire) once on each side twice a day. This may produce relief without administering an effective systemic dose and thereby avoid the undesirable side effects.

46. URTICARIA

Fred S. Kantor

DEFINITION. Urticaria, or hives, is an eruption of the skin characterized by elevated, erythematous, sharply demarcated wheals, usually intensively pruritic, lasting hours to days but often recurrent for weeks and sometimes years.

ETIOLOGY AND PATHOGENESIS. The characteristic lesion is produced by capillary dilation in the dermis, leading to loss of fluid into the tissues. Swollen collagen bundles, widening of the dermal papillae, and flattening of the rete pegs are seen microscopically. It is useful to divide the causes into immunologic, paraimmunologic, and nonimmunologic categories.

By far the most common *immunologic cause* of acute hives is food allergy. In this circumstance, vasoactive mediators such as histamine, kinins, and slow-reacting substance of anaphylaxis (SRS-A) are released from mast cells, basophils, and other tissues, producing capillary dilation. The release of mediators is typically due to interaction of antigen with circulating, or fixed, reaginic antibody, usually of the IgE variety. This antibody can be passively transferred by the serum of an affected individual to the skin of a volunteer. A wheal is produced at the transfer site upon ingestion of the offending food antigen. This is the classic Prausnitz-Küstner (PK) reaction. Reactions of IgE antibody with antigen are not complement dependent and produce no vascular necrosis. Complement-dependent IgG-antigen interactions may also cause mediator release by cytotoxic action on mediator-containing cells. These reactions may be produced by antibodies directed against cell antigens, such as isohemagglutinins, and may also be due to antibodies directed against foreign antigens in which the antigen or the complex is passively affixed to the cell surface. The urticaria of serum sickness (see Ch. 42) is such an example. The most frequent route of antigen presentation in the production of acute urticaria is oral ingestion. Inhalation uncommonly produces hives, and occasionally contact with allergen on the skin may suffice. People sensitive to animal dander often report that contact with the fur or saliva of the animal may cause hives; patients allergic to bees may develop hives of the lips and mouth upon contact with honey.

The *"paraimmunologic" causes* are likely to involve similar mechanisms to those of the first category, but the relationship of the antigens and antibodies involved is less apparent. Infection with viruses, bacteria, and fungi may present with hives; hepatitis is a common example. Intestinal parasites, particularly the roundworms, are often associated with hives and eosinophilia. Bites of common insects such as mosquitoes, bedbugs, lice, and other biting insects may produce not only local manifestations but generalized urticaria. Neoplastic diseases, particularly lymphomas of the Hodgkin's variety, and the myeloproliferative diseases are commonly associated with hives. Finally, in the paraimmunologic category are the diseases in which immune complexes have been demonostrated and are thought to play an important etiologic role. In this group, hives are most often associated with systemic lupus erythematosus and dermatomyositis, but the palpable purpura of leukocytoclastic angiitis (Henoch-Schönlein purpura) may first appear as urticaria and then become purpuric.

The nonimmunologic causes of urticaria include physical stimuli such as cold, heat, actinic energy (solar urticaria), and pressure. Cold urticaria may be a familial or sporadic disease in which areas exposed to cold develop urticarial wheals. In about 50 per cent of the sporadic cases, a factor in serum is capable of "sensitizing" normal skin so that a wheal develops when an ice cube is applied to the site. Cold urticaria may be symptomatic of an underlying systemic disease; multiple myeloma, cryoglobulinemia, and syphilis have been reported. The mediators responsible for cold urticaria are presumed to be similar to those released by allergic reactions, but the mechanism of release remains unclear.

Solar urticaria is produced by two spectra of actinic rays of 3100 to 3700Å and 4000 to 5000Å in wavelength. Marked sun exposure in a sensitive individual has led to generalized vascular collapse. Urticaria to sunlight can be passively transferred by serum from individuals who are sensitive to the lower spectrum. The mechanism of mediator release is unknown but, unlike cold urticaria, treatment with drugs and barrier creams is quite effective (see below).

Certain drugs and chemical compounds have the capacity to cause mast cell degranulation directly, resulting in mediator release without an antigen-antibody reaction. Surface-active materials such as saponin, highly negatively charged molecules like polylysines, and many drugs share this property. Common drug examples are morphine, quinine, polymyxin B, curare, decholin, hydralazine, and meperidine. Nonimmunologic release of histamine may be the basis of many "drug reactions" which have failed to yield immunologic mechanisms such as the rare reaction to radiographic contrast agents which are iodinated organic compounds. Indeed, the warm "glow" produced by good brandy is probably more a factor of mediator release than alcohol content, as any ethanol sampler can attest.

A special form of urticaria which consists of small, almost papular, wheals surrounded by a large axon flare is called cholinergic urticaria. Affected individuals will produce a similar eruption when injected with small amounts of mecholyl or acetylcholine. The mechanisms are obscure, but clearly emotional stress, exposure to heat, such as a warm bath, or exercise may bring out the eruption.

Urticaria pigmentosa, or systemic mastocytosis, is due to infiltration of the skin by mast cells; it is believed to be a true neoplasm of very slow growth in which the chemical manifestations are much more distressing to the patient than the invasive ones. Areas of infiltration are marked by freckle-like hyperpigmentation which, upon stroking, will produce a typical linear bumpy wheal, because the skin between the accumulation of mast cells does not urticate.

Chronic urticaria implies recurrent lesions for a period of six weeks or more. The clear causal relationship of certain foods to acute urticaria has led to the assumption that the chronic form is due to an extended exposure to an unidentified allergen or urticator. Investigation of such patients yields a single causal factor in very few, and the bulk of these patients defy elucidation of a specific etiologic factor. Many writers have emphasized psychologic factors in chronic urticaria, but these are difficult to assess.

CLINICAL MANIFESTATIONS. Typically, the wheal is 1 to 5 cm in diameter, often irregular, with a blanched center ("target" lesion) and surrounding erythema. The individual lesions are evanescent, often fading within hours. Successive crops appear for the duration of the disease. The lesions tend to appear at pressure points — e.g., the belt line, the brassiere straps, or the garters. Rarely are the soles and palms affected; but when they are, the patient may complain of difficulty in walking. Pruritus is common and sometimes so severe that the patient cannot wait to get home and fling off his or her clothes. When urticaria is due to a single exposure to a food or drug, it usually appears within minutes. An ingestant taken more than 24 to 48 hours before onset is rarely the cause. Occasionally summation of two allergic stimuli may be responsible; e.g., some patients may eat frozen strawberries in winter with impunity, but during the pollen season the same strawberries will cause hives.

TREATMENT. Acute or sporadic urticaria usually responds well to antihistaminics such as brompheniramine (Dimetane), 4 mg every four hours, or tripelennamine (Pyribenzamine) 50 mg every four hours. Long-acting preparations, containing 8 and 12 mg of brompheniramine respectively, are available and may be used in a twice-a-day regimen as opposed to giving 4 mg every four hours. If the patient is in acute distress, 0.3 ml of 1:1000 epinephrine subcutaneously will often provide relief until the antihistaminic effect is apparent. In severe or unresponsive cases of sporadic urticaria, four days of prednisone, 40 mg per day may be necessary and very helpful.

In chronic urticaria the cause is rarely evident and therefore hard to remove. Most patients have been treated with antihistaminics without benefit. The use of a rigid elimination diet may not only remove hidden allergens, but more likely may also remove foods such as spices which are direct releasers of histamine. In addition to the elimination diet, liberal doses of brompheniramine (Dimetane), 8 mg every four hours, and hydroxyzine, 10 to 25 mg three times a day, are helpful. After a period of relief, cautious reduction of the drug regimen and addition of selective foods in groups, such as eggs, milk, and milk products, one at a time every three to four days, will often result in cessation of symptoms. The result is frequently a grateful patient on a full diet; the doctor, however, remains perplexed. Recently attention has been drawn to a proportion (about 1:7) of patients with chronic urticaria in whom this is a manifestation of vasculitis. This should be suspected in patients with chronic urticaria associated with hypocomplementemia, arthralgia, elevation of erythrocyte sedimentation rate, or serum globulins.

Cold urticaria is often refractory to treatment with all the agents mentioned above, and often the patient has to adjust his life style to avoid the cold. In contrast, solar urticaria is readily treated with barrier creams that filter out the actinic energy of the appropriate wave length. Hydroxychloroquine (Plaquenil), 200 mg, once daily or even twice a week, may protect a sensitive person who anticipates sun exposure.

Mathison, D. A., Arroyave, C. M., Bhat, K. N., Hurewitz, D. J., and Marnell, D. J.: Hypocomplementemia in chronic idiopathic urticaria. Ann. Intern. Med., 86:534, 1977.

Matthews, K. P.: A current review of urticaria. Med. Clin. North Am., 58:185, 1974.

47.   ANGIOEDEMA

(Angioneurotic Edema)

Fred S. Kantor

DEFINITION. Angioedema is characterized by painless swelling in the subcutaneous tissues or submucosa, usually occurring about the face (eyes, lips, tongue), but any part of the body may be involved. Two types are now well recognized: sporadic, transient angioedema, related to giant urticaria but involving deeper vessels, caused primarily by food allergy; and hereditary angioedema, which is transmitted as an autosomal dominant trait and is marked by severe deficiency in function of an inhibitor to the activated first component of complement — C'1 esterase.

ETIOLOGY. The causes of the sporadic type are the same as in urticaria (see Ch. 46) and most frequently involve food allergy, although occasionally an inhalant or contactant may be incriminated. In some, emotional factors can trigger an attack. A definite relationship between aspirin ingestion and angioedema has been documented in some individuals. Often asthma and nasal polyps are also associated. Evidence does not favor an immunologic basis for this syndrome, and the mechanism is unknown; the recently reported effect of aspirin upon prostaglandins may provide an important lead.

The lesion of the familial variety is indistinguishable from the sporadic type but is not related to hypersensitivity. Serum from affected persons who are heterozygotes (the trait is dominant) has very low inhibitor activity between attacks and often none measurable during the attack. In a variant of the disease the inhibitor is present but in an inactive form. Deficiency of the inhibitor is due to impaired synthesis, because catabolic rates in affected patients are normal.

PATHOGENESIS. Sporadic angioedema may be thought of as a variant of giant urticaria, with dilation of subcutaneous instead of cutaneous vessels and leakage of fluid and colloid into the tissues. It is generally believed that interaction of ingested allergens with reaginic antibody causes release of vasoactive mediators, including histamine, slow-reacting substance of anaphylaxis (SRS-A), and, possibly, bradykinins. Because the affected capillaries are deep, redness and intradermal swelling are not features. Respiratory and gastrointestinal symptoms occur rarely; the latter should raise a strong suspicion of hereditary angioedema, because abdominal pain is a common feature of the familial disease.

The relationship of the deficiency of C'1 esterase inhibitor to the attacks of angioedema is a complicated one. Attacks are associated with the presence of active C'1, depletion of its natural substrates which are C'4 and C'2, and elevation of bradykinin levels. In addition to inhibiting C'1 esterase activity, the inhibitor is known to inhibit kallikrein and plasmin. Kallikrein converts a serum alpha globulin to bradykinin; plasmin is a broad tryptic-like enzyme which digests fibrin, may cleave C'3 to produce anaphylatoxin (a vasoactive mediator), and may digest Hageman factor into active fragments which can convert prekallikrein to kallikrein. C'1 esterase inhibitor also reduces the capacity of active Hageman factor or its fragments to convert prekallikrein to kallikrein and to convert plasminogen proactivator to the active form. To sum up: the C'1 esterase inhibitor acts at several places, and its deficiency favors the formation of vasoactive mediators from the complement sequence (C'2a, C'3a) and indirectly from the formation of active plasmin and kallikrein.

CLINICAL MANIFESTATIONS. The lesion is a tense, rounded, nonpitting swelling several centimeters in diameter which may last two or three days. In addition to the face, the hands, feet, and genitalia are often affected. In the familial form, laryngeal edema accounts for death in 30 per cent of the patients. Severe abdominal pain, vomiting, and the appearance of an acute intra-abdominal condition are common in the familial type and are important differentiating features from the sporadic variety. During abdominal attacks a characteristic pattern of bowel wall edema can sometimes be demonstrated in x-rays of the gastrointestinal tract. Attacks may be initiated after minor trauma such as tooth extraction, supporting the relationship to the clotting mechanism and the role of Hageman factor activation.

DIAGNOSIS. The sudden appearance of profound swelling without trauma or underlying infection is strongly suggestive of angioedema. Accompanying urticaria or a history of food allergy is helpful, but an inapparent insect bite can sometimes cause swelling of the eyelid or lip and must be considered. The familial form often presents with abdominal complaints accompanying the subcutaneous swelling, and laryngeal edema is also frequently noted. Symptoms of hereditary angioedema may rarely first appear in adult life, and the presence of active C'1 esterase inhibitor should be confirmed in any case involving laryngeal edema or abdominal complaints.

PROGNOSIS. The sporadic variety tends to recur either because all the causative factors are not identified, or, more likely, because the patient "cheats" and samples a forbidden food. The hereditary form of the disease is often fatal in early life, although not before reproductive age.

TREATMENT. Like urticaria, sporadic angioedema is treated with epinephrine, 0.3 to 0.5 ml, 1:1000, or an aqueous solution containing crystalline epinephrine 1:200 (Sus-Phrine), 0.6 to 0.8 ml, given in conjunction with antihistamines. Brompheniramine (Dimetane), 4 mg, tripelennamine (Pyribenzamine), 50 mg, or diphenhydramine (Benadryl), 50 mg, may be given every four hours. (Long-acting preparations, containing 8 and 12 mg of brompheniramine respectively, are available and may be used in a twice-a-day regimen as opposed to giving 4 mg every four hours.) Resolution is slow, because resorption of tissue fluid is required. Prednisone, 40 mg per day, may be given for three to four days in severe or prolonged cases. The patient should be carefully questioned about activities within the 12- to 24-hour period preceding the onset, with special reference to items passing the lips such as food, chewing gum, toothpaste, or aspirin. Usually the patient knows the culprit.

In the hereditary form of disease the aforementioned measures are useless. Poor responses to epinephrine, antihistamine, and corticosteroids are well documented. Highly encouraging results have been produced by treatment with androgen derivatives such as methyltestosterone and danazol, which not only prevent attacks of edema and abdominal pain but also cause a reversal of the biochemical defect. Danazol, 200 mg three times daily, is associated with rapid reappearance of the functional form of the serum C'1 esterase inhibitor and virtual absence of clinical attacks without virilizing side effects.

Gelfand, J. A., Sherino, R. J., Alling, D. W., and Frank, M. M.: Treatment of hereditary angioedema with danazol. Reversal of clinical and biochemical abnormalities. N. Engl. J. Med., 295:1444, 1976.

Ruddy, S., Gigli, I., and Austen, K. F.: The complement system of man. N. Engl. J. Med., 287:489, 1972.

48.   INSECT STINGS

Fred S. Kantor

Allergy to antigens contained in the venom of the Hymenoptera insects (bee, wasp, hornet, yellow jacket) may produce a fatal reaction when an otherwise healthy victim is stung. Often a history is obtained of a previous sting which produced local swelling more extensive and longlasting than usual. The patient may rapidly develop shock with or without respiratory difficulty, urticaria, or angioedema, and prompt treatment is vital. If the site of the sting is known, and on an extremity, a tourniquet should be placed above the site to delay further absorption of venom. Epinephrine, 1:1000, 0.3 to 0.5 ml, should be given subcutaneously. If the patient is in shock, the intravenous route must be used, despite the hazard of arrhythmia, to ensure absorption of the drug. Bees have barbed stingers and leave the stinger and venom sac at the site. These should be removed with a forceps or scraped off with the edge of a fingernail so that the venom remaining in the venom sac is not injected through the stinger into the patient. Antihistaminics and steroids are given as adjuncts to epinephrine as described in Ch. 47.

After the acute episode is controlled and before leaving, the patient should be given an emergency kit which contains two tourniquets (stings may be multiple), forceps, or an eyebrow tweezer, a syringe for epinephrine injection (1 ml, 1:1000), and antihistamine tablets. If restung, the patient is instructed to place the tourniquet above the site, take one antihistaminic tablet (diphenhydramine [Benadryl], 50 mg), and prepare the epinephrine syringe while obtaining help from others. Muscular activity enhances the rate of absorption of venom; the patient should be urged to walk, not run, toward help. Since a generalized reaction may lead to temporary skin-test refractoriness, the patient is urged to return in three weeks for testing and hyposensitization treatment. Venom rather than allergenic extracts of the whole insect's body are more efficacious for diagnostic testing and hyposensitization treatment. Until venom extracts are freely available for treatment, the physician should keep in mind and explain to the patient that the efficacy of whole body extracts is in question; they may be used until such time as venom is available.

Lichtenstein, L. M., Valentine, M. D., and Sobotka, A. K.: A case for venom treatment in anaphylactic sensitivity to hymenoptera sting. N. Engl. J. Med., 290:122, 1974.

Zeleznick, L .D., Hunt, K. J., Sobotka, A. K., Valentine, M. D., Tippet, M. M. S., and Lichtenstein, L. M.: Diagnosis of hymenoptera hypersensitivity by skin testing with hymenoptera venoms. J. Allergy Clin. Immunol., 59:2, 1977.

PART VI

CONNECTIVE TISSUE DISEASES ("COLLAGEN DISEASES") OTHER THAN RHEUMATOID ARTHRITIS

49. INTRODUCTION

K. Frank Austen

The connective tissue ("collagen") diseases or systemic rheumatic diseases are a group of clinicopathologic entities considered together because of common or overlapping clinical and histologic features. The term "collagen diseases" was introduced by Klemperer for such reasons and not because of any conviction about a common etiology. Each of the major entities within this grouping has prominent nonspecific constitutional manifestations coupled with patterns of organ involvement which determine the clinical designation, i.e., rheumatoid arthritis, rheumatic fever, systemic lupus erythematosus, scleroderma, dermatomyositis, and periarteritis nodosa (polyarteritis nodosa). Except for rheumatic fever (see Ch. 130), these entities are considered in this Part and in Part VII. The common histologic features of the group are widespread inflammatory damage to connective tissues and blood vessels, at times associated with deposition of fibrinoid material. Fibrinoid refers to an amorphous material, mainly fibrin, staining deeply eosinophilic with hematoxylin and eosin, which is deposited along connective tissue fibers and within vessel walls, and most probably represents a nonspecific response of connective tissue to injury. Clinical findings which have been invoked to support a common grouping include cardinal features of more than one entity in the same patient; transitions between one entity and another within the same patient; possible familial aggregation; and serologic abnormalities which may predominate in one entity but have an appreciable incidence in others.

Progressive systemic sclerosis (scleroderma), polymyositis alone or with cutaneous manifestations (dermatomyositis), and systemic lupus erythematosus (SLE) have distinct clinicopathologic and/or serologic features. By contrast, periarteritis nodosa has neither a characteristic morphologic, biochemical, or immunochemical abnormalty nor a clinical presentation that is easily distinguished from systemic necrotizing angiitis of other types, including those which may be associated with any of the other connective tissue diseases. It seems pertinent, therefore, to review historically the problem of necrotizing angiitis and to include an operational classification based almost entirely upon clinical considerations. A discussion of the structure and function of

the structural proteins, collagen and elastin, and the proteoglycan of the connective tissue matrix or ground substance is presented first.

CONNECTIVE TISSUE

Connective tissues are composed of various combinations of collagen, elastin, proteoglycans, and other less well characterized glycoproteins. The unique proportions and distribution of these individual components give different organs of connective tissue their particular qualities. The proteoglycans and the specific arrangement of collagen fibers at various layers give cartilage its smooth, translucent quality and its toughness with elasticity; in contrast, bone has a lesser amount of proteoglycans and a rigid structure related to mineralization within and around collagen fibers. The lens of the eye is transparent because of the precise orthogonal planes in which collagen fibrils are laid down. Skin and blood vessels are rich in elastin, which confers upon these tissues a capacity for distensibility. Basement membrane, a specialized form of collagen and glycoprotein, separates epithelium and endothelium from their environment in multiple tissues. Only in very rare diseases is a primary abnormality of the connective tissue responsible for symptoms or pathology. However, in all forms of arthritis or vasculitis the connective tissues are the site in which inflammation occurs. Although playing a passive, secondary role in pathophysiology, it is damage to connective tissue that results in the signs and symptoms of disease.

Collagen is synthesized by all mesenchymal cells and by some epithelial tissue as well. There are at least four genetic types of collagen distinguished by small but constant variations in amino acid composition: Type I collagen is found exclusively in bone, dentin, and tendon and is mixed in with other types of collagen in most other tissues; Type II collagen predominates in articular cartilage; Type III collagen (which contains an interchain disulfide bond within the helical portion of the molecule) is present in largest proportion relative to other types in skin and blood vessels; Type IV collagen, less well characterized, is an important component of basement membranes. Each collagen molecule has a biosynthetic precursor, or procollagen, which contains nonhelical peptide sequences at both NH_2^- and COOH-terminal ends of the molecule. After procollagen has been hydroxylated (hydroxyproline from proline and hydroxylysine from lysine) and glycosylated, it is released from the cell. The nonhelical ends of the molecules are cleaved off, and the collagen molecules aggregate with others to form fibrils. Each collagen molecule is formed of three α chains, each approximately 1010 amino acids in length, coiled about each other in a complex triple helical arrangement. It is this helical structure which confers upon the collagen stability, rigidity, and resistance to proteases.

This precise register of individual molecules in fibril form gives the 640 to 700 Å periodicity on electron microscopy characteristic of collagen fibrils. After fibril formation an additional change in primary structure of the molecule occurs to give cross-linking within and between different molecules. ϵ-Amino groups on lysine and hydroxylysine are oxidized to aldehydes. These reactive groups condense with other aldehydes or form a Schiff base with amino groups to create cross-links. These cross-links give stability through insolubility and resistance of fibrils to collagenolytic enzymes.

Recently synthesized collagen has a more rapid turnover than mature collagen. Since hydroxyproline is present only in collagen and elastin, and since collagen is the most abundant protein in the body, the excretion of urinary hydroxyproline serves as a rough index of collagen turnover. Collagen is degraded by collagenases present in mesenchymal tissues, certain epithelial tissues, and polymorphonuclear leukocytes; collagenases cleave through one site on each collagen triple helix. The reaction products uncoil, are thermally denatured at body temperature, and become immediately susceptible to multiple tissue proteases. In rheumatoid arthritis and certain skin and bone diseases, proliferation of cells which synthesize collagenase may result in excessive destruction of collagen.

Developmental abnormalities in the complicated sequence of collagen biosynthesis lead to expression of a number of diseases. For example, insufficient production of Type I collagen is found in some cases of *osteogenesis imperfecta*. Post-translational abnormalities include inadequate hydroxylation of lysine and proline in *scurvy*, inadequate hydroxylation of lysine in certain tissues in *Ehlers-Danlos* syndrome Type VI, insufficient procollagen conversion to collagen in Ehlers-Danlos *Type VII*, and inhibition of cross-link formation among collagen molecules in *homocystinuria* by the reactive sulfhydryl group in homocysteine.

Proteoglycans have a role in connective tissue not unlike that of cement in reinforced concrete. The proteoglycans are formed of subunits of disaccharides linked together (termed glycosaminoglycan chains) and joined to a protein core. In articular cartilage this core is a protein with a length of 20,000 to 50,000 Å. The disaccharide chains, many of which are sulfated, have a length of 15,000 to 36,000 Å. Each proteoglycan monomer (core protein plus disaccharide chains) is joined with others to form large aggregates with hyaluronic acid chains stabilized by a link glycoprotein. The physiologic implications of this macromolecular organization are probably related to the excluded volume effect; that is, in connective tissue, they control by virtue of size and domain the passage of other molecules to and from cells. The large net negative charge among proteoglycans serves to impart to tissues containing them in high concentration (e.g., cartilage) a resistance to compressive force. In the polysaccharide (glycosaminogly-can) component of proteoglycans one of the hexose residues of each disaccharide group is a hexosamine, and the other is a hexuronic acid moiety. Proteoglycans are synthesized by mesenchymal tissues by a complicated process involving assembly of the polysaccharide units, sulfation, and covalent linkage to the protein core.

Proteoglycans have a more rapid turnover than collagen and are degraded primarily by acid hydrolases found in lysosomes, such as cathepsin C and B. Factors such as vitamin A which destabilize lysosomal membranes can result in generalized depletion of proteoglycans from many connective tissues. Proteoglycan destruction is accentuated by an inflammatory response in the connective tissue.

Elastin has covalent cross-links, desmosine and isodesmosine, which are similar to cross-links in collagen and are formed from condensation of lysine residues on different parts of the same chain or other elastin polypeptides. Unlike collagen, which is a rigid rod, elastin is an amorphous random coil aggregate linked by these cross-links; this structure assures its return to an original configuration after it is distorted and gives rise to its elastic properties. Elastin fibers have two components: the amorphous elastin polypeptides containing a great quantity of nonpolar amino acids, and the glycoprotein microfibrils which may act as a template for amorphous elastin production. A proelastin has been described which, like procollagen, must have a COOH-terminal registration peptide cleaved away before insoluble elastic fibers can be formed.

HISTORICAL REVIEW OF ANGIITIS

The term *necrotizing angiitis* or *vasculitis* designates disorders in which there is segmental inflammation with fibrinoid necrosis of the blood vessels. Criteria that allow the definition of clinical syndromes include the gross and histologic appearance of the vascular lesions, the caliber of the affected blood vessels, the frequency of involvement of specific organs, and the absence or presence of hematologic and serologic abnormalities. Inasmuch as necrotizing angiitis is segmental and spotty in distribution, involvement of internal organs is generally not appreciated unless a partial or complete occlusion substantially compromises function. In contrast, this process is recognized visually in the skin without or with local or systemic symptoms.

The term *periarteritis nodosa* was aptly introduced by Kussmaul and Maier in 1866 to designate a morbid process manifested by numerous nodules along muscular-type arteries. Infiltration of the media with polymorphonuclear leukocytes and to a lesser extent eosinophils, plasma cells, and lymphocytes, disruption of the internal elastic lamina, fibrinoid necrosis, and extension to the adventitia and intima are characteristic. Proliferation of the intima leads to partial or total occlusion, and segmental scarring of the entire wall is responsible for the visible and/or palpable aneurysms. It is characteristic of the lesions to be in all stages of evolution from acute to healed. Additional characteristic features of periarteritis nodosa are the sparing of capillaries and veins except for involvement by spread from contiguous arteries, and the absence of involvement of pulmonary arteries despite the location of nodules in the bronchial arteries.

In 1923 Ophüls reported a patient with a periarteritis

nodosa–like illness with the additional features of pulmonary vessel lesions, extensive involvement of small arteries and veins, granulomatous vascular and extravascular reactions, and an intense eosinophilic infiltration of vascular and pulmonary parenchymal lesions. The granulomas often included an eosinophilic core of altered collagen and necrotic eosinophils surrounded by radially arranged macrophages, lymphocytes, plasma cells, and varying numbers of polymorphonuclear leukocytes, both neutrophilic and eosinophilic. A detailed study of similar patients in 1951 by Churg and Strauss emphasized the striking clinical feature of severe progressive asthma with peripheral eosinophilia followed by fever, and prompted these authors to term this entity *allergic angiitis and granulomatosis*. Rose and Spencer (1957) also appreciated these unique clinicopathologic features but preferred the term *polyarteritis with pulmonary involvement* to distinguish this group from classic polyarteritis.

In 1926 von Glahn and Pappenheimer considered that the *arteritis of rheumatic fever* could be distinguished from periarteritis nodosa by the absence of arterial thrombosis (or eosinophils), involvement of small arteries, and minimal fibrinoid necrosis. In the heart, Aschoff bodies represent a key extravascular histologic finding, although the clinical manifestations are predominantly related to rheumatic carditis.

Still another type of necrotizing vascular lesion, originally believed to be limited to the cranial arteries and characterized by the presence of multinucleated giant cells, was recognized by Horton, Magath, and Brown in 1934 and established as a clinical entity by Kilbourne and Wolff in 1946. The process usually involves the innermost layer of the media with predominantly a lymphocyte infiltration, the presence of multinucleated giant cells, fragmentation of the internal elastic lamina, and associated fibrinoid necrosis. The infiltration may extend to involve the adventitia and the intima, leading to intimal thickening with subsequent thrombosis. This entity, *giant cell arteritis*, can be predominantly local — presenting as cranial, especially temporal, or aortic arch (Takayasu's) arteritis — or it may be systemic. The syndrome of polymyalgia rheumatica seems to be associated with a local or systemic form of giant cell arteritis with or without arterial occlusion.

Necrotizing vascular lesions associated with the administration of horse antiserum and the development of clinical serum sickness were described by Clark and Kaplan in 1937. Rich observed similar lesions (1942) which he considered to be periarteritis nodosa not only in cases of serum sickness but also in circumstances of sulfonamide hypersensitivity. However, the more recent and prevailing view proposed by Zeek in 1952 is that hypersensitivity to drugs and serum, termed *hypersensitivity angiitis*, is distinguishable from periarteritis nodosa. Hypersensitivity angiitis involves small arteries, arterioles, and venules in a process of fibrinoid necrosis, occurring in the subendothelial ground substance and extending from the intima to involve the entire vessel wall; the accompanying cellular reaction is pleomorphic with polymorphonuclear neutrophil leukocyte predominance frequently including eosinophils. Hypersensitivity angiitis often involves the pulmonary system and is characterized by virtually all lesions of an episode being at a similar evolutionary stage.

Wegener's granulomatosis is distinguished from aller-

gic granulomatosis and angiitis as defined by Churg and Strauss. Wegener in 1936 described a disease characterized by necrotizing granulomatous lesions of the upper and lower respiratory tract, generalized focal necrotizing lesions of both arteries and veins, and a glomerulitis typified by fibrin thrombi, focal necrosis of tufts, and on occasion a granulomatous reaction. This complex is somewhat similar to allergic granulomatosis and angiitis, but is is noteworthy that Wegener's granulomatosis is not associated with progressive asthma and prominent peripheral eosinophilia and does not exhibit a prominence of eosinophils in the necrotizing lesions. Thus it seems reasonable to list this entity separately; lethal midline granuloma may be a related condition or a local variant. (See Ch. 68.) More recently, variants of Wegener's granulomatosis have been recognized in which the granulomatous reactions are predominantly lymphoid- and sarcoid-like, respectively.

OPERATIONAL CLASSIFICATION OF NECROTIZING ANGIITIS

Necrotizing angiitis is a convenient generic term for the entire group of syndromes in which vascular lesions, arterial or venous or both, may involve all three layers of the vessel wall with fibrinoid necrosis and various cellular infiltrates (see accompanying table). Zeek recognized five major syndromes in this group: periarteritis nodosa, allergic angiitis and granulomatosis, rheumatic fever, giant cell arteritis, and hypersensitivity angiitis. With some modification this tabulation continues to be operationally useful. The limitations of this classification, however, are becoming increasingly apparent with the demonstration of involvement of vessels of various sizes in the same clinical process.

Rheumatic fever can be placed under a category broadened to include those collagen diseases in which necrotizing vascular lesions are present but are not the most prominent aspect of the entity, i.e., rheumatoid arthritis, scleroderma, dermatomyositis, polymyositis,

---

Necrotizing Angiitis

Periarteritis nodosa (polyarteritis nodosa)
Allergic angiitis and granulomatosis of Churg and Strauss
  ("polyarteritis nodosa with pulmonary involvement")
Connective tissue disease ("collagen disease"), associated with
  Rheumatoid arthritis
  Scleroderma
  Poly- and dermatomyositis
  Rheumatic fever
  Erythema nodosum
  Sjögren's syndrome
Giant cell arteritis
Hypersensitivity angiitis
  Drug reaction
  Henoch-Schönlein purpura
  Systemic lupus erythematosus, rheumatoid arthritis, Sjögren's
    syndrome
  Mixed cryoglobulinemia
  Nodular vasculitis
  Hypergammaglobulinemic purpura
  C2 deficiency with vasculitis
  Australian antigenemia with vasculitis
  Subacute bacterial endocarditis and other infections
  Lymphoproliferative disorders
  Erythema elevatum diutinum
Wegener's granulomatosis and variants

Sjögren's syndrome, and erythema nodosum. The situation in rheumatoid arthritis is particularly instructive in that necrotizing angiitis presents with three syndromes: polyarteritis nodosa resulting from involvement of medium-sized muscular arteries; peripheral neuropathy, digital gangrene, and cutaneous ulcers secondary to disease of small arteries; and palpable purpura as a manifestation of cutaneous necrotizing venulitis.

The category of hypersensitivity angiitis is particularly diverse and contains a variety of clinical entities distinguishable on the basis of precipitating events (drugs, hepatitis B antigenemia, subacute bacterial endocarditis, and *Mycobacterium leprae* infection), serologic abnormalities (cryoglobulinemia, hypergammaglobulinemic purpura, homozygous C2 deficiency), underlying diseases (rheumatoid arthritis, systemic lupus erythematosus, Sjögren's syndrome, lymphoproliferative disorders), and characteristic clinical presentations (Henoch-Schönlein purpura, nodular vasculitis with its lower extremity distribution and predilection for females, and erythema elevatum diutinum appearing as erythematous plaques over articular surfaces).

The problems of any effort at classification are highlighted by the vasculitis associated with Australian antigenemia and designated periarteritis nodosa by some. The clinical manifestations of urticaria, arthralgia, fever, eosinophilia, and azotemia; the pathologic findings of fibrinoid necrotizing lesions of arterioles in liver and muscle and venules in skin with deposition of immunoglobulin, viral antigen, and complement; and the serologic presence of circulating immune complexes with hypocomplementemia are entirely consistent with hypersensitivity angiitis. The demonstration of abnormalities of the medium-sized muscular arteries by angiography emphasizes the continuum of lesions characteristic of periarteritis nodosa to hypersensitivity angiitis under these etiologic circumstances. In one study only a single patient out of nine with vasculitis and hepatitis B antigenemia presented the classic manifestations of polyarteritis nodosa alone, prompting the observers to propose the generic term generalized necrotizing vasculitis for this group.

An operational classification is nonetheless a justified interim measure because there are associated implications as to prognosis, treatment, and etiology. A classification based on etiology and pathogenetic mechanisms is a further goal. The fibrinoid in the lesions of systemic lupus erythematosus contains protein residues of nuclear origin, acid mucopolysaccharides derived from altered ground substance, and fibrinogen (or derivatives), immunoglobulins, and complement proteins. These findings are interpreted to mean the presence of immune complexes, consisting of nuclear antigen and antibody, complement fixation, and secondary deposition of fibrinogen and alteration of ground substance. In vasculitis associated with Australian antigenemia, immune complexes with specific antigen have been isolated from the plasma and recognized in tissues along with complement by immunofluorescent studies. Whereas in systemic lupus erythematosus, vasculitis with Australian antigenemia, and mixed cryoglobulinemia the specificity of the antibodies contributing to or responsible for the clinicopathologic manifestations of the disease is known, such is not the case for most of the other entities shown in the table. Studies of 1-μm-

thick sections stained with Giemsa's reagent have allowed the recognition of two cellular patterns in the skin of patients with cutaneous hypersensitivity angiitis. In individuals with serum hypocomplementemia the cellular infiltrate contains predominately neutrophils, whereas lymphocytes and activated lymphocytes are the predominant cells in the normocomplementemic group. Although the pathologic findings could represent different stages of a single process, transition from one to the other type of pathology in individual patients has not yet been reported, and the processes could reflect different host responses. Immunoglobulins and complement have been observed in the glomerular and cutaneous lesions of Henoch-Schönlein purpura, in the vascular lesions of rheumatoid arthritis and of periarteritis nodosa, and in the granulomatous response of allergic angiitis and granulomatosis (often with fibrinogen), but not in Wegener's granulomatosis. Such proteins could deposit nonspecifically owing to trapping, transudation or exudation, or because of aggregation of gamma globulin. It is also true, however, that deposition of immune complexes may be underestimated because of their rapid clearance. Studies should be directed toward determining the specificity of the deposited immunoglobulins. Arguments to favor specific deposition could be based on demonstration of antigen in the lesion, recognition of the antibody specificity following elution, and demonstration that the predominant L chain type or H chain subgroup in the deposit is different from the ratio observed in the circulation. Each of these criteria has been met with regard to the lesions of systemic lupus erythematosus.

Christian, C. L., and Sergent, J. S.: Vasculitis syndromes: Clinical and experimental models. Am. J. Med., 61:385, 1976.

Churg, J., and Strauss, L.: Allergic granulomatosis, allergic angiitis, and periarteritis nodosa. Am. J. Pathol., 27:277, 1951.

Frohnert, P. P., and Sheps, S. G.: Long-term follow-up study of periarteritis nodosa. Am. J. Med., 43:8, 1967.

Glass, D., Soter, N. A., and Schur, P. H.: Rheumatoid vasculitis. Arthritis Rheum., 19:950, 1976.

Gocke, D. J., Morgan, C., Lockshin, J., Hsu, K., Bombardieri, S., and Christian, C. L.: Association between polyarteritis and Australian antigen. Lancet, 2:1149, 1970.

Grant, M. E., and Prockop, D. J.: The biosynthesis of collagen. N. Engl. J. Med., 286:194, 242, 291, 1972.

Harris, E. D., Evanson, J. M., Dibona, D. R., and Krane, S. M.: Collagenase and rheumatoid arthritis. Arthritis Rheum., 13:83, 1970.

Kilbourne, E. D., and Wolff, H. G.: Cranial arteritis: Critical evaluation of syndrome of "temporal arteritis," with report of a case. Ann. Intern. Med., 24:1, 1946.

Klemperer, P.: The concept of collagen disease in medicine. Am. Rev. Respir. Dis., 83:331, 1961.

Kussmaul, A., and Maier, R.: Über eine bisher nicht beschreibene eigenthümlich Arterienerkrankung (Periarteritis nodosa), die mit Morbus Brightii and rapid fortschreitender allgemeiner Muskellähmung einhergeht. Deutsch. Arch. Klin. Med., 1:484, 1866.

Liebow, A. A.: Pulmonary angiitis and granulomatosis. Am. Rev. Respir. Dis., 108:1, 1973.

Silbert, J. E.: Biosynthesis of muco-polysaccharides and proteinpolysaccharides. *In* Perez-Tamayo, R., and Rojkind, M. (eds.): Molecular Pathology of Connective Tissues. New York, Marcel Dekker, Inc., 1973.

Soter, N. A., Mihm, M. C., Gigli, I., Dvorak, H. F., and Austen, K. F.: Two distinct cellular patterns in cutaneous necrotizing angiitis. J. Invest. Dermat., 66:344, 1976.

Wegener, F.: Über generalisierte, septische Gefässerkrankungen. Verh. Deutsch. Ges. Path., 29:202, 1936.

Wolff, S. M., Fauci, A. S., Horn, R. G., and Dale, D. C.: Wegener's granulomatosis. Ann. Intern. Med., 81:513, 1974.

Zeek, P. M.: Periarteritis nodosa: A critical review. Am. J. Clin. Pathol., 22:777, 1952.

50. SYSTEMIC SCLEROSIS

(Scleroderma)

Edward D. Harris, Jr.

GENERAL CONSIDERATIONS. *Scleroderma* is a disease involving blood vessels and connective tissue. The clinical picture is dominated by symptoms of vascular insufficiency caused by abnormalities in small arterioles and capillaries, and by progressive fibrosis in multiple organs. Most patients have involvement predominantly of the arms and hands with Raynaud's phenomenon and acrosclerosis. The face and upper chest may be affected as well, but it is interesting that the legs and feet are involved less often, and it is rare that diffuse involvement of the entire skin is seen. Associated with the cutaneous manifestations are dysfunctions of certain viscera, particularly the esophagus, lungs, and kidneys.

Localized scleroderma, a term which includes morphea and linear scleroderma, involves the skin exclusively.

The diagnosis of systemic sclerosis is made most often in patients between the ages of 35 and 55. Between three and five new cases per million population appear each year. Only 8 per cent of cases begin in the first two decades of life. The disease is three times more common in females than in males. There is some evidence that black women have a poorer prognosis than white women, and males a poorer prognosis than females.

PATHOGENESIS AND PATHOLOGY. Pathogenesis. Data are accumulating to indicate that abnormalities in the vascular system are primarily involved in the pathogenesis of this disease. Raynaud's phenomenon with its characteristic blanching and pain followed by suffusion is a very common initial complaint in systemic sclerosis. Patients with Raynaud's phenomenon have been shown to have significantly decreased cutaneous fingertip blood flow compared with that of normal controls when both are cooled to 18° C. In clinically unaffected muscle tissue, patients with scleroderma have been shown to have loss of 80 per cent of the normal amount of capillaries; those remaining capillaries have a diameter increased over normal, swollen endothelial cells, and reduplication of the basement membrane. Surface microvessels of the nail fold in systemic sclerosis are decreased in number, dilated, and tortuous. Digital arteriograms in patients with Raynaud's syndrome and scleroderma often have shown obstruction of the proper digital arteries, and plethysmography has demonstrated decreased amplitude of reflection of the pulse. There may be a common factor of altered vascular reactivity in the development of Raynaud's phenomenon, depressed sensitivity to cholinergic agonists of the lower esophageal sphincter, pulmonary hypertension, and reduced renal cortical blood flow — all abnormalities associated with systemic sclerosis.

Studies of the proliferative lesion of scleroderma (the appearance of excessive and inappropriate collagen deposition) have revealed no significant abnormality of physical properties, amino acid analyses, cross-linking, or solubility of collagen. Areas of rapid new collagen synthesis may have a higher ratio than normal of Type III to Type I collagen.

Numerous studies have indicated that there is an increased rate of collagen synthesis in scleroderma. Increased activity of protocollagen proline hydroxylase has been found in skin biopsies from scleroderma. Medium from cultures in vitro of some scleroderma skin fibroblasts has been found to contain significantly more collagen than does medium from control cells.

Association of fibrosis with the carcinoid syndrome has generated interest in study of amine metabolism. Some patients with scleroderma have been reported to have a decreased monamine oxidase activity in plasma, although measurements of plasma catecholamine concentrations and urinary catecholamine excretion patterns have been normal.

Interest has expanded in the possible involvement of the cellular immune system in pathogenesis of scleroderma. Lymphokines (e.g., soluble products of activated lymphocytes and monocytes) which stimulate collagen production by fibroblasts and which are chemotactic for dermal fibroblasts have been defined. Mononuclear cells from scleroderma patients produce a factor chemotactic for human monocytes when cultured in the presence of collagen.

Immunoglobulin and complement have been selectively localized in vascular lesions of the kidneys of patients with scleroderma, and antinuclear antibodies have been eluted from renal tissue, suggesting, but not proving, a role for immune complexes in pathogenesis of acute renal failure in this disease.

Pathology. The result of systemic involvement in scleroderma is sclerosis. Early findings in the *skin* in active scleroderma have revealed edema, plasma cell and/or lymphocyte infiltrates around eccrine sweat glands, loss of capillaries, and endothelial proliferation. Larger vessels may show fibromucinous accumulations in the intima. The *reticular dermis* is usually thickened. It may have a normal collagen-bundle pattern or may show broad, homogeneous, acellular deposits of collagen with indistinct bundle patterns. Other findings include atrophy of the rete pegs of the epidermis, atrophy of the hair follicles and sweat glands, perivascular lymphocytic infiltration, and hyalinization of arterioles. The subcutaneous tissue is replaced by thick collagen bundles which bind the dermis to deeper structures. Pathologic changes in the musculoskeletal system include acute and chronic inflammation in the *synovium* with no pannus formation but with more sclerosis than is found in rheumatoid synovium with an equivalent inflammatory response. Fibrin deposits are laid down around *tendons*, and in *muscles* there are a variety of abnormalities, the most common being fibrosis of the perimysium and epimysium, scattered cellular infiltrates, and atrophy and necrosis of muscle fibers similar to that seen in polymyositis.

In the internal organs, microvascular abnormalities (see Pathogenesis), mild inflammation, and edema in connective tissue are followed by increased deposition of fibrous tissue in both appropriate and inappropriate loci. This leads to distortion of the architecture of the tissues affected. In the *lungs*, a relatively low-grade interstitial pneumonitis is followed by interstitial fibrosis, most marked in lower lobes. After this, cyst formation and bronchiectasis may develop. Arteriolar thickening (concentric intimal proliferation or medial hypertrophy) is seen, particularly in those patients with clinical evidence of pulmonary hypertension. In the gastrointestinal tract, the *esophagus* is frequently involved with muscle atrophy and fibrosis. Lesions secondary to reflux of gastric contents are present in 20 per cent. Fibrosis around Brunner's glands in the submucosa of the *duodenum* occurs and can be recognized on specimens obtained by peroral biopsy. Involvement of the *small bowel* begins with patchy subserosal fibrosis and may progress to almost complete replacement of smooth muscle with fibrous tissue and marked thickening of the serosa. The small bowel may develop multiple sacculations, presumably at sites of weakness in the continuity of the wall. Dilation, muscle atrophy, and fibrosis are seen in the *colon;* the fibrosis is irregular, leading to the characteristic sacculations and diverticula. The *heart* is frequently enlarged and may be the only organ weighing more than predicted for the subject's body weight. Small patches of interstitial myocardial fibrosis are commonly found. In very severe cases, as much as 60 per cent of cardiac muscle is replaced by dense, relatively acellular and avascular fibrous tissue. Endocardial or valvular thickening is unusual and is rarely of hemodynamic significance. Fibrinous pericarditis is found quite often, even in the absence of uremia. *Kidneys* in scleroderma are normal in size when renal involvement has not been present clinically. In patients dying with uremia they may be small and frequently have small cortical infarcts. Histologically, fibromucinous intimal proliferation in the interlobular arteries, fibrinoid necrosis of small arteries and arterioles (including the glomerular tufts), and thickening of the basement membrane (the "wire-loop" lesion) may all be present. These changes are similar to those seen in kidneys from patients with malignant hypertension and occasionally may be present in the absence of renal failure or severe hypertension.

CLINICAL MANIFESTATIONS AND DIAGNOSES. The disease usually begins insidiously. Raynaud's phenomenon, vague weakness, weight loss, diffuse stiffness and aching, polyarticular arthritis, and diffuse edema of the hands are the most common initial symptoms. If the illness progresses, it generally does so slowly, and is marked by characteristic organ system changes. Rarely, rapid progression to severe cutaneous and visceral involvement may occur in less than six months.

Cutaneous System. The patient with classic, well-developed acrosclerosis presents with taut, thickened, or edematous skin bound tightly to subcutaneous tissues in the hands and fingers. Feet and toes are involved less often than hands, forearms, and neck. Normal skin folds at the knuckles disappear. Chronic recurrent painful ulcerations at the ends of the digits develop, and the fingers themselves may shorten through progressive resorption of the terminal phalanges. Joints become immobilized from tight encasement in thickened skin as well as from contractures of muscles and tendons and palmar fascia. Telangiectasia, increased or decreased pigmentation, and subcutaneous calcification are common. Hair becomes thin, and the skin of the face appears smooth and waxy. The skin around the mouth may constrict, restricting lip movement and preventing adequate dental hygiene. The normal sweating mechanism is often impaired; the involved skin feels leathery and dry and may scale and itch. The CREST syndrome (calcinosis, Raynaud's phenomenon, esophageal hypomotility, sclerodactyly, and telangiectasia) and the Thibierge-Weissenbach syndrome (diffuse deposition of insoluble calcium phosphates in subcutaneous tissue in the presence of acrosclerosis) are variants of the cutaneous expression of systemic sclerosis.

Musculoskeletal System. Almost half the patients with systemic sclerosis present with joint pain or develop it during the first year of their illness. Small joints are involved more often than large ones. Joint deformity and immobility in systemic sclerosis do not result from an invasive, erosive synovitis as in rheumatoid arthritis, but are the result of encasement as subcutaneous tissue is replaced by bundles of collagen. Muscle wasting is often severe in areas such as the hands, in which joint mobility is impaired by progressive tightening of the overlying skin.

Gastrointestinal Tract. Of the internal organ systems, the gastrointestinal tract is the one most often involved in systemic sclerosis. *Oral* symptoms include xerostomia and a progressive decrease in the size of the mouth. Sjögren's syndrome is seen often, and the frequency of its association with systemic sclerosis is probably underestimated. Symptoms referable to the *esophagus,* ranging from simple dysphagia to heartburn, nausea, and substernal fullness, are found in 45 to 60 per cent of cases. The dysphagia is related to absence of coordinated peristalsis, followed by loss of amplitude of esophageal body waves and incompetence of the lower esophageal sphincter. If reflex esophagitis becomes a persistent complication, stricture may develop. There is a very frequent association of Raynaud's phenomenon and decreased esophageal peristalsis, although this association is not limited to patients with scleroderma. Vomiting, abdominal distention, and pain or diarrhea may indicate involvement of the *small intestine.* As in the esophagus, motility of the small bowel is decreased, and there may be malabsorption secondary to intraluminal stagnation with concomitant bacterial overgrowth. Functional bowel complaints secondary to pathologic changes in the *colon* are common. Disease of both large and small bowel may produce a clinical picture identical to paralytic ileus with incomplete obstruction at any level. Pneumatosis cystoides intestinalis (air-filled cysts in the mesentery which may rupture, causing peritonitis) is a rare but striking complication of scleroderma bowel disease.

An association between primary biliary cirrhosis and scleroderma with CREST syndrome is now recognized.

Heart and Lungs. Dyspnea is the most common cardiorespiratory symptom in systemic sclerosis and is present in more than 50 per cent of patients. Fine, dry crackles at the bases of the lung are the first abnormality found on physical examination. In some patients, progression to respiratory insufficiency and death from hypoxemia is related to progressive pulmonary fibrosis. The earliest abnormality of pulmonary function is a decrease in pulmonary diffusion capacity. Those exposed in their occupation to silicate dust have a predilection to develop this form of the disease. Restriction of chest wall expansion by dermal fibrosis around the thorax rarely affects respiratory function. A few patients with severe cystic and fibrotic changes in the lungs have developed multifocal alveolar cell carcinomas.

Signs of elevated pulmonary vascular resistance may develop independent of parenchymal changes in the lungs and lead to cor pulmonale and congestive heart failure.

Replacement of myocardium with fibrous tissue on a primary basis ("scleroderma heart disease") is an occasional cause of heart failure. In addition, impaired cardiac function can be attributed to right ventricular failure secondary to pulmonary hypertension.

Kidneys. The sudden development of malignant hypertension resistant to therapy and uremia progressing rapidly to death is a dreaded complication of systemic sclerosis. Most patients have had skin changes before development of abnormal renal function. Renal arteriograms reveal narrowed interlobular arteries and afferent arterioles with focal or generalized loss of the cortical nephrogram. It is rare for patients with this complication to survive longer than four months unless nephrectomy and hemodialysis and/or transplantation are carried out.

Nervous System. Involvement of the nervous system is rare. Facial pain, questionably related to a trigeminal neuropathy, is seen in occasional patients and may be disabling. Significant reduction in mean conduction velocity of peripheral nerves has been reported.

LABORATORY FINDINGS. The erythrocyte sedimentation rate is elevated in most patients with systemic sclerosis, and a mild anemia of chronic disease may be present. In addition, iron deficiency anemia may result from bleeding from esophagitis, and vitamin B_{12} and/or folic acid deficiency from overgrowth of organisms in an atonic bowel. Hemolysis is unusual, although microangiopathic hemolytic anemia has been described in scleroderma (presumably related to fragmentation of erythrocytes from contact with diseased blood vessels and/or intravascular fibrin). A number of serologic abnormalities link systemic sclerosis to other connective tissue diseases. Mild hypergammaglobulinemia is present in 30 to 50 per cent of patients, rheumatoid factor in 25 to 35 per cent, antinuclear antibodies (often with a speckled or a nucleolar pattern) in sera of 30 to 40 per cent, and LE cells in less than 10 per cent of patients. There has been no correlation found between antinuclear antibody patterns and the course and activity of disease. DNA-binding activity in serum is absent.

The electrocardiogram shows nonspecific abnormalities in almost 50 per cent of patients. The pattern of conduction defects with very low voltage is seen only in those uncommon patients with marked myocardial replacement by fibrous tissue. Echocardiogram in these cases will reveal reduced ventricular wall motion. This technique is also useful in documenting small pericardial effusions. In general the electromyogram is normal; most patients have polyphasic waves of normal duration and size. Denervation potentials are seen only rarely.

Roentgenography. Roentgenograms are important for diagnosis and follow-up evaluation. The findings of soft tissue atrophy, subcutaneous calcinosis, and resorption of the tufts of the terminal phalanges without loss of apparent joint spaces between phalanges are virtually pathognomonic of systemic sclerosis when seen on hand films. The periodontal membrane is occasionally thickened. Upper gastrointestinal films reveal a dilated, atonic esophagus in about 60 per cent of patients. Small bowel studies may demonstrate segmental atony, dilation, and sacculation in the duodenum and jejunum. Linear or cystic pneumatosis (air in the wall of the gut) is occasionally seen in flat plates of the abdomen of patients with severe small bowel involvement. Barium studies of the colon reveal wide-mouth, asymmetrical diverticula in 20 to 40 per cent of patients; progression to a dilated, atonic megacolon rarely occurs. In patients with pulmonary involvement, chest roentgenograms reveal a diffuse reticular pattern with a honeycomb appearance in the lower lung fields. Serial films may document progression to a picture of dense interstitial fibrosis amid radiolucent cystic areas.

DIFFERENTIAL DIAGNOSIS. When systemic sclerosis presents as persistent symmetrical polyarthritis involving the hands without previous skin changes, it may be impossible to differentiate it from rheumatoid arthritis or systemic lupus erythematosus, or, if the overlying skin becomes edematous or red, dermatomyositis. In fact, "overlap" syndromes combining clinical or serologic manifestations of several of these entities are being described with increasing frequency, and one should avoid hasty classification of any clinical picture that is consistent with more than one of the connective tissue diseases.

Diseases or pathologic findings associated with Raynaud's phenomenon which must be differentiated from scleroderma include occupational trauma; anatomic lesions, e.g., scalenus anticus syndrome and cervical ribs; vasomotor syndromes resulting in disuse atrophy, e.g., Sudek's atrophy or the shoulder-hand syndrome; peripheral vascular arteriosclerosis; heavy metal or ergot poisoning; and hematologic abnormalities, e.g., polycythemia vera, paroxysmal cold hemoglobinuria, and presence of cold agglutinins or cryoproteinemia.

The atrophic changes in the skin in systemic sclerosis must be differentiated from those seen in Werner's syndrome, progeria (Hutchinson-Gilford syndrome), chronic hypostatic edema or myxedema, lichen sclerosus et atrophicus, porphyria cutanea tarda, and/or scleredema. Unlike systemic sclerosis, Werner's syndrome affects the feet more severely than the hands, and has associated with it a high-pitched voice, growth abnormalities, and premature cataracts, arteriosclerosis, and diabetes. Sclerodermatous changes have been reported in skin of patients with progeria, but the dwarf-like stature, characteristic facies, and premature death from coronary insufficiency set this syndrome apart. Porphyria cutanea tarda may have skin changes simulating scleroderma but can be differentiated on the basis of urinary or fecal porphyrin excretion. Scleredema (scleredema adultorum of Buschke) is a brawny edema which appears abruptly, involves skin of the neck and chest initially, and is characterized pathologically by the presence of a material resembling acid mucopolysaccharide diffusely interspersed among collagen bundles in the dermis. This is a self-limited process, perhaps related to a previous bacterial infection, and has a good prognosis. The cutaneous telangiectasia of scleroderma resembles Osler-Weber-Rendu disease (hereditary telangiectasia). Scleroderma-like reactions have been described in chronic graft-versus-host reactions in patients given renal allografts.

Involvement of viscera in systemic sclerosis can mimic many other illnesses. The abnormalities in pulmonary function and the roentgenographic findings seen are similar to those found in idiopathic pulmonary fibrosis (Hamman-Rich syndrome) and the pulmonary fibrosis of rheumatoid arthritis or advanced sarcoidosis. Scleroderma heart disease must be differentiated from infiltrative cardiomyopathies as well as fibrosis from diffuse coronary artery disease. The dysphagia of scleroderma is completely nonspecific, and disease of the bowel rarely can simulate sprue or any of the malabsorption syndromes, partial intestinal obstruction, or megacolon. Workers in vinyl chloride polymerization plants have an increased incidence of microvascular abnormalities, and some have scleroderma-like skin lesions or acro-osteolysis. The mechanism of this industrial disease is not known.

COURSE UNTREATED. The course of systemic sclerosis is variable. Those patients with primary acrosclerosis and decreased esophageal motility may have slowly progressive disease with no significant increased probability of early death. Others, particularly patients with pulmonary, cardiac, or renal involvement, may progress rapidly to early death. Renal failure is the cause of death of scleroderma in 20 to 40 per cent of patients. Recent data obtained using life-table methods suggest that there is a 50 to 70 per cent five-year survival. Chances for survival are worse if the patient is a black male, diagnosed over the age of 40 years, with cutaneous lesions of the trunk, pulmonary involvement, and an abnormal electrocardiogram or blood urea nitrogen greater than 40 mg per 100 ml.

TREATMENT. Patients with acrosclerosis can lead productive and useful lives. The most important goal in therapy is to preserve function in and prevent injury to the hands. Vocational and/or climatic change may be indicated. Hand care must be stressed, including instructions for active and passive exercises that the patient may do himself several times each day in order to prevent further deformity. Early signs of local infection in fingertips must be treated immediately before they progress to large ulcerations. Psychologic support can be of great value in helping a patient adjust to the discomfort and apparently inexorable progression of his disease.

Because so little is known about the underlying defect in scleroderma or its pathogenesis, no specific treatment is available. The one possible exception to this is the use of broad-spectrum antimicrobials (e.g., tetracycline, 0.25 gram twice a day, or erythromycin, 0.5 gram every day) in treatment of malabsorption associated with bacterial overgrowth in the upper small intestine. If esophageal motility is decreased, antacid therapy is used liberally to prevent secondary esophagitis and stricture. Surgical reconstruction of the esophagogastric junction has been effective in management of symptomatic reflux in selected patients. If stricture develops, bougienage will be needed. Salicylates in pharmacologic doses may decrease clinical signs of inflammation, e.g., elevated sedimentation rates, joint pain, and erythema, which is present in most patients at some time in the course of their disease.

Corticosteroids are ineffective in the treatment of systemic sclerosis; neither the vascular lesions nor the fibrosis are improved by their use. However, there is a subgroup of patients with an overlap syndrome called "mixed connective tissue disease" who present with a variety of symptoms, including Raynaud's phenomenon, arthritis, and skin changes consistent with scleroderma, but with features (including LE cells, leukopenia, inflammatory myositis, and lymphadenopathy) of other connective tissue diseases as well. Many of this group will have high titers of antinuclear antibody in a "speckled" pattern directed against an extractable nuclear antigen, a ribonucleoprotein distinct from Sm antigen. In general, this group of patients does not develop renal disease and responds to corticosteroid therapy.

Use of intra-arterial reserpine* has been advocated to decrease the frequency of Raynaud's phenomenon and potentiate healing of ulcers. Given intra-arterially (0.5 to 1.0 mg), benefit without side effects has often been prolonged. A decrease in finger vasoconstriction in response to cooling in patients with scleroderma given reserpine in the ipsilateral brachial artery has been documented. The placebo effect of this type of procedure and potential hazards of intra-arterial reserpine must be continually evaluated. Phenoxybenzamine (Dibenzyline, 20 to 100 mg per day) is an effective α-adrenergic blocking agent. The principal side effect of this class of drugs is postural hypotension. It may help relieve symptoms of Raynaud's phenomenon.

Potassium p-aminobenzoate, griseofulvin, vitamin E (1200 to 2000 IU per day), ethylenediaminetetraacetic acid, 6-aminocaproic acid infusions, and dimethyl sulfoxide applications have been employed by a number of investigators without firm proof of efficacy. D-Penicillamine,* capable of cleaving newly formed labile intermolecular cross-links of collagen in vitro, can inhibit the synthesis of collagen by active sclerodermatous skin. In doses of 750 to 1500 mg per day it may be effective in slowing progression of skin disease, although beneficial results have not been reported for visceral involvement and the toxicity of D-penicillamine is great. Pilot studies of immunosuppressive therapy are being evaluated; initial results show no clear-cut role for these drugs in systemic sclerosis. Colchicine (less than 1.5 mg per day), after initial promise, has not been proved effective in diminishing sclerosis.

Initial results in a few cases in which "scleroderma kidneys" were removed and hemodialysis and/or renal transplantation carried out have demonstrated that life of good quality can be prolonged by these aggressive approaches. Recurrence of vascular lesions in allografts has been described. To be effective, hemodialysis must be carried out relatively early in the accelerated, progressive renal failure, preferably while serum creatinine values are less than 6 to 8 mg per deciliter.

D'Angelo, W. A., Fries, J. F., Masi, A. T., and Shulman, L. E.: Pathologic observations in systemic sclerosis (scleroderma). Am. J. Med., 46:428, 1969.

Rodnan, G. P.: Progressive systemic sclerosis (scleroderma) and calcinosis. In Hollander, J. L., and McCarty, D. J. (eds.): Arthritis and Allied Conditions. 8th ed. Philadelphia, Lea & Febiger, 1972.

---

*Investigational drug for this use.

51. POLYMYOSITIS AND DERMATOMYOSITIS

H. Richard Tyler

GENERAL CONSIDERATIONS. The disorder termed polymyositis refers to an illness first described by Wagner in 1863 in which muscle weakness is the principal clinical feature. Inflammatory, degenerative, and regenerative changes can be seen in the muscles. When skin changes occur and are prominent, the cases are referred to as dermatomyositis. This subgroup was first delineated by Unverricht in 1887. The muscular lesions of dermatomyositis, however, are identical to those seen in polymyositis. Because of the dramatic skin lesions, dermatomyositis was more widely recognized. Appreciation that muscular syndromes are more common than dermatomyositis resulted from the increased use of muscle biopsy and the clinical awareness that an insidious onset and absence of muscle pain are common. If there are changes indicative of nerve damage, the term neuromyositis is occasionally used. Some authors prefer the nonspecific and noncommittal term polymyopathy and identify as separate entities only those cases whose specific cause is known. Others reserve the term polymyositis for cases with evidence of inflammatory changes in muscles. Until the cause of the majority of the cases is more clearly identified, one has to accept the need to re-evaluate nomenclature periodically. All these disorders form a large spectrum which ranges from the very acute cases with myoglobinuria to the very chronic localized disorders that mimic muscular dystrophy.

The incidence of the disease has been estimated between 0.1 and 0.6 per 100,000 population per year, with a prevalence of 6.3 per 100,000. As a cause of acute or subacute muscle weakness in an adult, polymyositis is much more common than muscular dystrophy.

The disease can appear at any age, but it is most common between the ages of 40 and 60. Females are affected about twice as frequently as males. In most instances, no precipitating cause is obvious, but some cases have followed a viral-like illness or the use of antimicrobial drugs. Virus-like particles have been noted in muscle in some cases. Their role in relation to the disease has not been defined. Hypersensitivity has been implicated by some because of the association with malignancy, the frequent relation to a previous infection, and the association with symptoms common to the other collagen diseases.

If one excludes obvious cases of collagen disease and childhood dermatomyositis, more than 10 to 15 per cent of cases are associated with malignancy. If one considers only cases above age 50, then the frequency of malignancy may double. It is important to recognize that the carcinoma may present up to three to five years after the onset of the polymyositis syndrome. The relationship between the two entities is not clear.

About 20 per cent of cases of polymyositis and dermatomyositis occur in the course of one of the other connective tissue disorders. This association favors females by 9:1.

In most instances, it is not possible to establish a definite etiology. Specific infections (such as toxoplasmosis) may cause a polymyositis, but in most cases there is no evidence of an infectious cause. It has not been possible to demonstrate antimuscle antibodies in these patients. The presence of antimyosin antibody and other antibodies in some patients is nonspecific, as it is also found in patients with muscular dystrophy and neuronal atrophy. It has been possible to produce a myositis in guinea pigs similar to human polymyositis by use of muscle plus Freund's adjuvant. In tissue culture preparations of rat skeletal muscle, "sensitized" lymph node cells from animals previously injected with muscle plus adjuvants destroyed the muscle cells when added to the culture, whereas unsensitized lymph node cells did not. The significance of these experiments for human disease remains uncertain.

The presence of particles resembling virus seen in electron microscope studies in a number of patients has raised the question of an altered reaction to a viral disease as a cause of some forms of polymyositis.

Lymphocytes or their products from affected patients have cytotoxic activity toward cells in 79 per cent of cases in one series, suggesting a cell-mediated immune response to muscle antigen. Intramuscular vascular deposits of immunoglobulin and C3 have been demonstrated, especially in the childhood form of dermatomyositis.

PATHOLOGY. Muscle biopsy may show inflammatory cells around vessels and in the interstitium frequently associated with individual muscle fiber necrosis. These necrotic muscle fibers are frequently in various stages of being phagocytized. Attempts at regeneration characterized by basophilic fibers having prominent sarcolemmal nuclei are usually impressive. It should be emphasized that histologic findings vary greatly in the same muscle and between different muscles so that sampling is important. The muscle tissue from the more chronic cases often shows surprisingly little change under the light microscope. This may consist of smaller muscle fibers, which vary significantly in cross-section diameter, associated with proliferation of sarcolemmal nuclei. In the polymyositis associated with Sjögren's syndrome, the muscle may be heavily infiltrated with plasma cells and lymphocytes. In the few studies utilizing the electron microscope, changes such as thickened basilar membranes, myofibrillary degeneration and, rarely, virus particles were seen. These studies have not contributed any new insight into the disease.

In the childhood form of dermatomyositis, there is intense perivascular inflammation with active arteritis and phlebitis. There is often occlusion of vessels with fibrin thrombi and infarction of muscles, nerves, and viscus (Banker and Victor). Other forms of more limited or less intense polymyositic syndromes in children have pathologic changes similar to those previously described.

The three useful laboratory tests, serum enzyme determinations, electromyography, and muscle biopsy, are not always abnormal. Any one or even two may yield normal findings in a particular case. In one series, electromyography was abnormal in 89 per cent and muscle biopsy was confirmatory in 63 per cent. Serum enzyme activities are usually elevated except in some slowly progressive or chronic cases.

CLINICAL MANIFESTATIONS AND DIAGNOSIS. The patient usually first notes the insidious development of *weakness in proximal muscles*. The weakness is more common at the hips than in the shoulders. Some weakness in the flexors of the neck is almost always present. Muscle discomfort or tenderness is common but can be completely absent. When present, it is more common in the shoulders, back, and arms than in the thighs. Muscular wasting is a late sign, and when it occurs it is usually in proximal muscles such as the quadriceps. The weakness is out of proportion to the loss of muscle bulk. Reflexes are depressed in proportion to muscle weakness.

The development and the rate of progression of the weakness may show great variations from patient to patient, and even in the same patient at different stages of the illness. Weakness can progress until the patient becomes bedridden, but this is unusual. Contracture of muscles may develop quickly.

A *skin rash* may or may not be present. It usually takes the form of an erythema over the face, shoulders, and arms. It can mimic erythema nodosum, eczema, or exfoliating dermatitis, or can manifest itself by thickened, brawny, edematous skin. On occasion, the skin lesions appear primarily in areas exposed to sunlight. Erythematous, slightly raised lesions occur over bony prominences, i.e., elbows, knuckles, knees, and medial malleoli. These lesions often become scaly and atrophic. Hyperemia around the nail beds is not uncommon. In childhood forms a violaceous suffusion of the upper eyelids, called a "heliotrope" rash, is diagnostic of this disorder. This may also be seen in adults.

Dysphagia, secondary to weakness of pharyngeal muscle and hypotonicity of the upper part of the esophagus, is frequent. About one third of the patients have arthralgias, Raynaud's phenomenon, or both. Other visceral manifestations are rare. Many patients have a tachycardia. Electrocardiograms may show nonspecific T wave changes. Interstitial fibrosis and pericarditis have been noted on histologic examination. A transitory pneumonitis has also been reported. Transitional cases with some features suggesting scleroderma have occasionally demonstrated severe gastrointestinal symptoms with malabsorption, severe myopathy, and only slight skin changes. If the muscle weakness comes on acutely with such muscle necrosis, myoglobinuria will occur. This can result in acute renal failure. Polymyositis may also be seen with Sjögren's syndrome.

The *childhood form of dermatomyositis* may be much more pernicious. It starts out with skin changes, anorexia, and fatigue. Weakness, stiffness, and pain in muscles customarily follow. Low-grade fever, dysphagia, contractures, and calcinosis usually develop. A perforated viscus or mediastinitis is often the immediate cause of death.

COURSE UNTREATED. The condition can progress to severe disability and death, but most patients either improve spontaneously or proceed to a chronic phase. In earlier series, including patients primarily recognized as having dermatomyositis, case fatality rates of 50 per cent were common. In a later series of adult patients with polymyositis, it was noted that about two thirds were alive after ten years. About 50 per cent of these had complete recoveries, and the rest had some degree of residual disability. Many of the patients in this series had received some steroid therapy.

In a survey by Sheard in which adult cases were accumulated from the literature, tumors were present in nearly 20 per cent, or five times the expected incidence. When polymyositis develops in an adult male, a greater than 50 per cent chance exists that a tumor will be discovered. In another series described by Shy, it was noted that when polymyositis appeared after the age of 50 a *cancer* was found in 71 per cent of males and 24 per cent of females. The muscular weakness may precede the detection of the tumor by two or three years despite diligent search, and in this series all nine males above 50 who were followed for three years or more had an associated neoplasm. In the male, the usual carcinoma is in the lung, stomach, intestine, or prostate; and in the female, in the ovary, uterus, or breast.

Childhood dermatomyositis appears to be a very specific subgroup of polymyositic disorders. It is severely disabling and is associated with a very high fatality rate.

LABORATORY FINDINGS. The sedimentation rate is usually elevated, and there may be mild leukocytosis, especially in the acute cases. A number of enzymes which derive from muscle are usually elevated in serum. Creatine phosphokinase and aldolase are the most specific, but lactic dehydrogenase and transaminase (SGOT) are usually elevated also. Serum protein changes occur in about 50 per cent of the patients. These most commonly consist of elevations of the $\alpha 2$ and γ globulins. Rheumatoid factors are positive in 10 to 50 per cent, depending on the series. About 5 per cent will have LE cells. Myoglobinuria is transient and is found only with acute and severe muscular degeneration.

In patients with dysphagia, the roentgenograms often reveal pooling of barium in the vallecular and pyriform sinuses. Hypomotility of the esophagus is present in about one third of the cases. The roentgenograms frequently reveal no abnormalities except the rare deposition of subcutaneous calcification in the childhood form of the disease. Electrocardiograms often show minor abnormalities.

Electromyography is almost always abnormal in the clinically affected muscles. There is excessive irritability of muscle when the needle is initially inserted. The motor units (which are made up of many muscle fibers supplied by a single nerve) often show a loss of amplitude, indicating a reduction in the number of functioning muscle fibers in each motor unit. The mean duration of the units is often shortened. Polyphasic discharges are common, indicating a loss of individual muscle fibers of the unit. Positive denervation waves of 20 to 50 msec and fibrillary potentials are seen, indicating some denervation or separation of a portion of the muscle from its afferent nerve supply. Repetitive discharges of pseudomyotonic firing are not uncommon. When the changes indicating denervation are prominent, the term "neuromyositis" has been used. The electromyogram is useful in indicating which muscles to biopsy. The site of biopsy should be selected to ensure that a proper sampling of abnormal muscle is being taken. It should not be taken at the site of previous electromyographic needle insertion.

DIFFERENTIAL DIAGNOSIS. The major causes of weakness, which must be differentiated from polymyositis, are those due to muscular dystrophy and disorders of the peripheral and central nervous system. Muscular dystrophy is usually a familial disorder which is longstanding and can often be traced to childhood. The involvement of proximal muscles and neck flexor weakness would be unusual in most adult forms of muscular dystrophy. In myotonic dystrophy, the only dystrophy which often demonstrates neck flexor weakness, there is a distal weakness of muscles in the extremities. There are also cataracts and myotonia to percussion. Fascioscapulohumeral muscular dystrophy and other proximal dystrophies usually spare neck flexors. All the dystrophies are characterized by family history, significant muscle wasting, and weakness; the deep tendon reflex loss is usually early and prominent. In polymyositis, reflexes are often relatively spared until severe weakness occurs. In some cases it may be impossible to distinguish a dystrophy from polymyositis. The family history may be difficult to verify, and the biopsy in chronic cases may not be characteristic. A few cases of familial polymyositis have been reported.

The weakness in peripheral neuritis tends to be distal, and careful examination usually enables one to find mild sensory loss, autonomic dysfunction, and distal areflexia. Weakness from spinal cord disease has characteristic reflex changes, such as extensor plantar responses and hyperreflexia. Occasionally, motor neuron disease (the primary muscular atrophy variant) presents as a myopathic disorder. Muscle biopsy and EMG usually distinguish between the two conditions. On occasion a subacute variety of Guillain-Barré disease can cause proximal weakness. Elevation of cerebrospinal fluid protein is helpful in establishing this entity and is not seen in polymyositis.

Of the muscular syndromes, the metabolic myopathies most closely mimic the distribution of muscle weakness and the weakness seen with polymyositis. Chronic thyroid myopathy is characterized by its involvement of proximal muscles with significant loss of muscle bulk. The reflexes are usually quite brisk. Although there are no distinctive features, the clinical signs of thyrotoxicosis and the presence of clinical tests to support hyperthyroidism usually make it easy to distinguish this group. The most common myopathy seen today is probably the one induced by excess or chronic use of corticotropin or steroids. This is especially true of the fluorinated steroids. It is identical to that seen with hyperadrenocorticism. The weakness is primarily proximal, most often involving the pelvic girdle. Early wasting of the quadriceps muscle is especially prominent. Pain and discomfort are unusual. Reflexes usually persist, and severe disabling syndromes are unusual. Muscle biopsy tends to show surprisingly little change, and then only very scattered and in single muscle fibers. These changes are usually much less than one would anticipate from the clinical status of the patients.

Since steroids are often used in the treatment of a number of clinical syndromes, it may be very difficult to establish whether progressive weakness is due to the underlying disease or the steroid treatment. Often one will have to either decrease the steroid dose sharply or increase it significantly to make such judgments. If pain is a significant problem, one must be cautious about the clinical evaluation of weakness or its disappearance with the use of high doses of steroids.

Hyperparathyroidism and hyperinsulinism have rarely been associated with syndromes of muscular weakness and must be separated from idiopathic polymyositis primarily by the associated laboratory findings. Muscle weakness is often associated with osteomalacia.

There are a number of parasitic diseases such as trichinosis and toxoplasmosis which should be considered in acute or subacute syndromes, especially when generalized symptoms and eosinophilia are noted. These are fully discussed elsewhere in this text.

Polymyalgia rheumatica is characteristically associated with significant muscular discomfort and a high sedimentation rate. Changes in serum enzymes or muscle biopsy are usually not present to any significant degree. There are noticeable short-term and even daily fluctuations of symptoms. Significant objective weakness is not common, although complaints of pain and fatigue and feelings of muscular weakness are often voiced by the patient. Although the findings in some are related to those seen with temporal arteritis, the findings in others are very similar to those of some patients seen with epidemic neuromyasthenia.

A newly described syndrome, *diffuse fasciitis associated with eosinophilia*, is easy to confuse with dermatomyositis. The biopsy specimen usually demonstrates pathology primarily in a thickened fascia rather than skin or muscle. The presence of eosinophilia in blood and bone marrow is a laboratory clue to the diagnosis.

Clinically, skin is often bound to the underlying tissue and contractions occur very easily. The cause of the syndrome is not clear. It appears to respond to steroids.

TREATMENT. The physician's obvious goal is to eradicate the active disease process, if possible, and improve the functional capacity of the patient. In almost all cases prolonged management and long-term follow-up will be necessary. Often the chronic nature and the severe disability caused by the illness make it essential for the physician to play an active role as a counselor and friend.

Many of these patients achieve significant symptomatic improvement of muscle function when treated with corticotropin, steroids, or salicylates. The use of immunosuppressive medication has been promising in a few cases. Methotrexate* has been used, especially in dermatomyositis. The disorder is rarely "cured," however, and relapses are common, especially if steroids are abruptly withdrawn. Patients may require medication for many years. The initial dose of corticotropin or steroids should be high (60 to 80 mg of prednisone) and tapered over months. It is useful to monitor serum enzymes during this period, as they often give an early indication of the patient's likely course. Relapses are common when steroids are withdrawn in the first two years, but less frequent if treatment lasts at least three years. When possible, steroids should be used on an alternate-day basis to decrease side effects. When steroid-treated and presteroid series of patients are compared in terms of long-range follow-up, as by Rose and Walton, the group receiving steroid treatment has fared better. Patients with some of the adult forms usually do well. Those with the childhood forms of dermatomyositis usually do not respond satisfactorily to steroids alone.

Banker, B. Q.: Dermatomyositis of childhood. J. Neuropathol. Exp. Neurol., 34:1, 1975.

Bohan, A., Peter, J. B., Bourman, R. L., and Pearson, C. M.: A computer-assisted analysis of 153 patients with polymyositis and dermatomyositis. Medicine, 56:255, 1977.

DeVere, R., and Bradley, W. G.: Polymyositis: Its presentation, morbidity and mortality. Brain, 98:637, 1975.

Pearson, C. M.: Polymyositis. *In* Milhorat, A. T. (ed.): Explanatory Concepts in Muscular Dystrophy and Related Disorders. Amsterdam, Excerpta Medica Foundation, 1967.

Schulman, L. E.: Diffuse fasciitis with eosinophilia: A new syndrome. Trans. Assoc. Am. Physicians, 88:70, 1975.

Shy, G. M.: The late onset myopathy. World Neurol., 3:149, 1962.

Walton, J. N.: Disorders of Voluntary Muscle. 3rd ed. London, J. A. Churchill, Ltd., 1974.

Walton, J. N., and Adams, R. D.: Polymyositis. Edinburgh, Livingstone, Ltd., 1958.

---

*Investigational drug for this use.

52. SYSTEMIC LUPUS ERYTHEMATOSUS

Peter H. Schur

GENERAL CONSIDERATIONS. Systemic lupus erythematosus (SLE) is a chronic, inflammatory disease of unknown cause affecting skin, joints, kidneys, nervous system, serous membranes, and often other organs of the body. The classic facial "butterfly rash" facilitates diagnosis, although the rash need not be present. The clinical course may be fulminant or indolent, but generally is characterized by periods of remissions and relapses. Patients with SLE develop distinct immunologic abnormalities, especially antinuclear antibodies. A diagnosis of SLE has frequently been confirmed by the finding of these antibodies, especially antibodies to DNA.

Lupus, which is Latin for wolf, has been used since about 1230 to describe cutaneous conditions which resemble the malar erythema of a wolf. Numerous publications in the nineteenth century by, among others, Bateman, Biett, Hebra, and Kaposi, described what we know now as lupus of the skin. In 1851, Cazenave first used the term "lupus erythemateux." Kaposi, in 1872, noted the systemic involvement in lupus, and in 1875 noted that the rash resembled a butterfly. Osler described the systemic complications of lupus and noted that they could occur in the absence of skin disease. The clinical recognition of SLE has changed greatly since Hargraves first described the LE cell test in 1948 and since the development of the immunofluorescent antinuclear factor test by Friou in 1957.

INCIDENCE AND ETIOLOGY. SLE is not a rare disorder. The prevalence rate is approximately 1 per 1000 population. The disease appears to occur more frequently in blacks than in whites and is rare among Asians. It occurs five to ten times more frequently among females than males and has been diagnosed in patients ranging from 2 to 97 years old. However, the majority of patients are first discovered to have SLE while in their third and fourth decades of life.

The cause of SLE remains unknown. Exposure to sunlight or ultraviolet radiation, viz., sunlamps, often leads to the prompt appearance of the facial butterfly rash or a rash on other exposed skin surfaces. Many other factors, including infections, surgery, and certain drugs, have been shown to be associated with exacerbations of SLE. Recent attention has focused on procainamide, hydralazine, hydantoins, and other drugs which may precipitate a lupus-like illness.

In view of the preponderance of the disease in females, endocrine factors have been thought to influence the development of SLE. The disease tends to remit during the last two trimesters of pregnancy and to relapse post partum. Inhibitors of ovulation may cause an exacerbation of SLE.

Genetic factors may influence the development of SLE in susceptible individuals. Much evidence supports this hypothesis. The high incidence of SLE among females might be considered an X-chromosome-related factor. Connective tissue disorders, including SLE, dysgammaglobulinemia, and autoimmune phenomena are observed frequently among relatives of many patients with SLE. There is a high concordance rate of SLE in twins. Immune deficiency, particularly of IgA and the second component of complement (C2), is noted with increased frequency among SLE patients. Additional evidence for a genetic role in SLE comes from studies in certain strains of inbred mice and dogs. NZB and NZW (New Zealand black and New Zealand white) mice develop an illness which includes hemolytic anemia, renal disease, and immunologic abnormalities, and is similar to human SLE. The F_1 hybrid generation, especially the females, develops the illness more frequently, at an earlier age, and with a much higher incidence of autoimmune phenomena.

Lupus erythematosus is characterized particularly by autoimmune phenomena. Patients develop antibodies to many of their own cells, cell constituents, and proteins. The origin of these autoantibodies is as obscure as is the cause of SLE. However, they do appear to represent a loss of tolerance to self antigens. Mice of the NZB strain have been found to lose their tolerance for foreign antigens much more rapidly than do other mice, possibly owing to a suppressor T cell defect.

A possible viral cause for SLE has also been proposed. Loss of tolerance may be influenced by viral infections. Structures resembling viral nucleocapsids — but shown not to be viruses — have been found much more frequently in endothelial cells in SLE patients than in normal persons. Antibody titers to certain viruses are elevated in SLE sera, but no one virus has been implicated. The presence, in many SLE patients, of antibodies to double-stranded RNA suggests reaction to an RNA virus (infection). "C" type RNA virus particles have been found in NZB mice; other viruses, including DNA and RNA viruses, can provoke the development of autoantibodies and nephritis in NZB mice. Cell-free filtrates, presumably containing a virus, have been prepared from spleens of dogs with lupus. These filtrates, when injected into normal dogs and mice, induce the formation of antinuclear antibodies; they also activate latent leukemia viruses in mice.

These data suggest that an abnormal immune response in genetically predisposed SLE patients may alter the delicate balance between immunity and tolerance and result in the development of antibodies to intracellular contents released during chronic viral infection or to new antigens to cells which result from viral infection or transformation.

PATHOGENESIS AND PATHOLOGY. Some of the manifestations of SLE appear to result from the deposition of antigen-antibody complexes in tissues. In laboratory animals, when immune complexes are formed in the circulation, serum complement levels falls and nephritis develops. In patients with SLE, especially in those with anti-DNA antibodies, a fall in complement levels is often associated with the development of nephritis. In addition, some patients with serum antibodies to DNA develop fever and nephritis as the antibody disappears and is replaced by free DNA, a sequence which presumably represents immune complex formation and deposition, followed by antigen excess. Furthermore, some sera from SLE patients with nephritis, when treated with deoxyribonuclease, have a rise in anti-DNA antibody levels. This fact suggests that DNA has been bound in vivo to the antibody as an immune complex. Also, cryoglobulins, which may represent immune complexes, have been isolated from SLE patients and shown on occasion to contain DNA and high specific activity antibodies against DNA. Immunoglobulins (especially IgG), complement components, and antigens (viz., DNA) have been detected in a granular and lumpy distribution along the renal glomerular basement membrane. After elution of the gamma globulin from the glomeruli, it has been possible to demonstrate that it consists primarily of antinuclear antibodies, including antibodies to DNA. Similar immune complexes have been demonstrated at the dermal-epidermal junction of lupus skin lesions, in nonlesional skin, and in the choroid plexus. It is hypothesized that, as the complement system is activated during immune complex formation and deposition, chemotactic factors are released and that damage to normal cells and extracellular tissue is caused both by activated terminal sequences of complement and by lysosomal enzymes released by polymorphonuclear leukocytes during phagocytosis.

The pathologic changes of SLE, even in clinically involved organs, are often minor when examined by routine histologic methods. Fibrinoid, an eosinophilic amorphous material, is commonly deposited along tissue fibers and in blood vessels. Fibrin and serum proteins (including immunoglobulins, complement, and DNA) have been detected in fibrinoid and possibly represent deposits of immune complexes. Synovium and serous membranes, including pleura and pericardium, may be edematous and contain deposits of fibrinoid. Vasculitis can involve venules, arterioles, and occasionally arteries. Hematoxylin bodies are rounded, hematoxylin-stained masses, roughly the size of nuclei, and are found in areas of inflammation. They are believed to represent in vivo LE bodies analogous to the cytoplasmic inclusions in LE cells.

Biopsies of skin lesions may show acute inflammation with liquefaction, degeneration of the basal layer with vacuolization of basal cells, edema of the dermis, and fibrinoid necrosis in the dermis and local blood vessels with cell infiltration. In chronic lesions, hyperkeratosis with follicular plugging is seen.

The spleen is the site of "onion skin lesions," which are characterized by concentric perivascular fibrosis around central and penicilliary arteries.

Libman-Sacks verrucous nonbacterial endocarditis consists of nonbacterial vegetations on the heart valves or chordae tendineae. Fibrinoid is deposited in the superficial connective tissue with infiltration of neutrophils, lymphocytes, and histiocytes. The myocardium may be involved by vasculitis.

Renal lesions are highly variable, from mild to severe. The mildest form of renal lesion consists of deposits of immunoglobulin and complement in the mesangium or along the glomerular basement membrane without any other observable histologic abnormality. The most common renal lesion is glomerulitis with minimal focal increase of cellularity, thickening of the capillary basement membrane, and fibrinoid change. In glomerulonephritis, these lesions are more generalized and severe and are usually a mixture of proliferative and membranous changes with hypercellularity of endothelial, mesangial, epithelial, and inflammatory cells, capsular inflammation leading to crescent formation, and focal thickening of the basement membrane. Some kidneys are found to have only a diffuse membranous glomerulonephritis with few cells but considerable thickening of the basement membrane. Basement membrane thickening, when associated with fibrinoid changes, results in the so-called "wire loop" lesions. There may also be hyaline thrombi in glomeruli, focal necrosis, and, occasionally, hematoxylin bodies and sclerosis in healed lesions. Tubular degenerative changes are common.

CLINICAL MANIFESTATIONS. The characteristic picture of a patient with well-advanced lupus is one of a young woman with fever, weight loss, arthralgia, a butterfly rash, pleural effusion, and nephritis. With better methods of detection (the antinuclear antibody tests), much larger groups of patients with less obvious and more varied symptoms and signs are being recognized. Most patients complain of some fatigue, arthralgia, rashes, and fever. When specific organs are involved, other symptoms may develop: pleurisy, pericarditis, edema, dyspnea and cough, Raynaud's phenomenon, bleeding, and purpura or seizures. The disease is now considered a chronic illness with periods of remission and activity.

TABLE 1. Frequency of Clinical Symptoms in Systemic Lupus Erythematosus*

	Per Cent
Weight loss	62
Fever	83
Arthralgia, arthritis	90
Skin	74
Butterfly rash	42
Photosensitivity	30
Mucous membrane lesions	12
Alopecia	27
Raynaud's phenomenon	17
Purpura	15
Urticaria	8
Renal	53
Nephrosis	18
Gastrointestinal	38
Pulmonary	47
Pleurisy	45
Effusion	24
Pneumonia	29
Cardiac	46
Pericarditis	27
Murmurs	23
EKG changes	39
Lymphadenopathy	46
Splenomegaly	15
Hepatomegaly	25
Central nervous system	32
Psychosis	15
Convulsions	15
Cytoid bodies	11

*Adapted from Dubois, E. L.: Lupus Erythematosus, New York, McGraw-Hill Book Company, 1966; Estes, D., and Christian, C. L.: Medicine, 50:85, 1971; and Fernandez-Herlihy, L.: Lahey Clinic Found. Bull., 21:49, 1972.

Musculoskeletal System. Most patients complain of pain in their joints (arthralgia) at some time. Commonly the fingers, hands, wrists, knees, ankles, and elbows are affected. Arthritis, i.e., inflammation, of joints is observed less frequently than is arthralgia. Although slight deformities at the metacarpophalangeal and proximal interphalangeal joints may occur, major joint swelling with synovial thickening, flexion deformities with subluxations, and deviation are uncommon. It is unusual for joint narrowing or cystic changes such as those seen in rheumatoid arthritis to be found on radiologic examination. The appearance of deformities or erosions on x-ray suggests a diagnosis of an overlap syndrome (rheumatoid arthritis–lupus). Muscle pain is a frequent complaint and is accompanied, occasionally, by proximal muscle atrophy. The bones are rarely affected, but an increased prevalence of aseptic necrosis of the femoral head or condyle has been noted, especially in those patients receiving corticosteroid therapy.

Mucocutaneous Manifestations. The classic "butterfly rash" is seen in less than half the patients with SLE. There may be only a blush and swelling or a scaly erythematous maculopapular rash on both cheeks and the bridge of the nose after exposure to the sun. This may clear spontaneously, only to recur. Other skin areas, particularly those exposed to the sun, may be involved. The lesions are called "discoid" when they scale, are associated with follicular plugging, and heal with atrophy, scarring (telangiectasia), hyperpigmentation, or hypopigmentation (vitiligo). Involvement may also occur on the forehead, pinna, and scalp, resulting in alopecia. Patchy hair loss is frequent and usually reversible, but discoid lupus with scarring can lead to permanent partial baldness. In these days of well-fitted hairpieces, alopecia is often undetected on cursory examination. Periungual erythema and telangiectasia are found in about 10 per cent of patients with SLE. Small ulcerations signifying an underlying vasculitis often develop on the fingertips and may progress to gangrene. Raynaud's phenomenon may occur in both fingers and toes. Painless ulcers are seen on the buccal mucosa, hard and soft palate, nose, and gums. Purpura and ecchymoses may reflect an underlying blood platelet and clotting problem, renal insufficiency, the side effects of corticosteroids, or vasculitis. Urticaria and angioedema may be present.

Renal Disease. Kidney involvement is found in about half of SLE patients and usually occurs within two years of the onset of symptoms. Acute nephritis or the nephrotic syndrome may be the presenting manifestation of SLE. The most common abnormality is a mild glomerulitis which is associated with minimal proteinuria or hematuria, or both. This lesion generally responds well to therapy initially, but may recur in mild form or as even more severe renal involvement. Acute lupus glomerulonephritis occurs less often and is associated with varying degrees of pyuria, hematuria, proteinuria, fluid retention, edema, hypertension, and azotemia. The nephrotic syndrome is associated with variable proteinuria, with fluid retention, and frequently with normal serum cholesterol levels. The finding of pyuria with fever in patients with SLE, especially in patients receiving corticosteroids, may reflect a urinary tract infection rather than lupus nephritis.

Most patients recover well from attacks of acute nephritis, with loss of edema and azotemia, but usually some proteinuria and decreased glomerular filtration rate (GFR) persist. Patients have recurrences, and some develop chronic glomerulonephritis with hypertension and proteinuria.

Cardiovascular Manifestations. The endocardium, myocardium, and pericardium are involved in nearly half the patients with SLE. Although electrocardiographic changes, such as nonspecific ST, T wave changes, are not uncommon, clinical myocarditis is seen less frequently. Myocarditis should be suspected when tachycardia is disproportionate to either fever or anemia. Cardiomegaly with congestive failure is rare. Precordial chest pain may be caused by either pleurisy or pericarditis. Careful, frequent auscultation may be rewarded by discovery of a pericardial friction rub. Tamponade or constrictive pericarditis is rare. Libman-Sacks or nonbacterial verrucous endocarditis usually occurs on the mitral valve and is recognized by murmurs which cannot be explained by fever or anemia; but generally this is a postmortem diagnosis. Bacterial endocarditis may develop on a previously damaged valve, especially in patients receiving corticosteroids. Recurrent thrombophlebitis may be the first manifestation of SLE. Occlusion of major arteries occurs rarely. Equally rare is pulmonary hypertension.

Pulmonary Involvement. Pleuritic pain is a common complaint and is often the first clue to the diagnosis of SLE. It is generally accompanied by a friction rub and a variable amount of fluid accumulation, but the effusions are often painless. There may be pulmonary infiltrates which are quite difficult to distinguish from those due to infections. The x-ray examination shows bilateral patchy infiltrations which may shift from lobe to lobe. The involvement can progress to atelectasis and to marked pulmonary insufficiency and cyanosis. Most pulmonary symptoms respond well to intensive corticosteroid therapy; but infections must be carefully considered as a cause of the infiltrate.

Neurologic and Psychologic Manifestations. Many patients have read in a dictionary or have heard that SLE is invariably a fatal illness; this understandably leads to great anxiety. Similarly the patient may be told that he or she has arthritis, which leads to ungrounded fears of disabling deformities. These natural fears and anxieties of a chronic illness are not to be confused with organic neurologic disturbances. The latter manifest themselves as behavioral disturbances, including hyperirritability, confusion, hallucinations, obsessional and paranoid reactions, and frank organic psychosis. The psychosis of SLE may easily be confused with, and in fact is difficult to differentiate from, a steroid-induced psychosis; other symptoms and signs of active SLE usually accompany the organic disease. The EEG is often abnormal in SLE with CNS involvement, but brain scans are usually normal. Organic brain damage most commonly manifests itself as convulsions, which occur in at least 15 per cent of patients. Other less frequent neurologic findings include peripheral neuropathy, hemiparesis, motor aphasia, ptosis, diplopia, and nystagmus.

"Cotton wool spots" are fluffy white exudates in the innermost layers of the retina, which may progress to cytoid bodies. They are usually present with other signs of active SLE, and are generally reversible.

Gastrointestinal Manifestations. Anorexia, nausea, vomiting, and abdominal pain are common. The cause is obscure, but may be from peritonitis, enteritis, pancreatitis, or a paralytic ileus. Diarrhea and hematochezia have been noted. The liver is often found to be enlarged because of chronic passive congestion, but this is usually transitory. Liver biopsy may be normal or show fatty infiltration and/or fibrosis.

These manifestations in SLE should not be confused with *lupoid hepatitis*, which is a condition primarily of young women with chronic active hepatitis leading to chronic liver disease and failure. Nephritis is said not to occur. Patients have high levels of gamma globulins, LE cells, and antinuclear antibodies; serum complement levels remain normal or elevated.

Lymph Nodes and Spleen. Lymph nodes, characteristically, are enlarged in SLE but are not tender. The enlarged nodes have been mistaken for lymphoma. Splenomegaly, considered very common years ago, is seen now in about 15 per cent of patients.

Menses and Pregnancy. Menses are frequently irregular or heavy, or both. In patients with circulating anticoagulants, bleeding may be profound. Although pregnancy carries some increased risk of miscarriage in the first trimester, most SLE patients without renal disease do well through term. It should be noted, however, that there is a considerable risk of postpartum exacerbation of the disease.

COURSE UNTREATED. Until recent years the natural course of untreated SLE was considered to be bleak. The average patient was considered to have but a few months or, at best, a few years to live. Since 1948, this situation has changed for the better. The reason for this improvement lies in the recognition of many cases of mild lupus through the development of very sensitive diagnostic tests (antinuclear antibodies), as well as in the development of improved forms of therapy. The

TABLE 2.   Laboratory Abnormalities in SLE*

	Per Cent
Anemia	71
Leukopenia	56
Thrombocytopenia	11
Hemolytic anemia	8
Circulating anticoagulant	2
Rheumatoid factor	19
Biologic false-positive test for syphilis	15
Hypoalbuminemia	50
Hyperglobulinemia	37
LE cell	82
Antinuclear antibodies	96
Anti-double stranded DNA	50
Anti-single-stranded DNA	62
Anti-double-stranded RNA	51
Anti-nucleoprotein	45
Anti-"Sm"	24
Anti-RNP	46
Hypocomplementemia	66
CH50	66
C4	64
C3	52

*Adapted from Dubois, E. L.: Lupus Erythematosus, New York, McGraw-Hill Book Company, 1966; Estes, D., and Christian, C. L.: Medicine, 50:85, 1971; and Fernandez-Herlihy, L.: Lahey Clinic Found. Bull., 21:49, 1972.

disease in most patients is characterized by periods of remissions and relapses, which may be protracted or brief. The same individuals usually have recurrences of the same symptoms they had previously, such as arthritis, pleurisy, nephritis, or rashes. However, variable symptoms and signs may develop years apart. If nephritis develops, it generally does so early in the course.

The prognosis for patients seems to improve each year, but mortality rates remain high during the first year after diagnosis. Whereas in 1956, patients were given only a 50 per cent chance of surviving four years, today they have a better than 90 per cent chance to survive at least ten years. Prognosis still remains somewhat poorer for patients with diffuse proliferative glomerulonephritis or with central nervous system involvement. Patients with only skin involvement have an excellent prognosis but a 15 per cent chance of eventually developing (mild) SLE.

LABORATORY FINDINGS. Hematologic.   Anemia occurs in many patients with SLE and is generally mild, normochromic, or normocytic. Anemia may also be due to infection, renal insufficiency, or bleeding. Autoagglutination of red blood cells may be observed. The Coombs test result is frequently positive, but severe hemolytic anemia is uncommon. Leukopenia occurs in about one half the patients. The differential cell count is usually normal, although mononuclear cells may be more suppressed than neutrophils. Complicating infections generally result in a rise of the white blood cell count either into the normal or elevated range. Corticosteroid therapy also causes leukocytosis. Thrombocytopenia, with or without purpura, may precede other manifestations of SLE by years or may disappear, leaving other manifestations of the disease. A circulating anticoagulant has been noted by some investigators in as many as 25 per cent of patients with SLE. This anticoagulant, either as antibody to factor VIII or, more commonly, as an inhibitor to the formation of "prothrombinase," results in prolonged clotting and pro-

thrombin times and may be associated with mild or, rarely, severe hemorrhages.

Renal.   Renal dysfunction occurs in over half the patients. Most patients have only some impairment of concentrating ability, a few red and/or white blood cells in the urine, and perhaps some proteinuria (< 0.5 gram per day). Active nephritis is defined when there is hematuria (> 5 rc per hpf), pyuria (> 5 wc per hpf), erythrocyte casts, increasing proteinuria, or a decreasing glomerular filtration rate. Hematuria and pyuria are rarely seen in lupus nephritis in remission.

Plasma Proteins.   The erythrocyte sedimentation rate is often elevated. Serum albumin levels are low, especially in the nephrotic syndrome. Gamma globulin levels which are elevated in many patients may be low in nephrotics. Cryoglobulins, consisting of immunoglobulins and complement components, have been noted frequently, especially in patients with renal disease.

Abnormal Immunologic Reactions.   Biologic false-positive test results (BFP) for syphilis have been noted in about 15 per cent of the patients with SLE, especially in those with circulating anticoagulants. The BFP may be the first laboratory clue to the diagnosis of SLE and may precede symptoms by years. Rheumatoid factors have been found in some patients with SLE, even in the absence of clinical rheumatoid arthritis.

Most characteristic of SLE are the large number of autoantibodies which react with cells and their nuclear and cytoplasmic constituents. Historically of greatest significance is the LE cell phenomenon. The LE cell is formed in vitro as follows: some leukocytes are traumatized and release nucleoprotein (DNA-histone); the nucleoprotein reacts with an IgG antibody; and the complex is phagocytized by the remaining viable leukocytes. The LE cell consists of a leukocyte with a large purple-red homogeneous globulin inclusion body which compresses the nucleus against the cell membrane, leaving only a thin rim of cytoplasm. Because LE cells are not always present in patients with SLE, more sensitive tests have been developed for the detection of various antinuclear antibodies (ANA). An immunofluorescent (IF) technique, employing rodent liver or kidney as the source of nuclei, detects ANA in over 99 per cent of SLE patients. The antibodies are usually of the IgG or IgM class. Circulating DNA and other antigens may rarely block the detection of the ANA. With this immunofluorescent technique, different patterns of nuclear fluorescence reflect antibodies to different nuclear structures. The "homogeneous" or "diffuse" pattern reflects antibodies to nucleoprotein. The "peripheral," "rim," or "shaggy" pattern reflects primarily antibodies to DNA. The speckled pattern reflects antibodies to a group of nuclear proteins (ENA, extractable nuclear antigen), including "Sm" and ribonucleoprotein (RNP). A nucleolar pattern has also been observed and appears to represent antibodies to a nuclear RNA.

Antibodies to some antigens, especially to DNA, may also be detected by other methods, including diffusion in agar, complement fixation, agglutination, and radioimmunoassays. The titers of antibodies to DNA and, to some extent, to nucleoprotein tend to be higher during periods of clinical activity, especially of active nephritis, than during clinical remissions.

Complement levels are depressed in most patients with SLE at some time during their illness, especially when disease activity is present. Markedly depressed complement levels are seen primarily in patients with

TABLE 3. Autoantibodies in SLE

Antinuclear	Nucleoprotein
	DNA
	Histone
	Sm
	RNA
	Ribonucleoprotein
	Residue
Anticytoplasmic	Mitochondria
	Lysosomes
	Microsomes
	Ribosomes
	Cytoplasmic sap glycoprotein ("Ro")
	RNA protein
Anti-RNA	Ribosomal RNA
	Double-stranded RNA (? viral)
	Single-stranded RNA
Anticell	Red cell
	White blood cell
	Platelet
Anticlotting factors	
Antithyroid	
Rheumatoid factor	
Biologic false-positive test for syphilis	

active lupus nephritis. The low levels reflect in vivo activation and fixation of complement components by circulating immune complexes. Serial determination of whole complement levels (CH50) or of individual complement components (especially C4 and C3) may be useful in following and managing patients with SLE. SLE has also been seen in some patients with congenital deficiency of complement components, particularly C2.

DIAGNOSIS. The diagnosis of SLE can be made if any four or more of the following manifestations are present, serially or simultaneously, during any interval of observation: butterfly rash, discoid lupus, Raynaud's phenomenon, alopecia, photosensitive rash, oral or nasopharyngeal ulceration, arthritis without deformity, LE cells, chronic biologic false positive test result (BFP) for syphilis, profuse proteinuria, cellular casts, pleuritis or pericarditis, psychosis and/or convulsions, or hemolytic anemia, leukopenia, or thrombocytopenia. SLE should also be suspected — especially in young females — with unexplained fever, purpura, easy bruising, diffuse adenopathy, hepatosplenomegaly, peripheral neuropathy, endocarditis, myocarditis, interstitial pneumonitis, peritonitis, or aseptic meningitis.

Patients are frequently first diagnosed as having rheumatoid arthritis, rheumatic fever (especially children), glomerulonephritis, tuberculosis, scleroderma, vasculitis, idiopathic thrombocytopenic purpura, lymphoma, anemia, or neutropenia. The LE cell is most specific for SLE, if rheumatoid arthritis, lupoid hepatitis, or drug reactions can be excluded. Although the LE cell test is quite often negative, the antinuclear antibody test result is positive in virtually all patients with SLE. Antinuclear antibodies have also been detected in 68 per cent of patients with Sjögren's syndrome, 40 to 75 per cent of patients with scleroderma, especially the speckled pattern, 16 per cent of patients with juvenile rheumatoid arthritis, and 25 to 50 per cent of patients with rheumatoid arthritis, especially the homogeneous pattern. However, antinuclear antibodies tend to be present in higher titers in patients with SLE than in those with other disorders. Antibodies to double-stranded DNA and to an RNA-ase resistant acidic nuclear protein, termed Sm antigen by some, are highly diagnostic of SLE. Antibodies to single-stranded DNA, nucleoprotein (NP), and RNP (an RNA-ase sensitive nuclear antigen) are frequently found in patients with SLE and RA; antibodies to RNP are frequently found in patients with scleroderma.

Some patients have clinical features of SLE, scleroderma, and dermatomyositis. The term *mixed connective tissue disease* (MCTD) has been applied to these patients, as they appear to have a unique combination of clinical and laboratory findings. Some authorities, however, maintain that MCTD represents a subgroup of SLE or scleroderma. MCTD is characterized by diffuse polyarthritis and polyarthralgias, myositis, Raynaud's phenomenon, swollen hands, abnormal esophageal motility, and decreased pulmonary diffusing capacity. These patients often have severe pulmonary disease, rarely have nephritis or CNS disease, and usually respond to treatment with steroids. The serologic abnormalities seen in MCTD include a positive ANA test result with a speckled pattern and a high titer of anti-ENA (extractable nuclear antigen) antibodies, particularly to RNP. Patients with MCTD may have low levels of anti-DNA-antibodies, but most do not.

DRUG-INDUCED LUPUS. Drugs that induce lupus can be divided into two categories: drugs that induce lupus in many individuals, and drugs associated with exacerbations of SLE. In the former group are hydrazides (hydralazine, isoniazid), anticonvulsants (Dilantin), and procainamide. Over 50 per cent of subjects taking procainamide develop antinuclear antibodies, including antibodies to RNP and single-stranded DNA; about 25 per cent develop symptoms and signs of lupus. Arthralgia, pleurisy with effusion, fever, and weight loss are common features, but renal disease, hypocomplementemia, and antibodies to double-stranded DNA are not seen. Symptoms generally clear in a few weeks after discontinuation of the drug, even though antinuclear antibodies persist for months. Antinuclear antibodies appear less frequently in subjects taking hydralazine. Patients with the hydralazine lupus syndrome may have arthritis, dermatitis, serositis, leukopenia, antinuclear antibodies, and anti-DNA antibodies, but rarely have renal or central nervous system disease. Symptoms usually stop after cessation of the drug. Patients with hydralazine lupus are slow acetylators of the drug. These studies suggest that certain subjects may have a genetic predisposition for developing drug lupus. Other drugs, including penicillin, sulfonamides, and oral contraceptives, are associated with exacerbations of SLE, and rarely cause lupus-like symptoms or antinuclear antibodies in other subjects.

THERAPY AND MANAGEMENT. As there are no specific remedies for the treatment of the underlying processes of SLE, the main goals of management must be limited to the treatment of acute relapses and prevention of exacerbations. Certain measures are helpful in prevention of relapses. Sunlight, ultraviolet radiation, blood transfusions, penicillin, and sulfonamides should be avoided when possible. Surgery or infections may lead to a relapse and may require more aggressive concurrent management of the lupus. In the long-term management of this illness, both patient and physician must learn to recognize those symptoms and signs that herald relapses. Although these symptoms may involve fever and arthralgia in some patients, they may appear as hair loss, mucosal ulcers, pleurisy, weight loss, or simply fatigue in others. Before frank clinical symptoms develop, many patients will develop abnormal laboratory tests such as a reduced level of hemoglobin or serum complement or a reduced white blood cell or platelet count; an abnormal urinalysis or creatinine clearance; or a rising titer of anti-DNA antibodies.

Many of the patients seen in the hospital by physicians or students have severe but not life-threatening disease. By contrast, many of the patients seen in the office have much milder disease. The patient fearing the unknown or having heard the worst must be reassured that a majority of patients have mild to moderate disease and that with proper management many of the more serious complications can now be controlled.

Active disease should be treated aggressively to prevent permanent tissue injury. The general measures to be taken include rest when the disease is active, sunscreens, and physical therapy for muscle weakness and deformities. For those patients on moderate to high dosages of corticosteroids, salt restriction and diuretics may be of benefit. Drugs used for the treatment of SLE include topical steroids, salicylates, antimalarials, corticosteroids, and immunosuppressives. The use of corticosteroids is indicated in most patients with SLE and has improved survival. Dosage should be individualized according to the activity of the disease and side effects. *Immunosuppressives* are best used according to the guidelines of Schwartz and Gowans, whose indications are life-threatening or seriously crippling disease; presence of reversible lesions; failure to respond to conventional therapy or intolerable side effects; no active infection; no hematologic contraindication; meticulous follow-up; and objective evaluation.

The acute erythematous maculopapular rash responds well to the avoidance of sunlight, local application of corticosteroid cream, and the systemic introduction of antimalarials such as hydroxychloroquine. Systemic corticosteroids are rarely warranted. The chronic lesion, or discoid lupus, responds to these same measures to a variable degree. Severe, extensive lesions have been treated with large doses of antimalarials when all else has failed. However, the patient should be cautioned about the relative risks of retinal damage when taking large doses of antimalarials. Arthralgia and arthritis respond well to rest, physical therapy, splinting, salicylates, and antimalarials. Steroids should not be needed.

Fever often responds to rest and salicylates. Antimalarials may be beneficial. Persistent fever not responsive to these measures usually coincides with other signs of activity and responds to moderate doses of corticosteroids. Infections must be excluded.

Pericarditis and pleurisy respond well to rest and corticosteroids. Pericardial fluid, if present in moderate amounts, is best removed. Myocarditis should be treated with moderate doses of steroids, fluid restriction, and careful administration of digitalis.

Hemolytic anemia and thrombocytopenia need not be treated unless symptomatic. They generally respond well to steroids. If not, immunosuppressives or a splenectomy may be necessary.

Involvement of the central nervous system responds poorly to treatment. Organic psychosis, in addition, may be difficult to differentiate from a steroid-induced psychosis. Because of the risk of permanent brain damage, large doses of steroids (2 to 3 mg of prednisone per kilogram of body weight per day) are recommended until maximal improvement is achieved, at which time the dosage of steroids is gradually tapered. Immunosuppressives may be helpful.

Mild focal glomerulitis with minimal urinary abnormalities may respond on occasion to bed rest; however, these patients generally require systemic corticosteroid therapy, 0.5 to 1 mg of prednisone per kilogram of body weight per day. Those patients with focal or diffuse proliferative glomerulonephritis generally require higher doses, 1 to 3 mg per kilogram, depending on the severity of the renal impairment. Patients unresponsive to these regimens may benefit from immunosuppressives. Medication is maintained until hematuria clears and serum complement levels return toward normal; this usually occurs within about three weeks. The LE cells, proteinuria, elevated sedimentation rate, and high titers of antinuclear antibodies may persist. The prednisone dosage is then tapered slowly — 10 mg every five days. Complete blood counts, urinalyses, serum creatinine levels, and serum complement levels are checked regularly to detect relapses; relapses usually respond either to maintaining the dosage at that level or increasing it by 5 to 10 mg of prednisone per day. Many patients can be maintained at a dosage of 5 to 10 mg per day; some can tolerate steroids on alternate days; a few can discontinue steroids and remain asymptomatic. Continued careful monitoring and early treatment of slight relapses may avoid more severe exacerbations.

Patients with chronic membranous glomerulonephritis and nephrotic syndrome respond less well to corticosteroids or immunosuppressives. Some, usually those with normal complement levels, may have fixed proteinuria.

Dubois, E. L., and Tuffanelli, D. L.: Clinical manifestations of systemic lupus erythematosus. JAMA, 190:104, 1964.
Estes, D., and Christian, C. L.: The natural history of systemic lupus erythematosus by prospective analysis. Medicine, 50:85, 1971.
Harvey, A. M., Shulman, L. E., Tumulty, A., Conley, C. L., and Schoenrich, E. H.: Systemic lupus erythematosus: Review of the literature and clinical analysis of 138 cases. Medicine, 33:291, 1954.
Rothfield, N. F., and March, C. H.: Lupus erythematosus. In Fitzpatrick, T. B., Arndt, K. A., Clark, W. H., Eisen, A. Z., Van Scott, E. J., and Vaughan, J. H. (eds.): Dermatology in Internal Medicine. New York, McGraw-Hill Book Company, 1971, pp. 1493–1518.
Schur, P. H., and Sandson, J.: Immunological factors and clinical activity in lupus erythematosus. N. Engl. J. Med., 278:533, 1968.

53. PERIARTERITIS NODOSA

(Polyarteritis Nodosa)

K. Frank Austen

DEFINITION. Kussmaul and Maier introduced the term periarteritis nodosa in 1866 to designate a morbid process manifested by numerous grossly visible or palpable nodules along the course of medium-sized muscular arteries. The lesions are segmental in distribution, have a predilection for the crotch of bifurcations and branchings, and involve all but the pulmonary arteries. The clinical manifestations are disparate and polymorphic, and result from partial or complete arterial occlusion, hemorrhage, and glomerulitis. In view of the necrotizing nature of the process, involving the entire arterial wall, Ferrari in 1903 suggested the alternative name of polyarteritis acuta nodosa.

The incidence, age distribution, and male-to-female ratio of periarteritis nodosa are difficult to determine because a diagnostic serologic procedure is lacking, and the spotty distribution of lesions makes biopsy uncertain. Nonetheless, the condition has been reported to occur from infancy to old age, with a peak incidence in the fifth and sixth decades of life, and the male to female ratio has been estimated at from 2 to 3:1.

Generalized necrotizing angiitis in association with hepatitis B antigenemia was first reported in 1970, and by 1976 the literature contained approximately 50 such cases. The incidence of hepatitis B antigenemia has been as high as one third in patients with generalized necrotizing angiitis, a generic term introduced to indicate that these patients have disease extending from the medium-sized muscular arteries to the venules. Serous otitis media and amphetamine abuse are major associated events in the hepatitis B negative group with generalized necrotizing angiitis. On clinical grounds no criteria have been identified to distinguish between the hepatitis B positive and negative patients except that all positive hepatitis B antigenemia patients had abnormal liver chemistries. These were, however, occasionally minimal and then not different from those of the hepatitis B negative group.

PATHOLOGY. The lesions of polyarteritis involve arteries of medium and small caliber, especially at bifurcations and branchings. The segmental process involves the media, with edema, fibrinous exudation, fibrinoid necrosis, and infiltration of polymorphonuclear neutrophils and varying numbers of eosinophils, and extends to the adventitia and intima. Thrombosis and infarction or hemorrhage occur at this stage. Subsequently, the regions of fibrinoid necrosis are replaced by cellular granulation tissue, and the intima proliferates. Finally the involved segment is replaced by scar tissue with associated intimal thickening and periarterial fibrosis. These changes produce partial occlusion, thrombosis and infarction, and palpable or visible aneurysms with occasional rupture.

The glomerulitis is characterized by capillary microthrombi, focal fibrinoid necrosis, polymorphonuclear neutrophil infiltration, and capsular proliferation. With progression, the necrotizing feature of the glomerulitis is less apparent, and the process is difficult to distinguish from glomerulonephritis of other causes.

CLINICAL MANIFESTATIONS AND DIAGNOSIS. The widespread distribution of the arterial lesions produces diverse clinical manifestations, which reflect the particular organ systems in which the arterial supply has been impaired. In addition, no study including a large number of living patients has or even can limit its patient population to those with classic periarteritis as defined by Kussmaul and Maier. The available studies are likely to include an admixture of patients with allergic angiitis and granulomatosis and hypersensitivity angiitis (see Ch. 49). Among the early general symptoms and signs of periarteritis nodosa are tachycardia, fever, weight loss, and pain in viscera and/or the musculoskeletal system so that the differential diagnosis is of fever of unknown origin. Striking and specific presenting signs may relate to abdominal pain, acute glomerulitis, polyneuritis, or myocardial infarction. Pulmonary manifestations, especially intractable bronchial asthma, would indicate allergic angiitis and granulomatosis rather than classic polyarteritis nodosa.

Renal. Renal involvement in two forms, renal polyarteritis and a glomerulitis, may occur separately or together. Renal polyarteritis was the most common lesion in the postmortem studies of Rose and Spencer (see accompanying table), and in the comparable analysis performed at the Armed Forces Institute of Pathology by Mowrey (1954). Manifestations of the renal involvement include intermittent proteinuria and microscopic hematuria with occasional hyaline and granular casts. The glomerulitis is manifested by marked microscopic and even macroscopic hematuria, proteinuria, cellular casts, and progressive renal failure; survival of the acute phase is followed by progressive hypertension. It is no longer the prevailing view that hypertension precedes or occurs in the initial phase of periarteritis nodosa, but rather that it reflects healing renal polyarteritis, progressive glomerulitis, or both. Such renal involvement is the cause of death in about two thirds of patients with classic periarteritis nodosa and about one third of those with allergic angiitis and granulomatosis.

Gastrointestinal. Characteristic arterial lesions are commonly found in one or more abdominal viscera. The principal manifestation is pain, especially in the umbilical region or right upper quadrant; anorexia, nausea, and vomiting are less prominent. Impaired arterial supply to the bowel can produce mucosal ulceration, perforation, or infarction with melena or bloody diarrhea. Involvement of appendix, gallbladder, or pancreas can stimulate appendicitis, cholecystitis, or hemorrhagic pancreatitis. Liver involvement can range from hepatomegaly with or without jaundice to the signs of extensive hepatic necrosis. Splenomegaly is uncommon. There has been no consistent relationship between the development of necrotizing angiitis and the appearance of liver disease in patients with hepatitis B antigenemia. Some of the observed combinations include necrotizing angiitis as the initial clinical finding, superimposed upon chronic active hepatitis, or appearing simultaneously with an acute hepatitis. Death in this group can occur from liver failure but is more commonly due to the generalized necrotizing angiitis.

Incidence of Necrotizing Angiitis in Various Organs at Necropsy*

	Polyarteritis Nodosa (Classic)	Allergic Angiitis and Granulomatosis ("Polyarteritis with Pulmonary Involvement")
	Per Cent	*Per Cent*
Lungs (pulmonary arteries)	0	47
Heart	35	60
Kidneys: Glomerulitis	30	57
Renal polyarteritis	65	60
Stomach and intestines	30	40
Liver	54	37
Pancreas	39	17
Spleen	35	43
Brain	4	3
Periadrenal connective tissue	41	40
Voluntary muscle	20	33

*Reproduced in modified form from Rose and Spencer: Quart. J. Med., 26:43, 1957. There were 54 cases in the periarteritis group and 30 with the diagnosis of allergic angiitis and granulomatosis.

Central and Peripheral Nervous System. Neurologic manifestations are generally late occurrences in the course of periarteritis nodosa, and their particular presentation reflects the specific brain area compromised. Headache, convulsive seizures, papillitis, and retinal hemorrhages and exudates occur with or without localizing signs referable to the cerebrum, cerebellum, or brainstem; meningeal irritation may occur as a result of subarachnoid hemorrhage. Multineuritis multiplex, that is, involvement of several or even many individual nerves at the same or different times, is a common finding and is attributed to arteritis of the vasa nervorum. The peripheral neuropathy is usually asymmetrical with both sensory and motor distribution. The former can be extremely painful, but the latter, with attendant muscular degeneration, has on occasion been so severe as to dominate the clinical presentation.

Articular and Muscular. Arthralgia and myalgia are frequent in polyarteritis nodosa. Arthralgia is migratory, generally without swelling, and apparently due to small localized arterial lesions rather than extensive synovitis. The interpretation of those rare instances of synovitis with deformity and arterial changes of periarteritis nodosa is difficult, but it seems preferable to consider such cases as rheumatoid arthritis. Muscle pain or weakness reflects either direct involvement of the arterial supply or a peripheral neuropathy from involvement of the vasa nervorum.

Cardiac. Polyarteritis of the coronary arteries and their branches has a frequency approaching that of renal polyarteritis, and heart failure is responsible for or contributes to death in one sixth to one half of the cases. An infantile form of periarteritis nodosa, affecting children mainly under 10 months of age, is manifested primarily by involvement of the coronary arteries. The clinical manifestations of cardiac involvement are those of partial or complete arterial occlusion as modified by the superimposition of renal hypertension and an appreciable incidence of acute pericarditis without effusion. Whereas the combination of infarction and hypertension commonly leads to left-sided failure, an occasional patient with allergic angiitis and granulomatosis will present with predominantly right-sided decompensation.

Genitourinary. Involvement of the ovaries, testes, and epididymis is frequent, though usually asymptomatic. Mucosal ulceration in the bladder can occasionally precipitate gross hematuria with dysuria.

Cutaneous. Cutaneous involvement of some form is believed to occur in over 25 per cent of those affected with periarteritis nodosa. The acute cutaneous manifestations of periarteritis nodosa include polymorphic exanthemata—purpuric, urticarial, and multiform in character—and severe subcutaneous hemorrhage, resulting from necrotizing arteritis, with secondary gangrene. Ulcerations and a persistent livedo reticularis are associated with the more chronic stage of the disease. A most characteristic but uncommon finding is cutaneous and subcutaneous nodules; these occur at any time in the disease course. The nodules tend to group, appear in crops, are usually movable, may regress in days or persist for months, range in size from a pea to a walnut, and may cause the overlying skin to become reddened or to ulcerate.

Allergic Angiitis and Granulomatosis ("Polyarteritis with Pulmonary Involvement"). Pulmonary lesions are absent in classic polyarteritis nodosa but almost always precede the onset of polyarteritic lesions in other organs in the process termed allergic granulomatosis and angiitis by Churg and Strauss. Such patients typically present with bronchitis, bronchial asthma, or the findings of pneumonia. The asthma is intractable and associated with a marked peripheral eosinophilia. The pneumonic episodes are transient or progressive and can include hemoptysis or pleuritic pain. The appearance and superimposition of polyarteritis nodosa in other organs is followed by a rapid deterioration, respiratory involvement accounting for half the deaths.

COURSE UNTREATED. The course of periarteritis nodosa is progressive with destruction of vital organs. Intermittent acute episodes resulting from thrombosis of vital or nonvital structures are prominent. Death is most frequently attributed to renal involvement in cases of classic periarteritis nodosa and to pulmonary lesions in those cases classified as allergic angiitis with granulomatosis. Cardiac failure caused by a combination of infarction and renal hypertension is an additional frequent cause of death in both groups, and acute vascular accidents in the gastrointestinal tract or central nervous system account for much of the remaining mortality. In the retrospective postmortem study of Rose and Spencer, the five-year survival rate was about 10 per cent in classic periarteritis nodosa, and about 25 per cent in allergic angiitis and granulomatosis if onset was dated from the start of respiratory symptoms. The more recent report of the British Medical Research Council in 1960 placed the 54 month's survival rate in polyarteritis nodosa at nearly 50 per cent. A similar survival rate attributed to early steroid treatment has been noted in a Mayo Clinic series in which pulmonary involvement did not appear to influence the prognosis. Rare patients with polyarteritis limited to nonvital sites have been reported to experience an unusually long course or even a lasting remission. The entire issue of prognosis will be influenced by the criteria for entry into a series until the entity of periarteritis is more definitively separated from the more favorable grouping of hypersensitivity angiitis.

LABORATORY FINDINGS. Leukocytosis, predominantly polymorphonuclear, is apparent in over 75 per cent of the cases of periarteritis nodosa or allergic angiitis and granulomatosis, eosinophilia often being marked in the latter group. The association of hepatitis B antigenemia with generalized necrotizing angiitis may be as high as one third of the cases, but probably this figure will prove to be smaller as experience widens. Hypocomplementemia, which has not been observed in classic periarteritis nodosa, has been present in patients with generalized necrotizing angiitis with or without hepatitis B antigenemia. The erythrocyte sedimentation rate is customarily elevated with or without some increase of the globulins. Abnormalities in the urine sediment, especially hematuria and proteinuria, reflect renal involvement. Abnormalities of the electrocardiogram and electroencephalogram are those expected on the basis of arterial occlusive disease or those secondary to the metabolic disturbances of uremia. Lesions apparent on chest roentgenograms are the rule in patients with allergic angiitis and granulomatosis. The findings range from transient or progressive infiltration to consolidation, cavitation, or scarring; upper and lower lobes are involved with equal frequency. As none of these findings is specific, antemortem diagnosis of polyarteritis depends upon biopsy. Since the arterial involvement is segmental and spotty in distribution, it is advisable to obtain tissue from a symptomatic site, and it is essential to section completely the entire specimen. A deep, open surgical biopsy, including subcutaneous tissue and underlying muscle, should be obtained whenever possible from a skeletal muscle exhibiting pain and tenderness. Involvement of the epididymis and testes is sufficiently common to make this a useful biopsy site, if palpation reveals the typical nodularity of segmental vascular lesions. Needle and surgical biopsies of internal organs with clinical involvement, such as liver or kidney, are gaining in favor. As an alternative or additional procedure, arteriography of several organs to detect aneurysms of medium-sized muscular arteries may be helpful.

DIFFERENTIAL DIAGNOSIS. The differential diagnosis of classic periarteritis nodosa includes all those conditions associated with necrotizing angiitis (see Ch. 49). The absence of pulmonary lesions distinguishes classic periarteritis nodosa from allergic angiitis and granulomatosis. Similarly, the relative absence of venular involvement, with or without hepatitis B antigenemia, may separate classic periarteritis nodosa from the more common generalized necrotizing angiitis. The hypocomplementemia in some patients with generalized necrotizing angiitis is more reminiscent of certain patients with hypersensitivity angiitis than of periarteritis nodosa. The other connective tissue diseases are recognized by their clinical characteristics even when necrotizing arteritis becomes prominent. For example, cases of rheumatoid arthritis with ulcerating cutaneous lesions and peripheral neuropathy often exhibit prominent rheumatoid nodules and a high titer of rheumatoid factor. Giant cell arteritis, in its limited form, cranial (especially temporal) or aortic arch (Takayasu's) arteritis, or in its disseminated state lacks the glomerulitis, peripheral neuropathy, and cutaneous manifestations notable in periarteritis nodosa. The drug-induced hypersensitivity angiitis group may be difficult to separate on purely clinical grounds, although the history of antecedent drug administration, the frequency of pulmonary involvement, infrequency of gastrointestinal manifestations, and absence of nodules along arteries are useful points. The clinical presentation in Henoch-Schönlein purpura, mostly in children and with a relatively good prognosis, is distinctive. The combination of progressive nephritis and pulmonary hemorrhage seen in Goodpasture's syndrome is unlike polyarteritis nodosa. The findings in the immunoglobulins which accompany active systemic lupus erythematosus or mixed cryoglobulinemia are distinctive; in addition, in the presence of active renal disease both entities manifest a reduced serum complement level not observed in periarteritis nodosa. Necrotizing vasculitis with or without renal disease in C2 deficiency, hypergammaglobulinemic purpura, and other syndromes listed under hypersensitivity angiitis (see Ch. 49) are differentiated by the unique features responsible for designating the entity.

The key morphologic differences between periarteritis nodosa and other causes of necrotizing angiitis are noted in Ch. 49 and include the absence of extravascular granulomas, sparing of the pulmonary arteries, failure of venous involvement except by contiguous spread, and predilection for medium-sized arteries. For allergic angiitis and granulomatosis the striking granulomatous response excludes all but Wegener's granulomatosis. The prominence of bronchial asthma, peripheral eosinophilia, and the usual absence of necrotizing lesions in the upper respiratory tract permit a tentative clinical distinction between allergic angiitis and gran-

ulomatosis (termed by some polyarteritis nodosa with pulmonary involvement) and Wegener's granulomatosis. Additional entities to be considered in the differential diagnosis are certain microbial and occlusive diseases with diverse manifestations, notably chronic meningococcemia, subacute infective endocarditis, trichinosis, certain rickettsial diseases, leptospirosis, and syphilis. A few vascular occlusive diseases, including Degos' disease and thrombotic thrombocytopenic purpura, must also be considered. Necrotizing papulosis of Degos, with its occlusive arterial lesions of the skin, gastrointestinal tract, and brain, is best characterized by the cutaneous manifestations. These lesions typically involve the trunk and extremities, begin as pink to gray papules, undergo central umbilication, and persist for variable periods with depressed (porcelain-like) centers covered with a removable scale and surrounded by a red elevated margin. The absence of both thrombocytopenia and intravascular hemolysis distinguishes periarteritis nodosa from thrombotic thrombocytopenic purpura. Additional points of help in the differential diagnosis of periarteritis nodosa in general are the rarity of Raynaud's phenomenon, the absence of the nephrotic syndrome, and the lack of lymphadenopathy.

TREATMENT. The therapy of periarteritis nodosa and allergic angiitis and granulomatosis is clearly unsatisfactory. Nonetheless, such patients can remain ambulatory and professionally active for periods of months to years after the clinical onset of the disease. The commonly employed anti-inflammatory agents such as salicylates or phenylbutazone have little or no clear effect, and thus corticosteroids have been employed most widely. Large doses, in the range of 40 to 60 mg of prednisone per day, afford symptomatic relief and apparently do improve the one-year survival statistics. On the other hand, the study by the Medical Research Council of England did not reveal a better 54 months' survival period in a steroid-treated group as compared with a control series, whereas early steroid treatment was considered efficacious in the Mayo Clinic series. The capacity of steroids in giant cell arteritis and of cyclophosphamide in Wegener's granulomatosis to produce convincing clinical responses and, apparently, even extended remissions has prompted an increased utilization of such agents in the treatment of other forms of necrotizing agiitis. Cytotoxic agents, generally accompanied by steroids, are certainly justified in the management of patients with periarteritis nodosa, generalized necrotizing angiitis, and allergic angiitis and granulomatosis.

Churg, J., and Strauss, L.: Allergic granulomatosis, allergic angiitis, and periarteritis nodosa. Am. J. Pathol., 27:277, 1951.

Collagen Diseases and Hypersensitivity Panel: Report to Medical Research Council. Br. Med. J., 1:1399, 1960.

Fink, C. W.: Polyarteritis and other diseases with necrotizing vasculitis in children. Arthritis Rheum., 20:378, 1977 (suppl.).

Gocke, D. J., Hsu, K., Morgan, C., Bombardieri, S., Lockshin, M., and Christian, C. L.: Association betwen polyarteritis and Australia antigen. Lancet, 2:1149, 1970.

Mowrey, F. H., and Lundberg, R. A.: The clinical manifestations of essential polyangiitis (periarteritis nodosa) with emphasis on the hepatic manifestations. Ann. Intern. Med., 40:1145, 1954.

Reza, M. J., Dornfeld, L., Goldberg, L. S., Bluestone, R., and Pearson, C. M.: Wegener's granulomatosis. Long-term follow-up of patients treated with cyclophosphamide. Arthritis Rheum., 18:501, 1975.

Rose, G. A., and Spencer, H.: Polyarteritis nodosa. Quart. J. Med., 26:43, 1957.

Sergent, J. S., Lockshin, M. D., Christian, C. L., and Gocke, D. J.: Vasculitis with hepatitis B antigenemia. Long-term observations in nine patients. Medicine, 55:1, 1976.

Trepo, G. C., and Thivolet, J.: Antigene Australien, hépatite à virus et periartérite nouveuse. Presse Méd., 78:1575, 1970.

PART VII

DISEASES OF THE JOINTS

Charles L. Christian

54. INTRODUCTION

Although the terms "arthritis" and "rheumatism" have similar connotations, the former is restrictive, denoting inflammatory disease of joints. "Rheumatism" embraces a wide variety of illnesses that affect components of the musculoskeletal system: joints, muscles, ligaments, tendons, and bursae. Rheumatic syndromes can be classified as either inflammatory or degenerative, but the pathologic processes are sometimes less distinct than the nomenclature implies. A joint damaged by inflammatory disease is more vulnerable to degenerative influences, and syndromes that appear to be primarily degenerative in nature may be associated with the cardinal signs of inflammation. Musculoskeletal pain and stiffness, although characteristic of rheu-

matic syndromes, can be significant manifestations of virtually every disease of man. Errors in diagnosis and management result from uncritical elicitation of the medical history, physical signs, and, probably most frequently, from unbalanced interpretations of laboratory data. Hyperuricemia, rheumatoid factors, and antinuclear factors are not disease specific; and radiographic evidence of degenerative joint disease does not constitute proof that pain in an extremity is due to that process.

The accompanying classification of rheumatic disease (table), condensed and somewhat amended from the American Rheumatism Association's recommended (tentative) nomenclature, indicates the diversity of illnesses that can cause manifestations of rheumatic disease.

Rheumatic Disease — Classification

1. Polyarthritis of unknown etiology:
   a. Rheumatoid arthritis
   b. Juvenile rheumatoid arthritis
   c. Ankylosing spondylitis
   d. Psoriatic arthritis
   e. Reiter's syndrome
   f. Others
2. "Connective tissue" disorders (acquired):
   a. Systemic lupus erythematosus
   b. Progressive systemic sclerosis (scleroderma)
   c. Polymyositis and dermatomyositis
   d. Necrotizing arteritis and other forms of vasculitis
3. Rheumatic fever
4. Degenerative joint disease (osteoarthritis):
   a. Primary
   b. Secondary
5. Nonarticular rheumatism:
   a. Fibrositis
   b. Intervertebral disc and low back syndromes
   c. Myositis and myalgia
   d. Tendinitis and peritendinitis (bursitis)
6. Diseases with which arthritis is frequently associated:
   a. Sarcoidosis
   b. Relapsing polychondritis
   c. Schönlein-Henoch purpura
   d. Ulcerative colitis
   e. Regional enteritis
   f. Whipple's disease
   g. Sjögren's syndrome
   h. Familial Mediterranean fever
   i. Others
7. Arthritis associated with known infectious agents:
   a. Bacterial
   b. Rickettsial
   c. Viral
   d. Fungal

   e. Parasitic
8. Traumatic and/or neurogenic disorders:
   a. Traumatic arthritis (the result of direct trauma)
   b. Neuropathic arthropathy (Charcot joints)
   c. Shoulder-hand syndrome
   d. Mechanical derangement of joints
   e. Others
9. Arthritis associated with known or strongly suspected biochemical or endocrine abnormalities:
   a. Gout
   b. Chondrocalcinosis articularis ("pseudogout")
   c. Alcaptonuria (ochronosis)
   d. Hemophilia
   e. Sickle cell disease and other hemoglobinopathies
   f. Agammaglobulinemia (hypogammaglobulinemia)
   g. Gaucher's disease
   h. Hyperparathyroidism
   i. Acromegaly
   j. Hypothyroidism
   k. Scurvy
   l. Hyperlipoproteinemia type II (xanthoma tuberosum and tendinosum)
   m. Hemochromatosis
   n. Others
10. Neoplasms
11. Allergy and drug reactions
12. Miscellaneous disorders:
    a. Pigmented villonodular synovitis and tenosynovitis
    b. Behçet's syndrome
    c. Erythema nodosum
    d. Avascular necrosis of bone
    e. Juvenile osteochondritis
    f. Erythema multiforme (Stevens-Johnson syndrome)
    g. Hypertrophic osteoarthropathy
    h. Multicentric reticulohistiocytosis

55. ARTHRITIS ASSOCIATED WITH KNOWN INFECTIOUS AGENTS

55.1. BACTERIAL ARTHRITIS

The great majority of cases of bacterial arthritis result from hematogenous spread of infections. Much less frequently, bacterial infection may result from joint aspiration or injection or by spread from contiguous osteomyelitis. In adults, gram-positive cocci (*Staphylococcus aureus, Streptococcus pyogenes, Diplococcus pneumoniae*) and *Neisseria gonorrhoeae* account for most cases. (Other areas of this text contain more detailed accounts of the problems and management of sepsis caused by specific bacterial organisms. The emphasis here is on principles of diagnosis and management that are common to all types of bacterial arthritis.)

Certain organisms appear to exhibit a tropism for joints: *N. gonorrhoeae, N. meningitidis, Hemophilus influenzae,* and *Streptobacillus moniliformis.* Host factors associated with debilitating chronic disease, rheumatoid arthritis, sickle cell anemia, hypogammaglobulinemia, and immunosuppressive therapy increase the risk of bacterial arthritis. A problem of increasing frequency is the development of low-grade infection complicating prosthetic joint placement. The recognition of infection may be delayed many months after joint replacement. Organisms of low virulence, especially *Staphylococcus albus,* predominate.

CLINICAL MANIFESTATIONS. Although inflammatory signs in a single joint should heighten one's suspicion of bacterial sepsis, the disease may be polyarticular, a pattern that predominates with gonococcal arthritis. Rigor and high temperature, common manifestations of bacterial arthritis, are rare in rheumatoid arthritis and other types of noninfectious joint disease. Inflammatory signs tend to be marked; but in the presence of debilitating disease or treatment with adrenocorticosteroids or immunosuppressive agents, pain, swelling, and erythema may be masked. In patients with chronic rheumatoid arthritis, a preponderance of inflammatory disease in one or a limited number of joints should arouse suspicion of complicating bacterial arthritis.

DIAGNOSIS. Since accurate diagnosis and effective management depend on isolation and characterization of the microbe, the highest priority is to be given to careful and complete bacteriologic studies. Although synovial fluid leukocyte counts in excess of 50,000 per cubic millimeter and reduced synovial fluid glucose content are common manifestations, no level of either is diagnostic of infection. Stained smears of joint fluid may demonstrate bacterial forms in the absence of a positive culture, especially when there has been chemotherapy. Synovial fluid and blood for microbiologic studies should be delivered without delay to the laboratory, preferably by someone involved in the patient's management. In addition to routine aerobic and anaerobic cultures, special media are needed for the isolation of *N. gonorrhoeae.* Obviously bacteriologic studies of other materials, such as sputum, urine, and cervical exudate, may help to identify the organism causing arthritis.

Radiographic signs indicating loss of articular cartilage or erosion of bone are uncommon during the first week of disease.

MANAGEMENT. Success in management, as in diagnosis, rests with identification of the pathogen. The selection of appropriate antimicrobial agents and recommendations regarding dose and duration of therapy are covered in other areas of this text (see Ch. 190). It should be remembered that bacterial arthritis is usually a part of systemic sepsis and that the involvement of the synovial bursae behaves like a closed space infection. Since there is adequate transport of the commonly employed antimicrobial agents from blood to joint fluid, there are rarely if ever indications for intraarticular therapy. When response to therapy is inadequate, measurement of bactericidal levels of drugs in synovial fluid may be indicated.

The decision whether to drain the joint bursae is influenced by the character of the exudate. When there is gross suppuration, and fluid cannot be easily aspirated with a large-bore needle, surgical incision and drainage are usually performed. When fluid can be aspirated with a needle and syringe, this is the preferred method for periodic decompression. The frequency of aspiration depends upon the extent and rate of reaccumulation. Gross joint destruction and the presence of contiguous osteomyelitis are indications for surgical drainage.

Physical therapy is inappropriate during the acute phase of bacterial arthritis. Maintenance of rest may be facilitated by removable splints. The rate at which gentle passive exercises can be graded into active motion should be tailored to each patient. Even in the absence of structural damage of weight-bearing joints, activity should be resumed until signs of acute inflammation have subsided. The prognosis for full recovery is good when effective therapy is initiated within a week of the onset.

Gonococcal Arthritis. Gonococcal infection is discussed in Ch. 139. Because of its frequency and characteristic manifestations, this form of bacterial arthritis deserves emphasis. It is most common in females and homosexual males whose primary infections, because they are often asymptomatic, are untreated. The manifestations vary, but the most common pattern is migratory polyarthritis associated with tenosynovitis (especially in the hand and foot), followed by a "settling" in one or two joints. Shaking chills often precede or accompany the synovitis. Erythematous skin lesions, which may be macular, vesicular, or pustular (often with a necrotic center), are common in gonococcemia. The same clinical pattern can be associated with *N. meningitidis* and *H. influenzae* infections, although the latter is rare in adults.

Tuberculous Arthritis. The general decline in the frequency of tuberculosis is reflected in the relative rarity of tuberculous bone and joint disease. During the past few decades tuberculous arthritis has been predominantly an adult disease with evidence of pulmonary or disseminated disease frequently lacking. It is usually manifest in a single joint, most commonly hip, knee, or wrist, but any articulation may be affected, and occasionally two or more may be involved. Tuberculous *spondylitis* (Pott's disease), predominantly a disease of children, has dramatically decreased in western countries.

Signs of acute inflammation are usually absent. Tuberculous arthritis is most commonly confused with monoarticular rheumatoid arthritis. The ultimate differentiation, in a tuberculin-positive subject, often requires synovial biopsy and subsequent histologic and bacteriologic studies. Modern chemotherapy (see Ch. 168.14) has made surgical procedures (drainage, synovectomy, or fusion) unnecessary except in a rare patient with severe joint destruction.

55.2. VIRAL ARTHRITIS

Prevailing theories regarding the pathogenesis of rheumatoid arthritis, systemic lupus erythematosus, and related syndromes implicate atypical microbial infection. Although evidence supporting such speculations is indirect, there are well-defined, common viral infections associated with polyarthritis, notably rubella and viral hepatitis. Other viral syndromes associated with arthritis include mumps, infectious mononucleosis, and several arborvirus infections. Polyarthritis resembling acute rheumatic fever or acute rheumatoid arthritis occurs in approximately one third of women with natural or vaccine *rubella* infection. Lower frequencies of this complication are seen in men and children. Rubella arthritis usually follows the onset, or the fading phase, of the characteristic rash. The virus has been isolated from affected joints. The duration of joint inflammation varies from a few days to two weeks, rarely longer. There has been no documentation of chronic arthritis resulting from rubella infection. The management of pain and stiffness, which may be severe, should require nothing more than salicylate therapy.

Transient polyarthritis—more commonly polyarthralgia—is a significant prodromal manifestation of viral *hepatitis*. As with rubella, the pattern of arthritis resembles that of acute rheumatoid arthritis. It is frequently associated with fever and an urticarial skin eruption. These antedate the signs and symptoms of hepatitis by a few days to a few weeks, and have generally receded by the time icterus is apparent. Persistent polyarthritis has not been observed as a complication of viral hepatitis, although a small percentage of individuals with chronic active hepatitis have mild chronic or recurrent synovitis. The role that hepatitis B (Australia) antigen plays in the pathogenesis of the arthritis is not known, but certain manifestations, i.e., depressed serum complement and urticarial rash, are consistent with the hypothesis that immune complexes may be involved. Treatment is symptomatic.

55.3. OTHER FORMS OF INFECTIOUS ARTHRITIS

SYPHILITIC ARTHRITIS. Syphilis is discussed in Ch. 171. Syphilitic arthritis, in its various forms, is now rare. A mild chronic synovitis, usually of the knees, may occur at about the age of puberty in patients with prenatal syphilis *(Clutton's joints)*. Earlier skeletal manifestation of prenatal syphilis are related to periostitis and osteochondritis. Rheumatic manifestations have been attributed to secondary syphilis, but these, along with gummatous involvement of bones and joints, have

more historical than current importance. The most common rheumatic expression of syphilis, neuropathic arthropathy or Charcot joint, is reviewed in Ch. 60.

MYCOTIC ARTHRITIS. Any of the invasive *mycoses* such as histoplasmosis, coccidioidomycosis, blastomycosis, and actinomycosis can affect joints, usually by extension from adjacent bone. Their manifestations generally resemble those of tuberculosis. Coccidioidomycosis can also cause the joint inflammation of erythema nodosum (see Ch. 179).

LYME ARTHRITIS. See Ch. 60.

Alpert, E., Isselbacher, K. J., and Schur, P. H.: The pathogenesis of arthritis associated with viral hepatitis: Complement component studies. N. Engl. J. Med., 285:185, 1971.

Davidson, P. T., and Horowitz, I.: Skeletal tuberculosis: A review with patient presentations and discussion. Am. J. Med., 48:77, 1970.

Keiser, H., et al.: Clinical forms of gonococcal arthritis. N. Engl. J. Med., 279:234, 1968.

Schmid, F. R.: Principles of diagnosis and treatment of infectious arthritis. In Hollander, J. L., and McCarty, D. J., Jr. (eds.): Arthritis and Allied Conditions. 8th ed. Philadelphia, Lea & Febiger, 1972.

Sharp, J. T.: Gonococcal arthritis. In Hollander, J. L., and McCarty, D. J., Jr. (eds.): Arthritis and Allied Conditions. 8th ed. Philadelphia, Lea & Febiger, 1972.

Smith, J. W., and Sanford, J. P.: Viral arthritis. Ann. Intern. Med., 67:651, 1967.

56. RHEUMATOID ARTHRITIS

DEFINITION. In 1858 Sir Alfred Garrod introduced the term rheumatoid arthritis for a syndrome which he recognized as distinct from gout and acute rheumatic fever. With only minor exceptions (Garrod included Heberden's nodes as features of rheumatoid arthritis) his description matches the modern definition. The American Rheumatism Association's criteria for "classical, definite, probable and possible rheumatoid arthritis" have led to more consistent reporting in clinical studies, but the diagnosis still rests mainly on exclusion of other causes of synovitis.

Rheumatoid arthritis is a systemic disease of unknown cause. The frequency of extra-articular manifestations justifies the concept of "rheumatoid disease," but in the majority of patients clinical and pathologic findings and disability are the result of chronic inflammation of synovial membranes. There is striking heterogeneity among patients regarding mode of onset, pattern of joint involvement, frequency of extra-articular manifestations, and clinical course. There is a tendency for symmetrical involvement of hands, wrists, and feet. Spontaneous remissions and exacerbations are characteristic. Ten to 20 per cent of patients have complete remissions,whereas the remainder have sustained fluctuating activity. Joint injury results from formation of chronic granulation tissue (pannus), products of proliferative and exudative synovitis; this is capable of altering articular and periarticular structures.

INCIDENCE AND EPIDEMIOLOGY. The frequency of rheumatoid arthritis, based on limited population surveys in Europe and North America, is in the range of 1 to 3 per cent. It is two to three times more common in females. The onset is most frequent in the fourth and fifth decades of life, but it may occur at any age. There are no consistent trends relating prevalence to geography, climate, or culture. The apparent relative rarity in tropical climates may reflect the age of indigenous populations and the level of available medical care. Multiple family members in selected kindreds may be affected; but in general, familial patterns (even in monozygotic twins) are not striking. An increased frequency of a histocompatibility antigen (HLA-DW$_4$) has been observed in rheumatoid arthritis subjects.

PATHOLOGY. The pathologic elements of chronic synovitis include exudation, cellular infiltration, and the proliferation of granulation tissue. Although polymorphonuclear leukocytes predominate in synovial fluid, the principal infiltrating cells in synovial membranes are lymphocytes. These are often arranged in nodular aggregates, occasionally as true lymphoid follicles with germinal centers. Rarely, the majority of infiltrating cells are plasmacytes. Multinucleated giant cells may be seen. None of the aforementioned histologic features are diagnostic of rheumatoid arthritis.

Pannus, presumably by its content of hydrolytic enzymes, is capable of eroding articular cartilage, subchondral bone, ligaments, and tendons. Products of exudation in synovial fluid may also contribute to cartilage injury. The variable pattern of joint disability (subluxation, loss of motion, or ankylosis) relates to destructive processes in articular and periarticular structures.

Extra-articular manifestations, although clinically evident in a minority of patients, may give rise to widespread pathologic features of rheumatoid arthritis. Many of these appear to result from focal perivascular inflammation. Ten to 20 per cent of patients with rheumatoid arthritis form *subcutaneous or periosteal nodules* over pressure or friction points. The histologic appearance of nodules (central areas of necrosis surrounded by palisading connective tissue cells and an envelope of granulation tissue) is characteristic. In rare instances, the same granulomatous process can occur in multiple organs. More commonly (probably in the range of 50 per cent of cases) there is a mild perivascular infiltration of mononuclear cells in *muscle and peripheral nerves.* An uncommon but significant complication of the disease is the development of diffuse *necrotizing arteritis* with visceral involvement indistinguishable from polyarteritis nodosa. Milder forms of vasculitis, manifested by peripheral neuropathy and *chronic skin ulcers* of the lower extremities, are much more frequent. In such patients chronic inflammation of the sclera is common.

Cardiac pathology is less evident clinically than it is histologically. At necropsy, between one third and one half of rheumatoid patients have evidence of pericarditis (usually healed). Granulomatous lesions resembling rheumatoid nodules rarely may be found in the epicardium, myocardium, valves, and proximal aorta.

Pulmonary lesions, although infrequent, are significant expressions of rheumatoid disease. They include (1) chronic *pleural effusion,* (2) *Caplan's syndrome* (exaggerated pulmonary nodule formation in rheumatoid patients exposed to silica dust), (3) involvement with *granulomatous lesions resembling rheumatoid nodules,* and (4) *interstitial fibrosis.*

The most common patterns of neurologic involvement are peripheral neuropathy and nerve root irritation or myelopathy secondary to vertebral involvement (especially at C1-C2).

PATHOGENESIS. The role of *inflammation* in the production of articular, periarticular, and extra-articular injury is evident. A variety of lysosomal enzymes, neutral proteases, and synovial collagenase are capable of hy-

drolyzing constituents of connective tissue, and the role of such enzymes in the induction of tissue injury seems explicit. A more basic question, however, is: What initiates and perpetuates the inflammatory response? In this regard, immunologic theories predominate.

Immunologic Features. Synovial tissue in rheumatoid arthritis often displays histologic features characteristic of lymphoid organs, with prominent collections of lymphocytes and plasma cells (sometimes in the form of germinal centers). Immunoglobulin synthesis has been demonstrated in rheumatoid synovial tissue by immunohistologic and tissue culture studies. There is evidence for a role of immune complexes in the induction of inflammation. Synovial fluid exudate cells and synovial lining cells contain deposits of immunoglobulin and complement. Complement levels in synovial fluid are reduced in a pattern consistent with immune activation, and complexes of immunoglobulins are detectable in joint fluid. Detailed characterization of these has not been accomplished, but in part they consist of rheumatoid factors.

Rheumatoid Factors. Rheumatoid factors are autoantibodies reactive with the Fc portion of IgG. Anti–gamma globulin activities are associated with the three major classes of immunoglobulins (IgM, IgG, and IgA), but, because of the enhanced agglutinating property of IgM antibodies, standard tests measure predominantly IgM rheumatoid factors. Rheumatoid factors form soluble complexes with their antigen (IgG). The complexes of IgM rheumatoid factor with IgG have a sedimentation coefficient of approximately 22S, whereas the complexes formed with IgG rheumatoid factors are very heterogeneous, sedimenting in the "intermediate" range between IgG and IgM. These intermediate complexes, which comprise at least part of the complexes measurable in rheumatoid synovial fluid, are capable of reacting with IgM rheumatoid factors to form insoluble aggregates. It is postulated that such complexes in joint fluid, perhaps augmented by their reactivity with IgM rheumatoid factor, activate complement-dependent mediators of inflammation and promote phagocytosis and subsequent release of hydrolytic enzymes. Although this hypothesis is attractive, there are a variety of reasons why one cannot assign an exclusive and primary role to rheumatoid factors in the induction of rheumatoid synovitis. On the basis of current evidence, it is more likely that rheumatoid factors are products of the host response to a more primary event. The nature of this postulated primary event is still unknown, but there is renewed interest in an old concept that microbial disease may underlie the development of rheumatoid arthritis.

Infectious Agents. A number of clinical and pathologic features of rheumatoid arthritis are mimicked by animal models of disease where microbial causes are explicit — in particular, chronic arthritis in swine induced by species of *Mycoplasma* and by *Erysipelothrix insidiosa.* An interesting aspect of these experimental models is that by the time chronic disease has developed, the inducing microorganism is often not demonstrable. By analogy, if the microbial hypothesis for rheumatoid disease is correct, the generally negative results of efforts to recover microorganisms may thus be explained. Although speculation regarding an infectious cause of rheumatoid disease has been augmented by modern concepts of viral persistence and by studies of animal models, direct evidence in its support is lacking. There have been periodic reports of the isolation of *Mycoplasma* and bacterial forms and of demonstrations that rheumatoid synovial cells are resistant to infection by exogenous viruses, but these observations still lack confirmation.

CLINICAL MANIFESTATIONS. Mode of Onset. Usually, rheumatoid arthritis has an insidious onset, often beginning with poorly localized arching and stiffness. These early symptoms may be attributed to "grippe," and the subsequent evolution of frank synovitis may be sufficiently slow that the patient does not seek medical attention for many weeks. A variety of "precipitating" factors have been entertained (trauma, environmental change, infections, and psychologic stress), but none of these is constant in the antecedent history. Most patiens manifest symmetrical polyarthritis early in the course of their disease, but a significant number (approximately one third) will have inflammation limited to one or two joints. Occasionally limited expressions of the disease, i.e., monarthritis or even tenosynovitis, may persist for many weeks or months. In contrast to the gradual onset of disease that characterizes the majority, the onset is precipitous in some patients, almost to the hour of a given day.

Symptoms. *Pain*, the dominant symptom, corresponds to the pattern and intensity of joint involvement, whereas *stiffness* is more generalized and is characteristically maximal after periods of physical inactivity. *Morning stiffness* is an almost invariable feature; its intensity and duration can guide one in assessment of disease activity.

The majority of patients experience *constitutional symptoms* such as weakness, increased fatigability, and diminished appetite. Temperature elevation in excess of 38° C is uncommon. Higher temperatures should prompt search for superimposed infection, but occasionally temperatures as high as 40° C have no other explanation than active rheumatoid arthritis. Many patients complain of coldness and hypesthesias and paresthesias in the hands and feet (in the absence of signs of nerve entrapment).

Physical Signs. The physical signs of rheumatoid arthritis vary enormously according to anatomic patterns, severity, and stage of disease. The "classic" articular and extra-articular expressions are features of *chronic* rheumatoid arthritis.

General Examination. Observations of gait and performance of simple tasks, such as removal of clothing, may reveal evidence of stiffness or specific anatomic patterns of disease. Many, but not all, patients appear chronically ill and undernourished. Generalized lymphadenopathy and splenomegaly are features in some subjects (approximately 10 per cent); rarely this picture is so striking that it mimics lymphomatous disease. Dependent edema not attributable to other causes is an infrequent but significant feature. Easy bruising and increased fragility of skin are common in patients with chronic disease; both are amplified by corticosteroid therapy. Nodules are most commonly found in subcutaneous tissue, but they can occur within the dermis and periosteum. Nodules are characteristically localized over points of pressure or friction, most commonly the extensor surfaces of the proximal forearms. In a bedridden patient they may be found over the posterior aspects of the head, trunk, and spine.

Skeletal Manifestations. The invariable signs of swelling, tenderness, and pain on motion in early cases

may seem poorly localized to joints. A common mode of onset, with symmetrical involvement of the distal upper extremities, is diffuse swelling of the hands and wrists. More discrete enlargement of articulations (Fig. 1) may not appear for weeks or months. Warmth is usually evident, especially over the large joints such as the knee, but skin erythema is infrequent. Swelling reflects varying degrees of synovial thickening and proliferation and increased volume of synovial fluid. From palpation and ballottement, the examiner can usually estimate the relative roles of effusion and synovial proliferation.

The characteristic deformities of joints which are products of sustained chronic disease are attributable to a variety of events: loss of articular cartilage, destruction or weakening of ligaments, tendons, and capsular structures, muscle imbalance, and the physical force associated with use of the affected joints (Fig. 2). In addition, there are biologic variations which in some patients favor joint subluxation and instability and in other patients result in bony or fibrous ankylosis.

Muscle atrophy of the affected extremities may be evident within weeks of onset of rheumatoid arthritis. Whether this relates to primary myopathic change or disuse is moot, but rarely an overt myopathy, indistinguishable from polymyositis, may be a feature of the disease.

Extensions or rupture of synovial bursae beyond the confines of joint capsules can result in features of special importance to the internist. The most common example of this is the communication of joints of the wrists with the tenosynovium of the finger extensors. Popliteal cysts associated with knee synovitis may rupture into the calf and produce an inflammatory reaction that very closely resembles deep vein thrombophlebitis. The sudden onset of this complication, often associated with forceful flexion of the knee, and the intense inflammation help distinguish it from phlebitis, but this differentiation is best accomplished by arthrography. Rarely, extensions from hip synovitis may result in the formation of pelvic or inguinal masses.

Extra-Articular Manifestations. Many of the features of rheumatoid arthritis that are associated with diffuse vasculitis have been discussed previously under

Figure 1. Early rheumatoid arthritis manifest as symmetrical swelling and slight flexion deformities of proximal interphalangeal joints of the hands. Roentgenograms were normal except for evidence of soft tissue swelling.

Figure 2. Hand deformities characteristic of chronic rheumatoid arthritis. *A*, Subluxation of metacarpophalangeal joints with ulnar deviation of digits. *B*, Hyperextension ("swan neck") deformities of proximal interphalangeal joints.

Pathology. The clinical expressions of vasculitis (neuropathy, chronic skin ulcers, digital gangrene, and rarely visceral arteritis) and the clinical patterns associated with disseminated granulomata (heart, lung, sclera, and dura mater) are invariably features of chronic "classic" disease and are rarely encountered in patients who lack the rheumatoid factor.

For reasons unknown, pulmonary involvement (pleural effusion, granulomatous pneumonitis, and diffuse interstitial fibrosis) is more common in males. Cavitating pulmonary nodules occasionally result in pneumothorax or chronic bronchopleural fistulas. The glucose content of rheumatoid pleural effusions is frequently less than 10 mg per 100 ml.

There are usually no problems in interpretation of neurologic signs related to peripheral neuropathy, nerve entrapment (median nerve involvement at the wrist is common), and radiculopathy. In contrast, the insidious progression of muscle weakness secondary to myelopathy from C1-C2 subluxation can mistakenly be attributed to "arthritis" and associated constitutional symptoms.

Other extra-articular manifestations of rheumatoid arthritis include amyloidosis, keratoconjunctivitis sicca, and Felty's syndrome.

CLINICAL COURSE AND PROGNOSIS. Statistics regarding the natural history of rheumatoid arthritis are based on studies in large rheumatic disease units where patients are not representative of the entire population of rheumatoid arthritics, i.e., they tend to be patients with more severe and sustained disease. Patients with more remitting patterns of disease are less apt to be entered into prognostic studies. However, even the published figures allow one to present a reasonably optimistic outlook to the patient. After 10 to 15 years of disease, over 50 per cent of patients remain fully employed and only about 10 per cent are completely incapacitated. Ten to 20 per cent of patients have virtually complete remissions; the course followed by the remainder is extremely varied. The average patient with episodic exacerbations and partial remissions will experience gradual progression of deformity and disability. The minority, with sustained disease activity and only slight remissions, may become completely disabled within a few years of onset. The *features associated with a poor prognosis,* in a statistical sense are (1) classic pattern of disease (symmetrical polyarthritis with subcutaneous nodules and high titers of rheumatoid factor), (2)

sustained disease of more than one year's duration, (3) onset below age 30, and (4) extra-articular manifestations of rheumatoid arthritis.

ROENTGENOGRAPHIC FINDINGS. Early in the disease roentgenograms of affected joints are usually negative except for evidence of soft tissue swelling and joint effusion. Osteoporosis, especially in juxta-articular locations, may be evident within weeks of onset of disease. Loss of articular cartilage, shown by reduction in the apparent "joint space," and bone erosions are rarely evident before several months of sustained disease. Subluxations, dislocations, and bony ankylosis, if they occur, are still later phenomena. Diffuse osteoporosis is common with chronic disease and is heightened with adrenocorticosteroid therapy. The frequency of avascular osteonecrosis, especially of the femoral heads, is also increased with such therapy.

LABORATORY FINDINGS. Mild *anemia*, similar to that associated with chronic infection, is common in rheumatoid arthritis. Serum levels of both iron and iron-binding protein are frequently depressed. Anemia is usually normocytic and normochromic, but if there is accompanying iron deficiency, the erythrocytes may be slightly hypochromic and microcytic. Leukocytosis, eosinophilia, and thrombocytosis are occasional laboratory features. (See Ch. 57.1 for discussion of neutropenia associated with Felty's syndrome.)

The *erythrocyte sedimentation rate* (ESR) is increased above the normal range is virtually all patients with active rheumatoid arthritis. There are a variety of other "acute phase reactants" in the serum which reflect inflammatory activity, but none of them match the simplicity of the ESR or exceed its sensitivity.

Rheumatoid *synovial fluid* is usually turbid with reduced viscosity, increased protein content, and slight reduction of glucose levels relative to the blood. Leukocyte counts (predominantly polymorphonuclear cells) vary between a few thousand and more than 50,000 cells per cubic millimeter. Cells containing inclusions are common, but these may be seen in other types of exudative synovitis. Complement in synovial fluid, relative to protein content, is commonly reduced, a finding usually associated with positive test results for rheumatoid factors.

There are no tests that are specific for rheumatoid arthritis, although the term "rheumatoid factors" has been applied to autoantibodies reactive with IgG (see Pathogenesis above). A variety of test systems are available, but more laboratories utilize the *latex fixation test*, in which polystyrene latex particles coated with IgG are agglutinated by rheumatoid factors. Less commonly applied systems include the *bentonite flocculation test* and a variety of *hemagglutination tests* employing erythrocytes coated with immunoglobulins. The latex fixation test result is positive (1:80 titer or higher) in approximately 70 per cent of rheumatoid subjects. Although test results are positive in less than 5 per cent of healthy control subjects, the rheumatoid factor is associated with other connective tissue syndromes, liver disease, and a variety of infectious diseases such as bacterial endocarditis, tuberculosis, syphilis, and leprosy. The frequency of positive test results for rheumatoid factor in the general population increases with age.

DIFFERENTIAL DIAGNOSIS. General. Differential considerations are numerous and vary according to the pattern of disease. There is seldom confusion in identifying "classic" rheumatoid arthritis, but symmetrical involvement of hand and wrist joints can be a feature of other syndromes (see below). Differentiation is more difficult and complex in patients with early acute polyarthritis or in those with arthritis limited to one or a few joints.

Chronic Polyarthritis. The most common form of chronic arthropathy, degenerative joint disease, is usually quite distinct from rheumatoid arthritis. Minimal inflammatory signs, absence of constitutional symptoms, ESR determinations in the range of normal, and the characteristic radiographic findings usually serve to identify degenerative joint disease. A clinical pattern of degenerative joint disease which has been termed "primary generalized osteoarthritis" (see Ch. 61) may be mistaken for rheumatoid arthritis, especially when there is symmetrical enlargement of interphalangeal joints in the hands. *Bouchard's nodes*, the bony enlargement of proximal interphalangeal joints of the hand (see Fig. 4B) are rather frequently misinterpreted as signs of rheumatoid arthritis.

Gout and *chondrocalcinosis* (see Ch. 535.1 and 60, respectively) may mimic chronic rheumatoid arthritis. The most definitive basis for their identification is polarized light microscopy of synovial fluid.

Other connective tissue syndromes such as *systemic lupus erythematosus* (SLE) and *progressive systemic sclerosis* are infrequently associated with chronic deforming joint change. Their differentiation from rheumatoid arthritis is based on characteristic multisystemic patterns of disease. Certain serologic features of SLE, especially hypocomplementemia and the antibodies to native deoxyribonucleic acid, are rare in rheumatoid arthritis. A few patients, with mixed clinical and laboratory features of two or more syndromes, defy classification.

The majority of patients with arthritis and *psoriasis* are indistinguishable from patients in the spectrum of rheumatoid arthritis. The designation psoriatic arthritis as a separate entity is in part arbitrary, but certain clinical and laboratory features of psoriatic arthritis (see Ch. 58.3) aid in its differentiation from rheumatoid arthritis.

Rheumatic manifestations of a wide variety of systemic diseases, including sarcoidosis, ulcerative colitis, regional enteritis, Whipple's disease, amyloidosis, acromegaly, chronic infection, and malignancies, can resemble rheumatoid arthritis. This list emphasizes the importance of exclusions in formulating a diagnosis of rheumatoid arthritis.

Acute Polyarthritis. The range of differential considerations for acute polyarthritis includes those listed above plus a variety of disorders that rarely if ever result in chronic joint disease. The most frequent set of diagnostic considerations for acute polyarthritis includes rheumatoid arthritis, acute rheumatic fever, infection, and drug hypersensitivity. Acute arthritis associated with chills and fever should be considered infectious until proved otherwise. The presence of carditis, evidence of recent streptococcal infection, fever, and prompt response to salicylate therapy contribute to the recognition of acute rheumatic fever. Important differentiating features of gonococcal arthritis are prominent tenosynovitis, the cutaneous manifestations, and, most important, isolation of the bacteria from blood or joint fluid. The common viral infections that can resemble acute rheumatoid arthritis are rubella and viral hepatitis. There are other remitting forms of polyarthritis in which viral causes are suspected but not established. A careful clinical history and the recognition of other allergic phenomena will help in the identification of drug hypersensitivity.

Monarthritis or Oligoarthritis. All the conditions listed above under Acute and Chronic Polyarthritis are appropriate to the differential diagnosis of arthritis affecting one or a limited number of joints; but when the pattern of joint involvement is restricted, the most important differential consideration is infection. A complete medical evaluation, including chest x-ray, tuberculin tests, and appropriate microbial studies, is indicated. When there is continued suspicion of bacterial or mycobacterial infection, synovial biopsy may be required.

MANAGEMENT. Basic Principles. In the management of rheumatoid arthritis, the physician should keep the following facts in mind: (1) in most patients the disease is chronic; (2) spontaneous remissions occur in almost all patients; (3) the majority of subjects can continue to lead active lives with varying degrees of restrictions; and (4) complications of drug therapy, most notably adrenocorticosteroids, can cause greater morbidity than the underlying disease.

The patient and the doctor must be educated not to expect and seek a short-term solution. The physician can present a reasonably optimistic prognosis, based on knowledge of the natural history of rheumatoid arthritis, and can assure the patient that there are conservative means of ameliorating symptoms and minimizing disability.

There are no specific dietary recommendations; rather, the general nutritional status of the patient and associated medical conditions influence diet selection. Weight reduction, in obese patients, should have high priority. Providing that the diet is well balanced, there are no indications for vitamin supplementation. The anemia of rheumatoid arthritis does not respond to hematinic therapy except to the extent that iron deficiency may be a complicating feature. Rarely the anemia may be so severe as to require transfusion.

Psychologic depression is a common consequence of chronic rheumatoid arthritis. From the physician, the patient needs sympathetic understanding of his problems and a willingness to help solve them. When depression is severe, these efforts may be facilitated by the use of antidepressive medication. If anxiety, restlessness, and insomnia are complicating features, the use of mild sedatives or tranquilizers may be indicated.

A basic program that is applicable to all patients includes (1) rest, (2) employment of salicylates for the relief of pain and suppression of inflammation, and (3) maintenance of joint function by physical measures. Some but not all patients will be candidates for medicinal therapy other than salicylates and/or orthopedic surgical procedures.

REST. Patients and physicians alike tend to be confused by the apparently conflicting goals of rest and exercise. They are not mutually exclusive (see Physical Measures below). It is clear that physical work, applied to an affected extremity, will intensify the synovitis of rheumatoid arthritis. The specific prescription of rest will vary according to the severity and pattern of involvement, but all patients should be directed to respect their symptoms of pain and fatigue and to restrict physical activities to the essentials. Any way that occupational duties can be modified to lighten the work load should be tried, and daytime rest periods are important. Occasionally when symptoms are very severe, hospitalization for attainment of more complete rest is indicated.

EMPLOYMENT OF SALICYLATES. All students of rheumatoid arthritis agree that salicylate therapy is part of the basic management. The majority of patients can tolerate acetylsalicylic acid in doses of 3.6 grams daily or more, if the physician is persistent in his recommendations. When gastrointestinal symptoms complicate therapy, ingestion of the drug with meals or the use of enteric-coated or buffered products may be helpful. When doses of acetylsalicylic acid in the range of 3.6 grams daily are tolerated but rheumatic symptoms are poorly controlled, gradual increase in the dose is warranted. It is too often concluded, on the basis of inadequate trials, that "aspirin was not effective." Measurement of blood salicylate levels is appropriate when there is a question of toxicity or absorption.

PHYSICAL MEASURES. The choice of various heat modalities (warm pool, tank, bath, shower, diathermy, or ultrasound) depends primarily on the areas affected and the availability of services. Diathermy and ultrasound treatments are contraindicated in patients with metal implants. A warm pool permitting exercise under water is optimal for the patient with very severe symptoms, but for most individuals a hot bath or shower will suffice. Morning stiffness and pain will be minimized by ingestion of salicylates followed by a hot bath.

The *goals of an exercise program* are (1) maintenance of motion of affected joints, and (2) prevention of muscle atrophy. Both of these can be achieved without submitting inflamed joints to the task of work. An active exercise program for the lower extremities can maintain motion and strength without heavy weight bearing, allowing the right combination of rest and exercise. The rate of progression from gentle passive exercises, required for the most symptomatic patient, to a more active program will vary according to the pattern of involvement and the response to therapy. In order that the patient avoid assuming a passive dependent role, it is crucial that emphasis be placed on what he or she can do independent of supervision. The average doctor is not sufficiently trained in physical medicine to write detailed prescriptions, but he should be very specific in what his goals are when referring the patient to a physical medicine service. Furthermore, he should review the program periodically with the patient and reinforce its importance in the total management. It is a moot point whether forceful active exercises are appropriate for the distal upper extremities; evidence suggests that heavy work will aggravate hand and wrist deformities. For a patient with acutely inflamed joints, removable splints to achieve rest are helpful, but there are no convincing demonstrations that such devices prevent development of chronic hand deformities.

The role of orthopedic surgery in the management of rheumatoid arthritis is discussed subsequently in this chapter.

Other Antirheumatic Therapy. For the patient whose response to salicylate therapy has not been adequate, several other anti-inflammatory agents can be employed. These include indomethacin, phenylbutazone (and oxyphenbutazone), antimalarial drugs (chloroquine and hydroxychloroquine), gold compounds, and several compounds (propionic acid derivatives and tolmetin) marketed in the United States after 1975 (see below). The adrenocorticosteroid drugs are the most potent anti-inflammatory medications available, but their value, for reasons stated below, is limited. Unfortunately all medications employed for the treatment of rheumatoid arthritis, except gold compounds, have in common the property of promoting peptic ulceration.

Among those who specialize in the management of rheumatic disease, there is no uniformity of habit regarding the employment of agents listed above, although the majority, at some time, will institute gold therapy for the patient with sustained rheumatoid arthritis. Codeine and related analgesics may be required on a temporary basis, but their chronic use should be discouraged.

Phenylbutazone is a reasonably potent anti-inflammatory agent, but there is limited enthusiasm for its use in long-term management of rheumatoid disease. In doses of 200 to 300 mg daily, this drug may be helpful in the treatment of intermittent exacerbations. The incidence of serious toxicity (exfoliative dermatitis and hematologic complications) is low but a source of concern. The occasional patient who is helped by long-term therapy should be under close medical supervision and should have periodic blood counts.

Indomethacin, although chemically unrelated to other analgesic and anti-inflammatory drugs, has a pattern of efficacy similar to that of phenylbutazone. Both are more effective in gout and ankylosing spondylitis than in rheumatoid arthritis. In the dose range of 50 to 200 mg per day, a few patients will experience sufficient benefit to warrant its continuation. Gastrointestinal symptoms and vascular headaches are common side effects, but serious complications are rare. Concomitant aspirin therapy appears to diminish gastrointestinal absorption of indomethacin.

Several *propionic acid derivative* drugs are available for treatment of rheumatoid arthritis, and others are under study. All these compounds have anti-inflammatory, antipyretic, and analgesic properties. Ibuprofen (1200 to 1600 mg daily), naproxen (500 to 750 mg daily), and fenoprofen (2400 mg daily) impart symptomatic control roughly equivalent to that achieved with acetylsalicylic acid in the dose range of 3.6 grams daily. Gastrointestinal intolerance appears to be less frequent than with salicylates.

Tolmetin (1200 mg daily) has a spectrum and level of efficacy similar to indomethacin, a chemically related drug.

Antimalarial compounds such as chloroquine and hydroxychloroquine have moderate anti-inflammatory activity in the treatment of rheumatoid arthritis. Because of the occasional association of irreversible retinopathy, the use of antimalarials has sharply declined.

Although soluble *gold compounds* have been employed in the treatment of rheumatoid arthritis since the 1930s, their mode of action is not known. There is no evidence that they have anti-inflammatory activity; rather, clinical impressions suggest that, in some unknown way, they increase the likelihood of remission. The level of enthusiasm for chrysotherapy varies considerably among rheumatic disease specialists. Some advocate such treatment within weeks of onset of disease; others reserve it for patients who have had sustained disease for several months or more in spite of more conservative therapy. There is a cumulative effect of gold compound administration. Sensitive assays can detect trace amounts many months after discontinuation of therapy. Gold is excreted primarily in the urine. The most common complications are dermatitis and stomatitis. Renal damage, manifested by proteinuria and microscopic hematuria, and hematologic dyscrasias (thrombocytopenia and granulocytopenia) are rare but significant complications of chrysotherapy.

The preparations employed are sodium aurothiomalate (Myochrysine) and aurothioglucose (Solganal). Both are administered by deep intramuscular injection at weekly intervals. It is common practice to use small doses (10 to 25 mg) for the first two or three injections, followed by 50 mg at weekly intervals thereafter. Complete blood count and urinalysis should be obtained prior to each injection for several weeks and every few weeks after that as long as therapy is continued. If there is any sign from these tests or from clinical assessment (pruritic rash or stomatitis) of gold toxicity, therapy should be interrupted. If unequivocal evidence of gold toxicity develops, such as severe stomatitis or exfoliative dermatitis or renal or hematologic complications, treatment should not be resumed. In the case of mild, transient skin reactions, it is common practice to reinstitute the medication at reduced levels after the rash has cleared. Experience indicates that remissions, if they occur on gold therapy, will occur during the course of 20 weekly injections (approximately 1 gram total dose). In the absence of improvement during this course, there is no point in continuing therapy. For the patient experiencing a remission, it is recommended that maintenance therapy be continued (50 mg at three- to four-week intervals). The decision as to maintenance therapy in patients who experience only partial remission is more difficult.

Mild gold-induced dermatitis may persist for several weeks or more, but usually requires no therapy other than topical corticosteroids. The most common presentation consists of several scattered, well-circumscribed pruritic lesions associated with mild scaling. The discomfort associated with severe dermatitis may warrant a course of systemic corticosteroid therapy (10 to 20 mg of prednisone daily) or the use of BAL (dimercaprol). Hematologic complications, most commonly thrombocytopenia, are also indications for dimercaprol therapy. Dimercaprol, 2.5 mg per kilogram of body weight, is given every four hours for two days, followed by the same dose twice daily for approximately a week. An alternative means of promoting gold excretion is the employment of penicillamine,* although there is less clinical experience to recommend it.

Adrenocorticosteroid Therapy. SYSTEMIC THERAPY. Since the early therapeutic trials of cortisone in 1949, several related compounds with potent anti-inflammatory activity have been introduced. These include prednisone, prednisolone, triamcinolone, methylprednisolone, dexamethasone, betamethasone, and paramethasone. Elec-

trolyte and water-retaining properties, associated with cortisone and hydroxycortisone therapy, are minimal with the newer drugs, but the more serious side effects are common to *all* adrenocorticosteroid preparations (see below). The approximate milligram equivalent of the various drugs that yield comparable pharmacologic effects are cortisone (25 mg), hydrocortisone (20 mg), prednisone (5 mg), triamcinolone (4 mg), methylprednisolone (4 mg), dexamethasone (0.75 mg), betamethasone (0.6 mg), and paramethasone (2 mg).

Because of frequent and potentially life-threatening complications of adrenocorticosteroid therapy, it should not be employed in the management of rheumatoid arthritis until there has been a sustained trial of more conservative therapy. In general, the more experienced the physician is in the management of rheumatoid disease, the more reluctant he is to begin adrenocorticosteroid therapy. The following facts should be pondered before initiating such treatment: (1) adrenocorticosteroid drugs suppress inflammation, but they do not correct or change the underlying process; (2) small doses, in the range of 5 to 10 mg of prednisone, often provide only partial and temporary gains; (3) over periods of months or years, there is a tendency for the dose to increase; (4) once instituted, it is very difficult to discontinue therapy; and (5) the morbidity and mortality associated with long-term adrenocorticosteroid therapy often exceed those of the underlying disease.

In the light of these facts, it is difficult to summarize indications for adrenocorticosteroid therapy of rheumatoid arthritis. If a conservative effort, employing less toxic drugs and physical measures, fails to check progressive disability and if the alternative to adrenocorticosteroid therapy seems to be chronic invalidism, such treatment may be indicated. In such cases the daily dose should not exceed 10 mg of prednisone or its equivalent; as little as 5 to 7.5 mg in divided doses may provide some benefit. Although pituitary-adrenal unresponsiveness and other complications of therapy are minimized by alternate-day or single daily dose regimens, most patients with rheumatoid arthritis do not tolerate such programs. Occasionally, sustained disease may be less severe but may compromise the occupational activity of a wage earner or mother of a household. A small dose (5 or 7.5 mg daily of prednisone or equivalent) may allow continuation of employment, but the physician and patient should make the decision deliberately and with full realization of the toxic potential of such therapy.

COMPLICATIONS OF ADRENOCORTICOSTEROID THERAPY. The frequency and severity of *osteoporosis*, a feature of rheumatoid disease regardless of therapy, are increased by adrenocorticosteroid treatment. Compression fractures of vertebral bodies are common. (Detailed discussions of the management of osteoporosis are presented in Ch. 557.) There are theoretic bases for employment of high calcium intake, vitamin D, fluorides, and anabolic steroids, but their efficacy in preventing or reversing osteoporosis is uncertain. Another frequent skeletal complication of adrenocorticosteroid therapy is *avascular osteonecrosis*, most commonly affecting the femoral head.

Although most antirheumatic drugs are associated with *peptic ulceration*, the frequency of this complication is probably highest in patients treated with adrenocorticosteroids. The problem is sometimes compounded, because the signs and symptoms of perforation and peritonitis may be masked by therapy.

Decreased host resistance to acquired or reactivated

---

*Investigational drug for this use.

infections is a well-documented feature of adrenocortico-steroid therapy. It is common practice to institute isoniazid prophylaxis in tuberculin-positive patients receiving steroid therapy.

Aggravation of latent or overt diabetes mellitus and psychic disturbances ranging from mild euphoria to frank psychosis are infrequent with the doses of adrenocortico-steroids used in the treatment of rheumatoid arthritis.

Any patient receiving daily adrenocorticosteroid therapy must be assumed to have an *inadequate pituitary adrenal response* to stress. With intercurrent illnesses, or with surgery, the dose should be increased and the patient observed closely for signs of adrenal insufficiency. The same precautions apply to those whose treatment has been discontinued up to two years prior to the stressful illness. The value of intermittent corticotropin therapy in the amelioration of pituitary adrenal unresponsiveness is un-proved.

INTRA-ARTICULAR ADRENOCORTICOSTEROID THERA-PY. Several adrenocorticosteroid preparations suitable for intra-articular therapy will temporarily suppress signs and symptoms of synovitis. This mode of therapy is help-ful for a patient whose disability relates primarily to disease in one or two joints. With rigorous antiseptic technique, the risk of infection is low. If there is any question of antecedent infection at the time of arthrocente-sis, intra-articular steroids should not be administered. The usefulness of intra-articular therapy is dependent upon the duration of symptomatic benefit. Because of clinical suspicions and experimental evidence that steroid compounds are deleterious to articular cartilage, most physicians will not inject a joint more frequently than every four to six weeks.

Immunosuppressive (Cytotoxic) Therapy. Several drugs initially developed for cancer chemotherapy have been applied in the treatment of rheumatoid arthritis. The categories of compounds include alkylating agents, purine and pyrimidine antagonists, and folic acid analogues. There is no basis for concluding that one compound is superior to another in immunosuppressive and anti-inflammatory properties, but the best data with regard to the treatment of rheumatoid arthritis derive from a con-trolled study of cyclophosphamide therapy. Patients re-ceiving up to 150 mg daily of cyclophosphamide sustained significantly fewer new bone erosions over the period of study. In spite of these observations, the use of immuno-suppressive agents is to be viewed as experimental thera-py. Acute toxicity, especially myelosuppression, is poten-tially fatal and, as well, there is concern that immunosuppressive therapy may foster the emergence of primary malignant tumors.

Other Experimental Drugs. *Penicillamine*, in a well-controlled study in England, had moderate efficacy in the suppression of severe chronic rheumatoid arthritis and resulted in reductions of rheumatoid factor titers. As an antirheumatic agent, penicillamine remains in the experi-mental category, primarily because of potentially serious toxicity (agranulocytosis and nephropathy).

Orthopedic Surgery. Orthopedic surgeons are playing an increasingly important role in the management of rheu-matoid arthritis. The value of reconstructive surgery in the rehabilitation of selected subjects is well established. Techniques of arthroplasty and prosthetic joint replace-ment have improved dramatically during the past decade. The rationale for synovectomy is sound, i.e., the removal of chronic pannus and its destructive potential, but proof of its efficacy is lacking. Disease frequently recurs in regenerated synovium, but the intensity of recurrent in-flammation tends to be less. On the basis of current experience, synovectomy is probably warranted for pa-tients with sustained (several months or more) prolifera-tive synovitis affecting knee, hand, and wrist joints.

Cooperating Clinics Committee of the American Rheumatism Association: A controlled trial of cyclophosphamide in rheumatoid arthritis. N. Engl. J. Med., 283:883, 1970.

Duthie, J. R. R., et al.: Course and prognosis in rheumatoid arthritis. Ann. Rheum. Dis., 23:193, 1964.

Freyberg, R. H., Ziff, M., and Baum, J.: Gold therapy for rheumatoid arthritis. *In* Hollander, J. L., and McCarty, D. J., Jr. (eds.): Arthritis and Allied Conditions. 8th ed. Philadelphia, Lea & Febiger, 1972.

Hollingsworth, J. W.: Local and Systemic Complications of Rheumatoid Arthritis. Philadelphia, W. B. Saunders Company, 1968.

Ruddy, S., and Austen, K. F.: The complement system in rheumatoid synovitis: I. An analysis of complement activities in rheumatoid synovial fluids. Arthritis Rheum., 13:713, 1970.

Short, C. L., Bauer, W., and Reynolds, W. E.: Rheumatoid Arthritis. Cambridge, Harvard University Press, 1957.

Winchester, R. J., Agnello, V., and Kunkel, H. G.: Gamma globulin complexes in synovial fluids of patients with rheumatoid arthritis: Partial characterization and relationship to lowered complement lev-els. Clin. Exp. Immunol., 6:689, 1970.

Zvaifler, N. J.: The immunopathology of joint inflammation in rheumatoid arthritis. *In* Dixon, F. J., and Kunkel, H. G. (eds.): Advances in Immunology. Vol. 16. New York, Academic Press, 1972.

57. VARIANTS OF RHEUMATOID DISEASE

57.1. FELTY'S SYNDROME

Splenomegaly is observed in approximately 5 per cent of patients with rheumatoid arthritis. Felty origi-nally described a syndrome consisting of rheumatoid arthritis, splenomegaly, and neutropenia. Anemia and thrombocytopenia are occasional features. This syn-drome is most common in older individuals who have had longstanding chronic rheumatoid disease. Other extra-articular manifestations of rheumatoid disease such as rheumatoid nodules, chronic skin ulcers, and keratoconjunctivitis sicca are common. Rheumatoid fac-tor test results are invariably positive, and antinuclear phenomena are more common than in uncomplicated rheumatoid arthritis. The indications for splenectomy are influenced primarily by the frequency and severity of infectious complications. Most patients experience hematologic remissions after splenectomy, but relapses occur in many of them.

57.2. SJÖGREN'S SYNDROME

In 1933 Sjögren called attention to the combination of rheumatoid arthritis, keratoconjunctivitis sicca, and xe-rostomia. The characteristic ocular and oral mucous membrane involvement may occur in the absence of rheumatic disease. In addition to its association with rheumatoid arthritis, it can be a manifestation of other connective tissue syndromes such as systemic lupus er-ythematosus, progressive systemic sclerosis, and poly-myositis. The sicca complex is clinically manifest in ap-proximately 10 to 15 per cent of patients with rheumatoid arthritis, but pathologic expressions, such as lymphoid infiltration of the minor salivary glands in the lip, are much more frequent. The diagnosis is most reliably established by lip biopsy. More than 90 per cent of affected patients are women, and most have had longstanding chronic arthritis. The frequency of a histocompatibility antigen (HLA-DW₃) in patients with sicca syndrome, in the absence of rheumatoid arthritis, was 84 per cent. (The frequency in control subjects was 24 per cent.)

The symptoms related to salivary insufficiency include difficulty with chewing and swallowing, dental caries, and ulcerations of the buccal mucous membranes. Dryness may also involve the upper respiratory tract, larynx, and tracheobronchial tree. In common with Felty's syndrome, patients with Sjögren's syndrome frequently manifest extra-articular features attributed to vasculitis. A small but significant number of patients with Sjögren's syndrome have developed reticulum cell sarcoma or a more benign lymphoproliferative disorder termed "pseudolymphoma." Because lymphomatous complications have occurred primarily in patients with a history of irradiation for parotid gland enlargement, this mode of therapy has been discouraged.

Rheumatoid factor test results are positive in the majority of patients, and antinuclear and a variety of other autoimmune reactants are associated with Sjögren's syndrome.

The treatment is symptomatic. Artificial tears of 0.5 per cent methylcellulose are helpful. Adrenocorticosteroid or immunosuppressive drugs are restricted to those patients with severe disability or life-threatening complications.

Barnes, C. G., Turnbull, A. L., and Vernon-Roberts, B.: Felty's syndrome: A clinical and pathological survey of 21 patients and their response to treatment. Ann. Rheum. Dis., 30:359, 1971.

Shearn, M. A.: Sjögren's Syndrome. Philadelphia, W. B. Saunders Company, 1971.

Whaley, K., Williamson, J., Chisholm, D. M., et al.: Sjögren's syndrome. I. Sicca components. Quart. J. Med., 42:279, 1973.

58. OTHER FORMS OF POLYARTHRITIS OF UNKNOWN ETIOLOGY

58.1. ANKYLOSING SPONDYLITIS

(Marie-Strümpell Spondylitis, von Bechterew's Syndrome, Rheumatoid Spondylitis)

In this syndrome there is prominent involvement of spinal articulations, sacroiliac joints, and paravertebral soft tissues. Because one third to one half of patients with ankylosing spondylitis manifest synovitis in peripheral joints (especially hips and shoulders), the syndrome was formerly viewed as a variant of rheumatoid arthritis. However, several features of ankylosing spondylitis are distinct from those of rheumatoid arthritis: (1) prominent ligamentous calcification and ossification with a tendency to bony ankylosis; (2) male preponderance; (3) impressive evidence of genetic transmission in selected kindreds; (4) symptomatic benefit with medications, notably phenylbutazone and indomethacin, that are minimally effective in rheumatoid arthritis; (5) absence of rheumatoid factor and rheumatoid nodules; and (6) the association of certain extra-articular manifestations such as iridocyclitis and aortitis.

ETIOLOGY. The cause of ankylosing spondylitis is unknown. The disease has been found to be 30 times more prevalent among the relatives of spondylitic patients than among relatives of controls. The striking association of ankylosing spondylitis with the histocompatibility antigen HLA-B27 has provided insight into the genetic transmission of the syndrome and, additionally, has helped define a group of spondylitic disorders. This category includes Reiter's syndrome, a subset of juvenile rheumatoid arthritis, psoriatic spondylitis, and inflammatory bowel disease that exhibits spinal involvement. The manner in which this histocompatibility antigen influences pathogenesis is unknown. Infectious causes have long been suspected but never established.

INCIDENCE AND PREVALENCE. Ankylosing spondylitis is a common cause of back pain in young men. The male-to-female ratio is approximately 8:1. In an English survey, the incidence of ankylosing spondylitis was 1 in 2000 among the population at large.

PATHOLOGY. On the basis of symptoms and early radiographic findings, the disease appears to begin in the sacroiliac joints, with subsequent involvement of zygapophyseal and costovertebral articulations, interspinous ligaments, and paravertebral tissues. The characteristic immobility of the spinal column results from bony ankylosis of zygapophyseal joints and ossification of paravertebral structures. Syndesmophytes, the bony bridges which unite adjacent vertebral bodies, form in the outer lamellae of the anulus fibrosus and adjacent connective tissue fibers. The pathologic character of synovial inflammation is not distinct from that of rheumatoid arthritis. Aortic involvement resembling syphilitic aortitis can result in aortic insufficiency. Iridocyclitis occurs in approximately 25 per cent of patients. The incidence of amyloidosis complicating ankylosing spondylitis is approximately 5 per cent. Rarely, a pattern of pulmonary fibrosis, sometimes associated with cavitation, has been described.

CLINICAL MANIFESTATIONS. In the majority of cases the onset of ankylosing spondylitis, usually in the second or third decade of life, is insidious. The initial symptoms are usually low back pain and stiffness; rarely, the first symptoms may relate to involvement of hip, shoulder, or peripheral joints. Symptoms may be sufficiently mild that the patient seeks no medical attention for months. At the other extreme, there may be debilitating pain at the outset, associated with fever, severe fatigue, and weight loss. In most patients, however, constitutional symptoms are not prominent. Pain and stiffness, which are maximal after periods of inactivity, often interrupt sleep in the early morning hours. Radicular and sciatic patterns of pain are common. The pattern and rate of spinal ankylosis are varied. The majority of patients experience gradual cephalad progression of spinal immobility, but the disease may remain confined to the sacroiliac joints and lumbar segments. The development of the poker back type of spinal deformity usually evolves gradually over a period of ten years or more. The majority of patients remain fully employed. Hip involvement, the most common cause of occupational disability, is now amenable to prosthetic surgery.

Physical signs are limited in the early stages of disease. Sacroiliac joint involvement may be evident from palpation of these joints or from orthopedic maneuvers which produce sacroiliac joint movement. Paravertebral muscle spasm and tenderness are common. Physical signs associated with the chronic phase of ankylosing spondylitis relate primarily to spinal immobility. The most accurate estimate of lumbar flexion is accomplished by comparing midline measurements from the sacrum to T-12 in flexion and extension. The normal difference in these two measurements is approximately 3 inches. The presence and progression of costovertebral joint involvement can be documented by measurements of chest expansion.

The most important extra-articular manifestations of ankylosing spondylitis are *iridocyclitis*, occurring in approximately one quarter of patients, and aortitis. The frequency of *aortic insufficiency* has been as high as 4 per cent in some series. *Cardiac conduction disturbances*, most frequently first degree A-V block, occur in about 10 per cent of cases. *Cauda equina involvement*, a rare but significant complication of longstanding spondylitis, is manifest as urinary or rectal sphincter incompetence and pain and sensory loss in the sacral distribution.

ROENTGENOGRAPHIC FINDINGS. Characteristic roentgenographic findings of ankylosing spondylitis involve the following structures: sacroiliac joints, zygapophyseal articulations, vertebral bodies, and paravertebral soft tissues. Changes in the sacroiliac joints are the earliest and most consistent findings. The margins of subchondral bone are blurred, followed by subchondral sclerosis and bony erosions. Progressive narrowing of the interosseous joint space and sacroiliac fusion develop slowly over a period of years. Sclerotic and erosive changes in zygapophyseal and costovertebral articulations are common but less readily demonstrated by x-ray. Alterations in vertebral bodies, loss of anterior concavity, and anterior marginal erosions are features of longstanding disease. Calcification and ossification of the anulus fibrosus and adjacent paravertebral ligaments give rise to the characteristic syndesmophytes that gradually bridge adjacent vertebral bodies. In advanced cases this results in the so-called *bamboo spine*. In addition to sacroiliac joints, other cartilaginous articulations such as the symphysis pubis and sternomanubrial joints may be involved. There is a tendency for ossification of ligaments and tendon insertions. Roentgenographic changes in the hips and shoulders, less commonly in more peripheral joints, are not distinct from those of rheumatoid arthritis, although the incidence of bony ankylosis of the hips is greater in ankylosing spondylitis.

The full set of roentgenographic findings, described above, is a product of many years of progressive disease. In a minority of patients with ankylosing spondylitis, the disease appears to go into remission after involvement of restricted segments of the spine.

DIAGNOSIS. Ankylosing spondylitis should be suspected in anyone, particularly a young male, with persistent or recurrent low back pain and stiffness or recurrent sciatic pain. Although associated phenomena such as elevation of erythrocyte sedimentation rate, thoracic girdle pain, arthritis in the lower limbs, and iridocyclitis will enhance the suspicion, early diagnosis should not be excluded on the basis of normal roentgenograms, because several months or, rarely, a few years may elapse before development of roentgenographic changes. Although degenerative joint disease

can result in back pain and loss of spinal motion, this is a problem of later decades of life, and the roentgenographic features are distinct from ankylosing spondylitis. Joint disease identical to ankylosing spondylitis can be a feature of *ulcerative colitis, regional enteritis, Reiter's syndrome*, and *psoriasis*.

TREATMENT. The highest priority goal in the management of ankylosing spondylitis is the maintenance of a functional posture. It is doubtful that any medication will prevent ankylosis of those spinal segments involved, but the suppression of pain and inflammation is essential before an appropriate physical medicine program can be instituted.

Indomethacin and phenylbutazone are usually more effective than other antirheumatic agents in the control of pain and stiffness, but an initial trial on salicylate therapy (3.6 to 4.5 grams daily) is recommended. For those patients who do not experience sufficient relief of symptoms with salicylates, indomethacin in doses of 100 to 150 mg daily or phenylbutazone (100 to 300 mg daily) is indicated. With control of symptoms, the dose of either indomethacin or phenylbutazone should be gradually reduced to the lowest level that will maintain improvement. With continuous use of phenylbutazone, the risk of hematologic complications should be kept in mind and periodic blood counts obtained. Adrenocorticosteroid therapy is rarely indicated for ankylosing spondylitis. If all other efforts to control progressive disability fail, such therapy may be indicated, as outlined under rheumatoid arthritis (see Ch. 56). Systemic adrenocorticosteroid therapy may be required for the control of iridocyclitis. Although roentgen therapy, directed at areas of involvement, is effective in control of symptoms, this mode of treatment is not recommended because of the demonstrations of chromosomal injury and an observed incidence of leukemia that is ten times greater in patients so treated than in the general population.

For the management of ankylosing spondylitis, emphasis should be given to the institution and maintenance of an exercise program. In order that flexion deformity of the spine be avoided, the patient should sleep on a very firm mattress, preferably without a pillow. There should be a twice daily performance of exercise directed at the maintenance of erect posture, strengthening of paraspinal muscles, and promotion of chest cage motion. A hot bath or shower will often facilitate exercise activity. If physical medicine measures fail to check the progression of flexion deformity, back splints or braces may be tried. In carefully selected individuals with advanced flexion deformity, spinal osteotomy can improve posture, but this is associated with significant risk of neurologic complications. For the patient with severe hip involvement, the most frequent cause of major disability, prosthetic hip replacement offers dramatic relief.

58.2. JUVENILE RHEUMATOID ARTHRITIS

Although the definition of juvenile rheumatoid arthritis is somewhat arbitrary (onset of disease under age 16), there are clinical features which tend to distinguish it from rheumatoid arthritis in adults. These include high fever, transient morbilliform rash, leukocytosis, uveitis, local growth disturbances, low frequencies of rheumatoid factor and subcutaneous nodules, and a higher incidence of monarticular disease than is observed in adults.

The discussions of etiology, pathogenesis, and pathology of rheumatoid arthritis (see Ch. 56) are relevant to juvenile rheumatoid arthritis except for speculations regarding a pathogenic role of rheumatoid factors.

In approximately 20 per cent of children with juvenile rheumatoid arthritis, the onset is acute and fulminating and is associated with systemic manifestations such as fever, rash, pericarditis, and splenomegaly (*Still's disease*). Occasionally these features may persist for several weeks before synovitis is evident. (A similar systemic pattern of disease has been observed, rarely, in adults.) In approximately half of patients, the onset is polyarticular, resembling rheumatoid arthritis in adults. In one third of juvenile rheumatoid arthritis patients, the onset is monoarticular. Several clinical subsets of juvenile rheumatoid arthritis have been recognized. One of these is pauciarticular (involvement of a few joints) in young girls, associated with positive antinuclear test results and chronic irridocyclitis. Boys with the pauciarticular pattern of disease have a high frequency of HLA-B27 and may manifest acute iridocyclitis. The latter group of patients appears to represent the juvenile form of ankylosing spondylitis. Abnormal skeletal growth adjacent to inflamed joints results from varied degrees of accelerated local growth and premature closure of epiphyseal plates.

Leukocytosis in the range of 15,000 to 25,000 is common. Serologic evidence of recent streptococcal infection is found in a third to a half of subjects, adding to the problem of differentiation from acute rheumatic fever. No more than 10 per cent of sera are positive in the commonly employed tests for rheumatoid factor. The frequency of antinuclear antibody is higher than in adults with rheumatoid arthritis. This is especially so in children with iridocyclitis.

Distinctive roentgenographic findings include local growth disturbances (noted above), abnormal periosteal bone accretion, and prominent involvement of cervical zygapophyseal joints.

Differential considerations vary according to the pattern of juvenile rheumatoid arthritis. The systemic form of disease resembles certain infectious syndromes. Recognition of the characteristic morbilliform rash, if it is present, is important in diagnosis. The polyarticular onset of disease, when accompanied by high fever and signs of carditis, is easily confused with acute rheumatic fever. Features of juvenile rheumatoid arthritis that may aid in this distinction are frequent onset of disease under age 5, nonmigratory pattern of polyarthritis, cervical spine involvement, marked leukocytosis, and rash. The immediate suppressive effect of salicylate therapy is less striking in juvenile rheumatoid arthritis than it is in rheumatic fever.

Fifty per cent or more of patients with juvenile rheumatoid arthritis experience complete remissions. The serious consequences of extra-articular involvement relate to carditis, chronic iridocyclitis, and amyloidosis.

Principles of management outlined for rheumatoid arthritis (see Ch. 56) apply to children with chronic arthritis. Contractures and restricted motion of articulations are more common in children than in adults. The patient's parents must be given important roles in the maintenance of a physical medicine program. Aspirin in the range of 90 to 130 mg per kilogram daily is the treatment of choice. Early in the course of the disease, adrenocorticosteroid therapy should be reserved for patients with severe systemic manifestations, such as carditis, that do not respond to salicylate therapy. Periodic ophthalmologic consultation, at approximately six-month intervals, is recommended, since iridocyclitis may be asymptomatic and missed by casual examination. Because of the threat of blindness from sustained iridocyclitis, systemic adrenocorticosteroid therapy may be indicated if this complication is severe and fails to respond to local treatment. In addition to the usual complications and limitations of adrenocorticosteroid therapy, growth retardation, a natural feature of the disease, is augmented by such treatment. The indications for the employment of gold therapy and doses are similar to those presented for rheumatoid arthritis (see Ch. 56).

58.3.   PSORIATIC ARTHRITIS

The recognition that psoriatic arthritis is a disease entity, as opposed to the coincidental occurrence of two common diseases, i.e., rheumatoid arthritis and psoriasis, is relatively recent. Based on population surveys, approximately 5 per cent of patients with cutaneous psoriasis have chronic arthritis. One quarter to one third of such patients manifest rheumatoid nodules or positive tests for rheumatoid factor, and probably represent cases of coexistence of two diseases. Patients with psoriasis and chronic arthritis are clinically heterogeneous, but some of them manifest sufficiently characteristic features to justify the term psoriatic arthritis.

Several clinical subtypes of psoriatic arthritis are recognized. The most common pattern is of a scattered asymmetrical involvement of interphalangeal joints of the hands and feet, frequently manifest as "sausage digits" (Fig. 3). Much less common, but recognized by all as "classic psoriatic arthritis" is the exclusive involvement of distal interphalangeal joints. In approximately one quarter of patients with psoriasis there is a symmetrical pattern of arthritis indistinguishable, apart from negative serology, from rheumatoid arthritis. In this group, there is a tendency for severe osteolytic involvement with resorption of bone and telescoping of digits (arthritis mutilans). Approximately 5 per cent of patients with psoriasis and arthritis manifest features identical to those of ankylosing spondylitis, although the roentgenographic character of syndesmophytes tends to differentiate the two syndromes. This pattern of disease has a striking association with the histocompatibility antigen HLA-B27.

It is important to recognize that there may be asynchronous onset of cutaneous involvement and arthritis and that a patient with typical psoriatic arthritis may have minimal or hidden cutaneous involvement. Psoriatic nail involvement occurs in over 80 per cent of patients with psoriatic arthritis, in contrast to only a 30 per cent incidence in patients with uncomplicated psoriasis. Typical psoriatic arthritis, especially spondylitis, may evolve after recurrent attacks of Reiter's syndrome.

The unique clinical patterns of psoriatic arthritis such as bone resorption, asymmetric involvement of interphalangeal joints, and spondylitis are represented in roentgenographic findings. An increased incidence of hyperuricemia in psoriatic patients probably reflects the

Figure 3. Common patterns of psoriatic arthritis in the hands. *A*, Asymmetrical enlargement of interphalangeal joints of right thumb and left ring finger. *B*, "Classic" involvement of distal interphalangeal joints and nails of digits two, three, and five of left hand.

increased metabolism of skin. Other than the absence of rheumatoid factor in patients with psoriatic arthritis, there are no immunologic, biochemical, or pathologic distinctions from rheumatoid arthritis.

Principles of management of psoriatic arthritis do not differ from those of rheumatoid arthritis. Antimalarial drugs are contraindicated, because they have been observed to provoke exfoliative dermatitis in psoriatic subjects. Reliance should be placed on a basic regimen of salicylates and physical therapy. Adrenocorticosteroid drugs should be employed only as a last resort. For the patient with very severe psoriatic arthritis, immunosuppressive therapy, in spite of its experimental status and considerable toxicity, is probably more appropriate than adrenocorticosteroid therapy.

For patients with severe psoriatic arthropathy that is not responsive to conventional antirheumatic therapy, methotrexate, in regimens that have proved efficacious for cutaneous psoriasis, may be employed. Intravenous or oral administration of methotrexate in doses of 10 to 25 mg once weekly (maximal dose, 50 mg per week) is usually successful in suppressing cutaneous and articular manifestations of psoriasis. A commonly employed oral regimen consists of a series of three doses (2.5 to 10 mg each) administered at 12-hour intervals each week. Close surveillance for evidence of myelosuppression is required. In addition, evidence for hepatotoxicity should be sought by periodic laboratory analyses.

58.4. REITER'S SYNDROME

Although the association of arthritis, urethritis, and conjunctivitis was recorded early in the nineteenth century, this triad of clinical manifestations bears the name of the German physician who, in 1916, described a patient with nongonococcal urethritis, conjunctivitis, and arthritis after an episode of diarrhea. Other common manifestations of the syndrome include fever, oral and genital mucous membrane lesions, cutaneous keratosis, and iritis. Most patients are young males; it is rare in women regardless of age.

ETIOLOGY. The cause of Reiter's syndrome is unknown, but most attention has focused on infectious causes. Venereal transmission seems apparent in many cases; in others the onset of Reiter's syndrome follows diarrheal illness. In several large epidemics of bacillary dysentery, a small percentage of patients have developed typical Reiter's syndrome, including genitourinary tract involvement. Mycoplasmal and chlamydial species are suspect as etiologic agents. The significance of sporadic isolation of such organisms from synovial fluid or synovial tissue is unknown. The frequency of HLA-B27 in Reiter's syndrome is close to that of ankylosing spondylitis.

CLINICAL AND LABORATORY MANIFESTATIONS. All the clinical features of Reiter's syndrome may appear simultaneously, but more commonly genitourinary or gastrointestinal symptoms precede the onset of ocular or rheumatic features by several days or a few weeks. Occasionally the classic pattern evolves slowly over weeks or months after the appearance of a single manifestation. Polyarthritis is frequently asymmetrical with predilection for involvement of articulations of the lower extremities, but the pattern of joint involvement can be varied. The majority of patients experience complete remissions within weeks or a few months of onset. A minority (range of 10 per cent) manifest persistence of synovitis in articulations of the extremities or spine and will have disability that parallels that of sustained rheumatoid arthritis or ankylosing spondylitis. Rarely, the clinical picture of chronic or recurrent Reiter's syndrome evolves into typical psoriatic arthritis.

There are no distinctive laboratory features. Peripheral blood leukocytosis is common. Properties of synovial fluid are similar to acute rheumatoid arthritis, although complement levels in joint fluid are invariably high. Roentgenographic abnormalities, equivalent to those associated with rheumatoid arthritis, are found in those patients with sustained synovitis. Periostitis, adjacent to involved joints, is a common but not distinctive feature of Reiter's syndrome.

The most common diagnostic alternative to Reiter's syndrome is *gonococcal arthritis*. The past literature is confusing because of the failure to distinguish these two syndromes and to recognize that gonococcal infection may be coincident to Reiter's syndrome. In a minority of patients, typical mucocutaneous lesions, particularly balanitis circinata and keratoderma blennorrhagica, leave no question regarding diagnosis, but the failure to isolate *N. gonorrhoeae* and the resistance of the manifestations to antimicrobial therapy are the main bases for differentiating Reiter's syndrome from gonococcal arthritis.

TREATMENT. The management of Reiter's syndrome is similar to that of rheumatoid arthritis. If salicylate therapy in the range of 3.6 to 4.5 grams daily fails to suppress synovitis or constitutional symptoms, phenyl-butazone or indomethacin (both in the range of 100 to 200 mg daily) may be beneficial. There is no experience to recommend gold therapy. There are a few reports describing remissions of very severe disease coincident to treatment with immunosuppressive agents; but in the light of their immediate and long-term toxicity, such therapy is considered experimental.

58.5. PALINDROMIC RHEUMATISM

This term has been applied to a recurring pattern of polyarthritis which results in no permanent joint deformity. The syndrome resembles gout in its acute onset and marked inflammatory signs. Rapid subsidence of signs and symptoms occurs within hours or a few days of onset. The frequency of episodes and the anatomic areas affected are variable, but for individual subjects the pattern of recurrent disease tends to be constant.

Since recurrent polyarthritis can be a feature of many rheumatic syndromes, the term palindromic rheumatism, if it is used at all, requires rigorous exclusion of other causes of synovitis. A significant number of patients, the majority in some series, with palindromic rheumatism eventually manifest typical features of rheumatoid arthritis. Systemic and constitutional symptoms are generally lacking. Since the brief episodes terminate spontaneously, there is no uniformity of opinion regarding response to therapy.

58.6. INTERMITTENT HYDRARTHROSIS

This term has been applied to the pattern of recurrent joint effusions, usually the knees, in which other inflammatory signs are minimal. The interval between episodes varies from one to a few weeks. In most reports of intermittent hydrarthrosis, there has been female preponderance. Occasionally recurrences correlate with menstruation. The diagnosis of intermittent hydrarthrosis, like palindromic rheumatism, should be restricted to individuals who have been followed long enough to exclude other causes of recurrent synovitis. A significant number of patients will eventually manifest chronic synovitis consistent with rheumatoid arthritis. When discomfort and restricted motion are attributable to joint space distention, simple arthrocentesis may be beneficial; there is no agreement regarding the efficacy of medicinal therapy in suppressing or preventing attacks.

Ansell, B. M., and Bywaters, E. G. L.: Rheumatoid arthritis (Still's disease). Pediat. Clin. North Am., 10:921, 1963.
Brewerton, D. A.: HLA-B27 and the inheritance of susceptibility to rheumatic disease. Arthritis Rheum., 19:656, 1976.
Calabro, J. J., and Marchesano, J. M.: The early natural history of juvenile rheumatoid arthritis. A ten year follow-up of 100 cases. Med. Clin. North Am., 52:569, 1968.
Kinsella, T. D., MacDonald, F. R., and Johnson, L. G.: Ankylosing spondylitis: A late re-evaluation of 92 cases. Can. Med. Assoc. J., 95:1, 1966.
Moll, J. M. H., and Wright, V.: Psoriatic arthritis. Semin. Arthritis Rheum., 3:55, 1973.
Ogryzlo, M. A.: Ankylosing spondylitis. In Hollander, J. L., and McCarty, D. J., Jr. (eds.): Arthritis and Allied Conditions. 8th ed. Philadelphia, Lea & Febiger, 1972.
Sharp, J. T.: Reiter's syndrome, In Hollander, J. L., and McCarty, D. J., Jr. (eds.): Arthritis and Allied Conditions. 8th ed. Philadelphia, Lea & Febiger, 1972.
Williams, M. H., et al.: Palindromic rheumatism: Clinical and immunological studies. Ann. Rheum. Dis., 30:375, 1971.

59. DISEASES WITH WHICH ARTHRITIS IS FREQUENTLY ASSOCIATED

Arthritis may be a significant feature of all of the syndromes listed in this chapter. Discussion here is brief and is limited to rheumatic manifestations of the various disorders. More detailed considerations will be found elsewhere in the chapters devoted to those diseases.

INFLAMMATORY BOWEL DISEASE

The reported incidence of arthritis complicating *ulcerative colitis* and *regional enteritis* (Crohn's disease) has varied, but it is generally in the range of 10 per cent. The most common rheumatic pattern is an asymmetric polyarthritis involving a few joints. In the majority of patients the disease is intermittent and results in minimal joint damage. The frequency and severity of arthritis are generally higher in those subjects with sustained and extensive bowel involvement, but occasionally rheumatic manifestations will antedate the recognition of enteric disease. *Erythema nodosum* and *uveitis* are three to four times more common in patients with enteritis and arthritis than in patients without rheumatic manifestations. In contrast to the generally benign character of rheumatic complications of enteritis, a small number (approximately 10 per cent of those with arthritis) experience a pattern of disease and disability equivalent to rheumatoid arthritis.

The incidence of *spondylitis*, which is indistinguishable from ankylosing spondylitis, in patients with ulcerative colitis and regional enteritis has varied between 2 and 6 per cent. This represents at least a twenty-fold increase in the frequency of spondylitis over that in the general population. Clinical, laboratory, or roentgenographic findings do not distinguish spondylitis complicating enteritis from ankylosing spondylitis unassociated with bowel disease, except that male predominance in the former is less striking and the incidence of HLA-B27 in subjects with enteropathic spondylitis, although increased relative to controls, is not as high as it is in ankylosing spondylitis.

There are no special recommendations regarding the management of arthritis associated with enteritis: the general principles outlined for the treatment of rheumatoid arthritis and ankylosing spondylitis (see Ch. 56 and 58.1) are appropriate. The main management effort is directed at the intestinal disease. Remissions of arthritis frequently follow surgical resection of diseased bowel, but rheumatic complications rarely affect the decision regarding surgical therapy.

Postinfectious arthritis complicating *Salmonella* and *Yersinia* enteritis shares with Reiter's syndrome and the spondylitis disorders a high association with HLA-B27.

WHIPPLE'S DISEASE

This is a rare syndrome, probably bacterial in cause, characterized by diarrhea, malabsorption, fever, anemia, increased skin pigmentation, and migratory polyarthralgia or polyarthritis. Permanent joint damage is rare.

FAMILIAL MEDITERRANEAN FEVER

Musculoskeletal pain occurs in approximately 7 per cent of patients with this heritable disease. The arthritis is usually monoarticular or limited to a few joints; most commonly involved are knees, ankles, hips, or shoulders. Severe pain and tenderness are out of proportion to other modest signs of inflammation. Arthritis, like other manifestations of this syndrome, is usually recurrent, but permanent damage to joints is rare. None of the anti-inflammatory medications have been found to be effective in the treatment of this form of arthritis. Management is limited to analgesics and local physical measures.

SARCOIDOSIS

The most common rheumatic manifestation of sarcoidosis is a transient acute polyarthritis associated with erythema nodosum and hilar adenopathy. Lower extremity joints are primarily involved. At times it is difficult to be certain whether inflammatory symptoms and signs reflect true synovitis or the cellulitis of erythema nodosum. Recovery is uniform. Most patients can be managed with salicylates but, if pain and disability are severe, a course of adrenocorticosteroid therapy may be indicated. Much less common than the acute rheumatic syndrome is chronic granulomatous synovitis that clinically resembles rheumatoid arthritis.

HYPOGAMMAGLOBULINEMIA

A mild polyarthritis, rarely deforming in character, has been observed in as many as one third of patients with congenital and acquired hypogammaglobulinemia. The pattern of joint disease resembles that of rheumatoid arthritis, although other connective tissue syndromes such as systemic lupus erythematosus, systemic sclerosis, and dermatomyositis have been associated with immune deficiency states. A variety of autoimmune phenomena and connective tissue syndromes have been observed in patients lacking IgA, the most common selective deficiency. Regression of arthritis frequently follows institution of gamma globulin therapy.

POLYCHONDRITIS

Relapsing polychondritis is a rare disorder characterized by inflammation and destruction of cartilage. In the majority of patients there is intermittent involvement of cartilage in ears, nose, trachea, pharynx, costochondral junctions, and peripheral joints. With subsidence of inflammation there may be collapse and deforming change of the ears, nose, and laryngotracheal structures. The pattern of joint involvement is usually that of recurrent polyarthritis associated with minimal residual deformity. Other manifestations include fever, iritis, episcleritis, cataracts, deafness, and aortic insufficiency. Aortic involvement, occurring in 14 per cent of reported cases, and involvement of cartilaginous structures of the respiratory tract are the two life-threatening complications of polychondritis. Pathologic studies demonstrate varying degrees of inflammation and loss of cartilage matrix. The cause is unknown. Adrenocorticosteroid therapy has been employed for life-threatening manifestations, but the generally remittent character of the disease makes it uncertain whether any mode of therapy changes its natural history. Aortic involvement has necessitated prosthetic valve replacement in a few reported patients.

BEHÇET'S SYNDROME

This syndrome was initially described as a triad (recurrent aphthous stomatitis, genital ulcerations, and iritis), but other manifestations are common: pyoderma, erythema nodosum, erythema multiforme, thrombophlebitis, and polyarthritis. Central nervous system involvement, in a minority of patients, may be fatal. Intermittent or chronic polyarthritis is usually limited to one or a few joints and rarely results in significant deformity. There is a strong suspicion that viral infection underlies the development of Behçet's syndrome, but attempts at microbial isolation have been equivocal or negative. Adrenocorticosteroid therapy is indicated if iritis is severe or if there are neurologic manifestations.

HEMOCHROMATOSIS

Joint involvement has been observed in as many as half of patients with idiopathic hemochromatosis. Joint swelling with bony enlargement is particularly common in the small joints of the hands, but other joints may be affected. The clinical and roentgenographic features resemble degenerative joint disease more than rheumatoid arthritis. There is narrowing of the joint space with subchondral erosions and sclerosis. Roentgenographic evidence of chondrocalcinosis is present in a third or more of patients with arthropathy and may account, via crystal-induced synovitis (see Chondrocalcinosis and Pseudogout in Ch. 60), for occasional acute inflammatory manifestations. The management of arthropathy is similar to that described for degenerative joint disease.

ACROMEGALY

The majority of patients with acromegaly develop an atypical form of degenerative joint disease. Increased levels of growth hormone result in hypertrophy of articular cartilage, subchondral bone, and periarticular tissues. Hypermobility of joints, a common manifestation, may contribute to degenerative change. The fingers and knees are most frequently affected. Radiographic features demonstrating overgrowth of bone are pathognomonic. Median nerve entrapment secondary to wrist synovitis is common.

HYPERPARATHYROIDISM

Patients with hyperparathyroidism are subject to a variety of associated rheumatic disorders which may occur singly or in combination. These include (1) hyperuricemia and gouty arthritis, (2) chondrocalcinosis with episodes of calcium pyrophosphate dihydrate crystal–induced synovitis, and (3) degenerative joint disease resulting from deformation of atrophic subchondral bone. Rheumatic symptoms, particularly those associated with chondrocalcinosis (see Chondrocalcinosis and Pseudogout in Ch. 60) may be the first manifestations of hyperparathyroidism.

SICKLE CELL DISEASE AND RELATED HEMOGLOBINOPATHIES

Severe polyarthralgia is a frequent manifestation of the crises of sickle cell disease. Occasionally pain is accompanied by transient joint effusion or other evidence of inflammation. The most common rheumatic symptoms result from avascular osteonecrosis of the femoral head, less commonly of other bony structures. This complication is also associated with sickle cell trait, hemoglobin C disease, SC disease, and sickle cell–thalassemia. In children, periostitis may result in transient diffuse swelling of the hands and feet. Sickle cell disease is associated with an increased incidence of bacterial arthritis and osteomyelitis, especially those caused by gram-negative organisms.

Bluestone, R., et al.: Acromegalic arthropathy. Ann. Rheum. Dis., 30:243, 1971.
Bywaters, E. G. L., Dixon, A. St. J., and Scott, J. T.: Joint lesions of hyperparathyroidism. Ann. Rheum. Dis., 22:171, 1963.
Ferguson, R. H.: Enteropathic arthritis. In Hollander, J. L., and McCarty, D. J., Jr. (eds.): Arthritis and Allied Conditions. 8th ed. Philadelphia, Lea & Febiger, 1972.
Hamilton, E., et al.: The arthropathy of idiopathic haemochromatosis. Quart. J. Med., 37:171, 1968.
McAdam, L. P., O'Hanlan, M. A., Bluestone, R., and Pearson, C. M.: Relapsing polychondritis: Prospective study of 23 patients and a review of the literature. Medicine, 55:193, 1976.
McEwen, C.: Arthritis accompanying ulcerative colitis. Clin. Orthop., 59:9, 1968.
McEwen, C., et al.: Ankylosing spondylitis and spondylitis accompanying ulcerative colitis, regional enteritis, psoriasis and Reiter's disease. A comparative study. Arthritis Rheum., 14:29, 1971.
O'Duffy, J. D., Carnery, J. A., and Deodhar, S.: Behçet's disease: A report of ten cases, three with new manifestations. Ann. Intern. Med., 75:561, 1971.
Spilberg, I., Siltzbach, L. E., and McEwen, C.: The arthritis of sarcoidosis. Arthritis Rheum., 12:126, 1969.

60.   MISCELLANEOUS FORMS OF ARTHRITIS

NEUROPATHIC JOINT DISEASE (CHARCOT JOINTS)

This chronic progressive degenerative arthropathy is a complication of a variety of neurologic disorders. Impairment of proprioceptive and pain sensation deprives the affected joint of the normal protective reactions when exposed to forces of weight bearing and motion. Although any neuropathic process which impairs sensory innervation may underlie neuropathic joint disease, syphilitic tabes dorsalis, in spite of its declining frequency, and diabetic neuropathy are the most common associated conditions. Syringomyelia, myelomeningocele, and congenital indifference to pain are less frequent neurologic bases for neuropathic arthropathy. The distribution of joints affected correlates with the pattern of neuropathy. In tabes dorsalis, the knees, hips, ankles, and vertebrae are frequently involved. In diabetic neuropathy, destructive changes are limited to the distal lower extremities, and in syringomyelia the shoulder and elbow joints are most commonly affected.

Although pain is generally present, discomfort tends to be disproportionately mild relative to signs of joint destruction. Clinical, pathologic, and roentgenographic features of chronic neuropathic joint disease reflect severe degrees of destruction and disorganization of affected joints. In the early cases, the differentiation from other causes of joint derangement depends upon the demonstration of sensory neuropathy.

Management includes immobilization of affected joints and restriction of weight-bearing activities with crutches, splints, and braces. Surgical arthrodesis, although frequently unsuccessful, is indicated in selected subjects. Depending on the anatomic pattern and extent of involvement, the application of prosthetic devices after amputation may improve function.

HEMARTHROSIS

Recurrent or chronic hemarthrosis is the most common manifestation of a group of heritable disorders of blood coagulation (see Ch. 520). Hemarthrosis can be a complication of anticoagulant therapy or trauma in an otherwise normal subject.

In hemophilia, joint bleeding usually begins before the age of five and tends to recur repeatedly during childhood in response to minor injury. The most commonly affected joints are the knees, elbows, and ankles, but any articulation may be involved.

Acute hemarthrosis usually results in marked local inflammatory signs and symptoms which recede within a few days. Approximately half the patients with hemophilia develop chronic deformities in one or more joints. Some of them suffer a chronic progressive synovitis, restricted to one or a few joints, which clinically and roentgenographically resembles rheumatoid arthritis. There may be marked synovial membrane hyperplasia, destruction of articular cartilage, and erosions of subchondral bone. This chronic progressive pattern probably results from a low level of continuous or intermittent bleeding into affected joints. Joint fluid, in the chronic cases, usually contains blood and very high levels of leukocyte-derived proteases. Other musculoskeletal manifestations of hemophilia result from bleeding into muscle and bone. The resolution of large hematomas may cause formation of chronic cysts.

The first principle in management is to prevent trauma, a goal not easily achieved in children. Acute hemarthrosis should be managed by immobilization, analgesic therapy, and the administration of plasma products which contain the appropriate coagulation factor. In the choice of analgesics, it is probably wise to exclude salicylates and other drugs which alter platelet function. If there is marked distention of the joint bursae, aspiration can be accomplished after the defect in coagulation has been corrected. When pain and acute inflammation have subsided, an exercise program directed at restoration of motion should be instituted. For the patient with chronic deforming joint disease, the availability of potent plasma products has permitted application of certain surgical procedures such as synovectomy and arthroplasty.

HENOCH-SCHÖNLEIN PURPURA

Nondeforming polyarthritis, most frequently affecting knees and ankles, is a common mainfestation of this syndrome, other features being nonthrombocytopenic purpura, abdominal pain, and glomerulonephritis. The syndrome is rare in adults.

MULTICENTRIC RETICULOHISTIOCYTOSIS
(Lipoid Dermatoarthritis)

This rare disorder usually begins in the middle decades of life and affects females three times more than males. It is characterized by the development of multiple histiocytic nodules in the skin and mucous membranes and severe polyarthritis which may simulate rheumatoid arthritis. The firm reddish-brown or yellow papular nodules are most commonly found on hands, forearms, head, neck, and chest. Mutilating joint destruction, especially in the distal interphalangeal joints, occurs in approximately half the patients with this syndrome. Diagnosis is by demonstration of histiocytes and multinucleated giant cells, containing PAS-positive material, in skin or synovium. Similar infiltrates have been observed in other organs. A few reports of apparent benefit from adrenocorticosteroid or immunosuppressive therapy are difficult to interpret because of the tendency for spontaneous remissions.

HYPERTROPHIC OSTEOARTHROPATHY

This term refers to a syndrome which includes clubbing of fingers and toes, periostitis with new osseous formation at the ends of long bones, arthritis, and signs of autonomic disorders such as flushing, blanching, and profuse sweating. The syndrome occurs with a wide variety of underlying disease states. Less commonly there are hereditary and idiopathic (pachydermoperiostosis) forms of disease. The fully expressed pattern is usually associated with intrathoracic disease: lung carcinoma, lung abscess, empyema, bronchiectasis, chronic interstitial penumonitis, or tuberculosis. Clubbing, usually without periostitis, may be seen with cyanotic heart disease, bacterial endocarditis, biliary cirrhosis, ulcerative colitis, regional enteritis, and thyroid disease.

The distal ends of metacarpals, metatarsals, and long bones of the forearms and legs are most frequently affected. There are inflammatory changes of periosteum, synovial membranes, and periarticular structures. The periosteum is "lifted" by the deposition of new bone matrix and subsequent mineralization. Clubbing results from edema, cellular infiltration, and connective tissue proliferation of the nailbeds.

The production of a humoral substance that mediates increased vascularity and/or connective tissue proliferation has long been suspected as the pathogenic factor in hypertrophic osteoarthropathy, but no such factor has been convincingly demonstrated. Evidence that neural factors are involved derives from observations of striking resolution of signs and symptoms after denervation of the hilum or vagotomy on the same side as the thoracic lesion. Regression of osteoarthropathy has also been observed after resection of pulmonary neoplasms.

Pain, tenderness, and enlargement of the distal portions of extremities may be accompanied by acute polyarthritis that resembles rheumatoid arthritis. The differentiation of the acute polyarthritis syndrome is aided by the recognition of clubbing and roentgenographic evidence of periostitis and intrathoracic disease.

Aside from therapy directed at the associated illness, there is no effective treatment of hypertrophic osteoarthropathy. Symptomatic benefit may be obtained from salicylates, other analgesics, or adrenocorticosteroids.

CHONDROCALCINOSIS AND PSEUDOGOUT

Chondrocalcinosis is defined as the presence of calcium-containing salts in cartilaginous structures of one or more joints. These salts include calcium pyrophosphate, calcium hydroxyapatite, and calcium orthophosphate. The term pseudogout refers to the acute and/or chronic synovitis associated with the appearance of calcium pyrophosphate dihydrate crystals in joint fluid.

There is a tendency to chondrocalcinosis in patients with hyperparathyroidism, alcaptonuria, hemochromatosis, Wilson's disease, and acromegaly, and perhaps with gout as well. There appears to be a significant association of diabetes mellitus with pseudogout, and a familial pattern of chondrocalcinosis has been described. Pseudogout, like true gout, appears to be an expression of crystal-induced synovitis.

The incidence of chondrocalcinosis increases with age. Several clinical patterns have been recognized. The most common is of a progressive arthritis of large joints, especially the knee and hip. This is usually indistinguishable from degenerative joint disease, although superimposed acute inflammatory episodes are common. The intermittent acute pattern of synovitis, which resembles gout, is less common. In a small percentage of patients there is a sustained progressive synovitis that resembles rheumatoid arthritis. Since many patients with calcification of articular cartilage manifest no rheumatic signs or symptoms, the terms chondrocalcinosis and pseudogout are not synonymous.

Attacks of *pseudogout* are usually monarticular; less commonly two or more joints may be involved simultaneously. The knee is the most frequently affected joint. The diagnosis rests on roentgenographic criteria, but proof requires the demonstration of calcium pyrophosphate dihydrate crystals under polarized light microscopy. These cystals usually have rod or rhomboid shapes and show weak positive birefringence.

Roentgenographic evidence of calcification of articular fibrocartilage may be found in many structures, including menisci, intervertebral discs, and symphysis pubis. Since punctate and linear radiodensities may be more evident in asymptomatic joints, suspicion of pseudogout should direct a survey of more than the affected articulation.

The metabolic basis for crystal deposition in chondrocalcinosis is not known. There are speculations regarding inhibition or deficiency of pyrophosphatases in cartilage, synovial tissue, or joint fluid.

Aspiration of an acutely swollen joint is often sufficient therapy in itself. If inflammatory signs are marked, aspiration may be followed by intra-articular adrenocorticosteroid therapy or the oral administration of phenylbutazone.

LYME ARTHRITIS

This inflammatory arthropathy was recognized because of an unusual geographic clustering of cases in three contiguous communities in eastern Connecticut. The syndrome is usually characterized by brief, recurrent episodes of asymmetric swelling and pain in large joints. The suspicion that the disease is transmitted by an arthropod vector was strengthened by recognizing an associated dermatologic lesion, erythema chronicum migrans, previously attributed to arthropod bites. In a prospective study during 1976, the peak onset of characteristic skin lesions was in June and July, and the majority experienced onset of arthritis during the months of July to September. Lyme arthritis followed the onset of skin lesion by four weeks (median), but this interval was highly variable, up to 22 weeks. Most patients had recurrent episodes of arthritis, but permanent joint deformity was not observed.

Symptoms and signs suggestive of aseptic meningitis were observed frequently. Two patients out of 27 studied prospectively had lymphocytic meningitis, and two had unilateral Bell's palsy.

Microbiologic and serologic studies seeking evidence of infection with bacteria, mycoplasmas, viruses, and a variety of agents that are transmitted by ticks were all negative.

Spontaneous variations in the natural course of the illness have made therapeutic evaluations difficult. Salicylate therapy has been recommended for symptomatic treatment of rheumatic symptoms. When visceral manifestations or severe systemic symptoms are present, corticosteroid therapy may be indicated.

SYNOVIAL TUMORS

Pigmented villonodular synovitis is the most commonly applied term for a syndrome characterized by villous or nodular growths affecting synovial linings of joints, bursae, or tendons, and a characteristic histopathological picture, i.e., presence of inflammatory granulomas containing hemosiderin and cholesterol crystals and multinucleated giant cells. There is dispute as to whether this condition should be classified as a form of synovitis or as a true neoplasm. Joint involvement is usually monoarticular. The knee is most frequently affected, less commonly the hip, elbow, ankle, or foot. Synovial fluid is usually hemorrhagic or xanthochromic. The inflammatory mass frequently invades cartilage, subchondral bone, and periarticular structures. Pigmented villonodular synovitis may affect extra-articular bursae and tendon sheaths or may occur as a localized tumor in only part of a joint. The treatment of choice is synovectomy. Recurrence is uncommon.

Synovial chondromatosis is an uncommon disorder characterized by the presence of multiple foci of cartilage metaplasia in synovial membranes. Bits of me-taplastic growths frequently detach and grow as loose bodies in the joint cavity and ultimately become ossified. In the latter state, this condition is referred to as synovial osteochondromatosis. The knee is most commonly affected; the disease is rarely polyarticular. Symptoms include pain, swelling, limitation in motion, and intermittent locking of the affected joint. The treatment is surgical synovectomy.

A variety of benign tumors (lipoma, chondroma, hemangioma, and xanthoma) may affect joints.

Primary malignant tumors are rare. Synovioma is a highly malignant fibroblastic sarcoma which probably originates in periarticular structures. This usually occurs in late childhood or early adult years. The recommended therapy is wide excision (frequently requiring amputation), regional lymph node dissection, and irradiation. With the most aggressive management the five-year "cure" rate is usually less than 50 per cent. Synovial chondrosarcoma is a rare neoplasm that may simulate synovial chondromatosis. Radical excision or amputation is the treatment of choice.

Barrow, M. V., and Holubar, K.: Multicentric reticulohistiocytosis. Medicine, 48:287, 1969.

Eichenholz, S. M.: Charcot Joints. Springfield, Ill., Charles C Thomas, 1966.

Howell, D. S.: Hypertrophic osteoarthropathy. *In* Hollander, J. L., and McCarty, D. J., Jr. (eds.): Arthritis and Allied Conditions 8th ed. Philadelphia, Lea & Febiger, 1972.

McCarty, D. J., Kohn, N. N., and Fares, J. S.: The significance of calcium phosphate crystals in synovial fluid of arthritic patients: The pseudogout syndrome: Clinical aspect. Ann. Intern. Med., 56:711, 1962.

Moskowitz, R. W., and Katz, D.: Chondrocalcinosis and chondrocalsynovitis (pseudogout syndrome): Analysis of 24 cases. Am. J. Med., 43:322, 1967.

Steere, A. C., Malawista, S. E., Harding, J. A., Ruddy, S., Askenase, P. W., and Andiman, W. A.: Erythema chronicum migrans and Lyme arthritis. The enlarging spectrum. Ann. Intern. Med., 86:685, 1977.

61. DEGENERATIVE JOINT DISEASE

(Osteoarthritis)

Early degeneration of articular cartilage probably begins in all subjects by the end of the second decade of life. In the pathologic sense, degenerative joint disease is a "normal" response to aging. If the incidence of degenerative joint disease is estimated by minimal roentgenographic criteria, approximately 90 per cent of the population by the age 40 is affected. Although only a small proportion of those with abnormal roentgenograms are symptomatic, degenerative joint disease is the most common cause of chronic disability.

Degenerative joint disease is sometimes classified as primary and secondary. The latter denotes the acceleration or augmentation of wear by abnormal stresses associated with injuries, obesity, and mechanical joint disturbances. Primary degenerative joint disease, in which there is no abnormal wear or forces, is probably influenced by one or more biochemical abnormalities that impair cartilage metabolism.

PATHOLOGY. The earliest lesions of degenerative joint disease are microscopic alterations of articular cartilage. These include diminution of metachromatic material, decreased numbers of chondrocytes, fatty degeneration, alteration of collagen fibrils, and surface irregularities. Later morphologic changes include localized softening of the cartilage with surface flaking and fibrillations. Abrasion of fibrillated cartilage results in progressive loss of carilaginous surfacing and exposure of subchondral bone.

Subsequent to ulcerations of cartilage, new bone formation occurs at the margin of articular cartilage. These marginal osteophytes are represented in roentgenograms as the characteristic "spurs." Other osseous changes include cysts of varying size beneath the joint surface and remodeling of subchondral bone.

Changes in synovial membranes, including fibrosis, hypertrophy, and occasionally synovitis, appear to be secondary to events affecting articular cartilage. Rarely the pathologic features of inflammation mimic those of rheumatoid arthritis.

ETIOLOGY AND PATHOGENESIS. Accepting the likely premise that primary changes in articular cartilage underlie the development of degenerative joint disease, etiologic considerations may relate to the reparative processes of cartilage. In response to injury, the metabolic activity of chondrocytes increases, but their capacity to replicate and form new matrix is limited. Secondary degenerative joint disease occurs when the forces of wear and tear exceed the restricted capacity for repair. When degenerative joint disease develops (frequently in familial patterns) in the absence of abnormal stresses, it is presumed that accelerated degeneration results from one or more biochemical abnormalities affecting cartilage metabolism. Chemical studies of degenerative cartilage have revealed several abnormalities: decreased water and chondromucoprotein contents and alterations in the profile of glycosaminoglycans. Some of these changes could be mediated by the action of lysosomal hydrolases, but the nature of the presumed biochemical defect in degenerative cartilage remains unknown.

Conditions which alter mechanical properties of joints or which affect the osseous support of articular cartilage are numerous. They include obesity, trauma, hypermobility of joints, neuropathy, acromegaly, Paget's disease of bone, hyperparathyroidism, and alterations of articular or periarticular structures by inflammatory joint disease.

CLINICAL PATTERNS OF DEGENERATIVE JOINT DISEASE. Pain is the dominant symptom of degenerative joint disease but, as noted earlier, disease which is roentgenographically moderate to severe may be asymptomatic. Pain is aggravated by joint motion or weight bearing. Transient stiffness after periods of inactivity is common. Loss of articular cartilage and osseous hypertrophy result in bony enlargement and malalignment of joints and crepitation on motion. Mild tenderness to palpation and effusions are common, but other inflammatory signs are usually absent.

The present discussion of clinical manifestations of degenerative joint disease is developed largely on anatomic lines, since signs and symptoms reflect regional patterns of involvement.

The Hand. *Heberden's nodes* are bony protuberances at the dorsal margins of distal interphalangeal joints. Early Heberden's nodes have a soft cystic consistency and may be associated with prominent inflammatory signs. The chronic stage of Heberden's nodes, characterized by bony enlargement and angular deformities (Fig. 4A), is usually minimally symptomatic. Heredity

Figure 4. Hand deformities of degenerative joint disease. *A,* Bony enlargement of distal interphalangeal joints (Heberden's nodes) and similar change in one proximal interphalangeal joint (Bouchard's node). *B,* Symmetrical degenerative changes in proximal interphalangeal joints (Bouchard's nodes), a pattern that is frequently mistaken for rheumatoid arthritis.

and sex are prominently involved in the development of Heberden's nodes. They are much more common in women. On the basis of family studies, it has been postulated that a single autosomal gene is involved which is dominant in females and recessive in males.

Patients with Heberden's nodes frequently show degenerative changes in other joints of the hands. The misinterpretation of proximal interphalangeal joint involvement (Bouchard's nodes) as rheumatoid arthritis is a common error (Fig. 4B). Metacarpophalangeal joint involvement is rare. Pain on the radial side of the wrist caused by degenerative disease in the first carpometacarpal joint is a frequent manifestation.

Coxarthrosis (Malum Coxae Senilis). Symptoms of *primary degenerative hip disease* usually appear in the later decades of life, but in as many as half the cases there is evidence of antecedent hip disease such as congenital dysplasia, slipped capital femoral epiphysis, or Legg-Calvé-Perthes disease. In addition, a variety of acquired disorders such as rheumatoid arthritis and avascular necrosis of the femoral head may lead to degenerative hip disease. Groin pain on motion or weight bearing is the dominant symptom, and this is often referred to the medial aspect of the thigh or knee. Over a period of months to a few years, the majority of patients become seriously disabled because of pain and restricted motion.

Degenerative Disease of the Knee. Involvement of the knees is the most common source of major disability in degenerative joint disease. Although mild synovitis and effusion may be present, joint enlargement primarily reflects bone proliferation. Crepitation on motion is a consistent finding. Degenerative changes are usually more prominent in the medial compartment of the knee, leading to varus deformity.

An early manifestation of degenerative change in the patellofemoral joint is termed *chondromalacia patellae*. This syndrome of knee pain and mild effusion, usually associated with trauma, is seen predominantly in young adults.

Vertebral Degenerative Joint Disease, Including Herniated Disc Syndromes. Two sets of articulations are present at all levels of the spinal column: the intervertebral discs and the posterior zygapophyseal joints. In addition to these, the cervical spine (between C2 and C7) has articulations between the lateral aspects of adjacent vertebral bodies, usually referred to as *joints of Luschka*. Degenerative changes in joints of Luschka are the most common cause of pain in the cervical area. In lumbar levels degeneration and herniation of the nucleus pulposus of intervertebral discs are usually the bases for symptoms.

CERVICAL SPINE. The close proximity of cervical nerve roots to the joints of Luschka makes them vulnerable to irritation or compression from any derangement in or about the joints. Since the greatest amount of stress in the cervical spine occurs at C4-C5 and C5-C6 levels, degenerative changes in the intervertebral discs and joints of Luschka are most common there. Osteophytic spurs at the margins of joints of Luschka may impinge upon nerve roots as they leave the intervertebral foramina. The pattern of pain and neurologic findings varies according to the level involved: pain is frequently in the supraclavicular and upper trapezius regions but can be referred into the occiput and more distal upper extremity. Discomfort is aggravated by motion of the neck, particularly rotation and lateral bending.

If there is degeneration of the intervertebral discs in the cervical spine, the joints of Luschka provide a barrier against lateral herniation of the nucleus pulposus. The protrusion and subsequent osteophytic reaction may therefore encroach directly on the spinal cord rather than nerve roots. The progression of the resulting cervical myelopathy may be insidious and painless.

LUMBAR SPINE. Symptoms of degenerative disease of the lumbar spine are nearly always attributable to involvement of intervertebral discs. Protrusion or extrusion of degenerated discs is directed posterolaterally, impinging upon nerve roots or the cauda equina. Although any of the lumbar discs can herniate, this most commonly occurs at L4-L5 and L5-S1. Patients with herniated lumbar discs frequently have a history of mild or recurrent backache prior to development of more acute discomfort. Pain radiates distally into one or the other lower extremity and is aggravated by spinal movement, particularly bending to the side of the pain. There is usually marked paravertebral tenderness and aggravation of pain by straight leg raising. Loss or suppression of the ankle jerk and sensory deficit in the lateral border and sole of the foot and toes suggest L5-S1 root compression. No reflex change, sensory deficit in the lateral leg and mediodorsal aspect of the foot, and weakness of the toe extensors suggest L4-L5 root compression.

Primary Generalized Hypertrophic Osteoarthri- tis. This is more a concept than a disease: it describes a polyarticular pattern associated with somewhat more inflammatory reaction than is customary with degenerative joint disease. There is usually involvement of the hands, including Heberden's and Bouchard's nodes, along with changes in the first carpometacarpal joints. Women in the middle years of life are most commonly affected, and a familial pattern is prominent. A closely related syndrome of degenerative joint disease has been termed *erosive osteoarthritis*.

LABORATORY FINDINGS. There are no specific laboratory abnormalities of degenerative joint disease. The erythrocyte sedimentation rate is usually normal. Synovial fluid is clear and exhibits high viscosity and normal mucin clot test. Leukocyte counts in synovial fluid vary in the range of 200 to 2000 per cubic millimeter. Fragments of cartilage are frequently identified in the fluid.

ROENTGENOGRAPHIC FEATURES. Osteophyte formation at the margins of affected joints is the basis for the most striking roentgenographic feature of degenerative joint disease, but earlier and more common findings, resulting from destruction of articular cartilage, are narrowing of the interosseous joint space and subchondral bone sclerosis. Radiolucent cysts, varying in size from a few millimeters to several centimeters, may be seen in periarticular bone.

Degeneration of cervical and lumbar discs results in interspace narrowing. Exostoses at the margins of vertebral bodies may coalesce with adjacent osteophytes, causing fusion at one or more levels. Roentgenographic documentation of intervertebral herniation requires contrast myelography. Disc degeneration is best observed by anteroposterior and lateral roentgenograms. For visualization of osteophytes encroaching on foramina, especially important in the cervical spine, oblique projections are required.

DIFFERENTIAL DIAGNOSIS. In their typical expressions, degenerative joint disease and rheumatoid arthritis are easily distinguished. The latter is usually associated with evidence of systemic disease, prominent signs of joint inflammation, and the characteristic symmetrical pattern of disease affecting the hands and wrists. When a patient presents with signs of mild inflammation in one or two weight-bearing joints of the lower extremities, the differentiation between these two syndromes is more difficult. In that setting a normal erythrocyte sedimentation rate, negative rheumatoid factor test result, and minimal abnormalities in synovial fluid support the diagnosis of degenerative joint disease. No test singly or in combination can be viewed as diagnostic; even the roentgenographic demonstration of marginal osteophytes may be a secondary change in rheumatoid arthritis. In the most experienced hands, there is a small percentage of patients in whom the diagnosis remains indeterminate.

A common diagnostic error is the interpretation of degenerative changes in proximal interphalangeal joints of the hands as evidence of rheumatoid arthritis (Fig. 4B). The deformities that characterize Heberden's and Bouchard's nodes may be marked, but this pattern of degenerative joint disease is not associated with prominent signs of inflammation, and the metacarpophalangeal joints and wrist joints are rarely or never affected.

Important aspects of differential diagnosis involve the recognition of syndromes in which secondary development of degenerative joint disease may occur. These include hemochromatosis, neuropathy, chondrocalcinosis, alcaptonuria, hypermobility of joints (including the Ehlers-Danlos syndrome), mechanical derangements of joints, and a variety of metabolic disorders that affect the support of articular cartilage by subchondral bone.

There should never be confusion in the differentiation of degenerative joint disease of the vertebral column from ankylosing spondylitis. Patients with the latter are almost invariably young men, and the roentgenographic features are distinct from those associated with degenerative joint disease.

TREATMENT. The management of degenerative joint disease is highly varied, depending upon anatomic patterns and the degree of joint deformity. An optimistic forecast is appropriate for most individuals. Patients should understand that disability can be minimized even though there is no specific remedy. The common statement that "nothing can be done for your kind of arthritis" is a false cliché.

Drugs. No medication has been shown to retard the development or progression of degenerative joint disease. The requirement for analgesic drugs is varied; many patients have so little pain that they require no medicinal therapy. Aspirin in moderate dosage (0.6 gram three to five times a day) is usually helpful for the patient with pain. Sustained salicylate therapy is superior to intermittent or erratic dosage. A common problem in degenerative joint disease, regardless of anatomic location, is the occurrence of intermittent episodes of increased pain which tend to subside spontaneously. For these recurrent episodes, phenylbutazone (100 to 300 mg daily) or indomethacin (75 to 150 mg daily) may be beneficial. Continuous use of drugs other than salicylates is rarely indicated in degenerative joint disease. Some patients with disabling hip pain, however, experience sufficient relief of symptoms with phenylbutazone or indomethacin to warrant maintenance therapy. It is common practice to prescribe muscle relaxants, such as diazepam or carisoprodol, for pain and muscle spasm of vertebral disease, but objective assessment of their efficacy is lacking.

Physical Measures. There are two general goals in the design of a physical medicine program for degenerative joint disease: minimizing the forces of work and weight bearing that apply to affected joints, and maintenance of normal joint alignment and motion. The patient with hip or knee disease should be instructed to avoid unnecessary walking or stair climbing. This recommendation is not inconsistent with the performance of an exercise program (in nonweight-bearing attitude) which can maintain muscle power and joint motion. Quadriceps isometric exercise for degenerative joint disease of the knees is particularly important. There is a powerful rationale for weight reduction for the obese patient with involvement of the spine or lower extremities. The use of a cane or a crutch can reduce forces of weight bearing applied to a symptomatic hip or knee by as much as 50 per cent. In selected patients with an unstable knee, fitting of a brace may be beneficial.

Certain physical measures are selectively relevant to degenerative joint disease of the spine. Patients need to learn to live with the altered mechanics of their spine. With cervical involvement, hyperextension and hyperflexion should be avoided. The patient should sleep supine with no more than one pillow. Most, but not all, patients with cervical radicular pain will be helped by intermittent traction. If this is beneficial, there are in-expensive devices for applying intermittent cervical traction at home. When symptoms are acute, wearing a cervical collar will restrict movement and minimize pain.

The patient with symptomatic degenerative disease of the lumbar spine should sleep on a hard mattress and avoid bending and lifting activities. A program of graded postural exercises is important when pain has subsided. External support provided by a lumbosacral corset will frequently minimize mild chronic symptoms. When lumbar disc herniation results in severe pain or nerve deficit, hospitalization is usually indicated. The majority of such patients will experience a remission of symptoms within a two- to three-week period. Consideration of surgical therapy is appropriate for those patients who fail to respond to conservative management.

Surgical Management. The main anatomic areas affected by degenerative joint disease that are amenable to orthopedic surgical therapy are the hip, the knee, and the vertebral column. Several surgical procedures are appropriate for the patient with debilitating hip pain. These include arthrodesis (if the disease is unilateral), mold arthroplasty, osteotomy, and total joint replacement. In most centers, the last is the preferred procedure. Operative procedures for the knee with degenerative joint disease include debridement, osteotomy, and a variety of prosthetic arthroplasties. If there is reasonable preservation of motion and stability of the malaligned knee, tibial or femoral osteotomy is frequently beneficial. When there is a serious disability attributable to malalignment and instability of the knee, one or another prosthetic procedure may be indicated. However, the successes, to date, of knee joint replacement have not been as predictable as have comparable procedures for the hip.

Virtually all orthopedic surgeons agree that surgical procedures for degenerative disease of the spine are appropriate *only* after there has been a systematic and sustained trial of conservative management. If radicular pain is relentless or if there are increasing neurologic deficits from nerve root involvement or myelopathy, surgical correction is warranted.

Armstrong, J. R.: Lumbar disc lesions. 3rd ed. Baltimore, Williams & Wilkins Company, 1965.

Friedenberg, Z. B., and Miller, W. T.: Degenerative disc disease of the cervical spine J. Bone Joint Surg., 45A:1171, 1963.

Kellgren, J. H., Lawrence, J. S., and Bier, F.: Genetic factors in generalized osteo-arthritis. Ann. Rheum. Dis., 22:237, 1969.

Mankin, H. J.: Biochemical and metabolic aspects of osteoarthritis. Orthop. Clin. North Am., 2:19, 1971.

Sokoloff, L.: The Biology of Degenerative Joint Disease. Chicago, University of Chicago Press, 1969.

62. THE PAINFUL SHOULDER

Because shoulder pain is frequent and due to diverse mechanisms, this subject deserves special attention. Of prime importance is recognition that pain in the shoulder may be referred from disease affecting cervical, intrathoracic, and diaphragmatic areas. Shoulder motion is affected by the action of muscles through a "joint complex" consisting of independent articulations — glenohumeral, acromioclavicular, and sternoclavicular, as well as the scapulothoracic surface relationship. In addition, shoulder function requires movement of gliding surfaces of periarticular structures — the musculotendinous cuff, the subdeltoid bursa, and the long head of the biceps. Any of the syndromes associated with synovitis may be responsible for shoulder pain. The primary concern in this chapter is a group of painful disorders which affect the periarticular soft tissues of the shoulder.

CALCIFIC TENDINITIS AND BURSITIS

The most common cause of shoulder pain results from degeneration of the supraspinatus and infraspinatus tendons. Approximately 3 per cent of people in their middle years have calcific deposits in these rotator tendons. Although the majority of such subjects have few or no symptoms, a significant percentage develop pain because of inflammation of the parietal surface of the overlying subdeltoid bursa. An inflammatory exudate containing calcareous matter may rupture into this bursa. The symptoms may be acute, subacute, or chronic. The acute syndrome is characterized by sudden onset of pain in the shoulder area, often with radiation into the neck and proximal arm. Any motion of the shoulder girdle elicits pain. There is frequently exquisite local tenderness over the anterior and anterolateral aspect of the shoulder joint. Night pain is a prominent feature. Roentgenographic studies usually demonstrate linear calcific deposits in the involved tendon or a more diffuse calcific pattern in the subdeltoid bursa. In most instances acute symptoms abate after a few days, but in a minority subacute discomfort persists for weeks.

The treatment is influenced by the severity and duration of symptoms. Anti-inflammatory agents, such as phenylbutazone or indomethacin, and analgesics are usually sufficient to control acute symptoms. In most patients there is a spontaneous remission of pain and a disappearance of calcific deposits. When the symptoms are very acute, aspiration of calcified material and injection of adrenocorticosteroid preparation may give prompt relief. The prospects of more chronic disability can be minimized by the institution of an active exercise program as soon as the level of discomfort permits. If the patient is not making progress toward regaining normal shoulder motion with a home exercise program, supervised therapy in a physical medicine department is important. A small percentage of patients with refractory pain and persistent roentgenographic findings may require surgical exploration for removal of calcific deposits.

BICIPITAL TENDINITIS

The long head of the biceps originates from the superior surface of the glenoid. It emerges from the glenohumeral bursa to lie in the bicipital groove of the humerus where it is covered by a synovial sheath. The shoulder pain of bicipital tendinitis frequently radiates along the biceps to the forearm, and is aggravated by abduction and internal rotation. Tenderness over the bicipital groove and accentuation of pain with resisted supination of the forearm, with the elbow flexed at 90 degrees, aid in the recognition of bicipital tendinitis. The management is similar to that described for calcific

tendinitis: local injection of adrenocorticosteroid preparations, systemic anti-inflammatory agents, and an exercise program. In refractory cases, surgical exploration with tendon transfer usually yields good results.

ROTATOR CUFF TEARS

The same degenerative changes that underlie the development of shoulder tendinitis can weaken the musculotendinous rotator cuff and predispose it to rupture. In most patients with this problem, there is acute onset of shoulder pain after trauma or performance of strenuous work. If the tear is complete, the patient is unable to abduct the arm, but it can be held in abduction, once elevated to 90 degrees, by the action of the deltoid muscle. With incomplete tears, the patient has only mild pain and moderate weakness. The diagnosis of rotator cuff tears can best be established by contrast arthrography. With complete rupture of the supraspinatus tendon, surgical repair is usually warranted. In patients with partial tears, partial immobilization followed by an exercise program is appropriate.

THE SHOULDER-HAND SYNDROME
(Reflex Neurovascular Dystrophy)

This is a poorly understood disorder characterized by pain and stiffness in the shoulder, together with pain, swelling, and vasomotor phenomena in the hand. Involvement of the distal upper extremity is frequently followed by dystrophic change that resembles·*Sudeck's atrophy*. The syndrome is presumed to result from reflex sympathetic stimulation analogous to that proposed for causalgia. It principally affects patients above the age of 50 and is often associated with acute illness such as myocardial infarction, trauma to the distal upper extremity, cerebrovascular accident, or pulmonary disease. The significance of associated degenerative change in the cervical spine is uncertain, because of its high frequency in the population at risk. When the disease is bilateral, the differentiation from acute rheumatoid arthritis may be difficult. Joint symptoms appear to result from periarticular involvement, but synovial biopsies, in a few cases, have disclosed mild histologic abnormalities: edema, proliferation, and disarray of synovial lining cells. There is marked variability in intensity and duration of acute symptoms and extent of dystrophic change. In a small percentage of patients the end result is "frozen shoulder" and dystrophic changes in the hands that resemble those of systemic sclerosis.

There is probably no condition for which aggressive physical therapy is more important than for the shoulder-hand syndrome. An active exercise program, facilitated by analgesic medication, should be instituted as soon as possible. When refractory pain impedes progress in the physical medicine program, a trial of systemic corticosteroid therapy (10 to 20 mg per day of prednisone or equivalent) or stellate ganglion block is warranted.

FROZEN SHOULDER

A minority of patients with any of the shoulder conditions discussed above develop chronic restriction of motion of the glenohumeral joint. When there is no apparent relationship of frozen shoulder to other shoulder disease, such as tendinitis or rotator cuff injury, the condition is sometimes termed *adhesive capsulitis*. This condition may be clincially indistinct from the shoulder-hand syndrome. Pain is generally less severe and less well localized relative to other conditions causing shoulder pain. The most important aspect of management of frozen shoulder is prevention. Early attention to the underlying cause of shoulder pain and the institution of an effective exercise program are nearly always successful in combating the progression of shoulder immobility. Management of the chronic frozen shoulder is much more difficult. Manipulation under general anesthesia followed by intensive physical therapy may be indicated when patients are not helped by conservative management.

DePalma, A. F., and Kruper, J. S.: Long-term study of shoulder joints afflicted with and treated for calcific tendinitis. Clin. Orthop., 20:61, 1961.

Kozin, F., McCarty, D. J., Sims, J., and Genant, H.: The reflex sympathetic dystrophy syndrome. 1. Clinical and histological studies: Evidence for bilaterality, response to corticosteroids and articular involvement. Am. J. Med., 60:321, 1976.

Steinbrocker, O.: The painful shoulder. *In* Hollander, J. L., and McCarty, D. J., Jr. (eds.): Arthritis and Allied Conditions. 8th ed. Philadelphia, Lea & Febiger, 1972.

63. NONARTICULAR RHEUMATISM

This term designates a group of painful disorders resulting from involvement of tendons, bursae, and other periarticular structures. Conditions causing shoulder pain are considered separately in Ch. 62.

BURSITIS

Bursae are closed synovial sacs located at sites of friction between skin, ligaments, tendons, muscles, and bones. Trauma is the most common cause of bursitis, but almost any illness characterized by joint synovitis may be associated with involvement of the lining of bursae. Bursae commonly involved include the following: subdeltoid, trochanteric, olecranon, and prepatellar. Septic or gouty bursitis can be documented by appropriate studies of aspirated fluid. Protection of an inflamed bursa from friction and trauma is the most important aspect of treatment, but moderate doses of salicylates, phenylbutazone, or indomethacin may be helpful. Local injection with an adrenocorticosteroid preparation is indicated if symptoms are severe or refractory to other treatments.

TENOSYNOVITIS

Tendon sheaths, like bursae, have synovial linings and can be involved by any process capable of inducing joint synovitis. Tenosynovitis in the hand or foot is a frequent manifestation of gonococcemia. Calcific tendinitis, a common source of shoulder pain (see Ch. 62), may be associated with marked inflammatory signs resembling acute gout. Focal thickening of the tendon sheath and adjacent tendon can result in "locking or

triggering" phenomena. This problem, termed stenosing tenovaginitis, is common in the flexor tendons of the fingers. Involvement of the abductor pollicis longus and extensor pollicis brevis tendons of the thumb (*de Quervain's syndrome*) results in pain and tenderness at the radial aspect of the wrist. There are no generalizations regarding management, since tenosynovitis may be a manifestation of various disease states, including rheumatoid arthritis and other connective tissue syndromes, infection, gout, and hypercholesterolemia. The common form of tenosynovitis, unassociated with systemic disease, will often subside with rest. If symptoms are severe or recurrent, local injections of adrenocorticosteroid preparations are usually effective. Surgical excision of the affected tendon sheath is indicated for those patients with persistent disability.

TENNIS ELBOW
(Epicondylitis)

This common condition is characterized by pain over the lateral aspect of the elbow. Tenderness is localized in the area of the common extensor insertion in the region of the lateral epicondyle. The problem, most common in middle-aged males, is related to sports or occupations that involve repetitive wrist extension or pronation-supination. Pain is accentuated by resisted wrist extension. If symptoms fail to respond to rest, injection of local adrenocorticosteroid preparations is usually successful. For the rare patient with persistent disability, surgical therapy may be needed.

CARPAL TUNNEL SYNDROME

This problem results from entrapment of the median nerve as it passes deep to the transverse carpal ligament of the wrist. Inflammation of the adjacent flexor tendon sheaths, the most common basis for median nerve entrapment, may be a feature of rheumatoid arthritis; but in most patients the tenosynovitis is localized and unassociated with systemic disease. The majority of patients are middle-aged women. The most consistent symptoms are dysesthesia, paresthesia, and hypesthesia in the middle three digits of the hand. Referred pain in the more proximal upper extremity is common. Symptoms are usually intermittent, occurring most frequently during the night. Forced flexion of the wrist or nerve compression locally may induce the characteristic symptoms. In a minority of patients, there is progressive wasting of the muscles of the thenar eminence. Conservative management consists of fitting a removable dorsal splint to hold the wrist in slight extension and the local injection of an adrenocorticosteroid preparation. Surgical release of the transverse carpal ligament is indicated for patients with persistent disability.

TIETZE'S SYNDROME

This mysterious benign disorder is characterized by painful enlargement of the upper costal cartilages. It is usually unilateral and limited to a single costochondral juncture. Occasionally the manubriosternal and sternoclavicular joints are affected. The disease may be recurrent, but remission is the rule. Some patients are concerned that they have cardiac disease; reassurance alone may be sufficient management. If discomfort is severe or recurrent, analgesics, heat, or local infiltration (adrenocorticosteroid or local anesthetic agents) may be beneficial.

FIBROSITIS

This term has been applied to a poorly defined symptom complex which is characterized by pain and stiffness in varying areas, most commonly in the neck, shoulder girdle, and posterior aspect of the trunk. Physical signs except for questionable nodules or thickening of the deep fasciae are lacking, and laboratory and roentgenographic studies are negative. The term fibrositis is based on vague hypothesis and common usage rather than on anatomic abnormalities. Localized areas of tenderness, commonly in the paravertebral areas medial to the scapula, have been termed "trigger points." The syndrome usually begins in the middle years of life. Because the majority of patients appear tense and anxious and have no recognizable objective basis for symptoms, the syndrome is often considered psychogenic. Since pain and stiffness can be manifestations of a variety of musculoskeletal, neurologic, and systemic disorders, the diagnosis of fibrositis requires the exclusion of more defined illnesses. The patient and his physician tend to share an unhappy experience in efforts to control symptoms. The results of strong reassurance that serious disease is lacking are variable, as are the results of therapy with salicylates, sedatives, tranquilizers, and muscle relaxants. Temporary relief is occasionally achieved by injection of local anesthetic into tender points or by chilling the overlying skin with ethyl chloride.

Levey, G. S., and Calabro, J. J.: Tietze's syndrome: Report of two cases and review of the literature. Arthritis Rheum., 5:261, 1962.

Phalen, G. S.: The carpal tunnel syndrome: Seventeen years' experience in diagnosis and treatment of 654 hands. J. Bone Joint Surg., 48A:211, 1966.

Swannell, A. J., Underwood, F. A., and Dixon, A. St. J.: Periarticular calcific deposits mimicking acute arthritis. Ann. Rheum. Dis., 29:380, 1970.

PART VIII

GRANULOMATOUS DISEASES OF UNPROVED ETIOLOGY

64. INTRODUCTION

Paul B. Beeson

The chapters to follow include a variety of rather uncommon and difficult-to-classify syndromes. These are characterized by long and fluctuating clinical courses, and the affected tissues show the picture of chronic inflammation, usually with formation of granulomas. Sarcoidosis is the most common and best known. The others are comparatively rare, and their natures and classifications are subject to controversy. For the purpose of textbook exposition, the best recognized clinical forms have been described as separate diseases. It should be noted, however, that there are shades of similarity and that each of these is thought by some students to be merely a variant expression of one of the other processes, e.g., panniculitis and retroperitoneal fibrosis. Some could well have been discussed with the diseases of connective tissue, as in fact they were in former editions. In the present state of knowledge — ignorance is more accurate — the editors have elected to place the descriptions of these syndromes under a heading with a noncommittal title.

65. SARCOIDOSIS

D. Geraint James

DEFINITION. Sarcoidosis is a multisystem granulomatous disorder of unknown cause most commonly affecting young adults and presenting most frequently with bilateral hilar lymphadenopathy, pulmonary infiltration, and skin or eye lesions. The diagnosis is established most securely when clinicoradiographic findings are supported by histologic evidence of widespread noncaseating epithelioid cell granulomas in more than one organ or by a positive Kveim-Siltzbach skin test. Immunologic features are depression of delayed-type hypersensitivity suggesting impaired cell-mediated immunity and raised or abnormal serum immunoglobulins suggesting lymphoproliferation. There may also be hypercalciuria with or without hypercalcemia. The course and prognosis correlate with the mode of onset: an acute onset with erythema nodosum usually heralds a self-limiting course and spontaneous resolution, whereas an insidious onset may be followed by relentless progressive fibrosis. Corticosteroids relieve symptoms and suppress inflammation and granuloma formation.

ETIOLOGY. The cause remains unknown. We do not know whether sarcoidosis is one disease or due to many contributing factors.

Infection. The various organisms claimed to be responsible for sarcoidosis have included human and anonymous mycobacteria, *Mycobacterium leprae,* fungi, viruses, and protozoa. Many organisms provoke a nonspecific granulomatous reaction, but this should not be misconstrued as multisystem sarcoidosis. Helminths provoke such reactions in the liver and central nervous system; anonymous mycobacteria cause swimming pool and fish tank granulomas, and *M. leprae* produces confusingly similar granulomas. Formerly, sarcoidosis was thought to be due to the human tubercle bacillus, but there are many important points differentiating sarcoidosis from tuberculosis.

Claims for a causal virus are longstanding, and at different times mumps, influenza, parainfluenza, Newcastle agent, and measles virus particles have been isolated.

There has been speculation concerning a transmissible agent from human sarcoid tissue into foot pads of mice, but similar changes occur with control nonsarcoid lymph node tissue. Attempts to demonstrate viruses by tissue culture of sarcoid lymph nodes have been unsuccessful.

High titers of antibodies to several viruses have been noted in sarcoidosis. This should not be misconstrued as indicative of a viral cause of sarcoidosis but rather as a reflection of lymphoproliferation by overactive B cells.

Genetic Factors. The occasional occurrence of familial sarcoidosis suggests a recessive mode of inheritance. We have observed 16 families, in whom 33 persons had sarcoidosis. The group comprised 11 brother-sister, 4 mother-offspring, and 1 uncle-niece relationships, and it was also noted once in husband and wife. The clinical, radiographic, and other features of the disorder are similar in familial and sporadic sarcoidosis, but the course of one sister was considerably worse than that of her brother, suggesting adverse hormonal factors. Four of these families were from the West Indies, suggesting a racial predisposition to familial sarcoidosis. Turiaf has also noted a greater incidence in French West Indians from Martinique; he finds familial sarcoidosis in 1 per cent of white Europeans but in 8 per cent of Martinicans living in Paris.

HLA Antigens. We have studied different clinical features individually. HLA-B8 (which was present in 27 per cent of controls) was found in 8 out of 13 with erythema nodosum alone (p < 0.015), 9 out of 11 with erythema nodosum and arthritis (p < 0.002), and 8 out of 9 with arthritis alone (p < 0.002). Thus B8 was present in 71 per cent of all patients with erythema nodosum and in 85 per cent with arthritis. It appears that there may be inherited susceptibility to arthritis and erythema nodosum in sarcoidosis, with B8 as a genetic marker for both disorders.

Allergy. Inhalation of pine pollen and peanut dust, clay-eating, and chewing pine pitch have all been incriminated as contributory regional factors in different areas.

Chemicals. Beryllium and zirconium are known to produce sarcoid granulomas in the sensitized individual, but other elements do not seem to be granulomagenic. Exhaustive skin testing with metals and other inorganic elements in sarcoidosis and controls has not revealed any peculiar hypersensitivity to chemicals. Skin tests for sarcoidosis, beryllium disease, zirconium hypersensitivity, and leprosy are very similar in that a sarcoid granuloma is present at the injection site one month after inoculation. Each skin test is individually specific for its own disorder, and there is no overlap.

Autoimmune Disorder. Sarcoidosis does not satisfactorily fulfill the criteria of an autoimmune disorder. There is one pattern of sarcoidosis that could conceivably fit — namely, erythema nodosum with hilar adenopathy, a syndrome which may be associated with a circulating immune complex; and these immune complexes have been shown to be present in sarcoidosis.

IMMUNOLOGY. Impaired Cellular Immunity. Depression of delayed-type hypersensitivity is reflected by T-cell anergy in vivo and in vitro (Fig. 1). Skin tests using tuberculin, fungal and viral antigens, and dinitrochlorobenzene are negative far more frequently than in control subjects. Sarcoid lymphocytes show diminished response to phytohemagglutinin (PHA). Quantitative tests for T cells are still crude and so results vary, but most reports indicate a reduction of the T cell subpopulation in the peripheral blood. It is likely that the number of peripheral blood sarcoid lymphocytes is most confusing and illusory to assess, for the plasma in which they are bathed may contain factors influencing

their behavior. With improved methods for assessing T cells, efforts should be directed to their enumeration within target organs and in sarcoid tissue, away from interfering T-cell antibodies.

Serum Inhibitors. Old theories of serum anticutins and procutins in sarcoidosis have been re-evaluated now that new techniques of lymphocyte morphology suggest that serum inhibitors are responsible for depression of cell-mediated immunity in sarcoidosis. Depending on the stimulus received, regulator T cells may suppress or amplify the immune response, producing lymphokines which affect the function of other T cells. In support of this concept is evidence of increased migration inhibition factors in sarcoid lymphocytes. When sarcoid serum has been removed, there is a return to normal function of these lymphocytes. Macrophages are active secretory cells which release potent enzymes perpetuating inflammation leading to granuloma formation, disturbing the traffic of re-circulating lymphocytes, and adding to this depression of cell-mediated immunity. This depression has been overcome by transfer factor both in vitro and in vivo, by blocking or otherwise overcoming serum inhibitors emanating from suppressor T cells. Levamisole may act similarly in overcoming depression of delayed-type hypersensitivity in vitro and in treatment.

Lymphoproliferation. Whereas there is cutaneous anergy and impaired cellular immunity, the reverse holds for humoral immunity. There is vigorous B cell activity with raised immunoglobulin levels; increased circulating antibody titers to Epstein-Barr virus, herpes simplex, rubella, measles, and parainfluenza viruses, and chlamydiae; increased antibody responses to mismatched blood; and occasional false-positive Wassermann reactions.

Circulating Immune Complexes. Various techniques have been employed to detect circulating immune complexes. They are most evident at the stage of erythema nodosum, iritis, polyarthralgia, and bilateral hilar lymphadenopathy in which C3 activation products have been found within the first six weeks. During this early stage of acute sarcoidosis, there is activation of the complement system due to circulating immune complexes. These tests for circulating complexes subside as the acute skin lesions disappear. At present, all tests for circulating complexes are crude, and it is necessary to use a battery of different techniques. When they are detectable, the sedimentation rate is very high, so this remains the cheapest bedside indicator of these complexes.

PATHOGENESIS. An antigenic insult, whether by an infective agent or by chemical or even vegetable matter, is met by a reticuloendothelial response in which both thymus-derived (T) cells and plasma (B) cells participate. The T cells are transformed, possibly by undergoing antigenic alteration on their cell surface, and become depleted. Serum inhibitors may block T cell function. Depletion may be due not only to T cell transformation but also to T cell interaction against transformed T cells. Depletion results in depression of delayed-type cutaneous and lymphocyte transformation tests. At the same time there is vigorous B cell proliferation, recognizable by an increase in circulating immunoglobulins. This phase of expansive lymphoproliferation with T cell eclipse is represented histologically by granuloma formation in many organ systems. During this same phase, circulating immune complexes may be

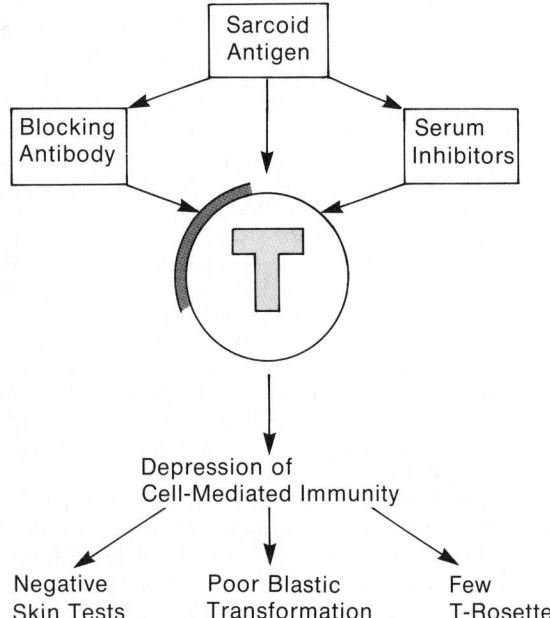

Figure 1. Depression of cell-mediated immunity is reflected by T cell anergy in bedside skin tests and in the laboratory.

responsible for such clinical phenomena as erythema nodosum and uveitis. The antigenic insult is probably airborne, for bilateral hilar lymphadenopathy is such a frequent mode of onset. The more acute the onset and the more active the reticuloendothelial response, the more likely will there be spontaneous remission with full restoration of T cell function. If this does not occur spontaneously, then it may be induced by corticosteroids, which may overcome T cell eclipse and restore normal T cell function.

The antigen responsible for lymphoproliferation, T cell transformation, and granuloma formation almost certainly resides in Kveim-Siltzbach antigen used in the sarcoidosis skin test. There is undoubtedly a complex interrelationship between the featureless null cell, the depressed T cell, and the B cell overactivity. Serum blocking factors may coat T cells so that they look like N cells and fail to produce the necessary lymphokines which recruit more T cells. T cell anergy means lack of suppressor control, thereby allowing B cell overactivity. It remains to be seen whether thymosin, levamisole, and BCG vaccine will transform N to T cells to correct the situation and whether therapeutic injections of transfer factor will recruit other T cells to repair the defect in cell-mediated immunity.

PATHOLOGY. High turnover granulomas are characterized by epithelioid and giant cells as seen in sarcoidosis, tuberculosis, Crohn's disease, and primary biliary cirrhosis. Epithelioid cells are large mononuclear cells about 20 μ in diameter with round or oval nuclei and are derived from macrophages. They are poorly phagocytic but highly secretory, and they indicate the constant arrival of macrophages into the granuloma pool. Giant cells up to 300 μ in diameter, containing as many as 30 nuclei, are usually arranged peripherally. They are also derived by fusion of macrophages, which are constantly arriving, dividing, and aging. Within these epithelioid and giant cells may be found three types of inclusion bodies — Schaumann, asteroid, and residual bodies — all of which are nonspecific end-products of the active metabolism and secretion which has taken place.

The sarcoid granuloma is surrounded by a peripheral rim of lymphocytes and contains macrophages, epithelioid and giant cells, and also T and B cells. Also within the granuloma are the various immunoglobulins which can be identified by immunofluorescence. As the lesion ages, reticulin fibers ramify between the epithelioid cells, which thicken and eventually become converted into collagen. The granuloma loses its outline and becomes a solid amorphous eosinophilic mass of hyaline material (Fig. 2).

So much for the morphology of the granuloma; what of its function? Macrophages are active secretory cells able to release a variety of potent enzymes, including lysozyme, glucuronidase, and angiotensin-converting enzyme. The last-named is useful for confirming the diagnosis of sarcoidosis (see Diagnosis).

EPIDEMIOLOGY. Sarcoidosis is worldwide in distribution, but is most frequently recognized in sophisticated communities with adequate diagnostic facilities. Mass chest roentgenography reveals an overall prevalence of 20 per 100,000 population, rising to a figure of 120 per 100,000 for Irishmen and 200 per 100,000 for Irishwomen in London. Although the overall prevalence is similar in men and women, it is twice as common in women of childbearing age. In the United States it is ten times more prevalent in blacks than in whites, regardless of birthplace or residence. This fact immediately raises the question of its frequency in the black population of Africa and the Caribbean. There is fresh information from South Africa indicating that sarcoidosis is ten times more frequent in the Bantu than in the white population — in fact, just as in the United States. It also afflicts the blacks in the same fashion, with gross skin lesions — including lupus pernio, papules, nodules, plaques in sites of old injury, and nail dystrophies — and a high frequency of intrathoracic involvement, bone cysts, and chronic uveitis. Of particular epidemiologic interest in the South African survey is that some of the patients had been in a leprosy institution. The diagnosis of sarcoidosis was entertained when patients had failed to improve on antileprotic, antituberculous, and antisyphilitic treatment. The South African Bantu is emerging from a scourge of tuberculosis, and sarcoidosis may follow in its wake.

Latent sarcoidosis will be found if sought in the right places. These include areas where tuberculosis has been eradicated; follow-up teams responsible for the eradication of tuberculosis should also look for sarcoidosis. It would be of interest to know the incidence of sarcoidosis in the Caribbean. Sarcoidosis is extremely common in the West Indian population in Britain and in Martinicans living in France, but is there the same preponderance in their home environments? It is possible that sarcoidosis bobs to the surface not only in the wake of tuberculosis but also after the eradication of leprosy.

CLINICAL MANIFESTATIONS. A recent worldwide re-

Figure 2. Features of a granuloma.

LYMPHOCYTE (T)

EPITHELIOID CELL 20 μ

GIANT CELL 300 μ

SCHAUMANN BODY 100 μ

ASTEROID BODY 5 μ

RESIDUAL BODY 1 μ

PLASMA CELL (B)

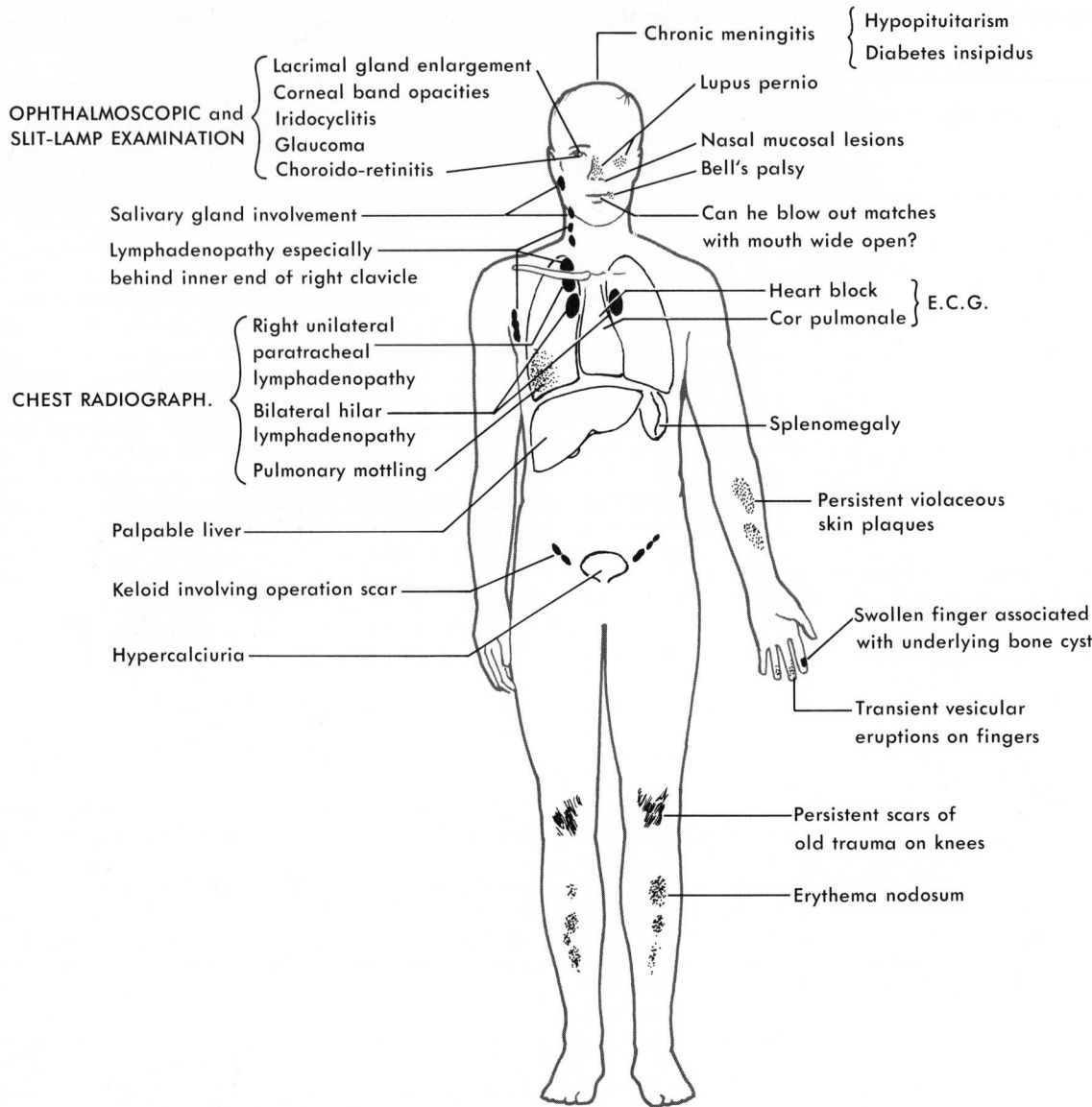

Figure 3. Clinical examination of a patient with suspected sarcoidosis.

view compares series of sarcoidosis in 11 cities. It comprises 3676 patients, 2082 (57 per cent) of whom were female and 2504 (68 per cent) of whom presented under 40 years of age (Table 1). The three common presentations were intrathoracic, dermatologic, and ophthalmic. An abnormal chest radiograph was the single most frequent presentation in 1475 patients (40 per cent), and another 783 (21 per cent) had respiratory symptoms. Seven hundred and thirty patients (20 per cent) presented with skin lesions; ocular lesions were observed in 539 (15 per cent).

Physical examination of the patient must be thorough (Fig. 3). It is incomplete unless accompanied by a chest radiograph, slit lamp examination of the eyes, and estimation of the 24-hour urinary calcium output. Multisystem involvement is a characteristic feature of sarcoidosis, with intrathoracic involvement in nine tenths of patients, ocular and skin involvement each occurring in about one quarter, and, depending on the series and country, erythema nodosum in up to one third of pa-

tients. Involvement of other tissues includes lymphadenopathy and splenomegaly in 28 per cent, neurosarcoidosis or salivary gland enlargement in 4 per cent, and bone cysts in about 3 per cent of patients (Table 1).

Sarcoidosis of the Upper Respiratory Tract. Sarcoidosis of the upper respiratory tract involves the nose, nasopharyngeal mucosa, and larynx. It is frequently associated with lupus pernio and may, in fact, precede and herald the onset of lupus pernio, a fact which is of practical clinical importance. It is a chronic manifestation occurring seven times more frequently in women and usually in the third decade, just as lupus pernio almost always occurs much more commonly in women in the fourth and fifth decades of life. A clinically significant point is that sarcoidosis may present to the nose and throat surgeon, who may perform a submucous resection for relief of nasal symptoms, with disastrous results including nasal septal perforation and progressive destruction of bone and cartilaginous septum.

Intrathoracic Sarcoidosis. Although only three fifths

TABLE 1. Data of a Worldwide Review of 3676 Patients with Sarcoidosis Followed in 11 Cities*

Features	Number of Patients	Per Cent
Total	3676	100
Women	2082	57
Age at presentation under 40 years	2504	68
Intrathoracic	3224	88
Lymph nodes and spleen	1031	28
Erythema nodosum	640	17
Other skin lesions	324	9
Ocular lesions	539	15
Parotid enlargement	160	4
Nervous system	134	4
Bones	109	3
Skin tests		
Positive Kveim-Siltzbach	1714/2189	78
Negative tuberculin	2093/3268	64
Hyperglobulinemia	808/1832	44
Hypercalcemia	200/1760	11
Treated with corticosteroids	1738	47
Mortality due to		
Sarcoidosis	84	2.2
Other causes	54	1.4

*London, New York, Paris, Los Angeles, Tokyo, Reading, Lisbon, Edinburgh, Novi Sad, Naples, Geneva. (From James, D. G., et al.: Ann. N.Y. Acad. Sci., 278:32, 1976.)

of patients have a respiratory presentation, a chest x-ray abnormality is evident at the onset in almost all patients; in the worldwide survey an abnormality was evident in 3377 (92 per cent) (Table 2).

STAGE 0. A clear chest radiograph in the presence of multisystem sarcoidosis was most unusual, occurring in only 277 patients (8 per cent).

STAGE 1. Bilateral hilar lymphadenopathy was noted in 1865 patients (51 per cent). Thus it was seen overall in half the series. Eventual resolution of this stage was noted in 65 per cent of the series overall.

STAGE 2. Hilar lymphadenopathy associated with pulmonary infiltration was the mode of presentation in 1066 (29 per cent). Chest x-ray resolution occurred in 49 per cent of these patients.

STAGE 3. It is unusual for the late stage of pulmonary infiltration with fibrosis to be a mode of presentation, and the overall resolution rate was only 20 per cent.

COURSE. When bilateral hilar lymphadenopathy alone is the initial chest x-ray appearance, the outcome is quite good, with clearance occurring in 65 per cent. When it is accompanied by erythema nodosum, the outcome is particularly favorable. Steroids are not usually necessary in these circumstances. The course of Stage 2 involvement is less favorable, and steroids are indicated to prevent progression to fibrosis. The course of Stage 3 involvement is poor, and steroids are mainly useful for relief of symptoms.

Skin Lesions. Erythema nodosum occurred in 640 patients (17 per cent). The incidence is higher in Britain and Scandinavia than elsewhere. It is infrequent in the black and the Asian.

Other skin lesions, including lupus pernio, maculopapular rashes, plaques, subcutaneous nodules, and scars, occurred in 324 patients (9 per cent) of the worldwide survey. Skin disease is almost always but one manifestation of multisystem involvement, in which there is also intrathoracic disease (in nine tenths of patients), uveitis, peripheral lymphadenopathy, parotid gland enlargement, neuropathy, and bone cysts.

Ocular Lesions. If slit lamp examination is routine, uveitis is seen in one fourth of patients with sarcoidosis; however, sarcoidosis is responsible for only about 7 per cent of instances of uveitis. Ocular sarcoidosis comprises anterior and posterior uveitis, conjunctival lesions, keratoconjunctivitis, scleral plaques, retinal vasculitis, papilledema, and secondary glaucoma and cataract formation. There are certain well-defined ocular syndromes. Heerfordt's or Waldenström's syndrome consists of uveitis, parotid gland enlargement, fever, and, commonly, seventh cranial nerve palsy. Other components include bizarre neurologic manifestations, hyperalgesia, papilledema, meningism, and spinal fluid pleocytosis. Löfgren's syndrome comprises erythema nodosum, bilateral hilar lymphadenopathy and acute iritis. Sjögren-like syndrome consists of keratoconjunctivitis sicca with or without parotid and lacrimal gland enlargement, mimicking Sjögren's syndrome but without the arthritis which is a feature of the latter. Chronic uveitis, lupus pernio, bone cysts, and pulmonary fibrosis make up another well-defined syndrome.

Neurosarcoidosis. This occurs in about 4 to 7 per cent of patients with sarcoidosis. Facial palsy is the most frequent presentation either alone or with other cranial nerve palsies or with papilledema. Other features include peripheral neuropathy, myopathy, meningitis, space-occupying brain lesions, epilepsy, cerebellar ataxia, hypopituitarism, and diabetes insipidus. Neurosarcoidosis has a mortality of 10 per cent, which is twice the overall mortality of sarcoidosis. The response to corticosteroids is more likely to occur in younger patients with an explosive onset of meningitis with erythema nodosum than in those with a space-occupying intracranial mass with chronic skin lesions, chronic uveitis, or pulmonary fibrosis.

Heart. Myocardial sarcoidosis is difficult to recognize clinically. It should be considered if a patient with florid multisystem sarcoidosis develops bundle branch block, arrhythmias, congestive cardiac failure, pericarditis, or clinical evidence of cardiomyopathy. Sudden death without previous evidence of a heart lesion may occur, particularly in patients over 40 years of age. Macroscopic changes are most evident in the posterior part of the ventricular septum. Microscopy discloses granulomas or fibrous tissue or both.

Bone Cysts. Sarcoidosis of bone is most frequent in hands or feet, but rarely it involves temporal or frontal bone or the hard palate. It is associated with soft tissue swelling, joint stiffness, and pain. Involvement of other

TABLE 2. Intrathoracic Disease in a Worldwide Review of 3654 Patients with Sarcoidosis

Features	Patients	
	Number	Per Cent
Total series	3654	100
Stage at presentation:		
0	277	8
1	1865	51
2	1066	29
3	446	12
Resolution of chest roentograms:		
Stage 1	1865	65
2	1066	49
3	446	20

systems includes lungs (in 77 per cent), lupus pernio and eyes (50 per cent), lymph nodes (32 per cent), parotids (23 per cent), liver (18 per cent), and spleen (14 per cent). There is no correlation between bone involvement and abnormal calcium metabolism. Three radiologic types of bone lesions are recognized:

PERMEATIVE. There is progressive cortical "tunneling" with remodeling of trabecular and cortical architecture.

LYTIC. Punched-out cysts are associated with pressure narrowing of the shaft, pathologic fractures, and residual cavities.

DESTRUCTIVE. Rapid destructive change may cause secondary joint surface involvement, and this may be followed by a periosteal reaction.

Pregnancy. Sarcoidosis is not a contraindication to pregnancy. In fact patients improve and are able to discontinue steroid therapy from the second trimester onward. Chest radiography is unnecessary until six months after delivery, which is the most likely time for recurrence. Excessive vitamin D intake during pregnancy must be avoided; it should be checked by determination of serum calcium level.

Childhood. In the Royal Northern Hospital, we have observed sarcoidosis in only one child under ten years of age, although we commonly see sarcoid granulomatous reactions which are mistakenly called sarcoidosis. Sarcoidosis should not be considered until the several other causes of granulomatous disorders — helminth infestation, mycobacterial infections, and chronic granulomatous disease of childhood — are excluded. We have noted sarcoidosis in 25 of 537 patients under 20 years of age (5 per cent). The main problem in management is that steroids are contraindicated in the growing child. Alternative treatments include corticotropin, oxyphenbutazone, indomethacin, and chloroquine.

DIAGNOSIS. Histology. The diagnosis is most secure when consistent clinical and radiographic findings are supported by histologic evidence of sarcoid tissue. The one without the other is commonly misconstrued. The clinical manifestations alone mimic many other disorders; conversely, histology of sarcoid granulomas alone is widely nonspecific. If there are skin lesions or peripheral lymphadenopathy, then biopsy will yield sarcoid tissue. *Fiberoptic bronchoscopy* with flexible forceps biopsy yields bronchial or lung tissue in four fifths of patients with intrathoracic disease. It is always positive in the early stage of hilar adenopathy and is least likely to be positive in those with pulmonary fibrosis.

Aspiration Liver Biopsy. This is invaluable for obtaining histologic confirmation, but it is important to establish the precise cause of the granuloma.

The histology of hepatic granulomas is similar, irrespective of the cause, so the cause is determined by collateral evidence. In Klatskin's series of 565 patients with epithelioid granulomas found on liver biopsy, the most common causes were sarcoidosis in 217 (38 per cent), underlying liver disease in 174 (31 per cent), tuberculosis in 70 (12 per cent), and schistosomiasis in 19 (3 per cent). These figures are very similar to those of our London survey, in which, of 138 patients with liver granulomas, 75 were found to have sarcoidosis (54 per cent), 26 had primary biliary cirrhosis (19 per cent), 23 had miscellaneous recognizable disorders (17 per cent), and 14 were undiagnosed (10 per cent). Ova are readily

recognizable in schistosomiasis when one is alert to the possibility, but acid-fast bacilli are demonstrable in only one tenth of patients with tuberculosis. The Kveim-Siltzbach test is of considerable value, for it is positive in about 70 per cent of patients with sarcoidosis but negative in patients with hepatic granulomas due to other causes. Likewise, the antimitochondrial antibody test is almost always positive in primary biliary cirrhosis but rarely positive in other disorders.

Kveim-Siltzbach Skin Test. This is a simple, specific outpatient skin test using human sarcoid tissue. It was found to be positive in four fifths of patients with sarcoidosis in a recent worldwide survey (Table 1). It is particularly helpful in delineating multisystem sarcoidosis from the numerous other granulomatous disorders which mimic sarcoidosis. Kveim-Siltzbach antigen is a saline suspension of human sarcoid tissue prepared from the spleen of a patient suffering from active sarcoidosis. The antigen, 0.15 ml, is injected intradermally very superficially into the flexor surface of the forearm, and the inoculation site is observed for the development of a visible and palpable nodule during the ensuing six weeks. Any palpable nodule is examined by biopsy, usually one month after the injection, using a Hayes-Martin drill. This core of tissue is serially sectioned for evidence of sarcoid tissue or of a foreign body giant-cell reaction; this decision is made blind, i.e., without knowledge of the clinical picture. A Kveim-Siltzbach test is reported as positive if the intradermally injected antigen produces a nodule in the course of three to six weeks and if this nodule shows evidence of sarcoid tissue, as distinct from a foreign body giant-cell reaction.

KMIF Test. Efforts are being made to develop in vitro Kveim tests by investigating the response of peripheral lymphocytes from patients with sarcoidosis and controls to stimulation by Kveim-Siltzbach antigen, using guinea pig macrophages as the indicator cells. The technique is termed the Kveim-induced macrophage inhibition factor (KMIF) test. Sarcoid lymphocytes, when stimulated in vitro with sarcoid material, produce a macrophage inhibition factor with a migration index of less than 0.8 in three fourths of subjects. Steroids make the KMIF test negative, as they do the skin test.

Serum Angiotensin–Converting Enzyme (SACE). Assay of serum ACE is useful for confirming the diagnosis of active sarcoidosis. It is elevated in the majority of patients with active disease, but normal levels are observed in burnt-out sarcoidosis, in those receiving steroids, and in lymphoma, leukemia, and other granulomatous disorders. Reduced values have been noted in asthma, emphysema, cystic fibrosis, lung cancer, and tuberculosis. It is likely that elevated serum ACE levels reflect enzyme secretory activity by epithelioid cells of the sarcoid granuloma.

Tuberculin Reaction. The tuberculin skin test was negative at a dilution of 100 units or its equivalent in two thirds of patients in the world survey. It reflects depression of delayed type hypersensitivity and incompetent T cells. With steroid therapy or with cure there is a tendency for the tuberculin reaction to revert to the sensitivity noted before the onset of sarcoidosis.

Physiology. Two useful practical tests of lung function are the single-breath diffusing capacity and the vital capacity. In the earliest stages of bilateral hilar lymphadenopathy (Stage 1) there may be reduction in the diffusing capacity and also in arterial oxygen tension. With radiographic evidence of pulmonary involvement, there is also reduction of vital capacity, airway resistance, maximum midexpiratory flow, and arterial oxygen tension on exercise. As might be anticipated, physiologic impairment correlates well with radiographic staging of pulmonary sarcoidosis. The worse the pretreatment impairment, the greater the temporary improvement in pulmonary function with steroids.

Unlike progressive systemic sclerosis and diffuse interstitial fibrosis, sarcoidosis rarely damages the pulmonary capillary bed even in the late fibrotic stage, so membrane diffusing capacity and pulmonary capillary blood volume provide prognostic information.

BIOCHEMISTRY. Hydroxyprolinuria. This is a feature of active sarcoidosis. It is not observed in chronic fibrotic burnt-out sarcoidosis, so hydroxyprolinuria neatly distinguishes acute exudative from chronic fibrotic sarcoidosis.

Calcium Metabolism. Hypercalcemia and hypercalciuria are such well-recognized components of sarcoidosis that they have been written into the definition of the disorder; despite this, the precise mechanism of the abnormal calcium metabolism is ill understood. In the world survey of sarcoidosis, hypercalcemia was noted in 200 of 1760 patients (11 per cent) examined in various centers. In a personal series of 75 patients with histologically confirmed sarcoidosis in whom simultaneous serum and 24-hour urine calcium levels were determined, calcium was raised in the serum or urine in 37 (49 per cent), in serum and urine in 10 (13 per cent), in urine only in 27 (36 per cent), and never in the serum alone. Three lessons were learned from this study: (1) The natural history of the calcium derangement follows that of sarcoidosis in other systems. It is transient and self-limiting in acute sarcoidosis and may indeed be missed if not sought early enough. Persistent hypercalciuria, when it occurs, is associated with persistent sarcoidosis. (2) Hypercalciuria is much more frequent than hypercalcemia. Urinalysis is the more sensitive method for detecting abnormal calcium metabolism, but unfortunately it is also the more cumbersome. We did not observe hypercalcemia in the absence of hypercalciuria. (3) Abnormal calcium metabolism is one feature of a multisystem disorder in which intrathoracic abnormalities were noted in 91 per cent, peripheral lymphadenopathy in 24 per cent, skin lesions in 21 per cent, and uveitis in 15 per cent of patients.

Uric Acid Levels. Hyperuricemia reflects renal failure in sarcoidosis; there is no particular association between it and bone and joint involvement. Its importance lies in the differential diagnosis of a patient with hyperuricemia and punched-out bone cysts resembling gout. The sarcoidosis profile under these circumstances will be that of a patient with chronic fibrotic sarcoidosis, raised blood urea nitrogen levels, probably intrathoracic changes, hypercalciuria, and possible chronic uveitis and skin lesions. These features are as a rule sufficiently distinctive for differentiation from gout.

Serum Immunoglobulins. We observed abnormal immunoglobulin levels in 57 of 71 patients (80 per cent) with sarcoidosis; IgG was increased in 40 (56 per cent), IgA in 19 (27 per cent) and IgM in 9 (13 per cent). IgG was increased in half of the white and two thirds of the West Indian patients. IgA was equally distributed between the two races, but IgM levels were elevated in one third of the white and two thirds of the West Indian patients. There was no significant difference when immunoglobulin levels were compared in acute and chronic sarcoidosis groups. Abnormal IgG levels bore no special correlation with organ systems involved. There was no significant correlation between serum immunoglobulin levels and changes in chest roentgenograms, Kveim-Siltzbach tests, depression of delayed-type hypersensitivity, and hypercalcemia.

SERUM IgD. IgD is less likely to be detected in the serum of sarcoidosis patients and more likely in tuberculosis. High levels of IgD occur predominantly in older patients with tuberculosis, whereas depression of IgD occurs in middle-aged patients with sarcoidosis; the age dependence of IgD seems highly significant. Elevated levels of serum IgM in patients with sarcoidosis may represent a compensatory change associated with low levels of serum IgD.

SERUM IgE. Although there is considerable overlap, significantly higher levels seem to occur in sarcoidosis compared with tuberculosis and control groups.

DIFFERENTIAL DIAGNOSIS. There are numerous unrelated granulomatous disorders. The chest physician must distinguish sarcoidosis from tuberculosis and extrinsic allergic alveolitis; the gastroenterologist, from Crohn's enteritis and primary biliary cirrhosis; the ophthalmologist, from other causes of uveitis; and the general physician, from Hodgkin's disease. Sarcoidosis is a multisystem disorder, so it should be considered when the patient is seen to attend many different outpatient clinics, particularly respiratory, ophthalmic, and dermatologic. The quickest ways of distinguishing active sarcoidosis are the Kveim-Siltzbach skin test, which is negative in all other granulomatous disorders, and the elevated serum angiotensin-converting enzyme.

COURSE AND PROGNOSIS. There are two distinct forms of sarcoidosis, acute and chronic, with clear-cut differences in onset, natural history, course, prognosis, and response to treatment (Table 3).

Acute Sarcoidosis. There is an abrupt explosive onset most common in patients 30 years or younger. Involvement of skin, eyes, and lymph nodes is acute and eruptive, and the histology is that of exudative sarcoid tissue rich in epithelioid and giant cells. In this phase of the disorder there is a positive Kveim-Siltzbach test, hydroxyprolinuria, raised serum angiotensin-converting enzyme, and abnormal calcium metabolism. Spontaneous remission rate is high, and prognosis is good.

Transient flitting polyarthralgia commonly precedes or accompanies erythema nodosum, probably reflecting a circulating immune complex at this phase of the disorder. If the process is particularly acute and exudative with considerable prostaglandin production into the joint or eye, an effusion or severe uveitis will develop. Bone cysts and persistent polyarthritis do not occur in this form of the disease.

Chronic Sarcoidosis. There is an insidious, ill-recognized onset and a persistent unrelenting course in all tissue systems, predominantly seen in patients aged 40 years and over. The histology is that of chronic fibrotic hyaline fibrosis with little evidence of mononuclear, epithelioid, and giant cells. Hydroxyproline excretion and serum angiotensin-converting enzyme levels are both normal. the Kveim-Siltzbach test is like-

TABLE 3.   Features Differentiating Acute from Chronic Sarcoidosis

Features	Acute (Transient)	Chronic (Persistent)
Age (years)	< 30	> 40
Onset	Abrupt	Insidious
Chest x-ray	Bilateral hilar lymphadenopathy	Pulmonary mottling
Eyes	Acute iritis, conjunctivitis, conjunctival nodules	Keratoconjunctivitis, chronic uveitis, glaucoma, cataract
Skin	Erythema nodosum, maculopapular rash, vesicular eruption	Lupus pernio, plaques, scars, keloids
Parotitis Lymphadenopathy Splenomegaly Bell's palsy	Usually transient	Rarely permanent
Bone cysts	No	Yes
Histology	Epithelioid and giant cells	Hyaline fibrosis
Lung biopsy	Positive	Negative
Calcium metabolism	Hypercalcemia, hypercalciuria	Nephrocalcinosis
Urinary hydroxyproline	Increased	Normal
Serum angiotensin-converting enzyme	Increased	Normal
Kveim-Siltzbach test	Positive	May be negative
Spontaneous remission	Frequent	Rare
Steroid therapy	Abortive effect	Symptomatic relief
Alternative drugs	Oxyphenbutazone	Chloroquine, potassium para-aminobenzoate
Recurrence after steroid therapy	Rare	Frequent
Prognosis	Good	Poor

ly to be negative, and calcium metabolism is unremarkable; all these parameters point to lack of activity in this chronic fibrotic form of sarcoidosis (see Table 3).

It is in this form that bone cysts are noted, with overlying soft tissue swelling, joint involvement, persistent painful polyarthritis, and deformities.

Treatment is directed toward symptomatic relief only. The prognosis is poor, for the mortality is significantly increased because of lung failure, cor pulmonale and cardiac failure, and nephrocalcinosis with renal failure.

COMPLICATIONS. Pulmonary fibrosis may be followed by cor pulmonale and both respiratory and cardiac failure. Abnormal calcium metabolism may lead to nephrocalcinosis and renal failure. Chronic uveitis may be complicated by secondary glaucoma and cataract formation with failure of vision. Corticosteroid eyedrops may cause a rise in intraocular pressure, which contributes to glaucoma, and prolonged oral steroids may contribute to posterior cortical cataract formation. Myocardial sarcoidosis may be a cause of sudden death.

The overall mortality is 3.6 per cent (2.2 per cent directly caused by sarcoidosis and 1.4 per cent resulting from unrelated causes).

TREATMENT. Corticosteroids are the sheet anchor of treatment; they are particularly indicated for uveitis, worsening chest roentgenogram, breathlessness, persistent hypercalciuria, disfiguring skin lesions, myocardial and neurologic involvement, involvement of salivary and lacrimal glands, and hypersplenism.

There are alternative treatments when steroids are contraindicated or have proved ineffective; the choice depends on the form of disease, i.e., acute or chronic sarcoidosis. Oxyphenbutazone controls acute exudative sarcoidosis, whereas chloroquine and potassium para-aminobenzoate are indicated for chronic fibrotic sarcoidosis. Azathioprine may be considered for its temporary steroid-sparing effect, when otherwise massive doses of steroids would be necessary. Persistent hypercalciuria may require a low calcium diet and drugs which chelate with calcium in the intestine, sodium phytate, and inorganic phosphate.

Studies are now being made to see whether levamisole can repair defective cellular immunity with benefit.

Certain treatments, formerly popular but now contraindicated, include radiotherapy, calciferol, and antituberculous drugs.

James, D. G., Neville, E., Siltzbach, L. E., Turiaf, J., et al.: A worldwide review of sarcoidosis. Ann. N.Y. Acad. Sci., 278:321, 1976.

James, D. G., Neville, E., and Walker, A. N.: Immunology of sarcoidosis. Am. J. Med., 59:388, 1975.

Lieberman, J.: Serum angiotensin-converting enzyme in sarcoidosis. Am. J. Med., 59:365, 1975.

Sharma, O. P., Neville, E., Walker, A. N., and James, D. G.: Familial sarcoidosis: A possible genetic influence. Ann. N.Y. Acad. Sci., 278:386, 1976.

Siltzbach L. E. (ed.): Seventh International Conference on sarcoidosis and other granulomatous disorders. Ann. N.Y. Acad. Sci., 278:1, 1976.

66.   POLYMYALGIA RHEUMATICA AND CRANIAL ARTERITIS

(Temporal Arteritis, Giant Cell Arteritis, Polymyalgia Arteritica)

Paul B. Beeson

66.1.   INTRODUCTION

The two clinical syndromes of cranial arteritis and polymyalgia rheumatica are described together, because they are often associated and because of the probability that they represent different expressions of one process. The age distribution of patients is almost unique, and the diseases seem to follow similar courses. Most persons affected are more than 60 years of age; occurrence before age 50 is exceedingly rare. These disorders are very rare in Oriental peoples, and appear to be unknown in blacks or American Indians. The distribution of HL–A haplotypes is not remarkable. Although symptoms may come on quite abruptly and may cause serious incapacity for a time, the natural tendency is toward gradual improvement, with complete subsidence after a period of several months to several years. The remarkable age incidence and self-limited course must figure prominently in any attempt to determine the nature of these disorders. A possibility to be considered is delayed recrudescence of an infection acquired early in life, as with varicella and herpes zoster or louse-borne typhus and Brill's disease.

66.2. POLYMYALGIA RHEUMATICA

Polymyalgia rheumatica is a distinctive kind of muscular rheumatism in old people, more frequent in women than in men. It is characterized by pain and stiffness in the neck, shoulders, and back, and sometimes in the pelvic girdle. Tenderness and true muscle weakness are usually lacking. The stiffness may be particularly troublesome in the morning so that patients are barely able to get out of bed. There may be headache or painful areas over the cranium. Systemic manifestations aside from occasional low-grade pyrexia are not prominent. The patients have a vague sense of malaise simply described as "feeling rotten." Unfortunately these people are too often dismissed with the assumption that symptoms are caused by degenerative processes about which little or nothing can be done.

The distinctive laboratory finding is marked elevation of the erythrocyte sedimentation rate, i.e., more than 80 mm by the Westergren method. Mild anemia is not uncommon, and some hematologists are reporting cases of unexplained anemia in old people which, like the muscular symptoms, respond promptly to steroid therapy. Other laboratory tests are of little help. Muscle biopsy generally reveals no significant inflammatory change even when the tissue is taken from areas which seem to be the site of much pain and stiffness. Blood enzymes which sometimes become elevated in other disorders of muscle are normal in this disease. There may be slight elevation of the alpha 2 globulin. Electromyographic findings are normal. Hepatic dysfunction may be reflected by moderately elevated blood alkaline phosphatase. A possible element of autoimmunity is indicated by the observation that lymphocyte transformation occurs in the presence of muscle tissue, especially during acute phases of the symptoms. The affected muscles do not atrophy.

Because of the frequent association of polymyalgia rheumatica with cranial arteritis, and especially because cranial arteritis may cause sudden blindness, some experienced clinicians believe that biopsy of a temporal artery should be carried out in all patients with polymyalgia rheumatica. When this has been done as a routine procedure, the artery has shown the characteristic changes in more than half the cases, regardless of clinical manifestations of arteritis. Others regard this as unnecessary because a trial of steroid therapy, which would be appropriate for cranial arteritis as well as for polymyalgia, will be carried out in any event. Visual disturbances are known to occur in this disorder, but their incidence is far lower than in patients with the clinical picture of cranial arteritis.

In the differential diagnosis, rheumatoid arthritis and degenerative joint disease may present problems; however, careful questioning and examination will show that polymyalgia is a disease of muscles, not joints. Various neoplastic diseases, including multiple myeloma, have to be considered in the differential diagnosis. Similarly the collagen diseases, especially polymyositis, may resemble polymyalgia rheumatica.

Therapy with adrenal steroids is remarkably effective, usually bringing about prompt amelioration of symptoms. It should be begun with a moderately large dose, e.g., 40 to 60 mg of prednisone daily for the first week, with gradual reduction over the next few weeks to a maintenance dose of 7 to 12 mg daily for a long time.

Some experienced observers recommend at least two years of this low-dose therapy for all patients. In one large study it was found that treatment had to be maintained for at least five years in 84 per cent of cases. There are cases on record in which the symptoms have persisted for as long as ten years. Usually, by occasional trials of reduced dosage and by following the sedimentation rate, the physician can determine when to terminate steroid therapy.

Coomes, E. N., Ellis, R. M., and Kay, A. G.: A prospective study of 102 patients with the polymyalgia rheumatica syndrome. Rheumatol. Rehab., 15:270, 1976.

Esiri, M. M., MacLennan, I. C. M., and Hazleman, B. L.: Lymphocyte sensitivity to skeletal muscle in patients with polymyositis and other disorders. Clin. Exp. Immunol., 14:25, 1973.

Hamrin, B.: Polymyalgia arteritica. Acta Med. Scand., Suppl. 533, pp. 1–131, 1972.

Von Knorring, J., and Wasastjerna, C.: Liver involvement in polymyalgia rheumatica. Scand. J. Rheumatol., 5:197, 1976.

66.3. CRANIAL ARTERITIS

This entity, like polymyalgia rheumatica, occurs only in people past middle age. In a substantial proportion of cases, symptoms resembling those of polymyalgia rheumatica are present weeks or months before the onset of the severe headache which characterizes cranial arteritis. Occasionally the only clinical presentation is that of fever of unexplained origin. The distinctive feature is a granulomatous arteritis, affecting large and medium-sized arteries of the upper part of the body, especially the temporal vessels. Histologic study reveals intimal thickening, and lymphocytic infiltration of the media and adventitia. In the media there are usually numerous giant cells, of the Langhans type. Eosinophils are not conspicuous. "Skip" areas do occur, and it is advantageous to make several sections of the vessel segment chosen for biopsy.

Cranial arteritis often has an abrupt onset, with severe pain usually in one temple but sometimes in the occipital area, face, jaw, or side of the neck. This may be associated with exquisite hyperesthesia so that the patient dislikes touching the scalp, combing the hair, or washing. The pain may have a throbbing character. Pain in the tongue, blanching of the tongue, and even gangrene of the tongue have been described in this disorder, doubtless ascribable to involvement of lingual arteries. Peripheral neuropathy with both sensory and motor components has also been described. The temporal artery may be tender, thickened, and nodular; conversely it may be pulseless and impalpable. The erythrocyte sedimentation rate is elevated, and there may be a substantial fever and polymorphonuclear leukocytosis.

The most feared complication of cranial arteritis is impairment of vision. It usually develops within three months of onset of other manifestations, and can be the first sign of the disease. This may consist of blindness in one or both eyes. The pattern of involvement may be uniocular, resulting from disease of the ophthalmic artery, or occipital, resulting from disease of the vertebral artery. Visual symptoms can also be caused by weakness of extraocular muscles. A precise estimate of the frequency of this complication cannot be made, because patients with visual symptoms receive special medical attention. Some articles state that visual impairment occurs in 50 per cent of cases, but this may be too high. The danger is real, and it is generally agreed that all patients with active cranial arteritis should receive steroid treatment, especially to prevent visual loss. There is also suggestive evidence that patients with cranial arteritis are at special risk of certain other vascular accidents, including brainstem strokes and coronary occlusion.

Although it cannot be doubted that the arteries most often affected are branches of the external carotid (accounting for the use of such names as cranial arteritis and temporal arteritis), it should be recognized that other arteries may also be the site of giant cell arteritis. Autopsy has disclosed arteritis in the aorta and even in the hepatic and renal vessels. Instances of aortic aneurysm thought to be due to giant cell arteritis are on record. These may result from an associated pathologic process described under a variety of names such as medial aortopathy.

Steroid therapy should be given according to the plan outlined for polymyalgia rheumatica.

Cullen, J. F., and Coleiro, J. A.: Review. Ophthalmic complications of giant cell arteritis. Surv. Ophthalmol., 20:247, 1976.

Ghose, M. K., Shensa, S., and Lerner, P. I.: Arteritis of the aged (giant cell arteritis) and fever of unexplained origin. Am. J. Med., 60:429, 1976.

Klein, R. G., Campbell, R. J., Hunder, G. G., and Carney, J. A.: Skip lesions in temporal arteritis. Mayo Clin. Proc., 51:504, 1976.

Swinson, D. R., Goodwill, C. J., and Talbot, I. C.: Giant cell arteritis presenting as subclavian occlusion. A report of two cases. Postgrad. Med. J., 52:525, 1976.

Wilkinson, I. M. S., and Russell, R. W. R.: Arteries of the head and neck in giant cell arteritis. Arch. Neurol., 27:378, 1972.

67. RELAPSING POLYCHONDRITIS

Paul B. Beeson

This is a rare but clinically distinctive disease characterized by inflammation and degeneration of cartilaginous structures. It occurs in persons of all ages, but most often in early and middle adult life. The sexes are about equally susceptible. Most of the reported cases have been in whites, but the disease has been observed in a few blacks and Orientals. The course is usually one of many years, with unpredictable fluctuations.

The pathologic lesion is primarily a loss of the mucopolysaccharide matrix in the affected cartilage. During acute flare-ups, neutrophil infiltration of the superficial portions of the cartilage is found; later, however, the inflammatory reaction is granulomatous in character, with predominance of lymphocytes; the end result is fibrosis.

The cause is unknown. Papain will cause similar changes in animals, and some metabolic disorder could be responsible. The prevailing conjecture is that the disorder has an immunologic basis. Both humoral and cellular reactions with cartilaginous antigens have been said to be demonstrable in patients with the disorder; perhaps the clearest evidence is lymphocyte transformation and macrophage migration inhibition by the cells of affected patients in reactions with purified cartilage matrix. It is also noteworthy that other "autoimmune" diseases have been present in about one third of the reported cases of relapsing polychondritis.

The most common site of inflammation is the cartilaginous structures of the ear. The lobe of the ear is spared, but the pinna becomes red or violaceous, tender, and swollen. Another common site of disease is the nasal septum, which, especially if subjected to ill-advised submucous resection, can cause a saddle-nose deformity resembling that seen in syphilis. Hoarseness may result from laryngeal injury, and life-threatening respiratory obstruction can be caused by degeneration of the cartilaginous rings of the trachea and bronchi. The cartilages of joints may be affected, so that monarthritis or polyarthritis may be prominent manifestations. The arthritis rarely progresses to bony destruction, and is not associated with subcutaneous nodules or rheumatoid factor in the blood. The sclera may become inflamed, and severe degeneration can lead to blindness. Involvement of inner ear structures or the eustachian tubes may cause deafness, tinnitus, or vertigo.

Other sites of damage, with potentially serious effects, are the aortic valve ring and the media of the aorta. Aortic incompetence and aortic aneurysms (either in the thorax or the abdomen) are found in approximately 10 per cent of patients. The "floppy mitral valve syndrome" has also been observed to develop during the course of this disease.

Standard clinical laboratory tests are unhelpful, except that the erythrocyte sedimentation rate is a useful index of activity.

Steroid therapy has been the main form of treatment and tends to damp down the intensity of the inflammatory manifestations. It may have to be continued over long periods of time, the dose being adjusted to the intensity of the symptoms. Immunosuppressive drugs have also been tried. Recently a few reports of dramatic "cure" of the disease by the use of dapsone (100 mg twice daily), have appeared; this treatment deserves further trial in view of its simplicity and small risk of toxicity. Surgery may be required for aortic valve incompetence or aortic aneurysm.

The course is unpredictable. Some patients have died as a result of respiratory or cardiovascular disease, many have continued to have low-grade and variable activity for years, and some have appeared to go into complete remission.

Arkin, C. R., and Masi, A. T.: Relapsing polychondritis: Review of current status and case report. Sem. Arth. Rheumatism, 5:41, 1975.

Barranco, V. P., Minor, D. B., and Solomon, H.: Treatment of relapsing polychondritis with dapsone. Arch. Dermatol., 112:1286, 1976.

Cipriano, P. R., et al.: Multiple aortic aneurysms in relapsing polychondritis. Am. J. Cardiol., 37:1097, 1976.

McAdam, L. P., et al.: Relapsing polychondritis: Prospective study of 23 patients and a review of the literature. Medicine, 55:193, 1976.

68. WEGENER'S GRANULOMATOSIS

Anthony S. Fauci

DEFINITION. Wegener's granulomatosis is characterized by the classic clinicopathologic features of necrotizing granulomatous vasculitis involving the upper and lower respiratory tracts, glomerulonephritis, and variable degrees of systemic, small vessel vasculitis.

ETIOLOGY. The cause is unknown, although it is generally considered to represent an aberrant hypersensitivity reaction to an unknown antigen. There have been no associations with allergic diatheses, geographic location, travel, or domestic or occupational exposure.

INCIDENCE AND PREVALENCE. Although an uncommon disease, Wegener's granulomatosis is no longer thought of as being extremely rare, as it is now recognized earlier and more frequently in clinical practice. The male:female ratio is approximately 3:2. The disease can be seen in any age group from infancy to old age. The peak incidence is in the fourth and fifth decades.

PATHOLOGY AND PATHOGENESIS. The characteristic histopathologic features of this disease are necrotizing vasculitis of small arteries and veins together with granuloma formation.

The upper airway disease most often is manifested by involvement of the paranasal sinuses and nasopharynx with necrotizing granuloma, with or without demonstrable vasculitis. Pansinusitis with erosion of adjacent bone may occur, as well as nasal septal perforation and saddle nose deformity.

Almost all patients have lung involvement (see Ch. 346.4). The infiltrates may take any form, but are usually multiple, bilateral, and nodular, with a tendency to cavitate.

Histopathologically, the renal lesion begins as a focal and segmental necrotizing glomerulitis which may lead to rapidly progressive glomerulonephritis and renal failure.

In addition to these classic features, virtually any organ can be involved with granuloma, vasculitis, or both.

The immunopathogenesis of the disease remains an enigma. Circulating immune complexes and immune complex–like renal deposits have been demonstrated in some patients. In contradistinction, the extensive granuloma formation in various organs is suggestive of delayed type hypersensitivity or cellular immune mechanisms. It is possible that there is an overlap of more than one type of immunologic mechanism, or that there is a granulomatous response to a particular type of immune complex in this disease.

CLINICAL MANIFESTATIONS. Wegener's granulomatosis is truly a multisystem disease manifesting a variety of signs and symptoms. However, in most patients the upper airway and, less frequently, the pulmonary symptoms dominate the presenting clinical picture.

Patients usually complain of severe upper respiratory symptoms and signs such as paranasal sinus pain, drainage, and purulent or bloody nasal discharge. Nasal mucosal ulceration and septal perforation may occur, as well as the classic saddle nose deformity. Serous otitis media commonly results from eustachian tube blockage, and variable degrees of hearing impairment may occur.

Eye involvement is seen at some time in up to 60 per cent of patients and may range from mild conjunctivitis to severe episcleritis, granulomatous sclerouveitis, ciliary vessel vasculitis, and proptosis.

Pulmonary manifestations may include cough, hemoptysis, chest discomfort, and shortness of breath. However, it is not uncommon that asymptomatic pulmonary infiltrates are discovered on chest x-ray during workup for other problems.

Nonspecific symptoms such as weakness, malaise, arthralgia, anorexia, and weight loss are common. Fever may result from the underlying disease, but often reflects secondary infection in paranasal sinuses.

Skin disease resulting from vasculitis with or without granuloma is seen in more than 40 per cent of patients.

Heart involvement is infrequent and usually appears as pericarditis or coronary vasculitis. Nervous system involvement, seen in up to 20 per cent of patients, may be exhibited in the form of cranial neuritis, mononeuritis multiplex, or cerebral vasculitis and/or granuloma.

Renal disease usually determines the course and ultimate outcome of generalized Wegener's granulomatosis. Proteinuria with variable degrees of hematuria, red blood cell casts, and other sediment abnormalities may indicate smoldering disease activity. However, once renal function abnormalities appear, evidence of rapidly progressive glomerulonephritis usually ensues, leading to renal failure if appropriate therapy is not instituted. A limited form of Wegener's granulomatosis without renal involvement has been described. However, it most likely constitutes part of the spectrum of the generalized disease.

There are no diagnostic laboratory findings in this disease. The erythrocyte sedimentation rate is invariably markedly elevated. Mild anemia and leukocytosis may be seen, but eosinophilia is not characteristic. Mildly elevated bentonite flocculation titers for rheumatoid factor are common, as is mild hypergammaglobulinemia, particularly of IgA.

DIAGNOSIS. Clinically, the diagnosis can be strongly suspected when the classic picture of upper and lower airway disease together with evidence of renal involvement is present. It is confirmed by the histopathologic demonstration of necrotizing granulomatous vasculitis in appropriate tissues such as nasal or sinus mucosa. The pulmonary infiltrates are the source of tissue with the highest diagnostic yield. Percutaneous renal biopsy is extremely important in documenting glomerulonephritis, particularly in early disease or when the diagnosis is unclear by other parameters.

Recognition of the classic clinicopathologic complex of Wegener's granulomatosis should make differentiation from other similar disorders relatively easy. However, differential diagnosis should include other vasculitides, connective tissue diseases, infectious and noninfectious granulomatous diseases, and tumors of the upper airway or lung. Goodpasture's syndrome is differentiated by the demonstration of antiglomerular basement membrane antibody. Idiopathic midline granuloma (see Ch. 69) is a localized destructive disease which mutilates the upper airway and facial tissues. Wegener's granulomatosis does not erode through facial tissue, and idiopathic midline granuloma does not include lung or renal disease. Of particular interest in the differential diagnosis is a disease called *lymphomatoid granulomatosis*. It involves predominantly lungs, skin, central nervous system, and kidney. It is clearly different from Wegener's granulomatosis. The vasculitis is really an invasion and destruction of vessels by atypical lymphocytoid and plasmacytoid cells resembling a lymphoma; the renal disease is not a glomerulonephritis but a nodular infiltration of the kidney by these bizarre lymphoid cells; and upper airway disease is quite uncommon.

TREATMENT AND PROGNOSIS. The treatment of choice in this disease is cytotoxic agents, and of the cytotoxic agents, cyclophosphamide is clearly the most effective. It should be given in daily oral doses of 1 to 2 mg per kilogram per day. In initiation of treatment in fulminant cases, the drug may be given intravenously in doses of 4 to 5 mg per kilogram per day for a few days, with subsequent change to the lower oral dosage regimen. It is important to emphasize that therapeutic response can usually be induced and maintained without causing severe leukopenia. Leukocyte counts should be closely monitored during therapy, and dosages of cyclophosphamide should be adjusted to maintain the leukocyte count above 3000 per cubic millimeter and the neutrophil count no less than 1000 to 1500 per cubic millimeter in order to avoid risk of infection. In patients who cannot tolerate cyclophosphamide, azathioprine in similar doses may be used.

Corticosteroids can be used initially, together with cyclophosphamide if disease activity is fulminant. Prednisone, 60 mg per day for a brief period of time, is recommended until the cyclophosphamide becomes effective (usually within 14 days). The prednisone should then be converted to an alternate day regimen, tapered, and discontinued. Serious eye involvement is a medical emergency and constitutes one of the only absolute indications for a limited course of corticosteroids. Other situations in which courses of adjunctive corticosteroids may be used are with serosal disease such as pericarditis or with central nervous system vasculitis.

The disease was formally universally fatal, usually within months after onset of renal disease. With cyclophosphamide use, the prognosis is quite good, and long-term remissions are induced in a high percentage of patients. Several patients have maintained remission for years following discontinuation of cyclophosphamide. It is recommended that the drug be continued for at least 1 year following induction of complete remission.

Carrington, C. B., and Liebow, A. A.: Limited forms of angiitis and granulomatosis of Wegener's type. Am. J. Med., 41:497, 1966.
Fauci, A. S.: Granulomatous vasculitides: Distinct but related. Ann. Intern. Med., 87:782, 1977.
Fauci, A. S., and Wolff, S. M.: Wegener's granulomatosis: Studies in eighteen patients and a review of the literature. Medicine, 52:535, 1973.
Liebow, A. A., Carrington, C. R. B., and Friedman, P. J.: Lymphomatoid granulomatosis. Hum. Pathol., 3:457, 1972.
Reza, M. J., Dornfeld, L., Goldberg, L. S., Bluestone, R., and Pearson, C. M.: Wegener's granulomatosis. Long-term followup of patients treated with cyclophosphamide. Arthritis Rheum., 18:501, 1975.
Wolff, S. M., Fauci, A. S., Horn, R. G., and Dale, D. C.: Wegener's granulomatosis. Ann. Intern. Med., 81:513, 1974.

69.   MIDLINE GRANULOMA

Anthony S. Fauci

DEFINITION.   Midline granuloma is a relentlessly progressive, localized destructive process that predominantly involves the nose, paranasal sinuses, and palate, with erosion through contiguous structures such as the orbit and face. It destroys soft tissue, cartilage, and bone, and is characterized by nonspecific acute and chronic inflammation and necrosis with or without granuloma formation. It is an uncommon disease which was first described in 1897 by McBride.

ETIOLOGY.   The cause of midline granuloma is unknown. Since the disease is characterized by a granulomatous inflammatory reaction suggestive of a hypersensitivity or immunologically mediated phenomenon, it has been hypothesized that this represents a localized hypersensitivity response to an unidentified antigen. Under certain circumstances the tissues of the upper airways can respond very intensely to the presence of an antigenic stimulation. It is this hyperreactivity to an unknown stimulus which leads to the inflammatory reaction and subsequent tissue destruction characteristic of this disease. Although some patients report histories of allergic rhinitis and chronic sinusitis, there is no evidence of these conditions being predisposing factors in this disease. Biopsy materials have been cultured for various microorganisms, and no etiologic connections have been found. Certain upper airway tumors can result in inflammatory and granulomatous responses which likewise can cause necrosis and destruction of tissue. The inflammatory response is often so intense that the underlying histopathology of the neoplasm can be masked and the process closely resembles midline granuloma. However, it is clear that true midline granuloma is a distinct entity in which no identifiable cause of the localized destructive inflammatory process can be found despite multiple deep biopsies, long term follow-up, and even postmortem examination. This entity should appropriately be referred to as idiopathic midline granuloma, as opposed to the inflammatory and even granulomatous responses associated with upper airway neoplasms.

PATHOLOGY.   The typical histopathologic features are nonspecific acute and chronic inflammation with necrosis. The tissue is infiltrated with neutrophils, monocytes, lymphocytes, plasma cells, and, in some cases, eosinophils. Although true granuloma formation with or without typical Langhans giant cells are considered the hallmark of the disease, this may not be present in every case and is often masked by the fulminant inflammation and necrosis. Thrombosis of small vessels, perivascular cellular infiltration, and secondary involvement of vessels resulting from the inflammatory process may occur, but true primary vasculitis is rarely seen. If neoplastic cells are identified, the process obviously can no longer be considered idiopathic midline granuloma. Secondary pyogenic infection of the involved tissue with its added inflammatory response is frequently found to a greater or lesser degree.

CLINICAL MANIFESTATIONS.   The disease can occur in all age groups, but most patients are in the fifth and sixth decades. It is slightly more common in women than men and occurs in all races.

The clinical presentation can vary from patient to patient, but in most cases symptoms can first be related to the nose and paranasal sinuses with rhinorrhea and nasal stuffiness. Symptoms persist and intensify, often followed by purulent nasal discharge resulting from superimposed infection. Nonhealing ulcerations of the nasal mucosa occur, and perforation of the nasal septum is frequently seen. Some patients present with disease in the oral cavity either alone or concomitant with nasal and paranasal sinus involvement. This usually occurs as ulcerations of the buccal mucosa, gums, or hard and soft palate. Some patients have presented with relatively painless perforation of the palate noted by the regurgitation of food or saliva into the nasal cavity. Occasionally, patients initially complain of symptoms related to the eye. The disease may be relatively indolent or fulminant, but it is always progressive. Relentless destruction of soft tissue, cartilage, and bone occur. Erosion of paranasal sinus walls occur, with spread into contiguous structures such as the orbit with subsequent eye involvement. Destruction of the soft and hard palate, the nasal septum, and even the entire nose occurs. If left untreated, the destructive process erodes through the skin of the face, resulting in dramatic mutilation of facial structures. This understandably leads to severe psychologic difficulties in some patients. The necrotic tissue as well as the paranasal sinus cavities frequently becomes infected, usually with *Staphylococcus aureus,* and this compounds the systemic symptoms of anorexia and malaise. The necrotic tissue can be quite malodorous, although the patients themselves frequently lose their sense of smell early in the course of the destructive process. It is of interest that local lymphadenopathy rarely occurs, and that when present it is suggestive of an underlying malignancy.

There are no characteristic laboratory findings except those related to the inflammatory process such as leukocytosis, elevated erythrocyte sedimentation rate, mild anemia of chronic disease, and hyperglobulinemia. Roentgenographic studies reveal pansinusitis with destruction of various cartilaginous and bony structures of the upper airways. The disease remains localized, and laboratory abnormalities related to other organ systems should prompt one to investigate other possible causes.

Although the disease may wax and wane in its progression, if left untreated, it is uniformly fatal. It has been reported that surgical procedures in the involved areas can lead to rapid acceleration of the disease, although, following appropriate treatment, debridement of necrotic areas may be beneficial to healing. Death usually occurs from secondary systemic infection or from inanition. Other causes of death are erosion into a major blood vessel with exsanguination or erosion into the central nervous system and subsequent meningitis.

DIAGNOSIS. The diagnosis of midline granuloma is made by the characteristic histopathologic findings in biopsies of the involved tissues together with the characteristic clinical presentation, but, most important, after other diseases with similar clinicopathologic findings have been ruled out.

Midline granuloma is sometimes confused with Wegener's granulomatosis. They are clearly distinct entities. Wegener's granulomatosis is a systemic disease characterized by necrotizing granulomatous vasculitis of the upper and lower respiratory tracts with glomerulonephritis (in the generalized form). Midline granuloma rarely manifests true primary vasculitis in the lesions and by definition is a localized disease without pulmonary or renal involvement. Furthermore, the destructive qualities of the upper airway lesions are different. Wegener's granulomatosis rarely or never causes palatal perforation and does not erode through facial tissues.

The greatest difficulty in differential diagnosis arises in distinguishing true idiopathic midline granuloma from neoplasms of the upper airways, particularly midline malignant reticulosis and certain lymphomas. Since these neoplasms can elicit destructive granulomatous reactions similar to those of midline granuloma, their true malignant histopathology can be masked by the intense inflammatory reaction. Careful search for disseminated malignancy as well as complete examination of multiple adequate biopsy specimens often reveals the neoplastic nature of these other disorders while confirming the true idiopathic nature of true cases of midline granuloma.

Other diseases which must be ruled out by appropriate cultures, special stains of tissue specimens, and/or other diagnostic laboratory tests are infectious diseases such as tuberculosis, syphilis, lepromatous leprosy, histoplasmosis, blastomycosis, coccidioidomy-

cosis, mucocutaneous leishmaniasis, and rhinoscleroma (caused by a *Klebsiella* species). Also included in the differential diagnosis is pseudotumor of the orbit.

TREATMENT. Surgical excision of the involved tissues has been attempted, only to result in continued progression and, in some cases, acceleration of the disease. Corticosteroid therapy likewise is ineffective and can cause worsening if infection is present. Cytotoxic agents have been used with reports of variable results, most of which were ultimately failures, or the diseases being treated were misdiagnosed as midline granuloma and were in reality midline neoplasms or Wegener's granulomatosis.

The treatment of choice clearly is local radiation therapy. It has been reported that low dose irradiation of 1000 rads or less induced remissions. However, relapses are common after such low doses, whereas high dose (5000 rads) radiotherapy to the involved areas has been shown to result in a high percentage of remissions.

PROGNOSIS. If left untreated, the disease is uniformly fatal. Since the use of high dose local radiotherapy, the prognosis for survival is excellent, with greater than 70 per cent remission rate and even cures after more than 10 years of follow-up. Hence the disease should no longer be referred to as "lethal" midline granuloma. It should be pointed out that high dose radiotherapy to this area is associated in some cases with serious complications and side effects. However, the risk is outweighed by the fatal alternative. The mutilation and disfigurement which result from far advanced disease are often a source of great psychologic difficulty now that survival is feasible. In this regard, reconstructive plastic surgery, as well as placement of prostheses, has resulted in dramatic functional and cosmetic improvements in patients in remission.

Blatt, I. M., Seltzer, H. S., Rubin, P., Furstenberg, A. C., Maxwell, J. H., and Schull, W. J.: Fatal granulomatosis of the respiratory tract (lethal midline granuloma — Wegener's granulomatosis). Arch. Otolaryngol., 70:7907, 1959.
Fauci, A. S., Johnson, R. E., and Wolff, S. M.: Radiation therapy of midline granuloma. Ann. Intern. Med., 84:140, 1976.
Fauci, A. S., and Wolff, S. M.: Wegener's granulomatosis: Studies in eighteen patients and a review of the literature. Medicine, 52:535, 1973.
Fechner, R. E., and Lamppin, D. W.: Midline malignant reticulosis. A clinicopathologic entity. Arch. Otolaryngol., 95:467, 1972.
Friedmann, I.: Midline granuloma. Proc. Roy. Soc. Med., 57:289, 1964.
Stewart, J. P.: Progressive lethal granulomatous ulceration of the nose. J. Laryngol., 48:657, 1933.
Walton, E. W.: Reticuloendothelial sarcoma arising in the nose and palate (granuloma gangrenescens). J. Clin. Pathol., 13:279, 1960.

70. WEBER-CHRISTIAN DISEASE

(Relapsing Febrile Nodular Nonsuppurative Panniculitis, Panniculitis)

Paul B. Beeson

In this chapter several unusual syndromes are described which may or may not be variants of the same disease. The feature shared by all is the occurrence of localized inflammatory lesions in adipose tissue.

The term *Weber-Christian disease* is usually applied to a clinical syndrome in which the principal involvement is in the panniculus adiposus. Young or middle-aged women are affected more frequently than men with this form of the disease. It is characterized by development of multiple tender nodules in the subcutaneous fat, from 5 mm to 10 cm in diameter. The lesions are located principally on the thighs and trunk and in the breasts. They are tender, and there may be some reddening of the skin. Occasionally necrosis of the skin leads to sinus formation with discharge of an oily liquid. The course is usually indolent; crops of lesions develop from time to time over periods of months or years. When the inflammation subsides, there often remains an area of loss of subcutaneous tissue which causes dimpling of skin. Systemic manifestations are usually mild, but may include malaise, low-grade fever, leukocytosis, and eosinophilia. Enlargement of the liver and spleen is reported in some cases. The illness may grumble along for months or several years and then cease.

A more serious expression of this pathologic process has been termed *systemic Weber-Christian disease*. Here there is widespread inflammation affecting not only the panniculus adiposus but also similar tissue within the abdominal and thoracic cavities. There may be parenchymatous inflammation, affecting thoracic or abdominal organs, including lungs, pericardium, pleura, bowel, spleen, kidneys, and adrenal glands. At least a dozen cases are recorded in which this form of disease has led to death.

The terms *mesenteric panniculitis* and *mesenteric lipodystrophy* have been applied to an obscure disease characterized by inflammation of the mesenteric fat. This has been encountered mainly in males, and reports of the syndrome have appeared principally in surgical journals. Symptoms include recurrent episodes of fever, abdominal pain, nausea, vomiting, and malaise. At operation the mesentery is found to be thickened, with red or yellow patches, and biopsy reveals the characteristic panniculitis or simply infiltration with lipid-laden macrophages, which may be indistinguishable from the histology of "Weber-Christian disease." Several writers have suggested that these forms of inflammation in the retroperitoneal adipose tissue may represent the initial lesion in at least some cases of retroperitoneal fibrosis. An association between some of the panniculitis syndromes and alpha$_1$-antitrypsin deficiency has been observed (Rubinstein et al., 1977). In a series of 54 cases from the Mayo Clinic, 8, or 15 per cent, were associated with malignant lymphoma. This seems more than coincidence.

An important differential diagnostic point arises in distinction of the fatty lesions in the syndromes described here from the syndromes associated with pancreatitis or acinar cell carcinoma of the pancreas. In these there may develop crops of discrete areas of inflammation in the subcutaneous fat, as well as in the fatty tissues of the body cavities, resulting from liberation of excessive quantities of pancreatic lipase. Undoubtedly this has led to confusion with other forms of lipodystrophy, such as the Weber-Christian syndrome or mesenteric panniculitis. Despite some statements to the contrary, it seems unlikely that the histologic changes found in various stages of these groups of conditions are sufficiently distinctive to permit differentiation on histologic grounds alone. In the pancreatic-

associated lesions elevation of blood lipase may provide the best clue.

Classically the pathologic findings in Weber-Christian disease are said to progress through three stages. In the early, symptomatic period, in which inflamed nodules are present, there is degeneration of fat cells, with a predominantly neutrophil infiltrate. The next stage shows a substitution of histiocytes and mononuclear cells for the neutrophils, and the histiocytes have a foamy appearance owing to ingested fat. In the third, atrophic stage fibrosis with lymphocytic cells is characteristic.

There is no specific therapy. It is difficult to evaluate any treatment because of the unpredictable remissions that characterize these diseases. Considerable relief of symptoms by use of large doses of steroids has been reported, but in other instances this has not proved helpful. Antimicrobial drugs should not be given. The use of immunosuppressive or cytotoxic agents could be considered, especially when there is evidence of systemic extension of the panniculitis, and benefit from treatment with cyclophosphamide has been reported. Other agents for which beneficial effects have been claimed include chloroquine (250 mg twice daily for one to three weeks), and thalidomide (100 mg twice daily for three or more weeks). Thalidomide is contraindicated in women of childbearing age.

Eravelly, J., and Waters, M. F. R.: Thalidomide in Weber-Christian disease. Lancet, 1:251, 1977.

Hallahan, J. D., and Klein, T.: Relapsing febrile nodular nonsuppurative panniculitis (Weber-Christian disease); review of literature and report of case. Ann. Intern. Med., 34:1179, 1951.

Kipfer, R. E., Moertel, C. G., and Dahlin, D. C.: Mesenteric lipodystrophy. Ann. Intern. Med., 80:582, 1974.

Lever, W. F., and Schaumburg-Lever, G.: Inflammatory diseases of the subcutaneous fat. In Histopathology of the Skin. 5th ed. Philadelphia, J. B. Lippincott Company, 1975, pp. 231–238.

Milner, R. D. G., and Mitchinson, M. J.: Systemic Weber-Christian disease. J. Clin. Pathol., 18:150, 1965.

Moore, S.: Syndromes resulting from dissemination of pancreatic enzymes. J. Rheumatol., 2:5, 1975.

Tannenbaum, H., Anderson, L. G., and Schur, P. H.: Association of polyarthritis, subcutaneous nodules, and pancreatic disease. J. Rheumatol., 2:14, 1975.

71.   FIBROSING SYNDROMES

(Multifocal Fibrosclerosis)

Paul B. Beeson

71.1.   INTRODUCTION

In rare instances the delicate fibrous areolar tissue in a certain anatomic region becomes the site of a chronic low-grade inflammatory process, leading to deposition of dense sclerotic plaques, which may obstruct or limit the movement of adjacent viscera. When the process is in the active phase, there are characteristic findings of chronic or granulomatous inflammation, featured by mononuclear cell infiltration and occasional giant cells. In the end-stages the pathologic lesion is simply that of scar tissue, so that by the time this process causes clinical manifestations there may be little evidence of the initial inflammatory reaction. As a general rule the process tends to originate in the midline, around the great vessels, and then to spread laterally. At the periphery of the lesion there appears to be an inflammation of fatty tissue; this is gradually converted to a dense fibrous mat, with little or no sign of inflammation. In at least some cases there is an accompanying vasculitis: a granulomatous inflammation in the walls of small and medium-sized veins. In most cases a clue to the inciting mechanism is lacking; hence the frequent use of the term "idiopathic" in describing the various syndromes. Indubitably this pattern of response may follow different kinds of injury. For example, there is an association between therapy with methysergide and some cases of retroperitoneal fibrosis, and the suggestion has been made that fibrosing mediastinitis can occur as a sequel to infection with *Histoplasma capsulatum*. In a number of instances the disease has developed concurrently with a neoplastic process such as reticulum cell sarcoma or carcinoid tumor.

Although most of these syndromes have been described as separate entities, depending on the clinical manifestations and the interests of the writers who have reported them, it should be emphasized that several anatomic areas may become affected in one person. For example, retroperitoneal fibrosis and sclerosing mediastinitis may be present at the same time. Even more interesting is the report by Comings and his associates of two brothers, offspring of a consanguineous marriage, who exhibited varying combinations of retroperitoneal fibrosis, mediastinal fibrosis, sclerosing cholangitis, Riedel's thyroiditis, and pseudotumor of the orbit. This remarkable constellation of syndromes in two siblings brings up the possibility of a genetic predisposition to disease of this character, but of course does not exclude other precipitating factors, e.g., common exposure to some chemical. The former possibility is given support by the recent description of an association between the occurrence of fibrosing syndromes and alpha$_1$-antitrypsin deficiency.

Alpert, L. I., and Jindrak, K.: Idiopathic retroperitoneal fibrosis and sclerosing cholangitis associated with a reticulum cell sarcoma. Gastroenterology, 62:111, 1972.

Comings, D. E., Skubi, K. B., Van Eyes, J., and Motulsky, A. G.: Familial multifocal sclerosis. Ann. Intern. Med., 66:884, 1967.

Meyer, S., and Hausman, R.: Occlusive phlebitis in multifocal fibrosclerosis. Am. J. Clin. Pathol., 65:274, 1976.

Palmer, P. E., Wolfe, H. J., and Kostas, C-I.: Multisystem fibrosis in alpha$_1$-antitrypsin deficiency. Lancet, 1:22, 1978.

Salmon, H. W.: Combined mediastinal and retroperitoneal fibrosis. Thorax, 23:158, 1968.

71.2. RETROPERITONEAL FIBROSIS
(Periureteral Fibrosis)

In retroperitoneal fibrosis the process usually begins over the promontory of the sacrum and extends laterally across the ureters and up as high as the level of the second or third lumbar vertebra. Less commonly the lesion develops in other extraperitoneal areas, for example, contiguous with the kidneys, duodenum, descending colon, or urinary bladder.

In some cases there has been an associated vasculitis in the skin and subcutaneous tissues, manifested by the formation of nodules, erythematous discolorations, and ulcerations. Similarly, inflammatory changes in small vessels at the sites of the sclerosis have been noted.

The occurrence of retroperitoneal fibrosis in patients taking methysergide for migraine has been reported with greater frequency than could be due to chance, i.e., 12 per cent of all cases reviewed by Koep and Zuidema. These authors also reported an association with some kind of neoplastic disease in 8 per cent of cases.

The disorder is about twice as common in males, and the peak age incidence is in the fifth and sixth decades. The manifestations are variable, depending on the anatomic location of the process. Pain is the most common symptom; it is vague, tends to be located in the low back, and may be accompanied by symptoms referable to the gastrointestinal tract. The patient is likely to lose weight and have low-grade fever. There may be some anemia and elevation of the erythrocyte sedimentation rate. Although the ureter is the structure most often affected, symptoms referable to the urinary tract are uncommon until obstructive uropathy has led to azotemia and other clinical manifestations of renal insufficiency. The fibrosing process may surround the inferior vena cava, but signs of obstruction of that vessel are uncommon; this contrasts with mediastinal fibrosis, in which the most common expression is superior caval obstruction.

Diagnosis of retroperitoneal fibrosis is difficult because of the lack of localizing manifestations. It is most often suggested by the findings at intravenous pyelography: displacement of the ureters toward the midline and evidence of obstruction, usually at the level of the pelvic brim. One or both ureters may be affected. Recent experience indicates that diagnosis by use of ultrasound may become very helpful. In rare instances a mass can be palpated in the pelvis or on the posterior abdominal wall. Once the presence of a mass has been disclosed, the main problem in differential diagnosis lies in distinguishing retroperitoneal fibrosis from retroperitoneal tumor, and, as already mentioned, retroperitoneal fibrosis can develop in response to various kinds of neoplastic disease. For that reason it is advised that multiple deep biopsies should be made at the time of laparotomy.

Surgical treatment, if employed before there has been severe renal damage, is often highly successful. Inasmuch as the fibrosing process is seldom invasive, the constricted organ can usually be freed by blunt dissection so that normal movement or flow is restored. Relief of ureteral obstruction is usually achieved simply by dissecting this structure free of its fibrous encasement and bringing it out on the anterior surface of the sclerotic mass. Occasionally, however, the obstruction recurs months or years after such treatment. The claim has been made that prolonged steroid therapy may be helpful, but the evidence for this is unconvincing, and prompt surgical relief should usually be attempted. Nevertheless, many people who have had experience with this disease recommend that steroid treatment be employed as an adjunct to surgical measures. When the inferior vena cava is obstructed, surgical relief is technically difficult and risky; here it may be preferable to temporize, in the hope that development of collateral pathways may alleviate the circulatory block.

The long-term outlook is fairly good if the disease is recognized and if its obstructive consequences can be treated suitably by surgical means. Prolonged observations of some successfully treated patients indicate that the disease tends to run its course and subside so that the life expectancy may not be shortened. Most deaths have been caused by renal failure.

Catino, D., Torack, R. M., and Hagstrom, J. W. C.: Idiopathic retroperitoneal fibrosis: Histochemical evidence for lateral spread of the process from the midline. J. Urol., 98:191, 1967.

Koep, L., and Zuidema, G. D.: The clinical significance of retroperitoneal fibrosis. Surgery, 81:250, 1977.

Ochsner, M. G., Brannan, W., Pond, H. S., and Goodlet, J. S., Jr.: Medical therapy in idiopathic retroperitoneal fibrosis. J. Urol., 114:700, 1975.

Usher, S. M., Brendler, H., and Ciavarra, V. A.: Retroperitoneal fibrosis secondary to metastatic neoplasm. Urology, 9:191, 1977.

71.3. MEDIASTINAL FIBROSIS

Taut bundles of collagenous tissue form in the superior and anterior mediastinum with impingement on the aorta, trachea, and pericardium, but the predominant manifestations are those caused by obstruction of the superior vena cava: puffy, suffused appearance of the face and conjunctivae; nonpitting edema of the face, neck, and upper extremities; and distended veins in the neck and upper extremities. The main task in differential diagnosis is to distinguish this relatively benign condition from obstruction caused by tumor. Roentgenographic examination of the chest may reveal little or no abnormality, but angiographic studies will show the obstruction of the superior vena cava and its large tributaries. Thoracotomy may be required for histologic diagnosis.

As already mentioned, histoplasmosis, and possibly tuberculosis too, may be a cause of mediastinal fibrosis; therefore these should be considered, and a trial of appropriate chemotherapy may be justified.

Some patients with this syndrome have shown gradual improvement over months or years, presumably because of development of collateral circulation. Attempts to remove the fibrosing tissues from the large veins are technically difficult and hazardous.

Goodwin, R. A., Nickell, J. A., and Dez Prez, R. M.: Mediastinal fibrosis complicating healed primary histoplasmosis and tuberculosis. Medicine, 51:227, 1972.

Schowengerdt, C. G., Suyemoto, R., and Main, F. B.: Granulomatous and fibrous mediastinitis: A review and analysis of 180 cases. J. Thorac. Cardiovasc. Surg., 57:365, 1969.

71.4. SCLEROSING CHOLANGITIS

A diffuse fibrous sheath sometimes envelops the common bile duct, hepatic ducts, and gallbladder. The clinical manifestation is usually that of insidious onset of jaundice, although there may be some discomfort in the right upper quadrant. Liver function tests give results compatible with extrahepatic biliary tract obstruction. The course is prolonged, with gradually deepening jaundice. Death may ensue after many months, and the findings may be those of biliary cirrhosis.

This clinical syndrome may be associated with inflammatory bowel disease (see Ch. 413 and 414), and in that situation progression to the clinical picture of biliary cirrhosis is rare.

Sclerosing cholangitis may also be associated with other forms of multicentric fibrosclerosis, e.g., retroperitoneal fibrosis, Riedel's thyroiditis. Cholangiography, by either the oral or intravenous route, usually fails to show the lesion, and even percutaneous transhepatic cholangiography may be technically difficult. On the other hand, endoscopic retrograde cholangio-graphy may be highly successful in demonstrating the ductal lesion.

The diagnosis is most often accomplished by laparotomy and biopsy. The latter may be needed to distinguish this disease from a sclerosing bile duct carcinoma.

Treatment is unsatisfactory. Steroids seldom help. Prolonged biliary tract drainage by T-tube may sometimes be useful.

Danzi, J. T., Makipour, H., and Farmer, R. G.: Primary sclerosing cholangitis. A report of nine cases and clinical review. Am. J. Gastroenterol., 65:109, 1976.

Ruskin, R. B., Katon, R. M., Bilboa, M. K., and Smith, F.: Evaluation of sclerosing cholangitis by endoscopic retrograde cholangiopancreatography. Arch. Intern. Med., 136:232, 1976.

71.5. FIBROSCLEROSIS IN OTHER ORGANS

Riedel's thyroiditis is a rare form of fibrotic disease affecting the structures in the anterior part of the neck (see Ch. 546.3). This differs from Hashimoto's thyroiditis in being equally common in males and females and in the tendency of the fibrotic process to involve not only the thyroid but also its neighboring structures.

Peyronie's disease is a sclerotic induration of the corpora cavernosa of the penis. This disease has been encountered in association with sclerosing processes in other parts of the body.

Pseudotumor of the orbit causes unilateral exophthalmos and is likely to be confused with tumor. It has been seen in association with Riedel's thyroiditis, as well as in other fibrosclerosing syndromes.

Früh, D., Jaeger, W., and Käfer, O.: Orbital involvement in retroperitoneal fibrosis (Morbus Ormond). Mod. Probl. Ophthalmol., 14:651, 1975.

71.6. PRACTOLOL PERITONITIS

An unusual fibrotic syndrome has been observed in more than 50 patients treated with the β-adrenergic blocking drug practolol. This drug closely resembles propranolol in chemical structure, but the risk of fibrotic reaction in the peritoneum is far smaller, perhaps nonexistent, with propranolol. Nevertheless, there is a little suggestive evidence that less severe disease may develop from prolonged use of propranolol.

Practolol peritonitis seldom manifests itself in less than 12 months after beginning treatment. Some cases have developed as long as a year after cessation of the therapy. It consists of a thick fibrous encasement of the small intestine, and the symptoms are those of subacute obstruction. It has usually been possible to relieve the symptoms by surgery, with blunt dissection to peel away the fibrous tissue. Some improvement can be anticipated in time simply by avoidance of further treatment.

This condition seems somewhat like the retroperitoneal fibrosis that is encountered in some patients who have taken methysergide for migraine relief.

Marshall, A. J., et al.: Practolol peritonitis. A study of 16 cases and a survey of small bowel function in patients taking β-adrenergic blockers. Quart. J. Med., 46:135, 1977.

72. EOSINOPHILIC SYNDROMES

Paul B. Beeson

72.1. INTRODUCTION

Many diseases characterized by eosinophilia are dealt with in other parts of this book, e.g., parasitic infestations, common allergic disorders, drug reactions, and skin diseases. This chapter contains a brief characterization of the cell and its behavior, with emphasis on the general pattern of diseases in which eosinophilia may or may not occur.

Although classed as a granulocyte because of certain morphologic and other similarities to the neutrophil, the eosinophil possesses some properties quite distinct from those of the neutrophil. For instance, eosinophils tend to disappear from the circulation after adrenal corticosteroids have been administered; neutrophils usually increase in number. By the same token, in acute inflammation, neutrophils predominate, locally and in the blood, whereas eosinophils recede from both areas. Conversely, in granulomatous inflammatory processes, in which neutrophils are inconspicuous, there may be both local and systemic eosinophilia. (It is partly for this reason that eosinophil behavior is dealt with in this part of the book.)

A major difference from the neutrophil is found in the fact that eosinophils behave like constituents of the immunologic apparatus. They congregate around certain kinds of antigen, especially in reactions involving immunoglobulin E. The eosinophil response becomes enhanced with repeated or continuous antigenic challenge, indicating the property of immunologic "memory." The response, which is mediated by T lymphocytes, can be ablated by administration of immunosuppressive agents, in a pattern remarkably similar to that characteristic of antibody production.

The eosinophil contains comparatively large quantities of certain enzymes, such as arylsulfatase, phospholipase, and histaminase. These are probably capable of interacting with pharmacologically active products of mast cells and basophils. It is therefore quite plausible to assume that one function of the eosinophil is to modulate the consequences of IgE-mediated allergic reactions in which mast cell and basophil products such as histamine are liberated. The eosinophil granule, when studied by electron microscopy, exhibits a crystalline substance which has been shown to be a protein, strongly basic in reaction, and undoubtedly capable of interacting with many humoral substances.

The weight of present evidence then indicates that the function(s) of the eosinophil lie mainly in interactions with endogenous products, such as those of the mast cell, and that it is comparatively unimportant in defense against bacteria, viruses, and protozoa. Whether it affords some protection against infestations by metazoan parasites is a field of active study at present.

72.2. EOSINOPHILIC PULMONARY SYNDROMES

It is notable that peripheral eosinophilia may be seen in association with many kinds of pulmonary disease. Possible factors in this include the presence of mast cells in lung tissue, the opportunity for repeated antigenic challenge by inhaled materials, and the frequency of granulomatous inflammation in pulmonary tissue. Some eosinophilic pulmonary syndromes are described in detail in Ch. 346.2. These include *Löffler's syndrome,* a benign illness usually lasting less than a month, characterized by transient pulmonary infiltrations, low fever, and peripheral eosinophilia. Some cases are undoubtedly manifestations of parasitic infestations, in which circulating parasites lodge in the lungs; however, a similar clinical picture can be observed in some drug sensitivity reactions. Steroid treatment usually causes prompt clearing and amelioration of symptoms.

An illness bearing some resemblance to Löffler's syndrome, but of longer duration and greater severity, has been called *pulmonary infiltration with eosinophilia,* or *PIE syndrome.* In this there can be marked disability, with high fever, cough, and shortness of breath persisting for months or a few years. Steroid therapy often controls the symptoms, but the disease tends to relapse when the treatment is terminated.

Tropical pulmonary eosinophilia is seen mainly in India, Southeast Asia, and the Pacific islands. The disease is characterized by fever, pulmonary infiltrates, and symptoms of asthma. As to etiology, present evidence points to filarial parasites for which man is not a natural host. Parasitemia cannot be demonstrated, but lung biopsies have revealed the presence of structures resembling filaria. The patients show antibodies to filaria and usually improve rapidly on treatment with the antifilarial drug diethylcarbamazine.

In addition to these, there are many other uncommon forms of pneumonia in which the inflammatory exudate contains eosinophils and there may or may not be blood eosinophilia. The cause of these is uncertain, and their response to steroid therapy is variable.

72.3. EOSINOPHILIC SYNDROMES AFFECTING OTHER ORGAN SYSTEMS

LÖFFLER'S EOSINOPHILIC ENDOMYOCARDITIS. This disorder is seen almost exclusively in males. It can lead to heart failure and is characterized by formation of mural thrombi, thickening of the endocardium on either side of the heart, and myocardial degeneration beneath the affected endocardium. This condition appears to be caused by presence of excessive amounts of some product of eosinophils. It can develop as a complication of any state in which there is high and prolonged blood eosinophilia, i.e., an absolute count higher than 2000 per cubic millimeter for longer than 12 months. It has been reported in association with eosinophilic leukemoid reactions, eosinophilic leukemia, eosinophilia in patients with solid tumors, and the so-called hypereosinophilic syndrome.

EOSINOPHILIC LEUKEMIA. Eosinophilic leukemia is a rare occurrence. Its existence has been disputed, but there are now on record a number of fatal illnesses characterized by the presence of immature eosinophils in the blood and marrow, blastic crises, thrombocytopenia, and anemia. In some of these, other markers of leukemia have been noted, including the Philadelphia chromosome and high levels of serum B_{12}.

HYPEREOSINOPHILIC SYNDROME. The hypereosinophilic syndrome is a name given to a disease exhibiting a myeloproliferative picture, with leukocytosis, eosinophilia, hepatomegaly, and splenomegaly. Most cases do not progress to a picture of eosinophilic leukemia, in that the eosinophils in blood appear to be mature, and that death does not result from blastic crises, thrombocytopenia, or anemia. Death may be due to heart failure, with the typical finding of Löffler's eosinophilic endomyocarditis. Another characteristic feature is high incidence of lesions in the central nervous system, not obviously caused by vascular disease. It is of interest that about 90 per cent of patients with this syndrome are males. It has recently been reported that a favorable clinical response can be obtained by treatment with hydroxyurea, whereas steroids and cyclophosphamide have had little effect.

EOSINOPHILIC COLLAGEN DISEASE. European clinicians have described a multisystem disease, with clinical features resembling dermatomyositis, in which there is marked eosinophilia. Chief complaints may be pains in the muscles and joints. The kidneys are seldom or never affected. This disease is considered by other writers simply to be a form of the hypereosinophilic syndrome described above.

EOSINOPHILIC GASTROENTERITIS. See Ch. 408.

72.4. DISEASES IN WHICH EOSINOPHILIA OCCURS OCCASIONALLY

NEOPLASTIC DISORDERS. Peripheral eosinophilia is encountered in a small proportion of patients with *carcinoma or sarcoma*, under 5 per cent. It is more likely to be present late in the disease when there has been extensive metastatic spread. Of the lymphomas, *Hodgkin's disease* is the principal form in which eosinophilia may be present. When present, it is usually just at the level of clinical recognition, but in occasional cases massive eosinophil leukemoid reaction has been observed. In the lymphoma-like syndrome called *immunoblastic lymphadenopathy*, about a third of the reported patients have had peripheral eosinophilia. Of unusual interest is a dermatologic tumor usually located in the tissues of the face or scalp, described under the term *angiolymphoid hyperplasia with eosinophilia*. The mechanism of eosinophilia associated with this small, usually nonmalignant tumor is of unusual interest.

RADIATION-RELATED EOSINOPHILIA. It has been reported that about 40 per cent of patients being treated for intra-abdominal neoplasm exhibit eosinophilia during the first few weeks after therapy has been begun.

RHEUMATOID ARTHRITIS. Perhaps 10 to 12 per cent of patients with rheumatoid arthritis may show a detectable peripheral eosinophilia at some time over the long course of their disease. In addition, in occasional cases, usually those of long standing with nodules and pleuropulmonary involvement, a substantial peripheral eosinophilia may be present.

IMMUNE DEFICIENCY SYNDROMES. Mild eosinophilia is often noted in the various kinds of immune deficiency syndromes observed in pediatric clinics. These include disorders of lymphocyte function as well as those in which there is defective neutrophil function. In any of the immune deficiency syndromes a fairly marked rise in eosinophils can accompany pneumocystis pulmonary infections.

CONGENITAL DEFECTS. Eosinophilia has been described in a significant proportion of patients with congenital heart disease, usually in forms featured by stenotic lesions. In the syndrome of thrombocytopenia with absent radius eosinophilia is frequently present.

INFLAMMATORY BOWEL DISEASE. Eosinophils are sometimes conspicuous in the inflammatory lesions of chronic ulcerative colitis, and a slight elevation of the blood eosinophils is occasionally seen in this disease. It is also reported by some observers that eosinophilia may be present during symptomatic phases of Crohn's disease and that this may be a helpful guide in the differential diagnosis between Crohn's disease and acute appendicitis.

PANCREATIC DISEASES. There is a distinctive clinical syndrome associated with acinar cell carcinoma of the pancreas, consisting of polyarthritis, areas of panniculitis in the subcutaneous fat, and blood eosinophilia. The panniculitis and arthritis are thought to be caused by pancreatic lipase affecting the subcutaneous fat or periarticular fatty tissue. There are also case reports describing symptoms similar to those just described for acinar cell carcinoma, occurring two to six weeks after acute pancreatitis.

CHRONIC ACTIVE HEPATITIS. Although not emphasized in standard clinical descriptions, reviews of reported cases of chronic active hepatitis mention eosinophilia in excess of 5 per cent in about one third of patients.

PERNICIOUS ANEMIA. Before there was a specific treatment of this disease, it was said that about one third of patients with pernicious anemia would exhibit eosinophilia at some time in the course of the disease.

ADDISON'S DISEASE. The assumption seems to have been made that Addison's disease may be characterized by eosinophilia. This must, however, be a rare event inasmuch as several fairly large series of cases of Addison's disease have not shown an elevation of the eosinophils.

SARCOIDOSIS. Prior to 1960, most reported series of cases of sarcoidosis indicated that eosinophilia was a clinical feature in an appreciable proportion of cases. Current writings about the disease deny eosinophilia as a feature. This unexplained change may be evidence to support the assumption that sarcoidosis is simply a pattern of response to a variety of environmental influences, and presumably the forms of the disease now prevalent do not seem to be those in which an eosinophil response is characteristic.

Beeson, P. B., and Bass, D. A.: The Eosinophil. Philadelphia, W. B. Saunders Company, 1977.

PART IX

MICROBIAL DISEASES

73. THE NATURE OF MICROBIAL DISEASES

Walsh McDermott

Microbial diseases are all those produced by a transmissible agent capable of multiplication in living tissue and sufficiently small in its individual units to be visible only by light or electron microscopy. One might question whether a useful purpose is served by including under the one label such diverse entities as diseases produced by protozoa and those caused by the smallest viruses. Certainly at one level of analysis a grouping of this sort is not particularly useful. For this reason, protozoa have been removed from the present Part and, with the helminths, form one of their own (Part X); general discussions of the rest of the microbial diseases have been placed with the individual subdivisions, such as viral or bacterial diseases. But there is a larger sense in which all these diseases are usefully regarded as a single group separate from and unlike all other diseases. For the nonmicrobial diseases, except for those resulting from undernutrition, are essentially individual, private affairs which, if uncontrolled, represent personal tragedies but seldom have wide public impact. By contrast, a society unable to employ contemporary technology to manage its microbial diseases is condemned to misery; infant and childhood deaths are a commonplace, pregnancy is virtually a permanent way of life for all women from their mid-teens to their mid-forties, and back-breaking toil is the lot of most people. To gain understanding of microbial disease in a scientific and technologic sense is thus an essential prerequisite to the building and maintenance of a modern society.

With that understanding of microbial disease is an appreciation of the tremendous adaptive plasticity of microbes — their great capacity for *change* both in themselves and in the conditions of their parasitism. This ability to adapt to change means that the microbial world is an enduring potential source of new diseases. It also means that there is no real prospect for a world free from microbial diseases, either those of man or of the plants and other animals. Thus if we are to continue our long record of successes in meeting microbial challenges to man, there can be no letup in our search for greater knowledge of the subject at the bedside, in the field, and in the laboratory. Our brilliant successes in the prevention and treatment of so many microbial diseases have not been founded on the extermination of the microbe. They have all been based on making the environment outside or within the human host a place in which the microbe cannot flourish to its full capacity. To exploit some weak link in the pathogenic chain in this way requires exact scientific and clinical knowledge. The incapacitation of the microbe thus affected may or may not jeopardize its survival as a species. Paleontology has taught us that species or genera have disappeared from this planet. Our systematic study of microbes is not yet of sufficient age to document such extinction of a disease-producing microbe, but there is no reason to doubt that it could occur. There is considerable reason to doubt, however, that it can be produced by the purposeful actions of man. A far greater body of knowledge would be necessary than is now available to produce such purposeful extinction of a microbial species. This is so not only because of microbial adaptability, but also because we have so little ability to identify and successfully interrupt *all* significant ecologic relationships involved. The story of the malaria eradication campaign (see Ch. 193) is a case in point. Whether the situation with smallpox will be any different remains to be seen. In the writer's judgment, it seems most unlikely. "Final victories" in the form of microbial extinction are not to be expected, but neither are they necessary or particularly desirable. Our existing conceptual base and pluralism of practical approaches have yielded an array of triumphs that make our current management of microbial disease one of the finest chapters in the whole history of science for man's benefit. To a considerable extent, however, these practical cures and preventives rely upon the change in hygienic habits in and around the home that come with, or are made possible by, improved socioeconomic status. What is needed now is not only a continued effort in the same direction but also a new massive effort of a different sort. This new effort should be devoted to reviewing those major microbial diseases for which we already have effective technologies, with the object of developing new and quite different methods suitable for wide application in economically underdeveloped regions.

Dubos, R. J.: Man Adapting. New Haven, Yale University Press, 1965, pp. 369–399.
McDermott, W.: Microbial Persistence. Harvey Lecture, Series 63, 1967–1968. New York, Academic Press.
Morrison, R. S.: The concept of eradication and public education. The Pharos, 23:3, 1963.

74. INTRODUCTION TO MICROBIAL DISEASES

Sheldon M. Wolff

Many remarkable advances have been made in our understanding of the pathogenesis, prevention, and therapy of a variety of microbial diseases. Nonetheless, infectious diseases are still the most common problems in ambulatory patients encountered by physicians in the United States, and this group of diseases continues to be the major cause of morbidity and mortality in the world. Despite the commonly held concept that important infectious diseases have been brought into check, there continue to be ominous signs that some are not as well controlled as many have hoped or expected. For example, the emergence of penicillin-resistant pneumococci could have major consequences. Conversely, the recent demonstration of the utility of polyvalent antipneumococcal vaccines may prove to be much more timely and important than originally considered (see Ch. 121). The continued eruption of cholera outbreaks in certain parts of the world must create apprehension because many had assumed that pandemics of this ancient illness were part of our historic past. Even the optimistic heralding of the eradication of smallpox may be premature. Aside from the problems concerning well-described illnesses, we continue to be confronted by the appearance of previously unrecognized diseases. A conspicuous example is legionnaires' disease (see Ch. 123).

Considerable progress continues to be made regarding the etiology and therapeutic approach to microbial diseases. For example, we are beginning to amass information pertaining to the causative agents of certain forms of viral gastroenteritis (see Ch. 104). The recognition and isolation of these agents will certainly lead to rapid improvement in our ability to diagnose and, ideally, to prevent and treat these common debilitating illnesses. The enormous increase in our knowledge of the etiology of both hepatitis A and B in the past ten years has already improved our ability to categorize, to diagnose, to prevent, and to alter the severity of these viral diseases. The development of vaccines for these conditions promises to be a fruitful outcome of this exciting research. The development of chemotherapeutic agents active in viral diseases, although not yet extensively applied, has provided some exciting advances; notably, adenine arabinoside has proved effective in the treatment of the dreaded encephalitic complication of herpes simplex infection.

Despite the development of new technology (such as laminar flow rooms) and the availability of blood products (including leukocytes for replacement therapy), opportunistic infections in susceptible hosts continue to be among the most serious problems facing medicine (see Ch. 124). In fact, these life-threatening infections will undoubtedly become far more frequent as chemotherapeutic and immunosuppressive therapy finds wider clinical use. We are thus facing a major problem, for all these patients are hospitalized and the majority require treatment in intensive care units. The expense of caring for such patients is great.

Microbial diseases provided the original models for early studies in immunology. In the past two decades, we have witnessed an extraordinary increase in the understanding of immunologic processes. This wealth of knowledge has continued to provide new information concerning the pathogenesis, prevention, and recovery from microbial diseases. The role of thymus-derived (T) lymphocytes in cell-mediated immunity, of bone marrow–derived (B) lymphocytes in humoral immunity, of the alternative complement pathway in the clearing of bacteria from the bloodstream, and of secretory immunoglobulins in defense against certain viral respiratory infections are only a few examples of the importance of this newly acquired information to our understanding of infectious diseases (see Ch. 38 to 40). In addition to this information, the rapidly expanding body of knowledge concerning the inflammatory response and cell functions such as chemotaxis, phagocytosis, and microbicidal activities has greatly improved our understanding of normal and abnormal host defenses. By virtue of these new data, many previously unrecognized syndromes have been described, and effective therapeutic approaches to several acquired and inherited defects have been formulated. Some new chapters and other extensively rewritten chapters attest to this profusion of knowledge.

All this new knowledge, in one way or another, represents change — change in our understanding of disease, change in our interventional skills, and change in the character and appearance of the very diseases themselves. The physician must keep up with these changes. One thing that helps in so doing is the unchanging nature of the logic involved in the approach to the patient whose illness may be a consequence of microbial disease. To outline precisely how to question and examine such a patient does not fit the scope of this chapter. Yet there are at least two questions that must be attacked and deserve mention here. The first is whether the process is indeed microbial in origin. Merely to ask the question may be enough to highlight the fact that the pneumonia is really an infarct or that the typhoid is really Hodgkin's disease. To see the major manifestation of a well-known microbial disease with no collateral evidences of infection should raise this question. At other times, in approaching the question every scrap of evidence must be carefully sifted, e.g., a high percentage of immature neutrophils within a normal total leukocyte count. On still other occasions the physician must examine the less quantifiable subtleties, such as the belief that patients with infection are generally sicker than those with the same degree of fever from other causes.

More often than not, however, the fact of infection will be clear. Indeed, the overwhelming majority of patients with microbial diseases will have self-limited and benign conditions. There will be some, however, who will have acute symptoms, and their condition could rapidly deteriorate. Such patients require immediate attention. This brings us to the answer to the second of the two major questions, namely, which of the infections conceivably present could kill this patient within the next 12 to 24 hours, and which of them could be so innocent-appearing at this stage. Most often the physician must rely on clinical knowledge and experience. Time may not permit the luxury of extensive and time-consuming laboratory examinations; yet certain key decisions must be made on how to best protect the patient until it is clear precisely what is present and to what extent steps should be taken to isolate the patient, examine contacts, and possibly start chemoprophylaxis of such contacts. Always in the forefront of the physician's thinking must be the need to ensure that proper diagnostic specimens are obtained just before whatever interventions are made.

One example of how this may be done is encountered in bacteremia due to gram-negative rods. Knowing something of the epidemiology, microbiology, and pathophysiology of this condition can sometimes be of crucial importance in the outcome of the patient's illness. If a patient with leukemia undergoing intensive chemotherapy suddenly develops chills and fever in the absence of any localizing physical findings, we must be prepared to act rapidly. Although this patient may have a localized infection, it is most likely that a generalized infection with bacteremia is present. It is useful to know that most gram-negative rod bacteremias are due to *Escherichia coli* but that in the leukemic patient *Pseudomonas aeruginosa* is the most common offender. Furthermore, it helps in deciding to institute therapy empirically to know that the mortality rate from bacteremia with this organism is higher than with other bacteria. In addition, patients with underlying rapidly fatal illnesses, such as acute leukemia, have the highest death rate from such infections. We should also realize that the risk of acquiring such an infection is greatest when the peripheral granulocyte count falls below 500 per cubic millimeter and, conversely, the replacement of granulocytes in such patients increases survival. Of crucial importance is the choice of the antimicrobial therapy to be employed early, as we cannot wait for the results of blood culture. Knowing these facts, such patients should clearly receive an aminoglycoside. Since these infections are often nosocomial, it is very helpful to know the drug-susceptibility patterns of the organisms being isolated in the hospital. Furthermore, in the granulocytopenic patients it would appear that the administration of carbenicillin with the aminoglycoside will improve the chance of survival. Needless to say, such patients may develop bacteremic shock, and, if this occurs, both monitoring and supportive measures must be instituted.

The advances of the past 30 years in prevention and care of microbial diseases are remarkable. The benefits to society of these endeavors are immeasurable. However, much remains to be done, and the study of microbial diseases should not only provide physicians with enormous pride in what their profession has accomplished, but also present the inquisitive with many still-to-be-solved riddles of immense importance.

Section One   VIRAL DISEASES

75. INTRODUCTION TO VIRAL DISEASES

Edwin D. Kilbourne

The thread that binds together such differing diseases as influenza, mumps, smallpox, and yellow fever for common consideration in this section is the tenuous one of viral etiology. All are the result of infection with viruses, and all viruses share in common submicroscopic size and complete and intimate dependence on the cells of the host that they infect. Yet these tiny packages of protein-coated nucleic acid are as different as the diseases discussed in these pages. They vary in size from the 30 mμ RNA-containing particle of yellow fever virus to the 250 mμ antigenically complex particle of smallpox virus, with its DNA core. The relation of design and function of viruses is now being appreciated. Certain myxoviruses, including the influenza and parainfluenza viruses, possess a potent neuraminidase that probably abets their release from the mucin-coated cells of the respiratory tract. The myxoviruses are fragile and unstable in the environment, whereas the enteroviruses, including poliovirus, can pass unscathed through the barrier of gastric acidity in their journey to the target cells of the small intestine.

Neither structural nor chemical similarity of viruses, however, is any sure guide to the diseases that they may cause. Mumps and parainfluenza viruses are indistinguishable by electron microscopy and even share antigens in common, but one invades the salivary glands, pancreas, or meninges, whereas the other produces mild upper respiratory tract infection or infantile croup. Nor does viral dissimilarity predict dissimilar disease. The structurally amorphous, genetically plastic RNA virus of influenza and the geometrically precise DNA-bearing adenovirus, with its potential for latency, both evoke clinical syndromes that may be difficult to differentiate.

With this caution in mind about the great dissimilarities among viruses and their associated diseases, the common features of viral infections can be considered as useful generalizations.

Most viral infections occur in childhood, at which time any of the 200 obligate human viruses ordinarily produce acute but benign disease or no disease at all. However, the unborn child may be peculiarly vulnerable to the effects of rubella, and the newborn — if unprotected by maternal antibody — may be severely damaged by infection with the ordinarily innocuous virus of herpes simplex. With the exception of the neonatal period, the severity of disease associated with primary or initial viral infections increases with the age of the patient. Poliomyelitis is more frequent and more severe in adult infection; varicella pneumonia is essentially limited to adults; the postpuberal complications of mumps are notorious; and jaundice occurs more frequently in older than in younger patients with infectious hepatitis. It is necessary to emphasize the evidence for greater potential susceptibility of the adult because it may *appear* that the adult is less vulnerable to viral disease, protected as he is by a legacy of immunity to many viruses from his childhood experience with them. This fact of age-related susceptibility is increasingly important as the epidemiologic patterns of viral infections change with changes in man's environment and with the introduction of new vaccines. If a vaccine induces impermanent immunity so that infection is merely postponed, the consequences might be disastrous.

Although firm and enduring immunity attended by persisting humoral antibody follows most viral infections, it is unlikely that antibody formation per se is the essential mechanism of recovery. Interferon, a nonspecific and nontoxic product of virus-infected cells, is more closely related temporally to the decline of virus in tissues and to recovery from infection, but its role in the self-termination of viral infections is still conjectural. Experimental evidence that corticosteroid hormones are inhibitory to interferon synthesis may explain the deleterious effect of these hormones or of stress on certain viral infections of man — notably on the extension of recurrent herpes simplex keratitis or on varicella in children already receiving steroid therapy.

The enduring immunity of viral infections has few exceptions. The frequency of common colds is now explicable as the result of multiple infections with multiple antigenically unrelated viruses; the seemingly transient immunity of influenza reflects the changing nature of the virus itself. For most viral infections there is no indication whether protracted immunity is maintained by recurrent subclinical infection or by persistence of the virus in the host. With a few — varicella-zoster, herpes simplex, and cytomegalic inclusion disease — all associated with herpesviruses which replicate in the cell nucleus, viral genomes undoubtedly persist throughout life in the tissues, integrated in host cell DNA, and may be reactivated there to produce recurrent disease in the partially immune host. In the growing number of patients who are immunologically crippled with cancer or subjected to chemical immunosuppression for transplantation surgery, such reactivations may occur as new and sometimes terminal diseases. Other "new" viral diseases (Lassa fever, Marburg disease) have emerged recently as the result of altered relationships of man and the animal carriers of the causative viruses.

Evidence is increasing that viruses are involved in a variety of mammalian cancers and also in chronic diseases of the central nervous system. In man, the association of the herpes-like Epstein-Barr virus (EBV) with Burkitt's lymphoma and cancer of the retropharyngeal space is striking, although an etiologic relationship has not been proved. The human papilloma virus (associated with the common wart) is a member of a group of mammalian viruses — the papovaviruses — two of which have been shown to be capable of genetic integration with the host cell chromosome in the manner of lysogenic bacteriophages. One such virus (JC) has been isolated from patients with progressive multifocal leukoencephalopathy (see Ch. 310.5).

The recent direct demonstration of a measles-like virus in patients with subacute sclerosing panencephalitis suggests the awesome potential of common agents of acute infection.

In contrast to the bacterial diseases of man, the viral diseases are relatively insusceptible at present to chemotherapy, but the efficient immunity of natural viral infection can be duplicated with vaccines. The coat proteins of all viruses are antigenic, and it is reasonable to conclude that vaccines could be made for all viruses that can be cultivated in the laboratory. The great number of viral pathogens limits the feasibility of this approach, however, as does our uncertain knowledge of the ultimate potential of these viruses for good or evil. The vaccine itself may be a two-edged sword: if a living virus, it may be contaminated with alien viruses or nucleic acid, or may retain virulence expressed only in certain individuals; if inactivated, it may be poorly antigenic. At its best, however, the vaccine may be the ultimate weapon if eradication of the virus can be effected by substitution in the community of vaccine virus for wild type. A trend in this direction is evident with poliomyelitis.

The intractability of viral infections to chemotherapy is a corollary of the intimacy of virus-host association. To the extent that the viral parasite subverts the host's cellular machinery to its own synthesis, it cannot be interrupted without compromising the host as well. But the presence of novel virus-coded enzymes in infected but not in normal cells suggests the possibility of employing highly selective antimetabolites specifically directed against virus synthesis. Indeed, this effect has already been realized in vitro, and in man limited success in arresting the progression of herpes simplex encephalitis has been achieved even with an antimetabolite not specific for the virus.

Man may never be free of viruses, but it is hoped that he may gradually replace the plagues of the past with more peaceful coexistence in the future.

VIRAL INFECTIONS
OF THE RESPIRATORY TRACT

76. THE COMMON COLD

(Acute Coryza)

George Gee Jackson

DEFINITION. The common cold is a symptom complex caused by viral infection of the upper respiratory passages. Most precisely, the term applies to afebrile, acute coryza of viral origin. In the broadest sense, the common cold refers to any undifferentiated upper respiratory infection. The terms rhinitis, pharyngitis, laryngitis, and "chest cold" are sometimes used to designate the principal anatomic site of infection. The main differences between the common cold and other viral or bacterial respiratory infections are the absence of fever, the nonexudative inflammation, and the relatively mild constitutional symptoms and signs.

ETIOLOGY. Many viruses can cause the common cold. No single strain of virus accounts for more than a

TABLE 1.   Viruses Associated with the Common Cold

Virus Class	Frequent	Infrequent
Picornaviruses	Rhinoviruses (numerous serotypes)	Enteroviruses (a few of many serotypes) Coxsackievirus A21, 24 (others) Coxsackievirus B3, 4, 5
Paramyxoviruses	Parainfluenza 1, 2, 3 Respiratory syncytial (RS)	Parainfluenza 4 Measles Mumps
Myxoviruses	Influenza A, B	Influenza C
Coronaviruses		>2 types
Reoviruses		Type 1
Adenoviruses		Types 1, 2, 5, 6 3, 4, 7, 14, 21

small proportion of the illnesses. Isolates have been made from about 70 per cent of acute coryzal illnesses in young adults and about 35 per cent of common colds in children. Among the viruses, rhinoviruses comprise the largest single etiologic group. The viruses listed in

Table 1 show the taxonomic groups that have been etiologically related to the common cold according to their frequency in most investigations. (The coxsackie- and echoviruses listed therein are also considered separately in Ch. 90 to 98.)

The increasing ability to recover viruses and better serologic means for the diagnosis of viral infections have shown that 5 to 10 per cent of common colds are associated with more than one virus, and definite evidence of simultaneous dual infection is not rare. The causative agents of some of the infections have not been revealed by tissue culture methods currently in use. Certain of the more labile or fastidious viruses have been grown only in unusual cultures of human cell strains or in organ cultures of human embryonic trachea. Other viruses can be shown only by the transmission of illness to volunteers. More than 90 antigenically different strains of rhinoviruses are known to cause the common cold syndrome. Many different types of viruses that can cause mild respiratory illnesses in man may be prevalent in the population at any one time.

EPIDEMIOLOGY. The common cold is spread by direct person-to-person contact and by self-inoculation from hands that have become contaminated with infectious virus. Under conditions of household association, 10 per cent of adults acquired the disease from an index case. From studies in volunteers, it was shown that some persons became infected and shed virus without having symptoms. This occurs in about one third of rhinovirus colds, two thirds of coronavirus infections, and a variable number of infections with other viruses.

It is a common observation that an increase in the frequency of colds occurs in the winter. Sometimes this has been correlated with sharp changes in the temperature, humidity, or pollution of the air, but the popular belief that cold weather causes common colds cannot be substantiated from epidemiologic observations in the Arctic or tropics or from studies in volunteers. Exposure of volunteer subjects to cold did not activate latent respiratory viruses. The reason for the apparent relation between the season and common colds remains unclear. In the United States, it is usual to observe three waves of common colds per year. One occurs in the autumn a few weeks after the opening of schools, another in midwinter, and a third wave in the spring. The separate epidemics have usually been shown to be due to different viruses, each of which may have its own seasonal epidemiology.

The *incidence* of common colds is related to age and environment. Preschool children have an average of six to twelve respiratory illnesses per year, most of which are common colds. Parents with young children have approximately six viral respiratory illnesses per year, and other adults have two to three per year. Statistics gathered by the United States Public Health Service show that in the winter quarter of the year at least one half of all persons acquire a common cold; 20 per cent of persons have a similar illness in the summer quarter.

The *prevalence* of common colds is approximately 15 per cent of persons per week during the winter months. Surveillance of a group of student nurses during one winter revealed that individuals had common cold symptoms on 10 per cent of the days. Among industrial employees in the United States, common colds account for one half of all absences and one quarter of the total time lost. Similarly, acute respiratory illness is highly prevalent among military forces, especially recruits, and is a major cause of disability. In a recent National Health Interview Survey, the common cold caused 116.2 days of restricted activity per 100 persons per year, or 1.16 days per individual each year.

PATHOLOGY. The pathologic changes in the mucous membranes of the respiratory passages are edema, hyperemia, transudation, and exudation. The severity of the cytopathic effect is related to the type and virulence of the infecting virus and the extent of infection. Picornaviruses (rhinoviruses and enteroviruses) have been observed to cause more metaplasia and degeneration in smears of exfoliated cells from the nasal turbinates than the myxoviruses. This generalization does not hold for infections of the lower respiratory tract. During the acute phase of infection, protein components of the respiratory secretions are altered, and serum proteins become more abundant. Abnormal soluble substances of cellular origin also can be found. The secretion is rich in glycoprotein. Repair is relatively rapid and, insofar as is known, occurs without residual pathologic damage. Recently, however, inquiry has been made regarding the role of repeated viral respiratory infections in the pathogenesis of later degenerative diseases, such as bronchitis and emphysema.

Viral infection induces swelling and some exudation, but it causes no significant change in the bacterial flora of the nasopharynx. When the inflammatory changes are of sufficient magnitude, channels connecting the paranasal sinuses and middle ear to the airway become obstructed. Suppuration can develop from secondary bacterial growth under these conditions.

MECHANISMS OF INFECTION AND IMMUNITY. Viruses from infected persons are airborne in droplet spray that is emitted during respiration, talking, sneezing, and coughing. Particles in the size range of 5 to 50 μ are probably the most infectious. Transmission can also be made by hand contact with virus acquired from contaminated surfaces. The nasopharynx and conjunctiva are the portals of infection. The incubation period is short, usually one to four days. Proliferation of virus can often be demonstrated within 24 hours after the infection of volunteers. Virus shedding usually precedes the onset of symptoms by one to two days, and the peak excretion occurs a few days later, during the symptomatic phase of the illness. Virus excretion decreases after several days, and symptoms decrease concomitantly. Later studies from the same person as well as attempts to recover viruses from well persons indicate that the carrier state after infection is transient, and asymptomatic chronic carriers are rare. Rhinoviruses have not been recovered from more than 1 to 2 per cent of well persons in populations where colds are occurring.

Host susceptibility or resistance to infection is determined primarily by the immunologic status resulting from recent previous infection with the same or related viruses. Some physiologic functions, such as menses and fatigue, and constitutional factors, such as an allergic diathesis and vasomotor rhinitis, are secondary determinants of host susceptibility. Emotional distress and overconcern with personal health increase symptoms, whereas stoical and ascetic personality traits decrease overt susceptibility. In controlled studies, chilling did not increase the susceptibility of volunteers to infection nor did ventilation with frigid air.

The nasal secretion is the first barrier against infection of the epithelial cells of the respiratory tract. In addition to the mechanical movement of mucus, the secretion contains glycoprotein inhibitors for some myxoviruses that can compete with cell receptors for the virus. Because virus union with inhibitors is reversible whereas cellular infection is not, these inhibitors probably do no more than delay and decrease the multiplicity of infection. Specific gamma globulins of low molecular weight, principally IgA and IgG, also are contained in nasal secretion. The former is primarily the result of local antibody production and plays an important role in immunity from prior infection. The activity of IgG is related to, but poorly correlated with, the height of specific antibody in the plasma. In one study, the gradient between nasal and serum antibody was 1 to 30. During the early stages of infection, before symptoms have begun, there is an easily demonstrable increase of globulins in nasal washings.

Infection with some respiratory viruses stimulates the local production of a protein or proteins referred to as interferon. Noninfected cells exposed to interferon are protected against viral infection. The mechanism offers an attractive thesis for the termination of infection and repair of the mucosa before specific antibody is formed.

A response in serum-neutralizing antibody against the infecting virus is not always sufficiently prompt or of great enough magnitude to permit diagnosis of the causative role of a virus in the infection. Specific immunity against illness from reinfection with the same strain of virus, however, is readily demonstrable in volunteers. This clinical immunity is apparent for a period of about two years after infection. Asymptomatic infections are not entirely prevented. Reinfection in the presence of serum antibody usually results in a modified illness. The specificity of the antibody and its concentration at the site of infection on the surface of the mucosa appear to be critical factors. Although serum antibody reduces infection and illness, it is possible for infection of the respiratory mucosa to occur. In such cases, the acute inflammatory response can be exaggerated, presumably as a result of the local antigen-antibody reaction or hypersensitivity of the persons resulting from earlier infection.

CLINICAL MANIFESTATIONS. The common cold is in large part a subjective symptomatic diagnosis. The major symptoms for any individual tend to be repetitive, but they differ appreciably from person to person. Some persons have only "head colds," whereas others complain regularly of pharyngitis or cough as characteristic principal symptoms of their colds. The occurrence of symptoms that 100 young adults described as characteristic of a naturally acquired common cold is shown in Table 2.

The same symptoms occur in volunteers challenged with an infectious virus, and their time of occurrence and duration have been observed. Sneezing, headache, and malaise are the initial symptoms, followed by chilly sensations, sore throat, rhinorrhea, and nasal congestion. The chilly sensations may be associated with some lowering of oral temperature that is sometimes interpreted as the initiating cause in natural colds. Fever of any significant degree is absent. The constitutional symptoms are transient, lasting only one or two days. There is sometimes a lull for a day between the early symptoms and the development of characteristic nasopharyngeal symptoms of a full-blown cold. The dry or sore throat tends to recede as the cold progresses.

TABLE 2.   The Syndrome of the Common Cold

Symptoms	Frequency
Severe:	
Nasal discharge	100
Nasal obstruction	99
Moderate:	
Sore or dry throat	96
Malaise	81
Postnasal discharge	79
Headache	78
Cough	76
Mild:	
Sneezing	97
Feverishness	49
Chilliness	43
Burning eyes and mucous membranes	28
Muscle aching	22

Nasal discharge is the hallmark of the common cold. At the onset, the secretion is clear, watery, and often profuse. Later, secretions thicken, become mucopurulent, yellow-green, and tenacious. Nasal obstruction is at first an intermittent symptom associated with an exaggeration of the rhythmic physiologic turgescence of the nasal turbinates. Later, the turbinates become swollen and boggy, encroaching on the nasal lumen, which contains increased secretions. These symptoms ordinarily run their course within a week. As the illness progresses, cough may appear as an increasingly prominent symptom, and persists for one to two weeks. It may be dry or productive of a variable amount of mucoid sputum.

Physical signs are limited to the nasopharynx, the surrounding sinuses, and middle ears. Usually, mild hyperemia, congestion, or both, are all that can be seen, and the deviation from normal may be insufficient to recognize as pathologic.

Hematologic changes have been observed in volunteers when the initial blood values and the time sequence of infection were known. Mild leukopenia with relative lymphocytosis is the initial response, followed after a day or two by a slight leukocytosis with some increase in polymorphonuclear leukocytes. A fall in the hematocrit and rise in the erythrocyte sedimentation rate can also occur. Although the aforementioned changes can be related to the infection in volunteers, their deviation from normal is not great enough to be useful in isolated cases.

Complications of a cold are usually bacterial in origin. They are infrequent and consist of suppuration in the nasopharynx and its contiguous passages. Serous effusion, however, may appear in the middle ear and perhaps in the sinuses. A recrudescence of symptoms, perhaps with fever, localized swellings and/or pus, and leukocytosis may be signs of a bacterial complication.

DIAGNOSIS. The diagnosis of a common cold is made on the basis of history and symptoms. At the peak of the illness, signs of the infection also are apparent. Examination is important for the recognition or exclusion of illnesses of more severe nature that patients may be prone to designate as a cold. The differential diagnosis includes prodromes of other infections and vascular, allergic, and neoplastic processes in the nose, pharynx, sinuses, or ears. Other serious diseases, such as bacterial endocarditis, tuberculosis, bronchitis, bronchiectasis, and lung abscess, have been called "chest colds" because of lack of characteristic symptoms and incomplete examination of the patient by a physician.

The diagnosis of common cold therefore should be avoided as a designation for a broad category of respiratory symptoms of diverse causes.

The clinical symptoms do not permit discrimination with regard to the specific viral cause of a cold. The overlap in the symptoms produced by infection with any one of many viruses that cause the common cold is so great as to preclude more than a judgment regarding the general group of viruses to which the etiologic agent might belong. Under the controlled conditions of studies in volunteers, different viruses cause appreciably different syndromes. For each, the clinical manifestations are also related to the dose, size of particle inhaled, and modifications by host factors. The diagnosis of the specific viral cause of a common cold is based on laboratory procedures. Virus isolation and/or the demonstration of a specific antibody rise in paired sera drawn several days apart are the methods most readily available. As a routine, specific viral diagnosis is not practical. It is recommended for academic reasons and in practice to determine the cause of local epidemics or to assist in the diagnosis of severe illnesses. Also, the differentiation of mycoplasmal and secondary bacterial pneumonias is essential for proper treatment.

TREATMENT AND PREVENTION. In considering treatment and prevention of the common cold, the following factors that have been discussed must be kept in mind: (1) The number of antigenically distinct viruses that cause the common cold is large. (2) Except for the time and economic loss, the infection is benign and the duration of severe symptoms is brief. (3) Viral infection does not significantly change the bacterial flora of the nasopharynx, and bacterial complications are infrequent. (4) Infection initiates production of interferon and antibodies that naturally limit the infection. (5) Specific immunity to illness with the same virus exists for one to two years after infection. (6) Reinfection can occur in the presence of antibody in the plasma.

At present there are no antimicrobial drugs of practical effectiveness in man against the viruses responsible for the common cold except for amantadine in influenza A. The use of antimicrobial drugs is thus not recommended. Carefully controlled trials with unlicensed drugs in volunteers indicate that effective chemoprophylaxis against the common cold is possible. The development of such products could initiate a more optimistic position regarding drug treatment. Suppurative complications are caused by obstruction more often than by the virulence of local bacteria. Purulent otitis or sinusitis should be treated with an appropriate antimicrobial. Group A streptococci, pneumococci, and *H. influenzae* are commonly associated with such complications and will usually respond to adequate doses of penicillin or, in the case of Group A streptococci, to erythromycin. Routine use of chemoprophylaxis selects drug-resistant strains and does not eliminate the development of suppurative complications with such strains; it is not advisable.

Supportive treatment is desirable and helpful. Additional rest in bed, warm clothing, and prevention of chilling increase the patient's comfort. If ventilatory insufficiency, stridor, and anoxemia that may accompany a cold are present, steam inhalation, a decongestant, a bronchodilator, or an expectorant may be indicated. Postural changes can help in the drainage of secretions and the raising of sputum. Because of the diverse causes and syndromes, there is no one regimen to be recommended. Aspirin in a dose of 0.6 gram for an adult or 10 mg per kilogram of body weight for children can reduce headache and malaise. However, it increases virus shedding and should generally be avoided. Oral phenylpropanolamine hydrochloride (15 to 50 mg), inhalation of hexamine vapor, or nose drops with 0.5 per cent ephedrine or phenylephrine shrink the vascular bed of the mucosa and provide temporary nasal decongestion. Nose drops in any oily vehicle should be avoided, and potent vasoconstrictors with transient action and physiologic rebound, such as epinephrine, are not desirable. Increased fluids or hard candy lozenges may be adequate for control of coughing. Cough syrups, such as elixir of terpin hydrate with codeine (64 mg per 30 ml), are more effective if necessary. Antihistamines have no effect on the common cold, except that a person prone to severe inhalant allergy may experience some reduction in the volume of nasal secretion. Large doses of vitamin C (ascorbic acid) have no significant protective effect against viral infections causing the common cold and no appreciable inhibitory effect on rhinoviral colds. Excessive amounts which have been recommended are rapidly excreted in the urine and can cause urinary symptoms owing to the increased acidity of the urine. The numerous compounded remedies, including those with vitamins, bioflavonoids, quinine, alkalinizers, multiple analgesics, antihistamines, decongestants, and tranquilizers, are developed for sales profit in a large market of uninformed and uncritical people. Their widespread and repeated use invariably leads to a few cases of hematologic disorders, eruptive or exfoliative dermatitis, and anaphylaxis or other severe idiosyncratic reactions.

Prevention of common colds by quarantine or isolation of cases is without effect because of the number of infected but asymptomatic persons and because virus excretion usually precedes the symptoms. The hygienic collection and disposal of respiratory secretions to reduce dissemination should be encouraged as common courtesy. Interruption of the airborne phase of transmission by increasing space, higher rates of air ventilation, alterations in temperature and humidity, vaporization of disinfectants, and ultraviolet irradiation of overhead air all have been given trials without clearly significant results.

Vaccines for protection against the common cold are not available. Former "cold vaccines" were bacterial suspensions and have no basis for effectiveness. The large number of antigenically distinct viruses augurs numerous difficulties in the production of an effective vaccine. Nevertheless, promising vaccines are being developed for specific groups of viruses.

Anderson, T. W., Reid, D. B. W., and Beaton, G. H.: Vitamin C and the common cold: A double-blind trial. Can. Med. Ass. J., 107:503, 1972.

Davis, D. J.: Measurements of the prevalence of viral infections. J. Infect. Dis., 133 Suppl.: A3–5, 1976.

Hendley, J. O., Wenzel, R. P., and Gwaltney, J. M.: Transmission of rhinovirus colds by self-inoculation. N. Engl. J. Med., 288:1361, 1973.

Jackson, G. G., Dowling, H. F., Anderson, T. O., Riff, L., Saporta, J., and Turck, M.: Susceptibility and immunity to common upper respiratory viral infections — the common cold. Ann. Intern. Med., 53:719, 1960.

Johnson, K. M., et al.: Role of enteroviruses in respiratory diseases. Am. Rev. Respir. Dis., 88:240, 1963.

Kaye, H. S., and Dowdle, W. R.: Seroepidemiologic survey of coronavirus (strain 229E) infections in a population of children. Am. J. Epidemiol., 101:238, 1975.

Lidwell, O. M., Morgan, R. W., and Williams, R. E. O.: The epidemiology of the common cold. IV. The effect of weather. J. Hyg. (Camb.), 63:427, 1965.

Monto, A. S., and Cavallaro, J. J.: The Tecumseh study of respiratory illness. II. Patterns of occurrence of infection with respiratory pathogens, 1965–1969. Am. J. Epidemiol., 94:280, 1971.

Tyrrell, D. A. J.: Common Colds and Related Diseases. Baltimore, Williams & Wilkins Company, 1965.

77. RHINOVIRAL RESPIRATORY DISEASE

George Gee Jackson

ETIOLOGY.   For many decades, attempts were made to isolate the common cold virus. On some occasions, propagation of infectious material was accomplished for a brief period, but the viruses could not be sustained. In 1954, the virus known as 2060 and the closely related JH strain were isolated from adults with acute coryza. These viruses were believed to be enteroviruses and were designated echovirus 28. Soon thereafter, several different workers isolated similar viruses that were designated in the early literature as Salisbury agents, ERC viruses, entero-like viruses, coryzaviruses, muriviruses, and unclassified common cold viruses. Because of common biologic properties, these are all designated now as rhinoviruses. More than 90 different serotypes of rhinoviruses have been recovered from infected persons. They comprise a subclass in the family of picornaviruses, which also includes the coxsackie-, polio-, entero- and echoviruses. These are all small viruses (10 to 30 mμ) of the ribonucleic acid (RNA) type that are not inactivated by ether. The acid lability (pH 3) of rhinoviruses is probably the reason for their absence from the intestine, and is the major property that distinguishes them from enteroviruses. Rhinoviruses characteristically grow best in tissue cultures held at a reduced temperature (33° C) similar to that found in the nose of man.

EPIDEMIOLOGY.   It is likely that rhinoviruses infect persons in all countries and climates. Nearly all adults have evidence of earlier infection with several different serotypes of rhinoviruses. Similar viruses have been recovered from cattle, but the transfer of infection from animals to man has not been shown. In human infections, some serotypes may occur annually, or commonly in different areas and at different times. Over the years since the methods for isolating rhinoviruses were developed, there has been a drift toward newer (higher numbered) types with fewer isolates of the serotypes that occurred earlier. Infections with rhinoviruses characteristically occur in the fall (September, October) and spring (April, May) as epidemiologic waves of acute respiratory illness; they also are the cause of a large proportion of summer colds. About 15 per cent of a young adult population will have neutralizing antibody against any one serotype. In persons with colds, one third of adults and 10 to 15 per cent of children have had rhinovirus recovered from the nasal secretion. However, children are the best transmitters of the disease. Rhinoviruses have been recovered in 1 to 3 per cent of well adults observed during epidemic disease. Infection is believed to occur by the airborne route, but transmission can also occur by hand transfer from contaminated surfaces.

CLINICAL MANIFESTATIONS AND DIAGNOSIS.   Rhinovirus infections begin with headache, malaise, chilliness, a dry, scratchy sore throat, and burning nasal membranes and eyes. Nasal discharge and obstruction of the upper air passages rapidly become the dominant symptoms. Cough is a variable and later symptom. Fever is absent or of slight degree and transient. No pharyngeal exudate is observed, but cervical adenopathy can occur. In children, rhinoviruses sometimes cause croup or lower respiratory tract disease, and viremia has been found. Adults occasionally develop symptoms of lower respiratory disease, and sensitive tests of bronchial clearance are abnormal even if lower respiratory symptoms are minimal or absent. In persons prone to asthma, wheezing is common. Also, rhinovirus infections have been observed to be associated with exacerbations of chronic bronchitis. The incubation period is one to three days, and the course of illness is about one week. Rhinovirus appears in the nasal secretion a day or two before the onset of nasal symptoms, and is shed during the period of illness; persistent virus shedding for 10 to 20 days is common. The pathologic findings and pathogenesis are described in Ch. 76. A rise in neutralizing antibody in the convalescent serum occurs in only about one half of the infections.

TREATMENT.   There is no specific treatment directed against propagation of the rhinovirus. Supportive measures are those given under treatment of the common cold. Quarantine is not necessary. Interferon produced by rhinovirus infection may be a principal factor in the amelioration of the disease. Pretreatment of volunteers by topical administration of high doses of interferon obtained from human leukocytes or with an interferon inducer was shown to reduce infection and illness. This is attractive, because interferon inhibits rhinoviruses without regard to serotype, but such treatment is not yet practical. In other studies, vitamin C (ascorbic acid) in doses of 3 grams per day by mouth failed to prevent infection and illness. No vaccine is available, but experimental vaccines have been effective against a single type of rhinovirus. The large number of distinct serotypes is discouraging to the prospects of developing an effective vaccine, but some strains produce heterotypic responses. Immunity to reinfection is quite specific and probably lasts only several months to two years after most infections, although detectable serum antibody may persist longer.

Beem, M.: Rhinovirus infections in nursery school children. J. Pediat., 74:818, 1969.

Blair, H. T., Greenberg, S. B., Stevens, P. M., Bilinos, P. A., and Couch, R. B.: Effects of rhinovirus infection on pulmonary function of healthy human volunteers. Am. Rev. Respir. Dis., 114:95, 1976.

Fox, J. P., Cooney, M. K., and Hall, C. E.: The Seattle virus watch. V. Epidemiologic observations of rhinovirus infections, 1965–1969, in families with young children. Am. J. Epidemiol., 101:122, 1975.

George, R. B., and Mogabgab, W. J.: Atypical pneumonia in young men with rhinovirus infections. Ann. Intern. Med., 71:1073, 1969.

Jackson, G. G., and Muldoon, R. L.: Viruses causing common respiratory infections in man. Rhinoviruses. J. Infect. Dis., 127:328, 1973.

Stanley, E. D., Jackson, G. G., Panusarn, C., Rubenis, M., and Dirda, V.: Increased virus shedding with aspirin treatment of rhinovirus infection. JAMA, 231:1248, 1975.

Stenhouse, A. C.: Rhinovirus infection in acute exacerbations of chronic bronchitis: A controlled prospective study. Br. Med. J., 3:461, 1967.

Urquhart, G. E. D., Path, M. R. C., and Stott, E. J.: Rhinoviraemia. Br. Med. J., 2:28, 1970.

78. VIRAL PHARYNGITIS, LARYNGITIS, CROUP, AND BRONCHITIS

George Gee Jackson

The same viruses that cause the common cold also cause other syndromes of respiratory illness. Pharyngitis, laryngitis, croup, or bronchitis may be even more characteristic of infection with some of the viruses than acute afebrile coryza. This clinical classification of the illnesses according to the anatomic site of predominant symptoms is the principal (although unreliable) way the physician has of differentiating diseases of different etiology. The mildest infections are those limited to the upper respiratory tract. As progressively more caudal sites are involved, the infections become more severe and cause more constitutional symptoms. *Acute rhinitis* (the common cold) and *nonexudative pharyngitis* nearly always occur without fever, whereas *exudative viral pharyngitis* is a febrile illness; type A coxsackieviruses are common causes of primary viral pharyngitis with exudate or ulcers, and herpes simplex virus can cause the syndrome. When adenovirus is the cause, *conjunctivitis* is very likely to be a prominent part of the syndrome. With viral pharyngitis the inflammation may extend into the eustachian tubes and cause *primary or secondary otitis media* and *sinusitis*. The lymphoid hyperplasia can include cervical adenitis. *Croup* is a distinctive clinical syndrome resulting from involvement of the larynx with resultant edema and stridor. It is a relatively common manifestation of respiratory viral infection in children. The classes of viruses most often causing croup are the myxoviruses and parainfluenza viruses. Bronchitis, bronchiolitis, and bronchopneumonia are severe manifestations of viral respiratory infection. They cause fever, respiratory difficulties, and symptoms that often require hospitalization of the patient. The course may be quite abrupt, including sudden unexpected death. More commonly it is acute but benign. Viral infections of the lower respiratory tract can mimic whooping cough or induce asthma or an exacerbation of chronic bronchitis. Similar nonviral infections of the lower respiratory tract with chlamydiae or mycoplasmas must be differentiated for proper therapy. The occurrence of these different clinical syndromes resulting from infection with some of the viruses responsible for the common respiratory infections is indicated in Table 3. Further details about the illnesses and their management are given in the discussions of the specific viruses.

The spectrum of diseases is caused not only by the fact that these viruses are relatively nonspecific in the clinical syndrome produced, but also because manifestations of infection are strongly influenced by age and season. Infants and children have a smaller airway and relative hypertrophy of lymphoid tissue. In them, croup and bronchitis are common symptoms of infections with the same viruses that may cause only coryza or undifferential upper respiratory infection in adults. Constitutional host factors such as allergies and proneness to asthma, bronchitis, or otitis are important determinants of the disease manifestations; sex and race and/or the socioeconomic level of the patient influence the incidence of infection and thereby, to some extent, the syndrome. The principal factor in the amelioration

TABLE 3. Spectrum of Clinical Syndromes Caused by Different Respiratory Viruses

Virus	Coryza	Pharyngitis	Croup	Bronchitis (Bronchiolitis)	Pneumonia or Systemic Disease
Influenza A, B	++		+++	++	++++
Influenza C	++			+	
Parainfluenza 1	+++	++	++++	+	
Parainfluenza 2	+		++++		
Parainfluenza 3	+++	++	+++		+++
Parainfluenza 4	+++	+			
Respiratory syncytial	+++		++	++++	+
Coronavirus	+++	+		+	
Reovirus 1	+				
Coxsackievirus					
A2, 3, 4, 6, 8, 10	+	++++	+		++
A21, 24	+++	+			
Coxsackievirus B2, 3, 4, 5	+	+	+	+	+++
Echovirus 7, 8, 11, 15, 19, 20 (others)	++	++	+		++
Rhinoviruses	++++	+	++		
Adenovirus 1, 2, 5	+	++			+
Adenovirus 3, 4, 7, 14, 21	++	++++		+	+
Herpes simplex		+++			
Nonvirus (filterable)					
Mycoplasmas		+			++++
Chlamydiae				+++	+

TABLE 4. Mechanisms that Contribute to the High Prevalence of Viral Respiratory Infection

Biologic Basis	Examples of Mechanism
New types of virus by mutation of recombination	Influenza A, B
Multiple serotypes simultaneously present	Rhinoviruses
Virus shedding before recognition of disease (and asymptomatic infections)	Influenza Parainfluenza Rhinoviruses
Latent infection with reactivation of virus	Herpes Adenoviruses 1, 2, 5, 6
Inconsistent antibody response to infection	Rhinoviruses Paramyxoviruses
Reinfection in presence of circulating antibody	Respiratory syncytial Parainfluenza 1, 3
Transient immunity after infection or vaccine	Rhinoviruses Influenza
Lasting immunity to disease but recurrent epidemics	Adenoviruses 4, 7 Measles

of viral respiratory illnesses is exerted by the preinfection immunologic status of the host owing to previous infections or vaccines.

FACTORS RELATED TO THE MANIFESTATIONS AND PREVALENCE OF VIRAL RESPIRATORY INFECTIONS

The initial infection with a virus may be resolved without establishing solid immunity to reinfection, or if immunity is established, it may be transient. The capacity of many of the respiratory viruses to cause reinfection has now been established. Reinfection in a partially immune host causes different illnesses from the initial infection. Usually the disease is milder on successive reinfections, but the dose of virus, manner of infection, season, presence of dual infection, and other factors may be of more importance. Sometimes, reinfection in the presence of antibody appears to increase the tissue response and exaggerate the symptoms.

In order for a viral infection to maintain a high prevalence of infection, one or more of several conditions is required. Some of these are virologic; others are epidemiologic or immunologic, as exemplified in Table 4. All these mechanisms are found in the case of one or another of the different viruses that cause common respiratory infections. The result is that we experience a continual endemic and cyclic epidemics of viral respiratory disease, with a large number of viruses infecting various sites of the respiratory tree and producing different anatomically designated clinical syndromes. The level of disease is exaggerated by new types of viruses or new exposures of susceptible hosts and is moderated by a progressive buildup of herd immunity developed by aging, naturally acquired infections, and vaccines. Likewise, the clinical syndrome is affected by these viral, epidemiologic, and host conditions. An appreciation of these factors is essential to the understanding of the problem of viral respiratory infections, their treatment, and control.

Beem, M. O., and Saxon, E. M.: Respiratory-tract colonization and a distinctive pneumonia syndrome in infants infected with chlamydia trachomatis. N. Engl. J. Med., 296:306, 1977.

Eadie, M. B., Stott, E. J., and Grist, N. R.: Virological studies in chronic bronchitis. Br. Med. J., 2:671, 1966.

Ferris, J. A. J., Aherne, W. A., Locke, W. S., McQuillin, J., and Gardner, P. S.: Sudden and unexpected deaths in infants: Histology and virology. Br. Med. J., 2:439, 1973.

Foy, H. M., Cooney, M. K., and Maletzky, A. J.: Incidence and etiology of pneumonia, croup, and bronchiolitis in preschool children belonging to a prepaid medical care group over a four-year period. Am. J. Epidemiol., 97:80, 1973.

Glezen, W. P., and Denny, F. W.: Epidemiology of acute lower respiratory disease in children. N. Engl. J. Med., 288:498, 1973.

Glezen, W. P., Fernald, G. W., and Lohr, J. A.: Acute respiratory disease of university students with special reference to the etiologic role of herpesvirus hominis. Am. J. Epidemiol., 101:111, 1975.

Minor, T. E., Dick, E. C., Baker, J. W., Ouellette, J. J., Cohen, M., and Reed, C. E.: Rhinovirus and influenza Type A infections as precipitants of asthma. Am. Rev. Respir. Dis., 113:149, 1976.

79. ADENOVIRAL INFECTIONS

George Gee Jackson

DEFINITION AND ETIOLOGY. The adenoviruses comprise a distinct group of viruses of the deoxyribose nucleic acid variety. The viral particle has a coat (capsid) consisting of 252 capsomeres arranged in an icosohedron, which is a structure with 20 equilateral triangular faces; it is 60 to 90 nm in size. Most of the capsomeres (240) are six sided, called hexons; the other 12, at the junctions of the triangles, are five sided, called pentons. The hexons have a common group-specific antigen characteristic of all adenoviruses. Each type has specific hexon and penton antigens. There are more than 31 specific serotypes among the strains of human origin. Only a few of them cause infections of the respiratory tract. The common types involved are 1, 2, 3, 4, 5, and 7. Types 14 and 21 also have caused acute respiratory illness. Type 8 is the principal cause of epidemic keratoconjunctivitis.

Some early isolates were recovered from surgically removed adenoids grown as tissue culture explants. These were reported as adenoidal degenerative or AD agents. The first strains from respiratory illnesses were designated RI agents. A later name, used briefly, was adenoidal-pharyngeal-conjunctival or APC agents. All the strains are now included under the term adenoviruses.

EPIDEMIOLOGY. Adenoviruses types 1, 2, and 5 infect virtually all persons early in childhood. They have been associated with febrile pharyngitis, with lower respiratory disease (sometimes fatal), and with gastrointestinal symptoms in infants. In older children and adolescents, adenoviruses, predominantly types 3 and 7 in the United States and 3, 4, 7, 14, and 21 in Europe, cause about 5 per cent of the viral respiratory illnesses. The incidence among college students may be as great as 8 per cent. At military recruit camps, infection with adenovirus types 4 and 7 is highly prevalent. It is often the predominant cause of respiratory illness, and 70 to 80 per cent of all incoming recruits become infected. Among civilian adults, adenoviruses cause only 1 to 3 per cent of respiratory illness.

Adenoviruses occur in all parts of the world. Man is the principal reservoir of infection. Many species of animals also are infected with adenoviruses, but these are of different serotypes, and cross-infection between man and animals either does not occur or is rare. Transmission is by person-to-person contact. The incubation period is three to eight days. In some investigations among civilians, respiratory infection occurred only with close or prolonged contact. However, as noted above, military inductees often become infected with adenoviruses 4 or 7 in the first few weeks of training. The syndrome called acute respiratory disease (ARD) has the highest incidence in the autumn and winter. Asymptomatic enteric infections are common. Conjunctivitis may be highly contagious and transferred by household items in common use, such as towels. Swimming pools have been an effective vehicle for the transmission of adenoviral conjunctivitis and of the disease pharyngoconjunctival fever.

PATHOGENIC MECHANISMS. During the acute infection and for a period of one to three weeks, virus is excreted in the respiratory secretions or in those of the eye, or in both. A high proportion of infected persons have virus in the stool, which may be a source for the spread of infection. Viruria also has been observed during the acute respiratory illness. Adenoviruses replicate in the nucleus of the cell and, when the concentration is high, form crystals of virus. The nuclear chromatin becomes clumped, and the cells may undergo lysis. A most remarkable aspect of adenoviral infections with types 1, 2, 3, and 5 is the capacity of the virus to persist as a latent infection in lymphoid tissue for years after the initial infection. Fifty to 90 per cent of surgically removed adenoids yield adenovirus of one of these types when cultured under conditions that will unmask latent virus. Whether this provides a source for infection of others or any harm to the host is unknown.

Some of the adenoviruses are capable of producing tumors when injected into newborn hamsters. Among the respiratory strains, some isolates of type 7 and type 3 have been oncogenic in baby hamsters. These studies on the tumorigenicity of adenoviruses also have shown the capacity of adenoviruses to combine within the same envelope (capsid) the oncogenic genome of some other tumor-producing viruses of DNA type, specifically the simian virus, SV-40. Thus under defined experimental conditions, adenoviruses can be oncogenic in their own right or act as a carrier for oncogenic material. There is no evidence that these properties give the virus any oncogenic capacity in man, but the phenomena are of basic biologic importance.

Some adrenoviruses have an associated smaller virus (AAV). It is a defective DNA virus which can multiply only in the presence of adenoviruses. The significance of AAV in the pathogenesis of adenoviral infections is not known.

CLINICAL MANIFESTATIONS AND DIFFERENTIAL DIAGNOSIS. Different clinical syndromes produced by adenoviral infections in older children and adults are characteristic. Fever and pharyngitis are the hallmarks; catarrhal otitis occurs frequently, cervical adenopathy is common, conjunctivitis may be present, and a few patients develop pneumonia. The syndromes have been given descriptive names, as follows: (1) acute febrile pharyngitis, (2) nonstreptococcal exudative pharyngitis, (3) acute respiratory disease of recruits, (4) pharyngoconjunctival fever, and (5) adenoviral pneumonia. Any single type of virus among those that cause natural respiratory infections in man can produce the entire spectrum of these clinical manifestations and also the common cold. The age of the patient and the route of inoculation are important. In newborn infants, giant cell pneumonia, myocarditis, and encephalitis have been described. In young children, mesenteric adenitis

and intussusception have been reported. Infection with adenovirus types 1, 2, 5, and 6 may occur in the preschool child without any overt illness, whereas type 7 causes severe illness in this age group, with 5 per cent fatality. The former types infect nearly all children, but type 7 infections are infrequent. The common adenoviruses have been associated in a possible interrelated role with *H. pertussis* in whooping cough. Type 11 has been found as a cause of acute hemorrhagic cystitis in children (girls).

Conjunctivitis, when present, is an acute follicular lesion, often unilateral, with marked erythema, suffusion, and narrowing of the palpebral fissure. Keratoconjunctivitis, caused by adenovirus type 8, is a serious infection of the eye with corneal infiltrates; it rarely occurs in pharyngoconjunctival fever. Pharyngeal exudate, if present, is more likely to appear on the pharyngeal wall than as follicular tonsillitis. Cervical lymph nodes are enlarged and firm but less tender than with streptococcal infections. A macular rash that is difficult to distinguish from rubella has been described in a few cases. The leukocyte count is normal or slightly elevated. A prompt antibody response usually accompanies the infection. It can be measured in the serum by complement fixation or virus neutralization tests.

TREATMENT AND PREVENTION. Treatment is supportive and with few exceptions recovery occurs without sequelae, excluding those of type 8 keratoconjunctivitis. Immunity to reinfection is demonstrable, but second infections have been observed with types 1, 2, 3, and 5. These types cause latent infections, and it is possible that later episodes represent an activation or recrudescence of the latent infection. Reinfection, if it occurs, usually causes mild illness.

Vaccine administration can elicit protective antibody and effectively prevent specific adenovirus infections. Live, enteric-coated, oral adrenovirus vaccines of types 4 and 7 have been extensively evaluated in military recruits at stations where the incidence of infection and disease is high. Given prophylactically, the vaccine stimulates antibody, prevents specific adenovirus illness, and reduces pharyngeal infection after natural exposure by about two thirds. In epidemic situations mass immunization with live virus vaccine promptly interrupts the epidemic. Use of the vaccine is not recommended for civilians because of the low incidence and sporadic occurrence of infection with adenovirus types 4 and 7 among them.

No adenovirus vaccines are available commercially.

Becroft, D. M.: Bronchiolitis obliterans, bronchiectasis, and other sequelae of adenovirus type 21 infection in young children. J. Clin. Pathol., 24:72, 1971.

Bell, J. A., Rowe, W. T., Engler, J. I., Parrott, R. H., and Huebner, R. J.: Pharyngoconjunctival fever. Epidemiological studies of a recently recognized disease entity. JAMA, 157:1083, 1955.

Brandt, C. D., Kim, H. W., Jeffries, B. C., Pyles, G., Christmas, E. E., Reid, J. L., Chanock, R. M., and Parrott, R. H.: Infections in 18,000 infants and children in a controlled study of respiratory tract disease. II. Variation in adenovirus infections by year and season. Am. J. Epidemiol., 95:218, 1972.

Chanock, R. S.: Impact of adenoviruses in human disease. Prev. Med., 3:466, 1974.

Chou, S. M., Roos, R., Burrell, R., and Gutman, L.: Subacute focal adenovirus encephalitis. J. Neuropathol. Exp. Neurol., 32:34, 1973.

Dudding, B. A., Top, F. H., Jr., Winter, P. E., Buescher, E. L., Lamson, T. H., and Leibovitz, A.: Acute respiratory disease in military trainees. The adenovirus surveillance program, 1966–1971. Am. J. Epidemiol., 97:187, 1973.

Fox, J. P., Brandt, C. D., Wasserman, F. E., Hall, C. E., Spigland, L., Kogon, A., and Elveback, L. R.: The virus watch program: A continuing surveillance of viral infections in metropolitan New York families. VI. Observations of adenovirus infections: Virus excretion patterns, antibody response, efficiency of surveillance, patterns of infection, and relation to illness. Am. J. Epidemiol., 89:25, 1969.

Jackson, G. G., and Muldoon, R. L.: Viruses causing common respiratory infections in man. Adenoviruses. J. Infect. Dis., 127:328, 1973.

Klenk, E. L., Gaultney, J. V., and Bass, J. W.: Bacteriologically proved pertussis and adenovirus infection. Possible association. Am. J. Dis. Child., 124:203, 1972.

Levy, J. L., Jr.: Etiology of "idiopathic" intussusception in infants. South. Med. J., 63:642, 1970.

Pereira, M.: Adenovirus infections. Postgrad. Med. J., 49:798, 1973.

80. RESPIRATORY SYNCYTIAL VIRAL DISEASE

George Gee Jackson

DEFINITION AND ETIOLOGY. Infection with respiratory syncytial virus (RS) causes epidemic acute respiratory disease. The illnesses are rather acute in onset and may be mild or severe. Since its recognition in 1956 as an infection of man, RS has produced regular epidemics of influenza-like respiratory disease.

Respiratory syncytial virus is a paramyxovirus that resembles influenza and parainfluenza viruses in its structure and many biologic characteristics. It is serologically distinct from them, does not agglutinate erythrocytes as they do, and does not cause lesions in eggs or common laboratory animals. The virus was first isolated from chimpanzees and was designated chimpanzee coryza agent (CCA). The name respiratory syncytial virus is descriptive of the cytopathic effect of the virus in infected tissue cultures. Only one type of the virus is known; some isolates have shown minor differences when tested against specific immune serum, but these appear clinically insignificant with regard to man.

EPIDEMIOLOGY. Respiratory syncytial virus has been recovered on different continents, suggesting that it has worldwide distribution. The epidemiologic pattern of infection lies somewhere between the epidemicity of influenza A and the endemicity of the parainfluenza viruses. Usually there are sharp, well defined limits to each epidemic. In the interepidemic period, the virus is detected much less frequently, but RS virus has been isolated from illnesses in every month of the year. Epidemics recur at intervals of 8 to 16 months. These have appeared simultaneously in geographically widely separated locations. During an epidemic, a large proportion of the population may experience infection, even persons who have had prior infection and have residual serum antibody. The pattern of the epidemic spread is characteristic of airborne or direct contact transmission. The incubation period is three to seven days.

The high prevalence of infection is indicated by the fact that 70 per cent of infants at birth have appreciable amounts of maternal antibody against RS virus. During the first few months of life this declines, and between 3 and 12 months about 35 per cent develop antibody as a result of natural infection. By five years of age, 95 per cent of children have been infected. The incidence of infection with RS virus varies because of its epidemicity, but it makes a significant contribution in the production of serious respiratory diseases of children. Among hospitalized pediatric cases, RS infection has been found to be etiologic in 10 to 20 per cent. In this respect, it ranks ahead of the parainfluenza viruses or adenoviruses and is also more prevalent than influenza as a cause of hospitalization in the first year of life. RS virus is the single most frequent clinical infection causing lower respiratory illness and is a major cause of death in this age group. Among adults, the incidence is less well documented because of the milder nature of the disease, but an increase in hospital admission of adults with lower respiratory disease occurs during periods of RS virus infection.

PATHOGENESIS. Infection causes inflammation of the respiratory mucosa with a tendency for necrotizing bronchiolitis, bronchiolar obstruction, focal atelectasis, and patchy pneumonia. Among people who become infected, 80 to 90 per cent are clinically ill. Infants and adults with chronic bronchopulmonary disease are especially at risk of fatal or severe illness. Ventilatory insufficiency, sometimes severe enough to cause elevation of the arterial Pco_2 as high as 60 to 70 mm Hg, can occur in infected infants. Bacterial pneumonia can be a complication. The annual epidemiologic recurrences of disease, the reisolation of virus from the same children in successive years, and investigations in adult volunteers have all emphasized the importance of reinfections with respiratory syncytial virus. The pathogenesis of the reinfections does not depend on antigenic differences among strains. Clinical investigations show convincingly that the presence of serum neutralizing antibody against the challenge strain does not prevent reinfection or illness. Neutralizing antibody (IgA) appears in the nasal secretion after infection and is protective but not persistent. The high prevalence and importance of RS virus in the causation of respiratory disease appears to reside in this capacity to produce reinfections with clinical symptoms.

CLINICAL MANIFESTATIONS. Fever and bronchiolitis are the characteristics of infection in children. Rhinitis and pharyngitis are usually present. Otitis may occur. In one study, pneumonia was shown roentgenographically in more than two thirds of the cases. Croup may develop, but it is relatively infrequent. The average maximal temperature is 39° C, but in individual patients it may reach 40.5° C. Ordinarily, fever lasts for three days. Dyspnea, cough, and wheezing are obvious symptoms. Tachypnea, rhonchi, and crepitant rales are present on examination. A few of the patients are cyanotic. The leukocyte count is elevated to between 10,000 and 20,000 per cubic millimeter in many cases. This clinical syndrome cannot be distinguished with certainty from epidemic influenza. Ordinarily, there is more rhinitis, and the onset is less abrupt. A fatality rate of 2.5 per cent has been estimated for hospitalized patients. Sudden death of infants and young children in their cribs at home after mild respiratory symptoms has been suspected by epidemiologic association to be of RS etiology.

In about two thirds of the documented cases there is a less severe syndrome, which has been diagnosed in outpatient clinics. These patients have fever, but they have fewer constitutional symptoms than those who are hospitalized. Rhinitis and pharyngitis are relatively more prominent. Cough is frequent, but rales and rhonchi are scarce.

Among adults with prechallenge antibody, the clinical manifestation of infection is acute coryza. However, age and antibody are independent factors in the prevention of severe disease. Serum antibody per se affords little protection. An analysis of proved cases in adults admitted to a hospital in one study indicated that persons with chronic bronchitis (one half of the cases studied) had an acute exacerbation of bronchitis; in one fourth of them infection caused bronchopneumonia, and in one fourth it produced the influenza syndrome with severe constitutional symptoms. Thus the entire spectrum of viral respiratory illness is produced in adults by RS virus.

DIAGNOSIS. The suspicion of RS virus infection is based upon clinical and epidemiologic observations. The diagnosis can be made by virus isolation from the respiratory secretions or by serologic tests. Respiratory syncytial virus is recovered by the inoculation of secretions into cultures of a human epithelial cell line or diploid cell strain. The specimens should be inoculated directly into susceptible cell layers, owing to the loss of virus infectivity by freezing and thawing specimens. Under these conditions virus identification can be made within a few days. The use of specific immunofluorescent antibody to recognize viral antigens in nasopharyngeal secretions has been recommended for rapid diagnosis.

Serodiagnosis can be made by either complement-fixation (CF) or neutralization tests, using paired sera collected as early as possible after the onset of illness and again after two to three weeks. A fourfold or greater rise in the serum antibody titer is regarded as diagnostic of infection.

TREATMENT AND PREVENTION. Careful assessment of respiratory competence, close observation, and supportive care are important, especially in children, in view of the relative severity of the involvement of the lower respiratory tract. Anticipation of the possible need for tracheostomy (to reduce respiratory dead air space and assist in the removal of secretions) and mechanical assistance with ventilation in occasional patients is wise. Antimicrobial drugs have no effect on the RS virus or on the outcome of the usual infection. Isolation of the patient from other susceptible contacts should be done during hospitalization. Nosocomial spread to susceptible contacts is common (30 to 50 per cent) and includes both the patients and the attending staff. However, the spread of infection in the community is not controlled by isolation procedures.

The annual occurrence of epidemic infection and the clear demonstration of reinfections, often with equally severe sequential episodes, might suggest that immunoprophylaxis would have little effect on the infection. On the other hand, the mildness and lower frequency of infections in adults are circumstantial support for the development of immunity. The antigens of the RS virus are labile and poorly antigenic. Use of investigational inactivated vaccine that produced nonprotective levels of serum antibody augmented the clinical severity and fatality of subsequent infection. Similarly, the high fatality among infected infants in the first few months of life, when maternal antibody is demonstrable, suggests that passively acquired antibody may have a paradoxical aggravating effect. Attenuated, temperature-sensitive mutants that can be given as live virus vaccines into the respiratory passages are being developed. Perhaps the larger amount of viral antigen and repeated doses that can be given in this way will induce protection.

Beem, M.: Repeated infections with respiratory syncytial virus. J. Immunol., 98:1115, 1967.

Berglund, B.: Respiratory syncytial virus infections in families. A study of family members of children hospitalized for acute respiratory disease. Acta. Paediat. Scand., 56:395, 1967.

Fransen, H., Sterner, G., Forsgren, M., Heige, Z., Wolontis, S., Svedmyr, A., and Tunevall, G.: Acute lower respiratory illness in elderly patients with respiratory syncytial virus infection. Acta Med. Scand., 182:323, 1967.

Gardner, P. S.: Respiratory syncytial virus infections. Postgrad. Med. J., 49:788, 1973.

Hall, C. B., Geiman, J. M., Biggar, R., Kotok, D. I., Hogan, P. M., and Douglas, R. G.: Respiratory syncytial virus infections within families. N. Engl. J. Med., 294:414, 1976.

Monto, A. S., Bryan, R. E., and Rhodes, L. M.: The Tecumseh study of respiratory illness. VII. Further observations on the occurrence of respiratory syncytial virus and mycoplasma pneumoniae infections. Am. J. Epidemiol., 100:458, 1974.

Parrott, R. H., Kim, H. W., Brandt, C. D., and Chanock, R. M.: Respiratory syncytial virus in infants and children. Prev. Med., 3:473, 1974.

Sommerville, R. G.: Respiratory syncytial virus in acute exacerbations of chronic bronchitis. Lancet, 2:1247, 1963.

Urquhart, G. E., and Gibson, A. A. M.: RSV infections and infant deaths. Br. Med. J., 3:110, 1970.

81.   PARAINFLUENZA VIRAL DISEASES

(Croup)

George Gee Jackson

DEFINITION. Infection with parainfluenza viruses is a common and recurrent cause of respiratory illness. Croup is a prominent syndrome in children, but the spectrum of illness varies from the common cold to pneumonia and systemic illness.

ETIOLOGY. Parainfluenza viruses are members of the family of paramyxoviruses. In structure they closely resemble influenza virus but differ from it serologically and in some biologic respects. Four distinct types of parainfluenza viruses are recognized that cause infections in man. They are closely related to one another and have some characteristics in common with mumps, measles, and respiratory syncytial virus. Types 2 and 4 differ somewhat from types 1 and 3 in the clinical illnesses produced and in their epidemiology.

Parainfluenza viruses were first designated as hemadsorption or HA viruses, owing to their property of causing erythrocytes to absorb and stick to infected cells in tissue cultures. Type 2 was recovered from cases of croup and initially was called the "croup-associated" or CA virus. A strain of parainfluenza type 1, the Sendai virus, was first isolated in mice and called influenza D. Mice and other rodents were then recognized to have natural infection with parainfluenza viruses. The Sendai and other animal strains of parainfluenza type 1 have slight serologic differences from strains of human origin. A simian myxovirus (SV-5) is commonly found in monkey kidney tissue cultures, occasionally in eggs and other tissues. It resembles parainfluenza type 2; virus isolates from cattle with shipping fever (SF-4) were found to be parainfluenza type 3.

EPIDEMIOLOGY. Few, if any, persons escape infection and reinfection with the different types of parainfluenza viruses. Most children develop antibody from infection with parainfluenza type 3 before the age of four years. By the time they enter school, 70 per cent of children have antibody against more than one type. Among older children and adults, nasopharyngeal reinfection with types 1 and 3 is common regardless of the presence of serum antibody. Reinfection with parainfluenza viruses accounts for an appreciable proportion of common colds and upper respiratory illnesses in adults. The annual rates of infection are inversely related to age with preschool children, principally those of ages two to five years, being highest at 80 to 95 per cent per year. The over-all rates are 30 to 45 infections per 100 persons per year. This accounts for about 5 per cent of all respiratory infections in children.

Parainfluenza types 1 and 3 are endemic and cause illness in all seasons of the year. A study in Glasgow, Scotland, indicated that infections in the autumn were usually type 1 and those in the summer type 3. The former tended to have a biennial epidemic cycle, occurring predominantly in even-numbered years. Parainfluenza type 2 may be reciprocal with type 1 in its times of occurrence. Type 3 is a more infectious virus, has annual endemicity, and is associated with a wide spectrum of respiratory infections, including viral pneumonia. Similar results have been obtained from most surveys. All types can cause epidemics of respiratory disease in the winter season. Together, the parainfluenza viruses cause about 40 per cent of all cases of croup. A greater proportion of infections with types 1 and 2 cause croup, but because of its greater prevalence and transmissibility, type 3 may be a more frequent cause of the croup syndrome. Type 3 virus spreads easily from person to person. It infects virtually all contacts who have no antibody and reinfects many persons with a demonstrable level of antibody in the serum. Type 1 virus does not spread as efficiently as type 3, but is nevertheless highly transmissible. Type 2 infection has been less prevalent and more episodic in its occurrence than either type 1 or type 3 and infects older children. Infections caused by type 4 have been entirely sporadic and infrequently recognized.

Although many animal species have a high incidence of infection with the parainfluenza viruses, spread to man from these sources has not been well established.

CLINICAL MANIFESTATIONS. The clinical syndrome of croup in children is the most common characteristic of infection with parainfluenza viruses. Involvement of the trachea and bronchi also increases the amount of mucous secretions, which can become inspissated and cause additional respiratory obstruction. Type 3 infections may be symptomatically more severe and cause more lower respiratory tract disease. Although croup is the most distinctive syndrome, parainfluenza virus infections cause rhinitis or pharyngitis more than twice as often as croup, and bronchitis, bronchiolitis, or pneumonia at least as frequently as croup. Over-all, croup is a symptom in fewer than 10 per cent of infections.

The initial infection with parainfluenza viruses produces more severe disease than reinfection and produces fever of 39 to 40° C in about three fourths of the cases. Among older children and adolescents only about two thirds of infections are symptomatic. Among adults, parainfluenza viruses cause mostly upper respiratory tract disease, predominantly the common cold or afebrile coryza. About one third of patients with reinfection will have fever, but many will be asymptomatic. In dual viral infections, a parainfluenza virus has been recognized as a common member of the pair with a resultant increase in the severity of the symptoms. Extrarespiratory manifestations are occasionally associated with parainfluenza infections, usually type 3. Associations that are presumed etiologic are myocardi-

tis, pericarditis, polyarthritis, meningoencephalitis, and rash.

DIAGNOSIS. Clinical differentiation of the type of parainfluenza viral infection and even the differentiation from other viral infections of the respiratory tract cannot be made with confidence. The virus can be isolated from nasopharyngeal secretions during the illness and for a brief period thereafter. This is the most certain and may be the only way to identify the specific type of parainfluenza virus involved. However, the sampling methods used are still relatively insensitive, and culture-negative infections are quite common. Serologic responses are often heterotypic owing to the nearly universal infection of persons with type 3 early in life and the common infection with types 1, 2, and mumps viruses. A rise in antibody against one of these viruses does not permit confidence in a strain-specific diagnosis.

TREATMENT. The treatment is supportive, as described for the common cold. The croup syndrome may be very acute, and cause respiratory insufficiency requiring urgent and decisive management. A comfortably warm, draft-free environment with high humidity (steam) is recommended for reducing laryngeal stridor. Maintenance of an adequate airway is essential. Antimicrobial drugs are usually contraindicated. Inactivated virus vaccines have been produced for types 1, 2, and 3, and their antigenicity has been shown, but their effectiveness in the prevention of natural infection has not been convincing.

Buchan, K. A., Marten, K. W., and Kennedy, D. H.: Aetiology and epidemiology of viral croup in Glasgow, 1966–72. J. Hyg. (Camb.), 73:143, 1974.

Cooney, M. K., Fox, J. P., and Hall, C. E.: The Seattle virus watch. VI. Observations of infections with and illness due to parainfluenza, mumps and respiratory syncytial viruses and *Mycoplasma pneumoniae.* Am. J. Epidemiol., 101:532, 1975.

Herrmann, E. C., Jr., and Hable, K. A.: Experiences in laboratory diagnosis of parainfluenza viruses in routine medical practice. Mayo Clin. Proc., 45:177, 1970.

Jackson, G. G., and Muldoon, R. L.: Viruses causing common respiratory infections in man. Enteroviruses and paramyxoviruses. J. Infect. Dis., 128:387, 1973.

Loda, F. A., and Glezen, W. P.: Parainfluenza virus infections. Prev. Med., 3:481, 1974.

Monto, A. S.: The Tecumseh study of respiratory illnesses. V. Patterns of infection with the parainfluenzaviruses. Am. J. Epidemiol., 97:338, 1973.

Starke, J. E., Heath, R. B., and Curwen, M. P.: Infections with influenza and parainfluenza viruses in chronic bronchitis. Thorax, 20:124, 1965.

Wenzel, R. P., McCormick, D. P., and Beam, W. E.: Parainfluenza pneumonia in adults. JAMA, 221:294, 1972.

82. INFLUENZA

Edwin D. Kilbourne

DEFINITION. Influenza is an acute, contagious disease that is usually attended by fever and prostration and is ordinarily benign in outcome. The headache, myalgia, and asthenia that characterize the disease are severe out of proportion to the symptoms originating from involvement of the respiratory tract — the primary and principal site of infection with the causative virus.

HISTORY. Epidemics of respiratory disease similar to modern influenza have been recorded through the centuries. Since the year 1510 there have been 31 pandemics described. The calamitous nature of these epidemics may have led to the naming of the disease by the Italians as an "influenza" or influence of the heavenly bodies or perhaps as an "influenza di freddo" (influence of the cold).

In 1933 the isolation of a virus in ferrets by Smith, Andrewes, and Laidlaw established the specific infectious etiology of the disease, and led rapidly to accurate definition of its epidemiology and clinical variations. The virus isolated in 1933 is now known as influenza A virus.

A second type of virus was isolated independently in 1940 by Francis and by Magill (influenza B virus). In 1950 influenza C was isolated from a patient in nonepidemic circumstances by Taylor, and later was shown by Francis and his associates to be the cause of epidemic disease.

Five pandemics of influenza have been recorded in the twentieth century (1900, 1918, 1946, 1957, and 1968). Of these, the pandemic of 1918 was most severe, accounting for at least 20 million deaths. Effective inactivated viral vaccines were introduced in the 1940's, but had never been employed in mass prophylaxis until 1976, when immunization of 50 million Americans was carried out in anticipation of a pandemic of swine influenza that never materialized.

ETIOLOGY. Influenza is a consequence of infection with certain *myxoviruses* that have common physical, chemical, and biologic properties. These viruses comprise three groups (A, B, and C), which are completely unrelated antigenically, do not induce cross-immunity to one another, and have different epidemiologic characteristics. Four major subgroups of influenza A viruses associated with human disease have been identified since discovery of the virus in 1933, each having replaced the other in chronologic succession. Serologic studies defined a virus that first appeared in swine in 1918 (HswN1) as the probable cause of the notorious human pandemic of that year. Influenza A virus subtypes are defined on the basis of antigenic analysis of their two outermost proteins. These biologically active glycoproteins (hemagglutinin [H] and neuraminidase [N]) are the primary determinants of immunity and mutate independently, as was clearly evident in the replacement of H2N2 by H3N2 (Hong Kong) virus in 1968 (see accompanying table). The hemagglutinin (H) is responsible for binding the virus to the cell; antibody to this protein therefore neutralizes the virus and is the major determinant of immunity. The viral neuraminidase (N) is instrumental in release of virus from cells; antineuraminidase antibody is not neutralizing, but limits viral replication and therefore the course of infection. As external spike-like projections from the viral envelope, H and N are in immediate contact with host antibody during infection and therefore are under selective pressure (see Epidemiology). Beneath these "spikes" the virus particle is bounded by a lipid bilayer derived from the host cell (Fig. 1). Just beneath the lipid layer the core of the particle is surrounded by

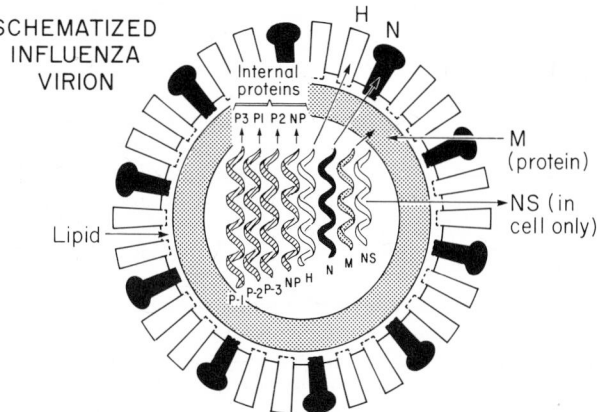

Figure 1. Schematic representation of influenza virion, indicating the eight viral genes and their polypeptide products. The relative sizes of the RNA genes are only approximate, and the structural details of their relationship to one another and to the internal proteins P1–P3 and NP are not known. (From Kilbourne, E. D.: The Harvey Lectures, series 73. New York, Academic Press, 1977–78.)

the M or membrane protein. The nucleoprotein (NP) occurs in helical form in association with the viral RNA. The internal M, NP, and three P proteins (of undefined location and function) are common to all influenza A viruses and do not differ significantly in antigenic nature from one subtype to the other. Type-specific A, B, or C categorization of virus thus depends on serologic reactions (usually complement-fixation) mediated by these internal antigens.

The viral genome within comprises eight segments of RNA (totaling 3.9×10^6 daltons) capable of reassortment during infection to provide an unusually high frequency of genetic recombination. Isolated viral RNA(s) is not infectious, because it does not constitute the message. Virus-coded transcriptase is necessary for viral replication. Thus the RNA segments code for monocistronic messages for each of the seven virion proteins and for a nonstructural protein detectable only in the host cell.

Influenza B and C viruses have been less thoroughly studied, but appear to be structurally similar to influenza A viruses. Little antigenic variation of influenza C virus has been remarked, and antigenic variation of influenza B virus has been of lesser magnitude than that observed with influenza A.

The influenza viruses are of medium size (approximately 850 Å in diameter), and by conventional electron microscopy they appear spherical or filamentous in form, with spike-like projections.

EPIDEMIOLOGY. The arbitrary designation of the three types of influenza virus as A, B, and C coincides fortuitously with their relative rank as causes of severe epidemic disease. Influenza B and C viruses have been associated chiefly with sporadic epidemics in children and young adults, notably in school or other institutional populations. Most adults carry antibodies to these viruses, probably as the result of recurrent subclinical infection. There is no evidence that pandemics of influenza B or C have occurred.

Discussions of influenza are usually concerned with the influenza A viruses, for these are the important and apparently more mutable viruses that cause widespread

Influenza Pandemics: Relation to Major Antigenic Change in Causative Viruses*

Pandemic, Year	Virus Isolation	Viral Antigens	Magnitude of Change	Pandemic	Severity†
1918	1930‡	Hsw1N1	...	Yes	Unequaled
1929	1933‡	H0N1	Moderate	?	Moderate
1946	Yes	H1N1	Moderate	Yes	Slight
1957	Yes	H2N2	Great	Yes	Great
1968	Yes	H3N2	Partial	Yes	Moderate

*From Kilbourne, E. D.: JAMA, 237:1225, 1977.

†Estimate based on excess mortality.

‡Year of isolation of probable agent. Virus not isolated in pandemic year.

epidemic and pandemic disease. The complicated and still puzzling epidemiology of influenza A is most conveniently considered by separate discussions of the *pandemic, epidemic,* and *endemic* infections — all attributable to the same virus under different conditions.

Pandemic Influenza. Pandemic or worldwide infection with influenza A viruses has occurred five times in the present century. Viruses isolated in the pandemics of 1946, 1957, and 1968 have proved to be antigenically very different with respect to their hemagglutinin antigens. The severity of pandemics can be roughly related to the magnitude of change in hemagglutinin and neuraminidase antigens (see table).

When such major antigenic changes in the virus occur — perhaps as a reciprocal of high immunity in the general population — the mutation may be so extreme that acquired immunity in the population to previously existing influenza A viruses is inadequate to prevent infection or disease initiated by the new virus, which replaces the older virus completely. Under these conditions, people of all ages and in all places are susceptible to influenza, and a worldwide epidemic or pandemic may ensue (Fig. 2). In 1976, the emergence of human infection with swine influenza virus at Fort Dix, New Jersey, was unusual in that a major epidemic did *not* follow, despite antigenic novelty of the virus. The replacement of the H3N2 subtype with the returning H1N1 ("Russian") subtype of the early 1950's appears to be in prospect.

The source of the markedly different strains of virus that suddenly appear to initiate pandemics is unknown. Direct mutation from the antecedent virus seems unlikely in view of the magnitude of change in H and N antigens. Therefore recombination in nature of human and animal influenza A viruses has been proposed to explain the recurrent decennial introduction of apparently novel viruses into the human population.

The incubation period of influenza is only 24 to 48 hours, so that, once progressive spread begins, the impact on the community is sudden and devastating. Both the incidence and the severity of illness are highly variable and are influenced by age, pregnancy, and pre-existing chronic disease and by such environmental factors as crowding and season of the year. Morbidity is usually first noted among schoolchildren, then in young adults, and finally in older, less active, and presumably less exposed members of the community. Infection of the aged is more frequently followed by bacterial pneumonia. As a consequence, a "second wave" of increased community mortality may coincide with the delayed appearance of influenza in this age group — *at a time when influenza is no longer apparent in the community* by the usual criterion of absenteeism from school or industry.

Specific immunity to influenza develops rapidly after infection, but it may decline within one or two years so that recurrence of infection and disease from the same antigenic type of virus may occur *under conditions of heavy exposure* as in military barracks or boarding schools. On the other hand, the steady decline in community morbidity after the initial pandemic wave obviously points to the acquisition of immunity of some durability by most of the population.

Interpandemic "Epidemic" Influenza. Influenza occurs in its characteristic acute epidemics in the early months of the year in the north temperate zone. In a particular community the epidemic usually comes and goes within a month, rising to a peak in 12 to 14 days, and subsiding almost as rapidly. Although the case fatality rate is less than 1 per cent, the presence of influenza may be detected by a sudden increase in unspecified total mortality in the community. This mortality occurs at both extremes of age, and is occasioned principally by the bacterial pneumonias that may complicate influenza in the very young and very old.

Epidemics of influenza A have been demonstrated to occur every year since discovery of the virus, but communities are usually spared recurrence for two or more years after an epidemic.

After a pandemic, the frequency and extent of epidemics gradually abate with the development of population immunity to the new virus. Minor antigenic variations of the virus may be detected during this time, but at least a decade seems to be required for change sufficient to establish a truly "new" subtype (Fig. 2).

Endemic Influenza. The interepidemic survival of influenza virus has long been a puzzle in view of the fragility of the virus and its apparently obligate restriction to human hosts. It has become increasingly clear,

INFLUENZA PANDEMICS OF THE PAST CENTURY
(Major antigenic variations)

Figure 2. Schematic representation of periods of prevalence of major hemagglutinin subtypes of influenza A viruses. The year of introduction of the "new" subtypes is indicated by arrows. The designations H0, H1, and so on refer to hemagglutinin subtype of the viruses without reference to their neuraminidase antigens. Subtypes Hsw, H0, and H1 are more closely related antigenically than they are to H2 or H3. Identification of viral subtypes prior to 1933 (marking the first isolation of a human influenza virus) is inferential on the basis of studies of human antibodies. The abortive appearance of Hsw in 1976 is shown. The future prevalence of H1 is conjectural. (From Kilbourne, E. D.: The Harvey Lectures, series 73. New York, Academic Press, 1977–1978.)

however, that influenza virus infections may occur continuously within the population, either as sporadic instances of disease that are not recognized as influenza or as clinically inapparent infections. As more and more members of the population develop immunity, infections without disease become more and more frequent and serve to maintain the virus in the community. Such infections are recognized by serologic studies.

PATHOLOGY AND PATHOGENESIS. The primary lesion of influenza is a necrosis of the ciliated epithelium of the respiratory tract. In the uncomplicated infection epithelial damage is probably confined to the upper and middle portion of the respiratory tract, the trachea being the most strikingly involved. Early in infection the necrotic ciliated cells are desquamated, leaving intact the basal cell layer. On about the fifth day of illness regeneration begins in the basal layer with the development of undifferentiated "transitional" epithelium, which may simulate metaplasia. After two weeks ciliated cells may again be seen.

When influenza is complicated by bacterial pneumonia, the pathologic findings are variable and depend on the nature of the secondary invader. However, *primary influenza virus pneumonia* presents a characteristic picture. The lungs are dark red, heavy, and edematous. The trachea and bronchi contain bloody fluid, and the mucosa is hyperemic. Microscopy shows ciliated epithelium to have been lost from the trachea, bronchi, and bronchioles, but evidence of epithelial regeneration may be seen. In the submucosa, focal hemorrhage, edema, and slight leukocytic infiltration may occur. Capillary thrombosis with focal leukocytic exudate has been described. The alveolar spaces contain neutrophilic and mononuclear cells admixed with fibrin and edema fluid. Intra-alveolar hemorrhage is common in the lower lobes. The alveolar septa may be thickened, and acellular hyaline membranes may line alveolar ducts and alveoli.

Pathologic changes attributable to influenza occur only rarely outside the respiratory tract. There are no physiologic or biochemical changes in the patient that are pathognomonic of influenza. Although "leukopenia" is often stated to be characteristic, total leukocytic counts in the uncomplicated disease may vary from 2000 to 14,000 cells per cubic millimeter, and are usually in the normal range. However, *lymphocytopenia* is commonly detectable, especially in the first four days of illness. The erythrocyte sedimentation rate may be moderately elevated or normal. No characteristic changes occur in the bacterial flora of the respiratory tract.

The Complicated Disease. In primary influenza virus pneumonia, *leukocytosis* is the rule, even in the absence of bacterial pathogens, although the erythrocyte sedimentation rate may not be elevated. *Serum glutamic oxaloacetic transaminase concentrations* are elevated in proportion to the severity of pulmonary involvement and may exceed 60 units per milliliter. *Oxyhemoglobin saturation* is reduced to 46 to 85 per cent. *Partial pressure of CO_2* is elevated, and the *pH of arterial blood* is lowered. The *proteinuria* and elevated *blood urea nitrogen* concentrations that may be noted are the results of fever and dehydration and do not reflect primary renal damage. No notable changes in *serum electrolytes* or in *blood clotting* occur.

CLINICAL MANIFESTATIONS. Infection with influenza virus may be asymptomatic, may be attended only by slight fever, or may result in the "typical" prostrating disease that identifies epidemics. This disease is remarkably constant in its expression from year to year, and the uncomplicated case of pandemic influenza does not differ from the "three-day fever" of nonpandemic outbreaks. The higher fatality rates associated with the 1918 pandemic were usually attributable to secondary bacterial pneumonia. Significant variations in the disease caused by any of the A or B subtypes of virus have not occurred. Influenza C appears to be a less severe disease, but it has not yet received adequate study.

Patients with influenza almost invariably *cough,* although this symptom may not be bothersome or even noted by the patient. The cough is brief and spasmodic, and usually not productive of sputum. Other symptoms related to the destruction of respiratory epithelium are *substernal burning pain* (from the trachea), *dryness or soreness of the throat,* and *nasal obstruction and discharge.* Neither sore throat nor evidence of rhinitis is particularly prominent in influenza. Slight *pharyngeal injection* may be noted. *Epistaxis* is rare, but is valuable diagnostically when it occurs. *Conjunctival burning and injection* are common.

In 5 to 10 per cent of patients with uncomplicated disease, crepitant or musical *rales, roughened breath sounds,* or *pleural friction rub* may be detected. Such signs rarely persist for more than one or two days. *Chest pain* may accompany the friction rub, or more often is substernal and referable to the trachea.

The prostrating effects of influenza are associated with *fever, chilly sensations* (seldom with rigors), *headache,* and *myalgia. Fever* usually exceeds 38° C. and may reach 41° C. It is usually abrupt in its onset and decline and lasts for only two to five days in the absence of complications. *Headache* is often frontal and is of the throbbing sort associated with fever; its severity is proportional to the degree of fever. *Extraocular myalgia* is a characteristic but not universal complaint that may be elicited only by examination. *Myalgia* may be generalized or confined to the back or lower extremities. *Gastrointestinal symptoms* are uncommon, and occur more often in patients with pre-existing gastrointestinal disease.

In sum, the picture of uncomplicated influenza is that of a patient with flushed face and reddened eyes who lies flat in bed and coughs occasionally with a dry spasmodic cough. He moves about fitfully, complaining of headache or backache. By contrast, the rare patient with influenza virus pneumonia (see below) sits erect, is extremely anxious and agitated, gasps for breath, and manifests *cyanosis* of the lips and nailbeds.

COURSE AND COMPLICATIONS. In both pandemic and epidemic influenza the disease, although acute and prostrating, is brief, so that it is uncommon for any symptom to last beyond seven to ten days, and fever usually subsides earlier (Fig. 3). A protracted *postinfluenzal asthenia* has been emphasized in some reports. It is not clear to what extent secondary bacterial infections or psychogenic factors contribute to the state. Nevertheless, the alerting of the patient to the possibility may save some apprehension during the convalescent period. *Encephalitis* and *myocarditis* have been described infrequently as complications of influenza, and have rarely been well documented or associated with virus isolation from the brain or heart.

The important and potentially lethal complications of

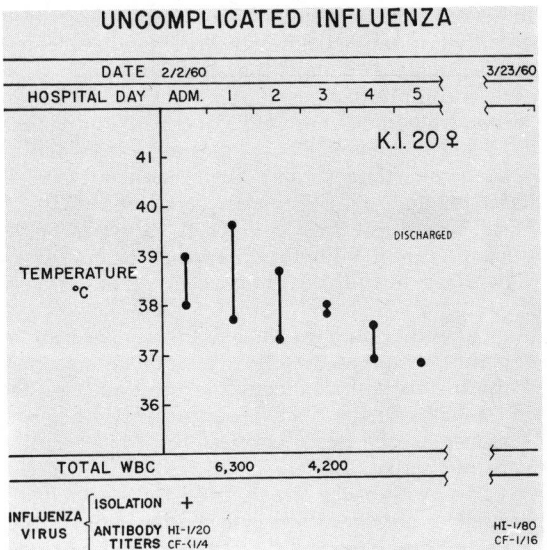

Figure 3. (From Kaye, D., et al.: Am. Rev. Respir. Dis., 85:9, 1962.)

influenza derive from infection of the lung, either with the influenza virus itself or with bacterial pathogens. The pulmonary complications of influenza may be considered as (1) *primary influenza virus pneumonia,* (2) *combined influenza virus and bacterial pneumonia,* and (3) *influenza complicated by secondary bacterial pneumonia.* All three types of complication are more frequent in patients with pre-existing cardiac or pulmonary disease or in women late in pregnancy. The aged, in whom apparent or inapparent chronic disease is more frequent, are also understandably more vulnerable to pulmonary complications of influenza. Neurologic complications have been temporally associated with influenza, as with other respiratory viral infections. Evidence for a clear-cut causative role of the virus in such sequelae is lacking. Recently, Reye's syndrome in children (see Ch. 309.4) has occurred with increased frequency after influenza epidemics, especially influenza B.

Primary Influenza Virus Pneumonia. Primary influenza virus pneumonia is a severe disease that is usually fatal. Within 24 hours of the onset of typical symptoms of influenza, the patient experiences high fever (39.5 to 40° C), a cough productive of bloody sputum, and profound dyspnea and anxiety. Cyanosis is notable, and poor air exchange is indicated by the generalized pulmonary findings, which include suppression of breath sounds, expiratory wheezing, and diffuse, moist rales. Signs of consolidation are absent. Chest roentgenograms disclose diffuse bilateral nodular infiltrates that radiate outward from the hilum, sparing the lung periphery.

The patient almost always dies within five to ten days of the onset of illness after a course characterized by unremitting fever, progressive pulmonary involvement, and terminal vascular collapse (Fig. 4). Antibacterial drugs, oxygen, bronchodilators, and corticosteroids are usually unavailing.

Pathogenic bacteria are not recoverable from the sputum, blood, or lung during life or post mortem, and influenza virus is demonstrable in high concentrations in the lung.

Primary influenza virus pneumonia ordinarily is restricted to patients with pre-existing cardiac or pulmonary disease or pregnancy. Still more specifically, the victim usually has rheumatic cardiovascular disease and mitral stenosis. The predilection of this complication for the patient with mitral stenosis suggests that hemodynamic factors such as pulmonary hypertension are more important in its pathogenesis than general debility or the absence of specific immune mechanisms.

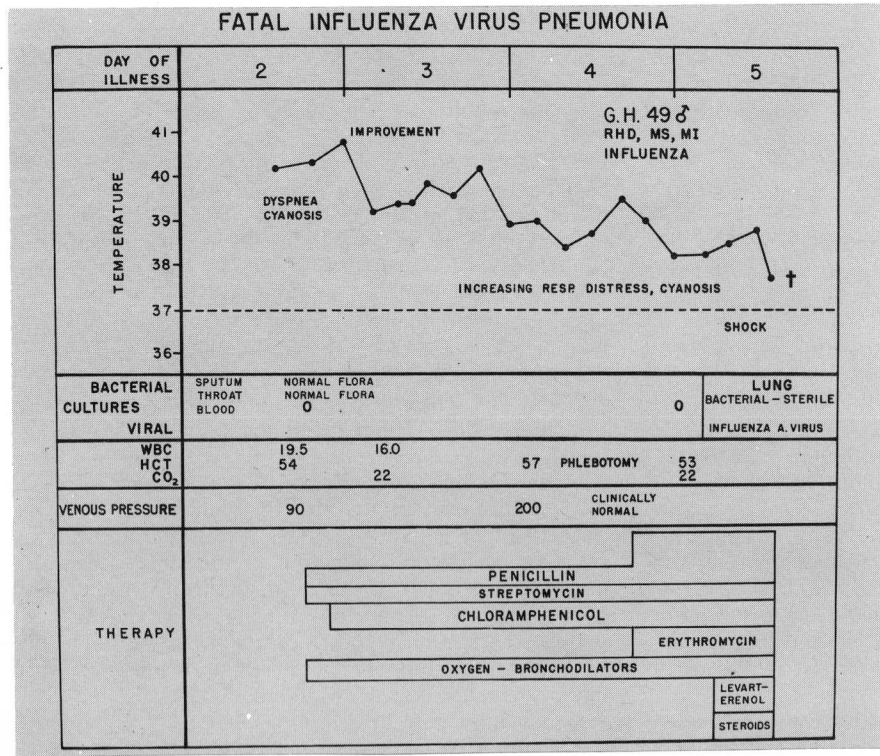

Figure 4. (From Kaye, D., et al.: Am. Rev. Respir. Dis. 85:9, 1962.)

There appears to be a graded spectrum of severity of the disease caused by influenza virus, so that, intermediate between the uncomplicated case with transient rales and the fatal virus pneumonia, occasional instances of "mild segmental influenza virus pneumonia" have been described.

Combined Influenza Virus and Bacterial Pneumonia. In patients with primary influenza virus pneumonia, infection with bacterial pathogens may supervene. In such patients the characteristic and dramatic onset of the virus pneumonia may be attended or closely followed by such symptoms of bacterial pneumonia as *productive cough, shaking chills,* or *pleuritic pain.* Signs of focal consolidation may be engrafted upon the diffuse pulmonary findings of the viral infection. Pneumococcus, *Staphylococcus, Hemophilus influenzae,* or, more rarely, group A streptococci may be demonstrated by culture of lung, blood, or sputum. In 1957–1958, pneumococcus and *Staphylococcus* were the most frequent bacterial invaders.

The host setting and course of the combined infection are basically the same as in the pneumonia associated with influenza virus infection alone.

Influenza Complicated by Secondary Bacterial Pneumonia. Bacterial pneumonia, characterized by focal consolidation, may occur after influenza in previously healthy persons as well as in the ill and infirm. This complication is further distinguished from influenza virus pneumonia by (1) the lag between influenzal symptoms and the appearance of pneumonia, sometimes with brief interval of freedom from symptoms; (2) the presence of focal and not diffuse pulmonary involvement; and (3) the absence of influenza virus in throat washings, but the presence of bacterial pathogens in the sputum. This "late" type of pulmonary complication is by far the most common.

DIAGNOSIS. In the context of an epidemic, influenza may easily be distinguished from other acute respiratory diseases, although diagnosis of the isolated case may be difficult. In its typical form influenza is characterized by relatively high fever, which sets it apart from the syndrome of the *common cold.* With the common cold, nasal symptoms predominate, but they are usually minor in influenza. *Adenoviral infections* are the most difficult to distinguish from influenza, but, in general, fever and prostration are less, onset is less sudden, and sore throat and laryngitis are more prominent in adenoviral disease. One of the clinical forms of respiratory syncytial viral disease may closely mimic influenza. The aching, febrile, minor illnesses associated with infection by various arbo- or enteroviruses may also simulate influenza but are notably unattended by cough, although sore throat may occur. In *streptococcal pharyngitis,* the greater frequency of vomiting, the predominance of sore throat, and the occurrence of cervical adenitis and leukocytosis are helpful in differential diagnosis. *Primary atypical pneumonia* is usually distinguishable clinically from influenza virus pneumonia by its more gradual onset, purulent sputum, and indolent, ordinarily benign course.

The *definitive diagnosis* of influenza depends upon isolation of the virus from throat washings or sputum and the demonstration of an increase in specific humoral antibodies. Viral isolation is most successful in the first two to three days of illness and is best accomplished by the intra-amniotic inoculation of chick embryos. Primary cultures of mammalian cells may also be used but are less satisfactory. If virus grows to high enough titer on the first passage, isolation and identification of the agent may be accomplished within 48 to 72 hours of inoculation of the specimen. Fluorescent antibody staining of exfoliated nasal epithelial cells, although infrequently used, can be applied as a quick and specific diagnostic test.

Antibody may be detected in the patient's serum by neutralization, hemagglutination-inhibition, or complement-fixation tests as early as eight to nine days after the onset of illness, but maximal response is evident only after 14 days. The diagnosis cannot be made with a single serum specimen because of the prevalence of antibody in the population; rather an *increase* in antibody titer of fourfold or more must be demonstrated by the study of two or more serum specimens obtained early in illness and in convalescence.

PROGNOSIS. The prognosis is ordinarily favorable in this brief and self-limited disease. However, the severity of the disease is a reciprocal of host susceptibility, and the outcome may be fatal in those with prior cardiac or pulmonary disease. The prognosis is also influenced by the prevalence of potential respiratory bacterial invaders in the community and the prospects for their control.

TREATMENT. There is no specific treatment for influenza. The general measures used in the symptomatic treatment of other infections are useful, including especially aspirin (0.3 to 0.6 gram) for the headache, malaise, and myalgia, and codeine sulfate (0.016 to 0.064 gram) for irritability, cough, and substernal pain. Diet may be regulated by the patient with the warning that high fat foods are not well tolerated. Fluids should be given in abundance.

Routine antibacterial prophylaxis is unnecessary and inadvisable, but may be considered for those with chronic disease with the view of forestalling the sequel of pneumococcal pneumonia. In this case, full therapeutic doses of penicillin should be given.

Treatment of primary influenza viral pneumonia is highly unsatisfactory, but oxygen therapy with positive pressure breathing devices has shown some promise.

PREVENTION. Influenza may be prevented by the parenteral injection of vaccines of influenza viruses that have been produced in the chick embryo and rendered noninfective (inactivated) by formalin or ultraviolet irradiation. The duration of protection usually does not exceed one year under conditions of epidemic exposure. Present vaccines are principally *bivalent* in that they contain the contemporary influenza A virus component and also lesser amounts of influenza B antigen. These newer vaccines have been purified by density gradient centrifugation or chromatography and are far less toxic than preparations of the past. So-called "split virus" vaccines contain antigens of the disrupted virus. They are of low reactogenicity, but may be less immunogenic than vaccines made from whole virus.

In experimental field trials amantadine hydrochloride has had a chemoprophylactic effect in influenza, as evidenced by lower infection rates and less severe illness in subjects who received the drug shortly before exposure to the infection. After infection, antibody titers were lower in drug-treated subjects, presumably reflecting a decreased antigenic stimulation from reduced viral replication. The drug is presumed to act by inhibiting virus penetration and not intracellularly on virus replication. Some evidence suggests that amantadine may have a slight therapeutic effect if given soon after the initiation of infection. Central nervous system toxicity may limit the usefulness of this compound in older people.

Because protection provided by inactivated influenza vaccine is transient, immunization of the general population is not usually indicated.

The objectives of vaccination differ in epidemic and pandemic years. In both situations, the prevention of *mortality* in the elderly and chronically ill is a major goal. In interpandemic periods, efforts to reduce morbidity have been restricted to those essential to the maintenance of community services or those particularly liable to epidemic disease such as military recruits and boarding school students. However, the wholesale morbidity associated with pandemics justifies consideration of mass immunoprophylaxis prior to or early in the course of such epidemics. An unanticipated increased risk of acquiring the Guillain-Barré syndrome was associated with the administration of almost 50,000,000 doses of swine influenza vaccine in 1976. It is not yet clear whether or not the enhanced risk is specifically related to influenza vaccine, or whether it might also be observed following mass administration of other antigens followed by similar prospective surveillance of the immunized population. Live virus vaccines offer promise of longer immunity, but have not yet been licensed in the United States.

Douglas, J. G., Jr.: Influenza in man. *In* Kilbourne, E. D. (ed.): The Influenza Viruses and Influenza. New York, Academic Press, 1975, p. 395.

Kilbourne, E. D.: Influenza pandemics in perspective. JAMA, 237:1225, 1977.

Louria, D. B., Blumenfeld, H. L., Ellis, J. T., Kilbourne, E. D., and Rogers, D. E.: Studies on influenza in the pandemic of 1957–1958. II. Pulmonary complications of influenza. J. Clin. Invest., 38:213, 1959.

Smith, W., Andrewes, C. H., and Laidlaw, P. P.: A virus obtained from influenzal patients. Lancet, 2:66, 1933.

VIRAL DISEASES
CHARACTERIZED BY CUTANEOUS LESIONS

83. MEASLES

(Morbilli, Rubeola)

Edwin D. Kilbourne

DEFINITION.   Measles is an extremely contagious, febrile disease of high morbidity characterized by rash and catarrhal inflammation of the eyes and respiratory tract. It is principally a benign disease of children, but may afflict with equal frequency persons of any age not previously immunized by infection or vaccination.

ETIOLOGY.   Measles is caused by a medium-sized RNA paramyxovirus approximately 1400 Å in diameter. The virus is of a single antigenic type and resembles other paramyxoviruses (e.g., parainfluenza and mumps viruses) in structure and biologic activity, except that it lacks a neuraminidase. Thus measles virus is an enveloped, lipid-containing virus that is released from the infected cell by budding evagination. The virus bears external spikes that contain a hemagglutinin capable of agglutinating erythrocytes of certain primates. Hemolytic and fusing activity is carried by another viral protein. In contrast to the genome of influenza viruses, the RNA is not segmented and high frequency genetic recombination of the virus does not occur. Antigenic variation of the virus has not been noted. Measles virus is antigenically and biologically related to the viruses of canine distemper and bovine rinderpest.

Measles virus replicates most readily in primary cultures of human embryonic tissue or primate kidney cells. However, adaptation of virus to a variety of primary or continuous mammalian and avian cell cultures has been achieved. (Vaccine viruses are propagated in chick embryo cells.)

Subhuman primates have long been known to be susceptible to measles; recently, propagation of the virus in the brains of mice, hamsters, and ferrets has been achieved, demonstrating its neurotropic potential.

EPIDEMIOLOGY.   Measles is a disease of cosmopolitan distribution, endemic in all but isolated populations. It may occur at any time of the year, but most outbreaks are in the late winter and early spring, with a peak at the end of April. The disease recurs in epidemic cycles at two- to three-year intervals in most civilized communities that have been studied. This epidemic periodicity is best explained as a result of the introduction of new susceptibles into the population by birth or ingress from other areas. When the proportion of nonimmunes reaches a certain crucial concentration (45 to 50 per cent), disease and coincident dissemination of virus may occur to produce an epidemic. It is likely that virus is introduced from sources external to the involved population, probably by incoming susceptibles. Isolated communities such as the Faröe Islands (Panum) are infrequently attacked by measles, at which times manifest illness appears in virtually all persons not previously infected. In Greenland, a country not known to have been invaded previously by the disease, an epidemic resulted in overt measles in 99.9 per cent of the indigenous population (Christiansen et al.).

Throughout most of the world, measles is a disease of children; most adults possess acquired immunity. Beyond the age of ten more than 90 per cent of the population have specific antibody. Although the peak attack rate coincides with the beginning of school (age six) in technologically advanced societies, it occurs between the ages of two and three in most developing countries. A recent trend of adolescent infection in the United States may have resulted from widespread but incomplete immunization that allows unimmunized children to escape infection until later as opportunity for natural infection has declined. Morbidity and mortality rates do not appear to be influenced by sex or race. Case fatality rates are highest in children less than five years of age, and are also relatively high in the aged. Congenital infection has occurred.

There is no evidence that the virus may vary in virulence in nature. The oft-cited and notorious virulence of the disease in primitive, isolated, or crowded populations may be explained as a corollary of (1) more prevalent infection of feeble and aged adults, (2) poor environmental conditions, (3) inadequate medical care, and (4) secondary bacterial infections. A strikingly increased mortality rate is observed in areas such as West Africa in which protein-calorie malnutrition is prevalent. Because measles virus per se rarely induces fatal disease, it is evident that fatalities attributable to measles may vary in incidence according to the prevalence of bacterial pathogens and the resistance of the population to their presence.

Communicability. Measles is one of the most contagious of infections. Demonstration of virus in nasopharyngeal secretions is in accord with epidemiologic evidence that infection is disseminated and acquired by the respiratory tract. Close physical proximity or direct person-to-person contact is the usual requisite for infection.

Immunity. An unmodified attack of measles is usually followed by lifelong immunity. This observation is in accord with the observed persistence of both complement-fixing and neutralizing antibodies after infection and the relatively high titer of antibodies present even in older persons. The mechanism of persistent immunity after measles is undefined. Although persistence of infective virus after infection seems not to occur, the internal nucleocapsid of measles virus or a closely related variant is demonstrable years after infection in the brain and peripheral lymph nodes of those rare individuals afflicted with subacute sclerosing panencephalitis (SSPE) (see Ch. 310.4). Thus the potential for viral persistence exists, and in those afflicted with SSPE, antibody levels to measles virus are higher than in those who have experienced uncomplicated measles.

A more likely explanation for the persistent immunity in measles is the maintenance of such immunity by subclinical exogenous reinfection. Careful studies of isolated or closed populations after administration of live virus vaccine have demonstrated a more rapid decline of antibody titer than in populations in which measles virus is circulating. Anamnestic antibody response in the absence of disease has been shown in immune contacts of patients with measles. Thus achievement of eradication of the virus may be compromised as vaccination (see below) is more and more effective in curtailing the circulation of the wild virus; then the booster immunization provided by natural reinfection will become inoperative, and repeated vaccination in the same subject may be required. Passively transferred maternal antibody protects the young infant from measles but also reduces the possibility of effective immunization by live virus vaccines at that age.

PATHOLOGY AND PHYSIOLOGIC RESPONSES. Pathologic changes in fatal measles usually represent the compound effect of viral and secondary bacterial infection. Pneumonia is almost invariably present; it is most frequently interstitial, but may produce purulent exudate within the alveoli. More representative are changes of the uncomplicated viral disease within the tonsillar, nasopharyngeal, and appendiceal tissue removed during the prodrome. These changes consist of subepithelial round cell infiltration and the presence of multinucleated giant cells. The latter are so characteristic that skilled pathologists have predicted the development of rash from their presence in surgical specimens. Similar cells are commonly observed in tissue cultures infected with measles virus. Cytoplasmic and nuclear inclusions may be seen in epithelial cells. The lesions clinically apparent as Koplik's spots derive from inflammatory mononuclear cell infiltration of buccal submucous glands and necrosis of focal vesicular lesions of the mucosa. Rash is the result of proliferation of capillary endothelial cells in the corium and the coincident exudation of serum, and occasionally erythrocytes, into the epidermis. Viral microtubular aggregates are found in the endothelium of dermal capillaries, but not in the epidermal layer. Therefore the rash may represent an Arthus reaction elicited by viral antigen within dermal capillaries. The contribution to disease and recovery of cytotoxic immunospecific lymphocytosis is under study.

No consistent or characteristic physiologic aberrations are observed with measles. The transient hemoconcentration and albuminuria found with other febrile diseases may occur. A normal total leukocyte count or leukopenia is observed throughout the febrile period. Initially, the leukopenia is occasioned by a decline in lymphocytes on the first day of fever; subsequently, granulocytopenia ensues as well. It has been demonstrated that measles virus replicates in lymphoid tissues (spleen, thymus, lymph nodes), can multiply in vitro in peripheral blood T and B lymphocytes and monocytes, and can be isolated from blood leukocytes during the course of the disease. The incubation period is characterized by neutrophilia, and convalescence by a relative lymphocytosis. Measles virus has been isolated from the leukocytic fraction of blood, and is propagable in suspensions of leukocytes in vitro. A false-positive serologic test for syphilis may be observed.

Immunosuppressive Effects of Measles. It has long been known that cell-mediated immunity is impaired during measles. There is transient suppression of the tuberculin reaction (observed also with measles vaccines), improvement in eczema and allergic asthma, delay in wound healing, and the induction of remissions in leukemia, Hodgkin's disease, Burkitt's lymphoma, and lipoid nephrosis. Actual infection of activated lymphocytes may explain the depression of cell-mediated immunity during the acute disease. In severe disease, the magnitude of depression of the total lymphocytes has been positively correlated with a lessened chance of recovery.

CLINICAL MANIFESTATIONS. After an incubation period that averages 11 days, measles becomes clinically manifest with symptoms of fever, malaise, myalgia, and headache. Within hours *ocular symptoms* of photophobia and burning pain are evidenced by conjunctival injection, tearing, and exudate in the conjunctival sac. Concomitantly, or soon thereafter, *catarrhal inflammation of the respiratory tract* is manifested by sneezing, coughing, and nasal discharge. Less commonly, hoarseness and aphonia may reflect laryngeal involvement. In this prodromal stage of one to four days' duration, petechial lesions of the palate and pharynx or tiny white spots on the buccal mucosa *(Koplik's spots)* may herald the appearance of skin rash. The white lesions described by Koplik characteristically occur lateral to the molar teeth, and typically are mounted on red areolae of injected mucosa, which may coalesce to form a diffuse red background. Not invariably present, they constitute a valuable, if not pathognomonic, diagnostic sign. The enanthem may involve other mucous membranes such as the vaginal lining. It may "overlap" the subsequent appearance of the cutaneous rash by one to

Upper: Early measles eruption. (Reproduction from Therapeutic Notes, by Courtesy of Parke, Davis & Company.) *Lower:* Koplik's spots in measles (Hecker, Trumpp, and Abt).

three days. Rarely, a transient, erythematous exanthema may occur in the prodromal period.

The *rash* of measles follows the prodromal symptoms by two to four days, occasionally as late as seven days. It first appears behind the ears or on the face as a blotchy erythema, spreads downward to cover the trunk, and finally is manifest on the extremities. The hands and feet may escape involvement. Initially, the eruption consists of discrete, reddish-brown macules that blanch with pressure. Subsequently, these lesions become slightly elevated, tend to coalesce, and may develop a hemorrhagic, nonblanching component. Rash is sometimes very extensive in children with protein-calorie malnutrition, and skin lesions associated with kwashiorkor may develop at the site of the exanthem. The rash fades in the order of its appearance; its disap-

pearance about five days after onset is attended by a fine, powdery desquamation that spares the hands and feet. At its maximum the exanthema usually marks the termination of malaise and fever in the uncomplicated illness.

The *fever* of measles is commonly of the typhoidal, progressively rising type, and falls by lysis. It persists for about six days, and frequently reaches 39.5° C. In the adult, fever may follow rather than antedate the catarrhal symptoms. Throughout the febrile period, productive *cough* and auscultatory evidence of bronchiolitis may be evident. These manifestations may persist after defervescence, and cough is often the last symptom to disappear. It is probable that bronchopulmonary symptomatology is an integral part of the primary viral infection; roentgenographic evidence of pulmonary involvement is frequently seen in the uncomplicated disease in the absence of leukocytosis and obvious bacterial infection.

COMPLICATIONS. It is difficult to distinguish between those complications directly attributable to the virus of measles and those resulting from secondary bacterial infections. The persistence or recurrence of fever and the occurrence of leukocytosis are presumptive evidence of the usual bacterial sequelae of *otitis media* or *pneumonia*. The pneumonia resembles other forms of viral pneumonia and is often caused solely by a specific reaction to the measles virus. Superimposed bacterial infection is common, however, and accounts for most of the severe or fatal cases. Pneumococcus, *Streptococcus hemolyticus, Staphylococcus aureus,* and *Hemophilus influenzae* are the usual secondary invaders. The incidence of bacterial complications is increased by crowding, debility, and the prevalence of bacterial pathogens in the population. Bacterially engendered sequelae may be unduly frequent in crowded contagious disease hospitals.

Serious complications directly related to the measles virus are rare. *Laryngitis* of sufficient severity to embarrass respiration has been observed, and may warrant tracheostomy. *Electrocardiographic abnormalities* may be found in as many as 30 per cent of children, but clinical evidence of cardiac disease is meager in such cases. *Abdominal pain* or *diarrhea* may be related to invasion of lymphoid tissue of the appendix or Peyer's patches. These symptoms may lead to unnecessary surgery before the appearance of the typical rash. The frequency of stomatitis and gastrointestinal symptoms is greater in malnourished children in tropical areas and may reflect coincident bacterial and parasitic infection.

Encephalomyelitis. A rare (0.1 per cent) but serious consequence of measles is a demyelinating encephalomyelitis that may appear from 1 to 14 days after the onset of infection. This complication is associated with a recurrence of fever, and headache, vomiting, and stiff neck. Stupor and convulsions occasionally follow. Localizing neurologic symptoms may or may not be present. Death ensues in about 10 per cent of patients; about half of survivors suffer permanent residuals of varying severity. Measles virus has been recovered from the brain of a patient with fatal measles "postinfectious" encephalitis six weeks after onset of measles. Recently, abnormal electroencephalograms were recorded in 51 per cent of children with measles *without evidence of encephalitis*. In some of the children the abnormal encephalographic findings were persistent. As noted above, the presence of virus has been demonstrated in patients with subacute sclerosing panencephalitis.

Other late sequelae of measles are thrombocytopenic purpura and exacerbation or activation of pre-existing pulmonary tuberculosis. The late complication of subacute sclerosing panencephalitis (see Immunity, above) is discussed in Ch. 310.4.

Giant-Cell Pneumonia. In children with severe disease involving the reticuloendothelial system (especially leukemia), measles virus may induce an interstitial pneumonia characterized by giant cells and intracellular inclusion bodies. The disease is usually fatal; if the patient survives, persistence of virus and poor antibody formation are evident in convalescence. The pneumonia may occur in the absence of rash so that its etiologic relation to measles may be unsuspected.

Measles Modified by Vaccine or Antibody Administration. Attenuation of the natural disease by antibody prophylaxis may result in an illness of lessened severity comparable with the milder infection of the maternally immunized newborn. Fever alone may be observed, but some degree of exanthema is usually apparent. Koplik's spots may not appear. In general, the course is truncated and relatively uncomplicated. Similar attenuated disease may occur in children partially immunized with inactivated viral vaccine.

Unfavorably Modified Measles—A New Disease. After administration of inactivated measles vaccine (no longer in general use), infection of vaccinees with either live measles vaccine or wild-type natural measles virus led to the development of a new syndrome characterized by dermal hypersensitivity to measles virus and an atypical (petechial, vesicular, or urticarial) rash atypical in distribution. In some cases pulmonary complications occurred. The mechanism of this reaction is unknown, but it may be a manifestation of delayed hypersensitivity to the viral proteins engendered by alum-precipitated inactivated viral vaccine. No such sequelae have followed primary immunization with live virus vaccine. Failure of inactivated vaccine to protect may be related to the absence of the hemolysin antigen of the viral envelope.

DIAGNOSIS. The experienced layman can diagnose typical measles. The querulous, bleary-eyed child, his face blotched and his nose crusted with exudate, presents a characteristic, if miserable, picture as he breathes open-mouthed between paroxysms of sneezing and coughing. The severity of the catarrhal symptoms distinguishes the disease from other eruptive fevers. In the prodromal period the diagnosis should be suggested by (1) fever higher than that of the usual common cold, (2) known measles in the community, and (3) Koplik's spots on the buccal mucosa.

Differential diagnosis (see accompanying table) includes consideration of rubella, scarlet fever, exanthema subitum, infectious mononucleosis, secondary syphilis, drug eruptions, and infection with certain coxsackie- and echoviruses. Of value in excluding these possibilities are the milder course and pinker rash of rubella, the sore throat and leukocytosis of scarlet fever, and serologic tests for infectious mononucleosis and syphilis. The rash of exanthema subitum does not appear until the termination of fever. Fever, enanthema, and catarrh are uncommon with the cutaneous manifestations of drug hypersensitivity.

Specific Diagnosis. Specific diagnosis depends on the isolation of measles virus from throat washings, blood, or urine by inoculation of various types of tissue culture with materials obtained during the first five days of illness. Increase in specific antibody may be detected as early as the first or second day of rash by the complement-fixation test. Antibody is also demonstrable by neutralization and hemagglutination-inhibition procedures. The latter is generally employed for serologic surveys and is correlated with susceptibility to infection.

Presumptive diagnosis may be made if giant cells are detected in stained smears of nasal exudate in the preeruptive period.

PROGNOSIS. Uncomplicated measles is rarely fatal, and complete recovery from the disease is the rule. Fatalities are almost always the result of secondary streptococcal or pneumococcal pneumonia, occurring principally in children below the age of five who become infected after the dissipation of passive neonatal immunity. Mortality in economically underdeveloped countries may be 250 times that observed in the United States or northern Europe. Case fatality rates are also high in elderly and tuberculous patients. Congestive cardiac failure is a common cause of death in patients over 50 years old.

Antimicrobial drugs effective against the usual secondary invaders have reduced the case fatality rate of measles sharply. The incidence of otitis media and pneumonia may be lowered by the prophylactic use of penicillin or a tetracycline early in illness.

Encephalitis occurs as frequently in mild as in severe measles (i.e., about one in a thousand cases). However, the incidence of neurologic sequelae after administration of attenuated live virus vaccine is only one in a million.

TREATMENT. There is no specific treatment for measles.

Symptomatic Therapy. In the absence of complications, bed rest is the essence of treatment in this usually benign, self-limited disease. Codeine sulfate (0.015 to

A Guide to the Differential Diagnosis of Measles

	Conjunctivitis	Rhinitis	Sore Throat	Enanthem	Leukocytosis	Specific Laboratory Tests Available
Measles	++	+	0	+	0	+
Rubella	±	±	±	±	0	+
Exanthema subitum	±	±	0	0	0	0
Enterovirus infection	0	±	±	0	±	+
Scarlet fever	±	±	++	0	+	+
Infectious mononucleosis	0	0	+	0	±	+
Drug rash	0	0	0	0	0	0

0 Not usually present; no test available.
± Variable in occurrence.

+ Present; test available.
++ Present and severe.

0.06 gram) is useful in the amelioration of headache and myalgia and is effective in the management of cough. Aspirin (0.3 to 0.6 gram) may be employed for its analgesic and antipyretic actions. Diet should be unrestricted. Bright light is not an ocular hazard, but photophobia may require darkening of the patient's room.

Antimicrobial Prophylaxis. The course of uncomplicated measles is not influenced by antimicrobial therapy. In common practice the incidence of serious bacterial infections is not sufficient to justify the routine prophylactic use of antimicrobials. Certain special circumstances may warrant full therapeutic dosage with penicillin or the tetracyclines in anticipation of the potentially fatal sequelae of pneumococcal or beta-hemolytic streptococcal infections. These circumstances include treatment of the chronically ill, the very young, or the aged, and the treatment of patients under crowded conditions that foster the increase and dissemination of pathogenic bacteria, as may occur in contagious disease hospitals. If careful observation of the patient is possible, rational therapy is based on the prompt recognition and etiologic definition of complications, followed by initiation of the appropriate antimicrobial drug in proper dosage.

PREVENTION. Vaccination. Highly effective vaccines are available for the prevention of measles. Most are derived from the Edmonston strain of measles virus isolated in the laboratory of Dr. John Enders. This strain, although it proved very effective in early trials as a live virus vaccine, produced febrile and other reactions (attenuated measles) with such high frequency that it has been supplanted by *"further attenuated" (live virus) vaccines* that are almost as effective as the original vaccine in inducing immunity. These live virus vaccines produce immunity by infection, and therefore need be given only as a single injection. They induce antibody response of somewhat lesser magnitude than that following natural infection. In children over one year of age, seroconversion after vaccination is 90 to 97 per cent. Although a gradual fall in antibody titer occurs in the absence of exposure to wild type virus (see Epidemiology: Immunity), serum antibody is demonstrable in most individuals 8 to 15 years after a single administration of vaccine. The occasional failure of live virus vaccine to protect has recently been related to vaccination at less than 12 months of age, at which time maternal antibody may inhibit replication of the vaccine virus. It is now recommended that measles immunization be deferred until after 15 months of age in technologically advanced countries in which infantile infection is uncommon. Reimmunization is not harmful and is recommended for those who have received vaccine before 13 to 15 months of age.

Contraindications to live virus vaccine include pregnancy, leukemia and other systemic malignant diseases, active tuberculosis, and administration of resistance-depressing drugs such as corticosteroids and antimetabolites.

Inactivated vaccine produces impermanent immunity and unfavorably alters response to later infection. It therefore is no longer recommended (see Complications, above).

Eradication of measles through administration of live virus vaccines is a scientifically reasonable possibility. The introduction of immunization in the United States in 1963 has led to a decrease in annual incidence of

from about 500,000 to 35,000 cases per year. However, subsequent resurgence of disease is undoubtedly attributable to underutilization of vaccine in susceptible groups, particularly populations in impoverished circumstances. The reinstitution of Federal funds for measles vaccine in 1971 reversed the upward trend of disease in the following year.

Christiansen, P. E., et al.: An epidemic of measles in southern Greenland, 1951. Acta Med. Scand., 144:313, 430, 450, 1952–53.

Enders, J. F., Katz, S. L., Milovanovic, M. V., and Holloway, A.: Studies on an attenuated measles-virus vaccine. I. Development and preparation of the vaccine: Technics for assay of effects of vaccination. N. Engl. J. Med., 263:153, 1960.

Kimura, A., Tosaka, K., and Nakao, T.: Measles rash. I. Light and electron microscopic study of skin eruptions. Arch. Virol., 47:295, 1975.

Koplik, H.: The diagnosis of the invasion of measles from a study of the exanthema as it appears on the buccal mucous membrane. Arch. Pediat., 13:918, 1896.

Panum, P. L.: Observations Made During the Epidemic of Measles on the Faröe Islands. Delta Omega Society, 1940.

Tyler, H. R.: Neurological complications of rubeola (measles). Medicine, 36:147, 1957.

Yeager, A. S., Davis, J. H., Ross, L. A., and Harvey, B.: Measles immunization. Successes and failures. JAMA, 237:347, 1977.

84. RUBELLA

(German Measles)

Edwin D. Kilbourne

DEFINITION. Rubella is an acute, benign, contagious disease of children and young adults. The cardinal manifestations of the illness are a pale pink rash and posterior cervical lymphadenitis. Paradoxically, this mild disease is one of the few viral infections convincingly associated with the genesis of fetal abnormalities. When infection is acquired in utero, it often results in generalized disease of the infant and protracted excretion of virus after birth. Accordingly, recognition and prevention of the disease are matters of far-reaching consequence.

ETIOLOGY. Rubella virus is a small, spherical RNA virus with a mean diameter of 550 to 600 Å. The particle is ether sensitive — an attribute of lipid-containing enveloped viruses. The virus develops by budding from marginal and intracytoplasmic membranes. On the basis of its structure and chemical characteristics, the virus has been classified as a separate genus (*Rubivirus*) of the togaviruses. Unlike other togaviruses, there is no evidence of its transmission by arthropods. The virus is clearly unrelated to the virus of measles.

The virus agglutinates the erythrocytes of newly hatched chicks — a characteristic that permits measurement of both virus and antibody. Rubella virus replicates with the production of cytopathic effects in a number of commonly employed cell culture systems, including African green monkey and human diploid cells. Virus replication and production of embryopathic effects similar to those in humans have been experimentally induced in rats.

EPIDEMIOLOGY. Precise information on the incidence of rubella is not available, but 82 to 90 per cent of young adults have specific hemagglutination-inhibiting (HI) antibodies against the virus. The mildness and brevity of clinical signs of rubella may confound the diagnosis and reporting of many instances of infection.

Studies of the experimental disease lend support to prior clinical evidence that infection may occur without rash, and indicate a further diagnostic pitfall. It can be said, however, that the disease is seen on every continent, may occur in epidemic form, and has its highest incidence in the early spring. The disease is less frequently acquired in childhood than measles, as is attested by serologic studies and by the fact that rubella is more common than measles in young adults. The higher incidence of infection in younger age groups in institutional outbreaks argues against a greater susceptibility of the adult. Prior to the introduction of rubella vaccination in the United States in 1969, the highest attack rates were observed in infants and children of less than nine years of age. Since 1972, a relative (but not absolute) increase in the number of cases in adolescents and young adults has occurred. It is probable that rubella is spread by the respiratory route by close and sustained personal contact. The usual infection is contagious during the period of prodromal symptoms and for as long as seven days after the appearance of rash. However, it is now recognized that the infant with congenitally acquired infection may excrete virus for months after birth and is contagious during this time. The epidemiologic implications of this fact — first established in the large epidemic of 1963–1964 — are yet to be determined. There is evidence that the newborn may be unusually contagious, and that although he may have no obvious stigmata of infection, yet he may be shedding virus. The relative contribution of children and young adults to the spread of infection is under debate. However, herd immunity is of little consequence in curtailing infection.

Immunity is lasting. HI antibodies have been demonstrated 30 years after initial infection. Authenticated second attacks are rare, and require serologic documentation because of the nebulous nature of the clinical syndrome. *Subclinical* reinfection demonstrated by increase in IgG serum antibody has been documented with increasing frequency as better serologic methods and increased surveillance have become available. Reinfection occurs most commonly in crowded populations in which the density of infection and probably of spread are high. It is important to note that most such reinfections are not associated with viremia and thus probably pose little threat in pregnant women. As in many other infections, IgM response serves to distinguish primary from reinfection. Presumably, as in measles, inapparent infections may boost immunity throughout life. Immunity that follows artificial immunization with live virus vaccine is of a lesser degree. (See Prevention, below.)

PATHOLOGY. Death from uncomplicated postnatally acquired rubella is unknown. Histologic changes characteristic of the disease have not been demonstrated. The onset of disease is attended by leukopenia resulting from a decrease in both lymphocytes and neutrophils. Rubella infection causes temporary suppression of response of lymphocytes to mitogens. After five days, absolute lymphocytosis is manifest. The total leukocyte count is normal at the tenth day.

Congenital Rubella. Necropsies of fetal and infantile victims of maternal infection have shown a variety of embryonal defects related to developmental arrest involving all three germ layers. Those defects most consistently associated with maternal rubella are microcephaly, cataract, patency of the ductus arteriosus, and

defects of the interventricular septum. However, recent studies have revealed a wide spectrum of tissue damage in association with virologically proved disease of varying severity. In some infants hepatic and renal degeneration and myocardial necrosis without inflammation have been noted, whereas in others thrombocytopenia and purpura may be the sole abnormality. It has been proposed that the generalized visceral involvement and characteristic residua of the disease may result from a sequence of platelet damage, intravascular coagulation, and thrombosis. Another theory holds that the smaller size of the rubella-infected infant and some abnormalities may reflect inhibition of multiplication of embryonic cells by the virus.

CLINICAL MANIFESTATIONS. Postnatally Acquired Rubella. Fourteen to 21 days after exposure to the infection, the onset of rubella is evidenced by symptoms variable in their occurrence and severity. Cough, sore throat, and coryza may initiate the illness, but are often absent; headache, malaise, and myalgia may precede the eruption, especially in young adults. Commonly, fever and obvious enlargement of posterior cervical nodes antedate the appearance of the rash. Fever, when present, rarely exceeds 38° C and seldom persists beyond 48 hours. Injection of the bulbar conjunctivae may be noted. Palpable, tender, and occasionally visible lymphadenopathy involves postauricular and suboccipital nodes with sufficient frequency to be an important diagnostic sign. Generalized peripheral lymphadenitis, and, more rarely, splenomegaly, may occur.

The exanthema of rubella is usually apparent within 24 hours of the first symptoms as a faint macular erythema that first involves the face and neck. Characterized by its brevity and evanescence, it spreads rapidly to the trunk and extremities, sometimes leaving one site even as it appears at the next. The pink macules that constitute the rash blanch with pressure and rarely stain the skin. Rubella virus has been isolated from the skin lesions. Diffuse erythema on the second day of rash may closely simulate scarlet fever. The eruption has vanished by the third day. Rubella may occur without rash. An enanthema has been described that is inconstant in form and occurrence, and lacks the premonitory significance of the Koplik spots of measles. The lesions consist of red macules that usually involve the soft palate.

COMPLICATIONS. Recovery is almost always prompt and uneventful, although relapse occurs with greater frequency than in most viral diseases (5 to 8 per cent). Secondary bacterial infections rarely occur. Rare complications are arthralgia, neuritis, gingivitis, thrombocytopenic purpura, and increased capillary fragility. Heart block has been described. A *meningoencephalitis* of short duration may occur one to six days after the appearance of rash. Its incidence is estimated at 1 in 6000 cases, and it is fatal in approximately 20 per cent of those afflicted. Rubella encephalopathy is not associated with demyelinization (in contrast to other postviral encephalitides). Survivors may have electroencephalographic abnormalities, but intellectual function seems to be preserved.

Congenital Rubella. The fortuitous coincidence of the development of cell culture systems for the isolation of rubella virus and the occurrence of a global epidemic of rubella (in 1963–1964) demonstrated that the classic ocular and cardiac "teratogenic" effects of rubella are but isolated manifestations of a continuing and persisting fetal infection. It is now clear that congenital trans-placental infection of the fetus occurs as a consequence of maternal infection (which may or may not be clinically evident), usually in the first trimester of pregnancy. Virus is demonstrable in placental and fetal tissues obtained by therapeutic abortion at that time. If pregnancy is not interrupted (and spontaneous abortion is uncommon), fetal infection persists, and upon delivery of the infant, virus is recoverable from the throat, urine, feces, conjunctivae, bone marrow, and cerebrospinal fluid of the living infant and from most organs at autopsy. About 10 to 15 per cent of infants born to mothers infected in the first trimester of pregnancy have stigmata of infection readily recognizable in the first year of life. These include *cardiac lesions, cataracts, glaucoma, microphthalmia,* and *esophageal atresia.* Most infants in whom virus is detectable do not have evidence of disease at birth or may simply have a lower than normal birth weight. In others, disease of intermediate severity occurs. Most prominent of these manifestations is *thrombocytopenic purpura,* which disappears soon after birth. *Hepatosplenomegaly* may persist for months. Other signs include *corneal clouding, fullness of the fontanels, lesions of the long bones,* and *electroencephalographic abnormalities.* A chronic erythematous rash associated with the presence of rubella virus in the skin has been reported in some patients. Recently, a progressive panencephalitis simulating subacute sclerosing panencephalitis has been observed in the second decade following congenital infection.

A striking finding has been the persistence of virus in the pharynx, gastrointestinal tract, and cerebrospinal fluid for as long as one year after birth (9 per cent). Infective virus was present in a congenital cataract after three years, and in the urine of a victim of congenital rubella 29 years after her birth. This evidence of continuing viral synthesis occurs coincidentally with circulating antibody (initially of maternal origin) and originally suggested a form of "immunologic tolerance" to the virus. However, it has been shown that the character of the antibody changes during the first year from IgG (presumably maternal) to IgM, indicating a primary response of the infant to the persisting viral antigen. Studies of older infants and children with stigmata of congenital rubella show them to be free of demonstrable virus and to possess the IgG immunoglobulins that characteristically persist after other viral infections. The defect in host response that is responsible for viral persistence has not yet been defined.

DIAGNOSIS. Rubella may be diagnosed clinically with assurance only during an epidemic. It may be difficult to distinguish from mild or modified measles, infectious mononucleosis, or scarlet fever. Distinction from measles may be made on the basis of pinker, nonstaining rash, the milder course, and the lesser catarrh of rubella. Sore throat is a more prominent complaint in scarlet fever; the course of infectious mononucleosis is often more protracted, and splenomegaly is more frequent than in rubella. Specific diagnosis of rubella is made by isolation of the virus in any of several cell culture systems, or by demonstration of neutralizing, hemagglutination-inhibiting, or complement-fixing antibody response during infection. The high incidence of dermatoglyphic abnormalities (50 per cent) and increased percentage of chromosome breaks described in patients following congenital rubella may prove to have diagnostic value when studied further.

PROGNOSIS. Complete recovery from postnatally acquired rubella is almost invariable. The rare deaths attributable to rubella follow the infrequent complication of meningoencephalitis. Infection in pregnancy constitutes a hazard to the fetus but not to the mother.

TREATMENT. There is no specific treatment for the disease. Few patients suffer discomfort severe enough to warrant symptomatic medication. Headache and myalgia may be controlled by aspirin; bed rest is advisable for the duration of the fever.

PREVENTION. Passive Immunization. *Administration of gamma globulin to the pregnant woman may only mask her symptoms of infection yet not protect the fetus from viral invasion.* Its use may thus only obscure the picture and confound decision about the need for therapeutic abortion. Hence the practice seems inadvisable unless continuation of pregnancy is elected.

Active Immunization. Rubella may be prevented in children and adults by the parenteral administration of attenuated live virus vaccines produced in cell cultures. Seroconversion rates after immunization are approximately 95 per cent. As with other live virus vaccines, serum antibody titers are lower than those that follow natural infection. However, antibody persists for at least eight years after vaccination, but the permanence of vaccine-induced immunity must still be established by further observation. Natural infection of individuals immunized with vaccine is not uncommon, although such infection is usually asymptomatic. In children, vaccination is attended by little or no reaction; but in women, rash, malaise, arthralgia, and mild, acute arthritis occur frequently, the incidence being directly related to age. For this reason, and in order to induce "herd immunity" to depress circulation of the virus, it is currently recommended in the United States that immunization be carried out principally in childhood. However, since the epidemic threshold—at least in semiclosed populations—is low (between 4.7 and 8.4 per cent), containment of the disease by childhood immunization has proved difficult. A high level of vaccine-induced immunity in elementary school children (83 per cent) failed to prevent the spread of rubella in one community. Despite the higher reaction rates in adults, it seems advisable to immunize adolescent girls or women of childbearing age for whose unborn children rubella may have tragic consequences. Of this population, only seronegative nonpregnant individuals should be immunized, and contraception (when appropriate) should be carried out for at least three months after vaccination. The inadvertent administration of vaccine to pregnant women has demonstrated that attenuated vaccine viruses can infect the fetus and thus have the *potential* for teratogenesis, although the risk is very low. The use of vaccine in the United States apparently has prevented a large epidemic of rubella expected in the early 1970's and has reduced the reported annual occurrence from 57,686 cases in 1969 to 16,343 in 1975.

Cooper, L. Z.: Rubella: A preventable cause of birth defects. *In* Bergsma, D. (ed.): Birth Defects: Original Article Series, Vol. IV, No. 7, Intrauterine Infections. The National Foundation, December, 1968, pp. 23–35.

Gregg, N. M.: Congenital cataract following German measles in the mother. Trans. Ophthal. Soc. Austral., 3:35, 1941.

Hayden, G. F., Modlin, J. F., and Witte, J. J.: Current status of rubella in the United States, 1969–1975. J. Infect. Dis., 135:337, 1977.

Proceedings of the International Conference on Rubella Immunization. Am. J. Dis. Child., 118, July 1969.

EXANTHEMS ASSOCIATED WITH ENTEROVIRAL INFECTIONS

See Ch. 95.

85. VARICELLA
(Chickenpox)
Sidney Kibrick

DEFINITION. Varicella is an acute infectious disease, characterized by a generalized vesicular eruption which appears in crops over several days. It is generally mild in children but may be severe in adults, newborns, and immunologically compromised patients.

Herpes zoster (shingles) is due to the same virus but is manifested by a localized eruption and primarily affects adults. It is thought to represent reactivation of a latent varicella virus in individuals with waning immunity to this agent (see Ch. 305).

ETIOLOGY. The agent responsible for these disorders is the varicella-zoster virus (V-Z virus), a member of the herpesvirus group. Weller isolated etiologic agents from both diseases in 1953 and subsequently established their similarity. Only one serotype is recognized. The virion, which is about 200 nm in diameter, has a DNA core, an icosahedral capsid, and a lipid-containing envelope. Man is the only known natural host. The virus is quite labile and loses its infectivity quickly (probably within hours) in the external environment. Complement-fixing antigens have been demonstrated in vesicle fluid and in cultures of the virus. When propagated in susceptible cells, V-Z virus produces a focal cytopathogenic effect similar to that induced in vivo, with multinucleated giant cells and intranuclear inclusions.

EPIDEMIOLOGY. The disease is spread by airborne droplets and by direct contact with infected lesions. It may also be spread from person to person by a third individual (i.e., by indirect contact) within a limited time and distance, as on a hospital ward. Varicella is communicable from one day before onset of the rash until all the vesicles have crusted — five or six days after the rash appears in the average case, somewhat longer in more severe cases. The prodrome and early stages of eruption represent the periods of greatest communicability.

Although V-Z virus may be spread by respiratory secretions, it has rarely been possible to isolate this agent from nasal or pharyngeal secretions. By contrast, infectious virus is easily recovered from vesicle fluid, and the communicability of this disease coincides with the period when virus can be recovered from the skin lesions.

Incidence and Prevalence. Varicella is primarily a disease of childhood. In temperate zones it is most common between two and eight years, with a peak on beginning school. Cases occur throughout the year but predominate in winter and spring. Inapparent infections are rare. Newborns of mothers who have had the disease are protected by maternal antibodies for up to about six months, but the degree of protection varies. Varicella is one of the most contagious of infectious diseases. Susceptible children exposed to cases in the same household had a secondary attack rate of 87 per cent. Histories of this disease in adults are often unreliable; in one study only 8 per cent of adults with supposedly negative histories acquired varicella from household contacts. Individuals with varicella usually develop lifelong immunity (but may subsequently develop zoster). Varicella may also be acquired by susceptible persons following close exposure to zoster; the attack rate has been estimated at about 15 per cent or less, however, which is considerably lower than that following similar exposure to varicella.

PATHOGENESIS AND PATHOLOGY. It is assumed but not proved that the virus enters and initially replicates in the respiratory tract. This is followed by a viremia which disseminates virus throughout the body. Focal lesions then appear in the skin and occasionally in the viscera and enlarge by virus spread from infected to contiguous cells. The occurrence of the lesions in crops is consistent with an intermittent viremia. With appearance of circulating antibody (about one to four days after onset of the rash) the viremia ceases and symptoms begin to subside.

The histopathology of the skin lesions in varicella, herpes zoster, and herpes simplex is identical. The initial skin changes occur in the endothelium of capillaries in the corium. Cells in the basal and prickle layers undergo ballooning degeneration, and edema fluid quickly accumulates, elevating the stratum corneum to form a clear vesicle containing large amounts of infective virus. The adjacent infected cells develop nuclear changes with margination of chromatin and appearance of an eosinophilic inclusion in each nucleus. In addition, multinucleated giant cells containing such inclusions begin to form at the edges and base of the lesions. As the vesicles begin to dry, they become cloudy with accumulated inflammatory cells and desquamated epidermal cells, and the viral content declines. Finally the lesions crust, the epithelial cells at their base regenerate, and the crusts are shed. In fatal cases, areas of focal necrosis associated with cells showing characteristic intranuclear inclusions may be found throughout the respiratory tract, kidneys, adrenals, liver, and other organs.

The pathologic changes associated with varicella encephalitis are nonspecific and are similar to those seen in the other viral postinfectious encephalitides (see Ch. 309).

CLINICAL MANIFESTATIONS. After an incubation period of 14 to 16 days (range, 10 to 23 days), the disease is usually manifested in young children by low-grade fever, malaise, and rash. In older patients, the eruption may be preceded by a one- or two-day prodrome consisting of fever and constitutional signs such as malaise, myalgia, and headache. The lesions, which first appear on the trunk and scalp, begin as small red macules and progress rapidly over 12 to 24 hours through stages to papules, vesicles, pustules, and crust formation. Pruritus is associated with the vesicular stage and may be quite marked. The vesicles are thin walled, superficial, and surrounded by prominent red areolae, which fade as the lesions dry. The crusts may fall off in a week or persist for several weeks, especially in lesions that become secondarily infected. Underlying areas generally heal completely over weeks to months; occasionally a pit or scar may persist.

The exanthem appears in successive crops over a

one- to six-day period. Thus, as the disease progresses, a characteristic feature is the presence of lesions in various stages of development in the same anatomic area. Those in the final crop may regress after reaching the maculopapular stage.

The varicella rash has a centripetal distribution, being most abundant on the trunk and face and relatively sparse on the extremities. It is usually increased, however, in areas of irritated, damaged, or inflamed skin.

Vesicles may also occur on the mucous membranes, especially in the mouth. Other sites which may be involved include the vaginal mucosa, conjunctiva, and pharynx. Lesions on mucous membranes break down to form shallow, generally painful ulcers, which heal without crusting.

Fever parallels the severity of the rash and persists while new lesions continue to appear. Prolongation or recurrence of fever is associated either with bacterial superinfection or with some other complication of the disease. As with many other viral infections, varicella is usually more severe in adults than in children, with higher fever, more marked rash, and more frequent complications.

About 16 to 33 per cent of adults, and uncommonly children, develop clinical or radiologic evidence of pneumonitis during their disease. Chest films show diffuse nodular densities throughout both lung fields with a tendency to concentrate at the bases and hilum. The changes subside quickly in mild cases but may persist for several months in severe cases, lagging behind clinical recovery. In some patients, fibrotic scars remain and gradually calcify over several years, resembling the radiologic changes in healed miliary tuberculosis.

Encephalitis may occur with both mild and severe cases of varicella and is responsible for 90 per cent of the neurologic complications of this disease. Its incidence is estimated at less than one per 1000 cases. The manifestations are similar to those associated with measles or vaccinial encephalitis and may be quite severe with coma, seizures, appreciable mortality, and permanent sequelae. In about one third of patients with encephalitis, especially in children, cerebellar dysfunction with ataxia is the most prominent feature, and such patients generally do well, recovering completely within one to three weeks (see Ch. 305).

Patients who are susceptible to varicella and who have leukemia, lymphoma, or congenital or acquired immunodeficiency or are on immunosuppressive medication represent a high risk group. Newborns whose mothers have developed varicella within the four days before delivery also fall into this category, presumably because they have received no maternal antibodies against this disease. In such high risk patients, varicella is generally more severe; pneumonia, disseminated visceral disease, secondary bacterial infection, central nervous system involvement, and hemorrhagic phenomena are more common, and mortality is significantly increased.

Additional manifestations which have been noted in varicella include *bullous rash, hepatitis, carditis, nephritis, orchitis, and arthritis.* About 10 per cent of cases of Reye's syndrome (acute encephalopathy and fatty degeneration of the viscera) have been associated with an immediately preceding varicella (see Ch. 309.4).

Maternal infection with V-Z virus during the first four months of pregnancy has been reported to result occasionally in a syndrome of severe congenital malformation with hypoplasia of body parts, neurologic deficits, and ocular lesions. The incidence of such cases is not known.

DIAGNOSIS. The typical case of varicella can be easily recognized on the basis of its characteristic clinical features. A history of exposure within the preceding several weeks is helpful. The demonstration of multinucleated giant cells in Wright- or Giemsa-stained scrapings of young vesicles (Tzanck smear) or in biopsies of affected tissues establishes the lesions as due to either V-Z or herpes simplex virus. Further differentiation between varicella, herpes zoster, and herpes simplex can then generally be made on the basis of associated clinical findings. Intranuclear inclusions, although also a feature of infection with these viruses, are best seen with stains which utilize acid fixatives such as Bouin's or Zenker's solution.

Viral isolation and/or serologic tests are generally necessary only to confirm unusual cases. The virus can be readily isolated from vesicle fluid and identified in appropriate tissue cultures, or the presence of viral antigen can be confirmed by immunofluorescence. The demonstration of a rising titer of complement-fixing antibodies to V-Z antigen is also useful but must be interpreted with care, as this virus shares some antigenic components with herpes simplex virus. Complement-fixing antibodies decline rapidly and may not be detectable after 6 to 12 months. Neutralizing antibodies persist, but their determination is technically difficult.

Other entities with a generalized vesicular eruption include smallpox, eczema vaccinatum, eczema herpeticum, rickettsialpox, disease due to certain coxsackieviruses, and some allergic rashes. None of these meet the criteria for diagnosis of varicella, and their differentiation from this disorder should present little difficulty.

TREATMENT. There is no specific therapy for varicella. Treatment is symptomatic and directed at relief of local discomfort and control of secondary infection. Supportive measures include aspirin for high fever and constitutional symptoms and lukewarm starch baths, calamine lotion, and/or antihistamines for pruritus. Nails should be kept clean and short to minimize skin infection from scratching. Patients with varicella pneumonia or encephalitis may need ventilatory support and attention to hydration, electrolyte balance, and nutrition. Bacterial or fungal superinfection may be important in the compromised host. There is no evidence that either prophylactic antimicrobial drugs or corticosteroids are of value in this disease. Patients who develop varicella while on immunosuppressive doses of steroids should have the dose of such medication reduced to one to one and a half times physiologic levels (0.7 to 1.0 mg of cortisone per kilogram per day or its equivalent) as rapidly as is consistent with safety, and should be maintained at this level until the disease has subsided. Patients receiving other immunosuppressive therapy should also have the dose of their medication reduced. There is no evidence that passive immunization may modify the disease in such patients.

PREVENTION. Human immune serum globulin in large doses, given to normal children within three days of exposure to varicella, does not prevent but will attenuate the disease. Zoster immune globulin (ZIG), prepared from convalescent zoster serum, is more potent and can prevent varicella under such circumstances. The ZIG does not prevent this disease in susceptible high risk children, but reduces both morbidity and mortality in this group if given within three days of exposure. *Information regarding the availability of ZIG for pediatric patients who meet high risk criteria and for high risk newborns may be obtained from the Division of Clinical Microbiology, Sidney Farber Cancer Institute, 44 Binney Street, Boston, Mass. Telephone: 617-732-3121.* Former ZIG consultants and officials from the CDC Immunological Division are available for consultation regarding alternative modes. Telephone: 404-633-311 (days) or 404-633-2176 (nights, weekends, or holidays). Exposed patients on immunosuppressive therapy should not only receive ZIG but also have the dose of their medication reduced until the risk of varicella is past.

An experimental live virus vaccine is currently being tested. Preliminary results are reported as promising.

Brunell, P. A., and Gershon, A. A.: Passive immunization against varicella-zoster infections and other modes of therapy. J. Infect. Dis., 127:415, 1973.

Cimons, I. M., Lacher, M. J., LaMonte, C. S., Levitt, L., Cady, B., and Beattie, E. J., Jr.: Treatment of varicella pneumonia. JAMA, 206:372, 1968.

Feldman, S., Hughes, W. T., and Daniel, C. B.: Varicella in children with cancer: Seventy-seven cases. Pediatrics, 56:388, 1975.

Kempe, C. H., and Gershon, A. A.: Varicella vaccine at the crossroads. Pediatrics, 60:930, 1977.

Weller, T. H.: Varicella-zoster virus. In Lennette, E. H. (ed.): Diagnostic Procedures for Viral and Rickettsial Infections. New York, American Public Health Association, 1969, pp. 733–754.

Williamson, A. P.: The varicella-zoster virus in the etiology of severe congenital defects. A survey of eleven reported instances. Clin. Pediat., 14:553, 1975.

86. VARIOLA AND VACCINIA

C. Henry Kempe

86.1. INTRODUCTION AND HISTORY

Immunization against the dread disease of smallpox was, until recently, perhaps the most widely applied immunization procedure. Over the past 150 years it has demonstrated its effectiveness beyond question. The vaccinia virus *(Poxvirus officinale)*, which is in effect a laboratory strain carried for many generations in a variety of laboratory animals, differs from the newly isolated virus of cowpox *(Poxvirus bovis)*, which was originally employed by Jenner (1798) and some of his fellow physicians for the immunization of man against the smallpox virus *(Poxvirus variolae)*.

Smallpox was described in detail by Rhazes in the tenth century, and had been described previously by Galen in the second century. Spread from Asia to Europe and North Africa occurred in the Middle Ages, and the disease was prevalent in the sixteenth century. At approximately the same time, the disease was introduced into the West Indies by African slaves and from there into Mexico and South America. The best studied epidemics are those in the eighteenth century in England, when over 90 per cent of the cases occurred in children under ten years of age and when smallpox accounted for one third of all deaths in children. Smallpox occurred in epidemic form less frequently in North America until 1752, when over 30 per cent

of the inhabitants of Boston, Massachusetts, were affected and the mortality rate was over 30 per cent (Creighton, 1894). In 1721, deliberate inoculation of smallpox (variolation) as protection against the natural disease was introduced in England from Turkey. It consisted of the inoculation of pustular material by puncturing the skin. This resulted in a febrile disease after an eight-day incubation and a general eruption on the ninth day. The mortality rate from this procedure was 1 to 2 per cent, and it is stated that 17 of 897 inoculated persons died from the disease (Woodville, 1796). Needless to say, modified infection did give rise to highly virulent natural disease in susceptible contacts. In 1738 variolation was successfully used in Charleston, South Carolina, with material that had been allowed to dry. With better care of the patients, the death rate was somewhat reduced. It was thought to be about one or two out of 500, whereas the mortality from the naturally acquired smallpox was 10 to 20 per cent. Variolation was replaced by inoculation of cowpox afer widespread acceptance of Jenner's studies published in 1798. Whether Jenner should be regarded as the originator of vaccination is not certain, but he did play a decisive role in popularizing this method of protection against smallpox, and variolation was outlawed in England in 1840.

86.2. VARIOLA
(Smallpox)

ETIOLOGY. Smallpox virus is readily visible with any microscope equipped with darkfield illumination or by phase contrast microscopy. With electron microscopy, the smallpox virus resembles elementary bodies of vaccinia virus. The elementary bodies are small, brick-shaped structures with a diameter of about 200 mμ. They can be demonstrated by direct examination of smears of early skin lesions. The virus is very resistant to drying, and living virus can be demonstrated in scabs kept at room temperature for over three years. Virulent virus has survived on clothing of patients, and has caused the disease in laundry workers who were not protected.

ERADICATION PROGRAM. In 1967, when an intensified eradication program was begun, there were 42 countries reporting a total of 131,000 cases of smallpox. As it is likely that only about 1 per cent of cases were actually reported, it is estimated that 10 to 15 million cases occurred in 1967 in 30 countries that had endemic smallpox and in 12 others that experienced importations. In contrast, in 1972, 19 countries reported 65,000 cases at a time when reporting had been vastly improved.

By 1977 only one country — Somalia — had endemic smallpox. Five cases occurred in Kenya as a result of importation.

In South America, Brazil was the last country to become smallpox free. Now, after 450 years, smallpox has been eliminated from the Western Hemisphere. Variola major was last seen on the subcontinent of Asia in 1975, whereas variola minor (alastrim) occurred in 1977 in Somalia.

EPIDEMIOLOGY. The only natural reservoir of smallpox is thought to be the patient suffering from the disease. The patient is not infective until the third day of the clinical disease, that is, one day before the maculopapular phase of the skin eruption is noted. Contacts may be allowed at large until they actually become ill, because patients are not infective during the early pre-eruptive febrile disease.

Intensive efforts are currently being made to determine a possible nonhuman host; among the possibilities are a nonhuman primate or a rodent. The surprising and significant animal reservoirs of yellow fever and malaria, which have materially affected the eradication campaign for those two diseases, have, understandably, also been of concern to those working in the field of smallpox.

Between 1970 and 1977, 28 cases of infection occurred in humans in areas of Africa which had been free of smallpox for two years or more. Only 2 of the 28 patients had been vaccinated. No human source of infection was discovered, but none of over 100 unvaccinated close contacts subsequently contracted the disease. Virus was isolated and appeared indistinguishable from monkeypox virus isolated among outbreaks in captive monkeys, but there was no illness among monkeys in the area (Ladnyr, 1973). Therefore, although it is possible that monkeypox can cause a clinical illness resembling smallpox in man, its infectivity appears to be low.

PATHOLOGY AND PATHOGENESIS. It is likely that the site of entry of the smallpox virus is the respiratory tract and, possibly, the eye. In the 12-day incubation period the virus probably multiplies in the regional lymphoid tissues. In the unmodified case, a massive viremia occurs at the onset of the fever, and continues during the first two or three days of the pre-eruptive phase. In this way the virus localizes in the mucous membranes and in the skin as well as in the internal tissues. After the virus disappears from the blood and the skin eruption appears, the patient feels better and the temperature tends to decrease. Antibodies are noted in the blood as early as the fourth day of the disease. The virus multiplies in the epithelial cells of the skin while relatively protected from the action of circulating antibody so that cell destruction continues for some time. When pustulation occurs, the temperature tends to rise again, probably because of the absorption of the toxic products of cell necrosis. It is of interest that patients become infectious on the third day of the disease, probably because saliva has been contaminated through the early mucosal lesions noted in the pharynx and mouth. Skin lesions become infective after the superficial cornified layer has been disrupted. Scabs remain infectious throughout the illness and until their separation during the third to fourth week of illness. The pitting is generally confined to the face and is due to destruction of sebaceous glands followed by organization and subsequent shrinking of granulation tissue and fibrosis. In cases of hemorrhagic smallpox numerous blood cells are present in the corium. Cytoplasmic inclusions are characteristic of infection with the vaccinia-variola group of viruses. Inclusion bodies can be shown best in epithelial cells, particularly of the involved skin and mucous membranes. Skin scrapings stained with hematoxylin and eosin show the inclusion to be round or oval homogeneous masses, either basophilic or acidophilic, located in the cytoplasm fairly close to the nucleus. The appearance of the inclusion bodies varies with the stage of infection but also with the method of fixation and staining, and this suggests that they consist of masses of elementary bodies. Intranuclear inclusions have also been described, but these are not invariably seen. With antimicrobial therapy, pathologic changes from bacteri-

al complications are not found, and bacterial cultures, in this situation, are usually sterile.

CLINICAL MANIFESTATIONS. The incubation period of smallpox is generally 12 days. The illness begins with severe malaise and high fever lasting for four to six days. There is intense prostration, and the clinical impression is often that of dengue. Severe headache, photophobia, and, occasionally, vomiting are noted. A small number of patients show a prodromal or "toxemic" rash, most easily noted in the groins, the axillae, and the flanks. On the fourth day the focal rash occurs, the fever diminishes slightly, and the patient feels better, just at a time when the first macular skin lesions begin to form. The focal rash usually occurs first on the mucosa of the mouth and pharynx, the face, or the forearms, and it then spreads to the trunk and legs. *A feature of variola is the fact that lesions in any one area are all at the same stage of development, whereas in varicella they are in all stages.* The initial rash is macular and quickly becomes papular. Within two days the papules have developed into vesicles, and these, within a few hours, become cloudy and pustular. On the eighth or ninth day from the beginning of the rash, drying and crusting begin. From three to four weeks from the onset of the disease, scabs have generally fallen off, leaving pigment-free skin. Subsequently, scarring or pitting develops. The eruption is characteristically more severe on the face and the distal parts of the arms and legs, and less severe over the trunk and abdomen. The groins and axillae may be entirely spared. This centrifugal distribution is distinct from the characteristic rash of varicella, which tends to be centripetal. Lesions are often found on the palms of the hands and the soles of the feet, a situation uncommonly seen in varicella of childhood, although these parts may be involved in the adult form. Varicella may also cause osteomyelitis and arthritis. Fever generally recurs during the pustular stage, but the temperature returns to normal as the lesions become encrusted. The characteristic pustular lesions of smallpox are round, raised, and tense, with a tendency to central depression as they begin to dry out. Clinical classification of disease from the mildest form (variola sine eruptione) to modified, to confluent, to malignant confluent, to hemorrhagic indicates degrees of severity of smallpox influenced in part by age, state of immunity, and state of hormonal balance. It is of great interest that women within a short time of term, either before or after delivery, tend to have a much more severe disease than those not pregnant.

In cases modified by vaccination or transplacental immunity in the first few months of life, the rash may be scant and the evolution of lesions may be very quick. Regardless of how mild an index case of smallpox may be, the susceptible infected contacts suffer unmodified disease, and overlooked mild cases are sometimes the cause of severe epidemics. Permanent scarring may result even in the absence of purulent infection of lesions with secondary bacterial pathogens (staphylococci and streptococci) in patients who have deep lesions and serious disease.

In previous years, the bacterial complications were incriminated as the principal cause of death, particularly after the pustular phase had commenced. It is now known that the mortality rate is chiefly related to the amount of virus present in the blood during the viremic phase that occurs in the first two days of the disease before any eruption is noted. It has been shown that if the amount of virus in the blood is so great that the whole blood of the patient in the viremic pre-eruptive phase can be used as the antigen in the complement-fixation test, the patient will almost surely die, although death may be delayed for nine or ten days. Patients who die in the first week of the illness often show evidence of heart failure and terminal pneumonia. Even in the absence of any antimicrobial therapy, the lungs are often sterile, indicating that the pneumonia is caused by the smallpox virus itself. The majority of deaths occur, however, in the pustular stage toward the end of the second week of the disease. Occasionally an encephalitis has been described that is indistinguishable from that associated with measles, varicella, or smallpox vaccination and tends to occur between the eighth and sixteenth days of disease.

INFECTION IN UTERO. No congenital anomalies have been described in infants of mothers infected with smallpox, but abortion is common because of the frequent bleeding that occurs during the toxemic phase. Infection of the fetus in utero may occur during the viremic phase in the mother; if this occurs near the end of the pregnancy, the child will show clinical disease within a few days after birth. Infection has also been shown to occur at the time of birth if the disease is still active in the mother. There are two reports of smallpox in babies infected in utero a few days before birth, although the mothers showed no signs of the disease (Bancroft, 1904; Lynch, 1932).

VARIOLA MINOR. In the twentieth century, a milder clinical form of smallpox became prevalent in the Western Hemisphere. It was recognized in Brazil in 1910, when a widespread outbreak of this mild form of the disease was recorded with a mortality of only 1 per cent. To this mild type of smallpox, the name alastrim — variola minor — was given. Similar mild forms of the disease were recognized in Africa.

The vast majority of epidemics seen in this century in North America and Europe have been due to variola minor. Thus there were 12,000 cases in 1927 in England and Wales and over 48,000 cases in 1930 in the United States. In the 1930's with the widespread application of smallpox vaccination in infancy, smallpox began to decrease in the United States. An important factor in this decrease was the better preservation of smallpox vaccine with the wider availability of refrigerators. It is likely that more potent vaccines and widespread improvement of health services also contributed to the decline in the number of cases. The two types of disease (variola major and variola minor) appeared to be distinct with a markedly different mortality for the two. At present there would appear to be no evidence that an outbreak of alastrim gives rise to cases of classic variola major, although the two types may produce coexistent separate outbreaks, as they apparently did in Detroit in 1924.

There is complete cross-protection for these two infections as there is from vaccinia. The clinical picture is similar in the prodromal or pre-eruptive phase to that of variola major, but hemorrhagic and toxic cases are almost never seen. The lesions tend to be more superficial and develop more rapidly; the total illness is shorter than in classic variola major. There may be no secondary fever during the pustular stage.

DIFFERENTIAL DIAGNOSIS. Smallpox is easily diagnosed, particularly during an epidemic period. More difficult to diagnose is the first and unsuspected case in those countries where smallpox is not endemic. This is particularly true if the first case is hemorrhagic. In this situation meningococcemia, a bleeding diathesis as part of a blood dyscrasia, or typhus may be the suspected diagnosis. Very mild smallpox, modified by previous vaccination or alastrim, may be thought to be varicella, a drug eruption, or erythema multiforme. Except after known exposure, the clinical diagnosis cannot be made with certainty during the febrile phase, because the picture is indistinguishable from that of dengue, enteroviral infections, and other febrile diseases. In the eruptive phase, the most useful clinical points to remember are (1) the centrifugal distribution of lesions; (2) the fact that in a given area all the lesions are at the same stage of development; (3) the presence of a severe, febrile, three-day pre-eruptive disease; and, on occasion, (4) a known contact at least 12 days previously.

LABORATORY TESTS. Laboratory diagnostic procedures are of great value in quickly establishing the diagnosis of smallpox in the first case that appears in a community. These consist of (1) electron microscopic demonstration of viral particles in stained smears of vesicular fluid, (2) serologic or fluorescent demonstration of viral antigen in materials from cutaneous lesions, (3) isolation of virus from such materials, and (4) detection of antibodies in the serum early in the eruptive phase. The results of such tests are particularly helpful in differentiating variola from varicella and the hemorrhagic forms of the disease from other conditions (see Ch. 85). A detailed description of these procedures may be found in the reference by Downie and Kempe.

TREATMENT. No specific treatment for smallpox is currently available, although a number of promising antiviral drugs are under study. Penicillin and broad-spectrum antimicrobials have been used in the prevention and treatment of bacterial complications. There is suggestive clinical evidence that secondary late bacterial complications, including pneumonia and staphylococcal involvement of skin and bones, are decreased by the use of antimicrobial therapy. But even with such therapy the mortality rates have not been reduced below 25 per cent in most outbreaks of variola major. Good nursing care and maintenance of fluid and electrolyte balance are essential. Convalescent smallpox serum and vaccinia-immune gamma globulin have been used in the treatment of severe cases without any evidence of success.

PREVENTION OF SMALLPOX. Management of Recently Exposed Persons. The use of vaccinia-immune gamma globulin (see below) has been successful in the prophylaxis of smallpox and has reduced the incidence after known contact fourfold in control trials (Kempe et al., 1956, 1961). The results among methisazone-treated* groups have been variable (Bauer et al., 1963, 1969; Do-Valle et al., 1965; Rao et al., 1969; Heiner et al., 1971). In Heiner's study only the vaccinated contacts showed a significant reduction in attack rates (twofold), and no difference in mortality or severity was noted between tested and placebo groups.

---

*Manufactured by Burroughs Wellcome. Available in England; not available commercially in the United States.

Community Control. There is no evidence that we owe our freedom from smallpox in the United States to routine vaccination. Compulsory routine vaccination was discontinued in Great Britain in the late 1950's, and 90 per cent of the population has either never been vaccinated or not vaccinated in the past ten years. Since 1969 there have been 12 smallpox importations into England, but the experience with secondary cases, deaths, and generations of cases until control has been no different in that country than in Germany, which has a far higher level of immunity in its population. Public health policy in the United States has long held that high immunity levels are vital. This has been thoroughly discredited, because importations have caused repeated outbreaks even though as many as 90 per cent of the population in an area were vaccinated. Individuals who have not had a recent successful vaccination can be infected and may have a difficult-to-diagnose case. They can, nevertheless, transmit the infection in its most virulent form. In 1973, this has been shown again in the case of the English laboratory worker who had a greatly modified case of smallpox but still was able to transmit the infection in a fatal form to two contacts. There has been no smallpox in the United States since 1949, because we have been fortunate in not having the virus introduced rather than because our population is adequately protected. If variola major had been introduced, secondary cases would have resulted. However, their number would have depended on early versus late diagnosis, prompt versus delayed vaccination of contacts, isolation of cases, surveillance of contacts and isolation of any who developed fever during the 14 days following exposure, careful case finding, as well as on the presence of a high level of immunity in our hospital staff personnel.

In 1964, because of the persistent concern with the number of serious complications of smallpox vaccination, the writer recommended the discontinuation of nonselective routine vaccination of American children. *Selective* vaccination as a general policy was endorsed in 1971 by all major public health and professional groups, except for the American Medical Association. Vaccination is now limited to (1) travelers to endemic areas, and (2) contacts of those with proved cases of smallpox. The global eradication programs have been successful in eradicating variola major. Until alastrim has also been eradicated, however, it will be necessary to remain constantly alert that foreign quarantine procedures and selected traveler surveillance are maintained at a high level, and that adequate measures are taken, from both the clinical and laboratory points of view, in making the proper diagnosis at the earliest possible time.

With currently available techniques, an importation of smallpox and the development of some secondary cases in an unprotected population will, even with failures in early diagnosis, not result in any greater number of deaths than have occurred in the past 40 years from universal infant vaccination itself.

Control of Infected Persons, Contacts, and Environment. All cases should be reported to the local health authority, and patients should be isolated in a hospital until all crusts have disappeared. All oral, nasal, fecal, and urinary discharges and articles associated with patients should be disinfected by burning, high-pressure steam, or boiling. All contacts at home, place of work, or elsewhere should be vaccinated or revaccinated with a potent product and kept under daily surveillance for 16 days from the time of last contact. Any fever during surveillance calls for prompt isolation until smallpox can be excluded. The patient's source case should be sought assiduously. Adults with chickenpox or patients with hemorrhagic or pustular lesions of the skin need careful review for possible errors in diagnosis.

Epidemic Measures. In an epidemic the measures to be taken are as follows: (1) All smallpox patients and suspects should be isolated in hospital until they are no longer infectious. (2) All contacts should be carefully listed, vaccinated, and kept under surveillance for 16 days. (3) A public statement of the situation should be made by all available methods, and all possible contacts should be urged to be vaccinated. Potent vaccine should be provided and arrangements made for early vaccination of inner-ring and outer-ring contacts. (4) The use of vaccinia immune gamma globulin for close household contacts should further decrease the number of secondary cases. (5) Mass immunization of the entire population of a community or larger area is an emergency measure to be used only when an outbreak has given evidence of uncontrolled spread.

International Measures. The World Health Organization and countries adjacent to the one in which an outbreak occurs should be notified by telegram of the existence of any cases of smallpox. At all times, the measures applicable to ships, aircraft, and land transport arriving from smallpox areas should be enforced, as specified in International Health Regulations. It should be noted that evidence of protection by successful vaccination or revaccination (within a period of three years) is a widely enforced requirement for entry to the United States for *travelers from endemic countries but no others.*

Vaccination vs. Chemoprophylaxis. Vaccination remains the best method of prevention for any individual likely to be exposed through travel in the smallpox-endemic regions. To be fully effective, successful revaccination every three years is recommended.

Upon exposure to a case of smallpox, vaccination and revaccination should be supplemented by vaccinia-immune gamma globulin. Vaccination after exposure is effective if done promptly but may not prevent disease. It should be done in any case, however, because in an epidemic situation subsequent repeat exposures may occur. The use of vaccinia-immune gamma globulin markedly reduces clinical incidence and severity when used in full doses of 10 ml intramuscularly once for adults and 5 ml intramuscularly once for children under 12 years. Vaccinia-immune globulin and methisazone* can and should both be given, when available, for a limited number of known close contacts.

WHO and health agencies of member countries in which there is endemic smallpox depend on vaccination alone and concentrate on the elimination of specific smallpox foci. One attempt is to break the transmission chain rather than to rely on mass vaccination campaigns, which had been the accepted method in the attempts at eradication in the past. It was shown that, particularly in Africa and Asia, it is much more efficient and economical to try to interrupt transmission at a time of low seasonal incidence of smallpox. Current strategy consists of an attempt to contain outbreaks of

---

*Manufactured by Burroughs Wellcome. Available in England; not available commercially in the United States.

smallpox by the early detection and containment of cases so as to reduce smallpox incidence as quickly as possible, rather than the institution of mass vaccination.

In an outbreak in central Java in 1969, when more than 95 per cent of the 23,000,000 inhabitants in the province bore vaccination scars, almost 1700 cases of smallpox nevertheless occurred, 85 per cent of them developing in persons who had never been successfully vaccinated. In other words, in a population in which only 5 per cent had not been successfully vaccinated, continued transmission was readily possible — definite evidence that "herd immunity" does not work. The incredible success obtained in West and Central Africa, Indonesia, Ethiopia, and the Indian subcontinent is entirely due to this change of strategy based on early detection of outbreaks and the establishment of trained teams to investigate and contain them. Case finding requires a reporting network which had to be developed. The use of freeze-dried potent vaccine replaced liquid vaccine in all WHO programs. A very useful tool for case finding is the WHO photo recognition card often given to schoolchildren, who proved to be one of the most fruitful sources of information in remote villages in Asia and Africa. The schoolchild through recognition cards, visits to the principal markets which are held every week in different locations, and searching out through walking from village to village and house to house are the bases for case finding which lead to case identification and subsequent vaccination.

86.3.   VACCINIA
(Vaccination)

Smallpox vaccine commonly in use is prepared from the vaccinia lesions on the skin of inoculated calves or sheep or from the allantoic membranes of chick embryos. All currently used smallpox vaccine contains infective virus, and all successful vaccinations are deliberately induced mild viral infections. The mortality in smallpox patients successfully vaccinated many years before is less than in the unvaccinated. There is no question that regular revaccination induces a high degree of immunity even with very massive exposure to the disease.

RECOMMENDED PROGRAM FOR VACCINATION IN THE UNITED STATES

We can look forward to the time when the present eradication program will have eliminated smallpox as a threat to man. At that time, vaccination will no longer be necessary, and jennerian vaccinations will then be a matter of only historic importance. Until this is achieved, however, smallpox vaccination will continue to be necessary for those travelers to endemic areas as well as those in the armed forces.

CONTRAINDICATIONS TO VACCINATION. Primary *routine* vaccination is no longer performed on North American infants, but even *selective* vaccination is contraindicated in infant patients who fail to thrive; in persons with dysgammaglobulinemia or blood dyscrasias; in those with eczema or other dermatitides; in the presence of radiation or other immunosuppressant therapy; in those exposed to infectious diseases; or in unvaccin-

ated siblings of children with eczema. If exposure is likely, elective vaccination of the eczematous child *should* be performed, because the incidence of eczema vaccinatum in this situation is only 1 in 150 and the mortality is zero. Vaccination or revaccination is absolutely contraindicated for adult patients with neoplastic diseases, including Hodgkin's disease, lymphomas, and other conditions involving the prolonged use of corticosteroids, nitrogen mustard, or radiation therapy.

When travel outside the limits of the United States to nonendemic areas is contemplated, vaccination is no longer required for re-entry into the United States. At most, telephonic health surveillance for 14 days after re-entry to the United States may be required. This is much to be preferred to life-threatening disease from vaccination. Vaccination has not been carried out by the Quarantine Service when the patient's physician has presented written evidence that the procedure should not be performed. If such a person must travel to an endemic area, the use of vaccinia-immune gamma globulin should be considered so as to provide temporary protection and to act as a substitute for the use of vaccination with live vaccinia virus.

RECOMMENDED VACCINATION TECHNIQUES. To minimize the risk of unnecessary complications, the following practices are recommended:

Age for Primary Vaccination. In nonendemic areas, primary vaccination is not routinely done. There are no conclusive data indicating the exact period when complication rates are minimal. The presence of some transplacental maternal immunity, provided that the mother has been vaccinated, may be desirable in modifying the primary vaccination reaction, and vaccination may be carried out in the first months of life. Vaccination of newborn infants has been done without complications (Kempe et al., 1952). However, in such cases in endemic areas, revaccination should be performed after an interval of six months. If primary vaccination is delayed for several months, children who are at increased risk, such as those suffering from the Swiss type of agammaglobulinemia, will have been readily identified by their clinical course and will therefore not become casualties of smallpox vaccination. The 1966 experience in the United States fails to show a higher risk of postvaccinial encephalitis for the two-to-ten age group (Neff et al., 1968), but some European authors have stressed that the first years of life may be a safer period. The case mortality for encephalitis is certainly highest among the youngest children (Berger, 1964; Coneybeare, 1948; Muller, 1946; Neff, 1968).

Site for Vaccination. Primary vaccination and revaccination are best performed on the outer aspects of the upper arm, over the insertion of the deltoid muscle, or behind the midline. Reactions are less likely to be severe on the upper arm than on the lower extremity or other parts of the body. With proper technique, resultant scars are small and unobtrusive.

Preparation of the Vaccination Site. With a clean skin, the best preparation is none at all. The use of chemical skin cleansers may leave a residue that contains virus-inactivating material, and vigorous physical cleansing of the site may create minute abrasions that then can become sites of secondary vaccinia eruptions, with resultant involvement of a comparatively large skin area.

Vaccination Technique. Regardless of age, primary vaccination should be performed with no more than two or three pressures with the side of a bifurcated needle. These pressure points should be as close together as possible, and should be made only at one site. With the highly potent vaccines currently in use, more numerous pressure points are not necessary and certainly should not be utilized for a nonimmune person. When children or adults are to be revaccinated after a lapse of more than five years, the same small number of pressure points should be used. For revaccination within a five-year period of those persons known to have had major reaction, the full complement of 30 strokes can safely be used (Leake, 1946).

VACCINATION REACTION. The description of the reactions after vaccination or revaccination should follow the criteria recommended by the Expert Committee on Smallpox of the World Health Organization. A successful primary vaccination is one that on examination after seven to ten days presents a typical jennerian vesicle. If this is not present, vaccination must be repeated with fresh vaccine and a few more pressures of the bifurcated needle. The successful revaccination is one that on examination one week (six to ten days) later shows a vesicular or pustular lesion *or* an area of definite palpable induration and congestion surrounding a central lesion; this lesion may be a scab or an ulcer. These reactions are termed *major reactions;* all others should be called *equivocal reactions*.

A major reaction indicates virus multiplication with consequent development of immunity. An equivocal reaction may merely represent an allergic response, which could be elicited by inactive vaccine or poor technique in someone who has been sensitized by earlier vaccination; or the equivocal reaction may result from sufficient immunity to prevent virus multiplication. Since the allergic response cannot be readily differentiated from the one caused by true immunity, another vaccination should be performed, using a different lot of vaccine if there is a possibility that the first was of weak potency, and the procedure should be completed with an additional number of pressures. The site should be examined one week later; if the result is again equivocal, revaccination should be repeated, using a full 30 pressures as recommended by Leake. For the sake of expediency, an equivocal reaction to revaccination with a minimal number of insertions may be followed by vaccination at two sites, not less than 2 inches apart, using known potent vaccine. This method will make a third return unnecessary in almost all instances.

To sum up: Successful smallpox vaccination consists of the production of a major reaction. When potent vaccine and good technique are used, repeated inability to produce a major reaction can be assumed to be due to solid immunity from previous immunization.

FREQUENCY OF VACCINATION. Revaccination is essential to reinforce the immunity conferred by previous vaccination. This not only maintains a high level of immunity against smallpox but also minimizes the risk of complications on revaccination. To maintain adequate immunity against smallpox, revaccination should be carried out at approximately three-year intervals.

COMPLICATIONS OF VACCINATION

With the abandonment of universal routine vaccination of infants in 1971, complications in the United States have markedly decreased. Life-threatening complications of primary vaccination include eczema vaccinatum, postvaccinial encephalitis, and vaccinia gangrenosa (progressive vaccinia). The principal danger after revaccination is vaccinia gangrenosa, a condition in which the impairment of the patient's immune mechanism permits the continuing multiplication of the vaccinia virus. Vaccinia gangrenosa is seen in seemingly normal subjects, as well as in those suffering from dysgammaglobulinemia, Hodgkin's disease, leukemia, blood dyscrasias, and other conditions in which corticosteroid therapy or ionized irradiation has been administered therapeutically. The presence of these conditions is an absolute contraindication to vaccination.

Human vaccinia-immune globulin has been shown to be effective in the prevention and treatment of eczema vaccinatum and has also been used extensively in the treatment of other complications, in which it also produces a significant reduction in mortality. Vaccinia-immune globulin reduces the incidence of postvaccinial encephalitis. In the Royal Netherland Army, 53,630 of 106,174 recruits received hyperimmune vaccinia-immune gamma globulin, and the remaining 52,544 recruits received a placebo. In the group treated with gamma globulin, 3 cases of postvaccinial encephalitis occurred in contrast to 13 cases in the control group. There was one fatality in each group. Gamma globulin failed to have an effect on the severity and duration of the encephalitis produced by the vaccination, and it was not effective in treatment. There is evidence that transplacental maternal immunity is also effective in modifying the course of primary vaccination; significant reactions are rarely reported in very young infants whose mothers have been vaccinated in the past. In cases of vaccinia gangrenosa, the use of vaccinia-immune globulin appears to be of value. Adequate early treatment of the complications of smallpox vaccination can materially reduce the morbidity and mortality. Through the Center for Disease Control in Atlanta, Georgia, a group of experts is available for telephone consultation (day: 404-633-3311; night: 404-633-2176). When such consultation is used in conjunction with vaccinia-immune globulin, effective diagnostic and therapeutic aids are available for all.

Bauer, D. J., St. Vincent, L., Kempe, C. H., Young, P. A., and Downie, A. W.: Prophylaxis of smallpox with methisazone. Am. J. Epidemiol., 90:130, 1969.

Downie, A. W., and Kempe, C. H.: Variola and vaccinia viruses. *In* Lenette, E. H. (ed.): Diagnostic Procedures for Viral and Rickettsial Diseases. New York, American Public Health Association, 1969, Chapter 25.

DoValle, L. A. R., DeMelo, P. R., DeSalles Gomes, L. F., and Proenca, L. M.: Methisazone in prevention of variola minor among contacts. Lancet, 2:976, 1965.

Heiner, G. G., et al.: Field trials of methisazone as a prophylactic agent against smallpox. Am. J. Epidemiol., 94:435, 1971.

Kempe, C. H.: Smallpox: Recent developments in selective vaccination and eradication. Am. J. Trop. Med. Hyg., 23:775, 1974.

Kempe, C. H., et al.: The use of vaccinia hyperimmune gamma globulin in the prophylaxis of smallpox. Bull. WHO, 25:41, 1961.

Kempe, C. H., et al.: Smallpox vaccination of eczema patients with a strain of attenuated live vaccinia (CVI-78). Pediatrics, 42:980, 1968.

Meiklejohn, G.: Maxwell Finland Lecture. Smallpox: Is the end in sight? J. Infect. Dis., 133:347, 1976.

Neff, J. M.: Complications of smallpox vaccination: I. National Survey in the United States, 1963. N. Engl. J. Med., 276:125, 1967.

Rao, A. R., et al.: Chemoprophylaxis and chemotherapy in variola major: I. An Assessment of CG 662 and Marboran in prophylaxis of contacts of variola major. Indian J. Med. Res., 57:477, 1969.

WHO Expert Committee on Smallpox: Second Report, Publication 393. World Health Organization Technical Report Series. Geneva, World Health Organization, 1968.

For more detailed lists of references see the following:

Dixon, C. W.: Smallpox. London, J. & A. Churchill, Ltd., 1962.

Downie, A. W.: Smallpox. *In* Horsfall, F. L., Jr., and Tamm, I. (eds.): Viral and Rickettsial Infections of Man. 4th ed. Philadelphia, J. B. Lippincott Company, 1965.

87. FOOT-AND-MOUTH DISEASE

(Aphthous Fever)

Walsh McDermott

Foot-and-mouth disease is a viral infection of animals, chiefly cattle, which occurs in man only with great rarity. Infection, when it does occur in man, presumably results from direct contact with the agent either in the laboratory or from handling the tissues or body fluids of infected animals. The disease in man is characterized by a short incubation period followed by the appearance of a febrile illness with vesicular lesions of palms, soles, and sometimes the oropharyngeal mucosa. Neurologic involvement has not been reported, and the disease is self-limited. It may occur in a totally asymptomatic form. The disease is unrelated to hand-foot-and-mouth disease caused by certain coxsackie-viruses, notably A16 (see Ch. 95). There is no treatment of established value; the tetracycline drugs have yielded inconclusive results in the treatment of laboratory animals. Prevention of the disease in man has not been extensively studied, for man generally has a high degree of resistance to the infection. Spread among cattle is presumably by the airborne route. An effective vaccine for use in cattle has been developed. As in influenza, however, there are many types and subtypes of foot-and-mouth (FMD) virus, and it is believed that for optimal effectiveness the homologous viral strain, i.e., the "epidemic" strain, should be present in the vaccine.

Annotations: Spread of foot-and-mouth disease. Lancet, 2:580, 1969.

Flaum, A.: Foot-and-mouth disease in man. Acta Pathol. Microbiol. Scand., 16:197, 1939.

Hyslop, N. St. G.: Transmission of the virus of foot-and-mouth disease between animals and man. Bull. WHO 46:577, 1973.

88. MUMPS

Dorothy M. Horstmann

DEFINITION. Mumps is an acute contagious viral infection, most commonly manifested by nonsuppurative swelling of the parotid glands. Other salivary glands, the testes, pancreas, and central nervous system are among the various organs that may also be involved.

HISTORICAL NOTE. Hippocrates described mumps and its association with orchitis in the fifth century B.C. Because of its characteristic manifestations, the disease was one of the earliest to be recognized as a clinical entity. A classic description was written by Hamilton (1790), who stressed the importance of orchitis as a complication. He also noted that central nervous system signs sometimes accompany the parotitis, but it was early in the twentieth century before clinicians recognized meningoencephalitis as a relatively frequent manifestation. In 1940 Wesselhoeft called attention to the occurrence of oophoritis and pancreatitis, and later others reported involvement of many organs and tissues. Not until 1934 did Johnson and Goodpasture prove the viral etiology of mumps by reproducing the disease in monkeys inoculated with filtrates of infective human saliva. The virus was adapted to growth in hens' eggs in 1945 by Habel, and by Levens and Enders, who demonstrated its hemagglutinating properties. Enders and his associates also described the appearance of dermal hypersensitivity and of complement-fixing (CF) antibodies after mumps. The availability of a skin test and of serologic tools allowed the demonstration that infection with mumps virus can occur without parotitis and not infrequently without any signs at all. Immunization with a killed virus vaccine was tried in the 1950's with limited success. In 1966 Bunyak and Hilleman developed a highly effective live attenuated mumps virus vaccine, prepared in chick embryo tissue culture, which is currently widely used.

ETIOLOGY. Mumps is an RNA virus, a member of the myxovirus family that includes the influenza and parainfluenza viruses. These agents all have the property of agglutinating chicken, human, and certain other erythrocytes. In nature mumps virus infects only man; in experimental infections it induces parotitis in monkeys and meningoencephalitis in hamsters and mice. The virus multiplies in embryonated chick embryos and in a variety of tissue culture cells. For primary isolation (usually from saliva), eggs or preferably cell cultures derived from monkeys or humans are used. In tissue cultures the presence of the virus is recognized either by the appearance of cytopathic changes or by means of the hemadsorption test, which depends on the ability of the virus-infected cells to adsorb guinea pig erythrocytes. Mumps virus is associated with soluble (S) and viral (V) antigens. Antibodies to the S antigen (complement fixing) appear one week after onset; those to the V antigen are delayed and develop after two to three weeks. Only antibodies to the V antigen appear to be protective; they are measured by neutralization, CF, hemagglutination-inhibition, and indirect immunofluorescence tests. A positive skin test indicative of delayed hypersensitivity develops in persons who have been naturally infected or have received mumps vaccine.

EPIDEMIOLOGY. Mumps is a common disease, endemic all over the world. It occurs throughout the year, but there is a seasonal incidence with a regular increase in cases in winter and spring, sometimes reaching epidemic levels. In the United States approximately 20,000 cases were reported in 1977, a marked reduction from the 88,000 median for the five years beginning in 1968 when the vaccine was introduced. Under-reporting is the rule, however, not more than 1 in 10 cases being recorded. The disease incidence is the same in both sexes, but males are more prone to develop central nervous system complications. Most cases occur between the ages of 5 and 15 years; young adults are sometimes susceptible, as evidenced by epidemics in military camps and schools. A far larger number of adults acquire mumps than either measles or chickenpox. There have been scattered case reports suggesting that mumps during pregnancy may have adverse effects on the fetus, but prospective investigations have not revealed differences in rates of abortion, stillbirths, or congenital anomalies in infected and matched control study groups.

The only known reservoir of infection is man. *Transmission* is by direct contact, air-suspended droplets, or fomites contaminated with saliva. The virus is present in saliva from two to seven days before to as long as nine days after parotid swelling appears, but contagiousness is greatest around the time of onset.

Although it is a common disease, only about half the adult population in the United States give a positive history, in contrast to more than 90 per cent for measles. The difference is due in part to the high rate (approximately 30 per cent) of inapparent mumps infections. Asymptomatic infections are particularly common in children under five years old. One experience with mumps virus — whether symptomatic or silent — appears to confer lifelong immunity.

PATHOGENESIS AND PATHOLOGY. The widespread involvement of glandular and other tissues in the body indicates that mumps is a systemic infection. The virus enters and multiplies first in the upper respiratory tract; it then invades the bloodstream, and localizes in the salivary as well as other glands and in the central nervous system. The parotids are one of many target organs, the greater frequency with which they are involved being simply a reflection of greater sensitivity.

Limited observations on pathologic specimens indicate that the reaction in the parotid gland is a nonspecific inflammatory one, which is not extensive. The testes and pancreas also demonstrate inflammatory and degenerative changes. In the rare cases of encephalitis, two types of central nervous system lesions are seen — those resulting from direct viral invasion producing primary encephalitic disease, and the demyelination characteristic of postinfectious encephalitis. Mumps virus has been shown to cause aqueductal stenosis and hydrocephalus in hamsters and mice; the same lesions have been reported as very rare sequelae of mumps encephalitis in man.

CLINICAL MANIFESTATIONS. The incubation period is 14 to 21 days, usually 18. In most cases, pain and swelling in the parotid region are the first signs of the disease, although occasionally in adults pain in the testicle may be the initial symptom. Rarely, meningitis appears first, followed later by parotitis. In more severe cases, there is often a prodromal period, sometimes lasting as long as two or three days, with fever, malaise, headache, chills, sore throat, earache, and tenderness along the region of the parotid ducts.

Parotid swelling is first observed below the ear, usually obliterating the hollow between the mastoid process and the ascending ramus of the lower jaw. The gland increases in size over a two- to three-day period, but there is great variation in the degree of swelling; in mild cases it may be scarcely apparent, but in severe ones the associated edema may eventually spread superiorly to the eyes, posteriorly to the mastoid region, and inferiorly below the chin and over the anterior aspect of the neck. For the first two days, unilateral involvement is the rule, but eventually both glands are affected in about 70 per cent of cases. The skin over the swollen parotids is not usually reddened, but is tense and tender on pressure. Not infrequently the submaxillary and sublingual glands are also affected. Involvement of the sublingual glands can result in swelling of the tongue, with attendant painful swallowing. Presternal pitting edema is also occasionally present, apparently because of obstruction of the lymphatics by the enlarged salivary glands.

The patient seldom suffers severe pain except on movement of the jaws, e.g., in talking or chewing. If Stensen's duct becomes partially occluded as the gland swells, there is sharp pain on taking food or an acid drink, which stimulates the secretory mechanism. Because this occurs only with partial occlusion of the duct, it is not a constant sign. The papillae at the opening of Stensen's or Wharton's duct may be reddened, but this also is inconstant.

Constitutional symptoms vary greatly and may be virtually absent. They are especially mild in children, but tend to be more severe in adults, in whom the incidence of extraparotid lesions is higher. Fever varies with the extent of involvement, ranging between 38 and 39.5° C in full-blown, uncomplicated cases, but going as high as 40.5 and 41° C if orchitis, meningoencephalitis, or both develop.

The duration of parotid swelling and fever is dependent upon the extent and severity of the process. Usually the temperature is normal within five days, and swelling has disappeared by seven to ten days. A peculiar tendency to relapse with recurrence of parotid swelling has been noted in buglers, horn players, and others whose occupations involve similar exertion.

Neurologic Manifestations. The incidence of *aseptic meningitis* varies widely in different epidemics, but can be as high as 25 per cent. Serial examination of the cerebrospinal fluid indicates that the cell count is elevated in approximately one half of all cases of mumps. Clinically evident neurologic involvements may occur preceding, simultaneously with, or after parotitis. It affects males three times more commonly than females, and may be the only manifestation of the infection. The clinical picture of headache, fever, stiff neck, and lethargy is similar to that in other forms of viral meningitis, but the cerebrospinal fluid findings may differ in several respects. Thus cell counts tend to be higher; 500 to 1000 cells, predominantly lymphocytes, are common, and occasionally even several thousand are present. The pleocytosis in mumps is also more prolonged, and may persist for several weeks. Glucose levels below 40 mg per 100 ml have recently been reported in up to 10 per cent of cases. The protein levels are moderately elevated. *Encephalitis,* whether resulting from direct attack by the virus or occurring as postinfectious encephalitis, is rare, but in the United States mumps is the most common cause of encephalitis for which an etiology is established.

Other rare neurologic complications include permanent nerve deafness, either unilateral or bilateral; labyrinthitis; polyneuritis, sometimes affecting the facial or trigeminal nerves; disturbances in accommodation; optic neuritis, iritis, and iridocyclitis; and possibly hydrocephalus.

Orchitis. Orchitis is rare before puberty. After puberty, its incidence varies, but it usually develops in about 25 per cent of cases; there is considerable variation in different epidemics. Testicular involvement is most often unilateral, but may be bilateral, one following the other by one to nine days. The onset is commonly between the fifth and tenth days of illness, as the parotid swelling is subsiding. In mild cases there may be nothing more than discomfort, with tenderness and slight fever. In others, onset is abrupt, with a chill, fever to 40° C or higher, nausea, vomiting, sweats, backache, prostration, and severe testicular pain. Swelling of the testicle may be moderate, or the gland may rapidly reach three to four times normal size, in which case it is excessively hard, tender, and so painful that even 0.030 gram of morphine is not always effective. Epididymitis frequently accompanies orchitis; the spermatic cord may also be involved, and occasionally the prostate.

In mild cases the testicle may be normal in four days, although in the most severe, it may require three or four weeks before all evidence of inflammation has disappeared. Some degree of atrophy, apparently caused by pressure necrosis, occurs in about a third to a half of all cases of orchitis, *but in most instances it is unilateral. Even when both testes are involved, the distribution of the inflammatory reaction and loss of functional tissue are apt to be spotty, and seldom result in sterility.*

Oophoritis. Oophoritis occurs occasionally in adult females, but it may be more frequent than suspected, as mild forms are difficult to recognize. High fever, chills, lower quadrant or back pain, and palpable ovarian enlargement have been described. Sterility resulting from mumps oophoritis is virtually unknown.

Pancreatitis. In the severe form there is sudden onset of epigastric pain and tenderness, vomiting, chills, fever, and prostration. This picture, which is rare, lasts three to seven days and is followed by complete recovery. Mild forms with only abdominal pain and discomfort are thought to be more common but are difficult to diagnose.

Diabetes mellitus has been occasionally reported as a sequela of mumps, leading to the hypothesis that there is a causal relationship between the virus and juvenile onset diabetes. Recent epidemiologic studies have not provided evidence to support this concept. The solution of the problem awaits further prospective investigation.

Other Organs. More rarely, other glands or organs are involved, particularly in adults. The following have been reported as complications of mumps: prostatitis, bartholinitis, and mastitis (in both males and females); involvement of the thyroid, thymus, and lacrimal glands; splenomegaly; and hepatitis. Transient abnormalities of renal function occur frequently, but persistent nephritis is unusual, although fatal cases have been reported. Polyarthritis, occurring ten days to two weeks after onset, is a rare complication. Myocarditis, accompanied by precordial pain or heart block, has been described. Serial electrocardiograms on patients with mumps have revealed some abnormality in as high as 15 per cent, although very few patients show clinical evidence of myocarditis. Several authors have suggested that endocardial fibroelastosis is a result of intrauterine infection with mumps virus. The evidence for this is conflicting, and the issue remains unresolved.

DIAGNOSIS. Sudden onset of parotitis in a previously healthy patient with a negative history of mumps presents no diagnostic problem. Another cause of parotid swelling is suppurative parotitis, an acute bacterial infection in which there is marked tenderness, the skin over the gland is red and hot, and pus can often be expressed from the duct. Salivary calculi obstructing the duct can give rise to recurrent parotitis. Chronic enlargement of the gland occurs with tumors, Mikulicz's disease, and uveoparotid fever of sarcoidosis. Preauricular and anterior cervical lymphadenopathy may simulate parotid involvement.

Mumps infection in the absence of parotitis is often difficult to recognize. Orchitis can be due in rare instances to infection with other viruses such as coxsackievirus B, echoviruses, and lymphocytic choriomeningitis virus. A variety of viral agents cause aseptic meningitis or meningoencephalitis that cannot be distinguished clinically from central nervous system involvement caused by mumps. In such situations specific laboratory tests are necessary to establish the etiology. Mumps virus can be isolated from saliva, urine, and, in meningitis, from the cerebrospinal fluid. More commonly, confirmation of the diagnosis is based on the demonstration of a significant rise in antibody titer when acute and convalescent serum samples are tested. If only a single convalescent specimen is available, the presence of a high titer is suggestive of recent infection. The *skin test* is of no value in diagnosis, because dermal hypersensitivity usually does not develop until three to four weeks after onset; it is less reliable than serologic tests in determining immune status.

Routine laboratory tests frequently indicate a relative lymphocytosis in uncomplicated parotitis; with orchitis, pancreatitis, or aseptic meningitis, the total leukocyte count often reaches 15,00 to 20,000, with a high percentage of polymorphonuclear cells. The blood amylase is usually elevated as a result of parotitis and is therefore not a reliable indication of pancreatic involvement.

PROGNOSIS. Complete recovery is the rule, and death is extremely rare. Fatalities have been associated with encephalitis, myocarditis, and nephritis. Permanent residua are also very uncommon; they include bilateral testicular atrophy (see above) and nerve deafness.

TREATMENT. Bed rest and symptomatic therapy are all that can be offered. For parotid pain, aspirin or codeine is effective. Some patients find an ice bag applied to the parotid region comforting, but others prefer heat. The headache associated with meningitis may be relieved by lumbar puncture. If orchitis is mild, no special treatment is required; if severe, meperidine (Demerol) (0.05 to 0.1 gram) or morphine (0.01 to 0.015 gram) may be necessary to control the pain. Local support and provision of warmth by means of a nest of absorbent cotton are more effective than an ice bag to the scrotum. Corticosteroids relieve the pain but do not appear to alter the duration of illness, nor do they protect against the subsequent development of atrophy. They are not indicated in mild cases, but in severe ones hydrocortisone, 10 mg per kilogram per day, may be given for three to four days.

PREVENTION. A live attenuated mumps virus vaccine, grown in tissue cultures of chick embryo cells, was licensed in 1968. It induces an inapparent infection which is noncommunicable. To date, more than 30 million persons have been immunized in the United States. The vaccine is available as a monovalent preparation or combined with measles and rubella vaccines. It is given subcutaneously, causes virtually no clinical reaction, and induces antibody conversions in more than 90 per cent of susceptibles. The serum titers are lower than those that follow natural infection, but they have persisted satisfactorily for the seven-and-one-half-year period over which antibodies have been tested. Vaccinees have been shown to be resistant to mumps when subsequently exposed to siblings with the disease.

The vaccine may be given to persons of any age over 12 months; it is not recommended for infants under one year because of the possible presence of residual maternal antibody which interferes with the development of active immunity. If the combined measles-mumps-rubella vaccine is used, it should not be given before 15 months of age, because the immune responses to measles antigen are often inadequate in younger infants. Immunization against mumps is recommended particularly for boys approaching puberty who give no history of the disease. If the vaccine is given after exposure, it is unlikely that it will protect. However, it may be given under these circumstances so that if contact infection failed to develop in a susceptible subject who was exposed, he will be protected when he next meets the virus.

Mumps vaccine should not be given to persons with allergy to egg proteins or to neomycin. It is contraindicated for those with any disease that results in compromised immune mechanisms and for patients on immunosuppressive therapy. Since the vaccine contains live virus, it should not be given during pregnancy.

Passive Immunization. Standard gamma globulin is ineffective; mumps hyperimmune globulin given after exposure is of questionable value in preventing parotitis, orchitis, or meningoencephalitis.

Beard, C. M., Benson, R. C., Kelalis, P. P., Elveback, L., and Kurland, L. T.: The incidence and outcome of mumps orchitis in Rochester, Minn., 1935–1974. Mayo Clin. Proc., 52:3, 1977.

Feldman, H. A.: Mumps. *In* Evans, A. S. (ed.): Viral Infections of Humans. New York, Plenum Publishing Corp., 1976, pp. 317–336.

Levitt, L. P., Rich, T. A., Kinde, S. W., Lewis, A. L., Gates, E. H., and Bond, J. O.: Central nervous system mumps. A review of 64 cases. Neurology, 20:829, 1970.

Reed, D., Brown, G., Merrick, R., Sever, J., and Feltz, E.: A mumps epidemic on St. George Island, Alaska. JAMA, 199:967, 1967.

Sultz, H. A., Hart, B. A., Zielezny, M., and Schlesinger, E. R.: Is mumps virus an etiologic factor in juvenile diabetes mellitus? J. Pediat., 86:654, 1975.

Weibel, R. E., Buynak, E. B., McLean, A. A., and Hilleman, M. R.: Persistence of antibody after administration of monovalent and combined live attenuated measles, mumps and rubella virus vaccines. Pediatrics, 61:5, 1978.

Wilfert, C. M.: Mumps meningoencephalitis with low cerebrospinal-fluid glucose, prolonged pleocytosis and elevation of protein. N. Engl. J. Med., 280:855, 1969.

VIRAL DISEASE OF LYMPHOID TISSUE

89. INFECTIOUS MONONUCLEOSIS

James C. Niederman

DEFINITION. Infectious mononucleosis is an acute infectious disease caused by Epstein-Barr virus (EBV). The infection is common in children, and the disease occurs frequently among adolescents and young adults. Identifying clinical features include fever, sore throat, lymphadenopathy, absolute lymphocytosis with an increased number of atypical lymphocytes, and the development of transient heterophil and persistent EBV antibody responses.

HISTORY. In 1889, Emil Pfeiffer described Drüsenfieber (glandular fever), characterized by fever, mild sore throat, adenopathy, and enlargement of liver and spleen in severe cases. Sprunt and Evans named the disease "infectious mononucleosis" in 1920 and called attention to implicative hematologic changes. A detailed description of the distinct mononuclear leukocytes was made by Downey and McKinlay in 1923. Paul and Bunnell established the association between mononucleosis and heterophil antibody in 1932, and shortly thereafter Davidsohn and Walker developed guinea pig kidney and beef cell absorption techniques for increasing the specificity of this antibody determination. EBV was reported as the causal agent of infectious mononucleosis in 1968 by Henle, Henle, and Diehl; and by Niederman, McCollum, Henle, and Henle.

ETIOLOGY. EBV, a member of the herpes group, was first recognized in electron microscopic studies of cell lines of Burkitt's lymphoma biopsies grown in tissue culture. This agent has been demonstrated in cultures of peripheral blood leukocytes from patients both during acute infectious mononucleosis and for years thereafter. In prospective clinical investigations, it has been shown that specific EBV antibodies are regularly absent before the onset of mononucleosis and develop during disease. IgG antibodies to EBV viral capsid antigen, measured by immunofluorescence techniques, are present early in clinical disease and persist for many years; in contrast, EBV-specific IgM antibodies disappear several months after acute illness.

Both heterophil and EBV antibodies develop in squirrel monkeys inoculated repeatedly with EBV autochthonous lymphoblasts. Infection of gibbons by direct pharyngeal injection of the virus has resulted in production of EBV antibodies and exudative tonsillitis. A spectrum of responses ranging from inapparent infection to lymphoid hyperplasia and malignant lymphoma has been observed in cotton-top marmosets following EBV inoculation. Atypical lymphocytes and heterophil antibody have not been demonstrated in experimentally infected marmosets; however, the EBV genome has been detected directly in tumor cell DNA by molecular hybridization techniques.

Inadvertent transmission of EBV to antibody-negative humans by blood transfusion has been associated with the development of EBV antibody and occasionally with the development of heterophil positive clinical infectious mononucleosis. EBV has been regularly demonstrated in the oropharynx of patients with infectious mononucleosis and is present in more than 80 per cent of patients during early disease; shedding persists for months and perhaps years after infection. Recent studies indicate that EBV is located extracellularly in oral fluids and suggest the existence of a cell in the oropharynx in which the full cycle of viral maturation occurs, including envelopment and release.

EPIDEMIOLOGY. Infectious mononucleosis and EBV infections occur worldwide. Antibody to this virus has been demonstrated in every population thus far studied, and the age at which infection is acquired is related to economic factors and hygienic conditions. Infection occurs early in life in economically underdeveloped countries and is usually subclinical or inapparent. In areas where exposure and infection are delayed until older childhood and young adult life, EBV infections are more often expressed as clinical infectious mononucleosis. Occurrence of the disease among young adults, especially in the 15- to 25-year age group, is the most characteristic epidemiologic feature.

No annual or seasonal variations have been observed in the general population. However, in college students periods of high frequency occur in early fall and spring. Among college-age susceptibles, the rate of EBV infections per year is approximately 12 per cent. Measurements of clinical:subclinical cases suggest a ratio of 1:2 to 1:3 in this age group.

Seroepidemiologic studies utilizing EBV-specific IgG antibody markers have regularly indicated that absence of antibody correlates with susceptibility to infectious mononucleosis and its presence with immunity. Prospective studies of over 5000 children and young adults have now been reported in various parts of the world to support this relationship. Antibody to EBV developed in 29 per cent of subjects previously negative to antibody who were observed over periods of four to eight years; the clinical attack rate was 2 per cent per year among these susceptibles.

EBV infections occur in all ethnic groups, and population surveys have indicated no differences in antibody prevalence rates by sex. Clinical infectious mononucleosis is also equally frequent in both sexes; in adolescence, females appear to develop the disease somewhat earlier than males. High EBV antibody prevalence rates among young children in economically underdeveloped countries suggest that the virus spreads rapidly under conditions of crowding and close interpersonal contact to infect almost all susceptibles.

PATHOLOGY AND PATHOGENESIS. Gross pathologic changes in this disease are confined almost exclusively to lymphoid tissues; lymphadenopathy, nasopharyngeal lymphoid hyperplasia, and splenomegaly are outstanding features. Widespread focal and perivascular aggregates of mononuclear cells develop throughout the body. Nonspecific hyperplastic changes occur in lymph nodes without infiltration of the capsule or surrounding tissues; atypical lymphocytes found in peripheral blood are also present in nodal tissues. Nonlymphoid organs, including liver, heart, lungs, central nervous system, and kidneys, are infiltrated, and these focal lesions may be associated with functional abnormalities. Hyperplasia and occasionally small granulomatous lesions have been described in bone marrow particle sections.

Recent observations that EBV is regularly present in saliva shed light on the pathogenesis of this infection. Prolonged excretion of small amounts of infectious virus into the oropharynx accounts for the moderate contagiousness of this virus and the difficulty in demonstrating case-to-case transmission. EBV is also found in throat washings of 15 to 20 per cent of healthy antibody-positive persons without a past history of infectious mononucleosis, indicating that oropharyngeal shedding is common among those who have experienced inapparent EBV infections. Demonstration of the extracellular location of EBV in the saliva elucidates some of the epidemiologic features of infectious mononucleosis. High rates of transmission of this agent in preschool children and young adults can be explained by the greater degree of salivary exchange characteristic of these age groups in comparison with others. The regular finding of EBV in saliva and buccal fluids collected from the orifices of Stensen's ducts points to the salivary glands as a probable major site of virus production. However, the specificity of the producer cell is unknown; it could be ductal or glandular epithelium, oropharyngeal and nasopharyngeal epithelium, or specialized lymphoid cells.

CLINICAL MANIFESTATIONS. Studies of contact infections have suggested an incubation period of 30 to 50 days in the adult. Clinical mononucleosis associated with production of both heterophil and EBV antibodies has developed five weeks after blood transfusion in several patients. Young children appear to have a shorter incubation period of 4 to 14 days, but existing information is scant on this point.

During a prodromal period of four to five days, mild symptoms, including malaise, fatigue, and headache, are frequent. Initial clinical symptoms are extremely variable in severity, but include fever, sore throat, and cervical lymphadenopathy in more than 80 per cent of cases. In adults, fever in the range of 38.3 to 39.4° C may persist for seven to ten days, and elevations to 40.5° C occur in some cases. Conversely, children experience little or no fever with this infection.

Sore throat develops during the first week of disease and is the most common clinical feature of infectious mononucleosis. Inflammation and edema of pharyngeal tissues are present, and an exudative tonsillitis with a thick, gray-white exudate occurs in approximately 50 per cent of patients and persists for seven to ten days. During early disease, the uvula and palatal arch have a gelatinous appearance. At the end of the first week of disease, petechiae are observed near the border of the hard and soft palates in about one third of patients. This palatal enanthem, consisting of crops of 5 to 20 circumscribed red petechiae, is highly suggestive, but not pathognomonic, of mononucleosis.

Lymph node enlargement is a hallmark of infectious mononucleosis. Anterior and posterior cervical nodes are commonly involved, and generalized adenopathy, including axillary, epitrochlear, mediastinal, and inguinal nodes, may develop during the course of disease. The lymph nodes, usually 5 to 25 mm in diameter, may be enlarged singly or in clusters; they are firm, tense, discrete, and distinctly tender on palpation. Lymphadenopathy gradually subsides over a period of several weeks, depending on the degree and extent of involvement.

Splenomegaly develops in approximately 50 per cent of patients. Commonly, the enlarged spleen extends several centimeters below the costal margin, and enlargement is greatest during the second and third weeks of illness.

Although hepatomegaly is demonstrable in only 10 per cent of patients, liver function tests, especially serum transaminase values, are abnormal for several weeks in most cases. Frank jaundice develops in 4 to 5 per cent of patients and occurs most commonly during the first two weeks of illness; it is probably caused by hepatocellular damage, is usually mild, and is rarely associated with acholic stools.

During early disease, about 10 per cent of patients manifest a transient, faint, erythematous, or maculopapular rash on the trunk and proximal extremities. This eruption often resembles rubella, but may be scarlatiniform, urticarial, or hemorrhagic in appearance. Bilateral supraorbital edema may also be a transient early clinical finding.

Less than 1 per cent of patients, usually in the adult age group, have symptoms referable to the central nervous system. In general, neurologic manifestations depend on the anatomic site and extent of involvement; these include aseptic meningitis, Bell's palsy, encephalitis, transverse myelitis, and the Guillain-Barré syndrome. Most patients experience complete recovery; however, a small number of fatalities have been reported in association with encephalopathy and severe paralysis.

A sharp increase of peripheral blood lymphocytes, including atypical lymphocytes, occurs at the end of the first week or ten days of illness. An increase of circulating B (bone marrow–derived) lymphocytes precedes that of T (thymus-derived) lymphocytes. Transient depression of cell-mediated immune responses exists during early disease; however, decreased lymphocyte responsiveness to a variety of antigens and mitogens usually returns to normal in three to six weeks.

DIAGNOSIS. Infectious mononucleosis is diagnosed on the basis of (1) clinical manifestations, (2) characteristic blood picture, and (3) elevated titers of heterophil and EBV antibodies.

The clinical features of this disease include fever, sore throat, lymphadenopathy, and splenomegaly. An absolute increase in the number of lymphocytes and atypical lymphocytes is an essential hematologic finding. Fifty to 60 per cent of peripheral blood leukocytes are of the lymphocyte series at some stage of the disease. Early in the first week of symptoms, there may be leukopenia, but often leukocytosis with a predominance of lymphocytes is present. During the second and third weeks the total count may rise to 20,000 and may occasionally range as high as 50,000 per cubic millimeter. Atypical lymphocytes usually represent more than 10 per cent of leukocytes during disease; also known as Downey cells, these lymphocytes vary in size, shape, and staining quality with round, indented, or lobulated nuclei and basophilic, vacuolated cytoplasm. Morphologically identical cells have been observed in other diseases, including viral hepatitis, rubella, rubeola, cytomegalovirus infections, mumps, and a variety of other infectious, immunologic, and lymphoproliferative disorders. However, in these conditions, unlike mononucleosis, the percentage of atypical lymphocytes is usually less than 10 per cent. Anemia is rare in infectious mononucleosis, and the platelet count is normal in the absence of complicating thrombocytopenia.

During the course of disease, patients develop elevated titers of sheep cell agglutinins (heterophil antibodies) in the serum. These agglutinins are often present during the first week of illness, but their appearance may be delayed. In one study of 166 mononucleosis patients, the heterophil antibody test was positive in 38 per cent of cases during the first week of disease, in 60 per cent during the second week, and in 80 per cent during the third week. Elevated heterophil titers usually persist for three to six months and occasionally longer. In general, the higher the antibody titer during acute illness, the longer it persists in convalescence. Adults usually have higher heterophil antibody levels than children.

The presence of sheep cell agglutinins is not specific for infectious mononucleosis; these occur in serum sickness, hepatitis, Hodgkin's disease, rubella, and leukemia; low titers may also be found in normal persons. However, sheep cell agglutinin titers are generally higher in infectious mononucleosis than in other conditions. Qualitative tests for heterophil antibodies have now been introduced, using formalin-treated horse erythrocytes, ox red blood cells, or enzyme-treated and untreated sheep erythrocytes; a titer above 1:128 is considered significant in many laboratories.

Absorption tests utilizing guinea pig kidney and beef red cells provide specific differentiation: (1) Infectious mononucleosis heterophil antibodies are removed by beef red blood cells, but not by guinea pig kidney; (2) heterophil antibodies present in normal serum are absorbed by guinea pig kidney, but not by beef erythrocytes; and (3) heterophil antibodies in patients with serum sickness are absorbed by both antigens. The sheep or horse red cell agglutination test after serum absorption with guinea pig kidney is widely used; a level of 1:40 or higher after absorption is considered diagnostic, and a rising titer indicates recent infection. The most sensitive determination is the absorbed horse cell test; elevated titers may persist over a year after onset. The beef hemolysin test is highly specific, but detectable antibody disappears several months after clinical illness.

Specific EBV antibody responses are absent before mononucleosis and appear during the course of disease. These are assayed in a number of ways: (1) immunofluorescence techniques which demonstrate viral capsid, early, membrane, and nuclear antigens; (2) complement fixation; (3) immunodiffusion; (4) enzyme-linked immunosorbent assay (ELISA); and (5) neutralization. The most widely used clinical antibody test is the indirect immunofluorescence technique demonstrating viral capsid antigen (VCA); titers of 1:80 to 1:320 occur during early illness, and significant antibody rises develop in 15 to 20 per cent of cases. Rarely, the appearance of both EBV and heterophil antibodies is delayed for several weeks after onset of clinical symptoms. EBV-specific IgM antibody is present in serum samples collected one to three weeks after onset of mononucleosis and, like heterophil antibody, usually disappears within three to six months; EBV-specific IgM antibody has also been found in mononucleosis cases in which heterophil antibodies have not been demonstrated. The time relationships between clinical features, hematologic findings, virus shedding from the oropharynx, EBV antibody titers, and heterophil antibody levels after guinea pig kidney absorption in a typical case of infectious mononucleosis are shown in the accompanying figure.

DIFFERENTIAL DIAGNOSIS. Infectious mononucleosis resembles a number of other disorders associated with fever, exudative tonsillitis, lymphadenopathy, and splenomegaly. Early after onset, it may be confused with other forms of febrile pharyngotonsillitis, such as streptococcal or viral pharyngitis and tonsillitis, diphtheria, and Vincent's angina. Differentiation depends on throat culture results, prompt response to penicillin in the case of streptococcal infection, and the development of characteristic hematologic and serologic features of infectious mononucleosis.

Blood dyscrasias, particularly leukemia, may be mistaken for mononucleosis. Laboratory studies, including demonstration of many immature leukocytes in peripheral blood and bone marrow, an associated anemia, severe thrombocytopenia, and absence of heterophil antibody distinguish these diseases.

Rubella is characterized by a two- to four-day prodromal stage associated with fever, malaise, and lymphadenopathy prior to appearance of the rash. A distinguishing feature of the rubella exanthem is its

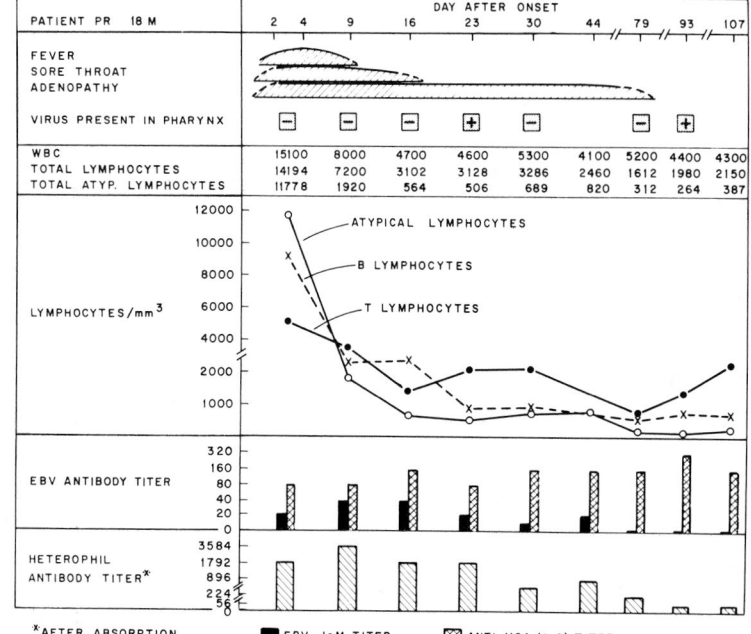

PATIENT PR 18 M	DAY AFTER ONSET									
	2 4	9	16	23	30	44	79	93	107
FEVER / SORE THROAT / ADENOPATHY										
VIRUS PRESENT IN PHARYNX	⊟	⊟	⊟	⊞	⊟		⊟	⊞	
WBC	15100	8000	4700	4600	5300	4100	5200	4400	4300
TOTAL LYMPHOCYTES	14194	7200	3102	3128	3286	2460	1612	1980	2150
TOTAL ATYP. LYMPHOCYTES	11778	1920	564	506	689	820	312	264	387

Sequence of clinical features, atypical lymphocytosis, EBV and heterophil antibody titers, and oropharyngeal virus shedding in a typical case of infectious mononucleosis.

*AFTER ABSORPTION   ■ EBV – IgM TITER   ▨ ANTI-VCA (IgG) TITER

regular presence on the face, whereas the less florid rash of mononucleosis is prominent on the trunk and usually spares the face. The presence of large numbers of atypical lymphocytes, EBV, and heterophil antibodies indicates infectious mononucleosis. Isolation of rubella virus from the pharynx and demonstration of a rise of rubella antibody titer confirm this diagnosis.

Cytomegalovirus mononucleosis usually involves an older age group than infectious mononucleosis and is characterized by fever, splenomegaly, hepatic involvement, and atypical lymphocytes. Pharyngitis and cervical adenopathy are not features of this infection; cases may be sporadic or may follow multiple blood transfusions. Cytomegalovirus can be isolated from urine, and a rise in specific complement-fixing antibody demonstrated.

Acquired toxoplasmosis infection is associated with fever, generalized lymphadenopathy, lymphocytosis, and splenomegaly. Differentiation from infectious mononucleosis is based on isolation of *Toxoplasma gondii* and on heterophil agglutination and dye test antibody determinations.

Aseptic meningitis may be the initial diagnosis in a patient having infectious mononucleosis with central nervous system signs and symptoms. Serologic tests are required for differentiation from other forms of viral meningitis.

Infectious lymphocytosis is a benign disease of obscure etiology in children, characterized by upper respiratory tract symptoms and occasionally by abdominal pain and signs of central nervous system involvement. Leukocytosis develops and small mature lymphocytes account for 60 to 90 per cent of the white blood cell differential; this blood picture may persist for several weeks or months. Heterophil antibody is not present, and an associated rise in EBV antibody level has not been demonstrated.

TREATMENT. Therapy of uncomplicated infectious mononucleosis is chiefly symptomatic and supportive. Antimicrobial agents are not effective and do not influence the course of infection. During the acute febrile stage of disease, bed rest is advisable. Salicylates are usually sufficient to control headache and sore throat; in severe cases, codeine or meperidine (Demerol) may be necessary. Gargling and throat irrigations with normal saline solutions provide symptomatic relief of pharyngitis and stomatitis.

In cases associated with severe toxic pharyngotonsillitis in which airway encroachment secondary to oropharyngeal edema is apparent, corticosteroids are useful to induce a prompt anti-inflammatory effect. A seven- to ten-day course of prednisone may be used, starting with 40 to 60 mg the first day and decreasing this amount 5 mg daily thereafter. Full doses of steroids should be utilized in the management of other complications, including (1) airway obstruction in which a tracheostomy may also be necessary, (2) neurologic sequelae, (3) thrombocytopenic purpura and hemolytic anemia, and (4) myocarditis and pericarditis.

Corticosteroid therapy is not recommended for treatment of usual cases of infectious mononucleosis. A well controlled study of steroid therapy in uncomplicated mononucleosis patients demonstrated a decrease in duration of fever to 1.4 days in steroid-treated patients, as compared with 5.6 days in matched control patients.

Splenic rupture, usually associated with severe abdominal pain, necessitates emergency surgery; transfusions, treatment for shock, and immediate splenectomy are required.

PROGNOSIS. In general, most cases of infectious mononucleosis are mild or moderately severe; after acute symptoms subside, patients usually recover uneventfully and return to normal activities within four to six weeks. In rare instances, symptoms persist for several months, and laboratory abnormalities, including liver function tests, are slow to resolve.

Severe hepatitis and toxic encephalopathy were recently reported in a fatal case of infectious mononucleosis and Reye's syndrome in a six-year-old child. Fulminating   lymphoproliferative   disease   following infectious mononucleosis has been described in several members of the same family, suggesting a genetically determined immune defect resulting in inability to contain an EBV infection.

Carter, R. L., and Penman, H. G.: Infectious Mononucleosis. Oxford, Blackwell Scientific Publications, Ltd., 1969.
Evans, A. S., Niederman, J. C., and McCollum, R. W.: Seroepidemiologic studies of infectious mononucleosis with EB virus. N. Engl. J. Med., 279:1121, 1968.
Henle, G., Henle, W., and Diehl, V.: Relation of Burkitt's tumor associated herpes-type virus to infectious mononucleosis. Proc. Natl. Acad. Sci. U.S.A., 59:94, 1968.
Joint Investigation by University Health Physicians and P.H.L.S. Laboratories: Infectious mononucleosis and its relationship to EB virus antibody. Br. Med. J., 4:643, 1971.
Niederman, J. C., Miller, G., Pearson, H. A., Pagano, J. S., and Dowaliby, J. M.: Infectious mononucleosis: EB virus shedding in saliva and the oropharynx. N. Engl. J. Med., 294:1355, 1976.

ENTEROVIRAL DISEASES

Nathaniel A. Young

90. INTRODUCTION

The picornavirus (*pico*, small; *rna*, nucleic acid type) family consists of two genera which commonly infect man: (1) the genus *Enterovirus*, found primarily in the gut, and (2) the genus *Rhinovirus*, whose members inhabit the respiratory tract and are the most important etiologic agents of the common cold (see Ch. 77). In addition there are picornaviruses whose natural hosts are other mammals, for example, foot-and-mouth disease virus of cattle and cardioviruses of rodents. Picornaviruses have common morphologic and biophysical properties, such as size of 20 to 30 nm, RNA genome, four structural polypeptides, and resistance to organic solvents. Human enteroviruses moreover share related nucleotide sequences. Historically, enteroviruses have been further subdivided into *polioviruses, group A and B coxsackieviruses,* and *echoviruses.* Sixty-three distinct immunotypes (species) were classified, based on differences in host range and antigenic relationships (67 immunotypes were originally recognized, but redundancies in numbering and changes in classification have reduced this figure to 63). Several enteroviruses had properties which straddled these arbitrary groupings. Because of this problem, newly discovered enteroviruses are no longer subclassified as coxsackieviruses A or B or echoviruses, but are simply numbered serially, beginning with enterovirus 68. Despite these difficulties, the older classification with its vast literature is clinically useful and has been retained for the original 63 immunotypes (Table 1).

DISTINCTIVE FEATURES OF NONPOLIO ENTEROVIRUSES

COXSACKIEVIRUSES. In contrast to polioviruses, which are readily isolated in susceptible primate cell cultures and are pathogenic only for primates, coxsackieviruses produce disease in suckling mice. Named for the village of Coxsackie in New York state, they were first recovered in 1948 from the feces of children who may have also suffered from paralytic poliomyelitis. Several related but immunologically distinct types were further categorized as *group A coxsackieviruses* when the histopathologic lesions induced in mice consisted of *generalized* myositis of skeletal muscle accompanied by flaccid paralysis. In contrast, *group B coxsackieviruses* produced *focal* myositis and widespread lesions of the central nervous system, myocardium, pancreas, and brown fat accompanied by spastic paralysis. Group B coxsackieviruses can be propagated readily in susceptible cell cultures as well as in mice, whereas most group A coxsackieviruses do not produce cytopathic effects in cultured primate cells. At present 23 immunotypes of group A and 6 of group B are recognized.

ECHOVIRUSES. These viruses were first isolated from feces of healthy children shortly after the discovery of coxsackieviruses. Unlike coxsackieviruses, they produce cytopathic effects in primate cell cultures and are nonpathogenic for mice. They differ from polioviruses immunologically and in their failure to produce disease in monkeys. Because at first no disease state in any host could be attributed to these "orphan" viruses, they

TABLE 1. Human Picornaviruses

Virus	Number of Immunotypes	Cytopathic Effect or Pathogenicity for		
		Cell Cultures	Suckling Mice	Primates
I. Enteroviruses				
A. Polioviruses	3	++	−	++
B. Coxsackieviruses A	23*	±†	++	−
C. Coxsackieviruses B	6	++	++	−
D. Echoviruses	30‡	++§	−	−
E. Enteroviruses	4	++	Variable; no longer used in classification	
II. Rhinoviruses (see Ch. 77)				

*Coxsackieviruses A1–A24; coxsackievirus A23 has been reclassified as echovirus 9.

†Most immunotypes of coxsackievirus A are not readily isolated in cell cultures, but exceptions exist.

‡Echoviruses 1–34; echoviruses 1 and 8 are identical; echovirus 10 has been reclassified as reovirus 1, and echovirus 28 as rhinovirus 1A; echovirus 34 is a variant of coxsackievirus A24.

§Except echovirus 21.

TABLE 2. Clinical Spectrum of Infection with Nonpolio Enteroviruses*

	Coxsackieviruses Group A	Coxsackieviruses Group B	Echoviruses	Enteroviruses
Illness associated with many enteroviruses	Asymptomatic infection Febrile illness with or without respiratory symptoms Aseptic meningitis (1, 2, 4–7, 9, 10, 14, 16, 22, 24) Paralysis (4, 7, 9) or encephalitis	Asymptomatic infection Febrile illness with or without respiratory symptoms Aseptic meningitis (1–6) Paralysis (1–5) or encephalitis	Asymptomatic infection Febrile illness with or without respiratory symptoms Aseptic meningitis (all except 24, 26, 27, 29, 32) Paralysis (1, 2, 4, 6, 7, 9, 11, 16, 18, 30) or encephalitis	Asymptomatic infection Febrile illness with or without respiratory symptoms (68) Aseptic meningitis (71) Paralysis (70)
Illness more characteristic of particular groups or immunotypes	Herpangina (2–6, 8, 10, 22) Hand-foot-and-mouth disease (5, 10, 16) Lymphonodular pharyngitis (10) Exanthem (9)	Pleurodynia (1–5) Pericarditis (1–5) Myocarditis (1–5) Orchitis Hepatitis Generalized disease of newborn	Exanthem (especially 9, 16 but also 1–8, 11, 14, 18, 19, 25, 30, 32) Neonatal "sepsis" Neonatal diarrhea (14, 18)	Acute hemorrhagic conjunctivitis (70)
Etiologic role undefined or uncertain	Diarrhea Hemolytic-uremic syndrome Chronic myopathy Guillain-Barré syndrome	Diarrhea Endocarditis Chronic cardiomyopathy Diabetes mellitus Hemolytic-uremic syndrome Mononucleosis-like syndrome	Diarrhea Reye's syndrome	

*The most commonly implicated immunotypes are designated in parentheses.

were named echoviruses (enteric cytopathic human orphan). Currently 30 immunotypes are recognized.

NEWER ENTEROVIRUSES. The four most recent additions, enteroviruses 68-71, have been given serial numbers because of difficulties in assigning them definitively to the older categories based on host range. Their pathogenicity for mice is inconstant even among different strains of a single immunotype. All can be isolated and propagated in cell cultures.

GENERAL ASPECTS OF NONPOLIO ENTEROVIRAL INFECTIONS

EPIDEMIOLOGY. Coxsackieviruses, echoviruses, and probably most of the newer enteroviruses are distributed worldwide. There is marked seasonal variation in their prevalence in temperate climates, most infections occurring in the summer and early autumn. Enteroviral illness is distinctly unlikely during the winter. In tropical climates, however, enteroviral infections commonly occur throughout the year. Usually only one or two immunotypes are prevalent in any city each year, and these may vary from one community to another. Virus replicates briefly in the oropharynx and for longer periods in the lower intestinal tract and is shed from these sites. Enteroviruses can regularly be isolated from urban sewage. Transmission is predominantly fecal-oral, and hence enteroviral infections tend to be associated with unsanitary environments, crowding, and low socioeconomic status. Marked clustering of infections in families is observed. When one family member is infected, secondary attack rates among susceptibles (i.e., those lacking type-specific immunity) are approximately 92 per cent for polioviruses, 75 per cent for coxsackieviruses, and less than 50 per cent for echoviruses. Virus is disseminated most efficiently by children less than two years old.

INFECTION AND ILLNESS. Approximately 50 to 80 per cent of enteroviral infections are asymptomatic, and many of the remainder are characterized by undifferentiated febrile illnesses lasting a few days, often accompanied by symptoms of upper respiratory tract infection. These illnesses may be caused by virtually any enterovirus immunotype and are clinically indistinguishable from infection by many other viral agents. In addition, enteroviruses have been established as the etiologic agents of a number of distinct, specifically recognizable clinical syndromes (Table 2), which may occur sporadically or in epidemics. Some of these syndromes are highly associated with a particular enterovirus group (e.g., herpangina with group A coxsackieviruses and myopericarditis with group B coxsackieviruses). Nevertheless the clinical diseases produced are not entirely specific; occasionally immunotypes from different groups may produce the same syndromes (e.g., herpangina caused by coxsackievirus B5 or carditis produced by an echovirus). Conversely, during a single epidemic one immunotype of group B coxsackievirus may cause pleurodynia, aseptic meningitis, or pericarditis in different individuals; or different strains of a single immunotype of echovirus may be associated with a high incidence of exanthem one summer but little or no exanthem in a different locality the following summer. The factors responsible for this diversity of manifestations are poorly understood.

LABORATORY DIAGNOSIS. The evidence establishing enteroviruses as the cause of specific disease syndromes has usually come from epidemics in which evidence of infection in patients with each syndrome is compared with matched controls. Establishing the etiologic role of an enterovirus in individual cases, however, is more difficult. Isolation of an enterovirus from throat secretions or feces, even when accompanied by a rising titer of type-specific antibodies, is not definitive etiologic proof of temporally associated illness because of the likelihood of intercurrent subclinical infection and prolonged (up to three months) fecal excretion of virus. On the other hand, if specimens are not collected until late in the course of illness, the intestine may be the only site from which virus is still being shed; under these circumstances fecal isolation of virus, although not definitive etiologic proof, may afford the only diagnostic clue. Isolation of virus from cerebrospinal fluid, vesicle fluid, pericardial fluid, or myocardium (as dictated by the clinical syndrome) provides convincing evidence of etiology. Measurement of type-specific neutralizing antibodies in serum is the most useful serodiagnostic test. Paired acute and convalescent sera, preferably separated by at least two weeks, are necessary, because the presence of antibodies even at high, stationary titers does not reliably distinguish recent infection from infection in the remote past. Serology has limited usefulness in the diagnosis of nonpolio enteroviral infections unless a virus has been isolated from the same patient. Without virus isolation it would be necessary, in the case of aseptic meningitis, to perform neutralization tests with more than 60 different enterovirus immunotypes. Requests to the laboratory for "viral antibody screens" are to be deplored, because it is generally feasible only to measure titers of antibody against the patient's own isolate or against one or two viruses known to be prevalent in the community at that time. A possible exception is in the case of myocarditis or pericarditis, in which measurement of antibodies against five immunotypes (coxsackieviruses B1–5) would detect the vast majority of these illnesses caused by enteroviruses.

PREVENTION AND TREATMENT. Specific chemotherapeutic agents are not available for enteroviral infections. Sanitation measures such as handwashing and containment of infectious excreta, particularly feces, should be practiced. Vaccines for nonpolio enteroviruses have not been developed, because permanent sequelae and death are rare and the immunologic diversity of the agents makes this approach unfeasible.

Kibrick, S.: Current status of Coxsackie and ECHO viruses in human disease. Prog. Med. Virol., 6:27, 1964.
Melnick, J. L.: Enteroviruses. *In* Evans, A. S. (ed.): Viral Infections of Humans. New York, Plenum Medical Book Company, 1976, p. 163.

POLIOMYELITIS AND ASEPTIC MENINGITIS DUE TO OTHER ENTEROVIRUSES

The most important enteroviral infections are poliomyelitis (see Ch. 307) and aseptic meningitis caused by coxsackieviruses and echoviruses, which are presented together with other causes of this syndrome (see Ch. 303).

91. PARALYSIS AND OTHER NEUROLOGIC COMPLICATIONS OF NONPOLIO ENTEROVIRAL INFECTIONS

Flaccid motor paralysis caused by enteroviruses other than polioviruses is extremely rare, but many coxsackieviruses and echoviruses have been incriminated in sporadic cases. The most commonly implicated immunotype, coxsackievirus A7, has been responsible for small outbreaks of paralytic disease in Scotland and the U.S.S.R. In general, paralytic disease caused by these viruses is transient and milder than that caused by polioviruses. A poliomyelitis-like syndrome, primarily occurring in adults, has been recognized increasingly as a complication of acute hemorrhagic conjunctivitis (see Ch. 96), which it generally follows by two to three weeks. Confirmation of the etiologic role of enterovirus 70 in this disease has been difficult, because titers of neutralizing antibodies are often maximal by the time paralysis occurs, and virus has not been recovered from the central nervous system.

Focal or generalized encephalitis accompanied by spastic paralysis may be seen in infants infected with coxsackieviruses and echoviruses. Coxsackievirus A9 has caused hemiconvulsions and hemiplegia followed by a chronic seizure disorder and porencephalic cyst. In other patients delirium, coma, cerebellar ataxia, and choreiform movements have occurred during infection with nonpolio enteroviruses.

Transverse myelitis and the Guillain-Barré syndrome have also been noted during enteroviral infections. Rarely virus has been recovered from the cerebrospinal fluid, but in most instances a firm etiologic relationship has not been established.

Grist, N. R., and Bell, E. J.: Enteroviral etiology of the paralytic poliomyelitis syndrome. Arch. Environ. Health, 21:382, 1970.
Kibrick, S.: Current status of Coxsackie and ECHO viruses in human disease. Prog. Med. Virol., 6:27, 1964.
Kono, R., Miyamura, K., Tajiri, E., Sasagawa, A., Phuapradit, P., Roongwithu, N., Vejjajiva, A., Jayavasu, C., Thongcharoen, P., Wasi, C., and Rodprassert, P.: Virological and serological studies of neurological complications of acute hemorrhagic conjunctivitis in Thailand. J. Infect. Dis., 135:706, 1977.

92. HERPANGINA

DEFINITION. Herpangina (*herpes*, vesicular eruption; *angina*, quinsy, or inflammation of the throat) is an infectious disease characterized by fever, sore throat, and a painful vesicular enanthem typically located on the anterior pillars of the tonsils and the soft palate.

ETIOLOGY. Group A coxsackieviruses (types 1–6, 8, 10, 16, and 22) are responsible for the great majority of cases. Uncommonly, other enteroviruses have been incriminated (coxsackieviruses B1–5 and echoviruses 3, 6, 9, 17, 25, and 30).

EPIDEMIOLOGY. Herpangina occurs predominantly in children during the summer months. Sporadic cases may occur, but most reports emphasize community outbreaks. Often multiple children within the same family are afflicted at intervals of two to five days; however, inapparent infections among contacts are more common.

CLINICAL MANIFESTATIONS. The illness begins with sudden fever of 37.7 to 40° C accompanied by sore throat and dysphagia, usually lasting two to three days. The pharynx and fauces are red but with little or no exudate. Headache and abdominal pain, occasionally accompanied by vomiting, may occur. The hallmark of the disease is the presence of vesicular lesions of the fauces. These begin as punctate macules which progress, over a period of 24 hours, to 2- to 4-mm gray papules and eventually to vesicles surrounded by an erythematous halo. They are located on the soft palate, especially on the free-hanging margin between the tonsils and the uvula, or on the anterior tonsillar pillar. Less commonly they are encountered on the buccal mucosa, posterior pharynx, or hard palate. The lesions are painful, but not exquisitely so, and are never numerous; two to six is usual, rarely a dozen. Late in the illness the vesicles ulcerate. Lesions generally persist two to three days after fever has subsided and are gone by one week. *Acute lymphonodular pharyngitis* is a variant of the syndrome in which the lesions having the characteristic distribution consist of tiny nodules of packed lymphocytes which do not vesiculate or ulcerate.

DIAGNOSIS. Herpangina is a disease of the posterior oral cavity. In contrast, the vesicular enanthems of primary herpetic gingivostomatitis and hand-foot-and-mouth disease involve the front of the mouth, particularly the anterior buccal mucosa and tongue or inner aspect of the lips. Moreover, primary herpes simplex infection typically is associated with prominent gingivitis, cervical lymphadenitis, greater systemic toxicity, and sometimes *exudative* tonsillitis and pharyngitis. Vesicles of the extremities are characteristic of hand-foot-and-mouth disease but are not seen in herpangina.

LABORATORY DIAGNOSIS. The white blood cell count and differential count in herpangina are normal. Virus may be isolated from throat secretions and feces.

TREATMENT AND PROGNOSIS. Children with herpangina are rarely very ill and recover without specific therapy in a few days. Antimicrobial drugs are ineffective and are not indicated. Parotitis has been reported as a complication but is not well documented.

Huebner, R. J., Cole, R. M., Beeman, E. A., Bell, J. A., and Peers, J. H.: Herpangina. Etiologic studies of a specific infectious disease. JAMA, 145:628, 1951.

Keuth, U., Esser, I., Wilhelmi, J., and Wilhelmi, I.: Die "herpangina" Epidemie 1967-68 (ECHO 30-6-3); Bericht über 590 klinisch beobachtete Fälle im Säuglings und Kindesalter. Dtsch. Med. Wochenschr., 94:1959, 1969.

Zahorsky, J.: Herpangina (a specific infectious disease). Arch. Pediat., 41:181, 1924.

93. EPIDEMIC PLEURODYNIA

(Bornholm Disease, Epidemic Myalgia, Devil's Grip, Sylvest's Disease)

DEFINITION. Epidemic pleurodynia (*pleura*, rib or side; *odyne*, pain) is an acute, febrile infectious disease characterized by sudden, sharp, spasmodic, often relapsing pain in the intercostal region of the chest or abdomen.

ETIOLOGY. The overwhelming majority of cases of epidemic pleurodynia are caused by group B coxsackieviruses. Outbreaks of illness consistent with pleurodynia have also been associated with echovirus 1 and sporadic cases with coxsackieviruses (types A4, 6, and 10) and echoviruses (types 1, 6, 9, and 19).

EPIDEMIOLOGY. Epidemic pleurodynia is predominantly a disease of children 5 to 15 years of age and their parents. The mean age is greater than that seen in aseptic meningitis caused by enteroviruses. Three fourths of patients are less than 30 years old. Males and females are attacked equally. Although Daae in 1872 described an epidemic involving 346 people in a Norwegian community of 1950 inhabitants, it was not until 1933 that Sylvest published his classic monograph describing the disease on the Danish island of Bornholm. Since then outbreaks have been recognized in many parts of the world. In different epidemics, from one third to two thirds of the cases have been in one member of a household, but multiple cases in a single family commonly occur either simultaneously or in rapid succession at intervals of two to five days. Unlike outbreaks of enteroviral aseptic meningitis, which are seen in urban areas during most summers, intervals of many years often elapse between epidemics of pleurodynia.

PATHOGENESIS AND PATHOLOGY. Despite its name, pleurodynia almost certainly results from infection of skeletal muscle rather than serosal surfaces. This is supported by the presence of palpable muscle tenderness at the site of symptoms in many cases. Although a pleural friction rub has been noted in up to 10 per cent of cases in some epidemics, this feature has been totally absent in other outbreaks, and even small pleural effusions are rare. Patients with abdominal pain have muscle spasm, but at laparotomy even localized peritonitis is absent. Neither isolation of group B coxsackieviruses from intercostal or other skeletal muscles nor histopathologic examination of these tissues has been reported in clear-cut cases of epidemic pleurodynia.

CLINICAL MANIFESTATIONS. Although about one quarter of cases of epidemic pleurodynia may have a prodome of a "head cold," headache, anorexia, or myalgia, the typical illness is ushered in by the onset of *spasmodic* pain typically occurring over the lower rib cage or upper abdomen. The pain varies from a mild "stitch" in the side to severe crushing, constricting, or band-like pain, which in adults may closely simulate the pain of myocardial ischemia. It is frequently described as smothering, stabbing, knife-life, catching, or vise-like, but it is the spasmodic nature of the pain which is nearly universal and is its hallmark. During each paroxysm lasting several hours or more, the patient is tachypneic, with visible splinting of the chest or abdominal muscles, and appears acutely ill. Auscultation of the chest reveals no signs of pneumonia. Paroxysms are separated by intervals of several hours, during which the patient may look entirely well. The pain, which the patient localizes with a vague area covered by a hand rather than a finger, is aggravated by breathing, coughing, turning over in bed, or in fact any motion. Adults typically complain of chest pain, which is usually unilateral, less often bilateral or subxiphoid. Young children more commonly have abdominal pain. In the Birmingham epidemic of 1951, 81 per cent of children had abdominal pain, 9 per cent had chest pain, and 11 per cent had both. In the Oxford epidemic of the same year, 9 per cent of patients experienced pain in neither the chest nor the abdomen, but instead in the neck or limbs; in these patients the diagnosis was made only by epidemiologic association with other family members. Abdominal pain is more common in the epigastrium or hypochondrium than around the umbilicus or right lower quadrant. Whatever the localization, thoracic or abdominal, the individual patient generally experiences severe pain in only one or two areas of the body. Localized tenderness to pressure occurs in about one quarter of cases, occasionally accompanied by palpable or visible muscle swelling or hyperesthesia of the overlying skin.

In addition to pain there is fever of 37.8 to 39.5° C, occasionally with profuse diaphoresis. Fever occurs simultaneously with pain and is diminished or absent during intervals between paroxysms. Headache, sore throat, nausea, and vomiting may occur, and mild cervical lymphadenopathy may be present.

The illness generally lasts one to four days, but in 20 per cent of patients paroxysms may persist up to two weeks. These recrudescent paroxysms usually occur a few days after the initial attack and are shorter in duration. However, as many as 10 per cent of individuals may re-experience symptoms one or more months after complete freedom from pain. The patient recognizes these late relapses as the same disease, often identical in all respects except duration to the original attack.

Laboratory tests typically reveal no abnormalities, although about 25 per cent of patients have a white blood cell count less than 5000 per cubic millimeter on the third or fourth day of illness. Assays of muscle enzymes in serum have not been reported.

COMPLICATIONS.   Most patients recover uneventfully. The two most common complications are aseptic meningitis (3 to 7 per cent), occurring 4 to 35 days after onset of pleurodynia; and orchitis (less than 5 per cent of postpubertal males), which often occurs late in the illness and may be followed by testicular atrophy. Pericarditis is rare.

DIFFERENTIAL DIAGNOSIS.   In a summer epidemic, the diagnosis is not difficult in children or young adults with characteristic spasmodic pain in the chest or upper abdomen, aggravated by breathing, in the absence of signs of pneumonia. However, in the Birmingham epidemic as many children were admitted to surgical wards as to medical wards, and 9 of 49 of the former were subjected to laparotomy before the diagnosis of epidemic pleurodynia was made. The protean character of the illness can mimic chest diseases such as pneumonia, pulmonary infarction, coronary insufficiency, and the pre-eruptive phase of zoster; and abdominal diseases such as appendicitis, pancreatitis, acute cholecystitis, and perforated peptic ulcer. The absence of auscultatory findings in the chest and negative roentgenograms are helpful in excluding pneumonia, as is the spasmodic and relapsing character of the pain. With abdominal pain and muscle spasm, signs of peritoneal irritation are lacking, but in some cases it may be difficult to exclude an abdominal catastrophe.

LABORATORY DIAGNOSIS.   Early in the illness, group B coxsackieviruses may be recovered from throat washings and feces, and rising titers of type-specific neutralizing antibodies can be detected in paired acute and convalescent sera. Virus has also been isolated from a testicular biopsy in a case complicated by orchitis.

PROGNOSIS AND TREATMENT.   Patients with pleurodynia may appear to be extremely ill, even in extremis. However, despite the tendency for relapses, eventual recovery is invariably complete. Profound asthenia occasionally persists for months after the illness. There is no specific treatment, but salicylates or narcotic analgesics may be required for relief of pain.

Finn, J. J., Jr., Weller, T. H., and Morgan, H. R.: Epidemic pleurodynia: Clinical and etiologic studies based on one hundred and fourteen cases. Arch. Intern. Med., 83:305, 1949.

Huebner, R. J., Risser, J. A., Bell, J. A., Beeman, E. A., Beigelman, P.
M., and Strong, J. C.: Epidemic pleurodynia in Texas. A study of
22 cases. N. Engl. J. Med., 248:267, 2953.

Pickles, W. N.: Sylvest's disease (Bornholm disease). N. Engl. J. Med.,
250:1033, 1954.

Warin, J. F., Davies, J. B. M., Sanders, F. K., and Vizoso, A. D.: Oxford epidemic of Bornholm disease. Br. Med. J., 1:1345, 1953.

94. PERICARDITIS AND MYOCARDITIS CAUSED BY ENTEROVIRUSES

Heart disease caused by enteroviruses in neonates is quite different from illness produced in older children and adults. In neonates the virus principally attacks the myocardium and the disease is fulminant, often fatal, with involvement of other organ systems. In contrast, in older children and adults, pericarditis usually predominates over myocarditis, and the illness is generally much milder.

ETIOLOGY.   Group B coxsackieviruses, types 1 to 5, cause a substantial majority of cases of pericarditis and myocarditis attributable to enteroviruses. Group A coxsackieviruses (types 1, 4, 9, and 16) and echoviruses (types 1, 3, 6–9, 19, and 22) have also been implicated in a few cases. The proportion of acute infections of the heart contributed by group B coxsackieviruses is unknown, but the best available studies suggest that they are responsible for only 13 per cent of cases of otherwise idiopathic acute pericarditis (range, 3 to 44 per cent) and 33 per cent of myocarditis. The causes of the remainder are largely unknown.

EPIDEMIOLOGY.   That coxsackieviruses can infect the heart was first recognized following catastrophic outbreaks of myocarditis in newborn nurseries in South Africa and Rhodesia during the early 1950's. In recent years only sporadic cases have been reported in neonates. Infection in nurseries is presumably nosocomial, transmitted by the fecal-oral route. Neonatal myocarditis may also be acquired during birth or in utero, in which case there is frequently a history of maternal illness consistent with cosackievirus infection in the two weeks preceding delivery. In older children and adults, even during epidemics of coxsackievirus infection, cases of pericarditis and myocarditis are sporadic, because involvement of the heart is an uncommon manifestation of infection. Only 3.5 per cent of group B coxsackievirus infections in 1966 to 1970 as reported by the World Health Organization had predominantly cardiac manifestations. Because of selective reporting of more serious illnesses, even 3.5 per cent is undoubtedly an overestimate.

PATHOGENESIS AND PATHOLOGY.   Coxsackieviruses and echoviruses have been isolated many times early in the illness or at autopsy from myocardium and pericardial fluid. Histologically there is focal muscle necrosis and inflammation with polymorphonuclear or round cells. These findings point to direct viral invasion of tissues as the factor responsible for the lesions. However, in laboratory animals myocardial inflammation and necrosis persist long after viral replication has ceased, and T lymphocyte function in mice appears to be necessary for both inflammation and a lethal outcome. An immunologic basis for myocardial injury is therefore suggested. Recrudescences of pericarditis reminiscent of Dressler's syndrome (see Ch. 365.2) also suggest the possibility of immunologically mediated disease.

CLINICAL MANIFESTATIONS. Myocarditis of the Newborn. The disease usually begins in the first week of life but occasionally up to three weeks or beyond. Typically the onset is abrupt. In one third of cases the illness is biphasic with one to three days of fever, anorexia, coryza, or loose stools followed by apparent recovery for one to seven days before the second phase begins. Circulatory failure then evolves rapidly over a period of a day or two. Only 70 per cent of infants are febrile during this phase. Most exhibit tachycardia (200 beats per minute or more), cardiomegaly, transitory systolic murmurs, and electrocardiographic changes of myocardial injury. In severely affected infants, respiratory distress, cyanosis, and the gray ashen pallor of circulatory collapse may follow, and progressive myocardial failure leads to edema, abdominal distention, and hepatomegaly. Myocarditis in fatal cases is often accompanied by disseminated viral infection involving other organs, particularly the central nervous system and the liver. In these infants liver enlargement and jaundice may reflect the combined effects of congestive heart failure and hepatocellular necrosis. Although most affected neonates are drowsy or stuporous, the presence of convulsions, bulging fontanelles, and cerebrospinal fluid pleocytosis is indicative of viral infection of the central nervous system. In fatal cases the interval from onset of illness to death is usually two to seven days, but a fulminant course with death in less than 24 hours is sometimes seen. The electrocardiogram is not of prognostic value during the acute phase. In survivors defervescence in approximately one week is accompanied by rapid improvement in cardiac function.

Myopericarditis of Older Children and Adults. Although the manifestations of coxsackievirus heart disease in older children and adults are predominantly those of pericarditis, the illness is more properly termed myopericarditis because involvement of the subepicardial myocardium is present in virtually all cases. A history of preceding upper respiratory infection is frequent. Fever, precordial pain, and a pericardial friction rub (often transient) are noted in 70 to 90 per cent of cases. Except for the common complaints of myalgia and arthralgia, noted in about 50 per cent, the symptoms and signs do not differ notably from acute serofibrinous pericarditis of other causes (see Ch. 365.2). Chest roentgenograms reveal enlargement of the cardiac silhouette in 40 to 75 per cent of patients, more commonly caused by pericardial effusion than cardiac dilatation. Pleural effusions, especially left sided, are seen in 20 to 50 per cent. The electrocardiogram is abnormal in all cases. In addition to S-T and T wave changes characteristic of pericarditis, Q waves and conduction disturbances, often accompanied by serum myocardial enzyme elevations, point to the existence of more severe myocardial involvement in occasional patients. Perhaps 10 to 15 per cent present initially with fever, gallop rhythm, and signs of severe congestive heart failure. The disease in these cases resembles myocarditis of other causes (see Ch. 366.4). Occasionally coxsackievirus myopericarditis is accompanied by aseptic meningitis; pleurodynia is rare.

LABORATORY ASPECTS. Most patients have a normal white blood cell count, but in nearly half there is a polymorphonuclear leukocytosis. Proof of enteroviral cause is made by isolation of virus from pericardial fluid or myocardium, but these specimens are not often available. Strong circumstantial evidence exists when virus is isolated from throat secretions or feces accompanied by a rising titer of type-specific neutralizing antibodies in serum. These specimens should be submitted for diagnosis whenever possible, but it is sometimes difficult to demonstrate seroconversion because many patients with coxsackievirus myopericarditis already have high, stable antibody titers within a few days of onset of illness. When no virus is isolated but a high, stable antibody titer to a group B coxsackievirus is present, the demonstration that these antibodies are of the IgM class is evidence of recent infection.

DIFFERENTIAL DIAGNOSIS. Coxsackievirus myocarditis of the newborn may resemble bacterial sepsis or pneumonia. When the liver and central nervous system are involved, the illness must be distinguished from neonatal herpes simplex without cutaneous lesions as well as from other viral infections. Although congenital heart disease may resemble neonatal myocarditis, fever or hypothermia and the nature of the electrocardiographic changes are helpful features pointing toward an infective etiology. The differential diagnosis in older individuals with pericarditis and myocarditis is found in Ch. 365.2 and 366.4.

PROGNOSIS. Although early reports indicated that coxsackievirus neonatal myocarditis was a highly lethal disease, accumulated experience now suggests that the mortality is considerably less than 50 per cent. There are few data on long-term follow-up of surviving infants. Most older children and adults recover uneventfully. In 11 of 12 adults with myocarditis caused by coxsackievirus B5, electrocardiographic abnormalities returned to normal by seven months, but the remaining subject had persistent T wave abnormalities. However, in another series 5 of 22 patients appeared to have permanent heart damage manifested by chronic congestive heart failure. The possible contribution of coxsackieviruses to chronic cardiomyopathy following unrecognized infection is unknown.

TREATMENT AND COMPLICATIONS. There is no specific treatment for the viral infection. During the acute illness pericardial pain, effusions, arrhythmias, and heart failure are managed as in patients having these disorders from other causes. Exercise and treatment with corticosteroids adversely affect the outcome of coxsackievirus myocarditis in laboratory animals. For these reasons bed rest is recommended and corticosteroids are not, although neither benefit nor harm has been clearly apparent in the few cases of steroid-treated disease in man. Constrictive pericarditis has been reported as a very rare sequel of coxsackievirus infection.

Grist, N. R., and Bell, E. J.: A six-year study of coxsackievirus B infections in heart disease. J. Hyg. (Camb.), 73:165, 1974.

Helin, M., Savola, J., and Lapinleimu, K.: Cardiac manifestations during a coxsackie B5 epidemic. Br. Med. J., 2:97, 1968.

Kibrick, S.: Current status of Coxsackie and ECHO viruses in human disease. Prog. Med. Virol., 6:27, 1964.

Koontz, C. H., and Ray, C. G.: The role of Coxsackie group B virus infections in sporadic myopericarditis. Am. Heart J., 82:750, 1971.

Sainani, G. S., Krompotic, E., and Slodki, S. J.: Adult heart disease due to the Coxsackie virus B infection. Medicine, 47:133, 1968.

95. EXANTHEMS CAUSED BY ENTEROVIRUSES

A variety of exanthems, occasionally associated with enanthems, are caused by coxsackieviruses, echoviruses, and the newer enteroviruses. In some patients they occur with aseptic meningitis, whereas in others they are associated with otherwise undifferentiated febrile summer illnesses. All occur more commonly in children than in adults with the same infection. The importance of these rashes is the clue they provide to the existence of enteroviral illness in the community, as well as their potential confusion with other childhood exanthems such as the rashes of meningococcemia, rubella, roseola infantum, varicella, and herpes simplex virus infections. The pathogenesis of enteroviral exanthems is poorly understood. In hand-foot-and-mouth disease, virus can be isolated from vesicle fluid, and the lesions are probably directly caused by hematogenously disseminated virus. Whether the maculopapular exanthems are also caused by direct viral invasion of the skin or are immunologically mediated is unknown. Whatever the mechanism, rashes may be caused by many different enteroviruses, and the type of rash elicited is with few exceptions not specific for a particular immunotype. Some, however, are distinctive:

HAND-FOOT-AND-MOUTH DISEASE
(Vesicular Stomatitis with Exanthem)

Most cases of this syndrome are caused by coxsackievirus A16, less commonly by A5 or A10, and rarely by coxsackievirus B2 or B5 or enterovirus 69. This disease is characterized by vesicular or mixed papulovesicular lesions on the dorsum, palms, or soles of the hands and feet, accompanied by vesicles or ulcers in the mouth. Children less than five years old account for 70 to 90 per cent of cases. Typically they refuse to eat and complain of a sore mouth. Oral lesions are present in nearly every case, but cutaneous lesions are seen in only about 70 per cent. The cutaneous lesions may occur in crops resembling varicella, but in hand-foot-and-mouth disease the lesions are far less numerous, do not pustulate or form scabs, and occur on the distal extremities rather than on the trunk. Vesicles are occasionally seen on the buttocks. Oral lesions are usually ulcerated and occur on the lips, tongue, anterior buccal mucosa, or hard palate, thus differentiating them from herpangina, in which the lesions occur more posteriorly. The lesions in the mouth may also resemble those of primary herpes simplex viral infection, but children with herpes generally appear more toxic, have gingivitis and prominent cervical lymphadenitis, and lack vesicles on the extremities. Patients with hand-foot-and-mouth disease do not appear very sick, and the lesions almost always disappear in less than one week.

RUBELLIFORM EXANTHEMS

A rubelliform rash caused by echovirus 9 is by far the most common enteroviral exanthem. In some epidemics as many as 50 to 70 per cent of children infected with this agent have had rash. Less commonly, indistinguishable exanthems have been associated with many other echovirus immunotypes, as well as coxsackieviruses A and B and enterovirus 71. The rash is typically maculopapular and involves the face in all cases, the neck and chest in three quarters, and the extremities in about half. It does not itch or desquamate. Fever characteristically occurs simultaneously with the rash. Unlike rubella, posterior cervical and postauricular lymphadenopathy is not prominent. The rash of echovirus 9 or coxsackievirus A9 may have a petechial component or may be exclusively petechial and is then easily confused with meningococcemia, especially when accompanied by signs of meningeal irritation. Occasionally the rash becomes confluent or produces large, blotchy violaceous lesions, particularly on the face. Both rash and fever usually clear in three to seven days.

ROSEOLA-LIKE EXANTHEMS

Most commonly caused by echovirus 16 ("the Boston exanthem"), this illness begins with fever of 38 to 39.5° C which lasts for 24 to 48 hours. The rash, consisting of salmon pink macules on the head and trunk, which appear only as the fever is declining or shortly after defervescence, lasts one to five days. This temporal sequence has also been noted with echoviruses 11 and 25 and coxsackieviruses B1 and B5.

Adler, J. L., Mostow, S. R., Mellin, H., Janney, J. H., and Mehsen Joseph, J.: Epidemiologic investigation of hand, foot, and mouth disease. Am. J. Dis. Child., 120:309, 1970.

Horstmann, D. M.: Viral exanthems and enanthems. Pediatrics, 41:867, 1968.

Lerner, A. M.: Exanthems caused by coxsackievirus, echovirus, and reovirus infections. In Demis, D. J., Dobson, R. L., and McGuire, J. M. (eds.): Clinical Dermatology, Vol. 3, unit 14-19. New York, Harper & Row Co., 1976, pp. 1-22.

Neva, F. A., Feemster, R. F., and Gorbach, I. J.: Clinical and epidemiological features of an unusual epidemic exanthem: JAMA, 155:544, 1954.

Sabin, A. B., Krumbiegel, E. R., and Wigand, R.: ECHO type 9 virus disease. J. Dis. Child., 96:197, 1958.

96. ACUTE HEMORRHAGIC CONJUNCTIVITIS

DEFINITION. Acute hemorrhagic conjunctivitis is a contagious disease occurring in explosive epidemics in Africa, the Indian subcontinent, and the Far East. It is characterized by conjunctival injection, tearing, and subconjunctival hemorrhages.

ETIOLOGY. A great majority of cases are caused by enterovirus 70. The disease has also been caused by coxsackievirus A24 or has occurred in mixed epidemics with adenovirus 11, which produces clinically indistinguishable disease.

EPIDEMIOLOGY. Acute hemorrhagic conjunctivitis emerged as an apparently new disease in West Africa in 1969 and appeared almost simultaneously in Vietnam and Indonesia. Since then the disease has spread to North Africa, the Indian subcontinent, and most of the

Far East. In the United Kingdom and the U.S.S.R., it appeared briefly in 1971 as circumscribed outbreaks of iatrogenic infection in eye clinics after introduction from abroad. Epidemics have continued in much of Africa and Asia in subsequent years. Secondary attack rates in families are high. Attack rates for clinical disease are greatest in young adults, whereas asymptomatic infection is more common in infants and children. Antibody surveys of sera collected prior to 1969 in affected countries reveal no clear evidence even in the elderly of previous infection with enterovirus 70, but following the epidemic as many as 40 to 50 per cent of the population had neutralizing antibodies. Neither clinical disease nor evidence of previous infection has been detected in the Western Hemisphere. Available evidence suggests that the disease is transmitted from hand to eye or by fomites, such as towels.

CLINICAL MANIFESTATIONS. Following an incubation period of 12 to 72 hours, the illness begins with sudden periorbital edema, severe pain, photophobia, blurred vision, lacrimation, and conjunctival suffusion. Disease typically begins in one eye but rapidly spreads to the other. Subconjunctival hemorrhages, present in 45 per cent of cases, may be small or massive and are the most distinctive feature of the infection. A scant purulent exudate is seen in 16 per cent. Punctate epithelial keratitis is frequent but transient. Conjunctival follicles and preauricular lymphadenopathy may be present. Systemic symptoms are variously reported as absent, or low-grade fever, malaise, headache, and symptoms of upper respiratory infection occur. Recovery is usually noticeable by the second or third day and is complete by ten days.

COMPLICATIONS. Discharge from the eye may become purulent when secondary bacterial infection supervenes. The most serious complication is the rare occurrence of a poliomyelitis-like motor paralysis (see Ch. 91).

LABORATORY DIAGNOSIS. Enterovirus 70 can be recovered from conjunctival swabs, but apparently cannot regularly be isolated from the intestinal tract during the acute stage of the illness. Rising antibody titers can be demonstrated in paired acute and convalescent sera.

TREATMENT AND PREVENTION. Treatment of conjunctivitis is symptomatic. Antimicrobial agents are not indicated unless there is secondary bacterial infection. Careful handwashing and use of separate towels are indicated to prevent contagion.

Acute hemorrhagic conjunctivitis. Lancet, 1:86, 1973.

Hierholzer, J. C., Hilliard, K. A., and Esposito, J. J.: Serosurvey for "acute hemorrhagic conjunctivitis" virus (enterovirus 70) antibodies in the southeastern United States, with review of the literature and some epidemiologic implications. Am. J. Epidemiol., 102:533, 1975.

Kono, R., Sasagawa, A., Ishii, K., Sugiura, S., Ochi, M., Matsumiya, H., Uchida, Y., Kameyama, K., Kaneko, M., and Sakurai, N.: Pandemic of new type of conjunctivitis. Lancet, 1:1191, 1972.

97. DIARRHEA ASSOCIATED WITH COXSACKIE- AND ECHOVIRUSES

Perhaps because of their name, enteroviruses are frequently cited as causes of epidemic or sporadic gastroenteritis and diarrhea. The preponderance of evidence, however, suggests that other viral and bacterial agents are far more important causes of these illnesses. Echovirus 18 and possibly other echoviruses have clearly been implicated in epidemic diarrhea of the newborn, but the role of enteroviruses in sporadic diarrhea, especially in older children and adults, is less certain. The consensus of several studies with well-matched controls is that there is a variable, usually small excess of enteroviral infections in children with diarrhea. Subsequent to these studies, rotaviruses and Norwalk-like agents (see Ch. 104), as well as toxigenic *Escherichia coli*, have emerged as major causes of gastroenteritis or diarrhea in children and adults. In light of this new knowledge, additional epidemiologic studies are needed before the contribution of enteroviruses in diarrheal illness can be assessed, but their role appears to be minor.

98. RESPIRATORY ILLNESS DUE TO ENTEROVIRUSES

Undifferentiated febrile illnesses with or without respiratory symptoms ("summer grippe") are far more common manifestations of enteroviral infections than the more specific syndromes usually associated with them. Although possibly all enteroviruses may be associated with respiratory disease, such illnesses are characteristic of certain immunotypes. Coxsackievirus A21 has been responsible for outbreaks of pharyngitis and "common cold syndrome" in military recruits as well as for sporadic cases in civilians. Less commonly it has produced influenza-like disease or atypical pneumonia. Many echoviruses, but especially echovirus 11, can cause common colds. Group B coxsackieviruses and enterovirus 68 have been associated in children 2 to 15 years old with pharyngitis, tracheobronchitis, bronchiolitis, and pneumonia. The respiratory illnesses produced by enteroviruses are not clinically distinguishable from similar disease caused by rhinoviruses, parainfluenza viruses, and other respiratory viruses.

ARTHROPOD-BORNE VIRAL FEVERS, VIRAL ENCEPHALITIDES, AND VIRAL HEMORRHAGIC FEVERS
(Arboviruses and Arenaviruses)

99. INTRODUCTION

Karl M. Johnson

Arthropod-borne viruses (arboviruses) are defined on an epidemiologic basis. Thus any virus is an arbovirus if it actually multiplies in one or more arthropods and if it is biologically transmitted to vertebrates with sufficient frequency by arthropods to make this an important means of virus survival. More than 300 distinguishable agents have been tentatively so classified. Many have similar physical and chemical properties and could reasonably be placed within families on this basis as well; others have fundamental properties relating them to animal virus groups not generally associated with recognized arthropod transmission.

Immunologic properties are currently used to cluster individual arboviruses. Viruses having such relationships are included in groups that historically began with A, B, and C; thereafter, the name of the first virus to be discovered was used to designate the group. Originally virus names were derived from antecedent diseases, e.g., yellow fever, dengue, and equine encephalitides. Later, geography in combination with disease syndrome was favored, providing names such as St. Louis encephalitis and Colorado tick fever. Finally, there are many geographically named arboviruses for which no clinical syndromes have been defined, either because they rarely infect man or because they have not been associated with morbidity of dramatic proportions.

About 90 arboviruses are known to infect man, and most of these have been shown to produce illness. With rare exceptions, such as dengue and urban yellow fever, these are zoonoses in which man is an accidental host of no apparent importance in the fundamental natural history of the virus.

Clinical syndromes produced by arboviruses share the common properties of fever and myalgia accompanied by viremia. Beyond that, classification is inevitably arbitrary, because the same virus can induce a wide variety of patterns in different patients, and different viruses have been linked to remarkably similar syndromes. Emphasis is given here to the often infrequent but spectacular severe diseases some of the agents evoke. Thus individual descriptions are placed in one of the following groups: (1) *fevers of a relatively undifferentiated type*, with or without rashes, usually benign; (2) *encephalitides*, often severe and with significant case fatality rates; and (3) *hemorrhagic fevers*, also frequently severe and fatal.

The largest number of viruses have been associated exclusively with milder, undifferentiated disease. The majority of these are encountered most commonly in tropical and semitropical countries (see table in Ch. 100.3). The classic clinical prototype is *dengue*. Those to be described represent but a small sample. Of these, *chikungunya, Mayaro, O'nyong-nyong,* and *Ross River*

are group A viruses, *dengue* and *West Nile* belong to group B, and the remainder are unclassified or are in the *sandfly fever* group. Although each gained entry to this book because of its proved epidemic disease potential for man, clinical differentiation even during epidemics is generally difficult; epidemiologic and laboratory methods are more important. When more than one such virus is simultaneously endemic, the latter techniques are essential.

All arboviruses conspicuously associated with encephalitis and hemorrhagic fever are included. In the case of the latter syndrome, all but one of the viruses belong to antigenic group B. Yellow fever is listed among the hemorrhagic fevers because many cases do not display the "classic" picture of jaundice, but manifest gastrointestinal hemorrhage (black vomit), epistaxis, and melena with fatal shock and thus fit this description better than either of the other two arbovirus clinical syndromes. Arenavirus-caused hemorrhagic fevers, although not arthropod borne, are described here because of their clinical similarity to those induced by arboviruses and because they are zoonotic infections.

It should be emphasized that all these viruses frequently provoke only mild clinically undifferentiated infections. Thus specific virologic diagnostic tests are of fundamental importance in sporadic infections as well as during epidemics. Specific diagnosis of all arboviral disease depends upon isolation of virus and/or detection of a homologous antiviral immune response. In many parts of the world malaria is first sought in acute febrile disease with or without neurologic manifestations. The findings of such parasites, however, may not solve the problem; it should be remembered that either a simultaneous arbovirus infection or a drug-resistant parasite may account for the lack of response to supposed specific chemotherapy.

Virus isolation, together with an antibody rise to that agent between acute and convalescent phase sera from the patient, provides nearly incontrovertible evidence for an etiologic association between virus and disease. Blood is the best source of virus for all the diseases here described except for Venezuelan equine encephalitis which may be gotten from pharyngeal swabs at least as readily. *Such specimens should be obtained on the very first day the patient is seen*, because viremia rarely persists for long into the encephalitic period. Since antibodies are often present at the end of the first week of symptoms, it is important to obtain the acute phase serum specimen for serologic diagnosis at this time. A convalescent serum obtained 10 to 30 days after onset will usually reveal an increase in specific antibodies when measured by the complement-fixation (CF), hemagglutination-inhibition (HI), or neutralization test. No more than 10 ml of blood need be obtained for any of these specimens unless special studies are contemplated. Materials for virus isolation should be kept chilled, or frozen at temperatures of at least $-60°$ C if shipment for testing involves great distances.

Berge, T. O. (ed.): International Catalogue of Arboviruses. 2nd ed. Department of Health, Education, and Welfare Publication 75–8301. Washington, D.C., U. S. Government Printing Office, 1975.

Hammon, W. McD., and Sather, G. E.: Isolation and identification of arthropod-borne-viruses. *In* Lennette, E. H., and Schmidt, J. J. (eds.): Diagnostic Procedures for Virus and Rickettsial Diseases. 4th ed. New York, American Public Health Association, 1969, pp. 227–280.

100. UNDIFFERENTIATED FEVERS

100.1. DENGUE

Karl M. Johnson

DEFINITION.   Dengue is an acute, febrile, self-limited infectious disease caused by an *Aedes* mosquito-borne dengue virus. Malaise, prostration, and pain of muscles and joints are characteristic, accompanied by lymphadenopathy, leukopenia, and one or two episodes of exanthem. Typically an illness of about one week is followed by one or more weeks of depression and weakness.

ETIOLOGY.   Four distinct immunologic subtypes of dengue virus have been recovered from patients. These agents produce partial cross-immunity such that a primary infection will protect against another subtype only for a few months, although homologous immunity is of long duration.

EPIDEMIOLOGY.   Man and certain *Aedes* mosquitoes are the essential links in the recognized natural virus cycle. Size of human populations and ecologic factors affecting the mosquito vector and multiplication of virus in that host are of prime importance. Thus the disease has occurred in all continents and many islands, but only in "summer-like" temperatures where there are large numbers of *Aedes aegypti, Aedes albopictus,* or *Aedes scutellaris* mosquitoes. Since infection is usually clinically apparent in adults and frequently inapparent in children, various combinations of human and *Aedes* ecology may produce nearly silent continuous endemic infection, repeated seasonal epidemics, or massive outbreaks affecting populations previously free of dengue for many years.

Viremia adequate for mosquito infection is present just prior to and for the first three days of illness. An infected mosquito requires eight to twelve days to become infective at warm temperatures. Such a mosquito is infective for life and may transmit the virus to one or more susceptible persons on whom it feeds or probes. The incubation period in man is five to six days.

Aedes aegypti, by far the most important vector, breeds, rests, and feeds in or near human habitations. It is primarily attracted to man, biting in daylight and twilight. These attributes make it an ideal virus vector and explain why dengue is principally an urban disease. In rural areas other *Aedes* species such as *A. albopictus* may transmit infection, but their habits and relatively sparse human populations render explosive epidemics uncommon.

No extrahuman virus reservoir has been conclusively documented, but there is suggestive evidence that monkeys and forest mosquitoes may be capable of virus maintenance.

PATHOLOGY.   Since dengue is rarely if ever fatal, the only information available is that from biopsy of the skin rash. Such lesions consist of endothelial swelling, perivascular edema, and mononuclear infiltration of small vessels. Petechiae are characterized by extravasation of blood without significant inflammatory reaction.

CLINICAL MANIFESTATIONS.   Dengue in adults is typically sudden in onset with rising temperature and only minor chilliness, headache, and fatigue. By the second day temperature is frequently 40° C, headache with ocular or retrobulbar pain is severe, and the patient complains of back pain, generalized myalgia, and aching joints. During this interval there is a diffuse blushing of the face and upper trunk, sometimes accompanied by a fleeting *erythematous macular* or *pinpoint rash* of the limbs. General lymphadenopathy is usually apparent, but hepato- or splenomegaly is rare. The leukocyte count at this stage is apt to be essentially normal.

At about the third to fifth day a *maculopapular* or *scarlatiniform rash* appears, beginning on the trunk and spreading in centripetal fashion. This generally lasts at least three days, becomes itchy as it fades, but rarely desquamates. The fever is generally of five to seven days' duration, sometimes with a fall at about the fourth day, giving a saddleback curve. The second bout of fever is often more severe, accompanied by relative or absolute bradycardia and by leukopenia. Monocytes, lymphocytes, and segmented leukocytes all decrease in absolute numbers, although there may be an absolute increase in immature polymorphonuclear cells. A few small petechiae may appear, especially on the lower extremities.

Dengue in young children is definitely a milder disease; recent longitudinal population studies in cities of endemic virus activity confirm an impression formed down the years by the paucity of description of pediatric cases during epidemics. Clinical manifestations may also vary with infecting subtype. Halstead retrospectively documented that volunteer studies done nearly 50 years ago in the Philippines employed subtype 1 and 4 viruses, the disease associated with the latter being milder and less "classic" than that caused by the former.

DIAGNOSIS.   During sharp epidemics occurring in places where ecologic factors are compatible, clinical diagnosis of many cases of average severity will usually be correct. But several other arboviruses as well as rubella may be the cause. Thus laboratory confirmation of a *few* cases during an epidemic and of *every* case when the pattern is sporadic is important. Travel history during the previous ten days is essential whenever dealing with a suspect case in areas where the disease is rare.

Virus may be isolated from blood or serum of patients early in the course of illness by inoculation of suckling mice, *Aedes* mosquitoes, or cell cultures. Serologic diagnosis is also possible, using acute and convalescent (two weeks) sera, but is frequently complicated by previous infection with one or more viruses of arbovirus group B. A laboratory competent to execute and interpret tests for a number of different arboviruses is required.

TREATMENT AND PROGNOSIS.   There is no specific therapy. Bed rest is indicated, as well as the usual supportive measures to maintain fluid and electrolyte balance and alleviate discomfort. Secondary bacterial infection is uncommon but should be anticipated and appropriately treated. Except in severely debilitated persons, the prognosis is uniformly excellent. Final recovery is complete, although temporary depression and lassitude are common during convalescence, and patients should not be rushed back to normal occupations.

PREVENTION. Vaccines for dengue viruses are not generally available, although experimental work on the problem continues. Individual protection is difficult, because mosquito attacks occur during daytime, and continuous use of repellent is not practical. Community protection is possible through effective control or eradication of the *Aedes* vector. Patients should be protected from mosquitoes during the first five days of illness in order to prevent further virus transmission, and space-spraying of buildings frequented by patients should be done to eliminate mosquitoes possibly infected prior to the diagnosis of the disease.

100.2. WEST NILE FEVER

Karl M. Johnson

DEFINITION. West Nile fever is an acute febrile mosquito-borne illness marked by headache, lymphadenopathy, and a macular skin eruption. It is generally self-limited, although rare cases of mortality caused by encephalitis occur in aged persons. The disease is caused by a group B arbovirus.

ETIOLOGY. West Nile virus is a small ribonucleic acid–containing virus belonging to an antigenic complex within the B group of arboviruses, which includes *Japanese B, Murray Valley,* and *St. Louis encephalitis* viruses, as well as *Ilheus* virus. Immunologic relationships are shared to a somewhat lesser degree with *yellow fever* and *dengue* viruses. Immunologic cross-protection is readily demonstrable experimentally among members of this antigenic complex. Despite the fact that such closely related viruses are frequently distributed geographically in a discontinuous manner, reflecting a long process of evolutionary segregation, West Nile and Japanese B viruses have been repeatedly recovered from the same mosquitoes in the same localities in southern India.

EPIDEMIOLOGY. Millions of people have been infected with West Nile virus, which is endemic in many parts of Africa, the Middle East, Southwest Asia, and southern Europe. Continuous human migration into Israel over the past 30 years has resulted in repeated epidemics among adults. Elsewhere the disease is mainly an affliction of children. Annual summer epidemics are correlated with seasonal peaks in populations of culicine mosquitoes. In Egypt and Israel, *Culex univittatus* is the principal epidemic vector. Much lower levels of virus transmission occur in winter when the suspected vector is *Culex pipiens.*

In ecologic terms, West Nile virus is one of the least evolved arboviruses. In addition to mosquitoes, it multiplies in, and can be experimentally transmitted by, the bite of various species of hard and soft ticks. It has been recovered from *Argas* and *Hyalomma* ticks in nature. Although the primary natural virus cycle appears

to comprise mosquitoes and wild birds, virus or antibody has been detected in rodents, camels, cattle, horses, and monkeys.

The incubation period in man is about three to six days. Most infections are clinically apparent. A number of documented laboratory infections suggest that the agent also can be transmitted by the respiratory route.

CLINICAL MANIFESTATIONS. Sudden onset of fever, lasting three to six days, is accompanied by photophobia, myalgia, and chilling. Nausea and vomiting may occur early in the febrile period. A saddleback fever curve is seen in a minority of patients, and there is usually a definite leukopenia with absolute reduction of polymorphonuclear cells by the third day of illness. At about this time a fine *maculopapular* rash is observed on the trunk and occasionally on the extremities. It is more common in children than in adults, is *nonirritating*, and fades rapidly without desquamation. Lymphadenopathy is often demonstrable at the time the patient is first seen.

Although mild meningismus is demonstrable in a minority of patients and may be accompanied by increased cells and protein in the cerebrospinal fluid, clinical encephalitis is not a feature of West Nile infection except in a handful of very old patients. Pathologic studies were not done in the few fatal cases reported. Convalescence is generally uneventful, although older patients may complain of generalized weakness for several weeks. No permanent sequelae have ever been observed.

DIAGNOSIS. Clinically this disease is so similar to dengue that laboratory diagnosis is essential in all cases. Virus isolation is by far the best hope, and blood specimens obtained as late as the fourth symptomatic day yield a reasonably high percentage of strains when inoculated into suckling mice or the yolk sacs of embryonated eggs. Serologic diagnosis may also be attempted with the usual paired serum samples, but previous infection with related group B arboviruses, including 17D live yellow fever vaccine, may render interpretation of results extremely difficult beyond the confirmation that infection was due to a mosquito-borne member of this large antigenic group.

TREATMENT AND PREVENTION. Management of patients is completely symptomatic. Complications are unusual, and the only reason to keep patients under observation after the rash has faded is to ensure the collection of appropriate diagnostic specimens in situations in which knowledge of the specific cause of illness may have public health implications.

Although there is an impression that prior infection with related group B viruses may lessen the symptomatology of West Nile fever, this has not been rigorously established. Inactivated or attenuated West Nile virus has been used in combination with other group B agents in experimental attempts to produce broad-spectrum immunity to this virus group. Such vaccines are not ready for general use. Thus mosquito control and individual protective measures against mosquito bite represent the only available means of prevention of this infection. Since the main epidemic mosquito vectors are not concentrated around human dwellings and since infection rarely causes severe human disease, expensive systematic mosquito control efforts have not often been mounted.

100.3. FEVERS CAUSED BY GROUP A ARBOVIRUSES: CHIKUNGUNYA, O'NYONG-NYONG, MAYARO, AND ROSS RIVER

Karl M. Johnson

DEFINITION. Chikungunya, O'nyong-nyong, Mayaro, and Ross River fevers are acute nonfatal diseases caused by an antigenically related, geographically dispersed complex of group A arboviruses. Maculopapular rashes and arthralgia are common features of these infections, which occur in Africa, Southeast Asia, tropical America, and Australia.

EPIDEMIOLOGY. Each of these viruses has caused epidemic disease in human populations. Perhaps the most dramatic was that due to O'nyong-nyong in East Africa from 1959 to 1962, when an estimated two million persons of all ages were affected. The important mosquito vectors of each disease are listed in the accompanying table. Chikungunya virus is often transmitted by *Aedes aegypti*; because of the rash and minor hemorrhagic phenomena associated with infection, this agent has at times been considered responsible for cases of hemorrhagic fever during outbreaks basically caused by dengue virus infection. O'nyong-nyong virus is the only known arbovirus transmitted principally by anopheline mosquitoes. Sylvan maintenance cycles involving arboreal mosquitoes and monkeys have been postulated for Mayaro and chikungunya viruses. Epidemic behavior of these agents is far from understood. Irregularly occurring outbreaks during warm rainy months are the rule. There is strong circumstantial evidence that chikungunya virus has moved steadily eastward into Asia from Africa during the last 25 years, employing a simple cycle composed of man and *Aedes*

aegypti mosquitoes. The incubation periods of these agents in man vary from about 2 to 12 days. Clinical attack rates are high in relation to those for infection, with the exceptions of Ross River and Mayaro viruses, which induce mild or inapparent infection in children.

CLINICAL MANIFESTATIONS. Onset is typically abrupt, and arthralgias or rashes are more likely to be the chief complaints than are headache and fever. Fever is usually mild, and is virtually absent with Ross River virus. Chikungunya virus frequently induces a saddleback fever curve, but the second episode, in contrast to dengue, is usually less severe. Arthralgias may or may not be symmetrical in distribution and usually involve terminal joints most severely. The maculopapular rashes are generally irritating, distributed over the trunk and extensor surfaces of the extremities, and may appear early or late in the course of the first week of symptoms. Leukopenia is a common feature of these diseases, and cervical lymphadenitis is frequently reported in cases caused by O'nyong-nyong and Ross River viruses.

DIAGNOSIS. All these viruses except Ross River can be recovered readily from the blood of patients during the initial three days of illness. Standard serologic techniques are highly reliable in making specific diagnosis, provided a second serum specimen is obtained 10 to 14 days after onset of symptoms. Differentiation of O'nyong-nyong and chikungunya viruses in East Africa may present problems. Malaria, rubella, enterovirus infection, and other nonviral causes of acute arthralgia must be considered in the differential diagnosis of individual cases.

TREATMENT AND PROGNOSIS. Treatment is symptomatic, and prognosis is uniformly excellent, although polyarthritis may persist or recur over an interval of several weeks to months. Corticosteroid therapy is contraindicated for joint pain in adults, at least until the

Etiologic and Epidemiologic Features of Undifferentiated Arbovirus Fevers

Fever	Virus	Vector(s)	Vertebrate Host(s)	Geographic Distribution	Human Epidemiologic Features
Dengue	Group B (4 types)	*Aedes aegypti*	Man	Tropics and subtropics; Old and New World	Varies from continuous endemic to repeated epidemic pattern based on human-*Aedes* population cycles
West Nile	Group B	*Culex* mosquitoes *Argas, Hyalomma* ticks	Wild birds	Mediterranean basin, Middle East, Soviet Union, Southwest Asia	Continuously endemic (tropics) to annually epidemic in Mediterranean climates
O'nyong-nyong	Group A	*Anopheles funestus, Anopheles gambiae*	Man	East Africa	Singular massive epidemic; malaria control may affect pattern
Chikungunya	Group A	*Aedes aegypti, A. africanus, Culex* mosquitoes	Man, monkeys?	Africa, Southern Asia, Philippines	Basically similar to dengue
Mayaro	Group A	*Haemagogus, Psorophora* mosquitoes	Monkeys, marsupials	Northern South America and Central America	Endemic, forest-associated infection; localized outbreaks during forest destruction
Ross River	Group A	*Culex, Aedes* mosquitoes	Wild mouse	Eastern Australia	Endemic infection in subtropical north; summer-fall epidemics farther south
Rift Valley	Ungrouped	*Aedes, Culex* mosquitoes	Large wild and domestic animals	East and South Africa	Sporadic rainy season transmission to man; mainly contact infections during livestock epizootics
Colorado tick	Bluetongue group	*Dermacentor andersoni* tick	Ground squirrels, chipmunks	Rocky Mountains of North America	Sporadic and focal summer infections during recreational and occupational activity
Sandfly	Phlebotomus fever group (20 types)	*Phlebotomus, Lutzomyia* sandflies	Man, monkeys, small wild mammals	Mediterranean basin, eastward to southern Asia; forests of tropical America	Annual seasonal transmission to children; epidemic whenever large numbers of susceptible adults introduced; forest-associated infections in American tropics

third week, when hormonal antibodies have appeared. Children possibly infected with chikungunya virus in areas where *Aedes aegypti* and dengue viruses are endemic should be hospitalized, because it is impossible to differentiate this disease from the prodrome of the dengue shock syndrome.

100.4.   COLORADO TICK FEVER

Theodore C. Eickhoff

DEFINITION.   Colorado tick fever is an acute, benign, tick-transmitted viral infection that occurs throughout the Rocky Mountain area, and is characterized by headache, back pain, a biphasic febrile course lasting about one week, and leukopenia.

ETIOLOGY.   Colorado tick fever virus is a member of the arbovirus group, in that it is transmitted to humans by the bite of the hard-shelled woodtick, *Dermacentor andersoni*. Human cases appear to be limited to the combined geographic distribution of the vector and the major mammalian reservoirs, ground squirrels and chipmunks. The virus, however, appears to be unrelated to other members of the arbovirus group. It is a double-stranded RNA virus (diplornavirus) that measures 35 to 50 nm in diameter, with a lipoprotein, hence ether-sensitive, outer coat.

EPIDEMIOLOGY.   The disease occurs during the spring and summer months, when tick exposure in the mountains is common. Disease activity appears to follow springtime in the mountains, for cases occur at lower altitudes during April and May and at higher altitudes during June and July, presumably reflecting the slower emergence of ticks at higher altitudes. Most patients give a history of having found attached ticks, but others will not be aware of the tick attachment and bite, even though they may have seen ticks on their body or clothing. Cases may occasionally be encountered in other areas of the country as a result of travel outside the endemic area during the incubation period, or from accidental transportation of infected adult ticks in clothing or bedding.

The virus has been recovered from as many as 14 per cent of *Dermacentor andersoni* collected in endemic areas. Replication of the virus within these ticks has been documented. It is not clear whether the virus is passed transovarially within the vector species. The reservoir of the disease probably resides in numerous small mammals, particularly golden-mantled ground squirrels and chipmunks, which have a prolonged viremia and infect nymphal ticks. Overwintering may thus occur in either nymphal ticks or hibernating small mammals. Adult ticks then transmit the virus to other small animals, humans being accidental hosts.

Incidence and Prevalence.   The disease has been reported from most states in the Rocky Mountain West and from western Canadian provinces, but the largest number of cases have generally been reported in Colorado. Several hundred cases are diagnosed annually in the endemic area, but it is likely that this represents but a small fraction of the total. Mild or wholly subclinical infections do occur, but their frequency has not been systemically evaluated.

The virus has been isolated from other species of ticks and from numerous species of small mammals, suggesting at least the possibility that the disease may occur over a wider geographic area than is presently appreciated.

PATHOGENESIS.   There is no unusual local reaction at the site of the tick bite inoculation, and the site of initial localization and replication of the virus is unknown. The onset of symptoms occurs three to seven days after tick exposure. Viremia can be demonstrated at the time of onset of fever, persisting not only during the febrile illness itself, but, remarkably, in red blood cells long after the virus has disappeared from serum and neutralizing antibody has appeared. The virus can be demonstrated within erythrocytes by fluorescent antibody staining for up to 120 days, and has been grown from washed erythrocytes 100 days after the original infection.

Few pathologic data in man are available, because only one fatal case has been recorded. In laboratory animals, the heart, lungs, spleen, bone marrow, and lymph nodes are important sites of viral replication. Occasional patients have clinical evidence of central nervous system or meningeal involvement, and Colorado tick fever virus has been recovered from cerebrospinal fluid.

CLINICAL   MANIFESTATIONS.   The   disease   begins abruptly, with chilly sensations, fever of 38 to 40° C, myalgias most prominent in the back and legs, headache, retro-orbital pain, and photophobia. Malaise and nausea may occur, but vomiting is uncommon. Physical findings during the first two to three days of illness are nonspecific. The patient may be flushed, with conjunctival and pharyngeal erythema. Lymphadenopathy is not prominent, although mild splenomegaly is sometimes present. Rashes have been reported in up to 12 per cent of patients, commonly macular or maculopapular and distributed over the entire body, sometimes petechial and involving primarily the extremities. Tachycardia is in proportion to the temperature elevation.

In approximately half the cases, a distinctly biphasic illness occurs, the so-called "saddleback" fever. Symptoms abate after two to three days, temperature becomes normal or nearly so, and the patient feels relatively well for one or two days, only to suffer an abrupt return of fever, headache, and back pain, often more intense than in the first phase. The second phase lasts two to four days and then subsides, leaving the patient with weakness and lassitude that disappear entirely during the succeeding week or two. Some patients do not exhibit the typical biphasic course and experience only one bout of fever, or have a typical illness but with a third phase of fever, or have a single prolonged febrile illness lasting five to eight days.

Evidence of central nervous system involvement has been seen in a few patients, invariably children. The presenting findings have been those of aseptic meningitis with nuchal rigidity and mononuclear pleocytosis or encephalitis with a depressed sensorium or stupor. Hemorrhagic manifestations have been described in a few children with encephalitis.

Laboratory findings very early in the illness are generally not helpful, but leukopenia is usually present by the third day of illness, and becomes even more pronounced during the second phase, reaching levels as low as 2000 per cubic millimeter. The most striking decrease is in the granulocyte series, with a relative lymphocytosis, and there is frequently an accompanying thrombocytopenia. Atypical, vacuolated lymphocytes are frequently observed. Bone marrow examination reveals a maturation arrest in the granulocyte series. The white blood cell count returns to normal during convalescence.

DIAGNOSIS. At the clinical level, the diagnosis should be suspected in any person with a history of tick exposure in the endemic area three to seven days prior to the onset of a febrile illness. Findings during the first phase, however, cannot be differentiated from those of many other acute febrile illnesses. A brief symptom-free interval followed by a second febrile illness should strongly suggest the diagnosis of Colorado tick fever. Profound leukopenia is usually present by that time, and lends support to the diagnosis.

The diagnosis is confirmed by isolation of the virus from serum or whole blood, via inoculation of suckling mice. More rapid diagnosis is possible by direct immunofluorescent staining of virus in the patient's erythrocytes. A diagnostic rise in both neutralizing and complement-fixing antibodies can generally be detected by examination of acute and convalescent sera.

The differential diagnosis can be troublesome, inasmuch as Rocky Mountain spotted fever is transmitted in the tick fever endemic area by the same vector, *Dermacentor andersoni*. Parodoxically, Rocky Mountain spotted fever has become an unusual disease in the Rocky Mountain area, and is outnumbered by Colorado tick fever in the state of Colorado by 20-fold. Nevertheless, differential diagnosis may be impossible early in the course of disease before the characteristic rash of Rocky Mountain spotted fever becomes apparent. A relatively symptom-free interval after two or three days would be most unusual in Rocky Mountain spotted fever, and strongly favors the diagnosis of Colorado tick fever.

TREATMENT. Therapy is entirely supportive, there being no specific therapy. Salicylates may be necessary to minimize headache and myalgias, but are neither required nor advisable in most patients.

PROGNOSIS. The disease is almost invariably benign, and the prognosis is excellent. Severe illness, complicated by central nervous system involvement, is rarely seen in children. The immunity derived is long-lasting.

PREVENTION. Both inactivated and live attenuated vaccines have been studied, but the modest number of cases and the benign nature of the disease suggest little need for active immunization.

The most effective means of preventing the disease is the use of protective clothing or repellents by people outdoors in endemic areas during the spring and summer months, together with frequent body inspection and prompt removal of ticks. Transfusion-associated disease can be prevented by exclusion of convalescent donors for a minimum of six months.

100.5.   RIFT VALLEY FEVER

Karl M. Johnson

DEFINITION. Rift Valley fever is a febrile illness of short duration characterized by headache, myalgia, prostration, photophobia, and leukopenia. It is the only such arbovirus infection accompanied by significant complications which are ocular. The virus is mosquito borne, enzootic in wild game animals, epizootic in domestic livestock, and restricted geographically to East and South Africa.

ETIOLOGY. Rift Valley virus is a 30 to 50 nm, ribonucleic acid–containing arbovirus antigenically unrelated to any other known agent. Historically it was the second disease-producing, mosquito-borne virus ever described, the first being yellow fever.

EPIDEMIOLOGY. The virus was initially recovered from sheep in East Africa. Subsequent investigations showed that infection was common among large wild mammals of the region, and that virus was naturally present in a variety of mosquito species of the genera *Aedes*, *Culex*, and *Erethmapodites*, many of which are now known to feed primarily on wild game. After seasonal rains which lead to high mosquito populations, the virus spills over from this wild cycle, causing epizootics with high mortality in sheep, cattle, and even fowl. The agent is pantropic in these animals, the most striking lesion being a severe necrotizing hepatitis, reminiscent of yellow fever in man.

Human infection can be acquired in at least two ways: by mosquito bite, which is usually associated with big-game hunting or with ranching activity, and by direct or aerosol contact with the virus through the handling of tissues of affected livestock, or working with the agent in the laboratory. More human disease has been associated with the "handling" mechanism than with mosquito transmission. This virus is so infectious to man, and of such potential economic hazard to the livestock industry, that it is now prohibited to bring it into the United States, even for experimental purposes.

CLINICAL MANIFESTATIONS. After an incubation period of three to six days, onset of symptoms is usually abrupt, with fever, photophobia, and severe generalized headache. There may be severe prostration, myalgia, nausea, and vomiting. Epigastric pain is a frequent complaint. Temperature oscillates between 38 and 40° C, is often "saddleback" in evolution, and may persist up to one week. Leukopenia is common, as is a relative bradycardia. Skin eruptions are almost never observed, although minor hemorrhages in skin and from mucous membranes are infrequently present. Several cases of frank hemorrhagic fever have been documented. Convalescence is usually, although not always, uneventful.

COMPLICATIONS. These consist of a *central serous retinopathy* with an associated *central scotoma*. The fundus shows exudates involving the macula that may be secondary to thrombosis of vessels. Whether such lesions represent direct viral damage or result from an immunopathologic reaction to infection is not known. The exudates usually shrink and disappear over the course of several weeks, but in a minority of patients *retinal detachment* has ensued.

DIAGNOSIS. This is above all a disease of place and of particular human activity. A history is more valuable than any other procedure. Blood obtained during the first three days of illness almost always contains virus which is lethal when inoculated into mice. Serologic diagnosis of this infection is also definitive, because interpretation of antibody responses in paired sera is never compromised by heterologous reactions with any other agent.

TREATMENT AND PREVENTION. Management of the illness, as for other arthropod-borne fevers, is symptomatic. Serial examination for retinal complications should be done, and continued rest is indicated for persons in whom such lesions occur. Since the ocular complications appear to have an acute episodic rather than a subacute or chronic allergic pathogenesis, corticosteroids are of no benefit in their management.

Prevention of infection is principally through individual anti-mosquito measures. A live attenuated vaccine has been used in animals and man in South Africa, but this has more recently been replaced for human use among persons at high risk of infection, such as veterinarians, by a formalin-killed preparation which appears to confer complete clinical protection for at least two years.

100.6. SANDFLY FEVER

Karl M. Johnson

DEFINITION. Sandfly fever is a self-limited viral disease consisting of fever, headache, and myalgia. Leukopenia and conjunctival injection are characteristic. It occurs during the warm season in the littoral of the Mediterranean Sea and eastward through Asia Minor, Pakistan, and northern India. Sporadic cases have been recognized in tropical America.

ETIOLOGY. Although the classic syndrome in the Old World is caused by two antigenically related viruses, Sicilian and Neapolitan, recent ecologic studies in various parts of the world have led to the recovery of at least 20 distinct but related agents from phlebotomine sandflies. These are now referred to as members of the phlebotomus fever group of arboviruses. Many can be isolated in suckling mice or hamsters, but cell cultures, especially an African green monkey continuous cell-line (Vero), appear to be uniformly susceptible to infection with cytopathic effect.

EPIDEMIOLOGY. The vector of classic sandfly fever is *Phlebotomus papatasii*, and the only known vertebrate host is man. The fly has a very short flight range, stays close to ground level, and breeds best during warm dry periods in small collections of organic debris beneath stones, in masonry cracks, and in other protected sites. It has a short life span, probably not more than three weeks, but because of its small size it can readily penetrate the usual barriers of screens or netting which exclude mosquitoes. Serial man-fly transmission probably accounts for much of the virus activity during the season of peak fly populations, but transovarial transmission by the vector appears to be an important mechanism for long-term virus survival in view of the repeated recovery of virus in nature from nonbiting male sandflies.

Although antibodies have been found in forest-dwelling rodents and especially arboreal mammals in tropical America, equivalent isolation rates of some serotypes from male and female flies strongly suggest that the transovarial mechanism is a basic biologic adaptation for maintenance of viruses of this antigenic group.

Human disease patterns are determined by geographic and ecologic distribution of vector and virus. In highly endemic areas most infections occur during childhood and are rarely recognized in epidemic form. Epidemics in such regions are generally the result of introduction of large numbers of susceptible adults, such as during wars and national immigration.

PATHOGENESIS. Since there are no fatalities, the pathology of this disease in man in unknown. Experimental studies in man, however, disclosed that after intracutaneous inoculation the incubation period is three to six days. Viremia is brief, usually being confined to the day prior to and that of the onset of symptoms. Postinfection immunity is type specific and is clinically complete for at least two years. It may be lifelong.

CLINICAL MANIFESTATIONS. Inapparent infection during experimental studies was rare. Onset is sudden, and peak fever is usually attained in the first 24 hours, subsiding after two to four days. It is accompanied by headache, myalgia, photophobia and ocular pain, and definite conjunctival injection. There may be erythema, but not a true eruption, over the face and upper trunk. Constipation and diarrhea sometimes occur. Bradycardia is not a feature of this disease, although the typical viral leukopenia is common. Cerebrospinal fluid remains normal. A few patients experience a second bout of fever and symptoms during the second week of evolution, but convalescence is otherwise uneventful and complete.

DIAGNOSIS, TREATMENT, AND PREVENTION. Epidemiologic history represents the best clue to diagnosis. Virus isolation and serologic procedures may be carried out but serve principally to exclude other possible causes such as dengue and influenza. Management of patients is purely symptomatic. No vaccine is generally available, but DDT and other insecticides have proved highly effective in control of the classic *Phlebotomus* vector.

Undifferentiated Fevers Exclusive of Colorado Tick Fever

Anderson, C. R., Downs, W. G., Wattley, G. H., Akin, N. W., and Reese, A. A.: Mayaro virus: A new human disease agent. II. Isolation from blood of patients in Trinidad, B.W.I. Am. J. Trop. Med. Hyg., 6:1012, 1957.

Barnett, H. C., and Suyemoto, W.: Field studies on sandfly fever and kala-azar in Pakistan, in Iran, and in Baltistan (Little Tibet). Trans. N.Y. Acad. Sci., Sec. II, 23:609, 1961.

Charris, B. J., Doherty, R. L., Fraser, J. R. E., French, E. L., and Muirden, K. D.: Epidemic polyarthritis: A cytological, virological and immunochemical study. Aust. N.Z. J. Med., 5:450, 1975.

Clarke, J. A., Marshall, I. D., and Gard, G.: Annually recurrent epidemic polyarthritis and Ross River virus activity in a coastal area of New South Wales. I. Occurrence of the disease. Am. J. Trop. Med. Hyg., 22:543, 1973.

Doherty, R. L., Barrett, E. J., Gorman, B. M., and Whitehead, R. H.: Epidemic polyarthritis in Eastern Australia, 1959–1970. Med. J. Aust., 1:5, 1971.

Halstead, S. B., Nimmannitya, S., and Margiotta, M. R.: Dengue and chikungunya virus infection in man in Thailand, 1962–1964: II. Observations on disease in outpatients. Am. J. Trop. Med. Hyg., 18:972, 1969.

Hotta, S.: Twenty years of laboratory experience with dengue virus. I. Epidemiology — past and present. *In* Sanders, M., and Lennette, E. H. (eds.): Applied Virology. Sheboygan, Wisc., Ellis Corporation, 1965, pp. 228–256.

Robinson, M. C.: An epidemic of virus disease in Southern province, Tanganyika Territory in 1952–1953. I. Clinical features. Trans. R. Soc. Trop. Med. Hyg., 49:28, 1955.

Sabin, A. B., Philip, C. B., and Paul, J. R.: Phlebotomus (pappataci or sandfly) fever. A disease of military importance. Summary of existing knowledge and preliminary report of original investigations. JAMA, 125:603, 693, 1944.

Schrire, L.: Macular changes in Rift Valley Fever. S. Afr. Med. J., 25:926, 1951.

Shore, H.: O'nyong-nyong fever: An epidemic disease in East Africa. III. Some clinical and epidemiological observations in the Northern province of Uganda. Trans. R. Soc. Trop. Med. Hyg., 55:361, 1961.

Spigland, I., Jasinska-Klingberg, W., Hofshi, E., and Goldblum, N.: Clinical and laboratory observations in an outbreak of West Nile fever in Israel. Harefuah, 54:275, 1958.

Taylor, R. M., Work, T. H., Hurlbut, H. S., and Rizk, F.: A study of the ecology of West Nile virus in Egypt. Am. J. Trop. Med. Hyg., 5:579, 1956.

Tesh, R.B., Chaniotis, B.N., Peralta, P. H., and Johnson, K. M.: Ecology of viruses isolated from Panamanian phlebotomine sandflies. Am. J. Trop. Med. Hyg., 23:258, 1974.

Weiss, K. E.: Rift Valley fever. A review. Bull. Epizoot. Dis. Afr., 5:431, 1957.

Wisseman, C. L., Jr.: The ecology of dengue. In May, J. M. (ed.): Studies in Disease Ecology. New York, Hafner Publishing Company, 1961, Chap. 2, p. 15.

Colorado Tick Fever

Eklund, C. M., Kohls, G. M., and Brennan, J. J.: Distribution of Colorado tick fever and virus-carrying ticks. JAMA, 157:335, 1955.

Emmons, R. W., Oshiro, L. S., Johnson, H. N., and Lennette, E. H.: Intraerythrocytic location of Colorado tick fever virus. J. Gen. Virol., 17:185, 1972.

Florio, L., Stewart, M. O., and Mugrage, E. R.: The etiology of Colorado tick fever. J. Exp. Med., 83:1, 1946.

Silver, H. K., Meiklejohn, G., and Kempe, C. H.: Colorado tick fever. Am. J. Dis. Child., 101:30, 1961.

Spruance, S. L., and Bailey, A.: Colorado tick fever. Arch. Intern. Med., 131:288, 1973.

101. ARTHROPOD-BORNE VIRAL ENCEPHALITIDES

Karl M. Johnson

101.1. INTRODUCTION

The arthropod-borne viral encephalitides comprise a group of clinically similar diseases induced by a variety of small viruses containing ribonucleic acid. Although infection usually occurs through the bite of an infectious arthropod, some of the agents are also transmitted by contact through mucous membranes, by aerosol, and by ingestion. In general, arthropods become infectious only after an extrinsic incubation period of one week or longer, which may be modified further by environmental temperature. Once infectious, however, such vectors remain so for long periods, in many cases for life. Encephalitis is usually an infrequent manifestation of human infection, but the agents to be considered all cause this dramatic and life-threatening syndrome with sufficient frequency that the term has been included as an integral part of viral nomenclature. This presentation is designed to provide the physician with the key clues necessary to aid him in sorting the variables involved in diagnosis and prognosis of infection, and to suggest areas in which ignorance rather than understanding characterizes the state of knowledge concerning these diseases and their clinical management. Because of the very real public health significance attached to the occurrence of even a single case of some of the encephalitides, the importance of specific diagnosis of arboviral encephalitis cannot be overstressed.

It is possible to subdivide these diseases in a variety of ways. They are distributed nearly worldwide, occurring in both temperate and tropical climates; they are caused by different viruses, some of which are antigenically related; they are transmitted by mosquitoes or ticks; they cause central nervous system (CNS) disease predominantly in adults or in children; and they may or may not clinically affect domestic livestock.

PATHOGENESIS AND PATHOLOGY OF ARBOVIRAL ENCE- PHALITIS. After deposition in the skin, virus may multiply locally and spread via lymphatics to cells of the reticuloendothelial system localized in lymph nodes, small vessels, and other organs such as spleen. In vitro studies suggest that macrophages are inherently susceptible to virus replication but that lymphocytes are resistant unless "blast transformed." Release of virus from such cells leads to viremia and widespread dissemination to other organs. Clinical symptoms and pathologic changes in many of these organs suggest that vascular endothelial cells are regularly damaged, but no direct or indirect visualization of virus in such cells in man has yet been achieved.

Although myocarditis, focal hepatic necrosis, and damage to lungs and kidneys may occur, the hallmark of these agents is their ability to induce damage to the brain. Despite some variation from virus to virus, a basic similarity exists in the gross and microscopic pathology of arbovirus-induced encephalitis. Brains are minimally edematous grossly with occasional small hemorrhages. Microscopic edema and hyperemia are present in the leptomeninges and cortex. There are small hemorrhages in many parts of the brain, sometimes with small arteriolar thrombi. Most striking of all are conspicuous collections of mononuclear, occasionally polymorphonuclear leukocytes around small vessels, the so-called "perivascular cuffs." Neuronal lesions are often focal and reveal nuclei and cytoplasm in various states of degeneration. Microglial and polymorphonuclear accumulations often present a picture of focal nodules. These lesions are most common in the gray matter, midbrain, basal nuclei, brainstem, and cerebellum, although some of the viruses induce destruction of anterior horn cells of the upper spinal cord.

Leukocytes and modest increases in protein concentration in cerebrospinal fluid are almost always seen. Although polymorphonuclear cells may be slightly more numerous early in the course of disease, there is always an evolution to a pleocytosis. It is of interest also that clinical encephalitis is almost always marked by a moderate leukocytosis rather than the leukopenia so characteristic of undifferentiated and primary hemorrhagic fevers produced by arboviruses.

A central question is how much of the CNS damage produced by these arboviruses is due to direct virus-induced destruction of neurons and how much may be the result of immunologically mediated injury to small vessels and/or neurons. In most instances virus is difficult to recover at autopsy from the brain, and it is not readily obtained from cerebrospinal fluid either. This has been explained in the past on the basis that antiviral antibodies are usually present at death in fatal encephalitis such that in vivo or in vitro neutralization obscures the real sequence of events. Although some neuronal destruction almost certainly occurs, the clinical course in the majority of patients who make rapid and nearly complete recovery and the pathognomonic *mononuclear* perivascular cuffs strongly point to an immune-induced inflammatory lesion as a major contributor to disease. What is wanted are new investigations of general and local immunologic reactions in patients with these diseases. The problem is of more than theoretical interest, because an elucidation of pathogenesis might well lead to a rationale for employment of therapeutic measures which present wisdom must continue to regard as potentially more harmful than helpful.

CLINICAL MANIFESTATIONS. The shifting, protean neurologic manifestations seen in arbovirus encephalitis suggest a mixture of permanent neuronal damage and temporary central dysfunction secondary to intermittent anoxia and edema. This pattern accounts also for the observed wide range of convalescent behavior and permanent sequelae.

The temperature course is frequently bizarre, indicating an anoxic effect on central thermoregulatory function. Indeed, persistent high fever is the most ominous clinical sign, and *external artificial control of temperature may be the most important measure available* for the management of the severely ill patient.

Although statistically significant differences in the frequency of specific neurologic symptoms and signs of encephalitis caused by individual arboviruses are slowly emerging, it remains evident that the range provoked by each agent is quite broad. Symptomatology in the individual patient rarely provides assurance as to the specific etiologic agent. Unexplained differences in patterns correlated with human age, however, are sometimes striking. Thus death caused by St. Louis encephalitis virus (SLE) is almost invariably restricted to the elderly, as though the vascular reserves available to cope with an acute inflammatory anoxia were compromised. By contrast, CNS disease and death caused by Venezuelan equine encephalitis virus (VEE) are observed almost exclusively in children. Major upper motor neuron destruction leading to permanent paralysis is largely attributable to Japanese B and Russian spring-summer encephalitis viruses. Sophisticated clinical investigation of all these diseases is nearly nonexistent. More work such as that of the Southwestern University Group in Dallas, who measured cerebral blood flow and certain hormonal functions in patients with St. Louis encephalitis virus, is urgently needed.

DIFFERENTIAL DIAGNOSIS. The most common disease clinically indistinguishable from arbovirus encephalitis is that caused by *herpes simplex* virus. Previous clinical herpetic infection and the fact that this disease occurs throughout the year may offer clues to its recognition (see Ch. 304).

Enteroviruses and *leptospira* may produce disease which mimics arboviral encephalitis, and the seasonal pattern is often coincident. Indeed mixed arboviral and enteroviral epidemics are not infrequently recognized.

Meningitis and rarely encephalitis caused by *mumps* virus may also be confused with that caused by arboviruses (see Ch. 88).

Postinfectious or *postvaccinal* encephalitis after measles, rubella, or varicella infection or inoculation with rabies or vaccinia vaccines must always be considered in such cases. History is the key to these diagnoses (see Ch. 83 to 86 and Ch. 309.3).

Rabies and *lymphocytic choriomeningitis* viruses can also resemble arboviral encephalitis. History of animal bite usually establishes the former diagnosis, but the latter must usually be separated by viral diagnostic procedures.

An assortment of acute febrile encephalopathies marked by hypoglycemia, diarrhea, convulsions, and coma, with or without visceral pathologic changes, has been described. These syndromes of undetermined etiology generally do not induce significant cerebrospinal fluid pleocytosis, nor do they display the marked central inflammatory changes so typical of arbovirus infection.

Bacterial and *fungal meningitides* can usually be distinguished by reduced sugar, high protein, and a mixture of cells, as well as by presence of stainable organisms in cerebrospinal fluid. Not uncommonly, however, incompletely treated bacterial meningitis may present a real diagnostic challenge.

Tumors and *abscesses* are usually separable by strong localization of neurologic signs, by absence of high fever unless septicemia is present, and by suitable tests to document abnormal space-filling lesions. *Toxic encephalopathies* must be thought of. History and chemical determinations are the best aids to establishment of such diagnoses.

It should thus be apparent that competent microbiologic diagnostic facilities are essential to establishing the specific diagnosis, and that such competence must extend beyond the arboviruses per se.

101.2. WESTERN EQUINE ENCEPHALITIS

ETIOLOGY. Western equine encephalitis (WEE) virus was the first such agent to be recovered from equines and humans. Isolated from an encephalitic horse in 1930 by Meyer, this agent represents the prototype for arboviruses immunologically collected into group A by Casals. The agent produces inapparent infection, mild febrile illness, or clinical encephalitis in both equines and humans.

EPIDEMIOLOGY. This virus, as well as its immunologic relative, Venezuelan equine encephalitis (VEE), is restricted to the Western Hemisphere. Eastern equine encephalitis (EEE), another group A agent of the New World, recently has been found to occur in Europe. Virologic and serologic studies have disclosed seasonal mosquito-bird activity cycles in many areas of the United States and Canada and in parts of southern and eastern South America as well. It is not present in tropical Middle America. In North America clinical infection of man has been recognized in the Mississippi drainage basin, the Great Plains, and the valleys between the western mountains. In most of these regions the mosquito vector is *Culex tarsalis,* and a variety of small birds appear to provide the principal blood virus source for mosquito infection. Equines and humans are frequently infected, as disclosed by population surveys for specific antibodies, but do not develop viremia of sufficient concentration to serve as hosts for further amplification of the basic cycle. Seasonal temperature fluctuations play a decisive role in disease transmission, exerting effects on mosquito population, on virus incubation period in mosquitoes, and on migratory behavior of birds. Thus WEE is a disease of summer and early fall.

Experimental work has shown that WEE virus may persist during winter in hibernating snakes and claims for such a mechanism in nature have been made but are as yet not generally accepted as valid. Human attack rates are highest in young adult males and in infants less than one year old. This pattern is due to the strong geographic localization of WEE virus and to the fact that agricultural irrigation projects vastly increase the breeding habitat available for *Culex tarsalis.* Incubation period of infection in man is generally five to ten days. Mortality among patients with encephalitis may reach 10 per cent.

CLINICAL MANIFESTATIONS. A two- to four-day prodrome of fever, headache, and myalgia commonly precedes the appearance of CNS signs in children; adults more often experience abrupt onset of stiff neck and drowsiness with fever and muscle aching. Clinically, CNS disease is almost always more severe in children, who, in addition to the hallmark signs of disorientation, somnolence, and coma, often suffer convulsions, abnormal reflexes, and flaccid or spastic paralyses. Fever lasts for a week or more, but rarely for two, and ranges from 39 to 40°C. Higher temperatures are prognostically ominous and should be reduced by external means.

Clinical improvement at the end of the febrile period is often dramatic in adults, most of whom make uneventful recoveries without residual motor or psychologic residua. Children, especially the very young, are not so fortunate; more than half of them are left with permanent damage, producing mental retardation, emotional instability, or spastic paralyses.

Although leukopenia may be present early in the course of illness, a mild leukocytosis with polymorphonuclear cells predominating is more common. Cerebrospinal fluid is clear, contains normal sugar concentration but moderately increased protein, and nearly always shows a mild pleocytosis.

DIAGNOSIS. Encephalitic signs occurring in both children and adults during summer should immediately raise suspicion of an arboviral causation. The major differential is similar disease caused by enteroviruses. Specific laboratory diagnosis is required in both instances.

Although WEE virus has been recovered on occasion from brain tissue of patients dying during the first week of disease, isolation of the agent from blood or cerebrospinal fluid is difficult even during the initial three days of symptoms. Specific diagnosis thus depends on demonstration of increasing anti-WEE antibody titers in sequentially collected sera. A specimen should be obtained and frozen as part of the initial examination of the patient, because such antibodies often appear during the first week of symptoms. The second serum can be taken 10 to 14 days later. Although single convalescent sera are of limited usefulness in areas where WEE infection is common, detection of specific antibodies of the IgM class is good evidence for very recent infection. This test is of proved utility in cases occurring among infants who have residual IgG from their immune mothers.

TREATMENT. Control of high fever and maintenance of water and electrolyte balance are the essential measures in management of patients. When necessary, reduction of fever should be by use of external chilling techniques rather than by use of analgesics such as aspirin. Continuous care should be taken to see that a patient's airway and normal respiratory function are maintained.

Convalescence is usually prolonged and should never be forced. Children should be thoroughly examined at intervals up to a year after acute encephalitis in order to detect those who may require psychiatric or special educational and motor therapy.

PREVENTION. During epizootics or epidemics the prime objective is to prevent mosquitoes from biting babies. Houses should be screened; cribs, bassinets, and carriages should be covered by fine mesh netting.

Transmission of WEE virus can also occur in utero; thus *pregnant women* should be especially protected against mosquito attack by restricting outdoor activity, by using repellents, and by use of residual and knock-down insecticides within and near their homes.

Community-wide organized control programs to reduce mosquito populations are important in areas where repeated epidemics have occurred. Based on combinations of insecticide and management of irrigation water, the value of such measures has been documented in California, Colorado, and Texas.

Epizootics of WEE in equines frequently precede human epidemics. An effective formalin-killed chick embryo virus vaccine is now used to protect horses, thus reducing the "sentinel" value of this species as a warning of an impending epidemic. The vaccine is not licensed for use in human medicine.

101.3. EASTERN EQUINE ENCEPHALITIS

ETIOLOGY. Eastern equine encephalitis (EEE) virus is a group A arbovirus which produces severe encephalitis and death in a high proportion of equine and human infections. It was first isolated in 1933 by Ten Broeck and Merrill and has been shown to be the most common cause of summertime epizootic-epidemic arboviral encephalitis in the eastern United States. Most outbreaks have occurred along the seaboard from northern Florida to Canada. Sporadic disease outbreaks also have been documented in some of the Caribbean islands during the fall. An antigenically distinguishable EEE virus variant is present in Middle and parts of South America. To date this variant has been associated with acute neurologic disease in equines but only rarely in man.

EPIDEMIOLOGY. Basic elements in the natural cycle of EEE virus in North America are the mosquito *Culex melanura* and a large number of species of small wild birds. Although reminiscent of WEE epidemiology, that of EEE differs significantly owing to the fact that *Culex melanura* distribution is strongly localized to a series of coastal fresh water hardwood swamps. Virus activity in these swamps occurs each summer, commencing later as one moves from south to north. Two possible mechanisms may account for this seasonal chain: either the virus overwinters in each swamp by infection of vertebrates (hibernating turtles as well as contact infections among rodents have been proposed), or the *Culex*-bird cycle is maintained through the winter in the most southerly swamps where frost is unusual. In the latter case spring migration of birds could provide the means for reintroduction of virus into northern swamps each year. Southward fall bird migration definitely seems to account for the Caribbean outbreaks because EEE-infected migrants have been detected in the southern United States and on the islands, and virus strains recovered during these autumnal epizootic epidemics were identified antigenically as North American rather than South American in origin.

Epizootics in equines and in exotic gallinaceous birds such as pheasants, chukar partridges, and Pekin ducks usually precede by one to three weeks the appearance of human encephalitis. Evidence has accumulated indicating that accessory mosquito vectors such as the salt-marsh *Aedes sollicitans* and the widely dispersed *Aedes vexans* may be important in transmission of virus to these abnormal hosts. As with WEE virus, equines and humans are of no or very limited significance as hosts for further mosquito infection. Disease patterns observed in game-bird farms strongly suggest, moreover, that direct contact infection is important in the epizootics which at times devastate these exotic species.

Although EEE infection of wild birds is usually not symptomatic, the reverse is true for horses and humans. More than half of equine infections are clinically overt, and mortality among such animals may approach 90 per cent. Serologic surveys among human populations resident very close to the fresh-water swamps have revealed individuals with specific antibodies and no history or stigmata of encephalitis. Nevertheless, it is probable that clinical encephalitis occurs in a high proportion of human North American EEE infections. Mortality among hospitalized patients runs to 50 per cent or higher, and many survivors have residual neurologic dysfunction regardless of age.

CLINICAL MANIFESTATIONS. The incubation period is assumed to be about seven to ten days, after which there is sudden onset of high fever, headache, conjunctivitis, nausea, and vomiting. This pattern, particularly common in adults, progresses rapidly from drowsiness to delirium and coma. There is stiff neck and irritability, at times accompanied by positive Kernig's sign, absent or hyperactive reflexes, and muscle spasticity in the extremities, often asymmetrical. Patients, if conscious, may be unable to speak or swallow. Excessive salivation is common. The disease terminates fatally within the first two weeks, usually within seven days, or shifting signs of deep CNS involvement may continue for several weeks, the patient gradually returning to consciousness. Serial neurologic examination usually discloses which centers and nerve supplies have sustained permanent damage.

Polymorphonuclear leukocytosis which can reach 50,000 cells per cubic millimeter is characteristic. During the first days of disease the CSF, usually under considerable pressure, also contains such cells in numbers up to 1000. Protein is elevated; as illness progresses, the cells become predominantly mononuclear.

A diphasic pattern of illness is often seen in children. After a day or two of fever, headache, and gastrointestinal upset, followed by two or three days of clinical improvement, there is fulminating onset of high fever, vomiting, delirium, convulsions, and coma. There may be intermittent or persistent opisthotonos, generalized rigidity, and localized paralyses. Circulatory stasis or mechanical obstruction leads to clinical cyanosis, especially in the very young.

Convalescence is slow, and during this time neurologic residua become apparent. There may be permanent damage to cranial nerves, as to those regulating muscle function of one or more extremities. Mental or emotional deterioration, or both, may be so severe as to require permanent institutional care.

DIAGNOSIS. Although EEE virus can be isolated from the brains of persons who die during the first week of illness, little success attends attempts to recover the agent from blood or CSF specimens during the acute illness. Sera taken during the first seven days of disease may contain neutralizing and hemagglutination-inhibiting antibodies for EEE virus. If so, the diagnosis is likely, because such substances are rarely found in the general population. A second serum obtained at about 14 days usually shows rising titers of specific antibodies.

TREATMENT. There is no specific chemotherapy, and there is no evidence that passively administered anti-EEE antibodies alter the course of clinically apparent disease. Thus management is that of any desperately ill patient: careful control of fluid and electrolyte balance, constant maintenance of a patient's airway, and external treatment of direct life-threatening hyperthermia. Secondary bacterial infections, if they occur, generally appear after the most acute primary phase of disease, and are those attendant to mechanical maintenance of respiratory and urinary function, physical inactivity, and bed sores. Physiotherapy to minimize paralytic contractures should begin after the febrile period.

PREVENTION. The principles are similar to those for WEE infection. There is a killed virus vaccine for equine, but not human, use. Since the ecology of EEE virus is centered in natural rather than man-modified habitats, organized mosquito-control efforts directed specifically at annual disease prevention are not economically feasible. Insecticides, however, are of some value both near residences and in accessible areas of mosquito-virus activity whenever a human epidemic exists or is threatened by the appearance of an epizootic.

Convalescent human plasma has been used to prevent disease after inadvertent direct exposure to EEE virus in laboratory workers. It is of unproved value and appears to be of no help unless given within 24 hours of the accident.

101.4. VENEZUELAN EQUINE ENCEPHALITIS

ETIOLOGY. Venezuelan equine encephalitis (VEE) virus is a group A arbovirus which causes fatal CNS disease in equines and an acute influenza-like syndrome in humans. During large epidemics cases of encephalitis are seen in young children, but the incidence of neurologic signs in this age group rarely exceeds 1 to 3 per cent of infections.

First isolated from horses by Kubes and Rios during a 1938 epizootic in Venezuela, the virus was not associated with human disease until several years later. Investigation of arbovirus ecology in tropical America during the past three decades has resulted in the recognition of several antigenic subtypes of VEE virus which differ in pathogenicity for equines and possibly humans and which have distinct cycles of maintenance and transmission. Taken together, VEE viruses have killed more equines and produced more human illness in the Western Hemisphere than any other arbovirus.

EPIDEMIOLOGY. Enzootic VEE virus cycles have been carefully studied in Trinidad, Colombia, Panama, Brazil, Mexico, and the United States (Florida Everglades). Virus activity was always focal, localized to shaded fresh-water swamps or to slow-moving bodies of water where floating water lettuce plants, *Pistia*, were common. The vector mosquitoes in each instance were members of the taxonomically complex subgenus *Culex melanoconion*. Small rodents, or in some cases water birds, are the principal vertebrate hosts. These animals develop high levels of virus in blood without significant mortality. Humans resident near or entering such enzootic foci suffer overt clinical infection, because the mosquito vectors are opportunistic rather than highly specialized blood feeders.

For some time it was thought that such enzootic foci were the sources for the periodic equine-human VEE outbreaks that swept large parts of Venezuela, Colombia, Ecuador, and Peru. But antigenic analysis of virus strains from all countries where VEE occurs together with experimental studies in horses has disclosed that enzootic VEE viruses were never involved in epizootics. Such strains, although capable of infecting and inducing cross-immunity, produced no encephalitis or sufficient viremia to infect mosquitoes when inoculated into equines. In contrast, antigenically distinct epizootic virus strains are highly pathogenic for equines, and induce truly dramatic viremias in them. Many genera and species of mosquitoes are thus infected and capable of further transmission of virus to equines, humans, and other vertebrates. Unlike the related WEE and EEE viruses, then, the equine is the single major host responsible for amplification and dissemination of the classic VEE strains. At present no mechanism has been discovered to account for interepizootic maintenance of such viruses in nature. Epizootics of VEE typically take place in rural tropical regions characterized by climates having a pronounced dry season. Cattle raising is the dominant land use, and outbreaks most often occur after the advent of the rainy season. Although human-mosquito transmission chains are possible, the timing of human disease one to two weeks after appearance of equine encephalitis suggests that epidemic VEE in man is mainly a spillover from the fulminant equine-mosquito cycle. At times nearly all equines and large fractions of rural human populations are infected during such outbreaks. Many thousands of human infections, most of them clinically apparent, can thus occur in a few weeks.

All subtypes of VEE virus are highly infectious for humans and other vertebrates when administered via the respiratory route. Thus many laboratory infections have been recorded.

CLINICAL MANIFESTATIONS. Onset of illness is typically abrupt, patients frequently reporting the exact time of appearance of severe headache, chills, fever, and explosive vomiting and diarrhea. These symptoms ensue two to four days after infectious mosquito bite but can occur within 24 hours after exposure to highly infectious aerosols. Conjunctival injection and mild sore throat are present early in the clinical course, and myalgia is usually intense. Fever often reaches 40° C. In general the first day of symptoms is the worst, and the fever curve shows daily evening peaks which regress to normal after three to five days. Mild somnolence is common, but severe neurologic signs are seen in only a small percentage of cases, nearly always among children. Individual cases may thus be readily confused with influenza, acute infectious or toxic gastroenteritis, or leptospirosis.

During the first day of illness blood leukocytes are usually normal or slightly increased in numbers, with a strong shift toward polymorphonuclear dominance and a conspicuous eosinopenia. There follows a definite leukopenia, and by the fourth or fifth day a relative lymphocytosis is usual. Normal total and differential values are re-established by about the tenth day.

Nuchal stiffness is unusual, and the CSF generally shows no cells or a very mild pleocytosis with normal protein. Children exhibiting more serious neurologic signs, including abnormal reflexes, spastic paralyses, convulsions, and coma, usually experience a biphasic febrile course with the second fever elevation associated with CNS signs. Epilepsy, paralyses, tremors, hallucinations, and emotional instability may persist as permanent sequelae of infection in children, and occasional cases of residual epilepsy and intention tremors have been cited among adults.

Most fatalities occur in children under five years of age. Autopsies revealed gross and histologic changes similar to those seen with other arboviruses causing encephalitis, but in addition were noteworthy for the presence of scattered gross focal hemorrhages in brain, heart, and lungs.

DIAGNOSIS. Since clinical presentation of VEE infection is rarely overtly encephalitic, the diagnosis will be missed unless it is considered in a patient with high fever, respiratory symptoms, and gastrointestinal upset who resides in or has recently visited either an enzootic focus or an epizootic area of tropical America. Virus can be recovered with ease, however, from either blood or throat swab specimens taken during the initial 72 hours of symptoms. Since patients are potentially infectious for humans and mosquitoes during this phase, the importance of establishing the cause is obvious. Paired serum samples obtained early in illness and about ten days later will reliably reveal rising levels of specific anti-VEE antibodies.

TREATMENT. There is no specific treatment. Analgesics and external chilling may be required to control hyperthermia. Life-threatening fluid and electrolyte imbalance may result from vomiting and diarrhea in children and must be alertly detected and corrected. Patients frequently complain of lassitude and inability to concentrate mentally for one to four weeks after fever has subsided, but convalescence is otherwise usually uneventful.

PROPHYLAXIS. Formalin-inactivated vaccines have been used to protect equines in South America for 30 years. The potency of these products is borderline at best, and the frequent persistence of live VEE virus in them may well have been the cause of subsequent major epizootics. An experimental live attenuated vaccine, strain TC-83, has been used with success in immunizing laboratory personnel at high risk of aerosol infection. This vaccine, which produces febrile reactions in up to 20 per cent of adult recipients, has not been tested in children or pregnant women. It has been associated with birth defects when inoculated into pregnant rhesus monkeys and seems unlikely ever to be generally safe for human protection.

Nevertheless, this vaccine is the single most important tool available for interdiction of human VEE epidemics. Most mosquitoes acquire virus from equines, and it has been shown that mass vaccination of equines prevents further viremic infection of these animals within three days. Once horse infections cease, transmission to man generally comes to an end within a short interval as infected mosquitoes die. Insecticides are useful in killing infected mosquitoes when temporally combined with equine vaccination.

Since patients are potentially infectious, precautions should be taken to prevent them from mosquito bite. Although medical personnel attending patients are potentially at risk of acquiring the disease by aerosol, the infrequent occurrence of significant coughing during VEE infection may explain the absence of well-documented instances of such transmission.

101.5. CALIFORNIA ENCEPHALITIS

DEFINITION. California encephalitis is an acute CNS disease which occurs during summer in many areas of the United States and is caused by one or more antigenically related viruses of the California arbovirus complex.

ETIOLOGY. The original virus strain of this antigenic complex was recovered from *Aedes dorsalis* and *Culex tarsalis* mosquitoes in the San Joaquin Valley of California in the 1940s. Serologic studies showed this agent to be associated with a few cases of childhood encephalitis previously thought clinically to be caused by WEE or St. Louis encephalitis viruses.

In 1960 the La Crosse strain was recovered from the brain of a six-year-old child who died of encephalitis. Although very few other isolates have been made from man, antigens prepared from the La Crosse agent have been used in recent years to document many cases of acute CNS disease in different regions of the United States.

At least six antigenically related California arboviruses have been recovered from a variety of mosquitoes and wild vertebrates in the United States. Related agents are known from tropical America, Europe, Africa, and Asia. One variant is annually active in the far north of western Canada and Alaska.

EPIDEMIOLOGY. Frequent epidemics of California encephalitis have been documented in Wisconsin, Indiana, Minnesota, and Ohio, and sporadic cases are on record from North Carolina and Florida. It is probable that the disease occurs over a much wider area of the midwestern and southern United States but is not diagnosed because specific serologic tests are not generally employed and because cases often appear sporadically in a large number of small rural communities.

The La Crosse virus is transmitted principally by tree-hole breeding mosquitoes of the genus *Aedes*. Small mammals such as rabbits, chipmunks, and squirrels provide sources of virus for new mosquito infection, but the basic mechanism of virus maintenance is probably transovarial transmission of virus through the various life stages of the mosquito. This behavior was recently proved for *Aedes triseriatus*, the first known instance of insect maintenance of a mosquito-borne arbovirus.

More than 90 per cent of human cases of encephalitis occur in persons 15 years old or under. Males are more often affected than females, probably because exposure to the virus is most frequently related to the outdoor recreational pursuits of camping, fishing, or hunting in woodlands where infected day-biting *Aedes* mosquitoes are present. Although mortality from California encephalitis has not been established, it is low, not exceeding 5 per cent. Serologic studies also show that human infection with these viruses is far more common than clinical encephalitis.

CLINICAL MANIFESTATIONS. Although not accurately known, the incubation period is probably between five and ten days. Onset of symptoms is typically insidious, with mild fever and headache for several days. As these symptoms increase, the headache usually becomes frontal, and the complaints are sometimes ascribed by patient or relatives to a minor traumatic incident. Mental confusion may or may not precede the sudden occurrence of convulsions, which may be the only overt sign of CNS disease on admission to hospital. Coma may supervene, and meningeal signs are occasionally seen, but shifting deep neurologic signs such as paralyses and reflex changes are rarely observed.

Mild to severe leukocytosis is characteristic of the acute stage of illness, counts sometimes reaching 30,000 per cubic millimeter. Cerebrospinal fluid is clear under moderate pressure and contains up to several hundred leukocytes, predominantly polymorphonuclear early, becoming mononuclear as illness progresses.

Fever generally subsides by lysis after a course of less than two weeks. Motor and sensory neurologic sequelae have not been observed, but emotional and learning dysfunction has been noted in children several months after physical convalescence is complete.

DIAGNOSIS. The differential diagnosis of importance is that between viral encephalitis and post-traumatic *subdural hematoma*. Favoring the former are season of occurrence, history of forest exposure, the presence of leukocytosis, a clear cerebrospinal fluid, and the absence of localizing neurologic signs.

Specific diagnosis of California encephalitis must be made serologically, no isolate having yet been obtained from blood or excretions of acutely ill patients. Thus a fourfold or greater increase in CF, HI, or neutralizing antibodies between acute and early convalescent serum specimens provides the only confirmation of etiology.

TREATMENT AND PROPHYLAXIS. Management of patients is completely symptomatic. Hyperthermia and respiratory failure, although unusual, are the dangerous signs that must be detected and corrected without delay. No vaccine is available, nor has any experimental work been reported in this direction. Mosquito control is virtually impossible on a large scale because of the specialized breeding habits of the vector species. Protective clothing, nets, and repellents are the only effective measures available to individuals entering the woodlands where infected mosquitoes are present.

101.6. ST. LOUIS ENCEPHALITIS

DEFINITION. St. Louis encephalitis (SLE) was the first recognized and is the most important arboviral encephalitis in the United States. It occurs sporadically and in major outbreaks during late summer and fall, afflicting rural populations in the West and urban-suburban communities elsewhere in the nation.

ETIOLOGY. St. Louis encephalitis virus is a group B arbovirus, most closely related antigenically to Japanese B and Murray Valley encephalitis viruses. It occurs only in the Western Hemisphere. A closely related virus, Rocio, was recently associated with a major epidemic of encephalitis in southern Brazil.

EPIDEMIOLOGY. The causative virus was first recovered from fatal cases during a major outbreak of encephalitis in St. Louis in 1933. Since that time sporadic cases and outbreaks of varying intensity have occurred in rural Washington and California, and in suburban and urban areas of Florida, Texas, Illinois, the lower Ohio and Mississippi Valleys, Pennsylvania, and New Jersey. Presence of virus is indicated by antibodies and/or isolation of virus strains from wildlife in Mexico, Central America, South America, and several Caribbean islands.

The basic virus cycle leading to human outbreaks involves birds and certain *Culex* mosquitoes. Although the possible mechanisms for virus survival during winter are not precisely known, they include reintroduction by northward migrating birds, recrudescent infection in nonmigratory birds, persistence of infected adult mosquitoes, and persistent infection in hibernating bats. The principal mosquito vector in the western United States is *Culex tarsalis*, especially abundant in irrigated agricultural areas. The vectors of urban-suburban epidemics elsewhere in the country are *C. pipiens, C. quinquefasciatus,* and *C. nigripalpus*. The virus has been recovered from many different mosquitoes in tropical America, many of them strongly arboreal in activity pattern, but it is not clear which are the most important in ecologic terms.

Although the distribution of SLE virus in the United States overlaps to a considerable degree with that of both EEE and WEE viruses, two important epidemiologic features distinguish the former from the latter group A viruses. First, although all three agents "spill over" from birds to horses, only EEE and WEE cause equine disease. Second, because the extrinsic incubation period in the mosquito is longer for SLE than for the equine viruses, St. Louis encephalitis always occurs later in the summer and is not found as far north as the group A encephalitides.

CLINICAL MANIFESTATIONS. Acute disease probably occurs in no more than 1 to 2 per cent of St. Louis encephalitis virus infections. Usually the course is benign, comprising a few days of fever and pronounced headache followed by complete recovery. More severe disease is occasionally seen in young children and occurs in a substantial number of adults more than 40 years of age. After an incubation period variously estimated at up to two weeks, there is acute onset of fever and altered sensorium. Convulsions are more common in children than in adults. The most common neurologic signs are stiff neck, tremors of the hands and face, dysdiadochokinesia, and nystagmus. Cranial nerve abnormalities are found in about 20 per cent of cases. Myalgia, photophobia, and conjunctival suffusion are common, and acute urinary symptoms with unexplained mild pyuria and increased blood urea nitrogen concentration occur in nearly one fourth of patients.

White blood cell counts are usually normal to moderately elevated, and increased numbers of immature polymorphonuclear leukocytes may be found early in the course. Although an occasional patient has no cells in the cerebrospinal fluid on admission to hospital, all eventually show a pleocytosis, the total number of leukocytes rarely exceeding 500. Although some polymorphonuclear cells may be present at the beginning, later examinations reveal only lymphocytes. Cerebrospinal fluid protein is typically increased, but rarely exceeds 100 mg per 100 ml.

DIAGNOSIS. Given appropriate season and place, the differential diagnosis of St. Louis encephalitis virus infection centers on other arboviruses and enteroviral meningitis in children and on *acute cerebrovascular accidents* in the elderly. An infectious cause may not even be considered in the latter group until a cluster of cases demands explanation. The virus itself has never been recovered from blood or cerebrospinal fluid of patients, and only rarely from brains of persons who die during the first week of illness. Specific diagnosis is thus dependent upon serologic testing of paired sera. The most practical technique is that of complement fixation, although the neutralization test provides the most definitive result if the early acute specimen is recovered before significant levels of antibody have been produced.

TREATMENT AND PROGNOSIS. Treatment is purely symptomatic. Persistent fever above 40° C is an ominous sign and should be vigorously combated. About 10 to 25 per cent of adults with acute encephalitis die, most of them from complications of underlying diseases. Such deaths generally occur after the first 10 days of illness when most of the neurologic manifestations have subsided. Hyponatremia is a frequent problem in management of the acute phase of disease, and in some cases has been ascribed to a partial persistent elaboration of antidiuretic hormone. Convalescence is often quite prolonged, and long-term examination of patients reveals frequent persistence of personality changes and emotional disturbance. Motor deficits are uncommon.

PREVENTION. There is no specific vaccine. Surveillance of seasonal mosquito-avian activity patterns of the virus in endemic regions is valuable as a guide to the timing of measures designed to reduce populations of vector mosquitoes. Emergency use of insecticides against adult mosquitoes during urban-suburban epidemics is probably of considerable help in reducing morbidity.

101.7. JAPANESE B ENCEPHALITIS

DEFINITION. Japanese B encephalitis is a severe arbovirus disease which occurs in eastern Asia. Summer-fall outbreaks occur in Siberia, Korea, Japan, Taiwan, and other Pacific islands. Continuous endemic virus transmission has been proved or is suspected in Southeast Asia, the Philippines, and East Indies.

ETIOLOGY. The causative agent is a group of B arbovirus closely related antigenically to St. Louis, Murray Valley, and West Nile viruses. Unlike these agents, however, Japanese B virus is pathogenic for certain monkeys and equines, and has been shown to induce abortion or stillbirth in pregnant sows, a fact of major economic significance to the porcine industry of Japan and Taiwan.

EPIDEMIOLOGY. The basic cycle of infection in both temperate and tropical areas is mosquito-vertebrate-mosquito. In temperate areas the primary vector is *Culex tritaeniorhyncus,* and the important vertebrate hosts are herons, egrets, and pigs. Virus is detected in a given locale annually, first in mosquitoes in July, and then in birds and pigs within a few weeks. Epidemics of encephalitis occur later, in August and September, and by November virus has apparently disappeared. Winter survival has not been elucidated. Epidemics tend to be larger in alternate years for reasons not clearly understood.

In tropical areas virus transmission is less strongly seasonal, and although the basic cycle is similar to that of temperate zones, other vectors such as *C. gelidus* in Malaysia, Thailand, and Vietnam and *C. annulirostris* on Guam are important. Regardless of area, the ratio of inapparent to disease-associated infections in man is very high. Annual infection rates in children may reach 10 per cent, but only 1 in 300 to 500 infections results in clinical disease. This ratio apparently declines with increasing age, one case of encephalitis occurring per 25 infections in United States troops.

CLINICAL MANIFESTATIONS. Japanese B infection is similar to that of St. Louis encephalitis virus in the high frequency of inapparent infection or mild illness, in onset, and in the signs or symptoms of central nervous system disease. But urinary tract symptoms and signs are less common, and the over-all severity of neurologic disease is more severe in Japanese B infections. Children commonly evidence paralysis of the face or extremities. Adults tend toward bilateral paresis without sensory changes. Sensorial changes, spastic rigidity, cerebellar signs, and coma are frequent in adults. The fever usually peaks four or five days after onset, then slowly subsides. Relative bradycardia is often seen, accompanied by a modest transient leukocytosis. Cerebrospinal fluid pressure is often increased moderately, and pleocytosis and increased protein are invariably present.

DIAGNOSIS. Although epidemiologic considerations may strongly suggest it, specific diagnosis requires a variety of virologic procedures. Isolation of virus from blood has been reported but is uncommonly achieved. Virus or, more often, fluorescent antigen can sometimes be demonstrated in brain tissue of fatal cases. Serologic diagnosis offers the best possibility of establishing the cause, but in many areas of Southeast Asia and India this is often confounded by the prior presence of antibodies to other related group B viruses. In Japan, where fewer such problems exist, it has been shown that primary infection induces early IgM antibodies reactive in neutralization and HI tests only, whereas IgG antibodies reactive in CF test are detectable eight or more days after onset of disease. Depending on the timing of serum specimens, diagnosis may thus require use of any or all three procedures. Detection of specific IgM HI antibodies has increased by precision of diagnosis in areas where related group B viruses are endemic.

TREATMENT AND PROGNOSIS. Intensive supportive care is mandatory and is all that is available. Artificial control of hyperthermia is frequently required. Anticonvulsant drugs may be needed, although prognosis in such cases is generally poor. The mortality rate varies from about 30 per cent for those under 20 years of age to nearly 80 per cent in older persons. Severity of clinical disease is directly correlated with quantitative antibody response. It has also been shown that early appearance of IgG antibodies was more common in persons who had received one dose of inactivated vaccine or who were more than 50 years old. Correlation of disease severity with early IgG immune response has not yet been reported.

Permanent sequelae are most common in children under age ten, severe residual damage generally being reserved for the very young. These changes run the gamut of upper motor paralyses, cerebellar syndromes, personality changes, and mental deterioration frequently requiring permanent institutional care.

PREVENTION. Formolized vaccine has been widely used in Japan and, providing that two or more doses are given, is credited with significant protection. A live attenuated vaccine has been tried in pigs in an effort to prevent annual amplification of the natural virus cycle; but although individual animals can be thus protected, the suppression of vaccine virus replication by passively acquired antibodies and the rapid turnover of this economically exploited species in Japan effectively preclude large-scale use of this measure. Specific vector control is not practical either, although modernization of rice culture techniques with attendant increased use of insecticides has apparently reduced peak mosquito vector populations in both Japan and South Korea, and is credited with significant reduction in epidemic disease transmission in recent years.

101.8. MURRAY VALLEY ENCEPHALITIS

Murray Valley encephalitis is similar to Japanese B encephalitis in pathogenesis and clinical features, and is caused by a very closely related virus. Diagnosis requires laboratory studies similar to those for other group B encephalitides.

The disease almost certainly was recognized in 1917–18 when an epidemic of 134 cases, then called *Australian X disease*, occurred in the Murray and Darling River valleys of Victoria and New South Wales. Virus strains isolated at the time were lost. Sporadic cases occurred during the next three decades, but the present designation was established during an outbreak of some 40 cases in 1951, more than a third of them fatal. This time the virus was recovered and completely characterized. Many inapparent human infections were detected. Endemic infection is maintained in a bird-mosquito cycle in Northern Australia and New Guinea, and it has been postulated that the virus is intermittently brought south by migratory birds, where an amplifying cycle involving domestic fowl, water birds, and *Culex annulirostris* mosquitoes produces epidemic disease, most commonly among children. Another epidemic in 1974 confirmed and extended these basic observations.

101.9. TICK-BORNE GROUP B ARBOVIRUS DISEASES: RUSSIAN SPRING-SUMMER ENCEPHALITIS, LOUPING ILL, KYASANUR FOREST DISEASE, OMSK HEMORRHAGIC FEVER

DEFINITION. The tick-borne complex of group B arboviruses cause mild to severe febrile illness with frequent neurologic abnormalities and in two instances (Kyasanur Forest disease [KFD] and Omsk hemorrhagic fever [OHF]) acute hemorrhagic manifestations. These agents are distributed throughout Eurasia (KFD, OHF, Russian spring-summer encephalitis [RSSE]) and Great Britain (louping ill). Powassan virus occurs in Canada and the northern United States but has so far caused only a few recognized cases of human disease.

ETIOLOGY. The group B tick-borne arboviruses constitute an antigenic complex readily distinguishable from most mosquito-borne group B agents, and separable into several closely related subtypes. With the exception of RSSE and OHF, which overlap geographically, these viruses are found in distinct regions of the world. Suckling mice and a variety of cell cultures have proved most satisfactory for virus isolation, and a complete range of serologic techniques is available for differential classification. Hemorrhagic pneumonia is induced in muskrats by inoculation of OHF virus, encephalitis with occasional hemorrhagic diathesis follows administration of KFD virus to langur and bonnet monkeys, and varying clinical encephalitis occurs upon intracerebral inoculation of monkeys, sheep, and goats with the remaining members of the complex.

EPIDEMIOLOGY. The viruses persist in discrete geographic foci by interchange between wild and domestic vertebrates and ixodid ticks, principally of the genera *Ixodes, Dermacentor,* and *Haemaphysalis.*

Many vertebrates, including rodents, birds, bats, sheep, goats, and cattle, experience clinically silent viremic infection. The capacity of the tick vectors to transmit virus transovarially has been experimentally documented, thus providing a fundamental mechanism for winter survival of some of the viruses. Persistent infection of hibernating species such as bats and hedgehogs has also been demonstrated. In the case of OHF and KFD viruses, respectively, viremia and overt fatal infection occur naturally in muskrats and monkeys, and major epizootics among these animals often precede or accompany outbreaks in man.

In addition to tick transmission, RSSE infection in man may be acquired through *raw milk* of infected goats and sheep. Tick-transmitted infection may result from factors affecting residence, occupation, or recreation. Residents of rural forested areas, particularly agricultural, veterinary, and forest workers, are at highest risk. Seasonal disease patterns reflect temperature-dependent tick activity, with peaks ranging from late spring to autumn, depending on the tick and the geographic locality. Some of the agents can also apparently infect man by the respiratory route, as evidenced by winter outbreaks among trappers and skinners of muskrats (OHF) and by aerosol-associated laboratory infections (OHF, KFD).

CLINICAL MANIFESTATIONS AND PATHOLOGY. Onset is typically abrupt after an incubation period of 3 to 12 days. The pattern is frequently diphasic except for OHF, the initial phase consisting of fever, headache, myalgia, gastrointestinal disturbances, and, in KFD, mild to moderate hemorrhages from the nose and intestines. Leukopenia is common during this phase, which lasts five to ten days.

The second phase usually begins with high fever and severe headache. Louping ill is usually mild to moderate in over-all severity, but RSSE infection tends to be progressively more severe from Europe to Far Eastern Asia. Although serous meningitis is the most common form over-all, infection in the easternmost part of the Soviet Union is frequently grossly encephalomyelitic, with transient or permanent flaccid paralysis, nystagmus, deafness, and somnolence. Bulbospinal disease is the most serious, resulting in neck and shoulder paralysis or even death. The second phase of KFD also is predominantly neurologic, although severity is usually moderate. Moderate leukocytosis and cerebrospinal fluid pleocytosis and elevated protein are characteristic of this phase. The latter abnormalities have been shown to persist in louping ill for weeks after apparent clinical recovery.

Pathologically the lesions produced by these viruses are generally similar to those observed with other arbovirus encephalitides or hemorrhagic fevers (inflammatory vasculitis in brain or focal capillary hemorrhages without inflammation). But not infrequently RSSE virus produces neuronal damage in the cervical cord reminiscent of poliomyelitis, and the viruses of OHF and KFD induce a focal hemorrhagic bronchopneumonia with occasional necrotic foci in the liver and gastrointestinal tract.

DIAGNOSIS AND TREATMENT. Specific diagnosis, in contrast to disease caused by most mosquito-borne encephalitides, can often be made by isolation of the virus from blood during the initial febrile phase, or from brain in rapidly fatal infection. Serologic diagnosis is even more reliable, although access to all three common techniques is necessary to establish the cause in some instances. With the exception of RSSE-OHF, anamnestic responses to infection with related agents are usually not a problem. Treatment is symptomatic. Blood loss in OHF and KFD is rarely sufficient to warrant transfusion.

PROGNOSIS AND PREVENTION. Louping ill virus infection has not caused fatalities or permanent neurologic sequelae. Far eastern RSSE, in contrast, has a fatality rate of more than 15 per cent and leaves many survivors with permanent paralysis of an arm or the shoulder girdle. Soviet workers also claim that 3 to 5 per cent of paralytic patients follow a chronic progressive course that develops into clonic spasms, epilepsy, and death. Strong indirect evidence for chronic virus persistence in the brain of one patient during a period of 14 years with final deterioration and death has been obtained by Japanese workers. Fatality rates do not exceed 5 per cent for KFD and OHF and there are no permanent sequelae associated with these diseases.

Soviet workers have administered formolized mouse brain RSSE vaccine to thousands of persons with reported good results. Work proceeds in that country on a live attenuated vaccine. Otherwise, protection is largely individual against tick bite, consisting of adequate clothing and insect repellents. Aerial spraying of insecticides has been tried on a large scale for tick control in parts of Russia but has been abandoned as too expensive.

Bennett, N. M.: Murray Valley encephalitis, 1974: Clinical features. Med. J. Aust., 2:446, 1976.

Blaskovic, D., and Nosek, J.: The ecological approach to the study of tick-borne encephalitis, In Melnick, J. L. (ed.): Progress in Medical Virology. Vol. 14. Basel and New York, S. Karger, 1972, pp. 275–320.

Feemster, R. F.: Equine encephalitis in Massachusetts. N. Engl. J. Med., 257:701, 1957.

Grabow, J. D., Mathews, C. G., Chun, R. W. M., and Thompson, W. H.: The electroencephalogram and clinical sequelae of California arbovirus encephalitis. Neurology, 19:394, 1969.

Hart, K. L., Keen, D., and Belle, E. A.: An outbreak of eastern equine encephalomyelitis in Jamaica, West Indies. I. Description of human cases. Am. J. Trop. Med. Hyg., 13:331, 1964.

Hilty, M. D., Haynes, R. E., Azimi, P. H., and Cramblett, H. G.: California encephalitis in children. Am. J. Dis. Child., 124:530, 1972.

Johnson, K. M., and Martin, D. H.: Venezuelan equine encephalitis. In Brandly, C. A., and Cornelius, C. E. (eds.): Advances in Veterinary

Science and Comparative Medicine. Vol. 18. New York, Academic Press, 1974, pp. 79–115.

Leon, C. A., Jaramillo, R., Martinez, S., Fernandez, F., Tellez, H., Lasso, B., and Guzman, R. de: Sequelae of Venezuelan equine encephalitis in humans: A four-year follow-up. Int. J. Epidemiol., 4:131, 1975.

Lincoln, A. F., and Sivertson, S. E.: Acute phase of Japanese B encephalitis. Two hundred and one cases in American soldiers, Korea, 1950. JAMA, 150:268, 1952.

Matthews, C. G., Chun, R. W. M., Grabow, J. D., and Thompson, W. H.: Psychological sequelae in children following California arbovirus encephalitis. Neurology, 18:1023, 1968.

Parkin, W. E., Hammon, W. McD., and Sather, G. W.: Review of current epidemiological literature on viruses of the California arbovirus group. Am. J. Trop. Med. Hyg., 21:964, 1972.

Quick, D. T., Thompson, J. M., and Bond, J. O.: The 1962 epidemic of St. Louis encephalitis in Florida. IV. Clinical features of cases occurring in the Tampa Bay area. Am. J. Epidemiol., 81:415, 1965.

Venezuelan Encephalitis: Washington, D.C., Pan-American Health Organization Publication Number 243, 1972, pp. 416.

Wallis, R. C.: Recent advances in research on the eastern encephalitis virus. Yale J. Biol. Med., 37:413, 1965.

Weaver, O. M., Haymaker, W., Pieper, S., and Kirland, R.: Sequelae of the arthropod-borne encephalitides. V. Japanese encephalitis. Neurology, 8:887, 1958.

Webb, H. E., and Rao, L.: Kyasanur Forest disease: A general clinical study in which some cases with neurological complications were observed. Trans. R. Soc. Trop. Med. Hyg., 55:284, 1961.

White, M. G., Carter, N. W., et al.: Pathophysiology of epidemic St. Louis encephalitis. Ann. Intern. Med., 71:691, 1969.

102. VIRAL HEMORRHAGIC FEVERS

102.1. INTRODUCTION

Karl M. Johnson

The viral hemorrhagic fevers form a group of acute diseases in which bleeding is a prominent clinical manifestation. These diseases occur in different parts of the world, are caused by ribonucleic acid–containing viruses, and may be transmitted to man by mosquitoes, by ticks, or by direct contact with excreta of virus-infected rodents (see accompanying table). Despite its longstanding fame as a cause of acute hepatocellular necrosis, *yellow fever* is included under this heading because of its recognized ability to induce gastrointestinal hemorrhage and a shock syndrome similar to that seen with other viruses of the group.

After a variable period of a few days to one to three weeks, during which virus multiplies in lymphoid cells and produces a viremia, hemorrhagic fever patients experience fever, myalgia, and other nonspecific symptoms. Bleeding ensues, generally near the end of the febrile period, and although usually not sufficient per se to account for it, such hemorrhage is the harbinger of a clinical crisis dominated by hypovolemic shock. In at least two instances, epidemic hemorrhagic fever and dengue hemorrhagic fever, there is evidence that shock is caused by a widespread capillary vascular lesion in which plasma protein escapes the circulation much faster than erythrocytes. Thrombocytopenia and deficits in various circulating hemostatic factors are frequently present, but it is not clear whether they are etiologically related to this condition.

How the hemorrhagic syndrome is produced thus remains a mystery. No evidence for a direct virus-induced lesion of capillary endothelium has been ob-

tained to date. Disseminated intravascular coagulation (DIC) has been shown in a few instances and postulated in others. But even assuming that DIC occurs, we have no clear idea about the vital pathophysiologic triggers for this chain reaction. Certain facts suggest, however, that altered immunologic function may be important in the pathogenesis of hemorrhagic fever. First, the pathology of such viral disease, unlike that associated with arboviral encephalitis, is characterized by the absence of inflammatory tissue reaction. Second, the high evidence of secondary bacterial infections and the delay of specific humoral antibody response observed in arenavirus-caused disease and Crimean hemorrhagic fever implies a direct suppression of B-cell lymphocyte function. Finally, there is the possibility that antigen-antibody complexes may be important in the genesis of some of these conditions. Available data include long incubation period, leukocytosis, and acute, reversible renal insufficiency in epidemic hemorrhagic fever; the temporal association between hemorrhagic disease and secondary dengue virus infection together with reduction of circulating complement components is even more suggestive. As for the arboviral encephalitides, elucidation of the operative variables is important. Clinical management of disease and vaccine development appear to offer more hope of averting fatal infection than does interruption of the nonhuman natural virus cycles.

102.2. YELLOW FEVER

Thomas P. Monath

DEFINITION. Yellow fever is an acute mosquito-borne viral infection characterized, in its severe form, by fever, jaundice, hemorrhage, and albuminuria. The disease is endemic-epidemic in tropical regions of the Americas and Africa, where it remains a major public health problem, but it does not occur in Asia.

ETIOLOGY. Yellow fever virus is the prototype of the flavivirus taxonomic group which is composed of a variety of other medically important, antigenically related viruses, including several which also cause hemorrhagic fevers (dengue, Omsk hemorrhagic fever, and Kyasanur Forest disease). Yellow fever virus (and other flaviviruses) are spherical, enveloped, RNA-containing particles of approximately 38 mμ in size; virions develop by budding from intracytoplasmic membranes of infected cells and accumulate in cisternae of the endoplasmic reticulum. Since the virus shares antigenic determinants with many other flaviviruses, some of which are common in the yellow fever endemic zone, serologic responses to infection are often nonspecific or difficult to interpret. Strains of yellow fever virus from Africa and South America are distinguishable in special serologic tests; strain variation in virulence markers for laboratory animals also occurs. However, no clear geographic differences have been shown in the clinical features of the human disease. Yellow fever virus is pathogenic for a variety of cell cultures, newborn mice, adult mice (when injected intracerebrally), and some monkey species. Rhesus monkeys have been used as an experimental model of the human disease.

EPIDEMIOLOGY. Two epidemiologic forms of yellow fever are classically distinguished on the basis of dif-

Viral Hemorrhagic Fevers: Etiologic and Epidemiologic Considerations

	Causative Agent	Vector(s)	Vertebrate Host(s)	Geographical Distribution	Epidemiologic Features of Involvement of Man	Control	Remarks
Yellow fever (urban)	YF virus—a group B arbovirus	*Aedes aegypti* in cities	Man	Human populations (usually urban) in tropics of South and Central America and Africa	Person-to-person passage by *Aedes aegypti*	*Aedes aegypti* control; vaccination	Sylvan YF can spread to cities
Yellow fever (sylvan)	YF virus—a group B arbovirus	*Haemagogus* mosquitoes in New World; *Aedes* species in Africa	Monkeys of several genera and species	Forests and jungles of South and Central American and West, Central, and East Africa	Man infected by exposure in jungle (i.e., woodcutters, hunters, etc.)	Vaccination	Human cases sporadic and unpredictable; disease often a "silent" endemic in forests
Dengue hemorrhagic fever	Dengue viruses of four types; group B arboviruses	*Aedes aegypti*	Man (involvement of other primates has been postulated)	Tropical and subtropical cities of Southeast Asia and Philippines	Small children usually involved in cities where *Aedes aegypti* densities are high	*Aedes aegypti* control; mosquito repellent, screens, etc.	Disease may represent an immunologic over-response to a sequential infection with a different dengue strain
Omsk hemorrhagic fever	Two distinguishable subtypes of HF virus	Ticks of genus *Dermacentor*	Small rodents and muskrats	Omsk region of USSR; northern Roumania	People exposed in fields and wooded lands.	Tick repellents and protective clothing	
Kyasanur forest disease	KFD virus—a group B arbovirus	Ticks of several species in genus *Haemaphysalis*	Monkeys (rhesus and langur) and small rodents and birds	Mysore State, India	People exposed in fields and wooded lands	Tick control; tick repellents and protective clothing	Monkey mortality signals epidemic activity
Argentine hemorrhagic fever	Junin virus, an arenavirus LCM-related	None proved; mites suspected	Small rodents: Akodon; *Calomys laucha, musculinus*	Argentina: NW of Buenos Aires extending west to Province of Cordoba	Field workers at harvest time are particularly at risk	Rodent control in fields	Infected rodents contaminate environment with urine
Bolivian hemorrhagic fever	Machupo virus, an arenavirus LCM-related	None recognized	Small rodent, *Calomys callosus*	Beni Province of Bolivia	Residents of small, rodent-infested villages and homes; 1971 nosocomial outbreak in Cochabamba, Bolivia	Rodent control in villages; full isolation in hospital patient care	High mortality in man
Lassa fever	Lassa virus, an arenavirus LCM-related	None required	Small rodent; *Mastomys natalensis*	West Africa: Nigeria, Liberia, Sierra Leone	Residents of small rodent-infested villages; dramatic nosocomial outbreaks	None known; possibly rodent control	High mortality in man
Crimean hemorrhagic fever	CHF-Congo virus; an ungrouped arbovirus	Ticks of several genera	Larger domestic animals implicated; also African hedgehog	Southern USSR, Bulgaria, East and West Africa	Cowhands and field workers in USSR; nosocomial outbreaks reported	Tick control relating to livestock; full isolation in patient care	Human disease important in USSR; importance to man in Africa not known
Korean hemorrhagic fever (hemor. nephroso-nephritis)	Not known; virus suspected	Not known	Possibly small mammals	Korea; northern Eurasia to and including Scandinavia	Rural or sylvan exposure (military, forest occupations, farmers)	None	A baffling epidemiologic and clinical entity

ferent mosquito vectors and vertebrate hosts involved in the cycle of virus transmission. These forms are clinically and pathoanatomically identical. In the *urban* form, yellow fever virus is passed from a viremic person to another, nonimmune individual by the agency of the peridomestic mosquito, *Aedes aegypti*. As with other arboviruses, a period of extrinsic incubation in the vector is required before virus can be transmitted; this interval (6 to 30 days in *Ae. aegypti*) is temperature dependent. *Jungle* (or sylvan) yellow fever is a zoonotic infection, incidentally acquired through the bite of one of a variety of forest mosquito vector species, which maintains the virus in a monkey-mosquito-monkey cycle. The epidemiology and epizootiology of the disease in the Americas and in Africa differ and must be considered separately. Despite years of intensive study,

many aspects of the ecology of yellow fever remain poorly understood.

Between 50 and 300 cases of *jungle yellow fever* are recognized annually in South America. The virus is active primarily in Brazil, Peru, Bolivia, and Colombia in forested and sparsely populated areas under limited cultivation, drained by tributaries of the Amazon, Orinoco, and Magdalena Rivers. Human cases reach a peak during the rainy months (in most areas, December through March). Human cases are often sporadic, but small epidemics (involving 20 to 50 cases) are not uncommon. In the past, large outbreaks have been associated with monkey epizootics which appear at 5- to 40-year intervals and spread through natural corridors into forested areas, such as Central America, normally outside the enzootic zone. In the forest canopy, the virus circulates in a primary cycle involving monkeys and marmosets and mosquitoes of the genus *Haemagogus*. The exact location of virus activity in the vast tropical forests of South America is difficult or impossible to ascertain at any point in time, and indeed the virus is constantly moving, thus assuring a supply of susceptible hosts adequate for maintenance of the cycle. Presence of the virus is, however, sometimes evident on the basis of monkey deaths, because some New World species succumb to the infection. Humans may accidentally acquire the disease during vocational activities, such as woodcutting, which bring them into contact with *Haemagogus* mosquitoes. Dramatic outbreaks have occurred when groups of unvaccinated laborers have penetrated jungle areas. Mosquito species of the drought-resistant genus *Sabethes* play a secondary role in the yellow fever cycle but may be important in maintaining transmission over the dry season.

In the Americas, *urban yellow fever* has not occurred since 1954 (in Trinidad), largely because of the eradication of *Aedes aegypti* mosquitoes from population centers of South America. Nonetheless, some *aegypti*-infested areas of northern South America remain in juxtaposition to the jungle cycle, and the risk of a viremic individual traveling to receptive regions of the Caribbean and southern United States is recognized. The recent occurrence of dengue epidemics in the Caribbean is prima facie evidence that this region is receptive to yellow fever.

The situation in Africa is considerably more complex. Relatively few sporadic cases are recognized annually, but this reflects under-reporting and inadequate surveillance and diagnostic facilities. Large epidemics, which occur at irregular intervals in areas of West, Central, and East Africa between 0 and 15 degrees N, have involved as many as 100,000 cases, with 30,000 deaths. Epidemics sustained by the peridomestic *Ae. aegypti* vector have occurred in both the urban and rural environments of West Africa. Epidemic yellow fever in the savannah and forest-savannah transition areas of West Africa has been transmitted by nondomestic *Aedes* species, including *luteocephalus* and *africanus,* with man acting as the probable intermediate host. Jungle yellow fever (transmission from monkey to man by wild *Aedes*) may occur but has not been documented in West Africa, where forested areas and nonhuman primate populations are now quite restricted. Enzootic transmission has nonetheless been documented in monkeys and wild *Aedes* (*africanus* and other species) inhabiting riverine forests.

In the more extensive forests of Central and East Africa, a jungle cycle analogous to that in the Americas operates, with *Aedes africanus* as the principal vector. Sporadic cases and epidemics in persons entering the forest or living at the forest fringe have resulted from exposure to this mosquito. In some areas, another vector, *Ae. simpsoni,* links the jungle cycle with human populations and has been responsible for intensive interhuman transmission.

All races are equally susceptible to yellow fever infection. The disease produced in native populations of Africa is thought to be milder than in whites, but this is probably a reflection of background immunity and cross-protection by related endemic flaviviruses; some outbreaks of yellow fever involving Africans have been severe, with high death rates. Nonimmune persons of all ages and both sexes are equally susceptible. The age and sex distribution is, however, determined by the rate of natural immunization in endemic areas, by vaccination campaign policies, and by occupational exposures. Adult males employed in woodcutting or agricultural pursuits are primarily affected by jungle yellow fever.

PATHOLOGY AND PATHOGENESIS. Gross pathologic lesions are relatively few; signs include icterus; hemorrhages or petechiae of the mucous membranes, stomach, duodenum, renal capsule, and urinary bladder; and small amounts of pleural and peritoneal fluid. Histopathologic changes of the liver may be characteristic, but even experienced pathologists may not be able to make an unequivocal diagnosis in atypical cases. Conditions with which yellow fever has been confused on the basis of liver pathology include Lassa fever, African (Marburg-Ebola virus) hemorrhagic fever, viral hepatitis, and leptospirosis. The typical yellow fever lesion is marked by cloudy swelling, then by coagulative necrosis of hepatocytes in the midzone of the liver lobule, sparing cells bordering the central vein. The centrilobular trabeculae show a degree of disorganization. Eosinophilic degeneration of hepatocytes results in the formation of *Councilman bodies;* intranuclear eosinophilic granular inclusions (Torres bodies) have also been described. Multi- and microvacuolar fatty change is nearly always present, especially after the eighth day of illness. An inflammatory response is absent or limited to a mild interstitial histiocytic infiltration late in the disease. The reticulin framework is preserved. Characteristic changes have been seen in biopsy specimens taken as early as the third day of illness; interpretation of biopsy or necropsy material obtained after the tenth day is often difficult. Histopathologic changes in other organs are variable and less specific. Renal glomerular changes are relatively insignificant compared to acute tubular necrosis and fatty metamorphosis, which may be marked. The myocardial fibers show moderate cloudy swelling, degeneration, and fatty infiltration. Lymphocytic elements in the spleen and nodes are depleted, and large mononuclear or histiocytic cells accumulate in the splenic follicles. The brain may show edema and petechial hemorrhages.

The *pathologic physiology* of yellow fever is poorly understood. Direct viral injury to the cells of major target organs, such as the liver, kidney, and heart, undoubtedly underlie the pathogenic process and may be mediated by activation of intracellular lysozymes. Immunopathologic mechanisms are also suspected but not proved. Hepatic coma has not been clinically or electroencephalographically defined, and the role of hepatic failure in the disease is uncertain. Some patients have prominent signs of acute renal failure, and deaths have been attributed to uremia. It is not known whether acute tubular necrosis is due to direct viral injury or is secondary to hemodynamic causes or hepatocellular necrosis. Deaths (especially late in the disease) have occurred because of cardiac failure or arrhythmia, but are rare. Hemorrhage undoubtedly exacerbates hypotension and oliguria and may precipitate vascular collapse and death, but it is usually minor and must be considered only a contributory problem; rhesus monkeys die in a fashion similar to humans, with little or no overt hemorrhagic manifestations. Evidence for disseminated intravascular coagulation as the basis for the hemorrhagic diathesis is conflicting. Acid-base and electrolyte imbalances have been poorly defined. At present, the complex pathophysiologic interrelationships of yellow fever cannot be specified, and directions for specific therapeutic interventions are consequently undetermined.

CLINICAL MANIFESTATIONS. Yellow fever infection produces a clinical spectrum varying from very mild, nonspecific, febrile illness to a malignant, sometimes fatal form with pathognomonic features. The precise frequency with which the various clinical forms occur is uncertain; however, it is clear that abortive infections are the rule and that the classic symptoms of severe yellow fever are found in only 10 to 20 per cent of cases. The incubation period (interval between bite of infected mosquito and onset of symptoms) is generally three to six days.

The typical or mild case will not be suspected or clinically diagnosed except in the setting of an epidemic. In its mildest form it is characterized by sudden onset of fever and headache, without other symptoms, lasting 48 hours or less. In other patients, the fever is higher, the headache more distressing, and the illness accompanied by a grippe-like syndrome with nausea, myalgia, slight albuminuria, and bradycardia in relation to the presence of fever (Faget's sign). The illness lasts several days, with uneventful recovery.

The severe forms of yellow fever begin abruptly with fever to 40° C, chills or chilliness, severe headache, and generalized myalgia often most acute in the lower back. The patient appears distressed and anxious, the conjunctiva congested, the face and neck flushed, the tongue reddened at the tip and edges, the breath foul smelling. Anorexia, nausea, vomiting, and constipation are present, and minor gingival hemorrhages or epistaxis may occur. Despite a persistent or rising temperature, the pulse may fall. This syndrome, persisting for approximately three days, corresponds to the "period of infection," during which yellow fever virus is present in the blood. It may be followed by a "period of remission," with partial or complete defervescence and mitigation of symptoms, usually lasting several to 24 hours. The fever and systemic symptoms then reappear with more *frequent vomiting, epigastric pain, prostration,* and the *appearance of jaundice* ("period of intoxication"). Viremia is generally absent, and antibodies appear during this phase. Hematemesis, coffee grounds or black (vomito negro), is a characteristic and frightening sign. It may be accompanied or followed by other hemorrhagic manifestations, including melena, metrorrhagia, petechiae, ecchymoses, and diffuse oozing from the mucous membranes. Dehydration resulting from vomiting and increased insensible losses is frequent. Renal damage is evidenced by the sudden appearance of albuminuria, which may rapidly increase, and by diminishing urine output. The pulse remains dissociated from fever, but may weaken as the blood and pulse pressures decrease. The patient recovers either rapidly after a period of intoxication of three to four days or over a protracted course of up to two weeks. Fatalities (occurring in up to 50 per cent of severe yellow fever cases) generally occur on the seventh to tenth day of illness, and are preceded by increasing albuminuria, hemorrhages, rising pulse, hypotension, oliguria, and azotemia. Hypothermia, a severe agitated delirium, intractable hiccup, stupor, and coma are terminal signs.

In individual cases hepatic, renal, or myocardial involvement predominates, with clinical signs of relatively pure hepatitis, acute renal failure, or hypotension and hypokinetic heart failure. Pre-eminent central nervous system involvement, producing meningoencephalitic signs, has also been described. Atypical, fulminant cases occur, with death on the second or third day in the absence of hepatic or renal signs.

Physical findings during the period of intoxication include scleral and dermal icterus, hemorrhagic manifestations, epigastric (rarely hepatic) tenderness without organomegaly, and the changes already noted in vital signs.

The convalescent stage is sometimes prolonged, with profound asthenia lasting one to two weeks. Late death, occurring at the end of convalescence or even weeks after complete recovery from the acute illness, is a rare but well documented phenomenon attributed to yellow fever myocardial damage, cardiac arrhythmia, or failure. Suppurative parotitis (resulting from dehydration) and secondary bacterial pneumonia are recognized complications.

CLINICAL LABORATORY FINDINGS. Leukopenia (neutropenia) occurs most often during the early phase of illness; the white blood count is, however, often normal or elevated. Prolongation of the clotting, prothrombin, and partial thromboplastin times is marked in cases with jaundice. The platelet count is usually normal, but may be decreased. The total and conjugated serum bilirubin rise together and may reach levels of 15 to 20 mg per deciliter in severe cases. Serum glutamic-oxaloacetic transaminase and serum glutamic pyruvic transaminase levels are markedly elevated in all icteric (but inconstantly and to lower levels in anicteric) patients, with peak values between days 5 and 10 of the illness, and return to normal by days 10 to 20. The alkaline phosphatase is generally normal, but other tests reflecting liver function (serum proteins, thymol turbidity, cholesterol) may be abnormal. In patients with severe hepatic damage, hypoglycemia has been occasionally noted.

During the period of infection, the urine may contain a small amount of albumin, which then increases suddenly on the fourth or fifth day, reaching levels of 3 to 5 (rarely as high as 40) grams per liter. The urine may coagulate in patients with massive proteinuria. The urine contains bile; the cell sediment may be abnormal but is not diagnostically helpful. The cerebrospinal fluid is clear, without cells, but it is often under increased pressure, and contains a mildly raised concentration of protein. ST-T wave electrocardiographic abnormalities have been described.

DIAGNOSIS. In endemic areas, recognition and diagnosis of a case are of great importance because it may indicate the presence of an epidemic and stimulate preventive or control measures. Because the incubation period is sufficiently long to permit an infected person to travel a long distance, the diagnosis should be suspected in all patients with fever and jaundice coming from tropical America or Africa. Specific diagnosis depends upon histopathologic study, isolation of the virus, or demonstration of a specific antibody response. The hemorrhagic diathesis renders liver biopsy hazardous, and pathologic diagnosis is thus a postmortem procedure. The virus is most readily isolated (by inoculation of mice or cell cultures) from serum obtained during the first three or four days of illness (period of infection), but it may be recovered from serum up to the twelfth day and occasionally from liver at death.

Serologic methods useful in the diagnosis of yellow

fever include hemagglutination-inhibition (HI), complement-fixation (CF), neutralization (N), and radioimmunoassay tests. The HI and N antibodies appear within a week of onset; the CF antibodies appear later. Paired, acute, and convalescent phase specimens are required to establish the diagnosis by rise in antibody titer. Cross-reactions with other flaviviruses and the high prevalence of background immunity to flaviviruses in tropical populations make serodiagnosis difficult in many cases.

Virus isolation and serologic tests are applicable to the diagnosis of all clinical forms of yellow fever and are the only means available of establishing the cause of abortive and mild infections.

DIFFERENTIAL DIAGNOSIS. Mild yellow fever cannot be clinically distinguished from a wide array of other infections. In the presence of jaundice and the other signs of severe yellow fever, conditions that must be differentiated include viral hepatitis, falciparum malaria, spirochetal infections (tick-borne relapsing fever and Weil's disease), Rift Valley fever, typhoid, Q fever, typhus, and surgical, drug-induced, and toxic causes. Other diseases (usually without jaundice) that may be confused with yellow fever include Lassa, African (Marburg-Ebola virus), Bolivian, and Argentine hemorrhagic fevers.

PROGNOSIS. Up to 50 per cent of patients with severe forms of yellow fever die; it should be recognized that patients in most reported series have been cared for under primitive conditions. The fatality rate of *all* patients with clinical illness is much lower (2 to 5 per cent). The prognosis should be guarded for the patient who, after a brief remission, enters a clear period of intoxication with rising fever, jaundice, and albuminuria. Certain clinical and laboratory features appear to correlate with a poor prognosis. These include early onset of bilirubinemia and albuminuria rising to high levels; prolongation of the prothrombin time beyond 25 per cent of normal; a rising and weakening pulse during the period of intoxication; and the appearance of coma, hypothermia, and intractable hiccup.

Relapses have not been described. The possibility of late death from myocardial or renal injury must be considered.

TREATMENT. No specific therapy exists at present. Complete bed rest, supportive care, and close monitoring of vital functions are essential. During the stage of infection, mild sedatives, analgesics, and antiemetics may be indicated, and attention should be given to fluid and electrolyte balance. Aspirin is contraindicated because of the bleeding diathesis. General and specific supportive measures are of critical importance during the period of intoxication if vomiting is severe, if hemorrhage appears, or if hypertension, hypokinetic heart failure, oliguria, azotemia, and electrolyte and acid-base imbalance become evident. In theory, these consequences of severe yellow fever might be lessened by intensive counter-regulation. Heroic measures (hyperalimentation, exchange blood transfusion) aimed at improving hepatic and neurologic function have been tried in experimentally infected rhesus monkeys, but without success.

Secondary bacterial infections or concurrent infections (in particular, malaria) should be treated by the usual appropriate means.

Return to activity should be gradual.

PREVENTION AND CONTROL. The patient with yellow fever should be isolated from possible contact with mosquitoes under netting or in a screened room.

Yellow fever 17D is one of the safest live, attenuated vaccines available and provides effective, longlasting immunity. For purposes of international certification, vaccination is considered valid for 10 years, but immunity has been documented to last 19 years and may be lifelong. Since yellow fever exists as a silent enzoosis over wide areas of the tropics and appears in epidemic form with little warning and without early recognition, vaccination of travelers is imperative. Immunity can be demonstrated within 10 days after vaccination. Mild vaccine reactions occur rarely, and serious complications have been exceedingly uncommon. No untoward consequences for the fetus have been recorded; but on theoretical grounds, pregnant women should not be vaccinated unless the risk of acquiring yellow fever is considered great. The vaccine is prepared in chicken embryos and should be used with caution in persons hypersensitive to egg proteins. The 17D vaccine available in the United States is presently contaminated with avian leukosis virus, but follow-up studies have not correlated this contaminant with any known human disease. Leukosis-free vaccine is commercially available in England and is under development in the United States. The French neurotropic viral vaccine is no longer produced or used anywhere in the world.

In the event of an epidemic, the disease may be controlled by mass vaccination and the use of insecticides to reduce infected vector populations.

102.3. HEMORRHAGIC FEVER CAUSED BY DENGUE VIRUSES

Karl M. Johnson

DEFINITION. These hemorrhagic fevers of Southeast Asia and India are acute, infectious, urban, mosquito-borne diseases caused by dengue viruses. Endoepidemic in pattern, dengue hemorrhagic fever is clinically defined as a dengue disease that worsens two or more days after onset, and is characterized by hypoproteinemia and one or more hemostatic abnormalities such as thrombocytopenia, prolonged bleeding time, or elevated prothrombin time. The dengue shock syndrome consists of hemorrhagic fever plus shock (hypotension or a pulse pressure of 20 mm Hg or less) and hemoconcentration (hematocrit at least 20 per cent greater than convalescent value). Chikungunya virus infections fulfilling these criteria are rarely encountered.

ETIOLOGY. All evidence suggests that these diseases are caused by each of the four recognized dengue virus subtypes. How they produce such disease is still not clear. A current hypothesis is that severe dengue disease is produced by an immunologic reaction that occurs in some individuals experiencing a second dengue infection. However, hemorrhagic fever has been unequivocally caused by primary dengue infection.

EPIDEMIOLOGY. These hemorrhagic fevers were first seen in epidemic proportions in Manila and Bangkok (1954) and in Singapore (1960). Other outbreaks have been reported from Malaysia, South Vietnam, India, Indonesia, and Oceania. In Bangkok age-specific rates in children have reached 7 to 8 per 1000. In most outbreaks cases occur only in children, principally below the age of 8 years; otherwise, the epidemiology of infection leading to dengue hemorrhagic fever is basically similar to that associated with ordinary dengue fever; outbreaks occur during the rainy season in large urban centers where *Aedes aegypti* is well established. Halstead has proposed that dengue hemorrhagic fever is an immune disease, brought on usually by a second (but not a third) dengue virus infection in a previously sensitized host. The syndromes have not been observed in many places where dengue is or has been prevalent, including the New World and many parts of Southeast Asia, Australasia, and Oceania.

PATHOLOGY. Autopsy data are scant. The chief abnormalities include generalized vascular congestion and dilatation with edema and multiple focal hemorrhages in most organs, mild to moderate pleural effusion and ascites, mononuclear cell infiltration of interstitial tissues and alveolar walls of lungs, focal myocardial congestion, and a decrease in mature lymphocytes with proliferation of mononuclear forms in the germinal centers of lymph follicles.

Necrosis is unusual, and no specific damage of the blood vessels has been observed. Perivascular infiltration by mononuclear cells is common, but there is no evidence for significant vasculitis or for platelet or thrombin thrombosis of vessel walls. About one third of cases show evidence of globulin on endothelial surfaces and the walls of arterioles. The bone marrow often shows maturation arrest of megakaryocytes, and sometimes there is marked generalized cellular hypoplasia with rapid restoration to normal after emergence from shock.

Pathologic change in the liver, although generally inconspicuous, consists of focal lesions and varies greatly in degree of severity. These lesions are of particular interest, because occasionally Councilman bodies and other changes characteristic of yellow fever are observed.

PATHOGENESIS OR MECHANISM OF DISEASE. The pathogenesis is as yet poorly understood. The vascular congestion, dilatation, and increased permeability lead to the extensive edema and hemorrhage observed in the gastrointestinal tract, the skin, and other tissues. The cause of these vascular changes is unknown, but they result in loss of plasma volume and associated electrolyte disturbances. Platelet deficiency probably plays a role in the hemorrhages. Bleeding time is usually prolonged, prothrombin times are somewhat prolonged, clot retraction is poor, and the blood fibrinogen is slightly reduced. None of these changes is very profound. The circulatory collapse and shock observed appear to be far in excess of what might be expected from the extent of loss of edema fluid and blood. The adrenal changes suggest exhaustion of steroid reserve. Death in some cases has been accompanied by severe hyperkalemia.

CLINICAL MANIFESTATIONS. The onset is that of a dengue infection, usually abrupt, with fever. Nausea and vomiting are common. The throat appears injected, and there may be a dry cough. About the second or third day petechiae appear, usually first on the face or distal portions of the extremities but sparing the axillae and chest. The tourniquet test may be conspicuously positive before petechiae appear. Purpura and large ecchymoses as well as other manifestations of bleeding tendency are occasionally prominent. There may be severe abdominal pain and tenderness. About the third or fourth day, vomiting may produce copious coffee-ground material. Melena also is not uncommon, but gross bleeding from the intestines is rare. Shock is likely to occur in severe cases about the fourth day, and this critical state lasts about 12 to 24 hours. At this time the temperature falls to normal, the blood pressure and pulse pressure are low or unmeasurable, and the limbs are cool and present a purple or brownish mottled appearance. Perspiration is frequently profuse. The face and hands appear edematous. Restlessness and apprehension are conspicuous as the patient enters shock. This state of shock is entirely out of proportion to the apparent loss of blood. Thrombocytopenia is noted during this period, and bleeding time is prolonged. Leukocytes remain at approximately normal levels, but are elevated in number in serious cases more frequently than they are depressed. The total and differential leukocyte counts are not those observed in dengue. Although the numbers of both immature and mature polymorphonuclear cells are decreased, there is an increase in lymphocytes and sometimes in monocytes.

DIAGNOSIS. Hemorrhagic fever begins as an extension of a classic dengue infection, and the early dengue syndrome intergrades into the milder and atypical manifestations of the later hemorrhagic syndrome. The diagnosis in a febrile child acutely ill for only two or three days is rendered highly probable by the presentation of petechiae, purpuric lesions, and unusual ecchymosis of the skin with most prominent distribution on the extremities and face, together with melena, thrombocytopenia, and a relatively normal leukocyte count. In a milder case or at an earlier stage, the tourniquet test may be of great assistance in detecting unusual capillary fragility. The rapid development of circulatory collapse and shock during the fourth to sixth day, associated with the aforementioned findings, differentiates this from most other exanthematous diseases. Meningococcemia and the Waterhouse-Friderichsen syndrome need careful consideration. Thrombocytopenic purpura can be expected to have an entirely different onset and is usually not associated with fever. Laboratory methods available for diagnosis are those described for dengue fever.

TREATMENT. There is no specific therapy, but case fatality rates can be greatly reduced by skillful management directed toward combating shock. Close monitoring of pulse, respiration, and blood pressure during the course of treatment is essential for at least 48 hours, because shock can occur and recur. Oxygen should be administered if there is cyanosis or labored breathing. Hypovolemia should be treated by administration of lactated Ringer's solution or 5 per cent glucose in normal saline, on the basis of 20 ml per kilogram of body weight, administered rapidly. In profound or unresponsive shock, plasma or a plasma expander (dextran in normal saline) can be given at the rate of 20 ml per kilogram of body weight. When signs improve, 5 per cent glucose in normal saline or in lactated Ringer's solution should be given at the rate of 10 ml per kilogram per hour, and continued until vital signs are normal. Acidosis should be corrected with sodium bicarbonate as necessary.

Whole blood should be given only if blood loss is known to be large. Administration of whole blood to a patient with elevated hematocrit may result in heart failure. Paraldehyde or chloral hydrate may be required for children who are markedly agitated. Salicylates administered during the febrile period may cause bleeding and acidosis, and they should not be given to febrile patients during a hemorrhagic fever outbreak. Pressor amines, alpha-adrenergic blocking agents, and steroids have not been demonstrated to be of value in treatment.

PROGNOSIS. Death is almost always associated with shock, and rarely occurs after the sixth day of illness. Case fatality rates among hospitalized patients have ranged from 5 to 50 per cent, depending to a large extent upon the condition of patients on admission and the facilities available for treatment. Careful management should be able to save all but the 5 or 10 per cent of patients admitted in a moribund state. Residual effects have not been observed, and, in contrast to primary dengue, recovery is usually prompt and complete seven to ten days after onset. Mental depression is seldom observed.

PREVENTION. The control of this hemorrhagic fever is the same as that for dengue, and consists of mosquito control or protection from mosquito bites and isolation of the patient from mosquitoes. No vaccine is available, and if the immunologic theory of causation is confirmed, vaccines as presently conceived would be specifically contraindicated.

102.4. CRIMEAN HEMORRHAGIC FEVER

Karl M. Johnson

DEFINITION. Crimean hemorrhagic fever (CHF) is an acute febrile disease, often marked by severe hemorrhage and high mortality, occurring in the Soviet Union, Bulgaria, and Pakistan.

ETIOLOGY. The CHF agent is an arbovirus first isolated from human blood specimens in 1967. It is pathogenic for suckling mice and grows in several types of cultured cells. This virus is indistinguishable from Congo virus of Africa in CF and neutralization tests. Strains from Eurasia and Africa are thus referred to as CHF-Congo virus.

EPIDEMIOLOGY. CHF-Congo virus is naturally transmitted by several species of hard ticks belonging to the genera *Hyalomma, Rhipicephalus, Amblyomma,* and *Boophilus.* Active foci of infection with transmission to man exist in the lower Don and Volga river basins, in the Central Asian republics of Kazakstan and Uzbekistan of the Soviet Union, and in Pakistan. Few human cases have been recognized in Africa. The disease occurs most frequently among adults who are heavily exposed to ticks while working among cattle. Cases begin to appear in April and reach a peak during summer months. Proved or presumed vertebrate hosts for the virus include cattle, goats, hares, rooks, and hedgehogs. Transovarial tick transmission is suspected but not yet proved. Nosocomial human infections have occurred repeatedly in Central Asia, suggesting transmission by aerosol. The incubation period is estimated at about one week.

CLINICAL MANIFESTATIONS. Onset is typically abrupt with high, unremittent fever, chills, headache, and myalgia. There may be hyperemia of the upper trunk and neck, conjunctival effusion, vomiting, and diarrhea. Hepatomegaly is noted in about half the cases; splenomegaly is uncommon. Pronounced panleukopenia is almost invariably present, as is thrombocytopenia.

Bleeding begins on about the fourth day of illness. Petechiae appear in the oral mucosa and skin, at times presenting as frank *purpura hemorrhagica.* Nose, gums, and intestinal tract are the most common sites of bleeding, and in this disease above all other viral hemorrhagic fevers, blood loss per se may be life threatening. Stiff neck, hyperexcitability, or coma occurs in about 10 per cent of cases and these are grave prognostic signs. The cerebrospinal fluid, however, contains no leukocytes or increased protein. There may be proteinuria and microscopic hematuria, but renal function is rarely compromised. The fever and bleeding generally resolve by lysis at about the eighth day. Hypovolemic shock with a paradoxical rising hematocrit may appear just prior to the end of fever and is the most common cause of death.

DIAGNOSIS. Virus can be easily obtained from blood of patients during the first few days of illness. Specific CF and neutralizing antibodies appear in the sera of most patients 30 to 60 days after onset of symptoms.

TREATMENT AND PROGNOSIS. Therapy is symptomatic. Management of fluid, electrolyte, and erythrocyte balance forms the continuous clinical challenge. Shock is a grave problem and should be anticipated and treated as outlined in Ch. 102.5 and 356. Whole blood transfusion may be necessary. Intercurrent bacterial infection is very common, especially pneumonia. Mortality in the Soviet Union ranges from 20 to 50 per cent. Patients surviving the acute illness generally recover completely, albeit quite slowly. Several instances of mono- or polyneuritis persisting for several months have been recorded.

PREVENTION. There is no vaccine yet available; thus avoidance of the disease in endemic foci depends on personal measures designed to prevent tick bites. Several nosocomial infections have occurred in the Soviet Union and Pakistan. Thus strict isolation of patients and use of protective clothing and respirators by medical personnel are indicated.

102.5. HEMORRHAGIC DISEASES CAUSED BY ARENAVIRUSES: ARGENTINE AND BOLIVIAN HEMORRHAGIC FEVERS AND LASSA FEVER*

Karl M. Johnson

DEFINITION. Argentine and Bolivian hemorrhagic fevers and Lassa fever are acute diseases caused respectively by Junin, Machupo, and Lassa viruses. Clinically, the diseases share the common features of fever, severe myalgia, leukopenia, hemorrhagic manifestations, shock, and (excluding Lassa fever) neurologic abnormalities.

ETIOLOGY. The three viruses are serologically and morphologically related, and related to lymphocytic choriomeningitis virus, in a grouping designated as arenaviruses.

GEOGRAPHICAL DISTRIBUTION, INCIDENCE, AND PREVALENCE. Argentine hemorrhagic fever is localized to the provinces of Córdoba and Junin in northern Argentina,

---

*The author wishes to express his thanks to Dr. Wilbur G. Downs for his considerable assistance in the preparation of this chapter, particularly with reference to the material on Lassa fever.

where several hundred to several thousand cases occur annually, principally in agricultural field hands, in the harvest months. Bolivian hemorrhagic fever has been reported only from Beni province of Bolivia, between the rivers Mamore and Branco, with the exception of a hospital outbreak in Cochabamba, Bolivia, in 1971, traceable to contact with a person from Beni province. Infections are seen in inhabitants of certain of the small towns, as well as in rural populations. Lassa fever has been reported from Nigeria, Liberia, and Sierra Leone, and hospital outbreaks account for most of the cases reported. Case fatality rates are estimates in the usual absence of prompt and specific diagnosis, but may be as high as 50 per cent in hospitalized cases of Lassa, and 10 to 20 per cent for the South American diseases.

EPIDEMIOLOGY AND PROBABLE MODE OF TRANSMISSION. The viruses have been isolated from wild rodents: Junin, most commonly from *Calomys musculinus, Calomys laucha,* and also *Akodon arenicola;* Machupo, from *Calomys callosus;* and Lassa, from *Mastomys natalensis.* An attractive current hypothesis is that infection is acquired by direct human contact (ingestion, inhalation, or entrance through mucous membranes or skin breaks) with virus-containing rodent excreta. For all three agents, persistent infection in rodents has been demonstrated, with viremia readily detectable for months. A similar pattern of chronic virus infection in rodents has been described for lymphocytic choriomeningitis virus.

PATHOLOGY. Few cases have received full study. Findings include irregularly focal diapedesis and capillary hemorrhage without much evidence of inflammatory reaction. Gross hemorrhages may be seen in the mucosa of the stomach and intestines and in the brain. Pulmonary infection, probably intercurrent, is frequently seen. Focal liver necrosis is prominent in Lassa fever.

CLINICAL MANIFESTATIONS. Although as many as half of all etiologically confirmed cases appear as acute undifferentiated fevers, the findings and clinical course of "full-blown" Argentine and Bolivian infections are so nearly identical as to justify joint description. The same holds for Lassa fever. Onset is usually gradual, with increasing fever, headache, diffuse myalgia, and anorexia. By the third day the temperature may be 39.5 to 40.5° C, with severe myalgia, particularly in the lumbar regions (or legs in Lassa fever). Conjunctival injection is present, a flush involving the upper trunk and face is frequently observed, and there may be a relative bradycardia. Beginning about the fourth day, scattered fine petechiae may appear on the face and neck, about the pectoral girdle, and/or in the buccal mucosa or palate. Aphthous ulcers of the oral mucosa and exudative pharyngitis have been a noteworthy feature of Lassa infections. The Rumpel-Leede test is frequently positive. Frank hemorrhages from one or more sites, including the stomach, intestines, nose, gums, and uterus, accompanied by microscopic hematuria, may occur. Hemorrhagic phenomena are not a common feature of Lassa infections. Although hemorrhage per se is rarely the precipitating cause, a hypotensive crisis frequently develops between the sixth and eighth days, coincident with a rapid return of temperature to normal after five or more days of sustained fever. Patients surviving this stress for 48 hours generally make slow but complete recovery.

Perhaps a fifth of the patients with the Bolivian or Argentine disease develop neurologic signs. These are quite characteristic, and begin on about the fifth or sixth day with a fine intention tremor of the tongue. This may become so severe as to render speech unintelligible and to preclude oral ingestion of solid or even liquid food. If so, gross intention tremors of the extremities usually appear, occasionally accompanied by an intermittent nystagmus. Such patients often become delirious, and may experience generalized clonic and tonic convulsions. The cerebrospinal fluid appears normal, however, and contains neither leukocytes nor virus. Convalescence is marked by weakness and signs of autonomic nervous system lability such as postural hypotension, spontaneous flushing and blanching of the skin, and episodes of diaphoresis.

In addition to delirium and occasional coma, 5 to 10 per cent of Lassa fever patients suffer significant permanent damage to one or both eighth cranial nerves. Some Lassa fever patients have shown electrocardiographic evidence of myocardial involvement.

Transient loss of scalp hair and typical Beau's lines in the nails, particularly those of the fingers, are observed in a majority of cases several weeks after subsidence of the high, sustained fever. Many patients are not able to resume full activity for at least one month after illness.

Leukopenia is almost invariably present, and cell counts may be as low as 1000 per cubic millimeter by the fourth or fifth day. All elements are reduced nearly equally, and there is often a mild to moderate thrombocytopenia during the first week. Usually the peripheral blood picture returns to normal rapidly after defervescence, although there may be transient relative lymphocytosis and mild anemia. During the latter portion of the febrile period, progressive increase in hematocrit similar to, but usually milder than, that of hemorrhagic nephrosonephritis (q.v.) is frequently observed. At about the same time, moderate proteinuria is common, although renal function is rarely compromised seriously, and frank azotemia and hyperkalemia are almost never present.

DIAGNOSIS. The presence of high fever, severe myalgia, and leukopenia should arouse immediate suspicion of viral hemorrhagic fever within the known endemic areas of its occurrence. Potential intimate contact with wild rodents in a rural or semirural setting serves to strengthen the likelihood of this diagnosis. Since these findings and all others described cannot be relied upon to differentiate the disease clinically from other infections such as yellow fever, typhoid and paratyphoid fevers, typhus, malaria, and leptospirosis, specific identification of cases depends upon laboratory confirmation. Virus can sometimes be isolated from blood, throat washing, and urine during the febrile period. At autopsy splenic tissue almost always yields the agent. Serologic detection of infection is a reliable method if paired acute and convalescent serums are employed. Both group-reacting complement-fixing antibodies and virus type-specific neutralizing antibodies appear in three to four weeks and reach peak values in seven to ten weeks after the onset of illness. Fluorescent antibodies appear in Lassa infections as early as seven days after the onset of symptoms.

These three agents have been responsible for several fatal laboratory infections, and work with the viruses should be carried out only with strictest precautionary measures, and complete isolation from other laboratory activities, in special high-risk laboratories.

TREATMENT. In the absence of any specific therapy,

successful treatment presents an acute challenge in the science and art of physiologic management. Patients require complete rest and maximal comfort. Mild sedatives and analgesics should be judiciously used. Careful measurement of fluid intake and output is mandatory. The electrolyte balance should be checked regularly; marked underhydration and overhydration are to be avoided, because these conditions appear to compromise the patient's ability to weather the hypotensive crisis. Daily hematocrit determinations and examinations of urine for protein are the most valuable tests for anticipating and managing this problem. Frequent measurement of blood pressure is also important, because many patients enter the shock phase with persistent relative bradycardia and warm, dry skin. Raising the foot of the bed may suffice to stabilize the pressure at levels adequate to preserve vital urinary output. If not, careful administration of human plasma or concentrated albumin (not whole blood) is indicated. In one instance of a Lassa infection, administration of plasma from a recovered patient appeared to be effective. Great care should be exercised in administering plasma or other fluids intravenously during shock, because intractable pulmonary edema is readily induced. Complications, particularly bacterial infections, should be anticipated and promptly treated. Convalescence should never be hurried.

PROGNOSIS. Although the case mortality may exceed 20 per cent, there is no single finding early in the disease that aids prognosis in the individual case. In general, the very young and the very old, as well as those who do not receive medical attention prior to the sixth day of disease, are subject to the highest risk. The onset of severe shock and neurologic abnormalities are both ominous prognostic signs, and at least half the patients exhibiting these signs succumb. The prognosis in Lassa fever is even poorer in diagnosed cases.

PREVENTION. Effective elimination of intimate human contact with certain wild rodents represents the only proved method for prevention of disease. This may be achieved by maintaining sound standards of personal and environmental hygiene. Campaigns to eliminate rodents, repair buildings, and clean rubbish near dwellings are highly successful when the disease is acquired mainly from peridomestic animals. There is insufficient evidence at present to warrant recommendation of systematic measures to control attacks by any potential arthropod vector.

Hospital outbreaks involving medical staff have provided most of the Lassa fever cases to date. A hospital outbreak of Machupo virus has occurred in Cochabamba, Bolivia. Such outbreaks can be extremely dangerous to personnel and demoralizing to hospital operation.

102.6.   AFRICAN HEMORRHAGIC FEVER

(Marburg Disease)

Karl M. Johnson

DEFINITION. African hemorrhagic fever is an acute, highly fatal disease characterized by fever, prostration, rash, proteinuria, major hemorrhagic manifestations, pancreatitis, and hepatitis.

HISTORY. The disease was first described in Ger-

many in 1967 and named Marburg disease. It was acquired through contact with green monkeys, *Cercopithecus aethiops,* imported from Uganda. Secondary nosocomial cases occurred. Three further cases occurred in South Africa in 1975, with origin postulated in Rhodesia. Major outbreaks with several hundreds of cases occurred in Sudan and Zaire in 1976.

ETIOLOGY. This syndrome is caused by morphologically identical viruses, Marburg and Ebola, which are immunologically distinct. These agents probably contain RNA, are about 100 nm in diameter, and have a helical capsid, but vary extremely in length. Particles as long as $14\,\mu m$ have been found.

EPIDEMIOLOGY. The ecology of Marburg and Ebola viruses is presently unknown. No evidence for Marburg infection was detected in green monkeys captured in Uganda subsequent to the original outbreak. The source of the index infection in Rhodesia and of the Ebola outbreaks in Sudan and Zaire remains a mystery. Transmission is person-to-person, associated with close contact with patients. In Zaire contaminated needles were the source of many infections. Incubation period is about one week.

PATHOLOGY. These viruses attack the lymphoreticular system, the liver, and possibly the pancreas. Prominent hepatocellular necrosis without inflammatory reaction is a hallmark of infection. Large eosinophilic inclusions are found in liver cells, but the over-all pattern of destruction is diffuse, rather than strongly midzonal as in yellow fever.

CLINICAL MANIFESTATIONS AND PATHOLOGIC PHYSIOLOGY. Onset is typically insidious with headache and progressive fever. There is severe myalgia, and often vomiting and/or diarrhea occur. About the fourth day of illness sore throat and abdominal pain appear, and a day or so later many patients develop a fine maculopapular rash over the trunk and back which spreads to the limbs and may fade in two or three days. Bleeding, principally gastrointestinal, begins on the fifth to seventh days and is associated with rapid decompensation, ending in shock and death. Leukopenia, thrombocytopenia, and proteinuria are almost invariably present. There are extreme elevations of plasma transaminases and of amylase. In the few cases studied, definitive evidence for disseminated intravascular coagulation was found.

DIAGNOSIS. High persistent viremia is the basis for establishment of the diagnosis in acute cases. Virus is recovered by inoculation of blood into Vero cell cultures or guinea pigs which undergo a febrile infection. No attempt at virus isolation should be made except in a specially protected facility. Immunofluorescent antibodies appear during the second week after onset and persist for several years. This method is more sensitive than the complement-fixation technique, which also has been used.

PROGNOSIS AND TREATMENT. With sophisticated medical management, mortality in Marburg infection is 25 to 30 per cent. Ebola virus infections treated in rural hospitals were 50 to 90 per cent fatal, the worst prognosis of any viral disease other than rabies. In addition to intensive supportive care, which should include continuous nasogastric aspiration to combat pancreatitis, two other forms of active intervention may be of value: continuous intravenous heparin therapy for intravascular coagulation, and *early* administration of plasma containing virus-specific antibodies.

PREVENTION. The secondary attack rate in African hemorrhagic fever rarely exceeds 10 per cent. Transmission can be interrupted by scrupulous isolation of patients, careful disposal of virus-contaminated excreta and fomites, and the use of protective clothing and full-face respirators by medical personnel.

102.7. EPIDEMIC HEMORRHAGIC FEVER: HEMORRHAGIC NEPHROSONEPHRITIS

Karl M. Johnson

DEFINITION. Epidemic hemorrhagic fever is an acute disease that occurs in northeastern Asia and, in milder form, in northern European U.S.S.R., Scandinavia, Czechoslovakia, Rumania, and Bulgaria. It is characterized by fever, prostration, vomiting, proteinuria, hemorrhagic manifestations, shock, and renal failure.

HISTORY. The disease was first described in the far east of the Soviet Union in the 1930's, with suggestive history as far back as 1913. An epidemic in United Nations troops in Korea, beginning in 1951, attracted much attention.

ETIOLOGY. The disease is caused by a filterable agent first recovered from the striped field mouse, *Apodemus agrarius*, in Korea. Strains also have been recovered from patients.

EPIDEMIOLOGY. The disease is rural, characterized by isolated cases widely separated in place. Environmental exposure in forests or fields near forests is invariably noted. Person-to-person transmission does not occur. Soviet workers believe that the disease is transmitted directly from asymptomatically infected rodents to man by means of virus-contaminated rodent excreta. Some outbreaks in Europe have coincided with population "explosions" of the redbacked vole (*Clethrionomys glareolus)*, involving invasion by rodents of fields, barns, and even houses.

PATHOLOGY. Profound, protein-rich retroperitoneal edema is characteristic of early death in shock, but not of later deaths. Changes in various organs apparently have a similar pathogenesis and consist of widespread, often focal, congestion and hemorrhage, sometimes accompanied by necrosis, without significant inflammatory response. The "pathognomonic" lesion is found in the kidneys, which appear swollen and, when incised, exhibit extreme hemorrhagic congestion sharply localized to the medulla. Gross congestion or hemorrhage derived from dilated, congested small blood vessels is also found frequently in the right atrium, the pituitary, and the stomach, and less often in intestines, adrenals, lungs, and central nervous system. Liver and spleen are usually not grossly involved. Petechial hemorrhages may occur in the skin, heart, adrenals, brain, and serous surfaces.

CLINICAL MANIFESTATIONS AND PATHOLOGIC PHYSIOLOGY. The following description is based on the minority of patients (about 20 per cent) who exhibit the more severe form of disease, which can be divided into five clinical phases. All patients, however, have fever, proteinuria, and isohyposthenuria.

The febrile phase lasts three to eight days and is characterized by fever, malaise, a flush over the face and neck, and injection of the eyes and palate. Toward the end of this period, petechiae occur, blood platelets decrease, traces of protein appear in the urine, and the hematocrit begins to rise.

The hypotensive phase develops suddenly during defervescence and lasts one to three days. Shock is insidious with warm dry extremities and initially no increase in pulse rate. The dominant feature is a reduction in effective blood volume owing to a loss of plasma from the vascular system. Hematocrit values may reach 70 per cent, and erythrocytes are sequestered in dilated capillaries. Nausea and vomiting are common, as are back and abdominal pain, the latter having occasioned ill-advised exploratory laparotomy in misdiagnosed cases. Heavy proteinuria and oliguria progressing to acute renal failure occur during this interval. Capillary hemorrhages are most prominent at this time also, and blood leukocytes, earlier normal or reduced, now show a leukemoid reaction.

The oliguric phase begins as the sequestered plasma returns to the vascular system and the hematocrit falls. Deaths during this three- to five-day interval are due to pulmonary edema, hyperkalemia, and shock secondary to dehydration or secondary pulmonary infections. Some patients become hypertensive and display a reactive hypervolemic syndrome that responds to phlebotomy. Biochemical abnormalities associated with renal failure appear at this time.

The diuretic phase, lasting for days or weeks, usually initiates clinical recovery but is fraught with problems in clinical management. Diuresis of 3 to 8 liters daily and isohyposthenuria lead to an extremely brittle situation with respect to hemodynamics and salt balance. Hypokalemia and hypernatremia can be problems. Shock may occur, and bacterial pulmonary infections are common. Nearly a third of all deaths occur during this phase.

Convalescence requires three to twelve weeks and is marked by gradual return of appetite, strength, and urinary concentrating ability.

DIAGNOSIS. Specific diagnosis is made by immunofluorescent technique, using lung sections from *Apodemus* rodents as source of antigen. Most patients already have low titers of antibody in acute phase sera, but diagnostic increases in titer regularly occur by the end of the second week of symptoms. The antibodies persist at least ten years. Retrospective serodiagnosis has now been confirmed in patients from the Soviet Union, Finland, and Japan, as well as Korea. Asymptomatic infections are unusual, but mild clinically apparent cases have been documented.

PROGNOSIS AND TREATMENT. Because antimicrobial drugs, convalescent serum, hormones, and other agents are entirely ineffective, the management of hemorrhagic fever must be supportive and based on an understanding of its physiologic and biochemical characteristics and on frequent clinical observations. Adequate sedation with barbiturates or opiates is frequently required for restlessness. Contrary to the practice in other febrile diseases, fluid intake must be limited because any excess will simply leak out of damaged capillaries and increase edema and symptoms. When intravenous fluid is required, it usually should be 10 per cent dextrose in water, and must be given very slowly. If shock fails to respond to simple measures such as shock blocks, then concentrated (salt-poor) human serum albumin to restore plasma volume may be required. Treatment in the oliguric phase is that of acute renal failure, with careful control of electrolytes and particular attention to hyper-kalemia. If oliguria persists, hemodialysis or peritoneal dialysis is indicated. Soviet workers have so treated 60 severe cases and report only three deaths. The chief problem of the diuretic phase is one of careful matching of fluid and electrolyte intake against the brisk urinary output, so as to avoid excessive dehydration and shock, on the one hand, and hypervolemia and pulmonary edema, on the other. Electrolyte abnormalities are still a problem, especially potassium deficiency. Overall mortality under optimal conditions seldom surpasses 5 per cent.

PREVENTION. Preventive measures are based on the assumption that the disease is transmitted by rodents with or without the aid of an associated arthropod vector. Vigorous rodent control measures, as well as dipping of clothing in acaricidal solutions and the individual use of insect repellents, are recommended in endemic areas during seasonal periods of disease activity.

Barnes, W. J. S., and Rosen, L.: Fatal hemorrhagic disease and shock associated with primary dengue infection on a Pacific island. Am. J. Trop. Med. Hyg., 23:495, 1974.
Bokisch, V. A., Top, F. H., Jr., Russell, R. K., Dixon, F. J., and Muller-Eberhard, H. J.: The potential pathogenic role of complement in dengue hemorrhagic shock syndrome. N. Engl. J. Med., 289:996, 1973.
Casals, J., Henderson, B. E., Hoogstraal, H., Johnson, K. M., and Shelokov, A.: A review of Soviet viral hemorrhagic fevers, 1969. J. Infect. Dis., 122:437, 1970.
Groot, H., and Bahia Ribiero, R.: Neutralizing and hemagglutination-

inhibiting antibodies to yellow fever 17 years after vaccination with 17D vaccine. Bull. WHO, 27:699, 1962.
Halstead, S. B., et al.: Observations related to pathogenesis of dengue hemorrhagic fever. Yale J. Biol. Med., 42:261, 1970.
International symposium on arenaviral infections of public health importance. Bull. WHO, 52:381, 1975.
Johnson, K. M., Halstead, S. B., and Cohen, S. N.: Hemorrhagic fevers of Southeast Asia and South America: A comparative appraisal. In Melnick, J. L. (ed.): Progress in Medical Virology, Vol. 9. Basel/New York, S. Karger, 1967, pp. 105–158.
Johnson, K. M., Webb, P. A., Lange, J. V., and Murphy, F. A.: Isolation and partial characterization of a new virus causing haemorrhagic fever in Zaire. Lancet, 1:569, 1977.
Lee, H. W., Lee, P. W., and Johnson, K. M.: Isolation of the etiologic agent of Korean hemorrhagic fever. J. Infect. Dis., 137:298, 1978.
Mertens, P. E., Patton, R., Baum, J. J., and Monath, T. P.: Clinical presentation of Lassa fever cases during the hospital epidemic at Zorzar, Liberia, March–April 1972. Am. J. Trop. Med. Hyg., 22:780, 1973.
Pantheir, R.: Yellow fever: In Debré, R., and Celers, J. (eds.): Clinicial Virology. Philadelphia, W. B. Saunders Company, 1970, pp. 299–315.
Sabattini, M., and Maiztegui, J. I.: Fiebre hemorrágica argentina. Medicina (Buenos Aires), 30: Suppl. 1, 111, 1970.
Simpson, D. I. H., Knight, E. M., et al.: Congo virus: A hitherto undescribed virus occurring in Africa. Part I. Human isolation — clinical notes. East Afr. Med. J., 44:87, 1967.
Smorodintsev, A. A., Kazbintsev, L. I., and Chudakov, V. G.: Virus Hemorrhagic Fevers (Y. Halperin, translator). Washington, D.C., Office of Technical Services, U.S. Department of Commerce, 1964.
Stode, G. K.: Yellow Fever. New York, McGraw-Hill Book Company, 1951.
Symposium on Epidemic Hemorrhagic Fever. Am. J. Med., 16:617, 1954.
Viral haemorrhagic fever. Weekly Epidemiol. Rec. WHO, 52:177, 1977.
WHO Expert Committee on Yellow Fever, Third Report. WHO Tech. Rep. Ser. No. 479, 1971.

VIRAL DISEASES CHARACTERIZED BY PROTRACTED, RECURRENT, OR LATENT INFECTION

These diseases are discussed in detail in Ch. 310.

VIRAL DISEASES (PRESUMPTIVE)

103. CAT SCRATCH DISEASE

(Benign Nonbacterial Regional Lymphadenitis, Inoculation Lymphoreticulosis)

Andrew M. Margileth

DEFINITION. Cat scratch disease is a benign, self-limited disease characterized by tender regional lymphadenopathy and frequently preceded by a primary skin lesion following cat contact or scratches, or both. The disease is being recognized more frequently in both children and adults. Persistence of the adenopathy for several months in a generally healthy patient with

gradual spontaneous resolution of the enlarged bubo is its natural course.

ETIOLOGY. Since 1967, when Warwick reviewed the etiologic investigations in cat scratch disease, little information regarding etiology has been published. A number of studies, including those of the writer and his associates, have not demonstrated any instance of complicity of fungi or bacteria, including rickettsiae or mycobacteria. It is presumed therefore that the etiologic agent is probably a virus. Particles that could represent viral particles have been detected (Kalter, 1970) in the cell cytoplasm of biopsied human lymph nodes. It appears that during acute illness patients with cat scratch disease have a transient state of lymphocyte unresponsiveness similar to that of patients with a variety of illnesses caused by viruses and mycoplasmas.

EPIDEMIOLOGY. Since the initial description by Debré (1950), more than 1500 patients with cat scratch disease have been reported in about 600 articles. An estimated 2000 unreported cases occur annually in the United States, primarily in children. The true incidence is unknown, because the number of reported cases varies greatly depending on the interest of the physician and the availability of the skin test antigen. The disease is worldwide, occurring in all races and apparently equally in both sexes. In temperate zones, most cases have occurred during fall and winter. Seasonal variation is minimal in warmer climates. Several epidemics in the same house or geographic locality have been recorded.

TRANSMISSION AND COMMUNICABILITY. The mode of transmission is presumably by direct contact, as the bubo usually follows a scratch, bite, or lick from a young cat. Cat contact occurs in 90 per cent of patients. The disease has also been thought to have developed through dog bite or scratch and, rarely, following a scratch from a thorn, wood splinter, or fish bone. An inoculation site may be detected in 55 to 96 per cent of patients. The disease has been transmitted experimentally to man, monkeys, baboons, and Hartley guinea pigs. There is no evidence that the disease can be transmitted from human to human. Regional lymphadenopathy was produced in each species following an intradermal injection of material aspirated from suppurative lymph nodes of human patients. Attempts to isolate virus from cat saliva or claws have been unsuccessful. The healthy cat — often a kitten — apparently acts as a mechanical vector for the infective agent, for skin tests with CS antigen on the implicated cats have been nonreactive. The writer's studies in family outbreaks have shown that the family cat usually transmits the causative agent no longer than two to three weeks.

PATHOGENESIS AND PATHOLOGY. No serologic test is available to measure antibodies to the causative agent. Fortunately, the cat scratch skin test is reliable and has a high degree of specificity; the reaction is a delayed hypersensitivity type. A positive reaction is usually detected at the time the clinical diagnosis is suspected; however, conversion may be delayed up to four weeks thereafter. Cutaneous reactivity lasts up to ten years. Second attacks have not been reported. A recurrence in the nodes originally involved has been observed, but is quite rare.

Biopsied lymph nodes may show distinct yet nonspecific stages, depending upon the interval between the time of onset and the time of biopsy. The early lesions reveal a reticulum cell hyperplasia followed by necrotizing granulomas, occasionally with giant cells, then multiple microabscesses, and, weeks to months later, frank abscess formation. Consequently, a presumptive histopathologic diagnosis of tularemia, brucellosis, tuberculosis, or sarcoidosis might be considered. Rarely a biopsy made early before suppuration has appeared has shown histologic changes, including reticulum cell hyperplasia and granulomas, which have been confused with those of Hodgkin's disease.

CLINICAL MANIFESTATIONS. The patient usually is not ill in spite of impressive lymphadenopathy; however, malaise, fever, and influenza-like symptoms may be present. Three to ten days elapse from the time of the scratch or contact until a primary skin papule or pustule forms. It may exhibit one or more erythematous papules. Rarely unilateral conjunctival granulomas occur. An inoculation site (a scratch or a primary lesion, or both) may be detected in more than half the patients, de-

pending upon the thoroughness of the examination and the duration of the bubo when first seen. Most primary lesions persist for one to three weeks; lesions rarely persist for seven weeks. The primary lesion usually heals without scar formation. Regional lymphadenopathy usually develops about two weeks after the scratch (observed range, 3 to 50 days). Lymphangitis has not been observed. Tender nodes, present in 80 per cent of patients for the first one or two weeks, are commonly found in the head, neck, or axilla. Epitrochlear, inguinal, femoral, or popliteal areas are involved less frequently. Multiple site involvement has occurred in about 10 to 20 per cent of cases in the writer's experience. Node size varies from 1 to 5 cm in the majority of cases. Enlargement persists for two to four months; lymphadenopathy rarely lasts for 6 to 24 months. Macroscopic node suppuration occurs in about one tenth of patients seen in office practice and in about one quarter of those admitted to hospitals.

No clinical signs other than lymphadenopathy occurred in approximately half of our 413 patients observed at various times throughout a 19-year period. In about one third of similar reported cases, patients had fever (38.3 to 41.2° C) lasting for 5 to 9 (1 to 30) days; 32 per cent of our 413 patients had malaise or an influenza-like syndrome lasting about 4 (1 to 21) days. Splenomegaly occurred in 16 per cent of the last 100 patients. Exanthems, i.e., maculopapular, petechial, or erythema nodosum or multiforme types, have been reported in 4 per cent of affected patients. The rash usually lasted 4 to 9 (3 to 14) days.

Unusual clinical manifestations reported include the oculoglandular syndrome of Parinaud (40 cases), presenting as an ocular granuloma or conjunctivitis with parotid area swelling caused by preauricular lymphadenopathy; encephalitis (41); thrombocytopenic purpura (7); osteomyelitis (4); and primary atypical pneumonia (4). In any patient with an ocular granuloma or conjunctivitis and parotid area swelling (preauricular lymphadenopathy), cat scratch disease should always be considered.

Children with central nervous system involvement may develop encephalopathy, meningitis, radiculitis, polyneuritis, or myelitis with paraplegia. Onset of neu-

TABLE 1. Clinical Features in 100 Patients with Cat Scratch Adenopathy and a Positive Skin Test (April 1975 to July 1977)

Category	Percentage of Patients
Animal contact	
Cat	88
Dog	9
None	3
Animal scratch	
Cat	72
Dog	3
None	23
Primary lesion	
Skin papule or pustule	53
Eye granuloma	3
Symptoms and signs	
None	66
Fever (38.3–42.1°C)	26
Malaise	17
Splenomegaly	16
Sore throat	7
Headache	5
Parotid swelling	2

TABLE 2.   Cat Scratch Lymphadenopathy in 100 Patients—Clinical Characteristics of Involved Nodes
and Duration of Adenopathy (April 1975 to July 1977)

Adenopathy (N = 100)	Per Cent	Size (cm) (N = 100)	Per Cent
Single node	46	1.0 to <3.0	46
Multiple nodes	54	3.0 to <5.0	39
Multiple sites	23	≥5.0	15
Tender nodes	81		
Suppuration	10		

Location (N = 120)	Per Cent	Duration (N = 100)	Per Cent
Head: total (N = 29)	24	Prior to diagnosis	
Submandibular	21	2 to <4 weeks	56
Preauricular	3	1 to <2 months	20
Neck: total (N = 44)	37	2 to <4 months	17
Posterior	20	4 to <6 months	4
Anterior	10	6 to <12 months	3
Supraclavicular	7	Regression (months, <1.0 cm)	
Extremities: total (N = 47)	39	1 to <2	24
Axillary	27	2 to <6	62
Epitrochlear	6	6 to <12	8
Inguinal	4	12 to <24	4
Femoral	2	≥24	1

rologic symptoms is sudden, usually with fever, and occurs within one to six weeks of the onset of adenopathy. Major symptoms and signs found in 41 cases of neurologic involvement were as follows: coma or convulsions in two thirds, neurologic abnormalities, noted above, in 25 per cent, and lethargy and/or confusion in one sixth. In 12 of 22 patients (55 per cent) with neurologic involvement, cerebrospinal fluid pleocytosis, elevated protein, or both were detected. Electroencephalograms were abnormal in most patients. Severe manifestations have lasted for one to two weeks, with gradual recovery to normal status in one to six months in most patients.

Recovery from thrombocytopenic purpura, osteomyelitis, pneumonitis, and Parinaud's syndrome has been complete.

DIAGNOSIS. Regional lymphadenopathy developing two weeks after cat contact and/or scratches, and especially if a primary inoculation papule or pustule followed the scratch, suggests a diagnosis of cat scratch disease. Three of the four following manifestations would confirm the diagnosis in a typical case, whereas all four would be necessary in an atypical case: (1) a history of animal (usually cat) contact or presence of a scratch and a primary dermal or eye lesion; (2) aspiration of sterile pus from the node (a presumptive diagnostic test) or negative laboratory studies excluding other etiologic possibilities; (3) a positive skin test to cat scratch antigen (5 per cent false positives occur; use of only one antigen may give a false negative result in 10 to 20 per cent of patients); (4) node biopsy revealing histopathology consistent with cat scratch disease.

If a negative skin test is found to one or two different cat scratch antigens applied simultaneously and again four weeks later, and if other studies are negative, a biopsy must be considered to rule out a benign tumor or lymphoma. The presence of tenderness favors cat scratch or a pyogenic or mycobacterial adenopathy rather than a neoplasm.

Skin Tests. A skin test using cat scratch antigen is positive in 90 per cent of patients who are clinically suspected of having cat scratch disease and have had cat scratches and/or contact. A negative skin test often occurs if the duration of illness is less than three or

four weeks, and about 10 per cent of patients with typical cat scratch disease will have negative skin tests with one or two different antigens. The positive reaction consists of a wheal or papule with 5 mm or more of induration, with or without erythema, occurring 48 to 72 hours after intradermal inoculation of 0.1 ml of antigen. Induration may persist for five to six days or longer. A positive test may be obtained for years (10 to 28) after the initial episode and hence does not necessarily indicate concurrent disease. False positive reactions have been reported in veterinarians (12 to 29 per cent), healthy persons (4 to 5 per cent), and family contacts; the over-all incidence is 5 per cent. Thus the limit of confidence for a positive reaction is about 95 per cent. If the reaction is negative at four-week intervals, the disease can be excluded with reasonable certainty, especially if two different antigens are used. Repeated skin testing with CS antigen in the same patients has not produced positive reactions. Skin tests with PPD-S and atypical PPD mycobacterium antigens have been rarely positive in patients with cat scratch disease; six patients with the disease had positive reactions to PPD Battey out of 413 patients tested. Dog contact and/or scratches were noted with greater frequency (8 per cent) in this period (1975 to 1977) than in the Margileth 1968 and 1971 studies.

Since CS antigen is not available commercially, all aspirated pus from affected nodes should be saved to prepare test antigen. This subject is treated in greater detail elsewhere (Margileth, 1968, 1971).

Laboratory Data. Laboratory tests are not diagnostic, but eosinophilia has been reported. At the onset the number of polymorphonuclear cells may be increased with a mild leukocytosis. A sedimentation rate, usually elevated during the first few weeks of adenopathy, suggests an inflammatory lymphadenitis, and is recommended.

DIFFERENTIAL DIAGNOSIS. Cat scratch disease should be considered in all patients with persistent lymphadenopathy (over three weeks), because it is the most common cause of chronic regional lymphadenitis in children or adolescents. The presence of an inoculation (dermal or ocular) lesion would strongly suggest cat scratch disease. Other, less common causes are sporotrichosis, primary syphilis, lymphogranuloma venereum, typical or atypical tuberculosis, other bacterial adenitis, tularemia, brucellosis, histoplasmosis, coccidioidomycosis, sarcoidosis, toxoplasmosis, infectious mononucleosis, and benign or malignant tumors. In atypical forms of cat scratch disease, one must consider benign recurrent parotid lymphosialadenopathy, Parinaud's oculoglandular disease, encephalitis, pneumonia, thrombocytopenic purpura, erythema nodosum, and osteomyelitis, as well as fluctuant lymphadenopathy simulating cystic hygroma or a thyroglossal duct cyst. If CS skin tests are negative, as well as appropriate cultures and serologic and other skin tests, a node biopsy will usually determine the cause.

TREATMENT. In the majority of patients the disease is self-limited. The best therapy is reassurance that the adenopathy is benign and in most cases will subside spontaneously within two or three months. Thus management consists of reassurance with appropriate follow-up examination, analgesics for pain, and aspiration if suppuration occurs. Lack of response to antimicrobials is the rule; if cat scratch disease is suspected, antimicrobial drugs are not recommended. In the child whose node suppurates, needle aspiration on an ambulatory basis is preferred to incision and drainage. Aspiration is performed, usually without local anesthesia. After washing with Betadine cleanser, a needle (18 or 20 gauge) is inserted through normal skin at the base of the mass in order to avoid a chronic sinus tract in the event that a tuberculous lesion is present. Aspiration provides material for skin test antigen, relieves painful adenopathy, and usually allows the patient to become symptom free within 24 to 48 hours. If fluid recurs, reaspiration may be necessary. Application of moist soaks to the primary lesion may facilitate drainage and shorten the duration of lymphadenopathy. The efficacy of steroid therapy in cat scratch disease is questionable, and it is not recommended. Excisional biopsy of the node may be necessary in selected patients because of persistent pain or for diagnostic purposes. Spontaneous drainage occurred in 6 per cent of our last 100 patients.

PROGNOSIS. The prognosis is excellent; lymphadenopathy usually regresses spontaneously in two to three months. One attack appears to confer lifelong immunity. Complications and sequelae are almost nonexistent and have not been seen or reported in typical cases. In France in one patient with encephalopathy, death apparently occurred during treatment of continued seizures with hypothermia. Rare patients have been reported to have had chronic adenopathy for two years; we have observed one such case in an adult in our most recent series. Only two patients have had a recurrence of the same adenopathy after a three-year period of well-being.

PREVENTION. Because of increasing numbers of household pets (50 million cats in the United States), cat scratch disease will be difficult to prevent. Disposal of the suspect cat is not recommended, because the cat involved is invariably well. Four to 9 per cent of family members scratched by the same cat may develop cat scratch disease. The patient with the disease does not require isolation or quarantine, as there is no evidence of disease spread from man to man. Active or passive protection is not available.

Altman, R. P., and Margileth, A. M.: Cervical lymphadenopathy from atypical mycobacteria — diagnosis and surgical treatment. J. Pediat. Surg., 10:419, 1975.

Margileth, A. M.: Cat-scratch disease in 65 patients: Evaluation of cat scratch skin test antigen in 109 subjects. Clin. Proc. Child. Hosp. D.C., 27:213, 1971.

Margileth, A. M., London, W. T., and Sever, J. L.: Cat scratch disease virus? Negative viral studies in mammals. Submitted for publication.

Warwick, W. J.: The cat-scratch syndrome; many diseases or one disease? Prog. Med. Virol., 9:256, 1967.

104. VIRAL GASTROENTERITIS CAUSED BY NORWALK-LIKE AGENTS AND ROTAVIRUSES

(Acute Infectious Nonbacterial Gastroenteritis, Epidemic Diarrhea, Winter Vomiting Disease)

Raphael Dolin

DEFINITION. The term "nonbacterial gastroenteritis," along with the descriptive phrases listed above, has referred to a group of acute, common, self-limited illnesses characterized chiefly by vomiting and/or diarrhea. An infectious cause for these diseases had been previously suspected, but it has been only recently that specific viral agents which cause at least a portion of such illnesses have been detected.

ETIOLOGY. Two groups of viral agents which induce acute gastroenteritis have been described. The first is the Norwalk-like agents, generally named after the location of the outbreak from which they have been derived (Norwalk, Hawaii, Montgomery County, "W," and Ditchling agents). These agents have not been cultivated in vitro and have been only partly characterized. They are small (26 to 27 nm in diameter), nonenveloped viral agents found in the stools of acutely ill patients. The biophysical properties of the best studied of these, the Norwalk agent, resemble those of parvoviruses. They have, thus, also been referred to as "parvovirus-like" agents. Among the Norwalk-like agents, at least three antigenic types have been detected thus far.

The second group, described in 1973, is the rotaviruses, also referred to earlier as "duovirus" or "reovirus-like" agents, which have been tentatively classified within the family of Reoviridae of mammalian viruses. They are 66 to 70 nm in diameter, contain double-stranded RNA, and have a characteristic double shell appearance. Although strain differences have not been fully analyzed, human rotaviruses appear to be of at least two antigenic types. Human rotaviruses can only be grown with difficulty in vitro, but can be detected directly in stool by a variety of techniques (see below).

It is of interest that other, previously described groups of viruses which infect the gastrointestinal tract (e.g., enteroviruses) do not appear to be major causes of acute gastroenteritis (see Ch. 97).

EPIDEMIOLOGY. Little is known about the specific epidemiology of the Norwalk-like agents because of the lack of suitable detection methods. Naturally occurring illnesses from which these agents have been derived appear to be exceedingly common and widespread and involve all age groups. Illness occurs most frequently between September and March in the Northern Hemisphere, and can present in distinct outbreaks with explosive patterns of spread.

Rotaviruses, on the other hand, have a well described epidemiologic pattern. Rotavirus-induced gastroenteritis occurs most frequently between 6 and 24 months of age, and occasionally up to 4 years of age. Disease also occurs in neonates. Illness in older children and adults is apparently unusual, although reinfection is common. Fifty-two to 90 per cent of individuals above two years of age have serum antibody against rotavirus. Rotavirus infections are seen primarily during the winter months in both Northern and Southern Hemispheres. Cases occur both sporadically and in distinct outbreaks during that time. Rotavirus infections have accounted for 42 to 55 per cent of hospitalized cases of gastroenteritis among infants and young children in studies carried out throughout the world.

PATHOGENESIS. *Acute infection with Norwalk and Hawaii agents* results in reversible histopathologic lesions which primarily involve the upper jejunum, with relative sparing of the stomach and rectum. The jejunal mucosa remains intact, but there is marked blunting of villi and shortening of microvilli. The lamina propria is infiltrated with both polymorphonuclear and mononuclear cells. Acute illness is also accompanied by malabsorption of d-xylose and fat. *Rotavirus infections* induce a similar pathology in the duodenum and jejunum, although inflammatory changes can on occasion be seen in the stomach and rectum.

The characteristics of immunity to infection with Norwalk-like agents and rotaviruses are not well defined. Such immunity does not correlate closely with serum antibody levels, and, in the case of the Norwalk agent, appears to wane after one to two years.

CLINICAL MANIFESTATIONS. *Illness induced by the Norwalk-like agents* consists of nausea, abdominal cramps, vomiting, and/or diarrhea, often accompanied by headache and myalgias. Onset of illness is often abrupt, and although both vomiting and diarrhea usually occur, either can be present alone. Low-grade fever ($< 38.9°$ C) can be found in approximately 50 to 60 per cent of patients. Incubation period for illness is generally from 18 to 48 hours, and disease manifestations last from 48 to 72 hours. Disease remits spontaneously and without known sequelae.

Rotavirus infections have clinical features which are similar to those described for the Norwalk-like agents. Incubation periods range from 24 hours to 96 hours, and among hospitalized children illness lasts for five to eight days. Even among hospitalized children, illness appears to be generally mild, although occasionally more severe and rarely fatal cases have been reported. Rotaviruses appear to be one of the causes of infantile diarrhea, which is a source of significant morbidity and mortality in economically underdeveloped countries.

DIAGNOSIS. Laboratory Tests. Norwalk-like agents, and antibody directed against them, currently can be detected only by immune electron microscopy, a spe-

cialized technique not suited for routine or large-scale investigations. Norwalk agent is found in stools during the first four to five days of illness, and serum antibody rises are noted two to six weeks later. Rotaviruses are easily detected in stools by a variety of techniques, including complement fixation (CF), immunofluorescence, and conventional electron microscopy. Virus can be found in stools for up to eight days and occasionally longer after onset of illness, and serum antibody (CF) rises are seen by two weeks after illness.

Clinical Diagnosis. Clinical diagnosis of infection with Norwalk-like agents or rotaviruses can be suspected on the basis of epidemiologic information (age, time of year, secondary cases). Although illness is generally milder than that observed with several bacterial pathogens, individual virus-induced cases cannot be differentiated from other causes of acute gastroenteritis on clinical grounds alone. Fecal leukocytes are absent in Norwalk-induced disease, and are usually absent in rotavirus infections, which may prove helpful for early differentiation from *Shigella* or *Salmonella* enteritis (see Ch. 153 and 155).

TREATMENT. Acute viral gastroenteritis is generally a benign, self-limited illness which requires no specific therapy. In severe cases, particularly in the very young, fluid replacement may be necessary, which can be generally provided in the form of clear liquids by mouth. In severe fluid loss, intravenous fluid and electrolyte replacement should be administered promptly. Occasionally, symptomatic treatment of headache or nausea may be required, and restriction of activity during acute illness according to the patient's own symptoms would appear to be prudent. Administration of inhibitors of intestinal motility may be considered in severe diarrhea, but their effect on these illnesses has not been studied.

PREVENTION. There are currently no available methods for prevention or control of these diseases, which represent major public health problems. In addition to the Norwalk-like agents and the rotaviruses, it is likely that other agents which induce acute gastroenteritis will be found in future studies.

Appleton, A. Z., Buckley, M., Thom, B. T., Colton, J. L., and Henderson, S.: Virus-like particles in winter vomiting disease. Lancet, 1:409, 1977.

Bishop, R. F., Davidson, G. P., Holmes, I. H., and Ruck, B. J.: Virus particles in epithelial cells of duodenal mucosa from children with acute nonbacterial gastroenteritis. Lancet, 2:1281, 1973.

Dolin, R., Blacklow, N. R., DuPont, H., Buscho, R. F., Wyatt, R. G., Kasel, J. A., Hornick, R., and Chanock, R. M.: Biological properties of Norwalk agent of acute infectious nonbacterial gastroenteritis. Proc. Soc. Exp. Biol. Med., 140:578, 1972.

Dolin, R., Levy, A. G., Wyatt, R. G., Thornhill, T. S., and Gardner, J. D.: Viral gastroenteritis induced by the Hawaii agent: Jejunal histopathology and serologic response. Am. J. Med., 59:761, 1975.

Flewett, T. H., Davies, H., Bryden, A. S., and Robertson, M. J.: Acute gastroenteritis associated with reovirus-like particles. J. Clin. Path., 27:608, 1974.

Kapikian, A. Z., Kim, H. W., Wyatt, R. G., Cline, W. L., Arrobio, J. O., Brandt, C. O., Rodriguez, W. J., Sack, D. A., Chanock, R. M., and Parrot, R. H.: Human reovirus-like agent as the major pathogen associated with winter gastroenteritis in hospitalized infants and young children. N. Engl. J. Med., 294:965, 1976.

Kapikian, A. Z., Wyatt, R. G., Dolin, R., Thornhill, T. S., Kalica, A. R., and Chanock, R. M.: Visualization of a 27 nm particle associated with acute infectious nonbacterial gastroenteritis. J. Virol., 10:1075, 1972.

Middleton, P. J., Szymanski, M. T., Abbott, G. D., Bortolussi, R., and Hamilton, J. R.: Orbivirus acute gastroenteritis of infancy. Lancet, 1:1241, 1974.

105. EPIDEMIC NEUROMYASTHENIA

(Iceland Disease, Benign Myalgic Encephalomyelitis)

Paul B. Beeson

Between 1934 and 1960, several epidemics were reported of symptoms resembling those of poliomyelitis. The acute phase was often followed by a prolonged period of disability, with headache, muscular weakness, fatigue, and mood depression.

Most outbreaks have occurred in summer, and about half of those reported have involved hospital personnel, especially student nurses. In all instances the attack rate has been much higher in women. Sporadic cases have been reported, but the diagnosis is difficult in the absence of an epidemic.

Severe generalized headache is nearly always a prominent complaint at the onset, and frequently there are pain and stiffness of the neck. Generalized tenderness of the muscles is common, and they frequently exhibit a characteristic of rapid fatigue and loss of motor power on repeated contraction. In perhaps 40 per cent of affected persons, areas of muscle weakness or paralysis appear during the first two weeks. These may be in the trunk or the extremities, and the pattern of involvement often changes from day to day. Cranial nerve signs, bladder dysfunction, and paresthesia may also be noted. In most cases complete recovery of neurologic function occurs within four to eight weeks, but relapses and exacerbations are common during the next few months.

Fever is inconspicuous or absent. The cerebrospinal fluid is usually normal, and routine tests of blood and urine reveal nothing of significance.

A striking feature of this illness is the prolonged period of disability after subsidence of the acute phase. Particularly troublesome are the behavioral manifestations of irritability and mood depression, which together with easy fatigue may interfere with normal living for months and even years after the acute episode. In this stage the subject may present a picture of hysteria or of simple neurasthenia.

Deaths have not been reported; therefore nothing is known of the pathology.

Extensive laboratory investigations failed to yield evidence of participation of any known pathogenic microorganism; nevertheless, the presumption had seemed warranted that it was an infectious disease. However, McEvedy and Beard have cast doubt on the likelihood of an infectious etiology. They carefully reviewed the reports of 15 recorded outbreaks, with special attention to the well-documented epidemic among nurses at the Royal Free Hospital, London. They suggest alternatively that these epidemics represented psychosocial phenomena: either mass hysteria among the subjects or altered medical perception. Their analysis and argument are persuasive, and the apparent lessening of the disease coincident with control of poliomyelitis further strengthens the case that some of the epidemics were indeed examples of mass hysteria.

Acheson, E. D.: The clinical syndrome variously called benign myalgic encephalomyelitis, Iceland disease and epidemic neuromyasthenia. Am. J. Med., 26:569, 1959.

Dillon, M. J., Marshall, W. C., Dudgeon, J. A., and Steigman, A. J.: Epidemic neuromyasthenia: Outbreak among nurses at a children's hospital. Br. Med. J., 1:301, 1974.

McEvedy, C. P., and Beard, A. W.: Concept of benign myalgic encephalomyelitis. Br. Med. J., 1:11, 1970.

Section Two   BACTERIAL DISEASES

106. INTRODUCTION

Walsh McDermott

In recent decades the term "bacterial diseases" has undergone considerable expansion for several reasons: (1) Certain organisms, the rickettsiae, the chlamydiae, and, for all practical purposes, the mycoplasmas, are now considered to be bacteria; (2) new organisms causing new conditions such as legionnaires' disease get discovered; and (3) there have been significant changes in the relation to man of bacterial species long known as "harmless." The first of these changes is of little consequence to most readers, for it is essentially a question of semantics. The second change likewise presents no real problems, for the emergence of recognizable entities such as legionnaires' disease does not happen every day, and, when they are recognized, their description can be easily included in an additional chapter. It is the third change — the continuing alteration in our relation to our own, or the "community," bacterial flora — that continues to significantly expand what the

physician should know. As so much of this changing relationship in bacterial disease is a consequence of our increasing capability to intervene, its degree of prominence is a crude indicator of the state of the health services available. Thus it is that for the past few decades the problems presented by bacterial and mycotic disease have presented themselves in two different forms, depending largely upon the nature of the society.

In the economically underdeveloped parts of the world, the individual diseases have presented in classic form, each occupying its traditional niche in the overall pattern. By contrast, in nations with highly developed health services, the familiar bacterial diseases have by no means disappeared, but their menace has been largely nullified by vaccines and by prompt and appropriate antimicrobial therapy. For example, one hears that lobar pneumonia "has largely disappeared." In actuality, it *has* become much less prominent, not because its major cause, pneumococcal infection, is any less frequent, but because with prompt chemotherapy the early pneumonic lesion is halted in its progress well short of the confines of the lobe. It is the same old pneumonia, but it is no longer "lobar." Expressed differently, without any change in the annual incidence of pneumococcal infection or disease, the annual incidence of *serious problems* from this cause has substantially diminished. Ideally they will be diminished still further by the appropriate use of the vaccine. In place of such clinical problems there are now essentially new menaces in the serious systemic disease produced by *E. coli, Proteus* species, *Pseudomonas, Candida,* and other microbes that were formerly regarded as basically harmless inhabitants of man. The diseases produced by staphylococci and tubercle bacilli can likewise be regarded as being partially of this sort, in that the microbes can subsist harmlessly in the tissues for considerable periods between eruptions as destructive disease. In effect these new clinical patterns represent *endogenous microbial disease* — clinical entities that appear almost exclusively in people with some temporary or sustained lowering of local or general defenses. Because of the resulting changes in the tissue environment, disease-producing microbes are evoked from the dormant or latent state. Generally speaking, these changes in the internal milieu represent a direct or indirect consequence of our modern therapies. They are the unsought-for effects of practical therapeutic gains that in themselves represent great scientific achievements. And because weakened hosts and powerful therapies tend to be congregated in hospitals, such infections are particularly prominent there — the so-called "nosocomial infections." The practices involved include the use of corticosteroids and immunosuppressants; the suppression of customary microbial flora by drugs, thus compromising the protection to the host afforded by *bacterial interference;* surgical procedures, e.g., subtotal gastrectomy or splenectomy that can reduce previously acquired host resistance; and the longer survival of many patients despite protracted, severe, and ultimately fatal illness. Sometimes, as elucidated in the studies by Pierce and Sanford, it is the equipment that is at fault.

The striking change in a large university center in just the first two decades of the "antibiotic era" may be seen from Rogers' study published in 1959 (see accompanying table). *Over-all* infections were either the major or a significant contributory cause of death in 28 per cent of patients hospitalized in 1938, in contrast to only 14 per cent of those hospitalized in 1958. In terms of the number of persons involved, therefore, great progress has been made. The nature of today's problem could be foreseen, however, by the observation that in 1938 most of the "28 per cent" *were admitted* to the hospital with infection; less than 10 per cent of the infections were hospital associated. Only 20 years later, when much of the current technology was available, over *half* of the "14 per cent" with serious infections had acquired them after having been admitted to the hospital for a nonmicrobial — usually life-threatening — disease problem.

Changing Pattern of Life-Threatening Microbial Disease at Necropsy (%) of 200 Consecutive Admissions in Each Period

Etiology	Year of Study	
	1938–1940	1957–1958
Pneumococci, streptococci, tubercle bacilli	20	2
Staphylococci	8	8
Gram-negative bacilli (aerobic)	4	11
Mycotic	1	4
"Hospital-associated infections"	7	54

The increasing ability to alter man's internal environment has had the effect that virtually no microbial species today can be considered nonpathogenic, for in appropriate circumstances virtually any can give rise to disease. All these mechanisms unleash what are, in effect, "new" microbial disease. There are other "new" diseases that may have been similarly unleashed or may have merely become easier to recognize by virtue of the selectivity of drug action. The separation of "atypical" pneumonia from bacterial pneumonia by the introduction of sulfonamide back in the 1930's and the importance of "atypical" mycobacteria as disease agents once antituberculous therapy was introduced are cases in point. What is happening was biologically predictable, and the changing nature of the situation may be expected to continue.

To be capable of staying with this change, the physician must know considerably more about the behavior of microbes, as they cause disease and are exposed to drugs with an otherwise normal or a compromised host, than he had to master only one or two decades ago. This knowledge is of two sorts: certain concepts and principles related to the microbe-drug-host interactions, and a body of knowledge sufficient to permit him to make microbiologically relevant diagnoses on clinical grounds. Knowledge of the latter sort is presented in the individual chapters that follow. For discussion of host defenses, see Ch. 41 and 119; for their behavior during administration of immunosuppressive drugs, the reader is referred to Ch. 38, 40, and 527. Endogenous microbial disease itself is discussed in Ch. 124, whereas the concepts and principles related to microbe-drug-host interactions are considered in Ch. 189 and 190.

McDermott, W.: Inapparent Infection. The Dyer Lecture. Public Health Rep., 74:485, 1959.

National Nosocomial Infections Study — United States, 1975-1976. MMWR, Vol. 26, No. 46, November 18, 1977.

Pierce, A. K., and Sanford, J. P.: Bacterial contamination of aerosols. Arch. Intern. Med., 131:156, 1973.

Rogers, D., et al.: Infections in the altered host. *In* Year Book of Medicine, 1978, Chicago, Year Book Medical Publishers.

Rogers, D. E.: The changing pattern of life-threatening microbial disease. N. Engl. J. Med., 261:677, 1959.

RICKETTSIAL DISEASES

107. INTRODUCTION

Charles L. Wisseman, Jr.

The diseases commonly referred to as the rickettsial diseases of man consist of several clinical entities, usually acute, self-limited fevers, caused by bacteria of the family Rickettsiaceae. They fall naturally into the typhus-like diseases (typhus groups, spotted fever group, and scrub typhus group), Q fever, and trench fever. The typhus-like diseases are caused by organisms of the genus *Rickettsia*; Q fever by *Coxiella burnetii*; and trench fever by *Rochalimaea quintana*. *Bartonella bacilliformis*, the cause of bartonellosis, belonging to the family Bartonellaceae, is included here for convenience because it is the only other member of the order Rickettsiales known to cause human disease and because there are certain selected superficial similarities (facultative intracellular parasite, arthropod transmission).

Organisms of the *Rickettsia, Coxiella*, and *Rochalimaea* genera, although very different in many respects, are very small bacteria (the former concept of intermediate between bacteria and viruses is no longer tenable) with a gram-negative bacterium-like cell wall, bacterial type internal structure (typical prokaryotic DNA arrangement with a genome size roughly equivalent to that of *Neisseria*; ribosomes), often a slime layer or microcapsule, and a substantially similar independent metabolic activity. Organisms of the genus *Rickettsia* and *Coxiella burnetii* are obligate intracellular parasites, i.e., they are known to date to grow only within eukaryotic host cells. *Rochalimaea quintana* can be grown on cell-free medium and grows extracellularly in the louse gut, but *may* be a facultative intracellular parasite in man. All organisms of the genus *Rickettsia* have the capacity to penetrate directly through the host cell plasma membrane into the cytoplasm, can cause host cell lysis from without, and multiply by binary fission free in the host cell cytoplasm not surrounded by a vacuolar membrane. Different species vary in their capacity to interact with other host cell membranes. Thus members of the spotted fever group can penetrate into the host cell nucleus, and these, as well as *R. mooseri*, can escape through the plasma membrane without requiring complete host cell destruction as does *R. prowazekii*. *Coxiella burnetii*, on the other hand, does not actively penetrate into host cells, is probably taken in by endocytosis, and grows within a membrane bound vacuole. These differences in action on host cell membranes are probably related to differences in disease patterns (host response) and immune mechanisms. Active penetration of host cells appears to be correlated with mouse lethal toxic action and hemolytic properties. On the other hand, members of the genus *Rickettsia* which have been studied and *Coxiella burnetii* have endotoxins similar in physiologic action to those of gram-negative bacilli.

All rickettsioses are transmitted by arthropod vectors, although Q fever is usually acquired from domestic animals. Many years ago, McGaw proposed an epidemiologically useful classification of rickettsial diseases based on arthropod vector — viz., louse-borne, flea-borne, tick-borne, and mite-borne. With the exception of louse-borne typhus and trench fevers, in which man is the key vertebrate host and reservoir, all the rickettsioses are zoonoses, existing in a natural cycle involving arthropods (vectors and in some cases reservoirs) and vertebrate (usually mammalian) hosts. In these, man acquires the disease by accidentally intruding into the natural cycle and is a "dead-end" host not sustaining the infection cycle. The reservoir mechanism varies considerably among the rickettsioses. The nonsterile immunity in the vertebrate host, with persisting infection and potential or proved capacity for recrudescence, appears to be important in louse-borne typhus and trench fever, in which the main reservoir is man, and in murine typhus in the rat. In these three infections, the vector (the human body louse in the first two and fleas in the last) does not transmit the organism transovarially to the next generation, and, in the case of louse-borne typhus, the infection in the louse vector is almost invariably fatal to the louse in a week or two. On the other hand, in the case of tick-, mite- and chigger-borne rickettsioses, the organism is efficiently transmitted transovarially to succeeding generations, a process which probably constitutes the main reservoir mechanism, whereas the vertebrate infection possibly only serves an amplifying role in some instances. *Coxiella burnetii*, possibly originally tick-borne, is sustained

TABLE 1. Selected Biologic Properties of Rickettsiae

| | DNA %GC | Slime Layer or Micro-capsule | Endo-toxin Action | Host Cell Membrane Actions | | | Replication Site | | | |
| | | | | Mode of Entry into Host Cells* | Mouse Lethal Toxin | Hemo-lysin | Cytoplasm | | | Type‡ in CE Cells |
							Free†	Vacuole	Nucleus	
Typhus group										
R. prowazekii	28–30	+	+	Active	+	+	+	0	0	1
R. mooseri	28–30	+	+	Active	+	+	+	0	0	2
R. canada	28–30	?	?	Active	+	?	+	0	+	?
Spotted fever group	32–33	+	?	Active	+	?	+	0	+	2
Scrub typhus group	?	Probably	?	Active	+	?	+	0	0	?
Coxiella burnetii	42.9	+	+	Passive	0	0	0	+	0	?
Rochalimaea quintana	38.8	?	?	?Passive	0	0	?	?	?	?

*Active = active penetration; passive = endocytosis by host cell.
†Free = free in cytoplasm with no surrounding vacuolar membrane.
‡Type 1 growth cycle = rickettsiae are retained within host cell until it breaks down. Type 2 growth cycle = in early stages, rickettsiae escape through plasma membrane without apparent host cell damage; rapidly spreading type of infection.

TABLE 2. Summary of Some Epidemiologic Features of Selected Rickettsial Diseases of Man

Disease	Organism	Natural Cycle		Usual Mode of Transmission to Man	Common Occupational or Environmental Association	Geographic Distribution
		Arthropod Vector	Reservoir/ Mammalian Host			
Typhus group						
Murine typhus	*Rickettsia mooseri* (*R. typhi*)	Flea	Rodents	Infected flea feces into broken skin or aerosol to mucous membranes	Rat-infested premises (shops, warehouses, grain elevators)	Scattered foci, worldwide
Epidemic typhus	*R. prowazekii*	Body louse	Man*	Infected crushed louse or feces into broken skin or aerosol to mucous membranes	Lousy human population with louse transfer	Worldwide
Brill's disease	*R. prowazekii*	Recrudescence months to years after primary attack of louse-borne typhus			Unknown; ?stress	Worldwide
Spotted fever group (selected examples)						
Rocky Mountain spotted fever	*R. rickettsii*	Ixodid ticks	Ticks, small mammals	Tick bite, mechanical transfer to mucous membranes, ?airborne	Tick-infested terrain, houses, dogs	Western Hemisphere
Boutonneuse fever	*R. conorii*	Ixodid ticks	Ticks, rodents, dogs	Tick bite	Tick-infested terrain, houses, dogs	Mediterranean, littoral, Africa, ?Indian subcontinent
Rickettsialpox	*R. akari*	Mouse mite	Mite, mice	Mouse mite bite	Unique mouse- and mite-infested premises (incinerators)	United States, U.S.S.R., Korea, ?Central Africa
Scrub typhus						
Tsutsugamushi disease	*R. tsutsugamushi* (multiple serotypes)	Chigger	Chigger, ?rodents	Chigger bite	Chigger-infested terrain; secondary scrub, grass airfields, golf courses	Asia, Australia, New Guinea, Pacific islands
Q fever†	*Coxiella burnetii*	?Ticks	Ticks, mammals	Inhalation of dried airborne infective material; ?tick bite	Domestic animals or products, dairies, lambing pens, slaughterhouses	Worldwide
Trench fever†	*Rochalimaea quintana*	Body louse	Man	Infected crushed louse or feces into broken skin; ?aerosol to mucous membranes	Lousy human population with louse transfer	Africa, Mexico, ?South America, ?Eastern Europe

*Recent isolations of putative *R. prowazekii* from flying squirrels in the eastern United States have not been evaluated as reservoirs for human infection. Previous claims of involvement of domestic animals are now largely discounted.

†Though *C. burnetii* and *R. quintana* are not strictly "rickettsiae" and Q fever and trench fever differ clinically from the others, they are conventionally considered with the rickettsiae.

by vertical passage in its vertebrate host (e.g., sheep, cattle) by virtue of its capacity to multiply to phenomenal levels in placental tissues and to be excreted in milk.

Thus, although they are commonly lumped together under the "rickettsial diseases of man," and possessing some points in common, it is apparent that there are major differences in the biologic properties of the organisms involved, in their interactions with host cells, and in their natural infection cycles and reservoir mechanisms. It is likely that organisms of diverse origin have acquired certain similar properties related to cell parasitism through a process of convergent evolution and that within groups diversification has occurred through divergent evolution. However, some similarities in cell tropism and the restricted ways in which man responds to injury have conspired to produce a group of clinical entities with many to few common features.

PATHOGENESIS, PATHOLOGY, IMMUNITY. Since the human diseases caused by members of the genus *Rickettsia* share many common features, although there are sufficient differences in detail to yield distinct clinical entities, it is convenient to consider here pathogenesis and immunity in a generalized framework.

The route of infection is frequently through the skin, injected through the vector mouth parts in the case of

tick-, mite-, and chigger-borne rickettsioses and by contamination of broken skin by infected louse or flea feces in the case of louse-borne typhus and murine typhus, respectively. Airborne rickettsiae in dried louse or flea feces may initiate airborne infection through the respiratory tract or conjunctiva. Aerosols of all rickettsiae are highly infectious via the respiratory tract.

Some local proliferation undoubtedly occurs at the inoculation site with all *Rickettsia* species. In some (e.g., scrub typhus, rickettsialpox, fièvre boutonneuse), a visible lesion (the *eschar*) develops at the inoculation site during the incubation period. The route or routes of dissemination of the infection from the inoculation site are not precisely known. However, regional lymphadenopathy (e.g., in scrub typhus) suggests lymphatic spread on the one hand, whereas on the other hand demonstration of rickettsiae in endothelial cells of small blood vessels at the inoculation site opens the possibility of hematogenous dissemination.

Some dissemination to, and proliferation in, distant sites must take place during the incubation period, but the organs or tissues involved have not been identified in man. Patent rickettsemia probably appears only late in the incubation period, e.g., only a few hours prior to the onset of clinical disease in volunteers infected with *R. tsutsugamushi*, is regularly present at onset, and persists throughout the febrile period of disease despite the appearance of humoral antibodies by the end of the first week of disease. It is unknown if this early wave of patent rickettsemia is fed and sustained by, or is responsible for, initiating the characteristic widespread infection of endothelial cells in small blood vessels. *Nevertheless, disseminated focal infection of the small blood vessels (capillaries, arterioles, and venules) of the skin, and, to a lesser but significant extent, in other organs such as brain, lung, heart, and kidneys, is the single most important known pathophysiologic feature of these diseases.* At focal points in the small blood vessels, rickettsiae infect, multiply in, and damage endothelial cells with cell necrosis, hypertrophy, and proliferation. Infection is limited to the endothelial cells in typhus and scrub typhus infections but may extend to all layers in Rocky Mountain spotted fever, causing necrosis of the media. At the sites of endothelial damage, platelet-fibrin thrombi tend to form, which, along with endothelial hypertrophy and proliferation, partially or completely occlude the vascular lumen. At these sites of infection and vascular damage there develops the typical perivascular inflammatory response, with polymorphonuclear and monocytic cells early and macrophages, lymphocytes, and occasional plasma cells later, coinciding approximately temporally with antibody response, suggesting the possibility of superimposition of a vascular immunopathologic component. This sequence suggests that perhaps a typical rickettsial infection evolves through an *early phase,* in which vascular damage is primarily the direct result of rickettsial infection, and a *late phase,* in which additional vascular damage is produced by immunologic mechanisms. The latter is unproved, but is consistent with the fact that in typhus and scrub typhus infections patients appear more "toxic" in this late phase and show greater vascular instability, and most deaths occur in the period *after* antibodies are demonstrable. On the other hand, the greater severity of vascular lesions, frequent early deaths, and often little perivascular cellular response and early unresponsiveness to antirickettsial therapy in early fatal cases of Rocky Mountain spotted fever suggest that direct rickettsia-induced vascular damage alone can initiate irreversible pathophysiologic changes.

The disseminated vascular lesions can account for many of the clinical and pathophysiologic abnormalities seen in these infections, viz., rash, edema and increased extravascular fluid space, hypotension, and gangrene (in louse-borne typhus and Rocky Mountain spotted fever), as well as the clotting abnormalities (up to disseminated intravascular clotting) which have been recognized recently to some extent in several rickettsial diseases but which are seen more regularly and in such a severe form in Rocky Mountain spotted fever that they may be a major problem contributing to death. The classic typhus nodules in the brain, most frequent in the midbrain and nuclear areas, are of the same vascular origin and help explain the mental changes and cranial nerve deficits. In Rocky Mountain spotted fever, discrete microinfarcts may occur in the central nervous system with persisting electroencephalographic changes. The heart often shows, in addition to the typical perivascular lesions, some edema, a diffuse mononuclear infiltrate of unknown origin, and a minor amount of muscle necrosis. Nonspecific electrocardiographic changes are common. Despite the dramatic histologic appearance of the heart, limited studies during World War II suggested that cardiac function was not impaired. This matter should be reinvestigated by modern methods. Typical perivascular lesions occur in the portal areas of the liver, along with nonspecific focal areas of fatty degeneration in hepatocytes. However, the origin of abnormal transaminase blood levels remains unknown. The kidneys also show focal interstitial vascular lesions and lesions involving a few nephrons. The characteristic oliguria and azotemia of typhus have been attributed in the past to prerenal causes, e.g., hypotension, tissue catabolism, but the occurrence of rickettsial antigen in the urine early, followed by its disappearance with antibody response, suggests that transient immune complex disease should be sought by modern methods. The lung shows a variable degree of interstitial type pneumonitis, on histologic examination and by x-ray, regardless of route of infection. Cough is a common early clinical manifestation, but physical signs are scant.

Immunity to the infecting rickettsial strain following recovery from infection tends to be solid and longlasting but of a nonsterile type, i.e., the rickettsiae are not entirely eradicated and may remain "latent" for at least many months to many years. The bases for immunity are not yet completely understood, although rapid advances are now being made in this field. An antibody response is detectable around the end of the first week of disease, but this does not cause an immediate control of rickettsemia. Cell-mediated immunity also develops, but the kinetics of its evolution in man have not yet been clearly documented. Laboratory studies suggest that both antibody-mediated and cell-mediated mechanisms contribute to immunity. Moreover, studies of murine typhus infection in guinea pigs showed a temporal correlation between the development of an immune response as measured by serum antibodies and the development of the typical mononuclear perivascular lesions, leaving open the possibility of a late immunopathologic component.

GENERAL CLINICAL CONSIDERATIONS. In classic form, the typhus-like rickettsial diseases (typhus group, spotted fever group, and scrub typhus group) display many common clinical features which may vary in degree and in detail, e.g., fever, headache, cough, prostration, rash, altered mental state, hypotension, normal to low white blood count. *Especially at the onset,* however, the signs and symptoms are those common to many acute infectious diseases, differential clinical diagnosis is difficult, and specific laboratory diagnostic methods are limited. Sometimes an early sign, such as an eschar, which is variable even in the rickettsioses in which it occurs, is helpful. Later, rash, hypotension, changes in mental state, and the like may give clues. But rickettsioses vary in severity, and not all cases are classic. Moreover, in many areas, other infectious diseases exist which are confusing clinically, especially in that early period when the correct choice of chemotherapy may be lifesaving (as with Rocky Mountain spotted fever, meningococcemia, or cerebral malaria). Hence, one must be acutely sensitive to the different possibilities in one's area of practice and must devise a kind of strategy for the diagnosis and management, sometimes empirically on the basis of probabilities, of a rickettsia-like disease, using all available bits of epidemiologic, clinical, and laboratory information. Simple observation of the patient for the development of diagnostic clinical or laboratory features is a hazardous practice. In the United States, the single major factor contributory to the continuing 5 to 10 per cent mortality in Rocky Mountain spotted fever is delay in institution of specific chemotherapy. Listed below are some practical considerations which have emerged from analysis of experiences of others and from the author's personal experience in several parts of the world.

The history of potential exposure (occupation, travel, recreational activities in wilderness areas), as well as of tick bite, is extremely important in alerting the physician to the possibility of a rickettsial disease. Modern air travel makes it possible to return from any part of the world within the incubation period of a rickettsial disease, e.g., scrub typhus and Kenya tick typhus in travelers returning to the United States.

In a given area, certain diseases commonly cause difficult clinical differential diagnostic problems. For example, in the United States, the two diseases most commonly confused with Rocky Mountain spotted fever are measles and meningococcemia. In central and east Africa, two diseases which cause major differential diagnostic problems with louse-borne typhus are cerebral falciparum malaria and typhoid fever. Milder cases of typhus may be indistinguishable clinically from influenza.

The most sophisticated modern laboratory diagnostic aids can sometimes help distinguish within hours between measles, meningococcemia, and Rocky Mountain spotted fever. Blood smears for malaria should be routine where malaria and rickettsial diseases coexist. Typhoid can be detected by cultures. (Only *early* diagnostic measures are stressed here. It is no victory to make a retrospective diagnosis!) Outside the United States and Europe, however, laboratory facilities may be unavailable, and an empirical therapeutic approach is often successful. For example, when it is not possible to distinguish between malaria, typhus, and typhoid, a combination of chloramphenicol and chloroquine often gives a satisfactory clinical response; or a "typhus suspect" not responding in 48 hours to a tetracycline drug can often be treated successfully with chloramphenicol.

Finally, outside the United States, a patient with a rickettsial infection may have another concurrent infection, e.g., typhus plus relapsing fever or trench fever; or typhus or scrub typhus plus malaria, bacterial pneumonia, or dysentery. These must also be diagnosed and treated specifically.

LABORATORY DIAGNOSIS. Methods for retrospective diagnoses (isolation of organism and serologic response) of rickettsial infections are reasonably well developed, although not universally available, and methods for specific diagnosis in the acute phase of disease, when crucial decisions about specific chemotherapy must be made, are generally unsatisfactory but are improving. The following paragraphs have been written specifically for the practicing physician, beginning with methods applicable to the early, acute phase and proceeding to more specific methods which sometimes tend to be only confirmatory or retrospective.

Exclusion of Diseases Which Present Common Differential Diagnostic Problems in a Given Locality. Examples include malaria smear, skin lesion smear for meningococci, demonstration of measles antigen in respiratory epithelial cells by fluorescence microscopy, and cultures for typhoid and other enteric fevers.

Direct Demonstration of Rickettsiae in Tissues or Rickettsial Antigens in Urine in Acute Phase of Disease. Attempts to demonstrate rickettsiae directly in tissues or cells of patients and to demonstrate rickettsial antigens in body fluids, such as urine, have been explored for many years with variable degrees of success, although none is yet available for routine diagnosis.

DIRECT MICROSCOPIC DEMONSTRATION OF RICKETTSIAE IN TISSUES. For diagnostic purposes, rickettsiae have been demonstrated in endothelial cells of skin biopsies, blood leukocytes (with or without a short period of in vitro incubation), and bone marrow smears in typhus and spotted fever infections of man or animals. The use of fluorescein-conjugated antisera permits identification of the organisms, specific at least to group. Refinement and standardization of these methods promise to yield practical routine methods for the early specific diagnosis of rickettsial infections and should be pursued vigorously. A different application of the general method is the direct demonstration by fluorescent antibody staining of R. rickettsii in attached ticks removed from a person (see Prevention and Control in Ch. 109).

DEMONSTRATION OF RICKETTSIAL ANTIGENS IN ACUTE PHASE URINE. Although theoretically feasible, demonstrable in certain experimental infections in animals, and sporadically reported in human disease, reliable demonstration of rickettsial antigens in acute phase urine has been fraught with difficulty. Application of modern immunologic methods (e.g., immunodiffusion, counterimmunoelectrophoresis, radioimmunoassay, enzyme-linked immunosorbent assay [ELISA] may improve sensitivity, specificity, and reliability and deserves concerted effort.

Isolation of Rickettsiae. The isolation of rickettsiae from the blood or tissues of a patient is hazardous, requires special laboratory facilities and trained personnel, usually does not yield results in time to influence patient management, and hence, was not encouraged as a routine procedure in the past. However, methods are improving, and moreover it is now urgent to change this position because serologic retrospective diagnoses are ill equipped to identify new species or variants of rickettsiae. A growing diversity of rickettsial agents (e.g., the flying squirrel agent and R. canada in the typhus group, new members of the spotted fever group) is being recognized in the United States and elsewhere, whose importance as causes of human disease remains unknown; this is partly because conventional serologic tests for retrospective diagnosis are largely *group* specific, might not recognize variants at the species level, and would not detect infections with totally new agents (e.g., the agent of "Kawasaki disease"). Isolation and characterization of the agent are the keystones of identification of new diseases.

Although isolation and identification of rickettsial agents are usually beyond the competence of the ordinary hospital laboratory, mechanisms do exist for accomplishing this. In the United States, properly collected and preserved (frozen at −70° C or lower) specimens can be sent through state health departments to the Center for Disease Control in Atlanta, Georgia, where specially trained personnel and special facilities exist to handle and characterize such agents. Moreover, the World Health Organization has established in this country and abroad a series of reference laboratories which are also capable of handling such agents.

Serologic Diagnosis. Serologic methods remain the mainstay of routine laboratory diagnosis of rickettsial infections and for epidemiologic purposes. However,

TABLE 3. Some Clinical Features of Selected Rickettsial Diseases

Disease	Usual Incubation Period (Days)	Rash				Usual Duration of Disease* (Days)	Usual Severity†	Fever After Chemotherapy (Hours)
		Eschar	Onset, Day of Disease	Distribution	Type			
Typhus group Murine typhus	12 (8–16)	None	5–7	Trunk → extremities	Macular, maculopapular	12 (8–16)	Moderate	48–72
Epidemic typhus	12 (10–14)	None	5–7	Trunk → extremities	Macular, maculopapular, petechial	14 (10–18)	Severe	48–72
Brill's disease	—	None		Trunk → extremities	Macular	7–11	Relatively mild	48–72
Spotted fever group Rocky Mountain spotted fever	7 (3–12)	None	3–5	Extremities → trunk, face	Macular, maculopapular, petechial	16 (10–20)	Severe	72
Boutonneuse fever	5–7	Often present	3–4	Trunk, extremities, face, palms, soles	Macular, maculopapular, petechial	10 (7–14)	Moderate	—
Rickettsialpox	?9–17	Often present	1–3	Trunk → face, extremities	Papular vesicular	7 (3–11)	Relatively mild	—
Scrub typhus (tsutsugamushi disease)	1–12 (9–18)	Often present	4–6	Trunk → extremities	Macular, maculopapular	14 (10–20)	Mild to severe	24–36
Q fever	10–19	None		None		6 (2–21)	Relatively‡ mild	48 (occasionally slow)

*Untreated disease.
†Severity can vary greatly.
‡Occasional chronic infections occur (e.g., hepatitis, endocarditis).

since an antibody response rarely occurs with any of the rickettsioses before the end of the first week of disease, and since a rise in antibody titer is more or less essential to a solid diagnosis, convincing serologic diagnosis may become available only *after* the critical point has been passed with respect to lifesaving decisions about chemotherapy. At present, serologic tests consist of (1) nonspecific (Weil-Felix) tests generally available to hospital laboratories through commercially produced antigens (a part of the "febrile agglutinin" package) and (2) more specific tests, generally available at State Health Departments, the CDC, and the WHO reference laboratories.

WEIL-FELIX REACTION. Based upon unique sharing of polysaccharide antigens between certain *Proteus* strains and some rickettsiae, this agglutination test performed with suspensions of rough *Proteus* OX-2, OX-19, and OX-K strains has an historical aura and the advantage of simplicity, ready availability of antigens, and sensitivity to early antibody response.

Proteus agglutinins tend to appear early (toward the end of the first week), attain peak titers between three and four weeks after onset, and then rapidly decline. The Weil-Felix test is not positive in all rickettsial infections, is variable in recrudescent typhus (Brill-Zinsser disease), will not distinguish between typhus and spotted fever group infections, is not positive in all scrub typhus infections (about 70 per cent positive in primary infections and fewer in second infections), and may yield "false positive" results in *Proteus* infections, relapsing fever, and leptospirosis. Nevertheless, properly applied and interpreted along with other information,

the test can be useful. Until more specific tests are generally available to physicians within a time frame useful for patient management, the Weil-Felix test, despite its deficiencies, will not die.

COMPLEMENT FIXATION (CF) TEST. For most of the rickettsioses, except for the scrub typhus group, the CF test remains the standard of serodiagnosis and seroepidemiology. With group ("soluble") antigens, sera can be screened for evidence of infection with any member of the typhus or spotted fever group and with the "specific" rickettsial body antigens; the offending organism can often be identified by titer differences, depending in part on the time of specimen collection, previous exposure to related organisms, and the like. By comparing titers obtained with low and high antigen doses or before and after treatment with ethanethiol or 2-mercaptoethanol, some information can be obtained on the presence of IgM and IgG antibodies. In a single serum specimen, such information allows one to judge if antibodies present are the result of recent or remote infection or to differentiate between primary louse-borne typhus (early IgM response) and recrudescent typhus (Brill-Zinsser disease) (secondary early IgG response). In the case of Q fever, persisting high titers with Phase I antigen suggest chronic infection (e.g., hepatitis, endocarditis).

There are some pitfalls. Spotted fever group antigens tend to be anticomplementary and are often unsatisfactory. Moreover, discrimination between infections of man caused by different members of the spotted fever group is not entirely satisfactory. Some cross-reactions may occur between typhus and spotted fever group in-

TABLE 4. Some Typical Serologic Responses in Rickettsial Infections of Man*

Rickettsial Infection	Weil-Felix Test†					Complement Fixation				Agglutination				Indirect Fluorescent Antibody Test‡			
	Agglutination with Proteus Strain			Kinetics		Specificity		Kinetics		Specificity		Kinetics		Specificity		Kinetics	
	OX-19	OX-2	OX-K	Day First Positive	Persistence	Group	Species or Strain	Day First Positive	Persistence	Group	Species or Strain	Day First Positive	Persistence	Group	Species or Strain	Day First Positive	Persistence
Typhus group	+++	+	0	5–9	Short	++	++	7–10	Long	++	+	5–7	Unknown	++	+	?	?
Brill-Zinsser disease	Variable, often negative	+		–	–	++	+	4–5	Long	++	+	Unknown	Unknown	++	Unknown	?	?
Spotted fever group	+++	+++	0	5–12	Short	++§	+§	8–14	Long	++	+	Unknown	Unknown	++	+	?	?
Rickettsialpox	+	0	0	5–12	Short	++§	+§	8–14	Long	++	+	Unknown	Unknown	++	++	?	?
Scrub typhus group	0	0	0–+++	10–14	Short	+	++	10–14	Unknown	Test not available				Single serotype		?	?
Q fever	0	0	0	–	–	Single serotype				Single serotype				Single serotype			
Phase I antigen												10–14				?	?
Phase II antigen								8–14	Inter-mediate¶			5–8	Inter-mediate			?	?

*Variations of microbial or host origin, early chemotherapy, etc., may alter "typical" responses.

†"False positives" may occur—viz., *Proteus* infections, relapsing fever, leptospirosis. "Significant" titer in single specimen is ≥ 1:160.

‡Experience is sufficient to establish utility in diagnosis but insufficient to establish precise patterns.

§Complement fixation test is of limited use in spotted fever group infections because antigens tend to be anticomplementary.

¶Phase I complement fixation antibodies ordinarily tend to be low and transient but may persist in high titer in chronic infections (e.g., hepatitis, endocarditis).

fections. Prior experience with a related organism may result in higher titers to that organism than to the current infecting agent. Thus, as with all serologic tests, interpretation requires care and knowledge of potential problems.

AGGLUTINATION TESTS. Agglutination tests with highly purified rickettsial suspensions are receiving increasing attention because they are simple to perform, are unaffected by anticomplementary factors in serum or antigen, are highly sensitive, and usually detect antibodies somewhat earlier in disease than does the CF test. Persistence of antibodies has not yet been thoroughly documented. Group specificity is good. Species specificity appears to be fair among the spotted fever group, but some problems have been encountered in distinguishing between murine and epidemic typhus infections of man (as opposed to high specificity in rodents). This test requires large amounts of antigen compared with the CF test. However, the original tube test has now been largely replaced with a highly satisfactory microtiter adaptation (MA test). (Note: The agglutination tests referred to here are not to be confused with the Giroud type of microscopic agglutination test, which is performed with relatively crude antigens and which is often unreliable).

INDIRECT FLUORESCENT ANTIBODY TESTS (IFA). IFA tests are undergoing rapid development for diagnostic and epidemiologic purposes. They are sensitive and useful with anticomplementary sera or blood collected on filter paper. IFA tests may be positive when blocking factors interfere with CF or MA tests. They can be made group specific. Methods for improved species differentiation are under study. IgG, IgM, and IgA antibody titers can be determined directly. Kinetics of antibody response have not yet been clearly defined. The IFA test is currently the most sensitive and reliable test available for the diagnosis of scrub typhus.

OTHER TESTS. Toxin neutralization tests, passive hemagglutination tests, and radioimmune precipitation tests have special uses. New tests, such as the ELISA type test, are under development and evaluation.

TREATMENT OF RICKETTSIAL DISEASES. The general principles of therapy are similar for all the common rickettsial diseases. Optimal management includes (1) specific antimicrobial therapy directed against the offending rickettsial agent; (2) supportive measures to correct physiologic abnormalities; (3) good nursing care to prevent serious complications; and (4) prompt, appropriate therapy of complications. In mild cases, patients treated early may require little more than the specific antimicrobial therapy. Vigorous supportive measures and good nursing may be lifesaving in severe cases.

Clinical Classification. A clinical classification system for efficient management of patients evolved during a large epidemic of louse-borne typhus fever is also useful in the sporadic, individual case of any of the rickettsioses. Thus the patient is evaluated immediately on admission according to duration and general severity of disease, neurologic involvement (coma, delirium, lucid state but inability to swallow), physiologic derangements (hypotension, shock, renal impairment, clotting derangement), state of nutrition and hydration, and presence or absence of complications. For practical management purposes, patients can then be classified as (1) mild or severe, (2) cooperative or uncooperative, and (3) uncomplicated or complicated. Even moderately severe but uncomplicated rickettsial infection in a cooperative patient is usually simple to manage with orally administered antibiotics, fluids, and nutriments. The uncooperative patient or the patient with complications requires added measures. Management is greatly simplified if the uncooperative patient can be brought quickly to the stage at which oral medications and fluids are possible (see below).

Antirickettsial Therapy. *Prompt adequate antirickettsial therapy is the single most important factor in shortening the disease, reducing mortality, and speeding convalescence.* In cooperative uncomplicated cases this may be the only medication required.

Antimicrobial drugs of the tetracycline series are the drugs of choice for the treatment of all rickettsial diseases. Although also highly effective, chloramphenicol is not recommended, unless tetracyclines cannot be used, because of the occasional complication of aplastic anemia. These drugs shorten the course of disease dramatically and reduce fatality rates virtually to zero except in neglected, complicated, or fulminating cases. The patient often begins to respond by 24 hours and is afebrile in one to four days, usually two to three days, depending on the specific rickettsia and the stage of disease at the time therapy is begun.

Penicillin, streptomycin, and sulfonamides are clinically ineffective. Practical concentrations of a wide range of aminoglycosides, semisynthetic penicillins, and cephalosporins do not inhibit *R. prowazekii* growth in vitro in cell cultures. *Note: Except for chloramphenicol,* none of the drugs (ampicillin, amoxycillin, co-trimoxazole) used for the treatment of typhoid fever, a serious differential diagnostic problem in some areas, gives clinical and/or in vitro evidence of effectiveness in typhus fever. Whether or not this applies to the other rickettsioses remains to be determined.

Tetracycline HCl is given orally in a total daily dose of 25 to 50 mg per kilogram of body weight. Two grams per day in divided doses at 4- to 6- or even 12-hour intervals usually suffices for adult patients. Chloramphenicol is given orally in amounts of 50 and 75 mg per kilogram of body weight per day for adults and children, respectively, usually in divided doses at 4- to 6- or even 12-hour intervals. (Caution: Doses larger than 25 mg per kilogram of body weight may be severely toxic for *newborn infants*.) Intravenous tetracycline is given in a dosage of 0.5 gram every 6 to 12 hours, to a maximum of 2 grams per day for adults. Although likely to cause pain or local reaction, up to 0.5 gram of the intramuscular tetracycline preparation can be given, if necessary, every 12 hours for a day or two until the patient can take the oral preparation. Chloramphenicol succinate, appropriately diluted, is given intravenously to adults in a dose of 1.0 gram every 8 to 12 hours. Parenteral therapy should be replaced with oral therapy as soon as the patient can swallow. When parenteral preparations are unavailable or intravenous drip therapy is impractical, oral preparations suspended in fluid may be administered by stomach tube.

Since neither tetracycline HCl nor chloramphenicol is rickettsicidal under ordinary circumstances, and since neither eradicates the organism from the body, ultimate freedom from clinical relapse (i.e., "cure") is probably dependent on an adequate immune response by the patient. Duration of therapy is dependent on the pharmacology of the particular drug employed; the susceptibility of the organism to, and rate of recovery from, the inhibitory effects of the drug employed, which may vary from one species of organism to another; and the stage of the disease at the time therapy is begun. Although not necessarily the minimal effective regimen, a practical conservative guide to duration of tetracycline or chloramphenicol therapy is to administer the drug until the patient has been afebrile for 48 hours and for an additional period until the total time elapsed from onset of disease is 12 to 14 days. Relapses respond to re-treatment with the same drug. The usual precautions are observed for administering antimicrobials, e.g., adjustment of dosage to compensate for problems of immaturity in infants and of renal or hepatic dysfunction of rickettsial or other origin, staining of developing teeth, changes in microbial flora and superinfection, pregnancy, drug susceptibilities, or blood dyscrasias.

The introduction of new lipotropic tetracycline derivatives which produce prolonged high blood and tissue levels after a single dose (viz., doxycycline and minocycline) has literally revolutionized the management of louse-borne typhus and perhaps scrub typhus. A *single* 100-mg dose of doxycycline will *cure* most adults, and a *single* 50-mg dose will cure most children, with only an occasional transient relapse which does not require additional therapy. A single 200-mg dose is rarely followed by relapse. Under extreme circumstances, single-dose doxycycline therapy, requiring only a single contact between patient and medical personnel, has been applied successfully on an outpatient basis. Unless in extremis from typhus or suffering from some unrelated disease, almost all patients will survive whether "hospitalized," at home, or transiently disoriented in the bush. Single-dose doxycycline is currently the treatment of choice for louse-borne typhus. Comparable results have been obtained with minocycline, but, because of its tendency to cause otitic complications, it is not recommended as a first choice drug.

Experience with single-dose doxycycline treatment of other rickettsioses is limited. However, some substantial evidence indicates that a single 200-mg dose of doxycycline will cure scrub typhus, with some transient recrudescences. On the other hand, very limited and uncontrolled observations suggest that a single dose will not suffice for the treatment of murine typhus or Rocky Mountain spotted fever, although a daily dose of 100 to 200 mg on a schedule described for tetracycline HCl is effective.

Antimicrobial Resistance. Antimicrobial resistance has not yet been encountered in naturally occurring rickettsial disease. However, in the laboratory, *R. prowazekii* strains have been selected that are resistant to erythromycin, chloramphenicol, penicillin, and certain other inhibitors. Moreover, it has been shown that therapeutic doses of antirickettsial drugs produce blood levels which transiently inhibit the growth of *R. prowazekii* in the louse gut, thereby creating potentially selective conditions. Since not all treated typhus patients are in fact effectively deloused, the possibility exists for the selection of antimicrobial-resistant strains of *R. prowazekii* which might emerge in either current epidemics or future epidemics through recrudescence of infection by antimicrobial-resistant strains.

Steroids. Although not rigorously controlled, studies have shown that corticosteroids given in conjunction with antimicrobial drugs may cause rapid defervescence, dramatic reversal of neurologic impairment (coma, difficulty in swallowing), and an apparent improvement in the general well-being of the patient without adversely affecting the infectious process. A comatose typhus patient given steroid therapy in the evening may be sitting up on the side of the bed in the morning, conversing with his fellow patients and able to take medication and fluids by mouth. Similar effects may be seen in patients unable to swallow. More limited observations with scrub typhus and Rocky Mountain spotted fever have shown similar apparently beneficial effects, although of course reversal of intravascular clotting in Rocky Mountain spotted fever will not be effected. This has been accomplished by giving 100 mg of hydrocortisone intravenously and 200 to 300 mg of cortisone acetate intramuscularly in addition to 500 mg of tetracycline intramuscularly upon admission. *(Falciparum malaria must be excluded by blood smear in patients at risk to both diseases.)* Often within 24 hours a typhus patient is able to swallow the final dose of antibiotic (100 mg of doxycycline), to take oral fluids, to attend to elimination, and to move spontaneously to reduce the chances of developing pressure necroses or thrombophlebitis. Usually no more therapy of any kind, antimicrobial or steroid, is required, and nutrition presents no problem. This therapy is reserved for seriously ill or "uncooperative" patients.

Fluid and Electrolyte Balance. Oral fluids sufficient to ensure a daily urine output of at least 1500 ml suffice for the conscious, cooperative patient. The comatose patient will require parenteral fluids to maintain an adequate urine output. Fluids should be given slowly so as not to tax the potentially labile cardiovascular system. Excess electrolytes contribute to the general edema and to cardiac load when the fluid re-enters the vascular compartment. Urine output, the presence of oliguria, and laboratory determinations will serve as guides to the proper volume and proportion of electrolytes, glucose and water.

Hepatic and Renal Systems. The cause of the disturbed liver (abnormal tests, rarely jaundice) and kidney (azotemia, albuminuria, oliguria) functions remains controversial, but these abnormalities are usually transient and disappear with convalescence. Hence management, if required, is guided by identification of the specific abnormalities present through appropriate tests and by the presence of other complicating abnormalities.

Cardiovascular System, Including Blood. The most prominent manifestations of the typhus, scrub typhus, and spotted fever groups of rickettsial diseases can be attributed to abnormalities of the cardiovascular system. Indeed, hypotension is common, and peripheral vascular collapse, frequently in the second week of disease, is a leading cause of death and has been difficult to manage. Its cause is only incompletely understood. However, the widespread focal lesions of the small vessels are assumed to be contributory to increased vascular permeability and collapse and may also account for some of the clotting abnormalities (thrombocytopenia, disseminated intravascular clotting as a result of endothelial damage, and defective synthesis from liver impairment) which have recently been recognized in certain rickettsioses. This in turn would help explain certain complications — hemorrhage, vascular occlusion (gangrene, hemiplegia, others), and thrombophlebitis — and would suggest more rational approaches to their prevention and management, especially when specifically identified by appropriate laboratory tests.

Accordingly, whole blood and plasma should be avoided. Albumin may be used to combat hypoproteinemia. Red cells are preferred to correct significant anemia. Heparin has been described as treatment for rickettsia-associated intravascular clotting, but others have failed to detect benefit in the intravascular clotting accompanying Rocky Mountain spotted fever.

The management of peripheral vascular collapse is empirical and largely of unproved benefit: (1) oxygen; (2) judicious use of salt-poor concentrated albumin as a plasma expander and to reduce edema; (3) vasopressor drugs, e.g., levarterenol bitartrate (Levophed); and (4) corticosteroids such as hydrocortisone.

Pulmonary edema and congestive heart failure, resulting from excessive intake of salt and water or from rapid resorption of edema fluid with vascular healing, are treated with digitalis. No guidelines are available for the use of diuretics, but if their use is contemplated, consideration should be given to the state of renal function.

Massive intravascular hemolysis, described in glucose-6-phosphate dehydrogenase–deficient subjects with murine or scrub typhus, has been managed successfully with peritoneal dialysis.

Other Complications. Bacterial pneumonia, still frequent in epidemic typhus, or other bacterial infections are treated with appropriate antimicrobial agents according to the causative organisms and their sensitivity patterns. Gangrene, decubitus ulcers, and thrombophlebitis are treated by the usual surgical and medical methods. Unless caused by a large destructive process (hemorrhage or thrombosis of a large vessel), neurologic abnormalities usually resolve with convalescence, although personality changes and deafness have been known to persist in some patients for months.

Nursing Care. Patients may be irrational or agitated and may injure themselves or even attempt self-destruction. Close observation and restraint may be required. Comatose patients should be turned frequently to prevent pressure necrosis, thrombophlebitis, and hypostatic pneumonia. Special skin care and protection of bony prominences may be desirable in view of the vascular damage associated with the disease. Good oral hygiene reduces the chances of suppurative parotitis.

Special Considerations. Although classic Q fever often responds promptly to chemotherapy with tetracycline drugs or chloramphenicol as outlined above, the response in some cases is slower and less dramatic. Treatment of chronic infection is less satisfactory. Chemotherapy of *C. burnetii* endocarditis is especially unsatisfactory, probably due to the fact that most antirickettsial drugs are only rickettsiostatic. There has been very limited success with combined chemotherapy administered over a period of many months. However, surgical replacement of the affected heart valve has been somewhat more successful.

Trench fever has been reported to respond to tetracycline drugs, but no information is available concerning the effects of brief chemotherapy on the persistence of the organism in the blood or on subsequent relapse rates.

General

Horsfall, F. L., Jr., and Tamm, I. (eds.): Viral and Rickettsial Infections of Man. 4th ed. Philadelphia, J. B. Lippincott Company, 1965.

Moulton, F. R. (ed.): Symposium on Rickettsial Diseases (Dec., 1946, Boston). Washington, D.C., American Association for the Advancement of Science, 1948.

Topping, N. H., et al.: Studies of typhus fever. National Institute of Health Bull. No. 183, 1945.

Weiss, E.: Growth and physiology of rickettsiae. Bacteriol. Rev., 37:259, 1973.

Wisseman, C. L., Jr.: Some biological properties of rickettsiae pathogenic for man. Zentralbl. Bakteriol. [Orig.] 206:299, 1968.

Wisseman, C. L. Jr. (ed.): Symposium on the spotted fever group of rickettsiae (Commission on Rickettsial Diseases, Armed Forces Epidemiological Board). Walter Reed Army Institute of Research Medical Science, Publication no. 7. Washington, D.C., Government Printing Office, 1960.

Zdrodovskii, P. F., and Golinevich, H. M.: The Rickettsial Diseases. New York, Pergamon Press, Inc., 1960.

Laboratory Diagnosis

DeShazo, R. D., Boyce, J. R., Osterman, J. V., and Stephenson, E. H.: Early diagnosis of Rocky Mountain spotted fever. Use of primary monocyte culture technique. JAMA, 235:1353, 1976.

Elisberg, B. L., and Bozeman, F. L.: Serologic diagnosis of rickettsial diseases by indirect immunofluorescence. Arch. Inst. Pasteur Tunis, 43:193, 1966.

Elisberg, B. L., and Bozeman, F. M.: Rickettsiae. In Lennette, E. H., and Schmidt, N. J. (eds.): Diagnostic Procedures for Viral and Rickettsial Infections. 4th ed. New York, American Public Health Association, 1969, pp. 826–868.

Fiset, P., Ormsbee, R. A., Silberman, R., Peacock, M., and Spielman, S. H.: A microagglutination technique for detection and measurement of rickettsial antibodies. Acta Virol. (Praha), 13:60, 1969.

Murphy, J. R., Wisseman, C. L., Jr., and Snyder, L. B.: Plaque assay for *Rickettsia mooseri* in tissue samples. Proc. Soc. Exp. Biol. Med., 153:151, 1976.

Murray, E. S., O'Connor, J. M., and Gaon, J. A.: Differentiation of 19S and 7S complement-fixing antibodies in primary versus recrudescent typhus by either ethanethiol or heat. Proc. Soc. Exp. Biol. Med., 119:291, 1965.

Ormsbee, R., Peacock, M., Casper, E., Plorde, J., Gabre-Kirdan, T., and Wright, L.: Serologic diagnosis of epidemic typhus fever. Am. J. Epidemiol., 105:261, 1977.

Philip, R. N., Casper, E. A., MacCormack, J. N., Sexton, D. J., Thomas, L. A., Anacker, R. L., Burgdorfer, W., and Vick, S.: A comparison of serologic methods for diagnosis of Rocky Mountain spotted fever. Am. J. Epidemiol., 105:56, 1977.

Robinson, D. M., Brown, G., Gan, E., and Huxsoll, D. L.: Adaptation of a microimmunofluorescence test to the study of human *Rickettsia tsutsugamushi* antibody. Am. J. Trop. Med. Hyg., 25:900, 1976.

Woodward, T. E., Pederson, C. E., Jr., Oster, C. N., Bagley, L. R., Romberger, J., and Snyder, M. J.: Prompt confirmation of Rocky Mountain spotted fever: Identification of rickettsiae in skin tissues. J. Infect. Dis., 134:297, 1976.

Clinicopathologic

Allen, A. C., and Spitz, S.: A comparative study of the pathology of scrub typhus and other rickettsial diseases. Am. J. Pathol., 21:603, 1945.

National Research Council Committee on Pathology: Pathology of epidemic typhus. Arch. Pathol., 56:397, 512, 1953.

Whelton, A., Donadio, J. V., Jr., and Elisberg, B. L.: Acute renal failure complicating rickettsial infections in glucose-6-phosphate dehydrogenase–deficient individuals. Ann. Intern. Med., 69:323, 1968.

Wolbach, S. B., Todd, J. L., and Palfrey, F. W.: The Etiology and Pathology of Typhus. Cambridge, Harvard University Press, 1922.

Wright, L. J., Barker, L. F., Mickenberg, I. D., and Wolff, S. M.: Laboratory-acquired typhus fevers. Ann. Intern. Med., 69:731, 1968.

Zarafonetis, C. J. D.: The typhus fevers. In Coates, J. B., and Havens, W. P. (eds.): Medical Department, United States Army. Internal Medicine in World War II. Vol. II, Infectious Diseases. Washington, D.C., Office of the Surgeon General, Department of the Army, 1963, pp. 143–223.

See Ch. 109 for selected references on coagulation abnormalities.

Chemotherapy/Treatment

Fabrikant, I. B., El Batawi, Y., and Wisseman, C. L., Jr.: Cortisone action at different stages of experimental *Rickettsia mooseri* infection in mice. Arch. Inst. Pasteur Tunis, 43:205, 1966 (review of corticosteroids).

Ley, H. L., Jr., and Smadel, J. E.: Antibiotic therapy of rickettsial diseases. Antibiot. Chemother., 4:792, 1954.

Sheehy, T. W., Hazlett, D., and Turk, R. E.: Scrub typhus: A comparison of chloramphenicol and tetracycline and its treatment. Arch. Intern. Med., 132:77, 1973.

Wisseman, C. L., Jr., et al.: Antibodies and clinical relapse of murine typhus fever following early chemotherapy. Ann. Intern. Med., 57:743, 1962.

Woodward, T. E.: Therapy of the rickettsial diseases with a discussion of chemoprophylaxis. Arch. Inst. Pasteur Tunis, 36:507, 1959.

108. THE TYPHUS GROUP

Charles L. Wisseman, Jr.

Three clinical and epidemiologic entities comprise the established diseases of the typhus group: (1) primary louse-borne epidemic typhus (*Rickettsia prowazekii*); (2) its recrudescent form, Brill-Zinsser disease (*R. prowazekii*); and (3) flea-borne murine typhus (*R. mooseri* [*R. typhi*]). These diseases are similar clinically and pathologically but differ in intensity of certain symptoms and signs, severity, and case fatality rate. This conventional listing of typhus group diseases has been complicated in the United States in recent years by (1) the isolation of a new species, *R. canada*, from ticks in Canada and its implication on serologic grounds as the possible cause of a Rocky Mountain spotted fever–like disease in Georgia; (2) the isolation of *R. prowazekii*–like rickettsiae from flying squirrels in the eastern United States and the growing suspicion of the occurrence of sporadic non–*R. mooseri* typhus cases in southern states; and (3) the strong one-way serologic cross-reactions between *R. canada* and *R. prowazekii*. Much more information, especially isolation and characterization of the agents from human cases, is needed for clarification.

108.1. EPIDEMIC LOUSE-BORNE TYPHUS FEVER

(Many Synonyms: Classic, Historic, European Typhus; Jail, War, Camp, Ship Fever; Fleckfieber [German]; Typhus Exanthématique [French]; Tifus Exantemático, Tabardillo [Spanish]; Dermotypho [Italian])

HISTORY. Typhus fever is one of the great epidemic diseases of mankind. It is best known in its epidemic form, which tends to emerge in association with wars, famines, and other forms of human misfortunes. Although it is probably ancient on an historical time scale and has been suggested as a possible cause of the plague of Athens in 430 B.C., the first reasonably accurate medical description of typhus is generally attributed to Fracastorius in 1546. In the ensuing four centuries it has changed the course of history, often being more decisive in military campaigns than the battles themselves, as Zinsser has recounted in his *Rats, Lice and History*. Typhus fever was an important factor in World War I and during the subsequent famine and sociopolitical unrest in Russia and eastern Europe between 1918 and 1922, when an estimated 30,000,000 cases of typhus with 3,000,000 deaths occurred. During World War II, millions of cases occurred in North Africa, Italy, Nazi prison camps, eastern Europe, and even Soviet Central Asia. At present, only sporadic cases are encountered in eastern Europe. The disease resurges from time to time in Afghanistan, probably occurs in the Himalaya Mountains, is epidemic to endemoepidemic in Central Africa and Ethiopia, and causes sporadic outbreaks in southern Africa. Typhus has a long history, dating from the Spanish conquistadores, in Mexico, Central America, and the Andean countries of South America, where it remains highly endemic with occasional sharp village outbreaks.

It was not until 1837 that Gerhard in Philadelphia clearly differentiated typhus from typhoid fever on clinical and pathologic grounds. Typhoid fever is still called *typhus abdominalis* in Europe, and the distinction between typhus and typhoid still poses practical problems of differential clinical diagnosis.

Louse transmission of typhus was demonstrated by Nicolle, Compte, and Consiel in 1909; da Rocha-Lima described the organism in the gut of the body louse and named it *Rickettsia prowazekii*. The classic work of Wolbach, Todd, and Palfrey (1922) clearly associated the clinical, pathologic, and etiologic aspects of typhus.

DEFINITION. Classic typhus fever is an acute infectious disease transmitted by the human body louse (*Pediculus humanus humanus*) and characterized clinically by sudden onset, sustained high fever of about two weeks' duration, a macular rash, and altered mental state.

ETIOLOGY (see Ch. 107). *Rickettsia prowazekii* is a small pleomorphic bacterium, ranging from coccobacillary to filamentous, with distinct tinctorial properties. Outer layers of the envelope possess group as well as specific antigens. No evidence has been obtained for significant variations in antigenic composition or virulence for man in strains from different areas, but attenuation has been observed as a laboratory phenomenon.

TRANSMISSION AND EPIDEMIOLOGY. The natural infection cycle is restricted to man and the human body louse (*Pediculus humanus humanus*), although the organism can also grow in the head louse (*Pediculus humanus capitis*). The louse acquires the rickettsia by feeding on the blood of a typhus patient during the rickettsemic phase. The organism multiplies in, and destroys, cells of the louse midgut, achieving numbers greater than 10^8 organisms per louse and causing death of the louse in one to two weeks. Large numbers of rickettsiae are excreted in the feces. The organism is not transmitted by bite. Instead, crushed infective lice or louse feces contaminate bite sites or other breaks in the skin, or airborne infective louse feces gain access through the respiratory tract.

The louse regularly dies of *R. prowazekii* infection, does not transmit the organism transovarially to the next generation, and is not a reservoir of typhus. Putative domestic animal reservoirs have largely been discounted as laboratory artifacts, but the role of the flying squirrel in the eastern United States has not yet been evaluated. Man, through the phenomenon of persisting infection and subsequent recrudescence (see Ch. 108.2) remains the most likely candidate for the major interepidemic reservoir.

One major key to epidemic typhus is the body louse vector. Typhus can occur anywhere when living conditions and political, socioeconomic, environmental, and cultural factors predispose to lousiness and the transfer of lice among people. These are currently supplied in mountainous parts of the Northern and Southern Hemispheres, as well as equatorial regions, in deserts (Sahara, Arabian deserts) where heavy clothing is worn continuously, and in tropical regions among nearly naked populations whose waistbands or arm and leg ornaments provide harborage for lice.

Depending upon many factors, louse-borne typhus can occur as a truly sharp epidemic disease, as a prolonged endemoepidemic disease (as in Ethiopia today), or as a highly endemic infection with sporadic, often unrecognized infections in young age groups but with sporadic sharp village outbreaks involving all age groups (as in Andean countries today).

PATHOLOGY. The general pathology and pathophysiologic features are described in Ch. 107.

CLINICAL MANIFESTATIONS AND COURSE. The following description applies to untreated full-blown classic typhus fever in adults. The incubation period usually is from 8 to 12 days but may be as short as 6 days or as long as 15 days. The disease may be divided into the prodromal, early, and late phases (see Pathogenesis in Ch. 107).

Prodromes of vague malaise and headache are not uncommon. The early phase is usually ushered in by the abrupt onset of fever, severe headache, myalgia of the back and legs, and chills or chilly sensations. The headache is intense and intractable, and persists day and night. Over the first two or three days the temperature attains a level of about 39 to 41° C, where it remains with only slight fluctuations until death or recovery. The skin is usually hot and dry. The face is flushed or dusky; the conjunctivae are suffused; photophobia is frequent. Deafness, tinnitus, and sometimes vertigo are prominent features. The mental state is dull. Weakness and prostration may be mild early, but after two or three days may become profound. Unproductive cough with sparse physical findings occurs in about two thirds of the cases. Nausea, vomiting, and diarrhea occur but are uncommon. Constipation is usually present.

The characteristic rash appears between the fourth and seventh days and ushers in the late phase of disease. In some instances, it is preceded by a diffuse, transient erythema. The lesions first appear on the trunk and axillary folds and spread to the extremities, sparing the face, palms, and soles, except in very severely ill patients. At first the lesions are pinkish red macules which blanch on pressure. The evolution of the rash depends on the severity of the illness. In mild cases it may fade completely in one or two days; in cases of moderate severity, it may become maculopapular, and may become hemorrhagic, changing to reddish brown and lasting for one to two weeks before fading; in very severe cases the lesions may be exceedingly numerous, almost confluent, quickly becoming hemorrhagic or even purpuric. The rash may be absent in 5 to 10 per cent of cases. With experience and proper lighting, it may be seen without too much difficulty in dark-skinned persons.

At first the pulse rate is slow in relation to the temperature, but by the end of the first week it becomes rapid (110 to 140), weak, and frequently undulating or irregular. The blood pressure is usually low, sometimes with a systolic pressure below 80 mm Hg, and there may be brief episodes of severe hypotension. Cyanosis may be present.

The mental state progresses from dullness to stupor, or occasionally to coma. The stupor may be interrupted by brief periods of delirium, excitement, or vigorous activity. Cranial nerves are selectively and variably involved (deafness, dysphagia, dysphonia). Coarse tremors may appear. Incontinence of urine and feces is encountered in moderately or severely ill patients.

Oliguria, proteinuria, and azotemia are common. Jaundice is rare, but elevations in serum transaminases may appear early. The white blood count may show a leukopenia early. In the second and third weeks of the disease it is normal or only slightly elevated unless complications ensue. Eosinophils are absent or rare in the early stages of typhus. Anemia may develop in the second or third week.

Death from typhus usually occurs between the ninth and eighteenth days of illness. The terminal period is usually characterized by a profound stupor, peripheral vascular collapse, and severe renal failure. When recovery is the outcome, the temperature begins to decline after 14 to 18 days and reaches a normal level by rapid lysis in two to four days. The mental and physical state of the patient improves strikingly as the temperature falls, but strength returns more slowly (two to three months).

Secondary bacterial bronchopneumonia, otitis media, and parotitis are common in untreated patients. Thrombosis may affect the large arteries with serious results (e.g., hemiplegia). Thrombosis of small vessels in the skin may lead to gangrene, particularly of the toes, fingers, or ear lobes. Necrosis of the skin may occur over the bony prominences, especially over the sacrum or greater trochanter.

Severity of disease and case fatality rate increase with age, being less severe and often uncharacteristic in younger children and increasing rapidly in those over the age of 40 years. In persons who contract typhus after having received killed typhus vaccine, the disease is greatly modified — with headache, fever of a few days' duration, and a transient rash but rare complications and negligible mortality.

PROGNOSIS. Depending on host factors, such as age, stress, nutritional state, other concurrent diseases, and perhaps the past typhus history of the population, case fatality rate in untreated typhus may range from 10 per cent or less to 60 per cent. Deep coma and severe hypotension and tachycardia associated with falling body temperature are signs of poor prognosis. Even such cases, however, often respond dramatically to appropriate chemotherapy and supportive measures. Appropriate treatment reduces the mortality rate in ordinary severe typhus fever virtually to zero.

TREATMENT. Treatment is described in Ch. 107. A single 200-mg oral dose of the long-acting tetracycline, doxycycline, is the treatment of choice under ordinary circumstances.

PREVENTION AND CONTROL. Infected lice and louse feces on a typhus patient present a special hazard to all nonimmune contacts, including physicians and attendants among whom infection is a common occupational hazard. Decontamination and delousing of the typhus patient and his clothing (including blankets and hats) are performed immediately upon hospitalization. Clothing and bedding are best decontaminated by heat, because this will kill the lice as well as the rickettsiae. After the patient is decontaminated and deloused, isolation and quarantine are not necessary.

Control of louse-borne typhus currently depends heavily upon control of the louse vector. When simple hygienic measures (e.g., bathing and laundering of clothes) cannot be followed, application of insecticide dusts (10 per cent DDT, 1 per cent malathion, 1 per cent lindane, or newer carbamates, depending upon local louse-resistance patterns) to fully clothed persons is very effective for reducing louse populations and controlling disease in acute outbreaks. Insecticides alone are less effective for long-term louse control in areas where conditions conducive to lousiness persist and where louse strains resistant to insecticides can be, and are, selected. The older methods of subjecting clothes and bedding to heat or fumigants (e.g., methyl bromide) are effective but cumbersome. It is possible but unproved that repellent-treated clothing (e.g., M-1960, diethyltoluamide) would reduce the chances of louse acquisition.

Vaccines composed of killed *R. prowazekii* are available, have been used extensively, definitely reduce the duration, severity, and mortality in vaccinated persons who acquire clinical typhus, and probably reduce the incidence of disease, although there are no quantitative controlled studies to assess accurately the degree of protection afforded. The attenuated E strain of *R. prowazekii*, when used experimentally as a living vaccine, has demonstrated substantial protection. The attenuated, immunizing infection occasionally is clinically overt, resembling an extremely modified typhus infection not requiring therapy. This vaccine is not yet generally available.

108.2.   BRILL-ZINSSER DISEASE
(Recrudescent Typhus)

HISTORY. In 1898 in New York, Nathan Brill reported a relatively mild typhus-like disease in immigrants from eastern Europe in the absence of body lice. Similar febrile illnesses were subsequently encountered in other cities in the eastern United States and were commonly referred to as Brill's disease. Then, in 1912, Anderson and Goldberger established the relationship between Brill's disease and typhus, and in 1931 murine typhus was recognized as a distinct entity. On the basis of an epidemiologic study, Zinsser in 1934 postulated that Brill's disease was in fact the late recrudescence of a latent infection following primary louse-borne typhus. This appeared to be confirmed, and the epidemiologic significance underlined in 1953, when Murray and Snyder infected body lice by allowing them to feed on Brill-Zinsser disease patients and then demonstrated that the organism was indistinguishable from fully virulent *R. prowazekii*.

DEFINITION. Brill-Zinsser disease is a recrudescence of typhus months to years after primary infection and clinically resembles a mild form of primary typhus.

ETIOLOGY. The etiologic agent is unmodified, fully virulent *R. prowazekii* that has persisted in tissues of the patient since his primary attack of typhus.

INTEREPIDEMIC SURVIVAL AND EPIDEMIOLOGIC CONSIDERATIONS. The nonsterile immunity and long persisting "latent" *R. prowazekii* infection that follows primary typhus constitutes, through rickettsemic recrudescence months to years later, the interepidemic reservoir for typhus and the mechanism by which the rickettsia is again made available to the louse vector. Neither the factors that precipitate recrudescence nor the precise rate of recrudescence among typhus convalescents is known. The efficiency with which lice become infected with *R. prowazekii* is apparently less during feeding upon Brill-Zinsser disease patients than upon primary typhus patients. Nevertheless, typhus outbreaks are known to have originated from Brill-Zinsser disease patients. This mechanism probably also plays a role in sustaining endemicity.

PATHOLOGY. The basic vascular lesions are similar to those of primary typhus.

CLINICAL MANIFESTATIONS AND COURSE. Recrudescent typhus is similar to primary typhus except that the fever is on the average lower and of shorter duration, the rash is less intense and often absent, and the case fatality rate is low. Nevertheless, it can be a serious and debilitating disease. Whether or not subclinical recrudescences occur is unknown.

DIAGNOSIS. The occurrence of a typhus-like disease of more than a few days' duration, with or without rash, in a patient who has no other stigmata of other bacterial infection and who has a history of previous primary typhus or residence in a typhus-endemic area should be considered as a potential candidate for Brill-Zinsser disease. In the laboratory, the organism can be demonstrated in vascular endothelial cells by skin biopsy. The Weil-Felix test is frequently negative. However, the diagnosis of *R. prowazekii* infection can be made with specific rickettsial serologic tests, and recrudescent typhus can be differentiated from primary typhus by the rapid appearance of dominantly IgG antibodies (secondary type of antibody response), as opposed to a somewhat slower antibody response, initially with a prominent IgM component, in primary typhus.

PROGNOSIS. Uncomplicated, untreated Brill-Zinsser disease has a low case fatality rate which should be reduced virtually to zero with specific antirickettsial treatment.

TREATMENT. Treatment is the same as for primary louse-borne typhus, as outlined in Ch. 107.

PREVENTION AND CONTROL. Prevention of primary louse-borne typhus infection is the only known reliable method for preventing Brill-Zinsser disease. None of the currently available antirickettsial chemotherapeutic agents are known to eradicate *R. prowazekii* from the infected person; hence, adequate antimicrobial therapy of primary louse-borne typhus probably will not prevent later recrudescence of infection. Since the factors leading to recrudescence are unknown, no specific manipulations of the host can be recommended. It is unknown, for example, if periodic vaccination of persons with a past history of primary louse-borne typhus will reduce the incidence of recrudescence. Prompt delousing of a patient with Brill-Zinsser disease will prevent the patient from becoming a source of primary louse-borne typhus infections in contacts.

108.3.   MURINE OR FLEA-BORNE
TYPHUS FEVER

HISTORY. In 1926, Maxcy's studies suggested a flea, mite, or tick vector and a rodent reservoir of the sporadic cases of typhus in the southeastern United States. In 1928 Mooser reported the distinctive characteristics of the microorganism; he suggested the term "murine typhus." In 1931, Dyer, Rumreich, and Badger obtained rickettsiae from rats in Baltimore, and in the same year Mooser, Castaneda, and Zinsser isolated a similar strain from the brains of rats in Mexico City. It was established that the infection is kept alive in a rat reservoir, is picked up from the rats by fleas, and is transferred by the flea vector to man. From rat to rat the infection can pass by both rat fleas and the rat louse, *Polyplax spinulosa*. Murine typhus was promptly found to be distributed all over the world, often existing in the same places where classic epidemic typhus fever occurs.

DEFINITION. Murine typhus fever is an acute, infectious disease communicable from rodent hosts to man sporadically by means of the rat flea (*Xenopsylla cheopis*). The disease is similar clinically to classic epidemic typhus except that it is much milder.

ETIOLOGY. The causative organism, *Rickettsia moo-seri (R. typhi)*, is similar to *R. prowazekii* in ultrastructure, metabolism, guanine and cytosine content of DNA, and staining characteristics and shares group antigens with *R. prowazekii* and *R. canada,* but it differs in specific antigens and host range. Significant cross-immunity between *R. mooseri* and *R. prowazekii* is produced by infection but not by killed vaccines.

TRANSMISSION AND EPIDEMIOLOGY. Murine typhus is not communicable from man to man. It is a zoonosis maintained in nature in a cycle involving rats and certain other small mammals as amplifying hosts and reservoirs and fleas and rat lice as vectors. In the rat flea (*Xenopsylla cheopis*) and perhaps other fleas infected by feeding upon rickettsemic rats, the organism grows in cells of the gut without killing the flea and is shed in the feces for the life of the flea. There is no transovarial transmission. It is transmitted to man, not by bite of the flea, but rather by contamination of broken skin with infective feces or by inhalation of dried infective feces.

Murine typhus is widely distributed over the world in the areas penetrated by *Rattus rattus* and *Rattus norvegicus* and where the vector fleas coexist. In some areas under appropriate conditions there may be spillover of *R. mooseri* from *Rattus* into other spatially closely associated small mammals and to man. Seasonal incidence of human infections appears to correlate with the periods of abundance of vector fleas, which in the United States is in the summer months. Rats are commensal animals closely associated with buildings or structures containing food (such as warehouses, markets, grain elevators, and godowns). Hence, acquisition of murine typhus by man is often associated with certain places and occupations.

PATHOLOGY. Although because of the low death rate few postmortem studies have been made, it is assumed that the lesions in man, as is the case in experimental infection of laboratory animals, are similar to those in louse-borne typhus.

CLINICAL MANIFESTATIONS AND COURSE. The incubation period of murine typhus lasts from 6 to 14 days. The symptoms are similar to those of louse-borne typhus, the principal differences being that murine typhus is a milder and shorter disease, the rash is less extensive and persists for shorter periods, there are fewer complications, and the case fatality rate is lower.

Although murine typhus is often referred to as mild, and truly mild cases do occur, this is mildness *relative* to louse-borne typhus. On an absolute scale, however, it can be severe and debilitating and may require two to three months for convalescence in untreated patients.

DIAGNOSIS. Clinical Diagnosis. The diagnosis of murine typhus may be suspected when a patient has sustained fever of several days' duration accompanied by headache, generalized aches and pains, and a macular or maculopapular rash appearing on the trunk on the fifth or sixth day after onset of fever. The patient with murine typhus may give a history of activities that have brought him into contact with places where rats are numerous. However, there is often no definite recollection of a flea bite. It is impossible on clinical evidence alone to distinguish an ordinary case of murine typhus from a case of Brill-Zinsser disease or a mild case of louse-borne typhus.

Laboratory Diagnosis. Diagnosis can often be made by specific rickettsial serologic tests or by isolation of the agent. (See Laboratory Diagnosis in Ch. 107.)

PROGNOSIS. The case fatality rate is usually less than 5 per cent in untreated patients and is virtually zero with rapid convalescence in uncomplicated murine typhus treated with appropriate antirickettsial drugs.

TREATMENT. Treatment follows the guidelines given in Ch. 107 with respect to the multiple dose antimicrobial regimen.

PREVENTION AND CONTROL. Individual preventive measures include avoiding endemic foci where rats and their fleas abound (e.g., warehouses, storage areas, grain elevators) or wearing repellent-treated clothing to prevent acquisition of fleas. A killed vaccine has been produced, but is unevaluated and is not now available.

General control measures are directed at reducing rat and flea populations. Among others, these include rat-proof construction and prevention of access of rats to food materials; reduction of rat populations by poison baits (e.g., warfarin, alphanaphthylthiourea), trapping, or poison gases into burrows; and reduction of the flea population through application of appropriate insecticides (such as DDT) to rat runs. When contemplating a rodent control program, it is important to plan insecticide application for flea control prior to, or simultaneously with, the rodent control measures to prevent increased exposure of man to fleas seeking alternative hosts.

Fox, J. P., Montoya, J. A., Jordan, M. D., Cornojo Ubillus, J. R., Garcia, J. L., Estrada, M. A., and Gelfand, H. M.: Immunization of man against epidemic typhus by infection with avirulent *Rickettsia prowazekii* (strain E). Arch. Inst. Pasteur Tunis, 36:449, 1959.

Gaon, J. A., and Murray, E. S.: The natural history of recrudescent typhus (Brill-Zinsser disease) in Bosnia. Bull. WHO, 35:133, 1966.

Hoeprich, P. D. (ed.): Infectious Diseases. New York, Harper & Row, 1972.

MacArthur, W. P.: The Athenian plague: A medical note. Classical Quarterly, 4:171, 1954.

Miller, E. S., and Beeson, P. B.: Murine typhus fever. Medicine, 25:1, 1946.

Murray, E. S., and Snyder, J. C.: Brill-Zinsser disease: The interepidemic reservoir of epidemic louse-borne typhus fever. Proceedings, Sixth International Congress of Microbiology, Rome; 4, Section 11, 31-44, 1953.

Price, W. H., et. al.: Ecologic studies of the interepidemic survival of louse-borne epidemic typhus fever. Am. J. Hyg., 67:154 1958.

Proceedings of the International Symposium on the Control of Lice and Louse-borne Diseases, Washington, D.C., December 4-6, 1972. Pan American Health Organization Scientific Publication No. 263, 1973.

Smadel, J. E.: Status of the rickettsioses in the United States. Ann. Intern. Med., 51:421, 1959.

Snyder, J. C.: The typhus fevers. *In* Horsfall, F. L., Jr., and Tamm, I. (eds.): Viral and Rickettsial Infections of Man. 4th ed. Philadelphia, J. B. Lippincott Company, 1965, Chapter 50.

Stuart, B. M., and Pullen, R. L.: Endemic (murine) typhus fever: Clinical observations of 180 cases. Ann. Intern. Med., 23:520, 1945.

Wisseman, C. L., Jr.: Problems of rickettsial diseases and vaccines: Desirable developments. Proceedings of the International Conference on the Application of Vaccines against Viral Rickettsial and Bacterial Diseases of Man, Washington, D.C., 14-18 Dec. 1970. Pan American Health Organization Scientific Publication No. 226, 1971, pp. 289-303.

Wisseman, C. L., Jr.: Concepts of louse-borne typhus control in developing countries: The use of the living attenuated E strain typhus vaccine in epidemic and endemic situations. *In* Kohn, A., and Klingberg, M. A. (eds.): Immunity in Viral and Rickettsial Diseases. New York, Plenum Publishing Co., 1972, pp. 97-130.

Wolbach, S. B., Todd, J. L., and Palfrey, F. W.: The Etiology and Pathology of Typhus. Cambridge, Mass., Harvard University Press, 1922.

Zdrodovskii, P. F., and Golinevich, H. M.: The Rickettsial Diseases. New York, Pergamon Press, 1960.

Zinsser, H.: Rats, Lice, and History. Boston, Little, Brown and Company, 1935.

109. ROCKY MOUNTAIN SPOTTED FEVER

(Spotted Fever, Tick Typhus [England], Fiebre Manchada [Mexico], Fiebre Petequial [Colombia], Febre Maculosa, São Paulo Typhus [Brazil])

Charles L. Wisseman, Jr.

DEFINITION. Rocky Mountain spotted fever is a mild to severe acute infectious disease of the Western Hemisphere caused by *Rickettsia rickettsii* and transmitted to man by several species of ticks. The disease is characterized by sudden onset with chills and headache, by fever of about two to three weeks' duration, and by a rash on the extremities and trunk beginning about the fourth day of disease.

ETIOLOGY. The disease is caused by *Rickettsia rickettsii*, the prototype species of the spotted fever group of rickettsiae with which it shares group antigens but from which it can be differentiated by more specific tests (see Ch. 107). It differs from the typhus and scrub typhus group organisms in its capacity to grow in the nucleus as well as the cytoplasm of host cells (see Ch. 107). Both mild and highly virulent strains coexist in many parts of the United States. Although several other species of the spotted fever group have been isolated from ticks in the United States (*R. parkeri, R. montana,* other recent isolates), to date only typical *R. rickettsii* has been isolated from infections of man. More intensive efforts to isolate and characterize rickettsiae from patients is needed to clarify the role, if any, of these other spotted fever group agents as causes of human disease.

DISTRIBUTION AND INCIDENCE. Although originally encountered in Rocky Mountain states (Montana and Idaho), Rocky Mountain spotted fever has been recognized in at least 46 states and is actually more prevalent in the south Atlantic states than in the west. In the eastern United States it extends from Cape Cod and some adjacent islands, through a focus on Long Island, to Florida, with almost half the cases in the United States occurring in Maryland, Virginia, North Carolina, and Georgia. The number of cases per year in the United States has risen steadily over the past several years to more than 700 in 1976. The reasons for this increase are not fully understood, but many include abundance of ticks, extension of suburbs into tick-infested rural areas, and increased recreational activities in wilderness areas. Rocky Mountain spotted fever has also been recognized in several provinces of Canada, Mexico, Central America (Panama, Costa Rica) and South America (Colombia, Brazil).

TRANSMISSION AND EPIDEMIOLOGY. Rocky Mountain spotted fever is a zoonosis maintained in a natural cycle between certain tick species and small (rodents, rabbits) and perhaps larger mammals. The ticks not only serve as vectors but also have an important reservoir function, because the infected female tick efficiently transmits the rickettsia transovarially to its progeny. Mammalian hosts probably serve more as an amplifying mechanism for infection of new ticks than they do as true reservoirs. Man, a dead-end host for *R. rickettsii*, becomes infected when he intrudes into this zoonotic cycle (as for recreational or occupational reasons) and is bitten by an infected tick. However, dogs can bring infected ticks into human dwellings.

Although multiple tick species (both hard and soft varieties) are known to become naturally infected and may play a role in transmission among animals, the main tick vectors for man are hard (Ixodid) ticks: the wood tick, *Dermacentor andersoni,* in the western United States; the dog tick, *Dermacentor variabilis,* in the eastern United States; *Amblyomma americanum* in Texas and Oklahoma; the brown dog tick, *Rhipicephalus sanguineus,* in northern Mexico (and introduced into the United States); and *Amblyomma cajennense* in Brazil and Colombia.

PATHOLOGY. The pathology of Rocky Mountain spotted fever conforms in general to the description in Ch. 107. Of special note is the fact that the vasculitis in Rocky Mountain spotted fever is not limited to the endothelium and is more severe than in typhus or scrub typhus, causing more pronounced thrombotic occlusion and necrosis of the muscular layers. Microinfarcts are seen with some frequency in the central nervous system.

CLINICAL MANIFESTATIONS AND COURSE. A history of tick bite can be elicited in the majority of, but not all, patients. Variation in incubation period (2 to 14, average 7 days) and severity of disease are seen in Rocky Mountain spotted fever, with a tendency for an inverse relationship between the two. Very severe disease often is preceded by a short (two- to five-day) incubation period. Prodromes, when present, consist of anorexia, irritability, malaise, feverishness, and chilly sensations. Attacks may be so mild that the patient remains ambulatory, or so severe that death may occur within three to six days of onset. The more typical infections are sudden in onset, with severe headache, chills, fever, prostration, myalgia (especially of the back and legs), nausea with occasional vomiting, conjunctival injections, and photophobia. There may be abdominal muscular pain, tenderness of muscles on palpation, and arthralgia.

Body temperature reaches 39 to 40° C in the first two days, is sustained at elevated levels for about 2 weeks, and declines by slow lysis over three or four days. Hyperthermia in the range of 41° C is a serious sign. Body temperature falling to near or below normal levels in the face of severe hypotension and tachycardia carries a grave prognosis.

The characteristic rash appears on about the fourth day (two to six days), first about the wrists and ankles, and then extends rapidly over all or most of the body, including palms, soles, face, and, occasionally, the mucous membranes of the mouth and throat. At first, the lesions are pink macules, 2 to 5 mm in diameter, which blanch on pressure. In two or three days, they become fixed, darker red, or purplish, maculopapular, and, about the fourth day, petechial. Hemorrhagic lesions may coalesce. The rash begins to disappear as the fever subsides but often remains as pigmented spots for weeks.

Early in the disease the pulse is full, regular, and elevated in proportion to fever. Later, it becomes more rapid and feeble, and some degree of hypotension develops. The electrocardiogram may show minor S-T deflections and prolonged P-R intervals. In some cases, hypotension may attain shock levels, and gangrene of fingers, toes, ears, nose, or genitalia may develop. Thrombosis of larger vessels may lead to loss of a portion of a limb or hemiplegia. The skin may become necrotic over body prominences. Hemorrhage from the nose, gastrointestinal tract, or kidney may occur. In recent years, disturbances in clotting mechanisms have been observed. Platelet counts are frequently low. Varying degrees of disseminated intravascular coagulation have been observed.

Central nervous system involvement is manifest by restlessness, insomnia, delirium, stupor, and, in severe cases, coma. Convulsions, muscular rigidity, tremors, and athetoid movements may occur. Cranial nerve involvement is variable. Transient deafness is common, but peripheral neuritis is uncommon. Electroencephalographic changes may persist for many months. Incontinence of urine and feces may be present in severe cases.

The liver may be enlarged and serum albumin depressed, but jaundice is not common. Oliguria and some azotemia are common in severe cases. Anuria and marked azotemia may be seen in critically ill patients. Complicating secondary bacterial infections (bronchopneumonia, otitis media, parotitis) occur but are uncommon.

Defervescence is usually by slow lysis. Convalescence may take weeks to months. Death, when it occurs in the nonfulminant variety, usually occurs late in the second week of disease (range about 9 to 18 days after onset).

DIAGNOSIS. An acute febrile illness with or without rash, in a person with a history of tick-bite, exposure to ticks (either in a tick-infested rural or suburban area or contact with a tick-infested dog), or, equally important, recreational or occupational activities which might have brought the patient into a potentially tick-infested area, should alert the physician to the possibility of Rocky Mountain spotted fever. Although other diseases, especially those with rash, may present transient early differential diagnostic problems, the two diseases which have consistently caused the greatest confusion are measles and meningococcemia. The most promising laboratory diagnostic method for providing a specific diagnosis early enough in the disease to permit effective specific therapeutic intervention is the demonstration by the fluorescent antibody technique of spotted fever group rickettsiae in skin biopsies. Isolation attempts, which are encouraged, and serologic diagnostic methods (see Laboratory Diagnosis in Ch. 107) are useful and important but rarely yield results in time for most efficient management.

PROGNOSIS. Although mild cases occur, the rapid, severe course in some patients makes it imperative to regard any suspected case of Rocky Mountain spotted fever essentially as a medical emergency. In untreated cases, the over-all case fatality rate was about 20 per cent, with areas of low ($\leqslant 10$ per cent) and high ($\geqslant 60$ per cent) rates. Prognosis depends on severity of infection, host factors (such as age, presence of other disease), and *the time after onset at which specific antirickettsial chemotherapy is started.* Even with effective antirickettsial drugs available, the case fatality rate has remained at 5 to 10 per cent. Analysis of fatal cases in recent years has shown that the single most important factor was *delay in institution of antirickettsial therapy,*

whatever the reason. With the time between onset and death as short as three to six days, the critical period when antimicrobial therapy can influence the outcome may be very short indeed and does not leave much latitude for correcting errors in clinical diagnosis.

TREATMENT. Prompt administration of a tetracycline antibiotic or chloramphenicol (see Treatment of Rickettsial Diseases in Ch. 107) is the single most important specific therapeutic measure. However, apparently serious physiologic derangements follow rapidly on the tissue damage produced by the rickettsial infection. Once initiated, these physiologic derangements do not respond directly to antimicrobial therapy and may require vigorous supportive measures and attempts at specific intervention. Shock and the consequences of disseminated intravascular clotting have been particularly resistant to correction in severe cases.

PREVENTION AND CONTROL. Individual preventive measures are directed primarily at prevention of tick bite. The chances of ticks attaching should be minimized by (1) avoiding places especially likely to harbor ticks (e.g., brush where livestock and game take refuge); (2) wearing boots and protective clothing designed to exclude ticks (preferably impregnated with a tick repellent, such as N-N-butylacetanilide); and (3) carefully inspecting the *entire* body once or twice daily to remove all ticks. Ticks usually crawl about on the body or in the clothing for some time prior to attaching. Thus frequent inspection usually discloses ticks before they attach. Moreover, since the chance of transmission of Rocky Mountain spotted fever appears to be a function of the duration of attachment, early removal of an attached tick probably reduces the chances of infection. Ticks should be removed (from man or dogs) with a pair of forceps, exerting gentle steady traction so that the mouth parts are released intact from the skin. Most other commonly recommended methods of tick removal are less satisfactory. Contact between tick and fingers should be avoided, because rickettsiae in tick feces or body fluids may enter a break in the skin or be transferred to mucous membranes and initiate infection.

For families living in tick-infested areas, an especially effective preventive measure is for parents to establish the routine of examining themselves and their children for ticks every evening at bath time during the tick season, and to teach the children to examine themselves as soon as they are old enough. In the author's own family, over the years this practice has detected many ticks, all still unattached.

The Rocky Mountain Laboratory of the United States Public Health Service has recently begun a service through state health departments to examine individual ticks for *R. rickettsii* (the "hemolymph" test). It is best practice today to place a person from whom a positive tick has been removed under close observation, recording morning and evening temperatures for two weeks, and instituting full antirickettsial chemotherapy only, but promptly, when a significant rise in temperature first appears. Attempts at chemoprophylaxis are likely only to delay onset of disease.

The current commercial killed *R. rickettsii* vaccine is of dubious value, and its manufacture may be discontinued. In a human vaccination-challenge study, it failed to protect against disease when minimal human infectious challenge doses were given intradermally, although the incubation period was lengthened. On the other hand, an uncontrolled retrospective study of potentially exposed laboratory personnel suggested protection against airborne infections. An experimental killed vaccine which may have greater potency has been developed but is not yet generally available.

Area control of ticks is still very difficult and is usually considered impractical. Ticks are unusually resistant to most insecticides. Yet, some measure of control may be achieved in time on small plots of ground, such as suburban lots, by intensive acaricidal treatment, the clearing of underbrush, intensive gardening or cultivation, and a reduction of the wild animal population. Changes in land use may affect tick populations. Some progress is being made toward identifying the specific habitat alterations that affect tick populations.

Atkin, M. D., Strauss, H. S., and Fisher, G. U.: A case report of "Cape Cod" Rocky Mountain spotted fever with multipe coagulation disturbances. Pediatrics, 36:627, 1965.

Graybill, J. R., Hawiger, J., and Des Prez, R. M.: Complement and coagulation in Rocky Mountain spotted fever. South. Med. J., 66:410, 1973.

Hand, W. L., Miller, J. B., Reinarz, J. A., and Sanford, J. P.: Rocky Mountain spotted fever. A vascular disease. Arch. Intern. Med., 125:879, 1970.

Harrell, G. T.: Rocky Mountain spotted fever. Medicine, 28:333, 1949.

Hattwick, M. A. W., O'Brien, R. J., and Hanson, B. F.: Rocky Mountain spotted fever: Epidemiology of an increasing problem. Ann. Intern. Med., 84:732, 1976.

Haynes, R. E., Sanders, D. Y., and Cramblett, H. G.: Rocky Mountain spotted fever in children. J. Pediat. 76:685, 1970.

Kurnick, J. E., Malinow, S. H. and Snyderman, M. C.: Disseminated intravascular coagulation in Rocky Mountain spotted fever. South. Med. J., 67:623, 1974.

Lackman, D. B., Bell, E. J., Stoenner, H. G., and Pickens, E. G.: The Rocky Mountain spotted fever group of rickettsias. Health Lab. Sci., 2:135, 1965.

Lennette, E. H.: Rocky Mountain spotted fever (editorial). N. Engl. J. Med., 297:884, 1977.

Miller, J. Q., and Price, T. R.: The nervous system in Rocky Mountain spotted fever. Neurology, 22:561, 1972.

Oster, C. N., Burke, D. S., Kenyon, R. H., Ascher, M. D., Harber, P., and Pedersen, C. E., Jr.: Laboratory-acquired Rocky Mountain spotted fever. N. Engl. J. Med., 297:859, 1977.

Ricketts, H. T.: Contributions to Medical Science by Howard Taylor Ricketts, 1870–1910. Chicago, University of Chicago Press, 1911, p. 278.

Sexton, D. J., Banks, P. M., Weig, S., and Roe, C. R.: Late appearance of skin rash and abnormal serum enzymes in Rocky Mountain spotted fever. J. Pediat., 87:580, 1975.

Wisseman, C. L., Jr. (ed.): Symposium on the Spotted Fever Group of Rickettsiae. Medical Science Publication No. 7, Walter Reed Army Institute of Research. Washington, D.C., U.S. Government Printing Office, 1960.

Woodward, T. E., and Jackson, E. B.: Spotted fever rickettsiae. In Horsfall, F. L., Jr., and Tamm, I. (eds.): Viral and Rickettsial Infections of Man. 4th ed. Philadelphia, J. B. Lippincott Company, 1965, p. 1095.

110. TICK-BORNE RICKETTSIOSES OF THE EASTERN HEMISPHERE*

Charles L. Wisseman, Jr.

DEFINITION. Three diseases, caused by three different members of the spotted fever group of rickettsiae, are currently the best recognized tick-borne rickettsioses of the Eastern Hemisphere and occur over distinct broad geographic areas: (1) African tick typhus (*R. conorii*), (2) North Asian tick-borne rickettsiosis (*R. sibirica*), and (3) Queensland tick typhus (*R. australis*). Each is a zoonosis, with man an accidental, dead-end

host, and is transmitted by the bite of one or more species of ixodid ticks. The three diseases, mild to moderate in severity, closely resemble one another with a short (average five- to seven-day) incubation period, a primary lesion (eschar, tache noire), a fever of a few days' to two weeks' duration, and a maculopapular to almost nodular rash which appears three to five days after onset.

As might be expected with a microorganism that shows distinct tendencies for geographic variants distributed over extensive and divergent land masses with enormous faunal variation, several lines of evidence, especially in the past few years, suggested that the tick-borne rickettsioses of the Eastern Hemisphere are probably more complex than is implied by the generally accepted classification given above. For example, a spotted fever group rickettsia, apparently distinct from *R. sibirica* and *R. conorii,* has been isolated from ticks in Slovakia. Two different, possibly new species of spotted fever group rickettsiae, probably not *R. conorii,* have been isolated from ticks from dogs and hedgehogs in Israel, and one of these was also isolated from a patient with clinical tick typhus. Moreover, some cases of tick typhus in this area differ from classic boutonneuse fever (*R. conorii*) by the absence of a primary lesion and possibly more fatalities. Early descriptions of "Indian tick typhus" suggested the possibility of more than one entity. The only strain of "Indian tick typhus" rickettsiae studied by modern methods and found to be identical with, or very similar to, *R. conorii* was isolated from a tick taken from a dog near the dwelling of a patient with Indian tick typhus in Kashmir. However, more recently multiple spotted fever group rickettsiae have been isolated from ticks in Pakistan, viz., *R. conorii*-like, *R. sibirica*-like, and one or two probable new species. Thus clinical tick typhus in south Asia may have multiple causes. Occasional human cases of tick typhus, with eschar, have been recognized in southeast Asia, viz., Indochina and Malaysia. Such infections are probably often misdiagnosed as scrub typhus. Serologic evidence has been presented for widespread spotted fever group rickettsial infection among small mammals in Malaysia. However, the rickettsial agent or agents responsible for the human and small mammal infections have not been isolated and identified. Only a single strain of spotted fever group rickettsiae, probably a new species, has been isolated from ticks in Thailand. Much work remains to be done to clarify the problem of the rickettsioses of the Eastern Hemisphere. It is especially important to isolate and fully characterize the rickettsiae from patients with tick typhus in order that the agents most commonly associated with human disease can be identified.

For lack of more comprehensive knowledge, the descriptions below are confined to the three established rickettsioses.

---

*My former colleague and author of this chapter in the previous edition of this book, Dr. Herbert Ley, left this chapter essentially unchanged from that originally written by our mutual mentor, friend, and colleague, Dr. Joseph E. Smadel, who masterfully and concisely unified concepts in a difficult area on the basis of the best information available at the time. Some of this chapter has been retained in its original form with minor editorial changes because it is difficult to improve upon excellence. Newer information, however, of the kind that Dr. Smadel would have strongly fostered, has reintroduced certain complexities and uncertainties, reflected primarily in the paragraphs on Definition and on History, Etiology, Distribution, and Epidemiology. I look forward to the time when sufficient information is available to permit a second generation of unification and simplification.   CLW Jr.

HISTORY, ETIOLOGY, DISTRIBUTION, AND EPIDEMIOLOGY. *Boutonneuse fever* was first recognized in 1910 in Tunisia by Conor and Bruch. During the next several decades similar diseases were recognized in other parts of Africa, in parts of Europe and the Middle East adjacent to the Mediterranian, Black and Caspian Seas, and in India where they were often given local names — e.g., Marseille fever, Indian tick typhus, Kenya tick typhus, South African tick typhus. Subsequent application of modern rickettsiologic methods led to the conclusion that all of these were in reality infection by *R. conorii* or closely related spotted fever group rickettsiae and could be classified under a single entity, African tick typhus. This probably is correct to a large degree. However, the serologic methods employed have limitations and cannot readily discriminate between infections caused by a new species and those caused by other members of this serologically cross-reactive group unless that new agent is included in the battery of specific antigens. The recent findings (see above) of a multiplicity of established and probable new species of spotted fever group rickettsiae along with *R. conorii* in some of the areas of presumed African tick typhus (*R. conorii*) distribution (e.g., Europe, Israel, India) suggest that considerable work must yet be done to clarify the question of distribution and nature of "African tick typhus." In the Mediterranean littoral, the main vector of fièvre boutonneuse is the dog tick, *Rhipicephalus sanguineus,* and the disease is often acquired in and around human habitations, i.e., a domesticated or urban pattern. In other areas, the causative agent of the local disease is transmitted by ticks which are parasitic on wild animals, and hence the disease is acquired in rural areas, e.g., certain stretches of the South African veldt.

North Asian tick-borne rickettsiosis (Siberian tick typhus), now known to be caused by *R. sibirica,* was first recognized as a clinical entity distinct from the other rickettsioses of the U.S.S.R. in the mid to late 1930's. It has since been found distributed from European Russia through Siberia to the Soviet Far East and, more recently, possibly to the Indo-Pakistan subcontinent. Several species of ixodid ticks have been implicated as vectors in different geographic regions. Its acquisition is characteristically in a sylvan or rural setting.

Queensland tick typhus is usually acquired in rural areas heavily infested with the tick, *Ixodes holocyclus,* and a history of tick bite and an eschar are common. The agent, *R. australis,* however, has only been isolated from the blood of patients. Antibodies have been detected in the blood of some small marsupials and a rat, suggesting a natural sylvan small animal–tick cycle.

PATHOLOGY. In fatal cases, which are few and usually limited to the aged and debilitated, the findings are similar to those in Rocky Mountain spotted fever except for the presence of the tache noire, the black button–like necrotic primary lesion that is generally found on the surface areas of the body ordinarily covered by clothing. The basic pathologic changes are found in the small blood vessels (see Ch. 107).

SYMPTOMS, LABORATORY FINDINGS, AND DIAGNOSIS. The three tick-borne rickettsioses that occur in different parts of the Eastern Hemisphere resemble one another closely. After an incubation period of about five to seven days, the disease begins with fever, headache, malaise, myalgia, and conjunctival injection. The primary lesion, which is present in most cases at the onset of fever, consists of a small ulcer 2 to 5 mm in diameter with a black center and a red areola; the regional lymph nodes are enlarged. The generalized erythematous maculopapular rash appears about the fourth day and quickly involves most of the body, including the palms and soles and often the face. In severe cases the rash becomes hemorrhagic. Fever abates during the second week. The prognosis is good except in the aged and debilitated. Complications and sequelae are unusual.

North Asian tick-borne rickettsiosis has been the subject of considerable laboratory and clinical observation by Soviet investigators. Mild hypotension, electrocardiographic changes, a reversal of the A/G ratio in serum (depressed albumin, early increased alpha globulins, followed by increase in gamma globulins), and abnormal liver function tests are noteworthy.

The laboratory findings of greatest importance are those derived from the serologic tests with Weil-Felix and rickettsial antigens (see Ch. 107). Agglutinins against *Proteus* OX-19 develop during the second week, and complement-fixing antibodies appear shortly thereafter.

Diagnosis is established by the clinical picture, including the tache noire, the geographic location, and positive serologic reactions. In the differential diagnosis the typhus fevers, meningococcal infections, and measles must be considered.

TREATMENT. Adequate information is available to indicate that treatment with the broad-spectrum antimicrobial drugs is as effective in patients with African tick typhus and North Asian tick-borne rickettsiosis as in those with other rickettsioses (see Ch. 107 for details of therapy). Presumably, these measures are also applicable to the other tick-borne rickettsioses of the Eastern Hemisphere. All the newly recognized strains display in vitro susceptibility to tetracyclines of the same order as *R. rickettsii* and presumably would respond to similar therapeutic regimens (see Ch. 107).

PROPHYLAXIS. Prevention of human disease is based on avoiding the bites of infected ticks. In Ch. 109 details are set forth regarding personal prophylaxis, including the use of protective clothing, chemical insect repellents, and reduction of tick population by measures involved in terrain control. Experimental vaccines prepared from formalin-treated yolk sac tissue infected with some of the three established Eastern Hemisphere rickettsiae under discussion are effective in animals, but commercial vaccines for human use are not available.

Bozeman, F. M., Humphries, J. W., Campbell, J. M., and O'Hara, P. L.: Laboratory studies of the spotted fever group of rickettsiae. *In* Wisseman, C. L., Jr. (ed.): Symposium on the Spotted Fever Group of Rickettsiae. Medical Science Publication No. 7, Walter Reed Army Institute of Research. Washington, D.C., U. S. Government Printing Office, 1960, p. 7.

Goldwasser, R. A., Klingberg, M. A., Klingberg, W., Steiman, Y., and Swartz, T. A.: Laboratory and epidemiological studies of rickettsial spotted fever in Israel. *In* Frontiers of Internal Medicine, Proceedings of 12th International Congress of Internal Medicine, Tel Aviv, 1974. Basel, Karger, 1975, pp. 270–275.

Hoogstraal, H.: Ticks in relation to human disease caused by *Rickettsia* species. Ann. Rev. Entomol., 12:377, 1967.

Lyskovtsev, M. M.: Tickborne rickettsiosis. Translation from the Russian in Miscellaneous Publications of the Entomological Society of America, 6:41, 1968.

Rehaček, I., Palonová, A., Zupancikova, M., Urvolgyi, J., Kovácová, E., Járábek, L., and Brezina, R.: Study of rickettsioses in Slovakia. I. *Coxiella burnetii* and rickettsiae of the spotted fever (SF) group in ticks and serological surveys in animals and humans in certain selected localities in the Lucenec and V. Krtis districts. J. Hyg. Epidemiol. Microbiol. Immunol., 19:105, 1975.

Robertson, R. G., and Wisseman, C. L., Jr.: Tick-borne rickettsiae of the spotted fever group in West Pakistan. II. Serological classification of isolates from West Pakistan and Thailand: Evidence for two new species. Am. J. Epidemiol., 97:55, 1973.

Woodward, T. E., and Jackson, E. B.: Spotted fever rickettsiae. In Horsfall, F. L., Jr., and Tamm, I. (eds.): Viral and Rickettsial Infections of Man. 4th ed. Philadelphia, J. B. Lippincott Company, 1965, p. 1095.

Zdrodovskii, P. I., and Golinevich, H. M.: The Rickettsial Diseases, New York, Pergamon Press, 1960, p. 191.

111.　RICKETTSIALPOX

Charles L. Wisseman, Jr.

DEFINITION. Rickettsialpox is a mite-borne rickettsial disease, mild and self-limited, which is characterized by an initial eschar-like lesion and a fever of a week's duration accompanied by headache, backache, and a generalized papulovesicular rash.

ETIOLOGY. Rickettsialpox is caused by *Rickettsia akari*, a member of the spotted fever group on the basis of shared group antigens but with unique specfic antigens and certain biologic properties.

DISTRIBUTION AND INCIDENCE. The disease has been reported from certain cities in the United States (New York, Boston, West Haven, Ct., Philadelphia, Pittsburgh, and Cleveland) and from the U.S.S.R. In the first three years after the disease was described in 1946, about 500 cases were reported in the United States, mostly from New York, but the number reported has since decreased markedly. Although the reasons for the decrease are not clearly established, it may be due to under-reporting of disease or to control measures.

TRANSMISSION AND EPIDEMIOLOGY. Although detailed information is sparse, it is clear that rickettsialpox is a zoonosis which can involve house mice (*Mus musculus*) and mouse mites (*Allodermanyssus sanguineus*). *R. akari* has also been isolated from rats in the U.S.S.R. and from voles (small field "mice") in Korea. It is unknown if the basic natural cycle involves field rodents and their ectoparasites with occasional spillover into the mouse-mite cycle or if the latter is in fact the basic sustaining cycle. Regardless, in the United States the mouse-mite cycle, greatly amplified and concentrated in discrete foci artificially created by, and frequented by, man himself (e.g., improperly fired apartment house incinerators), was responsible for bringing *R. akari* and man into effective contact with one another. The usually large mite population, which infested the walls and floors of the incinerator rooms, had access to people entering the foci with a frequency not usually encountered under natural circumstances. Transmission is presumably by bite of the mite. Simple control measures directed at the mice and mites have virtually eliminated the human disease.

PATHOLOGY. As no fatal cases have been encountered, studies of the pathology of rickettsialpox have been limited to an examination of skin biopsies. Histologically, the eschar of rickettsialpox resembles the eschars of scrub typhus and boutonneuse fever. The skin lesions composing the rash show a typical perivascular infiltration by mononuclear cells. Later, necrosis of the superficial epithelium leads to intraepidermal vesicle formation.

CLINICAL MANIFESTATIONS AND COURSE. The incubation period varies from about ten days to three weeks. An initial lesion (the eschar) appears at the site of the mite bite about a week before onset of fever in about 90 per cent of the cases, gradually enlarging and progressing from a papular lesion through vesicle formation, finally to form a dark encrusted lesion 0.5 to 1.5 cm in diameter. The onset of an intermittent fever is sudden and is accompanied by chills or chilly sensations, drenching sweats, headache, anorexia, and photophobia. The temperature ranges from about 38 to 40° C, lasts for about a week, is accompanied by headache, lassitude, and myalgia, and then gradually subsides. A sparse eruption appears on the trunk, extremities, and mucous membranes between the first and fourth days of fever, beginning as discrete maculopapular lesions and evolving into a vesiculopapular rash. The vesicles are firm, are sometimes surrounded by erythema, and, on drying, form a dark crust that falls off without leaving a scar.

DIAGNOSIS. Clinical Diagnosis. The clinical characteristics of the disease are so distinctive that in most patients a presumptive diagnosis may be made on clinical grounds. Chickenpox in adults poses the most difficult diagnostic problem. Important points in differentiation are as follows: the vesicles in rickettsialpox are seen to arise from the center of discrete papules; the lesions tend to appear at the same time instead of in crops; on the average, the number of lesions is fewer than in chickenpox; and there often is an initial lesion at the site of the mite bite. In smallpox, the lesions progress on to pustulation.

Laboratory Diagnosis. Laboratory diagnosis depends on isolation of the agent and on serologic response measured by rickettsial group and specific antigens. The Weil-Felix test is negative (see Ch. 107).

PROGNOSIS. Even without specific therapy, the course of the disease is benign, the prognosis excellent, and death unusual.

TREATMENT. Response to tetracycline drugs, given as outlined in Ch. 107, is rapid without relapse.

PREVENTION AND CONTROL. The transient emergence of rickettsialpox from a silent zoonosis to a human disease problem was an artifact of urban living, and its apparent disappearance is probably a result of minor changes in human behavior. The prevention and control of rickettsialpox depend on rodent and mite control by (1) the elimination of mice and mouse harborages, which should include proper care and firing of incinerators in dwellings, and (2) the application of residual acaricides to walls and other mite-infested areas. No vaccines have been developed.

Dolgopol, V. B.: Histologic changes in rickettsialpox. Am. J. Pathol., 24:119, 1948.

Greenberg, M., Pelliteri, O., Klein, I. F., and Huebner, R. J.: Rickettsialpox — a newly recognized rickettsial disease. II. Clinical observations. JAMA, 133:901, 1947.

Lackman, D. B.: A review of information on rickettsialpox in the United States. Clin. Pediat. 2:296, 1963.

Roueché, B.: The alerting of Mr. Pomerantz. In Roueché, B.: Eleven Blue Men. Boston, Little, Brown & Company, 1954, p. 48.

112. SCRUB TYPHUS (Chigger-Borne Rickettsiosis; Many Local Names: Tsutsugamushi Disease, Japanese River or Flood Fever, Mite-Borne Typhus, Tropical Typhus, Rural Typhus, Mossman Fever, Others)

Charles L. Wisseman, Jr.

DEFINITION. Scrub typhus is an acute, febrile, typhus-like disease of rural Asia transmitted by the bite of larval trombiculid mites (chiggers). The site of infection is often marked by an eschar accompanied by regional lymphadenitis.

ETIOLOGY. The disease is caused by infection with *Rickettsia tsutsugamushi* (*R. orientalis*). The organism, although an obligate intracellular parasite multiplying free in host cell cytoplasm, differs substantially from other members of the genus *Rickettsia* in ultrastructure, tinctorial properties, and certain biologic features, holds no known antigens in common with them, but shares an antigen with *Proteus* OX-K. Multiple serotypes exist which produce substantial homologous immunity but only transient cross-immunity in man. Virulence of strain for mice and man varies from low to very high.

DISTRIBUTION AND INCIDENCE. Scrub typhus is widely distributed in eastern and southern Asia and the islands of the western and southern Pacific. It is known as far north as the island of Hokkaido in Japan and the Primorye region of asiatic U.S.S.R., as far south as the northern tip of Australia, and as far west as Pakistan and Tadzhikistan. Endemic infection is unknown in the New World, Europe, and Western Asia; but cases imported during the incubation period following infection in an endemic area have been recognized in the United States.

Because of a general lack of diagnostic and medical facilities in endemic areas, scrub typhus is best known from its occurrence in substantial numbers when large groups of nonimmune persons enter an endemic area, such as in military operations, road building, land clearing, and certain agricultural settings such as rubber plantations. It is an important military disease, e.g., in World War II, Vietnam, the Indo-Pakistan war, and current campaigns against "insurgents" in Burma and Thailand. Application of modern epidemiologic and laboratory methods is currently revealing, as expected, that scrub typhus is a major cause of febrile disease in rural populations indigenous to endemic areas and thus promises to emerge as one of the major causes of febrile disease in Asia.

TRANSMISSION AND EPIDEMIOLOGY. Scrub typhus is a zoonosis whose main constant elements constitute a tetrad: (1) *R. tsutsugamushi;* (2) chiggers of the *Leptotrombidium deliense* group; (3) wild rats, especially of the subgenus *Rattus*; and (4) transitional vegetation. Man, not essential to maintenance of the infection cycle, is a dead-end host and acquires the disease when he intrudes into an endemic focus. The characteristic epidemiologic features of chigger-borne typhus, such as a marked focal distribution of cases and sudden outbreaks among field personnel, are explained by attributes of the vector chiggers. In temperate zones, most vector chiggers are active at some time during the warm months. On the Izu islands of Japan, *Leptotrombidium scutellare* transmits the disease in the winter. In tropical and subtropical regions, the disease may be more prevalent at one time of the year than another, depending on rainfall, flooding, and other factors. Chigger-borne rickettsiosis is transmitted by the bite of the infected larval mite. Since the chigger is the only parasitic stage of the mite and usually feeds only once, if infected, it must have acquired the organism transovarially from its mother. Naturally infected chiggers presumably constitute the main reservoirs of *R. tsutsugamushi* in nature. Chiggers of the *Leptotrombidium deliense* group are the main vectors to man and perhaps to other hosts as well; *L. deliense, L. akamushi, L. fletcheri, L. arenicola, L. pallidum, L. pavlovskyi,* and *L. scutellare* are known vectors. Infections also occur in areas where none of the known vectors is present. *Rickettsia tsutsugamushi*–infected chiggers often occur in very circumscribed foci or "islands." Rats, particularly wild rats of the subgenus *Rattus*, serve as prime hosts of *Leptotrombidium* throughout their native ranges. Other small mammals (e.g., field mice, voles, shrews) often serve as secondary hosts.

The rickettsiosis exists in a wide variety of habitats, ranging from semideserts to alpine meadows and subarctic scree in the Himalayas, and from disturbed rain forest to seashores. Some kind of transitional or secondary vegetation is characteristic of all terrain where outbreaks occur, and is present in some form in all known foci of chigger-borne rickettsiosis, even if only as fringe habitat along streams in deep forest. All known foci are characterized by changing environmental conditions, whether induced by man (e.g., clearing of forest) or by nature, either suddenly (e.g., landslides) or cyclically (tidal zones, spring floods, glacial runoff).

PATHOLOGY. The pathologic features of scrub typhus conform generally to those described in Ch. 107. Of special note in scrub typhus is the primary local ulcer with regional and, later, generalized lymphadenopathy. Vascular thrombosis is less frequent than in epidemic typhus and Rocky Mountain spotted fever, but inflammatory lesions of larger arteries are more common.

CLINICAL MANIFESTATIONS AND COURSE. The spectrum of clinical severity of untreated scrub typhus ranges from inapparent or mild to severe or mortal, with mortality rates varying from 0 to more than 30 per cent in different places and outbreaks. The following description pertains to a classic, relatively severe untreated case of scrub typhus.

The bite of the infecting chigger, which may· be on any part of the body, is usually unnoticed; but in roughly 60 to 70 per cent of the primary infections and substantially fewer in second infections, a small painless papule develops during the 6- to 18-day (usually 9-

to 12-day) incubation period. It enlarges, undergoes central necrosis, and crusts to form the eschar or primary lesion which is well developed at the onset of disease. The regional lymph nodes are enlarged and tender. Prodromes of headache, malaise, anorexia, and weakness may occur. The onset is usually acute. The fever rises progressively during the first few days, sometimes accompanied by chills after about the third day, to 39.5 to 40.5° C, accompanied by severe headache, ocular pain, conjunctival injection, anorexia, generalized aches, malaise, apathy, and cough. Interstitial pneumonitis is common. The pulse remains relatively slow. Toward the end of the first week, a macular rash, later sometimes papular, often appears, first on the trunk and then on the extremities. About this time there is generalized lymphadenopathy, soft splenic enlargement, and sometimes hepatomegaly.

During the second week of disease, the temperature remains elevated and signs of complex multiple organ system involvement appear. Apathy may give way to more pronounced signs of meningoencephalitis: delirium and restlessness, stupor, coma, convulsions, muscular weakness, hyperesthesias, and coarse intention tremors. Cranial nerves are selectively involved: varying degrees of nerve deafness and papilledema and congestion of retinal vessels are common; dysarthria and dysphagia are less frequent. Signs of diffuse and focal myocarditis may appear: soft first heart sound, systolic murmurs, ectopic beats, occasional cardiac enlargement, transient gallop rhythm, and minor abnormalities of the electrocardiogram (prolonged P-R interval, inverted T waves). Classic congestive failure is rare, but varying degrees of circulatory failure may appear: increasing pulse rate, falling blood pressure (commonly below 100 mm Hg systolic), rapid shallow respirations, cyanosis, sweating, and cold clammy skin. Gangrene is rare, but edema may be overt in severe cases. Clinical evidence for renal insufficiency is often absent, but oliguria or anuria occur in some. Spontaneous diuresis is fairly common late in the febrile course or in early convalescence.

In untreated cases, defervescence is by lysis usually after about 10 to 14 days (21 or more days in severe cases). Convalescence is prolonged. However, in nonfatal cases, all abnormalities appear to be completely reversible, although some, such as cardiovascular instability, personality changes, and deafness, may occasionally persist for weeks to months. Long-term (ten years or more) follow-up of United States servicemen who survived scrub typhus in World War II failed to reveal any significant residua.

An early leukopenia (1000 to 5000 white blood cells per cubic millimeter) gives way to slightly depressed or normal total white blood counts, which may become somewhat elevated late in the disease. Total serum proteins are usually normal or low, but the albumin-globulin (A/G) ratio is often reversed. Occasional clotting disturbances have been reported recently, including disseminated intravascular clotting syndrome. Jaundice is rare, but serum transaminase enzyme levels may be elevated. Albuminuria is common. Isosthenuria, oliguria, and azotemia may occur.

DIAGNOSIS. A typhus-like illness with a history of possible exposure in endemic areas and an eschar (in only about 40 to 70 per cent) with regional lymphadenitis should alert the physician to the possibility of scrub typhus. Differential diagnosis may be difficult in some endemic regions where the clinical picture may suggest other rickettsial infections (especially tick-borne typhus, which may also have an eschar) and other nonrickettsial infections (see General Clinical Considerations in Ch. 107). The Weil-Felix test with *Proteus* OX-K, not positive in all cases, is useful because of general availability. The indirect fluorescent antibody test is currently the serodiagnostic method of choice (see Laboratory Diagnosis in Ch. 107). Isolation can be accomplished by inoculating blood or tissue homogenates intraperitoneally into white mice.

PROGNOSIS. Untreated, the mortality ranges from essentially zero to over 30 per cent in different foci. Prompt antibiotic therapy reduces mortality virtually to zero.

TREATMENT. Tetracycline drugs, given as recommended in Ch. 107, and appropriate supportive measures are recommended treatment. A single dose of doxycycline may prove to be adequate for treatment.

PREVENTION AND CONTROL. Effective killed vaccines have not yet been developed to prevent scrub typhus. Transient cross-immunity among serotypes and more persistent homologous immunity can be induced by intentional infection with a virulent strain, followed by carefully timed chemoprophylaxis which permits subclinical immunizing infection, but this procedure is useful only under limited circumstances. Practical chemoprophylaxis with a long-acting tetracycline (doxycycline) is theoretically feasible and is currently under investigation. But practically, at this time, preventive measures against scrub typhus are directed primarily against the chigger vector. Mite-infested terrain should be avoided whenever possible. Individual prophylaxis against attack by larval mites consists of wearing protective clothing, impregnated with a mite repellent (benzyl benzoate, M-1960), and applying diethyltoluamide to exposed skin areas. The vector population in and around camp sites in endemic zones can be reduced (1) by treating the area intensively with acaricides (e.g., dieldrin), (2) possibly by reducing the rodent population through intensive poison bait campaigns, and (3) by destroying vegetation (bulldozing, power oil burners, herbicides). However, appropriate and relevant environmental, medical, and ecologic considerations must temper decisions on the use of persisting acaricides and herbicides.

Brown, G. W., Robinson, D. M., and Huxsoll, D. L.: Scrub typhus: A common cause of illness in indigenous populations. Trans. R. Soc. Trop. Med. Hyg., 70:444, 1976.

Deller, J. J., Jr., and Russell, P. K.: An analysis of fevers of unknown origin in American Soldiers in Vietnam. Ann. Intern. Med., 66:1129, 1967.

Ley, H. L., Jr., et al.: Immunization against scrub typhus. IV. Living Karp vaccine and chemoprophylaxis in volunteers. Am. J. Hyg., 56:303, 1952.

Smadel, J. E.: Influence of antibiotics on immunologic responses in scrub typhus. Am. J. Med., 17:246, 1954.

Smadel, J. E., and Elisberg, B. L.: Scrub typhus rickettsia. In Horsfall, F. L., Jr., and Tamm, I. (eds.): Viral and Rickettsial Infections of Man. 4th ed. Philadelphia, J. B. Lippincott Company, 1965, p. 1130.

Tamiya, T. (ed.): Recent Advances in Studies of Tsutsugamushi Disease in Japan. Tokyo, Medical Culture Inc., 1962.

Traub, R., and Wisseman, C. L., Jr.: Ecological considerations in scrub typhus. III. Methods of area control. Bull. WHO, 39:231, 1968.

Traub, R., and Wisseman, C. L., Jr.: The ecology of chigger-borne rickettsioses (scrub typhus) (review article). J. Med. Entomol., 11:237, 1974.

113. TRENCH FEVER
(Five-Day or Quintana Fever, Shin Bone Fever, Volhynian Fever)

Herbert L. Ley, Jr.

DEFINITION. Trench fever is a self-limited louse-borne rickettsial disease characterized by intermittent fever, generalized aches and pains, negligible mortality, and multiple relapses.

ETIOLOGY AND EPIDEMIOLOGY. The disease is caused by *Rochalimaea quintana,* a rickettsial agent that grows extracellularly in the louse intestine and is excreted in louse feces. Transmission takes place by rubbing louse feces into skin abrasions or into the bite wound left by the louse. The incubation period of the disease may vary from 5 to 38 days, but is usually two to four weeks. The disease was a major military problem during World War I, when an estimated 1,000,000 cases occurred in western Europe. It was not seen in epidemic form again until World War II when 80,000 cases were reported in eastern Europe. Recent studies have demonstrated the disease in endemic form in Mexico. During epidemics man is clearly the principal reservoir. He may also be the major long-term reservoir because the disease agent has been isolated from asymptomatic patients years after their initial infection.

PATHOLOGY AND CLINICAL MANIFESTATIONS. Because the disease has a negligible mortality, information on the histopathologic changes is limited. Biopsy studies reveal only perivascular inflammation, principally in the form of lymphocytic infiltrations. The presenting symptoms of the disease are recurrent fever, severe weakness, headache, dizziness, back and leg pains (particularly in the shins), and photophobia. Physical and laboratory examinations are not remarkable except for slight enlargement of the spleen and liver, areas of cutaneous tenderness distributed over the body, and a moderate leukocytosis. A transient rash of erythematous macules or papules occurs in about 70 per cent of patients. The patient's fever may rise as high as 40.5° C in an irregular fashion with intervals of nearly normal temperature between peaks of fever. The fever may last for only four or five days in the more fortunate patients. In others, the initial pyrexia may be followed after five or six days of normal temperature by one to eight relapses of fever similar to the initial episode. In still other patients, the initial fever may decline, shading into relapses without a true afebrile period, producing a "saddleback" or "typhoidal" fever curve.

DIAGNOSIS. The most important fact supporting the diagnosis of trench fever is a history of contact with lice within the incubation period of the disease. Xenodiagnosis — the feeding of clean uninfected lice on a patient suspected of having the disease — is a useful diagnostic aid. The lice are examined a week after feeding on the patient for the presence of rickettsiae in the lumen of the gut. The technique of cultivation of *R. quintana* on blood agar containing 10 per cent of fresh blood has also been used diagnostically. Recently developed serologic tests appear promising in the diagnosis of the disease. The differential diagnosis of the disease should include leptospirosis, dengue, malaria, relapsing fever, and the typhus fevers.

TREATMENT AND PROGNOSIS. Although the tetracyclines and other antimicrobials may be expected to be as effective in the treatment of trench fever as in the treatment of the other rickettsial diseases, in the absence of epidemics of trench fever no reliable information about their efficacy is available. Because the disease has a negligible mortality, the long-term prognosis is excellent. Even without treatment the majority of patients are able to return to full activity within one to two months after onset, although a few continue to experience recurrences of the symptoms of infection for months or years.

PREVENTION. The only practicable method of control of trench fever is the elimination of the louse vector of the disease by dusting clothing with residual insecticides. Ten per cent DDT powders proved highly effective for louse control during the World War II period, but the development of DDT resistance in lice in many parts of the world has forced the use of 1 per cent lindane or 1 per cent malathion powders. For additional comments on louse control, see Ch. 108.

Trench Fever: Report of Commission on Trench Fever. American Red Cross Medical Research Committee. London, Oxford University Press, 1918.

Varela, G., Vinson, J. W., and Molina-Pasquel, C.: Trench fever. II. Propagation of *Rickettsia quintana* on cell-free medium from the blood of two patients. Am. J. Trop. Med., 18:708, 1969.

Vinson, J. W., Varela, G., and Molina-Pasquel, C.: Trench fever. III. Induction of clinical disease in volunteers inoculated with *Rickettsia quintana* propagated on blood agar. Am. J. Trop. Med., 18:713, 1969.

Warren, J.: Trench fever rickettsia. *In* Horsfall, F. L., Jr., and Tamm, I. (eds.): Viral and Rickettsial Infections of Man. 4th ed. Philadelphia, J. B. Lippincott Company, p. 1161.

114. Q FEVER

Herbert L. Ley, Jr.

DEFINITION. Q fever is a self-limited rickettsial infection characterized by fever, headache, and constitutional symptoms, associated, in approximately half the patients, with a pneumonitis. It is unique among the rickettsial diseases of man in that human infection is most commonly acquired by inhalation of the agent rather than by contact with an arthropod vector.

ETIOLOGY. The disease is caused by *Coxiella burnetii,* a rickettsial agent having the general biologic characteristics of this class of microorganisms by possessing, in addition, a resistance to desiccation and to exposure in the dusts and soils that is unique among the rickettsiae. The organism may be propagated in embryonated eggs and in mice, hamsters, and guinea pigs, and has frequently infected laboratory personnel engaged in isolation studies on clinical material. Both patients and animals develop agglutinating and complement-fixing antibodies for the agent. On the other hand, *C. burnetii,* unlike most of the other rickettsiae, does not stimulate the production of Weil-Felix *Proteus* agglutinins in man.

EPIDEMIOLOGY. Incidence and Distribution. The true incidence of the disease in the human population is impossible to determine because the majority of infections are undiagnosed. Isolated serologic surveys have revealed that many persons exposed to infection in sheep and cattle ranches, abattoirs, meat packing plants, or wool processing plants present serologic evidence of past infection. More detailed investigation of animals and arthropods on a worldwide basis has shown *C. burnetii* to be ubiquitous in distribution except for the countries of Denmark, Finland, Ireland, the Netherlands, Norway, and Sweden. In the United States the disease, first recognized in the states of Montana and California, is now recognized as prevalent in most of the states in which sheep and cattle are produced. Small numbers of cases have been reported for most of the remaining states.

Transmission. The epidemiology of the disease is complex because it involves two major patterns of transmission. The first pattern, described in Australia, is a disease cycle in wild animals with transmission of the agent from animal to animal by a tick vector. Although the species of animal and arthropod vary from country to country, such a cycle has been demonstrated in Australia in two forms, bandicoot-tick-cattle and kangaroo-tick-sheep. In both these cycles the agent can be transmitted indefinitely as an inapparent infection in the wild reservoir (bandicoot and kangaroo) by ticks, but it may also be transmitted laterally by arthropod to a domestic animal in close contact with man. In these and similar cycles recognized in other parts of the world, *C. burnetii*, like the other rickettsial agents of human disease, is vector-transmitted.

However, Q fever patients rarely give a history of tick bite. Human infection with the agent has now been shown to occur almost exclusively by a second transmission pattern capable of sustaining itself independently of the wild animal cycle. The reservoirs of infection in the second pattern are animals domesticated by man, principally cattle, sheep, and goats, in which *C. burnetii* produces only an inapparent or mild infection. In sheep, Q fever organisms are excreted in very large numbers in placental tissue, and to a lesser degree in birth fluids, milk, and feces. In the cow, and probably the goat, excretion occurs mainly through the placenta and milk. *With all infected animals, the period of parturition is associated with the formation of a primary infectious aerosol, easily demonstrated by air-sampling studies.* Such aerosols infect other cattle in the herd and also the human population in direct contact with the animals. Further, because contaminated clothing, wool, hides, bedding, and soil may be the source of secondary aerosols, *the infections may be transmitted via these vehicles at considerable distances from the infected cattle;* in certain circumstances these distances are measurable in miles. The unique resistance of *C. burnetii* to prolonged exposure in nature contributes to the spread of the agent by such infectious microenvironments. Within California, where the local epidemiology of the disease has been studied in great detail, sheep are the major reservoir for human infection in the northern part of the state and cattle in the southern part. In the latter area milk may be a vehicle of infection if consumed raw. Although the pulmonary route is the most important portal of access of the agent to man, the transmission of the rickettsia from man to man by this method is rare, despite the occurrence of an infectious pneumonitis in some patients. Studies in Egypt, where the disease is endemic, have demonstrated that Q fever can be transmitted to the human fetus in utero without producing clinical signs of infection in the infant at birth.

PATHOLOGY. Because the mortality rate is low, postmortem studies have been limited. In those patients having a pneumonitis, the histopathology is similar to that seen in the viral pneumonias and psittacosis. Recent studies in patients have directed attention to hepatic pathology during the acute phase of the disease, demonstrable both in biochemical abnormalities of liver function (elevated cephalin-cholesterol flocculation, alkaline phosphatase, and thymol turbidity tests) and in histologic abnormalities in biopsy specimens (focal inflammation and granulomas). Q fever endocarditis, producing valvular vegetations from which rickettsiae may be isolated, has also been described. There is increasing evidence that Q fever can occasionally also cause myocarditis and paroxysmal ventricular tachycardia.

CLINICAL MANIFESTATIONS. After an incubation period of 9 to 20 days after respiratory exposure, most patients complain of an abrupt onset of fever, headache, muscle pains, and severe malaise. The temperature may rise as high as 40° C and remain elevated, with considerable fluctuation, for one to three weeks. Occasionally, patients may suffer a prolonged fever of several months' duration. In contrast to the other rickettsial infections, there is no rash. In approximately half the patients there is roentgenographic evidence of pneumonitis, manifested clinically as a slight, nonproductive cough developing in the second week of fever.

DIAGNOSIS. Q fever should always be suspected in a patient having a febrile illness for which no obvious cause can be found. If the patient's occupation brings him into contact with sheep, cattle, or goats, or byproducts such as wool or hides, particular care should be exercised to exclude Q fever from consideration. The presence of Q fever should be suspected in any patient in whom the differential diagnosis includes viral pneumonia, psittacosis, primary atypical pneumonia, pulmonary mycotic disease, or comparable infections. Furthermore, recent data would also support consideration of Q fever in the differential diagnoses of endocarditis and of hepatitis with or without jaundice.

Diagnostic laboratory studies usually must be limited to serologic studies because of the extensive history of accidentally acquired laboratory infections resulting from attempts at isolation. Either complement-fixation or agglutination tests may be employed, and with either test a fourfold or greater rise in titer of antibody may be expected to occur between the first and fourth weeks of illness. Recent reports have emphasized the importance of both strain and phase variation in the selection of antigens for diagnostic use.

TREATMENT AND PROGNOSIS. The tetracyclines or chloramphenicol are both effective in treatment of acute infections with *C. burnetii*, but because of the nature of chloramphenicol toxicity, the tetracyclines are definitely to be preferred. The dosage of antimicrobial given should be the same as that for epidemic typhus or Rocky Mountain spotted fever. The mortality is low (1 per cent or less), even in untreated patients, and is lower still in those treated with antimicrobial drugs. Therapy should be continued for approximately one week even though the patient usually becomes afebrile within 48 hours. Patients occasionally may experience relapses after treatment, and when this complication occurs additional drug therapy should be administered. No clinical data are available concerning the effectiveness of the lipotrophic tetracycline derivatives in the treatment of Q fever. Prognosis is less favorable for the rare patient in whom Q fever endocarditis develops. In some of these patients the disease has been reported to have been unresponsive to antimicrobial therapy, although favorable results have been reported in one patient treated with co-trimoxazole.

PREVENTION. Experimental lots of yolk-sac vaccines have been effective in prevention of clinical disease in volunteers experimentally infected via the respiratory route. Because this vaccine is not commercially available, control measures are limited to minimizing exposure to the agent. In particular, milk from cattle, sheep, and goats in endemic areas should be pasteurized or boiled before use. Because rickettsiae are excreted in the sputum and urine of patients, these materials should be disinfected by autoclaving to prevent secondary infection in hospitals.

Barraclough, D., and Papert, A. J.: Q fever presenting with paroxysmal ventricular tachycardia. Br. Med. J., 2:423, 1975.

Editorial: Chronic Q fever or Q fever endocarditis. Lancet, 1:1171, 1976.

Fiset, P., Wisseman, C. L., and el Batawi, Y.: Immunologic evidence of human fetal infection with *Coxiella burnetii*. Am. J. Epidemiol., 101:65, 1975.

Freeman, R., and Hodson, M. E.: Q fever endocarditis with trimethoprim and sulfamethoxazole. Br. Med. J., 1:419, 1972.

Ormsbee, R. A.: Q fever rickettsia. *In* Horsfall, F. L., Jr., and Tamm, I. (eds.): Viral and Rickettsial Infections of Man. 4th ed. Philadelphia, J. B. Lippincott Company, 1965, p. 1144.

Powell, O. W.: Liver involvement in "Q" fever. Aust. Ann. Med., 10:52, 1961.

Sheridan, P., MacCaig, J. N., and Hart, R. J. C.: Myocarditis complicating Q fever. Br. Med. J., 2:155, 1974.

Tigertt, W. D., and Benenson, A. S.: Studies on Q fever in man. Trans. Assoc. Am. Physicians, 69:98, 1956.

115. BARTONELLOSIS
(Carrión's Disease, Oroya Fever, Verruga Peruana)

Herbert L. Ley, Jr.

DEFINITION. Bartonellosis is an insect-borne microbial disease limited to South America. It is characterized by two distinctive clinical stages. The first of these (Oroya fever) presents a severe febrile infection associated with a marked anemia, bone and joint pains, bacteremia, and an appreciable mortality. The second stage (verruga peruana) is more benign and is distinguished by the appearance of a generalized eruption of hemangiomatous papules and nodules.

ETIOLOGY. The disease is caused by *Bartonella bacilliformis*, a small gram-negative pleomorphic bacillus that may be cultivated readily in enriched bacteriologic media. The disease is transmitted to man by the bite of sandflies of the genus *Phlebotomus*, with development of the characteristic symptoms of Oroya fever after an incubation period of two weeks to three months.

EPIDEMIOLOGY. Although a number of epidemics of the disease have been reported, it is more commonly seen as sporadic cases among populations of Peru, Colombia, and Ecuador, and is restricted within these countries to those who live at altitudes of 1500 to 9000 feet on both slopes of the Andes. In general, the distribution of the disease coincides with the ecologic zones supporting populations of *Phlebotomus*.

In Peru the disease is transmitted by *Phlebotomus verrugarum*, a night-biting sandfly. The biting habits of the vectors in the other countries are similar, although the species of *Phlebotomus* involved in transmission in the other areas are not conclusively identified. The principal reservoir of the disease appears to be man; no additional animal reservoirs have as yet been implicated in nature. Reports of cultivation of the agent from apparently healthy persons suggest that as much as 10 per cent of infections may be subclinical. Persons convalescent from the disease are known to have a low-level bacteremia for months or years, providing frequent opportunities for infection of the disease vector.

PATHOLOGY AND PHYSIOLOGIC RESPONSES. In the Oroya fever stage of illness the causative organism may be found in peripheral blood smears stained with Giemsa or Wright's stain as well as in the reticuloendothelial cells of the viscera and lymphatics. In the blood the parasite is found both free in the plasma and adhering to the erythrocytes. The parasitization of the erythrocytes causes an increased mechanical fragility and also an increased sequestration of the cells in the spleen and the liver. A hypochromic and macrocytic anemia develops rapidly during the febrile period, erythrocyte counts decreasing within a period of only a few days to levels of one million to two million cells per cubic millimeter. The bone marrow is hyperplastic, with an abundance of nucleated erythrocytes. The pathologic findings secondary to the anemia are present in the verruga stage of infection. The histopathology of the skin lesions is that of dilation of the capillaries and proliferation of the vascular endothelial cells that may be shown to contain the causative agent.

CLINICAL MANIFESTATIONS. The presenting symptoms of patients with Oroya fever are intermittent high fever, painful muscles and joints, tender enlarged lymph nodes, and the systemic symptoms and prostration of a severe anemia. These symptoms may persist from several weeks to several months in untreated patients, half of whom may die within the first three weeks of fever. If the patient survives, gradual convalescence is punctuated, after a few days to a month, by the appearance of the cutaneous lesions of the second phase of the disease. The verrugae may persist for a month to a year in untreated persons, but mortality is negligible. Occasional patients may experience only the fever and anemia without the skin manifestations or only the cutaneous lesions without the initial fever. Although these two aspects of the infection were once thought to be different diseases, there is no doubt that both syndromes are manifestations of infection with the same organism. The current interpretation that the skin lesions are an expression of developing immunity in the patient is supported by the observation that second attacks of the disease are exceedingly rare even in highly endemic areas and that the attacks are almost always caused by verruga rather than by Oroya fever.

DIAGNOSIS. In endemic areas the diagnosis can usually be made on the basis of clinical findings. In the acute stage of Oroya fever both blood smears and blood culture usually reveal the presence of the agent. As the patient progresses toward the verruga stage of infection, or with treatment, the organism becomes more difficult to demonstrate.

TREATMENT AND PROGNOSIS. The prognosis in the untreated patient depends upon both the nature and the severity of his infection. Mortality in the Oroya fever phase of the disease may exceed 50 per cent, particularly when the infection is complicated by concurrent attacks of malaria, amebiasis, tuberculosis, salmonellosis, or other diseases. The disease responds well to treatment with penicillin, streptomycin, and the tetracyclines. Chloramphenicol is favored by many South American clinicians because of the frequency of concurrent salmonella infections, but the risks of its potentially more serious toxicity must be weighed against the fact that the other drugs mentioned are therapeutically effective. In general, as in the rickettsial infections, the tetracyclines are the preferred form of antimicrobial therapy for bartonellosis. When the broad-spectrum antimicrobials have been used, oral doses of 1 to 2 grams per day have been used for a period of a week or more with excellent results. Patients become afebrile in 24 to 48 hours, and, if they receive transfusions, recover strength rapidly. Although the mortality of the verruga stage of infection is less than 5 per cent, antimicrobial therapy is desirable to hasten the disappearance of the skin lesions.

PREVENTION. Control measures are directed principally against the *Phlebotomus* vector. Because the insect is a night feeder and moves by a series of short "hops" between surfaces, the application of a residual insecticide to the exterior and interior of doorways, windows, and other avenues of entry to human habitation is effective. Where insecticide application is impracticable, bed nets or insect repellents provide significant protection. Control of breeding of the vector is difficult, but may be undertaken when it is otherwise impossible to prevent contact of the vector with man. No protective vaccine is available. Patients need not be isolated in hospital wards if the vector is absent because the disease is not transmitted by person-to-person contact.

Goldstein, E.: Bartonellosis. *In* Hoeprich, P. D. (ed.): Infectious Diseases. Hagerstown, Md., Harper & Row, 1972, p. 1159.
Reynafarje, C., and Ramos, J.: The hemolytic anemia of human bartonellosis. Blood, 17:562, 1961.
Weinman, D.: The Bartonella Group. *In:* Dubos, R. J., and Hirsch, J. G. (eds.): Bacterial and Mycotic Infections of Man. 4th ed. Philadelphia, J. B. Lippincott Company, 1965, p. 775.

DISEASES CAUSED BY CHLAMYDIAE

116. TRACHOMA AND INCLUSION CONJUNCTIVITIS

Ernest Jawetz

DEFINITION. Trachoma and "inclusion conjunctivitis" are chronic infectious diseases of the eye and genital tract, caused by closely related microorganisms and exhibiting overlapping spectra of clinical manifestations and epidemiologic patterns. These range from mild and self-limited to severe and blinding eye disease and a spectrum of involvement of the genital tract.

ETIOLOGY. The agents of *trachoma and inclusion conjunctivitis* are members of the psittacosis–lymphogranuloma venereum–trachoma group. Formerly these agents were considered viruses; now they are called *chlamydiae*. They are nonmotile, gram-negative, obligate intracellular parasites which multiply in the cytoplasm of their host cells by a distinctive developmental cycle. Chlamydiae differ from viruses in many important respects: they possess both RNA and DNA; they multiply by binary fission; they possess bacterial types of cell walls and ribosomes; they produce a variety of metabolically active enzymes; and their growth can be inhibited by several antibacterial drugs. It is probable that chlamydiae are closely related to gram-negative bacteria, but lack some significant mechanism for the production of metabolic energy so that they are restricted to an intracellular existence.

Chlamydiae fall into two distinct species: *C. psittaci* and *C. trachomatis*. The latter can infect epithelial cells of conjunctiva, cornea, urethra, and cervix of man and monkey, but does not replicate in most other tissues of the body. The infective particle ("elementary body") is a sphere with a diameter of 250 nanometers (millimicrons) and stains purple with Giemsa's or red with Macchiavello's stain. The infective particle is taken into the host cell by phagocytosis and, after replication, results in the development of an inclusion body. This is an oval or crescent-shaped mass of "elementary bodies" embedded in a matrix of glycogen, lying in the cytoplasm of an epithelial cell often adjacent to the nucleus. Inclusion bodies can be stained brightly with specific immunofluorescence.

Chlamydiae can be grown in the yolk sac of embryonated eggs and, by special techniques, in cell culture. The growth of chlamydiae is markedly inhibited by tetracyclines, erythromycins, and chloramphenicol, but not by aminoglycosides. Therefore aminoglycosides can be used to suppress bacterial contaminants in clinical specimens and to aid in isolation of chlamydiae in the laboratory.

All chlamydiae share a heat-stable group antigen. These are lipopolysaccharides detectable by complement-fixation tests. In addition, species- and type-specific antigens have been detected in the cell wall. Infected persons may develop antibodies to both types of antigens in serum and tears. By immunofluorescence tests specific antigens and antibodies can be identified. Thus genital chlamydial isolates usually fall within certain antigenic groups (D to K), whereas ocular isolates from endemic trachoma areas usually fall within other groups (A, B, C). At least 12 specific antigenic groups have been identified to date. There exist cross-reactions between the specific antigens of the chlamydiae of lymphogranuloma venereum and of trachoma and inclusion conjunctivitis. The immunologic labels are the only laboratory characteristics which differentiate different chlamydiae.

Chlamydiae can persist in man for years, with or without symptoms and signs of infection. Subclinical infection in the eye can be activated by trauma, corticosteroids, and bacterial superinfection. The development of scarring and blindness in some endemic trachoma regions is attributable to a large extent to recurrent bacterial infections of the eye, especially with *Hemophilus* or *Neisseria*.

EPIDEMIOLOGY. Since antiquity, trachomatous infection was recognized in the Mediterranean basin and in the Orient. Today, trachomatous eye disease is very prevalent in Africa and Asia. It has been estimated that up to 400 million persons may have eye infections with chlamydiae, and up to 20 million may be economically blinded as a result. Trachoma flourishes in areas that are hot and dry, and that have a shortage of available water and poor hygienic customs. In such areas endemic levels are high, and initial infection commonly occurs in early childhood. In certain parts of the world, e.g., in North Africa, virtually the entire population is infected with chlamydiae before reaching adulthood. The high prevalence of bacterial superinfection in such populations undoubtedly contributes to the severity of eye disease and to its causing widespread blindness. In parts of the United States, e.g., Indian reservations of the Southwest, endemic chlamydial infection is relatively common, but it rarely leads to major visual impairment, perhaps because bacterial superinfection is infrequent. Throughout the world sporadic cases of ocular chlamydial infection occur, often with a clinical picture resembling trachoma. It is probable that some of these originate in genital infections rather than in contact with ocular trachoma.

Active cases of ocular chlamydial infection shed the infective agent in desquamated conjunctival cells, conjunctival exudate, or tears. The infectious agent may be transmitted by fingers, fomites, and perhaps flies. Patients with early active infection probably shed more infective chlamydiae and thus are more infectious for contacts than are those with chronic infection. However, even patients with longstanding scarred eye disease, and without signs of current activity, may shed chlamydiae and thus serve as a source of infection.

These comments concern ocular chlamydial infection, particularly typical endemic trachoma. *Typical inclusion conjunctivitis* has a radically different epidemiologic pattern. Inclusion conjunctivitis is fundamentally an infection of the adult human genital tract, transmitted as a venereal disease. In the female the chlamydiae grow mainly in the transitional epithelium of the cervix. These cells may contain typical inclusions, and occasionally a mild cervicitis is present. In the male, genital infection may produce nongonococcal *urethritis*, as the chlamydial agent replicates in urethral epithelium. In both sexes, adult genital tract infection and proctitis are often asymptomatic. Adults may transfer genital secretions to their own or other eyes by fingers, by fomites, and — occasionally — in swimming pools. The infection may pass from the cervix of the infected mother to the eye of her newborn during passage through the birth canal. The newborn infant may then develop eye disease between 5 and 14 days after birth.

The epidemiologic patterns described for typical trachoma and typical inclusion conjunctivitis may be mixed. Thus the genital tract of women in endemic trachoma regions may harbor chlamydiae and these may produce either inclusion conjunctivitis or clinically typical trachoma in the offspring. Genital isolates from adults in nonendemic areas may, upon inoculation into the eye, give rise to disease resembling either inclusion conjunctivitis or trachoma.

PATHOLOGY AND PATHOGENESIS. *Chlamydia trachomatis* invades mainly the epithelium of the conjunctiva, cervix, and urethra. The earliest sign of infection is the appearance of inclusion bodies within epithelial cells and neutrophil infiltration of the epithelium of mucous membranes. Subepithelial infiltration with plasma cells and lymphocytes and the development of lymphoid follicles then follow. In the cornea, epithelial keratitis is often accompanied by the formation of subepithelial opacities. Blood vessels from the limbus, accompanied

by fibroblasts, may invade the cornea to form a pannus. Progression of the inflammatory process leads to necrosis and scar formation in the conjunctiva. In classic trachoma, these changes occur more markedly in the upper half of the conjunctival sac and cornea; in inclusion conjunctivitis, more markedly in the lower conjunctiva. Inflammatory changes, lymphoid infiltration, necrosis, and scar formation have also been observed in chlamydial infection of cervix and urethra.

Classic inclusion conjunctivitis of the newborn is an *acute purulent conjunctivitis*; in the adult it is a *follicular conjunctivitis*. However, all pathologic changes from limited follicular conjunctivitis to full-blown "trachoma" with scars and pannus may follow inoculation of genital isolates into the adult eye.

Classic, chronic, severe trachoma in hyperendemic areas progresses to marked lid deformation and loss of vision. As a result of cellular infiltration and scarring near the lid margins, the tarsal plate is bowed and the lid margins inverted (entropion), and some eyelashes turn inward (trichiasis), rubbing against the cornea with each lid movement, and aggravating corneal opacification. The scarring may destroy tear function, with resulting keratinization of corneal epithelium.

Chlamydiae exhibit a pronounced tendency to persist in infected tissues for years even in the absence of signs of active disease, and this predisposes to relapses and to chronicity.

CLINICAL MANIFESTATIONS. In experimental human infection with *Chlamydia trachomatis* the incubation period is from two to seven days. *Inclusion conjunctivitis* of the newborn usually begins between the fifth and fourteenth days of life (whereas gonococcal ophthalmia usually begins two days after birth). The incubation period of naturally occurring trachoma is uncertain because the onset is often insidious, particularly in children. Early symptoms of chlamydial infection are those of irritation, lacrimation, and mucopurulent discharge. The earliest physical signs are conjunctival hyperemia, mucopurulent discharge, papillary hypertrophy in infants, and follicular hypertrophy in adults. Newborns may develop pneumonitis.

Typical *trachoma* in children and adults begins as a follicular conjunctivitis, most noticeable in the conjunctiva of the upper lid and the tarsal plate. There are epithelial keratitis and subepithelial corneal infiltration, followed by gradual corneal vascularization from the upper limbus downward. This evolves into a dense fibrovascular pannus extending over part, or all, of the cornea, grossly impairing vision. Linear or stellate scars appear on the conjunctiva. Progressive scarring of the subepithelial tissues leads to deformation of the tarsal plate, resulting in entropion, trichiasis, and further corneal damage. These changes often follow secondary bacterial infection, which may also produce corneal ulceration and accelerate loss of vision. Typically there are no systemic symptoms or signs of infection, and the eye is the sole involved organ.

Typical *inclusion conjunctivitis* of the newborn presents as an acute purulent conjunctivitis with papillary hypertrophy but little involvement of the cornea. Over a period of weeks or months this tends to regress spontaneously and to heal with little scarring. In the adult, inclusion conjunctivitis is an acute mucopurulent conjunctivitis, often accompanied by preauricular adenopathy. Follicular hypertrophy is most noticeable in the conjunctiva of the lower lid, and tends to persist for weeks or months, occasionally accompanied by epithelial keratitis and subepithelial corneal infiltrates. Some adults with chronic inclusion conjunctivitis develop pannus and a few scars of conjunctiva and cornea.

Adult genital chlamydial infection usually precedes the eye involvement. Adult *cervicitis* and *urethritis* either are asymptomatic or produce only slight discharge and discomfort. This nongonococcal urethritis forms a substantial portion of the acute urethritis in the male seen in venereal disease clinics (see Ch. 139).

All intermediate stages between minimal self-limited inclusion conjunctivitis and typical progressive trachoma can occur as a result of infection with chlamydiae agents of either ocular or genital origin. The typical, severe trachoma that leads to blindness and is seen in hyperendemic areas occurs probably as a result of longstanding infection with many relapses of chlamydial activity, hypersensitivity reactions, and repeated bacterial superinfections. Conversely, the self-limited inclusion conjunctivitis of the newborn may be characteristic of a first infection, without hypersensitivity reaction, and without bacterial complications in an immunologically immature host. The basis for different clinical patterns of mild or severe disease seen in different areas of the world is not clearly understood.

DIAGNOSIS. The traditional criteria for the diagnosis of trachoma are the triad of follicular hypertrophy, most prominent on the upper tarsal conjunctiva, pannus, and conjunctival scars. The last two signs may be detected only by biomicroscopic examination (slit lamp).

The diagnosis of inclusion conjunctivitis rests on finding typical inclusions in a purulent conjunctivitis of the newborn or in a follicular conjunctivitis of the adult. There should be only minimal vascular invasion of the cornea. Examination of the adult genital tract may reveal cervicitis and urethritis with moderate discharge and inclusions in epithelial cells. Proctitis may be present.

Among laboratory tests for chlamydial infections, the demonstration of typical intracytoplasmic inclusions in conjunctival or genital epithelial cells is most widely used. Specific immunofluorescent stain is more sensitive than Giemsa stain. Polymorphonuclear leukocytes are often prominent in scrapings that contain chlamydial inclusions. Isolation of chlamydiae in embryonated eggs or in specially treated cell cultures remains a specialized laboratory procedure. Serologic tests can support the diagnosis only if a rise in complement-fixing or immunofluorescence antibodies occurs during acute disease.

DIFFERENTIAL DIAGNOSIS. In differential diagnosis of ocular chlamydial infections, adenovirus infections, herpetic keratoconjunctivitis, folliculosis of children, chronic follicular conjunctivitis (Axenfeld type), reactions to allergens and irritating chemicals, and certain bacterial infections must be considered. Some of these entities may coexist with chlamydial infections, and repeated competent ophthalmologic examinations and elaborate laboratory assistance may be required to establish a correct diagnosis. The demonstration of morphologically typical chlamydial inclusions by immunofluorescent or Giemsa stain is most helpful when combined with efforts to isolate viruses or bacteria of possible etiologic significance.

The differential diagnosis between ocular trachoma and oculogenital inclusion conjunctivitis requires epidemiologic considerations, clinical and laboratory examination of the genital tract, and a "typing" of the isolate by immunofluorescent tests. The eye lesions of trachoma and of oculogenital inclusion conjunctivitis in the adult cannot be distinguished. The most important differential diagnosis of inclusion conjunctivitis of the newborn is chemical or bacterial conjunctivitis.

TREATMENT AND PROGNOSIS. Chlamydiae are susceptible to several antibacterial drugs. Tetracyclines and sulfonamides have been most widely used in treatment. Tetracycline suspensions or ointments can cling to the conjunctiva for prolonged effect. Ophthalmic topical tetracycline preparations have been administered in various dosage schedules for several months in chronic endemic trachoma. In inclusion conjunctivitis of the newborn, there is a strong natural tendency toward healing. The administration of topical tetracycline two to four times daily for three weeks further accelerates healing.

Oral tetracycline hydrochloride, 1 to 2 grams in three divided daily doses, or doxycycline, 2.5 to 4.0 mg per kilogram in a single daily dose, or oral trisulfapyrimidines, 4 grams daily in divided doses for five to six weeks, can suppress signs of activity in chronic trachoma of adults. However, these treatment regimens often fail to eradicate the infectious agent. By contrast, in acute chlamydial infections these oral drug regimens alone, or combined with topical tetracycline, may result in permanent cure. This applies to acute infections of either the eye or the genital tract.

In areas of hyperendemic trachoma, mass treatment must be applied to early infection of children and must be repeated at intervals in order to control chlamydial infection before scarring occurs. Repeated courses of drug treatment are probably beneficial by reducing the reservoir of infection, by temporarily suppressing microbial and clinical activity in the patient, and by controlling bacterial superinfection. Even one monthly dose of 300 mg of doxycycline provides clinical benefit by converting severe to mild eye disease and preventing visual impairment.

Drug therapy has no influence on established scars or pannus. Surgical correction is required in serious entropion or trichiasis. Topical corticosteroids and caustics have no place in therapy.

PREVENTION. Endemic trachoma is favored by ignorance, poverty, and cultural patterns that oppose hygienic improvement and medical treatment. In addition, the sheer lack of water available for washing seems to be important.

The most potent preventive measures include efforts to increase the total supply of water, simple cleanliness such as frequent hand washing, avoidance of common towel or common eye pencil, and measures to reduce flies. It is also important to detect mild, early infection in young children in endemic areas and to apply effective drug treatment repeatedly. This prevents the blinding progression of the disease, and probably reduces the infective reservoir. Detection and treatment of adults who already suffer visual impairment can probably reduce the source of infection for children. Entire family groups or communities should be treated simultaneously.

Prevention of genital chlamydial infections requires the control of sexual promiscuity, early diagnosis and effective treatment of cases and sexual contacts, and prolonged follow-up to establish that the genital or ocular infection is not relapsing. Effective treatment of pregnant women with genital chlamydial infection can prevent inclusion conjunctivitis in the newborn. The usual instillations into the eye of the newborn (silver nitrate or penicillin) do not prevent inclusion conjunctivitis. A newborn baby with inclusion conjunctivitis should be isolated to prevent spread to others.

Experimental vaccines against chlamydial infections have failed to protect against infection or against progression of disease.

Natural infection engenders only minimal protection against reinfection. The most that could be expected of artificial immunization is an attenuation of the disease resulting from infection. The best current hope for control of chlamydial infections rests on a combination of public health measures and drug treatment.

Dunlop, E. M. C., Jones, B. R., Darougar, S., and Treharne, J. D.: Chlamydia and non-specific urethritis. Br. Med. J., 2:575, 1973.

Grayston, J. T., and Wang S. P.: New knowledge of chlamydiae and the diseases they cause. J. Infect. Dis., 132:87, 1975.

Holmes, K. K., Handsfield, H. H., Wang, S. P., Wentworth, B. B., Turck, M., Anderson, J. B., and Alexander, R. E.: Etiology of non-gonococcal urethritis. N. Engl. J. Med., 292:1199, 1975.

Jawetz, E.: Chemotherapy of chlamydial infections. In Garattini, S., Goldin, A., Hawking, F., and Kopin, I. J. (eds.): Advances in Pharmacology and Chemotherapy. Vol. 7. New York, Academic Press, 1969, pp. 253–282.

Jawetz, E., Hanna, L., Dawson, C., Wood, R., and Briones, O.: Subclinical infections with TRIC agents. Am. J. Ophthal., 63:1413, 1967.

Jones, B. R., and Darougar, S.: Communicable ophthalmia: The blinding scourge of the Middle East. Br. J. Ophthalmol., 60:492, 1976.

Moulder, J. W.: The relation of the psittacosis group (chlamydiae) to bacteria and viruses. Ann. Rev. Microbiol., 20:107, 1966.

Richmond, S. J., and Sparling, P. F.: Genital chlamydial infections. Am. J. Epidemiol., 103:438, 1976.

117. LYMPHOGRANULOMA VENEREUM

Ernest Jawetz

DEFINITION. Lymphogranuloma venereum (LGV) is an acute and chronic venereal disease with prominent systemic manifestations, caused by a chlamydial agent closely related to trachoma and inclusion conjunctivitis agents. LGV produces early genital lesions followed by enlargement and suppuration of regional lymph nodes and a variety of febrile systemic manifestations. Late results are prominent inguinal draining sinuses in men and fibrosing proctitis and rectal strictures in women and homosexual males.

ETIOLOGY. The chlamydiae of LGV are members of the species and share the characteristics of *C. trachomatis*, including the formation of compact intracytoplasmic inclusions with a glycogen matrix, inhibition of growth by sulfonamides, and antigenic features. All LGV chlamydiae carry the chlamydial group reactive antigen. Specific antigens have been defined by immunofluorescence, thus permitting classification of LGV isolates into three specific antigenic types. These antigens cross-react with type-specific antigens of other *C. trachomatis*. LGV chlamydiae differ from ocular isolates in growing more readily in cell cultures and in several animal tissues.

EPIDEMIOLOGY. LGV is transmitted almost exclusively by sexual contact. The genital tract and rectum of chronically infected persons serve as reservoirs of infection. The highest incidence of the disease has been reported from subtropical and tropical areas, but the in-

fection occurs all over the world. Definitive serologic surveys of LGV infection by appropriate specific methods have not been performed.

PATHOGENESIS AND PATHOLOGY. A primary vesicular or ulcerative lesion develops at the site of inoculation one to four weeks after infection. The chlamydiae spread rapidly to regional lymph nodes which become enlarged and inflamed. From the penis or vulva the spread is mainly to inguinal and iliac nodes. From the vagina or rectum the spread is mainly to perirectal and pelvic nodes. The involved nodes become matted and suppurate and may discharge pus through multiple sinus tracts.

During the stage of early, active lymphadenitis, the chlamydiae may become widely disseminated by the bloodstream and may reach various organs, including the central nervous system. In the late, chronic stages of infection, fibrosis, obstruction, and strictures develop. Lymphatic obstruction may lead to elephantiasis of external genitalia (penis, scrotum, vulva). Chronic proctitis may lead to progressive rectal strictures, with obstruction of the bowel lumen and fistula formation.

The histologic appearance of involved lymph nodes shows acute and chronic inflammation, suppuration, and fibrosis, but is not specific or diagnostic of LGV.

CLINICAL MANIFESTATIONS. Several days to several weeks after exposure, a small, evanescent papule or vesicle develops on any part of the external genitalia, anus, or rectum. The lesion may ulcerate, but usually — especially in women — it remains unnoticed and heals in a few days. Soon thereafter the regional lymph nodes enlarge and tend to become matted and often painful. In males, inguinal nodes are most commonly involved both above and below Poupart's ligament, and the overlying skin often turns purplish as the nodes suppurate and eventually discharge pus through multiple sinus tracts. In females, the perirectal nodes are prominently involved with proctitis and bloody mucopurulent anal discharge. This is also seen in homosexual males.

During the stage of active lymphadenitis, there are often marked systemic symptoms, including fever, headaches, meningismus, conjunctivitis, skin rashes, nausea and vomiting, and arthralgias. Rarely is there meningitis, arthritis, or pericarditis. Unless effective antimicrobial therapy is instituted at that stage, the chronic inflammatory process progresses to fibrosis, lymphatic obstruction, and rectal strictures. The lymphatic obstruction may lead to elephantiasis of the penis, scrotum, or vulva. The chronic proctitis of women or homosexual males may lead to progressive rectal strictures, rectosigmoid obstruction, and fistula formation.

DIAGNOSIS. LGV must be considered in every case of enlarged, matted, tender inguinal lymph nodes, active proctitis, draining inguinal or perianal fistulas, and rectal strictures. It must be distinguished from inguinal adenopathy of any cause, including pyogenic infection of lower extremities, plague, tularemia, chancroid, granuloma inguinale, syphilis, and inflammatory or neoplastic lesions of the rectum. A clinical impression of LGV can be supported by the demonstration of the chlamydiae, a skin test, or a meaningful serologic response, but histologic appearance of biopsied tissue is not specific.

Material from fluctuant suppurating nodes may be obtained by aspiration or biopsy. When inoculated into x-irradiated cell cultures, into embryonated eggs, or, by intracerebral injection, into mice, LGV chlamydiae can sometimes be isolated. Only rarely can chlamydial inclusions be seen in stained smears of such material.

The skin test (Frei test) consists of the intradermal injection of LGV antigens, prepared in embryonated eggs, and a suitable control of egg material. The test is considered positive if an indurated area or papule — at least 6 mm larger than the control site — develops in 48 hours. Reactivity to chlamydial group antigen develops within three to eight weeks after LGV infection and may remain positive for life. This delayed hypersensitivity reaction may be positive after *any* chlamydial infection. A negative skin test cannot exclude LGV infection. Skin tests with commercial antigens are sometimes negative even when LGV chlamydiae are isolated from pus, or when the serologic response unequivocally proves a chlamydial infection. Thus the Frei test is of only limited value in the diagnosis of suspected LGV infection. Early antimicrobial drug treatment may interfere with the development of a positive skin test and antibody response.

The complement-fixation (CF) test with heat-stable group reactive antigen is at present the most generally available test for LGV and other systemic chlamydial infections. In the presence of inguinal adenopathy or proctitis, a rise of antibody titer in sera taken two to three weeks apart strongly supports the diagnosis of LGV. In untreated LGV patients, the CF titer is often 1:64 or more, and such a high titer in a single serum from a patient with a compatible clinical picture also supports the diagnosis. With effective treatment the titer declines. Persisting high antibody titers suggest chronic persistent infection. Indirect immunofluorescence tests for antibodies to LGV antigens are as sensitive as and more specific than CF tests but are not generally available.

Other abnormal laboratory findings are less helpful. The white blood cell count is often elevated during lymph node suppuration or proctitis, sometimes with a relative monocytosis. Total serum proteins may be elevated with a reversed albumin-globulin ratio. Gamma globulin, cryoglobulin, rheumatoid factor, and IgM are sometimes significantly increased in serum.

TREATMENT. The growth of LGV chlamydiae can be inhibited by sulfonamides, tetracyclines, and some other antimicrobials. Full systemic doses of a soluble sulfonamide (e.g., trisulfapyrimidines USP, 6 to 8 grams on day one with 4 grams daily thereafter) or of a tetracycline (e.g., tetracycline HCl, 2 to 3 grams daily) are administered for three to four weeks as early in the course of LGV infection as possible. LGV acquired since 1967 in Southeast Asia has responded more regularly to tetracycline than to sulfonamides. In some patients, two or three courses of treatment are required. Supportive therapy consists of bed rest, compresses to inflamed areas, analgesics, and aspiration of fluctuant sites. Treatment is guided by the subsiding of constitutional symptoms and of lymph node swelling, closure of fistulas, and resolution of proctitis. If the infection is eradicated, the serum antibody titer drops markedly over a period of six to eight months.

PROGNOSIS. Although the acute illness in early LGV is usually self-limited, the chronic complications resulting from lymphatic blockade or rectal stricture are debilitating and often require surgical correction. It is important therefore to prevent these late complications by early diagnosis and prolonged or repeated treatment. Death from LGV uncomplicated by bacterial superinfection is very rare. There may be an increased incidence of anorectal carcinoma in persons with anorectal chronic LGV.

PREVENTION. Since LGV is generally acquired as a venereal disease, all measures applicable to the prevention of venereal diseases are pertinent. No active immunization is available.

Abrams, A. J.: Lymphogranuloma venereum. JAMA, 205:59, 1968.

Jawetz, E.: Chemotherapy of chlamydial infections. Adv. Pharmacol. Chemother., 7:235, 1969.

Schachter, J., Smith, D. E., Dawson, C. R., Anderson, W. R., Deller, J. J., Hoke, A. W., Smart, W. H., and Meyer, K. F.: Lymphogranuloma venereum. Comparison of the Frei test, complement fixation test, and isolation of the agent. J. Infect. Dis., 120:372, 1969.

Sowmini, C. N., Gopalan, K. N., and Chandrasekhara Roa, G.: Minocycline in the treatment of lymphogranuloma venereum. J. Am. Ven. Dis. Assoc., 2:19, 1976.

Thorsteinsson, S. B., Musher, D. M., Min, K. W., and Gyorkey, F.: Lymphogranuloma venereum, a cause of cervical lymphadenopathy. JAMA, 235:1882, 1976.

118.   PSITTACOSIS
(Ornithosis, Parrot Fever)

William Schaffner

DEFINITION. Psittacosis is a specific infection of birds produced by the obligate intracellular bacteria, *Chlamydia psittaci*. When transmitted to man, this agent can produce asymptomatic infection, a transient influenza-like illness, or serious pneumonic disease characterized by high fever, headache, cough, myalgia, pulmonary infiltrates, and a significant mortality. Because many species of birds other than the order Psittaciformes transmit psittacosis, *ornithosis* has been suggested as a more accurate title. Usage has made psittacosis the accepted term for the human disease.

HISTORY. In 1879, Ritter, a Swiss physician, described seven cases of an unusual pneumonia that occurred after contact with tropical birds. Morange, in 1894, established the parrot as a vector and termed the disease *psittacosis* after the Greek *psittakos* (the parrot). During 1929–1930 a serious epidemic of pneumonia occurred in Europe and America after shipments of infected South American parrots. This epidemic led to clearer recognition of psittacosis as a human disease. The etiologic agent was demonstrated to be a filterable agent by Bedson, Western, and Simpson in 1930. Subsequent studies have shown that over 90 species of birds can harbor the agent, and its worldwide distribution has been documented. Reported cases in the United States have declined since 1960, probably as a consequence of requiring tetracycline treatment of imported psittacine birds.

ETIOLOGY. *C. psittaci* is an obligate intracellular parasite. It is morphologically and serologically related to lymphogranuloma venereum, to trachoma, and to a number of mammalian agents that produce pneumonitis, meningoencephalitis, and abortion in their native hosts but that do not produce human disease. Because of their large size (250 to 400 mμ), possession of both RNA and DNA, a demonstrable cell wall containing muramic acid, division by binary fission, and their susceptibility to chemotherapeutic agents known to inhibit bacterial enzyme systems, these agents have recently been reclassified as specialized bacteria. Parrots and parakeets are common carriers and until recently represented the major source of human infection. With better control of psittacine disease in aviaries, other birds now contribute more human infections, and cases have resulted from contact with turkeys, pigeons, ducks, chickens, pheasants, finches, and other fowl. Although individuals of both sexes and all ages are susceptible, overt clinical infections in children are uncommon. Persons working with birds are at greatest risk of infection, and there is an increased incidence of psittacosis in pet shop employees, pigeon handlers, and poultry workers, especially in turkey processing plants. There is no risk associated with eating poultry products.

The agent is present in the blood, tissue, feathers, and discharges of infected birds. It is hardy and can withstand drying. Although the avian disease can be fatal, infected birds frequently show only minimal evidence of illness, such as ruffled feathers, lethargy, and failure to eat. Birds having active infections are most likely to transmit the disease, but asymptomatic carriers are common, and birds that recover can shed transmissible agent for many months. In general, human psittacosis acquired from psittacine birds or turkeys has been more severe than that acquired from pigeons, ducks, chickens, or pheasants. Bird ectoparasites can harbor the agent and may serve as a source of reinfection for domestic flocks. Antimicrobials incorporated in bird foodstuffs may not eradicate psittacosis from infected parrots or parakeets but can render them less infectious for man.

Psittacosis is generally acquired by the respiratory route through inhalation of infected dried bird excreta, more rarely by handling the feathers and the tissues of infected birds. On rare occasion the disease may be acquired through an open lesion or the bite of a bird. Mouth-to-beak intimacies have led to infection in man. Small epidemics have been attributed to aerosols of dust laden with dried excreta. Cases have been reported after only brief exposure to birds. There is some evidence that the incubation period may be shortened by a large inoculum. Person-to-person transmission of psittacosis, although rare, has been documented. These cases of "human" strain psittacosis have been severe, with high mortality.

PATHOLOGY. In birds, the principal sites of disease are the liver, spleen, and pericardium. In man, the lung is most commonly involved. The psittacosis agent generally gains access to the human body via the respiratory route, and then rapidly enters the blood and reaches the reticuloendothelial cells of the liver and spleen. After replication in these sites, invasion of the lung is by hematogenous spread. The agent can be isolated from the blood and sputum during the first two weeks of illness, and has been found in the spleen in fatal cases. The mature pulmonary lesion is a lobular pneumonitis. The process is initiated by inflammation and progressive edema of the alveolar cells. Exudation is often accompanied by small hemorrhages, accounting for clinical hemoptysis. Polymorphonuclear leukocytes appear early in the process. Later inflammatory exudates show lymphocytes and large numbers of mononuclear leukocytes within the alveoli and interstitial spaces. The mucosa of the trachea and bronchi generally remains intact but is edematous and invaded with mononuclear cells. Thick, gelatinous plugs of mucus may fill major and minor bronchi and account for the severe cyanosis and progressive anoxia seen in fatal cases. Foci of necrosis may occur in more severely affected areas of

the lung and are sometimes associated with capillary thrombi. The process is generally most severe in dependent bronchopulmonary segments. Vasculitis and thrombosis may account for many findings. Large monocytes and macrophages containing cytoplasmic inclusion bodies, which may represent the agent (LCL bodies), are characteristic of psittacosis infection. Hyperplasia and monocytic infiltration of pulmonary and hilar lymph nodes and splenic enlargement with occasional areas of focal necrosis may occur. Rarely the liver may show intralobular focal necrosis and swollen Kupffer cells containing the psittacosis elementary bodies. Changes in the myocardium, heart valves, pericardium, meninges, brain, adrenals, and kidneys have been reported.

CLINICAL MANIFESTATIONS. Wide variations can occur in the clinical picture. The incubation period ranges from 7 to 15 days but may occasionally be longer. Asymptomatic infection or mild influenza-like infections probably are the rule. Moderate or severe infections, although less frequent, are more commonly diagnosed. The onset of illness may be insidious, but it often starts with chills and a fever that rises slowly from initial levels of 38 or 39 to 39.5 to 40.5° C during the first week of illness. As with some other instances of intracellular infection, the pulse may be slow relative to the height of the fever. Headache is severe. Malaise, anorexia, severe myalgias, particularly in the neck and back, and arthralgias are common. Cough is generally prominent but may be delayed until late in the first week. Small amounts of mucoid sputum with occasional blood streaking are the rule, and pleuritic pain is rare. Changes in mentation are often seen. Delirium or stupor may occur in severe cases toward the end of the first week, and is usually associated with severe pulmonary involvement, cyanosis, and other evidences of anoxia. Other neurologic manifestations are uncommon. Nausea and vomiting are frequent. Epistaxis may occur early in the course of the illness. A macular rash (Horder's spots) resembling that seen in typhoid has occasionally been described. Jaundice and progressive nitrogen retention have been reported in severe cases. Severe dyspnea, tachypnea, tachycardia, cyanosis, jaundice, delirium, and stupor are all poor prognostic signs.

The physical findings of pneumonia are often sparse. Chest roentgenograms often reveal evidence of infiltrates not detected at the bedside. Examination may reveal only fever, painful muscle groups, an elevated respiratory rate, and a relative bradycardia. Fine, crepitant rales may be heard in localized areas over the lungs. Frank percussion or auscultatory changes suggestive of true consolidation are less common. Pleurisy with effusion can occur but is unusual. Mild hepatomegaly is frequent. A palpable spleen has been noted in a substantial number of patients. Splenomegaly in a patient with undiagnosed acute pneumonitis should raise the consideration of psittacosis. An erythematous pharynx may be noted. In rare instances there may be signs of pericarditis or myocarditis. In prolonged, severe illness, thrombophlebitis and pulmonary infarction have been reported as late complications.

Patients with mild cases may recover in seven to eight days. More severe infections may last 12 to 21 days without specific treatment. Fever is ordinarily sustained or remittent, and when accompanied by bradycardia, resembles the fever seen in untreated typhoid infections. Defervescence is generally slow, and a prolonged convalescence is common. Relapses have been reported even after appropriate treatment. Complicating bacterial infections are rare. Second attacks have been described. Recently, British physicians have reported occasional cases of endocarditis caused by *C. psittaci* in patients with sterile blood cultures.

LABORATORY FINDINGS. Simple laboratory studies are not helpful in establishing a diagnosis. The leukocyte count is usually normal, but leukopenia or low-grade leukocytosis ranging to over 20,000 cells per cubic millimeter may occur. The erythrocyte sedimentation rate is generally elevated. Proteinuria is common during the febrile period. Chest roentgenograms generally show soft patchy infiltrates radiating outward from the hilum, which tend to be more prominent in dependent lobes or segments. Occasionally diffuse miliary, nodular, or frank lobar distribution of infiltrates is seen.

A specific diagnosis can be made only by isolation of the agent or by serologic studies. The agent is present in the blood and sputum during the first two to three weeks, but isolation is hazardous, and should not be attempted except in special laboratories. Diagnosis is generally made by a fourfold rise in complement-fixing antibodies against a heat-stable group antigen prepared from psittacosis agent grown in eggs. Paired acute and convalescent sera should always be tested. A significant change in antibody titers is generally present by the twelfth to fourteenth day of disease; the titers are usually maximal by 30 days, then slowly disappear. Treatment can delay or suppress antibody response. A serum complement-fixation titer of 1:16 during the acute illness is presumptive evidence of psittacosis. There is considerable cross-reaction between antigens prepared from psittacosis and lymphogranuloma venereum agents. False positive complement-fixation tests may occur with Q fever or brucellosis. Cutaneous hypersensitivity to the Frei antigen may develop during psittacosis.

DIFFERENTIAL DIAGNOSIS. Specific diagnosis of psittacosis is of extreme importance because of its potential severity (reported case fatality rates show a wide range but have attained 40 per cent), its response to antimicrobials, and the public health significance of psittacosis infection. All cases should be reported to the local health department. The syndrome of viral pneumonia accompanied by protracted high fever, unusually severe headache, and relative bradycardia should suggest psittacosis. Often a history of contact with birds is the only clue to diagnosis and may be elicited only by repeated questioning of the patient and family. When pneumonic symptoms are prominent, psittacosis must be differentiated from viral pneumonias, mycoplasmal pneumonia, influenza, Q fever, tularemia, tuberculosis, fungal infection, and bacterial pneumonia distal to an obstructed bronchus. If pneumonic symptoms are not prominent, psittacosis can be confused with other systemic febrile illnesses such as typhoid fever, brucellosis, infectious mononucleosis, infectious hepatitis, miliary tuberculosis, or the viral meningoencephalitides.

TREATMENT. The tetracyclines are the drugs of choice, and early diagnosis and initiation of treatment may be lifesaving. After institution of therapy with 2 to 3 grams daily, both fever and symptoms are generally controlled within 48 to 72 hours, although the response may be indolent. Although the disease apparently responds to penicillin in doses above 2 million units daily, tetracycline remains the drug of choice. Treatment should be continued for at least 10 days after defervescence to prevent relapse. The high fever and progressive anoxia secondary to extensive pulmonary involvement in severe cases may require appropriate measures directed at these problems.

Harding, H. B.: The bacteria-like chlamydiae of ornithosis and the diseases they cause. CRC Crit. Rev. Clin. Lab. Sci., 1:451, 1970.

Meyer, K. F.: The ecology of psittacosis and ornithosis. Medicine, 21:175, 1942.

Schaffner, W., Drutz, D. J., Duncan, G. W., and Koenig, M. G.: The clinical spectrum of endemic psittacosis. Arch. Intern. Med., 119:433, 1967.

Ward, C., and Ward, A. M.: Acquired valvular heart-disease in patients who keep pet birds. Lancet, 2:734, 1974.

PNEUMONIA

119. INTRODUCTION TO PNEUMONIA

Herbert Y. Reynolds

Pneumonia is a general term denoting a group of clinically manifest diseases that result from microbial infection of lung parenchyma. It is a commonly encountered disease and, in one form or another, continues to be a leading cause of death in the United States. Histologically, the pneumonias represent an inflammatory reaction in the interstitium of alveoli and an accumulation of exudate in alveolar lumina. Consolidation and a degree of nonfunction may occur in affected lung tissue. With successful inactivation of the infecting agent, resolution occurs and normal lung structure is usually restored. Exceptions to the complete healing phase occur in certain necrotizing pneumonias, those caused by staphylococcal or gram-negative bacteria, after which lung scars or fibrosis may develop.

For the physician to discover that a pneumonia, i.e., an intrapulmonary process of some sort, is present in an adult patient is no very difficult feat; neither is that knowledge particularly helpful unless two further steps can be taken. These are detection of evidence that the disease is indeed microbial in origin and not an infarct or neoplasm, and identification of the specific microbe or kind of microbe that is involved. Every aspect of management — the choice of treatment, the complications to be watched for, and the hour-by-hour prognosis — depends on the nature of this information. To obtain it acccurately *and in proper time* requires the physician to be wholly familiar with the various ways in which each one of the microbial pneumonias expresses itself. Some of these — for example, plague pneumonia — he may never see. Yet he must know at least enough about plague pneumonia so that he could avert its terrible consequences for others should he ever encounter a case. Other forms of pneumonia encountered relatively rarely arise as complications of some familiar microbial disease such as measles or tuberculosis or streptococcal disease. Occasionally, well-known viruses such as influenza or chickenpox cause pneumonia, or the physician may be asked to see a patient with psittacosis. In the compromised host, necrotizing pneumonias caused by *Pseudomonas* and other gram-negative bacilli are commonplace. Most of the time, in an adult patient the physician is dealing with *mycoplasmal pneumonia* or with *one of three bacterial* pneumonias, pneumococcal, staphylococcal, or some other form of necrotizing pneumonia in an obviously altered host. This narrowing of the probabilities does not really lighten the seriousness of making the correct choice. The most effective treatment for pneumococcal pneumonia is utterly without value in *Klebsiella* pneumonia; a choice of therapy based on a diagnosis of mycoplasmal pneumonia when the patient actually has staphylococcal pneumonia could result in a fatality.

Mycoplasmal, pneumococcal, certain other primary bacterial pneumonias, and the necrotizing (frequently nosocomial) pneumonias are considered in Ch. 120 to 124. Because staphylococcal pneumonia is so closely related to influenza, it is discussed under influenza (see Ch. 82), as well as under staphylococcal disease (see Ch. 134). The pneumonias caused by viruses, rickettsiae, certain fungal species, i.e., *Histoplasma*, coccidioidomycosis, and *Aspergillus*) and other taxonomically less well defined species, such as *Pneumocystis carinii*, are considered in the individual chapters dealing with those infections.

Many microbial agents can infect the lungs and cause pneumonia, but bacteria do so most frequently. Although a common disease, bacterial pneumonia is a relatively rare occurrence in normal people, considering the burden of microorganisms in the ambient air and our frequent exposure to infectious respiratory droplets and secretions from sneezing and coughing fellow humans. This attests to the effectiveness of the lung host defense system. This defense system consists of a complex interrelationship of anatomic barriers and cleansing mechanisms present in the nasopharynx and upper airways and between local cellular and humoral factors operant in the terminal air-exchange units (alveoli). This might be described as the "natural defense system" of the respiratory tract. With respect to infectious agents, normal lungs are kept sterile beyond the first bronchial divisions.

Microorganisms reach lung tissue in several ways: (1) by direct inhalation of infectious particles from ambient air or by aspiration of secretions from the mouth and nasopharynx; (2) by deposition in lung vasculature following hematogenous spread from another site; and (3) by exogenous penetration of lung tissue. The last-named route includes trauma as well as iatrogenic inoculation of lung tissue with bacteria during chest surgery or from other kinds of diagnostic or therapeutic procedures, e.g., bronchoscopy. The inhalation-aspiration route is by far the most important. Also important are the size and configuration of inhaled particles and droplets which determine the site or level of deposition in the respiratory tract. For example, approximately 90 per cent of particles between 5 and 10 μ in diameter impact at some point along the trachea or in major bronchi, whereas those between 0.5 and 3 μ in size may escape filtration and be deposited in terminal air spaces or leave the body via expired air. Because many bacteria are in this small size range, they frequently plumb the airways to the alveoli. Of impor-

tance in pneumonia are the forces that can become operative to keep them there. Factors influencing the location of viral particles in the lungs are not so clear. Common to both viruses and mycoplasmas is their injury of the ciliary epithelium lining the trachea and lower respiratory tract. Such injury, caused in particular by viral infections, is a well-recognized predisposing factor to bacterial superinfection frequently with staphylococci. After viral infections, bacteria may not be cleared normally from the lower airways owing to damage in the ciliary clearing action of the respiratory epithelium. Subsequent stasis of mucus and respiratory secretions may inhibit phagocytosis and allows for bacterial multiplication; breaks in the lining surface permit submucosal penetration of bacteria. Pneumonia is a common aftermath.

In the upper respiratory tract and large airways, a combination of mechanisms excludes particulate material: (1) anatomic barriers such as the epiglottis, (2) frequent branching of the pulmonary tree (to affect aerodynamic filtration of inspired air), (3) mucociliary clearance of particulates which impact on the mucosa, (4) acute bronchial constriction, and (5) the cough response. When infectious agents, bacteria in particular, elude the physical or mechanical defenses described above and are deposited in the terminal airways and alveoli, another group of host factors takes over. These include phospholipid surfactant and proteins (immunoglobulins and complement factors) in the alveolar lining material and phagocytic cells, i.e., alveolar macrophages and polymorphonuclear neutrophils (PMN's). Anatomically, lung structure changes at the level of respiratory bronchioles and the terminal units (alveolar ducts and alveoli), in that ciliated epithelium and mucus-secreting cells (goblet cells and mucus glands), are no longer present. Therefore, mucociliary clearance does not exist, nor does coughing effectively clear material from the alveoli. Thus microbial clearance and removal of other antigenic material from alveoli are dependent entirely on cellular and humoral factors. Functionally, this portion of the airways from respiratory bronchioles to alveoli might be considered the lower respiratory tract.

If a bacterium of critical size is deposited in an alveolus (in the absence of edema fluid of either circulatory or inflammatory origin), the microbe may encounter at least three substances which conceivably might inactivate it, exclusive of its eventual inactivation by phagocytosis. First, surfactant, secreted by Type II pneumocytes, may have antibacterial activity against staphylococci and rough colony strains of some gram-negative rod bacteria. Second, immunoglobulins, principally of the IgG class and, in lesser concentration, monomeric and secretory forms of IgA, may have specific opsonic antibody activity for the bacterium. Although IgE is present and is considered to be a secretory immunoglobulin, no participation in the opsonic process has been identified for this immunoglobulin class. Third, complement components, especially properdin Factor B, might interact with the bacterium and trigger the alternative complement pathway. One or all of these possibilities described can prepare the bacterium for ingestion by an alveolar macrophage, or the activated complement sequence can lyse it directly. Although alveolar macrophages avidly phagocytose some inert particles, they ingest viable bacteria with considerably less enthusiasm. Coating or opsonizing the organisms will enhance phagocytosis approximately tenfold. However, immunoglobulin G appears to be the only substance capable of increasing alveolar macrophage phagocytosis. There is suggestive evidence that complement can function to enhance or amplify the process. Once phagocytosis has occurred, the alveolar macrophage can inactivate susceptible organisms. Intracellular killing proceeds but at an often slower rate than that measured in PMN's and along less well studied metabolic pathways. Whereas PMN's may kill ingested bacteria with one or a combination of four antimicrobial systems (H_2O_2, superoxide anion [O_2^-], myeloperoxidase, or halide anion), the process is less certain in alveolar macrophages.

Following containment of bacteria, the fate of alveolar macrophages is not certain. They are long-lived tissue cells which can survive at least several months and presumably are capable of handling repeated bacterial and other microbial challenges. Because they are mobile cells, they can migrate to other alveoli through the "pores of Kohn" or move to more proximal areas of the respiratory tract and get aboard the mucociliary escalator for elimination from the lungs. In addition, macrophages gain entry into lung lymphatics and can be carried to regional lymph nodes. This exit gives access to systemic lymphoid tissue and is important in initiating cellular immune responses. Undoubtedly, macrophages are instrumental in degrading antigenic material and presenting it to appropriate lymphocytes in these nodes.

Alveolar macrophages can usually inactivate microorganisms, and host defense surveillance is successful. Under this happy circumstance, clinical disease and pneumonitis never develop. However, if a sufficiently large bacterial inoculum reaches the lower respiratory tract, or if particularly virulent microorganisms are inhaled, the macrophage system can be overwhelmed. In such a situation, the lung parenchyma mounts an extensive inflammatory response that may be perceived as clinical illness. A chest roentgenogram usually reveals an infiltrate. The development of the inflammatory response and hence pneumonia is a deliberate and controlled reaction in the lungs. The ingredients of initiation, amplification, and, finally, suppression are present which make this sequence likely and will be reviewed.

The alveolar macrophage is the only resident phagocyte normally present in the alveoli. It is the bona fide first line of cellular defense on the airside of the lower respiratory tract. However, reserve phagocytic cells, the PMN's, are close by but located in the intravascular compartment. A plentiful supply of PMN's resides in the network of lung capillaries and by estimation may account for up to 30 per cent of the body's pool of marginated PMN's. Even though PMN's are in close proximity to alveolar spaces, they are nonetheless separated by several planes of tissue—capillary endothelium, interstitial space, and alveolar epithelium. Therefore granulocyte movement into the alveoli must be an orderly reaction initiated from the alveolar side. This is termed directed migration or chemotaxis. At least two mechanisms for chemotactic activity exist which can set in motion the inflammatory response in the alveoli: direct generation of chemotactic factors by microorganisms entering the alveoli, and release of chemotactic factors from alveolar macrophages following phagocytosis which might amplify the response. *The first* is best explained with the example of gram-negative rod bacteria

known to contain lipopolysaccharide substances termed endotoxins. Some complement components, particularly Factor B, are present in small amounts in brochoalveolar fluids as sampled by lavage of normal human lungs. Bacterial endotoxin can activate directly the alternative complement pathway, leading to the formation of fragments known to be potent stimulators of PMN chemotaxis, namely C5a and possibly C3a. Furthermore, endotoxin has the potential to convert Hageman factor, also a constituent of bronchoalveolar fluids, to an activated state which can subsequently initiate several pathways: coagulation, fibrinolysis, and kinin generation. In the fibrinolysis sequence, the enzyme plasminogen activator has chemotactic activity for PMN's and for mononuclear cells. In the kinin system, the enzyme kallikrein is chemotactic, and bradykinin is capable of increasing vascular permeability and may account for the accumulation of fluid and other humoral substances in alveoli that accompany pneumonia. Kinin activation is probably a nonspecific and nonimmune reaction (see Ch. 41). *The second mechanism* seems more specific and emanates from the alveolar macrophage itself. In vitro and in vivo studies with macrophages from monkeys and guinea pigs have shown that following phagocytosis of opsonized bacteria, a chemotactic factor is synthesized and secreted which will selectively attract PMN's. Such a factor is of small molecular weight (<5000 daltons), heat labile, and unaffected by antisera to complement components C3a and C5a, which neutralize their respective activities. Although this factor was identified first in macrophages of monkey and guinea pig origin, it has now been found in human cells as well. This mechanism would permit alveolar macrophages to recruit secondary phagocytes, PMN's, to help contain unruly bacteria in the alveoli. Once PMN's and other components of edema fluid have filled alveolar spaces, an exudative inflammatory reaction exists in lung parenchyma and pathologically pneumonitis is present. Ultimately lung tissues become consolidated.

Because of the inflammatory reaction, another quite significant mechanism of host defense — surface phagocytosis — assumes importance in pneumonia caused by well-encapsulated organisms. This phenomenon is of particular importance in patients who receive antimicrobial therapy early in the course of their disease. The reader should consult Ch. 121 for a presentation of this aspect of the subject.

After pneumonia has developed and pending successful containment of the infection, resolution and healing phases eventually occur. At present, however, little is known about the processes that turn off or limit the acute inflammatory reaction of pneumonia and initiate recovery. As in other disease situations, defects in immunoregulation of this part of host immunity are being exposed (see Ch. 41). Serum-derived chemotactic factor inactivator can inhibit immune-complex deposition in animal lung tissue and modify the ensuing inflammatory response. The identification of such inhibitors and the potential for manipulating them is a part of lung immunophysiology that is still in its infancy.

A number of patients with *recurrent bacterial pneumonia* as a major clinical problem have been found to be deficient in either granulocyte or mononuclear cell chemotaxis or both. Inability to mobilize phagocytes to the alveoli in response to an inoculum of bacteria may be a fundamental defect (see Ch. 41).

As indicated above, in most persons with pneumonia, the physician's opportunity for error comes not from overlooking altogether that respiratory disease is present, but from either falsely minimizing its importance ("a little bronchitis") or from lightheartedly mislabeling a quite serious *nonmicrobial* condition, such as pulmonary infarction, as "a viral pneumonia." The physician's two immediate assignments — to establish that a pneumonic process is present and to amass evidence that it is most probably microbial in origin — are met by sharp awareness of what it is that is being sought and the prompt use of the relevant clinical and the readily available and simple laboratory techniques. A urine examination, for example, might reveal that a young, previously well adult with a slight cough, sudden rigor, left-sided midback pain, and a temperature of 39.5° C had an acute infection of the urinary tract. Young adults often have the classic symptoms which can be readily pinpointed to the lower respiratory tract, whereas infants and the elderly may have so few respiratory symptoms as to cause concern that infection may be arising from another organ system. Elderly or severely ill patients may have an unimpressive amount of cough, scant sputum production, and little evidence of respiratory symptoms. Only after excluding infection systematically in other organ systems, such as the previously cited urinary tract, does the respiratory tract receive greater consideration. The onset of fever and agitation or altered mentation frequently ushers in an acquired or nosocomial lung infection in a hospitalized or immunocompromised patient (see Ch. 124). Obviously, a high index of suspicion is sometimes needed plus confirming evidence from the physical examination and other laboratory aids.

Once the nature of respiratory illness is determined, other problems come to mind which should be weighed appropriately. Will the patient require hospitalization versus outpatient management? Does the patient have any obvious risk factors or underlying illnesses which make him or her susceptible to a specific bacterial infection? Are there any special epidemiologic considerations, and — of special importance — are any other members of the immediate family ill? Is this a recurrent pneumonia? What other peculiar problems of the patient may complicate medical management, such as drug allergies, compromised renal or liver function, poor superficial arm veins which prevent easy intravenous access, and so on? Obviously, some of the considerations are not relevant for every case. The points for emphasis, however, are the use of a mental check list to cover most facets of the patient's presentation and initiation of an orderly plan for the management of the particular respiratory infection.

Three principles of patient management bear repeating and deserve emphasis: (1) obtain all the necessary specimens for appropriate bacteriologic cultures before antimicrobial therapy is begun so that there is a reasonable chance for laboratory recovery of the organism; (2) ensure that the drug therapy is as specific as one's certainty of the etiologic agent allows, yet sufficiently broad — temporarily at least — to cover the common yet unsuspected microorganisms as well; and (3) tailor or change the antimicrobial coverage in several days when the results of the cultures are available. A few days of a broad-spectrum antimicrobial coverage will usually not cause superinfections or selection of the drug-resistant bacteria, as long as the physician wisely

discontinues unnecessary drugs and appropriately narrows the antimicrobial spectrum as soon as possible.

It is of great importance to recognize that, if the chemotherapy of pneumonia is to be maximally effective, the correct drug or drug combination must be chosen quickly so that it can be given before irreversible changes have occurred. Yet to do this may be quite difficult, because periods of 24 hours or more are frequently necessary before laboratory techniques can reveal the particular microbe involved. Consequently, almost invariably the initial therapy must be chosen on the basis of the skillful interpretation of essentially *clinical* phenomena and must be heavily weighted toward protecting the patient against the most dangerous of the conceivable diagnoses in that particular set of circumstances. It is likewise of importance to make periodic (at least daily) reviews of the situation and to be quick to discontinue unneeded drugs once the identity of the microbe is known. For a discussion of this question, the reader is referred to Ch. 189.

Since the adequate examination and culture of respiratory secretions is so necessary for the rational treatment of pneumonia, the physician should be vigorous in his attempt to get adequate specimens. If the patient is not producing sputum, an attempt to induce secretions by nebulization of ultrasonic water particles is reasonable. Such particles (which may vary in size between 0.8 and 10 μ in diameter) serve as an irritant and stimulate most subjects to cough. Attempts to obtain lung secretions by passing a small rubber catheter through the nose or mouth — the red snake — rarely get beyond the vocal cords of an alert patient and should be recognized to accomplish little more than to greatly distress an already sick patient in order to obtain a sample of oropharyngeal fluids.

Within a few days of the start of therapy, the great majority of patients with a primary pneumonia can be assigned to one of three categories: a convincing bacteriologic diagnosis has been established by culture of the sputum, blood, or pleural fluid; absolute diagnostic proof is lacking but the patient is clearly recovering with antimicrobial therapy; or the patient is clearly recovering but without wholly convincing evidence that the pneumonia was bacterial in origin. There remains a fourth group, which is quite small. This consists of patients with impressive evidence of microbial pneumonia yet no real indication as to its cause. An appreciable number of these cases turn out to be fungal infections or caused by opportunistic organisms.

For this quite small group of pneumonias, the physician is justified in using various invasive methods to obtain material for microbiologic diagnosis, because to do so would be very much in the interests of the patient. This situation clearly differs from that obtaining in the usual patient with primary pneumonia, in whom such invasive procedures are seldom necessary. The nonprimary — the so-called nosocomial — pneumonias present a situation of their own. With them (see Ch. 124) the patient is usually suffering from at least one serious underlying disease, and the identity of the microbe causing the pneumonia can be considerably more difficult to establish than is the case with the primary pneumonias. At times, therefore, it seems proper on balance to use invasive procedures to establish the microbial agent in a nosocomial pneumonia. The point for emphasis, however, is that, as in primary pneumonia, the instances in which it is appropriate to do this are rare. Because such instances do occur, however, in the interest of completeness, the various techniques are set forth here:

Percutaneous transtracheal aspiration is a direct approach which eliminates much of the contaminating oral, microbial flora. The aspirate, performed through a plastic catheter (No. 14 or 16 size) and needle inserted through the cricothyroid membrane into the airway lumen, is obtained after a small injection of saline which makes the patient cough. If the head of the supine patient is placed below the level of the trachea and major bronchi, liquid injected through the transtracheal catheter may gravitate toward the larynx and possibly accumulate in the oropharynx. Under this circumstance, the patient may inhale oropharyngeal contents during coughing episodes which ensue. Thus transtracheal specimens can become contaminated with mouth flora and yield confusing results if shortcomings in the procedure are not recognized. Although this procedure is generally safe, occasionally some hazard accompanies it such as air leak, leading to subcutaneous or mediastinal emphysema, cardiac arrhythmia, or tracheal bleeding. The physician should use the procedure when indicated, with due caution and awareness of its complications. Anaerobic cultures should be planted as well as routine aerobic ones when a tracheal aspirate is obtained.

The availability of *fiberoptic bronchoscopy* with bronchial lavage and brushing provides another approach to lower respiratory secretions. The risk of bronchoscopy is small even in patients with extensive pneumonia; the administration of supplemental oxygen during the procedure is usually indicated. Often a direct view of the affected lung anatomy, particularly if a loss of volume in the lung lobe accompanies the infection, may provide evidence of an endobronchial obstruction. Removal of secretions or a mucus plug could make the procedure therapeutic as well as diagnostic.

Usually, the lavage fluid or brush culture will contain the offending pathogen; however, microbial cultures from the bronchoscopy specimens also contain contaminating flora from the nasopharynx. Interpretation of culture results is often confusing, and deciding what the predominant organism is may be difficult. To date, no one has perfected a completely reliable way to collect bronchoscopy lavage specimens to avoid this contamination. Several suggestions may improve specificity of the culture results somewhat. By using an area sampling technique to obtain oropharyngeal fluid and a nasal swab for nasal secretions, the nasopharynx can be cultured just prior to bronchoscopy. Then mouth organisms can be transiently suppressed by having the patient rinse the mouth and gargle with an antiseptic solution. Subsequent passage of the bronchoscope through an oropharyngeal tube or an endotracheal tube may reduce contamination even more. Final comparison between the oropharyngeal and nasal culture results and those obtained from lavage specimens may reveal differences that will be helpful in diagnosis. Quantitative bacterial cultures will not add much useful information in this setting and therefore are not recommended. Furthermore, if the patient has chronic bronchitis, for example, and already has colonization of the upper respiratory tract and tracheobronchial tree with *Streptococcus pneumoniae* or *Hemophilus* species, it is virtually impossible to localize or delimit the source of these bacteria in a meaningful way.

Direct examination and culture of affected lung tissue is often indicated. Physicians who care for adult patients with pneumonia generally do not think in terms of needle aspiration of lung tissue. Pediatricians, on the other hand, confronted with undiagnosed pneumonias in infants, feel more comfortable with the procedure and use it frequently. Precise indications for a needle aspirate in an adult cannot be formulated unequivocally; however, a localized, peripheral infiltrate which is "well situated" may lend itself to a needle approach with relatively small risk of complication. Spreading microorganisms along the needle track or soiling the pleural surface is always a consideration, but in actual practice it seems to occur rarely. A small pneumothorax may complicate a needle aspiration, but the frequency of this occurrence depends somewhat on the type and size of the needle used. Often the factor of most significance is the skill and experience of the physician doing the procedure; this usually dictates the frequency and success with which needle aspiration is used within a particular hospital or medical community. The need to do a *small open thoracotomy* to obtain lung tissue is often easier to agree upon. This approach gives the best piece of tissue and is tolerated surprisingly well by even the sickest patient. Generally thoracic surgeons are extremely skillful in managing this situation. Open lung biopsy is often necessary in the immunocompromised patient with an advancing, undiagnosed, pulmonary infiltrate and pneumonia. However, two failings often are observed with the procedure. Medical personnel procrastinate and wait too long to get the biopsy, thus delaying appropriate antimicrobial therapy, or they do not coordinate the handling of the tissue with the microbiologist and pathologist to ensure optimal analysis. A brief presurgical consultation with all the principals is most helpful. The pathologist can often suggest the best area of lung to biopsy, and having the microbiology laboratory prepared can ensure that the most appropriate cultures are quickly planted.

Each of the procedures, as noted above, carries with it some risk of producing a potentially serious complication in a patient who may be already quite sick. The use of any of these procedures should be carefully limited to those relatively rare situations in which the additional knowledge to be obtained could be of significant benefit to the patient.

Antimicrobial therapy — plus appropriate support with fluids, antipyretic drugs, oxygen, suction or postural drainage, and the other modalities employed to treat serious lung infection — remains the cornerstone of medical management. Intelligent use of antimicrobial drugs is not easy, and frequent reappraisal of their choice and patient response must be practiced. The perennial problem of emerging microbial resistance remains; therefore proper selection and use of new antimicrobials to meet the need require the continual education and attention of medical personnel. Although current drug use will be addressed in succeeding chapters, new patterns of microbial resistance must be carefully sought. Without constantly maintaining such vigilance, our accepted therapies could rapidly become obsolete.

Bartlett, J. G., Rosenblatt, J. E., and Finegold, S. M.: Percutaneous transtracheal aspiration in the diagnosis of anaerobic pulmonary infection. Ann. Intern. Med., 79:535, 1973.

Green, G. M., Jakab, G. J., Low, R. B., and Davis, G. S.: Defense mechanisms of respiratory membrane. Am. Rev. Respir. Dis., 115:479, 1977.

Haas, H., Morris, J. F., Samson, S., Kilbourn, J. P., and Kim, P. J.: Bacterial flora of the respiratory tract in chronic brochitis: Comparison of transtracheal fiberbronchoscopic and oropharyngeal sampling methods. Am. Rev. Respir. Dis., 116:41, 1977.

Hahn, H. H., and Beaty, H. N.: Transtracheal aspiration in the evaluation of patients with pneumonia. Ann. Intern. Med., 72:183, 1970.

Johanson, W. G., Pierce, A. K., and Sanford, J. P.: Area sampling technique for quantitative pharyngeal cultures. J. Appl. Microbiol., 18:276, 1969.

Kaltreider, H. B.: Expression of immune mechanisms in the lung. Am. Rev. Respir. Dis., 113:347, 1976.

Kazmierowski, J. A., Aduan, R. P., and Reynolds, H. Y.: Pulmonary host defense: Coordinated interaction of mechanical, cellular and humoral immune systems of the lung. Bull. Europ. Physiopath. Resp., 13:103, 1977.

Kazmierowski, J. A., Gallin, J. I., and Reynolds, H. Y.: Mechanisms for the inflammatory response in primate lungs: Demonstration and partial characterization of an alveolar macrophage–derived chemotactic factor with preferential activity for the polymorphonuclear leukocytes. J. Clin. Invest., 59:273, 1977.

Newhouse, M., Sanchis, J., and Bienenstock, J.: Lung defense mechanisms (medical progress). N. Engl. J. Med., 295:990, 1045, 1976.

Reynolds, H. Y., Atkinson, J. P., Newball, H. H., and Frank, M. M.:

Receptors for immunoglobulin and complement on human alveolar macrophages. J. Immunol., 114:1813, 1975.

Reynolds, H. Y., Kazmierowski, J. A., and Newball, H. H.: Specificity of opsonic antibodies to enhance phagocytosis of *Pseudomonas aeruginosa* by human alveolar macrophages. J. Clin. Invest., 56:376, 1975.

Reynolds, H. Y., and Newball, H. H.: Fluid and cellular milieu of the human respiratory tract. *In* Kirkpatrick, C. H., and Reynolds, H. Y. (eds.): Immunologic and Infectious Reactions in the Lung. New York, Marcel Dekker, Inc., 1976, p. 3.

Robertson, J., Caldwell, J. R., Castle, J. R., and Waldman, R. H.: Evidence for the presence of components of the alternate (properdin) pathway of complement activation in respiratory secretions. J. Immunol., 117:900, 1976.

The Human Mycoplasmas

Species	Usual Site of Occurrence
M. pneumoniae	Respiratory tract
M. salivarium	Oropharynx
M. orale 1	Oropharynx
M. orale 2	Oropharynx
M. orale 3	Oropharynx
M. fermentans	Oropharynx and genital tract (rarely detected)
M. hominis	Genital tract
Ureaplasma urealyticum (T-mycoplasmas)	Genital tract

120. MYCOPLASMAL DISEASES

Robert B. Couch

120.1. INTRODUCTION

The mycoplasmas (formerly called pleuropneumonia-like organisms, PPLO) are the smallest free-living organisms. Recent classification places them in the class Mollicutes, which is divided into two distinct families, Mycoplasmataceae and Acholeplasmataceae, and three genera, *Mycoplasma* (>40 species), *Acholeplasma* (five species), and *Ureaplasma* (one species). These organisms share a number of properties with bacteria, e.g., growth outside the host cell, susceptibility to antimicrobial drugs, generation of metabolic energy, reproduction by binary fission, and possession of both RNA and DNA. In contrast to bacteria, they do not possess a cell wall or the ability to synthesize cell wall precursors. The mycoplasmas are commonly confused with L-forms of bacteria, because L-forms also lack a cell wall and their colonial morphology resembles that of mycoplasmas. However, L-forms are related to their bacterial parents and are unrelated to the mycoplasmas.

Members of the genus *Mycoplasma* cause a variety of diseases in lower animals. These include sinusitis, pneumonia, arteritis, arthritis, and neurologic disease. Because of these varied pathologic states in animals, it has been proposed that many inflammatory diseases of man of unknown etiology are caused by mycoplasmas. In this regard, extensive efforts to incriminate mycoplasmas in the etiology of rheumatoid arthritis have thus far been inconclusive. At present, eight species of human mycoplasmas have been identified. Only one species, *Mycoplasma pneumoniae*, has been clearly shown to produce disease in man, and the disease is essentially limited to the respiratory tract. Two species are commonly cultured from the genitourinary tract; their role in disease there is not wholly clear, but probably at times they are the primary causative agent of disease. The other known species appear to be commensals. Nevertheless, because of the variety of animal diseases described, it would be surprising if some other human diseases are not caused by mycoplasmas.

The eight species of human mycoplasmas and their usual anatomic site of occurrence are shown in the accompanying table. *M. pneumoniae* is a significant cause of acute respiratory disease, including pneumonia. *M. salivarium* and *M. orale* 1 are common inhabitants of the oropharynx, particularly if oral hygiene is poor. *M.*

orale 2 and 3 are uncommon inhabitants of the oropharynx, and *M. fermentans* has on rare occasions been recovered from the oropharynx and genital tract. None of the latter five species have been shown to cause human disease. *M. hominis* and the T-mycoplasmas (so called because of the "tiny" colonies produced on agar medium) have been collectively called the genital mycoplasmas (see Ch. 120.3).

120.2. PNEUMONIA AND OTHER RESPIRATORY DISEASES CAUSED BY M. PNEUMONIAE

DEFINITION. Pneumonia is the most severe manifestation of respiratory infection with *Mycoplasma pneumoniae*. Bronchitis, pharyngitis, and asymptomatic infections are frequently seen, particularly in young children; pneumonia occurs predominantly among older children and young adults. The disease responds to treatment with the tetracyclines and erythromycins.

HISTORY. A pneumonia that was unlike lobar pneumonia of *Diplococcus pneumoniae* was recognized in the 1930's. Extensive bacteriologic studies failed to reveal a specific etiology in many of these cases, and Dingle and Finland in 1942 applied the term primary atypical pneumonia to this group of nonbacterial pneumonias. In 1943 the discovery that cold hemagglutinins developed in the sera of many of the patients provided a useful diagnostic test. During World War II the Armed Forces Commission on Acute Respiratory Disease described many of the clinical and epidemiologic characteristics of an atypical pneumonia, retrospectively identified by serologic tests as caused by infection with *M. pneumoniae*.

The causative agent was first isolated by Eaton in cotton rats, and subsequently was shown to infect hamsters and chicken embryos. It is filterable and for this reason was considered to be a virus for many years. In 1957, Liu reported an immunofluorescent test for antibody, using sections of infected chicken embryo bronchi for antigen, and Chanock in 1961 reported that the organism was the cause of most cases of pneumonia associated with the development of cold hemagglutinins. Subsequent to these studies and the demonstration that the organism was a *Mycoplasma,* it was given the name *Mycoplasma pneumoniae.*

ETIOLOGY. *Mycoplasma pneumoniae* can readily be distinguished from the seven other known human species of *Mycoplasma*. The organism is about 200 nm in size. It will grow aerobically or anaerobically on artificial media, but the medium must be enriched with 20 per cent horse serum and yeast extract. On solid medium, the small granular colonies grow embedded in the surface of the agar, and are best detected by microscopic examination. Tentative identification procedures utilize the fact that *M. pneumoniae* ferments glucose, exhibits hemadsorption, hemolyzes guinea pig and sheep red blood cells, and is resistant to methylene blue. Final identification requires serologic procedures.

Analysis of the lipids of *M. pneumoniae* has partially explained some of the serologic responses noted in this infection. The protective antigen appears to be a glycolipid contained in the membrane of the organism. A phospholipid which reacts with some Wassermann-positive sera has been identified, and cross-reactions with glycolipids of *Streptococcus* MG and the I antigen of human erythrocytes probably account for these occasional serologic responses. The anti-tissue antibodies noted in this infection may have a similar explanation.

EPIDEMIOLOGY. *M. pneumoniae* infection is endemic in large populations, but numerous localized outbreaks have occurred in schools and military populations. There is no periodicity such as occurs with influenza and no seasonal prevalence as with bacterial and viral respiratory illnesses.

The basic epidemiologic unit is the family, where the infection is often introduced by five- to nine-year-old schoolchildren. Infection spreads slowly but will ultimately involve 80 to 90 per cent of family members who are not immune. Though most common in young schoolage children, the very young, adolescents, and young adults frequently acquire the infection. It is uncommon after age 50, but may occur at any age.

Roentgenographic evidence of pneumonia occurs in 30 to 50 per cent of infected family members, but studies in the military have suggested that less than 10 per cent of infections result in pneumonia. Recent reports suggest that infection may be more common in infants and preschool children than was formerly thought, but pneumonia is uncommon. Thus an age relationship to the likelihood of occurrence of pneumonia exists, but the reasons for this are not clear.

PATHOGENESIS. *M. pneumoniae* is a primary pathogen of the respiratory tract that is spread by close and frequent contact between infected and susceptible persons. The organism can be recovered from sputum and throat swab specimens two to three days prior to onset of illness. Thereafter, the concentration of organisms in secretions rises to the time of occurrence of illness and remains high for four to six days. After illness subsides, the agent may persist in respiratory secretions for several weeks in a considerable percentage of cases, and positive cultures frequently occur after antimicrobial treatment.

The organism grows on the ciliated border and between respiratory epithelial cells. All evidence indicates that it does not invade lung parenchyma. It has been suggested that the peroxide produced by the organism might produce cell damage; more recently it has been suggested that the illness may be a result of hypersensitivity to the organism or one or more of its products as a result of prior mild or asymptomatic infection.

Resistance to infection has been shown to correlate with presence and magnitude of serum antibody. Antibody is detectable in respiratory secretions, and recent data suggest that resistance more closely correlates with this antibody than with serum antibody. The association between antibody and resistance probably accounts for prevalence of the infection in younger age groups, as most adults have higher levels of serum antibody. Nevertheless, reinfection may occur at any age and be accompanied by pneumonia.

PATHOLOGY. From the limited studies available, it is apparent that a great variety of pathologic findings may occur in pneumonia, including patchy or confluent bronchopneumonia, interstitial pneumonia, and lobar pneumonia. Pleuritis with a small pleural effusion may be present, but significant pleural effusion is rare. Macroscopic examination usually reveals patchy areas of lung infiltration and inflamed bronchial and bronchiolar lumina containing mucoid and occasionally purulent exudate. Microscopic sections reveal mononuclear peribronchial and peribronchiolar infiltrates with edema and mononuclear cell infiltration of neighboring alveolar septa. Mucosal cell lining of respiratory passages usually remains intact, and polymorphonuclear cell infiltration is prominent only if necrosis and sloughing of the mucosal cell lining occur. Pathology in other organs of the body has been described for a few patients with evidence of *M. pneumoniae* infection and death as a result of severe hemolysis, encephalitis, myocarditis, or pancreatitis. A predominance of mononuclear cells with edema and sometimes intravascular thrombosis and necrosis characterizes the pathology of involved organs.

CLINICAL MANIFESTATIONS. Infection may be manifested by pneumonia, tracheobronchitis, pharyngitis, or myringitis. Pneumonia is the most serious and best described syndrome. The incubation period to onset of illness is about three weeks, most cases occurring in 15 to 25 days.

Pneumonia. The onset of pneumonia is usually insidious, with malaise and headache as prominent symptoms. For a period of two to three days these symptoms increase in severity, and feverishness, myalgias, and sore throat may also occur. Cough is usually not prominent until two to three days after onset of illness. It is either nonproductive or productive of small amounts of mucoid sputum that occasionally contain flecks of blood. *Despite the delayed appearance of cough, it becomes the dominant respiratory symptom in mycoplasmal pneumonia, and its absence or the occurrence of only mild cough makes a clinical diagnosis questionable.* In some cases cough occurs early, and patients may exhibit the paroxysms, substernal discomfort, and tracheal tenderness characteristic of acute tracheobronchitis. Headache is commonly reported as the most distressing symptom in an adult. Ear discomfort, owing to myringitis, mild nasal symptoms, and prominent sore throat may also occur, especially in the younger age groups. Substernal or diffuse chest discomfort on inspiration is common, but typical pleuritic pain is rare. Arthralgias, anorexia, nausea, and vomiting may also be reported.

Patients usually do not appear seriously ill. Tachypnea, dyspnea, and cyanosis are rare and are not seen unless pulmonary involvement is extensive or other disease is present. Fever is present in virtually all cases of pneumonia; it varies between 37.7 and >40° C, although it is usually under 39° C.

Physical examination usually reveals mild nasal obstruction and discharge and mild to moderate injection of the posterior pharynx. Mild injection of the tympanic membranes is commonly seen, and about 15 per cent of patients will exhibit frank myringitis, some of whom will develop blebs or bullae. Hemorrhage into the blebs or bullae is common, and these patients usually complain of severe ear pain. Tender cervical lymphadenopathy is a common finding, particularly when pharyngitis is also present.

Findings on chest examination may be minimal, and

roentgenographic findings that seem out of proportion to physical findings frequently occur. Auscultation of the chest may reveal rhonchi and wheezes over the involved area of the lung owing to mucus in large bronchi and bronchioles, and fine to medium moist rales may also be heard. In the occasional patient with more extensive disease, signs of consolidation may be detected.

Tracheobronchitis. Tracheobronchitis alone may occur from infection with *M. pneumoniae* and is more common than pneumonia. The onset and clinical picture are little different from that described for pneumonia, and a significant proportion of cases clinically diagnosed as tracheobronchitis will exhibit infiltration when x-rays are obtained. The cases in which the chest x-rays are normal tend to be less severe.

Pharyngitis. Pharyngitis frequently accompanies the tracheobronchitis and pneumonia caused by *M. pneumoniae;* however, pharyngitis alone may also occur. The onset and constitutional manifestations are similar to those described for pneumonia, but sore throat appears early and persists as the predominant symptom. Mild nasal symptoms and some cough may also occur. Pharyngeal examination may reveal a diffusely erythematous pharynx with or without pharyngeal and tonsillar exudate, or only mild pharyngeal congestion may be present. Tender cervical lymph nodes frequently accompany pharyngitis.

Ear Disease. Myringitis, occasionally accompanied by blebs or bullae, is most commonly seen in association with disease of the respiratory tract; however, it has also been reported as an isolated disease occurrence. Such patients complain of ear pain which on occasion may be severe.

ROENTGENOGRAPHIC FINDINGS. No roentgenographic changes can be considered typical of mycoplasmal pneumonia. Infiltrates are usually unilateral, confined to a lower lobe, and more prominent near the hilum. Frequently a single segment is involved, but on occasion the infiltrate may be extensive and lobar or may involve more than one lobe. Small pleural effusions are not uncommon.

LABORATORY FINDINGS. In pneumonia and the other mycoplasmal respiratory diseases, the leukocyte counts are usually within normal limits and rarely exceed 10,000 to 15,000 per cubic millimeter. Differential counts usually reveal slight neutrophilia with counts of 60 to 85 per cent neutrophils. During the period of acute illness lymphopenia may be seen. The erythrocyte sedimentation rate is usually elevated. Urinalysis reveals normal findings except for occasional albuminuria, which may be attributed to fever. Gram stain of sputum may reveal neutrophils without a predominant bacterium, and culture of sputum usually reveals normal flora.

COURSE AND COMPLICATIONS. The clinical course is variable and is best described for pneumonia. Illness on occasion may be severe, but very few deaths from pneumonia have occurred. Fever is variable in duration, lasting from three days to two weeks. Fever usually subsides by lysis, and when this occurs, slow but progressive improvement in the cough, malaise, and lethargy ensues. However, symptoms may persist for three to six weeks. Roentgenographic abnormalities frequently persist for two to four weeks.

Recent reports of hospitalized patients with evidence of *M. pneumoniae* infection have emphasized the severe manifestations the pneumonia may exhibit and the occurrence of a variety of nonrespiratory complications. An accurate estimation of the incidence of these various complications is not available, but they are uncommon. The most common pulmonary *complication* is relapse soon after clinical recovery, and disease may involve the same or a different lobe of the lung. Patients with severe bilateral pneumonia, marked pleural effusions, lung abscess, pneumatoceles, and residual pleural abnormality have also been reported. Clinically apparent intravascular hemolysis in association with demonstrable cold hemagglutinins occurs in a small percentage of patients. Such patients usually exhibit cold hemagglutinin titers of 1:500 or greater and also have demonstrable hemagglutinins at room temperature. Hemolysis usually occurs when fever subsides or chilling of peripheral tissues occurs.

M. pneumoniae has been associated with nervous system and cutaneous disease, although respiratory disease is also usually present. Patients with nervous system disease have had psychosis, meningitis, meningoencephalitis, neuropathy, or cerebellar ataxia. Variable numbers and types of cells have been noted in the cerebrospinal fluid, although mononuclear cells are prominent. Skin manifestations have included urticaria, vesicular eruptions, maculopapular eruptions, erythema multiforme, and erythema nodosum, although many patients were simultaneously receiving drugs, so that causation is not certain. A reported association with Stevens-Johnson syndrome is perhaps of special significance, as these cases are frequently preceded by respiratory symptoms and accompanied by pneumonia. Evidence of *M. pneumoniae* infection should be sought in such cases.

Bronchiectasis, pericarditis, myocarditis, Guillain-Barré syndrome, arthritis, hepatitis, pancreatitis, and thrombocytopenic purpura have also been reported as complications of *M. pneumoniae* infection.

DIAGNOSIS. Early diagnosis can be made only by clinical means. The presence of marked headache, lassitude, myalgias, definite nasopharyngeal findings, and nonproductive cough suggests nonbacterial pneumonia. Absence of the usual features of bacterial pneumonia, such as sudden onset, shaking chlls, pleuritic pain, and purulent or bloody sputum, offers important support for the diagnosis. Other causes of pulmonary infiltration such as tuberculosis, mycotic infection, pulmonary infarction, and malignancy must be considered.

Among the causes of nonbacterial pneumonia that may mimic mycoplasmal pneumonia are psittacosis and Q fever, for which an exposure history should be sought, and adenoviral and influenzal pneumonias, which are usually more acute in onset and occur primarily during recognizable epidemics. If the age of the patient is 5 to 30 years and other similar cases have occurred in a family, diagnosis is more certain, but the only clinical finding that makes mycoplasmal pneumonia almost a certain diagnosis is the additional presence of myringitis with a bleb or bulla on the tympanic membrane.

Isolation of *M. pneumoniae* may be accomplished from sputum or throat swab specimens. Either enriched solid or special liquid medium may be used, although identifiable isolations are not usually detected for at least five days after inoculation, and 14 to 21 days of incubation may be required.

The cold hemagglutinin test is generally available and

useful. Sera of about 50 per cent of patients with *M. pneumoniae* pneumonia will develop a rise in titer of this autoantibody which agglutinates human red blood cells when reacted in the cold (4° C). It is more likely to occur in more severely ill patients, and usually appears toward the end of the first week or the beginning of the second week of illness. *Serum for this test should be separated from red blood cells before refrigeration.* Positive direct Coombs test and an occasional false positive serologic test for syphilis may occur.

A variety of serologic procedures have been described for detecting rise in specific serum antibody titer to *M. pneumoniae* between acute and convalescent sera. Complement fixation is the most available procedure and will demonstrate a rise in titer in 75 to 80 per cent of cases. Growth inhibition and mycoplasmacidal antibody assays are more sensitive but they require experience with cultivation techniques which is not widely available.

TREATMENT. Tetracycline and its derivatives and erythromycin have been shown to hasten the disappearance of fever, rales, and cough in treated cases of pneumonia. Since definitive diagnosis is not possible within the first few days after onset of illness, decisions regarding administration of antimicrobials must be made on clinical grounds. Patients presumed to have mycoplasmal pneumonia should receive tetracycline or its equivalent in doses of 0.25 gram every six hours. Erythromycin in doses of 0.5 gram every eight hours appears to be an acceptable alternative. Incomplete relief of cough, occasional relapse, and continued shedding of the organism frequently follow six- to eight-day courses of treatment with these antimicrobials. It is possible that continuing treatment for two to three weeks will provide more complete recovery, and therefore this duration of treatment is recommended. The additional use of antipyretics, antitussives, intermittent positive pressure breathing, oxygen, and the like is determined by individual needs.

It is recommended that all patients with bullous myringitis be treated with erythromycin or tetracycline for 10 to 14 days. Treatment of patients with pharyngitis and tracheobronchitis on a routine basis is not recommended unless the organism has been isolated, because these illnesses are indistinguishable by clinical techniques from the great majority of acute respiratory illnesses caused by viruses. However, if protracted illness occurs and *M. pneumoniae* has been isolated, the antimicrobials listed above may be used. An effect of antimicrobial therapy on the nonrespiratory complications of *M. pneumoniae* infections has not been shown; indeed, the occasional occurrence of these complications during adequate antimicrobial therapy raises questions regarding the role of the organism in their causation.

PREVENTION. No established method is presently available to prevent *M. pneumoniae* infection. Patients in the acute stage of pneumonia should probably be isolated and attempts made in the home to prevent close contact with ill individuals. There is no vaccine currently available.

Chanock, R.: *Mycoplasma* infections of man. N. Engl. J. Med., 272:1257, 1965.

Couch, R.: *Mycoplasma pneumoniae. In* Knight, V. (ed.): Viral and Mycoplasmal Infections of the Respiratory Tract. Philadelphia. Lea & Febiger, 1973, pp. 217–235.

Hayflick, L. (ed.): The Mycoplasmatales and the L-phase of Bacteria. New York, Appleton-Century-Crofts, 1969.

Mufson, M., Manko, M., Kingston, J., and Chanock, R.: Eaton agent pneumonia: Clinical features. J.A.M.A, 178:369, 1961.

Murray, H., Masur, H., Senterfit, L., and Roberts, R.: The protean manifestations of *Mycoplasma pneumoniae* infection in adults. Am. J. Med., 58:229, 1975.

120.3. MYCOPLASMAS IN GENITOURINARY DISEASE

ETIOLOGY. *Mycoplasma hominis* and *Ureaplasma urealyticum* (T-mycoplasmas) may cause genitourinary disease. *M. hominis* typically produces colonies on agar with the often-described "fried-egg" appearance. Colonies are usually 200 to 300 μ in diameter and are best visualized by microscopy. This colony size contrasts to that of the T-mycoplasmas, which is 10 to 30 μ in diameter. On agar medium *M. hominis* grows well under aerobic conditions, whereas T-mycoplasmas grow best anaerobically. Both grow well in broth, and tentative identification procedures employ the preferential metabolism of arginine by *M. hominis* and the fact that T-mycoplasmas possess a urease system and grow best in an acidic medium. The T-mycoplasmas are antigenically heterogeneous, and the number and significance of types or subtypes has not yet been delineated. A recent report suggests that *M. hominis* is also antigenically heterogeneous.

EPIDEMIOLOGY. The genital mycoplasmas may be recovered from the distal urethra of both the male and female and the vulva, vagina, and cervix of the latter. Presumably because of intimate association with mucosal surfaces, specimens that contain epithelial cells are superior to urine or secretion specimens for isolation tests.

Infants may become colonized with genital mycoplasmas at birth, presumably acquiring them from the birth canal. The frequency of recovery of organisms decreases for the first year or two of life, and most individuals then remain free of genital mycoplasmas until puberty. Mycoplasmas then reappear, and frequencies are directly proportional to extent of sexual activity and promiscuity, suggesting the possibility of infection being acquired venereally.

Despite the fact that genital mycoplasmas are commonly recovered from the urogenital tract, disease is uncommon. This suggests a low order of pathogenicity for these organisms.

CLINICAL MANIFESTATIONS.   **Nonspecific Urethritis.** The syndrome of dysuria, urgency, and frequency of urination with urethral discharge and without evidence of gonococcal infection has been called nonspecific or nongonococcal urethritis. A negative urine culture for bacteria and absence of prostatitis if the patient is a male are essential supportive findings. Patients with postgonococcal urethritis in which the gonococcus disappears but symptoms of urethritis remain are also included in this category of patients. The urethritis may be caused by a T-mycoplasma but apparently not by *M. hominis* (chlamydiae are the most likely alternative to T-mycoplasmas) (see Ch. 139).

Pelvic Inflammatory Disease. Patients with lower abdominal pain and fever who exhibit tenderness on movement of the cervix and in the adnexal areas are usually designated as having pelvic inflammatory disease. In most instances acute or subacute salpingitis is present, although tubo-ovarian abscesses or pelvic abscesses elsewhere may present similar findings. *M. hominis* may cause the disease in many of these cases.

Cervicitis and vaginitis as separate disease entities may occasionally be caused by *M. hominis,* although the data are inconclusive in this regard.

Mycoplasmal Disease in Pregnancy. Both *M. hominis* and the T-mycoplasmas have been recovered from the uterus, amnion, and fetus. Infection is more likely to occur with *M. hominis* than with T-mycoplasmas and to occur during therapeutic or spontaneous abortion, or when premature rupture of the membranes has occurred. Blood cultures are occasionally positive, and such patients exhibit fever and serum antibody responses. The frequency and significance of mycoplasmal infection of the uterus and products of conception are uncertain, but it seems probable that *M. hominis* is responsible for some cases of spontaneous abortion and puerperal infection. Infertility, infant low birth weight, and fetal death have been attributed to mycoplasma infection, but a causative relationship has not been established.

Postpartum fever in patients with normal pregnancy and delivery may occasionally be caused by invasion of the bloodstream with *M. hominis* or T-mycoplasma. The frequency of such cases attributable to mycoplasmas is apparently low.

TREATMENT. All mycoplasmas are susceptible to the tetracyclines. *M. hominis* is susceptible to lincomycin and resistant to erythromycin, whereas the converse is true for the T-mycoplasmas. Patients with nonspecific urethritis should receive tetracycline or its equivalent in doses of 0.25 gram every six hours for five to seven days. Although T-mycoplasmas are also susceptible to erythromycin, results of treatment have been somewhat better with tetracycline. Failure to respond may be attributable to resistance of the infecting strain to tetracycline, a recently reported finding of uncertain frequency. When erythromycin is used for therapy of nonspecific urethritis, patients should receive 0.5 gram every eight hours for five to seven days. Relapse and/or reinfection occurs in about 20 per cent of patients within three months. Second courses of the drug are frequently beneficial, but the sexual contacts of such patients should be examined for T-mycoplasmas. Unexplained recurrent nonspecific urethritis is an indication for urologic evaluation for structural abnormality of the urethra.

Since pelvic inflammatory disease may be caused by gonococci, *M. hominis,* and perhaps other bacteria, and since the site of disease is not accessible for obtaining culture specimens, antimicrobial therapy directed toward the specific cause is often not possible. In nonhospitalized patients tetracycline has been reported to be effective treatment. In most instances of postpartum fever associated with mycoplasmas, spontaneous cure without specific antimycoplasmal therapy occurs. Patients considered as candidates for treatment should receive tetracycline in doses noted above.

McCormack, W. M., Braun, P., Lee, Y. H., Klein, J. O., and Kass, E. H.: The genital mycoplasmas. N. Engl. J. Med., 288:78, 1973.

121. PNEUMOCOCCAL PNEUMONIA

Edward W. Hook

DEFINITION. Pneumococcal pneumonia is an acute bacterial infection of the lungs caused by *Streptococcus pneumoniae* (the pneumococcus) and characterized clinically by an abrupt onset, rigor, fever, chest pain, cough, and bloody sputum. Bacterial pneumonia occurring in otherwise healthy persons is usually caused by the pneumococcus.

BACTERIOLOGY AND IMMUNOLOGY. The somatic portion of the lancet-shaped pneumococcal cell is gram positive. In its virulent form (smooth, S), the pneumococcus has an outer capsule consisting of a high molecular weight polysaccharide polymer that is specific for each serologic type. In addition to the type-specific capsular antigen, there is a species-specific carbohydrate in the cell wall, known as the "C" substance. The capsule of pneumococcus acts as an armor against phagocytic cells and thus contributes significantly to the pathogenicity of the organism. Pneumococcal variants having no capsules (rough, R strains) are essentially avirulent. Antibody to the type-specific carbohydrate promotes phagocytosis by combining with the highly polymerized polysaccharide of the capsular gel. The pneumococcus also produces hyaluronidase, a hemolysin that causes greenish discoloration around colonies on blood agar, and autolytic enzymes that, when activated, render the organism gram negative and eventually cause its dissolution.

Pneumococci grow rapidly on a variety of bacteriologic media. Blood agar and beef infusion broth containing 0.5 per cent dextrose and 5 per cent blood or serum are the media most commonly used. On blood agar virulent strains form circular, glistening, dome-shaped colonies that are alpha hemolytic. Because of the great quantity of capsular polysaccharide formed by type 3 pneumococcus, its colonies are more mucoid and usually much larger than those of other types. Unlike other alpha-hemolytic streptococci, the pneumococcus is soluble in bile, sodium deoxycholate, and other surface-active agents, is highly sensitive to ethyl hydrocuprein chloride (optochin), and, with a few exceptions, is mouse virulent.

The extraordinary virulence of pneumococci for mice may be made use of in isolating the organisms from sputum. The technique usually used consists in injecting intraperitoneally 0.5 ml of sputum previously emulsified by having been drawn repeatedly into a tuberculin syringe. When virulent pneumococci are present, the mouse usually dies within 48 hours, and a pure culture of the organism can be isolated from the heart's blood. Since other bacteria in the sputum do not ordinarily produce fatal infections in mice, the animal serves as a convenient and highly sensitive differential "culture medium" for the isolation of pneumococci.

At least 85 different serologic types of pneumococci have been identified by agglutination tests with specific antiserums or by the quellung test. The latter is based upon the fact that when pneumococci come in contact with homologous capsular antibody, a capsular precipitin reaction and swelling occur, rendering the capsule easily visible under the microscope.

Specific polysaccharide, which has diffused away from the bacteria, can often be identified in the sputum, blood, or urine of patients with pneumococcal pneumonia. The lungs of patients with extensive pneumonia may contain up to 2 grams of capsular polysaccharide. The detection of these bacterial antigens in clinical specimens by counterimmunoelectrophoresis is gaining acceptance as a sensitive method for the rapid (e.g., two hours) diagnosis of infection.

Anticapsular antibody usually appears in the blood of patients with pneumococcal pneumonia between the fifth and tenth days of the disease. In some untreated patients, its appearance coincides with recovery; in others no such relation is demonstrable. The development of measurable type-specific antibody is delayed in patients with antigenemia detectable by counterimmunoelectrophoresis.

EPIDEMIOLOGY. Pneumococcal pneumonia may occur at any season, but it is most common during the winter and early spring, when viral respiratory infections are most prevalent.

The types of pneumococci that most commonly cause pneumonia in adults in the United States are types 1, 3, 4, 6, 7, 8, 12, 14, 18, and 19. Together, these ten types account for about three quarters of all cases. The most common types encountered in childhood pneumonias are 1, 6, 14, 19, and 23.

Pneumococci, particularly of the higher types, are frequently present in the respiratory tracts of normal subjects. Ordinarily the prevalence of carriers of highly pathogenic types is relatively low, except for type 3, which is a common inhabitant of the normal pharynx. Nevertheless, there is evidence that normal carriers play a more important role in the dissemination of infective types than do patients ill with pneumonia. Occasionally, in relatively closed communities, high carrier rates of pathogenic types are encountered. In such circumstances the occurrence of widespread viral disease of the respiratory tract may result in an epidemic of pneumococcal pneumonia. Except for these rare epidemics, most of which occur in hospitals or custodial institutions, the disease is sporadic.

PATHOGENESIS AND PATHOLOGY. The lung is the only major viscus of the body exposed to air. As the atmosphere, particularly in congested places, contains many pathogenic bacteria, it is remarkable that pneumonia is not more common. The failure of normal subjects to acquire acute bacterial pneumonia as an airborne infection is due to efficient defense barriers of the lower respiratory tract. These barriers include (1) the epiglottal reflex, which prevents aspiration of infected secretions; (2) the sticky mucus that lines the bronchial tree and to which airborne organisms adhere; (3) the cilia of the respiratory epithelium, which keep the mucus moving constantly toward the pharynx at the rate of 1 to 3 cm per hour; (4) the cough reflex, which serves to propel mucus or foreign bodies out of the lower tract; (5) the lymphatics that drain the terminal bronchi and bronchioles; (6) phagocytic cells, especially alveolar macrophages that are ever present in the normal alveoli; and (7) opsonins and specific antibody. In addition, the alveoli themselves are relatively dry and thus offer a poor medium for growth of bacteria that succeed in reaching them. Acute bacterial pneumonia results only when the defense barriers of the normal respiratory tract fail (see Ch. 119).

The thesis that bacterial pneumonia usually results from aspiration of infected secretions from the upper respiratory tract is strongly supported by both experimental and clinical observations. Rats infected with pneumococci in the nasopharynx regularly exhibit pulmonary lesions only when subjected to experimental procedures involving chilling of the body, anesthesia,

administration of morphine, or alcoholic intoxication, all of which are predisposing factors in human pneumonia and have been shown in laboratory animals to slow the epiglottal reflex and thus to facilitate aspiration. Experimental pneumonia can best be produced by intrabronchial inoculation of organisms suspended in mixtures of gastric mucin or starch having viscosities similar to that of mucus. Viral infection of the upper respiratory tract in man usually precedes the onset of acute bacterial pneumonia by several days. Not only is the volume of secretion from the nasopharynx greater than normal during viral infections such as the common cold, but also the number of pathogenic microorganisms in the secretions is significantly increased. Thus the stage is set for aspiration of infected mucus. That such aspiration often occurs at the onset of pneumonia in man is suggested by the usual sites of initial involvement of the lung. The earliest lesions of bacterial pneumonia usually appear in those parts of the lungs into which aspirated fluid is most likely to drain. Whereas most airborne bacteria are caught on the sticky surfaces of the bronchial tree and never reach the alveoli, organisms contained in thin nasopharyngeal secretions are readily carried into the alveoli by the liquid mucus. The latter, like Lipiodol, cannot all be ejected by ciliary action, and much of it penetrates to the farthest reaches of the bronchial tree, where it establishes the initial focus of infection.

Other factors known to predispose patients to acute bacterial pneumonia include exposure to noxious gases and anesthetics, cardiac failure, influenza viral infection of the lungs, and trauma to the thorax. A feature common to all these conditions is the accumulation of fluid in the alveoli. Harford (1950) has shown that the dry lungs of normal mice are able to rid themselves of large numbers of inspired bacteria, whereas lungs containing fluid are readily infected. This observation suggests that pulmonary edema, by providing a suitable culture medium for the bacteria, may facilitate the establishment of active infection within the alveoli. Influenza also causes destruction of the ciliated columnar epithelial cells lining the tracheobronchial tree, thus interfering with function of cilia. In addition, influenza virus also apparently inhibits phagocytosis.

Pneumococcal pneumonia may also occur as a complication of bronchogenic carcinoma, chronic pulmonary disease, such as bronchiectasis or lung abscess, or any process that produces obstruction of a bronchus.

Splenectomy carries an increased risk of severe bacteremic infections which are predominantly although not exclusively pneumococcal in etiology. The clinical course is often fulminant, frequently associated with evidence of diffuse intravascular coagulation and a high mortality rate. Although it appears that even healthy adults with post-traumatic splenectomies show increased susceptibility, the risk is greatest in infants and young children, in patients with underlying diseases which compromise reticuloendothelial function, and during the early postsplenectomy years. The mechanism of this relationship is unknown, but it appears that the spleen is important in removing encapsulated bacteria in the absence of antibody.

Persons with sickle cell anemia and other sickle hemoglobinopathies are especially vulnerable to severe pneumococcal infections, especially meningitis. The pneumococcus, not *Hemophilus influenzae*, is the most common cause of bacteremia and meningitis in children with sickle cell anemia. The factors accounting for this relationship are probably multiple and include deficiency of heat-labile opsonins which is secondary to a defect in the function of the alternative complement pathway (see Ch. 39), functional asplenia in some instances and actual splenic atrophy in others, and impaired phagocytic and killing capacity of reticuloendothelial cells.

In patients with severe pneumococcal infection with bacteremia and pneumonia or extrapulmonary sites of infection in cerebrospinal, pleural, or peritoneal fluids, the frequency of some other underlying disease exceeds 50 per cent. The incidence of pneumococcal pneumonia is increased in patients with hypogammaglobulinemia or multiple myeloma.

Early Lesion. Once the infection has gained a foothold within the alveoli, the lesion evolves in a characteristic manner. The first response of the lung to bacterial invasion is an outpouring of edema fluid into the alveoli which serves to "float" organisms into new alveoli through the pores of Kohn and terminal bronchioles. Centrifugal spread of infection occurs. After the outpouring of edema fluid, polymorphonuclear leukocytes and some erythrocytes accumulate in the infected alveoli, first in small numbers but later in such quantities as to fill each alveolus and thus render the area completely consolidated. Once the infected alveoli become crowded with leukocytes, phagocytosis of bacteria takes place, and the invading organisms are destroyed. Macrophages appear in the exudate, and resolution begins only after most of the organisms have been ingested.

Spreading Lesion. Three stages in the inflammatory reaction account for the distinguishing histologic features of the spreading pneumonic lesion. In the outermost portion there appears an "edema zone" in which the alveoli are filled with serous fluid containing only bacteria. Inside the edema zone a second zone may be identified in which there are signs of early consolidation with leukocytes in most of the alveoli. Here phagocytosis is often noted. Still more centrally a third transition to a "zone of advanced consolidation" is noted where the alveoli are packed with cells and where beginning resolution may be evident.

All stages of inflammation can be found in a spreading lesion. In the most recently invaded areas at the periphery, edema and hemorrhage predominate, causing "red hepatization," whereas in the older, more central parts of the lesion, dense consolidation with leukocytes accounts for the characteristic color of "gray hepatization."

Pneumococcal pneumonia may involve a lobe or segment of the lung, or lesions may be patchy in distribution and concentrated particularly about the bronchi. Bronchopneumonia is especially common in infants, the elderly, and persons with other lung diseases such as chronic obstructive pulmonary disease. Because a clearcut distinction between pneumococcal bronchopneumonia and lobar pneumonia cannot always be made even by the pathologist, and because management for the two conditions is the same, it is rarely important for the clinician to differentiate them. The etiology rather than the anatomy of the lesion determines therapy.

Interlobar Spread. The spread of the pneumonic process may be stopped by the pleural boundaries of the lobe. Often, however, the infection spreads to other lobes of the lungs by flow of infected edema fluid from bronchi of the involved lung into the bronchial tree of a new lobe.

Bacteremia. Bacteremia is common during the course of pneumococcal pneumonia, particularly when the infection is fulminating. The fact that organisms appear in the thoracic duct in experimental pneumonia before they appear in the systemic circulation suggests that the bacteria reach the bloodstream via the lymphatics. Blood cultures are positive in 20 to 30 per cent of patients with pneumococcal pneumonia. The prevalence of bacteremia increases with age, and is more common with type 2 pneumonia and less common with type 3 pneumonia than with other pneumococcal types.

Invasion of Pleura and Pericardium. The exact mechanism whereby pneumococci invade the pleura or pericardium is not known. As the lymphatics at the periphery of the lung drain outward toward the pleura, it is possible that the pleural invasion results from lymphangitic spread. When infection of a pleural or pericardial cavity occurs, there results an outpouring of serous fluid followed by the deposit of fibrin. Leukocytes accumulate in the infected cavity, and, if infection persists, a purulent focus results. The pus in such cavities is at first thin but later becomes thick and stringy as a result not only of fibrin formation but also of the presence of deoxyribonucleic acid derived from the nuclei of disintegrating leukocytes. Finally, the thick fibrinous pus becomes walled off, forming loculated foci of chronic suppuration.

Similar purulent foci may occur in the meninges, peritoneum, or joints, as a result of hematogenous spread. Acute vegetations on the endocardium of the heart valves are sometimes encountered. Children with nephrotic syndrome are more prone to pneumococcal peritonitis than normal children. Pneumococcal peritonitis also occurs as a complication of hepatic cirrhosis with ascites.

Mechanism of Recovery. Surface Phagocytosis. Owing to the antiphagocytic properties of their capsules, fully encapsulated, virulent pneumococci are resistant to phagocytosis when suspended in a fluid medium devoid of opsonins. In the presence of relatively immovable cellular surfaces, however, as in the alveoli, leukocytes are able to trap the encapsulated organisms and ingest them without the aid of opsonizing antibody.

Heat-Labile Opsonins. Leukocytes in vivo are also assisted, right from the start of infection, by heat-labile opsonins that are present in normal plasma. These opsonins, which gain access to acute inflammatory exudates, are immunologically polyspecific, i.e., they act on all sorts of bacteria, in contrast to the monospecific anticapsular antibody that is eventually generated. In nonimmune individuals the majority of serum opsonizing activity for pneumococci results from alternative pathway activation of C3 and C5 and fixation of the cleavage products C3b and C5b to the surface of the organism.

Anticapsular Opsonins. Most patients with pneumococcal pneumonia who survive long enough eventually generate an excess of monospecific anticapsular antibody. The process usually takes five to ten days. These newly formed immunoglobulins not only agglutinate the pneumococci in the edema zone of the lesion and thereby inhibit their spread, but also act as potent accessory opsonins and further increase the efficiency of phagocytosis.

a, Pneumococci in edema-filled alveoli at margin of spreading pneumonic lesion (×800).

b, Beginning stage of polymorphonuclear exudation in zone of early consolidation. Note leukocytes in alveolar capillaries, some in process of diapedesis (×800).

c, Leukocyte exudate (still predominantly polymorphonuclear) in inner zone of advanced consolidation. Pneumococci have been phagocytized and destroyed (×800).

d, Alveolar macrophage reaction characteristic of late stage of resolution (×800).

e, Pneumococci in edema fluid contained within lumen of a large bronchus. Such infected bronchial fluid causes spread of pneumonia to other lobes of the lungs (×1250).

f–i, Surface phagocytosis of encapsulated microorganisms in formalin-fixed rat lung (×1250). Bacteria shown in these photomicrographs are klebsiellae, but same results have been obtained with pneumococci.

f, Polymorphonuclear leukocyte is seen approaching bacteria near alveolar wall. Time 12:30.

g, Leukocyte has reached alveolar wall and is about to trap organisms against the tissue surface. Time 12:31.

h, Cell has trapped some of the encapsulated bacteria against the wall and is in the process of phagocytizing them. Time 12:32.

i, Having ingested several of the organisms, the leukocyte is moving up the alveolar wall. Time 12:35.

(Photomicrographs from studies on experimental pneumonia. W. B. Wood et al.: J. Exp. Med., Vol. 73; and Smith and Wood: *ibid.*, Vol. 86.)

MACROPHAGE REACTION. The exact role of the "macrophage reaction" in the recovery process is not entirely clear. Because the appearance of macrophages in the alveolar exudate coincides in general with the disappearance of organisms from the lesion, it has long been assumed that these large mononuclear phagocytes take an active part in destroying the bacteria, and in the final analysis tip the scales in favor of the cellular defenses of the host. Studies relating to experimental lymphadenitis cast some doubt upon this assumption. The "macrophage reaction" in a regional lymph node draining an area of active infection can be artificially initiated at any stage of the nodal inflammation by merely cutting the afferent lymph vessels bringing bacteria to the node. Thus it appears that macrophages accumulate in the exudate only when the active stimulus of direct bacterial invasion has been eliminated. If this interpretation is correct, the polymorphonuclear leukocytes may be looked upon as the "shock troops" that play the major role in controlling the infection, whereas the macrophages serve primarily to remove the particulate debris from the resolving exudate and thus promote clearing of the lesion.

RESOLUTION. One of the most remarkable features of pneumococcal pneumonia is the completeness with which it resolves. Even when several lobes are completely consolidated, recovery usually results in restoration of the entire pulmonary parenchyma to its normal state within a few weeks. Not all the processes that take part in this dramatic resolution have been identified, but they include (1) the action of cytolytic enzymes upon disintegrating leukocytes; (2) transport of cells from the lesion via lymphatics; and (3) phagocytosis and digestion of cellular debris by macrophages. The rarity with which tissue necrosis occurs in pneumococcal pneumonia, despite the violence of the inflammatory response, appears to account for the completeness of the healing. Occasionally recovery proceeds more slowly than usual and leads to "delayed resolution." The factors responsible for delaying the removal of exudate from the lesion in such cases are not known. In rare instances, as the result of irreversible damage to the pulmonary parenchyma, resolution fails to take place altogether, and the lesion becomes the site of intense fibroblastic activity that leads to permanent scarring or "organized pneumonia."

Infection with type 3 pneumococcus may occasionally lead to pulmonary necrosis and abscess formation. This pneumococcus has a large capsule that interferes with phagocytosis and accounts, at least in part, for its extraordinary pathogenicity.

SUPPURATIVE EXTRAPULMONARY FOCI. Suppurative pneumococcal lesions, which occur in such extrapulmonary sites as the pleura, pericardium, meninges, joints, mastoids, or accessory sinuses, resolve much less readily, even with intensive chemotherapy, than does uncomplicated pneumococcal pneumonia. In such areas of suppuration, phagocytosis appears to be relatively inefficient, because trapping of bacteria by leukocytes in the exudate is inefficient and many of the leukocytes in the exudate are not viable. Although a drug like penicillin may reach the organisms in a purulent focus, it may not destroy them, because pneumococci do not multiply rapidly in pus of long standing, and "resting" bacteria are not susceptible to the bactericidal action of penicillin. In fact, suppurative pneumococcal lesions may respond satisfactorily only when chemotherapy is combined with some form of drainage that removes the bulk of the necrotic exudate.

CLINICAL MANIFESTATIONS. Symptoms. Victims of pneumococcal pneumonia are often seriously ill when first seen. The degree of prostration may be such that an adequate history can be obtained only from the family. The story of a mild nasopharyngitis preceding by several days the onset of major symptoms is frequently elicited. The first distressing symptom is usually a shaking chill, lasting for several minutes to a half hour. More than 80 per cent of patients with pneumococcal pneumonia experience one or more chills during the earliest stages of the disease. The initial rigor is often so violent as to cause the bed to shake and the patient's teeth to chatter. It is followed in about one case in three by vomiting. The initial chill usually coincides with bacterial invasion of the lung and marks the onset of fever. Several chills may occur at the start of pneumococcal pneumonia, but repeated attacks of rigor late in the disease suggest an extrapulmonary complication such as empyema, pneumonia caused by some other bacterium, or administration of antipyretics.

CHEST PAIN. In approximately 70 per cent of cases, severe chest pain occurs at the onset and may even precede the rigor. The pain, which is "stabbing" in character and exaggerated by cough and respiration, is caused by inflammation of the pleura resulting from the characteristically peripheral location of the initial lesion. There may be local tenderness in the chest wall at the site of the pleurisy. When the diaphragmatic surfaces of the pleura are affected, the pain may be referred either to the corresponding side of the lower chest wall and upper abdomen or to the shoulder. The patient may gain some relief from the knifelike pain by lying on the affected side on a firm surface, thereby splinting that half of the thorax.

COUGH. A cough may be absent at the onset, but usually is a prominent symptom during the course of the disease. Stimulation of the cough reflex results from irritation of the lower respiratory tract and from accumulation of mucus and exudate within the bronchial tree. Approximately 75 per cent of patients raise diffusely bloody or "rusty" sputum in contrast to "blood-streaked" sputum. The thorough mixing of the blood appears to be due to the fact that bleeding occurs directly into the alveolar exudate and thus constitutes an integral part of the inflammatory response to the infection. When the sputum is particularly sticky or jelly-like, type 3 pneumococcus or *Klebsiella* should be suspected, because both these organisms produce an inordinate amount of capsular polysaccharide that causes the exudate to be highly viscous.

FEVER AND TOXEMIA. Constant features of the disease are fever and toxemia, with the temperature usually ranging between 39.5 and 41° C. During the febrile period complaints of malaise, anorexia, weakness, myalgia, and general prostration are extremely common. Pneumococcal pneumonia may occasionally progress with great rapidity, and the general condition of the patient may deteriorate alarmingly within a few hours.

Physical Signs. Patients with well-established pneumococcal pneumonia appear acutely ill. There is moderate to severe respiratory distress. The nostrils dilate with each inspiration. Paroxysms of hacking cough, often productive of bloody or rusty sputum, occur during the examination. The chest pain, which is usually unilateral, may be so severe as to interfere with the patient's breathing and coughing; in these circumstances grunting expiration results. The location of the pain indicates immediately the approximate site of at least part of the lesion. The patient occasionally appears apprehensive and may even be delirious.

The temperature, pulse rate, and respiratory rate are usually elevated by the time the patient seeks the aid of a physician. The temperature should be taken by rectum, because oral measurement with the subject breathing rapidly through the mouth is likely to be inaccurate. The pulse pressure is characteristically widened, as in any high fever.

The skin is usually hot and moist, with beads of perspiration visible on the face and forehead. Cold extremities may indicate impending shock. Herpetic blisters are frequently noted about the mouth. The lips, mucous membranes, and nail beds are often cyanotic as a result of blood passing through poorly aerated lung. The cyanosis may be exaggerated by lowered respiratory exchange associated with rapid shallow breathing, often resulting from pleural pain. Icterus of the sclerae should be carefully looked for because of the prognostic significance of overt jaundice in pneumonia.

The ears should always be examined with an otoscope to exclude the presence of active otitis. Tenderness over a mastoid process or over an accessory nasal sinus should also be noted. The presence of exudate in the pharynx or over the tonsils suggests the possibility of streptococcal or adenoviral pneumonia. Definite nuchal rigidity may indicate pneumococcal meningitis, a serious complication of pneumonia. The neck veins must be carefully examined to detect the presence of increased venous pressure caused by complicating congestive heart failure. Deviation of the trachea constitutes an important sign of either atelectasis (toward the involved side) or pleural effusion (away from the involved side).

EXAMINATION OF THE CHEST. Diminished respiratory excursion or a slight inspiratory lag of one side of the chest often reveals the side of the principal lesion. A localized area of tenderness in the chest wall, noted during percussion, may be one of the earliest signs of pleural invasion. Careful percussion and auscultation do not always reveal signs of consolidation. In early cases, particularly, there may be no conclusive physical signs. Lesions at a distance from the chest wall are difficult to outline by percussion. When consolidation is extensive, the typical findings of dullness to percussion, bronchial or tubular breath sounds, and fine crackling rales are easily elicited, except in the presence of complicating bronchial obstruction or extensive pleural effusion. A coarse "leathery" friction rub is frequently audible in the region of consolidation.

Examination of the heart may be difficult because of loud respiratory sounds. An apical systolic murmur is frequently heard during high fever and is often of no significance. Diastolic murmurs, on the other hand, arising from either the mitral or aortic valve, are usually indicative of underlying organic heart disease or complicating pneumococcal endocarditis. A pericardial friction rub often constitutes the first sign of spread of the pneumococcal infection to the pericardial cavity. Ventricular premature contractions are not uncommon in the presence of any moderate or severe infection.

ABDOMINAL DISTENTION. Distention of the abdomen is frequently encountered. When tympany is noted in the left axilla and left upper quadrant, acute gastrectasia should be suspected. Occasionally, the examiner will note rigidity and even tenderness in one or both upper quadrants of the abdomen, suggesting a subdiaphragmatic lesion. This sign is usually due to referred pain resulting from involvement of the parietal pleura over the outer part of the diaphragm.

Digital examination of the rectum may be postponed if the patient is acutely ill, but in women a sufficiently complete pelvic examination should be performed to exclude the possibility of an infected abortion, which may lead to metastatic bacterial pneumonia. The neurologic examination is rarely abnormal in pneumococcal pneumonia except in the presence of meningitis or brain abscess.

LABORATORY FINDINGS. As in most acute bacterial infections, the total leukocyte count in pneumococcal pneumonia is elevated, and there is a "shift to the left" in the differential count. The number of leukocytes in the peripheral blood during the active infection usually ranges from 10,000 to 25,000 per cubic millimeter; counts above 40,000 are occasionally encountered. Leukopenia (with a "shift to the left") is observed in fulminating pneumococcal infections, particularly in the presence of bacteremia and in alcoholics.

Although the presence and location of the pulmonary lesion can usually be determined by physical examination, confirmatory roentgenographic evidence is often helpful. Both posteroanterior and lateral views of the chest should be taken. Pneumococcal infection of the lungs usually begins in the right middle lobe or in one of the lower lobes. The pulmonary process is limited to a single lobe in the majority of patients. In fact, it is not unusual for the process to be limited to a single pulmonary segment. In the series of Austrian and Gold, collected since the introduction of antimicrobial drugs, fewer than one third of the patients with pneumococcal pneumonia and bacteremia had more than a single lobe involved. Bulging interlobar fissure may be observed occasionally in pneumococcal pneumonia, although it is much more characteristic of Friedländer's pneumonia.

Whenever the diagnosis of pneumococcal pneumonia is suspected, the patient's blood should be cultured. Anaerobic as well as aerobic cultures are recommended to aid detection of pneumonia caused by a microbe other than pneumococcus. A blood culture positive for pneumococci provides important information regarding both etiology and prognosis.

Pneumococci are usually present in sputum, nasopharynx, and material aspirated from the trachea. Sputum for smear and culture may be difficult to obtain, but this usually can be accomplished by urging the patient to cough, or a paroxysm of cough can be induced by passing a nasal catheter into the trachea. If a sputum specimen cannot be obtained, a nasopharyngeal culture should be collected, because there is a high positive correlation between specific pneumococci isolated from cultures of the nasopharynx and from the sputum of patients with pneumococcal pneumonia. Transtracheal aspiration or lung puncture is not indicated for the diagnosis of bacterial pneumonia in the usual patient.

The sputum in pneumococcal pneumonia shows large numbers of gram-positive, lancet-shaped diplococci in association with polymorphonuclear leukocytes. Gram-positive cocci which are not pneumococci are frequently observed in sputum smears and account for the poor correlation of results of studies to identify pneumococci on Gram-stained sputum smears and on sputum cultures. Omniserum, a pool of antibody against 84 of the known 85 pneumococcal types, can be used for definitive identification of pneumococci in sputum. The results of the quellung reaction with omniserum correlate with the results of cultures in about 90 per cent of cases. Because the carrier rate of pneumococci in the general population may be quite high, positive identification of pneumococci in sputum or nasopharynx does not establish a definitive diagnosis of pneumococcal pneumonia.

The technique of counterimmunoelectrophoresis for detection of specific polysaccharides in sputum, blood, or body fluids can be helpful in establishing definitive diagnosis, even in patients who have received antimicrobial therapy. Capsular antigens persist in secretions or fluids rendered sterile by antimicrobial drugs. Antigen can be detected in the sputum of the majority of patients with pneumococcal pneumonia, but positive results may also be obtained in patients with bronchitis without pneumonia. Circulating polysaccharide can be detected in the blood of at least one half of patients with pneumococcal bacteremia but much less often in the absence of demonstrable bacteremia. The concentration of polysaccharide in the circulation declines progressively during antimicrobial therapy, but circulating antigen remains detectable in two thirds of the patients with antigenemia for two weeks or longer.

Other laboratory examinations that may be of value in the management of the patient include hematocrit, blood electrolyte, and urea determinations.

CLINICAL COURSE. During the course of the disease the patient should be examined carefully once a day. More frequent physical examinations may unduly exhaust an acutely ill subject. The common complications of pneumococcal pneumonia should be specifically looked for during each examination, particularly when fever persists.

Defervescence. The fever of untreated pneumococcal pneumonia either may terminate abruptly by "crisis" five to ten days after onset or may gradually subside by lysis. When effective antibacterial therapy is used, a dramatic crisis may occur within 24 hours, or the fever may persist for several days. Physical signs in the chest may also change, coarse sticky rales of resolution replacing the fine crepitant rales and tubular breath sounds of consolidation. Complete clearing of the pulmonary lesion may occur within a few days, but usually the auscultatory signs of resolution persist for a week or more after defervescence. If resolution is not complete within 21 days, it is arbitrarily classified as delayed. The promptness of defervescence and the speed of resolution are in general inversely proportional to the age and extent of the lesion at the time treatment is begun. There is a high incidence of protracted illness and delayed resolution of pulmonary infiltrates in patients with polysaccharide antigenemia which persists for more than three weeks.

Crisis marking the start of recovery must be differentiated from the "pseudocrisis" occasionally noted at the onset of shock or at the time of interlobar spread of the infection. Although the temperature may fall precipitously during a pseudocrisis, the pulse rate remains elevated, and the patient's general condition fails to improve.

Relapse. Relapse may occur in pneumococcal pneumonia when chemotherapy is discontinued too soon. If fever, tachycardia, and other signs of active infection recur while the patient is still receiving penicillin therapy, it may usually be assumed that a previously unrecognized purulent complication of the pneumococcal infection (such as empyema) exists, that a drug-resistant secondary invader has gained a foothold in the lung, that hypersensitivity of the patient to penicillin has caused the development of drug fever, or that the diagnosis of pneumococcal pneumonia is incorrect.

COMPLICATIONS. Pleural Effusion. The most common specific complication of pneumococcal pneumonia is pleurisy with effusion. In somewhat less than 10 per cent of cases, fluid can be demonstrated in the pleural cavity by either physical or roentgenographic examination. Such effusions are usually small, and, when sterile, are rarely of significance. They result from inflammation of the pleura overlying the lesion in the lung. Occasionally they may be of sufficient volume to cause respiratory embarrassment and necessitate thoracentesis. Whenever pleural effusion is detected in a patient who has failed to respond promptly to treatment, a thoracentesis should be performed to determine whether the fluid is infected and thus represents an early empyema.

Empyema. Empyema, though less common than sterile pleural effusion, is far more serious. Before the advent of chemotherapy, the incidence of this complication was approximately 5 per cent. With the use of penicillin, empyema is much less common (less than 2 per cent). Its presence is indicated by continued fever (often irregular), persistent leukocytosis, and signs of pleural effusion. Localized tenderness is frequently noted in the chest wall overlying the site of the lesion. The exudate in the pleural cavity may become loculated by thick, fibrinous adhesions. When the lesion is confined to an interlobar fissure or is located in the thoracic "gutter" adjacent to the spine, it may be detectable only by roentgenographic methods. Repeated exploratory thoracenteses, done preferably with the help of fluoroscopy, may be required to prove the presence of empyema. Its detection is of the greatest importance, because, once discovered, it is amenable to proper therapy, whereas, if left untreated, it may eventually drain exteriorly through the chest wall (*empyema necessitatis*) or rupture into a bronchus and cause a bronchopleural fistula. Rarely, empyema heals spontaneously, causing calcification of the pleura.

Meningitis and Endocarditis. Two serious complications of pneumococcal pneumonia that are often associated with one another are endocarditis and meningitis. Pneumococci usually localize on the aortic valve, producing aortic insufficiency. The development of pneumococcal endocarditis is rare at present. Equally serious is *pneumococcal meningitis* resulting from blood-borne metastasis to the meninges. About 20 per cent of cases of pneumococcal meningitis develop secondary to pneumococcal infection of the lung. The meningitis is characterized by the presence in the pia-arachnoid of a heavily infected exudate, which may cause subarachnoid block or may lead to localized subarachnoid abscesses. Unless vigorous therapy is instituted promptly, the prognosis is hopeless. Even when treatment is intensive, the patient may fail to recover, or may sustain permanent damage to the brain.

Pericarditis. Like the other complications of pneumococcal pneumonia, pericarditis has also become relatively rare since the introduction of potent antimicrobial drugs. When the pericardium is invaded, the patient usually experiences precordial pain, and a leathery friction rub may be heard over the heart. Pericardial effusion usually results, causing a "dampening" of the heart sounds. If the fluid is sterile, the condition is benign, unless so large a volume accumulates as to cause cardiac tamponade. Empyema of the pericardium, on the other hand, is a serious complication requiring prompt and vigorous treatment. Pericardiocentesis is mandatory to establish the diagnosis of purulent pericarditis.

Other Specific Complications. Still rarer specific complications include peritonitis and pyogenic arthritis. Occasionally the pulmonary lesion of pneumococcal pneumonia fails to resolve even after many weeks, and finally is replaced by fibrous tissue.

Nonspecific Complications. *Acute dilatation of the stomach* (gastrectasia) and *paralytic ileus* occur particularly in patients suffering from anoxia and severe toxemia and give rise to gaseous distention of the abdomen (tympanites) that causes discomfort and often increases respiratory embarrassment. *Shock*, likewise, is a complication of severe toxemia and indicates a serious prognosis. *Congestive heart failure* occurs frequently as a complication of severe pneumonia in patients with underlying heart disease. As congestive heart failure is an important predisposing factor in bacterial pneumonia, it is not surprising that they are often associated, and obviously both must be treated. The diagnosis of congestive heart failure in the presence of pneumonia may at times be difficult, but it should be considered in any patient with abnormal distention of neck veins, peripheral edema, an enlarged tender liver, and elevated venous pressure. Pulmonary signs of congestion are difficult to interpret in patients with pneumonia.

Jaundice, the pathogenesis of which is controversial, may be related to lysis of erythrocytes in pneumonic lesions, depressed liver function resulting from anoxia, or focal hepatic necrosis consequent to the pneumococcal infection. Pneumococcal pneumonia may also precipitate hemolysis and jaundice in persons with glucose-6-phosphate dehydrogenase deficiency. The presence of prominent icterus usually indicates a poor prognosis, and may be associated with chronic liver disease, e.g., cirrhosis. As in any bedridden patient, *phlebothrombosis* may occur during pneumonia. Its early presence should suggest the possibility that the pulmonary lesion is due to infarction of the lung rather than to primary pneumonia. *Herpes labialis* occurs in at least 10 per cent of patients with pneumococcal pneumonia.

DIFFERENTIAL DIAGNOSIS. Pneumonia resulting from organisms other than pneumococcus may at times be difficult to differentiate from pneumococcal pneumonia. Only by bacteriologic study of the sputum can pneumonia caused by *Klebsiella pneumoniae* (Friedländer's bacillus), *Staphylococcus aureus,* or *group A Streptococcus* be identified. *Tuberculous pneumonia* rarely causes the acute prostration characteristic of coccal infection. *Mycoplasmal pneumonia* and other infections of the lungs, such as psittacosis and Q fever, do not often cause shaking chills, diffusely bloody sputum, severe pleural pain, or a marked leukocytosis, although they may at times be confused with acute bacterial pneumonia. *Tularemic pneumonia, legionnaires' disease,* and pneumonia caused by *H. influenzae,* especially common in young children, must also be considered. When the diagnosis

is in doubt, repeated examinations of the sputum should be made, using both the Gram and "acid-fast" stains.

The most important noninfectious processes that must be differentiated from pneumococcal pneumonia are pulmonary infarction and atelectasis. *Pulmonary infarction* may be exceedingly difficult to differentiate from pneumonia. The dyspnea, pleural pain, hemoptysis, fever, physical signs of pulmonary consolidation, roentgenographic findings, and leukocytosis are all in keeping with an acute infection of the lungs. Frequently, however, the initial symptom is intense pleural pain of sudden onset; shaking chills rarely occur; there is no preceding history of respiratory infection; the fever is usually not high; frank hemoptysis is common; pulmonary signs, when present, appear early; and the total leukocyte count rarely reaches 20,000 per cubic millimeter. Moreover, although the chest signs develop rapidly in pneumococcal pneumonia, they appear right away with a pulmonary infarct. Combination ventilation-perfusion radionuclide scanning reveals similar defects in pneumonia and pulmonary infarction. Perfusion defects without corresponding ventilation defects are evidence for pulmonary embolism; such perfusion defects in association with a matched ventilation-perfusion defect in the area of a pulmonary infiltrate suggest pulmonary infarction as the cause of the infiltrate.

When a pulmonary infarct becomes infected, as sometimes happens, differentiation from primary bacterial pneumonia may be extremely difficult. Although in such cases the patients should receive antimicrobial treatment as in pneumonia, recognition of the infarction is of importance because of the need for anticoagulant therapy.

Pulmonary atelectasis, resulting from bronchial obstruction, not only may simulate pneumonia but often leads to serious infection of the lung if the bronchial obstruction is not relieved. Aspiration of mucus during or after surgical anesthesia is a common cause of atelectasis. Dyspnea, cough, chest pain, splinting of one side of the thorax, dullness to percussion, and suppressed breath sounds may all suggest primary pneumonia. Fever and leukocytosis also are noted when infection is present. As pulmonary atelectasis may be relieved by forced coughing and postural drainage or, if necessary, by bronchoscopy, it is important to differentiate it from primary pneumonia. Occasionally, sufficient shift of the mediastinum occurs to make the diagnosis obvious. Collapse of a segment of the lung may also result from chronic bronchial obstruction caused by neoplasms, such as bronchogenic carcinoma, or by an aortic aneurysm.

Subdiaphragmatic infection may be confused with pneumonia. Subdiaphragmatic abscess, liver abscess, or other infections in the upper abdomen may extend to the diaphragm and produce local inflammation, small collections of pleural fluid, chest pain, and atelectasis secondary to decreased respiratory excursions. Conversely, pneumococcal pneumonia may simulate intra-abdominal disease. Pleurisy may result in pain referred to the abdomen so as to suggest acute appendicitis or cholecystitis.

Even when the diagnosis of pneumococcal pneumonia is established beyond doubt, the possibility of a second underlying lesion of the lung must be borne in mind. Chronic obstructive pulmonary disease or lung abscess may lead to repeated attacks of bacterial pneumonia and often becomes evident only after the pneumonic consolidation has resolved. Bronchogenic carcinoma or any lesion partially obstructing a bronchus may lead to recurrent pneumonia of the same pulmonary segment.

TREATMENT. The treatment of pneumococcal pneumonia may best be discussed under three headings: (1) antibacterial therapy, (2) supportive measures, and (3) the treatment of complications. Before the advent of effective antibacterial therapy, supportive treatment was of the greatest importance. The introduction, first, of antipneumococcal serum and, later, of sulfonamides, penicillin, and the other antimicrobial drugs has so altered the management of pneumococcal pneumonia that today supportive treatment is rarely crucial, and serious complications are only occasionally encountered.

Antibacterial Therapy. PENICILLIN. Penicillin is at present the drug of choice in the treatment of pneumococcal pneumonia. The vast majority of strains of the pneumococcus isolated in the United States and most other areas of the world are susceptible to penicillin, and most are inhibited in broth by concentrations of less than 0.02 μg per milliliter. However, a number of reports have appeared since 1967 which describe the isolation of pneumococci relatively resistant to penicillin G in Australia, New Guinea, England, Canada, and the United States. The minimal inhibitory concentration of benzylpenicillin for these strains is 0.1 to 2.0 μg per milliliter, although most strains isolated in the United States are inhibited by 0.2 to 0.4 μg per milliliter. Some of these strains have shown relative resistance to the penicillinase-resistant penicillins and cephalosporins, but most have been fully susceptible to antimicrobials other than benzylpenicillin.

The emergence of these relatively resistant strains of pneumococci in a number of different areas of the world has not altered our present over-all approach to the therapy of pneumococcal pneumonia. The dose of penicillin usually utilized in therapy of pneumonia is sufficient to inhibit or kill these strains. However, several reports of delayed response or failure of penicillin therapy of pneumococcal meningitis caused by these strains of "intermediate sensitivity" have been reported. Clinicians should consider the possibility that delay in response to therapy of pneumococcal infection, especially at sites where high concentrations of penicillin may be difficult to achieve, could be related to relative resistance of the infecting organism to penicillin.

A recent development in South Africa regarding the susceptibility of pneumococci to antimicrobials is of great potential importance. In May 1977, pneumococci highly resistant to multiple antimicrobial agents were isolated from pediatric patients and staff of several hospitals in Durban and Johannesburg, South Africa. These organisms are highly resistant to benzylpenicillin, penicillinase-resistant penicillins, ampicillin, cephalothin, erythromycin, clindamycin, tetracycline, and chloramphenicol, but are sensitive to rifampin, vancomycin, bacitracin, and fusidic acid. These organisms spread readily among patients in the hospital and, in addition to producing an asymptomatic carrier state, have also caused pneumonia, bacteremia, and meningitis unresponsive to conventional therapy. Physicians should be alert to the spread or emergence of these organisms in other areas of the world.

The effectiveness of antimicrobial treatment is due in part to the natural resistance of the host, which accounts for the destruction of a large proportion of the invading bacteria. Host resistance, which results primarily from the activity of phagocytic cells in the lung, when combined with the bacteriostatic and bactericidal effects of drug therapy, controls promptly all but the most malignant pneumonia. Even with no treatment at all, approximately seven of every ten patients with pneumococcal pneumonia eventually recover, but some will have experienced a very severe illness before recovery has occurred.

Antipneumococcal therapy should be initiated promptly, therefore, in order to halt the spread of the infection both locally and through the bloodstream. An effective method is to give aqueous procaine penicillin G intramuscularly in a dose of 300,000 units at 12-hour intervals. Some authorities recommend the administration of aqueous penicillin G by the intramuscular route in doses of 300,000 units several times during the first 24-hour period of observation in addition to the procaine penicillin. In the presence of shock, penicillin G should be given intravenously. Treatment should be maintained for at least one week or until the temperature has been normal for 72 hours; if treatment is discontinued too soon, relapse may occur.

Penicillin may also be given by mouth. However, in a serious infection such as pneumococcal pneumonia, it is inadvisable to rely on oral penicillin therapy in acutely ill patients. Parenteral therapy throughout provides the greatest margin of safety. If parenteral therapy is not feasible or advisable throughout the period of treatment, procaine penicillin G can be given parenterally initially and penicillin V can then be given orally after defervescence. When oral penicillin V is used, it should be given in a dosage of at least 250 mg every six hours.

Response to penicillin therapy is often dramatic. Bacteremia, when present at the start of treatment, clears within a few hours. A crisis, characterized by rapid defervescence and a striking subsidence of symptoms, occurs in less than 48 hours in approximately half the patients. The others experience a more gradual recovery, the temperature falling by lysis over a period of four to seven days. Frequently a secondary rise in temperature occurs after the crisis. This elevation is usually low-grade and subsides spontaneously within a few hours, or at most a few days.

When a patient's pneumonia fails to respond satisfactorily to penicillin therapy, four possible explanations should be considered: (1) that the patient is suffering from a serious complication such as empyema, endocarditis, meningitis, or pulmonary suppuration (possibly secondary to bronchogenic carcinoma); (2) that the primary infection is of nonpneumococcal origin and is due to an agent that is resistant to the action of penicillin, e.g., a penicillin-resistant strain of *Staphylococcus* or *Klebsiella;* (3) that drug fever has developed as a result of penicillin hypersensitivity; or (4) that the diagnosis of microbial pneumonia is incorrect and some other condition accounts for the fever and pulmonary lesions. Occasionally, patients will respond initially to treatment only to have unmistakable signs of persistent pneumonia subsequently develop in spite of continued therapy. This sequence of events is usually due to the presence of a mixed infection, the initial response to treatment resulting from control of penicillin-susceptible organisms, and the relapse occurring as a result of persistence of a penicillin-resistant species.

Re-examination of the sputum and modification of the antimicrobial therapy are immediately indicated. Patients with underlying chronic pulmonary disease are particularly prone to such mixed infections.

Persons giving a history of having had a penicillin reaction in the past should not be treated with penicillin.

OTHER ANTIMICROBIAL DRUGS. Cephalothin or cefazolin can be used as effective alternatives to penicillin for parenteral therapy in patients hypersensitive to penicillin. Patients hypersensitive to penicillin sometimes show cross-sensitivity to cephalosporins; a cutaneous scratch test with the cephalosporin to be used should probably be performed in these patients to determine whether the drug can be used as an alternative to penicillin. Cephalothin should be administered in doses of 1 gram every four hours by the intramuscular or intravenous route, and cefazolin should be given in doses of 0.5 gram every six hours. Cephalosporins should not be used in therapy of pneumococcal meningitis. Erythromycin in doses of 250 mg every six hours by the oral route is also adequate for treatment of patients with a history of penicillin allergy, provided they are not severely ill. Resistance of pneumococci to erythromycin has been reported but is quite rare. Methicillin, cloxacillin, and nafcillin are also effective in the treatment of pneumococcal pneumonia. Tetracyclines should not be used in treating pneumococcal infections unless the organism is known to be susceptible. The prevalence of tetracycline-resistant pneumococci has increased greatly in recent years, now exceeding 5 per cent in many areas of the world. Pneumococci are relatively resistant to gentamicin, and pneumococcal pneumonia has been shown to progress during the administration of this drug.

Supportive Treatment. Patients suffering from pneumococcal pneumonia should be kept at bed rest, and visitors to the sick room should be limited to the immediate family. Pleural pain, if mild, may be treated with codeine sulfate (30 to 60 mg) orally. A tight chest binder may relieve pain but is inadvisable because it inhibits effectiveness of cough. Hypoxemia should be treated with oxygen administered by nasal catheter or by mask. Acetylsalicylic acid should not be used, because it interferes with the utilization of the fever curve to evaluate response to therapy.

FLUID AND ELECTROLYTES. During the acute state of pneumococcal pneumonia, considerable fluid is lost from the body, chiefly through the skin as the result of high fever. Dehydration may develop rapidly and, if severe, may become a contributing factor in the development of shock. Intravenous fluids and electrolytes may be required to control dehydration. When hydration is adequate, the specific gravity of the urine should remain below 1.020. Pneumonia may occasionally lead to the syndrome of inappropriate secretion of antidiuretic hormone.

DIET. Many patients with pneumococcal pneumonia are too ill to tolerate a full diet and should receive only liquids during the height of the fever. Fruit juices, ginger ale, and soups are well tolerated. After the crisis a regular diet may be prescribed.

The patient should be kept in bed until the temperature is approximately normal and should be observed closely until the pneumonic lesion has resolved. As already emphasized, all patients should be subjected to a follow-up roentgenographic examination three to four weeks after recovery.

Treatment of Complications. SHOCK. Patients with peripheral vascular collapse (shock) resulting from severe pneumococcal pneumonia usually respond poorly to the accepted forms of antishock therapy. The prognosis is almost invariably grave when this complication develops. Oxygen therapy should be begun immediately, even if cyanosis is absent. Hemodynamic monitoring should be used as a guide for fluid replacement. The use of corticosteroids has not been demonstrated to be of value.

ABDOMINAL DISTENTION. Decompression is indicated if distention is severe. Acute gastric and ileal dilatation is best managed with the use of gastric suction; a rectal tube may be indicated if colonic distention is a problem.

DELIRIUM TREMENS. Delirium tremens may sometimes be difficult to control in patients with a history of chronic alcoholism. Restraints may be required. The safest sedative to control hyperactivity in these patients is diazepam (Valium) in a dose of 0.066 mg per kilogram every four to six hours.

EMPYEMA AND PERICARDITIS. The treatment of choice for empyema and purulent pericarditis is systemic antimicrobial therapy and surgical drainage. Injection of penicillin into the pleural or pericardial cavity is not required. Repeated needle aspirations are occasionally effective but do not provide effective drainage in most patients.

The treatment of the remaining two major complications of pneumococcal pneumonia, namely endocarditis and meningitis, is discussed in Ch. 131 and 140.

PROGNOSIS. The case fatality rate in untreated pneumococcal pneumonia ranges from 20 to 40 per cent. The widespread use of sulfonamide drugs in the late 1930's resulted in a lowering of the fatality rate among treated patients to approximately 10 per cent. Penicillin therapy has lowered the rate still further. At present approximately 95 per cent of patients with pneumococcal pneumonia recover when properly treated with penicillin.

The prognosis in pneumococcal pneumonia is influenced adversely by each of the following: (1) old age (and also infancy), (2) late treatment, (3) infection with certain types of pneumococci (particularly types 2 and 3), (4) involvement of more than one lobe of the lung, (5) leukopenia, (6) occurrence of bacteremia, (7) capsular polysaccharide detectable in blood by counterimmunoelectrophoresis, (8) jaundice, (9) the presence of complications (notably shock and meningitis), (10) pregnancy (particularly in the third trimester), (11) the presence of other disease such as heart disease or cirrhosis of the liver, and (12) alcoholic intoxication and delirium tremens. Through a consideration of these factors a rough estimate may be made of the severity of the infection in each case, and therapy may be modified accordingly.

Even with the most intensive penicillin treatment, a significant number of patients will die of pneumococcal pneumonia. A recent study, for example, has revealed that in patients destined, at the onset of illness, to die within five days (because of complicating disease, old age, etc.), penicillin therapy has little if any effect. Similarly, the case fatality rate in type 3 pneumococcal pneumonia with bacteremia still exceeds 50 per cent regardless of treatment.

PREVENTION. Because pneumococcal pneumonia is not highly contagious and usually responds promptly to early therapy, prophylaxis constitutes less of a problem than in many other infectious diseases. It is estimated that only one in every 500 persons of all ages in the United States may be expected to contract the disease in any one year.

Although pneumococcal pneumonia can undoubtedly be prevented (or at least aborted) in many patients by the intensive treatment of every upper respiratory tract infection with antimicrobial drugs, their use for this purpose should be avoided. The possible inconvenience to the patient of hypersensitivity reactions and the danger of favoring drug-resistant strains of bacteria outweigh the advantages to be gained in preventing such a relatively uncommon and readily treatable disease as pneumococcal pneumonia. Some authorities do recommend penicillin prophylaxis for children with sickle cell anemia less than three or four years of age whose circulating erythrocytes contain Howell-Jolly bodies as an indicator of splenic hypofunction.

During recent years Austrian has redirected attention to the possibility of specific immunization as a means of preventing pneumococcal infection. During World War II, MacLeod and colleagues showed in controlled experiments in man that pneumococcal polysaccharides are effective antigens, evoking the formation of antibody that persists for years and that confers type-specific immunity to pneumococcal infection. Austrian has proposed immunization of that portion of the population at greatest risk with the types of pneumococci that are most often responsible for disease. Austrian's data, reported in 1972, show that 62 per cent of 2000 cases of pneumococcal bacteremia in adults were caused by six types (1, 3, 4, 7, 8, 12), and that 70 per cent of 100 bacteremias in the pediatric age group were caused by six types (1, 6, 14, 18, 19, 23). Pneumococci of capsular types 6, 14, 19, and 23 are responsible for about 60 per cent of cases of otitis media in children. Since high risk groups can be identified and a large proportion of infections are caused by a few pneumococcal types, commercially available vaccine against those types was introduced in 1978. Vaccination is recommended for those over 2 years of age with a high risk of serious pneumococcal infection, especially patients with asplenia, sickle cell anemia, nephrotic syndrome, chronic cardiopulmonary diseases, or other deficiencies of host resistance. Whether effective immunization of certain groups by polysaccharide vaccines will be followed by an increasing occurrence of infections with other pneumococcal types is unknown but is a definite possibility.

Patient Isolation. The cross-infection rate in pneumococcal pneumonia is low, and patients receiving chemotherapy are probably not highly infectious. Isolation is not indicated in the usual patient.

Applebaum, P. C., et al.: *Streptococcus pneumoniae* responding to penicillin and chloramphenicol. Lancet, 2:995, 1977.

Austrian, R.: Current status of bacterial pneumonia with especial reference to pneumococcal infection. J. Clin. Path. (suppl.), 21:93, 1968.

Austrian, R., and Gold, J.: Pneumococcal bacteremia with especial reference to bacteremic pneumococcal pneumonia. Ann. Intern. Med., 60:759, 1964.

Austrian, R., Howie, V. M., and Ploussard, J. H.: The bacteriology of pneumococcal otitis media. Johns Hopkins Med. J., 141:104, 1977.

Blazevic, D. J., et al.: Penicillin-resistant *Streptococcus pneumoniae* — Minnesota. MMWR, 26: October 21, 1977.

Coonrod, J. D., and Drennan, D. P.: Pneumococcal pneumonia. Cap-

sular polysaccharide antigenemia and antibody response. Ann. Intern. Med., 84:254, 1976.

Coonrod, J. D., and Rytel, M. W.: Detection of type-specific pneumococcal antigens by counterimmunoelectrophoresis. II. Etiologic diagnosis of pneumonia. J. Lab. Clin. Med., 81:778, 1973.

Jay, S. J., Johanson, W. G., Jr., and Pierce, A. K.: The radiographic resolution of *Streptococcus pneumoniae*. N. Engl. J. Med., 293:798, 1975.

Kauffman, C. A., Watanakunakorn, C., and Phair, J. P.: Pneumococcal arthritis. J. Rheumatol., 3:409, 1976.

Kauffman, C. A., Watanakunakorn, C., and Phair, J. P.: Purulent pneumonococcal pericarditis. A continuing problem in the antibiotic era. Am. J. Med., 54:743, 1973.

Lerner, A. M., and Jan Kauskas, K.: The classic bacterial pneumonias. Disease-a-Month, February 1975, pp. 1–46.

Lukems, J. N.: Hemoglobin S, the pneumococcus and the spleen. Am. J. Dis. Child., 123:6, 1972.

Spencer, R. C., and Savage, M. A.: Use of counter and rocket immunoelectrophoresis in acute respiratory infections due to *Streptococcus pneumoniae*. J. Clin. Pathol., 29:187, 1976.

Wood, W. B.: Studies of the Cellular Immunology of Acute Bacterial Infections. The Harvey Lectures, Series 47, 1951–52.

122. PNEUMONIA DUE TO KLEBSIELLA PNEUMONIAE

(Friedländer's Pneumonia)

Herbert Y. Reynolds

Klebsiella may persist in the oropharynx of normal persons, although the prevalence is low, 1 to 6 per cent. There is no tendency for contacts to acquire the organism from a carrier, and it is difficult to implant organisms in the pharynx of healthy volunteers. As is the case with a number of other bacteria, the prevalence of *Klebsiella* in pharyngeal cultures increases (up to 20 per cent) in hospitalized subjects. Pulmonary infections arise most likely from the inhalation or aspiration of organisms from the oropharynx during circumstances in which the major pulmonary antibacterial defense mechanisms are compromised, but the demarcation is often indistinct, as classic primary *Klebsiella* pneumonia occurs in patients with underlying conditions such as alcoholism, chronic obstructive airways disease (emphysema-bronchitis) or diabetes mellitus. Operationally, infections may be considered as primary if *Klebsiella* organisms are isolated from specimens obtained when the patient first seeks medical aid. The designation "secondary" is then applied to those infections that either represent superinfection of an underlying infection or are opportunistic in origin. The present chapter is concerned with the primary pneumonia and hence includes the antimicrobial therapy of *Klebsiella* pulmonary disease. The management of the so-called "secondary" *Klebsiella* bronchopulmonary infections is essentially the same as for any nosocomial pneumonia (see Ch. 124).

In patients with primary pneumonia, males predominate heavily (80 to 90 per cent) and most infections occur in middle-aged and older patients. A common coexisting disease is alcoholism (66 per cent). Both chronic bronchopulmonary disease and, to a lesser extent, diabetes mellitus appear to predispose to *Klebsiella* pneumonia.

PATHOLOGY. The outstanding characteristic of *Klebsiella* pneumonia is its destructiveness; it is a necrotizing pneumonia. In fatal cases lobar involvement most often occurs, but infection may be lobular or may be a combination of both; an upper lobe is most frequently involved. The pleural surface is covered by a fibrinous exudate, and adhesions form early. Empyema is appreciably more frequent than in pneumococcal pneumonia and probably occurs in about one fifth of cases. Microscopically, in the acute stage the alveolar walls are congested. Usually the alveoli are filled with an exudate composed of a mixture of predominantly polymorphonuclear cells. There is abscess formation in association with the necrosis of the alveolar walls. Other findings at autopsy may include extrapulmonary sites of dissemination, e.g., pericarditis or meningitis. Evidence of alcoholic hepatitis and alcoholic cirrhosis is common.

CLINICAL MANIFESTATIONS. The onset is usually sudden (90 per cent), associated with cough productive of sputum (90 per cent), pleuritic chest pain (80 per cent), and true rigors (60 per cent). Early prostration is a usual feature. Occasionally the acute onset is preceded by a nondescript upper respiratory infection and cough. Rarely, epigastric pain and vomiting are the initial symptoms. Typically the sputum is described as a nonputrid homogeneous thick mixture of blood and mucus, often brick red in color. In some patients the sputum is sufficiently thick to be expectorated with difficulty. In others it is thin, resembling currant jelly. Almost always it is either blood tinged or rusty, and frank hemoptysis may occur. On examination, the patient appears acutely ill, febrile, dyspneic, and often cyanotic. Tachycardia is present in proportion to the fever. Chest examination usually reveals signs of pulmonary consolidation. There may be loss of lung volume as manifested by decreased size and expansion of the involved hemithorax and diaphragmatic elevation. Auscultation may reveal suppressed breath sounds with few rales, despite evidence of considerable consolidation. Involvement of more than one lobe is frequent (in two thirds of patients), with a predilection for upper lobes.

LABORATORY AND ROENTGENOGRAPHIC FINDINGS. Peripheral leukocyte counts vary from marked leukopenia to leukocytosis, but leukopenia (and neutropenia) is a poor prognostic sign. In one quarter of patients the total leukocyte count may be in the normal range. On sputum culture, other gram-negative bacilli may be isolated in addition to *Klebsiella*. A mixed sputum flora containing other gram-negative bacilli such as *Pseudomonas spp.* is especially common in secondary infections. A pulmonary source is often incriminated in patients with *Klebsiella* bacteremia. This is unusual, because in other types of gram-negative bacillary bacteremia the urinary tract usually represents the major primary source, followed by the gastrointestinal tract.

The roentgenographic features are variable and include massive lobar consolidation, lobular involvement, lung abscess formation with either multiple small thin-walled or large abscess cavities, and residual parenchymal fibrosis. Bulging of a fissure, sharp advancing borders of the infiltrates, and abscess formation occur with greater frequency than in other types of pneumonia. The pneumonic infiltrate is relatively dense, but shadows of similar density are seen with other types of pneumonia. Bronchopneumonic distribution is less characteristic but can occur, and even bilateral perihilar infiltrates are reported.

COMPLICATIONS. Rapid destruction of pulmonary tissue with suppurative or residual fibrosis occurs in as many as half of the surviving patients. Necrosis may occur within 24 to 48 hours, and abscess formation may be recognized within four days. Other less common pulmonary complications include pleural effusion and pneumothorax. In the past, activation of quiescent pulmonary tuberculosis has been reported. It is believed that some of these cases actually represent a slough of localized tuberculous disease by the necrotizing *Klebsiella* pneumonia.

The course of illness is not marked by frequent extrapulmonary manifestations, but they can occur and include pericarditis, meningitis, gastroenteritis, erythematous skin rashes, and nonsuppurative polyarthritis.

PROGNOSIS AND TREATMENT. In the preantimicrobial era, the case mortality of *Klebsiella* pneumonia ranged from 51 to 97 per cent. The use of antimicrobials has markedly decreased mortality, but in some series the mortality remains nearly 50 per cent. In these series there has been a predominance of severely ill, alcoholic patients, although good results have been reported even in this group. Analysis of the mode of death frequently reveals that inadequate removal of tenacious pulmonary secretions was a significant factor. The correlation of bloodstream invasion and fatality is frequently close.

The majority of strains of *Klebsiella* are susceptible in vitro to chloramphenicol, the cephalosporins, and the aminoglycosides. The antimicrobial regimen of choice varies according to the gravity of the acute clinical situation and the extent of the underlying problem. Because the necrosis of lung tissue can occur so rapidly, it is essential that maximally effective antimicrobial therapy be started immediately. In patients with life-threatening infection, which is at least potentially always the case, a two-drug regimen of cephalothin intravenously and gentamicin intramuscularly is recommended. After several days of such therapy, if the infection is clearly well under control, the cephalothin may be discontinued. Meticulous measures directed at supportive care — maintenance of clear airways, adequate but not excessive ventilation and oxygenation, adequate fluid and electrolyte replacement, and often control of delirium tremens — are essential.

An emerging problem is the developing resistance of *Klebsiella* to gentamicin. In such a clinical situation another aminoglycoside should be chosen, and, if possible, drug-susceptibility studies should be done. Streptomycin, amikacin, and tobramycin are the principal drugs from which a choice must be made.

CHRONIC CAVITARY KLEBSIELLA DISEASE

Occasionally a patient will be seen with a chronic cavitary disease of the lung resulting from infection with *Klebsiella*. In some cases this chronic disease is a known sequel to a primary pneumonia. In other cases, there is no convincing history of such an acute process and the disease appears to have been persisting in subacute or chronic form for many months. Because of the rarity of this form of *Klebsiella* disease, its natural history has not been well characterized. It should be treated initially with the drug-pairing regimen of cephalothin and gentamicin, which can be appropriately modified as improvement occurs. The general treatment should be that for any other lung abscess, including presumably the use of surgical excision in rare cases (see Ch. 347.1).

Bloomfield, A. L.: The fate of bacteria introduced into the upper air passages. V. The Friedländer bacilli. Bull. Johns Hopkins Hosp., 31:203, 1920.

Jervey, L. P., Jr., and Hamburger, M.: The treatment of acute Friedländer's pneumonia. Arch. Intern. Med., 99:1, 1957.

Knight, L., Fraser, R. G., and Robson, H. G.: Massive pulmonary gangrene: A severe complication of Klebsiella pneumonia. Can. Med. Assoc. J., 112:196, 1975.

Manfredi, F., Daly, W. J., and Behnke, R. H.: Clinical observations of acute Friedländer's pneumonia. Ann. Intern. Med., 58:642, 1963.

Pierce, A. K., and Sanford, J. P.: Aerobic gram-negative bacillary pneumonias. Am. Rev. Respir. Dis., 110:647, 1974.

123. LEGIONNAIRES' DISEASE

Herbert Y. Reynolds

In the late summer of 1976, a mysterious outbreak of severe respiratory illness occurred in Pennsylvania. Initially the disease developed among people who attended a State American Legion convention in Philadelphia at the end of July. Because a microbial agent was not readily identified and mortality initially appeared to be high, the outbreak received wide publicity and evoked concern that a new and virulent infection would become rampant. Public expectation was ripe for a sensational respiratory disease, for this was the year of the abortive swine influenza immunization program for the epidemic that failed to materialize. Later, when an etiologic agent was isolated from lung tissue of legionnaires' disease victims and a fluorescent antibody stain was developed, several interesting findings placed the legionnaires' disease outbreak in better perspective. It became apparent that this disease was not new, nor was the Philadelphia outbreak the first. In fact, based on serial changes in antibody titers, about 0.5 to 1.5 per cent of patients with an etiologically undiagnosed viral-like pneumonia may actually be infected with the legionnaires' agent. However, legionnaires' disease is usually a more serious infection than viral-like pneumonias. The Center for Disease Control estimates that there may be 45,000 cases annually in the United States.

The status of the disease is still in flux, and much is still not understood. Factual data about new outbreaks and recent developments in the drug susceptibilities of the putative bacterium are to be found in the daily newspapers rather than in the medical literature. As yet, the bacterium has not been classified taxonomically.

BACKGROUND. As mentioned, an outbreak of severe epidemic respiratory illness occurred chiefly among conventioneers who attended a State American Legion convention in Philadelphia between July 21 and 24, 1976. The outbreak had all the hallmarks of an infectious disease, with an onset of approximately six to eight days after the affected individual arrived at the convention in the Bellevue-Stratford Hotel. The illness, unfortunately dubbed legionnaires' disease, was not confined to participants in the American Legion convention, but included non-convention-goers as well. In one fatal case categorized as Broad Street pneumonia, the victim had been within a block of the Bellevue-Stratford but had not gone inside the hotel for three weeks prior to the convention. Other cases occurred among people who attended the Catholic Eucharistic convention during the first week in August. In total, 180 cases were recorded in Philadelphia, including 29 deaths.

Preliminary evidence indicated that neither food nor drink could be implicated as sources of the disease agent. Distribution of most cases at the headquarters hotel by room of occupancy showed no unusual pattern of occurrence. Illness in the American Legion conventioneers was associated with time spent in the hotel and clearly related to time spent in the lobby. The only other factor associated with illness was cigarette smoking. The illness was not contagious, and the hotel personnel were unaffected. Inhalation exposure to a list of toxins was entertained, especially to nickel carbonyl because nickel concentrations in lung tissues were found to be elevated. Apparently this cause and effect was not substantiated further. However, the presence of a significant pre-existing illness, such as cardiopulmonary disease, malignancy, or diabetes mellitus, was associated with a 29 per cent case-fatality ratio, compared with a 5 per cent ratio for those without. The actual number of cases of clinical disease was small compared to the several thousand legionnaires and guests who attended the convention and, for that matter, was very small when contrasted with the large number of tourists who visited Philadelphia for the Bicentennial celebration.

Approximately six months later, a presumptive etiologic agent (a gram-negative bacillus) was recovered from infected lung tissue. This bacterium provided an antigen source for an indirect immunofluorescent antibody staining test. With the availability of this assay some interesting developments occurred. First, previous outbreaks of undiagnosed pneumonia were solved. In 1965, 94 cases of unexplained pneumonia had occurred at St. Elizabeth's Hospital, a psychiatric hospital in the District of Columbia. Sixteen deaths occurred. Acute and convalescent sera were available from 14 patients, and 13 showed significant rises in antibody staining titers implicating the legionnaires' bacterium as the infecting agent. An equally baffling outbreak of respiratory illness in Pontiac, Michigan, in 1968 was also found to have been caused by the legionnaires' agent. In 1977, a number of outbreaks occurred, especially in the late summer. Clusters of cases have been found in Columbus, Ohio, Burlington, Vermont, Kingsport, Tennessee and Los Angeles, California; sporadic cases have been widely distributed across the country. In Burlington, Vermont, 32 cases of legionnaires' disease have been identified at this writing; 17 of the cases were fatal. The interesting twist to this outbreak was the development of disease in a number of patients requiring hemodialysis or renal homografting.

Clearly, this type of pneumonia is a nationwide phenomenon. The mortality rate appears to be about 15 to 20 per cent.

ETIOLOGY. The presumptive causative organism was finally isolated about six months after the index cases were discovered from lung tissues of one fatal case of legionnaires' respiratory disease and of one fatal case of "Broad Street pneumonia." Recovery of the microorganism was accomplished by inoculation of guinea pigs intraperitoneally. After a one- to two-day incubation period, the inoculated guinea pigs developed a febrile illness characterized in most animals by watery eyes and prostration. Spleen suspensions from these febrile guinea pigs were inoculated into yolk sacs of embryonated eggs from antibiotic-free chickens. The embryos died after four to six days, and microscopic smears of the yolk sacs (Gimenez stain) revealed pleomorphic gram-negative bacilli. The bacterial-like organisms proved difficult to grow on several artificial culture media but apparently did grow satisfactorily on Mueller-Hinton medium which was supplemented with 1 per cent hemoglobin and 1 per cent bacterial nutrients. Starch, iron, and cysteine seem to be essential ingredients for growth. Colonies could be detected in three to five days after inoculation with infected yolk-sac material or after transfer from other bacterial medium. Because most bacteria when inoculated into the yolk sac kill eggs in one to two days, it was thought that the organism's slow growth might imply that is was an unusual *Rickettsia*. However, the organisms were larger than *Rickettsia*, and they did not react with any standard rickettsial antigens in complement fixation tests. The organism was not acid fast.

The yolk-sac isolate is being called a bacterium on the basis of its size and morphology. The two yolk-sac isolates initially recovered appear similar. Both have been used as antigen in an indirect fluorescent antibody staining test. When both antigen preparations have been assayed with immune serum from selected patients with legionnaires' disease, comparable antibody titers have been found. Thus both yolk-sac isolates appear to be antigenically similar.

Antemortem cultures of respiratory secretions, blood, and lung tissue have not yielded growth of the organisms. However, the bacterium has been cultured from pleural fluid of at least two patients and the diagnosis substantiated. At present, the diagnosis of legionnaires' respiratory disease is usually made from fluorescent antibody staining titers in serum. Seroconversion ($\geq$4-fold titer increase) in paired sera, with one titer at least 1:128, and a typical clinical illness in the absence of an established microbial cause seem to be sufficient criteria for the diagnosis. Antibody titers are being performed by the Center for Disease Control at Atlanta and by a number of state health laboratories, as well. The availability of antibody testing will undoubtedly become more convenient in the near future. Direct fluorescent antibody technique and silver impregnation stains may be used to demonstrate organisms in tissues.

CLINICAL PRESENTATION. Many cases are clearly associated with institutions, including hospitals. Immunosuppressed hosts, particularly those receiving corticosteroids, and debilitated individuals are especially susceptible. The illness begins with headache, malaise, muscle pains, and a slight nonproductive cough; in some patients diarrhea is noted first. This rather mild illness may persist for two or three days, followed by the onset of rigors and high fever. True shaking chills occur, and fever is an impressive finding in most patients (39 to 40.5°C). The fever is usually nonremittent. Relatively slow pulse in relation to fever is common. The cough remains nonproductive or produces mucoid sputum. A chest x-ray can show either a diffuse patchy or scattered infiltrate with evidence of alveolar filling or a more discrete lobar infiltration. The total blood leukocyte count can be elevated to a range of 12,000 to 18,000 per cubic millimeter, with some left shift.

This is the extent and severity of the disease in some patients, and they gradually improve in a week or so, often without specific treatment. Other patients will progress in three to four days to a severe form of pneumonia with evidence of extensive three- to five-lobe infiltration or consolidation and marked obtundation and disorientation. The obtundation and disorientation are out of proportion to the extent of the lung involvement and hypoxia. The chest x-ray lags several days behind the fulminant respiratory and clinical picture. Some patients experience pleuritic chest pain, and hemoptysis

may occur. Shock occurs occasionally and is associated with a grave prognosis. A number of patients develop small pleural effusions; uncompromised patients seem to have larger effusions. As mentioned, cultures of pleural fluid have yielded the organism in several patients. The chest x-ray usually shows extensive air space filling and air bronchograms. However, a peculiar but distinctive x-ray pattern can be found with the disease and consists of the appearance of large fuzzy densities throughout the lung fields which almost have the appearance of widespread pulmonary metastases. Abnormal liver function tests (SGOT, alkaline phosphatase, LDH) are common, as are hyponatremia and hypophosphatemia. Renal function impairment, apparently directly attributable to the disease, may occur occasionally. Several clues which may tip one to the diagnosis of legionnaires' disease are extensive pneumonia without an obvious etiologic agent, predisposed host, nonproductive or mucoid cough, chills, high nonremitting fever, temperature-pulse dissociation, pleuritic chest pain, presence of diarrhea, myalgia, inappropriate obtundation, abnormal liver function tests, hypophosphatemia, failure of response to cephalosporins or gentamicin, and favorable response to erythromycin.

Postmortem examination of the lungs reveals an acute diffuse pattern of alveolar damage. Histopathologic changes include presence of hyaline membranes, regenerating alveolar epithelium, sparse interstitial round cell infiltrate, and intra-alveolar proteinaceous debris. Organisms may be demonstrated within macrophages or polymorphonuclear leukocytes among the intra-alveolar debris. This pattern of injury is nonspecific and may be caused by many infections and toxic agents. Focal bacterial pneumonia is often present, suggesting that a superimposed infection has occurred.

TREATMENT AND PROGNOSIS. Full supportive respiratory care is often required, including supplemental oxygen and mechanical ventilatory support with tracheostomy or endotracheal intubation. Details for pulmonary care will not be reviewed here (see Ch. 351). Prompt antimicrobial therapy is important, and erythromycin, given as 2 to 4 grams per day in divided doses intravenously, seems to be an effective drug. Antimicrobial susceptibility of the legionnaires' disease bacterium was evaluated in protection studies in embryonated hens' eggs and in vitro by agar dilution. Erythromycin was effective. Moreover, erythromycin has proved to be effective treatment in the guinea pig model of the disease. Tetracycline may also be effective. Recent information indicates that rifampin may be an effective drug as well, but its use is not advocated as a single drug regimen.

Chandler, F. W., Hicklin, M. D., and Blackmon, J. A.: Legionnaires' disease: Demonstration of the agent in tissue. N. Engl. J. Med., 297:1218, 1977.

Chen, J. R., Francisco, R. B., and Miller, T. E.: Legionnaires' disease: Nickel levels. Science, 196:906, 1977.

Fraser, D. W., et al.: Legionnaires' disease: Description of an epidemic. N. Engl. J. Med., 297:1189, 1977.

Keys, T. F.: A sporadic case of pneumonia due to legionnaires' disease. Mayo Clin. Proc., 52:657, 1977.

Legionnaires' disease. Lancet, 2:1265, 1977.

McDade, J. E., et al.: Legionnaires' disease: Isolation of a bacterium. N. Engl. J. Med., 297:1197, 1977.

124. PNEUMONIA AND NOSOCOMIAL RESPIRATORY INFECTIONS CAUSED BY AEROBIC GRAM-NEGATIVE BACILLI

(Pseudomonas, Escherichia Coli, and Serratia)

Herbert Y. Reynolds

Bacterial species that belong to the families Enterobacteriaceae and Pseudomonadaceae are considered together because of (1) similarities in the pulmonary infection they produce and (2) common circumstances in which they cause disease. Only a few of the bacteria that are frequently encountered as respiratory pathogens will be discussed individually. Others may be inportant in special instances, but statistically are less of a problem. Specialized texts on microbial diseases and the periodical literature can supply more detailed information about rare or unusual infections.

The family Enterobacteriaceae is composed of numerous interrelated bacilli, all of which are gram-negative, are nonsporing, grow on ordinary media, and rapidly ferment glucose. The following genera are included in the family: *Shigella, Escherichia, Salmonella, Arizona, Citrobacter, Edwardsiella, Klebsiella, Enterobacter, Serratia, Proteus, Providencia,* and *Erwinia.* The nonfermenting aerobic gram-negative bacilli are recognized with almost equal frequency. Organisms in this category include *Pseudomonas aeruginosa, P. maltophilia, P. pseudomallei, P. cepacia, P. stutzeri, Acinetobacter lwoffi* (previously *Mima polymorpha*), *Acinetobacter anitratus* (previously *Herellea vaginicola* and *Achromobacter anitratus*), *Alcaligenes spp., Achromobacter spp., Flavobacterium spp., Moraxella spp.,* and *Aeromonas hydrophilia.* Infections caused by *Pseudomonas pseudomallei* (melioidosis) are presented in Ch. 159.2.

Pulmonary infections associated with the small aerobic gram-negative bacilli belonging to the genera *Bordetella, Brucella, Hemophilus,* and *Yersinia,* as well as nonsporulating anaerobic gram-negative bacilli, e.g., *Bacteroides* and *Fusobacterium,* are discussed in the individual chapters dealing with each of these infections. Pneumonia caused by *Klebsiella* is the subject of Ch. 122.

Aerobic gram-negative bacilli are frequently the cause of respiratory infection in two groups of patients: those who develop a superinfection or acquire an infection in the hospital (nosocomial) and those who are immunocompromised. Many patients become infected with their endogenous bacterial flora. These clinical conditions are not necessarily distinct, but will be separated for convenience of discussion. For example, primary *Klebsiella* pneumonia (see Ch. 122) may be associated with a number of underlying of perhaps predisposing conditions in the patient, such as alcoholism, chronic obstructive airways disease (emphysema), and diabetes mellitus. By contrast, nosocomial, i.e., hospital-acquired, infections can occur from environmental bacteria or from an organism considered to be part of the normal bacterial flora of the gut or oropharynx.

NOSOCOMIAL PNEUMONIA

Mechanisms and Prevalence

Many common aerobic gram-negative bacteria normally inhabit the human gastrointestinal tract. Moreover, a significant number of healthy, normal people have oropharyngeal colonization with a small number of these bacteria. Certain species such as *Pseudomonas aeruginosa* can be isolated from various skin sites (hands and axillae) in some instances. Since these bacteria are part of the normal microbial flora, they rarely cause primary infection. However, an unwanted byproduct of modern medicine, which can manipulate so many facets of human physiology to salvage and restore health, is the development of iatrogenic and drug-induced infections. The magnitude of this infectious disease problem is large in terms of patient morbidity and mortality, and the financial burden to the health care system. Hospital-acquired infections developed in approximately 3.5 per cent of hospitalized patients (range, 2.6 to 5.8 per cent) reported for 1975–1976 in the National Nosocomial Infections Study of the Center for Disease Control. Urinary tract and surgical wound infections were most common, but lower respiratory tract infections were reported for 21 per cent of the infections of medical patients and 15 per cent of the infections of surgical patients. Perhaps more disturbing than the frequency of respiratory infections is the poor success generally cited for treatment and control. Serious underlying disease is usually present and, despite antimicrobial therapy, the case mortality from nosocomial pneumonia may approach 50 per cent, depending somewhat on the specific causative bacterium and the clinical setting of the patient. The statistics become even worse in patients immunocompromised by acute bone marrow failure and leukemia. In such a group reported from the National Institutes of Health, Bethesda, Maryland, deaths were caused by systemic infections in 46 per cent, in most cases from a gram-negative bacterium and/or fungal species. In the other half of the group, death was attributed to pneumonia caused most frequently by fungal species but closely followed by gram-negative rod bacteria. In the past bacterial deaths accounted for an even higher percentage. The early administration of drug combinations having a broad antibacterial spectrum in febrile, granulocytopenic cancer patients has more effectively controlled some bacterial infections. However, the emergence of drug-resistant strains of *Klebsiella pneumoniae, Pseudomonas aeruginosa,* and others to commonly used aminoglycosides (gentamicin, for example) could alter tremendously the prospects for bacterial control. Superinfection of the respiratory tract with fungi (*Aspergillus* frequently) and other opportunistic organisms (*Pneumocystis carinii*) continues to gain in importance at a time when gram-negative bacterial ones seem to be coming under better control. The therapy for fungal and other opportunistic infections is not usually started as promptly as is the rule for bacterial infections because of the persistent difficulty in obtaining an early and reliable diagnosis. Invasive procedures to obtain lung tissue for a histologic diagnosis are sometimes necessary, thus adding to the delay in instituting appropriate therapy.

Predisposing Factors

Conditions which lead to nosocomial pneumonia are well defined and are usually obvious. Susceptible patients invariably have one or a combination of the following: (1) chronic debilitating illness often requiring prolonged hospitalization; (2) prior therapy with antimicrobial drugs having a broad spectrum; (3) a breach of the airway by tracheostomy or endotracheal tube; and (4) impaired host immunity (cellular and/or humoral) owing to a primary disease or as a consequence of immunosuppressive therapy.

The hospital environment itself has been implicated as a prime source of opportunistic microorganisms, and to some extent it is. Certainly it is a good repository for some hardy drug-resistant strains; but this may vary, as with staphylococci, which may exhibit more drug resistance among community strains than hospital-associated ones. In this context, however, it is well to remember the point emphasized by Feingold (1970) that *hospitalization itself does not predispose the patient to infection; rather, the hospitalized patient is often an altered host with enhanced susceptibility to infection because of either the disease or the therapy.* For this reason the term "nosocomial," strictly defined as an infection originating in a hospital or as one which is not clinically evident or incubating at the time of hospital admission, does not differentiate the etiology and site of infection or the circumstances inducing it. Other descriptions such as iatrogenic or autogenic infection and superinfection are often more appropriate. Thus it is important to remember that these infections may not be acquired from the hospital environment or hospital personnel but may arise from the indigenous microbial flora of the patient.

Hospitalization per se is associated with some striking changes in patterns of bacterial colonization of the respiratory tract which seem significant. As mentioned, the isolation of a variety of potentially pathologic species of gram-negative rods from the oropharynx occurs in a significant percentage (18 per cent) of normal people. Other studies (Johanson et al., 1969, 1972) have reported a lower incidence of gram-negative rod recovery (2 to 12 per cent), but these did not utilize a broth culture medium, which seems to facilitate bacterial recovery. Generally the oropharynx of a normal person is not a very suitable environment for growth of aerobic gram-negative bacteria. Yet colonization developed rapidly in patients admitted to a medical intensive care unit and occurred in about 40 per cent of them within four days of admission to the unit. Such colonization of the respiratory tract apparently plays a major role in the pathogenesis of nosocomial respiratory infections. In the study by Johanson, Pierce, and Sanford, 22 of 95 patients (23 per cent) who were colonized with gram-negative bacilli developed respiratory infections with these bacteria. By comparison, only 4 of 118 patients (3.3 per cent) who were never colonized with these bacteria developed infections. There is additional evidence that susceptibility to oropharyngeal colonization of the hospitalized patient with gram-negative bacilli is related to the severity of the primary underlying disease and is therefore greatest in the moribund subject. The

precise mechanism for such colonization in the chronically or severely ill patient is unknown, but undoubtedly it is related to altered upper airway clearance mechanisms to be discussed. It is noteworthy that when pharyngeal and sputum cultures become positive for Enterobacteriaceae or Pseudomonadaceae and other pathogenic bacteria, it is likely that the respiratory tract is also colonized with these microorganisms. Such a pattern should alert one to impending respiratory infection. New techniques to assess adherence of bacteria to the patient's in vitro cultured buccal mucosa cells may prove important in selecting patients who are more susceptible to bacterial colonization. Consequently, such susceptible persons might profit from prophylactic use of a tropical antimicrobial drug in the oropharynx to prevent colonization with potential pathogens. The future will decide the usefulness of this approach.

The importance of prior antimicrobial therapy as a determinant of oropharyngeal colonization with gram-negative bacilli is not as obvious as might be expected. Several of the cited studies which recorded development of colonization in hospitalized patients failed to find strong evidence that prior or concomitant antimicrobial use was a requisite factor, although such therapy did indeed increase the occurrence of colonization (Pierce and Sanford). On the contrary, in principle, broad-spectrum antimicrobial therapy that reduces a proportion of the normal bacterial flora of the gastrointestinal tract and naso-oropharyngeal area should improve the opportunity for more drug-resistant strains to emerge. Perhaps of greater significance nowadays is the emergence of fungal strains in the wake of a bacterial void so that colonization with these opportunistic organisms presages respiratory infection.

An interruption in the continuity of the airway with a tracheostomy, for example, is often associated with bacterial colonization of the tracheobronchial tree and with recurrent respiratory infections. Obviously, important mechanical barriers which guard entry into the lungs are bypassed and microorganisms have direct access. The situation is compounded if ventilatory equipment is attached which may itself contain a source of bacteria and, in fact, forcefully aerosolize them into the airways. In the time since it was demonstrated that contaminated inhalation respiratory equipment could be the source of nosocomial pneumonia, significant improvement has occurred in the general care and handling of this equipment in many respiratory therapy programs, with the pleasing result that this form of iatrogenic infection is less frequent.

The immunocompromised patient presents a complex array of disordered host defenses, and the lungs are but one organ system at risk for infection. Predisposition to pneumonia with gram-negative bacilli occurs because a number of cellular components in the respiratory tract are either vulnerable to the direct effects of various antineoplastic chemotherapy drugs and anti-inflammatory agents, or may have been depleted because renewal from the bone marrow, for example, is inadequate. (See Ch. 41 and 527.)

Granulocytopenia is the most common abnormality in patients who have ineffective granulocytopoiesis or are receiving cytotoxic chemotherapy. This results from an inadequate systemic supply of circulating phagocytic cells; subsequently, a lack of reserve or marginated granulocytes develops in capillary storage areas. The lung capillary vasculature is but one such involved site.

The effect is to deplete the lower respiratory tract of secondary phagocytes that can be attracted to alveolar areas and to diminish the cellular inflammatory response.

Available evidence indicates that bone marrow–derived circulating monocytes are the precursors of tissue macrophages in the lungs. After the monocyte enters the pulmonary lymphoreticular system, it undergoes further development into a mature phagocytic macrophage which has a life span of several months. Alveolar macrophages obtained by lung lavage from leukemia patients who have been leukopenic (monocytopenic) for several months are functionally and morphologically normal, despite intensive chemotherapy. Such findings indicate longevity of alveolar macrophages. Moreover, some human pulmonary macrophages are capable of a slow rate of replication, which suggests that the number of lung macrophages can be maintained in part by local cell proliferation when the usual influx of cells from peripheral blood and from bone marrow is absent. Although it is difficult to demonstrate that alveolar macrophages are readily depleted in immunosuppressed subjects, in contrast to short-lived polymorphonuclear granulocytes, it is probable that subtle metabolic effects from cytotoxic drugs impair the phagocytic and bactericidal capacity of lung macrophages. This would help account for the greater susceptibility to respiratory infections in these patients. For example, it has been demonstrated that corticosteroids, experimentally, impair the release of lysosomal enzymes from macrophages and granulocytes, impede the migration of cells into inflammatory sites, diminish phagocytosis by macrophages, block the response of macrophages to migration inhibition factor produced by immune lymphocytes, and interfere with granulocyte chemotaxis (Fauci et al., 1974, 1976).

Lymphoid tissue is extensive along the airways, and its alteration could directly affect the lung's handling of antigenic substances contained in respired air. Cell-mediated immune responses could be blunted, and development might be impaired of immunoglobulin-producing lymphocytes and plasma cells which secrete local secretory antibodies onto respiratory mucosal surfaces. However, assessment of the integrity of lymphoid tissue in the lungs of normal people or the immunosuppressed is difficult, because suitable methods are lacking. Customary techniques such as skin testing or antigenic stimulation of peripheral blood lymphocytes are not necessarily representative of immunologic events occurring in vivo in lung tissue. Thus the demonstration of abnormal lymphocyte function in the respiratory tract remains a theoretic consideration. Yet certain populations of lymphocytes are sensitive to radiotherapy (T cells) and may be eliminated when various forms of irradiation therapy are given. Cytotoxic drugs such as cyclophosphamide have various effects on both major subpopulations of lymphocytes (B and T cells).

The consequence of injury to other cell-types in the lung, such as surfactant-secreting Type II alveolar epithelial cells, various mucus-producing cells, and ciliated epithelial cells, are largely conjectural, because the deleterious effects of immunosuppressive agents on these cell-types have not been established. Yet it seems plausible that drastic regimens of immunosuppressive therapy may impair the function of these cells. The cumulative effects of diminished surfactant production promoting lung atelectasis, altered mucus secretion, and reduced ciliary clearance all could contribute to stasis and accumulation of lung secretions which promote local bacterial growth and subsequent pneumonia.

Possible Future Management of Nosocomial Pneumonia

What is the future of therapy in the immunocompromised host? Without question, the cornerstone of the medical treatment for bacterial respiratory infections is antimicrobial therapy. This is likely to remain the situation in the forseeable future, and other forms of therapy will be at best adjuncts. Although the antimicrobial drugs have provided splendid therapy for many infections, the increasing prevalence of many bacteria resistant to them necessitates constant re-evaluation of drug dosages and drug combinations and the continual development of new antimicrobial agents.

As mentioned, granulocytopenia is usually present when an immunosuppressed patient develops a serious bacterial infection. The absence of granulocytes may allow bacteria to become established in lung tissue. Moreover, should bacteremia develop, death of the patient from sepsis can occur quickly. Logically, the replacement of these phagocytic cells by transfusion is a reasonable mode of therapy. A number of clinical trials using granulocyte transfusions show the usefulness of this therapy for certain patients with bacteremia. The rationale is to prevent or contain the infection with chemotherapy and granulocyte transfusion support until there is a return of indigenous bone marrow function and circulating granulocytes. Whether such therapy would prove useful in specific organ infections such as pneumonia remains to be determined.

Alveolar macrophages are not depleted in immunosuppressed patients, despite many weeks of peripheral blood leukopenia and monocytopenia which would be expected to remove precursor cells. Although lung macrophages may undergo some local cellular replication in the immunosuppressed patient, this is judged to be insufficient to maintain the quota of lung phagocytes. Despite the longevity of the macrophage, the high incidence of pulmonary infections in the immunosuppressed patient suggests that it does not function well. Conceivably the situation might be ameliorated by a stimulus such as BCG and perhaps someday by infusion of purely monocytic preparations into leukemic hosts.

The delivery of a specific antibody is generally agreed to be desirable for an immunocompromised patient. The appropriate way to give such therapy is not established and reflects persisting inadequacies in antibody technology. Questions remain about the best route of immunization, the appropriate antigens to use, and the level or quantity of circulating antibody which is protective. In the immunodeficient host, active primary or booster immunization does not reliably provide high or lasting antibody titers, and a supplemental form of passive immunization is usually necessary. Yet loss of body tissue mass from cachexia and/or thrombocytopenia limits the use of parenteral gamma globulin, making intravenous preparations in the form of hyperimmune plasma desirable. The class of immunoglobulin antibody delivered is also important. IgG would appear to be the preferable form of opsonic antibody for established lower lung infections, whereas secretory IgA agglutinating antibody might be preferable to prevent bacterial adherence and colonization in the upper respiratory tract. Currently available parenteral gamma globulin preparations and plasma will both supply IgG antibody adequately, but neither contains a suitable form of IgA (see Ch. 40.8).

Perhaps the most critical decision is selection of the appropriate antigen for immunization of the patient or the donor. In the case of pneumococcal prophylaxis, a multivalent polysaccharide vaccine containing antigens to a limited number of common clinical strains is now available (see Ch. 121). For the gram-negative bacteria, which so frequently cause pulmonary infections in immunosuppressed hosts, the selection of appropriate antigens is not so evident. The variety of infecting strains of Enterobacteriaceae is so large that a comprehensive vaccine, including even the most commonly incriminated strains, is impractical. The alternative approach is to select an antigen which will elicit an antibody that is broadly reactive with many strains and will offer protection against a large number of similar infecting bacteria. In fact, this solution has been achieved experimentally (McCabe; Young et al.) A similar approach has been taken for *Pseudomonas*. Immunization with a J_5 mutant (^Rc glycolipid antigen) of *Escherichia coli* 0:111 induces antibody that protects against *P. aeruginosa* and Enterobacteriaceae organisms. The protein moiety of the endotoxin (OEP) from *P. aeruginosa* has been used for experimental immunization; it affords protection from *P. aeruginosa* infection regardless of the serotype of the organisms. Thus the most important factor in devising practical immunization for the immunodeficient host — the proper selection of antigens that evoke cross-reactive antibodies — is being addressed and should improve the prospects for antibody immunoprophylaxis.

PNEUMONIA CAUSED BY PSEUDOMONAS

Pseudomonas, which is a distinct genus of bacteria and is not included in the family Enterobacteriaceae, is widespread in the environment and is generally part of the usual bacterial flora of hospitals and intensive care units. *Pseudomonas* organisms are frequently carried on the skin (axillary and anogenital areas) of normal people and transiently may be part of the intestinal flora in a significant number (up to 20 per cent). Almost any alteration in normal health status, such as hospitalization or antimicrobial or immunosuppressive therapy, is associated with increased carriage of *Pseudomonas* organisms. People with cystic fibrosis usually have persistent colonization of their respiratory tract with these bacteria.

For this discussion, *Pseudomonas* respiratory infection refers to those caused by *Pseudomonas aeruginosa*, which is the most important pathogen of the genus. The reader should remember, however, that other *Pseudomonas* species can cause serious infections (*P. pseudomallei* [melioidosis] and *P. mallei* [glanders]). Moreover, other less frequently encountered species are being implicated in human infection. *P. cepacia* has the distinction of being the only one in this group of clinical pathogens that is generally not susceptible to gentamicin, hence making drug-susceptibility testing necessary for proper drug selection.

PREDISPOSING FACTORS. *Pseudomonas* rarely produces infection in a normal person but is a frequent cause of sepsis and pneumonia in the abnormal host. Currently it is the second most frequent organism isolated from patients with nosocomial pneumonia (*Klebsiella* now has assumed first place in many recent series). In the past, chronic lung or heart disease was an associated condition that apparently increased susceptibility to *Pseudomonas* pneumonia; now the presence of leukopenia (granulocytopenia) and other evidence of immunosuppressive disease or treatment is more common. *Pseudomonas* infection is likely to be an acquired or secondary pneumonia following any one of the predisposing causes already outlined. As a form of primary pneumonia, it is essentially limited to patients who are receiving inhalation therapy that incorporates reservoir nebulization. Following *Pseudomonas* bacteremia, pulmonary complications are well described, consisting of nodular areas of lung infarction with massive bacterial infiltration of arterial and venous walls. Such bacteremia produces a form of necrotizing pneumonia. This presentation may occur in illicit intravenous drug users who develop *Pseudomonas* tricuspid endocarditis.

PATHOLOGY. On microscopic section, the intraalveolar inflammatory exudate is a mixture of polymorphonuclear leukocytic and mononuclear cells, or the cellular infiltrates may consist predominantly of mononuclear cells admixed with fragmented pyknotic nuclei of necrotic neutrophils. At a later stage, alveolar spaces are filled with a deeply basophilic granular material containing large macrophage-like cells and dense colonies of gram-negative bacilli. In the areas of an abscess there is often focal hemorrhage. The dominant microscopic lesion is that of alveolar septal necrosis. In association with these necrotizing lesions, necrosis of arterial walls and secondary thrombosis of vessels have been encountered when the *Pseudomonas* pneumonia is of bacteremic origin or associated with nebulizing therapy equipment. In primary *Pseudomonas* pneumonia, as reported by Tillotson and Lerner (1968), the vascular involvement is not a feature. *Pseudomonas cepacia* is also associated with a necrotizing granulomatous pneumonia.

CLINICAL FEATURES AND COURSE. In patients with *Pseudomonas* pneumonia, apprehension, toxicity, confusion, and progressive cyanosis are characteristic; hemoptysis is unusual. Relative bradycardia may occur. Alteration in diurnal temperature patterns, with the peak temperature in early morning, was noted by Tillotson and Lerner. The physical signs over the thorax are not characteristic. The development of empyema is common (30 to 50 per cent). Roentgenograms reveal bilateral pneumonic infiltrates, usually in the lower lobe, that are often nodular and may undergo necrosis with abscesses that may be small but are often greater than 1 cm is diameter. A pattern of interstitial infiltration may be seen. With resolution of pneumonia, areas of lung with poor expansion and residual "scarring" may be noted on follow-up chest films.

LABORATORY FINDINGS. The usual laboratory tests such as leukocyte counts are of little help, being either normal or moderately increased and often reflecting the bone marrow status of an underlying disease. Cultures of sputum are of only moderate help, because *Pseudomonas* organisms are frequently present as commensals in patients who are receiving antimicrobial therapy or in those who are critically ill. In the relatively rare situations in which it becomes necessary to establish with certainty the organism involved, specimens could be collected by the transtracheal technique. With empyema, thoracentesis with staining and culture of the fluid will help confirm the diagnosis and facilitate the selection of optimal therapy.

PROGNOSIS AND TREATMENT. Prognosis varies with the underlying condition of the patient. Case mortality rates in the range of 80 per cent are not uncommon with *Pseudomonas* pneumonia, especially if bacteremia develops. However, in recent years, the mortality seems to be distinctly less and appears to be about 35 per cent. Several important things have occurred. First, better antimicrobial drugs are available. The use of an aminoglycoside, gentamicin, and carbenicillin in combination for *Pseudomonas aeruginosa* infections has had a dramatic impact. (It should be remembered, however, that the gentamicin can be inactivated by carbenicillin when the two remain long in the same solution [see Ch. 190].) Second, medical personnel are much more aware of their role in the transmission of this ubiquitous microorganism, and appropriate changes in patient care techniques have been made. Third, meticulous cleanliness of respiratory ventilation equipment and use of disposable endotracheal or tracheostomy suctioning devices are routine. Sadly, however, microbial resistance to one or both of these mainstay antibiotics is now seen on occasion. In 1976, two other aminoglycosides became available, tobramycin and amikacin. Both are effective against many gentamicin-resistant *P. aeruginosa*. Tobramycin appears to be the drug of choice for nonresistant strains of this organism. Undoubtedly, it will be necessary to have additional antimicrobials in the future to keep ahead of the adaptable *Pseudomonas* strains.

Clinical experience and experimental results in leukopenic animal models indicate that a single aminoglycoside (i.e., gentamicin) is usually insufficient to eradicate and cure an extensive *Pseudomonas* pneumonia. Tobramycin appears no better in this situation and probably offers a measurable advantage only when a gentamicin-resistant organism is the cause. The two drugs give slightly different degrees of oto- or nephrotoxicity and other side effects which may dictate the choice of drugs in some patients. The combined use of an aminoglycoside and carbenicillin does offer an improvement in therapy and outcome. Carbenicillin, which seems an especially effective drug in leukopenic patients, should not, however, be relied upon as a single drug, because drug resistance may develop quickly in this setting. Other forms of supportive care are very essential also. Because *Pseudomonas* organisms are difficult to clear from infected lung tissue, patients will frequently relapse after drug therapy is discontinued, despite what is considered an adequate course of therapy. Re-treatment is usually necessary and should be done in conjunction with drug-susceptibility testing of the bacterium to confirm appropriate drug selection. With successful treatment, *Pseudomonas* may still reappear in the sputum, making it necessary to distinguish between relapse and persistent colonization of the respiratory tract. Changing lung infiltrates and clinical signs help to separate the two. As discussed above, current experimental work might lead to other therapies in practical form, such as passive antibody administration of anti-*Pseudomonas* gamma globulin or prophylactic immunization of high-risk patients with *Pseudomonas* lipopolysaccharide antigens. Granulocyte transfusion therapy in appropriate patients could be considered a reasonable possibility at present and does offer hope for improving current therapy.

PNEUMONIA DUE TO OTHER AEROBIC GRAM-NEGATIVE BACILLI
(E. Coli, Serratia Marcescens, and Proteus sp.)

The large number of bacterial species other than *Klebsiella pneumoniae* that belong to the families Enterobacteriaceae and Achromobacteraceae may produce pulmonary infection. In addition, in many hospitals other gram-negative organisms such as *Serratia marcescens* are being encountered, especially in hospital-associated secondary pneumonia.

Primary *E. coli* pneumonia tends to be present as a scattered pneumonic process in the lower lobes. The pulse is proportional to the temperature. Early findings include rales without consolidation. Empyema formation is less common than with *Klebsiella* or *Pseudomonas*. *E. coli* bacteremia from a urinary source more commonly results in lung infection than does that from other gram-negative bacilli.

Proteus species also produce a clinical picture similar to that of *Klebsiella* (see Ch. 122), with fever, chills, dyspnea, pleuritic chest pain, and cough productive of purulent sputum. Signs of consolidation are usual. Roentgenograms reveal dense infiltrates in the posterior segment of an upper lobe or superior segment of the right lower lobe. Progression to lung abscess or empyema is common.

Serratia infections, which are always secondary, have been associated with the clinical oddity "pseudohemoptysis" owing to a red pigment produced by some strains of *Serratia marcescens*. Other features may include abscess formation, empyema, or both.

Clinical experience with the other bacterial genera such as *Flavobacterium* and *Acinetobacter* is limited, but suggests that their clinical manifestations are similar to those of secondary *Klebsiella* infections.

The antimicrobial regimen of choice may be selected according to the physician's knowledge of the epidemiologic pattern of drug resistance to be anticipated in a given community, but should be confirmed, when possible, by tests on an individual patient's organism.

Brachman, P. S.: Nosocomial respiratory infections. Prev. Med., 3:500, 1974.

Gilardi, G. L.: Infrequently encountered *Pseudomonas* species causing infection in humans. Ann. Intern. Med., 77:211, 1972.

Johanson, W. G., Pierce, A. K., and Sanford, J. P.: Changing pharyngeal bacterial flora of the hospitalized patients. N. Engl. J. Med., 281:1137, 1969.

Johanson, W. G., Pierce, A. K., Sanford, J. P., and Thomas, G. D.: Nosocomial respiratory infections with gram-negative bacilli: The significance of colonization of the respiratory tract. Ann. Intern. Med., 77:701, 1972.

McCabe, W. R.: Immunization with R mutant of *S. minnesota*. I. Protection against challenge with heterologous gram-negative bacilli. J. Immunol., 108:601, 1972.

National Nosocomial Infections Study—United States, 1975–76. MMWR, Vol. 26, No. 46, November 18, 1977.

Pennington, J. W., Reynolds, H. Y., Wood, R. E., Robinson, R. B., and Levine, A. S.: Use of *Pseudomonas aeruginosa* vaccine in patients with acute leukemia and cystic fibrosis. Am. J. Med., 58:629, 1975.

Pierce, A. K., and Sanford, J. P.: Aerobic gram-negative bacillary pneumonias: State of the art. Am. Rev. Respir. Dis., 110:647, 1974.

Reynolds, H. Y.: Prevention and future control of hospital-associated infections commonly caused by gram-negative bacteria. Prev. Med., 3:507, 1974.

Reynolds, H. Y., Levine, A. S., Wood, R. E., Zierdt, C. H., Dale, D. C., and Pennington, J. E.: *Pseudomonas aeruginosa* infections: Persisting problems and current research to find new therapies. Ann. Intern. Med., 82:819, 1975.

Rosenthal, S., and Tager, I. B.: Prevalence of gram-negative rods in the normal pharyngeal flora. Ann. Intern. Med., 83:355, 1975.

Westwood, J. C. N., Legace, S., and Mitchell, M. D.: Hospital acquired infection: Present and future impact and need for positive action. Can. Med. Assoc. J., 110:769, 1974.

Williams, D. M., Krick, J. A., and Remington, J. S.: Pulmonary infection in the compromised host. Part 1. Am. Rev. Respir. Dis., 114:359, 1976.

Young, L. S., Stevens, P., and Ingram, J.: Functional role of antibody against "core" glycolipid of Enterobacteriaceae. J. Clin. Invest., 56:850, 1975.

STREPTOCOCCAL DISEASES

125. INTRODUCTION

Gene H. Stollerman

Streptococci constitute a large heterogeneous group of gram-positive bacteria that are very common parasites of man. Their name derives from their growth in liquid media as chains of globular bacteria. Classification of streptococci has been confusing, because a single species may cause a variety of diseases and because several kinds of streptococci can often be cultured from the same site of infection.

CLASSIFICATION

The modern classification of streptococci is based upon Lancefield's identification of the group-specific cell wall "C" carbohydrate antigens which are present in beta-hemolytic streptococci and in some nonhemolytic species as well.

GROUP A INFECTIONS. The most important human streptococcal pathogen, *Streptococcus pyogenes*, can be identified as containing group A carbohydrate with specific rabbit antiserum to the carbohydrate cell wall antigens, and thus can be distinguished from other beta-hemolytic streptococci which are also frequently isolated from the respiratory tract of man. Diseases caused by group A streptococci will be considered in detail in Ch. 126 to 130 and in Ch. 374.3. Streptococci belonging to other serogroups that are of importance to man will be mentioned briefly here.

The traditional classification of streptococci by their properties of hemolysis on the surface of blood agar plates is clinically useful. It helps to distinguish hemolytic streptococci, to which the more virulent species belong, from the alpha-hemolytic viridans streptococci ("green" streptococci), the predominant normal flora of the upper respiratory tract, and the nonhemolytic streptococci which include the enterococci, a common inhabitant of the gastrointestinal tract.

Beta-hemolytic streptococci are those that produce a completely clear zone around the colony as a result of the formation of either extracellular hemolysin, streptolysin O and streptolysin S, or both. Classification of streptococci based on the type of hemolysis they produce, however, is unsatisfactory for many reasons. Many species belonging to specific serologic groups may be nonhemolytic, such as group D. On the other hand, some enterococci belonging to the usually nonhemolytic group D may produce beta hemolysis, or some apparently nonhemolytic colonies may become alpha

hemolytic upon prolonged incubation. Beta hemolysis is therefore primarily useful in the first step of the identification of group A organisms which are, with only rare exceptions, consistently hemolytic.

GROUP B INFECTIONS. The group B organisms are classically represented by the species *Streptococcus agalactiae*. They were well known for many years as the cause of bovine mastitis but produced human disease rarely. Until recently, little attention was paid to group B organisms in man, although it was known that they could colonize the vagina and genitourinary tract and were occasionally found in the upper respiratory tract as well. In fact, between 5 and 10 per cent of hemolytic streptococci isolated from man were identified in many studies as group B. In the past two decades, however, group B streptococci have been reported with increasing frequency as a cause of perinatal infections. In the preantimicrobial era, group A streptococci were the common agent of puerperal fever. Since the early 1960's, however, group B streptococci have emerged as a major cause of puerperal infection and as a cause of neonatal sepsis, with or without meningitis. These organisms have been subdivided into five serotypes — Ia, Ib, Ic, II, and III — based on their polysaccharide capsular antigens and minor protein determinants. Types Ia and III are the strains most often isolated from septic infants in the first week of life, and type III is predominantly associated with meningitis. Transplacentally acquired opsonic antibodies appear to be important as a mechanism of neonatal host defense, and considerable interest now exists in the possibility of immunizing against what is currently the most common serious neonatal bacterial infection in the United States.

The frequency with which group B streptococci are recovered from the female genital tract (and the male genitourinary tract as well) appears to be increasing, and cervicovaginal carrier rates in normal pregnant women vary from 3 to 6 per cent. In some studies, approximately one third of infants born to such carriers have contracted serious group B infections. Group B organisms also seem to be causing bacteremic complications of pyelonephritis in both men and women more often than heretofore, especially in diabetics and other compromised hosts. These infections have remained susceptible to penicillin so far.

GROUP D INFECTIONS. This group includes *Streptococcus faecalis*, often referred to as enterococcus because of the frequency with which it is found in the human gastrointestinal tract. Enterococci may also be cultured from the oropharynx and, although usually nonhemolytic, some strains can produce beta or alpha hemolysis.

S. faecalis is an exceptionally hardy organism which can resist heat (62° C for 30 minutes), grow well at room temperature, multiply in hypertonic media (6.5 per cent sodium chloride), and grow in the presence of 0.05 per cent sodium azide.

Enterococci are often isolated from the blood in bacterial endocarditis and from the urine in urinary tract obstruction. The precise role of these organisms in the pathogenesis of pyelonephritis has not been fully evaluated. They can be associated with suppurative abdominal lesions, especially after bowel surgery.

The failure of some laboratories to distinguish the enterococci from other streptococci often leads to inappropriate therapy in serious infections. These organisms may also be recovered from the respiratory tract and may be regarded mistakenly as penicillin-resistant group A streptococci. This error occurs most often during the post-treatment follow-up study of cases of group A streptococcal sore throat and may lead to needless overtreatment in an attempt to eradicate the organisms from the pharynx. Enterococci do *not* cause pharyngitis and tonsillitis.

STREPTOCOCCI OF OTHER GROUPS. Strains of groups C, E, G, H, K, and O are isolated from the respiratory tract of man but are of little clinical significance. "Human" group C strains may occasionally cause illnesses that resemble those of group A, but such infections are relatively rare. Moreover, as far as is known, only group A organisms cause rheumatic fever. Group G may occasionally cause mild infections, but these are relatively infrequent and are uncomplicated. Groups A, C, and G all elaborate in vivo antigenically similar streptolysin O, streptokinase, hyaluronidase, and erythrogenic toxin.

ALPHA-HEMOLYTIC STREPTOCOCCI ("GREEN" STREPTOCOCCI). The alpha-hemolytic streptococci are often referred to collectively as the *viridans group*. They have never been satisfactorily classified. Their colonies are surrounded by a narrow zone of incompletely hemolyzed red cells (some red cells are spared for unknown reasons). Green discoloration of the colonies occurs owing to the formation of an unidentified reductant of hemoglobin. The degree of "greening" varies with the animal source of blood and is best brought out by sheep red blood cells which differentiate most clearly beta from alpha hemolysis.

Viridans streptococci make up the predominant normal flora of the upper respiratory tract and are generally nonpathogenic except as a cause of subacute bacterial endocarditis. *Streptococcus salivarius* is one of the most commonly encountered of these species. The importance of the streptococci that colonize the oral cavity in the pathogenesis of caries is now well recognized. Species in saliva, such as *Streptococcus mutans, sanguis,* and *mitis,* have remarkable affinity for the enamel of teeth. When the diet is rich in sucrose, the bacteria produce particular long chain polysaccharides which stick to enamel. The formation of lactic acid by the adherent bacteria dissolves enamel and thus causes caries. Bacterial adherence of this kind seems to be due to surface substances with specific affinities for host cell membranes (see Ch. 126). Variations in host susceptibility to caries may be related to factors in saliva and in diet that affect bacterial adherence.

The term *nonhemolytic Streptococcus* is confusing because it is often used to include any *Streptococcus* that is not beta hemolytic, and because many nonhemolytic species (including the common *Streptococcus faecalis*) possess the same group specific cell wall antigens as certain hemolytic strains. The organisms of the nonhemolytic group are generally of low pathogenicity for man and, like alpha-hemolytic streptococci, are of concern to physicians primarily as causative agents of subacute bacterial endocarditis. They may multiply and cause inflammation in traumatized or diseased structures and wounds and in obstructed sinuses, bronchi, and urinary and biliary tracts.

ANAEROBIC STREPTOCOCCI. The varieties of streptococci considered above are facultative anaerobes. Microaerophilic streptococci which are *obligate* anaerobes do exist, however, and cause human disease. They are usually nonhemolytic and have not been systematically classified. One of the most ubiquitous genera of these is the *Peptostreptococcus,* a major component of the anaerobic intestinal flora. These organisms are found in the mouth, bowel, and female genital tract. Their virulence is low and they tend to multiply in necrotic or frankly gangrenous lesions, producing a foul odor such as may be noted in lung abscesses or intra-abdominal or intrauterine infections. They may cause very extensive necrotizing wound infections. Although most anaerobic streptococci are susceptible to antimicrobial drugs, usually penicillin, the lesions in which they are found often require adequate surgical drainage as well as chemotherapy. Peritonsillar, brain, lung, liver, and intra-abdominal abscesses resulting from mixed anaerobic bacterial infections may contain peptostreptococci. *Peptostreptococcus* is also involved in the pathogenesis of necrotizing fasciitis, producing, in synergy with aerobic streptococci or staphylococci, a fulminant, often fatal wound infection (Meleney's synergistic gangrene).

126. GROUP A STREPTOCOCCAL INFECTION

Gene H. Stollerman

HISTORY. Many of the clinical syndromes caused by group A streptococcal infection were recognized for many years before the discovery of *Streptococcus pyogenes* by Rosenbach in 1884. Thus Sydenham is often stated to have described scarlet fever, but the early accounts are inadequate and inexact. Certainly clinical recognition of scarlet fever, of tonsillitis and pharyngitis without a skin rash, of erysipelas, and of puerperal sepsis date back for many centuries before the modern era of bacteriology. Significant understanding of streptococcal infections, however, began with the discovery by Schottmüller, in 1903, that certain strains produce hemolysis on blood agar. Brown, in 1919, defined this reaction in greater detail and coined the descriptive terms that are still in use.

The streptococcal cause of scarlet fever and tonsillitis was known by 1895. The more modern work of the Dicks and of Dochez (1925) resolved the temporary issues raised concerning the possible role of other pharyngeal bacteria in scarlet fever, and Bloomfield clearly defined the streptococcal etiology of most cases of tonsillitis. The serologic classification of the organism into groups by Lancefield and into types by Lancefield and Griffith by 1935 and the introduction of the antistreptolysin O titer by Todd (1932) to identify streptococcal infection immunologically led to the modern era of the clinical bacteriology, immunology, and epidemiology of streptococcal infections and their nonsuppurative sequels, acute rheumatic fever (ARF) and acute glomerulonephritis (AGN).

The great epidemics of streptococcal disease in the armed forces in World War II supplied an enormous volume of clinical material for the clearer definition of the epidemiology of group A streptococcal disease and of the effect of penicillin therapy and prophylaxis upon the prevention of rheumatic fever and glomerulonephritis. The current era has been one of precise chemical definition of the structure and antigenic composition of *Streptococcus* and the pathophysiologic effects of the cellular and extracellular antigenic and nonantigenic products it produces. Of particular interest has been the demonstration of immunologic cross-reactivity of streptococcal products with tissues of the heart and of the skin and the demonstration of complement-fixing immune complexes in the glomeruli of patients with acute nephritis.

The recent intensive studies of group A streptococcal skin infections have clarified the roles of these organisms in impetigo and secondary pyodermas and have pointed out the difference in the serotypes that produce such infections from those that produce pharyngitis alone. Such studies have sharpened the distinction between three populations of group A streptococci: (1) those that infect the throat but not the skin and that cause acute rheumatic fever (ARF) but not acute glomerulonephritis (AGN); (2) the streptococcal pharyngeal strains that cause AGN; and (3) the pyoderma strains that primarily affect the skin but may also be found in the throat, and that cause AGN but apparently little or no ARF. The persistent enigma of the pathogenesis of ARF and of AGN continues to stimulate studies that unfold the remarkable complexity and variation of *Streptococcus pyogenes*.

PATHOGENESIS. The two most common sites of infection with streptococci in man are the nasopharynx and the skin. Most of our knowledge of the host-parasite relation is based on studies of the former, whereas streptococcal skin infection received little attention until recently. A growing interest in the role of streptococcal pyoderma in acute glomerulonephritis has led to increasing awareness of many distinctive features that set skin infections apart from those of the upper respiratory tract. In the ensuing discussion, some of these will be pointed out, and the specific clinical features of skin infections will be considered separately.

Strains of group A streptococci may vary greatly in infectivity or virulence. During epidemics of pharyngitis, most strains isolated from the throats of patients who are acutely ill contain relatively large amounts of the type-specific surface antigen, M protein. More than 70 antigenically distinct types of M protein have been differentiated so far. This substance has particular importance in the pathogenesis of group A streptococcal infection because immunity is type specific, that is, dependent upon antibody to the homologous type of M protein. Such antibodies tend to persist for many years after infection. For this reason, repeated infections with strains of different M types occur during the lifetime of most persons, but reinfection with the same M serotype is very rare unless the type-specific immune response is suppressed by penicillin therapy.

The production of large amounts of M protein is correlated with the ability of *Streptococcus* to resist phagocytosis. A hyaluronic acid capsule, which may attain very large size in some epidemic strains and produce large mucoid colonies, also contributes to the organism's resistance to phagocytosis, particularly in certain laboratory animals such as mice. Rapid passage of group A streptococci through mice usually results in increase in M protein production by group A strains and

frequently in an increased size of the capsule. Interestingly, strains that form mucoid colonies (large capsules) are rarely if every found in the skin. In the presence of homologous anti-M antibody, virulent group A streptococci are rapidly and efficiently destroyed by human blood phagocytes. This phenomenon forms the basis for the so-called bactericidal test for the presence of circulating type-specific anti-M antibody.

Despite the location of the type-specific M protein on the surface "hairs" or "fimbriae" that project from the streptococcal cell wall and the envelope of hyaluronic acid that surrounds them, the factor responsible for the *adherence* of streptococci to mucosal cells has been shown recently to be a lipoteichoic acid (LTA), a bacterial cell wall substance with high affinity for cell membranes. The same LTA is found also in other serogroups of streptococci, viridans streptococci, and staphylococci. The role of LTA in the localization of streptococcal infections and its possible role in the deposition of streptococcal antigens in various organs is currently receiving considerable attention.

It is not yet clear to what extent cross-immunity exists to strains of streptococci less virulent than those that are rich in M protein and that are highly encapsulated. Strains of group A organisms lacking both these virulence factors are readily phagocytized and destroyed by human and animal blood. It is possible that with increasing age and number of previous streptococcal infections, the human host acquires greater resistance to all but the most virulent strains of group A streptococci. This may account, in part, for the striking age incidence in the epidemiology of human group A streptococcal pharyngitis and streptococcal pyoderma. It also may account for the progressive tendency, between infancy and childhood, for nasopharyngeal inflammatory reactions to become more and more focalized and intense. Certainly, immediate and delayed skin allergy to streptococcal products becomes increasingly frequent and severe during childhood and adolescence. Indeed, the widespread incidence of immediate and delayed allergy to streptococcal products has seriously hampered the development of effective vaccines against streptococcal M protein preparations.

The portion of highly purified M protein which is not the type-specific determinant is, instead, one or more determinants common to most if not all M proteins and has been called "M-associated" or "non-type-specific M" protein. Both cellular and humoral hypersensitivity to these antigens are intense in man, and antibodies prepared to them can cross-react with streptococcal protoplast membranes and with the sarcolemma of myocardial tissues.

Recently the type-specific M determinant has been separated and purified in T24 streptococci by extraction with dilute pepsin at suboptimal pH. This purified M protein fraction has been shown to be free of cross-reactivity with other M proteins, molecularly homogeneous by amino acid sequencing, immunogenic in laboratory animals, and far less toxic in human skin than any previously studied M protein preparation. Such progress in the immunochemical definition of the type-specific determinant and its separation from the stubbornly associated cross-reactive and toxic moieties has again encouraged prospects for human immunization against group A streptococci.

Other somatic protein antigens of the streptococcal surface that are of clinical significance are the so-called

T proteins of group A streptococci. Although these play no part in virulence, they are useful antigenic markers of streptococci, particularly when the latter have dissociated to less virulent strains with the loss of their M protein marker. The T antigens include a number of immunologically distinct proteins which resist digestion by proteolytic enzymes. Antisera prepared against these antigens can identify the T type of trypsin-digested whole streptococci by a slide agglutination method. This method has proved particularly useful in identifying pyoderma streptococci (see below) which could not be serotyped with available anti-M sera because these organisms contained M proteins of hitherto unidentified types. Thus the T type pattern of a streptococcal strain is a useful marker in following its epidemiology, especially when its M protein marker is unknown or not present. There is little difficulty in M-typing the strains isolated from most outbreaks of acute streptococcal respiratory infection, but it is seldom possible to identify an M antigen in more than 50 per cent of any large and unselected collection of cultures. This is generally not due to the absence of M antigen but to the difficulty of preparing anti-M antisera to some types and the apparent large number of M proteins which still remain unidentified.

No definite biologic property has been defined for the *"C"-carbohydrate group A antigen*. The antigenic determinant of group A polysaccharide has been shown to be composed of repeating units of a dimer of N-acetyl glucosamine and rhamnose. Antibodies against this somatic antigen are not readily demonstrated in man by conventional antibody tests, but recent studies employing radioactive-labeled antigen have identified very persistent antibodies to group A polysaccharide in the sera of patients with rheumatic heart disease. The *mucopeptide* (peptidoglycan) which forms the backbone of the streptococcal cell wall cross-reacts with the structurally similar mucopeptides of many other bacteria and produces many of the same biologic reactions as the endotoxins of gram-negative bacteria.

In the course of human infections, group A organisms produce a great variety of antigenic extracellular products, such as streptolysin O, streptokinase (fibrinolysin), hyaluronidase, nicotinamide adenine dinucleotidase (NADase), several deoxyribonucleases (DNAses), and proteinases. The antibody responses to many of these substances are useful in diagnosis (see below), and some of these products undoubtedly contribute to the pathologic features of streptococcal infection. For example, the breakdown of fibrin and nucleic acids by streptokinase and the DNAases, respectively, produces the characteristic thin pus of streptococcal infections and, with hyaluronidase, may aid the organisms' rapid spread through tissues, as observed in streptococcal cellulitis and lymphagitis. The erythrogenic toxin causes the typical erythema of scarlet fever (see below). The pathogenic role of other toxins is not yet clearly understood.

A streptococcal product receiving attention recently for its possible biologic significance is a type-specific lipoprotein lipase which causes opalescence in serum. This "serum opacity reaction" (SOR) has been used to identify strains of certain M protein serotypes. SOR⁺ strains appear to produce less intense anti-M immune responses and seem to be rarely associated with rheumatic fever.

With the virtual disappearance of diphtheria in the United States, the group A *Streptococcus* is the only significant bacterial organism that commonly causes primary sore throat, that is, that can invade the normal tissues of the pharynx. Because nasal and throat carriage of these organisms is very common, virulent streptococci may be inoculated into open wounds or skin abrasions, producing rapidly spreading *cellulitis* and *lymphangitis* or *erysipelas;* they may contaminate the denuded postpartum endometrium to produce puerperal sepsis; they may secondarily infect the lungs to produce a *streptococcal pneumonia* after viral respiratory diseases such as influenza. Therefore group A streptococci have always been a major cause of sepsis and suppurative complications. In addition, certain so-called *nonsuppurative complications* such as *rheumatic fever* and *glomerulonephritis* may follow streptococcal infection by pathogenic mechanisms that are not yet clear. The relation of streptococcal antigens to the pathogenesis of ARF and AGN is discussed in Ch. 130 and 374.3.

EPIDEMIOLOGY. Quantitatively, upper respiratory infections, including scarlet fever, pharyngitis, and tonsillitis, are the most important forms of group A streptococcal infection. Illness in these categories occurs most frequently in children from 5 to 15 years of age, but younger and older persons are also highly susceptible to infection. The key to the understanding of the epidemiology of streptococcal infection is an appreciation of its mode of transmission. Transmission of group A streptococcal infections occurs as a result of direct contact between infected persons or healthy carriers and susceptible persons. Significant extrahuman or animal reservoirs of these organisms do not exist, although occasional outbreaks caused by contamination of an article of food, often milk, have occurred. In general, however, streptococci dissociate rapidly outside the human host, and organisms recovered from clothing, bedding, or house dust, although identifiable as group A, have been found to be noninfective when inoculated into the throats of human volunteers. Children, among whom infection is commonplace and healthy carriers are abundant, are primarily responsible for the spread of streptococcal disease. The introduction of an untreated, infected five-year-old into a family will be followed by pharyngeal infection of more than half of his siblings and a significant number of adults in the household. The spread of an M-typable, virulent strain of group A *Streptococcus* through a family occurs much more readily than that of non-M-typable organisms. The problem of control of hemolytic streptococcal disease is complicated by the fact that a very large proportion of infections by these organisms is either exceedingly mild or completely inapparent. Persons with this type of "subclinical" infection are fully capable of disseminating the streptococci, but will not necessarily come under the care of a physician who could apply modern chemotherapy, eradicate streptococci from the pharyngeal tissues, and eliminate the possibility of transmission of the disease.

Epidemiologic factors such as climate, season, and geography are important primarily as they affect close contact of individuals. For example, military recruit populations, particularly when mobilized in large camps in cold climates and crowded housing conditions, provide the most ideal circumstances for the rapid passage of the organism from individual to individual, and such populations give rise to some of the most severe epidemics on record. Streptococcal disease is most severe in civilian populations when poverty and poor housing promote the most crowded living conditions.

In the northern cities of the United States pharyngeal streptococcal infections vary strikingly with the season of the year. The peak incidence occurs between December and May, and only sporadic infections appear during the hot summer months. In family studies of a large metropolitan area in the northern part of the United States, it was estimated that a streptococcal infection occurs approximately once every three to four years during childhood and adolescence, and that in a middle class population in this metropolis only about 2 per cent of all respiratory illnesses that occurred were due to group A streptococcal infection.

The epidemiology of *scarlet fever* is the same as that of other group A streptococcal infections except that the strains producing the infection seem to be lysogenized by a bacteriophage that induces the production of erythrogenic toxin in a manner analogous to diphtheria organisms that produce diphtheria toxin. Thus the epidemiology of scarlet fever is essentially that of any other strain of group A *Streptococcus* that does not produce the erythrogenic toxin. This explains the mild sporadic cases of scarlet fever, the severe epidemics of streptococcal pharyngitis *without* any scarlet fever cases, and the localized outburst of scarlet fever in a single concentrated population such as a school or institution.

The epidemiology of streptococcal *pyoderma* is strikingly different from that of streptococcal pharyngitis in several respects. Seasonal occurrence of the two is quite disparate in temperate climates: pharyngitis is more common and intense in cold weather, whereas streptococcal pyoderma occurs often in the late summer and early fall. The close indoor contact during the colder months may facilitate respiratory spread, whereas increased exposure of the uncovered skin to minor trauma and insect bites may favor skin infection during the warmer months. Although, geographically, epidemic streptococcal pharyngitis is more common in temperate or cold climates and streptococcal pyoderma in hot or tropical climates, exceptions are not uncommon in both diseases.

Streptococcal pyoderma affects an even younger age group than pharyngitis, occurring most often in children of preschool age and in infants. Transmission of streptococcal pyoderma may be aided mechanically by insects, particularly flies, that are attracted to skin lesions. Poverty and filth, as well as crowding, are major predisposing factors. Patients with streptococcal pyoderma often harbor the same organisms in the throat that colonize the skin.

The Contrasting Epidemiology of Acute Rheumatic Fever and Acute Glomerulonephritis (see accompanying figure). Students of the nonsuppurative sequels of group A streptococcal infection have long been impressed with the extreme rarity with which ARF and AGN occur in the same patient at the same time, and the antecedent infection is considered, therefore, to be due to a strain that is *either* "rheumatogenic" *or* "nephritogenic," but not both. Simultaneous appearance of both sequelae has not been a feature of the reported experience of large numbers of patients with either disease in severe epidemics in which a single streptococcal strain could be identified as the cause. The route of infection also seems to differentiate rheu-

Seasonal distribution of acute rheumatic fever (ARF) and acute glomerulonephritis (AGN) admissions at City of Memphis Hospitals, September 1965–August 1968. (After Bisno, A. L., Pearce, I. A., Wall, H. P., Moody, M. D., and Stollerman, G. H.: N. Engl. J. Med., 283:561, 1970.)

matogenic from nephritogenic strains. Acute rheumatic fever seems to be almost always, if not exclusively, a complication of a pharyngeal infection. Acute glomerulonephritis occurs after *either* skin or pharyngeal infection. Although skin strains often parasitize the throat, the best known rheumatogenic pharyngeal strains do not seem to parasitize the skin.

The strains which belong to the M serotypes that have clearly caused pharyngitis followed by rheumatic fever are those commonly encountered in the throats of children in the cities of the temperate zones of the United States and western Europe and include, among others, 1, 3, 5, 6, 14, 18, 19, and 24. *All* strains containing these M antigens are not necessarily nonnephritogenic, and from time to time sporadic cases of AGN have appeared which seemed to be due to strains representing some of these serotypes (types 1, 3, and 6).

The identification of M type 12 organisms as the major pharyngeal serotype that has been associated with AGN (Rammelkamp et al., 1952) is of interest because this M serotype is one of the most common ones encountered in the throats of schoolchildren, and yet AGN does not appear consistently in populations harboring this strain. Thus not all members of a given M serotype are necessarily nephritogenic.

The recent attention to the bacteriology of skin strains of steptococci has revealed them to contain M and T proteins of types hitherto unrecognized. Since the identification of the nephritogenic type 49 (Red Lake) skin strain, a seemingly endless procession of new M types has been identified, and the number accepted by international reference laboratories now exceeds 70. Although AGN has occurred in association with most of the strains in these categories, no specific M or T antigen per se has been related to this complication.

The factors of infection determining the attack rate of rheumatic fever are also quantitative. The attack rate may vary from as low as 0.3 per cent after very mild, sporadic streptococcal infections associated with strains of low virulence to as high as 3 per cent or greater after infections with highly virulent strains of group A streptococci. The two factors that appear to have most influence on the frequency with which rheumatic fever follows a streptococcal infection are (1) the duration of convalescent carriage of the strain after the infection, and (2) the magnitude of the immunologic response associated with the infection. Thus patients with relatively feeble antistreptolysin O responses may show an attack rate of rheumatic fever of considerably less than 1 per cent, whereas those with the most vigorous streptococcal antistreptolysin O responses may suffer attack rates of rheumatic fever as high as 5 to 10 per cent. The acquisition of streptococci in the throat and their subsequent carriage *without* immunologic response has not been associated with reactivation of rheumatic fever in rheumatic subjects, nor do primary attacks of rheumatic fever occur very often without a well defined immune response. The epidemiology of rheumatic fever is therefore a reflection of the prevalence and severity of group A streptococcal pharyngitis.

127. CLINICAL SYNDROMES OF GROUP A STREPTOCOCCAL INFECTION

Gene H. Stollerman

127.1. STREPTOCOCCAL SORE THROAT

The classic syndrome described as most typical of group A streptococcal infection in older children and adults is as follows:

SYMPTOMS. There is a sudden onset of sore throat, sometimes associated with abdominal pain and nausea, especially in children, accompanied by constitutional symptoms of malaise, headache, and feverishness.

SIGNS. Redness and edema of the throat are present, particularly an *exudate* on the tonsils or tonsillar fossae; enlargement and particularly *tenderness* of the anterior cervical nodes, and fever of 38.2° C or greater. Helpful laboratory data, other than results of throat culture, include leukocytosis greater than 12,000 leukocytes per cubic millimeter.

Although this classic syndrome is, indeed, associated with group A streptococcal infection, the full clinical picture develops in a minority of patients with pharyngitis, except during epidemics. Much more common in clinical practice is the patient with some, but not all, of the aforementioned signs and symptoms. It is not unusual for mild streptococcal disease to be associated with *nonexudative* pharyngitis, and, conversely, for viral infections, particularly adenovirus and Epstein-Barr virus, to produce purulent tonsillar exudate and a syndrome indistinguishable from streptococcal tonsillitis. Hemolytic streptococci are the only common *bacterial* cause of nonexudative pharyngitis. Many viral infections may mimic this clinical state, making the study of upper respiratory infection without bacteriologic control most difficult.

Streptococcal respiratory infection is not accompanied by significant cough or by coryza. The presence of either of these manifestations should suggest a different cause. *Rhinorrhea* does occur in young children, who may develop suppurative sinusitis.

SCARLET FEVER. The disease is clinically similar in almost all respects to tonsillitis and pharyngitis caused by nonscarlatinal strains of group A streptococci. Its name, however, comes from the presence of a skin rash caused by the erythrogenic toxin produced by scarlatinal strains. The erythrogenic effect of the toxin on the skin can be neutralized by antitoxin. This is the basis of the diagnostic *Schultz-Charlton reaction*. The injection of 0.1 ml of scarlet fever antitoxin, or of 0.2 to 0.3 ml of convalescent human serum, into an area where the rash is florid will be followed by blanching around the site of injection in 8 to 12 hours. Streptococcal antitoxin is no longer readily available, and usually clinical and bacteriologic studies suffice for diagnosis.

The enanthem of scarlet fever includes a tongue that may be bright red with large papillae (raspberry tongue) or coated with the red papillae protruding (strawberry tongue). These manifestations of the disease are rarely seen in adults. The rash usually appears on the second day of the disease. It consists of a diffuse, bright scarlet erythema with many points of deeper red. The distribution is variable, but the trunk and inner aspects of the arms and thighs are most often affected. In many cases the rash is clearly seen only in the axillae and groins. The face is flushed and red, but a pale area, the *circumoral pallor*, is often seen around the mouth. The palms and soles are not erythematous. Petechiae and occasionally ecchymoses are observed, especially in severely ill patients. The application of a tourniquet to the arm for five minutes will be associated with the appearance of large numbers of petechiae distal to the obstruction in nearly all cases. This is the *Rumpel-Leede* sign; it is not specific for scarlet fever. The erythema disappears usually by the sixth to the ninth day of infection in association with the return of the temperature and the throat to normal. *Desquamation of the skin* is characteristic of scarlet fever, and it begins as a fine scaling of the face and body that is usually completed during the second week. About this time the extensive and characteristic desquamation of the palms and soles starts and continues for one to two weeks. Often the diagnosis is made retrospectively in patients who show this desquamation after a sore throat and in whom the scarlatinal rash may have been overlooked. *Eosinophilia* may be a feature of scarlet fever, especially during desquamation, and is sometimes striking (up to 20 per cent).

The course and clinical features of scarlet fever vary greatly with the severity of the disease. Many mild cases are observed in which constitutional symptoms and sore throat are minimal, fever is low grade and of short duration, and the rash is evanescent. A florid eruption is sometimes seen in persons in whom all other evidences of the disease are slight, indicating that the reaction to the erythrogenic toxin per se is not primarily responsible for the systemic manifestations of scarlet fever. Again, the situation is comparable to that in diphtheria. A mild sore throat with a strain that is a potent toxin-producer may result in a clinical picture dominated by the effects of the exotoxin. Conversely, severe pharyngeal infection may be present with a strain that is a relatively mild toxin-producer, and the clinical manifestations resulting from the toxin may be slight.

COURSE OF STREPTOCOCCAL PHARYNGITIS. The course of untreated hemolytic streptococcal pharyngitis in older children and adults is benign. Seventy-five per cent of patients are afebrile within 72 hours after onset, but sore throat, abnormal signs in the pharynx, and tender adenitis may persist for two or three days after the return of the temperature to normal. Although the whole process is shortened 24 to 48 hours by appropriate antimicrobial therapy, it is not always easy to distinguish the treated from the untreated patient. An acute pharyngitis that *fails to respond* to adequate penicillin therapy is virtually never due to group A streptococcal infection. On the other hand, the course of viral pharyngitis is often also very brief, and a spontaneous defervescence in 24 to 48 hours may mislead the clinician who has treated the patient into believing the patient has had a therapeutic response to penicillin therapy. In severe streptococcal infections, leukocytosis, when present in the acute stage, may persist in more than one half of untreated patients for a week or more, but this disappears more quickly after the institution of antimicrobial therapy. The erythrocyte sedimentation rate returns to normal in 80 per cent of patients by the third week.

Group A streptococci tend to persist in the pharynx for long periods after recovery if antimicrobial therapy has not been employed. In general, the more virulent the strain, the longer and more consistent is the duration of convalescent throat carriage. Under epidemic conditions, 80 per cent of untreated patients may carry the infecting strain for as long as four weeks. On the other hand, sporadic and mild streptococcal infections among schoolchildren studied in recent years have not been as frequently associated with such prolonged throat carriage.

Streptococcal pharyngitis in infants and small children lacks an acute and well defined onset, has *rhinorrhea* as a dominant manifestation, is rarely associated with high fever, and runs a protracted and indeterminate course. The physical signs in the throat are nondescript, and usually do not permit an accurate clinical diagnosis. Suppurative complications such as otitis media and cervical lymphadenitis occur frequently.

The change of the pharyngeal response after the first few years of life to an explosive onset with fever, sore throat, and exudative pharyngitis may be a reflection of the sharp increase in delayed hypersensitivity (cellular immunity) that appears after the first or second year of life as a result of repeated infection with different types of group A streptococci. It is noteworthy that rheumatic fever is very rare before heightened cellular and humoral immunity to the *Streptococcus* occurs, whereas acute glomerulonephritis is common.

DIAGNOSIS OF STREPTOCOCCAL PHARYNGITIS. Streptococcal tonsillitis and pharyngitis in its typical form needs to be differentiated from diphtheria, nonstreptococcal exudative pharyngitis (usually adenovirus), and infectious mononucleosis. When streptococcal infection is nonexudative, however, it cannot be differentiated (in the absence of scarlet fever) from a variety of viral agents producing an identical clinical picture. Cough, coryza, and rhinorrhea (in adults) make a nonbacterial disorder more likely. Unfortunately therefore the clinical diagnosis of the kind of streptococcal pharyngitis that now occurs most commonly as a sporadic infection in civilian communities is usually a crude guess. It is possible, however, to *exclude* the diagnosis of streptococcal disease in considerably more than half the patients studied for sporadic pharyngitis by the use of throat cultures. The incidence of throat cultures positive for beta-hemolytic streptococci decreases progressively with age in patients with sporadic acute respiratory diseases in civilian communities. In several large cities in the northern sections of the United States, surveys have shown that less than 5 per cent of adults who had routine cultures for upper respiratory infections harbored group A streptococci in their throats. It is obvious therefore that without bacteriologic confirmation, the clinical diagnosis of viral versus streptococcal pharyngitis is quite unsatisfactory.

Before any antimicrobial therapy is administered, swabs should be passed through the mouth under direct vision, using a good light, and rubbed over the tonsils and posterior pharynx. The swab should be streaked directly, with a minimum of delay, on sheep blood agar plates of low dextrose content. After incubation overnight, the number of hemolytic streptococci present should be recorded in a roughly quantitative manner. These organisms will be very numerous in nearly all cases if they are the cause of the infection. The presence of a few does not provide convincing evidence that they are responsible for the illness, because 5 to 10 per cent of the general population are nasopharyngeal carriers of these organisms. Serologic grouping and typing of the isolated organisms are usually not necessary for routine clinical diagnosis. Because all group A streptococci are susceptible in vitro to discs containing less than 0.02 unit of bacitracin, some laboratories determine the bacitracin susceptibility of hemolytic streptococci routinely. A hemolytic *Streptococcus* resistant to such low concentrations of bacitracin is virtually never a group A *Streptococcus*. On the other hand, approximately 5 per cent of non-group A hemolytic streptococci are also susceptible to this low concentration.

Immunologic Diagnosis of Streptococcal Pharyngitis. The immunologic diagnosis of group A streptococcal infection is of no value in the treatment of the acute illness, because an antibody response will not usually be detected until 10 to 20 days after the onset of the disease. Measurement of antistreptolysin O, anti-DNAse B, antihyaluronidase, antistreptokinase, or anti-NADase is of great value in determining whether or not there has been preceding streptococcal pharyngitis in patients with possible rheumatic fever or glomerulonephritis. The presence of low titers of such antibodies during convalescence virtually excludes recent streptococcal disease except in patients who have been intensively treated early in the illness.

It should be noted that streptococcal pyoderma does not produce an equally strong immune response to all streptococcal antigens. In particular, antistreptolysin O and anti-NADase are increased relatively infrequently, whereas anti-DNAse B and antihyaluronidase, particularly the former, are better indicators of streptococcal pyoderma.

Recently, a sensitive hemagglutination test has been devised for detecting an increase in streptococcal antibodies in human serum following group A infections. The test depends on the detection of one or more extracellular antigens that adhere to the membrane of red blood cells. The extracellular substance or substances have not been clearly identified but do not appear to be any one of the aforementioned extracellular products. They have been called "streptozyme" and the hemagglutinating antibodies to them, "antistreptozyme." Although the test is not yet immunologically standardized and not yet proved to be entirely specific for group A streptococci, the frequency with which this system reflects antecedent group A streptococcal infection is very high, approaching 100 per cent in rheumatic fever and in poststreptococcal glomerulonephritis. A low antistreptozyme titer therefore in a patient with migratory polyarthritis or acute glomerulonephritis helps to exclude a streptococcal cause for either condition.

The clinician should be aware that elevated serum levels of streptococcal antibodies may persist for long periods of time after an immune response has occurred. Such elevated serum levels do not necessarily imply an unfavorable prognosis, and are not an indication for additional prolonged antimicrobial therapy.

The Value of Throat Cultures in Deciding When to Treat. There may be some difficulty in interpreting the significance of a throat culture weakly positive for hemolytic streptococci when streptococcal disease is mild and sporadic. Such a positive culture may represent the acquisition of a strain temporarily in the pharynx that does not actually invade the deeper tissues of the host, does not produce a significant immune response, and does not lead to acute rheumatic fever. Such a positive culture may also represent the convalescent carriage of an infection that occurred several weeks previously and may bear no relation to subsequent acute symptoms of viral pharyngitis from which the patient may now be suffering. The physician's problem in deciding which patient with pharyngitis to treat with antimicrobial drugs will be clarified if he obtains throat cultures routinely in all such patients whom he examines. By doing this he becomes alert to the epidemiology of the infections he encounters. A throat culture negative for beta-hemolytic streptococci will exclude a great many patients from unnecessary and promiscuous use of expensive antimicrobial drugs. In outbreaks of exudative pharyngitis, negative throat cultures in a succession of patients will immediately reveal the nonstreptococcal nature of the disease encountered. Conversely, a succession of strongly positive cultures leaves little doubt that a local outbreak of streptococcal pharyngitis is in progress.

When exudative pharyngitis is associated with a throat culture heavily seeded with beta-hemolytic streptococci, there is little argument with the general recommendation for prompt and adequate antimicrobial therapy. Moreover, when a succession of such cases is observed, the practitioner is immediately alerted to the need to culture material from the throats of asymptomatic contacts to prevent the spread of an epidemic. It is with the sporadic cases of nonexudative pharyngitis that are associated with positive throat cultures that some argument has been raised as to the need to employ intensive penicillin therapy in the regimens recommended for the prevention of rheumatic fever (see below). In some populations and under some conditions, such intensive treatment may not be necessary. At present, however, these conditions have not yet been sufficiently defined to justify broad generalizations. Until further studies define more precisely the risk of withholding or modifying chemotherapy of such infections, it is safer to err on the side of overtreatment

and thus to ensure the prevention of passage of streptococcal strains through a population. Indeed, with the assistance of the throat culture, all contacts of patients with well diagnosed exudative streptococcal pharyngitis may be studied for acquisition of potentially dangerous strains, and those identified as carriers may be treated. The consequence of such practice would undoubtedly have a profound influence on the epidemiology of streptococcal infection and therefore upon the incidence of rheumatic fever and glomerulonephritis.

COMPLICATIONS OF PHARYNGITIS. Suppurative and nonsuppurative complications may follow untreated streptococcal tonsillitis and pharyngitis.

Suppurative Complications. *Peritonsillar abscess* or *quinsy sore throat* is an interesting and infrequent complication of streptococcal tonsillitis. Its exact pathogenesis is unknown. Suppuration extends through the capsule of the palatine tonsil into the loose connective tissue of the neck. This is associated with formation of brawny edema of the affected side with movement of the tonsil toward the midline of the throat. An abscess eventually forms and drains in untreated cases, *but the pus does not regularly contain streptococci.* It is probable that the initial streptococcal infection does not cause this lesion directly, but may permit commensal organisms such as anaerobic gram-negative bacilli of the oropharynx and anaerobic nonhemolytic streptococci to gain a foothold in the affected tissues. The onset of this complication is marked by an abrupt increase in soreness and swelling of the neck, and often by increased fever and malaise. The involved tonsil and anterior pillar are greatly swollen, the cervical nodes are large and tender, and eventually a fluctuant mass may be felt in the affected area with the gloved finger. Complications of peritonsillar abscess arise when the infection extends further into the neck or leads to the development of suppurative thrombophlebitis. Peritonsillar abscess is only rarely seen today, because severe hemolytic streptococcal tonsillitis is often treated early in its course with effective antimicrobial agents.

Direct extension of hemolytic streptococci from the locus in the throat to the surrounding tissues may result in certain suppurative complications. *Paranasal sinusitis, otitis media, mastoiditis, suppurative cervical adenitis,* and *impetigo* are the most common, and will occur most frequently in untreated children less than four years old. It has been demonstrated that otitis media occurring early in the course of streptococcal respiratory infection is caused by the same serologic type that was present in the throat at the onset. A similar complication that develops after the first week is likely to be the result of a reinfection, and a different type will be recovered from the purulent exudate. Bacteremia was once observed rather frequently during the course of streptococcal respiratory infection and was often associated with metastatic lesions in the joints, bones, and elsewhere. Such cases are now almost unknown, even if antimicrobial therapy is withheld. Similarly, there has been a nearly complete disappearance of group A streptococcal meningitis. Pneumonia has always been a surprisingly uncommon complication of streptococcal upper respiratory infections. Tender cervical adenitis is regularly present and is not to be regarded as a complication unless the lymph nodes become very large and fluctuant. All the various suppurative streptococcal complications may be prevented by early and adequate antimicrobial therapy. Response to similar management is excellent if any such complications should develop in an untreated patient.

Nonsuppurative Complications. The principal non-suppurative complications of streptococcal disease, acute rheumatic fever (ARF) and acute glomerulonephritis (AGN), are discussed in Ch. 130 (ARF) and in Ch. 374.3 (AGN).

127.2. STREPTOCOCCAL SKIN INFECTIONS

STREPTOCOCCAL PYODERMA

CLINICAL FEATURES. Aside from secondary infections of wounds or burns, group A streptococci can cause at least two kinds of skin infection, *pyoderma* and *erysipelas*. These differ markedly in clinical appearance, in epidemiology, in pathogenesis, and perhaps in the strains of streptococci causing infection. The term streptococcal pyoderma includes all kinds of streptococcal skin infections, other than erysipelas, many of which are secondary infections. The term *impetigo,* or *impetigo contagiosa*, describes what often appears to be a *primary* infection, is initially and transiently vesicular, and presents as crusted, nonscarring lesions in its later stages.

The initial lesion of streptococcal impetigo is a papule that develops rapidly into a vesicle with a small surrounding area of erythema. The vesicles are often missed clinically because of their evanescence and rapid transformation into pustules with thick, amber-colored crusts that appear to be "stuck on" the skin. Aside from occasional itching and burning, the lesions are not painful unless they become deep seated. Regional lymph nodes are commonly involved even without extensive local cellulitis. Often an apparently innocuous lesion may yield large numbers of group A streptococci in cultures taken beneath dried crusts, and such indolent-appearing lesions can produce full-blown acute glomerulonephritis. Bacteremia, which is rare in streptococcal pharyngitis, occurs more frequently with skin and wound infections, and occasionally scarlet fever has been reported. Superficial streptococcal skin infections often pursue a chronic course of weeks or months, and their onset is often difficult to establish. A deeply ulcerated form is known as *ecthyma*.

Contagiousness of streptococcal skin infections is evident from the tendency of multiple cases to occur in a family and from their tendency to occur in epidemics. The importance of antecedent skin trauma is apparent in the epidemiology of streptococcal pyoderma (see above). Its preponderance in the summer when insect bites and trauma to exposed parts of children are most common, especially in populations in which poverty results in poor hygiene, neglect, flies, and crowding, suggests the conditions for maximal opportunity of invasion of the skin by virulent strains. Because of the frequency, especially in children, of such minor skin trauma as mosquito bites, abrasions, burns, eczema, scabies, and pediculosis, it is often difficult to determine whether or not group A streptococci invade the unbroken skin. In epidemic conditions owing to particularly virulent strains, the clinical appearance of the lesions often suggests direct invasion, but it is virtually impossible to exclude minute and transient antecedent trauma.

DIAGNOSIS. The frequency with which staphylococci colonize the skin makes contamination of skin lesions with these organisms almost the rule. Cultures of lesions more clearly considered streptococcal pyoderma are frequently also associated with staphylococci, and the relative role of each organism in the etiology of impetigo has caused much confusion and controversy. Although the issue is not entirely settled, current evidence suggests that impetigo can be divided on clinical, bacteriologic, and epidemiologic grounds into two basic forms: *a bullous type,* in infants, which forms thin, varnish-like crusts and is primarily staphylococcal in origin, and *a vesicular type,* which develops thick "stuck-on" crusts and is primarily streptococcal in etiology. Whereas the classic bullous impetigo caused by staphylococci yields a pure culture of phage Type 71 organisms, the early vesicular stage of streptococcal impetigo may yield pure cultures of group A streptococci, but in the purulent and crusted stages large numbers of staphylococci may be present also. The latter are of a variety of phage types suggesting secondary colonization.

Skin cultures of pyodermas should be made after careful cleansing of the surface of the lesions with gauze soaked in sterile warm water, avoiding antiseptics, soaps, and detergents that kill or suppress the more fastidious streptococci and favor the survival of the more adaptable *Staphylococcus*. Often the removal of crusts and careful culture of the serous exudate beneath will yield large numbers of hemolytic streptococci in almost pure culture. Sheep blood agar plates incubated anaerobically or in 10 per cent CO_2 favor the growth of streptococci.

The higher numbered M and T serotypes associated with pyoderma strains of group A streptococci set them apart from the primarily pharyngeal strains, although it should be noted that throat carriage of the "skin strains" may be high in populations in which much pyoderma is present, especially during the summer months.

The weak antistreptolysin O response to pyoderma strains should be borne in mind, and anti-DNAse B, antihyaluronidase, or antistreptozyme titers should be measured when studies of the immune response to these streptococcal infections are indicated (see above), as in the diagnosis of poststreptococcal AGN.

ERYSIPELAS

This form of group A streptococcal skin infection has special characteristics and may be considered in greater detail. Erysipelas usually involves the face and head, but may affect any area of the body. Other than an occasional case of a group C strain that has been recognized, erysipelas is caused by group A streptococci. The precise way in which the bacteria are introduced into the skin in primary facial erysipelas has not been determined. Large numbers of group A streptococci are fairly constantly present among the nasopharyngeal flora of patients with early erysipelas. It may be that the primary infection is a nasopharyngitis from which the organism is transferred to the skin.

After reaching the face, the streptococci may enter

the skin through minute abrasions that are not recognizable after the disease is well established. In surgical and wound erysipelas, it is probable that streptococci are introduced into the traumatized areas from external sources, usually the nose and throat of attendants and other patients. The epidemiology of facial erysipelas differs somewhat from that of group A streptococcal infection in the affected age groups. This disease, when large numbers of cases were observed in the past, was rather common in infancy, rare between the ages of six and thirty, and predominantly a disorder of middle age. There had been no explanation for this discrepancy in age distribution.

Erysipelas usually begins as an abrupt onset of fever with a shaking chill. A history of preceding acute or subacute upper respiratory infection is obtained in about one third of adult cases and more frequently in infants. Very early in the disease a definite zone of redness and edema of the skin appears, most frequently around the birdge of the nose or around a surgical incision, traumatic wound, area of dermatitis, or the newly severed umbilical cord. Facial erysipelas is usually self-limited if no antibacterial therapy is administered. Under these circumstances, the temperature remains at a high level for four to ten days and then falls by lysis or crisis. During this interval a local process involves a large part of the face. As the lesion develops and spreads from the central focus, the skin is red, hot, edematous, and glistening. Blebs are frequently formed. The advancing edge of the lesion is sharply defined and slightly elevated. Great swelling occurs when the infection involves the eyelids.

The disease may involve one or both sides of the face, and usually remains active and spreading until the cheeks and eyelids are affected. Very often the inflammatory process does not extend over the bony prominences, and is limited to the area between the mandible, the malar eminence, and the hairline. In certain cases the ear is included, but spread to the scalp and trunk is rare except in infants.

Untreated *erysipelas of the trunk or extremities,* which usually occurs in infants or persons who have undergone surgery or have been injured, is a more malignant disease. Large areas of skin are often involved rapidly, prostration frequently occurs, and death is a common event. In this form of the disorder it is often possible to observe the characteristic recovery of the skin first affected while the process advances elsewhere. Healing of the skin requires one to two weeks after the temperature has returned to normal.

127.3. HEMOLYTIC STREPTOCOCCAL PNEUMONIA

Group A hemolytic streptococci were once responsible for 3 to 5 per cent of cases of bacterial pneumonia, but this form of disease is now rarely seen. It usually appears as a complication of influenza or other viral respiratory infection or in persons with underlying pulmonary disease. It is almost never observed as a sequel to streptococcal tonsillitis and pharyngitis or scarlet fever.

The pneumonic process is lobular in distribution in the lung. Empyema develops in 30 to 40 per cent of untreated cases. It is present early in the illness and is characterized by the formation of large amounts of thin fluid. Bacteremia is demonstrable in 10 to 15 per cent of the cases of streptococcal pneumonia. The demonstration of large numbers of hemolytic streptococci in the sputum by cultural methods, or the isolation of these organisms from the blood or pleural fluid, is required for diagnosis. (See Ch. 119 to 124.)

128. TREATMENT OF GROUP A STREPTOCOCCAL INFECTION AND CHEMOPROPHYLAXIS OF NONSUPPURATIVE COMPLICATIONS

Gene H. Stollerman

The management of the various group A streptococcal illnesses should include those general measures that are applied in all acute infections. Bed rest, light or liquid diet if pharyngeal discomfort is present and severe, and adequate but not excessive fluid intake are indicated.

Most important is the prompt institution of appropriate antimicrobial therapy, which has four goals: (1) the prompt control of the acute suppurative process in the respiratory tract or elsewhere, (2) the prevention of suppurative complications, (3) the prevention of nonsuppurative complications, and (4) the elimination of the carrier state and the prevention of transmission of the organism to others. The third and fourth goals will be fully attained only if the organism is permanently eradicated from the tissues. This can best be accomplished by the administration of penicillin. Sulfonamides are not effective either in eradicating the carrier state or in preventing an immunologic response, and thus do not prevent nonsuppurative complications. Erythromycin is an acceptable second choice to penicillin in the presence of allergy to penicillin. Tetracycline-resistant group A streptococci have been described with increasing frequency, and this drug is therefore an unreliable choice. It is essential that treatment in full doses be given over a period of at least ten days, regardless of which of the effective drugs is used.

Group A streptococci are among the most susceptible of all bacteria to the action of penicillin. The range of susceptibility for all strains of this serologic group is extremely narrow, between 0.01 and 0.04 unit per milliliter of culture. Moreover, no penicillin-resistant strains of group A streptococci have been demonstrated.

Duration of exposure to penicillin is the most important factor in therapy. Prolonged exposure to small concentrations of pencillin therefore is just as effective as a more intensive form of treatment of group A streptococcal pharyngitis. A single intramuscular injection of 600,000 units of benzathine penicillin provides blood levels that are barely detectable but that persist for about ten days; 1.2 million units results in levels that persist for at least two to four weeks or more. Such doses cure streptococcal pharyngitis, terminate carriage in the throat, and prevent rheumatic fever with optimal efficiency. Shorter-acting penicillin salts, such as aqueous procaine pencillin, must be administered still more often (usually daily for ten days) in a dose of 300,000 or 600,000 units intramuscularly to accomplish the same results. In the treatment of streptococcal pharyngitis, combinations of aqueous, procaine, and benzathine penicillin have no advantage over a single injection of benzathine penicillin G alone if a dose of at least 600,000 units or, preferably, 1.2 million units of the latter is employed.

If given orally, penicillin G must be administered in doses of 200,000 to 250,000 units four times daily for ten days. Thus, penicillinemia of about ten days' duration, regardless of the choice of preparation, is necessary to ensure the highest rates of bacteriologic cure. Sulfonamides are ineffective in preventing rheumatic fever when used to treat streptococcal pharyngitis. They do not suppress the immune response, do not terminate pharyngeal carriage of streptococci, and thus do not reduce the attack rate of subsequent rheumatic fever. They may be used, however, as continuous prophylaxis to *prevent* new infections (see below).

PREVENTION OF RHEUMATIC FEVER

Treatment of streptococcal sore throat should be started as soon as a definite diagnosis of streptococcal infection is made. It has been shown, however, that a short delay (even for several days) in initiating antimicrobial therapy while awaiting throat culture results does not significantly interfere with rheumatic fever prevention. One exception to this statement involves the patient with a history of rheumatic fever. In such a patient, the prevention of rheumatic recurrence is not always possible unless treatment is instituted at the first clinical sign of streptococcal infection. In such a patient, any delay of therapy entails the risk of reactivation of the disease. Certain features of the chemoprophylaxis of rheumatic fever are also presented in Ch. 130.

Patients with more serious streptococcal infections, such as streptococcal pneumonia, severe wound infections with sepsis, or suppurative complications of ordinary respiratory infection, should receive 600,000 units of procaine penicillin G per day intramuscularly for several days until the illness is well controlled, when a shift to a single dose of benzathine penicillin or to oral penicillin may be made. The response of extrapharyngeal suppurative complications of streptococcal infection to penicillin is good, and recovery without surgical intervention is the rule, with one exception. Sterilization of abscesses in well-established suppurative cervical adenitis is most difficult. Incision and drainage is usually required in such cases unless spontaneous rupture occurs. As in all situations of antimicrobial therapy in the presence of pus and necrosis, prolonged therapy for as long as several weeks may be required when adequate debridement is not possible. For patients allergic to penicillin, erythromycin is recommended in doses of 1 gram per day, which may be given in four divided doses for a period of ten days. Severely ill patients may receive 500 mg of erythromycin twice daily intravenously for a short time until they are able to accept the drug by month.

PREVENTION OF GLOMERULONEPHRITIS

Unlike the situation in rheumatic fever, treatment of streptococcal sore throat after the infection is well established will often fail to prevent acute glomerulonephritis. The latent period of this complication is much shorter than that of rheumatic fever. However, the spread of a nephritogenic strain through a family, school, or community can be stopped with effective antimicrobial therapy. In the case of pyoderma, the onset of the infection is not sharp and the symptoms are often not severe enough to make the patient seek treatment. Even when he does, the infection may be too well established to prevent glomerulonephritis in the patient himself. *Awareness of the presence of an index case of acute glomerulonephritis in the population he attends is therefore of great importance to the physician.* It will help him determine how promptly and vigorously he identifies, cultures, and treats patients with streptococcal infections and their contacts.

The treatment of streptococcal pyoderma has been studied far less methodically than pharyngitis and has varied widely in practice. The principles guiding the treatment of pyoderma may be somewhat different from those of pharyngitis in which prevention of rheumatic fever requires thorough eradication of group A streptococci. Unlike pharyngeal infections, topical treatment of skin infections may be adequate for mild cases of impetigo. Whether or not parenteral antimicrobial drugs are used, the removal of crusts and cleansing of the affected skin surfaces with soap seems to be an important part of the treatment of streptococcal pyoderma. In patients with extensive, persistent, or recurring impetigo, intramuscular benzathine penicillin is the treatment of choice.

Again, the decision to treat pyoderma with penicillin may depend upon, in addition to the severity of the infection, the appearance of an index case of acute glomerulonephritis in the population. In such instances, it is prudent to use an injection of benzathine penicillin G, which is the most effective measure. Where hygienic conditions are not improved, however, skin infections may recur after penicillin treatment, and it may be difficult to eradicate a nephritogenic strain from the population by penicillin therapy of infected individuals alone.

Obviously, the decision of when and how to treat a patient with a streptococcal infection, and whether or not to identify and treat his contacts, will vary with the severity of the infection, with the epidemiologic setting in which the infection occurs, and with the awareness of the presence or absence of index cases of rheumatic fever or acute glomerulonephritis in the community.

129. PROPHYLAXIS OF STREPTOCOCCAL INFECTION

Gene H. Stollerman

MASS PROPHYLAXIS. Mass prophylaxis is the term applied to the treatment of an entire population, both healthy and affected persons, to interrupt or prevent an epidemic, impending or in progress. This has been done frequently in military populations when epidemic streptococcal pharyngitis and its aftermath of rheumatic fever or glomerulonephritis have appeared. Occasionally, similar measures have been taken against local epidemics in schools or institutions. A single injection of 1.2 million units of benzathine penicillin G intramuscularly has proved extremely effective for this purpose because it (1) is therapeutic in those actually infected, (2) terminates pharyngeal carriage, and (3) protects against the acquisition of new infections for four to five weeks.

Unfortunately, no form of immunization is available. However, alert medical practitioners who will promptly detect and adequately treat streptococcal infections, a good system of public health reporting of rheumatic fever and acute glomerulonephritis, and good facilities for routine use of throat cultures should reduce extensive epidemics of streptococcal disease to a rarity. This should so alter the spread of streptococcal infections as to diminish the virulence and epidemicity of the *Streptococcus* and thereby continue the present trend in the decline of nonsuppurative complications of streptococcal disease.

Tonsillectomy has been employed prophylactically in the past, but is now known to be useless for this purpose, as it does not prevent infection by hemolytic streptococci. Subsequently acquired streptococcal respiratory illnesses may be less severe, but the frequency of occurrence of nonsuppurative complications is not reduced.

CONTINUOUS CHEMOPROPHYLAXIS. Continuous chemoprophylaxis against group A streptococci has proved to be highly effective in preventing recurrences of rheumatic fever (see below) and may be attained by one of three regimens listed here in order of their apparent efficacy and practicability:

1. Benzathine penicillin G in a single injection of 1.2 million units will provide protection for about 30 days. The disadvantages and discomfort of this regimen have to be weighed against the susceptibility to rheumatic recurrences of the individual patient. Those with rheumatic heart disease, those who have had a recent attack of rheumatic fever, and those exposed to an environment in which the incidence of streptococcal infection is frequent deserve the most effective protection. For such patients, benzathine penicillin by injection monthly is recommended.

2. Sulfonamide in daily administration by mouth of 1.0 gram of sulfadiazine or one of the other sulfapyrimidines provides satisfactory prophylaxis, but failures will occur. Toxic reactions may be observed during the first 60 days of continuous treatment. These have been rare, however, with the small doses of sulfadiazine that have been employed extensively.

3. Oral penicillin in doses of 200,000 (125 mg) units of penicillin G has been employed widely for prevention of streptococcal infections. This regimen has not been any more effective, however, than the daily dose of 1.0 gram of sulfadiazine. Indeed, 200,000 units of penicillin *twice* daily has not proved as yet to be clearly superior to the single dose. It is possible that the oral dose of penicillin may have to be increased to nearly therapeutic proportions to be more effective than sulfonamides, and this would increase further its expense and impracticability.

Baker, C. J., and Kasper, D. L.: Correlation of maternal antibody deficiency with susceptibility to neonatal group B streptococcal infection. N. Engl. J. Med., 294:752, 1976.

Beachey, E. H., and Ofek, I.: Epithelial binding of group A streptococci by lipoteichoic acid on fimbriae denuded of M protein. J. Exp. Med., 143:759, 1976.

Beachey, E. H., Stollerman, G. H., Chiang, E. Y., Chiang, T. M., Seyer, J. M., and Kang, A. H.: Purification and properties of M protein extracted from group A streptococci with pepsin: Covalent structure of the amino terminal region of type 24 M antigen. J. Exp. Med., 145:1469, 1977.

Bisno, A. L., and Ofek, I.: Serologic diagnosis of streptococcal infection: Comparison of a rapid hemagglutination technique with conventional antibody tests. Am. J. Dis. Child., 127:676, 1974.

Bisno, A. L., and Stollerman, G. H.: Streptococcal antibodies in the diagnosis of rheumatic fever. *In* Cohen, A. S. (ed.): Laboratory Diagnostic Procedure in the Rheumatic Diseases. 2nd ed. Boston, Little, Brown & Company, 1974, pp. 207–263.

Gibbons, R. J., and Van Houte, J.: Bacterial adherence in oral microbial ecology. Ann. Rev. Microbiol., 29:19, 1975.

Rammelkamp, C. H., Jr.; Epidemiology of Streptococcal Infections. Harvey Lectures, Series 51, 1955–56. New York, Academic Press, 1957, p. 113.

Rheumatic Fever Committee, American Heart Association: Prevention of Rheumatic fever. Circulation, 55:S1, 1977.

Seegal, D., and Seegal, B. C.: Facial erysipelas: A study of 281 cases treated at the Massachusetts General Hospital from 1870–1927. JAMA, 93:430, 1929.

Stollerman, G. H.: The relative rheumatogenicity of strains of group A streptococci. Mod. Concepts Cardiovasc. Dis., 44:35, 1975.

Stollerman, G. H.: Rheumatic Fever and Streptococcal Infection. New York, Grune & Stratton, 1975.

Stollerman, G. H.: Streptococcal vaccines revisited. J. Lab. Clin. Med., 91:872, 1978.

Wannamaker, L. W.: Infections of the throat and skin. N. Engl. J. Med., 282:23, 78, 1970.

Wannamaker, L. W., and Matsen, J. M. (eds.): Streptococci and Streptococcal Diseases. New York, Academic Press, 1972.

Wood, H. F., Feinstein, A. R., Taranta, A., Epstein, J. A., and Simpson, R.: Rheumatic fever in children and adolescents. III. Comparative effectiveness of three prophylaxis regimens in preventing streptococcal infections and rheumatic recurrences. Ann. Intern. Med., 60 S5:31, 1964.

130. RHEUMATIC FEVER

Richard M. Krause

DEFINITION. Rheumatic fever is an uncommon, but by no means rare, delayed sequel of an upper respiratory tract infection caused by group A hemolytic streptococci. The pathogenesis remains obscure. Multiple focal aseptic inflammatory lesions are the basis for the acute manifestations, which may include migratory arthritis, carditis, chorea, erythema marginatum, and subcutaneous nodules, as well as a number of less prominent signs and symptoms. Recurrences of rheumatic fever are common after an untreated streptococcal infection in patients with a previous history of this disease. The acute disease is of limited duration, but the carditis may lead to permanent valvular damage. It is for this reason that extensive studies have been concerned with methods to prevent first attacks as well as recurrences of rheumatic fever. Prevention can be achieved only by the prompt detection, diagnosis, and treatment of streptococcal pharyngitis set forth in the immediately preceding chapters.

ETIOLOGY AND PATHOGENESIS. Despite the decline in recent years in the incidence of rheumatic fever, interest in the disease is unabated because of its unique relationship to streptococcal infections. All the available evidence indicates that only group A streptococcal infections of the upper respiratory tract lead to rheumatic fever. Further, the two episodes are separated by a latent period during which the signs and symptoms of either illness are commonly absent. Although streptococci may be present in the throat from the onset of pharyngitis to the onset of rheumatic fever, there is no satisfactory evidence that foci of living streptococci contribute to the occurrence of rheumatic inflammatory lesions. Thus rheumatic fever appears to be a *reaction* to the streptococcal infection, and not a continuation of the infectious process.

The epidemiologic, clinical, and laboratory evidence for the association between streptococcal infections and rheumatic fever deserves special comment. Numerous epidemiologic studies have described a temporal relationship between these two diseases. Prior to the days of penicillin, an epidemic of scarlet fever in a closed population, such as a boarding school, was followed in two to four weeks by an uncommonly high incidence of rheumatic fever. But the certain relationship between the two diseases was only established once there had been major advances in the bacteriology of streptococci. The advent of methods to delineate the antigenic structure of the group A *Streptococcus* and the immune response to the various streptococcal antigens permitted the identification of the group A *Streptococcus* as the only pathogen that causes the pharyngitis leading to rheumatic fever. The serologic methods to detect antibodies to streptococcal antigens played an especially important role in establishing this relationship. With such methods, it was possible to determine for the first time that nearly every patient with rheumatic fever had a preceding streptococcal sore throat. This was not always evident from the results of throat cultures taken at the onset of rheumatic fever. Although group A streptococci may persist in the throat during the interval between streptococcal pharyngitis and rheumatic fever, it is not uncommon for repeated cultures of the pharynx to be negative for these organisms.

The most persuasive argument in favor of a relationship between streptococcal pharyngitis and acute rheumatic fever stems from the treatment schedules that have been devised to prevent primary as well as recurrent attacks of rheumatic fever. In brief, it is clear that adequate antimicrobial therapy of streptococcal pharyngitis will prevent a subsequent attack of rheumatic fever.

Once the bacteriology of streptococcal pharyngitis was clarified, the recurrent nature of rheumatic fever was no longer a mystery. Group A streptococci are classified into more than 70 serologic types on the basis of serologically distinct M proteins. Almost all serologic types are apparently capable of causing a pharyngitis that can lead to rheumatic fever (the possible exceptions to this rule are some of the recent new types of streptococci that have been most prominently isolated from skin lesions, some of which are associated primarily with the occurrence of acute nephritis). Because immunity to streptococcal infections is M-type specific, infection with one type results in no significant protection against the many other types. Thus it is common for a child to experience several different streptococcal infections during the school years, and this, in turn, makes possible repeated attacks of rheumatic fever. A child who has had an attack of rheumatic fever retains a special susceptibility to repeated attacks in subse-

quent years. However, the reason for this special susceptibility remains to be explained.

Most, if not all, serologic M types of group A streptococcal infections of the pharynx can lead to rheumatic fever. Although the attack rate of rheumatic fever is as high as 3 per cent following untreated streptococcal pharyngitis during epidemics, the rate is 0.5 per cent or less following sporadic infections. Epidemiologic evidence indicates that rheumatic fever occurs only after streptococcal pharyngitis, but not in association with streptococcal skin infections, e.g., impetigo. It is conceivable that the response to the pharyngeal infection is qualitatively and quantitatively different from the response to skin infections. It is known, for example, that the antibody response to streptolysin O is more likely to be elevated after pharyngeal infections than after skin infections, whereas the antibody response to DNAse B occurs with high frequency after infection at either site. Thus it is conceivable that the special consequences of a pharyngeal infection set the stage for the occurrence of rheumatic fever.

The selective occurrence of rheumatic fever in only a few people with pharyngitis argues for the importance of host factors in addition to the infectious process in the pathogenesis of rheumatic fever. It is possible that the accumulative effects of repetitive streptococcal infections in any one individual are a factor that increases the risk. Young children under the age of three have streptococcal pharyngitis, but rheumatic fever is uncommon in this age group. Throughout the remainder of childhood repetitive streptococcal infections lead to delayed hypersensitivity to streptococcal products, but such hypersensitivity is not commonly present in children less than three years of age. It is after the age of four that rheumatic fever is most common in children. The possible importance of genetic factors in predisposition has been suggested. Although it has been observed that rheumatic fever may occur in families, no clear-cut genetic pattern has been found. In a study of monozygotic twins, less than one fifth were concordant for rheumatic fever. Unsatisfactory and inconclusive though these studies are, the selective occurrence of rheumatic fever in only a few of all those infected with streptococci suggests that predisposing factors work in conjunction with the infectious process to produce rheumatic fever, but the nature of such contributory causes has remained obscure.

Although the central role of streptococcal infections in the etiology of rheumatic fever is now established beyond question, the mechanism by which the hemolytic streptococci initiate the disease process is unknown. For convenience, evidence can be marshaled for the support of three different theories of pathogenesis. Each of these theories is less than satisfactory.

The most currently attractive hypothesis is that rheumatic fever is a consequence of an immunologic response or hypersensitivity reaction, or both, to streptococcal antigens. An immunologic mechanism is suggested by the intriguing parallel between the latent period of serum sickness and rheumatic fever. Patients who develop rheumatic fever appear to have an exaggerated antibody response to streptococcal antigens. Such patients commonly, but not always, have a higher antistreptolysin O response than those who do not develop this complication after streptococcal pharyngitis.

The arguments suggesting that autoimmunity may be

of importance in pathogenesis cannot be recorded in detail here. The occurrence of autoantibodies that react with mammalian muscle in the sera of patients with rheumatic fever in concentrations greater than in the sera of patients who do not develop this complication has been emphasized. What remain to be determined are the source of antigenic stimulus for this autoantibody and the pathologic significance of such autoantibody. Because this autoantibody cross-reacts with a streptococcal antigen, it has been argued that these antibodies are only another manifestation of the immune response to the preceding streptococcal infection. It is also possible, however, that the host's own tissues were so altered by the toxic processes at the time of infection that altered tissue antigens became the stimulus for autoantibody production. In addition to the controversy over the source of the stimulus that gives rise to these autoantibodies, there is the additional controversy over their pathologic significance. It is unknown if they participate in the genesis of the inflammatory lesions in a manner similar to the autoantibodies to nucleic acid which appear to be intimately associated with the inflammatory lesions of lupus erythematosus.

Another possible explanation for the pathogenesis of rheumatic fever is that the inflammation is a direct consequence of the deleterious effects of streptococcal toxins produced at the time of the infection. Despite the marked toxicity of certain streptococcal products, such as streptolysin O and S, there is little evidence for or against the importance of toxins in pathogenesis.

It remains to mention the possible role of persistent foci of the infecting *Streptococcus* in the pathogenesis of rheumatic fever. Aside from several earlier bacteriologic reports prior to the era of antimicrobial drugs, there is little bacteriologic evidence for a direct infection of the heart valves, the myocardium, or other organs involved in rheumatic fever. Nevertheless, because the prevention of rheumatic fever requires the successful and complete eradication of the infecting *Streptococcus* from the pharynx by drug therapy, the view lingers that persistence of the infecting *Streptococcus* in some form may be a factor in the disease process.

EPIDEMIOLOGY. It is obvious from what has been said that the epidemiology of acute rheumatic fever and the epidemiology of streptococcal pharyngitis are clearly interrelated. The incidence of the two diseases is related. Any environmental or host factor that enhances the occurrence of streptococcal pharyngitis will enhance the occurrence of rheumatic fever. Streptococcal disease is most common between the ages of five and fifteen years, with a peak incidence between six and eight years, and this is the age group with the highest attack rate of rheumatic fever. Although adults have fewer streptococcal infections than children because of acquired immunity and less exposure to streptococci, the special circumstances of military service or close association with children enhance the risk of higher attack rates for adults.

As is the case for most other respiratory diseases, the occurrence of streptococcal pharyngitis fluctuates widely with the seasons. The occurrence of acute rheumatic fever parallels such fluctuations. The peak occurrence falls in the late winter and early spring months, although not uncommonly the number of cases increases sharply for a brief period shortly after the onset of school in the early fall.

Classic epidemiologic studies indicate that rheumatic fever occurs most commonly in the temperate zones. But recent reports from Africa, India, and countries of Southeast Asia suggest that rheumatic heart disease is by no means rare in these areas. This has prompted a search for acute rheumatic fever in economically underdeveloped countries of the world. A recent clinical study in Egypt has revealed that rheumatic fever there has the same characteristics as the disease which occurs in the United States and Europe.

Socioeconomic factors such as overcrowding, either in tenement areas or in army barracks, that favor the spread of streptococcal disease also favor the occurrence of rheumatic fever. There is no evidence for differences of susceptibility because of race or sex, although chorea and mitral stenosis are more common in females, and aortic insufficiency is more common in males.

A number of factors have undoubtedly been responsible for the decline in the occurrence of rheumatic fever and rheumatic heart disease in the past several decades. Not the least of these are improvements of socioeconomic conditions and the treatment of streptococcal infections with penicillin. Certainly antimicrobial therapy has had a major impact on the prevention of recurrent attacks of rheumatic fever, and such cases have shown a precipitous decline. Less well documented is the decline in first attacks. Indeed, long-time students of the disease have commented on the persistent occurrence of first attacks in the large cities of the United States, and suggest that the over-all decline in cases stems from the prevention of recurrences as well as from the prevention of first attacks.

For the United States at large, the yearly incidence of first attacks of rheumatic fever has been estimated at about 50,000 to 100,000 children, but for a variety of reasons such estimates are unsatisfactory. The disease is not reportable in all states and, in addition, without unequivocal pathognomonic signs and symptoms that clearly establish diagnosis, the disease is both over- and underreported. Some idea of the continued occurrence of rheumatic fever in the population can be obtained by the examination of schoolchildren, college students, and military recruits for the prevalence of rheumatic heart disease. Among schoolchildren, the prevalence is between 0.7 and 1.6 per 1000. The prevalence for freshmen college students and servicemen is between 6 and 9 per 1000.

CLINICAL MANIFESTATIONS. The most striking clinical manifestations are due to arthritis, carditis, and chorea. Each sign and symptom of rheumatic fever may be either mild or severe, and the severity of each may vary independently. Thus severe carditis may be associated with minimal or no evidence of arthritis, and vice versa. Because the manifestations of rheumatic fever at first glance appear so variable, and because no single set of manifestations is typical for rheumatic fever, the Jones criteria have been devised as a guide to aid in the differential diagnosis. The signs and symptoms that comprise the Jones criteria are listed in the accompanying table. Use of these criteria for guidance in differential diagnosis will be discussed later.

Although a history of a preceding streptococcal pharyngitis is common, this infection may have been so mild as to have escaped medical attention. Indeed, a number of patients can recall no recent sore throat. The interval between the pharyngitis and the onset of rheu-

Clinical and Laboratory Manifestations of Acute Rheumatic Fever

Major Manifestations	Minor Manifestations
1. Carditis	1. Clinical
2. Polyarthritis	a. Previous rheumatic fever or
3. Chorea	rheumatic heart disease
4. Erythema marginatum	b. Arthralgia
5. Subcutaneous nodules	c. Fever
	2. Laboratory
	a. Acute phase reactions, elevated
	erythrocyte sedimentation rate,
	C-reactive protein, leukocytosis
	b. Prolonged P-R interval

plus

Supporting evidence of preceding streptococcal infection (increased ASO or other streptococcal antibodies, positive throat culture for group A Streptococcus, recent scarlet fever)

The Jones criteria (revised) have been employed as a guide in the diagnosis of rheumatic fever, but this scheme has not received universal acceptance. The presence of two major manifestations, or of one major and two minor manifestations, indicates a high probability of the presence of rheumatic fever *if supported by evidence of a preceding streptococcal infection.* The absence of the latter should make the diagnosis doubtful, except in situations in which rheumatic fever is first discovered after a long, latent period from the antecedent infection, e.g., Sydenham's chorea or low-grade carditis.

Adapted from the recommendations of the Committee of The American Heart Association (Circulation, 32:664, 1965.)

matic fever has been termed the latent period. This is a period of one to five weeks, and during this time the patient usually appears entirely well. On some occasions, however, laboratory examination will reveal evidence of disease activity.

The onset of rheumatic fever, with characteristic signs and symptoms, is usually sudden, but it may be insidious. In the latter case, diagnosis depends on observation of the clinical course and the interpretation of laboratory data. Usually the first symptoms are fever and joint pain. Fever may be high and sustained in severe cases, but more frequently it is moderate and often low grade. Sore throat is not uncommon, even though examination reveals minimal evidence of acute inflammation. Epistaxis occurs commonly both at the onset and throughout the acute stage of the disease, and in some cases results in serious loss of blood. In children, severe abdominal pain is not uncommon, and vomiting may occur. Localization of such pain in the right lower quadrant with fleeting signs of peritoneal inflammation may suggest the diagnosis of appendicitis.

Arthritis. The arthritis in rheumatic fever may involve multiple joints, but a characteristic feature is that the inflammation occurs and subsides in the joints first affected, only to occur in others that were initially spared. This phenomenon has been termed migratory polyarthritis. The large joints of the extremities are most frequently affected, but all are potentially susceptible. Arthritis can occur in the hands, feet, or spine, or in such joints as the sternoclavicular and the temporomandibular.

The manifestations of arthritis may be either mild with vague discomfort in the joints of the extremities, or severe. Acutely inflamed and swollen joints are commonly very painful. In mild cases there may be no objective evidence of arthritis. When arthritis is severe, the skin over the joint shows local redness and heat, the joint is swollen, and fluid is obviously present within the joint cavity. Passive or active movement of

the joint is extremely painful. The fluid in such cases is turbid and contains leukocytes, indicating an inflammatory reaction, but is sterile on bacteriologic culture.

Although uncommon, the arthritis may not affect multiple joints. Experienced clinicians have observed the occasional case in which arthritis may persist for prolonged periods in only one joint, with minimal evidence of arthritis in the others.

There is usually a difference between the pattern of arthritis in children and that in adults. Frank arthritis is less common in children between four and six years of age. Only mild joint pains may be noted, or merely vague localized aching in the extremities. It is this type of complaint that has been referred to in the past as "growing pains." Such symptoms and low-grade fever suggest a mild illness, but examination of the heart may reveal severe carditis. It bears repetition that rheumatic fever can occur without any evidence of joint involvement whatever.

Carditis. Palpitation and precordial chest pain or discomfort are common symptoms. If the carditis is severe, symptoms of cardiac failure may occur in addition to those of rheumatic fever. The final and definitive diagnosis of carditis depends upon the physical, roentgenographic, and electrocardiographic examinations.

The carditis may be mild or severe. In mild cases, tachycardia, persistent during sleep, may be the only sign suggesting carditis. Bradycardia has been well documented in rheumatic fever, particularly during the recovery process. In the more severe cases, generalized cardiac enlargement frequently occurs, often associated with a diffuse precordial impulse.

On auscultation, the heart sounds in the apical area may be muffled, indistinct, and of poor quality. The second sound in the pulmonic area is usually greatly accentuated in comparison with the second aortic sound. Gallop rhythm may occur, and is usually an indication of serious myocardial disease. The sounds may seem distant if precordial effusion is present, and the pericarditis may produce a to-and-fro friction rub (see Ch 365).

Cardiac murmurs may be present at the initial examination, or they may develop during the first few weeks of the illness. Several characteristic murmurs, occurring alone or in any combination, are indicative of carditis. These are a holosystolic apical murmur due to relative or actual mitral regurgitation; a diastolic murmur along the left sternal border at the third and fourth interspaces, due to relative or actual aortic regurgitation; and an apical mid-diastolic rumble often associated with mitral regurgitation during acute carditis and referred to as a Carey-Coombs murmur. As the murmurs may disappear permanently on recovery, their final significance cannot be determined except by repeated examinations during and after convalescence. Mitral stenosis and aortic stenosis are late manifestations of cardiac damage that do not develop until months or years after the initial or repeated attacks.

Disturbances of the conduction system are a common feature of rheumatic carditis. Although certain irregularities, such as second-degree heart block, can be recognized clinically, the electrocardiogram is the best method to detect all potential conduction system disturbances. One of the most commonly observed electrocardiographic changes is the prolongation of the P-R interval. In some cases, the Wenckebach phenomenon is observed. Further delay in conduction may lead to drop beats, with the occurrence of couplets and triplets. Finally, complete dissociation is indicated by an independent rhythm for both the ventricles and the atria. Atrial fibrillation is uncommon during the acute attack.

In addition to these conduction abnormalities, the electrocardiogram may show T wave changes, such as inversion of the T wave in one or more leads. When pericarditis is present, elevation of the S-T segment is observed initially. Late in the course, the configuration of the T wave stimulates that seen in coronary disease.

Although cardiac enlargement, when present, is usually detectable on physical examination, the dilatation of the various chambers of the heart is more accurately determined by roentgenography of the chest. It is not uncommon for dilatation to arise rapidly when severe myocarditis is present.

The recurrence of active rheumatic fever should be suspected in patients with chronic rheumatic heart disease when the character of the murmurs changes over a short period of time. Cardiac failure may occur, but in carditis associated with recurrent rheumatic fever in such cases poses several diagnostic problems, because the manifestations of acute rheumatic carditis are superimposed on those of chronic valvular disease. Furthermore, the status of the pre-existing heart disease is often unknown. When there is evidence of advanced valvular deformity, all final assessment of the extent of cardiac damage must await convalescence from the acute attack.

Erythema Marginatum. *Erythema marginatum* or *circinatum* of the skin is one of the characteristic manifestations of acute rheumatic fever and occurs in 10 to 20 per cent of the childhood cases. Because it comes and goes, it is frequently missed, particularly if the patients are not examined *completely*. It is a multiform type of erythema, and consists of roughly circular lesions that may be distributed over the extremities, the trunk, and sometimes the face, and that spread centrifugally, leaving a clear center. The lesions tend to coalesce so that, although individual areas are iris-like, the larger areas are serpiginous in outline. The erythema blanches on pressure and may be evanescent, disappearing and later reappearing at the same sites. The lesions are usually not elevated, although in some cases a slight papular quality may be detected. Most commonly, no discomfort is associated with the lesions. Erythema marginatum is uncommon in other diseases.

Subcutaneous Rheumatic Nodules. These lesions are one of the physical findings that lend strong support to the diagnosis of rheumatic fever, but in recent years they have occurred less commonly than was the case in the past. They are firm, insensitive nodules that occur over the bony prominences of the various joints and tendons of the extremities, the spine, and the back of the head. They are loosely attached to the underlying tissue, and the skin is freely movable over them. If the joint can be flexed without undue pain, the nodules are more readily apparent because of the tension of the skin. If nodules are numerous, they may occur in a symmetrical distribution. The nodules are more frequently encountered in the more severe cases of rheumatic fever with serious cardiac involvement.

Sydenham's Chorea. Chorea may occur in combination with other symptoms of rheumatic fever, but it is commonly seen as the sole manifestation of the disease. This phenomenon is explained by the fact that chorea tends to make its appearance late in the course of rheu-

matic fever. The onset may be delayed for as long as six months after the initiating streptococcal infection, although the delay is usually less than this. Patients with chorea may have had an easily recognizable preceding attack of arthritis and carditis, and, indeed, may have been hospitalized with it, only to have the chorea occur as a late manifestation at a time when all other evidence of any inflammatory process had disappeared. When the onset of chorea is delayed and the other manifestations of rheumatic fever have abated, the laboratory findings are often normal. It is not uncommon for chorea to occur in patients who can recall no earlier illness. It seems likely that such individuals had an attack of acute rheumatic fever in the recent past which was so mild that it escaped clinical detection. It is for this reason that patients with so-called "pure chorea" may develop rheumatic heart disease.

The onset of chorea is usually insidious, and the parents of the child with chorea may first note increased awkwardness and a tendency to spill food or drop objects that is attributed to carelessness. Even the appearance of involuntary purposeless movements of the extremities may be discounted as nervousness. However, with further progression of the disease, the irregular and uncontrollable movements become obvious. They may become extensive, and may involve not only the hands, feet, arms, and legs, but the tongue and facial muscles. The severity may range from no more than minimal involuntary movements observed only by close inspection, to violent, continual activity, totally incapacitating the patient and requiring protection from self-injury. In moderate cases, interference with all coordinated activity, such as writing and eating, is common. On occasion, chorea may be limited to one side of the body. The disease appears to affect females somewhat more frequently than males.

Miscellaneous Clinical Manifestations. Rheumatic pneumonitis may occur, but this is difficult to detect clinically, particularly if there is superimposed heart failure. Rheumatic pneumonia has seldom been seen in recent years, probably because the disease process itself appears to be much milder than in former times. Such few cases as do occur are in patients with severe rheumatic fever.

LABORATORY FINDINGS. Hematology. There are no characteristic abnormalities of the leukocyte differential count that are indicative of rheumatic fever. Leukocytosis is common, but not always present, with a total count from 12,000 to 24,000 per cubic millimeter. This is associated with an increase in the percentage of polymorphonuclear cells.

A moderate degree of anemia is generally seen, which is normochromic with proportional decreases in the hemoglobin concentration and the erythrocyte count. The anemia usually persists for as long as the rheumatic process is active. The most severe anemias are obviously encountered in patients who have an associated blood loss owing to epistaxis.

Urinary Findings. Some proteinuria and an increase in the number of red and white cells in the urine are common during the acute phase of the disease. However, it is seldom that these abnormalities are as great as those characteristically encountered in acute glomerulonephritis. When this is the case, simultaneous acute nephritis and rheumatic fever must be considered, but such a combination is a most uncommon event.

Evidence for a Prior Streptococcal Infection. The

most important laboratory information for establishing the diagnosis of rheumatic fever is data that substantiate the prior occurrence of streptococcal pharyngitis. The detection of group A beta-hemolytic streptococci by a throat culture is helpful in this regard, but of greater usefulness is the serologic detection of antibodies that are indicative of a previous streptococcal infection.

Because the streptococci that caused the initial infection may persist for many weeks in the pharynx in those instances in which antimicrobial therapy was not given or was inadequate, a throat culture may detect the infecting group A streptococci at the time of the onset of rheumatic fever. But such a finding is only suggestive of a preceding streptococcal pharyngitis and is not an unambiguous indication of it. This stems from the fact that 5 to 30 per cent of the healthy population may carry group A streptococci in the pharynx during the respiratory disease season. Thus the recovery of this organism from a patient may be an inadvertent finding and not indicative of a preceding streptococcal sore throat. Nevertheless, the throat culture is helpful, and should be obtained in all cases. When the patient has a negative throat culture, it is frequently possible to isolate the group A streptococci from other members of the family. Such a finding is indicative of a recent intrafamilial spread of streptococci.

The most helpful information that is indicative of a recent streptococcal infection is obtained with tests that detect serum antibodies to streptococcal antigens. The most widely employed test is the antistreptolysin O determination. As with all antibody tests, the detection of an antibody rise over a one- to three-week interval is the only unequivocal evidence for the recent occurrence of a streptococcal infection. If a patient is seen in the first few days after the onset of rheumatic fever, the antistreplysin O titer at that time may be less than the titer seen several weeks after onset of rheumatic fever. Not uncommonly, however, the titer has reached a maximal plateau so that it is not possible to detect a progressive increase in titer. When this is the case, the antistreptolysin O titer should be at least 250 units in adults and at least 333 units in children over five years of age to be acceptable as an indication of a previous streptococcal infection. Obviously, a certain proportion of the individuals in the normal population have had a recent streptococcal infection at any one time, and they will have antistreptolysin O titers similar to these.

Approximately 15 to 20 per cent of the patients with rheumatic fever and nearly all patients who exhibit only chorea have a low or borderline low antistreptolysin O titer. In such instances, it is helpful to employ another antibody test. The anti-DNAse B test is becoming widely accepted as a second antibody test, and it is a useful means to obtain additional evidence for the occurrence of a previous streptococcal infection. When both these antibody tests are used, it is possible to obtain antibody evidence for a preceding streptococcal infection in almost all cases of rheumatic fever.

One other serologic test should be mentioned because it may be used more widely in the future. It has been noted that nearly all patients with rheumatic fever have readily detectable serum autoantibodies that react with muscle tissue, including heart, whereas the concentration of these antibodies is very much less or absent in sera of patients with other rheumatic diseases. Such findings suggest that this antibody test may have clinical usefulness for the differential diagnosis of rheumatic fever.

Other Laboratory Tests. An elevated sedimentation rate and a positive C-reactive protein are present in rheumatic fever, but these findings are nonspecific indicators of inflammation, and they cannot be used to differentiate rheumatic fever from other diseases. However, a normal C-reactive protein and a normal sedimentation rate are helpful in excluding active rheumatic fever. The sedimentation rate, when properly done, is strikingly elevated in all cases of *acute* rheumatic fever, exclusive of patients with chorea, and other concomitant diseases such as sickle cell disease or fibrinogenemia. If the sedimentation rate and the C-reactive protein are normal, active rheumatic fever is unlikely in patients with mild symptoms, such as vague arthralgia and lassitude.

DIAGNOSIS AND DIFFERENTIAL DIAGNOSIS. A history of severe sore throat in the recent past, migrating polyarthritis, carditis, fever, and an elevated antistreptolysin O titer is such a classic combination of signs and symptoms that the diagnosis can seldom be questioned. But the problem is often not as straightforward as this. *Furthermore, it cannot be emphasized too strongly that there is no specific diagnostic laboratory test for rheumatic fever.*

The various major manifestations of rheumatic fever that have been described above are considered to be part of the same disease because they occur together with a frequency that far exceeds chance. Because they may occur singly or in various combinations in any individual patient, the diagnostic criteria originally proposed by Jones have been suggested as a guide to diagnosis. These criteria are listed in the table. Any combination of these criteria can occur in patients with other disorders. It is for this reason that stress is placed on supporting evidence for a preceding streptococcal infection. When this is the case, the diagnosis is weighed in favor of rheumatic fever and against the other connective tissue disorders that may mimic it. The footnote to the table should be especially noted.

The designations major and minor for the various criteria are based on the diagnostic importance of the particular findings. The major ones are more indicative of rheumatic fever than the minor. The occurrence of two major manifestations is strong presumptive evidence for rheumatic fever. Only one major manifestation and any combination of the minor suggest possible rheumatic fever. In any case, if evidence is lacking for a preceding streptococcal pharyngitis, the possibility of other diseases must be kept in mind.

In many ways the most useful purpose of the criteria is their value in reducing overdiagnosis. For example, not uncommonly, patients, after streptococcal infections, may have vague pains in the extremities, an increased sedimentation rate, and a borderline temperature elevation. Careful follow-up of such patients has not revealed the delayed occurrence of rheumatic heart disease. Therefore the diagnosis of rheumatic fever should be made with caution and only with clear evidence of one or more of the major manifestations. When the diagnosis is in doubt, because the symptoms are of such a mild nature, treatment with aspirin and steroids should be withheld until the signs and symptoms are unmistakable. Early treatment of a questionable case may so depress the disease activity that clear-cut clinical signs and symptoms do not develop.

In the early stages, during the acute onset, *rheumatoid arthritis* and *systemic lupus erythematosus* may mimic rheumatic fever. Indeed, if the streptococcal antibody tests are elevated, the diagnosis may be in question unless the special diagnostic tests for the other diseases are clearly positive. Usually as time progresses, the special distinctive clinical features of rheumatoid arthritis and lupus serve to exclude the diagnosis of rheumatic fever. On occasion, at the onset, Still's disease may be confused with rheumatic fever, but again the clinical course will aid in differentiating the two.

Subacute bacterial endocarditis can occur in persons with valves previously damaged by rheumatic fever, and it often presents a clinical picture that is not readily distinguishable from a rheumatic recurrence. Vague pains in the extremities are more common than overt arthritis, but these symptoms together with fever and debility in a known rheumatic patient are sufficient to suggest a rheumatic recurrence. The difficulties are increased by the fact that in some cases it is not possible to recover the offending organism in a blood culture. The characteristic petechiae and painful septic emboli of endocarditis are helpful in differential diagnosis (see Ch. 131).

The so-called *benign idiopathic pericarditis* is not rheumatic in origin and has been observed with coxsackievirus infection. It is indistinguishable in the acute phase from those cases of rheumatic fever in which pericarditis is the major detectable manifestation. The diagnosis of idiopathic pericarditis is dependent primarily on elimination of other possibilities and on the subsequent course of the disease, which is characterized by complete recovery without residual damage. Thus the final conclusion is often reached only in retrospect, and must remain somewhat uncertain because rheumatic pericarditis with minimal involvement of the myocardium and endocardium could conceivably behave in a similar fashion.

Fever, arthritis, and positive acute phase reactants may also occur in bacterial arthritis, serum sickness, subacute bacterial endocarditis, sickle cell anemia, and acute aleukemic leukemia. In such cases in which confusion exists, only a careful assessment of the clinical course, physical examination, and laboratory findings will exclude rheumatic fever.

Persistent monarticular arthritis, without other major manifestations of rheumatic fever, is usually not due to rheumatic fever, and osteomyelitis or local injury must be considered.

THERAPY. There is no specific treatment for rheumatic fever. Therapeutic measures are devised to promote, or at least ideally not to hinder, the natural healing processes. Bed rest is always prescribed, and most students agree that it should continue until the acute manifestations of arthritis and carditis are under control. It is not at all clear that absolute bed rest without bath privileges is essential. A program for a progressive increase in recreational and occupational therapy has important psychologic value and should be an integral part of the long-term bed rest management. Schooling should not be neglected during this time. Hospital or home visit teaching programs, or both, are available in many cities, and instruction should be begun as soon as the acute manifestations of the disease are brought under control by anti-inflammatory therapy.

After the first few weeks of bed rest, gradual ambulation can be started. During the period of bed rest, the patient is permitted a number of activities in increasing amounts, such as sitting up in a chair, occupational therapy, and schoolwork. In some patients with pronounced tachycardia, as well as evidence of severe myocarditis, the period of bed rest should be prolonged.

The period of bed rest is a good time for patients of all ages to be informed about the nature of the illness and the optimistic prospects for an active, long life. The need for a continuous program to prevent streptococcal pharyngitis should be discussed in detail. It is at this time, also, that patients with more severe forms of heart disease should be advised that some curtailment of normal physical activity may be necessary during convalescence. But pessimism is not warranted. All too often, patients are left with the impression that their useful, active life is at an end. This is almost invariably not the case.

If there is no evidence of rheumatic carditis or heart disease following the termination of therapy, full physical activity can be gradually resumed. Any long-term restrictions on physical activity in patients with persistent rheumatic heart disease will depend on an assessment of valvular disease.

It is recommended that all patients with acute rheumatic fever be treated with a course of penicillin to eliminate the hemolytic *Streptococcus* from the pharynx. This is recommended even if the throat culture does not reveal group A beta-hemolytic streptococci, because these organisms may persist in areas where they remain undetected, such as the crypts of the tonsils. Parenteral penicillin is the drug of choice unless there is a history of allergy to it. Three hundred thousand units of procaine penicillin G once a day in children and twice a day in adults for ten days is an effective dose. A single dose of 1.2 million units of long-acting benzathine penicillin is preferred by many, as the one injection facilitates administration. Oral penicillin, 200,000 units four times a day, also for ten days, is acceptable therapy, but requires careful supervision in order to be sure that all doses are taken without fail. If there is a history of penicillin allergy, the drug of choice is erythromycin. The dose is 250 mg four times a day for ten days. Sulfonamide in any form should never be used. After completion of the ten-day course of penicillin or erythromycin, a continuous prophylaxis regimen should be started to prevent reinfection with group A streptococci and to reduce the risk of recurrent attacks of acute rheumatic fever (see Ch. 128). Prevention of infective endocarditis is an important aspect in the management of patients with rheumatic heart disease. This is discussed in Ch. 131.

Aspirin and Steroid Therapy. Most patients respond rapidly to either steroid or aspirin therapy. After one or two weeks, arthritis and fever have disappeared, and the acute phase reactants frequently have returned to normal, or nearly so. On occasion, neither fever nor arthritis responds to full aspirin dosage, and steroids are required to control the disease. Many, but not all, clinicians favor use of steroids in nearly all patients with carditis. It is certainly indicated in patients with severe carditis and pancarditis. Some prefer to withdraw the steroid treatment after several weeks and continue treatment by substituting aspirin. Others continue steroid therapy for the full course. The arthritis in nearly all patients responds readily to aspirin alone. The evidence remains equivocal for the beneficial effect of steroid therapy in preventing the development of permanent rheumatic heart disease, even though there is apparent clinical improvement in the acute carditis when steroids are used.

It should be stressed again that when full and adequate treatment eliminates all the clinical manifestations of the disease, including laboratory abnormalities, the underlying disease process is still continuing unabated for its natural course. If the drugs are withdrawn before the process is at an end, the disease with all its clinical manifestations will recur. Duration of therapy is discussed below.

The daily dose of aspirin is 60 mg per pound of body weight. The actual dose per day varies from 3 grams in young children to 10 grams in adults. It is preferable to give this total amount in at least six divided doses. Aspirin should be given throughout the 24-hour day, at least during the early stages of the disease. Individual variation in the efficacy of absorption or excretion of the drug and in its therapeutic effectiveness requires readjustment of the dose in many cases. The aim is to give the minimal dose that results in full control of symptoms and to avoid serious toxic side reactions because of overdosage. Studies on the concentration of salicylates in the blood have shown that optimal therapeutic effect usually requires at least 25 mg per 100 ml of serum. The optimal therapeutic range is between 25 and 35 mg per 100 ml of serum. Levels greater than the upper limit are associated with toxicity. When aspirin is given in conjunction with the prednisone, it is frequently necessary to give a daily dose of aspirin larger than that recommended above in order to achieve the therapeutic salicylate level. Furthermore, as aspirin is continued upon the withdrawal of prednisone, less aspirin is frequently required to maintain an adequate serum salicylate level.

The most common toxic manifestations of aspirin therapy are nausea, vomiting, and gastric distress. Tinnitus and partial but temporary impairment of hearing usually occur only at full therapeutic dosage. Hyperpnea frequently results from central stimulatory action in respiration and can lead to alkalosis. It is uncommon to see the more severe metabolic disturbances of acute salicylate toxicity.

In practice, nausea and vomiting are the most frequent complications that result from starting aspirin. This can be minimized if the initial daily dosage is below the optimum and then is gradually increased over a period of a few days. Attempts to achieve full and optimal salicylate levels within 24 hours often result in severe nausea and vomiting. In such cases it may be difficult to reach an effective therapeutic level of salicylate, and in such instances steroids afford an alternative therapeutic approach. The use of sodium bicarbonate to reduce gastric irritation is not recommended, as it increases the excretion of salicylate and interferes with the maintenance of an anti-inflammatory concentration of the drug in the blood. If a portion of the aspirin is given as enteric-coated pills, some degree of gastric irritation can be eliminated.

Prednisone is the recommended steroid because a low salt diet and added potassium are usually not required. There is no firm agreement on the dosage of this drug. The usual procedure is to begin with a relatively large daily dose until activity of the disease appears to be under control, and then to reduce the dosage to the minimal amount that will maintain the full effect. In the experience of many, the total daily dosage of 0.3 to 0.5 mg per pound given in divided doses is adequate to bring the signs of inflammation, including fever, rapidly under control. Almost all signs and symptoms are suppressed in two or three days. It is at this point that the daily dose may be reduced. After two or three weeks of steroid therapy, some prefer to shift to aspirin, particularly for those patients without carditis. The advantage of this is that most side effects of prolonged steroid therapy, such as the mild manifestations of Cushing's disease, are avoided. Prolonged use of steroid therapy may lead to complications, such as infections, growth retardation, gastric ulcers, and toxic psychoses.

The treatment of chorea is symptomatic. There is no evidence that either steroids or aspirin have any influence on the symptoms of chorea. The usual case lasts from two weeks to several months, but in rare instances it may persist longer. Nevertheless, almost without exception, complete recovery is the rule. Many patients show improvement when bright light, noise, and undue activity are eliminated from their bedroom. In some cases, measures must be taken to prevent self-injury from violent chorea movements, including tongue-biting. Phenobarbital and other sedatives may be helpful.

Duration of Therapy. The duration of therapy bears some relationship to the severity of the acute manifestations. The disease process in the typical mild case without carditis subsides in three to four weeks. When severe arthritis and carditis are present, the natural course lasts two to three months. Such estimates for the duration of the disease can be used to determine the termination of therapy, recognizing, however, that disease activity in the occasional case may persist for many months. Laboratory tests such as determination of the sedimentation rate and the C-reactive protein assume normal values during the course of adequate therapy. For this reason, they cannot be used to determine the duration of therapy.

Many clinicians prefer to withdraw either aspirin or steroid therapy gradually over a period of one or two weeks. After withdrawal, a clinical "rebound" is commonly seen. This may be so mild that only the acute phase reactants indicate its occurrence, but not uncommonly clinical manifestations are present. These may be mild or severe, and include fever, arthritis, and tachycardia. Usually the rebound subsides in five to ten days without use of anti-inflammatory drugs. The occurrence of positive C-reactive protein, an elevated sedimentation rate, and an elevated white count, without significant clinical manifestations, is not sufficient grounds for reinstituting therapy. But progressive clinical severity and particularly the emergence of severe carditis may require reinstitution of therapy. In such instances, it is assumed that the natural duration of the disease has yet to run its course. In practice, if therapy must be reinstated because of the emergence of carditis, the drugs are continued for another three to four weeks.

If no significant rebound occurs, ambulation should begin, and usually full activity, except vigorous exercise, may be permitted three to four weeks after the termination of therapy. If persistent rheumatic heart disease is present, the permissible level of physical activity is determined by an assessment of its severity.

PREVENTION. Prior to the days of antimicrobial drugs, measures were not available to prevent recurrences of rheumatic fever. Now properly supervised continuous chemoprophylaxis is effective in preventing these recurrences, and it should be employed for all patients with a well-documented history of rheumatic fever or unequivocal evidence of rheumatic heart disease. Prophylaxis prevents streptococcal pharyngitis and therefore the recurrences of rheumatic fever.

A detailed consideration of drug regimens for prophylaxis has been presented in Ch. 128. Intramuscular benzathine penicillin, 1.2 million units each month, is the preferred drug and route of administration. Such a route of administration does not leave open to question the degree of patient compliance, as is the case with orally administered penicillin.

The duration of antimicrobial prophylaxis should be extended through childhood. In the case of adolescents and adults, it should not be terminated as long as the patient is associated with population groups that have high attack rates of streptococcal infections, such as military recruits, schoolchildren, medical personnel, and school teachers. Because of the risk of additional valvular damage during a recurrence, *prophylaxis should be continued for life for all patients with definite rheumatic heart disease.* Contrary to popular belief, people in late middle age can have a recurrence of rheumatic fever after streptococcal pharyngitis.

Epidemiologic studies clearly indicate that streptococcal disease spreads in the home and in the school. The physician must be alert to the occurrence of streptococcal pharyngitis in the family and the school of the patient on prophylaxis. This is a potential risk to the patient, and strict compliance with the prophylaxis must be urged. If streptococcal disease occurs in the family, it should be treated with adequate antimicrobial drugs.

For a number of reasons, the prevention of first attacks of rheumatic fever is difficult to achieve. Prompt recognition and treatment of streptococcal pharyngitis is hampered in a number of cases by the fact that the symptoms are so mild that the patient does not see a physician. Not uncommonly, when the patient is seen by a doctor, the disease is misdiagnosed or the antimicrobial therapy prescribed is inadequate. For example, the tetracyclines should never be used to treat streptococcal pharyngitis, because 25 to 40 per cent of all group A streptococci are now resistant to this family of drugs.

The occasion arises when special measures are needed to control epidemics of streptococcal pharyngitis in a school or a community or in an army recruit camp. Several unexpected cases of rheumatic fever in a short period of time in a small population group should alert the physician to the possibility that there is a serious streptococcal epidemic in the community in question. Methods to curtail such epidemics have been described in Ch. 129.

PROGNOSIS. Recovery from the acute attack is the rule. Death at this stage is very rare, even in cases of severe carditis, because of the anti-inflammatory effects of steroid therapy. The disease process in mild cases of rheumatic fever without carditis usually subsides in two to four weeks, and the patient usually makes a complete recovery. When carditis is present, the disease usually persists for six weeks to three months. Patients with carditis during the acute attack may progress to valvular rheumatic heart disease. This is less common in patients without carditis, but absence of carditis during an acute attack is unfortunately not an absolute guarantee against the development of subsequent valvular deformity. Approximately one third of the rheumatic fever patients develop valvular heart disease.

Chronic disability and death owing to rheumatic heart disease are related to recurrent attacks. In former years, before antimicrobial therapy, patients who had had rheumatic fever usually suffered recurrences. Additional valvular deformity was the frequent outcome of each recurrence. As a result, a progressive severity of rheumatic heart disease was common. In current times the prognosis is more optimistic. Progressively severe valvular deformity after an initial attack, if recurrences are prevented, appears to be much less common than in former times, but this point requires further epidemiologic study. The efficacy of adequate chemoprophylaxis in the prevention of recurrences is clearly documented. In one study more than two thirds of the patients with a history of rheumatic fever who were not on prophylaxis had one or more recurrences over an eight-year follow-up period. If prophylaxis is adequately supervised and the drug is taken without fail, a recurrence is an extremely uncommon event.

Kuttner, A. G., and Mayer, F. E.: Carditis during second attacks of rheumatic fever: Its incidence in patients without clinical evidence of cardiac involvement in their initial rheumatic episode. N. Engl. J. Med., 268:1259, 1963.

Lendrum, B. L., Simon, A. J., and Mack, I.: Relation of duration of bed rest in acute rheumatic fever to heart disease present 2 to 14 years later. Pediatrics, 24:389, 1959.

Markowitz, M., and Gordis, L.: Rheumatic Fever. 2nd ed. Philadelphia, W. B. Saunders Company, 1972.

McCarty, M.: Missing links in the streptococcal chain leading to rheumatic fever: The T. Duckett Jones Memorial Lecture. Circulation, 24:488, 1964.

United Kingdom and United States Joint Report: The natural history of rheumatic fever and rheumatic heart disease: Ten-year report of a co-operative clinical trial of ACTH, cortisone, and aspirin. Circulation, 32:457, 1965.

Wood, H. F., and McCarty, M.: Laboratory aids in the diagnosis of rheumatic fever and in evaluation of disease activity. Am. J. Med., 17:768, 1954.

Zabriskie, J. B., Hsu, K. C., and Seegal, G. C.: Heart-reactive antibody associated with rheumatic fever: Characterization and diagnostic significance. Clin. Exp. Immunol., 7:147, 1970.

ENDOCARDITIS

131. INFECTIVE ENDOCARDITIS

Donald Kaye

acute and subacute forms is useful, it is more important to classify by infecting organism (e.g. enterococcal endocarditis, *S. aureus* endocarditis, and so on). The identity of the organism has implications for the course (i.e., acute or subacute), but more important, has therapeutic implications for the antimicrobial regimen.

DEFINITION

Infective endocarditis is defined as infection on the endocardium. Most commonly a heart valve is involved, but infection may be on a septal defect or mural endocardium. Infection of an arteriovenous shunt or coarctation of the aorta is more properly called endarteritis. However, the clinical syndrome of endarteritis is similar to that of endocarditis, and therefore the discussion of endocarditis relates to both endocarditis and endarteritis.

CLASSIFICATION

For many years infective endocarditis has been classified by course into acute and subacute disease. *Acute endocarditis* is most frequently caused by *Staphylococcus aureus* (and occasionally by pneumococci, group A streptococci, gonococci, or other organisms); it often occurs on a normal heart valve and results in rapid severe destruction. Metastatic foci of infection are common. Untreated, the infection will kill in days to weeks. However, the mortality rate is high even with appropriate therapy. *Subacute endocarditis* is usually caused by streptococci of the viridans group and occurs on already damaged valves, producing additional damage slowly. Metastatic foci of infection are rare, and results of treatment are good. Without therapy the infection will take six or more weeks and even up to years to kill. The correlations between infecting organism, rapidity of the course, and underlying valvular disease are not perfect. For example, endocarditis caused by streptococci of the viridans group can occasionally cause endocarditis with an acute course on a normal valve, and *S. aureus* can cause subacute disease.

Although the division of infective endocarditis into

MICROBIOLOGY

Almost any species of bacteria is capable of producing infective endocarditis. However, streptococci and staphylococci account for the vast majority of cases (over 90 per cent) in which an infecting organism can be identified.

STREPTOCOCCI. In most reported series, streptococci are the causative microorganisms in 60 to 80 per cent of cases of endocarditis with demonstrated bacteremia. Viridans streptococci (most commonly *S. sanguis* and *S. mitis*) are numerically the most important of the streptococci, accounting for about 50 per cent of the cases of streptococcal endocarditis. Enterococci are the next most frequent streptococci and cause about 15 per cent of cases. The remaining streptococci, including microaerophilic and anaerobic streptococci, nonhemolytic streptococci, group A beta-hemolytic streptococci, and streptococci of other groups, are isolated in the remainder of the cases. There has been a trend during the past 30 years toward an increasing incidence of enterococcal endocarditis and a decreasing incidence of viridans streptococcal endocarditis.

Enterococci and group A beta-hemolytic streptococci can attack normal or previously damaged heart valves and may cause rapid destruction. The other streptococci are much more likely to cause endocarditis on already damaged heart valves and rarely cause rapid destruction. Enterococci also can cause abscesses, e.g., in the spleen, which are uncommon with other streptococci.

STAPHYLOCOCCI. Staphylococci are the causative microorganisms in 10 to 30 per cent of cases of infective endocarditis with positive blood cultures. *S. aureus* is isolated much more frequently than *S. epidermidis*. If patients with acute endocarditis only are considered, *S. aureus* is the causative agent in the vast majority. In patients with subacute disease, *S. epidermidis* is found more often than *S. aureus*. The incidence of staphylococcal endocarditis has risen over the past 30 years, and part of the increase is attributable to the high frequency of staphylococcal endocarditis in narcotic addicts and in patients following cardiac surgery.

S. aureus attacks either normal or previously damaged heart valves and causes rapid destruction. The course is often fulminant, leading to death from overwhelming bacteremia within days or from heart failure within weeks. Abscesses are common at multiple sites (e.g., kidneys, lungs, brain, and heart). *S. epidermidis* usually attacks abnormal heart valves without causing rapid destruction.

S. PNEUMONIAE. The pneumococcus, which was responsible for 10 per cent or more of cases of endocarditis before the advent of antimicrobial therapy, is now an uncommon cause. This organism can attack normal or previously damaged heart valves and can cause rapid destruction with a fulminant course. The coexistence of

Differences Between Acute and Subacute Infective Endocarditis*

	Acute	Subacute
Causative agent	Capable of primary invasion (e.g., *S. aureus*)	Normally noninvasive, usually viridans streptococci
Pre-existing valve damage	Often not present	Usually present
Metastatic foci of infection	Common	Rare
Duration if untreated	Days to weeks	Months to one to two years
Response of infection to appropriate chemotherapy	Cure rate of 50% or less	High cure rate

*Modified from Beeson, P. B.: Infective endocarditis. *In* Beeson, P. B., and McDermott, W. (eds.): Textbook of Medicine. 14th ed. Philadelphia, W. B. Saunders Company, 1975.

endocarditis in patients with pneumococcal meningitis and pneumonia is common (up to one third of cases).

N. GONORRHOEAE. Neisseria (notably gonococcus), once a common cause of endocarditis (5 to 10 per cent of cases), now rarely causes the disease. It can attack and rapidly destroy normal or previously damaged heart valves. Gonococcal endocarditis was a common cause of endocarditis involving the right side of the heart; 25 per cent of patients with gonococcal endocarditis in the older series had right-sided involvement. About 50 per cent had double daily temperature elevations, and jaundice was common. Both these manifestations are rare in other types of endocarditis.

OTHER BACTERIA. Almost all species of bacteria are reported as occasionally causing endocarditis, including the enteric gram-negative bacilli, *Salmonella, Streptobacillus, Serratia marcescens, Bacteroides, Hemophilus, Brucella*, meningococci, *Listeria*, and even diphtheroids. Gram-negative bacilli account for less than 5 per cent of cases of endocarditis but are common causes in drug addicts and patients with prosthetic heart valves.

FUNGI. *Candida, Aspergillus*, and *Histoplasma* species are the most common causes of fungal endocarditis, with *Candida* endocarditis occurring most frequently. In addition, *Blastomyces, Cryptococcus, Mucor, Torulopsis*, and other fungi can cause endocarditis. *C. albicans* is the most common candidal organism isolated, but *C. tropicalis, C. krusei, C. parapsilosis*, and other candidal species have also caused endocarditis. *Candida*- and *Aspergillus*-induced endocarditis often occur in patients with intravascular catheters who frequently have received corticosteroids, broad-spectrum antimicrobial drugs, or cytotoxic agents. Fungal endocarditis is common in narcotic addicts (*Candida*) and in patients following cardiac surgery (*Candida* and *Aspergillus*).

The course of fungal endocarditis is usually subacute. Large friable vegetations are common and give rise to large emboli, often to the lower extremities. In patients with prosthetic cardiac valves, malfunction of the valve may occur because of the size of the vegetations. The prognosis is grave in fungal endocarditis, partly because of the relatively poor activity of the available antifungal agents and their toxicity for man, features that make their use difficult.

OTHER MICROORGANISMS. Spirochetes (e.g., *Spirillum minus*), cell wall–deficient bacteria, rickettsiae (*Coxiella burnetii*), and the psittacosis agent have all been reported as rare causes of endocarditis.

EPIDEMIOLOGY

SEX AND AGE. The proportion of males is somewhat higher than that of females in most reported series. The mean age of patients with endocarditis has increased during the past 30 years: at present, mean ages in most series range from the mid 40's to the 50's, with 50 per cent or more being 50 years or older. The mean age of males with endocarditis is about six or seven years higher than the mean age of females. Endocarditis is uncommon in children.

UNDERLYING HEART DISEASE. *Rheumatic valvular disease* is the underlying cardiac disease in about 40 to 60 per cent of patients with infective endocarditis. The mitral valve is most commonly involved. Aortic valve infection is also common. Right-sided endocarditis occurs in fewer than 10 per cent of patients with endo-

carditis superimposed on rheumatic heart disease and usually involves the tricuspid valve.

Congenital heart disease is the underlying lesion in about 10 per cent of patients with endocarditis. Some of the congenital lesions that predispose to endocarditis are patent ductus arteriosus, ventricular septal defect, tetralogy of Fallot, coarctation of the aorta, pulmonary stenosis, and bicuspid aortic valve. In contrast, atrial septal defects of the secundum type rarely serve as an underlying lesion in endocarditis.

Degenerative heart disease can be a predisposing cardiac lesion in endocarditis. For example, endocarditis has been reported on a calcified mitral annulus and on valves with degenerative changes. Calcific aortic stenosis resulting from degenerative aortic valve disease or a bicuspid aortic valve is being seen with increasing frequency in the elderly and can serve as an underlying lesion for endocarditis. Infective endocarditis has also been reported in patients with *hypertrophic subaortic stenosis*, the *systolic click syndrome* (mitral valve prolapse), *Marfan's syndrome*, and *syphilitic aortic valve disease*.

A new and important cardiac lesion which serves as an underlying abnormality for production of endocarditis is the *prosthetic cardiac valve*. Similarly, intravascular sutures, pacemaker wires, and Teflon-Silastic tubes serve as predisposing factors to development of endocarditis or endarteritis. Arterioarterial or arteriovenous fistulas also predispose to endocarditis.

In 20 to 40 per cent of patients with infective endocarditis, *no underlying heart disease* can be recognized. It is likely that some of these patients have underlying lesions that are difficult to recognize (e.g., degenerative heart disease, hypertrophic subaortic stenosis, systolic click syndrome). Others probably have no underlying lesions at all.

PATHOGENESIS AND PATHOLOGY

The characteristic lesions of infective endocarditis are vegetations on the valve leaflets or elsewhere on the endocardium. The disease usually arises secondary to localization of microorganisms on a sterile thrombotic vegetation. This type of sterile vegetation is termed nonbacterial thrombotic endocarditis and may form as a result of trauma to the endothelial cells (e.g., from intracardiac foreign bodies). Thrombi also may form over a subendothelial inflammatory reaction, such as in acute rheumatic fever or myocardial infarction. Vegetations commonly on the mitral and aortic valves (marantic endocarditis) are found at autopsy in patients with wasting disease, particularly from malignant tumors. Infective endocarditis has complicated sterile thrombus formation in all these circumstances.

When bacteremia occurs, the surface of the vegetation can become secondarily infected and converted to the typical vegetation of infective endocarditis. This results from deposition of platelets and fibrin over the bacteria. The vegetation then becomes a "protected site" into which phagocytic cells penetrate poorly. Although healthy valves may develop the lesions of nonbacterial thrombotic endocarditis, damaged valves appear to be much more frequently affected.

HYDRODYNAMIC FORCES. Sites of involvement suggest an important role for hydrodynamic forces. Endocarditis occurs where blood flows through a narrow orifice at a high velocity from a high- to a low-pressure chamber. Lateral pressure is lowest and the velocity of blood greatest a short distance downstream from the opening between the two chambers. A decrease in lateral pressure lowers perfusion of the intima, perhaps resulting in an area more susceptible to infection. This is the location where infective endocarditis initially develops in patients with congenital heart defects or valvular insufficiency. For example, endocarditis is found immediately distal to the constriction in coarctation of the aorta, on the pulmonary artery immediately beyond the junction with the ductus in patent ductus arteriosus, and on the right side of the defect in ventricular septal defect.

Endocarditis does not usually occur when there is only a small pressure gradient, as in artrial septal defects, or when a congenital defect is large enough practically to abolish the pressure gradient. Valvular endocarditis occurs more frequently in valvular incompetence than in pure stenosis and is characteristically on the atrial side of the incompetent mitral valve and the ventricular surface of the incompetent aortic valve. A high velocity stream of blood can produce satellite-infected lesions at distant points of impact. The reported cures of endocarditis at the sites of patent ductus arteriosus and arteriovenous fistulas with surgical ligation alone emphasize the role of hydrodynamic factors in both the initiation and maintenance of the infective process.

Experimental observations suggest that a hyperdynamic state of the cardiovascular system alone can initiate nonbacterial and subsequently infective endocarditis. Spontaneous endocarditis of the mitral and aortic valves occurs in dogs following surgical production of large arteriovenous fistulas and has been described in patients with traumatic arteriovenous fistulas and in patients undergoing hemodialysis with surgically produced arteriovenous fistulas or shunts.

INHERENT PATHOGENICITY. Microorganisms that possess little pathogenicity in other situations, e.g., alpha-hemolytic (viridans) streptococci, usually implant on heart valves deformed by pre-existing disease, although more virulent microorganisms, e.g., *S. aureus* and pneumococci, can implant on apparently normal valves. Infective endocarditis is found at autopsy in as high as 65 per cent of patients with *S. aureus* bacteremia and in one-third of patients with both pneumococcal pneumonia and meningitis.

INVASION OF CIRCULATION. Organisms must gain access to the circulation in sufficient numbers for a sufficient interval for endocarditis to result. Invasion of the bloodstream occurs in many infections. For example, transient bacteremia is found in about 30 per cent of patients with early pneumococcal pneumonia and is seen following compression of infected foci (e.g., bones, gums, tonsils, boils, prostate, diverticula, and endometrium).

BACTEREMIA. Transient bacteremia is common during traumatic procedures involving the epithelial surfaces normally laden with an indigenous bacterial flora (oropharynx, genitourinary and gastrointestinal tracts, and skin). Surgical incision of the skin, ordinarily inhabited by staphylococci and diphtheroids, is often associated with bacteremia, usually staphylococcal (either *S. aureus* or *S. epidermidis*). Bacteremia occurs in about 25 per cent of patients after toothbrushing, chewing hard candy, or use of an oral irrigation device. Streptococci of the viridans group are the most common bacteria isolated from the blood, either alone or more often mixed with other bacteria, after trauma to the tissues of the mouth. In one study, following tooth extraction, over 90 per cent of patients had mixed bacteremia, which included viridans streptococci in 74 per cent and *Bacteroides melaninogenicus* in 61 per cent of bacteremic patients. Many other bacterial species are occasionally isolated from blood after dental procedures (peptostreptococci, diptheroids, peptococci, staphylococci, fusobacteria, actinomyces, veillonella, bacteroides, spirillum, and vibrios). The frequency of bacteremia is related to the degree of periodontal disease and to the amount of trauma.

PORTAL OF ENTRY. Although the portal of entry for the initiating episode of bacteremia in endocarditis is often not apparent, oral cavity infection or operative or manipulative dental procedures appear to be the most common clinically apparent portals of entry, especially in endocarditis caused by viridans streptococci. Endocarditis caused by viridans streptococci has also occurred in edentulous patients in association with oral ulcers from poorly fitting dentures.

The incidence of bacteremia after sigmoidoscopy and barium enema has been reported to be about 10 per cent, with one half caused by enterococci. Similarly, bacteremia occurs in up to one third of patients after transurethral prostatic resection, cystoscopy, urethral dilatation, and urethral catheterization. The organisms are usually enterococci and gram-negative bacilli.

Endocarditis, especially enterococcal endocarditis, has developed after urinary tract surgery or instrumentation, prostatic massage or resection, delivery, abortion, pelvic infection, operative intervention or instrumentation of the female reproductive tract, and placement of a contraceptive uterine device. Instrumentation of the gastrointestinal tract has occasionally been implicated as a portal of entry for microorganisms in patients with endocarditis.

Endocarditis has also followed intravenous injection in drug addicts and has occurred with the prolonged use of plastic intravenous catheters.

MECHANISMS IN PRODUCTION OF LESIONS. The pathogenesis of the manifestations of endocarditis is both a result of the vegetations themselves, and an *immue reaction* to the infection. The vegetations may become so extensive, especially in fungal endocarditis, that the valve orifice is occluded. There may be rapid, massive destruction of tissue with consequent valvular insufficiency, especially in *S. aureus* endocarditis. Areas of healing may cause scar formation and consequent valvular stenosis or insufficiency. Infection may extend along the chordae tendineae or into the myocardium from the periphery of the valve, e.g., into the mitral annulus or along the sinus of Valsalva into the aortic ring, producing burrowing abscesses. Conduction abnormalities, fistulas (between a chamber of the heart and either another chamber or the pericardium or major vessels), or rupture of the chordae, a papillary muscle, or the ventricular septum may result. Valve ring abscesses with conduction abnormalities carry a grave prognostic significance.

The vegetations, containing necrotic calcified infected debris, are friable, and pieces break off and are swept into the circulation. Multiple emboli occlude the blood supply both to the heart itself and to the brain, kidney, spleen, liver, extremities, and lung (in endocarditis of the right side of the heart). Infarcts and perhaps abscesses (with *S. aureus* endocarditis) result at these sites. Septic embolization to the vasa vasorum or direct bacterial invasion of the arterial wall may result in formation of mycotic aneurysms which may rupture. Aneurysms involve medium or large arteries frequently at bifurcations. They most often develop in the cerebral arteries, abdominal aorta, sinus of Valsalva, ligated ductus arteriosus, and superior mesenteric, splenic, coronary, and pulmonary arteries. Vessels within the head are involved in about 50 per cent of the cases, vessels within the abdomen and chest in about 40 per cent, and vessels in the limbs in about 10 per cent of cases.

In addition, vasculitis on an immunologic basis is thought to contribute to the findings. Patients with infective endocarditis usually have high circulating antibody titers against the infecting microorganism. This contributes to the formation of immune complexes. Complexes composed of immunoglobulin and complement have been demonstrated in the glomeruli of patients with endocarditis and diffuse glomerulonephritis. In addition to glomerulonephritis, Roth's spots, petechiae, and Osler's nodes are thought to usually be due to allergic vasculitis. In contrast, Janeway's lesions are thought to be on an embolic basis.

Myocarditis is an important complication of endocarditis. Although its exact pathogenesis is still undetermined, present theories include ischemic damage secondary to coronary artery occlusion by emboli, damage produced by microbial toxins, myocardial invasion by organisms, or the result of immune complex deposition in blood vessels. Myocardial abscesses or myocardial infarction secondary to an arterial embolus may occur.

In addition to emboli or abscess formation, the kidneys may be involved with focal embolic glomerulitis or diffuse glomerulonephritis. The diffuse glomerulonephritis has been shown to be related to immune complex deposition, and it is likely that the focal type has the same cause. Focal glomerulitis occurs in over half of patients with subacute endocarditis. Diffuse glomerulonephritis is less common.

CLINICAL MANIFESTATIONS

In most patients with infective endocarditis, no event can be identified as the etiologic factor in the endocarditis. A history of a dental procedure can be elicited in only 15 to 20 per cent of patients with endocarditis caused by streptococci of the viridans group. About 50 per cent of patients with enterococcal endocarditis have had a preceding urologic or genital tract procedure, and about 35 per cent of patients with staphylococcal endocarditis have a history of a preceding staphylococcal infection. Symptoms of endocarditis generally start within two or three weeks of the procedure. The onset is usually gradual, with mild fever and malaise with endocarditis caused by streptococci of the viridans group and other organisms of low pathogenicity. With *S. aureus*, pneumococci and other organisms of high pathogenicity, the onset is often acute with high fever.

For purposes of orientation, it may be helpful to present prototypes of patients with the syndromes of subacute and acute bacterial endocarditis.

SUBACUTE ENDOCARDITIS. A 44-year-old white man with rheumatic heart disease was admitted to the hospital with four weeks of malaise, weakness, and anorexia without any cardiac symptoms. Erythromycin had been given from 12 to 7 days prior to admission, during which time the patient felt better. However, symptoms returned several days after stopping the drug. During the illness he had lost 10 pounds. There was no recent history of a dental procedure. Although he denied fever, a rectal temperature was found to be 38.4° C. Murmurs of mitral stenosis and mitral insufficiency were heard. There were no petechiae, but an enlarged spleen was palpated. He was started on antimicrobial therapy, and subsequently five blood cultures, taken at time of admission, were positive for viridans streptococci (*S. mitis*).

ACUTE ENDOCARDITIS. A 60-year-old female who had been in good health was admitted to the hospital with a history of sudden onset of high fever and recurrent shaking chills starting five days before and dyspnea starting on the day of admission. There was no history of heart disease. The rectal temperature was 40° C, and the blood pressure was 160/40 mm Hg. Bibasilar rales and a loud murmur of aortic insufficiency were present. There were no petechiae or splenomegaly. Although antimicrobial therapy was promptly initiated on the night of admission, she developed severe pulmonary edema, had a cardiac arrest, and died. Five of five blood cultures, taken at time of admission, were subsequently positive for *S. aureus*.

FEVER. Fever is present in almost all patients during the course of endocarditis. Most exceptions are elderly patients or patients with renal failure, congestive heart failure, or severe debility. The temperature is usually low grade (less than 39.4° C) except with acute disease.

CARDIAC MURMUR. Cardiac murmurs are almost always present except with acute endocarditis or in intravenous narcotic addicts. Those who develop endocarditis secondary to intravenous drug abuse often have vegetations on the tricuspid valve, and murmurs are frequently absent. True changes in murmurs or the appearance of a new murmur is uncommon except in acute endocarditis in which a new murmur (particularly aortic insufficiency) is a frequent occurrence. Changes in the intensities of murmurs during the course of endocarditis are often due to changes in heart rate and/or cardiac output such as occur with development of anemia and do not necessarily indicate progressive valvular damage.

SPLENOMEGALY. Splenomegaly is present in 25 to 60 per cent of reported cases of endocarditis and is most common in disease of long duration (i.e., less common in acute endocarditis).

PETECHIAE. Petechiae are present in 20 to 40 per cent of patients, most commonly in patients with more prolonged illness. Petechiae are most frequently found in the conjunctivae, palate, buccal mucosa, and extremities. Care must be taken in the interpretation of petechiae in areas of the body where they may have been induced by local trauma, such as the hard palate in patients with poorly fitting dentures or the lower conjunctival sac in women who wear eye makeup. Petechiae may also be found in elderly persons in whom there is no evidence of infection.

OTHER SIGNS. *Splinter hemorrhages* are subungual, linear, dark red streaks that may appear in endocarditis, but are also commonly the result of local trauma. What are commonly called *Roth's spots* are oval, retinal hemorrhages with a clear pale center. These are seen in less than 5 per cent of patients with endocarditis and may also occur in collagen vascular diseases and in severe anemia. *Osler's nodes* are small tender nodules most frequently found on the finger or toe pads which persist for hours to days. They are found in 10 to 25 per cent of patients with endocarditis, but also occur in other diseases such as typhoid fever and collagen vascular disease; they are uncommon in acute endocarditis. *Clubbing of the fingers* is present in some patients, usually those with longstanding disease. *Janeway's lesions* are nontender, macular, hemorrhagic areas on the palms and soles most commonly seen in acute endocarditis.

EMBOLIC EPISODES. Clinically apparent embolic episodes are recognized in about one third of patients with endocarditis and may occur early (as the first symptom) or late (after successful therapy). Splenic emboli with infarction may cause left upper quadrant pain radiating to the shoulder. Retinal emboli cause blindness, and coronary artery emboli can cause myocardial infarction. Emboli to large arteries such as the femoral or brachial arteries are often the result of fungal endocarditis with its large friable cardiac vegetations. Pulmonary emboli often occur in right-sided carditis, especially common in narcotic addicts, in whom the emboli may be the presenting symptoms. Pulmonary emboli may also be seen in endocarditis in patients with congenital heart disease with left-to-right shunts.

MYCOTIC ANEURYSMS. Mycotic aneurysms occur in about 15 per cent of patients with infective endocarditis, most commonly with less virulent organisms such as viridans streptococci. The aneurysms are most often found in the brain, where they tend to be small. Symptoms from mycotic aneurysms are usually lacking but may be those of an expanding mass until rupture occurs. These lesions can rupture at any time before, during, or even years after therapy for endocarditis.

NEUROLOGIC MANIFESTATIONS. Neurologic manifestations are present in about one third of patients with endocarditis. Major cerebral emboli occur not infrequently and usually involve the middle cerebral artery system. Mycotic aneurysms also most often involve this system. Rupture results in hemorrhage into the brain, ventricle, or subarachnoid space. Patients with endocarditis can also develop toxic encephalopathy and/or personality changes. Brain abscess and purulent meningitis are most common with *S. aureus* endocarditis.

CONGESTIVE HEART FAILURE. Congestive heart failure is a frequent complication of endocarditis and may occur at any time during the course of the disease, including long after cure. It carries a bad prognosis. Some of the factors which contribute to heart failure are valve destruction, myocarditis from vasculitis, coronary artery emboli with infarction, and myocardial abscesses.

RENAL DISEASE. Renal disease is present in most patients with infective endocarditis. Up to 50 per cent of endocarditis patients have microscopic hematuria, and proteinuria is even more common. These findings may be due to renal emboli, focal embolic glomerulitis, or diffuse glomerulonephritis. Renal insufficiency may occur in diffuse glomerulonephritis but is rare as a consequence of emboli or focal embolic glomerulitis.

SPECIAL SYNDROMES

ENTEROCOCCAL ENDOCARDITIS. Enterococci (*S. faecalis* varieties *zymogenes* and *liquefaciens*, *S. faecium*, and *S. durans*) are alpha-, beta-, or gamma-hemolytic streptococci that are normal inhabitants of the gastrointestinal tract, the anterior urethra, and occasionally the mouth of man. Enterococci may be distinguished from other streptococci by their ability to grow in media containing sodium azide, 0.1 per cent methylene blue, 40 per cent bile, or 6.5 per cent sodium chloride and to grow at 45° C. All enterococci are in Lancefield's group D, although all organisms in group D are not enterococci.

Two other group D streptococci, *S. bovis* and *S. equinus*, should be separated from the enterococci, because endocarditis caused by these two species can be treated like endocarditis caused by viridans streptococci. To separate *S. bovis* and *S. equinus* from the enterococci, biochemical tests must be performed, such as the ability to grow in 6.5 per cent sodium chloride broth. For all practical purposes *S. bovis* and *S. equinus* can be demonstrated not to be enterococci by the fact that they are highly susceptible to penicillin G (inhibited by 0.1 μg per milliliter), whereas enterococci are much more resistant.

Enterococcal endocarditis is more common in men than in women. The average age for males is near 60 years, whereas in women it is just under 40 years. This age distribution is probably closely related to the suspected portal of entry of the organism. About 50 per cent of patients give a history of genitourinary tract manipulation, trauma, or disease within three months of their admission to the hospital. For men this usually means cystoscopy, urethral catheterization, or prostatectomy, thus explaining the older age in males. For women the genitourinary factors are abortions, pregnancy, cesarean section, and urethral catheterization. Since many of these manipulations occur mainly during the childbearing years, this explains the lower age of female patients.

About one half of the patients with enterococcal endocarditis have no prior history of heart murmurs, indicating the ability of enterococci to attack normal heart valves. There is a tendency to form metastatic abscesses.

ENDOCARDITIS IN DRUG ABUSERS. Infective endocarditis is a complication of parenteral narcotic addiction. In these patients bacteremia may result from cellulitis or phlebitis at sites of injection or from drug contamination with virulent microorganisms. The skin is probably the most common source of microorganisms responsible for endocarditis in the addict. *S. aureus* is responsible for over 50 per cent of cases, and fungi (mainly *Candida*) and gram-negative bacilli (about one-third of which are *Pseudomonas* species) cause most of the remaining cases. Viridans streptococci are uncommon infecting agents in endocarditis in addicts.

Only about 20 per cent of narcotic addicts presenting with their first episode of endocarditis appear to have previously damaged heart valves. The tricuspid valve is infected in over 50 per cent of addicts, the aortic in 35 per cent and the mitral in about 30 per cent. There is a striking association of *S. aureus* endocarditis with tricuspid valve involvement; over 75 per cent with *S. aureus* infection have endocarditis on the tricuspid valve. Gram-negative bacilli also commonly involve the tricuspid valve (about 50 per cent of gram-negative bacillary cases), whereas fungi and streptococci (often enterococci) usually involve the left side of the heart.

Signs and symptoms of pulmonary emboli or pneumonia related to septic pulmonary emboli are common presentations in addicts with tricuspid valve endocarditis, and murmurs are frequently absent.

PROSTHETIC VALVE ENDOCARDITIS. The widespread use of prosthetic heart valves (and other intracardiac foreign bodies such as sutures or pacemaker wires) has created a new form of endocarditis. An intracardiac prosthesis predisposes to the development of endocarditis and makes eradication of the infection extremely difficult.

Endocarditis occurs at least two or three times more frequently after insertion of a prosthetic heart valve than after other open-heart operations and has been reported to occur in 1 to 3 per cent of patients with prosthetic valves. Endocarditis is much more likely to occur on aortic than mitral valve prostheses. The infection is usually found on the suture line.

Prosthetic valve endocarditis is usually divided into early endocarditis (onset within two months of valve replacement) and late endocarditis (onset after two months). Early endocarditis is a consequence of contamination during the surgical procedure or bacteremia in the postoperative period, whereas late endocarditis is probably related to episodes of transient bacteremia associated with dental, skin, and genitourinary tract trauma or infections.

The causative microorganisms in prosthetic valve endocarditis differ from those usually seen in other patients with endocarditis. About one third of both early and late endocarditis episodes are caused by staphylococci, with S. epidermidis occurring as a more frequent infecting organism than S. aureus. Gram-negative bacilli cause up to 25 per cent of early cases and are less common in late endocarditis. Fungi (most commonly Candida) are responsible for up to 25 per cent of early cases and are much less common in late endocarditis. Streptococci are the most frequent single causes of late endocarditis (about 40 per cent of cases) but are uncommon infecting organisms in early endocarditis. Diphtheroids have been the infecting organisms in up to 20 per cent of early cases and are less common in late endocarditis.

Early prosthetic valve endocarditis is often associated with valve dysfunction or dehiscence and a fulminant course. Although late endocarditis may have a similar clinical course, it is commonly characterized by a clinical syndrome indistinguishable from that occurring in patients without prosthetic valves. This is especially likely when the infecting organism is a streptococcus.

LABORATORY FINDINGS

Anemia is an almost constant finding in infective endocarditis except in acute cases. The anemia is usually normocytic and normochromic. Most patients with endocarditis have normal white blood cell and differential counts. However, in acute disease, leukocytosis may be present. Proteinuria, gross or microscopic hematuria, or both are present in most patients. The erythrocyte sedimentation rate is almost always elevated except in the presence of congestive heart failure. In those with severe renal complications (usually diffuse glomerulonephritis), the blood urea nitrogen or serum creatinine may be elevated.

About 50 per cent of patients with endocarditis of at least several weeks' duration have a positive serum test for rheumatoid factor. This tends to disappear with cure of endocarditis. The serum complement may be decreased, especially in patients with glomerulonephri-

tis. Large mononuclear cells have been described in the first drop of blood obtained after massage of the ear lobe ("ear lobe histiocytes") in about 25 per cent of patients with endocarditis. These cells are found in other chronic infections such as typhoid fever and malaria.

The demonstration of serum antibodies to teichoic acid (a major cell wall antigen in S. aureus) may be helpful in suggesting the possibility of endocarditis in a patient presenting with staphylococcal bacteremia. Bacteria can be seen inside leukocytes in buffy coat preparations of blood in about 50 per cent of patients with bacterial endocarditis.

The single most important finding in patients with endocarditis is bacteremia or fungemia. Blood cultures should be obtained promptly in anyone with suspected endocarditis and should be positive in over 95 per cent of patients. The bacteremia of endocarditis is constant; if any cultures are positive, it is likely that all will be positive. Therefore there is no advantage to obtaining cultures at any particular time or level of body temperature. Culture of arterial blood or marrow offers no advantage over culture of antecubital vein blood.

In patients with subacute disease who have not received previous antimicrobial therapy, five blood cultures should be obtained over a period of 12 to 24 hours and therapy initiated. If previous therapy has been given, treatment may be expeditiously delayed in an attempt to obtain positive blood cultures. In general, in acute disease therapy should not be delayed for more than two to three hours while obtaining cultures. Proper technique of blood culture involves thorough cleansing of the skin with a bactericidal disinfectant (e.g., 70 per cent alcohol and iodine), obtaining only one culture from each venipuncture, using anaerobic as well as aerobic techniques, keeping cultures for three weeks, and making periodic blind Gram stains and subcultures. In selected patients (especially those who have received previous antimicrobial therapy), cultures in hypertonic media may be helpful in an attempt to isolate cell-wall deficient forms.

Blood cultures have usually been negative in those rare cases of endocarditis caused by Aspergillus, Histoplasma, and Coxiella burnetii. In fungal endocarditis, large emboli to the lower extremities are common, necessitating embolectomy. Histologic examination and culture of the embolus may be diagnostic. Serologic tests for C. burnetii are positive in patients with endocarditis caused by this organism. Blood cultures may be sterile in patients with Brucella endocarditis unless special techniques are used.

Echocardiograms, although not diagnostic, may suggest the location of a vegetation. Serial phonocardiography and cineradiography are useful in evaluating patients with prosthetic valve endocarditis for valve dysfunction or dehiscence. Disappearance of an opening or closing click suggests presence of a vegetation on the valve; this is especially likely to occur with large vegetations, as are seen in fungal endocarditis. Cineradiography of the valve will show abnormal motion if the sutures are pulling out.

DIFFERENTIAL DIAGNOSIS

The possibility of infective endocarditis should be suspected in any patient with a heart murmur and unexplained fever present for at least one week. However, many other diseases can present with these same manifestations. A definitive diagnosis can be made only in the presence of positive blood cultures. In the small percentage of patients with sterile blood cultures, the differential diagnosis can be very difficult.

Some of the clinical entities which can exactly duplicate the syndrome of infective endocarditis (including fever, murmur, and emboli) are atrial myxoma and nonbacterial thrombotic endocarditis. Acute rheumatic fever, lupus erythematosus, and sickle cell disease can also produce fever and heart murmur. Any patient with an existing heart murmur can develop fever related to another illness such as infectious mononucleosis, toxoplasmosis, multiple pulmonary emboli, miliary tuberculosis, or lymphoma. Drug fever is another important possibility. Therefore in the absence of positive blood cultures, a search must be made for other causes of fever.

Following cardiac surgery, fever may be related to bacterial infection at sites other than the prosthetic valve, to the postcardiotomy syndrome, or to a "post-pump syndrome" (e.g., cytomegalovirus infection).

TREATMENT

Principles of Therapy

In order to achieve cure of infective endocarditis, it is necessary to eradicate essentially all microorganisms from the vegetation. Unlike other infections, inhibition of growth of the microorganism is not adequate for cure, because the cellular and humoral host defense mechanisms that normally eliminate organisms from other sites are not very effective in the vegetation of endocarditis. Therefore *bactericidal drug regimens are necessary in therapy of endocarditis, and treatment must be continued for a long enough period of time to achieve sterilization of the vegetation.* In addition, sufficient concentrations of antimicrobial agents must be reached in the serum to guarantee penetration of antibacterial concentrations into the vegetation. Available evidence indicates that if peak serum concentrations are bactericidal for the infecting microorganism at a 1:8 dilution in normal serum, therapy is probably adequate. Except for unusual circumstances, the route of administration should be parenteral to guarantee adequate absorption of drugs.

Different regimens have been used in therapy of infective endocarditis. One fact that seems incontrovertible is that therapeutic regimens, including penicillins and cephalosporins (and perhaps vancomycin), give far better results than regimens in which these drugs cannot be used either because of resistance of the organisms or because of drug reactions.

Drug susceptibility tests using disks are usually not very helpful in management of patients with bacterial endocarditis; more precise determinations of bacteriostatic and bactericidal end-points by broth dilution tests are necessary. These tests are critical when infection is caused by organisms other than gram-positive cocci, treatment has failed, or drug regimens other than penicillins or cephalosporins must be used. In vitro tests are also helpful in selecting appropriate drug combinations and in determining the dilution at which the patient's serum is bactericidal for the infecting organism. Once the infecting microorganism is isolated, it should be saved for future testing (e.g., serum antibacterial activity, evaluation of different antimicrobial drugs, or comparison with a strain obtained during relapse).

Intravascular catheters are to be avoided in treatment of endocarditis, as their use increases the risk of superinfection of the vegetation. This does not seem to be a problem with intravascular needles. Anticoagulants were used at one time to reduce the size of the vegetation in conjunction with antimicrobial drugs. However, the increased risk of hemorrhage (especially intracranial) far outweighs any advantage.

Specific Antimicrobial Regimens

The initial treatment of subacute infective endocarditis while awaiting culture results should be directed at the most common infecting organism, the streptococcus. As enterococci require the most vigorous therapy, the regimen is directed against the enterococcus. However, if the course is acute, if the patient has an intracardiac foreign body, or if the patient is a parenteral drug abuser, therapy for staphylococcal endocarditis must be added. This is the principle of initially treating for the most resistant infecting organism likely to be present. However, once the infecting organism is isolated, the regimen should promptly be altered. For example, if a streptococcus highly susceptible to penicillin is isolated, there would be no need for antistaphylococcal agents, and the dose of streptomycin would be decreased or stopped to avoid ototoxicity. In the event that cultures remain sterile and culture-negative endocarditis is felt to be present, treatment for enterococcal endocarditis is continued for six weeks, provided that the response is adequate.

STREPTOCOCCI. *Streptococci inhibited by 0.1 μg per milliliter penicillin G:* (These are classified as *penicillin-susceptible* and include over 90 per cent of viridans streptococci but no enterococci.) Although penicillin alone is highly active in vitro against these strains, the combination of penicillin and streptomycin exerts a more rapid bactericidal action than does penicillin alone. Three regimens have been widely used: (1) penicillin alone for four weeks in doses of 4 to 5 million units daily, which results in a low relapse rate (e.g., 1 per cent) after therapy is stopped; (2) penicillin and streptomycin in combination for two weeks, which results in a relapse rate of about 5 per cent; and (3) penicillin plus streptomycin for two weeks with penicillin therapy extended another two weeks, which results in essentially no relapses.

The writer's preferred regimen is procaine penicillin, 1.2 million units administered intramuscularly every six hours for four weeks, plus streptomycin, 0.5 gram given intramuscularly every 12 hours for the first two weeks. If the patient prefers intravenous infusions, penicillin G can be given intravenously in doses of 10 to 20 million units each day rather than by intramuscular injections. If penicillin is contraindicated because of hypersensitivity, cephalothin or cefazolin can be given instead in doses of 2 grams every four hours or 1 to 2 grams every six hours, respectively. Cephalosporins should be administered for four weeks, together with streptomycin for the first two weeks. Patients who are hypersensitive to penicillin may also be hypersensitive to the cephalosporins. If neither penicillin nor a cephalosporin can be used, vancomycin can be given intravenously in a dose of 0.5 gram every six hours for four weeks, together with streptomycin for the first two weeks.

In these regimens, streptomycin should be discontinued if vestibular toxicity occurs and should not be used if renal insufficiency is present.

Streptococci resistant to 0.1 μg per milliliter penicillin G: (These are classified as *relatively resistant to penicillin* and include all enterococci and up to 10 per cent of viridans streptococci.) Larger doses of penicillin must be used in these patients than are used for the therapy of endocarditis caused by penicillin-susceptible streptococci. Penicillin or ampicillin alone is inadequate therapy for enterococcal endocarditis, and an aminoglycoside must be added. In vitro, streptomycin combined with penicillin provides a more rapid and more complete bactericidal effect than penicillin alone against the majority of strains of enterococci. Some strains of enterococci do not demonstrate this in vitro effect with penicillin and streptomycin but do with penicillin and gentamicin. The enterococci that demonstrate a more rapid and complete bactericidal effect in the presence of streptomycin are inhibited by 2000 μg per milliliter, and those that do not are resistant to 2000 μg per milliliter of streptomycin. Thus this simple in vitro test can help predict which strains will or will not demonstrate the penicillin-streptomycin potentiation.

The therapy recommended for *enterococcal endocarditis* is aqueous penicillin G, 20 million units daily intravenously by continuous drip for six weeks, plus streptomycin, 1 gram every 12 hours intramuscularly for the first two weeks, followed by 0.5 gram every 12 hours for the remaining four weeks. The serum antibacterial activity should be determined, and if a 1:8 dilution does not inhibit the infecting enterococcus, the dose of penicillin should be doubled.

Although it is clear that penicillin plus gentamicin is bactericidal against more strains of enterococci in vitro than penicillin plus streptomycin, there are no clinical data to suggest that penicillin plus gentamicin is superior treatment. However, some investigators advocate the use of penicillin plus gentamicin (1.0 to 1.5 mg per kilogram of body weight every eight hours) as initial therapy in enterococcal endocarditis until in vitro studies are complete. Others prefer to use penicillin plus streptomycin, because renal toxicity is a more serious problem with gentamicin than with streptomycin. Once in vitro tests are completed, penicillin plus gentamicin may be used if there is an apparent advantage of gentamicin. If relapse occurs following a course of penicillin and streptomycin, the penicillin-gentamicin combination should be tried if tests in vitro demonstrate an advantage of this combination.

Vertigo or disturbances of balance develop in 20 to 30 per cent of patients who receive streptomycin for six weeks. If ototoxicity develops, the streptomycin may be terminated at four weeks, although penicillin is continued for the full six-week course. In patients with renal insufficiency, serum levels of streptomycin should be measured and the doses of streptomycin adjusted to maintain peak serum concentrations (one hour after dosage) between 10 and 15 μg per milliliter.

In contrast to endocarditis caused by penicillin-susceptible streptococci, *cephalosporins have no place in the treatment of enterococcal endocarditis*. Enterococci are highly resistant to cephalosporins in vitro, and the clinical results have been unsatisfactory. No alternative drug has been extensively tested for efficacy in the treatment of enterococcal endocarditis. Therefore an effort should be made to use penicillin in most patients who have a history of allergy to penicillin or in patients developing minor reactions during the course of therapy. In a patient with a history of a rash to penicillin, a "desensitization" procedure should be tried. This involves a scratch test through a drop of penicillin G (100 units per milliliter). This is followed in 30 to 45 minutes by graded amounts of penicillin intradermally, beginning at 0.001 unit per 0.1 ml of test solution and continued in tenfold increments every 30 to 45 minutes; with increasing amounts, administration is changed to the subcutaneous, intramuscular, and finally intravenous route. Epinephrine and diphenhydramine should be on hand for emergency use during the procedure if needed for an anaphylactic reaction. It is important to maintain continuous intravenous administration of penicillin throughout the course of treatment. If the intravenous infusion is stopped, it may be necessary to repeat the entire "desensitization."

Patients with a history of anaphylaxis to penicillin or those who develop severe reactions can be treated with vancomycin in a dose of 0.5 gram intravenously every six hours for four to six weeks. Streptomycin combined with vancomycin provides a more rapid and complete bactericidal effect against most enterococci than vancomycin alone and probably should be included in the therapeutic program. Vancomycin is difficult to administer intravenously because of the occurrence of phlebitis. On occasion it is nephrotoxic and ototoxic. A decision to use vancomycin in therapy should be made only after careful deliberation.

Endocarditis caused by streptococci that are not inhibited by 0.1 μg per milliliter penicillin G in vitro, i.e., relatively resistant, should probably be managed in the same manner as enterococcal endocarditis. However, with these nonenterococcal, relatively resistant streptococci, a cephalosporin can often be used as substitute therapy in the penicillin-allergic patient, provided that adequate serum bactericidal activity is achieved. Obviously, in such instances, the fact that the organism is *not* an enterococcus must be clearly established (see Laboratory Findings, above).

STAPHYLOCOCCI. *S. aureus* endocarditis is frequently a fulminant disease, requiring immediate antimicrobial therapy. It should be suspected when endocarditis occurs either in narcotic addicts or after the insertion of prosthetic heart valves or in the presence of the clinical syndrome of acute endocarditis. More than 50 per cent of community-acquired and over 80 per cent of hospital-acquired *S. aureus* produce penicillinase and are therefore resistant to penicillin. Only penicillinase-resistant penicillins (nafcillin, methicillin, or oxacillin) or cephalosporins may be relied on in initial treatment of staphylococcal endocarditis. Therapy must be given for four to six weeks. The doses are 2 grams of nafcillin, methicillin, oxacillin, or cephalothin intravenously every four hours or 1 to 2 grams of cefazolin intramuscularly or intravenously every six hours. Only when staphylococci are exquisitely susceptible to penicillin G (i.e., inhibited by 0.1 μg per milliliter) can penicillin G be used and then only in high doses (e.g., 20 million units daily by continuous intravenous infusion). If a penicillin or cephalosporin cannot be used, vancomycin, 0.5 gram intravenously every six hours, is the drug of choice.

Penicillins and gentamicin have been shown to result in a more rapid bactericidal effect against *S. aureus* than penicillins alone, both in vitro and in an animal model of endocarditis. Because of the high mortality of *S. aureus* endocarditis, some investigators have recommended the use of the combination in infection in man. At present, there is no clinical evidence to suggest that the combination has any advantage over the penicillin or cephalosporin alone. Furthermore, the additional toxicity of the aminoglycoside is sufficient to warrant further investigation before recommending routine use of the combination.

Resistance of *S. aureus* to methicillin has been noted elsewhere in the world, but it is not a major problem in the United States. Methicillin-resistant strains of *S. aureus* are resistant to other penicillinase-resistant penicillins such as nafcillin or oxacillin, and to the cephalosporins as well. Endocarditis caused by methicillin-resistant *S. aureus*, although rare, requires vancomycin therapy.

S. epidermidis endocarditis, which is often associated with prosthetic valves, should initially be treated with a cephalosporin. These organisms are often resistant to penicillin G and occasionally to methicillin but usually are susceptible to the cephalosporins. *S. epidermidis* endocarditis caused by a cephalosporin-resistant strain will require therapy with vancomycin.

OTHER ORGANISMS. *Pneumococcal, gonococcal,* and *meningococcal* endocarditis should be treated with 20 million units of penicillin G intravenously daily for four weeks. However, if a case of endocarditis should occur with one of the recently described strains of gonococci that produce penicillinase, penicillin G will not be appropriate therapy, and a regimen would have to be chosen on the basis of in vitro bactericidal tests.

The therapy of endocarditis caused by *gram-negative bacilli* must consist of bactericidal antimicrobials, preferably a penicillin or cephalosporin with or without an aminoglycoside, and must be given in sufficient doses to achieve peak concentrations in the serum that are bactericidal for the infecting organism at a 1:8 dilution. Penicillin G or ampicillin (for *E. coli, Proteus mirabilis,* or *Salmonella*), cephalosporins (for *E. coli, Proteus mirabilis,* or *Klebsiella* species), and carbenicillin (for *Enterobacter* species, *Pseudomonas aeruginosa*, or *Proteus* species other than *P. mirabilis*) are the drugs most likely to be effective but must be selected on the basis of in vitro bactericidal tests. An aminoglycoside such as gentamicin is often added to achieve a greater bactericidal effect; this is particularly important in *Pseudomonas* endocarditis. The usual doses are as follows: penicillin G, 20 million units or more intravenously daily; ampicillin, 2 grams or more every four hours intramuscularly or intravenously; cephalothin, 2 grams or more every four hours intravenously; cefazolin, 1 to 2 grams every six hours intramuscularly or intravenously; carbenicillin, 500 mg per kilogram of body weight daily intravenously in divided doses every four hours; and gentamicin, 1 to 1.7 mg per kilogram intramuscularly every eight hours. The adequacy of therapy must be monitored by testing serum bactericidal activity. Therapy is continued for four to six weeks.

If the gram-negative bacillus is resistant to the penicillins and cephalosporins, either an aminoglycoside as sole therapy or bacteriostatic antimicrobials may have to be used. The results of therapy with these alternatives are usually poor. Surgical management to remove the vegetation and replace the valve may be necessary for cure.

If *other infecting bacteria* are found, the susceptibility to antimicrobial agents must be determined in vitro. If the organism is susceptible to a penicillin or cephalosporin, therapy with one of these agents in high doses plus streptomycin (unless streptomycin does not increase the bactericidal activity in vitro) should be given for four to

six weeks. Serum bactericidal activity should be monitored. If the organism is resistant to all penicillins and cephalosporins, vancomycin with (or without) streptomycin should be used if in vitro studies indicate susceptibility. If the organism is resistant to penicillins, cephalosporins, and vancomycin, therapy will probably be unsuccessful. Under these circumstances, treatment should be initiated with the bactericidal drug grouping that demonstrates the best activity in vitro; if the patient does not respond, or if relapse occurs after four to six weeks of therapy, antimicrobial therapy plus cardiac surgery to remove the vegetation and replace the valve will probably be necessary.

Results of therapy of *fungal endocarditis* have been very disappointing. Amphotericin B, the only fungicidal agent available for parenteral use, is very toxic and difficult to use. It is difficult to achieve adequate fungicidal serum levels with amphotericin without causing profound toxicity. Another agent, flucytosine, is fungistatic but may increase the fungicidal activity of amphotericin B in vitro. Amphotericin B is generally administered intravenously in a dose of 0.5 mg per kilogram daily; flucytosine is given orally in a dose of 75 to 150 mg per kilogram each day. Although some cures have been reported with antifungal therapy alone, surgical intervention with valve replacement is usually necessary to achieve a cure.

ENDOCARDITIS WITH STERILE BLOOD CULTURES. Most experts favor treating these patients as they would patients with enterococcal endocarditis. If there is no clinical response to the penicillin plus aminoglycoside regimen within three to five days, the dose of penicillin should be doubled to 40 million units daily. When the course is acute and fulminant, antistaphylococcal therapy with a penicillinase-resistant penicillin or cephalosporin should be added.

ENDOCARDITIS ON INTRACARDIAC PROSTHESES OR SUTURES. These patients probably require longer courses of therapy than patients without intravascular foreign bodies. Treatment is usually continued for at least six weeks for streptococci inhibited by 0.1 μg per milliliter of penicillin and eight weeks for all other microorganisms. With the exception of streptococcal endocarditis, results of medical therapy of prosthetic valve endocarditis have been very poor. Therefore in patients with endocarditis caused by organisms other than streptococci, valve replacement should be carefully considered.

Untoward Effects of Antimicrobial Therapy

Hypersensitivity reactions are common during therapy with penicillins. If a rash develops, therapy can be continued and antihistamines or even corticosteroids given to suppress the reaction. If the reaction is severe, requiring discontinuation of a penicillin, a cephalosporin can be tried if appropriate therapy. When neither penicillins nor cephalosporins can be used, vancomycin is the best alternative for endocarditis caused by gram-positive organisms.

The large amounts of penicillins used daily are accompanied by significant cation loads that may be of clinical significance. Twenty million units of potassium penicillin G contains approximately 34 mEq of potassium; 10 grams of nafcillin contains about 30 mEq of sodium; and 30 grams of carbenicillin contains about 141 mEq of sodium. Streptomycin, gentamicin, and vancomycin are all potentially nephrotoxic and ototoxic and must be used in reduced doses in patients with renal insufficiency; serum levels should be monitored during therapy to achieve therapeutic but nontoxic serum concentrations.

Surgery in the Management of Endocarditis

When appropriate microbicidal therapy is not available and positive blood cultures continue on therapy or relapse occurs after therapy is discontinued, removal of the vegetation and replacement of the valve with a prosthesis should be considered. The surgical repair should ideally be performed after several days or more of the best available antimicrobial therapy. The therapy should then be continued for two weeks or longer in the case of organisms that tend to produce metastatic foci. Some investigators have found it unnecessary to replace the tricuspid valve after removal. *Immediate valve replacement (even after only hours of therapy) is essential in patients developing congestive heart failure secondary to severe valvular insufficiency.* Surgery should also be strongly considered in patients with recurrent emboli despite adequate antimicrobial therapy.

Current evidence indicates that to achieve cure in fungal endocarditis surgical intervention is almost always required in addition to treatment with antifungal agents. Because of the toxicity of antifungal agents and the complications of continued infection (e.g., large emboli), early valve resection is best.

Patients with prosthetic valve endocarditis often require valve replacement for cure. The indications for valve replacement are valve dysfunction, continuation of embolization, organisms resistant to bactericidal antimicrobials, infection with fungi, and continuing bacteremia during or relapses after an appropriate course of therapy. Surgery is most often required in early prosthetic valve endocarditis both because of the microorganisms involved (fungi and other resistant organisms) and because of valve dysfunction.

RESPONSE TO THERAPY AND PROGNOSIS

RESPONSE. Defervescence and an increased sense of well-being usually occur within several days to a week of initiation of appropriate antimicrobial therapy. Blood cultures should be obtained periodically during treatment and generally become negative within several days of onset of therapy. Lack of response of fever (at times accompanied by persistently positive blood cultures) may be associated with metastatic abscess formation (especially in *S. aureus* endocarditis).

The most common cause of persistent or recurrent fever during therapy with an appropriate drug regimen is a reaction to the antimicrobial agents, either true drug fever or inflammation at the site of administration. Another cause of febrile episodes is emboli. Superinfection of a heart valve, although rare, is especially likely when intravascular plastic catheters are used.

Weight gain, a fall in erythrocyte sedimentation rate, and disappearance of rheumatoid factor follow the fall in temperature, but may be delayed in some patients for as long as several weeks after therapy has been discontinued. Regression of clubbing occurs after many weeks. Hematuria, proteinuria, and changes in renal function tend to disappear with therapy. Splenomegaly may persist for months. Although anemia may respond within weeks, the rise in hemoglobin may be very slow and may not occur until weeks after discontinuation of therapy.

Petechiae, Osler's nodes, and emboli may occur during and for weeks after successful antimicrobial therapy. Mycotic aneurysms may regress on drug therapy or may become clinically evident by rupture weeks to months after successful therapy.

Heart failure may occur at any time during or after therapy and is a poor prognostic sign. Patients with aortic insufficiency are especially likely to develop heart failure and have a high mortality. Even with mild heart failure, aortic insufficiency may be associated with sudden death. In addition to valvular insufficiency, vegetations (especially in fungal endocarditis) may become large enough to cause obstruction of the valvular orifice.

The vast majority of relapses should be detected with blood cultures obtained one, two and four weeks after discontinuation of therapy.

PROGNOSIS. The factors that tend to make the prognosis relatively bad are (1) nonstreptococcal disease, (2) development of heart failure, (3) aortic valve involvement, (4) prosthetic valve, and (5) old age. The cure rate in streptococcal endocarditis is about 90 per cent. The failures are not due to uncontrolled infection but to death from heart failure, an embolus, rupture of a mycotic aneurysm, or renal failure. The cure rate in staphylococcal endocarditis is about 50 per cent, most deaths being due to early overwhelming infection or to heart failure. Results in endocarditis caused by fungi and gram-negative bacilli have been poor. Early cardiac surgery for heart failure or for cases refractory to antimicrobial therapy should improve these results.

Following cure of infective endocarditis, there is an increase in morbidity and mortality as compared with those in the normal population. This increase is in part related to the pre-existing underlying heart disease and in part to the consequences of the endocarditis. The mortality rate without cardiac surgery is about 5 per cent per year for the first four years and then 2 to 3 per cent annually thereafter. The prognosis is much poorer in the presence of aortic insufficiency, with only about 70 per cent alive in two years; thereafter the mortality is less than 4 per cent annually. With cardiac surgery, the survival rates should be higher.

About two thirds of the deaths are due to heart failure, with embolic phenomena, renal failure, and rupture of a mycotic aneurysm accounting for most of the remainder. The onset of heart failure can occur early in endocarditis or may be delayed for weeks, months, or even years after successful therapy. Emboli can occur months (and perhaps years) after cure of endocarditis. Mycotic aneurysms can rupture months or years after cure of infective endocarditis. Renal failure resulting from the glomerulonephritis of endocarditis is usually reversible with cure of endocarditis. About 5 to 8 per cent of patients who have been cured of one episode of endocarditis will have one or more additional episodes over a period of years.

PROPHYLAXIS OF ENDOCARDITIS

An apparent portal of entry for the infecting organism can be demonstrated in only a minority of patients with infective endocarditis. However, it seems clear that the oropharynx serves as the site of origin for most patients, with the genitourinary tract next. It is obvious that oral hygiene should be optimal in patients with underlying cardiac lesions that predispose to endocarditis, especially those who are to have prosthetic cardiac valves implanted.

Although the risk of endocarditis is small and there is no proof of efficacy, antimicrobial prophylaxis is recommended for patients with predisposing cardiac lesions who are to undergo procedures known to result in transient bacteremia. The cardiac conditions for which prophylaxis is recommended are valvular or congenital heart disease (except for uncomplicated atrial septal defect), intracardiac prostheses, and previous episode of infective endocarditis. The antimicrobial therapy is directed at the bacteria which lodge at an endocardial site and therefore is analogous to treatment of very early endocarditis.

DENTAL MANIPULATIONS AND OTHER PROCEDURES IN THE MOUTH, NOSE, OR THROAT. Prophylaxis is directed against viridans streptococci and is recommended for all procedures likely to cause gingival bleeding and for tonsillectomy and bronchoscopy. Based on data in laboratory animals, regimens likely to be effective are (1) aqueous penicillin G, 1 million units, mixed with procaine penicillin, 600,000 units, *plus* streptomycin, 1 gram, both intramuscularly 30 minutes before the procedure; (2) aqueous penicillin G, 1 million units, mixed with procaine penicillin, 600,000 units, intramuscularly 30 minutes before the procedure, followed by penicillin V, 0.5 gram orally every six hours for eight doses; (3) vancomycin, 1 gram intravenously over a 30- to 60-minute period starting 30 to 60 minutes before the procedure; or (4) penicillin V, 2 grams orally 30 minutes before the procedure and then 0.5 gram every six hours for eight doses. The penicillin-plus-streptomycin regimen is preferred for patients with prosthetic heart valves, and vancomycin should be used in the patient who is hypersensitive to penicillin. Erythromycin, 1 gram orally one and one half hours before the procedure and then 500 mg every six hours for eight doses, is probably less effective. The American Heart Association recommends continuation of therapy after penicillin plus streptomycin (penicillin V, 500 mg orally every six hours for eight doses) and after vancomycin (erythromycin, 500 mg orally every six hours for eight doses), but this additional oral treatment is probably unnecessary except in the case of a prolonged procedure.

GENITOURINARY AND GASTROINTESTINAL TRACT PROCEDURES OR SURGERY. Prophylaxis is directed against enterococci and is recommended for procedures that cause significant trauma to the genitourinary or gastrointestinal tracts (e.g., urethral catheterization, prostatic surgery, and colonic or gallbladder surgery). Regimens likely to be effective are (1) ampicillin (1 gram intramuscularly or intravenously) plus gentamicin (1.5 mg per kilogram intramuscularly or intravenously) or streptomycin (1 gram intramuscularly) 30 minutes before the procedure, and then two additional doses every eight hours for ampicillin plus gentamicin and every 12 hours for ampicillin plus streptomycin; or (2) vancomycin, 1 gram intravenously over a 30- to 60-minute period starting 30 to 60 minutes before the procedure, plus streptomycin, 1 gram intramuscularly 30 to 60 minutes before the procedure.

CARDIAC SURGERY. Prophylaxis is directed against staphylococci and consists of 2 grams of methicillin, oxacillin, nafcillin, or cephalothin intravenously every four hours starting one hour before the procedure and continuing for several days. Vancomycin in a dose of 0.5 gram intravenously every six hours can be used in patients hypersensitive to penicillins and cephalosporins. Because of an extremely low risk of endocarditis, prophylaxis is not recommended in association with cardiac catheterization.

A. H. A. Committee Report: Prevention of bacterial endocarditis. Circulation, 56:139A, 1977.

Bayer, A. S., Theofilopoulos, A. N., Eisenberg, R, Dixon, F. J., and Guze, L. B.: Circulating immune complexes in infective endocarditis. N. Engl. J. Med., 295:1500, 1976.

Dreyer, N. P., and Fields, B. N.: Heroin-associated infective endocarditis. A report of 28 cases. Am. Intern. Med., 78:699, 1973.

Duma, R. J.: Infections of Prosthetic Heart Valves and Vascular Grafts. Baltimore, University Park Press, 1977.

Kaye, D.: Infective Endocarditis. Baltimore, University Park Press, 1976.

Mandell, G. L., Kaye, D., Levison, M. E., and Hook, E. W.: Enterococcal endocarditis. An analysis of 38 patients observed at the New York Hospital–Cornell Medical Center. Arch. Intern. Med., 125:258, 1970.

Rubinstein, E., Noriega, E. R., Simberkoff, M. S., Holzman, R., and Rahal, J. J., Jr.: Fungal endocarditis: Analysis of 24 cases and review of the literature. Medicine, 54:331, 1975.

Wolfe, J. C., and Johnson, W. D., Jr.: Penicillin-sensitive streptococcal endocarditis: In vitro and clinical observations on penicillin-streptomycin therapy. Ann. Intern Med., 81:178, 1974.

STAPHYLOCOCCAL INFECTIONS

F. Robert Fekety, Jr.

132. INTRODUCTION

Staphylococci are the most common cause of suppurative skin infections of man. They also cause bacteremia and serious infections of lungs, pleura, endocardium, meninges, muscles, bones, joints, and other viscera. Staphylococcal infections became more frequent and troublesome after antimicrobial drugs were introduced. Staphylococci are ubiquitous in our environment and are constituents of our normal flora. They are resistant to some of our most useful antimicrobial drugs and increase in prevalence when these agents are used. Hospitalized patients are frequently exposed to staphylococci as well as being highly susceptible to them. Such patients are most likely to develop serious staphy-

lococcal infections and to have difficulty in handling them. Hospital-acquired staphylococcal infections are still an important problem even though we have developed several good drugs for treating them.

BACTERIOLOGY. Staphylococci are spherical gram-positive cocci that grow well either aerobically or anaerobically on simple laboratory media. Grapelike clusters of organisms are seen in stained smears of cultures; small irregular clusters, pairs, and short chains are seen in smears of pus. When gram-positive cocci are seen *within* leukocytes, it is very likely that they are staphylococci, as other cocci are usually killed and digested soon after phagocytosis, but pathogenic staphylococci are not.

Staphylococci are the most important pathogens in

the genus *Micrococcus*, which includes many saprophytes. Pathogenic staphylococci are noteworthy for their metabolic and biochemical versatility. Two species can be tentatively identified by pigment production: *S. aureus* is characteristically golden yellow on agar, and *S. epidermidis* (formerly *S. albus*) is white. *S. aureus* often grows as white colonies on primary isolation; cream-colored, orange, or lemon-yellow colonies of *S. aureus* are also seen. *S. aureus* is the most important pathogenic *Staphylococcus*.

Pathogenic staphylococci can produce a variety of exotoxins with hemolytic, necrotizing, leukocidal, vasospastic, or lethal properties. They are capable of fermenting mannitol and other sugars, and produce other possibly important substances, including lysozyme, catalase, enterotoxin, epidermolysin, fibrinolysin, hyaluronidase, lipase, thermonuclease, beta-lactamase, phosphatase, deoxyribonuclease, protease, and coagulase (a plasma-clotting substance). The pathogenetic role of these toxins and enzymes is still uncertain. Coagulase and thermonuclease production and mannitol fermentation correlate well with pathogenicity for man. By convention, coagulase-positive, mannitol-fermenting staphylococci are called *S. aureus*. The tube coagulase test is more reliable than the slide test, which measures bound coagulase (clumping factor).

Coagulase-negative and mannitol-negative isolates are called *S. epidermidis*. *S. epidermidis* does not often cause infection of man unless susceptibility is increased or there is a nidus of infected foreign material, such as an intracardiac prosthesis or an intravascular plastic catheter or shunt. These opportunistic organisms are being recognized more and more frequently as the etiologic agents in endocarditis, bacteremia, and other serious infections, and *they can no longer be dismissed automatically as contaminants whenever they are isolated from cultures of blood or other specimens.*

Nonhemolytic, coagulase-negative staphylococci that ferment mannitol under certain conditions have been classified recently as *Staphylococcus saprophyticus.* They can also be recognized by their resistance to novobiocin. These organisms can cause urinary tract infections, especially in young women. This is the primary reason for calling attention to them and for attempting to distinguish them from *S. epidermidis*, which often is a contaminant in urine cultures.

PATHOGENESIS. Suppuration and abscess formation are the characteristic features of staphylococcal infection. When staphylococci lodge in susceptible tissues, multiply, and produce their exotoxins, an acute inflammatory reaction ensues. Small blood vessels thrombose, and fibrin is deposited about the lesion, which becomes avascular, necrotic, and surrounded by fibroblasts. The tissues become hypertonic, edematous, tense, and painful. The center of the lesion gradually liquefies, forming the characteristic thick, creamy yellow pus which is slightly acidic, hypoxic, and composed of dead organisms, leukocytes, and proteinaceous substances. Further evolution of the lesion is slow even when antimicrobials are given unless it drains, after which it usually begins to heal. Antimicrobial drugs do not affect undrained abscesses very much, (1) because the drugs may not diffuse into abscesses very well, (2) because they may be destroyed or inactivated there, or (3) because the organisms in abscesses may not be multiplying and thus are in a relatively insusceptible state. Granulomatous reactions are

occasionally seen at sites of chronic staphylococcal infections.

Very little that is conclusive has been established about the mechanisms of the pathogenicity of staphylococci. Virulence probably is the result of multiple mechanisms acting together. There are obvious clinical implications for the dermonecrotic, lethal, and leukocidal toxins, but their true importance is unknown. Fibrin products of coagulase activity may help wall off the lesion and protect the organism from granulocytes, but the resultant fibrin network may also enhance surface phagocytosis. Lipases may nullify the bactericidal action of cutaneous lipids. Capsular structures and cell wall teichoic acids may be antiphagocytic.

Some of the substances that may be important in pathogenesis have been used as antigens in experimental vaccines, but immunization as a means of enhancing resistance to staphylococci has met with little success. Most adults possess serum antibodies to a number of staphylococcal antigens, but high titers of these antibodies have not correlated well with protection from disease. The factors important in promoting phagocytosis and intracellular killing of the organism are incompletely understood. Protein A, a component of staphylococcal cell walls, nonspecifically binds antistaphylococcal (and other) antibodies at the Fc fragment instead of appropriately at the Fab fragment. This reverse attachment of immune globulins appears to render them functionally ineffective, and may be the explanation for the observation that neither vaccination nor the disease seems to result in immunity despite the production of large amounts of antibody. In addition, there is some evidence that hypersensitivity reactions to antigenic products of the microorganism may lower local resistance to infection. Additional studies are required if safe and effective vaccination against staphylococci is to become possible.

EPIDEMIOLOGY. Pathogenic staphylococci are normally acquired by a high percentage of healthy infants within a few days or weeks of birth. They may be responsible for epidemics in nurseries. Most healthy humans harbor virulent staphylococci in the anterior nares or on the skin, either occasionally or consistently. Clinical disease occurs in exposed persons or asymptomatic carriers when local or general resistance is decreased or when exposure is heavy. Staphylococci are abundant in our environment and can survive in dust for long periods, but implantation of large numbers of staphylococci derived from air and other exogenous sources seems an uncommon explanation for disease. To produce skin infections experimentally in healthy persons more than a million pathogenic staphylococci must be inoculated, and no significant differences have been demonstrated between strains derived from lesions or from healthy mucous membranes. In the presence of a silk suture, the infective dose is reduced to less than 100 organisms. The evidence that certain strains of pathogenic staphylococci are especially virulent is inconclusive, but the epidemiologic evidence suggests that enhanced virulence may be responsible for nursery outbreaks. Factors that increase host susceptibility to relatively small numbers of ordinary staphylococci seem of greatest importance in explaining the development of staphylococcal disease.

Although numerous conditions are known to predispose to staphylococcal infection, the mechanisms causing staphylococci to become invasive are not well understood. Skin infections usually begin about hair follicles, sebaceous glands, or at sites of wounds, abrasions, or foreign bodies such as intravenous catheters. Greasy substances, oils, sunburn, and other conditions causing blockage of the ducts of cutaneous glands predispose to infection. In some cases infection results from multiplication of the organism within serous exudates, hematomas, or devitalized tissues. Burns, surgical wounds, and chronic dermatitic lesions frequently become secondarily infected with staphylococci. Diabetics seem to have an increased frequency of cutaneous staphylococcal infections, possibly because their acute defensive inflammatory responses may be delayed and deficient (especially during ketoacidosis), because of vascular disease and gangrene, and because of the frequent exposure that diabetics have to hospitals and to medical procedures that increase the risk of infection. The chronic granulomatous disease of childhood is characterized by refractory infections with catalase-positive organisms such as staphylococci, because the granulocytes of the affected individuals are unable to generate sufficient hydrogen peroxide to permit intraleukocytic bactericidal mechanisms to operate normally. Other congenital or acquired conditions associated with frequent staphylococcal infections have been described; eczema, elevated serum IgE or depressed IgM levels, and depressed leukocyte chemotaxis are often documented. Malnutrition and a variety of chronic debilitating diseases predispose to serious staphylococcal infection. In some cases this association may be attributable to treatment with antimicrobial drugs that encourage overgrowth of drug-resistant, pathogenic staphylococci. In others, it may be the consequence of therapeutic efforts or disease processes that adversely affected cellular or humoral defense mechanisms. Neoplasms, uremia, lengthy operations, and treatment with adrenal steroids and cytotoxic or immunosuppressive agents predispose to staphylococcal infection. Influenza, measles, diabetes mellitus, and cystic fibrosis predispose to staphylococcal pneumonia. Newborn infants are hypersusceptible to this organism and are subject to severe spreading skin infections and primary staphylococcal pneumonia with pneumatocele formation.

Because of their ubiquity, versatility, and resistance to antimicrobial drugs, staphylococci have become a major cause of serious infections in highly susceptible persons who tend to congregate in hospitals (see Ch. 124). Bacteriophage typing of staphylococci has contributed to understanding the modes of transmission of these infections. Man is the major source of the organism. Patients and personnel in hospitals are more commonly asymptomatic carriers of the organism than are those without hospital contact. The organism is most often found in the anterior nares, in intertriginous areas and hair, and on the hands. Carriers and infected patients readily contaminate their environment, and staphylococci can be isolated from air, dust, floors, mops, blankets, clothing, dressing carts, and other fomites. Heavily colonized or clinically infected patients tend to shed more organisms than do asymptomatic carriers. The usual habitat of *S. epidermidis* is the skin and mucous membranes of man and animals.

Studies in nurseries for the newborn have shown that transmission of the organism occurs primarily via the hands of personnel who either are carriers or have recently handled infected or colonized newborns. The spread of organisms from heavily colonized infants ("cloud-babies") via the airborne route may occur, but this seems much less frequent than transmission via hands. Postoperative wound infections are more frequent in nasal carriers of staphylococci and often appear to be attributable to strains carried by the patient prior to operation (endogenous infection). Infected patients or personnel are also important sources of strains causing wound infections (exogenous infections); the usual mechanism is contact spread via hands. Air, environment, or fomites are less common sources of the organism. All these mechanisms contribute to the perpetuation of the reservoir of staphylococci in the hospital and to the spread of organisms to personnel and highly susceptible patients, especially those treated with antimicrobial drugs.

Most authorities believe that special attention to measures such as isolation and frequent handwashing in order to prevent the spread of staphylococci is worthwhile. Infected patients can shed large numbers of bacteria into the environment and should be isolated unless the infection is at a closed site (e.g., blood, meninges). Personnel with clinical infections should not have contact with susceptible patients. The indiscriminate use of antimicrobial drugs favors the transmission and survival of drug-resistant strains. Few surgical procedures are indications for prophylactic antimicrobials, for there is little evidence that such agents are capable of preventing staphylococcal infection. Because so many persons are asymptomatic carriers of pathogenic staphylococci, it is not practical to exclude all of them from contact with susceptible persons in hospitals. Actually, healthy carriers of ordinary strains seem unlikely to acquire new and potentially more dangerous strains, which is probably an example of *bacterial interference*. However, it may be necessary during outbreaks to exclude carriers of *especially dangerous* staphylococcal strains (as demonstrated by both bacteriophage typing and clinical experience) from nurseries, delivery rooms, and operating rooms.

TREATMENT. Although antimicrobial therapy has markedly improved the prognosis in serious staphylococcal infection, it must be emphasized that surgical drainage of abscesses and removal of infected foreign bodies are not only equally important but may be the only way to achieve a cure. Patients with staphylococcal infections usually respond relatively slowly to therapy, and despite optimal treatment the mortality rate is high in persons with compromised defense mechanisms. Although antimicrobial therapy is considered in detail in Ch. 187 and 188, there are certain points that should be stressed here.

Appropriate cultures and drug susceptibility tests should always be obtained to confirm the diagnosis of serious staphylococcal disease and to guide therapy. Although many antimicrobial drugs are now available for treating these infections, the unpredictable susceptibility of the organism narrows the initial choice to only a few. Bactericidal penicillin analogues are preferred unless the patient is allergic to them. Because most isolates causing infection in the hospital and in the community are resistant to penicillin G and ampicillin, the choice should be limited to drugs that are not significantly inactivated by staphylococcal beta-lactamase. Toxic-appearing patients with serious infections are best treated parenterally. Methicillin, oxacillin, nafcillin, cephalothin, cefazolin, and cephapirin are recommended for serious infection. Used properly, they seem to produce equally good therapeutic results. Many experts still prefer methicillin, but nafcillin has become increasingly popular because it is the most active derivative and rarely causes nephritis or other serious side effects. The cephalosporins are especially useful with mixed infections because of their relatively broad spectrum. Cephaloridine should rarely be used because it is nephrotoxic when used in doses greater than 4.0 grams per day. Cefazolin is a well tolerated new cephalosporin preparation providing good serum antistaphylococcal activity, and is preferred over the other cephalosporins for intramuscular use. Cephalosporins should be avoided in treating central nervous system staphylococcal infections unless intravenous therapy is supplemented with intrathecal cephaloridine (50 mg daily).*

For oral therapy of less serious infections, cloxacillin, dicloxacillin, and the more expensive cephalexin are suitable and equally efficacious when given properly. Oxacillin and nafcillin are not recommended for oral use because their absorption is too erratic.

The penicillinase-resistant penicillin analogues are adequate for the treatment of infections caused by more susceptible organisms such as penicillin-susceptible staphylococci, pneumococci, and group A beta streptococci when the dosages commonly recommended for staphylococcal disease are used. Consequently, it is *not* necessary to add penicillin G to the regimen when these organisms are suspected of playing a role in the illness. However, many persons prefer to use both penicillin G and methicillin or nafcillin initially and to switch to the more active drug when the nature of the etiologic agent becomes clear. If the organism is susceptible to it, penicillin is preferred because it is usually the most active drug as well as the most convenient and inexpensive one to administer. Penicillin V is better than penicillin G for oral therapy of staphylococcal infections because of its better absorption.

If the patient is allergic to penicillin, all the semisynthetic penicillins should be avoided. Vancomycin (0.5 gram intravenously every six hours), clindamycin, cephalothin, cefazolin, or cephalexin are suitable substitutes, but allergic cross-reactions between penicillin and the cephalosporins have been observed. Tetracyclines, including minocycline, and chloramphenicol are less frequently employed because of drug resistance, fear of toxicity, or lack of bactericidal action.

Because there are several suitable antimicrobial agents and many different clinical situations, only general guidelines for dosage and duration of treatment can be given here. A delay in initiating appropriate therapy for these necrotizing infections is often deleterious. These infections respond slowly and often require high doses of antimicrobial drugs for long periods. Relapses are common if therapy is terminated too early, especially if the lesion has not drained or foreign bodies are not removed. It is unusual for staphylococci to become resistant to penicillin derivatives *during therapy of closed infections*, such as endocarditis. Endocarditis and other serious infections are usually treated for at least four to six weeks. In serious infections, parenteral therapy is preferred because of the desirability of ensuring high concentrations of the antimi-

crobial in blood and tissues. In order to maintain adequate serum antistaphylococcal activity, the interval between intravenous doses of penicillins and cephalosporins should not exceed four hours in critically ill patients; also, the drugs should not be given rapidly as an intravenous bolus in order to avoid neurotoxic reactions and the rapid renal elimination of the drug.

Although methicillin-resistant strains of *S. aureus* have been encountered frequently in Europe, they are not common in the United States. Faulty testing disks occasionally are responsible for their spurious detection. Methicillin-resistant organisms usually show resistance to other semisynthetic penicillins and cephalosporins. Resistant strains grow better at 30° than at 37°C and in high concentrations of sodium chloride. They may be recognizable only after prolonged incubation (48 hours) in the presence of methicillin or oxacillin, presumably because the isolates contain only a small proportion of resistant clones. Most laboratories do not employ these special conditions routinely. Resistant organisms seem less virulent than methicillin-susceptible staphylococci, but they have occasionally been of clinical importance. Wide misuse of the new penicillins will probably result eventually in an increase in the prevalence of these strains. Vancomycin, gentamicin, clindamycin, or a combination of kanamycin or gentamicin with cephalothin or methicillin has been recommended for treatment of infections with these organisms.

Attention has been directed to the observation that certain drugs (including methicillin, oxacillin, gentamicin, vancomycin, or cephalosporins) that are ordinarily considered bactericidal may be primarily bacteriostatic for some staphylococci. In a few instances of serious infection with such isolates, responses to treatment have been slow or unsatisfactory. In the hope of increasing the rapidity and frequency of response, there has been a growing tendency to treat serious staphylococcal sepsis with a combination of bactericidal drugs such as a penicillin and gentamicin. In vitro studies have shown a more rapid killing effect with such combinations, and experimental infections in animal models also have been controlled more rapidly with them. However, there is no proof as yet that therapeutic results in humans are better with combination therapy.

Cephalosporins, vancomycin, gentamicin, and the macrolides are the most active antimicrobials against *S. epidermidis*. These coagulase-negative organisms are often surprisingly resistant to methicillin and the other semisynthetic penicillins.

133. CUTANEOUS STAPHYLOCOCCAL INFECTIONS

133.1. FURUNCLES

A furuncle (boil) is an acute circumscribed staphylococcal abscess of the skin and subcutaneous tissues. The term folliculitis refers to pustular furuncles involving hair follicles. Folliculitis is common in persons with

---

*Intrathecal use is not mentioned in the manufacturer's package insert approved by the U.S. Food and Drug Administration. Therefore its use in these circumstances must be considered investigational.

oily skin, poor hygiene, or occupational exposure to cutting oils. Deep folliculitis of the beard area is known as *sycosis barbae*. Patients with multiple or recurrent furuncles are said to have furunculosis; otherwise normal adults commonly experience an average of five or six furuncles per year. Furunculosis is an important problem in the newborn.

Furuncles are most common on the face, neck, buttocks, thighs, perineum, breasts, and axillary skin. Most furuncles begin at the base of a hair follicle and take three to five days to evolve. Itching or pain may be the earliest symptom. As the center of the lesion becomes necrotic and hypertonic, fluid is drawn into the furuncle and it swells, thinning the overlapping erythematous skin. Spontaneous drainage usually occurs soon thereafter. A hard core of necrotic debris is sometimes extruded from the center of the abscess. Relief of pain and onset of healing are usually rapid after drainage occurs, although erythema and swelling may persist for several weeks. A furuncle may regress without draining and form a "blind boil" that is indolent and prone to exacerbation following minor local trauma.

When the sebaceous glands of the face and upper back are extensively involved with furuncles, the condition is referred to as *pustular acne vulgaris. Juvenile acne* is not caused by staphylococci, but these organisms may secondarily infect acne lesions.

Furuncles involving blocked apocrine sweat glands (*hidradenitis suppurativa*) frequently become chronic. This troublesome infection tends to spread to other local sweat glands and hair follicles and leads to interconnecting draining sinuses and extensive scarring. Lesions occur in the axillary, perianal, and genital areas. Various organisms can be responsible. Hidradenitis is difficult to cure solely with antimicrobial therapy and drainage. Excision of the involved tissues and skin grafting are frequently necessary and usually successful.

Although systemic symptoms and bacteremia are unusual with an ordinary furuncle unless the lesion is squeezed or manipulated, asymptomatic bacteremia secondary to a furuncle is probably fairly common. Furuncles are believed to be important in the pathogenesis of endocarditis, osteomyelitis, pyarthrosis, and other metastatic infections developing after hematogenous dissemination. Septic thrombophlebitis resulting from local extension of infection is another serious complication of furuncles. Lesions in the middle third of the face are especially dangerous, because they may spread intracranially via emissary veins and cause cavernous sinus thrombophlebitis.

133.2. CARBUNCLES

A carbuncle is a large furuncle or an aggregate of interconnected furuncles. Carbuncles often drain through multiple skin openings. They represent an acute suppurative inflammation of subcutaneous tissues extending between hair follicles in clefts along fibrous and adipose tissues. They occur where the skin is especially thick and tough (such as the back of the neck). Carbuncles may attain the size of lemons, and can be associated with extreme pain, chills, fever, leukocytosis, malaise, prostration, and bacteremia. They are serious and sometimes fatal infections.

133.3. IMPETIGO

Impetigo is a superficial primary pyoderma caused by group A beta streptococci, *S. aureus,* or both (see Ch. 127.2). Most common in infants and children, it begins as macules and progresses to vesicles and bullae which rupture, releasing a cloudy yellow fluid that forms crusts and reveals a weeping denuded area. The lesions may become chronic and resemble fungal infections. They are superficial, are rarely larger than 2 cm, and spread by autoinoculation. Streptococci are usually responsible for impetigo, but there is good evidence that staphylococci of bacteriophage type 71 may be involved in some cases.

133.4. THE SCALDED SKIN SYNDROME

An association of bacteriophage group II staphylococci with exfoliative dermatitis has been recognized in three distinct but related clinical entities: (1) *Generalized exfoliative dermatitis (scalded skin syndrome, pemphigus neonatorum, Ritter's disease, staphylococcal toxic epidermal necrolysis)* is severe and characterized by generalized painful erythema, formation of large flaccid bullae, a positive Nikolsky sign (epidermis is detached easily by the examining finger), and shedding of the upper epidermis in large sheets. The focus of infection may be at a distant site. The disease is usually seen in newborns but has been recognized in adults, and is often confused with pemphigus. (2) *Bullous impetigo* is a localized form of the scalded skin syndrome in which the infection occurs at the site of the lesion. (3) *Staphylococcal scarlet fever* is a mild variant of the generalized scalded skin syndrome and is clinically similar to streptococcal scarlet fever. A localized infection is the usual focus.

These three clinical variants appear to represent the spectrum of a disease process with a common etiology — the epidermolytic exotoxin produced usually by group II staphylococci (especially types 3A, 3C, 55, and 71). Antibodies to the streptococcal erythrogenic toxin do not seem to be cross-reactive. The disease has been duplicated in an experimental model. The characteristic lesion consists of intraepidermal cleavage through desmosomes of the stratum granulosum. Other forms of toxic epidermal necrolysis can be distinguished easily because they show necrosis of the entire epidermis with a deeper cleavage plane near the dermoepidermal junction. Frozen sections of peeled skin or cytologic studies of cells from the denuded base of a lesion can yield a diagnosis rapidly.

133.5. TREATMENT OF CUTANEOUS INFECTIONS

Some authorities believe that furuncles and pustules can be aborted at early stages by the administration of an antimicrobial drug or by the local application of an antiseptic such as alcohol. Once drained, small lesions require no further therapy, but they should be kept covered with a dressing or zinc oxide ointment to prevent spread of organisms. More severe lesions require both local and systemic therapy. Rest, heat, and elevation of the affected site relieve pains and hasten resolution. Warm compresses hasten maturation of the lesion, but care should be taken to prevent maceration. Incision should be delayed until frank suppuration and fluctuance are detectable, as early incision is ineffective and may promote bacteremia.

Antimicrobials should be given for large furuncles, for those on the face or neck, or for those accompanied by lymphadenitis, fever, or other systemic reaction. They should also be given if the patient has diabetes, congenital or valvular heart disease, or another underlying disease predisposing to complications, or if surgical incision is to be performed. Oral therapy with penicillin, erythromycin, or clindamycin is usually satisfactory. Therapy should be continued until signs of active inflammation have disappeared; a week is usually sufficient. Gamma globulin, adrenal steroids, and vaccines are of no proved value.

Impetigo responds rapidly to treatment with appropriate antimicrobials given systemically; topical bacitracin ointment may be adequate in mild cases.

133.6. PREVENTION OF CUTANEOUS INFECTIONS

Furuncles are difficult to prevent because the resistance of the patient usually cannot be influenced and the organism is ubiquitous. However, measures that protect the skin and minimize contact with the organism may be worthwhile. Predisposing conditions should be treated or eliminated. Skin irritants and abrasive tight clothing should be avoided. The fingernails should be kept short, and frequent handwashing should be stressed. Draining lesions should be considered highly contaminated and kept covered. Daily bathing and shampooing with antiseptic soap may be useful. Very rarely it may be possible to treat carriers with antimicrobials for several weeks or months and to eliminate the organism and thus prevent recurrences. Antimicrobial ointments (gentamicin or neomycin-bacitracin) or 2 per cent hexachlorophene cream may be applied several times daily to susceptible areas or to the anterior nares to suppress the organism. A short course of treatment with both dicloxacillin and rifampin may eradicate the organism. It is sometimes possible to get rid of a troublesome organism by intentionally inducing nasal carriage with a relatively nonpathogenic species after the more virulent staphylococcal strain has been suppressed by drug therapy (bacterial interference). The 502A strain of *S. aureus* has been employed for this purpose in patients with recurrent furunculosis. Small numbers of organisms of the 502A strain have been used to intentionally colonize the umbilicus and nares of newborn infants in order to prevent acquisition of more dangerous strains. Outbreaks in nurseries have been terminated in this way. Infections have been caused in infants and adults by strain 502A, and its use is still experimental. Staphylococcus vaccines, toxoids, and bacteriophage lysates are of no proved value in prevention, and irradiation to produce atrophy of cutaneous glands is not recommended.

134. STAPHYLOCOCCAL PNEUMONIA

Staphylococci cause less than 5 per cent of all bacterial pneumonias, except during influenza epidemics, but the disease is especially important because of its high mortality rate (up to 50 per cent) (see Ch. 119 to 124).

In so-called *primary staphylococcal pneumonia*, the organisms gain access to the lung via the tracheobronchial tree. Primary staphylococcal pneumonia is most often seen in infants; in children with cystic fibrosis or measles; in adults with influenza; or in debilitated, hospitalized persons being treated with antimicrobials, steroids, cancer chemotherapy, or immunosuppressants.

The diagnosis of primary staphylococcal pneumonia in adults with serious underlying diseases is often difficult. High remittent fever, multiple chills, cyanosis, rapidly progressive dyspnea, chest pain, and the production of thick, creamy yellow, salmon-colored, or reddish-yellow sputum should lead to the suspicion of staphylococcal pneumonia. Peripheral vascular collapse and marked signs of toxicity should also cause one to suspect the diagnosis in patients with pulmonary filtrates. Staphylococcal pneumonia developing in association with influenza or an underlying debilitating illness characteristically begins with a sudden and marked worsening of the illness, accompanied by prostration, cyanosis, tachypnea, bloody or purulent sputum, and high fever. Fever, cough, sputum production, dyspnea, and chest pain may be minimal during early stages of staphylococcal pneumonia. In infants the sudden development of pneumothorax, pneumatoceles, or empyema is characteristic. Necrosis with formation of multiple abscesses is characteristic in adults, but pneumothorax can occur, particularly in patients treated with adrenal steroids.

Hematogenous or secondary staphylococcal pneumonia is seen most frequently in narcotic addicts with endocarditis and in others with bacteremia from a focus elsewhere. Secondary staphylococcal pneumonia is characterized by multiple peripheral infiltrates that resemble embolic lesions and progress to necrosis and abscess formation, with a high frequency of pleuritic pain and empyema. Pneumothorax may occur, characteristically in young children. The signs of septicemia frequently overshadow the pulmonary disease in these patients.

The physical findings in patients with staphylococcal pneumonia are highly variable. A toxic appearance and low-grade fever may be the only detectable manifestations, particularly when the pneumonia is early and in a central location or interstitial, which is common. Patchy pneumonia with multiple small abscesses is another common presentation, and can be detected by the presence of either coarse or fine rales. Dullness to percussion is not an early sign, and signs of frank consolidation are rarely found. Pleural effusion and empyema are frequent, but the fluid is commonly loculated in interlobar fissures and may not be readily detected or aspirated.

The leukocyte count is usually elevated to between 15,000 and 25,000 per cubic millimeter. A leukocyte count greater than 15,000 in an adult with influenza should raise the question of a secondary bacterial pneumonia. The Gram-stained smear of the sputum usually shows polymorphonuclear leukocytes and large numbers of clustered gram-positive cocci. When cocci are seen within leukocytes in sputum, staphylococcal pneumonia is the presumptive diagnosis. The blood culture is *not* often positive unless the pneumonia is secondary to staphylococcal bacteremia originating at some other site.

DIFFERENTIAL DIAGNOSIS. All other forms of pneumonia must be considered. The distinction from pneumonia caused by gram-negative organisms is especially important in patients developing pneumonia in the hospital. A carefully performed Gram stain of a good sample of sputum is the keystone of choosing initial therapy, and may be helpful in interpreting subsequent culture reports. Abscess formation, salmon-colored sputum, and an appropriate host for the development of staphylococcal pneumonia are helpful clues.

As drug-resistant staphylococci frequently colonize the respiratory tract soon after the administration of antimicrobial drugs, one should not diagnose staphylococcal pneumonia solely on the basis of a sputum culture revealing rare or moderate numbers of the organism in someone under treatment for other pulmonary infections.

PROGNOSIS. Even under the best of circumstances, the case fatality rate for pneumonia is 15 to 20 per cent. Higher fatality rates are seen in very young infants and in elderly or debilitated patients. As this pneumonia is characterized by necrosis of lung parenchyma, recovery is usually slow. Improvement following the initiation of therapy is often not evident for 48 to 72 hours, and the illness usually lasts three to four weeks. Convalescence may be prolonged when empyema is present. Bronchiectasis can be a consequence of staphylococcal pneumonia.

TREATMENT. Once the diagnosis is tentatively established, vigorous parenteral antimicrobial therapy should be initiated promptly. Methicillin, oxacillin, nafcillin, cephalothin, or cefazolin, in doses of at least 1 gram every four to six hours, are preferred and equally good. The organism should be considered resistant to penicillin and ampicillin until it is demonstrated to be susceptible. If the organism is susceptible, penicillin G (20 million units intravenously per day) is the drug of choice. If the patient is allergic to penicillin, vancomycin (0.5 gram intravenously every six to eight hours) or clindamycin (600 mg four times per day) may be used. Therapy should be continued for 10 to 14 days or more after the patient shows a definite clinical response. The clinical response is usually very gradual. When empyema is present, it may be helpful to administer antimicrobial drugs directly into the pleural cavity, and proteolytic enzymes may be instilled to help thin the exudate. Because the pus is often loculated or too thick for needle aspiration, surgical drainage of empyema with a chest tube is usually required. Oxygen, bronchodilators, expectorants, fluids, and other supportive measures are important.

135. STAPHYLOCOCCAL OSTEOMYELITIS

Staphylococcus aureus is the etiologic agent in the majority of instances of *primary or hematogenous osteomyelitis*. The disease is becoming uncommon and is readily cured if treated early with appropriate antimicrobials. Bacteremia occurring from a skin infection which may be no more serious than a furuncle is the usual inciting event. *Secondary staphylococcal osteomyelitis* is usually related to penetrating trauma, surgery, or a contiguous focus of infection. It is also seen in patients with diabetes mellitus or peripheral vascular disease following local cutaneous infections.

Hematogenous staphylococcal osteomyelitis is primarily a disease of children, adolescents, and intravenous drug abusers. It is more frequent in males. It usually begins in the metaphyseal area of the diaphysis near the epiphyseal plate, and is uncommon following epiphyseal closure. The metaphysis is a weak spot in growing bones. It has a terminal blood supply subject to bacterial embolization and thrombosis. The capillary and venous networks in this area are extensive, and minor injuries may result in hematomas that afford a nidus for bacteria. Furthermore, the capillaries in this area are deficient in phagocytic lining cells. The most common sites of involvement are the lower femur, upper tibia, ankle, wrist, or hip, but any metaphyseal area can be involved. The vertebrae are more commonly involved in adults, particularly narcotic addicts. As the infectious process develops in the metaphysis, the arterial blood supply is usually compromised, because it is terminal and encased in rigid bony canals. Thromboses and vascular insufficiency develop and lead to necrosis of bone. Early radiologic signs of osteomyelitis include decalcification or rarefaction of bone due to hyperemia and injury to osteoblasts, and periosteal elevation. If the infection is untreated, a sequestrum of necrotic bone will separate in six to eight weeks. Treatment with antimicrobial drugs has practically eliminated this result. In pyogenic osteomyelitis it is characteristic for the periosteum to react to the infection by forming a layer of reparative bone (osteosclerosis) called the involucrum. Reactive bone formation is much less common in tuberculous osteomyelitis, unless the process has been going on for more than six months.

The infection tends to spread along the diaphysis or outward to the subperiosteal space, where an abscess often forms, particularly in children. From there the infection may extend and involve nearby joints. This is seen in about 10 per cent of cases, and is more frequent when the hip or shoulder bones are infected. It is uncommon for the infection to enter the joint by crossing the epiphyseal plate barrier in children, but this is not unusual in adults. In addition, sterile joint effusions are not uncommon when there is an osteomyelitic focus nearby.

If not treated early or adequately, the infection tends to become chronic, with recurrent exacerbations, formation of draining sinuses, and extensive scarring eventually requiring surgical debridement and saucerization of bone. Amyloidosis occasionally develops after longstanding osteomyelitis.

Staphylococcal infections of vertebrae and intervertebral discs are especially frequent in intravenous drug abusers. They are also seen following pelvic and urinary tract infections, but other organisms are more frequent in these settings. The patients usually complain of back pain accentuated by straining or coughing, pain radiating down the leg, or abdominal pain. Paravertebral abscesses are a frequent complication. Narrowing of the disc space, erosion of the vertebral end-plates, and bridging of the disc space by new bone formation are important radiologic findings. The condition may be mistaken for tuberculous spondylitis, but osteophytic bridging or isolated involvement of the vertebral arches or processes is unusual in tuberculosis. Acute endocarditis is an occasional complication of staphylococcal vertebral osteomyelitis.

High fever, chills, throbbing bone pain, local tenderness, muscle spasms, splinting, or limping are the early manifestations. Redness, swelling, and warmth are seen later. Bacteremia is frequent in osteomyelitis, and the patient may appear delirious and critically ill. The systemic signs and symptoms may overshadow the local manifestations. Leukocytosis and anemia are common. Rarefaction of bone is the earliest radiologic sign, but may not appear until 10 to 14 days after onset. Periosteal reaction with new bone formation is seen after the disease has been present for at least a month. Bone scans using radioactive technetium, strontium, fluorine, or gallium can localize the lesion prior to x-ray changes. They are particularly useful in drug addicts who present with fever and vague complaints referable to the lower back.

Rheumatic fever, traumatic lesions, leukemia, scurvy, pyogenic arthritis, hemoglobinopathies, Ewing's tumor, and other neoplasms should be considered in the differential diagnosis of osteomyelitis.

TREATMENT. With appropriate treatment, death from acute osteomyelitis is rare, and progression to chronic osteomyelitis is not likely. Mixed infection with other organisms, such as *Pseudomonas,* is seen fairly often. Empirical treatment without the aid of exudate or aspirated or operative specimens for culture and Gram stain is hazardous and should be avoided. Since early treatment is important, therapy directed against staphylococci should be started as soon as cultures have been obtained when this organism appears likely. Parenteral bactericidal drugs should be given initially. One of the penicillins, cephalosporins, or clindamycin is recommended. Gentamicin is useful in addicts when *Pseudomonas* as well as *Staphylococcus* is suspected. Immobilization is important for relief of pain and for clinical improvement. Some evidence of a clinical response should be noted within four days. It may be necessary to aspirate a subperiosteal abscess, or to surgically drain it. Vigorous parenteral treatment should be continued for at least four weeks. Subsequent oral therapy is not needed in most cases. Radiologic signs of the infection may never become apparent if treatment is given early. Although small sequestra usually absorb spontaneously, larger pieces of dead bone require surgical removal, especially if there is a slow or incomplete clinical response. Operative removal of foreign bodies is frequently necessary to achieve a cure in secondary osteomyelitis.

With chronic osteomyelitis, antimicrobial therapy should be given, and sequestrectomy, saucerization of infected bone, and removal of sinus tracts should be performed. Only rarely will such patients respond to drug therapy alone. Closed irrigation with antimicrobial agents is occasionally a useful adjunct to surgery.

136. STAPHYLOCOCCAL BACTEREMIA AND ENDOCARDITIS

Bacteremia may occur with any localized staphylococcal infection, but is relatively uncommon with minor postoperative wound infections and pneumonia, unless of hematogenous origin. Carbuncles, skin infections, infected intravascular shunts, catheters, and other foreign bodies, endocarditis, and osteomyelitis are the most common foci causing bacteremia. Staphylococcal bacteremia is frequent in patients with marked granulocytopenia or serious chronic debilitating diseases. It is usually associated with hectic fever, repeated shaking chills, and marked systemic toxicity. Widespread metastatic abscesses may develop in kidneys, lungs, bone, skin, brain, meninges, myocardium, and other viscera.

Bacteremia with coagulase-negative staphylococci sometimes pursues an indolent course for many weeks with remarkably few clinical manifestations. Bloodstream infections with these organisms are usually seen following ventriculoatriostomy shunting or cardiac surgery with insertion of prostheses. A proliferative and membranous glomerulonephritis and the nephrotic syndrome may be seen as a result of chronic *S. epidermidis* bacteremia in patients with infected shunts, and prompt improvement in the renal disease may follow removal of the shunt.

Endocarditis frequently complicates staphylococcal bacteremia from another site. The disease is usually of the acute, malignant, or ulcerative type with *S. aureus,* but a form indistinguishable from that caused by *S. viridans* is occasionally seen, especially when *S. epidermidis* is responsible. The illness usually has an acute onset with shaking chills, high fever, changing cardiac murmurs, cutaneous pustules and petechiae, splinter hemorrhages, metastatic abscesses, hematuria, progressive anemia, and marked leukocytosis. Thrombocytopenia and disseminated intravascular coagulation may be seen. Normal heart valves may be destroyed in just a few days. Abscess of the myocardial valve ring occurs frequently and should be suspected when arrhythmias develop.

Acute staphylococcal endocarditis in heroin addicts is often characterized by involvement of the tricuspid valve. Multiple septic pulmonary emboli and infarcts with abscess formation and empyema are the usual presenting manifestations. The classic peripheral cutaneous manifestations of endocarditis, such as splenomegaly, Osler's nodes, and splinter hemorrhages, may be lacking in right-sided endocarditis, but blood cultures are usually positive. Antibodies to staphylococcal teichoic acid are usually present, and tests for rheumatoid factor are often positive. Cerebral manifestations relative to abscess formation, embolization, meningitis, and subarachnoid hemorrhage are frequent. Panophthalmitis is occasionally a complication. A murmur from the tricuspid lesion is usually present but is often overlooked initially until pulmonary emboli call attention to its presence. Other clues to tricuspid involvement are atrial or ventricular diastolic gallops along the lower left sternal border and the external jugular vein, or a short soft systolic murmur along the lower left sternal border which is increased with inspiration (Carvallo's sign), and with the patient standing.

Acute proliferative glomerulonephritis of the immune complex type may develop during the course of staphylococcal endocarditis and is sometimes confused with an allergic reaction to drugs used in treatment.

The distinction between endocarditis and bacteremia originating from another focus may be difficult. Continuous bacteremia suggests endocarditis or other intravascular focus; intermittent bacteremia suggests an extravascular focus.

TREATMENT. Even with appropriate therapy, staphylococcal bacteremia still has a mortality rate of about 40 per cent. Patients over the age of 50 or with underlying diseases have a mortality rate of more than 60 per cent. Parenteral therapy is necessary, and the regimen must be bactericidal. Therapy for endocarditis should be continued for four to eight weeks. A clear-cut clinical response to treatment may not be seen until the end of the first week. Surgical treatment of the focus of infection is always important to consider. When the site of infection is an intravascular foreign body, the infection is rarely cured until the foreign material is removed. However, infected cardiac prostheses are not usually replaced until at least one course of intensive treatment has proved unsuccessful, because 5 to 10 per cent of these infections may be cured with medical therapy alone. Early replacement of damaged valves may be necessary if there is severe or intractable heart failure.

If there is a removable focus of infection, no evidence of heart disease or metastatic infection, no serious derangement of host defenses, no teichoic acid antibodies, and a prompt clinical response, treatment of staphylococcal bacteremia can be terminated at the end of two or three weeks. In doubtful cases in which endocarditis remains a good possibility, therapy should be given for at least four weeks.

137. MISCELLANEOUS INFECTIONS

Staphlyococci are commonly found in *nose* or *throat* cultures, but they do not cause pharyngitis or tonsillitis, except in patients with agranulocytosis or leukemia. Their presence in healthy persons usually represents nothing more than colonization, and does not by itself justify treatment with antimicrobial therapy. Staphylococci have been recognized as a cause of cervical lymphadenitis in infants.

Staphylococcal pyarthrosis represents a diagnostic and therapeutic challenge in adults. It may occur following orthopedic surgery or in association with osteomyelitis. Infected skin ulcers or contaminated intra-articular injections or aspirations are often responsible. Rheumatoid factor may bind antistaphylococcal antibodies and contribute to lowered resistance. Joint infection should be suspected in all patients with rheumatoid arthritis who show an apparent exacerbation of joint disease with fever, pain, effusion, and leukocytosis. Chills favor the diagnosis of septic arthritis over rheumatoid disease. Joint fluid aspiration is essential for early diagnosis. Immobilization, repeated aspiration, surgical drainage when indicated, and appropriate antimicrobial drugs given for two to four weeks are the treatment.

Staphylococcal meningitis is uncommon. It is usually the result of penetrating trauma, local surgery, or bacterial endocarditis. Therapy must be vigorous. If the organism is known to be susceptible to penicillin G, 24 to 30 million units should be given daily by the intravenous route. If it is resistant to penicillin G or of unknown susceptibility, nafcillin (12 grams per day), oxacillin (12 grams per day) or methicillin (12 to 24 grams per day) may be used. Cephalosporins are not recommended unless they are supplemented with intrathecal cephaloridine* (50 mg daily).

---

*Intrathecal use is not mentioned in the manufacturer's package insert approved by the U.S. Food and Drug Administration. Therefore its use in these circumstances must be considered investigational.

Primary spinal epidural abscess is a neurosurgical emergency in which prompt recognition and treatment are indicated to prevent permanent spinal cord damage. It is sometimes seen in narcotic addicts in association with vertebral osteomyelitis. The process is usually acute, located dorsally in the lower thoracic or lumbar regions, and most often caused by staphylococci. Fever, localized spinal tenderness, and rigidity of the spine are followed by root pain, localized weakness, progressive paresthesias, sphincter changes, and evidence of spinal cord compression. The lumbar spinal fluid usually is under reduced pressure and shows pleocytosis, but may be normal. Myelography localizes the lesion but *is seldom necessary*. Antimicrobials are merely adjuncts to treatment, for total recovery depends on early diagnosis followed by *prompt* surgery, usually laminectomy and drainage (see Ch. 299).

Staphylococcal pericarditis usually occurs following bacteremia, often in association with osteomyelitis or endocarditis, with formation of focal myocardial abscesses and spread to the pericardium. The staphylococcus is the most frequent cause of purulent pericarditis. Treatment consists of antimicrobial therapy and pericardiocentesis, but if rapid improvement is not noted, open surgical drainage should be instituted.

Staphylococcal parotitis is seen in debilitated adults, especially those who become dehydrated and receive inadequate mouth care. Extensive edema, erythema, and tenderness are seen in the parotid area, and pus may be seen oozing from Stensen's duct. The patient usually has a high fever and disorientation. Shock and death are common. Irradiation of the gland may be a useful therapeutic adjunct, but appropriate antimicrobial therapy and supportive care are more important.

Staphylococcal (tropical) pyomyositis is a relatively common disease of indigenous residents of hot, humid tropical areas. It is occasionally seen in temperate climates, where it is usually misdiagnosed. Bacteremia resulting from minor superficial lesions is followed by abscess formation beneath the deep fascia of skeletal muscles, especially in the upper leg. Local trauma may be important in determining the site. There is diffuse swelling of the limb, but usually no fluctuance or regional adenopathy. The skin may become tense and cellulitic, but is often normal. Fever may be minimal during the first week of illness. The diagnosis is usually made at operation, when multiple abscesses are found to have coalesced and extended between muscle fasciculi and within fascial compartments. It is uncommon for osteomyelitis to coexist. Staphylococci of bacteriophage group II are usually implicated. Surgical drainage and antimicrobial drugs are efficacious.

138. STAPHYLOCOCCAL GASTROENTERITIS AND ENTEROCOLITIS

The enterotoxins produced by staphylococci are an important cause of acute epidemic gastroenteritis or food poisoning. The toxin is formed prior to ingestion of contaminated and usually improperly refrigerated or stored food (see Ch. 22.2).

Staphylococci are normal inhabitants of the intestines, although they are not usually detected unless selective media are used. They may increase during antimicrobial therapy, and patients may concomitantly experience mild diarrhea. Much more rarely the organisms cause acute necrotizing pseudomembranous enterocolitis. Most common following abdominal surgery, shock, or antimicrobial therapy, or in leukemia, this syndrome has a high mortality rate. Locally produced enterotoxin is thought to be responsible for the manifestations of the disease, but the pathogenesis is still uncertain. Staphylococci are implicated in only a relatively small proportion of total cases. Recent data suggest that toxigenic *Clostridium difficile* is the most important cause of the disease. Symptoms include abdominal pain, distention, ileus, fever, diarrhea, bloody stools, electrolyte depletion, dehydration, and shock. Gram stain of the stool reveals leukocytes and large numbers of cocci in sheets and clumps, and establishes the diagnosis of staphylococcal enterocolitis. Vancomycin given by *mouth* is useful in treatment. The usual dose is 0.5 gram every six hours. Parenteral therapy with another appropriate drug may also be given. Oral neomycin is no longer recommended, as many staphylococci in hospitals are resistant to it. Shock and electrolyte imbalance should be treated vigorously with appropriate fluids.

Andriole, V. T., and Lyons, R. W.: Coagulase-negative staphylococcus. Ann. N. Y. Acad. Sci., 174:533, 1970.

Banks, T., Fletcher, R., and Ali, N.: Infective endocarditis in heroin addicts. Am. J. Med., 55:444, 1973.

Barrett, F. F., McGehee, R. F., and Finland, M.: Methicillin-resistant *Staphylococcus aureus* at Boston City Hospital. N. Engl. J. Med., 279:441, 1968.

Boyle, J. D., Pearce, M. L., and Guze, L. B.: Purulent pericarditis: Review of literature and report of eleven cases. Medicine, 40:119, 1961.

Cluff, L. E., Reynolds, R. C., Page, D. L., and Breckenridge, J. C.: Staphylococcal bacteremia and altered host resistance. Ann. Intern. Med., 69:859, 1968.

Cohen, J. O. (ed.): The Staphylococci. New York, Wiley-Interscience, 1972.

Elek, S. D.: Staphylococcus Pyogenes. Edinburgh, E. and S. Livingstone, Ltd., 1959.

Elias, P. M., Fritsch, P. and Epstein, E. H.: Staphylococcal scalded skin syndrome. Arch. Dermatol., 113:207, 1977.

Fekety, F. R.: The epidemiology and prevention of staphylococcal infection. Medicine, 43:593, 1964.

Iannini, P. B., and Crossley, K.: Therapy of *Staphylococcus aureus* bacteremia associated with a removable focus of infection. Ann. Intern. Med., 84:558, 1976.

Karten, I.: Septic arthritis complicating rheumatoid arthritis. Ann. Intern. Med., 70:1147, 1969.

Keys, T. F., and Hewitt, W. L.: Endocarditis due to micrococci and *Staphylococcus epidermidis*. Arch. Intern. Med., 132:216, 1973.

Levin, M. J., Gardner, P., and Waldvogel, F. A.: "Tropical" pyomyositis. N. Engl. J. Med., 284:196, 1971.

Mailbach, H. I., Strauss, W. G., and Shinefield, H. R.: Bacterial interference: Relating to chronic furunculosis in man. Br. J. Dermatol., 81: Suppl. 1:69, 1969.

McCloskey, R. V.: Scarlet fever and necrotizing fasciitis caused by coagulase-positive hemolytic *Staphylococcus aureus*, phage type 85. Ann. Intern. Med., 78:85, 1973.

Pollack, N., Spinner, M., and Richman, R.: Hematogenous pyogenic spondylitis. N.Y. J. Med., 64:2870, 1964.

Rahal, J. J., MacMahon, H. E., and Weinstein, L.: Thrombocytopenia and symmetrical peripheral gangrene associated with staphylococcal and streptococcal bacteremia. Ann. Intern. Med., 69:35, 1968.

Shinefield, H. R., Ribble, J. C., Boris, M., and Eichenwald, H.: Bacterial interference: Its effect on nursery acquired infection with *Staphylococcus aureus*. Am. J. Dis. Child., 105:646, 1963.

Smith, D. T.: Autogenous vaccines in theory and practice. Arch. Intern. Med., 125:344, 1970.

Stickler, G. B., Shin, W. H., Burke, E. C., Holley, K. E., Miller, R. H., and Segar, W. H.: Diffuse glomerulonephritis associated with infected ventriculoatrial shunt. N. Engl. J. Med., 279:1077, 1968.

Tu, W. H., Shearn, M. A., and Lee, J. C.: Acute diffuse glomerulonephritis in acute staphylococcal endocarditis. Ann. Intern. Med., 71:335, 1969.

Tuazon, C. U., and Sheagren, J. N.: Teichoic acid antibodies in the diagnosis of serious infections with *Staphylococcus aureus*. Ann. Intern. Med., 84:543, 1976.

VanProhaska, J., Mock, F., Baker, W., and Collins, R.: Pseudomembranous (staphylococcal) enterocolitis. Surg. Gynecol. Obstet., 112:103, 1961.

Waldvogel, F. A., Medoff, G., and Swartz, M. N.: Osteomyelitis: A review of clinical features, therapeutic considerations and unusual aspects. N. Engl. J. Med., 282:198, 260, 316, 1970.

Watanakunakorn, C., Tan, J. S., and Phair, J. P.: Some salient features of *Staphylococcus aureus* endocarditis. Am. J. Med., 54:473, 1973.

Wentworth, B. B.: Bacteriophage typing of staphylococci. Bacteriol. Rev., 27:253, 1963.

Williams, D. N., Lung, M. E., and Blazevic, D. J.: Significance of urinary isolates of coagulase-negative Micrococcaceae. J. Clin. Microbiol., 3:556, 1976.

DISEASES CAUSED BY NEISSERIA

139. GONOCOCCAL DISEASE

Donald Kaye

DEFINITION. Gonorrhea is an infection of the mucous membrane of the urethra and genital tract caused by *Neisseria gonorrhoeae*. Involvement of the pharynx and anal canal is common. Infection is almost always the result of sexual contact. After invasion of mucosal sites, gonococci may spread and cause infections such as arthritis, tenosynovitis, perihepatitis, endocarditis, and meningitis.

ETIOLOGY. *N. gonorrhoeae* is a gram-negative coccus that was first described by Neisser in 1879 in exudates from patients with gonorrhea. In stained smears of exudates the organisms appear as diplococci with flattened or slightly concave adjacent sides and resemble a pair of kidney beans. A considerable portion of the organisms in exudates are within polymorphonuclear leukocytes. Gonococci grown in laboratory media assume an oval or spherical form, and single cocci and clumps of cocci may be found in addition to diplococci. *N. gonorrhoeae* can be distinguished from other *Neisseria* by its ability to ferment glucose but not maltose or sucrose.

Primary isolation of the gonococcus is difficult. The organism is fastidious in its growth requirements, and is susceptible to toxic substances that are present in many media. Blood, serum, ascitic fluid, or other agents must be added for enrichment, as growth will usually not occur on plain agar. Blood is commonly used, and the medium is heated (chocolate agar) to reduce the deleterious effect exerted by certain amino acids toxic to the gonococcus. Commercial media are available that satisfy the various growth requirements of *N. gonorrhoeae*. Most strains require an atmosphere of 2 to 10 per cent carbon dioxide. Overgrowth with other bacterica occasionally occurs in cultures of exudate from the urethra, vagina, and cervix and is frequent in cultures from the pharynx and anal canal if nonselective media are used.

Colonies of N. gonorrhoeae are round, gray-white, and translucent. On subculture on special media, four morphologically different colonial variants can be recognized: T_1, T_2, T_3, and T_4. T_1 and T_2 colonies are virulent, and the gonococci in the colonies are covered with tiny hairlike projections called pili. T_3 and T_4 colonies are much less virulent, and the gonococci do not have pili. Pili may be important for attachment of gonococci to mucosal cells in the pathogenesis of infection.

All Neisseria produce an oxidase that can be used for tentative identification of colonies of N. gonorrhoeae (colonies turn purple on exposure to 1 per cent paraaminodimethylaniline monohydrochloride). With cultures from the genital tract, the combination of colonies of typical morphology composed of gram-negative diplococci and a positive oxidase test is strong presumptive evidence of the presence of N. gonorrhoeae. However, confirmation by fermentation reactions or by fluorescent antibody techniques is necessary for definitive identification.

Thayer-Martin selective medium, containing a mixture of antimicrobials, permits growth of N. meningitidis and N. gonorrhoeae but inhibits growth of many other bacteria frequently found in specimens from urethra, cervix, vagina, anal canal, and pharynx.

EPIDEMIOLOGY. N. gonorrhoeae is a parasite of man; it does not cause disease in animals in nature. Gonorrhea is almost always acquired from sexual contact. Exceptions are gonococcal conjunctivitis (which occurs primarily in infants) and vulvovaginitis. Conjunctivitis results either from passage of the infant through an infected genital tract (ophthalmia neonatorum) or from contamination after birth. Vulvovaginitis is an infection of the genital tract of infants and preadolescent girls that results from direct contact with infected adults or, rarely, can be spread by contact with towels or linens contaminated with gonococci.

Repeated attacks of gonorrhea are common; therefore individual attacks seem to confer little or no immunity. However, individual variation in susceptibility to infection has been demonstrated after inoculation of N. gonorrhoeae into the urethras of male volunteers. Trauma to the urethra probably increases susceptibility to gonorrhea. After an episode of acute gonorrhea, N. gonorrhoeae may remain in the genital tract for months. Chronic asymptomatic carriers of the gonococcus are important in the epidemiology of gonorrhea because they are difficult to detect and therefore are rarely treated. It has been common knowledge that most women with gonorrhea are relatively asymptomatic, but only recently has it been reported that as many as 10 per cent of males with gonorrhea seen in a venereal disease clinic may be asymptomatic and that up to 40 per cent of asymptomatic male contacts of women with symptomatic gonorrhea have positive urethral cultures.

There has been an increase in the reported incidence of gonococcal infections in recent years. However, the true incidence and prevalence of gonorrhea are unknown because of problems in diagnosis, antimicrobial therapy by nonmedical persons, incomplete reporting by physicians, and the presence of many undetected asymptomatic carriers. It has been estimated that over 2 million new cases of gonorrhea occur annually in the United States. The magnitude of the problem of asymptomatic gonorrhea may be demonstrated by the fact that there is about a 5 per cent prevalence of asymptomatic gonorrhea in pregnant women.

Gonorrhea is a disease of the sexually active, and most cases occur in patients 15 to 24 years of age. Gonorrhea rates are higher among military personnel, migrant groups (such as itinerant laborers and seafarers), homosexuals, and prostitutes. In surveys 10 to 33 per cent of prostitutes have gonorrhea.

PATHOGENESIS AND PATHOLOGY. In males the urethra is attacked first, resulting in purulent urethritis and involvement of the urethral glands. Direct spread of infection may result in prostatitis, epididymitis, or seminal vesiculitis (all rare conditions currently). During stages of healing, stricture formation may occur. Gonococcal proctitis in the male is almost always the result of rectal intercourse.

In the female, urethritis is mild and transient. Bartholin's and Skene's glands and glands of the cervix may become infected with or without involvement of the urethra. Contiguous spread of infection can cause acute salpingitis, which is said to occur in about 10 per cent of women with genital tract gonorrhea. Proctitis may result from contiguous spread or rectal intercourse. Gonococcal salpingitis is usually bilateral and may cause pyosalpinx and formation of a tubo-ovarian abscess. The inflammation tends to heal with fibrosis and adhesions that may produce obstruction of the fallopian tubes and sterility. Subsequent secondary infections with other microorganisms (chronic pelvic inflammatory disease) may play a major role in the destructive process. Ascent of infection to the fallopian tubes often occurs during or just after menstruation. Although endometrial infection is usual when N. gonorrhoeae invades the fallopian tubes, it is not serious and tends to subside promptly. The vagina does not become infected in adults, probably because of the presence of squamous epithelium with many layers of cells and the lack of glands.

Conjunctivitis is the most common manifestation of gonococcal disease in infants. It is a destructive inflammation of the eye and before the use of antimicrobial agents frequently caused blindness. Between one year of age and pubescence, gonococcal infection is rare in males but causes vulvovaginitis in females. The increased susceptibility to gonococcal infection of the immature vaginal mucous membrane in contrast to the resistance of the mucosa of adults is probably explained by the thin mucous membrane present prior to adolescence.

Gonococcal infection of the pharynx is common and results from oral-genital contact. Gonococcal pharyngeal infection has been demonstrated in up to 20 per cent of homosexual men and 20 per cent of women practicing fellatio who had gonococcal infection at any site. In 3 to 8 per cent of these patients, only pharyngeal cultures are positive for gonococci.

N. gonorrhoeae have been found to produce a protease that cleaves human IgA. This destruction of IgA may play a role in the ability of gonococci to produce infection on mucosal surfaces.

Occasionally invasion of the blood occurs and N. gonorrhoeae may disseminate and produce infection at distant foci. Joints are the most frequent extragenital sites of localization, but tenosynovitis, endocarditis, meningitis, skin lesions, and infection at other foci may also occur.

Dissemination of gonoccocal infection is about twice

as common in women as in men and is probably more common in homosexual males than in heterosexual males. This is probably explained by the fact that men with gonococcal urethritis are usually symptomatic (90 to 95 per cent) and therefore are treated promptly, greatly decreasing the chances of dissemination of infection. In contrast, women with gonorrhea and males with gonococcal proctitis or pharyngitis (almost always homosexuals) are usually asymptomatic and are therefore unlikely to be treated. There is also a disproportionately high incidence of men with asymptomatic urethral gonorrhea among males with disseminated gonococcal infection. The source for dissemination may be the genital tract, rectum, or pharynx. It has been estimated that dissemination of gonococcal infection occurs in up to 3 per cent of women with gonorrhea and is most prone to occur during pregnancy or during or just after menstruation. Strains of *N. gonorrhoeae* that disseminate have usually been found to be highly susceptible to penicillin G and to require arginine, hypoxanthine, and uracil for growth.

CLINICAL MANIFESTATIONS. **Gonorrhea in the Male.** The incubation period of gonococcal urethritis in the male is usually two to eight days. There is sudden onset of dysuria, urgency, and frequency associated with mucoid urethral discharge that rapidly becomes purulent and profuse. Gonococcal urethritis usually does not cause fever, but prostatitis, seminal vesiculitis, or epididymitis is frequently associated with fever. Acute urinary retention may result from involvement of the prostate. Rectal examination reveals tenderness of the affected organ in the presence of prostatitis or seminal vesiculitis. Epididymitis causes severe pain and tenderness of the epididymis.

Untreated gonorrhea subsides over a period of weeks, but a small amount of mucoid discharge from the urethra may continue to be found each morning for months. Urethral stricture is a common sequela of untreated urethritis, especially after recurrent attacks of gonorrhea. Epididymitis can result in sterility.

About 5 to 10 per cent of men who develop urethral infection remain asymptomatic, do not seek therapy, and become an important vector for spread of infection.

Gonorrhea in the Female. In females the disease may begin with dysuria, urgency, and frequency after an incubation period of two to eight days. However, the urethritis is frequently of short duration and often is mild or completely asymptomatic. Cervicitis gives rise to a mucopurulent discharge that varies from scant to profuse. Involvement of Skene's ducts or Bartholin's glands is common, and abscess formation may occur. Gonococci can be isolated from the anal canal in 20 to 50 per cent of women with gonorrhea, and occasionally can produce symptomatic proctitis. In 5 per cent of women with gonococcal infection only the anorectal culture contains gonoccoi. The duration of symptoms from an untreated infection that remains localized in the lower genital tract is usually no longer than a month or two. However, the patient may remain a carrier of the disease for many months.

Salpingitis is manifested by acute onset of fever and lower abdominal pain. Physical examination usually reveals lower abdominal tenderness, pain on movement of the cervix, and tenderness of the adnexa (with or without palpable masses). Subsequently pelvic inflammatory disease with pelvic pain and fever may recur and is usually caused by bacteria other than gonococci. Sterility is common.

Extragenital Gonococcal Infection. PROCTITIS. Gonococcal proctitis is usually asymptomatic but may be manifested by anal discharge, burning rectal pain, blood and pus in the stools, and pain on defecation.

PHARYNGITIS. Gonococcal infection in the oropharynx can probably cause symptomatic pharyngitis, tonsillitis, and gingivitis but is usually asymptomatic.

ARTHRITIS. Arthritis is the most common form of clinically recognized disseminated gonococcal infection; it usually occurs within one to three weeks after initial infection in the genital tract or may follow pharyngeal or rectal infection. Onset may be gradual with migratory polyarthalgias leading to frank arthritis in one or more joints, or it may be sudden with hot, swollen, and extremely painful joints. Fever and leukocytosis are usually present. Over 75 per cent of patients have polyarthritis. The joints that are most commonly involved are the knees, ankles, and wrists, but any joint may be involved, including the spine and sternoclavicular and temporomandibular joints. *Tenosynovitis,* which is rarely observed in other types of pyogenic arthritis, is common in gonococcal arthritis and most often occurs about the wrists and ankles. The skin lesions associated with gonococcal bacteremia are also frequently present.

N. gonorrhoeae can be isolated from joint fluid in only 25 to 50 per cent of cases. The fluid ranges from serous to frankly purulent, has the protein content of an exudate, and usually contains increased numbers of leukocytes that are mainly polymorphonuclear. Muscle wasting about the joint and permanent deformity may result. Some authorities have described two types of arthritis produced by the gonococcus: (1) polyarticular arthritis, usually with no or small effusions that tend to be sterile, often associated with bacteremia and skin lesions, and (2) frank pyogenic arthritis (often involving one joint from which gonococci can frequently be isolated) without bacteremia or skin lesions. The first type has been attributed by some to hypersensitivity, but it seems more likely that it represents the initial or bacteremic phase during which organisms localize in joints. Frank pyogenic arthritis may occur after a clinically apparent or inapparent bacteremic phase. Sterility of the joint fluid in patients during the bacteremic phase may be due to taking cultures early in disease, before microorganisms in the joint have sufficient time to proliferate.

GONOCOCCAL BACTEREMIA. Gonococcal bacteremia can produce a syndrome with recurrent episodes of fever, skin lesions, tenosynovitis, arthralgia or arthritis, mild to severe constitutional symptoms, and intermittently positive blood cultures. This syndrome occurs with infection in the genital tract, anal canal or pharynx, and, if untreated, can recur over a period of months or even years. The rash usually appears during the first day of symptoms and may recur with each episode of fever. The rash is found on the distal part of the extremities and consists of scanty pin-point erythematous macules that rapidly become maculopapular, vesiculopustular, and frequently hemorrhagic. Bullae can form. The mature lesion is elevated, has a dirty gray necrotic center, and is surrounded by erythema. It heals in three to four days. Gram-negative cocci can often be seen in stains of fluid from the lesions, but cultures for *N. gonorrhoeae* are usually negative. Immunofluorescent studies on the exudate from the pustules demonstrate *N. gonorrhoeae* in a high percentage of patients. Identical skin lesions may be seen in patients with meningococcemia, which can present an indistinguishable clinical sydrome.

GONOCOCCAL ENDOCARDITIS. Gonococcal endocarditis is extremely rare at present. In most patients, previously normal valves are attacked. The valves on the left side of the heart are involved most often, but valves on the right side are affected with a higher frequency than with endocarditis caused by other bacteria. A double daily temperature elevation (double quotidian) is common in patients with gonococcal endocarditis.

PERIHEPATITIS (FITZ-HUGH–CURTIS SYNDROME). Perihepatitis is a rare complication in women with gonococcal pelvic inflammatory disease and results from direct spread of gonococci from the pelvis to the upper abdomen. It is manifested by fever, upper quadrant pain (usually right upper quadrant), tenderness and spasm of the abdominal wall, and occasionally a friction rub over the liver. During the acute stage the gallbladder temporarily may not be visualized on cholecystography; this can lead to an erroneous diagnosis of cholecystitis. The patient often has a recent history of pelvic pain or vaginal discharge, and physical examination may reveal evidence of pelvic inflammatory disease. *N. gonorrhoeae* can frequently be demonstrated in the cervical or vaginal discharge.

The symptoms respond to antimicrobial therapy. The untreated disease subsides after one to four weeks of fever and abdominal pain, leaving "violin-string" adhesions between the anterior surface of the liver and the anterior abdominal wall. This syndrome has been reported in a male, probably caused by lymphatic or hematogenous dissemination.

DIAGNOSIS. In the male the combination of urethritis and the presence of intracellular gram-negative diplococci in smears of exudate from the urethra is strong presumptive evidence of gonorrhea. Confirmation is obtained by culture or, if available, fluorescent antibody studies. Cultures of the anal canal should be obtained in homosexual males. Urethral cultures in asymptomatic males are made by inserting a wire tipped with a calcium alginate swab into the urethra.

For routine screening, cervical cultures will detect the vast majority of females with asymptomatic gonorrhea. Gonorrhea should be suspected in any female contact of an infected male. Similarly the asymptomatic carrier state should be suspected in asymptomatic male contacts of symptomatic females or asymptomatic females detected by routine cultures. In the female with suspected gonorrhea, cultures of exudate from the cervix and anal canal should be obtained in addition to urethral cultures.

Pharyngeal cultures for *N. gonorrhoeae* should be obtained from homosexual males and females practicing fellatio. In all patients with suspected disseminated gonococcal infections, cultures of the pharynx and anal canal should be obtained in addition to genital tract cultures.

Gonococci die within hours if allowed to dry. Therefore exudates should be inoculated as soon as possible on Thayer-Martin medium or on a suitable transport medium for *N. gonorrhoeae* such as Transgrow, which is available commercially.

With use of fluorescent antibody it is frequently possible to make a definite identification of *N. gonorrhoeae* in exudate within one hour of obtaining a specimen.

A substantial portion of the cases of urethritis in men in the United States today are nongonococcal. A substantial portion of these are caused by *Chlamydia trachomatis*. Although the evidence is not conclusive, many of the remaining cases may be due to *Ureaplasma urealyticum*. *Trichomonas vaginalis* can also cause

urethritis. The urethral discharge in gonorrhea is usually profuse and yellow, whereas in nongonococcal urethritis the discharge is usually white and scanty. However, Gram stain and culture are necessary for definitive differentiation. The chlamydial form of urethritis is discussed in Ch. 116.

Salpingitis. Acute salpingitis must be differentiated from appendicitis and tubal pregnancy. The presence of bilateral tenderness in the adnexa with or without masses, a history of recent sexual intercourse followed by urethritis or vaginal discharge, and demonstration of gonococci in the cervical exudate are strongly suggestive of gonococcal salpingitis. When it is impossible to differentiate acute salpingitis from appendicitis or tubal pregnancy, the diagnosis must be established at laparoscopy or laparotomy.

Bacteria indigenous to the female genital tract (e.g., anaerobic gram-positive cocci) are also responsible for cases of acute salpingitis and for continuing infection following an episode of gonococcal salpingitis (chronic pelvic inflammatory disease). The risk of pelvic inflammatory disease seems to be increased by intrauterine devices.

Arthritis; Blood-Borne Lesions. The diagnosis of gonococcal arthritis or bacteremia with skin lesions should be suspected in a patient with the appropriate clinical syndrome, especially if there is a recent history of urethritis or vaginal discharge. Tenosynovitis is suggestive of disseminated gonococcal infection. Isolation of *N. gonorrhoeae* from the genital tract, rectum, or pharynx is supportive evidence, and demonstration of gonococci in skin lesions, blood, or joint fluid is confirmatory. The serum complement-fixation test for gonococci may be of aid in suggesting gonococcal arthritis, especially if titers are rising. However, this test is not generally available. Other serologic tests which look promising are currently under investigation.

When stains and cultures of joint fluid are negative for gonococci (50 to 75 per cent of cases), it is frequently difficult to differentiate gonococcal arthritis from Reiter's syndrome (nonbacterial urethritis, conjuctivitis, and arthritis) (see Ch. 58.4). The problem in differential diagnosis is compounded by the fact that patients with Reiter's syndrome may have concomitant gonococcal urethritis. Urethritis and arthritis in a female suggest gonococcal arthritis, because this disease is more common in females, whereas Reiter's syndrome is rare in females. The presence of tenosynovitis and response to antimicrobial therapy strongly imply gonococcal arthritis. Patients with Reiter's syndrome frequently have prolonged courses with recurrences, do not respond to antimicrobial therapy, and develop keratodermia blennorrhagica (a symmetrical eruption with a predilection for the soles, palms, and genitals).

Gonococcal arthritis can often be differentiated from acute rheumatic fever, rheumatoid arthritis, and gout by the absence of carditis, lack of rheumatoid factor in serum, and failure to respond to colchicine, respectively.

When *N. gonorrhoeae* cannot be isolated from the joint, the response to penicillin therapy is often the strongest confirmatory evidence of gonococcal arthritis.

TREATMENT AND PROGNOSIS. Prior to 1954, all gonococci were highly susceptible to penicillin, and a single injection of 300,000 units of penicillin cured almost all cases of gonorrhea. Subsequently, gonococcal strains of increased resistance to penicillin (requiring up to 2.0 μg per milliliter for inhibition) have constituted as much as 50 per cent or more of all isolates. Concomitantly there has been a striking increase in the frequency of failure of therapy with 600,000 to 2,400,000 units of penicillin, requiring larger doses for cure.

N. gonorrhoeae have also been becoming more resistant to tetracycline. The same strains of N. gonorrhoeae that are relatively resistant to penicillin also tend to have increased resistance to tetracycline and ampicillin but not to spectinomycin.

In 1976, for the first time, strains of gonococci were isolated that produced penicillinase and were therefore highly resistant to penicillin in vitro and against which penicillin was totally ineffective clinically. These gonococci also tend to be relatively resistant to tetracycline. Many of these strains seem to have originated in Southeast Asia, where they are widely disseminated. Cases have been reported from various areas (Australia, Belgium, Canada, Denmark, Hong Kong, Japan, Korea, the Netherlands, New Zealand, Norway, the Philippines, Singapore, Sweden, Switzerland, and Great Britain) and from many states within the United States. Because these strains are not yet widely disseminated within the United States, the recommendations for initial treatment of gonorrhea assume that the infecting organism is not a penicillinase producer. However, if the patient or contact has had any relationship with Southeast Asia, the infecting organism is assumed to be a penicillinase producer.

The recommendations of the Venereal Diseases Branch of the Center for Disease Control for treatment of uncomplicated gonorrhea (urethral, cervical, pharyngeal, or anal canal) or *for patients with known exposure* to gonorrhea are as follows: The regimen of choice is aqueous procaine penicillin (4.8 million units) administered intramuscularly at one visit (two sites of injection), together with 1 gram of oral probenecid just before the penicillin. An alternative regimen is 3.5 grams of oral ampicillin simultaneously with 1 gram of probenecid. When penicillin or ampicillin is contraindicated, spectinomycin, 2 grams in one intramuscular injection, or tetracycline hydrochloride orally, 1.5 grams initially, followed by 0.5 gram four times a day for four days (total 9.5 grams), can be used. If the infection is caused by a strain suspected to be a penicillinase producer, initial treatment should be with spectinomycin. However, spectinomycin should not be used indiscriminately as rare isolates of gonococci are resistant to spectinomycin and widespread use of the drug may encourage spread of these strains.

If a penicillin cannot be used in a pregnant patient because of hypersensitivity, since tetracycline is contraindicated, one of the following regimens is suggested: erythromycin, 1.5 grams orally, followed by 500 mg four times daily for a total of 9.5 grams; cefazolin, 2 grams intramuscularly, together with 1.0 gram of probenecid orally; or spectinomycin, 2 grams intramuscularly. Each of these regimens has problems: (1) the efficacy of the erythromycin regimen has not been established; (2) cefazolin should not be used in a patient with a history of anaphylaxis to pencillin because of the danger of cross-reactions; and (3) the safety of spectinomycin for the fetus has not been established.

Spectinomycin and ampicillin do not seem to be effective in eliminating N. gonorrhoeae from the pharynx. With this exception, the cure rates with these regimens in the United States before the introduction of penicillinase-producing gonococci were 97 per cent for procaine penicillin, 93 per cent for ampicillin, 96 per cent for tetracycline, and 95 per cent for spectinomycin. Aqueous procaine penicillin and spectinomycin have the important advantage of one-visit parenteral therapy which guarantees absorption of the total course of treatment. A major advantage of the procaine penicillin regimen (although clearly more painful) is that it will cure incubating syphilis. A disadvantage of the penicillin regimen in addition to the possibility of hypersensitivity is the possibility of neurotoxicity from the procaine (procaine reaction). The advantage of the tetracycline regimen is that it will usually prevent postgonococcal urethritis in males (see below).

Urethritis should subside within two to three days after therapy. A watery urethral discharge may persist in males for weeks despite elimination of gonococci. This is frequently due to so-called postgonococcal urethritis, which is actually nongonococcal urethritis (e.g., chlamydial) acquired at the same time as the gonorrhea. Postgonococcal urethritis can usually be prevented by use of tetracycline for therapy of gonorrhea. If severe enough to require therapy, postgonococcal urethritis will usually respond to 500 mg of tetracycline four times a day for seven days; the sexual partner should be treated simultaneously to avoid reinfection.

Relapse of gonorrhea occurs most commonly during the first week after treatment. Therefore to evaluate cure, a culture should be obtained seven days after completion of therapy. In homosexual males and in females, anorectal cultures should be obtained as well as cervical cultures. If relapse occurs (and relapse is often difficult to differentiate from reinfection), the patient should be retreated with spectinomycin.

Causes of apparent failure of therapy, other than infection with gonococci resistant to penicillin, are failure to distinguish between relapse and reinfection, failure to identify nongonococcal urethritis, and possibly the presence of other penicillinase-producing bacteria at the site of infection.

Patients with gonococcal prostatitis, seminal vesiculitis, epididymitis, salpingitis, or perihepatitis should be hospitalized and treated with 20 million units of aqueous penicillin G intravenously each day. Following clear-cut improvement, therapy can be changed to 0.5 gram of ampicillin orally four times a day to complete ten days of treatment. Patients who are allergic to penicillin or who are treated as outpatients can be given 1.5 grams of tetracycline orally, followed by 0.5 gram four times a day for ten days. Outpatients can also be treated with the procaine penicillin plus probenecid or ampicillin plus probenecid regimens for uncomplicated gonorrhea, followed by 0.5 gram of ampicillin orally four times a day for ten days. Because of the possibility of polymicrobial infection in pelvic inflammatory disease, aminoglycosides (for enteric gram-negative bacilli), often along with clindamycin or chloramphenicol (for *B. fragilis*), are frequently added to the regimen in the severely ill patient with salpingitis.

Recent evidence indicates that gonococci that are relatively resistant to penicillin are less likely to cause bacteremia and disseminated infection, i.e., are less pathogenic. Consequently, in the treatment of disseminated infection, after several days of intravenous penicillin therapy the course can be completed with oral ampicillin. Patients with gonococcal arthritis or bacteremia with skin lesions (arthritis-dermatitis syndrome) should be treated with aqueous penicillin G, 10 million units intravenously each day for three days or until there is clear-cut improvement. Therapy can then be changed to oral ampicillin, 0.5 gram four times a day, to complete at least seven days of therapy. Other effective regimens are ampicillin, 3.5 grams orally, plus 1.0 gram probenecid, followed by 0.5 gram of ampicillin four times a day, or tetracycline, 1.5 gram orally, followed by 0.5 gram four times a day for at least seven days. In the penicillin-allergic pregnant patient (in whom tetracycline is contraindicated) erythromycin, 500 mg intravenously every six hours for at least three days, can be used.

There has been little experience with treatment of salpingitis or disseminated gonococcal infection caused by penicillinase-producing gonococci. Although not approved for repeated doses, spectinomycin intramuscularly in a dose of 2 grams every six to twelve hours for seven to ten days would probably be the most effective therapy. Other regimens that probably would be effective are cefazolin in doses of 2 grams every six hours intramuscularly or intravenously or trimethoprim-sulfamethoxazole in a dose of about 3200 mg of sulfamethoxazole and 640 mg of trimethoprim daily orally.

Response of gonococcal infections to therapy usually occurs within two to three days. However, arthritis frequently responds more slowly, and it may take seven to ten days for the patient to become afebrile.

In acute gonococcal disease in the genital tract, surgery is indicated only for drainage of abscesses. However, in the chronic state in some female patients it may become necessary to remove involved pelvic organs. In gonococcal arthritis, pus should be aspirated by needle when possible. With the exception of the hip, open drainage of the joint is rarely necessary. Injection of penicillin into the joint is not indicated. Physiotherapy should be started during the period of convalescence to promote return of function of the joint.

For gonococcal endocarditis or meningitis, 20 million units of aqueous penicillin G should be administered intravenously each day for four weeks in the case of endocarditis and for two weeks for meningitis. Chloramphenicol would probably be the agent of choice in meningitis caused by penicillinase-producing gonococci; in endocarditis, drug susceptibility tests would be necessary to select effective bactericidal therapy.

About 3 per cent of patients with gonorrhea may be in the incubation period of syphilis. The doses of procaine penicillin recommended for therapy of uncomplicated gonorrhea will cure incubating syphilis but will not cure established syphilis. Therefore serologic tests for syphilis should be performed prior to initiation of therapy in all patients treated for gonococcal infections. If the serologic test is positive, therapy for syphilis must be initiated. If the serologic test is negative, no follow-up tests are required if procaine penicillin is used to treat the gonorrhea. Ampicillin, spectinomycin, and tetracycline in the doses recommended for gonor-

rhea have not been shown to abort incubating syphilis. Therefore serologic tests for syphilis should be obtained three months after therapy for gonorrhea with these regimens.

PREVENTION. Use of a condom provides a high degree of protection for the uninfected partner. Past experience has indicated that prophylactic use of oral penicillin in a dose of 250,000 units within two to three hours after exposure markedly decreases the incidence of infection. *Sexual partners of patients with gonorrhea should be identified and treated as quickly as possible to prevent further spread of disease.*

The instillation of 1 per cent silver nitrate (Credé method) or an antimicrobial drug into the eyes of the newborn has largely eradicated gonococcal ophthalmia neonatorum.

Barr, J., and Danielsson, D.: Septic gonococcal dermatitis. Br. Med. J., 1:482, 1971.

Blankenship, R. M., Holmes, R. K., and Sanford, S. P.: Treatment of disseminated gonococcal infection. N. Engl. J. Med., 290:267, 1974.

Danielsson, D., Juhlin, L., and Mardh, P.: Genital Infections and Their Complications. Uppsala, Almqvist and Wiksell International, 1975.

Eschenbach, D. A., Buchanan, T. M., Pollock, H. M., Forsyth, P. S., Alexander, E. R., Lin., J., Wang, S., Wentworth, B. B., McCormack, W. M., and Holmes, K. K.: Polymicrobial etiology of acute pelvic inflammatory disease. N. Engl. J. Med., 293:166, 1975.

Handsfield, H. H., Lipman, T. O., Harnisch, J. P., Tronca, E., and Holmes, K. K.: Asymptomatic gonorrhea in men: Diagnosis, natural course, prevalence and significance. N. Engl. J. Med., 290:117, 1974.

Handsfield, H. H., Wiesner, P. J., and Holmes, K. K.: Treatment of the gonococcal arthritis-dermatitis syndrome. Ann. Intern. Med., 84:661, 1976.

Jaffe, H. W., Biddle, J. W., Thornsberry, C., Johnson, R. E., Kaufman, R. E., Reynolds, G. H., Wiesner, P. J., and The Cooperative Study Group: National gonorrhea therapy monitoring study: In vitro antibiotic susceptibility and its correlation with treatment results. N. Engl. J. Med., 294:5, 1976.

Kaufman, R. E., Johnson, R. E., Jaffe, H. W., Thornsberry, C., Reynolds, G. H., Wiesner, P. J., and The Cooperative Study Group: National gonorrhea therapy monitoring study: Treatment results. N. Engl. J. Med., 294:1, 1976.

McCormack, W. M., and Finland, M.: Spectinomycin. Ann. Intern. Med., 84:712, 1976.

Oriel, J. D., Reeve, P., Thomas, B. J., and Nicol, C. S.: Infection with *Chlamydia* group A in men with urethritis due to *Neisseria gonorrhoeae.* J. Infect. Dis., 131:376, 1975.

Penicillin-resistant gonorrhea: New strain spreading worldwide. Science, 194:1395, 1976.

Recommended treatment schedules for gonorrhea — 1974. Arch. Intern. Med., 135:615, 1975

Vickers, F. N., and Maloney, P. J.: Gonococcal perihepatitis. Report of three cases with comments on diagnosis and treatment. Arch. Intern. Med., 114:120, 1964.

Wiesner, P. J.: Gonococcal pharyngeal infection. Clin. Obstet. Gynecol., 18:121, 1975.

MENINGOCOCCAL DISEASE

See Ch. 141.

BACTERIAL MENINGITIS

140. BACTERIAL MENINGITIS

Morton N. Swartz

Meningitis is an inflammation of the arachnoid, the pia mater, and the intervening cerebrospinal fluid. The inflammatory process extends throughout the subarachnoid space about the brain and spinal cord, and regularly involves the ventricles. Pyogenic meningitis, considered in this chapter, is usually an acute infection due to bacteria which evoke a polymorphonuclear response in the cerebrospinal fluid (CSF). One of its major forms, that caused by meningococci, is considered in Ch. 141; less acute forms of bacterial meningitis, characterized by a mononuclear cell response in the CSF, are discussed in Ch. 168.8 and 301.

ETIOLOGY AND INCIDENCE. *Streptococcus pneumoniae, Neisseria meningitidis,* and *Hemophilus influenzae* type b are the three most common causes of pyogenic meningitis, accounting for approximately 70 per cent of cases. The relative frequencies with which the different bacterial species cause meningitis are age related (see accompanying table). In the newborn, gram-negative bacilli (most frequently *E. coli* strains containing K1 capsular antigen, but also other enteric bacilli and *Pseudomonas*) and group B streptococci are the principal causes. Beyond the first month of life and extending through childhood, *H. influenzae* and *N. meningitidis* are the most frequent causes of bacterial meningitis. In adults *S. pneumoniae* and *N. meningitidis* are responsible for most cases. Meningococcal meningitis is the only type which occurs in outbreaks; its relative frequency among the meningitides will depend on whether statistics have been gathered during an epidemic period. In about 10 per cent of patients with pyogenic meningitis the bacterial cause cannot be defined. Simultaneous mixed meningitis is rare, occurring in the setting of neonatal meningitis, penetrating head injury, or intraventricular rupture of a cerebral abscess; the isolation of anaerobes should strongly suggest the last of these.

CLINICAL SETTINGS. The clinical setting in which meningitis develops may provide a clue as to the specific bacterial cause. Meningococcal disease, including meningitis, may occur sporadically and in cyclic outbreaks; military recruits are particularly susceptible, but large urban outbreaks also occur, as in Brazil in 1971 (see Ch. 141).

Certain predisposing factors are frequently associated with the development of *pneumococcal meningitis. Acute otitis media* and *mastoiditis* occur in about 30 per cent of patients. *Pneumonia* is present in about 25 per cent of patients with pneumococcal meningitis, a much higher frequency than in meningitis caused by *H. influenzae* or *N. meningitidis. Acute pneumococcal sinusitis* is occasionally the initial focus from which infection spreads to the meninges. A significant head injury (recent or remote) has occurred in about 10 per cent of patients with pneumococcal meningitis. CSF rhinorrhea (usually caused by a defect or fracture in the cribriform plate) is present in about 5 per cent of patients with pneumococcal meningitis. Among patients with recurrent bacterial meningitis, a pneumococcal cause is found about ten times as frequently as any other. Meningitis occurring in young children with sickle cell anemia is most likely to be due to *S. pneumoniae.* A variety of defects in host defenses (primary or acquired immunoglobulin deficiencies, the asplenic state) may predispose to pneumococcal disease, particularly meningitis. Alcoholism is an underlying problem in 10 to 25 per cent of adults with pneumococcal meningitis in urban hospitals.

S. aureus meningitis is seen most commonly as a complication of a neurosurgical procedure, following penetrating skull trauma, or secondary to staphylococcal bacteremia and endocarditis. Meningitis caused by *gram-negative bacilli* is usually a nosocomial infection, occurring principally in neonatal and neurosurgical patients. Among the latter, *Klebsiella, Enterobacter,* and *Pseudomonas aeruginosa* have been the organisms most frequently involved. *Bacteremic Klebsiella meningitis* is sometimes seen in patients with diabetes mellitus. The most frequent causes of bacterial meningitis in patients with neoplastic disease are gram-negative bacilli, *Listeria monocytogenes, S. pneumoniae,* and *S. aureus.* Meningitis caused by *group A streptococci* is uncommon, but occasionally occurs following acute otitis media, mastoiditis, or sinusitis. *Clostridium perfringens* is a rare cause of meningitis usually secondary to a penetrating injury.

The age-related incidence (children under five years) of *H. influenzae* type b meningitis is so striking that the occurrence of this disease in an adult should raise the question of the presence of an underlying anatomic or immunologic defect, circumventing the usual barrier interposed by serum bactericidal mechanisms.

PATHOLOGY. The purulent exudate is distributed widely in the subarachnoid space, most abundant in the basal cisterns and about the cerebellum initially, but also extending into the sulci over the cerebrum. The exudate in pneumococcal meningitis tends to be more evident over the convexities of the brain than in the basilar region. There is no direct invasion of cerebral tissue by the infecting organism or the inflammatory exudate, but the subjacent brain becomes congested and edematous. The effectiveness of the pial barrier accounts for the fact that cerebral abscess does not complicate bacterial meningitis. Indeed, when these two processes coexist, the sequence usually has been that of

Bacterial Causes of Meningitis

	Adults (>15 years) (%)	Children (1 month to 15 years) (%)	Neonates (<1 month) (%)
S. pneumoniae	30–50	10–20	0–5
N. meningitidis	10–30	30–40	0–1
H. influenzae	1–3	35–45	0–1
Streptococci	5–10	2–4	10–25
Staphylococci	5–15	1–2	5
Listeria	5	1–2	2–10
Gram-negative bacilli	1–10	1–2	55–60

an initial abscess subsequently leaking its contents into the ventricular system, producing meningitis. Structures adjacent to the meninges may show a variety of pathologic changes secondary to bacterial meningitis. *Cortical thrombophlebitis* results from venous stasis and adjacent meningeal inflammation. Infarction of cerebral tissue may follow. *Involvement of small pial arteries* with peripheral aneurysm formation and vascular occlusion occurs occasionally in bacterial meningitis. In fulminating cases (particularly meningococcal meningitis), *cerebral edema* may be marked even though the CSF pleocytosis is only moderate. Rarely such patients develop temporal lobe and cerebellar herniation, resulting in compression of the midbrain and medulla. *Damage to cranial nerves* occurs in areas where dense exudate accumulates; the third and sixth cranial nerves are also vulnerable to damage by increased intracranial pressure. *Ventriculitis* probably occurs in most cases of bacterial meningitis; rarely this progresses to the accumulation of pus, *ventricular empyema. Hydrocephalus* can develop during meningitis from obstruction to CSF flow within the ventricular system (obstructive hydrocephalus) or extraventricularly (communicating hydrocephalus). *Subdural effusions* are sterile transudates which develop over the cerebral cortex in about 15 per cent of infants with bacterial meningitis. Rarely such effusions become infected, producing a subdural empyema. In the past the diagnosis has been made almost exclusively in infants, in whom abnormal transillumination or increasing head size can be detected. Its frequency in adults is not known. Cerebral CAT scanning techniques may provide an answer.

PATHOGENESIS. Bacteria may reach the meninges by several routes: (1) systemic bacteremia, (2) direct ingress from the upper respiratory tract or skin through an anatomic defect (e.g., skull fracture, eroding sequestrum, meningocoele), (3) passage intracranially via venules in the nasopharynx, or (4) spread from a contiguous focus of infection (infection of the paranasal sinuses, leakage of a brain abscess). Bacteremic spread to the meninges is probably the most frequent path of infection. Bacteremia is common in meningitis and suggests this route; but bacteremia also can be a consequence of meningitis as suggested by its occurrence in experimental meningitis following bacterial inoculation into the subarachnoid space of animals and by its occurrence in about 30 per cent of patients with posttraumatic pneumococcal meningitis. The primary focus initiating the bacteremia is usually in the upper respiratory tract or lung (pneumonia), but may be in the heart (endocarditis) or the gastrointestinal or urinary tracts. Once established in any part of the meninges, infection quickly extends throughout the subarachnoid space.

CLINICAL MANIFESTATIONS. History. An acute onset of fever, generalized headache, vomiting, and stiff neck is common to many types of meningitis. Although some patients develop bacterial meningitis in the absence of respiratory symptoms, the majority of patients with pyogenic meningitis of the three common causes have had an antecedent or accompanying upper respiratory tract infection, acute otitis (or mastoiditis), or pneumonia. Myalgias (particularly in meningococcal disease), backache, and generalized weakness are common symptoms. The illness usually progresses rapidly with development of confusion, obtundation, and loss of consciousness. Rarely the onset may be less acute,

with meningeal signs present for several days to a week prior to hospitalization.

General Physical Findings. Evidences of meningeal irritation (drowsiness and decreased mentation, stiff neck, positive Kernig's and Brudzinski's signs) are usually present. In certain patients the findings of meningitis may be easily overlooked; obtunded elderly patients with congestive failure or pneumonia may develop meningitis without prominent meningeal signs. Their lethargy should be investigated carefully and meningeal signs should be sought; if any doubt exists, examination of the CSF is indicated.

The presence of a petechial, purpuric, or ecchymotic rash in a patient with meningeal findings almost always indicates meningococcal infection and requires prompt treatment because of the rapidity with which this infection can progress (see Ch. 141). Rarely, extensive petechial and purpuric lesions occur in meningitis caused by *S. pneumoniae* or *H. influenzae*. Very rarely skin lesions almost indistinguishable from those of meningococcal bacteremia occur in patients with acute *S. aureus* endocarditis who also have meningeal signs and a CSF pleocytosis (secondary either to staphylococcal meningitis or to embolic cerebral infarction). Usually one or two of the lesions in such a patient are those of purulent purpura; aspiration of material reveals staphylococci on Gram stain. In the summer months viral aseptic meningitis (particularly caused by echovirus 9) may produce meningeal signs, macular and petechial skin lesions, and a CSF pleocytosis of several hundred to 1000 cells.

Neurologic Findings and Complications. *Cranial nerve abnormalities*, involving principally the third, fourth, sixth, or seventh nerves, occur in 10 to 20 per cent of patients with bacterial meningitis. These usually disappear shortly after recovery. Partial or complete sensorineural hearing loss (sometimes irreversible) occurs in about 20 per cent of patients with bacterial meningitis over the age of three years, and is not correlated with coincident otitis media. Hearing loss occurs more frequently after meningitis caused by *N. meningitidis* than after that caused by *H. influenzae* or *S. pneumoniae*.

Seizures (focal or generalized) occur during the acute phase of bacterial meningitis in 20 to 30 per cent of patients and may be due to readily reversible causes (high fever in infants; penicillin neurotoxicity when large doses are administered intravenously in the presence of renal failure) or to focal cerebral injury. Seizures can occur during the first few days, or can appear with associated focal neurologic deficits caused by cortical vein phlebitis seven to ten days after the onset of the meningitis.

Brain swelling and increased CSF pressure are associated with seizures, third nerve dysfunction, abnormal reflexes, coma, hypertension, and bradycardia. Papilledema is rare in bacterial meningitis even with high CSF pressures. Its presence should raise the possibility of some other associated or independent suppurative intracranial process (subdural empyema, brain abscess). Marked central hyperpnea sometimes occurs in patients with severe bacterial meningitis; CSF acidosis (principally caused by increased lactic acid levels) provides much of the respiratory stimulus.

Focal cerebral signs (hemiparesis, dysphasia, visual field defects) occur in about 15 per cent of patients with bacterial meningitis. They may develop during early meningitis secondary to occlusive vascular processes or some days later. It is important to distinguish lateralizing findings resulting from postictal changes (Todd's paralysis) which usually persist for no more than several hours.

Prompt treatment of bacterial meningitis usually results in rapid recovery of neurologic function. Persistent or late onset of obtundation and coma without focal findings suggests the development of brain swelling, subdural effusions (in the infant), hydrocephalus, loculated ventriculitis, or cortical thrombophlebitis. The last two are commonly associated with fever and a continuing CSF pleocytosis.

Residual neurologic damage remains in 10 to 20 per cent of patients who recover from bacterial meningitis.

LABORATORY DIAGNOSIS. Cerebrospinal Fluid Examination. Initial CSF pressure is usually moderately elevated (200 to 300 mm H_2O). Striking elevations (over 400 mm) occur in occasional patients with acute brain swelling complicating meningitis in the absence of an associated mass lesion.

GRAM-STAINED SMEAR. By the time of hospitalization, most patients with pyogenic meningitis have large numbers (at least 10^5 per milliliter) of bacteria in the cerebrospinal fluid. Careful examination of the Gram-stained smear of the spun sediment of CSF reveals the etiologic agent in 70 to 80 per cent of cases. In most instances when gram-positive diplococci (or short-chaining cocci) are observed on stained CSF smear they are pneumococci. In certain clinical settings it is important to distinguish the organism from the relatively penicillin-resistant enterococcus, which would require the addition of an aminoglycoside to penicillin in treatment. If sufficient organisms are present in the CSF, prompt identification of a pneumococcus can be made by the quellung reaction, employing pooled pneumococcal antisera. Culture of the cerebrospinal fluid reveals the etiologic agent in 80 to 90 per cent of patients with bacterial meningitis.

SPECIAL IMMUNOLOGIC AND SEROLOGIC PROCEDURES. In patients in whom the etiologic agent is not identified on Gram-stained smear of the CSF, rapid diagnosis may sometimes be made by detection of specific bacterial antigens by countercurrent immunoelectrophoresis (CIE). This technique has been employed most extensively in the rapid diagnosis of meningitis caused by H. influenzae type b, but has also been used in the diagnosis of meningococcal and pneumococcal meningitis; identification of the pathogen can be accomplished in 55 to 80 per cent of cases of meningitis resulting from these three common pathogens. Failure to detect these antigens does *not* exclude bacterial meningitis. The reliability of the test depends on the activity and specificity of the antisera employed; false-positive results may occur because of cross-reactivity of some antigens (e.g., E. coli K1 with group B meningococcus). Since the bacterial cause can be found on Gram-stained smear in most cases of bacterial meningitis, the role of CIE appears to be as an adjunct in rapid diagnosis when no organisms are observed or in providing a specific rather than a morphologic (Gram stain) diagnosis.

The limulus gelation assay for endotoxin is positive in the CSF of patients with meningitis caused by gram-negative bacteria but not in the case of meningitis caused by gram-positive organisms.

CELL COUNT. The cell count in untreated meningitis usually ranges between 100 and 10,000 per cubic millimeter, with polymorphonuclear leukocytes predominating initially (80 per cent or more) and lymphocytes appearing subsequently. Extremely high cell counts (>50,000 per cubic millimeter) may occur rarely in primary bacterial meningitis, but should also raise the possibility of intraventricular rupture of a cerebral abscess. Cell counts as low as 10 to 20 may be observed early in bacterial meningitis (particularly that caused by N. meningitidis and H. influenzae). Occasionally, in granulocytopenic patients or in the elderly with overwhelming pneumococcal meningitis, the cerebrospinal fluid may contain very few leukocytes and yet may appear grossly turbid just because of the presence of myriads of organisms. Meningitis caused by several bacterial species (M. tuberculosis, T. pallidum) characteristically produces a lymphocytic pleocytosis. Listeria monocytogenes meningitis in infants may produce a primarily lymphocytic response in the CSF; in the adult there is usually a polymorphonuclear response, but rarely lymphocytes predominate.

GLUCOSE. The CSF glucose is reduced to values of 40 mg per deciliter or below (or less than 50 to 60 per cent of the simultaneous blood level) in over 50 per cent of patients with bacterial meningitis; this finding can be very valuable in distinguishing bacterial meningitis from most viral meningitides or parameningeal infections. A normal CSF glucose does not exclude the diagnosis of bacterial meningitis. The simultaneous blood glucose level should be determined, because patients with diabetes mellitus (or who are receiving intravenous glucose infusions) will have an elevated level of glucose in the CSF, and its significance can be appreciated only on comparison with the simultaneous blood level. However, it may take 90 to 120 minutes for equilibration to occur after major shifts in the level of glucose in the circulation. The hypoglycorrhachia characteristic of pyogenic meningitis appears to be due to interference with the normal carrier-facilitated diffusion of glucose.

PROTEIN. The level of protein in the cerebrospinal fluid is usually elevated above 100 mg per deciliter, and the higher values are more commonly observed in pneumococcal meningitis. Extreme elevations, up to 1000 mg per deciliter or more, indicate impending or actual subarachnoid block secondary to the meningitis.

OTHER ABNORMALITIES IN THE CSF. Elevated levels of lactic acid occur in pyogenic meningitis. Lactic dehydrogenase levels (particularly isozymes 4 and 5 derived from granulocytes) are commonly elevated in patients with bacterial meningitis. Although the levels of lactic dehydrogenase are higher in patients with bacterial meningitis than in those with viral infections of the central nervous system, these alterations are not of help in determining the specific etiologic agent involved.

Other Laboratory Tests. BLOOD AND RESPIRATORY TRACT CULTURES. Bacteremia is demonstrable in about 80 per cent of patients with H. influenzae meningitis, 50 per cent of those with pneumococcal meningitis, and 30 to 40 per cent of those with meningococcal meningitis. Cultures of the upper respiratory tract have not proved helpful in establishing an etiologic diagnosis. Determination of serum creatinine and electrolytes is important in view of the gravity of the illness, the occurrence of specific abnormalities secondary to the meningitis (syndrome of inappropriate secretion of antidiuretic hormone), and problems in therapy in the presence of renal dysfunction (seizures and hyperkalemia with high-dose penicillin therapy). In patients with extensive petechial and purpuric skin lesions, evaluation for coagulopathy is indicated.

RADIOLOGIC STUDIES. In view of the frequency with which pyogenic meningitis is associated with primary foci of infection in the chest, nasal sinuses, or mastoid, roentgenograms of these areas should be taken at the appropriate time after institution of antimicrobial therapy. If a mass lesion (cerebral abscess, subdural empyema) is suspected by history, clinical setting, or physicial findings (papilledema), then radionuclide or CAT scans should be performed.

DIAGNOSIS. The diagnosis of bacterial meningitis is not difficult in a febrile patient with meningeal symptoms and signs developing in the setting of a predisposing illness. The diagnosis may be less obvious in the elderly, obtunded patient with pneumonia or the confused alcoholic patient in impending delirium tremens. Examination of the cerebrospinal fluid should be carried out promptly under these circumstances or whenever there is any question of meningitis.

Headache, fever, vomiting, stiff neck, and CSF pleocytosis are features of meningeal inflammation and are common to many types of meningitis (e.g., bacterial, fungal, viral) and also to some parameningeal processes. The cerebrospinal fluid findings are most helpful in distinguishing among these processes (see Ch. 298). In the patient with meningitis whose cerebrospinal fluid does not reveal the etiologic agent on examination of Gram-stained smear, particularly when the CSF glucose is normal and the polymorphonuclear pleocytosis is atypical, certain treatable processes which can mimic bacterial meningitis should be considered in differential diagnosis: (1) *Parameningeal infections.* The presence of infections (chronic ear or nasal accessory sinus infections, lung abscess) predisposing to brain abscess, epidural (cerebral or spinal) abscess, subdural empyema, or pyogenic venous sinus phlebitis should be sought. Neurologic findings may appear in the course of primary bacterial meningitis, but their presence should alert the physician to the need for close scrutiny for the presence of a space-occupying infectious process in the central nervous system. Neurologic symptoms or findings antedating the onset of meningeal symptoms should raise the question of a parameningeal infection. The isolation of an anaerobic organism should suggest the possibility of intraventricular leakage of a cerebral abscess. (2) *Bacterial endocarditis.* Bacterial meningitis may occur during bacterial endocarditis caused by pyogenic organisms such as *S. aureus* and enterococci. In subacute bacterial endocarditis sterile embolic infarctions of the brain may occur and produce meningeal signs and a CSF pleocytosis containing several hundred cells, including polymorphonuclear leukocytes. A history of dental manipulation, fever, and anorexia antedating the meningitis should be sought; careful examination for heart murmurs and peripheral stigmata of endocarditis is indicated. (3) *"Chemical" meningitis.* The clinical and CSF findings (polymorphonuclear pleocytosis and even reduced glucose level) of bacterial meningitis may be produced by chemically induced inflammation. Acute meningitis following a diagnostic lumbar puncture or spinal anesthesia may be due to bacterial (usually *Pseudomonas* species or coliform organisms) or chemical contamination of equipment or anesthetic agent. Endogenous chemical meningitis resulting from leakage into the subarachnoid space of material from an epidermoid tumor or a craniopharyngioma can produce

a polymorphonuclear pleocytosis and hypoglycorrhachia. Birefringent material may be seen on polarizing microscopy of the CSF sediment.

NON-NEUROLOGIC COMPLICATIONS. Shock. When shock occurs in pyogenic meningitis it is usually a manifestation of an accompanying intense bacteremia, as in fulminant meningococcemia, rather than of the meningitis itself. Shock is the result both of the bacteremia (and possible associated endotoxemia) and of cardiac injury (myocarditis). Management is guided by the principles of septic shock therapy with appropriate modifications for myocardial failure. (See Ch. 141.)

Coagulation Disorders. Coagulopathies are frequently associated with the intense bacteremias (usually meningococcal, occasionally pneumococcal) and hypotension which can accompany meningitis. The changes may be mild such as thrombocytopenia (with or without prolongation of prothrombin and partial thromboplastin times) or more marked with clinical evidences of disseminated intravascular coagulation (see Ch. 521.5).

Septic Complications. ENDOCARDITIS. Previously, 5 to 10 per cent of patients with pneumococcal meningitis, particularly those with bacteremia and pneumonia as well, developed acute endocarditis, most commonly on the aortic valve. The incidence is currently much lower, as a result of earlier treatment of the initiating infection. The early diagnosis of simultaneous pneumococcal endocarditis in a patient with meningitis may be difficult, because treatment of meningitis may control the manifestations of endocarditis. However, in such patients, febrile relapse and a new murmur may appear shortly after completion of antimicrobial therapy for meningitis.

PYOGENIC ARTHRITIS. Septic arthritis may result from the bacteremia associated with pyogenic meningitis. Most commonly it occurs with pneumococcal meningitis, but it may complicate meningitis caused by *N. meningitidis, H. influenzae,* or *S. aureus.*

Prolonged Fever. With appropriate antimicrobial treatment of meningitis of the three most common bacterial causes, patients become afebrile within two to five days. Sometimes fever persists beyond this or recurs after an afebrile period. In the patient with persisting headache, obtundation, and cerebral findings, inadequate drug therapy or neurologic sequelae (cortical venous thrombophlebitis, ventriculitis, subdural collections) are important considerations. Re-evaluation of the cerebrospinal fluid, particularly Gram-stained smear and culture, is essential under these circumstances. Drug fever may be responsible in the patient who continues to show clinical improvement in all other respects. Metastatic infection (septic arthritis, purulent pericarditis, thoracic empyema, endocarditis) may be the cause of continuing or recurrent fever.

A syndrome consisting of fever, arthritis, and pericarditis three to six days after initiation of effective antimicrobial therapy of meningococcal meningitis occurs in about 10 per cent of patients. Synovial and pericardial fluids are characteristically serosanguineous and sterile, unlike the purulent fluid which can occur in both sites early in the course of meningococcal infection. The clinical features are reminiscent of those of serum sickness. Immunopathologic study of skin and synovial lesions implicates immune complex formation in their genesis. Pericardial effusions usually do not become hemodynamically significant, but close observation is indicated. Symptomatic relief is provided by salicylates.

RECURRENT MENINGITIS. Repeated episodes of bacterial meningitis generally indicate a host defect, either in local anatomy or in antibacterial and immunologic defenses. *S. pneumoniae* is by far the most frequent cause of recurrent meningitis. Eleven per cent of patients with pneumococcal meningitis have had more than one episode, whereas 0.5 per cent of patients with meningitis caused by other organisms have had recurrent attacks. A history of head trauma is much more frequent in patients with recurrent meningitis. Organisms may directly enter the subarachnoid space, through a defect in the cribriform plate (the most common site), via a basilar skull fracture, through an erosive sequestrum of the mastoid, through congenital dermal defects along the craniospinal axis (usually evident before adult life), or as a consequence of penetrating cranial trauma or neurosurgical procedures. The anatomic defect may produce a frank CSF leak (rhinorrhea or, less commonly, otorrhea) or may entrap a vascular cuff of meninges which might subsequently serve as a direct route for organisms to reach the meninges. CSF rhinorrhea may be intermittent, and meningitis may occur months or years after head injury.

Any patient with bacterial meningitis, particularly if meningitis is recurrent, should be evaluated carefully for any congenital or post-traumatic defects. The presence of CSF rhinorrhea should be sought at admission and subsequently (rhinorrhea may clear during active meningitis only to recur when inflammation has resolved). Demonstration of glucose in nasal secretions with glucose oxidase "sticks" (Dextrostix) suggests the presence of cerebrospinal fluid. Quantitative determination of glucose and chloride content of nasal secretions can definitively establish the presence of CSF rhinorrhea.

Recurrent pneumococcal meningitis may occur without apparent predisposing circumstances, and cryptic CSF leaks should be sought actively in such patients by polytomography of the frontal and mastoid regions and by radioisotope techniques. (Radioiodine-labeled albumin is introduced intrathecally, and pledgets of cotton placed in the nares are subsequently examined for the radionuclide.) Surgical closure of CSF fistulas should be carried out to prevent further episodes of meningitis.

In most patients with CSF otorrhea and rhinorrhea following an acute head injury, the leak ceases in one or two weeks. *Persistent rhinorrhea for more than four to six weeks is an indication for surgical repair.* Prolonged administration of penicillin will not prevent pneumococcal meningitis and may encourage infection with more drug-resistant species.

Rarely, recurrent meningitis of nonbacterial etiology may mimic bacterial meningitis. *Mollaret's meningitis* consists of repeated febrile episodes of mild meningeal symptomatology, usually without neurologic abnormalities. Initially, large "endothelial" cells may be seen in the CSF along with polymorphonuclear leukocytes, which subsequently are replaced by lymphocytes. *Behçet's syndrome,* characterized by relapsing oral and genital ulcers and ocular lesions (hypopyon), may exhibit a variety of neurologic abnormalities, including recurrent meningitis.

PROGNOSIS. The introduction of antimicrobial agents has converted bacterial meningitis from a disease that was almost always fatal to one in which the majority of patients survive without significant neurologic residua. The mortality rate for bacterial meningitis varies with the etiologic agent and the clinical circumstances. With current antimicrobial therapy the mortality rate for *H. influenzae* meningitis is below 5 per cent and that for meningococcal meningitis is about 10 per cent. The highest mortality is with pneumococcal meningitis, in which the rate is about 20 per cent. Poor prognostic factors include advanced age, presence of other foci of infection, underlying diseases (leukemia, alcoholism), coma, and delay in instituting appropriate therapy.

TREATMENT. Antimicrobial Agents. *Antimicrobial therapy should be begun promptly in this life-threatening emergency.* If the etiologic agent is observed on Gram-stained smear of the CSF sediment, specific therapy can be initiated. If the etiologic agent is not observed on smear (or not detected by counterimmunoelectrophoresis), treatment for bacterial meningitis of unknown cause should be started, aiming at the most likely possibilities based on available clinical clues (age of the patient, presence of a purpuric rash, a recent neurosurgical procedure, CSF rhinorrhea).

With the exception of chloramphenicol, the commonly employed antimicrobial agents do not readily penetrate the normal blood-brain barrier; but the passage of penicillin and other antimicrobials is enhanced in the presence of meningeal inflammation. Antimicrobial drugs should be administered intravenously throughout the treatment period; reduction in dosage as the patient improves should be avoided, because normalization of the blood-brain barrier during recovery reduces the CSF levels of drug that are achievable. Bactericidal drugs (penicillin, ampicillin) are preferred whenever possible in the treatment of meningitis caused by susceptible bacteria. Several antimicrobial drugs (cephalosporins, clindamycin) which do not provide effective levels in the cerebrospinal fluid should not be used.

MENINGITIS OF SPECIFIC BACTERIAL CAUSE. The treatment of choice for pneumococcal meningitis in the adult is penicillin (24 million units daily in divided doses every two hours) or ampicillin (12 grams daily in divided doses every two to three hours). Chloramphenicol (4 to 6 grams intravenously daily) is a suitable alternative in the patient with a major penicillin allergy. The recent emergence in South Africa of pneumococcal strains significantly resistant to most antimicrobial drugs, including penicillin and chloramphenicol, indicates a need for determining antimicrobial susceptibilities of pneumococcal isolates from cerebrospinal fluid and blood.

The treatment of meningococcal meningitis is the same as for pneumococcal meningitis (see Ch. 141).

The recent appearance of *H. influenzae* strains highly resistant to ampicillin has dictated a change in initial management of this form of meningitis. Chloramphenicol (100 mg per kilogram intravenously daily for a child; 4 grams intravenously daily for an adult), either alone or in combination with ampicillin (300 to 400 mg per kilogram intravenously per day for a child; 12 grams intravenously per day for an adult), is the preferred treatment until drug susceptibilities are determined. If the organism is proved susceptible to ampicillin, then this drug can be used alone in treatment.

Adult meningitis caused by *S. aureus* should be treated with a penicillinase-resistant penicillin (oxacillin or nafcillin in a dosage of 10 to 12 grams intravenously per day). In occasional cases, particularly when staphylococcal meningitis complicates a craniotomy, adjunctive intrathecal therapy (5000 to 10,000 units of bacitracin)* may be considered. Vancomycin (2.0 grams intravenously daily in the adult) has been used as an alternative in the penicillin-allergic patient, and adjunctive therapy with intrathecal bacitracin may be indicated.

Treatment of enterococcal meningitis in the adult involves the use of intravenous penicillin (24 million units daily) or ampicillin (12 grams daily), supplemented with parenterally administered gentamicin (3 to 5 mg per kilogram daily in divided doses every eight hours). In the patient who fails to respond promptly to parenteral therapy, adjunctive intrathecal therapy with gentamicin* (3 to 5 mg) should be considered.

Initial treatment of adults with gram-negative bacillary meningitis involves the use of chloramphenicol (4 grams intravenously daily) as well as intravenous gentamicin (5 mg per kilogram daily in divided doses every eight hours) and intrathecal gentamicin* (3 to 5 mg administered at intervals of 24 hours for the first few days). Intrathecal (or intraventricular) therapy is particularly important in patients with meningitis after neurosurgical procedures. Following identification of the specific infecting species and determination of its drug susceptibilities, alterations in antimicrobial therapy may be indicated; if the organism is *Pseudomonas aeruginosa*, parenteral and intrathecal gentamicin would be continued but carbenicillin (30 to 40 grams intravenously daily) would be substituted for chloramphenicol.

Initial treatment of meningitis when the etiologic agent cannot be identified on Gram-stained smear of cerebrospinal fluid is based on available clinical clues. *In the neonate*, a wide range of gram-positive (group B streptococci, *Listeria*) and gram-negative organisms (*E. coli, Klebsiella, H. influenzae*) may be the cause, indicating the use of combined therapy with drugs such as ampicillin and gentamicin. *In children*, therapy is directed at the three most frequent pathogens: *H. influenzae, S. pneumoniae*, and *N. meningitidis*. The appearance of ampicillin resistance among strains of *H. influenzae* has necessitated the shift from single drug therapy (ampicillin) to a two-drug approach (ampicillin-chloramphenicol or penicillin-chloramphenicol) in the treatment of meningitis of unknown cause in this age group, pending results of culture. *In adults*, therapy with ampicillin or penicillin is directed at the most common pathogens (*S. pneumoniae* and *N. meningitidis*). However, because *H. influenzae* type b infections appear to be increasing in adults, and because of the increased incidence of gram-negative bacillary meningitis in certain clinical settings, broader initial therapy may be indicated if clinical features suggest unusual organisms.

Duration of Therapy. The frequency of cerebrospinal fluid examinations depends on the clinical course, but a repeat examination should be done in 48 hours if there has not been satisfactory improvement. Meningococci are rapidly eliminated from the circulation and cerebrospinal fluid with appropriate antimicrobial therapy, which should be continued for at least five to seven days after the patient becomes afebrile. *H. influenzae* meningitis should be treated for a minimum of

ten days (at least for seven days after the patient becomes afebrile); re-examination of the CSF at that time usually shows cell counts of less than 60 (over 90 per cent mononuclear). Since pneumococcal meningitis produces a more intense inflammatory response, antimicrobial treatment should be continued for 10 to 14 days and follow-up examination of the cerebrospinal fluid should show resolution. More prolonged therapy is indicated with concomitant parameningeal infection or mastoiditis. Treatment of gram-negative bacillary meningitis with parenteral antimicrobials is prolonged, usually for a minimum of three weeks, in order to prevent relapse.

Other Aspects of Treatment. Occasional patients with acute bacterial meningitis develop marked brain swelling (CSF pressure exceeding 400 mm H_2O), which may lead to temporal lobe or cerebellar herniation following lumbar puncture. To reduce this increased pressure, an intravenous infusion of 20 per cent mannitol solution (1.5 to 2.0 grams per kilogram) is administered over 20 to 60 minutes. Continued control of increased intracranial pressure, if needed therafter, may be effected with mannitol, dexamethasone (10 mg intravenously, followed by 4 mg every six hours), or both. Brain swelling is about the only indication for the use of corticosteroids in the treatment of pyogenic meningitis; they should be employed only when the appropriate antimicrobial drugs are administered. Fluid restriction (1200 to 1500 ml daily in adults) is advisable during the first 24 to 48 hours to minimize brain swelling.

Patients with acute bacterial meningitis should receive constant nursing attention to ensure prompt recognition of seizures and to prevent aspiration. If seizures occur, they should be treated acutely with diazepam (Valium) administered slowly intravenously in a dose of 5 to 10 mg in the adult. Maintenance anticonvulsant therapy can be continued thereafter with intravenous diphenylhydantoin (Dilantin) until the medication can be administered orally. Sedation should be avoided because of the danger of respiratory depression and aspiration.

Bayer, A. S., Seidel, J. S., Yoshikawa, T. T., Anthony, B. F., and Guze, L. B.: Group D enterococcal meningitis. Arch. Intern. Med., 136:883, 1976.

Carpenter, R. R., and Petersdorf, R. G.: The clinical spectrum of bacterial meningitis. Am. J. Med., 33:262, 1962.

Chernik, N. L., Armstrong, D., and Posner, J. B.: Central nervous system infection in patients with cancer. Medicine, 52:563, 1973.

Colding, H., and Lind, I.: Counterimmunoelectrophoresis in the diagnosis of bacterial meningitis. J. Clin. Microbiol., 5:405, 1977.

Finland, M., and Barnes, M. W.: Acute bacterial meningitis at Boston City Hospital during 12 selected years, 1935–1972. J. Infect. Dis. 136:400, 1977.

Hand, W. L., and Sanford, J. P.: Posttraumatic bacterial meningitis. Ann. Intern. Med., 72:869, 1970.

Hermans, P. E., Goldstein, N. P., and Wellman, W. E.: Mollaret's meningitis and differential diagnosis of recurrent meningitis. Am. J. Med., 52:128, 1972.

Hyslop, N. E., and Swartz, M. N.: Bacterial meningitis. Postgrad. Med., 58:120, 1975.

Levin, S., Nelson, K. E., Spies, H. W., and Lepper, M. H.: Pneumococcal meningitis: The problem of the unseen cerebrospinal fluid leak. Am. J. Med. Sci., 264:319, 1972.

Mangi, R. J., Quintiliani, R., and Andriole, V. T.: Gram-negative bacillary meningitis. Am. J. Med., 59:829, 1975.

McCracken, G. H.: Rapid identification of specific etiology in meningitis. J. Pediat., 88:706, 1976.

Swartz, M. N., and Dodge, P. R.: Bacterial meningitis—a review of selected aspects. N. Engl. J. Med., 272:725, 779, 842, 898, 954, 1003, 1965.

Tugwell, P., Greenwood, B. M., and Warrell, D. A.: Pneumococcal meningitis: A clinical and laboratory study. Quart. J. Med., 45:583, 1976.

---

*Intrathecal use is not mentioned in the manufacturer's package insert approved by the U.S. Food and Drug Administration. Therefore its use in these circumstances must be considered investigational.

141. MENINGOCOCCAL DISEASE

Harry A. Feldman

DEFINITION. Meningococcal infections may affect the upper and lower respiratory tracts, blood (meningococcemia), central nervous system (meningococcal meningitis, cerebrospinal fever, spotted fever, or epidemic cerebrospinal meningitis), joints (arthritis), heart, pericardium, eyes, skin, urethra, cervix, and rectum, singly or in any combination in a given patient. First recognized in 1805 by Vieusseux in Geneva and in 1806 by Danielson and Mann in Massachusetts, *meningococcal meningitis*, the best known form, occurs sporadically and as localized or widespread epidemics.

ETIOLOGY. *Neisseria meningitidis*, a variable sized gram-negative coccus which may be seen singly or as biscuit-shaped diplococci, was established to cause meningitis by Weichselbaum in 1887. Metabolically fastidious, the organism grows best on enriched culture media at 37° C in an atmosphere of increased CO_2 concentration. Mueller-Hinton or meat infusion broths or agar containing 10 per cent of blood (rabbit, sheep, or horse) or human ascitic fluid are excellent. Chocolate agar is very good for initial isolation. The addition of vancomycin and colistin with or without nystatin (modified Thayer-Martin agar) is especially useful for isolation from throats or other areas of marked contamination. Meningococci are very susceptible to chilling or drying, so all cultures should be inoculated and incubated promptly. Since some meningococcal strains are exquisitely susceptible to sulfonamides, media inoculated with specimens from patients receiving such drugs should contain para-aminobenzoic acid (5 mg per 100 ml).

Identification of meningococci is based on morphology, Gram staining, oxidative utilization of glucose and maltose but not sucrose, and immunologic reactions. The following serogroups are recognized: A, B, C, D, X, Y, Z, 29-E, and W-135. Those which most commonly cause illness are A, B, C, and Y. Group D is exceedingly rare. The groups are identified through their specific polysaccharide antigens. A and C organisms have prominent capsules so young cultures or organisms in cerebrospinal fluid quell (capsular swelling) with specific antisera. Groups B and C have been further subdivided on the basis of protein antigens, some of which are shared. Group A strains can be subdivided similarly within the group. At present these characteristics appear to be useful for epidemiologic studies, but their role in protection remains undefined.

Lipopolysaccharides or "endotoxins" in purified form have been prepared from meningococci. These are toxic for animals and are increasingly being demonstrated to play significant roles in the pathogenesis of human disease.

EPIDEMIOLOGY. The epidemiology of meningococcal infections is complicated by the multiplicity of their serogroups. Sporadic infections may be seen almost constantly in all areas. Major epidemics are generally caused by group A organisms and seem to occur in 20- to 30-year cycles. For example, during World Wars I and II there were massive civilian and military outbreaks which persisted for several years. Groups B and C produce most cases in the intervening years. The remaining groups are usually detected in carriers and sporadic cases. Group Y is the most frequent disease producer after A, B, and C. Thus the over-all picture is that of high waves about every 20 to 30 years and lower ones in the interims. There are localized exceptions to this generalization. Detroit had a major group A epidemic in 1929, with 724 cases reported in an eight-month period and a general mortality rate of 50 per cent (no specific treatment available). In infants, however, the mortality rate was 84 per cent, and in those over 40 years, 72 per cent. Santiago, Chile, had a severe group A epidemic in 1941 to 1942 with 5885 cases; of these, 15.9 per cent were fatal (sulfonamides used).

In recent years the most devastated areas have been that portion of Africa which lies below the Sahara and north of the Equator, and Brazil. The African "meningitis belt" now averages about 10,000 cases per year with about 1200 deaths, but from 1939 to 1962 it reported 593,738 cases with 102,956 (17 per cent) deaths! In earlier outbreaks in the same area, as many as 85 per cent of cases were fatal. Here, as in South Africa, group A organisms continue to predominate. The Brazilian epidemic was centered in São Paulo but occurred in other areas as well. It began unusually as a group C epidemic in 1971, which in 1973 became a predominately group A outbreak. It began to die out in 1975 and faded drastically in 1976. The great mystery here is the unanswered question as to what conditions made it possible for two epidemics to overlap in the same general area.

Other recent epidemics, all caused by group A, have occurred in Canada, Finland, Outer Mongolia, and Morocco. Group A infections remain rare in the United States, except for a localized nidus in the "skid row" area of Seattle and, to a lesser extent, among a similar population in Anchorage.

About 60 per cent of cases occur in those less than 15 years of age. Military recruits for some unknown reason are especially vulnerable. About 80 per cent of their cases are seen within the first 90 days of service, most often in the first month. The incidence of both cases and carriers is usually higher in males. Race and color (except for those with sickle cell disease) do not seem to influence either incidence or susceptibility, but socioeconomic level does. The higher rates reported among blacks in certain urban areas probably reflect increased poverty with its concomitant crowding. The exact incubation period is often nondeterminable, but the range is probably one to ten days. There are a few instances reported in which this may have been a long as three weeks.

The portal of entry of meningococci is the upper respiratory tract, and transmission from person to person may result from direct or intimate contact, airborne droplets, or articles contaminated with fresh secretions from the respiratory tract. Mouth-to-mouth resuscitation has resulted in several cases in physicians. In one instance, nasopharyngeal carriage followed a kidney transplant from a donor who had died of unrecognized meningococcemia; in another, meningococcal pneumonia also followed a kidney transplant. Yet even during severe epidemics, the majority of clinical infections seems to be unrelated to others, so that case-to-case spread is almost impossible to trace. Posterior nasopharyngeal culture surveys during outbreaks may demonstrate carrier rates as high as 90 per cent, constantly or intermittently, without clinical evidence of disease. Although the carrier rate often is less than 5 per cent during interepidemic periods, much of the population may harbor meningococci at some time.

Until 1963, meningococci of all serogroups were highly susceptible to sulfonamides so that such drugs were exceedingly effective for both the treatment of cases and mass prophylaxis. Unfortunately, sulfonamide-resistant group B meningococci were found to be prevalent in that year. Markedly resistant group C strains were detected soon after. Recently, and perhaps even more disturbing, sulfonamide-resistant group A strains first were isolated during an epidemic in North Africa, and subsequently in the "belt" below the Sahara, South Africa, Australia, Brazil, Canada, Finland, Greece, Mongolia, Norway, and Southeast Asia. This phenomenon is now so widespread that all cases caused by organisms of *any* serogroup must be considered to be the result of sulfonamide-resistant strains unless specifically proved otherwise. The same holds for carrier strains.

The physician is often concerned with the question of whether family members or other contacts of meningococcal patients are at excessive risk from this disease. Fortunately, secondary cases are unusual, but they do occur. In the Detroit epidemic of 1929, 4 per cent of cases were in affected households. In the Santiago epidemic of 1941–1942, the over-all secondary attack rate was 2.5 per cent. Because most of these follow within ten days (many four days) of the index case, they are often considered to be co-primaries. Acceptance of this concept leads to another control approach which will be dealt with subsequently (see Prevention). Household carrier rates, on the other hand, generally are high. In several studies of families of meningococcal patients, 45 to 50 per cent were found to be carrying organisms of the same serogroup as the patient, providing some justification for the anxieties of both families and physicians over household cases. Unfortunately, these no longer can be resolved by the relatively simple procedure which was possible when sulfonamide-susceptible strains were the rule.

PATHOGENESIS AND PATHOLOGY. In meningococcemia the essential lesion is vascular, with endothelial damage, inflammation of vessel walls with necrosis and thrombosis, and focal hemorrhages into cutaneous, subcutaneous, submucosal, and synovial tissues. In rapidly extending meningococcemia the Waterhouse-Friderichsen syndrome is often present. This is usually but not necessarily accompanied by bilateral adrenal hemorrhages.

Involvement of the central nervous system is characterized by *acute purulent meningitis,* although, if suspected early, there may be only hyperemia. Some degree of encephalitis usually accompanies the meningitis. When treatment is delayed or ineffective, permanent cranial nerve damage may be anticipated.

The pathogenesis of meningococcal infections is usually initiated by the colonization of the posterior nasopharynx and adjoining structures by organisms entering through the upper respiratory passages. Symptoms and signs of an acute upper respiratory infection may result, although this is not accepted by all observers. If invasion of the bloodstream follows, this may be relatively asymptomatic in some, but in others there may be metastatic lesions in skin, meninges, joints, eyes, lungs, pericardium, urethra, and other organs and tissues. The sites and extent of these localizations determine the symptoms and signs that follow.

We are totally at a loss to explain why meningococcal infections are so limited and innocuous in some individuals and so extensive and overwhelming in others. No microbe can kill more quickly; deaths have been observed within several hours after the first symptom.

Chemical alterations reflecting the severity of the meningococcal infection may be profound. Their cause is not known, but to some degree they are endotoxic in origin and furthered by the release of various substances from damaged tissue cells. Hemorrhagic manifestations may result from direct vascular damage because of a Schwartzman-like reaction, thrombocytopenia, or both. Other changes are those found in acute sepsis: fever, dehydration, reduction in blood volume, and altered acid-base and negative nitrogen balances. In severely ill patients, cyanosis, circulatory collapse, and other signs of shock appear, probably the result of the combined actions of bacterial endotoxins and tissue anoxia. Alterations suggestive of acute adrenal insufficiency, low serum sodium, elevated potassium, low chloride, and hypoglycemia may be present and are consistent with absent or diminished cortical secretion by damaged adrenal glands. There is no evidence that adrenal insufficiency as judged by the degree of excretion of corticosteroids in fulminating infections per se occurs independently of glandular destruction.

CLINICAL MANIFESTATIONS. A sequential development of clinical manifestations of meningococcal infections can be discerned from a number of cases, but any one patient may present with symptoms and signs of advanced diffuse illness. The usual sequence consists of infection of the upper respiratory tract, bacteremia, septicemia, meningitis, and/or other metastatic localization. One stage may be dominant, giving the appearance of mild illness, grave illness, or none.

Infection of the Upper Respiratory Tract. The upper respiratory tract is the most frequent site of meningococcal infection. Most patients have no or inconsequential symptoms so that the organism is detectable only by culture of the posterior nasopharynx. Whether symptoms result from such colonization is contested by many observers, because descriptions of this stage usually have been derived from military recruits at a time when they are subject to many viral and mycoplasmal respiratory infections. On the other hand, many but not all patients with meningococcal illnesses give histories of preceding or concurrent nasopharyngitis.

Meningococcemia. Bacteremic meningococcal infections may vary from acute fulminating illnesses of a few hours' duration to indolent, chronic infections lasting days, weeks, or, rarely, months. Symptoms may be relentlessly progressive or intermittent, with relapses and recrudescences at different times.

MILD OR SUBACUTE MENINGOCOCCEMIA. The most common form of meningococcemia is that of a relatively mild, acute, or subacute infection. Prodromal symptoms are frequently absent except for those of a mild upper respiratory infection in some. Onset is usually sudden, with fever, chilliness or frank chills that may be recurrent, malaise, myalgia, and apathy. The presenting symptoms may be any combination of these, but frequently the initial complaints are those of recurrent fever, rash, arthralgia, acute mono- or polyarthritis, conjunctivitis, nausea, and vomiting. Symptoms may regress or persist if the disease progresses. Fever may be remittent and irregular with elevations to 39 or 39.5° C. The pulse rate is proportionate to the fever. Respirations are usually normal or only slightly increased except when pneumonia or pleurisy is present.

The most striking feature on physical examination is the rash, which occurs often. It appears soon after onset, is variable (the severest is petechial or purpuric), measuring from 1 or 2 mm to 1 cm or more in diameter, and is pink to reddish blue (see accompanying figure). Early in the disease there may be a generalized, mottled erythema which appears dusky in slightly cyanotic patients. Light pink macules resembling the "rose spots" of typhoid, wheals, or nodules like erythema nodosum may appear before petechiae and ecchymoses. Careful search in good daylight may be necessary to detect early lesions. Occasionally, vesicular, pustular, or bullous lesions are present. Superficial or deep ulcerations may result from petechiae, especially when coalescent. These are sometimes very extensive and ultimately may require grafting. The rash often appears first on the wrists and ankles, but any area may be involved, including the conjunctivae and the mucous membranes. Hemorrhagic lesions fade to a brown, rusty color three or four days after their appearance; if new crops appear, often after chills, a variety of skin lesions may be present at the same time. This is more likely when treatment is delayed or unsuccessful.

Other physical findings, including splenomegaly, are inconstant. Herpetic lesions of the lip are found in about 10 per cent of the cases. Unless meningismus develops, symptoms referable to the central nervous system are absent, although those resulting from metastatic localizations are usually self-evident, depending upon their site.

The firm diagnosis is established with laboratory aids. Leukocytosis up to 40,000 cells per cubic millimeter with 80 to 90 per cent neutrophils is almost always present. In overwhelming cases, leukopenia may be profound and gram-negative intracellular diplococci may be seen within leukocytes in stained smears from capillary blood, buffy coat, or skin lesions. A blood culture positive for meningococci furnishes final etiologic proof. It should be emphasized that several cultures of the blood may be necessary to detect meningococci and that growth of the organism in liquid medium may be slow. Other laboratory examinations are either normal or compatible with any febrile illness.

The subsequent course is dependent on therapy, although some patients with very mild disease recover spontaneously after several weeks or months. Any of the complications and sequelae of meningococcal infections may develop.

ACUTE FULMINATING MENINGOCOCCEMIA. This differs from the milder form in the rapidity with which it progresses and in its overwhelming character. The onset is usually abrupt and quite dramatic, with a shaking chill, severe headache, dizziness or vertigo, collapse, and unconsciousness. Patients with massive purpura, low blood pressure, rapid, quiet respiration, and overwhelming bacteremia are said to have the Waterhouse-Friderichsen syndrome. They are often clear mentally. Their extensive rash (see figure) involves skin and mucous membranes as well as internal organs such as skeletal muscle and, classically, the adrenal glands. Leukopenia is another indicator of the gravity of the patient's condition. Body temperature may be subnormal, normal, or elevated. Within a few hours there may be circulatory collapse with intravascular coagulation. Often there is a consumptive coagulopathy (see Ch. 140).

Others may have the encephalitic form, which is characterized by rapidly developing coma, rapid stertorous breathing, a petechial but not massive purpuric rash, and normal blood pressure. Some may present with a combination of encephalitis and adrenal involve-

Skin lesions in fulminating meningococcemia. (Courtesy of Dr. Worth B. Daniels.)

ment with early deep coma, low blood pressure, and purpura. Occasionally, the pituitary gland, like the adrenals, is damaged by hemorrhage. These severe illnesses are often rapidly fatal. It is in the attempt to prevent or to reverse this rapid course that so much emphasis is placed upon early, intensive treatment.

CHRONIC MENINGOCOCCEMIA. Chronic meningococcemia is an uncommon form of meningococcal disease in which episodes of fever of a few days' duration recur at intervals of days, weeks, or, more rarely, months. Chills and arthralgic symptoms are frequent, but rash may be absent or evanescent. Repeated cultures of the blood may be necessary before meningococci are recovered. Failure to suspect, recognize, and treat chronic meningococcemia may result in meningitis or endocarditis.

Meningitis. Although meningitis constitutes only a relatively small percentage of the total number of meningococcal infections, it is the most characteristic and important manifestation. The onset and symptoms are often indistinguishable from those of a generalized infection; in some, meningeal involvement seems to predominate. In others, both groups of symptoms appear almost simultaneously, but there may be great variations in their intensity and severity. In addition to the signs of sepsis and the rash, patients with meningitis have evidence of inflammation of the meninges: pain in the neck and back on forward flexion of the head, stiff neck, retraction of the head or severe opisthotonos, positive Kernig's and Brudzinski's signs, hyperesthesia, hyperirritability, and exaggerated reflexes. Unequal reflexes are unusual, but may be present. Involvement of the cranial nerves, when present, may result in strabismus and deafness. The increased intracranial pressure may lead to severe headache, nausea, vomiting, dilated or irregular pupils, engorgement of the fundal veins, choking of the discs, irregular slow pulse, and moderately elevated blood pressure. Cheyne-Stokes or Biot's respiration may appear. As the disease progresses, restlessness and irritability may be followed by delirium or by generalized or jacksonian type convulsions; the patient may become greatly depressed, somnolent, and finally stuporous and comatose. The signs of meningitis in infants may be no more than refusal of feedings, vomiting or regurgitation, diarrhea, irritability, and fever. Convulsions and bulging of the fontanelles may be noted in more severely ill young infants.

LABORATORY FINDINGS IN MENINGITIS. The cerebrospinal fluid is under increased pressure and varies from clear to frankly purulent. The cell count is elevated, often to thousands per cubic millimeter, mostly neutrophils. Gram-negative intra- and extracellular diplococci can be seen in variable numbers in stained smears of the sediment. The total protein in the cerebrospinal fluid is increased, and its sugar content is usually reduced. Meningococci may be grown from the fluid by proper cultural methods. Although fluid obtained early in meningitis may have few or no cells and no reduction of its glucose content, cultures often are positive.

COURSE OF MENINGITIS. Extremely variable, the course is greatly influenced by therapy. In untreated cases the temperature is erratic, and symptoms progress to early death or to chronic meningitis with severe sequelae or delayed death.

COMPLICATIONS OF MENINGOCOCCAL INFECTIONS. The complications of the different forms of meningococcal infections include intercurrent infec-

tions, metastatic localizations, and permanent damage to the central nervous system. These may appear during the acute stage or subsequently. Intercurrent infections of the respiratory tract with other agents may occur. Bacteremic or metastatic complications include conjunctivitis, panophthalmitis, otitis, purulent mono- or polyarthritis, pneumonia, pleurisy, pericarditis, myocarditis, endocarditis, orchitis, epididymitis, jaundice, hepatorenal failure, transient albuminuria and hematuria, and adrenal hemorrhage with necrosis. Infection of the central nervous system may produce convulsions, transient or permanent paralyses, hemiplegia, neuroradiculitis, encephalitis, encephalomyelitis, altered cerebration, cranial nerve damage, cerebral thrombosis, and brain abscess. Organization of exudate in the ventricular channels and the subarachnoid space may mechanically obstruct the flow of cerebrospinal fluid, producing hydrocephalus. The accumulation of subdural fluid of high protein content, which when encapsulated resembles a subdural hematoma, is fairly frequent in infants and young children. *Recurrent meningitis* caused by meningococci or other bacteria is usually due to structural defects of bone resulting from trauma or other causes which sometimes require surgical repair. Complications resulting from therapy can be avoided or minimized, if anticipated.

Permanent sequelae may result from almost any complication; the most frequent are deafness, ocular palsies, blindness, hydrocephalus, diminished intellectual capacity, and psychoses.

DIAGNOSIS. The specific diagnosis of meningococcal disease depends primarily upon differentiation from other acute systemic infections. Final confirmation of the diagnosis requires identification of a meningococcus as the causative organism. During an epidemic, especially in a recruit military camp or a closed population, all cases of fever with abrupt onset, of prostration with or without fever, of petechial or purpuric rash, of drowsiness or coma, and of meningitis should be treated vigorously as meningococcal infections whether or not organisms are found in initial smears and cultures.

Meningococcal infections in their early stages may resemble any acute systemic infection. In sepsis caused by pyogenic organisms such as staphylococci, streptococci, or pneumococci, there may be a preceding upper respiratory infection, recurrent fever, malaise, arthralgia, and leukocytosis. A rash similar to that of severe meningococcemia and even signs of the Waterhouse-Friderichsen syndrome may be present in such cases. Final proof of cause is accomplished by isolation of the offending organisms from the blood, joint fluid, sputum, and so forth. Meningococcal infections also must be differentiated from the acute exanthems, typhus (both endemic and epidemic), typhoid and other enteric fevers, subacute bacterial endocarditis, rheumatic fever, brucellosis, and others.

Diagnosis of Meningitis. The diagnosis of meningococcal meningitis requires differentiation from meningismus, other bacterial meningitides, viral meningoencephalitis, myeloencephalitis resulting from bacterial toxins (tetanus, botulinus) or chemicals, and noninfectious illnesses such as subarachnoid or cerebral hemorrhages or thrombosis, diabetic coma, and uremia. In most cases of meningococcal meningitis, the diagnosis is readily established by the specific identification of the organism; in others the cause may not be determinable when the patient is first seen, but a number of helpful procedures can be carried out. The usual medical history should be obtained with a careful inquiry into recent localized infections, especially of the ear. Trauma to the head should be investigated, because this predisposes to secondary bacterial meningitides, more likely to be caused by *H. influenzae* or pneumococci.

Physical examination should include a thorough search for diseases of the eyes and upper respiratory passages, sinuses, and ears, and for evidence of injury to the head, in addition to careful general and neurologic examinations. A complete blood count should be made and cultures of the blood and posterior nasopharynx obtained. Any suspected localized areas of infection likewise should be cultured. Urinalysis and determinations of serum electrolytes and the blood nonprotein nitrogen may aid in the differential diagnosis and help to indicate precautions to be observed in therapy. In seriously ill, or perhaps all, patients, blood coagulation analyses should be performed to determine the presence of a consumptive coagulopathy. Bleeding from the upper gastrointestinal tract ("stress ulcers") should be suspected in the very sick, especially those in shock.

Lumbar puncture should be performed as soon as possible and before specific treatment is instituted. After determining the initial pressure, fluid should be removed slowly until the pressure is reduced to an approximately normal level. The dynamics of the cerebrospinal fluids can then be estimated by jugular compression for evidence of block or sinus thrombosis. Examination of the cerebrospinal fluid should include the following: gross appearance, total and differential cell counts, determination of sugar (compare with blood level) and protein, and cultures and examination of Gram-stained smears. If organisms are seen, they can often be identified tentatively from their appearance and precisely with proper and *potent* antisera by a positive direct quellung test if of group A or C. Where the technique is available, counterimmunoelectrophoresis can be used, often successfully even when organisms are not seen on smear.

A *presumptive diagnosis* can usually be made from the Gram-stained smear, the differential cell count, and the sugar content of the cerebrospinal fluid. Caution should be exercised in the interpretation of smears, because even experienced observers may be misled by overdecolorized or dead gram-positive diplococci or other bacteria. Final identification depends on serogrouping organisms from culture. The leukocytes are almost entirely neutrophils in purulent meningitides, except for those caused by tubercle bacilli. In the latter, as in viral infections (mumps, herpes, coxsackieviruses, echoviruses and others), mononucleated cells predominate except in their early stages. The sugar content is usually decreased in bacterial meningitis and normal or elevated in viral infections. In meningismus the fluid is usually normal. The proportion of erythrocytes to leukocytes is similar to that in whole blood in cases of subarachnoid hemorrhage. The history, other physical findings, and special laboratory tests should help to differentiate myeloencephalitides resulting from toxins or chemicals.

TREATMENT. During the past 30 years, groups A, B, C, and, less often, Y meningococci have been responsible for almost all meningococcal infections regardless of their clinical forms. Until about 1963, practically all meningococcal strains were exquisitely susceptible to the sulfonamide drugs, whether in carriers or cases. For these reasons, the sulfonamides were the agents of choice for both treatment and prophylaxis. They are still excellent, but only when specific tests have demonstrated that the patient or carrier has a sulfonamide-susceptible organism.

Since sulfonamide-resistant group A, B, C, and Y strains are now commonplace, the treatment of choice is penicillin G in massive dosage. For adults, this means 20,000,000 units per day intravenously or 1,000,000 units every two hours intramuscularly. The latter route should not be used for patients in or on the verge of shock, because of possible failure of absorption. When the 20,000,000-unit dose is used intravenously, it is best to divide it into four or more doses per day rather than to administer it by continuous drip. Doses in children should be reduced in accordance with pediatric therapeutic principles.

Ampicillin may be used as an alternative, although an occasional patient does not seem to respond adequately to this drug. Close observation of the patient's course will alert the physician to this problem should it arise. The dose should be at least 150 mg per kilogram per day for children and 10 to 12 grams per day for adults, parenterally, divided into six to eight doses.

In patients known to be truly allergic to penicillin, and ill with sulfonamide-resistant strains of meningococci, chloramphenicol is the alternative drug of choice. The use of this drug imposes precautions of its own. These can be managed but close watch should be kept on the hematopoietic system and the drug withdrawn immediately if a complication appears. Thus far, no meningococci resistant to penicillin or chloramphenicol have been identified. If the patient's organism is found to be susceptible to sulfonamide, treatment can be altered accordingly. Cephalothins and lincomycin should not be used, because therapeutic failures have followed their administration.

Patients with meningococcal disease are usually more dehydrated than they appear. Care should be taken to ensure a daily urine output of more than 1000 ml. Treatment should be continued at least until all signs and symptoms have been normal for a minimum of two days and preferably for five. It may be stopped abruptly. Relapse occurs occasionally and requires prompt treatment.

Patients with fulminating meningococcemia or meningitis, or both, should be started on therapy as soon as the diagnosis is suspected and specimens obtained without waiting for bacteriologic confirmation. Penicillin should be given by vein. (Patients allergic to penicillin are best treated with chloramphenicol.) The central venous pressure should be monitored and corrected as necessary. Disseminated intravascular coagulation, when diagnosed, should be managed as in any other disease state (see Ch. 521.5). Norepinephrine, intravenously, may be required to maintain blood pressure. Steroids are clearly required if there is evidence of adrenal collapse; such patients are managed as are those with acute adrenal insufficiency. Otherwise, there is no good evidence that steroids are of any positive value. These severely ill patients are the most likely ones to bleed from gastric lesions ("stress ulcers") which require special handling, contraindicating steroids. Intravenous infusions will be required to correct dehydration, but an excess should be avoided. Oxygen therapy should be instituted and maintained as long as cyanosis or dyspnea is present. Blood transfusions have not been shown to be of significant value in this type of circulatory failure.

Certain laboratory tests such as *hematologic examinations* should be repeated as aids in monitoring the patient's course. This is especially true for patients admitted with severe leukopenia or thrombocytopenia. Their reversal is of considerable positive prognostic significance. *Blood cultures* should be repeated if the fever persists or returns, for continued bacteremia suggests the presence of endocarditis or other metastatic localization. *Repeat lumbar punctures* are indicated if there is persistent increased intracranial pressure, failure to respond to adequate therapy, or relapse of meningitis.

Symptomatic and supportive treatment is essential for patients with meningococcal infections. Sedation should be minimal, yet sufficient to assure adequate rest but not to interfere with the assessment of the patient's course. Approximately one month of convalescence is required for complete recovery in most cases and even more for those who had severe illnesses.

The treatment of complications of meningococcal infections is primarily that of the underlying disease. Should fever or signs of meningeal irritation reappear, then the most probable causes are recurrence of infection with the meningococcus because of inadequate treatment, drug fever, or superinfection with another organism. In such circumstances, the cerebrospinal fluid and blood should be re-examined and cultured. If the meningococcal infection has relapsed, intensive treatment should be reinstituted and maintained until the patient has fully recovered.

PROGNOSIS. The prognosis in meningococcal infections has improved enormously since the sulfonamides and penicillin became available. In untreated cases of meningococcemia and meningitis, the mortality formerly varied from 20 to 90 per cent, averaging about 70 per cent. The introduction of serum therapy reduced this to about 50 per cent. With the sulfonamides, the case fatality rate was reduced to 5 to 10 per cent, depending upon age and complicating conditions. The recent recognition of sulfonamide-resistant meningococci has not altered this significantly, because cases can be treated as successfully with penicillin. Age is perhaps the most important factor in prognosis, for the greatest mortality, despite adequate therapy, occurs in those less than 2 or more than 40 years old. In the U.S. Army during World War II, the over-all mortality was slightly less than 5 per cent and, in some series, even below 1 per cent. More than 90 per cent of these cases were caused by sulfonamide-susceptible group A strains. In addition to a most favorable age distribution in the Army, the excellent physical condition of patients, early diagnosis, and the prompt institution of effective therapy were probably responsible for this remarkable recovery rate. The prognosis is still poor in fulminating cases with abrupt onset, extensive cutaneous lesions, and circulatory collapse. In spite of rapid, intensive therapy, such cases frequently terminate fatally. Relapses, recurrences, and complications have been greatly reduced by specific treatment so that the prognosis for total recovery is generally good. The most frequent permanent sequelae despite adequate treatment are deafness, cranial nerve paralyses, mental deficiency, and, less often, blindness and hydrocephalus. These are all relatively

uncommon and usually result from treatment delays for whatever cause.

PREVENTION. Prophylaxis as applied to meningococcal infections during the past 30 years represented an outgrowth of the World War II experience, which indicated not only that sulfadiazine rapidly cured meningococcal disease but also that the nasopharyngeal carrier state was reversed (not true of penicillin) soon after such treatment was begun. After several successful trials in military recruits, a policy was adopted whereby small amounts of sulfadiazine were administered simultaneously to all members of recruit training centers, schools, ships, and similar groups upon the recognition of a predetermined number of cases. This resulted in an immediate reduction in carriers and a sharp decrease in cases, reflecting the interaction of a susceptible organism with an effective drug when administered to a total population at risk. Because of the fears often generated by the diagnosis of meningitis, the same sulfadiazine regimen was adopted for general use by physicians and health departments to treat family and hospital (staff) contacts of sporadic cases. But the "secondary" cases which occasionally occur in households usually begin within 96 hours or less of that of the index patient, suggesting that they may be co-primary rather than secondary. Less often, this interval may be as long as seven to ten days. It would seem then that if disease is to be prevented under such circumstances, therapeutic rather than "prophylactic" medication is needed. Unless the causative strain is known to be sulfonamide susceptible, it must be assumed to be resistant, requiring penicillin dosage in the therapeutic range. If taken orally, this will require 8 million or more units per day in young or older adults. Suitably reduced doses should be prescribed for children. Either oral or parenteral regimens for *streptococcal prophylaxis* provide *no* protection for meningococcal infections.

The recommendation for meningococcal disease is really for intervention rather than prevention. Alternatively, one can observe closely (including nasopharyngeal cultures) and treat immediately upon the appearance of any symptoms. But over-all, the risk is very low and should not induce the hysteria which so often accompanies the hospital admission or diagnosis of a case of meningococcal meningitis. The isolation of patients after 24 to 48 hours of adequate therapy is not indicated.

Although the foregoing is suitable for the immediate contact or family, it is not applicable to a population group such as in a camp, school, or mental institution. In such instances the objective is to rapidly reduce the over-all carrier level to a point at which transfer is impeded, decreasing the case rate. Again, sulfonamides are the most effective drugs for this purpose, but only when the causative organisms are susceptible. Penicillin, in contrast to sulfonamides, often fails to eliminate the carrier state, even in therapeutic doses. Rifampin (600 mg daily for five days) has been used for this purpose in military and civilian populations. Meningococcal carrier rates are reduced quite effectively by rifampin, but resistance does occur and increases with reuse. Recent experience has indicated considerable toxicity with minocycline so that it has been all but discontinued for meningococcal prophylaxis. The widespread use of rifampin in populations with high tuberculosis rates probably should be exercised with some caution because of possible increased resistance among tubercle bacilli. At no time should rifampin be used for the treatment of cases of meningococcal disease.

Vaccines. There is considerable reason for optimism regarding meningococcal vaccines. Potent group-specific polysaccharides have been prepared from meningococci of groups A, C, and Y but not yet from B. After very careful graduated trials, group C meningococcal polysaccharide vaccine, in single subcutaneous doses of 50 μg, was made routine for all American military recruits. Disease caused by this serogroup has all but been eliminated from that population. Group A polysaccharide vaccine has been found to be equally effective in a Finnish epidemic and among South African miners, and combined group A and C vaccine also was efficacious in the massive Brazilian epidemic which was caused by organisms of both serogroups. The duration of protection has not yet been established, although it would appear likely to be of long duration. Measurable responses to polysaccharide vaccines are quite different and diminished in children (especially under 18 months of age) than adults. Although group A and C polysaccharide vaccines have been licensed in the United States and elsewhere, they are not available for general use in the United States.

Artenstein, M. S., Gold, R., Zimmerly, J. G., Wyle, F. A., Schneider, H., and Harkins, C.: Prevention of meningococcal disease by group C polysaccharide vaccine. N. Engl. J. Med., 282:417, 1970.

Evans, R. W., Glick, B., Kimball, F., and Lobell, M.: Fatal intravascular consumption coagulopathy in meningococcal sepsis. Am. J. Med., 46:910, 1969.

Feldman, H. A.: Neisseria infections other than gonococcal. In Bodily, H. L., Updyke, E. L., and Mason, J. O. (eds.): Diagnostic Procedures for Bacterial, Mycotic and Parasitic Infections. 5th ed. New York, American Public Health Association, Inc., 1970.

Feldman, H. A.: Meningococcal infections. In Stollerman, G. H. (ed.): Advances in Internal Medicine, Vol. 18. Chicago, Year Book Medical Publishers, 1972, pp. 117–140.

Makela, P. H., Kayhty, H., Weckstrom, P., Sivonen, A., and Renkonen, O.-V.: Effect of group-A meningococcal vaccine in army recruits in Finland. Lancet, 2:883, 1975.

142. HEMOPHILUS INFECTIONS WITH SPECIAL EMPHASIS ON HEMOPHILUS INFLUENZAE TYPE B

John B. Robbins

Pfeiffer, in 1892, identified the genus *Hemophilus* from the sputum of individuals with respiratory disease during an influenza pandemic. The requirement of the microbe for whole blood prompted his designation *Hemophilus influenzae*. Studies, especially during the influenza pandemics of 1917 and 1918, revealed that this organism was not the etiologic cause of influenza. Subsequently, other bacterial species have been designated *Hemophilus* because of similar morphology, physiology, and growth requirement for blood-enriched media (see accompanying table). All *Hemophilus* species are facultatively aerobic, nonmotile, and nonsporeforming. *H. influenzae* is the most important for its potential for serious human disease.

Clinical Differentiation of *Hemophilus* Species

Species	Normal Habitat	Growth Factor Requirement		Hemolysis
		X	V	
H. influenzae	Upper respiratory tract	+	+	−
H. parainfluenzae	Upper respiratory tract	−	+	−
H. aegyptius	Upper respiratory tract, eye	+	+	−
H. hemolyticus	Upper respiratory tract	+	+	+
H. parahemolyticus	Upper respiratory tract	−	+	+
H. ducreyi	Genital	+	−	+

ETIOLOGY. *H. influenzae* exists in the encapsulated form (opalescent colonies) with raised mucoid appearance and the uncapsulated form (flat bluish translucent colonies). On optimal media, the organisms appear as comparatively small uniform coccobacilli (1 to 1.5 by 0.3 μ). However, under less than optimal conditions, especially in body fluids, *H. influenzae* exhibits polymorphism and may be long slender filaments, often attaining a length of 20 to 30 μ. Its bipolar bodies may retain the gram-positive stain under certain conditions, and *H. influenzae* has often been mistaken for pneumococci or meningococci. *H. influenzae* requires V factor (heat labile, NAD) and X factor (hemin). These nutritive factors are the basis for differentiation among *Hemophilus* species (see table).

Occasionally, mistakes may be made by the exuberant transfer of colonies from chocolate agar (containing both growth factors) to a differential medium. In this case, the small amounts of nutrients carried over on thick swabs may be sufficient to allow other *Hemophilus* species to grow, resulting in confusion, such as has occurred between *H. parainfluenzae* and *H. influenzae*. *H. influenzae* will grow in any enriched nonselective medium. Complex mixtures, such as brain-heart infusion plus hemolyzed blood, provide the most effective medium in the author's experience. Enriched media, such as chocolate agar, lose their nutritive activity because of the factor V decay. Further, if the blood supplement is not carefully prepared (extensive heat may destroy its enriching properties), laboratories may fail to report *H. influenzae* isolates. Quality control measures, such as growing standardized *H. influenzae* strains, should be practiced. The "satellite" phenomenon is often used to accelerate the growth of *H. influenzae* on blood agar. In this technique, the formation of NAD and hemin mediated by *Staphylococcus aureus* provides a local environment that favors *Hemophilus* growth.

As defined by Pittman, there are six chemically and serologically distinct capsular polysaccharide antigens. With the use of the appropriate antisera, these capsular polysaccharides may be visualized on fresh isolates or bacteria grown under optimal conditions by a variety of techniques, including the quellung reaction and immunoprecipitation. Although the over-all chemical and physical properties of the six capsules are similar, virtually all serious human disease is caused by type b.

ECOLOGY. *H. influenzae* is usually found in the upper respiratory tract. The nonencapsulated form can be recovered from nasopharyngeal cultures of about 80 per cent of healthy individuals. In contrast, encapsulated organisms, especially type b, are found in comparatively few individuals (1 to 3 per cent) during infancy and early childhood and only rarely in healthy adults. In cases of severe systemic *H. influenzae* type b disease, case contacts, including siblings and parents, usually have positive cultures.

PATHOGENICITY AND IMMUNITY. The relation of the type b capsule to systemic disease with *H. influenzae* resembles that observed for pneumococcal and meningococcal capsular polysaccharides. The presence of the capsule inhibits effective phagocytosis. However, the mechanism by which *H. influenzae* type b invades the nasopharyngeal mucosa of only some individuals is not known. It has been suggested that toxic substances in this organism may inhibit ciliary action or that simultaneous infection with some viruses may predispose to septicemia. Pathogen-free infant rat models suggest that the escape of one organism into the blood in a nonimmune individual is sufficient to cause septicemia. When concentration of organisms in the blood reaches a critical level (approximately 10^3 per milliliter), the chance of penetrating the meninges increases considerably.

Immunity to systemic disease is mediated by serum antibodies. Serum concentrations of 0.15 to 0.2 μg of anti-type b antibodies have been shown to be protective. However, complete protection against this disease with currently available *H. influenzae* type b capsular polysaccharide vaccines in infants up to 18 months has not yet been achieved because of poor immunogenicity in this high-risk age group. Antibodies to other surface bacterial components, such as outer membrane proteins and lipopolysaccharides, may also confer protection. Their use as potential vaccines is also under study. Other host resistance mechanisms are important, as shown by the extreme susceptibility of individuals who have splenic dysfunction, such as is seen in excessive hemolytic states as sickle cell anemia or its variants, in splenectomy, or in congenital absence of the spleen. Individuals with deficient immunoglobulin synthesis, including highly specialized defects such as that of IgG 2, are extraordinarily susceptible to repeated and severe *H. influenzae* type b disease. Passive immunization of X-linked hypogammaglobulinemia patients with pooled immunoglobulin is highly effective preventive therapy.

Meningitis is the most important and frequent of serious systemic disease with *H. influenzae* type b. This organism is the leading cause of all bacterial meningitis in the United States. Other important *H. influenzae* type b diseases include epiglottitis, pyoarthrosis, and pneumonia and its complications, including empyema, osteomyelitis, and pericarditis. Occasionally, superficial and deep cellulitis in the buccal area may occur. This may be recognized by a bluish hue to the surrounding tissues and is usually accompanied by a septicemia. The over-all incidence in the United States is 4.5 per 100,000, but in children up to five years of age the incidence is 50 to 80 per 100,000. The incidence is also much higher in adults with acquired immunologic defects. In one survey, *H. influenzae* type b was found to be the most common cause of bacterial meningitis in adults in New York City. Some have suggested that the frequency of *H. influenzae* type b diseases has recently increased, but improved laboratory facilities and increasing awareness of this organism as a pathogen may have contributed to these figures. Unusually high attack rates of systemic *H. influenzae* type b diseases, including meningitis, occur in certain communities and closed populations such as day care nurseries.

DIAGNOSIS. Systemic disease with *H. influenzae* type b is most accurately diagnosed by identification of the organism in body fluids, such as the blood, cerebrospinal fluid, or pleural fluid. Care must be taken that the medium used for cultivation of the organism is fresh and can sustain *H. influenzae* growth. The use of 5 per cent carbon dioxide and high humidity environment increases the rapidity with which the organism can be identified and recovered from fluids with low concentration of organisms or in patients treated with antimicrobials.

Immunochemical identification of the capsule may be accomplished by the quellung reaction of fresh isolates and by the demonstration of the capsular material in body fluids. The use of concentrated urine samples from patients with systemic disease with *H. influenzae* type b is very productive. There are many bacterial antigens cross-reactive with the type b capsular polysaccharide, including one *E. coli* capsular type, K100; also, gram-positive bacteria containing ribitol phosphate as a component of their cell wall teichoic acid, including pneumococcus types 6B, 29, and 34, some *Bacillus* species, and *S. aureus,* could yield false-positive reactions. In addition, circulating type b antigen may be masked by host antibody. In this case, dissociation techniques for measuring type b antigen have been reported. The determination of trace and unique *H. influenzae* type b metabolites by more sophisticated techniques seems promising, but such techniques are not yet available in most centers.

Meningitis caused by *H. influenzae* type b does not present any distinctive clinical features (see Ch. 140).

Epiglottitis caused by this organism presents an acute clinical emergency in any age group. The appearance of upper respiratory obstruction associated with a clinical infection, especially with fever, pain, and no external swelling, should alert the physician to the possibility of *H. influenzae* type b epiglottitis. Direct visualization of the inflamed, cherry red epiglottis is diagnostic. In many cases, the simple maneuvering of the tongue may acutely increase the respiratory obstruction, and tracheal intubation or tracheostomy may be necessary. Thus facilities must be at hand if this acute infectious upper respiratory obstruction is suspected.

Fever of unknown origin in children is often due to *H. influenzae* type b. Such individuals respond rapidly to proper therapy without evidence of localized disease. However, complications or blood-borne infections such as meningitis and osteomyelitis may occur.

TREATMENT. Prior to the availability of effective therapeutic agents, systemic *H. influenzae* diseases, particularly meningitis and epiglottitis, had at least a 95 per cent mortality. Currently, highly effective antimicrobial drugs, including ampicillin and chloramphenicol, are available. However, the use of ampicillin has been curtailed because of the widespread emergence of beta lactamase–producing *H. influenzae* type b disease isolates. Surveillance studies in many communities indicate that at least 10 per cent of disease isolates produce this inactivating enzyme. The diagnosis of ampicillin resistance is achieved by acid liberated from penicillin or a chromogen for a cephalin derivative synthesized for penicillinase detection. Chloramphenicol, despite its bone marrow toxicity, provides a highly effective agent for the treatment of all systemic *H. influenzae* type b diseases, including meningitis and arthritis. However, some disease isolates have shown resistance to chloramphenicol and tetracycline. It is now recommended that all *systemic* diseases with

H. influenzae type b be treated with chloramphenicol until their drug resistance patterns can be determined. Ampicillin remains the drug of choice for susceptible organisms. Surveillance is necessary to assess the frequency of the drug resistance patterns.

Antimicrobial therapy for meningitis has been recommended for approximately seven to ten days (see Ch. 140). Cellular and protein levels may require more than two weeks to return to normal. In children, persistent fever with meningitis may signify localized collections of fluid. Signs of increasing intracranial pressure or localizing signs may warrant further diagnostic studies to identify such complications as subdural empyema or intracortical abscess formation. Endocarditis or pericarditis caused by *H. influenzae* type b has been treated successfully by approximately four to six weeks of therapy. The other aspects of treatment of meningitis, mentioned in Ch. 140, apply to the treatment of *H. influenzae* type b diseases at all ages.

Other H. Influenzae Diseases. Nonencapsulated *H. influenzae* organisms are frequently found in the respiratory tracts of individuals with chronic lung disease. Their pathogenic role has been incompletely defined, but it seems probable that high sputum populations of *H. influenzae* in those with chronic lung disease exert a deleterious effect. The finding of *H. influenzae* in the sputum of patients with chronic lung disease poses a therapeutic problem. Most physicians feel that when this finding is accompanied by signs of respiratory infection, antimicrobial therapy is indicated. Treatment resulting in diminution or disappearance of *H. influenzae* from the sputum of such patients often results in marked relief of symptoms such as fever, cough, and dyspnea. *H. influenzae* is often found in the exudate of infants and children with middle ear infection. In most cases, these are nonencapsulated organisms and the response to antimicrobial therapy is rapid. In about 3 to 4 per cent of cases, however, type b organisms may be isolated directly from middle ear aspirants. This finding may be accompanied by *H. influenzae* type b systemic disease, including meningitis. Accurate etiologic diagnosis of otitis media with nasopharyngeal cultures is not possible. Accordingly, in most instances, acute otitis media is treated with the antimicrobial drugs designed to combat the agents most often responsible for this infectious disease in the appropriate age group.

PREVENTION. It has been reported with increasing frequency that secondary cases of *H. influenzae* type b disease, especially meningitis, may occur under certain unusual conditions, such as day care nurseries or chronic care institutions. In this case, there have been reports of trials with various antimicrobial agents and immunization with the purified capsular polysaccharide. The latter, in its present form, prevents disease in individuals for more than two years. Various antimicrobials, including ampicillin for the treatment of drug-susceptible organisms, sulfonamides, and others, have been used without any clear definition of their effectiveness in preventing further disease in outbreak situations. It should be realized that secondary cases occur among families, especially when there are siblings of susceptible age in close contact with the affected patient. Indeed, the secondary attack rate under certain circumstances is comparable to that for meningococcal disease. Attempts at disease prevention of siblings should include antimicrobial regimens designed to treat meningitis. The morbidity (fixed central nervous deficits) remains high even after optimal therapy, and vaccine development for prevention is under active research.

Other Human Hemophilus Species. *H. influenzae* types a, c, d, e, and f, as well as *H. parainfluenzae, H. aphrophilus*, and *H. hemolyticus*, occasionally are isolated from individuals with systemic bacterial infections. There is yet no known predisposing lesion to identify the pathogenic processes involved in infection with such unusual organisms. The treatment of these *Hemophilus* infections requires no unusual therapy except for the caution that their isolation may be impeded by the use of conventional or outdated media. *H. aegyptius* is the cause of a severe form of conjunctivitis. This form of conjunctivitis may occur in epidemic form, especially in the summer among crowded communities such as those seen in summer camps. Its diagnosis can be achieved by direct smear of the purified fluid or by cultivation on appropriate media. Therapy with antimicrobials is successful. Drug resistance among these *Hemophilus* species has been reported, but its frequency is not well characterized.

H. ducreyi is the cause of chancroid. This venereal disease is characterized by a one- to two-week incubation with centrally ulcerating lesions of about 2 to 20 ml on or in the immediate genital area. There is usually painful nonindurated lymphadenopathy accompanying these lesions. Suppuration of the regional lymph nodes may make the diagnosis of simultaneous syphilis difficult. Sulfadiazine remains the treatment of choice for chancroid, but it should be realized that the symptoms of chancroid may obscure simultaneous infection with syphilis, which requires a different therapy (see Ch. 171).

Peltola, H., Kayhty, H., Sivonen, A., and Makela, P. H.: *Haemophilus influenzae* type b capsular polysaccharide vaccine in children: A double blind field study of 100,000 vaccinees 3 months to 5 years of age in Finland. Pediatrics 60:730, 1977.

Pittman, M.: Variation and type specificity in the bacterial species *Haemophilus influenzae*. J. Exp. Med., 53:471, 1931.

Robbins, J. B., and Hill, J. C. (eds.): Current status and prospects for improved and new bacterial vaccines. A symposium held at the National Institutes of Health, Bethesda, Maryland, March 29–April 1, 1976. J. Infect. Dis., *136* (suppl.), August 1977.

Robbins, J. B., Schneerson, R., Argaman, M., and Handzel, Z. T.: *Haemophilus influenzae* type b: Disease and immunity in humans. Ann. Intern. Med., 78:259, 1973.

Schneerson, R., and Robbins, J.: Induction of serum *Haemophilus influenzae* type b capsular antibodies in adult volunteers fed cross-reacting *Escherichia coli* 075:K 100:H5. N. Engl. J. Med., 292:1093, 1975.

Smith, D. H., Ingram, D. L., Smith, R. L., Gilles, F., and Bresnan, M. J.: Bacterial meningitis. A symposium. Pediatrics, 52:586, 1973.

WHOOPING COUGH

143. WHOOPING COUGH

(Pertussis)

Stephen I. Morse

DEFINITION. Whooping cough is an acute respiratory illness that classically affects infants and young children. The etiologic agent is usually *Bordetella pertussis;* occasionally *B. parapertussis* and rarely *B. bronchiseptica* produce a similar syndrome. The descriptive name derives from a distressing, prolonged inspiratory effort that follows paroxysmal coughing. Whooping cough is still responsible for a significant number of deaths in infants in areas where pertussis immunization is not practiced.

HISTORY. The disease was first recorded in the middle of the sixteenth century by Moulton and by DeBaillou. Whether whooping cough was indigenous to Europe or had been transported there in the preceding century is uncertain. Sydenham applied the name "pertussis" to any illness accompanied by violent coughing, but the term became restricted to the epidemic disease that was a well-recognized clinical entity by the middle of the eighteenth century. In 1900 Bordet and Gengou observed coccobacilli in the sputum of a child with whooping cough, but it was not until 1906 that they were able to culture the organism. Many years passed before the Bordet-Gengou bacillus was universally accepted as the etiologic agent of whooping cough was indigenous to Europe or had been transmorphologic changes on prolonged cultivation, thereby accounting for the difficulties in establishing the etiologic role of the agent and the inconstant protective effect of immunizing preparations. Although the mortality rate of whooping cough in the United States began to decline in the early part of this century, the incidence in young children did not significantly decrease until after the use of prophylactic vaccines became widespread.

ETIOLOGY. When first isolated, *Bordetella pertussis* is a minute, nonmotile, weakly staining, gram-negative coccobacillus, 0.5 to 1.0 μ in length. Capsules can be demonstrated by special procedures, and bipolar metachromatic granules are present. The complex medium containing blood originally employed by Bordet and Gengou is still often used for cultivation. *Primary isolates, phase I organisms, will not grow on conventional laboratory media,* but will do so after prolonged passage. At the same time colonial morphology changes, marked pleomorphism of individual cells is evident, and there is an alteration in antigenic composition. This occurs in a series of phases, and the change from phase I to phase IV has been likened to the smooth to rough transition of other microbes. Only phase I organisms are virulent, and *only phase I organisms* provide effective immunizing material.

Members of the *Bordetella* genus were formerly regarded as species of *Hemophilus.* However, the *Bordetella* group does not have the strict requirement for X and V growth factors, and they are antigenically distinct. The addition of blood to Bordet-Gengou medium is required for the growth of phase I organisms, but the blood acts to neutralize bacterial substances, probably fatty acids, rather than to provide nutrients. Charcoal, starch, or ion exchange resins can be substituted for blood.

B. pertussis produces a heat-stable toxin (endotoxin) and a heat-labile toxin. A role of toxins in the development of disease has not been demonstrated. A hemagglutinin has also been isolated. The capsular material does not swell in the presence of antiserum. A species agglutinogen has been recognized as well as agglutinating factors that differ between strains. Serotyping is therefore a useful epidemiologic tool. The role of the interaction between the organism and phagocytes has not been defined, although the presence of antisera appears to increase uptake of *B. pertussis* by leukocytes.

Remarkable biologic effects are induced in laboratory animals by the injection of killed phase I organisms. These include development of heightened sensitivity to histamine and serotonin; increased susceptibility to anaphylaxis and to experimental allergic encephalomyelitis; increased antibody production, including reaginic antibody, in response to heterologous antigens; and hyperleukocytosis and hyperlymphocytosis. The factors responsible for these reactions have not been characterized fully.

It should be emphasized that none of the cellular components or products of *B. pertussis* have been shown to be of central importance in the pathogenesis of whooping cough.

Approximately 5 to 10 per cent of clinical whooping cough is caused by *B. parapertussis.* The animal pathogen *B. bronchiseptica* is responsible for a very minor percentage of cases. These organisms can be differentiated from *B. pertussis* by appropriate further bacteriologic or serologic procedures. It has recently been suggested that adenoviruses, along or in concert with *B. pertussis,* may play an etiologic role in some cases of whooping cough.

EPIDEMIOLOGY. In communities of susceptibles the family attack rate is 80 to 90 per cent, which is extremely high for a bacterial disease, approaching that seen in varicella or measles. Transmission is by droplet infection. Carriers of *B. pertussis* are found infrequently, and the reservoir is therefore unknown. Disease usually occurs in late winter in the northern climates and in late spring in southern zones, but there is great variation.

The mortality rate from whooping cough has fallen since the turn of this century owing to improved supportive therapy. The incidence of whooping cough, however, did not change until after the 1940's, when immunization of young children became standard practice. In the five-year periods 1926–1930, 1936–1940, 1956–1960, and 1965–1969, the fatality rate per thousand cases in the United States was 39.1, 19.4, 6.8, and 5.9 respectively. In the same time frames, the number of reported cases was 909,705; 956,262; 146,989; and 32,329, respectively. The majority of deaths, over 70 per cent, occur in children under one year of age, with the preponderance in infants under the age of six months.

Neither immunization against pertussis nor natural disease provides lifelong protection. In the case of artificial immunization, an attack rate greater than 50 per cent has been reported when the interval after immunization exceeds 12 years, a rate no different from that in unimmunized individuals of the same age. Thus in the face of routine immunization, it is possible that pertussis will become primarily a disease of older children and adults.

PATHOLOGY. Interpretation of pathologic material obtained at autopsy is difficult because of the common presence of complicating respiratory infections. Lesions caused by *B. pertussis* are found principally in the bronchi and bronchioles, but changes are also seen in the nasopharynx, larynx, and trachea. Masses of bacteria are intertwined with the cilia of the columnar epithelium together with mucopurulent exudate. There is also necrosis of the midzonal and basilar epithelium with infiltration of polymorphonuclear leukocytes and macrophages. Peribronchial accumulation of lymphocytes and granulocytes produces the picture of interstitial pneumonitis. Secondary atelectasis and localized emphysema are common. The alveoli in uncomplicated whooping cough do not contain exudate.

CLINICAL MANIFESTATIONS. After an incubation period of 7 to 16 days, symptoms appear. It is customary to divide the clinical course into three stages, each of two weeks' duration, but variation is frequent, particularly in the immunized community.

Catarrhal Stage. Whooping cough begins with symptoms indistinguishable from those of a mild viral upper respiratory infection or common cold. Sneezing is frequent, the conjunctivae are injected, and a nocturnal cough appears. The temperature may be slightly elevated at this time. Infectivity is greatest during the catarrhal stage.

Paroxysmal Stage. Seven to 14 days after onset, the cough becomes more frequent, diurnal, and then paroxysmal. In a typical paroxysm there is a series of 15 to 20 short coughs of increasing intensity, and then with a deep inspiration the air is drawn into the lungs, making the "whoop." A tenacious mucus plug is usually expelled, and vomiting frequently follows the spasmodic episode. Paroxysms may occur as often as every half hour, and are accompanied by signs of increased venous pressure. The conjunctivae are deeply engorged; there is periorbital edema; and petechial hemorrhages, particularly about the forehead, as well as epistaxis are common. During the attack the infant may be cyanotic until the crowing whoop occurs. In between paroxysms the child usually feels well though justifiably apprehensive.

Physical examination of the chest is usually unremarkable, although scattered rhonchi may be heard. The chest roentgenogram sometimes reveals hilar and mediastinal nodal enlargement. The presence of fever immediately suggests the development of a secondary infectious process.

Convalescent Stage. Gradually the paroxysms become less frequent and less intense, vomiting ceases, and slow recovery ensues. Often for many months even a mild, unrelated respiratory infection will be manifested by a return of paroxysmal cough and whoop.

It is important to recognize those patients with whooping cough in whom variation from the pattern frequently occurs. In young infants the paroxysms and the whoop are often absent; instead, choking spells and apneic periods may be the major manifestations. Second attacks of whooping cough as well as disease occurring in previously immunized individuals often present simply as an upper respiratory illness or bronchitis.

Complications. Complications may be related to the primary disease or to secondary events. Alterations in acid-base balance occur as a result of metabolic alkalosis when vomiting is severe. Recurrent vomiting can also lead to malnutrition. Anoxemic manifestations are seen when ventilation is markedly impaired. Central nervous system changes can result from cerebral anoxia or hemorrhages consequent to the elevated venous pressure. Rarely, cortical degeneration occurs, but the exact pathogenesis of the encephalopathy is unknown. A serous meningitis with lymphocytosis of the cerebrospinal fluid has been described. Localized areas of emphysema and atelectasis generally return to normal after the disease has run its course, and pneumothorax and interstitial emphysema are infrequently seen.

The major cause of death in whooping cough is complicating pneumonia or bronchopneumonia caused by other bacteria or viruses. In addition, secondary bacterial otitis media occurs frequently.

DIAGNOSIS. There is little difficulty in making the clinical diagnosis of whooping cough in a patient who, after a variable period of coryzal symptoms, develops paroxysmal coughing with a terminal inspiratory whoop. Toward the end of the catarrhal stage, or early in the spasmodic phase, leukocytosis often occurs. In contrast to the leukocytosis found in most bacterial diseases, the predominating cell type is the mature small lymphocyte. Characteristically the leukocyte count ranges from 15,000 to 30,000 per cubic millimeter, and 80 per cent of the cells are small lymphocytes. However, the leukocyte count either may be normal or may reach a level greater than 100,000 per cubic millimeter. Polymorphonuclear leukocytosis suggests a secondary bacterial complication.

Difficulty in recognizing whooping cough occurs in the catarrhal stage, in abortive or mild cases, and in young infants. Epidemiologic awareness may suggest the possibility, but microbiologic identification of the organisms is required. During the early stages of whooping cough *B. pertussis* can be isolated from approximately 90 per cent of patients. By the third or fourth week of illness the organism can be recovered in only 50 per cent of cases, and in the convalescent stage it is unusual to obtain a positive culture.

Adequate specimens and appropriate media are essential if bacteriologic diagnosis is to be efficient. *Specimens are best obtained by pernasal swab rather than by the cough plate method.* A sterile cotton swab wrapped about a flexible copper wire is passed through the nares, and mucus is obtained from the posterior pharynx. The swab must not be allowed to dry out because *B. pertussis* is readily killed by desiccation. As quickly as possible the specimen is plated onto fresh Bordet-Gengou medium, to which penicillin has been added to prevent overgrowth of adventitious organisms. Incubation is at 35° C, and although the trained observer can recognize the small, bisected pearl colonies of *B. pertussis* within 48 hours, at least 72 hours of growth is usually required. Presumptive identification can be made by agglutination tests with appropriate antisera. It is virtually impossible to distinguish between *Bordetella* species on primary isolation except by serologic means.

A fluorescent antibody staining procedure that can be applied directly to clinical specimens as well as to organisms grown in culture is now in more general use.

Serologic procedures are of little help in the diagnosis of whooping cough because a rise in titer of most antibodies does not occur until at least the third week of illness.

It is difficult to distinguish abortive or mild cases of pertussis from tracheobronchitis caused by other agents except by bacteriologic means. On the other hand, paroxysmal coughing may be associated with pulmonary lesions such as allergic bronchitis, atypical pneumonia, or cystic fibrosis.

TREATMENT. Mild cases of pertussis require only supportive treatment. Specific therapy of severe whooping cough has been disappointing despite the in vitro susceptibility of *B. pertussis* to various antimicrobial agents and the protective effect of passively administered antibody in experimental disease.

Antimicrobials. A number of antimicrobial drugs have significant in vitro activity against *B. pertussis*. Agents that readily eradicate the organisms in human disease may shorten the course of the illness if given in the catarrhal or early paroxysmal stages. In the established paroxysmal stage the organisms can also be readily eliminated by antimicrobials, but the course of the illness is unaltered. Even in the paroxysmal stage the use of drugs is justified in order to render the patient noninfectious.

Erythromycin, oxytetracycline, and several other drugs are effective in eliminating organisms. Erythromycin is the drug of choice. The daily dose is 50 mg per kilogram of body weight given in four divided doses. The organism is eliminated after a few days of therapy, but because bacteriologic relapse may occur, treatment should be continued for 10 to 14 days.

Immunotherapy. Hyperimmune human gamma globulin is used in therapy of unimmunized patients, particularly small infants, but its effect is controversial. The usual dose is 1.25 or 2.5 ml intramuscularly for three successive days.

Supportive Therapy. Particularly in the young infant, supportive measures combined with careful nursing care are of paramount importance. Specific attention must be devoted to the maintenance of proper water and electrolyte balance, adequate nutrition, and sufficient oxygenation. Constant alertness for the presence of secondary infectious complications such as pneumonia is required, and appropriate therapy should be promptly instituted upon discovery.

PREVENTION. The great communicability of whooping cough, particularly during the first few weeks of illness, makes it desirable to isolate the patient for four to six weeks, or, ideally, until cultures are negative. Unfortunately, the diagnosis is usually not made until the end of the catarrhal stage, and by then spread of the disease has already occurred. Exposed susceptibles should receive erythromycin prophylaxis, and contacts under four years of age who have been previously immunized should receive a booster dose of vaccine in addition to erythromycin. Booster doses of vaccine have been used to protect adults, such as hospital staff, but side effects tend to be frequent, and erythromycin chemoprophylaxis may be preferable.

Active Immunization. The fall in incidence of whooping cough in the very young is directly related to widespread immunization with suitable, killed suspensions of *B. pertussis*. The highest risk of serious morbidity and mortality is in the young infant. Women of childbearing age generally do not have significant levels of protective antibody in their sera, and consequently the newborn are not protected by maternal antibodies. Therefore active immunization is begun as early as is commensurate with the production of a satisfactory immune response. At present, it is recommended that the infant receive three injections of pertussis vaccine at one-month intervals beginning at 6 to 12 weeks of age. Each injection provides four NIH* units. The NIH unitage is based upon the ability of a vaccine to protect mice against a standard intracerebral infection. The pertussis suspension is usually incorporated into a triple vaccine with alum-precipitated diphtheria and tetanus toxoids (DPT). Booster injections are given one and five years after completion of the initial course. Administration of pertussis vaccine to those over six years of age is not generally recommended because of an apparent increased incidence of untoward reactions. However, low doses have been administered to adults without incident. There is no protection against parapertussis.

As previously noted, immunization does not confer lifelong protection. Approximately 80 per cent of those vaccinated within four years of exposure will be protected, whereas 80 to 90 per cent of a matched unimmunized group with similar exposure will contract pertussis. However, as the time after immunization increases, the attack rate in both groups approaches 50 per cent.

Instances of "vaccine failure" have usually been shown to be due to the use of preparations of low potency. However, it has been suggested that a change in the dominant serotype causing disease, unrepresented in certain vaccine preparations, may be of importance. This controversial point is under study.

Local reactions as well as fever may occur after injection of pertussis vaccine. The exact incidence of the more severe complication of encephalopathy is uncertain, but both fatalities and residua have been reported. The occurrence of neurotoxicity appears to be decreasing as more refined immunizing suspensions are used, and certain soluble extracts of *B. pertussis* may prove to be effective without engendering serious side effects. Despite the small, but real, incidence of neurologic complications of pertussis immunization, the risk still seems far less than the hazards of whooping cough in the young child. Nevertheless, in infants with a personal or family history of convulsions or other neurologic disorders, pertussis immunization should be deferred, or very small doses should be cautiously administered. Care should also be exercised in the immunization of children with a family history of an allergic diathesis.

Linneman, C. C., Jr., Ramundo, N., Perlstein, P. H., Minton, S. D., Englender, G. S., McCormick, J. B., and Hayes, P. S.: Use of pertussis vaccine in an epidemic involving hospital staff. Lancet, 2:540, 1975.

Morse, S. I.: Biologically active components and properties of *Bordetella pertussis*. Adv. Appl. Microbiol., 20:9, 1976.

Nelson, K. E., Gavitt, F., Batt, M. D., Kallick, C. A., Reddi, K. T., and Levin, S.: The role of adenoviruses in the pertussis syndrome. J. Pediat. 86:335, 1975.

Olson, L. C.: Pertussis. Medicine, 54:427, 1975.

Steigman, A. J. (ed.): Report of the Committee on Infectious Diseases. 18th ed. Evanston, Ill., American Academy of Pediatrics, 1977.

*National Institutes of Health.

GRANULOMA INGUINALE

144. GRANULOMA INGUINALE

Walsh McDermott

Granuloma inguinale is an indolent granulomatous and ulcerative disease usually localized to the genitalia or perianal region and caused by a pleomorphic coccobacillus, *Donovania granulomatis*, the so-called "Donovan body." When grown on artificial medium, the presumed organism, *Calymmatobacterium granulomatis*, develops a large capsule that reacts immunologically with klebsiella capsular material. It also resembles *K. pneumoniae* in morphology. The infection appears to be customarily transmitted during coitus or other close body contact, and the degree of communicability appears to be relatively low. The lesion tends to be single, and may rarely appear on surfaces of the body other than the genitalia. Systemic infection, notably with the production of arthritis or osteomyelitis, has been reported. Usually the lesion appears on the genitalia or in the perianal area as a relatively painless nodular infiltration that soon breaks down, leaving a sharply demarcated ulcer with friable granulation tissue at the base. On histologic examination, the lesion appears well vascularized and is the site of considerable cellular infiltration, especially with polymorphonuclear leukocytes and monocytes. In appropriately stained tissue scrapings (Wright-Giemsa), the microbe *C. granulomatis* may be seen situated principally within the monocytes, although smaller numbers of extracellular microorganisms can usually be identified. The lesion spreads by direct extension, it is highly destructive to the skin and subcutaneous tissue, and secondary infection with other microorganisms is common. Rarely, if sufficiently extensive, the process may cause elephantiasis of the genitalia.

There is nothing particularly characteristic about the lesions of granuloma inguinale, and the early lesion is indistinguishable from those produced by *T. pallidum*, *H. ducreyi*, or other processes that involve the genitalia. The diagnosis can be established only by appropriate microbiologic techniques, and these should be employed whenever the physician encounters a genital lesion (or an indolent ulceration elsewhere) that is not clearly caused by some other process. Microscopy of deep scrapings or impression smears from the lesion of granuloma inguinale stained by the Wright-Giemsa method usually reveals the microbe within the monocytes. The ease with which the microorganisms can be detected varies to some extent with the age of the lesion. In a relatively old lesion, the scrapings should be made from the depth of the lesion, and an extensive search of the smears may be necessary. The microorganisms can also be cultured in medium containing chick embryo yolk by methods originally developed by Anderson and her associates. Antigen prepared from capsular material of *C. granulomatis* has been employed in a complement-fixation reaction and in a cutaneous reaction, but these have not had wide application.

Granuloma inguinale was initially treated successfully with streptomycin and tetracycline, but this is no longer the case. Ampicillin has become the drug of choice. In all but 2 of 31 patients treated by Breschi et al. with ampicillin, the lesions healed completely. The two failures were successfully treated by a second course of ampicillin in one and by a two-week course of lincomycin following a dorsal slit in the other. Ampicillin should be given in individual doses of 500 mg orally every six hours for two weeks. With extensive lesions, the chemotherapy should be extended for one or two weeks more. In uncircumcised men, a dorsal slit may be necessary if the ulceration is beneath a partial phimosis. Lincomycin in the same dosage as recommended above for ampicillin has been used successfully in patients known to have shown allergy to penicillin, and should be employed in such circumstances.

No detailed studies are available concerning the prevention of granuloma inguinale. It seems likely, however, that thorough washing of the genitalia with soap and water immediately after sexual intercourse has a significant influence in reducing the probability of infection.

Anderson, K., Goodpasture, E. W., and DeMonbreun, W. A.: Immunologic relationship of *Donovania granulomatis* to granuloma inguinale. J. Exp. Med., 81:41, 1945.

Breschi, L. C., Goldman, G., and Shapiro, S. R.: Granuloma inguinale in Vietnam: Successful therapy with ampicillin and lincomycin. J. Am. Vener. Dis. Assoc., 1:118, 1975.

Davis, B. D., Dulbecco, R., Eisen, H. N., Ginsberg, H. S., and Wood, W. B., Jr.: Microbiology. New York, Hoeber Medical Division, Harper & Row, 1970, Chap. 36.

DIPHTHERIA

145. DIPHTHERIA

Heonir Rocha

Diphtheria is an acute infectious disease caused by a bacillus, *Corynebacterium diphtheriae*. The infection usually localizes in the pharynx, larynx, and nostrils and occasionally in the skin, and gives rise to both local and systemic signs. The latter are related to the production of a potent soluble exotoxin elaborated by the microorganisms multiplying at the site of infection.

ETIOLOGY. *Corynebacterium diphtheriae* is a gram-positive, nonsporulating, nonmotile pleomorphic bacillus, which grows best aerobically and does not form gas. In stained smears diphtheria bacilli are frequently club shaped in appearance and are arranged in palisade form. The most common media used to isolate the bacilli are Löffler's and potassium tellurite agar. By the appearance on tellurite agar and the ability to ferment starch and glycogen, three distinct types of colonies can be idenfitied: *gravis*, *mitis*, and *intermedius*. All three types can produce the same powerful toxin, which is a heat-labile polypeptide, with a molecular weight of 62,000, produced by bacterial cells infected with a lysogenic bacteriophage. In so-called avirulent diphtheria strains no parasitism with bacteriophages can be demonstrated, and the bacilli fail to produce toxin. Thus acquisition of phage leads to toxigenicity, and the amount of toxin produced depends on genetic and nutritional factors. The ability to produce toxin under laboratory conditions is not entirely related to potential for causing severe disease, because several virulent strains are poor toxin formers. Around 10 per cent of *Corynebacterium diphtheriae* isolated from clinically typical cases were nontoxigenic when tested by the Eleck-plate method or by guinea pig inoculation. It should be mentioned that nontoxigenic *Corynebacterium diphtheriae* can cause symptomatic infection in humans. Diphtheria caused by nontoxigenic strains, however, is mild and behaves as localized disease caused by toxigenic strains.

It is usually said that the *gravis* strain is more frequently associated with epidemic diphtheria; also, that the case fatality rate associated with any epidemic is determined by the proportion of cases infected with the *gravis* or *mitis* types. However, these views are not generally accepted. Although there seems to be a trend toward more severe infection with the *gravis* and *mitis* types, without question the same clinical picture can be produced by all three types.

EPIDEMIOLOGY AND IMMUNITY. Diphtheria has a world-wide distribution, its natural incidence being greatest in temperate climates. The disease occurs predominantly in poor socioeconomic conditions where inadequately immunized hosts and crowding are common. It exhibits a tendency to be most prevalent in autumn and winter but can give rise to epidemics at any time of year.

The human host is the only significant reservoir of *Corynebacterium diphtheriae,* which is transmitted directly or indirectly from one person to another. The usual habitat of *Corynebacterium diphtheriae* is the respiratory tract. The organism can multiply in the mucous membranes of the respiratory tract (pharynx or nares) of immunized hosts without giving rise to clinical disease. The transmission of diphtheria is mainly via droplets, although fomites and dust may have a minor role. Milk has been shown to be a vehicle of infection in rare instances. Duration and closeness of contact are the important factors in transmission. In some tropical areas the skin has been implicated as a major reservoir of *Corynebacterium diphtheriae* infection.

Immunity against the disease depends basically upon the existence of antitoxin in the blood of the host, which is formed in response to direct stimulation of diphtheria toxin either by artificial immunization or by clinical or subclinical infection. Infants under the age of six months are normally protected by passive immunity received through the placenta from immune mothers. Adults are usually protected by artificial immunization or subclinical infection. It has been suggested that undiagnosed cutaneous diphtheria may be the main way whereby natural immunization is acquired in tropical countries.

A relatively simple method to gain valuable information concerning a patient's immune status is to observe the local reaction after the intradermal injection of 0.1 ml of diluted, highly purified diphtheria toxin (Schick test). A positive reaction is interpreted to mean that the patient is susceptible to the disease; a negative reaction indicates that the levels of antitoxin exceed 0.03 unit per milliliter and that the host is not likely to acquire the clinical disease. It should be mentioned, however, that immunization status does not appear to reduce the likelihood of acquiring disease from nontoxigenic strains and has no discernible effect on the severity of clinical illness associated with those strains.

The maximal age incidence of diphtheria lies in the period of two to six years. The disease is an unusual occurrence in adults in endemic areas. However, recently in the United States, approximately 25 per cent of the cases occurred in persons 15 years of age or older.

PATHOGENESIS. The most serious consequences of *Corynebacterium diphtheriae* infection are the result of production and absorption of an extremely active and damaging exotoxin. The organisms multiply on epithelial cells at the infected site (usually pharynx), secreting the specific toxin which produces local signs and is absorbed, resulting in a systemic illness. The initial cytotoxic effect of the toxin is in tissues immediately adjacent to the bacterial growth, resulting in necrotic changes. As a consequence, an exudate which tends to coalesce is formed during the initial 24 to 48 hours. This fibrinous exudate contains leukocytes, necrotic epithelial cells, red blood cells, and the growing diphtheria bacillus. The exudate forms a tough membrane (so-called pseudomembrane) which is firmly attached, with a white shiny center and a gray or brownish periphery. If this membrane is forcibly removed, bleeding occurs. Occasionally it extends throughout the tracheobronchial tree, forming a cast. In the trachea and larynx, probably because of mucus production, this membrane tends to be adherent. Edema of soft tissues subjacent to the membrane may be intense. These local lesions when present in the larynx can result in encroachment of the airway with varying degrees of respiratory obstruction. Tracheal and bronchial obstruction can also result from detachment of the pseudomembrane.

From the local site of production the soluble toxin is disseminated by the blood and lymphatics and can produce degenerative changes in the heart, nervous system, and kidneys. The diphtheria toxin is regularly lethal to the affected cells. It becomes absorbed to the cell membrane, penetrates into the cell, and alters the protein synthesis by interfering with the transfer of amino acids from RNA to the growing polypeptide chain. By breaking disulfide bonds, the molecule can be split into two fragments; fragment B has no independent activity, but is required for the transport of fragment A into cells. Fragment A inactivates the EF-2 (elongation factor), which is required for translocation of polypeptidyl–transfer RNA from the acceptor to the donor site on the eukaryotic ribosome. This results in abrupt arrest of protein synthesis, presumably bringing about degeneration and death of the cell. Specific antitoxin may neutralize even adsorbed toxin, but does not prevent the chain of events once the toxin penetrates the cell.

Diphtheria infection may be localized infrequently in wounds, buccal mucosa, vagina, and conjunctiva. These extrarespiratory locations usually give rise to milder disease with much less systemic illness.

CLINICAL MANIFESTATIONS. The incubation period of diphtheria varies from one to seven days, but is most commonly two to four days. The clinical picture depends upon the anatomic location of the lesions and the severity of the toxic process.

Faucial diphtheria is the most common clinical presentation and includes the most toxic forms. In a typical case the onset is usually sudden, with low-grade fever (37 to 38° C), malaise, and mild sore throat. The pharynx is only moderately injected, and a thick tonsillar whitish exudate is frequently seen. This exudate usually spreads from one tonsil to the other and may invade the pillars, uvula, soft palate, and pharyngeal wall. Moderate tonsillar as well as cervical lymph node enlargement is usually present.

In some cases the membrane or exudate is limited to the tonsils *(tonsillar diphtheria),* and toxic manifestations are inconspicuous. In other cases, there is spread of the original process to the uvula, posterior pharyngeal wall, and posterior nasal mucosa *(nasopharyngeal diphtheria),* sometimes with massive cervical lymphadenopathy (bullneck appearance) and signs of toxemia. In this clinical form the child is pale, lethargic, prostrated, restless at times, and extremely weak. The pulse is rapid and thin; heart beats become muffled; respiration is labored and frequently noisy. This state of toxemia may result in death within a few days if the condition remains untreated. Finally, in some patients the infection spreads downward to the larynx, producing a clinical picture of progressive laryngeal obstruction *(laryngeal diphtheria).* When the larynx is involved, the first symptoms are hoarseness, dyspnea, a brassy cough, and an increasing expiratory and inspiratory stridor. In a few instances laryngeal involvement may be the first sign of infection. As the obstruction progresses, dyspnea becomes more severe, bronchial secretions accumulate, the accessory muscles of respiration come into full play, and there are supra- and infrasternal retraction at each stridulous breath. If obstruction is not relieved, the patient becomes extremely restless, anxious, and cyanotic, and the condition then merges into severe exhaustion and a comatose stage.

In some cases the infection is basically localized in the anterior nasal area *(anterior nasal diphtheria).* Clinically it is manifested by bilateral or unilateral serous or serosanguineous discharge which erodes the skin around the nostrils and the upper lips, occasionally resulting in small crusted lesions. Small rounded ulcers, some of them covered with a whitish exudate, are usually seen in the anterior part of the nasal septum. Constitutional symptoms are lacking, and this process is chiefly important because of its epidemiologic implications. It is frequently undiagnosed in an endemic area, and may be an important source of spreading the disease.

Other parts of the body may be the site of primary or secondary diphtheric lesions, the most commonly described being the skin. *Cutaneous diphtheria* takes the form of chronic nonhealing ulcers, sometimes covered with a grayish membranous exudate. It seems probable that these ulcers, mainly described in the tropics, have a complex etiology. Treatment with antitoxin alone usually gives disappointing results. Involvement of the conjunctiva, vagina, or ear by *Corynebacterium diphtheriae* has been rarely reported. These uncommon localizations are practically always secondary to faucial infection.

DIAGNOSIS. In most instances of diphtheric oropharyngeal infection, a presumptive diagnosis must be made on clinical grounds, without awaiting laboratory confirmation, because therapy should be started at once.

The clinical manifestations which should arouse suspicion of *nasopharyngeal diphtheria* are (1) insidious onset of a painless pharyngitis associated with an exudate (usually localized or predominantly in one tonsillar area); (2) association of a faucial exudate with insidious and progressive signs of laryngeal obstruction or with a serous or serosanguineous nasal discharge; and (3) the presence of faucial exudate with marked cervical adenopathy and signs of toxicity (prostration, tachycardia, marked pallor).

For laboratory diagnosis, a swab from the suspected site (usually a pharyngeal and a nasal swab are taken) should be promptly inoculated on a Löffler slant, a tellurite plate, and a blood agar plate. Identification of the etiologic agent can be made after overnight incubation on the basis of colony formation, cellular morphology, and sometimes fermentation reactions. Immunofluorescence techniques have been tried for the rapid diagnosis of diphtheria. For reliable results the specimen has to be incubated four hours before applying the fluorescent antibody technique. Slides prepared directly from throat swabs are unsatisfactory. The fluorescent antibody technique is not of value for the identification of toxigenic strains. Tests to detect the toxigenicity of diphtheria-like organisms cultured (guinea pig skin reaction, in vitro test on agar plate or Elek-plate method, and tissue culture test) are usually performed days after therapy has been started, because they require the isolation of *Corynebacterium diphtheriae;* two to three days thereafter are necessary for correct reading.

Several conditions may be confused with diphtheria, especially during an epidemic bout. This is the case, for instance, with streptococcal pharyngitis. In this condition there is usually high fever (39 to 40° C) with frequent chills, the throat is fiery red, the exudate is thin and easily removable, and swallowing is painful. Other pharyngeal infections which may be accompanied by an exudate are adenoviral exudative pharyngitis, infectious mononucleosis, Vincent's angina, and angina of agranulocytosis. Rhinitis associated with diphtheria must be differentiated from rhinitis of simple colds and from foreign bodies in the nostrils. The distressful laryngeal manifestations of diphtheria should be differentiated from acute obstructive laryngitis, either infectious (viral, *Hemophilus*) or allergic.

COMPLICATIONS. The most important complications of diphtheria are related to the cardiovascular and nervous systems. They are most frequently associated with the severe forms of the disease.

Although electrocardiographic changes have been described in a high percentage (25 per cent) of cases of diphtheria, clinically manifest myocarditis is less common. The onset of myocarditis is often insidious, appearing in the second or third week of the infection. Characteristically, the patient exhibits a weak rising pulse with distant heart sounds and a profound weakness and lethargy. When heart failure ensues, the patient becomes dyspneic, with marked pallor and epigastric pain, and he develops cardiac enlargement and an apical diastolic gallop. The most common electrocardiographic changes are T wave flattening or inversion, bundle branch block or intraventricular block, and several types of disorders of rhythm (premature contractions and atrial fibrillation).

Diphtheria myocarditis, particularly when associated with heart block, carries an extremely poor prognosis. Despite vigorous treatment, including steroids and digitalis, the mortality rate is very high. Glucagon has also been tried but is ineffective.

Nervous system involvement is manifested by cranial nerve or peripheral nerve paralysis. The most common form of cranial nerve palsy is paralysis of the soft palate, which is suspected by the development of nasal regurgitation of fluid upon attempted swallowing. Nasal speech may be present but is frequently slight. This condition is mild, and recovery usually occurs within two weeks. Ciliary paresis and oculomotor paralysis (affecting both sides) make up the next most common form. Rarely, facial, pharyngeal, or laryngeal paralysis is observed.

Peripheral neuritis, usually affecting the limbs, may appear from about the fourth to the eighth week. It varies greatly in extent but is frequently manifested by weakness in the dorsiflexors of the feet, accompanied by decreased or absent tendon reflexes in the lower extremities. Less commonly, the upper limbs, the neck, and the trunk may be involved. The prognosis is good. Diphtheric polyneuritis has been described after cutaneous diphtheria.

It must be emphasized that recovery from the complications of diphtheria is nearly always complete insofar as can be determined by clinical examination. It has been suggested that a lowering of cardiac reserve can persist in some cases, but this assumption needs further documentation.

TREATMENT. The most important act in the treatment of diphtheria is to administer antitoxin as soon as the diphtheria is suspected on clinical grounds without awaiting laboratory confirmation. Admittedly this practice will result in the unnecessary use of antitoxin in some cases. But this is of little consequence in view of the considerable improvement in prognosis in severe forms of the disease when antitoxin is administered early and in adequate amounts.

Opinions vary as to what constitutes an efficient dose. It is usually accepted that in mild or moderate cases a dose of 30,000 to 50,000 units, injected intramuscularly, is enough. In severe cases, 60,000 to 100,000 units is the recommended dose, half of it being given by slow intravenous infusion in critically ill patients. As the antitoxin is a horse protein, precautions should be observed to avoid severe hypersensitivity reactions (anaphylaxis). It is mandatory to inquire if allergy to horse serum is known, and to perform a conjunctival or intracutaneous skin test with a 1:10 saline dilution of the antitoxin. If a positive reaction is obtained by either method, desensitization with increasing doses of antiserum is recommended. Epinephrine must be at hand before antitoxin is administered by any route.

As the *Corynebacterium diphtheriae* is susceptible to several antimicrobials, these drugs have been used routinely, in addition to antitoxin, in cases of diphtheria. Penicillin G is still the drug of choice, and is usually given as procaine penicillin, 400,000 units intramuscularly every 12 hours, for a period of 8 to 12 days. Erythromycin, also very active against the diphtheria bacillus, is an alternative drug and is recommended in a dosage of 30 to 40 mg per kilogram of body weight for a similar period. In suspected cases, these drugs must not be administered without the antitoxin, because they may mask the infection and thus may make it impossible to establish a laboratory diagnosis.

Bed rest is essential in all patients during the acute phase of the disease; this can vary in completeness and duration, depending on the degree of toxicity and the presence of cardiac involvement. In any event, the patient's return to activity should be carefully guided by the physician. Complications such as dehydration, shock, and congestive heart failure should be promptly diagnosed and properly treated.

In cases exhibiting marked toxicity and in patients with severe laryngeal involvement and/or shock, corticosteroids (prednisone, 3 to 5 mg per kilogram of body weight per day) have been advocated along with the antitoxin and antimicrobial. Cases of laryngeal obstruction may require emergency tracheostomy and careful postoperative aspiration to avoid complications. Such patients need special nursing for safety.

Patients with diphtheria should be isolated, preferably in hospital. Before their discharge from isolation, cultures from throat and nose (or local lesion) should be taken, and at least two consecutive negative cultures should be obtained.

PREVENTION. Diphtheria may be effectively prevented by *active immunization.* The primary course of immunization should be administered within the first year of life, preferably between the third and sixth months. Of the preparations available, *fluid toxoid* and *alum-precipitated toxoid* are the most commonly used. The primary course of fluid toxoid consists of three intramuscular injections (0.5 ml, 1.0 ml, and 1.0 ml) at weekly intervals (one to three weeks). For immunization with the alum-precipitated toxoid, two 1-ml intramuscular injections administered at intervals of one to two months are enough. Despite its greater antigenic potency, the alum-precipitated toxoid also has a greater sensitizing ability, and may induce sterile local abscesses at the injection site owing to the irritating effect of the alum upon tissues. Both fluid and alum-precipitated toxoid are excellent immunizing agents, conferring immunity to at least 90 per cent of those receiving a primary course. After this immunization in infancy, one stimulating dose should be given one or two years later, and another given at the time the child enters school.

Diphtheria toxoid has been combined with immunizations against tetanus and pertussis and should be given within the first year of life. All children under six years of age who are not immunized are susceptible to diphtheria and should be actively immunized without preliminary Schick testing. In older children and adults, before immunization with toxoid, a sensitivity test should be done. The development of a local reaction within 48 hours of the intracutaneous injection of 0.1 ml of 1:10 dilution of toxoid in normal saline *(Moloney test)* is a warning that toxoid should be administered cautiously in multiple small diluted doses.

Passive immunization against diphtheria may be rapidly conferred by subcutaneous inoculation of 1500 units of diphtheria antitoxin. This procedure should be limited to persons peculiarly at risk of infection, such as nonimmunized children heavily exposed to an infected case. The protection is limited to a period of two to three weeks, and active immunization with a toxoid preparation should be started at the same time. Human diphtheria antitoxin is not yet available.

Treatment of Diphtheria Carriers. Whenever diphtheria is common, carrier rates are high. In approximately 15 to 20 per cent of cases, the cultures will remain positive for as long as one month after the disease, but they will subsequently become negative in most instances. Erythromycin in a dosage of 30 to 40 mg per kilogram of body weight has been found effective for treatment of carriers. Benzathine penicillin could be used (600,000 units for children of ages one to five years, and 1,200,000 units for older patients) only when patients cannot be relied upon to complete a seven-day course of oral therapy. Tonsillectomy and adenoidectomy have also been advocated to eliminate the carrier state.

Barksdale, L., Garmiese, L., and Horibata, K.: Virulence, toxigeny, and lysogeny in *Corynebacterium diphtheriae.* Ann. N.Y. Acad. Sci., 88:1093, 1960.

Bray, J. P., Burt, E. G., Potter, E. V., Poon-King, T., and Earle, D.: Epidemic diphtheria and skin infections in Trinidad. J. Infect. Dis., 126:34, 1972.

Collier, R. J.: Diphtheria toxin: Mode of action and structure. Bact. Rev., 39:54, 1975.

McCloskey, R. V., Eller, J. J., Green, M., Mauney, C. V., and Richards, S. E. M.: The 1970 epidemic of diphtheria in San Antonio. Ann. intern. Med., 75:495, 1971.

McCracken, A. W., and Mauney, C. V.: Identification of *Corynebacterium diphtheriae* by immunofluorescence during a diphtheria epidemic. J. Clin. Pathol., 24:641, 1971.

Naiditch, M. J., and Bower, A. A.: Diphtheria: Study of 1433 cases observed during 10-year period at Los Angeles County Hospital. Am. J. Med., 17:229, 1954.

Scheid, W.: Diphtherial paralysis. An analysis of 2292 cases of diphtheria in adults, which included 174 cases of polyneuritis. J. Nerv. Ment. Dis., 116:1095, 1952.

CLOSTRIDIAL DISEASES

146. INTRODUCTION

Emanuel Wolinsky

The clostridia are spore-forming anaerobic grampositive bacilli that for the most part lead a saprophytic existence in nature. They may be found in large numbers in the intestinal tracts of humans and animals, and in the soil. They are capable of producing disease by virtue of their elaboration of powerful exotoxins, but special conditions must be present in the tissues to allow the organisms to germinate, proliferate, and elaborate toxins. The mere presence of clostridia in the wound or on the surface of the body is not significant. Most clostridial disease is caused by *C. perfringens*, although occasionally *C. novyi (oedematiens), septicum, sordellii (bifermentans), histolyticum,* and *fallax* may be human pathogens.

The pathologic states attributable to clostridial infection cover a wide range of severity and localization, from the relatively benign wound infection to the highly fatal gas gangrene; from transient bacteremia to life-threatening septicemia; from relatively mild food poisoning to necrotic enteritis; and from pleural empyema to purulent meningitis. The neurotoxic disease caused by *C. tetani* is discussed below, and that caused by *C. botulinum* is discussed in Ch. 22.3.

BACTERIOLOGY

All the clostridia owe their pathogenicity to the elaboration of exotoxins that have enzymatic activity. Four major toxins and eight minor ones have been described and given Greek letters. The most important of them is the alpha toxin, which is a lecithinase capable of splitting lecithin in the red cell envelope and causing severe hemolysis. Many of the species of clostridia have been separated into types according to their ability to elaborate specific exotoxins. *C. perfringens* may be divided into five or six toxigenic types; Type A elaborates more alpha toxin than any other type or species and is by far the most important variety of *Clostridium* in human disease, particularly gas gangrene.

147. CLOSTRIDIAL MYONECROSIS

(Gas Gangrene)

Emanuel Wolinsky

The clostridial gas gangrene is best called *clostridial myonecrosis* because the outstanding feature is rapidly progressive muscle necrosis with relatively little inflammatory reaction, and because other organisms can produce skin and subcutaneous gangrene, and myositis, with gas formation. The disease most often arises from traumatic or surgical wounds in which anoxic conditions prevail as a result of ischemia or crushed muscle. Battle wounds of World Wars I and II supplied plentiful case material for study; gas gangrene occurred in approximately 10 per cent of World War I wounds and in 1 per cent of those that occurred in World War II. In civilian practice the rate of gas gangrene among 188,000 major open wounds has been estimated to be 1.8 per cent. The rate of contamination or local infection of open wounds, on the other hand, amounts to 30 to 80 per cent. The soil is the usual source of the clostridia in exogenous infection, the intestine or biliary tract in autogenous infection.

PATHOGENESIS. The factors that predispose to the invasion of muscle by the bacilli with the subsequent elaboration of exotoxins are related to lack of oxygen and lowering of the oxidation-reduction potential of the tissues. These factors are (1) impaired local vascular supply owing to vessel trauma or pressure from foreign bodies, casts, or tourniquets; (2) presence of metallic bodies, clothing, or dirt in the wound; (3) presence of necrotic tissue or hemorrhage; and (4) growth of aerobic microorganisms in the wound.

Under these circumstances the bacilli can multiply anaerobically and elaborate toxins, which diffuse out and damage surrounding muscle, which in turn becomes colonized with the bacilli. Thus the disease spreads rapidly to surrounding muscles and gains momentum. The severe generalized toxemia remains poorly explained. Alpha toxin is not found in the blood, and it is postulated that a toxic factor that acts on certain vital centers or enzymes is produced by the interaction of clostridial toxin with necrotic muscle.

CLINICAL MANIFESTATIONS. The clinical picture of gas gangrene is dominated by rapidly progressive toxemia and shock. After a relatively short incubation period of one to four days the patient suddenly exhibits restlessness and anxiety; the temperature and pulse rate begin to rise and the blood pressure to fall. He is noted to be pale and sweating. The wound becomes painful and markedly swollen. Some hours later, after progression of the signs and symptoms, a thin brownish exudate begins to ooze from the wound, and a small amount of crepitus may be noted in the surrounding tissues. A bronze discoloration starts at the edge of the wound and progresses outward. Blebs filled with purplish fluid may appear. An odor characterized as "mousy" or "sickly sweet" is described by many observers. By this time the patient may be anuric and in irreversible vascular collapse. When the muscle is exposed by incision, it appears to be "cooked" or dead — it does not bleed when cut or retract when pinched. Smears from *involved muscle* show many large gram-positive rods and no other organisms, but very few pus cells. Smears and cultures from the *wound exudate* at the surface may reveal other organisms in addition to the clostridia, especially in grossly contaminated wounds. Roentgenograms reveal the presence of gas in and around muscle bundles in the form of fernlike, lacy patterns. Untreated, fully developed clostridial myonecrosis is almost always fatal.

Myonecrosis must be differentiated from clostridial and nonclostridial *crepitant cellulitis*, from *anaerobic streptococcal myonecrosis*, and from *physical* and *chemical* causes of gas in the tissues. *Clostridial cellulitis* (anaerobic cellulitis, local gas gangrene, epifascial gas gangrene, or gas-forming fasciitis) is a gas-forming infection of connective tissue mainly localized to subcutaneous areas with spread in fascial planes, but healthy muscle is not involved. It arises as a result of clostridial infection of tissue already necrotic from ischemia or trauma. The onset is gradual, and toxemia, pain, and swelling are less than in gas gangrene. A large amount of gas is distributed in the form of large bubbles along the fascial planes, but not in the muscle. Incision will show that the muscle is viable, and smears from muscle tissue away from the open wound will not reveal organisms.

Nonclostridial crepitant cellulitis is similar to clostridial cellulitis, except that the infection is associated with other organisms, usually in a mixed flora consisting of two or more of the following: aerogenic coliforms (*E. coli, Klebsiella, Enterobacter*), anaerobic streptococci, *Bacteroides*, and gamma streptococci. In many cases this mixed bacterial flora in gas-forming cellulitis includes clostridia; these cases do not appear to differ in prognosis from those in which clostridia are absent. It is not clear how often cellulitis progresses to myonecrosis, but varying degrees of muscle gangrene may be seen in patients who present with classic anaerobic cellulitis, especially of the nonclostridial variety. Thus a sharp distinction between cellulitis and myonecrosis is not always possible, although one or the other condition usually predominates.

Anaerobic streptococcal myonecrosis was described by MacLennan in infected war wounds from the Middle East in 1948, but there have been few reports since then. Other organisms, especially group A streptococci and *Staph. aureus,* were always found with the primary agent, and 3 of 19 patients had anaerobic streptococcal bacteremia.

Simple contamination of wounds with clostridia is not uncommon. The organisms, usually in association with a mixed flora, exist as saprophytes on necrotic tissue and debris and do not invade further. Clostridia may also be found in localized collections of purulent material in wounds, or in foul-smelling brownish fluid known as a "gas abscess" or a "Welch abscess." Drainage will usually suffice to bring these conditions under control.

DIAGNOSIS. The diagnosis of gas gangrene is essentially a clinical one. Upon first suspicion of the disease, dressings and casts must be removed and the wound or suspected area thoroughly inspected. Roentgenograms may help to show the fine bubbles of gas distributed in and around muscle bundles. Incision should be made into the muscle so that the characteristic appearance may be appreciated. At the same time a specimen of muscle may be examined by Gram stain of imprint slides and by anaerobic cultural techniques. Smears and cultures from the exudate around the wound surface may be misleading. Tables 1 and 2 summarize the most important findings for the differential diagnosis.

TREATMENT. Treatment must be prompt and vigorous. Most important is thorough *debridement* and *excision* of all devitalized tissue and dead muscle. Hopelessly involved extremities usually need to be amputated except perhaps under the influence of hyperbaric oxygen. It is said that if any infected muscle is left behind, it will prevent cure. General *supportive measures* should include intravenous fluids and blood, other measures to combat vascular collapse and shock, and peritoneal dialysis when necessary. *Antimicrobial* treatment is given to prevent bloodstream invasion and to suppress further spread of infection. Penicillin is the drug of choice given in large doses of 10 to 20 million units per day intravenously. A cephalosporin or clindamycin may be substituted in patients allergic to penicillin. Approximately 20 per cent of *C. perfringens* strains are resistant to tetracycline, and erythromycin is not suitable because of poor activity at low redox potential and in acidic environment. *Antitoxin* is recommended, especially during the first few hours of the disease, in the hope of neutralizing any free toxin in

TABLE 1.　Classification of Histotoxic Clostridial Disease

Traumatic
　　A. Wound infection (war and civilian)
　　　　1. Simple contamination
　　　　2. Localized (purulent or "gas abscess")
　　　　3. Gas-forming cellulitis
　　　　4. Myonecrosis
　　B. Uterine infection (postabortion and postpartum)
　　C. Burns, panophthalmitis, brain abscess, etc.

Nontraumatic
　　A. Postoperative (abdominal, amputation)
　　B. Postinjection
　　C. Spontaneous
　　　　1. Localized (pneumonia, empyema, cholecystitis, myonecrosis)
　　　　2. Septicemic (malignant disease, intestinal lesion)
　　D. Bacteremia without hemolysis or sepsis (from decubitus ulcer, gangrenous extremity, uterus)

TABLE 2. Gas-Forming Soft Tissue Infections

	Clostridial Myonecrosis	"Anaerobic" Cellulitis	Streptococcal Myonecrosis
Onset	Sudden	Gradual	Gradual
Toxemia	Extreme	Slight	Slight
Pain	May be severe	Slight	Gradually increasing
Swelling	Marked	Slight	Marked
Skin color	Bronze	No change	Erythematous
Exudate	Thin, brown	Thin, bloody; later purulent	Profuse, thin seropurulent
Gas	Little, in muscle	Profuse, large bubbles in fascial planes	Little, in muscle
Muscle	Dead, "cooked," healthy muscle invaded	Not involved	Initially edematous, then hemorrhagic
Bacteriology	Mixed flora from exudate or open wound; from muscle aspirate pure gram-positive rods	May be pure clostridia or mixed flora from exudate or subcutaneous tissue; no organisms in muscle aspirate	Anaerobic streptococci, along with Group A *Streptococcus, Staph. aureus, etc.,* from exudate and muscle
Prognosis	Serious	Good	Good
Treatment	Radical surgery, penicillin, antitoxin, hyperbaric oxygen	Surgical drainage and debridement, appropriate antimicrobials	Surgical drainage and debridement, penicillin

the body fluids, although its usefulness is doubtful because the exotoxins are very rapidly bound to cells. The recommended dose is 40 thousand units of trivalent or pentavalent antitoxin intravenously at once and 20 to 40 thousand units repeated at four- to six-hour intervals. The usual precautions for horse serum must be observed. *Hyperbaric oxygen* at 3 atmospheres has been recommended by some as a dramatically successful mode of therapy that should take precedence over immediate surgical treatment and antitoxin. It is said that debridement may be deferred until systemic toxicity has been relieved and demarcation between necrotic and viable tissue is clear. In this way loss of tissue may be minimized and amputation sometimes avoided. If a suitable chamber is not available locally, it is probably unwise to delay surgical extirpation in favor of a long journey (see Ch. 31).

Treatment of "anaerobic" cellulitis and streptococcal myonecrosis need not be so radical. Usually wide excision and debridement along with supportive measures and appropriate antimicrobials will suffice. A Gram-stained smear of wound exudate and muscle aspirate will help one to decide whether penicillin alone should be given (for pure *Clostridium* or *Streptococcus*) or whether antistaphylococcal, antibacteroides, or anticoliform agents should be added or substituted. Reasonable drug regimens for mixed anaerobic cellulitis are gentamicin plus clindamycin, or chloramphenicol alone. A penicillinase-resistant penicillin or cephalosporin should be included if staphylococci are recognized.

PREVENTION. The prophylactic use of antitoxin and antimicrobials at the time of injury does not prevent gas gangrene. Careful attention to good surgical technique is most important. All devitalized tissue must be excised and vascular supply left intact. Care must be taken with tourniquets and casts to prevent undue ischemia. Plaster of Paris itself may be contaminated with clostridia.

UTERINE INFECTION

Postabortion and postpartum clostridial infections of the uterus are still important causes of serious disease in obstetrics. At least 5 per cent of women harbor clostridia in the vagina as simple contaminants. Fulminant infection usually follows criminal abortion or prolonged and difficult labor, and presents a clinical picture similar to that seen in traumatic gas gangrene. Unlike wound gas gangrene, however, uterine infection is frequently accompanied by clostridial sepsis leading to jaundice, hemolysis, hemoglobinemia, hemoglobinuria, and renal shutdown. As in wound infection, there may be various grades of clostridial involvement, from simple contamination to secondary invasion of necrotic matter in the uterus or a dead fetus to true invasion of intact uterine muscle producing myonecrosis or "physometra." Clostridial infection must be differentiated from the more slowly progressive uterine infection produced by anaerobic streptococci and *Bacteroides* which commonly leads to pelvic thrombophlebitis and septic pulmonary infarcts.

Treatment is essentially the same as that outlined above, except that a decision must be made quickly on whether to do a hysterectomy or merely to empty the uterus. Evidence of uterine perforation or necrosis will call for the more radical procedure. Antimicrobial therapy should probably include clindamycin or chloramphenicol in addition to penicillin to control *Bacteroides*.

POSTOPERATIVE GAS GANGRENE

Nontraumatic gas gangrene that follows surgical operations is probably the most common variety of the disease in civilian hospitals today. Of 42 cases of *C. perfringens* infection reported from a single hospital, 18 followed operations and 10 were secondary to trauma (Pyrtek and Bartus, 1962). Most of these infections involve the abdominal wall after biliary or intestinal surgery, or the leg or hip after amputation or correction of hip fractures, although the complication has been described after many other kinds of surgical procedures. Recent investigation in England indicated that most of these infections were sporadic and autogenous in origin, probably as a result of fecal contamination of the skin. Parker called attention to the importance of adequate preoperative sterilization of the skin with sporicidal agents and the advisability of giving prophylactic penicillin from a few hours before operation to one week after to those patients at greatest risk from postoperative clostridial infections — elderly patients who will have hip surgery or thigh amputations.

Altemeier, W. A., and Culbertson, W. R.: Acute non-clostridial crepitant cellulitis. Surg. Gynecol. Obstet., 87:206, 1948.

Ayliffe, G. A. J., and Lowbury, E. J. L.: Sources of gas gangrene in hospital. Br. Med. J., 2:333, 1969.

Darke, S. G., King, A. M., and Slack, W. K.: Gas gangrene and related infection: Classification, clinical features and aetiology, management and mortality. A report of 88 cases. Br. J. Surg., 64:104, 1977.

Holland, J. A., Hill G. B., Wolfe, W. G., Osterhout, S., Saltzman, H. A., and Brown, I. W.: Experimental and clinical experience with hyperbaric oxygen in the treatment of clostridial myonecrosis. Surgery, 77:75, 1975.

MacLennan, J. D.: The histotoxic clostridial infections of man. Bact. Rev., 26:177, 1962.

Parker, M. T.: Postoperative clostridial infections in Britain. Br. Med. J., 3:671, 1969.

Roding, B., Groenveld, P. H., and Boerema, I.: Ten years' experience in the treatment of gas gangrene in hyperbaric oxygen. Surg. Gynecol. Obstet., 134:579, 1972.

Schwartzman, J. D., Reller, L. B., and Wang, W. L.: Susceptibility of Clostridium perfringens isolated from human infections to twenty antibiotics. Antimicrob. Agents Chemother., 11:695, 1977.

VanBeek, A., Zook, E., Yaw, P., Gardner, R., Smith, R., and Glover, J. L.: Nonclostridial gas-forming infections. A collective review and report of seven cases. Arch. Surg., 108:552, 1974.

Weinstein, L., and Barza, M. A.: Gas gangrene. N. Engl. J. Med., 289:1129, 1973.

148.   OTHER CLOSTRIDIAL DISEASES

Emanuel Wolinksy

SEPTICEMIA

Clostridial septicemia occurs rarely from traumatic wound gangrene, occasionally from postoperative gas gangrene, and commonly from uterine infection. In addition, nontraumatic or spontaneous clostridial septicemia has been described from such conditions as acute cholecystitis, perforated peptic ulcer, ulcerating carcinoma of the colon, acute pancreatitis, diverticulitis, appendiceal abscess, decubitus ulcer, and gangrenous limbs. Septicemia may occur in terminal cancer patients from portals of entry such as ulcerations of the respiratory or alimentary tracts. A study of 21 patients suffering from various malignant diseases who had septicemia caused by *C. septicum* has been reported. As a result of septicemia, infection may localize in the pleura, myocardium, endocardium, and meninges. Benign clostridial bacteremia without hemolysis was observed in a series of 20 patients, all of whom survived (Rathbun, 1968). Neonatal omphalitis and septicemia occur rarely.

MISCELLANEOUS FORMS

Pneumonia and empyema may be associated with clostridial infection, usually as a result of aspiration of contaminated material from the mouth or the stomach, but occasionally by way of the bloodstream. Penetrating injuries may lead to serious clostridial infections of the eye, brain, and meninges. Severe gas gangrene may result from injections into the buttock or thigh, presumably from inadequately sterilized skin. In at least one instance the organism was also isolated from cotton sponges soaked in alcohol.

Alpern, R. J., and Dowell, V. R., Jr.: Nonhistotoxic clostridial bacteremia. Am. J. Clin. Path., 55:717, 1971.

Bogdan, J. C., and Rapkin, R. H.: Clostridia infection in the newborn. Pediatrics, 58:120, 1976.

Cabrera, A., Tsukada, Y., and Pickren, J. W.: Clostridial gas gangrene and septicemia in malignant disease. Cancer, 18:800, 1965.

149.   CLOSTRIDIAL GASTROENTERITIS

Emanuel Wolinsky

Clostridial food poisoning has been the second most common variety reported to the Communicable Disease Center, representing 16 per cent of the total outbreaks and 34 per cent of the cases. It is discussed in Ch. 22.2.

A similar disease, called "pig-bel," is endemic in Papua, New Guinea, and has been attributed hypothetically to lack of proteolytic activity resulting from low protein diet and trypsin inhibitors in the dietary staple, sweet potato. Without protease, the beta toxin of Type C organisms may initiate the disease.

Lawrence, G., and Walker, P. D.: Pathogenesis of enteritis necroticans in Papua, New Guinea. Lancet, 1:125, 1976.

150.   TETANUS*

John H. Kerr

Tetanus, often called "lockjaw," is a disease of the nervous system characterized by intense activity of motor neurons resulting in severe muscle spasms. It is caused by an exotoxin of *Clostridium tetani*.

HISTORY. Tetanus has caught the imagination of physicians since Hippocrates, and this is probably due in part to the horrifying nature of the clinical picture in the established untreated case. The presence of the causative organism in soil was demonstrated by Nicolaier, who produced tetanus in animals by soil injections. The *Clostridium* was isolated in pure culture in 1899 by Kitasato, and in 1892 Nocard immunized horses by injections of antitoxin horse serum. Passive immunization after wounding saved many lives in World War I, and active immunization with toxoid almost eliminated tetanus in the allied armies in World War II. Curare was first suggested as having an application in the treatment of tetanus in 1811, but as curare in sufficient dosage to abolish the spasm of severe tetanus will certainly paralyze the muscles of ventilation, the large-scale use of curare had to wait almost 150 years until intermittent positive pressure ventilation (IPPV) through a cuffed tracheostomy tube was introduced into the treatment of tetanus in Denmark in 1953 (Bjørnboe et al.).

ETIOLOGY AND PATHOGENESIS. *Clostridium tetani* is a gram-positive actively motile bacillus which in its spore-bearing form has a characteristic "drumstick" appearance. Spores may develop at either end of the bacillus, giving a "dumbbell" appearance. It is a strict anaerobe, and spores will not germinate in the presence of even the smallest amount of oxygen. An oxidation-reduction potential of $+0.01$ volt or less at pH7 is required if germination is to take place. The *Clostridium* grows well on laboratory media at $37°$ C, and growth occurs slowly at $22°$ C. Vegetative bacilli are readily killed by antiseptics and by heat, but spores are highly resistant to antiseptics and, to a certain extent, are resistant to heat. To kill most spores, boiling for one hour is necessary, but the most resistant may require boiling for four hours. Autoclaving for ten minutes at $120°$ C

---

*This chapter is based on the one contributed to the previous edition by Professor A. Crampton Smith, with whom the author has worked for many years.

may, however, be relied on to sterilize contaminated objects. *Clostridium tetani* is commonly found in soil and in the feces of domestic animals and humans. Presumably by contamination with soil and feces, spores can be recovered from dust and clothing; in suitable surroundings such as dried earth, spores will survive for many years.

Clostridium tetani produces two exotoxins, tetanospasmin and tetanolysin, and of these tetanospasmin is the neurotoxin which produces the typical muscle spasm of tetanus. It is extremely potent, each milligram of crystallized toxin containing 50 to 75 million mouse-lethal doses. This extreme toxicity may be the reason why an attack of tetanus does not confer immunity, as it is postulated that the fatal dose of tetanus toxin is less than the amount required to provoke an immune response. Tetanolysin can cause hemolysis on blood agar plates, but does not seem to play any significant part in the pathologic process caused by the *Clostridium*.

There have been differences of opinion about the site of action of tetanospasmin and about the route by which it spreads, but it now seems firmly established that the toxin acts in the spinal cord and in the brainstem and that it spreads centrally along motor nerve trunks and up the spinal cord. Tetanus will follow the intravenous injection of toxin into animals, but the route by which toxin in the blood enters the nervous system is not clear. Toxin injected intramuscularly apparently spreads not only by passing up motor nerves but also by absorption into the blood, and it has been suggested that vascular spread is the more important route in generalized tetanus.

EPIDEMIOLOGY. The incidence of tetanus is difficult to establish because it is not a notifiable disease in many countries. The total world deaths each year, however, probably exceed 400,000. If the average crude fatality rate is about 45 per cent (and it may be higher), there must be nearly 1 million cases in the world every year. Tetanus is thus still a major public health problem in economically underdeveloped countries. The disease is common in warm climates and in rural areas that are highly cultivated and consequently have a large population of men and animals. Agricultural workers, in whom injuries may easily be contaminated with the *Clostridium*, are particularly at risk. *Clostridium tetani* can also be found in urban areas, but the degree of contamination is not high, and it is likely that the increased standard of living and hygiene which urbanization implies also contributes to a lower incidence of tetanus in cities. It remains a common, and usually lethal, complication of drug addiction. Further evidence of the importance of education and hygiene is the absence of neonatal tetanus in countries where obstetric hygiene is good, compared with the high incidence in countries where dung is sometimes used as a dressing for the umbilical stump.

PREVENTION OF TETANUS. Before Injury. ACTIVE IMMUNIZATION. The United States Public Health Service Advisory Committee has stated that the need for active immunization against tetanus is universal and that such immunization is the only way by which tetanus may be eliminated as an important health problem. There is little doubt that active immunization with adsorbed tetanus toxoid will convey a remarkably high degree of immunity. La Force et al. (1969) calculated that the incidence of tetanus in the under-ten age group in the United States of America was about 3.8 per 100 million. This underscores the excellent results obtained by active immunization of American and British military personnel in World War II.

In the United Kingdom, the recommended course of injections is three doses of adsorbed toxoid in a mixed vaccine, one injection at six months of age, and two others, with six to eight weeks between first and second and six months between second and third. A booster is advised at school entry and another at age 15 to 19. Thereafter, booster doses should be given at ten-year intervals. The American Academy of Pediatrics suggests three injections of toxoid no less than one month apart in infancy, a reinforcing dose about 12 months later, and a fifth or booster injection on entering school. Subsequent routine toxoid boosters should be administered at intervals of approximately ten years. Placental transfer of maternal tetanus antibodies appears to take place so that at least temporary passive immunity can be conferred on the neonate. Active immunization in pregnancy has proved to be an effective method of reducing the incidence of neonatal tetanus.

After Injury. PREVENTION OF CONTAMINATION. Simple measures that prevent contamination can contribute significantly to the prevention of tetanus, and the effect of attention to treatment of the umbilical stump on the incidence of neonatal tetanus is a good example of the effectiveness of simple hygiene. The aim of surgery in prophylaxis is to remove all dead tissue and foreign bodies from a wound. This will not only remove spore-bearing material but will also deny the spores the anaerobic conditions necessary for their growth. Tetanus occurs significantly often in patients in whom no wound is found, so that a precise definition of a "tetanus-prone" wound is difficult, although it is generally agreed that certain features increase the likelihood of tetanus. These features include an interval of more than six to eight hours between injury and treatment, heavy contamination of the wound with soil or manure, the retention of devitalized tissue or foreign bodies within the wound, and deep puncture wounds in which anaerobic conditions may occur.

Active Immunization. The protection against tetanus conferred by a full course of three injections of adsorbed toxoid lasts for at least ten years, and the reactivation provided by a booster dose of toxoid is equally long lived. Since the incidence of local reactions to toxoid is considerable, both United States and United Kingdom authorities recommend that a booster dose of toxoid is required after injury only if the patient is known, or suspected, not to have been actively immunized at all, or if more than ten years has elapsed since immunization or the most recent toxoid booster. If the wounds are of the "tetanus-prone" type described above, it is suggested that a toxoid booster be given if there has been an interval of more than five years since immunization or the most recent booster.

Passive Immunization. The use of passive immunization by means of antitoxin has probably saved many lives. The absence of a controlled trial precludes certainty, but circumstantial evidence is very strong. Experiments in laboratory animals show that antitoxin given soon after inoculation with tetanus will protect against the disease, and Bruce (1920), reviewing 1458 cases of tetanus occurring in World War I, showed that the incidence of tetanus, after prophylactic antitoxin was available in large quantities, fell from 9 per 1000 wounded to 1.4 per 1000 wounded. Other improvements in surgical care could have been contributory, but it seems likely that antitoxin was an important factor in the decrease in incidence.

Although antitoxin produced by the active immunization of horses has been widely employed since 1894, methods for the production of human tetanus antitoxin have been developed recently, and this agent is now widely available. Human tetanus immune globulin has two great advantages over equine antitetanus serum and should be employed whenever available. The first advantage is that the severe and sometimes fatal anaphylactic reactions which were relatively common after injection of horse serum are extremely rare after human antitoxin, so that it is not believed necessary to recommend a small test dose of human tetanus immune globulin before administration of the full dose. Epinephrine should, however, be available whenever either human or equine antitoxin is to be given. The second advantage is that human tetanus immune globulin shows less tendency than equine antitoxin to form the immune complexes which are excreted rapidly. An intramuscular injection of 250 units of human tetanus immune globulin maintains a blood level at or above that recommended for prophylaxis (0.01 unit per milliliter) for a period of four weeks, whereas 1500 units of equine antitoxin is required to produce a comparable but shorter-lived protection.

Tetanus antitoxin need not be given after clean, minor wounds; but if a wound with "tetanus-prone" features is present, a prophylactic dose of 250 units of human tetanus immune globulin should be administered intramuscularly unless the patient has been fully immunized against tetanus. United States recommendations are that two previous toxoid injections provide adequate immunization unless the wound is more than 24 hours old, whereas the United Kingdom recommendations suggest that tetanus antitoxin should be given unless a full course of three toxoid injections or a booster dose of toxoid has been received within ten years. If tetanus antitoxin is to be given, active immunization should be commenced immediately with an injection of adsorbed toxoid into another limb.

Chemoprophylaxis. Antimicrobial drugs can inhibit the multiplication of *Clostridium tetani* and kill the vegetative form of the organism. By killing aerobic organisms coexisting with the *Clostridium*, antimicrobial drugs can prevent multiplication by denying the *Clostridium* the conditions favorable to its growth; they have no effect, however, on tetanus toxin. Although data have been presented showing no increase in the incidence of tetanus after the substitution of chemoprophylaxis for passive immunization with equine antitetanus serum, the less toxic human antitoxin is currently recommended for tetanus prophylaxis if indicated after injury.

If human antitoxin is not available and chemoprophylaxis is to be employed, the drug chosen must be one to which the organism is susceptible and also one to which the patient is not sensitive. *Clostridium tetani* is susceptible to a variety of drugs, including penicillin, tetracycline, and erythromycin, so that it is probably not difficult to make a suitable choice for a particular patient. Smith (1964) has shown that in mice inoculated with tetanus spores, chemoprophylaxis was effective if it was started four hours after inoculation but not if started eight hours after inoculation. The time interval in humans is not established, but it is suggested that in

injuries seen later than six hours after infliction, some other form of prophylaxis should be chosen. Antimicrobial therapy must be continued for a sufficient time to ensure that tetanus spores cannot survive, and this means for at least five days.

PATHOGENESIS. If tetanus is to supervene, the *Clostridium* must be introduced into human tissue, and the disease may follow a trivial or a serious injury. In countries with good medical services, serious wounds receive effective treatment and tetanus is usually avoided. Apparently minor wounds then become a common cause of the disease, and in quite a high proportion of cases no responsible injury can be identified. The site of action and method of spread of the exotoxin have been mentioned, but it is rather surprising that no unequivocal evidence of recognizable pathologic lesions caused by tetanus has yet been forthcoming even after careful postmortem studies.

CLINICAL FEATURES AND CRITERIA OF SEVERITY IN TETANUS. The criteria of severity may be established in two ways: from the history, and from the symptoms and signs.

From the History. The severity of an attack of tetanus is related to the incubation period (the period from injury to the first sign of tetanus) and the onset period, described by Cole (1940) as the period from the first sign to the first generalized spasm. If the former is less than nine days and the latter less than 48 hours, the attack of tetanus may be expected to be severe. The length of the onset period is, in general, the more reliable guide to the expected severity of the attack.

From the Symptoms and Signs. In *the mild case*, tetanus usually presents with rigidity of muscles, and this rigidity may be severe enough to cause pain. The patient with mild tetanus may have "local tetanus," in which rigidity affects only one limb, or the patient may have mild generalized rigidity. Stiffness of the jaw muscles causes trismus, and stiffness of the facial muscles may cause a change of expression. Stiffness of the muscles of the neck and back may cause discomfort or even pain on attempted flexion of the spine.

In *the moderate case*, the patient has more severe generalized rigidity. Trismus is pronounced, the mouth can hardly be opened, and rigidity of the muscles of the face may cause the sneering "risus sardonicus." Opisthotonos may be pronounced, but more typically the stiffness of the antagonist muscles makes the patient lie "at attention" in bed, and the muscles of the back and abdomen are hard to the touch. Patients with moderate tetanus may show mild exacerbations of this generalized rigidity as "reflex spasms." These spasms may arise spontaneously or more commonly as a result of stimuli. The important difference, however, between the patient with mild and the patient with moderate tetanus is the presence or absence of dysphagia. Spasm of the pharyngeal muscles makes swallowing difficult, and the patient coughs or splutters while drinking. This will predispose to the inhalation of pharyngeal contents and is the diagnostic characteristic of the moderate case.

The patient with *a severe case* is distinguished from the patient with a moderate case by the presence of reflex spasms that may be of appalling intensity. If the spasms are untreated, opisthotonos becomes extreme and the intense muscle spasm may fracture vertebrae. Spasm of the laryngeal muscles, the diaphragm, and the intercostals prevents ventilation and cyanosis occurs. The occurrence of reflex spasms that cause cyanosis and cannot be controlled except by powerful relaxants such as curare is the characteristic feature of the severe case of tetanus.

Autonomic Disturbances. Disturbances of the autonomic nervous system occur frequently in severely affected tetanus patients and may prove fatal, particularly when the disease occurs in drug addicts. Younger patients often develop a fluctuating hypertension and increasing tachycardia after a few days of treatment, and cardiovascular responses to stimuli such as the aspiration of secretions from the respiratory tract become exaggerated so that systolic blood pressures of over 300 mm Hg are not uncommon. Patients sweat profusely, and may become extremely vasoconstricted peripherally with a sharp line of demarcation between warm and cold skin. Hyperpyrexia occurs in the absence of significant secondary infection and probably reflects the inability of the vasoconstricted patient to lose heat. High metabolic rates have been measured in spite of muscular paralysis, and the cardiac output is often disproportionately high in relation to tissue oxygen utilization, suggesting increased neurogenic drive to the heart. Raised plasma and urine catecholamine levels occur in association with these disturbances, and it seems likely that the sympathetic nervous system is grossly overactive and incoordinate. Prolonged overactivity has been followed by supraventricular tachycardia and multifocal ventricular ectopic beats, unresponsive hypotension, sudden bradycardia, and cardiac arrest.

Perhaps fortunately, patients with severe tetanus often remember little of their illness, but many recall weird and sometimes frightening dreams. Electroencephalography usually shows a sleep pattern with activation during stimulation such as tracheal aspiration.

DIAGNOSIS. The diagnosis of the established case of tetanus is all too easy, and strychnine poisoning is the only condition which is truly similar to established tetanus. Trismus may occur from dental infections, and the author has seen one case of hysterical tetanus. Overdose with or sensitivity to the phenothiazine group of drugs can be confused with tetanus, but the movements in these conditions usually include grimacing and jaw movements in which the jaw is opened widely.

CAUSES OF DEATH IN TETANUS. One of the most remarkable features of tetanus is that when patients recover, even from the most severe forms of the disease, they recover completely. It would therefore seem reasonable to study the causes of death carefully in tetanus so that by avoiding them the natural tendency of the disease toward recovery may be exploited. In a survey in Oxford, the causes of death in 20 of 110 patients were as follows: bronchopneumonia, 4; pulmonary embolus, 3; technical failure, 2; coincidental causes, 6; and no identifiable cause of death, 5.

Bronchopulmonary complications of tetanus are becoming less common now that the management of patients receiving intermittent positive pressure ventilation (IPPV) through a tracheostomy tube is better understood, and it is likely that chest complications will become still less common in the future. In general on the writer's service, pulmonary embolus is not a common cause of death in patients with other diseases treated by tracheostomy and IPPV. However, the difference in the incidence of pulmonary embolus between patients with tetanus requiring treatment with curare and IPPV and patients with other diseases similarly treated is so striking that anticoagulants are now used in patients with tetanus severe enough to merit treatment in this way. The incidence of technical failure underlines the complexity of treating the fully paralyzed patient; the coincidental causes of death apparently had nothing to do with the main disease. No identifiable cause of death could be found in five patients who had all displayed the pattern of clinical features suggestive of sympathetic overactivity.

TREATMENT. Treatment in tetanus is essentially symptomatic, but all patients with the disease should receive antimicrobial drugs and active and passive immunization, and should undergo wound excision. To allow the earliest possible detection of possibly lethal manifestations of the disease such as severe muscular or laryngeal spasms, the treatment of tetanus should be conducted in a well lighted intensive care unit rather than in isolation in a darkened side room. Treatment with penicillin (1 million units six hourly intramuscularly) or tetracycline (100 mg six hourly intramuscularly) should be commenced to ensure that all clostridia are killed. Human antitetanus immunoglobulin (3000 to 10,000 units) should be administered intravenously to produce a high blood level as early as possible. Investigations are under way in several parts of the world to assess the efficacy and dangers of administering a much smaller dose of the expensive human tetanus immunoglobulin via the intrathecal route. If a focus of infection is found, surgical debridement should be carried out shortly after administration of the antitoxin so that any toxin released into the circulation at surgery is neutralized. Because an attack of tetanus does not confer immunity, active immunization with adsorbed toxoid should be started and a full course of injections given during the recovery period.

Symptomatic Measures. MUSCULAR HYPERTONICITY. The trismus and increased muscle tone of the mild case of tetanus can usually be controlled adequately with small doses of diazepam (10 mg. three to four hourly orally or parenterally). Barbiturates and chlorpromazine have also been widely and effectively employed against these symptoms.

DYSPHAGIA AND AIRWAY MANAGEMENT. Trismus is a common early symptom in tetanus and is frequently accompanied by incoordination of the swallowing and laryngeal protective reflexes. Correct management of the airway is of vital importance, because laryngeal spasm may occur spontaneously or may be induced by attempts to swallow saliva or to pass a nasogastric tube. In addition, dysphagia may allow inhalation of infected material and saliva from the mouth so that atelectasis and pneumonia can follow; the latter remains a common cause of death in tetanus.

To minimize pulmonary complications, protection of the airway by intubation with a cuffed tube is advocated as soon as dysphagia is suspected. The symptom may be demonstrated as a tendency to cough and clear the throat after swallowing a mouthful of water, and, in more advanced form, as an inability to swallow saliva so that the patient drools or spits it out. Orotracheal intubation should be performed under general anesthesia and after muscle paralysis, allowing an elective tracheostomy with a cuffed tube. Meticulous pulmonary care should be instituted and maintained until normal pharyngolaryngeal function returns.

MUSCLE SPASMS. Muscle spasms in tetanus can be

either localized or generalized and of varying severity. Sustained contraction of the muscles is exhausting, painful, and, if the respiratory muscles become involved, dangerous. When large doses of diazepam or chlorpromazine are employed in attempts to control severe spasms, oversedation may lead to hypoventilation between spasms. In this situation, and when muscle spasms themselves interfere with ventilation, therapeutic paralysis should be induced with curare and the resultant ventilatory failure treated with intermittent positive pressure ventilation. Curare is given intramuscularly or intravenously and with sufficient frequency to allow ventilation to proceed freely and to keep the patient comfortable. This method of treatment has proved most satisfactory when used early in the disease rather than after prolonged attempts to manage the patient with sedative agents. Smythe et al. have reported remarkable success in neonates with similar techniques.

Once curarization and IPPV have commenced, anxiety in the conscious but paretic patient should be minimized by frequent reassurance from the nursing staff and by mild hypnosis from diazepam or a barbiturate. Some of the most severely affected patients, however, become unresponsive and appear comatose for periods of one to three weeks during the critical phase of their illness, and in this situation sedative agents and muscle relaxants should be administered only if clearly indicated. These patients usually regain consciousness during the recovery phase and appear normal apart from amnesia. After one to four weeks of treatment, curare requirements decrease and diazepam may be reinstituted to reduce muscle stiffness during weaning from IPPV.

NUTRITION. Patients with mild tetanus may be fed orally, but once dysphagia develops a nasogastric tube should be inserted while the patient is anesthetized for tracheostomy. The considerable caloric (2500 cals per day) and fluid requirements of the tetanus patient can be satisfied effectively over the two- to four-week period of dysphagia by nasogastric feeding; since tube feedings normally contain milk, the chance of gastrointestinal bleeding is reduced. Paralytic ileus occurs fairly frequently in severe tetanus but usually responds to intermittent gastric drainage followed by the instillation of antacids and gut stimulants (e.g., metoclopramide).

FLUID BALANCE. The maintenance of a balanced fluid status in the severe tetanus patient is complicated by the considerable insensible fluid losses produced by profuse sweating and by unswallowed saliva. If reliance is placed entirely upon measured fluid input and output, fluid losses may be seriously underestimated, and dehydration may result.

Underhydration in an immobilized patient increases the possibility of deep venous thrombosis and of pulmonary embolism, and the latter has already been mentioned as a common cause of death in tetanus. Although anticoagulation started 24 hours after tracheostomy and continued until remobilization has been practiced without significant complication in several centers, protection against pulmonary embolism has not been complete, and it is likely that avoidance of dehydration is equally important.

Insensible fluid losses are best monitored by weighing the patient each day, and dehydration is avoided by measuring the specific gravity (or osmolality) of the urine regularly. Enough fluid should be given parenterally or by nasogastric tube to produce a daily urine flow of 1.5 to 2 liters and to maintain the urine specific gravity below 1.015. Particular care must be taken to react promptly to the severe hypovolemia which may develop rapidly when overactivity of the sympathetic nervous system causes excessive sweating in association with paralytic ileus.

Cardiovascular Disturbances. In some of the tetanus patients who show severe muscular symptoms, cardiovascular changes in the form of tachycardia, hypertension, and increased responses to therapeutic maneuvers, such as tracheal aspiration, may appear after two to five days of treatment by curarization and artificial ventilation. These changes are probably produced by overactivity of the sympathetic nervous system and have been controlled successfully with adrenergic blocking agents. To reduce the tachycardia resulting from the intense sympathetic stimulation of the heart, a beta-adrenergic blocking agent such as propranolol (10 mg three to six hourly via the nasogastric tube) should be administered until the heart rate averages less than 100; if hypertension persists, an antihypertensive (e.g., bethanidine, 10 mg two to six hourly) should be added.*

Although other combinations of antiadrenergic agents might be more effective, short-acting drugs are preferred, because, particularly in drug addicts and in elderly patients, the pattern of autonomic disturbance may change very rapidly. In these groups of patients, episodes of profound hypotension and bradycardia may suddenly occur and, on occasion, lead to cardiac arrest. Provided that resuscitation is prompt, the cardiovascular status may be restored rapidly and repeatedly by measures such as tracheal aspiration and mildly painful stimuli which result in the release of endogenous catecholamines. These sudden and readily reversible episodes, during which the circulation appears unstimulated and dilated, must be contrasted with the unresponsive preterminal hypotension accompanied by tachycardia, vasoconstriction, and hyperpyrexia which has followed prolonged and unrelieved sympathetic overactivity. In view of the varying patterns of cardiovascular disturbance, continuous direct monitoring of heart rate and of arterial and central venous blood pressures has proved of considerable benefit in guiding therapy.

In summary, in a *mild case* the patient needs (1) wound excision, (2) human or equine antitoxin, (3) penicillin or another appropriate antimicrobial drug, and (4) a centrally acting relaxant and sedative drug, such as diazepam.

In the *moderate case* the patient needs in addition (5) tracheostomy and the insertion of a cuffed rubber tracheostomy tube to separate the pharynx from the trachea and to make inhalation of foreign material impossible, and (6) nasogastric tube feeding.

In the *severe case* the patient needs in addition (7) virtually complete paralysis with curare or another powerful relaxant and IPPV, (8) anticoagulant drugs, and (9), if sympathetic overactivity is present, treatment with alpha- and beta-adrenergic blockers.

PROGNOSIS. The patient with mild tetanus will almost certainly survive whether treated or not. The patient with moderate tetanus, if untreated, is at risk

---

*Bethanidine is not available in the United States; guanethidine might be substituted.

from inhalation of foreign material, and repeated episodes of this kind may lead to fatal pneumonia. The patient with moderate tetanus, if treated, should not die except from causes unrelated to the primary disease. The patient with severe tetanus who is having reflex spasms severe enough to cause cyanosis will certainly die if untreated, but even with treatment the severity of the illness and the complexity of the therapeutic regimen make the outlook uncertain. In the United Kingdom in 1967, even in the best centers, the mortality in patients with tetanus severe enough to indicate treatment with curare and IPPV varied between 10 and 40 per cent. Over-all mortality in the best hands is often still as high as 20 per cent, and at the extremes of age the mortality may be higher. It is paradoxical that in advanced countries where the immunization programs are efficient, mortality in the cases that do occur is high, not only because unimmunized patients are generally at the extremes of age, but also because patients who escape the immunization programs tend to have a poor physical status.

Adams, E. B., Laurence, D. R., and Smith, J. W. G.: Tetanus. Oxford, Blackwell Scientific Publications, 1969.

Bjørnboe, M., Ibsen, B., and Johnson, S.: Et tilfaelde af tetanus behandlet med curarisering, tracheostomi of overtryksventilation med kvaelstofforilte og ilt. Ugeskr. Laeger., 115:1535, 1953.

Fraser, D. W.: Preventing tetanus in patients with wounds. Ann. Intern. Med., 84:95, 1976.

Sanders, R. K. M., Martyn, B., Joseph, R., and Peacock, M. L.: Intrathecal antitetanus serum (horse) in the treatment of tetanus. Lancet, 1:974, 1977.

Smythe, P. M., Bowie, M. D., and Voss, T. J. V.: Treatment of tetanus neonatorum with muscle relaxants and intermittent positive pressure ventilation. Br. Med. J., 1:223, 1974.

Tsueda, K., Oliver, P. B., and Richter, R. W.: Cardiovascular manifestations of tetanus. Anesthesiology, 40:588, 1974.

ANAEROBIC BACTERIA

151. DISEASE DUE TO NONSPOREFORMING ANAEROBIC BACTERIA

Sydney M. Finegold

DEFINITION. Essentially every type of infection may be caused by nonsporeforming anaerobes. No organ or tissue of the body is immune to infection with these organisms. The majority of anaerobic infections involve two or more anaerobes, but infection with a single species of anaerobe does occur. Aerobic or facultatively anaerobic organisms may also be present in mixed infections. In mixed anaerobic infections, clostridia may be found together with nonsporeforming anaerobic bacilli and cocci. There are a number of unique features associated with certain clostridial infections, however, and it is convenient to consider these infections separately (see Ch. 146 to 150). Actinomycosis may also show distinctive clinical features; this disease (also often a mixed infection) is discussed in Ch. 163.

ETIOLOGY. The nonsporulating anaerobic bacteria are distributed widely throughout the body as indigenous flora. Numerically, they are the dominant flora on the various mucosal surfaces.

The anaerobic gram-negative bacilli and the anaerobic cocci are the major etiologic agents in anaerobic infections. They are encountered at least 15 times as frequently as clostridia. Gram-positive nonsporeforming anaerobic bacilli are encountered less commonly.

Anaerobic Gram-Negative Bacilli. The anaerobic gram-negative bacilli found in human infections belong to the genera *Bacteroides* and *Fusobacterium*, the former being encountered with much greater frequency. The *Bacteroides fragilis* group (five closely related species) is the most commonly seen of all anaerobes. It is of added importance because it is the most resistant of the anaerobes to antimicrobial compounds. The species of the *B. fragilis* group recovered most often from infections are, in order, *fragilis*, *thetaiotaomicron*, and *vulgatus*.

The *B. fragilis* group, like other gram-negative anaerobic rods, stains poorly. The staining is usually irregular. There is a variable amount of pleomorphism. Two other *Bacteroides* species seen relatively often, though rarely as single infecting agents, are *B. melaninogenicus* (coccobacilli) and *B. oralis* (morphologically similar to *B. fragilis*). *Fusobacterium nucleatum*, the fusiform bacillus, is the most frequently found of the fusobacteria. This organism is long and thin, with tapered ends; it is seen often in pairs end to end. Long filaments may also be noted. Granules (sometimes gram-positive) may be seen. *F. necrophorum*, formerly commonly encountered, is now seen much less. Other species of *Fusobacterium* seen include *F. mortiferum* and *F. varium*, the latter being relatively resistant to antimicrobials. Medically important fusobacteria other than *F. nucleatum* tend to be highly pleomorphic, with long filaments containing central swellings, large, free round bodies, and considerable irregularity of staining.

The spirochetes of the genus *Treponema*, also gram-negative anaerobes, which are part of the indigenous flora, are very likely not pathogenic, judging from experimental studies. The old terms "fusospirochetal infection" and "Vincent's infection" are therefore no longer appropriate.

Anaerobic Cocci. The anaerobic cocci include gram-positive streptococci (*Peptostreptococcus*), gram-positive cocci in pairs or masses (*Peptococcus*), and gram-negative cocci (*Veillonella, Megasphaera, Acidaminococcus*). The gram-negative cocci are not important pathogens. The anaerobic cocci are not usually pleomorphic, but many are smaller than facultative streptococci. *Veillonella* are tiny cocci in masses. As a group, anaerobic cocci are found in human disease almost as often as are the gram-negative anaerobic bacilli. The most commonly encountered species include *Peptostreptococcus anaerobius, intermedius* (this organism is actually microaerophilic), and *micros*, and *Peptococcus magnus, asaccharolyticus*, and *prevotii*.

The microaerophilic cocci and streptococci are a very poorly characterized heterogeneous group. They are best defined as organisms which tolerate reduced oxygen tension (18 per cent oxygen) — with or without added carbon dioxide. Most of these are actually facultative streptococci. These organisms are encountered in serious infections with some frequency, not uncommonly in pure culture. They are considered with the obligate anaerobes because they will often be overlooked unless good anaerobic techniques are used for transporting and culturing clinical specimens.

Gram-Positive Nonsporeforming Anaerobic Bacilli. The most commonly encountered gram-positive anaerobic nonsporeforming bacilli belong to the genus *Eubacterium*, particularly *E. lentum, E. alactolyticum,* and *E. limosum.* Gram-positive anaerobic bacilli in general destain readily and may appear gram-negative. *Eubacterium* strains may be filamentous. *Propionibacterium* strains, chiefly *P. acnes,* are seldom involved in infections of significance other than endocarditis (in patients with pre-existing valvular disease or artificial heart valves) or other infections related to implanted artificial prostheses. *Bifidobacterium eriksonii* is another well-established pathogen. *Actinomyces* may also be involved in infections without the distinctive clinical features of actinomycosis.

Features of Infections Due to Various Organisms. There are differences in the types of infection involving various anaerobes related to differences in their distribution in the body as normal flora. Thus the anaerobic cocci are encountered more often in oral and pulmonary infections and in female genital infections than in intra-abdominal disease. *Bacteroides fragilis,* which is the dominant member of the colonic flora, is involved in intra-abdominal infection commonly but is less frequently involved in dental infections or lung abscess. Aside from these differences, all the nonsporeforming anaerobes may be involved in any of the infections to be discussed in this chapter. Furthermore, the clinical picture is basically the same in these conditions regardless of the specific flora involved. Minor exceptions include distinctive odors related to end-products of metabolism (e.g., butyric acid produced in large amounts by *Fusobacterium* strains), the occasional formation of soft granules resembling sulfur granules by *Fusobacterium,* and the production of black color in blood-containing exudates by *B. melaninogenicus.*

Relative Importance of Various Organisms in Mixed Infections. It is difficult to determine the role of each species recovered from a mixed anaerobic infection and to assess the relative importance of the anaerobes and aerobic or facultative bacteria in mixed infections. Quantitative culture techniques may help. A small number of patients with pulmonary and intra-abdominal mixed infections of mild to moderate severity have been treated with agents active only against the anaerobes and have done well. This suggests that the anaerobes may have been the key pathogens.

EPIDEMIOLOGY. Anaerobic infections are the most frequently overlooked or misdiagnosed of all bacterial infections. Fortunately, the introduction of simplified anaerobic cultural procedures and an increased awareness of anaerobes and their importance on the part of bacteriologists and clinicians are beginning to overcome the problem.

Good data on the incidence of anaerobes in various infections are not always available. One big problem has been a tendency to overlook anaerobes in mixed cultures when one or more aerobic or facultative forms are present. Problems in specific identification have interfered with accurate determination of the involvement of particular organisms in various anaerobic infections.

There are now a number of studies supporting the view that anaerobes are common causes of infection. Some years ago Stokes (1958) found anaerobes in over 10 per cent of 4737 positive cultures of clinical specimens. Lodenkämper and Stienen (1955) detected 690 anaerobic infections in an eight-year period. Mattman et al. (1958) found anaerobic cocci in 45 per cent of 437 positive cultures from hospitalized patients. Martin (1974) isolated 10,998 anaerobes from clinical specimens in a two-year period.

A number of studies have combined good clinical and bacteriologic analysis to yield reliable information on the incidence of anaerobes in certain infections. Thus Heineman and Braude (1962) have shown that anaerobes are the dominant cause of brain abscess. Frederick and Braude (1974) noted an important role for anaerobes in chronic sinusitis. Bartlett and coworkers (1972, 1973, 1974) have established that lung abscess and aspiration pneumonia are most often due to anaerobes and that these organisms are important causes of necrotizing pneumonia and of empyema. Several groups have data to indicate that 85 to 95 per cent of cases of intra-abdominal abscess and of peritonitis involve anaerobes. Very likely well over half of all cases of pyogenic liver abscess also involve these organisms. A number of workers have documented the importance of anaerobes in a variety of obstetric and gynecologic infections. Other types of infections in which anaerobes play an important role include chronic otitis media, gingivitis and other oral infections, dental infections, bronchiectasis, other pulmonary infections, breast abscess, appendicitis, diverticulitis, abdominal and other wound infections, puerperal sepsis, ischiorectal and perirectal abscess, infected pilonidal sinuses, gas-forming cellulitis, necrotizing fasciitis, human and animal bite infections, and septic thrombophlebitis.

PATHOGENESIS OR MECHANISMS. Anaerobic bacteria basically are saprophytic members of the indigenous flora. Under certain conditions, however, they may invade and produce disease.

A simplistic definition of anaerobic bacteria would be bacteria which cannot survive in the presence of air. However, it is well known that a number of anaerobes generally regarded as fairly fastidious will tolerate 2 to 8 per cent oxygen in the atmosphere, and a number of these organisms will tolerate considerably more. Another factor determining whether or not the environment is suitable for growth of anaerobic bacteria is the oxidation-reduction potential of the medium. This is a measure of the tendency of the system to give up electrons and is usually expressed as the Eh value in millivolts. The Eh of a system is a function not only of its inherent reducing tendency but also of its hydrogen ion concentration, the Eh becoming more negative as the hydrogen ion concentration decreases.

One of the major defenses of the body against infection by anaerobes is the normal Eh (+120 mv). Lowering of the redox potential permits anaerobic growth in tissues, even those exposed to air. Lowered oxidation-reduction potential results from impaired blood supply, tissue necrosis, and growth of facultative bacteria in a wound. Thus vascular disease, epinephrine injection, cold, shock, edema, trauma, surgery, presence of a foreign body, malignancy, gas production by microorganisms, and aerobic infection all may predispose to anaerobic infection. The predisposition of diabetics to anaerobic infection is undoubtedly related at least partially to impaired blood supply and lowering of Eh. The association of malignancy (particularly of the colon, the bronchus, and the uterus) and anaerobic infection is well established; at times, anaerobic infection may be the first clue to the malignant process.

Certain toxins such as collagenase, hyaluronidase, deoxyribonuclease, and proteinases account for the virulence of some anaerobic infections.

The septic thrombophlebitis seen commonly in anaerobic infections may relate to production of heparinase by anaerobic bacteria and to acceleration of coagulation by gram-negative anaerobic rods. This lesion may lead to metastatic infection and helps account for the difficulty in eradicating anaerobic infections. Tissue destruction and abscess formation are also common manifestations of anaerobic infection.

Previous antimicrobial therapy is a not uncommon background for anaerobic infection. Preoperative "bowel preparation" with oral neomycin often results in a residual anaerobic flora, as many anaerobes tolerate even the very high concentrations achieved in the bowel lumen with such therapy. The popular combination of an aminoglycoside plus a cephalosporin (given parenterally) may lead to anaerobic superinfection, particularly with *Bacteroides fragilis*.

Conditions which predispose to infection in general (malnutrition, severe debilitating disease, corticosteroid and other immunosuppressive therapy, granulocytopenia) also facilitate anaerobic infection.

Aspiration and poor dental hygiene are common background factors in anaerobic pulmonary infection.

The unique involvement of only certain species of the *B. fragilis* group in infection is probably related to capsule formation (Kasper, 1976) and to resistance to normal serum bactericidal factors (Casciato et al., 1973). Under anaerobic conditions the granulocyte phagocytic bactericidal system may not function efficiently.

CLINICAL MANIFESTATIONS. For the most part the manifestations of anaerobic infection are those of the basic process (e.g., peritonsillar abscess, cholangitis, endometritis). Tissue necrosis, abscess formation, and septic thrombophlebitis are common with anaerobic infection, as are a foul odor and gas in tissues or in discharges.

Tonsillitis, Ludwig's Angina. Exudative tonsillitis (Vincent's angina) used to be a common anaerobic infection, usually caused by *Fusobacterium necrophorum*. The local tonsillar infection undoubtedly still occurs but is rarely recognized as an anaerobic process. The dreaded Ludwig's angina (cellulitis of the submandibular space), probably an anaerobic infection in most cases, is also uncommon now.

Bacteremia, Endocarditis. In recent years, bacteremia caused by anaerobes has dominated clinical reports on anaerobic infections. Most likely this is because anaerobes are much more likely to be present in pure culture in bacteremia than in other types of anaerobic infection, and consequently it is much easier to isolate the offending organism. On the other hand, it is clear that anaerobic bacteremia is relatively common, accounting for 10 to 15 per cent of all bacteremias. The primary sources of anaerobic bacteremia at present are the gastrointestinal and gynecologic tracts. Less common sites include infected decubitus ulcers and other wounds. Septic shock and disseminated intravascular coagulation have been described in the course of anaerobic bacteremia.

In large series of endocarditis, only 1 to 2 per cent of positive blood cultures have yielded anaerobes as a rule. As high as 15 per cent, however, were sterile in the presence of strong clinical or pathologic evidence of endocarditis. Our experience is that approximately 10 per cent of cases of endocarditis are caused by anaerobic or microaerophilic cocci. The main portals of entry for anaerobes in bacterial endocarditis are the mouth, the gastrointestinal tract, and, to a lesser extent, the genitourinary tract. The incidence of pre-existing heart disease is lower in the case of anaerobic endocarditis, and there is evidence to indicate that embolization may be more common in the case of the disease involving anaerobes.

Pleuropulmonary Infection. Anaerobic pulmonary infection is commonly overlooked. Unfortunately, even when suspected, it has often not been confirmed by proper culture of appropriate specimens. Coughed sputum culture is unsatisfactory because of the presence of anaerobes as normal upper respiratory tract flora. The clinical course of anaerobic pulmonary infection ranges from incidentally discovered infection to fulminant infection. Most patients present with a smoldering illness. The most common underlying condition is a predisposition to aspirate caused by altered consciousness or dysphagia. Important clues to anaerobic etiology are aspiration, pulmonary necrosis, indolent course, and foul-smelling sputum or pus. The principal types of anaerobic pulmonary infection are lung abscess, necrotizing pneumonia, and pneumonia without necrosis; many patients have an associated empyema.

Anaerobes are probably second only to the pneumococcus as causes of pneumonia in hospitalized patients, because aspiration pneumonia is a common event.

Intra-abdominal Infection. Anaerobes are a prime cause of peritonitis and intra-abdominal abscess and are involved in virtually all cases of complicated appendicitis or diverticulitis.

Anaerobes (especially nonsporeformers) play a relatively minor role in gallbladder infection.

Genitourinary Tract Infection. Various urinary tract infections may involve anaerobes, but these organisms are not common causes of such infection. Factors predisposing to anaerobic urinary tract infection are stones, malignancy, obstruction, and previous renal tuberculosis.

A large variety of female genital tract infections involve anaerobic bacteria. Clostridia cause the most serious female genital tract infections, but infections in this system are much more commonly produced by nonsporeforming anaerobic bacteria. Predisposing conditions include pregnancy, the puerperium (particularly with premature rupture of the membranes, prolonged labor, or postpartum hemorrhage), abortion (spontaneous or induced), malignancy, radiation, surgery, cauterization, stenosis, uterine fibroids, and old gonococcal salpingitis.

Skin, Soft Tissue, and Muscle Infection. These infections include such entities as cellulitis, pyoderma, infected cysts, infection of decubitus and other ulcers, abscesses, bacterial synergistic gangrene, chronic undermining ulcer of Meleney, necrotizing fasciitis, bite infection, noma, and tropical ulcer. Anaerobes are common infecting agents in hidradenitis suppurativa. Subcutaneous abscesses involving anaerobes are seen in narcotic addicts who are "skin-poppers."

Anaerobic (gas-forming) cellulitis is an acute soft tissue infection, seen particularly in diabetics and commonly ascribed to coliforms. Although gas-producing nonanaerobes may be involved, it is our experience that anaerobes predominate. Muscle is usually not involved, but it is essential that clostridial myositis be ruled out. This differentiation may require surgery, which, in any case, is important therapeutically.

Anaerobic streptococci may produce a myositis simulating "gas gangrene," but the infection is much less severe. Bacteroides and anaerobic cocci may be involved in a milder form of myositis known as synergistic anaerobic cellulitis, as well as in necrotizing fasciitis.

Bone and Joint Infection. Osteomyelitis caused by anaerobes is probably overlooked often. Anaerobes are relatively common in infected diabetic ulcers of the foot with bony involvement.

There are a number of well-documented cases of purulent arthritis caused by anaerobes, chiefly gramnegative bacilli. Predisposing factors include underlying joint disease and local or systemic corticosteroid therapy. Any joint may be affected, but there is a peculiar susceptibility of the sternoclavicular and sacroiliac joints.

DIAGNOSIS. Clues Suggesting Anaerobic Infection. Features indicating the likelihood of anaerobic infection include foul or putrid odor, infection located near mucosal surfaces (particularly with manipulation of the associated organs), tissue necrosis, gas in tissues or discharges, infection associated with malignancy or other tissue-destructive process, endocarditis with negative routine blood cultures, infection related to the use of aminoglycoside antimicrobials (by any route) and/or broad-spectrum penicillins or cephalosporins, septic thrombophlebitis, infection after bites, black coloration or red fluorescence under ultraviolet light of discharges or lesions (*B. melaninogenicus* infection), unique morphology on Gram stain of exudate, and failure to obtain growth on routine culture (particularly when organisms are seen on Gram stain of exudate).

Specimen Collection. The major consideration is to avoid "contaminating" a specimen with normal flora, because anaerobes are prevalent as indigenous flora.

Expectorated sputum is not suitable for anaerobic culture. Bronchoscopically obtained specimens are also not suitable, although it is possible that quantitative culture of material obtained via a sheathed fiberoptic bronchoscope may prove useful. This is not established. Transtracheal needle aspiration or direct lung puncture is the optimal method of obtaining specimens from patients with suspected anaerobic pulmonary infection, unless empyema fluid is available.

In the case of uterine infection, there is no satisfactory method for obtaining reliable bacteriologic data unless there is an accompanying bacteremia. However, quantitation of growth from carefully obtained intrauterine cultures may be of some value.

In the case of abscesses, the unbroken skin or mucosal surface is decontaminated, and pus is removed with a syringe. This is preferable to using a swab on a portion of an exposed lesion.

Voided midstream urine may contain anaerobes from the urethral flora; therefore percutaneous suprapubic bladder aspiration is necessary.

Specimen Transport. Proper transport of specimens to the laboratory is crucial for recovery of anaerobes which may be present. Since some anaerobes are tolerant to oxygen contact, a laboratory which isolates such organisms as *B. fragilis* and *C. perfringens* may not realize that it is overlooking more demanding anaerobes. Many anaerobes responsible for clinical infections do not tolerate oxygen exposure well, so that special transport methods are needed to ensure their survival. Various means for proper anaerobic transport include the following:

1. Syringe technique — eliminate all air from specimen in syringe and needle and then stick needle into a sterile rubber stopper (for transport time of 30 minutes or less).
2. Gassed-out tubes — inject specimen into butyl rubberstopped tube which has been gassed out with oxygen-free CO_2. Commercial vials of this type are available.

TREATMENT. General Aspects. Surgical aspects of therapy are extremely important. Drainage of collections of pus and excision of necrotic tissue are commonly necessary, and in minor infections they may be all that is required. Obstructions must be relieved and tissues decompressed when this is indicated.

Anticoagulant therapy or venous ligation may be indicated in patients with septic phlebitis. Treatment of shock and disseminated intravascular coagulation, when they occur, and general supportive measures are important aspects of therapy.

Local use of hydrogen peroxide or zinc peroxide is useful. Hyperbaric oxygen therapy is not indicated in infection with nonsporeforming anaerobes.

Antimicrobial Therapy. In vitro susceptibility tests, properly performed, serve as a good guide to drug therapy of anaerobic infections. Standardized disc susceptibility tests are available for most anaerobic bacteria but are most satisfactory with organisms which have been identified. Use of a disc test without measurement of zones of inhibition, or application of standards which were developed for aerobic and facultative organisms, yields completely undependable results. Conventional tube or plate dilution tests with incubation in an anaerobic jar are reliable. Patterns of susceptibility to selected drugs are noted in the accompanying table.

Penicillin is active against most anaerobes other than *Bacteroides fragilis;* however, this organism is the anaerobe most commonly isolated from infection. Certain strains of anaerobic cocci require as much as 16.0 to 32.0 μg per milliliter for inhibition, and occasional strains of *Fusobacterium varium* are resistant to penicillin. Dosage of penicillin G should be at least 8 to 12 million units daily in the case of seriously ill adults or infection with relatively resistant strains. Ampicillin and cephaloridine are usually comparable to penicillin G, but several other penicillins and cephalosporins are less active. Some agents in these classes may be useful because very high blood levels are achieved safely or because of their resistance to beta lactamases.

Tetracycline is no longer valuable in many geographic areas, because many strains of anaerobes of all types are now resistant. Two new tetracycline derivatives, doxycycline and minocycline, are more active, but susceptibility testing is required because a number of strains of most types of anaerobes are resistant.

Lincomycin, erythromycin, and vancomycin are active against certain anaerobes; more information is needed, however, on the validity of in vitro tests with these drugs, and they are not approved by the Food and Drug Administration for use in anaerobic infections.

Susceptibility of Anaerobes to Selected Antimicrobial Agents

	Microaerophilic and Anaerobic Cocci	Bacteroides fragilis	Bacteroides melanino-genicus	Fuso-bacterium varium	Other Fusobacterium Species	Eubac-terium
Penicillin G	+++ to ++++	+	++++*	+++*	++++	++++
Clindamycin	++ to +++	+++	+++	++	+++	++ to +++
Metronidazole†	++	+++	+++	+++	+++	++
Chloramphenicol	+++	+++	+++	+++	+++	+++

++++ Drug of choice.   ++ Moderate activity.
+++ Good activity.   + Poor or inconsistent activity.

*A few strains are resistant.
†Experimental for anaerobic infections.

Chloramphenicol is active against all anaerobes, with only rare strains resistant, and is very effective clinically. It penetrates the central nervous system well. However, because of its serious and unpredictable toxicity, it should be reserved for seriously ill patients and used only until bacteriologic data indicate that a less toxic drug would be suitable. Nevertheless, chloramphenicol is the drug of choice for serious anaerobic infection of uncertain cause. Initial dosage of chloramphenicol in such a patient should be 40 to 50 mg per kilogram of body weight daily; once the patient has shown a good response, 30 mg per kilogram per day should be adequate.

Clindamycin (7-chlorolincomycin) has broad activity against anaerobes, with only *Fusobacterium varium*, among the nonsporeformers, commonly resistant. However, a number of strains of *Clostridium* other than *C. perfringens* are not uncommonly resistant; this is also true for a number of *Peptococcus* strains and occasional strains of *B. fragilis*. Clindamycin is one of the drugs of choice for nonsporeforming anaerobic infections, except in central nervous system infections and in very serious infections in which the nature of the infecting organism and its susceptibility to clindamycin are not yet known. Colitis caused by clindamycin is an uncommon but sometimes serious complication; it is now known to be caused primarily or exclusively by *Clostridium difficile*. Oral dosage for adults is 150 to 450 mg every six hours, and parenteral dosage is 600 to 2700 mg per day (in two to four equal doses), depending on the severity of the infection. Daily doses as high as 4.8 grams have been given intravenously to critically ill patients.

Metronidazole has broad activity against anaerobic microorganisms and is consistently bactericidal versus *Bacteroides fragilis* and other anaerobes. It is very effective in anaerobic infections, but it has not yet been approved by the U.S. Food and Drug Administration for this purpose.

Although it is true that *Bacteroides fragilis* infections are more common below the diaphragm and that most anaerobes recovered from infections above the diaphragm are penicillin susceptible, there is too much overlap for practical application of this knowledge in the individual case — particularly if the patient has a serious infection. For example, *B. fragilis* is part of the infecting flora of 10 to 20 per cent of anaerobic pulmonary infections. It has also been recovered from such infections as sinusitis, mastoiditis, and brain abscess.

Therapy with antimicrobial agents in anaerobic infections must be intensive and prolonged. These infections have a considerable tendency to relapse.

PROGNOSIS. In general, infection with nonsporeforming anaerobes carries a relatively good prognosis, provided the diagnosis is suspected and confirmed early and appropriate therapy instituted promptly. To some extent, of course, the prognosis varies with the site and extent of the lesion. Brain abscess is still a very serious infection with a significant mortality (50 per cent). The over-all mortality in anaerobic pulmonary infections is 15 to 20 per cent, with a distinctly higher mortality in the case of necrotizing pneumonia (30 per cent). The mortality in liver abscess varies greatly from series to series, depending primarily on whether or not cases were discovered ante mortem and on how early they were picked up. On the whole, the mortality is in the range of 25 to 50 per cent. The mortality in sepsis caused by nonsporeforming anaerobes is 30 per cent. In patients with endocarditis caused by gram-negative anaerobic bacilli, mortality is also 30 per cent, but it is higher in cases caused by *Bacteroides fragilis* than in those caused by other, more sensitive gram-negative anaerobic bacilli. The mortality in endocarditis caused by anaerobic cocci is not significantly different from that caused by facultative streptococci. The availability of a number of effective drugs has permitted a reduction in mortality and morbidity resulting from anaerobic infection.

PREVENTION. The major principles in prophylaxis are avoidance or early correction of conditions which reduce the redox potential of the tissues and avoidance of the introduction of anaerobes from the indigenous flora into sites where they may set up infection. Discriminate use of antimicrobial drugs will minimize anaerobic superinfection.

Early appropriate therapy of anaerobic infections will prevent metastatic infection.

Precautions to minimize the possibility of aspiration will be helpful in preventing anaerobic pulmonary infection. Good surgical technique (e.g., minimal devitalization of tissue, use of closed methods of resection) will prevent postoperative anaerobic infections.

Bartlett, J., and Finegold, S. M.: Anaerobic pleuropulmonary infections. Medicine, 51:413, 1972.

Finegold, S. M.: Anaerobic Bacteria in Human Disease. New York, Academic Press, 1977.

Gorbach, S. L., and Bartlett, J. G.: Anaerobic infections. N. Engl. J. Med., 290:1177, 1237, 1289, 1974.

Ledger, W. J.: Infection in the Female. Philadelphia, Lea & Febiger, 1977.

Marcoux, J. A., Zabransky, R. J., Washington, J. A., II, Wellman, W. E., and Martin, W. J.: Bacteroides bacteremia: A review of 123 cases. Minn. Med., 53:1169, 1970.

Saksena, D. S., Block, M. A., McHenry, M. C., and Truant, J. P.: Bacteroidaceae: Anaerobic organisms encountered in surgical infections. Surgery, 63:261, 1968.

TYPHOID FEVER AND SALMONELLOSIS

152. TYPHOID FEVER

Sherwood L. Gorbach

Typhoid ("cloudy") fever is a febrile illness of prolonged duration which is marked by hectic fever, delirium, enlargement of the spleen, abdominal pain, and a variety of systemic manifestations. Although caused primarily by *Salmonella typhi*, typhoidal disease occasionally is produced by other types of salmonellae. The portal of entry is the gastrointestinal tract, but typhoid fever is not truly an intestinal disease, having more systemic symptoms than those related to the bowel. There is a mortality of 1 to 5 per cent in drug-treated patients; the causes of death are intestinal perforation, hemorrhage, and severe toxemia.

EPIDEMIOLOGY. Improvements in environmental sanitation have reduced the incidence of typhoid fever in the industrialized nations. Approximately 500 cases occur each year in the United States, with the greatest occurrence in young people. Most cases are sporadic, but are invariably related to a human carrier. The organism is essentially confined to humans, either in a disease state or as a carrier. Large-scale epidemics of typhoid occur on a regular basis, usually traced to contaminated food which may be imported from an endemic area or to contaminated water supplies. A recent epidemic in Mexico has been associated with bottled beverages.

Typhoid fever is a classic food- and water-borne pathogen. The major routes of passage are by the five F's: flies, fingers, food, feces, and fomites. *S. typhi* is extremely hardy and can survive for extended periods in polluted waters, contaminated foods, and soiled bedclothes. In earlier times, typhoid fever was considered "morbus medicorum," being capable of spread within hospitals to cause a high mortality among doctors and nurses. With effective chemotherapy and intelligent isolation procedures, intrahospital spread is extremely uncommon.

Since *S. typhi* cohabits exclusively with man, the occurrence of a single case means the presence of a carrier. An investigation by public health authorities should be instituted to determine the source and the presence of other cases. Chronic carriers, as they are discovered, are registered with the health authorities, and the microorganism is phage typed so that it can be traced in the event of an outbreak. However, the registered carriers represent only a minority of the potential reservoir, and do not take account of the "imported" cases of typhoid, which include nearly half of the acute infections in the United States.

PATHOGENESIS AND PATHOLOGY. The pathologic events of typhoid fever are initiated in the intestinal tract following oral ingestion of typhoid bacilli. The organism penetrates the small bowel mucosa, sparing the stomach, and makes its way rapidly to the lymphatics, the mesenteric nodes, and, within minutes, to the bloodstream. There is a paucity of local inflammatory findings, which explains the lack of intestinal symptoms at this stage. This sequence of events is in marked contrast to that of other forms of salmonellosis and to shigellosis in which the intestinal findings are prominent at the onset.

The organism must survive passage through the stomach, warding off the destructive action of gastric acid. Food and beverages, the classic vehicles of typhoid fever, also serve as an excellent buffer to acid. The number of bacilli ingested is a critical determinant of infection. An inoculum of 10^9 bacilli produces disease in 95 per cent of apparently healthy people, whereas 10^3 organisms rarely cause symptoms. The incubation period is inversely related to inoculum size; an inoculum of 10^9 bacilli is associated with a five-day latent period, which is extended to nine days or longer in those receiving a smaller dose.

Following the initial bacteremia, the organism is sequestered in macrophages and monocytic cells of the reticuloendothelial system. It undergoes multiplication, and re-emerges several days later in recurrent waves of bacteremia, an event which initiates the symptomatic phase of infection. Now in great numbers, the organism is spread throughout the host, infecting many organ sites. The intestinal tract may be seeded by direct bacteremic spread, as, for example, to Peyer's patches in the terminal ileum. Alternatively, the gallbladder contains a large number of bacilli, and contaminated bile is another method of infecting the gut.

Hyperplasia of the reticuloendothelial system, including lymph nodes, liver, and spleen, is characteristic of typhoid fever. The liver contains discrete, micronodular areas of necrosis, surrounded by macrophages and lymphocytes. Inflammation of the gallbladder is common, and may lead to acute cholecystitis. Patients with pre-existing gallbladder disease have a penchant for becoming carriers, because the bacillus becomes intimately associated with the chronic infection and may be incorporated within the gallstones themselves. Lymphoid follicles in the gut, such as Peyer's patches, become hyperplastic, with infiltration of macrophages, lymphocytes, and red blood cells. Subsequently, a follicle may ulcerate and penetrate through the submucosa to the intestinal lumen, discharging in its wake large numbers of typhoid bacilli. As the bowel wall is progressively involved, it becomes paper-thin, and is susceptible to transmural perforation into the peritoneal cavity. This occurs most commonly in the distal ileum, 25 cm from the ileocecal sphincter. Erosion into blood vessels produces severe intestinal hemorrhage.

An analogy has been drawn between the biologic effects of endotoxin and typhoid fever. Both cause chills, fever, headache, nausea, and vomiting, as well as the laboratory findings of leukopenia and thrombocytopenia. With endotoxin, however, increasing doses produce a state of tolerance in which further administration has no effect. By contrast, typhoid fever is a relentless and sustained state of illness. Administration of viable typhoid organisms to volunteers rendered tolerant to endotoxin still produces symptoms. Thus typhoid fever cannot be explained merely as a reaction to endotoxin, although this material may play some role in the disease state.

CLINICAL MANIFESTATIONS. Typhoid fever lasts about four weeks, evolving in a manner consistent with the pathophysiologic events. Classically, the illness is described as a series of one-week stages. Although in general the illness follows such a pattern, individual cases may deviate significantly, and the illness may persist (with accompanying bacteremia) with only slight improvement for four weeks or more. The *incubation period* is generally 7 to 14 days, with wide variations on either extreme. During the *first week*, the triad of fever, headache, and abdominal pain is commonly encountered. The onset usually is insidious with a stepladder rise of fever which later becomes persistent. It is accompanied by a dull headache. The pulse is often slower than would be expected for the degree of temperature elevation. Abdominal pain is localized to the right lower quadrant in most instances, although it can be diffuse. In approximately 50 per cent of patients, there is no change in bowel habits; in fact, constipation is more common than diarrhea in children. Near the end of the first week, enlargement of the spleen is noticeable. An evanescent and rather classic rash, "rose spots," becomes manifest at this time. It is observed in approximately 70 per cent of whites, but considerably less frequently in dark-skinned persons. Rose spots are deeply red, 2- to 4-mm macules, often present in clusters, blanching on pressure; they occur most often on the upper anterior abdominal wall and lower thorax. During the *second week*, the fever becomes more continuous. The patient looks sick and withdrawn, although he may be fully responsive. In some, marked deterioration in the mental condition, lassitude, delirium, and even coma may develop. Cough is commonly present and epistaxis is not infrequent. During the *third week*, the patient's illness continues in the "typhoidal state." There may be disoriented mentation and, in some cases, extreme toxemia. In this period there may be intestinal involvement, manifested clinically by greenish "pea-soup" diarrhea and the dire complications of intestinal perforation and hemorrhage. The *fourth week* usually but not invariably brings slackening of the fever and improvement in clinical status. The patient becomes more interested in the surroundings. There is significant weight loss, anemia, and profound fatigue. Typhoid fever is among the longest and most debilitating of microbial diseases.

The clinical course is altered by many factors, such as the pathogenicity of the infecting strain, the immune and nutritional status of the host, the size of the infecting dose, and antimicrobial therapy.

COMPLICATIONS. Since the typhoid bacillus is widely disseminated through recurrent waves of bacteremia, many organ sites are involved. Pneumonia occurs in 10 per cent of patients, although cough, without radiographic findings, is encountered in approximately two thirds. Rarely there is a small pleural effusion. During the severe toxemic phase, patients may aspirate gastric contents and develop a suppurative pneumonia. Severe headache, delirium, and even coma are often noted, but suppurative disease of the brain and meninges is quite uncommon, being seen in less than 1 per cent of patients. Typhoid pyelonephritis associated with renal pain, hematuria, and pyuria is occasionally encountered. The gallbladder and liver are often involved with inflammatory changes. Acute cholecystitis can occur during the initial period of typhoid fever. Jaundice, on the basis of diffuse hepatic inflammation, has been observed in some patients. The microorganism may spread to bone, especially ribs and spine, and to the large joints. Nerve deafness, conjunctivitis, keratitis, and optic neuritis have all been seen on rare occasions.

Although the litany of organ site involvement is long, the pre-eminent complications are intestinal hemorrhage and perforation. These events are most apt to occur in the third week and during convalescence and are not closely related to the severity of the disease. However, they tend to occur in the same patient, with the bleeding serving as a warning of a possible perforation to come. Bleeding may be sudden and severe, or a slow ooze. Prior to chemotherapy, the incidence of hemorrhage was 7 to 20 per cent in various series; it is somewhat less frequent since specific treatment has been available. The ileum is the main site of bowel perforation. The onset may be sudden with signs of acute abdomen. Or there may be a leak of intraluminal contents to form an abscess in the lower quadrant or pelvis, producing a more chronic, insidious course. Approximately 3 per cent of patients with typhoid fever will experience intestinal perforation.

RELAPSE. After defervescence has occurred and the patient has apparently "ridden through the storm," there remains a potential for recurrence. The relapse generally occurs eight to ten days after cessation of drug therapy and consists of a re-enactment of the major manifestations such as fever, chills, skin rash, and bacteremia. Early chemotherapy of the initial infection may increase the potential for relapse because it prevents the development of natural immunity, an important feature in eventually controlling the organism within the host.

CARRIERS. The disappearance of typhoid bacilli from the bowel has a prolonged and unpredictable course. After six weeks, approximately 50 per cent of typhoid victims are still shedding the organism in their feces. This figure progressively declines so that after three months only 5 to 10 per cent are excreters. A chronic carrier is defined as a person with stool cultures positive for *S. typhi* at least one year following an episode of typhoid or, in some cases, positive stool cultures without a documented history of disease. The possibility of spontaneously aborting the carrier state is very unlikely after this time. Chronic carriers are more common in older age groups, in women (a 3:1 ratio of women to men), and in people with gallbladder disease. The organism usually is harbored in the gallbladder, often forming part of gallstones, and persists in a noninflammatory symbiotic relationship with the host, causing neither local inflammation nor systemic symptoms. Occasionally, the gallbladder is free of the organism, and it is apparently carried in the large bowel. In the usual case, the bile contains enormous numbers of bacilli, up to 10^9 per milliliter, and they are discharged in the feces in varying concentrations. The organisms are viable and fully infective, so the carrier may be a source of new infection.

LABORATORY FINDINGS. Many laboratory features of typhoid fever are consistent with prolonged sepsis. A normochromic, normocytic anemia persists throughout the infection; it may be made worse by intestinal blood loss or a reaction of the bone marrow to agents such as chloramphenicol. Thrombocytopenia occurs during the initial hectic period of the disease. Leukopenia is characteristic of the first week of illness, with the major depression in polymorphonuclear leukocytes.

The definitive diagnosis of typhoid fever is established by isolating the organism. During the first week, blood cultures are positive in 90 per cent of patients. As bacteremia abates during the subsequent weeks, other sites become colonized. It is not always appreciated, however, that, if the clinical illness persists essentially unimproved, the bacteremia likewise persists. As a consequence, the blood culture may be positive for several weeks or more. The blood culture thus is the primary diagnostic test. Stool cultures usually become positive in the second and third weeks when the organisms are shed from the lymphoid follicles of the intestinal wall. During the third week, urine culture yields typhoid bacilli in approximately 30 per cent of patients. Rose spots harbor the organism, and they can be sampled by small skin snips of the lesion which are cultured in nutrient broth. These are positive in two thirds of patients. A most useful source is the bone marrow, which is positive for *S. typhi* in 90 per cent of patients, even when they have received some antimicrobial therapy.

The titer of agglutinins (Widal test) against somatic (O) and flagellar (H) antigens rises during the third week of illness. An O titer of 1:80 or more in nonimmunized individuals is suggestive of typhoid fever. Higher initial titers or a fourfold rise provides stronger evidence. The H antigen is more nonspecific, and is likely to be elevated from prior immunization or infection by other enteric bacteria. There are many false-positive and occasional false-negative Widal reactions so that a diagnosis based on titer rises alone is rather tenuous.

DIAGNOSIS. In endemic regions the most perplexing diagnosis is between typhoid fever and malaria, because both diseases can cause fever, chills, splenomegaly, and neutropenia. Travelers to such areas may acquire either disease so that they present with the same diagnostic dilemma. Blood smears usually are positive in malaria, and typhoid is identified by isolating the organism in culture or, as an early clue, a positive Widal reaction. In certain parts of the world, Lassa fever or dengue is a diagnostic alternative. Other salmonellae can mimic typhoid fever. Among bacterial infections which may be confused with typhoid, tuberculosis, shigellosis, leptospirosis, and bacteremias associated with cholecystitis and pyelonephritis should be given consideration. Viral agents such as infectious mononucleosis and infectious hepatitis can present with similar symptoms. Patients having delirium or coma with normal cerebrospinal fluid may be thought to have viral encephalitis rather than typhoid fever. Rickettsial diseases may be considered, but the absence of a characteristic rash would militate against this diagnosis.

TREATMENT. Drug resistance, mediated by plasmids, can occur among typhoid bacilli. Most strains are susceptible to chloramphenicol and ampicillin, although notable epidemics with strains resistant to either of these drugs have been reported in recent years. Hence, a great effort should be made in each case to isolate the organism and to perform drug susceptibility tests. Chloramphenicol remains the standard therapy because of its proved efficacy and its high activity against most clinical isolates of typhoid bacilli. The response to therapy is remarkably constant, as defervescence regularly occurs three to five days after initiating treatment. The clinical condition improves within one to two days, with decreased toxemia and slowly declining fever. In adults, chloramphenicol should be given in a total daily dose of 3 to 4 grams, administered in four equally divided doses. Occasionally in very sick patients it may be necessary to give the drug by the intravenous route, and the same total daily dose of 3 to 4 grams should be used. Oral medication can then be given after improvement in the clinical status. Chloramphenicol is well

absorbed from the intestinal tract, but is rather poorly absorbed from intramuscular sites. Thus the intramuscular route is to be avoided. The duration of treatment is two weeks; prolongation of this treatment does not reduce the incidence of complications or carriers. Intestinal perforation and hemorrhage can occur during what is apparently successful treatment. Relapse may follow an otherwise uneventful course, and should be treated with the same drug.

Ampicillin has been recommended as alternative therapy, but it has been somewhat disappointing in comparison with chloramphenicol. The dose is 6 grams per day, intravenously, in four to six divided doses. Amoxicillin, a closely related drug, provides better absorption and increased efficacy. Several studies have shown that amoxicillin, in doses of 4 grams per day in four divided doses, has good activity, but is somewhat less effective than chloramphenicol. Co-trimoxazole has also been used in the therapy of typhoid fever, and the initial results are promising.

Corticosteroids are administered for severe toxemia and fever, and may produce a dramatic response in the patient with profound sepsis. The treatment should be given in high doses, 60 mg per day of prednisone divided in four doses, and rapidly tapered over the next three days. The wide experience with steroid treatment has failed to show any adverse effects, although the potentiality for masking intestinal perforation is still present. Thus steroids are best reserved for patients with severe toxicity.

Intestinal perforation is managed by standard surgical practices. All patients should be treated with nasogastric suction. Indications for operation are progressive peritoneal signs or localization of an abscess. Simple closure of the perforation is the treatment of choice. However, the ileum may be riddled with multiple perforations, and resection or exteriorization of the intestinal loop may be required. Intestinal perforation can lead to secondary infection with enteric bacilli, so it is advisable to initiate treatment with a broad-spectrum antimicrobial such as an aminoglycoside, in addition to continuing chloramphenicol.

Good nursing care plays a major role in the recovery from typhoid fever. The pyrexia can be managed with tepid baths and sponging. Salicylates and antipyretics should be avoided, as they cause severe sweating and may lower the blood pressure.

A chronic carrier, who has been discharging *S. typhi* for longer than one year, can be treated with antimicrobials in an attempt to eliminate the infection. One regimen which works in approximately two thirds of patients is 6 grams of ampicillin per day in four divided doses for six weeks. Reappearance of the carrier state following such treatment is generally associated with gallbladder disease. In persons with gallstones or chronic cholecystitis, cholecystectomy eliminates the carrier state in 85 per cent. This procedure, however, is recommended only for those whose profession is not compatible with the typhoid carrier state, i.e., food handlers and health care providers.

PROGNOSIS. Prior to antimicrobial therapy, the case mortality of typhoid fever was around 10 to 15 per cent. The introduction of chloramphenicol has reduced this to 1 per cent, and most patients now succumb to either perforation or hemorrhage. However, in areas of the world with poor nutrition and limited medical facilities, the mortality may be higher. Factors which influence a lethal outcome are severity of the disease at time of admission (coma is a poor prognostic sign); age, with the very young and the very old being at greatest risk; and prior infection, because a second attack, although uncommon, is less severe than the primary episode.

PROPHYLAXIS. For control of intrahospital spread, enteric precautions should be initiated; fecal, urine, and blood specimens should be disposed of by double-bag techniques and always handled with gloves. Additional precautions are unwarranted.

Typhoid vaccine affords 70 per cent protection. This relative immunity can be overcome by a large inoculum of bacilli. The most active vaccine is the acetone-dried product which is administered in two doses of 0.5 ml, subcutaneously, at four-week intervals. The phenol-inactivated product has somewhat reduced immunogenicity, but it produces less local discomfort, a problem which is prominent with the acetone-dried vaccine. There is no relationship between serum antibody levels measured against O, H, or Vi antigens and resistance to disease, relapse, or reinfection. It is apparent that the major forces of immunity act at the intestinal mucosa surface. Oral live vaccines, theoretically the most attractive approach, have not proved successful, because either they have failed to colonize the intestine or the mutated vaccine strain has reverted to a pathogen. Despite its limitations, typhoid vaccine is recommended for travelers to endemic regions; revaccination should be done every three years with a single 0.5-ml dose.

Hornick, R. B., Greisman, S. E., Woodward, T. E., DuPont, H. L., Dawkins, A. T., and Snyder, M. J.: Typhoid fever: Pathogenesis and immunologic control. N. Engl. J. Med., 283:686, 739, 1970.

Johnson, W. D., Jr., Hook, E. W., Lindsey, E., and Kaye, D.: Treatment of chronic typhoid carriers with ampicillin. Antimicrob. Agents Chemother., 3:439, 1973.

Kim, J-P., Oh, S-K., and Jarret, F.: Management of ileal perforation due to typhoid fever. Ann. Surg., 181:88, 1975.

Pillay, N., Adams, E. B., and North-Coombes, D.: Comparative trial of amoxycillin and chloramphenicol in treatment of typhoid fever in adults. Lancet, 2:333, 1975.

Snyder, M. J., Gonzalez, O., Palomino, C., Music, S. I., Hornick, R. B., Perroni, J., Woodward, W. E., Gonzalez, C., DuPont, H. L., and Woodward, T. E.: Comparative efficacy of chloramphenicol, ampicillin, and co-trimoxazole in the treatment of typhoid fever. Lancet, 2:1155, 1976.

Wicks, C. B., Holmes, G. S., and Davidson, L.: Endemic typhoid fever. Quart. J. Med., 159:341, 1971.

Woodward, T. E., and Smadel, J. E.: Management of typhoid fever and its complications. Ann. Intern. Med., 60:144, 1964.

153. SALMONELLA INFECTIONS OTHER THAN TYPHOID FEVER

Edward W. Hook

DEFINITION. The genus *Salmonella* consists of more than 1700 serotypes and variants. These organisms with a few exceptions are primary pathogens for animals that are readily transmitted to man. The outstanding exception is *S. typhi*, which is a parasite only of man and does not cause disease in lower animals in nature.

Human infection with *Salmonella* may be expressed as *acute gastroenteritis*, *enteric fever* (paratyphoid fever), *bacteremia*, or *localized metastatic infection* at almost any site. The clinical syndromes resulting from *Salmonella* infection cannot always be sharply differentiated and sometimes overlap.

Transient *asymptomatic infection* of the intestinal tract is also common with most serotypes. A *chronic carrier state* may occur occasionally after infection with *Salmonella* other than *S. typhi*, and is characterized by prolonged excretion of the organism in feces or urine.

Typhoid fever is considered in a separate chapter (see Ch. 152) because of its historical identity, the host specificity of the pathogen, and the wealth of data on basic and clinical aspects of the disease. This separation is unrealistic to the extent that an illness closely resembling typhoid fever can result from infection with other salmonellae, and *S. typhi* can on occasion produce all the clinical syndromes described for the other *Salmonella* serotypes.

ETIOLOGY. Salmonellae are gram-negative, aerobic, nonsporing rods that grow readily on simple culture media. Presumptive identification of salmonellae involves relatively simple biochemical tests and agglutination reactions performed with group-specific antisera. The majority of strains isolated from man fall into groups A through E. Definitive identification of serotype depends on precise analysis of the somatic (O) and flagellar (H) antigens of the organism. Subdivision of certain serotypes, for example *S. typhimurium*, can be achieved by bacteriophage typing. Specific identification of all isolates is desirable, especially for epidemiologic reasons, and can be obtained through local, state, or federal health agencies.

Salmonella serotypes most frequently isolated from human infections in the United States during 1975 were, in descending order of frequency, *S. typhimurium*, *S. newport*, *S. enteritidis*, *S. heidelberg*, *S. agona*, *S. infantis*, *S. saint-paul*, *S. typhi*, *S. oranienburg*, and *S. javiana*. These ten serotypes accounted for about 70 per cent of the total *Salmonella* isolates from man during 1975. *S. typhimurium* is the serotype most frequently isolated year after year, usually accounting for 20 to 30 per cent of the total.

EPIDEMIOLOGY. Salmonellae are widespread among members of the Animal Kingdom in all parts of the world. Virtually all domestic and many wild animal species have been shown to harbor these organisms, and infection rates range from 1 per cent to more than 40 per cent. For example, in certain studies salmonellae have been isolated from 41 per cent of turkeys, 7 to 50 per cent of swine, and 24 per cent of apparently healthy cattle.

In 1975, 23,445 isolations of *Salmonella* from humans were reported in the United States. The annual incidence of reported isolations has remained approximately constant since 1963, the first full year of operation of the Salmonella Surveillance System in the United States. The true incidence of human salmonellosis is probably much higher than the number of reported cases. It is estimated that only about 1 per cent of cases are reported.

The prevalence of asymptomatic human carriers of salmonellae in the general population has been estimated to be about 0.2 per cent. The carrier state in the vast majority of these people is transient and probably represents persistence of organisms in the stools after asymptomatic or mild intestinal infection. The transient carrier state is more frequent in persons whose occupations provide opportunity for contact with *Salmonella* in foods, such as professional food processors or abattoir workers, than in the general population.

Man almost always acquires *Salmonella* infection by the oral route. Any item of food or drink can be contaminated directly or indirectly with viable bacilli from infected animals or man and can serve as a source of infection. Although the role of human carriers in the spread of salmonellosis must not be minimized, the majority of infections of man in the United States are related to the enormous reservoirs of salmonellae in lower animals.

The greatest single source of human disease is poultry products, including chickens, turkeys, ducks, and eggs. Other animal meats, especially pork, beef, and lamb, also serve as sources of infection. Salmonellae on meats or other foods contaminate utensils, tables, and other items in the processing plant, market, or kitchen, and may be transferred from these items to previously uninfected foods. A significant proportion (1 to 58 per cent) of raw meat purchased in retail markets is contaminated with salmonellae.

Eggs or egg products are common sources of *Salmonella* infection. The bacilli may be found on the external surface of the eggshell, between the shell and the shell membranes, or in yolks of eggs from hens with ovarian infection. The incidence of infection of eggs is low, but pooling of large numbers for freezing or drying increases the possibility of contamination of large quantities of materials. Prepared food mixtures containing dried eggs have been implicated many times in outbreaks of *Salmonella* infection.

Sterilization of contaminated foods is not always achieved by cooking. Viable salmonellae contaminating large birds such as turkeys, especially if the fowl is stuffed, may persist despite the baking process, and organisms in eggs occasionally survive frying, scrambling, or boiling in the shell.

The numerous byproducts of the meat-packing industry, such as bone meal, fertilizer, domestic animal food, and fish meal, often contain salmonellae and may serve as sources of infection, especially among lower animals. Finally, in considering potential sources of infection, household pets, including dogs, cats, birds, and turtles, should not be overlooked; all have been shown to harbor salmonellae.

Direct transmission from man to man without food as the intermediate source does occur. Transmission by person-to-person contact appears to be a relatively common mode of spread in hospital outbreaks, especially those occurring in nurseries or pediatric wards. For example, salmonellae may be introduced into a nursery by a newborn infected at birth from an infected mother and then spread to other babies by nursery attendants. Several nursery and hospital outbreaks have also been described in which infection appeared to be perpetuated by airborne spread of salmonellae.

S. choleraesuis bacteremia has been reported in immunologically compromised patients who received platelet transfusions from a donor with chronic intermittent bacteremia secondary to minimally symptomatic osteomyelitis.

The incidence of *Salmonella* infection shows a seasonal pattern. In the United States, the largest number of infections are reported in July through November and the smallest number in February through April. Chil-

dren under two years of age have the highest incidence of infection.

PATHOLOGY. Death from *Salmonella* gastroenteritis occurs primarily in infants, the aged, and persons with underlying diseases. The intestinal mucosa is red and swollen and often shows petechial hemorrhages. The pathologic findings in paratyphoid fever are qualitatively similar to those of typhoid fever, although the involvement of Peyer's patches is less prominent and ulcerations are much less frequent. Intestinal lesions are usually absent in patients with *Salmonella* bacteremia, and the findings are similar to those of any acute generalized infection. Blood-borne salmonellae may localize in almost any organ, producing single or multiple suppurative lesions.

PATHOGENESIS. Multiplication of salmonellae in the intestinal tract is associated with invasion of mucosal cells of the small intestine, inflammation of the intestinal mucosa, and symptoms of gastroenteritis. Gastroenteritis is a true infection of the mucosa; ingestion of a large number of dead bacilli will not produce the disease. The mechanism of the production of diarrhea is unknown. However, certain salmonellae have been reported to cause ileal secretion in experimental infections by stimulating adenylate cyclase.

Salmonellae multiplying in the intestinal tract occasionally gain access to the blood, producing transient bacteremia or localized infections that can serve as sources of persistent bacteremia. The pathogenesis of enteric or paratyphoid fever is similar to that of typhoid fever.

The prevalence of salmonellae in foods for human consumption makes it almost inevitable that man come in contact with these organisms relatively frequently. The outcome of such exposures depends on many factors, especially the characteristics of the *Salmonella* serotype, the number of bacteria ingested, and the status of the host.

Almost every serotype of *Salmonella* has the capacity to produce asymptomatic infection, acute gastroenteritis, bacteremia with or without localized infection, or paratyphoid fever. However, some serotypes are much more likely to produce certain of these clinical syndromes than others. For example, *S. anatum* usually produces inapparent infection or gastroenteritis and only rarely invades the blood. In contrast, *S. choleraesuis* only occasionally produces gastroenteritis or inapparent infection but is a common cause of bacteremia or metastatic infection. Differences in pathogenicity are observed not only between serotypes but also between strains of the same serotype.

Limited information is available on the number of organisms required to produce salmonellosis in man. Experiments in volunteers suggest that a large number (approximately 10^5 to 10^6) of viable salmonellae are usually required to produce gastroenteritis in normal adults. However, several outbreaks have been described in which as few as 100 to 1000 cells were apparently responsible for illness. A transient carrier state may follow ingestion of inocula 10 or 100 times smaller than those required to produce disease.

The resistance of the host also plays a major role in determining the wide range of responses from no disease to rapidly fatal illness observed in human salmonellosis. Local factors in the stomach and intestine may be the first lines of defense. It is known that salmonellae are rapidly killed at a pH of 2, a level readily attained in the stomach, and that concomitant administration of certain antacids reduces the challenge dose of organisms required to initiate infection under experimental conditions. It has been established that major gastric surgery, including subtotal gastrectomy, gastroenterostomy, and/or vagotomy, predisposes to *Salmonella* gastroenteritis. The mechanism of this effect is unknown, but may be related to reduced bactericidal activity of gastric juice or altered intestinal flora. It has been shown in experimental *Salmonella* infections of mice that the microbial flora of the normal intestine exerts a protective action by suppressing multiplication of salmonellae. In these studies alteration of intestinal flora by antimicrobial drugs increased susceptibility to infection with *S. typhimurium* 100,000 times, and resistance was restored by re-establishing the normal enteric flora. Prior antimicrobial therapy also enhances susceptibility of man to symptomatic intestinal infection with salmonellae.

The incidence of severe *Salmonella* infections is increased in patients with certain underlying diseases. Another process, such as hepatic cirrhosis, lupus erythematosus, leukemia, lymphoma, or neoplasm, is present in one third to one half of patients with *Salmonella* bacteremia. These conditions are associated with a general depression of resistance to microbial invasion, and secondary infection is not unexpected. However, in a few diseases — acute bartonellosis, sickle cell anemia, and, perhaps, malaria — there appears to be a predisposition to infection with salmonellae that exceeds any general susceptibility to other bacterial species. The acute hemolytic phase of bartonellosis is complicated by the development of *Salmonella* bacteremia in as many as 40 per cent of cases. Patients with sickle cell anemia and other sickle hemoglobinopathies are unusually susceptible to invasion of the blood by *Salmonella*, and there is a strong tendency for localization of infection in bone. In fact, *Salmonella* species, not staphylococci, account for the vast majority of instances of osteomyelitis in patients with sickle cell anemia. Osteomyelitis is probably related to the localization of organisms in the areas of ischemia and necrosis of bone so common in sickle cell anemia; this is but one example of the striking tendency of salmonellae to localize at sites of pre-existing disease. Localization of salmonellae has been reported in vascular aneurysms, bone compressed by aortic aneurysms, hematomas, areas of infarction, and a variety of cysts and neoplasms.

CLINICAL MANIFESTATIONS. Salmonella Gastroenteritis. Symptoms of gastroenteritis develop 8 to 48 hours after ingestion of contaminated food. The relatively long incubation period represents the time required for multiplication and invasion by the organism. Nausea and vomiting are common initial manifestations and are rapidly followed by colicky abdominal pain and persistent diarrhea, occasionally with mucus or blood. Nausea and vomiting are rarely severe or protracted. An initial chill is not unusual, and fever of 38 to 39° C is common. Symptoms usually subside in two to five days, and recovery is uneventful.

Considerable variation in the severity of *Salmonella* gastroenteritis is observed, even among patients infected at the same meal. Some patients have a mild afebrile disease with a few loose stools, whereas others have high fever and 30 to 40 liquid stools per day. Severe diarrhea occasionally occurs in an afebrile patient. Abdominal pain may be intense, localized, and associated with rebound tenderness, suggesting appendicitis or some other acute intra-abdominal process. Symptoms of gastroenteritis persist in some patients for as long as two weeks. Active proctitis and colitis may occur and play a role in the tenesmus and small-volume bloody stools seen in some patients.

The leukocyte count is usually normal, and blood cultures are sterile in almost all cases. Stools of patients with diarrhea may contain large numbers of polymorphonuclear neutrophils. The causative organism can be isolated from the feces of almost all patients during the acute illness. About 50 per cent of the patients continue to have stool cultures positive for salmonellae at two weeks after onset of gastroenteritis, but only 15 per cent remain positive at the end of the fourth week. A small proportion of patients continue to excrete organisms after two months, but in most of these the cultures become negative in the next six months. The period of excretion of organisms in stool tends to be longer in infants than in older children or adults. The term "chronic enteric carrier" should be reserved for the patient shown to have persistently positive stools with the same *Salmonella* species for one or more years.

Enteric (Paratyphoid) Fever. Salmonellae other than *S. typhi* may produce an illness with all the features of typhoid fever, including prolonged sustained fever, respiratory and gastrointestinal symptoms, rose spots, leukopenia, and positive blood, stool, and urine cultures. Although paratyphoid fever may be clinically indistinguishable from typhoid fever, it is usually milder with a shorter course and a lower mortality rate. The organisms most likely to produce this syndrome are *S. paratyphi A, S. paratyphi B,* and *S. choleraesuis.* Paratyphoid fever is occasionally preceded by manifestations of *Salmonella* gastroenteritis.

Bacteremia. Salmonellae also produce a clinical syndrome that is characterized by chills, prolonged intermittent fever, anorexia, and weight loss. The characteristic features of typhoid or paratyphoid fever, such as rose spots, sustained fever, and leukopenia, are absent. Patients with this form of illness usually have no gastrointestinal complaints, and, indeed, stool cultures are usually negative for the causative organism despite its presence in blood. The leukocyte count is normal in most cases.

A prolonged febrile illness lasting weeks or months and characterized by weight loss, anemia, hepatosplenomegaly, and bacteremia with salmonellae, including *S. typhi,* has been described in South America and the Middle East in patients with schistosomiasis. The organisms apparently find a protected environment for multiplication within the gut of the worm. Eradication of the worms may also result in cure of the bacterial infection (see Ch. 210).

Localized Disease. Signs of localized infection appear in many cases of *Salmonella* bacteremia. Abscess formation may occur at almost any site, or bronchopneumonia, empyema, endocarditis, pericarditis, pyelonephritis, osteomyelitis, or arthritis may develop. Meningitis is a focal manifestation more common in newborns and infants than in adults. Patients with localized infections usually have striking polymorphonuclear leukocytosis as high as 20,000 to 30,000 cells per cubic millimeter of blood.

DIAGNOSIS. *Salmonella* gastroenteritis must be differentiated from other acute diarrheal diseases, especially shigellosis, invasive and enterotoxigenic *Escherichia coli* infection, staphylococcal food poisoning, and enteritis produced by *Vibrio parahaemolyticus, Yersinia enterocolitica,* and viral agents. A short incubation period, absence of fever, and prominence of nausea and vomiting are characteristic of staphylococcal food poisoning, whereas tenesmus, dysentery, and numerous fecal leukocytes suggest a diagnosis of shigellosis. However, differentiation on the basis of clinical information alone is difficult, especially in sporadic cases, and definitive diagnosis depends on isolation of the causative organism from the stool.

In patients with enteric fever, blood cultures are usually positive early in the course of the disease, and feces and urine become positive somewhat later. In patients with *Salmonella* bacteremia, the organisms can be isolated from blood, or in some cases from pus or exudate from localized infection.

Patients with salmonellosis may show during the course of illness a fourfold or greater increase in titer of agglutinins against the causative organism or closely related species. However, agglutination tests performed in the ordinary clinical laboratory are usually not helpful in diagnosis.

TREATMENT. The most important aspect of the management of patients with *Salmonella* gastroenteritis is prompt correction of dehydration and electrolyte disturbances. Diphenoxylate hydrochloride with atropine (Lomotil), paregoric, or small doses of morphine may be used to relieve abdominal cramps and diarrhea if contraindications do not exist. Some authorities feel that administration of such agents is not indicated. Inhibition of gut motility does enhance susceptibility to intestinal infection in laboratory animals. There is no convincing evidence that antimicrobial drugs, including chloramphenicol, ampicillin, or co-trimoxazole, reduce the duration of illness or the period of excretion of organisms in the stool. In fact, the period of excretion of salmonellae in the stool during convalescence after symptomatic intestinal infection is actually longer in patients who have been treated with antimicrobial drugs during the acute illness than in patients who have received no antimicrobial therapy.

In *Salmonella* bacteremia, paratyphoid fever, or localized infections of bones, joints, meninges, and other sites, chloramphenicol is the drug of choice and should be administered in divided doses of about 50 mg per kilogram per day for at least two weeks. Four to six days may be required for defervescence in favorable cases and even longer in patients with localized infection. In patients with localized infections, it may be necessary to continue antimicrobial therapy for four to six weeks, and surgical drainage of collections of pus may be required. Salmonellae persisting in tissues during chloramphenicol therapy may be responsible for relapse after the antimicrobial is discontinued. Relapse is not related to the emergence of chloramphenicol-resistant strains during therapy, and clinical response to a second or third course of therapy usually differs in no way from the first.

Ampicillin has also been shown to be effective in treating paratyphoid fever, but the response to ampicillin is slower than the response to chloramphenicol.

Ampicillin is also often effective in the treatment of other systemic *Salmonella* infections if the causative organism is susceptible to this drug. Ampicillin is preferred over chloramphenicol for patients requiring prolonged therapy. Ampicillin resistance is common among *Salmonella* serotypes. In a recent study in the United States, about 30 per cent of strains of *S. typhimurium, S. heidelberg,* and *S. newport* were found to be resistant to ampicillin. Resistance to the aminoglycosides, sulfonamides, or tetracyclines is also common, but resistance to chloramphenicol or co-trimoxazole is uncommon. Resistance is usually to multiple antimicrobials and is transferable by R-factors. Nosocomial outbreaks with serotypes resistant to ampicillin, chloramphenicol, and co-trimoxazole have been described.

Co-trimoxazole appears to be of some value in the therapy of enteric fever, but its relative position among effective antimicrobials has not been established at present.

Excretion of salmonellae in stool after clinical or subclinical infection ceases spontaneously in almost all patients; the convalescent carrier state is not an indication for antimicrobial therapy. Chronic enteric carriers of salmonellae other than *S. typhi* are managed as are typhoid carriers.

PROGNOSIS. The case fatality rate in *Salmonella* gastroenteritis rarely exceeds 1 or 2 per cent, and probably averages about 0.3 per cent. Fatalities occur almost entirely in infants, the aged, and persons with major underlying disease. The case fatality rate in the more serious systemic infections is high; it approaches 20 per cent in *S. choleraesuis* bacteremia.

PREVENTION. Every effort should be made to prevent the spread of salmonellae among the population by the excreta of patients with acute illness and convalescent or chronic carriers. Patients with acute illness should be isolated, and convalescent or chronic carriers should not be employed as food handlers and should practice strict personal hygiene.

The control of salmonellosis among animals and prevention of spread of infection to man present many problems. Progress is being made in developing methods of detection and control of salmonellosis in domestic animals and in improving hygienic conditions in food-processing and food-dispensing establishments.

Aserkoff, B., and Bennett, J. V.: Effect of therapy in acute salmonellosis on salmonellae in feces. N. Engl. J. Med., 281:636, 1969.

Bennett, I. L., Jr., and Hook, E. W.: Infectious diseases (some aspects of salmonellosis). Ann. Rev. Med., 10:1, 1959.

Center for Disease Control: Salmonella Surveillance Annual Summary, 1975. Issued September 1976, Atlanta, Georgia.

D'Aoust, J. Y., and Pivnick, H.: Small infectious doses of *Salmonella.* Lancet, 1:866, 1976.

Hornick, R. B.: *Salmonella* infections — newer perspectives of an old infection. Trans. Am. Clin. Climatol. Assoc., 85:164, 1973.

Lintz, D., Kapila, R., Pilgrim, E., Tecson, F., Dorn, R., and Louria, D.: Nosocomial *Salmonella* epidemic. Arch. Intern. Med., 136:968, 1976.

Musher, D. M., and Rubenstein, A. D.: Permanent carriers of nontyphosa salmonellae. Arch. Intern. Med., 132:869, 1973.

Neu, H. C., Cherubin, C. E., Longo, E. D., Flouton, B., and Winter, J.: Antimicrobial resistance and R-factor transfer among isolates of *Salmonella* in the northeastern United States. A comparison of human and animal isolates. J. Infect. Dis., 132:617, 1975.

Rhame, F. S., Root, R. K., MacLowry, J. D., Dadisman, T. A., and Bennett, J. V.: Salmonella septicemia from platelet transfusions. Study of an outbreak traced to a hematogenous carrier of *Salmonella choleraesuis.* Ann. Intern. Med., 78:633, 1973.

Wahab, M. F. A., Robertson, R. P., and Raasch, F. O.: Paratyphoid A fever. Ann. Intern. Med., 70:913, 1969.

OTHER BACTERIAL INFECTIONS

154. ENTERIC BACTERIAL INFECTIONS

Calvin M. Kunin

DEFINITION. The wide variety of microorganisms commonly found in the gastrointestinal tract, particularly the gram-negative, nonsporulating bacilli, have become increasingly important in clinical medicine. They are the principal organisms found in infections of the abdominal viscera, peritoneum, and urinary tract, as well as being frequent secondary invaders of the respiratory tract, burned or traumatized skin, and sites of decreased host resistance and instrumentation. Currently, they are the most frequent cause of life-threatening bacteremia. Infections with these organisms will be considered together because of their common habitat in the gut and on mucous surfaces, the similarity of epidemiologic and pathogenic characteristics, and the common approach used in diagnosis, treatment, and prevention.

BACTERIOLOGY. The gastrointestinal flora is exceedingly complex. The large intestine contains about 10^{10} to 10^{11} organisms per gram of contents. Of these, 90 to 95 per cent are obligate anaerobes. Most common are the gram-negative bacilli, *Bacteroides* and *Fusobacterium*, gram-positive bacilli, including *Bifidobacterium, Eubacterium,* and *Corynebacterium* species, and a wide variety of anaerobic streptococci. Other anaerobes include the gram-positive spore-forming rods of the clostridia species and gram-negative cocci, *Veillonella* (see Ch. 151). Enterococci are also present. The well-known aerobic gram-negative rods, which are members of the family Enterobacteriaceae, account for only 5 to 10 per cent of the total flora. These include the most common, *E. coli,* as well as the *Klebsiella-Enterobacter* group, *Proteus, Providencia, Edwardsiella, Serratia,* and, under pathologic conditions, *Salmonella* and *Shigella. Pseudomonas* is an entirely unrelated species, and is usually found in only small numbers in the bowel. Various yeasts are also found in lesser numbers in the normal large intestine.

Although the human gastrointestinal tract is usually considered to be colonized in the anatomic regions proximal to the cardia of the stomach and distal to the ileocecal valve, recent studies have demonstrated organisms in the jejunum and almost always in the ileum. Moderate changes in the diet do not affect the ratio of predominant bacteria in the feces, but antimicrobial therapy has a strong selective effect and is the single most important reason for the increasing emergence in human infection of these heretofore unusual organisms.

All the microorganisms of the gastrointestinal tract are potentially pathogenic under conditions of altered host resistance. The major diagnostic problem is to differentiate superficial colonization from actual tissue invasion.

ENDOTOXIN. The gram-negative bacteria of the gastrointestinal tract produce disease by invasion of tissue and by release of a pharmacologically active lipopolysaccharide from the cell wall, known as endotoxin. Endotoxins from a wide variety of unrelated species behave quite similarly, regardless of the inherent pathogenicity of the microorganism from which they are derived or their antigenic structure.

In the intact microorganism they exist as complexes of lipid, polysaccharide, and protein. The biologic activity seems to be a property of a lipid and carbohydrate portion. The cell wall of gram-negative bacteria may be roughly divided into three regions. The outermost region contains the chains of specific sugars which characterize the O-specific antigens and determine individual serotypes within a species. This is linked to a core polysaccharide which is of similar structure among related groups of bacteria. This is in turn linked through 2-keto-3-deoxyoctonate trisaccharides to the major lipid component termed lipid A. Evidence has now accumulated to indicate that all the properties of endotoxin may be accounted for by this complex lipid substance. Lipid A is a polymer containing glucosamine disaccharide units linked through pyrophosphate bridges and esterified with lauric, palmitic, and myristic acids. Perhaps the most important finding in recent years is that lipid A is immunogenic and will induce antibodies which cross-react among the gram-negative bacteria. Animal studies reveal that antibody prepared against the active component of endotoxin will protect against challenge from heterologous gram-negative bacteria; however, better protection is obtained by immunization with specific O antigens which induce opsonizing antibodies. The frequency of shock and death in patients with gram-negative bacteria appears to be lower in individuals with initially high titers of cross-reacting antibody to the Re or core lipopolysaccharide (lipid A) component. These findings hold promise for development of immunoprophylaxis and therapy.

When inoculated intravenously, the endotoxins cause fever, leukopenia, circulatory collapse, capillary hemorrhages, necrosis of tumors, and the Shwartzman phenomenon. Noteworthy is the remarkable tolerance that develops after repeated injections of endotoxin. For example, the first intravenous injection in man of as little as 0.01 ml of typhoid vaccine will give rise to a violent response, with chill and high fever; yet after 10 to 14 daily injections of increasing quantities, the subject can accept 25 ml or more without symptoms and with only a slight rise in temperature. This state of tolerance is not obviously dependent on specific antibodies; it extends to endotoxins of unrelated bacterial strains. The clinical features of gram-negative bacteremia resemble the reaction of laboratory animals or man to intravenous injection of purified endotoxic preparations, and may well represent a direct "pharmacologic" response to bacterial endotoxin. In other types of infectious process there is reason to doubt that such phenomena as fever, leukocytosis, and leukopenia are direct effects of endotoxin liberation.

The phenomenon of endotoxin tolerance may explain the remarkable tendency of the symptoms of pyelonephritis to subside spontaneously. By contrast, endotoxin tolerance is not a feature of experimental typhoid fever, but, rather, volunteers infected with this organ-

ism have been shown to be hypersensitive to its effects. Endotoxin tolerance is currently under intensive
study because of the presumed important pathologic effect of this substance. The often conflicting observations on tolerance to the fever-producing property of
endotoxin now appear to be due to the fact that multiple phenomena are operating simultaneously. Endotoxin is believed to be pyrogenic by inducing macrophages (monocytes, Kupffer and related cells) to release
a protein, termed endogenous pyrogen. This protein is
carried in the circulation to the temperature-regulating
nuclei in the hypothalamus, producing an alteration in
thermoregulation. Frequent, repeated doses of endotoxin are thought to exhaust the cells' capability of releasing this substance. More prolonged exposure is believed to induce antibodies which block the action of
endotoxin.

ANTIBODIES. Antibodies reacting with most Enterobacteriaceae can be demonstrated in sera of normal animals and man, probably because of the continual production of antigen in the gastrointestinal tract.
Gram-negative bacteria contain a wide variety of antigenic determinants. The best studied include the H or
flagellar antigens which are heat-labile proteins present
in motile strains. They have not been shown to be of
pathogenetic significance. Some of the enteric bacteria
contain K or capsular polysaccharides. They constitute
the Vi antigens of *S. typhi* and are particularly prominent in *Klebsiella*, but are not confined to these groups.
These surface slime layers interfere with phagocytosis
and may be important in imparting virulence to encapsulated strains. They appear to account for invasiveness
but not toxicity. *E. coli* K_1 capsular antigen, which is
immunochemically identical to meningococcal Group B
polysaccharide, appears to be the most important property of strains that are associated with neonatal meningitis. The K antigens also have been linked to invasiveness of *E. coli* in pyelonephritis. The Enterobacteriaceae
share a common antigen (CA). Antibody to core lipopolysaccharide, described above, is currently thought to
be the key determinant of resistance to endotoxin damage. Antibodies to the O or somatic antigens of *E. coli*
have been most extensively studied. Very low titers are
present in human newborns, presumably because they
are mostly of the high molecular weight IgM variety,
and do not readily pass the placenta. Human colostrum
is rich in O antibody, but this is not absorbed during
breast feeding. Colonization of the digestive tract, however, is soon accompanied by appearance of a wide variety of antibodies in serum, which contains virtually
all the *E. coli* O antibodies by one year of age.

As a rule, most strains are susceptible to lysis by the
combined effects of antibody and complement. Invasive
strains are often found to be insusceptible to lysis in
vitro. This system may be of great importance in preventing strains from invading and persisting in the
blood.

TESTS FOR ENDOTOXEMIA. A remarkably sensitive
test for endotoxemia has been developed, based on the
finding that small amounts will cause gelation of lysates
of amebocytes of the horseshoe crab. The test must be
currently considered primarily as a research test, because, although it is commonly positive in gram-
negative bacteremia, this is not always true, and a positive test does not correlate well with the outcome of

infection. Since endotoxemia does not require living organisms, the test may be positive in the absence of detectable bacteremia.

THE ROLE OF ENTERIC BACTERIA IN PYOGENIC INFECTIONS OF THE ABDOMINAL CAVITY

The mixed flora of the intestinal tract participates in
infections that originate from lesions of the bowel, such
as appendicitis, cholangitis, diverticulitis, and perforation (from ulcerative colitis, ileitis, or carcinoma). These
may lead to subdiaphragmatic, hepatic, and pelvic abscesses, which are frequent causes of fever of unknown
origin in the patient recovering from abdominal surgery or trauma to this region. Because enteric bacteria
grow luxuriantly in both aerobic and anaerobic media
and therefore are likely to predominate in cultures,
their relative importance tends to be exaggerated. There
is good reason to believe that anaerobic bacteria — bacteroides, clostridia, and anaerobic streptococci — play
important roles in this process. It should be pointed
out here that a "fecal" odor of pus, though often
ascribed to coliforms, is doubtless caused by associated
anaerobic bacteria. Anaerobic bacteria are usually present as mixtures of two or more species. They should be
suspected when there is foul pus and when organisms
can be visualized microscopically but fail to grow under
routine conditions.

OTHER INFECTIONS CAUSED BY THE ENTERIC BACTERIA

GASTROENTERITIS. A significant proportion of cases
of gastroenteritis occurring in the neonatal period of
life appear to be caused by *E. coli* as well as *Salmonella*
and *Shigella*. Outbreaks of diarrhea among adults, particularly travelers abroad, have been associated with
enterotoxigenic strains of *E. coli*. It was formerly
thought that enteropathic *E. coli* were limited to a small
number of serotypes. It is now clear that the pathogenetic properties of these strains are due to a surface factor that permits colonization and the ability to secrete
one or both of two enterotoxins (a heat-labile protein
resembling that of *V. cholerae* or a heat-stable toxin).
These properties may be transmitted by plasmids to
other *E. coli*. Thus the presence of a common serotype
in an outbreak is more likely to be an epidemiologic
marker than to denote virulence. Sporadic epidemics
with invasive strains have been reported after ingestion
of imported cheese. Certain strains of *Proteus* and *Pseudomonas* have at times also been held responsible for
similar illness.

MENINGITIS AND BRAIN ABSCESS. During the first
four weeks of life, purulent meningitis is frequently
caused by members of the enteric group of bacteria.
Such cases occur sporadically in nurseries, and may be
associated with infection of any other tissue of the
body (see discussion of K antigens, above). Infants
with meningoceles are especially liable to enteric bacterial meningitis. In adults, such infections are rare, but
may occasionally be seen as complications of gram-
negative bacteremia or in association with other diseases affecting host resistance, e.g., diabetes mellitus or
lymphoma (see Ch. 140). Nontraumatic brain abscess is

frequently due to infection by multiple species of anaerobic organisms similar to those found in the gastrointestinal tract. The sites of origin include chronically infected ears, sinuses, lung, abdomen, and pelvis.

BACTEREMIA IN HEPATIC CIRRHOSIS. Occasionally persons with cirrhosis of the liver develop an acute febrile illness and are found to have bacteremia caused by one of the enteric organisms, usually *E. coli*. Occasionally patients with ascites develop "spontaneous" peritonitis, but in most of these cases the bacteremia comes "out of the blue" without evidence of localized sepsis anywhere. The illness is short and self-limited or responds to appropriate chemotherapy. Speculation as to its pathogenesis has included the possibility of shunting bacteria away from the filtering action of the liver, impairment of humoral or cellular defense mechanisms, or complement inactivation owing to high blood ammonia. In actuality a satisfactory explanation is lacking at present.

SURFACE INFECTION. Enteric bacteria, particularly *Proteus* and *Pseudomonas*, are commonly recovered from the surfaces of burns, varicose ulcers, decubitus ulcers, tracheostomy sites, and the like. Generally, these organisms appear to play no pathogenic role, and satisfactory healing may proceed regardless of their presence. They can at times result in fulminant gram-negative sepsis, particularly in the patient with severe burns. The exudate from the sinus of a chronic osteomyelitis or chronic otitis media often contains *Proteus* as the dominant organism. Otitis of the external auditory canal owing to *Pseudomonas* may give troublesome local symptoms, especially in swimmers.

PERIRECTAL ABSCESS. Perirectal abscess is an important complication in patients with marked granulocytopenia. Rectal examination should be carefully performed in such patients, particularly when they develop fever and perianal pain.

ABSCESSES AT SITES OF SUBCUTANEOUS INJECTIONS. Rarely, enteric bacilli cause abscesses in subcutaneous tissue at sites of hypodermic injections, notably in diabetic subjects who inject their own insulin. These are sometimes characterized by gas formation, and they thus arouse fear of more serious clostridial infection, whereas, in fact, they are usually of minor clinical importance.

METASTATIC INFECTIONS. Despite the frequency with which enteric bacteria succeed in invading the blood, metastatic localization of infection is rare. There are, however, occasional instances of such suppurative lesions as arthritis and panophthalmitis in patients with bacteremia originating in acute pyelonephritis. Of special interest in this regard is osteomyelitis of the spine. This is usually seen in men with prostatic disease, chronic cystitis, and posterior urethritis. Possibly the method of spread here is by way of septic emboli to the spine through the vertebral venous plexus.

SUPERINFECTION. Enteric bacteria frequently predominate in the bronchial secretions of patients who are chronically ill or are treated with antimicrobial agents. In most instances, this is not of significance and simply represents emergence of bacterial strains after the suppression of the primary pathogens. Transtracheal aspiration, followed by Gram stain and culture of the secretions, is a useful method to distinguish between colonization of the pharynx versus true infection of the lower respiratory tract. Pharyngeal colonization is not an indication for antimicrobial therapy unless there is clinical evidence of tissue invasion by the newly emergent organism. Primary gram-negative bacterial pneumonia often superimposed on viral influenza, however, does occur and may be exceedingly difficult to manage.

GRAM-NEGATIVE BACTEREMIA

Bacteremia caused by gram-negative bacilli has become a problem of greater relative importance since the advent of penicillin and better control of gram-positive coccal infections. Urinary tract infection accounts for about one half of all cases of blood invasion by the enteric bacteria. Other causes include surgical disease of the gastrointestinal tract, infections developing at the site of "cut-downs" and intravenous catheters, postpartum or postabortal sepsis (including the so-called "placental bacteremia"), and infection of wounds, ulcers, burns, and internal prosthetic devices such as heart valves. Sometimes there is a clearly apparent precipitating factor such as cystoscopy, surgical or obstetrical procedure, or manipulation of an infected wound.

These bacteremias have clinical characteristics closely resembling the recognized biologic effects of gram-negative bacterial endotoxins. Onset of symptoms may occur with a shaking chill and rise in temperature to 38 to 40.5° C. There is an initial leukopenia, but after 6 to 12 hours usually there is leukocytosis. An *important and highly significant accompaniment is circulatory embarrassment with lowering of the blood pressure.* This may be manifested only by some alteration in the patient's state of consciousness, and the skin may continue to feel warm, although sometimes the skin is cold and clammy. Occasionally patients slip into a shocklike state without much elevation of temperature; hence infection of this kind must always be taken into consideration in evaluation of peripheral circulatory failure. Some patients, however, do develop the syndrome of disseminated intravascular coagulation (DIC). This phenomenon is not unique to gram-negative bacteremia and may be due to such diverse causes as rickettsial and gram-positive bacterial infections. The most common findings are reduced platelet count, low factor V levels in plasma, and fibrin split products in serum. Serum complement is low only in the most seriously ill patients (see Ch. 140). With so-called "gram-negative shock" there is diminution in urine output, increase in proteinuria, and often a rise in nonprotein nitrogen of the blood. The cardiac output may be unpredictably low, normal, or elevated. Some patients show shifts in acid-base balance in the direction of metabolic acidosis, whereas others have compensatory hyperventilation. The pH of the blood, however, often remains normal. Lactic acidosis is common in severely ill patients. It is characterized by a marked anion gap with low levels of both serum bicarbonate and Pco_2. These findings are often confusing, particularly if they occur in patients with complicating problems such as pulmonary or renal insufficiency or congestive heart failure. Serum lactate levels are helpful in sorting out these factors. Much depends on the nature of the underlying disease and the renal reserve. The outlook is grave, being influenced by age, associated disease, and evidence of shock. When obvious signs of circulatory collapse are present, the fatality rate may be as high as 75 per cent.

UNIQUE FEATURES OF PSEUDOMONAS INFECTIONS

Pseudomonas infections, although often similar to those caused by other gram-negative bacteria, sometimes have unique characteristics. As already mentioned, this organism frequently appears in necrotic tissue, as in ulcers, burns, or draining sinuses. Usually such colonization is of little clinical significance, and mere removal of necrotic tissue may cause it to disappear. Nevertheless, under certain circumstances, especially in chronically debilitated persons or in patients with agranulocytosis or acute leukemia, severe sepsis may be produced by this class of bacteria. In addition to endotoxin, *Pseudomonas aeruginosa* produces several enzymes, including collagenase, proteases, elastase, and a recently described exotoxin (PA toxin) whose mode of action is similar to that of diphtheria toxin.

Pseudomonas is notoriously resistant to antimicrobial therapy; hence it tends to emerge as the dominant microorganism after eradication of other bacteria by drugs. It may then be responsible for the phenomenon of superinfection, as in the bronchopulmonary infections that may complicate prophylactic chemotherapy of chronic lung disease.

Because *Pseudomonas* commonly occurs in tap water, and because it may be resistant to antiseptics used in sterilizing instruments, it is likely to be carried into the body by such procedures as cystoscopy. Furthermore, meningitis after lumbar puncture has been associated with this organism.

Tissue invasion, most often seen in patients with leukopenia or relapse in leukemia, is characterized by necrotizing vasculitis with bacterial invasion of the walls of arteries and veins. This leads to a distinctive necrotic skin lesion (called ecthyma gangrenosum) that is found most commonly along the axillary folds or in the anogenital area, but may also develop on any part of the body. It may begin as a vesicle that later becomes necrotic. The typical lesion of ecthyma gangrenosum is a round, indurated ulcer with a black center that varies from a few millimeters to several centimeters in diameter.

TREATMENT OF ENTERIC BACTERIAL INFECTIONS

GENERAL PRINCIPLES. The major clinical problems in management of enteric bacterial infections are (1) differentiation of superficial contamination that often requires no treatment from true or potential tissue invasion, (2) early recognition and drainage of abscesses, (3) anticipation of the role of anaerobic bacteria that cannot be readily cultured, and (4) early recognition of bacteremic shock. *Many of these infections are preventable*, particularly those arising from instrumentation of the urinary tract, intravenous catheters and contaminated fluids, suction, and ventilation equipment. *Every physician must consider elimination of such sources of contamination as one of his prime responsibilities.*

GRAM-NEGATIVE BACTEREMIA. The presence of gram-negative organisms in the blood should alert the physician to search for a site of origin such as intravenous or urinary catheters and abdominal, pelvic, or perirectal abscesses. Removal of devices and drainage of abscesses should be done as soon as possible. It should be remembered that gram-negative bacteremia is more common than is usually suspected and is often transient and without complication. For example, bacteremia may occur after gastrointestinal endoscopy, urinary instrumentation, and manipulation of the bowel during surgery. These events often go undetected, or there is a single temperature rise and no further complications. Antimicrobial therapy probably plays little role in management of these transient episodes. The main problem is caused by the release of endotoxin, which is not affected by antimicrobial drugs. Judgment will therefore have to be made to determine whether there is an infected site which requires treatment.

The site of origin of the infection, the underlying illness of the patient, and prior receipt of antimicrobial agents are key determinants in planning therapy. The response to antimicrobial agents and the mortality from gram-negative bacteremia are closely related to whether the patient has rapidly fatal, ultimately fatal, or nonfatal underlying diseases. Consequently, the nature and status of the underlying disease is a major determinant in selecting appropriate treatment. The treatment must often be begun in the rapidly and ultimately fatal group before organisms are isolated and their drug susceptibility patterns are determined.

In rapidly fatal conditions (severe leukopenia, acute leukemia, extensive burns, and immunosuppressed patients), gram-negative bacteremia often occurs in hospital settings where there are organisms with multiple-drug resistance such as *Pseudomonas, Klebsiella, Serratia, Providencia,* and *Proteus.* In the febrile patient, after obtaining blood and other cultures from suspected sites of infection, therapy should be begun with an aminoglycoside (gentamicin, tobramycin, or amikacin) and either carbenicillin or ticarcillin. The addition of a parenteral or antistaphylococcal agent such as a penicillinase-resistant penicillin (methicillin, oxacillin, or nafcillin) or cephalosporin (cephalothin, cefazolin, or cephapirin) should also be considered. The choice of a specific aminoglycoside drug, such as amikacin, will depend on whether the hospital has a high frequency of endemic strains resistant to gentamicin or tobramycin. Once the organism is isolated from the blood or suspected site of infection, therapy should be altered, if needed, to the most appropriate, least toxic agent(s).

In ultimately fatal conditions (severe obstructive pulmonary disease, end-stage renal failure, obstructive uropathy, or carcinomatosis), there is usually a determinable site of infection. After obtaining blood and other cultures of the suspected site (transtracheal aspiration, urinary catheterization, thoracentesis, paracentesis, lumbar puncture, subcutaneous aspiration of an abscess) and gram-negative bacilli are seen on Gram stain in association with polymorphonuclear leukocytes, therapy should be begun. Until drug susceptibility tests are available, treatment should be started with an aminoglycoside drug as described above. Gram-negative meningitis often requires intrathecal injection of aminoglycosides. When *Klebsiella* is strongly suspected (such as in pneumonia), a cephalosporin may be added. When anaerobic organisms are suspected in the lower respiratory tract, penicillin should be added; when they are suspected in the abdomen, pelvis, or anogenital area, clindamycin or chloramphenicol should be added. Once drug susceptibility data are available, therapy may be changed to the most appropriate agent(s).

In nonfatal conditions, such as urinary tract infections, osteomyelitis, cholecystitis, or abdominal, pelvic, or wound infections in an otherwise healthy patient, therapy will depend on the urgency of the patient's condition, the most likely invasive organism, and the local pattern of drug susceptibility to common organisms, such as *E. coli.* In the acutely ill hospitalized patient, a parenteral form of an aminoglycoside or cephalosporin or ampicillin may be used. Clindamycin or chloramphenicol should be added in abdominal, pelvic, or decubitus infections when anaerobes are suspected. Acute cholecystitis is usually associated with *E. coli* and may be treated with ampicillin, tetracycline, or a cephalosporin. Acute urinary infections are most likely to respond to oral agents such as co-trimoxazole or nitrofurantoin. Alternative agents, such as ampicillin, tetracycline, nalidixic acid, a sulfonamide, or an oral cephalosporin may be used, depending on drug susceptibility tests. *Pseudomonas* infections occurring in nonfatal conditions often can be treated with an aminoglycoside antimicrobial when the organism is susceptible. Carbenicillin or ticarcillin need only be added or used when the organism is resistant to an aminoglycoside or when the patient has severe renal failure or fails to respond to other agents. Oral carbenicillin should be reserved for treatment of *Pseudomonas* urinary infections outside the hospital because of the danger of selecting resistant organisms. *Antimicrobial therapy is ineffective for more than a few days in the patient with an indwelling urinary catheter and should be reserved for acute episodes of sepsis.*

Management of bacteremic shock is complex, requiring corrective measures designed to improve cardiac function, tissue perfusion, and electrolyte imbalance, particularly acidosis. This requires monitoring of the central venous pressure by a well-placed catheter in the superior vena cava or right atrium in an attempt to achieve a pressure of about 8 to 12 cm of water, and following the dynamics of pressure changes as fluid replacement is given. Replacement fluids include blood, dextran, and saline solutions. Drugs such as dopamine may be used to increase cardiac output and improve tissue perfusion; vasopressors such as metaraminol should be used sparingly except in severe shock. High doses of corticosteroids are widely used, but their efficacy has not been established by controlled studies. Heparin may be useful in the syndrome of disseminated intravascular coagulation (see Ch. 356).

Finegold, S. M.: Anaerobic Bacteria in Human Disease. New York, Academic Press, 1977.

Fried, M. A., and Vosti, K. L.: Importance of underlying disease in patients with gram-negative bacteremia. Arch. Intern. Med., 121:418, 1968.

Mangi, R. J., Quintiliani, R., and Andriole, V. T.: Gram-negative bacillary meningitis. Am. J. Med., 59:829, 1975.

Young, L. S., Martin, W. J., Meyer, R. D., Weinstein, R. J., and Anderson, E. T.: Gram-negative rod bacteremia: Microbiologic, immunologic and therapeutic considerations. Ann. Intern. Med., 86:456, 1977.

155. SHIGELLOSIS

Charles C. J. Carpenter

DEFINITION. Shigellosis is a specific acute bacterial infection of the intestinal tract of man, with predominant involvement of the distal colon, sigmoid, and rectum, caused by bacteria of the genus *Shigella.* It most commonly presents as a clinically nonspecific diarrhea. In the more severe cases, the initial mild diarrhea is accompanied by fever and followed by true dysentery, with cramping abdominal pains, tenesmus, and frequent stools in which mucus, leukocytes, and erythrocytes are abundant.

ETIOLOGY. Shigellae (dysentery bacilli) are nonmotile, gram-negative, rod-shaped bacilli belonging to the family Enterobacteriaceae. Four species of shigellae are recognized, based on antigenic and biochemical properties: *S. dysenteriae* (Group A), *S. flexneri* (Group B), *S. boydii* (Group C), and *S. sonnei* (Group D). Among these species there are 39 serotypes, each of which is designated by the species name followed by a specific Arabic number. With the exception of *S. flexneri* 6, they do not ferment lactose. The most common species in the United States until 1965 was *S. flexneri,* but this species has now largely been replaced by *S. sonnei. S. sonnei* is now the most commonly reported shigella in Western Europe and Japan, as well as North America. *S. boydii* is so rarely encountered in the United States that its isolation usually indicates exposure during foreign travel. *S. dysenteriae,* the most virulent shigella, is now unusual in the more developed countries, but is currently prevalent in Central America.

EPIDEMIOLOGY. Incidence and Prevalence. Despite generally high standards of hygiene in the United States, there were over 16,000 cases of shigellosis reported to the Center for Disease Control in 1976. *S. sonnei* was the predominant etiologic agent, and the great majority of patients were children. The few cases caused by *S. dysenteriae* could generally be traced to contact with individuals from infected areas in Central America. The true incidence is undoubtedly severalfold higher than the number of reported cases.

The same general pattern of infection has been observed throughout Western Europe and Japan in the past ten years. In Eastern Europe and Russia, where the over-all incidence of shigellosis is greater, *S. flexneri* has continued to be the predominant microorganism. *S. flexneri* is also the most commonly isolated species in most of the economically underdeveloped nations of the world. *S. dysenteriae* 1 (Shiga bacillus), which has nearly disappeared as a major cause of dysentery in most parts of the world, re-emerged as a major epidemic problem throughout Central America from 1969 to 1973; imported cases of dysentery caused by the Shiga bacillus continue to be reported sporadically from the southwestern United States.

Spread of Infection. Shigellosis is found throughout the world. Although seasonal patterns vary in different regions, the incidence of shigellosis characteristically peaks in the late summer and early autumn in the United States. Man remains the only known reservoir of *Shigella* infection. During clinical illness and for a variable period (up to six weeks) following recovery, shigellae excreted in the stools may be transmitted to other persons. Although the organisms are quite sensitive to desiccation, they may survive for long periods in foods and water. Transmission most often occurs by close person-to-person contact involving contaminated hands. Children in the one- to four-year age group are at highest risk of developing shigellosis, and young males are affected more often than young females. In young adults the incidence is higher in women than in men, probably reflecting the fact that many young adult women are in close contact with ill children, either in the home or in an institutional setting. Intrafamilial spread is especially likely to occur when the initial case has occurred in a preschool child. Attack rates in affected families range from 10 to 80 per cent.

Custodial institutions, especially those caring for the retarded, are frequent settings for large epidemics. Because of the difficulty in maintaining adequate hygiene among residents in these settings, endemic shigellosis is often a nearly intractable problem. Up to 30 per cent of admissions to certain custodial institutions experience an episode of shigellosis within a year of arrival. Nursery schools and day care centers, because of the young age group and the close contact of the populations, have especially high attack rates whenever shigellae are introduced.

Since shigellae are transmitted primarily by the fecal-oral route, crowded living conditions, poor housing, poor water supply, and inadequate sewage facilities all correlate significantly with increased risk of infection. Therefore, within the United States, the urban ghetto areas and Indian reservations are settings in which incidence of shigellosis is excessively high. By the same token, rural villages in the economically underdeveloped nations are areas of high rates of shigellosis. The recent pandemic spread of *S. dysenteriae* 1 (Shiga bacillus) from Guatemala and El Salvador throughout Central America and Mexico was a matter of grave concern. This pandemic has, however, subsided without major spread to either South America or the United States. As has been true of pandemics in the past, the reason for the development of the 1969–1973 Central American Shiga bacillus pandemic remains obscure.

PATHOGENESIS AND PATHOPHYSIOLOGY. Although moderately resistant to acid, shigellae have less difficulty than other enteric pathogens in passing the human gastric barrier. In volunteer studies, as few as 200 ingested bacilli regularly initiate disease in 25 per cent of healthy volunteers. This contrasts strikingly with the much larger numbers of typhoid bacilli and the strikingly greater number of cholera bacilli which must be ingested to produce disease in man. During the incubation period, which is usually 36 to 72 hours, the organisms traverse the small bowel and proliferate in the lower ileum and colon. In the colon shigellae reach concentrations of 10^6 to 10^{10} organisms per gram of stool. Unlike the case with certain other enteric pathogens (*V. cholerae* and enterotoxigenic *E. coli*), epithelial cell penetration is essential to the pathogenesis of shigellosis. Multiplication of bacteria occurs within the epithelial cells of the colon, predominantly in the villi, and this is followed by an acute inflammatory response in the subjacent lamina propria. This results in destruction of the villous tips, distortion of the mucosal architecture, and the formation of superficial microabscesses. In the more severe cases, long segments of colon may be affected with a diffuse inflammatory process which,

however, remains confined to the lamina propria. The altered mucosa is friable and is covered with an exudate of polymorphonuclear leukocytes. Stool therefore contains large numbers of erythrocytes and leukocytes. Since the inflammation is superficial, bacteremia is rare and colonic perforation seldom occurs as a complication of shigellosis.

S. dysenteriae and certain strains of *S. flexneri* and *S. sonnei* produce an enterotoxin which causes secretion of isotonic fluid by the small bowel. The role of this enterotoxin in the pathogenesis of clinical shigellosis is not certain, but it has been suggested that the enterotoxin is responsible for the mild watery diarrhea which often precedes full-blown bacillary dysentery. It is possible that the enterotoxin is entirely responsible for the clinical manifestations in those mild cases characterized by only short-lived, nonbloody diarrhea.

CLINICAL MANIFESTATIONS. Shigellosis is often a biphasic disease, beginning with cramping abdominal pain and watery diarrhea, sometimes accompanied by fever (up to 40° C) and generalized myalgias. Fluid and electrolyte losses are greatest during this phase of the illness; such losses are rarely voluminous enough to be life threatening except in very young children and in the elderly. This first phase usually lasts for one to three days; in the more severely ill patients, it is followed by a second phase, which, in the absence of treatment, may last for weeks. The second phase is that of true dysentery; the character of the stool changes with a decrease in the quantity of each bowel movement and the appearance of bright red blood and mucus in the feces. During this phase, tenesmus may become a vexing feature, and anorexia and weight loss are common. Fever is not prominent during the second phase of the illness.

It is important to emphasize that many patients who are infected with shigellae, especially *S. sonnei*, are entirely asymptomatic, and an additional large number simply have mild cramping abdominal pain and watery diarrhea which cannot clinically be differentiated from the illnesses caused by several other microorganisms. Only the more severe cases, presenting with the classic bacillary dysentery pattern, can readily be diagnosed clinically as shigellosis. Of the *Shigella* strains now encountered in the United States, *S. dysenteriae* is the most virulent and by far the least common. *S. flexneri* is intermediate in both virulence and frequency, and *S. sonnei*, which accounts for 80 per cent of cases in the United States, presents the mildest clinical picture.

The onset of shigellosis is often more fulminant in children, who may present with unexplained high fever with or without convulsions. Neurologic symptoms and signs, including delirium, headache, nuchal rigidity, and lethargy, rarely occur in adults, but are quite common in children in the one- to four-year age group. Roughly 25 per cent of children hospitalized for shigellosis experience convulsions. The basis for the convulsions is unknown; it seems unlikely that the neurologic manifestations are caused by *Shigella* neurotoxin, as similar neurologic manifestations may be seen in children with salmonellosis.

DIAGNOSIS. Shigellosis should be considered in any patient with the acute onset of fever and diarrhea. Diagnosis is more likely, however, in the high-risk groups delineated above. Examination of the stool is quite useful in the diagnosis. Blood, pus, and mucus may be seen grossly in severe bacillary dysentery; even in milder forms of the disease, microscopic examination of the stool reveals numerous leukocytes and erythrocytes. The fecal leukocyte examination should be performed with a portion of liquid stool, preferably containing mucus. A drop of stool is placed on a microscopic slide and mixed thoroughly with two drops of methylene blue solution. A cover slip is placed over the mixture for microscopic examination. The presence of abundant polymorphonuclear leukocytes helps in distinguishing shigellosis from salmonellosis (in which leukocytes are present but are predominantly mononuclear) and from diarrheal syndromes caused by enterotoxigenic *E. coli* and *Vibrio cholerae* (in which fecal leukocytes are characteristically absent). The peripheral white cell count is of little diagnostic value, in that the white cell count may range from less than 3000 to more than 30,000, with a mean value in the high-normal range. Sigmoidoscopic examination characteristically reveals diffuse erythema and a friable mucosa, with shallow ulcers which are characteristically 3 to 7 mm in diameter.

Definitive diagnosis depends on isolating shigellae by use of selective media. A rectal swab, a swab of a colonic ulcer obtained by sigmoidoscopic examination, or a freshly passed stool specimen should be inoculated immediately on culture plates or into carrying media. If a delay of more than a few hours is anticipated before appropriate culture media are available, the stool should be placed in a buffered glycerol-saline solution for preservation. Since isolation rates of shigellae from freshly passed stools of patients known to have shigellosis may be as low as 67 per cent, culturing for three successive days is recommended in order to maximize the chance of isolation. Stool cultures are generally positive within 24 hours after the onset of symptoms and may remain positive for several weeks in the absence of antimicrobial therapy. Blood cultures are so rarely positive as to be of no diagnostic value.

Appropriate culture media include blood, desoxycholate, and salmonella-shigella (S-S) agars. Selected colonies suggestive of shigellae should be placed on triple sugar-iron agar and lysine-iron agar. Colonies showing an alkaline slant and acid butt without gas or hydrogen sulfide in either agar should be definitively diagnosed by agglutination with polyvalent shigella antisera. It is important to recognize that the commonly used S-S agar is inhibitory for the most virulent of the *Shigella* species, *S. dysenteriae* 1.

Definitive bacteriologic diagnosis becomes of critical importance in distinguishing the more severe and prolonged cases of shigellosis from ulcerative colitis, with which it may be confused both clinically and by sigmoidoscopic examination. Occasional patients with shigellosis have been subjected to colectomy with the mistaken diagnosis of ulcerative colitis; a positive culture for shigellae could clearly prevent such a therapeutic misadventure.

TREATMENT. The three steps in the treatment of shigellosis include correction of fluid and electrolyte balance, antimicrobial therapy, and symptomatic relief. Although voluminous diarrhea is unusual in shigellosis, fluid loss may be lethal in the very young and the very old. Fluid losses in shigellosis are qualitatively similar to those in other bacterial diarrheal diseases, and the patient should be treated with appropriate intravenous fluids (lactated Ringer's solution is a generally available and adequate solution) in quantities adequate to correct clinical signs of saline depletion. The requirement for intravenous fluids is generally brief, but will be lifesaving in exceptional cases.

The efficacy of antimicrobial agents in treating shigellosis has been well established. Although infections with *Shigella sonnei, flexneri,* and *boydii* are generally self-limited except in the very young and very old, appropriate antimicrobial therapy may decrease the duration of symptoms by 50 per cent and decrease the duration of excretion of shigellae (an important epidemiologic factor) by a far greater percentage. Infection by *S. dysenteriae* 1 may result in a 10 to 20 per cent mortality rate in the absence of antimicrobial therapy, and appropriate antimicrobials are therefore mandatory with this pathogen. Ampicillin is currently the drug of choice for shigellosis in the United States. It should be administered orally in four divided doses for a total of 2 grams a day to adults and 100 mg per kilogram per day to children for a five-day period. Because of the increasing frequency of plasmid-mediated antimicrobial resistance to *Shigella* infections, drug susceptibility testing is important. For patients with ampicillin-resistant isolates, tetracycline is sometimes effective. It is important to recognize that certain drugs which appear effective in vitro, especially orally administered, nonabsorbable antimicrobials such as neomycin or kanamycin, are *not* effective in vivo, and that sulfonamide resistance is so widespread as to nullify the value of these chemotherapeutic agents when used alone. However, cotrimoxazole is an alternative drug to which significant resistance has not yet been demonstrated.

Agents which decrease intestinal motility should *not* be used. Such preparations as diphenoxylate and paregoric may exacerbate symptoms, presumably by retarding intestinal clearance of the microorganisms. There is no convincing evidence that the pectin- or bismuth-containing preparations are of any positive value.

PROGNOSIS. The mortality rate in untreated shigellosis is dependent upon the infectious strain, and ranges from greater than 20 per cent in certain outbreaks of infection caused by *S. dysenteriae* 1 to less than 1 per cent in many outbreaks caused by *S. sonnei.* Even with infection caused by *S. dysenteriae* 1, the mortality rate should approach zero if appropriate fluid replacement and antimicrobial therapy are initiated early in the course of the disease.

PREVENTION. Individuals excreting shigellae, whether symptomatic or not, should be excluded from all phases of food-handling until cultures of stool specimens collected on three consecutive days, after antimicrobial therapy has been discontinued, are reported as negative. In outbreaks in custodial institutions or day care centers, strict and early separation of those with illness from those who are unaffected is mandatory. Targeted antimicrobial chemoprophylaxis in this setting has generally been disappointing. The most important control measure is scrupulous handwashing by all individuals involved in handling food.

Recognition, reporting, and investigation of epidemics in schools and institutions remain important, and reporting of shigellosis cases to health authorities should be considered mandatory.

For the traveler to countries with major *Shigella* problems, no chemoprophylactic agent is an adequate substitute for good personal hygiene and the avoidance of contaminated water, fruits, and vegetables. No effective vaccine is yet available.

DuPont, H. L., and Hornick, R. B.: Adverse effect of Lomotil therapy in shigellosis. JAMA, 226:1525, 1973.

DuPont, H. L., Hornick, R. B., Dawkins, A. T., Snyder, M. J., and Formal, S. B.: The response of man to virulent *Shigella flexneri* 2a. J. Infect. Dis., 119:296, 1969.

Haltalin, K. C., Kusmiesz, H. T., Hinton, L. V., and Nelson, J. D.: Treatment of acute diarrhea in outpatients. Am. J. Dis. Child., 124:554, 1972.

Harris, J. C., DuPont, H. L., and Hornick, R. B.: Fecal leukocytes in diarrheal illness. Ann. Intern. Med., 76:697, 1972.

Keusch, G. T., and Jacewicz, M.: The pathogenesis of *Shigella* diarrhea. VI. Toxin and antitoxin in *Shigella flexneri* and *Shigella sonnei* infections in humans. J. Infect. Dis., 135:552, 1977.

Neisman, J. B., Martin, K. I., Lewis, J. N., Friedman, C. T. H., and Gangarosa, E. J.: Impact in the United States of the Shiga dysentery pandemic of Central America and Mexico; a review of the surveillance data through 1972. J. Infect. Dis., 128:574, 1973.

Ogawa, H.: Experimental approach in studies on pathogenesis of bacillary dysentery — with special reference to the invasion of bacilli into intestinal mucosa. Acta Pathol., 20:261, 1970.

156. CHOLERA

(Asiatic Cholera)

Charles C. J. Carpenter

DEFINITION. Cholera is an acute specific infectious disease of man caused by *Vibrio cholerae*. All manifestations of the disease are caused by an enterotoxin elaborated by *Vibrio cholerae* which have colonized the small bowel of the susceptible individual. In its most severe form the disease is characterized by voluminous diarrhea, with rapid loss of fluid and electrolytes from the gastrointestinal tract, resulting in hypovolemic shock, metabolic acidosis, and, if untreated, death. Cholera is endemic in the Gangetic Delta of the Indian subcontinent, and has been responsible for seven major pandemics during the past 150 years.

ETIOLOGY. In his classic study in 1857, John Snow carefully described an outbreak of cholera in London, and clearly incriminated contaminated water as the source of the disease. In 1883, Koch identified *Vibrio cholerae* as the etiologic agent of this disease by identifying this microorganism in the feces of large numbers of patients with cholera. *Vibrio cholerae* are short (0.2 to 0.4 μm by 1.5 to 4.0 μm), slightly curved, gram-negative rods and may readily be seen in the gram-stained smears of the watery excreta of patients with cholera. Vibrios grow aerobically on a variety of nutrient media at 37° C, preferentially at an alkaline pH. There are two biotypes of *Vibrio cholerae*, the "classic" and the eltor. The eltor biotype is hardier than the classic strain, persists longer in nature, and is more likely to cause a carrier state in man; the eltor biotype can be readily distinguished from the classic biotype by its resistance to polymyxin B. The distinction between the two biotypes is important for epidemiologic purposes. *Vibrio cholerae* can be differentiated from noncholera vibrios by antigenic and fermentative reactions, as well as by biologic testing.

EPIDEMIOLOGY. Incidence and Prevalence. For the past century and a half, cholera has remained endemic in the common delta of the Ganges and Brahmaputra

Rivers. The disease has caused seven worldwide pandemics since 1817, and the three major North American epidemics of 1832, 1848, and 1867 have shown that the potential distribution of cholera is worldwide. The period 1961 to 1976 witnessed a seventh pandemic spread of cholera from Indonesia westward through South and Central Asia to Western Europe and to the entire African continent. Serious outbreaks of cholera occurred in Israel in 1970, in Spain in 1972, in Italy in the summer of 1973, in Portugal and Guam in 1974, and in Syria in 1977. Isolated cases have been identified in travelers returning to most of the nations of Western Europe, as well as to Canada and Japan. An isolated case was identified in Port Lavaca, Texas, in 1973. Although there has been no further geographic spread of the disease in 1977, cholera appears to have become endemic in several Central and Western African nations which had been previously free of this disease for at least four decades. Fewer than 70 thousand cases of cholera were reported to the World Health Organization in 1977, representing a sharp decrease from 148,000 cases at the peak of the seventh pandemic in 1971.

Spread of Infection. Man is the only natural host and victim of *Vibrio cholerae*. Most major epidemics of this disease have been water borne, and water plays the major role in the transmission of *Vibrio cholerae* in the endemic rural areas in the Gangetic Delta. During major pandemics, however, the direct contamination of food with infectious excreta may be important. Contaminated fresh vegetables appeared to have been a major factor in the transmission of cholera in Israel in the outbreak in 1970, and shellfish may have been a significant factor in the spread of cholera in Naples in 1973. Persons with mild or asymptomatic infections (contact carriers) may play a significant role in the dissemination of epidemic disease. The clinical case-to-infection ratio with infection by the classic *V. cholerae* biotype is about 1:6; with infection by the eltor biotype, this ratio may be as low as 1:50. A prolonged gallbladder carrier state may develop in 3 to 5 per cent of adult patients convalescing from cholera caused by the eltor biotype. The gallbladder carrier state is more common in older convalescents and has never been observed in the pediatric age group. The role of such convalescent carriers in the transmission of the disease has not been clarified. *Vibrio cholerae* does not survive well in fresh water, but may survive for long periods in sea water; this has recently been reaffirmed in association with the 1973 outbreak of cholera in Portugal.

In the cholera endemic areas of Bangladesh and West Bengal, cholera is predominantly a disease of children. Attack rates are ten times greater in the one- to five-year age group than in those over 20 years of age. When the disease spreads to previously uninvolved areas, the attack rates are initially at least as high in adults as in children. As the disease becomes endemic in new locations, as has occurred in the Philippines over the past 15 years, the endemic epidemiologic pattern develops, with the disease becoming far more common in young children than in adults.

PATHOGENESIS. *Vibrio cholerae* causes disease when a large number of viable organisms are ingested, survive passage through the stomach, colonize the small bowel, and produce enterotoxin. The incubation period may vary from 12 hours to as long as 6 days. Because of the remarkable susceptibility of *Vibrio cholerae* to gastric acid, an enormous number of microorganisms must be ingested to cause this disease in a previously healthy individual. Volunteer studies have indicated that ingestion of even 10 billion organisms will not consistently produce clinical disease in healthy adults. If, however, gastric acid is neutralized by sodium bicarbonate, ingestion of 1 million viable organisms produces clinical disease in roughly 50 per cent of normal individuals. The individual with relative or absolute achlorhydria is therefore abnormally susceptible to cholera, and this susceptibility has been demonstrated by the very sharp increase in incidence of cholera in individuals with total or subtotal gastrectomy in the recent outbreaks of cholera in Israel and Italy.

Once vibrios have colonized the small bowel, an enterotoxin, with a molecular weight of 84,000, is produced. The binding unit of this enterotoxin combines rapidly, and apparently irreversibly, to a monosialoganglioside in the small bowel epithelial cell wall, allowing the active toxin subunit to stimulate adenyl cyclase in the intestinal epithelial cells. The resultant increase in intracellular levels of cyclic adenosine 3',5'-monophosphate leads to rapid excretion of electrolytes into the small bowel lumen. The action of the cholera toxin on the small bowel mucosa causes no visible morphologic damage to the gut mucosa, and this is reflected in the very low protein content, and the virtual absence of leukocytes, in the cholera stool.

All signs, symptoms, and metabolic derangements in cholera result directly from the rapid loss of fluid and electrolytes from the gut. All segments of the small bowel participate in the increased secretion of isotonic fluid. Precise studies have demonstrated that, in the adult, cholera stool is nearly isotonic with plasma, with sodium and chloride concentrations slightly less than those of plasma, bicarbonate concentration approximately twice that of plasma, and potassium concentration three to fives times that of plasma.

CLINICAL MANIFESTATIONS. The clinical onset of cholera is generally that of abrupt, painless, watery diarrhea. Stool volumes vary greatly, and in all epidemics there are large numbers of mild cases in which the fluid loss is not severe enough to require hospitalization. In the more severe cases, however, the initial stool volume may exceed 1500. At variable intervals after the onset of diarrhea, vomiting ensues; this is also characteristically effortless and productive of rice-watery material. In fulminant cases, severe muscle cramps, most commonly involving the gastrocnemius group, almost invariably develop. Prostration occurs at varying intervals following the onset of symptoms, in direct relationship to the magnitude of the fluid loss.

When first seen by the physician, the severely ill cholera patient presents a characteristic appearance: collapsed, cyanotic, with no palpable peripheral pulses, pinched facies, and scaphoid abdomen. The voice is very weak, high-pitched, and often nearly inaudible. Vital signs include tachycardia, varying degrees of tachypnea, hypopyrexia, and hypotension, often with no obtainable blood pressure. Heart sounds are faint or inaudible, and bowel sounds are hypoactive or entirely absent. Major alterations in mental status are not common in adults; the adult usually remains well oriented, although apathetic, even in the face of severe hypovolemic shock. As many as 10 per cent of small children, however, may have central nervous system abnormalities that range from stupor to convulsions.

Laboratory abnormalities are those which would be expected to result from a massive gastrointestinal loss of an isotonic, alkaline, virtually protein-free fluid (see accompanying table). These include increased plasma and whole blood specific gravity, elevated plasma protein, decreased plasma bicarbonate, low arterial pH, normal plasma sodium, slightly increased plasma chloride, and moderately elevated plasma potassium. Since the bicarbonate loss is proportional to stool volume, the decrease in whole blood pH is roughly proportional to the increase in plasma protein concentration at all stages of the untreated disease.

The illness may last from 12 hours to 7 days, and later clinical manifestations depend on adequacy of therapy. With adequate fluid and electrolyte repletion, recovery is remarkably rapid. If therapy is inadequate, the case mortality rate may exceed 50 per cent. The important causes of death are hypovolemic shock, uncompensated metabolic acidosis, and renal failure. When renal failure occurs, the characteristic pathologic findings are those of acute tubular necrosis secondary to prolonged hypotension.

DIAGNOSIS. The working diagnosis of cholera should be made on the basis of the clinical picture; appropriate fluid and electrolyte replacement therapy, as indicated by the physical findings, should be initiated immediately. Although a cholera-like illness may be caused by microorganisms other than *Vibrio cholerae*, most frequently by enterotoxigenic *Escherichia coli*, the resulting physiologic and metabolic abnormalities are the same, so that identical intravenous and oral electrolyte therapy may be used in all such cases.

Once appropriate therapy has been initiated, a geographic history should be obtained. The diagnosis of cholera is unlikely if the patient has not recently been in a known endemic or epidemic area. Stool examination should then be performed. Since the cholera enterotoxin causes neither inflammation nor destruction of intestinal mucosa, no leukocytes or erythrocytes are usually seen on microscopic examination of a fresh cholera stool stained with methylene blue. This dictum is, however, not absolute, as cholera may occasionally be superimposed on other acute or chronic inflammatory bowel disease. With *darkfield microscopy*, rapid tentative diagnosis can be made by direct observation of the characteristic rapid motility of the comma-shaped bacilli in fresh stool. Group- and type-specific antisera immobilize homologous strains and clearly distinguish them from other vibrios. *Fluorescent microscopy*, using fluorescein-labeled type-specific antibody, when available, also provides a rapid and accurate means of diagnosis.

Diagnostic culture techniques are relatively simple. A reliable and practical method consists of direct plating of feces on thiosulfate–citrate–bile salt–sucrose (TCBS)

Serial Blood Chemical Determinations in Cholera; Average Values in 40 Consecutive Patients

	On Admission	Four Hours	24 Hours
Sodium*	152	156	153
Chloride*	117	118	113
Potassium*	5.7	3.3	3.1
Bicarbonate*	7.4	21.0	24.5
Arterial pH	7.21	7.43	7.46
Plasma specific gravity	1.043	1.026	1.026

*Plasma electrolyte values are expressed in milliequivalents per liter of plasma H_2O.

agar. On TCBS agar typical opaque yellow colonies appear in 18 hours. Distinction between the two major serotypes, Inaba and Ogawa, requires agglutination with type-specific antisera. Identification of the eltor biotype of *Vibrio cholerae,* which is important for epidemiologic purposes, can be simply determined on the basis of the resistance of this biotype to polymyxin B.

TREATMENT. Successful therapy demands only prompt replacement of gastrointestinal losses of fluid and electrolytes. A "diarrhea treatment solution," recommended for intravenous therapy by the World Health Organization, is uniformly effective in both adult and pediatric patients; this solution may be simply prepared by adding 4 grams of sodium chloride, 6.5 grams of sodium acetate, 1 gram of potassium chloride and 10 grams of glucose to a liter of sterile distilled water. Alternatively, lactated Ringer's solution may be administered. Either of these intravenous fluid preparations should be infused intravenously and rapidly, 50 to 100 ml per minute, until a strong radial pulse has been restored. Subsequently the same fluid should be infused in quantities equal to gastrointestinal losses. If these losses cannot be measured accurately, intravenous fluid should be given at a rate sufficient to maintain a normal pulse volume and normal skin turgor. Overhydration can be avoided by careful observation of the neck veins and by auscultation of the lungs. Close observation of the patient is mandatory during the acute phase of the illness, as an adult patient can lose as much as 1 liter of isotonic fluid per hour during the first 24 hours of the disease. Inadequate or delayed restoration of electrolyte losses results in a very high incidence of acute renal insufficiency.

In children, complications are both more frequent and more severe. The most serious include stupor, coma, and convulsions (unique to pediatric patients), pulmonary edema, and cardiac arrhythmias. The central nervous system complications may be due to hypoglycemia (observed only in pediatric patients); hypernatremia resulting from the administration of isotonic fluid to the pediatric patient (who, unlike the adult patient, produces feces with a sodium concentration significantly less than that of plasma); or cerebral edema, presumably secondary to rapid fluid shifts during the administration of intravenous fluids. Pulmonary edema may result if fluids are given intravenously at too rapid a rate prior to the correction of the metabolic acidosis. Serious cardiac arrhythmias may result from potassium depletion in children, but rarely occur in adults with cholera. Each of these complications can be avoided by the careful administration of intravenous fluids that are carefully designed to replace the fecal electrolyte losses. The "diarrhea treatment solution," recommended by the World Health Organization for cholera as well as for other acute diarrheal diseases, has been used successfully to correct the acidosis, hypokalemia, and hypoglycemia without provoking hypernatremia. If lactated Ringer's solution is used in the pediatric patient, peroral supplementation of potassium and glucose is needed. The outcome in pediatric cholera should be essentially as favorable as that in the adult disease, with an over-all mortality rate of less than 1 per cent.

Peroral replacement of water and electrolytes is also remarkably effective in adults, and in children who are alert. This development of peroral therapy has greatly increased the capability to treat cholera in field conditions and thus represents a major achievement in the effort to use modern science and technology for the health problems of economically underdeveloped countries. An oral glucose-electrolyte solution (prepared by the addition of 20 grams of glucose, 3.5 grams of sodium chloride, 2.5 grams of sodium bicarbonate, and 1.5 grams of potassium chloride to 1 liter of drinking water) can be given in mild cholera cases throughout the course of illness, and is also satisfactory in more severe cases once the hypovolemic shock has been corrected by the initial rapid intravenous fluid therapy. When oral therapy is employed, about 1.5 volumes of oral solution must be given to replace each volume of stool lost. Glucose is an essential component of this solution in that the success of oral therapy in cholera depends upon enhanced intestinal absorption of sodium in the presence of intraluminal glucose.

Although adequate fluid therapy results in rapid recovery in virtually all cholera patients (table), adjunctive therapy with antimicrobials dramatically reduces the duration and volume of diarrhea and results in rapid eradication of vibrios from the feces. Tetracycline, in a total daily dose of 40 to 50 mg per kilogram of body weight divided into four equal portions and given perorally every six hours for two days, has been uniformly successful. Furazolidone and chloramphenicol are also of value, but are slightly less effective than tetracycline.

PROGNOSIS. Without treatment, mortality rates in cholera epidemics have exceeded 50 per cent. With adequate therapy, however, the mortality rate approaches zero. Largely because of the mechanical problems inherent in the administration of large amounts of fluid to small children, a mortality rate of 1 to 2 per cent still obtains in pediatric patients despite the best current therapy. A single attack of cholera confers only relatively short-lived, type-specific protection against subsequent infection by *V. cholerae.*

PREVENTION. Immunization, using two injections of standard commercial vaccine (containing 10 billion killed bacteria per milliliter), provides 60 to 80 per cent protection for three to six months to adults in cholera endemic areas. In recent field trials, immunization with toxoid proved to be no more effective than the standard whole-cell vaccine. Since immunization against cholera has not proved to be effective in altering the transmission of this disease, administration of cholera vaccine is no longer a requirement for entrance into the United States from cholera endemic areas. At present, careful hygiene provides the only certain protection against cholera.

Barua, D., and Burrows, W.: Cholera. Philadelphia, W.B. Saunders Company, 1974.

Carpenter, C. C. J., Mitra, P. P., and Sack, R. B.: Clinical studies in Asiatic cholera. Parts I-VI. Bull. Johns Hopkins Hosp., 118:165, 1966.

Holmgren, J., Lonnroth, I., Mansson, J. E., and Svennerholm, L.: Interaction of cholera toxin and membrane GM-1 ganglioside of small intestine. Proc. Natl. Acad. Sci. U.S.A., 72:2520, 1975.

Hornick, R. B., Music, S. I., Wenzel, R., Cash, R., Lebonati, J. P., Snyder, M. J., and Woodward, T. E.: The Broad Street pump revisited: Response of volunteers to ingested cholera vibrios. Bull. N.Y. Acad. Med., 47:1181, 1971.

Mahalanobis, D., Choudhuri, A. B., Bagchi, N. G., Bhattachrya, A. K., and Simpson, T. W.: Oral therapy of cholera among Bangladesh refugees. Johns Hopkins Med. J., 132:197, 1973.

Pierce, N. F., Sack, R. B., Mitra, R. C., Banwell, J. G., Brigham, K. L., Fedson, D. S., and Mondal, A.: Replacement of water and electrolyte losses in cholera by an oral glucose-electrolyte solution. Ann. Intern. Med., 70:1173, 1969.

Wallace, C. K., Anderson, P. N., Brown, T. C., Khanra, S. R., Lewis, G. W., Pierce, N. F., Sanyal, S. N., Segre, G. V., and Waldman, R. H.: Optimal antibiotic therapy in cholera. Bull. WHO, 39:239, 1968.

157. PLAGUE

Jay P. Sanford

DEFINITION. Plague is an infection caused by *Yersinia pestis* which in man usually presents in either of two major clinical patterns: acute lymphadenitis (bubonic plague) or acute severe pneumonia (pneumonic plague). Plague is primarily an infection of rodents caused by *Y. pestis* with transmission by a flea vector. Man usually acquires bubonic plague through the aberrant bite of plague-infected rodent fleas. With the occurrence of bacteremia, secondary pulmonary involvement may occur, which in turn may be followed by subsequent human-to-human respiratory transmission. In the fifteenth century, plague, which was known as the black death, assumed catastrophic proportions, killing an estimated one quarter of the population of Europe. The pathophysiology underlying the clinical features of black death appear to be multiple, but would appear to include the occurrence of profound cyanosis and disseminated intravascular coagulation with purpura and extensive symmetrical peripheral gangrene.

ETIOLOGY. *Y. pestis* is a gram-negative, nonmotile, aerobic coccobacillus which in smears from tissues or secretions stains in a bipolar "safety pin" pattern. This classic appearance is best demonstrated with Wayson's (methylene blue and carbofuchsin) or Giemsa's stain rather than with Gram's stain. The organism grows readily on most culture media, ordinary nutrient agar, blood agar, or deoxycholate agar with optimal growth at 28° C, although it will grow at temperatures of 1 to 43° C. However, growth is slow, requiring 48 hours before colonies are readily discernible. *Y. pestis* may remain viable for weeks in dry sputum or flea feces at room temperature. *Y. pestis* produces a number of antigenic components, several of which are of major importance in the pathogenesis of disease. These include a capsular antigen, which is a heat-labile protein designated as Fraction 1 (F1), and the VW antigens, which include a protein V and lipoprotein W. The F1 and VW antigens which render the organism resistant to phagocytosis are produced during growth at 37° C, but are not produced during growth at 28° C. *Y. pestis* contains an endotoxin, which may be less lethal than endotoxins extracted from Enterobacteriaceae, and exotoxins which are lethal (cardiotoxic) for the mouse and rat but against which other species appear to be resistant.

EPIDEMIOLOGY. Geographic Distribution and Prevalence. Plague is endemic in Vietnam, other parts of Indochina, India, Burma, Java, and South Central and East Africa, including Madagascar. The disease also has been reported sporadically in Egypt, Saudi Arabia, North Africa (Tunisia and Morocco), South America (Argentina, Bolivia, Brazil, Ecuador, Peru, and Venezuela), and the western and southwestern United States (Arizona, California, Colorado, New Mexico, Oregon, and Texas). In 1967, at the peak of an outbreak which subsequently declined, over 5000 cases were reported to the World Health Organization from South Vietnam. In the United States during the past ten years, an average of 7.4 cases per year (1 to 20) has been reported. In the United States since 1950, 60 per cent of cases have been in persons less than 20 years old, with a predominance of males (55 per cent). The over-all fatality-to-case ratio has been 20 per cent.

Transmission and Host Range. Plague is a natural disease of both domestic and wild rodents. Rats are the primary reservoir in urban areas. The oriental rat flea (*Xenopsylla cheopis*) becomes infected when it feeds on the blood of a bacteremic rat, which usually dies a short time after becoming bacteremic. Levels of *Y. pestis* in the rat may reach 10^7 bacilli per milliliter of blood. With the death of its host, the hungry flea seeks another host. The transmission from rat to rat by fleas is not primarily mechanical but involves biologic transmission, which is dependent upon the "blocking" of the flea proventriculus with plague bacilli. The extrinsic incubation period required for *X. cheopis* to become "blocked" varies, but on the average it requires two weeks. The ingested blood, which contains *Y. pestis*, is coagulated in the flea stomach by a coagulase produced by the organism embedding the bacilli in a matrix of fibrin. This fibrin anchor serves to retain *Y. pestis* in the proventriculus until the organ is occluded by a mass of multiplying bacilli. The "blocked" flea, which undergoes progressive desiccation, makes repeated attempts to feed; at each attempt, being unable to pass the blood meal past the blocked proventriculus, the flea regurgitates, thereby inoculating 25,000 to 100,000 bacilli into the site of the bite. It has been observed that flea-borne bubonic plague cannot exist in epidemic proportions when the mean ambient temperature is above 27.5° C. This observation seems particularly enigmatic, because the F1 and VW antigens which are antiphagocytic are not elaborated at these lower temperatures. Cavanaugh has elucidated the enigma by showing that when temperatures are elevated to about 27° C, fibrin is rapidly destroyed by a fibrinolytic factor elaborated by *Y. pestis* and a trypsin-like enzyme of the flea stomach. In the absence of the fibrin anchor, *Y. pestis* is eliminated from the stomach and proventriculus and fleas become noninfective. In the rat-flea-rat cycle, if another rodent is not available, the flea will accept a human host as a blood source; man then becomes an accidental host in the usual rat-flea-rat transmission cycle.

Epizootic plague occurs when *Y. pestis* is introduced into rodent or small mammal populations (e.g., prairie dogs) that are more highly susceptible to the lethal effects of infection than is the rat. The risk of exposure is high when man interfaces with epizootic plague. Transmission from animal hosts to man is termed zootic plague, whereas transmission from man to man is termed demic plague.

In recent years in the United States all but one case have resulted from exposure in rural or suburban settings. The principal animals involved have been ground squirrels, prairie dogs, marmots, wood rats, rabbits, and hares. Human infection from rabbits and hares usually results from direct tissue contact rather than flea bites. Carnivorous animals — including cats, dogs, and coyotes — in areas of enzootic and epizootic plague regularly show serologic evidence of infection. Recently, several human cases have been associated with handling of sick or dead dogs, coyotes, or cats. The communicability of plague pneumonia varies with the extent of cough and character of sputum, which often is thick and tenacious. Secondary cases have occurred most frequently in household contacts and medical personnel. Fortunately, no spread to contacts in the United States has been observed since 1925. The introduction of air travel requires that physicians throughout the world consider the occurrence of plague and recognize that air travel increases the danger of transmission. The index of clinical suspicion of plague outside endemic areas (e.g., the Southwest) is unfortunately low, as reflected in the occurrence of plague in a geologist who was infected in New Mexico but developed disease which was unrecognized and fatal in New England, or in a soldier who returned from Vietnam.

Y. pestis has been isolated from the throats of healthy persons who are in contact with pneumonic and presumably uncomplicated bubonic plague infections. Experimental evidence suggests that persons with plague infections of the upper respiratory tract, including asymptomatic pharyngeal "carriers" of *Y. pestis,* probably are incapable of respiratory transmission to other persons.

PATHOGENESIS. *Y. pestis* may enter the body via the blood, skin, conjunctiva, or mucous membranes of the respiratory or digestive tracts. The organisms which enter the body through the bites of fleas lack F1 and VW antigen, and hence are readily phagocytized by neutrophils and promptly killed. However, some organisms are phagocytized by mononuclear cells. Cavanaugh and associates have shown that at 37° C the organisms produce F1 and VW antigens and are able to kill the mononuclear cell. The organisms released from mononuclear cells are able to resist phagocytosis by neutrophils and reach lymph nodes. A local vesicle or pustule may form at the site of inoculation. If *Y. pestis* passes the local pustule, organisms reach lymph nodes which acutely enlarge and become embedded in a gelatinous periglandular edema. Infection may be contained at this stage, and is designated as pestis minor. If bacilli escape from the regional nodes, they pass into the bloodstream with the potential for involvement of multiple organs: lungs, spleen, meninges, and liver. In 42 patients studied by Butler and associates, 40 per cent had positive blood cultures. Endotoxemia as measured by the limulus gelation test has been demonstrated in some patients with negative blood cultures. A strong association has been demonstrated between axillary location of buboes and the development of meningitis and pneumonia.

CLINICAL MANIFESTATIONS. Bubonic plague is the more common form. The incubation period may vary from a few hours to 12 days, but is usually two to five days. The onset is abrupt, often associated with chills, and the temperature rises to 39.4 to 41.4° C. The pulse often is rapid and thready and hypotension occurs. Painful, enlarged lymph nodes appear simultaneously with or even shortly before the fever. Usually, there is no primary lesion at the site of the bite, but occasionally a primary cutaneous lesion, varying from a small vesicle with slight local lymphangitis to an eschar, may be seen. The most commonly involved lymph nodes are femoral or inguinal (50 per cent), followed by axillary (22 per cent), cervical (10 per cent), or multiple nodes (14 per cent). The nodes are usually tender and vary in size from 1 to 5 cm. The overlying skin often is smooth and reddened. In addition, headache and gastrointestinal complaints, anorexia, vomiting, and abdominal pain are common (about one fourth of patients). Restlessness, delirium, confusion, and incoordination may occur. The liver and spleen may be palpable.

Benign forms of bubonic plague, such as pestis minor with lymphadenitis, fever, headache, and prostration, may subside within a week. This is usually seen only in endemic areas. Recently, the occurrence of asymptomatic pharyngeal carriers of *Y. pestis* has been recognized.

Primary pneumonic plague has an incubation period usually lasting only two to three days, followed by the abrupt onset of high fever, chills, tachycardia, and headache, which is often severe. Initially, cough is not a prominent symptom. Within 20 to 24 hours a productive cough develops. Sputum is mucoid but rapidly shows blood specks, then uniformly becomes pink or bright red (resembling raspberry syrup) and foamy in character. There is associated tachypnea and dyspnea but no pleurisy. Signs of consolidation are rare; rales may be absent. Chest radiographs show a rapidly progressing pneumonia. Most untreated patients die one and one half to two days after onset of symptoms.

Primary septicemic plague, which usually occurs in association with the bubonic form, presents as an acute fulminant illness which may be fatal before either lymph node or pulmonary manifestations predominate. Other, less classic forms are pharyngeal plague and plague meningitis.

LABORATORY FEATURES. Hematocrit determinations have been normal or reflect other causes of anemia. Leukocyte counts are elevated in over 90 per cent of patients when initially seen. In patients with bubonic plague whose clinical conditions are stable, the usual leukocyte counts are 15,000 to 20,000 per cubic millimeter, with a marked neutrophilia. In patients who appear "septic" or who are hypotensive, leukocyte counts are usually 30,000 per cubic millimeter or higher. Peripheral blood smears will often (approximately 10 per cent) show *Y. pestis*. Patients commonly develop disseminated intravascular coagulation (86 per cent in a group of patients studied by Butler and associates), as manifested by elevated titers of fibrinogen-fibrin degradation products, thrombocytopenia, and hypofibrinogenemia, although none showed overt bleeding. Electrocardiograms have usually been normal, although STT segment depression consistent with ischemia associated with marked tachycardia may be seen. Liver function tests usually are normal, although elevations in SGOT have been seen. In patients with plague meningitis, endotoxin may be demonstrated in cerebrospinal fluid, using the limulus lysate gelation test.

DIAGNOSIS. This is based on recovery of *Y. pestis*, which may be cultured from blood (almost half of patients have positive cultures), sputum, or lymph node aspirate. Prompt smears of lymph node aspirate stained with Wayson's stain (or methylene blue) usually provide a rapid presumptive diagnosis. Surgical drainage of a bubo may disseminate organisms: hence needle aspiration is preferable. *Y. pestis* can be grown on ordinary culture media or isolated by animal inoculation. Since most pyogenic bacteria grow within 24 hours, a "negative" culture at 24 hours should raise suspicion of tularemia and plague. Serologic tests include complement fixation, passive hemagglutination, and immunofluorescent staining of a node, secretions, or tissues. Since clinical illness occurs in vaccinated individuals, a vaccine history does not exclude plague in the differential diagnosis.

Differential diagnostic considerations in the patient with buboes include tularemia, lymphogranuloma venereum, impetigo with lymphadenitis, and erysipelas, whereas such considerations in the patient with pneumonic involvement must include the spectrum of acute, viral, bacterial, fungal, and parasitologic causes. It is noteworthy that several of the patients seen in the southwestern United States have been admitted with diagnoses of incarcerated hernias.

THERAPY AND MANAGEMENT. Treatment, which should be immediate upon suspicion of plague, includes general supportive measures and specific therapy. Prompt treatment will reduce mortality to 5 per cent. In the septicemic or pneumonic forms, treatment must begin within 24 hours to afford protection. The tetracyclines, chloramphenicol, and streptomycin are highly effective against naturally transmitted forms of plague. Streptomycin, 0.5 gram intramuscularly every three hours for 48 hours, followed by 1.5 to 2.0 grams per day for seven to ten days, is preferred. Occasional (about 1 per cent) strains of *Y. pestis* encountered in Vietnam were resistant in vitro to streptomycin. These strains were susceptible in vitro to kanamycin, which has been shown to be effective. Gentamicin has not been proved to be effective and should not be relied upon as an alternative. As an alternative, tetracycline or chloramphenicol, 500 mg intravaneously every three hours for 48 hours, 4 grams per day orally for the next two days, and then 3 grams per day orally for an additional four to five days, may be used, and is preferred by some authorities. Patients with plague meningitis should receive chloramphenicol as well as streptomycin. Recent studies suggest that co-trimoxazole is effective, but the duration of fever and incidence of complications were greater than occurred in patients treated with streptomycin. Penicillins are not effective. Some authors have advised against the use of streptomycin because of possible Herxheimer reactions. Such reactions were not encountered in patients treated in Vietnam. Despite laboratory evidence of disseminated intravascular coagulation based upon extrapolation from other infections, heparin therapy would not seem indicated. Routine aseptic precautions are adequate for patients with bubonic plague. In contrast, primary or secondary plague pneumonia demands strict isolation. Response to streptomycin treatment usually is prompt, most patients becoming afebrile within the first week (median, four days). Buboes usually become nontender concomitantly with defervescence and either resolve or become smaller. Occasional nodes become fluctuant and require incision. It should be noted that positive cultures may be obtained from such nodes after seven to ten days of therapy.

PREVENTION. Prevention is based upon rodent control and use of repellents to minimize attacks by fleas. There is indirect evidence from Vietnam that the killed plague vaccine used in the United States is highly effective in preventing plague. Although vaccination against plague is not required by any country as a condition for entry and is not recommended for travelers to most countries, it is advisable for all persons traveling to the interior regions of Indochina. Immunization is also recommended for persons whose occupation brings them into frequent contact with wild rodents in plague enzootic areas.

Butler, T., Bell, W. R., Linh, N. N., Tiep, N. D., and Arnold, K.: *Yersinia pestis* infection in Vietnam. I. Clinical and hematologic aspects. J. Infect. Dis. (Suppl.), 124:5, 1974.

Butler, T., Levin, J., Linh, N. N., Chau, D. M., Adickman, M., and Arnold, K.: *Yersinia pestis* infection in Vietnam. II. Quantitative blood cultures and detection of endotoxin in cerebrospinal fluid of patients with meningitis. J. Infect. Dis., 133:493, 1976.

Cantey, J. R.: Plague in Vietnam. Clinical observations and treatment with kanamycin. Arch. Intern. Med., 133:1380, 1974.

Cavanaugh, D. C.: Specific effect of temperature upon transmission of the plague bacillus of the oriental rat flea, *Xenopsylla cheopis*. Am. J. Trop. Med. Hyg. 20:264, 1971.

Cavanaugh, D. C., and Randall, R.: The role of multiplication of *Pasteurella pestis* and mononuclear phagocytes in the pathogenesis of flea-borne plague. J. Immunol., 83:348, 159.

Pollitzer, R.: Plague. WHO Monograph No. 22, Geneva, 1954.

Reed, W. P., Palmer, D. L., Williams, R. C., and Kisch, A. L: Bubonic plague in the southwestern United States: A review of recent experience. Medicine, 49:465, 1970.

Schwade, J., and Sanford, J. P.: Hepatic granulomata due to "benign" plague imported from Vietnam: Case report. Milit. Med., 139:554, 1974.

158. TULAREMIA

Theodore E. Woodward

DEFINITION. Most cases of tularemia are characterized by the formation of a focal ulcer at the site of entry of the causative bacillus, enlargement of regional lymph nodes, and a constitutional reaction of fever, prostration, myalgia, and headache. There may be pneumonia, which is occasionally accompanied by pleurisy or a typhoid-like illness.

Francisella tularensis, the microbial agent, is transmitted to humans by insect vectors such as ticks or deer flies, by the handling or ingestion of infected animal tissues, or by inhalation of infected aerosols. The clinical diagnosis is confirmed by demonstration of bacteremia, by isolation of the bacillus from the sputum, tissue exudates, or gastric washings, and by demonstration of serum agglutinins in early convalescence.

HISTORICAL FEATURES. The knowledge of the ecology and clinical features of tularemia has been developed in the United States through the pioneering work of Francis and other Public Health Service investigators. McCoy described the disease in 1911 while studying a plaguelike illness in ground squirrels in Tulare County, California. The first clinical description and bacteriologic proof of illness is attributed to Wherry and Lamb in 1914. In a series of studies conducted in Utah and elsewhere, Francis (1928) incriminated rabbits as important animal hosts and established the transmissibility of disease by deer flies.

ETIOLOGY, SPECIFIC LABORATORY DIAGNOSIS, AND EPIDEMIOLOGY. Tularemia is caused by a pleomorphic, nonmotile, small gram-negative rod. There is only one serologic group of all *F. tularensis* isolates. However, there are two varieties recognized which vary in virulence. One variety is highly virulent for rabbit and man (Jellson type A) and is found only in North America. It ferments glycerol and has citrulline ureidase activity. The second variety is avirulent for the rabbit but causes mild tularemia in man (Jellson type B). It is found in Europe, Asia, and North America. This variety lacks glycerol-fermenting enzymes and also citrulline ureidase.

CULTURE. Blood-glucose cysteine agar is the basic medium needed for propagating the organism. All culturing and animal inoculations should be done in an appropriate contagion hood to minimize laboratory-acquired infections. The routine inoculation of animals (mice or guinea pigs) is not generally recommended because of the risk of infecting personnel and also initiating an epizootic. Organisms can be recovered from ulcers and draining regional lymph nodes during the first few weeks in patients with ulceroglandular tularemia. Patients with pneumonic disease or symptoms of a bronchitis may have organisms isolated from bronchial secretions and gastric washings. Bacteremia does occur, but few organisms are present and are difficult to isolate. Bone marrow aspirations may yield *F. tularensis.* The organisms should be identifiable within two to four days in the culture media.

Serologic Diagnosis. The conventional serum agglutination reaction is a very useful diagnostic test, because specific agglutinins appear within eight to ten days from the onset of illness. Maximal titers are reached in about four weeks. Demonstration of a rise in titer through examination of serial specimens is confirmatory evidence of infection, although single titers of 1:160 or more are usually significant. Sera from patients with brucellosis or tularemia may show cross-agglutination, although the titer is usually higher with the homologous antigen.

Cutaneous Test. Foshay described a diagnostic skin test that consists of the intradermal inoculation of a purified antigen consisting of a killed suspension of *F. tularensis.* The reaction is of the delayed tuberculin type, becoming positive in 48 hours. The test is highly specific and becomes positive during the first week of tularemia either prior to or coincident with the development of agglutinins. The test remains positive for years.

EPIDEMIOLOGY. Tularemia has been detected in many areas of the Northern Hemisphere, including Japan, Central Europe, Asian and European Russia, and Scandinavia. Man can be infected by as few as 50 organisms injected intradermally, and that number and probably fewer *F. tularensis* delivered as a small particle (<5 microns) aerosol will cause pneumonic disease. This unique infectiousness of these bacilli for man points up the need for caution when culturing or inoculating animals as well as when handling infected animals. The organisms are found in many species of animals. In North America, the cottontail rabbit is associated with many cases of ulceroglandular and typhoidal forms of tularemia. These animals will have large numbers of tularemia organisms in the liver and bloodstream. In the process of eviscerating an infected animal, there is ample opportunity for direct hand contamination as well as generation of an infectious aerosol. Tiny puncture wounds of the skin, hair follicles, or cracks around nail beds can serve as portals of entry for the initiation of ulceroglandular tularemia. Restricted sale of wild rabbits in metropolitan areas has resulted in a sharp decline of the disease.

Many cases have their origin from infected arthropods such as ticks, deer flies, or mosquitoes. In North America the ticks *Dermacentor andersoni, Dermacentor variabilis,* and the Lone Star tick are important reservoirs and vectors. Infected female ticks transmit *F. tularensis* transovarially. A primary ulcer often forms at the site of tick attachment.

Tularemia occurs in all seasons: among hunters and trappers in the fall and winter, and during the spring and summer when ticks and deer flies are active. All ages and both sexes are susceptible. Since 1967, fewer than 200 cases have been reported annually in the United States.

MECHANISM OF INFECTION AND PATHOLOGY. The disease may present in a variety of forms with two major subdivisions, depending on whether or not the initial site of entry can be visualized. In all forms there is lymph node involvement. In most instances there is a primary ulcer, variable in size, which may be located on the skin (ulceroglandular), in the eye (oculoglandular), or in the nasopharynx with necrotizing lesions. Sometimes the cutaneous lesion may be insignificant, so that the picture is that of "glandular tularemia" without an overt primary lesion. The entry also may be through the intestinal tract (enteric or typhoidal) or via the lungs (pulmonary).

After infection, *F. tularensis* reaches the blood via the lymphatics and nodes; the microbe, although phagocytized, resides intracellularly without loss of viability. Granulomatous lesions develop within the reticuloendothelial system, particularly in lymph nodes, liver, and spleen. These lesions, usually hyperplastic, bear some resemblance to tuberculosis and may caseate or form small local abscesses. The macrophage is the predominant cell type that surrounds an area of caseous necrosis. Langhans' cells are observed occasionally, and the larger lesions are liable to central abscess formation.

Pneumonia is a common development in tularemia, occurring in approximately 30 per cent of patients who acquire the disease, regardless of the type of infection. Histologically, the early lesion is edematous, and consists of fibrin and leukocytes associated with necrosis of alveolar walls. In non-necrotic areas the exudate consists of the large mononuclear type. The gross lesions resemble the pneumonia of tuberculosis, although histologically there is less epithelioid cell transformation. Tubercle-like nodules are more common in lymph nodes than in the lungs. Mediastinal nodes are involved frequently.

CLINICAL MANIFESTATIONS. The incubation period of tularemia ranges from two to ten days. Headache, fever, and toxic signs characterize all forms of the illness and are in no way dissimilar to those in other infectious illnesses. The pertinent historic and epidemiologic features are often helpful clues, and in approximately three fourths of all patients there is a primary lesion associated with adenopathy.

Ulceroglandular Tularemia. The initial lesion begins as a reddish papule, which is often undermined and more extensive than the small area of superficial induration indicates. Neighboring and draining lymph nodes are enlarged, tender, and discrete. Fluctuation of these nodes occurs later in the illness, after two or more weeks, when other acute signs may have partially abated. Such diseased nodes may subsequently require incision and drainage. The lymph nodes during the early stages are laden with *F. tularensis* and, if incised, may provoke bacteremia and toxemia. Fluctuant buboes four or more weeks old are usually sterile. Generalized lymphadenopathy occurs. Systemic signs of toxemia may be severe in ulceroglandular tularemia, although most cases are mild or moderate in severity. Pneumonia of all gradations may accompany this type of infection.

Occasionally, tularemia referred to as the glandular type may occur as generalized adenopathy and toxemia but without cutaneous lesions.

Enteric Form of Tularemia (Typhoidal or Cryptogenic). Man is not readily infected by the oral route. Aerosols consisting of large particles or the swallowing of huge numbers of tularemia bacilli will cause illness characterized by symptoms of abdominal pain, high fever, and toxicity, which can be confused with the symptoms of typhoid fever. Usually there are prominent enlarged cervical lymph nodes. This typhoidal systemic reaction may typify any of the clinical varieties of tularemia regardless of the presence of a cutaneous lesion. The term "cryptogenic" has often been used to connote the absence of an obvious portal of entry.

Pulmonary Tularemia. Lung involvement occurs in all forms of tularemia, subsequent to the bacteremia. Available evidence suggests that primary tularemic pneumonia is an entity, particularly in those persons such as laboratory workers who are exposed to infected aerosols. The incubation period varies from two to five days, depending upon the number of viable bacteria inhaled. In addition to headache, fever, malaise, and prostration, there is a nonproductive harassing cough and a sensation of substernal discomfort. Later the sputum may be mucoid or bloody and, in severely ill patients, pleural pain, dyspnea, tachycardia, and cyanosis occur.

In spite of extensive pulmonary involvement, there may be a paucity of physical signs. The early roentgenographic signs, seldom evident before the second to the fourth day of fever, consist of small irregular oval lesions with hilar adenopathy. Later in the illness, the infiltrate may be annular. True abscess formation is rare, although during resolution and convalescence, which in untreated patients or in those treated late may be prolonged, shadows suggesting abscess formation may be noted. Pleuritis with effusion is not uncommon.

Oculoglandular Tularemia. After ocular contamination there may be pain, photophobia, intense congestion, itching, lacrimation, chemosis, and a mucopurulent discharge. Small yellowish granulomatous lesions may appear on the palpebral conjunctivae or cornea and may eventually ulcerate. The preauricular and other regional lymph nodes may enlarge and ultimately suppurate. In untreated patients, serious ocular complications, including corneal perforation or optic atrophy, may ensue.

Other General Manifestations. Initially, in severely ill patients, there is a rigor followed by pyrexia that persists for a month or more. The fever may be continuously high or remittent, and defervescence is usually gradual. Hepatomegaly and splenomegaly with tenderness over the respective organs are relatively common. Toxic signs in all cases include fever, headache, myalgia, and nausea. Rashes are very uncommon; when present, they consist of localized papular lesions along the peripheral lymphatics or maculopapular body eruptions. In untreated patients or in those first given antimicrobial therapy late in the course of illness, convalescence may be prolonged with sporadic episodes of fever, weakness, muscular pains, and chronic respiratory signs.

NONSPECIFIC LABORATORY FINDINGS. The erythrocyte sedimentation rate and C-reactive protein are elevated during the active stages. In contrast, the total blood leukocyte count is usually normal or low. Occasionally there may be moderate leukocytosis. Mild albuminuria may occur at the height of illness.

DIFFERENTIAL DIAGNOSIS. Ulceroglandular tularemia is recognized readily in endemic areas. Punctate lesions with surrounding erythema at the site of prior arthropod attachment suggest *Rocky Mountain spotted fever*, particularly when associated with fever, headache, and toxic signs. The absence of a rash would favor tularemia, because patients with rickettsial disease develop a characteristic exanthem. *Meningococcemia* is recognized by its fulminant character, the typical exanthem, leuko-

cytosis, and the bacteriologic findings. Fever, toxic signs, pharyngitis, adenitis, hepatomegaly, and splenomegaly are common to tularemia and *infectious mononucleosis*. The hematologic and serologic findings are usually distinctive. *Cat scratch disease* is characterized by peripheral ulceration and regional adenopathy; a history of contact with cats, the cutaneous reaction to specific antigens, and the absence of agglutinins for *F. tularensis* are distinguishing features. *Ecthyma* and *furunculi* are similar in some respects to this form of tularemia, although lymphadenitis and systemic signs are less likely to develop.

The lesions of *sporotrichosis* are multiple, occur along the course of lymphatics, attach themselves firmly to the skin, and are freely movable.

Certain forms of tularemia may present with clinical features similar to those of psittacosis, Q fever, and mycoplasmal pneumonia. Broad-spectrum antimicrobial drugs are effective in each of these conditions. Appropriate serologic tests or viral isolation may be required to define the precise cause. Influenza with associated pneumonia is similar but does not respond to specific drugs, and its clinical course is short. Fungal diseases, such as *histoplasmosis* and *coccidioidomycosis*, may be acute and may simulate pulmonary tularemia. Consideration of the history, the epidemiologic data, and the cutaneous manifestations, as well as the bacteriologic and serologic findings, usually will permit proper identification.

The presence of unexplained pleural effusion, similar to tuberculous fibrinous pleurisy, requires differentiation. The results of cultural and serologic tests will aid in differentiation.

COMPLICATIONS. Pericarditis and meningitis are distinctive but unusual complications of tularemia. Pericardial involvement may develop by direct extension from the pulmonary lesions or lymph nodes, and is characterized by a fibrinous or fibrocaseous exudate. In untreated patients constrictive pericarditis may ensue. Tularemic meningitis is characterized by a lymphocytic pleocytosis in the cerebrospinal fluid, and was usually fatal prior to the availability of specific antimicrobial drugs. Rare instances of tularemic peritonitis, perisplenitis, osteomyelitis, and endocarditis have been reported.

TREATMENT. Specific Therapy. Tularemia is very amenable to treatment with antimicrobial drugs. Streptomycin is preferable, but the broad-spectrum antimicrobials are equally beneficial in ameliorating the active manifestations. They are less effective, however, in eradicating the organism, primarily because of their bacteriostatic mode of action. With the latter drugs, relapses are liable to occur if treatment is initiated within the first week of illness.

AMINOGLYCOSIDES. Streptomycin, when given in doses of 1.0 gram daily to adults for about one week, results in prompt recovery. Most patients are improved within 24 hours, and are afebrile within 48 hours. Relapses are uncommon with streptomycin except when insufficient drug is given during the very early stages of illness. Strains resistant to streptomycin have been induced in vitro but have not been isolated from patients with naturally acquired disease. Kanamycin and gentamicin are equally effective, but the experience with these drugs is meager, and kanamycin carries with it a greater risk of ototoxicity.

TETRACYCLINE AND CHLORAMPHENICOL TREAT-

MENT. Broad-spectrum antimicrobials are very effective in rendering the patient afebrile and free from toxicity within 48 to 72 hours. Relapses are uncommon when therapy is initiated 10 to 12 days after the onset of illness, but are frequent if it is given during the first week. *F. tularensis* does not develop resistance to chloramphenicol or tetracycline; hence, retreatment leads to prompt response.

The following dosage schedule is considered optimal: for tetracycline, an initial oral dose of 25 mg per kilogram of body weight; and for chloramphenicol, 50 mg per kilogram of body weight. Subsequent daily doses are calculated on the same basis as the initial loading dose, dividing the requirement equally and giving it at six- to eight-hour intervals. Antimicrobial therapy is continued until the patient is improved and has been afebrile for about five to seven days.

No supplementary chemotherapy is necessary with any of the aforementioned regimens. Tetracycline is preferred solely because reactions to it are potentially less serious.

General Management. An adequate diet with appropriate protein intake is advisable. Oxygen treatment is indicated for all severely ill patients with pneumonia whether or not cyanosis is present. Other supportive measures useful for treating patients with pneumonia, such as frequent turning and the performing of a tracheostomy to provide a proper airway, are indicated. Thoracentesis for removal of fluid will allay respiratory embarassment.

The local ulcer requires no special measures. During the early several weeks of illness, lymph nodes should not be manipulated unduly or incised. Later, fluctuant buboes, which are usually sterile, may require incision and drainage. Recovery ensues rapidly.

PROGNOSIS AND POSTINFECTION IMMUNITY. In untreated patients, the case fatality rate in ulceroglandular tularemia was formerly approximately 5 per cent. However, of those patients with typhoidal tularemia or with pulmonary manifestations, about 30 per cent succumbed. With the advent of streptomycin and later the broad-spectrum antimicrobials, death from tularemia has been virtually eliminated and the morbidity shortened drastically to several days after institution of treatment, even among severely ill patients.

Second attacks of tularemia with systemic complications are uncommon, because recovery from the initial episode usually confers immunity. However, it is not unusual for patients to develop primary lesions when reinfected long after the initial systemic infection. Viable *F. tularensis* may be isolated from such recurrent primary ulcers, which resemble a Koch reaction. Under these conditions, systemic manifestations are unusual.

Under test conditions in volunteers, when streptomycin is given soon after intradermal infection (before the onset of clinical illness), an attack may be aborted fully. Immunity does not develop, agglutinins fail to appear, and such subjects are prone to further infection. This phenomenon is of little practical significance, as patients are usually encountered after a week or more of active clinical illness. Partial to complete resistance to infection follows such antigenic stimulation.

CONTROL MEASURES. General. In infected areas those measures designed to repel ticks, mosquitoes, or deer flies should be employed. Gloves should be used for handling all potentially infected animals, particularly rabbits, and animals to be consumed should be cooked thoroughly. Laboratory workers exposed to infected aerosols should exercise care by wearing suitable masks and utilizing other protective devices.

Vaccination. The available killed vaccines afford only partial protection to man against tularemia. Viable attenuated preparations have been used with considerable success in the Soviet Union. The vaccine is administered intradermally and provokes a reaction similar in severity to that which follows smallpox immunization. Significant protection has been demonstrated in volunteers in the United States vaccinated with a similar viable product and who subsequently were exposed to virulent strains of *F. tularensis* by the respiratory or cutaneous routes. In those subjects who have developed clinical illness after immunization, the disease has been mild.

Foshay, L.: Tularemia. Ann. Rev. Microbiol., 4:313, 1950.
McCrumb, F. R.: Aerosol infection of man with *Pasteurella tularensis*. Bact. Rev., 25:262, 1961.
Meyer, K. F.: Pasteurella and franciscella. In Dubos, R., and Hirsch, J. G. (eds.): Bacterial and Mycotic Infections of Man. 4th ed. Philadelphia, J. B. Lippincott Company, 1965, Chap. 27, p. 659.
Young, L. S.: Tularemia epidemic, Vermont, 1968. Forty-seven cases linked to contact with muskrats. N. Engl. J. Med., 280:1253, 1969.

159. DISEASES CAUSED BY MALLEOMYCES

Leighton E. Cluff

159.1. GLANDERS

(Farcy)

DEFINITION. Glanders, or farcy, is an infectious disease of horses, mules, and donkeys caused by *Malleomyces mallei*. The infection is occasionally transmitted to man, and is characterized by an acute fulminant febrile illness or a chronic indolent disease with abscesses of the respiratory tract or skin. Farcy refers to the nodular abscesses observed in skin, lymphatics, and subcutaneous tissues.

ETIOLOGY. Glanders was described by Aristotle about 330 B.C., and the occurrence of the disease in horses was observed by Apeyrtos about 375 A.D. Royer's (1837) monograph on glanders in man remains the classic description of the disease. The microorganism responsible for glanders was isolated in 1882. It is a gram-negative bacillus culturable aerobically on ordinary nutrient media. It is variously called *Malleomyces mallei*, *Bacillus mallei*, or *Pfeiferella mallei*. *M. mallei* is nonmotile. It elaborates a specific antigen (mallein) upon lysis that is used as a skin test material for diagnostic purposes. The bacillus is antigenically separable from *M. pseudomallei*, which causes melioidosis. When grown on potato slices or potato infusion agar, *M. mallei* produces a brown pigment resembling that of *Pseudomonas aeruginosa*. The bacillus produces fatal infection experimentally in guinea pigs and hamsters but will not cause disease in rats, cattle, hogs, or fowl.

EPIDEMIOLOGY. Glanders has probably never been a common disease in man. It occurs almost exclusively in persons handling horses. It has been reported from all parts of the world. It has been eradicated in the United

States and the United Kingdom, but may still occur in Asia and South America.

Glanders is a communicable disease among horses, and it may occur sporadically in other animal species in contact with horses. In horses, glanders is manifested by nasal symptoms and abscesses and by cutaneous nodules or abscesses (farcy). The bacillus preferentially invades areas of abraded or injured skin. Experimental infection can be induced in animals by inhalation of the bacillus, and certain laboratory-acquired infections indicate that infection may develop in man after inhalation of the microorganism. *Unlike melioidosis, glanders can be transmitted from person to person.*

PATHOLOGY AND PATHOGENESIS. Characteristically glanders is associated with cellulitis, necrosis, abscess, and thromboses with septic embolization. Healing occurs by fibrosis, and, rarely, by calcification.

CLINICAL MANIFESTATIONS. Glanders may occur as a fulminant acute febrile disease, as a chronic indolent and relapsing disease, or as a subclinical occult infection detectable incidentally at postmortem examination or by serologic test. The two principal features of glanders are (1) nasal cellulitis and necrosis-producing septal perforation and palatal and pharyngeal ulceration; or (2) cutaneous cellulitis, vesiculation, and ulceration at the site of inoculation of the bacillus into the skin, followed by lymphangitis with nodular abscesses along the lymphatics and lymphadenopathy (farcy).

Pulmonary involvement is common in glanders, producing pneumonia, abscesses, pleural effusion, and empyema. Occasionally, in chronic indolent glanders, small nodular granulomatous lesions may be found in the lungs. Hilar lymph node enlargement is common in pulmonary glanders.

When glanders becomes disseminated, destructive polyarthritis, subcutaneous and muscular abscesses, osteomyelitis, meningitis, and pustular skin lesions, particularly over the joints and face, are seen. Prostration and stupor may develop, and are followed by death in two to three weeks.

Chronic glanders may be punctuated by recurrent acute relapses with bacteremia, often resulting in a fulminant course and death. Amyloidosis may be a complication of chronic glanders.

Fever and chills, headache, and backache are common in acute glanders. Leukopenia or a normal leukocyte count is the rule, but leukocytosis has been observed.

DIAGNOSIS. There are no pathognomonic chronic clinical features of glanders. The nodules along lymphatics resemble those seen in sporotrichosis. The respiratory lesions may be difficult to distinguish from other ulcerative infections of the nose and mouth. The cutaneous lesion often resembles streptococcal cellulitis. The multiple abscesses mimic many mycotic and staphylococcal infections and are difficult to distinguish from those of melioidosis. The acute fulminant illness may resemble typhoid fever or disseminated tuberculosis. The diagnosis of glanders can be established by combination of a history of exposure to horses, isolation of *M. mallei*, serologic tests (agglutination, complement-fixation), and skin test with sterile culture filtrate (mallein). Inoculation of infected material into guinea pigs may facilitate identification of the microorganism.

TREATMENT. There are reports of successful treatment of glanders with sulfonamides. Sulfadiazine, administered in divided doses by mouth for a total daily dosage of 100 mg per kilogram for a three-week period, is recommended. Tetracycline, chloramphenicol, and streptomycin may be useful, but there is little clinical experience with these drugs in glanders. Because of the serious prognosis and the lack of documented experience with drug therapy, it is advisable to administer daily streptomycin (1.0 gram) or tetracycline in association with a sulfonamide until all evidences of disease have disappeared. Incision, drainage, and excision of abscesses must be done with caution, for the infection may be disseminated by such manipulation.

PROGNOSIS. Although a few patients have been cured with chemotherapy, the effect of treatment on the mortality rate is not known. *More than 90 per cent of patients with glanders will die from the disease if untreated.* However, the frequency of occurrence of occult or subclinical glanders is not known.

PREVENTION. Infected horses have been identified by skin tests with mallein and by serologic tests. Destruction of infected animals has eliminated glanders as a public health problem in the United States and most other countries.

Howe, C., and Miller, W. R.: Human glanders. Report of six cases. Ann. Intern. Med., 26:115, 1947.

Howe, C., and Miller, W. R.: The pseudomallei: A review. J. Infect. Dis., 124:598, 1971.

Mendelson, R. W.: Glanders. U.S. Armed Forces Med. J., 1:781, 1950.

159.2. MELIOIDOSIS

DEFINITION. Melioidosis is a rare disease of man caused by *Malleomyces pseudomallei*. It has been observed most frequently in Malaysia, the People's Republic of China, Burma, India, and other parts of the Far East and Southeast Asia, but has only rarely been observed in North and South America. It is a disease of wild rodents and some domesticated animals, and probably is transmitted to man by contact with diseased animals or animal excreta and possibly by contact with contaminated soil. The disease in man appears in a subclinical (detectable only by serologic tests), pulmonary, septicemic, or extrapulmonary form. The septicemic and pulmonary disease may be acute and fatal. The pulmonary and extrapulmonary infection with abscesses may be chronic and debilitating.

ETIOLOGY. Melioidosis was first identified by Whitmore and Krishnaswami (1912) in Rangoon. The disease was recognized as similar to glanders and attributable to a gram-negative bacillus resembling but differing from *Malleomyces mallei*. The microorganism causing melioidosis has been variously called *Malleomyces pseudomallei*, *Bacillus whitmori*, and *Pfeiferella whitmori*. It is a motile bacillus that grows aerobically on nutrient agar. Culturally it may resemble *Klebsiella* and *Pseudomonas aeruginosa*. *M. pseudomallei* is antigenically distinguishable from *M. mallei*. It produces fatal infection in guinea pigs, rabbits, and other laboratory animals.

EPIDEMIOLOGY. *M. pseudomallei* has been found to cause disease sporadically, endemically, and epidemically among a wide variety of animal species, including rats, rabbits, goats, hogs, dogs, cats, and horses. In addition, the bacillus has been found to be harbored by mosquitoes and fleas. Frequently, the initial manifestations of melioidosis in man are cutaneous abscesses, diarrhea, and pneumonia; therefore it is probable that the disease is transmitted by direct contact with infected animals or by ingestion or inhalation of contaminated material. All these routes of inoculation can produce the disease experimentally in animals. It is unlikely that melioidosis is ever transmitted from man to man. Infection has been observed in narcotic addicts, and in infants, or in patients with diabetes mellitus, renal or liver disease, and pregnancy as predisposing factors.

CLINICAL MANIFESTATIONS. Melioidosis may appear acutely or insidiously, and most often follows a fulminant course with septicemia or a chronic indolent course with multiple abscess formation. The incubation period of the disease is not known. The acute illness is often associated with fever, chills, cough, production of bloody and purulent sputum, diarrhea, or abdominal pain. Physical examination may reveal signs of pneumonia, empyema, lung abscess, hepatomegaly, jaundice, and splenomegaly. *A subacute or chronic illness may follow the acute disease or may develop in the absence of an acute illness.* In this situation the patient often has osteomyelitis, suppurating lymphadenopathy, subcutaneous abscesses, psoas abscess, lung abscess, pyelonephritis, or liver or spleen abscess. Bronchocutaneous and other types of fistulas may appear. Patients with this chronic illness may survive for many months, and occasionally may recover.

DIAGNOSIS. Inapparent infection has been recognized by serologic tests in 6 to 8 per cent of adult men in some parts of Southeast Asia. Only 1 per cent of adult women have been similarly infected. Melioidosis may resemble typhoid fever, malaria, mycotic infection, and occasionally acute staphylococcal septicemia or staphylococcal pneumonia. The chronic pulmonary disease most resembles tuberculosis. Melioidosis can be differentiated from these diseases only by bacteriologic identification of the bacillus from blood, sputum, urine, or pus. Hemagglutination and complement fixation tests may be useful when acute and convalescent serologic titers are compared. A single positive test may only indicate previous clinical and subclinical infection.

The leukocyte count of the peripheral blood often is normal in melioidosis, but may rise to levels of 20,000 per cubic millimeter. Urinalysis may show pyuria and hematuria.

TREATMENT AND PREVENTION. There is no available antigen for active immunization against melioidosis. Prevention of the disease is possible by controlled sanitation and improved standards of living. Patients have been successfully treated with chloramphenicol, sulfonamides, or tetracycline, given over long periods of time. The drug susceptibility of *M. pseudomallei*, however, is variable. In adults, 3 grams of tetracycline a day orally for 90 days or, alternatively, in septicemia, large doses of chloramphenicol are preferred. Surgical drainage of abscesses is essential for proper management.

Buchman, R. J., Kmiecik, J. E., and LaNove, A. M.: Extrapulmonary melioidosis. Ann. J. Surg., 125:324, 1973.
Howe, C., and Miller, W. R.: The pseudomallei: A review. J. Infect. Dis., 124:598, 1971.
Khaira, B. S., Young, W. B., and Hart, P. DeV.: Melioidosis. Br. Med. J., 1:949, 1959.
Prevatt, A. L., and Hunt, J. S.: Chronic systemic melioidosis. Review of literature. Am. J. Med., 23:810, 1957.
Spotnitz, M., Rudnitsky, A., and Rambaud, J. J.: Melioidosis pneumonitis. JAMA, 202:950, 1967.

160. ANTHRAX

Leighton E. Cluff

DEFINITION. Anthrax is an infectious disease of wild and domesticated animals caused by *Bacillus anthracis*. Occasionally it is transmitted to man. A necrotic ulcer of the skin or mucous membranes is the most common feature of the disease, but hemorrhagic mediastinitis and disseminated infection with hemorrhagic meningitis may also develop. Depending upon the most prominent feature of the disease, anthrax has been variously referred to as *malignant pustule, splenic fever, woolsorters' disease, milzbrand,* and *charbon.*

ETIOLOGY. *Bacillus anthracis* was identified in 1849 by Davaine, and was further characterized by Koch in 1877. It is a gram-positive, sporeforming, encapsulated, hemolytic, aerobic microorganism. It resembles *B. subtilis* and *B. cereus* but can be differentiated from these organisms by its virulence for laboratory animals such as the mouse and rabbit, by its lack of hemolytic activity on blood agar, and by lysis of *B. anthracis* with specific bacteriophage. In broth, the bacillus elaborates an antigen that can be used for specific immunization ("protective antigen"). The spores of *B. anthracis* are killed by boiling for ten minutes but survive for long periods of time in soil, in animal carcasses, and after aerosolization.

EPIDEMIOLOGY. Anthrax has occurred sporadically and in epidemics throughout the world. Cattle, sheep, goats, horses, and swine are most commonly found to have anthrax; outbreaks of the disease in these animals rarely occur in the United States. Although the disease has been acquired by butchering, skinning, or dissecting infected carcasses, human infection in the United States is observed almost exclusively in persons handling imported contaminated hides, wool, goat hair, or other animal products. Epidemics of anthrax occurred in cattle in Texas and in horses in the state of Washington during 1974, attributed to contaminated saddle packs containing goat hair imported from Pakistan. No human infections were known to have been contracted during these outbreaks, although cats fed carcass meat developed anthrax. Three human infections occurred in the United States in 1975–1976. The infection may be transmitted to man by direct contact, inhalation, and ingestion of infected material.

PATHOLOGY AND PATHOGENESIS. Anthrax is characterized by edema, hemorrhage, necrosis, and various degrees of inflammation. *B. anthracis* possesses a glutamyl polypeptide capsule that interferes with phagocytosis, and this contributes to its pathogenicity. The gelatinous edema of anthrax infection contains large amounts of bacterial capsular material. The serum of many animals has lytic activity against the bacillus, but this anthracidal substance seems to bear little or no relationship to natural resistance. It is probable that *B. anthracis* initiates infection in the skin only through abrasions, cuts, or other types of injury. During the course of lethal anthrax infection in laboratory animals, Smith and Keppie demonstrated a bacterial toxin in blood which is responsible for death. This lethal toxin can be neutralized by specific antitoxin.

CLINICAL MANIFESTATIONS. The skin lesion of anthrax usually begins as a small erythematous papule that becomes vesicular, necrotic, and covered with a dark crust or eschar. Intense nonpitting edema, which may not be erythematous, often surrounds and may extend a considerable distance from the eschar. Characteristically the lesion is pruritic but not very tender or hot. The skin lesion is commonly on exposed areas of hands, arms, neck, or face; and there may be mild regional lymph node enlargement. Lymphangitis is not usually observed. Constitutional symptoms and fever are frequently absent unless the skin disease is severe or the infection becomes disseminated, when high fever, prostration, and death may occur.

Infrequently anthrax may develop without a lesion, possibly after inoculation into the skin, but probably more commonly after inhalation of spores of the bacillus in contaminated air. Characteristically, this form of anthrax is severe and is associated with disseminated infection. *Hemorrhagic mediastinitis,* often without pneumonia, and *hemorrhagic meningitis* may occur. Death is common in this form of anthrax; the illness may begin abruptly, be of short duration, and terminate rapidly. Dyspnea and cyanosis are indicative of respiratory or ventilatory insufficiency. Roentgenographic examination of the chest in inhalation anthrax reveals widening of the mediastinum. Leukocytosis is ordinarily not pronounced. Pleural effusion may complicate pulmonary anthrax. Anthrax in man from ingestion of bacilli is rare.

DIAGNOSIS. Anthrax is most readily diagnosed in persons known to have been exposed to animals or animal products potentially contaminated with *B. anthracis*. Cutaneous anthrax can be differeniated from many other bacterial infections of the skin by the insignificance of regional adenopathy, lymphangitis, and cellulitis in relation to the severity of the eschar and edema. Furthermore, pruritus, lack of tenderness, and intense nonpitting edema are characteristic of anthrax. Small skin lesions, however, may be more difficult to recognize. Pulmonary anthrax can be identified by a history of occupational exposure and acute widening of the mediastinum shown by roentgenographic examination. Anthrax meningitis is confused with subarachnoid hemorrhage or cerebrovascular accident, but is usually associated with prominent signs of infection, and gram-positive bacilli can be seen in the cerebrospinal fluid.

In disseminated anthrax infection, blood cultures are often positive. Occasionally, the bacilli may be identified in the centrifugal sediment of blood treated with 3 per cent acetic acid solution and stained with Wright's stain.

In cutaneous anthrax, the bacilli can usually be cultured from the lesions, or typical encapsulated bacilli will be seen when stained with a polychrome eosin–methylene blue stain (Wright or Giemsa). Their direct cultivation on peptone agar should always be attempted. If the specimen has to be shipped, the specimen should be dried on silk threads or on a sterile glass slide. In view of the occurrence of anthrax-like bacilli on the skin, it is imperative that diagnoses be confirmed by animal inoculations, preferably in guinea pigs or mice or by specific bacteriophage lysis. In pulmonary anthrax, the bacillus has been found microscopically in the sputum and in the pleural exudate.

An agar-gel precipitin serologic test has been useful in epidemiologic studies of anthrax. This test, however, is of no value in diagnosing the acute disease.

PROGNOSIS. Cutaneous anthrax is often a self-limited disease, but dissemination of the infection and death may occur in 20 per cent of patients. A fatal outcome in cutaneous anthrax can be averted by appropriate treatment, but treatment of disseminated infection is often unsuccessful in preventing death.

TREATMENT. *B. anthracis* is susceptible to the action of penicillin, the tetracyclines, chloramphenicol, erythromycin, and streptomycin. Penicillin G should be given in total daily doses of at least 1.2 million units, starting as soon as anthrax is diagnosed or seriously suspected. The effectiveness of the tetracyclines is probably not quite so great as that of penicillin; nevertheless, they are effective in cutaneous anthrax and may be administered in a total daily dose of 2.0 grams. Therapy with penicillin or the tetracyclines should be continued for seven days. It should be emphasized that in patients with disseminated anthrax, the progressive course may be so rapid that antimicrobial drugs may not save the patient's life.

PREVENTION. Anthrax can be prevented in man by control of infected animals or animal products. Autoclaving or treatment of imported goat hair with 5.25 per cent sodium hypochlorite (Chlorox) is often impracticable, although this is the means employed to prevent infection from clothing, rugs, and other products, such as shaving brushes, made of potentially infected materials. Vaccination with "protective antigen" is effective in preventing infection in persons likely to be occupationally exposed.

Brachman, P. S.: Human anthrax in the United States. *In* Hobby, G. L. (ed.): Antimicrobial Agents and Chemotherapy. Baltimore, Williams & Wilkins Company, 1965.
Brachman, P. S., Plotkin, S. A., Bumford, F. H., and Atchison, M. M.: An epidemic of inhalation anthrax. II. Epidemiologic investigation. Am. J. Hyg., 72:6, 1960.
Gold, H.: Anthrax: Report of 117 cases. Arch. Intern. Med., 96:387, 1955.
Hughes, M. H.: Anthrax. Br. Med. J., 1:488, 1973.
Plotkin, S. A., Brachman, P. S., Utell, M., Bumford, F. H., and Atchison, M. M.: Epidemic of inhalation anthrax, first in twentieth century. I. Clinical features. Am. J. Med., 29:992, 1960.

161. LISTERIOSIS

Leighton E. Cluff

DEFINITION. Listeriosis is an infectious disease of animals and man with exceptionally protean manifestations, including meningitis, disseminated granulomas, lymphadenopathy, respiratory symptoms, and ill-defined acute febrile illness. It can produce abortion and fetal or neonatal death. The infection is caused by a gram-positive bacillus called *Listeria monocytogenes* and is worldwide in distribution.

ETIOLOGY. Infection of the human being with *Listeria monocytogenes* was identified in 1929 by Nyfeldt. The microorganism was first characterized, however, by Murray, Webb, and Swann in 1926, during an epizootic among rabbits and guinea pigs. Subsequently the microorganism has been identified as a cause of disease in fox, raccoon, goat, lemming, mouse, rat, hamster, pig, horse, cow, dog, domestic fowl and wild birds, and other animals. *L. monocytogenes* is a gram-positive, nonsporeforming, aerobic or microaerophilic, motile bacillus. It ferments a number of sugars, with formation of acid but no gas. It can be grown on nutrient agar or broth, preferably containing 1 per cent glucose, and produces beta hemolysis on blood agar. *L. monocy-*

togenes resembles *Erysipelothrix rhuziopathiae* and diphtheroids, but can be differentiated from these bacteria by its motility (best at 20 to 30° C), its specific antigenicity, and its animal pathogenicity. *Listeria* regularly — and *Erysipelothrix* occasionally — produces purulent keratoconjunctivitis in rabbits after inoculation into the conjunctival space, whereas diphtheroids do not.

EPIDEMIOLOGY. Listeriosis in man and animals has been observed throughout the world. It has been recognized more frequently in humans in recent years, but its true incidence is not known. Confusion in bacteriologic differentiation accounts largely for inadequate recognition of listeriosis. In addition, the diverse manifestations of the disease render it difficult to identify clinically.

Listeriosis may develop after inhalation, ingestion, or direct contact with contaminated food or animal products. The disease is most common in persons living in rural areas. Although infection with *Listeria* occurs in many domesticated and wild animals, there are only rare instances of epizootics or outbreaks in animals other than man. Transmission of infection from person to person probably occurs under some circumstances, notably in nursery outbreaks. Women can carry *Listeria* in the vagina, and infection may be transmitted venereally. Whether or not man can be an asymptomatic carrier of *Listeria* under other conditions is not known.

PATHOLOGY AND PATHOGENESIS. Human listeriosis is characterized by disseminated granulomas and focal necrosis or suppuration in involved tissues. Lesions may develop in liver, intestinal tract, gallbladder, skin, mucous membranes of the respiratory tract, lung, heart, spleen, lymph nodes, placenta, and brain. The fetus may be infected transplacentally through the umbilical vein, with production of septicemia. Debilitating diseases such as chronic infection and cancer predispose to the occurrence of listeriosis. Pregnancy may increase susceptibility to infection, but the disease in pregnant women may be less severe than in other persons. Administration of adrenal cortical steroids may also increase susceptibility to listeriosis. Infection also occurs in persons with no underlying disease.

CLINICAL MANIFESTATIONS. *Meningitis* is the most commonly recognized form of listeriosis in the United States. It is characterized at onset by symptoms of headache, myalgia, fever, chills, nausea, vomiting, and photophobia, followed by the development of stiff neck, stupor, convulsions, somnolence, and, finally, death. The onset may be abrupt or gradual, and the initial symptoms may be those of gastrointestinal or respiratory illness. Examination reveals manifestations of meningitis or encephalitis in varying degrees of severity. There may be pharyngitis, rhinitis, otitis media, neck rigidity, ocular palsy, and signs of depressed cerebral function. Leukocytosis is common, with granulocytosis and, occasionally, monocytosis, in the early phase of the disease. The cerebrospinal fluid, with decreased sugar, elevated protein, and cell counts of 150 to 3000 per cubic millimeter, is indistinguishable from that in many purulent meningitides. Early, the cells in the fluid may be principally granulocytes, but later there may be a predominance of mononuclear cells.

Febrile pharyngitis with cervical and generalized lymphadenopathy can be caused by *Listeria*, and may be difficult to differentiate from *infectious mononucleosis*.

Patients with this type of illness, however, may have an abrupt onset of fever, chills, headache, myalgia, conjunctivitis, macular rash, and sore throat. Lymph nodes in the neck and elsewhere may enlarge, and there may be hepatosplenomegaly. Blood leukocytes occasionally increase in number with a more or less pronounced monocytosis. The absorbed heterophil serologic test for infectious mononucleosis is negative, *Listeria* can be isolated from blood and pharynx, and there will be a rising serum agglutinin titer for *Listeria*.

Lymph node enlargement in the neck and elsewhere without respiratory symptoms may also be attributed to listeriosis. In addition, lymph node enlargement associated only with conjunctivitis may occur. Isolated acute upper respiratory illness may be attributable to listeriosis, although for obvious reasons this diagnosis is seldom established. Chronic urethritis in men has been described, and possibly may be responsible for subclinical or occult infection, demonstrable by culture of the bacillus from bone marrow.

Papular skin lesions associated with disseminated listeriosis have been seen in infants, but adults may acquire primary cutaneous infection after direct contact with infected animal tissues.

Disseminated listeriosis in infants has been reported frequently in Europe, but infrequently in the United States. The disease may arise by transplacental infection of the fetus, causing abortion, fetal death, or serious illness within several days after birth. Outbreaks of infection may develop in newborn nurseries, probably by person-to-person transmission. The disease is characterized by disseminated visceral granulomas and abscesses. When it manifests itself in infants a few weeks old, it often begins as a mild febrile illness with cough, coryza, gastrointestinal symptoms, and pneumonia. Granulomas may be formed on the posterior pharyngeal wall. Granulocytosis and occasionally mononucleosis are present. Pleural and pericardial effusions may develop. Listeriosis has been reported as a common cause of neonatal death and fetal damage in Europe.

Listeriosis in pregnancy may be subclinical or may be associated with an acute febrile illness resembling influenza and occasionally pyelonephritis; it is rarely severe. Its occurrence after the fifth month of pregnancy, however, is likely to affect the fetus seriously. A woman may become a vaginal carrier of *Listeria* and may possibly infect her infant at birth.

Disseminated listeriosis in adults has an abrupt onset with chill and fever. Meningitis can occur, as well as bacterial endocarditis. Blood cultures are usually positive, and there may be a consumptive coagulopathy. This type of listeriosis is observed most often in patients with carcinoma or debilitating disease, and its development may have been facilitated by adrenal steroid therapy.

DIAGNOSIS. There are no pathognomonic clinical features of human listeriosis. The diagnosis rests on isolation of the microorganism or rising agglutinin titers in the serum. It is likely that the recognition of listeriosis has been difficult because of the failure to differentiate *Listeria* from diphtheroid bacilli in culture. The isolation of microorganisms resembling diphtheroids from infectious material or blood should alert one to the necessity for further bacteriologic characterization.

Listeriosis may resemble influenza, miliary tuberculosis, typhoid fever, mycotic infections, and several bacterial infections with septicemia. *Infectious mononucleosis* is most often confused with listeriosis in adults, for the two diseases may be clinically alike. However, listeriosis is infrequently associated with monocytosis, it does not produce a positive absorbed heterophil serologic test, and in systemic disease the bacillus can be isolated from blood, bone marrow, urine, or upper respiratory tract.

TREATMENT. *Listeria monocytogenes* is susceptible in vitro to sulfonamides, penicillin, tetracycline, chloramphenicol, erythromycin, novobiocin, and occasionally streptomycin. Penicillin is the drug of choice, but the tetracyclines and erythromycin are also effective. Some have recommended use of the aminoglycosides, but most strains of *Listeria* are susceptible to less toxic antimicrobial drugs, and these are preferred unless in vitro resistance is demonstrated. Penicillin G should be administered in a dose of 250,000 units per kilogram of body weight each day and should be continued for about seven days after the patient with meningitis becomes afebrile. In other types of infection, treatment should be given for a period of several days, depending upon the course of the disease.

PROGNOSIS. Listeria meningitis has a fatality rate of 70 per cent in untreated patients. The fatality rate in treated patients is considerably lower. The prognosis in adults with pharyngitis and lymph node enlargement is good, whether treated or not, but meningitis may supervene. Recovery from meningitis may leave residual symptoms of central nervous system damage. Infection of the newborn is very serious; the fatality rate and the incidence of congenital defects are high. Untreated, disseminated listeriosis is usually a fatal disease.

PREVENTION. Listeriosis must be regarded as primarily a contagious disease of animals; prevention of human infection would require elimination of animal reservoirs, but this would not prevent person-to-person transmission. Pasteurization prevents transmission of the disease by contaminated milk. Animal products, including meat, should be declared unfit for consumption if the disease is found in slaughtered animals. Better recognition of the disease should clarify its epidemiology and indirectly facilitate control measures. There are no effective agents for immunization.

Gray, M. L., and Killinger, A. H.: *Listeria monocytogenes* and listeric infections. Bact. Rev., 30:309, 1966.

Hoeprich, P. D.: Infections due to *Listeria monocytogenes*. Medicine, 37:143, 1958.

Lowenstein, M. S., Fox, M. D., and Martin, S. M.: Human listeriosis in the U.S. J. Infect. Dis., 123:328, 1971.

Medoff, G., Kunz, L. J., and Weinberg, A. N.: Listeriosis in humans: An evaluation. J. Infect. Dis., 123:247, 1971.

Moore, R. M., and Zehmer, R. B.: Listeriosis in the U.S., 1971. J. Infect. Dis., 127:610, 1973.

162. ERYSIPELOID OF ROSENBACH

Leighton E. Cluff

Erysipeloid of Rosenbach is a specific infectious disease attributable to *Erysipelothrix rhuziopathia*. It occurs in man after contact with infected animals or animal products, particularly swine, cattle, sheep, fish, birds, dogs, horses, reindeer, rabbits, mink, rats, and mice. The disease in man therefore usually arises in abattoir employees, butchers, kitchen workers, those handling fish, those handling animal hides and pelts, and those working with bone or bone meal. Most infections in human beings can be related to skin injury. The causative microorganism is a gram-positive bacillus, nonsporeforming, that can be grown aerobically or anaerobically on nutrient broth containing 1 per cent glucose or upon blood agar. It produces death in laboratory animals, particularly mice, causing focal abscesses in the liver or cutaneous cellulitis. The bacillus is susceptible in vitro to tetracycline, penicillin, chloramphenicol, cephalosporins, erythromycin, and clindamycin.

Erysipeloid in man occurs seasonally, usually in summer and early fall, and is worldwide in distribution. Most commonly it is characterized by a nonsuppurative violaceous lesion of the hand or fingers that is swollen, is very slightly tender, and has a sharply defined margin rarely extending above the wrist. In contrast to streptococcal cellulitis, there are usually burning, tingling, and itching, but little pain in the involved area; rarely does the patient have systemic symptoms of fever, chills, malaise, or headache. Lymphangitis is infrequent, and when it develops it is often attributable to secondary infection with staphylococci or streptococci. The localized disease is self-limited, lasting a few days, and resolution is rapid, associated with brownish discoloration of the involved skin and rarely desquamation. A bacteriologic diagnosis can be made by culture of material aspirated or biopsied from the margin of the lesion, but isolation of the bacillus is not invariable. Ordinarily, the lesion is sufficiently distinctive to permit a clinical diagnosis when the microorganism is not cultured.

Infrequently *Erysipelothrix* infections may become disseminated, causing a diffuse involvement of skin. Rarely, bacteremia may develop, and bacterial endocarditis can occur.

Erysipeloid continues to occur frequently in exposed persons. The ubiquitousness of the bacillus has made it difficult to eradicate the disease. The ordinarily benign character of the infection, however, has made it an insignificant public health problem. Treatment of erysipeloid with penicillin in a dose of 1.2 million units of benzathine penicillin G shortens the localized illness. Disseminated infection should be treated with penicillin G in a dose of 6 to 12 million units each day for four to six weeks. Relapses of the disease have occurred in persons who are untreated or who receive inadequate treatment.

Ewing, M.: Erysipeloid. Med. J. Aust., 1:449, 1957.

Klauden, J. V.: Erysipeloid as an occupational disease. J.A.M.A., 111:1345, 1938.

Price, J. E. L., and Bennett, W. E. J.: The erysipeloid of Rosenbach. Br. Med. J., 2:1060, 1951.

Sneath, P. H. A., Abbott, J. D., and Cunliffe, A. C.: The bacteriology of erysipeloid. Br. Med. J., 2:1063, 1951.

163. ACTINOMYCOSIS

John P. Utz

DEFINITION. Actinomycosis is a chronic, systemic disease characterized by multiple indurated abscesses and sinus tracts characteristically in the face, neck, chest, and abdomen.

HISTORY. Lebert is credited with the first report, in 1857, of actinomycosis in man. Bollinger described the disease in cattle in 1876. In 1877 Harz named the causative organism *Actinomyces bovis*. In 1878 Israel clearly defined the disease in man by a summary of the clinical and pathologic characteristics observed in 38 patients. The same author in collaboration with Wolff in 1891 succeeded in growing the microorganism in anaerobic culture. In 1910 Lord observed *A. bovis* in and about carious teeth and tonsillar crypts in the mouths of otherwise normal persons.

ETIOLOGY. Actinomycosis in man is caused by *A. israelii* and in cattle by *A. bovis,* but species characteristics overlap. In the normal mouth *A. israelii* grows as a pleomorphic rod-shaped bacterium and in tissues as a granule. In draining pus, mycelial clumps measuring 1 to 2 mm in diameter and colored white to yellow have been termed "sulfur" granules. Microscopically these are composed of 0.5 to 1.0 μ filaments which stain gram-positive. On agar media under strictly anaerobic conditions, *A. israelii* grows as a white spherical or lobulated colony. Laboratory animals are generally not susceptible to experimental infection. Although long considered to be a fungus, the microbe is now classified under the bacteria, a designation that more closely fits certain of its major characteristics, including susceptibility to penicillin.

EPIDEMIOLOGY. The disease is worldwide in distribution. During the first part of the twentieth century it was viewed as being the most common of the "systemic mycoses," but the incidence has been decreasing of late. Males are affected almost twice as frequently as females, and the illness seems most common among farmers and in rural areas. Disease is produced by direct invasion of contiguous tissues by *A. israelii* commonly present in the mouth or bowel. There is virtually always concurrent infection with other anaerobic bacteria. Disease in the brain, heart valves, or extremities may be exceptional instances of hematogenous dissemination. Disease in cows, dogs, or swine has no contagious relation to that in man.

PATHOLOGY. In tissues the characteristic and classic findings are the actinomycotic granules. These are usually found in abscesses and are surrounded by polymorphonuclear leukocytes. Chronic granulomatous reactions are also seen with giant cells, especially about granules.

CLINICAL MANIFESTATIONS. Cervicofacial Form. The cervicofacial form occurs in less than half of all cases. Infection probably spreads secondarily to trauma or to carious teeth or infected tonsils. The subcutaneous tissues at the angle of the mandible and of the neck have a characteristic "woody" or indurated feeling, and the skin over these areas is reddened and may have single or multiple draining sinus tracts. Pain is seldom prominent even with osteomyelitic or periosteal lesions of bone.

Thoracic Form. This form of disease arises from aspiration into the bronchi of *A. israelii* or in a few instances from extension of disease from the esophagus to mediastinal tissues and secondarily to pleura and lung. Fever and cough are minimal early in the illness. As disease progresses to consolidation, pleurisy, and draining sinuses, prominent symptoms are weight loss, night sweats, and high fever. Rib involvement occurs occasionally, pleural effusion rarely. Pericarditis (with effusion) and multiple systemic to pulmonary artery fistulas have recently been described.

Abdominal Form. Actinomycosis of the abdomen generally follows appendicitis, appendiceal abscess, a perforating lesion of the stomach, or a diverticulum of the large bowel. An abdominal mass is usually palpable, and may be extensive; and there may be burrowing sinus tracts, some of which may open to the skin in the inguinal or other regions. Pelvic actinomycosis can occur in patients with an intrauterine contraceptive device. Retroperitoneal and thoracic spread through the diaphragm are common.

Other Forms. Approximately 10 per cent of patients have lesions in the brain, heart valves, anorectal area, or subcutaneous tissue of the extremities. Rare instances of actinomycosis of the finger have been attributed to injury to the hand by an adversary's tooth.

DIAGNOSIS. The diagnosis of actinomycosis is supported by the finding in pus of granules that microscopically are composed of gram-positive, branching, often beaded filaments. It should be emphasized that granules may be expressed from otherwise normal tonsils and may not be found in cerebrospinal fluid in cases of central nervous system disease. The diagnosis is confirmed by the isolation of the microorganism in anaerobic culture from a lesion.

Skin test and serologic methods of confirmation are unreliable and are generally unavailable.

Cervicofacial forms of actinomycosis must be distinguished from Ludwig's angina, tuberculosis, osteomyelitis, and malignancy. The thoracic form of disease is suggestive of tuberculosis, other fungal infections, and malignancy. Abdominal actinomycosis is often suspected of being tuberculosis, malignant disease, and, occasionally, amebiasis.

TREATMENT. Penicillin, first used for actinomycosis in 1944, continues to be the best drug in treating all forms of the disease. Although most strains are inhibited in vitro by levels of 0.1 unit per milliliter, the nature of the pathologic process leads often to treatment failures and necessitates prolonged therapy. Doses of 10 to 20 million units parenterally daily for at least six weeks or until lesions have healed are recommended. In penicillin-allergic patients, alternative agents are tetracycline, clindamycin, or chloramphenicol.

Surgical resection and incision and drainage of chronically infected tissues are important adjunctive therapeutic measures.

PROGNOSIS. Prior to antimicrobial therapy, prognosis for life was poor in all forms. With penicillin therapy, the approximate recovery rates are as follows: cervicofacial, 90 per cent; abdominal, 80 per cent; and thoracic, 40 per cent.

Cope, V. Z.: Actinomycosis. London, Oxford University Press, 1938.
Lerner, P. I.: Susceptibility of pathogenic actinomycetes to antimicrobial compounds. Antimicrob. Agents Chemother., 5:302, 1974.
Slack, J. M., and Gerencser, M. A.: Actinomyces and Filamentous Bacteria. Minneapolis, Burgess, 1975.

164. NOCARDIOSIS

John E. Bennett

DEFINITION. Nocardiosis is an uncommon acute or chronic suppurative infection, most often originating in the lung, with a marked tendency to spread to brain and other organs.

HISTORY. Eppinger described the first case in 1890 and isolated the etiologic agent.

ETIOLOGY. *Nocardia asteroides* is the etiologic agent in most cases of nocardiosis. *N. brasiliensis* and *N. caviae* cause an occasional case of nocardiosis. *N. brasiliensis* more typically is responsible for mycetoma or, rarely, a lymphocutaneous disease resembling sporotrichosis. *Nocardia* species are aerobic, higher bacteria with branching hyphae less than 1 μ wide. Hyphae are weakly gram-positive and weakly acid fast. On Gram stain of pus, *Nocardia* often appear beaded and refractile. *Nocardia* grow readily at 25 or 37° C on many drug-free culture media. Colonies are initially smooth and white or cream colored, later becoming chalky with an orange or yellow hue. Growth is often apparent in the first week of incubation. Identification of an isolate as *N. asteroides*, *N. caviae*, or *N. brasiliensis* is a complex task, best assigned to a reference laboratory.

EPIDEMIOLOGY. *Nocardia* organisms are soil saprophytes. Portal of entry is the lung or, rarely, through trauma to the skin or gastrointestinal tract. Man-to-man transmission is unknown. Nocardiosis is infrequent but worldwide. Infection in males is two to three times as common as in females. Disease occurs at any age but is more frequent in older adults. No occupational predisposition is known. Many patients have pre-existing debilitating conditions, such as neoplasia, immunosuppressive therapy, alveolar proteinosis, or chronic granulomatous disease of childhood.

PATHOLOGY. The lung lesion is a bronchopneumonia, with a tendency to suppuration, empyema, and abscess formation. Brain lesions are poorly encapsulated abscesses, often multiple. Purulent meningitis may result from rupture of a brain abscess into the cerebrospinal fluid. Neutrophils are the most prominent inflammatory cell in all sites, but lymphocytes and plasma cells also occur. Giant cells or epithelioid cells are infrequent. Branching filaments of *Nocardia* are scattered in the lesion, with no granule formation. Hyphae are best demonstrated histologically by a tissue Gram stain, such as Brown and Brenn. An overstained Gomori methenamine silver procedure can also be used.

CLINICAL MANIFESTATIONS. Presenting symptoms usually refer to the lung, brain, or subcutaneous tissue, in that decreasing order of frequency. Pulmonary infection may be acute or of many months' duration. Symptoms include fever, cough, purulent sputum, weight loss, anorexia, fatigue, dyspnea, and chest pain. Radiologic appearance of the lung lesion is variable, but typically there are one or more areas of dense pneumonia. Lesions tend to cavitate with time. Infection sometimes extends from the lung into the chest wall, forming a subcutaneous abscess. The central nervous system is infected in 30 per cent of cases. This may be the initial or sole manifestation of the disease or may be a late complication of pulmonary nocardiosis. Clinically the neurologic disease presents as a brain abscess or purulent meningitis. Skin or subcutaneous abscesses also occur in about 30 per cent of cases, usually in the presence of pulmonary nocardiosis. Dissemination to many other organs may occur, particularly heart, kidney, spleen, and liver.

DIAGNOSIS. A refractory, suppurative pneumonitis should suggest the possibility of nocardiosis, particularly in the presence of immunosuppression, brain abscess, or skin abscesses. Sputum, bronchoscopic washings, pleural fluid, percutaneous lung aspirates, and pus aspirated from other sites should be Gram stained and cultured for *Nocardia*. Cultures of blood, bone marrow, urine, or cerebrospinal fluid are rarely positive.

Branching, gram-positive filaments on smear raise the possibility of actinomycosis or nocardiosis. *Nocardia* can usually, but not always, be distinguished from *Actinomyces* on smear by the absence of granules and weak acid-fastness of the former. Acid-fastness is best demonstrated by a modified Ziehl-Neelsen stain or in tissue by a modified Fite-Faraco stain. Use of dilute sulfuric acid rather than acid-alcohol during destaining is critical. Diagnosis of nocardiosis by culture alone is fraught with problems. *Nocardia* organisms are difficult to isolate from heavily contaminated specimens, such as sputum, and accurate culture identification of *Nocardia* requires both time and expertise.

Occasionally *Nocardia* is isolated from a specimen, usually sputum, either as a contaminant or as the cause of a mild, self-limiting disease. It is much more common, however, for subsequent developments to indicate that the *Nocardia* had been the cause of symptoms incorrectly ascribed to tuberculosis, neoplasm, or another disorder.

TREATMENT. Treatment of choice is enough sulfadiazine to give serum concentrations of 10 to 15 mg per 100 ml. Six to nine grams per day is usually required for an adult. Copious fluid intake and urine alkalinization with oral sodium bicarbonate are necessary to prevent crystalluria. After about a month, if the patient is improving, sulfadiazine dosage may be reduced to 4 to 6 grams per day, or an equivalent amount of sulfisoxazole or trisulfapyrimidines may be used instead. Therapy is usually continued at this dose for 12 to 18 months. Pus in the brain, pleura, or soft tissues should be drained. Whether or not drugs other than sulfonamides are useful is an open question. Only a few patients not receiving sulfonamides have survived. It is common practice for patients responding poorly to sulfonamides to be given an additional drug, particularly ampicillin, 150 mg per kilogram per day. Cycloserine, erythromycin, minocycline, and co-trimoxazole also have their advocates.

PROGNOSIS. Clinically apparent nocardiosis is usually fatal without treatment. With appropriate therapy, nocardiosis confined to the lung has the best prognosis (50 to 60 per cent survival) and central nervous system infection the worst (13 per cent survival). The occurrence of nocardiosis in the presence of immunosuppressive therapy portends a poor prognosis.

Frazier, A. R., Rosenow, E. C., and Roberts, G.: Nocardiosis. A review of 25 cases occurring during 24 months. Mayo Clin. Proc., 50:657, 1975.

Krick, J. A., Stinson, E. B., and Remington, J. S.: *Nocardia* infection in heart transplant patients. Ann. Intern. Med., 82:18, 1975.

Palmer, D. L., Harvey, R. L., and Wheeler, J. K.: Diagnostic and therapeutic considerations in *Nocardia asteroides* infection. Medicine, 53:391, 1974.

Young, L. S., Armstrong, D., Blevins, A., and Lieberman, P.: *Nocardia asteroides* infection complicating neoplastic disease. Am. J. Med., 50:356, 1971.

165. BRUCELLOSIS

Thomas M. Buchanan

DEFINITION. Brucellosis is an infectious disease characterized by fever, sweats, weakness, malaise, and weight loss that is transmitted to man from animals or animal products containing bacteria of the genus *Brucella*.

ETIOLOGY. *Brucella suis*, *Brucella abortus*, *Brucella me-*

litensis, and *Brucella canis* may all cause human brucellosis. Brucellae are small, nonmotile, nonsporeforming, gram-negative rods. The four species are differentiated by biochemical and serologic reactions. Hogs are generally infected with *Br. suis,* cattle with *Br. abortus,* sheep and goats with *Br. melitensis,* and dogs with *Br. canis.* However, infections of swine with *Br. abortus* or of cattle with *Br. suis* may occur, and *Brucella* infection of caribou, deer, horses, moose, cats, and chickens has been reported. Animal-to-animal transmission is usually venereal or via ingestion of infected tissue or milk. Human infection most commonly results from ingestion of infected animal tissue or milk products, or through skin wounds directly bathed in freshly killed infected animal tissues, as in abattoir workers. Human infection via inoculation of the conjunctival sac has also been documented (for example, with strain 19, an attenuated *Br. abortus* used to vaccinate cattle), and there is epidemiologic evidence to suggest rare infection via inhalation of aerosols containing *Brucella* organisms. In recent years, approximately 57 per cent of patients in the United States have been infected with *Br. suis,* 33 per cent with *Br. abortus,* and 10 per cent with *Br. melitensis* or an unidentified *Brucella* species.

EPIDEMIOLOGY. Since 1970, cases of human brucellosis in the United States have ranged from 175 to 328 per year, with 328 cases in 1975 and 271 in 1976. Worldwide, the disease is more common and closely correlates with the extent of animal brucellosis in any country. States with the highest incidence of brucellosis during the past ten years were Iowa, Virginia, Illinois, Minnesota, Nebraska, California, Tennessee, North Carolina, Georgia, Florida, Mississippi, Arkansas, and Louisiana. Texas, Oklahoma, Missouri, and Pennsylvania each reported more than 40 cases during this same period, and all states except Nevada and the District of Columbia experienced one or more cases of human brucellosis during this interval.

Brucellosis most frequently occurs in persons with high rates of exposure to *Brucella*-infected tissues, milk, or milk products. This includes slaughterhouse workers (some persons handle 3000 freshly killed hogs or 800 freshly killed cattle per day), livestock producers, veterinarians, and persons who ingest unpasteurized milk or milk products. In 1976 in the United States, brucellosis patients by occupation were packing house employees (54 per cent), livestock producers (11 per cent), veterinarians and meat inspectors (9 per cent), and farmers, students, children, and other miscellaneous categories (18 per cent). The number of organisms required to produce infection via different routes is least for penetration through broken skin; considerably more for exposure to *Brucella* organisms through the conjunctival sac or by ingestion of contaminated materials; and still more for inhalation of infected aerosols. Brucellae may remain viable in unpasteurized milk or cheese for approximately 10 or 90 days, respectively. Isolation of *Brucella* from infected meat markedly decreases over a few days with refrigeration, and particularly with the curing and smoking processes used for ham and bacon. In the abattoir setting, persons with a combination of both high accidental cut rates and considerable exposure to the blood and lymph of freshly killed animals are most likely to develop *Brucella* infections. *Brucella* infections are often controlled by the patient's immune response, and asymptomatic infections are up to ten times more common than symptomatic disease and the

clinical syndrome of brucellosis. Approximately 90 per cent of patients are immune to developing subsequent clinical brucellosis following recovery from their first infection. Therefore in populations with high exposures to potentially infected tissues (e.g., abattoir workers), most cases are seen in younger persons who have been exposed for shorter periods to potentially infected tissues and are less likely to have developed immunity. Also, brucellosis affects men more commonly than women; in 1975, brucellosis was nearly six times more frequent in men than in women.

PATHOGENESIS AND PATHOLOGY. *Brucella* organisms penetrate the epithelial cells of the human skin (i.e., hands), oropharynx, conjunctivae, or lung. In the submucosa they interact with polymorphonuclear leukocytes (PMN) and/or tissue macrophages. Many are phagocytized, and, if the inoculum is sufficient, some spread via the lymphatics to regional lymph nodes. The most common sites of lymphadenitis in brucellosis are in the axillary, cervical, and supraclavicular locations, perhaps reflecting the high frequency of the hand-wound or oropharyngeal routes of infections. If the inoculum is sufficient to overcome host immune attempts at localization of *Brucella* organisms within the lymph nodes, bacteremia follows. The usual incubation period between infection and bacteremia with associated symptoms is 10 to 11 days with a heavy inoculum, and two to three weeks with a smaller inoculum. Incubation periods as short as seven days or as long as three months have been reported. Bacteremia is usually accompanied by phagocytosis of nearly all free *Brucella* organisms within a few hours by circulating PMN. These phagocytized brucellae are further localized most commonly to the spleen, liver, and bone marrow. The patient's fever, chills, and sweats may in part result from endogenous pyrogen release from PMN that have phagocytized *Brucella* organisms. Brucellae are located with phagocytic vacuoles within PMN, and transient intracellular survival and even multiplication of *Brucella* organisms within phagocytes have been reported. In most instances, the inoculum is not large, the human host defenses prevail, granuloma formation does not occur, and the patient recovers. Similarly, even with a large inoculum, prompt (within three to four weeks of onset of symptoms) treatment of sufficient duration (four to eight weeks) results in rapid healing of the small granulomas and complete recovery. However, if the inoculum is large and the patient is not treated, small granulomas may fuse to form large granulomas that may eventually suppurate and serve as a source for recurrent bacteremia. Persistent bacteremia may lead to multiple system involvement, including most commonly infections and abscesses of the skeletal system (spine and joints), genitourinary tract (kidneys, bladder, epididymis, testes, urethra), optic nerve, lung, liver (abnormal liver function tests, jaundice), and cardiovascular system (endocarditis, myocarditis, pericarditis). *Br. suis* and *Br. melitensis* are more virulent than *Br. abortus* and more readily form abscesses.

CLINICAL MANIFESTATIONS. Over 90 per cent of patients experience chilly sensations, sweats, and fever, accompanied by weakness and general malaise. The fever ranges from 38.3 to 40° C, and approximately 70 per cent of patients experience body aches. Over half of patients with brucellosis complain of anorexia and experience weight loss, averaging 15 to 20 pounds. Nearly 45 per cent of patients complain of headaches. Cough and/or arthralgias are present in approximately 20 to 25 per cent of patients. Diarrhea, constipation, visual disturbance, eye pain, dizziness, tinnitus, or genitourinary disturbance may occur, although less frequently. The most common signs of brucellosis in addition to fever are lymphadenopathy (up to 40 per cent), splenomegaly (up to 40 per cent), hepatomegaly (up to 8 per cent), and tenderness over the spine (up to 6 per cent), with the prevalence of each sign reflecting the chronicity of infection in the patient population studied. The average number of work days lost for an abattoir worker with brucellosis varies from 30 to 50 days. One third to one half of patients experience a sudden onset of symptoms; in the remainder the onset is gradual, over several days to weeks.

Observed complications in patients with untreated and longstanding brucellosis have included pleurisy, pleural effusion, lung abscess, millet-seed pulmonary calcification, empyema, pneumonia, chronic pulmonary granuloma, spondylitis, suppurative arthritis, osteomyelitis, hydroarthrosis, epididymitis, orchitis, cystitis, pyelitis, nephritis, optic neuritis, keratitis, uveitis, retinopathy, meningitis, encephalitis, neuritis, hemolytic anemia, thrombocytopenia or pancytopenia associated with hypersplenism, cholecystitis, pericholecystic or subdiaphragmatic abscesses, chronic cutaneous ulcers, endocarditis, myocarditis, thrombophlebitis, pulmonary embolization, and cardiac rupture. Many diseases more common than brucellosis have signs and symptoms that partially or almost totally mimic brucellosis. It is therefore important to exclude other more common illnesses and to obtain objective evidence of *Brucella* infection before making a diagnosis of brucellosis. Diseases that may resemble brucellosis include influenza; infectious mononucleosis; toxoplasmosis; viral hepatitis; acute pyelonephritis; ankylosing spondylitis; thyrotoxicosis; disseminated gonococcal infection; rheumatic fever; systemic lupus erythematosus; malaria; tuberculosis; sarcoidosis; leptospirosis; typhoid fever; Hodgkin's disease; lymphoblastic and lymphocytic leukemia; myeloblastic and myelocytic leukemia; metastatic carcinoma of the lung, colon, prostate, pancreas, stomach, or liver; and thiamin deficiency. If the patient has had recent exposure to animal tissue or products potentially infected with *Brucella* organisms, the clinical suspicion of brucellosis should be increased. However, even abattoir workers experience influenza or influenza-like viral syndromes more frequently than brucellosis.

Objective findings useful for evaluation of possible brucellosis in a patient include physical signs, cultures, serologic data, and x-rays. The absence of at least intermittent fever of 38.3° C or higher makes a diagnosis of brucellosis extremely unlikely (less than 5 per cent of patients). Weight loss is present in approximately half of patients, and lymphadenopathy and splenomegaly are other common signs.

The definitive evidence of *Brucella* infection is the isolation of *Brucella* organisms from the patient. *However, culturing Brucella organisms may be dangerous to laboratory personnel. All cultures should be clearly marked "possible brucellosis" and should be processed with sterile techniques in a biohazard hood certified for handling class III infectious agents. Culturing for Brucella organisms is not recommended for hospitals and clinics without these facilities.* Early in the course of illness, particularly in association with fever and chills, the patient is likely to have *Brucella* bacteremia. Approximately 50 to 75 per cent of these patients who have not received antimicrobial drugs will yield *Brucella* organisms from their blood when one or two samples are cultured in standard blood culture bottles (containing trypticase soy broth) for one to three weeks in the presence of 5 to 10 per cent CO_2. Later in the course of the illness, bacteremia is less frequent and organisms are more likely to be isolated from infected lymph nodes, or from granulomas involving the spleen, liver, or skeletal system (most frequently, spine). During the past ten years only 15 to 20 per cent of brucellosis cases in the United States have been confirmed by culture. Most cases (80 to 85 per cent) were diagnosed serologically.

The most reliable and standardized *serologic screening test* for brucellosis is the standard tube *Brucella* agglutination test. A four-fold or greater rise in titer for sera drawn one to four weeks apart is indicative of recent exposure to *Brucella* or *Brucella*-like antigens. Separate sera should be tested on the same day, in the same laboratory, and under identical conditions to examine for seroconversion. Significant seroconversion is defined as fourfold or greater rise in titer from an initial titer of at least 40 or higher to eventual titer of 160 or higher. The titer is the reciprocal of the maximal serum dilution that produces 50 per cent or more agglutination of the *Brucella* organisms under the test conditions. Most patients develop rising agglutination titers to *Brucella* antigens within one to two weeks of illness, and approximately 80 per cent of persons have an eightfold or higher rise in their agglutinins during the acute illness. Within three weeks of illness, approximately 97 per cent of patients with brucellosis will have serologic evidence of their infection if a single serum sample is tested. With repeat testing, less than 0.7 per cent of all patients will remain seronegative (titer <160). The maximal *Brucella* agglutination titers in sera from persons with asymptomatic *Brucella* infections may reach as high as titers in patients with clinical brucellosis. It should be noted that the *Brucella* skin test, cholera vaccination, or infection with *Vibrio cholerae, Pasteurella tularensis,* or *Yersinia enterocolitica* may cause seroconversion to elevated *Brucella* agglutination titers and not represent *Brucella* infection. Provided that these "cross-reactive" causes of seroconversion are ruled out, a fourfold rise in titer of *Brucella* agglutinating antibodies is indicative of current *Brucella* infection. If such a patient has signs and symptoms compatible with brucellosis, then it is likely that the patient has a symptomatic *Brucella* infection known as brucellosis.

The standard *Brucella* agglutination test is performed as follows: (1) Serial twofold dilutions of the patient's serum are prepared in normal saline, beginning with a 1:10 dilution. (2) Antigen consisting of a standardized diluted suspension of *Brucella abortus* strain No. 1119 (available from the Department of Agriculture, National Animal Diseases Laboratory, Ames, Iowa) is added to each serum-containing well. The tubes containing antigen and serum are mixed and incubated at 37° C for 48 hours. The serum titer is the reciprocal of the maximal serum dilution that produces 50 per cent or more agglutination of the bacterial suspension. This agglutination is accomplished by divalent (IgG) or multivalent (IgM) antibodies bridging two or more *Brucella* organisms. The latticework produced forms a clump that can be seen by observing each agglutination test tube with a fluorescent light against a dark background. A titer of 160 or higher is very rare in persons with no exposure to *Brucella* organisms and is considered indicative of past or present antigenic stimulation with *Brucella* organisms or antigens "cross-reactive" with *Brucella* species. If the clinical suspicion of brucellosis is strong, the patient's serum should be tested in dilutions as high as 1:1280, because prozones — falsely negative tests for agglutination due to "blocking" IgA or nonagglutinating IgG antibodies — have been reported in titers as high as 640.

Significance of Elevated Antibody Titer. During the first one to two weeks of illness, the primary agglutinating antibody response to *Brucella* is of the IgM immunoglobulin class. Thereafter, IgG antibodies are formed in addition to IgM antibodies. Both IgG and IgM agglutinating antibodies are detected in the standard *Brucella* agglutination test. However, with early diagnosis and prompt treatment of sufficient duration, IgG agglutinating antibodies rarely persist beyond 6 to 12 months following onset of the disease. However, if the diagnosis is delayed for many months to years and no treatment is received, some patients (fewer than 15 per cent) will develop continuing *Brucella* infection with potentially serious complications. These patients will maintain elevated IgG *Brucella* agglutinins until diagnosed and treated. This information is useful to the clinician, because the *Brucella* agglutination performed in the presence of 0.05 M 2-mercaptoethanol (2-ME) recognizes only IgG agglutinating antibodies to *Brucella*. Thus in the absence of a rising agglutination titer, a single elevated 2-ME *Brucella* agglutination test titer is the most objective evidence that the patient has a current or recent infection. A titer of 160 or higher in the 2-ME test suggests either a current or recent asymptomatic infection or, if the patient is symptomatic, active infection with disease and the need for treatment. Titers of 40 to 80 in the 2-ME *Brucella* agglutination test are rarely associated with significant recent infections. In a patient with symptoms of three or more weeks' duration, a 2-ME *Brucella* agglutination titer of 20 or lower essentially eliminates the possibility that the patient's symptoms are due to brucellosis. A significant proportion of patients maintain elevated IgM agglutinating antibodies and consequently have elevated standard *Brucella* agglutination titers for many years, even after presumed complete cure of their brucellosis. In fact, standard *Brucella* agglutination titers of ≤160 are very common in completely asymptomatic abattoir workers. For this reason, the 2-ME *Brucella* agglutination test that measures only IgG agglutinating antibodies is the most useful indicator of whether the patient was cured (negative test).

The Brucella skin test is not recommended for diagnostic purposes, because it may remain positive for many years following symptomatic or asymptomatic *Brucella* infection and it may interfere with interpretation of serologic tests by causing a rise in titer of the standard tube agglutination test.

TREATMENT. The combination of streptomycin and tetracycline is superior to tetracycline alone, and tetracycline therapy should be maintained for a minimum of six weeks. These antimicrobials quickly kill *Brucella* organisms in vitro, but during brucellosis some organisms survive the antimicrobial therapy, perhaps by being located within cells, granulomas, or abscesses. The long duration of chemotherapy permits mobilization of the humoral and cellular immunity that is required for eventual complete elimination of infecting *Brucella* organisms. A regimen used successfully to treat more than 200 workers who acquired brucellosis in a midwest slaughterhouse was streptomycin, 1 gram daily intramuscularly during days 1 to 6 and 8 to 13; and tetracycline, 500 mg orally four times daily during

days 1 to 45. One of these patients developed significant complications of his brucellosis that lasted six to eight months, and none developed chronic disease (illness ≥1 year's duration) or death. Relapses occurred in approximately 2 per cent of the patients, and these responded to retreatment. Nearly all were able to return to their former work in the abattoir. Variations on the streptomycin-tetracycline regimen have been reported, e.g., substitution of another aminoglycoside, gentamicin, for the streptomycin, use of a tetracycline with prolonged action (doxycycline), or use of co-trimoxazole as a supplement. However, at present the efficacy of these alternatives to the streptomycin-tetracycline therapy is unproved, and further investigations are warranted before their value can be established. After six weeks of treatment, if the patient is without signs or symptoms of brucellosis and has evidence of decreasing agglutination titers, antimicrobial therapy may be discontinued. Relapses occur in less than 5 per cent of cases when the patient receives treatment early in the course of illness and for six weeks' duration. Relapse is more frequent when treatment is delayed or of insufficient duration. Most relapses occur within three months, and nearly all develop within ten months of completing initial therapy. Nearly all relapses rapidly respond to a repeat course of therapy.

PROGNOSIS. Brucellosis diagnosed within one month of onset of illness and treated with appropriate antimicrobial therapy for a sufficient period is a completely curable illness. Even before antimicrobial therapy was available, 85 per cent of patients recovered within three months. With chemotherapy, chronic brucellosis (illness lasting more than one year) or severe complications have become extremely rare. When either of these situations is found, it is almost invariably associated with a prolonged delay before diagnosis and/or failure to take prescribed medications. Acute brucellosis produces substantial malaise, weakness, fever, and weight loss and is frequently associated with an inability to work for one to two months, even with antimicrobial therapy. Without therapy, complications such as *Brucella* abscesses of the liver, spleen, vertebral column, heart valve, skin, meninges, lung, or bone marrow may occur; but with therapy, these complications are rare (less than 1 per cent). They almost invariably occur only in patients with continuous or intermittent fever of 38.3° C or higher and positive standard and 2-ME *Brucella* agglutination test results (titer greater than 160).

A febrile patient with chronic symptoms suggestive of a complication of brucellosis or of chronic brucellosis should be screened with a standard agglutination test. If this is positive, a 2-ME *Brucella* agglutination test should be performed. A titer of lower than 40 in the 2-ME *Brucella* agglutination test is strong evidence against chronic brucellosis or a complication of brucellosis. The absence of fever, a localized lesion, and elevated 2-ME resistant *Brucella* agglutinins essentially eliminate the possibility that the patient may have chronic brucellosis or a complication of brucellosis. When complications of brucellosis are demonstrated, they usually respond to a combination of surgical removal of the localized lesion and antimicrobial therapy. Hypersensitivity to *Brucella* antigens may occur, but in recent years it has been very unusual even among abattoir workers who are maximally exposed to potentially infected animal tissue. Therefore patients should be allowed to return to their former work, even if it means re-exposure to *Brucella* antigens, as development of hypersensitivity is unlikely. Also, immunity to reinfection follows the first *Brucella* infection in most (92 per cent) cases, and thus patients returning to work following treatment are less likely to acquire brucellosis than are previously uninfected employees. However, if symptoms resembling hypersensitivity occur, it should be determined whether small amounts of *Brucella* antigens can induce these symptoms. If so, these patients should avoid *Brucella* antigens, and this may require changing occupations.

PREVENTION. Infection with *Brucella* confers an impressive immunity. Reinfection occurs but is uncommon (fewer than 5 per cent of patients). Effective prevention of brucellosis in cattle results from a live attenuated *Brucella* vaccine. No vaccine is presently available for humans. The risk of acquiring brucellosis may be reduced by decreasing one's exposure to freshly killed animal tissue from potentially infected animals, and by drinking pasteurized milk and milk products. Slaughterhouse workers, meat inspectors, and veterinarians who occupationally examine large numbers of cattle and hogs may reduce their risk of infection by wearing protective gloves and goggles or eyeglasses and by avoiding hand or arm cuts that might provide a route of entry for *Brucella* organisms. Complete elimination of brucellosis in humans will first require elimination of *Brucella* infection in animals.

Alton, G. G., et al.: Laboratory Techniques in Brucellosis. Geneva, World Health Organization, 1975.

Buchanan, T. M., et al.: Brucellosis in the United States, 1960–1972: An abattoir-associated disease. I. Clinical features and therapy. II. Diagnostic aspects. III. Epidemiology and evidence for acquired immunity. Medicine, 53:403, 415, 427, 1974.

Morales-Otero, P.: *Brucella abortus* in Porto Rico. Porto Rico J. Public Health Trop. Med., 6:3, 1930.

Reports of the Commission for the Investigation of Mediterranean Fever. London, Harrison & Sons, Part 1 to 7, 1905–1907.

Reddin, J. L.: Significance of 7S and macroglobulin *Brucella* agglutinins in human brucellosis. N. Engl. J. Med., 275:1263, 1965.

Smith, C. C.: Treatment of human brucellosis. Scott. Med. J., 21:132, 1976.

Spink, W. W.: The Nature of Brucellosis. Minneapolis, University of Minnesota Press, 1956.

Zoonoses Surveillance, Annual Brucellosis Summaries. Atlanta, Center for Disease Control, published yearly.

DISEASES DUE TO MYCOBACTERIA

166. TUBERCULOSIS

Roger Des Prez

GENERAL CONSIDERATIONS

Tuberculosis is a chronic infection, potentially of lifelong duration, caused by two species of mycobacteria, *M. tuberculosis* and, rarely, *M. bovis*. It is almost always initiated by inhalation of infectious material, rarely by ingestion, and more rarely still by cutaneous inoculation (prosector's wart). Early in infection a silent bloodstream spread seeds the lymphatic system and other organs throughout the body, leaving foci which may cause clinical illness after long periods of latency. Tuberculosis must be differentiated on bacteriologic grounds from chronic infections caused by other species of mycobacteria.

Although paleopathologic evidence indicates that humans were infected with tuberculosis in neolithic times, the infection became epidemic with the Industrial Revolution, which produced the crowded living conditions most favorable to its spread. In the mid-nineteenth century, it is said to have accounted for one quarter of adult deaths in Europe. During that century three great strides led to an accurate conception of the disease and its cause. In 1804, Laennec published the opinion that the many different forms of tuberculosis in the lungs and elsewhere, previously regarded as different diseases, were actually different manifestations of one disease. By 1839, the term *tuberculosis* had come into use, reflecting the unifying anatomic feature of tubercle formation. In 1865, Villemin established the contagious nature of the process by infecting laboratory animals with diseased tissue. In 1882, Koch reported isolation and culture of the tubercle bacillus and successful production of disease in animals by these isolates.

The sanatorium movement, which began because of emphasis on climate in treatment, received further impetus from the demonstration of the infectious nature of the process. As a result, phthisiology became a distinct and sophisticated medical specialty but one which was separated from the mainstream of medicine. The development of diagnostic radiology led to an appreciation of the pivotal importance of cavity formation. Treatment, other than general supportive measures and bed rest, became directed almost entirely at the goal of cavity closure, utilizing methods such as pneumoperitoneum, therapeutic pneumothorax, and collapse of the chest wall by surgical measures (thoracoplasty).

By 1947, it had become established that streptomycin (SM) was a truly effective antituberculous drug, initiating the chemotherapy era. Soon after, it was shown that combination of SM with para-aminosalicylic acid (PAS) tended to prevent treatment failures associated with development of bacterial resistance to SM, establishing the principle of combined drug therapy. The availability of effective drug treatment also made it possible for the first time to resect diseased tissue, a procedure which had previously frequently resulted in spread of infection. Some form of pulmonary resection became a part of treatment of many if not most cases. This attitude persisted for some 15 years until it became clear that resection added very little to the long-term results of effective and extended drug therapy.

In 1952, isoniazid (INH) was established as an antituberculous drug of a different and higher order than SM, and tuberculosis became a medically curable illness in most cases. Since patients on treatment became rapidly noninfectious and required little bed rest or specialized therapeutic methods aimed at cavity collapse, the need for sanatoriums disappeared, and tuberculosis became, perhaps for the first time, the legitimate province of the general physician and general hospital. Treatment began to be applied not only to patients with demonstrably active cases but also to individuals in whom active disease seemed only reasonably likely to develop (chemoprophylaxis). Finally, the more meticulous bacteriologic techniques required to determine drug susceptibility of infecting strains was, more than anything else, responsible for the recognition and eventual definition of many other pathogenic mycobacteria, all of which are less susceptible to isoniazid.

BACTERIOLOGY

Mycobacteria are acid-fast, nonmotile, nonsporulating, weakly gram-positive rods classified in the order Actinomycetales. Until recently, only *M. tuberculosis*, the human tubercle bacillus, and *M. bovis* were regarded as pathogenic for man. *M. avium*, which causes tuberculosis in poultry and swine, is thought to produce human disease only rarely. Recently other mycobacteria, previously either unrecognized or regarded as saprophytes, have become recognized as human pathogens. The clinical importance of these "atypical" mycobacteria is discussed in Ch. 169.

Such distinguishing characteristics as slow growth rate, resistance to chemical disinfectants, and the ability to survive within phagocytic cells are attributed to the hydrophobic, lipid-rich (60 per cent of dry weight) mycobacterial cell wall. Its composition accounts for the typical diagnostic staining characteristics. In the Ziehl-Neelsen method, staining with carbolfuchsin is facilitated by steaming the smear. Subsequent treatment with acid-alcohol elutes carbolfuchsin from other bacteria and organic material, but "acid-fast" mycobacteria resist decoloration.

When pulmonary tuberculosis is sufficiently advanced to cause symptoms, most patients will demonstrate acid-fast bacilli in the sputum. Because it facilitates a more rapid scanning of a sputum smear, an auramine-rhodamine fluorescent stain is now commonly used. The first sputum raised in the morning is the best material to submit for culture. When sputum is not produced, respiratory secretions can be obtained by gastric aspiration or stimulated by inhalation of heated, hypertonic aerosols (10 per cent saline). The aerosol is inhaled for 15 minutes, and all sputum raised then and for a 15-minute period thereafter is collected. Gastric aspiration has been largely abandoned. The procedure, however, is effective for culture purposes when accomplished immediately upon awakening in the morning before the overnight gastric contents have passed from the stomach.

Differentiation of Clinically Important Myobacterial Species

Definitive identification of mycobacteria is usually accomplished by reference laboratories, but good species identification can be achieved by a few simple observations. Rate of growth and production of pigment were used by Runyon to classify the so-called "atypical" mycobacteria into four groups: Group I is characterized by formation of yellow colonies after brief exposure to light (photochromogens), Group II by production of yellow or orange colonies without light stimulation (scotochromogens), Group III by nonpigmented colonies, and Group IV by growth within seven days. These characteristics, together with nonsusceptibility to isoniazid, lack of production of niacin, and production of the enzyme catalase, suffice for tentative identification of those mycobacteria known to be of pathogenic importance in man. *M. tuberculosis* usually requires two or three weeks for visible growth. Colonies are rough, and no pigment is produced. It is the only species which produces a positive niacin test. Isoniazid-susceptible strains of *M. tuberculosis* produce catalase, whereas isoniazid-resistant strains are usually catalase negative. *M. bovis* resembles *M. tuberculosis* but does not produce niacin. The *photochromogenic* property of *M. kansasii* (Runyon Group I) is its most distinguishing characteristic. Growth is slow, colonies are either rough or smooth, moderate isoniazid resistance is usual, catalase production is marked, and niacin is not produced. *M. marinum* (Runyon Group I) resembles *M. kansasii* except that growth is poor at 37° C and good at room temperature. *M. avium* and *M. intracellulare* (the Battey bacillus) grow slowly, produce smooth, thin, nonpigmented colonies, are highly resistant to isoniazid, produce catalase, and do not produce niacin. They are serologically closely related and differ

only in that *M. avium* grows well at 45° C and *M. intracellulare* does not. They are classified in Runyon's Group III. *Scotochromogenic mycobacteria* (Runyon Group II) produce yellow to orange pigment in the dark, grow slowly, have smooth colonies, are highly resistant to isoniazid, produce catalase, and do not produce niacin. *Rapid growers* (Runyon Group IV) produce colonies within seven days and are catalase positive, niacin negative, and very resistant to isoniazid.

EPIDEMIOLOGY

In much of the world, bovine tuberculosis remains a significant problem and infection by mouth is frequent. In Western nations, however, infection is almost always by inhalation. Most importance is attached to the dried residue of droplets aerosolized by cough, called *droplet nuclei*, which may remain suspended in air for prolonged periods and are sufficiently small to reach terminal air passages where removal is difficult and bacterial multiplication can begin. Well-studied epidemics in certain closed environments such as naval vessels and boarding schools indicate that one person with cavitary disease may "poison" the environment with droplet nuclei and infect virtually all susceptibles in the same environment, even in the temporary absence of the infectious person himself. A tuberculosis ward is probably not a place of great risk when care is taken, because persons receiving chemotherapy become rapidly noninfectious. Infected urine may rarely be contagious for young children using the same toilet facilities, owing to droplet nuclei formed from urine aerosolization. Transmission of tuberculosis by the genital route is rare. Inoculation of abraded skin by contaminated tissues at autopsy examination may produce a primary skin infection in tuberculin-negative individuals (prosector's wart). Fomites are of no importance in the spread of infection.

INCIDENCE AND PREVALENCE. The decline in tuberculosis mortality which began in the middle of the last century was probably due to improved living conditions and heightened social awareness. In the past 20 years of drug treatment, mortality has declined somewhat more rapidly but the incidence of new cases has fallen less, suggesting a residue of older individuals infected in earlier years. In the young, it is clear that the new case rate has drastically fallen in urban United States. In 1928, 53 per cent of 16-year-old schoolchildren in Philadelphia were tuberculin positive. By 1968, this had decreased to 1.4 per cent. At present, less than 10 per cent of cases of active tuberculosis represent new infections, the remainder developing in persons infected years previously, and succumbing to host-dependent factors, such as age and intercurrent illness, favoring progression of the infection. In the United States active disease is now most frequently diagnosed in nonwhite older males.

IMMUNOLOGIC RESPONSE AND PATHOLOGIC FEATURES

Tuberculosis is the prototype of infections which require cellular immune responses for control. Infection induces a rich antibody response, but what role, if any, these antibodies play in control of infection is not clear. In the first few weeks after established infection, the previously unexposed host has virtually no defense against multiplication of the infectious inoculum either at the initial site or at various metastatic foci established by lymphohematogenous dissemination. During this silent period, lymphocytes genetically coded to react with antigens of the tubercle bacillus proliferate and circulate throughout the lymphatic system. At some interval, usually three to six weeks after infection, the population of specifically reactive lymphocytes usually reaches sufficient size and dissemination to bring the infection under control. The mechanism by which this is accomplished is the elaboration, by reactive lymphocytes in contact with antigen, of a series of lymphocyte products which attract or entrap macrophages at the site of the lymphocyte-antigen interaction, stimulate them to a metabolically more active state in which their mycobactericidal activity is greatly enhanced, and cause some macrophages to differentiate into epithelioid cells and fibroblasts. This sequence of events results in a quite efficient control of infection. However, activated lymphocytes may also elaborate cytotoxic materials which in some instances, particularly when large concentrations of antigen interact with large populations of reactive lymphocytes, may cause cellular necrosis, an event of central importance in the progression of the infection. Although the details of these antigen-lymphocyte-macrophage interactions are by no means clear, *in a general sense tissue hypersensitivity, as manifested by the tuberculin reaction and by cellular necrosis, and cellular immunity, as manifested by successful containment of the infection, are parallel consequences of the appearance of a population of specifically reactive lymphocytes.*

The pathologic response to tuberculous infection is determined in large part by interaction of these two factors, the population of specifically reactive lymphocytes present in the host and the mass of antigen present in the lesion, as modified by structural characteristics of the tissue involved. Small numbers of bacilli in a host with well established lymphocyte reactivity to tuberculosis antigens induce *tubercle formation,* characterized by central multinucleated giant cells surrounded by a cluster of epithelioid cells. More peripherally, lymphocytes are seen admixed with fibroblasts and, in older lesions, fibrosis. Visible bacilli are few or absent. Lesions of this histologic character are termed *productive* and represent successful local containment of infection. When large bacterial concentrations coexist with high levels of lymphocyte reactivity, an exudate rich in fibrin and a nonspecific inflammatory reaction containing polymorphonuclear leukocytes, monocytes, and small numbers of epithelioid and giant cells results; such lesions, termed *exudative,* may progress to *caseous necrosis.* In contrast to many other infections, tissue autolysis in tuberculosis is initially incomplete. The term caseous depicts its cheesy, semisolid, or solid consistency, which appears microscopically as amorphous, homogeneous, eosinophilic material. When specific lymphocyte reactivity has waned because of age or intercurrent illness, and breakdown of a previously quiescent chronic focus leads to extensive bacteremia, the cellular response may be minimal or lacking entirely in the presence of large concentrations of multiplying bacteria in the miliary foci. This histologic picture has been termed *nonreactive tuberculosis.*

Since the histopathologic response is determined in part by local factors, quite different patterns may occur simultaneously in the same individual and even in different parts of the same lesion, some representing progression and some successful containment. In pulmonary caseous foci, for instance, the histologic response at increasing distances from the caseous center (where antigen concentration is greatest) comes more and more to resemble that associated with successful containment of infection, with tubercle formation and fibrosis predominating. It is important to emphasize that these histologic features are not diagnostic of tuberculosis and may be seen in some combination in a wide variety of other conditions.

PATHOGENESIS

The tubercle bacillus requires ready access to oxygen for growth, and even under the most favorable circum-

stances cell division occurs no more frequently than every day or two, explaining the chronic character of tuberculous disease. In unfavorable circumstances it may become metabolically dormant and persist in necrotic tissue for years. Infection by inhalation requires very few bacilli contained in a particle small enough to escape the mucociliary clearance mechanism of the conducting airways and lodge in the air-exchanging portion of the lung (respiratory bronchioles, alveolar ducts, or alveoli). Bacterial multiplication proceeds with little or no reaction, spreads to regional nodes in the hilum of the lung, and thence gains access to the bloodstream. *It is important to emphasize that asymptomatic lymphohematogenous dissemination of the primary infection before the acquisition of tuberculin hypersensitivity probably occurs in all instances; it is this event which sets the stage for the development of chronic pulmonary and extrapulmonary tuberculosis at a later time.* The metastatic bacterial colonies throughout the body also multiply in unimpeded fashion prior to development of tuberculin reactivity. Circulating bacilli are most efficiently cleared from the bloodstream by reticuloendothelial organs, but bacterial multiplication is favored in those areas known to be associated with clinical tuberculosis, most importantly the apices of the lungs, and to a lesser degree the kidneys, richly vascularized skeletal areas, and lymph nodes. The fact that the lung apices provide a particularly favorable environment for metastatic foci of infection has been attributed to the high oxygen tensions in these areas, but this is conjectural.

As mentioned, the subsequent development of *tuberculin hypersensitivity* and *cellular immunity* greatly alters the balance in favor of the host. Activated macrophages reduce the bacterial population at both initial and metastatic foci, and further bacterial growth is inhibited. It is likely, however, that slowly metabolizing viable bacilli persist at most foci. When antigen concentration at the site of initial infection and in the regional lymph nodes is sufficiently large, cellular necrosis may develop and eventually calcify, producing the so-called *Ghon complex.* This roentgenographic finding, for years considered pathognomonic of tuberculosis, is now known to be caused also by certain fungi, notably histoplasmosis and coccidioidomycosis, and other mycobacteria.

FATE OF THE PRIMARY INFECTION. In most people, the infection remains quiescent after the development of tuberculin hypersensitivity and is of no further clinical significance. In an appreciable number, however, infection may evolve into clinical tuberculosis in a number of ways. In some, particularly the very young, the preallergic bacteremia (early hematogenous dissemination) may progress directly into *generalized acute hematogenous tuberculosis.* The resemblance of the resulting disseminated tubercles to millet seeds led to the designation *miliary tuberculosis.* At times it is the strategic location of miliary tubercles rather than progression of the bacteremia which is critical, particularly with respect to development of *tuberculous meningitis,* because subependymal foci in brain or spinal cord may rupture into the subarachnoid space and produce spread of the infection via the subarachnoid fluid. Meningitis may occur in the setting of obvious, progressive bloodstream infection but also may be due to a nonprogressive and otherwise asymptomatic bacteremia.

Local rather than hematogenous events may also determine the outcome. The initial focus may directly evolve into progressive pneumonia (*progressive prima-*

ry); rarely cavitation may result. Large hilar nodes may become necrotic, liquefy, discharge into the bronchial tree, and produce tuberculous pneumonia in this fashion, or, particularly in the young, often partially compress the major bronchi, producing bronchial obstruction and collapse of a pulmonary segment or lobe. When the site of the initial infection is subpleural in location, rupture into the pleural space may occur, producing the clinical picture of *serofibrinous pleurisy with effusion*. A hematogenous focus located near the pleural surface can also produce this syndrome.

Numerically, the most frequent serious sequel of the preallergic bacteremia is chronic pulmonary tuberculosis. Pulmonary sequestration of blood-borne bacteria occurs in a distribution proportional to blood flow, but conditions in the superior and posterior aspects of the lungs greatly favor bacterial multiplication. Over the years it has been a matter of controversy whether chronic apical pulmonary tuberculosis of the so-called *reinfection type* results from breakdown of latent residua seeded at the time of the initial infection (*endogenous reinfection*) or from acquisition of new infection from the environment (*exogenous reinfection*). Many authorities assume that both can occur. However, it now seems likely that exogenous reinfection is considerably less important, and that pulmonary tuberculosis is almost always a direct consequence of the primary infection, with progression (then or later) in that area caused by local factors favoring bacterial growth, whereas the initial focus, when located in the mid or lower lung fields, almost always regresses.

The time at which apical pulmonary tuberculosis appears depends on three factors: first, the period of life in which infection occurs; second, normal, age-dependent factors favoring or inhibiting growth of the apical lesion; and third, non-age-related factors altering resistance. All mortality curves from urban populations in the early part of this century, in which infection in childhood was the rule, demonstrate a peak in the first three years of life owing to the relative deficiency in cellular immunity which characterizes this period of life. In very young children, progressive hematogenous tuberculosis, particularly miliary and meningeal disease, constituted a large part of the over-all mortality. Older prepubertal children (roughly between 5 and 15), although in no way resistant to *infection*, very seldom manifested progressive *disease*. After puberty a second mortality peak was seen, which continued through the second and into the third decade and was more pronounced in females than in males. Thereafter, the death rate continued at a lower level until old age, when a third, less dramatic mortality peak was seen. At present, in countries with low prevalence, clinical tuberculosis is becoming more a disease of the elderly, particularly the older male, presumably caused in part by waning immunologic competence in old age.

As mentioned, persons infected during the disease-resistant period of childhood (roughly 5 to 15) are prone to develop clinical tuberculosis in the postpubertal and early adult period of life, presumably owing to age-dependent host factors favoring evolution of the infection. In contrast, apical pulmonary tuberculosis caused by infection after childhood most often becomes manifest within two years of initial infection. Beyond this period of maximal jeopardy, quiescent foci in the lungs and elsewhere may evolve to produce clinical disease at any time when a combination of local and systemic factors favors reactivation.

The importance of local factors in reactivation of previously quiescent foci is illustrated by development of tuberculous arthritis after joint injury, activation of pulmonary tuberculosis by destructive lung disease such as lung abscess or carcinoma, and the appearance of late hematogenous dissemination after trauma. Thus any tuberculin-positive individual is at risk to develop any form of tuberculosis, often as a result of a remote and clinically undetectable primary infection. The role of immunologic senescence or other processes altering cellular immunity needs to be emphasized; reactivation of tuberculosis becomes progressively likely as individuals become more aged.

ENDOBRONCHIAL SPREAD OF CHRONIC PULMONARY TUBERCULOSIS: THE IMPORTANCE OF CAVITY FORMATION. In contrast to the earliest stages of tuberculous infection in which lymphohematogenous dissemination is the rule, once chronic pulmonary tuberculosis has become established, further spread occurs for the most part via the bronchial tree. The cavity, which is responsible both for progression of pulmonary disease in the individual and for infection of others, has provided the environment which has nurtured the tubercle bacillus through so many centuries of coexistence with the human species. *Especially in the era prior to the availability of effective drugs, cavity formation was the pivotal event in the course of pulmonary tuberculosis, to the prevention or treatment of which most forms of therapy were directed.*

LATE HEMATOGENOUS DISSEMINATION. Foci seeded at the time of the preallergic bacteremia may, after prolonged quiescent periods, break down and liberate bacteria into the bloodstream. Chronic pulmonary foci may cause late bacteremia in this manner, but extrapulmonary and often clinically inapparent foci, particularly in lymph nodes, bones, and the urogenital system, cause most instances of miliary tuberculosis in older individuals.

THE TUBERCULIN TEST

The tuberculin test is best performed by intracutaneous injection of 0.1 ml of purified protein derivative (PPD of Seibert). Proper introduction will be indicated by a raised white area that persists for some minutes after injection. Dosage is expressed in terms of tuberculin units (1 TU is 0.00002 mg; 5 TU is 0.0001 mg; 250 TU is 0.005 mg). In children or in persons with ocular involvement, the 1 TU dose is used. In adults a 5 TU dose is employed first. *Production of visible and palpable induration over 10 mm in diameter after 48 to 72 hours is considered virtually diagnostic of infection with M. tuberculosis.* A smaller reaction is of uncertain significance, because it may be due to other mycobacterial infections. If the test is negative, retesting with 250 TU is carried out. A positive reaction to this larger (second-strength) dosage is also of uncertain significance, because it may reflect cross-reactivity. A negative reaction in a *nonfebrile, relatively well individual* in whom generalized cutaneous anergy can be ruled out by a positive skin test to candida or mumps antigen is strong evidence against tuberculosis. However, as many as 15 per cent or more of persons constitutionally ill with proved tuberculosis may fail to react to 250 TU when first tested, becoming reactive again as health returns. Associated illnesses such as Hodgkin's disease, sarcoidosis, less commonly other neoplasias, and acute infections, notably the viral exanthems, may also cause false negatives. False positives are almost always due to infections with other mycobacterial species. Repeated testing may recall sensitivity to 250 TU in remotely infected individuals in whom reactivity had waned.

FACTORS MODIFYING THE COURSE OF TUBERCULOSIS

Nutritional status, mental and physical stress, and exhaustion modify the course of tuberculosis, as is well illustrated by the peak in mortality statistics observed during the major wars in both belligerent and nonbelligerent nations. *Pregnancy, delivery, and the puerperium,* long regarded as risk periods, have probably been overemphasized. Although statistical evidence is lacking, there is little doubt that *prolonged therapy with corticosteroids* predisposes to exacerbation of tuberculosis, as does *therapy with oncolytic or immunosuppressive agents. Diabetes* predisposes to clinical tuberculosis, and the disease tends to be more fulminant, particularly in young, poorly controlled diabetics. *Silicosis* or *anthracosilicosis* alters host response to tuberculosis in important ways. Instances of infection with the usually nonpathogenic *M. avium* and other mycobacteria of usually decreased virulence is observed in silicotics. Once established, silicotuberculosis may produce massive conglomerate fibrosis with little potential for resolution and little response to antituberculous drugs. Moreover, conglomerate fibrosis often contains quite small bacterial populations held fast within the fibrotic masses, making bacteriologic diagnosis difficult. In times past, *sarcoidosis* was thought to predispose to the progression of tuberculosis, but this no longer appears to be the case. *Hodgkin's disease, leukemia, and other lymphatic neoplasms* are often confused with tuberculosis and may also be complicated by active tuberculosis caused presumably by the detrimental effects of these diseases on cellular immune mechanisms. *Carcinoma* and *destructive infections* such as histoplasmosis, other mycobacterial infections, and lung abscess may erode an old tuberculous focus, releasing tubercle bacilli which may or may not produce disease. Severe viral illness, notably rubella and influenza, may have detrimental effects on the course of tuberculosis. *Gastric resection,* for unknown reasons, favors the progression of previously inactive pulmonary foci, and as many as 4 to 6 per cent will develop active disease. *Pulmonary surgery* may also cause progression of quiescent pulmonary foci. The role of various types of trauma in activating latent foci has been mentioned previously.

PREVENTION OF TUBERCULOSIS

Vaccination

BCG (bacille Calmette Guérin) is a strain of *M. bovis* with attenuated virulence for man. Several large studies have produced convincing evidence that vaccination with an effective strain of BCG in high-risk groups will prevent approximately four of every five cases of active tuberculosis which otherwise would have developed. Also of benefit is the fact that vaccinated persons who do become ill develop less progressive forms of tuberculosis. Miliary and meningeal disease in young children, for instance, is rare after BCG vaccination, a major advantage, considering the gravity of these conditions in the very young. (Disseminated infection with BCG itself is so rare as to be of no importance.)

BCG vaccination programs have been carried out with substantial success in some European countries and the United Kingdom. In the United States the falling rates of infection and disease make vaccination valuable only in specialized circumstances (see below). Tuberculin positivity is induced by BCG, thus destroying the major indicator of early infection, an important consideration weighing against vaccination in areas of low prevalence; the success of isoniazid prophylaxis (see below) is another. Almost all authorities advise the use of BCG in tuberculin-negative children in areas in which 20 per cent or more of secondary schoolchildren are tuberculin positive. (Vaccination is, of course, of no use in tuberculin-positive persons.) Vaccination may also be appropriate for missionary or government personnel prior to assignment to areas of known high prevalence, in groups of health professionals with high (over 20 per cent) incidence of infection, and even in some military personnel. Vaccination of infants born to tuberculous mothers or who must live in known high-risk environments is the procedure of choice, but is compromised somewhat by the problem of keeping the infant isolated for the four- to ten-week period required for development of tuberculin hypersensitivity in response to BCG vaccination.

Chemoprophylaxis

The term chemoprophylaxis has been applied to two distinct situations: first, the treatment of tuberculin-negative individuals in the hope of preventing infection in high-risk situations; and second, treatment of tuberculin-positive persons in the hope of preventing evolution of infection into disease. In a practical sense, it means treatment with isoniazid.

Circumstances in which *infection prophylaxis* (primary prophylaxis) is indicated are few. When an infant cannot be isolated from a mother with active tuberculosis long enough to establish tuberculin hypersensitivity with BCG, isoniazid may be administered to the child until and for a few months after the mother stops discharging tubercle bacilli in the sputum under treatment. When the period of risk cannot be defined, such as in households with recalcitrant infectious patients or in geographic pockets of known high risk, it may be useful to continue therapy for two years or more, because the morbidity associated with meningitis is less in older children. Alternatively, it may be reasonable to stop chemoprophylaxis at some point for a period long enough to achieve vaccination and tuberculin conversion and then to resume therapy for another year, assuming that the conversion might be due to either vaccination or infection, and that in either case protection would result. Prophylactic treatment of tuberculin-negative household contacts of newly discovered patients with active cases, particularly children and young adults, is advised by many. Two and one-half per cent of untreated household contacts will develop active tuberculosis within the next year regardless of tuberculosis status at the time of testing.

Certain exposure to highly contaminated material, as in laboratory accidents or in mouth-to-mouth resuscitation of positive patients, may be covered with prophylactic isoniazid for a period of several months. In the latter situation, attention should be given to the possibility of isoniazid resistance if these data are available, and therapy adjusted accordingly. The status of the tuberculin test during and after treatment should be monitored.

In certain conditions, notably sarcoidosis and Hodgkin's disease, cutaneous anergy may make it impossible to determine whether or not infection has occurred, the roentgenographic and histologic abnormalities may resemble those produced by tuberculosis, and both may require corticosteroid therapy (see below). For these reasons, some persons with sarcoidosis, Hodgkin's disease, and related lymphomas are treated with isoniazid without certain knowledge whether or not infection has in fact occurred. Similarly, prolonged corticosteroid therapy in gravely ill individuals is ordinarily accompanied by isoniazid regardless of tuberculin status.

In contrast, *disease prophylaxis* (secondary prophylaxis) is a frequently employed and well established procedure. Its greatest use is in the *recent tuberculin converter*, which in point of fact represents treatment of an early and active infection. Treatment of children under five years with a positive reaction to a 5 TU dose of tuberculin is recommended without exception. This may also be the case in older persons in whom tuberculin conversion is known to be a relatively recent (within two years) event. Early studies of isoniazid prophylaxis in known recent converters demonstrated an incidence of 5 per cent active tuberculosis within the first year in the nontreated controls. Household contacts of newly discovered patients who are tuberculin positive at the time of contact study and not treated demonstrate a similar incidence of overt disease. This figure probably represents the morbidity of large infections in susceptible age groups, and it is likely that quantitatively smaller inocula in less susceptible age groups produce considerably less disease; nevertheless, the morbidity of a tuberculous infection is substantial during the first 12 to 18 months after infection, and continues to carry some risk throughout life. The protection afforded by treatment of the tuberculin converter persists for many years.

Individuals under 35 with positive (greater than 10 mm induration) reactions to 5 TU in whom prior tuberculin status is not known should in most instances receive chemoprophylaxis. Over that age, the risk of isoniazid-induced hepatitis exceeds the risk of development of active tuberculosis. Reactions requiring large (250 TU) concentrations of tuberculin to be elicited in the well population have entirely different implications and are not taken as evidence of possible recent conversion or indication for treatment.

In addition to treatment of the preclinical infection, as defined above, a number of situations known to be prejudicial to the course of tuberculous infection constitute sufficient reason for chemoprophylaxis in tuberculin-positive individuals. These include *silicosis, severe and poorly controlled diabetes, the postgastrectomy state, progressive neoplastic disease of the lung or of the myeloid or lymphatic systems* (particularly when treatment with oncolytic agents is employed), and *prolonged treatment with corticosteroids.* The occurrence of severe viral illness in a tuberculin-positive individual is regarded by some as an indication for chemoprophylaxis. Persons with an *undiagnosed pulmonary infiltrate and a positive tuberculin reaction*, in whom for one reason or another definitive diagnosis is not indicated, should be given prophylaxis, as the risk for the development of manifest active disease is approximately 1 per cent per year in such individuals. It is essential in such circumstances, however, to ensure that the period of prophylaxis does not serve to postpone appropriate diagnostic approaches for more serious diseases. Similarly, *patients with known presumably inactive tuberculosis who had received either inadequate or no chemotherapy in the past* will demonstrate a similar (approximately 1 per cent per year) rate of relapse and should receive chemoprophylaxis.

Chemoprophylaxis in adults consists of isoniazid in dosage of 300 mg once daily for a period of a year. In children, the dose is 6 to 8 mg per kilogram. The indications for the use of isoniazid in uncertain situations should be balanced against the real risk of hepatotoxicity, particularly in older persons. The incidence of *isoniazid hepatitis* is negligible in those under 20 years of age, 0.3 per cent between 20 and 35, 1.2 per cent between 35 and 50, and 2.3 per cent over 50. In older age groups women are more frequently affected than men. The symptom complex is identical to that of viral hepatitis (nausea, malaise, fever, vomiting, dark urine, and jaundice in some combination), and the histologic picture is also indistinguishable, ranging from mild hepatocellular disease to severe hepatic necrosis or chronic active hepatitis. Prolonged reactions may lead to cirrhosis. Most cases develop within the first two months of treatment, but may occur at any time. Everyone receiving isoniazid should be told of the symptoms of isoniazid hepatitis, and ideally should be seen monthly by a knowledgeable medical worker. If careful surveillance of symptoms is maintained, periodic liver function testing is probably not necessary. The great majority of fatalities have occurred in persons who continued to take isoniazid in spite of recognizable symptoms and signs of liver dysfunction. The presence of established unrelated liver disease complicates the picture. There is no evidence that liver disease predisposes to isoniazid hepatotoxicity, but its detection is more difficult in the presence of unrelated liver disease, and the consequences of hepatotoxicity might be more serious in the presence of an already damaged liver.

167. PULMONARY TUBERCULOSIS

Robert A. Goodwin, Jr.

SYMPTOMATIC PRIMARY INFECTION

The primary infection consists of a small parenchymal focus or cluster of small infiltrates with regional hilar and mediastinal lymphadenitis of varying degrees usually attended by few or no recognizable symptoms. It is more often symptomatic in infants and young children because of an age-related tendency to more extensive lymphadenitis and lymphohematogenous spread, and accordingly has traditionally been termed childhood tuberculosis. At the time of tuberculin conversion, fever and lassitude may be present; rarely *erythema nodosum* or symptomatic inflammation of the eye *(phlyctenular keratoconjunctivitis)* will develop. Hilar lymphadenitis may partially compress the major bronchi, producing a brassy cough and occasionally sputum and localized bronchial obstruction. The chest roentgenogram will often reveal hilar adenopathy, usually unilateral, and at times a small parenchymal infiltrate.

Diagnosis is based on a positive and usually strongly reactive tuberculin test. Acid-fast bacilli may occasionally be found in sputum smears, and cultures positive for *M. tuberculosis* can probably be demonstrated in most patients if obtained repeatedly. Syndromes based on hilar adenopathy, pleural effusion, and, rarely, direct progression of the initial pulmonary infiltrate may be seen.

Hilar adenopathy may compress the small and relatively flaccid bronchi in the very young, producing partial or complete bronchial obstruction and obstructive pneumonitis. Involvement of the bronchial wall and mucosa by direct extension from contiguous tuberculous lymphadenitis can seed tuberculous foci distally. Prolonged obstruction and endobronchial scarring may result in distal bronchiectasis. Occasionally a node will rupture into a bronchus, producing intense bronchitis and pneumonitis which may go into caseation. (This may also occur in the adult [see below].) *Tuberculous pleurisy and effusion* (see Ch. 350.1) is an important and not uncommon complication occurring soon after infection in both children and young adults. Although this syndrome is itself usually self-limited, two thirds of patients will subsequently develop progressive pulmonary or extrapulmonary tuberculosis; accordingly, tuberculin-positive patients with unexplained pleural effusion should be treated as having active tuberculosis unless another cause can be definitely established. The term *progressive primary* connotes direct evolution of the initial infiltrate into a pneumonic, caseous process. It differs from apical chronic pulmonary tuberculosis in that hilar adenopathy is prominent and the process most often involves the middle or lower lung fields.

Features characteristic of childhood tuberculosis may occasionally be seen in young adults, and prominent hilar adenitis may be confused with lymphoma.

TREATMENT. Children are usually given a larger dosage of isoniazid (10 to 15 mg per kilogram) than adults, because the risks of isoniazid toxicity are negligible in the young. An uncomplicated infection is usually treated with isoniazid alone except when drug resistance seems likely on epidemiologic grounds (contact with a known drug-resistant patient). Symptoms resulting from bronchial compression may be benefited by brief corticosteroid treatment (prednisone, 20 to 40 mg daily). Treatment of progressive caseous pulmonary parenchymal disease requires more than one drug.

CHRONIC PULMONARY TUBERCULOSIS

Pulmonary tuberculosis in adults is predominantly an apical parenchymal process almost always caused by evolution of hematogenous foci seeded during the preallergic phase of the initial infection. This may occur fairly promptly or after long periods of quiescence. Whether or not a latent period intervenes, these metastatic foci gain largest size and are therefore most unstable in the superior areas of the lung in which local factors favor bacterial growth.

Chronic pulmonary tuberculosis begins as a small patch of pneumonia surrounding a growing bacterial colony, most commonly in the posterior or apical segment of an upper lobe or the apical segment of a lower lobe. The inflammatory response in the sensitized host produces fibrin-rich alveolar fluid containing a mixture of inflammatory cells. Intense inflammation may progress to caseous necrosis which, while solid, is an effective mechanism of host defense, causing the death of most organisms. (Invariably, however, a few metabolically dormant organisms persist.) However, caseous foci

in upper lung zones have a marked tendency to liquefy and discharge into the bronchial tree, producing a cavity in open communication with inspired air, from which infectious secretions spread via the bronchi to other areas of the lung and to the outside environment. *Once reactivation occurs, the progressive nature of tuberculosis in the sensitized host is largely due to the combination of these factors: (1) the tendency of apical caseous foci to liquefy; (2) the access of liquefied infectious material to the bronchial tree; and (3) the aerobic nature of the organisms, resulting in huge bacterial populations within open cavities.*

Bronchogenic spread of infectious material is enhanced by coughing, which aerosolizes infectious material and then on inhalation distributes it widely throughout the lung. Sooner or later new foci of disease develop, which then may undergo caseous necrosis and then heal, or liquefy, slough, and produce another cavity. New lesions usually appear first in the segment or lobe initially involved, producing scattered, patchy disease. The apical posterior areas of the contralateral lung are quite apt to become involved. In addition to the exudative response, some associated productive tissue reaction is usually found, characterized by giant cells and epithelioid cells forming tubercles and leading eventually to fibrosis and healing. This is particularly true in the anterior and basal portions of the lung, areas which respond to continual bronchogenic seeding from apical cavities with granuloma formation, fibrosis, and scarring but very rarely become necrotic or cavitary. Almost all lesions will contain some mixture of exudative and productive tissue responses, with progression in one area and regression in another. The pace and tempo of progressive disease is highly variable in different individuals and in the same individual at different times. Intercurrent or genetic factors, vigorous hypersensitivity reactions, and large numbers of organisms favor acute and rapidly progressive reactions which may produce confluent pneumonia (*tuberculous pneumonia or phthisis florida*). At the other end of the spectrum, relatively effective immunity and low bacterial populations favor predominantly productive lesions with a greater tendency to spontaneous healing.

Mechanisms of healing are basically the same whether spontaneous or after drug treatment. The exudative component of the early infiltrate may resolve with preservation of normal lung architecture. More often it is replaced with fibrous tissue. Solid caseous foci may become encapsulated by fibrosis. An open cavity occasionally may become obstructed by granulation tissue at the bronchocavitary junction, and become inspissated and encapsulated, producing a tenuous form of healing. An open cavity probably always remains infectious except after prolonged antimicrobial therapy, which may eliminate all necrotic and infectious tissue and result in a clean fibrotic cavity wall. Regardless of the type and extent of healing, however, it is probable that dormant organisms capable of renewed growth and reactivation of disease persist in all cases.

SYMPTOMS. Small apical infiltrates may persist for months or even years in tenuous balance, undergoing minor extensions and regressions and producing no symptoms. Discovery of such cases by chest roentgenogram is a fortunate event. When the infection reaches a certain size, however, absorption of antigenic substances results in entirely nonspecific *constitutional symptoms* such as anorexia, fatigue, fever, chilliness, night sweats, and wasting. Constitutional symptoms usually begin insidiously and progress slowly. Weight loss and fatigue are more likely to lead to medical attention than is fever, usually in the afternoon, which is often unrecognized.

Symptoms resulting from local pulmonary inflammation are also variable in degree and in time of onset. *Cough* and *sputum* are the most consistent, due both to secretions draining from a cavity and to superficial bronchial mucosal and submucosal disease caused by these highly infectious secretions. Their presence indicates advanced disease. Cough may vary from mild to severe, and sputum may be scant and mucoid or copious and purulent.

Hemoptysis and *chest pain* are unpredictable symptoms which cause the patient great concern and are likely to lead to medical attention. Hemoptysis may be due to slough of a caseous lesion or bronchial ulceration. It usually is minor in degree but nevertheless connotes advanced disease. Particularly in late chronic disease, bleeding may be copious and sudden, owing to rupture of an artery within the fibrous walls of a cavity (Rasmussen's aneurysm). Exsanguination is unusual, but, particularly in extensive disease, there may be a real threat of drowning, requiring prompt positioning for drainage (prone or Trendelenburg) and avoidance of drugs which suppress cough. (Hemoptysis may also be due to an aspergilloma in an old healed cavity and so does not necessarily connote reactivation of inactive tuberculosis.) *Pleural pain* usually is due to extension of inflammation to the pleural surface with involvement of the parietal pleura without production of pleural fluid (*dry pleurisy*). Much less commonly, pleural pain will be associated with serofibrinous pleurisy with effusion (which usually occurs prior to established apical pulmonary tuberculosis), and rarely tuberculous empyema will be discovered. Rarely, medical attention is not sought until disease in other tissues bathed in highly infectious pulmonary secretions occurs, such as painful pharyngeal ulcers, hoarseness and dysphagia resulting from laryngeal involvement, tuberculous otitis media, or anal pain caused by a tuberculous perirectal abscess. Shortness of breath is common in pneumonic or extensive destructive disease.

PHYSICAL EXAMINATION. Physical findings usually underestimate the extent of involvement and may be entirely negative even with advanced disease. However, the physical examination provides some information not obtainable in any other way, such as asymmetry in respiratory excursion, contraction of the hemithorax, and deviation of the trachea. Dullness to percussion and increased tactile fremitus are usual over the side of the lesion. Dullness associated with decreased fremitus may detect pleural thickening or pleural fluid. Auscultation may reveal rales, very frequently detected only during quick inspiration following a short cough (posttussic rales). (Interestingly, rales may persist for years after disease has become inactive, presumably because of permanent distortion of small bronchi.) Tubular breath sounds and whispered pectoriloquy may be heard. Distant, hollow tubular breath sounds heard over cavities are termed *amphoric*, as they resemble sounds made by blowing across the mouth of a jar (amphora). Forced hyperventilation may detect local stenosis and obstruction of a bronchus. Scrotal examination may uncover an asymptomatic epididymal nodule. Careful funduscopic examination may reveal choroidal tubercles. Physical findings must be correlated with the chest roentgenogram. Neither is adequate without the other.

ROENTGENOLOGIC FINDINGS. The chest roentgenogram is central to diagnosis, determination of extent and character of disease, and evaluation of response to treatment. Although not diagnostic, the finding of a patchy infiltrate located in the apical posterior area is highly suggestive of tuberculosis. Cavities can usually be seen on the standard posteroanterior chest roentgenogram, but may be missed, and are much more clearly seen with planigrams. Certain histopathologic characteristics of the infiltrates can be estimated from the chest roentgenogram. Exudative lesions tend to have soft indistinct margins. Increased density suggests caseation. Productive lesions tend to be small and nodular with sharply defined margins. Scar tissue produces quite sharp margins and tends to contract. Healing exudative lesions first become smaller and less dense and then, as scarring develops, become more sharply defined. Roentgenographic stability, except for slow further contraction, is one criterion indicating achievement of quiescent or inactive status.

OTHER LABORATORY FINDINGS. A normocytic, normochromic anemia is usual and may be severe. The white blood count is usually normal; a monocytosis of 8 to 15 per cent may be seen. Prolonged and severe infections may cause hyperglobulinemia and hypoalbuminemia. Hematuria or pyuria may disclose coexisting renal tuberculosis; marked albuminuria may indicate amyloidosis. A low serum sodium is sometimes found in extensive chronic pulmonary tuberculosis, more often due to abnormal retention of water (inappropriate secretion of antidiuretic hormone) than to coexistent Addison's disease. It is important to rule out diabetes.

DIAGNOSIS. A strong presumptive diagnosis of tuberculosis may often be made on the basis of roentgenographic characteristics alone. A stained sputum smear positive for acid-fast bacteria on microscopy — a finding usual in extensive disease — will in the proper setting provide nearly conclusive evidence. It must be remembered, however, that any destructive process in the lung, particularly in the apical posterior area, may erode an inactive focus and cause appearance of acid-fast bacilli in the sputum with or without development of new, active tuberculosis. A positive tuberculin test, although of great use in children, has limited diagnostic significance in older age groups. A negative reaction to 250 TU when a positive reaction to candida or mumps antigen indicates that anergy is not present is very strong but still not completely conclusive evidence against active tuberculosis. *Histologic demonstration of granulomatous disease* provides only presumptive evidence of tuberculosis, and even demonstration of acid-fast bacteria is not definitive in that they may represent mycobacteria other than *M. tuberculosis*. Definitive diagnosis requires culture and speciation of the organism.

DIFFERENTIAL DIAGNOSIS. Although tuberculosis may be confused with virtually any intrathoracic condition, certain diseases are frequently considered in differential diagnosis. *Fungal disease,* particularly histoplasmosis, and disease caused by other mycobacteria can be indistinguishable from chronic cavitary or fibroid tuberculosis. (Coexistence of histoplasmosis and tuberculosis in the same individual is not rare.) *Bronchiectasis* may present with symptoms suggesting tuberculosis, and bronchiectatic and emphysematous areas surrounded by infiltrate may mimic cavitation roentgenographically. *Cavitary lung abscess* often involves the dorsal segments of the lower lobes and posterior segments of the upper lobes owing to patterns of aspiration during unconsciousness. Typically lung abscess causes little in the way of physical findings, may have a fluid level, and is not associated with patchy bronchogenic infiltrates; in contrast, physical findings are prominent over tuberculous cavities, fluid levels are rare, and patchy infiltrates elsewhere are the rule. *Acute bacterial pneumonias* may resemble florid tuberculosis in all particulars except for the sputum examination and response to antimicrobial drugs. *Neoplasm* may resemble tuberculosis, as in an isolated coin lesion, an obstructing and inconspicuous endobronchial tumor causing distal chronic inflammation, or a caviting neoplastic mass. (An irregular cavity wall suggests necrotic neoplasm.) The association between neoplasm and tuberculosis is complex: first, in that cancer may erode into and reactivate a latent tuberculous focus; second, in that saprophytic mycobacteria may be found in association with a destructive neoplasm; and third, in that chronic scarring in a tuberculous focus may induce neoplastic degeneration. New roentgenographic progression of a previously stable, fibrotic tuberculous focus may be due to "scar cancer" rather than progressive infection.

LOWER AND MIDDLE LOBE TUBERCULOSIS IN OLDER INDIVIDUALS. As tuberculosis in young adults becomes less frequent, certain atypical presentations in older individuals are being recognized. A progressive infiltrate in the lower or mid-lung field may rarely be due to a progressive primary infection, presumably because of deficient immune mechanisms in the elderly. Also, tuberculous hilar lymph nodes from a remote infection may rupture into a bronchus, causing tuberculous pneumonia in the associated lobe or segment. For some unexplained reason, middle lobe tuberculosis is not uncommon in diabetics.

CLASSIFICATION OF PULMONARY TUBERCULOSIS. Previous classifications included the following description of the extent of disease. *Minimal:* the total area of disease, taken in the aggregate, is less than the area from the second chondrocostal junction and the fifth vertebral body to the apex of the lung on one side, and no cavity is demonstrable (planigrams usually required). *Moderately advanced:* The aggregate total area of scattered, small lesions is less than one lung field, or of dense, confluent lesions less than the equivalent of one third of one lung field. The total diameter of cavitation, if present, is less than 4 cm. *Far advanced:* Disease greater in extent than moderately advanced.

The present classification (American Thoracic Society, 1974) is as follows:

0. No tuberculosis exposure, not infected (no history of exposure, negative tuberculin skin test).
I. Tuberculosis exposure, no evidence of infection (history of exposure, negative tuberculin skin test).
II. Tuberculous infection, without disease (positive tuberculin skin test, negative bacteriologic studies (if done), no roentgenographic findings compatible with tuberculosis, no symptoms due to tuberculosis). Chemotherapy status (preventive therapy), dates, if given.
III. Tuberculosis: infected, with disease.

The current status of the patient's tuberculosis shall be described by the following characteristics:

A. Location of disease (e.g., pulmonary, pleural, lymphatic).
B. Bacteriologic status (microscopy and culture with dates).
C. Chemotherapy status (give dates).

TREATMENT OF PULMONARY TUBERCULOSIS

Treatment of pulmonary tuberculosis, long the province of specialized physicians in special hospitals, now is properly the responsibility of the general internist. Although in most instances treatment is best initiated in a hospital setting, providing easier accomplishment of laboratory studies and perhaps more importantly a period in which education of the patient and the family

can be accomplished, it is perfectly acceptable in individuals who are not in poor health otherwise to initiate and complete therapy entirely in an outpatient setting. It is well established that individuals on treatment very promptly become noninfectious for others in the environment even when sputum smears and cultures remain positive. If the patient can be taught to cough into tissue and to maintain a brief period of modified separation from the rest of the family, it is probable that serious infectiousness ceases entirely with initiation of therapy, or a week or two thereafter, and even the minor risk of infectiousness within that initial period is hardly of consequence compared to the risk already undergone by those in the patient's environment prior to diagnosis. The crux of tuberculosis control is diagnosis and treatment of the patient and proper investigation and treatment of contacts (see Chemoprophylaxis in Ch. 166) and not patient isolation. It should be restated that tuberculosis is communicated by aerosolized secretions and not at all by fomites. Competent treatment requires knowledge of the antituberculosis drugs, an understanding of the principles of combined and prolonged drug therapy, and an appreciation of how cases should be followed, particularly with regard to monitoring of patient compliance and the development of drug resistance. Effective use of drugs now available should provide cure in 95 to 100 per cent of previously untreated cases. In actual practice, results are less satisfactory. In part this may reflect poor medical direction, but much more important is the often carefully obscured failure of the patient to follow his drug regimen.

THE ANTITUBERCULOSIS DRUGS. *Isoniazid* (INH) remains the keystone of original treatment of pulmonary tuberculosis. It is highly effective (bactericidal against actively metabolizing cells, bacteriostatic against metabolically dormant cells), well absorbed, distributed throughout all tissues in effective concentrations, of low toxicity, and inexpensive. Drug resistance may emerge in the presence of very large bacterial populations such as are associated with pulmonary or renal cavities, and one or more companion drugs must be added to prevent this. However, INH, in contrast to all other antituberculosis drugs, may retain some in vivo effectiveness even when in vitro studies indicate resistance, probably owing in part to a slightly decreased pathogenicity of INH-resistant strains. Accordingly, it is advisable *in all regimens not continuing rifampin* to continue administration of INH in spite of development of in vitro resistance, while adding other effective drugs. The marginal benefit of continuing INH when rifampin is added to INH-resistant infections does not at present justify the increased risk of hepatotoxicity of INH-rifampin in combination. The incidence of INH-resistant isolates from previously untreated patients has remained for some years at approximately 2 per cent in the United States and England, although in other areas this figure may be higher. Allergic reactions to INH are uncommon. Transient elevations of SGOT occur in 10 per cent of patients, and INH-related hepatitis, reversible in its early stages, occurs in less than 1 per cent. (See Chemoprophylaxis in Ch. 166.) INH depletes body pyridoxine stores and may induce peripheral neuritis, particularly in nutritionally compromised patients such as alcoholics. Pyridoxine (50 mg a day) is often given with INH and is mandatory with doses greater than 300 mg daily and in severe alcoholics. INH dosage is 5 mg per kilogram of body weight, which in most adults usually is rounded off to 300 mg in a single daily dose. Larger doses (10 to 15 mg per kilogram) may be given at cost of greater toxicity (pyridoxine always added) in extensive caseous disease and in INH-resistant infections, particularly when supporting drug therapy is weak.

Rifampin (RMP) is a new antituberculosis agent of the same order of effectiveness, low incidence of toxicity, and high degree of patient acceptance as INH. It is expensive. Its effectiveness (with companion drugs) in INH-resistant treatment failures has radically changed the prognosis in such cases from uncertain at best to favorable in the majority. Its role in initial treatment has yet to be established. Clinical evidence in studies of short-term (six- to nine-month) chemotherapy indicates that RMP plus INH is more effective than any other regimen, resulting in fewer relapses after discontinuation of therapy than is the case with any other regimen administered for this period of time. However, when therapy is continued for 18 months, as is routinely recommended although at times hard to achieve, there is no advantage to the combined use of these two most potent agents. Further, hepatotoxicity is increased by the use of INH and RMP together in comparison to regimens containing only one or the other. Finally, in contrast to INH, RMP loses all effectiveness when resistant strains emerge. At present it seems justifiable to employ both agents in treatment of cases of extraordinary gravity such as extensive miliary or caseous pulmonary tuberculosis associated with marked debility. At the time of this writing, however, it is the author's practice to reserve RMP for retreatment in the usual case of pulmonary tuberculosis when it seems likely that compliance with 18 months of drug treatment can be achieved.

RMP is excreted by the liver and should be used cautiously in the presence of liver disease. Rarely it may cause bilirubinemia, usually with larger than ordinary dosage. Thrombocytopenic purpura and a serum sickness type of reaction have been observed. These allergic phenomena are rare at conventional daily dosage but are not uncommon when larger than usual dosage and intervals greater than 24 hours are employed. Therefore use of RMP in intermittent courses is not recommended. The recommended dosage is 450 to 600 mg administered by mouth in a single daily dose given at least an hour before or after meals, as food delays absorption. At the beginning of treatment RMP colors the urine a reddish orange, a somewhat alarming finding to which the patient should be alerted.

Streptomycin (SM) is substantially less effective than INH or RMP but more effective than any other agent. It is often administered for a few months as the third drug in three-drug therapy (INH ± ethambutol + SM) of severe disease. In conjunction with INH, it offers a strong two-drug regimen for hospitalized patients. In the unusual situation in which neither INH or RMP can be used, SM in combination with two other drugs, optimally including pyrazinamide (see below), provides acceptable therapy. SM is excreted by the kidneys, and toxic levels may develop when renal function is compromised. Eighth nerve toxicity (especially the vestibular branch) is a troublesome complication, more serious in those over 50 in whom the ability to compensate for loss of vestibular function is less effective. SM is administered intramuscularly in a dose of 1 gram daily during the first few months of treatment, but may be reduced to 1 gram two or three times weekly thereafter.

Ethambutol * (EMB) is the most useful oral companion drug for INH (replacing PAS) in original treatment cases, and, if not previously used, for RMP in retreatment (INH-resistant) cases. A tendency to induce optic neuritis (loss of visual acuity, field constriction, and loss of green color discrimination) limits dosage. An acceptable incidence of 2 per cent allows the use of 25 mg per kilogram of body weight in hospitalized patients, but 15 to 20 mg per kilogram is recommended for outpatient treatment, at which dosage the incidence of optic neuritis is negligible.

Para-aminosalicylic acid (PAS), the principal companion drug to INH for years, has now been replaced by the much less toxic EMB. PAS is difficult to take and poorly tolerated because of gastric irritation. In addition, it causes serious hypersensitivity reactions more frequently than any other antituberculosis drug. PAS is now used mainly as a companion drug in retreatment cases with limited drug options. It is usually administered as the sodium salt in a dose of 5 grams three times daily with meals or 10 grams in a single daily dose given on a full stomach.

Pyrazinamide (PZA) follows SM in antimicrobial effectiveness, but its value is limited by early development of drug resistance (as early as six weeks in an active infection). This may be offset by its use with multiple drugs, with a strong drug, or in an already fairly well controlled infection. SM plus PZA is a good combination. Hepatotoxicity is a limiting factor, with 15 per cent showing altered liver function tests and 3 per cent frank jaundice, and with reported fatal hepatitis as high as 1 per cent. The usual oral dosage is a total of 2 to 3 grams daily given in two to three divided doses.

Ethionamide (ETH) is moderately effective in retreatment cases as a companion drug with a strong agent or as one of three or more weak drugs. Patient intolerance is moderately high due to central nervous system mediated nausea. It is administered by mouth in a dose of 500 to 1000 mg daily, most often as 250 mg three times daily.

Cycloserine * (CS) is a toxic and rather ineffective drug used in retreatment with a strong drug or as a member of a three or more drug combination. Its tendency to induce a variety of central nervous system symptoms, including convulsions, limits the dosage to 0.5 to 1.0 gram daily, the lower being of questionable effectiveness and the higher a dose that few tolerate. A regimen of 250 mg three times daily is a reasonable compromise.

Capreomycin * (CM) is an aminoglycoside approaching SM in effectiveness, with similar dosage requirements and toxicity. There is no cross-resistance with SM and in general it can be substituted for that drug, but it is best to include it in a three-drug regimen.

Viomycin * (VM) and *kanamycin* (KM), aminoglycosides less effective and more toxic than SM or CM, are used only in retreatment with quite limited antimicrobial drug resources. The aminoglycosides have additive toxicities, and only one can be used at a time.

COMBINED DRUG THEAPY. Drug resistance may be *primary* (in previously untreated patients) or may emerge during treatment. Although a matter of continuing concern, primary resistance is not yet a major problem in most areas. Continuing surveys in the United States and Great Britain indicate a rather stable level of 2 to 3 per cent of previously untreated infections primarily resistant to either INH or SM, and less than 1 per cent to both drugs. However, some careful studies have demonstrated a higher incidence of primary drug resistance in children in urban areas of known high prevalence.

Drug resistance emerging during treatment is a major problem recognized ever since earliest drug trials. Canetti's detailed studies provide insight into the mechanisms of this phenomenon. Naturally occurring mutants resistant to INH appear at a predictable rate of 1 per 10^5 or 10^6 bacterial cells. This is true with respect to SM and in general other antituberculosis drugs. When INH is administered alone and the bacterial population is large, drug-susceptible cells are killed or suppressed and resistant mutants may in time repopulate the site of infection. This is of little practical importance in closed (noncavitary) lesions with a low bacterial population (10^3 to 10^5 cells per gram tissue), but is extremely important in open cavitary lesions associated with huge bacterial populations. Pulmonary cavities usually contain 10^7 to 10^9 but occasionally 10^{10} or more organisms; therefore as many as 10^3 or more INH-resistant bacteria might be present from the outset, providing an ample nidus for establishment of a drug-resistant infection once the larger susceptible population is suppressed. Under these circumstances, significant numbers of resistant organisms may appear in the sputum in a few weeks, and after three to four months the major portion

---

*Conditions for safe use in children have not been established. The Editors.

*Conditions for safe use in children have not been established. The Editors.

of the bacterial population may be INH-resistant. If two effective drugs are used at the same time and organisms resistant to each are present in a ratio of 1 to 10^5 bacterial cells, then the population of organisms resistant to both would be approximately 1 in 10^{10} bacteria, making emergence of resistance unlikely. This is the basis of the principle of combined therapy in which two or more effective drugs are used, each active against organisms resistant to the other (see Ch. 189).

If in the course of treatment the development of drug resistance appears to be threatening (continued presence of significant numbers of tubercle bacilli in the sputum after three to four months), caution should be exercised in introducing a single new drug without ensuring (recent drug susceptibility studies) the presence of at least one other drug to which the organisms are known to be susceptible. When in doubt, it is best to add two new drugs in compliance with the principle of combined therapy.

PROLONGED THERAPY. The principle of prolonged therapy was also established early by the occurrence of relapse when treatment was terminated too soon because of limited supplies of drug. Such relapses were ordinarily due to organisms still susceptible to the agents administered. Since the antituberculosis drugs are bacteriostatic for dormant organisms, suppressive therapy must be continued until the slow processes of host healing mechanisms secure control of residual infection. This usually means a treatment course of at least 18 months, and in advanced disease 24 months. As discussed below, the exceptions to this rule are drug regimens containing both INH and RMP. As brief a period as nine or even six months' treatment with these have produced results comparable to 18 months' treatment with standard, INH-containing regimens, but at a cost of greater hepatotoxicity and the disadvantage of not having RMP in reserve should treatment fail.

INITIAL TREATMENT. In the initial treatment of pulmonary tuberculosis, the most generally used *all-purpose* drug regimen is *SM (two months) + INH + EMB* for 18 months (SM, 1 gram daily first two months; INH, 300 mg, and EMB, 25 mg per kilogram, first three months, then 15 mg per kilogram thereafter — all given in a single daily dose). However, a more individualized approach is recommended when feasible, taking into account first the character of the disease and then patient response in order to minimize drug toxicity by reducing drug coverage on the one hand and giving added drug support when needed on the other. Based on the character of the disease, the following drug regimens are recommended for initiation of therapy: *(1) Double therapy, INH + EMB in usual mild or moderate disease with small infiltrates and thin-walled cavities, and (2) triple therapy, SM (until sputum conversion) + INH + EMB in extensive and severe disease, particularly when large areas of caseation or thick-walled cavities are identified.*

The rate of disappearance of tubercle bacilli from the sputum is an important prognostic event during the course of drug therapy. Although there is some correlation of severity of disease and persistence of organisms in the sputum, this is not predictable, and some as yet not understood biologic relationship between host, organisms, and drugs also determines whether patients are "rapid converters" or "slow converters." Slow sputum conversion favors drug resistance and a greater tendency to relapse if drug therapy is terminated too soon. Tubercle bacilli may disappear from the sputum by smear and culture as early as one month into drug treatment even in extensive disease, but more often sputum conversion takes place between the first and third months of treatment. Beyond this point the continued presence of organisms in the sputum defines the slow converter (if lapse in drug taking can be excluded), and after four to six months of continued discharge of tubercle bacilli in the sputum drug resistance is very likely to have developed.

The better prognosis of those who show prompt sputum conversion on either the two- or three-drug regimen allows safe termination of treatment in 18 months, and, in addition, drug coverage may be reduced to INH alone during the suppressive phase of treatment beginning six months after tubercle bacilli have disappeared from the sputum. On the other hand, the continued presence of tubercle bacilli in the sputum four months or more into drug therapy (even in the absence of drug resistance) indicates the need for more prolonged and vigorous therapy. Consequently, it is recommended that drug therapy be continued for a total of 24 months and that at least two drugs (INH and EMB) be used throughout (in the triple-drug regimen SM is best continued at least until reversal of infectiousness has been demonstrated).

Because of the threat of drug resistance when tubercle bacilli persist in the sputum well beyond four months into drug therapy, drug susceptibility studies are critically important at this time. The introduction of *two new drugs* (SM + PAS or RMP + SM) is advisable in a threatening situation pending report of drug susceptibility studies. Further therapy for a total of 24 months should be based on at least two drugs to which the organism is shown to be susceptible (or to which it has not previously been exposed), including one strong drug (INH, RMP, or SM).

Ordinarily a bacteriologic diagnosis is established at least by microscopy before institution of drugs. If smears are negative on microscopy, five or six adequate sputum specimens should be submitted for culture before initiating drug therapy. In severely ill patients, drugs should be started immediately, because a few days of antituberculosis drugs will not interfere with demonstration of tubercle bacilli on sputum smear or culture. Monthly chest roentgenograms allow adequate monitoring of the active course of the disease, and three monthly intervals suffice during healing stages. After the first month and before reversal of infectiousness, it is best to obtain sputum specimens at fortnightly intervals in order to detect either disappearance of the bacilli or early evidence of drug resistance. Drug susceptibility studies for the commonly used drugs should be obtained before treatment, and again in three or four months if sputum remains positive, or at any time of bacteriologic relapse.

All patients receiving INH should be instructed regarding symptoms suggestive of hepatitis and questioned concerning these at monthly intervals (see Chemoprophylaxis in Ch. 166). Patients receiving EMB should be questioned regarding visual symptoms; if they are receiving high doses, visual acuity (Snellen chart) and green color perception should be tested regularly. Patients receiving SM should be questioned concerning hearing and vestibular function and tested regularly for high frequency loss if over 50 years of age.

In patients with marked debility and severe constitutional symptoms, *corticosteroid therapy* in relatively low doses (30 mg daily of prednisone) will usually effect prompt symptomatic improvement, decrease fever, and promptly repair serious anemia when this is present. It is usually possible to taper the dose by 2.5-mg decrements every four or five days. In the rare instance of hypoxia resulting from a diffusion defect, usually in severe miliary tuberculosis but also observed in extensive bronchogenic dissemination, a larger dosage of corticosteroids (60 to 80 mg of prednisone daily) may be necessary for a few days before quickly decreasing to 30 mg of prednisone daily and then tapering. The unusual coexistence of Addison's disease and active pulmonary tuberculosis should be borne in mind. The adverse effect of steroids on tuberculous infection can be disregarded in the presence of effective antituberculosis drug therapy.

TREATMENT OF THE NONCOMPLIANT PATIENT. Patient failure to take drugs is the most frequent and important cause of treatment failure. There are many reasons such as simple forgetfulness, the illusion of health associated with the disappearance of symptoms, and the always underestimated reluctance of almost all persons to subject themselves to any discipline for prolonged periods. Alcoholics are almost predictably noncompliant and should probably be always regarded as potentially so. It is impossible to overemphasize the importance of a suspicious attitude regarding compliance with therapy. Every physician who treats tuberculosis has often observed relapse in a patient who indignantly maintains that he has taken his drugs faithfully — only to find that the infection is still drug susceptible and that the disease promptly responds to the same drugs given under supervision.

Two treatment methods have been applied successfully to the management of tuberculosis in alcoholics and other noncompliant patients. *Short-term chemotherapy,* using INH (300 mg) plus RMP (600 mg) daily, possibly with the addition of SM (1 gram) or PZA (1 gram twice a day), or both, is given under supervision for a period of six months. This ordinarily requires hospitalization. If completed successfully, this short-term vigorous course is thought to be comparable to 18 months of standard therapy. Continued suppressive therapy with INH is recommended for another 6 to 12 months, but in this circumstance noncompliance is less important. *Intermittent chemotherapy,* usually provided by a public health clinic and usually requiring some means of bringing the patient to the clinic or the medications to the patient, has been successful throughout the world. In the United States, an initial period of intensive hospital treatment as outlined above (usually two to three months) is followed by an intermittent twice weekly drug regimen of either (1) INH, 15 mg per kilogram orally, plus EMB, 50 mg per kilogram orally,* or (2) INH, 15 mg per kilogram orally, plus SM, 25 to 30 mg per kilogram intramuscularly, given for a total of 18 months. RMP is not recommended in intermittent therapy because of the tendency to allergic reactions under these circumstances.

RETREATMENT. In most retreatment circumstances it is very important that the patient be managed in a hospital experienced with tuberculosis. Expert judgment is particularly important in drug-resistant tuberculosis in order to attain maximal effectiveness from limited drug resources. The determination of the susceptibility of the organism to all available drugs is critical to proper management.

In drug-resistant infections, RMP, if it has been held in reserve, offers an excellent chance for final successful treatment when combined with one other drug to which the organism is susceptible and under circumstances guaranteeing uninterrupted drug ingestion for at least 24 months. An infinite variety of circumstances attends each retreatment case. Some of these, along with certain principles of retreatment, are tabulated here: (1) A relapse following prompt reversal of infectiousness almost always indicates that drugs have been stopped too soon, usually by the patient. If drugs were stopped completely, most will harbor drug-susceptible strains and respond again to the initial drug regimen. (2) If lapse in treatment and relapse are followed by irregular drug ingestion, resistant organisms will probably be present. (3) A patient with tubercle bacilli in the sputum after more than four to six months of treatment is probably excreting drug-resistant organisms. (4) Under circumstances of suspected or presumed drug resistance, a two- or three-drug combination, including an unused strong drug (INH, RMP, SM) and an unused companion type drug (EMB, PZA, ETH, PAS, CS), may be added to drugs previously given while awaiting drug susceptibility studies. (5) CM can replace SM in the aforementioned regimens. VM and KM are less effective and more toxic, and their use is limited to last-resort situations. (6) SM, CM, VM, and KM have similar and additive toxicities, and no more than one should be used at the same time. (7) If only drugs of limited effectiveness remain available (ETH, CS, PAS, and either VM or KM), three or four should be used at the same time and INH also given in high dosage (15 mg per kilogram). INH-resistant strains are less pathogenic and more susceptible to the weaker drugs, and INH should therefore be given in high dosage even though drug resistance is already established.

OTHER FORMS OF TREATMENT. Bed Rest. Modified bed rest is beneficial during symptomatic disease, but its effect is insignificant compared to drugs in over-all therapy. In treatment failures resistant to all drugs, modified bed rest and continued use of INH may together in time salvage many apparently hopeless cases. In retreatment cases with resistance to all but the weakest drugs, modified bed rest will improve chance of success.

Surgery. Surgery is now rarely used in the treatment of pulmonary tuberculosis. However, surgical resection may still occasionally have a place in treatment failures with residual cavities and meager drug resources or when lack of patient cooperation compromises the prospects of successful use of limited drug resources. Here experienced judgment is critically important.

DURATION OF OBSERVATION. The incidence of relapse following adequate antimicrobial therapy of tuberculosis is of such a low order that the time-honored custom of long-term or lifelong follow-up of patients with tuberculosis is no longer considered necessary by many authorities. Therefore, routine follow-up chest roentgenogram and sputum examinations after successful treatment are no longer considered important. However, exception should be made in the case of unusually extensive disease, unusually slow bacteriologic response to treatment, patients in whom there is reason to question faithfulness of drug taking, and certain high-risk patients such as diabetics.

---

*See p. vi, Dosage Notice, immediately following Preface.

168. EXTRAPULMONARY TUBERCULOSIS

Roger Des Prez

168.1. INTRODUCTION

Extrapulmonary tuberculosis falls into two groups on the basis of pathogenesis. The first comprises conditions resulting from *lymphohematogenous dissemination,* (*miliary tuberculosis, tuberculosis of bone and joints, renal tuberculosis,* most cases of *tuberculous lymphadenitis, female genital tuberculosis, peritonitis, pericarditis, meningitis,* and some instances of *pleural effusion and tuberculous laryngitis).* These illnesses may coexist with tuberculosis elsewhere or *may be isolated clinical manifestations.* The second comprises conditions which complicate pulmonary tuberculosis caused either by bronchial or gastrointestinal spread of infectious secretions *(intracanalicular spread),* or by direct contiguous invasion (pleura, pericardium, esophagus). Urogenital tuberculosis may represent a combination when a hematogenous renal focus cavitates and seeds the lower urinary tract via the ureter.

168.2. PRINCIPLES OF DRUG THERAPY

Most extrapulmonary tuberculosis responds more readily to drugs than does advanced pulmonary tuberculosis, because the bacterial populations are small. The exception is cavitary renal tuberculosis, which may contain large bacterial populations requiring combined drug therapy. In the remainder, the likelihood of drug resistance developing on therapy is negligible, and the choice of a drug regimen depends on how life threatening the illness is judged to be. Those conditions carrying a threat of early mortality (miliary and meningeal tuberculosis, and probably spondylitis and pericarditis) are treated with maximal drug therapy (isoniazid and daily streptomycin, or isoniazid and rifampin) at least until response is established, thus increasing antimicrobial potency and eliminating the small possibility of a primarily isoniazid-resistant infection. Less threatening conditions such as involvement of serous membranes, lymph nodes, the skeletal system (excluding the spine), and genital tuberculosis are treated with isoniazid and ethambutol for 18 to 24 months. Although not widely accepted, some authorities treat these conditions with isoniazid alone. As a rule, response is good. When it is not, other drugs may be added without significant loss (see Treatment in Ch. 167).

168.3. TUBERCULOSIS OF THE PLEURA

Subpleural foci established during the preallergic bacillemic phase of the primary infection may, when tuberculin hypersensitivity develops, rupture into the pleural space, evoking a brisk allergic reaction and the clinical syndrome of *primary serofibrinous pleurisy with effusion.* This occurrence, of itself usually unilateral and self-limiting, is important in identifying rather extensive initial (primary) infections which are very likely to result in progressive tuberculosis elsewhere at a later time. Unilateral or bilateral pleural effusion, occasionally with concurrent tuberculous peritonitis or pericarditis, may also result from subpleural foci established as a part of acute or subacute hematogenous (miliary) tuberculosis. Established chronic pulmonary tuberculosis more frequently causes local inflammation and visceral-parietal pleural adhesions (dry pleurisy), precluding sudden delivery of large amounts of antigenic material into the pleural cavity. However, uncommonly, serofibrinous pleurisy with effusion can complicate chronic pulmonary foci, and, rarely, rupture of a necrotic chronic focus into the pleural space may produce tuberculous empyema and bronchopleural fistula (see Ch. 350.1 for a more complete discussion).

168.4. ENDOBRONCHIAL TUBERCULOSIS

Cavitary tuberculosis inevitably produces bronchial mucosal infection in the immediate vicinity of the cavity and usually in spotty distribution elsewhere. In the days before drug therapy, such involvement at times obstructed the bronchocavitary junction or even a whole segment or lobe, with subsequent inspissation, fibrosis, and contraction, an important although tenuous healing mechanism. Superficial bronchial lesions respond promptly to chemotherapy, and now usually require little attention. However, partial degrees of bronchial cicatrization may cause nontuberculous complications such as atelectasis and obstructive pneumonitis, and rarely may produce complete obstruction of a bronchus even during the course of chemotherapy. Some degree of permanent bronchial distortion probably occurs in all moderately extensive pulmonary tuberculosis. Tuberculosis of the trachea, now rare, is an extension of florid endobronchial tuberculosis. The consequences of bronchial involvement in childhood are discussed in Ch. 167.

168.5. TUBERCULOSIS OF THE LARYNX

Prior to drug therapy, tuberculosis of the larynx was a dread late complication of extensive pulmonary tuberculosis. The onset of hoarseness, dysphagia, and perhaps pain, sometimes referred to the ear, often initiated a downhill course, with extensive bronchogenic spread throughout both lung fields from copious, thin, laryngeal secretions. This is now almost never seen, even in patients with a drug-resistant strain and highly infectious sputum. Rarely isolated tuberculous ulcers or nodules with intact mucosa, resembling carcinoma, are diagnosed either by biopsy or by association with active pulmonary tuberculosis. Laryngeal lesions are now more commonly seeded via the bloodstream, usually accompanied by hematogenous involvement of the lung as well, but rarely as a clinically isolated focus. Pain, often accentuated by swallowing, and hoarseness are prominent symptoms. Response to drug therapy is excellent and surgery usually unnecessary.

168.6. GASTROINTESTINAL TUBERCULOSIS

Gastrointestinal tuberculosis frequently complicated extensive pulmonary tuberculosis in years past, and also was caused by ingestion of contaminated milk. It is now rare, but occasionally complaints related to a gastrointestinal focus may lead to recognition of pulmonary tuberculosis; even more rarely, gastrointestinal tuberculosis presents in the absence of recognizable active pulmonary disease.

Tuberculosis of the tongue and mouth may present as painful ulcers or as a nonhealing tooth socket after dental extraction. Untreated, the process is indolently progressive, but response to chemotherapy is rapid. Extension of oropharyngeal disease via the eustachian tube may produce *tuberculosis of the middle ear and mastoid bone. Tuberculosis of the tonsil and pharyngeal lymphatic tissue* was common when bovine tuberculosis was epidemic; draining regional nodes were termed *scrofula. Tuberculosis of the esophagus* may very rarely result from penetration of an adjacent node, leading to bronchoesophageal fistula or to ulcerative or hyperplastic disease on the esophageal wall. *Tuberculosis of the stomach,* rare even when untreated pulmonary tuberculosis was common, has been described as resembling diffuse neoplastic involvement (linitis plastica type) or nonhealing ulcers, and may, if caused by extension from an adjacent lymph node focus, present as an isolated clinical manifestation. Hyperplastic or ulcerative *duodenal tuberculosis* may resemble peptic or neoplastic obstructive disease. Tuberculosis of the intestine may produce ulceration with bleeding and a tendency to perforation and fistula formation, hyperplasia with obstructive symptoms, or a combination of the two. *Tuberculosis of the small intestine* is more liable to produce perforation than disease elsewhere in the bowel. *Ileocecal tuberculosis* is the most frequently observed form of bowel involvement, presumably because of cecal pooling of infectious fecal material producing mucosal disease, occult bleeding, obstruction, or fistula formation. *Tuberculosis of the ascending and transverse colon* is much less common, and may present as a concentric, hyperplastic lesion producing obstruction. *Tuberculosis of the sigmoid colon* may resemble carcinoma, atypical ulcerative colitis, or diverticulitis. All these lesions may perforate and produce *tuberculous perirectal and pelvic abscesses and fistula in ano.* Diagnosis is now almost always an unexpected finding at surgery, but if it is established by nonsurgical means, the effects of chemotherapy should be determined. Even advanced lesions usually respond satisfactorily, but occasionally death results in spite of chemotherapy and surgery.

168.7. MILIARY TUBERCULOSIS

The term *acute miliary tuberculosis* was coined to describe the appearance of lungs and other organs from fatal cases of progressive tuberculous bacteremia in which the disseminated small tubercles suggested millet seeds. It is at present applied to the more extensive and acute form of hematogenous (bloodstream) dissemination. The hematogenous phase of the primary infection is especially liable to evolve into miliary tuberculosis in very young children and, together with the

associated meningitis, accounts for most tuberculosis deaths in this age group. In adults miliary tuberculosis may be an early sequel of the primary infection as in children, or may be due to old residua of remote infections which reactivate, undergo necrosis, and seed the circulation. A pulmonary focus may be responsible, but more frequently a previously undetected or clinically undetectable lymphatic, genitourinary, or skeletal focus is the cause. Such foci may cause multiple bacteremic episodes, and the process may be protracted, intermittent, and low grade (chronic hematogenous tuberculosis). Host factors such as debility; advanced age; intercurrent therapy with oncolytic agents, immunosuppressives, or corticosteroid hormones; malignant disease, particularly of the lymphatic and hematopoietic systems; and occasionally local injury are frequently associated with activation of latent foci.

CLINICAL FEATURES AND DIAGNOSIS. **Acute Miliary Tuberculosis.** In the very young, the illness is usually an acute and severe illness, with high intermittent fevers, night sweats, and occasionally rigors. Complications such as pleural effusion, peritonitis, or meningitis occur in as many as two thirds, usually developing several weeks after the onset of constitutional symptoms. A similar acute illness may occur in adults as well. The onset, although perhaps not actually abrupt, can nevertheless be dated. The patient is prostrated, frequently had a moderately severe headache, and, although conscious and oriented, usually seems to wish to be left alone. A leukopenia is present, sometimes as low as 3500 to 4000 cells per cubic millimeter, and there is a considerable increase of immature forms. Although meningeal signs may be absent, eventually meningitis appears in about two thirds of patients. However, in some, miliary tuberculosis may be covert and subtle, with weeks or months of nonspecific, slowly progressive constitutional symptoms such as weight loss, weakness, and low-grade or absent fever. This clinical picture, ascribed to small, intermittent bacteremic episodes and designated *chronic hematogenous tuberculosis,* is more common with increasing age. As in the more acute form, the initial clinical manifestation may be serous membrane involvement, meningitis, or, less commonly, disseminated lymphatic involvement. Choroidal tubercles are often absent. Splenomegaly is unusual in both acute and chronic miliary disease. In an appreciable number, particularly older individuals (see below), specific symptoms may be entirely lacking. *Accordingly, the diagnosis of miliary tuberculosis should be entertained in any wasting illness with or without fever.* Often a therapeutic trial of isoniazid will be diagnostic. Very uncommonly the tissue response to hematogenous dissemination is atypical, consisting of foci containing myriads of acid-fast organisms, nonspecific tissue necrosis, and a sparse polymorphonuclear cellular infiltrate. This histologic picture has been termed *nonreactive tuberculosis.* The usual clinical course is acute overwhelming sepsis; less commonly a more protracted fever of unknown origin is observed. Splenomegaly and a variety of hematologic disorders (see below) are the rule in patients with this histologic picture.

Diagnostic studies are usually initiated because of the appearance of a typical miliary infiltration on chest roentgenogram. However, *individuals may succumb to miliary tuberculosis before the miliary pulmonary infiltrate has become roentgenographically detectable.* The tuberculin test is of little help, because *as many as one fourth of patients with proved cases may be initially tuberculin negative,* reactivity returning when treatment results in improvement. Anemia is usual. The white blood count is usually normal or depressed initially (see below). Gastric and urine cultures, although frequently positive, are of little immediate diagnostic help. *Culture of spinal fluid may be positive without pleocytosis, protein elevation, or meningeal signs.* Evidence of associated tuberculosis is helpful but often lacking. In many, a tentative diagnosis is made when granulomatous lesions are discovered on bone marrow aspiration or liver biopsy. Culture of these tissues may be positive without histologic evidence of disease, and negative findings do not exclude the diagnosis.

Primary Hepatic Tuberculosis. Rarely miliary tuberculosis may present as fever and a pattern of hepatic functional derangement, suggesting disseminated hepatic infiltration of neoplastic or nontuberculous granulomatous origin (elevation of serum alkaline phosphatase, less elevation of serum bilirubin, and little indication of hepatocellular damage), resembling at times extrahepatic obstruction with ascending cholangitis. Diagnosis is made by liver biopsy.

Primary Splenic Tuberculosis. Even more rarely miliary tuberculosis may present as clinically isolated splenomegaly with or without the hematologic consequences of splenic enlargement (hypersplenism).

Miliary Tuberculosis and Hematologic Disease. Many hematologic illnesses may be mimicked by miliary tuberculosis (leukemoid reaction, leukopenia, thrombocytopenia, aregenerative anemia, hemolytic anemia, myelofibrosis, and even polycythemia). This is particularly the case with the histologic picture of *nonreactive tuberculosis.* The confusion is compounded by the fact that, particularly when steroid therapy has been employed, miliary tuberculosis may complicate, as well as mimic, serious hematologic illnesses. Some authorities state that miliary tuberculosis may present the clinical picture of leukemia as well. However, probably all such cases actually represent coexistent leukemia and hematogenous tuberculosis, and the hematologic abnormality is not reversed by antituberculous chemotherapy.

Electrolyte Abnormalities. A surprising number of patients with miliary tuberculosis, especially but not exclusively those complicated by meningitis, will demonstrate hyponatremia. Although the possibility of coexistent adrenal insufficiency should always be entertained, the syndrome of inappropriate secretion of antidiuretic hormone is a much more frequent cause.

TREATMENT AND PROGNOSIS. Treatment of miliary tuberculosis with regimens containing isoniazid should be successful in virtually all except those dying within the first few weeks or with serious underlying disease. The prognosis with concurrent meningitis is less favorable. Maximal drug therapy with isoniazid, 300 mg, and rifampin, 600 mg once daily, is recommended. When a good response has been established and the infecting strain is known to be isoniazid susceptible, rifampin may be discontinued. Isoniazid should be continued for a total of at least two years. (A good response to isoniazid in a therapeutic trial of unproved disease makes it unnecessary to add another drug.) Response to treatment may be dramatic or may require some weeks. Adjunctive therapy with corticosteroids is advisable in severe cases with extensive pulmonary involvement and serious hypoxemia, and also in cases with poor response resulting from severe debility. It is, of course, mandatory in the rare instance of coexistent adrenal insufficiency. Other causes for poor response to treatment, such as miliary disease caused by mycobacteria other than *M. tuberculosis,* are rare, presumably owing to the decreased virulence of these organisms.

168.8. TUBERCULOUS MENINGITIS

Tuberculous meningitis is invariably fatal when untreated and often produces incapacitating neurologic damage, particularly in the very young, even with prompt therapy. It was long regarded as primarily a children's disease, but at present one half or more of cases are observed in adults. Meningitis complicates the majority of untreated cases of miliary tuberculosis. The infection reaches the subarachnoid space by direct extension from a subjacent focus, most frequently a small, subependymal tubercle, less frequently a tuberculoma or parameningeal focus in the spine, middle ear, or elsewhere. Since the critical factor is location, extensive bacteremia merely enhances the probability of a strategically placed subependymal tubercle, but such a lesion may be also seeded during a small, transient, otherwise inapparent hematogenous phase, as in the preallergic bacteremia of the primary infection, and may remain latent for years. Once infectious material ruptures into the subarachnoid space, an allergic inflammatory response spreads infection via the spinal fluid, implanting bacilli elsewhere on the meningeal surfaces. Involvement is usually most marked at the base of the brain and may produce a grossly thickened, space-occupying exudate, causing pressure injury to adjacent cranial nerves and long tracts. Obstructed basilar foramina may cause hydrocephalus. Vascular thrombosis and ischemic brain damage may also occur.

CLINICAL FEATURES AND DIAGNOSIS. The usual case of tuberculous meningitis is an illness of one to six weeks' duration, beginning with a nonspecific febrile prodrome and followed in many with focal neurologic signs, particularly oculomotor palsies, pupillary changes, and other cranial nerve abnormalities, and then the development of meningeal signs and symptoms associated with mononuclear pleocytosis and a low sugar concentration in the cerebrospinal fluid. However, the illness may be abrupt and severe, resembling pyogenic meningitis, or subtle and chronic. In some instances defects in mentation or affect may develop with little to suggest infection. Extrameningeal tuberculosis is clinically apparent in one half and the tuberculin test is positive in three fourths, *but the absence of both does not exclude the diagnosis.* A variety of neurologic abnormalities may develop, including pupillary abnormalities, cranial nerve palsies, blindness, deafness, long tract signs, subarachnoid block, disorders of consciousness ranging from mild confusion to dementia or coma, and, as mentioned, the syndrome of inappropriate secretion of antidiuretic hormone.

An increase of cells in the cerebrospinal fluid, more than half mononuclear cells, is the rule. Cell counts are rarely over 1000 per cubic millimeter, more frequently in the 50 to 200 range, and may be as low as only a few lymphocytes. Uncommonly, in acute severe disease cerebrospinal fluid may, early on, contain predominantly polymorphonuclear leukocytes resembling pyogenic meningitis. The cerebrospinal fluid protein is almost always elevated and glucose usually depressed in comparison with simultaneously determined blood glucose. Smears of the spinal fluid sediment will reveal acid-fast bacilli on microscopy in less than 25 per cent; this return may be improved if the pellicle which forms on the top of the fluid specimen, if it is allowed to sit for several hours, is stained and examined. Culture will eventually be positive for *M. tuberculosis* in 75 per cent of cases. Of the spinal fluid abnormalities, only the degree of pressure elevation has prognostic import, higher pressures being associated with a tendency to herniation at the base of the brain. Accordingly, fluid should be removed cautiously and slowly.

TREATMENT AND PROGNOSIS. Therapy should always include isoniazid and either rifampin or streptomycin, probably the former. Early in the course, isoniazid should be administered in larger than conventional dosage (8 to 12 mg per kilogram in the adult, and 15 to 20 mg per kilogram in children) with pyridoxine (100 mg per day). If response is favorable, these dosages may be reduced after four weeks or so. Isoniazid may be given by mouth or by intramuscular administration if oral therapy is not possible (equal total dose). Rifampin is administered as described for pulmonary tuberculosis. Intrathecal therapy is not indicated.

Bacteriologic cure should be achieved in three fourths or more, but permanent neurologic residua (weakness, paralysis, blindness, or deafness, other cranial nerve palsies, hydrocephalus, compromised intelligence, and rarely, symptoms and signs of pituitary or hypothalamic dysfunction such as precocious puberty, obesity, diabetes insipidus, and panhypopituitarism) may result in as many as 25 per cent. These are local complications of the inflammatory response, and accordingly adjunctive anti-inflammatory therapy should be advantageous. Use of *corticosteroid hormones or corticotropin* has received wide acceptance. Although evidence is conflicting, most studies reveal a slight but definite survival advantage in groups receiving adjunctive corticosteroid therapy, particularly in prevention of brainstem herniation. The response to corticosteroid therapy may be dramatic, with rapid clearing of sensorium, regression of abnormalities in the cerebrospinal fluid, defervescence, and loss of headache. Even if long-term benefits are slight, this symptomatic improvement justifies corticosteroid therapy. Prednisone (60 to 80 mg per day) is recommended in all cases of established tuberculous meningitis complicated by altered consciousness, neurologic abnormality, subarachnoid block, or spinal fluid pressures in excess of 300 ml of water. This will include most cases. The corticosteroid therapy may be tapered rapidly in the second or third week to a level of 30 mg, then decreased at a slower rate every third or fourth day, using the signs and symptoms of meningeal inflammation as a guide to dosage reduction, and usually discontinued entirely after six to eight weeks.

168.9. TUBERCULOMAS

Tuberculomas, once the most frequent cause of intracranial mass lesions in children, are now rare. Except in cases in which meningitis develops as a result of extension to the subarachnoid space, the symptoms are those of an expanding cerebral or cerebellar mass. Diagnosis is usually made at surgery. Antimicrobial therapy

should be administered when the diagnosis is made, both in hope of some resolution and to prevent development of meningitis. In the spinal cord *epidural granulomas* may behave clinically exactly like metastatic neoplasm, causing paraplegia with no evidence of infection or spinal fluid abnormalities and diagnosed at laminectomy.

168.10. TUBERCULOUS PERICARDITIS

The subject of pericarditis is covered in Ch. 365.2, and this discussion concerns only aspects unique to tuberculous pericarditis. The pericardium is most often contaminated by an adjacent mediastinal node, less frequently by a pulmonary focus, and rarely as a part of generalized hematogenous tuberculosis, evoking an allergic effusion which disseminates the infection over the entire pericardial surface. Associated pleural effusion is present in approximately half the patients, and peritoneal involvement may also occur, a syndrome termed *tuberculous polyserositis*. Although always associated with other tuberculosis foci, frequently pericarditis is the only clinically apparent manifestation. Prior to the era of chemotherapy, tuberculous pericarditis was fatal in 90 per cent or more of cases, with deaths caused both by progressive infection and by acute and chronic cardiovascular complications such as tamponade, constriction, restriction, and myocardial and coronary artery involvement.

Features tending to differentiate tuberculosis from other causes of pericarditis are a somewhat chronic course, less prominent pain, decreased frequency and prominence of a pericardial friction rub, and symptoms of chronic systemic infection. At times a symptom complex resembling progressive right heart failure leads to the diagnosis. Etiologic diagnosis of tuberculous pericarditis, once the anatomic process has been established, is always difficult. The tuberculin test is usually positive (over 90 per cent) but may be negative. *Pericardiocentesis* is often employed for both diagnosis and relief of tamponade. *This procedure is associated with significant morbidity and mortality and, if done, should always be preceded by unequivocal evidence of pericardial fluid.* It is not only risky, but also provides meager diagnostic information. The character of the fluid will not differentiate tuberculous disease from other causes of pericardial exudate (with the possible exception of pyogenic pericarditis). The fluid is rarely positive for acid-fast bacilli on microscopy, and culture (positive in approximately 40 per cent) requires too much time to be of immediate therapeutic assistance. It is the writer's preference to advise pericardiocentesis only for temporary relief of tamponade or to exclude the possibility of a pyogenic process when associated clinical manifestations (high remittent fever, marked leukocytosis, associated nontuberculous infection) make this uncommon process a serious consideration. Pericardiocentesis is best carried out in association with right heart catheterization and only after arrangements for prompt thoracotomy have been made, should this become necessary. When the presence of documented tuberculous disease elsewhere makes tuberculous pericarditis likely and little hemodynamic compromise is present, therapy may be initiated with isoniazid, 300 mg, and rifampin, 600 mg, in a single daily dose, and the course carefully followed. If, because of uncertain diagnosis, unfavorable hemodynamic conditions, or less than prompt improvement, this approach becomes unsatisfactory and the general condition of the patient is otherwise fairly good, we advise thoracotomy and anterior pericardial stripping. The advantages of this approach are (1) accurate diagnosis; (2) relief of tamponade and very probably prevention of some instances which would otherwise progress to constrictive or restrictive disease; (3) a favorable surgical technical situation prior to the development of chronic inflammation, scarring, and fibrosis; and (4) relief of right atrial hypertension which favors fluid retention, venous thrombosis, and pulmonary embolization. Our personal experience with patients succumbing to pulmonary embolic disease had led us to this rather prompt and decisive diagnostic and therapeutic approach.

Some authorities advise the use of corticosteroids to favor resolution of the inflammatory process. Although this is acceptable when the diagnosis is certain and the inflammatory reaction is particularly intense, in most cases therapy is initiated before mycobacterial diagnosis has been established. In these the risk of an infectious process not susceptible to antituberculous drugs, although minor, is always present.

168.11. TUBERCULOUS PERITONITIS

Tuberculous peritonitis usually results from rupture of an adjacent caseous lymph node, fallopian tube, or subserosal tubercle into the peritoneal cavity, or as a component of generalized hematogenous tuberculosis. It frequently may be the only clinical manifestation of infection. Peritoneal involvement from a bowel focus is rare. The most frequent clinical picture is the relatively abrupt onset of unexplained ascites, usually associated with some fever and abdominal discomfort. The syndromes of chronic fibroid peritonitis (doughy abdomen) and of localized abdominal tumor are rare. The process may be loculated and hyperplastic with gelatinous exudate tending to fibrosis and caseation, but much more frequently involves the entire peritoneal surface with development of clear or slightly cloudy ascites containing several hundred to several thousand mononuclear cells per milliliter. Erroneous initial diagnoses, which are almost the rule, include peritoneal carcinomatosis, unexplained ascites, fever of unknown origin, bowel obstruction, or, in unusual cases of abrupt onset, bacterial peritonitis or perforated viscus. Some fever is the rule, and the tuberculin test is most often positive. Recognition of tuberculous peritonitis in cirrhotics may be difficult, because the symptoms may resemble those of uncomplicated cirrhosis with ascites, requiring paracentesis for detection (ascitic fluid in uncomplicated cirrhosis usually contains less than 800 cells). Fever, abdominal pain, or both in the cirrhotic with ascites should raise the question of some other complicating abdominal condition, including tuberculous peritonitis.

Diagnosis may be made on the basis of clinically detectable tuberculosis in the chest or elsewhere, but frequently is the result of laparotomy or response to specific antituberculous chemotherapy. The peritoneal fluid resembles that found in tuberculous pleurisy with effusion, but is indistinguishable from that which may occur in peritoneal carcinomatosis. In acute cases the ascitic pleocytosis may be predominantly polymorphonuclear, at least early on, suggesting a pyogenic process. Acid-fast stain of the fluid sediment is rarely positive, and tubercle bacilli can be cultured in fewer than 20 per cent of cases. Needle biopsy of the parietal peritoneum (Cope or Abrams needle) will be diagnostic in most patients, but has resulted in death from occult intraperitoneal bleeding. Accordingly, if tissue is required, a limited exploratory laparotomy is safer. When the therapeutic implications of tissue diagnosis are limited to the question of whether or not to treat for tuberculosis, a trial of isoniazid is often an acceptable alternative. Multiple drug therapy, at present isoniazid and ethambutol, is advised by most authorities, but single drug therapy with isoniazid for a period of 24 months has produced completely satisfactory responses in all cases known to the writer.

168.12. TUBERCULOUS LYMPHADENITIS

Prior to the control of bovine tuberculosis, cervical tuberculous lymphadenitis or *scrofula* was commonplace due to local infection of the oropharynx and draining cervical lymphatics. This mode of acquisition of tuberculous cervical lymphadenitis is now extremely rare in areas with no bovine tuberculosis problem. In contrast, in children, cervical granulomatous lymphadenitis caused by mycobacteria other than *M. tuberculosis* and *M. bovis* is almost certainly acquired by the oral route (see Ch. 169).

The term tuberculous lymphadenitis is now used to describe superficial lymph node involvement either caused by extensive lymphatic spread from a primary pulmonary focus or as a part of a generalized lymphohematogenous dissemination. The cervical and mediastinal nodes are most frequently involved. Clinical evidence of associated tuberculosis is lacking in more than half the cases. Painless or, less frequently, painful unilateral cervical node enlargement is the usual presenting complaint, but multiple areas of lymphadenopathy may be present. The nodes may become fluctuant and drain. Systemic symptoms are frequent but may be lacking completely or so subtle as to have gone unnoticed.

Drug therapy (isoniazid and ethambutol) may produce complete resolution, but, in as many as one half in some series, response to drugs, especially when fluctuant areas are present, may be inadequate, requiring repeated aspiration or surgical excision. In some cases cervical lymphadenitis may locally progress or develop de novo while coexisting pulmonary disease is responding well to chemotherapy. This does not represent bacterial resistance to the antimicrobials but rather the fact that tuberculous nodes, especially when necrosis has taken place, may be very slow to resolve or actually enlarge even when the infection is well controlled. Prolonged rest or hospitalization is not necessary once treatment has been initiated. Careful bacteriologic investigation is mandatory in view of the frequency of granulomatous lymphadenitis caused by other mycobacteria which are more drug resistant and more frequently require surgical removal.

168.13. GENITOURINARY TUBERCULOSIS

RENAL TUBERCULOSIS

Renal tuberculosis develops from foci in the cortex seeded via the bloodstream. Although it is usually unilateral when detected, 50 per cent of cases will become bilateral in the absence of treatment, because of progression of contralateral hematogenous foci which are probably always present. The bacilli lodge in the cortex, but infection does not become progressive until it reaches the medulla (via the renal tubules), where the environment is much more favorable to bacterial multiplication. Foci in the renal papillae may cause obstruction and retrograde involvement of the obstructed segment, or may undergo necrosis, excavate, and seed the ureteral and vesical mucosa. Papillary obstruction with infection may cause segmental renal obstruction; scarring in the renal pelvis and ureters may cause obstructive hydronephrosis; and the contaminated urine may cause bladder irritability, contracture, and scarring as well as infection of the male genitalia. The interval between the initial infection and active renal tuberculosis, when this can be dated by some early manifestation such as pleural effusion, is usually quite long, often many years.

Symptoms are usually subtle and often lacking entirely even with advanced cavitary renal tuberculosis. Sterile pyuria should suggest tuberculosis, especially with frequency and dysuria, but it should be kept in mind that infection with conventional urinary pathogens may coexist with renal tuberculosis. Pyuria may be intermittent and low grade (10 WBC per high power field). Intermittent hematuria may be the only recognizable abnormality. Fever and backache are uncommon and probably late symptoms. Male genital tuberculosis (epididymitis or orchitis) is often the first clue to renal involvement. Some evidence of intrathoracic tuberculosis, usually healed but at times active, will be present in as many as one half. Hypertension and renal insufficiency, when present, are almost always due to some coexistent process other than tuberculosis.

Culture of several early morning urine specimens will yield the diagnosis in 80 per cent or more of active cases; diagnosis in the remainder is based on evidence of tuberculosis elsewhere together with pyelographic abnormality or persistent pyuria. Demonstration of acid-fast bacilli by microscopy of concentrated sediment should be regarded with suspicion, although the smegma bacillus may be responsible. Intravenous pyelography, which is abnormal to some degree in two thirds or more, may provide the first evidence of disease and is necessary to assess the degree of involvement and whether or not ureteral stricture is present. However, unless calcification is present, the findings are nonspecific.

Treatment with a two-drug regimen including isoniazid for a period of at least two years will arrest the disease in most instances. Relapse is usually associated with emergence of drug resistance, and retreatment with two drugs to which the infection is susceptible is advised. Intravenous pyelograms at three-month intervals to detect and treat ureteral strictures complicating the healing process are recommended by some authorities. Very rarely obstruction with complicating pyogenic infection or pain may require partial or complete nephrectomy, but this is unnecessary in the absence of symptoms regardless of the degree of renal destruction. Hypertension is not an indication for nephrectomy.

MALE GENITAL TUBERCULOSIS

Male genital tuberculosis affects the *prostate*, the *seminal vesicles*, the *epididymides*, and more rarely the *testes*; it may be secondary to recent or remote renal tuberculosis or to lymphohematogenous spread. Most instances present as an epididymal lesion, varying from a firm, painless, small nodule to an inflamed and draining mass. Diagnosis is usually made by prostatic or epididymal biopsy. Some instances may be detected because of poor healing and fistula formation complicating prostatic or scrotal surgery; in these, diagnoses may require a therapeutic trial of isoniazid, because culture of the draining material is often unrevealing. Response to drug therapy with isoniazid and ethambutol is excellent in most patients, and surgery usually is not required except for diagnosis.

FEMALE GENITAL TUBERCULOSIS

Female pelvic tuberculosis begins as a hematogenous endosalpingeal focus. Infection may spread to the ovary, the endometrium, and, rarely, the cervix, producing an ulcerating granuloma resembling carcinoma. Local or generalized peritonitis may also develop. The most common symptoms are menstrual disorders and abdominal pain. Most patients are sterile. In a small number, pregnancy and delivery appear to activate a previously latent focus. When conception does occur, tubal disease favors ectopic pregnancy. Pelvic inflammatory disease unresponsive to antimicrobial therapy may lead to the recognition of tuberculosis. In the majority, however, local and constitutional symptoms are mild or absent. Diagnosis is made by histologic study and culture of endometrial scrapings, culture of menstrual blood, and often by exploratory laparotomy. Response to a drug regimen containing isoniazid is usually excellent, and surgery is only rarely necessary to remove large tubo-ovarian abscesses.

168.14. TUBERCULOSIS OF BONES AND JOINTS

Blood-borne tubercle bacilli tend to lodge in the anterior aspects of vertebral bodies and in the metaphyseal areas of long bones. Evolution of foci in bone may produce cystic areas of osteomyelitis without joint involvement but often erode the end plate and involve the adjacent joint space. At present, bone and joint tuberculosis is not common in the United States, but several cases are seen each year on most medical services. It remains a major problem in some other areas of the world.

TUBERCULOUS SPONDYLITIS

The most grave form of skeletal tuberculosis is *tuberculous spondylitis* or *Pott's disease*. The originating focus is usually in the anterior aspect of the vertebral body near an intervertebral disc. The developing infection may erode the cortex, destroy the intervertebral disc, and involve the adjacent vertebral body. The roentgenographic picture of rarefaction and destruction of adjacent areas of two vertebral bodies, loss of the intervening disc space, and a tendency to anterior wedging or collapse is typical of tuberculous spondylitis, but is also caused by other infectious processes. The anterior foreshortening and angulation of the spine may result in a visible and tender posterior bony prominence or gibbus. Less frequently, the infection may begin in the center or posterior aspect of the vertebral body. The thoracic, thoracolumbar, cervical, and lumbosacral areas are involved in order of decreasing frequency. More than one area may be involved with intervening normal vertebrae. Characteristically, the infection dissects anterolaterally from the vertebral body, producing a paraspinal abscess. In the thoracolumbar area, this may be seen as mediastinal widening or a pear-shaped retrocardiac density on chest roentgenogram. In the lumbar area, the psoas shadow may be lost. In the cervical area, the abscess may cause anterior displacement or even obstruction of the esophagus or trachea. Pus dissecting under the firm paraspinal ligamentous structures may result in very high pressures in the abscess and produce ischemic paralysis in the subjacent spinal cord. This high abscess pressure also may cause the pus to dissect along ligamentous planes and present as a fluctuant or firm mass in the groin, the gluteal area, or the supraclavicular space.

CLINICAL FEATURES AND DIAGNOSIS. Symptoms are usually insidious and prolonged, and may not include fever, although weight loss is common. Local back pain is frequent, and referred pain imitating renal colic or abdominal disorders occurs. Walking may be painful, and the gait may become stilted. Miliary, meningeal, or pulmonary tuberculosis may develop and dominate the picture in the untreated patient. Severe anterior angulation of the spine may eventually produce a hunchback deformity. Frequently, however, it is the development of *weakness or paralysis* of the sphincters or legs which leads to medical attention. Paralysis, now the most serious consequence of Pott's disease, may develop owing to pressure from abscess fluid, to generalized inflammatory edema, or to intrusion of bony sequestrum or granulation tissue on the anterior aspect of the cord. Paralysis resulting from angulation and displacement is unusual, as the anatomic abnormality develops slowly, but violent movement may produce sudden cord transection when spine instability is marked.

In prior years most infectious spondylitis was tuberculous. However, it is now clear that entirely similar roentgenographic and clinical pictures can be produced by several other organisms, notably staphylococci, gram-negative enterobacteria, fungi, and rarely mycobacteria other than *M. tuberculosis*. Accordingly, in the absence of strong ancillary evidence for tuberculosis, aspiration or open biopsy of the vertebral body is indicated for microbiologic diagnosis.

TREATMENT. The most important aspect of the treatment of Pott's disease is antimicrobial therapy. Usually isoniazid and streptomycin or rifampin for a period of two years or more are recommended. Some period of bed rest during the first month or two is usually recommended, but its usefulness in the uncomplicated case, except to relieve pain or in patients with marked instability of the spine, is not established. Body casting is generally not indicated except as an adjunct to surgical procedures. When paralysis develops or fails to improve on therapy, surgery is required; the procedure, whether abscess evacuation, debridement of granulation tissue, or removal of sequestra, is dictated by the findings at operation. Usually some form of spinal fusion will also be carried out. Although orthopedic opinion tends to favor prompt surgical intervention with debridement, spinal fusion, and casting, experienced internists prefer to assess the effects of drug therapy and bed rest while maintaining close surveillance of the neurologic status, and many individuals will achieve stable spines and remission of neurologic symptoms without operative intervention or casting.

TUBERCULOUS ARTHRITIS

CLINICAL FINDINGS AND DIAGNOSIS. Tuberculous arthritis involves the hips, knees, elbows, shoulders, and small joints of the hands and feet in roughly that order. The initial symptoms are pain on motion or weight bearing, usually with some swelling. The process is usually monarticular, chronic, and associated eventually with considerable muscle wasting, pain, and stiffness, although low grade and trivial symptoms may have been present for months or even years at the time of diagnosis. A history of trauma to the involved joint can frequently be obtained. In the absence of proved associated tuberculosis, diagnosis requires biopsy, histologic study, and culture. The need for verification by culture as well as histology has been emphasized by reports of cases of granulomatous arthritis caused by mycobacteria other than *M. tuberculosis* (see Ch. 169).

TREATMENT. Isoniazid and ethambutol provide effective drug therapy; isoniazid alone is adequate in most cases. Intra-articular injection of drugs is not recommended. Many and perhaps most instances of tuberculous arthritis will heal with preservation of joint function when treated with mild immobilization, bed rest until pain is gone in the case of weight-bearing joints, and chemotherapy. When progress is not entirely satisfactory, joint exploration and removal of hypertrophied and fragmented synovial granulation tissue may be required. Casting and procedures to effect joint fusion are rarely necessary and often detrimental.

OTHER FORMS OF SKELETAL TUBERCULOSIS

Cystic tuberculosis of bone (tuberculous caries or *tuberculosa multiplex cystica*) is a rare condition in which osteolytic cystic areas of long and flat bones, particularly the ribs, and occasionally the tubular bones of the hands or feet are caused by tuberculosis. *Tuberculosis of the costochondral junction* may present as a cold abscess overlying the area of involvement. *Tuberculosis of the tendon sheaths and bursae* is usually secondary to involvement of the adjacent joint bone, but may be present in the absence of bony involvement. These usually respond readily to chemotherapy, but chronic lesions may require surgical evacuation of fibrinous material referred to as rice bodies.

168.15. RARE FORMS OF TUBERCULOSIS

Ocular tuberculosis is one of the causes of *granulomatous intraocular infection. Phlyctenular keratoconjunctivitis* is a rare allergic external ocular inflammation observed in children at the time of the primary infection and characterized by small blisters (phlyctenules) at the junction of conjunctiva and cornea. *Choroidal tubercles* often provide a clue to the presence of disseminated tuberculosis. They produce no symptoms and are difficult to differentiate from other retinal exudates.

Cutaneous tuberculosis, once important but now only rarely seen, is usually grouped into two categories. The first, in which organisms are present, includes *lupus vulgaris, tuberculosis verrucosa cutis* (anatomic or prosector's wart), *scrofuloderma* (the skin changes surrounding a draining tuberculous sinus or overlying a tuberculous node), and *tuberculosis orificialis* (nodular and ulcerated lesions around the mouth or other orifice through which highly infectious material passes). These are all very responsive to isoniazid. The second group comprises the *tuberculids* (including *erythema induratum* or Bazin's disease). These reactions are thought to be allergic and comprise a variety of erythematous, papular, and ulcerative forms. Their relationship to tuberculosis is poorly understood. *Tuberculosis cutis miliaris acuta disseminata* is a rare complication of overwhelming miliary tuberculosis, usually in children.

Tuberculosis of the adrenals is important only as a now uncommon cause of adrenal insufficiency. Tuberculosis of the *thyroid, pancreas,* and *breast* may all occur and mimic other infections or neoplastic change in these organs.

American Lung Association: Preventive therapy of tuberculous infection. Am. Rev. Respir. Dis., 110:371, 1974.

Berger, H. W., and Mejia, E.: Tuberculous pleurisy. Chest, 63:88, 1973.

Black, M., Mitchell, J. R., Zimmerman, H. J., Ishak, K. G., and Epler, G. R.: Isoniazid-associated hepatitis in 114 patients. Gastroenterology, 69:289, 1975.

Brown, A. B., Gilbert, R. A., and Telinde, R. W.: Pelvic tuberculosis. Obstet. Gynecol., 2:476, 1953.

Canetti, G.: Present aspects of bacterial resistance in tuberculosis. Rev. Respir. Dis., 92:687, 1965.

Christensen, W. I.: Genitourinary tuberculosis: Review of 102 cases. Medicine, 53:377, 1974.

Davidson, P. T., and Horowitz, I.: Skeletal tuberculosis. A review with patient presentations and discussion. Am. J. Med., 48:77, 1970.

Diagnostic Standards and Classification of Tuberculosis and other Mycobacterial Diseases. 13th ed. New York, American Lung Association, 1974.

Fox, W., and Mitchison, D. A.: Short-course chemotherapy for pulmonary tuberculosis. Am. Rev. Resp. Dis., 111:325, 1975.

Gelb, A. F., Leffler, C., Brewin, A., Mascatello, V., and Lyons, H. A.: Miliary tuberculosis. Am. Rev. Respir. Dis., 108:1327, 1973.

Goyette, E. M.: The treatment of tuberculous pericarditis. Prog. Cardiovasc. Dis., 3:141, 1960.

Huhti, E., Brander, E., Paloheimo, S., and Sutinen, S.: Tuberculosis of the cervical lymph nodes: A clinical, pathological and bacteriological study. Tubercle, 56:27, 1975.

Johnston, R. F., and Wildrick, K. H.: The impact of chemotherapy on the care of patients with tuberculosis. Am. Rev. Respir. Dis., 109:636, 1974.

Kocen, R. S., and Parsons, M.: Neurological complications of tuberculosis: Some unusual manifestations. Quart. J. Med., 39:17, 1970.

Konstam, P. G., and Blesovsky, A.: The ambulant treatment of spinal tuberculosis. Br. J. Surg., 50:26, 1962.

Newman, R., Doster, B. E., Murray, F. J., and Woolpert, S. F.: Rifampin in initial treatment of pulmonary tuberculosis. A United States Public Health Service tuberculosis therapy trial. Am. Rev. Respir. Dis., 109:216, 1974.

O'Brien, J. R.: Non-reactive tuberculosis. J. Clin. Path., 7:216, 1954.

Rich, A.: The Pathogenesis of Tuberculosis. 2nd ed. Springfield, Ill., Charles C Thomas, 1951.

Singh, M. M., Bhargava, A. N., and Jain, K. P.: Tuberculous peritonitis. An evaluation of pathogenetic mechanisms, diagnostic procedures and therapeutic measures. N. Engl. J. Med., 281:1091, 1969.

Smith, D. T.: Diagnostic and prognostic significance of the quantitative tuberculin tests. Ann. Intern. Med., 67:919, 1967.

Smith, D. T.: Isoniazid prophylaxis and BCG vaccination in the control of tuberculosis. High-risk groups. Arch. Environ. Health, 23:235, 1971.

Wales, J. M., Mumtaz, H., and MacLeod, W. M.: Gastrointestinal tuberculosis. Br. J. Dis. Chest, 70:39, 1976.

169. DISEASES DUE TO MYCOBACTERIA OTHER THAN M. TUBERCULOSIS AND M. LEPRAE

Robert A. Goodwin, Jr.

The term tuberculosis traditionally refers to infection associated with *M. tuberculosis* (var. *hominis* and var. *bovis*). It has long been known that other mycobacterial species exist in nature, some of which cause disease in animals. For years their role in human disease was unappreciated due largely to the overwhelming prevalence of *M. tuberculosis.* When found, their significance was denied because of the notion that mycobacteria were human pathogens only if they produced disease in the guinea pig (these did not). In recent years modern culture methods and drug susceptibility studies stimulated by the chemotherapy era have identified many mycobacterial species other than *M. tuberculosis* in human disease tissue. Much of the most important bacteriologic work on these "atypical" mycobacteria has been carried out by Runyon, who classified them into four groups primarily on the basis of the presence and type of pigment production and growth rate. (See Bacteriology in Ch. 166.) Most recently most of the known human pathogens have received tentative species designations, which will be employed herein. The relationship of these to the Runyon classification is as follows: *M. kansasii* and *M. marinum* — Runyon Group I (photochromogens); *M. scrofulaceum* — Runyon Group II (scotochromogens); *M. intracellulare* (Battey bacilli), *M. avium,* and *M. xenopi* — Runyon Group III (nonpigmented species); *M. fortuitum* — Runyon Group IV (rapid growers).

Human infection with many of these opportunistic mycobacteria is found throughout most of the world. Many of the organisms involved are widespread in nature, being found particularly in the soil and in water. *M. kansasii* has been recovered from milk in Dallas and tap water in California, but its source in nature is not clear. *M. intracellulare* is readily found in soil and in house dust, and has been demonstrated in throat swabs of normal individuals. *M. avium,* also of widespread distribution, is found in chickens and other birds as well as in household mammals. *M. scrofulaceum* has been isolated from soil and water, and is frequently found in oropharyngeal secretions of healthy men. *M. fortuitum* has widespread distribution in nature, may be found in saliva of normal persons, and is probably a frequent skin contaminant. *There is no evidence of man-to-man transmission of any of these, and no source case has ever been identified in human disease.*

The diseases produced by these organisms have

roentgenologic, pathologic, and, to some extent, clinical similarities to tuberculosis, but there are distinct differences in virulence, treatment, and prognosis. The term *mycobacteriosis* has been suggested to differentiate them from tuberculosis. However, species orientation is preferable, because there are differences in organ susceptibility, treatment, and prognosis. It is convenient from a clinical standpoint to group these infections according to organ involvement. Pulmonary disease, mainly in older white men with chronic bronchitis and emphysema, is the most common clinical manifestation. Lymphadenitis in children and granulomatous skin lesions in all age groups are next in frequency. Injection abscesses are not uncommon. Rarely, disseminated disease, meningitis, renal or skeletal involvement, penetrating wound infection, and corneal ulcers following trauma are reported.

PULMONARY DISEASE

M. kansasii and *M. intracellulare* (Battey bacilli) and, less frequently, *M. avium* and *M. fortuitum* may produce a chronic granulomatous pulmonary disease in susceptible individuals, as may rarely *M. xenopi* and *M. chelonei* (subsp. chelonei) and even more rarely *M. aquae, M. szulgai, M. scrofulaceum,* and *M. simiae.*

PREVALENCE. In the United States and Europe, 1 to 5 per cent of hospital admissions for tuberculosis are due to infection with either *M. kansasii* or *M. intracellulare*. There are geographic variations, particularly in the United States. The incidence of *M. intracellulare* infections is relatively high in Georgia and northern Florida, and *M. kansasii* infection is much more frequent in the central United States. In some localities the incidence is as high as 7 to 15 per cent of hospital admissions for tuberculosis.

CLINICAL MANIFESTATIONS. Pulmonary disease caused by *M. kansasii, M. intracellulare, M. avium, M. fortuitum,* and other "atypical" mycobacteria primarily affects white males over the age of 45; less frequently, by roughly a factor of 1 to 10, females and blacks; and rarely or never, children. Chronic bronchitis, emphysema, bullous disease, silicosis and other pneumoconioses, and, in *M. fortuitum* infection, lipoid pneumonia and achalasia are commonly present singly or in combination, and pre-existing chronic pulmonary disease in all probability is prerequisite to colonization with these saprophytic organisms. In this and other respects these pulmonary infections are more akin to that of *H. capsulatum,* a fungus of low human pathogenicity known to colonize abnormal pulmonary spaces, than to the much more virulent *M. tuberculosis* to which they are commonly compared. The earliest stages of these infections have not been described. The later stages are characterized by the presence of multiple thin-walled cavities, inconspicuous exudative and caseous disease, slowly progressive fibrosis, and a course marked by periods of stability and regression but, in general, slow progression.

Clinical symptoms when present tend to be mild. At least 50 per cent are said to be asymptomatic, and disease is often discovered on routine chest roentgenogram. Cough with expectoration to some extent probably occurs in all and is the most common complaint when recorded. Hemoptysis is not uncommon and occurred in 30 per cent in one series. Aching chest pain is an occasional complaint. Constitutional symptoms when present are mild and nonspecific and include malaise, fatigue, mild weight loss, and occasionally feverishness. Fever when found is low grade; chills and night sweats are rare. Constitutional symptoms usually disappear on rest. Remission and spontaneous healing may occur, but usually there is gradual progression over a period of many years. The infected individual usually dies of some other cause, and in only 15 per cent or less can death be attributed to the pulmonary disease and then as a result of pulmonary insufficiency. None of these opportunistic infections are contagious, and isolation is unnecessary.

DIAGNOSIS. Diagnosis is dependent upon bacteriologic identification of the specific organisms. With the exception of *M. kansasii,* mycobacteria other than *M. tuberculosis* may be found in oropharyngeal secretions of normals; therefore diagnosis of disease required repeated demonstration of the organism in significant numbers in the presence of compatible pulmonary disease. A tuberculosis-like disease that does not respond to antimicrobial therapy or the demonstration that the infecting organisms are highly drug resistant should suggest the possibility of another mycobacterial species.

TREATMENT. Only *M. kansasii* shows significant *in vitro* susceptibility to the antituberculosis drugs, although the degree of susceptibility is not always comparable to that of *M. tuberculosis.* Although no controlled studies have been done, it appears that a regimen of streptomycin (1 gram), isoniazid (300 mg), and ethambutol (25 mg per kilogram, reduced in two or three months to 15 mg per kilogram) given daily for 18 months will result in healing in 90 to 95 per cent of cases. Rifampin (600 mg daily) is probably the most effective drug, but rifampin-containing regimens have not been shown to exhibit any superiority, and some prefer to reserve this drug for the few patients requiring retreatment. This drug does have the advantage of oral administration, and a full oral regimen of rifampin, isoniazid, and ethambutol is reasonable and practical but carries greater hazard of liver toxicity. Whether two-drug regimens are effective has not been determined. Surgery is no longer considered necessary or advisable except for the few instances of drug failures.

M. intracellulare, M. avium, M. fortuitum, and all other saprophytic mycobacteria causing pulmonary disease are highly resistant in vitro to all the antituberculosis drugs. Some may show in vitro susceptibility to rifampin at levels unattainable in treatment of human disease. In spite of demonstrated in vitro resistance, many physicians use antituberculosis drugs in various combinations, and some report improvement, particularly with combinations including three or more drugs. However, there have been no controlled studies and no firm evidence of benefit. It has long been observed that significant improvement occurs with rest therapy, although relapse usually takes place in the presence of residual cavities. Surgical resection has been successful in controlling 75 per cent of *M. intracellulare* infections, and this would probably apply to the other pulmonary mycobacterioses as well. The incidence of surgical complications in these infections of low virulence is remarkably low even without effective drug coverage. A decision for or against surgery must be individualized, taking into account pulmonary function status, the severity of symptoms, evidence of progression, and other factors. Rest therapy for several months with or without a rifampin-containing drug regimen (such as rifampin, ethambutol, and streptomycin) is recommended for significant disease without prominent cavitation, and surgical excision (if not contraindicated) for localized extensive cavitary disease.

LYMPHADENITIS

Infants and young children may respond to a primary infection with certain atypical mycobacteria with the clinical manifestations of scrofula. Reports from the United States, Europe, and Australia in recent years indicate that 75 per cent of granulomatous cervical adenitis suggestive of tuberculosis is actually caused by mycobacteria other than *M. tuberculosis*. *M. scrofulaceum*, a scotochromogen, *M. avium*, *M. intracellulare*, and, less commonly, *M. kansasii* are the responsible agents. Each of these may be the predominant cause of adenitis in certain geographic areas and not found at all in others. In the vast majority the adenitis is cervical, occasionally preauricular, and rarely inguinal, axillary, or epitrochlear. Cervical adenitis most commonly occurs in the submaxillary and submandibular areas and is almost always unilateral, in most instances representing a regional component of a primary infection. Submaxillary and submandibular involvement suggests that the buccal mucosa is the portal of entry; involvement of the preauricular node implies conjunctival infection. In the extremities the infection usually follows a puncture wound. The pathology of the lesion is similar to that of tuberculosis, as are the clinical manifestations. Enlarged, firm, and nontender single nodes or groups of nodes may appear and persist unchanged or progress to fluctuation, drainage, and sinus formation, sometimes quite rapidly. Surgical excision is usually employed for both diagnosis and treatment. Infections with *M. kansasii* may be an exception, and a trial of drug treatment is indicated (see Pulmonary Disease, above). Isoniazid treatment of granulomatous cervical adenitis is recommended prior to cultural identification because the infection may be due to *M. tuberculosis*. If antigens are available, the demonstration of skin hypersensitivity to some other mycobacterial species and a negative or smaller reaction to PPD-S (*M. tuberculosis*) is regarded as diagnostic. PPD-B (Battey) may be used for this purpose. Although recurrence may develop in an adjacent lymph node, surgical excision of grossly involved nodes is usually curative.

SUPERFICIAL SKIN DISEASE

In addition to *M. leprae* (leprosy) and *M. tuberculosis*, two other mycobacteria, *M. marinum* and *M. ulcerans*, occasionally produce skin infections. Both have temperature requirements below 37° C, accounting for limitation of infection to superficial areas of the skin. *M. marinum*, previously referred to as *M. balnei*, is a photochromogenic saprophyte first described in marine fish. It is widely distributed in nature, occurring in soil, water, and freshwater fish as well. The temperature for optimal growth is 30 to 32° C. It has been implicated in epidemics of granulomatous skin disease traced to infected swimming pools, beaches of several of the Hawaiian Islands, and, more rarely, tropical fish aquariums. The granulomas occur at the site of minor abrasions, most commonly on the elbows, but also on the knees, toes, fingers, dorsum of the feet, and bridge of the nose, appearing two to three weeks after exposure as papules or nodules which increase slowly in size and may ulcerate. A line of granulomatous nodules may follow the draining lymphatics. Spontaneous healing is to be expected after several months. Diagnosis may be established by culturing a biopsy of the lesion at 30° C. Histologically, the tissue usually suggests a tuberculosis-like granuloma, but may appear to be a nonspecific chronic inflammatory reaction. Rifampin may speed spontaneous healing.

Disease caused by *M. ulcerans* is relatively rare in most areas of the world but strangely is quite common in the Buruli district of the upper Nile in Africa. This organism has a limited temperature requirement in the range of 32 to 33° C. Disease begins as a painless nodule, usually on the extremities, which may grow rapidly and ulcerate. The ulcers (Buruli ulcers), seldom less than 5 cm in diameter and often much larger, have characteristic undermined margins. They tend to be persistent and progressively destructive. Surgical excision is curative and much simpler when the lesion is recognized in the preulcerative stages.

OTHER INFECTIONS

Several hundred cases of *injection abscesses* have been reported, mostly caused by the common saprophyte, *M. fortuitum*, but also by *M. chelonei* (subsp. abscessus). These have occurred mostly in adults and usually respond to incision and drainage but occasionally require excision. The same organisms, and more rarely *M. kansasii*, have occasionally caused penetrating wound infections. *M. fortuitum* infection may result in corneal ulceration following trauma.

A dozen or so usually fatal cases of *disseminated* infection have been reported in young children and more rarely in immunologically deficient adults. Many different mycobacteria have been implicated, including *M. kansasii*, *M. avium*, *M. intracellulare*, *M. scrofulaceum*, and *M. fortuitum*. Rare cases of multiple and single *bone and joint* lesions have been reported, mostly in children, caused by the same organisms implicated in disseminated infection with the addition of *M. triviale*. Rare cases of *meningitis* in children and adults are reported with *M. avium*, *M. kansasii*, and *M. fortuitum*. One case of renal infection caused by *M. kansasii* has been found. A single case of *pleural effusion* caused by *M. fortuitum* has been reported.

Bates, J. H.: A study of pulmonary disease associated with mycobacteria other than *Mycobacterium tuberculosis*: Clinical characteristics. Am. Rev. Respir. Dis., 96:1151, 1967.

Corpe, R. F.: Clinical aspects, medical and surgical, in the management of Battey-type pulmonary disease. Dis. Chest, 45:380, 1964.

Harris, G. D., Johanson, W. G., and Nicholson, D. P.: Response to chemotherapy of pulmonary infection due to *Mycobacterium kansasii*. Am. Rev. Respir. Dis., 112:31, 1975.

Lincoln, E. M., and Gilbert, L. A.: Disease in children due to mycobacteria other than *Mycobacterium tuberculosis*. Am. Rev. Respir. Dis., 105:683, 1972.

Pfuetze, K. H., and Hubble, R.: Nontuberculous mycobacterial diseases. Disease-a-Month, September 1968.

Schaefer, W. B., and Davis, C. L.: A bacteriologic and histopathologic study of skin granuloma due to *Mycobacterium balnei*. Am. Rev. Respir. Dis., 84:837, 1961.

170. LEPROSY
(Hansen's Disease)
M. F. R. Waters

DEFINITION. Leprosy is a chronic inflammatory disease of man caused by *Mycobacterium leprae*, which displays a wide clinical "spectrum" related to host ability to develop specific cell-mediated immunity (CMI). In high resistant "tuberculoid" leprosy, the localized signs are restricted to skin and nerve. Low resistant "lepromatous" leprosy is a generalized disease involving many systems, with widespread lesions of skin, peripheral nerves, upper respiratory tract, eyes, testes, and the reticuloendothelial system. Common complications include more acute, immunologically mediated, inflammatory episodes ("reactions"), secondary inflammation in the anesthetic areas which result from nerve damage, and deformity of hands, feet, and face.

ETIOLOGY AND MICROBIOLOGY. Although Hansen recognized the leprosy bacillus in 1873, as yet *M. leprae* has not been cultured in vitro. Past attempts to infect human volunteers were unsatisfactory, and successful experimental transmission was not achieved until 1960, when Shepard reported limited infection in mouse footpads. Since that date, leprosy has been one of the fastest growing points in medical research. In 1967, Rees and his colleagues obtained lepromatous leprosy in thymectomized-irradiated mice. In 1971, Kirchheimer and Storrs described lepromatous leprosy developing in a proportion of immunologically normal nine-banded armadillos inoculated with leprosy bacilli. Subsequently, the only known animal reservoir, a small focus in armadillos, was discovered in Louisiana.

M. leprae is an intracellular, rod-shaped, acid-fast organism, 1 to 7 μ long and 0.25 μ in width; morphologically it resembles *M. tuberculosis*. However, in suspensions prepared from lepromatous tissues, bacilli are frequently arranged in characteristic "cigar-bundle" groups and in larger aggregates or "globi" derived from multinucleate Virchow giant cells. The cytoplasm of many bacilli is fragmented; such bacilli are dead. The percentage of solid-staining, presumed viable bacilli is known as the morphologic index (MI). Dead organisms are only slowly broken down, and may remain in tissues for many months or years.

In normal mice, a footpad inoculum of 5000 or 10,000 bacilli yields 10^6 after about six months, but no subsequent increase occurs. During the log phase of multiplication, the generation time is 12 to 13 days, the longest of any known bacterium. In thymectomized-irradiated mice, yields of 10^9 bacilli per footpad are not uncommon and systemic spread occurs, but the generation time remains unchanged. The footpad technique has been applied to studying the effect of drugs in leprosy, the detection of drug resistance, and the immunology and pathogenesis of the disease.

M. leprae is most easily detected in patients by Wade's "scraped incision" method. After cleansing, the skin is pinched to exclude blood, and a small cut made in the skinfold some 2 to 3 mm deep. One side of the cut is then scraped with the back of the scalpel point. The tissue pulp collected on the blade is spread on a glass slide, dried, fixed, and stained by the Ziehl-Neelsen method, care being taken never to overheat the carbolfuchsin. Leprosy bacilli are very scanty in tuberculoid lesions, and are often not detected by routine methods. They become more numerous as the spectrum is crossed and are present in huge numbers in lepromatous lesions. A lepromatous patient may have more than 10^{12} bacilli in the body. The density of bacilli in smears or tissues is termed the bacterial index (BI).

A standardized, autoclaved suspension of *M. leprae* is used as a prognostic intradermal skin test, the "lepromin test," which gives an accurate assessment of specific CMI in leprosy patients; it is negative in lepromatous and positive in tuberculoid leprosy. However, the test is often positive in nonleprosy patients, including those who have never visited leprosy-endemic areas, and shows some cross-reactivity with tuberculin. Therefore it is of no diagnostic or epidemiologic value.

EPIDEMIOLOGY. Incidence and Prevalence. Although governmental returns indicate a world total of 12 million leprosy patients, many consider that 15 million is a more accurate estimate, and that 1 million new patients will arise over the next five years. The importance of leprosy lies not only in numbers but also in the chronicity of the disease, which frequently disables but now seldom kills. Therefore it makes disproportionate demands on the health services and economies of developing countries.

Leprosy occurs in almost all tropical and warm temperate regions, including Japan and Korea, and is endemic in several states of the United States. It has only recently died out in certain northern European countries and Canada. It seems to be related particularly to overcrowding, so that as living standards rise, the disease becomes less common.

Transmission. Because *M. leprae* cannot be cultured, and because there is no simple, specific immunologic test of past or present infection, epidemiologic studies have hitherto been restricted to clinical cases. These have been further hampered by the long incubation period of three or more years. Close (household) contacts of lepromatous patients may show a tenfold higher incidence of leprosy and those of tuberculoid patients a twofold higher incidence than the general population. Lepromatous patients are thought to form the main source of infection in the community.

The lepromatous dermis is full of bacilli, but these are not shed in significant numbers through the intact epidermis. However, leprosy bacilli are excreted freely in lepromatous nasal secretions, so that 24-hour smears are comparable in numbers to those of *M. tuberculosis* coughed up in cavitary pulmonary tuberculosis. Bacilli from dried nasal secretions remain viable after being kept in the dark for at least 24 hours, and thus could be largely responsible for the spread of leprosy. The possibility of insect spread is also being reinvestigated. It has been assumed that *M. leprae* gains entry through the skin or the respiratory tract.

Studies in twins and other subjects suggest that lepromatous disease is a host-determined characteristic possessed by a fixed proportion of all people. Godal (1971) has developed a specific lymphocyte transformation test (LTT) which may help to clarify the epidemiology of leprosy.

PATHOLOGY AND CLINICAL MANIFESTATIONS. Leprosy has two special features. One is the invasion by *M. leprae* of certain superficial nerves, which may become thickened and firm. The other is the wide range of clinical and histologic manifestations, reflecting the intricacies of the host-parasite relationship. Skin lesions, which are best seen in good oblique light, may occur anywhere, although rarely on the hairy scalp and perineum. Nerves of predilection, which should always be palpated, include the ulnars at and above the medial humeral epicondyle, the superficial radials and medians at the wrist, the great auriculars at the edge of the sternocleidomastoid muscle, and the lateral popliteals (common peroneal) at the neck of the fibula. Appropriate muscle weakness and wasting may occur, resulting in claw hand (ulnar and/or median), foot drop, claw toes, and facial nerve paralysis, the last-named usually incomplete but including lagophthalmos. Wrist drop is comparatively rare.

The spectrum of leprosy has been particularly well defined by Ridley and Jopling, who proposed a five-group system of classification according to certain immunologic features, principally *the cytology* of the host cells of the macrophage-histiocyte series (whether histiocytic or epithelioid), *the bacterial density,* and *the degree of infiltration by lymphocytes.* Their classification enables the majority of patients to be diagnosed accurately from the clinical features, although the intermediate "borderline" (dimorphous) groups are relatively unstable, and tend to move toward lepromatous in the absence of treatment and toward tuberculoid after institution of effective chemotherapy. The five groups are, in order across the spectrum, *tuberculoid* (TT), *borderline-tuberculoid* (BT), *borderline* (BB), *borderline-lepromatous* (BL), and *lepromatous* (LL). Their distinctive clinical manifestations are now described, and these, with their corresponding pathologic, bacteriologic, and immunologic features, are summarized in the accompanying table.

Tuberculoid (TT). The typical tuberculoid lesion is large and annular, with a sharply raised outer edge and a thin erythematous rim which slopes gradually to a hypopigmented, flattened center. In profile, it resembles a saucer the right way up. The surface is dry, hairless, and sometimes scaly, with loss of sweating and marked anesthesia. Sometimes the lesion is a plaque with a dry, pebbly surface, or a macule. The lesion is usually single — at most two or three may be present — and, frequently, running to it may be palpated a thickened cutaneous sensory nerve in which caseation may occur. Sometimes, one of the nerves of predilection in the region of the skin lesion may be enlarged; rarely the only sign is a thickened nerve. Tuberculoid leprosy appears to be related to delay in the development of adequate cell-mediated immunity, and it forms a stable group.

Borderline-Tuberculoid (BT). The skin lesions resemble those of TT leprosy, but are usually multiple, though asymmetrical, and smaller in size, or else small "satellite" lesions may be present near the periphery of larger lesions. Sharp-edged papules may also occur. Enlarged cutaneous sensory nerves are less commonly found, but frequently one or more nerves of predilection are thickened. Therefore BT leprosy is often associated with deformity of one or both hands and/or feet; a patient may present with, or later develop, a plantar ulcer in an anesthetic foot or burns or infection of anesthetic fingers. Lagophthalmos may result in exposure keratitis.

Borderline (BB). The rather numerous, though asymmetrical, skin lesions are erythematous or hyperpigmented, and vary markedly in size. They occur as papules, plaques, and most characteristically as annular

Summary of the Clinical, Histologic, Bacteriologic and Immunologic Findings of the Five Groups of the Leprosy Spectrum

	TT	BT	BB	BL	LL
Skin lesions					
Numbers	1 to 3	Very few to moderate	Moderate	Moderate to many	Very many
Symmetry	Very asymmetrical	Asymmetrical	Asymmetrical	Slightly asymmetrical	Symmetrical
Anesthesia	Very marked	Marked	Marked to moderate	Slight to nil	Nil
Nerve enlargement					
Cutaneous sensory	Common	May occur	0	0	0
Peripheral nerves*	0 or one	Common; asymmetrical	Common; asymmetrical	Moderately asymmetrical	Symmetrical
Skin histology					
Granuloma cell	Epithelioid	Epithelioid	Epithelioid	Histiocyte	Foamy histiocyte
Lymphocytes	+++	+++	+	± or ++	±†
Dermal nerves	Destroyed	Mostly destroyed	Some visible	Visible	Easily visible
Bacilli numbers (routine examination)	0	0, + or ++	+, ++ or +++	++++	+++++
Lymph nodes					
Paracortical infiltrate	Nil; immunoblasts	Sarcoid-like	Diffuse epithelioid	Diffuse histiocytes	Massive infiltrate with foamy histiocytes and Virchow cells
Germinal centers	Normal	Normal	Normal	Some hypertrophy	Gross hypertrophy
Lepromin test	+++	++	± or 0	0	0
Reactions					
ENL	0	0	0	Rare	Very common
Lepra	?	Common	Very common	Very common	(Rare)‡

*Nerves of predilection, i.e. ulnar, median, lateral popliteal, facial, great auricular, and posterior tibial.

†In LL leprosy, the peripheral blood shows an absolute decrease in T and an absolute increase in B lymphocytes.

‡Lepra reactions are occasionally seen in treated LL patients who have developed from borderline (BT, BB, or BL) in the absence of treatment.

lesions with broad rims. The outer edge is often flattish and irregular; it rises to a thick inner edge, and the anesthetic, hypopigmented center is always sharply "punched out." The profile resembles a saucer the wrong way up, except that where the cup should sit is a deep central depression. Satellite lesions are common. Moderate and widespread, though asymmetrical, enlargement of the nerves of predilection may occur with or without associated muscle weakness and wasting.

Borderline-Lepromatous (BL). The skin lesions are numerous, but are not usually bilaterally symmetrical. They consist of erythematous or hyperpigmented papules, nodules, or plaques which appear moist and succulent, and which possess normal sensation or show only mild hypoesthesia. Small, indefinite-edged, hypopigmented macules may also be present. Some nodules may be dimpled, and often one or two lesions, usually the first to appear, have punched-out, hypopigmented, anesthetic centers, indicating progression from BB leprosy. Nerves of predilection close to the latter are often markedly thickened; elsewhere they may be only slightly enlarged. Ear lobes may appear normal, or be asymmetrically (more rarely symmetrically) enlarged. The eyebrows, nasal cartilage, and eyes are unaffected. Although bacilli are very numerous in the lesions, they are often undetected in normal-looking skin.

Lepromatous (LL). Lesions show marked bilateral symmetry. Skin lesions are very numerous, with erythematous, smooth, shiny surfaces, and are neither anesthetic nor anhidrotic. Early cases may have numerous, small, hypopigmented macules with vague edges and small papules with indefinite edges; nerves may be but slightly thickened at this stage, although significant involvement of the nasal mucosa is frequently detected. With time, plaques and nodules develop, and the skin progressively thickens as lepromatous infiltrate increases; rarely, but especially in Central America, infiltrate alone occurs. The ear lobes enlarge, and the lines of the face coarsen and deepen (leonine facies). The lips often swell, and the eyebrows and eyelashes become scanty and are lost. Iritis and keratitis are common. Nasal blockage occurs, with ulceration and bloodstreaked discharge, and in time the nasal cartilage and bones may be gradually destroyed, resulting in saddle-nose deformity. Lepromatous laryngitis may cause hoarseness. Edema of the extremities may occur, lymph nodes often enlarge, and testicular involvement frequently leads to atrophy and occasionally to gynecomastia. Dermal nerve damage leads to a progressive pseudo- "glove-and-stocking" anesthesia; light touch, pain, and temperature sensation are eventually lost over most of the body except scalp and flexures, but position sense is well preserved. Very numerous bacilli are present not only in the skin, in the draining lymph nodes, and in nerves of predilection, but also in the liver, spleen, bone marrow, and blood; there are relatively few in the kidney, and the lungs, heart, and central nervous system are not clinically involved in the infection.

In some peoples, such as the Chinese, many of the lepromatous cases originate as borderline, and a small number of residual BB-type lesions may be found; otherwise the signs are consistent with LL. In treated LL patients whose disease relapses, the new lesions are usually asymmetrical initially, but otherwise retain lepromatous characteritics.

Indeterminate Leprosy. Some child contacts of adult cases develop a single (occasionally two or three) hypopigmented macule, 2 to 5 cm in diameter, which shows hypoesthesia and decreased sweating. Histologically, there is lymphocytic infiltrate around the dermal appendages and neurovascular bundles. If left untreated, about one quarter later develop leprosy which may be of any type on the spectrum.

Reactions. Erythema Nodosum Leprosum (ENL)— Lepromatous Lepra Reaction. More than 50 per cent of treated LL patients, and the occasional untreated LL or treated BL patient, suffer from episodes of erythema nodosum leprosum. Over the course of a few hours, a crop of painful erythematous papules develops, typically on the extensor surfaces of the body except the scalp. The papules last for two to three days, becoming more purple, and then gradually subside, leaving dark staining of the skin. The episodes are usually associated with fever and general malaise. They may be isolated or may occur continuously over months or years, leading, if untreated, to gross prostration, weakness, and occasionally death. In severe ENL, the papules may form sterile pustules and ulcers. A frequent complication is painful neuritis, usually of the ulnar, median or lateral popliteal nerves, and muscle weakness may increase. Lymphadenitis, iritis, and orchitis may also occur, and more rarely nephritis and large-joint arthritis. The ENL is due to immune complex formation, resulting in vasculitis and polymorphonuclear infiltrate. The antigen is probably derived from the cytoplasm of dead leprosy bacilli, and serum immunoglobulin levels are markedly elevated in LL leprosy.

Nonlepromatous Lepra Reactions. These occur very frequently in BT, BB, and BL leprosy. The leprous lesions themselves become markedly swollen, erythematous, and often scaly, and new lesions may appear. The reaction lasts for many weeks or months. Systemic upset and fever are uncommon, but neuritis may occur, and ulceration of the friable skin may lead to unsightly scarring. The reaction is often associated with change in specific CMI and therefore of a patient's leprosy classification, so that untreated patients become more lepromatous and treated patients more tuberculoid.

DIAGNOSIS AND DIFFERENTIAL DIAGNOSIS. It is essential to consider leprosy in all patients with skin or peripheral nerve lesions who have resided in endemic areas. The three most helpful findings are (1) thickening of one or more nerves, either of predilection or cutaneous sensory; nerve enlargement is found in some TT, many BT, and the great majority of BB, BL, and LL patients; (2) anesthetic skin lesions, which are found in almost all TT, BT, and BB patients, in many BL patients, and in those LL patients who have evolved from borderline; and (3) acid-fast bacilli (AFB) in skin smears, which are positive in many BT and in all untreated BB, BL, and LL patients. Smears are usually taken from both ear lobes and up to six typical skin lesions. Leprosy should be suspected when skin or nasal symptoms persist despite routine treatment; in chronic, painless, plantar ulceration; in foot drop unassociated with trauma; or in unusual presentations of arthritis and erythema nodosum. Confirmation should be obtained by skin biopsy or, in neural leprosy without skin lesions, by biopsy of a thickened sensory nerve.

Lack of anesthesia differentiates vitiligo, mycotic infections, lupus erythematosus, and psoriasis from TT and BT leprosy. Nerves are not enlarged in neurologic conditions such as syringomyelia, motor neuron disease, and Friedreich's ataxia; they are enlarged in hereditary sensory neuropathy of Dejerine and Sotta, which can be differentiated by the absence of skin lesions and of AFB and by the familial history. Dermal leishmaniasis, yaws, secondary syphilis, and neurofibromatosis may resemble LL leprosy, but there is no nerve thickening, and smears for AFB are negative.

TREATMENT. Treatment is made difficult by the excessive prejudice and outdated fear of leprosy persisting in many cultures, and by the extreme chronicity of the infection and slowness of response to treatment which is related in part to the unique generation time of *M. leprae*.

Treatment of the Infection. The drug of choice remains DDS (dapsone, 4-4' diaminodiphenyl sulfone), which is as cheap as aspirin and may be administered by mouth or parenterally. In LL and BL patients, clinical improvement is detected from about three months after starting DDS (often earlier in TT, BT, and BB leprosy), and around this time bacilli from nose and skin will no longer infect mice. The MI reaches zero by six months, but the BI takes many years to become negative. Small numbers of viable, probably dormant, bacilli have been shown to persist in a number of tissue sites, in LL patients treated continuously for at least ten years; such patients may relapse if treatment is stopped. Therefore it is recommended that DDS be given for the following minimum periods:

Indeterminate and TT	3 years
BT	5 years
BB	7 years
BL	15 years
LL	20 years or for life

Although the minimal effective dose of DDS is less than 1 mg, the recommended standard adult dose in LL and BL leprosy is 100 mg daily by mouth or 300 to 400 mg twice weekly by injection. This results in an incidence of drug resistance of only 2.5 per cent, whereas the incidence may be many times higher on lower dosage, especially if irregularly taken. Secondary (emergent) resistance to DDS has not yet been reported from the other types of leprosy (TT, BT, BB, and indeterminate), in which bacillary loads are so much lower. In these, a dosage of 50 mg DDS daily is acceptable.

Sulfone resistance has been detected 4 to 25 years after the start of treatment, sometimes long after the patient has become smear negative. New active lesions, usually asymmetrical papules and small plaques with high BI and MI, are found on a background of old, resolving, or resolved lepromatous leprosy. Bacilli from these lesions will grow in the footpads of mice treated with DDS mixed in their diet (Pettit and Rees, 1964). Clinically, resistance must be distinguished from relapse off treatment by a therapeutic trial of DDS, 400 mg given regularly twice weekly by injection. In drug-susceptible relapse, uninterrupted improvement occurs. In resistant patients, some initial improvement may occur if there is a mixed bacterial population of partially and highly resistant organisms, but the MI is unlikely to fall to 0, and further new lesions, with raised MI, will sooner or later appear.

Toxic effects of DDS include dose-related sulfhemoglobinemia and hemolytic anemia, the latter especially in glucose-6-phosphate dehydrogenase–deficient patients. Drug allergy, which occurs in one in several

hundred cases, may be serious and even fatal; three to seven weeks after starting DDS the patient develops fever, pruritus, and dermatitis, which may become exfoliative, and jaundice and psychosis sometimes occur. DDS must be stopped immediately and prednisolone given for several weeks.

To reduce the risk of DDS resistance, it is now recommended that a second antileprosy drug should be given with DDS during an initial intensive course of treatment in LL and BL leprosy for a duration of up to six months. Available drugs include rifampin, clofazimine, and ethionamide (or prothionamide). Alternative treatment is also required in sulfone allergy and in proved cases of sulfone resistance. Clofazimine (B663, Lamprene), a rimino-phenazine dye, is both antimycobacterial and, in high dosage, anti-inflammatory. It is relatively nontoxic, its chief disadvantage being that it causes a reddish-brown pigmentation of the skin which is objectionable to most light-skinned patients. In a dose of 100 mg daily, it appears clinically and bacteriologically approximately as effective as DDS. Clofazimine resistance has not yet been reported, although the drug has been given for over 14 years to sulfone-resistant patients. It is used widely in dark-skinned races, in a dose of 100 mg three times a day (a dose level that should not usually be maintained for longer than about three months) to control ENL and lepra reactions, although several weeks elapse before its full anti-inflammatory effect is produced.

Rifampin is bactericidal. It kills leprosy bacilli faster than any other drug tried hitherto, so that patients may be rendered minimal public health risks within a few days; clinical improvement is seen in about three weeks, and the MI falls to zero within six weeks. It has been used for more than a decade in the treatment of DDS-resistant leprosy, usually in combination with the second-line drug thiambutosine, or with ethionamide, with excellent results, although the BI falls no faster than with clofazimine. Dosage is 600 mg daily, and intermittent therapy is under trial. Rifampin combined with DDS is of particular value in the initial therapy of sulfone-susceptible LL leprosy, when a rapid therapeutic effect is especially desirable.

Treatment of Reactions. In mild erythema nodosum leprosum, paracetamol or aspirin may suffice. Somewhat more severe episodes often respond to two or three courses of stibophen,* 2 ml daily parenterally for five days. In severe continuous ENL, or in all episodes complicated by significant neuritis or iritis, there are three alternative regimens. Prednisone, given in addition to DDS, rapidly suppresses ENL, but in the long term severe steroid toxicity is common. Therefore steroids are best reserved for short-term cover for operations, childbirth, and similar situations. The drug thalidomide is equally effective in controlling reactions, but its use is contraindicated in women because of its teratogenic potential. The dosage is initially 200 mg twice daily; subsequently it is progressively lowered to a maintenance dose, usually of 50 to 100 mg nightly, which may be continued for years. DDS must not be discontinued. The third alternative is clofazimine in high dosage. In light-skinned males and postmenopausal females thalidomide is probably the drug of choice; in dark-skinned patients and premenopausal women clofazimine is the safest drug, provided that a rapid action is not required. *Lepra reactions* can often be con-

---

*Discontinued by manufacturer in May 1977.

trolled with paracetamol, with or without stibophen. But whenever neuritis occurs or when there is risk of skin ulceration, the signs of inflammation should be suppressed with prednisone. Although steroids may be required for some months, toxicity is rare, because the dosage is usually less than for ENL and the total duration of the reaction is shorter. In dark-skinned patients, clofazimine can be commenced with the prednisone, and the latter drug slowly withdrawn. Thalidomide is useless in this type of reaction.

Other Treatment. Patients must be educated to protect their anesthetic limbs. The healing of plantar ulcers is aided by rest and plaster splints. Reconstructive surgery and physiotherapy are valuable in the rehabilitation of deformed patients. The use of transfer factor in LL and BL leprosy is being assessed.

PROGNOSIS. Even without treatment, patients with TT leprosy and three quarters of those with "indeterminate" disease eventually cure themselves; however, the patients with BL, most BB, and many BT forms of disease tend to lose cell-mediated immunity, and their disease becomes more lepromatous. Widespread nerve damage may develop in the BT and BB groups. Patients with the LL form used to die from uncontrolled leprosy, intercurrent infection, or amyloid nephritis, and blindness was common. With correct treatment, the prognosis now is good. Death from leprosy is rare, although amyloidosis is still seen occasionally, especially in inadequately treated ENL. Patients who fail to care for anesthetic extremities may suffer from repeated trauma or infection, resulting in gradual absorption of digits, or amputation may become necessary for chronic osteomyelitis. Even with careful management, reactional neuritis may sometimes cause increased deformity, and ENL may also, if rarely, result in blindness or significant renal damage.

PREVENTION. Because *M. leprae* cannot be grown in vitro, there is no specific vaccine. The precise value of BCG in protecting against early leprosy is being further assessed. Prophylactic DDS or acedapsone (diacetyl DDS) may be justified in special local situations. Otherwise prevention rests on early diagnosis of cases, and annual examination of known contacts may be rewarding.

Committee on Experimental Chemotherapy: Experimental chemotherapy in leprosy. Bull. WHO, 53:425, 1976.

Pearson, J. M. H., Rees, R. J. W., and Waters, M. F. R.: Sulphone resistance in leprosy. A review of one hundred proven clinical cases. Lancet, 2:69, 1975.

Ridley, D. S., and Jopling, W. H.: Classification of leprosy according to immunity. A five-group system. Int. J. Lepr., 34:255, 1966.

WHO Expert Committee on Leprosy. Fifth Report. Technical Report Series 607. Geneva, World Health Organization, 1977.

TREPONEMAL DISEASES

171. SYPHILIS

P. Frederick Sparling

DEFINITION. Syphilis is a subacute to chronic infectious disease caused by the bacterium *Treponema pallidum*. It is usually acquired by sexual contact with another infected individual. Syphilis is remarkable among infectious diseases in its large variety of clinical presentations. It progresses, if untreated, through primary, secondary, and tertiary stages. The early stages (primary and secondary) are infectious. Spontaneous healing of early lesions occurs, followed by a long latent period. In about 30 per cent of untreated patients, late disease of the heart, central nervous system, or other organs ultimately develops. At one time this disease was termed "the great imitator." Although the disease is less common now than previously, it still remains a great challenge to the clinician because of its protean manifestations, and is of great interest to biologists as well because of the long and tenuous balance between the host and the invading spirochete.

ETIOLOGY. The etiology of syphilis was first discovered in 1905 by Schaudinn and Hoffman when they visualized spirochetal organisms in early infectious lesions. The causative agent of syphilis, *Treponema pallidum*, is closely related to other pathogenic spirochetes, including those causing yaws (*Treponema pertenue*) and pinta (*Treponema carateum*). *T. pallidum* is also related in a more distant manner to other pathogenic spirochetes, including *Leptospira* (cause of leptospirosis) and *Borrelia* (cause of relapsing fever).

T. pallidum is a thin, helical cell approximately 0.15 μ wide and 6 to 50 μ long. Ordinarily there are approximately 6 to 14 spirals. The organism is tapered on either end. It is too thin to be seen by ordinary Gram stain but can be visualized in wet mounts by darkfield microscopy (see below), or by silver stains or fluorescent antibody methods.

The organism bears considerable structural resemblance to gram-negative bacteria. A peptidoglycan cell wall is closely adherent to the cytoplasmic membrane. The exterior surface of the cell is made up of a trilaminar lipoprotein outer envelope. This is structurally similar to the outer membrane of gram-negative bacteria, but no biologically active endotoxin has been identified in *T. pallidum* or in any other pathogenic spirochete. Between the outer envelope and the cell wall are six axial fibrils. The axial fibrils are attached three at each end and overlap in the center of the organism. They are structurally and biochemically similar to flagellae, and may be in part responsible for the motility of the organism. The spiral shape of the cell is primarily determined by the peptidoglycan cell wall. Microtubular structures have been seen in the cytoplasm of many treponemes, including *T. pallidum;* treponemes are apparently the only bacteria with microtubules.

It has not been possible to culture *T. pallidum* in vitro. Motility is prolonged under microaerophilic to anaerobic conditions. *T. pallidum* was formerly considered a strict anaerobe, but recent evidence shows that it is a microaerophilic to aerophilic organism. It can be maintained by serial passage in rabbits without loss of virulence. The Nichols strain of *T. pallidum* has been maintained in the laboratory in this manner for over 50 years. Only a few strains of *T. pallidum* have been isolated in rabbits and carefully studied, and little evidence is available regarding the genetic diversity of the organism. All studied isolates have been susceptible to penicillin and are similar antigenically. Immunity to the homologous strain develops readily in rabbits, but protection is often not conferred against heterologous isolates of *T. pallidum*. The only known natural hosts for *T. pallidum* are man and certain monkeys and higher apes. A related organism, *T. paraluis-cuniculi*, is a pathogenic spirochete of rabbits.

HISTORY. A great epidemic of syphilis occurred throughout Europe in the late fifteenth century. Because of the severity of the infection it was termed the "great pox" in contrast to another prevalent infection, smallpox. Severe morbidity and sometimes death occurred during the secondary stage of syphilis at that time; in later periods secondary syphilis has usually not been so severe. The pandemic started soon after Columbus returned from the West Indies, and one school holds that the disease was imported into a nonimmune population by the returning sailors. However, there is evidence in the Old Testament and also in ancient Chinese writings of similar diseases, and there are other reasons for disbelieving the Columbian origin of syphilis. Among these are the extensive knowledge of the course of the disease and the effectiveness of mercurial therapy in writings published only a relatively few years after Columbus and his men returned. It seems more likely that syphilis was endemic in Europe, but rose to particular prominence in the late fifteenth century because of the wartime conditions which prevailed. It will probably never be possible to settle the precise point of origin of syphilis.

The disease was recognized to be sexually transmitted in the early sixteenth century. Its name is derived from the sixteenth century poem by Fracastorius about the mythical shepherd, Syphilis, who was afflicted with the disease. The major cardiovascular and neurologic complications were recognized later in the eighteenth and nineteenth centuries. Many great figures of Western civilization had syphilis of the central nervous system, with untold effects on the course of history. The disease was confused with gonorrhea for some time, in part because of experiments by the great eighteenth century physician and surgeon John Hunter. He inoculated himself with pus from a patient with gonorrhea, and subsequently (and unfortunately) developed both gonorrhea and syphilis. The latter was eventually fatal. He concluded that both infections had a single cause. A clear distinction between syphilis and gonorrhea was finally made by Ricord in the mid 1800's.

Syphilis was treated for centuries with various heavy metal preparations. Until 1910, inunctions of mercury were the mainstay of therapy which was apparently moderately effective, although extremely toxic. In 1910, Ehrlich introduced arsphenamine, the "magic bullet." This and subsequent arsenical compounds were more effective and less toxic than mercurial compounds and were revolutionary at the time. They had to be administered for periods of up to two years to be effective. Bismuth salts also were effective and were frequently used in combination with arsenicals between World War I and World War II. The final revolution occurred in 1943, when penicillin was introduced for therapy of syphilis. It was so effective and exhibited so little toxicity that many thought that this ancient disease would soon be eradicated. Although syphilis did decline rapidly in incidence after World War II, it has proved to be a resilient foe and continues to be a significant problem.

PATHOGENESIS AND HOST RESPONSE. *T. pallidum* may penetrate through normal mucosal membranes and also may penetrate through minor abrasions of epithelial surfaces. In experimental rabbit syphilis, spirochetes can be found in the lymphatic system within 30 minutes of inoculation and are found in blood shortly thereafter. There have been occasional instances in man of transfusion syphilis using blood from a donor who was in the incubation stage of his disease. Therefore it seems clear that syphilis is a generalized disease from the onset in man as well. However, the first lesions to appear are at the site of primary inoculation, presumably because of the large numbers of treponemes implanted at this site. In laboratory animals, there is an inverse relationship between numbers of treponemes inoculated and time required for development of the primary cutaneous lesion. The minimum number of treponemes required to establish infection is not known, but may be as low as one treponeme. Multiplication of organisms is very slow, with a division time in rabbits of approximately 33 hours. Similarly slow growth of treponemes in man probably accounts in part for the protracted nature of the illness, and for the relatively long incubation period of 10 to 90 days before appearance of the primary chancre (average time, 21 days).

T. pallidum is not known to produce any toxins. Although the outer membrane structurally resembles those of gram-negative bacteria, there is no biologically active endotoxin in *T. pallidum*. Hyaluronic acid has been seen in experimental lesions, and it has been postulated that the hyaluronic acid slime layer may serve to protect treponemes against host defenses. No true capsule of treponemes is known. Recent evidence shows that treponemes are capable of specific attachment to host cells, but it is not known whether attachment results in damage to host cells. Most treponemes are found in intercellular spaces, but occasional treponemes can be seen within phagocytic cells. However, there is no evidence for intracellular survival of treponemes.

The primary pathologic lesion of syphilis is a focal endarteritis. There is an increase in adventitial cells, endothelial proliferation, and presence of an inflammatory cuff around affected vessels. Lymphocytes, plasma cells, and monocytes predominate in the inflammatory lesion, and in some cases polymorphonuclear cells are seen as well. The vessel lumen is frequently obliterated. With healing there is considerable fibrosis. Treponemes may be seen in most early lesions of syphilis, and in some of the late lesions such as the meningoencephalitis of general paresis.

Granulomatous reaction is also frequently seen in secondary syphilis and in late syphilis. The granuloma is histologically nonspecific, and more than a few cases of syphilis have been incorrectly diagnosed as sarcoidosis or other granulomatous diseases. There is evidence from human inoculation studies that the pathogenesis of the gumma, which is a granulomatous lesion, involves hypersensitivity to small numbers of virulent treponemes introduced into a previously sensitized host.

Intracutaneous inoculation of patients with syphilis in various stages with partially purified antigens of *T. pallidum* showed that delayed cellular hypersensitivity developed only in late secondary syphilis but was uniformly present in latent syphilis. Recent studies have shown that there may be temporary hyporesponsiveness of lymphocytes from patients with primary and secondary syphilis to treponemal antigens; some studies have suggested that this partial inhibition of lymphocyte transformation in primary and secondary syphilis is due to a factor which appears in plasma. It is possible but not yet proved that the explanation for the unusual waxing and waning of lesions in early syphilis depends on the balance between development of effective cellular immunity and suppression of thymus-derived lymphocyte function.

The host also responds to infection with production of numerous antibodies, and in some instances circulating immune complexes may be formed. The nephrotic syndrome has been recognized occasionally in secondary syphilis, and renal biopsies from such cases have shown membranous glomerulonephritis characterized by focal subepithelial basement membrane deposits. The deposits contain both IgG and C3, and treponemal antibody.

Rarely patients may develop paroxysmal cold hemoglobinuria. This is due to production of an IgG antibody which binds to the red cell at 4° C and which, upon rewarming of the blood in the presence of complement, results in hemolysis. Thus patients may develop massive hemolysis and hemoglobinuria after cold exposure. This was formerly usually due to congenital syphilis but is now almost always due to other infections. Treatment with penicillin usually stops the attacks.

Antibodies useful in diagnosis are discussed under Serologic Tests, below.

EPIDEMIOLOGY. Syphilis, with the exception of congenital syphilis, is acquired almost exclusively by intimate contact with the infectious lesions of primary or secondary syphilis (chancre, mucous patches, condylomata lata). This is usually through sexual intercourse, including anogenital and orogenital intercourse. Health workers have sometimes been infected during unsuspecting examination of patients with infectious lesions. Infection by contact with fomites is extremely uncommon.

Syphilis is most common in large cities, and in young sexually active individuals. The highest rate in both men and women occurs at ages 20 to 24, followed by ages 25 to 29 and 15 to 19 years. Among predominantly rural areas in the United States the disease is most prevalent in the southeast.

Syphilis spares no class, race, or group, but is more prevalent in the United States among the poorly educated and economically deprived than among more economically prosperous groups. Studies of patients with repeat venereal disease, who are probably representative of syphilis patients, show increased rates of broken families and mental illness, as well as earlier age of onset of sexual activity and greater promiscuity. Increased numbers of different sexual partners and perhaps indiscriminate choice of partner increase the risk of acquiring sexually transmitted disease. Patients with primary and secondary syphilis name on the average nearly three different sexual contacts within the previous 90 days. A cornerstone of syphilis control is epidemiologic investigation of sexual contacts of patients with primary or secondary lesions, and of patients with early latent disease.

In recent years male homosexuals have apparently accounted for an increasing proportion of the total cases of infectious syphilis. The ratio of male:female cases of primary and secondary syphilis in the United States rose from 1.6:1.0 in 1965 to 2.5:1.0 in 1975. In many large cities over 50 per cent of all infectious syphilis occurs in male homosexuals. In 1975, more than half of all white males with infectious syphilis named at least one male sexual partner during the recent past. In contrast only 2 per cent of primary and secondary syphilis in females occurred in women who named a sexual contact of the same sex. Similar trends have been noted in other countries.

Another important method of case detection is routine serologic testing. Of the approximately 38 million blood specimens examined annually in the United States, approximately 1 million are reactive. Almost 14 per cent of all primary and secondary syphilis is initially detected through tracing of a reactive serology. Approximately 35 per cent of primary and secondary syphilis and 75 per cent of early latent syphilis are detected annually by either serologic screening or contact treating.

The annual incidence of syphilis has generally declined worldwide for approximately 100 years with the exception of periods of extensive war. Reported annual rates of all stages of syphilis were approximately 200 per 100,000 in the 1930's in the United States, and peaked at approximately 430 cases per 100,000 in 1943. Reported cases of infectious primary and secondary syphilis in the United States peaked in 1947 at approximately 73 cases per 100,000 population. With introduction of penicillin there was a rapid decline in primary and secondary syphilis after World War II, to annual rates of approximately 4 cases per 100,000 in 1957. This resulted in declining federal expenditure for syphilis control, however, and there was a subsequent resurgence in infectious primary and secondary syphilis in the United States, reaching peaks of over 12 cases per 100,000 in 1965 and again in 1975. Intensified epidemiologic control efforts have recently resulted in renewed decline in rates of early syphilis. Total reported cases of primary and secondary syphilis in 1976 were 23,731. Over 71,000 cases of syphilis (all types) were reported in the United States in 1976, ranking syphilis third in incidence behind gonorrhea and varicella among reported infectious diseases.

The reported figures are considerably less than the true incidence of the disease. Surveys of private physicians who treat most cases of early syphilis showed that they report less than 20 per cent of cases to public health authorities. It has therefore been estimated that over 80,000 new cases of primary and secondary syphilis occurred in the United States in 1974, and that there may currently be 360,000 untreated cases of syphilis in all stages in the United States.

Reported deaths from syphilis declined from 2434 in 1965 to 200 in 1976. Infant deaths from syphilis and first admissions for syphilitic psychoses have fallen by 98 to 99 per cent since 1940. Less than 800 total cases of congenital syphilis were reported in 1976 in the United States, of which only 170 were among infants less than one year of age. Patients with clinically manifest late syphilis, particularly gummas, are becoming less common, perhaps as a result of the effectiveness of penicillin therapy for early syphilis. However, surveys indicate that there still are significant numbers of patients with untreated cardiovascular and neurologic syphilis, especially among older age groups. There is suggestive evidence that neurosyphilis may be presenting with atypical clinical manifestations, and therefore not easily recognized.

NATURAL COURSE OF UNTREATED SYPHILIS. The incubation period from time of exposure to development of the primary lesion at the place of initial inoculation of treponemes averages approximately 21 days, but ranges from 10 to 90 days. A painless papule develops, and gradually breaks down to form a clean-based ulcer with raised indurated margins. This persists for several weeks (two to six weeks) and then heals spontaneously.

Several weeks after disappearance of the chancre the patient characteristically develops a secondary stage characterized by low grade fever, headache, malaise, generalized lymphadenopathy, and a mucocutaneous rash. There may be involvement of visceral organs. The secondary eruption may occur while the primary chancre is still healing or may occur several months after the disappearance of the chancre. The secondary lesions heal spontaneously within two to six weeks, and the infection then enters latency. Some patients may later develop relapsing lesions similar to those of the secondary stage; rarely the relapse will take the form of recurrence of the primary chancre. About one third of untreated patients eventually develop late destructive tertiary lesions involving one or more of the eyes, central nervous system, heart, or other organs. These may occur at any time from a few years after initial infection to as late as 25 years following infection.

The course of untreated syphilis has been extensively studied in two large groups of patients. In the Oslo Study (1891–1951), over 2000 untreated patients diagnosed clinically (without serologic tests or lumbar punctures) were followed for the ultimate course of the disease. None of these patients received treatment with arsenicals or other compounds. A smaller prospective study was also done in the United States among black Afro-American males in rural Alabama (the Tuskegee Study, 1932–1972). This study, which was initiated in the arsenical era because of uncertainty that the beneficial effects of treatment outweighed the toxicity of prolonged exposure to arsenical compounds, extended into the penicillin era. It has been subjected to much criticism because curative penicillin therapy was not given when it became available in the mid 1940's, although antimicrobial drugs given for other purposes may have influenced the course of the disease in some patients.

In the Oslo Study, relapsing secondary lesions developed in the first four years after infection in nearly 25 per cent of patients. Twenty-eight per cent of patients eventually developed tertiary syphilis. The most common late lesions were benign tertiary gummas of the skin, mucous membranes, and skeleton. Cardiovascular syphilis was diagnosed in slightly over 10 per cent and symptomatic neurosyphilis in 6.5 per cent of patients. Syphilis was the primary cause of death in 50 per cent of males and 8 per cent of females. Pregnancy had a beneficial effect on the disease. Among autopsied patients cardiovascular syphilis was proved in 35 per cent of men and 22 per cent of women. Serious late complications were more common in men than in women.

The Tuskegee Study showed that among men aged 25 to 50 years, death rates were 75 per cent greater in syphilitics than in appropriately matched noninfected control subjects. Cardiovascular or central nervous system syphilis was the primary cause of death in 30 per cent of syphilitic men. Among autopsied patients aortitis was found in about 50 per cent of syphilitics with a persistently positive serologic test. Central nervous system syphilis was found in only 4 per cent. There was no definite anatomic basis for some of the excess mortality among syphilitics noted in the Tuskegee Study. Thus the incidence of cardiovascular syphilis was higher but the incidence of neurological syphilis was lower in the Tuskegee Study than in the Oslo Study. On the basis of these data, plus other uncontrolled clinical observations, it has been suggested that black patients are particularly prone to development of cardio-vascular syphilis, and white patients to central nervous system syphilis, but the evidence is not definitive. The reasons for the possible racial differences are unknown.

CLINICAL MANIFESTATIONS. Primary Syphilis. The typical lesion of primary syphilis is the chancre, a painless, clean-based, indurated ulcer occurring 10 to 90 (average, 21) days after exposure to a sexual contact with infectious primary or secondary lesions. The chancre starts as a papule, but then superficial erosion occurs, resulting in the typical ulcer. The borders of the ulcer are raised, firm, and indurated. Occasionally, secondary infections change the appearance, resulting in a painful lesion. Most chancres are single, but multiple ulcers are sometimes seen, particularly when skin folds are opposed ("kissing chancres"). The untreated chancre heals in several weeks, leaving a faint scar. The chancre is usually associated with regional adenopathy, which may be either unilateral or bilateral. The regional nodes are movable, discrete, and rubbery. If the chancre occurs in the cervix or in the rectum, the affected regional iliac nodes are not palpable.

It was formerly taught that 90 per cent of chancres occurred in the genital region. Presently a much higher proportion of nongenital chancres are observed, particularly among male homosexuals, in whom chancres in or near the rectum are common. Rectal chancres may have an atypical appearance mimicking rectal fissures or other more benign lesions, and are frequently overlooked. Conversely, they have also been mistaken for malignant disease. In general it is reasonable to assume that any ulcer occurring in the genital area or, in male homosexuals, around the rectum is syphilitic until proved otherwise. Chancres may also be seen in the pharynx, on the tongue, around the lips, on the fingers, on the nipples, or in many other diverse areas. The morphology depends in part on the area of the body in which they occur and also on the host immune response. Chancres in previously infected individuals may be small and may remain papular. Chancres of the finger may appear more erosive and may be quite painful.

The *differential diagnosis* of a genital ulcer should include lesions caused by herpesvirus hominis type II. Herpetic ulcers can usually be distinguished because they are multiple, superficial, and, if seen early, vesicular. They are often painful. Herpetic ulcers, unlike syphilitic ulcers, have a positive Tzanck test—multinucleated giant cells in the base of the ulcer. The ulcers of chancroid are usually painful, often multiple, and frequently exudative and nonindurated. Lymphogranuloma venereum may produce a small papular lesion associated with a regional adenopathy. Other conditions which must be distinguished include granuloma inguinale, drug eruptions, carcinoma, superficial fungal infections, traumatic lesions, and lichen planus. Of these, the one most likely to cause difficulty is the ulcer of granuloma inguinale, which is usually redder and more granular in appearance (see Ch. 144). Final distinction in most cases is made on the basis of darkfield examination which is positive only in syphilis.

Secondary Syphilis. Approximately four to eight weeks following the appearance of the primary chancre, patients typically develop lesions of secondary syphilis. They may complain of *malaise, fever, headache, sore throat,* and other systemic symptoms. Most patients have generalized lymphadenopathy, including the epitrochlear nodes. Approximately 30 per cent of patients

A, Primary syphilis, chancre. *B,* Secondary syphilis, mucous patch. *C,* Secondary syphilis, papulosquamous rash. *D,* Secondary syphilis, condylomata lata.

will have evidence of the healing chancre, although many patients, including male homosexuals and women, give no history of a primary lesion.

At least 80 per cent of patients with secondary syphilis have cutaneous lesions or lesions of the mucocutaneous junctions at some point in their illness. The diagnosis is usually first suspected on the basis of the cutaneous eruption. The rash is often minimally symptomatic, however, and many patients with late syphilis do not recall either primary or secondary lesions. The rashes are quite varied in their appearance, but have certain characteristic features. The lesions are usually widespread and are symmetrical in distribution. They often are pink, coppery, or dusky red, particularly the earliest macular lesions. They usually are nonpruritic, although occasional exceptions have been noted, and are almost never vesicular or bullous in adults. They are indurated except for the very earliest macular lesions and frequently have a superficial scale (papulosquamous lesions). They tend to be polymorphic and rounded, and on healing they may leave residual pigmentation or depigmentation. The lesions may be quite faint and difficult to visualize, particularly on dark-skinned individuals.

The earliest pink macular lesions are frequently seen on the margins of the ribs or the sides of the trunk with later spread to the rest of the body. The face is often spared except around the mouth. Subsequently a papular rash appears which is usually generalized but is *quite marked on the palms and soles.* These frequently are associated with a superficial scale and may be hy-

perpigmented. When the rash occurs on the face, it may be pustular, resembling acne vulgaris. On occasion the scale may be so great as to resemble psoriasis. Ulceration may occur, producing lesions resembling ecthyma. In malnourished or debilitated patients extensive destructive ulcerative lesions with a heaped-up crust may occur, the so-called rupial lesion. Lesions around the hair follicles may result in a patchy alopecia of the beard or of the scalp.

Ringed or annular lesions may occur, especially around the face, particularly on black individuals. Lesions at the angle of the mouth or the corner of the nose may have a central linear erosion (the so-called "split papule").

In warm, moist areas such as the perineum, large pale flat-topped papules may coalesce to form condylomata lata. These may also be seen in the axilla and rarely in a generalized form. They are extremely infectious. They are not to be confused with the common venereal warts (condylomata acuminata), which are small, often multiple, and more sharply raised than condylomata lata.

Other lesions of the mucous membranes are common. The palate and pharynx may be inflamed. Approximately 30 per cent of patients develop the so-called mucous patch. This is a slightly raised oval area covered by a grayish-white membrane, which when raised reveals a pink base that does not bleed. These may be seen on the genitalia, in the mouth, or on the tongue, and, like condylomata lata, are highly infectious.

Other manifestations of secondary syphilis include hepatitis, which has been reported in up to 10 per cent of patients in some series. Jaundice is rare, but an elevated alkaline phosphatase is common. Liver biopsy reveals small areas of focal necrosis and mononuclear infiltrate or periportal vasculitis. Spirochetes can often be visualized with silver stains. Periostitis with widespread lytic lesions of bone has been reported occasionally; use of bone scans appears to be a sensitive test for early syphilitic osteitis. An immune complex type of nephropathy with transient nephrotic syndrome has been rarely documented. There may be iritis or an anterior uveitis. From 10 to 30 per cent of patients have pleocytosis in the cerebrospinal fluid, but symptomatic meningitis is seen in less than 1 per cent of patients. Symptomatic gastritis may be present.

Differential diagnosis of secondary syphilis includes a large number of diseases. The cutaneous eruptions may be mimicked by pityriasis rosea, which can be differentiated by the occurrence of lesions along lines of skin cleavage and frequently by the presence of a herald patch in pityriasis rosea. Drug eruptions, acute febrile exanthems, psoriasis, lichen planus, scabies, and other diseases must also be considered in some cases. The mucous patch may superficially resemble oral candidiasis (thrush). Infectious mononucleosis may appear very similar to secondary syphilis, with sore throat, generalized adenopathy, hepatitis, and a generalized rash. Infectious hepatitis may also cause confusion. A high index of suspicion is required to make the diagnosis of syphilis in some cases. Unfortunately even classic cases with widespread, hyperpigmented, papulosquamous lesions involving the palms and the soles are not infrequently misdiagnosed in the current era. Fortunately, if the serologic tests for syphilis are obtained, they will be found to be positive in 99 per cent of patients. The condylomata lata and mucous patches contain large numbers of treponemes as seen on darkfield examination. Aspiration of lymph nodes may occasionally reveal motile *T. pallidum*. Hardly in any other disease is it of such importance as in suspected syphilis to make a careful and complete examination of the entire skin, mucous membranes, and body systems.

Relapsing Syphilis. Condylomata lata are likely to recur. The skin manifestations tend to be unilateral, the eruptions more dense, marked, with fewer lesions, and sometimes solitary. They are also more infiltrated and of somewhat longer standing, and have some characteristics that resemble the skin lesions in late syphilis. This reflects the increasing immunity with the duration of the early disease. Neurorecurrences, as well as ophthalmic and other relapsing manifestations, may occur. If the patient has been inadequately treated, relapses may be delayed.

Latent Syphilis. By definition latent syphilis is that stage in which there are no clinical signs of syphilis and the cerebrospinal fluid is normal. Latency begins with the passing of the first attack of secondary syphilis and may last for a lifetime thereafter. It is usually detected by positive specific treponemal antibody tests for syphilis. The test must be shown to be reactive on more than one occasion to rule out technical errors. Diseases known to cause occasional false-positive treponemal tests for syphilis, such as systemic lupus erythematosus, must be excluded. In addition, congenital syphilis must be excluded before the diagnosis of latent syphilis can be made. Patients may or may not have a history of earlier primary or secondary syphilis, although such history is obviously helpful in making a firm diagnosis of latent syphilis.

Latency has been divided into two stages: *early* and *late latency*. Early latency is ordinarily considered infection of less than four years' duration, based upon evidence in the Oslo Study that mucocutaneous relapse could occur at any time during the first four years. However, more recent evidence suggests that most relapses occur in the first year, and epidemiologic evidence shows that most infectious spread of syphilis occurs during the first year of infection. *Therefore early latency in the United States is now defined as the first year after infection.* Late latent syphilis is ordinarily not infectious except for the case of the pregnant woman, who may transmit infection to her fetus after many years. Approximately 30 per cent of untreated patients with latent syphilis eventually develop late (tertiary) complications of syphilis. Since treponemal antibody tests usually remain reactive for life, it is likely that small numbers of treponemes persist throughout latency even if the patient shows no ill effects of the disease.

Late Syphilis. Late or tertiary syphilis is the destructive stage of the disease and can be crippling. It has affected many prominent figures in history, and until the advent of penicillin it was a dread complication of this infection. Late syphilitic complications are still important medical problems, but newly recognized cases of late syphilis have been declining steadily in the United States since World War II.

Late syphilis is usually very slowly progressive, although certain neurologic syndromes may have sudden onset due to endarteritis and thrombosis in the central nervous system. Late syphilis is noninfectious. Any organ of the body may be involved, but three main types of disease may be distinguished: late benign (gummatous), cardiovascular, and neurosyphilis.

LATE BENIGN SYPHILIS. Late benign syphilis or gumma was the most common complication of late syphilis in the Oslo Study. In the penicillin era gummas are quite rare. They typically develop from one to ten years after the initial infection and may involve any part of the body. Although they may be very destructive, they respond very rapidly to treatment and therefore are clinically relatively benign. Histologically the gumma is a granuloma. The histology is nonspecific and may be associated with central necrosis surrounded by epithelioid and fibroblastic cells and occasionally giant cells. There is sometimes vasculitis. *T. pallidum* is ordinarily not demonstrable by silver stains but can sometimes be recovered by inoculation of rabbits.

Clinically gummas may be solitary or multiple. They are usually asymmetrical, and are often grouped. They may start as a superficial nodule or as a deeper lesion which breaks down to form punched-out ulcers. They are ordinarily indolent and slowly progressive with curving or polycyclic borders. They are indurated on palpation. There often is central healing with an atrophic scar surrounded by hyperpigmented borders. Cutaneous gummas may resemble other chronic granulomatous ulcerative lesions caused by tuberculosis, sarcoidosis, leprosy, and other deep fungal infections. Precise histologic diagnosis may not be possible. However, the syphilitic gumma is the only such lesion to heal dramatically with penicillin therapy. Another form of gumma is papulosquamous, and may mimic psoriasis.

Gummas may also involve deep visceral organs, of which the most common are the respiratory tract, the gastrointestinal tract, and bones. In earlier centuries gummas of the nose and palate commonly resulted in septal perforations and disfiguring facial lesions. Gummas may also involve the larynx or the pulmonary parenchyma. Gumma of the stomach may masquerade as carcinoma of the stomach or lymphoma. Gummas of the liver were once the most common form of visceral syphilis, presenting often with hepatosplenomegaly and anemia, occasionally with fever and jaundice. Skeletal gummas typically produce lesions in the long bones, skull, and clavicle. A characteristic symptom is nocturnal pain. Radiologic abnormalities when present include periostitis and either lytic or sclerotic destructive osteitis.

CARDIOVASCULAR SYPHILIS. The primary cardiovascular complications of syphilis are aortic insufficiency and aortic aneurysm, usually of the ascending aorta. Less commonly other large arteries may be involved, and rarely involvement of the coronary ostia results in coronary insufficiency. These complications in all cases are due to obliterative endarteritis of the vasa vasorum with resultant damage to the intima and media of the great vessels. This results in dilatation of the ascending aorta and eventually in stretching of the ring of the aortic valve, producing aortic insufficiency. The valve cusps remain normal. Death may eventually result from congestive heart failure. Recently there has been some success with placing prosthetic heart valves in patients with syphilitic aortic insufficiency. Even in the present era, aneurysms are seen presenting as a pulsating mass bulging through the anterior chest wall. Occasionally syphilitic aortitis may involve the descending aorta, but this is almost always proximal to the renal arteries, unlike atherosclerotic aneurysms, which typically involve the descending aorta below the renal arteries.

The disease usually begins within five to ten years after initial infection but may not become clinically manifest until a total of 20 or 30 years after infection. Cardiovascular syphilis is thought to be more common in men than in women and possibly in blacks than in whites. Conceivably this could represent an effect of mechanical stress on a damaged aorta and the relative frequency of chronic hard physical exertion by various groups. The effects of genetic and nutritional factors on development of this and other complications of late syphilis are unclear. Cardiovascular syphilis does not occur after congenital infection — a phenomenon that remains unexplained.

Asymptomatic aortitis is best diagnosed by visualizing linear calcifications in the wall of the ascending aorta by x-ray. The signs of syphilitic aortic insufficiency are the same as for aortic insufficiency of other causes. Syphilitic aneurysms may be fusiform but are more typically saccular, and do not lead to aortic dissection. Approximately 10 to 25 per cent of patients with cardiovascular syphilis have coexistent neurosyphilis, and it is therefore mandatory to do a lumbar puncture in all patients with cardiovascular syphilis.

At present, syphilis is a relatively more common cause of aortic insufficiency among the elderly than among younger patients; this is due to the progressively decreasing incidence of new cases of late cardiovascular syphilis.

NEUROSYPHILIS. Neurosyphilis may be divided into four groups: asymptomatic, meningovascular, tabes dorsalis, and general paresis. Division is not absolute and there may be considerable overlap between syndromes. There is limited evidence that currently occurring cases of neurosyphilis are more likely than heretofore to be variants of the classic syndromes, possibly as a result of use of antimicrobials for other diseases.

Asymptomatic Neurosyphilis. Asymptomatic neurosyphilis is diagnosed when there is a positive VDRL* in the cerebrospinal fluid (CSF) in the absence of signs and symptoms of neurologic disease. False-positive VDRL tests do not occur in CSF in the absence of a traumatic tap. The CSF usually shows an increased total protein and a lymphocytic pleocytosis, but some of these findings may be absent. If the CSF is normal two or more years after the initial infection, the patient is not likely to develop a positive CSF later. Although up to 30 per cent of patients with untreated secondary syphilis have an abnormal CSF, studies show that penicillin therapy prevents progression to late symptomatic neurosyphilis. Because of this, routine lumbar punctures for examination of CSF are not indicated in early syphilis. Unfortunately, it has become common practice to avoid lumbar punctures in later stages of syphilis as well, electing instead of treat with doses of penicillin which are thought to be effective for neurosyphilis, if present. As a result, there are few data on the present frequency and course of asymptomatic neurosyphilis.

Many laboratories perform an FTA-ABS* test on spinal fluid. Admittedly, there are published reports of positive FTA-ABS tests in the CSF of patients with otherwise normal spinal fluid, in whom there were clinical signs and symptoms compatible with neurosyphilis. However, the CSF FTA-ABS test has not been standardized, and there is some evidence that positive CSF FTA-ABS tests are the result of passive transfer of serum antibody into spinal fluid. At present no diagnosis of asymptomatic (or symptomatic) neurosyphilis should be based on the CSF FTA-ABS* test.

Meningovascular Syphilis. An acute to subacute aseptic meningitis may occur at any time after the primary stage but usually within the first year of infection. It frequently involves the base of the brain and may result in unilateral or bilateral cranial nerve palsies. In about 10 per cent of cases, the onset of meningitis coincides with the rash of secondary syphilis. The spinal fluid shows a lymphocytic pleocytosis with increased protein and usually normal glucose concentration. The CSF VDRL is nearly always positive. Rarely CSF glucose concentration is decreased. This syndrome can mimic tuberculous or fungal meningitis or nonpurulent meningitis of various causes.

In other patients, the meningeal involvement may be less prominent but there is sufficient endarteritis and perivascular inflammation to result in cerebrovascular thrombosis and infarction, with signs and symptoms typical of those of cerebrovascular accidents of any cause. This usually occurs five to ten years after the initial infection and is more common in males. There often is an associated aseptic meningitis as well. Most cerebrovascular accidents are not due to syphilitic ar-

---

*See Serologic Tests, below. Also refer to Table 1.

teritis even in patients with a positive serologic test for syphilis. However, syphilis should be considered as the cause in young patients with a history of syphilis and without other causes for cerebrovascular accidents.

A variety of other meningeal syndromes may rarely be seen, including transverse myelitis and radiculitis. A rare syndrome of meningomyelitis may involve the lateral regions of the cord, resulting in anterior horn damage and paralysis of one or more extremities.

Tabes Dorsalis. Tabes dorsalis is a slowly progressive degenerative disease involving the posterior columns and posterior roots of the spinal cord, resulting in progressive loss of peripheral reflexes, impairment of vibration and position sense, and progressive ataxia. There may be chronic destructive changes in the large joints of the affected limbs in far advanced cases (Charcot's joints). Incontinence of the bladder and impotence are common. Sudden and severe painful crises of uncertain cause are a characteristic part of the syndrome. These may involve the larynx, vagina, rectum, or other organs. Not infrequently severe sharp abdominal pains lead to exploratory surgery. Lightning pains in the extremities are severe and may require opiates for relief. These may be triggered by exposure to cold or other stresses, or may arise with no obvious precipitating cause.

The eyes are frequently involved as well. Optic atrophy is seen in 20 per cent of cases. The pupils are abnormal in 90 per cent of cases, with bilaterally small pupils which fail to constrict further in response to light but which do constrict normally to accommodation (Argyll Robertson pupils).

The cause of tabes dorsalis is unclear. Spirochetes cannot be demonstrated in the posterior column or dorsal roots.

Onset of the disease is usually delayed, often not being seen until 20 to 30 years after initial onset of infection. It is thought to be more common in whites and in males. Typical cases presenting with lightning pains, ataxia, Argyll Robertson pupils, absent deep tendon reflexes, and loss of posterior column function are easy to diagnose. Atypical cases may be more troublesome, particularly because the VDRL test in the serum is normal in as many as 30 to 40 per cent of cases, and 10 to 20 per cent of cases (even before the advent of penicillin) have normal CSF as well. The FTA-ABS test in serum is nearly always positive.

Treatment is unsatisfactory. Penicillin does not reverse the symptoms, although it does usually result in clearing of the abnormal spinal fluid. Carbamazepine in doses of 400 to 800 mg per day has been reported to be effective in treatment of the lightning pains.

Tabes dorsalis is now thought generally to be quite uncommon, although a recent survey of newly diagnosed late syphilis in Denmark in the decade 1961 to 1970 showed that in approximately 10 per cent of all persons with late syphilis and 40 per cent of all with clinical neurosyphilis there was evidence of tabes dorsalis.

General Paresis. This form of neurosyphilis is a chronic meningoencephalitis resulting in gradually progressive loss of cortical function. It typically occurs 10 to 20 years after the initial infection. Pathologically there is a perivascular and meningeal chronic inflammatory reaction with thickening of the meninges, a granular ependymitis, degeneration of the cortical parenchyma, and abundant spirochetes in the tissues.

The most devastating effect of general paresis is on the mind. This was formerly a common cause of insanity and was one of the first diseases for which a definite cause of insanity was found. With effective penicillin therapy this disease has become much less common; in the United States, first admissions to mental hospitals because of syphilitic psychosis have declined from 7694 in 1940 to 154 in 1968, the last year for which definite figures are available.

Symptomatically in its early stages general paresis results in nonspecific symptoms such as irritability, fatigability, headaches, forgetfulness, and personality changes. Later there is impaired memory, defective judgment, lack of insight, confusion, and often depression or marked elation. The patients may be delusional, and seizures are sometimes seen. There may also be loss of other cortical functions, including paralysis or aphasia.

Physical signs of the illness are primarily those of the altered mental status. Cranial nerve palsies are uncommon. Optic atrophy is rare. The complete Argyll Robertson pupil is also uncommon, but irregular or otherwise abnormal pupils are not infrequent. Peripheral reflexes are often somewhat increased.

The cerebrospinal fluid is nearly always abnormal with lymphocytic pleocytosis and increased total protein. The VDRL is nearly always reactive in both spinal fluid and serum. The disease responds well to penicillin therapy if administered early, although as many as a third of treated patients may develop progressive neurologic decline in later years. Fever therapy induced with malaria was formerly an effective adjunct to treatment with arsenicals, but has now been abandoned.

Classic general paresis is now infrequently seen in the United States, but there is increasing evidence that variant forms of paresis may be occurring in significant numbers. Nearly 4 per cent of a recent series of over 200 elderly patients with dementia or psychiatric illness, most of whom were not hospitalized, had evidence of inadequately treated or untreated syphilis. Some investigators believe that small doses of antimicrobial drugs given for other reasons may be modifying the expression of late neurologic syphilis. Further investigation is needed before clear conclusions can be drawn, but it remains reasonable to suspect syphilis as the cause of undiagnosed neurologic illness. Since the VDRL may be negative in patients with late neurologic syphilis, the FTA-ABS test on serum must be performed before syphilis can be excluded.

Congenital Syphilis. Congenital syphilis results from transplacental hematogenous spread of syphilis from the mother to the fetus. The incidence of congenital syphilis among newborns or infants under one year of age in the United States rose from 180 cases in 1957 to 422 cases in 1972, but has since declined to less than 200 cases annually. Each case of congenital syphilis represents a tragedy which possibly could have been prevented by better case reporting and by proper prenatal care. A VDRL should be obtained in all expectant mothers at the beginning and near the end of pregnancy.

It has generally been held that maternal syphilis cannot be transmitted to the fetus until the sixteenth to eighteenth week of pregnancy. However, recent data show that spirochetes can be found in abortuses of as little as nine to ten weeks' gestation. The risk of fetal infection is greatest in the early stages of untreated maternal syphilis and declines slowly thereafter, but the mother may infect her fetus during at least the first five years of her infection. Adequate treatment of the mother prior to the sixteenth week will usually prevent manifest clinical illness in the neonate. Later treatment may not prevent late sequelae of the disease in the child. Untreated maternal infection may result in stillbirth, neonatal death, prematurity, or syndromes of early or late congenital syphilis among surviving infants.

Manifestations of early congenital syphilis are often seen in the perinatal period, but may not develop until the infant has been discharged from the hospital. The disease resembles secondary syphilis of the adult except that the rash may be vesicular or bullous, which is extremely rare in adults. There often is rhinitis, hepatosplenomegaly, hemolytic anemia, jaundice, and pseudoparalysis (immobility of one or more extremities) due to painful osteochondritis. There may be thrombocytopenia and leukocytosis. The early stages of congenital syphilis must be differentiated from rubella, cytomegalovirus infection, toxoplasmosis, bacterial sepsis, and other diseases.

Late congenital syphilis is defined as congenital syphilis of more than two years' duration. The disease may remain latent with no manifest late damage. Cardiovascular alterations have not been observed in congenital syphilis. Neurologic manifestations are common, and there may be eighth nerve deafness and interstitial keratitis. The latter occurs in over 10 per cent of patients but may not be manifest until the tenth year of life or later. Periostitis may result in prominent frontal bones, depression of the bridge of the nose ("saddle nose"), poor development of the maxilla, and anterior bowing of the tibias ("saber shins"). There may be late onset arthritis of the knees (Clutton's joints). The permanent dentition may show characteristic abnormalities known as Hutchinson's teeth; the upper central incisors are widely spaced, centrally notched, and tapered in the manner of a screwdriver. The molars may show multiple poorly developed cusps (mulberry molars). Some of the late manifestations such as interstitial keratitis and Clutton's joints may be due to hypersensitivity responses, and are benefited by corticosteroids in some cases.

DIAGNOSIS. Darkfield Examination. The most definitive means of making a diagnosis is finding spirochetes of typical morphology and motility in lesions of early acquired or congenital syphilis. The darkfield examination is almost always positive in primary syphilis and in the moist mucosal lesions of secondary and congenital syphilis. It may occasionally be positive in aspirates of lymph nodes in secondary syphilis. Problems arise, however, because of false-negative examinations in primary syphilis owing to application by the patient of soaps or other toxic compounds to the lesions. A single negative examination is therefore insufficient to exclude syphilis. Patients with suspicious lesions but with an initially negative darkfield examination should be instructed to avoid washing the lesion and to return daily for two successive examinations. Confusion may also arise because of presence of spirochetes which are morphologically indistinguishable from *T. pallidum* in the mouth, particularly around the gingival margins. For lesions in these areas therefore diagnosis often depends upon clinical appearance, history, and serologic testing.

To perform the darkfield examination, the surface of the suspected ulcerative lesion should be cleaned with saline and gauze without production of bleeding. Presence of red cells in the specimen makes it difficult to visualize small numbers of *T. pallidum*. Squeezing of the lesion (with gloves on!) may help produce serous fluid, which is picked up on a glass slide, covered with a coverslip, and examined with the darkfield microscope. Living *T. pallida* demonstrate gradual motion to and fro, rotational movement around the long axis, and rather sudden 90 degree bending near the center of the organism. Since most physicians do not have the proper equipment and are not familiar with the techniques of darkfield microscopy, the state public health authorities can be called for assistance. A mail-in darkfield test, in which lesion fluid is drawn up in a capillary tube, sealed, and mailed to a state laboratory for fluorescent antibody identification of treponemes, is under investigation but not readily available.

T. pallidum may also be demonstrated in biopsies or pathologic specimens by fluorescent antibody stains or by silver stains.

Serologic Tests. Two basic types of humoral antibody are stimulated by infection with *T. pallidum*: nonspecific antibody directed against diphosphatidyl glycerol (cardiolipin), which is a normal component of many tissues; and specific treponemal antibodies. Nonspecific antibodies against cardiolipin were formerly designated "reagin," a term which should be discarded to avoid confusion with another "reagin," IgE. The kinds of tests used in syphilis are summarized in Table 1.

NONSPECIFIC TESTS. Anticardiolipin antibodies were first discovered by Wassermann in 1907, using extracts of congenitally syphilitic livers as the antigen for a complement fixation test. Subsequently it was shown that normal livers contained the same antigen as do many other tissues; the antigen for this class of test is now extracted from beef heart. As yet there is no convincing explanation for why patients infected with *T. pallidum* develop increasing titers of antibody against a normal tissue component.

The Wassermann test has now been replaced by related tests. The standard test in use today for detection of anticardiolipin antibody is the Venereal Disease Research Laboratories (VDRL) test, which is an easily quantitated slide flocculation test. Many similar tests,

TABLE 1. Serologic Tests for Syphilis

Type	Use
Nonspecific (anticardiolipin) antibodies:	
VDRL (slide flocculation)	Screening, quantitation, following response to treatment
RPR (agglutination)	Screening
Kolmer (complement fixation)	Limited
Specific treponemal antibodies:	
FTA-ABS (immunofluorescence with absorbed serum)	Confirmatory, diagnostic, not for routine screening
MHA-TP (microhemagglutination)	Similar to FTA-ABS but can be quantitated and automated
TPI (immobilization)	Most specific but not generally available

VDRL = Venereal Disease Research Laboratories test.
RPR = Rapid plasma reagin test.
FTA-ABS = Fluorescent treponemal antibody absorption test.
TPI = *Treponema pallidum* immobilization test.
MHA-TP = Microhemagglutination assay for *T. pallidum*.

including the rapid plasma reagin (RPR) test and the unheated serum reagin (USR) test, are frequently used for screening for syphilis.

The VDRL and related tests are simple, well standardized, cheap, and easy to perform and are the screening tests of choice. The VDRL is the test of choice for following response of patients to treatment. Since the VDRL detects antibody against a normal tissue component, it may be falsely positive in a significant number of patients. The relative proportion of patients with a false-positive VDRL depends on the prevalence of syphilis in the community; the lower the prevalence of syphilis, the higher the proportion of positive VDRL tests which are due to nonsyphilitic causes.

The VDRL test begins to turn positive a week or two after the onset of the chancre. In large series of patients with primary syphilis, approximately two thirds have had a positive VDRL test. Obviously then a negative VDRL test does not exclude primary syphilis, particularly if the lesion is less than two weeks old. The VDRL is positive in 99 per cent of patients with secondary syphilis, the only exceptions being patients with such high titers of antibody that they are in antibody excess; dilution of the serum will then paradoxically result in conversion of a negative test to positive. VDRL reactivity tends to diminish in later stages of the disease, and only about 70 per cent of patients with cardiovascular or neurosyphilis have a positive VDRL test.

The *quantitative titer* of the VDRL test is somewhat useful in diagnosis and quite useful in following therapeutic response. The titer is reported as the highest dilution which gives a positive response. Most patients with secondary syphilis have titers of at least 1:16. Most patients with false-positive VDRL tests have titers of less than 1:8. No single titer is in itself diagnostic. Significant rises (fourfold or greater) in paired sera, however, are strongly indicative of acute syphilis.

TREPONEMAL TESTS. There are many varieties of specific treponemal antibody tests. The first and still perhaps best test is the *Treponema pallidum* immobilization (TPI) test, which when properly performed is nearly completely specific for infection by *T. pallidum* or related pathogenic spirochetes. Unfortunately it is cumbersome and expensive and therefore is not routinely done in the United States at present. The most widely used treponemal antibody test is the fluorescent treponemal antibody absorption (FTA-ABS) test. Patient serum is absorbed with extracts of nonpathogenic cultivable treponemes to remove cross-reacting group treponemal antibody. The absorbed serum is reacted with dried *T. pallidum* on a glass slide, and specific antitreponemal antibodies are detected by subsequent addition of fluorescein-labeled anti-human gamma globulin. Other treponemal tests are based on agglutination of red cells to which *T. pallidum* antigens have been fixed. The most commonly used hemagglutination test is the microhemagglutination assay for *T. pallidum* (MHA-TP).

The precise nature of the antigens involved in these tests is not known. Characterization of the antigens of *T. pallidum* has been greatly hindered by inability to grow the organism in cell-free culture. Antibodies reactive in the various tests are found in all major immunoglobulin classes (IgG, IgM, IgA). A modification of the FTA-ABS test has been developed using fluorescein-labeled anti-human IgM (IgM FTA-ABS). The IgM FTA-ABS test is of some use in diagnosis of early congenital syphilis but is of no use in distinguishing acute disease from old infections in adults.

The FTA-ABS test is best used as a confirmatory test. It is somewhat more difficult to perform than the VDRL test and cannot be easily quantitated. It is sensitive and has a high degree of specificity, being positive in only approximately 1 per cent of normal individuals. It is positive in 85 per cent of patients with primary syphilis, 99 per cent with secondary syphilis, and in at least 95 per cent with late syphilis. It may therefore be the only test positive in patients with cardiovascular or neurologic syphilis. In late syphilis the FTA-ABS test usually remains positive for life despite adequate therapy. It (as well as the TPI and MHA-TP) is positive in other treponemal diseases such as pinta, yaws, and bejel.

The FTA-ABS test is reported in terms of relative brilliance of fluorescence, from borderline to 4+. Borderline reactivity has the same meaning as nonreactive for clinical purposes. Most laboratories report 1+ positive tests as reactive, but some studies have shown that such tests may be relatively difficult to reproduce. Occasional laboratories therefore only report as positive tests with 2+ or greater reactivity. In patients lacking historical or clinical evidence of syphilis but with a reactive FTA-ABS test, one should repeat the FTA-ABS test. Use of another treponemal test such as the MHA-TP may be helpful in certain problem cases.

The MHA-TP test is less sensitive than either the VDRL or the FTA-ABS test in primary syphilis. Its sensitivity and specificity otherwise are nearly identical to those of the FTA-ABS test, being positive in nearly all patients with secondary syphilis and in 95 per cent or more of patients with late syphilis. An automated version of the MHA-TP test is now being developed for widespread use. The reactivity of serologic tests for syphilis in various stages of disease is shown in Table 2.

False-Positive Serologic Tests for Syphilis. The VDRL or RPR test may be positive in a variety of diseases other than syphilis. A false-positive test is defined as a reproducible positive test in a patient with no clinical or historical evidence of syphilis, and whose serum FTA-ABS or MHA-TP test is negative.

"Acute" (less than six months) false-positive VDRL tests occur with low frequency in atypical pneumonia, malaria, and other bacterial or viral infections, and may occur after smallpox or other vaccinations as well. *Chronic false-positive VDRL tests* (lasting longer than six months) are relatively common in autoimmune disorders such as systemic lupus erythematosus, in narcotic addicts, in leprosy, and in aged persons. From 8 to 20 per cent of patients with systemic lupus erythematosus have been reported as having false-positive VDRL test, and the false-positive test may develop many years prior to the onset of other manifestations of the disease. A chronic false-positive VDRL test in females age

TABLE 2.   Frequency of Positive Serologic Tests in
Untreated Syphilis

Stage	VDRL (%)	FTA-ABS (%)	MHA-TP (%)
Primary	70	85	50-60
Secondary	99	100	100
Latent or late	70	98	98

TABLE 3. Penicillin Treatment Practice in Syphilis as Recommended by
United States Public Health Service (1976)

Indications for Syphilis Therapy†	Dosage and Administration*		
	Benzathine Penicillin G	Aqueous Benzyl Penicillin G or Procaine Penicillin G	Procaine Penicillin G in Aluminum Stearate Suspension (PAM)
Primary, secondary, and early latent syphilis (<1 year); epidemiologic treatment	Total of 2.4 million units; single IM dose of two injections of 1.2 million units in one session	Total of 4.8 million units IM in doses of 600,000 units daily for eight consecutive days	Total of 4.8 million units IM; first dose 2.4 million units and 1.2 million units at each of two subsequent injections three days apart (over nine days)
Late latent (>1 year) or when cerebrospinal fluid was not examined in "latency"; asymptomatic neurosyphilis, symptomatic neurosyphilis, cardiovascular syphilis, late benign (cutaneous, osseous, visceral gumma)	Total of 7.2 million units IM in doses of 2.4 million units at seven-day intervals, over 21 days	Total of 9 million units IM in doses of 600,000 units daily over 15 days; in selected cases of symptomatic CNS syphilis, 2 to 4 million units of aqueous (crystalline) penicillin G intravenously every four hours for at least ten days	No recommendation by USPHS; total dose of 9 million units over 15 to 21 days is effective
Congenital Early Up to two years of age	If CSF is normal: Total of 50,000 units per kilogram IM in a single or divided dose at one session	If CSF is abnormal: Total of 50,000 units per kilogram IM per day for ten consecutive days‡	No recommendation by USPHS
Late Two to 12 years, weight 32 kg (71 lb) or less	Same as for early congenital syphilis	Same as for early congenital syphilis	Same as for early congenital syphilis
Over 12 years, or over 32 kg	Same as for adult late latent syphilis	Same as for adult late latent syphilis	Same as for adult late latent syphilis

*Individual doses can be divided for injection in each buttock to minimize discomfort.

†In *pregnancy*, treatment is dependent on the stage of syphilis.

‡For aqueous penicillin, give in two divided doses per day; for procaine penicillin, give as one daily dose.

20 or younger carries a significant risk of future development of systemic lupus erythematosus, thyroiditis, or other autoimmune disorders, and such patients should be followed carefully for a considerable period of time. As many as one third of patients with narcotic addiction have a false-positive VDRL test. Over 1 per cent of patients aged 70 and 10 per cent of patients over age 80 have a low titer false-positive VDRL test. Most false-positive VDRL tests have a titer of 1:8 or less, although occasional patients with lymphoma and other diseases have been described with very high titer false-positive VDRL tests.

A positive FTA-ABS test is usually indicative of recent or past syphilis. However, there is an increased incidence of false-positive FTA-ABS tests in systemic lupus erythematosus and in other chronic diseases associated with hyperglobulinemia, including rheumatoid arthritis, biliary cirrhosis, and others. False-positive tests are of two kinds in systemic lupus erythematosus: the most common is one with a beaded pattern of fluorescence, which has been shown to be due to anti-DNA antibodies; there also may be homogeneous fluorescence of the treponeme indistinguishable from a true positive test in syphilis. Patients with systemic lupus who have a false-positive FTA-ABS test almost always have a negative VDRL test (and conversely, patients with SLE with a positive VDRL usually have a negative FTA-ABS).

Occasionally one encounters reproducible positive FTA-ABS tests in patients with no clinical or historical evidence of syphilis, and in whom there is no evidence of diseases associated with false-positive FTA-ABS tests. It may be wise to obtain cerebrospinal fluid for examination of total protein, cells, and VDRL reactivity in order to rule out neurosyphilis. If in doubt and if the patient is not allergic to penicillin, it is often wisest to treat such patients for possible syphilis.

IgM FTA-ABS Test for Congenital Syphilis. Mothers with a positive VDRL or FTA-ABS test will deliver infants with a positive VDRL and FTA-ABS test because of passive transfer of the IgG antibodies reactive in these tests. Since many infants with congenital syphilis are clinically normal at birth but develop serious symptomatic disease some weeks later, it is important to determine whether a newborn with a positive VDRL or FTA-ABS test has passively transferred maternal antibody or is actively infected. Since maternal IgM antibodies are not passively transferred to the fetus, an IgM FTA-ABS test has been developed to test for syphilis in the newborn. Unfortunately there is approximately a 35 per cent incidence of false-negative IgM FTA-ABS tests in delayed-onset congenital syphilis. There also is a false-positive rate of approximately 10 per cent. For these reasons the IgM FTA-ABS test is of limited use in diagnosis of neonatal syphilis.

If the mother has been adequately treated for syphilis during pregnancy and the infant is clinically normal at birth, one may elect to follow the infant carefully by serial examination and VDRL titers. If the positive VDRL in the infant is due to passively transferred maternal antibody, the titer of reactivity will fall markedly in the first two months of life. A rising titer indicates active disease and the need for treatment. Many physicians are unwilling to risk failure of proper follow-up of VDRL-positive but clinically normal neonates, and instead administer effective therapy immediately. The risk of penicillin allergy in neonates is very low.

TREATMENT. There have been many therapies for syphilis in the past, including mercurial, arsenical, and bismuth compounds, as well as induced fever. All of these have been replaced by penicillin because it is more effective, simple, and safe.

T. pallidum is highly susceptible to penicillin, being inhibited by less than 0.01 μg of penicillin G. Since treponemes divide slowly, and since penicillin acts only on dividing cells, it is necessary to maintain serum levels of penicillin for many days. Studies in animals and in man show that more therapy is required as the length of infection increases. Current recommendations for treatment of syphilis are summarized in Table 3.

Early (Less Than One Year) Infectious Syphilis. Early syphilis may be treated with a single injection of 2.4 million units of *benzathine penicillin G*, which provides low but effective serum levels for over two weeks. Extensive studies in the 1940's and 1950's with regimens which provided similar serum levels and duration of therapy showed that approximately 95 per cent of patients were cured by such treatment. Many of the remaining 5 per cent who had clinical or serologic evidence of relapse may actually have been reinfected. It is not necessary to examine the cerebrospinal fluid at this stage, because penicillin prevents development of later neurosyphilis. Motile treponemes disappear from primary lesions in 24 hours.

A single injection of 2.4 million units of *aqueous procaine penicillin*, which provides relatively high serum levels for a brief period, is ineffective in established early syphilis, but is curative if the disease is still in the incubating stage (e.g., in a patient who is being treated for gonorrhea and who happened to acquire syphilis simultaneously). Other regimens currently useful for gonorrhea have uncertain effects on incubating syphilis, and careful follow-up for syphilis is indicated in gonorrhea patients treated with regimens other than procaine penicillin. The incidence of incubating syphilis in gonorrhea patients is 2 per cent or more in several series.

For patients allergic to penicillin, tetracycline hydrochloride may be given in a total dose of 30 grams over 15 days, or erythromycin base may be given in a total dose of 30 grams over 15 days. Particularly careful follow-up is necessary in patients treated with drugs other than penicillin, because patients may not be fully compliant with these prolonged courses of oral therapy and these regimens have been less fully evaluated clinically. Cephaloridine or other cephalosporins may be effective but have not been well studied. Chloramphenicol is of equivocal efficacy and for this reason, as well as because of the risk of toxicity, should not be used. Spectinomycin has essentially no effect on syphilis.

Syphilis of More Than One Year's Duration. Larger doses of penicillin are needed for *neurosyphilis* (see Ch. 301) than for syphilis of less than one year's duration. In general, patients with general paresis respond better to treatment than do patients with tabes dorsalis, although patients with paresis should be expected to show residual effects of the infection. This is particularly true in advanced cases. Meningovascular syphilis usually responds well, except for residual damage to cranial nerves or cortical function resulting from ischemic infarcts. Published studies show that a total of 6.0 to 9.0 million units of penicillin G results in a satisfactory clinical response in approximately 90 per cent of patients with neurosyphilis.

Currently used benzathine penicillin regimens have received relatively little study in neurosyphilis. Benzathine penicillin G in a total dose of 7.2 million units given as 2.4 million units weekly for three successive weeks is effective in most patients. However, there are reports of patients who have failed standard penicillin therapy for neurosyphilis but who responded to intensive intravenous therapy which provided high serum levels of penicillin. Benzathine penicillin does not provide measurable levels of penicillin in the spinal fluid or aqueous humor of the eye. *Therefore in cases of symptomatic central nervous system syphilis, which is a serious disease, there is considerable rationale to treatment with aqueous penicillin G, 600,000 units daily for 15 days, or for intensive intravenous therapy with penicillin G (20 million units per day for at least 10 days in hospital).* Therapy of neurosyphilis not infrequently results in increased CSF pleocytosis for seven to ten days after starting treatment, and may transiently convert a normal CSF to abnormal.

Limited evidence suggests that treating *latent syphilis* with 7.2 million units total dose of benzathine penicillin is curative even if the patient has asymptomatic neurosyphilis. However, because of the possible lack of the efficacy of benzathine penicillin in some patients with central nervous system syphilis, it is desirable to examine cerebrospinal fluid in all patients with latent syphilis to exclude asymptomatic neurosyphilis. Alternatively, one may reasonably elect to perform a lumbar puncture at the conclusion of the follow-up period (two years); if the CSF is normal, the patient can be reassured that neurosyphilis will not develop.

There is no evidence that therapy with antimicrobial drugs is clinically beneficial to patients with *cardiovascular syphilis*. Nevertheless, treatment of cardiovascular syphilis is recommended in order to prevent further progression of disease and because approximately 15 per cent of patients with cardiovascular syphilis have associated neurosyphilis.

There is no evidence as to the efficacy of other antimicrobials in treatment of late syphilis. Therefore if patients are allergic to penicillin, it is mandatory that the cerebrospinal fluid be examined before therapy is undertaken. Either tetracycline, 2 grams daily for 30 days, or erythromycin, 2 grams daily for 30 days, is probably effective.

Syphilis in Pregnancy. All pregnant women should be examined with a VDRL or RPR test during pregnancy; if they are at high risk for syphilis, a second test should be obtained before delivery. Because of the risk of infection to the fetus, evaluation and treatment of the VDRL-positive patient should be done as rapidly as possible, particularly for patients first seen in the later stages of pregnancy. If a confirmatory FTA-ABS test is positive and the patient has not been treated, penicillin (or erythromycin for patients who are allergic to penicillin) should be administered in doses appropriate for early or late syphilis as outlined above. For patients who are VDRL positive but FTA-ABS negative and who have no clinical signs of syphilis, treatment may be withheld. In such patients a quantitative VDRL test and another FTA-ABS test should be repeated in four weeks. If the VDRL titer has risen by fourfold or more, or if clinical signs of syphilis have developed, the patient should be treated. If after repeat examination the diagnosis remains equivocal, the patient should be treated to prevent possible disease in the neonate. After treatment a quantitative VDRL titer should be followed monthly; if it rises fourfold, the patient should be treated a second time.

Congenital Syphilis. Proper treatment of the mother usually prevents active congenital syphilis in the neonate. However, infected infants may be clinically normal at birth, and the infant may be seronegative if the mother's infection was acquired late in pregnancy. The infant should be treated at birth if the mother had received no or inadequate treatment, or had been treated with drugs other than penicillin, or if the infant cannot be carefully followed up for several months after birth. Cerebrospinal fluid should be examined before treatment of the infant. If the cerebrospinal fluid is normal, treatment may be with a single injection of 50,000 units per kilogram of benzathine penicillin G. If the fluid is abnormal, treatment should be with aqueous penicillin G, 50,000 units per kilogram intramuscularly or intravenously daily, given in two divided doses, for a minimum of ten days. Alternatively, a single daily intramuscular injection of procaine penicillin G, 50,000 units per kilogram, may be given for ten days. These recommendations are based upon the failure of benzathine penicillin to provide adequate treponemicidal levels in spinal fluid, and on evidence that aqueous or procaine penicillin does provide adequate cerebrospinal fluid levels of penicillin.

Tetracycline should not be used to treat children of less than eight years of age. Antimicrobial agents other than penicillin are not recommended for treatment of congenital syphilis.

Follow-up Examinations. All patients with early syphilis or congenital syphilis should return for quantitative VDRL titers and clinical examination 3, 6, and 12 months after treatment. Patients with late latent syphilis should be examined also at 24 months after therapy; if cerebrospinal fluid was not examined prior to therapy, a lumbar puncture should be done prior to discharge to rule out inadequately treated asymptomatic neurosyphilis.

The quantitative VDRL titer should return to normal within 12 months after therapy of primary syphilis or 24 months after therapy of secondary syphilis. In a small percentage of patients with early syphilis, the VDRL will remain reactive in low titer for long periods of time. Chronic low titer VDRL reactivity after therapy is much more common in late syphilis and should not be viewed with alarm. A progressively rising VDRL titer after therapy (a fourfold or greater rise) is sufficient evidence for retreatment. Patients with treated early syphilis are fully susceptible to reinfection, and many clinical and serologic relapses after therapy are probably reinfections. As such they represent failures of proper epidemiologic case finding and preventive therapy of the patient's sexual contacts.

Patients with neurosyphilis should be followed with serologic tests for at least three years and with repeat examination of cerebrospinal fluid at six-month intervals. The cerebrospinal fluid pleocytosis is the first abnormality to disappear, but cell counts may not be normal for one to two years. The elevated cerebrospinal fluid protein falls more slowly, followed by the positive cerebrospinal fluid VDRL test, which may take years to become negative. Rising cerebrospinal fluid cell counts, protein, and VDRL titer obtained at follow-up are an indication for retreatment.

Epidemiologic Investigation and Treatment. All patients with syphilis should be reported to public health authorities. In the absence of an effective vaccine, control of syphilis depends on finding and treating persons with infectious lesions of primary and secondary syphilis before they can further transmit the disease, and on finding and treating persons with incubating syphilis before they have developed infectious lesions. All patients with early syphilis (less than one year) should be carefully interviewed by qualified persons to determine the nature of their recent sex contacts. Approximately 16 per cent of the named recent contacts of patients with early syphilis will be found to have active untreated syphilis on examination, and a similar proportion of

individuals named as suspects or associates will also have active syphilis. Approximately 20 per cent of cases of early syphilis seen in the United States at present are found by epidemiologic investigation of index cases with syphilis.

Most authorities, particularly in the United States, recommend treatment of sexual contacts of patients with early syphilis even if the contacts are clinically and serologically normal on examination. This is justifiable, because 30 per cent of clinically normal individuals named as contacts of persons with infectious lesions of syphilis within the previous 30 days will go on to develop syphilis if untreated. In general, preventive treatment is given to all sexual contacts of the past 90 days, although nearly all cases of syphilis in contacts will have developed within 60 days of exposure.

Jarisch-Herxheimer Reaction. Up to 60 per cent of patients with early syphilis, and a significant proportion of patients with later stages of syphilis, experience a transient febrile reaction after therapy for syphilis. This usually occurs in the first few hours after therapy, peaks at six to eight hours, and disappears within 12 to 24 hours of therapy. Temperature elevation is usually low grade, and there is often associated myalgia, headache, and malaise. The skin lesions of secondary syphilis are often exacerbated during the Herxheimer reaction, and cutaneous lesions which were not visible may become visible. It is usually of no clinical significance and may be treated with salicylates in most cases. In patients with syphilis of the coronary ostia or of the optic nerve, there is a theoretical risk that local inflammation coincident with the Herxheimer reaction could precipitate serious damage. This is the subject of much discussion in the old literature, but there is little current evidence that "local Herxheimer reactions" constitute a significant risk to the patient. Corticosteroids have been used to prevent adverse effects of the Herxheimer reaction, but there is no evidence that they are clinically beneficial (other than reducing fever) or necessary. Institution of treatment with small doses of penicillin does not prevent the Herxheimer reaction.

The pathogenesis of the Herxheimer reaction is unclear. It may be due to liberation of antigens from the spirochetes. There is evidence of activation of the complement cascade, including transient consumption of C3, C4, C6, and C7, and of transient decrease in treponemal antibodies coincident with the Herxheimer reaction. There is also evidence for endotoxemia, obtained by positive limulus amebocyte gelation tests, at the time of the Herxheimer reaction, although *T. pallidum* does not contain biologically active endotoxin. These seemingly contradictory observations could be explained if the reaction resulted in release of endogenous endotoxin from the gut.

Persistence of Treponemes After Treatment. Studies in man and in rabbits have shown that spiral forms may be visualized by silver stains in lymph nodes after effective treatment. Living virulent treponemes have occasionally been recovered by rabbit inoculation from lymph nodes, cerebrospinal fluid, or ocular fluids after effective treatment has been given. These documented cases of treponemal persistence are very rare, however. There are many other reports of spiral forms in various body tissues and fluids which stain with fluorescent treponemal antibodies; the significance of these is difficult to assess, as infectivity tests in rabbits were not performed in the majority of these reports. At present there is little reason to worry about persistence of virulent treponemes after therapy with penicillin, with the possible exception of central nervous system syphilis, which needs further evaluation. There is no evidence for selection of penicillin-resistant mutants of *T. pallidum* to date.

PROSPECTS FOR PREVENTION. Solid immunity develops in rabbits following prolonged infection with virulent *T. pallidum*. It has not yet been possible to passively transfer immunity in laboratory animals by either immune serum or immune lymphocytes alone, suggesting that both cellular and humoral systems are necessary for immunity. Rabbits have been effectively immunized with multiple injections of treponemes which have been rendered avirulent by irradiation or by exposure to cold. However, a very large number of injections and a large mass of treponemes are necessary to effect immunity in the laboratory animal. For this reason and since *T. pallidum* cannot yet be grown in a virulent state in cell-free medium, there is no immediate prospect for a vaccine. However, significant immunity does develop in man after prolonged infection, and it should be possible to develop an effective vaccine after successful cultivation of *T. pallidum* has been accomplished. There is reason for optimism that this may happen in the foreseeable future. For the present, control depends entirely on clinical awareness on the part of physicians, adequate reporting to public health authorities, and vigorous application of epidemiologic investigation and preventive treatment of sexual contacts.

There is a real need for better health education, starting in the schools. It is not unreasonable to educate about sexually transmitted disease as early as the sixth grade. The public needs to be reminded that condoms will help to prevent disease, and that soap and water may possibly avert an infection if used immediately after exposure. Many contraceptive foams are treponemicidal. Patients can be educated to report to a physician upon the earliest signs of disease. It is difficult to alter patterns of sexual behavior, but proper education and case reporting will help control the incidence of syphilis. Each physician bears a portion of the over-all responsibility for this task.

Bryceson, A. D. M.: Clinical pathology of the Jarisch-Herxheimer reaction. J. Infect. Dis., 133:696, 1976.

Drusin, L. M., Singer, C., Valenti, A. J., and Armstrong, D.: Infectious syphilis mimicking neoplastic disease. Arch. Intern. Med., 137:156, 1977.

Fehér, J., Somogyi, T., Timmer, M., and Józsa, L.: Early syphilitic hepatitis. Lancet, 2:896, 1975.

Fischer, A., Kristensen, J. K., and Husfelt, V.: Tertiary syphilis in Denmark 1961–1970. A description of 105 cases not previously diagnosed or specifically treated. Acta Dermatovener., 56:485, 1976.

Fulford, K. W. M., Johnson, N., Loveday, C., Storey, J., and Tedder, R. S.: Changes in intra-vascular complement and anti-treponemal antibody titres preceding the Jarisch-Herxheimer reaction in secondary syphilis. J. Clin. Exp. Immunol., 24:483, 1976.

Gamble, C. N., and Reardan, J. B.: Immunopathogenesis of syphilitic glomerulonephritis: Elution of antitreponemal antibody from glomerular immune-complex deposits. N. Engl. J. Med., 292:449, 1975.

Gjestland, T.: The Oslo study of untreated syphilis: An epidemiologic investigation of the natural course of the syphilitic infection based upon a re-study of the Boeck-Bruusgaard material. Acta Derm. Venereol., 35: Suppl. 34, 1955.

Kaufman, R. E., Olansky, D. C., and Wiesner, P. J.: The FTA-ABS (IgM) test for neonatal congenital syphilis: A critical review. J. Am. Vener. Dis. Assoc., 1:79, 1974.

Magnuson, H. J., Thomas, E. W., Olansky, S., Kaplan, B. I., De Mello, L., and Cutler, J. C.: Inoculation syphilis in human volunteers. Medicine, 35:33, 1956.

Musher, D. M., Schell, R. F., Jones, R. H., and Jones, A. M.: Lympho-
cyte transformation in syphilis: An in vitro correlate or immune suppression in vivo? Infect. Immun., 11:1261, 1975.

Prewitt, T. A.: Syphilitic aortic insufficiency. JAMA, 211:637, 1970.

Raskind, M. A., and Eisdorfer, C.: Screening for syphilis in an aged psychiatrically impaired population. West. J. Med., 125:361, 1976.

Schroeter, A. L., Turner, R. H., Lucas, J. B., and Brown, W. J.: Therapy for incubating syphilis: Effectiveness of gonorrhea treatment. JAMA, 218:711, 1971.

Sparling, P. F.: Diagnosis and treatment of syphilis. N. Engl. J. Med., 284:642, 1971.

Syphilotherapy 1976: Position papers for the current USPHS recommendations. J. Am. Vener. Dis. Assoc., 3:98, 1976.

Tramont, E. C.: Persistence of *Treponema pallidum* following penicillin G therapy: Report of two cases. JAMA, 236:2206, 1976.

Turner, T. B.: Syphilis and the treponematoses. *In* Mudd, S. (ed.): Infectious Agents and Host Reactions. Philadelphia, W. B. Saunders Company, 1970.

Wilner, E., and Brody, J. A.: Prognosis of general paresis after treatment. Lancet, 2:1370, 1968.

172. NONSYPHILITIC TREPONEMATOSES

Thorstein Guthe

172.1. YAWS

(Frambesia Tropica, Pian, Bouba, Parangi, Patek)

DEFINITION. Yaws is produced by a spirochetal microorganism, *T. pertenue*, which causes a chronic human infection, most often with onset in childhood. An initial cutaneous lesion usually appears, followed by relapsing infectious secondary nondestructive lesions of the skin, periosteum, and bones, frequently interspersed with symptom-free periods. Late manifestations include destructive and deforming lesions of skin, bones, and joints. Hyperkeratosis, notably of the soles, may develop in secondary and late yaws. There is no evidence of cardiac or nervous system involvement or of prenatal manifestations. Infected persons slowly develop relative immunity, and humoral antibodies can be detected by serologic tests reactive also in other treponematoses (syphilis, pinta).

HISTORY. Yaws probably existed in Africa from remote times. Early accounts suggest that it was brought to the West Indies with the slave trade in the sixteenth century. By the eighteenth century it had become a serious health problem of the Antilles, Central America, and South America, as well as in areas of Oceania and Southeast Asia. Savages (1778) proposed the name frambesia for the disease because of the raspberry-like appearance of its papillomatous secondary lesions. Moseley (1800) observed its clinical course, notably that yaws ends in enlarged nodes and destructive lesions. Maxwell (1839) determined its incubation period to be three to four weeks after inoculation of lesion material into humans. Castellani (1905) identified *T. pertenue* as the causative microorganism of yaws. Lambert (1923) first attempted community-wide treatment with arsenicals in the Pacific Isles. The advent of long-acting penicillin preparations and single injection therapy revolutionized case treatment and made possible important reduction of yaws by mass penicillin campaigns (World Health Organization, 1950–1970) in the tropics.

The author wishes to acknowledge the valuable advice of his colleagues Drs. J. Ridet and G. Causse, Medical Officers, Communicable Diseases Division, World Health Organization, Geneva, concerning this chapter.

ETIOLOGY. The causative agent, *T. pertenue,* is a helical cell 8 to 12 μ in length and about 0.2 μ in diameter, with several closely set spirals. It resembles *T. pallidum* (syphilis) and *T. carateum* (pinta) morphologically in dark-field illumination and structurally in electron microphotographs. *T. pertenue* has not been grown in vitro, but will survive in special media for several days without multiplication. Strains stored in glycerin remain virulent for many years at $-70°$ C (CO_2 ice) or lower temperatures, e.g., liquid nitrogen or helium. *T. pertenue* is pathogenic for the same animal species as *T. pallidum.* The latter causes subclinical "silent" infection in the hamster, whereas *T. pertenue* causes a specific dermatitis — a procedure sometimes used to differentiate between treponemes in the laboratory (Vaisman, 1969). Pathogenic treponemes closely resembling or identical with *T. pertenue* have been isolated from wild cynomolgous African monkeys (Fribourg-Blanc et al.; Sepetjian et al., 1968).

EPIDEMIOLOGY AND PATHOGENESIS. Despite mass penicillin campaigns in recent years, yaws has remained a disease of many rural communities in the intertropical zone in Africa, the Americas, Southeast Asia, and Oceania. Areas of high prevalence of active yaws sometimes lie within a few miles of communities where the disease is rarely observed, depending on the ecologic situation, the evolutionary stage of endemicity, and the number of susceptibles at any given time. There is also a higher frequency of early yaws lesion in the rainy than in the dry season (Harding, 1947). Moreover, skin lesions are less frequent in cooler climates in mountainous tropical communities where they also become less moist and where papillomas tend to erupt in sweaty, mucocutaneous junctions and skin folds rather than involving the flat body surfaces (Ramsey, 1925). Furthermore, the occasional yaws lesions encountered after mass penicillin campaigns appear to be less extensive and less moist. In areas where no further lesions are encountered after such campaigns, continued specific seroreactivity (TPI) in a small proportion of children born after the campaigns could suggest the possibility of asymptomatic infection taking place in the new circumstances.

T. pertenue is incapable of penetrating unbroken skin. It is also unable to pass the placenta and cause congenital yaws. Transmission usually occurs through contact of skin abrasions, cuts, or lesions, e.g., trauma, injury, dermatoses, with infectious yaws lesions of another person. Indirect transmission via contaminated hands is believed to occur among children. Nursing mothers are sometimes infected directly by their infants. In addition to early infectious lesions, untreated latent yaws cases — which are liable to relapse with active lesions — form an important part of the reservoir maintaining the disease in rural communities. Humidity, moisture-holding soil, and mean annual temperatures of 27° C or more are also necessary for the spread of yaws. Moreover, transmission is favored by scant clothing, bare feet, crowded dwellings, and deficient personal hygiene. The gradual improvement of environmental and socioeconomic conditions will reduce the attack rate of yaws (Saxena and Prasad, 1963).

No true vector has been found in which *T. pertenue* actually multiplies, but it has been shown that disease can be transmitted by experimentally infected gnats. In some areas *Hippelates pallipes* may serve as mechanical carriers (Kumm and Turner, 1936). Geographic coexistence of foci of human yaws and natural treponematoses of wild cynomolgous monkeys has been observed in Africa (Baylet et al., 1970).

The age distribution of yaws depends on the rate of transmission and level of endemicity. In hyperendemic communities, e.g., the former Netherlands New Guinea (Kranendonk), the highest incidence of infectious lesions was in the two- to five-year-olds, with a seroprevalence of more than 90 per cent, pointing to an early almost complete epidemic "saturation" of the community with yaws. In areas of moderate or low endemicity the highest seroprevalence is in older age groups. For example, this has been observed among the pygmies in the Cameroons and in Zaire, where FTA/ABS seroreactivity was found to be 45 to 50 per cent in those more than 30 years of age (Pampligione and Wilkinson). After mass penicillin campaigns in areas of high endemicity, maximal seroprevalence was in the 45- to 59-year-olds, e.g., Nigeria, signaling regression of a hyperendemic situation many years ago. In the latter instance many more young individuals are susceptible to yaws in the new generation, but there are also more barriers to impede renewed spread of the infection, e.g., education, health consciousness, chemotherapy, and health services. On the other hand, the greater number of serologically nonreactive young people in the new generation have, when reaching puberty, less protective cross-immunity to infection with venereal syphilis. This, in turn, has been reported to be among the reasons for the increased incidence of syphilis noted in tropical countries in the last decade.

PATHOLOGY. A main pathologic feature of yaws is the involvement of the skin. In early lesions the epidermis is thickened. There is cell infiltration ("plasmocytoma") of the dermis, hyperplasia, edema, and the presence of many treponemes. The papillae are elongated, often with thickening of the interpapillary pegs. Proliferation of vascular endothelium and obstruction of vessels are less characteristic of yaws than of syphilis. The epithelium may show hyperkeratosis, become superficially eroded, and be covered by dried exudate. The acanthotic epidermis and the papillary proliferation give rise to a fungating, frambesiform, crust-covered lesion. Diffuse periostitis and cortical rarefaction of the long bones are common in early yaws and are more marked than in venereal syphilis. The late lesions of yaws are due to a different tissue response, and endarteritis is observed histopathologically. Late lesions include ulcerating granulomatous nodules and gumma of the skin and bones. The gumma is built of elements similar to syphilitic lesions. Late skeletal affliction is mostly characterized by periosteal proliferation, rarefaction, or destruction of multiple areas of the long bones which can lead to extensive deformities.

CLINICAL CHARACTERISTICS. At the site of entry of *T. pertenue* an initial lesion usually develops after an incubation period of three to four weeks. The implantation is facilitated by previous breaks in the skin (abrasion, injury, vaccination). The lesion is a papule situated on the legs in more than half the cases. In babies and toddlers it often appears on the buttocks or in the perineum. The papule grows into a round, broad-based granulomatous lesion ("mother yaw") covered by a serous crust from which *T. pertenue* can be recovered. The regional lymph nodes are frequently enlarged, not

A, Initial lesions in early pinta. *B*, Late pigmented blue variety pinta. *C*, Early papillomatous yaws. *D*, Osteoperiostitis of yaws. *E*, Deep ulcerated late yaws of arm before therapy with long-acting penicillin. *F*, Same patient after treatment.

"shotty," and do not suppurate. An initial lesion will heal spontaneously within three to six months; ulcerating initial lesions require more time to heal.

As a result of early treponemia a generalized secondary eruption appears before or after the healing of the initial lesion. The most frequent and characteristic eruptions are roundish, raised, rough, granulomatous papules ("yaws" or frambesides), often covered by a brownish crust. These lesions appear anywhere on the skin, but rarely on the scalp. They sometimes show arciform arrangements. Secondary lesions may last for more than six months. A new crop may appear before the preceding lesions heal. Relapsing crops tend increasingly to become localized, e.g., to periaxillary, perianal, or circumoral areas. Sometimes the papilloma may be solitary. Plantar papules appear late, often after the generalized eruption, and are modified by a thick keratotic layer characteristic of barefoot people: a cherry-like granuloma appears in a well of cracked horny layer, frequently giving rise to painful disability ("crab yaws"). On the body, micropapular as well as various forms of macular or desquamative macular ("pian dartre") lesions may also appear. Lesions of mucous membranes are rare, but occur. Desquamatous macules can develop in the palms and notably on the soles, which are sometimes covered by a thick hyperkeratotic layer. In addition to skin eruptions in early yaws, there is superficial lymph node enlargement. In many cases there are pain and tenderness of the tibial shaft and other long bones owing to early periostitis. Such periostitis sometimes leads to saber tibia and polydactylitis. In many cases the general health of the patient appears little affected; in others there are systemic manifestations, with irregular fever, loss of appetite, and weight loss.

The secondary lesions begin to regress after several months, but relapses may occur on and off for four to five years before true latency is reached. The latter can be interrupted by late lesions of several types. (1) *Superficial ulcerations* of the skin with central healing tendency are observed, and *cutaneous and subcutaneous nodules* with ulceration and marginal healing may leave markedly dyspigmented atrophic scars, sometimes with deforming contractures. (2) *Diffuse or more localized hyperkeratosis* of the soles — less frequently of the palms — with fissuring and pitting can result in a characteristic mottled pattern, occasionally complicated by ulceration and sometimes developing more than 15 years after the infection. (3) *Osteal or periosteal gummatous lesions* of the tibia and other long bones may penetrate subcutaneous and cutaneous tissues, resulting in chronic ulcerations. These may also affect tarsal and carpal bones, the scapula, the sternum, and the skull. Affliction of palatonasal structures may lead to gangosa (rhinopharyngitis mutilans), a spectacular condition similar to that in syphilis. The osteitis and periostitis can occur both in association with generalized skin lesions and after these have receded.

Other yaws lesions are less common and include painless subcutaneous fibromatous juxta-articular nodes, paranasal egg-shaped swelling of the superior maxillary bone (goundou), chronic late macular or hyperkeratotic lesions of palmar surfaces, and volar aspects of wrists and insteps of soles, frequently followed by depigmentation.

DIAGNOSIS. Typical early yaws lesions are generally not confused clinically with other conditions. Ulcerated initial leg lesions may sometimes be mistaken for other ulcerations, e.g., tropical ulcer. Also, spirochetes found in tropical ulcers resembling *Borrelia vincentii* may be mistaken for *T. pertenue*. Facial yaws papules may look like crusted impetigo. Individual lesions may resemble those of secondary syphilis or cutaneous leishmaniasis. Demonstration of treponemes by microscopic darkfield examination of exudate from the lesion and seroreactivity in reagin and treponemal antibody tests (VDRL, FTA-ABS, TPI, TPHA) serve to distinguish yaws from other conditions except those of the treponematosis group. Differential tests using *T. pertenue* as antigen have not given uneqivocal findings (Garner et al.). Reagin tests become positive in serum about a month after the initial lesion (Li and Soebekti, 1955), and TPI titers can be very high (1:2560) in early yaws (WHO, Eastern Nigeria, 1968). Ulcerating contractures and mutilating lesions may present differential diagnostic problems in relation notably to leprosy and tuberculosis. Hyperkeratosis of the soles is often confused with other plantar conditions, mainly keratoma plantare sulcatum, plantar pitting, and tropical hyperkeratotic conditions of unknown origin (Hackett and Lowenthal).

PROGNOSIS. In infected persons the prognosis is favorable when early treatment is provided. Otherwise, periodic infectious recurrences over many years give rise to months of incapacity. An undetermined number of infected persons develop late lesions. Others go on to spontaneous clinical cure; some also become serologically nonreactive ("burnt-out yaws"). Among those developing late chronic lesions, extensive invalidism, deformities, and functional impairment often result.

TREATMENT AND CONTROL. The aim of treatment of individual patients is cure of the early disease and prevention of late manifestations. Intramuscular injection of 1.2 million units of benzathine penicillin (DBED) or 2.4 million units of PAM (procaine penicillin G in oil and 2 per cent monosterate)* in adults and half doses for children suffices to cause disappearance of early lesions and prevent relapses. The response is dramatic. The early lesions usually become darkfield-negative within 48 hours, and healing takes place within one to two weeks. Serologic titers decline, but many retain low-titer reagin seroreactivity, depending on the duration of the infection (D'Mello and Krag, 1955). Penicillin sometimes causes a Herxheimer reaction. The usual safeguards against hypersensitivity reactions to penicillin should be taken (see Ch. 43). Persons with late yaws lesions may require repeated therapy. Oxytetracycline and chloretetracycline are reported to be useful in cases of deforming osteoperiostitis, indolent gummas, or ulcerations. A minimum of two grams daily for five to ten days in adults and proportionately less for children are given. Ulcerations of late yaws may also require application of local antiseptic dressings. Deformities caused by chronic osteitis and contractures may necessitate local surgery in addition to drug therapy.

In the efforts to achieve community-wide control of yaws, the previous work of the Jamaica Yaws Commission (1936) was in recent years extended under the auspices of the World Health Organization. Since 1950, more than 210 million people in 49 countries were examined, and some 53 million treated with long-acting penicillin in large-scale control programs. The aim was

---

*Not available in United States of America.

(1) to survey entire area populations so as to control the reservoir of infection; (2) to interrupt the spread of yaws through mass treatment, rendering early cases noncontagious, preventing infectious recurrences, and aborting incubating disease; and (3) to undertake post-campaign yaws surveillance by periodic resurveys to detect and promply treat overlooked cases or new infections that might arise. Untreated early cases free of clinical symptoms between outbreaks form an important part of the reservoir of infection and contribute to maintain the disease in rural communities. Accordingly, mass treatment criteria in these campaigns were based on a certain association in the population between the occurrence of clinically active lesions and of seroprevalence owing both to such lesions and to clinically symptom-free infections (Hackett and Guthe). The criteria for mass treatment are as follows: (1) When the prevalence of active yaws cases is 10 per cent or higher (hyperendemic areas), more than 50 per cent of the population is seroreactive, and all members of the community are to be treated. (2) When there are 5 to 10 per cent of active cases (mesoendemic area), all children and their obvious contacts are treated, because most contagious cases occur in the lower age groups. (3) Where there are less than 5 per cent active cases (hypoendemic areas), solely case and contact treatment is provided. This wide use of penicillin results in rapid regression of active lesions. The prevalence thus declined within a few years from more than 20 per cent to less than 1 per cent after mass campaigns in many areas. Examples of reduction in *infectious* yaws are: in N. Nigeria from 4.2 (1954) to 0.1 per cent (1964); in W. Samoa 3 per cent (1955) to nil (1965).

Indifference must be anticipated in rural populations toward long-term surveillance after mass campaigns that resulted in "disappearance" of community-wide diseases. In the case of yaws, seroepidemiologic studies have shown continued low-level transmission with tendency to focal outbreaks ten to fifteen years after mass campaigns (Guthe). Using cardiolipin serology, 40 per cent of children in areas of Indonesia remained seroreactive four to eight years after treatment, and 13 per cent of the seroreactive children still had high seroreactivity titers. A potential for clinical relapses therefore remains. It is really not possible to drive a community disease out of existence by the use of a drug alone even if the population coverage in mass campaigns is nearly complete. Broader measures are needed, notably development of basic health services, into the functions of which the continued surveillance of communicable diseases can be integrated following mass campaigns, e.g., against yaws. (World Health Organization, 1970).

PROPHYLAXIS. Prevention of yaws depends on avoidance of minor injuries to the skin, and of shielding of open wounds and abrasions from contamination by insects. Open infectious lesions should be protected. Health eduation should aim at improvement of personal hygiene (soap) and community hygiene (water). Children with infectious lesions should be treated and excluded from school until noninfectious. Mass therapy represents an important control measure. No method of artificial immunization is available.

Fluker, J. L., and Hewitt, A. B.: Late yaws. Br. J. Vener. Dis., 46:264, 1970.

Garner, M. F., Backhouse, J. L., Daskalopoulos, G., and Walsh, J. L.: Use of *T. pertenue* in the fluorescent and immobilization tests. Investigation of sera from yaws areas found reactive only in the TPHA test. Br. J. Vener. Dis., 50:264, 1974.

Guthe, T.: Clinical serological and epidemiological features of framboesia tropica (yaws) and its control in rural communities. Acta Dermatovener. (Stockholm) 49:343, 1969.

Hackett, C. J., and Guthe, T.: Some important aspects of yaws eradication. Bull. WHO, 15:869, 1956.

Hackett, C. J., and Lowenthal, L. J. A.: Differential Diagnosis of Yaws. WHO Org. Monograph Series No. 45, Geneva, 1960.

Kantor, I., et al.: Test patterns of yaws antibodies in New Zealand. Arch. Dermatol., 103:226, 1971.

Pampiglione, S., and Wilkinson, A. E.: A study of yaws among pygmies in Cameroon and Zaire, Br. J. Vener. Dis., 51:165, 1975.

Turner, L. H.: Notes on the Treponematoses with an Illustrated Account of Yaws. Kuala Lumpur, Government Press (Institute for Medical Research, Federation of Malaya, Bulletin No. 9), 1959.

Turner, T. B., and Saunders, G. M.: Yaws in Jamaica: 1. An epidemiological study of two rural communities. Am. J. Hyg., 21:483, 1935.

World Health Organization: Bibliography on yaws 1905–1962. Geneva, 1963.

World Health Organization: Scientific Group of Treponematoses Research. WHO Techn. Rep. Ser., No. 455, 1970.

172.2.   BEJEL

(Endemic Syphilis, Nonvenereal Childhood Syphilis, Belesh, Dichuchwa, Njovera, Skerljevo)

DEFINITION. Bejel is a chronic, inflammatory childhood disease of the treponematosis group. The early disease is characterized by infectious mucocutaneous lesions and osseous manifestations resembling those of secondary syphilis. After disappearance of early lesions and an undetermined latency period, late manifestations may develop. There are skin and bone lesions similar to those of late "benign" venereal syphilis. If they occur at all, cardiovascular, nervous system, and prenatally acquired manifestations are extremely rare.

ETIOLOGY. The bejel treponeme is morphologically indistinguishable from *T. pallidum, T. pertenue,* and *T. carateum.* It is present in early lesions or lymph node aspirate. The organism has not been cultivated in vitro. In laboratory animals Turner and Hollander showed consistent differences in cinical reaction as compared with that of yaws and venereal syphilis treponemes. The bejel treponeme is apparently an intermediate between the two (Paris-Hamelin et al., 1968). Like other treponematoses, bejel is accompanied by antibody formation with seroreactivity in reagin, e.g., VDRL, and treponemal antibody (TPI-FTA) tests. Childhood infections with bejel protects against later infection with syphilis.

EPIDEMIOLOGY. Humans are the reservoir of bejel. Treponemes are most likely transmitted directly among children by skin-to-skin contact, or by hands moistened with treponeme-containing saliva, or indirectly via drinking flasks, the spouts of which have been demonstrated to contain treponemes (Grin). Treponeme implantation is generally facilitated by labial and oral fissures, occurring in dry climates, or by small mucosal lesions. Bejel is a household disease. In some instances 60 to 70 per cent of rural community populations have been reported to be infected. Narrow huts, crowded dwellings, unhygienic living conditions, and low socioeconomic standards favor transmission.

There are many scattered endemic centers of bejel in backward rural areas north and south of the tropics.

Bejel occurs along the Kalahari and Sahara deserts in Africa, in the countries of the Balkans and the Eastern Mediterranean region, on the Arabian peninsula, in central Asian countries, and in Australia. It prevails in arid areas in contrast to yaws, which is encountered in moist, tropical jungle regions. Bejel was first described as a disease of nomadic people, subsequently to occur in settled rural populations, e.g., among the Dogons of Mali, the Islamic descendants of Bosnia, and the Bakwenas of Botswana. Previously it was widespread in the Middle East and Europe. Bejel has not been observed in the Western Hemisphere, where pinta and yaws are the prevailing childhood treponematoses. Bejel is in regression from its higher prevalence of two to three decades ago as a result of extensive mass penicillin campaigns and some improvement of health services. In certain areas the prevalence of bejel has remained higher than that of yaws because of occurrence in nomadic tribes, on account of geographic inaccessibility of endemic foci, and inadequacy of health services (Basset, 1963). It is likely to recur when mass treatment has been incomplete. Thus in Niger infectious lesions (5 per cent) and seroreactivity (30 to 40 per cent) were found some years after a mass treatment campaign.

CLINICAL MANIFESTATIONS AND DIAGNOSIS. The experimental incubation period is approximately three weeks. Initial lesions are rarely encountered. The earliest lesions are mucous patches of the secondary type localized to the oral and faucial mucosa. "Split papules" occur at the oral angles. Local papular condylomata lata or anal, genital, or other intertriginous skin areas were observed in 25 per cent of infected children in Iraq (Guthe and Luger). Generalized secondary rashes and alopecia are relatively rare. Regional lymphadenopathy is common. Polyadenitis is rare. The early disease is followed by a latency period of undetermined duration, with seroreactivity as the sole sign of infection. Late "benign" manifestations of the skin develop in some patients. They do not differ in character from those in late venereal syphilis. Superficial tuberoulcerative skin lesions and characteristic serpiginous nodular ulcers occur. Nasopharyngeal ulcerations may occur and range from palate perforation to rhinopharyngitis mutilans as in yaws and syphilis (gangosa). Gummatous ulceration of the breast may occur in women previously infected with bejel who are suckling a child with oral lesions, a phenomenon which supports the concept that gummas may be delayed hypersensitivity reactions from repeated exposure (see Ch. 171). Juxta-articular nodes have been described in some geographic areas.

Bone lesions are the most frequent manifestations of late bejel, affecting the clavicle, the frontal bones, the tibias, and other long bones (Goldstein et al.), giving rise to swelling, tenderness, and pain. There is periosteal and endosteal proliferation, and deformities may result. Isolated cases of cardiovascular and neurologic system involvement have been described in Bosnia (Grin) and Botswana (Murray et al.). Incidental cases of prenatally acquired disease have also been reported. No case of prenatal or systemic disease was observed in several thousand examinations in a WHO project in Syria which included radiologic and cerebrospinal fluid examinations. When observed, the systemic manifestations may be due to the occurrence also of venereal syphilis in the geographic area concerned.

DIAGNOSIS. The diagnosis of early bejel is established on epidemiologic and clinical grounds. It may be confirmed by darkfield demonstration of treponemes in the lesions or in node aspirate and by serologic tests (VDRL), reactive in nearly 100 per cent of cases. Serodiagnostic tests cannot differentiate latent bejel from latent yaws or syphilis. Because late clinical lesions are similar to those of yaws and syphilis, the local epidemiologic situation is an important diagnostic consideration. As distinct from the manifestations of late prenatal syphilis, dental deformities and interstitial keratitis are not observed in bejel.

TREATMENT AND PREVENTION. Penicillin is as effective against bejel as it is against yaws, syphilis, and pinta. In the control campaigns initiated by the World Health Organization in several countries, one dose of 1.2 million units of long-acting penicillin PAM* or benzathine penicillin G (DBED) was given intramuscularly in early cases, with two further doses at three- to seven-day intervals to patients with late manifestations. Half doses are used for contacts. The longer acting benzathine penicillin is preferred in contact treatment among nomadic tribes. Rapid healing of early lesions was followed by seroreversal in a large proportion of cases. Late destructive lesions required more time. Healing with scars progressed slowly but definitely and with some reduction in reaginemia, but with little or no effect on treponemal antibody tests (TPI-FTA), as in venereal syphilis.

Seroepidemiologic studies undertaken in Bosnia, Yugoslavia, 20 years after the penicillin mass campaign — which was followed by systematic periodic surveillance over ten years — showed that childhood infection had been reduced to nil, the community seroimmunologic profiles indicating complete interruption of transmission. During this period adequate basic health services were provided, health education promoted, and general socioeconomic development took place. Bosnia remains the only example of eradication of endemic treponematoses. However, eradication of childhood infection has resulted in a population susceptible to venereal syphilis in later life. The absence of protective cross-immunity has thus created a new epidemiologic situation in which sporadic cases of the sexually transmitted treponematosis occurs.

Goldstein, M. S., Arensburg, C., and Natan, H.: Pathology of Bedouin skeletal remains from two sites in Israel. Am. J. Phys. Anthropol., 45:891, 1975.

Grin, E. I., and Guthe, T.: Evaluation of previous mass campaigns against endemic syphilis in Bosnia and Herzegovina. Br. J. Vener. Dis., 49:1, 1973.

Guthe, T., and Luger, A.: Epidemiological aspects of non-venereal "endemic" syphilis. Dermatologica, 115:248, 1957.

Hudson, E. H.: Non-venereal Syphilis. Edinburgh and London, E. & S. Livingstone, Ltd., 1958.

Turner, T. B.: Syphilis and the treponematoses. In Mudd, S. (ed.): Infectious Agents and Host Reactions. Philadelphia, W. B. Saunders Company, 1969.

Turner, T. B., and Hollander, D. H.: Biology of the Treponematoses. WHO Monograph series no. 35, Geneva, 1957.

*Not available in United States of America.

172.3. PINTA

(Mal del Pinto, Carate)

DEFINITION. Pinta is a skin infection with a chronic course. It is caused by *Treponema carateum*, giving rise to an initial lesion and a generalized secondary rash, both containing treponemes. Late skin manifestations comprise extensive dyschromic (treponeme-containing) and achromic (treponeme-free) conspicuous splotches. Antibodies are produced, detectable by serologic tests reactive also in syphilis and yaws. Organ systems are not involved, physical health is not impaired, and prenatal disease is not known.

HISTORY. Manifestations of pinta were described by Muciño (1798) and by Berecochea and Corona (1811). Frequent seroreactivity (Wassermann complement fixation test) in pinta patients led Menck (1926) to imply association with syphilis and made Herrejon (1927) assume a treponeme to be the causative microorganism. Armenteros and Triana (1938) identified *T. carateum* in Cuban pinta. Leon Blanco (1939) obtained early generalized eruptions by self-inoculation of darkfield-controlled material from lesions. In therapy Corona (1811) showed the usefulness of mercury, Maria Graz (1913) of arsenobenzoles, and Varela (1944) of penicillin.

ETIOLOGY. The etiologic agent, *T. carateum*, is a slender helical cell, 8 to 35 μ long and 0.2 to 0.3 μ wide. It has regular spirals, performs characteristic movements in microscopic darkfield examination, and is morphologically indistinguishable from the treponemes causing syphilis and yaws. *T. carateum* has not been cultivated in vitro.

EPIDEMIOLOGY. Pinta is an endemic treponematosis of large rural populations in tropical forest and valley regions of Central and South America. For example, in rural areas of Mexico the prevalence of pinta varied from 1.3 to 9 per cent (1964) of the census population. Pinta cases occasionally reported from Pacific islands, India, Indonesia, and West Africa have not been verified and may have been "pintide" yaws. Unlike yaws, pinta is not a disease of earliest childhood. Community data (Mexico) indicate age-specific prevalences of early pinta lesions to be 2.5 per cent below five years of age, 8.8 per cent between five and ten years, and 12.2 per cent between ten and fifteen years. In late life some early lesions occur also after 40 years of age.

Transmission presumably takes place by person-to-person contact and is facilitated by poor hygiene, low economic standards, and limited health services. Treponemes are present in early lesions as well as in extensive late dyschromic lesions, where they can be found up to 40 years after the infection. Pinta does not appear to be very contagious, because an infected spouse with treponeme-containing lesions may sometimes not infect a serologically nonreactive partner or other family members. Scratches and insect bites may provide portals of entry for the agent. Blanco found 63 per cent of 257 initial lesions located on the legs and dorsum of feet. Arthropods (Simuliidae, *Hippelates*, or *Ornithodorus*) have not been convincingly demonstrated

The author wishes to acknowledge the valuable advice of his colleague Dr. S. Christiansen, Scientific Adviser, WHO Reference Centre for Treponematoses, State Serum Institute, Copenhagen, Denmark, concerning this chapter.

to be reservoirs of treponemes or biologic vectors, although mechanical transmission cannot be excluded.

Host-Treponeme Relationship. Laboratory animal infection has been achieved in the chimpanzee (Kuhn et al., 1968). Man is the only known natural host of *T. carateum*.

As in syphilis, two types of antibody are formed during the human infection: (1) *Reagin*, detectable by cardiolipin antigen tests (VDRL), appears two to six months after the infection. (2) *Treponemal antibody*, identified in treponemal tests (fluorescent [FTA], hemagglutinating [TPHA] and immobilizing [TPI] antibody tests), is produced notably during dyschromic late manifestations but possibly before this stage. In untreated pinta the antibodies persist for many years. Asymptomatic seroreactors in communities affected by pinta are rare or absent. Superinfection can be achieved experimentally during the early generalized erythrosquamous stage of disease, but not after establishment of dyschromic late lesions. Varying degrees of cross-immunity between pinta, syphilis, yaws, and bejel have been reported (Medina, 1965). However, knowledge of humoral and cell-mediated immunity mechanisms is lacking. The same applies to immunologic (immunopathologic) processes possibly concerned in the genesis of lesions. Related aspects are discussed in Ch. 171.

The histopathology of pinta is characterized by a perivascular infiltrate of inflammatory cells composed of lymphocytes, some plasma cells, histiocytes, and macrophages. Swollen endothelial cells show no proliferation, arterioles and capillaries are not obliterated (as is the case in syphilis), and granulomatous tuberculoid structure is not observed. In dyschromic lesions accumulation of melanin-filled chromatophores in the upper corium is characteristic, and is caused by pigment "fall-out" from the epidermis. This might be a consequence of the primary process. In achromic lesions the picture is quite different — epidermis is atrophic with flattened rete pegs, melanocytes and melanin are lacking, elastic fibers are destroyed, and there is collagenic sclerosis, which explains the porcelain whiteness of achromic lesions. The pigment changes may result from direct action of *T. carateum* on the epidermal "melanin unit" (a melanocyte with a pool of associated malpighian cells [Duchon et al., 1968]). Pinta lesions are localized to skin areas exposed to sunlight. This is unrelated to the number and distribution of melanocytes. A photosensitization process is therefore unlikely.

CLINICAL MANIFESTATIONS AND DIAGNOSIS. The incubation period in experimental pinta is 7 to 21 days. In man, the initial manifestation is a small papule developing by extension or by coalescence with satellite lesions into a scaly maculopapular lesion. There is regional lymphadenopathy. A generalized erythrosquamous rash develops three to nine months after infection, and can be of the "wandering" type. Palpable polyadenitis is not a feature of secondary pinta in contrast to secondary syphilis. One to three years after the initial lesion, sizable dyschromic macules develop. These late lesions develop from secondary pintides or independently, and pass from slate blue through violet to brown and white — the final achromic phase of the pathogenic process. The time required to pass through these stages varies for different patches in the same individual, and the coexisting colored and white skin areas present a mottled appearance. Dyschromic lesions are usually located on frontal skin, cheeks, ears, forearms, back of hands, and dorsum of feet, but never the scalp. Blue lesions may be punctate, but most often appear as smudges on the brow, cheeks, and side of nose, and may last for one to two years. Brown lesions last much longer, and white elements are of lifelong duration. The achromic lesions are porcelain white and exhibit a "geographic coast" appearance; the skin is not supple and has no skin lines or lanugo. A different clinical course of pinta has been described in Cuba (Pardo-Castello, 1942), where the early phase is limited to palms and soles, with hyperpigmented spots turning into keratotic elements. The hyperpigmentation extends to the backs of hands and forearms. In Cuba implication of the cardiovascular and nervous systems has also been suggested. Such systemic involvement has not been verified in other pinta-affected areas of Central and South America. For instance Mazotti (1966) found nonreactive treponemal antibody tests (TPI) in the cerebrospinal fluid of a series of advanced pinta patients in Mexico. Neither were abnormalities found in the cerebrospinal fluid of pinta patients in Venezuela (Lawton-Smith and Medina, 1971).

Early pinta may be difficult to differentiate from *neurodermatitis* (darkfield examination is decisive even if there is seroreactivity); *trichophytosis of the glabrous skin* (pinta does not have vesicles or pustules); *pityriasis alba* (early pinta is more infiltrated); *tinea versicolor* (secondary pintides are more sharply delineated and infiltrated); or *psoriasis* (on removal of scales in pinta no bleeding points appear on a smooth surface). In *late pinta* the leukoderma may closely resemble similar lesions in *syphilis* and *yaws* (scarring); *vitiligo* (supple skin in scalp and perianal areas); *chloasma* (pregnancy and disorders of female genitals); *melanosis* (telangiectasis and poikiloderma are not features of pinta); or *incontinentia pigmenti* (urticaria prior to spots in infancy, pattern of splotches different, concomitant retinal and organ disease).

LABORATORY METHODS. A diagnosis of pinta depends on microscopic darkfield demonstration of *T. carateum* in fluid from early initial and secondary generalized lesions and late dyschromic lesions, as well as on serologic reagin and treponemal antibody tests. Methodologic considerations and interpretations concerning these are related to those in syphilis.

TREATMENT. The treatment of choice is repository, long-acting penicillin, notably procaine penicillin G in oil with aluminium monostearate (PAM)* and benzathine penicillin G (DBED). The considerations regarding time-dose relationship, oral therapy, and alternative antimicrobial drugs in persons hypersensitive to penicillin are the same as are discussed in Ch. 171. Rein et al. obtained highly satisfactory treatment results with 2.4 to 4.8 million units of PAM in early and late pinta. Injections of 2.4 million units of the longer-acting benzathine penicillin G can be effectively applied in a single dose or two injections of 1.2 million units in each buttock in one session.

PROGNOSIS. Pinta neither endangers life nor gives rise to prenatal disease. It has little appreciable effect on general health of patients. Treatment causes treponemes to disappear rapidly from the lesions, which sometimes regress very slowly, depending on their extent. Achromic patches in which atrophy of the epidermis has occurred do not change. However, the disfigurement from pinta, notably of younger persons, is sometimes associated with psychologic misery and social ostracism. Freedom of choice of habitat, mate, and employment is curtailed.

PREVENTION. Pinta prevention consists in examination and treatment with long-acting penicillin, of all patients and their contacts, along with improvement of rural health services, hygiene, and economic standards. In the frame of the international treponematoses program of the World Health Organization (WHO) and the Pan-American Health Organization (PAHO), extensive penicillin treatment campaigns have been undertaken in rural endemic pinta areas by several national health administrations in Central and South America during the last two decades. For instance, in Mexico more than 350,000 pinta patients and contacts have been treated since 1959. Prevalence was reduced from 5.9 to 0.4 per cent in nine main states. In 1974 only 248 cases were discovered. The age pattern and the stages of the disease indicated the effectiveness of the campaign (Lopez de Nava).

Chandler, F. W., Kaufman, A. F., and Kuhn, U.S., III: The histopathology of experimental pinta in the chimpanzee. J. Invest. Dermatol., 58:103, 1972.

Lopez de Nava, G.: Eradication of pinta disease in Mexico. Activities and results. Sal. Publ. Mex., 18:383, 1976.

Mazotti, L.: Negatividad de la prueba de inmovilizaciom de treponemas (TPI) en el liquido cefalorraquideo de 10 enfermos de pinto (carate). Rev. Inst. Salubr. Enferm. Trop., 22: Nos. 1 and 2, 1962.

Rein, C. R., Kitchen, D. K., Marquez, F., and Varela, G.: Repository penicillin therapy of pinta in the Mexican peasant. J. Invest. Dermatol., 18:137, 1952.

Smith, J. L., et al.: Neuro-ophthalmological study of late yaws and pinta. II. The Caracas project. Br. J. Vener. Dis., 47:226, 1971.

---

*Not available in United States of America.

SPIRILLARY AND LEPTOSPIRAL DISEASES

173. RELAPSING FEVER

Anthony D. M. Bryceson

173.1. INTRODUCTION

DEFINITION. Relapsing fever is a systemic infection with spirochetes of the genus *Borrelia* that are transmitted from man to man by the body louse, *Pediculus humanus,* or by soft-backed ticks of the genus *Ornithodoros.* Many species of tick-borne borreliae that infect man are zoonotic and so have an animal reservoir. Other species are of veterinary importance.

The disease is characterized by an abrupt, severe, self-limiting infection lasting several days with one or more relapses of diminishing duration and severity. The brunt of the infection is borne by the spleen, liver, brain, and myocardium, and there may be profound disturbance of the coagulation system. Treatment may be complicated by a severe Jarisch-Herxheimer reaction.

ETIOLOGY AND PATHOGENESIS. Borreliae are helical organisms 3 to 25 μ long with 4 to 30 coils. The body of the organism is 0.2 to 0.5 μ thick. They divide transversely. Borreliae contain endotoxin-like activity, but it is not known whether they contain lipopolysaccharide. Borreliae are susceptible to drying and to most chemical disinfectants, but survive for three months in citrated blood in the refrigerator, and much longer at $-70°$ C. They do not grow readily on artificial culture medium, but do so in chick embryos. Tick-borne species may be maintained in rodents or in ticks.

Epidemic or *louse-borne relapsing fever* is caused by *B. recurrentis.* Organisms circulate in the patient's bloodstream, are taken up by the louse when it feeds, and develop in the coelomic cavity. The louse becomes infective five to eight days later and remains so throughout its few weeks of life. Infected coelomic fluid is spilled on the skin when the louse is crushed during scratching. Spirochetes can penetrate broken skin, intact mucosa, and possibly intact skin, and so infect man.

Tick-borne disease may be caused by one of a wide range of spirochetes which are more or less specific for their vector. The tick becomes infected by feeding on human blood, and is infective three to four days later when spirochetes may be found in saliva and coxal fluid, which carry the organism into the bite of the tick when it next feeds. The tick remains infective for life, which is on average two years but may be as long as 25 years. Ticks are hardy and need not feed more than once a year. In addition, the ovaries of the tick become infected and the spirochete is transmitted to larvae and nymphs, which are infective for man. Up to 100 per cent of eggs of the most efficient vector, *O. moubata,* are infected. This tick is the only reservoir of *B. duttonii.* Borreliae transmitted by other species of ticks have, in addition, another reservoir, usually a rodent, whose burrow the tick shares. In nature a wide range of animals have been found infected with borreliae capable of infecting man. Lice can transmit tick-borne borreliae, but ticks cannot transmit *B. recurrentis.*

Borreliae circulate in the blood during the febrile periods and disappear during the remissions. They produce a *relapsing* infection because of antigenic variation. Spirochetes isolated from the blood during a relapse can be shown serologically to be distinct from the previous isolate. In louse-borne disease up to eight antigenically distinct isolates have been recognized. They tend to follow a regular pattern of variation and to revert to their original identity on passage through the vector. During each febrile episode variant specific antibodies are formed which immobilize and, in the presence of complement, lyse the organism. It is not clear to what extent spontaneous remission and antigenic variation are inherent properties of borreliae or are mediated by the patient's immune response.

173.2. LOUSE-BORNE RELAPSING FEVER

(Yellow Plague, Yellow Famine Fever, Vagabond Fever, Bilious Typhoid, Recurrent Fever)

EPIDEMIOLOGY. Man is the only reservoir of infection. In times of peace and prosperity, as now, louse-borne disease is restricted to a few endemic foci where it smolders ready to break out into epidemics in times of war, the movement of refugees, famine, and the breakdown of medical services.

The most important focus is the Ethiopian highlands, where about 10,000 cases occur annually, and whence it has spread into Sudan. Other foci may be found in the high Andes, in Afghanistan, in Cambodia, and possibly in the People's Republic of China. Important characteristics of endemic foci are cold, which discourages washing, and poverty, which encourages overcrowding and movement of laborers. These conditions favor the multiplication and spread of lice. Microfoci of disease are found in jails, army camps, and orphanages. Transmission is greatest in the winter months.

Louse-borne relapsing fever is one of the classic epidemic diseases of history. In ancient times it ravaged Europe as one of the famine fevers. After World War I it killed 5 million people in Europe and hundreds of thousands in Africa. During World War II there were 1 million cases in north Africa, besides many other lesser outbreaks, and from 1945 to 1947 there were over 1 million cases in Egypt alone with a case mortality of 8 per cent. Epidemic typhus (see Ch. 108.1) has often accompanied outbreaks of louse-borne relapsing fever, and the two diseases have been confused in the past. The present state of unrest in Africa threatens the epidemic spread of this disease within and beyond that continent. Nomads, pilgrims, seasonal laborers, traders, and dealers in old clothes may spread the disease, as well as soldiers and refugees. All are susceptible to infection, but the highest incidence is in young men. Immunity after an attack lasts at least one year.

PATHOGENESIS. Severity of illness bears little relationship to density of spirochetemia, which commonly ranges between 5000 and 500,000 microorganisms per milliliter during the febrile episodes. Most tissues of the body are invaded by the spirochete. Hepatocellular damage is present in all patients, and biochemical tests of hepatic function are deranged. Hyperbilirubinemia, mainly unconjugated, is present in three quarters of patients, and the urine contains an excess of urobilinogen and frequently bile. Histologically, parenchymatous cells are degenerate, sinuses congested, and endothelial cells prominent. In the spleen spirochetes accumulate in the sinuses, and there are miliary foci of necrosis and sometimes larger infarcts which may become secondarily infected. Perisplenitis is common. Dehydration is common and renal function is impaired, over half the patients having protein or cells in their urine; blood urea nitrogen is raised in four fifths of patients. Histologic examination shows tubular damage. There is no gross electrolyte disturbance. Heart failure with pulmonary edema develops in a few patients; prolonged Q-Tc interval is present in two fifths of electrocardiograms and prolonged P-R interval in a smaller proportion. Autopsy specimens show petechial hemorrhages on the serosal surfaces and, on microscopy, interstitial myocarditis with focal myocardial necrosis. There is no defect of pulmonary ventilation, but pulmonary venous admixture may exceed 20 per cent of cardiac output and lowers arterial oxygen saturation to 85 per cent. The high metabolic rate is reflected in the tachycardia (90 to 160 beats per minute), tachypnea (20 to 70 breaths per minute), and increased cardiac output (8 to 14 liters per minute). Systemic vascular resistance is low.

Borreliae, especially the tick-borne species, are neurotropic. Cerebrospinal fluid contains a moderate excess of polymorphonuclear leukocytes, lymphocytes, and protein; meninges may be inflamed, and cranial nerve palsies occasionally develop.

Bleeding occurs in half the patients. The early petechial rash is due to clumps of circulating spirochetes impacted in capillaries and is associated with thrombocytopenia, which is present in 85 per cent of patients. Later in the infection severe bleeding is associated with hepatocellular damage, and prolonged prothrombin and partial thromboplastin times are found in half the patients. Epistaxis may be profuse and prolonged, and there may be bleeding in the brain, meninges, subdural space, gut, urinary tract, and serosal surfaces.

In most patients fibrinogen levels are elevated; but in a few who develop widespread bleeding and shock, a low fibrinogen level is accompanied by other evidence of disseminated intravascular coagulation.

CLINICAL MANIFESTATIONS. After an incubation period of 2 to 15 days, the illness starts with chills, repeated several times during the day, and high fever. Few other diseases make the patient so ill so quickly. During the first two or three days chills and fever are accompanied by profound malaise, severe headache, dizziness, and nightmares. A bitter taste, thirst, and dysphagia are followed by anorexia, nausea, and vomiting in one third of the patients. Generalized aches and pains are common, especially in muscles and lower back. Two thirds complain of upper abdominal pain and of pain on breathing and, more rarely, of pain in the left shoulder. Half the patients cough, with mucoid frothy sputum. One quarter have epistaxis.

By the third day the patient is apathetic, with glazed expression, dull or confused mind, hot forehead, and cold hands. He is shivering and breathless. The presence of epistaxis, a petechial or purpuric rash, jaundice, or tenderness over the liver or spleen strongly suggests

the diagnosis. The rash is most commonly over the shoulders, sides of the trunk, and inner aspects of the arms and thighs. The incidence of physical signs varies from one outbreak to another. All patients have fever and tachycardia. Systolic blood pressure is often low, and one quarter of patients have a gallop rhythm. Respiration is rapid, but added breath sounds are rarely heard. The liver or spleen is palpable in half the patients. In addition to confusion, two fifths of patients have signs of meningism, iritis, or cranial nerve palsies. Deafness or blindness occasionally develops. Delirium and coma may follow. Half the patients have tender muscles. Abortion or miscarriage is common.

Complications from secondary bacterial infection include pneumonia, endocarditis, and diarrhea. Concomitant infections such as typhus, malaria, typhoid, and dysentery are common in epidemics.

Throughout the illness the temperature remains around 39 to 40° C; sweating is slight. After 3 to 13 days the temperature falls by crisis. This is accompanied by physiologic changes similar to, but less severe than, those which characterize the Jarisch-Herxheimer reaction after treatment (see below) and may be fatal. If he survives, the patient remains exhausted for several days.

In the untreated patient there is an afebrile remission of five to seven days, rarely longer, during which he still feels unwell; it is followed by a second attack of fever. This relapse seldom lasts more than four days. Its features are those of the first attack, although less severe and without a rash. Second and third relapses may follow, rarely more, after which the patient makes a gradual but complete recovery.

DIAGNOSIS. Diagnosis is suggested by the typical clinical picture in the appropriate environment, and is confirmed by demonstrating spirochetes in peripheral blood taken from the first or second day of the illness onward. Thick and thin films are prepared and stained with Field's stain or Leishman's stain as for the diagnosis of malaria (see Ch. 193), and examined under the oil immersion objective. In the thick film tangled clumps of spirochetes are seen, whereas in the thin film individual spirochetes lie between the erythrocytes. Platelets are scanty. During remission spirochetes are difficult or impossible to find in the blood. There is no place for serologic tests which are technically difficult and hazardous, or for the inoculation of laboratory animals. In up to 30 per cent of patients anticardiolysin antibody (detectable by VDRL tests) is present transiently, and Weil-Felix OXK or OX19 titers may be raised.

There is usually a mild normocytic normochromic anemia, moderate polymorpholeukocytosis, and marked thrombocytopenia. Biochemical evidence of hepatocellular and renal damage is usual. The cerebrospinal fluid may contain a slight excess of cells, lymphocytes more than polymorphonuclear leukocytes, and of protein.

DIFFERENTIAL DIAGNOSIS. Relapsing fever, once suspected, is easy to diagnose or exclude. Clinical differentiation is from other causes of febrile jaundice, of meningism, of abdominal or chest pain with fever, and of septicemia.

Of the causes of febrile jaundice, malaria is the most important to differentiate, as specific therapy for it may be lifesaving. Severe *Plasmodium falciparum* infections may have most of the features of relapsing fever, but the rash is absent and hemorrhage is rare; muscle tenderness is unusual. Leptospirosis has many features in common with relapsing fever; it is often an occupational hazard (see Ch. 176). Rat-bite fever, especially that caused by *Spirillum minus,* is a less severe relapsing fever, with its own epidemiologic setting. Yellow fever may be suspected on epidemiologic as well as clinical grounds and is diagnosed by animal inoculation, serologically or at autopsy. Viral hepatitis (A or B) is seldom as severe or hemorrhagic and is a diagnosis of exclusion. A sickle crisis, presenting in someone flying in from a relapsing fever area, may show fever, jaundice, and generalized pains.

TREATMENT. The objectives of treatment are to support failing organs and systems, to kill the spirochete, to mitigate the effects of the ensuing Jarisch-Herxheimer reaction, and to prevent relapse.

The patient must be put to bed until at least three days after the first dose of an antimicrobial drug. Drinking is encouraged; but if there is vomiting, intravenous rehydration with 0.18 per cent saline in 4.3 per cent dextrose may be needed. Jugular or central venous pressure should be monitored. Nursing care for the febrile debilitated patient is needed, and sometimes for restlessness, delirium, unconsciousness, convulsions, and incontinence during the reaction. Pain may be relieved by oral paracetamol (acetaminol), known as acetaminophen in the United States, 1 gram every four hours.

Borrelia recurrentis is susceptible to penicillin, erythromycin, streptomycin, tetracycline, and chloramphenicol. The faster the organism is killed, the worse the reaction. Oral medication is often vomited. A slowly released preparation of penicillin given by intramuscular injection is the best compromise. Procaine penicillin in a dose of 300,000 units clears the blood of spirochetes in eight to nine hours. Penicillin aluminium monostearate,* 600,000 units, induces a less severe reaction and is considered by some to be safer, but the blood is not cleared of spirochetes for 17 hours (Warrell et al., 1976). Intravenous tetracycline, which clears the blood in one to two hours, in dangerous because it induces the most severe reaction. In an epidemic or when diagnostic facilities are poor, a single dose of 100 mg of doxycycline by mouth has the advantage of curing louse-borne typhus as well as relapsing fever. Penicillin is not completely effective in clearing borreliae from the brain, and the relapse rate after its use is 3 per cent. Relapse is prevented by giving the patient tetracycline, 500 mg, or doxycycline, 100 mg, by mouth the following day.

Petechial hemorrhage is unimportant. Severe hemorrhage is treated by blood transfusion. Vitamin K, 20 mg, may be given, but the prothrombin time returns to normal within three days of treatment regardless. There has been little experience with use of heparin to treat disseminated intravascular coagulation in relapsing fever. Liver and kidney function return rapidly to normal after treatment, and there is seldom need for specific support. Intercurrent infection should be sought and treated, especially typhoid.

JARISCH-HERXHEIMER REACTION. As spirochetes are killed, either during the natural crisis or following an antimicrobial drug, they are phagocytosed and removed from the circulation, and the Jarisch-Herxheimer reac-

tion begins. The characteristic feature is the chill, just before which the patient becomes uncomfortable, restless, or delirious and may pass urine or stool or may vomit. The chill lasts 10 to 30 minutes. After the chill, the patient suddenly feels hot and soon breaks out into a profuse sweat, after which he feels comfortable and falls asleep exhausted. During and after the chill the temperature rises to 40 to 42° C.

The metabolic rate rises sharply and attains a peak during the chill, and the cardiac output reaches 10 liters per minute. Ventilation is stimulated to cope with the demand for oxygen, and the respiratory rate may rise above 80 breaths per minute. Despite this, arterial oxygen saturation remains low and lactic acidosis develops. Arterial blood pressure rises sharply immediately before the chill, falls abruptly after it to dangerously low levels, and remains low for at least eight hours and often for two or three days. During this period the systemic vascular resistance falls and peripheral vessels dilate. The first eight hours after the chill are critical: the cardiac output is strained to its limit, the circulatory volume is falling, death of spirochetes in the myocardium precipitates or aggravates myocarditis (in about one third of the patients treated with tetracycline), and cardiac failure may follow. There is also evidence suggesting accelerated defibrination.

It is not certain whether the reaction is due primarily to endotoxin release, massive intravascular phagocytosis, or immune complex deposition.

Management of Jarisch-Herxheimer Reaction. HYPERPYREXIA. The oral temperature is taken every 30 minutes after treatment is given. If, after the chill, the oral temperature rises above 40° C, the patient should be sponged with tepid water and fanned vigorously until the temperature falls to 38.5° C.

SHOCK. After the profuse sweating, the patient is deceptively quiet and warm, and the pulse may feel full, but the blood pressure and pulse rate should be recorded every 30 minutes. If the systolic pressure falls below 60 mm Hg, the foot of the bed is raised and oral fluids are encouraged. If this is inadequate, intravenous fluid is given, with monitoring of the central venous pressure and listening for evidence of pulmonary edema. A peripheral vasoconstrictor drug such as metaraminol bitartrate, 10 mg by intramuscular injection, may be helpful.

MYOCARDIAL FAILURE. This responds to sitting the patient upright and giving digoxin, 1 mg intravenously, followed by 0.5 mg twice daily for a few days.

CEREBRAL EDEMA. Prolonged coma may be due to intracranial hemorrhage or to cerebral edema; mannitol, 2 grams per kilogram of body weight, may be given as 20 per cent solution intravenously.

LACTIC ACIDOSIS. Lactic acidosis may be prevented by letting the patient breathe 100 per cent oxygen during the reaction. This seems to speed convalescence, but its benefit during the reaction is uncertain.

Corticosteroids in large doses, such as hydrocortisone, 1 gram hourly, reduce fever before the reaction but do not mitigate any of the changes of the reaction.

PROGNOSIS. The case mortality of louse-borne relapsing fever has varied markedly (4 to 40 per cent) in different outbreaks, depending upon age, nutrition, underlying disease, residual immunity, variations in the virulence of the organism during an epidemic, and the availability, nature, and timing of treatment. In the

---

*No longer available in the United States.

individual case deep jaundice, coma, and shock are bad prognostic signs. Early treatment improves the prognosis, but treatment late in the attack may induce a reaction which is more severe than the natural crisis. The disease tends to kill during the first attack, or just after the crisis, rather than during the relapses.

PREVENTION. During an outbreak, anti-louse measures are instituted in the population at risk. Clothes are treated by dry heat or insecticide powder, such as carbaryl 5 per cent or malathion 5 per cent, which are superseding gammexane 1 per cent and DDT 10 per cent, to which lice are resistant in many parts of the world. Personal hygiene and cleanliness are important, and this may be helped by shaving body and head hair. Mass prophylaxis with penicillin aluminium monostearate,* 1 million units, or doxycycline, 100 mg, would seem sensible but has not been tried. Patients and their clothes should be deloused with insecticide, and medical attendants should wear gloves while performing venipuncture or handling blood samples. If blood is spilled on the skin, tetracycline, 500 mg orally, should be taken once. International Sanitary Regulations require notification of cases and may direct disinfection of persons arriving from infected areas. There is no vaccine.

173.3. TICK-BORNE RELAPSING FEVER

(Tick Fever; Many Local Names in Endemic Areas)

EPIDEMIOLOGY. The patterns of endemic or tick-borne relapsing fever depend upon the habits of their vectors and animal reservoirs and of man's contact with the ticks. The patterns vary from place to place.

In the far western United States and Texas, ticks live in caves; in Kansas, in prairie dog burrows; in Washington state, in owl burrows; in southwest Texas, in rodent burrows. Hunters and vacationers tend to become infected. *Ornithodoros turicata* inhabits caves frequented by goats and sheep, but is becoming domesticated in Central Mexico. *O. hermsi* lives in or near cabins at high altitude where it is associated with hibernating rodents. Early summer visitors acquire the disease. *O. erraticus* inhabits a wide range of animal burrows on the Mediterranean coast, and the disease affects both settled and nomadic peoples. *O. tholozani* inhabits caves and burrows and is attracted to fowls and camels and so reaches a large human population. It travels on sheep and camels on long caravan routes.

O. moubata has the closest association with man. It is found throughout the savanna of Central, East, and South Africa but not in the deserts, forests, or mountains. It prefers to live in and near human huts in cracks and crevices in the earthen floor, but is also found in animal burrows. It emerges at nightfall to feed on the inhabitants. The disease is therefore truly endemic, and sporadic cases occur throughout the year, most commonly in children. Visitors of any age are susceptible.

PATHOGENESIS. This is essentially the same as for the louse-borne disease, but tick-borne borreliae are more neurotropic, which alters slightly the clinical pattern and increases the liability to relapse. During remissions borreliae survive principally in the brain and seem relatively resistant to antimicrobial drugs and possibly to antibodies. The infection may cross the placenta.

CLINICAL MANIFESTATIONS. In endemic areas where people are repeatedly exposed to infection, the disease is commonly mild and brief. In nonimmunes it may be severe, and in general it follows the same course as the louse-borne infection.

The duration of the febrile periods and remissions is less regular than in the louse-borne disease, and the number of relapses tends to be greater. *B. duttonii* causes the most severe infection, and in the untreated nonimmune patient ten relapses of ten days each are not uncommon. Mediterranean and Middle Eastern infections are less severe and the American ones least so.

Neurologic complications are common. Iridocyclitis occurs in up to 15 per cent of patients and presents with eye pain, ciliary injection, and dim vision. Up to 30 per cent develop other complications, including coma, convulsions, cranial nerve lesions, hemiplegia, peripheral neuritis, and transverse myelitis. Nightmares, hallucinations, and severe anxiety and depressive states may develop. Most neurologic and psychiatric changes eventually disappear. Neurologic signs may be the sole feature of a late relapse.

DIAGNOSIS. Ticks emerge at night and their bite is often painless, so there may not be a clear history of bite. Sometimes their bites give rise to a local allergic response. Spirochetemia is often scantier than in louse-borne disease. Repeated examination of blood slides may be necessary. A concentration technique that has been used successfully in animals is to examine the buffy coat of blood centrifuged in a microhematocrit tube. Alternatively, 2 ml of blood may be inoculated intraperitoneally into mice; tail blood is examined for spirochetes from the second to fourteenth days. Occasionally during a relapse, only the cerebrospinal fluid may contain spirochetes.

PROGNOSIS. The initial attack of tick-borne relapsing fever is not usually so severe as the louse-borne variety, but, untreated, the disease is far more prolonged and debilitating, and death usually occurs in one of the relapses. The mortality is in general less, being very low in the United States, Middle East, and Asia and rising to 5 per cent in Africa, but a mortality of 27 per cent has been reported from Venezuela.

TREATMENT. Some strains of tick-borne Borreliae are not susceptible to penicillin; therefore tetracycline is commonly used. The dose is 250 mg orally every six hours until the patient is afebrile. Relapse is prevented by giving 500 mg six hourly for seven days, or 2 grams weekly for four weeks. In patients who are vomiting, 250 mg of tetracycline can be given intravenously, but a severe reaction can be expected within two hours. Alternatively, an initial dose of procaine penicillin may be tried, as for the louse-borne disease.

PREVENTION. In areas where the disease is endemic and the tick is associated with houses or frequents caves, as in Africa with *O. moubata* and parts of central Asia with *O. tholozani*, an insecticide should be sprayed, preferably in an oily base, on the lower part of the walls of the huts, on their floors, and at their entrances. A suitable preparation is 3 per cent benzene hexachloride in diesoline, which keeps huts free of ticks for over two years. Powders have a much shorter effect. Travelers should sleep under mosquito nets and inspect their clothing in the morning. A light kept burning at night discourages ticks. In the long run, better housing controls the disease. In areas where the disease is sporadic and ticks live in caves or burrows,

---

*No longer available in the United States.

anti-tick measures are impracticable, and personal prophylaxis is advised. It is best to avoid entering caves or
using old camp sites; second best is the use of insect
repellents. Clothes may be impregnated with 5 per cent
dimethylphthalate in a 2 per cent oil emulsion. Washing with 10 per cent carbol soap is also effective. Insect
repellent creams may be applied to the skin. Summer
cabins in the Rocky Mountains should be rodent proof,
and wooden walls and floors treated with creosote. In
the spring, bedding should be treated with insecticide.
There is no vaccine.

Bryceson, A. D. M., Parry, E. H. O., Perine, P. L., Warrell, D. A.,
    Vukotich, D., and Leithead, C. S.: Louse-borne relapsing fever.
    Quart. J. Med., 39:130, 1970.
Coffey, E., and Eveland, W. C.: Experimental relapsing fever initiated
    by B. hermsi. J. Infect. Dis. 117:28, 1967.
Felsenfeld, O.: Borrelia. Strains, Vectors, Human and Animal Borrelio-
    sis. St. Louis, W. H. Green, 1971.
Parry, E. H. O., Warrell, D. A., Perine, P. L., Vukotich, D., and Bryce-
    son, A. D. M.: Some effects of louse-borne relapsing fever on the
    function of the heart. Am. J. Med., 49:472, 1970.
Perine, P. L., Krause, D. W., Awoke, S., and McDade, J. E.: Single
    dose doxycycline treatment of louse-borne relapsing fever and epi-
    demic typhus. Lancet, 2:742, 1974.
Warrell, D. A., Pope, H. M., Parry, E. H. O., Perine, P. L., and Bryce-
    son, A. D. M.: Cardiorespiratory disturbances associated with in-
    fective fever in man: Studies of Ethiopian louse-borne relapsing
    fever. Clin. Sci., 39:123, 1970.

174. TROPICAL PHAGEDENIC ULCER

Anthony D. M. Bryceson

DEFINITION. Tropical phagedenic ulcer is an acute
specific ulcer of skin and subcutaneous tissue, associated in its early stages with infection with *Borrelia vincentii* and anaerobic bacteria of the genus *Bacteroides*.
The ulcer is usually situated below the knee, has certain
typical characteristics, and commonly becomes chronic.

ETIOLOGY AND PATHOGENESIS. *B. vincentii* is a loosely coiled spirochete 5 to 10 μ long; it is a common oral
commensal. *Bacteroides* is a curved, cigar-shaped rod 5
to 14 μ long, often beaded when stained; it, too, is an
oral commensal and is common in moist soils. Either or
both of these organisms are present in the acute stage
of the ulcer. They gain entry through a tiny wound in
the skin. Experimentally, they will cause ulcers only in
malnourished subjects or animals. Other organisms,
especially cocci, may also be found in established
ulcers.

EPIDEMIOLOGY. The condition is common and widespread in the tropics and rare elsewhere. It may be
found in all climates and at any altitude. In some countries hot wet areas are especially affected. In parts of
some countries, active ulcers have a prevalence of 2 per
cent and scars of 15 per cent. It is often the most common complaint of hospital outpatients, representing up
to one third of new patients, and may be the most
common cause of surgical admissions.

Tropical ulcer is typically a sporadic disease, especially affecting adolescent males. It is most common in the
lower socioeconomic groups. Although the patient may
not appear grossly malnourished, there is a clear clinical and experimental association with malnutrition. No
specific nutritional deficiency has been identified, but
tropical ulcer is rare in those who eat adequate animal
protein and is especially common in labor gangs, ill-

kept prisoners of war, and other physically deprived
groups, among whom it can appear as an epidemic.
This association with malnutrition and deprivation is
also found in two other infections with the same organisms, cancrum oris and trench mouth.

**PATHOGENESIS, CLINICAL MANIFESTATIONS, AND
PROGNOSIS.** The lesion starts at the site of a minor
wound or insect bite, which the patient can usually recall. Often the site is neglected or treated with a native
remedy, or sucked by mouth to clean it. A small blister
appears, containing serosanguineous fluid, and ruptures, exposing an ash gray slough which has a characteristic foul smell. The ulcer spreads rapidly to involve
subcutaneous tissue and often muscle and tendon
down to bone. It reaches its final diameter of 1 to 40 cm
in a few days. The central slough liquefies, exposing a
gray-brown base. The ulcer is circular, with a raised
edge and surrounding edema, and may encircle the
limb. It is painful and bleeds easily. Regional lymph
nodes may be enlarged and tender. The most common
sites of tropical ulcers are over the bony parts of the leg
at the level of, or just above, the ankle.

Histologic examination shows three layers: a superficial layer of coagulation necrosis in which organisms
are abundant, a layer of granulation tissue, and a highly vascular base. The edge of the ulcer shows pseudoepitheliomatous hyperplasia.

Fifty per cent of ulcers heal spontaneously within
three months, and 80 per cent within six months.

Chronic ulcers become less painful and lose their
odor. They become irregular with a rigid base and edge
and are filled with pink granulation tissue. Histologically there is much surrounding fibrosis. Squamous cell
carcinoma develops in 9 per cent of chronic ulcers after
a period of three months to 50 years. Tetanus and gangrene are rarer complications.

DIAGNOSIS. In the acute stage the appearances and
smell are typical. The specific organisms can be demonstrated in a drop of fluid aspirated from the ulcer, either by darkfield microscopy or by Gram stain or staining with 1 per cent carbolfuchsin. Histologic
examination is seldom needed. It is more difficult to
identify the cause of chronic ulcers. The differential
diagnosis includes yaws (serology and radiology), cutaneous diphtheria (climate, culture), Buruli ulcer (undermining, acid-fast bacilli), squamous cell carcinoma and
melanoma (histology), and varicose ulcers (age group,
venous abnormality).

TREATMENT. In the acute stage the patient is put to
bed and the limb elevated. The ulcer is dressed with
sterile saline or resorcinol monoacetate (Euresol). Hydrogen peroxide may be used for a few days to help slough
out. Strong antiseptics are contraindicated. Penicillin is
given by intramuscular injection for seven days; procaine
penicillin, 600,000 units twice daily, or penicillin aluminium monostearate,* 1,200,000 units daily, is suitable.
Metronidazole, 200 mg thrice daily by mouth, is a suitable alternative to penicillin. The synergistic effect of the
two drugs has not been tested.

This treatment controls the infection and cleans the
ulcer. Ulcers under 5 cm in diameter should now heal
satisfactorily. Ulcers over 5 cm should be grafted with
split skin.

Chronic ulcers are treated initially in the same way,
and are then completely excised and grafted. A walking

---

*No longer available in the United States.

plaster may then be applied, and healing is complete within three weeks.

PREVENTION. Good nutrition and physical health are the best preventives. Legs should be covered while walking in country where thorns or sharp grass may scratch them. Minor cuts and scratches should be washed and treated with local antiseptic.

Edington, G. M., and Gillies, H. M.: Tropical ulcers. In Pathology in the Tropics. London, Arnold, 1976, p. 726.

Lindler, R. R., and Adeniyi-Jones, C.: The effect of metronidazole on tropical ulcers. Trans. R. Soc. Trop. Med. Hyg., 62:712, 1968.

Lowenthal, L. J. A.: Tropical phagedenic ulcer: A review. In Lincicome, D. R. (ed.): International Review of Tropical Medicine. New York, Academic Press, 1963, p. 267.

175. RAT-BITE FEVER

Jay P. Sanford

Rat-bite fever represents two clinically somewhat similar but etiologically distinct diseases which usually follow the bite of a rat or other rodent. Streptobacillary rat-bite fever is caused by the pleomorphic gram-negative bacillus *Streptobacillus moniliformis*, whereas spirillary rat-bite fever is caused by *spirillum minus*. In the United States, streptobacillary rat-bite fever is far more common.

Rat-bite fever occurs throughout the world, with a higher incidence in urban areas where sanitation is poor and the rat population is great. In the United States, approximately half of the reported cases have occurred in children under 12 years of age. Rat-bite fever is said to follow about 10 per cent of rat bites; however, with an estimated 14,000 persons bitten by rats annually in the United States, this estimated frequency appears excessively high.

STREPTOBACILLARY RAT-BITE FEVER

EPIDEMIOLOGY. *Streptobacillus moniliformis* is found in the oropharynx of healthy rats. Although several epidemics have apparently been associated with the ingestion of raw milk, Haverhill fever, the portal of entry is usually an animal bite. Animals incriminated include rats, mice, weasels, dogs, and cats. Currently rat-bite fever represents a particular hazard to biomedical laboratory workers.

CLINICAL MANIFESTATIONS. Following a bite, the primary wound usually heals promptly. After an incubation period of 1 to 22 (usually less than 10) days, the patient abruptly develops severe chills, fever, vomiting, headache, and pains in the joints and back. The fever tends to remit in two to five days. About the third day, a morbilliform, petechial rash appears over the feet and hands in more than 90 per cent of patients. After remitting briefly, the fever recurs and is characteristically (70 per cent of patients) associated with arthralgia and arthritis. In most patients, multiple joints, especially the wrists and elbows, are involved. Untreated, the joint findings may persist for several days to several months.

Cases have been reported of patients who develop infective endocarditis caused by *Streptobacillus moniliformis*. In such instances there are usually no aspects of the history, such as that of rat bites or clinical features, to lead one to suspect *Streptobacillus moniliformis* as the etiologic agent.

LABORATORY FEATURES. Leukocyte counts may range between 6000 and 30,000 per cubic millimeter. There are no other distinctive features. False-positive serologic tests for syphilis have been reported in 25 per cent of cases.

DIAGNOSIS. Diagnosis is confirmed by culturing the organism from blood or joint fluid on ordinary nutrient media, although growth is enhanced by addition of 20 per cent horse serum to the medium and incubation under 5 to 10 per cent CO_2.

The differential diagnosis includes the following viral diseases: rubella with associated arthralgia-arthritis (however, the rash in rubella is centripetal); hepatitis B virus infection with arthralgia-arthritis, although the rash is usually urticarial; and dengue, although a diphasic febrile course is typical, a maculopapular rash appears on the third to fifth day, severe arthralgia is characteristic, and arthritis is not a feature (also, in dengue the peripheral leukocyte count usually is less than 5000 per cubic millimeter by the third to fifth day). In Africa, other arboviral causes which are associated with rash and arthritis include Chikungunya, O'nyong-nyong, and Sindbis virus; in Australia, epidemics of polyarthritis associated with rashes occur with Ross River virus. The rash of streptobacillary rat-bite fever may resemble that seen with Rocky Mountain spotted fever in character, distribution, and time of occurrence. Other bacterial diseases to be considered in the differential diagnosis include disseminated gonococcal infection, chronic meningococcemia, and leptospirosis, especially in children, in whom peripheral rash is more frequent.

THERAPY. The organisms are susceptible to penicillin, the tetracyclines, and most other antimicrobial drugs. Penicillin V (phenoxymethyl penicillin, 2.0 grams per day divided into three or four doses, or procaine penicillin, 600,000 units intramuscularly every 12 hours for 10 days, is recommended. In patients with hypersensitivity to penicillins, tetracycline, 2.0 grams per day orally divided into four doses, is an effective alternative.

PROGNOSIS AND SEQUELAE. Mortality is low except with endocarditis. Treatment will shorten the febrile course.

SPIRILLARY RAT-BITE FEVER
(Sodoku)

EPIDEMIOLOGY. *Spirillum minus* is a cause of ocular infection in rats, the organism apparently reaching the rat's mouth by way of the nasolacrimal ducts. Occasionally, the bites of cats have been incriminated.

CLINICAL MANIFESTATIONS. Following a bite, the initial wound usually heals promptly. After an incubation period of 4 to 28 (usually greater than 10) days, inflammation recurs at the primary wound site, with associated fever and regional lymphadenitis. A roseolar-urticarial rash may occur, but it is less evident than with streptobacillary rat-bite fever. Arthritis is rare. An episode lasts three to four days and then subsides. Recurrence is usual after a few days.

LABORATORY FEATURES. The leukocyte count usually is 5000 to 30,000 per cubic millimeter. False-positive serologic tests for syphilis occur in about one half of patients.

DIAGNOSIS. *Spirillum minus* has not been cultured on

artificial medium; hence diagnosis is established by demonstrating *Spirillum minus* in a darkfield preparation of exudate from an infected site or lymph node. Alternatively, inoculation of material intraperitoneally into mice and examination of the mouse blood 5 to 15 days later by Giemsa stain or darkfield microscopy may enable demonstration of the spirillum.

THERAPY. Response to treatment with penicillin or with the aminoglycoside streptomycin is prompt.

Cole, J. S., Stoll, R W., and Bulger, R. J. Rat-bite fever: Report of three cases. Ann. Intern. Med., 71:979, 1969.

Place, E. H., and Sutton, L. E.: Erythema arthriticum epidemicum (Haverhill fever). Arch. Intern. Med., 54:659, 1934.

Roughgarden, J. W.: Antimicrobial therapy of rat-bite fever. Arch Intern. Med., 116:39, 1965.

Watkins, C. G.: Rat-bite fever. J. Pediat. 28:429, 1946.

176. LEPTOSPIROSIS

Jay P. Sanford

DEFINITION. Leptospirosis is an inclusive term applied to disease caused by all leptospires regardless of specific serotype. Correlation of clinical syndromes with infection by differing serotypes indicates that a single serotype of *Leptospira* may be responsible for a variety of clinical features; likewise, a single syndrome, e.g., aseptic meningitis, may be caused by multiple serotypes of leptospires. Hence, the general term leptospirosis is preferred rather than the synonyms such as Weil's disease or Canicola fever.

ETIOLOGY. The genus *Leptospira* contains only one species, *L. interrogans,* which may be subdivided into two complexes, interrogans and biflexa. The interrogans complex includes most of the pathogenic strains, whereas the biflexa complex includes mainly saprophytic strains with no recognized hosts. Despite contrary common usage, an example of the correct designation of leptospira is as follows: pomona serogroup of *L. interrogans,* not *L. pomona.* The interrogans complex now contains about 130 serotypes arranged in 16 serogroups (the number in parentheses refers to number of serotypes within the serogroup): Icterohemorrhagiae (13), Hebdomadis (28), Autumnalis (13), Canicola (11), Australis (10), Tarassovi or Hyos (10), Pyrogenes (9), Bataviae (8), Javanica (6), Pomona (6), Ballum (3), Cynopteri (3), Celledoni (2), Grippotyphosa (2), Panama (2), and Shermani (1). At least 22 serotypes of *Leptospira* occur naturally in the United States.

EPIDEMIOLOGY. Leptospirosis, although not a common disease, has been reported from all regions of the United States. Between 1960 and 1976, 50 to 90 cases were reported annually. Occasional upswings in the number of cases have been the result of common source outbreaks.

Infection in man is incidental and is not essential to the maintenance of leptospirosis. Infection occurs in a wide range of domestic and wild animal hosts. In many species, such as opossums, skunks, raccoons, and foxes, infectivity ratios in the range of 10 to 50 per cent are not unusual. Interspecies spread of specific serotypes of leptospires between animal hosts is frequent, e.g., *pomona*, a serotype principally associated with livestock, has been demonstrated in dogs. The infection in animals may vary from inapparent illness to severe fatal disease. The carrier state may develop in many animals wherein the host may shed leptospires in its urine for months to years.

It has not been established that pathogenic leptospires are capable of multiplication outside a host. Survival in nature is governed by factors including pH of the urine, soil, or water into which they are shed and ambient temperature. Acid urine permits only limited survival; however, if the urine is neutral or alkaline and is shed into a similar moist environment which has low salinity and is not badly polluted with microorganisms or detergents, and with a temperature above 22° C, leptospires may survive for several weeks. Human infections can occur either directly by contact with urine or tissue of an infected animal or indirectly through contaminated water, soil, or vegetation. The usual portals of entry are abraded skin, particularly about the feet, and exposed mucous membranes, conjunctival, nasal, and oral. The concept that organisms can penetrate intact skin has been questioned. Although leptospires have been isolated from ticks, they appear to be unimportant in transmission.

With the ubiquitous infection of animals, leptospirosis in man can occur in all age groups, at all seasons, and in both sexes. However, it is primarily a disease of teenage children and young adults (at least 50 per cent of patients are between ages 10 and 39 years), occurs predominantly in males (75 per cent), and develops most frequently in hot weather (in the United States two thirds of infections occur from June to October). The wide spectrum of animal hosts results in both urban and rural human disease. Leptospirosis has been considered an occupational disease; however, improved methods of rat control and better standards of hygiene have reduced the incidence among occupational groups such as coal miners and sewermen. Currently only 10 per cent of patients in the United States have direct contact with animals, i.e., farmers, abattoir workers, or veterinarians. The majority of patients have incidental exposure, two thirds being children, students, or housewives. Swimming or partial immersion in contaminated water has been implicated in one fifth of patients and has accounted for most of the recognized common source outbreaks.

PATHOLOGY. In patients who have died with hepatic involvement (Weil's syndrome), renal involvement, or both, the significant gross changes include hemorrhages and bile-staining of tissues. The hemorrhages, which vary from petechial to ecchymotic, are widespread but are most prominent in skeletal muscle, kidneys, adrenals, liver, stomach, spleen, and lungs.

In skeletal muscle, focal necrotic and necrobiotic changes thought to be rather typical of leptospirosis occur. Biopsies early in the illness demonstrate swelling, vacuolation, and subsequently hyalinization. Leptospiral antigen has been demonstrated in these lesions by the fluorescent antibody technique. Healing ensues by the formation of new myofibrils with minimal fibrosis.

The renal lesion in the acute phase involves the tubules predominantly and varies from simple dilatation of distal convoluted tubules to degeneration, necrosis, and basement membrane rupture. Interstitial edema and cellular infiltrates, consisting of lymphocytes, neutrophilic leukocytes, histiocytes, and plasma cells, are uniformly present. Glomerular lesions either are absent or consist of mesangial hyperplasia and focal foot process fusion, which are interpreted as representing non-specific changes. Microscopic alterations in the liver are not diagnostic, and correlate poorly with the degree of function impairment. The changes include frequent double nuclei and cloudy swelling of hepatocytes, disruption of liver cords, enlargement of Kupffer cells, and bile stasis in biliary canaliculi. The changes in the brain and meninges are also minimal and are not diagnostic. Microscopic evidence of myocarditis, including focal hemorrhages, interstitial edema, and focal infiltration with lymphocytes and plasma cells, has been recorded. Pulmonary findings consist of a patchy, localized hemorrhagic pneumonitis. Special staining techniques utilizing silver impregnation methods have demonstrated organisms in the lumina of renal tubules but rarely in other organs.

CLINICAL MANIFESTATIONS. General Features. The incubation period after immersion or accidental laboratory exposure has shown extremes of 2 to 26 days, the usual range being 7 to 13 days and the average, 10 days.

Leptospirosis is typically a biphasic illness. *The leptospiremic or first phase* is characterized by the presence of leptospires in the blood and cerebrospinal fluid. The onset is typically abrupt (75 to 100 per cent of patients). Initial symptoms include headache, which is usually frontal, less often retro-orbital, but occasionally may be bitemporal or occipital. Severe muscle aching occurs in most patients, the muscles of the thighs and lumbar areas being most prominently involved and often accompanied by pain on palpation. The myalgia may be accompanied by extreme cutaneous hyperesthesia (causalgia). Chills followed by high fever are prominent. The leptospiremic phase typically lasts four to nine days. Features during this interval include recurrent chills, high spiking temperature curve (usually reaching 39° C or greater), headache, and continued severe myalgia. Anorexia, nausea, vomiting, and abdominal pain are encountered in about one half of patients. Occasional patients have diarrhea (7 to 29 per cent). Pulmonary manifestations, usually either cough or chest pain, have varied in frequency of occurrence from less than 25 to 86 per cent. Hemoptysis occurs but is rare. Examination during this phase reveals an acutely ill febrile patient. A relative bradycardia may be noted. The blood pressure is usually normal in adults. In children hypertension is common. Disturbances in sensorium may be encountered in up to 25 per cent of patients. The most characteristic sign is conjunctival suffusion which usually appears on the third or fourth day. It may be lacking in some patients, but more often it is overlooked because of its benign nature. This may be associated with photophobia, but serous or purulent secretion is unusual. Less common findings (in 10 to 50 per cent of patients) may include pharyngeal injection, nuchal rigidity, lymphadenopathy, cutaneous hemorrhages, and skin rashes that are usually macular, maculopapular, or urticarial, and usually occur on the trunk. Uncommon findings (usually less than 10 per cent) are erythema nodosum, splenomegaly, hepatomegaly, or jaundice. Defervescence and improvement in symptoms coincide with the disappearance of leptospires from the blood and cerebrospinal fluid.

The second phase has been characterized as the "immune" phase and correlates with the appearance of circulating antibodies which are predominantly IgM class.

The clinical manifestations of this phase exhibit greater variability than those during the first phase After a relatively asymptomatic period of one to three days, the fever and earlier symptoms recur and meningismus may develop. The fever rarely exceeds 39° C and is usually of one to three days' duration. It is not uncommon for fever to be absent or quite transient. Even when symptoms or signs of meningeal irritation are absent, routine examination of cerebrospinal fluid after the seventh day has revealed pleocytosis in 50 to 90 per cent of patients. Less common features include iridocyclitis, optic neuritis, and other nervous system manifestations, including encephalitis, myelitis, and peripheral neuropathy.

Some clinicians recognize a third or convalescent phase, usually between the second and fourth weeks, when fever and aching may recur. The pathogenesis of this stage is poorly understood.

Leptospirosis during pregnancy may be associated with an increased risk of fetal loss.

Specific Features. WEIL'S SYNDROME. Weil's syndrome, which may be due to serotypes other than *icterohemorrhagiae*, is defined as severe leptospirosis with jaundice, usually accompanied by azotemia, hemorrhages, anemia, disturbances in consciousness, and continued fever. There is uncertainty as to the pathogenesis of the syndrome, i.e., whether it represents direct toxic damage caused by leptospires or whether it is the consequence of immune response to leptospiral antigens. The consensus favors toxic damage.

The onset and first stage are identical with the less severe forms. The distinctive features of Weil's syndrome appear from the third to the sixth day but may not reach their peak until well into the second stage. As in the other forms of leptospirosis, there is a tendency for the fever to lyse about the seventh day; however, with its recurrence it is marked and may persist for several weeks. Either renal or hepatic manifestations may predominate. Hepatic disturbances include tenderness in the right upper quadrant and hepatic enlargement, both of which are common when jaundice is present. SGOT values are rarely increased more than fivefold regardless of the degree of hyperbilirubinemia, which is predominantly conjugated (direct). The mechanism of hyperbilirubinemia appears to be an intracellular block to bilirubin excretion.

Renal manifestations consist primarily of proteinuria, pyuria, hematuria, and azotemia. Dysuria is rare. The maximal level of blood urea nitrogen is usually reached on the fifth to seventh day. Serious renal damage usually occurs in the form of acute tubular necrosis associated with oliguria. Hemorrhagic manifestations include epistaxis, hemoptysis, gastrointestinal bleeding, hemorrhage into the adrenal glands, hemorrhagic pneumonitis, and subarachnoid hemorrhage. These have been explained on the basis of capillary injury. In addition, in some patients hypoprothrombinemia and thrombocytopenia have been observed.

ASEPTIC MENINGITIS. A leptospiral cause has been incriminated in 5 to 13 per cent of patients with aseptic meningitis. The pleocytosis is not present before the immune phase, when it develops rapidly. There are usually tens to hundreds of cells, occasionally 1000 per cubic millimeter, which may be neutrophils or mononuclear cells. The cerebrospinal fluid glucose level is almost always normal, but occasional instances of lowered glucose levels have been recorded. With leptospirosis the cerebrospinal fluid protein may exceed 100 mg per 100 ml early in the course. Xanthochromic cerebrospinal fluid has been observed in the presence of jaundice. Each of the serotypes of leptospires that are pathogenic for man is probably capable of association with this syndrome. The most prevalent serotypes have been *Canicola, Icterohemorrhagiae,* and *Pomona.*

PRETIBIAL (FORT BRAGG) FEVER. An illness was observed in the summer of 1942 that had an onset identical with that of the first phase of leptospirosis. The most distinctive feature was the development of a rash on about the fourth day, characterized by 2 to 5 cm slightly raised erythematous lesions that were usually symmetrically distributed over the pretibial areas. In contrast to other leptospiral syndromes, splenomegaly occurred in 95 per cent of these patients. This outbreak, which related to exposure while swimming, was caused by the Autumnalis serogroup. Subsequently Pomona has been observed in association with rashes, which are usually truncal in distribution but have also been pretibial in location.

MYOCARDITIS. Cardiac arrhythmias, including paroxysmal atrial fibrillation, atrial flutter, and ventricular tachycardia, have been described, but are usually of little clinical significance. However, on rare occasions definite cardiac dilatation with acute left ventricular failure has been observed. Associated manifestations have included jaundice, pulmonary infiltrates, arthritis, and skin rashes. The serogroups thus far incriminated have included Icterohemorrhagiae and Pomona.

CHILDREN. Several clinical features occur in children which are not seen or are very rare in adults: acalculous cholecystitis (five of nine children in one series), pancreatitis, abdominal causalgia, peripheral desquamation of rash which may be associated with gangrene, and cardiopulmonary arrest. The features of desquamation, myocardial involvement, and hydrops of the gallbladder suggest the recently described "mucocutaneous lymph node syndrome."

LABORATORY FEATURES. Leukocyte counts vary from leukopenic levels to mild elevations in the anicteric patients. In patients with jaundice, leukocytosis as high as 70,000 per cubic millimeter may be present. However, regardless of the total leukocyte count, neutrophilia of greater than 70 per cent is very frequently encountered during the first stage.

Hemolytic substances have been demonstrated in cultures of pathogenic leptospires. In contrast to many hemolysins of bacterial origin, which are not hemolytic in vivo, the leptospiral hemolysins appear active in vivo. In patients with jaundice, anemia may be severe and is most characteristically due to intravascular hemolysis. Anemia owing to leptospirosis is unusual in anicteric patients.

Rarely thrombocytopenia sufficient in magnitude to be associated with bleeding is encountered. The erythrocyte sedimentation rate is elevated in more than one half of patients but is usually less than 50 mm per hour.

Urinalyses during the leptospiremic phase reveal a high frequency of abnormalities, including mild proteinuria, casts, and an increase in cellular elements. In anicteric infections, these abnormalities rapidly disappear after the beginning of illness. Proteinuria and abnormalities in urine sediment are usually not associated with elevations in blood urea nitrogen values. Since the

anicteric form of the disease has often gone undiagnosed, estimates of the frequency of azotemia and jaundice are probably high. Azotemia has been reported in approximately one fourth of patients. In three fourths of these patients the blood urea nitrogen is less than 100 mg per 100 ml. Azotemia is usually associated with the occurrence of jaundice. The serum bilirubin levels may reach 65 mg per 100 ml; however, in two thirds of patients the levels are less than 20 mg per 100 ml. During the first phase one half of patients have increased serum creatine phosphokinase (CPK) values. In contrast, increases are not seen in viral hepatitis. Mean transaminase values in leptospirosis approximate five times normal. A slight increase in transaminase with a definite increase in CPK suggests leptospirosis rather than viral hepatitis.

DIAGNOSIS. Diagnosis is based upon either cultural or serologic studies. The most common initial diagnostic impressions in patients with leptospirosis are meningitis, hepatitis, nephritis, "FUO," and influenza. Leptospires may be isolated quite readily during the first phase from blood and cerebrospinal fluid or during the second phase from the urine. Leptospires may be excreted in the urine for up to 11 months after the onset of illness. Whole blood should be inoculated immediately into tubes containing semisolid medium, such as Fletcher's. If culture medium is not available, leptospires reportedly will remain viable up to 11 days in blood anticoagulated with sodium oxalate. Animal inoculation (preferably of either suckling hamsters or guinea pigs) may also be used and is of particular value if specimens, e.g., urine, are contaminated. Direct examination of blood or urine by darkfield methods so frequently results in failure or misdiagnosis that it should not be employed as the only diagnostic test. Antibodies appear from the sixth to the twelfth day of illness. Four serologic tests are available: the macroscopic plate agglutination test (the easiest to perform but a relatively insensitive technique), hemolytic test (complex in performance but requiring only a single antigen), microscopic agglutination test (complex in performance but most specific), and complement-fixation test. Serologic criteria for diagnosis include a fourfold or greater rise in titer during the course. Cross-agglutination reactions between various serotypes commonly occur so that the infecting serotype often cannot be determined with certainty without isolation of leptospires.

PROGNOSIS AND SEQUELAE. Between 1966 and 1975, a case fatality ratio of 9.8 per cent has been reported in the United States. Age is the most significant host factor related to increased mortality. In a representative series, the mortality rose from 10 per cent in men less than 50 years of age to 56 per cent in those over 51 years of age. In anicteric patients, mortality is essentially unknown. With the occurrence of jaundice, mortality in various series has ranged from 15 to 40 per cent. The long-term prognosis after the acute renal lesion of leptospirosis is good. However, a few patients exhibit residual tubular dysfunction, e.g., a defect in renal concentrating ability, and a patient with permanent renal damage has been recorded.

THERAPY AND MANAGEMENT. A variety of antimicrobial drugs, including penicillin, streptomycin, the tetracycline congeners and erythromycin, have been effective in vitro and against experimental leptospiral infections. The data obtained from controlled observations in man are conflicting as to over-all efficacy. If antimicrobial drugs have any beneficial effect, they must be administered within four days, and preferably within two days, of the onset of illness. This means that the decision to start chemotherapy must be made mainly on clinical suspicion (see Ch. 189). The agents most studied have been penicillin G and the various tetracycline congeners. Turner states that large doses of penicillin G or tetracycline are beneficial. Within four to six hours after initiation of penicillin G therapy, a Jarisch-Herxheimer type reaction may occur, which suggests antileptospiral activity. There is general agreement that antimicrobials administered after the fifth day have no beneficial effect. Since diagnosis within the first five days requires a very high index of suspicion, management is primarily supportive. The clinical impression exists that early bed rest may minimize the subsequent morbidity. The presence of azotemia and jaundice requires meticulous attention to fluid and electrolyte therapy.

Alston, J. M., and Broom, J. C.: Leptospirosis in man and animals. Edinburgh and London, E. S. Livingstone, Ltd., 1958.

Edwards, G. A., and Domm, B. M.: Human leptospirosis. Medicine, 39:117, 1960.

Feigin, R. D., and Anderson, D. C.: Human leptospirosis. C.R.C. Crit. Rev. Clin. Lab. Sci., 5:413, 1975.

Heath, C. W., Jr., Alexander, A. D., and Galton, M. M.: Leptospirosis in the United States. Analysis of 483 cases in man. 1949–1961. N. Engl. J. Med., 273:857, 915, 1965.

Johnson, R. C.: The Biology of Parasitic Spirochetes. New York, Academic Press, 1976.

Johnson, W. D. Jr., Silva, I. C., and Rocha, H.: Serum creatine phosphokinase in leptospirosis. JAMA, 233:981, 1975.

Turner, L. H.: Leptospirosis. Br. Med. J., 1:537, 1973.

Wong, M. L., Kaplan, S., Dunkle, L. M., Strechenberg, B. W., and Feigin, R. D.: Leptospirosis: A childhood disease. J. Pediat., 90:532, 1977.

Section Three   THE MYCOSES

177. INTRODUCTION

John P. Utz

Increased awareness by physicians, continuing improvement in cultural techniques and in their use by laboratory technicians, and the existence of a valuable (and difficult) antifungal agent, amphotericin B, have led to an increased importance of the systemic mycoses in human disease. The fact that infection occurs with fungi that are free-living forms in soil, decaying vegetation, and bird excreta poses a difficult problem of control. The deliberate impairment of immune response, e.g., to decrease host-versus-graft reactions in patients with organ transplants, has created still another setting for infection by "opportunistic" fungi.

Although the chapters that follow are devoted to the mycoses per se, it should be pointed out that fungi have other pathways through which they can produce disease. P. K. C. Austwick has well summarized these phenomena:

Fungi cause three main types of animal and human disease:

Mycoses: diseases resulting from the invasion of living tissues by the fungus.

Allergies: diseases resulting from the development of hypersensitivity to fungal antigens.

Mycotoxicoses resulting from the ingestion of toxic fungal metabolites formed in food, and *mycetisms* resulting from the ingestion of toxic fungal fruiting bodies.

There are also three indirect ways in which fungi can be involved in pathogenic processes in animals, viz., by inducing the formation of toxic substances (including estrogens) by a host plant which is then eaten by an animal; by so degrading a foodstuff that macronutrient deficiencies appear in animals feeding on it; and by forming substances such as enzymes, which, although not acting directly on metabolic processes themselves, affect the availability of growth substances to the animal, e.g., vitamins, which may lead to micronutrient deficiency.

Fungal pathogenicity thus covers a much wider range of activity than that seen in other pathogenic microorganisms, and its height of complexity may be realized when it is possible for all three types of disease to be present in one individual animal, each caused by the same species of fungus playing three different roles at one time. Infection and allergy due to *Aspergillus fumigatus* are not uncommon together in man.

Further complications arise in the existence of two types of fungal thallus morphology in vivo. Firstly, apical hyphal growth leads to spherical or disc-like colonies whose spread is by peripheral extension and by fragmentation, a process compensating for its slowness of dissemination by the provision of relatively large inocula for its extension, and so of more certainty of success. Secondly, the self-replication of single cells either as yeast cells or endosporulating spherules can more readily play a leading role in the dissemination of infection in the body, but for this the fungus is generally dependent upon phagocytosis. It may be said that, in the first instance, the fungus is essentially active, making its own way through the tissues and, in the second, passive and dependent on the bloodstream or blood cells for transport. The latter type of growth is also directly comparable to that in many bacterial and viral infections, being frequently accompanied by acute pyrexial symptoms, while the former is generally associated with a chronic inflammatory process extending sometimes over many years.

Failure to understand this fundamental difference in the behavior in vivo of fungi has led to much confusion in the classification of fungal disease, and it still remains a major problem when trying to generalize on the pathogenesis of the mycoses. The ability of fungi to adopt a wide range of vegetative morphology according to their environment is being increasingly observed, and a number of filamentous saprophytic fungi are now known to be capable of budding as yeast cells under defined experimental conditions, e.g., *Mucor rouxii* and *Aspergillus parasiticus* (Bartnicki-Garcia and Nickerson, 1962; Detroy and Ciegler, 1971). The possession of hyphae or of a unicellular state therefore bears no relationship to the classification or to the potential pathogenicity of the species.*

The systemic mycoses have important properties in common in addition to their point of origin in nature. With few exceptions, they are not contagious from animal to man or man to man, and epidemics or outbreaks arise from a common source. Infection is acquired by inhalation or, in a few instances, by traumatic implantation. The primary focus is usually the lung, and infection spreads hematogenously or, less commonly, by direct extension. The gross and microscopic appearance of infected tissue is that of a granulomatous process. The immunologic response is generally effective (reinfection is rare), and cellular and serologically mediated immune mechanisms have been demonstrated (see Ch. 38 and 40).

178. HISTOPLASMOSIS

John P. Utz

DEFINITION.   Histoplasmosis is a systemic fungal disease, respiratory in origin, that spreads to the pulmonary lymphatics and by the blood to the mediastinal lymph nodes, spleen, liver, adrenals, gastrointestinal tract, kidneys, skin, central nervous system, heart, and other organs. It may be asymptomatic, acute and benign, or progressive and eventually fatal.

HISTORY.   Darling in Panama in 1905 reported three fatal cases of disseminated disease, which he considered to be due to a *"plasmodium"* with a *"capsule,"* in *histiocytes* which he termed *Histoplasma capsulatum*. In a study of tissue section, da Rocha Lima concluded in 1913 that the agent was a fungus. In 1934 De Monbreun correctly identified the fungus in cultural and in laboratory animal studies. Ten years later Christie and Peterson recognized the benign form of human disease with pulmonary calcification and associated skin hypersensitivity to histoplasmin. Subsequently, Palmer showed widely varying rates of hypersensitivity according to geographic areas in this country.

ETIOLOGY.   *H. capsulatum* has two morphologic forms, *yeast* and *hyphal*, dependent upon a variety of environmental factors. The yeast form seen in tissues measures 2 to 3 by 3 to 4 μ and has a clear area resulting from skrinkage of cytoplasm from the rigid cell wall. In artificial media or natural substrate the yeast form is converted readily at room temperatures to the hyphal form with the production on Sabouraud's glucose medium of a white to brown cottony mold. On microscopic examination this is composed of branched hyphae, characteristic spherical forms with spiny projections (tuberculate macroconidia) 8 to 14 μ in diameter, and smaller forms (microconidia) measuring 2 to 5 μ. Conversion of the hyphal to the yeast form occurs characteristically after inoculation into animals or less readily on enriched media at 37° C. Skin hypersensitivity, complement-fixing, and other antigens have been demonstrated. Mice and guinea pigs are susceptible to experimental infection.

EPIDEMIOLOGY.   Histoplasmosis occurs with highest frequency in infancy and old age and equally in the

sexes except more often in the male in old age. It has been reported in more than 30 countries in both temperate and tropical zones. Skin hypersensitivity rates are as high as 80 to 90 per cent in some parts of the eastern and midwestern United States. Rates of skin reactivity increase rapidly with age to young adulthood and then more slowly thereafter. Man and animals are infected by inhalation of the fungus in dust. Soil from chicken houses or from areas contaminated or composted by bat or bird dung is especially rich in fungi. Massive exposure through such activities as destruction of chicken houses, exploration of caves, or community "clean-up" activities has resulted in outbreaks. Fifty per cent of dogs and cats in some areas and many species of wild animals are known to be infected. *Histoplasma duboisii*, a closely related fungus, produces in African patients a disease marked by lymphadenopathy and bone, joint, and skin involvement.

PATHOLOGY.   The tissue reaction is characteristically engulfment of yeast forms by histiocytes or macrophages derived from organs of the reticuloendothelial system. Epithelioid or histiocytic granulomas are formed, with tubercle-like nodules, caseation necrosis, and calcification in the lung, lymph nodes, liver, spleen, adrenals, and other organs. The organism can best be identified in tissues by culture or by use of special stains (periodic acid–Schiff, Gridley, or Gomori methenamine silver methods). However, fungal cells may be few, crowded, and not differentiated with certainty from those of *H. duboisii, Blastomyces dermatitidis, Torulopsis glabrata,* or *Candida albicans*.

CLINICAL MANIFESTATIONS.   On the basis of delayed cutaneous hypersensitivity studies, it appears that primary infection with *H. capsulatum* is usually asymptomatic or produces a respiratory illness that is not distinctive.

Primary Acute Form.   The primary acute form is characterized by respiratory symptoms of cough, shortness of breath, pleuritic chest pain, hoarseness, hemoptysis, and cyanosis in that order. Associated generalized symptoms are commonly fever, chills, myalgia, malaise, and weight loss. In focal outbreaks, where there is exposure to large numbers of spores, sudden onset and pleuritic pain are common. Pleural effusion, however, is rare. The chest film may show bilateral disease with the characteristic diffuse miliary type of lesion from hematogenous seeding, or, more commonly, localized infiltrations, especially in the lower lobes. There may be hilar and peritracheal lymphadenopathy unaccompanied by other lesions. That infection is not localized to lungs alone is attested by the frequent splenic calcification seen later and the occasional isolation of *H. capsulatum* from urine during the acute illness. In many patients lesions resolve completely, but in others calcification or fibrotic scarring persists. Calcified peribronchial nodes may compress the bronchus, leading to bronchiectasis, or may erode and result in broncholithiasis. A distinctive residue of primary infection is the solitary nodule of the lung, located just beneath the pleura, appearing roentgenographically as a "coin lesion." Mediastinal histoplasmosis with esophageal abscess or superior vena cava syndrome is being increasingly reported.

Progressive Disseminated Form.   Rarely the disease progresses and resembles that form originally described by Darling. Pulmonary findings are often not prominent; illness is characterized instead by fever, enlarge-

---

*From Austwick, P. K. C.: The pathogenicity of fungi. *In* Microbial Pathogenicity in Man and Animals. Twenty-second Symposium of the Society for General Microbiology, Imperial College, London. Cambridge, England, Cambridge University Press, 1972.

ment of the liver and spleen, generalized lymphadenopathy, weight loss, anemia, and leukopenia. One particular feature may predominate, and the illness then appears as endocarditis, pericarditis, meningitis, adrenal insufficiency, or multiple ulcerations of mouth, pharynx, larynx, stomach, or small or large bowel. Belief in *H. capsulatum* uveitis persists despite the extraordinary rarity of isolation of the fungus from any material derived from patients.

Chronic Cavitary Form. In older adult males especially, a chronic, cavitary pulmonary disease occurs that closely simulates and is often labeled tuberculosis. This form is characterized by cough, weight loss, dyspnea, low-grade fever, chest pain, and hemoptysis. This form is most likely a reactivation of a previously quiescent primary infection.

DIAGNOSIS. The isolation in culture and microscopic identification of the fungus establish the diagnosis. In suspected cases of acute primary disease both sputum and urine should be cultured. In the widely disseminated forms, the fungus may be cultured from blood, bone marrow, cerebrospinal fluid, ulcer swabs, urine, sputum, lymph nodes, and material from liver biopsy. Conversion of a skin test from negative to positive and a titer of the complement-fixing antibodies that rises and falls or is in excess of 1:32 only support the clinical impression. A single positive histoplasmin skin test indicates only recent or remote exposure to this or related antigen. Frequently, both skin and complement-fixation tests are negative in a patient with severe or early disease. Careful microscopic study of properly stained tissue sections may reveal characteristic fungal forms, providing additional supporting evidence for the clinical diagnosis (see Pathology).

Acute primary histoplasmosis should be considered in the differential diagnosis of any persistent febrile respiratory disease, especially those occurring after exposure to chicken or other bird excreta and in any pneumonia without appropriate bacteria in sputum. Hepatosplenomegaly, lymphadenopathy, anemia, and leukopenia of the severe disseminated form may closely simulate Hodgkin's disease and leukemia. Mucosal alterations so closely resemble cancer that repeated biopsies for tissue study have been performed, all with negative results, before cultures were done. As a general rule, histoplasmosis should be suspected in any patient with findings suggestive of tuberculosis but without supporting laboratory data.

TREATMENT. Amphotericin B is the most active of the presently available antifungal drugs for the treatment of the disease in man. The drug is customarily given intravenously; 1.0 mg dissolved in 500 ml of a 5 per cent glucose solution is recommended as the first dose. Dosage should be increased daily by increments of 5 to 10 mg. At present there are many recommendations and no consensus as to optimal daily dosage (from 0.5 to 1.0 mg per kilogram), duration of therapy (from 6 to 14 weeks), or total dosage (from irrelevant to about 2 grams). Each infusion should be administered over at least a two-hour period and preferably longer, e.g., four to six hours. Such undesired side effects as local thrombophlebitis, fever, chills, nausea, vomiting, anorexia, rise in serum urea nitrogen, hypokalemia, and anemia may occur in approximately 80 per cent of patients but should not require abandonment of the therapy. After treatment is stopped, most indices of renal function return toward normal, but in about 80 per cent of patients on higher drug doses the values are never again the same as before treatment. Salicylates, antihistamines, and corticoids reduce the severity or frequency of such side effects of treatment as nausea, chills, and fever.

A few patients with localized disease in the lungs have been helped by surgical excision of lesions.

PROGNOSIS. Except in localized outbreaks with inhalation of large numbers of fungi, acute primary histoplasmosis is almost always a benign illness from which the patient recovers rapidly. Therapy usually has not been administered.

Since progressive disseminated disease is fatal in 80 to 90 per cent, and the chronic cavitary form in 30 per cent of cases, chemotherapy is indicated. Approximately 80 to 90 per cent of patients with severe disease have recovered with amphotericin B treatment.

Corticoid treatment has been associated with deleterious effects in experimental infections of animals and with relapse after amphotericin B therapy in man.

Austwick, P. K. C.: The pathogenicity of fungi. *In* Microbial Pathogenicity in Man and Animals. Twenty-second Symposium of the Society for General Microbiology, Imperial College, London, April 1972. Cambridge, England, Cambridge University Press, 1972.

Butler, W. T.: Pharmacology, toxicity and therapeutic usefulness of amphotericin B. JAMA, 195:371, 1966.

Drutz, D. J., Spickard, A., Rodgers, D. E., and Koenig, M. G.: Treatment of disseminated mycotic infections: A new approach to amphotericin B treatment. Am. J. Med., 45:406, 1968.

Goodwin, R. A., Jr., and Des Prez, R. M.: Histoplasmosis. Am. Rev. Respir. Dis., 117:929, 1978.

Vanek, J., and Schwarz, J.: The gamut of histoplasmosis. Am. J. Med., 50:89, 1971.

179. COCCIDIOIDOMYCOSIS

(Valley Fever)

Demosthenes Pappagianis

DEFINITION. Coccidioidomycosis is a fungal infection usually acquired by the respiratory route. In most cases it is arrested in the lungs, but it may spread to virtually all organs or tissues. Chronic persistent infection may ensue. Infrequently the infection is fatal.

HISTORY. The disease we recognize as coccidioidomycosis was first described in 1892 by Alejandro Posadas in an Argentinian man in Buenos Aires. In the infected tissues a cystlike organism thought to be a protozoan was observed. The second case was reported in 1894 by Rixford in California, the place of origin of the succeeding several hundred recognized cases. The resemblance of the organism to the protozoon *Coccidia* led to the name *Coccidioides*. Ophuls and Moffitt in 1900 recognized the causative organism to be a cultivable mold in vitro. Most early recognized cases of coccidioidal infection were severe, often with widespread cutaneous and visceral lesions, and frequently fatal, but Gifford and Dickson in the early 1930's established that San Joaquin or valley fever was a mild infection caused by *Coccidioides immitis*. Introduction of amphotericin B in 1956 led to successful therapy in coccidioidal infections with an otherwise dismal outlook.

ETIOLOGY. In the infected host, *C. immitis* exists as a spherule (sporangium), 20 to 100 μm in diameter, and reproduces by formation of few to several hundred endospores. These endospores are released and in turn enlarge to mature spherules. The filamentous septate *mycelial* form usually found in cultures and in nature produces chains of *arthrospores*. These arthrospores (about $2 \times 5 \mu m$) are readily airborne and constitute the inhaled infectious form of the organism. Confirmation of the identity of *C. immitis* requires demonstration of the spherule form of the organism in the patient or by animal inoculation, and constitutes the single best diagnostic procedure.

EPIDEMIOLOGY. Coccidioidomycosis is usually encountered in the southwestern United States (California, Arizona, New Mexico, Texas, southern portions of Nevada and Utah), Mexico, Central America, Argentina, Paraguay, Venezuela, and Colombia. These areas correspond to location of *C. immitis* in the soil. Travelers may acquire the infection during brief visits to these areas. Rarely exportation of the fungus on some product of the endemic region can lead to infection elsewhere. The true *incidence* is likely greater than the 300 to 400 cases reported per year in California, or the more than 500 per year in Arizona. Some 50 deaths per year caused by coccidioidomycosis are reported in the United States. It has been estimated that 25,000 to 35,000 new infections occur per year in California. About a fifth of those so affected will have symptomatic infections that bring them to a physician. The *prevalence* of coccidioidomycosis increases during the dry, dusty summer and fall. An occupational risk of infection exists in agricultural or other disturbers of the soil. In some endemic areas the proportion of the population which has been infected increases with time of residence and may exceed 85 per cent. *C. immitis* survives for months at -20 to $42°$ C and a pH of 4 to 9. It can be found in rodent burrows and elsewhere, persisting for years in the soil. Rodents, dogs, cattle, sheep, and other animals are also infected by inhalation of arthrospores. The infection is not spread from animals to man or from man to man (although one case of in utero infection has been reported).

Humans from a few weeks to 85 years of age have been infected. In general, infection may be milder in children. In adults, about 60 per cent of infections are asymptomatic. Of the 40 per cent with symptomatic infections, most will recover. Approximately 1 in 100 adult white males with symptoms will develop disseminated coccidioidomycosis. Filipinos and blacks have higher rates of dissemination. Adult white females less frequently develop disseminated coccidioidomycosis, perhaps associated with their greater tendency to develop the prognostically favorable erythema nodosum.

PATHOGENESIS AND PATHOLOGY. The nature of the response to infection with *C. immitis* appears related to the morphologic states of the organism and to the development of delayed hypersensitivity. Endospores appear to induce a granulocytic response, spherules a macrophagic response. Lesions may resemble closely the granulomatous lesion of tuberculosis or sarcoid, but frequently there is juxtaposed suppuration. The mixed inflammatory reaction may yield amorphous necrosis, hyalinization, fibrosis, and calcification. The contribution of delayed hypersensitivity to pathogenesis is not clear, but anergy to coccidioidin is prognostically unfavorable.

Primary infection usually presents as a pneumonitis. (Fewer than 20 cases of primary cutaneous coccidioidomycosis have been reported.) The infection is usually arrested in the pulmonary parenchyma and regional nodes. Occasionally the organisms spread lymphogenously and hematogenously to virtually any tissue (the gastrointestinal mucosa has not been involved, and the brain and the endocardium only rarely). Such dissemination usually ensues early after the primary infection, but occasionally the pulmonary lesion has cleared by the time dissemination is apparent. In about 5 to 10 per cent of patients with primary pulmonary coccidioidomycosis, a chronic cavity or granuloma will develop. Viable *C. immitis* may persist for years in such lesions, although the patient's clinical status remains favorable. Pulmonary cavities occur and recur more frequently in patients with diabetes mellitus. Prognostically more serious but less frequent is an apical chronic progressive fibrocavitary disease.

CLINICAL MANIFESTATIONS. Clinically apparent primary pulmonary coccidioidomycosis will develop in 7 to 28 days (average, 10 to 16 days) after inhalation of the spores, presenting with fever, malaise, pleuritic pain, dry cough, night sweats, anorexia, headache, and weight loss. Chest pain is common and may be severe. Early after onset of symptoms, a macular, urticarial, scarlatiniform or morbilliform rash may develop transiently. It may be seen particularly in the inguinal areas and on the palms and soles, even before coccidioidin sensitivity develops. Such a rash is seen more frequently in children.

Along with the respiratory component, "valley fever" classically includes erythema nodosum of the anterior tibia or erythema multiforme of the extensor aspects of the upper extremities, palms, and upper thorax and neck. This may be seen in about 40 per cent of adult white females and 5 per cent of adult white males who have symptomatic infections, and is accompanied by arthralgia and swelling of ankles and knees. Erythema nodosum indicates marked sensitivity to coccidioidin and is not likely to be coccidioidal in cause if the skin test is negative. Initially primary coccidioidomycosis may be bronchial or peribronchial. The chest x-ray may reveal pneumonitis resembling acute bacterial, mycoplasmal, viral, or other fungal pneumonias with lobar, lobular, or scattered patches of infiltrate. Hilar densities (parenchymal and adenopathy) and pleural effusion are common. Infrequently there is pericardial effusion. A transient cavity occasionally develops during the acute phase. Primary infection of the skin yields an ulcerative lesion and regional adenopathy. Resolution of primary pulmonary coccidioidomycosis usually occurs within several weeks, although asthenia and easy fatigability may last for several months. There may be persistent and unexplained chest pain despite recovery from the acute infection.

Dissemination of the infection to metapulmonary tissues, including the meninges, may also be recognized only after the primary pulmonary lesion has faded. The progression is sometimes difficult to discern clinically until an overt lesion of bone, skin, lymph node, or meninges is detected. It may be suspected from deterioration of the patient with persistent fever, weight loss, marked bronchomediastinal adenopathy, or mental deterioration (in meningitis), or from laboratory parameters to be discussed below.

Chronic cavities, coccidioidomas, or *bronchiectasis* may remain after apparent clearing of the primary pneumonitis, or they may be detected on routine roentgenograms years after the primary infection. Hemoptysis may be the first indication of a pulmonary cavity.

DIAGNOSIS. Awareness of the extreme variability of clinical patterns offered by coccidioidomycosis is essential. It may resemble influenza; bacterial, mycoplasmal, or other mycotic pneumonia; acute or chronic tuberculosis or histoplasmosis; or neoplasms. The hilar or bronchomediastinal adenopathy may resemble that of sarcoid or lymphomas. The chronic pulmonary cavity is characteristically thin-walled on x-ray, but may resemble a pulmonary abscess or be partially filled with fluid. Coccidioidal fibrosis or bronchiectasis may resemble that of other causes. Lesions of bones or soft tissues may resemble those of blastomycosis, tuberculosis, or other bacterial infections. The erythrocyte sedimentation rate is elevated, and there is often a moderate leukocytosis, sometimes with eosinophilia. Sustained eosinophilia is unfavorable.

Coccidioidal meningitis may resemble tuberculosis or other mycotic meningitis. Decrease in the cerebrospinal fluid (CSF) glucose is often an early significant change. Occasionally in the early stages there may be a polymorphonuclear pleocytosis, but the onset is usually more insidious and the CSF changes in cell and protein are suggestive of chronic or "aseptic" meningitis. A "paretic" colloidal gold curve often accompanies these changes.

Coccidioidomycosis is confirmed by direct demonstration of endosporulating spherules in biopsied tissue or exudates utilizing special fungal stains. *Cultures* from lesions or sputum also yield a diagnosis, provided that animal inoculation or special culture methods are used to confirm the production of spherules. The CSF should be cultured but often fails to yield *C. immitis.*

The time involved and hazard of working with *C. immitis* cultures require that appropriate skin test and serologic studies be carried out. The coccidioidin (mycelial phase antigen) skin test may become positive in three days to three weeks after onset of symptoms. (A newly developed antigen, spherulin, appears more reactive in detecting sensitivity.) A positive coccidioidin skin test means past or present infection. A negative test does not exclude a coccidioidal cause, for the test is often negative in disseminated infections or with old pulmonary lesions (cavities or coccidioidomas). The skin test should be repeated in following the course of the illness, for anergy is unfavorable. The skin test does not interfere with coccidioidal serologic studies. Precipitins (IgM) are produced early and assist in diagnosis of primary infections. These are detected by a tube test and by a latex particle agglutination test. They fade within the first few weeks but may persist in severe infections and may reappear, e.g., with a bronchopleural fistula or in reinfection via ventriculoperitoneal or ventriculoatrial shunt. Complement-fixing (CF) antibodies (IgG) appear later and may persist for many months or years after recovery. They are readily detected by immunodiffusion. The CF antibody titer rises proportional to severity (extent of involvement). Thus metapulmonary dissemination is usually reflected in an elevated titer (usually above 1:16, but this level may vary between laboratories), and declining titer indicates improvement. Pleural, joint, and cerebrospinal fluids may contain CF antibody, although usually at lower titer than in the serum. In coccidioidal meningitis the CSF infrequently is seronegative but the serum positive. The basilar meningitis may yield CF-positive cisternal and lumbar fluids even though the ventricular fluid is negative. Complement fixation by the CSF is usually diagnostic of coccidioidal meningitis, although an extradural (paravertebral) abscess can yield CF antibody in the CSF. In this instance the CSF protein is elevated, with glucose and cells normal.

The CF test is positive in about 60 per cent of cases (immunodiffusion is more often positive) with chronic coccidioidal cavities, but is often negative in patients with asymptomatic coccidioidomas. Thus diagnosis of the latter often is not assisted by serologic tests. Cross-reactions occur between *C. immitis, Histoplasma capsulatum,* and *Blastomyces dermatitidis* in serologic and skin tests. Primary coccidioidal infections are sometimes accompanied by higher CF titers with *Histoplasma* and *Blastomyces* antigens. Sequential sera should yield higher homologous titers.

TREATMENT. Symptomatic therapy is indicated for primary coccidioidomycosis. Amphotericin B, the most extensively used antifungal agent, should be applied in most cases of disseminated disease, although miconazole has been effective in some cases. Occasionally, as with a small single cutaneous lesion, excision may be curative. In the absence of overt evidence of dissemination, systemic amphotericin may be administered for severe primary coccidioidal infection or when the clinical or laboratory picture indicates likelihood of dissemination. Amphotericin may be administered intravenously on alternate days, with the dose gradually raised to 1.0 mg per kilogram of body weight. The MIC in vitro of most strains of *C. immitis* is approximately 1 μg per milliliter. Prolonged therapy is often needed in coccidioidomycosis, increasing the risk of nephropathy, hypokalemia, anemia, phlebitis, and other side effects. Meningitis can be treated preferably by intracisternal administration of up to 1.0 mg, usually three times a week. Arachnoiditis has frequently complicated lumbar administration. The use of 10 per cent (hyperbaric) glucose with amphotericin, with the patient's head lowered, may lessen but does not eliminate arachnoiditis. Under some circumstances amphotericin may be given by the intraventricular route via the Ommaya reservoir and catheter. The total dose required must be determined by the progress of the patient. Therapy of meningitis should be continued for at least three months after the CSF becomes normal, but continued vigilance for years is required because of the possibility of relapse.

Excisional therapy may also be needed for osseous, articular, or soft tissue lesions. Pulmonary cavities, although generally benign, may be resected if complicated by progressive enlargement, rupture into the pleural space, hemorrhage, or secondary infection. Pre- and postoperative therapy with amphotericin is advisable, although some thoracic surgeons have had few complications without such coverage. Treatment of chronic pulmonary cavities or fibrocavitary disease with amphotericin B is usually without benefit. The usually benign solitary pulmonary nodule may have to be resected for differentiation from other lesions.

Immunotherapy with Lawrence's leukocyte transfer factor from coccidioidin-sensitive donors has had limited trials. This may provide an important additional therapeutic modality, particularly in anergic patients who have not responded to amphotericin or who may be at risk of recurrence of cavities, e.g., diabetics.

PROGNOSIS. Prior to amphotericin therapy, more than half the patients with disseminated infections and all with coccidioidal meningitis died. With amphotericin therapy, patients with coccidioidal meningitis have survived for 15 to 20 years, some apparently cured.

Nonmeningeal disseminated infections have also been successfully treated, although infections involving joints may be recurrent despite treatment with amphotericin B. Recovery from infection leads to resistance to reinfection (exogenous reinfection has occurred only in a very few laboratory workers). Immunosuppressive therapy of intercurrent disease such as Hodgkin's disease with accompanying cytotoxic therapy may reactivate old arrested coccidioidomycosis.

PREVENTION. A vaccine prepared from killed spherules has provided good protection of laboratory animals and has appeared safe in humans. However, it has not had a field trial in humans exposed to infection. Avoidance of exposure to the arthrospores would prevent infection, but the widespread distribution of the organism and impracticality of eradicating it from the soil make avoidance difficult in those who are occupationally tied to the soil. The use of lightweight masks or other measures to reduce inhalation of spores during overt dusty exposures is justified.

Ajello, L. (ed.): Coccidioidomycosis. Tucson, University of Arizona Press, 1967.

Ajello, L. (ed.): Coccidioidomycosis. Miami, Fla., Symposia Specialists, 1977.

Drutz, D., and Catanzaro, A.: Coccidioidomycosis. Am. Rev. Respir. Dis., 117:559, 727, 1978.

Fiese, M. J.: Coccidioidomycosis. Springfield, Ill., Charles C Thomas, 1958.

Huntington, R. W., Jr.: Coccidioidomycosis. In Baker, R. D. (ed.): Human Infection with Fungi, Actinomycetes and Algae. New York, Springer-Verlag, 1971, Chap. 6.

Smith, C. E., Saito, M. T., and Simons, S. A.: Pattern of 39,500 serologic tests in coccidioidomycosis. JAMA, 160:546, 1956.

180. BLASTOMYCOSIS

(North American)

John P. Utz

DEFINITION. Blastomycosis is a chronic systemic fungal disease, respiratory in origin, which, classically, disseminates to the skin and occasionally to subcutaneous tissue, bone, and other organs.

HISTORY. In 1894 Gilchrist and in 1898 Gilchrist and Stokes reported the first two cases and named the responsible fungus *Blastomyces dermatitidis.*

ETIOLOGY. *B. dermatitidis* is a dimorphic fungus existing in tissue as a yeastlike form (8 to 15 μ, rarely 30 μ), with a characteristic thick wall (0.5 to 0.75 μ). The yeast form reproduces by budding, and the typical bud is characterized by its large size and attachment to the parent cell by a persistent wall and a wide pore. On Sabouraud's glucose medium *B. dermatitidis* grows as a white mycelium composed of slender hyphae to which are attached, either directly or by lateral slender stalks (conidiophores), smooth spherical 2 to 10 μ forms (conidia). The perfect, sexual state, *Ajellomyces dermatitidis,* has recently been defined. Skin hypersensitivity, complement-fixing, and other antigens have been demonstrated. Mice and other laboratory animals are susceptible to experimental infection.

EPIDEMIOLOGY. Blastomycosis was at first exclusively American in distribution: Canada, Mexico, Central America, northern Latin America, and, in 98 per cent of reported cases, the United States. However, cases have now been reported from widely separated sites in Africa. The disease affects all ages, but there is a slightly higher frequency in the third and fourth decades. Men are affected six to nine times more frequently than women. Infection results from inhalation of conidia, but the saprophytic source of the fungus in nature is not known. In one reported instance, genital infection was acquired conjugally. Benign, subclinical cases have been reported, but the skin test studies do not support a high incidence of infection in certain areas similar to that of histoplasmosis and coccidioidomycosis. Common source epidemics have been reported in Big Fork, Minnesota, and Pick County, North Carolina.

PATHOLOGY. The characteristic tissue response to *B. dermatitidis* is a combination of suppuration and epithelioid and giant cell granulomas. In the lung the disease may be localized or may spread as a pneumonia. Cavitation and circumscribed, calcific nodules are rarely encountered. The skin lesions reveal characteristically pseudoepitheliomatous hyperplasia and microabscesses in which *B. dermatitidis* may be seen. In bone, subcutaneous tissue, meninges, prostate, epididymis, and other organs the histologic appearance is again a combination of suppuration and granulomas.

CLINICAL MANIFESTATIONS. **Primary Pulmonary Form.** Primary pulmonary blastomycosis begins usually as a mild respiratory infection (rarely as a fulminant pneumonia) with cough, pleuritic chest pain, and, occasionally, hemoptysis. As the disease progresses, generalized symptoms of fever, night sweats, anorexia, and weight loss appear. Physical signs may not be prominent. However, there may be dullness, bronchial breath sounds, and rales characteristic of consolidation. Roentgenographically, manifestations vary from those of a consolidated lobar pneumonia to multiple infiltrations. Hilar adenopathy is common, localized nodules are less so, and cavitation is rare. Although pleural disease is common, effusion is characteristically extremely rare.

Cutaneous Form. Although cutaneous blastomycosis represents spread from a primary pulmonary infection, the presenting complaint of many patients is a cutaneous lesion, either solitary or multiple. The initial papule or pustule progresses within weeks or months into an ulcerated or warty lesion. The advancing border of this lesion is serpiginous, dusky red, or violaceous, elevated 1 to 3 mm, and has an outer edge that slopes abruptly. The base of the lesion contains small abscesses, from which characteristic budding yeast cells can be demonstrated. The central area may become crusted, or, in older lesions, may heal with a thin atrophic scar. In contrast to the skin lesion that follows accidental laboratory implantation, regional lymphadenopathy does not occur.

Other Systemic Forms. A subcutaneous form of the disease consists of single or more often multiple soft to firm nodules, palpable deep beneath the skin. These may enlarge to become bulging abscesses, but in various stages contain pus. The skin over the nodules may have a slightly reddish hue.

Osteomyelitis or periostitis of long bones or spine occurs frequently. The first manifestation of disease may be a psoas abscess. A septic arthritis may occur either alone or by extension from bone.

Genitourinary blastomycosis is frequently seen in men and is manifested by pain and swelling of the epididymis, prostate, or seminal vesicles.

There may also be involvement of the central nervous system, eye, adrenals, thyroid, and larynx. In contrast to histoplasmosis, the gastrointestinal tract is almost never involved.

DIAGNOSIS. Although skin lesions may be strongly suggestive, the diagnosis of blastomycosis is confirmed by the finding of typical budding yeast cells in direct preparations or by the culture and identification of *B. dermatitidis* from pus or lesions. When appropriate, sputum, urine, cerebrospinal fluid, bone marrow, or other biopsy and autopsy tissue should also be cultured. Skin tests are almost always negative, especially in earlier stages of the disease, and serologic procedures may show a higher titer or a positive reaction only to *Histoplasma capsulatum.*

The pulmonary form of the disease is rarely diagnosed clinically or roentgenographically and is usually thought to be tuberculosis or, less frequently, sarcoidosis, acute bacterial pneumonia, malignancy, or other fungal infections more common in the geographic area. Skin lesions are suggestive of basal cell carcinoma, tuberculosis, nodulo-ulcerative syphilid, pyoderma, or other fungal infections. Other systemic manifestations mimic those of tuberculosis or other chronic bacterial infection.

TREATMENT. Amphotericin B has been used extensively for all forms of blastomycosis. Details of administration are given in Ch. 178. Rather less drug is necessary, however, and for involvement of organs and tissues other than bones, 1 to 2 grams is usually sufficient.

2-Hydroxystilbamidine, administered intravenously, is probably less toxic than amphotericin B. It is a satisfactory alternative only in nonprogressive cutaneous disease. The usual dosage has been 225 mg per day and 8.0 grams per course of therapy.

Surgical drainage of abscesses is frequently indicated. Chemotherapy before and after surgery is advisable.

PROGNOSIS. Pulmonary infection of an inapparent or benign form occurs only rarely. Blastomycosis is, if untreated, a chronic and usually progressive disease. Cutaneous and other disseminated disease is eventually fatal in 10 to 30 per cent of cases.

Except with moribund patients chemotherapy usually effects a prompt recovery. Relapse requiring additional therapy has occurred, however, in at least 10 to 15 per cent of patients.

Lockwood, W. R., Allison, F. L., Batson, B. E., and Busey, J. F.: The treatment of North American blastomycosis: Ten years' experience. Am. Rev. Respir. Dis., 100:314, 1969.
Witorsch, P., and Utz, J. P.: North American blastomycosis. A study of 40 patients. Medicine, 47:169, 1969.

181. PARACOCCIDIOIDO-MYCOSIS

(South American Blastomycosis)

John P. Utz

DEFINITION. Paracoccidioidomycosis is a chronic systemic fungal disease, probably respiratory or gastrointestinal in origin, with dissemination to the lymph nodes, skin, lung, and other organs.

HISTORY. Lutz in 1908 first described the disease and the organism observed in tissues of a Brazilian patient. In 1909 and 1912, Splendore described more fully the characteristics of the disease and the fungus.

ETIOLOGY. The disease is caused by a dimorphic fungus, *Paracoccidioides brasiliensis,* which appears in tissues and exudates as a multiple-budding yeast 2 to 60 μ in diameter. The bud is characterized by a thin wall (0.2 to 1.0 μ) and narrow pore. At temperatures less than 30° C on Sabouraud's glucose medium, a white (later brown) membranous or wrinkled mycelium appears that microscopically is composed of branching hyphae and oval forms (conidia). Delayed cutaneous hypersensitivity and complement-fixing antigens have been demonstrated. Guinea pigs and mice can be experimentally infected.

EPIDEMIOLOGY. Except for reports of occasional immigrants to North America, the disease occurs exclusively in residents of Central and South America and is especially prevalent in Brazil. It is approximately ten times more frequent in males, and is slightly more frequent in persons 40 to 50 years of age. Manual laborers and farmers seem especially susceptible. Infection is probably acquired by the respiratory route, but a saprophytic, environmental source of fungi is not known. Disease in animals and animal-to-man or man-to-man spread are unknown. Widespread infection of a benign form has been suggested by skin test surveys.

PATHOLOGY. The histopathologic reaction to *P. brasiliensis* may be suppurative with abscess formation; in other sites it may be granulomatous with fibroblasts, macrophages, lymphocytes, caseation, and giant cells containing organisms. Lesions are seen in the mucosa of the gastrointestinal tract, lymph nodes, spleen, lungs, and liver.

CLINICAL FORMS. Primary. The primary lesion is commonly on the oral or nasal mucosa. Rarely, the conjunctival or anorectal mucosa may be involved. The earliest lesion is a papule that ulcerates and spreads to adjacent tissue.

Cutaneous Form. A variety of skin lesions may be seen, most of which progress to an ulcerative, crusted form suggestive of blastomycosis. In contrast, however, regional lymphadenopathy frequently accompanies skin lesions only in paracoccidioidomycosis. A keloidal form (Lobo's disease) of milder nature, without lymphadenopathy and caused by a different species (*Loboa loboi*) may be another type of paracoccidioidomycosis.

Lymphangitic Form. In this form there are lymphangitis and enlargement of regional lymph nodes, which suppurate and drain. Cervical and submandibular nodes are most commonly affected.

Visceral Form. The gastrointestinal tract is frequently involved as a primary site of infection. The spleen, adrenals, lungs, and liver may be affected by hematogenous spread. Bone, myocardium, and central nervous system involvement are less frequently seen.

DIAGNOSIS. The diagnosis is established by the culture and identification of *P. brasiliensis* and is only supported by positive skin and complement-fixation tests.

The disease must be differentiated from syphilis, tuberculous adenitis and skin disease, yaws, leishmaniasis, and other fungal infections.

TREATMENT. Amphotericin B (see Ch. 178) is the

drug of choice. Continuous sulfonamide therapy, still employed today, results in remission but not cure.

PROGNOSIS. All forms of the disease are fatal if untreated. Over 90 per cent of cases are cured by amphotericin B.

Emmons, C. W., Binford, C. H., Utz, J. P., and Kwon-Chung, K. J.: Medical Mycology. 3rd ed. Philadelphia, Lea & Febiger, 1977.
Paracoccidioidomycosis. Scientific Publication No. 254. Washington, D.C., Pan American Health Organization, 1972.

182. MADUROMYCOSIS

(Mycetoma, Madura Foot)

John P. Utz

DEFINITION. Maduromycosis is a chronic systemic fungal disease that follows traumatic or imperceptible implantation of the skin. It is characterized by swelling, induration, suppuration, and draining sinuses of the skin, subcutaneous tissue, and bone, typically of the foot.

HISTORY. The disease was first recognized and described in 1712 by Kaempfer in India, and was called Madura foot, after the city of that name. It has been suggested, however, that Madura foot was described by Sophocles in the hero of *Philoctetes*.

ETIOLOGY. Many species of ten genera have been reported as etiologic agents; the most common of these have been *Madurella mycetomi, Nocardia brasiliensis,* and, in the United States, *Allescheria boydii*. In tissues or pus these fungi, except for *Nocardia* (see Ch. 164), are characterized by the appearance of "grains" of oval or irregular shape measuring 0.5 to 2.0 mm, and of white, red, black, or yellow color. Microscopically they are composed of 2 to 4 μ segmented, branched hyphae or round encysted forms (chlamydospores).

A. boydii grows rapidly on Sabouraud's glucose medium, forming a white (later gray or brown) cottony, aerial mycelium, which microscopically consists of thin hyphae to which are attached short or long stalks (conidiophores) bearing a single 8 to 10 by 5 to 7 μ pyriform or ovoid form (conidium). Large (50 to 200 μ) flask-shaped vessels containing asci and spores (4 to 7 μ) can be seen when material from the surface of agar is crushed and examined.

When inoculated intraperitoneally into mice, *A. boydii* is pathogenic, but progressive disease similar to that in humans has not been produced.

EPIDEMIOLOGY. Although occasionally reported from temperate areas, the disease is seen most often in those tropical zones where few people wear shoes. The disease occurs chiefly in adults and more often in males. Most causative organisms are saprophytes of soil or plants. The disease has been reported in the dog, cow, and horse, but animal-to-man or man-to-man spread has not been reported.

PATHOLOGY. The typical swollen foot has numerous draining sinuses communicating with abscesses of the skin, subcutaneous tissue, or bone. Drainage sites have characteristic collars of fibrous or epithelial tissues. Suppuration with epithelioid, plasma, and giant cells is intermingled with areas of fibrosis, and one or the

other reaction may predominate. With Gram, hematoxylin and eosin, or periodic acid–Schiff stains, fungal cells may be seen either in pus or within macrophages or giant cells.

CLINICAL FORMS. Although lesions have been reported on the leg, torso, hand, and face, the characteristic site of disease is the foot. The first manifestation consists of a papule, small nodule, indurated area with a vesicle, or an abscess that ruptures with sinus tract formation. Infection spreads and new nodules appear, leading to generalized swelling and distortion of the toes. Pain is infrequent, and there are few generalized symptoms. Roentgenographic examination may show lytic lesions with reaction and proliferation of the bone.

DIAGNOSIS. Diagnosis is confirmed by the demonstration of granules in draining material, but the specific cause is dependent on isolation of the fungus in culture. Serologic and skin tests have not been developed for most of the responsible fungi. Maduromycosis must be distinguished from other fungal infections and from tuberculosis, yaws, neoplasms, and elephantiasis.

TREATMENT. With the variety of antimicrobial agents available, each with specific activity, it is essential that definitive mycologic studies be done prior to treatment to determine the identity and, if feasible, the drug susceptibility of the causative fungus. The failure to do so in many past reports is undoubtedly a factor in the generally pessimistic attitude toward treatment and the early resort to amputation.

The drug of choice for infections caused by *Nocardia brasiliensis* is a sulfonamide (see Ch. 164), whereas for those caused by *Aspergillus,* amphotericin B is indicated (see Ch. 187). Tetracycline and diaminodiphenylsulfone have been reported to be successful in a few cases of *M. mycetomi* infections. Amphotericin B has been reported ineffective in two cases of *A. boydii* infection.

PROGNOSIS. The disease is usually progressive and rarely self-limited.

Butz, W. C., and Ajello, L.: Black grain mycetoma. Arch. Dermatol., 104:197, 1971.
Rippon, J. W.: Medical Mycology. Philadelphia, W. B. Saunders Company, 1974.
Zeisler, E. B.: A case from Sophocles. Arch. Dermatol., 84:136, 1961.

183. CHROMOMYCOSIS

John P. Utz

DEFINITION. Chromomycosis is a chronic systemic fungal disease, acquired in the cutaneous form by traumatic or imperceptible implantation, and characterized by wartlike, ulcerated, crusted lesions of the skin and subcutaneous tissues.

HISTORY. Although rare in this country, chromomycosis was first reported from Boston in 1915, separately by Lane and Medlar, and the organism responsible was named *Phialophora verrucosa* by Thaxter. Subsequently, cases caused by other genera of fungi were described by Brumpt and Carrion.

ETIOLOGY. A number of fungi have been incriminated, but chiefly *Phialophora verrucosa, P. pedrosoi, P. compactum,* and *Cladosporium carrioni*. In tissues these fungi resemble each other and appear as single or clustered, round, thick-walled, 6 to 12 μ budding cells of a striking brown color, from which the disease draws its name. On culture, mycelia are produced that vary according to genus and species. Skin hypersensitivity and complement-fixing antigens have been demonstrated in some fungal species. Laboratory animals are susceptible to experimental infection, but the equivalent of natural disease in man is not produced.

EPIDEMIOLOGY. The disease is seen more often in adult males in the rural areas of the tropics, especially in Brazil, Puerto Rico, and Cuba. The responsible fungi are saprophytes of soil, but are found more often in decaying wood and vegetation. Infection in animals has not been reported, and animal-to-man or man-to-man spread is unknown.

PATHOLOGY. Varying degrees of hyperkeratoses, acanthosis, and pseudoepitheliomatous hyperplasia are seen. In the cutis the reaction may be granulomatous with mononuclear, epithelioid, and Langhans' giant cells. Fungal cells are seen readily with hematoxylin and eosin stains.

CLINICAL FORMS. Chromomycosis is a disease of the skin and subcutaneous tissue.

The first patient reported had lesions of the buttock. The most common site is the lower extremity. The disease appears also, in descending order of frequency, on the hand, forearm, arm, neck, and shoulders. The earliest lesion is a nodule or pustule that, over a period of weeks to months, ulcerates, drains, enlarges, dries, and becomes violaceous and wartlike. There is rarely pain, but itching is common. Lesions do not spread generally, but scratching results in autoinoculation and satellite or secondary distal lesions.

DIAGNOSIS. Although older typical skin lesions may be clinically and histologically suggestive, the diagnosis is confirmed by the culture and identification of the causative fungus.

Early lesions may be confused with blastomycosis, tuberculosis, leprosy, yaws, and syphilis.

TREATMENT. Surgical resection of early skin lesions has been the most common and efficacious therapy. Amputation has been required in a small number of cases. Most of the fungi causing chromomycosis are resistant to amphotericin B, but successful treatment has been reported in two cases when the drug was injected locally into the skin. This drug needs further trial in this disease.

PROGNOSIS. The cutaneous form of chromomycosis is chronic and compatible with long life (in one case, 40 years).

Al-Doory, Y.: Chromomycosis. Missoula, Montana, Mountain Press, 1972.

184. CRYPTOCOCCOSIS

(European Blastomycosis, Torulosis)

John E. Bennett

DEFINITION. Cryptococcosis is a systemic fungal infection, its most common and most lethal manifestation being meningoencephalitis.

HISTORY. Busse, who reported the first case in 1894, observed the fungus in tissue and isolated the causative agent. That same year Sanfelice isolated from peach juice the same fungus, naming it *Saccharomyces hominis*. The fungus received no less than 37 additional names until 1952, when Lodder and Kreger-Van Rij's monumental taxonomic study of yeast gave the fungus its current name, *Cryptococcus neoformans*. The fungus was rarely isolated from natural sources until 1955, when Emmons demonstrated that *C. neoformans* was a frequent saprophyte in weathered pigeon droppings. This lent support to the emerging concept that the disease was acquired by inhalation of fungus-laden dust. The discovery of amphotericin B, reported by Gold and co-workers in 1956, was to provide the first successful chemotherapy of cryptococcosis.

ETIOLOGY. Cryptococcosis is caused by *Cryptococcus neoformans*, a round or oval yeastlike fungus measuring 4 to 7 μ in diameter. It reproduces by budding. This fungus is unique among systemic mycoses of man in that it is highly encapsulated in tissue. The polysaccharide capsule releases into the host the soluble antigen which provides a means of serologic diagnosis. The fungus can be isolated as a smooth, creamy white colony on a variety of common laboratory media. Culture identification is by gross and microscopic appearance, biochemical reactions, and growth at 37° C.

EPIDEMIOLOGY. The disease is sporadic throughout the world, with no clear focal outbreaks in man or sharply defined areas of high endemicity. Disease occurs occasionally in warm-blooded feral and domestic animals, excluding birds. Cryptococcal mastitis may spread through dairy herds, probably by way of milking machines, and contaminate unpasteurized milk. No spread of infection from animal to man or man to man has been reported. Reservoir of infection is probably saprophytic sources in nature, such as weathered pigeon droppings. Presumed portal of entry is the lung, although this site is often clinically inapparent. The fungus is not a part of the normal flora of man or animals, although occasionally it appears to colonize a patient's damaged bronchial tree. No occupational group is known to be predisposed to cryptococcosis. Infection is uncommon before puberty and is more frequent in males. Predisposing factors include Hodgkin's disease, lymphoma, leukemia, sarcoidosis, and supraphysiologic doses of adrenal corticosteroids.

PATHOLOGY. The most frequent and characteristic abnormality on gross examination occurs in the brain, which shows basilar arachnoiditis and focal collections of small, glistening, gelatinous cysts, particularly in the cortical gray matter and basal ganglia. Microscopic examination reveals the cysts to be clumps of cryptococci, with little surrounding inflammation. A dense inflammatory response to the fungus may be noted in meninges or brain but is more characteristic of extraneural lesions. Cellular response consists of macrophages, giant cells, and lymphocytes. Necrosis is seen occasionally at the center of a dense inflammatory response, particularly in the lung. Features notable for their infrequency include polymorphonuclear leukocytes, calcification, extensive scarring, and hemorrhage.

CLINICAL MANIFESTATIONS. **Meningoencephalitis.** Symptoms begin with the insidious onset of headache, followed by nausea, vomiting, blurred vision, or decreased mental acuity. Less frequent symptoms include photophobia, diplopia, and gait ataxia. Gradually the patient becomes lethargic and prefers to remain undisturbed. Somnolence or irritability may appear. Fever is low grade or absent. Although no one physical finding is highly frequent or characteristic, examination may disclose papilledema, mild to moderate nuchal rigidity, cranial nerve palsies, or extensor plantar response.

Extraneural Cryptococcosis. Pulmonary cryptococcosis is the second most common clinical manifestation. Even patients with no clinically apparent pneumonitis but with cryptococcosis elsewhere in the body are often found to have a pulmonary focus on careful postmortem examination or sometimes on sputum culture. Chest symptoms and radiologic findings, when present, commonly mimic primary or metastatic carcinoma in the lung. Pleural effusions, cavitation, and hilar adenopathy are not common. Skin lesions occur in 10 per cent of patients with cryptococcosis, and bone lesions occur in about 5 per cent. Either may be the sole clinical manifestation of the infection or may be associated with disease in other organs. Skin lesions begin as asymptomatic papules, pustules, or soft subcutaneous nodules. They tend to become painful as they slowly enlarge, ulcerate, and drain glary pus. Osteolytic lesions may appear in almost any bone and present as a cold abscess. Rare clinical manifestations include prostatitis, hepatitis, endocarditis, pericarditis, renal abscess, and endophthalmitis.

DIAGNOSIS. Lumbar puncture in patients with symptomatic cryptococcal meningoencephalitis usually reveals one or more of the following abnormalities: elevated opening pressure, pleocytosis predominantly composed of mononuclear cells, increased protein concentration, and hypoglycorrhachia. A smear of cerebrospinal fluid sediment, mixed with India ink, reveals encapsulated yeast in about half the cases. The smear may be difficult to interpret and provides only a tentative, albeit useful, diagnosis. Another rapid diagnostic aid is serologic detection of cryptococcal antigen in serum and cerebrospinal fluid. With current techniques, about 90 per cent of patients with cryptococcal meningitis have detectable antigen if both sites are tested. Extraneural cryptococcosis may result in serum antigen if infection is extensive. A falling antigen titer during recovery is a favorable prognostic sign.

Final diagnosis depends upon culture or biopsy. Several milliliters of cerebrospinal fluid should be cultured for cryptococci in cases of indolent meningoencephalitis and also in every case of documented extraneural cryptococcosis, in order to detect subclinical extension to the central nervous system. The frequency of subclinical renal infection in disseminated cryptococcosis makes urine culture useful. Sputum, blood, prostatic fluid, and pus from cutaneous lesions may also yield the fungus. Biopsy may be required to diagnose cryptococcosis in the lung, skin, or bone. Histologic diagnosis can usually be made with accuracy by those experienced in this area.

THERAPY. Intravenous amphotericin B is the treatment of choice for cryptococcosis of the central nervous system. Treatment should be continued for at least four weeks after all weekly cultures become negative. 5-Fluorocytosine therapy cures some cases of cryptococcosis, but drug resistance often arises during therapy. Combination therapy, using 5-fluorocytosine and low-dose intravenous amphotericin B, is probably better than amphotericin B alone in cryptococcal meningitis, but experience is required to avoid serious toxic reactions to 5-fluorocytosine. Intrathecal amphotericin B may be a useful adjunct in patients failing an adequate trial of intravenous therapy or with such poor renal function

that reduced doses of intravenous amphotericin B are obligatory. Development of communicating or noncommunicating hydrocephalus may require neurosurgical intervention.

Intravenous amphotericin B is the usual treatment of choice for extraneural cryptococcosis. A probable exception is the patient without either hematologic malignancy or immunosuppressive therapy who, on thorough study, has infection confined to one focus in lung, skin, or bone. Surgical excision of skin or lung lesions, curettage of bone lesions, or simply prolonged observation may be warranted if the lesion is not extensive and is stable or regressing.

PROGNOSIS. Cryptococcal meningoencephalitis is invariably fatal unless treated. With currently available therapy, the case fatality rate is about 25 per cent. Patients with Hodgkin's disease, lymphoma, or leukemia or who require continued immunosuppressive therapy fare less well. Death usually results from the sequelae of coma or from brainstem compression. Despite successful therapy, patients may be left with optic atrophy, hydrocephalus, personality changes, or decreased mental acuity.

Diamond, R. D., and Bennett, J. E.: Prognostic factors in cryptococcal meningitis. Ann. Intern. Med., 80:176, 1974.

Fetter, B. F., Klintworth, G. K., and Hendry, W. S.: Mycoses of the Central Nervous System. Baltimore, Williams & Wilkins Company, 1967.

Salfelder, K.: Cryptococcosis. *In* Baker, R. E. (ed.): Human Infections with Fungi, Actinomycetes and Algae. New York, Springer-Verlag, 1971, pp. 383–464.

185. SPOROTRICHOSIS

John P. Utz

DEFINITION. Sporotrichosis is a chronic systemic fungal disease, acquired usually by traumatic implantation and localized to cutaneous lymphatic tissues, or rarely by the respiratory route with dissemination throughout the body.

HISTORY. From a patient at Johns Hopkins Hospital, in 1896 Schenck isolated a fungus that was identified by E. F. Smith as *Sporotrichum*; it was named *Sporotrichum schenckii* by Hektoen and Perkins in 1900. A great number of cases were seen subsequently in France, and more than 2800 cases in a single epidemic in the gold mines of South Africa.

ETIOLOGY. *Sporothrix schenckii*, a dimorphic fungus, is occasionally observed in tissues as round to cigar-shaped yeast- or bacteria-like forms. On Sabouraud's glucose medium at room temperature, a white, cottony, aerial mycelium appears that in three to seven days becomes wrinkled and changes in color from cream to black. Microscopically, branching, septate hyphae are seen, 2 μ in width, bearing directly or on lateral branches ovoid to spherical bodies (conidia) measuring 2 to 4 by 2 to 6 μ in diameter. Mice are susceptible to experimental infection. Delayed cutaneous hypersensitivity and agglutinogen antigens have been demonstrated.

EPIDEMIOLOGY. The disease is worldwide in distribution; it has appeared epidemically in South Africa and in localized outbreaks in Mexico and Florida. It is more common in men. It frequently affects laborers, farmers, and florists and is considered a true occupational disease. The fungus exists in its saprophytic form in soil, peat moss, and decaying vegetation and on thorns. In the cutaneous lymphatic forms, infection results from accidental implantation into the skin. In disseminated forms, the mode of entry is probably respiratory. Spontaneous sporotrichosis has been reported in dogs, horses, mules, cats, and other animals, and human disease has resulted from animal contact. Direct transfer from man to man is not known to occur.

PATHOLOGY. The histopathologic reaction to *S. schenckii* is varied, frequently acute and suppurative, but also subacute or chronic. In some instances granulomas are seen with epithelioid and giant cells either diffusely distributed or localized in a typical tubercle. Fungi may be seen more readily after staining with a modified Schiff-MacManus technique.

CLINICAL FORMS. **Cutaneous Lymphatic Form.** The earliest lesion is a pustule, papule, or nodule of the skin appearing characteristically on a finger and at a site where the patient may recall an earlier, seemingly insignificant scratch or prick. The nodule enlarges, becomes red to violaceous, and is followed by a chain of subcutaneous nodules along regional lymphatics. These are at first freely movable, but become attached to the skin, and may ulcerate and drain a thin gray to yellow pus. Streaking and pain characteristic of acute lymphangitis are not present. Generalized symptoms are rare.

Other Forms. Other forms may appear secondary to the cutaneous lymphatic lesion either by direct extension to contiguous, subcutaneous tissue, bone, and joint or by hematogenous spread to distant sites. Sometimes the original site of infection is inapparent, and the disease presents as a septic arthritis or osteomyelitis. Less frequently, there may be involvement of the eye, gastrointestinal tract, central nervous system, or skin. In disseminated disease, systemic symptoms of fever, weight loss, inanition, malaise, pain at sites of lesion, anemia, and leukocytosis are commonly present. Two forms of pulmonary disease are now recognized. The more common is chronic cavitary, resembling tuberculosis. The other is less chronic, resolves spontaneously, and is characterized by hilar lymphadenopathy with a sparing of lung parenchyma.

DIAGNOSIS. Although the diagnosis may seem readily apparent in the cutaneous lymphatic form of disease, the clinical impression is confirmed by the culture and identification of the fungus. Agglutination or complement-fixation serologic and skin tests may be helpful, but are not generally available.

Cutaneous lymphatic sporotrichosis must be distinguished from tularemia, pyoderma of bacterial origin, and other fungal infections. Disseminated disease resembles tuberculosis, staphylococcal osteomyelitis, or neoplastic disease.

TREATMENT. The cutaneous lymphatic form of disease responds slowly but progressively to the oral administration of iodides in the form of a saturated solution (1 gram per milliliter) of potassium iodide given in dosage of 4 to 5 ml three times daily. Treatment should be prolonged one to two months beyond the time of apparent healing.

Disseminated disease, especially of bone and joints, is frequently resistant to iodide therapy. Dramatic improvement has been seen in a few patients treated with amphotericin B, and for this form of disease this drug is recommended.

PROGNOSIS. Untreated cutaneous lymphatic sporotrichosis may persist for many months to years. Treated lesions respond slowly but completely. Disseminated disease is progressive and usually fatal unless treated.

Baum, G. L., Donnerberg, R. L., Stewart, D., Mulligan, W. J., and Putnam, L. R.: Pulmonary sporotrichosis. N. Engl. J. Med. 280:410, 1969.

Crout, J. E., Brewer, N. S., and Tompkins, R. B.: Sporotrichosis arthritis. Ann. Intern. Med., 86:294, 1977.

Wilson, D. E., Mann, J. J., Bennett, J. E., and Utz, J. P.: Clinical features of extracutaneous sporotrichosis. Medicine, 46:265, 1967.

186. MUCORMYCOSIS

John E. Bennett

DEFINITION. Mucormycosis is an acute, often fatal infection caused by fungi of the order Mucorales. Phycomycosis is a term which encompasses mucormycosis and several other mycoses.

HISTORY. Two cases of pulmonary mucormycosis reported by Fürbringer in 1876 were probably the first cases described with enough clarity to permit any confidence in the diagnosis. It was not until 1943 that Gregory described mucormycosis originating in nose and paranasal sinuses.

ETIOLOGY. *Rhizopus* and *Mucor* species are the principal pathogens of mucormycosis. These fungi appear in tissue as hyphae 6 to 50 μ wide, rarely septate, irregular in contour, and tending to branch at nearly right angles. Hyphae may be demonstrated histologically by staining with hematoxylin and eosin, Gomori methenamine silver, or periodic acid–Schiff. Growth at 25 or 37° C is profuse and rapidly spreading on most media. Identification of the culture is based largely on microscopic appearance. Only very specialized laboratories are competent to pursue identification beyond a tentative designation of genus.

EPIDEMIOLOGY. Mucormycosis is uncommon and sporadic around the world, usually afflicting patients with serious pre-existing disease. *Mucormycosis of the paranasal sinuses and contiguous structures occurs predominantly in patients with poorly controlled diabetes mellitus.* Pulmonary and disseminated mucormycosis also occurs occasionally in diabetics but is most prevalent in immunosuppressed patients, particularly treated leukemics. Among the varied underlying disorders present in patients with gastrointestinal mucormycosis, uremia, severe malnutrition, and diarrheal diseases seem prominent. Mucormycosis occurs at any age, with no strong predilection for race or sex. It does not spread from man to man. Disease is probably acquired by inhalation of fungal spores. Mucorales are ubiquitous in the environment, growing on decaying vegetation, dung, and foods of high sugar content.

PATHOLOGY. Necrosis is the predominant gross and microscopic finding. This is accounted for in part by the propensity of hyphae to proliferate within small and medium-sized arteries, producing thrombosis. Infarcted areas may be ischemic or hemorrhagic. Neutrophils predominate in the inflammatory response.

CLINICAL MANIFESTATIONS. Mucormycosis originating in the nose and paranasal sinuses produces a characteristic clinical entity. Initial symptoms mimic bacterial sinusitis, with low-grade fever and sinus pain. However, nasal discharge is not purulent but is thin and sometimes blood streaked. Over the next few days, infection spreads to contiguous structures. Invasion of the orbit may lead to reduced range of ocular motion, proptosis, chemosis, or blurred vision. Direct invasion of the globe or thrombosis of the ophthalmic artery may occur. Nasal turbinates or hard palate develop areas which are black, friable, and bloodless. Frontal or temporal lobes of the brain may be infected by direct extension, producing headache and deepening stupor. Invasion of the carotid artery within the cavernous sinus may cause embolization, mycotic aneurysm, or thrombosis. Without treatment, the patient usually dies in coma a few days to a few weeks from onset.

Pulmonary mucormycosis presents as a rapidly progressive dense bronchopneumonia, accompanied by high fever, toxicity, and tachypnea, but with little cough or sputum. The necrotic central portion of a lesion is sometimes expectorated, producing hyphae in sputum and a cavity on chest x-ray. Gastrointestinal lesions of mucormycosis begin as one or more shallow ulcerations in esophagus, stomach, or intestine. The ulcer tends to enlarge, deepen, and perforate the viscus. Disseminated mucormycosis may originate in nasal area, lung, or gastrointestinal tract. Sometimes no portal is evident. Hematogenous spread may involve brain or other organs. Pulmonary and disseminated mucormycosis are clinically indistinguishable from invasive aspergillosis.

DIAGNOSIS. *Cranial mucormycosis* is easily mistaken for bacterial sinusitis with cavernous sinus thrombosis. The diagnosis requires biopsy of infected mucosa in the nose or sinus. Hyphae are often abundant on histologic section or wet smear of crushed tissue. Hyphae seen in cross-section may be mistaken for yeast. Occasionally hyphae are confused with capillaries, or vice versa.

Pulmonary and disseminated infections caused by Mucorales, *Aspergillus,* and *Pseudomonas aeruginosa* have many similarities. Diagnosis of mucormycosis, like that of aspergillosis, requires biopsy. In the proper clinical setting, demonstration of broad, nonseptate hyphae in bronchial brush specimens or sputum would be strongly suggestive. Culture of biopsy specimens is certainly of interest, but isolation of a ubiquitous organism like Mucorales must be interpreted with caution. Blood cultures are very rarely positive for the fungus.

TREATMENT. Mucormycosis originating in the nose and paranasal areas should be treated by optimal regulation of diabetes mellitus, extensive surgical debridement, and intravenous amphotericin B. After debridement, sinus cavities can be irrigated daily with amphotericin B, 1 mg per milliliter. Although good guidelines for dose and duration of intravenous amphotericin B are not available, it has been customary to treat vigorously at least until disease progression halts. Treatment should probably continue for another month beyond that. Tomograms of the orbit and sinuses can be very helpful in evaluating disease progression. Carotid arteriogram may demonstrate extension to the ophthalmic artery or carotid siphon. Electroencephalogram and lumbar puncture provide late evidence of intracranial extension.

Intravenous amphotericin B is probably useful in other forms of mucormycosis, but too few patients have been treated for this question to be answered.

PROGNOSIS. A substantial number of cures have been reported recently in mucormycosis of the nose, sinus, and orbit. Prognosis is poor once central nervous system signs appear. Other forms of mucormycosis have largely been diagnosed post mortem.

Baker, R. D.: Mucormycosis. *In* Human Infection with Fungi, Actinomycetes and Algae, New York, Springer-Verlag, 1971, pp. 832–918.

Bartrum, R. J., Watnick, M., and Herman, P. G.: Roentgenographic findings in pulmonary mucormycosis. Am. J. Roentgenol., 117:810, 1973.

Meyer, R. D., and Armstrong, D.: Mucormycosis — changing status. Crit. Rev. Clin. Lab. Sci., 4:421, 1973.

Price, D. L., Wolpow, E. R., and Richardson, E. P.: Intracranial phycomycosis: A clinicopathological and radiologic study. J. Neurol. Sci., 14:359, 1971.

187. ASPERGILLOSIS

John E. Bennett

DEFINITION. The term aspergillosis embraces a variety of diseases which have in common growth of the fungus *Aspergillus* in tissue or within air-containing spaces of the body, such as bronchus or pulmonary cavity.

HISTORY. Micheli first described the genus *Aspergillus* in 1729. The first case of aspergillosis in man was probably observed by Sluyter in 1847, although disease in birds had been reported before then. In 1856 Virchow reviewed the literature and reported four autopsied cases. Renon's classic paper of 1897 attracted attention to the disease.

ETIOLOGY. The etiologic agent *Aspergillus* is a fungus largely composed of septate hyphae about 4 μ in diameter. Sporulating structures, called conidial heads, may be seen when the fungus is growing in nature, on artificial medium, or within air-containing spaces of the body. The most frequent pathogen for man is *Aspergillus fumigatus.* However, many other species can clearly cause either invasive or noninvasive disease in man, particularly *Aspergillus flavus.* Aspergilli grow rapidly on many routine laboratory media and, because of their ubiquity, are encountered in the laboratory as airborne contaminants. Identification is by gross and microscopic appearance.

EPIDEMIOLOGY. Aspergilli are often found growing on decaying vegetation. Under proper conditions millions of spores, about 2 to 4 μ in diameter, may be released into the air. Inhalation of these spores must be a common event, but disease is infrequent. Both insects and animals may acquire aspergillosis. The disease is an economically important cause of mycotic abortion in cattle and horses. In man the disease is sporadic and worldwide, with no clear occupational predisposition. Transmission from animal to man or man to man has not been encountered.

PATHOLOGY. The fungus is capable of eliciting a wide variety of tissue responses, depending upon site and host. A ball of hyphae may be situated within an ectatic bronchus or epithelialized lung cavity and provoke little or no histologic response. During invasion of tissue in a markedly immunosuppressed host, blood vessel invasion by hyphae, thrombosis, necrosis, and hemorrhagic infarction are prominent features. In invasion of more normal tissue, a pyogenic necrotic reaction is common, but epithelioid granulomas with giant cells may be observed instead. Chronic, fibrosing, nonnecrotizing granulomatous inflammation has typically been seen in the paranasal sinus and orbit.

Inhalation of *Aspergillus* spores may provoke an allergic response without invasion of the body, but this condition will not be considered here. Certain aspergilli, given proper growth conditions, produce proteolytic enzymes or toxins. As far as is known, these substances play no important role in aspergillosis.

CLINICAL MANIFESTATIONS. Pulmonary Aspergillosis. *Aspergillus* can colonize ectatic bronchi, cysts, or cavities in the lung. Colonization is usually a sequel of a chronic inflammatory process, such as tuberculosis, bronchiectasis, histoplasmosis, or sarcoidosis. A ball of hyphae may form within an air-containing space, particularly in the upper lobes, and is termed an aspergilloma. The fungus rarely invades the wall of the cavity, cyst, or bronchus in such patients. During bacterial pneumonia, lung abscess, or empyema in a colonized patient, *Aspergillus* may appear in the inflammatory process, although its role is uncertain. In most patients it is difficult to determine clinically whether specific symptoms or signs of disease progression are due to the underlying condition or to some allergic, inflammatory, or obstructive process caused by *Aspergillus*. The most common symptoms are chronic productive cough and hemoptysis. *Aspergillus* can cause chronic pneumonia in patients with chronic granulomatous disease of childhood or, rarely, in previously healthy persons. In a few instances, acute bilateral pneumonia has occurred in normal persons, usually after a presumed massive inhalation of spores. However, the majority of patients with invasive aspergillosis now being encountered are markedly neutropenic or are receiving immunosuppressive therapy, or both. A patch of pneumonia appears and steadily becomes larger and denser. The lesion may remain focal or, at any time, may spread hematogenously to one or more sites in the lung, brain, or other organs. The lung lesion may also erode directly through the diaphragm or pericardium.

Lesions of Extrapulmonary Origin. Necrotizing lesions originating in the palate, paranasal sinuses, epiglottis, or gastrointestinal tract may occur in the immunosuppressed patient. *Aspergillus* may infect intracardiac or intravascular prostheses. Chronic granulomatous inflammation may originate in the paranasal sinuses and spread to orbit or brain. Progressive mycotic keratitis caused by *Aspergillus* may follow corneal trauma. Growth of *Aspergillus* on cerumen and detritus within the external auditory canal is termed otomycosis.

DIAGNOSIS. Culture of *Aspergillus* from sputum usually has no clinical significance. Repeated isolation of *Aspergillus* from sputum or demonstration of hyphae on sputum smear suggests endobronchial colonization. Precipitins to *Aspergillus* antigens are often demonstrable in the sera of such colonized patients. Radiologic appearance of an aspergilloma is distinctive. In the severely immunosuppressed patient, isolation of *Aspergillus* from even a single sputum should raise suspicion of possible invasive infection. Biopsy is usually required to diagnose invasive aspergillosis in lung, paranasal sinus, orbit, or brain. Histology may provide evidence of tissue invasion and permit a presumptive diagnosis of aspergillosis. For absolute confirmation and determination of species, the biopsy should be cultured. Neither serologic tests nor cultures of blood, cerebrospinal fluid, or urine are helpful in most forms of invasive aspergillosis.

TREATMENT. Surgical excision may be helpful in fungus ball of the lung or in aspergillosis of the parana-sal sinus and orbit. Measures to improve bronchopulmonary drainage may assist the patient with endobronchial colonization. Intravenous amphotericin B is not helpful in endobronchial or endocavitary aspergillosis, but in invasive pulmonary aspergillosis a prolonged course of treatment will occasionally arrest progression. Ultimate cure of invasive pulmonary aspergillosis requires not only intravenous amphotericin B but also significant restoration of the host's defense mechanisms.

PROGNOSIS. Endobronchial or endocavitary aspergillosis rarely becomes invasive or disseminated. Although the condition is not usually the sole cause of death, it may contribute problems to an already damaged lung. Cure is infrequent in invasive aspergillosis of the lung, heart, paranasal sinus, orbit, or brain.

Green, W. R., Font, R. L., and Zimmerman, L. E.: Aspergillosis of the orbit. Arch. Ophthalmol., 82:302, 1969.
Kilman, J. W., Ahn, C., Andrews, N. C., and Klassen, K.: Surgery for pulmonary aspergillosis. J. Thorac. Cardiovasc. Surg., 57:642, 1969.
Young, R. C., Bennett, J. E., Vogel, C., Carbone, P. P., and DeVita, V. T.: Aspergillosis. Spectrum of the disease in 98 patients. Medicine, 49:147, 1970.

188.   CANDIDIASIS

(Candidosis, Moniliasis, Thrush)

John E. Bennett

DEFINITION. Candidiasis is an infection of the skin, mucous membranes, or viscera caused by species of *Candida*, a yeastlike fungus. Thrush refers to candidiasis of mucous membranes, as in the mouth or vagina.

HISTORY. Thrush as a clinical entity has been appreciated for centuries, but its relationship to fungi was unknown until Langenbeck isolated the pathogen from a patient's throat in 1839. Among the many names applied to this fungus, the most significant have been *Oidium albicans* (given by Robin in 1853), *Monilia albicans* (Zopf, 1890), and *Candida albicans* (Berkhout, 1923).

ETIOLOGY. *Candida albicans* is the usual cause of candidiasis. A substantial number of cases of disseminated candidiasis have been caused by other species of *Candida*, particularly *C. tropicalis* and *C. parapsilosis*. The size and shape of *Candida* cells are variable, but most commonly the cells are oval and 4 to 6 μ in their longest axis. Growth usually appears within a few days of incubation at 25 or 37° C. Deep inoculation into certain media, such as corn meal Tween 80 agar, causes *Candida* to grow as long tubules called pseudohyphae. Individual species of *Candida* are distinguished by their ability to utilize or ferment certain sugars. For routine laboratory purposes, *C. albicans* can be identified by its ability to form chlamydospores or, in the presence of serum, to form germ tubes. *Candida* species look very similar in infected tissue, but usually can be distinguished from other fungi. *Candida* generally, but not always, grows in tissue as both budding yeast and pseudohyphae. Both tissue forms are well demonstrated by Gomori methenamine silver, periodic acid–Schiff, or tissue Gram stains.

EPIDEMIOLOGY. *C. albicans* is a frequent commensal in the human mouth, gastrointestinal tract, and vagina.

Candida is also commonly isolated from the gut of animals. Isolation of this fungus from the environment is unusual, and most of the exceptions could have represented contamination by animals or man. This leads to the presumption that the fungus is spread from man to man and animal to animal. It is usually impossible to trace this spread, because colonization is asymptomatic. A probable exception is the newborn infant, in whom colonization usually leads to oral thrush. Later in life, disease seems to occur when a previously colonized patient becomes more vulnerable to tissue invasion. A wide variety of conditions predispose to candidiasis, particularly diabetes mellitus and therapy with either broad-spectrum antimicrobials or adrenal corticosteroids. Chronic maceration predisposes to cutaneous candidiasis, as in paronychia of bartenders and housewives, intertrigo of obese patients, or diaper rash. Women in the later months of pregnancy are particularly susceptible to vulvovaginal candidiasis. Patients with acute leukemia are prone to gastrointestinal and systemic candidiasis. An important route for acquiring systemic candidiasis is through unsterile intravenous injections of narcotics or through use of plastic intravenous catheters. When the infusion through the catheter is designed to meet the patient's total caloric requirement, the risk of systemic candidiasis goes even higher.

PATHOLOGY. In mucocutaneous candidiasis, pseudohyphae and yeast tend to be confined to the epithelium. Leukocytes infiltrate the epithelium as well as the submucosa or corium. Parakeratosis is usual. Ulceration and hyphal invasion of the submucosa is a more frequent characteristic of gastrointestinal candidiasis. In systemic candidiasis, abscesses may be found in almost any organ, but kidney, brain, spleen, heart, and liver are frequent sites. Such abscesses on gross inspection may appear as small, white, firm, cheesy nodules. Histologically these foci show necrosis, leukocytes, pseudohyphae, and yeast. Giant cells are seen occasionally. In the immunosuppressed patient, inflammatory cells may be scanty or absent. Patients with plastic intravenous catheters may develop at the catheter tip an endovenous fibrin sleeve containing *Candida*. Presumably, this can continue to seed the bloodstream for several days after withdrawal of the catheter.

CLINICAL MANIFESTATIONS. The mouth is the most common site of candidiasis. *Oral thrush* is usually an acute, self-limiting disease which presents as discrete and confluent white plaques on the oral and pharyngeal mucosa. The plaque is a pseudomembrane which can be scraped off with difficulty, exposing a red base. *Candida denture stomatitis* is characterized by well-circumscribed areas of erythema and edema in the mucosa under the upper dentures. *Candida* also appears to cause chronic hyperplastic oral lesions resembling leukoplakia. All the aforementioned oral lesions tend to be asymptomatic. *Cutaneous candidiasis* can present as diaper rash, red macerated areas in large skin folds, fissuring and desquamation in interdigital areas, angular cheilitis, paronychia, balanitis, or pruritus ani. *Chronic mucocutaneous candidiasis,* also called *Candida granuloma,* is an uncommon disease, usually beginning in early childhood, in which hyperkeratotic lesions wax and wane in the skin and mucous membranes for many years. The most severe skin lesions occur on the face, scalp, and hands. Involvement of mouth, vagina, and nails is usual. Children with this disorder frequently seem to have defective function of thymus-derived lymphocytes and tend to develop hypofunction of the parathyroid, thyroid, and adrenal glands.

The most common symptom of *Candida vaginitis* is pruritus. Other frequent symptoms include discharge and burning pain, the latter being worse on urination or intercourse. Speculum examination reveals an inflamed vaginal mucosa and a thin exudate, sometimes with white curds. Within the gastrointestinal tract, the *esophagus* is the most common site of candidiasis and the only site likely to be symptomatic. Substernal burning and either pain or a sense of obstruction on swallowing may occur. Blood-borne *Candida abscesses* are usually manifest only as fever and toxicity. Hematogenous dissemination to the choroid is detected on funduscopic examination as fluffy white retinal exudates. The abscesses gradually enlarge and extend into the vitreous humor, which becomes increasingly hazy. Cells and flare may also appear in the anterior chamber. The most common symptoms are orbital or retro-orbital pain, blurring, scotoma, and opacities floating across the visual field. *Candidiasis of the endocardium* or around the edges of an intracardiac prosthesis resembles bacterial infections in these sites. *Candida meningitis* clinically mimics cryptococcosis. *Pulmonary and renal candidiasis* are usually hematogenous in origin and cause no focal symptoms. Extensive renal cortical abscesses may cause azotemia. *Candidiasis in the lining of the bladder or renal pelvis* usually appears in a diabetic patient with chronic or recurrent bacterial urinary tract infections or after instrumentation or surgery on the urinary tract. Dysuria, pyuria, and passage of pseudohyphae in the urine are frequent findings. Rarely, pseudohyphae will be found packed in a necrotic renal papilla. A sloughed papilla, largely then a ball of fungus, may obstruct a ureter.

DIAGNOSIS. Demonstration of pseudohyphae on smear with confirmation by culture is the procedure of choice for diagnosing candidiasis of epithelial surfaces. Scrapings for this purpose may be made of skin, oral mucosa, vagina, or nails. Cerebrospinal fluid and joint fluid cultures are helpful in diagnosing *Candida* meningitis or arthritis. Progression of funduscopic findings usually permits an operational diagnosis of *Candida* endophthalmitis. Esophagram and esophagoscopy can aid the diagnosis of *Candida* esophagitis. Biopsy is required to diagnose candidiasis of lung or liver. Blood cultures are very useful in diagnosing *Candida* endocarditis but are less commonly positive in other forms of systemic candidiasis. The fungus can be isolated from blood, using the same routine media employed for bacteria, but one to three weeks of incubation are often required and the bottles should be vented. Rarely, *Candida* is seen on blood smear. Skin tests with *Candida* antigens are so commonly positive in normal people that they are not useful in diagnosing candidiasis. Diagnostic interpretation of serologic tests for candidiasis remains controversial.

TREATMENT. Oral thrush is best treated by rinsing the mouth with and then swallowing nystatin suspension, 100,000 units four times daily. Painting the lesions with 1 per cent aqueous gentian violet is a messy but effective alternative. Vaginal thrush usually responds to deep insertion of a nystatin vaginal suppository once or twice daily for two weeks. Cutaneous candidiasis of macerated areas requires measures to keep the skin dry plus topical nystatin or amphotericin B. Mild symptoms of *Candida* esophagitis may respond to the patient's sucking on a nystatin suppository three or four times daily. With pronounced esophageal symptoms, a short course of intravenous amphotericin B is more beneficial. Bladder thrush may be eradicated by bladder irrigation with amphotericin B, 50 μg per milliliter. If a Foley catheter is not in place, oral 5-fluorocytosine is an alternative. Isolation of *Candida* from blood may or may not indicate the need for intravenous amphotericin B. If the patient is febrile and severely immunosuppressed, a single positive blood culture for *Candida* is generally an indication for prompt chemotherapy. All too often the patient dies before additional blood cultures are reported positive. In the patient who is not immunosuppressed, significance of candidemia depends upon the number of positive cultures and the presence or absence of a plastic intravenous catheter. Multiple positive blood cultures in the absence of such a catheter indicate the need for chemotherapy. In the presence of such a catheter, discovery of candidemia should prompt removal of the catheter and culturing of its tip. If the patient is not seriously ill and is improving, treatment may be postponed to await clinical progress and the results of subsequent blood cultures. The species of *Candida* isolated is irrelevant to the decision about therapy. Temporization is inappropriate when endocarditis, endophthalmitis, arthritis, or other hematogenous lesions are detect-ed. Systemic candidiasis is treated with the same daily doses of intravenous amphotericin B as are used with other systemic mycoses. Adequate guidelines for judging duration of therapy are not known. There is also inadequate information to judge whether 5-fluorocytosine has a role in the treatment of systemic candidiasis.

PROGNOSIS. Most forms of mucocutaneous candidiasis are benign and respond to local treatment, although relapse is not rare. Chronic mucocutaneous candidiasis of children responds to intravenous amphotericin B, but relapse is virtually inevitable. For some reason these children rarely develop systemic candidiasis. The ability of treatment to prevent death from most forms of systemic candidiasis and to eradicate candidiasis of the urinary and gastrointestinal mucosa depends largely on the severity of the underlying condition. Candidiasis of the endocardium or around an intracardiac prosthesis is usually fatal despite treatment.

Edwards, J. E., Jr., Foos, R. Y., Montgomerie, J. Z., and Guze, L.: Ocular manifestations of *Candida* septicaemia. Review of 76 cases of haematogenous *candida* endophthalmitis. Medicine, 53:47, 1974.

Eras, P., Goldstein, M. J., and Sherlock, P.: Candida infection of the gastrointestinal tract. Medicine, 51:367, 1972.

Kirkpatrick, C. H., Rich, P. R., and Bennett, J. E.: Chronic mucocutaneous candidiasis. Ann. Intern. Med., 74:955, 1971.

Young, R. C., Bennett, J. E., Geelhoed, G., and Levine, E.: Fungemia with compromised host resistance. Ann. Intern. Med., 80:605, 1974.

Section Four   CHEMOTHERAPY OF MICROBIAL DISEASE

189.   DRUGS AND MICROBES

Walsh McDermott

In choosing the initial therapy for a patient with a presumed microbial disease, the physician is confronted with a formidable dilemma. On the one hand, if therapy is to be maximally effective, the correct drug or drug-pairing must be chosen quickly so that it may be administered before significant tissue damage or irreversible physiologic changes have occurred. On the other hand, if the choice is to be made quickly, it is difficult to make it exactly; for there are still only a few techniques by which the cause of an infection can be positively identified during the early hours of acute illness. Thus the physician is in the uncomfortable position of knowing that if he is to obtain the greatest advantages of antimicrobial therapy for his patient, he must make the correct choice of drugs one to five days before solid evidence of the identity of the infection will be forthcoming. An obvious way out of the dilemma would be by the introduction of rapid diagnostic methods illustrated by techniques such as the quellung test or the use of fluorescent-tagged antibody to swiftly identify organisms. However, surprisingly little effort has been devoted to developing a better, more rapid diagnostic technology. Given this situation, the physician has to rely on his *clinical* acumen and a full knowledge of all the microbial diseases that might reasonably be expected to institute threats to his patients. In actuality, to make this choice of the initial drug regimen from evidence obtained at the bedside is not as difficult as it sounds once the physician realizes what it is that he should be trying to do. While doing it, he can also be comforted by the thought that the expert consultant must go through exactly the same exercise; for he, too, seldom has any secret diagnostic weapons, and is equally hampered by the slowness of the available diagnostic tests. Attempts should be made to differentiate, on clinical grounds, those situations or syndromes that require immediate and intensive action from those that properly may be left to unfold until precise identification becomes possible. Moreover, when a choice of therapy is made, it should be made on the basis of careful consideration of the most serious threats to the patient that are likely. The drug or drugs chosen should be the ones that do most to protect the patient overnight or for a somewhat longer interval against the reasonably likely threats, while at the same time do the least to mask the identity of other infections that might conceivably be present. Above all, once the identity of the infecting microbe *is* established, the physician should be quick to discontinue all but the scientifically relevant therapy.

An example of the exercise involved is as follows:

A young man was first seen with a high fever, a cough, and obviously excruciating pleural pain. His systolic blood pressure was 90 mm of mercury; his leukocyte count was 4000 per cubic millimeter, with a marked increase in immature neutrophils. Less than four hours previously, he had been enjoying himself at the theater, although he had had a mild respiratory infection for the preceding five or six days.

It was apparent that he had an infection, that it was progressing rapidly, and that it involved lung and pleura. What reasonable inferences could be drawn concerning the identity of the infection and hence both its relative threat to him and the appropriate choice of therapy?

At least four microbial species, pneumococcus, *Streptococcus*, *S. aureus*, and *Klebsiella* (Friedländer's bacillus), are capable of producing this particular situation, and faced with the individual case there is absolutely no way of differentiating one from another at the bedside. Nevertheless, the clinician knows that this syndrome occurs in such a severe fulminating form in less than 5 per cent of pneumococcal pneumonias, whereas such severity is the characteristic picture of the rapidly necrotizing pneumonias caused by staphylococci, klebsiellae, or, in some instances, streptococci. He also knows that primary staphylococcal pneumonia is extremely rare in the absence of viral influenza, but that as a complication of viral influenza it is by no means uncommon. Here his day-to-day "community epidemiologic knowledge" can stand him in good stead, for he should know whether viral influenza "is around" or has not been seen for some time; in this case, it has been "around." He likewise has discovered that his patient is a medical student, and he knows that staphylococci acquired from hospitalized patients are even more apt to be penicillinase producers than in the world at large, where, to be sure, they are by no means uncommon. He knows that primary streptococcal pneumonia of this severe type is a rarer phenomenon than primary staphylococcal pneumonia except in the middle of an outbreak of viral influenza. By contrast, *Klebsiella* pneumonia, although a not unlikely possibility in such a severe pneumonia syndrome, characteristically occurs in middle-aged weakened hosts and would be a most unlikely happening in an otherwise healthy young man.

In this situation as described, the amount of immediately useful knowledge that was produced is considerable. Armed with this knowledge, the physician who knows that he must start drug therapy right away actually has a pretty good idea of the nature of the problem. Indeed, the assembled information made it seem most likely that the patient had a primary staphylococcal pneumonia. Be that as it may, the physician knows the drug regimen he chooses must provide maximal protection against pneumococcus and *Streptococcus* (penicillin); maximal protection against *Klebsiella* (an aminoglycoside such as gentamicin or streptomycin); and maximal protection against *Staphylococcus*, including penicillinase producers (methicillin or a similar drug, along with gentamicin or streptomycin). Eighteen to 24 hours later when the identity of the infection presumably would become known, the therapy could be modified appropriately. It so happened that the cause of the illness was discovered to be a penicillinase-producing strain of *S. aureus* which was well controlled by the therapy. It should be stressed that once the microbe is identified, the physician's responsibility to modify the therapy is great. Almost invariably the patient has been receiving one or more drugs that are now known to be unnecessary, and the risks of their toxicities should be terminated promptly.

The body of knowledge from which selectivity of the sort described can be obtained is presented in the various chapters on bacterial and mycotic diseases and in Ch. 41. There are other sorts of knowledge also necessary to the clinician — knowledge about antimicrobial therapy and the drugs themselves (see Ch. 190) and information about some of the microbial mechanisms whereby the impact of drug therapy could be withstood and the microbe survive. One form of survival, viewing the microbial world as a whole, is the "new diseases" that emerge as *endogenous microbial diseases*, so-called nosocomial infections (see Ch. 124). These "new diseases" are a form of microbial survival of drug challenge, because they ensure that *some* mi-

crobes will endure. To ensure the survival of a particular microbial species and hence a particular disease, however, there are two other and quite different survival patterns, *microbial persistence* and *microbial drug resistance*. The latter phenomenon, under the name "drug-fastness," has been recognized since the early days of this century. Microbial persistence, on the other hand, was not recognized — indeed could not be recognized — until the development of penicillin, because it was only then that a powerful antimicrobial drug could be given in virtually any dosage and thus permit exclusion of the obvious possibility that the microbial survival was only a consequence of underdosage.

MICROBIAL PERSISTENCE. Microbial persistence can be defined as the phenomenon whereby a microbial strain that is susceptible to a drug in the test tube is nevertheless capable of surviving long-term exposure to that drug in the body. Persistence is thus sharply distinguished from drug resistance, which is a heritable property of a microbial strain and is demonstrable in the test tube as well as in the body. In numerical terms, microbial persistence is of the greater importance, because it is the phenomenon that is responsible for most instances of post-treatment relapse, that interferes with the effectiveness of chemoprophylaxis, and that balks attempts to use drugs for the "eradication" of microbes (see Ch. 190). Once recognized and studied, it became clear that microbial persistence — the drug-related phenomenon — was only one aspect of the larger phenomenon of latent microbial infection with its potentiality for evocation as endogenous microbial disease. As our knowledge accumulates, it is likewise beginning to appear that microbial persistence and genotypic drug resistance are veering toward each other, and may eventually come to overlap. Persistence thus serves as a link between the other two phenomena, and indeed all three may ultimately be seen to shade into each other. However, we are not yet at that point. Recognition of the present clearly visible difference among the three has been most valuable in that it has made it possible for each to be recognized, reasonably well defined, and isolated for study. For more detailed consideration of these phenomena, the reader is referred to the references at the end of this chapter. Certain aspects of microbial persistence and heritable drug resistance deserve mention at this point.

Until microbial persistence was recognized in the 1940's, the conceptual base of antimicrobial therapy was *therapia sterilisans magna* as originally conceived by Ehrlich; namely, the goal was to effect a total eradication of the infecting microbes from the host. With penicillin and the subsequently introduced drugs, it was discovered that such total eradication did not occur uniformly and predictably. In a significant number of cases of virtually any bacterial disease, drug-susceptible cells of the infecting strain could be isolated well after completion of drug therapy. At times these persisters would increase and produce clinical relapse, which was then easily treatable by the appropriate drug. At other times they would persist in the carrier state or might ultimately disappear either into latency or presumably by leaving the host altogether. Evidence was obtained that this microbial survival could not be explained by failure of drug delivery, namely, that the microbes were located in some sanctuary such as a body compartment or the center of a necrotic area where they could not be reached by the molecules of drug in the extracellular fluid; nor could the phenomoneon be explained on the basis that the drug molecules were deviated from making contact with the microbes because the inflammatory-necrotic lesion either chemically degraded the drug or wholly bound it in some way. On the contrary, convincing evidence exists that the capacity to persist is a nonheritable property of a minority of the microbial population, and it is mediated by the ability to assume a metabolic state that has been termed "drug indifference" or "physiologic" spore formation. To what extent bacterial pleomorphism, including such forms as protoplasts, plays a role in persistence is not known. Another phenomenon of penicillin survival demonstrated in vitro has been designated *tolerance* (Sabath et al.). This may represent a fifth form of drug resistance (see below); an aspect of persistence; or, most likely, another phenomenon linking the two together. Whatever may be the mechanism or mechanisms of microbial persistence, it is also clear that even though an infecting microbial population may be wholly drug susceptible in the conventional sense, actual therapy with that drug will not be uniformly or predictably *eradicative*. This is the case irrespective of whether the drug is classified as "bacteriostatic" or "bactericidal." It is this capacity of drug-susceptible bacteria to survive and outlast periods of drug administration that is responsible for most clinical relapse, failures to eliminate the carrier state, and certain failures of chemoprophylaxis. It is not generally known that Ehrlich in his late years came to perceive that *magna sterilisans* conceived as eradication was untenable. He then subtly changed the *concept* of the "sterilisans" without changing the *word*, and offered the idea that the bacteria in the tissues were in effect rendered sterile, i.e., incapable of having progeny. In the last analysis all that is added to this "latter-day Ehrlich" by the present concept of microbial persistence is the point that the sterile state is reversible.

DRUG RESISTANCE. Strictly speaking, any microbial strain that is unaffected by appropriate concentrations of a drug in vitro could be called drug resistant. In actual practice, however, the designation is reserved for the drug-resistant representatives of bacterial species that are customarily susceptible to the drug in question. *Primary resistance* refers to situations in which the infecting bacterial strain is already drug resistant at the time it initiates the infection. *Emergent resistance* refers to the emergence to predominance of a drug-resistant population during the treatment of a microbial disease that was drug susceptible when treatment was started.

All drug-susceptible bacterial species possess the capability to show emergent resistance—that is to say, to escape during therapy — to *some* drug or drugs. But *all drugs* are not associated with emergent resistance. Specifically, no instance of emergent resistance to penicillin has been observed,* and all penicillin resistance is primary. Whether drug resistance can emerge or not thus *depends not so much on the bacterial species as on the drug*. This clearly indicates that there exists a phenomenon of drug action on a microbe wherein the emergence to predominance of drug-resistant forms is a great rarity. The existence of such a phenomenon in drug action is of obvious importance in considerations

of the possible mechanisms involved in multiple drug regimens, as discussed below. Although still important, this distinction between primary and emergent resistance is diminished by virtue of the relatively abrupt appearance of pneumococci highly resistant to penicillin among patients and staff of an inpatient pediatric service in South Africa (see Ch. 121). The speed with which this situation became evident created a problem not too far removed from that facing the physician when a patient's disease responding well to antimicrobial therapy "escapes" because of emergent resistance. The issue really comes down to the precise nature of the change in the pneumococcal cell. If it is a process that can occur speedily, as with pneumococci and sulfonamide, emergent resistance presumably will occur, and the physician will have to be alert for the occurrence of either form of penicillin resistance in his patients with pneumococcal pneumonia. Conceivably, with another type of process, only primary resistance has to be feared; whether it is likely to be present or would constitute a great rarity is a judgment in which the physician would be guided by his up-to-the-minute knowledge of "community epidemiology."

Four Different Forms of Drug Resistance. The pluralistic nature of this broad phenomenon called "drug resistance" can readily be seen by examining different drugs or drug-microbe pairings. At least four distinct forms are identifiable. There is the *sulfonamide-streptomycin form,* in which the resistant bacteria maintain full pathogenic potential and are otherwise altered little, if at all, except for their loss of susceptibility to the drug. There is the *major isoniazid form,* in which certain enzymes have been lost (catalase and peroxidase), and the pathogenicity for laboratory animals, including primates, has been significantly reduced. (There is another, much less frequently encountered form of isoniazid resistance in which full pathogenicity is maintained.) There is a form characterized by *episomal or plasmid transfer,* exemplified by enteric bacteria but also by staphylococci. There is also a form seen most clearly with penicillin and staphylococci in which the critical element in producing the resistance is the *presence of a beta-lactamase,* so-called penicillinase. In some strains of staphylococci the enzyme is inducible; in other strains and species it can be constitutive. Combinations of these various forms of phenomena occur. For example, some strains of isoniazid-resistant tubercle bacilli are of the sulfonamide-streptomycin form, although these are rare; the genetic capability of staphylococci to elaborate penicillinase can be passed from one cell to another by episomal transfer, and the actual enzymatic process of synthesizing penicillinase is induced by exposure to the substrate penicillin.

Episomal transfer is an example of nonchromosomal inheritance, for bacteria not only have chromosomal genes but also have what are in effect free-floating genes that can pass from one cell to another as if they were a virus. The particles are of two sorts: *the episomes* and *the plasmid*. The difference between them is that the plasmid does not attach itself to the chromosome at any time, whereas the episome can either exist freely in the cytoplasm or at times attach itself to the chromosome. Synergism between an episomal gene and a chromosomal gene can occur. In one such experiment, two genes, one present in the episomal factor and the other in the chromosomal, each of which singly conferred resistance to streptomycin concentrations of 25 mg per

---

*The penicillin-resistant pneumococci reported from Australia (Hausman et al., 1971) were not isolated in a situation of *emergent* resistance. This also appears to have been the case with the strains isolated by Tempest et al. (1974) at the Navajo Medical Center.

milliliter, *cooperated* to yield organisms to 1000 mg per milliliter. It is believed that the synergism was acquired as a direct result of genetic recombination between the chromosome and the episomal factor. The "infection" of the strain of *E. coli* in the form of the episomal factor could be removed by treatment with an acridine dye — in effect, a form of drug therapy in vitro. The last-named observation is of considerable theoretic significance when one attempts to analyze the ways in which two-drug therapy can be more effective than the more powerful drug used alone.

Aid to the Clinician. In what way is the clinician benefited by acquaintance with this expanding body of knowledge on the multiple forms of what can only loosely be called "drug resistance"? The principal gain—and it is by no means a minor one—is that he is able to perceive that *the results of testing a microbial strain for drug susceptibility in vitro represent only one bit of information, and one that is not always relevant to the therapeutic problem presented by his patient.* The identity of the microbial species, its probable source, e.g., whether acquired in hospital or acquired from a drug-treated household contact, and the *history* of drugs received earlier in the illness and their observed effects usually represent a body of evidence of greater reliability and predictive value than drug-susceptibility tests as they are frequently performed. For example, the highly successful streptomycin-penicillin treatment of enterococcal endocarditis would never have been instituted had the results of the streptomycin-susceptibility tests been the controlling factor. Likewise, a patient's pulmonary tuberculosis may respond well to isoniazid despite isoniazid resistance of the patient's strain when subjected to conventional drug-susceptibility tests. But this is not always the case, which merely reflects that there is obviously more than one form of isoniazid resistance. What is clear is that the clinician should be very wary of abandoning a particular drug therapy that appears to be working satisfactorily and introducing a substitute *solely* on the basis of drug-susceptibility tests. Like many laboratory procedures, drug-susceptibility tests have a place, but their results should seldom be the sole factor in determining the choice of therapy.

DRUG PAIRINGS. Consideration of the mechanisms of drug resistance leads to scrutiny of the use of two antimicrobial drugs together. One of the avowed goals of such multidrug therapy is to postpone or prevent drug resistance of the emergent type; the other is to obtain greater antimicrobial effectiveness per unit of time. Conceivably the same process could be responsible for both effects, although this is not the customary way of looking at the matter. With respect to drug resistance, the orthodox explanation dates from Ehrlich's day and is based on the notion that emergent resistance is prevented or postponed because drug A is effective against those bacterial mutants that are resistant to drug B, and vice versa. By this concept it would be possible for a two-drug regimen to affect emergent resistance without exerting an enhanced antimicrobial effectiveness per unit of time. The enhanced effectiveness phenomenon, which is seen, for example, in the penicillin-streptomycin treatment of enterococcal endocarditis, presumably would have to be explained on some other basis. The issue here is not whether, in appropriate circumstances, two-drug therapy can affect emergent resistance or increase total antimicrobial effectiveness.

The question is *how* these phenomena are brought about. If the combined drug action is exerted independently, with drug A acting on cells resistant to drug B, virtually any two-drug regimen would be expected to be effective. Contrariwise, if the respective drug actions are dependent, it would presumably represent a highly specialized phenomenon. To settle this issue would thus be a matter of considerable practical importance. Unfortunately, a reasonably complete and authoritative answer cannot be given at this time.

It can be said from the relatively few sets of observations available (see McCune et al.) that enhancement of antimicrobial effectiveness by concurrent administration of two drugs appears to be a *dependent* phenomenon, *with both drugs generally acting on the same microbial cell.* The phenomenon seems to have considerable specificity in terms of drugs and microbial species involved; hence superior drug pairings are relatively rare, and are not to be expected with just any pairing and any drug-susceptible parasite. Whether the "dependent" mechanism is also the major way by which two-drug regimens influence emergent resistance is less clear. In the writer's judgment, there is considerable reason to believe that this is indeed the case and that *when a drug pairing does exert an influence on emergent resistance, it does so by the action of both drugs on the microbes susceptible to both drugs.* Hence in large measure the action would consist of both drugs acting on the same microbial cell. As in the situation with enhancement, such effective drug pairings would represent highly specialized sets of circumstances.

The indication that drug pairings superior to the more powerful drug alone are special affairs is in agreement with the rarity with which multiple drug regimens are of demonstrated value in clinical medicine. Indeed to all intents and purposes, the examples are largely limited to infections with enterococci, tubercle bacilli, and viridans streptococci. Conceivably it might be possible to add *Pseudomonas aeruginosa* infections and the drug pairing of gentamicin and carbenicillin to the list. The problem here, as in general, is that most microbial infections do not produce *human disease* in a form that lends itself to comparative measurements of drug effectiveness, even when it is ethically permissible to do so. It is important for the physician to keep reminding himself therefore that, except for these few microbial diseases, the solid justification for the use of more than one antimicrobial drug at a time is largely limited to situations in which an etiologic diagnosis has not yet (or never) been established. Usually, as discussed above, this occurs only during the early hours of treatment, and the physician should be quick to change to single drug therapy as the situation is clarified.

NEED FOR SELECTIVITY. The day has gone by when the physician could prescribe all two or three of the available antimicrobial drugs to an acutely febrile patient and relax with the comforting thought that all that modern science could do was being done. With today's multiplicity of drugs, the emergence of "new" microbial diseases, and our considerably expanded knowledge about mechanisms of microbial survival, the physician must be highly selective in his drug choices, and hence must have mastery of a considerably greater body of clinical and laboratory-derived knowledge than was needed even a few decades ago. The physician's "comforting thought" today is of quite a different sort. It consists of the knowledge that, however difficult modern science is making things for *him* in the management of infections, it is making things ever so much better for his patients.

Applebaum, P. C., et al.: *Streptococcus pneumoniae* responding to penicillin and chloramphenicol. Lancet, 2:995, 1977.

Blazevic, D. J., et al.: Penicillin-resistant *Streptococcus pneumoniae*–Minnesota. MMWR, 26: October 21, 1977.

Davis, B. D., Dulbecco, R., Eisen, H. N., Ginsberg, H. S., Wood, W. B., Jr., and McCarty, M. (eds.): Microbiology. 2nd ed. New York, Harper & Row, 1973.

Dubos, R. J.: Man Adapting. New Haven, Yale University Press, 1965.

McCune, R. M., Feldman, F. M., and McDermott, W.: Microbial persistence. II. Characteristics of the sterile state of tubercle bacilli. J. Exp. Med., 123:469, 1966.

McDermott, W.: Microbial Persistence. Harvey Lecture Series No. 63, 1969, pp. 1–31.

McDermott, W.: Microbial drug resistance. Barnwell Lecture. Am. Rev. Respir. Dis., 102:855, 1970.

Sabath, L. D., et al.: A new type of penicillin resistance of *Staphylococcus aureus*. Lancet, 1:443, 1977.

190. ANTIMICROBIAL THERAPY

Richard B. Roberts

The announcement of the first sulfonamide in 1935 ushered in the modern era of antimicrobial therapy, an era characterized by the dramatic reduction in incidence, morbidity, and mortality of many infectious diseases. The most outstanding examples include the reduction in disease incidence or death caused by pneumococcal pneumonia, microbial endocarditis, tuberculosis, and syphilis. The impact by this class of agents on medical, public health, and economic factors related to disease states has been unparalleled in the history of drug therapy.

The abuse of these therapeutic agents, however, is alarming. In the United States, production of antimicrobial agents and the use of these drugs by physicians has steadily increased in the past two decades. Antimicrobial agents are a commonly prescribed medication in office practice (about 15 per cent of all drugs), and approximately one third of hospitalized patients receive such drugs. Surveys have suggested that two thirds of these patients receive the incorrect agent or an inappropriate dose. Indiscriminate use of these drugs may be accompanied by such complications as adverse reactions (allergic or dose related), superinfection, emergence of resistant organisms, and delay in identifying the causative organism.

Since many clinical situations dictate that antimicrobial therapy be instituted prior to identification of the specific etiologic microbe, intelligent use of these drugs requires a thorough knowledge of the suspected infectious process as well as of the changing patterns of microbial resistance. (see Ch. 189). In addition, an understanding of the physical and chemical properties of antimicrobial agents is important, because these properties determine adequate drug levels and toxicity, depending on absorption, distribution, and excretion of these drugs.

SELECTION OF ANTIMICROBIAL AGENTS

Host Determinants

AGE AND WEIGHT. The dose of an antimicrobial drug is usually calculated on the basis of body weight and, less commonly, body surface (Table 1). The route of administration, dosage, and the incidence of adverse reactions may also vary, depending on the age of the patient. For example, in the neonate and aged patient, renal function may be compromised, and the dosage of drugs excreted by the kidney should be adjusted accordingly. *Tetracycline* should not be used in pregnant women, infants, or young children, because this drug may cause enamel hypoplasia, tooth discoloration, and disturbance in bone growth. *Sulfonamides* should not be given to newborns because of possible elevated serum levels owing to abnormalities in acetylation or kernicterus owing to displacement of bilirubin from serum albumin. Similarly, the liver of premature and newborn babies produces only small amounts of glucuronyl transferase, the enzyme necessary to inactivate *chloramphenicol*. High levels of the biologically active drug may cause the "gray baby syndrome," characterized by abdominal distention, progressive pallor and cyanosis, vasomotor collapse, and death.

SITE OF INFECTION. The anatomic location of an infectious process often determines the choice of the antimicrobial and the route of its administration. Clinical studies have shown that adequate levels of most antimicrobial agents except the polymyxins are achieved in inflamed joints, making intra-articular instillation unnecessary. Antimicrobial drugs also penetrate inflamed pleura. Aminoglycosides should not be instilled into a body cavity (i.e., pleural or peritoneal), because neuromuscular blockade and respiratory paralysis may occur. Adequate drainage in addition to effective drug levels in the blood is necessary in infections associated with obstruction in the respiratory, biliary, or urinary tracts. Adequate levels of an antimicrobial agent in the cerebrospinal fluid are determined in part by the pharmacologic properties of the drug and meningeal inflammation. The penicillins, because of their low toxicity, can be given in sufficient dosage parenterally to achieve adequate levels in the cerebrospinal fluid. Chloramphenicol and sulfonamides cross the blood-brain barrier and are effective in bacterial meningitis. However, therapeutic levels of cephalothin and clindamycin in the cerebrospinal fluid are not achieved in the presence of normal or inflamed meninges, and these drugs should not be used in bacterial meningitis. Gentamicin and polymyxin B cross the blood-brain barrier poorly and should be given intrathecally as well as parenterally to patients with gram-negative bacillary meningitis.

UNDERLYING DISEASE. Serious and life-threatening infections in the compromised host present as one of the most difficult diagnostic and therapeutic challenges in medicine. A variety of microbes, including bacteria, viruses, fungi, and protozoa, infect patients who have malignant disorders or who receive immunosuppressive and cytotoxic therapy for cancer, rheumatic diseases, and renal transplantation. These patients often require antimicrobial therapy before the etiologic agent or agents are identified. Since infections in the compromised host are usually severe and are caused by a number of diverse microorganisms, an aggressive diagnostic approach, often culminating in invasive biopsy procedures, may be necessary. Initial antibacterial therapy should include a penicillinase-resistant penicillin or a cephalosporin and gentamicin. Carbenicillin is added if the clinical or laboratory findings are consistent with *Pseudomonas* bacteremia. Clindamycin should be given if anaerobic organisms, especially *Bacteroides fragilis*, are suspected. These drugs should be given in maximal doses parenterally. If the initial bacterial cultures are negative after three to five days, the patient should be re-evaluated. If diagnostic studies are negative, the drug therapy should be discontinued, because superinfection with resistant gram-negative bacilli and fungi may occur. Even with appropriate therapy, clinical response may be delayed and may ultimately depend on remission of the underlying disease or reduction of immunosuppressive therapy.

Function of the liver and kidneys may be affected by many underlying diseases. Since these are the major excretory organs for antimicrobial drugs, either many antimicrobial drugs should not be used or their dosage should be modified in the face of compromised hepatic or renal function. These precautions are discussed subsequently under the heading Excretion.

GENETIC FACTORS. The genetic background of patients may play a determinant part in the use of some antimicrobial agents. Although there may be other examples as yet unrecognized, the following known phenomena are important in determining, in part, the response to therapy as well as the risk of adverse reactions.

The rate at which isoniazid and sulfapyridine are conjugated and biologically inactivated in the liver is genetically determined. These drugs are inactivated in the liver by acetylation. Studies have shown that certain groups of patients receiving a sulfonamide or isoniazid acetylate the drug rapidly and others slowly. The rate of acetylation determines the concentration and duration of biologically active drug in the serum. Although sulfapyridine is not commonly used, salicylazosulfapyridine, which is often administered to patients with mild ulcerative colitis, is metabolized by the microbial flora of the colon to sulfapyridine and 5-aminosalicylic acid. The former metabolite is rapidly absorbed into the systemic circulation and is responsible for the adverse reactions that accompany the use of salicylazosulfapyridine.

Acute hemolytic anemia is associated with the administration of certain antimicrobial agents in patients with glucose-6-phosphate dehydrogenase deficiency. This enzyme abnormality is transmitted as a sex-linked partially dominant characteristic with full expression in homozygous males. Affected females are usually heterozygous. The antimicrobial agents that may precipitate acute hemolysis in these patients are chloramphenicol, niridazole, nitrofurantoin, primaquine, and sulfonamides. Sulfonamides may also be responsible for acute hemolysis in patients with certain hemoglobinopathies.

DRUG SUSCEPTIBILITY. One of the most important determinants in the selection of an antimicrobial agent is the susceptibility of the causative organism. It is imperative that appropriate stains and cultures of blood, secretions, cavity fluids, and the like be obtained prior to the institution of antimicrobial therapy. Once the organism has been isolated, drug-susceptibility determinations may be performed by either one of two methods: the disc (agar) diffusion technique, or the tube (broth) or plate (agar) dilution technique. The former method is routinely used in most clinical laboratories. Because of the many factors which may influence drug-susceptibility determinations, standardization of this method must take into account the growth of the organism, the inoculum size, the type and quantity of media employed, the size and concentration of drug-

impregnated discs, and the duration and environmental conditions of incubation. If these conditions are adhered to, the diameter of the area of growth inhibition about the impregnated disc distinguishes resistant from susceptible strains. In addition, precautions concerning specific bacteria or drugs must also be taken into consideration. Resistance of *Staphylococcus aureus* to methicillin is reliable only if the zones are measured within 20 hours of incubation, because methicillin deteriorates rapidly at incubating temperatures. Fastidious and slow-growing organisms such as *Bacteroides* and certain streptococci may not produce visible colonies within 24 hours, and reports of susceptibility may not be reliable. Disc susceptibility tests performed in anaerobic jars may give misleading results. Colistin and polymyxin B diffuse poorly in agar, and the drug-susceptibility results may be inaccurate. The standarized disc test is not recommended for gonococci or for *Mycobacterium tuberculosis*.

In certain clinical settings, namely patients with endocarditis and osteomyelitis, a more precise method for determining the susceptibility of an organism may be indicated. The *dilution method* — that is, twofold dilutions of the drug in broth or agar containing a standardized inoculum of the infecting organism — is the technique commonly employed in many laboratories. Results are expressed as the minimal inhibitory concentration, or MIC, which is the smallest amount of drug that will inhibit growth after 18 to 24 hours of incubation.

The serum antibacterial activity may also be determined. At a specified time after the drug is given (usually one hour after parenteral administration), serum is collected and serially diluted in a medium inoculated with the organism. A serum dilution of 1:8 or greater that inhibits the growth of the test organism is indicative of an adequate blood level for serious and life-threatening infections. Accurate serum concentrations can be determined by impregnating discs with known concentrations of a drug and other discs with serum dilutions from the patient. These discs are placed on agar previously inoculated with the organism, and zones of growth inhibition are compared after incubation. More recently, radioimmunoassay procedures have been developed for determining the serum levels of certain aminoglycosides.

Knowledge of the drug-susceptibility patterns of bacteria is important for the intelligent use of antimicrobial agents. For example, despite the common use of penicillin G, group A streptococci, pneumococci, and meningococci have remained generally susceptible to it. Methicillin-resistant *Staphylococcus aureus* strains, however, have been reported especially from Denmark and less commonly from England and the United States. These strains are also resistant to the cephalosporins. Patterns of susceptibility and resistance of gram-negative bacilli vary from hospital to hospital as well as temporally within the same institution. This phenomenon is principally due to the widespread use of antimicrobial agents active against gram-negative bacilli and the development of emergent resistance. Because of the changing patterns of susceptibility and resistance of bacteria, continuous laboratory surveillance of the incidence and susceptibility of isolates by hospital epidemiologists and clinical laboratories is extremely important. The antimicrobial susceptibilities of various microbes are discussed later in this chapter.

BACTERICIDAL AND BACTERIOSTATIC DRUGS. Bactericidal agents are drugs that kill organisms at or near the minimal inhibitory concentration. Examples of bactericidal agents include the penicillins, cephalosporins, vancomycin, aminoglycosides, and polymyxins. In general, patients with severe infections should receive bactericidal drugs. This is especially true in patients with abnormal host defense mechanisms involving antibody function, phagocyte function, or cellular immunity. Bacteriostatic drugs inhibit the growth of organisms and include erythromycin, lincomycin, clindamycin, chloramphenicol, tetracycline, and the sulfonamides. Erythromycin, lincomycin, and clindamycin may have bactericidal activity at high concentrations against certain organisms. An intact immunologic system is an important determinant in the response of patients receiving bacteriostatic drugs. In many clinical situations, such as upper respiratory tract infections, anaerobic infections, and uncomplicated urinary tract infections, bacteriostatic drugs are as effective clinically as bactericidal agents.

COMBINATION THERAPY. The administration of more than one antimicrobial agent at the same time is indicated for (1) initial therapy in a critically ill patient when the causative organism is not known, (2) polymicrobial infection in which the organisms are not susceptible to one antimicrobial agent, (3) reducing or postponing the emergence of resistance to one or both agents, such as in the therapy for tuberculosis, and (4) synergism. Synergism is best exemplified by the penicillins, the cephalosporins, vancomycin, and the aminoglycosides. In vitro studies suggest that this enhanced antimicrobial effect by bactericidal agents may be due to the inhibition of cell wall synthesis by the penicillins or vancomycin resulting in increased permeability and penetration of the aminoglycosides. The combination of penicillin or vancomycin with streptomycin or gentamicin should be used in patients with enterococcal endocarditis. Limited clinical studies suggest that carbenicillin and an aminoglycoside may be more effective than either drug alone in severe *Pseudomonas aeruginosa* infections. (For additional discussion of multiple drug therapy, see Ch. 189.)

Antagonism between two antimicrobial agents can be demonstrated in vitro. Since bactericidal drugs such as penicillin inhibit cell wall synthesis or rapidly multiplying bacteria, the simultaneous use of a bacteriostatic drug may interfere with bactericidal activity. It is uncommon, however, to detect adverse effects clinically with combined bactericidal and bacteriostatic therapy.

Absorption and Distribution

Pharmacologic properties differ markedly between classes of antimicrobial agents and between agents within the same class. Knowledge of these properties is important for the intelligent use of these drugs. Antimicrobial drugs may be administered by various routes, including topical, oral, and parenteral (intramuscular and intravenous). *Topical administration* should be restricted to special circumstances whenever possible because of possible absorption into the systemic circulation, allergic reactions, and the development of microbial resistance. Examples of appropriate local administration include severe burns, intravenous catheter sites, and purulent conjunctivitis. The *oral route* is used chiefly in initial therapy for mild to mod-

erately severe infections and for the completion of therapy in patients with severe infections. Because of the variable absorption of antimicrobial agents in the presence of gastric acidity, oral medications should be given in the fasting state, i.e., 1 to 2 hours before or after meals. *Parenteral administration* of antimicrobial drugs is indicated for severe infections that require high and sustained blood levels. Many drugs cannot be administered intramuscularly because of severe pain. These include cephalothin, vancomycin, erythromycin, chloramphenicol, and tetracycline. *Intravenous administration* is indicated in patients with severe infections or hypotension, or when appropriate levels cannot be achieved by the intramuscular route. Intravenous appliances must be changed every 24 to 48 hours to avoid thrombophlebitis and local infection with or without bacteremia. In general, medications should be diluted in 50 to 100 ml of solution and allowed to run in over a period of 15 to 30 minutes. Adverse reactions, especially associated with the aminoglycosides and polymyxins, may occur with rapid intravenous administration. Intrathecal and intra-articular therapy may be necessary in gram-negative infections. Complications associated with intrathecal administration include arachnoiditis with severe pain, paresthesias, and transient to permanent paralysis. The intrapleural or intraperitoneal administration of antimicrobial drugs is not recommended.

The distribution of a drug is a complex phenomenon and depends on many factors, including (1) molecular size, (2) electrical charge at pH 7.4, (3) lipid solubility, (4) plasma protein binding, and (5) presence of inflammation. If adequate blood levels are present, most antimicrobial agents will enter infected synovial and serous fluids. However, even in the presence of inflamed meninges, therapeutic levels of cephalothin, clindamycin, polymyxin, or gentamicin may not be achieved.

Excretion

The liver and the kidneys are the two principal excretory organs for antimicrobial agents. Renal clearance, by either glomerular filtration or tubular secretion, or both, is a major determinant of serum levels. Probenecid increases and prolongs the serum level of those antimicrobials excreted by tubular secretion (i.e., the penicillins and cephalosporins). Repeated evaluation of hepatic and renal function must be performed when antimicrobial agents are given in high doses for a prolonged period of time. Ampicillin, nafcillin, erythromycin, tetracycline, chloramphenicol, lincomycin, clindamycin, and novobiocin should be used with caution in patients with liver disease. In the face of impaired renal function, the following agents should be administered with caution, and the dosage reduced accordingly: amphotericin B, cephaloridine, colistimethate, flucytosine, methenamine mandelate, neomycin, nitrofurantoin, penicillins, polymyxin B, the aminoglycosides, sulfonamides, tetracycline, and vancomycin. Many of these agents not only are excreted largely by the kidney but also are nephrotoxic. Although the initial loading dose is the same, subsequent doses are reduced or the duration between doses is prolonged. Formulas for drug dose and interval between doses have been derived based on renal function, i.e., serum creatinine or creatinine clearance. These guidelines are useful but cannot be relied upon alone. Adjustments are best guided by repeated determinations of the serum concentration of the drug. In addition, knowledge of the dialyzability of antimicrobial agents with hemodialysis and peritoneal dialysis is necessary for the management of patients with acute and chronic renal failure.

Adverse Reactions

The administration of antimicrobial agents may be associated with toxic or allergic reactions. Adverse reactions are widely variable, as shown by the following examples: (1) local irritation at the site of administration; (2) hypersensitivity reactions; (3) dose-related hepatic, renal, and bone marrow toxicity; and (4) adverse reactions caused by the composition of the drug preparation (i.e., hyperkalemia with potassium penicillin G, fluid retention with disodium carbenicllin). The adverse reactions associated with specific antimicrobial agents are discussed below.

SPECIFIC ANTIMICROBIAL AGENTS

Antimicrobial agents may be classified as to their chemical structure, mechanism of action, antimicrobial spectrum of activity, and bactericidal versus bacteriostatic properties. Table 1 lists the common antibacterial agents with their route of administration, dosage, and mechanism of action. More detailed descriptions of the indications of each drug are included in the chapters dealing with specific organisms or infectious diseases.

TABLE 1. Antimicrobial Agents for Bacterial, Fungal, and Viral Infections

	Adult Daily Dosage (Time Interval of Divided Doses)	Route	Mechanism of Action
Adenine arabinoside		Local	Inhibition of nucleoprotein synthesis
Amantadine hydrochloride	200 mg/day	PO	Unknown
Amikacin	15 mg/kg/day (q. 8–12 hours)	IM, IV	Inhibition of protein synthesis (30S ribosomal binding)
Aminosalicylic acid	12 grams/day (t.i.d.)	PO	Replacement of para-aminobenzoic acid
Amphotericin B	1.0 mg/kg/day or every other day (total dose: 2–3 grams) or 15–50 mg/day × 10 weeks	IV	Interaction with sterols of cell membrane
Bacitracin	t.i.d.	Local	Inhibition of cell wall synthesis
Capreomycin	1 gram/day	IM	Unknown
Cephalosporins			Inhibition of cell wall synthesis
Cephalothin	4–12 grams/day (q. 4–6 hours)	IV	
Cephapirin	4–12 grams/day (q. 4–6 hours)	IM, IV	
Cephaloridine	2–4 grams/day (q. 6 hours)	IM	
Cefazolin	2–6 grams/day (q. 6–8 hours)	IM, IV	
Cephradine	2–6 grams/day (q. 4–6 hours) 1–2 grams/day (q.i.d.)	IM, IV, PO	Inhibition of cell wall synthesis
Cephalexin	1–4 grams/day (q.i.d.)	PO	
Chloramphenicol	2–4 grams/day (q. 6 hours) 1–2 grams/day (q.i.d.)	IV PO	Inhibition of protein synthesis (50S ribosomal binding)
Clindamycin	0.6–4.5 grams/day (q. 6–8 hours) 0.4–1.2 grams/day (q.i.d.)	IM, IV PO	Inhibition of protein synthesis
Co-trimoxazole (trimethoprim-sulfamethoxazole)	4 tablets/day (q. 12 hours) (1 tablet = T80 mg/S400 mg)	PO	Sequential inhibition of folic acid reduction
Cycloserine	500–750 mg/day (q. 12 hours)	PO	Inhibition of cell wall synthesis
Cytarabine	10–100 mg/square meter/day	IV	Inhibition of nucleoprotein synthesis
Erythromycins			Inhibition of protein synthesis (50S ribosomal binding)
Erythromycin ethylsuccinate	1–4 grams/day (q. 6 hours) 400 mg/day (q. 6 hours)	PO IM	
Erythromycin stearate	1–4 grams/day (q. 6 hours)	PO	
Erythromycin gluceptate	1–4 grams/day (q. 6 hours)	IV	
Erythromycin lactobionate	1–4 grams/day (q. 6 hours)	IV	
Ethambutol	15 mg/kg/day	PO	Unknown
Ethionamide	500–750 mg/day (q. 12 hours)	PO	Unknown
Flucytosine	150 mg/kg/day × 6 weeks (q. 6 hours)	PO	Inhibition of nucleoprotein synthesis (competition with cytosine)
Gentamicin	3–6 mg/kg/day (q. 8 hours) 4–6 mg/day	IV, IM IT	Inhibition of protein synthesis (30S ribosomal binding)
Idoxuridine	100 mg/kg/day	IV Local	Inhibition of nucleoprotein synthesis (competition with thymidylic acid)
Isoniazid	300 mg/day	PO	Inhibition of enzymes requiring pyridoxal as cofactor
Kanamycin	15 mg/kg/day (q. 8–12 hours) 4–8 grams/day (q. 4–6 hours)	IV, IM PO	Inhibition of protein synthesis (30S ribosomal binding)
Lincomycin	2–8 grams/day (q. 6 hours) 0.6–2.4 grams/day (q. 6–12 hours) 2 grams/day (q.i.d.)	IV IM PO	Inhibition of protein synthesis (50S ribosomal binding)
Methenamine mandelate	4–12 grams/day (q.i.d.)	PO	Unknown
Methisazone	1.5 grams/day × 2 days	PO	Inhibition of nucleoprotein synthesis
Nalidixic acid	2–4 grams/day (q.i.d.)	PO	Unknown
Neomycin	4–8 grams/day (q. 6 hours) t.i.d.	PO Local	Inhibition of protein synthesis (30S ribosomal binding)
Nitrofurans			Unknown
Nitrofurantoin	5–10 mg/kg/day (q.i.d.)	PO	
Novobiocin	2–4 grams/day (q. 6 hours) 1–2 grams/day (q. 6 hours)	PO IV	Unknown

The antituberculous drugs (isoniazid, rifampin, strep-tomycin, para-aminosalicylic acid, pyrazinamide, cap-reomycin, cycloserine, ethambutol, ethionamide, and viomycin), the antiviral drugs (adenine arabinoside, amantadine hydrochloride, cytarabine, idoxuridine, and methisazone), and the antifungal agents (ampho-tericin B, flucytosine, and nystatin) are included in Table 1 and are discussed in detail in the chapters deal-ing with the respective diseases for which they are used. Table 2 lists the antiprotozoan and antimetazoan drugs with their clinical indications, dose, route of ad-ministration, and toxicity. The following antiparasitic drugs are not approved by the Food and Drug Admin-istration for general use in the United States: antimony sodium gluconate, bithional, melarsoprol, niclosamide, niridazole, pentamidine, and suramin. These agents, however, may be easily obtained for therapy of the in-dicated diseases by calling the Parasitic Diseases

Branch of the Center for Disease Control in Atlanta, Georgia, at 404–633–3311.

PENICILLINS.   Penicillinase-Sensitive Penicillins. The penicillins that are susceptible to penicillinase are penicillin G (benzyl penicillin), phenoxymethyl penicillin, amoxicillin, ampicillin, carbenicillin, and ti-carcillin. Penicillin G has three intramuscular forms which differ in the rate of absorption, thus affecting the concentration and duration of drug in serum. *Aqueous crystalline penicillin G* is well absorbed but is painful and is therefore usually given intravenously. *Procaine penicillin G* is well tolerated intramuscularly and is slowly absorbed so that injections are only necessary every six to twelve hours. *Benzathine penicillin G* is also given intramuscularly and is slowly released from the site of injection over three to four weeks. Procaine pen-icillin G and benzathine penicillin should not be admin-istered intravenously. Penicillin G is unstable in the

TABLE 1.   Antimicrobial Agents for Bacterial, Fungal, and Viral Infections *(Continued)*

	Adult Daily Dosage (Time Interval of Divided Doses)	Route	Mechanism of Action
Nystatin	1.5–3 million units (t.i.d.)	PO	Interaction with sterols of cell membrane
Penicillins, penicillinase-sensitive			Inhibition of cell wall synthesis
Aqueous crystalline penicillin G	0.6–20 million units/day (q. 2–6 hours)	IV, IM	
Procaine penicillin G	600,000–4.8 million units/day (q. 6–12 hours)	IM	
Benzathine penicillin G	600,000–2.4 million units (q. 4 weeks)	IM	
Phenoxymethyl penicillin	1–4 grams/day (q.i.d.)	PO	
Penicillins with gram-negative bacillary activity			Inhibition of cell wall synthesis
Amoxicillin	0.75–1.5 grams/day (q. 8 hours)	PO	
Ampicillin	4–12 grams/day (q. 4–6 hours)	IV, IM	
	1–4 grams/day (q. 6 hours)	PO	
Carbenicillin	4–35 grams/day (q. 4 hours)	IV, IM	
	2–4 grams/day (q.i.d.)	PO	
Ticarcillin	4–20 grams/day (q. 4 hours)	IV, IM	
Penicillins, penicillinase-resistant			Inhibition of cell wall synthesis
Cloxacillin	2–4 grams/day (q. 6 hours)	PO	
Dicloxacillin	1–2 grams/day (q. 6 hours)	PO	
Methicillin	6–12 grams/day (q. 4–6 hours)	IV, IM	
Nafcillin	4–8 grams/day (q. 4–6 hours)	IV, IM	
Oxacillin	4–8 grams/day (q. 6 hours)	IV, IM	
	2–4 grams/day (q. 4–6 hours)	PO	
Polymyxins			Disruption of cell wall–membrane complex
Polymyxin B	2.5 mg/kg/day (q. 8 hours)	IV, IM	
	5.0 mg/day	IT	
Polymyxin E			
Colistimethate sodium	5.0 mg/kg/day (q. 6 hours)	IV, IM	
Colistin sulfate	5.0 mg/kg/day (q. 6 hours)	PO	
Pyrazinamide	25 to 30 mg/kg/day in 3 or 4 divided doses	PO	Unknown
Rifampin	600 mg/day	PO	Inhibition of DNA-dependent RNA polymerase
Spectinomycin	2.0 grams/day	IM	Inhibition of protein synthesis (30S ribosomal binding)
Streptomycin	1–2 grams/day (q. 12–24 hours)	IM	Inhibition of protein synthesis (30S ribosomal binding)
Sulfonamides			Competition with para-aminobenzoic acid
Sulfisoxazole	4–6 grams/day (q. 6 hours)	PO, IV	
Sulfasalazine	4–8 grams/day (q. 3–6 hours)	PO	
Tetracyclines			Inhibition of protein synthesis
Tetracycline HCl	IV: 0.5–1.0 gram/day (q. 12 hours)	IV, PO	
Chlortetracycline		IV, PO	
Oxytetracycline	PO: 1–2 grams/day (q. 6 hours)	IV, PO	
Demeclocycline	0.6–1.2 grams/day (q. 6 hours)	PO	
Methacycline	0.6–0.9 grams/day (q. 6–12 hours)	PO	
Doxycycline	0.1–0.2 gram/day (q. 12 hours)	IV, PO	
Minocycline	0.1–0.4 gram/day (q. 12 hours)	PO	
Tobramycin	3–6 mg/kg/day (q. 8 hours)	IM, IV	Inhibition of protein synthesis (30S ribosomal binding)
Vancomycin	2 grams/day (q. 6 hours)	IV	Inhibition of cell wall synthesis
Viomycin	1 gram twice weekly	IM	Inhibition of protein synthesis

Table 2. Antimicrobial Agents for Protozoan and Metazoan Infections

Protozoan Infections	Infecting Organism	Antimicrobial Agent	Adult Dose	Route	Adverse Reactions (Most Frequent Are *Italicized*)
Amebiasis Asymptomatic cyst	*Entamoeba histolytica*	Diiodohydroxyquin	650 mg t.i.d. × 3 weeks	PO	*Iodine toxicoderma*, rash, slight thyroid enlargement, nausea
Intestinal disease		Metronidazole	750 mg t.i.d. × 5–10 days	PO	*Nausea*, vomiting, diarrhea; *headache*, vertigo, insomnia, ataxia
Hepatic disease		Diiodohydroxyquin	650 mg t.i.d. × 3 weeks	PO	See above
		Metronidazole and	750 mg t.i.d. × 10 days	PO	See above
		Chloroquine	500 mg q.d. × 10 days	PO	*Vomiting, headache, pruritus*, ocular damage, convulsions, psychosis, rash; hair, nail, and mucous membrane discoloration
Giardiasis	*G. lamblia*	Quinacrine	100 mg t.i.d. × 5 days	PO	*Vomiting, vertigo, headache*; psychosis, blood dyscrasia, ocular damage, rash, hepatic necrosis
		or Metronidazole	250 mg t.i.d. × 10 days	PO	See above
Leishmaniasis Visceral	*L. donovani*	Antimony Na gluconate*	600 mg q.d. × 10 days	IM	Similar to antimony potassium tartrate but less severe
Cutaneous	*L. tropica*	Antimony Na gluconate*	600 mg q.d. × 10 days	IM	See above
Mucocutaneous	*L. brasiliensis*	Antimony Na gluconate*	600 mg q.d. × 10 days	IM	See above
Toxoplasmosis Moderate–severe illness	*T. gondii*	Pyrimethamine and	75 mg first day, then 25 mg q.d. × 4 weeks	PO	*Folic acid deficiency*, blood dyscrasia, rash, vomiting, convulsions, shock
Immunosuppressed host		Sulfadiazine plus	1 gram q.i.d. × 4 weeks	PO	*Rash*, photosensitivity, hepatic and renal toxicity, blood dyscrasia, vasculitis
		Folinic acid	6 mg q. 2 days	IM	
Malaria	*Plasmodium vivax, malariae, ovale*	Chloroquine followed by	1 gram, then 500 mg in 6 hours, then 500 mg q.d. × 2 days	PO	See above
		Primaquine	26.3 mg q.d. × 14 days	PO	*Hemolytic anemia* in G-6-PD deficient patients, neutropenia, nausea, hypertension
	P. falciparum Chloroquine-susceptible	Chloroquine	1 gram, then 500 mg in 6 hours, then 500 mg q.d. × 2 days	PO	See above
	Chloroquine-resistant	Quinine and	650 mg t.i.d. × 14 days	PO	*Cinchonism, hypotension, arrhythmias*, blood dyscrasias, photosensitivity, blindness
		Pyrimethamine plus	25 mg b.i.d. × 3 days	PO	See above
		Sulfadiazine	500 mg q.i.d. × 5 days		See above
	Comatose patient	Quinine†	600 mg/300 ml saline q. 8 hours until PO tolerated	IV	See above
Trichomoniasis	*T. vaginalis*	Metronidazole	250 mg t.i.d. × 10 days	PO	See above
Trypanosomiasis	*T. gambiense* and *T. rhodesiense*	Suramin*	1 gram on days 1, 3, 7, 14, and 21 after 100 mg test dose	IV	*Rash, pruritus, paresthesias, vomiting*, peripheral neuropathy, shock
		followed by Melarsoprol*	2.0–3.6 mg/kg q.d. for 3 days; repeat after 1 week and, if necessary, after an additional 10–21 days	IV	*Encephalopathy*, vomiting, neuropathy, rash, myocarditis, hypertension
	T. cruzi	Nifurtimox*	8 mg/kg q.d. × 120 days	PO	Nausea, dizziness, insomnia, peripheral neuropathy
Pneumocystosis	*P. carinii*	Pentamidine* or	4 mg/kg/day × 12–14 days	IM	See above
		Co-trimoxazole	20 mg/kg and 100 mg/kg q.d.	PO	See above (i.e., sulfadiazine)

*Available from Center for Disease Control (404-633-3311, Ext. 3670).

†If parenteral preparations of quinine are not available locally, they may be obtained from the Parasitic Disease Drug Service, Center for Disease Control (404-633-3311, Ext. 3670).

presence of gastric acid. *Phenoxymethyl penicillin*, although ten times less active than benzyl penicillin, is acid stable and is preferred for oral therapy. Renal clearance of the penicillins is by glomerular filtration and tubular secretion, and the simultaneous administration of probenecid will increase and prolong serum levels. However, probenecid may cause such adverse reactions as nausea, vomiting, hypersensitivity reactions (rash and fever), and rarely the nephrotic syndrome, hepatocellular injury, and aplastic anemia. Acute gout as well as the development of uric acid stones may be precipitated by probenecid. Penicillin G is active against streptococci of groups A, B, C, and G, viridans streptococci, pneumococci, nonpenicillinase-producing staphylococci, *Corynebacterium diphtheriae, Listeria monocytogenes*, anaerobic streptococci, *Fusobacterium, Clostridia*, treponemes, *Leptospira* species, *Neisseria, Pasteurella multocida*, and *Actinomyces*.

Penicillins with gram-negative bacillary activity include ampicillin and carbenicillin. *Ampicillin* differs from penicillin G only in the presence of an amino group on the side chain. This minor alteration is responsible for the difference in antimicrobial activity. Ampicillin is active against enterococci, *Hemophilus influenzae, Shigella, Salmonella, Escherichia coli*, and *Proteus mirabilis*. Indole-positive *Proteus* species (i.e., *P. rettgeri, P. morgani, P. vulgaris*) and *Pseudomonas* species are resistant. Ampicillin may be given either parenterally or orally, and the serum half-life is twice as long as that of penicillin G. *Amoxicillin*, an analogue of ampicillin and available only in oral form, has several pharmacologic advantages over ampicillin. It is more stable in the presence of gastric acid and thus better absorbed. Serum levels are higher and more prolonged than those of ampicillin. Both drugs have the same spectrum of antibacterial activity.

Carbenicillin is also similar in structure to penicillin G except for a carboxyl group on the side chain. It is active in vitro against *E. coli, Pseudomonas* species, *Proteus* species, and some strains of *Enterobacter*. The minimal inhibitory concentrations for *Pseudomonas* are very high when compared to other drug susceptibilities (i.e.,

TABLE 2. Antimicrobial Agents for Protozoan and Metazoan Infections (*Continued*)

Metazoan Infections	Infecting Organism	Antimicrobial Agent	Adult Dose	Route	Adverse Reactions (Most Frequent Are *Italicized*)
Intestinal nematodes	*Ascaris lumbricoides* (roundworm)	Pyrantel pamoate	11 mg/kg (maximum 1 gram), single dose	PO	*GI disturbance,* headache, dizziness, rash, fever
	Enterobius vermicularis (pinworm)	Pyrantel pamoate	11 mg/kg, single dose; repeat after 2 weeks	PO	
	Necator americanus (hookworm)	Mebendazole	100 mg b.i.d. × 3 days	PO	*GI disturbance*
	Ancylostoma duodenale (hookworm)	Mebendazole	100 mg b.i.d. × 3 days	PO	
	Trichuris trichiura (whipworm)	Mebendazole	100 mg b.i.d. × 3 days	PO	
	Strongyloides stercoralis	Thiabendazole	25 mg/kg b.i.d. × 2 days	PO	*Nausea, vomiting, vertigo, rash,* leukopenia, color vision disturbance, tinnitus, shock
Tissue nematodes Filariasis	*Wuchereria bancrofti*	Diethylcarbamazine	2 mg/kg t.i.d. × 14 days	PO	*Allergic and febrile reactions* due to worm disintegration; encephalopathy
	Loa loa	Diethylcarbamazine	2 mg/kg t.i.d. × 14 days	PO	See above
River blindness	*Onchocerca volvulus*	Diethylcarbamazine plus	2 mg/kg t.i.d. × 14 days	PO	See above
		Suramin*	1 gram per week × 5 weeks	IV	See above
Trichinosis	*Trichinella spiralis*	Thiabendazole and/or	25 mg/kg q.d. until symptoms subside	PO	See above
		Prednisone	40 mg q.d. for 3–5 days	PO	
Cestodes (tapeworms)	*Taenia saginata* (beef tapeworm)	Niclosamide*	2 grams in a single dose	PO	Nausea, abdominal pain
	Diphyllobothrium latum (fish tapeworm)	Niclosamide*	2 grams in a single dose	PO	
	Taenia solium (pork tapeworm)	Niclosamide*	2 grams in a single dose	PO	
Trematodes (flukes) Schistosomiasis	*S. mansoni*	Niridazole*	25 mg/kg q.d. × 5–7 days	PO	*Vomiting, diarrhea, dizziness, headache,* EKG changes, rash, insomnia, paresthesias, convulsions, psychosis, hemolysis
	S. haematobium	Niridazole*	25 mg/kg q.d. × 5–7 days	PO	See above
	S. japonicum	Niridazole*	25 mg/kg q.d. × 5–7 days	PO	See above
Paragonimiasis	*P. westermani*	Bithionol*	50 mg/kg q.o.d. × 15 doses	PO	*Photosensitivity, urticaria, abdominal pain, vomiting, and diarrhea*

*Available from Center for Disease Control (404-633-3311, Ext. 3670).

75 to 100 μg per milliliter). However, carbenicillin is a relatively nontoxic agent which can be given in doses of 30 to 40 grams per day intravenously with serum levels of 200 to 400 μg per milliliter. One half this dose is usually adequate for *E. coli, Proteus,* and *Enterobacter* infections. Carbenicillin is principally excreted by the kidneys, and very high urine levels are present after 0.5 or 1.0 gram is given parenterally (1000 μg per milliliter of urine or more). Thus a dose of 4 to 6 grams per day is adequate for uncomplicated urinary tract infections. Since *Pseudomonas aeruginosa* may develop resistance during therapy, especially if the drug is given in suboptimal doses, carbenicillin should not be used alone in patients with severe infections, cystic fibrosis, or chronic urinary tract obstruction when prolonged therapy may be indicated. In addition, superinfection, especially with *Klebsiella* species and *Serratia* species, is not uncommon. An oral form of carbenicillin, the indanyl salt of the sodium ester, is indicated only in uncomplicated urinary tract infections caused by susceptible organisms. Whereas serum levels are low after 0.5 to 1.0 gram orally, urine levels are in excess of the minimal inhibitory concentration of susceptible gram-negative bacilli.

Ticarcillin, now available for general use, is two to four times more active against *Pseudomonas aeruginosa* than carbenicillin. Otherwise, the spectrum of activity and pharmacologic properties of the two drugs are similar.

Penicillinase-Resistant Penicillins. The semisynthetic penicillins that resist penicillinase are methicillin, nafcillin, oxacillin, cloxacillin, and dicloxacillin. The principal indication for using these penicillins is infections caused by *Staphylococcus aureus* which produce penicillinase. These drugs are also active against group

A streptococci and pneumococci. Cloxacillin and dicloxacillin are acid stable and are the preferred agents for oral therapy. Nafcillin is the only penicillinase-resistant penicillin excreted primarily by the liver, and the dose need not be significantly altered in patients with renal failure.

Adverse Reactions to the Penicillins. In general, severe adverse reactions to the penicillins are uncommon, and a wide range exists between therapeutic and toxic serum levels. Hypersensitivity reactions occur in 2 to 5 per cent of patients. These reactions may take two clinical forms: (1) immediate reactions, including anaphylaxis, accelerated urticaria, and angioneurotic edema; and (2) delayed reactions, which are more common and include delayed urticaria, morbilliform eruption, and serum sickness. Hypersensitivity reactions have been reported with all the penicillin derivatives. Patients allergic to one penicillin are allergic to all congeners. Drug fever is not uncommon. Coombs-positive hemolytic anemia may result from the formation of antibody to penicillin-coated red cells. This is most likely to occur when large parenteral doses are given over a long period of time. Central nervous system toxicity, characterized by myoclonus and generalized seizures, may be seen when high doses of parenteral penicillins are administered to patients especially with renal insufficiency. Hyperkalemia may be seen in patients with renal insufficiency, because the potassium salt of penicillin G has 1.6 mEq of K+ per million units. Diarrhea is common in patients receiving oral ampicillin. Skin rashes have been reported to be more common in patients with infectious mononucleosis who receive oral ampicillin. Carbenicillin must be used with caution in patients in whom sodium restriction is important, because 1 gram of carbenicillin contains 4.7 mEq of sodium. Carbenicillin may cause elevated hepatic enzymes, neutropenia, and increased clotting and prothrombin times with bleeding in patients with renal insufficiency. Methicillin and, less commonly, penicillin G have been reported to cause interstitial nephritis and reversible azotemia. Bone marrow depression with anemia and leukopenia has also been associated with methicillin therapy.

CEPHALOSPORINS. Six cephalosporins are currently marketed in the United States: cephalothin, cephapirin, cefazolin, cephaloridine, cephradine, and cephalexin. The cephalosporins are active against most organisms susceptible to the penicillins, i.e., group A streptococci, viridans streptococci, pneumococci, *Staphylococcus aureus*, and *C. diphtheriae.* Susceptible gram-negative bacilli include *Escherichia coli, Klebsiella,* and *Proteus mirabilis. Enterobacter* species, indole-positive *Proteus* strains and *Pseudomonas* species are resistant to the cephalosporins. Cephalothin, cephapirin, cefazolin, and cephaloridine are used parenterally; cephaloglycin and cephalexin, orally. *Cephalothin* is usually given intravenously, because intramuscular injections of greater than 0.5 gram are painful. Renal clearance is rapid, and the drug should be given every four hours. *Cephapirin* has antibacterial spectra and pharmacologic properties similar to cephalothin. *Cefazolin* has several pharmacologic advantages over cephalothin. Because of its low renal clearance and longer half-life, serum levels are two to three times higher and more sustained. Cefazolin may produce less thrombophlebitis than cephalothin and may be given intramuscularly. *Cephaloridine* should be given only by the parenteral route and must be avoided in patients with renal insufficiency. *Cephalexin* is acid stable and well absorbed. Urine levels are within the therapeutic range after a 0.5 to 1.0 gram oral dose. Since the excretion of the cephalosporins is by tubular secretion, serum levels may be increased and prolonged with the simultaneous administration of probenecid. Since the cephalosporins do not achieve therapeutic levels in the cerebrospinal fluid, these agents should not be used in patients with bacterial meningitis. *Cephradine* is available in both parenteral and oral forms.

At the time of this writing, two new compounds, cephamandole, a cephalosporin, and cefoxitin, a cephamycin, appear to be more resistant to the action of cephalosporinase and therefore more active than other cephalosporins against certain gram-negative bacilli.

Adverse reactions to the cephalosporins are relatively uncommon. The question of cross-allergenicity between the penicillins and the cephalosporins remains controversial. The incidence of cross-sensitization must be low, because cephalosporin compounds have been given successfully to many patients with prior penicillin reactions. However, the cephalosporins should probably not be administered to patients with a documented history of an immediate hypersensitivity reaction to penicillin. Thrombophlebitis is commonly seen with the intravenous use of large doses of cephalothin and cephapirin, and frequent changes of the intravenous site are necessary if these drugs have to be given over an extended period of time. A positive Coombs test without hemolysis may occur with large doses of cephalothin; leukopenia is rare and usually responds to discontinuing the drug. Cephaloridine is nephrotoxic, especially if the dose is greater than 4 grams per day or if patients are receiving ethacrynic acid or furosemide.

Acute tubular necrosis has also been reported in patients receiving cephalothin and gentamicin. The specific role of either drug or the combination in this complication is unknown. Nausea and vomiting may accompany the administration of the oral cephalosporins. The presence of cephalexin in the urine may give a false positive test for glucose with Benedict's solution or Clinitest tablets.

VANCOMYCIN. Vancomycin is active against penicillinase-producing *Staphylococcus aureus* and *S. epidermidis,* viridans streptococci, and enterococci. It is an important alternative drug in patients allergic to the penicillins and the cephalosporins who have severe staphylococcal infections or endocarditis caused by penicillin-resistant viridans streptococci and enterococci. Methicillin-resistant *Staphylococcus aureus* strains are usually resistant to the cephalosporins but susceptible to vancomycin. All gram-negative bacilli are resistant to this antimicrobial. Vancomycin can only be administered intravenously. Pain at the site of injection is frequent and thrombophlebitis common. Chills, fever, and urticaria may also accompany its administration. The more severe adverse reactions include reversible nephrotoxicity with albuminuria, casts, and azotemia, and ototoxicity with deafness when very high blood levels are achieved.

ERYTHROMYCIN, LINCOMYCIN, AND CLINDAMYCIN. *Erythromycin* is one of two macrolide antimicrobials. It should be classified with lincomycin and clindamycin, because all three drugs have a similar mechanism of action (inhibition of protein synthesis by binding the 50S ribosomal unit). The spectrum of activity of these drugs, with a few exceptions, is similar. Erythromycin is active against group A streptococci, pneumococci, and *Staphylococcus aureus. Mycoplasma pneumoniae* and *T. pallidum* are also susceptible to it. Erythromycin may be used in patients allergic to penicillin who have respiratory tract or soft tissue infections caused by pneumococci and group A streptococci, respectively. It may be used as the primary drug in *M. pneumoniae* infections. Erythromycin should not be used for serious *Staphylococcus aureus* infections. Local irritation at the site of parenteral administration is common, and gastrointestinal disturbance may be associated with oral therapy. Erythromycin estolate may produce reversible cholestatic hepatitis, and other preparations of erythromycin should be used. Hypersensitivity reactions, such as rash and eosinophilia, and drug fever are uncommon.

Triacetyloleandomycin is also a macrolide antimicrobial, but it is used infrequently because of adverse reactions.

Lincomycin and clindamycin (a chloro-derivative of lincomycin) are also active against group A streptococci, pneumococci, and penicillinase-producing staphylococci. Enterococci, gram-negative bacilli, and *Mycoplasma pneumoniae* are resistant. Many strains of *Staphylococcus aureus* resistant to erythromycin are also resistant to lincomycin and clindamycin. Staphylococci resistant to erythromycin but susceptible to lincomycin or clindamycin may rapidly develop resistance to the latter drugs during lincomycin-clindamycin therapy (dissociated cross-resistance). Clindamycin is well absorbed from the gastrointestinal tract and produces higher serum levels than oral lincomycin. Clindamycin is also more active against many anaerobes, especially *Bacteroides fragilis,* and has become the drug of choice in the initial therapy of severe anaerobic infections. Erythromycin crosses the blood-brain barrier, but lincomycin and clindamycin do not, and therefore the latter agents should not be used in bacterial meningitis. Gastrointestinal disturbances such as nausea, vomiting, abdominal cramps, and diarrhea occur with clindamycin and lincomycin. Pseudomembranous colitis has been observed with both drugs. Rapid intravenous administration may be associated with cardiopulmonary arrest. Reversible hepatocellular toxicity and bone marrow depression (leukopenia) have been reported after clindamycin therapy. Hypersensitivity reactions such as rash and generalized pruritus are rare.

NOVOBIOCIN. The antibacterical spectrum of novobiocin is similar to that of penicillin G and erythromycin; *Staphylococcus aureus* and pneumococci are susceptible to this antimicrobial. It is well absorbed from the gastrointestinal tract and may also be given intravenously. However, the high incidence of adverse reactions precludes the routine use of this drug, and it is rarely prescribed at present. Toxic reactions include gastrointestinal disturbances (nausea, vomiting, diarrhea, and bleeding), bone marrow depression (pancytopenia), hypersensitivity reactions (eosinophilia, rash, fever, angioedema, exudative erythema multiforme), alopecia, and yellow discoloration of the skin and sclera caused by a degradation product of the drug.

BACITRACIN. Bacitracin is a polypeptide antimicrobial agent for topical use only. *Staphylococcus aureus*, *Staphylococcus epidermidis*, enterococci, viridans streptococci, and group A streptococci are susceptible to it. Gram-negative bacilli are resistant to bacitracin. The antibiotic is stable in ointments only when it is incorporated in petrolatum. Bacitracin is indicated in open superficial skin infections such as eczema, dermal ulcers, and minor wounds infected with drug-susceptible bacteria. Purulent conjunctivitis and infected corneal ulcers may also respond to topical bacitracin when caused by similar organisms. Furunculosis, impetigo, pyoderma, and subcutaneous abscesses should not be treated with topical bacitracin alone. Adverse reactions are rarely seen with this topical drug.

AMINOGLYCOSIDES. The six drugs that belong to this class of antimicrobial agents are streptomycin, neomycin, kanamycin, gentamicin, tobramycin, and amikacin. *Streptomycin*, one of the first aminoglycosides available for parenteral administration, was widely used in the 1940's and 1950's, because *Mycobacterium tuberculosis* and gram-negative bacilli, especially *Escherichia coli*, *Klebsiella-Enterobacter* species, and *Proteus* strains were susceptible. However, with the development of other drugs for these infections and because adverse reactions, notably vestibular toxicity, are a risk, the use of intramuscular streptomycin is now limited to a few specific diseases. Most strains of enterococci are resistant to streptomycin in vitro. Nevertheless, streptomycin in combination with penicillin or vancomycin is the therapy of choice in patients with penicillin-resistant viridans streptococcal and enterococcal endocarditis. These drug combinations should also be used for prophylaxis against enterococcal bacteremia in patients with underlying congenital or valvular heart disease who have urogenital or gastrointestinal manipulation. Streptomycin has substantial activity against *M. tuberculosis*, and the indications for its use in this disease are discussed in Ch. 167. Streptomycin may also be used in the therapy of plague, tularemia, and brucello-

sis. *Neomycin,* also discovered in the 1940's, has limited clinical application because of nephrotoxicity and neurotoxicity. The drug is poorly absorbed from the gastrointestinal tract and is therefore useful in patients with severe hepatic disease with impending or frank coma, inhibiting bacterial growth in the intestinal tract and reducing absorption of nitrogenous compounds. Unfortunately, neomycin is widely used in topical antimicrobial preparations, many of which are available without a prescription. There is no evidence from controlled studies that neomycin is effective in healing or preventing skin infections. Indeed, topical neomycin frequently causes contact dermatitis. Injudicious use of neomycin in patients with extensive wounds or burns or instillation into body cavities may result in absorption of the drug and life-threatening adverse reactions.

Kanamycin is closely related to neomycin but is less toxic. It is active against most gram-negative bacilli, including *E. coli, Klebsiella-Enterobacter* species, and *Proteus* species. The drug is also active in vitro against *Shigella, Staphylococcus aureus,* and *M. tuberculosis,* but is not indicated for clinical use in these infections, because less toxic agents are available. *Pseudomonas aeruginosa* strains are universally resistant to kanamycin. Ampicillin plus kanamycin has been the initial therapy of choice in suspected neonatal sepsis. However, if it is known that kanamycin-resistant gram-negative organisms have been isolated from the nursery, ampicillin plus gentamicin is recommended.

Gentamicin is widely used for serious gram-negative bacillary infections. It is active against *Pseudomonas* species as well as *E. coli, Klebsiella-Enterobacter* species, and *Proteus* species. *Staphylococcus aureus* strains are also susceptible to gentamicin; however, less toxic antistaphylococcal agents are available, and gentamicin should not be used for this purpose. Gentamicin may be given by either the intramuscular or the intravenous route. Therapeutic levels in the cerebrospinal fluid are usually not achieved with parenteral administration, and intrathecal injections are indicated in patients with gram-negative bacillary meningitis. In patients with urinary tract infections, the urine should be alkaline for maximal antimicrobial activity. Carbenicillin when mixed with gentamicin in the same solution will inactivate the latter drug over a prolonged period of time.

Recently, two additional aminoglycosides have become available for general use. *Tobramycin* is two to six times more active against *P. aeruginosa* than gentamicin and is the drug of choice for infections caused by this microbe. The spectrum of gram-negative bacillary activity and pharmacologic properties of the two drugs are similar. *Amikacin,* despite a chemical structure similar to that of kanamycin, has excellent activity against *P. aeruginosa*. Since amikacin is a poor substrate for many of the enzymes produced by gram-negative organisms that inactivate gentamicin and tobramycin, this drug should be reserved at present for infections caused by gentamicin- and tobramycin-resistant organisms.

Adverse reactions are commonly seen with administration of the aminoglycosides. These agents are excreted principally by the kidneys and should be avoided or the dose adjusted in patients with compromised renal function. Furthermore, the therapeutic serum level often approximates the toxic level, and adverse reactions may be unavoidable in patients with life-threatening infections. Since gentamicin has such a wide spectrum of activity against aerobic gram-negative bacilli, it is often used in conjunction with a penicillinase-resistant penicillin or a cephalosporin for the initial therapy in patients with malignancies or who are on immunosuppressive or cytotoxic agents. If the infecting organism proves to be susceptible to a less toxic drug, gentamicin should be discontinued and that agent instituted for the remainder of the patient's therapy. The aminoglycosides should never be injected into body cavities or given rapidly by vein, because neuromuscular blockade with respiratory arrest may ensue. This curare-like effect may be reversed with neostigmine or calcium gluconate. All the aminoglycosides are nephrotoxic and neurotoxic. Neomycin, kanamycin, and amikacin cause auditory toxicity with deafness. Deafness is more commonly seen in patients with renal insufficiency or in patients receiving ethacrynic acid or furosemide. Streptomycin, gentamicin, and tobramycin usually cause vestibular damage which may be irreversible. Occasionally deafness may also occur. During long-term therapy, patients must be closely followed with daily tandem-walking and weekly caloric reactions and audiograms. Paresthesias, peripheral neuropathy, and optic neuritis are rarely observed. Hypersensitivity reactions have been reported with each of the aminoglycosides.

POLYMYXINS. Polymyxin B and polymyxin E are polypeptide antimicrobials that are active against *E. coli*, *Klebsiella-Enterobacter* species, and *Pseudomonas* species. *Proteus* species are resistant to these drugs. Polymyxin B is given parenterally and may also be administered intrathecally. The polymyxins do not cross the blood-brain barrier and must be given both parenterally and intrathecally in patients with gram-negative bacillary meningitis. Polymyxin E has two forms, parenteral colistimethate sodium and oral colistin sulfate, a nonabsorbable antimicrobial. Although active in vitro against many species of gram-negative bacilli, polymyxin is most useful in the therapy of *Pseudomonas aeruginosa* infections. Since the polymyxins are excreted by the kidneys, caution must be used when these agents are given to patients with renal insufficiency. Serious adverse reactions are dose related. Neurotoxic reactions include circumoral or fingertip paresthesias that are usually reversible. Ataxia, slurred speech, and blurred vision are uncommon. Respiratory paralysis may occur with rapid intravenous administration or in patients receiving succinylcholine and may be reversed by intravenous calcium gluconate but not neostigmine. Azotemia and impaired renal function are seen with high doses. Hypersensitivity reactions have been reported and include eosinophilia and rash.

SPECTINOMYCIN. Spectinomycin is active against *Neisseria gonorrhoeae* and has been approved only for use in uncomplicated gonorrhea. The drug does not have treponemicidal activity. It should be considered for use in patients with gonococcal urethritis and cervicitis who are allergic to penicillin, because it can be given as a single dose intramuscularly. There is no cross-resistance between spectinomycin and penicillin. Although spectinomycin inhibits protein synthesis by binding 30S ribosomal subunits (similar to the aminoglycosides), adverse reactions, except for fever and urticaria, have been uncommon to date.

CHLORAMPHENICOL. Chloramphenicol has a broad spectrum of activity against the rickettsiae, gram-positive bacteria, gram-negative bacteria, including *Salmonella* and *Shigella,* and anaerobic bacteria. The drug is well absorbed from the gastrointestinal tract. It is metabolized by the liver and can therefore be used in patients with renal insufficiency. Adequate levels in the cerebrospinal fluid are present after intravenous injection. Chloramphenicol causes bone marrow aplasia and fatal pancytopenia in 1 of every 40,000 or more courses of therapy or 1 of 25,000 to 50,000 people exposed. This severe toxic reaction is a form of hypersensitivity or idiosyncratic reaction which cannot be predicted before therapy. For this reason, chloramphenicol should be used only for certain specific, severe infections. These indications include (1) typhoid fever or other *Salmonella* infections, (2) initial therapy for *Hemophilus influenzae* meningitis, (3) as an alternative drug for penicillin G in pneumococcal and meningococcal meningitis, (4) severe anaerobic infections for which clindamycin is not effective, (5) gram-negative bacillary infections that do not respond to other antimicrobial agents, and (6) severe rickettsial infections when tetracycline is not effective.

Anemia which is dose related and not a hypersensitivity reaction may occur with prolonged use. This form of bone marrow depression is reversible and is characterized by interference with iron metabolism, with increased serum iron and saturation of iron-binding globulin, decreased reticulocyte count, and vacuolization of red cell precursors. Patients receiving chloramphenicol must have repeated complete blood counts and serum iron and saturation determinations. This type of anemia is most commonly seen in patients with liver disease or renal insufficiency and in those receiving high doses. Fatal toxicity may develop in neonates ("gray baby syndrome"). Optic neuritis and peripheral neuropathy are rarely seen with prolonged therapy. Hypersensitivity reactions have been reported.

TETRACYCLINES. The tetracyclines have a broad spectrum of activity. *Rickettsia, Chlamydia, Mycoplasma pneumoniae,* gram-positive and gram-negative bacteria, certain anaerobic organisms, and *T. pallidum* are susceptible to the tetracyclines. At present, 25 to 50 per cent of group A streptococci, 5 to 10 per cent of pneumococci, and most *Staphylococcus aureus* isolates are resistant. In addition, many aerobic gram-negative bacilli and *Bacteroides* species are also resistant. These changing susceptibility patterns since the introduction of tetracycline in the 1940's have made it necessary to restrict the use of these drugs to the following indications: (1) *Rickettsia* infections; (2) *M. pneumoniae* infections; (3) *Chlamydia* infections, including psittacosis, trachoma, lymphogranuloma venereum, and nongonococcal urethritis; (4) granuloma inguinale and chancroid; (5) alternative therapy for gonorrhea and syphilis; and (6) urinary tract infections caused by susceptible gram-negative bacilli.

Tetracycline has replaced *chlortetracycline* and *oxytetracycline* as the agent of choice. It may be given orally or intravenously, although thrombophlebitis often accompanies the latter route of administration. Tetracycline should be avoided in patients with renal insufficiency. Four long-acting tetracyclines are available: *demethylchlortetracycline, methacycline, doxycycline,* and *minocycline.* The rate of renal excretion of these agents is less and oral absorption greater than those of tetracycline, resulting in prolonged serum levels. Minor variations in the degree of antibacterial activity exist among the four preparations which are reflected in the amount of drug recommended per dose. Doxycycline does not accumulate in the serum of patients with renal insufficiency and may be advantageous when the status of renal function is unknown. However, because of the low renal clearance of both doxycycline and minocycline, their usefulness in urinary tract infections may be limited by low urinary concentrations. With few exceptions all the tetracycline compounds produce the same adverse reactions. These include gastrointestinal disturbances such as nausea, vomiting, and diarrhea, thrombophlebitis with intravenous administration, staining and hypoplasia of dental enamel and disturbed bone growth in neonates and young children, pseudotumor cerebri with bulging fontanelles and increased cerebrospinal fluid pressure in infants, and acute fatty degeneration of the liver in pregnant women and patients with renal insufficiency. Photosensitivity reactions are not infrequently seen with the long-acting tetracyclines. A variant of the Fanconi syndrome caused by toxic products may occur with administration of outdated tetracycline preparations. Superinfections with resistant gram-negative bacilli, *Staphylococcus aureus,* and *Candida* may occur with prolonged therapy.

SULFONAMIDES. For four decades, sulfonamides have been widely prescribed for a variety of clinical infections. However, their present use is limited because of resistance of gram-positive and gram-negative organisms, the availability of more active antimicrobial agents, and adverse reactions. The major indications are (1) nocardiosis; (2) suppressive therapy for paracoccidioidomycosis; (3) prophylaxis in sulfadiazine-susceptible meningococcal infections; (4) alternative prophylaxis for acute rheumatic fever in patients allergic to penicillin; (5) uncomplicated urinary tract infections caused by susceptible organisms, especially *E. coli*; (6) salicylazosulfapyridine therapy in patients with mild ulcerative colitis; (7) certain protozoal infections (toxoplasmosis, *Pneumocystis carinii*, and chloroquine-resistant *P. falciparum* malaria); and (8) when administered in combination with antifolate compounds, chronic urinary tract infections and typhoid fever.

Sulfisoxazole is well absorbed from the gastrointestinal tract and may also be administered parenterally if necessary. The drug is chiefly excreted by glomerular filtration and thus is not affected by probenecid. *Sulfamethoxazole* is a congener of sulfisoxazole, but is absorbed less and the renal excretion is delayed. The more potent *sulfadiazine*, once widely used, is less soluble and tends to cause crystalluria. The incidence of crystalluria is decreased by increasing fluid intake and maintaining an alkaline urine. The risk of precipitation of the drug in the renal tubules is appreciably increased if the sulfadiazine is administered intravenously. Long-acting sulfonamides, such as *sulfamethoxypyridazine* and *sulfadimethoxine*, although widely used in the past, have no place in clinical antimicrobial therapy because of their toxic effects. The poorly absorbed sulfonamides, *succinylsulfathiazole* and *phthalylsulfathiazole,* are principally used to decrease bacterial counts in the intestine prior to surgery. These agents are of doubtful value. *Salicylazosulfapyridine* may decrease the severity of disease in patients with mild ulcerative colitis. This effect may be due to the antibacterial action of sulfapyridine or the anti-inflammatory effect of 5-aminosalicylic acid.

Adverse reactions caused by the sulfonamides include the following: hypersensitivity reactions with fever, rash, photosensitivity, and rarely vasculitis; nephrotoxicity with crystalluria and renal tubular necrosis; kernicterus in the newborn; hepatitis (occasion- ally with noncaseating granuloma); agranulocytosis and aplastic anemia; and acute hemolytic anemia in patients with G-6-PD deficiency. Long-acting sulfonamides may cause Stevens-Johnson syndrome and myocarditis.

TRIMETHOPRIM-SULFAMETHOXAZOLE (CO-TRIMOXAZOLE). This drug combination sequentially inhibits the utilization of para-aminobenzoic acid by bacteria in the synthesis of folic acid. A double sequential blockage is thus produced, and relatively low concentrations of each drug are required for antimicrobial activity. At present, the drug combination (trimethoprim, 80 mg; sulfamethoxazole, 400 mg) has been approved in the United States only for chronic urinary tract infections and pneumocystis infections. Clinically trials suggest that it may be useful in patients with bronchitis, gonorrhea, and possibly typhoid fever resistant to both chloramphenicol and ampicillin. Adverse reactions are the same as those described for the sulfonamides, including the Stevens-Johnson syndrome, and those caused by trimethoprim, including nausea, vomiting, skin rashes, and macrocytic anemia resulting from folic acid deficiency. Serious nephrotoxicity has been reported in patients with diminished renal function.

NITROFURANTOIN. Nitrofurantoin is an oral antibacterial agent that is excreted in the urine by both glomerular filtration and tubular secretion. The drug is most active against *E. coli, Klebsiella-Enterobacter* species, and some strains of enterococci. The susceptibility of *Proteus* strains is variable, and *Pseudomonas* species are resistant. Nitrofurantoin should be used only for uncomplicated urinary tract infections or suppressive therapy in patients with chronic urinary tract infections. The drug is most active in the presence of an acid urine, and emergent resistance has not been noted. It should not be prescribed in pregnant women, because it crosses the placenta, or in patients with renal insufficiency. Adverse reactions include nausea and vomiting, hypersensitivity reactions (fever, rash, allergic pneumonitis), paresthesias which may progress to severe polyneuropathy if the drug is not discontinued, acute hemolytic anemia in patients with G-6-PD deficiency, and cholestatic hepatitis.

NALIDIXIC ACID. Nalidixic acid is also an oral antimicrobial agent used in the therapy of uncomplicated urinary tract infections. The drug is active against strains of *E. coli, Klebsiella-Enterobacter* species, and *Proteus* species; *Pseudomonas* species are resistant. Gram-negative bacilli may rapidly develop resistance to this agent, and repeated urine cultures with drug-susceptibility determinations should be performed during therapy. Adverse reactions include nausea, vomiting, hypersensitivity reactions (rash, eosinophilia, photosensitivity), and rarely cholestatic jaundice, blood dyscrasias, visual disturbances, toxic psychosis, and convulsive seizures. Severe headache associated with papilledema has been observed in children.

METHENAMINE MANDELATE AND HIPPURATE. These antimicrobial compounds are the salts of methenamine and mandelic acid and hippuric acid, respectively. They are well absorbed from the gastrointestinal tract and rapidly excreted in the urine. They are bactericidal in acidic urine (pH less than 5.5). An acidifying agent is necessary if the infecting organism forms ammonia. Methenamine mandelate or hippurate may be used for chronic suppression of urinary tract infections. *Escherichia coli* is susceptible to these drugs. *Proteus* species and *Pseudomonas* species are usually resistant. Adverse reactions are uncommon and include epigastric pain, dysuria, crystalluria, and metabolic acidosis, especially in patients with renal insufficiency.

FAILURE OF ANTIMICROBIAL THERAPY

The failure of a patient to respond to antimicrobial therapy may be due to factors related to the host and the nature of the disease or to an error in the choice, dosage, or route of administration of the drug. The following causes are most common: (1) incorrect diagnosis; (2) impaired host defense mechanisms; (3) inadequate dose, route of administration, or distribution of drug; (4) closed space infection; (5) presence of a foreign body; (6) superinfection; and (7) microbial drug resistance.

Resistance of microorganisms to antimicrobial agents may be classified as primary (natural) or emergent (acquired) (see Ch. 189). Microorganisms acquire resistance by either mutation or episomal transfer. Mutation patterns may be multi-step, involving a number of genes, or large-step, involving one gene. The efficiency of mutation is increased in the presence of low-dose antimicrobial drug administration. Both gram-positive and gram-negative bacteria develop resistance by mutation. Recognition of episomal transfer of resistance is presently restricted to gram-negative bacilli and *Staphylococcus aureus*. The transfer of cytoplasmic DNA (R factor) requires cell-to-cell contact and is termed conjugation. The transfer of resistance may be single or multiple, and occurs most commonly in the gastrointestinal tract. It is often designated infectious drug resistance.

CHEMOPROPHYLAXIS

Antimicrobial agents are often administered to individuals who are believed to be at some increased risk of acquiring a bacterial infection.

Prophylaxis is usually successful only when a single drug is given for a specific organism. The antimicrobial drugs and their clinical indications which are considered to be of value are summarized in Table 3. Except for the use of amantadine in influenza A infection (see Ch. 82), antimicrobial prophylaxis is not effective in either viral respiratory diseases or viral exanthems. In addition, prophylaxis is not indicated in clean abdominal surgery or congestive heart failure. Unlike the therapeutic situation in which the identity of the offending microbe might be in doubt and there is urgency in selecting therapy, with chemoprophylaxis there is usually no urgency, and the microbe in question is known. Consequently, the use of antimicrobial drugs in chemoprophylaxis should be more rational than in therapy. Unfortunately, this is not always the case, and in many

TABLE 3. Recommendations for Antimicrobial Prophylaxis

Disease or Clinical Setting	Etiologic Agent	Antimicrobial Drug
Acute rheumatic fever (recurrent)	Group A streptococcus	Penicillin, erythromycin, sulfonamide
Meningococcal infections	*Neisseria meningitidis*	
	Sulfonamide-susceptible	Sulfisoxazole
	Sulfonamide-resistant	Rifampin
Microbial endocarditis		
Oral cavity instrumentation	Viridans streptococcus	Penicillin, erythromycin
Urogenital and gastrointestinal instrumentation	Enterococcus	Penicillin or vancomycin plus streptomycin
Open heart surgery	*Staphylococcus aureus* and *epidermidis*	Penicillinase-resistant penicillin, cephalosporin
Newborn nursery epidemics	Enteropathic *E. coli*	Neomycin, Colistin
	Staphylococcus aureus	Penicillinase-resistant penicillin
	Group A streptococci	Penicillin
Tuberculin reactors of certain sorts	*Mycobacterium tuberculosis*	Isoniazid
Malaria	Plasmodia	
	Chloroquine-susceptible	Chloroquine followed by primaquine
	Chloroquine-resistant (*P. falciparum*)	Pyrimethamine and sulfadoxine *or* Chloroguanide and sulfone
Ophthalmia neonatorum	*Neisseria gonorrhoeae*	Silver nitrate, penicillin
Burns		Silver sulfadiazine, silver nitrate
Bronchitis (chronic)	Pneumococcus or *Hemophilus influenzae*	Ampicillin, tetracycline

instances the prophylactic use of antimicrobial agents is unwarranted, ineffective, and often dangerous because of toxic reactions, superinfection, and emergent resistance. The matter of drug toxicity requires comment. Selection of a drug is a matter of weighing offsetting risks. It is easy to forget that a degree of drug toxicity that is acceptable when weighed against an instance of a particular disease may be unacceptable when weighed against the chance that someone *might* acquire that disease. Finally, although one must emphasize the need for caution in chemoprophylaxis, it is fitting to remember that in terms of the number of people benefited, the use of the drugs in this way represents one of the greatest achievements of modern biomedical science and technology.

Balows, A.: Current Techniques for Antibiotic Susceptibility Testing. Springfield, Ill., Charles C Thomas, 1974.

Goodman, L. S., and Gilman, A.: The Pharmacological Basis of Therapeutics. 4th ed. New York, Macmillan, 1970.

Handbook of Antimicrobial Therapy. The Medical Letter on Drugs and Therapeutics (revised ed.), 1977.

Kunin, C. M., et al.: Use of antibiotics. A brief exposition of the problem and some tentative solutions. Ann. Intern. Med., 79:555, 1973.

Lowbury, E. J. L., and Ayliffe, G. A. L.: Drug Resistance in Antimicrobial Therapy. Springfield, Ill., Charles C Thomas, 1974.

Pratt, W. B.: Chemotherapy of Infections. New York, Oxford University Press, 1977.

Weinstein, L., and Dalton, A. C.: Host determinants of response to antimicrobial agents. N. Engl. J. Med., 279:467, 1968.

PART X
PROTOZOAN AND HELMINTHIC DISEASES

191. INTRODUCTION

Philip D. Marsden

With rapid air travel, so-called parasitic infections are becoming more important in temperate climes. They have always been important in the tropics.

Parasitic disease is usually taken to imply infections caused by protozoa and helminths, although, in their relationship to the host, bacteria, viruses, and rickettsiae equally fulfill the general criteria used to describe an organism as parasitic. The reason for this nomenclature is historic; because they are bigger organisms, helminths and protozoa were discovered relatively early by medical investigators. *Ascaris* and tapeworms are dramatic enough to have been recognized in ancient times, and protozoa were seen with the first crude microscopes.

A knowledge of where the infection occurs in the world is important, and this information is included in the succeeding chapters. For example, schistosomiasis would not be considered as a cause of portal hypertension in a patient from the Indian subcontinent, and malaria caused by *Plasmodium vivax* is rare in West Africa.

For the correct diagnosis of parasitic disease the physician must be as competent at the microscope and in using the laboratory procedures to find parasites as he is at defining the clinical presentation at the bedside and interpreting it. As with other infectious diseases, a firm diagnosis rests on finding the infectious agent. Recently serologic tests have been used much more to aid diagnosis, and, interpreted wisely, they are valuable. Broadly speaking, they mean that a patient has developed antibodies of a certain type to a parasitic antigen. Rarely do they give any confirmation about the status of the parasite in the body of man in terms of numbers present or whether they are multiplying. Positive serologic findings should often be an indication for redoubling one's efforts to find the parasite.

Whether a complement fixation test, hemagglutination test, fluorescent antibody test, or gel diffusion test is positive at a significant titer must be decided in the light of known facts about the specificity of the tests.

Many of the drugs used are toxic to man but more toxic to the parasites. We know little of the mechanisms of drug action in many cases, e.g., Pentostam in leishmaniasis. With some drugs such as heavy metal containing compounds and emetine the toxic dose for man is near the therapeutic dose. Physicians should be especially careful to check their prescriptions of these drugs, especially if they are not used to prescribing them often.

The Center for Disease Control, Atlanta, Georgia, offers unique services to the physician in the United States for the management of parasitic disease. Not only is there a laboratory for diagnostic serology, but a number of rare drugs previously not available in the United States and mentioned in this book have become available through the Parasitic Disease Drug Service in the Epidemiology Program. These include drugs for the treatment of both types of human trypanosomiasis, leishmaniasis, amebiasis, pneumocystis infection, and schistosomiasis.

With regard to diagnostic serology, Dr. Irving G. Kagan has kindly provided the information on serologic tests available for parasitic diseases in the United States (see accompanying table).

Immunodiagnostic Tests for Parasitic Infections

	Complement Fixation	Precipitin	Particle Agglutination Tests				Fluorescent Antibody	ELISA
			Bentonite Flocculation	Hemagglutination	Latex Agglutination	Cholesterol Flocculation		
Trichinosis	+	+	+*	±*	+*	+*	+*	0
Echinococcosis	+	+	+*	+*	+*		+	0
Schistosomiasis	+*		±*	±*		+*	+*	0
Ascariasis/toxocariasis			+*	+*			0	±*
Filariasis	±		+*	+*	0		0	0
Cysticercosis	+	0		+*	±		0	±*
Chagas' disease	+*	±	0	+*	0		0*	0
Leishmaniasis	+			+*			0	0
Toxoplasmosis	+*			+*	0		+*	±*
Amebiasis	+*	+	±*	+*	±		±*	0
Malaria				±*			+*	0

*Tests available in the United States.
ELISA = Enzyme-linked immunosorbent assay.
0 = Under experimental investigation.
± = Used for diagnosis, but requires further evaluation for routine use.
+ = Generally accepted useful routine diagnostic test.
Adapted from data supplied by Dr. Irving Kagan, Center for Disease Control.

Section One   PROTOZOAN DISEASES

192.   INTRODUCTION

Philip D. Marsden

Malaria remains the greatest challenge in parasitic disease both in terms of prevalence (over 500 million people still live in malarious areas) and in the amount of morbidity and mortality it causes. In many tropical countries, notably Africa, malaria has a profound influence on the pattern of clinical medicine.

Trypanosomiasis is a good example of geographically restricted disease. *Trypanosoma brucei* infections are restricted to Africa because tsetse flies (*Glossina* species) are not found elsewhere. African sleeping sickness demands attention because human infections once established are so frequently fatal. Also, this same group of trypanosomes are responsible for widespread fatal disease in cattle, profoundly influencing animal husbandry. South American trypanosomiasis (Chagas' disease) is restricted to the Americas because again the great majority of reduviid bugs occur in this location. The significance of this infection as a public health problem is a matter of current concern. One estimate suggests that 7 million people are infected and 30 million exposed to the risk of infection. Permanent cardiac damage often ensues, and at the time of writing there is no cure.

Also in the family Trypanosomatidae, the genus *Leishmania* is responsible for considerable human suffering. Visceral leishmaniasis is a debilitating infection, and without treatment the terminal event is usually a secondary bacterial infection, often a pneumonia. Cutaneous and mucocutaneous leishmaniasis can be disfiguring infections. Therapy is far from satisfactory.

Amebiasis ranks fourth in this consideration, because, although bowel infections are widely prevalent, invasive disease is less common. Then come a miscellany of rarer protozoal disease entities.

The reader will appreciate that the first three groups of diseases caused by protozoa all have arthropod vectors: *Anopheles* for malaria, *Glossina* and Reduviidae for trypanosomiasis, and *Phlebotomus* for leishmaniasis. It is relevant and important for medical people to have some knowledge of these vectors. A few examples of why this is so will suffice. At the time of writing there have been a few cases of indigenous vivax malaria recognized in the United States. Epidemiologic work has revealed vector *Anopheles* in the area. Xenodiagnosis using clean Reduviidae is the best way of finding *Trypanosoma cruzi* parasites in a patient with a chronic infection, and because of this these insects are most important, as they are used in diagnostic medicine. *Phlebotomus* remains very susceptible to DDT, and spraying of this insect's habitats will result in the control of human leishmaniasis.

Another medical consideration worth emphasizing is that blood protozoa can be transmitted by blood transfusion. Particularly important in this respect are malaria and *Trypanosoma cruzi* infections. Suitable selection of donors in temperate countries is necessary to avoid this complication in nonimmune persons exposed to the risk of malaria parasites in transfused blood. *Trypanosoma cruzi* infections transmitted by blood transfusion are said to be particularly acute. It is of interest that recent advances in immunology enable us to screen blood donors for malaria with the indirect fluorescent antibody test, whereas for *Trypanosoma cruzi* the valuable complement-fixation test or an indirect fluorescent antibody test is available.

Belding, D. L.: Textbook of Parasitology. 3rd ed. New York, Appleton-Century-Crofts, Inc., 1965.

Faust, E. C., and Russell, P. F.: Clinical Parasitology. 8th ed. Philadelphia, Lea & Febiger, 1970.

Hunter, G. W., Swartzwelder, J. C. and Clyde, D. F.: Tropical Medicine. 5th ed. Philadelphia, W. B. Saunders Company, 1976.

Wilcocks, C., and Manson-Bahr, P. E. C.: Manson's Tropical Diseases. 17th ed. Baltimore, Williams & Wilkins Company, 1972.

Woodruff, A. W.: Medicine in the Tropics. New York, Longman, 1974.

193.   MALARIA

Thomas C. Jones

GENERAL CONSIDERATIONS.   Malaria is characterized by shaking chills, relapsing fever, prostration, splenomegaly, and anemia. After the initial illness, the disease may follow a chronic or relapsing course. It is caused by four species of the genus *Plasmodium (P. vivax, P. falciparum, P. malariae,* and *P. ovale)*. The infection is maintained in nature by the feeding habits of female mosquitoes of the genus *Anopheles,* in which sporogony occurs, feeding on blood of humans, in which schizogony and gametocytogony occur. Malaria remains a common cause of morbidity and mortality in the world. Delay in diagnosis or inappropriate therapy may lead to severe complications which include coma, acute renal failure, severe anemia, pulmonary edema, or shock. Recognition of the association between malaria and hemoglobinopathies, persistent hypergammaglobulinemia, and the tropical splenomegaly syndrome has emphasized the often subtle but significant influence of malaria on populations living in endemic areas.

HISTORY.   The term malaria originated in the seventeenth century in Italy where the death of patients after intermittent or so-called Roman fevers was attributed to the bad air (mal'aria) of the marsh and swamp lands. These fevers were recognized in ancient times in China, India, and Mesopotamia, but the earliest record of quotidian, tertian, and quartan fevers was that of Hippocrates in the fifth century B.C. The Greeks and Romans were aware of the association of these fevers with marsh lands and conducted one of the earliest public health campaigns by draining the stagnant water. Cinchona bark was recognized as being effective against fevers in 1600 in Peru, after which it was widely used in Europe. Torti, in 1712, clearly distinguished the fevers that responded to cinchona from those that did not.

The protozoan was first described in the blood of a patient

by Charles Laveran in 1880, who observed the parasite in an unstained smear of fresh blood. In 1891 Romanowsky developed a technique for staining blood smears for accurate study of the erythrocytic stage of malaria. In 1897, William MacCallum observed penetration and fertilization of the female gamete, documenting that a sexual cycle occurred in malaria. The role of the mosquito as a vector in malaria was postulated by Sir Patrick Manson after he documented that filaria could develop in the mosquito. The careful studies of Sir Ronald Ross in 1898 documented that in avian malaria the protozoan developed in the stomach of infected mosquitoes and migrated to the salivary glands, from which it could infect healthy birds. Several months later Bignami, Bastianelli, and Grassi documented the transmission of malaria to man by *Anopheles* mosquitoes. Our present knowledge of the malaria cycle was completed in 1948 when Shortt, Garnham, Bray, and others confirmed the presence of the pre-erythrocytic stage in man.

A decrease in the prevalence of malaria during this century has resulted from campaigns to control mosquitoes and the widespread use of drug therapy directed against malaria. The systematic approach to mosquito control organized by Col. William Gorgas in the Canal Zone in 1906 was one of the outstanding achievements in preventive medical science. Effective insecticides were first introduced in 1939, and a number of synthetic antimalarial drugs were developed. The global program of malaria eradication was instituted during the 1950's. It has become clear recently, however, that various biologic, technical, and socioeconomic problems in some countries have required that careful methods of malaria control be substituted for attempts at eradication of the disease.

EPIDEMIOLOGY. Malaria is an endemic disease in parts of Africa, Asia, and Central and South America, where environmental factors, including temperature, humidity, and standing water, support the breeding of mosquitoes and where there is close contact between the mosquitoes and man. The disease in these areas contributes to a high infant mortality and syndromes of chronic malaria. The prevalence of malaria in endemic areas is usually determined by documenting the proportion of people with large spleens (spleen rate) or the proportion of people with blood smears positive for malaria parasites (parasite rate). It has been estimated that 100 million cases of malaria occur each year. Approximately 1 per cent of these patients die of the disease, although this figure can vary from less than 1 per cent to over 10 per cent, depending on the species of *Plasmodium* most prevalent, the level of immunity of the host, and the availability of prompt medical care.

Acute disease caused by malaria often occurs when nonimmune persons enter endemic areas. Through the centuries the most impressive effects of malaria have been recorded during time of war when large numbers of nonimmunes are placed in malarious areas. This has certainly been the major factor contributing to the incidence of malaria in American citizens in the past 35 years. The number of cases of malaria in the United States rose from less than 100 in 1960 to 4000 in 1970 as a direct result of the exposure of nonimmune military personnel to the disease in Vietnam.

Epidemics of malaria may occur when the parasite is introduced into a region with a large nonimmune population. This occurred in the Soviet Union after World War I when more than 5 million cases were reported in 1923; and in Ethiopia in 1958 when 3 million cases and 150,000 deaths caused by malaria were reported. Such epidemics are reminders of the potential threat to localities where effective malaria eradication has created a large nonimmune population but where mosquito vectors persist in large numbers. Vectors for transmission

of plasmodia, primarily *A. quadrimaculatus* and *A. freeborni,* persist in parts of the United States. In the past 25 years there have been a dozen outbreaks of malaria resulting from mosquito transmission within the United States.

Falciparum and vivax malaria are widely spread throughout the tropics and subtropics, particularly in hot, humid regions. Malariae malaria is also widespread, but it is of lower prevalence, and it tends to be less evenly distributed. Ovale malaria is primarily seen in West Africa.

During the past decade malaria has been found to be associated geographically with several other conditions, including various erythrocyte abnormalities and Burkitt's lymphoma. Patients with sickle hemoglobin have been shown to acquire falciparum malaria as frequently as those with normal hemoglobin, but their disease is less severe. The malaria parasite appears less able to divide in these abnormal erythrocytes. Other hemoglobinopathies and inherited enzyme defects, including hemoglobin C, D, E, K, O, b-thalassemia, and glucose-6-phosphate dehydrogenase deficiency, have also been shown to occur more commonly in areas endemic for malaria. These defects appear to provide a selective advantage for survival in malarious areas. Correlation of the prevalence of Burkitt's lymphoma with prevalence of malaria has led to suggestions that chronic malaria suppresses mechanisms for immunologic surveillance, leading to expression of this tumor. Some work in laboratory animals chronically infected with malaria supports this view, but the relationship needs further clarification.

The epidemiology of malaria is inseparable from the epidemiology of its mosquito vectors. Entomologists must document different and changing characteristics of the numerous species of anopheline mosquitoes, including their flying and resting habits, feeding habits, and degree of resistance to insecticides. For example, a change in mosquito living habits from domestic to sylvatic in Central America has rendered the usual technique of household DDT residual spraying less effective. Several instances have been recorded in which mosquito feeding habits changed from cattle to man, resulting in epidemic malaria.

Although the mosquito is the primary vector for malaria, direct transfer of infected erythrocytes from one individual to another by blood transfusion or syringe usage in common by addicts will cause malaria. In these cases the sexual cycle in the mosquito and the pre-erythrocytic stages of malaria in man are bypassed. In the past 20 years, over 50 cases of malaria transmitted by transfusions were reported in the United States. The American Association of Blood Banks has recommended that blood not be taken from anyone who has emigrated from an endemic area or had malaria during the preceding three years, or who has visited a malarious area during which antimalarial prophylaxis was taken in the preceding two years. Travelers to malarial areas who remained symptom free and who did not take antimalarials may donate blood after six months. An epidemic of vivax malaria (which affected 47 persons) was reported from California after the sharing of heroin injection equipment by drug addicts. In the past, malaria was transmitted intentionally by physicians as a method of causing fever in patients for treatment of neurosyphilis and other diseases. Congenitally acquired malaria probably occurs more commonly in

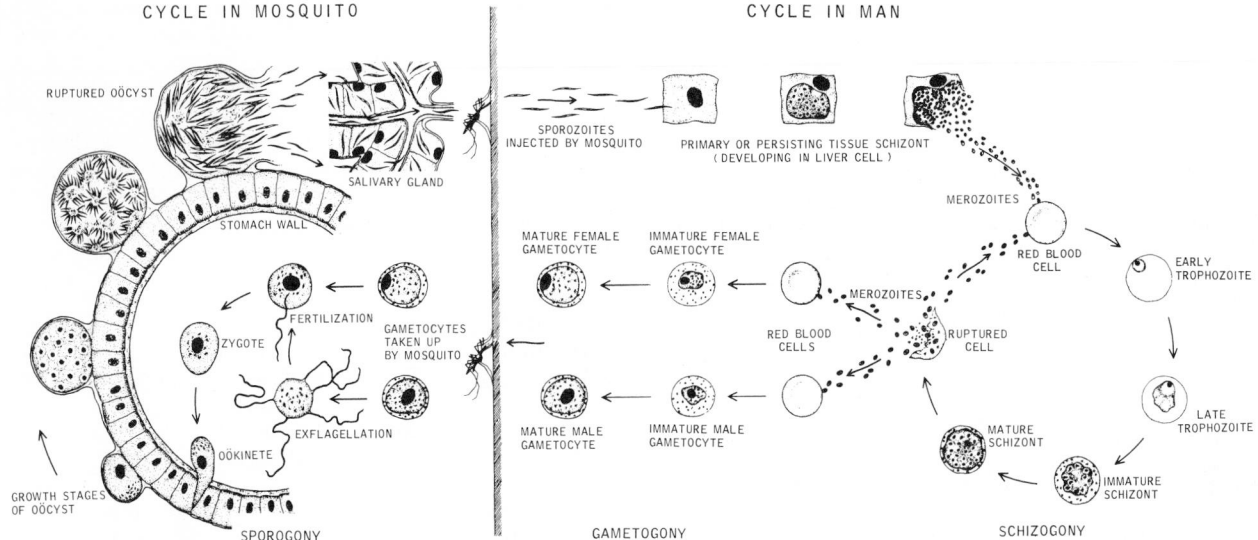

Figure 1. Life cycle of *Plasmodium* in mosquito and man. (Adapted from Alvarado, C. A., and Bruce-Chwatt, L. J.: Scientific American, Vol. 206, May, 1962. Copyright © 1962, by Scientific American, Inc. All rights reserved.)

endemic areas than has been recorded. Transmission of malaria of monkeys, *P. knowlesi* and *P. cynomolgi*, from monkey to man has been demonstrated in the laboratory and rarely documented in nature.

The major thrust against malaria has been the worldwide cooperative program of malaria eradication begun approximately 25 years ago. The program was a unified approach divided into four carefully defined phases: preparatory, attack, consolidation, and maintenance. The techniques included concentrated spraying with residual insecticides, use of antimalarial drugs, and case-detection surveys. Recently, a number of problems have challenged the completion of malaria eradication using these techniques: inadequate finances in some regions; social disorganization during war and natural disaster; resistance of mosquitoes to insecticides; and resistance of plasmodia to antimalarial drugs. Realization of these limitations has led to programs concentrating on malaria control rather than eradicaton. There has been an increased interest in malaria immunity, both to define mechanisms of natural or acquired resistance and to develop potentially useful vaccines.

THE PROTOZOAN. Over 100 different species of *Plasmodium* are capable of infecting the red blood cells of mammals, birds, and reptiles. There are several hundred species of *Anopheles* mosquitoes which can be infected by the protozoan and therefore transmit the disease. Male anopheline mosquitoes feed on nectar and therefore do not transmit the infection. The female requires products of a blood meal for egg production. Female mosquitoes vary in their feeding habits so that only 50 species participate in transmission of human malaria. During the process of feeding, the mosquito injects fluid from the salivary glands. Sporozoites may be released with the salivary fluid if the mosquito ate a blood meal two to four weeks previously which contained male and female malaria gametocytes (Fig. 1).

The sporozoites enter the circulation immediately, and a transient parasitemia occurs which lasts less than one hour. During this period the sporozoites enter hepatic parenchymal cells, initiating the *pre-erythrocytic* stage of plasmodium infection by forming a primary

hepatic schizont. The duration of this pre-erythrocytic stage is usually short in *P. falciparum* (5.5 to 7 days) and *P. vivax* (6 to 8 days) but somewhat longer in *P. ovale* (9 days) and *P. malariae* (13 to 16 days). Merozoites are then released from the hepatic cells and enter circulating erythrocytes. Occasionally, when the number of sporozoites inoculated is very low, the period from infection to onset of erythrocyte infection lasts for months or even years. In falciparum malaria the tissue phase terminates at the beginning of the *erythrocyte cycle*; in vivax and ovale malaria, the hepatic forms persist.* This species variation necessitates different therapeutic approaches in treating malaria. The species also differ in the number of merozoites released after primary hepatic schizogony: *P. falciparum*, about 40,000 from each infected cell; *P. ovale*, 15,000; *P. vivax*, 10,000; and *P. malariae*, 2000. The large number of merozoites released into the cirulation in *P. falciparum* may contribute to the high levels of parasitemia seen in this infection and perhaps to the increased frequency with which erythrocytes are observed to contain multiple organisms.

The merozoite attaches to specific receptors on the red blood cell and then enters by inducing erythrocyte endocytosis, and the organism begins to develop within a vacuole in the erythrocyte. Using Giemsa or Wright stains, the parasite is first identified with light microscopy as a characteristic "ring-form," an early *trophozoite* (Figs. 2A and 2B). The organism increases in size, partially filling the red blood cell; this is termed the late *trophozoite*. Later the nuclear material is segregated by schizogony, and the red cell becomes partially filled with the cytoplasm and the multiple nuclei of the *schizont* (Fig. 2C). The erythrocyte cycle is completed when the red blood cells rupture, releasing the merozoites formed from the schizont, which then invade other erythrocytes. This cycle takes 48 hours in *P.*

*The exoerythrocytic state is described in this chapter as "persistent" rather than cyclic, based on the arguments presented by Coatney et al. in the first cited reference. It is recognized that not all malariologists agree with this change in terms or the implied change in the nature of tissue schizogony and the mechanism of relapse.

falciparum, P. vivax, and *P. ovale* malaria, and 72 hours in *P. malariae* infection. Symptoms of fever and chills coincide with the release of merozoites; hence the clinical descriptions of tertian malaria (fevers on days one and three) and quartan malaria (fevers on days one and four). The number of merozoites formed during erythrocyte schizogony is helpful in species diagnosis. Examination of a mature schizont of *P. malariae* will reveal 6 to 12 developing merozoites, *P. ovale* 6 to 16, and *P. vivax* 12 to 24.

By mechanisms which remain unknown, some merozoites do not continue the cycle of schizogony but develop into female and male gametocytes (Fig. 1). These first appear in the peripheral blood several days after the onset of the erythrocytic cycle, and they may persist for weeks after schizogony has been suppressed. During the blood meal of an *Anopheles* mosquito, the gametocytes are ingested. Conditions exist in the stomach of the mosquito for the male gametocyte to form motile male gametes (exflagellation) which then fertilize the female gamete. After fertilization, the *zygote* becomes a motile *ookinete*, penetrates the stomach wall, and multiplies in an enlarging *oocyst.* Rupture of this cyst allows release of sporozoites which are distributed throughout the mosquito and accumulate in the salivary gland. The formation of sporozoites completes the process of *sporogony,* the sexual or mosquito cycle of malaria.

PATHOGENESIS AND IMMUNITY. There has been no documentation of generalized or significant host injury or response during the periods of sporozoitemia or hepatic schizogony, although antisporozoite antibodies have been demonstrated. After release of merozoites from the hepatic cells into the circulation, however, marked changes occur. Parasitized and nonparasitized red blood cells undergo alterations. In *P. falciparum* infection the erythrocytes develop electron-dense knoblike projections, take unusual shapes, and become less deformable. They also become more adhesive to vascular endothelium and more permeable to sodium, and demonstrate increased osmotic fragility. During the erythrocyte cycle, red blood cells are damaged at the time merozoites are released, leading to intravascular hemolysis and progressive anemia. Damage to vascular endothelium also occurs. B lymphocytes begin to produce immunoglobulin M and G antibodies directed against the merozoites, and excess antibody is seen in the plasma in several days. These antibodies coat merozoites, after which they do not enter uninfected red cells, and they are removed from the circulation by phagocytic cells in the bone marrow, spleen, and liver. T lymphocytes release materials which stimulate increased metabolic and phagocytic activity of macrophages. This series of events produces the clinical and pathologic changes observed in acute and chronic malaria.

In acute falciparum malaria a number of complications result from alteration of the red blood cells and the vascular endothelium. The severe anemia and the adherence of red cells to capillary endothelium decrease oxygen supply to the tissues. The anoxia causes serious functional impairment of the brain and kidneys, less commonly of the liver, myocardium, and bone marrow. In fatal cases of falciparum malaria the brain is edematous, and blood vessels are occluded by parasitized erythrocytes, and surrounded by areas of hemorrhage and necrosis. The kidney may show ischemia of the renal cortex and diffuse glomerulitis, as well as tubular necrosis. The liver may show centrilobular degeneration and necrosis. These changes in the kidney and liver are believed related more to ischemia secondary to severe anemia and hypovolemia than to vascular obstruction by erythrocytes. In patients who die in pulmonary edema unrelated to fluid overload, the cardiac and pulmonary vessels are filled with parasitized red cells. Impaired bone marrow function in man is manifested by thrombocytopenia, absence of reticulocytes, and varying degrees of leukopenia.

Accelerated intravascular coagulation can be documented in patients with malaria; that is, factors V, VII, VIII, X, fibrinogen, and platelets are decreased, prothrombin and partial thromboplastin times are prolonged, and fibrin degradation products are increased. However, disseminated intravascular coagulation is not a prominent feature at autopsy of patients who die of malaria.

During the acute attack of falciparum malaria, most patients develop vasodilation, just as in other acute febrile diseases. This results in decreased effective circulating blood volume and orthostatic hypotension. Changes secondary to this include increased aldosterone levels, increased plasma volume, hyponatremia, and reversal of the urinary sodium to potassium ratio.

Some of the clinical and pathologic features of malaria are related to the host immune response. Patients occasionally have a Coombs-positive hemolytic anemia. This may partially explain the rapid intravascular hemolysis which exceeds that attributable to the level of parasitemia alone. "Blackwater fever," the complication of falciparum malaria characterized by rapid hemolysis and acute renal failure, occurs both in patients who have received quinine and in patients who have a history of previous exposure to the *Plasmodium* and who have not received quinine. Antibody damage to red cells has been postulated in both situations. The pathologic changes seen in blackwater fever include renal ischemia and tubular necrosis. Recent evidence has suggested that the glomerulitis seen in some patients with falciparum malaria may be induced by immune complexes.

The pathologic picture in malaria of long duration is in large part that due to the immune response. Marked elevation of the serum immunoglobulins (IgG and IgM) is seen, and the liver and spleen are enlarged consistent with continued stimulation to the reticuloendothelial system. Anemia is common. A number of patients in an area hyperendemic for malaria develop marked splenomegaly (tropical splenomegaly syndrome). Parasites may not be demonstrable in peripheral blood smears, but elevated fluorescent antimalarial antibody titers are present, and the patients respond to prolonged therapy with antimalarials. Liver biopsy frequently shows hepatic sinusoidal lymphocytosis. In *P. malariae* infection of long duration, nephrotic syndrome is not uncommon. There is good evidence that this is related to immune complex injury to the glomerulus. Preliminary evidence has suggested that patients with chronic malaria have depressed cellular immune responses.

Host Resistance. Resistance to malaria involves numerous complex metabolic and immunologic factors. As mentioned previously, certain hemoglobinopathies and enzyme defects of the erythrocytes render patients less vulnerable to the severe complications of malaria. Blacks are less susceptible to *P. vivax* infection than

Figure 2. *See opposite page for legend.*

whites. This has recently been shown to be associated with the absence of Duffy blood group substance in a majority of blacks. *Acquired immunity* to malaria requires both humoral and cellular defense mechanisms. Circulating antibodies are of primary importance in control of the acute infection, documented by studies in which antimalaria IgG was transferred to infected hosts and found to be protective. This protection was species specific. The role of antibody has been shown by the transfer of immunity from mother to fetus, with protection of the neonate during the period in which maternal IgG persists. Whether decreases in immunoglobulin levels contribute to relapse of malaria has not been clearly shown. The importance of cellular defense mechanisms has been suggested by the intense phagocytic activity of cells of the reticuloendothelial system during malaria infection.

CLINICAL MANIFESTATIONS. The patient with malaria experiences chills and fever, often associated with frontal headache and myalgias. In the early period of the illness the fever may be persistent for several days before developing into a synchronous periodicity, the hallmark of tertian or quartan malaria. When the typical pattern has been established, the patient has a chill, a rise in temperature to 40 to 41° C, headache, and myalgias. This is followed in several hours by diffuse sweating and a fall in temperature. In vivax and ovale malaria these paroxysms occur every 48 hours (benign tertian malaria) and in malariae malaria every 72 hours (quartan malaria). In falciparum malaria the temperature is usually persistently elevated, but it may occasionally progress to a 48-hour cycle (malignant tertian malaria). Between the paroxysms of chills and fever, the patient often feels well except for some weakness or fatigue.

The illness may occasionally begin with nonspecific symptoms such as *malaise, dry cough,* and *abdominal pain.* Most patients have *nausea* and *anorexia; vomiting* is less common. These symptoms may mislead the physician into making a diagnosis of pharyngitis, influenza, or gastroenteritis. Occasionally, the only sign of malaria is fever. In the postoperative surgical patient, fever caused by malaria is frequently confused with that caused by drug allergy. Rarely fever may be absent.

Physical examination reveals a tachycardia, and the skin is warm and flushed. *Jaundice* is not common, but occasionally it can be a prominent feature of the illness. *Hepatomegaly* is commonly found, and the liver may be moderately tender. The spleen is often palpable in acute malaria and is usually quite soft and occasionally tender. Attempts to palpate the spleen should be made carefully in view of the relative ease with which splenic rupture can occur. *Splenomegaly* is more commonly found in the early stage of vivax and ovale malaria than in falciparum malaria. Orthostatic hypotension can be documented in falciparum malaria. Lesions of herpes simplex virus may be seen.

Examination of peripheral blood after several days of illness reveals a normochromic, normocytic anemia which is usually mild, but it may be severe in prolonged infections or in those presenting with high parasitemia or acute hemolysis. The number of reticulocytes is usually normal until several days after therapy has been begun; then reticulocytosis is seen. The white blood cell count is normal or low. Monocytosis may be present, but eosinophilia is not a feature of malaria. Thrombocytopenia of a moderate degree is usually present. Serum α1 glycoproteins are increased, whereas α2 glycoproteins (containing haptoglobin) are decreased. A false-positive serologic test for syphilis (VDRL) may occur. The serum transaminases are almost always elevated to moderate degrees and total bilirubin is often elevated. This is predominantly indirect bilirubin, but occasionally increased conjugated bilirubin is seen. Severe cases of malaria may be associated with sufficient liver dysfunction to be misdiagnosed as infectious hepatitis. Tests for determining intestinal absorption have been shown to be abnormal in some malaria patients. Urinalysis reveals trace amounts of albumin and bilirubin in uncomplicated cases, and rarely marked proteinuria has been documented. In falciparum malaria hyponatremia, reversal of the urinary sodium/potassium ratio, and transient increases in serum creatinine and blood urea nitrogen can frequently be recorded.

Fever and related symptoms gradually subside over several weeks in untreated vivax, ovale, and malariae malaria. However, relapse of vivax or ovale infection may occur months or even years later. The illness at the time of relapse is usually milder and of shorter duration than the initial illness. Death caused by infection with these species is very uncommon.

Complications. In falciparum malaria high levels of parasitemia and serious complications may develop rapidly. The most important of these complications are *coma, severe hemolytic anemia, acute renal failure,* and *acute pulmonary edema.* The patient may first demonstrate confusion with increasing lethargy, and within a few hours be unconscious. Focal neurologic signs are uncommon, but hyperreflexia and Babinski signs may be seen. Examination of the cerebrospinal fluid will reveal increased pressure and increased protein, without

---

Figure 2. *A to D* show various erythrocyte forms of falciparum or vivax malaria ($\times$ 1500).

A, "Ring forms" of *Plasmodium falciparum.* Note the delicate rings and an erythrocyte containing two organisms.

B, Trophozoite of *Plasmodium vivax.* The red cell is enlarged, Schüffner's dots are seen, and the parasite is large and ameboid.

C, Schizont of *Plasmodium vivax* with at least 18 merozoite nuclei.

D, Gametocyte of *Plasmodium falciparum.* The crescent or banana shape is characteristic.

E, Trypanosoma rhodesiense in the peripheral blood. It has a nucleus, posterior kinetoplast, an undulating membrane, and flagellum ($\times$ 1500).

F, Spleen smear showing a cell filled with *Leishmania donovani.* The rod-shaped kinetoplast and large round nucleus appear as two adjacent red dots.

G, Methenamine silver nitrate stain of clump of *Pneumocystis* cysts. They appear as black circles against the blue background ($\times$ 800).

H, Stool sample observed by light microscopy, showing a motile *Entamoeba histolytica* moving in a straight line across the field. The ameba contains lucent vacuoles and shows a pseudopod directed to the upper right ($\times$ 500).

(*A, C, D,* and *F* are photographs taken by T. C. Jones from the Cornell Parasitology teaching slides; *B* is from the collection of H. Zaiman, originally photographed by M. Wittner; *E* and *G* were provided by R. B. Roberts; *H* is a photograph of fresh material provided by T. C. Jones.)

pleocytosis. *Massive intravascular hemolysis* may result from high levels of parasitemia, quinine therapy, drug administration to patients with glucose-6-phosphate dehydrogenase deficiency, or hypersensitivity after previous malaria infections. Hemoglobinuria, acute tubular necrosis, and renal failure may result. *Hemolysis, hemoglobinuria,* and *renal failure* make up the striking clinical picture of severe malaria known as "blackwater fever." Acute renal failure may occur in the absence of signs of intravascular hemolysis and can be detected early only by careful monitoring of the urine volume and serum creatinine or urea nitrogen levels. Acute pulmonary edema is an uncommon complication, but it may develop rapidly and be particularly refractory to therapy. Pulmonary edema may be due to excessive fluid administration, but a number of cases have been reported in which intravascular volume was normal. Patients may present with signs and symptoms of vascular collapse — so-called algid malaria. A rare complication of malaria is splenic rupture, the only complication which is probably more common in vivax than falciparum malaria. Patients who survive untreated falciparum malaria may have recurrences of symptoms for a number of months, but thereafter they remain asymptomatic.

Syndromes Associated with Chronic Malaria. Syndromes associated with chronic malaria are most likely the result of repeated exposure of immune patients to *Plasmodium* and occur predominantly in hyperendemic areas of malaria. The patients may be asymptomatic, but they have intermittently detectable parasitemia, hypergammaglobulinemia, elevated antimalaria antibody titers, anemia, and splenic enlargement. Some patients develop marked splenomegaly—the tropical splenomegaly syndrome. Patients infected with *P. malariae* may develop nephrotic syndrome (quartan nephrosis). This is most common in children. It is associated with a poor prognosis and does not respond well to corticosteroid administration.

DIAGNOSIS. The diagnosis of malaria must be suspected in every patient with fever, coma, or shock who has lived or traveled in a malarious area, has received a blood transfusion, or may be a drug addict. The only technique for confirming the clinical suspicion of malaria is the identification of plasmodia in fixed, stained blood smears. The diagnosis may be made by an alert technician during examination of a differential white count. However, it is usually only when a high suspicion of the possibility of malaria exists that the proper smears will be done and the necessary time taken to make the diagnosis.

Thin blood smears are made by placing a drop of blood on the end of a glass slide, touching the drop with another slide, and rapidly moving the edge of the second slide along the surface of the first. A thick blood smear is made by placing a drop of blood on a slide, then spreading it to fill a diameter of about 1 cm. The slides are allowed to dry. The thin blood smear is fixed in methanol and stained with Giemsa, or fixed and stained with Wright's. The thick blood smear is first dipped in water to lyse the red blood cells, then fixed and similarly stained. For the inexperienced observer the thin smear is easiest to examine and most likely to yield the diagnosis in the nonimmune patient with malaria. Careful examination of several thousand red blood cells on a properly stained smear will usually reveal the protozoan. When malaria is suspected but smears do not reveal the organism, smears should be repeated several times a day. The highest level of parasitemia is said to be demonstrable several hours *after* a chill. A thick smear can be particularly helpful for finding the characteristic gametocyte of falciparum malaria (Fig. 2D), but it may also reveal organisms when they are too infrequent to be easily identified on a thin smear.

The correct diagnosis of the species of *Plasmodium* is critical in determining therapy and prognosis in malaria. The following brief description and the photomicrographs in Figure 2 were selected to aid in differentiating *P. vivax* and *P. falciparum* in peripheral blood.

Differentiation of P. Vivax and P. Falciparum in Blood Smears. The following characteristics can be used to identify *P. falciparum*. Only the ring forms are usually seen in the peripheral blood; they are small and delicate, often with two chromatin dots (Fig. 2A). The erythrocytes containing these protozoa are not conspicuously enlarged, and red dots (Schüffner's dots) are not present. The level of parasitemia may be high (more than 5 to 10 per cent of the erythrocytes infected), and some erythrocytes may contain several parasites. Organisms may appear to be on the surface of the erythrocyte (appliqué forms). *P. vivax* ring forms are often larger than falciparum rings and in later stages appear quite pleomorphic (Fig. 2B). The infected erythrocytes are usually larger than normal, and if properly stained, Schüffner's dots can be identified. By examining blood films at various times, the maturation of *P. vivax* in the peripheral blood can be documented. The mature schizont (Fig. 2C) contains 12 to 24 chromatin dots, and the parasite cytoplasm almost fills the red blood cell. The gametocyte of *P. falciparum* is very characteristic (Fig. 2D) and should be looked for carefully since it substantiates the diagnosis. It has a crescent or banana shape, whereas the shape of *P. vivax* gametocytes is globular.

Mixed Infection. Even after one species of malaria is identified, it must be kept in mind that the patient could have a mixed infection (1 to 2 per cent of cases). Mixed infection can best be diagnosed by careful review of several thin blood films. Repeated blood films for one to two days after the start of treatment should show decreasing levels of parasitemia. If a *P. vivax* infection is diagnosed and treated with chloroquine but parasitemia is seen to be increasing, a mixed infection with chloroquine-resistant *P. falciparum* should be suspected. At present, *P. falciparum* infection acquired in Asia and parts of Central and South America is resistant to chloroquine (see below). All patients diagnosed as having *P. falciparum* should have repeated smears during therapy to ensure that the parasitemia is decreasing.

Chloroquine Susceptibility Test. A technique for documenting whether *P. falciparum* is susceptible or resistant has been developed. At the time of initial diagnosis and before therapy is instituted, a sample of the patient's blood is defibrinated and added to vials (1 ml each) containing varying concentrations of chloroquine and 5 mg of glucose per 100 ml. During 24 hours of incubation, *P. falciparum* will mature to the schizont stage in the vials containing insuffcient levels of chloroquine. Chloroquine susceptibility can be calculated from these data.

Antibody Tests. Antibody tests for malaria are not useful in the diagnosis of the acute illness. The indirect fluorescent antibody and hemagglutination tests are of value in testing populations to determine the prevalence of malaria and in screening blood donors when tracing cases of transfusion-induced malaria. They have also been of help in confirming recent malaria and supporting morphologic diagnosis of malaria species.

Differential Diagnosis. The differential diagnosis of malaria is lengthy and varies, depending upon the area of the world, the dominant malaria species, and whether the disease is acute or chronic. The fever of malaria must be separated from fever caused by dengue and other arboviruses, typhus, amebiasis, typhoid, relapsing fever, heat stroke, drug allergy, influenza, bacterial pneumonias, and wound infections. Intermittent chills secondary to antipyretics may simulate the chills and fever of malaria in all these conditions. Cerebral malaria must be distinguished from viral encephalitides, drug overdose, and other causes of coma. The jaundice of malaria must be distinguished from viral hepatitis and leptospirosis. In more chronic malaria infection in which splenomegaly and anemia are prominent, one must also consider infective endocarditis, schistosomiasis, visceral leishmaniasis, and lymphoma.

THERAPY. Elimination of Parasitemia. The initial therapeutic goal in the treatment of malaria is to eliminate the erythrocytic stage of the infection, because all the acute symptoms are due to this hematogenous process. Chloroquine, a 4-aminoquinoline, is the drug of choice to accomplish this purpose. It can be given orally, or parenterally if the patient is vomiting. Chloroquine diphosphate is given orally as follows: 1 gram initially (600 mg of base), followed by 500 mg (300 mg of base) at 6 hours, 24 hours, and 48 hours after the initial dose (total dose 2.5 grams; 1.5 grams of base). Children should receive a loading dose of 17 mg per kilogram, followed by 8.5 mg per kilogram at 6, 24, and 48 hours.* Chloroquine hydrochloride is available for intramuscular or intravenous injection. It is important to note that the hydrochloride salt contains a different quantity of chloroquine base than the diphosphate salt. Chloroquine base, 300 mg, is given intramuscularly every six hours for three doses (total of 900 mg base). On the second and third days therapy may be changed to oral medication, or single intramuscular injections can be continued until a total dose of 1.5 grams chloroquine base is reached. Intravenous medication with chloroquine is seldom indicated, because the patient in shock or coma will usually be given quinine realizing the possibility of a drug-resistant infection (see below). If intravenous chloroquine is considered necessary, 300 mg of base is diluted in 300 ml of saline and given over 30 to 60 minutes. It can be given every six to eight hours, but not in excess of a total daily dose of 1000 mg of base.

The exact mechanism of action of chloroquine remains unknown. It interrupts the vacuolar digestive mechanisms of protozoa, and it binds strongly to nucleic acids. Higher concentrations of the drug are found in infected erythrocytes than in uninfected cells or plasma. This enhanced uptake of chloroquine by parasitized cells may be very important, as suggested by the observation that chloroquine-resistant strains do not enhance the concentration of chloroquine by erythrocytes. In spite of the fact that chloroquine is also concentrated in the liver, it is ineffective in inhibiting tissue schizogony. Chloroquine is absorbed rapidly from the gastrointestinal tract. Fifty per cent becomes bound

to plasma proteins, and only about 10 per cent of the active compound is excreted in the urine. Most of the drug is concentrated in tissue, and degradation probably occurs in the liver. It disappears from tissue over a period of several weeks after the drug is stopped. Chloroquine is usually well tolerated, but it can cause transient headache, visual disturbances, nausea, and vomiting. At toxic levels it can cause delirium, psychotic reactions, and convulsions. Its use is not contraindicated during pregnancy for treatment of malaria. When given for prolonged periods in doses higher than that used in malaria chemoprophylaxis, punctate keratitis and retinitis have been recorded. Amodiaquine is as effective as chloroquine for treating malaria.

Drug-Resistant Plasmodia. When falciparum malaria is diagnosed, a careful history must include the country where the infection was acquired. If the illness was acquired in South America or Central America, and the level of parasitemia is greater than 2 per cent of erythrocytes, or if it was acquired in any part of Asia, regardless of the level of parasitemia, or if the source of the infection is unknown (such as in transfusion malaria) and parasitemia is high, then quinine sulfate should be used instead of chloroquine. *P. falciparum* acquired in the areas cited has been documented to show varying degrees of resistance to chloroquine.

Resistance of plasmodia to antimalarial drugs has been recognized for many years. Shortly after pyrimethamine and proguanil were introduced, strains resistant to these drugs were identified. This was not unexpected, because protozoa have been known to rapidly develop resistance to inhibitors of folate metabolism. Strains of *P. falciparum* which required higher than standard doses of quinine for inhibition were recorded many years ago. Only in the past decade, however, has the problem of drug resistance been brought to particular attention by appearance of resistance of *P. falciparum* to previously accepted therapeutic levels of chloroquine. Resistant strains apeared in several parts of the world at about the same time, unrelated to whether chloroquine had been commonly used in the area or not.

Resistance of *P. falciparum* to chloroquine has been divided, based on response in level of parasitemia after initiation of therapy: no reduction (termed RIII level of resistance), and partial reduction (termed RII). The first level of chloroquine resistance (RI), to be considered in more detail below, is one in which *patent* parasitemia is eradicated but parasitemia and clinical symptoms recur in a few days to several weeks; i.e., recrudescent malaria. At present, quinine is effective in removing patent parasitemia in these cases; however, a number of other drugs are necessary to prevent recrudescence. Careful attention to the diagnosis of chloroquine-resistant malaria is now an integral part of the management of patients with malaria (see Diagnosis).

To eradicate parasitemia in cases suspected to be caused by chloroquine-resistant strains, quinine is given orally, 650 mg every eight hours for 10 to 14 days. Quinine dihydrochloride is used intravenously in patients unable to take the drug orally. Quinine, 600 mg, is dissolved in 100 to 200 ml of 5 per cent glucose and water and administered over 30 minutes. This is repeated every eight hours. The mechanism of action of quinine against the malaria parasite is unknown. It has been shown to block protein synthetic and glycolytic pathways. It is absorbed readily from the gastrointesti-

---

*See p. vi, Dosage Notice, immediately following Preface.

nal tract, and over 70 per cent is bound to plasma proteins. Like chloroquine, it is concentrated in tissues, including erythrocytes. Only 5 per cent of administered quinine is excreted unchanged in the urine. The most common side effects of quinine are tinnitus, vertigo, nausea, and vomiting. Although these symptoms are annoying, they are not indications to discontinue medication. Since deafness and blindness have been reported due to quinine, blood levels should be checked and decreased dosage should be considered in those with signs of significant nerve toxicity. A Coombs-positive hemolytic anemia is a rare complication of quinine therapy.

Prevention of Recrudescent Falciparum Malaria. Recrudescence of falciparum malaria occurs frequently in patients whose infection was acquired in Asia, Central America, or South America. Recrudescence is due to persistence during an asymptomatic period of erythrocytic stages of *P. falciparum* at undetectable levels, followed by increased parasitemia and symptoms several days to six weeks after apparently successful control of the illness by chloroquine or quinine. This is the first level of chloroquine resistance (RI). To prevent this, several drugs have been added to the initial therapeutic program for treatment of falciparum malaria acquired in the areas previously mentioned. Most commonly, pyrimethamine is given, 50 mg orally per day for three days in combination with sulfadiazine, 1 gram every six hours for five days. A long-acting sulfonamide, e.g., sulfadoxine,* is frequently used in place of sulfadiazine. These drugs act by blocking folate metabolism at the paraminobenzoic acid and the dehydrofolate reductase steps. They can cause bone marrow suppression and allergic reactions. Difference of opinion exists over whether these drugs should be started on the first day of chloroquine or quinine therapy or several days later. We recommend that the drugs be started at the end of chloroquine treatment or on the fourth day of quinine therapy. This reduces the possibility of complicating the clinical picture by potential side effects of the drugs. Clindamycin or tetracycline has been found effective in combination with quinine against recrudescence of falciparum malaria. In cases in which recrudescence has occurred repeatedly, intravenous quinine has been used in place of oral quinine in combination with these drugs.

Gametocytes usually disappear from the peripheral blood within a few days after schizogony is interrupted, and no specific therapy is needed. Primaquine is an effective gametocidal drug and can be used in the rare patient with prolonged asymptomatic gametocytemia.

Prevention of Relapse Due to Persistent Hepatic Schizonts. Relapse of *P. vivax* and *P. ovale* malaria is caused by the persistence of hepatic schizogony.† Primaquine, an 8-aminoquinoline, is usually effective in preventing relapse (approximately 90 per cent of patients are cured). Since relapse is common in these infections, chloroquine therapy should always be followed by a course of primaquine. The adult dose is 15 mg of base daily for 14 days. Children should be given 0.25 mg per kilogram of body weight per day for 14 days. If relapse occurs after a full course of primaquine, a second 14-day period of therapy is usually successful.

The mechanism of action of primaquine is unknown, but it does appear to block glycolysis.

Primaquine can induce hemolysis in patients whose erythrocytes are deficient in glucose-6-phosphate dehydrogenase. Therefore patients should be tested for this deficiency before therapy is started, and if glucose-6-phosphate dehydrogenase deficiency is documented, red blood cell counts should be monitored carefully during treatment.

Supportive Therapy. Treatment of malaria is often accomplished with ease even in cases of falciparum malaria. However, since the course of falciparum malaria is unpredictable and complications may develop rapidly, all cases should be approached as medical emergencies. The management of a patient with malaria includes complete bed rest during the period of orthostatic hypotension. In the occasional patient with very high fever, this should be controlled by continuous antipyretic administration, sponging, and cooling. Frequent determinations of hematocrit, electrolytes, creatinine, urine volume, bilirubin, and transaminases are necessary. The level of consciousness should be carefully monitored.

The patient with falciparum malaria should receive transfusions with packed erythrocytes if severe anemia develops. The vascular volume and cardiac function should be monitored carefully by following the blood pressure, and in severe cases monitoring the central venous pressure may be necessary. Intravenous fluids should be given judiciously with full knowledge of the vascular volume, renal function, and serum electrolytes.

If cerebral malaria develops, the patient should be managed according to procedures used in the care of any comatose patient (see Ch. 219). Corticosteroids have been advocated in these cases to reduce cerebral edema. Heparin therapy should be considered in the rare patients documented to have clinically significant intravascular coagulation.

If the patient develops oliguria, a trial of furosemide or mannitol may be given. However, when acute renal failure is present, judicious administration of fluids associated with hemodialysis or peritoneal dialysis is indicated (see Ch. 372). The dose of quinine should be reduced to half in patients with renal failure, but maintained at therapeutic levels once hemo- or peritoneal dialysis is instituted.

If signs of pulmonary edema develop, standard therapeutic approaches are indicated, including digitalis preparations and methods to reduce the central venous pressure. This complication, however, has been quite refractory to treatment.

PREVENTION. An individual entering an area where malaria remains endemic must avoid contact with mosquitoes and systematically take drug prophylaxis. Use of mosquito netting, screens, insecticides, and mosquito repellents are the main mechanisms for avoiding contact with mosquitoes. The best repellent available at present is N,N-diethyltoluamide. It remains effective for up to 18 hours, a considerable advance over the odor repellents which are of value for only two or four hours.

The best means of malaria prevention is chemoprophylaxis. This is a cumbersome method, requiring intelligence, compulsiveness, and often willingness to tolerate the mild side effects of the medicaton. Travelers should check with medical officials in the area they visit for up-to-date advice on malaria chemoprophy-

---

*This ultralong-acting sulfonamide is not available in the United States, but is available in the United Kingdom.
†See footnote, page 568.

laxis. The primary drug recommended for prophylaxis for travelers from the United States is chloroquine diphosphate or sulfate. Five hundred milligrams (300 mg of chloroquine base) is taken once a week. Children of ages 8 to 12 should receive 250 mg; ages 4 to 7, 200 mg; and ages 1 to 3, 125 mg; infants should receive 75 mg weekly. Where malaria is hyperendemic, 500 mg twice weekly has been recommended. Chloroquine should be started one to two weeks before entering the malarious area and continued for six weeks after departure from the area. Chloroquine does not prevent the hepatic infection, but simply suppresses the erythrocytic stage; *therefore the period of prophylaxis after leaving the malarious area is very important.* It is this period which travelers most often ignore and which leads to their illness several weeks after leaving the endemic area. After chloroquine prophylaxis, primaquine (15 mg of base per day) should be given for 14 days to eradicate the hepatic stages of plasmodia infections.

A single tablet containing 300 mg of chloroquine base and 45 mg of primaquine base was used for chemoprophylaxis by the U.S. military during the Vietnam war. This tablet is not recommended for use in preference to chloroquine alone. However, if primaquine is unavailable, this drug combination may be used after the traveler leaves the endemic area; it will prevent chloroquine-sensitive falciparum malaria and relapsing malaria. One tablet is taken per week for eight weeks. It is important that this combination *not* be used in the treatment of malaria, because the dose of primaquine base is at toxic levels when 1.5 grams of chloroquine base is given.

Prophylaxis When Chloroquine Resistance Is Present. Chloroquine prophylaxis may be ineffective in areas such as Asia and parts of Central and South America where chloroquine-resistant falciparum malaria is encountered. Travelers to these areas must balance their likely level of exposure to infected mosquitoes with the dangers of more vigorous chemoprophylaxis. The Center for Disease Control has recommended that travelers to these countries take chloroquine in the dose usually recommended for other areas of the world (500 mg once weekly). Chloroguanide hydrochloride (100 to 200 mg per day) is an effective alternative to chloroquine chemoprophylaxis. The travelers must be told that these drugs may not be effective, and they should seek medical care promptly if fever occurs. A drug combination which at present is completely effective in preventing chloroquine-resistant falciparum malaria is pyrimethamine, 25 mg, plus sulfadoxine,* 500 mg, taken once a week. This combination is not available in the United States, but it can be obtained in many other countries. Another effective drug combination is chloroguanide hydrochloride, 100 mg per day, plus dapsone, 25 mg daily. However, an increased risk of agranulocytosis caused by dapsone makes it less desirable as chemoprophylaxis for civilian travelers unless heavy exposure to infected mosquitoes is anticipated.

Prevention in a Community. Prevention of malaria in communities in endemic areas requires a coordinated effort directed at reducing the number of *Anophleles* mosquitoes and identifying and treating human cases of malaria. *Anopheles* are reduced in the environment by draining or filling breeding areas and by the use of larvicides. Effective campaigns against adult mosquitoes usually include spraying of all buildings with residual insecticides twice a year. DDT has been particularly effective for this purpose in the past; however, because of mosquito resistance and potential unacceptable side effects of DDT, other drugs such as hexachlorocyclohexane, dieldrin, malathion, and carbamates are now being used.

In areas endemic for malaria, use of chemoprophylactic drugs is usually reserved for children or pregnant women (to prevent congenital transmission of malaria). In some areas entire populations are treated by including the drug in the salt distribution for daily use. These approaches are used to reduce morbidity and mortality before adequate immunity is acquired. It is hoped that some form of active immunization will replace this method in the future.

Coatney, G. R., Collins, W. E., Warren, M., and Contacos, P. G.: The Primate Malarias. U.S. Department of Health, Education, and Welfare, National Institutes of Health. Washington, D.C., U.S. Government Printing Office, 1971.

Hall, A. P.: The treatment of malaria. Br. Med. J., 1:323, 1976.

Inter-American Malaria Research Symposium. Am. J. Trop. Med. Hyg., 21:613, 1972.

Jeffery, G. M.: Malaria control in the twentieth century. Am. J. Trop. Med. Hyg., 25:361, 1976.

Maegraith, B., and Fletcher, A.: The pathogenesis of mammalian malaria. Adv. Parasitol., 10:49, 1972.

Miller, L. H.: Malaria. *In* Hoeprich, P. D. (ed.): Infectious Diseases. 2nd ed. Hagerstown, Md., Harper & Row, 1977, p. 1075.

Miller, L. H., Mason, S. J., Dovorak, J. A., McGinniss, M. H., and Rothman, I. K.: Erythrocyte receptors for (*Plasmodium knowlesi*) malaria: The Duffy blood group determinants. Science, 189:561, 1975.

Neva, F. A., Sheagren, J. N., Shulman, N. R., and Canfield, C. J.: Malaria: Host-defense mechanisms and complications. Ann. Intern. Med., 73:295, 1970.

World Health Organization: Chemotherapy of Malaria and Resistance to Antimalarials. WHO Tech. Rep. Series No. 529, 1973.

194. TRYPANOSOMIASES

194.1. INTRODUCTION

Philip D. Marsden

Some differences between the four species of trypanosomes which can be found in the bloodstream of man are listed in the accompanying table. *Trypanosoma rangeli* is nonpathogenic but may be mistaken for *T. cruzi* in bug feces during xenodiagnosis. In contrast to *T. cruzi*, *T. rangeli* can be found in the hemolymph and salivary glands of reduviid bugs. In areas where the two species coexist, dissection of such bugs is necessary.

There are similarities as well as differences between Chagas' disease and African sleeping sickness. Essentially both infections have three phases. There is an initial phase of local multiplication following inoculation and a secondary phase of bloodstream dissemination with reticuloendothelial activation; together, these constitute the acute phase of Chagas' disease and first and second stages of sleeping sickness. The blood trypanosome can be found in blood films at this time.

The prolonged tertiary phase is one of organ localization and damage, involving tropisms that are still poorly understood. With the development of immunity the trypanosome is no longer visible in blood films, and

---

*This ultralong-acting sulfonamide is not available in the United States, but is available in the United Kingdom.

Some Differences Between the Human Trypanosomiases

	Trypanosoma gambiense, rhodesiense	Trypanosoma cruzi	Trypanosoma rangeli
Geographic distribution	Africa	South and Central America	Central and South America
Insect vector	Glossina	Reduviidae	Reduviidae
Pathogenicity for insect vector	Low	Low	High
Pathogenicity for man	High	High	Low
Method of transmission by insect	Saliva (bite)	Contamination with feces	Saliva (bite)
Site of dominant human pathology	Brain	Heart muscle, smooth muscle of gut	No pathology
Multiplying form of organism in man	Trypanomastigote	Amastigote	Trypanomastigote
Size of kinetoplast of blood trypanosome	Small	Large	Small

special diagnostic techniques are necessary to demonstrate it. Serology becomes important as a diagnostic aid. During the dissemination phase trypanosomes come in contact with all body tissues, but chronic inflammatory processes proceed principally in the cerebrum in African trypanosomiasis and in the heart and smooth muscle in Chagas' disease. In both diseases evidence of autoimmune mechanisms responsible for this pathology has begun to appear in the literature. Both diseases are notoriously difficult to treat, and to date vaccine production has been impossible. The best hope for control lies in breaking the contact between man and the infected insect vector.

Cancado, J. R.: Doenca de Chagas. Belo Horizonte. Imprensa Oficial do Estado de Minas Gerais, 1968.
D'Alessandro, A.: Biology of Trypanosoma (Herpetosoma) rangeli. Tejera, 1920. In Lumsden, W. H. R., and Evans, D. A.: Biology of the Kinetoplastida. Vol. I. London, Academic Press, 1976, pp. 327–403.
Mulligan, H. W., and Potts, W. H. (eds.): The African Trypanosomiases. London, Allen and Unwin, 1970.

194.2. AFRICAN TRYPANOSOMIASIS (Sleeping Sickness)

B. M. Greenwood

DEFINITION AND ETIOLOGY. *Trypanosoma brucei*, the causative agent of African trypanosomiasis, is named after Sir David Bruce, who, in 1894, demonstrated that this organism caused the cattle disease nagana. Eight years later it was shown that the same trypanosome caused human sleeping sickness, a disease that occurs in two forms — West African or Gambian sleeping sickness and East African or Rhodesian sleeping sickness. Trypanosomes causing these diseases cannot be distinguished morphologically, but differentiation of strains that are pathogenic for man from those that are not is often important. In the past this has been achieved by infecting human volunteers, but safer methods are now available. Nonpathogenic strains (*T. b. brucei*) lose their infectivity for laboratory animals when incubated in human serum, whereas the two strains pathogenic for man (*T. b. gambiense* and *T. b. rhodesiense*) do not. These two strains can usually be differentiated by the electrophoretic pattern of two of their component enzymes, alanine aminotransferase and aspartate aminotransferase.

On light microscopy *T. brucei* is seen to be an elongated trypanosome with a prominent nucleus, kinetoplast, and flagellum. Its length varies from 10 to 40 μ, slender and stumpy forms being found in the patient at the same time. Electron microscopy has revealed the detailed structure of the trypanosome. It is coated with an amorphous material which contains the variant antigens which are of vital importance to its survival.

EPIDEMIOLOGY. Distribution and Prevalence of Sleeping Sickness. Sleeping sickness is restricted to tropical Africa where it has probably occurred in scattered foci for many centuries. The disease was described in the ancient kingdom of Mali in the fourteenth century, and sleeping sickness was well known to the West African slave traders. Around 1890, major epidemics broke out in the Congo basin, around Lake Victoria, and in Nigeria, perhaps because the early colonial explorers and traders carried the disease into areas where it had not previously occurred. At least half a million people died in these epidemics. In the 1930's, the disease again became very active in West Africa, 300,000 cases occurring in Nigeria alone. Since 1950, the incidence of the disease has declined, with the exception of a major outbreak in Zaire in the early 1960's which followed a breakdown in surveillance measures. Zaire still accounts for most of the 5000 to 10,000 cases of sleeping sickness reported annually. Small outbreaks still occur intermittently in nearly all West and Central African countries south of the Sahara. In East Africa the disease is most active in Tanzania and Zambia, a few cases occurring in neighboring countries. In 1968, a new focus of sleeping sickness was discovered in Ethiopia. When present in cattle, trypanosomiasis also affects human health indirectly through its role in contributing to protein malnutrition. In large areas of tropical Africa it is not possible to rear cattle because of trypanosomiasis; in other areas the infection produces sickly animals giving a poor yield of meat.

Pathway of Infection. Tsetse flies are the natural vector of African trypanosomiasis, but it is possible that the disease may occasionally be transmitted mechanically by other biting flies. Intrauterine transmission has been recorded. Infections have followed accidental inoculation with trypanosomes in the laboratory.

When a tsetse fly bites an infected host, trypanosomes are sucked into the midgut with the blood meal. Here they pass through the peritrophic membrane, migrate forward between it and the gut wall, penetrate the gut wall, and reach the salivary glands where development into new infective forms occurs. When a new host is bitten, trypanosomes pass down the proboscis with the saliva to start a new infection. Development within the fly takes two to five weeks.

Epidemiology of Gambian Sleeping Sickness. Man is the only known natural host of *T. b. gambiense*. Pigs, rodents, and other animals can be infected experimentally, but the existence of an important natural reservoir has never been established. Gambian sleeping sickness is spread mainly by two species of tsetse fly, *Glossina palpalis* and *G. tachinoides*. These flies inhabit the shaded areas alongside rivers and streams, areas where their human victims can often be found as they come to the stream for water. In some areas these flies will also rest and bite within a village. Contact between man and these species of tsetse flies is often very close, providing ideal conditions for transmission of the disease.

Epidemiology of Rhodesian Sleeping Sickness. *T. b. rhodesiense* differs from *T. b. gambiense* in being primarily a parasite of wild game, man acting only as an occasional and accidental host. Rhodesian sleeping sickness is spread by tsetse flies of the *G. morsitans* group, flies that can live in open savanna with enough vegetation to provide shade and resting places. Rhodesian sleeping sickness is an occupational disease, occurring mainly in those whose work takes them into areas of bush where wild game, especially the bushbuck, survives. Hunters, fishermen, honey-gatherers, and tourists are all at risk. This form of trypanosomiasis is usually a sporadic infection, but epidemics can occur. In the epidemic situation direct man-to-man transmission probably takes place.

PATHOLOGY.   Few studies of the pathology of African trypanosomiasis have been made since the classic work of Mott published in 1906. In the early stage of the disease the lymph nodes and spleen are enlarged and infiltrated with plasma cells and macrophages. Later, lymph nodes shrink and patchy fibrosis occurs. Lymphocytic infiltration of the pericardium and myocardium may be found, especially in the Rhodesian form of the disease. Characteristic changes are found in the brain and meninges once invasion of the central nervous system has occurred. These changes are most marked in longstanding cases of Gambian sleeping sickness. The meninges are thickened and infiltrated with lymphocytes, plasma cells, and morular cells. Morular cells are large cells with an eccentric nucleus displaced by numerous cytoplasmic vesicles which contain IgM. As the disease progresses, chronic inflammatory changes extend along the perivascular spaces to produce prominent perivascular cuffing. Finally, infiltration of the brain substance with lymphocytes, plasma cells, and morular cells takes place with accompanying neuronal degeneration and microglial proliferation.

PATHOGENESIS AND IMMUNITY.   The immune response of the host probably plays an important part in the pathogenesis of sleeping sickness. Stimulation of the reticuloendothelial and humoral immune systems contributes to the lymphadenopathy and splenomegaly of the early phase of the disease. Vessel damage is an important feature of the advanced stage of the infection and may be due to immune complex deposition, for patients with sleeping sickness have high levels of circulating immune complexes and have laboratory features indicating activation of the complement and kinin pathways.

T. brucei possesses surface and core antigens which both induce a humoral immune response. Little is known about the role of cell-mediated immunity in this infection. In the presence of antibody, trypanosomes are lysed or taken up by cells of the reticuloendothelial system, but successful eradication of the parasite is prevented by the phenomenon of antigenic variation. By progressive alteration of the structure of its surface antigens, the trypanosome is able to keep continually one step ahead of the host's immune response and thus to persist until the host eventually dies. The mechanism of antigenic variation is not known, but contact with antibody probably initiates the antigenic switch.

Large amounts of IgM are produced in the serum and cerebrospinal fluid of patients with sleeping sickness. Only a small proportion of this immunoglobulin is parasite-specific antibody; the rest contains antibodies with a wide variety of specificities, including autoantibodies. The mechanism of this polyclonal B lymphocyte activation is not understood and is currently being studied. Humoral and cellular immune responses are suppressed in patients with sleeping sickness, and this immunosuppression may underlie their increased susceptibility to secondary infections such as pneumonia.

CLINICAL FEATURES.   Sleeping sickness passes through three pathologic and clinical phases: an initial phase in which trypanosomes are localized to the site of the tsetse fly bite; an early or systemic phase in which trypanosomes are widely distributed throughout the body; and a neurologic or advanced stage in which trypanosomes are largely restricted to the central nervous system. Rhodesian sleeping sickness is usually a much more rapidly progressive illness than Gambian sleeping sickness with less distinction between systemic and neurologic stages. However, this distinction is not an absolute one; in some outbreaks Gambian sleeping sickness has progressed rapidly, whereas occasionally Rhodesian sleeping sickness follows a more benign course.

Gambian Sleeping Sickness.   Ten days after a bite by an infected tsetse fly, a small nodular lesion, a chancre, may develop at the site of the bite and persist for two to three weeks. This lesion, if it occurs, frequently passes unnoticed.

Months or even years after an infected bite, systemic invasion with trypanosomes occurs. Fever and lymphadenopathy are the main features of this early stage of the infection. Fever is usually intermittent and may be mild.

Some Contrasting Features of Gambian and Rhodesian Sleeping Sickness

	Gambian Sleeping Sickness	Rhodesian Sleeping Sickness
Causative organism	*Trypanosoma brucei gambiense*	*Trypanosoma brucei rhodesiense*
Distribution	West and Central Africa	East Africa
Source of infection	Man	Wild game (man)
Vector	*Glossina palpalis* or *tachinoides* (riverine tsetse)	*Glossina morsitans* (savanna tsetse)
Clinical features		
Lymphadenopathy	++	+
Heart failure	0	++
Neurologic	++	+
Disseminated intravascular coagulation	0	+
Diagnosis	Trypanosomes in lymph node juice or CSF	Trypanosomes in blood or CSF
Course of infection	Slow	Rapid

Lymphadenopathy may be general, but the posterior cervical nodes are nearly always involved. Enlarged nodes are firm but not usually tender. Moderate splenomegaly may occur. Urticarial rashes, erythematous rashes, and localized edema may be seen. A variety of eye lesions have been recorded, but these are rare. Electrocardiograms are often abnormal, but clinical signs of heart disease are unusual. Mild normocytic anemia and mild thrombocytopenia are common. The serum IgM level is nearly always raised.

Months or years after the first appearance of symptoms, the clinical features of the early phase of the disease regress to be replaced by new symptoms and signs indicating invasion of the nervous system. Mild behavioral and personality changes are often the first sign of central nervous system involvement. Later, more florid psychologic changes may occur with hallucinations and delusions. Headache and backache are common complaints. Drowsiness during the day, the feature from which the disease takes its name, may occur but is not invariable, and some patients are manic. If no treatment is given, the patient's level of consciousness progressively deteriorates until finally he lapses into stupor. Convulsions occasionally occur. Chorea and athetosis are the most frequently encountered localizing neurologic signs. Pyramidal tract involvement is less frequent, and cranial nerve lesions are rare. Obesity and impotence or amenorrhea probably follow from damage to the hypothalamus. Severe itching is a frequent but unexplained symptom that may lead to skin changes. The cerebrospinal fluid shows an increase in cells and protein, much of which is IgM. Most of the cells are lymphocytes, but a few plasma cells and morular cells may be seen. Trypanosomes may be present.

Rhodesian Sleeping Sickness. The clinical picture of Rhodesian sleeping sickness is similar to that described above, but on presentation the patient is usually more acutely ill than a patient with Gambian sleeping sickness, and the disease progresses more rapidly. Heart failure and jaundice occur more frequently than in Gambian sleeping sickness, but lymphadenopathy is usually less prominent. Neurologic features similar to those described above may be present, but sometimes death occurs before these have had time to develop. Anemia and thrombocytopenia are usual, and disseminated intravascular coagulation may occur. Liver function tests are often abnormal, and an abnormal electrocardiogram is usually obtained. Cerebrospinal fluid changes are the same as those described above.

DIAGNOSIS. The chancre of trypanosomiasis has no special features and is unlikely to be recognized unless there is a strong reason for suspecting trypanosomiasis. It must be differentiated from an allergic reaction to a tsetse fly bite. Trypanosomes are present in juice obtained from the lesion.

The clinical features of the early phase of sleeping sickness are similar to those of many infectious, neoplastic, and connective tissue diseases. Trypanosomiasis must be considered in the differential diagnosis of unexplained pyrexia or lymphadenopathy in any patient who has visited an endemic area. Diagnosis of Rhodesian sleeping sickness can usually be made by the demonstration of trypanosomes in a thick blood film. However, trypanosomes are rarely found in the blood of patients with Gambian sleeping sickness even when concentration, culture, or animal inoculation is used. Diagnosis is most readily made in the early stage of this form of sleeping sickness by the detection of trypanosomes in the juice

obtained on puncturing an enlarged lymph node with a venipuncture needle.

Once invasion of the central nervous system has occurred, clinical diagnosis of sleeping sickness is usually not difficult. However, tragic misdiagnoses have been made in patients with predominantly psychologic features. Chorea may be so marked as to suggest Sydenham's chorea, and confusion with other extrapyramidal syndromes may occur occasionally. Diagnosis of the advanced stage of sleeping sickness is confirmed by examination of the cerebrospinal fluid. Trypanosomes can be found in most patients provided both that the cerebrospinal fluid is examined immediately after collection and that scrupulously clean glassware is used. Measurement of the cerebrospinal fluid IgM level is often of great diagnostic help in patients in whom trypanosomes cannot be found. A high cerebrospinal fluid IgM in the presence of a modest increase in total protein is a characteristic feature of sleeping sickness very rarely found in other diseases, such as tuberculous meningitis and neurovascular syphilis, with which it might be confused.

Many different serologic tests have been used to diagnose sleeping sickness; the recently developed ELISA test is especially promising. These tests have proved of great value in survey work but are of less value in the investigation of individual patients, as false-positive and false-negative reactions can occur.

TREATMENT. General Measures. Whenever possible, patients with sleeping sickness should be treated in hospital. Lumbar puncture to determine the stage of the disease must be carried out before treatment is started. If abnormalities are found (a raised cell count or protein), the patient must be treated as having a case of advanced disease, even if there are no clinical signs of central nervous system involvement. Poorly nourished patients may require dietary supplements. A search should be made for any associated infections, and these should be treated. Malaria prophylaxis should be given if malaria is endemic.

Many different drugs and dosage regimens have been used in the treatment of sleeping sickness, but few controlled trials have been undertaken and the treatment schedules currently in use were largely established empirically. All the drugs used in the treatment of sleeping sickness were developed many years ago, and all are toxic; there is still a great need for safer effective drugs.

Chemotherapy of Early Disease. Suramin is an effective treatment for early Gambian and Rhodesian sleeping sickness, but it is ineffective in advanced disease as it penetrates poorly into the cerebrospinal fluid. Suramin* is a white powder which is made up in an aqueous solution immediately before use and given intravenously in a dose of 20 mg per kilogram of body weight. Occasionally it causes vomiting and collapse, so it is customary to start with a test dose of one fifth of this amount. A course comprises five to ten injections given at two- to five-day intervals. The drug can cause renal damage; because of this, it should not be given in more than a single course and the urine should be tested for protein and casts before each injection. Mild proteinuria can be ignored; but if heavy proteinuria develops or if casts are found, treatment should be stopped. Three injections of melarsoprol (see below) is an effective alternative form of treatment which is considered by some to be the treatment of

---

*Available from the Center for Disease Control (404-633-3311, Ext. 3670).

choice. Berenil is also effective but has been less widely used.

Chemotherapy of Advanced Disease. Melarsoprol (Mel B) is the treatment of choice for both Gambian and Rhodesian sleeping sickness once involvement of the central nervous system has occurred, even though the drug is very toxic. It is possible that toxicity is reduced by a prior course of suramin, but melarsoprol should be started right away in patients who are very sick. Mel B is dispensed as a 3.6 per cent solution in polyethylene glycol. This is very irritating and is liable to produce thrombophlebitis. The full dosage of Mel B* is 3.6 mg (0.1 ml) per kilogram of body weight given intravenously up to a maximum of 5.0 ml. The following is an effective schedule of treatment for an adult: 2.5 ml on day 1 and 3, followed by 5.0 ml on day 5; rest for one to two weeks; 5.0 ml on days 8, 10, and 12; rest for a further week; and then 5.0 ml on days 15, 17 and 19 (total dose, 40.0 ml). Other schedules employ a more gradual build-up to full dosage. Treatment schedules should be kept flexible and slowed down if reactions occur. Febrile reactions are common after the first injection of Mel B, especially if suramin has not been given. Mel B can produce rashes, marrow depression, and renal damage, but its most serious side effect is an encephalopathy which occurs in about 5 per cent of patients. Encephalopathy occurs most frequently at the time of the third or fourth injection; it may develop very rapidly and is sometimes fatal. Dimercaprol (BAL) has been used to treat this complication of Mel B treatment, but its value has not been clearly established. It has been suggested that corticosteroids protect patients from Mel B encephalopathy, but no protection was demonstrated in a recent controlled trial.

Follow-up and Treatment of Relapses. The results of treatment of patients with early disease with suramin are excellent, but occasional patients subsequently develop neurologic disease and require treatment with a full course of Mel B. Regular follow-up with clinical examination and lumbar puncture is therefore necessary for at least a year after treatment.

Patients with neurologic disease also require regular follow-up, for treatment failures and relapses occasionally occur. Patients with a relapse of advanced disease should receive another full course of Mel B* (total dosage, 40.0 ml for an adult) together with nitrofurazone, for, despite the toxicity of this drug, there is an impression that patients treated with melarsoprol and nitrofurazone do better than those receiving melarsoprol alone. The adult dosage of nitrofurazone* is 0.5 gram given by mouth every six hours for five days, this course being repeated on two or three occasions. Nitrofurazone is a toxic drug causing peripheral neuropathy and hemolytic anemia, especially in those with glucose-6-phosphatase deficiency.

PROGNOSIS. Many patients with early Gambian sleeping sickness remain relatively well for months or years, and it is possible that a few recover spontaneously. Once central nervous system involvement has occurred, death is inevitable unless treatment is given. Death frequently follows a secondary infection, often pneumonia, in a stuporous and malnourished patient. Patients with Rhodesian sleeping sickness may die from heart failure.

The results of treatment of patients in the early phase of sleeping sickness are excellent, over 90 per cent making a complete recovery. However, a few patients subsequent-ly develop central nervous system involvement and require further treatment. Mel B achieves a parasitologic "cure" in at least 90 per cent of cases of advanced disease, and many patients make a complete recovery. Unfortunately some patients are left with irreversible neurologic damage. These patients must be differentiated from those who have had a true relapse and require further treatment. About 5 per cent of patients die as a result of Mel B treatment.

An attack of sleeping sickness does not induce protective immunity, and reinfection may occur.

CONTROL AND PROPHYLAXIS. Many different approaches have been made to the control of sleeping sickness. In West Africa, survey teams have been used extensively to detect and treat asymptomatic patients early in the course of their disease, thus reducing the reservoir of infection. In East Africa, attempts have been made to reduce the reservoir of infection in wild game. Man-fly contact can be reduced by encouraging farmers to live in villages rather than in scattered hamlets. Tsetse flies can be destroyed by hand catching, trapping, or destruction of their natural habitat, but most control programs now rely on insecticides sprayed either by hand or from the air. Several large aerial spraying projects are now in progress aimed mainly at destruction of the tsetse flies responsible for cattle trypanosomiasis, but the vectors of human sleeping sickness are also being destroyed.

Pentamidine* has been successfully used as a chemoprophylactic in Gambian sleeping sickness when given by a single intramuscular injection of 4 mg per kilogram every three to six months. However, its use carries the risk of producing cryptic infections, and the drug can cause diabetes. It should therefore be used only in those who are in great danger of being infected.

The occurrence of antigenic variation has been a major obstacle to the development of a successful vaccine. However, recent progress in culture of *T. brucei* in vitro and in analysis of the detailed chemical structure of its variant antigens holds out hope for the future.

Apted, F. I. C.: Clinical manifestations and diagnosis of sleeping sickness. *In* Mulligan, H. W. (ed.): The African Trypanosomiases. London, George Allen and Unwin, 1970, p. 661.

Ford, J.: The Role of the African Trypanosomiases in African Ecology. Oxford, Clarendon Press, 1971.

Goodwin, L. G.: The African scene; mechanisms of pathogenesis in trypanosomiasis. *In* Trypanosomiasis and Leishmaniasis with Special Reference to Chagas' Disease. Ciba Foundation Symposium, 20. Amsterdam, Associated Scientific Publishers, 1974, p. 107.

Mott, F. W.: Histological observations on sleeping sickness and other trypanosome infections. Reports of the Sleeping Sickness Commission of the Royal Society, 7:3, 1906.

Vickerman, K.: Antigenic variation in African trypanosomes. *In* Parasites in the Immunised Host: Mechanisms of Survival. Ciba Foundation Symposium, 25. Amsterdam, Associated Scientific Publishers, 1974, p. 53.

194.3. CHAGAS' DISEASE
(American Trypanosomiasis)

Vanize Macedo

DEFINITION. Chagas' disease, an infection caused by *Trypanosoma cruzi* and named after its Brazilian discoverer, Carlos Chagas, is found only in the Western Hemisphere. A distinction must be made between in-

---

*Available from the Center for Disease Control (404-633-3311, Ext. 3670).

*Available from the Center for Disease Control (404-633-3311, Ext. 3670).

fection and disease. The majority of infected patients develop no signs of clinically detectable disease. Chagas himself described the two main disease forms occurring years after the initial infection: a chronic cardiomyopathy often with intracardiac conduction defects, and dilatation of the esophagus or colon (the mega syndromes).

ETIOLOGY. The trypanomastigote is visible in peripheral blood films of man and the multitude of naturally or experimentally infected animals studied in the early or acute phase of the disease. It is polymorphic, 15 to 25 μ long, and has a large subterminal kinetoplast. The proportion of narrow, broad, and intermediate forms appears to vary with the strain. Multiplication takes place only in an amastigote phase in host cells. The trypanomastigote penetrates a host cell (frequently a cardiac or smooth muscle cell), rounds up, and commences to replicate by binary fission every 12 hours. The time of rupture of this host cell will depend on its size. The amastigotes change into trypanomastigotes, which are released to circulate in the peripheral blood and penetrate new cells. Experimentally, myotropic, neurotropic, and reticulotropic strains have been identified, and it is possible that different strains of *T. cruzi* are responsible for geographic variations in the human disease. After a period of weeks, the host immune response suppresses the trypanomastigote parasitemia to subpatent levels. Small numbers continue to circulate for years.

EVOLUTIONARY CYCLE. The insect vector of *T. cruzi* is a hemipteran, a reduviid bug of the subfamily Triatominae, of which about 100 species have been described. They are obligate blood suckers and withdraw a large blood meal rapidly by directly tapping a subcutaneous capillary with their stylet mouth parts. The great majority of these are sylvatic and maintain cycles among wild animals. Such bugs are found from within 200 miles of New York to the south of Argentina. For reasons that are unclear, a small number of species have become highly domesticated, and those cohabiting with man are the transmitters of Chagas' disease. The most important species in this respect are *Triatoma infestans, Panstrongylus megistus,* and *Rhodnius prolixus.*

T. cruzi probably originated as a parasite of these insects which remain extraordinarily susceptible to infection with the protozoan. All stages of the bug are easily infected after ingestion of blood from an infected mammalian host, even one in which circulating trypanosomes cannot be detected by any other means. *T. cruzi* undergoes a complex cycle of morphogenesis as it passes down the intestines of the bug. Infective trypanomastigotes can be found in the rectum after 20 to 30 days, and these will penetrate cells to replicate and initiate the infection in mammalian hosts.

EPIDEMIOLOGY. Transmission is usually at night, when the bugs are active. They feed mainly on the face and arms, the uncovered parts of sleeping man. As they engorge with blood, the rise in intra-abdominal pressure promotes defecation, and the trypanomastigotes in the feces can penetrate mucous membranes or small skin abrasions. The three main species of transmitting bugs all tend to defecate soon after feeding.

Congenital transmission and infection by blood transfusion can occur. More rarely, transmisson may occur as a result of a laboratory accident. There exists the possibility of contamination by the digestive tract.

Chagas' disease has been described in all the countries of South America and Central America with the exception of Guyana and Surinam. In Mexico it is rare. Two autochthonous acute cases have been reported in Texas. The high standard of housing and the discrete nature of the sylvatic cycles makes transmission to man a very rare event in North America. Chagas' disease is a serious public health problem in South America, principally in Argentina, Brazil, Chile, Uruguay, and Venezuela. There are geographic differences in the disease; for example, cardiomyopathy is rare in Chile, and the mega syndromes are unknown in Venezuela. From some countries (e.g., Bolivia) there is little information on the status of Chagas' disease.

It is estimated that the prevalence of trypanosomiasis may reach 20 per cent in the rural zones of the countries where it is endemic. Socioeconomic conditions are bad in these areas and dwellings are of poor construction with mud and sticks, building materials which favor bug colonization. Chagas' disease is intimately linked with economic underdevelopment.

The medicosocial importance of the disease has not been determined, and we do not know for certain the role American trypanosomiasis plays in the economy of countries where it is endemic. Cardiopathy is the most important form of the disease, causing a significant mortality and inability to work in the most productive phase of life. Many employers in Brazil will not hire a worker with positive serology.

PATHOGENESIS. The local tissue inflammation promoted by rupture of nests of amastigotes of *T. cruzi* was the first interpretation of the pathology of the disease. This view explains the alterations that occur in the acute phase but not all those that occur in the chronic phase. In this phase amastigotes are rarely found. Early workers introduced theories of allergic or hypersensitivity reactions to hypothetical toxins of *T. cruzi* to explain the chronic inflammation in the absence of a parasite. A neurotoxin was said to be responsible for degeneration of parasympathetic ganglia. Although such denervation goes far to explain the genesis of the mega syndromes, it is only one factor in the development of cardiac disease.

There is evidence suggesting that an autoimmune process is at work in the chronic cardiomyopathy of Chagas' disease. Santos, Buch, and Teixeira have demonstrated that sensitized lymphocytes from rabbits chronically infected with *T. cruzi* are cytotoxic to normal cardiac cells. Cossio and colleagues have identified circulating autoantibodies to heart tissue in patients with chronic cardiomyopathy.

The importance of strains of the parasite or reinfection in the pathogenesis of Chagas' disease is still not clear.

PATHOLOGY. In the acute phase the infection is generalized, and amastigotes of *T. cruzi* can be found in cells of the reticuloendothelial system. Initially reticular cells are parasitized, and in a short time smooth and striated muscle cells, including cardiac muscle, glial and nerve cells, and fat cells are invaded.

The inoculation lesion shows inflammation with infiltration of lymphocytes and plasma cells and fibroblastic proliferation. The heart is enlarged and flabby, with predominance of dilatation over hypertrophy. Hemorrhagic foci may be seen on the endocardium. Microscopically there is diffuse edema, both intestinal and interfibrillar congestion, and the presence of amastigotes in the cardiac fibers. The cardiac fibers show hyaline necrosis and degeneration (lesions of Margarino Torres). In the central nervous system there is mononuclear infiltration of the leptomeninges, congestive perivascular inflammation, and hemorrhage with glial proliferation and neurophagia. Amastigotes may be encountered in the cells of the central nervous system.

In the chronic cardiac form the heart is enlarged with both hypertrophy and dilatation so that the apex is formed by the terminations of both ventricles. The epicardium is congested, and there may be a small pericardial effusion. There are no organic valvular lesions. The thinned myocardium of the apex may distend to form an apical aneurysm, a characteristic lesion of Chagas' disease. Mural thrombosis is frequent on the endocardium, particularly in the right atrium and the apex of the left ventricle. Thrombosis at the apex is an important finding in Chagas' myocarditis. These intracardiac thrombi are the source of emboli principally to the lungs, kidneys, cerebrum, and spleen. There is chronic passive congestion of the organs.

Microscopy demonstrates an intense diffuse myocarditis with focal areas of cellular infiltration containing mononuclear cells, lymphocytes, and plasma cells. There is hypertrophy of the cardiac fibers with small areas of focal necrosis, hemorrhage, and granular degeneration. A variable degree of fibrosis is associated with edema and vascular dilatation and congestion. Tissue amastigotes are rarely seen in chronic cases.

Andrade has shown that these inflammatory changes directly involve the conducting system of the heart, particularly the sinoatrial node, the interior third of the atrioventricular node, the right half of the main bundle, the right bundle branch, and the anterior ramification of the left bundle branch. He established a good correlation between the electrocardiogram in life and these pathologic changes.

In the indeterminate form of Chagas' disease, active myocarditis with granuloma formation and neuronal destruction of Auerbach's plexus has been found, but in lesser degree than established cardiomyopathy. In megaesophagus and megacolon the organ is dilated with focal myositis associated with a diminution in the number of nerve cells in Auerbach's plexus.

In the congenital form a chronic placentitis with ischemia of the chorionic villi occurs. Edema and a histiocytic inflammatory infiltrate are present with small foci of necrosis in these villi. Amastigotes are visible in the cytoplasm of macrophages.

CLINICAL PRESENTATION. Chagas' disease has an acute and chronic phase. It is noteworthy that in endemic areas discrepancies exist between the prevalence of the chronic phase and the small number of cases diagnosed as acute disease.

Acute Phase. In areas endemic for Chagas' disease, the acute phase is diagnosed in about 1 per cent of patients. Probably in the majority of individuals the initial phase of the infection is inapparent. Seventy per cent of patients in this phase are children under ten years of age. Acute Chagas' disease is rare in adults.

The incubation period is 4 to 12 days. The signs at the portal of entry often call the attention of the physician to the possible diagnosis of the disease. Romaña's sign is present in half the patients in the acute phase. This is a unilateral, bipalpebral, firm, violaceous edema, frequently with conjunctivitis and enlargement of the preauricular gland. An inoculation chagoma may occur in exposed areas, such as the face or arms, where

the bug has an opportunity of biting. This also is characterized by erythema and infiltrative tumefaction of the skin with satellite ganglion reaction, which, when it disappears, leaves hyperpigmentation. It is found in 25 per cent of patients in the acute phase. A minority of patients do not present signs of a portal of entry.

The disease is characterized by prolonged fever, asthenia, enlargement of lymphatic glands, edema of the face and legs, and hepatosplenomegaly. Tachycardia is frequently present even in the absence of temperature. This is a sign of myocarditis which is benign in the majority of cases and only diagnosed on electrocardiogram.

The signs of the acute phase disappear in two to four months. The so-called schizotrypanides are skin rashes that rarely occur in the acute phase. They may take the form of erythematous indurated plaques or may be morbilliform or urticarial in type, suggesting an allergic nature. Meningoencephalitis is also a rare complication, often occurring in children under one year of age and usually fatal. Clinical evidence of encephalitis may be complicated by convulsions.

Congenital Disease. Since this is rarely diagnosed, its prevalence in endemic areas cannot be estimated. Such newborns are underweight and afebrile, and have hepatosplenomegaly and often edema. Petechiae, bruising, and frank hemorrhage may be noted. Meningoencephalitis may produce convulsions and tremors of the face and limbs. If jaundice is present, it disappears in the third week. Metastatic chagomas have been described, with skin infiltration, infection, and even necrosis.

The Chronic Phase. INDETERMINATE FORM. After the acute phase, individuals can stay for many years or all their lives in a latent or indeterminate phase. These subjects do not have clinical, radiologic, or electrocardiographic signs. In endemic areas, approximately half of those infected show this form. It is probable that this number will diminish as more sophisticated methods for detecting disease are developed.

CARDIAC FORM. This is the most important clinical form of the chronic phase, and its prevalence can reach 30 per cent of individuals in an endemic area. The majority of patients have no cardiac symptoms or signs but only electrocardiographic evidence of disease.

Palpitations, usually the result of extrasystoles, are a frequent initial symptom. They may be accompanied by dizziness and precordial pain. Right-sided ventricular failure predominates, and dyspnea is infrequent.

Physical examination shows an irregular pulse and distant heart sounds, fixed splitting of the pulmonary second sound, gallop rhythm, and a functional regurgitant murmur in the mitral area. In advanced cases, tricuspid regurgitation can occur and cyanosis is present. Thromboembolic phenomena are very frequent and may precede symptoms of cardiac insufficiency. Total atrioventricular block is rare but is frequently accompanied by Stokes-Adams attacks.

DIGESTIVE FORM. The digestive form is characterized by dilatation and alteration in motility of the esophagus or colon. Rarely the stomach or small intestine shows similar changes.

In megaesophagus the principal symptom is longstanding dysphagia, which begins with difficulty with solid food and progresses until the patient can swallow only soft foods with the aid of frequent sips of water. In advanced cases, patients have pain on swallowing, regurgitation, and pyrosis with a sensation of suffocation. Hiccup, sialorrhea, and nocturnal cough are associated symptoms. Hypersalivation is accompanied by parotid gland enlargement. Marked weight loss is present, and aspiration pneumonias may occur in advanced cases.

Megacolon is evidenced by retention of feces and gas and often progresses to fecaloma formation. Volvulus and intestinal obstruction are frequent complications. The majority of cases of megacolon are associated with megaesophagus. Half of the patients with digestive forms of Chagas' disease have abnormal electrocardiograms.

OTHER CLINICAL FORMS. Rare complications are megaureter, megabladder, megagallbladder, and bronchiectasis. The forms of central nervous system involvement in chronic infection, described by Chagas himself, are still debatable. The denervation process has been implicated in the dysfunction of various exocrine and endocrine glands.

DIAGNOSIS. Acute Phase. The acute phase is usually diagnosed by finding the trypanomastigote in the peripheral blood on direct examination of thick films. This is the best criterion for diagnosing the acute phase. Should this fail, simple concentration methods are usually positive, such as examination of the leukocyte cream after centrifugation or allowing the blood to clot and examining the supernatant (Strout's method). Biopsy of the calf muscle shows myositis and frequently nests of amastigotes.

The *xenodiagnostic test* is often positive before 30 days owing to the high number of circulating trypanosomes. Similarly, cultures (NNN) and subinoculation of mice recover the organism. The serologic reactions, usually positive in this early stage, are precipitins and agglutinins. There is a raised IgM. The complement fixation test becomes positive four to six weeks after infection. The indirect immunofluorescent test becomes positive earlier than the hemagglutination and complement fixation tests. The white cell count shows leukocytosis caused by an intense lymphocytosis with atypical lymphocytes. The erythrocyte sedimentation rate is increased, as are the mucoproteins. Heterophil antibodies may appear in the serum, and the Paul Bunnell reaction may be positive. Protein electrophoresis reveals a slight hypoalbuminemia with a rise in gamma and alpha 2 globulins. The transaminases are slightly elevated. The electrocardiogram may show sinus tachycardia, low voltage complexes, first degree atrioventricular block, increased QT space, primary alterations in ventricular repolarization, and sometimes subepicardial ischemia. Alterations in cardiac rhythm are rare at this stage and a bad prognostic sign.

On x-ray examination, there may be enlargement of the cardiac shadow, which may be transitory. At times such enlargement is due to a pericardial effusion. Marked cardiomegaly indicates a bad prognosis.

Chronic Phase. Evidence of infection is established mainly by serologic tests such as complement fixation, hemagglutination, and immunofluorescence. Xenodiagnosis, using 40 bugs, will isolate an organism in about 50 per cent of cases. In the indeterminate phase, only these investigations will be positive.

A chest x-ray may be normal, but frequently a degree of cardiomegaly is seen progressing to marked global enlargement of the heart. The electrocardiogram is valuable, as conduction defects are common. In the endemic area of São Felipe, Brazil, the following abnormalities were present in a frequency of 15 to 20 per cent: complete right bundle branch block with anterior hemiblock, ventricular extrasystoles, first degree atrioventricular block, and alterations in ventricular repolarization. Total atrioventricular block or complete left bundle branch block occurred in only 0.2 per cent. There may be evidence of septal fibrosis. Digestive tract involvement is revealed by radiologic studies in a patient with a suggestive history. Both the esophagus and colon are dilated, with abnormal peristalsis and evidence of retained food residues.

Rezende has proposed the following classification of megaesophagus based on radiologic findings:

Group I — The caliber of the esophagus is normal, but there is slow transit and retention of barium.

Group II — The caliber of the esophagus is slightly or moderately enlarged with marked retention of contrast. Tertiary waves are present.

Group III — The esophagus is greatly enlarged and hypotonic with marked barium retention.

Group IV — Dolichomegaesophagus occurs, with massive retention capacity, atonia, and doubling of the esophagus on top of the diaphragm.

DIFFERENTIAL DIAGNOSIS. Romaña's sign must be distinguished from conjunctivitis, orbital cellulitis, cavernous sinus thrombosis, insect bites, and trauma, all of which produce unilateral orbital edema. Clinically the acute phase may resemble typhoid fever, infectious mononucleosis, kala-azar, brucellosis, toxoplasmosis, and acute glomerulonephritis. Other types of acute myocarditis must be considered.

Congenital infections must be distinguished from syphilis, toxoplasmosis, and cytomegalic inclusion disease.

Chronic cardiomyopathy involves a differential diagnosis from the cardiomyopathies associated with alcohol, pregnancy, idiopathic cardiomyopathy, endomyocardial fibrosis, and ischemic heart disease. The absence of organic valvular lesions usually permits a distinction from rheumatic valvular disease. Carcinoma of the esophagus may mimic megaesophagus. The presence of positive serology and electrocardiographic changes assist in the differential diagnosis from megaesophagus and megacolon not caused by Chagas' disease.

EVOLUTION AND PROGNOSIS. Chagas' cardiomyopathy is variable in its course and of uncertain prognosis. In the acute phase only 10 per cent of patients die of myocarditis or acute meningoencephalitis. The latter condition usually occurs in children under one year of age. The indeterminate phase can last a lifetime. The factors influencing the evolution of the disease are not clear. There is some evidence that reinfections could play a role in an endemic area. The strain of parasite and the host's response to it could be important. Cardiomyopathy begins in the second to fifth decade. Heart failure in these age groups leads to death one to five years after its initial appearance. The prognosis is poor if cardiac failure appears before 30 years of age.

A longitudinal study in São Felipe, Brazil, showed that each year the disease made a detectable progression in 5.5 per cent of patients. The mortality was 0.7 per cent per year. The principal cause of death was cardiac failure in 58.3 per cent. Sudden death from conduction defects occurred in 37.5 per cent. The following electrocardiographic changes were associated with a 50 per cent mortality in five years: total atrioventricular block, atrial fibrillation, left bundle branch block, multifocal extrasystoles, and septal fibrosis.

TREATMENT. Two drugs appear to kill circulating trypanosomes and may have value in the specific treatment of Chagas' disease. These are nifurtimox, a nitrofuran derivative (Bayer 2502 [Lampit]), and benznidazole, a nitroimidazole RO7–1051 Rochagan).

Nifurtimox* is used in a dose of 8 mg per kilogram of body weight per day for a period of 120 days. With regard to eradicating parasitemia, it has given good results in patients in the acute and chronic phases in Chile, Argentina, and southern Brazil. In other areas of Brazil, such as Bahia, Goiás, and Minas Gerais, the results have been less satisfactory, only 40 per cent of individuals being uniformly negative on repeated xenodiagnosis after treatment. Experiments in animals infected with different strains of *T. cruzi* demonstrated different susceptibilities to nifurtimox. This reinforces the hypothesis that different strains of *T. cruzi* may be responsible for these variations in response to treatment. Benznidazole* is used in a dose of 5 mg per kilogram per day for 60 days and also eradicates parasitemia in a proportion of patients. Both these drugs have serious side effects and should be used only under direct medical supervision. The side effects include polyneuritis, dizziness, loss of weight, nausea, and insomnia. With use of benznidazole, exfoliative dermatitis and thrombocytopenic purpura have also been seen.

It is not known how important such specific treatment is in arresting the disease. If parasitemia is an important factor in the evolution of the disease, then certainly the acute phase should be treated. In the acute phase, both serologic tests and xenodiagnosis may remain negative after treatment. In the chronic phase, those in whom xenodiagnosis becomes negative remain positive serologically. It is still not clear whether such treatment is of value in the chronic phase.

When chronic myocarditis is associated with heart failure, the treatment is symptomatic. Digitalis must be used with care because of sensitivity of the damaged cardiac fiber, and the response is poor in relation to other cardiomyopathies. Extrasystoles, the most frequent arrhythmia, may be helped by procainamide. In ventricular tachycardia, procainamide and lidocaine are the drugs indicated. Beta-adrenergic blocking agents are dangerous in acute arrhythmias in Chagas' myocarditis, as they may produce bradycardia and shock. Deaths have been reported after the use of propranolol. In Stokes-Adams crises, isopropyl norepinephrine is useful. In patients with total atrioventricular block and a normal or slightly enlarged heart, implantation of the pacemaker is indicated. When there is marked cardiac enlargement, this measure carries a poor prognosis, because either the weak cardiac muscle cannot support the new rhythm or an intramural clot may become dislodged.

Initially megaesophagus is treated by balloon dilatation; in more advanced cases cardiotomy is often successful. Operations consisting of excision of the aperistaltic esophagus and replacement with a segment of colon or small intestine have been developed. In megacolon evacuation of a fecaloma may be an emergency procedure. It has to be carried out with care, for rupture of the colon and septicemia can follow the procedure. Resection of the aperistaltic segment may relieve persistent constipation.

PROPHYLAXIS. Since transmission usually occurs in a domestic setting in poor-quality housing, Chagas' disease is a direct reflection of poverty. The important prophylactic measures in the control of Chagas' disease are better housing, public health education, and application of insecticides in the house and its environs. Benzene hexachloride (BHC), the insecticide of choice, is applied in a suspension of 500 mg of the gamma isomer per square meter every six months.

In blood banks in endemic areas of Chagas' disease, 1:4000 gentian violet is added to stored blood 24 hours before use in order to kill the trypanosomes. To date no results that can be applied to humans have been obtained with immunoprotection for Chagas' disease.

American Trypanosomiasis Research. PAHO Scientific Publication 318, 1975.

Andrade, Z., and Andrade, S. G.: Chagas' disease (American trypanosomiasis). *In* Marcial-Rojas, R. A. (ed.): Pathology of Protozoal and Helminthic Disease. Baltimore, Williams & Wilkins Company, 1971.

Chagas, C.: Processos patojênicos da tripanosomiase americana. Memórias do Instituto Oswaldo Cruz, 8:5, 1916.

Köberle, F.: Patologia y anatomia patológica de la enfermedad de Chagas. Bol. Sanit. Panam., 51:404, 1961.

Laranja, F. S., Dias, E., Nóbrega, G., and Miranda, A.: Chagas' disease — a clinical epidemiologic and pathologic study. Circulation, 14:1035, 1956.

Prata, A., Andrade, Z., and Guimarães, A.: Chagas' heart disease. *In* Shaper, A. G., Hutt, M. S. R., and Fejfar, Z. (eds.): Cardiovascular Disease in the Tropics. London, British Medical Association, 1974.

Romaña, C.: Enfermedad de Chagas. Buenos Aires, Lopez Liberos, 1963.

World Health Organization: Chagas' Disease: Report of a Study Group. Technical Report Series No. 202, 1960.

195. LEISHMANIASIS

Anthony D. M. Bryceson

195.1. INTRODUCTION

DEFINITION. Leishmaniasis is an infection with parasites of the genus *Leishmania*. It is usually a zoonosis transmitted by phlebotomine sandflies between wild or peridomestic animals, especially rodents or canines. Man is infected when he interrupts the natural cycle.

In man the infection is either visceral or cutaneous. Visceral leishmaniasis is a severe chronic infection of the reticuloendothelial system, characterized by fever, chills, weight loss, splenomegaly, leukopenia, anemia, and a high natural mortality. It is caused by *L. donovani*. Cutaneous leishmaniasis is characterized by single or several chronic sores which usually heal spontaneously. In parts of South and Central America, severely mutilating metastatic lesions of the mouth and nose are seen. Cutaneous leishmaniasis is caused by *L. tropica* in the Old World, and by members of the *L. mexicana* and *L. brasiliensis* groups in the New World.

ETIOLOGY. *Leishmania* exist in two forms, one in the vertebrate host, including man, and the other in the sandfly and in artificial culture. In the vertebrate host the parasite is in the amastigote (Leishman-Donovan body) stage, so called because it has no free flagellum.

---

*Available from Center for Disease Control (404-633-3311, Ext. 3670).

It is a round or oval body 2 to 3 μ across, containing a nucleus and a smaller kinetoplast which stain respectively red and purple with Giemsa, Wright's or Leishman's stain, and stand out against the pale blue cytoplasm. *Leishmania* are strict intracellular parasites and are found in macrophages in which they multiply by binary fission. Heavily parasitized host cells rupture, and fresh cells are invaded. Sandflies become infected when they feed on an infected person or animal and take up parasites from blood or skin. In the sandfly the parasite is in the promastigote (leptomonad) stage, so called because of the anterior origin of its flagellum. Promastigotes are supple, highly motile, spindle-shaped organisms, 15 to 25 μ long and 1.5 to 3.5 μ broad. Promastigotes are found in the hindgut or midgut of the sandfly, where they divide and whence they migrate forward into the pharynx and buccal cavity, rendering the sandfly infective. The cycle of development in the sandfly takes about seven days. Once inoculated into man, the promastigote rapidly penetrates macrophages, flagellum first, and transforms into an amastigote.

Biochemical taxonomy of *Leishmania* (isoenzymes, DNA analysis) has proved a valuable adjunct to the traditional epidemiologic and serologic methods of species differentiation.

IMMUNOLOGY. The patterns of disease in man are partly determined by the species of parasite (tropism for skin or viscera, differences in immunogenicity and allergenicity) and partly by man's response to the parasite. Resistance to *Leishmania* depends upon the development of specific cell-mediated immunity. The capacity of individuals to mount such a response varies, and consequently leishmaniasis presents a spectrum of disease in the same way that leprosy does. At one end of the spectrum lie visceral leishmaniasis and diffuse cutaneous leishmaniasis, characterized by abundance of parasites, absence of lymphocytes in lesions, insensitivity to leishmanin, and poor prognosis. At the other end lie the self-healing sores, with relatively scanty parasites, marked lymphocytic infiltration, and leishmanin sensitivity. Accompanying cell-mediated immunity is delayed hypersensitivity to numerous parasite antigens, which causes the destructive pathology of leishmanial ulcers, especially in the chronic conditions of mucocutaneous leishmaniasis (see below) and leishmaniasis recidiva (see below) in which the normal balance between immunity and hypersensitivity has been lost. The mechanisms underlying these abnormal immune responses are not understood.

Antibody, which is produced in large quantities in visceral leishmaniasis, is not protective, and it has been suggested that it may even contribute to the pathogenesis of hemolytic anemia, nephritis, and amyloidosis. Healing is usually accompanied by long-lasting immunity to the particular species of *Leishmania* involved, but not to other species.

Leishmanin (Montenegro) Test. Leishmanin is a suspension of 10^6 promastigotes in 1 ml of 0.5 per cent phenol saline. The test is performed by injecting 0.1 ml intradermally into the volar surface of the forearm. A palpable nodule, 5 mm or more in diameter after 48 to 72 hours, is considered positive. The test is an index of delayed hypersensitivity, but not necessarily of immunity to *Leishmania*. It is not species specific. It is used to map out the extent of past infection in a community and may be of help in diagnosis in individual patients.

195.2. VISCERAL LEISHMANIASIS
(Kala-Azar, Ponos)

EPIDEMIOLOGY. It has been suggested that the zoonotic origin of *L. donovani* was among jackals in the steppes of Central Asia, where sporadic cases of visceral leishmaniasis are still sometimes seen among nomads and in settlers in the outskirts of rapidly expanding towns. From here the disease spread and developed three distinct epidemiologic patterns.

Visceral Leishmaniasis with a Canine Reservoir. This is the pattern in a belt which stretches from Portugal to Peking between latitudes 30 and 48 degrees North, the most important areas being the Mediterranean littoral, including North Africa, the shores of the Caspian Sea, central Soviet Asia, and northeast China. The main vectors are *Phlebotomus perniciosus* and *P. ariasi* in Western Europe, *P. major* in Eastern Europe, *P. papatasii* in the Middle East, and *P. chinensis* in China. In the Mediterranean and Chinese foci, the host-parasite relationship is relatively stable, and the disease is most common among children between one and four years of age. For this reason the parasite is sometimes called *L. infantum*, although adults in areas into which the disease has newly been introduced or visitors of any age are highly susceptible. Domestic dogs and foxes are the reservoir.

Portuguese and Spanish settlers possibly introduced *L. donovani*, also called *L. chagasi*, into the New World and initiated a zoonosis among foxes and dogs, although man may still be an occasional reservoir. The likely vector is *Lutzomyia longipalpis*. Visceral leishmaniasis is epidemic in northeast Brazil and sporadic in Amazonia, northern Argentina, and Paraguay and extends up through Venezuela and Colombia as far as Guatemala and Mexico. In Brazil male children are most commonly affected.

Visceral Leishmaniasis with a Rodent Vector. This is the pattern in Africa south of the Sahara from Lake Chad in the west to Somalia in the east, sparing the highlands of Ethiopia. The apparent absence of the disease in West Africa and south of the equator is unexplained. In the Sudan the zoonosis is between the Nile rat (*Arvicanthus niloticus*) and *P. orientalis* on the flood plains of the Nile and its tributaries. Visceral leishmaniasis is found among nomads who occupy temporary villages in riverine acacia woodland and migrant workers from adjoining countries.

In Kenya the disease is associated with termite hills where the vector *P. martini* rests and around which village men gather in the evenings. The reservoir is probably the gerbil *Tatara vicina*. The disease is usually sporadic, but epidemics have occurred. Males are affected four times as often as females, and the disease is most common in teenagers.

Visceral Leishmaniasis with a Human Reservoir. This is true epidemic kala-azar and is the pattern of the disease in northeast India, Bangladesh, Assam, and Burma. Classically the disease spreads along the Brahmaputra valley every 20 years or so. Transmission is by the highly anthropophilic, domestic sandfly *P. argentipes*. Often, many cases are found to have originated from one house. The age and sex pattern is the same as in Africa. Man is the only reservoir, and *P. argentipes* is readily infected from blood or from the lesions of post-kala-azar dermal leishmaniasis. The disease virtually disappeared over large areas as a result of DDT spraying for malaria control, but returned in epidemic form in Bihar in 1975.

FACTORS AFFECTING TRANSMISSION. Opportunities for contact with infected sandflies largely determine the pattern of disease in a given area. This is modified by the level of immunity of the population or individual. An attack of visceral leishmaniasis confers lifelong immunity, which determines the periodicity of epidemics. Subclinical infections with *L. donovani* or possibly even lizard and rodent species of *Leishmania* affect the pattern of spread in Africa and around the Mediterranean.

PATHOLOGY. The organs most severely affected are the spleen, liver, bone marrow, lymph nodes, intestines, and skin. The patient suffers from hyperplasia within and damage to these organs and from effects secondary to splenomegaly, reticuloendothelial blockage, and chronic parasitemia. Histologically the disease is characterized by massive proliferation of parasitized macrophages with little or no lymphocytic response. In Africa and Central Asia a cutaneous nodule or leishmanioma commonly develops at the site of parasite inoculation. Parasites multiply within histiocytes which may become the focus of a tuberculoid granuloma that heals spontaneously, and the infection proceeds no further. In the majority of cases, however, after a period of months, the infection disseminates.

The spleen is grossly enlarged, smooth, and firm and the capsule thick. The pulp is friable and infarcts are usual. There is massive hyperplasia of reticuloendothelial cells which are heavily parasitized. In the liver, Kupffer cells are hyperplastic and contain parasites. Occasionally parenchymal cells are parasitized. In chronic untreated cases there is parenchymal cell degeneration which may be followed after several years by fibrosis and even cirrhosis with clinical and biochemical evidence of hepatic dysfunction.

The bone marrow is heavily infiltrated with parasitized macrophages. Erythropoiesis and granulopoiesis are normal in the early stages of the disease, but may be depressed later. The peripheral blood shows anemia and leukopenia. The anemia is probably due to increased plasma volume, sequestration of erythrocytes in the spleen, and hemolysis. Leukopenia is due to splenic pooling and is said to predispose the patient to secondary infections. Lymph nodes and lymphoid tissue of the nasopharynx and gut are enlarged and contain many parasitized cells.

Kidneys may show cloudy swelling of tubular cells. Immunoglobulin and complement are deposited in the glomerular basement membrane. In fatal cases hyaline thickening of the glomerular mesangium has been found, and in chronic cases amyloidosis can develop. The skin, although normal in appearance, contains many intracellular parasites. In *post-kala-azar dermal leishmaniasis* there is variable infiltration with lymphocytes, histiocytes, and parasites.

In visceral leishmaniasis there is an enormous overproduction of IgG, only a small fraction of which is specific antibody. Some of it is autoantibody.

CLINICAL FEATURES. The incubation period is normally two to six months, but may be as short as ten days or as long as nine years. The onset is usually insidious, especially in indigenous peoples who may feel well and have a good appetite despite daily bouts of fever; however, in those who are poorly nourished and have several underlying parasitic infections, the disease may then progress rapidly. In Africa a primary cutaneous nodule may be noticed for a few months before there are any systemic symptoms. The earliest symptom is fever. This is usually gradual in onset and accompanied by sweats, often without preceding chills. Alternatively, the onset is sudden with high fever and chills. This is common in Americans and Europeans who have contracted the disease while visiting an endemic area. Associated with fever there may be dizziness, weakness, and weight loss. Other common early symptoms include cough, diarrhea, pain, or discomfort in the left hypochondrium and symptoms of complicating secondary infections.

The important physical findings are fever, splenomegaly, lymphadenopathy, and skin changes. Fever at first is often inconstant, with apyrexial periods of several days or weeks. In over 80 per cent of cases, however, the fever eventually develops a characteristic pattern with twice daily elevations reaching 38 to 40° C, and may then undulate as in brucellosis. In the most acute cases fever and toxemia may be the only signs. Splenic enlargement is not necessarily rapidly progressive, nor does the size of the spleen correlate with the duration of the disease. In many instances, however, it reaches the right iliac fossa. It is firm and not tender unless there has been a recent subcapsular infarct. The liver enlarges more slowly and becomes palpable in about 20 per cent of cases and is likewise firm and not tender. Generalized lymphadenopathy is common in patients from Mediterranean countries, Africa, or China. Various changes have been reported in the skin. Classically there is hyperpigmentation of hands, feet, and abdomen. This may be missed in black Africans; in lighter-skinned Indians it looks gray or black (kala-azar means black sickness). In Africans warty eruptions or ulcers of the skin and oronasal lesions are occasionally seen (Abdalla et al, 1975).

COURSE AND COMPLICATIONS. As the disease progresses, anemia becomes clinically apparent. There may be bleeding from the nose or gums. In longstanding cases jaundice and signs of hypoalbuminemia may develop, namely, brittle hair, opaque nails, subcutaneous edema and ascites. Finally, after a course which may run for a few months or for five years, the patient becomes emaciated and exhausted. Intercurrent infections are the cause of death in 90 per cent of fatal cases. The most common are cancrum oris, pneumonia, pulmonary tuberculosis, bacillary dysentery, amebic dysentery, and, in Africa, brucellosis. Massive gastrointestinal hemorrhage accounts for another 1 to 2 per cent.

Post-Kala-Azar Dermal Leishmaniasis. About 20 per cent of Indian patients develop a rash one to two years after treatment or spontaneous recovery. The lesions develop slowly and may last for several, even 20, years. In Africa the rash develops in 2 per cent of cases, usually during treatment, and does not persist. It commonly starts as hypopigmented or erythematous macules on the face and sometimes on the arms, legs, and trunk. On the face the rash gradually becomes papular or nodular, especially on the forehead, cheeks, and earlobes, and closely resembles lepromatous leprosy. In 25 per cent of cases the lesions resolve spontaneously.

DIAGNOSIS AND LABORATORY FINDINGS. The diagnosis must be suspected in any person living in, or having visited, an endemic area who has a prolonged fever. The diagnosis is likely in the presence of splenomegaly, granulocytopenia, anemia, and hyperglobulinemia and is made by isolation of the parasite or by characteristic immunologic changes.

ISOLATION OF PARASITE. This is best done by needle aspiration of bone marrow, spleen, liver, lymph nodes, or blood. Material obtained is:

1. Used to make a thin film on a glass microscope slide, stained, and examined under oil immersion for amastigotes, which must be distinguished from platelets. Parasitized macrophages usually rupture on smearing and free parasites must be looked for (see Fig. 2F, Ch. 193). Bone marrow aspiration is the procedure of choice. However, splenic puncture is safe so long as the tip of the spleen is well below the costal margin and the prothrombin and bleeding times are normal. A hypodermic needle on a syringe is inserted into the spleen, allowed to rest a moment, and withdrawn without suction. Organisms are seen in about 90 per cent of splenic aspirates and rather less often from other tissues. Buffy coat preparations show parasites in over 90 per cent of cases in India, but in only about 1 per cent in Africa.

2. Inoculated onto NNN (Novy-MacNeal-Nicolle) medium overlaid with balanced salt solution, containing streptomycin and penicillin (but not amphotericin). Cultures are kept in the dark at 22 to 25° C (not at 37° C), and every three to four days a drop of fluid is taken and examined wet for promastigotes. If after four weeks no parasites are seen, the fluid overlay is reinoculated onto a fresh NNN slope. Culture greatly improves the chances of making a diagnosis.

3. Inoculated intraperitoneally into hamsters, which are susceptible to a single amastigote. Though sensitive, this method is slow and seldom valuable.

IMMUNOLOGIC TESTS. Antileishmanial antibodies can be demonstrated by indirect immunofluorescence of promastigotes in over 90 per cent of cases and by precipitation in gel in 95 per cent. Cross-reactions with *Trypanosoma cruzi* antibodies can be absorbed out. Complement fixation is positive in 65 per cent, but if the older antigen made from Kedrowsky's bacillus is used, reactions may be expected in some patients with mycobacterial disease. Serum obtained by eluting blood dried onto filter paper in the field can be used satisfactorily in all these techniques. The leishmanin test is *negative* in cases of active visceral leishmaniasis, but becomes positive after recovery, being most intense after one to two years, after which it fades slowly.

Total serum proteins are raised up to and over 10 grams per 100 ml. This increase is due almost entirely to the IgG fraction of gamma globulin. On immunoelectrophoresis the IgG pattern is characteristically skewed. In some cases IgM is also slightly increased, but this is said to be transient and to revert rapidly to normal on treatment. In advanced cases serum albumin levels fall. This disturbed globulin pattern underlies the older diagnostic aldehyde test which is also positive in other diseases with a grossly disturbed globulin pattern.

LABORATORY FINDINGS. The principal laboratory findings have to do with the blood and with the plasma proteins.

Blood Changes. Leukopenia is the most characteristic finding. The total count is below 2000 cells per cubic millimeter in 75 per cent of cases. There are an absolute neutropenia and eosinopenia and a relative lymphocytosis and monocytosis. Agranulocytosis occasionally develops. Anemia is slower in onset but becomes severe. It is normocytic and normochromic unless complicated by bleeding or deficiency states. There is often a mild reticulocytosis, and erythrocyte half-life is reduced. Thrombocytopenia is usual and progresses with the disease. Early on, tests of clotting are normal but later

the prothrombin, partial thromboplastin, bleeding, and clotting times are prolonged. There are no characteristic findings in the urine.

DIFFERENTIAL DIAGNOSIS. In Europeans, Americans, and others who are not immune, malaria must be excluded by examination of thick and thin blood films. In immunes, the presence of malarial parasites in the blood film does not exclude the additional diagnosis of leishmaniasis. In many parts of the tropics where malaria and schistosomiasis are endemic, a palpable spleen is commonplace and is usually unrelated to a recent febrile illness. Diseases which can be confused with visceral leishmaniasis include aleukemic leukemia and lymphomas, tropical splenomegaly syndrome (serum IgM, liver biopsy), cirrhosis of the liver with portal hypertension and hypersplenism, miliary tuberculosis, histoplasmosis, acute schistosomiasis, brucellosis, typhoid, and other septicemias, including bacterial endocarditis.

PROGNOSIS. Studies of an epidemic of visceral leishmaniasis in Italy suggest that subclinical infection is four times as common as classic kala-azar (Pampiglione et al., 1974, 1975). Untreated, 75 to 90 per cent of patients with established disease die. Treated, in all early cases, patients should recover. The mortality of late or severe disease in malnourished patients treated under difficult conditions can be over 25 per cent. Bad prognostic signs include extreme emaciation and toxemia, agranulocytosis, and the absence of the lymphocytosis which usually appears during treatment.

TREATMENT. Chemotherapy. Pentavalent antimony is the drug of choice, and, of the available preparations, sodium stibogluconate* (Sb) (Pentostam, Solustibostam) is probably the best. This is marketed as a solution containing 100 mg Sb per milliliter. The dose is 0.1 to 0.2 ml per kilogram of body weight daily by intravenous or intramuscular injection, not exceeding 10 ml per dose. In India six injections are usually adequate, but elsewhere 30 are considered necessary. Alternative preparations include the following: (1) Meglumine antimoniate (Glucantime, 30 mg per ml), 0.4 ml per kilogram of body weight daily for 14 days. (2) Ethyl stibamine (Neostibosan), which must be freshly prepared as a 5 per cent solution. The adult dose is 0.1 gram the first day, 0.2 gram the second day, and 0.3 gram daily thereafter for 8 to 16 doses by intravenous injection. (3) Urea stibamine, 100 to 200 mg intravenously on alternate days for 15 doses. Side effects of pentavalent antimony are cumulative but rare. They are nausea, vomiting, urticaria, bradycardia, and electrocardiographic changes. The response to antimonial treatment varies in kala-azar from different parts of the world. It is excellent in India and Brazil but less satisfactory in patients from East Africa or the Mediterranean. The choice then lies between two toxic drugs, pentamidine isethionate* (Lomidine, 40 mg per milliliter) and amphotericin B (Fungizone). The dose of pentamidine is 0.1 ml per kilogram of body weight by intramuscular injection every three to four days for ten doses, or less frequently if side effects develop. If the drug is accidentally injected intravenously, the patient will collapse, but recovers quickly if the feet are raised. Cumulative side effects include fatigue, anorexia, nausea, abdominal pain and, in 2 per cent of cases, prolonged hypoglycemia. Ten per cent of patients develop diabetes whose onset is not related to

*Available from Center for Disease Control (404-633-3311, Ext. 3670).

the duration of treatment. If this drug has to be used, a glucose tolerance test should be performed weekly. Amphotericin B is given by slow intravenous infusion in 5 per cent dextrose in a dose of 1 mg per kilogram of body weight on alternate days to a total of 2 grams for a 50-kg adult. Side effects include rigors, thrombophlebitis, nausea, vomiting, fatigue, anemia, and uremia. This drug is more difficult to administer than pentamidine but is preferable.

Supportive Treatment. Bed rest, good nursing care, oral hygiene, an adequate fluid intake, and sufficient food are all desirable. Complicating infections must be sought and treated. Anemia responds as the patient recovers, but if severe, and especially if there is bleeding, blood transfusion should be given. Deficiencies of iron, folate, and other vitamins need treating.

Response to Treatment. Little improvement may be seen until the course of treatment is nearly over. The patient then continues to improve steadily. Lymphocytosis and reticulocytosis develop. No criterion of cure has been established. The patient should be seen monthly for six months and at a year. At each visit blood is cultured for *Leishmania*, spleen size is measured, and hemoglobin and serum IgG estimated. Complement-fixing antibody should not be detectable after six months. The spleen does not always become impalpable, and may indicate that cirrhosis has developed.

Relapses and Post-Kala-Azar Dermal Leishmaniasis. These usually respond to a further course or courses of antimony. If not, one of the other drugs may be used. One month should elapse before repeating a course. Rarely, if repeated courses of drugs fail to eliminate the parasite, the spleen remains huge, and the patient suffers from hypersplenism, splenectomy may be indicated. It must be followed by a course of chemotherapy, and in malarial areas by antimalarial prophylaxis for life.

PREVENTION. On a mass scale the detailed epidemiology of the local disease must be known. This will enable reservoir control (destruction of stray dogs, early detection and treatment of cases) and vector control (insecticide spraying in the right places) to be carried out, and people may be able to avoid contact with infected flies, e.g., Kenyan termite hills. In some areas insecticide spraying against malarial mosquitoes reduced or eliminated kala-azar. Personal prophylaxis depends on wearing protective clothing in the evenings, the use of insect repellents, and sleeping under fine mesh netting.

195.3. CUTANEOUS LEISHMANIASIS OF THE OLD WORLD

(Oriental Sore)

EPIDEMIOLOGY. The innumerable names of this disease (Delhi or Bagdad boil, Biskra button, Aleppo evil, bouton de Crete, little sister) testify to its extent and familiarity throughout the Mediterranean basin, the Near and Middle East, and parts of India. Four epidemiologic situations are recognized.

"Rural" leishmaniasis throughout these areas is caused by the subspecies *L. tropica major*. The disease is a zoonosis among the desert gerbils (*Rhomobomys opimus*) and is transmitted to man by *Phlebotomus papatasii*. Where village settlements are close to gerbil colonies, up to 100 per cent of the population become infected, usually in early childhood. Travelers, hunters, and soldiers also get the disease. In "urban" leishmaniasis, the parasite *L. tropica minor* is adapted to dogs and to man, either of whom can act as reservoirs. *P. sergenti* is the main vector. This disease was the scourge of Middle Eastern cities; every adult inhabitant bore the scar, and few visitors were spared.

In Africa two distinct zoonoses exist. In West Africa the situation is "rural." Human cases are uncommon and sporadic. The vector and reservoir are not definitely established, but rodents and dogs are probably involved. In Ethiopia and Kenya the disease is confined to the highlands, where the reservoir is the rock hyrax (*Procavia*). The vector is *P. longipes*, which bites villagers at night in their houses. The parasite has recently been designated *L. aethiopica*.

PATHOLOGY. At the site of inoculation there is a massive infiltration with monocytes and histiocytes which take up the parasites and support their growth. The lesion then becomes surrounded by or mixed with lymphocytes and a few plasma cells. Macrophages develop into epithelioid cells, and parasites diminish. In later cases loose tubercles composed of loosely packed cells may develop. The overlying dermis ulcerates. The epidermis shows hyperkeratosis, acanthosis, pseudoepitheliomatous hyperplasia, intraepidermal necrosis, and ulceration. Healing is accompanied by fibrosis and is followed by lifelong immunity. Second infections are seen in only about 2 per 1000 cases, and then often in association with a generalized depression of immunity.

If cell-mediated immunity fails to develop, the patient gets diffuse cutaneous leishmaniasis, the disease spreading to other parts of the skin. Histologic study shows masses of heavily parasitized macrophages with little or no lymphocytic infiltration or epidermal change. The leishmanin test is negative.

In leishmaniasis recidiva, failure to heal is associated with exquisite delayed hypersensitivity, extreme chronicity, a tuberculoid histology with epithelioid giant cells but without caseation, and scanty or undetectable parasites.

CLINICAL MANIFESTATIONS. The earliest lesion is a small erythematous papule, appearing two to eight weeks after the sandfly bite. It may itch slightly. The typical "urban" sore grows slowly into a nodule 1 to 2 cm across, and after a period of weeks or months forms a central crust under which is a shallow ulcer. The edge of the lesion is characteristically studded with small satellite papules. The sore usually remains in this state for a few more months and then heals gradually, leaving a depressed mottled scar. The whole process takes from three months to two years. The most common site is the face, followed by the arms and legs. There may be one or several sores. Immunity after healing is usually lifelong, but second infections may develop in old age or in patients taking corticosteroid drugs. About 1 per cent of urban sores develop *leishmaniasis recidiva (lupoid leishmaniasis)*. The ulcer fails to heal completely, scarring centrally but spreading peripherally, or heals and recrudesces at the edge of the scar. The lesion lasts for many years and resembles cutaneous tuberculosis.

There are many variants of the typical pattern of Oriental sore. "Rural" sores are commonly multiple, rapid

Early diffuse cutaneous leishmaniasis in an Ethiopian. Post-kala-azar dermal leishmaniasis may also look like this.

in evolution, and more florid, and produce more scarring. Ethiopian lesions are solitary, facial, milder, and slower in evolution, although lesions affecting the mucocutaneous border of the nose are extremely chronic and disfiguring.

Ethiopia and Kenya are the only Old World countries where *diffuse cutaneous leishmaniasis* is found. It is a rare condition, occurring in perhaps 1 in 100,000 cases. The primary nodule does not ulcerate, but after a period of months or years starts to spread locally, and

the disease disseminates to other parts of the skin, notably on the face and the extensor surfaces of the limbs, producing infiltrative and nodular lesions which may resemble lepromatous leprosy and do not heal spontaneously. The viscera are not involved, and the patient feels well.

DIAGNOSIS. Leishmaniasis must be suspected as the cause of any chronic nodule or ulcer in a person living in or having recently visited an endemic area. Typical sores are diagnosable on sight. Diagnosis is confirmed by finding parasites in stained slit skin smears taken from a nonulcerated part of the lesion. The slit must reach the dermis, and the smears must contain tissue juice, not blood or pus. If unsuccessful, the crust is removed, the ulcer cleaned of all debris, and smears made of tissue scraped from the base of the ulcer. These methods are simpler and more likely to show parasites than is histology. In healing lesions and lupoid leishmaniasis, parasites are scanty and culture of juice or biopsy tissue may be necessary.

The leishmanin test becomes positive as the lesion ulcerates and is of diagnostic value in patients who do not live in endemic areas; it also may help to distinguish lupoid leishmaniasis from cutaneous tuberculosis, late syphilis, and fungal granulomas, which may be histologically similar.

There are no characteristic blood changes, and antibodies are difficult to demonstrate by usual techniques.

TREATMENT. Treatment remains unsatisfactory, but, as almost all cases heal spontaneously, the systemic use of toxic drugs is seldom justified. Fortunately most cases respond to a course of pentavalent antimony* Failure to respond is usually due to inadequate dosage or duration of treatment. Local infiltration with 0.5 ml 2 per cent berberine sulfate or 15 per cent mepacrine is often effective. Indolent sores may respond to heating to 50° C by coned infrared rays, to curettage and skin grafting, or to intralesional injections of corticosteroids combined with a course of antimony. Secondary infection is treated with the customary antimicrobial drugs.

PREVENTION. Detailed epidemiologic knowledge has permitted attacks on the reservoir in Central Asia and in Middle Eastern cities, where demolition of mud

---

*Available from Center for Disease Control (404-633-3311, Ext. 3670).

Cutaneous Leishmaniasis of the New World: Epidemiology

Parasite	Vector to Man	Reservoir	Geography	Human Disease
L. mexicana mexicana	*Lutzomyia olmeca*	Numerous rodents	Yucatan, Central America	"Chicle ulcer, bay sore" in forest workers; single skin lesions, healing in six months; diffuse cutaneous leishmaniasis
L. mexicana amazonensis	*Lutzomyia flaviscutellata*	Numerous rodents	Brazil, Trinidad; ?= *L. pifanoi*, Venezuela	Rare, single skin lesions; diffuse cutaneous leishmaniasis
L. brasiliensis brasiliensis	*Psychodopygus wellcomei*, *Lutzomyia spp.*	Uncertain	All Amazon forests, esp. Brazil	"Espundia"; single or few large persistent destructive skin ulcers; oronasal metastases common
L. brasiliensis guyanensis	*Lutzomyia anduzei*	Unknown	Guyanas, into Brazil, Venezuela	"Forest yaws, pian bois"; multiple, widespread, deep skin ulcers, with nodular lymphatic metastases; ? oronasal metastases
L. brasiliensis panamensis	*Lutzomyia trapidoi*, *Psychodopygus pana-mensis*, and others	Rodents, sloths, dogs	Panama	Single or few deep skin ulcers with nodular lymphatic metastases; ? oronasal metastases
L. peruviana	*Lutzomyia verrucarum*, ? *Lutzomyia peruensis*	Dogs	Peru, west slopes of Andes to 3000 meters	"Uta"; single or few skin lesions, healing in one year

buildings and antimalarial spraying have reduced the number of sandflies. Immunization with live, virulent organisms is practiced on a mass scale in Russia and traditionally in the Middle East (see R. A. Neal, 1968).

195.4. CUTANEOUS LEISHMANIASIS OF THE NEW WORLD

(Including American Mucocutaneous Leishmaniasis or Espundia)

EPIDEMIOLOGY AND PARASITOLOGY. Cutaneous leishmaniasis is endemic in Central and South America as far south as the Parana Estuary in the east and the Peruvian Andes in the west. In this extensive and varied terrain many different zoonoses exist, each associated with its own reservoirs and vectors and a particular pattern of human disease. Two main groups of parasites are now distinguished, those of *L. mexicana* and of *L. brasiliensis*. The former, which grows easily in NNN medium and in the hamster, is responsible for most of the cutaneous leishmaniasis in Central America and a little in Brazil. The latter, which grows poorly in NNN medium and in the hamster, is responsible for most of the disease in South America, including mucocutaneous leishmaniasis. Epidemiologic details are summarized in the accompanying table.

Cutaneous leishmaniasis presents a formidable obstacle to the development of the Central and South American forests, in large areas of which transmission of the infection is extremely high. This is particularly true in Brazil, where many workers on the trans-Amazonian highway become infected and run the risk of developing mutilating oronasal metastatic lesions. Amerindians, on the other hand, commonly develop transient mild infections so that by the age of 40 years up to 100 per cent are sensitive to leishmanin. They rarely develop mucocutaneous lesions.

PATHOLOGY. The pathology of cutaneous lesions is similar to that of Oriental sore. Metastatic lesions of *L. brasiliensis* arise in the mucosa of the nose and mouth and show at first a typical leishmanial granuloma with numerous parasites, which later become scanty, and can be seen also in cells in cartilage, which is rapidly invaded and destroyed. There is vasculitis with edema, necrosis, and fibrosis.

CLINICAL MANIFESTATIONS. Cutaneous lesions develop and heal in the same way as Oriental sores, but tend to be less nodular and more ulcerative and destructive. Lesions of *L. mexicana* on the pinna may last for many years and slowly destroy the cartilage. Regional variations are given in the table.

In espundia, from 2 per cent (Panama) to 80 per cent (Paraguay) of primary cutaneous sores are followed after a period ranging from a few days to 25 years by metastatic lesions of the nose or mouth, most commonly on the mucocutaneous borders, but sometimes on the palate or larynx and rarely on the conjunctiva or external genitalia. Nasal obstruction is the most common early symptom. These lesions may arise many years after the primary lesion has healed. At first there is crusting or polyp formation, and then ulceration and perforation of the septum. Alternatively, large protruding granulomas of the nose and lips develop. The lesion heals slowly, if at all, after many years. Scarring

may constrict the nose or mouth, producing gross deformity and making eating difficult. Secondary sepsis is common and increases the patient's debility.

Diffuse cutaneous leishmaniasis is a rare disease described mainly from Venezuela and northern Brazil. Its clinical features are the same as in Ethiopia.

DIAGNOSIS. The approach to diagnosis is set forth in Ch. 195.2 and 195.3. In late cases of espundia it may be impossible to isolate the parasite, but geographic history, clinical pattern, and leishmanin sensitivity make the diagnosis likely. Antibodies are detectable by immunofluorescence in over 90 per cent of patients with cutaneous or oronasal lesions, and disappear when the disease has been successfully treated. Blastomycosis is added to the list of differential diagnoses.

TREATMENT. The milder varieties of solitary sores seldom need treatment, unless they are disfiguring. If there is any suspicion that a sore has been caused by *L. brasiliensis,* it must be treated by a course of pentavalent antimony (see Ch. 195.2). Established oronasal lesions frequently do not respond to antimony, or are liable to relapse. Amphotericin B (see Ch. 195.2) is then the drug of choice. Diffuse cutaneous leishmaniasis responds initially to antimony, but becomes resistant in relapse. Amphotericin B should then be tried.

PREVENTION. Prevention in South America is difficult. Intensity of transmission in the forest and lack of detailed epidemiologic information make mass prophylaxis a hopeless approach at the moment. People who are obliged to enter the forest could attempt to follow a regimen of the application of insect repellents every few hours and of sleeping under a fine mesh netting, but admittedly both these procedures can produce considerable discomfort.

Chance, M. L., Peters, W., and Shchory, L.: Biochemical taxonomy of *Leishmania*. Ann. Trop. Med. Parasit., *68*:307, 317, 1974.
Lainson, R., and Shaw, J. J.: Leishmaniasis of the New World: Taxonomic problems. Br. Med. Bull., 28:44, 1972.
Manson-Bahr, P. E. C., and Winslow, D. J.: Cutaneous leishmaniasis. *In* Marcial-Rojas, R. A. (ed.): Pathology of Rickettsial and Helminthic Diseases. Baltimore, Williams & Wilkins Company, 1971, p. 97.
Marsden, P. D., and Nonata, R. R.: Mucocutaneous leishmaniasis: A review of clinical aspects. Rev. Soc. Bras. Med. Trop., 9:309, 1975.
Most, H., and Lavietes, R. H.: Kala-azar in American military personnel. Medicine, 26:221, 1947.
Symposium on leishmaniasis. Bull. WHO, 44:477, 1971.
Turk, J. L., and Bryceson, A. D. M.: Immunological phenomena in leprosy and related diseases. Adv. Immunol., 13:209, 1971.
Walton, B. C., Brooks, W. H., and Arjona, I.: Serodiagnosis of American leishmaniasis by indirect fluorescent antibody test. Am. J. Trop. Med. Hyg., 21:296, 1972.
Wilcocks, C., and Manson-Bahr, P. E. C. (eds.): Manson's Tropical Diseases. 17th ed. Baltimore, Williams & Wilkins Company, 1972.
Winslow, D. J.: Visceral leishmaniasis. *In* Marcial-Rojas, R. A. (ed.): Pathology of Rickettsial and Helminthic Diseases. Baltimore, Williams & Wilkins Company, 1971, p. 86.

196. AMEBIASIS

Richard Knight

DEFINITION. Amebiasis is caused by infection with *Entamoeba histolytica*. This species normally lives as a commensal within the large bowel lumen, where it may persist for several years. Symptoms of the disease may be produced if there is bowel wall invasion or subsequent blood-borne spread to the liver.

ETIOLOGY. Noninvasive trophozoites of *E. histolytica* measure 10 to 20 μ in diameter and live adjacent to the mucosa of the proximal colon, where they feed upon bacteria and exfoliated epithelial cells. They multiply by binary fission every eight hours; some of them round up, eliminate their cytoplasmic inclusions, and secrete a rigid cell wall to become uninucleate spherical cysts (10 to 16 μ in diameter); immature cysts contain a large glycogen vacuole. The cysts mature either within the bowel lumen or outside the body. Most mature cysts have four nuclei resulting from two nuclear divisions, and cigar-shaped chromatoid bars that constitute a ribosome store. When these mature cysts are ingested, they undergo one additional nuclear division. The cyst wall is destroyed in the small intestine, releasing eight motile uninucleate amebae or trophozoites.

Invasive *E. histolytica* are larger than noninvasive forms, up to 50 μ, and move much more actively by unidirectional pseudopodial movement. They contain ingested erythrocytes — hence the term hematophagous — and few or no bacteria.

Freshly isolated strains of *E. histolytica* behave differently when inoculated intracecally into weanling rats, those from patients with dysentery often being the most pathogenic. Strain virulence is relatively unstable and in culture often decreases quite rapidly, although it may usually be restored by animal passage. A few strains have been isolated that differ from *E. histolytica* antigenically and by their ability to grow at room temperature and in hypotonic media. These atypical or *E. histolytica*–like amebae are probably never pathogenic; *all other strains of E. histolytica are potentially virulent.*

EPIDEMIOLOGY. About 10 per cent of the world's population harbor *E. histolytica.* In the United States the prevalence is 2 to 5 per cent, in some tropical countries over 40 per cent. Poverty and poor sanitation encourage infection. Cysts may survive a month in water but are killed by drying. Rats, dogs, and certain monkeys are sometimes infected, but almost all human infections are from cysts passed by human carriers. *Encystment does not occur outside the body,* so patients passing only trophozoites in their stools are not infectious. Food is the most common vehicle of transmission; it may be contaminated by infected food handlers or flies. Direct contamination with human feces used as fertilizer is most common with salad vegetables. Direct fecal spread is important among children or the mentally handicapped in institutions, where infection rates may be very high.

Water-borne infection occurs, occasionally in epidemic form, as in the famous Chicago epidemic in which there were 1400 known cases and more than 100 deaths. Epidemics are probably not often recognized because the incubation period is so variable and many infections asymptomatic. Cysts may appear in the stool as early as four days after infection. The rate of spontaneous loss of infection is perhaps 15 per cent per year, so persons coming to temperate countries from the tropics may remain infected for five years or more. In countries where there is continuous transmission, prevalence rates remain stable from year to year. In certain parts of the world, such as Mexico, parts of South America, the West Coast of Africa, Natal, and Southeast Asia, invasive disease is especially common. The incidence of disease does not necessarily correlate with the prevalence of infection.

PATHOGENESIS AND PATHOLOGY. Commensal trophozoites thrive adjacent to the colonic mucosa where the oxygen tension is moderately low and the pH between 6.0 and 6.5. Host tissues are damaged only by direct contact with amebae, when membrane-bound cytolytic enzymes are released from dendritic plasmalemmal processes. The relatively anoxic and acid conditions of cell necrosis favor further penetration of amebae into the tissues. Although some amebic bowel lesions are secondarily infected, the role of intestinal bacteria in pathogenesis is still uncertain. They may act mainly by creating a milieu suitable for amebic growth.

Amebic ulceration is most common in the cecum and rectosigmoid, but may affect any part of the large bowel, appendix, and terminal ileum. The initial lesions are small, discrete superficial mucosal erosions which may then extend more deeply through the muscularis mucosae and spread laterally, producing ulcers that are flask shaped in cross-section. Lesions may coalesce, causing extensive mucosal loss. Blood vessel involvement usually results in local thrombosis. Penetration may extend through the muscle coats, causing *peritonitis,* the most dangerous complication of intestinal amebiasis. Microscopically, tissue necrosis is the main change; amebae occur throughout the lesion, but particularly at the advancing edge, and even beyond into healthy tissue. In tissue sections, amebae may appear shrunken and be surrounded by a clear space. They stain rather indistinctly with ordinary hematoxylin and eosin but stand out clearly as bright red bodies with periodic acid–Schiff stain; iron hematoxylin staining is necessary to show the nuclear structure clearly. The lymphocytic inflammatory response is slight or moderate; some neutrophils are also present, especially if there is secondary bacterial infection.

Ulcers heal rapidly after treatment, and persistent scarring is uncommon. Sometimes localized bowel lesions show a more vigorous host response, with edema and a marked inflammatory reaction producing an amebic granuloma or ameboma. These are most common in the cecum and rectosigmoid and may be multiple.

Although strain virulence may influence the probability of tissue invasion, host factors are also important. Women in late pregnancy and the puerperium are especially susceptible, as are patients on cytotoxic or corticosteroid therapy. Colonic cancers may be secondarily invaded by *E. histolytica.* *Trichuris trichiura* infections and intestinal schistosomiasis may also encourage invasion. The low protein diets of developing countries may enhance susceptibility, especially in children.

Hepatic Involvement. In many patients with invasive intestinal disease, amebae probably reach the liver via the portal vein, but most are destroyed. Hepatomegaly is frequent in acute amebic dysentery because of products of colonic tissue destruction or bacteria reaching the liver. Established amebic infection of the liver usually causes progressive cytolytic lesions that extend in all directions, with trophozoites proliferating near the advancing edge. Perhaps these lesions begin at the sites of venous embolism or thrombosis. Secondary bacterial infection is rare, and the content of such a "liver abscess" is necrotic liquefied liver tissue. The abscess is sharply demarcated from surrounding liver, which shows edema, hyperemia, and a narrow zone of lymphocytic and polymorphonuclear infiltration; a fibroblastic reaction occurs in longstanding lesions. Most liver abscesses are solitary and occur long after any clinically evident bowel ulceration; but both solitary and the rarer multiple abscesses may develop during or shortly after a bout of dysentery. The term *amebic hepatitis* has been used by clinicians, but there is no pathologic basis for a diffuse lesion of this kind. In adults, 80 to 90 per cent of amebic liver abscesses occur in men, but before puberty both sexes are similarly affected. No other host factors have been definitely identified, although pre-existing liver disease and alcoholism may be relevant. Most complications of liver abscess are due to direct spread to adjacent structures.

Antibody Response. Tissue invasion provokes a humoral antibody response, mainly IgG, and a skin sensitivity to injected amebic antigen. It is not known whether this response has any protective function. Using sensitive techniques, antibodies can be detected in 25 per cent or more of apparently healthy carriers, suggesting that mild self-limiting bowel invasion is more common than has been supposed.

CLINICAL MANIFESTATIONS. Intestinal Amebiasis. Most persons with *E. histolytica* in the stool have no symptoms, and many will remain symptomless carriers for the whole duration of their infection. Invasive bowel disease begins most commonly between one and six months after infection but sometimes much later, especially in an immunologically compromised host.

The disease spectrum is wide, and the clinical picture depends on the severity and extent of bowel wall involvement. Most commonly, ulceration is localized and not severe enough to produce dysentery. The patient complains of colicky pains in the right or left iliac fossa, flatulence, and an altered bowel habit, often with some diarrhea. A little blood or mucus may be noted in the stool; there is little constitutional upset. The cecum or sigmoid colon may be tender or feel abnormal on palpation. Symptoms may persist intermittently for months thereafter, and spontaneous cure is not uncommon.

Widespread colonic or rectosigmoid ulceration produces amebic dysentery with frequent bloody stools. Dysentery may begin abruptly, but often follows a varied period of the milder colonic symptoms noted above. Initially, many patients remain ambulant, but later, fever, colicky abdominal pains, and tenesmus appear. The illness is usually less acute than bacillary dysentery and dehydration less evident. There may be colonic tenderness and some hepatomegaly. The stool is often offensive and contains some fecal matter; much of the blood present is altered unless there is rectal ulceration. Sigmoidoscopic appearances are not pathognomonic, but the procedure is useful for initial assessment and follow-up; scrapings should be examined immediately for hematophagous trophozoites. In the rare fulminating form of the disease, toxic megacolon occurs with progressive abdominal distention, vomiting, dehydration, and electrolyte loss; some very ill patients have relatively few bowel actions. Sigmoidoscopy and barium enema examination should not be carried out in patients with severe dysentery; when the diagnosis is in doubt, a limited endoscopy may be justified.

Amebomas may present as a tender abdominal mass, sometimes with fever and constitutional upset. Partial bowel obstruction may occur, especially when the lesion is annular. The appendix may be affected primarily, or secondarily by a cecal lesion. This may resemble simple appendicitis, except that pain begins in the right iliac fossa, and guarding and rigidity are slight unless perforation has occurred.

COMPLICATIONS. A grossly diseased and atonic large bowel may perforate at several points. Absent bowel sounds with relatively little pain, rigidity, or tenderness should suggest this very dangerous possibility. Free gas in the peritoneum confirms it. Less commonly, when perforation is localized, classic signs of peritonitis are produced. Local perforation can also lead to pericolic abscess or retroperitoneal fecal cellulitis. *Fibrous strictures* of the colon rarely follow amebic dysentery or amebomas, but may require surgical relief. Serious hemorrhage is uncommon, but can be life threatening. Amebic ulceration or an ameboma may rarely initiate a cecocolic intussusception. Irritable bowel syndrome may follow amebic colitis and persist for several months. Much rarer is the syndrome of postdysenteric colitis which can continue for several years despite eradication of the amebic infection. It is distinct from simple ulcerative colitis and is associated with very high amebic antibody titers; endoscopy shows a reddened edematous mucosa, sometimes with superficial erosions. Barium enema examination will exclude the rare possibility of internal fistulas.

Cutaneous amebiasis takes the form of deep, painful, and rapidly spreading ulceration. The most common sites are the perianal area, perineum, laparotomy incisions, and colostomy stomas. Rarely, the uterine cervix is affected, giving lesions that may resemble carcinoma. Penile lesions may follow anal coitus.

Hepatic Amebiasis. About half of all patients with liver abscess have a history suggestive of amebic dysentery between a week and many years previously. Solitary lesions are most common in the upper part of the right lobe; multiple lesions are often associated with coexistent dysentery. The illness begins insidiously with fever, sweating, and pain in the liver region. If the diaphragm is involved, there may be right pleuritic or shoulder pain. Most patients present within a few weeks of onset; as the disease progresses, weight loss and anemia develop. *Those developing the condition in temperate countries after returning from the tropics rarely have bowel symptoms.* Hepatomegaly is always present, but if enlargement is mainly upward, it may not be very evident on abdominal palpation. Left lobe lesions are palpable as an epigastric mass. Liver tenderness is mainly localized to the site of the lesion, and, in suspected cases, all the lower right intercostal spaces should be carefully palpated. Pain on heavy percussion or compression of the liver is not a very specific sign, because many types of liver and chest disease will be painful with these procedures. Crepitations and signs of lung consolidation or pleural fluid in the lower right chest are quite common. Jaundice occurs only when lesions are very large or numerous. The blood sedimentation rate is raised, and normally there is polymorphonuclear leukocytosis and some normocytic normochromic anemia. Levels of serum transaminase and alkaline phosphatase are variable and of little diagnostic value. *The most suggestive roentgenographic finding* is an immobile, raised, or bulging right hemidiaphragm; lung or pleural involvement may also be visible. Liver scans help considerably to show the site, size, and number of lesions present; radioisotope scans are probably most useful, but ultrasound and computerized axial tomography may also be helpful.

COMPLICATIONS. Rupture through the diaphragm can produce amebic lung abscess or empyema and sometimes a bronchohepatic fistula so that the patient coughs up amebic pus. Extension to the body surface may lead to sinus formation and cutaneous lesions. Amebic peritonitis follows rupture into the peritoneum, and the primary source may be evident only at laparotomy. The gut, stomach, vena cava, spleen, and right kidney can also be involved by direct spread. A dangerous complication of left lobe lesions is *amebic pericarditis;* urgent aspiration may be necessary to relieve tamponade, and fibrous constrictive pericarditis is a rare late sequel. More than 100 cases of *amebic brain abscess* have been reported. All have been associated with liver abscess and, so far, all patients have died. This condition should not be confused with primary amebic meningoencephalitis caused by free-living amebae *(Naegleria).* Hematogenous lesions also occasionally occur in the lung and perhaps elsewhere.

DIFFERENTIAL DIAGNOSIS. Intestinal Amebiasis. Amebic dysentery may resemble bacillary dysentery, nonspecific ulcerative colitis, intestinal salmonellosis, and, more rarely, heavy infection with intestinal schistosomiasis or *Trichuris trichiura.* Patients with nondysenteric colitis are often suspected of having irritable bowel syndrome, and blood in the stool may be attributed to hemorrhoids. Diverticulitis, carcinoma, and Crohn's disease of the colon may require exclusion by barium enema and sigmoidoscopy. *The finding of E. histolytica should not delay the search for another disease, especially because amebic ulceration may be superimposed upon a carcinoma.* Amebomas may mimic neoplastic, infective, and granulomatous conditions of the large bowel, including lymphogranuloma venereum when the rectum is involved. The interpretation of therapeutic trials with tissue amebicides may be difficult, and the delay can make a tumor inoperable.

Hepatic Amebiasis. In the differential diagnosis of hepatic amebiasis, it is necessary to exclude primary and secondary neoplasms of the liver, subphrenic abscess, and pyogenic liver abscesses, including those caused by migrating *Ascaris* worms. Other conditions to be considered are hydatid cyst, the painful or tender hepatomegaly of viral or alcoholic hepatitis, and various pleural or lung lesions of the right lower chest. Liver scans and amebic serology have made *diagnostic needle aspiration* less often necessary, but the finding of relatively odorless brownish or pink material with no bacteria on Gram staining is almost pathognomonic. An 8-cm pleural aspiration needle 1.5 to 2.0 mm in diameter connected to a large syringe via a three-way tap is normally used. When there is no definite clinical evidence as to the site of the lesion, the eighth or ninth right intercostal space should be explored in the midaxillary line.

LABORATORY DIAGNOSIS. Microscopy and Culture. The finding of hematophagous trophozoites in fresh stools or material obtained at endoscopy confirms the presence of invasive colonic amebiasis. Symptomless carriers and those with mild ulceration of the proximal colon pass only cysts in their stools. Liver abscess patients pass cysts or, less commonly, hematophagous trophozoites; sometimes, however, no bowel infection can be demonstrated.

Hematophagous trophozoites should be sought in temporary wet mounts of dysenteric stools, bowel wall scrapings, material from suspected skin lesions, and in the last portion of pus obtained at liver aspiration. If necessary, the material should be diluted with buffered saline (ideally, pH 6.8). In nondysenteric stools, flecks

of mucus or pus should be looked for and examined. Trophozoites remain active and recognizable for about 30 minutes above 18° C (see Fig. 2, Ch. 193). If delay will inevitably be longer than this, the specimen should be kept cool as activity is restored, even after several hours at 4° C. If necessary, amebae may be preserved in polyvinyl alcohol and identified after staining with Heidenhain's iron hematoxylin or Gomori's trichrome stain; alternatively, a smear may be fixed in Schaudinn's fixative and stained later. In wet mounts, the definitive identification of nonhematophagous *E. histolytica* is not possible, and even in stained preparations, it is not easy; for this reason purged stool specimens are of no help unless hematophagous amebae are obtained. On the other hand, *E. histolytica* cysts can be readily recognized in wet mounts, using dilute Lugol's iodine to define nuclear and chromatoid morphology. Cyst concentration techniques using formol ether sedimentation or zinc sulfate flotation give a diagnostic sensitivity of about 70 per cent per specimen compared with 30 per cent without concentration. Examination of concentrates from stools obtained on three separate days is normally sufficient to exclude an intraluminal amebic infection. Cysts in stool may be preserved in 10 per cent formalin, but this reduces the effectiveness of concentration procedures. Besides *E. histolytica,* three nonpathogenic species of *Entamoeba* may infect man; they are never hematophagous and may be recognized by their cystic stages.

E. hartmanni is closely related to *E. histolytica* but is smaller, the peripheral nuclear chromatin is more clumped, and the quadrinucleate cysts are less than 10 μ in diameter (mean, 8 μ). *E. coli* is another common commensal, whose sluggish trophozoites (20 to 30 μ) have coarse granular endoplasm. The karyosome is eccentric and the peripheral chromatin coarser than that of *E. histolytica.* Mature cysts (12 to 20 μ) have eight nuclei and thin-pointed chromatoids. *E. polecki* is primarily a pig parasite and is rare in man except in parts of New Guinea where pigs and man live in close association. The mature cyst has only one nucleus and resembles an immature *E. histolytica* cyst.

Cultivation of *E. histolytica* from fresh stool is not difficult with appropriate media, and is sometimes helpful in confirming the diagnosis. Stained preparations of isolates must be made for accurate identification. If amebic liver pus is to be cultured, the medium should be preconditioned with *Escherichia coli.*

Serologic Tests. The most sensitive tests for the detection of amebic antibodies are indirect hemagglutination, indirect immunofluorescence, and counterimmunoelectrophoresis. Latex agglutination and gel diffusion precipitation tests are also used. Over 90 per cent of patients with liver abscess normally have positive serologic tests, compared with 60 to 80 per cent of those with invasive intestinal disease. Results must be interpreted with caution, as antibody may persist for several years, and in endemic areas some asymptomatic carriers and noninfected persons will have positive reactions. However, negative serologic tests are quite strong evidence against a diagnosis of liver abscess. Serologic tests are also valuable in suspected amebomas and other localized colonic lesions beyond the reach of sigmoidoscopy.

TREATMENT. Clinical Pharmacology. TISSUE AMEBICIDES. Metronidazole (Flagyl) is a potent and safe oral ambicide that is rapidly absorbed by the small bowel to reach all tissues. It is also useful in the treatment of intraluminal infections, because some is excreted in the bile in modified form and some directly into the colon. A five- or eight-day course of 750 or 800 mg thrice daily is effective in all forms of invasive amebiasis. Paradoxically, higher doses are required to eliminate a bowel infection than to destroy all tissue-invading amebae. Side effects very rarely necessitate stopping treatment; they include dizziness, nausea, abdominal pain, a metallic taste in the mouth, brownish discoloration of the urine, and a confusional state if alcohol is taken. The effectiveness of metronidazole has greatly simplified the chemotherapy of amebiasis, but its action is slightly less rapid than that of emetine, and a few treatment failures have been reported. A parenteral preparation of metronidazole has recently become available and may find a place in the treatment of amebic peritonitis.

Intramuscular emetine hydrochloride and the synthetic compound dehydroemetine dihydrochloride* are the most rapidly acting tissue amebicides, but both are toxic and cumulative. Emetine is given in a dose of 1 mg per kilogram of body weight daily (maximum, 60 mg daily) for up to ten days. *Serious cardiotoxicity* is suggested by hypotension, dyspnea, precordial pain, tachycardia, and palpitations, but is unusual until at least six doses have been given. Electrocardiographic changes include T wave inversion, prolongation of P-R interval, widening of the QRS complex, and arrhythmias. Less serious side effects are weakness, nausea, and vomiting, local myositis at the site of injection, and, rarely, a more generalized myositis. A course of treatment should not exceed ten days and should not be repeated without an interval of at least two weeks. Complete bed rest is essential. The drug should not be given to patients with cardiovascular disease, and is not generally recommended for pregnant women or for children. Dehydroemetine is excreted more rapidly in the urine than emetine, and a daily dose of 1.25 mg per kilogram of body weight (maximum, 90 mg daily) is necessary; it is probably less cardiotoxic.

The only indication for chloroquine is hepatic amebiasis, because the drug is concentrated by, and accumulates within, the liver. The usual regimen for adults consists of 150 mg base twice daily for three weeks. Some toxicity may occur with this regimen, including T wave changes on the electrocardiogram. *Patients being treated for invasive intestinal amebiasis with drugs other than emetine or metronidazole should be given a two-week course of chloroquine to prevent the development of hepatic lesions.*

LUMINAL AMEBICIDES. Tetracycline can be very useful in some patients with invasive intestinal disease; it acts upon bacteria within the lesions, but also has some direct amebicidal activity. Tetracycline is used in situations when a parenteral drug is needed, and when metronidazole or emetine is contraindicated or not available. It should not be used for long-term treatment (four weeks or more) in those under the age of puberty. If the drug is used alone, parasitic cure is uncommon, and there may be clinical relapse. For adults, the dosage is 250 or 500 mg every six hours for five to ten days.

Numerous substances have been used to eliminate the bowel infection in symptomless carriers and in patients with invasive disease who are not given metro-

nidazole. The most effective are diiodohydroxyquin, diloxanide furoate (Furamide),* and paromomycin (Humatin). The adverse effects of diiodohydroxyquin are mild diarrhea, pruritus ani, rashes, and rarely iodism. The related compound clioquinol (iodochlorohydroxyquin) has been incriminated as a rare cause of myelo-optic neuropathy.

Management. INTESTINAL AMEBIASIS. Amebic dysentery and nondysenteric colitis should be treated with emetine, metronidazole, or tetracycline, depending upon drug availability and contraindications. If emetine is given, only a three- to six-day course is normally required to control the acute phase of the disease. It should be combined with or followed by metronidazole or tetracycline with chloroquine. Tetracycline should probably be given to all patients with severe dysentery. Amebic peritonitis should be treated medically with gastric suction and intravenous fluid and electrolytes, together with emetine and parenteral tetracycline. If the diagnosis is made at laparotomy, surgical repair may be difficult because the bowel wall is so friable. Amebomas may be successfully treated with a full course of metronidazole or a ten-day course of emetine. In all forms of intestinal disease, if metronidazole is not used, a luminally active drug must also be given to eradicate the infection.

In countries where transmission rates are low, such as the United States and Western Europe, it is generally recommended that all detected symptomless infections should be treated to prevent later invasive disease or transmission to others. Suitable regimens for adults are diiodohydroxyquin, 650 mg thrice daily for 21 days; entamide furoate, 500 mg thrice daily for 10 days; or paromomycin, 500 mg thrice daily for seven days. Alternatively, a full course of metronidazole can be given, particularly if there is suspicion of tissue invasion or concurrent infection with *Giardia lamblia.*

HEPATIC AMEBIASIS. Liver abscess may be successfully treated with a ten-day course of emetine plus chloroquine for three weeks and a luminal amebicide. Alternatively, a five- or eight-day course of metronidazole may be used; 400 or 500 mg thrice daily will cure the liver lesion, but 750 or 800 mg should be given to eliminate the coexistent gut infection which must be assumed to be present. Being better tolerated, metronidazole will usually be the treatment of choice; however, unless the lesion is drained, resolution may be slower with this drug, and a few therapeutic failures have been reported.

Aspiration of the liver is sometimes necessary for therapeutic purposes as well as for diagnosis. Consequently, if it is at all possible, the patient with liver abscess should be treated in association with a surgeon. This is easily accomplished in a large metropolitan center. By contrast, in a remote rural area it may be necessary for the physician to perform needle aspiration. However, if drainage of the abscess is necessary and satisfactory facilities are available, it is preferable that this procedure, whether by needle or through laparotomy, be conducted as a surgical procedure. There is some risk of spreading the infection within the peritoneal cavity, but this is greatly lessened by preaspiration chemotherapy.

The indications for surgical drainage are as follows: (1) when aspiration is strongly indicated on clinical

---

*Available from Center for Disease Control (404-633-3311, Ext. 3670).

*Available from Center for Disease Control (404-633-3311, Ext. 3670).

grounds, but attempts by percutaneous route have failed to locate or adequately drain the lesion; (2) when the lesion continues to refill despite chemotherapy and several percutaneous aspirations; and (3) in the presence of left lobe lesions when not superficial or when the diagnosis is uncertain. An indwelling soft rubber drain is rarely required after surgical drainage; if used, it must be connected to a sterile underwater seal and removed early.

The principal indications for percutaneous aspiration are: (1) very large lesions and those in the left lobe, especially when there is clinical or radiologic evidence that rupture is imminent; (2) after rupture, if this has occurred into the pleural cavity or pericardium (these also must be aspirated); and (3) poor clinical response after five days of medical treatment. Sometimes the procedure may have to be repeated two or three times. The principal complications are hemorrhage and introduction of bacterial infection; the latter is suggested if the aspirate changes color, becomes very liquid or offensive, or contains gas. Bleeding is less common than might be expected, because in liver abscess the right hemidiaphragm rarely moves with respiration.

Amebic lung lesions will respond to treatment given for the associated liver lesion. Cutaneous lesions respond to either emetine or metronidazole.

PROGNOSIS. Despite a normally rapid response to treatment, invasive intestinal disease may relapse if the infection is not eliminated. Host factors may be relevant in some persons, including perhaps those with mild nonspecific colitis. If symptoms recur, care must be taken to exclude other colonic disease. There is so far no evidence of drug resistance by any strain of *E. histolytica*. Amebic peritonitis, especially when there are multiple gut perforations, carries a grave prognosis; but permanent sequelae after any form of amebic colitis are rare. Hepatic scanning suggests that filling defects normally disappear within two or four months after treatment of liver abscess. Failure to aspirate large lesions adequately may lead to clinical relapse or much slower resolution. Healing occurs with little scar formation, but if the lesion was secondarily infected, bizarre hepatic calcification may be seen years afterward. Published reports of unselected patients suggest that a 10 per cent mortality is not unusual in liver abscess, but the prognosis can be much better with early diagnosis and adequate treatment.

After successful treatment for amebiasis, there is no reason why a person from a temperate country should not return to the tropics.

PREVENTION. Chlorination of water supplies does not destroy *E. histolytica* cysts, but proper filtration is effective. A weak solution of iodine is a more potent cysticide than chlorine. Salads and vegetables may be soaked in vinegar or potassium permanganate solution; these are procedures of doubtful benefit, and for some they render the food inedible. A solution of sodium hypochlorite has been found useful. Visitors to the tropics should avoid purchasing food from street vendors and from premises where flies are evident. Fruit that can be skinned should be safe. Boiling water for five minutes kills cysts. Members of domestic staffs involved in food handling should have their stools examined.

Intermittent mass chemotherapy with entamide furoate and metronidazole has been successfully attempted in Mexico and elsewhere where invasive disease is common; it may also be useful in mental institutions in temperate countries. *Personal chemoprophylaxis* by visitors to the tropics is not recommended, and it is better for such persons to avoid eating uncooked foods and to have their stools examined on return.

Amoebiasis: Report of a WHO Expert Committee. WHO Technical Report Series No. 421, 1–52, 1969.

Barbour, G. L., and Juniper, K., Jr.: A clinical comparison of amebic and pyogenic abscess of the liver. Am. J. Med., 53:323, 1972.

Biagi–F., F., and Beltran, H. F.: The challenge of amoebiasis: Understanding pathogenic mechanisms. Int. Rev. Trop. Med., 3:219, 1969.

Elsdon-Dew, R.: The epidemiology of amoebiasis. Adv. Parasitol., 6:1, 1968.

Krogstad, D. J., et al.: Amebiasis: Epidemiologic studies in the United States, 1971–1974. Ann. Intern. Med., 88:89, 1978.

Powell, S. J.: New developments in the therapy of amoebiasis. Gut, 11:967, 1970.

Sepulveda, B., and Diamond, L. S.: Amebiasis. Instituto Mexicano del Seguro Social, Mexico, 1976.

Wilmot, A. J.: Clinical Amoebiasis. Oxford, Blackwell, 1962.

197. TOXOPLASMOSIS

Thomas C. Jones

GENERAL CONSIDERATIONS. Toxoplasmosis is a common infection of mammals and birds which occasionally results in protean disease. It is caused by the protozoan *Toxoplasma gondii*. In man, tissue parasitism during the proliferative phase may occur without signs or symptoms; it may lead to a transient illness characterized by lymphadenopathy, fever, and fatigue; or it may cause extensive damage to the brain, eyes, muscle, heart, liver, or lungs. Severe manifestations of the disease most commonly occur when a fetus is infected (congenital toxoplasmosis) or when infection occurs in patients with impaired immunity. Chronic infection may lead to a recurrent inflammatory process usually recognized by progressive ocular damage. When members of the cat family ingest *Toxoplasma* organisms, infection of epithelial cells in the intestinal tract results in production of oocysts which, when excreted, provide an important means by which the infection is transmitted in nature. Viable organisms within cysts in muscles and brain of infected animals provide a continued source of infection to carnivores.

HISTORY. In 1907 *Toxoplasma gondii* was recognized as a distinct protozoan and named by Nicolle and Manceaux. The first human case of congenital infection was recorded in 1923 by Janku in Prague, and in 1938 Wolf, Cowen, and Paige described the first cases from which the parasite was isolated. Toxoplasmosis in adults was first described by Pinkerton and Henderson in 1941. Eye damage caused by *Toxoplasma* in adults was first suggested by Frenkel and confirmed after observations made by Wilder in 1952. The present realization that 500 million humans are infected with the protozoan evolved from the extensive epidemiologic studies of Feldman, Desmonts, Thalhammer, and Jacobs, and from the recognition by Siim and others of the varied, often mild clinical patterns of acquired infection. In 1967, Hutchison first suggested that the cat played a role in the life cycle of *Toxoplasma gondii*, a cycle which was subsequently delineated in 1970.

THE PROTOZOAN. When mammals or birds ingest either infective oocysts or cysts in muscle or brain of other animals, an *intermediate* or asexual cycle of *Toxoplasma* infection is initiated. This consists of an obligate intracellular *proliferative stage* and a *cyst* stage. In the proliferative stage, *trophozoites*, which are ovoid or arc shaped, 3 to 4 μ in diameter, 6 to 7 μ in length, enter host cells by endocytosis and then divide by endodyogeny; two daughter cells are formed within each parent. Division continues until the host cell ruptures, releasing organisms which in turn infect adjacent cells. As the host develops immunity, parasite proliferation gradually slows, and a firm wall (cyst) forms around the organism allowing the *Toxoplasma* to persist for years in this cyst stage.

When *cats* ingest cysts or oocysts of *Toxoplasma gondii*, however, an addition process can occur, i.e., the *definitive* or sexual cycle initiated within the cat's intestinal epithelial cells. Parasites released from cysts or oocysts penetrate the epithelial cells where they first enter a proliferative stage and then mature by gametogony into *macro-* or *microgametocytes*. A *zygote*, formed by union of the gametocytes, matures in one to four days into an infective *oocyst*. The mature infective oocyst is oblong, 9 by 13 μ, and it contains two *sporocysts*, each of which contains four *sporozoites*. Oocysts are excreted by the cat for one to three weeks, beginning three to five days after ingestion of the *Toxoplasma*-containing tissue. Cats generally also acquire a systemic infection (intermediate cycle) at the time of first exposure to *Toxoplasma*, just as other mammals do. They occasionally repeat the sexual cycle after reinfection, although the period of oocyst shedding may be shorter.

EPIDEMIOLOGY. *Toxoplasma gondii* infects almost all mammals and birds. The usual life cycle in nature is among cats, small mammals, and birds, but man has intruded on this cycle with his taste for uncooked meats and his close association with cats. In some areas, such as Tahiti and the Easter Islands, the prevalence of *Toxoplasma* infection is near 100 per cent. In most parts of the world the prevalence ranges between 20 and 60 per cent of the population. Only in very dry areas, such as Arizona, and in very cold areas, such as northern Alaska, are low prevalence rates found. A few small islands in the Pacific, where cats have never been introduced, have remained free of toxoplasmosis.

The means by which the parasite is transmitted varies from one area to another: in one, oocyst ingestion seems more likely; in another, cyst ingestion. For instance, the very high rates in certain parts of the tropics are believed to be due to close contact with cat feces. In these areas infection is often acquired in childhood. The oocysts are resistant to drying and to a wide range of temperatures, and may remain infectious in moist soil for a year. Ingestion of oocysts is made more likely by the demonstration that cockroaches and flies can disseminate them to various exposed foods. In the United States the population appears to acquire the infection more commonly by ingesting uncooked infected meat. The infection is acquired at a rate of 1 per cent of the population per year of life from age 15 to age 50. Mutton and pork have been found to be more frequently infected than beef. Rarely, transmission of infection has followed accidental inoculation of trophozoites by laboratory workers, organ transplantation, and leukocyte transfusion from immunosuppressed donors. Blood transfusions from healthy donors have not been shown to be a means of transmitting toxoplasmosis.

Transplacental Transmission. Transplacental transmission in humans occurs only at the time of parasitemia, during the acute infection. The frequency of this secondary form of transmission therefore follows the frequency of acquisition of infection during childbearing years. In the United States and Europe 0.5 to 1.0 per cent of women have been demonstrated to have rising or very high antibody titers to *Toxoplasma* during pregnancy. Forty per cent of these adult infections are transmitted to the fetus. This may result in abortion or stillbirth, or an infant with clinical signs of toxoplasmosis (one third to one half of infected infants). Alternatively, infected infants may be completely asymptomatic but may show an antibody response to *Toxoplasma* antigens as evidence of transplacental infection. These infected asymptomatic infants are believed to make up a population which later in life may show signs of recurrent retinochoroiditis. There is no significant relationship in humans between chronic *Toxoplasma* infection and either recurrent abortion or prematurity.

PATHOGENESIS AND IMMUNITY. Multiplication of *Toxoplasma* organisms within cells causes little obvious disturbance to host cell function until the dividing parasites cause the cell to rupture. Adjacent cells are then infected, resulting in progressive tissue necrosis and an acute inflammatory response (edema and infiltration with mononuclear cells and a few polymorphonuclear leukocytes). Organisms are disseminated hematogenously throughout the body. New sites of necrosis and inflammation are initiated, particularly in myocardium and skeletal muscle. In those patients who develop severe generalized toxoplasmosis significant encephalitis, myocarditis, myositis, pneumonitis, hepatitis, and skin rash have been documented.

Generalized lymph node enlargement, along with other signs of systemic infection such as fever and malaise, develops one to two weeks after ingestion of infectious tissue. These lymph nodes show histocytic hyperplasia rather than follicular hyperplasia, giving the hematoxylin-eosin–stained section a rather typical appearance of containing predominantly eosin reactive cells. The architecture of the lymph node is preserved. Necrosis and giant cells are not seen, and only rarely can groups of *Toxoplasma* organisms be identified. Occasionally, even in relatively mild infections, myositis or myocarditis can be demonstrated.

Associated with the development of marked lymphoreticular activity, both humoral and cellular immunity can be demonstrated. Antibodies against various *Toxoplasma* antigens can be demonstrated in the peripheral blood. Later *Toxoplasma* antigen induces lymphocyte proliferation and lymphokine production, and mononuclear cells no longer support division of intracellular *Toxoplasma*. The acute infection resolves, but *Toxoplasma* organisms remain viable within cysts in the infected tissue for the lifetime of the host.

Congenital Infection; Immunologic Deficiency. Although the healthy adult usually deals effectively with the *Toxoplasma* infection, the immunologically deficient patient does not. The best example of this is the pathologic changes of congenital toxoplasmosis. The infected placenta may show areas of necrosis, inflammatory cells, and parasites, more frequently on the fetal than on the maternal side of the placenta. The fetal brain shows necrosis, glial cell proliferation, and perivascular lymphocytic infiltration. *Toxoplasma* can be identified in these lesions. High ventricular fluid protein, aqueductal obstruction, and hydrocephalus are often seen. If the infant survives several months, calcification of these areas occurs. Necrotic lesions in the retina are also seen. Organisms can be isolated from numerous organs of the body, but extensive inflammation is most often identified as pneumonitis, myocarditis, hepatitis, and splenitis.

About half the infections which occur in utero are caused by a sufficiently low number of organisms or are of low enough virulence that infection is manifest only by the appearance of humoral and cellular immune responses. Cysts develop and persist in brain, retina, and cardiac and skeletal muscle. Rupture of these cysts, many years later, can lead to transient episodes of inflammatory response and scarring. These inflammatory lesions are usually well localized, but in the retina they lead to significant organ impairment. The enucleated eye may show areas of necrosis in the retina often associated with proliferating *Toxoplasma* organisms, as well as a granulomatous inflammation of the choroid and sclera. The eye damage is the result of proliferation of organisms released at the time of cyst rupture which invade other cells, combined with damage caused by the vigorous hypersensitivity reaction.

In the patients with abnormal or suppressed immune responses, primary infection or cyst rupture may lead to symptomatic myositis, myocarditis, retinochoroiditis, or encephalitis.

CLINICAL MANIFESTATIONS. Manifestations of toxoplasmosis can be divided into four clinical patterns: acquired disease in otherwise healthy individuals, congenital infection, retinochoroiditis, and disease in the altered host.

Acquired Toxoplasmosis. Patients with acquired toxoplasmosis usually present with lymphadenopathy (90 per cent), fever (40 per cent), or malaise (40 per cent). Lymph node enlargement may be the only sign, and since cervical lymph node enlargement is particularly common, the patient may seek medical attention only because of concern about a neck mass. The nodes are usually nontender and rubbery in consistency. Generalized lymphadenopathy occurs in over half the cases, and transient splenomegaly has been recorded in approximately one third. The fever is usually low grade, but occasionally it may be high and of prolonged duration. Fatigue is often rather marked and may be associated with generalized muscle discomfort. Less commonly recorded signs or symptoms have included sore throat, headache, and a maculopapular rash. The pharynx is usually hyperemic; exudative pharyngitis is not seen. Specific organ involvement in this form of the disease includes myocardium (rarely pericardium), skeletal muscle, brain, rarely liver, and skin. When such organ involvement occurs, the abnormalities in organ function may dominate the clinical picture. Retinochoroiditis in association with the acute acquired disease is unusual.

The course of the illness is quite variable. Occasionally fever, malaise, and specific organ involvement are marked and the illness prolonged. More commonly, fever lasts only a few days or weeks, although fatigue and lymphadenopathy may persist for several months. Lymph nodes will occasionally fluctuate in size during the recovery period.

Laboratory tests usually reveal a normal total leukocyte count with a slight monocytosis or lymphocytosis. Atypical lymphocytes may be described, but they are usually not present in large numbers. Hematocrit and hemoglobin are usually normal; however, a Coombs-negative hemolytic anemia has occasionally been reported. Serum transaminases are usually normal, but early in the illness they may be slightly elevated (less than 100 U). The Paul-Bunnell test for heterophil antibodies is negative. The electrocardiogram may show ST and T wave abnormalities in cases in which myocarditis is prominent. The chest film is usually normal; hilar adenopathy is very rare. Lymph node biopsy shows histocytic hyperplasia. Antibodies against *Toxoplasma* antigens are present in high or rising titers.

Congenital Toxoplasmosis. Cases of congenital toxoplasmosis may be manifested as micro-ophthalmia, microcephaly, seizures, retardation, hepatosplenomegaly, pneumonitis, rash, and fever. If aqueduct of Sylvius obstruction has occurred, hydrocephalus will be prominent. Occasionally, signs may not be obvious at birth, but they may progress during the first months of life. Cerebral calcification may be seen after several months. The infant will show progressive signs of failure to thrive, followed by death. Cases of congenital toxoplasmosis may be mild, demonstrating only mental retardation, a seizure disorder, or retinochoroiditis. Laboratory tests reflect the severity of the specific organ involved. *Toxoplasma* antibody titers are elevated and will show a persistent or rising titer as maternal antibody disappears.

Toxoplasmic Retinochoroiditis. This form of toxoplasmosis is usually a late sequela of otherwise asymptomatic congenital infection, though infection of the eye during adult acquired illness has been recorded. Symptoms are usually first noted in the second or third decade of life. Patients have recurrent episodes of ocular pain and decreased vision associated with progressive loss of vision. The lesion is retinal, with an associated posterior uveitis. *Toxoplasma* infection probably does not cause an isolated anterior uveitis. Systemic signs of *Toxoplasma* infection are not usually present. *Toxoplasma* antibody titers are frequently low and tend not to change.

Toxoplasmosis in the Altered Host. Toxoplasmosis may present as a disseminated disease in patients with neoplasms of the lymphatic system, particularly Hodgkin's disease, or in patients being treated with immunosuppressive drugs. The clinical manifestations of the systemic disease are variable. Fever, encephalitis, myositis, hepatosplenomegaly, or myocarditis may occur. Pneumonitis has been described rarely in this setting. Lymphadenopathy may or may not be present. The primary difficulty is in separating the numerous other causes of these signs or symptoms from those caused by toxoplasmosis. At present one clinical pattern seems dominant, that is, progressive signs of encephalitis (confusion, headache, coma). In a patient with altered cellular immunity, these signs should lead to a consideration of and probably treatment for toxoplasmosis. If untreated, this illness is almost always progressive and fatal. *Toxoplasma* antibody titers are usually elevated; but changing titers are often not seen.

DIAGNOSIS. The diagnosis of toxoplasmosis rests on the presence of changing or elevated titers of antitoxoplasma antibodies and on isolation of the parasite from infected tissue. The antibody tests available include the indirect fluorescent antibody test (IFA), the Sabin-Feldman dye test, and a complement fixation test. The IFA and dye test show high antitoxoplasma antibody titers usually from the time of earliest symptoms (one to two weeks after infection). A titer of 1:1024 or higher, or evidence of a rising titer, is suggestive of active infection. The high titers will decrease during the subsequent months and after two to four years reach low levels (1:16 to 1:256) for the lifetime of the individual. An IgM-IFA test has been developed which demonstrates immunofluorescence of IgM-coated organisms at titers of patient serum greater than 1:20 during the first few months after infection. An indirect hemagglutination test is available; however, the rise in antibody titer is too slow to be helpful clinically.

The complement fixation test becomes positive later than the dye test, three to six weeks after infection, when symptoms are often present. Thus one is often able to see a changing titer over several weeks by using this test in a patient whose dye test is elevated. A significant complement fixation test is a titer of 1:8 or greater or a fourfold increase in titer. This test usually becomes negative within a few years after infection. In conjunction with the dye test it can help separate those patients with persistently high dye test antibody titers from those with recent infection. This may help in deciding if symptoms which began weeks or a few months previously are due to recent *Toxoplasma* infection or, in an asymptomatic pregnant female, whether the infection was recently acquired. Treatment may transiently decrease complement fixing antibody titers.

In congenital toxoplasmosis the contribution of transferred maternal IgG antitoxoplasma antibody must be excluded. This is done by performing several tests over the first few months; if positive titers are due to maternal antibody, the titer will fall about 50 per cent per month over four to six months. If the infant had been infected, the titer would remain stable, dip transiently, or increase. One may also test for IgM antitoxoplasma antibodies by using an IFA test to determine if the observed antibodies are fetal or maternal in origin. Since IgM antibodies do not cross the placenta, their presence indicates fetal antibody synthesis. In some infected infants this test may be falsely negative.

The diagnosis of *Toxoplasma* retinochoroiditis by serologic means is difficult. Since the infection is chronic, dye test and IFA titers are usually positive in low titer, and complement fixing antibodies are absent. The diagnosis of toxoplasmic retinochoroiditis may be suggested by finding higher antibody titers in the anterior chamber fluid than in the serum, or by isolating the organism at the time of enucleation. A negative dye test or IFA excludes *Toxoplasma* as the cause of retinochoroiditis.

The use of serologic tests in the immunodeficient patient to determine "activity" of the infection has also been difficult. Some patients with repeatedly low antibody titers have demonstrated a sudden rise in titer associated with a moribund state and death; however, at autopsy, disseminated toxoplasmosis could not be implicated as a factor contributing to death. Elevated antibody titers, plus progressive encephalitis, should be sufficient to warrant antitoxoplasma therapy in an immunodeficient patient. Evidence of the organism on biopsy of organs such as muscle, kidney, lung, and liver should also be an indication for therapy in these patients.

The diagnosis of toxoplasmosis can be substantiated by isolation of the organism. Biopsy material (particularly lymph node or muscle), tissue at the time of autopsy, or blood, sputum, or cerebrospinal fluid can be inoculated intraperitoneally into *Toxoplasma*-free laboratory animals. Smears of peritoneal fluid can be made at seven to ten days, stained by Giemsa technique, and examined for the protozoa. If the smear is negative, the peritoneal fluid should be injected intraperitoneally into another animal. If the infected animals survive for three weeks, they are sacrificed and their brains examined for *Toxoplasma* cysts and their serum for *Toxoplasma* antibody. Isolation of *Toxoplasma* organisms from human tissue should be correlated with histopathology of the tissue and antibody titers.

The differential diagnosis in a patient with lymphadenopathy and fever usually rests between lymphoma and infectious mononucleosis, although numerous infections, such as tuberculosis, brucellosis, tularemia, cat scratch disease, and certain systemic viral and rickettsial illnesses, must be considered. Toxoplasmosis can be distinguished from infectious mononucleosis by absence of marked atypical lymphocytosis and heterophil antibodies and normal or nearly normal hepatic transaminases; and from lymphoma by absence of anemia, hilar adenopathy, and a lymph node biopsy which shows histocytic hyperplasia rather than neoplastic cells. The other numerous causes of lymphadenopathy and fever must be excluded by appropriate serologic and skin tests, biopsy, and cultures. *Toxoplasma* encephalitis may resemble the localized necrosis of herpes infection.

Congenital toxoplasmosis must be distinguished from cytomegalovirus infection. Microcephaly is more common in cytomegalovirus infection than in toxoplasmosis. Ventricular fluid protein content is often higher in toxoplasmosis than in cytomegalovirus infection. Bacterial and fungal meningoencephalitis must be excluded by appropriate cultures. Viral encephalitis, particularly the rubella syndrome, must be considered. Congenital malformations are unusual in toxoplasmosis.

Toxoplasmic retinochoroiditis must be distinguished from cytomegalovirus, herpes, tuberculosis, histoplasmosis, and sarcoidosis by appearance of the retinal lesion and appropriate serologic and skin tests.

TREATMENT. A combination of pyrimethamine (Daraprim) and sulfadiazine has been shown to be effective in controlling *Toxoplasma* during the proliferative stage. There is no known therapy for eradicating organisms in the cyst stage. Pyrimethamine is given orally, 75 mg the first day, followed by 25 mg per day for one month. Infants are given 1 mg per kilogram per day for the first three days, and then 0.5 mg per kilogram per day thereafter. An intramuscular preparation is not commercially available. Sulfadiazine is given orally, 4 grams daily in divided doses for one month. Infants can be given 100 mg per kilogram per day. Sufficient fluid intake to maintain good urine flow should be assured during sulfadiazine therapy. Whether the drug combination co-trimoxazole will be a useful, less toxic agent in treating toxoplasmosis requires further study. Other sulfonamides such as the triple sulfonamides can be substituted for sulfadiazine; however, sulfisoxazole (Gantrisin) has been found ineffective. Other drugs such as spiramycin, clindamycin, and sulfones are less effective than the aforementioned drugs. Since pyrimethamine and sulfonamide inhibit folate synthesis, folinic acid (leucovorin), 6 mg per day, should be used in conjunction with the aforementioned therapy to prevent potential bone marrow toxicity. Platelet counts and white blood cell counts should be performed twice weekly during therapy.

Study of the effectiveness of these drugs in acquired human toxoplasmosis has been limited by the marked variability and spontaneous improvement without therapy. However, in some cases there has been evidence that this treatment shortens the period of fever and malaise, although lymphadenopathy may persist. It has therefore been recommended that only patients with fever, myalgias, or malaise be considered for therapy. Asymptomatic adults should be considered for treatment (1) after accidental laboratory infection and (2) when a pregnant female demonstrates serologic evidence of recent infection, only after appropriate consultations and considerations have led to a rejection of therapeutic abortion and have weighed potential fetal damage from the drugs. There is no adequate evidence to recommend treating dye-test-positive women who wish to become pregnant or who abort habitually, or in treating asymptomatic women after delivery of a congenitally damaged infant.

Congenital toxoplasmosis should be treated whether asymptomatic or symptomatic, because the proliferative stage may continue for several months before adequate immunity has developed to control the infection. Treatment will not be effective when given late in the course of the disease or when severe central nervous system damage has already occurred.

In toxoplasmic retinochoroiditis, the primary therapy should be directed at controlling the hypersensitivity response with corticosteroids. Pyrimethamine and sulfadiazine should be used in conjunction with this therapy to prevent dissemination of infection and to limit local damage caused by proliferating organisms.

In patients with altered immunity and toxoplasmosis, good therapeutic response to this drug combination has been recorded. Fever has been controlled, and evidence of progressive encephalitis has been reversed. In these patients long-term therapy has to be considered because appropriate immunologic responses do not occur, making relapse of the disease likely.

PREVENTION. Toxoplasmosis is commonly transmitted by consumption of undercooked meat or *Toxoplasma* oocysts. Thus, dye-test-negative pregnant women or patients with depressed cellular immunity should avoid both these sources of infection. Meat should be cooked at a temperature in excess of 60° C for at least 15 minutes. Susceptible individuals should avoid soil or sand boxes where cats may defecate, because oocysts may survive in these places for months. If cats are kept in the house, they should not be fed raw meat or allowed access to wild rodents or birds. Baseline antibody testing should be done in patients who are to receive immunosuppressive drugs, who have lymphatic malignancies, or who are to act as organ or leukocyte donors.

Beverley, J. K. A.: Toxoplasmosis. Br. Med. J., 2:475, 1973.
Feldman, H. A.: Toxoplasmosis. N. Engl. J. Med., 279:1370, 1431, 1968.
Frenkel, J. K.: Toxoplasma in and around us. Bio. Science, 26:343, 1973.
Frenkel, J. K.: Toxoplasmosis. *In* Marcial-Rojas, R. D. (ed.): Pathology of Protozoal and Helminthic Diseases. Baltimore, Williams & Wilkins Company, 1971, p. 254.
Kean, B. H.: Clinical toxoplasmosis — 50 years. Trans. R. Soc. Trop. Med. Hyg., 66:549, 1972.
Remington, J. S.: Toxoplasmosis — recent developments. Ann. Rev. Med., 21:201, 1970.
Ruskin, J., and Remington, J. S.: Toxoplasmosis in the compromised host. Ann. Intern. Med., 84:193, 1976.
Wallace, G. D.: The role of the cat in the natural history of *Toxoplasma gondii*. Am. J. Trop. Med. Hyg., 22:313, 1973.

198.   PNEUMOCYSTOSIS

Thomas C. Jones

Pneumocystosis is an acute pulmonary disease characterized by fever, tachypnea, dyspnea, and cyanosis which occurs in immunodeficient patients and malnourished or premature infants. It is caused by species of the genus *Pneumocystis*, organisms of uncertain classification, but probably protozoa. The organisms cause asymptomatic infection in healthy mammalian hosts and are seen extracellularly in the pulmonary alveoli.

HISTORY. In 1909 Carlos Chagas described what he thought was a stage of sporogony of *Trypanosoma cruzi* occurring in the lungs of experimentally infected guinea pigs. The next year Carini observed the same forms in rats infected with *T. lewisi*. In 1912 Delanoe and Delanoe recognized that the "cyst of Carini" was not part of the life cycle of trypanosomes, but was a different organism. The first reports of such an organism in humans appeared in 1938 when Ammich and Beneke independently described them in the lungs of infants dying during the first year of life. Epidemics of the disease in institutionalized children were subsequently described throughout Europe. In 1953 Vanek, Jirovec, and Lukes recognized the relationship between *Pneumocystis* and the pathologic entity interstitial plasma cell pneumonia. Reports of pneumocystosis have increased since that time, associated with the increased use of corticosteroids and antimetabolites as therapy in malignant disease or in patients undergoing organ transplantation, and with the increased life span of patients with congenital immunodeficient syndromes.

ORGANISM. The life cycle of *Pneumocystis* is unknown. At present, one can only postulate that the life cycle in lungs of infected mammals includes an extracystic body or trophozoite which changes to a cyst followed by the development of oval bodies (sporozoites) within the cyst. These are then released to initiate another cycle. A trophozoite-to-trophozoite cycle may also occur. Both cyst and trophozoite stages of the organism are found in exudate within the alveoli. The cyst is the form commonly demonstrated in clinical specimens. It is 5 to 6 μ in diameter, and its outer wall stains well with methenamine silver nitrate (see Fig. 2G, Ch. 193), Gram-Weigert stains or periodic acid–Schiff reagents. Using Giemsa stain, the sporozoites (1 to 2 μ in diameter) can be recognized within the cyst and are usually eight in number. After release from the cyst, the organisms are termed trophozoites. They move freely about the alveoli, and gradually undergo changes, including loss of internal structure, appearance of villous microprojections on the outer membrane, and development of an unusual trilaminar membrane, characteristics which identify it as a new cyst.

EPIDEMIOLOGY. *Pneumocystis* species are widely distributed, affecting rodents, rabbits, sheep, dogs, and other mammals, in addition to humans. It is unlikely that animals serve as a reservoir for infection of humans, since organisms of different mammals appear to be host specific. Evidence at present best supports the thesis that infection is transmitted by the respiratory route by droplet spray. In a few cases congenital infection has been considered the most likely route of infection. The disease is principally one of immunodeficient subjects.

Epidemiologic data suggest that the organism is quite infectious, that infection is usually asymptomatic, and that apparently healthy, infected individuals can transmit the disease to immunodeficient patients. This is supported by observations in animals that healthy rats and rabbits when caged communally acquire the infection, and when the animals are rendered immunodeficient by corticosteroid administration, disease may be manifest. It is supported in humans by the increased prevalence of antibodies to *Pneumocystis* in personnel working in medical institutions (7 to 15 per cent), the epidemics of disease in the institutionalized infants, and the sporadic clusters of cases in hospitalized immunodeficient patients.

Disease that follows recent infection or reactivation of latent infection has been seen most commonly in patients with hypogammaglobulinemia of immunoglobulins G or M, in malnourished infants in the second to fourth months of life (when passively transferred maternal antibodies first reach low levels), or in patients receiving corticosteroids or antimetabolites. A few patients not on immunosuppressive drugs and with normal immunoglobulin levels and a few patients with isolated defects in cellular immunity have acquired the disease. Organisms reach high numbers in the lungs of infected persons showing clinical disease, and it is likely that these patients can more readily spread the disease than asymptomatic carriers.

PATHOLOGY AND PATHOGENESIS. When conditions exist in the alveoli for the multiplication of *Pneumocystis*, an inflammatory response is elicited which includes transudation of fluid into the alveoli and thickening of alveolar interstitial spaces. The alveoli become filled with foamy, proteinaceous material in which trophozoite nuclei are found along with clumps of the *Pneumocystis* cysts. The interstitial spaces have been noted to contain predominantly plasma cells and alveolar epithelial cells when pathologic material was studied in malnourished or premature infants; hence the origin of the pathologic description, interstitial plasma cell pneumonia. However, in the immunodeficient child or adult, this pattern is not seen. The inflammatory response in these patients has been described as primarily lymphocytes, macrophages, and occasionally eosinophils. Polymorphonuclear leukocytes are not seen. The lung is usually diffusely involved with this process, although localized disease has occasionally been described. The lung is firm and rubbery in consistency. Other organisms, such as cytomegalovirus or bacteria, are frequently found in association with *Pneumocystis*. Less commonly, *Pneumocystis* is found in lungs which also contain mycobacteria, fungi, or toxoplasma. Rarely, pneumocystis may become generalized, involving lymph nodes, spleen, and bone marrow.

CLINICAL MANIFESTATIONS. The major symptoms of pneumocystosis are tachypnea and a nonproductive cough. These symptoms often develop insidiously over a period of several weeks and may be associated with fever, dyspnea, and cyanosis. It has been noted that these symptoms may first appear during the period when corticosteroids are being withdrawn. The disease may also present with an abrupt onset (over two to three days) of high, spiking fever, cough, dyspnea, and cyanosis, with the patient reaching a moribund state within a few days. Most of the patients presenting with this rapid course have been on continuous high doses of corticosteroids. In the United States at present the disease which presents with an abrupt onset may be more common than the more insidious onset characteristic of the illness seen in institutionalized infants in Europe. After renal, bone marrow, or cardiac transplantation, pneumocystosis is an important cause of pneumonia occurring three to four months later.

On physical examination the patient shows signs of respiratory distress (tachypnea and dyspnea) associated with fever and cyanosis. Auscultation of the lungs may reveal no abnormalities, although scattered rales and rhonchi may be heard.

There are no diagnostic laboratory tests. *The white blood cell count* may reflect the underlying disease of the patient or other complications, but leukocytosis may be seen. Significant eosinophilia has occasionally been reported, particularly in children with humoral immune deficiency. *The blood gases* will usually indicate hyperventilation and decreased oxygen saturation even while the patient is on continuous oxygen, consistent with an alveolar capillary block syndrome. Some have reported associated mild respiratory acidosis. *The chest radiograph* usually shows diffuse mixed alveolar and interstitial pneumonitis. This appears as a granular haziness beginning in the hilar region, which progresses to a frank alveolar pattern with air bronchograms. Atypical features such as asymmetrical involvement, segmental infiltrates, and pleural effusions occur in up to half the cases.

Course. In immunodeficient patients the course of pneumocystosis will usually be one of progressive deterioration unless improvement occurs in the underlying immune defect. Increasing pulmonary consolidation, cyanosis, and death are the natural history of the disease. After institution of specific therapy against pneumocystis, improvement begins in five to ten days. The roentgenographic findings may become transiently worse after institution of therapy, but will then show gradual improvement over one to three weeks. Some have suggested that pneumocystosis of long duration may lead to interstitial fibrosis or emphysema. This has been difficult to document in view of the many factors leading to pulmonary changes in these patients.

DIAGNOSIS. Once the suspicion of pneumocystosis is raised by the clinical setting of immune deficiency and progressive pulmonary symptoms, pulmonary secretions should be examined by methenamine silver, Gram-Weigert, or Giemsa stains. If these examinations are negative, the patient should be considered for lung biopsy. Most centers now recommend transbronchial or open lung biopsy rather than percutaneous needle biopsy, because the latter provides no visualization of the lung and a greater risk of lung collapse or bleeding. Biopsy is required to distinguish pneumocystosis from drug-induced interstitial fibrosis, cytomegalovirus infection, *Aspergillus* or other fungi, unusual forms of bacterial bronchopneumonia, toxoplasmosis, or leukemic infiltration. Impression smears of the biopsy specimen at the time of surgery can be fixed in methanol and stained with Giemsa, methenamine silver, or Gram-Weigert stains and carefully examined for the presence of *Pneumocystis* cysts. Specimens are also preserved for bacterial and fungal cultures. If the biopsy must be delayed, or if surgery is believed to be contraindicated for other reasons, then a therapeutic trial with specific drugs against *Pneumocystis* should be instituted. Immunofluorescent antibody tests are now being evaluated. However, they show significantly elevated titers in only about 30 per cent of cases of pneumocystosis. Although measurement of antibody response using fluorescent antibody techniques is relatively insensitive, it appears to be specific. Thus a change in titer from negative to positive adds support to the diagnosis, whereas the absence of such a change does not exclude it.

TREATMENT. Therapy for pneumocystosis, if started early in the disease, has proved to be quite successful. During the past decade pentamidine isethionate has been used. This has reduced mortality from *Pneumocystis* infection from near 100 per cent to below 50 per cent and considerably lower in some circumstances. The drug is made rapidly available by calling the Parasitic Disease Drug Service, U.S. Public Health Service (404–633–3311). The patient is given 4 mg per kilogram per day intramuscularly for 12 to 14 days. The mechanism of action of the drug remains unknown, but it does cause megaloblastic cell changes, inhibits incorporation of nucleotides into DNA and RNA, and inhibits oxidative phosphorylation. Folinic acid therapy can be used in patients who develop signs of folate deficiency without interfering with action of the drug against the organism. Pentamidine may also cause hypoglycemia, hyperglycemia, and nephrotoxicity. When given intravenously, hypotension can occur. The possibility that pentamidine causes pulmonary interstitial fibrosis has been raised by studies in animals. Because of these observed and potential toxic effects, another drug combination, co-trimoxazole, the fixed combination of trimethoprim and sulfamethoxazole, has been tested for treatment of pneumocystosis. Although there have been fewer patients treated with this combination than with pentamidine, it appears to be effective and less toxic. This drug combination interferes with the synthesis of folinic acid. For treatment of adults, 20 mg per kilogram per day of trimethoprim and 100 mg per kilogram per day of sulfamethoxazole, divided into four doses, can be given by mouth. An intravenous preparation is available as an investigational drug from the manufacturer. Since inadequate levels of the drug have been documented in the serum of critically ill patients after oral therapy, serum concentrations should be checked. If levels of trimethoprim are less than 4.6 μg per milliliter, parenteral therapy should be used.

Because of the relationship between the occurrence of pneumocystosis and hypogammaglobulinemia, gamma globulin administration has been recommended. However, commercially available gamma globulin has proved to be of little value when given alone for treatment of pneumocystosis. In general, attempts should be made to reduce the dose of corticosteroids when signs of pneumocystosis appear; however, in some patients whose respiratory symptoms developed during tapering of corticosteroids, a transient *increase* in the dose of these drugs while pneumocystosis therapy is started should be considered. Supportive measures such as oxygen therapy, assisted ventilation, and careful fluid and electrolyte balance are important parts of the management.

PREVENTION. In order to interrupt spread of *Pneumocystis* infection, a great deal must be learned about its life cycle. Since the diseased patient may be able to spread the organism to other patients, healthy person-

nel, and relatives, appropriate respiratory precautions should be considered when the diagnosis is suspected. Attention to preventing contact between susceptible patients and diseased patients in open wards and in clinics may reduce the spread of the disease. For certain highly susceptible patient populations, prophylactic treatment with co-trimoxazole has been found to be beneficial. The disease will be better controlled when the relationships between certain types of immune deficiency or corticosteroids and rapid proliferation of the organism are better understood.

Burke, B. A., and Good, R. A.: *Pneumocystis carinii* infection. Medicine, 52:23, 1973.
Norman, L., and Kagan, I. G.: Some observations on the serology of *Pneumocystis carinii* infections in the United States. Infect. Immun., 8:317, 1973.
Robbins, J. B., DeVita, V. T., and Dutz, W.: Symposium on *Pneumocystis carinii* Infection. National Cancer Institute Monograph 43. U.S. Department of Health, Education and Welfare, October 1976.
Rosen, P., Armstrong, D., and Ramos, C.: *Pneumocystis carinii* pneumonia. A clinicopathologic study of twenty patients with neoplastic diseases. Am. J. Med., 53:428, 1972.
Walzer, P. D., Perl, D. P., Krogstad, D. J., Rawson, P. G., and Schultz, M. G.: *Pneumocystis carinii* pneumonia in the United States. Epidemiologic, diagnostic, and clinical features. Ann. Intern. Med., 80:83, 1974.

199.   BABESIOSIS

(Babesiasis, Piroplasmosis)

Thomas C. Jones

Babesiosis is an acute febrile illness characterized by myalgias, fatigue, and hemolytic anemia caused by species of the intraerythrocytic protozoa, *Babesia*, transmitted by infected ticks. Animal infection with *Babesia* has long been recognized; however, significant transmission of disease to man has been documented only recently. In asplenic patients the disease is likely to be serious and may be fatal.

HISTORY. Babès, in 1888, identified the organism in the peripheral blood of cattle with anemia and fever. Smith and Kilborne in 1893 observed a similar organism as the cause of Texas cattle fever, described it as a protozoan, and documented the role of the tick as vector — the first demonstration that arthropods could transmit protozoan diseases. In 1904, Wilson and Chowning described blood smears from several patients in Montana which looked like piroplasmosis of cattle; they termed the organism *Piroplasma hominis*. These cases were identified in the midst of another tick-borne disease, Rocky Mountain spotted fever, and were therefore considered to be examples of this rickettsial disease. In retrospect, these cases may have been the first descriptions of babesiosis in man. Svkrabalo reported in 1957 a fatal case of babesiosis presenting with fever, anemia, and hemoglobinuria in a splenectomized man. Twenty additional cases have been identified in the past decade, 16 of which have occurred on Nantucket and Martha's Vineyard islands and on the tip of Long Island.

ORGANISM. *Babesia* is a protozoan with asexual multiplication (shizogony) occurring in mammalian erythrocytes and a sexual cycle (sporogony) in the tick. The organism is introduced during the bite of the tick, when sporozoites in salivary glands enter the bloodstream and invade erythrocytes. In the erythrocyte stained with Romanowsky stains, organisms are 2 to 3 μ in diameter with blue-staining, irregularly shaped cytoplasm and a red nucleus. They may appear as ring, binucleate, or quadrinucleate forms. *Babesia* does not produce pigment within the red cell, a feature clearly distinguishing it from *Plasmodium*. A period of prolonged parasitemia occurs. When a tick ingests parasitized red blood cells, the sexual cycle occurs in the digestive tract of the tick with formation of zygotes and ookinetes. A systemic infection of the tick allows transmission of the organism at the time of its next blood meal as well as infection of the tick eggs, leading to vertical transmission to larvae, another source of mammalian infection. Congenital transmission of infection in ticks complicates the epidemiology by allowing long periods of tick infection in the absence of contact with mammalian blood cells.

PATHOLOGY AND IMMUNITY. Babesiosis leads to red cell destruction (hemolytic anemia, hyperbilirubinemia, hemoglobinuria, splenic enlargement) and capillary obstruction associated with parasitized red blood cells (leading to tissue anoxia). In those patients who have been autopsied, findings have included generalized hyperemia and hemorrhage. The liver revealed parasitized red cells, many within phagocytic cells, but no pigment deposition as seen in malaria. The kidneys showed the changes of tubular nephrosis consistent with intravascular hemolysis and hemoglobin damage. In animals a proliferative glomerulitis has been demonstrated and glomerular deposits of IgG and C3 documented.

A delicate balance between progressive infection and host immune response leads to prolonged parasitemia with variable signs of tissue injury. The severe illness which has been described in humans without spleens (three of four patients died) and the documented severe illness in experimentally splenectomized animals gives strong support for the role of this organ in the immune response to *Babesia*.

Hamsters infected with *B. microti* of human origin demonstrated excess antibody in the serum by two weeks after infection, which reached a peak titer of 1:1280 by eight weeks. In these animals, parasitemia persisted until the sixth week. Marked splenic enlargement occurred during this period. Parasitemia recurred in hamsters splenectomized three to four months after infection. In infected animals *B. microti* have been shown to undergo degenerative changes within the red cells. This observation and cross-immunity between *Babesia* and *Plasmodium* suggest that an immunologically nonspecific substance could be important in the immune response. Antibody may contribute to control of the infection by agglutination or opsonization of organisms and by inhibiting the entry of *Babesia* into red cells.

EPIDEMIOLOGY. A number of species of Babesia have been described. These have been characterized as host specific: *B. bigemina* and *B. bovis* in cattle, *B. ovis* in sheep, *B. canis* in dogs, *B. equi* in horses, and *B. microti* in rodents. It is now clear both from cross-species animal infections and the emergence of disease in humans that these zoonoses can infect and cause disease in more than one animal species. Infection in splenectomized man has been due to *B. bovis* acquired from ticks feeding on cattle and one case possibly due to *B. equi*. The disease in man on Nantucket island has been caused by the rodent species, *B. microti*, and has led to illness in immunologically normal humans.

Infection with *B. microti* in those exposed to infected ticks is probably frequent. On Nantucket island, of 133 persons with a history of tick bite, 10 had significant antibody titers against *B. microti* (>1:64) consistent with recent infection. Infection of rodents with *B. microti* has been recognized in many parts of the world for decades. Recent studies on Nantucket confirmed a very high rate of parasitemia (82 per cent) in field and white-footed mice. The deer tick, *Ixodes scapularis*, has become abundant in the past few decades and has replaced the rodent tick, *Ixodes muris*, as the dominant tick. This change in the ecology of ticks may have contributed to the emergence of infection in man. A change in the organism itself rendering it more adaptable to infection in man is possible, but comparative studies have not been done.

CLINICAL MANIFESTATIONS. The clinical manifestations of babesiosis are undoubtedly quite varied. The following description is based on detailed observations on only a few patients. The first signs of illness have occurred one to six weeks after a tick bite, although only a few patients have recalled such a bite. There may be absence of a history of tick bite because the small tick larvae may go unnoticed.

The first symptoms include fatigue, general malaise, and anorexia, followed in a few days by fever. The fever may be high (40° C), and drenching sweats, chills, myalgias, and arthralgias may accompany it. Nausea and vomiting may occur. Several of the patients have had symptoms of depression, emotional lability, and transient hyperesthesias. The illness may be sudden in onset or quite indolent and prolonged, lasting a month before diagnosis. On physical examination, splenomegaly has been noted in two of eight patients. No rash or lymphadenopathy has been recorded. In the fatal cases in asplenic patients, signs of massive hemolysis (pallor, icterus, and dark urine), prostration, dehydration, and renal insufficiency were most prominent.

Patients demonstrate a low hemoglobin and a moderate reticulocytosis. Leukocyte counts are normal, but some patients have thrombocytopenia. Urinalysis usually shows proteinuria. Liver function tests may be slightly abnormal. Peripheral blood smears show 1 to 10 per cent of erythrocytes infected with *Babesia* organisms.

DIAGNOSIS. The diagnosis of babesiosis should be suspected in any patient with fever and unexplained hemolytic anemia. This should be considered particularly if the laboratory reports identify malaria parasite on smear. Diagnosis can usually be made by observing the nonpigmented organisms in erythrocytes on thick and thin peripheral blood smears. In suspected cases in which the smear is equivocal, inoculation of laboratory rodents will allow confirmation of the diagnosis. The Center for Disease Control has developed a serologic test using *B. microti* antigen which appears specific and which will be helpful in both clinical diagnosis and epidemiology.

THERAPY. Treatment with chloroquine phosphate, 1500 mg initially, followed by 500 mg daily or every other day until symptoms subside and parasitemia decreases, has been recommended. Parasitemia may continue for many weeks even while the patient is on therapy. Malaise and fatigue may also persist for several weeks. Pentamidine, 4 mg per kilogram per day, may be more effective and should be used in severely ill patients. Supportive therapy for acute renal failure with dialysis and for anemia with blood transfusion may be necessary in severe cases.

PREVENTION. No chemoprophylaxis is available. Avoiding tick-infested areas will decrease likelihood of acquiring the disease. Removal of ticks present on the skin, use of clothing impregnated with tick repellents, and use of insecticide sprays all have value in limiting transmission of tick-borne diseases. Patients who have had splenectomy should avoid occupations and vacations which might bring them in contact with infected ticks.

Anderson, A. E., Cassaday, P. B., and Healy, G. R.: Babesiosis in man. Am. J. Clin. Pathol. 62:612, 1974.

Annable, C. R., and Ward, P. A.: Immunopathology of the renal complications of babesiosis. J. Immunol., 112:1, 1974.

Healy, G. R., Spielman A., and Gleason, N.: Human babesiosis: Reservoir of infection on Nantucket island. Science, 192:479, 1976.

Ruebush, T. K., II, Cassaday, P. B., Marsh, J. H., Lisker, S. A., Voorhees, D. B., Mahoney, E. B., and Healy, G. R.: Human babesiosis on Nantucket island. Ann. Intern. Med., 86:6, 1977.

Svkrabalo, Z.: Babesiosis (piroplasmosis). In Marcial-Rojas, R. A. (ed.): Pathology of Protozoal and Helminthic Diseases. Baltimore, Williams & Wilkins Company, 1971, p. 225.

200. OTHER PROTOZOAN DISEASES

200.1. INTRODUCTION

Philip D. Marsden

Apart from *Entamoeba histolytica,* at least four genera and seven species of amebae have been established as living in man. Common stool amebae are *Entamoeba coli, Endolimax nana,* and *Iodamoeba bütschlii.* They are nonpathogenic, but such protozoa have a double importance. First, they must be distinguished from the pathogenic *E. histolytica* by the available clear morphologic criteria. Second, they provide an index of fecal contamination. If any stool protozoan is encountered, it is wise to examine a further specimen, for, because of the variable appearance of protozoa in the stool, the second specimen may reveal a pathogen. *Dientamoeba fragilis* has a delicate ameba form without a cystic stage. Some clinicians believe it is a cause of mild diarrhea, but the evidence is not convincing.

Several flagellates are also found in the stool, among them the nonpathogenic *Trichomonas hominis* and *Chilomastix mesnili.* Information on the differential diagnosis of these intestinal protozoa can be found in texts of parasitology. Here we will consider briefly the clinical significance of six pathogenic types of protozoa: *Giardia lamblia* and *Trichomonas vaginalis* (both flagellates), *Balantidium coli* (a ciliate), *Naegleria* and *Acanthamoeba* (amebae), and *Isospora* and *Sarcocystis* (sporozoa).

Knight, R.: Giardiasis, isosporiasis, and balantidiasis. Clin. Gastroenterol., 7:31, 1978.

200.2. GIARDIASIS

Philip D. Marsden

Abdominal pain, distention and flatulence, and recurrent diarrhea may be associated with *Giardia lamblia* infection, especially in children. Inhabiting the duodenum and upper jejunum, the parasite is a pear-shaped flagellate, anteriorly broad and rounded and tapering to a point not unlike a tennis racket. It is convex dorsally with a ventral attachment disc. There are sets of identical structures on either side of the median line. When stained, there are two nuclei, four pairs of flagella, and a parabasal body. In fresh stool this trophozoite is actively motile with an irregular characteristic progression. It reproduces by longitudinal binary fission.

The thick-walled cysts are 10 to 14 μ by 6 to 10 μ and have two to four nuclei with curved rods or axostyles. In some infections several million cysts per gram of feces may be passed. Only in patients with very rapid bowel transit times do trophozoites appear in the stool, although they may be found in duodenal samples obtained by duodenal aspiration, biopsy, or, preferably, Beal's string test. Cultivation of *Giardia* in vitro has been achieved but is not a practical diagnostic procedure.

The infective cysts are transmitted in food and drink, and the infection is cosmopolitan. The great majority of patients are asymptomatic, but there is no doubt that heavy infections are associated with symptoms. There is an association between symptomatic giardiasis and the immunodeficiency syndrome of nonselective variable hypogammaglobulinemia. Diarrhea is the most common symptom, and the stools are pale and contain mucus. *Giardia* is in fact a cause of steatorrhea, and patients have abnormal fat balances and D-xylose tests which return to normal after successful treatment. The hypothesis that this malabsorption is the result of a mechanical barrier produced by large numbers of parasites attached to the microvillar surface is attractive, but effects on digestive enzyme activity and microvillar function are possible. Villous flattening with inflammatory infiltration has been demonstrated.

Diarrhea may alternate with constipation, and apart from these symptoms epigastric pain resembling a peptic ulcer may be a disabling symptom. Anorexia, meat intolerance, and loss of weight may occur. Although *Giardia* may be found in the gallbladder, the evidence that it is responsible for cholecystitis is unsatisfactory. Giardiasis must be distinguished from other causes of malabsorption and peptic ulcer.

Giardiasis, symptomatic or not, should always be treated. Two drugs are equally effective. Metronidazole (Flagyl), 250 or 400 mg three times a day for five to ten days, has few side effects. Good cure rates have been obtained with single doses of 2 grams. It is the drug of choice for children and when *Giardia* coexists with *Entamoeba histolytica.* Quinacrine hydrochloride (Atabrine, mepacrine), in an *adult* dose of 100 mg three times a day after food for seven days, is an established therapy, but the drug has a bitter taste, and nausea and vomiting may result. It may also stain the skin yellow, but psychosis does not occur at this dosage level. Both drugs have about an 80 per cent cure rate, and in the event of failure of one drug the other can be tried. The follow-up procedures are similar to those in amebiasis.

Hoskins, L. C., Winawer, S. J., Broitman, S. A., Gottlieb, L. S., and Zamchek, N.: Clinical giardiasis and intestinal malabsorption. Gastroenterology, 53:265, 1967.

Yardley, J. H., Takano, J., and Hendrix, T. B.: Epithelial and other mucosal lesions of the jejunum in giardiasis: Jejunal biopsy studies. Bull. Hopkins Hosp., 115:389, 1964.

200.3. TRICHOMONIASIS

Thomas C. Jones

Another group of lumen-dwelling protozoa with flagella are the trichomonads. Three species of the genus *Trichomonas* frequently inhabit man: *Trichomonas hominis, Trichomonas tenax,* and *Trichomonas vaginalis.* Only the last-named is considered pathogenic.

T. vaginalis is a pear-shaped, colorless, single-celled

organism 10 to 20 μ in size with two pairs of anterior flagella, an eccentrically located nucleus, an undulating membrane, and a structure termed an axostyle leading to a posterior flagellum. The flagella and undulating membrane move the organism rapidly through exudative material in a jerky, rotating manner. Its survival on mucosal surfaces is dependent on certain environmental conditions. For instance, activity of the organism decreases rapidly at a pH below 5.

The organism can persist in endocervical or uethral glands without causing symptoms, or it can induce inflammation on the mucosal surfaces of the vagina, urethra, urinary bladder, or prostate. The inflamed area takes on a characteristic "strawberry-like" appearance owing to vasodilation. Exudate filled with polymorphonuclear leukocytes and mononuclear cells covers the surface. *Trichomonas* infection can make interpretation of cervical Papanicolaou smears more difficult, but there is no evidence that infection contributes to carcinoma of the cervix.

Patients usually present with symptoms of vaginal itching or burning and a yellow blood-tinged discharge. These symptoms are more commonly associated with menstruation. If the urethra is involved, symptoms of dysuria and a mild urethral discharge are seen. Approximately 20 per cent of females with documented *Trichomonas* infection are asymptomatic.

Diagnosis is made by observing the motile organisms in fresh specimens of vaginal discharge. A drop of warm saline containing methylene blue is mixed with the exudate and examined immediately, using low-power microscopy. *T. vaginalis* can also be cultured. Nitroimidazoles, such as metronidazole, provide effective therapy. One gram of metronidazole should be given in a single dose to both sexual partners. If this is ineffective, the more traditional therapy of 250 mg three times daily for ten days can be used. Because of potential drug side effects, only patients documented to have *Trichomonas* vaginitis and their sexual partners should be treated. Failure to treat both partners results in reinfection, so-called "Ping-Pong" vaginitis. The infection is usually acquired by sexual intercourse. It can be transmitted to infants at the time of birth, and may survive on nonmucosal surfaces for a sufficient time to be spread in places such as mental institutions where personal hygiene is poor. In severely immunocompromised patients, trichomonads have been identified in pleural and cerebrospinal fluids consistent with communication between these sites and mucosal surfaces.

Dykers, J. R.: Single dose metronidazole for trichomonal vaginitis: A follow-up. N. Engl. J. Med., 295:395, 1976.
Trussell, R. E.: *Trichomonas Vaginalis* and Trichomoniasis. Springfield, Ill., Charles C Thomas, 1947.

200.4. BALANTIDIASIS

Philip D. Marsden

Balantidium coli is the largest protozoan of man, measuring 50 to 70 μ in length by 30 to 60 μ in width. It infects the colon of man and may produce diarrhea and dysentery. When viewed under the low power of the microscope in a saline smear of stool, the grayish-green trophozoite can be seen gliding across the field powered by spiral longitudinal rows of cilia. There is a large oval macronucleus and a smaller micronu-

cleus. A cytostome or mouth ingests organic matter that circulates as food vacuoles. Erythrophagocytosis has been observed. Reproduction is by binary fission or conjugation. A resistant cyst form is passed in formed stools, and this is the infective form. *Cosmopolitan in distribution, it is a rare infection of man although common in pigs.* When man and pig share shelter, human infections are common, and this accounts for the high incidence of human infection in parts of New Guinea (20 per cent) and Peru. *B. coli* of man can be transmitted to monkeys, cats, guinea pigs, and rats, but the importance of these animals as reservoirs is minor. Handling pigs in slaughterhouses may be an occupational risk.

This ciliate can be a tissue invader, and similar factors to those mentioned for *E. histolytica* may well determine this behavior. Proteolytic secretions produce necrosis and ulceration of the mucosa. Columns of balantidia may be seen lying in the submucosa. Secondary infection with bacteria results in an accompanying inflammatory reaction. The ulcers are often quite large and deep, with a broad, indurated base. A liver abscess with *B. coli* in situ has been described, and balantidia have been found in the lung and heart in isolated cases.

Less than one fifth of infected persons have symptoms. Severe infections are associated with diarrhea and the passage of blood and mucus in the stools. Constitutional symptoms of fever, nausea, vomiting, and asthenia are described. Examination of fresh stools reveals the trophozoite or cyst. Culture of the stools on media similar to those used for amebiasis may reveal an infection when conventional microscopy has failed; in symptomatic patients this is usually not necessary. Balantidiasis must be differentiated from amebic dysentery and ulcerative colitis. Although arsenical preparations have been used in the past, oxytetracycline is the drug of choice in an adult dose of 500 mg three times a day for ten days. Paromomycin (Humatin) is also effective. The value of metronidazole is still uncertain. Spontaneous recovery has been noted. The infection may be fatal if bowel perforation occurs.

Arean, V. M., and Koppisch, E.: Balantidiasis: A review and report of cases. Am. J. Path., 32:1089, 1956.
Garcia Laverde, A., and De Bonilla, L.: Clinical trials with metronidazole in human balantidiasis. Am. J. Trop. Med. Hyg., 24:781, 1975.
Van der Hoeven, J. A., and Rijpstra, A. C.: Intestinal parasites in the central mountain district of Netherlands, New Guinea. An important focus of *Balantidium coli*. Docum. Med. Geog. Trop., 9:225, 1957.

200.5. PRIMARY AMEBIC MENINGOENCEPHALITIS

Philip D. Marsden

Recently it has been realized that *free-living amebae* are capable of producing severe brain lesions in man. Several species are implicated, but *Naegleria gruberi* had been the species usually identified when cultures are made. They can be cultured on plain agar plates with *Aerobacter aerogenes* as a nutrient source, but we need to know more about their cultural requirements. The *Naegleria* amebae possess the capacity to transform in culture from ameboid trophozoites to highly mobile flagellates. Another organism, *Acanthamoeba castellani,* was among the first to be recognized. An ameba 6 to 8 μ long, with foamy cytoplasm, a nucleus of 2 μ, and a 1 μ darkly staining central karyosome, it is present as a commensal in human mouths and throats and was shown to be pathogenic for mice and monkeys before the first cases were reported in man. An initial report from Australia in 1965 described a rapidly progressive meningitis that proved fatal. Early symptoms in the first two days or so are fever, severe frontal headache, defects of olfactory sense, lethargy, sore throat, and obstructed nostrils. By the third day vomiting and impaired consciousness may be present, progressing to deepening coma and death on the fourth day. At postmortem, destruction of the inferior surface of the frontal lobes and olfactory bulbs was seen, associated with a purulent exudate. Histologic examination revealed columns of amebae extending into the brain substance, especially via the perivascular spaces.

This clinical entity has now been reported from several parts of the United States (Florida, Virginia, Texas) and from Great Britain and Czechoslovakia. It is usually found in children and young people, and is invariably fatal. It appears to be acquired by swimming, diving, or water skiing in lakes known to contain large numbers of free-living amebae. Pressure changes under water probably force the amebae through the cribriform plate. *Naegleria* has repeatedly been found in the cerebrospinal fluid of man. The CSF also shows an increased protein level, decreased sugar, neutrophils, and red cells, but is bacteriologically sterile. Most of the patients to date have died, usually because the diagnosis has been missed.

Emetine, arsenicals, sulfonamides, tetracyclines, and metronidazole have been used without success. Amphotericin B therapy has resulted in recovery of a patient in whom *Naegleria* organisms were recovered from the CSF, and in vitro studies show that therapeutic concentrations are amebicidal. In one fatal case *Naegleria gruberi* was recovered from the lungs, liver, spleen and heart blood, as well as from the central nervous system. In patients with persistent eye inflammation *Acanthamoeba polyphaga* has been isolated. Since such free-living amebae are ubiquitous, doubtless reports from other countries will appear in the future

Carter, R. F.: Primary amoebic meningo-encephalitis. Trans. Roy. Soc. Trop. Med. Hyg., 66:193, 1972.

Culbertson, C. G.: Pathogenic acanthamoeba (Hartmannella). Am. J. Clin. Path., 35:195, 1961.

Dumar, R. J., Helwig, W. B., and Martinez, A. J.: Meningoencephalitis and brain abscess due to a free-living amoeba. Ann. Interno. Med., 88:468, 1978.

Duma, R. J., Rosenblum, W. I., McGehee, R. F., Jones, M. M., and Clifford, N. E.: Primary amoebic meningoencephalitis caused by Naegleria. Ann. Intern. Med., 74:923, 1971.

Visvesvaka, G. S., Jones, D. B., and Robinson, N. M.: Isolation, identification and biological characterization of Acanthamoeba polyphaga from a human eye. Am. J. Trop. Med. Hyg., 24:784, 1975.

200.6.   ISOSPORIASIS
(Coccidiosis)
Philip D. Marsden

Isospora have alternate asexual and sexual generation in the same host, and the nature of the cycle is not dis-

similar to plasmodia in the forms produced. There is probably only one human species, *Isospora belli*, which parasitizes the small intestinal epithelium. The cycles of schizogony and gametogony have now been described in small bowel mucosal biopsies from symptomatic patients, and it has been suggested that this organism causes a malabsorption syndrome. Until recently the case for the pathogenicity of *Isospora* rested mainly on laboratory infections that resulted in diarrhea lasting about three weeks, accompanied by the passage of the diagnostic form of the parasite in the stool. This is a thick-walled oocyst 25 to 35 μ × 12 to 16 μ in size. Both ends are rounded, and one is contracted to form a neck. This stage is the zygote. Further development in two to four days results in the formation of two sporoblasts, which mature into oval sporocysts. Each sporocyst ultimately contains four sporozoites. These oocysts are very resistant to physical and chemical insult and will readily sporulate in potassium dichromate. Many instances of spurious parasitemia have been reported in man when oocysts of various animals and fish coccidia have passed unchanged through the bowel to appear in the stool and pose a diagnostic problem. The mild persistent diarrhea during the active phase of the infection is usually accompanied only by nausea and abdominal discomfort. In a report cited below, the patients had severe diarrhea and steatorrhea unresponsive to therapy, and three died.

Brandborg, L. L., Golberg, S. B., and Breidenbach, W. C.: Human coccidiosis — a possible cause of malabsorption. The life cycle in small bowel mucosal biopsies as a diagnostic feature. N. Engl. J. Med., 283:1306, 1970.

Smitskamp, H., and Oey-Muller, E.: Geographical distribution and clinical significance of human coccidiosis. Trop. Geogr. Med., 18:133, 1966.

200.7.   SARCOSPORIDIOSIS
Philip D. Marsden

The genus *Sarcocystis*, like *Isospora*, *Toxoplasma*, and *Plasmodium*, belongs to the subphylum Sporozoa, parasites which show alterations of generations, one sexual (sporogony) and the other asexual (schizogony). Unlike *Isospora*, however, in *Sarcocystis* these two cycles occur in different hosts. The parasite previously designated *Isospora hominis* has been renamed *Sarcocystis hominis* because sporocysts appear in the stools of man following the ingestion of sarcocysts in uncooked beef or pork. Man also acts as an intermediate host for *Sarcocystis lindemanni* which may cause polymyositis sometimes associated with eosinophilia. Both these parasites are rarely reported, but their true prevalence in man is unknown.

Jeffrey, H. C.: Sarcosporidiosis in man. Trans. Roy. Soc. Trop. Med. Hyg., 68:17, 1974.

Rommel, M., and Heydorn, A. O.: Beiträge zum Lebenszyklus der Sarkosporidien. III. Isospora hominis (Raillet and Lucet, 1891) Wenyon, 1923, eine Dauerform der Sarkosporidien des Rindes und des Schweins. Berl. Münch. Tieraerztl. Wochenschr., 85:143, 1972.

Section Two HELMINTHIC DISEASES

201. INTRODUCTION

Philip D. Marsden

Compared to protozoans, helminths are very large organisms with a complex cellular structure. As they feed on host tissue, their metabolism results in various protein secretions and excretions; and because they themselves largely consist of complex protein, it is not surprising that invasion of the body by worms is frequently associated with an eosinophilic response. Thus, in the invasive stage of schistosomes, hookworm, ascaris, and similar parasites, an eosinophilia is usual. Yet when these worms have matured and settled at their site of election, eosinophilia often is not found. It might be argued in the case of intestinal nematodes that this is because they are in the gut and in a strict sense outside the body, but because the phenomenon also occurs with schistosomiasis and tissue filariae this is too facile an explanation. At present the mechanisms and course of eosinophilia produced in a host in response to a foreign protein are not clearly understood (Beeson and Bass).

With regard to immunology, understandably, complex helminths produce complex crude antigens of low specificity. At the moment, with a few exceptions, group-specific reactions with antigens for schistosomes, hermaphroditic flukes, nematodes, and cestodes are all that are available using tests such as complement fixation or indirect hemagglutination. Skin tests on the whole are much less satisfactory than those based on serology. Many of these helminths are recognized by the presence of characteristic progeny in the form of either eggs in the stools, sputum, or urine, or larvae in the tissues.

The concept of the over-all population or load of worms is important in human disease, as *the parasitic load* is one of the factors determining the extent of pathology (another would be the host response). Today many helminthic infections can be quantitated, and these methods will be mentioned under diagnosis. Another important aspect of worm infections is their relatively long life. Many flukes live for decades after the infection has been acquired, and similarly many filarial species are long lived. This illustrates the importance of obtaining a very detailed history of the patient's move-

TABLE 1. Prevalence of Common Helminth Infections in Man*

Parasite	Source of Infection	Approximate Locality	Estimated Incidence in U.S. and Canada	Estimated World Incidence
Trematodes (flukes):				
Schistosoma japonicum	Water through skin	Far East	—	46,000,000
Schistosoma haematobium	Water through skin	Africa, Middle East	—	39,200,000
Schistosoma mansoni	Water through skin	Africa, South America, Caribbean	—	29,200,000
Clonorchis sinensis	Fish	Far East	—	19,000,000
Opisthorchis felineus	Fish	Far East	—	1,100,000
Paragonimus westermani	Crabs, crayfish	Africa, South America	—	3,200,000
Fasciolopsis buski	Water nuts	Far East	—	10,000,000
Cestodes (tapeworms):				
Diphyllobothrium latum	Fish	Around Arctic Circle, N. Europe, Russia, America	†	10,400,000
Taenia saginata	Beef	Cosmopolitan	10,000	38,900,000
Taenia solium	Pork	Cosmopolitan	†	2,500,000
Echinococcus granulosus	Dog feces	Cosmopolitan	†	†
Nematodes (roundworms):				
Intestinal nematodes				
Strongyloides stercoralis	Human feces	Cosmopolitan	400,000	34,900,000
Hookworm	Human feces	Cosmopolitan	1,800,000	456,800,000
Ascaris lumbricoides	Human feces	Cosmopolitan	3,000,000	644,400,000
Trichuris trichiura	Human feces	Cosmopolitan	400,000	355,100,000
Enterobius vermicularis	Human feces	Cosmopolitan	18,000,000	208,800,000
Tissue nematodes				
Trichinella spiralis	Pork	Cosmopolitan	21,100,000	27,800,000
Wuchereria bancrofti and *Brugia malayi*	Mosquitoes	Africa, South America, South Asia	—	189,000,000
Loa loa	*Chrysops*	Equatorial Africa	—	13,000,000
Dipetalonema perstans	*Culicoides*	Africa, South America	—	27,000,000
Mansonella ozzardi	*Culicoides*	South America	—	7,000,000
Onchocerca volvulus	*Simulium*	Equatorial Africa, Central America	—	19,800,000
Dracunculus medinensis	*Cyclops*	Middle East, India, Africa	—	48,300,000

*Based on data calculated by N. R. Stoll (J. Parasit., 33:1, 1947). Since the world population has subsequently increased by more than 50 per cent, all the figures given can be regarded as extremely conservative. For instance, it is said that 180 million people in the world are infected with one of the three species of schistosomes that infect humans.

†Represents less than 100,000 infections.

ments around the world, because a visit to an endemic area 20 years ago may be connected with a current clinical problem.

It must be remembered that there are a large number of helminths that rarely infect man, and many cannot be included in this book. For information on these a standard textbook on parasitology (see references in Ch. 192) should be consulted. An important topical point is that we are now beginning to realize that for every worm adapted to man there are many others which gain access to man's tissues but fail to mature because they are natural parasites of other mammals or birds. These may cause very puzzling clinical problems. An increasing proportion of unexplained eosinophilia encountered in clinical practice is being explained on a basis of invasion of the body by a worm that will not mature in man because he is not the definitive host.

By a simple classification, worms may be separated into trematodes or flukes, cestodes or tapeworms, and nematodes or roundworms. A check list adapted from H. W. Brown's table in the twelfth edition of this text is given here in Table 1, together with information on the source of infection and the main areas of occurrence in the world. The most important helminthic infections in terms of disease in man and incidence are schistosomiasis, hookworm, and filariasis.

Beeson, P. B., and Bass, D. A.: The Eosinophil. Philadelphia, W. B. Saunders Company, 1977.

Marcial Rojas, R. A. (ed.): Pathology of Protozoal and Helminthic Diseases with Clinical Correlations. Baltimore, Williams & Wilkins Company, 1971.

Marsden, P. D. (ed.): Intestinal Parasites. Clinics in Gastroenterology, Vol. 7, No. 1. Philadelphia, W. B. Saunders Company, 1978.

Muller, R.: Worms and Disease. London, Heinemann, 1975.

THE CESTODES
(Tapeworms)

Philip D. Marsden

202. INTRODUCTION

The cestodes are endoparasitic flatworms, the hermaphroditic adults of which are flat and ribbonlike and inhabit the intestinal tract of vertebrates. *Taenia* species and the fish tapeworm may have a life of 25 to 30 years if left alone. The larval forms may require more than one intermediate host and develop in the tissues of vertebrates, and in some instances invertebrates. Most adult tapeworms consist of a scolex or head equipped for attachment with suckers, hooks, or grooves and a strobila or tapelike chain of progressively developing segments or proglottides. The neck is the site of segment generation, and mature segments are complete hermaphroditic units with both sets of sex organs. There is no digestive system, food being absorbed directly through the cuticle. There are longitudinal primitive excretory systems and a nervous system. In gravid segments the uterus is loaded with eggs, and these pass out of the bowel either in the segment or free in the stool. The delicate outer membrane of the eggs is often lost, but the thick-walled inner membrane contains a form infective for the intermediate host.

When eggs are ingested by the appropriate intermediate host, larvae (termed oncospheres) are released which are capable of penetrating the intestinal mucosa. The method by which the larvae develop into encysted forms differs among the cestodes and leads to different clinical patterns. Oncospheres in *Taenia solium* each develop into a small (0.5 to 1.0 cm) fluid-filled structure containing a single inverted "head." These are called *cysticerci*, or bladder worms, and many such larvae distributed in various organs cause the disease cysticercosis. The oncospheres in *Hymenolepis nana* penetrate only into the intestinal mucosa. They develop similarly to those just described; however, fluid is usually not present in the larva, and hence it is termed a *cysticercoid*. In the case of *Echinococcus granulosus*, usually only one oncosphere is able to develop (unilocular) within the intermediate host. However, this larva develops an internal germinating membrane capable of producing an entire population of daughter and granddaughter cysts within the primary cyst. This cyst is called an *echinococcal* or *hydatid* cyst. It continues to enlarge as the population of scolices within increases and will commonly reach a diameter of 20 to 30 cm after many years.

The clinical pattern of disease reflects these various methods of development; the cysticercoid of *H. nana* presents as intestinal irritation; the cysticercus of *T. solium* leads to multiple small lesions, often in the brain, causing seizure disorders; the *Echinococcus* produces a single large space-occupying lesion which often because of its size interferes with liver, lung, or cardiac function.

In the following chapters, we will deal with only the six most common of the 30 or more species of tapeworm which have been found in man. These are listed in Table 2. They will be discussed in the order cited in

TABLE 2. Common Important Tapeworms

Official Name	Intermediate Host(s)	Stage in Man
Diphyllobothrium latum	Water fleas, freshwater fish	Adult worm
Taenia saginata	Cattle (beef)	Adult worm
Taenia solium	Pigs (pork)	Adult worm and larval stage
Hymenolepis nana	Man	Adult worm and larval stage
Echinococcus granulosus	Man, sheep, cattle	Larval stage
Echinococcus multilocularis	Man, sheep, cattle	Larval stage

the table: first those in which man is the definitive host, then those in which he serves as both definitive and intermediate host, and finally those in which only the larval stage can develop in man.

Jones, T. C.: Cestodes. Clin. Gastroenterol., 7:105, 1978.

203. DIPHYLLOBOTHRIUM LATUM
(The Fish Tapeworm)

Infection with the fish tapeworm is most common in temperate areas such as Scandinavia and around the Baltic Sea. It also occurs in Canada and in the northern United States, notably Alaska. Central Europe is an endemic focus. In the tropics relatively few reports have appeared from the Philippines, Madagascar, Botswana, Uganda, and Chile. A human parasite, *Diphyllobothrium pacificum*, has been described from Peru. The adult is the largest tapeworm of man, reaching 10 meters and having 4000 segments. (The spatulate head has two deep sucking grooves for attachment to the wall of the ileum.) The gravid segment disintegrates, and operculated ova are passed in the feces.

From the egg a ciliated embryo is eaten by a freshwater flea (*Cyclops* or *Diaptomus* species) in which it develops to a *procercoid*. When the infected flea is swallowed by freshwater fish, e.g., salmon, pike, further development takes place in the muscles of the fish to the *plerocercoid*, the form infective to man. The plerocercoid on being liberated into the small intestine grows to an adult in three to six weeks. Although the adult worm causes no pathologic lesion, there is a very important complication to this infection, namely a megaloblastic anemia. This appears to be due to the avidity of the worm for vitamin B_{12}. Forty-four per cent of a single dose of Co^{60} labeled vitamin B_{12} has been absorbed by a worm, the radioactivity being concentrated in the proximal growing part. Also, the nearer the worm is to the jejunum, the greater the chance of developing megaloblastic anemia. It is not clear why the worm needs so much vitamin B_{12}. The worm also appears to require folic acid in the same way. Thus the full range of neurologic symptoms of subacute combined degeneration of the cord may appear, particularly in severe cases of multiple parasitism. Peripheral neuritis appears very early in the parasitism, and recently optic atrophy has been reported.

The *diagnosis* is made by direct examination of the stools, because the eggs are present in very large numbers. Yellowish-brown and operculated, they have to be distinguished from fluke eggs such as *Paragonimus*, but the large number in the stool favors the diagnosis of fish tapeworm even to the uninitiated. The operculum is actually less conspicuous in *Diphyllobothrium*, and there is a small knob at the anopercular end (mean size, 70 by 45 μ). Because the treatment for the tapeworms of this group and of the *Taenia* genus is the same, they are considered together later.

Prophylaxis is readily accomplished by thoroughly cooking fish before consumption. Freezing of fish for 48 hours at $-10°$ C will also prevent infection. The infection is not uncommon in New York among Jewish housewives who make their own gefilte fish and sample it in the process.

SPARGANOSIS

This condition requires mention here, because it is the name of an infection caused by the migrating larvae or spargana of several species of tapeworm related to *D. latum* but requiring final hosts other than man. It presents as a migrating subcutaneous painful swelling suggesting a cellulitis. Marked eosinophilia is usually present. The eye may be involved with orbital swelling or even actual penetration of the globe. In China this results from applying infected frogs on poultices to the eye. Biopsy reveals inflammatory tissue reactions and an immature cestode, many of which are quite impossible to identify. *Diphyllobothrium mansonoides* (*Spirometra mansonoides*) is a common offender. So-called *Sparganum proliferum* is unknown in the adult stage, but may distribute thousands of larvae throughout the body, and in contrast to other forms carries a poorer prognosis. This type of infection is rare, but occurs in many tropical countries, diagnosis being made by finding the plerocercoid larvae in tissues.

Bjorkenheim, G.: Neurological changes in pernicious tapeworm anemia. Acta Med. Scand., 140 (Supplement): 260, 1971.
Swartzwelder, J. C., Beaver, P. C., and Hood, M. W.: Sparganosis in the southern United States. Am. J. Trop. Med. Hyg., 13:43, 1964.
Vik, R.: The genus *Diphyllobothrium*. Exp. Parasitol., 15:361, 1964.
Von Bowsdorff, B.: Diphyllobothriasis in man. New York, Academic Press, 1977.

204. TAENIA SAGINATA
(The Beef Tapeworm)

The beef tapeworm has a cosmopolitan distribution, being particularly common in the Middle East, Kenya, and Ethiopia. In the last-named country many people habitually take a monthly purge of herbs to get rid of an impressive length of worm, but rarely get rid of the head. Beef tapeworm is also common in parts of South America, Mexico, and Russia. In all these countries it is acquired by eating undercooked or raw beef — a delicacy in Ethiopia. It is doubtful whether *T. saginata* causes any symptoms, although epigastric pain, appetite disturbances, and general malaise have been ascribed to the presence of the worm. It is possible that multiple worms may be associated with symptoms. Very rarely the worm may block the pancreatic or cystic duct or appendix, producing acute inflammation (16 such cases have been reported). The 5- to 10-meter adult worm has four suckers on the head to attach it to the wall of the small intestine. The gravid segments are usually recognized in the stool, but, being muscular, they can traverse the anal sphincter and appear in the underclothing. They contain more than 12 uterine branches, which distinguish them from *T. solium*, although recently some doubt has been cast on the reliability of this criterion. Characteristic *Taenia* eggs may be found in the stool or on the anal margin. When the eggs are swallowed by cattle, llamas, or buffaloes, the hatched embryos gain the skeletal muscles by the bloodstream after bowel penetration and develop into the encysted bladder-like larval forms or cysticerci which are infective for man.

Man is the only definitive host in which the adult worm can develop. The larval cysticercus form has been reported only three times in man, so host specificity seems to be strict. Treatment will be discussed later; prevention consists in not ingesting beef containing cysticerci.

Pawloski, Z., and Schultz, M. G.: Taeniasis and cysticercosis (*Taenia saginata*). Adv. Parasitol., 10:269, 1972.

205.   TAENIA SOLIUM
(The Pork Tapeworm Causing Human Cysticercosis Due to Cysticercus Cellulosae)

In contrast to *T. saginata*, both larval and adult forms of this species can develop in man. Again this worm is cosmopolitan in distribution although relatively rare in North America and western Europe; cysticercosis is the most common identifiable cause of epilepsy in the Durban African population and is a serious disease because of the frequency of brain involvement. It is common in Mexico and parts of Central and South America. Man, again the only definitive host of importance, acquires the infection by eating undercooked measly pork containing cysticerci. Pigs and wild boars are the usual intermediate hosts.

The adult worm usually causes no symptoms in the small intestine. For attachment the head has four suckers and two rows of hooklets on a prominent rostellum. It is smaller than *T. saginata* (2 to 4 meters). Its segments are more delicate than *T. saginata* and there are usually less than twelve branches to the uterus in the gravid segment. The eggs are indistinguishable from *T. saginata*, both being approximately 35 μ, thick-walled, brown, and containing an embryonic oncosphere with six hooklets. In *T. solium* infection, however, these eggs are infective to man, but must pass through the stomach and undergo tryptic digestion before hatching occurs. The usual way in which man is infected with eggs is by external autoinfection, transferring eggs from the anus to the mouth or to food fecally contaminated by a carrier of the worm. Internal autoinfection by regurgitating segments of the worm into the stomach is a theoretic possibility, but has not been recorded.

Once free from the egg in the intestine, the oncosphere penetrates the intestinal wall with its hooklets and, as in the pig, settles in the body tissues. The invaded organs in order of frequency are subcutaneous tissue, brain, eye, muscles, heart, liver, lung, and peritoneum. The cysticercus matures in four months to an ellipsoidal translucent cyst, 10 to 20 by 5 to 10 mm, with an opaque invaginated scolex with suckers and hooks. It is gradually surrounded by a thick fibrous capsule and may live for years. Death is frequently associated with calcification. Some authors distinguish *Cysticercus cellulosae*, in which a scolex is present, from *Cysticercus racemosus;* the latter is a degenerate cyst in which the scolex is absent.

The invasive phase may be associated with fever, headache, muscle pain, and high eosinophilia. Usually years after this stage more serious symptoms occur owing to brain involvement, with the onset of epilepsy, personality changes, signs of raised intracranial pres-

sure, or long tract signs. In every patient with epilepsy of late onset coming from an endemic area, especially if eosinophilia is present, this possibility should be excluded by (1) taking a detailed history, especially in relation to a past history of tapeworm infection; the stool should be examined for *Taenia* eggs and segments, because rarely the worm may still be in situ; (2) having a full physical examination, especially for subcutaneous nodules containing cysticerci; biopsy will establish the diagnosis; (3) taking roentgenograms of the skull, buttocks, and thighs for calcified cysticerci which have a characteristic size and shape; and (4) performing either a complement-fixation test or an indirect hemagglutination test, using antigen from lyophilized pig cysticerci. The cerebrospinal fluid may be under increased pressure, show an excess of eosinophils, and demonstrate a positive complement fixation test. More rarely the globe of the eye is involved, as well as the heart and skeletal muscle. A cysticercus may be visible on the tongue. Sometimes the cysticerci become secondarily infected. In the brain, inflammation around them may produce internal hydrocephalus. Although the adult worm can be eradicated easily, there is no medical treatment for *Cysticercus cellulosae* save palliative anticonvulsants. Mebendazole has been shown to kill cysticerci in mice. Rarely surgical intervention may be necessary in cases of raised intracranial pressure. Again prophylaxis rests on avoiding opportunities of eating infected meat and the inspection and thorough cooking of pork.

Campbell, W. C., and Blair, L. S.: Prevention and cure of hepatic cysticercosis in mice. J. Parisitol., 60:1049, 1974.
Marquez-Monter, H.: Cysticercosis. *In* Marcial Rojas, R. A., (ed.): Pathology of Protozoal and Helminthic Diseases. Baltimore, Williams & Wilkins Company, 1971.
Powell, S. J., Procter, E. M., Wilmot, A. J., and McLeod, I. N., Cysticercosis and epilepsy in Africans: A clinical and serological study. Ann. Trop. Med. Parasitol., 60:152, 1966.

206.   TREATMENT OF INFECTIONS WITH ADULTS OF THE FISH, BEEF, AND PORK TAPEWORM

Niclosamide (hydroxychlorobenzamide, Yomesan)* is safe, effective, and easy to administer. When the patient wakes in the morning, two tablets of 0.5 gram each are chewed thoroughly and swallowed with a little water. The same procedure is repeated one hour later. No fasting or purgation is necessary, and children receive a proportionately smaller dose. Alternatively, paromomycin can be used in the adult. The dosage for niclosamide and for paromomycin is the same: 1 gram every four hours, for a total of 4 grams. The worm disintegrates so that unfortunately the head cannot be sought as proof of cure. For this reason follow-up at six months is desirable.

Quinacrine hydrochloride (Atabrine, mepacrine) is indicated in cases in which the aforementioned therapy had been unsuccessful. The rationale is that a single comparatively large dose of this drug causes the worm

---

*Available from Center for Disease Control (404-633-3311, Ext. 3670).

to release its hold and it can then be voided. The most successful technique for adults is as follows: Admit the patient to hospital and give only fluids for 36 to 48 hours. Then pass a tube into the duodenum and, with the patient resting quietly, inject 1 gram of quinacrine hydrochloride down the tube in 40 ml of water, using a 20-ml syringe. Half an hour later a saline purge is injected down the tube, and all feces saved for the next 24 hours. Long lengths of the worm stained yellow with the drug are passed, and the head should be identified. If the head is not dislodged, the worm will regenerate in two to three months, and segments will reappear in the stools. The duodenal tube reduces the chances of vomiting the drug. If the head of the worm is found, one can usually reassure the patient that the worm is eliminated unless it is a rare case of multiple infection. It must be remembered that feces from patients harboring *T. solium* are an infectious risk. The patient should scrub his hands after defecation and pass his feces into disinfectant.

Keeling, J. E. W.: The chemotherapy of cestode infections. *In* Goldin, A., Hawking, F., and Schnitzer, R. J. (eds.): Advances in Chemotherapy. New York, Academic Press, 1968, Vol. 3, pp. 109–152.

207. HYMENOLEPIS NANA (Dwarf Tapeworm)

H. nana is less important as a cause of symptomatic disease than the other tapeworms described here. However, since it is spread directly by contact with contaminated stool, the infection can reach epidemic proportions in institutions where fecal-oral exposure is difficult to control, such as in mental hospitals or schools for young children. In one study of children in a school for the mentally retarded (Willowbrook, New York), almost 8 per cent were found to be infected.

Clinical manifestations of this infection include anorexia, diarrhea, and abdominal pain secondary to irritation of the intestinal mucosa. In addition, systemic signs and symptoms such as headache, dizziness, and occasionally seizures are not infrequent. The treatment of choice is hydroxychlorobenzamide (niclosamide),* 2 grams daily for three days, followed a week later by a second course of therapy. This treatment schedule has been developed because relapse occurred when shorter courses of therapy were used. Relapse is thought to occur for two reasons: first, the chlorobenzamide is effective only against the adult; and second, the cysticercoid stage may persist in the mucosa for several weeks before developing into an adult.

Yoeli, M., Most, H., Hammond, J., and Scheinesson, G. P.: Parasitic infections in a closed community. Results of a 10-year survey in Willowbrook State School. Trans. R. Soc. Trop. Med. Hyg., 66:764, 1972.

208. ECHINOCOCCOSIS (Hydatid Disease)

There are two species of the genus *Echinococcus* which infect man, *Echinococcus granulosus* and *Echinococcus multilocularis*. They are the most important ces-

*Available from Center for Disease Control (404-633-3311, Ext. 3670).

todes producing serious disease in man because of the size and location of their larval form, the hydatid cyst. Man is only one of a number of intermediate hosts, other important ones being sheep, cattle, and deer. The definitive hosts for these very small adult tapeworms are canines such as dogs, wolves, jackals, and foxes.

Hydatid disease is cosmopolitan because infected stock have been distributed all over the world for breeding purposes. The incidence of human infection is low in many countries, but where the triad of man, dog, and sheep or cattle is common, hydatid disease is relatively frequent. Examples are countries such as Australia, Argentina, Chile, Kenya, New Zealand, and the United Kingdom (Wales). It has been reported from 15 states in the United States. A distinct variant, *E. granulosus var. canadensis*, is present in Alaska and is also found in Canada.

Human infection follows ingestion of the eggs excreted by infected dogs. The adult tapeworm measures only 2.5 to 9.2 mm and has a head with hooklets and suckers, a growing neck, and only three segments: immature, sexually mature, and gravid. Heavy infections of dogs are common, but the worm lives for only about six months in the upper jejunum. The eggs produced are indistinguishable from *Taenia* eggs and like them produce an oncosphere with six hooklets. On reaching the intestine of the intermediate host such as man, they pass through the intestinal wall and circulate in the blood and can develop in any body tissue. It may take 20 to 30 years before the slowly growing hydatid cyst causes symptoms. Often they remain small (less than 10 cm), but they may grow as large as the human head. The host parasite factors determining growth are not clearly understood, but growth is variable from 0.25 to 1 cm a year. The structure of a developed hydatid cyst is complex. Briefly, it really consists of a whole colony of infective larval forms, for inside the laminated, defined cyst wall is a germinal layer that is constantly budding off new infective individuals. The cyst is filled with fluid, and second and third generation cysts containing thousands of infective forms or scolices are suspended in this fluid. There is little wonder that when a dog eats an infected sheep's liver he acquires many adult *Echinococcus* organisms.

When the infective embryo or oncosphere passes into the portal circulation of man, it is first held up in the liver where more than half (58 per cent) of those that survive develop. Many are destroyed by phagocytic cells. The next tissue filter is the lungs, where 27 per cent lodge. Finally, 15 per cent escape into the general circulation to involve the abdominal cavity, muscle, kidney, spleen, bone, heart, and brain.

ECHINOCOCCUS GRANULOSUS

Echinococcus granulosus is the common species; there are several types of cysts, as follows: (1) The classic unilocular cyst is usually fertile and surrounded by a false capsule of host tissue fibrosis. Rupture of such a cyst will cause dissemination of daughter cysts with secondary hydatids. (2) Alveolar hydatids have a reticulated irregular outline resulting from uneven growth of the germinal membrane. They resemble those of *E. multilocularis*, but there is no metastatic growth. This cyst usually occurs in the liver and is difficult to remove. It is often sterile, and its contents degenerate. (3) Osseous hydatid. The nature of bone does not permit a host or parasite capsule to form. Daughter cysts form in the bone medulla, erode the cortex, and produce a pathologic fracture. If they escape from the bone, the cysts grow in their normal spherical shape with the usual capsules in the extraosseous tissues.

Clinically, the hydatid cysts may produce signs of a space-occupying lesion in relation to the organ in which they occur. In the liver abdominal pain and vomiting may be presenting symptoms, a mass being visible or palpable. Usually the cysts are too tense to show fluctuation. In the lung they are usually detected on routine chest films as spherical, well-defined shadows. They are more common in the right lung, and rarely are associated with cough and hemoptysis. Those of the brain are indistinguishable from a cerebral tumor. In the kidney, hematuria or loin pain may be the first sign, whereas hydatid cyst of bone may present as a pathologic fracture.

The *complications* of hydatid disease are important. The most serious is rupture and dissemination of further infective larvae. Patients with suspected hydatid disease should always be gently palpated — a leaking cyst may present as anaphylactic shock with an urticarial rash and high eosinophilia. The cyst may become secondarily infected with bacteria and present similarly to a liver or lung abscess.

A suggestive tumor in a patient from an endemic area demands the following investigations. An eosinophilia may be present. Plain roentgenograms may show calcification in the cyst wall, although this does not mean that the cyst is not infective. An isotope scan of the liver reveals the extent of the tumor, but gives no clue as to its nature. In the chest film the round, uniformly dense shadow is suggestive. A skin test using cyst air in the cyst means communication with a bronchus and possibly secondary infection. A skin test using cyst fluid is positive in the majority of patients, but it has been shown that the reaction depends on the concentration (nitrogen content) of protein in the fluid injected. A cross-reaction occurs in patients with schistosomiasis. Until there is universal acceptance of a standard skin test antigen, a negative result is meaningless. Hydatid complement-fixation tests, hemagglutination tests, and bentonite flocculation tests are all practicable and are helpful. A scolex antigen is probably the best (Bull. WHO, 1968). Rarely cyst fragments, such as scolices, may be found in the sputum or urine. It must be recalled that one in five patients has multiple cysts, so that if a cyst is located in one site, especially if it is not the liver, there may be others. *A liver scan should be done in every patient with an extrahepatic cyst. Diagnostic aspiration is never indicated because of the risk of rupture.* In the liver and lung, carcinoma and abscess are often difficult differential diagnoses.

It should be emphasized that many hydatid cysts never get very large (5 to 10 cm) and never cause symptoms. Until recently there was no medical treatment for human hydatidosis. Now limited studies suggest that fluoromebendazole in an oral adult dose of 2 grams daily for six months to a year may kill the organism. The suggestion that specific antibodies and immune complexes are useful in assessing treatment requires confirmation. Surgery is indicated only in cysts that are enlarging, producing pressure symptoms, or developing complications. The physician should consult a surgeon who has experience with this problem. If possible the cyst should be removed entirely. To prevent spillage and dissemination, the cyst is usually aspirated at operation after packing off the site; 20 ml of fluid is withdrawn, and an equal quantity of 1 per cent iodine or 30 per cent sodium chloride is introduced to kill the scolices. Injection of a 1 per cent aqueous solution of iodine in a volume amounting to one twentieth of the whole cyst volume is lethal to scolices within one minute. Anaphylactic reactions resulting from spillage during operation may require corticosteroids.

E. granulosus var. canadensis is common in Alaska and Canada where it has a sylvatic cycle in deer and wolves. It produces smaller and more delicate cysts in man than the classic *E. granulosus;* the latter are more frequent in the lung, are usually asymptomatic, and almost never cause serious complications so that the distinction is important.

ECHINOCOCCUS MULTILOCULARIS

The medical importance of distinguishing between these two species is that *Echinococcus multilocularis* does not produce large single cysts with endogenous growth and well-defined fibrous tissue encapsulation but rather an aggregate of innumerable small cysts that multiply by exogenous budding to produce the so-called alveolar or malignant hydatid. More than 90 per cent occur in liver, which is progressively honeycombed by a multitude of small cysts. They may become confluent and even metastasize like a malignancy. Intrahepatic or portal hypertension develops with splenomegaly, and biliary obstruction may produce icterus. The hepatic infection may be difficult to differentiate from a malignancy. As surgical techniques improve, this infection may become an indication for a total liver transplant. This species of cestode occurs in south central Europe, Russia, and Alaska. Rarely cases have occurred in Australia, England, and Argentina.

Prevention of infection with both these species entails elimination of the infection from dogs by worming with arecoline hydrobromide regularly and preventing their eating infected offal. Contamination of the hands, food, and drink with dog feces should be avoided.

Arana Iniguez, R.: Hydatid echinococcosis of the nervous system. *In* Spillane, J. D. (ed.): Tropical Neurology. New York, Oxford University Press, 1973, p. 408.

Bouree, P., and Molimard, R.: Treatment of trichinococcosis. Br. Med. J., 1:307, 1978.

Danis, M., Brücker, G., Gentilini, M., et al.: Treatment of hepatic hydatid disease. Br. Med. J., 2:1356, 1977.

Dew, H. R.: Hydatid Disease. Sydney, Australian Publishing Co., Ltd., 1928.

Echinococcosis. Bull. WHO, 39: No. 1, 1968.

Jalayer, T., and Askavi, I.: A study of the effect of aqueous iodine on hydatid cysts in vitro and in vivo. Ann. Trop. Med. Parasitol., 60:169, 1966.

Katz, A. M., and Pan, C.: *Echinococcus* disease in the United States. Am. J. Med., 25:759, 1958.

Wilson, J. F., Diddams, A. C., and Rausch, R. L.: Cystic hydatid disease in Alaska. A review of 101 cases of *Echinococcus granulosus* infection. Am. Rev. Respir. Dis., 98:1, 1967.

209.   OTHER TAPEWORMS

Two other species of adult tapeworms that parasitize the human intestine are usually mentioned; but in comparison with those discussed above, they are of little importance in human disease. The rat tapeworm *Hymenolepis diminuta* is acquired by swallowing insects carrying the *Taenia* eggs from rats. *Dipylidium caninum* is the common tapeworm of cats and dogs throughout the world, and is transmitted by their fleas to children handling the pets. The gravid proglottids are shaped like melon seeds and may be seen in the stool. For these parasites niclosamide or paromomycin can be used.*

Coenurus infections of man, like hydatid, take the

---

*Available from Center for Disease Control (404-633-3311, Ext. 3670).

form of cystlike larvae in the tissue; 64 cases have been recorded to date. Infection in temperate regions is probably due to the larval cyst *Multiceps multiceps* (a dog tapeworm) and usually occurs in the central nervous system. Similar cysts are found in the brain of sheep, producing a fatal disease known as gid, which is characterized by somnolence, loss of weight, visual disturbance, and ataxia. In Africa *Taenia brauni* seems to be responsible for similar "hydatid-like" cysts in the subcutaneous tissues of man.

Templeton, A. C.: Anatomical and geographical location of human *Coenurus* infection. Trop. Geogr. Med., 23:105, 1971.

DISEASES CAUSED BY TREMATODES
(Flukes)

210. SCHISTOSOMIASIS
(Bilharziasis)

Kenneth S. Warren

DEFINITION. Schistosomiasis, a chronic infection of more than 200,000,000 people in Asia, Africa, the Caribbean region, and South America, is caused by three different worm species, *Schistosoma mansoni, S. japonicum,* and *S. haematobium.* Infection occurs during immersion in fresh water containing schistosome cercariae. These larval forms penetrate the skin and migrate via the lungs and liver to the final habitat of the half-inch-long adult worms: the veins of the intestines and urinary bladder. The worms themselves do not multiply within man, but produce large numbers of eggs, many of which remain in the body, damaging primarily the intestines, liver, and urinary tract. Eggs that are excreted in the urine and feces and that reach fresh water hatch into ciliated miracidia. These organisms penetrate into snails, multiply, and develop into cercariae, the infective form for man.

ETIOLOGY. Although the cercariae of many different schistosome species penetrate human skin, there are three major species that complete their life cycles in man and are thus capable of causing systemic disease: *Schistosoma mansoni, japonicum,* and *haematobium.* The life cycles of these schistosomes are essentially similar, all being digenetic trematodes alternating a sexual phase of reproduction in man (definitive host) with an asexual reproductive phase in snails (intermediate host). Nevertheless, at each phase of the life cycle there are differences among the species that play crucial roles in the epidemiology, pathogenesis, and clinical picture of the disease.

The adult worms or schistosomes are members of the class Trematoda of the phylum Platyhelminthes or flatworms. The male worms (10 to 20 × 0.5 to 1 mm) have cleft bodies within which the longer and thinner females reside, *S. japonicum* being the largest of the three species. The worms may live in man for as long as 30 years, but recent evidence suggests that their mean life span is five to ten years. The habitats of the adult *S. mansoni, japonicum,* and *haematobium* worms are, re-

spectively, the veins of the large intestine, small intestine, and urinary bladder.

The worms absorb metabolites through both their intestines and integument. Their energy processes depend on anaerobic catabolism of carbohydrates; the schistosomes utilize an amount of glucose equivalent to one fifth of their dry body weight each hour and convert 80 per cent of it to lactic acid. In addition, the ingestion of red blood cells appears to be of nutritional significance, as the worms contain a proteolytic enzyme that breaks down globin; the remaining insoluble hematin-like pigment is regurgitated because the schistosome intestine terminates blindly. The rapid metabolic rate of these worms may in part be related to their continual output of large numbers of eggs, estimated at 1400 to 3000 per day for *S. japonicum* and one tenth that number for *S. mansoni.* The eggs of the last-named species are released singly, whereas those of the other two species are deposited in large aggregates. They embryonate over a period of six days and increase in size, reaching a mean of 66 by 155 μ for *S. mansoni,* 60 by 143 μ for *S. haematobium,* and 67 by 89 μ for *S. japonicum.* The shape of the eggs is distinctive, *S. mansoni* being ellipsoidal and having a lateral spine; *S. haematobium,* also ellipsoidal but with a terminal spine; and *S. japonicum,* spheroidal with a tiny knob. The eggs remain viable for approximately 21 days after laying, during which time they must pass out of the body if their life cycle is to be completed. Passage from the blood vessels through the tissues and into the lumen of the excretory organs is apparently facilitated by enzymatic secretions of the eggs plus muscular movements of the gut or bladder. A large proportion of the eggs, however, either remain in the intestinal and vesical tissues or break free in the bloodstream and are carried into the liver and lungs.

The eggs that pass out of the body in feces or urine and reach fresh water hatch rapidly into free-swimming ciliated miracidia. The miracidia of *S. mansoni* are negatively geotropic and positively phototropic, although those of *S. haematobium* appear to be the opposite. Their average life span is about six hours. If during this time a snail is encountered, the organisms may penetrate it, and if it is of the genus *Biomphalaria* for *S. mansoni, Bulinus* for *S. haematobium,* or *Oncomelania* for

S. japonicum, the organism can complete its life cycle. The former two snail genera are aquatic, the latter amphibious. The miracidium remains close to the site of penetration, developing into a mother sporocyst. After about ten days daughter sporocysts begin to migrate into the digestive gland of the snail, and at about five weeks from the inception of the process cercariae produced from the daughter sporocysts begin to be shed by the snail. Maximal stimulus for shedding of *S. mansoni* and *haematobium* cercariae is provided by light, but darkness seems to favor the output of *S. japonicum* cercariae. The average daily output of *S. mansoni* and *S. haematobium* cercariae is about 700, but that of *S. japonicum* cercariae is only about two. These organisms may live for two to three days under ideal conditions, but their infectivity is lost by 20 hours; under field conditions both their life span and their infectivity are usually greatly reduced. The fork-tailed schistosome cercariae are about 125 to 200 μ in length by 50 to 75 μ in width. *S. mansoni* and *haematobium* cercariae alternate periods of rest, during which they sink slowly, with periods of movement, during which they rise toward the surface of the water. In contrast, *S. japonicum* cercariae attach themselves to the surface film where they tend to remain at rest. When cercariae encounter mammalian skin, they attach themselves with suckers, and by mechanical means, aided by enzymatic secretions, the heads penetrate, leaving the tails behind. This process occurs during immersion in water or while the skin remains moist (drying kills the organism), and takes four to ten minutes for *S. mansoni,* but only a few seconds to three minutes for *S. japonicum.*

As the worms do not multiply in the mammalian host, each cercaria that penetrates the skin can develop into only one worm. Many cercariae die in the skin, however, and in the best of experimental hosts only about 60 per cent of the *S. mansoni* organisms reach maturity. Within a few hours to days the schistosomula (the cercariae are completely changed both biochemically and physiologically immediately after penetration) migrate to the lungs by either the bloodstream or lymphatics. After a few days in the pulmonary vessels the schistosomula migrate to the liver, largely by the bloodstream. This phase takes ten to twelve days for *S. mansoni,* a somewhat shorter period for *S. japonicum,* and a longer one for *S. haematobium.* Once in the intrahepatic portal venules the worms rapidly reach maturity, mate, and move against the blood flow to their final habitats. Egg output is detectable at five to six weeks for *S. japonicum,* seven to eight weeks for *S. mansoni,* and ten to twelve weeks for *S. haematobium.*

EPIDEMIOLOGY. Initial infection in schistosomiasis usually occurs in childhood, and reinfection may continue as long as there is contact with fresh water. It must be remembered that the worms do not multiply in the human body, that complete immunity apparently does not occur, and that the worms may live for decades. Under these circumstances the incidence of schistosomiasis in endemic areas is low and occurs principally in children, but the prevalence of the disease may build up to massive proportions.

The worldwide prevalence of schistosomiasis is now estimated at over 200,000,000 cases. It is known to be endemic in 71 countries that have a total population of 1,362,635,000.

In Africa, *S. haematobium* and *S. mansoni* are widespread. Only the former species occurs in Tunisia, Algeria, Morocco, Mauritania, Guinea-Bissau, Niger, the Congo Republic (Brazzaville), Somalia, and the island of Mauritius. Both species are found in all other countries, including the Malagasy Republic. Sixty per cent of Africans live in areas where exposure to schistosomes is possible, and 40 per cent of these (about 75,000,000 people) are infected.

In Southwest Asia, *S. haematobium* is endemic in Aden, Saudi Arabia, Yemen, Israel, Iraq, Iran, Syria, Turkey, and Lebanon. *S. mansoni* occurs in the first four of these countries, and is particularly prevalent in Yemen, where half the 3,500,000 population are thought to be infected. The highest prevalence rate for *S. haematobium* occurs in Iraq, where 20 per cent of the exposed population of 5,000,000 are infected. Of the 87,003,000 population of Southwest Asia an estimated 10,745,000 are exposed to infection.

In the Orient, *S. japonicum* occurs in China, Japan, the Philippines, and the Celebes. The prevalence in China was estimated at 32,000,000, but it is reported that this number has been substantially reduced by a recent massive control campaign. Schistosomiasis is under control in Japan, but seems to be spreading in the Philippines. Small foci of schistosomiasis japonica have recently been discovered in Thailand and Laos. Of the 868,531,000 population of Southeast Asia, 337,051,500 are estimated to be exposed. A small focus of *S. haematobium* infection was found in India, in Maharashtra State, but it is now believed that transmission there has ceased.

In endemic areas of the New World (population 98,339,000) where only *S. mansoni* is found, 18,199,750 people are estimated to be exposed. Brazil has the largest number of cases, estimated at 8,000,000, and the infection seems to be spreading. Schistosomiasis also occurs in Venezuela, where it is apparently on the wane, and in Surinam. It is endemic in the following Caribbean islands: Puerto Rico, Vieques, Dominican Republic, Antigua, Guadeloupe, Martinique, and St. Lucia. The parasite has not been found in any of the Central American countries.

The one tiny focus of schistosomiasis in Europe, *S. haematobium* in southern Portugal, has now been eliminated.

The life cycle of schistosomiasis will become established only in areas where there is a susceptible snail species. Thus the infection is prevalent on the West Indian island of St. Lucia, although St. Vincent, 30 miles away, is completely free of the parasite. There are 1,450,000 Puerto Ricans now living on the mainland of the United States, and 100,000 immigrants from other areas endemic for schistosomiasis entering this country each year, but the presence of susceptible snails in the continental United States has not been established. Prevalence rates within endemic areas may be exceedingly variable, ranging from close to 100 per cent in some localities to almost none in others. This is governed by the interaction of multiple local ecologic factors relating to both the snail and human populations. Another important factor in the epidemiology of schistosomiasis is the variation in geographic strains of the species; for example, *S. japonicum* on Formosa is highly infective to domestic and wild animals but not to man, and *S. mansoni* in Africa south of the Sahara appears to be relatively avirulent.

Animal reservoirs are undoubtedly of significance in maintaining the life cycle of *S. japonicum* — in particular, cows and dogs. Natural *S. mansoni* infections have been found in rodents, baboons, insectivores, and dogs in Africa, but it is generally believed that animal reservoirs do not play a significant role in the life cycle of this species. *S. haematobium* is rarely encountered in animals.

Although *transmission patterns* differ among the three species of schistosomes, *there is little question that for each species agricultural development, particularly irrigation, may lead to a marked increase in the prevalence of schistosomiasis.* A major epidemic occurred in Egypt after the construction of the low Aswan dam, and in Rhodesia after development of large scale irrigation schemes.

In regard to morbidity and mortality, precise demographic figures are not available, particularly because schistosomiasis is such an insidious disease. The few investigations of morbidity now available show little or no effect of schistosomiasis on educational attainment or work capacity. Most studies suggest, however, that disease and death in schistosomiasis are correlated with intensity of infection. As the worms do not multiply in man, the number of parasites in a given individual is related to the degree of water contact and perhaps the occurrence of partial immunity. Under these conditions, schistosomes have an overdispersed distribution in which most members of the host population bear low worm burdens. As far as has been determined, little or no morbidity occurs in the large majority of the population carrying infections of low intensity. Though the proportion of heavily infected individuals is small, when this figure is multiplied against the vast number of people with schistosomiasis, it becomes obvious that this helminthic infection constitutes a major medical problem. In addition, there is no question that in all its forms schistosomiasis is potentially lethal — Katayama fever in *S. japonicum* infections, portal hypertension with hematemesis in both schistosomiasis japonica and mansoni, uremia in *S. haematobium* infection, and cor pulmonale in all three. Schistosomiasis may also potentiate the development of other diseases such as hepatitis, hepatoma, cirrhosis, and cancer of the urinary bladder.

PATHOGENESIS AND CLINICAL MANIFESTATIONS. Basic to an understanding of the disease processes in schistosomiasis are these facts: the schistosomes do not multiply in man; complete immunity does not follow initial infection; repeated infections usually occur; the worms are relatively long lived; most individuals have low worm burdens, but large numbers of worms may accumulate; and a large proportion of schistosome eggs are not excreted but remain within the body. Disease is correlated with the intensity of infection and is related not only to the presence of the various stages of the schistosomes in the body tissues and their secretions and excretions, but to the inflammatory responses of the host as well.

Clinically, three distinct syndromes occur at different stages of schistosome infection. Within one day of cercarial penetration, swimmer's itch, a pruritic papular rash, may appear. Several weeks later Katayama fever, a self-limited but possibly fatal illness resembling serum sickness, may develop. Finally, after many years, during which the infection may be either asymptomatic or associated with relatively mild intestinal or urinary tract symptoms, fibrosis of the liver may result in the signs and symptoms of portal hypertension in schistosomiasis mansoni and japonica; fibrosis of the ureters and bladder in schistosomiasis haematobia may result in changes associated with urinary tract obstruction.

Schistosome Dermatitis. Schistosomiasis begins with penetration of the skin by cercariae. These organisms are not discriminating and will penetrate the skin of most animals whether they are susceptible or insusceptible, living or dead. When nonhuman schistosomes, those that complete their life cycle in animals or birds, enter the skin of man, they die. Even in highly susceptible experimental hosts many *S. mansoni* cercariae die in the skin and perhaps in the lung; in the hamster almost 40 per cent are lost in this manner. In the highest primate thus far studied, the chimpanzee, 4 to 8 per cent of *S. mansoni* cercariae, 14 to 40 per cent of *S. haematobium* cercariae, and 1 to 48 per cent of *S. japonicum* cercariae were recovered as adult schistosomes. In most laboratory animals the recovery rate for *S. japonicum* is higher than that for the other two species.

The death of cercariae in the skin leads to the development of a pruritic papular rash known as swimmer's itch. This syndrome occurs in its most severe form after exposure to animal schistosomes, and has been shown to be a sensitization phenomenon, rarely occurring on primary exposure. Papules appear in sensitized persons at 5 to 15 hours, and there is massive round cell invasion of the dermis and epidermis, suggesting a delayed hypersensitivity response. Swimmer's itch has been demonstrated in infected patients experimentally re-exposed to *S. mansoni* and *S. haematobium* cercariae. A mild form of swimmer's itch appears to occur in patients exposed to *S. japonicum* cercariae, but the rice paddy dermatitis of the Far East is caused mainly by avian schistosomes.

Katayama Fever. The next clinical phase of schistosomiasis begins 20 to 60 days after exposure and has been known in Japan as Katayama fever since the mid-nineteenth century. This syndrome occurs most frequently and is most severe in *S. japonicum* infections; in schistosomiasis mansoni it is usually found only in patients with very heavy initial infection; it is rarely if ever seen in schistosomiasis haematobia. In addition to fever, the patient suffers from chills, sweating, anorexia, headache, diarrhea, and cough. Hepatosplenomegaly is frequent, and generalized lymphadenopathy and urticaria are often seen. Eosinophilia occurs in most cases, averaging about 40 per cent. The fever may last for several weeks; when it subsides the other signs and symptoms also disappear. Death may occur in the Katayama fever stage of schistosomiasis japonica, but rarely does so in *S. mansoni* infection. At autopsy, massive infection is almost invariably found, with large numbers of eggs in the liver and intestines; 1608 worm pairs were demonstrated at autopsy in a Brazilian child. Katayama fever, which usually appears on initial infection, begins at about the time of onset of egg-laying by the worms; thus large amounts of antigen are suddenly added to moderate levels of cross-reacting antibody formed in response to the developing worms. It is possible, therefore, that this serum sickness–like syndrome may be a form of immune-complex disease.

Chronic Schistosomiasis. A correlation between the number of worms and the development and extent of chronic disease (except for patients with advanced liver fibrosis) was recently demonstrated by techniques quantitating human worm burdens at surgery and at autopsy. Heavy worm burdens were apparently a prerequisite for the development of severe disease, whereas light infections appeared to be of little consequence pathologically. *Thus patients with few worms may never show any signs or symptoms related to schistosome infection.*

It is said that patients with chronic schistosomiasis mansoni or japonica may complain of fatigue, abdominal pain, and intermittent diarrhea or dysentery. Although this may be true in selected hospital populations, recent controlled field studies have revealed few such signs and symptoms, even in heavily infected individuals. On sigmoidoscopy, particularly in Egypt, granulomatous nodules or polyps may be observed. In *S. haematobium* infection, terminal hematuria, and, occasionally, dysuria and frequency are found. Mild chronic blood loss has been measured by radioisotope labeling in both *S. mansoni* and *S. haematobium* infections, but anemia is not usually seen in areas where there is normal iron intake. All the aforementioned signs and symptoms are related to the passage of eggs through the mucosa of the intestine and the urinary bladder.

Many eggs do not, however, leave the body; in laboratory animals less than half of them are excreted. Over a period of 20 years, for each *S. mansoni* worm pair producing eggs at a rate of 300 per day, at least 1,000,000 eggs will remain in the body. This figure can be multiplied by 10 for each *S. japonicum* worm pair.

In *S. mansoni* and *S. japonicum* infections, some of the eggs remain in the intestinal walls, but many of them enter the circulation and are carried into the liver. In schistosomiasis haematobia many eggs remain in the tissues of the bladder and adjacent organs, but some (usually too few to cause significant disease) enter the lungs via the inferior vena cava as well as the liver via the portal system. *Granulomatous inflammation* develops around the eggs trapped in the tissues; in the case of *S. mansoni* this has been demonstrated to be an immunologic response of the delayed hypersensitivity type. Both the eggs and the reactions to them are being constantly resorbed, but if large numbers of eggs gather together, the fibrosis subsequent to inflammation may remain. In schistosomiasis mansoni and japonica this leads to hepatic portal fibrosis, and in schistosomiasis haematobia, to fibrosis of the ureters and bladder.

Hepatosplenic Schistosomiasis. As the liver parenchyma is relatively unharmed by the pathologic processes involved in hepatic schistosomiasis japonica and mansoni, the clinical consequences of the disease relate primarily to granulomatous inflammation and portal fibrosis. Pathophysiologically this results in an intrahepatic block to portal blood flow and the development of portal hypertension and portal-systemic collateral circulation. The lesion is presinusoidal; thus intrasplenic and portal pressures are markedly elevated, whereas wedged hepatic vein pressure is normal. Total liver blood flow tends to remain within normal limits owing to a compensatory increase in arterial flow.

Clinically, the earliest sign of significant liver involvement is hepatomegaly. With progression, the spleen enlarges and becomes firm in consistency. Eventually it may extend to well below the umbilicus. At this point the patient tends to be in good general health, but may consult a physician because of a dragging feeling in the left upper abdominal quadrant.

The other major factor bringing the patient to the physician is a sudden hematemesis because of bleeding esophageal varices. Such an episode may not reappear for many years or may recur at fairly frequent intervals. The consequences of hematemesis in schistosomiasis are very different from those in cirrhosis of the liver: the blood ammonia concentration tends to remain normal, hepatic coma rarely occurs, and mortality is very low, being primarily due to exsanguination. This is consistent with relatively normal liver function. Jaundice is almost never seen in uncomplicated schistosomiasis, and the levels of both conjugated and unconjugated bilirubin are usually normal. Serum albumin concentration is normal or only slightly decreased, and globulin is somewhat elevated. As a consequence, ascites and edema are rarely encountered. Even sulfobromophthalein retention is often normal in these patients. Stigmata of chronic liver disease such as palmar erythema, spider angiomas, altered hair distribution, and gynecomastia are rare. Patients may suffer multiple severe hatemeses; but aside from temporary changes, liver function tends to remain relatively normal.

In spite of moderate chronic and occasional severe acute intestinal blood loss, a significant degree of anemia rarely occurs in uncomplicated schistosomiasis. The white blood count is usually within normal limits, but there is a moderate eosinophilia. Splenomegaly, however, may result in hypersplenism, the patient developing leukopenia, thrombocytopenia, and anemia with decreased red blood cell life span.

Patients with decompensated hepatic disease characterized by liver parenchymal malfunction and all the physical stigmata of this state, including jaundice and ascites, are seen in localities in which schistosomiasis is endemic. This is particularly common in the case of schistosomiasis japonica, and may, perhaps, be related to overwhelming embolization of the liver with the large numbers of eggs produced by this parasite. Pathologists have stated, however, that *it has not been possible to prove the transformation of advanced schistosomal fibrosis into true cirrhosis.* In Egypt it has been suggested that patients with schistosomiasis might concomitantly have other forms of liver disease. Finally, it must be recognized that all those infected with *S. mansoni* and *S. japonicum* perforce have some degree of liver involvement, and that the effect of malnutrition, hepatotoxins, and hepatitis may be potentiated; such interrelationships have been demonstrated in laboratory animals.

Pulmonary Schistosomiasis. Pulmonary schistosomiasis, which in its most severe state is characterized by signs and symptoms of cor pulmonale, is a complication of hepatosplenic schistosomiasis. Portal-systemic collateral circulation enables the eggs to bypass the liver, and they are trapped in the pulmonary capillary bed. Arteritis with angiomatoid formation occurs, and there is obstruction to pulmonary blood flow. Pulmonary hypertension is found in every case, but cardiac output usually remains within the normal range. Arterial oxygen saturation is usually normal, and cyanosis is rare. The lungs are often involved in schistosomiasis haematobia because of the passage of eggs from the vesical plexuses into the inferior vena cava, but egg embolization appears to be relatively light, and significant disease is uncommon.

Urinary Tract Schistosomiasis. Severe urinary tract disease may occur in both the early and late phases of *S. haematobium* infection. Initially there may be ureteral obstruction owing to florid granulomatous inflammatory reactions to the eggs in both the ureters and the bladder; these lesions appear to be highly reversible after antischistosomal therapy. Later in the course of the disease irreversible fibrosis may supervene. Bladder fibrosis and calcification lead to frequency and dysuria. On cystoscopy, so-called sandy patches may be seen on the bladder walls; these are made up of large numbers of schistosome eggs. The disease may progress through hydronephrosis, secondary infection, and finally uremia. An association between cancer of the bladder and urinary schistosomiasis has been demonstrated.

In the past decade there has been a growing impression among Brazilian clinicians and pathologists that there is an increased frequency of renal disease in patients with schistosomiasis mansoni. Initially proteinuria was noted in patients with hepatosplenic schistosomiasis, and then, at autopsy, the renal glomeruli of similar patients were found to have pathologic changes. This was followed by ultrastructural and immunocytochemical studies which revealed electron-dense deposits in the glomerular basement membranes which contained immunoglobulins. Similar deposits have been observed in laboratory animals. It should be pointed out, however, that specific schistosomal antigen has not been demonstrated as yet, and comparable lesions have been found in the kidneys of patients with cirrhosis of the liver.

Central Nervous System Schistosomiasis. Schistosomiasis of the central nervous system, although relatively rare, is an important complication of the infection. *S. japonicum* usually involves the brain, whereas *S. mansoni* and *S. haematobium* tend to affect the spinal cord. Schistosomiasis japonica is reputed to be one of the important causes of focal epilepsy in the Far East. The disease may also present as a space-occupying lesion or occasionally as a generalized encephalitis. Cerebral schistosomiasis japonica may appear at any time in the course of infection from the first three weeks on. At autopsy the lesions almost always consist of large collections of eggs in the venous circulatory system, suggesting the presence of adult worms, although they have never been found. *S. mansoni* and *S. haematobium* in the spinal cord may be associated with a transverse myelitis-like syndrome; at surgery or autopsy large granulomas made up of eggs are usually found.

The development of chronic salmonellosis has been described in schistosomiasis in both man and laboratory animals. In the latter, schistosomiasis has also been associated with increased severity of viral hepatitis and intestinal amebiasis.

DIAGNOSIS. When schistosomiasis is considered as a diagnosis in nonendemic areas, the first question that should be asked is: "Where have you been?" It must then be determined whether there was contact with fresh water, whether transient pruritus was observed soon thereafter, and if there was a febrile episode several weeks later. For schistosomiasis mansoni and japonica, abdominal symptoms and signs might be considered, and for *S. haematobium* infection, terminal hematuria, dysuria, and frequency are important. The presence of eosinophilia is a useful sign of schistosome infection. A wide variety of serologic tests (e.g., complement-fixation, flocculation, fluorescent antibody,

and circumoval precipitin) and a skin test of the immediate type are available. *These immunologic methods, which are all based on detection of circulating antibody, essentially have no place in the diagnosis of the individual case,* as cross-reactions with other parasitic infections providing false-positive results are relatively common; false-negative reactions also occur.

Definitive diagnosis can be made only by finding schistosome eggs in the excreta (feces or urine) or in a biopsy specimen — usually rectal. Eggs may not be present in the early stages of acute schistosomiasis. Schistosome eggs are relatively large, and are easy to identify because of their distinctive shape. Direct fecal smear is too insensitive, but techniques which provide both concentration and quantitation of eggs in the feces have been developed. This is important, because correlations between egg output and intensity of infection have been made. The Kato thick smear technique is a simple and highly effective method for fecal egg counting. A small portion of stool (schistosome eggs are distributed randomly in feces) is passed through 105-mesh stainless steel bolting cloth (W. S. Tyler Co., Cleveland, Ohio) and 50 mg is added to a tared glass slide and covered with a cellophane cover slip (no. 124PD, E. I. DuPont de Nemours, Inc., Film Department, Wilmington, Delaware) impregnated with 50 per cent glycerin. The slides are inverted and pressed onto a bed of filter paper, turned face up, and left for a period of at least 48 hours during which the fecal matter clears. Although the embryo within the egg also clears, the characteristic shape of the egg shell can be easily seen. After counting all the eggs in the sample, multiplication by 20 provides the number of eggs per gram of feces.

Rectal biopsy is a highly efficient method for the diagnosis of *S. mansoni* and *japonicum* infection, and will often help detect *S. haematobium* eggs. Through a proctoscope, snips are taken from the valves of Houston (8 to 10 cm from the anus), pressed between glass slides, and examined immediately under a microscope. Sometimes only opaque dead eggs are observed, suggesting a burnt-out or successfully treated infection. Liver biopsy has been suggested as a means of diagnosis, but will only rarely detect an infection not revealed by the aforementioned methods.

For the diagnosis of schistosomiasis haematobia, urine is collected at midday, because a diurnal variation in egg output has been demonstrated. The urine specimen is centrifuged and the sediment examined. For quantitative data a 10 ml aliquot of urine collected between 1100 and 1300 hours is passed through a Nuclepore Filter (13 mm in diameter with a pore size of 10 μm) held in a PT-013 chamber (Nuclepore Corp., Pleasanton, California). The filter is removed, placed face down on a microscope slide, and examined immediately at $\times$ 40 magnification, and the terminal-spined eggs are counted. *S. mansoni* eggs are occasionally found in urine.

For determining the severity of intestinal disease, sigmoidoscopy and barium enema are of value. The extent of liver disease may be estimated by liver biopsy, barium swallow, esophagoscopy, and especially splenoportography with measurement of intrasplenic pressure. In schistosomiasis haematobia, cystoscopy and intravenous pyelography are useful techniques.

TREATMENT. Antischistosomal treatment should never be instituted without proof of infection by the demonstration of living eggs in excreta or biopsy specimens, except in the rare case of suspected schistoso-miasis of the central nervous system. A positive sero-logic or skin test does not provide a definitive diagnosis. Complete cure is not necessary and indeed is not always desirable in schistosomiasis (particularly in endemic areas where reinfection may occur), because disease is related to intensity of infection, surviving worms do not multiply, and immunity may be premunitive, i.e., dependent on the presence of living organisms. The recent use of quantitative egg counts has shown that in cases in which cure is not achieved by the full course of treatment with an established drug, egg output is usually reduced by over 90 per cent. Thus striving for cure by increasing the drug dosage or repeating the course of treatment is rarely necessary and, because of the toxicity of the antischistosomal drugs, may actually be harmful.

None of the drugs now available for human use have any effect on the schistosomes during their early migratory phases in the body (the first three to six weeks), thus rendering it difficult to treat Katayama fever; steroids have been used to suppress the clinical manifestations during this stage of the infection. The three schistosome species vary considerably in their response to drugs, S. haematobium being the most susceptible and S. japonicum the most resistant. Under these circumstances it is generally stated that it is still necessary to treat schistosomiasis japonica with the highly toxic antimony potassium tartrate (tartar emetic). In a 1972 report of a World Health Organization consultant group, however, it was noted that the cure rates in S. japonicum infections with tartar emetic, stibocaptate (Astiban), and niridazole (Ambilhar), respectively, ranged between 40 and 75, 40 and 75, and 40 and 70 per cent. Thus it can be recommended that those infected with any of the three species of human schistosomes be treated with niridazole or stibocaptate, the latter when there are signs or symptoms of liver or cerebral disease. Both these drugs may be obtained from the Parasitic Disease Drug Service of the Center for Disease Control, Atlanta, Georgia 30333. Particularly in the case of S. mansoni infections, it would not be unreasonable to withhold treatment with these drugs in asymptomatic individuals with very low egg counts.

Niridazole is administered orally in two divided doses totaling 25 mg per kilogram of body weight daily, for a period of five to seven days. Vomiting, diarrhea, cramps, and dizziness may occur. Side effects are greatly exacerbated in patients with signs and symptoms of liver or cerebral disease. Under these circumstances stibocaptate can be substituted; this antimony compound is administered intramuscularly in a dose of 8 mg per kilogram once per week for five weeks. Antimony compounds are cardiotoxic; stibocaptate is also associated with anorexia, vomiting, abdominal pain, headache, and pain at the site of injection. Recently good success has been reported in treating human Schistosoma mansoni infections in Brazil with a new drug, oxamniquine. Relatively nontoxic, it is given in a single oral dose for adults of 15 mg per kilogram of body weight. Further research will establish the importance of this compound.

Utilizing a combination of surgery and a single dose of antischistosomal drug, many of the worms can be sieved out of the bloodstream. Although such extracorporeal hemofiltration is a valuable research tool, it should never be used as a form of treatment.

In general, the surgical treatment of schistosomiasis should be approached with caution. Many of the apparently irreversible lesions of urinary tract schistosomiasis will resolve completely after antischistosomal treatment, particularly in young patients. Cerebral schistosomiasis japonica is frequently cured or markedly ameliorated by drug therapy. Finally, prophylactic portacaval shunts should never be performed in hepatosplenic schistosomiasis, because hematemesis is not invariable and is unpredictable in onset, and, when it occurs, mortality is low. If the creation of shunt by surgery is necessitated by repeated bleeding episodes, splenorenal anastomosis is preferable to portacaval shunt because of a much lower incidence of chronic portal systemic encephalopathy. Prior to shunting, however, antischistosomal therapy is necessary to prevent prolonged passage of eggs into the lungs which may lead to the development of cor pulmonale.

PROGNOSIS. The prognosis is usually good. Many patients with schistosomiasis never have symptoms or signs of disease, or have only relatively mild ones. Epidemiologically, both the infection and the disease reach their peak in early adult life and decline with age. Disregarding the factor of death among heavily infected patients, this may be due to decreased exposure to infection, gradual death of the worms, slow development of immunity, and diminution in the inflammatory response to the parasite and its products.

The early stages of hepatic or urinary tract disease appear to be reversible after antischistosomal therapy. Although late disease seems relatively irreversible, progression may be halted and gradual improvement may follow drug therapy. In hepatosplenic schistosomiasis the prognosis in patients suffering a hematemesis is far better than in those with cirrhosis, because the former do not tend to go into hepatic coma. Patients with cerebral schistosomiasis japonica may show remarkable improvement after antischistosome therapy.

PREVENTION. On the individual level, schistosomiasis may be prevented by avoidance of contaminated waters. If this is not possible, boots should be worn; if contaminated water reaches the skin, rapid drying or rubbing with alcohol will prevent infection. Storage of water for several days will ensure the death of cercariae, as will the boiling of drinking water. Sea water is safe for swimming, although the mouths of rivers and streams should be avoided; chlorination of swimming pools will prevent infection. Repellents are of no great value, and vaccines or prophylactic drugs are not available.

There are three approaches to the control of schistosomiasis on a mass basis: (1) destruction of the snail intermediate host, (2) prevention of snail infection by the treatment of human infection and the construction of privies, and (3) elimination of contact with contaminated water by the provision of safe water supplies. Destruction of the snail is primarily based on the use of molluscicides such as the various copper salts, sodium pentachlorophenate, Bayluscide, and n-trityl-morpholone. Molluscicides, however, are quickly inactivated by sunlight and adsorption to mud and organic matter; they pass rapidly through running water or are diluted in vast bodies of still water, and they often destroy other aquatic fauna and flora. Also, although molluscicides may appear to be highly effective, only a few surviving snails can rapidly repopulate an area. Many biologic control measures have been advocated, including the use of nonsusceptible snail species which may compete for miracidia, food, and space; snail-eating fish and ducks; and snail pathogens. None of these measures has shown outstanding promise. The snails that transmit *S. japonicum* are amphibious and are frequently found along the banks of water courses; their eradication can necessitate the use of earth-moving equipment and flame throwers. When the snails are "buried" in this way, as in the campaigns in the People's Republic of China, it appears to reduce the infectivity of the environment.

An attempt to break the life cycle at the stage of transmission from man to the snail has been hampered by the lack of practical mass therapy. The recent development of effective oral drugs and of a single-dose intramuscular drug offers great promise for the future. An important adjunct to this approach is the construction of privies. Breaking the cycle at the stage of transmission from the snail to man can be accomplished by the provision of safe water supplies for washing and recreational purposes.

Control measures based on the destruction of snails are an end in themselves, and in addition may be inimical to the environment. In contrast, mass antischistosomal treatment coupled with the construction of privies or the provision of safe water supplies should contribute greatly to the general health of the population.

Arap Siongok, T. K., Mahmoud, A. A. F., Ouma, J. H., Warren, K. S., Muller, A. S., Handa, A. K., and Houser, H. B.: Morbidity in schistosomiasis mansoni in relation to intensity of infection: Study of a community in Machakos, Kenya. Am. J. Trop. Med. Hyg., 25:273, 1976.

Cheever, A. W., Kamel, I. A., Elwi, A. M., Mosimann, J. E., and Danner, R.: *Schistosoma mansoni* and *S. haematobium* infections in Egypt: II. Quantitative parasitological findings at necropsy. Am. J. Trop. Med. Hyg., 26:702, 1977.

Clark, W. D., Cox, P. M., Jr., Ratner, L. H., and Correa-Coronas, R.: Acute schistosomiasis mansoni in 10 boys. An outbreak in Caguas, Puerto Rico. Ann. Intern. Med., 73:379, 1970.

Lehman, J. S., Jr., Farid, Z., Smith, J. H., Bassily, S., and El-Masry, N. A.: Urinary schistosomiasis in Egypt: Clinical, radiological, bacteriological and parasitological correlations. Trans. R. Soc. Trop. Med. Hyg., 67:384, 1973.

Warren, K. S.: Regulation of the prevalence and intensity of schistosomiasis in man. Immunology or ecology? J. Infect. Dis., 127:595, 1973.

Warren, K. S.: Schistosomiasis: A multiplicity of immunopathology. J. Invest. Dermatol., 67:464, 1976.

Warren, K. S., Rebouças, G., and Baptista, A. G.: Ammonia metabolism and hepatic coma in hepatosplenic schistosomiasis. Patients studied before and after portacaval shunt. Ann. Intern. Med., 62:1113, 1965.

WHO Reports on Schistosomicidal Drugs. II. Report of a WHO consultant group on the comparative evaluation of new schistosomicidal drugs for use in treatment campaigns. Bol. Of. Sanit. Panam. (English), 6:89, 1972.

211. HERMAPHRODITIC FLUKES

Philip D. Marsden

211.1. INTRODUCTION

The hermaphroditic flukes, unlike *Schistosoma* flukes, have both sets of sex organs in the same worm, and frequently self-fertilization occurs. These flukes are flat leaflike worms with oral and ventral suckers. They have a complex life cycle. The egg hatches to produce a motile ciliated *miracidium*, which penetrates the soft tissue of a snail and undergoes a cycle of development similar to that in schistosomiasis. *Cercariae* are produced by the snail after a few weeks, but unlike schistosomes these cercariae encyst in a second intermediate host, either fish, crab, or plant. These encysted cercariae or *metacercariae* are a relatively resistant form which can survive adverse conditions. If the metacercaria is then ingested by man, it hatches to produce an immature fluke which migrates through the body tissues to gain its site of final development. This varies with the species concerned, being the liver for *Clonorchis* and *Fasciola,* the lung for *Paragonimus,* and the intestine for *Fasciolopsis buski.* None of these trematodes are principally human parasites, and they show different degrees of adaptation to man.

Initial invasion is often accompanied by eosinophilia, but it takes a month or longer before the characteristic eggs are produced. All the eggs have an operculum or lid through which the miracidia escape, unlike *Schistosoma* eggs. Some of these flukes live for a long time, producing progressive damage in the tissues of the host. When searching for the ova of trematodes in the biliary tree, duodenal aspiration may be more rewarding than stool examination. Therapy, especially in the hepatic hermaphroditic trematodes, is unsatisfactory.

Skah, S. K. K.: Digenetic trematodes. Clin. Gastroenterol., 7:87, 1978.

211.2. HEPATIC HERMAPHRODITIC FLUKES

CLONORCHIASIS (CLONORCHIS SINENSIS). Man is infected by eating the flesh of undercooked or raw freshwater fish in which the metacercariae are encysted. More than 40 species of fish, mainly of the carp and salmon (cyprinoid) group, have been found to harbor metacercariae. The natural definitive hosts other than man are fish-eating mammals, including cats, dogs, mink, and rats. Widespread in the Far East, the main endemic areas of human infection are Japan, Korea, China, and Vietnam. As the flukes live for decades (20 to 30 years) in the biliary tree, immigrants from Asia have been found infested in many countries. A portion of the Chinese in New York and San Francisco are infected. Infections recorded in Hawaiians are attributed to imports of infected frozen, dried, or pickled fish from Japan.

It appears that most of the larval flukes ascend the biliary tree directly from the duodenum, but some may pass via the portal circulation to the liver. They mature in the bile ducts, and the grayish-brown adults, measuring 10 to 20 mm by 2 to 4 mm, move sluggishly around by means of their suckers in the distal biliary passages. They feed on secretions from the mucosa of the bile duct and possibly also on cellular elements. Occasionally they gain access to the gallbladder and pancreatic ducts. In effect they cause a chronic cholangitis with inflammation of the biliary tree, proliferation of the biliary epithelium, and progressive portal fibrosis. The severity of these changes depends upon the load of flukes.

After ingesting the metacercariae, the patient may present with epigastric pain, malaise, and tender hepatomegaly. An eosinophilia is usually present in the early stages, but no eggs can be found until about one month has passed and the flukes have matured. Light infections are often asymptomatic, but a firm liver edge is often discovered within the costal margin on routine examination. In an Asian, this finding should prompt a careful search for ova in the stool. In heavy infections (10,000 to 20,000 flukes), more serious sequelae occur. The marked portal fibrosis may be associated with signs of portal hypertension. Extension of the fibrosis into the liver parenchyma may be associated with liver cell death and fatty change. Jaundice is more likely to be associated with biliary obstruction owing to a mass of flukes or stone formation. Cholangiocarcinoma is a late complication of severe clonorchiasis, a metaplastic change occurring in the irritated biliary epithelium. In Hong Kong there is a high incidence in males after the fourth decade, the adenocarcinomas showing varying degrees of differentiation. Suppurative cholangitis and chronic pancreatitis are other complications.

The diagnosis is made by finding the eggs in the stool. Unfortunately they are not characteristic and can be easily confused with a number of other trematodes producing small, similar eggs (*Heterophyes, Opisthorchis, Metagonimus*). The eggs average 29 by 16 μ; they are light brown and ovoid. There is a definite shoulder in the shell wall near the operculum and a boss at the anopercular end.

The invasive stage must be distinguished from that of other fluke infections, *visceral larval migrans*, and *hepatic amebiasis*. The last-named condition is not associated with eosinophilia. The late stages may resemble cirrhosis and uncomplicated cholecystitis. Hypoglycemic coma can also be a manifestation of a hepatocellular carcinoma. In the elderly, repeated nonparasitic cholangitis is sometimes a difficult diagnosis to establish in patients with pyrexia of unknown origin.

Treatment and Prevention. Most investigators agree that the drugs available for treating this infection are often ineffective and disappointing. In those patients who have no symptoms, no treatment is advised. Prolonged chloroquine therapy is chiefly suppressive; however, it is still the drug of choice. Chloroquine diphosphate in a dose of 300 mg base (two 250 mg tablets) three times a day for three to six weeks is a standard course. Some workers have increased this dose or used it for periods of up to a year. Various percentages of cures are claimed, but it depends on the criteria used and especially on what stool concentration technique is employed and how frequently. At the higher dosage levels the more severe side effects of chloroquine toxicity may be seen, namely, corneal deposits and retinopathy, central nervous system changes (a parkinsonian-like syndrome), dyspigmentation, cardiac arrhythmias, and peripheral myopathy and neuropathy. The compound hexachloroparaxylol proved effective, but alarming toxicity tests in studies in laboratory animals have resulted in its withdrawal. Biliary obstruction may require surgical relief, and at surgery as many flukes as possible should be removed from the biliary tree. Prevention of this infection relates to the competent cooking of freshwater fish.

OPISTHORCHIASIS (OPISTHORCHIS VIVERRINI AND FELINEUS). *Opisthorchis felineus* is prevalent in the Philippines, India, Japan, and Vietnam, as well as in the U.S.S.R. and parts of Eastern Europe, whereas *Opisthorchis viverrini* is common in north Thailand and Laos.

The life cycles of these flukes are similar to that of *Clonorchis sinensis* and are completed in about four months under favorable conditions. Snails are infected by fecal contaminants of water from infected persons or animal reservoirs, e.g., cats. In northeast Thailand 90 per cent of people more than ten years of age are infected with *O. viverrini*, and 3.5 million in the whole country. With all infections of this type, as might be expected, the incidence rises with age. The source of infection is a popular dish of raw fish, rice, vegetables, and spices.

The pathologic findings are similar to those in *Clonorchis sinensis*, although stone formation is said to be unusual. Cholangiocarcinoma has also been reported to be associated with this infection. The eggs are indistinguishable from *Clonorchis*. This emphasizes the importance of a geographic history, for the only other way of distinguishing the parasite would be by examination of the adult flukes. Percutaneous transhepatic cholangiography may reveal radiologic changes such as a single cystic cavity or mulberry-like dilatation of the intrahepatic bile ducts.

DICROCOELIASIS. *Dicrocoelium dendriticum* is acquired by eating ants in which the metacercariae have developed following ingestion by the ant of slime balls containing cercariae secreted by the snail. Infections are generally uncommon, but occur in Europe and Asia and around the Mediterranean basin. Being light infections, their main importance is for the physician to recognize the small, fully embryonated thick-shelled eggs (40 μ by 25 μ) for what they are. Spurious parasitism, in which nonhuman species ingested in liver pass through the bowel unchanged, is well documented.

FASCIOLIASIS (FASCIOLA HEPATICA). This is also a biliary fluke, but it is less well adapted to man than is *Clonorchis sinensis*. It is a common parasite of sheep, producing marked liver damage. Worldwide in distribution in sheep, it is prevalent in low wet pastures where suitable species of snails are indigenous. The metacercariae encyst on plants, and man is infected mainly as a result of eating wild watercress and other plants gathered in these pastures. Human infections are more common where such salad is favored, e.g., Europe, Cuba, and Chile. In England outbreaks are associated with particularly wet summers.

The adult fluke is large, 2 to 3 cm in length by 0.8 to 1.3 cm in breadth, and may occlude the *common bile duct*. Indeed, many human infections have been first recognized at surgery for biliary obstruction. Again an invasive stage of fever, eosinophilia, and hepatomegaly is associated with larval flukes moving through the liver substance to gain the biliary tract, for the larval flukes produced from the metacercariae in the jejunum pass across the peritoneal cavity to pierce Glisson's capsule and move through the liver substance. Far fewer flukes than *Clonorchis* are found in man, but again hyperplasia, necrosis, and cystic dilation of the biliary tract, accompanied by leukocytic infiltration and eventually periportal fibrosis, can ensue if the load of flukes is heavy enough. The differential diagnosis is similar to that of clonorchiasis.

The *diagnosis* depends on finding large yellowish operculate eggs 130 to 150 μ in length in the feces or aspirated bile. Liver should be excluded from the patient's diet in areas where raw liver is eaten, because eggs in such livers will pass through the intestinal tract unchanged. A complement-fixation test using an extract of the adult fluke as antigen is a useful diagnostic aid, especially in infections in which the flukes are ectopic. A hemagglutination test has also been developed.

Unlike the other hepatic hermaphroditic flukes. *Fasciola hepatica* and the closely allied *Fasciola gigantica* are occasionally found in sites other than the liver. This could be related to man's being a relatively poor host species. Thus a migrating subcutaneous swelling associated with intense eosinophilia may contain such an immature fluke, and there are records of occurrences in many sites, including the brain.

A further oddity associated with *Fasciola hepatica* infection is the parasitization of the pharynx by young post-metacercarial flukes which are acquired by eating raw liver in which the young flukes are actively migrating. This occurs in Lebanon, where such raw sheep and goat livers are eaten; the patient complains of intense inflammation of the back of the throat. This syndrome of parasitic pharyngitis, known as halzoun, can also be produced by a leech or a pentosomid (a worm-like arthropod).

Bithionol,* a drug used for *Paragonimus,* has replaced emetine and chloroquine for initial therapy. It is given in an oral dose of 30 to 50 mg per kilogram on alternate days for 10 to 15 doses.

Ectopic flukes are removed surgically.

Clonorchiasis

Hou, P. C.: The relationship between primary carcinoma of the liver and infestation with *Clonorchis sinensis.* J. Pathol., 72:239, 1956.
Komiya, L.: Clonorchis and clonorchiasis. *In* Dawes, B. (ed.): Advances in Parasitology. London, Academic Press, 1966, Vol. 4, pp. 53–106.
Viranuvatti, V., and Stitnimankarn, T.: Liver fluke infection and infestation in South East Asia. *In* Popper, H., and Schaffner, F. (eds.): Progress in Liver Disease, Vol. 4. New York, Grune & Stratton, 1972, pp. 537–547.
Weng, H. C., Chung, H. L., Ho, L. Y., and Hou, T. C.: Studies in *Clonorchis sinensis* in the past 10 years. Chin. Med. J. (Peking), 80:441, 1960.

Opisthorchiasis

Harinasuta, C.: Opisthorchiasis in Thailand: A review. *In* Harinasuta, C. (ed.): Proceedings of the Fourth Southeast Asian Seminar on Parasitology and Tropical Medicine: Schistosomiasis and Other Snail-Transmitted Helminthiases. Manila, 1969, pp. 177–199.

Fascioliasis

Hardman, E. W., Jones, R. L. H., and Davies, A. H.: Fascioliasis — a large outbreak. Br. Med. J., 3:502, 1970.
Khalil, G. M., and Schacher, J. F.: *Linguatula serrata* in relation to halzoun and the Marrara syndrome. Am. J. Trop. Med., 14:736, 1965.
Neghume, A., and Ossandan, M.: Ectopic and hepatic fascioliasis. Am. J. Trop. Med., 23:545, 1943.
Pantelouris, E. M.: The Common Liver Fluke. Oxford, Pergamon Press, 1964.

211.3. LUNG HERMAPHRODITIC FLUKES

(Paragonimiasis)

Although *Paragonimus westermani* is the most common species of this group infecting man, recently a number of other human pathogens have been recognized in the genus *Paragonimus,* which to date numbers more than 31 species. These include *P. africanus* found in Nigeria, the Cameroons, and the Congo, and two new Chinese flukes, *P. skrjabini* and *P. heterotremus. P. westermani* is widely distributed in the Far East, occur-

*Available from Center for Disease Control (404-633-3311, Ext. 3670).

ring as an important human infection in China, Japan, Vietnam, Korea, Formosa, the Philippines, and Thailand. Species also occur in South America in Peru, Colombia, Ecuador, and Venezuela.

Paragonimiasis is a chronic lung infection of man caused by this group of flukes, the adults living in cystic spaces in the lung. Reddish-brown plump oval flukes, they resemble in size a coffee bean (0.8 to 1.6 cm long by 0.4 to 0.8 cm wide). They are covered with little spines and live singly or in pairs in the lung parenchyma, feeding on host exudates. They live five to six years usually. Oval yellowish-brown operculated ova (85 μ by 35 μ) are coughed up in thick, blood-stained sputum. These hatch to produce a miracidium which invades specific snails. The cercariae subsequently produced by these snails encyst as metacercariae in the muscles and viscera of freshwater crabs. Man acquires the infection by eating the crabs raw or partly cooked. The larval flukes released from the metacercariae usually migrate to the lung via the peritoneal cavity, penetrating the diaphragm, but may mature in the abdomen or brain.

For many species man is not the definitive host, felines being preferred. For instance, other hosts apart from man for *P. westermani* are cats, tigers, leopards, mink, badgers, dogs, lions, and rats. *P. westermani* was discovered by Westerman in 1877 in a tiger in the Amsterdam zoo.

PATHOGENESIS AND PATHOLOGY. The larval fluke tunnels into the lung at the periphery. There is an inflammatory reaction around it with many eosinophils. Later it forms a cystic space with a fibrous tissue wall. These cysts usually communicate with a bronchus and often become secondarily infected with abscess formation. Death of the fluke is often followed by calcification. Ova may be reaspirated, with an eosinophilic inflammatory response and the formation of small lung granulomas.

Although the target organ for *Paragonimus* is the lung, it must be realized that often adults go astray, and if the invading species is one less adapted to man, this is more liable to happen. Thus a characteristic feature of *P. skrjabini* infection is migrating subcutaneous nodules that contain active flukes. Such granulomas in the subcutaneous tissue may require excision as in fascioliasis.

In the brain the temporal and occipital lobes are occasionally the site of an eosinophilic granuloma containing flukes and, in a few cases, ova. A transverse myelitis is known. Flukes in the peritoneal cavity produce adhesions and abscesses, and ulceration of the intestine occurs with ova in the stool. Adult and mature flukes have been found in many other organs, including intestine, spermatic cord, testis and scrotum, vagina, and muscles.

CLINICAL MANIFESTATIONS. Lung infections are encountered with symptoms of persistent hemoptysis, breathlessness on exertion, pleural pain, and recurrent pulmonary infections. The condition is known as endemic hemoptysis. Clubbing of the fingers is common, and persistent rales may be heard over the affected lung segments as in nonparasitic bronchiectasis. A lung abscess may be present. Pneumothorax, pleural effusion, and empyema are rarer complications. Chest films early in the disease show infiltrations, but later dense nodular opacities or ring shadows indicate the site of the cysts. Pleural adhesions and calcification are late signs. Coexistent pulmonary tuberculosis occurs in some patients. There are rarely more than 20 parasites in the lungs.

It has been estimated that there were 5000 cases of cerebral paragonimiasis in South Korea in January 1968. Cerebral paragonimiasis may present signs of a space-occupying lesion with epilepsy and paresis of varying degrees. Ophthalmic signs are optic atrophy associated with papilledema or direct involvement with the inflammatory process. The cerebrospinal fluid shows a raised protein, and eosinophils are present. There may be calcifications present on skull roentgenograms; pneumoencephalography may show the site of a pseudotumor. Abdominal paragonimiasis is a difficult condition to diagnose, but an abdominal mass in a patient with lung disease should raise this suspicion.

DIAGNOSIS. This rests mainly on finding ova in the sputum. One third of patients also have ova in the stools because of swallowed sputum or a coincidental intestinal lesion. Complement-fixation tests are useful, and positive results correlate closely with an active infection. Yokogawa has treated patients on this basis alone. The intradermal test remains positive for a long while after active infection and is not a reliable guide. Work goes on defining the antigenic structure of the parasite. The extent to which the *Paragonimus* antigen cross-reacts with other flukes is not clear.

Pulmonary paragonimiasis may resemble bronchiectasis, lung abscess, bronchial carcinoma, or — most important of all — pulmonary tuberculosis. Cerebral paragonimiasis mimics other space-occupying lesions but especially other helminths in the brain. These include *Fasciola, Schistosoma japonicum, Angiostrongylus cantonensis,* and hydatid.

PROGNOSIS. Fatalities are rare, and lung lesions resolve spontaneously in five to ten years. Cerebral involvement may be associated with persistent epilepsy. Two per cent of the cases of lung paragonimiasis are complicated by pulmonary tuberculosis.

TREATMENT. Bithionol* (Actamer, Biton) is 2,2'-thiobis(4,6-dichlorophenol) and is given orally in a dose of 30 to 50 mg per kilogram of body weight on alternate days for 10 to 15 doses. Skin reactions and gastrointestinal irritation are rarely severe enough to interrupt treatment. Results are far superior to those obtained with chloroquine or emetine drugs used in the past. Granulomas containing *Paragonimus* adults and ova may require surgical removal from the skin, testis, abdominal organs, or brain.

PREVENTION. It might be thought that it would be a simple matter to dissuade people from eating raw, fresh salted, pickled, or imperfectly cooked crabs and crayfish, but such local delicacies are not easily relinquished. Drunken crab, a favorite dish, involves immersing live crabs in alcohol prior to consumption. In Korea and West Africa, fresh crab juice is used as a home remedy in the treatment of measles.

Chang, H. T., Wang, C. W., Yü, C. F., Hsü, C. F., and Fang, J. C.: Paragonimiasis, a clinical study of 200 adult cases. Chin. Med. J., 77:3, 1958.

Grados, O. B., Cuba, C. C., Morales, F. N., and Mazabel, T. C.: Epidemiologia de la paragonimiasis en el Peru. Arch. Peruanos Pat. Clin., 26:33, 1972.

Miyazaki, I.: Lung Flukes in the Western Hemisphere. Tokyo, Overseas Technical Cooperation Agency, 1972.

Nwokolo, C.: Endemic paragonimiasis in Eastern Nigeria. Clinical fea-

tures and epidemiology of the recent outbreak following the Nigerian Civil War. Trop. Geogr. Med., 24:138, 1972.

Yokogawa, M.: Paragonimus and paragonimiasis. In Dawes, B. (ed.): Advances in Parasitology. London, Academic Press, 1969, Vol. 7, pp. 375–387.

Yokogawa, S., Cort, W. W., and Yokogawa, M.: Paragonimus and paragonimiasis. Exp. Parasitol., 10:81, 139, 1960.

Yokogawa, M., Okawa, T., Tsuji, M., Iwasaki, M., and Shigeyasu, M.: Chemotherapy of paragonimiasis with bithionol. III. The follow-up studies for 1 year after treatment with bithionol. Jap. J. Parasit., 11:103, 1962.

211.4. INTESTINAL HERMAPHRODITIC FLUKES

FASCIOLOPSIASIS
(Fasciolopsis Buski)

Fasciolopsis buski is a large fleshy fluke, 3 cm long and 1.2 cm wide. It is found mainly in China but also in India, Indonesia, Thailand, Malaya, and Taiwan, normally as an intestinal parasite of pigs. The eggs are passed in the feces, and miracidia are released to penetrate a snail. The cercariae subsequently produced encyst as metacercariae on edible water plants called water caltrop or water chestnuts. The tubers and fruits of these plants are eaten fresh and raw from July to September and as they are peeled with the teeth, people are easily infected. The ponds are often fertilized with night soil or contaminated by pigs.

Most infections are asymptomatic, but foci of inflammation may occur at the site of attachment of the worms in the small intestine. In heavy infections abdominal pain may simulate a peptic ulcer, and there may be alternating diarrhea and constipation. A recent investigation does not suggest that malabsorption occurs. Intestinal stasis, ulceration, and even obstruction have occurred. Several thousand worms may be harbored by the patient, and in severe cases, especially in children, edema of the face and trunk has been described. The mechanism of this edema may be complex, as anemia and hypoproteinemia from blood loss in the bowel are possible. Definite allergic edemas do not appear to be reported in the literature, but there is a variable eosinophilia with heavy loads. Ascites and death from exhaustion are rare.

DIAGNOSIS. Diagnosis depends on finding the characteristic eggs in the stool. These are large, 130 to 140 μ by 80 to 85 μ, yellowish, and rather similar to *Fasciola* but with a smaller operculum. Occasionally an adult fluke may be vomited or passed in the stool. Facial edema may raise the question of differentiating fasciolopsiasis from trichinosis or the nephrotic syndrome.

THERAPY. The old cheap anthelmintics are effective, such as tetrachloroethylene* in a dose of 0.1 ml per kilogram body weight or hexylresorcinol in an adult dose of 1 gram. Since these are difficult to obtain now, piperazine (see Ch. 213.8) or bephenium hydroxynaphthoate (5-gram oral dose for adults) can be used. Not all flukes may be eradicated, but the therapy can be repeated after a few days. Prevention entails cooking the offending plants, eradicating snails with molluscicides, and preventing fecal contamination of ponds.

---

*Available from Center for Disease Control (404-633-3311, Ext. 3670).

*Not available in the United States except as a veterinarian product, Nema worm caps.

OTHER INTESTINAL HERMAPHRODITIC FLUKES

Two very small intestinal flukes—*Heterophyes heterophyes* and *Metagonimus yokogawai*—deserve mention. The former is found in Egypt, Tunisia, South China, India, and the Philippines, and the latter occurs in the Far East and Indonesia. Both are acquired by eating raw or inadequately cooked fish that contain the respective metacercariae. The adult flukes, 2 to 3 mm long, are attached to the mucosa of the small intestine and are alleged to produce superficial inflammation and ulceration. Usually they are not present in sufficient numbers to produce symptoms. Very rarely eggs may gain access to the circulation and be found in internal organs. Usually they are passed in the stool and closely resemble *Clonorchis* eggs, which is perhaps their main importance. Both species can be treated with tetrachloroethylene as used for hookworm. Many species of the genus *Echinostoma* can also infect man in the Far East, but again rarely produce symptoms. Their eggs resemble those of *Fasciola* but are smaller. *Gastrodiscoides hominis* is a fascinating fluke with a large ventral sucker. Like the others, it can produce diarrhea. It occurs in Assam, Indochina, India, and Malaysia. In Canada the eggs of *Metorchis conjunctus* are occasionally found in the stools of man.

Barlow, C. H.: The life cycle of the human intestinal fluke *Fasciolopsis buski* (Lankester). Amer. J. Hyg., Monograph 4, 1925.

Cross, J. H.: Fasciolopsiasis in South East Asia and the Far East: A review. *In* Harinasuta, C. (ed.): Proceedings of the Fourth Southeast Asian Seminar on Parasitology and Tropical Medicine: Schistosomiasis and Other Snail-Transmitted Helminthiases. Manila, 1969, pp. 177–199.

Plaut, A. G., Kampanort-Sanyakorn, C., and Manning, G. S.: A clinical study of *Fasciolopsis buski* in Thailand. Trans. Roy. Soc. Trop. Med. Hyg., 63:470, 1969.

THE NEMATODES
(Roundworms)
Philip D. Marsden

212. INTRODUCTION

Roundworms have an intestinal tract and a large body cavity bordered by a complex cuticle and containing the reproductive, nervous, and excretory systems. They have elongated, cylindrical, bilaterally symmetrical, smooth, nonsegmented, translucent, flesh-colored bodies, often filiform, with a pointed posterior and rounded anterior end. The Nematoda constitute the second largest class in the Animal Kingdom, with 500,000 species. Many are free living. They are unisexual, and the female is usually bigger than the male. There is a great variation in size among the common species infecting man. For example, in the intestinal nematodes a female *Ascaris* may reach 18 cm whereas a female *Strongyloides* is smaller than 1 mm. Their bodies are muscular and require high carbohydrate reserves.

The common nematodes infecting man can be roughly divided into the *intestinal nematodes,* of which the common ones in order of importance are hookworms, *Ascaris, Strongyloides, Trichuris,* and *Oxyuris,* and the *tissue nematodes.* The latter group includes *Trichinella* and the various filarial worms. Heyneman has suggested that the life cycles of the intestinal nematodes of man can be shown to demonstrate an increasing dependence upon the host and a decrease in the proportion of metabolically active time in the free-living stages if they are arranged in a certain sequence. This sequence reflects different degrees of adaption by the parasite to the host and is presented in Table 1.

Rhabditis, a free-living nematode which rarely infects man, is but one step away from the relatively common *Strongyloides stercoralis. Strongyloides* represents the first stage in parasitic adaption. Hookworms are obligate parasites with no free-living stage. Both these nematodes and *Ascaris* have a phase of lung migration by immature larvae in the host, the explanation of which is not known. *Ascaris, Trichuris,* and *Enterobius* have progressively shorter oval maturation times. *Trichinella spiralis* is viviparous; the intestinal phase is transient, and the larvae persist in the host muscle.

Although the adult *Trichinella* organisms are intestinal nematodes, from a clinical viewpoint trichinosis can be considered as a tissue parasite infection, as it is the larvae that produce the disease syndrome. The final break from the free-living state is illustrated by the filariae, in which the adult worms live in the host tissue, specific arthropods serving as the intermediate hosts. Whether filariae evolved from insect parasites or arose by adaption of intestinal parasites to insects after ingestion of eggs by coprophagic insects is a matter for speculation.

As in schistosomiasis, the number of worms present in the host determines the clinical manifestations, and many mild infections are asymptomatic. Quantitative techniques to determine adult worm load are commonly used in some nematode infections. Among the intestinal nematodes, *Strongyloides* and *Oxyuris* infections

TABLE 1.   Sequence for Common Human Intestinal Nematodes (Heyneman)

Species	Details of Life Cycle
Strongyloides stercoralis	Most primitive since parasitism is irregular and exists in free-living adult stage in soil
Necator americanus *Ancylostoma duodenale*	Regular parasitism; no free-living adults, only larvae in soil
Ascaris lumbricoides	All hatched larval stages as well as adults in host; only eggs in soil
Trichuris trichiura	Similar to *Ascaris*, but newly hatched larvae do not migrate through host's body; all development confined to the intestine
Enterobius vermicularis	Eggs infective shortly after being laid; soil phase for eggs rarely involved
Trichinella spiralis	No eggs laid; larvae hatch within female, are deposited in mucosa, which they penetrate, and migrate via blood stream to encyst in tissues

cannot be quantitated owing to the variability in excretion of progeny. *Ascaris* produces so many eggs that quantitative techniques are usually not worthwhile, but hookworms and *Trichuris* eggs can be quantitated by a stool-dilution technique. For example, in Stoll's method 3 grams of stool is emulsified in 42 ml of water in a special flask. Tenth normal sodium hydroxide may be used to soften hard feces. Glass beads and shaking after standing produces a uniform fine emulsion; 0.15 ml volume of this is pipetted onto a glass slide, and all the eggs counted in this volume are equivalent to 0.01 gram of feces. Knowing the number of eggs per gram of stool, the total volume of stool, the egg output per female worm, and the usual sex ratio of the species population, it is possible to calculate the approximate worm load. The Kato technique has gained popularity as a quick quantitative method. All the eggs are counted in 50 mg of stool cleared under a glycerin-soaked cellophane cover slip. Tissue helminths can also be quantitated in terms of larval output by expressing results in *Trichinella spiralis* infections as the number of larvae per gram of skeletal muscle or the number of microfilariae per milliliter of blood at a certain time of day. *Onchocerca* infections are likewise expressed as number of microfilariae per milligram of skin.

Multiple infections with intestinal nematodes often occur, especially in the tropics (for example, *Ascaris,* hookworm, and *Trichuris* in conjunction). Broad-spectrum anthelmintics have been developed to facilitate single dose oral treatment. Notable among these are the benzimidazoles, of which thiabendazole was the first broad-spectrum drug; the latest, mebendazole, shows great promise, although it is expensive.

Another important feature of nematode infections is the frequency with which infections with nonhuman parasites are encountered as abortive infections, with larvae only rarely maturing to adults, thus suggesting helminths in a process of adaption into man. A number of such parasites will be mentioned in the text that follows, including the genera *Oesophagostomum, Toxocara, Anasakis, Angiostrongylus, Dirofilaria,* and others of clinical importance.

Heyneman's sequence is followed in the present discussion of the nematodes, although it is important to point out that, in terms of human suffering, hookworm and Bancroftian filariasis are by far the most serious infections.

Beaver, P. C.: The nature of visceral larva migrans. J. Parasitol., 55:3, 1969.

Davis, A.: Drug Treatment of Intestinal Helminthiases. Geneva, World Health Organization, 1973.

Heyneman, D.: The life cycle of the nematodes parasitic in man: An evolutionary sequence. Med. J. Malaya, 20:249, 1966.

Knight, R., Schultz, M. G., Hoskins, D. W., and Marsden, P. D.: Intestinal parasites, a progress report. Gut, 14:145, 1973.

Stevens, D. P.: Quantitative techniques. Clin. Gastroenterol., 7:231, 1978.

213. INTESTINAL NEMATODES

213.1. STRONGYLOIDIASIS
(Cochin-China Diarrhea)

DEFINITION. Strongyloidiasis is an infection of the small intestine with the invasive small nematode *Strongyloides stercoralis.* Most infections are asymptomatic, but a few can be life threatening; because of this, treatment is always necessary.

ETIOLOGY AND TRANSMISSION. The parasitic female worm is small (2.2 mm long) and lives in the mucosa of the intestinal villi. The parasitic male has rarely been observed, and experimental work suggests that parthenogenesis is the rule. The eggs produced by the female hatch rapidly, producing larvae in the small intestine, and these may reinvade the bowel mucosa before being voided in the feces (internal autoinfection). On the other hand, they may invade immediately after voiding via the perianal skin (external autoinfection). Other larvae become infective within hours of contact with the soil, and invasion of a fresh host occurs via the skin. Alternatively, voided larvae may develop into *free-living adults in the soil.* These adults produce further generations of infective larvae in the soil. These alternative cycles make the life history of *Strongyloides* the most difficult one to grasp.

After skin penetration, the infective larvae undergo the same curious migration as hookworms via the venous system to the lungs (in 24 to 48 hours). Autoinfective forms may take a peritoneal or lymphatic route to the same site. From the lungs the developing larvae ascend the trachea, drop down into the stomach, and mature in the small intestine. Because of the frequency of autoinfection this nematode is self-perpetuating, and infections can last for 30 to 40 years. Man is the only common host, although primates and dogs can be experimentally infected.

DISTRIBUTION. The parasite is cosmopolitan, but it is more frequent in the tropics. Local habitats where warmth, moisture, and lack of sanitation favor the free-living existence are endemic sites. Curiously enough, in nearly all populations, however, the infection seems to be sporadic and an incidence comparable with that seen in hookworm infection is not encountered. This infection, like all intestinal parasitic infections, has been reported in high incidence from some mental institutions. Resistance to reinfection has been suggested by animal studies.

PATHOLOGY AND PATHOGENESIS. The adult female worms burrow through the intestinal submucosa above the muscularis mucosae, depositing eggs as they go. They cause a chronic inflammatory cell infiltrate with many eosinophils. The rapidly hatching larvae are responsible for most of the pathologic findings, and their powers of penetration are such they can be distributed widely throughout the body. For reasons not clearly understood, the whole process may be accelerated (the so-called hyperinfective syndrome). Debility on the part of the host, malnutrition, or corticoid administration favors the development of this syndrome. Obviously prolonged bowel transit time would increase the possibility of internal autoinfection. Inflammation of the small bowel may be so intense as to cause malabsorption, thickening, and edema visible roentgenographically. The mesenteric lymph nodes enlarge, and ulceration and necrosis of the mucosa may occur. The lungs and liver may also show abscess formation, and fatty changes in the liver may indicate primary or secondary malnutrition. In recent years several series of fatal cases have been described from the West Indies, Brazil, and Africa. Acute small bowel obstruction has been described, as well as *E. coli* bacteremia with meningitis, the latter perhaps arising from bacteria being introduced from the bowel on migrating larvae. The gut may be invaded at any level by larvae, and gastric and colonic involvement are well documented. Rarely larvae are found in other abdominal organs. Involvement of the kidney, heart, and endocrine glands is described.

CLINICAL MANIFESTATIONS. Dermal invasion, either as a result of primary exposure or by external autoinfection, may be characterized by linear, erythematous, urticarial wheals, which are the sites of migrating larvae. Particularly common around the buttocks, they may occur anywhere, and are often recognized for what they are, as they are relatively fast moving. It is a form of cutaneous larva migrans (see Ch. 213.4). Lung invasion may be associated with signs of bronchospasm or pneumonia. These may be short-lived or recurrent if several waves of larvae arrive in the lung. Hemoptysis is not uncommon as the larvae burst through the pulmonary alveoli. They may be found in the sputum, and there is usually a marked eosinophilia. Bowel involvement may give rise to a variety of clinical manifestations, but again it must be stressed that many light infections are asymptomatic. The most common gastrointestinal symptom is epigastric pain, which is often to the right of the midline, constant, and of a dull, aching character, mimicking peptic ulcer. Tenderness may be present on abdominal palpation over the duodenum. In heavy infections diarrhea is common; it may not be just the result of inflammation but may also reflect the coexistent malabsorption. Upper abdominal pain and vomiting from the involved upper gut are frequent, but intestinal obstruction is rare. Marked large bowel involvement may resemble ulcerative colitis. In the hyperinfective syndrome an eosinophilia is often present and death may result from disseminated inflammatory lesions, often with superimposed bacterial infection.

DIAGNOSIS. Strongyloidiasis must always be thought of in patients with unexplained eosinophilia. The high eosinophilia is probably associated with recurrent larval invasion. The diagnosis is made by finding the larvae in the stool, preferably by using a concentration technique. Unfortunately there are a number of difficulties. In warm climates fresh stool should be examined, as hookworm larvae hatch quickly from the eggs; they can be differentiated, but only by an expert. The excretion of larvae in strongyloidiasis is intermittent, and multiple stool specimens should be examined. The Baermann funnel technique, filter paper culture technique, and Beal's string test have facilitated diagnosis. Sometimes larvae are demonstrated in the duodenal aspirate or sputum when other techniques have failed. Jejunal biopsy may show larvae and adult parasites in section in the mucosa. The filarial complement-fixation test is often positive and of diagnositc help in difficult cases. Barium studies may show thickening and deformities of the small bowel owing to inflammatory edema.

TREATMENT. As so little is known about the conditions governing development of serious infections, all patients should be treated with thiabendazole, 25 mg per kilogram twice daily for three days. The tablets should be chewed; they have an orange taste. Common side effects are nausea, vomiting, and vertigo. It is said not to kill larvae or eggs, so treatment may have to be repeated. Rarely cases are resistant to repeated thiabendazole therapy. Recently cambendazole, a related compound, has been used with success. Assessment of parasitologic cure requires repeated stool examinations using special techniques. The eosinophilia should fall within eight weeks. The prognosis is good in otherwise healthy subjects, but may be poor in the exceptional circumstances described above. Prophylaxis involves avoiding unsanitary conditions when infection is likely. Strongyloides of nutria and raccoons have caused transient creeping eruptions (cutaneous larva migrans) in Louisiana trappers. The position of *Strongyloides fulleburni* as a human pathogen is unclear at this time.

Bras, G., Richards, R. C., Irvine, R. A., Milner, P. F. A., and Ragbeer, M. M. S.: Infection with *Strongyloides stercoralis* in Jamaica. Lancet, 2:1257, 1964.

Carvalho Filho, E.: Strongyloidiasis. Clin. Gastroenterol., 7:179, 1978.

Rodrigues, L. D., Martirani, J., Cabeca, M., Soares, W., and Brandao, J. A.: Cambendazol: Nova antihelmitico na terapeutica da estrongiloidiase. Rev. Inst. Med. Trop. São Paulo, 19:57, 1977.

Stemmerman, G. N.: Strongyloidiasis in migrants. Pathological and clinical considerations. Gastroenterology, 53:59, 1967.

Tanaka, H.: Experimental and epidemiological strongyloidiasis of Amaini Oshima Island. Jap. J. Exp. Med., 28:159, 1958.

213.2. CAPILLARIASIS

Until recently the genus *Capillaria* appeared to infect man so rarely that it would not have merited inclusion in a general work of this kind. The most common form, *Capillaria hepatica* (less than 20 cases reported), was recognized by finding *Trichuris*-like eggs encapsulated in the liver. Species of the genus had also been reported in the lungs and skin of man.

Recently, however, a new parasite of man *Capillaria philippinensis*, has been described from the northern Philippines, where more than 1000 cases and 100 deaths have been confirmed. Patients with intestinal capillariasis have colicky abdominal pain, chronic diarrhea, muscle wasting, and edema, which may lead to debility and death in four months. Clinical studies have shown the presence of a severe protein-losing enteropathy in these patients with malabsorption of fats and sugars.

A tiny nematode (3 to 4 mm by 0.03 to 0.04 mm), *C. philippinensis* is confined to the small intestine, particularly the jejunum. The eggs detected in the stool are similar to *Trichuris trichiura* (to which the *Capillaria* are closely related) but are smaller, are more oval, and have less prominent bipolar plugs. There is evidence that hatching may occur in the small intestine, and tissue invasion of the bowel similar to strongyloidiasis has been noted at postmortem examination. The mode of transmission of the disease is not fully worked out, but three species of fish have been found to contain infective larvae. It is still uncertain whether interhuman transmission occurs.

Intravenous feeding is necessary in severe cases. Mebendazole is the treatment of choice in an oral dose of 100 to 400 mg per day for 10 to 30 days.

Cross, J. H., Banzon, T., Clarke, M. D., Basaca Servilla, V., Watten, R. H., and Dizon, J. J.: Studies on the experimental transmission of *Capillaria philippinensis* in monkeys. Trans. R. Soc. Trop. Med. Hyg., 66:819, 1972.

Singson, C. N., Banzon, T. C., and Cross, J. H.: Mebendazole in the treatment of intestinal capillariasis. Am. J. Trop. Med. Hyg., 24:932, 1975.

Watten, R. H., Beckner, W. M., Cross, J. H., Gunning, J. J., and Jarmillo, J.: Clinical studies of *Capillaria philippinensis*. Trans. Roy. Soc. Trop. Med. Hyg., 66:828, 1972.

213.3.   HOOKWORM DISEASE
(Ancylostomiasis, Miner's Anemia)

DEFINITION.   The two common hookworms of man, *Ancylostoma duodenale* and *Necator americanus,* attach themselves to the small bowel by their buccal capsules and suck blood, thereby causing chronic blood loss. Depending on their number and the iron stores of the host, a variable degree of anemia often results. A distinction is made between hookworm infection when the load is too light to produce symptoms and hookworm disease.

PATHOGENIC CHAIN. Etiology.   The human hookworms measure about 1 cm in length, the female being slightly longer than the male, which is recognizable by an expanded posterior end, the copulating bursa. *A. duodenale* is larger than *Necator americanus,* and the two species are differentiated most easily by the fact that *A. duodenale* has two pairs of teeth in its buccal capsule, whereas *N. americanus* has a pair of cutting plates only. The eggs of the two species are indistinguishable and are passed in the feces. In warm moist soil the larva hatches within 48 hours. The rhabditiform larva has a free-living cycle in the soil, feeding on bacteria, during which time it molts twice. The filariform larvae resulting from the second molt are the infected stage for man and can survive several months in favorable conditions. They tend to migrate up grass stems or gain any elevation up to 3 feet, and on coming into contact with the skin of man, quickly penetrate it, enter the bloodstream, and are transported to the lungs. Like *Strongyloides,* there they leave the vascular system and emerge into the alveoli, migrate up the bronchi and trachea, and down the esophagus to reach the small intestine where maturity is attained. In contrast to *N. americanus,* with *Ancylostoma duodenale* a duodenal infection is easily acquired in the mucosa of the upper intestinal tract, and the migrating larvae in the body tissues can remain dormant for nine months before completing development. Usually eggs appear in the stool five or more weeks after invasion, and the adults live one to nine years. A dog hookworm, *Ancylostoma ceylonicum,* has been described as an occasional human pathogen in the Orient.

Epidemiology.   Over 400 million people have hookworm infections, but in the majority the worm load is small. *Ancylostoma duodenale* is the Old World hookworm, being prevalent in Europe, North Africa, and the Middle and Far East. *Necator americanus* is found more in the New World and tropical Africa. During the past 30 years both parasites have become widely distributed, and rigid geographic demarcations are not possible.

The survival of larvae is favored by a damp sandy soil, high in humus content at a temperature of 24 to 32° C. Promiscuous defecation and the absence of shoes are the chief factors responsible for infections. Such conditions occur in mines as well as on the surface of the ground. Urban people tend to have less hookworm than agricultural rural workers at locations where night soil is often used as fertilizer. Infection can be acquired by ingesting or handling contaminated vegetables. Coffee, banana, sugar cane, rice, and sweet potato fields are ideal for the growth and development of larvae. Often one locality is used as a communal latrine in the area, and people reinfect themselves by visiting these sites again and again. *The distinction between hookworm infection and hookworm disease is important.* Methods of estimating the intensity of the infection show that in endemic areas most patients have few worms and no significant anemia. Those who have hookworm anemia have more worms, and these heavy infections could be the result of repeated exposure or a failure of immunity on the part of the host. With canine hookworm, small repeated infections give almost complete immunity. Antibodies have been demonstrated in sera of infected patients, but this degree of immunity to reinfection seen in the dog does not seem to occur.

Pathology and Pathogenesis.   Inflammatory cell infiltration is seen at the site of penetration of the hookworm larvae, and in the lungs small hemorrhages occur with eosinophilic and leukocytic infiltration. An eosinophilia is present during the invasive phase. The main feature of the established disease is the active sucking of blood by the worms. They create a negative pressure in the buccal capsule and suck in a piece of mucosa which acts as both an anchorage and a source of blood. It is still not clear what hookworms abstract from the blood. Vital preparations in vitro show red cells being vigorously expelled from the posterior end. *Ancylostoma* sucks between 0.16 and 0.34 ml of blood per day and *Necator,* 0.03 to 0.05. The development of anemia depends upon three factors: the iron content of the diet, the state of the iron reserves, and the intensity and duration of infection.

When iron intake is high, a heavy worm load is needed to produce a significant anemia. Up to 60 per cent of the iron from the hemoglobin extracted by the hookworm is reabsorbed in the intestine. At open operation small punctate hemorrhagic spots are encountered at the site of attachment. In addition to anemia, hypoalbuminemia occurs owing to a combination of blood loss and a low rate of albumin synthesis, possibly associated with anoxia affecting liver cell function. Malabsorption is said to occur in a few cases with partial villous atrophy and chronic inflammatory cell infiltration of the lamina propria.

CLINICAL MANIFESTATIONS.   The site of skin penetration by the larvae is associated with pruritus and the development of an erythematous papular eruption (ground itch) which may last several days or even longer, depending on the host's immune response. Within a week after penetration the patient may have a transient asthmatic attack, but this is not as commonly seen as in invasive ascariasis.

Established hookworm disease is associated with general symptoms of anemia, weakness, fatigue, dyspnea, palpitation, and mental and physical retardation. Pica may be noted. On examination the skin and mucus membrane are pale. Peripheral edema is due possibly to a variety of factors, namely, hypoalbuminemia, a rise of capillary venous pressure, and tissue anoxia. In severe cases there is evidence of congestive cardiac failure. The pulse is rapid with a high pulse pressure. On auscultation of the enlarged heart, a third heart sound and an ejection type of systolic murmur are commonly heard; regurgitant systolic and even diastolic murmurs may occur and disappear when the anemia is corrected. For this reason it is very unwise to diagnose a valvular lesion clinically in such anemic patients until that anemia has been corrected. The hemoglobin may be very low (2 grams per 100 ml) and the patient still ambulant.

The patient may complain of upper abdominal pain, and radiologic changes suggestive of a duodenitis have been reported.

DIAGNOSIS AND DIFFERENTIAL DIAGNOSIS. Stool microscopy, either by a direct smear or by a concentration technique, reveals hookworm ova. Quantitation of the egg excretion enables the physician to decide whether the patient has a significant worm load. This is done by diluting a known volume of stool and counting a sample (Stoll technique) or by using a Kato thick smear, which must be read promptly or else the eggs will clear beyond recognition. Hookworm ova are 60 to 70 μ long by 35 to 40 μ wide and have a characteristic morphology with a clear shell and developing embryo inside. They must be distinguished, however, from both *Trichostrongylus* and *Ternidens deminutus,* both of which have larger eggs. Test tube cultivation of ova and differentiation of the resultant larvae are of value in doubtful cases. A skin test using an extract of *Necator americanus* larvae of standard nitrogen content has proved useful in screening a hookworm-infected population. Fluorescent antibody, complement-fixation, and hemagglutination tests have been developed but have little clinical application.

The anemia of hookworm disease is a classic iron deficiency anemia with a low hemoglobin, mean corpuscular hemoglobin concentration and serum iron, and a high iron-binding capacity. On the film the red cells are microcytic and hypochromic. Folic acid deficiency may sometimes be superimposed on macrocytosis. The serum albumin is low, and liver function tests may be abnormal. In the edematous patient there may be confusion with kwashiorkor, wet beriberi, or the nephrotic syndrome. The anemia has to be differentiated from other iron deficiency anemias.

TREATMENT. Tetrachloroethylene* and bephenium hydroxynaphthoate (see previous edition) are being replaced by newer less toxic drugs. Mebendazole in an oral dose of 100 mg twice a day for three days can be used for adults and children over two years of age. Pyrantel pamoate or embonate in a single oral dose of 11 mg per kilogram of body weight (maximum dose, 1 gram) is also accompanied by few side effects and is effective. These drugs also act on coexistent *Ascaris* infections. Both drugs will remove a large number of worms at the first dose, but to get rid of the last 5 to 10 per cent is often very difficult. In many areas total eradication may not be desirable or necessary.

The anemia responds well to ferrous sulfate, 200 or 300 mg three times daily. Occasionally the hemoglobin is so low, or there is an associated acute infection, that the patient presents in extremis owing to heart failure. Pregnancy may also precipitate acute heart failure. Intraperitoneal blood transfusion or exchange transfusions have been lifesaving. The prognosis is good in most cases. It is wise to delay treating the hookworm infection until the hemoglobin is above 50 per cent after oral iron. Without treatment of the worm infection, the anemia will relapse when iron therapy is discontinued. *Prevention* involves the sanitary disposal of human excreta and the prevention of soil pollution. The wearing of shoes cuts down the opportunities for infection.

*Available in the United States only as a veterinarian product, Nema worm caps.

Banwell, J. G., and Shad, G. A.: Hookworm. Clin. Gastroenterol., 7:129, 1978.
Gilles, H. M., Williams, E. J. W., and Ball, P. A. J.: Hookworm infection and anemia. Quart. J. Med., 33:1, 1964.
Roche, M., and Layrisse, M.: Nature and causes of hookworm anemia. Am. J. Trop. Med., 15:1031, 1966.
Stoll, N. R.: On endemic hookworm, where do we stand to-day? Exp. Parasitol., 12:241, 1962.
Stoll, N. R.: For hookworm diagnosis is finding one egg enough? Ann. N.Y. Acad. Sci., 98:712, 1962.

213.4. CUTANEOUS LARVA MIGRANS
(Creeping Eruption)

Cutaneous larva migrans is considered at this point because its most common cause is *Ancylostoma braziliense,* although it may be produced by a variety of other helminths. It is characterized by an erythematous, serpiginous, intracutaneous track or burrow, the anterior end of which is observed to migrate at the rate of 1 to 2 cm per day. There is often intense irritation, and secondary infection may result from scratching. This migration is due to the infective larva of *A. braziliense* (the cat and dog hookworm), which does not visceralize in man but wanders around in the skin. This migration may last for 2 to 50 weeks before the larva dies. Rarely some larvae reach the lungs, causing high eosinophilia and patchy pulmonary infiltration.

Patients are often infected by lying on beaches contaminated by dog or cat feces. The feet, legs, and hands are the most common sites, and the appearance of the lesion is usually diagnostic. It is virtually impossible to remove the larva from the skin.

Ancylostoma braziliense is found in the southern United States, Central America, the Caribbean, and tropical South America, as well as in tropical Africa and parts of the Far East, especially the Malay peninsula. There have been several reports of the worm maturing in the gut of man and eggs appearing in the feces, so there is not an absolute host specificity. Two other dog hookworms, *Uncinaria stenocephala* and *Ancylostoma caninum,* can produce similar lesions. Occasionally the ground itch of the two common human hookworms may persist and resemble creeping eruption in immune subjects.

The larva migrans track of *Strongyloides stercoralis* tends to be a short line, erythematous and rapidly moving (larva currens). Rodent *Strongyloides* may produce similar lesions but no mature worms. A form of myiasis with the horse botfly maggot (*Gasterophilus*) can produce a larger deeper migrating form of cutaneous larva migrans.

TREATMENT. Thiabendazole by mouth, 25 mg per kilogram per day for two days, is usually effective. If not, the dose can be doubled and repeated. Alternatively, the advancing end of the burrow can be treated with topical thiabendazole sprinkled on elastoplast or in a cream containing 15 per cent thiabendazole powder in a hydrosoluble base. This drug has completely superseded the other, more unsatisfactory treatments such as ethyl chloride spray and Hetrazan.

Battistini, F.: Treatment of creeping eruption with topical thiabendazole. Tex. Rep. Biol. Med., 27 (Supplement 2):645, 1969.
Beaver, P. C.: Larva migrans. Exp. Parasitol., 5:587, 1956.
Stone, O. J.: Systemic and topical thiabendazole for creeping eruption. Tex. Rep. Biol. Med., 27 (Supplement 2):659, 1969.

213.5. TRICHOSTRONGYLIASIS

The adult worms of the genus *Trichostrongylus* are much smaller than hookworms, being under 100 mm long. They lie embedded in the mucosa of the duodenum and jejunum, where they suck a small quantity of blood. Eight species have been reported in man. Infections are most frequent in the Far East, especially in Japan, China, Korea, and Indonesia. High infection rates have been reported in Iran and south and western Asia. Worm loads in man are usually light and asymptomatic. Infection is acquired by ingesting salad contaminated with infective third-stage larvae. The importance of *Trichostrongylus* lies in the fact that the egg is frequently mistaken for hookworm. These "hookworm eggs" appear to persist after therapy and are termed drug resistant. Frequently, these so-called drug-resistant hookworms turn out to be *Trichostrongylus*. The eggs of *Trichostrongylus* are larger and more sharply pointed at one end and have more advanced embryonation than hookworm ova. They are from 73 to 94 μ in length and 40 to 50 μ in width. Larvae recovered from fecal culture of the ova can also be distinguished from hookworm. Treatment is seldom needed, but pyrantel pamoate or thiabendazole is effective in the majority of cases.

Ghadirian, E., and Arfaa, F): Present status of *Trichostrongylus* in Iran. Am. J. Trop. Med. Hyg., 24:935, 1975.

Marcial Rojas, R. A.: Trichostrongyliasis. *In* Marcial Rojas, R. A. (ed.): Pathology of Protozoal and Helminthic Disease with Clinical Correlation. Baltimore, Williams & Wilkins Company, 1971, p. 753.

Wolfe, M. S.: Oxyuris, trichostrongylus and trichuris. Clin. Gastroenterol., 7:201, 1978.

213.6. GNATHOSTOMIASIS

Although *Gnathostoma* species are more closely related to *Ascaris*, this group is mentioned at this point because it also presents as *creeping eruptions* or, more commonly, as *migratory swelling in the subcutaneous tissues*. More than 100 human infections with the immature stages of *Gnathostoma spinigerum* have been reported from the Far East, particularly Thailand. Normally a parasite of wild felines, dogs, and foxes, *Gnathostoma* infects man when he eats the larvae in undercooked fish (fermented fish is a Thai delicacy). The larva causes a migratory swelling, often in the subcutaneous tissues, associated with an intense eosinophilia. Occasionally the larva comes to the skin surface and resembles cutaneous larva migrans, but the area of involvement is larger. Sometimes the larva burrows deep into the internal tissues and may lodge in the gut wall or elsewhere and produce an abscess. Indeed, secondary infection frequently occurs. Brain involvement in fatal cases with eosinophilic meningitis has been reported. Eye involvement with iritis and orbital cellulitis is also described. If the worm does not reach the body surface, the symptoms can persist for months. Some recommend extraction of the worm, but Hetrazan has been said to be useful. There is insufficient experience with thiabendazole thus far to permit a definite statement of its value, but its trial seems reasonable.

Miyazaki, I.: On the genus *Gnathostoma* and human gnathostomiasis with special reference to Japan. Exp. Parasitol., 9:338, 1960.

213.7. OESOPHAGOSTOMIASIS

Oesophagostomiasis is more closely related to hookworm and *Strongyloides* than to *Gnathostoma*, but like *Gnathostoma* it may rarely form a tumor in the human gut wall. Again, man is not the definitive host. The infection is often carried by pet monkeys, and the clinical picture is usually one of intestinal obstruction. Bacterial infection of the tumor nodule is common. Surgical excision of the tumor shows it to contain worms of *Oesophagostomum* species.

Anthony, P. P., and McAdam, I. W. J.: Helminthic pseudotumours of the bowel: Thirty-four cases of helminthoma. Gut, 13:8, 1972.

213.8. ASCARIASIS

DEFINITION. Ascariasis is infection with *Ascaris lumbricoides*, the large roundworm of man. The adults mature in the small intestine and can produce disease by intestinal obstruction or migration. The passage of larvae through the lungs may result in pneumonitis.

ETIOLOGY. *Ascaris* is a large whitish nematode; the female (20 to 35 cm) is larger than the male (15 to 30 cm), which often has a curly tail. The vulva of the female is situated ventrally at the junction of the anterior and middle thirds of the worm. Frequent copulation is necessary to ensure the continuous production of fertile eggs. A female worm has a reproductive capacity of 26 to 27 million eggs and a daily output of 200,000. The life span of the adult worms is relatively short (12 to 24 months). They are not attached to the wall of the jejunum, but bridge themselves across the lumen and by their muscle tone maintain themselves against the fecal stream. In a largely anaerobic environment they obtain nourishment from the semidigested food of the host and possibly from epithelial cells of the intestinal mucosa. The high protein and vitamin content of the parasite suggests that they deprive the host of nutrients.

The brownish eggs with a thick shell and albuminous coat become infective ten days after being passed in the stool. Fertile and infertile eggs have a different morphology. On ingestion of infective eggs by man, the larvae hatch in the small intestine, and, penetrating its wall, are carried by the blood and lymphatic system to the lungs. It has been suggested that this migration is necessitated by the need for oxygen, which is not available in the intestine, at this stage of the life cycle. Here, like hookworm and *Strongyloides*, the larvae migrate up the respiratory passages to the epiglottis and down to the esophagus. A new generation of eggs appears in the feces approximately two months after the ingestion of embryonated eggs.

EPIDEMIOLOGY. Although cosmopolitan, this worm is most abundant in the tropics, where sanitation is poor. One in every four people in the world is infected with *Ascaris lumbricoides*. The eggs are killed by direct sunlight and temperatures above 45° C; nevertheless, under optimal conditions they may remain viable for ten years. The eggs pass unchanged through the intestine of animals with the possible exception of the pig. The pig *Ascaris*, *Ascaris suum*, is morphologically identical to the human *Ascaris*, and there is some evidence that cross-infections can occur. The susceptibility to infection is greatest in childhood, reaching a peak at puberty, and transmission is by fecal contamination of food and drink. Circulating antibodies appear to play some role in host immunity.

PATHOLOGY AND CLINICAL MANIFESTATIONS. Light infections of a dozen or so worms often pass unnoticed, especially in adults. During the phase of larval migration, especially if many eggs have been ingested, respiratory symptoms may appear 4 to 16 days after infection. The pulmonary migration of larvae is associated with fever, cough, occasionally hemoptysis, and either crepitations or more rarely the signs of consolidation on auscultation of the chest. The sputum contains larvae and eosinophils, and there is a high blood eosinophilia. Sections of the lungs at this stage would show larvae in the bronchioles with patchy infiltration of alveoli with polymorphs and eosinophil leukocytes. Aberrant larvae may lodge in the liver, producing granulomatous lesions and hepatomegaly. More rarely such larvae, which fail to re-enter the circulation, are found in other abdominal organs.

When adult worms are present in the intestine, the established infection is often associated with occasional colicky abdominal pain and some abdominal distention. These adults may produce complications by mechanical effects within the gastrointestinal tract, or by wandering outside it, or more rarely by producing allergic manifestations in a sensitized host.

Heavy loads of worms may particularly be associated with intestinal obstruction, intussusception, volvulus, appendicitis, and hernial strangulation. A bolus of *Ascaris* may be a common cause of intestinal obstruction in childhood in an endemic area. Before undertaking bowel surgery, an *Ascaris* infection should always be excluded, because these worms are difficult to control once the bowel is opened, and considerable peritoneal soiling may result. Migration of adult worms may occur spontaneously or as a result of some stimulus such as fever or tetrachloroethylene. The *Ascaris* adults may perforate a suture line or cause a bile or pancreatic duct obstruction. Occasionally they migrate into the stomach and are vomited up, or pass down into the large bowel and out with the stool. Adult worms have been described issuing from umbilical fistulas, and even from the nose or ear. Obstruction of the bile duct is associated with cholangitis, and eggs may be deposited in the liver. *A. lumbricoides* has been said by some to be second only to *E. histolytica* in producing liver abscesses. Blockage of the pancreatic duct results in acute pancreatitis. Once the adult worm has left the bowel, it often dies, releasing foreign protein that may produce a reaction in a sensitized host. These reactions range from facial edema and giant urticaria to acute local necrosis and anaphylaxis. Laboratory personnel who work with *Ascaris* invariably become sensitized to the worms. Young pigs infected with *Ascaris* do not gain weight normally, and it is possible that heavy loads of human *Ascaris* may affect children similarly, as the worms will consume much food in the actively growing phase.

DIAGNOSIS. Examination of the feces reveals the characteristic ova. Usually in view of the number of ova produced, they can be found in ordinary direct smear. Although fertilized eggs are easy to recognize, unfertilized eggs assume bizarre shapes and may be mistaken for debris. Rarely one encounters infections of immature worms or only male worms. Sometimes an infection is diagnosed in barium meal examination, as the barium can be seen in the *Ascaris* gut. Although many serologic tests have been developed for *Ascaris*, including complement-fixation, hemagglutination, and gel diffusion, they are seldom used for diagnostic purposes.

TREATMENT. Although piperazine is still widely used, it is being replaced by new, less toxic drugs such as levamisole, pyrantel, and mebendazole. Levamisole is given in a single oral dose of 15 mg for adults and 5 mg per kilogram for children. Pyrantel embonate is also given in a single oral dose 11 mg per kilogram of body weight (maximum dose, 1 gram). The dose of mebendazole is the same as that given for hookworm (see Ch. 213.3). Piperazine salts act by blocking the neuromuscular junctions of the worm. The paralyzed worm can no longer bridge itself across the intestinal lumen and is carried along in the fecal stream and passed in the stool. Piperazine citrate is given in a dose of 75 mg per kilogram to a maximal single dose of 4 grams. This will clear 75 per cent of patients of their worms, but the dose can be repeated the following day with safety. No special preparation or purgation is necessary. Neurotoxic effects from piperazine have been reported in patients with renal failure who cannot excrete the drug. Being a cheap drug, piperazine is still widely used in the tropics. In multiple intestinal helminthic infections, *Ascaris* should always be treated first.

When examining stools for ova after therapy, it must be remembered that eggs may be passed in the stool for up to a week after the worms have been eradicated owing to the delay in the colonic circulation of feces.

The following regimen is suggested to deal with *intestinal obstruction* caused by *Ascaris*. Initially conservative treatment with nasogastric suction, intravenous fluids, and piperazine therapy should be tried for 48 hours. If no improvement follows, at laparotomy it is often possible to manipulate the bolus of worms into the large bowel through the terminal ileum. Only if this is not possible should enterotomy and worm extraction be performed.

PREVENTION. This consists of disposal of human excreta in sanitary privies and toilets. Children must be taught to use these facilities and avoid contamination of food with ova.

Blumenthal, D. S., and Schultz, M. G.: Incidence of intestinal obstruction in children infected with *Ascaris lumbricoides*. Am. J. Trop. Med. Hyg., 24:801, 1975.

Chang, C. C., and Han, C. T.: Biliary ascariasis in childhood. A clinical analysis of 788 cases. Chin. Med. J. (Peking), 85:167, 1966.

Gelpi, A. P., and Mustafa, A.: Seasonal pneumonitis with eosinophilia: A study of larval ascariasis in Saudi Arabia. Am. J. Trop. Med. Hyg., 16:646, 1967.

Lejkina, E. S.: Research in *Ascaris* immunity and immunodiagnosis. Bull. WHO, 32:699, 1965.

Pawlowski, Z. S.: Ascariasis. Clin. Gastroenterol., 7:157, 1978.

Piggott, J., Hansbarger, E. A., and Neafie, R. G.: Human ascariasis. Am. J. Clin. Path., 53:223, 1970.

The Control of Ascariasis. World Health Organization Technical Report, Series No. 379, 1967.

213.9. TOXOCARIASIS
(Visceral Larva Migrans)

Toxocariasis is an accidental human infection with the cat and dog *Ascaris* (*Toxocara cati* and *Toxocara canis*). The eggs of these species are infective two to three weeks after being passed, and if ingested by man the second stage larvae emerge. These penetrate the intestinal wall and reach the liver. The majority remain in the liver but others migrate to other organs, particularly the brain and the eye. Rarely they complete their cycle of development in man and produce adult worms in the bowel. Children are particularly susceptible because of more frequent soiling of the fingers and habits of playing with puppies, in which the incidence of infection is very high. Initially reported from the southern United States, these parasites are common in dogs and cats in many parts of the world. Although many reports have come from North America and Europe, it is likely that this syndrome also occurs in other parts of the world.

The migrating larvae produce "eosinophilic trails" and tissue inflammation in the affected organ. Usually a granuloma forms with epithelial cells, fibroblasts, lymphocytes, plasma cells, and occasional giant cells. A fibrous capsule eventually encloses the larva, which may remain alive for months. The granulomas can be seen macroscopically as small grayish-white spots. Such granulomas have been found in the lungs, eyes, brain, heart, kidney, and striated muscle.

The most common clinical form is that of a patient with a mild fever and tender hepatomegaly. Routine investigation reveals a marked eosinophilia (50 to 60 per cent), and further questioning often brings to light a history of contact with dogs. These signs and symptoms may persist for 18 months. The serum globulins may be elevated and anti-γ globulins are found. Another clinical form is as an *endophthalmitis* with a space-occupying granuloma visibly distorting the contour of the retina on funduscopy. In the past such granulomas were often mistaken for retinoblastomas, and the eye was removed. Several such series of "retinoblastomas" have been examined, and many of the tumors were found to consist of granulomas containing *Toxocara* larvae. Many mild infections are asymptomatic.

The syndrome of tender hepatomegaly and eosinophilia must be distinguished from invasive schistosomiasis or fascioliasis. A variety of nematodes can produce visceral larva migrans in special circumstances, among them *Ascaris lumbricoides*, *Necator americanus*, and *Strongyloides stercoralis*. Other nonhuman nematodes such as *Gnathostoma*, *Capillaria*, and *Dirofilaria* may be involved in granuloma formation in the liver. Sarcoidosis and periarteritis nodosa may mimic this disease. Blind liver biopsy is seldom helpful, but where facilities exist, direct visualization of surface granulomas of the liver with a peritoneoscope may enable biopsy of a granuloma to be made. A definitive diagnosis can often be made by examination of this granuloma. A diagnosis of second-stage *Toxocara* larva can be made on a section at mid-gut level, showing a maximal width of 12 to 20 μ and lateral alae. A variety of serologic tests are available but lack specificity, as they cross-react with other helminthic infections. However, in areas where such infections are rarely encountered, a fluorescent antibody test or an indirect hemagglutination test may be helpful.

TREATMENT. Diethylcarbamazine (see Bancroftian Filariasis in Ch. 214.3) has been used and does kill some larvae in the tissues of infected mice. A resolution of symptoms has followed the use of thiabendazole in one case in a dose of 25 mg per kilogram twice daily for seven days. The prognosis is good if the source of infection is removed by treating the dog with piperazine. Care must be taken to worm pets regularly, especially puppies, if they are in contact with children.

Huntley, C. C., Costas, M. C., Williams, R. C., Lyerly, A. D., and Watson, R. G.: Anti-γ-globulin factors in visceral larva migrans. JAMA, 197:552, 1966.
Kagan, I. G.: The serological diagnosis of visceral larva migrans. Clin. Pediat. (Phila), 7:508, 1968.
Mok, C. H.: Visceral larva migrans: A discussion based on a review of the literature. Clin. Pediat. (Phila.), 7:565, 1968.
Nelson, J. D., McConnell, T. H., and Moore, D. V.: Thiabendazole therapy of visceral larva migrans: A case report. Am. J. Trop. Med. Hyg., 15:903, 1966.
Woodruff, A. W.: Toxocariasis. Br. Med. J., 3:663, 1970.

213.10.　ANISAKIASIS

Although the full life cycle is still unknown, it appears that man is occasionally infected by the ascarid *Anisakis marina*, which has its larval stages in herrings. The adult worms develop in marine mammals such as seals, dolphins, porpoises, and whales. Man is infected by eating raw or undercooked herrings, and infection has occurred where such food is considered a delicacy, namely, northeastern Europe (particularly the Netherlands) and Japan. The larvae appear to burrow into the wall of the stomach or small bowel to produce an eosinophilic granulomatous mass that may be mistaken for a malignancy. Perforation of the bowel wall has been reported, as has stenosis following granuloma formation. Usually the correct diagnosis is not made until the specimen is examined after surgical resection. Government regulations in the Netherlands require that all raw herring be frozen at −20° C for 24 hours to kill the larvae. This has practically abolished the disease.

Van Thiel, P. H.: The present state of anisakiasis and its causative worms. Trop. Geog. Med., 28:73, 1976.
Yokogawa, M., and Yoshimura, H.: Clinicopathologic studies on larval anisakiasis in Japan. Am. J. Trop. Med. Hyg., 16:723, 1967.

213.11.　TRICHURIASIS
(Whipworm Infection, Trichocephaliasis)

In trichuriasis, the adult worms are shaped like a whip. The long anterior threadlike portion of the worm consists of a cellular esophagus buried deep into the submucosa of the colon, making it difficult to dislodge. These adults are pinkish-gray and are 30 to 50 mm long. The male is distinguished from the female by its coiled caudal extremity. The female produces 5000 to 10,000 eggs per day. The eggs are 50 to 55 μ long, golden brown with prominent characteristic bipolar plugs. Under favorable conditions they become infective in three to five weeks, and when ingested by man the first stage larva hatches in the small intestine and spends three to ten days in the intestinal villi. Then it passes down to the large bowel where it matures in 30 to 90 days. The adult worms live for three to five years.

Of worldwide distribution, trichuriasis is most frequently encountered in the tropics. Often in a particular endemic locality, the infestation has a patchy distribution because of dense shade, heavy rainfall, and the clay soils that hold water as well as fecal pollution, thus facilitating transmission. In the United States, whipworm infection is found in the southern Appalachians and southwestern Louisiana; it is not infrequent in Puerto Rico.

The great majority of infections are asymptomatic; only heavy loads of worms cause clinical illness. The worms are distributed throughout the colon and rectum, and heavy infections may be associated with colic and diarrhea with blood. *Trichuris trichiura* abstracts 0.005 ml of blood per worm from the host each day. In children in precarious iron balance a load of over 800 worms may be associated with an iron deficiency anemia. Up to 5000 worms have been recovered from heavily infected children. In such infections rectal prolapse may complicate the diarrhea, and the appearance of the congested mucosa associated with the whitish bodies of the worms has been described as the "coconut cake" rectum. Early infections may be associated with a mild blood eosinophilia. *Trichuris* has been implicated as a predisposing factor to acute amebic dysentery by causing an initial breach of the mucosa, this suggestion being based on finding a higher incidence of *Trichuris* in patients with acute bowel amebiasis than is normal for the area. *Trichuris* is often associated with other helminthic and protozoal infections. Appendicitis and peritonitis with the presence of worms in the peritoneal cavity have been described.

Diagnosis is made by finding the eggs in the feces, either on direct smear or by concentration methods. In the rare *Trichuris* dysentery the eggs may appear in aggregates in the mucoid stools, together with eosinophils and Charcot-Leyden crystals. Egg counts below 10,000 per gram are unlikely to be associated with symptoms.

Treatment should be confined to heavily infected individuals presenting with symptoms and to those employed as food handlers, nurses, and so forth. Mebendazole, in an oral dose of 100 mg twice a day for three days, gave a cure rate of 64.3 per cent in one trial. It is well tolerated and has a direct ovicidal effect. A second or even a third course can be given. Thiabendazole in a similar dose to that used in *Strongyloides* (25 mg per kilogram of body weight twice daily for two days) eradicates the infection in one third of cases, and the course can be repeated after one week.

Boon, W. H., and Hoh, K. K.: Severe whipworm infection in children. Singapore Med. J., 2:34, 1966.

Franz, K. H., Schneider, W. J., and Pohlman, M. H.: Clinical trials with thiabendazole against intestinal nematodes infecting humans. Am. J. Trop. Med. Hyg., 14:383, 1965.

Jung, R. C., and Jelliffe, D. B.: The clinical picture and treatment of whipworm infection. West Afr. Med. J., 1:11, 1952.

Layrisse, M., Apariedo, L., Martinez Torres, C., and Roche, M.: Blood loss due to infection with *Trichuris trichiura*. Am. J. Trop. Med. Hyg., 16:613, 1967.

Sargent, R. G., Savoury, A. M., Mina, A., and Lee, P. R.: A clinical evaluation of mebendazole in the treatment of trichuriasis. Am. J. Trop. Med. Hyg., 23:375, 1974.

Wagner, E. D., and Chavarria, A. P.: In vivo effects of a new anthelmintic, mebendazole (R 17,635), on the eggs of *Trichuris trichiura* and hookworm. Am. J. Trop. Med. Hyg., 23:151, 1974.

213.12. ENTEROBIASIS
(Oxyuriasis, Pinworm or Seatworm Infection)

Infestation with the pinworm, *Enterobius vermicularis*, is not limited to rural communities and the poor as with many intestinal nematodes, but occurs also in urban communities. Reportedly worldwide in distribution, it appears to be rarer in the tropics. Children are more commonly infected than adults.

The adult female worm is 8 to 13 mm long, and the male, which is rarely seen, 2 to 5 mm. Both live in the cecum and adjacent large and small bowel. The females migrate at night to the anal orifice, where they deposit their eggs. Within a few hours larvae develop in the eggs, which are then infectious and on ingestion hatch in the duodenum and migrate to the large bowel where they mature in 15 to 28 days. The ova can be transferred from the anal margin to the mouth by contamination of the hands, and ova lodge under the nails after scratching of the anal margin. The eggs also become widely disseminated in the environment, notable in bedclothes and dust samples. It has been suggested that hatching of larvae on the anal margin may result in the colon's being colonized from below as a form of autoinfection. Fortunately the eggs are relatively susceptible to drying, and in a warm dry environment survive only a few days.

Usually pinworm infestation is harmless and is often asymptomatic. Pruritus ani is the chief complaint caused by the migrating female worms. Numerous other symptoms have been described, including enuresis, irritability, and insomnia, which may result from the pruritus. Less convincing reported manifestations are abdominal pain, teeth grinding, nausea, and weight loss.

Rarely the female worm may penetrate into the mucosa of the bowel, where it has been a primary cause of appendicitis. Occasionally female worms migrate into the vagina, causing an intense vulvitis. Prostatitis is a rare complication in the male, and secondary ischiorectal abscesses may follow perianal eczema. Granulomas may form around worms that enter tissues, and such granulomas have been described in the uterus, fallopian tubes, and peritoneum, presumably associated with migration of worms up the female genital tract. A rare case not reported in the literature occurred in a mentally deficient child who developed pulmonary eosinophilic granulomas owing to massive inhalation of *Enterobius* eggs present in the dust of the mental institution.

The best method for finding *Enterobius* eggs is by means of the sealing tape (Scotch tape) swab. A piece of Scotch tape 2 inches long is folded, sticky side out, over the end of a wooden tongue depressor and pressed firmly against the perianal region. The tape is then stuck to the slide, acting as a coverslip, and the specimen is scanned for the typical eggs, which are 50 to 60 μ in length, are flattened on one side, and contain a developing embryo. The patient can be given six such swabs, and he does the examination every morning for six mornings on rising and before taking a bath. All can then be examined at the laboratory. Adult worms are rarely observed in feces or on the perianal skin, or seen with the sigmoidoscope. All members of the family should be examined in view of the frequency with which whole families are infected. The eosinophil count is rarely elevated in this infection.

Single-dose treatment is practical with either mebendazole, a 100-mg tablet for all ages, or pyrantel pamoate, 1 ml per 5 kilograms of body weight to a maximal dose of 15 ml. Pyrvinium pamoate, in a dose of 5 mg per kilogram, should be repeated after two weeks.

This drug turns the stool red, and may occasionally be associated with vomiting, diarrhea, and skin rashes. The methods of transmission should be explained to the patient, and care of personal hygiene (short nails, frequent baths, and clean underclothes) instituted before treatment. Follow-up tape swabs are necessary. There is a tendency for some patients to become overanxious about this infection, occasionally with the development of a "worm neurosis." They should be strongly reassured.

Chandrasoma, P. T., and Mendis, K. M.: Enterobius vermicularis in ectopic sites. Am. J. Trop. Med. Hyg., 26:644, 1977.
Cram, E. B.: Studies on oxyuriasis, xxviii. Summary and conclusions. Am. J. Dis. Child., 65:46, 1943.
Most, H., Gellin, G. A., Yager, R., Aron, B., Friedlander, M., and Quarfordt, S.: Enterobius (pinworm infection): A study of 951 Puerto Rican and 315 non-Puerto Rican children in New York City. Am. J. Trop. Med. Hyg., 12:65, 1963.

214. TISSUE NEMATODES

214.1. TRICHINOSIS*

(Trichiniasis, Trichinellosis)

DEFINITION AND ETIOLOGY. Trichinosis is a self-limited infection of the intestine (by the adult parasite) and of the striated muscle (by the larvae) produced by a small nematode, *Trichinella spiralis*. The same animal host thus acts as both the final and the intermediate host, harboring the adults temporarily and the encysted larvae for long periods. When infected meat containing larvae is ingested, these larvae are released into the upper small intestine by the action of digestive juices. They become adult in five to seven days, the males and females mate, and the fertile female begins to deposit larvae into the mucosa. These larvae pass into the circulation through the hepatic and pulmonary filters, and are carried to all parts of the body. They burrow into the muscles and encyst and complete their development in striated muscle. In other tissues such as the myocardium, brain, and eye, the larvae disintegrate and are absorbed. Among the muscles heavily parasitized are the diaphragmatic, masseteric, intercostal, laryngeal, extraocular, nuchal, pectoral, deltoid, gluteus, biceps, and gastrocnemius. A total of 1500 larvae are liberated by each female worm, usually in four to eight weeks but up to 16 weeks, after which the females die.

Larvae attain a size of 0.4 by 0.025 mm in a cyst in the muscle by the thirty-fifth day. The capsule is complete in three months, and calcification occurs within six months to two years. Recent evidence suggests that there may be strain differences in relation to host susceptibility. The parasite is chiefly found in man, hogs, rats, bears, foxes, walruses, dogs, and cats, but any carnivorous or omnivorous animal may be infected.

EPIDEMIOLOGY. Generally of worldwide distribution, the parasite has not been reported from the islands of the Pacific, Brazil, or Australia. It occurs more frequently in the Northern Hemisphere than in the tropics. It is common in Europe and the United States. Fatal cases have recently been described from Kenya and Chile. It is rare east of the Suez Canal. In the United States there has been a marked reduction in the incidence of the infection, owing to laws requiring the cooking of garbage fed to hogs, storage of meat at low temperature, and education of the public resulting in thorough cooking of pork.

Until quite recently, trichinosis was relatively common in New York City, as pork was being obtained from garbage-fed hogs in New Jersey. However, hog-rearing in this way has substantially declined. Pigs become infected by eating infected meat and occasionally infected rats. Rats are infected in the same way. One of the main methods of transmission is in sausages, wursts, or hamburgers in which the beef is diluted (or actually contaminated in mechanical grinders) with a little pork. Infections from bear and walrus meat have been reported. The low incidence in the tropics is probably due to the fact that meat of any kind is a luxury to many people. Hindus, Jews, and Moslems eschew pork, and the Chinese cook it very well.

PATHOLOGY AND PATHOGENESIS. Three to four days after invasion of the muscle, the fiber becomes edematous, loses its cross striations, and undergoes basophilic degeneration. The nuclei increase in number and size, and there is interstitial inflammation around the muscle with a chronic inflammatory cell infiltrate. The severity of the disease depends on the adult worm load, the age of the patient, and the degree of host resistance as well as the numbers of organs involved.

In the heart a focal interstitial myocarditis may occur. Acute nonsuppurative meningitis may be associated with larvae in the cerebrospinal fluid. Larvae may cause lesions in the choroid and retina. Catarrhal enteritis, pulmonary edema, and pneumonia may occur in the early stages of the disease.

CLINICAL MANIFESTATIONS. The cardinal features of trichinosis are fever, orbital edema, myalgia, and eosinophilia. Only a small percentage of infected patients have sufficient parasites, however, to produce such clinically recognizable disease. The clinical picture can be divided into distinct stages in a symptomatic infection. First, there is the stage of adult maturation during the first weeks after infection associated with transient gastrointestinal symptoms. From the seventh to the fourteenth day larviposition begins, and muscle penetration commences. This is usually associated with an irregular persistent fever (37.8 to 40.5° C), urticarial rash, and occasionally respiratory symptoms in the form of cough and bronchospasm. Muscle pains become prominent and unusual, but the characteristic physical signs are bilateral orbital edema and subungual and subconjunctival hemorrhages. A severe infection may result in death four to eight weeks after infection from toxemia, secondary pneumonia, myocardial failure, or trichinous encephalitis. Severe muscle involvement may render breathing, masticating, swallowing, or locomotion painful. An eosinophilia beginning seven days after the infection may rise to very high levels (70 per cent) and persist for months. Serum transaminases are also elevated in the invasive stage.

DIAGNOSIS AND DIFFERENTIAL DIAGNOSIS. Although the rising eosinophilia together with a suggestive clinical picture leads one to suspect this diagnosis, it is proved by finding the larvae in a muscle biopsy. This should be done in the fourth week of infection when a small piece of

---

*The present chapter is based on the article on trichinosis prepared by Dr. Harold W. Brown for the twelfth edition of this book. Little new clinical information has developed in the interval; what has appeared has been incorporated in the basic article. P.D.M.

muscle is removed from the deltoid or gastrocnemius. Crushed between two microscope slides and examined under the low-power objective of the microscope, the living coiled larvae can be seen. In light infections when the direct examination is negative, the biopsy specimen can be incubated overnight in an acid-pepsin mixture and the centrifuged deposit examined for larvae.

Calcified cysts and calcified larvae represent older infections, as calcification usually takes 18 months, but the larva may live inside the calcified cyst for many years. Calcified cysts appear as tiny white spots in fresh muscle, but are too small to be detected radiologically.

A variety of serologic tests are available. The bentonite flocculation test is as sensitive as the complement-fixation test and much easier to perform. It is usually positive four weeks after infection, but may be present earlier. A change from a negative to a positive test during the illness is significant. The indirect fluorescent antibody test detects some infections at an earlier stage. Few other parasitic infections are associated with such persistent fever or generalized muscular aches and tender muscles. Polymyositis of nonparasitic cause may present like this and be associated with eosinophilia. Periarteritis nodosa may also mimic trichinosis.

TREATMENT. Congestive cardiac failure should be searched for and, if present, should be treated. Mild analgesics can be given for the muscle pain. Anti-inflammatory steroids (prednisone, dexamethasone) relieve fever, edema, and muscle pain in severe acute cases but are said not to affect the adult worms' fecundity or the number of larvae settling in the muscle. In patients with central nervous system involvement this effect of steroids is dramatic.

Thiabendazole, in a dose of 25 mg per kilogram of body weight for five to seven days, has also produced a marked resolution of the symptoms of fever and muscle pain, but living larvae have still been recovered on muscle biopsy after much larger courses of the drug. In severe infections the use of corticosteroids and thiabendazole may be life-saving, but when the parasite load is not considerable, the prognosis is good even without treatment.

PREVENTION. The ultimate prevention of trichinosis is dependent on its elimination in hogs, and the incidence in these animals can be greatly reduced by heat-sterilizing garbage. Freezing meat at $-32°$ C for a few hours (or -15 to $-30°$ C for several weeks) kills larvae, as does gamma radiation of the meat. Pigs fed on a diet containing 0.1 per cent thiabendazole fail to incubate *T. spiralis* on challenge. Routine meat inspection does not detect the infection, and serologic and skin tests on pigs have not been helpful in detecting infected animals. The chief safeguard at present is the thorough cooking of pork at $60°$ C for 30 minutes for each pound of meat.

Gould, S. E.: Trichinosis in Man and Animals. Springfield, Ill., Charles C Thomas, 1970.
Hennekeuser, M. H., Pabst, K., Poeplau, W., and Gerok, W.: Thiabendazole for the treatment of trichinosis in humans. Tex. Rep. Biol. Med., 27 (Supplement 2):581, 1969.
Kim, C. W.: Trichinellosis. New York, Intext Educational Publishers, 1974.
Maynard, J. E., and Kagan, I. G.: Trichinosis (serology). Practitioner, 191:622, 1963.
Moser, R. H.: Trichinosis from Bismarck to polar bears. JAMA, 228:735, 1974.
Proceedings of the International Commission in Trichinellosis: No. VI. Wiad, Parazyt., 14:127, 1968.
Zimmerman, W. J., Steele, J. H., and Kagan, I. G.: The changing status of trichiniasis in the U.S. population. Public Health Rep., 83:957, 1968.

214.2. ANGIOSTRONGYLIASIS

ANGIOSTRONGYLUS CANTONENSIS. Eosinophilic meningoencephalitis, a syndrome caused by *Angiostrongylus cantonensis* (the rat lung worm), was first recognized in New Caledonia in 1950, and has since been reported from Hawaii, Tahiti, other Pacific Islands, Indonesia, and Thailand. The human disease has only been reported from the Far East and the Pacific to date, although infected rats have been found in Madagascar, Mauritius, Ceylon, and Sarawak.

The life cycle was described by workers in Australia in 1955 before the importance of the worm as a human pathogen was known. A delicate filiform nematode, 17 to 25 mm in length, the adult lives in the lungs of rats, and the eggs are coughed up, swallowed, and pass out in the feces as first-stage larvae. Further development occurs in slugs and snails to the third-stage infective larvae. These larvae are ingested by man either while in this intermediate host or after they have been shed by it onto some other article of food, e.g., lettuce. Crabs and freshwater prawns have also been found to be infected with these metastrongyloid larvae, but probably act as paratenic hosts. The dispersal of the giant African land snail *Achatina fulica* may have assisted the spread of the infection. When infective larvae are ingested by the rat, they migrate to the brain and reach young adulthood in four weeks. They then migrate to the pulmonary arteries and after two more weeks start laying eggs. Unfortunately if man accidentally ingests these infective larvae, they migrate to the brain (as in the rat), and there produce the clinical picture of a meningoencephalitis associated with fever, signs of cerebral irritation, mental deficit, and varying degrees of loss of consciousness. Mild blood eosinophilia is present, and lumbar puncture reveals a fluid under increased pressure with increased protein and many eosinophils (from 100 to 3000 per cubic millimeter). Occasionally patients present with a facial nerve lesion or complaints of diplopia and paresthesia. A complement-fixation test using an extract of adult worms as antigen has been developed. The illness usually persists for some weeks or months and then the patient recovers spontaneously.

Young adult worms have been found in the brain and cerebrospinal fluid of man, and experimental infection of monkeys produces a similar syndrome. The pathology of the brain in fatal cases is one of focal areas of softening, the meninges and subarachnoid space being infiltrated with plasma cells, lymphocytes, eosinophils, and neutrophils. There is perivascular cuffing with chronic inflammatory cells in the brain substance. Careful sectioning of the brain is necessary to find the 0.16 to 8 mm nematodes.

This condition must be differentiated from a variety of other parasitic infections involving the central nervous system. In Thailand cerebral gnathostomiasis and *Angiostrongylus* infections occur. Cerebral paragonimiasis could be an important differential diagnosis in parts of the Far East. In other situations the syndrome of eosinophilic meningitis could be produced by cysticercosis, hydatid, schistosomiasis, fascioliasis, trichinosis, and possibly strongyloidiasis. Refinements of serologic diagnostic techniques will help in this sometimes difficult clinical problem.

The author has been able to trace no references to treatment with thiabendazole, although this would seem to be the drug to try. Prevention entails education regarding dangerous foods such as raw crabs and prawns and undercooked snails, and making sure that lettuce is free of slugs and snails. Freezing of crustaceans and molluscs at $-15°$ C for 12 hours has been found to be effective in destroying the infective larvae of *A. cantonensis*.

MORERASTRONGYLUS COSTARICENSIS. Human disease caused by this parasite has been described from Costa Rica where 130 cases have been studied. The worm also occurs in Honduras and Panama. Patients, usually children, present with right iliac fossa pain, fever, and blood eosinophilia, and often an abdominal mass is palpable. At operation an eosinophilic granulomatous cecal pseudo-tumor is found to contain adult worms and eggs.

The intermediate host is a slug, *Vaginulus (Sarasinula) plebius,* and the definitive host is the cotton rat *Sigmodon hispidus.* Infected slugs contaminate lettuce leaves with infective third-stage larvae, and man acquires the disease by ingesting the slug itself on contaminated salad. In the rodent host — and probably in man — the cycle occurs in the abdominal cavity. The third and fourth larval molts occur in lymph vessels. After three months the young adults move to radicles of the mesenteric arteries, mate, mature, and oviposit. Arteritis and thrombosis may be followed by macro- or microinfarcts of the gut, with ulceration and necrosis of the gut wall. Fistulization or generalized peritonitis may ensue. Neither larvae nor eggs are usually detected in the stools of man.

In *Morerastrongylus costaricensis* infection of man, sexually mature adult worms develop, and as such this species is better adapted to man than *Angiostrongylus cantonensis.*

Alicata, J. E.: Present status of *Angiostrongylus cantonensis* infection in man and animals in the tropics. J. Trop. Med. Hyg., 72:53, 1969.
Mackerras, M. T., and Sanders, D. F.: The life history of the rat lungworm *Angiostrongylus cantonensis* (Chen) (Nematoda; Metastrongylidae). Aust. J. Zool., 3:1, 1955.
Morera, P.: Life cycle and redescription of *Angiostrongylus costaricensis* (Morera and Cespedes 1971). Am. J. Trop. Med. Hyg., 22:613, 1973.
Schollhaminer, G., Aubry, P., and Rigaud, J. L.: Quelques réflexions sur la méningite à éosinophiles à Tahiti. Étude clinique et biologique de 165 observations, à propos d'un cas atypique. Bull. Soc. Pathol. Exot., 59:341, 1966.

214.3.   FILARIASIS

GENERAL CONSIDERATIONS

To talk of filariasis as such is to use a general term like anemia, for there are seven types of nematodes found in man belonging to the superfamily Filarioidea, as well as one member of the superfamily Dracunculoi-dea (the guinea worm), which is usually included in a consideration of this group. Of these Filarioidea, the embryos or microfilariae are found in the blood in five and in the subcutaneous tissues in two species. The adults are viviparous, and the blood microfilariae demonstrate a periodicity in the peripheral blood, depending on the species. They may remain ensheathed in their elongated egg shell or have no sheath. These microfilariae are distinguished on their criteria as well as on the pattern of distribution of nuclei seen in stained specimens in their tails. Giemsa stain can be used, but better results of sheath staining are obtained with Delafield's hematoxylin or Mayer's acid hemalum.

In Table 2 the various species are listed and the characteristics of their microfilariae are shown. The adult worms live for many years, whereas blood microfilariae have a life of three to six months. After being bitten by an infected arthropod it may take 1 year to 18 months before microfilariae are present in the peripheral blood, a long prepatent period. The controlling mechanism for periodicity has never been satisfactorily explained for many of these human species. However, Hawking's work suggests that at least two circadian rhythms are involved, one mechanism within the microfilariae themselves, and the other some physiological tide in the host (body temperature for certain animal species). This periodicity fits the habits of the insect vector; for instance, the *Loa* insect vector flies by day, but most bancrofti infections are transmitted nocturnally. The geographic distribution of these species is of particular importance, because in some it is markedly restricted. For instance *Loa loa* is a filarid of Equatorial Africa, and *Mansonella ozzardi* is found only in South America.

Not all the species listed are significantly pathogenic. Few symptoms have been ascribed to *Mansonella ozzardi* infections, and the case for the pathogenicity of *D. perstans* is very shaky. Two of these filarial infections are notable in terms of their importance in man. These are the *Wuchereria-Brugia complex,* which produces bancroftian filariasis with lymphatic obstruction and elephantiasis, and *onchocerciasis,* which is a common cause of blindness in endemic areas. Multiple infections occur in endemic areas; for instance, in parts of West Africa a patient may be seen infected with *Loa loa,* bancrofti, perstans, and onchocerciasis.

This final group of the most modified nematodes will be considered in the order in which they are listed in Table 2, except that the guinea worm will be considered first. Dirofilariasis and pulmonary tropical eosinophilia will then be reviewed.

TABLE 2.   Common Filarioidea of Man as Distinguished by Characteristics of Microfilariae

	Periodicity of Microfilariae	Sheathed or Unsheathed	Tail Morphology
Microfilariae in blood:			
Wuchereria bancrofti	Majority nocturnal	Sheathed	Nuclei not to tip of tail
Brugia malayi	Majority nocturnal	Sheathed	Two distinct nuclei in tail tip
Loa loa	Diurnal	Sheathed	Nuclei to tip of tail
Mansonella ozzardi	Nonperiodic	Not sheathed	Nuclei not to tip of tail
Dipetalonema perstans	Nocturnally subperiodic	Not sheathed	Nuclei to tip of tail
Microfilariae in subcutaneous tissues:			
Onchocerca volvulus	Nonperiodic	Not sheathed	Nuclei not to tip of tail
Dipetalonema streptocerca	Nonperiodic	Not sheathed	Nuclei to tip of tail, which is crooked

Hawking, F.: Advances in filariasis. Trans. R. Soc. Trop. Med. Hyg., 59:9, 1965.

Hawking, F., Moore, P., Gammage, K., and Worms, M. J.: Periodicity of microfilariae. XII. The effect of variations in host body temperature on the cycle of *Loa loa, Monnigofilaria setariosa, Dirofilaria immitis*, and other filariae. Trans. R. Soc. Trop. Med. Hyg., 61:674, 1967.

Sasa, M.: Human Filariasis. Baltimore, University Park Press, 1976.

Muller, R.: Dracunculus and dracunculiasis. *In* Dawes, B. (ed.): Advances in Parasitology, Vol. 9, New York, Academic Press, 1973, p. 73.

Pardanani, D. S., Trivedi, V. D., Joshi, L. G., Daulatram, J., and Nandi, J. S.: Metronidazole (Flagyl) in dracunculiasis: A double blind study. Ann. Trop. Med. Parasitol., 71:45, 1977.

Raffier, G.: Efficacy of thiabendazole in the treatment of dracunculiasis. Texas Rep. Biol. Med., 27(Supplement 2):601, 1969.

DRACONTIASIS
(Guinea Worm)

Infection with the guinea worm (*Dracunculus medinensis*) usually presents as a skin ulceration at the site of emergence of the female adult worm. Man is probably the only reservoir, although monkeys and dogs can be experimentally infected. Human infections are widespread in the tropics, occurring in local distribution in West Africa and the Nile Valley, the Middle East, India and Pakistan, the Caribbean Islands, and Guyana. Infection occurs on ingesting infected water fleas (*Cyclops*) present in drinking water from shallow wells or ponds. The infective larvae in the *Cyclops* penetrate the intestinal walls and mature in the loose connective tissue under the skin, especially that of legs and feet. The male worm is small and dies after copulation. The female requires a year to become gravid, and then measures up to a meter long and is 2 mm in diameter. When ready to discharge larvae, she approaches the skin surface, and a blister is produced by secretion of a toxic substance from the anterior end of the worm. The blister breaks down to form an ulcer a few centimeters across, and the anterior end of the worm protrudes into this ulcer. On contact with water the head of the worm ruptures, and the uterus periodically discharges the tightly coiled larvae infective to the water flea. Secondary infection of the ulcer with resultant cellulitis is common. Generalized allergic symptoms may occur prior to the blister formation or when surgical removal of the worm is attempted. Multiple infections are common. The lesion is usually on the lower leg, but may occur on the genitalia, buttocks, or upper limbs. In water carriers lesions have been observed on the back, suggesting that the worm is positively hydrotropic. Alternatively, the mature female may never reach the surface of the body and may be absorbed or calcify in the tissue. The radiologic appearance is pathognomonic because the worm is so large. If a gravid worm dies in situ or is broken during extraction, cellulitis and secondary infection often occur. This may give rise to contractures. Also *Clostridium tetani* may contaminate the wound and tetanus may result. Rarely the adult worm involves serous cavities, the extradural space, or joints. Guinea worm arthritis appears to be due to the presence of the adult worm or larvae in the joint. A microscopic diagnosis can be made by finding embryos in the exudate from the guinea worm ulcer after exposure to a few drops of water.

Gradually winding the worm out of the ulcer by turning it on a stick a few centimeters a day is still common practice. Surgical extraction is also practiced. Metronidazole (Flagyl) in an adult dose of 400 mg three times a day for 10 to 20 days rapidly reduces symptoms. Thiabendazole is also effective. Prevention involves constructing water sources that cannot be contaminated and killing *Cyclops* by chlorination or boiling water to be used for drinking.

BANCROFTIAN FILARIASIS

ETIOLOGY. Bancroftian filariasis is caused by the filarial worm *Wuchereria bancrofti*. The adult worms reside in the lymphatic system and produce recurrent lymphangitis with fibrosis and obstruction. The infection is transmitted by culicine and anopheline mosquitoes.

The threadlike adult worms are 4 to 10 cm long and live for decades. The female worm is viviparous, producing microfilariae 130 to 320 μ long which are found in the peripheral blood; in some forms this occurs only at night, whereas during the day the microfilariae are in the lungs. If ingested by a suitable mosquito, these microfilariae develop in the thoracic muscles of the insect and are present in the mouth parts after two weeks. They enter the skin through the puncture wound when the mosquito next feeds, and, finding their way to the lymphatics of the host, the males and females mate and mature. More than a year after infection microfilariae appear in the peripheral blood.

EPIDEMIOLOGY. Man is the only definitive host of this common type of filariasis. Periodic bancroftian filariasis is found throughout tropical Africa and North Africa, as well as in the tropical coastal borders of Asia and Queensland. It is endemic in the West Indies and the northern countries of South America. In the northern Pacific bancroftian filariasis exhibits nocturnal periodicity, but in the Pacific Islands east of 160 degrees of longitude (including New Caledonia, Fiji, Samoa, the Ellis and Cook Islands, Society Islands, and the Marquesas) the microfilariae are nonperiodic, being present in the peripheral blood throughout the 24-hour period. The term *W. bancrofti var. pacifica* has been applied to this strain.

PATHOLOGY. The severity of the lesions probably depends on the adult worm load and their site of development and the susceptibility of the host. Light infections are often asymptomatic, and microfilariae are detected on incidental blood examinations. Maturing adults in the lymphatics are associated with endothelial thickening, fibrin deposition, and infiltration with eosinophils, histiocytes, and lymphocytes. Giant cells occur. Fibrotic and inflammatory changes tend to obstruct the lymphatics, and this process is exacerbated by death of the worms, which may calcify. There is reactive hyperplasia in the lymph nodes, and small granulomas are seen. An eosinophilic endophlebitis of the small veins is present in the lymph nodes. The testicles and epididymis often show similar changes with evidence of chronic inflammation. Worms may not be present at the site of inflammation. Secretions of the worm, especially after molting, are thought to be responsible for some of these changes. As lymphatic obstruction becomes more extensive, chronic edema develops in the infected areas. Recently lymphedema has been produced in laboratory animals with longstanding brugia infections.

CLINICAL MANIFESTATIONS. Attacks of fever, headache, and lymphadenopathy sometimes associated with urticarial rashes are known as filarial fever and occur in the acute phase of the disease. Often, however, no history of this early phase can be obtained. Epididymitis may occur as a lone lesion. Lymphatics most affected are those of the inguinal region, upper arms, and spermatic cord. Chronic lymphadenopathy is often the only sign of infection for years. Retrograde lymphangitis may be noted. In a small proportion of infected individuals, with increasing lymphatic obstruction over the years, all degrees of chronic edema occur, affecting especially the lower limbs and scrotum. Initially the edema is pitting, but as organization of collagen occurs in the edematous subcutaneous tissues, it becomes nonpitting. Eventually the giant limbs of elephantiasis are produced. The skin over the affected part, at first smooth, later becomes scaly and is fissured at the points where the fascia is attached to the skin. Hyperkeratosis produces warts and nodules. Varicose nodes in the groin are the result of lymphatic dilatation and may lead to scrotal lymphedema. Infection may supervene in any of these lesions with formation of a chronic discharging sinus. Chronic inflammatory disease of the testicle and epididymis with or without hydrocele occurs.

Chyluria may be renal or vesical in origin, depending on the level at which the lymph varix communicates with the urinary tract. Cystoscopy and intravenous or retrograde pyelography help to establish the site of communication.

DIAGNOSIS. In the early stages and when lymphadenopathy only is present, microfilariae are usually present in night blood films. Although the motile microfilariae are easily seen in fresh films, staining is necessary for identification. Microfilariae may be absent in the late stage; thus they were found in only 4 per cent of patients with elephantiasis, and 30 per cent of patients with hydrocele had microfilariae in one series. Concentration techniques are available for microfilariae, and they may be found in the chylous urine or hydrocele fluid. A millipore filtration concentration technique has shown that small numbers of microfilariae are circulating during the day in periodic infections. Eosinophilia is not a constant finding. The filarial complement-fixation test and skin test, although only group specific, are useful in suggesting a filarial cause for a lymphedema. Lymphangiograms reveal the extent of the lymphatic obstruction and may be a useful preoperative measure. It is rarely justified to remove an enlarged lymph node to find the adults because this still further prejudices the lymphatic circulation. In an endemic area surgeons frequently encounter adult worms when operating on the groin.

The differential diagnosis depends on the type of clinical syndrome. Lymphadenopathy caused by other infections and neoplasms must be considered. Elephantiasis may be associated with congenital defects of the lymphatic drainage as well as tuberculous inguinal lymphadenitis. Tuberculosis, *Schistosoma haematobium,* and gonorrhea produce epididymitis, and relatively few hydroceles are filarial. Lymphatic obstruction caused by many other agents may produce lymphedema and chyluria.

TREATMENT. Diethylcarbamazine (Banocide, Hetrazan) is believed to kill a large proportion of adults as well as microfilariae. It is usually given in an oral dose of 6 mg per kilogram, in three divided doses after meals. This dose is then given for 14 days. Reactions are mild in comparison with those seen in onchocerciasis, but fever, nausea and vomiting, and skin rashes may occur as with any drug. The arsenical Mel W and the antimonial Astiban (sodium dimercaptosuccinate) kill adult filariae, but are too toxic for general use. All patients with microfilaremia should receive an adequate course of treatment.

The management of lymphedema depends on its severity. Mild degrees are best treated with elevation of the foot of the bed and an elastic stocking. Careful instructions regarding foot care should be given, as ascending streptococcal cellulitis is common in the edematous tissues and further prejudices the lymphatic circulation. Some workers believe the *Streptococcus* to be more important in producing lymphangitis than the worms themselves. Any foot sepsis requires early and vigorous treatment with antimicrobial drugs. Tinea infections should be eradicated. Banocide therapy is often given in elephantiasis on the ground that it may prevent further lymphatic damage, but clinical improvement is seldom observed.

A variety of surgical operations have been devised to remove the edematous subcutaneous tissue from the leg, scrotum, and breasts. Success depends on the type of operation and the skill of the surgeon. In scrotal elephantiasis care must be taken to preserve the testicles. Hydroceles can be treated by the injection of sclerosing agents. Chyluria of bladder origin can be terminated by fulgurating the leaking bladder lymphatics. Renal chyluria is best left alone, although in the past kidneys have been wrapped in cellophane with the subsequent production of renal hypertension.

PREVENTION. Diethylcarbamazine, 3 mg per kilogram per month for 12 to 18 months, has been effective in mass treatment for preventive purposes. Residual DDT or dieldrin is effective against many of the mosquito vectors, and systematic destruction of mosquito-breeding sites has also met with success. Biologic control of mosquito vectors is receiving intensive field trials, but thus far they have not resulted in methods for mass application.

MALAYAN FILARIASIS

A disease similar to bancroftian filariasis is produced by a closely related filarial worm, *Brugia malayi*. The sheathed microfilariae of this species have two distinct caudal nuclei. Transmitted by *Mansonoides* mosquitoes, it is the only filarial infection of man in Malaya and Borneo, whereas in India, Ceylon, and tropical China it coexists with *W. bancrofti. Brugia malayi* is responsible for only mild lymphedema in man, usually below the knee, with enlargement of the popliteal and femoral nodes. In contrast to bancroftian filariasis, the microfilaremia rates in the Malayan form are quite high in children younger than five years. In this infection, also, there are two types of organisms, one with nocturnal periodicity, and another subperiodic form. The latter is found in many animals (primates, carnivores, and rodents) and is a true zoonosis.

Galindo, L., Von Lichtenberg, F., and Baldison, C.: Bancroftian filariasis in Puerto Rico: Infection pattern and tissue lesions. Am. J. Trop. Med., 11:739, 1962.

Nelson, G. S.: The pathology of filarial infections. Helminth. Abst., 35:Pt. 4, 311, 1966.

Schacher, J. F., and Sahyoun, P. F.: A chronological study of the histopathology of filarial disease in cats and dogs caused by *Brugia phangi* (Buckley and Edeson, 1956). Trans. R. Soc. Trop. Med. Hyg., 61:234, 1967.

Turner, L. H.: Studies on filariasis in Malaya: the clinical features of filariasis due to *Wuchereria malayi*. Trans. R. Soc. Trop. Med. Hyg., 53:154, 1959.

Wilson, T.: Filariasis in Malaya — A general review. Trans. R. Soc. Trop. Med. Hyg., 55:107, 1961.

LOIASIS

Loa loa infection is characterized by the appearance of transient swellings mainly on the limbs; these are thought to be the site of the migrating adult worms in the subcutaneous tissue. Occasionally a worm will traverse the conjunctiva of the eye.

The male adult worm is 30 mm long and the female 70 mm. They live for many years, and gain access to the body through the proboscis of biting flies (deer flies of the genus *Chrysops*). These worms appear to be in a state of continuous migration in the subcutaneous tissues of the body. It is not clearly understood how the sexes locate each other, but they meet and mate, and the female produces microfilariae that appear in the blood during the day and are infective to the insect vector.

Man is the only reservoir host, with the possible exception of monkeys. Human loiasis is restricted to Africa, mainly the West Coast. It occurs from Sierra Leone to the Cameroons and extends into the heart of Africa in the region of the Congo basin.

CLINICAL MANIFESTATIONS. The main clinical manifestation is the repeated occurrence of hot erythematous swellings (5 to 10 cm or more) called Calabar swellings after the endemic area of Calabar. These occur in the upper limbs particularly, are painful, and subside in a few days. They are associated with the presence of an adult worm. A similar swelling occurs around the eye when the adult worm crosses the eye beneath the conjunctivae. The patient notices the worm in his line of vision ("like a submarine, doctor") and it is worth inquiring for such a history. Calabar swellings seem to occur more frequently in the extremities. Why this is so is not known. Routine roentgenography in endemic areas often reveals calcified dead worms lying between the metacarpals. Rarely, neurologic symptoms may be associated with the infection if the Calabar swelling involves a peripheral nerve. Also the parasite has been found in the cerebrospinal fluid associated with a meningoencephalitis.

DIAGNOSIS. The initial diagnosis is usually based on a history of Calabar swellings in a patient coming from an endemic area. Examination of the daytime blood reveals sheathed microfilariae with a characteristic distribution of caudal nuclei. In early loiasis, microfilariae may not be detected even by concentration techniques. Very high eosinophil counts are encountered at this stage (50 to 70 per cent). A positive filarial complement-fixation test is usually present. Occasionally the adult worm can be extracted as it crosses the eye.

TREATMENT. Diethylcarbamazine (Hetrazan) kills both adults and microfilariae. One course of 6 mg per kilogram of body weight for 14 days is all that is necessary. Reactions are rare.

Woodruff, A. W.: Loiasis, *In* Fairley, N. H., Woodruff, A. W., and Walters, J. H. (eds.): Recent Advances in Tropical Medicine. London, J. & A. Churchill, Ltd., 1961, pp. 178–194.

MANSONELLA OZZARDI

Mansonella ozzardi is found only in the New World, occurring in South America and certain foci in the Caribbean. *Culicoides* midges are the vectors in Trinidad; in Brazil, *Simulium amazonicum* has been implicated. The adult worms are embedded in visceral adipose tissue. Although they are usually regarded as nonpathogenic, fever, headache, lymphadenitis, and erythematous irritant skin rashes have been reported in association with their presence. Cold extremities, the result of peripheral vasoconstriction caused by a postulated filarial toxin, have been reported. The microfilariae show no particular periodicity and are about twice the size of perstans and have a different caudal morphology. A recent survey, cited below, showed that of 810 Colombian Indians, 96.2 per cent harbored microfilariae of *Mansonella ozzardi*. Diethylcarbamazine (Hetrazan) is ineffective.

Marinkelle, C. J., and German, E.: Mansonelliasis in the Comisaría del Vaupes of Colombia. Trop. Geog. Med., 22:101, 1970.

Undiano, C.: Importance and present-day concepts of the pathogenicity of *Mansonella* infections. Fev. Fac. Cienc. Med. Univ. Cordoba, 24:183, 1966.

DIPETALONEMA PERSTANS

Filariasis caused by *Dipetalonema perstans* has an extensive distribution in Equatorial Africa, the Caribbean, and South America, where it sometimes overlaps with *Mansonella ozzardi*. The adult worms are found in association with the serous cavities of the body, usually behind the limiting membrane. They may be seen at postmortem examination moving behind the peritoneum or pleura. The small (100 μ) unsheathed microfilariae are found in the blood throughout the 24 hours, but there is a peak in the peripheral blood population at night. A *Culicoides* species, a small balck midge, is responsible for transmission.

The vast majority of patients exhibiting microfilaremia have no symptoms, but there have been recent reports of clinical symptoms associated with this infection. These reports include fever, Calabar swellings, arthritis, and upper abdominal pain associated with hepatomegaly. A high eosinophilia is often present in cases with scanty embryos, and such a finding in a patient from an endemic area should prompt a careful search for these. Diethylcarbamazine (Hetrazan) has little effect on the adults or on the microfilariae.

Wiseman, R. A.: *Acanthocheilonema perstans:* A cause of significant eosinophilia in the tropics. Comments on its pathogenicity. Trans. R. Soc. Trop. Med. Hyg., 61:667, 1967.

ONCHOCERCIASIS
(River Blindness)

River blindness is a form of cutaneous filariasis caused by infection with *Onchocerca volvulus* and is characterized by skin irritation, corneal opacities, and skin nodules.

ETIOLOGY. The threadlike adult worms lie tangled together in fibrous nodules in the subcutaneous tissues or fascial planes. Microfilariae produced by the females become widely distributed in the surrounding skin. Female black flies (buffalo gnats) of the genus *Simulium* ingest these larvae while taking a blood meal. After development in the fly for one week, the larvae are infective for man and are deposited when the fly next bites. They take more than a year to mature, mate, and produce microfilariae. Adult worms live 7 to 15 years.

EPIDEMIOLOGY. Human onchocerciasis is found on the West Coast of Africa from Sierra Leone to the Congo and in the east from the Sudan to Nyasaland. It also occurs in Guatemala, Mexico, Eastern Venezuela, Northern Brazil, and Surinam. *Simulium* larvae and pupae are usually found in rapidly running highly oxygenated water. Small insects (3 mm long), the flies bite low on the legs in Africa, but more around the head in Central America, which may account for the high incidence of nodules on the head in the latter locality. In East Africa *Simulium naevi* larvae and pupae evaded detection for many years until they were found on the shells of fresh-water crabs.

PATHOGENESIS AND PATHOLOGY. An initial inflammatory reaction around the adult worm is followed by a foreign body granulomatous reaction and fibrous capsule formation. The nodules are literally the graveyards of the adult worms, for these eventually die and degenerate, sometimes with secondary abscess formation. The microfilariae in the surrounding subcutaneous tissues produce a low-grade inflammatory reaction with lymphocytes, plasma cells, and eosinophils. Thickening of the epidermis and dermis owing to fibrosis eventually occurs, with destruction of elastic fibers and sometimes reduction in pigmentation.

Microfilariae migrate into the tissues of the eye to produce important inflammatory lesions which may result in blindness. Punctate keratitis is associated with death of microfilariae in the cornea, and such multiple corneal opacities may result in permanent corneal scarring. A low-grade iritis and iridocyclitis result in pupillary distortion and even occlusion. Choroidoretinitis also occurs.

CLINICAL MANIFESTATIONS. Any patient who has a persistent irritating skin rash or visual disturbances and has been in one of the endemic areas may have onchocerciasis. More rarely, the presenting complaint takes the form of deep-seated muscular pains. The early skin lesions consist of an erythematous papular irritant rash. In heavy infections definite thickening and hyperkeratosis of the skin occur (craw-craw or crocodile skin). Rarer late complications are depigmentation and pendulous bags in the groins containing sclerosed lymph nodes.

Nodules vary much in size from a few centimeters to as big as a tennis ball. They are frequently detected over bony prominences such as the greater trochanter, the iliac crest, the olecranons, ribs, and occiput. Often the adult worms are located deep in the fascial planes, and no nodules are palpable. To detect the small milky dots of punctate keratitis near the limbus the eyes should be examined with a strong pencil torch, the beam directed obliquely across the cornea. Signs of iritis may be present. With a slit lamp, microfilariae may be visible in the aqueous humor. Funduscopic examination may reveal the much rarer posterior segment lesion.

DIAGNOSIS. Skin shavings are used to demonstrate microfilariae. Thin sections of the superficial skin are removed with a razor blade, mounted in saline, teased out, and examined. Many motile microfilariae emerge from those snips within an hour after they have been made. Blood contamination can be avoided if the shavings are superficial, and this is important if there is coexistent blood microfilaremia. If there is a definite site of skin irritation, shavings should be taken from this area. In lightly infected patients multiple shavings may be necessary to detect microfilariae, and quite often they are not found. The reaction to a test dose of 50 mg of diethylcarbamazine (Mazzotti's test) in the form of an exacerbation of the itching rash is suggestive, as are an eosinophilia and a positive filarial complement-fixation test. In up to 35 per cent of cases microfilariae can be found in the urine.

Scabies and superficial mycoses are the most common irritant skin rashes of the tropics and are important differential diagnoses. Although an infection with no mortality, the recurrent irritation of onchocerciasis can be most distressing. Severe ocular lesions may induce total blindness, and this is the blinding filarid.

TREATMENT. When practicable, all nodules should be excised; this simple measure will reduce the load of adult worms. Suramin* is effective in killing adult worms and is more suitable for mass treatment programs. The side effects and method of administration of this drug are mentioned under African Trypanosomiasis (see Ch. 194.2), which should be consulted before its use. A suitable course for onchocerciasis is 1 gram weekly for six weeks. As the drug is nephrotoxic, treatment should be stopped if more than 30 mg per 100 ml of protein appears in the urine.

Diethylcarbamazine is effective in killing microfilariae but does not kill the adult worms. In sensitized individuals, reactions occur when the microfilariae die in the tissues. Skin irritation becomes more intense, and there may be edema of the skin with fever, headache, and malaise. More serious is acute inflammation of the eye which may prejudice sight. As these reactions are dose related, it is usual to start therapy with a small dose of the drug (0.25 mg per kilogram) and increase gradually to a maximum dose of 6 mg per kilogram of body weight per day for three weeks. Eye reactions can be controlled with 1 per cent cortisone acetate eye drops and the general reactions controlled with antihistamines and, in severe cases, with systemic steroids.

PREVENTION. *Simulium* larvae and pupae are very sensitive to small concentrations of DDT in the river water (less than 1 part per million), and this has been the most effective form of control of the insect vector. Personal prophylaxis is possible to a limited extent by avoiding places where biting *Simulium* are numerous.

---

*Available from Center for Disease Control (404-633-3311, Ext. 3670).

Buck, A. A. (ed.): Onchocerciasis. Symptomatology, Pathology, and Diagnosis. Geneva, World Health Organization, 1974.

Duke, B. O. L.: Onchocerciasis. Br. Med. J., 4:301, 1968.

Nelson, D. S.: Onchocerciasis. In Dawes, B. (ed.): Advances in Parasitology. Volume 8. New York, Academic Press, 1970, p. 173.

Onchocerciasis in the Western Hemisphere. PAHO Sc. Pub. No. 298. Washington, D.C., 1974.

WHO Expert Committee on Onchocerciasis. World Health Organization Technical Report Series No. 335, 1–92, 1966.

STREPTOCERCIASIS

Dipetalonema streptocerca is carried by midges of the genus *Culicoides*. It occurs in Central Africa, particularly in the Congo and neighboring countries. The adult worms are found in the region of the shoulder girdle, and the microfilariae produced in the skin cause a reddish brown irritant rash which may be associated with some degree of edema. Skin shavings reveal the unsheathed microfilariae with the crooked tails and the nuclei going down to the tip. Treatment with diethylcarbamazine is effective.

Meyers, W. M., Connor, D. H., Harman, L. E., Fleshman, K., Moris, R. and Neafie, R. G.: Human streptocerciasis: A clinicopathologic study of 40 Africans (Zairans), including identification of the adult filaria. Am. J. Trop. Med. Hyg., 21:528, 1972.

DIROFILARIASIS

Several dirofilariae have been reported to occasionally cause symptoms in man, particularly in the United States. Such infections have also been reported from the Mediterranean basin, South America, and Africa. In Louisiana and Texas a subcutaneous filarid of raccoons (*Dirofilaria tenuis*) occasionally invades man, but does not mature. It produces a painful subcutaneous nodule, consisting of an eosinophilic inflammatory reaction around the worm; this may be a granuloma or may be located in a lymph node. This diagnosis is usually made after biopsy. Mosquitoes transmit the infection.

Other species found in man include *D. conjunctivae*, *D. repens*, and *D. immitis*. Adult worms have been detected in the heart and great vessels and in the eye. They have also caused infarcts in the lung and "coin" lesions at the hila which may be mistaken for a bronchial carcinoma and excised before the nature is known. In sections the worm is seen in cross-section in the center of an infarcted area infiltrated with eosinophils.

Beaver, P. C., and Orihel, T. C.: Human infection with filariae of animals in the United States. Am. J. Trop. Med. Hyg., 14:1010, 1965.

Beskin, C. A., Colvin, S. H., Jr., and Beaver, P. C.: Pulmonary dirofilariasis, cause of a pulmonary nodular disease. JAMA, 198:665, 1966.

POSSIBLE HUMAN MENINGONEMIASIS

Orihel has pointed out that microfilariae recovered from patients with neurologic disorders in Rhodesia and thought to be *Dipetalonema perstans* more closely resemble *Meningonema peruzzii*. The adults of this species inhabit the leptomeninges of the brainstem in African monkeys.

Orihel, T. C.: Cerebral filariasis in Rhodesia — a zoonotic infection. Am. J. Trop. Med. Hyg., 22:596, 1973.

PULMONARY TROPICAL EOSINOPHILIA
(Eosinophilic Lung, Weingarten's Syndrome)

Since the early part of this century Indian physicians have recognized a syndrome of paroxysmal cough and nocturnal bronchospasm associated with high eosinophilia, and have called it pulmonary tropical eosinophilia. Low fever, dyspnea, and malaise may be accompanying symptoms. The absolute eosinophil count is above 3000 per cubic millimeter, and may reach very high levels. Chest films may show increased reticulation, prominence of bronchovascular markings, or diffuse miliary mottling of the lung fields. In Ball's series of 1000 cases the great majority were Indian; the condition is much more common among Indians in Singapore. It is now generally accepted that this syndrome is caused by occult filarial infections. The evidence that this is so can be listed as follows: (1) Patients have a consistently high titer of filarial complement-fixing antibodies in the absence of evidence of microfilariae in the blood. (2) There is a clinical, hematologic, and serologic response to therapy with the antifilarial drug diethylcarbamazine. (3) The syndrome has been produced in a volunteer by inoculation of *Brugia malayi* infective larvae and *Brugia pahangi* (a feline filaria). (4) Microfilariae have been demonstrated in lung granulomas in such cases by several groups of workers.

It is possible that eosinophilic lung results from an alteration in host immunity to the filarial parasite, giving rise to allergic phenomena manifested by persistent hypereosinophilia and pulmonary symptoms. What is not yet settled is the precise identification of the parasite. It is likely that several species of filaria of the genera *Wuchereria* and *Brugia*, some human, some animal, may be involved, depending on the locality in which the syndrome occurs. The high incidence in Indians is noteworthy and may suggest a genetic predisposition in certain racial groups. The course of diethylcarbamazide recommended is similar to that for bancroftian filariasis. Often the symptoms get temporarily worse after starting the drug, but invariably they resolve, and a second course of the drug or the use of carbarsone as an alternative is seldom necessary.

The question of occult filariasis has been reviewed, and it has been pointed out that in many instances it has not been possible to identify the helminth responsible because of the difficulty of interpreting the microfilariae in tissue sections even if they are found. Quite apart from the well defined clinical entity of pulmonary tropical eosinophilia there are patients presenting with signs of reticuloendothelial activation (enlarged lymph nodes, hepatosplenomegaly) and eosinophilia for which it is difficult to find a cause.

Ball, J. D.: Tropical pulmonary eosinophilia. Trans. R. Soc. Trop. Med. Hyg., 44:237, 1950.

Donohugh, D. L.: Tropical eosinophilia, an etiologic enquiry. N. Engl. J. Med., 269:1357, 1963.

Danaraj, T. J., Pacheco, G., Shanmugaratnam, K., and Beaver, P. C.: The etiology and pathology of eosinophilic lung (tropical eosinophilia). Am. J. Trop. Med. Hyg., 15:183, 1966.

Islam, N.: Tropical eosinophilia. East Pakistan, Islam A. Chittagong, 1964.

Lie Kian, J., and Shandosham, A. A.: The pathology of clinical filariasis due to *Wuchereria bancrofti* and *Brugia malayi* and a discussion of occult filariasis. In Shandosham, A. A., and Zaman, V. (eds.): Proceedings of Seminar on Filariasis and Immunology of Parasitic Infections, and Laboratory Meeting. Kuala Lumpur, Malaysia, Rajiv Printers, 1969, p. 125.

DISORDERS WITH SOME RELATION TO HELMINTHS

Philip D. Marsden

215. EOSINOPHILIA IN RELATION TO HELMINTHIC INFECTIONS

Hypereosinophilic states are considered elsewhere in this book, and conditions such as periarteritis nodosa, eosinophilic leukemia, and allergic diseases are discussed in the appropriate chapters. However, the author believes that a number of the cases of unexplained eosinophilia seen today in diagnostic units will in time be explained on the basis of helminthic infections, and it is worthwhile making one or two general points in relation to such infections.

As can be seen from the preceding chapters, almost all helminthic infections in contrast to protozoal infections are at some time or other associated with eosinophilia. In terms of the parasites for which man is the definitive host, the eosinophilia often coincides with the invasive phase of a trematode, cestode, or nematode infection, and the diagnosis may not be apparent until several weeks or months later when the adults begin to produce progeny. For this reason patients with obscure eosinophilia should always be kept under observation, and stool or tissue specimens examined after an interval. Some parasites are notorious in presenting a problem of eosinophilia for diagnosis, notably *Strongyloides* and *Trichinella* infections. After effective treatment of helminthic infections, particularly those in close contact with body tissues, there is often a pronounced rise in circulating eosinophils.

Perhaps more interesting is the clinical situation in which a patient has a significant human helminth load and yet little or no expected eosinophilia in the absence of cortisone therapy. Recent work suggesting that sensitized lymphocytes play an important role in the genesis of eosinophilia may throw some light on this problem.

Eosinophilia is a prominent feature of infections with nonhuman helminths, e.g., *Angiostrongylus*, and situations in which there is an abnormal host response, e.g., pulmonary tropical eosinophilia. It appears that a small number of nonhuman helminths passing through man's tissues may engender marked eosinophilia and even hypergammaglobulinemia, e.g., toxocariasis, gnathostomiasis. To find the helminths responsible is impossible in many patients, and when found they may be very difficult to identify. Our elucidation of this clinical problem appears to rest on the elaboration of more specific and sensitive serologic tests, and the techniques of indirect hemagglutination, gel diffusion, indirect fluorescent antibody tests, and similar procedures are useful here to detect host response to helminthic antigens. However, much difficult work will be needed to characterize these complex antigens.

Finally, in a clinical consideration of this problem, common things occur commonly. A survey of a series of patients with occult eosinophilia in a large teaching hospital in New York City revealed a few cases of strongyloidiasis, but eosinophilia was most frequently one of the signs of a reaction to drug therapy.

Beeson, P. B., and Bass, D. A.: The Eosinophil. Philadelphia, W. B. Saunders Company, 1977.

216. TROPICAL PYOMYOSITIS

This is a condition of a large deep-seated abscess, single or multiple, occurring in any voluntary muscle. Strange lumps for diagnosis in the tropics sometimes turn out to be deep-seated abscesses. By far the most frequent organism isolated is *Staphylococcus aureus*. Histologically there are areas of focal muscle necrosis with inflammatory cell infiltration. The regional lymph nodes are rarely affected, and there may be no fever or leukocytosis in the peripheral blood. The cause is unknown. Subcutaneous helminthic infection, particularly filaria, and sickle cell disease have been suggested as predisposing conditions, but as yet there is no convincing evidence to this effect. Treatment consists of antimicrobial therapy (initially with penicillin) and surgical drainage.

Elebute, E. A.: Pyomyositis. *In* Schwartz, S. I., Adesola, A. O., Elebute, E. A., and Rob, C. G. (eds.): Tropical Surgery, New York, McGraw-Hill Book Company, 1971.
Marcus, R. T., and Foster, W. D.: Observations on the clinical features, aetiology and geographical distribution of pyomyositis in East Africa. East Afr. Med. J., 45:167, 1968.
Tropical myositis. Lancet, 1:862, 1978.

PART XI
DISORDERS OF THE NERVOUS SYSTEM AND BEHAVIOR

217. INTRODUCTION

Fred Plum

The scientific revolution has begun to invade if not yet fully conquer the fields of neurology and psychiatry. The 12 years that have elapsed since I first had the privilege of writing this introductory chapter have spawned pharmacologic treatments for depression and mania, the knowledge of the infectious nature of Creutzfeldt-Jakob disease, the realization that slow or latent viral infections can cause neurologic disease, a specific and rational treatment for parkinsonism, the awareness that myasthenia gravis is an immunologic disorder and can be treated as such, and much of our understanding of how the hypothalamus specifically regulates the pituitary gland. Since the last edition of this textbook appeared, medicine has learned that man's nervous system not only contains specific receptors to which opiates bind to produce their extraordinary effects, but that brain-made endogenous peptides, the enkephalins or endorphins, attach to these natural sites to modify intrinsic sensations and behavior. Also since the last edition, computerized transaxial (CT) scanning has transformed diagnostic neurology, seemingly making obsolete many of the physician's traditional slow and imprecise approaches to the patient.

The aforementioned discoveries have meant marvelous advances in clinical care. Unfortunately, however, new diagnostic machines and new drugs to treat symptoms can sometimes leave untouched many of the complex, human needs of patients, and this can be especially true of individuals with neurologic complaints. The neurologic and psychiatric patient, perhaps more than most, requires a physician who not only sees a symptom or disease but looks beyond that to see who is sick and asks why.

Most diseases express themselves, sooner or later, through nervous system symptoms, and this fact sometimes makes neurology complicated and also places limitations on the information to be gained from the diagnostic machines that neurologists use. Pain, sensory loss, weakness, disturbed thinking, and impaired mood or alertness can reflect a systemic disorder as often as a primary neurologic illness. Perhaps even more frequently, such symptoms derive from man's faulty adjustment to his environment. Unless they specifically remind themselves to do otherwise, physicians educated to respond predominantly to the diagnostic accuracies of blood tests, CT scans, contrast radiographs, electrical nerve and muscle studies, and electroenceph-

alographic tracings may overlook the fact that none of these tests or machines can detect most of the miseries which bring most patients to seek the help of their doctors. Most patients consult physicians because they are afraid — afraid of pain, of cancer, of heart disease, of losing their memories and minds, of humiliation, of loneliness — ultimately, of death. It takes clinical experience and wisdom to separate symptoms born of these fears from complaints which arise from a diseased structure or function. The descriptions and approaches included in Part XI attempt to give the physician a framework for making that separation in patients with neurologic problems.

A word of reassurance may be in order about how to approach the patient with a neurologic complaint or a suspected neurologic lesion. If one is logical, systematic and thorough, the seeming complexities of such patients will be found rapidly to become analyzable. The most reliable approach to neurologic patients lies in the full, thorough, and educated application of clinical method, emphasizing neither the laboratory nor the bedside examination at the expense of the other. A recent analysis of diagnostic accuracy in medical illnesses indicates that a careful history provides 80 per cent of diagnoses and that the laboratory adds no more than another 10 per cent. Obviously, the history, physical examination, and laboratory all offer important confirmations of each other. But all evidence still indicates that a careful history contributes the largest share of neurologic diagnosis even when all the new technical diagnostic procedures are fully utilized. Accurate diagnosis in neurology still depends mainly on the thorough understanding of the pathologic physiology of signs and symptoms.

Part XI is organized in two main categories. The first considers the more general functions of the nervous system: how it is organized, how it handles certain normal activities, and how it expresses psychologic and somatic symptoms in response to either real or symbolic threat or injury. The second takes the more traditional approach, and discusses neurologic diseases according to anatomic and causative categories. Heavy emphasis is placed on the mechanism of disease and, when known, the biochemistry of its treatment.

As the following chapters regrettably illustrate, many neurologic and neuromuscular diseases still lack satisfactory specific treament. Yet this shortcoming should not becloud the principle that much of the practice of medicine directs itself at protecting or recouping brain function, sometimes at the necessary, temporary expense of other organs. Man's brain makes him human.

Damage it and life loses its meaning in direct proportion, no matter what other physiologic benefits may accrue in the process. The brain cannot be regenerated, repaired, or homotransplanted. It accumulates no metabolic debts and, unless supplied continuously by an effective circulation carrying large amounts of oxygen and glucose, it digests itself irreparably. One cannot "let the brain go" while solving other medical problems. If an elderly man with severe anemia suffers an ischemic stroke while awaiting accurate blood studies, there is no satisfaction later in a correct hematologic diagnosis. If an adolescent girl suffers permanent dementia from hypoglycemia while having her diabetes regulated, the perfect control of glycosuria seems hardly worth it. To maintain the integrity of the nervous system remains the first goal in therapeutics.

Section One   CONSCIOUSNESS AND ITS DISTURBANCES

218.   INTRODUCTION

Fred Plum

From the medical standpoint, consciousness includes two interdependent but separate functions, namely, wakefulness and psychologically recognizable mental activity. Dementia, apathy, amnesia, and aphasia are conditions in which the content of consciousness is reduced but, as long as enough appropriate responses remain in other behavioral functions, consciousness is considered to be preserved. Obtundation and drowsiness describe states of impaired alertness or wakefulness, often with an excessive tendency to sleep. Stupor is a state wherein subjects arouse when vigorously stimulated, but immediately sink back again as soon as external stimuli are withdrawn. Coma is complete unresponsiveness with eyes closed and no evidence of psychologically appropriate responses to stimulation.

The present physiologic concept of consciousness is that it depends upon a close functional interaction between the intact cerebral hemispheres and the central gray matter of the upper brainstem. The hemispheres contribute most of the specific components of consciousness, including language, memory, intellect, and learned responses to sensory stimuli. But in order for the cerebrum to function, the organism must be aroused or activated by more caudally placed mechanisms that reside in the thalamus, hypothalamus, midbrain, and upper pons. An important component of this arousal mechanism is located within what Magoun and his colleagues called the ascending reticular activating system; other brainstem systems also influence cerebral cortical activity and the state of consciousness.

The relation of the cerebral cortex to consciousness is more quantitative than qualitative: All hemispheric lesions undoubtedly reduce, at least to some degree, the content of man's consciousness, and the total loss of the cortex causes at least several weeks of coma even if the brainstem is intact. Between the extremes of an injury so small that it is clinically almost undetectable and so large that it causes coma lies a continuum along which the size of the lesion and the impairment of mind, memory, wit, and personality are roughly proportional.

219.   THE PATHOGENESIS OF STUPOR AND COMA

Fred Plum

As noted in Ch. 218, consciousness depends on the integrity of the sum of the physiologic activity of the two cerebral hemispheres and an activating system located in the central core of the upper brainstem. It follows that to produce an alteration of consciousness, a disease or dysfunction must damage or depress either the two hemispheres or the brainstem core or both. A potentially bewildering series of individual maladies can have one or both of these effects, as may be seen in the accompanying table. However, if one examines the mechanisms by which neurologic diseases cause coma, all these maladies fall into three categories that can be distinguished by their signs and symptoms: (1) supratentorial mass lesions, (2) subtentorial compressive or destructive lesions, and (3) metabolic brain diseases.

The Common Causes of Stupor and Coma

Supratentorial lesions (causing upper brainstem dysfunction)
    Cerebral hemorrhage
    Large cerebral infarction
    Subdural hematoma
    Epidural hematoma
    Brain tumor
    Brain abscess (rare)

Subtentorial lesions (compressing or destroying the reticular formation)
    Pontine or cerebellar hemorrhage
    Infarction
    Tumor
    Cerebellar abscess

Metabolic and diffuse lesions (see also Table 1 in Ch. 220)
    Anoxia or ischemia
    Hypoglycemia
    Nutritional deficiency
    Endogenous organ failure or deficiency
    Ionic and electrolyte disorders
    Exogenous poison
    Infections
        Meningitis
        Encephalitis
    Concussion and postictal states

SUPRATENTORIAL MASS LESIONS

Supratentorial masses are rarely so large that they produce coma by directly destroying or replacing the cerebral hemispheres. Rather, they interfere with consciousness because they shift and squeeze the contents of the supratentorial compartment and, in so doing, compress the diencephalon. The expanding process can originate anywhere in the hemisphere and ultimately produce this reaction because the fibrous tentorium and the bones of the base of the skull resist movement except toward the tentorial opening. As a result, when supratentorial masses demand room for expansion, the diencephalic tectum and adjacent midbrain are likely to be compressed, and the diencephalon may be displaced downward through the tentorial notch (transtentorial herniation).

How do supratentorial masses progress so that these reactions occur? The brain has certain common responses to injury, including edema, vascular dilatation, and the invasion of leukocytes and proliferation of glial cells. The intensity, tempo, and exact contribution of each of these responses varies according to the nature of the original lesion and the rate at which it appears, but each shares in the brain's defenses against neoplasms, infections, infarcts, and irritants. Thus the original lesion gradually enlarges and, ripple-like, tends to impair structures ever more remote from itself in the inexpansible intracranial cavity. The remote effects are due partly to edema spreading away from the edges of the primary lesion and partly to an actual shift of the brain within the skull, compressing normal tissues and blood vessels against rigid structures such as the falx cerebri and the tentorium. At this stage, clinical signs of increased intracranial pressure are common and imply that an intracranial lesion is already exerting generalized deleterious effects.

The clinical picture of supratentorial mass lesions producing stupor or coma has several distinctive features. If a history is available, localizing symptoms such as frontal headache, focal seizures, or other changes consistent with hemispheric disease will usually be found to have preceded unconsciousness. Physically, most patients demonstrate a combination of *focal* hemispheral signs, e.g., sensorimotor defect, aphasia, and visual field defect, reflecting the site of the original pathologic process, plus *diffuse* signs of supratentorial dysfunction, indicating that the lesion is exerting remote effects on the opposite hemisphere and the deep diencephalon. An important negative finding is that, unless the patient is in the terminal stages of illness, no evidence of direct subtentorial brainstem dysfunction can be found: pupillary and oculovestibular reflexes remain intact. As a supratentorial lesion progresses, the neurologic signs and symptoms evolve in a characteristic, orderly, rostral-caudal pattern. The more rostrally located neurologic functions first disappear, followed by more caudal impairment, first in the diencephalon and then down the brainstem almost as if the structures were being progressively transected from above downward, each plane of function being removed almost completely before the next is impaired.

The aforementioned description needs amplification to be complete. Some supratentorial masses begin and enlarge in neurologically silent areas such as the frontal lobes or the subdural space and lack a focal signature.

Lesions of this type may be revealed only when the patient develops signs of diffuse forebrain dysfunction plus, perhaps, headache and evidence of increased intracranial pressure.

Stupor or coma with supratentorial lesions is ominous because it implies that the deeply located upper brainstem is already compressed or distorted and that the much more serious complication of herniation of the forebrain downward into the tentorial notch is about to occur. Such herniation begins either with direct downward displacement of the diencephalon (central herniation) or with the uncus of the temporal lobe squeezing into the tentorial notch and against the midbrain (uncal herniation). Either way, if the hernia develops fully, it usually impacts itself upon the midbrain and nearly always results in permanent brain damage or death. A characteristic constellation of symptoms heralds each of these patterns of transtentorial herniation. With impending *central* herniation, stupor becomes gradually deeper, and the subjects sigh, yawn, or develop periodic respirations. The pupils shrink to 1 to 2 mm in diameter, but retain their light reflexes. Oculovestibular reflexes are brisk, and the extremities stiffen into bilateral rigidity or spasticity, combined with extensor plantar responses. With *uncal* herniation, signs are in many ways similar to the above except that as the uncus slides over the tentorial edge, it often compresses the third nerve ahead of it, even before the diencephalon is squeezed. The result is that the pupil on the side of the herniation begins to dilate more than its fellow. Eventually, the pupil dilates widely and becomes light-fixed, and the patient becomes stuporous. Shortly afterward, oculomotor functions of the third nerve are usually impaired, and the involved eye turns outward. If the herniating process continues, the opposite third nerve becomes involved as well, and then the brainstem. To initiate effective treatment one must recognize the process before this advanced stage and halt it with osmotic decompressing agents or surgical treatment. Otherwise, when conditions progress this far, few subjects recover without substantial, permanent neurologic injury.

SUBTENTORIAL MASS OR DESTRUCTIVE LESIONS

These conditions cause stupor or coma if they destroy or compress the centrally located activating systems in the brainstem anywhere above approximately the midpons. Expanding lesions of the posterior fossa have the same effect if they compress the midbrain upward. Compression against the medulla oblongata with an ensuing cerebellar pressure cone produces stiff neck, along with respiratory and cardiac irregularities, but does not directly cause loss of consciousness.

The characteristic clinical feature of subtentorial destruction or compression causing coma is the presence of restricted and usually asymmetrical signs of focal brainstem dysfunction, which frequently can be anatomically pinpointed to a single locus by the clinical findings. Seldom do the signs indicate complete brainstem transection. This restricted, discrete localization is unlike metabolic lesions causing coma in which the signs commonly indicate incomplete dysfunction at several different levels of the brain, and also is unlike the secondary brainstem dysfunction and coma that follow supratentorial herniation, in which *all* function at any given level tends to be lost as the process progresses from rostral to caudal along the neuraxis.

Purely compressive lesions of the posterior fossa rarely cause coma until late in their course when the patient is near death. The pathologic process involved is usually a hemorrhage, abscess, or tumor of the cerebellum or fourth ventricle. As a result, occipital headache, nystagmus, diplopia, nausea, vomiting, cranial nerve signs, and ataxia usually precede unconsciousness. Important points in distinguishing both destructive and compressive posterior fossa lesions from metabolic depression of the brainstem are that in metabolic depression oculovestibular responses are generally preserved until the advanced stages, and pupillary light reflexes are nearly always preserved. By contrast, structural brainstem lesions causing coma always disrupt the oculovestibular responses, and those involving the midbrain also interrupt the pupillary reflexes.

METABOLIC DEPRESSION OF THE BRAIN CAUSING COMA

Primary metabolic encephalopathies are intrinsic to the neuron, the glial cell, or the white matter, respectively. They often produce dementia, but rarely cause coma except terminally. *Secondary* metabolic encephalopathies are those in which brain function is disrupted either because the brain is not supplied with a required substance, e.g., thiamine, oxygen, or glucose, or because it is poisoned by an ingested or endogenous toxin, e.g., depressant drugs or the products of uremia. The secondary metabolic encephalopathies are frequent causes of delirium as well as of stupor and coma; their relationship to the normal metabolism of the brain is discussed in detail in Ch. 220.

Experimental evidence conflicts as to whether most metabolic agents causing coma depress mainly the brainstem reticular formation or the cerebral cortex. Clinically, most patients with metabolic encephalopathy appear to suffer depression of the forebrain more than of the brainstem. The remarkable finding with most metabolic encephalopathies, however, is the uneven degree to which they affect different parts of the brain without regard for simple anatomic levels. Thus metabolic encephalopathy characteristically depresses certain susceptible functions at several different brain levels, but at the same time spares other functions that emanate from identical levels. For example, nearly all metabolic poisons spare the pupillary light reflex so that reactive pupils persist into the deepest stages of metabolic coma until asphyxia intervenes. (Poisoning with glutethimide or parasympathomimetics provides the only exception to this rule, both drugs blocking the light reflex in large, coma-causing doses.) Most of the metabolic encephalopathies cause delirium before stupor or coma, and many of them are accompanied in their early stages by asterixis, a flapping irregular tremor of the outstretched hands, or by random myoclonic muscle twitches. Although the metabolic encephalopathies occasionally produce asymmetrical motor signs, they more characteristically impair body movement symmetrically, and they never impair central sensory pathways except as an accompaniment to the over-all depression of the sensorium.

To epitomize, diseases causing stupor or coma fall into three categories:

1. Supratentorial mass lesions present with asymmetrical neurologic signs of hemispheral dysfunction combined with evidence of intact subtentorial brainstem function. As supratentorial lesions evolve, the signs indicate progressive rostral-caudal neurologic deterioration, almost as if the brain were being serially sectioned from top to bottom.

2. Subtentorial compressive and destructive lesions present from the outset with either cranial nerve abnormalities or other focal brainstem signs, including pupillary and oculovestibular reflex abnormalities. Long tract motor signs are usually present and asymmetrical.

3. Metabolic brain diseases present a picture of either diffuse cortical depression or, more often, of impaired function in both the hemispheres and the brainstem accompanied by retained pupillary light reflexes. The multifocal distribution of metabolic encephalopathy is usually symmetrical and not accompanied by sensory impairments.

APPROACH TO THE PATIENT IN STUPOR OR COMA

The physician must ensure that the brain and other vital organs receive no further injury while he obtains whatever history, examinations, and laboratory data are required. Before anything else he must provide a free and open airway and determine that the subject is breathing deeply enough to oxygenate his lungs and eliminate carbon dioxide. Next, the heart and blood pressure should be examined, and possible sources of bleeding checked to be certain that cardiac output and blood volume are sufficient to supply the metabolic needs of the brain and kidney. In all patients in coma an intravenous infusion or central venous pressure line should be started, using a large-bore needle. Blood samples for typing and cross-matching, as well as for other appropriate laboratory determinations, can be obtained at this time. Whenever the cause of coma is doubtful, and particularly when the clinical signs suggest a metabolic disorder, blood should be taken for sugar determination, and then 50 ml of 50 per cent glucose given intravenously. Hypoglycemic encephalopathy can take many forms, some of which mimic other diseases. If glucose is given promptly, no further cerebral damage occurs while the doctor awaits definitive laboratory diagnosis. Intravenous sugar harms nothing if the coma has another cause.

Beyond these immediate, lifesaving measures, it requires considerable restraint to approach a patient in a coma methodically, for the urge to act without delay is understandably strong but potentially dangerous. Inquiry into both the past medical history and the circumstances under which the patient lost consciousness generally discloses more of diagnostic value than any other maneuver. Is there any suggestion that head trauma could have occurred recently? Has there been renal, hepatic, or myocardial disease? Could a seizure have preceded the present unconsciousness? Has the subject been taking insulin? Have there been recent changes in mood, behavior, or neurologic function to suggest an evolving intracranial process? Was the subject "blue," depressed, or moody, and did he have access to depressant drugs? Is he a "spree" drinker? These and other questions must be covered comprehensively with relatives, past physicians, friends, police, or ambulance personnel.

One must perform both a meticulous neurologic examination and a thoughtful physical review of every body system, because disease in remote organs often causes or accentuates dysfunction in the brain.

Fever implies infection, inflammation, or neoplasm. On the other hand, hypothermia (30 to 36° C) in a patient not severely exposed to cold suggests depressant drug poisoning, hypoglycemia, or severe lower brainstem injury, as by infarction. Hypertension may be the cause of hypertensive encephalopathy or the underlying cause of cerebral hemorrhage. Conversely, an elevated blood pressure can be a symptom of subarachnoid hemorrhage in a subject not previously hypertensive. Hypotension in a supine patient implies low blood volume (hemorrhagic or traumatic shock; severe nutritional and fluid depletion), low cardiac output (myocardial infarction), or low peripheral resistance (depressant drug poisoning). Tachycardia (over 160 per minute) can mean that unconsciousness is the result of lowered cardiac output from a supraventricular cardiac arrhythmia. Bradycardia suggests heart block and the Adams-Stokes syndrome or a myocardial infarct.

The pattern and depth of respiration are often informative in evaluating both neurologic function and acid-base balance, so much so that the evaluation of breathing is discussed more fully in Ch. 220.

The skin should be searched for petechiae (thrombocytopenic or nonthrombocytopenic purpura, meningococcemia, and bacterial endocarditis), bruises, evidence of nutritional deficiency, icterus, angiomatous spiders, and the bright pinkness of carbon monoxide poisoning. Fleshy or clubbed fingertips suggest carcinoma of the lung, or, less often, lung abscess or congenital heart disease (with brain embolism or abscess). A meticulous examination of the optic fundi is imperative but should be completed without cycloplegics, the use of which destroys the potential diagnostic value of pupillary reactions in coma. In the fundus oculi, the pathologic changes of many diseases causing coma can be viewed directly: increased intracranial pressure, hypertensive vascular disease, diabetes, blood dyscrasia, tuberculosis, sarcoidosis, bacterial endocarditis, cryptococcosis, collagen vascular disease, and even subarachnoid hemorrhage producing subhyaloid bleeding.

Chest examination has two potentially rewarding findings: cardiac murmurs suggest bacterial endocarditis with consequent focal, embolic encephalitis; the wheezes and obstructive sounds of the pulmonary cripple suggest CO_2 retention causing narcosis. In the abdominal examination, the presence of masses suggesting polycystic kidneys increases the chances that subarachnoid hemorrhage has occurred, whereas liver enlargement (hepatic coma is common with hepatomas) or splenic enlargement (both blood dyscrasias and infectious mononucleosis can cause encephalitis-like illnesses) can provide valuable leads.

During the neurologic examination, certain potentially informative steps are sometimes overlooked. The skull should always be palpated and inspected meticulously. Edema of the scalp commonly overlies fresh fracture lines, and basal skull fractures predispose to blood pigment stains behind the ear (Battle's sign) and about the orbit (raccoon eyes). Blood also may escape from basal fractures into the ear canals, the middle ears, or the nostrils. The skull should be percussed, because focal or unilateral skull tenderness, manifested by grimacing or withdrawal in a stuporous subject, often overlies an intracranial mass lesion. The neck should be tested carefully: stiff neck can reflect meningitis, cerebellar tonsillar herniation or, occasionally, simply skeletal muscle spasticity. The stiff neck of acute bacterial meningitis is rarely equivocal; that of impending herniation is commonly less severe and lacks accompanying signs of infection or a prominent Kernig sign. It usually requires several hours or a day or more for stiff neck to develop after subarachnoid bleeding.

It is useful to watch the unconscious patient for a time, observing whether or not the extremities move equally and whether tremor, myoclonus, or single or repetitive seizures involve any part of the body. Status epilepticus with focal continuous epilepsy is not uncommon, but is often overlooked.

Laboratory Examination of the Patient in Coma

Patients should be subjected to a skull roentgenogram (looking for fracture lines, densities, and pineal shifts), a blood count and smear, and a urinalysis. When the clinical findings are consistent with metabolic encephalopathy but the cause is uncertain, the blood glucose and serum sodium, potassium, and bicarbonate should be obtained promptly. Knowledge of the arterial pH greatly helps diagnosis in metabolic coma (see Table 3 in Ch. 220).

When to do a lumbar puncture is always a serious question. All physicians are aware that in patients with increased intracranial pressure the procedure sometimes induces fatal herniation of the brain through the tentorium or foramen magnum. For this reason, lumbar puncture is best avoided if the physician strongly suspects his patient of having an expanding intracranial mass, particularly in the posterior fossa. Such forbearance is particularly advisable when CT scanning is immediately available. There are certain treatable diseases such as meningitis, however, that can be diagnosed only by lumbar puncture, and many others in which the procedure yields valuable preliminary diagnostic information. When the advice of neurologic specialists is unavailable, the doctor has no choice but to proceed with lumbar puncture if the diagnosis is in doubt and he believes the procedure has a reasonable chance of offering valuable information. Certain steps minimize the risk. One is to use a small (No. 20), sharp needle. Another is to fill the manometer with saline and attach it to the needle before releasing fluid, a technique that prevents sudden subarachnoid pressure shifts. Jugular manometrics should *never* be performed, for they offer little useful data and increase the risk of impacting potential intracranial herniations.

Magoun, H. W.: The Waking Brain. 2nd ed. Springfield, Ill., Charles C Thomas, 1963.

Plum, F., and Posner, J. B.: The Diagnosis of Stupor and Coma. 2nd ed. Philadelphia, F. A. Davis Company, 1972.

220. DELIRIUM AND EXOGENOUS METABOLIC BRAIN DISEASE

Jerome B. Posner

INTRODUCTION

There are few situations in clinical medicine that confuse and distress the physician so much as when he confronts a patient whose state of consciousness is rapidly deteriorating. The physician's task in such a situation is both enormous and exacting. First he must decide which of three major categories of disease is responsible for the patient's condition: (1) structural brain disease (e.g., brain tumors, subdural hematomas, cerebral infarctions); (2) "functional" brain disease (e.g., schizophrenia, manic-depressive psychosis); or (3) metabolic brain disease or delirium (see definitions below). If the patient's disorder falls into one of the first two categories (discussed elsewhere in this book), the physician can obtain help from highly skilled specialists in those areas (neurologists, neurosurgeons, or psychiatrists). If the patient's behavioral change is due to metabolic brain disease, the general physician must then determine himself which of a bewildering variety of metabolic defects is responsible (Table 1) and must rapidly begin treatment to assure that the metabolic defect does not produce irreversible brain damage. While he is carrying out these exacting tasks, he is often impeded by the fact that the patient is noisy, obstre-

TABLE 1.   Causes of Metabolic Brain Disease

I. Deprivation of oxygen, substrate, or metabolic cofactors
   *A. Hypoxia (interference with oxygen supply to the entire brain—cerebral blood flow normal)
      1. Decreased oxygen tension and content of blood
         Pulmonary disease
         Alveolar hypoventilation
         Decreased atmospheric oxygen tension
      2. Decreased oxygen content of blood—normal tension
         Anemia
         Carbon monoxide poisoning
         Methemoglobinemia
   *B. Ischemia (diffuse or widespread multifocal interference with blood supply to brain)
      1. Decreased cerebral blood flow resulting from decreased cardiac output
         Stokes-Adams syndrome, cardiac arrest, cardiac arrhythmias
         Myocardial infarction
         Congestive heart failure
         Aortic stenosis
         Pulmonary embolus
      2. Decreased cerebral blood flow resulting from decreased peripheral resistance in systemic circulation
         Syncope: orthostatic, vasovagal
         Carotid sinus hypersensitivity
         Low blood volume
      3. Decreased cerebral blood flow due to generalized increase in cerebrovascular resistance
         Hyperventilation syndrome
         Increased blood viscosity (polycythemia), cryo- and macroglobinemia
      4. Decreased local cerebral blood flow due to widespread small vessel occlusion
         Disseminated intravascular coagulation
         Systemic lupus erythematosus
         Subacute bacterial endocarditis
         Cardiopulmonary bypass
      5. Alterations of blood flow due to failure of autoregulation
         Hypertensive encephalopathy
   *C. Hypoglycemia
         Resulting from exogenous insulin
         Spontaneous (endogenous insulin, liver disease, etc.)
   D. Cofactor deficiency
         Thiamin (Wernicke's encephalopathy)
         Niacin
         Pyridoxine
         B_{12}
         Folate

II. Diseases of organs other than brain
   *A. Diseases of nonendocrine organs
         Liver (hepatic coma)
         Kidney (uremic coma)
         Lung (CO_2 narcosis)
   *B. Hyper- and/or hypofunction of endocrine organs
         Pituitary

         Thyroid (myxedema-thyrotoxicosis)
         Parathyroid (hyper- and hypoparathyroidism)
         Adrenal (Addison's disease, Cushing's disease, pheochromocytoma)
         Pancreas (diabetes, hypoglycemia)
   C. Other systemic diseases
         Diabetes
         Cancer
         Porphyria
         Sepsis
         Fever

III. Exogenous poisons
   *A. Sedative drugs
   B. Acid poisons or poisons with acidic breakdown products
         Paraldehyde
         Methyl alcohol
         Ethylene glycol
   C. Other enzyme inhibitors
         Heavy metals
         Organic phosphates
         Cyanide
         Salicylates
   D. Psychotropic drugs
         Tricyclic antidepressants and anticholinergic drugs
         Amphetamines
         Lithium
         Phenothiazines
         LSD-mescaline
         Monoamine oxidase inhibitors
   E. Others
         Penicillin
         Anticonvulsants
         Steroids
         Cardiac glycosides

IV. Diseases producing toxins or enzyme inhibition in CNS
   A. Meningitis
   B. Encephalitis
   C. Subarachnoid hemorrhage

V. Abnormalities of fluid, ionic or acid-base environment of CNS
   A. Water and sodium (hyper- and hyponatremia) (hypo- and hyperosmolality)
   B. Acidosis (metabolic and respiratory)
   C. Alkalosis (metabolic and respiratory)
   D. Magnesium (hyper- and hypomagnesemia)
   E. Calcium (hyper- and hypocalcemia)
   F. ? Trace metal deficiency or excess

VI. Miscellaneous diseases of unknown cause
   A. Seizures and postictal states
   *B. "Postoperative" delirium
   C. Concussion
   *D. "Sensory deprivation"
   E. Drug withdrawal states

*Alone or in combination, the most common causes of delirium seen on medical or surgical wards.

perous, and uncooperative, and by his own knowledge that appropriate treatment is essential and inappropriate treatment (e.g., injudicious use of sedative drugs in patients with incipient respiratory failure) potentially deleterious or even fatal. To deal with metabolic brain disease, the physician must understand some pathophysiologic aspects of cerebral metabolism and must undertake a systematic and thorough physical and laboratory examination of the patient.

DEFINITIONS

Metabolic encephalopathy is a term applied to the behavioral changes which result from diffuse or widespread multifocal failure of cerebral metabolism. When the cerebral disorder arises from an intrinsic failure of neuronal or glial metabolism, it is referred to as *primary or endogenous encephalopathy*. The primary disorders usually begin insidiously, progress inexorably, and produce a clinical picture of dementia, as discussed in Ch. 226 to 231. When the encephalopathy results from interference with brain metabolism by extracerebral disease, it is called *secondary or exogenous metabolic encephalopathy*. The secondary encephalopathies usually begin acutely or subacutely and often subside with time and/or treatment. They produce a clinical picture in which confusion, thinking errors, behavioral abnormalities, disorders of consciousness, and abnormal motor activity predominate. The causes of secondary metabolic encephalopathy are as many and varied as the illnesses that disturb body chemistry. Some causes of metabolic encephalopathy are listed in Table 1.

In some instances, the distinction, both clinically and pathophysiologically, between primary and secondary metabolic encephalopathies is blurred. For example, both vitamin B_{12} deficiency and hypothyroidism interfere with brain metabolism, causing an exogenous metabolic encephalopathy. The usual clinical findings in these disorders, however, resemble dementia (see definition below) rather than delirium, although on occasion either can produce a subacute delirium. The brain dysfunction is reversible by appropriate treatment in each of these disorders, and in this respect both resemble exogenous encephalopathy rather than endogenous encephalopathy. On the other hand, some primary disorders of the central nervous system, such as encephalitis, meningitis, concussion, and seizure disorders, appear acutely, are reversible with appropriate treatment, and clinically resemble delirium rather than dementia. For this reason, these disorders are grouped with the secondary metabolic encephalopathies in Table 1.

Metabolic brain disease is common and often misdiagnosed. When mild, it produces intellectual dullness, social indifference, and vague perplexity easily mistaken by observers for psychogenic depression or simply low intelligence. More severe encephalopathy elicits either a florid picture of tremulous agitation, rich and frightening hallucinations, and periods of seemingly complete loss of contact with the environment, or a more quiet, withdrawn, akinetic state which may fade into stupor or coma. The former, often called *delirium* or *toxic psychosis*, may be confused with a functional psychosis, and the latter, often called *acute* or *subacute confusional state*, is likely to be mistaken for structural brain disease. Although certain specific systemic disorders characteristically cause one or another

of the aforementioned syndromes, each can occur with any of the metabolic brain diseases; thus the terms "delirium," "toxic psychosis," and "confusional state" are used interchangeably in this chapter to describe the wakeful stage of metabolic encephalopathy. A patient who is drowsy but can be coaxed to respond to verbal stimuli is *obtunded*. When he no longer responds to verbal stimuli but responds appropriately to noxious cutaneous stimuli, he is *stuporous*. If he does not respond appropriately to noxious stimuli, he is *comatose*.

The term *dementia* is used operationally to describe an irreversible loss of memory and cognitive functions, usually insidious in onset, irreversible, and often, but not always, due to intrinsic disease of the brain. Demented patients usually do not have the clouding of consciousness associated with delirium. However, an insidiously developing, quiet delirium may be clinically indistinguishable from the early stages of dementia.

SOME PATHOPHYSIOLOGIC ASPECTS OF METABOLIC BRAIN DISEASE

Pathologic changes in metabolic brain disease depend upon the nature and severity of the illness. The brains of some patients delirious during life are entirely normal at postmortem examination. In some cases, however, at least microscopic pathologic changes can be identified if the process causing delirium has lasted for some hours or days prior to death. The pathologic changes, if present, are bilateral, symmetrical, and usually diffusely or multifocally distributed in the cerebral hemispheres. Lesions may be present in the neurons, the glial cells, or the white matter, depending on the nature of the primary illness.

Perhaps the most common pathologic cerebral changes are observed after anoxia, ischemia, or hypoglycemia. The mildest abnormalities are visible only microscopically and consist of "microvacuoles" in neuronal cytoplasm of neocortex and hippocampus. The microvacuoles are swollen mitochondria, and this change is probably reversible. With more severe insults there is dissolution of the Nissl granules (particles of ribonucleic acid) and generalized pallor of staining. Finally, the nuclei shrink and become hyperchromatic, and irregular basophilic rings and granules appear in the swollen cytoplasm. These changes are not reversible. After severe and prolonged insults, all neurons in the cerebral cortex may disappear, and the third layer of the cortex may completely degenerate so that the naked eye detects a thin line of spongy necrosis (laminar necrosis). Anoxic changes also affect the basal ganglia to cause grossly visible focal necrosis of the globus pallidus. Occasionally, there may be diffuse demyelination of the subcortical white matter. Characteristically, the brainstem and spinal cord are spared unless the process has been overwhelmingly severe.

A nonspecific but common pathologic change in patients who have died with uremia, hyponatremia, diabetic coma, or CO_2 narcosis is cerebral swelling, recognized grossly by flattened gyri, narrowed sulci, and small ventricles. Microscopically, large perivascular and perineuronal spaces attest to the presence of edema.

Unusual glial cells with ballooned, lobulated nuclei are found in the cortex and basal ganglia of patients who die in hepatic coma, and are relatively specific for this disorder. Widespread perivascular "cuffs" of lymphocytes or polymorphonuclear leukocytes indicate an inflammatory lesion of the brain and meninges from viral or bacterial invasion.

In most cases of metabolic brain disease, the cerebral oxygen uptake declines in rough proportion to the degree of brain dysfunction observed clinically. So far, we understand in only a few instances how systemic illnesses interfere with cerebral metabolism, but these few serve as models to suggest the possible mechanisms for the others. The following material outlines some of our knowledge of normal and abnormal cerebral metabolism.

GLUCOSE. Glucose is the brain's only substrate under physiologic conditions, and is transferred across the blood-brain barrier by facilitated transport. Other substances can serve as substrates of brain in extraordinary circumstances (e.g., ketone bodies during starvation). Under normal circumstances, each 100 grams of brain utilizes about 31 μmol (5.5 mg) of glucose per minute, which represents almost the body's entire basal glucose consumption. Under aerobic conditions, 85 per cent of brain glucose uptake is oxidized to form CO_2, water, and energy; the remainder is probably accounted for by production of lactate, pyruvate, and other intermediates of glucose metabolism, and by synthesis of some chemicals. Under anaerobic conditions, lactic acid is the end product of glucose metabolism, but the energy so produced is insufficient to maintain neuronal function. There are about 2 grams of reserve glucose (as such and as glycogen) in the brain, an amount that allows the brain of a hypoglycemic patient to survive (although not to function at a normal metabolic rate) for about 90 minutes without suffering irreversible damage. The blood glucose concentration at which cerebral metabolism fails and clinical symptoms develop is variable from patient to patient, but, in general, levels below 30 mg per 100 ml cause confusion, and below 10 to 15 mg per 100 ml, coma.

OXYGEN. Oxygen, the other substance vital for normal cerebral function, is not stored by the brain, and a few seconds of anoxia is sufficient to cause coma. After a variable period of time, usually minutes, both hypoxia and ischemia cause irreversible neuronal damage. The normal brain consumes about 156 μmol (3.5 ml) of oxygen per 100 grams per minute and produces an equal amount of carbon dioxide (R.Q. = 1). Cerebral oxygen consumption represents about 20 per cent of the total body oxygen consumption at rest and is remarkably constant in normal man, whether awake or sleeping. However, significant deviations in oxygen consumption occur with brain dysfunction. For example, seizures increase the brain's demand for oxygen and usually are associated with an increased cerebral blood flow and oxygen uptake. Sedative drugs decrease the brain's metabolic demands; an overdose is usually associated with decreased blood flow and oxygen uptake. Clinically, delirium usually accompanies oxygen uptakes below 2.5 ml and when the uptake falls below 2.0 ml per 100 grams per minute, most patients are unconscious. The degree of hypoxia necessary to cause clinical symptoms depends not only on the blood oxygen tension but also on hemoglobin concentration, cerebral blood flow, and serum pH. In general, Pa_{O_2} values below 50 mm Hg cause delirium, and below 25 mm Hg, coma.

Blood brings both glucose and oxygen to the brain. Under resting conditions, each 100 grams of the brain receives 55 ml of blood each minute; the total brain blood flow of 800 ml per minute is about 15 per cent of the cardiac output. If the flow falls, the brain compensates by extracting more oxygen and more glucose from the blood it receives. Increased extraction of oxygen maintains normal metabolism in the face of a decreased cerebral blood flow up to the point where so much oxygen has been extracted that the oxygen tension of the brain's venous blood falls to about 20 mm of mercury (a level at which hemoglobin is about 35 per cent saturated). At this point, which is reached when cerebral blood flow falls to about half of normal, the oxygen tension is too low to maintain normal metabolism, and the patient loses consciousness. With hemoglobin concentrations below about 8 grams per 100 ml, cerebral blood flow must increase to assure an adequate oxygen supply. Profound anemia thus becomes a potential contributor to cerebral hypoxia.

OTHER SUBSTANCES. In addition to glucose and oxygen, the brain requires other substances (e.g., enzymes, vitamins, amino acids, electrolytes) to maintain metabolism, synthesize transmitter substances, preserve cellular structure, and maintain membrane potentials. Abnormalities of any of these essential substances lead to metabolic brain disease. The unique function of nervous tissue is to transmit electrical impulses, both within cells and by synaptic transmission between cells. The integrity of intracellular transmission depends not only on energy from oxidative metabolism (to maintain the sodium pump) but also on finely controlled intra- and extracellular electrolyte balance. Thus, for example, alterations of extracellular sodium, an ion necessary for propagation of the action potential, produce behavioral changes and delirium. Lithium, a cation with properties similar to both sodium and potassium, changes behavior in manic patients and, in overdose, can lead to severe delirium and coma. The integrity of intercellular transmission is regulated by the synthesis, release, re-uptake, and breakdown of transmitter substances and by maintenance of postsynaptic transmitter receptor sites. Several substances have been identified as putative transmitters in the nervous system, including norepinephrine, dopamine, serotonin, acetylcholine, and amino acids, especially glycine, gamma-aminobutyric acid, and glutamic acid. Most psychotropic drugs are believed to exert their behavioral effects by altering the activity of biogenic amines in the central nervous system, and in overdose most of these drugs produce delirium and sometimes coma. By the same token, severe alterations in amino acid metabolism lead to delirium. Interference with transmitter function may occur when the synthesis, breakdown, or release of the transmitter is inhibited, or when a foreign substance having a structure similar to the transmitter competes for sites on the postsynaptic receptor. Such a "false transmitter" may be the mechanism by which hallucinogenic drugs act, and may also be responsible for the production of "hepatic coma." However, despite these considerations, in no instance is the exact mechanism of delirium in either electrolyte or putative transmitter abnormalities clearly understood.

The biochemical common denominator of metabolic brain disease is decreased oxygen uptake: Is there an anatomic common denominator? Two concepts have arisen delineating a principal locus of metabolic brain disease. One is that the neurons of the cerebral cortex are affected first and, as the process becomes more severe, subcortical structures are affected from the rostral end downward, the phylogenetically oldest and most caudal structures resisting most strongly. This view is supported by the pathologic distribution of cerebral anoxic and hypoglycemic changes and by physiologic studies of hypoglycemic animals in which abnormal electrical activity was recorded from the cortex before it appeared in the hypothalamus.

The second concept is that the neurons of the brainstem reticular formation are the most susceptible to metabolic change and, at least at first, the cortical neurons cease to function only because they lose their reticular stimulation. This concept is supported by physiologic experiments on animals, demonstrating that moderate degrees of hypoxia, hypoglycemia, anesthesia, and cyanide poisoning all block electrical conduction through the reticular formation before they block the ability of cortical neurons to receive messages via other afferent pathways (the lemniscal system).

Neither of these experimental concepts fully explains the several human disease states in which metabolic lesions clinically affect several different levels of the neuraxis simultaneously, with the major locus of early dysfunction differing not only from patient to patient but sometimes from one attack to the next in the same patient. This phenomenon is exemplified by the varied picture of hypoglycemia: Some patients first suffer loss of consciousness and have bilaterally synchronous slow waves in the EEG, suggesting an initial reticular involvement. Others first experience restricted cerebral motor or sensory signs unaccompanied by either EEG abnormalities or impaired consciousness. Still other patients convulse with one attack of hypoglycemia but suffer only quiet coma in the next. It appears that in the clinical situation, regional factors such as blood flow and energy requirements must vary from moment to moment to predispose first one part of the brain and then another to metabolic insult.

CLINICAL FEATURES OF METABOLIC BRAIN DISEASE

The purpose of the physical and laboratory examination in a patient with suspected metabolic brain disease is twofold: first, to determine if the observed changes in consciousness are due to metabolic brain disease (i.e., to rule out structural brain disease or psychiatric dysfunction); and second, to determine exactly the type of metabolic defect causing the delirium. In general, evaluation of the state of consciousness, motor activity, and autonomic activity, as detailed below, helps to answer the first question, whereas the general physical examination, examination of ventilation, and laboratory examination (the latter two detailed below) help to answer the second question. It cannot, however, be overemphasized that, despite the difficulties of examining a delirious patient, a thorough and systematic general physical, neurologic, and laboratory examination *must* be undertaken if a definitive diagnosis is to be established and definitive treatment to be applied. Some principles of the examination are outlined in Table 2.

STATE OF CONSCIOUSNESS AND MENTAL CONTENT. Mental changes are the earliest and most subtle sign of metabolic brain disease. Restlessness or lethargy, emotional lability, insomnia or drowsiness, and vivid nightmares may appear before other mental changes. Patients often appear fearful and anxious, or depressed, and may express the fear that they are "going crazy." They may be restless, irritable, and easily distracted. Conversely, they may lie quietly or sleep when left alone, and rarely read or tend to the world around them. With more severe metabolic disturbances, patients become drowsy and finally stuporous or comatose. The particular affect that prevails in patients with metabolic encephalopathy depends partly on the nature of the illness and partly on the rapidity of its development; previous personality often has surprisingly little influence. Thus, barbiturate- or alcohol-withdrawal syndromes, acute liver necrosis, and porphyria often cause an agitated delirium, whereas uremia, pulmonary encephalopathy, and anoxia usually produce a more quiet illness. Rapidly developing metabolic abnormalities are more likely to produce agitated delirium than those that develop more slowly.

Disturbances in cognition appear along with altered alertness and awareness and are characterized by difficulties with immediate recall and the ability to abstract. Normal subjects readily recall and repeat 6 or 7 digits forward and 5 or 6 backward and can identify the common denominator between such pairs as an apple and an orange or a fly and a tree, but delirious patients cannot. However, innate intelligence and education also determine cognitive abilities and, unless the physician has examined the patient previously, it is difficult to attribute mild disturbances to a metabolic defect. An early sign of delirium, although usually not as early a sign as altered alertness and cognition, is impairment of memory and orientation. Loss of memory for recent events is a hallmark of metabolic and other organic brain disease and is tested by asking the patient about the names of his doctors, some important current events, and his recent activities. Orientation to place

TABLE 2. Physical Examination of Patients with Suspected Metabolic Brain Disease

History (from relatives or friends)
    Previous medical illnesses (diabetes, uremia, heart disease)
    Previous psychiatric history
    Access to drugs (sedative, psychotropic drugs)
    Recent complaints (headache, depression)

General physical examination
    Evidence of trauma
    Evidence of chronic or acute systemic illness
    Ventilation

Neurologic examination
    Mental status
        Affect (agitated, depressed, apathetic)
        Alertness (delirium, obtundation, stupor, coma)
        Memory (recent events, recall of objects)
        Orientation (time, place, person)
        Perceptual abnormalities (illusions, delusions, hallucinations)
        Psychomotor activity
    Motor examination
        Focal weakness
        Tremor
        Asterixis
        Myoclonus
        Seizures
    Autonomic examination
        Pupillary size and responses
        Temperature
        Heart rate and rhythm
        Diaphoresis

and time should be specifically tested by asking the date and year, the day of the week, and the present location. Orientation for time, particularly the year, is lost early in patients with delirium and orientation for place a little later.

Perceptual errors, e.g., mistaking the physician for an old friend or family member, illusions, and hallucinations are common accompaniments of delirium. They frighten and agitate some patients, but are quietly tolerated by others. The nature of the illusions and hallucinations seems to reflect the individual's personality, and often the same hallucinations accompany separate episodes of delirium. A quiet, withdrawn patient must be specifically asked about hallucinations, because he often fails either to volunteer the information or to behave as if he were hallucinating. Hallucinations of metabolic origin are usually visual, contrasting with those of schizophrenia, which are usually auditory.

Fluctuations of the mental status are common in metabolic encephalopathy. Patients may be totally out of contact one moment and lucid the next. Lucid intervals appear unpredictably and last for minutes or hours. Some of the fluctuation is environmentally related. Thus delirious patients characteristically become more disoriented at night, in unfamiliar surroundings, and in situations in which restraints and background noise and unfamiliar activity replace familiar sensory stimuli. One study demonstrated a significantly higher incidence of postoperative delirium in patients treated in a windowless intensive care unit than in those treated in a similar one with windows.

MOTOR ACTIVITY. Tremor, asterixis, and multifocal myoclonus are characteristic of metabolic brain disease, and the specificity of the latter two makes them the most important physical signs that distinguish metabolic encephalopathy from psychiatric illness or from structural brain disease.

The *tremor* of delirious patients is coarse and irregular at a rate of about eight to ten per second. It is usually absent at complete rest. It is best seen in the fingers of the outstretched hands. It is less specific than asterixis and multifocal myoclonus, and may be seen in patients with psychiatric disease as well as systemic illness not associated with delirium.

Asterixis is an abnormal, involuntary jerking movement elicited in the hands by asking patients to dorsiflex the wrist and spread the extended fingers. In its mildest form there are irregular random lateral jerking movements of the fingers at the metacarpal phalangeal joints. With fully developed asterixis there is sudden palmar flexion of the fingers at the metacarpal phalangeal joint and of the wrist. The movements are asynchronous in the two hands and are nonrhythmic. They occur every 2 to 30 seconds, recover quickly, and cannot be controlled by the patient, even when he is aware of their presence. Asterixis may also involve the feet and tongue. In the obtunded patient the same movement can sometimes be evoked by passively dorsiflexing the wrist or the ankles. Bilateral asterixis almost universally accompanies metabolic encephalopathy at some stage of the illness. It is absent in patients with psychiatric disorders unless they are taking large amounts of drugs, and is encountered rarely, and then unilaterally, in patients with gross structural brain disease such as decompensating subdural hematomas or deep hemispheral infarcts, especially involving the basal ganglia.

Multifocal myoclonus consists of sudden nonrhythmic, nonpatterned gross muscle contractions in a resting person. The movements are most common in the face and shoulders but occur anywhere in the body. Multifocal myoclonus can often be elicited, if not present at rest, by passive movements of the shoulder and upper arm. It occurs in a later and more severe stage of metabolic illness than does asterixis, and may physiologically represent a more intense and widespread manifestation of that abnormal movement. Multifocal myoclonus makes its most frequent appearance in uremia, hypercarbic-anoxic encephalopathy, and penicillin overdose, but can occur in virtually all metabolic encephalopathies.

Psychomotor activity ranges from extreme hyperactivity to total immobility. Delirious patients may be unwilling or unable to stay in bed, pacing the halls, in constant movement, with outbursts of aggressiveness which may culminate in attacks on others. With more severe delirium, there may be groping movements, picking at the bedclothes, and constant tossing and turning. Such patients may fall out of bed and injure themselves. Increased psychomotor activity is typically observed in acute deliria such as delirium tremens and drug withdrawal states. More commonly, delirium is manifested by reduced activity, with the patient lethargic, drowsy, and generally bradykinetic. The same patient may run the gamut from psychomotor overactivity to reduced activity during the course of the same delirium. *Speech* is often abnormal. Patients with increased psychomotor behavior often speak rapidly, with a muttering or slurred speech which, because of its speed, is incomprehensible. Patients with reduced psychomotor activity may speak slowly, monotonously, and so softly as not to be clearly heard.

Seizures, weakness, and *hyperactive stretch reflexes* frequently accompany severe metabolic brain disease. The seizures are usually generalized, and the motor abnormalities are usually symmetrical. Focal paresis and focal seizures are by no means rare, however, especially with anoxia, hypoglycemia, or hyperosmolality. Signs of focal disturbance make it more difficult to distinguish between metabolic and structural brain disease. However, in metabolic brain disease the focal signs are usually mild and fleeting, and they are accompanied by more widespread neurologic dysfunction than occurs with gross structural disease.

AUTONOMIC ACTIVITY. *Pupillary light reactions are always preserved in metabolic coma with the few exceptions to be mentioned, and absence of the pupillary light reaction strongly suggests a structural lesion.* The exceptions are glutethimide intoxication, which may produce mid-position or slightly dilated fixed pupils; anticholinergic drug administration, which produces fixed, dilated pupils; and exposure to severe anoxia, or asphyxia, which produces fixed dilated pupils and, if sustained, probably implies irreversible brain damage. The pupils, whatever their size and reaction to light, are usually symmetrical in patients comatose from metabolic brain disease, but often asymmetrical in patients comatose from structural brain disease.

Hypothermia is common in delirious patients with myxedema, hypoglycemia, and barbiturate intoxication. Hyperthermia with profuse perspiration and tachycardia accompanies most agitated deliria and is especially common with delirium tremens. Hyperthermia without perspiration suggests anticholinergic drug ingestion or infection. Hyperthermia also marks salicylate and occasionally phenothiazine overdosage.

VENTILATION. The clinical features of delirium that have been described are common to many metabolic disorders and aid little in the differential diagnosis of specific types of metabolic coma. Ventilation is an exception. A rapid evaluation of the patient's ventilatory status, coupled with an estimate of blood acid-base balance, frequently narrows the range of possible causes of metabolic coma. A careful clinical examination of the respiratory rate and depth usually allows the physician to estimate whether his patient is hyperventilating, eupneic, or hypoventilating. Caution must be exercised in evaluating patients with severe emphysema whose respiratory effort is increased and who may be tachypneic but nevertheless hypoventilating because of ineffective lungs. Caution must also be used in evaluating patients poisoned with depressant drugs who appear to be hypoventilating but are actually eupneic because their metabolic needs are so low. Unexplained abnormalities in the respiratory pattern demand rapid determination of blood gas and acid-base status. A delirious and clinically *hyperventilating* adult with a low serum pH probably has diabetic ketosis, uremia, lactic acidosis, or poisoning with an acidic product. Severe metabolic acidosis, if not treated, is rapidly lethal. Uremia, diabetes, and Addison's disease can be treated specifically (see Ch. 371, 531.1, and 547.3), and the others often respond to prompt and urgent treatment of the acidosis by infusion of bicarbonate. If, however, the serum pH is elevated in the delirious and hyperventilating adult, pulmonary disease, cardiac disease, hepatic coma, or neurogenic hyperventilation are the probable causes. Pneumonia is probably the most common cause of mild respiratory alkalosis in unconscious patients; the others can be evaluated by appropriate laboratory tests. When the serum pH is elevated and the bicarbonate is between 10 and 15 mEq per liter (mixed respiratory alkalosis and metabolic acidosis), sepsis, especially with gram-negative organisms, salicylism (which causes acidosis in children, alkalosis in adults), and severe hepatic coma are the probable causes.

A similar analysis can be applied to *hypoventilating* patients. In these, the severe problems are depressant drug poisoning, which produces a low serum pH with a normal bicarbonate, and chronic pulmonary failure, which produces a low serum pH and usually a high serum bicarbonate. (The serum bicarbonate level indicates the duration of hypoventilation.) Both situations demand ventilatory support.

ELECTROENCEPHALOGRAM (EEG). The EEG is useful in evaluating patients with metabolic brain disease because it is usually slower than in normal subjects and because it is symmetrical. The slowing indicates that there is neural dysfunction, and the bilateral symmetry suggests a diffuse process. The degree of slowing roughly parallels the severity of the encephalopathy. Patients with agitated deliria are often exceptions in that such patients, particularly those suffering from drug withdrawal, may have rapid rather than slow EEG's. Normal 8 to 13 Hz activity, however, is usually absent. The normal EEG has a basic frequency of 8 to 13 Hz. In metabolic disease, bilateral, synchronous, paroxysmal bursts of 1 to 3 Hz activity are frequently superimposed upon a background of mildly slow 5 to 7 Hz activity. A normal EEG is incompatible with severe delirium. An EEG with focal or unilateral slow activity strongly suggests a structural and not a metabolic brain disorder.

OTHER LABORATORY TESTS. The causes of metabolic coma are legion, and a final diagnosis usually depends on extensive laboratory tests. The tests which should be performed immediately to establish the presence of life-threatening metabolic defects are listed in Table 3, along with those whose results are not available immediately but should be done as soon as possible if the diagnosis is unclear.

DIAGNOSIS OF METABOLIC ENCEPHALOPATHY

The physician should consider metabolic encephalopathy as the possible diagnosis for every patient whose thinking, behavior, or state of consciousness has recently become disordered. The diagnosis requires, first, that one establish that metabolic encephalopathy rather than psychiatric disease, a structural brain lesion, or dementia is causing the abnormal behavior and, second, that one identify the specific metabolic illness responsible.

Psychiatric disease is distinguished in the awake patient by examination of the mental status and motor function. Psychotic patients are oriented and usually have normal cognitive function if one can enlist their cooperation. Delirious patients are disoriented and confused. Some patients with psychogenic amnesia claim to be confused about who they are as well as to the place and time; patients with metabolic brain disorders always know who they are. Hallucinations in psychiatric illness are usually auditory; in metabolic illness they are usually visual. Recent memory and cognitive abilities are generally preserved in psychiatric patients but are lost early in patients with metabolic illness. Tremor plagues anxious patients, and occasionally generalized seizures wrack those with catatonic schizophrenia, but asterixis and multifocal myoclonus are never present in psychiatric disease. Asterixis, if carefully searched for, is present in most patients with metabolic brain disease. Rarely, a patient with "hysterical coma" will present a diagnostic problem. Such patients are quietly unresponsive, and all their limbs are flaccid, but they often strongly resist passive eye opening. If the diagnosis is doubtful, irrigating the tympanum with 50 ml of cold water is informative; this procedure produces

TABLE 3. Laboratory Evaluation of Metabolic Brain Disease

Test	Reason for Test
Immediate:	
Glucose	Hypoglycemia, hyperosmolar coma
Na$^+$	Osmolar abnormalities
Ca^{++}	Hyper- or hypocalcemia
BUN	Uremia
pH, P_{CO_2}	Acidosis, alkalosis
P_{O_2}	Hypoxia
Lumbar puncture	Infection, hemorrhage
Later:	
Liver function tests	Hepatic coma
Sedative drug levels	Overdose
Blood and CSF culture	Sepsis, encephalitis, meningitis
Full electrolytes, including Mg^{++}	Electrolyte imbalance
Coagulation profile	Intravascular coagulation
EEG	

physiologic nystagmus in the patient with "hysterical coma," but only tonic eye deviation in the comatose patient with metabolic disease. The EEG in "hysterical coma" shows a normal awake record; it is always abnormal in metabolic coma. The EEG is less helpful in distinguishing agitated delirium from affective psychosis. The EEG in patients with an agitated delirium (e.g., alcohol withdrawal) is often not slow but instead marked by low voltage fast activity with no normal 8 to 13 Hz waves, a pattern seen at times in normal or psychotic patients.

Supratentorial mass lesions that encroach on the diencephalon produce diffuse brain dysfunction (see Ch. 219). However, supratentorial lesions produce focal motor and/or sensory signs early in the illness, often before mental changes, and these focal signs either persist or grow worse. Hemiparesis or hemisensory defects, although occasionally present in metabolic disease, are usually mild, often fleeting, and generally appear only after consciousness is lost. Late in the course of mass lesions, when transtentorial herniation has impaired midbrain function, bilateral decorticate or decerebrate rigidity usually replaces unilateral motor signs. These motor signs of midbrain dysfunction may also be present in metabolic coma, but in metabolic coma the pupillary light reflexes are retained, thereby ruling out a structural lesion. The EEG of a patient with a supratentorial mass lesion is usually slow either focally in one area or laterally over one hemisphere; that of a patient with metabolic brain disease, even when focal neurologic abnormalities are present, is usually symmetrically slow. Computerized transaxial tomography (CT scanning) (see Ch. 267) is the best single laboratory test to identify mass lesions in the brain and should be performed whenever the cause of an encephalopathy is in doubt.

Subtentorial structural lesions are distinguished from metabolic brain disease by the presence in the former of signs of cranial nerve and focal brainstem dysfunction. In patients with subtentorial lesions causing changes in consciousness, the pupils are almost always abnormal, either because pontine and medullary sympathetic pathways are involved or because the third nerve nuclei or fibers are destroyed. Both pupillary light reflexes and the ciliospinal reflex (pupillary dilatation to noxious cutaneous stimuli) are preserved in metabolic disease. Dysconjugate eye movements are common with subtentorial lesions, rare with metabolic disease. Unilateral facial weakness involving both the brow and lower face, unilateral facial anesthesia, absent caloric responses to one side, or eye deviation toward a paralyzed arm and leg all suggest a subtentorial lesion and are against the diagnosis of metabolic disease.

Dementia is the expression of irreversible metabolic brain disease in which the primary metabolic error usually resides in the brain rather than affects the brain secondarily. For this reason, the incipient signs of dementia can resemble delirium, and distinction may sometimes be difficult. In general, dementia begins gradually, whereas delirium begins either acutely or subacutely. Recent memory loss, cognitive difficulties, and disorientation to place occur early in dementia and precede any change in consciousness, whereas lethargy, apathy, decreased awareness, and disorientation in time are early marks of delirium. Tremor, asterixis, and myoclonus are rare in dementia (except myoclonus in Creutzfeldt-Jakob disease). Mild or moderate dementia

reduces the brain's defenses against metabolic insults, and thus it is common for a fully reversible delirium to complicate mild systemic illnesses in demented patients. In these cases only treatment of the systemic disorders will separate the delirious component from the dementia (see Ch. 226 to 231).

DIFFERENTIAL DIAGNOSIS. Delirium means that a metabolic illness is so advanced that it not only threatens brain function but may threaten life itself unless promptly diagnosed and reversed by treatment. Since the neurologic manifestations of the various metabolic encephalopathies are often similar, specific diagnosis by physical examination is often impossible, so some systematic approach to the problem is needed.

In Table 1 are listed all of the common and many of the less frequent causes of metabolic brain disease. Those marked with an asterisk either alone or in combination account for most of the delirium encountered on general medical wards. The table is designed as a checklist; the specific symptoms, signs, and management of each of the systemic disorders causing delirium can be found elsewhere in this book. Table 3 lists the laboratory tests most helpful in achieving a definitive diagnosis.

When the cause of delirium is unclear, the first conditions to consider are *hypoxia, hypoglycemia,* and *metabolic acidosis.* Unless promptly treated, all three are potentially rapidly lethal, and the first two very quickly damage the brain irreversibly.

Certain physical signs, such as respiratory abnormalities, convulsions, and fever, suggest specific diagnoses. The examination of respiration aids in the diagnosis of pulmonary encephalopathy, sedative drug poisoning, "gram-negative sepsis," and hepatic coma. Often an early clue to the diagnosis of hepatic coma is the presence of respiratory alkalosis, which then prompts liver function tests or a blood ammonia determination to support the diagnosis. *Generalized convulsions* occur in many metabolic brain disorders, especially with hypoxia and hypoglycemia. Repeated seizures are dangerous since they create the risk of brain damage and should be treated even before their cause is clear. If hypoxia and hypoglycemia are not the cause, repeated seizures suggest sedative drug withdrawal, uremia, hyponatremia, hypocalcemia, or penicillin encephalopathy.

Agitated delirium accompanied by fever prompts immediate consideration of intracranial infection. Often the patient with meningitis is so combative that nuchal rigidity cannot be adequately assessed, and only lumbar puncture confirms the diagnosis. A lumbar puncture should be performed on any patient who is delirious without obvious cause and who lacks evidence of chronically increased intracranial pressure (e.g., papilledema, history of chronic progressive headache and/or focal neurologic signs). If one suspects that a mass lesion is the cause of delirium, a CT scan should be performed before lumbar puncture. Encephalitis and subarachnoid hemorrhage often present initially with delirium accompanied by little or no fever and no nuchal rigidity, and may not be diagnosed unless the cerebrospinal fluid is examined. In any delirious patient with nystagmus or ocular palsies, thiamin deficiency encephalopathy (see Ch. 285 to 287) should be immediately considered, because if this condition is untreated, cardiovascular collapse and death may follow.

Once the dangerous and potentially lethal illnesses detailed above are excluded, there is time to consider the many other causes of metabolic brain disease and to make the tests appropriate to their diagnosis. In most cases, a single cause for delirium is not found. Instead, the patient has multiple metabolic defects, no one of which is sufficient to produce delirium, but the sum total of which in a susceptible patient is responsible. A common example is an *elderly* patient with mild *congestive heart failure, anemia,* and *hypoxia* being given *sedative drugs* for agitation and diuretics which have caused an electrolyte imbalance. The dismay caused by the multiplicity of diagnostic possibilities is partially offset when the physician makes the happy therapeutic discovery that treatment of any one of the metabolic disorders may substantially improve his patient's delirium.

PROGNOSIS AND TREATMENT OF METABOLIC BRAIN DISEASE

Metabolic brain disease can be definitively treated only by correcting the systemic disorder responsible for the delirium, and the effectiveness of this correction, in turn, determines the prognosis of the delirium. With the exception of severe hypoxia, hypoglycemia, or thiamin deficiency, all of which can cause neuronal death, delirium clears as the systemic disorder causing it improves. Often, however, the encephalopathy improves much more slowly than the systemic illness so that severe encephalopathy may persist four to five days or more after the systemic disorder has been fully reversed. Such a delay need not portend an unfavorable outcome, and vigorous efforts to prevent infections and other complications of delirium and coma are indicated during this period, for full recovery of cerebral function still is possible.

Certain general therapeutic measures apply to all delirious patients (Table 4). An adequate *airway* and *oxygenation* of the blood must be assured. For stuporous or comatose patients, this may require an endotracheal tube or tracheostomy. *Blood volume, cardiac output,* and *blood pressure* must be maintained at near normal levels to assure adequate cerebral blood flow. If the cause of coma is not known, a blood glucose should be obtained; but even before the results are reported, intravenous glucose (50 ml of 50 per cent solution) should be given to assure that hypoglycemia will not cause irreversible brain damage. Abnormalities of *acid-base balance* and of *electrolyte balance* should be corrected. Correction should be carried out over several hours, because too rapid correction often leads to other metabolic abnormalities. Infection should be treated and fever lowered. If the diagnosis is unclear and narcotic overdose is a potential cause of the patient's delirium, a diagnostic test of naloxone should be considered. However, it must be remembered that naloxone will cause acute withdrawal symptoms in patients tolerant to narcotics and may reverse narcotic encephalopathy but wear off before the narcotics are fully metabolized.

The awake, delirious patient should be kept in a quiet room, away from the unfamiliar noises and bustle of the general ward. The room should be well lighted, especially at night, because darkness accentuates disorientation and hallucinations. Physicians and nurses can reassure the patient by introducing themselves at each contact and quietly apprising him of his whereabouts. All procedures must be carefully and often repetitively explained before they are done. Drugs not essential for treatment of the patient's systemic illness should be withdrawn. This applies particularly to sedatives, narcotics, and tranquilizers, all of which commonly cause or accentuate delirium; it also applies to extensive use of diuretics, antihypertensive drugs, anticonvulsants, and even digitalis, medications that are less widely recognized to cause or accentuate delirium. If the patient is agitated and hyperactive, small doses of diazepam, starting with 5 mg orally and increasing as necessary, can be given to quiet him but not to render him unresponsive.

Careful attention is required to other systemic disorders that, although not of themselves sufficiently severe to cause delirium, may increase an already present encephalopathy. Oxygen should be given to mildly hypoxic patients, and transfusions should be administered to those with significant anemia. Mild electrolyte disorders such as hypokalemia and hyponatremia are diagnosed by periodic serum electrolyte determinations and are corrected by appropriate fluid control. Such measures often improve a patient's delirium considerably, even if the primary cause cannot be treated. Fluid losses should be routinely measured and replaced parenterally if the patient is not eating. Vital signs and the state of consciousness must be checked frequently to ensure that sudden worsening does not go undetected.

Jacobs, J. W., Bernhard, M. R., Delgado, A., and Strain, J. J.: Screening for organic mental syndromes in the medically ill. Ann. Intern. Med., 86:40, 1977.

Metabolic and deficiency diseases of the nervous system, Part II. *In* Vinken, P. J., and Bruyn, G. W. (eds.): Handbook of Clinical Neurology, Vol. 28. Amsterdam, Elsevier North-Holland Biomedical Press, 1976.

Plum, F., and Posner, J. B.: The Diagnosis of Stupor and Coma. 2nd ed. Philadelphia, F. A. Davis Company, 1972.

Sokoloff, L.: Circulation and energy metabolism of the brain. *In* Siegel, G. J., Albers, R. W., Katzman, R., and Agranoff, B. W. (eds.): Basic Neurochemistry. 2nd ed. Boston, Little, Brown & Company, 1976, Chap. 19, pp. 388–413.

221. SLEEP AND ITS DISORDERS

William R. Shapiro

The average adult sleeps 7½ to 8 hours out of every 24. Despite the fact that a third of life is spent sleeping, little is understood of its function. Sleep is an active state. Cerebral metabolism diminishes hardly at all during sleep, and although sleeping individuals often appear quiescent, they are known to go through a series of contortion-like movements as many as 20 times in the course of a given night. Twenty-five per cent of the

---

TABLE 4. Immediate Treatment of Metabolic Brain Disease

1. Assure oxygenation
2. Maintain circulation
3. Give glucose
4. Restore acid-base balance
5. Treat infection
6. Control body temperature
7. Stop seizures
8. Consider naloxone

night is spent dreaming, and a large body of literature, both scientific and mythological, has been devoted to explaining dreams. Sleep is essential, but studies in man and animals do not, as was once thought, indicate that sleep deprivation produces permanent physiologic damage in adults, although temporary neurologic and psychologic changes can be demonstrated. Recently neuroendocrinologic research has shown that some hormonal secretions have cyclic rhythms which may relate to sleep. Growth hormone output is increased during the early hours, and prolactin output increases during the morning hours of sleep. Disturbances of sleep represent a major source of distress to patients and a cause for the consumption of enormous quantities of sleep-related medications.

PHYSIOLOGY AND PHARMACOLOGY OF SLEEP

Studies from several sources have identified sleep not merely as a cessation of contact with the environment, but also as an active state in which cerebral metabolism does not diminish and in which several active processes can be identified. Two sleep states can be defined. One, called slow wave (SW) sleep, consists of gradual slowing of the electroencephalographic (EEG) rhythms, with increasing amplitude and synchronization through four stages from mild drowsiness (stage 1) to profound somnolence (stage 4). A second sleep state, called rapid eye movement (REM) sleep, is characterized by EEG activity which is low voltage, fast, and desynchronized and is associated with, respectively, rapid eye movements (hence its name), profound hypotonicity of the skeletal muscles with an associated low voltage electromyogram, and absent reflexes. Other phasic components identifiable in REM sleep include abrupt changes in respiration, pupil diameter, blood pressure, and pulse rate, muscle twitching, and penile erection. In electrical recordings abrupt spike activity in the pons and geniculate and occipital cortex (PGO waves) are detected. The two sleep states characteristically cycle during normal sleep. SW sleep occurs early, with the subject progressing through the four stages and returning back toward stage 2 in the course of the first 90 to 100 minutes. This is followed by REM sleep lasting 15 to 20 minutes, after which the subject returns again to SW sleep. REM sleep gradually occurs more often during the night, but on average makes up about 25 per cent of adult sleep time. Much of dreaming occurs during REM sleep, and subjects awakened during this state have described vivid, colorful, frequently uninhibited dreams. Dreaming of a more prosaic nature occurs also during SW sleep, but it tends to be related more to the subject's daily activities than does the imaginative introspective dreaming of REM sleep. The cycling between SW sleep and REM sleep varies with age, there being a greater proportion of REM sleep in infants and young children than in adults. There is evidence that human beings have a specific biologic need for a certain minimum of REM sleep as well as total sleep, and humans deprived of REM sleep experience a rebound in which extra REM sleep periods occur.

The mechanism by which sleep-wake cycles occur has been an active area of investigation. It has been determined that the brainstem contains structures identifiable both anatomically and neuropharmacologically which can cycle sleep-wake patterns in the absence of cerebral connections. On the other hand, it is possible to sever the connections between brainstem and cerebrum in animals and still demonstrate sleep-wake cycles in the cerebral cortex by EEG. Although inconsistencies still exist in the experimental evidence, a working model of the sleep-wake cycle system can be constructed which is based primarily on Jouvet's work with the decerebrate cat. In Jouvet's model, sleep-waking cycles are regulated by two antagonistic ascending monoaminergic systems that operate tonically. One system involves serotonin (5-hydroxytryptamine) containing neurons lying primarily in the raphe nuclei that are important in inducing SW sleep and priming REM sleep. The other includes catecholaminergic neurons (mostly noradrenergic) and acetylcholinergic neurons occupying the nucleus locus ceruleus and nucleus locus subceruleus that appear to induce cortical arousal and the waking state and also subserve elements of REM sleep. It is possible to isolate regions of these nuclei that specifically mediate the components of the REM state.

DISORDERS OF SLEEP

There are three major disorders of sleep. *Insomnia* means too little sleep; *hypersomnia*, an excess of sleep, usually during the day. *Disturbed sleep* occurs during otherwise normal sleep and includes enuresis, sleepwalking, and night terrors.

When considering the diagnosis of a sleep disorder, it is important to bear in mind the variable nature of sleep. Some individuals require more than eight hours of sleep, whereas a few get along well on three or four. Women usually sleep longer than men. Children require more sleep than young adults, and less sleep is needed with advancing age. In most people a few nocturnal awakenings normally occur; they become of medical concern only when they increase in number or duration so much that they substantially reduce total sleep time. Similarly, many individuals normally nap during the day; hypersomnia implies excessive somnolence, especially an increase over the subject's usual level.

Insomnia

According to Kales, insomnia is the sleep disturbance most frequently treated by the general physician. It may consist of difficulty of falling asleep, difficulty in staying asleep, too early awakenings, or a combination of these. Insomnia may be a symptom associated with medical disorders. Chronic pain may produce difficulty in sleeping throughout the night. Pulmonary insufficiency may cause frequent nocturnal awakenings. Insomnia may accompany acute infectious illness and is common in Sydenham's chorea and in bulbar poliomyelitis. More often no specific medical disorder is present and the complaint is treated symptomatically, usually by hypnotic medications. It is estimated that 7 to 10 per cent of the population uses hypnotics, including alcohol, minor tranquilizers, and nonprescription sleeping medications. Psychologic factors probably contribute to insomnia in most such patients. In direct testing, over three fourths of insomniacs evaluated on the Minnesota Multiphasic Personality Inventory (MMPI) showed high scores on the depression scale. At least one MMPI scale was abnormal in 85 per cent of insomniac patients. Further, many chronic insomniacs are described as tense, complaining individuals who are oversensitive to minor discomforts and unable to relax easily. The advent of sleep laboratory research has disclosed that the degree of sleeplessness is frequently overestimated by patients. The Sleep Disorders Clinic at Stanford University found that compared with laboratory recordings of 122 drug-free subjects who complained of chronic insomnia, most subjects consistently underestimated the amount of time they slept and overestimated the latency in falling asleep. On the other hand, most patients had more arousals during the night than they reported. *Drug treatment does not alleviate insomnia for more than a few days.* In direct sleep laboratory studies, Kales found that compared to drug-free insomniacs, those chronically habituated to hypnotics have more awakenings during the night, less stage 3 and 4 SW sleep, the same degree of prolonged sleep latency, and a marked reduction in REM sleep. If patients attempt to reduce hypnotic medications abruptly, there is profound REM rebound with excessive dreaming and increased insomnia. Patients continue to take hypnotics, and may increase the dose, because of the REM rebound. The problem of chronic use of sleeping medications is complicated by the patients' failure to recognize the psychologic components of their insomnia, denying depression and focusing on the somatic complaint of poor sleep.

It is apparent that the evaluation of chronic insomnia requires special attention to the patient's psychologic needs. Since psychologic testing indicates that the majority of patients with chronic insomnia are depressed, the physician must inquire into associated symptoms of depression, including poor appetite, early awakenings, sadness, crying spells, significant weight loss, changing bowel habits, and personal loss. If the physician determines that the patient's major problem is depression, referral for psychotherapy may be indicated.

Treatment of chronic insomnia depends on the results of evaluation: specific medical disorders should be treated directly. Symptomatic treatment of the insomnia requires attention to general measures and specific pharmacologic considerations. Helpful measures in the general treatment of chronic insomnia include reduction of stimulant drugs, i.e., caffeine or amphetamines, regulation of bedtime and wake time, elimination of daytime naps, relaxation exercises, and recommendation for moderate daily exercise. Some persons simply need the reassurance that they require less sleep than others.

Pharmacologic therapy for insomnia requires an awareness that many drugs affect sleep. Some are designed specifically to induce or ward off sleep. Others not designed to alter sleep do so as a side effect. For example, L-dopa, used to treat Parkinson's disease, and exogenous corticosteroid hormones regularly produce insomnia. Drug effect depends on host circumstances and previous exposure. Many sedative drugs under certain circumstances actually produce excitement; barbiturates given to elderly patients may cause an agitated confusion. Conversely, amphetamine and methylphenidate, both stimulants, can quiet hyperactive children. Chronic administration of both sedative and analeptic drugs can rapidly lead to tolerance; abrupt withdrawal can lead to profound physiologic disturbance. The following points should be observed when prescribing such drugs. Barbiturates lead to tolerance within two weeks. They then become ineffective after a short while, and, because they profoundly depress REM sleep as tolerance develops, there is marked REM rebound and restlessness on withdrawal. Benzodiazepines are similar to barbiturates, although Kales has reported that flurazepam does not lose its effectiveness in two weeks. Less REM rebound is reported following cessation of benzodiazepines than occurs with barbiturates. Tricyclic antidepressants and monoamine oxidase (MAO) inhibitors reduce REM sleep during chronic therapy; REM rebound occurs after drug withdrawal. Amphetamines tend to decrease REM sleep, but withdrawal effects have not been studied. Variable effects on sleep have been produced by analgesics and alcohol and by antipsychotic agents. In part the effects depend on the subjects; normal healthy volunteers differ more in their response to single doses of opiates than do subjects addicted to such compounds.

Pharmacologic therapy for insomnia should be limited, whenever possible, to occasional use of sleeping medications for acute episodes. Most hypnotics may be used safely for up to three days; typical bedtime doses are secobarbital, 100 mg; pentobarbital, 100 mg; and chloral hydrate, 1 gram. Glutethimide has been reported as a cause for suicide in a sufficient number of patients to suggest replacement by another hypnotic. Chronic use of hypnotics does not relieve insomnia. If therapy must extend for more than a few days, flurazepam is the drug of choice because it surpresses REM sleep less than barbiturates and does not produce tolerance after two weeks. Flurazepam, 15 mg, is administered at bedtime to be increased after a week to 30 mg if sleep is not improved. For drug-withdrawal insomnia and hypnotic drug dependency, very slow drug withdrawal is recommended to avoid REM rebound. The therapeutic dose should be reduced no more frequently than once every five or six days, and the patient must be informed that increased dreaming, vivid dreams, and even nightmares may occur. Insomnia often improves after withdrawal. Because of the REM rebound special care must be taken in withdrawing hypnotics too quickly from those patients who suffer from coronary artery disease or duodenal ulcer, as both of these conditions are potentially made worse by excessive REM sleep.

Hypersomnia

NARCOLEPSY. Narcolepsy is a chronic disorder characterized by irresistable episodes of sleep occurring from a few to many times a day, between which the patient may be alert or drowsy. Narcolepsy may be accompanied by cataplexy, sleep paralysis, and/or hypnagogic hallucinations. *Cataplexy* is a sudden decrease or loss of muscle tone that may be generalized or confined to individual muscles. When mild, cataplexy consists of a sense of weakness, a tendency to drop things, or of having one lower limb give way; when severe, the patient may fall in a heap. Such attacks generally last less than a minute and occur from one to 12 to 25 times in 24-hour period. They may be precipitated by heightened emotional tone — e.g., laughter or anger — but when severe they occur spontaneously or with any kind of movement. *Sleep paralysis,* like cataplexy, is also characterized by the inability to move but occurs when the patient is either falling asleep or just coming out of a sleep spell. *Hypnagogic hallucinations* are vivid, visual, or auditory dreamlike states which occur while dozing or while being aroused. They are so vivid that patients may act out the dream state on awakening and are surprised to discover that they have been dreaming. These four symptoms constitute the narcoleptic tetrad. Twenty-five per cent of narcoleptic patients have sleep attacks only, whereas 70 per cent have both narcolepsy and cataplexy. Approximately 12 per cent of patients experience all four symptoms. The incidence in men and women is approximately equal. A family history is present in half the patients. Although the disease commonly begins in the teens and twenties, the diagnosis is frequently delayed for five to eight years because neither the patient nor the physician recognizes the nature of the attacks.

The pathogenesis of narcolepsy is unknown, but two theories have been proposed. Yoss and Daly suggested that narcolepsy represents one end of a continuous spectrum from full wakefulness to deep sleep. Narcoleptic patients are thought to have a genetically determined greater incidence of otherwise normal drowsiness (reduced vigilance), and the degree of such sleepiness can be determined by pupillographic studies. The second theory was advanced after the two different sleep states, SW and REM, were recognized. In most normal subjects an interval of an hour to an hour and a half elapses between falling asleep and the first appearance of REM sleep in the EEG tracing. In the patients with narcolepsy, especially those with cataplexy, the sleep syndrome may begin abruptly with a period of REM sleep. Narcoleptic patients without cataplexy may have non-REM onset sleep attacks. The thesis that narcolepsy-cataplexy is associated with REM onset sleep patterns explains cataplexy as the sudden loss of motor tone that occurs with REM. Hypnagogic hallucinations represent the dream component of the REM state, and sleep paralysis is also associated with loss of motor tone occurring during sleep. Amphetamines inhibit both SW sleep and REM sleep but only to a moderate degree, whereas tricyclic antidepressants profoundly inhibit REM sleep but do not influence SW sleep and have no effect on the sleep attacks of narcolepsy. It is the REM inhibiting property of the antidepressants which makes them effective in treating cataplexy. They appear to suppress the tonic components of REM sleep, apparently by action on brainstem structures responsible for inhibition of muscle activity and reflexia. It is likely that the narcoleptic disorder involves both the REM and SW systems, because methysergide is mildly effective against narcoleptic sleep attacks, suggesting an effect on the SW serotonergic system.

Narcolepsy is distinguished from other causes of hypersomnia, for example, structural brain lesions, because the latter occur more acutely and with greater severity. Narcoleptic patients are easily aroused, whereas patients with structural lesions causing lethargy become progressively unarousable and have associated respiratory, cranial nerve, and motor signs. In structural brain disease there is usually impaired cognition. Narcolepsy dates to early life with a stable course over many years. Late onset hypersomnia may occur in sleep apnea or other syndromes associated with hypoventilation (see below). Occasionally narcolepsy itself may be associated with sleep apnea.

Treatment of narcolepsy is difficult, both because it requires stimulants whose side effects are difficult to control and because it requires a regulated, almost rigid life style usually unacceptable to young patients. Dextroamphetamine sulfate in the form of sustained release capsules or tablets at doses of 15 to 50 mg per day is generally effective against the sleep attacks, especially in the first years of use. Tolerance develops, however, and the drug becomes less effective. Methylphenidate has the advantage that tolerance develops more slowly than with the amphetamines, and it has a reduced excitatory potential. Methylphenidate is used in doses up to 200 mg per day but must be administered on an empty stomach. It is the drug of choice in narcoleptic patients who are also hypertensive. Unfortunately methylphenidate does not prevent cataplexy, and the amphetamines are only minimally effective. The tricyclic antidepressants, including imipramine and desmethylimipramine, are effective in moderately high doses, but the most effective drug to treat cataplexy is clomipramine. Clomipramine may be used in doses of 25 to 75 mg a day according to the number and severity of cataplectic attacks. A troublesome side effect of the tricyclic antidepressants is the tendency to produce impotence in men. They also exaggerate the natural tendency of narcoleptic patients to overeat and increase the difficulty in controlling weight. Monoamine oxidase inhibitors and L-dopa have been used to treat narcolepsy, but their side effects preclude general use. Although narcolepsy is a benign disorder, its course may be gradually progressive, the patient becoming refractory to therapy. Whether this constitutes progression of the disease or increasing tolerance to the medication produced by weight gain or other factors is not known.

SLEEP APNEA. The specific association of hypersomnia and chronic alveolar hypoventilation in the presence of extreme obesity, polycythemia, and excessive appetite is called the pickwickian syndrome. Cessation of respiration while sleeping was first described in patients with severe bulbar poliomyelitis. A similar disorder may follow surgery of the high spinal cord or brainstem in which patients become apneic upon falling asleep. This is called "Ondine's curse," a literary illusion to the revenge that Ondine, a river nymph, takes upon a deceitful mortal who jilted her; the curse requires him to attend consciously to his autonomic functions, and when he falls asleep he stops breathing and dies. More common than any of these is the disorder characterized by hypersomnia with obstructive periodic apneas during sleep, so-called *sleep apnea.*

The patient with sleep apnea usually presents with excessive daytime sleepiness of subacute or chronic duration. A history is obtained from family members that the patient snores loudly and excessively through the night. The spouse may report that the patient's sleep is often disturbed by sudden starts and violent arm swings which sometimes produce injury and occasionally necessitate separation of sleeping arrangements. A minority of the patients have known narcolepsy. Constitutionally, sleep apnea patients often complain of morning headaches, are frequently hypertensive, and may have cardiac arrhythmias. Most patients with sleep apnea are obese middle-aged men, but a few have the severe obesity and hypercapnia of the pickwickian patients, and the syndrome can occur in nonobese individuals, women, and children. It may also be related to the sudden infant death syndrome. Nocturnal sleep recordings in these patients are characterized by up to hundreds of episodes of apnea with abrupt awakenings. The Po_2 falls during apnea, the Pco_2 rises, and both are reversed as the patient awakens and takes four or five breaths. The cycle repeats as the patient lapses into sleep. Apnea occurs during both REM and SW sleep but has been observed to be more specifically associated with REM sleep. Three types were initially described: a central apnea, in which there was cessation of diaphragmatic excursions; upper airway apnea, characterized by obstruction to airflow past the oral pharynx but with persistent diaphragm movement; and a mixed apnea, defined by cessation of air flow and absent respiratory effort early in the episode, followed by unsuccessful attempts at respiration later in the episode. It is now recognized that most patients have intermittent upper airway obstruction as the cause of their apnea. The pathogenesis of sleep apnea remains obscure. Functional obstruction in the oral pharynx seems to be caused by recurrent closure of the upper pharyngeal wall and posterior movement of the tongue. There is secondary downward movement of the soft palate and hypopharyngeal closure from abortive thoracic and diaphragmatic respiratory movements. The questions of the cause of the upper pharyngeal collapse and the pathogenesis of the daytime somnolence remain to be explained.

Sleep apnea sometimes responds to vigorous weight reduction. Otherwise, treatment of sleep apnea secondary to upper airway obstruction is tracheostomy, although weight reduction and tricyclic antidepressants may reduce daytime somnolence. The presence of associated cardiovascular abnormalities requires that the patient be treated promptly. Following tracheostomy, most patients improve remarkably, the daytime somnolence disappears, nocturnal sleep is uninterrupted, and constitutional symptoms, including hypertension and the arrhythmias, usually improve.

OTHER CAUSES OF HYPERSOMNIA. With the recent rise in amphetamine abuse, occasional patients are seen with hypersomnolence secondary to amphetamine addiction or abrupt withdrawal. Tolerance and dependency paradoxically increase daytime sleepiness; the diagnosis depends on the history of chronic use of stimulant medication. A rare condition of recurrent hypersomnia combined with excessive eating is sometimes observed in adolescent males and is known as the *Kleine-Levin syndrome*. The cause is unknown, but the attacks last several days to a week or more, during which the patient eats voraciously and often develops disturbed behavior. Intervals of months to years of normal behavior separate the attacks. There is no treatment, and the attacks tend to disappear as the patient reaches adulthood.

Disturbed Sleep

Somnambulism or sleepwalking has been reported to occur in 15 per cent of children at least once between ages 5 and 12. Most reports describe aimless wandering usually without falls. Somnambulism may occur in isolation or in association with *enuresis*. The latter, bedwetting at night with daytime continence, occurs in 10 per cent of children between ages 4 and 14 and is more common in boys. Its cause is thought to be functional, but only rarely does it indicate severe psychopathology. Both sleepwalking and enuresis occur during stages 3 and 4 of SW sleep. Both tend to disappear with age. They should be treated with reassurance. Enuresis has been reported to respond to tricyclic antidepressants.

Night terrors (pavor nocturnus) also occur in children, usually associated with stage 3 and 4 of SW sleep. The child suddenly awakens, intensely afraid, with tachypnea and tachycardia. The attack lasts only minutes and is rarely recalled in the morning. Most children grow out of the episodes. Night terrors can be distinguished from nightmares, in that the latter are less intense, tend to occur during the dreaming of REM sleep, and are usually remembered.

Physiology and Pharmacology

Petre-Quadens, O., and Schlag, J. D. (eds.): Basic Sleep Mechanisms. New York, Academic Press, 1974.
Williams, R. L., and Karaccen, I.: Pharmacology of Sleep. New York, Wiley, 1976.

Insomnia

Carskadon, M. A., Dement, W. C., Mitler, M. M., Guilleminault, C., Zarcove, V. P., and Spiegel, R.: Self-reports versus sleep laboratory findings in 122 drug-free subjects with complaints of chronic insomnia. Am. J. Psychiat., 133:1382, 1976.
Kales, A., and Kales, J. D.: Sleep disorders. Recent findings in the diagnosis and treatment of disturbed sleep. N. Engl. J. Med., 290:487, 1974.
Regestein, Q. R.: Treating insomnia: A practical guide for managing chronic sleeplessness, circa 1975. Compr. Psychiatry, 17:517, 1976.

Hypersomnia

Guilleminault, C., and Dement, W. C.: 235 cases of excessive daytime sleepiness. J. Neurol. Sci., 31:13, 1977.
Guilleminault, C., Dement, W. C., and Passouant, P. (eds.): Narcolepsy. Advances in Sleep Research, Vol. 3. New York, Spectrum, 1976.
Guilleminault, C., Elridge, F. L., Tilkian, A., Simmons, F. B., and Dement, W. C.: Sleep apnea syndrome due to upper airway obstruction. A review of 25 cases. Arch. Intern. Med., 137:296, 1977.
Parkes, J. D.: The sleepy patient. Lancet, 1:990, 1977.

Section Two FOCAL DISTURBANCES OF HIGHER NERVOUS FUNCTION

Norman Geschwind

222. LANGUAGE, APHASIA, AND RELATED DISORDERS

Language is one of the most striking biologic attributes of man. Recent evidence suggesting that some potential for language exists in chimpanzees may open up new possibilities for investigation of the neurologic foundations of linguistic behavior. At present, however, nearly all our knowledge of the neural substrate of language is based on man. Detailed postmortem studies of well-described patients have provided the majority of the information, but useful data have been accumulated from patients with other types of disorders and from studies of the effects of stimulation of the brain during operations.

A striking feature of the human brain is dominance, i.e., the superiority of one hemisphere in the performance of certain functions. Dominance is not known definitely to exist in any mammal other than man. There is, however, left-brain dominance for singing in birds. About 93 per cent of people are right-handed, and at least 99 per cent of right handers have left hemisphere dominance for speech.

The situation is more complex and less well defined in the non-right-handed, i.e., the left handers and those with varying degrees of ambidexterity. Such patients become aphasic as a result of a lesion in *either* hemisphere, although left hemisphere lesions generally produce more lasting disability. A third group, *pathologic left handers*, who have suffered early childhood injury to the left hemisphere, are usually right-brained for speech.

The cause of dominance was in dispute for many years. We now know that the temporal speech region on the left is generally larger than the corresponding area on the right. The nondominant side is, however, endowed genetically with the capacity to develop language. Thus if the dominant hemisphere is damaged before age nine, there is nearly always excellent recovery of language over a period of months or even years, although the over-all degree of mental development is slowed. Spontaneous recovery from aphasia also occurs in later life but less frequently. Dominance in the intact human can be studied by two recently developed techniques. The *Wada test* consists of the injection of sodium amytal into the internal carotid artery. This causes a hemiplegia on the side opposite the injection, but aphasia results only from injection on the dominant side, especially in non-right-handed patients. Another technique, the *Kimura test*, is that of dichotic listening, in which different words are simultaneously presented to the two ears. Normal individuals tend to report first the words presented to the ear opposite the dominant hemisphere.

223. APHASIA

The aphasias may be defined as disorders of language secondary to lesions of the brain. In most cases there is disorder of the output of speech. In the experience of the author, aphasia in spoken speech is invariably accompanied by similar abnormalities in writing. Aphasia in spoken language is of two major types: (1) *Nonfluent aphasia*, in which few words are produced slowly and with great effort, and sounds are incorrectly articulated. Production of grammatical words is relatively more affected so that sentences tend to be ungrammatical, e.g., "Weather sunny." (2) *Fluent aphasia*, in the more extreme forms of which the patient produces runs of well-articulated speech, which has the rhythm and melody of normal language and a basically normal grammatical structure, but which tends to convey little information, e.g., "I was at the other one and then I was at this one," a fluent aphasic's circumlocutory manner of explaining that he was in another hospital previously. The speech of these patients usually contains many incorrect words, called *paraphasias*. Literal (or phonemic) *paraphasias* are substitutions of well-articulated but incorrect sounds, e.g., "spoot" for "spoon," and *verbal paraphasias* are incorrect usages of words, e.g., "knife" for "fork," or "department" for "hospital."

The terms *expressive* and *receptive* aphasia should be avoided, as they have been used with different meanings in the literature. Thus some authors use expressive aphasia to describe only the nonfluent forms, whereas others use it to describe both nonfluent and fluent forms. Receptive aphasia has been used to describe pure word deafness by some; others use it for the full syndrome of Wernicke's aphasia, in which all modalities of language are affected.

In differential diagnosis, one must be wary of describing *mutism* as aphasia, because even severe aphasics are usually not mute. Causes of mutism are (1) uncooperativeness; (2) psychiatric disorders, e.g., severe depression or schizophrenia; (3) widespread disorders of brain, such as trauma, subarachnoid hemorrhage, or metabolic disorders; (4) lesions of mesencephalic and pontine tegmentum; and (5) bilateral lesions of the cranial nerves serving the speech organs, their nuclei, or their supranuclear pathways.

Dysarthria should not be confused with aphasia. Dysarthric speech is incorrectly articulated, but, if transcribed, shows correct grammar and word usage. A helpful clue is that if a patient who is mute or has completely unintelligible speech can produce fully normal language (not just his own name) in writing or on a typewriter, he is almost certainly not aphasic.

A common error is to misdiagnose a fluent aphasia as *schizophrenic word-salad*. Several clues help to make the differential diagnosis. Fluent aphasia is much more common than schizophrenic word-salad. The schizophrenic speech disorder usually develops in chronic "back ward" schizophrenics. By contrast, fluent aphasia may come on abruptly as the result of a stroke in a previously well person. Finally, fluent aphasia from vascular disease usually occurs in older people, whereas schizophrenia almost always is manifest before the age of 30.

APHASIC SYNDROMES AND THEIR LOCALIZATIONS. *Broca's aphasia* is the result of a lesion of Broca's area, i.e., the portion of the frontal lobe just anterior to the face, lip, tongue, and mouth area of the motor cortex. This produces a nonfluent aphasia, and writing is also involved. Repetition is impaired. The patient's greatest difficulty in repetition is with phrases consisting of small "grammatical" words (e.g., "If he were here I would go there") rather than with long words. Comprehension of language is intact. There is nearly always a right hemiplegia. *Wernicke's aphasia* results from a lesion of Wernicke's area, the posterior portion of the superior temporal gyrus. The aphasia is typically fluent. Written language is equally impaired. Comprehension of spoken and written language is severely impaired. Repetition of spoken language is poor. There is usually no hemiplegia, and other elementary neurologic signs are usually lacking. *Conduction aphasia* results from a lesion of the parietal operculum, i.e., the region lying above the sylvian fissure. There is fluent aphasia involving speech and writing, with severely impaired repetition but intact comprehension. Elementary neurologic signs are usually absent, with the occasional exception of cortical sensory loss on the opposite side. Some patients with Wernicke's area lesions may recover comprehension and are therefore left with the same syndrome. *Anomic aphasia* is characterized by fluent aphasia in speech and impairment of written language, but with intact comprehension and repetition. The components of Gerstmann's syndrome (discussed in Ch. 224) are often present. In this syndrome the lesion, if focal, is at the region of the parietotemporal junction, but a similar syndrome is produced in nonfocal widespread disease of the brain, such as is caused by metabolic disease or by large masses with raised intracranial pressure regardless of their location. It is also the most common form of aphasia in patients with closed head injury. Anomic aphasia may also be seen in the recovery stage from almost any other form of aphasia. Thus, in contrast to Broca's, Wernicke's, and conduction aphasia, anomic aphasia is much more difficult to localize.

These four syndromes are the most common, and although overlapping forms are common, relatively pure forms are not rare. Certain other syndromes are much less common.

Isolation of the speech area is caused by a large lesion involving the cortex and underlying white matter in a C-shaped configuration that spares Broca's area, Wernicke's area, and their interconnections, but destroys the cortex and underlying white matter that surround the speech region. These patients either may show little spontaneous speech or may have fluent abnormal speech. The most striking characteristic of this disorder is that, despite an almost total lack of comprehension, the patient can repeat well without dysarthria. This lesion is usually the result of anoxia or of carotid insufficiency. *Alexia without agraphia* is a syndrome in which the patient speaks and writes normally but cannot comprehend written language. The lesion, almost always the result of infarction in the distribution of the left posterior cerebral artery, consists of destruction of the left visual cortex and the splenium, i.e., the posterior portion, of the corpus callosum. In *alexia with agraphia* the patient can neither write nor comprehend written language, but other language functions are normal. Other components of Gerstmann's syndrome (see Ch. 224) may be present. The lesion involves a portion of the left angular gyrus. A right visual field defect may occur if the lesion extends deeply into the white matter but is often absent. *Pure word-deafness* described a syndrome in which there is dense incomprehension of language in the presence of intact hearing, although other language functions are intact. Two types of lesion produce this; either a single lesion lying subcortically in the posterior temporal lobe or bilateral lesions of the middle portion of the first temporal gyrus. *Pure agraphia* is extremely rare as the result of any focal lesion, but is common in patients with confusional states of toxic, metabolic, or traumatic orgin.

Aphemia is an uncommon syndrome in which the patient has speech which is slow, effortful and dysarthric, but without significant disorder of grammar or word choice. The patient's written language is essentially normal. A right hemiplegia is often present at the onset but usually disappears. Aphemic patients usually improve markedly, but it may take up to three years. It is likely that this syndrome results from small lesions in Broca's area, whereas larger lesions produce the typical Broca's aphasia with a right hemiplegia.

Aphasic syndromes in children are more difficult to localize. Mutism is more common in childhood aphasia. Fluent aphasia occurs very rarely in childhood even with lesions that usually lead to fluent forms in adults. Older adults are more likely than younger adults to have grossly fluent aphasias.

Aphasias in left handers have some special properties. Left handers appear to become aphasic with lesions in either hemisphere, although those occurring after right hemisphere lesions are more likely to be transient. Most permanent severe aphasias in left handers result from left-sided lesions. Comprehenshion difficulty is less common in left handers, and apraxia (see below) is also less common as an accompaniment of aphasia. Recovery is better not only in left handers but also, according to Luria, in right handers with left-handed parents, siblings, or children.

At present the evidence is that most *recovery in adult aphasics* takes place spontaneously. Although speech therapy has not been proved to produce major changes, it can be very useful in mobilizing the patient's residual language capacities for most effective communication.

224. OTHER DISORDERS OF THE HIGHER FUNCTIONS

APRAXIA. Apraxia is the inability to perform a learned act in response to a stimulus which would normally elicit it, and which cannot be accounted for by weakness, incoordination, reflex change, sensory loss, incomprehension, inattention, or uncooperativeness. Three lesions may produce apraxia. With lesions of the corpus callosum there will be apraxia of the left side of the body, but not of the right or of the face. Patients with Broca's aphasia (who usually have a right hemiplegia) will show apraxia that is usually most marked in the face and is also often present in the left limbs. With lesions in the left parietal operculum, producing a conduction aphasia, there is usually apraxia in the face (where it is most marked) and in the limbs of both sides of the body. In all forms of apraxia, axial movements, i.e., movements in which the muscles of the trunk or neck are involved, e.g., "stand up," "sit down," "turn around," and movement of eye-closing and eye-opening as well as movements of the eyes (e.g., "look up") are preserved. In all forms of apraxia the defect is most marked to verbal command (although the patient comprehends), usually somewhat less marked on imitation of the examiner, and least marked in the handling of objects, although in some patients even this latter category is impaired.

AGNOSIA. Agnosia is a failure of recognition of complex stimuli in the face of preserved elementary perception. The most common form is visual agnosia, in which there are usually bilateral posterior occipital lobe lesions. The agnosias are less well understood than the aphasias or apraxias.

CALLOSAL SYNDROMES. These were first brilliantly described by Hugo Liepmann in the early 1900's, but have been rediscovered only in recent years. In some cases of anterior cerebral artery occlusion there is infarction of the anterior four fifths of the corpus callosum. The patient will carry out verbal commands with the right hand but not the left. He will name objects held (concealed from vision) in the right hand but not the left. He can, however, with the left hand draw or select from a group of objects the one previously held in the left hand. He manifests, in brief, inability to transfer information between the two hemispheres. Involvement of the splenium of the corpus callosum plays a role in alexia without agraphia (see Ch. 223).

GERSTMANN'S SYNDROME. This consists of agraphia, right-left disorientation, acalculia (difficulty in carrying out calculations), and finger agnosia (inability to name fingers or to identify them). The patient almost invariably also shows constructional disorder, i.e., a difficulty in drawing or copying designs, especially three-dimensional ones. When all the components of this syndrome are present, the lesion almost invariably lies in the left posterior parietal region. It should, however, be kept in mind that a single component has little localizing value.

RIGHT HEMISPHERE SYNDROMES. Lesions of the right parietal region produce constructional difficulty that is more severe on the average than that produced from any other site. It should be recalled, however, that constructional difficulty is common with left hemisphere lesions. Patients with right hemisphere lesions may also show a dressing disorder manifested by great difficulty in putting on clothes. Milder degrees of the difficulty may be brought out by such maneuvers as putting one sleeve of the bathrobe inside out; the patient may be unable to get the bathrobe on properly.

A striking feature of acute lesions of the right hemisphere is *anosognosia*, i.e., a tendency to deny or neglect disability or, when admitting its presence, to be unconcerned with it. It is a common experience that the patient with an acute left hemiplegia will show this type of behavior, although by contrast the patient with an acute right hemiplegia will, even if aphasic, usually show appropriate awareness of disability and will be depressed. These disorders in right hemisphere lesions are always accompanied by a curious mental state, in which the patient shows apathy, poor attention, and often jocularity. These states (and the accompanying unconcern with illness) are usually transient, but are sometimes permanent in cases of large right parietal lesions. These curious mental states probably reflect the fact that the right hemisphere has a special role in many aspects of subjective emotional response and emotional expression.

Not all patients who deny illness suffer from right hemisphere disease. Weinstein has shown that a patient with any disability may deny illness if he is sufficiently obtunded. Thus a patient may deny blindness resulting even from disease of the eyes if he develops a confusional state from metabolic disorder or drugs.

225. MEMORY

Memory describes the processes by which past experience is stored and retrieved. Disorders of memory include *anterograde amnesia*, i.e., the failure to store new memories, or *retrograde amnesia*, i.e., disorders of storage or retrieval of memories laid down in the past.

Certain separable stages in memory storage have become clear from clinical observation. There is a stage of *immediate* memory, which is the ability to retain material presented as long as attention is not distracted. This is examined by such tests as digit span, i.e., the ability to repeat a series of digits spoken by the examiner. Most normal persons can immediately repeat a series of seven such digits. The next step is *transfer* to the long-term memory store. The first step in this is *intermediate memory* storage, and the later step is called *remote memory*. The reason for separating these steps will become clear when we discuss the clinical syndromes.

ANATOMY OF MEMORY

Memories are probably held in short-term store simply by continuation of nervous activity. The transfer to the long-term store probably involves some molecular change either in nerve membrane or in intracellular organelles. The neural structures most involved appear to lie in the limbic system, especially the hippocampal region, mammillary bodies, and, according to some authors, the dorsomedial nuclei of the thalamus (Victor et al.). The intactness of these structures appears to be important, in some as yet undefined way, in the transfer of memories from the intermediate to the long-term stores. The memories are probably not laid down in these limbic structures, because their destruction does not lead to loss of remote memories. They must therefore act on the structures which are the sites of storage. The limbic structures are also important, as will be seen below, in retrieval from the intermediate store.

CLINICAL DISORDERS OF MEMORY

Memory disorder may be evidence in widespread disorder of the brain such as may be produced by drugs or metabolic disorders. On the other hand, memory may be relatively or dramatically spared in many of the dementias. Thus memory is much less impaired than such functions as calculation and abstraction in general paresis. By contrast, in Alzheimer's disease, in which involvement of hippocampus is prominent, memory disorder is a salient feature of the initial states in most but not all cases. In Pick's disease, which is much less common, memory is frequently spared.

Disease processes predominantly affecting the hippocampal-mammillary system will produce significant memory disorder with little or no effect on other intellectual functions. This clinical state is called *Korsakoff's syndrome.* When caused by thiamin deficiency, the most striking lesions are in the mammillary bodies. The hippocampus may be involved in Alzheimer's disease, head injury, or tumors. Disease of the posterior cerebral artery may cause infarction of the hippocampus. Herpes simplex encephalitis has a predilection for all the structures of the limbic system. Occasional cases of severe memory loss have been reported after bilateral removal of the medial temporal structures surgically.

In order to produce a permanent memory deficit, bilateral lesions of the mammillo-hippocampal system are required. However, a unilateral lesion of the *left* hippocampus will produce a transient memory disorder, which may last as long as three months (Geschwind and Fusillo).

The memory disorder that sometimes follows head injury illustrates well the different states of the memory process outlined above. A patient who shows this disorder, let us say a week after the episode, may exhibit the following picture. He will be alert, awake, and cooperative and may, on a standard I.Q. test, score in a normal or even superior range. In addition his immediate memory, as shown, for example, by digit span, will be normal. By contrast he shows an anterograde amnesia, i.e., an inability to learn new material. He also shows a retrograde amnesia extending back from 3 to 20 years. More remote memories, in particular most of what was learned before the age of 12, are usually but not invariably much better preserved. Over the next two or three months the condition improves. The ability to learn new material reappears (but the patient will have a permanent gap in his memory for the period in which he lacked this ability). The retrograde amnesia gradually shrinks until it reaches its permanent form, with a duration of seconds to minutes. The long retrograde amnesia must therefore have been a disorder of retrieval rather than storage. It thus appears that the integrity of the limbic structures is necessary for the retrieval from intermediate but not remote memory. In cases of persistent Korsakoff's syndrome, such as occur frequently with other forms of disorders that produce permanent bilateral limbic system damage, the retrograde amnesia does not improve significantly.

A prominent feature of many but not all cases of Korsakoff's syndrome, especially in the early stages, is *confabulation,* i.e., the tendency of the patient to invent fanciful replies to questions whose answers he does not know. Confabulation usually becomes less marked with the passage of time. Some patients with Korsakoff's syndrome show distinct improvement, although not to normal, over periods of months or even several years.

Functional amnesia occurs in hysteria (usually in young people) or in older patients who are depressed. A similar clinical picture seen in malingerers is usually easy to recognize. The patient may show either a highly selective memory disorder, e.g., denying that he is married, although all other recent and remote facts are preserved, or a global disorder, e.g., professing total amnesia for all events of his life. Failure of a patient without aphasia to state his own name is invariably not organic in orgin. Another common syndrome is the fugue state in which the patient denies any memory of his activities for a period of time ranging from hours to weeks, during which his external activities appeared normal or during which he disappeared and traveled extensively. Although some short-lasting fugue states may occasionally be the result of temporal lobe epilepsy, the author's experience has been that these are nearly all functional in origin.

Kral, on the basis of study of several hundred aging subjects, has pointed out that the finding of true Korsakoff's syndrome leads to a poor prognosis for psychologic function and survival. He has distinguished another syndrome of *benign forgetfulness* with onset usually in middle life. Patients with this disorder have difficulty remembering specific details, especially proper names, although they recognize the correct answer, and on other occasions recall the same data without difficulty. These patients are very embarrassed by these failures to recall. The senile Korsakoff patient is more likely to forget recent events in more global fashion, often fails to recognize the correct data, and is often unconcerned. The benign disorder tends to remain delimited over many years, and is compatible with the highest levels of professional activity. It is more common in men, whereas senile dementia is more common in women.

In some patients *mid-life depression* is associated with distinct memory impairment. When this is the presenting symptom the correct diagnosis may be overlooked. When the depression is successfully treated, the memory disorder clears.

Recovery from memory disorder: Post-traumatic Korsakoff's syndromes typically improve, as pointed out above. A seemingly permanent metabolic amnestic syndrome also may improve slowly over many years. There is no evidence that any therapy is effective in treating memory disorders, but active research is now going on in this field.

Geschwind, N.: Disconnexion syndromes in animals and man. Brain, 88:237, 585, 1965.

Geschwind, N.: The organization of language and the brain. Science, 170:940, 1970.

Geschwind, N., and Fusillo, M.: Color-naming defects in association with alexia. Arch. Neurol., 15:137, 1966.

Kral, V. A.: Senescent forgetfulness: Benign and malignant. Can. Med. Assoc. J., 86:257, 1962.

Victor, M., Adams, R. D., and Collins, G. H.: The Wernicke-Korsakoff Syndrome. Philadelphia, F. A. Davis Company, 1971.

Zangwill, O. L.: Cerebral Dominance and Its Relation to Psychological Function. Springfield, Ill., Charles C Thomas, 1960.

Section Three   DEMENTIA
Paul R. McHugh

226.   INTRODUCTION

GENERAL CONSIDERATIONS. Dementia means deterioration in intellectual capacity. The condition is distinguished from mental retardation, in which subnormal intellectual ability has been lifelong and may or may not be caused by brain injury; and from aphasia and Korsakoff's psychosis, in which specific intellectual skills (language and memory, respectively) have deteriorated without a proportional disturbance in other cognitive functions.

Dementia is a clinical entity. Any pathologic process affecting the cerebral hemispheres can lead to an impairment in intellectual capacity. The extent of the brain injury and not its location or the nature of the neuropathology determines its severity. Treatment and prognosis, however, depend on the nature of the pathologic process. Some pathologies and the dementias they produce are relentlessly progressive. Others are curable. Therefore the diagnostic task consists of two steps: first, the recognition of dementia; and second, the identification of the cerebral pathology producing it. The first step requires skill in the assessment of mental function; the second, an appreciation of the clinical features, course, and diagnostic laboratory data that characterize various cerebral pathologies.

CLINICAL MANIFESTATIONS. The earliest symptoms of dementia can pass almost unrecognized. They appear as disturbances in the patient's capacities for problem solving, grasp of situation, and agility of thought. He may carry out his daily routines at home and at work adequately, but he becomes less efficient and may fail in tasks that are demanding or require his special skills. The changes may be hard to distinguish from fatigue or boredom. The appreciation of their importance will depend on how well the examiner knows the patient and on how much the patient's livelihood depends upon mental capacity. Thus relatives and fellow workers usually notice a change before doctors can be sure of it; and professional, managerial, or skilled workers are more quickly brought for help than are individuals with unskilled occupations.

As a dementia progresses, however, the disability will be obvious to all because its symptoms are defects in basic mental functions. Memory failure is often the first definite symptom. The patient becomes forgetful particularly of the events of the day, overlooks appointments, fails to remember conversations, or forgets the purpose of his errands.

Other symptoms reflect the patient's bewilderment in the face of complexity. He becomes lost in attempting to find his way in the city. He fails to understand a conversation, particularly if several people are involved, as at a meeting. He cannot follow directions that involve a series of steps.

Language presents special difficulties. He is unable to use words with facility and pertinence, but depends on clichés and habitual forms of expression. His conversation becomes rambling and repetitious, his letters long and vague, his directions to others involved and obscure. Defining a word or a proverb for his examining physician is very difficult because he is unable to call up the meaning of abstract words and concepts.

At this stage in a dementing illness, habit often sustains the patient's social behavior. He can for example take part in superficial, polite conversation giving appropriate replies. But if a mental status examination is carried beyond casual interchange to test memory, orientation, or grasp of situation, this façade of customary manners and speech cannot hide the deficits in mental capacity.

The dementing patient often suffers from emotional disturbances. Sudden outbursts of emotion, taking the form of anger, tears, or aggressiveness, may occur when the patient is attempting a task that is beyond his present mental skill. These *catastrophic reactions* are usually of short duration, but their repeated appearance may be a prominent feature of the illness almost from its onset.

More sustained and chronic emotional disorders, such as depression and anxiety, are also seen in dementing illness for reasons that are not immediately obvious. They may represent a response of a patient who comprehends his growing difficulties but may also represent injury to central nervous system mechanisms mediating emotional expression.

A symptom seen in some dementing patients and easily confused with depression is a progressive apathy or mental inertia. This may be just a loss of sparkle or liveliness of character, but progresses to involve initiative and physical energy. Such apathy can result in much poorer performance in daily affairs than can be explained at first by the cognitive disabilities, but worsens as the dementia progresses and can reach such a state of unresponsiveness that the patient is inaccessible to examination.

Finally, if the dementing disorder is relentlessly progressive, the patient will lose all his mental powers. He loses his remote memories, now failing to recognize his closest relatives. He cannot care for any of his physical needs. He becomes bedridden, unaware of his situation, and dependent, and soon dies of intercurrent infection or malnutrition.

DIAGNOSIS. It is not difficult to recognize advanced intellectual impairment. More taxing is the recognition of intellectual impairment when it is slight and potentially reversible. The tests of cognitive function that are part of the neurologic examination of every patient are intended to accomplish this, but they must be interpreted with care.

It is customary to test (1) orientation to time, place, and person; (2) language skills, by naming common objects and comprehending commands; (3) fund of knowledge, such as the names of some capital cities and of presidents; (4) recent memory, by setting three objects to be remembered for 5, 10, and 30 minutes; (5) attention span, by asking for a serial subtraction of 7 from 100 or any other arithmetic task that requires "carrying over"; (6) abstract reasoning power, by asking for definitions of proverbs or the similarity of words such as apple-orange, ear-eye, poem-statue; and (7) constructional capacity, by asking the patient to draw simple objects such as a clock or to copy an abstract design.

As a means of scoring cognitive impairment and following its progress, the Mini-Mental Status of Folstein et al. has proved useful. It employs several of these standard clinical tests to derive a quantitative assessment that is sensitive, reliable, and brief enough to be part of every bedside examination.

The results of these tests must be interpreted in the light of other knowledge about the patient. If the patient was a gifted professional person whose family has noted a decline in his judgment and an increasing forgetfulness, the discovery that he cannot hold three words in mind for five minutes and that he interprets proverbs clumsily provides some evidence that he is suffering from a disturbance to his intellectual power. On the other hand, if the patient was not a person with intellectual achievements in the past and has received a poor education, difficulties in proverb interpretation or fund of knowledge are less likely to represent brain disease. Although it is possible to find all the intellectual functions disturbed in dementia, the tests for recent memory, for attention, and for constructional capacity are most useful. Deficiencies here are easy to document; these functions are affected early in the course of many brain diseases, and they are little dependent on education. Also, tests for recent memory are useful in differentiating a patient with mental retardation from an individual of limited intelligence who is developing a brain disease, since memory function is intact in the mildly retarded individual.

It is important to differentiate Korsakoff's syndrome and aphasia. The patient with Korsakoff's syndrome will fail the test of recent memory. He will be disoriented to time and place, but he will be able to name objects, obey commands, and accomplish tasks of abstract reasoning and drawing if he can hold the question in mind. His disorder is in memory. The rest of his intellectual function is relatively spared. The aphasic patient will have severe problems in naming objects and comprehending words. But if this difficulty can be surmounted, it will be evident that language is specifically disturbed, and other mental functions such as memory, orientation, and constructional capacity are relatively intact.

It is sometimes useful to supplement the bedside tests of mental function with standardized examination of intellectual skills. The Wechsler Adult Intelligence Scale as described in Ch. 236 is most often employed.

DIAGNOSTIC ISSUES IN DEMENTIA. As mentioned previously, the symptoms of dementia appear with an injury to the cerebral hemispheres, and are not specific for a particular pathology. It is the course of their development, the associated neurologic signs, and the laboratory findings that permit diagnosis of the pathologic entities producing the dementia.

Since the same symptoms can be produced by curable, reversible pathology as by incurable and progressive disorders, the first diagnostic consideration should reflect a search for the treatable pathologic entities. All the following conditions represent potentially treatable disorders that should be considered and excluded in every patient: general paresis, myxedema, intracranial mass lesions such as tumors, hematomas and abscesses, hepatolenticular degeneration (Wilson's disease), avitaminosis B (particularly niacin deficiency [pellagra] and

B_{12} deficiency), occult hydrocephalus, and a depressive illness in advanced age. Many of these conditions can be diagnosed by evidence derived from the clinical examination; others demand clinical laboratory studies. A group of laboratory tests are required in the diagnostic evaluation. As a routine, all patients should have a lumbar puncture to measure intracerebral pressure and to obtain a sample of cerebrospinal fluid for analysis. Cell count, protein content, and a test for the antisyphilis antibodies will be needed in cerebrospinal fluid. Blood serologic examination for syphilis, analysis for protein-bound iodine, and serum B_{12} analysis are also indicated. An electroencephalogram may reveal a local lesion or a severe generalized slowing of the rhythms characteristic of delirium. Skull roentgenograms can also reveal a local lesion. The recently developed brain CT scan (see Ch. 267) has become the radiographic procedure of choice in the diagnosis of dementia, providing information that can be critical in the diagnosis of many different cerebral pathologies.

The onset and course of a dementing disorder must be carefully analyzed when considering the likely pathologic entities. Was the onset abrupt or insidious, was the subsequent course a gradual and relentless loss of mental faculties, or was it a series of sudden losses producing a steplike decline? Did it require months or only a few weeks to develop? Different pathologic entities produce different clinical histories in these respects.

Thus the typical dementia produced by arteriosclerotic disease of the brain (*multi-infarct dementia*) will take the course of occlusive vascular infarctions. The mental decline will come with "strokes." It will be a steplike decline with each step sudden in onset, varying in extent, intermittent and unpredictable in timing, and usually associated with some motor-sensory deficits on neurologic examination. The dementia of the degenerative disorders such as Alzheimer's disease appears insidiously rather than suddenly, progresses slowly but steadily rather than irregularly and intermittently, and is free of motor-sensory features until the condition is advanced. The dementia of general paresis or pellagra tends to be subacute and steadily progressive.

An occasional elderly patient with a depressive illness will present with a dementia syndrome quite responsive to treatment of his depression. The course of such depressions is helpful in diagnosis, since, in contrast to Alzheimer's disease, the dementia appears and progresses in a subacute fashion (days to a few weeks). Helpful as well is the recognition of a depression of mood, a change in self-attitude, and a previous history of attacks of mania or depression. Treatment is discussed in Ch. 233 3.

Folstein, M., Folstein, S., and McHugh, P. R.: "Mini-mental state." A practical method for grading the cognitive state of patients for the clinician. J. Psychiat. Res., 12:189, 1975.
Wells, C. E. (ed.): Dementia. 2nd ed. Philadelphia, F. A. Davis Company, 1977.

227. ALZHEIMER'S DISEASE

Alzheimer's disease is a progressive degenerative process of the brain that produces a dementia in middle to late life. It is the most common specific pathologic entity provoking dementia in the United States. Autopsy diagnoses vary from 1 to 10 per cent in mental hospitals, the particular figure depending on whether the observers make a distinction between Alzheimer's disease and senile dementia. Its defining characteristics are its pathologic features.

The brain in Alzheimer's disease very gradually atrophies, nerve cells disappearing from the cortex. The major brunt of the atrophic process appears to be in the frontal and temporal regions of the brain, but microscopic examinations demonstrate pathologic changes throughout the cortex.

The atrophic cortex contains many "senile plaques," microscopic collections of granular argyrophilic particles which tend to form in a halo around an indefinite center containing sudanophilic fat and an amyloid-like substance. These plaques are collections of neuron particles, degenerative synaptic boutons, surrounding a central core of amyloid fibrils. In the cortex many of the neurons that remain show a peculiar alteration of their neurofibrils, which are thickened and twisted into distinctive "neurofibrillary tangles."

The dementia of Alzheimer's disease parallels the pathologic features. In fact the severity of the cognitive symptoms has been directly correlated with the quantity of plaques and tangles in a clinicopathologic study by Blessed et al. The dementia, as the pathology, is slowly but relentlessly progressive. The onset is insidious, and for a considerable period into the course only psychologic symptoms are found. Motor or sensory neurologic signs appear late, if at all.

A disturbance in memory for recent events is usually the first symptom. This amnesic difficulty is accompanied by some disorientation in time and place but may be otherwise the only symptom for some time. Usually within one or two years other cognitive difficulties, as in judgment, comprehension, or abstract reasoning, appear and gradually worsen.

With the development of these cognitive symptoms, emotional unrest can appear. This at first may take the form of anxiety and depression related to the patient's self-awareness of his difficulties. But usually after three or four years of illness, emotional reactions are prompted by delusionary false beliefs that develop in 30 to 40 per cent of these patients. Auditory and visual hallucinations are found in a smaller number of patients.

At approximately the same time in the progression of the illness, symptoms related to focal cortical injury such as aphasia, apraxia, and agnosia often become prominent. The aphasia begins as a naming problem, but quickly dysphasic jargon appears and severely disrupts communication.

By three or four years of the illness, when these intellectual and emotional disturbances are well advanced, neurologic functions begin to deteriorate. The first symptom of this sort is a disorder of gait. This takes the form of difficulty in starting the rhythmical movements of walking. A synchronous activation of agonists and antagonist muscles results in a locking of the legs and a hesitant shuffle. Focal or generalized seizures occur in approximately 15 per cent of patients in the far advanced stages of the illness. Within five to eight years of the onset of symptoms the patient reaches a terminal stage. Here there is a profound dementia and a decerebrate physical state with flexion contractures of all limbs. Death comes from an intercur-

rent infection or some other complication of the bedfast condition.

The age of onset varies. Because this disorder was first recognized among relatively young people, the term "presenile dementia" has been applied to Alzheimer's disease. But the cerebral pathology and the clinical course of patients who develop symptoms before or after age 65 are the same. Alzheimer's disease, defined as it is by the cerebral pathology of atrophy with senile plaques and neurofibrillary tangles, is a disorder appearing with increasing frequency as people age. A distinction between Alzheimer's disease and senile dementia is argued, but pathologically they are identical.

The cause of Alzheimer's disease is unknown. Most examples occur sporadically, but a few patients have a family history. It is not certain whether Alzheimer's disease is a specific response to one noxious biologic process or whether it is a more general response of the brain to many injurious processes. The latter possibility is suggested by the occasional appearance of Alzheimer pathology in such different situations as the punch-drunk syndrome of boxers, Down's syndrome (trisomy 21), and postencephalitic parkinsonism. Experimental neuropathology has produced intriguing results such as the occasional but far from regular production of a neuropathic condition in primate hosts following injections of tissue from Alzheimer patients, the recognition of a deficit in the cortical cholinergic system in Alzheimer's disease, and the discovery of an increase in aluminum in Alzheimer brains. But as yet no confirmation has been provided of what might constitute a primary cause and what the secondary effects.

Blessed, G., Tomlinson, B. E., and Roth, M.: The association between quantitative measures of dementia and senile changes in the cerebral grey matter of elderly subjects. Br. J. Psychiatry, 114:797, 1968.

Corsellis, J. A. N.: Mental illness and the Ageing Brain. London, Oxford University Press, 1962.

Sjogren, T., Sjogren, H., and Lindgren, A. G. H.: Morbus Alzheimer and morbus Pick: A genetic clinical and pathological study. Acta Psychiat. Scand. (Suppl. 82), 1952.

Wolstenholme, G. E. W., and O'Connor, M. (eds.): Alzheimer's Disease and Related Conditions. Ciba Foundation Symposium. London, Churchill, 1970.

228. PICK'S DISEASE

Pick's disease is also a degenerative disorder of the cerebral cortex that produces dementia in middle and late life. It is distinguished from Alzheimer's disease by its morbid anatomy.

In contrast to Alzheimer's disease, in which the cerebral atrophy is diffuse, in Pick's disease, the relatively severe atrophy is confined to the frontal and temporal lobes. The microscopic pathology is distinctive and includes individually degenerating neurons characterized by the accumulation close to the nucleus of a globular argyrophilic mass that distends the cell body into a swollen ballooned form. This "Pick cell" is usually found widespread in the atrophying areas of cortex. There are usually neurofibrillary tangles and senile plaques as well in the atrophic parts of brain.

It is difficult to distinguish an example of Pick's disease from Alzheimer's disease on clinical grounds. Patients with Pick's disease may have less difficulty in gait than patients with Alzheimer's disease. Otherwise, the conditions seem clinically identical. Pick's disease is considerably less common than Alzheimer's disease, but, as in that condition, no definite cause has been identified. Some examples of Pick's disease appear to be transmitted by an autosomal dominant trait, but many examples lack a family history.

229. CREUTZFELDT-JAKOB DISEASE

The dementia in Creutzfeldt-Jakob disease is rapidly progressive, advancing noticeably day by day from its onset to a fatal termination, usually within a year. The dementia is accompanied by a variety of neurologic symptoms such as ataxia, aphasia, paralysis, and visual disturbances and by prominent myoclonic jerking of the limbs and body at some stage in the disorder. The EEG is abnormal early in the disturbance, its normal rhythms lost and replaced with a distinctive mixture of slow and sharp waves useful for diagnosis. The condition is the result of a degeneration of cerebral cortex thought to be caused by a transmissible agent of the latent or slow virus variety. It is more thoroughly discussed in Ch. 310.3.

230. HUNTINGTON'S CHOREA

Huntington's chorea is a distinctive disease entity in which a dementia associated with chorea appears usually in the fourth or fifth decade of life. Its neuropathology is characteristic, and the disease is transmitted as an autosomal dominant trait. The condition is discussed more fully in Ch. 277.3.

231. TREATMENT OF THE DEMENTED PATIENT

With the exception of the specific treatments for curable diseases, the issue of treatment for the demented patient is most often that of management of particular symptoms rather than reversal of a pathologic process. Often, a treatment based on some research finding is proposed for the degenerative disorders only to prove of little value when employed in a clinical trial. Thus the discovery that cerebral oxygen consumption is reduced in Alzheimer's disease led to treatments with both oxygen inhalation and hyperbaric chambers. But these treatments failed to produce significant improvement, almost certainly because the observed reduction in oxygen consumption is due to a reduction in the number of viable neurons rather than to an inadequate oxygen supply. Any treatment that is proposed for these distressing conditions is liable to be uncritically acclaimed, with eventual disappointment. The importance of the clinical trial with double-blind technique in assessing these treatments cannot be exaggerated.

Some general principles of management of the demented patient can be emphasized. First, complicating medical conditions such as congestive heart failure, dehydration, iron deficiency anemia, infections, and electrolyte imbalance can, even if not severe in themselves, make the mental condition of a patient with degenerative brain disease much worse and should be corrected. Second, much of the emotional unrest in demented patients is due to fear produced by their disorientation, misidentifications, and misinterpretations. Great relief of these symptoms can come from a willingness of nurses and doctors to explain repeatedly to the patient his situation and the proper interpretation of what is happening. Changes in surrounding and in nursing personnel should be minimized; well lighted rooms, preferably with familiar possessions, serve best, and an attitude that is accepting and supportive does much to assist the patient. Any situations that require effort beyond his capacity and so produce catastrophic reactions must be avoided. Third, considerable help for individual symptoms can be gained by the use of pharmacologic measures. Sleep disturbances in demented patients are best treated with chloral hydrate, up to 1.0 to 1.5 grams at night.

The agitated states associated with delusions, misinterpretations, and *catastrophic* reactions can be among the most disruptive features of these disorders. They can be considerably ameliorated by a combination of the supportive management described above and modest amounts of phenothiazine or butyrophenone medication. Thioridazine, in doses of 50 to 100 mg three to four times daily, or haloperidol, 2 to 5 mg three times daily, has proved helpful. Depressive symptoms respond to antidepressant medication (imipramine, 50 mg three to four times per day).

All these drugs should be used sparingly, as the patient with cerebral degeneration may demonstrate toxic signs at much lower doses than normal patients. Drug toxicity can worsen the condition severely.

In general, the management of the demented patient rests on an appreciation of the nature of his psychologic disabilities and the application of psychosocial medical and nursing principles. The response to this management is often gratifying.

Miller, E., and Pearce, J.: Clinical Aspects of Dementia. London, Bailliere Tindall, 1973, pp. 98–124.

Post, F.: Clinical Psychiatry of Late Life. New York, Pergamon Press, 1965.

Section Four PSYCHOLOGIC ILLNESS IN MEDICAL PRACTICE

Paul R. McHugh

232. THE CONCEPT OF DISEASE IN PSYCHIATRY

Any general hospital can provide an experience in psychiatry, because an example of every psychologic disorder will eventually appear among patients admitted to its services. However, many thoughtful physicians feel unsure of their ability to manage these disorders. They are apt to contrast their knowledge of somatic illness founded firmly in morbid anatomy and pathophysiology with their understanding of psychologic medicine in which classifications seem based on confusing mixtures of symptomatology and speculative theories, and the most effective treatments are empirical. Such physicians will continue uncertain until they grasp how the basic concept of disease can bring order to aspects of psychiatry as it does in all of medicine. This they must accomplish before they can profit from a review of the clinical facts of particular psychiatric conditions; hence this chapter.

The term "disease" is difficult to define, because it is a concept and not something concrete or given in nature. As a concept it focuses on patients as organisms and conveys the idea that among all the morbid changes in physical and mental health it is possible to recognize groups of abnormalities as distinct entities or syndromes separable from one another and from the normal and that these separations will prove to have some biologic explanation when the entities have been thoroughly investigated.

Abnormalities can as logically be viewed as quantitative changes merging imperceptibly into one another and into the normal, and can then be explained as consequences of disturbed interactions of a few vital processes. The Galenic concept of "humors" is just such a view. In fact the concept of disease based on qualitatively distinct syndromes is a convention championed by Sydenham, and remains but a convention today. However, this has been one of the most useful conventions in the natural sciences. It has become so indispensable in medical thinking that it is taken for granted in most discussions. Neglect of this convention explains much of the difficulty faced by students in psychiatry. Its logic thus needs review here.

The concept of any given disease passes through several stages as knowledge increases. At each stage attention focuses on certain features of the condition which are the "defining characteristics." At the first stage a "clinical disease entity" is recognized and defined as a constellation of symptoms and physical signs running a more or less predictable course or natural history. Dropsy, hemophilia, and epilepsy are typical clinical disease entities. But these entities are not pure species.

Each can be the expression of any one of several different pathologic conditions: glomerulonephritis, congestive heart failure, constrictive pericarditis. Thus the second stage is the division of the clinical disease entity into several "pathologic disease entities." When a disease can be conceived as a pathologic entity, the defining characteristics on which concept and diagnosis rest are results of laboratory tests that reveal pathologic function or morbid anatomy. Again, by way of example the demonstration of an elevated blood urea nitrogen and albumin and casts in the urine of a patient with dropsy leads to a presumptive opinion that the pathologic disease entity responsible for his condition is glomerulonephritis. This presumptive diagnosis is confirmed by studying the histopathology of the kidney. The third and final stage in the concept of a disease is the recognition of a particular etiologic agency. This recognition can derive from any aspect of biologic knowledge: genetics, microbiology, and biochemistry have all made their contributions. For glomerulonephritis the etiologic agency is the phenomenon of autoimmunity, and it will be from investigations of this phenomenon that physicians can expect to gain a complete understanding of glomerulonephritis as well as a treatment that can prevent and cure it.

For many medical diseases the mark of the twentieth century has been the discovery of etiologic agencies and their action. This is less so for psychiatry. For most psychiatric disorders knowledge has not passed the first stage on the traditional path, and for many even the hold on this stage is insecure. This insecurity arises in part from the difficulty of the subject matter, but also from a lack of consensus over the applicability of the disease concept in this field. It implies a distinction between those mental disturbances that arise in the mind of a subject coping with conflict and those that are a result of disease in the organism. This is a distinction some would deny, holding the opinon that *all* psychologic disturbances are to be viewed as emotional reactions to some form of environmental distress, and thus are quantitative abnormalities differing from normal in a continuous and smooth fashion rather than grouping into qualitatively distinct entities with separable pathologies and etiologies.

One objection to this view has to be the practical one that it discards for no obvious advantage a convention that has ordered other abnormalities successfully. Another is that it oversimplifies mental disturbances to make them all expressions of a few psychologic mechanisms. A consideration of the forms of disorder for which psychiatry assumes responsibility will demonstrate the utility found in the concept of disease for some of them.

Three groups of disturbances fall into manageable

psychiatric categories. *The first holds all those disturbances in mind and behavior that are a result of observable brain pathology.* Represented here are the clinical disease entities of delirium, dementia, and mental retardation. The conceptual and investigative approach to these conditions is indistinguishable from that for other somatic diseases. Such pathologic disease entities as Alzheimer's disease and such etiologic agencies as perinatal hypoxia, infections, and metabolic changes have been discerned.

The second group holds the two functional psychoses in which no obvious brain pathology is evident: schizophrenia and manic-depressive disorder. That these conditions are not unlike somatic disorders and should be conceived as clinical disease entities defined by symptoms and course is impossible to prove at this time. But this view was first prompted by the alien form of the psychologic symptoms such as hallucinations and delusions that appear in these disorders. It has been strengthened by the discovery of pharmacologic treatments specific to each entity and by the recognition of a few morbid conditions of the central nervous system leading to identical clinical conditions — amphetamine toxicity leading to a schizophrenia-like disorder, and the reserpine reaction that mimics a depressive disorder. It is now more conceivable that we are on the threshold of discoveries that will provide pathologic disease entities and etiologic agencies for these conditions than that they will be explained as quantitative exaggerations of emotional reactions.

The third group of disturbances in mind and behavior are the personality disorders and neurotic symptoms. The concept of disease with its logical extension from clinical entity through pathology to etiology does not fit these conditions. To seek, for example, a neuropathology provoking grief would seem an obvious category error — mistaking a subject's problem for an organism's disease. A different method is needed to explain problems. This method rests on the assumption that many expressions of distress in mood and behavior (neurotic reactions) can be understood from an appreciation of an individual's personality traits and his life experiences. His personality traits are the relatively stable features of temperament that distinguish him from others. They are quantitative distinctions and no more diseases than would be shortness of stature, plainness of face, or dullness of wit. Through an appreciation of his temperament, we can comprehend the meaning to him that links his past experiences, present events, mood, and behavior.

Psychiatry is the medical discipline that must consider both the subject and the organism in man. The concept of disease assists this consideration by organizing some clinical phenomena in a fashion similar to that of general medicine. In the following chapters the application of this concept to particular conditions as well as its distinction from methods for appreciating a subject's problems will be described.

Jaspers, K.: General Psychopathology. Translated by J. Hoenig and M. Hamilton. Manchester, Manchester University Press, 1963.

Scadding, J. G.: Diagnosis: The clinician and the computer. Lancet, 2:877, 1967.

Taylor, F. K.: Psychopathology. Its Causes and Symptoms. London, Butterworth and Co., Ltd., 1966.

Wightman, W. P. D.: The Emergence of Scientific Medicine. Edinburgh, Oliver and Boyd, 1971.

233. FUNCTIONAL PSYCHOSES

233.1. INTRODUCTION

The psychoses form a loose category that gathers together several different clinical entities. To be placed within the category an entity must produce disturbances in thinking and perception that are inexplicable solely as responses to experience and are severe enough to distort the patient's appreciation of the real world and the relationship of events within it. The category psychosis has no uniform foundation as in somatic pathology nor any more objective aspects of psychopathology to mark its distinction from other collections of psychiatric symptoms. It is thus a term difficult to use with precision. Sometimes psychosis is used as a euphemism for insanity, sometimes as a synonym for schizophrenia, one of the entities within the category, and sometimes to draw an elusive distinction as between neurotic and psychotic depression.

The unmodified term can be qualified by a differentiation into organic psychoses and functional psychoses. Here the term psychosis means only severe mental illness. The organic psychoses, delirium, dementia, and Korsakoff's syndrome, are produced by a variety of cerebral pathologies. The functional psychoses, schizophrenia and manic-depressive disorder, lack a recognizable neuropathology.

This differentiation is practical. It draws a distinction in kind that affects treatment and prognosis, and it indicates the character of the clinical problem. For the organic psychoses the central problem is the cause of the pathologic changes. For the functional psychoses the central problem is consistent diagnosis.

Schizophrenia and manic-depressive disorder are clinical disease entities. The criteria for their diagnosis are their symptoms alone. There are no objective tests verifying a diagnosis. Only the natural history or response to empirically discovered treatments can confirm a diagnostic opinion. Since they lack a recognized neuropathology and are by definition inexplicable as responses to experience, there are no comprehensive etiologic explanations for these disorders. Treatment therefore is symptomatic rather than fundamental. Both prevention and radical cure await a chance discovery or a major scientific advance in understanding the biologic foundations of human behavior.

233.2. SCHIZOPHRENIA

Schizophrenia is a most devastating mental illness. It is a disturbance of mind and personality appearing in clear consciousness and characterized by several distinctive alterations in mental experiences, modes of thinking, and mood that are seldom completely resolved. The most characteristic features occur during the active phases of the disturbance, and take the form of hallucinations, delusions, and altered behavior toward others. Specific intellectual and affective disabilities varying from minimal to severe can develop insidiously or remain after an attack. A crucial element of the definition is that all these symptoms occur in a patient free of any relevant and discernible pathologic change in his nervous system.

CLINICAL MANIFESTATIONS. The symptoms of schizophrenia can begin at almost any stage in life, but most commonly occur during adolescence and early adulthood and then either insidiously or as an acute attack followed by a series of attacks, each leaving behind personality defects of increasing severity.

In some patients it is possible to recognize a particular premorbid personality. They may have seemed more timid or seclusive than others. They may have been bookish, unsociable, and preoccupied with philosophic and religious ideas to the exclusion of friendships and community experiences. But this so-called *schizoid personality* is not found in most patients who develop schizophrenia. *At least half of schizophrenic patients had premorbid personalities indistinguishable from normal.*

Among the mental changes that mark the onset of a schizophrenic illness, only some are specific to this disorder. Emotional unrest, uncertainty, perplexity, and confusion can be found in many disorders other than schizophrenia, and therefore a diagnosis of schizophrenia cannot rest on them. There are, however, a number of mental changes that are more or less diagnostic. These can be usefully divided into abnormal mental experiences and disturbed modes of expression. The abnormal mental experiences are somewhat more reliable evidence of the illness simply because they are easier to elicit with confidence and less dependent upon interpretation than disturbances in expression.

Hallucinations and delusions are the outstanding schizophrenic mental experiences. Although hallucinations can occur in many disorders such as delirium, dementia, and occasionally manic-depressive disorder, certain forms of hallucinations are more specific for schizophrenia. Thus auditory hallucinations are the most common hallucinations in schizophrenia, and certain kinds of auditory hallucinations are almost diagnostic. Thus hearing one's thoughts aloud or hearing voices commenting about one's every action or several voices engaged in a conversation in which derogatory and praising remarks are passed with the patient discussed in the third person are the most typical schizophrenic hallucinations.

Although delusions, i.e., false beliefs that are incorrigible, idiosyncratic, and preoccupying, can be found in many disorders other than schizophrenia, in this illness delusional experiences are dramatic and well developed. They can begin as vague, fearful interpretations and "half-beliefs" and develop into firm incorrigible convictions. A delusion coming on suddenly, not prompted by any hallucination or previous delusion, nor related in any obvious way to the patient's mood, is called a "primary delusion" and is highly suggestive of schizophrenia. Many other schizophrenic experiences are of delusional form, but have such individual characteristics that they have been named for themselves.

Commonly schizophrenics have delusions about bodily control, the so-called passivity experiences. The patient feels as though he were under the control of some outside force or power making him behave as an automaton without a will of his own. He may feel hypnotized and feel forced to make particular movements, speak with a special voice, or walk to certain areas. The patient may believe these feelings come to him as penetrating waves from electronic or telephonic equipment.

The schizophrenic patient may experience changes in his thinking. Particularly he may feel that his thoughts are disrupted by some outside agency, that his thoughts are withdrawn from his mind, or that other thoughts are inserted into it. He may believe that people can hear his thoughts, which are leaving his mind as waves broadcast to others.

In contrast to these abnormalities of experience are the disturbances in the patient's mode of expression. Particularly noticeable is his abnormal language. Characteristically, he is difficult to understand. His thinking is expressed in a vague and awkward fashion with words poorly chosen and ideas poorly related to one another. Strikingly, the patient makes no effort to correct the vagueness of his thinking or to improve the clarity of his talk. Often, asking a question of the patient, the examiner receives a reply that is off the point and that goes into unnecessary details. Although the questions of the interview seem to start the patient toward a particular answer, it is never reached, but the patient takes up abstract and unnecessary ideas and must be redirected toward his goal. The examiner, laying the responsibility for the confusion on himself, may work to express himself more clearly, and only after considerable effort recognize that the difficulty in communication rests with the odd replies from the patient.

Another prominent disturbance is emotional expression of these patients. They seem distant, unresponsive, and cold. On some occasions the patient's emotional attitude seems incongruous, particularly for the thoughts he is expressing. Thus he may laugh while saying that he is in mortal danger. This cold or incongruous attitude and manner give the schizophrenic patient his most striking features, and even when at their mildest can be baffling and distressing symptoms to his family.

Other abnormal modes of expression of the schizophrenic patient are disturbances in stance and mobility called catatonic symptoms. Gestures may seem stiff, slow, and mannered. Some schizophrenic patients make repetitive movements or facial grimaces. Others may become totally immobile and mute. Still others may assume unnatural postures and hold them for long periods.

During the active phases of the schizophrenic illness the flamboyant subjective experiences are most prominent. During the chronic phase of schizophrenic illness expressive disturbances in thought and emotion are more evident, varying from mild to severe. Although at times some patients seem free of symptoms, whether a careful examination does reveal mild residual disturbances in thinking and emotional responsiveness is debated and difficult to disprove.

DIAGNOSIS. The diagnosis of schizophrenia rests on recognition of the distinctive clinical symptoms of this disorder and the exclusion of other conditions which may produce similar symptoms.

Many disorders of brain function can imitate schizophrenic symptoms; but with the exception of the three schizophrenia-like disorders to be discussed, patients with the other brain disturbances also manifest disturbed consciousness, disorientation, and disruption of cognitive abilities, particularly recent memory function, that are not found in schizophrenia.

Mania or depression can be confused with schizophrenia (to the considerable embarrassment of the diagnostician when the patient recovers completely on receiving treatment appropriate for these conditions). A source of difficulty is the occurrence of delusions, which are common enough in mania and depression but usually spring directly from the mood and the attitudes of self-confidence or self-blame that are so prominent in those disorders.

In schizophrenia disturbances in experience, including the auditory hallucinations and delusions just described, form the most secure basis for diagnosis. Thus, in a person free of brain disease or drug intoxication, recognition of auditory hallucinations with voices commenting on the patient in the third person, primary delusional experiences, passivity experiences, or disturbances in "thought control" permit the diagnosis of schizophrenia to be made with some confidence. In fact, Kurt Schneider has referred to these as "first rank symptoms" of schizophrenia because of the diagnostic confidence their discovery brings.

If these symptoms cannot be found, then diagnosis must rest upon recognition of manifest disturbances in thought and emotional expression. It should be pointed out, however, that opinion holding a person's thought to be illogical and vague, or his affective responses to be inadequate or incongruous, is an evaluative judgment and must be held with somewhat less confidence, if the difficulties are minimal or inconstant, than opinion resting on recognition of delusions and hallucinations.

Catatonic symptoms of immobility, posturing, and grimacing, along with the disturbances in behavior described as negativism or reluctance to cooperate, must be carefully interpreted. Only in those patients in whom no evidence of a prominent mood change can be found should a diagnosis of schizophrenia be made. Motility changes in the direction of psychomotor retardation are prominent features of depressive disorder, a condition as common as schizophrenia and more common than the catatonic variety of schizophrenia.

Symptoms of emotional unrest, anxiety, withdrawal, and hostility can be found in schizophrenic patients, but these are common to many other psychiatric disorders, and therefore can never form the basis for a secure diagnosis of schizophrenia. However, that diagnosis is rendered more likely if it can be established that the patient was developing normally without an apparently vulnerable personality, and if these symptoms appeared without a change in the patient's mood or the pattern of his life. Since these more general symptoms can be found in both schizophrenia and many other psychiatric disturbances, it is important to search carefully for the more basic symptoms of hallucinations and delusions from which emotional unrest and unpredictable behavior may stem. Often repeated efforts are required to gain cooperation of the patient so that he will divulge the existence of those basic symptoms that make a diagnosis of schizophrenia certain.

ETIOLOGY. There is no neuropathology or consistent pathophysiology that can be observed to develop with progression of the disorder and that might give some hint of causation. An approach to a consideration of etiology has to be more circuitous and the opinions derived held with somewhat less assurance than is true of other clinical entities. Two aspects of etiology can be conveniently separated for the purpose of organizing the information we have. One aspect is "cause," that is, any prerequisite element needed to set in motion a train of events leading to the entity. The other is "mechanism," that is, the particular nature of the train of events, be they psychologic, neurologic, or biochemical, that produce the symptoms. For schizophrenia there is some information relating to "cause" and also to "mechanism," but it is far from conclusive.

"Cause" or Prerequisite Elements in Schizophrenia. The genetic constitution has been decisively demonstrated to be one of the "causes" of schizophrenia. The risk of schizophrenia increases with the closeness of genetic relationship to a schizophrenic patient. Thus only 1 per cent of very distant relatives of a schizophrenic patient will themselves suffer from the disorder. This is no higher than the risk in the general population. But 5 to 6 per cent of siblings and 40 to 50 per cent of monozygotic twins of schizophrenic patients will have schizophrenia.

The possible objection that these data merely reflect the increasingly common environment of progressively closer relatives has been refuted by observations on monozygotic twins brought up apart who continue to show an identical high risk. Heston made the same point in a different fashion by studying a group of offspring of schizophrenic mothers. These particular children were raised from earliest infancy in foster homes by normal, nonschizophrenic mothers and fathers. The incidence of schizophrenia in these children was exactly the same as that reported for children raised by a schizophrenic parent. They thus resembled their biologic mother although reared apart from her.

It has nevertheless been impossible to fit schizophrenia into a clear mendelian pattern of dominant or recessive inheritance. Some students of the disease would describe the hereditary contribution to schizophrenia as polygenic, i.e., the sum of a number of contributions from the genes no one of which is solely responsible. The polygenic concept might permit environmental factors to play a larger role in causation. Thus a mild genetic vulnerability might express itself in a schizophrenic phenotype only in those who face stressful environments, whereas those carrying a more severe genetic vulnerability might show the disorder in any environment. It is difficult at the moment to propose a test that would exclude the polygenic hypothesis as a possibility.

Some studies that have established a genetic contribution to the etiology of schizophrenia have also given evidence of the inadequacy of genetics as a sufficient cause for the disorder. That 50 per cent of monozygotic twins of schizophrenic patients are free of this illness means one of the following: (1) Although the genetic constitution is necessary and sufficient to produce schizophrenia, the symptoms employed to define a case fail to provide an adequate means of recognizing all examples of the disorder, and 50 per cent are mistakenly called normal. (2) The defining symptoms encompass a mixed group of disorders, and in only 50 per cent of these disorders are genetic features necessary and sufficient causes for the symptoms. (3) A genetic vulnerability for schizophrenia is necessary but not sufficient. It must be combined with certain life experiences that need not be common for genetically identical individuals.

The present inadequacy of the genetic hypothesis to provide a complete description of the "cause" for schizophrenia reinforces a search for environmental and experiential causes. It has proved just as difficult to determine an environmental contribution as to define the genetic contribution. Thus the experiences of being raised by a cold and distant mother, or of receiving insistent, simultaneous, but incompatible directions from the parents, or of simply living in a disharmonious family incapable of providing a healthy environment for psychologic growth have all been considered causes of schizophrenia.

Such disturbed experiences have been found in the lives of some schizophrenic patients when viewed retrospectively after the onset of the illness. But none has proved to be a common experience in all schizophrenic people. Nor has it been possible to predict an increased incidence of schizophrenia among individuals living in comparably disturbed situations. Presently the most economical view of the role of life experiences in the "cause" of schizophrenia holds that *any* adversity, be it a psychologic shock, abnormality in critical relationships, or physical injury (particularly brain injury) may provide a partial contribution in causing schizophrenia, but that most of these adversities are exerting their causal effects upon a genetically vulnerable individual.

"Mechanism" of the Schizophrenic Syndrome. This is the other aspect of etiology. Given that some combination of genetic and environmental attributes is probably prerequisite for the illness, by what derangements are the symptoms produced? Are they produced by some change in a psychologic function that might have been learned or developed through experience, or are they produced by some morbid change in the nervous system that alters the normal capacity to perceive, integrate, and respond? There have been proposals for each of these "mechanisms."

It has been proposed that the mechanism of the disturbance has been through the production of a particular psychologic change fundamental to the whole syndrome and from which all the symptoms can be explained. Thus Federn has proposed a "loosening of ego boundaries" as the essential feature mediating this illness, whereas Bleuler proposed a basic disturbance in associational thinking. A crisis of identity has been proposed by exponents of existential psychiatry. These views have a ring of plausibility perhaps derived from their resemblance to experiences common to all men, part of which can seem to be reflected in the behavior of schizophrenic patients. But they depend on concepts that are difficult to define except in terms of what they purport to explain.

Other studies have attempted to demonstrate the possibility that the mechanism is a change in the central nervous system. No such change has been demonstrated in schizophrenia as yet, so supporters of this possibility have had to reason by analogy.

Three well documented conditions affecting the brain can give rise to a mental disturbance resembling schizophrenia. The most familiar is the syndrome found with *chronic amphetamine intoxication.* In this condition the patient is alert and oriented but preoccupied by auditory hallucinations and delusional ideas indistinguishable from those seen in schizophrenia. The disturbance may last from several days to a few weeks, but disappears eventually after the withdrawal of the stimulant.

Slater, Beard, and Glithero have demonstrated that among patients suffering from *psychomotor epilepsy,* caused by an irritative lesion in the limbic portions of

the temporal lobe, a certain number develop a paranoid schizophrenia-like syndrome after 10 to 15 years of epilepsy. This condition displays all the classic delusional and hallucinatory symptoms of schizophrenia, but there is less tendency toward deterioration of thinking and personality.

Finally, certain patients, *withdrawing from excessive alcohol ingestion,* suffer from a period of auditory hallucinations. Although in most of these patients the hallucinatory experience clears within 24 to 48 hours, in a small proportion a chronic condition of persisting auditory hallucinations associated with delusional beliefs, incongruous affect, and disturbed thought develops. This chronic condition may be indistinguishable from the schizophrenic syndrome, and may persist for many years.

For all these schizophrenia-like conditions the possibility exists that the pertinent features might be the expression of a latent predisposition for schizophrenia in the affected individuals. But there is no evidence of a predisposition. The relatives of these patients do not have an increased incidence of schizophrenia, and the patients themselves do not have schizoid traits in their premorbid personalities.

The existence of these conditions demonstrates that the symptoms of schizophrenia are capacities of the damaged human brain. Yet we are ignorant of any common pathologic feature of these brain disorders that could by implication be the fundamental mechanism for schizophrenia. One possibility is that each of these disorders represents an extraexcitatory arousal of the brain, particularly of the reticular formation and limbic system, either directly via amphetamine or epileptic discharge or in rebound from long-continuing action of the depressant ethanol. It may be that the condition of schizophrenia itself is thus produced by some excessive activity in these or related brain regions evoked by the genetic-environmental "causes" discussed above. Mednick and Schulzinger have also found some evidence suggestive of hyperarousal in children of schizophrenic mothers who go on to develop the disease themselves.

Another proposed mechanism for producing schizophrenia is through some change in body metabolism or chemistry that could itself alter cerebral and psychologic functions. Many students have been prompted to consider this alternative because of the remarkable growth in biochemical methodology. In fact the difficulties in establishing a role for biochemistry in the etiology of schizophrenia rest not with the chemical methodology but with such issues as defining the group bing studied, avoiding chemical artifacts related to dietary habits or medications given chronically hospitalized people, and deciding what biochemical change to look for with little knowledge of what kinds of change might produce symptoms. The papers of Kety should be consulted for a more thorough discussion of these difficulties. A rare condition, periodic catatonia, has been documented by Gjessing to be associated with a phasic change in nitrogen balance, but no relationship between this disorder and schizophrenia in general has been found.

Snyder has proposed that a functional excess of cerebral dopamine may be the critical feature in schizophrenia. He based this suggestion mainly on the observation that the therapeutic potency of the phenothiazines parallels their relative capacities to block dopamine receptors. Although this evidence is indirect, the hypothesis has provided a specific focus to research efforts that seem close to providing some confirmatory evidence.

Thus our knowledge of "mechanism," as much as our knowledge of "cause," is still fragmentary and provisional. But on the bits of evidence at hand, the view that seems easiest to defend is that schizophrenia will prove to be due to some deranged neural mechanism that can occasionally be produced by coarse brain disease but more often is the outcome of an anomaly of the genetic constitution.

TREATMENT. The treatment for any schizophrenic patient is complex and should not be attempted by the inexperienced. A period of hospitalization will usually be required. There a program to include drug therapy, psychologic treatment, and social evaluation can be planned.

The sheet anchor of treatment now for schizophrenia is the *phenothiazine* drugs, discovered in the 1950's almost by accident. To date there is no secure explanation for their effectiveness. Clearly they are not simply acting by virtue of their sedative effect, since their remarkable action is not mimicked by other sedatives. They can remove the symptoms of schizophrenia, including the delusions, hallucinations, and disordered thought, and are not restricted to relieving excitement or anxiety as the term tranquilizer might imply.

The most versatile phenothiazine preparation is the original: chlorpromazine. The dose required to treat acute symptoms varies widely from patient to patient, and amounts from 200 to 2000 mg per day may be necessary. Maintenance dosage is similarly an individual matter, but 100 to 200 mg per day is usually an effective range. Since cessation of treatment results in the reappearance of symptoms in 60 to 70 per cent of patients within six months, drug therapy is often given over years. This practice, however, must be evaluated in light of a movement disorder (tardive dyskinesia) that may appear with prolonged use of phenothiazines. Tardive dyskinesia is a chronic choreoathetotic disorder affecting primarily the faciobulbar musculature but in some examples the extremities as well. It is resistant to most pharmacologic treatment with the exception of giving larger doses of the phenothiazines that provoked it originally. Since it is a particular danger of chronic high dose phenothiazine treatment, the attempt should be to employ as small a dose as possible in chronic administration. The report of Crane gives details.

The *psychotherapy* suitable for the schizophrenic patient has been a subject of intense controversy. The more radical approaches based on psychologic and particularly psychoanalytic views of the genesis of schizophrenia have not achieved their optimistic goals of curing the patient by relieving some basic psychologic conflict. More modest psychotherapy is indispensable when it is intended to help the patient in his everyday affairs, taking advantage of those personal assets that persist despite his illness, and establishing a relationship of friendly rapport in order to guide him in his management of personal and social issues, which, if mishandled, can lead to distress and further illness. A particularly pressing issue for the schizophrenic patient is the social situation into which he is placed after hospitalization. His psychiatrist, usually at first with the help of a psychiatric social worker, must strive to find a job that is regular and well within the patient's power but not excessively challenging, a domestic arrangement that is calm and supportive but not too emotionally demanding, and a daily routine that combats the tendency to withdraw from all social contacts into an isolated and perhaps fantasy-ridden existence. To accomplish these goals is one of the most challenging exercises in medical treatment. The growth of "halfway houses" as residences for previously hospitalized schizophrenic patients has been prompted by recognition of the need for stable and structured social environments for schizophrenic patients once they have improved enough to leave the hospital.

PROGNOSIS. Prognosis for any patient diagnosed as schizophrenic is always guarded. Certain features carry a good prognosis: high intelligence, a normal premorbid personality, an acute onset, catatonic features in the illness, and a family history of affective disorder. Other features carry a poor prognosis: low intelligence, schizoid premorbid personality, insidious onset of the illness, symptoms of thought disorder, affective blunting in the illness, and a family history of schizophrenia.

The use of phenothiazines has considerably improved the prognosis of schizophrenia, 30 to 50 per cent of patients having complete remissions on follow-up over five years. Another 30 to 40 per cent show some residual symptoms but are able to live in the community, and only 10 to 20 per cent require further hospitalization if phenothiazine treatment is begun and maintained after their first attack of the illness.

Connell, P. H.: Amphetamine Psychosis. Maudsley Monographs, No. 5. London, Chapman and Hall, Ltd., 1958.

Crane, G. E.: Persistent dyskinesia. Br. J. Psychiatry, 122:395, 1973.

Fish, F. J.: Schizophrenia. Bristol, John Wright & Sons, 1962.

Heston, L. L.: Psychiatric disorders in foster home reared children of schizophrenic mothers. Br. J. Psychiatry, 112:918, 1966.

Kety, S. S.: Biochemical theories of schizophrenia, I and II. Science, 129:1528, 1590, 1959, 1969.

Klein, D. F., and Davis, J. M.: Diagnosis and Drug Treatment of Psychiatric Disorders. Baltimore, Williams & Wilkins Company, 1969.

Mednick, S. A., and Schulzinger, F.: Some premorbid characteristics related to breakdown in children of schizophrenic mothers. J. Psychiat. Res., 6:267, 1968.

Schneider, K.: Clinical Psychopathology. Translated by M. W. Hamilton. New York, Grune & Stratton, Inc., 1959.

Shields, J.: The genetics of schizophrenia in historical context. *In* Coppen, A. J., and Walk, A. (eds.): Recent Developments in Schizophrenia. Brit. J. Psychiat., Special Publication No. 1, pp. 25–41, Ashford Kent, 1968.

Slater, E., Beard, A. W., and Glithero, E.: The schizophrenia-like psychoses of epilepsy. Br. J. Psychiatry, 109:95, 1963.

Snyder, S. N.: The dopamine hypothesis of schizophrenia: Focus on the dopamine receptor. Am. J. Psychiatry, 133:2, 1976.

233.3. MANIC-DEPRESSIVE PSYCHOSIS

The essential feature of this psychosis is an excessive disturbance of mood and self-appraisal from which its other mental symptoms seem to arise. This disturbance can be in the direction of elation and self-confidence or sadness and self-blame. The course tends to be episodic, even periodic, with attacks of elation (mania) or sadness (depression) interspersed with periods of apparent mental health varying in length from weeks to years. Individual patients may suffer attacks of only one kind throughout their lifetime. Single or repetitive attacks of depression seem to be the most common manifestation, but attacks alternately manic and then depressive or even repetitively manic are not unusual.

CLINICAL MANIFESTATIONS. Depression. During an

attack of depression the patient complains of feeling miserable and uncertain of himself. He may give evidence of his sadness by a dejected appearance and by restlessness and distractibility. Some patients are slowed in their activity, and this can progress to a psychomotor retardation of such severity that the patient seems totally unresponsive.

Mental examination of the depressed patient usually brings to light not only his feelings of sadness or misery but also a lowered self-esteem that can vary in intensity from feelings of inadequacy and incompetence to convictions of personal worthlessness, blameworthiness, and evil. This combination of depressed mood with self-blame is the diagnostic sign of this condition. It will also explain most of the other symptoms, modes of behavior, and dangers faced by the depressed patient.

Other symptoms include delusional extrapolations of the attitudes of self-blame. These can increase to a belief that the patient's guilt is notorious, that he is to be arrested, and that he will be condemned to die or to suffer some extraordinary punishment either in this world or the next. Suspiciousness and fear of mistreatment based on these delusional beliefs may be difficult to distinguish from similar attitudes in the paranoid schizophrenic patient. A useful if not cast-iron distinction is the depressive's belief that the suspected ill treatment comes as a justified punishment and not, as with the schizophrenic, as an undeserved persecution.

In some severely depressed patients delusional ideas can become bizarre and even grandiose in concept. Thus they come to believe that they have been the cause of cosmic disasters, that the sun is darkened by them, that whole cities have been deserted because of their presence, or that they and their progeny are accursed in the sight of the Divinity. Delusions of bodily change may take the form that their brains are rotting, their bowels totally blocked, or their bones fractured and dislocated.

Delusional ideas may concern the relationship of the patient to the world and to others. He may believe that he has lost all his money, that he has become a burden to others, that he is universally despised, or even that he gives off such a bad odor that people cannot stand his presence. Again, these beliefs are usually reflective of the patient's inner attitude of self-blame, self-contempt, and hopelessness.

The point about these opinions is that they are delusional and not just false. They are unshakable opinions held in the face of all contrary evidence. Only treatment of the depressive disorder will remove them.

The most worrisome symptom of the depressed patient is *inclination to suicide*. It is easily appreciated that attitudes of such hopelessness and despair as have been described could prompt self-destruction. But it is not necessary to have such exaggerated delusions for suicide to be a distinct risk. Vigilance for suicidal intentions must be maintained throughout the course of the depressive disturbance. The physician should ask any depressed patient about thoughts of self-injury. A series of questions useful in estimating suicidal risk is provided in Ch. 234.3. Often this simple action will reveal both the severity of the mood disturbance and the need to bring the patient into hospital for his own protection.

Homicide is also a possibility for the depressed patient, and is particularly likely in those who harbor beliefs that their family shares in their guilt and accursed characteristics. Any suggestions by the patient that he might prefer death should be most seriously believed.

Along with these psychologic symptoms the depressed patient will often suffer from disturbances in his sleep, particularly waking early in the morning and being unable to return to sleep. Other physical disturbances include bodily aches and pains, loss of appetite, constipation, and weight loss. These features may combine with the retardation to give the appearance of chronic physical ill health. In fact, many depressed patients will first consult internists complaining of such physical symptoms. Helpful to the differentiation of the patient whose somatic symptoms are part of a depressive illness is a discovery of the features of depressed mood, and attitudes of self-blame or hopelessness when these features are combined with complaints of poorly localized pains, with loss of appetite or weight loss, or even with preoccupations about the state of the inner organs.

Mania. Symptoms that are almost the exact opposite of those seen during an attack of depression appear during an attack of mania. Now the patient says that he is in excellent spirits, that he feels well, and in fact has never felt better. He is active and restless, and appears energetic, confident, and quick-witted. These characteristics tend to worsen, and it is in their more extreme form that they become recognized as symptoms. The restlessness and energy become overactivity, with the patient moving constantly and planning progressively less plausible projects. His speech becomes incessant, rapid, and disjointed, one idea following another with little connection between them. His attitude of confidence becomes grandiose self-satisfaction. He may be overbearing and pompous. He often will be irritated by his surroundings, easy to anger, and perhaps suspicious that the efforts being made to control him are unjust.

Although a manic patient can usually be recognized by his overactivity, ebullience, and great self-confidence, he can develop as well ideas of resentment and feelings that he is being in some way unfairly noticed or persecuted. These ideas, on investigation, are found to derive from his own delusional opinion that he is so important that he must be under scrutiny by forces such as foreign powers. Occasionally, these persecutory ideas are so prominent that a diagnosis of schizophrenia is entertained. It is, however, the direct connection of these ideas to the attitude of self-confidence that allows a diagnosis of mania to be made.

With the mental changes manic patients exhibit disturbed social behavior. They may have increased sexual interest and may become promiscuous. They tend to overspend and be reckless with money. They may insult their employers and so be fired from their jobs. In the first attack of mania and before the severe restlessness and disorganization of thought appear, these activities may not be recognized as the products of mental illness, but may be construed as actions for which the patient can be held accountable. Thus the patient can be subjected to severe losses, to legal actions, or to moral criticism that can hamper his life long after his manic attack is over. To protect him from these consequences hospitalization of the manic patient may be required.

ETIOLOGY. **"Cause" or Prerequisite Elements in Manic-Depressive Disorder.** As with schizophrenia, an important genetic contribution to the etiology of the manic-depressive disorder seems certain. There is a progressive frequency of incidence with increasing blood relatedness so that with monozygotic twins the concordance rate is over 50 per cent. It is likely that genetic constitution is a necessary but not sufficient cause for this disorder. Certain other features of the illness require consideration. First, the illness does appear in attacks interspersed with periods in which the person appears to be normal. Second, the attacks are somewhat seasonal, appearing more frequently in the spring and fall than in summer and winter. Third, although many attacks occur spontaneously, many seem to be precipitated by some disturbing event. Presumably some other elements must combine with the genetic vulnerability to explain these features. Again, the most easily defended position would hold that a necessary cause for manic-depressive disorder is the genetic constitution of the patient, but that any of a large number of environmental disturbances can bring out the disorder.

Mechanism in Manic-Depressive Disorder. As with schizophrenia, a pharmacologically induced disorder has enhanced confidence that, whatever the "cause," the mechanism for affective disorder is a neural one. Treatment with reserpine for hypertension produced depression in up to one of four patients, and this depression was accompanied by the typical delusional attitudes of the manic-depressive psychosis. The discovery that reserpine depleted brain neurons of biogenic amines, particularly norepinephrine and serotonin, has prompted a variety of hypotheses that propose some lack of norepinephrine, serotonin, or other biogenic amines at synaptic sites in the brain for emotional control. That many effective antidepressant agents also influence these same amines has been a further support to these hypotheses.

TREATMENT. The first rule in managing either manic or depressed patients is that most of them should be in a hospital. Their conditions can bring catastrophe to themselves and their families in the form of financial mismanagement in mania and suicide in depression. If these diagnoses are strongly suspected, then psychiatric opinion should be immediately sought so as to determine whether hospitalization should be imposed. It is critical to have expert help, because the patient can often hide the severity of the disorder in a mass of explanations which may appear quite plausible. In the hospital the suicidal patient must be closely supervised and definitive treatment should not be long deferred.

It is crucial to diagnose these patients and separate them from those with other conditions, because new drug treatments have proved effective for them and are specific to the affective disorders. Two classes of pharmacologic agents are effective in *depression*. Seemingly more effective are the so-called *tricyclic antidepressants*, the prototype of which is imipramine. This drug, given in doses of from 75 to 300 mg per day, will relieve a depressive attack in 50 per cent of patients. The recent development of the means for measuring plasma levels of tricyclic antidepressants has revealed a partial explanation for failures to respond. A narrow range (50 to 170 ng per milliliter) encloses therapeutic plasma nortriptyline levels. The failure to reach this level or the exceeding of it inhibits a full response. A rational pharmacology for these medications will soon require plasma measurements to be available as a routine. The

technologic advances to achieve this ideal seem near at hand. Maintenance therapy of 100 to 150 mg per day should be continued for six to eight months after recovery. If tricyclics are ineffective, the logical practice should be to switch to the other class, which includes the drugs that have as their primary action the capacity to inhibit the enzyme monoamine oxidase. These drugs, in doses of 45 to 75 mg per day, have also proved useful in depression.

If *monoamine oxidase inhibitors* are used, the patient must be warned to avoid foodstuffs such as cheese, broad beans, and some yeast extracts, which have pressor amines of the phenyl-ethyl-amine group that includes tyramine. If absorbed by patients whose monoamine oxidase enzyme is depleted, they can cause sudden elevation of blood pressure with headache, blurred vision, and even cerebrovascular hemorrhage.

The mainstay of treatment for severe depression is *electroconvulsive treatment* (ECT). In contrast to the drugs which relieve the symptoms of depression, ECT will terminate an attack of depression usually in four to eight treatments. This treatment can produce the most dramatic and quick recovery from the depths of a life-threatening depression, and should not be withheld from a delusional patient or any seriously depressed patient who has failed to respond to drug treatment after three to four weeks. Maintenance with imipramine, 100 to 150 mg per day for six months, is recommended after ECT for the avoidance of relapse shortly after successful treatment.

The *treatment of mania* is often very difficult, particularly if the patient is suspicious about medicines. Haloperidol in doses of 2 to 10 mg thrice daily taken orally has proved effective. This compound is liable to produce severe extrapyramidal side effects which can be combated with antiparkinsonian drugs and with Benadryl. Chlorpromazine in doses of 300 to 1000 mg per day can also be tried.

A recent and effective measure for controlling mania has been the use of lithium ion in the form of lithium carbonate. This compound is available in 300 mg tablets, and daily intake of 900 to 2400 mg per day can relieve manic excitement. It is, however, essential to follow plasma lithium concentration in these patients, because toxic signs of disorientation, tremor, anorexia, and diarrhea can appear if plasma lithium concentration rises above 2 mEq per liter. The therapeutic level and the toxic level of lithium are close, and therefore the medication must be started when the patient can be carefully supervised in a hospital. Maintenance lithium treatment can be recommended, because there is fair clinical evidence that in this fashion some further attacks of mania may be avoided.

PROGNOSIS. The prognosis for a single attack of mania or depression is excellent. Even without treatment patients tend to recover completely within six months. With antidepressant treatment the medication can be withdrawn after six to eight months with fair assurance that symptoms will not recur at this time.

The longer-range prognosis is not so favorable. Eighty per cent of people who have suffered one attack of affective disturbance will have another at some time in their lives, but this may not be for many years. Some patients, however, will have recurrent attacks of mania or depression interrupted by only brief intervals of normal behavior.

The best advice to give patients who have suffered from their first affective attack is that they will very likely be quite well for years, but that they and their family should be aware that their mood changes are to be considered seriously, and they should seek psychiatric attention promptly if such a mood change tends to persist or worsen. Prien's work indicates that individuals who suffer recurrent attacks of any form of manic-depressive disorder are best maintained on lithium for an extended, even an indefinite, period.

Astrup, C., Fossum, A., and Holmboe, R.: A follow-up study of 270 patients with acute affective psychoses. Acta Psychiat. Scand. (Suppl. 135), 1959.

Kragh-Sorensen, P., Hasen, C. E., and Asberg, M.: Plasma levels of nortriptyline in the treatment of endogenous depression. Acta Psychiat. Scand., 49:444, 1973.

Lewis, A.: Melancholia. J. Ment. Sci., 80:277, 1934.

Prien, R., and Caffey, E., Jr.: Relationship between dosage and response to lithium prophylaxis in recurrent depression. Am. J. Psychiatry, 133:567, 1976.

Prien, R., Klett, J., and Caffey, E., Jr.: Lithium prophylaxis in recurrent affective illness. Am. J. Psychiatry, 131:198, 1974.

Schildkraut, J. J.: The catecholamine hypothesis of affective disorders: A review of supporting evidence. Am. J. Psychiatry, 122:509, 1965.

234. PERSONALITY DISORDERS AND NEUROTIC SYMPTOMS

234.1. INTRODUCTION

GENERAL CONSIDERATIONS. The concept of disease entities that supports our understanding of the functional psychoses does not suit all psychologic disturbances and particularly those that are described as personality disorders or neurotic symptoms. There is uncertainty both in terms and in concept here. For example, the designation neurosis is ambiguous in that it seems a name for a clinical entity with some sharp distinction from normal, but a cardinal symptom of one neurosis, *anxiety,* is an experience of all people at some time and is an appropriate mood in certain circumstances. What then is abnormal in *anxiety neurosis?* Is this abnormality of a quantitative or a qualitative nature? To what kind of patient can the term anxiety neurosis be applied? Should we use it only for patients in the emotional "state" of anxiety, or is it suitable regardless of the present state if a patient has "traits" that make him prone to this emotion?

The term *personality* and particularly its extension, *personality disorder,* can be just as troublesome. Personality seems a word similar to such terms as character or temperament, words intended to describe aspects of human psychologic variation distributed in a smoothly graded fashion in the population. But if that is true, then the distinction personality disorder can seem an arbitrary, socially contrived, or judgmental decision, since no sharp dividing line is to be expected in smoothly graded characteristics. In Ch. 234.2 to 234.4, an attempt is made to dispel some of these ambiguities while considering several emotional disturbances often called neurotic that occur in a general medical setting.

Although many mental changes and emotional disturbances in patients can be ascribed to known or presumed pathologic changes in brain function, certain varieties of human psychologic constitution and certain life experiences can themselves provoke emotional disturbance and disrupted behavior. The terms personality disorder and neurotic symptoms are intended to describe the disturbances that result from variation in human constitution and experience by invoking the concepts of potential and response. Personality always means *potential.* It encompasses and describes the abiding and distinctive traits or tendencies of an individual to react to circumstances in a particular fashion. Thus by "optimistic personality" is meant an individual who can be expected to respond with cheerfulness and optimism in situations in which others are less likely to do so. An individual's personality is the sum of numerous traits, and a comparison with others is implicit in the description of each trait. Thus every trait can be conceived as a dimension of variation along which people can be dispersed in a fashion similar to their dispersal along the dimensions of height, weight, or intelligence. Any definition of an individual's personality is an attempt to place him in relationship to others in respect to one or more traits. An individual can be said to have a disorder of personality if he deviates to such an extreme along the range of variation for some trait that either he or others complain of its effects.

Whereas personality and personality disorder indicate potential, the neurotic symptoms are emotional *responses* displayed when the individual is troubled by circumstances. For anyone certain environments and life events are conducive to anxiety, others to depression, and still others to suspiciousness. People with a disorder of personality have an increased potential for these responses and are provoked to them by less extreme circumstances and less specific stimuli. Thus paranoid personality disorder is a term used to describe an individual who tends to show attitudes of suspiciousness and feelings of persecution (the neurotic symptoms) in settings so minimally threatening that they will seldom provoke such attitudes in others. If, however, his life is relatively free of threatening features, these feelings will be diminished and, despite his personality traits, symptoms may be avoided.

Before such concepts can be used in the evaluation and management of a particular patient, that patient must be well known to the doctor, and the possibility of other conditions that could produce similar symptoms must be excluded. For this a detailed psychiatric history, mental status, and physical examination are needed. The latter two can be obtained during the first interview, but historical information about the patient's family background, developmental milestones, sexual adjustment, scholastic and occupational achievement, habits, and medical problems may require several hours of examination. Observations from his relatives improve the accuracy of such information, and their descriptions of his personality are indispensable. All these data, combined with the knowledge of the patient's present condition, form the basis for diagnosis, treatment, and prognosis, and to embark on such matters without this information is to commit a capital error. The result is often failure of treatment, because the patient has been misunderstood and emphasis given to minor rather than major features of his problem.

As it becomes clear that a given patient's disturbance is the outcome of the kind of person he is and the situations that he faces, the data of the psychiatric history and the mental status examination can usually be divided into three categories which, although closely related, are usefully distinguished: (1) the predisposing factors for the disturbance, including personality traits and formative life experiences; (2) the precipitating factors; and (3) the symptoms themselves and their effect on the patient.

PREDISPOSING FACTORS. Predisposing factors are those features special to an individual that make him vulnerable to emotional disturbance. The most critical factor is personality, the traits of which are distinguished in the patient's temperament, attitudes, and predictable responses. But personality is the outcome of genetic constitution, intellectual endowment, and lifetime experiences, and each of these is a predisposing factor in itself. As intriguing examples of studies in these issues, the work of O'Connor on the role of intellectual subnormality in emotional instability and the study of Granville-Grossman on the relationship of parental loss to depression in adulthood can be recommended. Predisposing factors often overlooked are the patient's social status and cultural situation. The scholarly study of Dr. Beatrice Berle, *80 Puerto Rican Families in New York City*, and the recent work of the Dohrenwends in social psychiatry are excellent examples of empirical work in these areas.

Finally, the state of health is an important predisposing feature, because physical illness, through the distress it produces or by direct effects on the central nervous system, interferes with a person's capacity to cope with circumstances and thus leads to psychologic symptoms.

PRECIPITATING FACTORS. The precipitating factors are events or experiences that have disrupted emotional equilibrium and bear a close temporal relationship to the disturbance for which the patient seeks help. The common-sense expectations that personal illness, or conflict produced by changes in family or occupational circumstances, could precipitate psychologic distress have been confirmed in studies such as those of Brown and Birley. Holmes has attempted to grade life events in a hierarchy of emotional stressfulness, and many workers have found his scale useful for estimating the relative distress different patients have endured. Some psychologic precipitants are more recondite, because they depend on a special meaning an individual gives events, perhaps a symbolic meaning derived from the particular patient's early life experiences. Before emphasizing these more abstruse precipitants of a unique character, it is usually wise to consider the more immediate and obvious ones that may be present.

SYMPTOMS. In Ch. 234.2 to 234.4, the symptoms of anxiety, depression, and hysterical reaction are discussed, because they are common in the general practice of medicine.

All these neurotic symptoms emerge as complaints either of the patient himself or of others who must deal with him. They are symptoms in the sense that they disturb the patient's sense of well-being or they interfere with his behavior and his adaptability to circumstances. They can vary from mild to severe, and they can be acute or chronic.

In the assessment of these symptoms the patient should be encouraged to describe how he feels, how the symptoms developed, what seems to make them worse or better, what they are like when compared to previous emotional reactions, and how they disturb him now. *The aim is to come to appreciate these symptoms as understandable responses of this particular person to his particular circumstances.* The over-all principle is that we are considering here not classes of patients suffering from distinct disease entities, but individuals troubled by their special life circumstances and needing assistance tailored to their particular personal nature and situation. The specific symptoms, their characteristic predisposing and precipitating factors, their effects on behavior, and modes of treatment will be considered in the balance of this chapter.

Berle, B. B.: 80 Puerto Rican Families in New York City. New York, Columbia University Press, 1958.

Brown, G. W., and Birley, J. L. T.: Social precipitants of severe psychiatric disorders. *In* Hare, E. H., and Wing, J. K. (eds.): Psychiatric Epidemiology. New York, Oxford University Press, 1970.

Dohrenwend, B. P., and Dohrenwend, B. S.: Social Status and Psychological Disorder. A Causal Inquiry. New York, John Wiley & Sons, 1969.

Holmes, T. H., and Rahe, R. H.: The social readjustment score. J. Psychosom. Res. 11:213, 1967.

Jaspers, K.: General Psychopathology. Manchester, Manchester University Press. 1962.

O'Connor, N.: Psychology and intelligence. *In* Shepherd, M., and Davies, D. L. (eds.): Studies in Psychiatry. New York, Oxford University Press, 1968.

234.2. ANXIETY

DEFINITION. Anxiety is an unpleasant mood of tension and apprehension. It is fear's first cousin and, like fear, has prominent autonomic effects when severe. But fear is an emotion sharply focused on immediate dangers, whereas anxiety is usually imposed by the anticipation of future danger, distress, or difficulties. As an emotional response common to men, anxiety is useful. Activities that arouse it are avoided and those that diminish it are sustained. Although anxiety may spur people to perform difficult tasks skillfully and admirably, when excessive it is a hindrance, as some well prepared students demonstrate when facing a critical examination. *Anxiety is a medical problem when it is excessive, inappropriate, or without obvious cause.*

PREDISPOSING AND PRECIPITATING FACTORS. Anxiety is the psychologic response to anticipated troubles, real or imagined, dimly or accurately perceived. But men and troubles vary. Some persons, the timid, the inexperienced, the excessively conscientious, are frequently anxious in situations that seem not to affect others. Most people are at least mildly anxious whenever they seek medical advice, and when threatening dangers are intense or prolonged, as in chronic painful illness or in battle, even the most resistant individuals can develop incapacitating anxiety.

Resistance to anxiety varies with physical condition, and when tired, sick, or injured, people are more easily threatened. Also, they are more vulnerable to anxiety when their powers of analysis and discrimination are failing or underdeveloped. Thus, because of inadequate comprehension or imprecise perception, the immature, the elderly, or the person with brain damage may become anxious in situations in which a person with a healthy, mature brain is comfortable. In fact, one of the first indications of a dementia can be an attack of severe anxiety without obvious provocation.

Common precipitants of anxiety in daily life are circumstances of conflict in which an action is demanded but the correct action may be difficult to discern. Thus a person may be anxious over difficult decisions on which rest his economic and social success or because the decisions produce an unpredictable response in an inconsistent superior. Laboratory models for this kind of situation and its effects on the emotional state have been easy to produce. Pavlov trained dogs to respond to the picture of a circle by rewarding such responses with food. He did not reward responses to an ellipse. Then, by simply compressing the ellipse so that it gradually approached a circle in shape, he made the discrimination progressively more difficult. The emotional response of these dogs was remarkable. They became ferocious and violent when put into harness for the experiment. They tore at their restraints, barked uncontrollably, and refused to attempt the discrimination. In this state, not only did they make many mistakes, but they became unable to make discriminations that had previously been easy. It is not difficult to see analogies in both situation and behavior between Pavlov's dogs and men with emotional conflicts.

An emotional state of anxiety can be produced in other ways than as an understandable response to anticipated difficulties. A prolonged irritable anxiety state can follow a head injury as one of the symptoms of the so-called *postconcussional syndrome*. Gronwall and Wrightson demonstrate that it may be caused by a mild disturbance in cognitive capacity subjectively evident to the patient but demonstrable objectively only with difficulty. Similarly, a mood of tension and agitation with tremulousness can occur in the delirious states, such as those that follow withdrawal of alcohol or barbiturates and are sometimes produced by the hallucinogenic drugs such as LSD-25. In these situations, it may be disturbed perceptions and misinterpretations that arouse anxiety, but often the anxiety is independent of anything that the patient definitely experiences or understands. Roth describes a peculiar and chronic anxiety state that can follow a calamitous emotional experience. This condition, referred to as the *phobic anxiety syndrome*, occurs in mildly obsessional persons after a severe fright. The disturbance can last for many months. These patients are in a state of considerable anxiety, mostly unformulated, and, associated with this, they have an unwillingness to leave their homes because of vague fears. The peculiar psychologic response of *depersonalization*, which is a change in the awareness of self such that the person feels unreal, is present in many of these patients. In the phobic anxiety syndrome the mood of anxiety follows rather than precedes difficulty, demonstrating that anxiety, normally an anticipatory psychologic response, may take on a self-sustained activity after certain experiences such as severe frights or sudden disasters.

The role of learning and of conditioning has too often been neglected in considerations of anxiety. This probably derived from attempts to explain all anxiety in terms of basic instinctive drives. That a fear-provoking situation could train an individual to experience symptoms of anxiety in circumstances that resembled these situations is very likely, and is indicated by research on emotion in animals. The capacity to develop anxiety via conditioning mechanisms seems the probable explanation for certain cases of phobic anxiety focused on specific objects.

MANIFESTATIONS OF ANXIETY. The manifestations of anxiety are divisible into three groups. *First* are the inner feelings of tension, apprehension, and dread that form the anxious mood itself. *Second* are disturbances of the intellectual power of the anxious patient. He is unable to think clearly, to use proper judgment, to learn efficiently, or to remember accurately. *Third* are the autonomic, visceral, and endocrine changes that have been analyzed by Walter B. Cannon and his followers as the companions of emotional excitement and particularly of anxiety or fear. These include tremor, tachycardia, hypertension, increased perspiration, dilated pupils, and reduced salivation and gastric secretion. Increased activity of the sympathetic nervous system and of the adrenal medulla mediates the majority of these visceral responses to anxiety.

A model anxiety state is to be seen among front-line soldiers. The infantryman is a prepared subject for anxiety. He is always threatened with death or mutilation. He must go without sleep, remain exposed to the weather, and often be hungry. He is usually unable to understand what is happening around him. He is repeatedly frightened by gun fire and distressed by the death of comrades. If he is exposed long enough, he develops a severe and persisting anxiety state sometimes called "battle fatigue." He becomes tense and easily startled. His judgment is poor, and he cannot efficiently sustain a complex offensive action. Among other physical complaints, he suffers from headache, anorexia, and diarrhea. He is usually convinced that death is imminent. Almost all men develop this condition if exposed to battle long enough. Wolff reports that the average man in the army of the United States reached this point after 85 days of combat; 75 per cent could be expected to break down by combat day 140, and 90 per cent by combat day 210. These figures vary little among nations, although few are willing publish them. They make the point that, in his resistance to crippling anxiety, even the bravest man has a "breaking point." On reaching it, he does not betray his group or run from the enemy, but rather he becomes less efficient in protecting himself and runs a high risk of death.

The symptoms of anxiety that physicians see in patients are not different. The patients all have the same three groups of symptoms, but, depending in part on the cause, these symptoms can appear as a relatively brief attack or as a more prolonged, chronic disturbance of mood.

Anxiety attacks may be single episodes or may be periods of exacerbation in a chronic state of tension. They are short periods of tension, varying in severity from mild apprehension to severe panic. An anxiety attack can occur at any time. A favored time is when the patient is traveling in a plane, bus, or train. Most commonly, though, an attack develops at night when, with the disappearance of daytime distractions, a patient begins to ruminate on his troubles. The apprehensions grow to preoccupy his thoughts, and he develops visceral responses of fear. Clear thinking becomes impossible, as does sleep. The heart pounds. A common complaint in an anxiety attack is the sensation of tightness in the chest as though the lungs could not be adequately filled. The patient responds to this sensation by deep and sighing respirations. Sometimes he may produce in this way a respiratory alkalosis with feelings of giddiness and vertigo, tingling of his fingertips, and even tetany with carpopedal spasm. This is the *hyperventilation syndrome*, and the resulting symptoms may add to anxiety.

Full-blown anxiety attacks have an hysterical flavor and may, in part, depend on personal tendencies to self-dramatization and suggestibility. But they also can be the results of a psychic chain reaction, the initial apprehensions and anxiety stirring up cardiac and respiratory changes that are themselves frightening. Granville-Grossman and Turner have provided more evidence that visceral responses to anxiety can increase the subjective symptoms of anxiety by demonstrating that these latter symptoms are improved when an anxious patient is treated with propranolol, a drug that blocks the adrenergic beta-receptors of the sympathetic nervous system and slows the heart rate.

Chronic anxiety may be punctuated by or may begin with an acute attack, but it may be just a steady and distressingly prolonged disturbance of mood. The symptoms are less intense although not different in quality from those of acute anxiety. The patient is tense and "on edge." He may also report some feelings of sadness or hopelessness along with his anxiety. It can be difficult to differentiate his condition from an agitated depression. His intellectual powers are diminished, and he has considerable difficulty in concentration and in thinking. He will score poorly on intelligence tests, particularly on the performance subtests, just as does a patient with dementia. He will have a number of somatic complaints: frontal or occipital headache, anorexia, diarrhea, and weight loss, among other things. On examination, he may have the physical signs of tension, a fine tremor of the extended arms and brisk tendon reflexes, rapid heart beat, increased blood pressure, and pupillary dilatation. More extensive laboratory studies may reveal other visceral and endocrine disturbances, such as reduced gastric acid secretion or increased adrenocortical activity.

DIAGNOSIS. Usually diagnosis is not difficult. In both acute and chronic anxiety, the patient's major complaint is the distressing emotional state. Associated disturbances in thinking and autonomic function serve to confirm the diagnostic impression. For these patients, the major issue is not the diagnosis of anxiety, but rather the question of why they have become anxious now. This question must be answered from knowledge of the circumstances and personality of the patient.

An occasional patient focuses his complaints on his physical symptoms, such as irregularities in the beat of his heart, the change in bowel habits, weight loss, anorexia, or easy fatigability. From these symptoms a more severe illness such as a hidden malignancy, a chronic infection, or some endocrine disorder like hyperthyroidism of Addison's disease may be suspected. Although these conditions are usually seen to be only remote possibilities, laboratory studies may be required to exclude them. As with all psychologically disturbed patients, laboratory studies should not be delayed or protracted but should be decided upon, and this phase of the examination should be finished as promptly as possible.

TREATMENT. Treatment will vary with the cause and severity of anxiety. Many mildly anxious patients can be helped by a physician who is willing to listen carefully to their difficulties and offer some support and occasional advice. Most patients with anxiety have this mild type. Their disturbances are transient and are based on some particular problem or self-doubt that has developed acutely and is eventually resolved.

Those with more severe anxiety can be aided by a combination of pharmacologic treatment and repeated compassionate discussions of their troubles. Barbiturates have been the preferred agents for relief of anxiety in the past. However, barbiturates can be addictive, and there is the ever-present danger that they may be used in a suicide attempt by an anxious patient who is also depressed. In several double-blind clinical trials, chlordiazepoxide (Librium) has been found as effective as barbiturates for treating anxiety, and can be recommended. Dosage of 10 mg three to four times a day is usually effective. Up to 20 to 25 mg three times daily can be given to severely disturbed patients.

Patients with persisting anxiety can be referred with some confidence to specialists in psychotherapy. The effectiveness of psychotherapy seems to depend on the comfort provided by frequent sympathetic discussions and an increased recognition by the patient of the irrational aspects of his anxiety. The particular school of psychotherapeutic theory subscribed to by the therapist seems less important.

Only the most severely anxious patients need hospitalization and then usually only for an acute attack of anxiety. They are treated best with sedation; chlordiazepoxide in doses of 25 to 30 mg three times daily can be used. The somatic symptoms from the respiratory alkalosis of the hyperventilation syndrome can be treated by placing a bag over the nose and mouth that will retain the expired CO_2 for rebreathing.

Careful consideration should be given to any evidence that the anxious patient may be depressed. Agitated depression can be easily confused with simple anxiety. If depression is thought to be the diagnosis, then antidepressant medication, such as imipramine, 75 to 300 mg per day, should be given rather than sedatives.

For those individuals with restricted anxieties prompted by particular stimuli, i.e., phobias, there is growing evidence that deconditioning techniques based on learning theory may have an important place in therapy. Certainly some impressive controlled trials have been published indicating a faster response to this mode of management than to interpretive therapy for individuals suffering from a single phobia. This treatment, like any other, should not be attempted without experience and guidance.

Granville-Grossman, K. L., and Turner, P.: The effect of propranolol on anxiety. Lancet, 1:788, 1966.

Gronwall, D., and Wrightson, P.: Delayed recovery of intellectual function after minor head injury. Lancet, 2:605, 1974.

Roth, M.: The phobic anxiety-depersonalization syndrome and some general aetological problems in psychiatry. J. Neuropsychiatry, 1:293, 1960.

Wolff, H. G.: Every man has his "breaking point." Milit. Med., 125:85, 1960.

234.3. DEPRESSION

DEFINITION. Depression is a term for a mood of sadness and gloom. It can be a symptom of manic-depressive psychosis, and Ch. 233.3 should be consulted for a complete consideration of the subject. Here we are dealing with depression that occurs as a response to troubled life circumstances. Such depression can usually be given a more specific name, such as discouragement, demoralization, or grief — terms that carry specifically the connotation of an emotional reaction.

The troubled mood is usually not hard to recognize. The patient appears miserable, his face expressive of sadness and perhaps tension. He may move without confidence or purpose and report that his energy is decreased and his thinking slow and difficult. Appetite is usually lessened, often with weight loss, and sleep is restless and diminished. Sexual interest will be greatly reduced. The patient may also say that he is irritable and fearful. Depending on the severity of his depression, the patient will seem socially disorganized, proving inefficient in work, failing in duties, and neglectful of appearance. His acknowledged inadequacies in these respects may add to his sense of misery and may prompt thoughts of resigning from work, leaving his family, or even committing suicide.

Although various troubles can provoke depression, there is a specific response that illustrates features common to many depressive reactions. That response is *grief*, well studied by Dr. C. M. Parkes.

Grief is an experience in almost every lifetime and is the response that follows the loss, usually by death, of some relative or friend. The severity of the reaction and its duration depend upon many factors, but the most important is the closeness of the relationship and degree of dependence of the mourner on the lost individual.

Grief is a state that follows a pattern of development in which certain stages can be recognized even though the transition from one to the next is not possible to define exactly and features from one can persist in the others. *The first stage*, which lasts several days, begins upon learning of the death. The mourner feels stunned and appears bewildered, does not seem to grasp his loss fully or to relate its implications to his feelings coherently. He may appear irritable, tearful, or anxious, but can also seem calm and capable. Although his emotions and behavior may be unpredictable, they are often culturally modified as he carries out such customs as funeral rituals. He himself will usually report afterward that his emotions were blunted and his thinking uncertain, and that his depressed mood was not fully experienced. Parkes refers to this period as the stage of numbness, blunting, or shock.

This stage ends gradually but usually within one week of the bereavement, when there is an increase in the emotion of sadness and the appearance of an intense sense of loss that comes in waves, called pangs of yearning or pining by Parkes. In this *second stage*, between these surges of distressing feelings, which are so frequent at first as to be almost continuous, the patient is usually irritable and sad, with sleep and appetite diminished. Activity, which often takes the form of aimless moving about rather than productive work, may be increased, particularly so during a depressive surge, a point Parkes uses to support his analogy of this stage of grief to the searching behavior of animals separated from their mates. It is the phenomenon of *surges of misery*, however, that is most characteristic of grief and usually aids in its recognition. With time these occur less often, but it is common experience to have such a wave of depressive feelings sweep over a person following a reminder of the loss years after the bereavement.

The third period of grief appears with a diminution in the attacks of yearning and the anxious restlessness. This phase, usually entered into within several weeks of bereavement, customarily lasts the longest. It is a stage of depressed feelings with apathy and a disinclination to find purpose or interest in work. The patient is no longer restless, sleepless, or without appetite, but his emotional state is one of gloom and discouragement and his capacity for enjoyment or for physical or intellectual work is greatly reduced. Parkes refers to this as the stage of disorganization when the patient seems withdrawn, may complain of ill health, and fails to plan ahead. This state may last over a year and only gradually be replaced with more customary feelings. Recovery may be brought about in part by the natural but chance occurrence of new integrative activities and friendships, and can be facilitated by efforts of the mourner to expose himself to the opportunities for these restorative experiences.

Depressions that are responses to difficulties in life other than bereavement are very similar to this third stage. Symptoms like those in the first two stages of grief can appear briefly in distressing situations that have a sudden onset, such as being informed of an unexpected personal misfortune. But these are usually transient features and are soon replaced by a mood of sadness and discouragement very like that of the third stage.

PRECIPITATING FACTORS. In this form of depression it is usually not difficult to recognize the change as a response to some difficulty, for the patient is often preoccupied with the trouble itself and is ready to draw the link between it and his present mood. Precipitating situations can be of many kinds. They can be sudden and specific events in which something is lost, such as a relationship or a job. Other provocations are situations chronically thwarting to the sense of achievement and self-esteem, as in an education program in which students are confronted with their errors but given little effective teaching to overcome them. Moving away from home can provoke the very unpleasant depressive reaction, homesickness, especially in persons who depend a great deal on the support of friends and family. In general, circumstances that disturb a person's sense of stability, security, effectiveness, or worth provoke depressive responses.

The more such a precipitant is prolonged or accompanied by a growing realization of his difficulties, the more likely the person is to show a depressive response. A paradigm of these features for a precipitant is found in debilitating physical illnesses such as cancer. Here the protracted and continually worsening clinical situation provides constant reminders of losses suffered and brings more each day. That depression is a universal occurrence in such circumstances has been demonstrated by Hinton in his study of the dying.

For reasons not fully understood, there are some physiologic states and physical illnesses that commonly provoke depressive moods. Patients with hepatitis or any severe viral illness are particularly prone to report a depressive mood and to find reasons for it in trifles that did not trouble them when they were well. Endocrine alterations such as the postpartum state, Cushing's disease, or Addison's disease are also precipitants of depressive feelings that can be very distressing to the patient and of such profound degree as to occasionally promote a suicidal action. Certain brain diseases, particularly stroke, may also precipitate a prolonged and distressing depressive state. In all these circumstances the mood of depression may rest on some disturbed physiologic mechanism in the central nervous system as yet unknown. Their possible relationship to manic-depressive disorder is discussed in Ch. 233.3.

PREDISPOSING FACTORS. Given that situations of difficulty can lead to depression, there are features of personality that can make an individual more vulnerable to this response, perhaps by making him assess losses and difficulties more acutely and by inhibiting his power to resolve them. Especially vulnerable are those insecure and sensitive individuals who perceive criticism when none is intended and find a source of depressive feelings in their self-doubting.

Another depressive predisposition is that of the self-dramatizing and emotionally unstable and immature individual who tends to amplify emotional reactions of all sorts. When such an individual finds himself in situations of discomfort in which his feelings may be neglected, he seems more prone than others to develop a sense of dissatisfaction, distress, and depression. Slavney and McHugh present empirical evidence of this predisposition in their report of depressive symptoms in 80 per cent of patients hospitalized with the diagnosis of hysterical personality.

Finally, individuals limited in their capacity to cope with difficulties are predisposed to depressive responses. Particularly vulnerable for this reason are the mentally retarded. Even modest impairment in intellectual endowment will interfere with the person's ability to find solutions to situations that present him problems, and his failure and uncertainty tend to provoke a depressive mood. Borderline mental retardation is often overlooked in the search for predisposing factors, and a history of poor occupational and scholastic performance in a depressed patient warrants formal intelligence testing.

DIFFERENTIAL DIAGNOSIS. The differential diagnosis of depressive states can be difficult, particularly if it is not carried out methodically. The most important distinction to draw is that between depression as a response to troubled circumstances and depression as a symptom of manic-depressive disorder. This important discrimination rests on clinical grounds and cannot be made with certainty in all situations. Thus, although the depressions of the widow, the homesick, and the patient with a fatal illness can all be recognized as responses, the trap is in making this understandable connection with every depression and explaining it always as being due to some recent difficulty. If the family of the patient says he is more depressed than they would expect him to be under the circumstances, the diagnosis of a depressive response might be questioned. Also, the presence in the patient of remarkable changes in self-attitude such as the appearance of beliefs that he is a criminal or deserves punishment for minor transgressions, or that he is infectious and filled with physical corruption, are not seen in the usual depressive response and should lead to the consideration of manic-depressive psychosis. Finally, a previous history of mania or of depression, or a family history of affective disorder, should influence the interpretation of depression and sway the diagnosis away from the depressive response (see Ch. 233.3).

TREATMENT. Although the depressive response is characteristic enough to be recognized easily again and again, the particular predispositions, precipitants, and interactions are never the same from one patient to another. Treatment is based on these particulars and is thus unique to some extent to each occasion. It is therefore hard to describe the treatment of depression without some sense of dissatisfaction because, although the principles are simple, no list of them applies to every patient.

An important early decision in treatment is the need for hospitalization. This is usually determined by how severely the mood disturbance interferes with self-care, by the availability of a supportive and protective environment at home, and particularly by the presence of suicidal features. To assess the last, the patient must be asked if he has been considering self-injury. Although judgment is required in evaluating his answers, a sequence of questions probing for suicidal thoughts should be routine for every patient with depression. A proportion of the patients will deny all thought of self-injury and can be assumed to be of lesser suicidal risk. Those who admit to such thoughts should be asked if they have any means in mind. To that question still more patients will reassure the doctor that their thoughts on suicide have not reached so severe an intensity. Those patients, however, who admit to having considered a means (pills, gas, shooting) must be considered of higher risk, and thought must be given to protecting them, perhaps by hospitalization or by guaranteeing that they are under the supervision of friends or relatives. Finally, the patients should be asked if they have acquired any means or done anything to try them out. Again a proportion of patients will say that they have not been that despondent, but those who say that they have done such things are at very high risk and should in most cases be hospitalized.

Once a decision is made about the site of treatment, in a hospital or on an outpatient basis, the act of reaching a secure diagnosis of a depressive reaction in a patient is the first step in its treatment, because this judgment requires that the doctor has come to understand the patient and his predicament. To gain this understanding the doctor's first meetings should be devoted to listening to the patient's description of his circumstances, of his emotional changes, and of the connections he draws between his experiences and his depressive mood. If appropriate, other informants such as relatives can amplify on the patient's statements and give details of his past modes of coping with trouble. All these efforts are intended to bring the doctor an appreciation of this particular individual and the circumstances that he faces. Such knowledge, combined with the relationships of trust, respect, and empathy that develop naturally in its acquisition, provides the resources for treatment.

The therapeutic efforts from this foundation are directed toward re-engaging the patient in life experiences in which success can be found, replacements for losses enjoyed, and a sense of integrity and control regained. Usually the first need of the patient is some help in simple tactics for the management of his current troubles and for the avoidance of their repetition in the future.

At this stage a sense of helplessness often prompts the patient to abandon many of his activities and efforts, but if at all possible he must be encouraged not to give in to these promptings, because doing so tends to perpetuate the disturbed mood by holding him from opportunities to reassess his situation and to try out solutions. His daily work, even when less efficiently performed, is often helpful in directing his attention to matters other than his troubles.

With assistance in simple matters of personal management, the patient can be helped to some success in his circumstances, bringing him encouragement and promoting a willingness to maintain his efforts and to plan for the future. Educating the patient in how certain circumstances strike his particular vulnerabilities and so provoke depressive responses can be helpful.

The most useful ingredient of the treatment is the support and interest of the doctor. This encourages the patient to express his feelings and discuss his circumstances. In this way not only is the physician provided with more information about assets and vulnerabilities of the patient, but often there is spontaneous recognition by the patient of causal features for his difficulties that brings both relief to his mood and self-perceived tactics for their resolution. If this supportive relationship can be maintained and developed, improvement of depression can be expected. For the occasional patient with whom such a relationship fails or who succumbs frequently to depressive reactions because of some intractable predisposition, more prolonged treatment by specialists in psychotherapy can be recommended.

Finally, treatment with pharmaceutical agents may help. Chlordiazepoxide, 10 mg three times daily, may relieve agitation somewhat in the bereaved or otherwise relatively depressed. A sleeping medication, flurazepam hydrochloride (Dalmane), is helpful for the sleeplessness. *The antidepressant medications*, although most useful in the manic-depressive psychoses, can be tried in some patients with a prolonged depressive response. Imipramine in a dose of 150 to 250 mg a day or the monoamine oxidase inhibitor phenelzine, 15 mg three times daily, has helped individual patients, but this symptomatic relief should be considered a minor part of the treatment plan in patients with this form of depression.

Granville-Grossman, K. L.: The early environment in affective disorder. *In* Coppen, A., and Walk, A. (eds.): Recent Developments in Affective Disorder. Br. J. Psychiatry, Special Publication No. 2, 1968.

Hinton, J. M.: Physical and mental distress of the dying. Quart. J. Med., 32:1, 1963.

Parkes, C. M.: The first year of bereavement. Psychiatry, 33:444, 1970.

234.4. HYSTERIA

DEFINITION.   Hysteria is a disturbance of behavior in which symptoms and signs of physical ill health are imitated more or less unconsciously for some personal advantage. As the phrase "more or less unconsciously" implies, hysteria may be hard to distinguish from "malingering," in which the imitation of illness is a well-appreciated fraud. Frank malingering is rare, though, because the power of human self-deception is usually adequate to persuade a person of the validity of his own symptoms. The only ones who can be called malingerers with any confidence are some self-mutilating patients and the remarkable pathologic liars, picturesquely called examples of the *Munchausen syndrome*, who travel from hospital to hospital gaining admission by means of dramatic acts of illness.

PREDISPOSING AND PRECIPITATING FACTORS.   Hysterical symptoms are to be seen as responses to distressing experiences. They can occur in almost any person facing danger or difficulty, especially if, as with soldiers in battle or prisoners, the distress is intense and prolonged and physical symptoms can provide a viable escape. Dull-witted or immature persons with inadequate powers of introspection and self-control may produce transparently hysterical symptoms in response to milder distress, such as school difficulties or family problems. Some of the exaggerations and elaborations of medical symptoms common in hospitalized patients may be similarly interpreted as responses to the distress of illness by persons whose capacity for self-control has been weakened by somatic illness. Hysterical symptoms can be the first manifestations of a dementing illness or of a depressive or schizophrenic psychosis, and these disorders must be considered when a previously well balanced adult develops a suspiciously hysterical symptom.

Commonly, though, hysteria is a disturbance in the be-

havior of a person predisposed by an attention-seeking, emotionally unstable, and egocentric personality. In fact, these characteristics form what has become known as the "hysterical personality" even though hysteria can occur in other types of people, and these characteristics do not invariably produce hysterical symptoms. Most easily recognized in such people is their flair for the dramatic. They show this tendency in flamboyant dress and in exaggerated, even melodramatic, responses to questions about their symptoms. They are never so happy as when they are the center of attention. Karl Jaspers characterized the hysterical personalities as those who "crave to appear, both to themselves and others, as more than they are and to experience more than they are ever capable of." The zeal of these patients for exaggeration and drama renders them more liable to hysterical symptoms. But other kinds of people can have these symptoms. In all of them usually a discouraged, depressive mood has been prompted by difficulties in life, and the hysterical symptoms then emerge from this mood state.

SYMPTOMS AND SIGNS.   Many of the phenomena of somatic illness can be imitated by hysteria. The accuracy of the imitation depends on the medical sophistication of the patient. A doctor or nurse is more likely to produce a convincing imitation than is an unqualified person.

Common hysterical symptoms are vague subjective disorders, such as generalized weakness, dizziness, indigestion, or pain. Hysterical pain can occur in any part of the body, but the head and neck, the region over the heart, and the low back are particularly favored. Hysterical pain can be of any character, from dull aching to sharp and stabbing pain, but it is often described by the patient in vivid similes such as "like a bullet," "like a bolt of lightning," "aches like an abscessed tooth," or "sore as a hot boil." Usually, hysterical pain is not confined to a local area as around a pathologic lesion, nor is it referred into the distribution of a particular nerve or dermatome. Rather, hysterical pain is felt in a general region of the body and spreads, sometimes in bizarre ways, into contiguous areas without regard to neuroanatomic boundaries. Thus pain beginning in the face may spread along the side of the head and into the back, crossing from the region of the trigeminal nerve into the upper cervical nerve regions. Hysterical pain often varies in its character, intensity, and distribution, changing considerably with attention or suggestion. Occasionally it can be remarkably improved by a small amount of intravenous amobarbital sodium when analgesics do not help.

Although vague symptoms of a subjective kind such as pain or dizziness are the present vogue in hysteria, crude and gross symptoms are still seen. These may be psychologic, such as the amnesia or fugue states, in which memory is partially lost, often in situations in which the patient is depressed or anxious. Other psychologic symptoms shown occasionally include auditory and visual hallucinations and even flamboyant delusions. These must be carefully judged, but appear most commonly in young people who have read popular books on psychology and psychiatry and are apparently suggested into these symptoms by their reading at a time when they are distressed over other matters.

Motor disturbances in the form of abnormal movement, disturbed gaits, seizures, or paralyses are occasionally hysterical symptoms. Hysterical seizures can usually be distinguished from epileptic ones. The patients only rarely injure themselves, bite their tongues, or lose their urine. They do not have the typical tonic and then clonic phases of a seizure, but tend to show a dramatic flailing of the limbs. Consciousness is partially retained, and seizures hardly ever occur when the patient is alone. The EEG is normal.

Sensory disturbances are particularly favored hysterical symptoms. Thus, *blindness* or *deafness* is common, often developing dramatically at a time of emotional distress. Loss of sensation over one side of the body to pin prick or light touch is frequently found after a susceptible patient has been examined by a neurologist.

DIAGNOSIS. Diagnosis of hysteria is seldom easy and never popular. Ideally, it should rest on three supports: first, the *form* of the hysterical manifestation; second, the *personality* of the patient; and third, the *setting* in which the symptoms developed. Often it is not possible to find all three supports to a diagnosis, but all should be sought.

Commonly, hysterical symptoms are vague and variable. In fact, the more definite and consistent a patient's description of the onset, location, nature, and duration of his symptoms, the less likely the symptoms are to be hysterical. Hysterical symptoms and signs are also usually incompatible with what is known of anatomy and physiology. Thus sensory losses do not conform to patterns of nerve distribution; reflexes remain intact and unchanged in the palsies of arm and leg; seizures of the entire body do not disturb consciousness; total blindness appears without a disturbance of pupillary reflex or of opticokinetic nystagmus. The hysterically mute person can phonate on coughing. The hysterically deaf person speaks louder to be heard over increased ambient noises. Many other hysterical symptoms have been analyzed for such inconsistencies by Head.

Knowledge of the personality and past history of the patient is helpful to a diagnosis of hysteria. The recognition that the symptoms are occurring in an hysterical personality should prompt an observer to look very closely at the symptoms before embarking on extensive laboratory tests or upon surgery. Similarly, knowlege of a previous vague and poorly understood medical disturbance can lend weight to an opinion that a new symptom that has eluded diagnosis is occurring in an individual prone to hysteria. Conversely, hysteria can usually be eliminated as an explanation for symptoms in an emotionally stable, middle-aged person. People who have passed through adolescence and young adulthood without resorting to hysterical behavior are unlikely to employ it when older.

The setting in which the symptoms develop should be carefully scrutinized, and a search made for a distressing event that may have provoked an hysterical reaction or for any purpose that the hysterical symptoms may serve. Occasionally, a clear association between the symptoms chosen and a particular recent disturbance in the life of the subject can be found, such as an amnesia developing in a person who has done something shameful or criminal, or weakness and pain persisting in a person who is seeking financial compensation for an injury. Often, though, motivations behind hysterical symptoms are vague and uncertain. It is usual to find that the patient is unhappy or anxious about some aspect of his life circumstances and that the hysterical symptoms serve to call attention to his distress. Also, it may be possible to demonstrate that the development of particular symptoms has been prompted by suggestion: weakness of legs, for example, developing in a nurse caring for a paraplegic patient, or peculiar falling attacks after the patient has witnessed an epileptic seizure.

Guzé and his associates have pointed out a subgroup of patients with a chronic hysterical disorder who have had recurrent complaints of symptoms involving almost every bodily system. These patients, with what Guzé terms Briquet's syndrome, present diagnostic difficulties to many specialists as their complaints change, worsen, and improve in unpredictable ways. They usually have undergone multiple medical and surgical procedures. The same criteria that lead to the diagnosis of single hysterical symptoms can be applied to this group. Additionally they can be reliably differentiated from most medical patients by the sheer number of systems that have been involved in their past complaints. The role of particular personality traits in Briquet's syndrome has been explored by Kaminsky and Slavney.

A careful study of the symptoms, the personality, and the life setting of a patient usually allows a reasonably certain differentiation of hysterical symptoms from those of a medical illness. There are, however, certain medical problems that are notoriously easily confused with hysteria. These are the diseases that produce vague and changing symptoms that seem to vary with the patient's motivation and, at least in their early phases, lack convincing physical signs. If such an illness occurs in a patient who has features of the hysterical personality and who will therefore describe the symptoms in a dramatic and flamboyant fashion, physicians may be even more persuaded to believe that the illness is only deceptively physical. Examples of diseases frequently confused with hysteria because of their subtle clinical features are the first attack of multiple sclerosis, particularly if sensory changes alone are produced; the weakness of arms and legs seen early in acute idiopathic polyneuritis of the Guillain-Barré type; the difficulty in swallowing of bulbar myasthenia gravis; the attacks of muscular weakness in periodic paralysis; the tonic posturings and oculogyric crises of postencephalitic parkinsonism; the pain of a cauda equina tumor; and the abdominal pain of acute intermittent porphyria.

MANAGEMENT OF HYSTERIA. The management of hysterical patients is difficult. No one method can be recommended unqualifiedly. But there are certain principles that can be followed. To help hysterical patients it is essential to have sympathy for them. Many doctors find these patients irritating. It is just as possible to see them as individuals displaying an intriguing aspect of human behavior that has profound implications in their lives. It is pointless to argue with these patients about the validity of their symptoms. A useful approach is to agree that they have had an illness producing their symptoms, but that they are now improving even though total recovery has not arrived.

It is important to diagnose hysteria promptly. Hesitation in diagnosis leading to several hospital admissions for extensive laboratory investigations is a good way to solidify hysterical symptoms in a patient. Among other things, the uncertainty of doctors helps persuade a patient that the symptoms are real. Repeated examinations increase the consistency with which symtpoms are reported. Long hospitalization, mounting bills, and the inconvenience caused to others make it difficult for a patient to abandon symptoms without embarrassment. The gratifying attention given to the patient in the hospital, perhaps as an example of an intriguing diagnostic problem, can feed the self-dramatizing tendencies and so encourage the behavior.

There is always risk of error in any diagnosis, because diagnosis is only a weighing of probabilities. The diagnosis of hysteria, though, depends purely on a physician's judgment and, before relief of symptoms is accomplished, can be confirmed in the laboratory only by evidence of health. Physicians, for obvious reasons, fear more the error of calling a physically sick patient hysterical than the error of mishandling hysteria. They often prefer to exclude, by laboratory examination, progressively more unlikely diseases than to study carefully the symptoms and the individual who has produced them, even though this would lead more directly to a definite diagnosis as well as an understanding of the response. It may be unwise to counsel too strongly against this behavior because medical diagnosis is never easy. A compromise can be found in the admonition to perform immediately the laboratory tests that seem necessary for a patient, but when hysteria is suspected, to bring the period of investigation as quickly as possible to a close so that management of the specific symptom can be begun.

Treatment of the specific symptoms rests basically upon persuasion. The doctor is persuading the patient to perform the functions that the patient claims are disabled. Intravenous amobarbital sodium given to the point where the patient is mildly intoxicated and his speech slurred is particularly helpful in making and establishing a persuasion. Usually, some ingenuity is required for success. The hysterically blind person can, for example, be persuaded first that he can distinguish light from dark and then gradually to distinguish forms, to read large print, and, finally, small newspaper type. The person who claims he cannot walk can be encouraged first to move his legs in bed, and then to stand, to make a few tentative shuffles, and finally to stride out. The hysterically deaf person can be persuaded to hear through a stethoscope and then gradually that he can hear without it. A dramatic show of some kind is often helpful in removing these symptoms. If a physician has success in partially removing hysterical symptoms, he should persist in his treatment without interruption in order to bring about as much improvement as possible and even to restore full function. When there is recovery of function, the patient should perform his recovered skills in public — before his family, other patients, and several doctors — to prevent his relapsing immediately into his former state.

The fear that sudden removal of hysterical symptoms will result in a disastrous psychologic colllapse is exag-gerated. Rarely, a depressed patient with hysterical symptoms has an increase in depression, but it is clear that in those situations a depression was overlooked and the more secondary hysterical symptoms were emphasized.

Some hysterical disorders are refractory to treatment. Among these are the disorders assumed for some material gain, such as compensation. They usually are not improved until some settlement is made. Episodic disorders such as hysterical seizures can be hard to control. Sometimes, however, a statement to the patient that they will not recur, given with full authority by a physician whom the patient trusts and respects, may eliminate these symptoms. The longer the patient has hysterical symptoms, the harder they are to remove. This is a corollary to the aforementioned observation that hysterical symptoms produced for transparent reasons and bordering on malingering are more difficult to eliminate than are the ones produced by an attention-seeking personality in some emotional distress. Symptoms held for a long time cannot be easily abandoned without embarrassing the patient.

Simultaneously with treatment of the specific symptoms, the emotional state and present life of the patient should be studied to discover any distress that may have precipitated the hysterical symptoms. Then advice, social assistance, or guidance can be offered to aid the patient in resolving these difficulties. This aspect of their psychologic treatment depends on developing a relationship of friendship and mutual respect identical to that found necessary in treating an anxious or depressed person.

Long-term management of hysterical patients is much more difficult than treatment of individual symptoms. It is not wise to have the average hysterical patient embark on depth psychotherapy, because he tends to produce more symptoms and to recount involved sexual and other fantasies in order to maintain the interest of his doctor. If possible, these patients should be followed by one physician who understands them and the behavior that they are liable to produce and is also competent to recognize physical illness should it arise. This physician can save these patients from needless surgery and long hospitalization. He can remove hysterical symptoms promptly by being alert to the diagnosis and providing help for the difficulties that precipitate them.

Guzé, S.: The validity and significance of the clinical diagnosis of hysteria (Briquet's syndrome). Am. J. Psychiatry, 132:138, 1975.

Head, H. The diagnosis of hysteria. Br. Med. J., 1:827, 1922.

Kaminsky, M. J., and Slavney, P. R.: Methodology and personality in Briquet's syndrome: A reappraisal. Am. J. Psychiatry, 133:85, 1976.

Slavney, P. R., and McHugh, P. R.: The hysterical personality: A controlled study. Arch. Gen. Psychiatry, 30:325, 1974.

Walters, A.: Psychogenic regional pain, alias hysterical pain. Brain, 84:1, 1961.

Section Five PSYCHOLOGIC TESTING IN CLINICAL MEDICINE

Paul R. McHugh

235. INTRODUCTION

Psychologic tests are intended to assist clinical evaluation of behavioral disorders by bringing accurate measurement to the mental examination. Physicians are familiar with instruments, such as the thermometer or sphygmomanometer, that bring accurate measurement to observations in the physical examination. They are so easy to employ that knowledge of the normal readings in the human population and implications of deviations from normal have been established. Although psychologic tests are aimed at more abstract phenomena such as intelligence or personality, they similarly attempt to bring precision through numerical or graphic measurements and provide a means by which an individual can be compared in these features with others.

The mere provision of a numerical expression does not prove a test useful, as the numbers may not be meaningful. Often in our fascination with a new test and its intriguingly plausible scales for measurement, we overlook its failure to satisfy the criteria of *reliability* and *validity*.

The reliability of a measuring instrument, whether it be for a physical or a psychologic function, is an expression of the accuracy and reproducibility of its findings. No instrument is perfectly reliable, but the range within which it is unreliable must be a small fraction of the potential range of measurement if it is to be capable of detecting a genuine deviation in the variable under study. The validity of an instrument is an expression of its capacity to measure what it claims to measure.

How can we be sure that psychologic tests are actually measuring the psychologic variables that they claim to measure? How can we be sure that intelligence tests, for example, measure intelligence? The only proof that a psychologic test is valid is the demonstration that scores on it predict behavior in life thought to be the expression of the trait it claims to measure. For example, results on a valid intelligence test should correlate to some extent with scholastic performance.

The issues of reliability and validity are fundamental to all test evaluation. For more thorough consideration the reader is directed to Zubin's review and Messick's article.

236. INTELLIGENCE

The quantitative measurement of the mental attribute, intelligence, was first attempted by Binet at the turn of the century. His success and the Stanford-Binet battery of tests developed from his work brought such predictive power to the study of intelligence that they provide an impetus to the development of tests to examine other mental functions. But the tests of intelligence have through their revisions, particularly the *Wechsler Bellevue Intelligence Scale* published in 1939 and the *Wechsler Adult Intelligence Scale (WAIS)* of 1955, remained the most secure and useful tests of mental function.

Intelligence is difficult to define. It is the abstract concept used to explain the observation that individuals vary in their mental capacities and in the effectiveness with which they employ them. Intelligence is more easily defined in practice by pointing to instances of its action. This way is in fact used in our daily life. We judge a man's intelligence by observing his bearing, his speech, his apparent grasp of situations, his judgments, and his emotional control. Then in the light of our past experience of watching other men, we call an individual bright or dull. We are doing nothing conceptually different when we estimate intelligence at the bedside or by means of psychologic tests. We organize the testing so that a series of observations can be made within a reasonable period of time. We add scope to our examination by asking for performance in several different kinds of mental activity. We bring accuracy to the observations by scoring the performance.

The questions on orientation, memory, attention and concentration, fund of knowledge, and capacity to reason abstractly that constitute the test of cognition routinely carried out at the bedside in the course of the physical and mental examination provide a doctor an estimate of his patient's intellectual functioning. In the light of knowledge of the patient's past life and demonstrated abilities, the doctor makes a judgment whether there has been damage to intellectual functioning. Psychologic tests are able to give a more accurate estimate of the intelligence of a patient at the moment of testing than do these bedside examinations, because these tests have proved both reliable and valid.

All these approaches, from the casual observations to the most refined test, are applications of a fundamentally identical method: an assessment of a performance thought on practical grounds to be a reflection of intelligence. However, any performance will be influenced by other factors, particularly the factors of education and experience. *Since these factors derive from opportunities and social heritage of the subject, every one of these assessments must be qualified and interpreted in the light of the subject's cultural and educational background.*

Subcultural differences that are obvious on bedside examination, being recognized as modifications in expression and in experience, *are allowed for almost automatically in that assessment but are sometimes forgotten when formal intelligence test scores are displayed.* Just as there is no culture-pure bedside examination, there is no culture-pure intelligence test. Test scores must be interpreted in relationship to all that is known about the patient. Particular care in the interpretation is demanded if he is a member of a subculture different from the standard criterion group employed in the development of the formal tests: urban, school-educated whites. The greater his divergence in this respect, the greater the allowance needed in interpreting the scores of his tests. Emotional disturbances or other preoccupations that interfere with the patient's concentration or cooperation will also obviously affect these performances. Allowances must be made for any of these features in assessing test scores, just as allowance is made for these features on bedside examination.

The *Wechsler Adult Intelligence Scale* is the most reliable and valid instrument we have for measuring the intellectual function of the adult. Its reliability has been demonstrated by the close correlation of test scores given on separate occasions to the same individuals and by the similarity of scores when one half of a test is compared with another half (split-half method). Its validity has been demonstrated by its correlation with life performances of individuals it scores as intelligent or dull.

In its present form the WAIS consist of 11 subtests of mental skill. Six of these subtests are "verbal tests." In these the patient is requested to define words, to recognize similarities between words, to do arithmetic, to remember numbers forward and backward, to answer questions on his fund of knowledge, and to judge and interpret proverbs. These tests are followed by five "performance tests," in which a patient is asked to work with rather unfamiliar material and solve problems set to him by that material. Tests here include the putting together of puzzles, work with symbols, the setting out of logical stories from pictures disorganized for the test, construction of patterns from multicolored blocks, and the recognition of things missing from drawings. The performance tests seem somewhat less related to the education of a person than are the verbal tests. All the subtests that have been chosen for the WAIS have a long history of investigation. They are combined together to produce a thorough and accurate instrument.

The scoring of the WAIS is in the form of the *Intelligence Quotient (I.Q.)*. In fact, the WAIS derives a verbal I.Q. from the verbal tests and a performance I.Q. from the performance tests. A full-scale I.Q. is derived from the combination of all 11 subtests.

The I.Q. compares an individual with others. Historically it was developed for children. I.Q. then was the ratio of mental age over chronologic age times 100 when mental age was defined in terms of a child's ability to succeed on tests which the average child of a given age could do. Thus a child solving problems which the average nine-year-old could solve had a mental age of nine. If he, himself, was nine years old at the time of the test, he had an average ability and an I.Q. of $^9/_9 \times 100$, or 100; if his chronologic age was six, he would be an advanced child with an I.Q. of $^9/_6 \times 100$, or 150. Terman demonstrated the constancy of I.Q. in the growing child.

But a ratio of mental to chronologic age is unlikely to be useful in adults because tested intelligence does not increase after the late teens. The WAIS and many other tests for adult intelligence continue to use the term I.Q. This is possible because of the fact that tests of intelligence appear to distribute individuals in a "normal" or gaussian fashion. This curve has a mean at I.Q. 100 and a standard deviation of ±15 I.Q. points. It is possible to divide the curve into percentiles of the population. The WAIS score of any person places him in the percentile of the population with similar scores, and his I.Q. can be extrapolated from percentile by means of the distribution curve. Thus an individual whose performance on the WAIS is equal to 50 per cent of the population is said to have an I.Q. of 100, whereas individuals whose test performances exceeded 98 per cent of the population will be said to have an I.Q. of 135 or above.

The WAIS has found its greatest clinical utility in the study of patients with brain disease. Any damage to the cerebral hemispheres will injure intellectual ability and disturb the scores on the WAIS. An intriguing observation is that early in the course of brain disease performance tests are disturbed before the verbal test scores change. This may indicate that verbal tests measure more what an indivdual has learned and practiced, whereas performance tests measure his capacity to meet new problems. The verbal and performance scores of normal individuals are usually comparable. The verbal I.Q. can be considered a fair estimate of the original intellectual endowment of an individual suffering from a brain injury. The decline of the performance I.Q. is a useful measure of the degree of injury to the cerebral tissue the patient has endured. With an advancing brain disease verbal I.Q. will fall eventually, but a patient will usually continue to demonstrate higher verbal than performance scores.

Emotional unrest such as anxiety or depression will also interfere with WAIS scores. Here, as with cerebral disease, the performance I.Q. will fall below the verbal I.Q., demonstrating that the capacity to work with unfamiliar material is disturbed more than tests of what has been well learned. But because these findings are identical to those in persons with brain disease, the differentiation of an emotional disturbance from dementia cannot come from WAIS results. It must rest on other information such as is derived from the history, physical examination, and mental status.

The WAIS is useful not only in demonstrating deterioration of intellectual function; when done serially, it can also document recovery of function with treatment. Since it is so simple to employ, its increasing utility in clinical research is assured.

237. PERSONALITY

By personality is meant all the abiding traits of character that constitute an individual's potential to respond in particular ways to circumstances. All physicians are aware of how much information they must acquire through several interviews with the patient and from independent sources before they can have much confidence in their diagnostic opinion on personality. Tests that could elucidate personality more accurately and more rapidly would be useful. Two alternative approaches have been developed, "projective" tests and questionnaires, and each approach has raised particular problems.

In the so-called projective tests of personality ambiguous situations are set before the patient, and his responses are recorded. Thus he is presented with sentences to complete or a picture to interpret, or, in the most well known projective test, the Rorschach test, he is presented with a standardized set of ink blots and asked to describe the forms that he can recognize within them. Since there is nothing in the situations themselves that forces any particular response, the responses of the patient are thought to derive from his personal predilections and inner needs, drives, and conflicts. This seems logical. But logic is not the essential criterion for a test intended to aid the clinical examination. It must be demonstrated that the responses on projective tests provide measurements that are reliable and valid. This remains to be done.

Certain features of a patient can be expected to be seen in any set of his responses. For instance, overly conscientious persons will tend to be fixed on details, the schizophrenic patient with his disordered thought will demonstrate this feature in distorted expression, and the depressed patient will speak of unhappy themes as he discusses any matter. These features will appear whether the patient is being examined by his doctor or doing a projective test. Until the reliability and validity of projective tests can be demonstrated, it cannot be known whether they are superior to the clinical examination, and if they are not superior to the clinical examination, they are of doubtful utility to the physician. The question of their value is shrouded in controversy.

The other approach to personality measurement is the questionnaire. This was developed from the clinical examination. Since questions are used there to gain information from the patient, it seemed logical that a questionnaire including these and many other questions would improve on the clinical examination. It came as a surprise when tests developed in this fashion proved to be unreliable and invalid. This was demonstrated when different questionnaires intended to probe similar features of personality, such as introversion, did not correlate well with one another, and in fact could give quite opposite impressions of the same person. Questionnaires developed in this fashion proved so misleading that the method fell into disrepute. It was, however, eventually recognized that these early tests gratuitously assumed that questions would be accurately answered by patients. Consider the question, Do you lack self-confidence, yes or no? To presume that a person will understand this question exactly the same way as the examiner intends and that his criterion for a yes or nor answer is the same as that of all other people is to presume too much. Also these early tests failed to consider that many individuals might attempt to show themselves in some more favorable light and therefore not answer questions truthfully.

The most intriguing conceptual advance in the study of personality was the recognition that an objectively truthful answer to questions was not needed for a valid, useful test. In fact, more information can be obtained from observing the patient's replies to questions than from any belief that the statements they agree to or reject are in themselves accurate descriptions of their personality. The task of building questionnaires changed from finding questions that would display the inner feelings of people to finding questions that would be answered differently by different personality types.

To build such a questionnaire the first step was to gather together specific groups of people for study: normal people, anxious patients, hysterical patients, depressed patients, for as many groups as could be differentiated. These patients, the criterion groups, were asked a large number of questions, and the replies were compared from group to group. The questions which differentiated the groups best were then collected for the questionnaire. This questionnaire then given

to an individual was interpreted not from the content of questions rejected or affirmed but from the number of questions replied to in the same fashion as in one or more of the criterion groups.

The most useful questionnaire that has been developed is the *Minnesota Multiphasic Personality Inventory (MMPI)*. The questions in that test have been carefully studied and chosen so that they differentiate the groups to the greatest degree possible with it. Because of the complexity of issues of personality, the numbers of questions needed to derive a profile with this test is 550. It was possible in the MMPI to fit in many questions that give an indication of the tendency of the patient to lie, exaggerate, or misunderstand questions.

The results of the MMPI are expressed as a series of ten scales or dimensions along each of which an individual is placed by means of his responses that correspond to responses of nine criterion groups. These scales were originally derived from clinical groups and given clinical names, i.e., hypochondriasis, depression, hysteria, psychopathic, masculine-feminine dimension, paranoid, psychaesthenic, schizophrenic, manic, and social introversion. Three so-called reliability scales are also scored for each test.

The MMPI is a reliable instrument, the accuracy and reproducibility of its readings having been demonstrated in repeated testing of individuals over many years. The validity of its scales varies. Some of the scales measure the personality characteristics for which they are titled. Scores on the psychopathic and manic scales do correlate with the clinical features intended by these terms. Scores on the schizophrenic and hysterical scales do not correlate well with these clinical disorders but with aspects of bizarreness and self-dramatization, respectively, features not specific to schizophrenia or hysteria. In an effort to avoid these invalid implications, the MMPI scales are no longer referred to by clinical titles, but by numbers of letters derived from the original names.

The tendency to look at specific scales for diagnostic impressions has been replaced by consideration of the "profile," or pattern of the several scales together, hoping to derive in this way a more global view of personality structure. This approach emphasizes the multidimensional character of personality. It takes advantage of the features of reliability found in this test. But, once again, the establishment of validity for these profiles must be accomplished. This is being attempted by matching the life course of individuals with predictions from the profiles, but work is still in progress.

Current practice is to find the MMPI useful as a screening and probing instrument that often suggests aspects of personality difficulty that might well be more carefully studied. However, its validity for the differentiation of clinical psychiatric entities or specific personality types is uncertain, and thus it must not be regarded as the arbiter in differential diagnosis.

Anastasia, A.: Psychological Testing. New York, Macmillan, 1976.

Butcher, H. J.: Human Intelligence, Its Nature and Assessment. London, Methuen & Co., Ltd., 1968.

Messick, S.: The standard problem — meaning and values in measurement and evaluation. Am. Psychol., 30:955, 1975.

Terman, L. M., and Oden, M.: The Gifted Group at Mid-Life. Genetic Studies of Genius, Vol. V. Stanford, California, Stanford University Press, 1959.

Welsh, G. S., and Dahlstrom, W. G.: Basic Readings on the MMPI. Minneapolis, University of Minnesota Press, 1956.

Zubin, J.: Classification of behavior disorders. Ann. Rev. Psychol., 18:373, 1967.

Section Six MEDICAL ASPECTS OF SEXUALITY

Harold I. Lief

238. THE PHYSICIAN'S ROLE

PREVENTION AS WELL AS THERAPY

In dealing with sexual problems, the physician has a splendid opportunity to practice preventive as well as therapeutic medicine. By aiding a young person to overcome sexual anxieties and inhibitions, he is helping to prepare that young person for satisfactory relationships and, eventually, marriage itself. By counseling a married couple, enabling them to obtain greater sexual pleasure and mutuality, the physician prevents increasing marital discord, perhaps even divorce itself, and the consequent emotional and physical sequelae for the couple and their children. Marital unhappiness and frustration have been implicated in a variety of illnesses, perhaps the most prominent of which is depression, which, in turn, is often a contributing factor to a variety of diseases. Helping patients with sexual problems is good medical care. It is more than the enrichment of life, important as that is, because sexual counseling reduces one of the most frequent sources of human suffering and thus aids in preventing individual illness, family uprooting, and resultant social disorganization.

Most sexual problems presented to physicians are in the context of a marital relationship, either as primary causes of marital dysfunction or as consequences of other areas of marital discord, but which nevertheless augment and maintain marital unhappiness. It seems reasonable then to make sex and marriage counseling a "package" in the training of the physician and in the delivery of medical care. Even in the case of the pediatrician, it is still logical, for he soon comes to recognize the direct connection between the marital relationship of the parents and the sexual problems of the child.

Although marriage counseling is important, it is not the only way the physician can practice effective preventive medicine. Early intervention can occur in a number of other clinical situations, e.g., premarital counseling, family-planning services during pregnancy, postpartum care, and family-life education for teenagers and young adults. The pediatrician and obstetrician have especially significant points of entrance into the system of health care, enabling these specialists to practice effective prevention.

PHYSICIAN COMFORT

Not only are marital and sexual problems frequent in medical practice, but they are often overlooked or avoided — either because of the physician's lack of training and his feeling of incompetence in this area, or because these problems impinge on his own marital and sexual conflicts or values and make him uncomfortable. Even if he consciously or unconsciously avoids the issue by failing to follow cues, changing the subject by responding with a trite and stereotyped form of reassurance, e.g., "this is just a phase — your problem will disappear in time," he is carrying out counseling of sorts. Vincent has stated it well: "The theoretical position that the physician cannot or should not engage in any marriage or sexual counseling becomes meaningless when the patients expect this role of their physician and when their illnesses have sexual and marital implications — if not origins. The majority of physicians literally have no choice; even to do and say nothing in response to the patient's questions and/or presentation of symptoms in the sexual and marital areas is, by default, one form of counseling."

To be competent in handling the therapeutic and preventive aspects of the sexual, marital, and family problems he sees almost daily in his practice, the physician must not only have a store of *information*, but must also develop a set of *skills* and *attitudes* that facilitate his making optimal use of his information. Surely the key factor in competent sex and marital counseling is the degree of comfort of the counselor. His skill in interviewing, in eliciting salient data about the most intimate, personal dimension of patients' lives, will depend directly on his capacity to react not with anxiety, anger, or self-righteousness, but with openness, ease, and a clear desire to achieve an atmosphere of genuine communication of feelings as well as thoughts. Lacking these skills and attitudes, his quantity of information, even if vast, is of little use.

LEVELS OF INTERVENTION

Four levels of intervention are possible for the physician treating patients with sexual dysfunctions, namely, (1) diagnostician, (2) educator, (3) counselor, or (4) therapist.

Diagnostician

Sexual problems fall into the following categories: overt, covert, associated with physical illness, associated with mental illness, and false or pseudosexual problems.

OVERT. Presenting complaints may be overtly sexual, e.g., impotence or anorgasmia. The physician has the task of discovering the meaning and importance of the symptom, whether it has been lifelong or acquired (following a period of adequate functioning prior to the onset of the symptom), generalized (with all partners in all situations), or situational (with one partner or in one situation). If it is situational, for example, limited to one partner, it will usually call for couple counseling rather than individual treatment.

COVERT. By contrast, with covert problems, the physician has to be on the lookout for the presence of sexual or marital problems that lie behind a host of physical symptoms — headache, backache, fatigue, menstrual irregularities, or dysmenorrhea. Osler said of syphilis that it was "the great imitator" of other disease states. Today it may be said more accurately that sexual dissatisfaction plays that role.

ASSOCIATED WITH PHYSICAL ILLNESS OR DRUG THERA-PY. Although diabetes is the illness most often implicated in sexual dysfunction, other diseases, especially chronic ones not necessarily related to the neurologic or vascular pathways subsuming sexual responsivity, often have sexual connotations. Most physicians do not even discuss sex with their postcoronary patients, and when they do they may offer vague, uncertain advice such as "Take it easy." Patients who have a chronic illness or who have had an organ ablation such as hysterectomy *are* concerned about their sexual functions: How often? Under what circumstances? Am I still virile or attractive? Those are questions many patients are too embarrassed to ask. One study showed that only 10 per cent of women who had undergone mastectomy had discussed with their physicians their concerns about sexual behaviors, body-image, and the impact of the surgery on their husbands. The physician must be sensitive to when and how he can initiate such discussion with his patients. Antihypertensive drugs are frequently implicated in impotence, retrograde ejaculation, or diminished capacity for vaginal vasocongestion. Other medications, certainly the psychotropic drugs, may be similarly related to a decrease in sexual adequacy.

ASSOCIATED WITH MENTAL ILLNESS. Among the major mental illnesses, depression is the disorder most often found to have an adverse effect on sexual competence. The most frequent sexual consequence of depression is inhibition of sexual desire usually found in conjunction with a generalized anhedonia. This disturbance is found even more frequently than impotence; indeed, impotence often follows a decrease in sexual desire.

FALSE OR PSEUDOSEXUAL COMPLAINTS. Occasionally a patient will complain of a sexual problem as a primary reason for the consultation when, in fact, the primary difficulty may be a marital problem or depression. The sexual problem is used as a "calling-card" to gain entry into the health-care system, meanwhile avoiding some other problem that may be even more painful to face or to deal with.

Educator

As an educator, the physician can pass on to the patient correct information about sexual anatomy and physiology; he can discuss with the patient the range of sexual behaviors, including what is normative. He should always be mindful of the influence of society on what is judged "normal," for in today's changing sexual scene, yesterday's perversions and deviations are tomorrow's variations. Examples are masturbation, oral sex, premarital intercourse, and homosexuality. The physician has the opportunity to dispel sexual myths and misconceptions, e.g., anxiety about penis size, the effects of hysterectomy on sexual functioning, the frequency of coital orgasm in women, or the alleged effects of aging on sexual capacities. As an educator, a physician may point out to the patient the relations of

the adverse or painful emotions ("emergency" emotions) — anxiety, anger, guilt — to the inhibition of sexual functioning. The physician-educator may convey appropriate information on psychosexual development to adolescents or to the parents of younger children.

Counselor

The educator role merges into the counselor role, and often there is more overlap than discontinuity. An example will illustrate this. The man recovering from a myocardial infarction can be told that the exertion in coitus is no more strenuous than climbing two flights of stairs; these comments constitute education. In the role of counselor, however, the physician would inquire into the patient's concerns about sexual capacity and, through the role of "inquirer" (expert listening is a crucial facet of counseling), would convey caring and understanding. In response to the patient's questions, the physician would be able to assume the role of educator more effectively, imparting more relevant information. The physician could counsel more precisely concerning resumption of sexual activity, the amount of activity, coital positions, and the like. By being precise, the physician will reduce the patient's anxiety and prevent the appearance of impotence or premature ejaculation. The physician-counselor may wish to discuss the situation with the patient's wife, elicit her cooperation, and reduce her fear that sexual activity will damage her husband. Anxiety is "contagious," and to reduce anxiety in one partner is not enough if the titer of anxiety is high in the other partner. In such a case, the anxiety of the spouse will spread to the patient, undermining the counseling efforts directed at the patient.

The physician who is too busy to set aside the time or who shies away from marital therapy may have to treat the couple by dealing with one patient only. Many situations can be handled in this fashion, e.g., the urologist who cures male dyspareunia by clearing up the patient's prostatitis, the internist who helps restore his patient's potency by reassuring him that sexual activity will not result in another coronary occlusion, the gynecologist who reassures his patient that she will suffer no loss of sexual drive after hysterectomy. *Yet sexual behavior involves a relationship; hence, in most instances therapy should also be directed toward the relationship.*

Therapist

The sex therapist is a specialty role requiring specialized training currently available in only a few first-rate training centers in the United States. The sex therapist should be competent in marital therapy and in individual psychotherapy and should be able to employ, as well, the specific behavioral techniques first set forth by Masters and Johnson. The sex therapist's greatest skill is in making an appropriate appraisal on the basis of which he can decide the form of treatment apt to be most effective in a given situation.

An encouraging sign is that more training centers in medical schools are being developed. A recent survey demonstrated that 39 per cent of United States medical schools now have separate sex therapy clinics; approximately 50 per cent carry out some form of sex therapy in their outpatient settings.

Of the four levels of intervention, most physicians will restrict their activities to the first three, namely,

TABLE 1. The Sexual System (Sexuality)

1. Biologic sex: chromosomes, hormones, primary and secondary sex characteristics
2. Core gender identity: sense of maleness and femaleness
3. Gender identity: sense of masculinity and femininity
4. Gender role behavior:
   a. Nonsexual gender role behavior: behavior that is often associated with masculinity and femininity
   b. Sexual behavior: behavior motivated by desire for sexual pleasure, ultimately orgasm (physical sex)
      (1) Proceptive behavior
      (2) Acceptive behavior
      (3) Conceptive behavior

diagnostician, educator, and counselor. A good rule of thumb for the physician-counselor is to arrange for his individual or couple patients to come in for six sessions. At the end of six sessions, if the physician feels that he is not making sufficient progress, he should refer patients to a sex therapist.

239. SEXUALITY

Sexuality refers to the totality of one's sexual being, of which physical sex is only one part. One's sense of being male and masculine, female and feminine, and the various roles these self-perceptions engender or affect are important ingredients of sexuality. Cognitive, emotional, and physical sex all contribute to the totality. In this sense, our sexuality is what we *are*, rather than what we *do*. Sexuality may be described in terms of a system somewhat analogous to the circulatory or respiratory system. The components of the sexual system are set forth in Table 1.

The brain is apparently programmed during fetal life for later sexual behavior. Fetal androgens during a critical period of fetal life (between the sixth and twelfth weeks) are necessary for an XY fetus to develop normally into a male. A deficiency of fetal androgens or androgen-insensitive tissues will interfere with normal male development. Similarly, excessive androgens in an XX fetus will bring about masculine changes. Chromosomal or hormonal abnormalities may create problems of intersexuality which may, if not corrected early in life, lead to conflicts in core gender or gender identity. The assigned sex is, with rare exceptions, more important in determining gender identity than is biologic sex. Sex-change procedures are usually unwise after the age of 18 months, when the sense of maleness and femaleness is far advanced. Some of the intersex patients and some without evident biologic defect have grave difficulties in developing a core gender identity of the same biologic sex. These are transsexuals. If they are biologic males, they think of themselves as "a female trapped in a male body." Transsexual biologic females consider themselves to be "a male trapped in a female body." With those relatively rare exceptions, development of sexuality leads to a secure sense of maleness or femaleness which is generally complete by the age of three. However, in our culture doubts and conflicts about masculinity and femininity are ubiquitous. Serious disturbances lead to paraphilias such as transvestism, fetishism, voyeurism, and exhibitionism.

SEXUAL SYSTEM AND PERSONALITY. Much more often the physician is called upon to deal with less overt conflicts about gender identity that create significant marital problems with sexual connotations; examples are the Don Juan who has to prove his masculinity by sexual conquests, the promiscuous housewife who tries to prove to herself her femininity by finding the elusive orgasm or by demonstrating her attractiveness, the woman who cannot respond sexually because she is afraid of being completely dominated or possessed by a male, and the husband who cannot have sexual intercourse with his wife on top because it seems unmanly. The "battle of the sexes" is carried out not only in bed but in every area of marital interaction, generally by people who are uncertain of their masculinity or femininity and who fight to gain self-respect by derogating the partner. Several generations ago these sexually related social roles were handed down or "assigned" by tradition; today, roles are negotiable, and problems become serious when negotiation is impossible to attain because of faulty communication, or when it breaks down because of disturbed perception or the fear of compromise. The sexual system develops as such an integral part of personality development that sexuality and personality are inseparably interwoven. The physician who wishes to be an effective sex counselor, therefore, must deal with sexual relations in the context of human, especially marital, relations.

GENDER ROLE BEHAVIOR. Gender role refers to the entire spectrum of roles for a particular sex, male or female, in a particular cultural system. The culture has orientations as to, for example, whether that sex should place primary emphasis on an occupational career or on a family; whether that sex should develop attributes of aggressiveness or of nurture; whether members of that sex should be leaders of a political party or of a religious group, or teach in a primary school or in a university system. The culture defines in sometimes clear and sometimes not so clear terms the expectations of society for males and females and the expectations of the males and females in each institution in society. There is a reciprocal relationship between gender identity and gender role behavior. How one feels about oneself as masculine or feminine affects one's behavior in institutional settings; conversely, one's behavior in a variety of institutional settings affects the way one feels about one's sex.

Sexual role behavior may be thought of as *proceptive*, *acceptive*, and *conceptive*. The proceptive is the phase of initial, erotic interaction between the couple — of attraction and attractiveness, solicitation and courtship. It may be initiated by either partner serially or by both reciprocally. In the absence of a partner, it may be initiated in imagery and fantasy. Whether alone or with a partner, the subjective experience includes anticipatory sexual drive, interest, or desire. The proceptive phase may be viewed in its longitudinal aspects, as part of psychosexual development, and it may be seen, as well, as part of a single sexual encounter, or of an ongoing relationship.

Proception is followed by acception, the phase of bodily interaction and potential genital union. This phase subdivides into stages of excitement, plateau, orgasm, and resolution. Excitement involves a subjective sense of sexual pleasure accompanying physiologic changes. The major change in a male consists of penile tumescence (erection). The major changes in the female consist of vasocongestion generalized in the pelvis with lubrication of the vagina and swelling of the external genitalia. Plateau consists of sustained sexual excitement and progressive physiologic changes. In the male there is the appearance of Cowper's gland secretion. In the female there is the development of the orgasmic platform, which is the swelling of the outer third of the vaginal vault, vasocongestion of the labia minora, breast tumescence, and ballooning of the inner two thirds of the vaginal vault. Orgasm consists of a subjective sense of ecstatic peaking of sexual pleasure with which sexual tension is resolved. The male has a sensation of ejaculatory inevitability preceding ejaculation of semen, propelled by spasmodic contractions of the prostate, seminal vesicles, and urethra. The female has spasmodic contractions of the outer third of the vaginal vault which may be subjectively experienced as either pulsatile or diffuse. Both male and female undergo generalized muscular contractions, usually including involuntary pelvic thrusting. Resolution consists of general muscular relaxation and a sense of well being and contentment. During this phase men are physiologically refractory to responding to additional sexual stimulation for a variable period of time. In women the refractory period may be very brief, depending on the intensity of the erotic stimulation and response.

Sexual inhibition may occur at the proceptive stage, leading to anxiety-ridden or neurotic forms of pair-bonding. Inhibition at this phase may also lead to inhibition of sexual desire. Inhibition in the acceptive phase may occur at any of the four subphases, although rarely is an inhibition of the resolution phase of primary clinical significance.

The conceptive phase is the phase of conception, pregnancy, childbirth and, eventually, parenthood. Pregnancy and parenthood usually have important repercussions on sexual behavior. The life-cycle changes often usher in sexual problems demanding the attention of the physician.

240. CLASSIFICATION OF SEXUAL DYSFUNCTIONS

The major sexual dysfunctions are listed in Table 2.

INHIBITED SEXUAL DESIRE

In most cases, a persistent inhibition of sexual desire is situational and acquired and is usually a result of marital conflicts and disappointments. If lifelong, it is a consequence of the early association of sexual pleasure with anxiety and/or guilt, occasionally resulting from sexual trauma such as rape or incest. Generalized inhibited sexual desire can occur as a defense against impulses (homosexual and sadomasochistic are the most common) that the patient is trying to ward off. Much more frequently it is caused by depression. Not uncommonly, one finds inhibited sexual desire as a consequence of chronic illness, even in the absence of depression. In men inhibition of desire may on rare occasions be associated with low levels of plasma testosterone, perhaps 250 nanograms per 100 ml, warranting a trial of replacement hormone; but usually there is no direct correlation between testosterone levels above 300 ng per 100 ml and sexual desire or capacity for erection. (In women there seems to be a more direct relationship between testosterone levels and sex drive and responsivity.) However, the relationship between the husband's sexual initiation and his wife's sexual responsivity, defined as the "sexual compatibility ratio," over a three-month period correlates significantly ($P < 0.05$) with the husband's average testosterone levels over the same period of time, indicating that biologic factors play a role in the frequency and responsivity of sustained sexual relationships.

INHIBITED SEXUAL EXCITEMENT

One of the most frequent sexual dysfunctions is the recurrent and persistent inhibition of sexual excitement during sexual activity with another person or alone. The inhibition is manifested by either (1) partial or complete failure to attain or maintain erection until completion of the sexual act (impotence), or (2) partial or complete failure to attain or maintain the lubrication-swelling response of sexual excitement until completion of the sexual act (frigidity). The term "frigidity" can be used if we narrow the definition to make it synonymous with "inhibited sexual excitement." In the past the term "frigidity" has been of little use, because it has been used to mean "inhibited sexual desire," "inhibited excitement," or "inhibited orgasm," or even the lack of pleasure in the presence of normal psychophysiologic responsivity. The diagnosis of "inhibited sexual excitement" should be made only if the clinician judges that the individual engages in sexual activity which is adequate in focus, intensity, and duration with the desired partner or means. Often, the failure to respond with adequate vasocongestion of either the penis or the vagina is a consequence of inadequate sexual stimulation due to either ignorance or selfishness.

IMPOTENCE. Impotence may be secondary to an inhibition of sexual desire. In the face of failure to attain or maintain an erection, the man's frustration is generally much more intense if there is adequate desire. The most common cause of impotence is anxiety with a particular partner, in which case marital-sexual therapy is the treatment of choice. If impotence is generalized and does not seem to be a consequence of marital conflict, the clinician should look for depression or some organic factor such as diabetes, and should also inquire about medication being used by the patient, e.g., antihypertensive drugs or psychotropic agents. Chronic alcoholism is often associated with impotence because testosterone metabolism seems to be adversely affected, with resultant low levels of plasma testosterone. This usually occurs in the presence of liver disease.

If the man gives a history of absent or infrequent morning or nighttime erections, or the inability to attain good erections with masturbation, rapid eye move-

TABLE 2. Types of Sexual Dysfunctions

Inhibited sexual desire
Inhibited sexual excitement (frigidity, impotence)
Inhibited female orgasm
Inhibited male orgasm
Premature ejaculation
Dyspareunia
Vaginismus
Other psychosexual dysfunctions

ment (REM) sleep studies are indicated, since the normal man has about 90 minutes of "erection time" associated with REM sleep during a nighttime of sleeping. It is possible to measure nocturnal penile tumescence (NPT) with special recording devices. If organic factors are present, there will be absent or inadequate erections during REM sleep.

FRIGIDITY (AS FORMERLY DEFINED). With either impotence or frigidity, lifelong inhibition of sexual excitement results from the association of adverse emotions, namely, anxiety, shame, and guilt, with sexual pleasure. In those cases, individual psychotherapy is often the treatment of choice, but only after a trial of conjoint couple therapy. However, most cases of inhibited sexual excitement in the female are acquired and are a consequence of the same negative emotions operating within the context of marriage. If the woman has been responsive earlier with her husband, or is now responsive with other partners, conjoint marital-sexual therapy is indicated, provided she is sufficiently committed to her marital relationship. This, in conjunction with specific behavioral techniques by which the woman is able to re-experience the sexual pleasure she has now lost, may be curative. However, if there is a great deal of hostility toward the spouse, marital therapy aimed at reducing anger and resentment must be carried out prior to specific sexual behavioral therapies. If frigidity is generalized, i.e., even with self-stimulation and/or with other partners, the clinician should search for organic causes. Here again, diabetes and medication are the most common causes of frigidity.

INHIBITED FEMALE ORGASM

This syndrome is characterized by the recurrent and persistent inhibition of the female orgasm, as manifested by delay or absence of orgasm following a normal sexual-excitement phase during sexual activity which is judged by the clinician to be adequate in focus, intensity, and duration. The majority of women are able to experience orgasm during clitoral stimulation but are not able to experience orgasm during coitus. There is evidence that suggests that in some instances this represents a symptomatic inhibition, justifying this diagnosis. In other women, failure to achieve orgasm during coitus represents a normal variation of the female sexual response. This is based on surveys which indicate that only approximately 30 per cent of women are able to achieve coital orgasm fairly frequently. If 70 per cent of women cannot achieve coital orgasm at all, or do so infrequently, it is probable that coital anorgasmia may be a normal variation, rather than a consequence of psychopathology. This difficult diagnosis can be made only by a thorough sexual evaluation, which may even require a trial of treatment. It is an important distinction clinically, since many women still ask for professional assistance because of this complaint.

The woman who is unable to achieve orgasm at all through *any* source of stimulation (about 10 per cent) can be helped in about 80 per cent of the cases by behavioral techniques. The use of sensate-focus as described by Masters and Johnson and the use of a vibrator have been helpful aids, at least in attaining noncoital orgasm. It is generally more difficult, even for the experienced sex therapist, to decrease a woman's inhibitions so that she is able to obtain coital orgasms fairly regularly. Referring back to the levels of intervention and the various roles of the physician, the physician-counselor is usually able to treat a woman who is completely anorgasmic, whereas it is generally necessary to refer a woman who wishes to achieve coital orgasm to a sex therapist.

INHIBITED MALE ORGASM

A relatively infrequent complaint compared with other types of sexual dysfunction is the recurrent and persistent inhibition of the male orgasm as manifested by a delay or absence of either the emission or ejaculation phases, or more usually both, following an adequate phase of sexual excitement. Although the vast majority of these cases are psychogenic, occasionally one finds this difficulty as a sequela of antihypertensive medication. Retarded ejaculation must be differentiated from retrograde ejaculation, which occurs most commonly after prostatectomy. Treatment of retarded ejaculation usually requires a combination of psychotherapy and couple-oriented behavioral techniques.

PREMATURE EJACULATION

It is impossible to use a normative length of time for the plateau phase of the sexual response cycle, i.e., the time between erection and ejaculation. Thus the diagnosis of premature ejaculation depends entirely on the man's distress over the recurrent and persistent absence of reasonable voluntary control of ejaculation and orgasm during sexual activity. Stated more simply, ejaculation occurs before the individual wants it. This dysfunction, with rare exceptions, is psychogenic and is a consequence of anxiety. The natural biologic sequence would be for rapid ejaculation after erection, and the male has to learn through experience to extend the plateau phase. Fortunately, there are excellent behavioral techniques for overcoming this frequent disorder. Use of the so-called "stop-and-start" technique during stimulation of the penis by his partner allows the male to recognize the sensations *prior* to ejaculatory inevitability. At the point when sensation will soon merge into ejaculatory inevitability, he signals his partner to cease stimulation for about 30 seconds, after which stimulation can be resumed. The same technique can be learned during copulatory pelvic thrusting. In this fashion over 95 per cent of men with premature ejaculation are reported to be cured of this distress. This technique is a simple one that can be easily taught to the patient; it thus comes under the province of the physician-counselor. The rare patient refractory to this method of therapy should be referred to a sex therapist.

"IMMEDIATE" CAUSES OF SEXUAL DYSFUNCTION

Every patient with inhibited excitement or orgasm or with premature ejaculation is adversely affected by "immediate" causes of sexual dysfunction. These are fear of failure, or anxiety over performance, which increases the underlying source of anxiety; the monitoring of one's own performance, called "spectatoring" by Masters and Johnson, that puts distance between the patient and his participation in the sex act; often an inordinate need to please the partner, providing another significant cause of increased anxiety; and the failure to talk about one's sources of anxiety, a reparative device which generally tends to accentuate anxiety. These dimensions of dysfunction can be dealt with by the physician-counselor, provided he is aware of them and is skillful enough to get his patient to discuss them. Reducing these immediate causes of sexual dysfunction is the first therapeutic task of any counselor or therapist. In many instances the immediate causes of sexual dysfunction turn out to be the only ones. For example, a man may lose his erection two or three times in the course of a week or two because of fatigue or preoccupation with business or because of some animosity toward his wife or because of too much drinking. This starts a vicious cycle of fear of failure or anxiety about performance, monitoring his own behavior, and being too exquisitely tuned to the reactions of his female partner. The anxiety increases into panic, and the inhibition becomes definite and pronounced. Indeed, anxiety can be differentiated from panic by the following quip: *"Anxiety is the first time a man cannot get an erection twice, and panic is the second time he cannot get it once."*

DYSPAREUNIA

Recurrent and persistent genital pain associated with coitus is not restricted to the female, although it is much more common in women than in men. Organic factors are frequent, so that adequate gynecologic and/or urologic examination is mandatory. Despite this, the most frequent cause of dyspareunia in the female is the relative absence of lubrication during the sexual response cycle. Coitus with a dry vagina often produces dyspareunia. A test of this can be made by having the woman use artificial lubrication. Dyspareunia may or may not be accompanied by vaginismus.

VAGINISMUS

Vaginismus can be diagnosed if there is a history of recurrent and persistent involuntary spasm of the musculature of the outer one third of the vagina that interferes with sexual activity. The diagnosis can be confirmed during a pelvic examination. If the vaginismus has been preceded by a history of dyspareunia, the underlying causes of dyspareunia must be discovered and treated first. If the vaginismus is psychogenic, the disorder can be readily overcome by a combination of psychotherapy and the use of graduated Hegar dilators. Very frequently the woman can be taught to dilate her own vagina in the so-called "sexological" examination. Techniques of doing this are demonstrated in the presence of her husband, as his cooperation is enlisted. Many but not all so-called "unconsummated" marriages are due to vaginismus. The treatment of the unconsummated marriage is then directed toward the treatment of vaginismus. (It should not be overlooked that a significant number of unconsummated marriages are due to either impotence on the part of the husband or to an inhibition of sexual desire in either or both husband and wife.)

OTHER SEXUAL DYSFUNCTIONS

In the absence of a specific sexual dysfunction, distress can come from a variety of other reasons. An individual may feel that he or she is not meeting some fantasied standard of sexual performance, or there may be feelings of inadequacy related to self-imposed standards of masculinity or femininity such as bodily habitus or size or shape of the sex organs. Sometimes a patient may express distress over the inability to respond sexually in certain specific situations in ways that are desired. Although the patient is desirous of sexual activity, there may be a marital conflict leading to avoidance of sexual activities, which in turn increases conflict. Sometimes the very intensity of sexual excitement can create anxiety and discomfort. Occasionally one finds a patient engaging in a variety of sexual behaviors, but who feels very little or no pleasure in the activity (sexual anhedonia). A very frequent couple conflict results when there are discrepant sexual desires for frequency, forms of foreplay, or coital positions, or when partner is exerting deliberate control of sexual expression over the other.

As has been discussed earlier, the physician-educator who is comfortable in dealing with sexual problems can clear up many sexual concerns by giving appropriate information. Sexual misunderstanding and misinformation are extensive; only a few examples are given here: the adolescent boy who thinks his penis is too small, or the teenage girl who thinks she is abnormal because of her sexual urges; the notion that oral-genital sex is a perverse activity; the frequent concept that coital orgasm is the only form of orgasm that is normal; that masturbation is abnormal and may even lead to mental illness; that direct clitoral stimulation must be continued until penetration occurs; that waxing and waning of sexual excitement is abnormal; that sexual activity during pregnancy or weeks after recovery from a coronary occlusion is dangerous; or that after the age of 50 or 60 or 70 a person is sexually "over the hill."

241. ADDITIONAL PROBLEM AREAS

When any of the specific sexual dysfunctions occur in a marital relationship, they may be the result of (1) sufficient psychopathology on the part of one or both spouses, (2) a poor relationship of "fit" between the spouses, or (3) relative ignorance of one or both partners. An example of the first category is the wife whose life experience taught her that sex is nasty and sinful and who cannot experience sexual pleasure, for the pleasure would increase her guilt inordinately. Patients in this category with longstanding sexual dysfunction are generally referred to psychiatrists. Patients whose difficulties stem largely from a poor marital relationship may be seen by the nonpsychiatric physician, who, unless he has had special training in sex and marriage counseling, must be mindful of his own capacities and limitations.

In evaluating any sexual problem, it is necessary to determine how much weight to attach to the three factors contributing to the problem. Often, all three are represented. The woman who has the concept of sex as a sinful activity and who inhibits her responsivity may have only a hazy idea of what pattern of stimulation is best suited to increase her sexual excitement, and may make all sorts of excuses to her husband ("I'm tired" or "I have a headache" or "It's my period") to avoid sex, or she may grant or withhold sex as a weapon to punish her husband or in bargaining for something she wants.

Although the sexual problems that arise in marriage constitute the most frequent and most important need for professional intervention, additional characteristic sexual problems arise during the life cycle. Including marital sexual problems, some of the more frequent problem areas are the following:

Helping children and their parents deal with problems of sexual development includes concerns about masturbation, sex play among children, menstruation, wet dreams, sexual fantasies, and coital activity among teenagers. "How do I, as a parent, talk to my children about sex?" is a question often asked of physicians.

Concerns of teenagers may include masturbation, penis size, how far to go during petting, the relation of sex to the relationships between sexes (how does sex relate to love?), erotic arousal for members of the same sex, contraception, and sexual performance. Unwanted pregnancy creates a need for abortion or "problem pregnancy" counseling. Venereal disease may occur at any age level, but it is increasing rapidly among teenagers.

Among young adults contemplating marriage, concerns include sexual performance and compatibility, as well as family planning.

Separation, such as occurs with divorce or death in the middle-aged or elderly, creates very special sexual problems. The loss of companionship and affection may be even more important than the decrease in sexual opportunities, although the interest in sex itself among the elderly is characteristically unrecognized or minimized by the physician.

Although *childhood sex play and masturbation* are now recognized as part of normal psychosexual development, parents are frequently concerned enough to ask their physicians about these behaviors. In most instances reassurance is all that is needed. If the sexual activity is "excessive" (and this is often subject to varying interpretation), it indicates a narrowing of the range of healthy social activities of the child rather than the abnormality of the sexual behavior per se. The basic points in talking to children or teenagers is to be as comfortable as possible, and to be brief, concise, and factual once the real concerns are elicited, by gently encouraging the child to talk and, above all, to avoid lecturing in a pontifical fashion. The physician is more apt to be "heard" if he discusses the pros and cons of sexual decision-making, rather than expressing his own value position in a forceful manner.

The problem of premarital coitus is characteristically presented by the unmarried girl who asks her physician for the "pill." If freedom of the physician is not restricted by his own set of values, this provides him with an opportunity to discuss with the young patient her feelings and expectations about her relationship with her actual or intended partner. Physicians are often concerned that prescribing contraception for the unmarried girl will be a license for sexual activity, and some still refuse to do so. Actually, the young girl usually asks for contraception *after,* rather than before, the initial coital experience. A study of over 500 unwed never-pregnant teenagers aged 13 to 17, who for the first time sought professional help to obtain contraception, showed that 96 per cent of those teenagers who asked for contraception were previously sexually active; most of them had been having intercourse for more than a year; few were using any contraceptives, and still fewer were using one of the most effective methods. It should be clear that if a minor requests contraception, she needs it. This study and others suggest that contraceptive information and educational programs directed at minors will not be a significant factor in their decision to become sexually active.

A special area of increasing concern to physicians is called *"problem pregnancy" counseling.* This is not restricted to teenagers, as the majority of abortions are performed on married women. The unmarried pregnant teenager, however, is in a highly vulnerable position, because pregnancy and childbearing may seriously interfere with her educational and economic status, while the negative social sanctions against abortion that still persist make her face difficult choices. The various options — e.g., continuing with the pregnancy and giving up the baby for adoption or keeping the baby, whether to marry or not, or whether to terminate pregnancy — must be discussed thoroughly, and outside pressures for decision-making should be separated from internal conflict. The availability of legal abortion for those who can afford it has greatly eased the situation. However, the decision for abortion should never be made lightly, because the physician should be fairly certain that the patient will not be in the small minority who suffer from depression or remorse after the abortion. This applies to married women as well as to the unmarried. Most patients (who are not harmed by the abortion procedure per se) would derive special benefits by more intensive contraceptive, sex, and family counseling than is ordinarily provided to women seeking abortion.

Family-planning counseling gives the physician an unparalleled opportunity for exploring the connections between sexual attitudes and behavior and contraceptive concerns. The choice of the appropriate method of contraception is influenced by the frequency of coitus, attitudes toward responsibility and decision-making, fears of bodily damage, and desires for greater sexual spontaneity, as well as religious and moral values. Contraceptive failures are related to risk-taking, to the failure to learn how or under what conditions conception occurs, or to the individual's being under stress so that "contraceptive vigilance" is reduced. Adequate communication with the partner about contraceptive planning is an important consequence of appropriate counseling. Family planning is much more than the prescription of a contraceptive method. It includes the timing of marriage, timing of the first child, child-spacing, the total number of children desired, and sex- and marriage-counseling, as well as counseling in contraception, problem-pregnancy, and sterilization methods. Genetic counseling may also be a significant dimension of family planning. In this sense, family-planning counseling is an essential feature of premarital counseling, but should be available throughout the childbearing years.

Patients frequently misperceive *the spouse's desired frequency of intercourse;* most often the wife overestimates her husband's desired frequency. In one sixth of the cases studied, there was a gross underestimation of the wife's desires. The perception of the problem is usually more significant than the reality. The physician can often help by asking each spouse separately how often each wants intercourse, and each one's perception of the spouse's desires. Better communication is the first step toward relieving this problem and, in many instances, may be all that is required. The physician also has to bear in mind that the sex drive in the male is at a peak between the ages of 15 and 25, whereas in the female it peaks a decade later.

242. HOMOSEXUALITY

The etiology of homosexuality — preferential or exclusive sexual activity with a member of the same sex — is not known. At present an intense debate among psychiatrists is raging whether to regard homosexuality as a normal sexual variant or as a psychopathologic development — in other words, a deviation. The American Psychiatric Association has removed homosexuality from its list of disorders (Diagnostic and Statistical Manual No. 2) and has established a category called "sexual orientation disorder" for those who are distressed by their homosexual desires or behavior and seek help to resolve this conflict.

Although homosexuality is found in virtually every society and culture around the world, there is no society in which it is the dominant or preferred mode of sexual activity. (If there were, it is clear that that particular society would eventually vanish.) It is also known that if, in a given society, repression of sexual behaviors — including homosexual play — is absent during prepubertal development, adult homosexuality is extremely rare. This implies, but is by no means a proven fact, that childhood repression of sexual behavior is the principal cause of adult homosexuality.

Sexual programming of the brain, principally the hypothalamus, during a critical period of fetal life prepares the individual for later sexual behavior. This occurs in every mammalian species studied, including man. It is conceivable but still highly conjectural that some as yet unknown mechanism interfering with this brain programming may be an important contributing factor in the etiology of homosexuality. It may take a combination of brain programming and certain types of social learning in childhood to bring about preferential same-sex behavior in the adults.

If called upon to give counsel to a homosexual, the physician's approach should in no way differ from the approach to a heterosexual. No attempt should be made to try to direct him into heterosexual behavior unless he specifically requests such help. If his motivation is high, if he still has heterosexual dreams or fantasies, if he has had one or more successful heterosexual encounters, and if his first homosexual experience occurred after the age of 16, the prognosis for changing to bisexuality or even preferential heterosexuality is reasonable. About one in three with these good prognostic indicators can be helped to become successfully heterosexual. This generally requires the skillful help of a competent and experienced psychotherapist.

LESBIANISM

The young woman who discovers that she is attracted to members of her own sex and who gradually develops an erotic interest in other females faces two major problems. One is the definition of her own gender identity; the other is a sense of isolation. Such women often remain uncertain of their sexual preferences for several years, and their resulting intense internal struggle is heightened by actual or anticipated parental and societal disapproval or rejection. Strong feelings of alienation accompany the self-condemnation of this internal conflict, and the affected woman may regard herself as unique with problems shared by few others, especially not by her friends or peers.

The physician or school counselor who is called upon to help these young women has to set a neutral, non-condemnatory, nonjudgmental course. Too quick an acceptance of the patient's lesbianism with facile reassurance may increase the young woman's anxiety, for she may be far from certain of her sexual preferences, whereas obviously a judgmental, censorious attitude will make her too uncomfortable to remain in treatment. The counselor's task is to help the patient reach some sort of closure (and this may take considerable time) about which direction she wishes to take, and then to help her with the social skills necessary to achieve a degree of intimacy, either heterosexually or homosexually. If the young woman decides that her preference is for lesbianism, the counselor also has to help the patient deal realistically with her parents and possibly with school authorities.

This is often a delicate matter, involving ethical decisions by the counselor, and tact, sensitivity, and good judgment are essential. Many schools have peer counseling adjuncts which, along with group counseling, may be useful in overcoming the woman's loneliness and feelings of inferiority. Although social condemnation for homosexual men and women is decreasing and "gay" groups are organized in many communities, most young people are afraid to identify themselves as being homosexual, and the adjustment to that special subculture, although ultimately helpful, is almost never without apprehension and even anguish.

SUMMARY

If the physician is interested in helping his patients with sexual problems, and if he is reasonably comfortable and tactful and has an appreciation of the role his own feelings and attitudes play in interviewing and treatment, he will be able to establish a feeling of confidence and hope in his patient. This empathic relationship, coupled with the physician's growing fund of information and skills in interviewing, makes possible the competent management of marital and sexual problems that heretofore have been either neglected or mishandled. In no other area of his practice can the physician derive greater reward and satisfaction from his efforts.

Abse, D. W., Nash, E. M. and Louden, L. M. R. (eds.): Marital and Sexual Counseling in Medical Practice. New York, Harper & Row, 1974.

Gadpaille, W. J.: The Cycles of Sex. New York, Scribners, 1975.

Kaplan, H. S.: The New Sex Therapy. New York, Bruner-Mazel, 1974.

Lief, H. I.: Sexual counseling. *In* Romney, S., Gray, M. J., Little, B., Merrill, J., Quilligan, T., and Stander, R. (eds.): Gynecology and Obstetrics: The Health Care of Women. New York, McGraw-Hill Book Company, 1975, Chap. 31, pp. 526–548.

Mandel, T., and Oline, P.: Counseling the lesbian. *In* Money, J., and Musaph, H. (eds.): Handbook of Sexology. Amsterdam, Excerpta Medica, 1977, Chap. 101, pp. 1279–1288.

Money, J., and Musaph, H.: Handbook of Sexology. Amsterdam, Excerpta Medica, 1977.

Vincent, C. E.: Sexual and Marital Health: The Physician as Consultant. New York, McGraw-Hill Book Company, 1973.

Section Seven   DRUG ABUSE, DEPENDENCE, AND INTOXICATION

243. INTRODUCTION

Robert B. Millman

Drug abuse is behavior that results from the complex interaction of an individual, his social and cultural environment, and the pharmacology and availability of particular drugs. There is frequently no sharp line that distinguishes appropriate use from misuse of any drug. Drug abuse may therfore be defined as the use of any substance in a manner that deviates from the accepted medical, social, or legal patterns within a given society. This section will consider the abuse of drugs that are primarily used to induce alterations in mood, perception, and behavior. These may be grouped into six major classes: (1) opiates; (2) central nervous system depressants, including alcohol, hypnotics, and tranquilizers; (3) central nervous system stimulants, including the amphetamine group and cocaine; (4) cannabis; (5) psychedelics; and (6) miscellaneous inhalants.

Abuse of some drugs may be intermittent and lead to little physical, psychologic, or social deterioration. In other cases, the user may become dependent on the drug in order to function at what he perceives to be a satisfactory level. This *psychologic dependence,* or habituation, varies in intensity and may culminate in *compulsive drug abuse,* in which the supply and use of particular drugs become primary concerns of living. In addition, certain drugs have the capacity to produce *physical dependence.* This is an altered physiologic state induced by the repeated administration of a drug that requires the continued administration of the drug to prevent the appearance of a syndrome characteristic for each drug, the *withdrawal,* or *abstinence, syndrome.* The term *"addiction"* has been used in the literature to refer to either behavioral or pharmacologic events. As used herein, it refers to a pattern of compulsive drug use that includes both physical dependence and an overwhelming involvement with the supply and use of a drug. Neither a diabetic who is on insulin nor a well adjusted patient in methadone maintenance treatment is an addict in this sense of the term, although both are physically dependent on their medication.

ETIOLOGY AND PATTERNS OF ABUSE. No single factor is the basis of all drug-taking experience, and no person's drug taking has a single cause. Initially, drugs may be taken to satisfy curiosity, to reduce pain, to influence mood, to change activity levels, to reduce tension and anxiety, to decrease fatigue and boredom, to facilitate social interaction, to heighten sensation and awareness, and for many other reasons. If caffeine, nicotine, alcohol, and prescription and over-the-counter depressants and stimulants are included, few people in the United States would be found who take no psychoactive drugs. Patterns of abuse vary from the experimental or intermittent use of a particular drug or combination under defined circumstances, such as the use of marijuana and alcohol at a party, to a compulsive "polydrug-abuse" pattern, in which a variety of drugs are taken in a disorganized and dangerous manner on a daily basis.

SOCIOLOGIC FACTORS. Social and cultural factors determine which drug-abuse patterns are acceptable for a given group; and in some cases, groups derive their identity from particular drug-using behavior. The use of alcohol is condoned and even encouraged in many segments of society. Cannabis and psychedelic use are an integral part of membership in some white middle class groups. Heroin use, until recently, was considered an involving, exciting pursuit in inner-city ghetto areas. Given the limited opportunities to experience pleasure, satisfaction, or pride in certain underprivileged groups, moreover, the aggressive, goal-oriented life of a heroin addict may appear attractive to a young boy or girl. Social factors also determine the availability of particular drugs. Heroin is easily available in the inner city, whereas the suburban dweller may have to travel long distances to obtain the drug. The extent and patterns of abuse change rapidly in response to a variety of social and cultural factors. Accurate epidemiologic information is difficult to obtain because of the illegal or covert nature of the behavior and the necessarily indirect surveying methods. Currently (1978), the prevalence of heroin, alcohol, and polydrug abuse in this country appears to be increasing; amphetamine and psychedelic use are decreasing. Cocaine and marijuana appear to be more frequently used, and the patterns of abuse of these drugs have changed considerably over the last decade.

PSYCHOBIOLOGIC FACTORS. Personality and constitutional factors, in part, determine the psychoactive effects that drugs elicit in individual users and influence the choice of drugs and patterns of abuse. Amphetamines may produce tranquility in some people. Alcohol and barbiturates impair behavior control in others and may permit certain personality types to act in a hostile and violent manner. Genetic factors have been strongly implicated in the development of alcoholism.

Controversy exists as to whether drug abuse implies a personality disturbance that antedates drug use and that can be classified in distinct groups according to the drug and pattern of abuse. Some workers describe well defined addictive or alcoholic personality types, characterized by a mixture of neurotic traits and character disorders, although present evidence suggests that personality characteristics in drug-abusing populations vary considerably and that psychologic factors play a markedly variable role in the etiology of drug abuse. Although premorbid personality disturbances are crucial in the etiology of some cases of compulsive drug use, the psychopathology noted in other cases may be a reaction to the behavioral patterns of compulsive abuse in a society that condemns the drug-dependent life. *Moreover, no predictive test or system has been developed that will determine whether or not a person will become a compulsive user, nor which people will use which drugs.* It is generally agreed that the experimental or intermittent abuse of drugs is not necessarily an indication of psychopathology. Compulsive drug use *is* frequently associated with psychopathology. In some people the drug use may be an attempt at *self-medication* of painful feelings of anxiety, shame, inadequacy, loneliness, guilt, and depression. Others may be seeking to allay unacceptable aggressive or sexual drives or to control psychotic symptoms. At the same time, some severely disturbed people have experimented with alcohol, opiates, and other drugs and have not become compulsive users. The more aberrant an individual's drug-abuse behavior pattern is for his particular social or cultural milieu, the more likely there is a significant degree of psychopathology.

Conditioned learning is an integral part of the development and maintenance of compulsive drug-abuse patterns. The feelings of dysphoria that the drug-taking behavior allayed or some of the situations attendant to the behavior become, in time, the conditioned stimulus for the experience of drug craving and the persistence of drug-seeking behavior. This may occur in the presence or absence of physical dependence. The drug-craving and withdrawal syndrome that long abstinent ex-addicts experience when they return to a site of former drug use is, in part, a reflection of this conditioning process. Learning also influences the nature of the drug experience.

Various disease states are treated with psychoactive drugs for prolonged periods. The drug use of a small percentage of patients may come to exceed medically recommended dosages or indications and eventuate in drug dependence in some cases. Psychologic and sociologic factors should be considered in the etiology of these behavior patterns in addition to the physical and pharmacologic determinants.

PHARMACOLOGIC FACTORS. The nature of the psychic and physical effects of particular drugs is a determinant of their abuse potential. Considerations of physical dependence and tolerance influence the pattern of abuse. *Tolerance* refers to the decreased effect obtained from repeated administration of a given dose of a drug or to the need for increased amounts to obtain the effects that occurred from the first dose. Tolerance may be either *drug disposition* (metabolic) in type, in which there is more rapid inactivation or excretion of a drug, or *pharmacodynamic* (cellular), in which cells in the nervous system adapt to drug concentrations. Both may occur with the same drug. The physical dependence that develops concurrently with tolerance to opiates, barbiturates, and alcohol is poorly understood and may be related to pharmacodynamic tolerance mechanisms. *Cross-dependence* refers to the ability of one drug to suppress abstinence symptoms produced by withdrawal of another. Cross-dependence may be complete or partial, as with alcohol and the barbiturates.

DIAGNOSIS. To provide adequate treatment, it is necessary to characterize the specific problems of drug abuse and dependence in each patient as well as the psychologic set and the social situation attendant to the use of the psychoactive substances. The nature and degree of drug-induced psychoactive effects and any abstinence symptoms and signs should be assessed. This requires careful history taking when possible, including information on the type, amount, and pattern of chemical use, and a complete physical examination. Drug abusers are often poor historians and may minimize or exaggerate the extent of their drug use, depending on their perception of the situation, their needs, and the attitude of the examiner. It is likely that an opiate user will exaggerate the extent of his use so as to obtain more opiates during the detoxification process and perhaps suffer decreased abstinence symptoms. A college student may minimize his diazepam dependence, since the extent of his use might be considered evidence of weakness or serious psychopathology. Pressing social or legal needs should be identified with a view toward providing realistic, often necessarily short-term solutions.

Evaluation of the mode of administration and the adverse effects of the drugs of abuse is important in establishing a diagnosis. Signs of repeated intravenous injections ("tracks") suggest heroin, amphetamine, or cocaine abuse. These drugs are also "sniffed," whereby the material is inhaled and absorbed through the mucous membranes of the nasopharynx and respiratory tract. Chronic sinusitis or perforation of the nasal septum may suggest this mode of administration. Personal hygiene and patterns of behavior and dress may further define the clinical picture.

Routine qualitative procedures for the detection in urine of morphine (the major metabolite of heroin), methadone, amphetamines, cocaine, and the most frequently abused general depressants are currently available in many laboratories. Results will generally be positive if a dose sufficient to produce pharmacologic effects has been taken within 24 hours prior to the urine sample. Since results are not immediately available ordinarily and since false positives occur, these tests should be used to confirm the clinical impression. They are most useful as an adjunct to the long-term evaluation of patients already in treatment. In emergency situations, blood levels of suspected drugs can usually be obtained immediately.

TREATMENT AND PREVENTION. Treatment procedures should vary according to the individual and his social set, the pattern and extent of abuse, and the pharmacology of the abused drugs, as well as the goals of treatment. As distinct from most other patients, drug abusers frequently know more about the behavior and disability incident to drug taking than do their physicians. Serving to further complicate therapeutic efforts, drug abusers are often faced with prejudice and hostility on the part of treatment personnel, e.g., "They did it to themselves." Since many of their personality characteristics and behavior patterns occur in response to the attitudes of society, an inquiring, compassionate attitude is crucial in the treatment of this group of patients.

These patients commonly do not show consistent progress, often resuming the use of drugs after detoxification and varying periods of abstinence. This tends to frustrate the efforts of the physician or the treatment team, who may be provoked to give up on particular patients. The problem here may be a conceptual one;

physicians often regard substance abuse as an acute illness, not unlike pneumonia, and liable to complete cure after detoxification. This is an unrealistic assumption given the chronic nature of most psychologic and social difficulties. Then, too, the character of the pharmacologic dependence may be more protracted than previously imagined. Since the clinical course in some of these patients may be reminiscent of diabetes or schizophrenia, with remissions and exacerbations, treatment should be seen as consisting of both immediate and long-term measures. Patience and continuing enthusiasm are as essential as in most other branches of medicine.

Drug-abuse prevention programs have focused on educational efforts in which the risks of drug abuse are publicized, and on legal sanctions. Both approaches have serious deficiencies. Perhaps more important than either of these would be the provision of reasonably attractive vocational, recreational, and educational alternatives to drug abuse in those most at risk, namely, the young and psychosocially disadvantaged. Physicians must be extremely prudent in their prescribing practices with respect to potentially abusable drugs.

244. THE OPIATES

Robert B. Millman

Opiates or narcotic analgesics refer to natural or synthetic drugs that have pharmacologic actions similar to those of the derivatives of opium. Opium is obtained from the poppy plant *Papaver somniferum* and contains more than 20 alkaloids, of which morphine and codeine are relevant to this discussion. Heroin, the principal opiate of abuse in the United States, is converted from morphine by the addition of two acetyl groups (diacetyl-morphine). Meperidine and methadone are synthetic narcotic analgesics. Pentazocine is a synthetic analgesic compound that has actions similar to both the opiates and the narcotic antagonists.

INCIDENCE. People have used opium for medical, religious, or recreational purposes since ancient times. Marked changes have occurred in the characteristics of the opiate-abusing population in the United States during the past 100 years. The use of patent medicines containing opiates was widespread in the middle class during the period from 1850 to 1906, when the labeling requirements of the Pure Food and Drug Act caused many preparations to be withdrawn. The Harrison Narcotics Act of 1914 and Supreme Court decisions in the 1920's made possession of narcotics without a prescription a crime and created a climate in which addicts were considered to be criminals and in which physicians could not prescribe narcotics to addicts. The number of oral opiate users declined, and the primary remaining group were those who injected heroin or morphine. Illegal dealers became the only source of opiates. Prices rose precipitously, and addicts frequently resorted to criminal activity to finance their addiction. The addict population from the 1930's to World War II predominantly consisted of white individuals involved in criminal activity or the entertainment professions who used intravenous heroin as well as morphine, cocaine, and other drugs. The growth of urban black ghettos and the development of efficient production and delivery systems ushered in the present era of extensive heroin use associated with a pervasive street culture that supports the heroin-dependent life.

Heroin use reached epidemic proportions in the United States in the mid- to late 1960's. The majority of users were members of ethnic minority groups and lived in major urban areas. Males predominated over females, and the population was quite young. In New York City in 1971, heroin was the major cause of death in males aged 15 to 35. Large numbers of affluent white suburban youths were also becoming addicted. During the early 1970's, the incidence of heroin addiction declined owing to a multiplicity of factors, including changing social and cultural styles, the proliferation of effective treatment programs, and decreased availability of heroin. More recently there appears to be a resurgence of the problem, with a shift in the highest rates of incidence to smaller cities and more rural areas. The total number of heroin addicts in this country in 1975 was estimated to be between 500,000 and 600,000.

PATTERNS OF ABUSE. People initially experiment with heroin for many reasons, including a search for pleasure, curiosity, anxiety, immaturity, sexual problems, psychopathology, and peer pressure. In some urban ghetto areas, given the lack of attractive alternatives, using and selling heroin appears to be a rewarding, involving "career" that carries with it the illusion of wealth and significance. Users are generally introduced to the drug by a friend or acquaintance already using the drug. The majority of first-time users have already had drug-abuse experience, particularly alcohol and marijuana. The role of the nonaddicted drug dealer ("profiteer") is minimal in exposing new users to the drug. Street heroin ("smack," "scag," "junk," "dope") is adulterated ("cut") with quinine, lactose, mannitol, maltose, and other substances as it passes from the importer to the street user. The final amount of heroin in a street package costing from two to ten dollars may vary from 2 to 20 mg.

Initial street use is generally by "sniffing," in which the material is absorbed through the mucous membranes of the nasopharynx and respiratory tract. A user's first experience with the drug is often characterized as somewhat unpleasant because of nausea, vomiting, and anxiety; these symptoms abate with subsequent use. Effects may then be perceived as a sense of relaxation and peace with relief of worry and tension, a euphoric state in which all things are as they should be. At the outset, use may be intermittent and separated by weeks or months. It is not known how many people experiment with the drug and do not continue its use. Those who do continue to use heroin develop tolerance to its euphoric effects. In an attempt to maximize the euphoric effects of a given street amount, users will begin to inject the drug subcutaneously ("skin-popping") and eventually intravenously ("mainlining"). Intravenous injection produces a warm flushing of the skin and pleasurable sensations in the entire body, described as similar to sexual orgasm and called a "rush" or "kick." Many years of intravenous use of opiates and other drugs may result in obliteration of patent, available veins, necessitating a return to the subcutaneous mode of injection.

As tolerance increases and the awareness of physical dependence becomes manifest, more drug must be used more often. The urban street addict with little access to legitimate sources of money or drug must devote all his time and energy to the acquisition of heroin to support his addiction ("habit"). Involvement in the "junkie" subculture, with its own language and behavioral systems, ensures his supply of drug and provides for the transmission of skills, information, and ideology that make it possible to live as an addict. Any source of money is acceptable; males frequently engage in theft and forgery, whereas females will be prostitutes and shoplifters. Every user is a potential "dealer" of drugs, because this is the most efficient way of making money. Food, clothing, sexual desires, and dignity may become subordinate to the ever-present need for opiates. An unknown number of heroin addicts, particularly those in the entertainment professions, are able to maintain their employment and their families and do not become immersed in the behavior patterns of the street "junkie."

If heroin is not available or is in poor supply, addicts will use other opiates, particularly illicitly obtained ("street") methadone because of its long duration of action, to allay their withdrawal symptoms. Compulsive use of illicit methadone occurs, although usually after an initial period of heroin dependence. Primary methadone addiction is rare, because the drug is commonly available in oral form only and the intensity of its euphoric properties is less than that of heroin. Concurrent use of alcohol, sedatives, and marijuana occurs in up to 75 per cent of narcotic addicts, and mixed addictions in this group are frequently seen. Use of stimulants in association with narcotics is also quite common.

Opiate addicts are a heterogeneous group. They demonstrate a significant amount of psychopathology, including high levels of neurotic, personality, and psychotic characteristics, although no common pathologic pattern is apparent. Personality characteristics and behavior patterns frequently result from the interaction of the addict and the drug in the sociocultural environment of addiction. The incidence of premorbid psychopathology is controversial and depends in part on how deviant the behavior is relative to a given social milieu and how difficult it is to get the drugs. Inner-city minority-group addicts are often remarkably stable given their difficult living situations and the high degree of personality integration and intelligence required to survive as a street addict. Middle-class people are often more severely disturbed, and the drug use represents an attempt at self-medication for the symptomatology incident to borderline or psychotic personality disorders. The ability of the drugs to control severe symptomatology may derive from their anxiety-relieving qualities, direct antipsychotic effects, as well as the very structured existence street-heroin addiction often mandates. Some of these people are able to function effectively as street addicts but decompensate acutely or chronically when the heroin is withdrawn or when methadone is substituted. Under these circumstances, patients often will abuse other drugs, particularly those in the sedative-alcohol group.

PHARMACOLOGY. Opiates are absorbed from the gastrointestinal tract or the nasal mucosa, and after subcutaneous, intramuscular, or intravenous injection. Morphine and heroin lose much of their analgesic potency when taken orally, whereas codeine and meperidine remain quite active, and methadone retains most of its analgesic efficacy after oral administration. Heroin is hydrolyzed to morphine in the body and, except for its greater potency and more rapid onset of action, has pharmacologic properties similar to those of morphine. Morphine is concentrated in parenchymatous tissues, skeletal muscle, and, to a lesser extent, brain. It is conjugated with glucuronic acid and excreted primarily in the urine and secondarily in the feces. Traces of morphine can be found in urine for 48 hours, although 90 per cent or more is excreted within the first 24 hours.

Administered subcutaneously, methadone and morphine exert approximately equal analgesic effects; heroin is three times stronger, whereas meperidine and codeine are approximately one tenth as potent. Morphine or heroin taken intravenously is effective almost immediately; duration of action varies from three to six hours. Oral administration prolongs the action of all the opiates, particularly that of methadone, in which the onset of effect occurs within 30 minutes and the duration of action in nontolerant individuals is four to ten hours.

Morphine or heroin administered to a nontolerant individual induces analgesia through a reduction in the anxiety and tension that result from the perception of pain. Related to this is a positive feeling of well-being or euphoria. Somnolence, characterized by an inability to concentrate, sleepiness, or "nodding," also occurs. Opiates cause pupillary constriction, depression of respiration by decreasing the responsiveness of the brainstem to carbon dioxide, depression of body temperature, and stimulation of central nervous system centers to produce nausea and vomiting. Other acute effects include decreased motility of the stomach, diminished pancreatic and biliary secretions, decreased propulsive contractions of the small and large intestine, and increased tone of the anal sphincter, leading to constipation. Increased tone of the detrusor muscle leads to a sensation of urgency accompanied by increased tone of the vesical sphincter, resulting in urinary retention. An acute release of antidiuretic hormone is effected, as well as inhibition of release of ACTH, corticotropin-releasing factor, and gonadotropin. Peripheral vasodilatation occurs, resulting in pruritus and possibly causing the observed increase in perspiration. Histamine release occurs, frequently resulting in a wheal-and-flare reaction, or "hive," at the site of injection and in a "pins-and-needles" sensation.

ADDICTION AND WITHDRAWAL PROCESSES. Repeated use of narcotic analgesics produces tolerance to most of the acute narcotic effects, and the lethal dose is markedly increased. Whereas a 10-mg dose of morphine may produce euphoria in a nontolerant individual, the daily use of 5 grams has been reported in addicts. The rate at which this tolerance develops depends on the frequency and magnitude of use. Street addicts may spend from $20 to $200 or more daily on heroin and may inject themselves every three to six hours. Tolerance to all the opiate effects does not occur equally, because highly tolerant users will continue to demonstrate pupillary constriction and constipation. Cross-tolerance occurs with all narcotic analgesics. Tolerance to narcotics is primarily due to some form of cellular adaptation to the drug's action, with increased metabolism of lesser importance.

Physical dependence develops concurrently with tolerance and has been demonstrated after only a few exposures on succeeding days. It is marked by the development of an acute abstinence syndrome upon withdrawal of opiates, the "cold-turkey" process. This syndrome is quite variable in severity and characteristics and depends upon the particular drug, the dose, the interval between doses, and the duration of narcotic use, as well as on the personality and immediate environment of the narcotic addict. With heroin, the first withdrawal signs are generally seen shortly before the next scheduled dose. They are purposive in nature and include feelings of anxiety, restlessness, irritability, and drug craving. Lacrimation, rhinorrhea, yawning, and perspiration become apparent 8 to 15 hours after the last dose of narcotic. A restless sleep may intervene, the so-called "yen sleep," from which the addict awakens with more severe withdrawal symptoms and signs, including dilated pupils, sneezing, coryza, anorexia, nausea, vomiting, diarrhea, abdominal cramps, bone pains, myalgias, tremors, weakness, insomnia, goose flesh, and, very rarely, convulsions or cardiovascular collapse. With morphine and heroin, withdrawal symptoms peak at 36 to 48 hours, and most observable symptoms gradually subside over the next five to ten days. With methadone, the onset of withdrawal symptoms is more gradual, the peak is less pronounced and later, and the duration may be more than two or three weeks. The abstinence syndrome may be precipitated within minutes in opiate-dependent persons by administration of a narcotic antagonist such as nalorphine, levallorphan, or naloxone, although there are no medical indications for this diagnostic procedure.

Pentazocine (Talwin), a drug with weak opiate-antagonist effects and moderate opiate-agonist effects, elicits morphine-like subjective effects in nontolerant individuals. Higher doses produce dysphoric effects, including nervousness, anxiety, and, infrequently, bizarre alterations in perception and behavior. Tolerance and physical dependence occur, and cases of addiction to this drug are reported. Abrupt withdrawal of the drug from persons taking 500 to 700 mg daily results in an abstinence syndrome marked by irritability, abdominal cramps, nausea, vomiting, hyperthermia, lacrimation, and drug-seeking behavior. When pentazocine is administered to opiate-dependent patients, its antagonistic actions may precipitate withdrawal symptoms.

Subsequent to the termination of abstinence symptoms or after a course of detoxification with decreasing doses of opiates, most addicts experience recurrent urges for narcotics and generally resume their use of these drugs. The traditional psychologic theory of relapse presumes that, after withdrawal, the physiologic causes of drug taking have been removed, but that addicts have an "addictive personality" disorder that causes them to return to opiate addiction to escape reality. Psychologic factors play a role, although no predictive test has been developed to distinguish future addicts from future nonaddicts; nor are addicts able to be distinguished from nonaddicts by psychologic evaluation when they are observed under the same abstinent conditions. Evidence is accumulating that metabolic and neurophysiologic changes persist long after the detoxification process is completed, as does some tolerance. Protracted abstinence signs, as indicated by alterations in blood pressure, pulse rate, body temperature, respiratory rate, and pupillary size, and symptoms, including the depression and anxiety, have been documented for up to 30 weeks, and may relate to the chronic drug craving reported and the high incidence of relapse. The conditioned associations abstinent ex-addicts experience when they are exposed to their old neighborhoods and friends are also involved in the persistence of drug craving.

Narcotic addiction with its implicit relapses after periods of abstinence should be viewed as a disease of complex etiology in which *a persistent neurochemical disturbance*, as well as profound psychologic and social factors, contributes to the dominance of drug-seeking behavior.

MECHANISM OF OPIATE ACTION. The recent discovery of structurally and sterically specific receptors for the opiates in brain, spinal cord, and other nervous tissue in all vertebrates studied, including man, may shed light on the mode of action of the opiates and on the dependence-withdrawal cycle. These receptors seem to be localized in the areas of the nervous system associated with the integration of sensory information and emotion, particularly the limbic system. The presence of these receptors in species that have little or no contact with opiates led to the discovery of naturally occurring morphine-like peptides in the brain and gastrointestinal tract (enkephalins) and pituitary gland (endorphins) of many animal species. These endogenous morphine-like compounds elicit analgesia, produce tolerance and physical dependence, and compete with radioactive opiates for the receptor. It is of considerable interest that all the peptides so far identified except one have amino acid sequences present in the pituitary hormone, β-lipotropin. The function of these substances is not clear, but certain of them may be neurotransmitters and implicated in the control of pain, affective states, and appetitive drives. A model that includes a neurohumoral feedback mechanism has been postulated to play a part in the opiate addiction syndrome. If, under resting conditions, opiate receptors are exposed to a basal level of the morphine-like substances, when exogenous opiate is administered, the overloading of the opiate receptors might suppress the release of endogenous opioid. Termination of the exogenous opiate administration might produce a deficiency of the endogenous opioid at the receptor, which could be implicated in the immediate or protracted abstinence syndrome.

MEDICAL COMPLICATIONS. When a known dose of an opiate is administered under aseptic conditions, either occasionally or chronically, medical complications are almost unkown. There are well-documented cases of long-term opiate addiction in physicians and others in whom no adverse physical effects were found. The patterns of use, including life style, unknown and markedly variable opiate dose, lack of hygienic administration techniques, and the variety of adulterants used to dilute the opiate, are responsible for the extensive morbidity and mortality (estimated to be about 1 per cent per year) associated with opiate abuse and dependence.

Acute heroin reactions secondary to intravenous use of street drug are responsible for one half to three quarters of all fatalities from narcotics. Formerly thought of as true pharmacologic overdoses with respiratory depression, these reactions may also be due to opiate-induced cardiac arrhythmias or hypoxia by unexplained mechanisms. Acute reactions to adulterants, including quinine, allergic reactions, and synergistic effects from multiple-drug use, may also be implicated. The syndrome is marked clinically by the rapid development of cyanosis, pulmonary edema, respiratory distress, and varying levels of consciousness progressing to coma. Increased intracranial pressure and occasionally convulsive seizures are seen. Fever to 40° C may occur initially and may persist for 48 hours in association with leukocytosis. The pupils are usually pinpoint, although dilated, nonreactive pupils may occur in the presence of hypoxia or multiple-drug use. The pathologic picture includes pulmonary congestion and edema and frequently cerebral edema.

Skin abscesses, cellulitis, and *thrombophlebitis* are the most frequent complications of heroin addiction. Skin manifestations are particularly noted after the subcutaneous injection of heroin and its adulterants. Pentazocine injection causes characteristic chronic ulcers in areas of severe "woody" induration. *Septicemia* and *acute* and *subacute bacterial endocarditis* with involvement of either or both sides of the heart are seen. *Staphylococcus aureus* is frequently the causative organism in right-sided lesions. Peripheral and pulmonary embolic phenomena occur. Osteomyelitis occurs infrequently. Malaria was a frequent complication in the 1930's. The introduction of quinine as an adulterant and the eradication of malaria in this country have decreased the incidence of this complication.

Viral hepatitis transmitted by the communal use of contaminated needles is a frequent complication of intravenous drug use. Abnormal liver function tests, hypergammaglobulinemia, and increased serum immunoglobulins that persist for long periods of time after the acute episodes and that occur in addicts with no history of hepatitis are due in some cases to variants of chronic hepatitis, but may also be due to effects produced by alcohol, malnutrition, allergic phenomena, adulterants, and recurrent or chronic infections. False-positive serologic tests for syphilis are due to these factors, although there is a high incidence of syphilis and other venereal diseases in this population. The nephrotic syndrome has been seen in association with street heroin use as well.

Pulmonary complications include pneumonia, abscess, infarction, and tuberculosis. Disseminated extrapulmonary tuberculosis has been reported. Angiothrombotic pulmonary hypertension and granulomatosis result from the intravenous injection of foreign bodies, including talc or cotton. Vascular lesions include local arterial occlusion, phlebitis, mycotic aneurysms, and necrotizing angiitis.

Neurologic complications of street heroin use include transverse myelitis, peripheral nerve lesions, toxic amblyopia secondary to quinine, and muscle disorders, including acute rhabdomyolysis with myoglobinuria and a fibrosing chronic myopathy. Septic states may lead to bacterial meningitis and brain, subdural, and epidural abscesses. In this country, narcotism is a leading cause of tetanus, particularly when the drugs are injected by the intramuscular route. The course is generally more severe relative to a non-drug-using population, with mortality rates in the 50 to 75 per cent range.

Menstrual irregularities in addicted women have been described, although it is unknown whether these can be ascribed to narcotic-induced suppression of adrenocorticotropic hormone and gonadotropic release or to malnutrition, frequent infections, and the general life style of female addicts. There is a high incidence of toxemia and of prematurity in infants born to addicted mothers, probably because of these life-style factors and the lack of prenatal care. Withdrawal symptoms are noted in a variable percentage of these newborn. Sexual difficulties, including decreased libido, impotence, and delayed ejaculation, are frequent in male heroin addicts, although the etiology is unclear.

Homicide, suicide, and *accidents* account for between 20 and 40 per cent of all narcotic-related deaths. It is often difficult to distinguish these.

TREATMENT. Methods of treatment of narcotic dependence vary considerably, depending on the treatment goals, the factors that are thought to be most significant in the etiology of a patient's addiction, and the characteristics of individual patients. The magnitude of the addict's desire to stop using opiates is an important factor in the selection of the appropriate treatment modality as well as in the outcome. These motivational factors are difficult to assess, since, within one or two years after the onset of the addiction, most addicts express the wish to terminate it. Nevertheless, many continue the compulsive use of heroin for many years and suffer repeated treatment failures. Approaches are primarily psychosocial, pharmacologic, or combinations of these. Since addiction has physical, psychologic, and social determinants, treatment is best provided by a well-organized team approach. Individual practitioners should be prepared to make an accurate diagnosis, treat the acute and chronic sequelae of the drug use, and effect the appropriate referral.

WITHDRAWAL TECHNIQUES. Withdrawal of narcotics is most effectively accomplished by inpatient or outpatient substitution of oral methadone for any of the natural or synthetic narcotic analgesics (detoxification). Doses ranging from 20 to 40 mg daily are instituted, followed by a gradual reduction of dosage over the course of 10 to 14 days or more. Detoxification with decreasing doses of propoxyphene napsylate, a mild analgesic, has been effective, particularly when the degree of dependence is minimal or methadone is not available. In some cases, patients are withdrawn in a drug-free environment without opiate substitution, although this has proved less justifiable on medical and moral grounds. The chronic nature of this disease necessitates the provision of psychologic, legal, and vocational supportive services throughout the detoxification process and continuing into the drug-free period.

METHADONE MAINTENANCE

In this country, methadone maintenance has been the most widely used approach in the treatment of opiate dependence. This mode of therapy emphasizes social and emotional rehabilitation rather than abstinence. The treatment is based on the two major properties that distinguish methadone from other narcotics: good oral efficacy and long duration of action. After oral ingestion in tolerant individuals, the duration of action of methadone is extended to 24 to 36 hours owing to a reservoir of drug in tissues. Initially, oral methadone is administered daily in doses that will allay symptoms of abstinence. The dose is gradually increased until a stabilization level is reached at which patients will be tolerant to the euphoric effects of the drug and will experience no persistent craving for opiates. If the stabilization level is high enough (80 to 100 mg), there is a good degree of cross-tolerance to the effects of other narcotics, such that the effects of even large doses of intravenous opiates will not be felt ("narcotic blockade"). Approximately 65 per cent of patients in well-run programs remain in treatment. Improvement has been noted in the work and school records of patients retained in the program, and their criminal activity has declined markedly. Long-term methadone maintenance has been shown to be medically safe, with no toxicity when properly administered. Side effects include increased sweating, constipation, and some impairment of sexual function. Performance and learning are normal in methadone-maintained subjects. Medication should be dispensed in a clinic situation that provides medical care and extensive rehabilitative services so as to facilitate satisfactory re-entry into non-drug-dominated ("straight") society.

The effort to treat large numbers of people with limited budgets and space has produced overcrowded treatment programs that provide few ancillary services. A significant percentage of patients, although they may be heroin free, are unable to acquire the necessary skills and education to alter their life styles and continue to compulsively abuse alcohol and other drugs. Illicit diversion of methadone doses by clinic patients has led to the availability of the drug for the street-addict population.

Programs using methadone maintenance for varying periods of time followed by a slow-detoxification process are being evaluated, although the majority of adult patients with long-term addiction histories have been unable to remain drug free for extended periods of time. Clinical trials are presently under way with levo-alpha acetyl methadol (LAAM), a synthetic congener of methadone that extends opiate effects for 72 hours. Treatment might be rendered more efficiently if certain patients were required to attend clinics only three times weekly to ingest medication, and the risk of narcotic diversion would be minimized.

Various programs that would provide heroin under supervision are also being considered (heroin maintenance). The short-acting nature of the drug, the rapid development of tolerance, and the necessity to inject it render this form of treatment less potentially useful.

NARCOTIC ANTAGONISTS

Narcotic antagonists such as cyclazocine and naltrexone are being evaluated for the treatment of detoxified addicts. These agents block or attenuate the euphoriant effects of narcotics and prevent the development of physical dependence in patients who continue to use narcotics. Drug-seeking behavior might be extinguished insofar as it depends on conditioned associations to euphoric drug effects or abstinence symptoms. Prevention of the development of physical dependence might also minimize the continuation of narcotic use after a spree, and increase periods of abstinence. These drugs do not relieve the chronic opiate-drug hunger, and patients are prone to omit their dose of antagonist and relapse to heroin. A major advance would be the discovery of a medicine that relieves all symptoms of physical dependence, blocks the opiate-induced euphoria, does not itself produce physical dependence, and is not subject to abuse.

PSYCHOSOCIAL APPROACHES — ABSTINENCE PROGRAMS

A diverse array of programs exist that emphasize abstinence from opiates and other drugs as a primary component of treatment. These take the form of either voluntary groups or supervised institutionalization.

Voluntary groups are generally communities that are self-regulatory in nature and staffed predominantly by former drug users. The individual remains in the closed, drug-free environment for variable periods of time, frequently one to two years, and is encouraged to develop a new set of social and living skills that will enable him to remain drug free upon completion of the program. Outpatient programs are also under way. Intensive therapeutic techniques are utilized to eliminate the social and personality deficiencies of residents that led them to drug use. These facilities serve to reduce the sense of isolation felt by many drug users and attempt to provide role models for responsible behavior. Some of the well-known groups are Synanon, Daytop Village, and Phoenix House. Although sharing many common methods and doctrines, these communities vary considerably in the nature of the therapeutic milieu created and in the complex system of rewards and punishments provided residents. Therapeutic communities are valuable for many people, although only a small percentage of heroin addicts are motivated to enter a community, and follow-up studies of individuals who have returned to society are not presently available.

An alternative approach is programs which involve the nonpunitive incarceration of an addict for the purposes of rehabilitation (civil commitment). These programs generally include a period of enforced abstinence in a prison, hospital, or other locked facility, followed by a careful supervision of the individual in the community. If renewed drug abuse or other antisocial behavior is noted, the addict is reinstitutionalized. To date, these programs have met with meager success. If adequate rehabilitative services and facilities are made available in the future, the efficacy of these programs might be increased.

Results of traditional psychotherapeutic techniques, other than to enhance motivation, have been disappointing for the majority of compulsive opiate abusers. Specialized forms of group psychotherapy may be useful for some patients. After variable and sometimes prolonged periods of addiction, an unknown number of addicts spontaneously cease opiate use. This "maturing-out" process may be related to advanced age and the difficulty of obtaining drugs, a decline of internal psychologic conflicts, and the cumulative effect of various treatment programs.

245. CENTRAL NERVOUS SYSTEM DEPRESSANTS

Robert B. Millman

All central nervous system depressants are subject to abuse. The most frequently abused drugs in this category are the short-acting barbiturates, particularly pentobarbital (Nembutal) and secobarbital (Seconal), assorted other hypnotics such as glutethimide (Doriden), methyprylon (Noludar), and methaqualone (Quāālude), and tranquilizers, particularly diazepam (Valium) and chlordiazepoxide (Librium), and amitriptyline (Elavil), an antidepressant with sedative properties. Bromide abuse has become rare. Since many of the characteristics of these drugs are similar, this discussion will center on the barbiturates, with other agents considered when relevant.

INCIDENCE AND PATTERNS OF ABUSE. There is a continuum of depressant use that extends from appropriate use to compulsive abuse and addiction. Depressants in general and the benzodiazepines in particular have become the most widely prescribed drugs throughout the world. In 1971 alone, in the United States there were 50 million prescriptions for diazepam and 24 million for chlordiazepoxide. The medical indications are quite broad and include insomnia, depressive and anxiety states, convulsive disorders, and alcohol withdrawal. The pattern of use may begin as intermittent use at night to decrease anxiety and ensure sleep, progress to nightly use with increased doses, and culminate in prolonged daily use to maintain an adequate level of function. An individual may obtain drugs from several physicians at one time, none of whom are aware of the magnitude of their patient's depressant use. In this group there may be no illicit drug use, although alcohol is frequently used in association with the depressants.

Hypnotic and tranquilizer use is also present in urban drug subcultures. Heroin addicts use depressants ("downs") to supplement the poor quality of heroin available. Alcoholics will also use hypnotics when they are available, since the quality of the intoxications is similar. Although some people abuse depressants preferentially, concurrent physical dependence on alcohol or opiates is more common than pure depressant dependence in these groups. Illicit sources of drugs are most often employed, and a wealth of street names have evolved for the most popular hypnotics, including "reds" (secobarbital), "yellows" (pentobarbital), and "double trouble" (amobarbital and secobarbital). Most abuse is oral, although some individuals inject their drugs intravenously or intramuscularly. The amounts taken vary markedly, but some individuals have ingested as much as 30 hypnotic doses of the short-acting barbiturates or benzodiazepines daily over many months.

Recently, a marked increase in the use of illicitly obtained depressants has been noted in some adolescent and preadolescent populations. Patterns and extent of use vary markedly, but generally multiple-drug use occurs and is considered appropriate behavior within these groups. Intermittent users may take several times the therapeutic dose, possibly in addition to marijuana, alcohol, and amphetamines if they are available, to get "high" enough to enjoy a concert or party.

The "high" that obtains from abuse of depressant drugs has been characterized as the sense of tranquility or peace that occurs just prior to sleep in normal individuals. The world is seen as limited to the immediate. Inhibitions and anxiety are blunted, and there may be a feeling of aggressiveness, freedom, and pleasant numbness. Sexual pleasure and ability are said to be enhanced at low doses of these drugs; higher doses lead to a decreased ability to perform sexually. Violent and antisocial behavior occurs, frequently serving to isolate depressant abusers ("down heads") from other groups of drug abusers.

There appears to be a high incidence of serious psychopathology in compulsive abusers of the depressant drugs. Users may be seeking obtundation in attempts to cope with anxiety arising from a variety of sources.

PHARMACOLOGY. Barbiturates and related hypnotics are rapidly absorbed after oral administration and are distributed throughout the body. They are general depressants of nerves and of skeletal, smooth, and cardiac muscles, although at low doses the central nervous system is primarily affected. Central nervous system effects vary from mild sedation to coma, depending on the particular drug, the dose, the route of administration, the degree of excitability of the nervous system, and tolerance. In some individuals under certain circumstances, small doses produce an initial stimulation not unlike that produced by alcohol. Barbiturate-induced sleep is similar to physiologic sleep except for a reduction in the proportion of rapid eye movement (REM) sleeping time. Duration of action varies with the particular barbiturate. Aftereffects, including drowsiness, depression, impairment of judgment and performance, and occasionally hyperexcitability, may persist for many hours.

Both drug-disposition and pharmacodynamic tolerance to the barbiturates and related hypnotics develop rapidly with repeated administration. Drug-disposition tolerance in the short-acting barbiturates and some other depressants results from the activation of drug-metabolizing liver-enzyme systems and is characterized by the more rapid degradation of the drug and a decrease in sleeping time. The range of tolerance is narrow, and individuals tolerant to the sedating and intoxicating effects of 1 gram of pentobarbital may become intoxicated for prolonged periods upon the addition of 0.1 gram. Although the lethal dose of barbiturates varies in individuals, in distinction to the opiates, tolerance does not increase this dose significantly from that of nontolerant individuals. Severe poisoning is likely to occur when more than ten times the hypnotic dose is ingested at one time. Acute barbiturate poisoning may thus be superimposed on chronic intoxication at any time. The combination of sublethal doses of depressants with opiates or alcohol may also result in acute poisoning. Cross-tolerance develops to all barbiturates as well as to paraldehyde, meprobamate, and benzodiazepines. Partial cross-tolerance between alcohol and the depressants occurs.

CLINICAL MANIFESTATIONS. Acute depressant poisoning may occur either accidentally or incident to a suicide attempt. Accidental overdoses may be due in some cases to "drug automatism"; an individual may fail to fall asleep after several hypnotic doses, become confused, and ingest an overdose. Upon recovery, there may be no memory of the excessive drug ingestion. The clinical manifestations and treatment of poisoning are discussed in Ch. 251. The acute and chronic signs and symptoms of mild hypnotic intoxication resemble those of intoxication with alcohol. The individual shows general sluggishness, difficulty in thinking, slowness of speech and comprehension, poor memory, faulty judgment, emotional lability, and narrowed attention span. Neurologic signs of depressant intoxication include thick, slurred speech, nystagmus, diplopia, strabismus, vertigo, ataxic gait, positive Romberg sign, hypotonia, dysmetria, and decreased superficial reflexes. Sensation, deep-tendon reflexes, and pupillary responses are unaltered. Skin rashes have been reported. Unexplained seizures in adults should always prompt one to consider chronic depressant drug abuse.

With compulsive users, clothing may be unkempt and nutrition poor; needle marks and abscesses from intramuscular or intravenous use may be present. Adverse effects of chronic depressant use are poorly documented, but may be similar to those of alcohol on organ systems and the brain.

ABSTINENCE SYNDROME. Physical dependence, as indicated by abstinence signs and symptoms, develops to all the central nervous system general depressants. A characteristic *general depressant withdrawal syndrome* occurs and is similar to the symptoms of withdrawal from alcohol. It varies in severity, depending on the drug, dose, and frequency of use. *In contrast to the opiate withdrawal syndrome, that from depressants may be life-threatening.* The first manifestation of this syndrome might be considered the rebound increase in nightly rapid eye movement sleep, associated with nightmares and a sense of having slept badly, that occurs after discontinuation of use of only therapeutic doses of barbiturates for several nights. After a daily dose of 0.4 gram of pentobarbital for three months, abrupt withdrawal produces paroxysmal EEG changes without other significant symptoms. After 0.6 gram per day for one to two months, 50 per cent of patients experience insomnia, tremors, and anorexia. Sudden withdrawal from long-term daily use of only therapeutic doses of the benzodiazepines (45 mg of diazepam per day) will produce abstinence symptoms; withdrawal from higher doses may produce seizures and delirium. In general, the time required to produce physical dependence is shorter with the short-acting barbiturates and the withdrawal symptoms are more abrupt in onset and more severe than with the longer-acting sedatives.

When short-acting hypnotics are abruptly withdrawn, signs and symptoms of the intoxication clear over the initial 12 to 16 hours, and the patient appears to improve. Increases in restlessness, anxiety, tremulousness, and weakness then occur, which may be accompanied by cramps, nausea, vomiting, and orthostatic hypotension. These symptoms progress, and coarse hand tremors, muscle twitching, hyperactive deep reflexes, and increased blink reflex appear within 24 hours. Symptoms generally attain their peak during the second and third days, and convulsions may occur then or before. Some patients who have seizures may begin to show improvement, but 50 per cent develop a delirium that is marked by sensorial clouding, visual and auditory hallucinations, and disorientation to time and place. During the delirium, which usually occurs between the fourth and seventh days, hyperthermia, tachycardia, and agitation can lead to exhaustion and sometimes to fatal cardiovascular collapse. The abstinence syndrome generally clears by about the eighth day, and there is usually no residual physical damage. Clearing is frequently preceded by a period of prolonged sleep. With longer-acting barbiturates and benzodiazepines, seizures may not occur until the seventh or eighth day. Psychotic symptoms may persist for many months, but these may be related to pre-existing psychopathology.

TREATMENT. Treatment procedures include withdrawal and rehabilitative phases. Compulsive abusers of depressants are often considered more difficult to treat than any other class of drug abusers. Outreach and educational programs aimed at intermittent abusers of depressants before they become addicted may be important in this regard. The pattern of use and extent of physical dependence should be evaluated by means of a careful history and physical examination. Depressant abusers frequently distort or are unaware of the magnitude of their use, particularly those with a concurrent addiction to heroin.

If physical dependence is suspected, close observation or hospitalization is indicated. When the diagnosis is established, a suitable general depressant should be administered after the intoxication clears but before major withdrawal symptoms have begun. Phenobarbital orally is a suitable substitute for most of the general depressants. Its long duration of action provides for more constant blood levels and added protection against the development of either withdrawal symptoms or dangerous intoxication. Other barbiturates or benzodiazepines may be used as well if the pharmacology of both the drug of abuse and the withdrawal regimen are known. Patients who are taking large amounts of lesser known sedatives should probably be withdrawn from the original drug of abuse if it is known. If the patient will not tolerate the oral administration of phenobarbital or more rapid sedation is required, intramuscular injections of the same doses may be used. Patients may usually be switched to oral drugs after a few intramuscular injections. Sufficient phenobarbital should be given to produce a mild but manageable level of intoxication marked by inconstant slow nystagmus on lateral gaze, slight dysarthria, and ataxia. A rough approx-imation of the dosage of phenobarbital to be given daily is calculated by substituting 30 mg of phenobarbital for each 100 mg of the short-acting barbiturate the patient reports using. Most patients will require between 100 and 300 mg daily for stabilization, to be given in four divided doses; a total of 600 mg daily should not be exceeded. This "stabilization dose" should be carefully controlled to prevent signs of increased intoxication, such as dysarthria, emotional lability, constant nystagmus, or gross ataxia. Patients should be maintained on this dose for 24 to 48 hours, after which the dose of phenobarbital should be reduced by 30 mg or less daily. The patient should be observed carefully for signs of insomnia, tremulousness, and orthostatic hypotension, at which time the withdrawal should be suspended for one to two days. If symptoms are severe, the patient should be given 100 mg of phenobarbital intramuscularly immediately, which will usually suppress them. Delirium, convulsions, or fever should be treated as emergencies with increased doses until the patient is able to sleep for 8 to 12 hours, after which the stabilization dose is determined, as described above. Once a withdrawal delirium develops, increased doses of phenobarbital may fail to restore equilibrium; agitation and disorientation may persist for several days.

Fluid and electrolyte losses must be replaced, and complicating medical and surgical conditions treated. Increasing fever without evidence of infection necessitates additional sedation, antipyretics, sponging, or cooling blankets. Phenothiazines, butyrophenones, and diphenylhydantoin are not indicated. In general, the use of the phenobarbital substitution technique may take from ten days to three weeks. It should not be hurried. During the process, patients should be encouraged to be as active as possible, eating regularly and taking part in group activities. Patients who are concurrently dependent on opiates should be withdrawn from the general depressant first, while being maintained on suitable doses of methadone. Opiate withdrawal procedures may then be effected.

After withdrawal is completed, provision must be made for high-frequency supportive counseling. Patients are frequently withdrawn and depressed, and the danger of relapse or suicide is great. The inclusion of patients in therapeutic programs, either on an inpatient or on an ambulatory basis, should be assured.

Physicians must be cautious when prescribing depressants for the relief of anxiety and insomnia. Attempts should be made to diagnose and treat the source of these symptoms without medication. If necessary, benzodiazepine tranquilizers may be used in low doses for well-defined, short periods or on an intermittent basis.

BROMIDES. Chronic bromide intoxication (bromism) has become rare, because bromide has been supplanted in modern medicine with more effective and less toxic sedative and analgesic compounds. The daily ingestion of small doses will result in an accumulation of this long-acting drug to toxic levels over a period of weeks. Central nervous system symptoms and signs are the most common features and include drowsiness, impaired thought and memory, dizziness, and irritability, leading in more severe cases to delirium, hallucinations, lethargy, and coma. Neurologic disturbances include tremors, thick speech, motor incoordination, and decreased superficial reflexes. The diagnosis of chronic bromide intoxication is established by serum bromide levels above 9 mEq per liter in association with the aforementioned clinical picture.

Treatment consists of the daily administration of 200 mEq of either sodium or ammonium choride, together with sufficient fluids to ensure a large urine output. This reduces the half-life of bromide to three or four days. Diuresis with chloruretic drugs may be useful if more rapid displacement of bromide is indicated. Hemodialysis rapidly clears bromides and may be indicated in treating comatose patients.

246. CENTRAL NERVOUS SYSTEM STIMULANTS

Robert B. Millman

Central nervous system stimulants or sympathomimetics that are subject to abuse include the *amphetamines, cocaine, methylphenidate* (Ritalin), *phenmetrazine* (Preludin), and *diethylpropion* (Tepanil). This discussion will consider the amphetamine group primarily, including amphetamine, dextroamphetamine, and methamphetamine, which are synthetic derivatives of ephedrine, and cocaine, an alkaloid of the coca plant which grows in the Andes in South America.

INCIDENCE AND PATTERNS OF ABUSE. *Amphetamine abuse* has been widespread in industrial societies, particularly in Japan, Sweden, Great Britain, and North America. Enormous quantities were prescribed by physicians for the treatment of a variety of conditions, including obesity, depressive syndromes, behavior disorders, narcolepsy, and the reduction of fatigue. Many patients, frequently middle-class women, became dependent on these drugs when they found that they had to continue to ingest the drug to prevent depression and to perform optimally. The advent of tolerance necessitated increased doses, occasionally five to ten times the original 5- or 10-mg amount prescribed. Amphetamine abuse by students, athletes, truck drivers, and others who want to increase their efficiency or productivity is common. In both these patterns, oral preparations are used. Hypnotics are often used by this group to ensure sleep, and concurrent dependence on both classes of drugs is not unusual. A decline in use and abuse has occurred recently as a result of federal and state regulations that severely limit prescribing and manufacturing practices with respect to the amphetamines.

Another category of amphetamine abuser is composed of multidrug users, primarily young, who use these drugs for their mood-elevating properties. Any amphetamine may be used, although methamphetamine ("speed," "crystal," or "meth") is preferred, because it has more pronounced central effects and less peripheral ones. The drugs are taken orally on occasion, although "sniffing" or intravenous use is common in drug-dominated groups. Most methamphetamine is manufactured in illegal laboratories, but commercially available oral preparations are also dissolved for intravenous use.

Upon "sniffing," or particularly after intravenous use, the user experiences a "flash" or "rush" that is described as a sense of increased mental capacity and physical strength, with little need for food or sleep, and a feeling of power and intensity that is quite distinct from the feeling of satiation induced by the opiates. Increased activity, planning, and talking occur. Dissipation of the drug effects after three to six hours is experienced as an unpleasant sense of fatigue and depression ("crashing"). Use may be intermittent and limited to special occasions such as a party or journey, or may be more regular. Rarely, chronic amphetamine abusers report that the daily, controlled use of these drugs decreases the anxiety and tension they experience normally, and enhances their ability to eat, sleep, and generally function.

Some individuals use the drug continuously, to maintain the "high" or stave off the "crash" for several days or even longer (a "run"). As tolerance develops, the dose is increased and the drug taken more frequently, such that 1 gram may be injected every two to four hours. At this stage, the compulsive user, or "speed freak," is usually nervous, irritable, and suspicious. There may be intense involvement in complicated and often unnecessary tasks such as disassembling a television set or reorganizing a room. When the supply of drug is depleted or the user becomes too disorganized or debilitated to continue, the "run" ends. Cessation of amphetamine use is usually followed by a prolonged deep sleep. Hypnotics or alcohol are often used to minimize the duration of the "crashing" phase and facilitate the induction of sleep. Upon awakening, although much of the paranoid ideation may be gone, a feeling of lassitude, apathy, and depression may be present. Intravenous users frequently inject other drugs alone or in combination with amphetamines. The combination of amphetamines or cocaine and heroin is known as a "speed ball."

Most of the psychoactive effects of *cocaine* are similar to those of the amphetamines with regard to elevation of mood, decreased need for food or sleep, and hyperactivity. Supply is always through illicit channels; it is more expensive than the amphetamines, with a variable "gram" costing between $60 and $100, and it is much shorter acting. After intravenous administration, the primary mode in this country until recently, effects last 5 to 15 minutes. Intravenous use is generally seen in the same population that abuses heroin. Psychologic dependence and compulsive use occur, such that during a "run" of varying druation, 1 to 10 grams may be used during the course of a day via injections every half hour. In contrast to the amphetamines, there has been a recent marked increase in cocaine abuse in all sectors, particularly by affluent and middle-class people in urban areas. Use in this group, by sniffing the much-adulterated white powder, is generally intermittent; it is regarded as luxurious punctuation for a variety of occasions, to be used in conjunction with alcohol, hypnotics, and marijuana.

PHARMACOLOGY. Systemic effects of amphetamines and cocaine include increased cardiac contraction, increased blood pressure and heart rate, relaxation of the bronchial musculature, increased contractility of the urinary bladder sphincter, increased venous pressure, pulmonary arterial pressure, and renal blood flow. Central effects include stimulation of the cerebrospinal axis and the medullary respiratory center. In low doses these drugs increase alertness and physical and cognitive ability, particularly when performance has been compromised by lack of sleep. The significant appetite depression seen is probably due to a combination of factors, including an inhibitory effect on the feeding center in the lateral hypothalamus as well as the improvement in mood that occurs. Cocaine is an effective topical local anesthetic and vasoconstrictor of mucous membranes.

Tolerance develops to both the peripheral and central effects of the amphetamines. Tolerance to cocaine is not thought to occur; there may be some degree of psychologic tolerance to the euphoric effects of this drug, although it apparently dissipates rapidly. Cross-tolerance exists between the amphetamines, but no cross-tolerance has been demonstrated between the amphetamines and cocaine.

Cessation of amphetamine or cocaine use does not generally produce major physiologic symptoms. The depression, anxiety, increased appetite, lassitude, and prolonged sleep that ensue might be considered an abstinence syndrome and evidence of some physical dependence. Moreover, during this sleep, a characteristic electroencephalographic pattern is produced that shows a marked increase in the percentage of REM sleep, and nightmares may occur. In some cases, withdrawal has been marked by headaches, profuse sweating, muscle cramps, disorientation, and confusion.

ADVERSE EFFECTS. Adverse physical effects in intermittent users of amphetamines or cocaine by the sniffing route may be limited to irritation of the nasal mucosa or perforation of the nasal septum. Chronic users may be markedly debilitated and subject to numerous infections as a result of lack of sleep and poor nutrition. A sensation of something crawling under the skin is described ("cocaine bugs"), such that chronic users will frequently have excoriations and open sores from constant scratching and pinching. The intravenous use of these drugs is fraught with the numerous complications that result from nonsterile conditions, which are detailed in Ch. 244. Reports of necrotizing angiitis and moderate-to-severe occlusion of cerebral vessels resulting from the direct toxic effect of chronic methamphetamine use require further clarification, but may be implicated in brain damage and cerebrovascular accidents in youthful populations. *Acute amphetamine toxicity* is marked by extensions of the sympathomimetic effects, including tachycardia, hypertension, and arrhythmias culminating in convulsions, cerebrovascular accidents, and coma. *Acute cocaine toxicity* is characterized by initial sympathomimetic effects followed by cortical depression and anesthetization of the midbrain and medulla, leading to respiratory failure and cardiovascular collapse. The incidence of sudden fatalities due to amphetamines or cocaine is unknown. The lethal dosage of amphetamines is variable, depending on the extent of tolerance; that of cocaine is estimated to be about 1.2 grams.

There is a high incidence of pre-existing psychopathology in compulsive amphetamine and cocaine abusers, and the abuse itself engenders severe psychologic complications. The most frequent complications of amphetamine and cocaine abuse are paranoid ideation and stereotyped compulsive behavior. Chronic users are frequently aware of these characteristics of the drugs and will not act on ideas of persecution. Antisocial or violent behavior may occur when this insight is lacking. Continued use frequently leads to a well described *amphetamine or cocaine psychosis* that is often indistinguishable from acute paranoid schizophrenia. These reactions appear to be inevitable if the dose and frequency of use of amphetamines and cocaine are continually increased or high doses maintained. Psychotic episodes have also been precipitated in some individuals after only one small dose. The syndrome is marked by paranoid ideation; stereotyped compulsive behavior; visual, auditory, and tactile hallucinations; and loosening of associations occurring in a setting of clear consciousness and correct orientation. The etiology of these disorders may be related to actions of amphetamines and cocaine in inhibiting the re-uptake inactivation of the catecholamines, dopamine, and norepinephrine, thus potentiating their synaptic effects. The psychotic episodes invariably appear while the patients are under the influence of the drug, and generally abate within a few days to several weeks after cessation of drug use. Prolonged psychotic episodes occur and may relate to the premorbid personality of the user.

TREATMENT. Amphetamine and cocaine abusers are a heterogeneous group who demonstrate markedly diverse patterns of drug use. Accordingly, treatment must be flexible. Treatment of the acute and chronic physical complications of abuse are considered in the appropriate chapters of this textbook. Treatment of sympathomimetic stimulation may be accomplished with diazepam or other depressant drug. Withdrawal from these drugs requires a safe, supportive atmosphere, much reassurance, and benzodiazepines when necessary for extreme anxiety. Detoxification with decreasing doses of the sympathomimetics is not generally indicated. Treatment of paranoid ideation or the overt psychotic episodes may necessitate short-term hospitalization. Phenothiazines or other major tranquilizers may be necessary for prolonged psychotic reactions.

After recovery, depressive symptoms should be sought and the possibility of suicide must be considered. The compulsive abuser may require long-term supportive care under close supervision, with provision for psychiatric and social rehabilitation.

Physicians would do well to prescribe amphetamines and related drugs with great caution. Some authorities suggest that the childhood hyperkinetic disorders and narcolepsy are the only indications for their use.

247. CANNABIS
(Marijuana and Hashish)
Robert B. Millman

Marijuana and hashish are derived from *Cannabis sativa*, the hemp plant, an herbaceous annual which grows readily in many parts of the world and reaches maturation in four to five months. All parts of both the male and female plants contain varying amounts of the major psychoactive principle, delta-9-tetra hydrocannibinol; its active isomer, delta-8-THC; and numerous other cannabinoids. The concentration of delta-9-THC in the flowering tops of these plants is a function of genetic and environmental factors and varies from less than 0.2 per cent in the fiber-type plants to more than 4 per cent in those plants grown for drug content. In the United States, *marijuana* refers to the dried mixture of crushed leaves and flowering tops with or without the inclusion of stems and seeds. The flowering tops of the plants secrete a clear, varnish-like resin, which when collected and compressed is called *hashish* and is thought to be four to eight times more potent than marijuana. Cannabis or its products are also called *kif*, *bhang*, *ganga*, *charas*, and *dagga* in various parts of the world.

INCIDENCE AND PATTERNS OF ABUSE. Cannabis has been used extensively in many societies since antiquity as a form of folk medicine, as a work adjunct, in association with religious practices, and for recreational purposes. The prevalence of cannabis use increased explosively in the United States and Western Europe during the past 20 years, in association with the changing styles of youth culture. Several recent surveys suggest that use continues to increase and that the number of people in the United States who have ever used cannabis is 36 million. Users fall heavily into the teenage and young adult group; more than 50 per cent of people from 18 to 25 are estimated to have used the drug. Increased use is being noted in older age groups as well. Whereas geographic, social, and cultural considerations are determinants of whether a person will use cannabis, personality characteristics are important in determining the frequency and pattern of use. Many people experiment with the drug and do not continue its use; over half are estimated to use the drug one or more times per month; about one in four who use it that often do so three times or more a week. The present trend toward the reduction or elimination of legal sanctions against cannabis possession and use may further broaden the demographic base of users and increase prevalence.

The drug is peripheral to the life of the occasional user, and frequently there is no other drug use. Others demonstrate a compulsive abuse pattern, in which their lives are dominated by the acquisition and use of cannabis and other drugs. Occasional users generally smoke in groups, where the ritual of preparation and sharing of the cigarette is an integral part of social interaction. Chronic smokers will also frequently smoke alone.

Marijuana is usually smoked in homemade cigarettes ("joints"). Hashish is smoked in a wide variety of small pipes. Both preparations may be ingested in combination with food or drink, although this is less common. The weight of a marijuana cigarette on the street may vary from 0.5 to 1 gram. The delta-9-THC content may vary from less than 1 per cent in domestic material to much more in imported varieties.

PHARMACOLOGY. Cannabis preparations are three to four times more potent when smoked than when taken orally. After inhalation, effects begin within minutes, peak within one hour, and are dissipated within three hours. After ingestion, effects begin in 30 minutes to two hours, peak at three hours, and persist for four to six hours. The effects of cannabis correlate with the appearance in plasma of active polar metabolites of delta-9-THC. Kinetic interactions have been described between several of the cannabinoids in marijuana, suggesting that, in accordance with popular belief, the pharmacologic and psychoactive effects of different strains may vary apart from the differences in delta-9-THC content.

The acute physiologic effects of cannabis are dose related and include an increase in heart rate, conjunctival vascular congestion, decreased intraocular pressure, bronchodilatation, increased airway conductance, and peripheral vasodilatation. Dryness of mouth and throat, fine tremors of fingers, ataxia, nystagmus, nausea, and vomiting have been noted. Orthostatic hypotension and loss of consciousness occur infrequently. Sleep patterns may be altered.

Psychoactive effects are highly variable and depend on the dose, the route of administration, the personality of the user, his prior experience with the drug, his personal expectations, and the environmental and social setting in which the drug is used. Enhanced perception of colors, sounds, patterns, textures, and taste is common. Mood changes are complex; a sense of increased well-being is frequently experienced, although anxiety and depression may be increased by the drug as well. Drowsiness or hyperactivity and hilarity may occur. Ideas may seem disconnected, rapid flowing, and associated with altered importance. Time seems to pass slowly, and short-term memory may be impaired. Motor performance is variably impaired, as is reaction time. Although attention can be maintained in certain situations, it is probable that alterations in attention are responsible for some of the reported decrements in performance and cognitive function. *Driving performance is significantly impaired by marijuana intoxication.*

Inexperienced users of cannabis report fewer subjective effects, but demonstrate more decrement in perceptual and psychomotor performance than experienced users. A learning process may be involved in the initial perception of psychoactive effects, although enzymatic induction with more rapid conversion of delta-9-THC to active metabolites is also possible. A varying degree of tolerance develops to some of the psychologic and

physiologic effects of the drug. Physical dependence on cannabis does not occur in man.

ADVERSE EFFECTS. There are no documented reports of human fatalities caused by an overdose of cannabis in any form. Decreased pulmonary function has been reported in chronic users, with an increased incidence of bronchitis, sinusitis, and nose and throat inflammations. The reported in vitro reduction in thymus-dependent lymphocytes and inhibition of DNA, RNA, and protein synthesis require clarification. Reduced testosterone levels and altered cellular characteristics of sperm in chronic cannabis users have been reported, but the functional significance of these findings is unclear.

Adverse reactions are generally psychologic in nature, infrequent, and dependent on dose, the personality of the user, and the setting. The most common adverse effects are simple depression, acute panic reactions, and paranoid ideation. These symptoms usually abate in several hours. An acute toxic psychosis, transient in nature, with confusion, disorientation, and auditory and visual hallucinations, occurs infrequently and is thought to be related to high doses of the drug. There is disagreement as to whether cannabis may precipitate a psychotic episode in a stable, well-structured personality. It is agreed that the drug may trigger a prolonged psychotic episode in people with borderline psychologic adjustments. Larger doses are associated with an increase in these reactions, though in a nonlinear way. "Flashback" phenomena similar to those seen with psychedelic use occur rarely.

There is no evidence that the chronic heavy use of marijuana causes diminished goal-directed activity, apathy, inability to master new problems, or poor social and work adjustment ("amotivational syndrome"), although it is possible that the drug may inhibit the output of workers who have complex tasks or for whom mental operations usually predominate. There is no evidence that cannabis use leads to criminal activity. Socially or psychologically predisposed individuals may experiment with other drugs as a result of positive experience with cannabis.

TREATMENT. Treatment of the frequently seen depressive and panic reactions should be personal, supportive, and reassuring. The patient must be continually reminded of the drug-induced nature of his difficulty. Tranquilizers are sometimes indicated in violent or aggressive states. Psychotherapy and hospitalization may be indicated in more severe or chronic disorders. The chronic use of marijuana may be associated with a subculture that rejects conventional mores and orientation. To be effective, treatment efforts should be sensitive to these value systems.

248. PSYCHEDELICS
Robert B. Millman

The distinguishing characteristics of the psychedelics is their ability to reliably produce distinctive alterations in perception, thought, feeling, and behavior. They are among the oldest known psychoactive drugs, having been used as an adjunct to religious practices in some societies. They are sometimes classified as hallucinogens, psychotogens, or psychotomimetics. In this country, the most frequently abused drugs in this category are related either to the indolealkylamines such as the synthetic *lysergic acid diethylamide (LSD, "acid")*, *psilocybin ("magic mushrooms")*, *psilocin, dimethyltryptamine (DMT)*, and *diethyltryptamine (DET)*, or to the phenylethylamines such as *mescaline*, which is derived from the peyote cactus, and the substituted amphetamines such as 2,5-dimethoxy-4-methylamphetamine *(DOM, "STP")*. Since the pattern of physiologic and psychologic effects produced by other agents is similar to that seen with LSD, this discussion will center on LSD. By virtue of their ability to produce bizarre alterations in behavior, anticholinergic compounds and *phencyclidine* ("angel dust," "PCP") a drug with anesthetic properties, will be considered in this chapter. Their psychoactive effects are distinct from the other psychedelics.

INCIDENCE AND PATTERNS OF ABUSE. LSD became available through illicit channels in 1960, and use apparently peaked in the 1967–1968 period, when the new styles of youth culture and its leaders were being popularized by the mass media. Estimates varied from 500,000 to 1 million users at that time, and have been lower since then.

Use has been primarily among middle-class, white, educated youth in this country who are seeking an enriching, ecstatic, mystical, or transcendental experience. A complex set of metaphysical and religious beliefs and social styles often distinguish the user.

Use is generally intermittent, frequently less than one "trip" monthly, separated by periods in which marijuana is used. Rarely, individuals may take the drug more often ("acid heads"), and some remain in intoxicated states for prolonged periods. Opiate and excessive alcohol use are not often seen in this population, although intermittent amphetamine and hypnotic use are not unusual in the intervening periods. The drug is generally taken in groups so that support is available in the event of a "bad trip." A naive user will frequently be attended by a guide who has previously had the psychedelic experience. As in the case of cannabis, a supportive, safe environment is sought for the experience to minimize the effects of unpleasant reactions.

LSD is generally synthesized in illegal laboratories and made available in a variety of forms, including impregnated paper or sugar cubes, capsules, and tablets. Users are often unaware of the dose they ingest or of whether the preparation is actually LSD or another of the psychedelics.

In contrast to LSD, abuse of illicitly produced phencyclidine has increased recently. It is available in a variety of forms and is used in a fashion similar to the other psychedelics.

PHARMACOLOGY. LSD is the most potent psychedelic known. It is more than 100 times more potent than psilocybin and 4000 times more potent than mescaline in producing psychologic effects. The usual illicit street dose is probably around 200 μg, but doses as low as 20 μg produce psychologic effects in susceptible individuals. It is generally taken orally, although it has been injected on occasion. Central sympathomimetic stimulation occurs within 20 minutes after ingestion, characterized by mydriasis, hyperthermia, tachycardia, elevated blood pressure, piloerection, increased alertness, and facilitation of monosynaptic reflexes. Nausea and occasionally vomiting occur.

Psychoactive effects are fully evident within one to two hours; these are quite variable from subject to subject and in the same subject under different conditions of dose, mood, expectation, setting, and time. Perceptions are heightened and may become overwhelming. Afterimages are prolonged and overlap with ongoing perceptions. Objects may seem to move in a wavelike fashion or melt. Illusions and synesthesias, the overflow of one sense modality to another, are common.

There may be a sense of unusual clarity, and one's thoughts may assume extraordinary importance. Time may seem to pass very slowly, and body distortions are commonly perceived. True hallucinations with loss of insight may occur in susceptible individuals. Mood is highly variable and labile, and may range from expansive reactions characterized by euphoria and self-confidence to a constricted reaction marked by depression and panic.

The syndrome begins to clear after 10 to 12 hours, and fatigue and tension may persist for an additional 24 hours. The duration of action of mescaline is about 12 hours, that of psilocybin is four to six hours, that of DOM is six to eight hours, and that of phencycline is two to four hours. DMT must be injected or sniffed, and effects last less than two hours.

Tolerance to LSD develops rapidly, repeated daily doses becoming ineffective in three to four days. Recovery is equally rapid, so weekly use of the same dose is possible. Cross-tolerance has been demonstrated between LSD, mescaline, psilocybin, and the amphetamine-based psychedelics, but not between LSD and amphetamine. Physical dependence does not occur with LSD or any of the psychedelic drugs.

Mechanisms of action of LSD are unknown, but may depend on a complex interaction of serotonin and norepinephrine systems in the central nervous system. LSD lowers the threshold for reticular arousal via sensory input and may influence the processes concerned with the filtration and integration of sensory information.

ADVERSE EFFECTS. Acute physiologic toxicity of the LSD-related psychedelic drugs is low at doses that produce marked psychologic effects. In man, no deaths directly attributable to the use of these drugs have been reported. Controversy exists as to whether the illicit use of LSD increases the rate of chromosome breakage in users and leads to an increased incidence of congenital defects in children born to parents who had taken this drug. Evidence suggests that pregnant women exposed to illicit LSD had an elevated rate of spontaneous abortions. LSD may inhibit antibody formation and disrupt the body's immune system. Additional study of these adverse effects are necessary because illicit users of LSD frequently take other drugs and may be malnourished and debilitated.

The acute panic reaction ("bad trip," "freak-out") is the most frequent complication of psychedelic use. These vary in intensity and have led to suicide attempts and accidents on rare occasions. Fear of death or insanity and sensations of breathlessness or paralysis are commonly reported. In most cases, this acute reaction subsides as drug effects are dissipated. Other complications include prolonged psychotic disorders, acute and chronic paranoid reactions, and depressive states. "Flashback" phenomena, the recurrence of some aspect of the drug experience when the individual is not under the influence of the drug, have been reported. The intensity, frequency, and duration of these episodes are quite variable. Adverse psychologic reactions are most frequent in emotionally disturbed individuals in crisis situations or insecure environments who take the drug in unsupervised settings. High doses of psychedelic drugs lead to an increased incidence of these complications. Whether the psychedelics cause prolonged adverse reactions in emotionally stable people is not clear.

Acute toxic effects of phencyclidine are frequent, and a

significant number of deaths have been reported. It may produce either depression or stimulation of the central nervous system, depending on the dose and the route of administration. Common features include emotional lability, excited intoxication, nystagmus, elevated blood pressure, and increased deep-tendon reflexes which may progress to a state of extreme muscular rigidity. High doses may lead to arrhythmias, convulsions, and coma. A chronic organic brain dysfunction has been described in phencyclidine abusers, marked by memory gaps, some disorientation, and visual and speech disturbances.

ANTICHOLINERGIC COMPOUNDS. Ingestion of the alkaloids *atropine, hyoscyamine,* and *scopolamine* in their natural plant forms is increasing incident to the ingestion of "herbal teas" or leaves, and several deaths have occurred. Excessive use of *antihistaminic* compounds with anticholinergic effects also occurs. Symptoms of the potent peripheral effects of intoxication with these drugs include dilated, fixed pupils, dry skin and mouth, flushing, hyperthermia, and tachycardia. Psychoactive effects are those of an acute toxic psychosis, with clouding of consciousness, delirium, and loss of memory for the period of intoxication. Vivid sensory phenomena are not prominent, although hallucinations may occur.

TREATMENT. Treatment of the acute panic reaction may usually be accomplished by ensuring a warm, supportive environment with someone in constant attendance and with a minimum of other external stimuli. The user should be reminded continually that the effects he is experiencing are due to the drug and will pass in time. In particularly agitated patients, phenothiazines or diazepam orally or intramuscularly may be used. In the event of precipitation of prolonged psychosis, hospitalization with supportive care may be required. Flashbacks are treated with reassurance and/or psychotherapy when these are severe. In general, the duration and severity of these decrease with time if psychedelic drug use ceases. Treatment of the acute intoxication caused by low doses of phencyclidine is similar to that for the other psychedelics, particularly with respect to reduction of external stimuli and tranquilization. Toxic reactions from higher doses may require hospitalization and intensive supportive care.

Treatment of anticholinergic poisoning is symptomatic and consists of protecting the patient from self-injury, providing fluids, and reducing the fever. Administration of cholinesterase inhibitors and suitable tranquilizers may be indicated, although phenothiazines are contraindicated because of their anticholinergic effects.

249. MISCELLANEOUS INHALANTS

Robert B. Millman

NITROUS OXIDE. Recreational inhalation of nitrous oxide alone or in combination with oxygen is a rarely reported phenomenon that occurs in some youthful populations. Psychoactive effects occur in 15 to 30 seconds and persist for less than five minutes. The experience is described as one of intoxication, euphoria, and hilarity. Adverse effects have not been reported.

ORGANIC SOLVENTS. The inhalation of a wide range of organic solvents, particularly the toluene in glue, has

received a good deal of attention from the mass media and law-enforcement agencies. It is likely that this publicity has contributed significantly to the incidence of this practice in the adolescent and preadolescent population. The material is usually squeezed into a plastic bag and the vapors inhaled. Prolonged exposure, as in the case of industrial workers, may have serious adverse effects on a variety of organ systems. As used recreationally, these solvents produce intoxication and dizziness not unlike that experienced with alcohol. Few side effects have been reported, although suffocation caused by the plastic bag has apparently occurred. A number of deaths have been reported secondary to the inhalation of the anesthetic agent halothane, a halogenated hydrocarbon. The inhalation of aerosol sprays containing fluorocarbon propellants is also occurring. The mechanism of toxicity and death may be the induction of cardiac arrhythmias or upper-airway obstruction and hypoxia.

AMYL NITRITE. Amyl nitrite ("amies," "poppers") inhalation occurs in some youthful drug-abusing populations, notably among homosexual men. A recent phenomenon is the similar use of other volatile nitrites that are marketed as deodorizers or "aromas" under a variety of exotic brand names. Use is intermittent and characterized by an instantaneous feeling ("rush") of flushing, dizziness, hilarity, and activity. Effects persist for minutes. Adverse effects include palpitations, postural hypotension occasionally proceeding to loss of consciousness, and headache. Chronic use is rare, and more severe adverse effects have not been reported.

Brecher, E. M., and the Editors of Consumer Reports: Licit and Illicit Drugs. The Consumers Union Report on Narcotics, Stimulants, Depressants, Inhalants, Hallucinogens, and Marijuana, Including Caffeine, Nicotine and Alcohol. Mount Vernon, N. Y., Consumers Union, 1972.

Dishotsky, N. I., Loughman, W. D., Mogar, R. E., and Lipscomb, W. R.: LSD and genetic damage. Science, 172:431, 1971.

Dole, V. P.: Narcotic addiction, physical dependence and relapse. N. Engl. J. Med., 286:988, 1972.

Dole, V. P., and Nyswander, M.: A medical treatment for diacetylmorphine (heroin) addiction. JAMA, 193:646, 1965.

Grinspoon, L., and Bakalar, J. B.: Cocaine: A Drug and Its Social Evolution. New York, Basic Books, 1976.

Isbell, H., Altschul, S., Kornetsky, C. H., et al.: Chronic barbiturate intoxication. An experimental study. Arch. Neurol. Psychiat., 64:1, 1950.

Jaffe, J.: Narcotic analgesics and drug addiction and drug abuse. *In* Goodman, L. S., and Gilman, A. (eds.): The Pharmacological Basis of Therapeutics. 5th ed. New York, Macmillan, 1975, p. 245.

Kales, A., Bixler, E. O., Tan, T-L., et al.: Chronic hypnotic-drug use: ineffectiveness, drug-withdrawal insomnia, and dependence. JAMA, 227:513, 1974.

Kreek, M. J.: Medical safety and side effects of methadone in tolerant individuals. JAMA, 223:665, 1973.

Peterson, R. C. (ed.): Marijuana Research 1976, NIDA Research Monograph No. 14. U. S. Department of Health, Education, and Welfare, July 1977.

Snyder, S. H.: The opiate receptor and morphine-like peptides in the brain. Am. J. Psychiat., 135:645, 1978.

Stimmel, B.: Heroin Dependency: Medical, Economic and Social Aspects. New York, Stratton Intercontinental Medical Book Corporation, 1975.

250. ALCOHOL ABUSE AND ALCOHOL-RELATED ILLNESS

Jack H. Mendelson

DEFINITION. The most widely accepted operational definition of alcohol abuse is excessive drinking which adversely affects an individual's health, impairs social function, or both. Although it is not difficult to assess the impact of alcohol abuse on biologic function, it is often impossible to quantify alcohol-related social impairment. Experts disagree about both the type and the severity of problem drinking which cause social dysfunction because of wide variations in societal norms for characterizing deviant drinking behavior. Attempts to establish criteria for normative drinking behavior based upon volume and consumption frequency indices have not been satisfactory because of conflicting social, cultural, religious, and even political perceptions of how individuals in various societies may consume alcohol.

The frequently used term "alcoholism" is ambiguous. "Alcoholism" is often not synonymous with alcohol abuse, but denotes a series of problems ranging from deviant drinking behavior (as defined by the society in which it occurs) to alcohol addiction. Some of the phenomena which are reported to occur during the progression of *alcohol abuse* to *alcohol addiction* include excessive drinking in normal social situations; drinking in isolation; drinking to reduce anxiety, apprehension, or anger; drinking to facilitate the induction of sleep during conditions of insomnia; early morning drinking; and alterations in memory function (blackout) during heavy episodic alcohol intake. All or none of these phenomena may be reported by individuals who demonstrate evidence of addiction to alcohol, and no specific pattern of events is pathognomonic of behavior attributes for transition of alcohol abuse to alcohol addiction.

Addiction to alcohol is characterized by both tolerance and physical dependence. Tolerance occurs when an individual consumes progressively larger quantities of alcohol over a period of time in order to induce changes in feeling states or behavior which previously were induced by smaller doses of alcohol. Physical dependence occurs when an individual develops subjective discomfort and/or overt withdrawal signs after partial or complete cessation of drinking. It is important to emphasize that withdrawal signs and symptoms may occur in alcohol addicts when they reduce drinking but do not completely cease all alcohol intake. Relatively small decrements in sustained high blood alcohol levels may be associated with precipitation of the withdrawal syndrome.

As with most behavior disorders, it is often impossible to establish a precise definition of clinical status, e.g., alcohol abuse versus alcohol addiction. The physician must make a judgment about the presence and severity of an alcohol-related problem on the basis of careful determination of physical and mental status, occupational performance, social interaction, and — not least important — the patient's own perception of how alcohol consumption enhances or compromises his or her health and well-being.

ETIOLOGY. No specific biologic, psychologic, or social variable has been shown to have high predictive value for determining which individuals are at high risk to develop and sustain problem drinking behavior. There are no known psychologic tests which can reliably differentiate alcohol abusers from normal drinkers. Many theories have purported to explain the causation of alcoholism in terms of psychodynamic factors, personality profiles, psychosocial developmental and growth characteristics, nutritional idiosyncrasies, allergic disorders, and specific and nonspecific metabolic derangements. To date, none of these theories of the causation of alcohol abuse or alcohol addiction have significant support from well-controlled laboratory and clinical investigations.

The contribution of specific genetic and environmental factors which may enhance the risk for development of alcohol-related problems has not been clarified. Many patients who develop alcohol-related problems have no family history of alcohol abuse or alcohol addiction. But it is also known that individuals with a family history of alcohol abuse, particularly those who report that both parents had alcohol problems, may be at very great risk for developing alcohol abuse themselves. It is likely that this enhanced risk occurs, in part, as a function of growing up in an environment where excessive drinking is employed for coping with or modifying social stress. Moreover, there are recent data which indicate that a genetic component may be associated with the causation of alcohol problems. Studies of adoptees in Denmark have demonstrated that these individuals are more likely to develop alcohol problems if their biologic parents were alcohol abusers than if the adopted parent had abused alcohol. Thus at present it appears reasonable to conclude that both genetic and developmental factors may contribute to the genesis of alcohol-related illness.

INCIDENCE AND PREVALENCE. Surveys of American drinking practices reveal that approximately two thirds of the adult population of the United States use alcohol at least occasionally. It is estimated that about 12 per cent of the American population are heavy drinkers, i.e., individuals who drink almost daily or who once a week consume five or more drinks per occasion. It is obvious that this definition of heavy drinking may be associated with a number of ambiguities, and it is difficult to rate relative degree of drinking (heavy versus light) from self-written reports about the volume and frequency of alcohol consumed. Thus, individuals may consume the same quantity of alcohol during a given interval of time, but variations in the spacing or the concentrating of the drinking may indicate vastly different drinking patterns. For example, alcohol addicts who are spree drinkers may consume enormous amounts of alcohol in a two- or three-day interval during a month and remain relatively abstinent the remainder of the time.

A recent survey of American drinking practices and problems revealed that the largest population of problem drinkers were city-dwellers of low socioeconomic status. The highest rates of alcohol-related problems were found in young (under 25) urban men; the number of heavy drinkers among white and black males was similar (22 and 19 per cent, respectively). However, black women reported a significantly higher rate of drinking (11 per cent) than white women (4 per cent). American Indians and Eskimos have high reported rates of alcohol abuse and addiction.

Repeated surveys have shown that alcohol problems can be found in anyone who drinks alcohol to excess and that individual variations obliterate the significance of any group, ethnic, or cultural qualities. Case finding in alcoholism is difficult because of the stigma associated with the disorder. However, most agree that alcoholism represents the major drug problem in America today. It has been estimated that about 5 million adults in the United States have significant alcohol-related problems. It is also estimated that an additional

4 million abuse alcohol to the extent that they are at high risk for the development of alcohol addiction. These figures imply that 7 per cent of the adult population have a significant alcohol-related problem.

PHARMACOLOGIC ASPECTS. After the consumption of alcohol, absorption occurs primarily from the small intestine, but gastric emptying and the rate of absorption from the intestine are influenced by a number of factors. The rate of absorption is accelerated with increasing concentrations of alcohol up to a maximum of 40 per cent. Concentrations of ingested alcohol above 40 per cent may be absorbed more slowly as a consequence of delayed gastric emptying. Similarly, high concentrations of congeners in beverage alcohol delay absorption because they impede gastric emptying by inducing pyloric spasm. The ingestion of food along with beverage alcohol also reduces the speed of absorption by delaying the emptying time of the stomach.

After absorption, ethanol is distributed to all portions of the body and achieves equilibrium with body water compartments. Blood alcohol levels are dependent upon the total body water concentration. No impermeable or semipermeable membranes impede the diffusion of alcohol into any body organ or tissue.

Alcohol is removed from the body primarily by metabolism in the liver, and only 2 to 10 per cent is excreted directly by the kidneys and the lungs. Alcohol is catabolized in the liver by well-known enzymatic mechanisms involving the enzyme alcohol dehydrogenase and the cofactor NAD. The rate of alcohol metabolism in normal drinkers and in abstinent alcohol addicts is not significantly different. However, the rate of ethanol metabolism may increase in alcohol addicts during the course of spree drinking, and it is believed that this increase is due to an ethanol-induced increase in rate of hepatic metabolism.

There are no known pharmacologic agents which may be utilized in clinical practice to enhance the rate of ethanol catabolism in man. Although it has been shown that high dosage administration of fructose may accelerate rates of ethanol metabolism, the clinical use of this is impractical.

Blood alcohol levels depend upon the amount of alcohol ingested and the weight of the individual. For the average man, it has been estimated that the consumption of 180 ml of distilled spirits on an empty stomach will produce a blood alcohol level of approximately 100 mg per 100 ml. Values around 100 mg per 100 ml have been established by most jurisdictions as the legal limit of sobriety for operating a motor vehicle. Blood alcohol levels achieved in usual social drinking situations average about 50 to 75 mg per 100 ml. At this blood level a subjective state of pleasant tranquility and a mild degree of sedation may occur. Overt signs of intoxication usually occur in social (nontolerant) drinkers between 100 and 200 mg per 100 ml. Severe intoxication is observed in social drinkers at levels above 200 mg per 100 ml, but alcohol addicts who are tolerant to the effects of ethanol may appear relatively intact and nonintoxicated with such blood alcohol levels. Regardless of the degree of tolerance, blood alcohol levels above 400 mg per 100 ml produce stupor and/or coma, and concentrations above 500 mg per 100 ml are frequently fatal.

ALCOHOL AND BEHAVIOR. Acute Intoxication. Although the concomitants of acute intoxication are well known and easily recognized (dysarthria, ataxia, and emotional lability), there is no simple correlation between the volume of alcohol consumed and an individual's ability to carry out cognitive and motor tasks successfully. Indeed, some individuals actually show improved performance on perceptual and psychomotor tasks with low to moderate doses of alcohol. This paradox obtains because small to moderate doses of ethanol may act in a manner similar to a minor tranquilizer, i.e., to reduce anxiety which may affect skill and performance. Individuals who demonstrate little impairment in performance of cognitive and motor tasks with high blood ethanol concentrations (150 to 200 mg per 100 ml) have probably developed tolerance for alcohol as a consequence of recurrent heavy drinking.

Moderate dosage of alcohol usually impairs visual-motor coordination in most social drinkers. In particular, brightness discrimination and visual adaptation after exposure to bright lights are often markedly reduced. Auditory and tactile sensation are usually unchanged. The integration and evaluation of sensory information, rather than the impairment of sensory input itself, are most severely compromised during acute intoxication. An individual's ability to initiate or maintain sustained attention to stimuli and to judge the qualities of stimuli is usually significantly diminished after moderate alcohol intake. Individuals under such conditions tend to underestimate the speed and distance of objects as well as to show impairment in making judgments regarding the passage of time.

Impairments of behavior associated with acute intoxication are also determined by factors related to the setting. If a person consumes alcohol in a situation in which drunkenness is both expected and tolerated, this anticipation may influence his behavior more than the dosage of alcohol ingested. Similarly, individuals who fear the consequences of intoxicated behavior may successfully mask the manifestations of acute inebriation even though they consume relatively large amounts of alcohol.

Alcohol, Aggression, and Accidents. Although it is well known that alcohol ingestion and acute intoxication are significant factors in accidents, the causal relationship is not a simple one. Alcohol intoxication may effect a number of patterns of behavior which combine to produce enhanced risk for an accident. These include compromised judgment, enhanced emotional lability, and inability to suppress expression of aggression. Acute alcohol intoxication also contributes to situations which result in death and injury as a function of violence and aggressive behavior. Homicide, armed robbery with aggravated assault, and other crimes of violence are frequent in perpetrators or victims who are acutely intoxicated.

Acute alcohol intoxication has been frequently implicated in fatal accidents. For example, over half of the nonhighway accident fatalities involve alcohol addicts or abusers. A recent survey carried out in a general hospital emergency room in which blood alcohol values were determined in accident victims showed that 30 per cent of the individuals involved in highway accidents, 22 per cent involved in home accidents, and 16 per cent involved in occupational accidents had elevated blood ethanol levels.

Alcohol abuse is a significant contributing factor to over 50 per cent of motor vehicle fatalities, and it was estimated during a recent 12-month period that 28,000 highway deaths were associated with alcohol intoxication. Increasing evidence suggests, however, that alcohol-related automobile fatalities may not be simply associated with episodic acute intoxication in social drinkers, but rather are phenomena related to chronic intoxication and alcohol addiction. Statistics obtained from studies of blood alcohol levels in individuals involved in single vehicle fatalities indicate that a majority had blood ethanol values above 150 mg per 100 ml. Such high blood levels are more characteristic of alcohol addicts than of social drinkers.

Alcohol and Sexual Function. The effect of acute intoxication on sexual behavior and function is poorly understood. The classic reference is Shakespeare's perception that intoxication increases desire but impairs sexual performance. Although the effects of acute alcohol intoxication on sexual behavior in moderate drinkers may be quite variable, sexual function and behavior are often markedly impaired in alcohol addicts. Male alcohol addicts often report sexual impotence and diminished heterosexual desire. A tendency to initiate or increase alcohol intake has been reported by female alcoholics during premenstrual periods. Gynecomastia and testicular atrophy have been reported in male alcohol addicts, particularly those who also show evidence of alcohol-related liver disease. Recent studies have demonstrated that alcohol administration to alcohol addicts is associated with suppression of plasma testosterone levels. Alcohol also suppresses plasma testosterone levels in normal males when blood ethanol levels are between 50 and 100 mg per 100 ml. Alcohol-induced suppression of testosterone is probably due to inhibition of testosterone biosynthesis in the testes. There is also evidence that chronic alcohol intake induces enzymes which enhance the rate of testosterone biotransformation in the liver.

The "Hangover." A well-known consequence of acute alcohol intoxication is a syndrome of generalized somatic discomfort, headache, nausea, agitation, and mild tremulousness which has been termed the "hangover." The physiologic mechanisms related to the hangover have not been determined. Current evidence indicates that the hangover may be the equivalent of a mild withdrawal syndrome. There is no evidence that any specific characteristic of beverage alcohol, such as its congener content, or any unique pattern of drinking, such as mixing different beverages, is the causal basis for the hangover. No specific form of pharmacotherapy is available for treatment of the problem, and there is little evidence that the plethora of popular remedies have any efficacy.

ADDICTION TO ALCOHOL. Addiction to alcohol is characterized by the presence of both tolerance and physical dependence. Although many individuals may frequently abuse alcohol, not all become physically dependent. Moreover, it is difficult to predict addiction liability on the basis of dosage of alcohol and frequency of consumption alone. There is no question, however, that physical dependence on alcohol is analogous to physical dependence induced by a number of other centrally acting drugs and is not caused by intercurrent illness or by vitamin or nutritional disorders. Withdrawal signs and symptoms have been observed in otherwise healthy alcohol addicts exclusively as a concomitant of cessation of drinking. Physical dependence has also been induced in a number of species of laboratory animals without producing derangements in nutritional or metabolic function.

Tolerance appears to develop more rapidly than physical dependence for alcohol and other drugs which affect the central nervous system (i.e., narcotics, barbiturates, and psychotropic drugs). Three forms of tolerance may be observed in the alcohol addict: behavioral tolerance, pharmacologic tolerance, and cross-tolerance to certain other drugs which have their primary effect on central nervous function.

Behavioral tolerance is manifest when the alcohol addict can consume relatively large amounts of ethanol without impairment in social behavior or psychomotor coordination. It has been observed clinically and demonstrated in research ward studies that some alcohol addicts can consume as much as 1 quart of beverage alcohol per day without evidence of gross intoxication. It has also been shown that many alcohol addicts can perform relatively complex tasks without error when their blood alcohol levels are twice the legal limit of intoxication for many state jurisdictions.

Pharmacologic tolerance reflects a metabolic adaptive change in the alcohol addict as a consequence of long-term drinking. Evidence of pharmacologic tolerance was originally inferred from the finding of low blood alcohol levels in alcohol addicts who had consumed large amounts of alcohol (up to 1 quart of bourbon per day for 20 consecutive days). Subsequent studies demonstrated an enhanced rate of ethanol metabolism in alcohol addicts during protracted episodes of drinking. The pharmacokinetics of alcohol-induced enhancement of ethanol metabolism have not been clarified, but they appear not to persist after long periods of sobriety. Pharmacologic tolerance may contribute to some small aspect of behavioral tolerance, but adaptive processes in the central nervous system are probably far more important for behavioral tolerance than alcohol-induced enhancement in rates of ethanol metabolism.

Clinical reports have stressed that alcohol addicts may show reduced sensitivity and responsivity to a number of other drugs: *cross-tolerance.* There are reports that alcohol addicts require significantly higher doses of both the barbiturate and volatile anesthetics for induction and maintenance of appropriate levels of surgical anesthesia. Alcohol addicts frequently show cross-tolerance for barbiturates, hypnotics, and psychotropic agents such as the minor tranquilizers. However, cross-tolerance and cross-dependence have not been demonstrated between alcohol and the opiates. It is important to point out that cross-tolerance occurs in alcohol addicts when they are temporarily abstaining from drinking. When alcohol addicts are intoxicated, both synergism and potentiation with narcotics, opiates and analgesics, barbiturates, and a variety of other psychotropic agents may occur. In fact, there is some evidence which indicates that the consumption of drugs such as barbiturates during heavy alcohol intake is associated with a decreased catabolic degradation of both agents.

Although tolerance for ethanol may appear to be very great for some alcohol addicts, the degree of tolerance which can be developed for ethanol is much smaller than that which can potentially occur in opiate or barbiturate addiction. Barbiturate addicts may ingest as much as 2 grams of secobarbital or pentobarbital daily without gross impairments of behavior. Heroin addicts may eventually employ a dosage 50 times larger than their initial intake. On the other hand, blood alcohol levels exceeding 450 mg per 100 ml for any drinker, social or addicted, are rarely observed, because this level is almost invariably associated with a comatose state. Moreover, the lethal level of 500 to 600 mg per 100 ml is no different for alcohol addicts as opposed to normal drinkers, because such blood alcohol levels cause severe and often irreversible respiratory depression.

Physical dependence upon alcohol is characterized by the appearance of withdrawal signs and symptoms after cessation of drinking. Tremulousness, delirium, and seizure disorders were first reported by Hippocrates to accompany alcohol abuse, and detailed descriptions of the abstinence syndrome are reported in the medical literature of the late eighteenth century. Systematic studies by Victor and Adams in 1953 are the basis for the classification of the withdrawal syndromes currently identified in clinical practice. Three types of withdrawal states have been differentiated: tremulous states, seizure disorders, and delirium tremens.

Tremulousness is the most frequent and benign type of abstinence syndrome. Although the onset of tremulousness usually occurs 12 to 48 hours after reduction of alcohol intake or initiation of abstinence, this sign may be observed as early as six hours after cessation of drinking. Tremor is usually mild with involvement of the hands, but in some instances it may be generalized with involvement of all extremities as well as the tongue and trunk. Tremor may be increased when the patient extends the arms with the palms upright and the fingers separated. Tremulousness usually remits or is significantly diminished by 72 hours after cessation of drinking, but in rare instances it may persist for five days.

Hallucinosis may be associated with a tremulous state or may occur independent of tremor. Hallucinations also may occur in alcohol addicts during conditions of severe intoxication as well as during conditions of complete or partial cessation of drinking.

Seizure disorders usually occur 12 to 24 hours after cessation or reduction of drinking. Seizures may be associated with tremulousness, but may be present without any other evidence of withdrawal signs. The seizure disorder is of the grand mal type, usually not preceded by auras but almost always followed by postictal stupor and even residual focal signs. Seizures may be observed in patients who have no overt evidence of a neurologic disorder and who have no abnormalities of the electroencephalogram. Victor and Adams have emphasized that approximately one third of all patients who have seizure disorders after cessation of drinking progress to develop delirium tremens.

Delirium tremens is the rarest form of the alcohol withdrawal syndrome. Delirium tremens is characterized by confusion, disorientation, delusions, hallucinations, psychomotor agitation, and autonomic dysfunction. The peak incidence of this syndrome is 72 to 96 hours after cessation of drinking. The severe confusional states and delirium which are the hallmark of delirium tremens are rarely observed in the more frequent instances of tremulousness after cessation of drinking. Patients who develop delirium tremens also often have profuse sweating, tachycardia, hypertension, and fever. Delirium tremens is a potentially lethal illness which requires hospitalization and intensive medical care.

Although the basic mechanisms underlying the alcohol withdrawal syndrome remain to be determined, a number of associated disorders affect the severity of the disorder. Significant disturbances in acid-base, water,

and electrolyte homeostasis may be associated with the abstinence syndrome. After cessation of alcohol intake, many alcohol addicts develop transient hyperventilation which may produce respiratory alkalosis and elevations in blood pH. This condition is usually associated with hypomagnesemia. The low serum magnesium levels observed in alcohol addicts during the withdrawal syndrome are probably caused both by poor dietary intake of magnesium during heavy drinking and by magnesium shifts from the intravascular to the intracellular fluid compartments associated with the pH shift of respiratory alkalosis. It is also important to remember that alcohol addicts who develop withdrawal syndromes may be not dehydrated, but in fact, overhydrated.

INTERCURRENT ILLNESS AND ASSOCIATED DISORDERS. Alcohol addicts are at high risk for developing a number of disorders which are observed frequently in general medical practice. These are discussed individually in other chapters of this text, but a few merit mention here.

Alcohol-related hepatic disease is a leading cause of morbidity and mortality in adult males. It has been demonstrated that alcohol intake alone without concomitant nutritional deficiency may induce hepatic disorders such as fatty metamorphosis, alcoholic hepatitis, and Laennec's cirrhosis (see Ch. 465.2). However, since many people consume large quantities of alcohol without developing these disorders, the crucial determinants of the interrelationships between heavy alcohol consumption and hepatic disease remain to be determined. Gastritis and pancreatitis (see Ch. 402 and Ch. 410.2 and 410.3) are also frequently seen in those who abuse alcohol. A variety of malabsorption syndromes may be associated with heavy alcohol intake (see Ch. 408).

The most severe neurologic disorders seen in alcohol addicts are peripheral neuropathies (see Ch. 335 to 337) which are characterized by motor and sensory impairments in the upper and lower extremities. Pain, paresthesia, motor weakness, and paralysis may occur as a consequence of poor dietary intake in conjunction with heavy ethanol intake.

Diseases of the central nervous system may also be associated with chronic alcohol abuse. Wernicke's disease and Korsakoff's psychosis (see Ch. 287) are characterized by derangements of memory function and disorders of thought processes. The genesis of many "organic brain diseases," which at present constitute the majority of first admissions to state mental hospitals, may be related to nutritional and metabolic derangements associated with alcohol abuse.

There is accumulating evidence that alcohol abuse may be a factor in the development of coronary artery disease and hypertension. Individuals who have a familial Type IV hyperlipidemia (see Ch. 532.5) are at high risk for developing elevations in blood triglyceride levels with even moderate alcohol intake. Studies carried out in the United States and France suggest that alcohol abusers are at higher risk for developing carcinoma of the oral cavity and esophagus. A number of cardiomyopathies have been found in alcohol addicts. Finally, it has been shown that chronic alcohol abuse may cause derangements in hematopoiesis, produce muscle wasting, and suppress immune mechanisms with consequence of higher risk for infection.

AFFECTIVE DISORDERS AND PSYCHOSIS. Some individuals with neurotic and psychotic affective disorders drink excessively, but many others with severe depression never abuse alcohol. In manic-depressive illness patients are more prone to drink excessively during the manic phase of their disorder than when they are depressed. There is also evidence to indicate that chronic alcohol abuse enhances rather than reduces feelings of depression.

Approximately 25 per cent of all suicide victims have detectable amounts of alcohol in body fluids on necropsy examination. It is estimated that one third of all suicides are associated with chronic alcohol abuse, but these findings may relate mainly to white middle-aged males. Suicide rates for black males over 35 are low, even though drinking problems may be high.

TREATMENT AND PREVENTION. Although there are occasional reports of children who die of respiratory failure associated with ethanol overdosage, death from *acute ethanol poisoning* is rare. Rapid ingestion of large amounts of ethanol usually induces vomiting. Those who consume large amounts of ethanol slowly usually become stuporous before they can ingest a dose necessary to produce significant respiratory depression. The rate of ethanol catabolism in man ranges from 15 to 22 mg per 100 ml per hour, and there are no clinically useful or efficacious methods for rapidly decreasing blood alcohol levels.

Acute ethanol intoxication may be complicated by concurrent intoxication with other centrally acting drugs. There appears to be an increasing degree of polydrug abuse in the United States, particularly drugs which act synergistically with or potentiate the actions of ethanol. Alcohol abusers also frequently abuse barbiturates and minor tranquilizers. The most commonly reported form of drug abuse in narcotic addicts maintained on methadone is with alcohol. In hospital practice it is advisable to obtain blood determinations for other possible central nervous system depressants when a severe depression of consciousness is noted in patients who appear only to be intoxicated with ethanol.

Many persons who seek a physician's aid during conditions of acute ethanol introxication have other medical disorders. These patients should receive the most careful physical examination and diagnostic workup. Most states have adopted legislation requiring that patients with alcohol-related illness, including acute intoxication, should not be denied admission to hospitals and medical facilities. In addition, the American Medical Association and the American Hospital Association have endorsed resolutions against discriminatory policies for patients with alcohol-related problems who seek admission to general medical facilities. Some patients may request hospital treatment for detoxification after chronic alcohol intake when there is no evidence of any significant intercurrent illness. If the patient's motivation for receiving medical assistance appears good, the physician should attempt to provide the best available hospital care. However, involuntary commitment of patients with alcohol problems is not legal in most jurisdictions if hospitalization is initiated only on the basis of a diagnosis of alcoholism without evidence of a serious psychotic disorder.

Treatment of the *alcohol withdrawal syndrome* has improved significantly during the past decade. Less than 15 years ago many hospitals reported a 15 per cent mortality in patients with delirium tremens. The current mortality rate associated with delirium tremens is less than 1 per cent. The major factor affecting reduction in both mortality and morbidity is the application of good general medical care. Patients requiring treatment for the withdrawal syndrome should have the following procedures carried out on a systematic basis: (1) a careful physical and roentgenologic examination to identify any traumatic injuries (especially trauma to the skull); (2) a search for infection of the pulmonary and genitourinary systems; (3) a search for hepatic, gastrointestinal, and cardiac disorders; and (4) an evaluation of the state of hydration, electrolyte, and acid-base status, with appropriate measures instituted to correct any derangements. It should not be assumed that patients exhibiting the withdrawal syndrome are dehydrated or have any particular derangement in electrolyte or acid-base balance status unless demonstrated by appropriate clinical and laboratory examinations.

Chlordiazepoxide is the best drug for reducing pyschomotor agitation in patients who have withdrawal syndromes, provided the agent is used judiciously. In general, the dosage employed should permit reduction of tremor and anxiety without compromising the patient's ability to tolerate fluid and foods orally. Patients exhibiting the withdrawal syndrome should not be sedated deeply simply to produce long periods of sleep. Whenever possible, medication should be given orally, although at the initial stages of the withdrawal syndrome it may be necessary to use the intramuscular route. The routine use of corticosteroids is contraindicated, and the efficacy of diphenylhydantoin (Dilantin) in controlling seizure disorders is questionable. Administration of multivitamins orally or intravenously should be based upon judgment of the patient's nutritional status.

The *treatment of chronic alcohol abuse* is often difficult because most patients with alcohol-related problems tend to deny the severity of their illness and to avoid or reject assistance by physicians and other health care professionals. It has been postulated that the patient's acceptance of treatment can be greatly improved if initial contacts with the physician and the hospital are sympathetic and positive. The point has often been made that treatment for the alcohol abuser and alcohol addict should have limited goals and that alcohol-related illness should be considered as a chronic disease analogous, in some ways, to chronic pulmonary and cardiac conditions. For the most part, physicians treating such illnesses strive to alleviate suffering and to induce compensation rather than achieve absolute cure. A reasonable treatment goal is to restore physical and behavioral status after decompensation in alcohol abusers, even if recidivism is expected. Multimodality therapy suited to the needs of the individual and his resources should be offered. However, the question of which treatment will maximally benefit the patient with alcohol problems remains unanswered.

At present there is no uniformly effective, specific treatment for alcohol abuse. A number of treatment techniques have been employed singly or in combinations which have proved effective for some patients. These include individual and group psychotherapy, Antabuse therapy, referral to self-help groups such as Alcoholics Anonymous, and a number of behavioral modification techniques. It is discouraging that the few relatively well controlled therapy evaluation studies have demonstrated a low rate of alcohol abstinence after therapy. But since these evaluations were carried out in specialized clinic treatment settings, it remains likely that the individual counseling and relationship offered by the family physician will offer a greater degree of success.

The spontaneous recovery rate for alcohol abusers has been estimated to be about 20 per cent over a three-year period. Thus physicians should not assume that alcohol-related disorders are intractable. Since all variants of alcohol abuse are multiply determined, alcohol problems present the treatment challenge of any complex behavioral disorder. Although there is no evidence to indicate that alcohol abuse is invariably associated with a predisposing psychiatric illness, the development of problem drinking rarely occurs in isolation from emotional, interpersonal, and job-related problems.

The physician should employ a multifaceted program of treatment which can be best determined from assessing the patient's motivation, resources, and ability to sustain treatment relationships. For some individuals, self-help groups such as Alcoholics Anonymous may be useful, but one must first explore whether any given patient can effectively utilize this form of assistance. The physician should familiarize himself with all available resources which exist in the patient's community for assistance with alcohol-related problems. It is often essential that the physician involve other members of the family in cooperating with some form of treatment program.

Adequate techniques for *prevention of alcohol-related disorders* have yet to be devised. Although significant emphasis has been placed upon public education and information concerning the responsible use of alcohol, the impact of such programs is difficult to evaluate. Since there are relatively poor incidence and prevalence data for alcohol abuse, it is impossible to argue that public education programs or attempts to shape attitudes have had any impact on alcohol abuse and alcohol addiction. Increased programs of public education and information may appear logical, but it should be remembered that problem drinking usually occurs in situations in which behavior is not determined by logical thinking but rather by internal and external stresses which are not highly amenable to rational persuasion.

Kalant, H.: Absorption, diffusion, distribution and elimination of ethanol: Effects on biological membranes. *In* Kissin, B., and Begleiter, H. (eds.): The Biology of Alcoholism, Vol. 1. New York, Plenum Press, 1971.

Mello, N. K.: Behavioral studies of alcoholism. *In* Kissin, B., and Begleiter, H. (eds.): The Biology of Alcoholism, Vol. 2 New York, Plenum Press, 1972.

Mendelson, J.H., and Mello, N. K.: Alcohol, aggression and androgens. Proc. Assn. Res. Nerv. Ment. Dis., 52:225, 1974.

Mendelson, J. H., and Mello, N. K.: Behavioral and biochemical interrelations in alcoholism. *In* Creger, W. P., Coggins, C. H., and Hancock, E. W. (eds.): Annual Review of Medicine. Palo Alto, Annual Reviews, Inc., 1976.

Wolfe, S., and Victor, M.: The physiological basis of the alcohol withdrawal syndrome. *In* Mello, N. K., and Mendelson, J. H. (eds.): Recent Advances in Studies of Alcoholism. Washington, D. C., U. S. Government Printing Office, Publ. No. (HSM) 71-9045, 1971.

251. ACUTE DRUG POISONING

Fred Plum

Almost any physician may be called upon to treat accidental or intentional drug overdose. Suicide produces a high death rate among all adolescent and adult age groups, and its incidence climbs steadily with age in single white males. Furthermore, psychologically engendered drug abuse plagues many countries, with fatal or near-fatal "accidents" often affecting youngsters of secondary school age as well as adults. No social stratum enjoys immunity. The physician's job is made harder by the fact that the mentally unbalanced or those just seeking new sensations have an ever-expanding roster of pharmaceutical or industrial chemicals to draw from. Nevertheless, changing fashions affect the minority, and the most frequent agents causing drug poisonings will undoubtedly continue to resemble those listed in Table 1.

Table 2 lists the most common drug poisonings presently encountered in the United States, gives their principal signs of toxicity, and outlines their treatment. Clinical appraisal still must be used to diagnose the agent causing several of these reaction patterns, specific chemical tests being either unavailable or impractically slow. Blood levels or size of the dose are generally unreliable guides to the potential danger with almost any of the drugs listed because tolerance develops to their chronic ingestion, making individuals react differently to similar doses. Also, the mixing of drugs with each other and with alcohol adds to the unreliability of blood levels as a guide to treatment or prognosis of the drugs listed in Table 2. Only the opiates and the sedatives create any appreciable risk of death; concurrent alcohol ingestion enhances both these risks. Opiate poisoning is discussed in more detail in Ch. 244. The rest of this chapter gives details of the management of sedative drug overdose. For the diagnosis and treatment of suspected drug or chemical poisonings not covered in these pages, physicians should consult the *Physicians' Desk Reference* or the Poison Control Center of a large city.

SEDATIVE OVERDOSE

PATHOGENESIS. All the sedative drugs depress the central nervous system, although not equally on a gram-molecular weight basis, and not to the same degree so far as different central structures are concerned. The duration of action varies widely and depends largely on how the particular drug is detoxified or eliminated. The short-acting barbiturates, pentobarbital, secobarbital, and amobarbital, are detoxified by the liver, as is methaqualone. They exert their maximal effects promptly after being absorbed and, even in huge doses, seldom cause neurologic depression lasting longer than three to five days. Barbital and phenobarbital are partially detoxified by the liver and partially excreted in the urine. Severe poisoning with the latter

TABLE 1. Drugs Used, in Order of Frequency, Among Severe Overdose Subjects, New York Hospital, 1969–1973

Alcohol	Lithium
Barbiturates, glutethimide	Salicylates
Heroin or methadone	Phenothiazines
Methaqualone	Diphenylhydantoin
Meprobamate	Bishydroxycoumarin, Coumadin
Scopolamine	Tolbutamide, phenformin
Amphetamine	Insulin
Imipramine	

TABLE 2. Common Drug Poisonings, Signs of Toxicity, and Treatment

Drug	Mild Toxic Signs	Tissue for Diagnosis	Treatment	Severe Overdose Signs	Treatment
Opiates: Heroin Morphine Demerol Methadone	"Nodding" drowsiness, small pupils, urinary retention, slow and shallow breathing; skin scars and subcutaneous abscesses; duration 4–6 hrs; with methadone, duration to 24 hrs	Urine	Levallorphan 1 mg IV, naloxone 0.4 mg IV or IM; repeat at 15-min intervals not more than twice; repeat in 3 hrs if necessary	Coma; pinpoint pupils, slow irregular respiration or apnea, hypotension, hypothermia, pulmonary edema	Levallorphan, nalorphine, naloxine; if no response by second dose, suspect another cause; treat shock; find and detect infection
Depressants: Alcohol	Confusion, rousable drowsiness, delirium, ataxia, nystagmus, dysarthria, analgesia to stimuli	Blood, urine, breath	Alcohol excitement: diazepam or chlorpromazine None needed for acute toxicity; withdraw drug under supervision if patient is a chronic user	Stupor to coma; pupils reactive, usually constricted; oculovestibular response absent; motor tonus initially briefly hyperactive, then flaccid; respiration and blood pressure depressed; hypothermia; with glutethimide, pupils moderately dilated, can be fixed; with meprobamate, withdrawal seizures common; with methaqualone, coma, occasional convulsions, tachycardia, cardiac failure, bleeding tendency	Intubate, ventilate, gavage; drainage position; antimicrobials; keep mean blood pressure above 90 mm Hg and urine output 300 ml/hr; avoid analeptics; hemodialyze severe phenobarbital poisoning
Barbiturates Glutethimide (Doriden) Meprobamate (Equanil)		Blood Blood Blood			
Methaqualone (Quaalude, Sopor, Mandrax)	Hallucinations, agitation, motor hyperactivity, myoclonus, tonic spasms	Blood			As above; diuresis of little help
Chlordiazepoxide (Librium) Diazepam (Valium)	Usually taken with another sedative if poisoning the attempt	Blood			
Stimulants: Amphetamines Methylphenidate	Hyperactive, aggressive, sometimes paranoid, repetitive behavior; dilated pupils, tremor, hyperactive reflexes; hyperthermia, tachycardia, arrhythmia Acute torsion dystonia	Blood	Reassurance if mild Chlorpromazine if intense	Agitated, assaultive and paranoid excitement; ocasionally convulsions; hypothermia; circulatory collapse	Chlorpromazine
Cocaine	Similar but less prominent than above; less paranoid, often euphoric	None: clinical appraisal only	Chlorpromazine Reassure	Twitching, irregular breathing, tachycardia	Sedation
Psychedelics (LSD, mescaline, psilocybin, STP)	Confused, disoriented, perceptual distortions, distractable, withdrawn or eruptive, leading to accidents or violence; wide-eyed, dilated pupils; restless, hyperreflexic; less often, hypertension or tachycardia		Reassure; "talk down"; do not leave alone	Panic	Reassure; diazepam satisfactory; avoid phenothiazines
Atropine-scopolamine (Sominex)	Agitated or confused, visual hallucinations, dilated pupils, flushed and dry skin		Reassure	Toxic disoriented delirium, visual hallucination; later, amnesia, fever, dilated fixed pupils, hot flushed dry skin, urinary retention	Reassure; sedate lightly; (1) avoid phenothiazines; (2) do not leave alone
Antidepressants: Imipramine (Tofranil), amitriptyline (Elavil)	Restlessness, drowsiness, tachycardia, ataxia, sweating	Clinical	Physostigmine for arrhythmias	Agitation, vomiting, hyperpyrexia, sweating, muscle dystonia, convulsions, tachycardia or arrhythmia	Symptomatic; gastric lavage
MAO inhibitors: tranylcypromine (Parnate), phenelzine (Nardil), pargyline (Eutonyl)	Hypertensive crises, agitation, drowsiness, ataxia	Clinical	Withdrawal	Hypotension; headache; chest pain; agitation; coma, seizures and shock	Symptomatic; gastric lavage
Phenothiazines	Acute dystonia, somnolence, hypotension	Clinical	Benadryl 0.05 gram 3–4 times daily; withdrawal	Coma; convulsions (rare); arrhythmias; hypotension	Symptomatic; gastric lavage

agent can cause coma lasting 10 to 14 days. Glutethimide has a short duration of action comparable to that of secobarbital, but it is poorly absorbed from the gut and may generate more long-lasting neurotoxic metabolites. Meprobamate has an intermediate duration of effect lasting for days. Bromide rarely causes full coma, but, once it reaches high levels, it replaces chloride in the blood and tissues, and persists for weeks to cause symptoms without further ingestion. Chemical autoanalyzers in hospital use do not differentiate these halide ions and report falsely high chloride levels in bromide poisoning.

Although the sedatives have few important effects outside the nervous system, glutethimide and meprobamate in toxic doses tend to produce hypotension. Also, glutethimide possesses anticholinergic properties and is the only sedative that predictably produces light-fixed pupils in toxic doses.

A withdrawal syndrome consisting of tremulousness, agitation, and sometimes delirium and convulsions can develop after prompt withdrawal of any of the hypnotic sedatives. Convulsions seem to be a particular problem after withdrawal from meprobamate and methaqualone.

CLINICAL MANIFESTATIONS. Stupor or coma caused by depressant drug poisoning presents the characteristic picture of severe metabolic brain disease. The depression of the central nervous system tends to be bilateral and symmetrical, and the drug affects simultaneously many levels, including the spinal cord. Respiratory and circulatory controlling mechanisms in the lower brainstem are affected only with very high doses or not at all, and, except with glutethimide, the pupillary light reflexes are preserved. Early in the course of poisoning, patients can demonstrate muscular hypertonus or even spasticity as the result of uneven depression of different neurologic levels. Within a short time, usually an hour or less, flaccidity supervenes, and the stretch reflexes tend to disappear. Even moderate degrees of drug depression depress or block the oculovestibular reflexes.

Four grades of coma have been described in order to aid in estimating the severity of poisoning and the effects of treatment. *Grade I* is light coma in which vigorous noxious stimulation evokes withdrawal or groaning. *Grade II* is deep coma in which only minimal grimacing or reflex responsiveness can be evoked by a noxious stimulus. In *grade III* subjects fail to respond in any way to a noxious stimulus. In *grade IV* unresponsive patients remain in deep coma for over 36 hours and, in addition, have serious respiratory or circulatory depression. As mentioned above, a relationship between the blood level of a sedative drug and the depth of coma is only approximate. Generally speaking, however, blood levels of short-acting barbiturates of more than 2.5 mg per 100 ml and phenobarbital blood levels of more than 12 mg per 100 ml are associated with grades III and IV coma.

DIAGNOSIS. The combination of unresponsiveness, preserved or sluggish pupillary reactions, absent oculovestibular reactions, motor areflexia, hypothermia, and depression of respiration and circulation is clinically diagnostic of sedative-anesthetic drug poisoning. Only pontine infarction resembles this clinical state, and with lesions of the pons the pupils are usually small or pinpoint, the stretch reflexes are generally preserved or hyperactive, and the plantar responses are extensor. Specific chemical tests will detect barbiturates, glutethimide, meprobamate, methaqualone, and bromides in blood or urine, and are readily done as emergency measures.

MANAGEMENT OF COMA. There are no specific antidotes. Treatment consists of physiologic support and preventing complications until the drug is detoxified and is excreted. Proper management saves all but a very few patients if they survive to reach the hospital. Among the writer's very large series of patients with drug coma, fewer than 2 per cent have died. To achieve this low rate required meticulous attention to the airway and ventilation, to the circulation, and to the potential complications of the comatose state.

AIRWAY AND VENTILATION. Several mechanisms threaten to obstruct the airway of patients in coma from sedative drugs. If the subject lies on his back, the tongue and pooled secretions occlude the hypopharynx, with the result that secretions are aspirated into the lungs. The cough reflex and the ciliary action of the tracheobronchial mucosa are depressed. Many subjects aspirate stomach contents into the lungs, particularly if gastric lavage is attempted before tracheal intubation.

An oropharyngeal airway is sufficient to manage patients in light coma who cough when the larynx is stimulated. A cuffed endotracheal tube should be placed in more deeply anesthetized patients who lack a cough reflex. It is wise to precede intubation with atropine, 0.0008 gram intravenously, to reduce the danger of cardiac arrest. How long to leave the endotracheal tube in place in an unresponsive subject is often a difficult question. One practice is to deflate the cuff hourly for 5 minutes, to replace the tube at 24 hours, and to perform a tracheostomy at somewhere between 36 and 48 hours if the cough reflex has not returned or if no other signs indicate a lessening of coma.

To drain the lungs and improve oxygenation, patients should be placed in the prone position, as illustrated in the accompanying figure, and suctioned gently through the endotracheal tube every half hour, or more often if pulmonary secretions accumulate. It is desirable to administer low concentrations (25 per cent) of moistened oxygen, but not to occlude the tube with a large catheter. Tubes are removed when active coughing or bucking returns.

Hypoventilation should be treated with artificial respiration. Shallow breathing in a deeply comatose patient frequently reflects no more than the subject's depressed metabolism, but if the rate falls below 12 per minute or if the physician entertains serious doubts as to the adequacy of ventilation, artificial respiration is indicated. Ideally, arterial blood gases should be measured in deeply comatose patients and artificial respiration initiated if the arterial Pco_2 climbs above 45 mm of mercury. High concentration (>30 per cent) oxygen therapy should be avoided for patients not receiving artificial respiration, for its use increases the risk of hypoventilation and CO_2 retention.

Circulation. Severe shock is rare with depressant drug poisoning unless the patient has been asphyxiated. However, moderate hypotension is common and significantly reduces glomerular filtration and renal clearance of the barbiturates. Fluids should be given liberally to restore blood volume and promote urine flow, and pressor agents, such as dopamine or isoproterenol, are indicated to keep the diastolic blood pressure above 60 mm of mercury and the systolic above 90 mm of mercury. Digitalis or similar compounds are useful only in patients with heart disease. Cardiac arrhythmias induced by tricyclic antidepressant ingestion should be treated with physostigmine. Corticosteroids are unnecessary.

Prevention of Complications. As long as he remains unconscious, the patient should be kept semiprone in the drainage position and changed from side to side in the semiprone position, but never placed on his back. Since the duration of unconsciousness is to be measured in days, the emergence of drug-resistant bacteria is of less concern than is pneumonia caused by already aspirated material. Thus it is useful to administer penicillin or tetracycline.

The blood pressure, pulse, and respiration should be recorded each half hour, and any abnormalities should be met appropriately. Body temperature elevations imply an infection if stimulants have not been given. Hypothermia above 32° C requires no special treatment. To evaluate the rate of urine flow, most physicians prefer to insert an indwelling catheter.

Other Measures. *Gastric lavage* is desirable for any patient who has ingested depressant drugs within the preceding few hours. A large Ewald tube must be used to remove capsular material. The procedure should be done gently to avoid producing pulmonary aspiration, and is best preceded by tracheal intubation with a cuffed tube in deeply comatose subjects. Subjects too lightly anesthetized to tolerate intubation should be turned prone before being lavaged. Care is required to avoid misplacing the tube and irrigating the lungs.

Forced diuresis and alkalinization of the urine have been recommended as adjuncts in treating barbiturate poisoning. Forced diuresis increases the renal clearance of both short- and long-acting barbiturates, and the quantity cleared increases proportionately to the volume of urine. Phenobarbital has a relatively high pK value, and raising the urine pH appears to increase its dissociation and excretion. Several programs have been employed to achieve diuresis. The first step is to assure an adequate blood pressure; the second, to infuse a hypotonic electrolyte solution. The infusions are given at

hourly rates up to 600 ml, depending upon urine flow. Close attention must be given to hour-by-hour fluid balance and 12-hour electrolyte balance. If urine flow does not match the infusion rate by the second or third hour, infusions should be slowed and more attention given to raising the blood pressure. Chemical and osmotic diuretics are contraindicated. Hypokalemia is a greater risk than hyperkalemia.

For treating bromide intoxication, diuresis should be combined with a high intake of sodium chloride to displace bromide from blood and tissues.

Hemodialysis is not necessary to treat poisoning with the short-acting hypnotics. However, hemodialysis is indicated to shorten the duration of coma for patients who have ingested large amounts of long-acting barbiturates such as barbital or phenobarbital, or who are in grade IV coma from glutethimide overdose. Dialysis also is indicated for severe lithium or bromide poisoning.

Analeptics and pharmacologic stimulants are contraindicated for coma caused by depressant drug poisoning. Most carry the risk of overstimulating or producing convulsions in lightly poisoned patients.

RECOVERY AND PROGNOSIS. Patients recovering from coma require close medical supervision. Severe pneumonitis can develop as late as three to four days after recovery. If antimicrobial drugs were started during coma, they are best continued for at least 48 hours after it ends. Permanent physical sequelae to coma are rare. Among 356 cases, residual brain injury was observed only once (in a patient who suffered an acute cardiac arrest). Peripheral nerve injuries from pressure developed in 6 subjects, and 14 subjects had pressure skin lesions leaving scars. There were no other residua.

Later management varies according to the patient's underlying psychiatric disorder and his attitudes upon recovery. Serious suicide attempts are never accidents, and reports of near-fatal ingestion caused by misunderstanding the dose or forgetting previous doses carry little validity. The expert opinion of a psychiatrist should be sought before deciding whether to release a patient or to institutionalize him. The immediate prognosis is good, but there is a high incidence of recurrent attempts at self-destruction over the years.

Bourne, P. G.: Acute Drug Abuse Emergencies. New York, Academic Press, 1976.
Douglas, W. D., Rehder, K., Beyner, F. M., Sessler, A. D., and Marsh, H. M.: Improved oxygenation in patients with acute respiratory failure: The prone position. Am. Rev. Respir. Dis., 115:559, 1977.
Physicians' Desk Reference to Pharmaceutical Specialties and Biologicals. Published annually by Medical Economics Co., Oradell, N. J.

Section Eight THE HYPOTHALAMUS AND NEUROLOGIC DISORDERS

Fred Plum

252. INTRODUCTION

The hypothalamus links the emotional forebrain, the autonomic nervous system, and the endocrine system. Diseases involving this tiny spot not only produce protean symptoms but often develop insidiously and progress slowly, making early recognition difficult. Hypothalamic dysfunction must often be considered as a possible cause of emotional, autonomic, or endocrine disorders, and the following chapters should be read in conjunction with the description of the endocrine hypothalamus in Ch. 542.

253. FUNCTIONAL ANATOMY

The hypothalamus is made up of a diffuse reticulum of neurons richly traversed by fiber pathways. Only the paraventricular and supraoptic nuclei have sharp anatomic definition, other neuronal collections being defined better as regions or areas than as specific nuclei. Similarly, only a minority of the conduction pathways are collected into discretely identifiable tracts. This imprecise anatomy reflects itself in the localization of hypothalamic functions, many of which overlap several of the region's anatomic subdivisions (Table 1). Afferent connections come from the limbic forebrain, from the cerebral cortex of the frontal and temporal lobes, from the thalamus, and from the midbrain reticular formation. The hypothalamus, in turn, sends direct neural connections to the thalamus, the brainstem reticular formation, the brainstem autonomic nuclei, and the posterior lobe of the hypophysis.

From the standpoint of clinical medicine, ventromedian and posterior hypothalamic lesions tend to produce greater functional changes than ones elsewhere in the structure. Except for sympathetic activities, bilateral damage is required to produce discernible changes in hypothalamic function. Ventromedian lesions not only interfere bilaterally with hypothalamic functions localized in that area but commonly interrupt the flow of hypothalamus-to-pituitary neurosecretion as well. Posterior hypothalamic lesions both destroy local functions and interrupt descending common paths to the more caudal brainstem. Table 2 lists the most common causes of hypothalamic disease.

254. SLEEP AND AROUSAL

Sleep and arousal are active behavioral states influenced by nervous structures that extend from the anterior hypothalamus down to the mid pons. The hypothalamic components of this system appear to influence both sleeping and waking behavior more specifically than do the nuclei of the midbrain and pons. In animals, stimulation of the anterior hypothalamus produces a state that behaviorally and physiologically resembles true sleep; destruction of this region results in sustained insomnia. Conversely, posterior hypothalamic stimulation produces arousal, whereas its destruction results in sustained sleep-like unresponsiveness. In human beings, hypothalamic insomnia is rare, and has been observed only acutely with anterior hypothalamic injury. Posterior hypothalamic lesions, on the other hand, are a well established cause of lethargic behavior, hypersomnolence, or sleep-like coma and should be specifically searched for when these symptoms arise.

TABLE 1.   Regional Functions of the Hypothalamus*

	Preoptic Anterior Hypothalamus	Tuberal and Ventromedian Hypothalamus	Posterior Hypothalamus
Receptor:	Thermal, osmotic	Caloric	Thermal set-point
Integrates:	Endocrine, thermal, autonomic	Cognition; endocrine; autonomic; caloric balance; fluid balance	Consciousness; cognition; complex endocrine; autonomic; thermal
Contains:	Sleep-inducing mechanism; forebrain parasympathetic paths	Thermoregulatory paths; final common endocrine paths	Reticular activating system; thermoregulatory effectors
Acute lesions:	Insomnia? diabetes insipidus; hyperthermia; diabetes insipidus; inappropriate ADH	Hyperthermia; diabetes insipidus; hypothalamic-endocrine disorders	Hypersomnia; emotional disorders; poikilothermia; autonomic storm
Chronic lesions:	Insominia; complex endocrine changes (e.g., precocious puberty); final common path endocrine changes; hypothermia; hypodipsia	Medial: memory loss; emotional disorders; hyperphagia and obesity; final common path endocrine disorders. Lateral: emotional disorders; emaciation; loss of thirst	Memory loss; emotional disorders; poikilothermia; incoordination of autonomic reflexes; complex endocrine disorders (e.g., precocious puberty)

*As indicated in the text, functional localization is more precise for some activities than others.

TABLE 2. Principal Causes of Hypothalamic Diseases in Adolescents and Adults

Congenital midline brain defects, e.g., agenesis of corpus callosum
"Familial" disorders, e.g., diabetes insipidus
Chronic hydrocephalus or increased intracranial pressure
Tumors: craniopharyngiomas, glioma, hamartoma, dysgerminoma, dermoid, lipoma, lymphoma or leukemia, meningioma
Encephalitis: various viral encephalitides, exanthematous demyelinating encephalitides, disseminated encephalomyelitis
Granulomas: sarcoid, tuberculosis, histocytosis X
Trauma
Subarachnoid hemorrhage; aneurysms; arteriovenous malformation
Wernicke's polioencephalopathy (thiamin deficiency)
Progressive idiopathic degeneration

255. MEMORY AND EMOTION

The ventromedian hypothalamus stands in the pathway that links the limbic forebrain to the thalamus and the brainstem reticular formation. Damage to this region in man impairs recent and intermediate term memory, the severity of the defect roughly paralleling the anatomic extent of the damage. Present research leaves unsettled whether the critical anatomic structures include the mammillary bodies or the immediately more anterior hypothalamic region which contains projections from both the amygdala and fornix. Diseases that bilaterally invade or destroy this ventromedian area can produce a severe dementia, marked by memory loss, withdrawn and confused behavior, and, sometimes, aggressive outbursts. Loss of libido accompanies ventromedian hypothalamic disease but most probably reflects gonadal hypotrophism rather than a direct neural effect.

256. HEAT REGULATION

The question of hypothalamic dysfunction repeatedly arises in patients with cryptogenic fever. In fact, hypothalamic disease rarely or never produces subacute or chronic fever, although several kinds of hypothalamic damage reduce body temperature. Experimental evidence indicates that the preoptic anterior hypothalamus contains separate receptors for warmth and cold as well as for pyrogens. The hypothalamus integrates information generated by these receptors with stimuli arriving directly from peripheral thermoreceptors as well as from nonspecific sources, such as the subject's general level of arousal. Diurnal changes in central nervous system excitability and in the level of circulating ovarian hormones provide additional nonspecific stimuli. In turn, the hypothalamus activates varying combinations of behavioral, autonomic, and endocrine responses that conserve or dissipate the body heat.

Gross stimulation of the anterior hypothalamus activates mainly the more abundant warm receptors located in that region and leads to heat dissipation and a fall in body temperature. Conversely, acute anterior or lateral hypothalamic destruction causes transient hyperthermia that subsides gradually over several days to weeks as more caudally placed and peripheral thermoreceptors take charge.

The posterior hypothalamus integrates thermoregulation and generates the signals that initiate the physiologic, affective, and behavioral adjustments that guarantee the stability of body temperature. Selective stimulation of dorsomedial-caudal hypothalamic and rostral mesencephalic sites activates heat production mechanisms. In contrast, ventrolateral-caudal hypothalamic stimulation inhibits heat production and activates heat dissipation. Large posterior hypothalamic lesions destroy both heat loss and heat production mechanisms and result in poikilothermia.

HYPOTHERMIA. Relative Poikilothermia. Poikilothermia, defined as the fluctuation in body temperature of greater than 2° C with changes in ambient temperature, is the most common central abnormality of heat regulation in man. Most such cases are detected by a lowered body temperature. Poikilothermia results from degeneration or metabolic dysfunction of the final integrator and effector sites for thermoregulation located in the posterior hypothalamus and rostral mesencephalon. Lesions in this area impair not only autonomic heat regulating pathways but those that control thermal discomfort, and the behavioral regulation of body temperature as well. As a result, many patients with poikilothermia are unaware of their condition and do little to avoid it. At ordinary ambient temperatures of 20 to 25° C, the degree of hypothermia tends to be proportional to the degree of functional hypothalamic impairment. Relative poikilothermia resulting from impaired hypothalamic-autonomic function is frequent in the elderly, making them dangerously susceptible to lowered environmental temperatures. Chronic poikilothermia accompanies several degenerative disorders of the brain in children and adults. Metabolic causes of poikilothermia include acute or chronic sedative drug ingestion, hypoglycemia, and myxedema. Poikilothermia regularly accompanies extensive damage to the posterior hypothalamus or midbrain by stroke, trauma, or neoplasm.

Paroxysmal Hypothermia. *Sustained hypothermia* (as opposed to relative poikilothermia) is rare in man. Somewhat less uncommon is *paroxysmal hypothermia*, consisting of attacks of lowered body temperature that vary widely in frequency from daily to more than a decade apart. Such attacks usually begin abruptly, last from minutes to days, and are characterized by sweating, flushing of the skin, and a fall in body temperature, usually to 32° C or lower. Fatigue, decreased mental responsiveness, hypoventilation, hypotension, cardiac arrhythmias, ataxia, lacrimation, and asterixis may accompany the lowered body temperature. The attacks subside either slowly (hours to days) or rapidly with shivering and peripheral vasoconstriction. During hypothermia, mechanisms for both heat production and heat dissipation respond normally, but around a lower temperature set-point. Most of the patients have had direct evidence for hypothalamic disease; several have had agenesis of the corpus callosum.

HYPERTHERMIA. Hyperthermia resulting from central nervous system damage occurs only with acute pathologic processes, and rarely lasts for more than two weeks following the initial event. The most frequent causes include gross head injury, either surgical trauma or bleeding into the region of the anterior hypothalamus, or hemorrhage in the adjacent meninges or the third ventricle. With neurogenic hyperthermia, the body temperature can rise to potentially fatal levels of 42° C or higher as a result of active heat production unbalanced by heat dissipation. The cardiovascular changes that normally accompany fever are disproportionately lacking. Small (2 mg) doses of morphine can be useful in ameliorating dangerously high neurogenic fevers.

257. SYMPATHETIC AND PARASYMPATHETIC FUNCTIONS

Symptoms of sympathetic and parasympathetic dysfunction figure prominently in many medical and psychophysiologic illnesses. Nearly all these responses are mediated through hypothalamic pathways, and their presence repeatedly leads physicians to question whether these structures play a primary role.

Autonomic influences originating in the cerebral hemispheres converge on the hypothalamus and are integrated there to be transmitted down the neuraxis. Generally speaking, stimulation of the anterior hypothalamus evokes primarily parasympathetic responses, whereas posterior hypothalamic stimulation elicits sympathetic activity. Destructive lesions have the opposite effect. The evoked sympathetic responses occur mainly ipsilaterally and represent the only example of a unilateral localization and projection of a hypothalamic function.

Experiments of recent years have disclosed that the autonomic functions of the hypothalamus are specific to the degree that stimulation of an isolated fiber can engender a predictable response in specific peripheral organs. A similar precision applies to afferent pathways. Despite its capacity for individual autonomic responses, however, the predominant autonomic role of the hypothalamus is integrative. Without the hypothalamus, one can still obtain individually normal baseline autonomic activities, but the complex coordination of autonomic and behavioral responses that assures homeostasis is impaired or lost.

Central neurogenic autonomic abnormalities in man accompany acute disease of the hypothalamus and its efferent pathways. With the exception of partial sympathetic paralysis, however, chronic hypothalamic lesions rarely produce clinically detectable abnormalities in autonomic control systems.

CARDIOVASCULAR EFFECTS. An extensive clinical literature describes changes in cardiovascular function accompanying acute disease of the brainstem and hypothalamus. The abnormalities include hypertension, cardiac arrhythmias of various types, and a number of electrocardiographic abnormalities, some of which can simulate acute myocardial infarction. Many affected patients have no evidence of previous cardiovascular disease. Subarachnoid hemorrhage and acute diseases of the brainstem can induce multifocal myocardial necrosis, possibly due to coronary arteriolar vasoconstriction in response to the outpouring of catecholamines that accompanies the acute event. The specific relationship of such changes to hypothalamic damage has not been proved, and they may equally well reflect the effects of excitation of descending autonomic pathways.

Pulmonary edema and hemorrhage can be a sudden and striking accompaniment to acute hypothalamic injury in animals. Many observers believe that a similar process occurs in man, perhaps causing the wet lungs often observed after acute intracranial injury, infection, or hemorrhage. The response probably is nonspecific, however. Some patients develop pulmonary edema in association with anterior hypothalamic compression, intraventricular hemorrhage, or rupture of an anterior communicating arterial aneurysm. Others develop similar lung changes in association with lesions involving intracranial sites remote from the hypothalamus.

Theories of the pathogenesis of "neurogenic" pulmonary edema have centered on the excitation of an adrenergic cardiovascular mechanism producing acute hypertension and a shift of blood from the systemic to the pulmonary vascular beds. Direct studies in humans with acute neurogenic pulmonary edema, however, have failed to demonstrate either an elevated blood pressure or an elevated central venous pressure. Whatever its cause, acute pulmonary congestion accompanying acute central nervous system injury often requires urgent attention to minimize hypoxemia and the deleterious effects of overvigorous breathing efforts.

GASTROINTESTINAL FUNCTIONS. In laboratory animals, acute lesions placed anywhere from the level of the preoptic hypothalamus rostrally to the region of the vagal nuclei in the medulla caudally can result in gastrointestinal hemorrhage. Posterior hypothalamic lesions can result in ulceration, but anterior hypothalamic lesions generally confine their effects to producing hemorrhagic gastromalacia.

Hemorrhage and acute ulceration are the major gastrointestinal complications of central nervous system dysfunction in man, and they can affect the gastrointestinal tract anywhere from the lower esophagus to the large bowel. Intracranial surgery, head trauma, encephalitis, cerebral hemorrhage and infarction, acute multiple sclerosis, brain abscess, meningitis, and a variety of intracranial tumors all may precipitate acute gastrointestinal ulceration or hemorrhage. The common denominator of all these lesions is the acute nature of their onset. The most frequent specific gastrointestinal abnormality seems to be lower esophageal ulceration, an otherwise rare lesion. Gastric and duodenal ulcerations account for an even greater association, but much of this reflects their high non-neurogenic incidence. Neurogenic ulcers occur in all age groups from neonates to those over 80 years old. The ulcers themselves are morphologically identical to those that accompany the acute stresses of burns, pneumonia, and general body trauma. Acute gastrointestinal ulceration and hemorrhage in association with intracranial disease thus arises as a manifestation of nonspecific damage or an imbalance in descending central autonomic pathways rather than of any specific hypothalamic effect. Sympathetic hyperactivity elevating the systemic levels of catecholamines and parasympathetic hyperactivity producing elevated gastrin levels have been noted in affected patients. No one knows which of these is more important.

258. FEEDING BEHAVIOR AND CALORIC BALANCE

Forebrain and especially limbic system influences assume such an importance in feeding behavior in man that primary hypothalamic error accounts for no more than a tiny fraction of human obesity or emaciation.

In animals, stimulation of the ventromedian region inhibits feeding, whereas lesions destroying this region produce hyperphagia and a weight gain which later stabilizes at a new elevated set-point, after which time the hyperphagia subsides. The critical damage influencing feeding may be to the catecholaminergic pathways that lie in close proximity to the ventromedian nucleus as they traverse the hypothalamus toward the forebrain. Stimulation of the lateral hypothalamus in animals induces feeding behavior, whereas damage to the region results in a temporarily severe aphagia that slowly recovers to maintain a lowered body weight that represents a new set-point. The critical site affecting feeding behavior may be the paths traversing this lateral hypothalamic region, and not intrinsic hypothalamic neurons themselves.

HYPOTHALAMIC OBESITY.   Most patients with hypothalamic obesity have shown at autopsy diffuse or large lesions involving the greater part of the structure, although frequently sparing the posterior hypothalamus. A few have had precisely placed abnormalities destroying the ventromedian hypothalamus with the size of the destructive lesion at least roughly corresponding with the degree of obesity. Occasional examples have been due to leukemic infiltration of the periventricular hypothalamus, with the most severe damage localized in the ventromedian region; others have been discrete tumors in this area.

These lesions in patients with hypothalamic obesity provide the most discrete localization of any disorder of the human hypothalamus. The patients have experienced remarkable combinations of food-seeking behavior, including hyperphagia, finickiness in food selections, decreased activity, and obesity, just as in the laboratory animal with medial tuberal damage.

The hypothalamus evidently contains a set-point mechanism that roughly regulates body weight. When one encounters a patient with hypothalamic obesity, the presence or absence of continued hyperphagia depends on whether or not the neurologic process is stable and the body weight set-point has been attained. Patients with obesity following upon surgical or blunt head trauma to the hypothalamus illustrate this principle. Characteristically, such individuals initially display a ravenous hyperphagia and gain weight quickly following the injury until they reach their new set-point, at which point they become normophagic and their weight stabilizes. After six months or so, many such patients then become hypophagic and their weight declines to reapproach the pretrauma level.

Emaciation sometimes accompanies hypothalamic disease in man, but in such instances the lesions usually have been large and their specificity uncertain. A causative association between hypothalamic disease and anorexia nervosa has not been established.

259. WATER BALANCE

Homeostatic control of body water and osmolality depends heavily on the hypothalamic coordination of affective thirst, drinking behavior, and antidiuretic hormone (ADH) release. Hypothalamic disease or dysfunction can produce four principal disorders of water balance. The syndromes of ADH deficiency (diabetes insipidus) and inappropriate ADH excess are dis-

cussed in Ch. 544.2 and 530, respectively. The syndromes of essential or central hypernatremia and of episodic hyperdipsia are often related to central nervous system dysfunction and are discussed in this chapter.

PHYSIOLOGY.   The osmoreceptors that most influence thirst, water drinking behavior, and the osmotic control of ADH release lie within the preoptic anterior hypothalamic region. In laboratory animals, one can identify in this area cells that respond to both local sodium concentration and circulating levels of angiotensin, a polypeptide released during systemic dehydration. Osmoreceptors in other hypothalamic regions possess more limited functions.

Peripheral receptors influence water balance less strongly than do the hypothalamic receptors. Thirst is stimulated by osmoreceptors lying in the systemic interstitial fluids, as well as by receptors in the mouth responsible for the sensation of dryness. Excitation of volume receptors in the left atrium of the heart and in the large capacitance systemic veins tends to inhibit drinking behavior and ADH release. Baroceptor influences, ascending through the brainstem, exert a similar effect. Thermal stress, eating, psychic stress, and other influences all can activate drinking and ADH release so as to influence water balance.

The magnocellular neurons in the supraoptic and paraventricular nuclei of higher animals produce ADH and transport it to the median eminence and neurohypophysis, whence it passes into the blood. These neurosecretory cells maintain a low baseline firing rate that is increased by stimulation from excitatory osmoreceptors or decreased by stimuli from inhibitory volume receptors. All evidence indicates that the threshold for ADH release depends on the set-point of the associated osmoreceptor. Once above threshold, further changes in ADH release in response to changes of osmolarity appear to depend on the integrated sum of the various inputs. Under normal conditions, osmoreceptors are the most influential determinant of ADH release.

Most human disorders of water balance can be reproduced experimentally. Diabetes insipidus is the most easily obtained and requires a 90 per cent or greater loss of the magnocellular neurons of the supraoptic and paraventricular nuclei. Such a high percentage of cell loss requires direct hypothalamic damage, explaining why hypophysectomy (which spares the neurons secreting into median eminence vessels) usually causes only a temporary diabetes insipidus.

Lesions that impinge on the supraoptic nucleus but do not destroy it result in an inappropriately high secretion of ADH, presumably by interrupting inhibitory pathways to the nucleus. Destruction of the receptor-containing preoptic region produces a permanent hypodipsia or adipsia accompanied by loss of the ADH response to osmotic stress.

Electrical stimulation of the lateral hypothalamus or nonspecific arousal in animals results in polydipsia, whereas destructive lateral lesions cause a temporary adipsia. Stimulation of higher limbic system structures tends most often to inhibit drinking and ADH release. Ventromedian hypothalamic stimulation inhibits drinking, whereas lesions of the ventromedian region may produce hyperdipsia.

THE SYNDROME OF ESSENTIAL HYPERNATREMIA.   Four features characterize essential hypernatremia in man: (1) hypernatremia unaccompanied by a corresponding extracellular fluid deficiency, (2) a preserved renal tubular responsiveness to ADH, (3) an inadequate secretion of ADH in response to osmotic stimuli, and (4) the absence or deficiency of thirst with otherwise fully conscious behavior. True essential hypernatremia is rare; most cases of serum hyperosmolarity accompanying intracranial disease result from a nonspecific combination of dehydration and stupor.

Essential hypernatremia in its milder and more chronic forms often elevates the serum sodium only modestly, and such patients characteristically have no symptoms except for a remarkable lack of thirst. When sodium levels climb to the 160 to 170 mEq per deciliter range, however, most patients develop weakness and some, fever, as well as muscle tenderness and cramping that may progress to fatigue, ataxia, and even myoglobinuria. Mental symptoms include lethargy, anorexia, depression, and irritability. With elevations of serum sodium above 180 mEq per deciliter, most patients become confused or stuporous, and some will die. All patients with essential hypernatremia fail to demonstrate thirst, but many retain persistent habitual drinking, although at a volume insufficient to maintain a normal serum osmolality.

For poorly understood reasons, patients with essential hypernatremia lack clinical evidence of dehydration; only mild hypovolemia or even normovolemia can accompany serum sodium levels as high as 200 mEq per deciliter or more. An associated hypokalemia usually contributes to the muscular symptoms. Urine volumes may be low or normal but are always more dilute than appropriate for the serum hyperosmolarity. The administration of exogenous ADH induces a much more concentrated urine. Further evidence of abnormal ADH release to naturally occurring stimuli comes from the observation that either an acute water load or a hypertonic saline load can produce an increase in free water clearance.

The hypothalamic defect producing essential hypernatremia in man is poorly localized. Almost all affected patients have associated neurologic abnormalities, but many have lacked radiographic evidence of morphologic central nervous system abnormalities. Others have had diffuse head trauma or space-occupying lesions destroying the entire hypothalamic region by the time of death. In a few affected patients restricted lesions have involved the preoptic and tuberal region. The mechanisms of essential hypernatremia remain unsettled and may not be the same in all instances. The absence of thirst is critical, and this, along with the lack of ADH response to changes in serum osmolality, indicates that osmo- and volume receptor function is uncoupled from the behavioral and hormonal control of water balance. Baroreceptor influences on ADH secretion may remain intact. The presence of normovolemia accompanying the hypernatremia remains difficult to explain.

Treatment consists of lowering the serum sodium and raising the potassium by manipulating the diet and conditioning the patient to drink several liters of water each day regardless of thirst. Spirolactone, chlorpropamide, and the thiazide diuretics contribute to achieving these ends. More vigorous treatment of hypernatremic crises must be initiated slowly. Becuse their intracellular osmolality has climbed to a new high steady state, patients with essential hypernatremia can develop symptoms of water intoxication if rapidly hydrated, even when the serum remains hyperosmolar compared to normal.

HYPERDIPSIA AND WATER INTOXICATION. Excessive water drinking in the absence of either hypovolemia or serum hyperosmolality is termed primary hyperdipsia and must be differentiated from the compensatory hyperdipsias of conditions such as diabetes insipidus, polyuric renal failure, or diabetes mellitus. In the absence of inappropriate ADH secretion, symptoms of severe hyperdipsia, i.e., hypervolemia, hyponatremia, and clinical water intoxication with stupor, delirium, and convulsions, are infrequent. These usually develop only in patients with renal dysfunction or those who imbibe greater than 15 liters per square meter per day of water, the quantity necessary to overcome the diluting capacity of the normal kidney. Because of the ability of the kidney to excrete large amounts of free water, almost all patients with water intoxication recover with fluid restriction and proper supportive care. Some, however, convulse, and a substantial proportion of these may suffer permanent brain damage.

Causes of primary hyperdipsia include habitual drinking and drinking in response to excessive thirst. Patients with *beer drinker's hyponatremia* drink up to 6 liters or more of beer per day, slowly developing chronic hyponatremia which predisposes them to symptoms from the acute water load associated with a binge. Other examples of habitual hyperdipsia produce their symptoms simply because of a tremendous ingestion of water over a brief period. Most such patients have acute psychiatric disorders and drink excessively to overcome delusional fears. Occasionally, acute water intoxication occurs in systematically healthy persons trying to quell the epigastric burning of gastritis or in youngsters drinking huge amounts of fluids on a dare, or during tea-party games.

Martin, J. B., Reichlin, S., and Brown G. M.: Clinical Neuroendocrinology. Philadelphia, F. A. Davis Company, 1977.
Plum, F., and Van Uitert, R.: Non-endocrine diseases and disorders of the hypothalamus. Res. Publ. Assoc. Res. Nerv. Ment. Dis., Vol. 56, 1977.

Section Nine PROMINENT NEUROLOGIC SYMPTOMS AND THEIR MANAGEMENT

260. PAIN

Jerome B. Posner

INTRODUCTION

Pain is the most common symptom for which patients seek medical assistance, and chronic pain is among the most vexing problems which physicians face. Pain can have no precise definition because only the individual suffering it, not the observer, perceives it. Sir Thomas Lewis described the situation exactly when he said pain is "known to us by experience and described by illustration." Pain always has two aspects: the first is an emotionally neutral perception of a stimulus which is usually sufficiently strong to produce tissue damage; the second is an affective response to the perception of that stimulus. Pain implies damage to the organism, either physical or psychologic, and chronic pain, if untreated, will itself damage the organism. It is the physician's twofold therapeutic task to discover and treat the cause of pain and also to treat the pain itself, whether or not the underlying cause is treatable. To meet this twofold task, the physician must know something of the anatomy, physiology, and biochemistry of pain pathways.

PAIN PATHWAYS

ANATOMY AND PHYSIOLOGY. The accompanying figure outlines schematically our current understanding of pain pathways. Pain receptors in the skin and other tissues (nociceptors) are believed to be the free nerve endings of small myelinated and unmyelinated fibers. "Free nerve endings" have never been identified microscopically, nor is there complete agreement on the adequate stimulus for discharging these receptors. Current studies suggest that nociceptors are stimulated either by strong mechanical deformation or by extremes of hot or cold. It is believed that tissue damage from mechanical or thermal injury liberates chemical substances which lower the firing threshold of the mechano- and thermonociceptors so that previously innocuous mechanical or thermal stimuli produce pain. Substances liberated by tissue damage which lower the threshold of pain receptors include potassium, acetylcholine, histamine, serotonin, prostaglandins, and bradykinin. There is some evidence that the lowering of nociceptor threshold is mediated by prostaglandins. Some investigators suggest that aspirin analgesia results from that drug's ability to inhibit prostaglandin synthesis.

The nociceptors are connected to two sets of peripheral fibers: small (6 μ), thinly myelinated, "A delta" fibers which conduct at about 35 meters per second, and unmyelinated "C" fibers (1 to 2 μ) which conduct at about 0.5 meter per second. This dual set of fibers explains the phenomenon of "double pain." A noxious stimulus elicits first a sharp, pricking, well-localized pain mediated by the more rapidly conducting

fibers, and the C fibers mediate a burning, poorly localized, exceedingly unpleasant "second pain." C fiber stimulation in man at a rate of 3 per second causes almost unbearable pain. Not all A delta and C fibers are "pain fibers"; a considerable number are low threshold mechanoreceptors which presumably subserve other sensory modalities.

All primary sensory afferents have their cell bodies in the dorsal root ganglion. Pain fibers enter the spinal cord via the dorsal root, lateral to the large myelinated (touch and proprioception) fibers. Experimental section of the lateral portion of the dorsal root decreases the perception of pain but leaves large fiber modalities intact. Nociceptive fibers enter the cord, and then ascend or descend for one or two segments in the medial portion of Lissauer's tract to enter the more ventrally placed dorsal horn. Lesions of the medial portion of Lissauer's tract contract the dermatomal field of a single root, indicating that it carries excitatory fibers from adjacent roots, and lesions in the lateral portion expand the dorsal root dermatome, indicating that it carries inhibitory fibers.

The dorsal horn consists of six laminae, with lamina 1 being the most dorsal. Laminae 2 and 3 taken together are often referred to as the substantia gelatinosa, but the functional boundaries of this area are not clearly defined. Fibers subserving pain probably end in all six laminae, with laminae 1 and 5

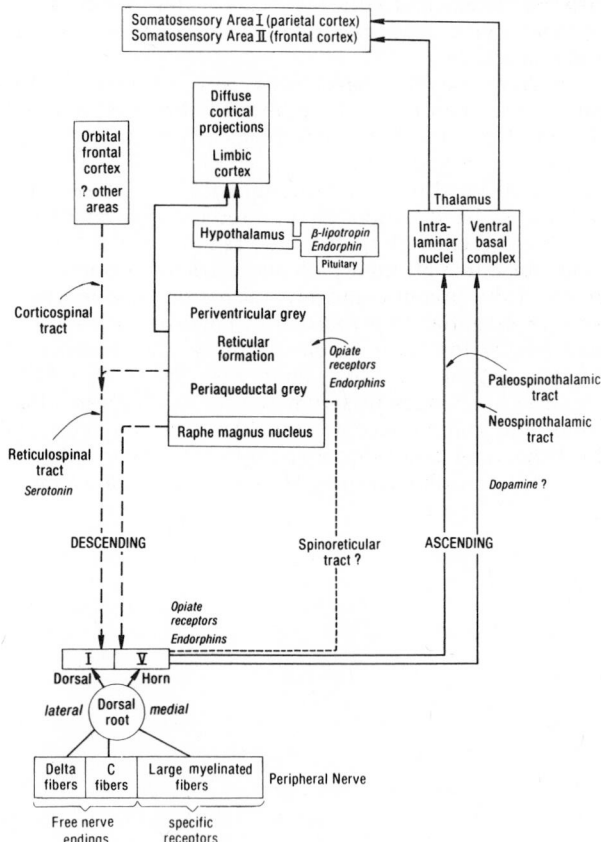

being most important. Interaction between neurons in the dorsal horn is an important site for modulating sensory input. These interactions in the substantia gelatinosa of the dorsal horn are the subject of the "gate control theory of pain," which, although highly controversial, has generated much experimentation. Melzack and Wall hypothesize that sensory fibers have two functions: (1) to carry patterned information, depending upon the specialized properties of each unit, and (2) to modulate the effectiveness of synaptic transmission between peripheral nerve and ascending spinal fibers. The first site of the putative modulating action is in the substantia gelatinosa of the spinal cord, where large fibers are presumed to activate an inhibitory system and small fibers stimulate an activating system. If large fiber stimulation is sufficient, synaptic transmission is inhibited and pain fiber activity which arrives later is less effective in exciting ascending spinal pathways. If the larger fiber stimulus is insufficient or absent, small fibers excite an action system and carry pain messages to higher centers. Descending fibers from cerebral cortex or lower structures also modulate this system.

The ascending pain pathways in the spinal cord are characteristically divided into two groups: the neospinothalamic tract, which is believed to subserve the perception of intensity and localization of pain, and the phylogenetically older paleospinothalamic tract, which is believed to subserve the arousal and emotional components of pain. The axons of the neospinothalamic tract arise from the dorsal horn (cell origin unknown), cross in the anterior commissure, and ascend in the anterolateral quadrant of the spinal cord. The axons terminate in the ventral basal complex of the thalamus, principally within the posterolateral ventral nucleus (VPL) ipsilateral to the side of their ascent. The thalamic terminations of these fibers coincide to a large extent with those of the dorsal column, and the pathway shows somatotopic localization at the thalamic level, the face and upper body being represented most medially. Third order neurons from the thalamus project to somatosensory area I (sensorimotor cortex), with the same somatotopic localization as other sensory modalities. Lesions made in the neospinothalamic pathway at either the thalamus or the cortex rarely relieve pain, and in fact lesions in this pathway at the thalamic level often lead to chronic so-called "thalamic pain." The paleospinothalamic tract, whose cells of origin in the dorsal horn receive C fiber input, also crosses in the anterior commissure and ascends in the spinal cord closely applied to but more ventral than the neospinothalamic tract. Many of the fibers of the paleospinothalamic tract give collaterals to the reticular formation of the brainstem, but some reach the thalamus, terminating in several nuclei, particularly the nucleus centralis lateralis and the intralaminar nuclei. None of these fibers project to center median despite the fact that lesions in this nucleus have been reported to relieve pain. The intralaminar nuclei of the thalamus project to somatosensory area II both ipsilaterally and contralaterally with some degree of somatotopic localization. The intralaminar nuclei also project diffusely, affecting large regions of both the frontal and parietal lobes. There is no somatotopic localization in projection. A third spinal ascending pathway which may play some role in nociception is the spinoreticular pathway, also referred to as the archispinal-lemniscal pathway, and phylogenetically the oldest of the nociceptive pathways. The pathway consists of projections from small myelinated and unmyelinated fibers. It originates in the dorsal horn and ascends via multiple synapses in the dorsal horn, mostly ipsilaterally, but to a lesser degree contralaterally, to terminate in the brainstem reticular formation, particularly that of the pons and medulla. The role this pathway plays in the conscious perception of pain in man is unclear, but it is unlikely to be major because spinal cord hemisection in humans usually completely eliminates pain contralaterally, thus ruling out a significant contribution by ipsilateral pathways. Such a multisynaptic ipsilateral pathway may explain, however, why some anterolateral cordotomies fail.

Fibers originating in the brainstem reticular formation receive input from several sources, including almost certainly the paleospinothalamic and spinoreticular pathways, and ascend in a polysynaptic projection to wide areas of the thalamus. The anatomy and physiology of the reticular formation is becoming increasingly important in our understanding of pain perception, because recent evidence (see below) suggests that electrical stimulation of this area produces analgesia and that the site of the action of narcotic drugs is here.

Descending pathways from fibers which originate in the orbital-frontal cortex and probably descend via corticospinal tracts, and fibers which originate in the midbrain reticular formation and raphe nucleus of the medulla and descend via polysynaptic pathways, both reach the dorsal horn to modulate input to all the laminae of the dorsal horn, particularly lamina 5. These descending fibers may influence activity at the dorsal horn level via either pre- or postsynaptic contacts and may be either facilitory or inhibitory. Electrical stimulation of the ventrolateral portion of a central gray substance of the mesencephalon and periventricular gray matter of the hypothalamus produces a profound analgesia in both animals and man, reversed by the opiate antagonist naloxone. There is no interference with motor function or the organism's responsiveness to other sensory stimuli. The anatomic substrate for these descending neural inhibitory systems is unclear, but their potency is striking.

BIOCHEMISTRY AND PHARMACOLOGY. A stereospecific receptor for narcotics has been identified in brain. This "opiate receptor" exists in highest concentrations in brainstem reticular formation, thalamus, and limbic system, the areas where narcotic analgesics are believed to act. The receptor binds both narcotic agonists and antagonists. In addition, several peptides called collectively the endorphins, which have morphine-like properties, have been isolated from brain. These analgesic peptides, enkephalin and β-endorphin, are smaller molecules of the pituitary hormone β-lipotropin and are believed to be neurotransmitters in pathways of pain or other behavior. The highest concentrations of both substances are in the same area as the opiate receptor. These substances bind to the opiate receptor, and can be displaced by opiate antagonists. They increase in concentration following electrical stimulation of the brainstem.

Another recent discovery has been the ability to dissociate biochemically opiate analgesia from opiate tolerance. Cyclohexamide, a protein synthesis inhibitor, blocks the development of tolerance to morphine in animals when given at doses that do not affect the acute response to morphine. Cyclic AMP and gamma-aminobutyric acid (GABA) accelerate the development of tolerance and physical dependence but at the same time decrease morphine analgesia. The ability to dissociate these two aspects of opiates biochemically suggests the possibility that a substance may be developed which will produce analgesia without the unwanted side effects of physical tolerance and dependency.

Other neurotransmitters, especially dopamine and serotonin, also appear to be important in pain biochemistry. Dopamine enhances the effect of both morphine analgesia and brainstem stimulation and may be the transmitter which subserves ascending inhibitory pathways to the brainstem reticular formation. Serotonin also has an inhibiting effect on pain perception and is probably the transmitter of descending inhibitory pathways which arise in the raphe nucleus of the medulla. GABA may be an inhibitory transmitter modulating pain at the level of the dorsal horn of the spinal cord.

DIAGNOSIS OF PAINFUL DISORDERS

Pain is either "acute" or "chronic." The point at which acute pain becomes chronic pain varies, but pain of over six months' duration is usually considered chronic. Several clinical features differentiate acute from chronic pain. In patients suffering severe acute pain, the autonomic nervous system is hyperactive, with tachycardia, hypertension, diaphoresis, mydriasis, and pallor. These autonomic signs serve as objective evidence of the patient's pain. In patients suffering from chronic pain, however, the autonomic nervous system adapts and the signs of autonomic hyperactivity disappear. The lack of such objective evidence forces the physician to rely upon the complaints of the patient and may lead the physician to believe that the patient's complaints are exaggerated. Since there are no reliable objective tests to assess chronic pain, the physician *must* believe the patient's report, taking into consideration his age, his cultural background, his environment, and other psychologic circumstances known to alter reaction to pain. *In general, the physician is wise to accept at face value the patient's report of the severity of his pain unless there is overwhelming evidence to the contrary.*

A thorough history, general physical examination, and careful neurologic examination are imperative in any patient complaining of pain. Often the description of the nature and distribution of the pain is so characteristic (e.g., trigeminal neuralgia or tabetic lightning pains) (see below) that it allows no other diagnosis. At times the history is so vague and bizarre and the distribution of pain so unanatomic as to suggest that the pain is a somatic delusion and not due to structural or even physiologic abnormality. Inquiry should be made concerning (1) the temporal pattern of pain, (2) its distribution, (3) exacerbating factors, and (4) relieving factors.

For example, headache beginning early in the morning before arising suggests increased intracranial pressure, whereas headache occurring late in the day is more suggestive of tension. Back pain and sciatica made worse by sitting or walking suggest disc disease, whereas back pain and sciatica which are worse while in bed suggest intraspinal tumor. Pain limited to a specific area is usually due to organ disease, whereas pain distributed in the distribution of a peripheral nerve or nerve root suggests that the nerve itself is diseased. Back pain and sciatica exacerbated by cough or sneeze suggest intraspinal disease, whereas similar pain not exacerbated by cough or sneeze suggests disease in the pelvis. Pain in the back or legs exacerbated by straight leg raising suggests disease of the nervous system, whereas a similar pain exacerbated by rotating the hips suggests pelvic or hip disease. Most pain caused by structural disease is relieved at least to some degree by analgesic drugs, whereas psychogenic pain often is not. Skeletal muscle relaxants or local heat may relieve pain of musculoskeletal origin. Both psychogenic and organic pain are relieved to some extent by distraction and a pleasurable environment. Both are exacerbated by anxiety or stress.

A careful psychiatric history, looking particularly for signs and symptoms of depression, should be elicited from all patients. Specifically, physicians should inquire about the degree to which pain has interfered with the patient's activities, whether he is having difficulty sleeping, and whether there is a change in appetite or bowel habits. Early morning awakening, anorexia, and constipation are somatic manifestations of depression, and either may be caused by chronic pain or may exacerbate the effects of the pain.

A general physical examination must be performed. Both the physical and laboratory examination should begin with the assumption that the site of pathologic change is at the site of pain. The painful areas should be examined for swelling and redness as well as for any obvious deformity. (The pain of herpes zoster usually precedes the rash, and occasionally on examination one may note only the faintest reddening of the skin in a dermatomal distribution.) The areas reported as painful should be palpated, the temperature estimated, and points of tenderness sought. (If the site of pain is in a soft tissue, bone, or joint, it should be tender to palpation as well as spontaneously painful.) Joints should be taken through a full range of motion and the effect of movement on the pain assessed. Nerve trunks going to the extremities should be palpated and stretched by movement of that extremity (e.g., straight leg raising; abduction and extension of the arm). Inflamed and compressed nerve roots and nerve plexuses are more painful when stretched. A careful neurologic examination must also be performed. If there are neurologic abnormalities (e.g., weakness, sensory loss, reflex changes) in the painful part, one can infer that nervous system disease is responsible for the pain. The absence of specific neurologic abnormalities on first examination does not guarantee, however, that the nervous system is free of disease, because the process may simply not have advanced beyond the stage of selectively involving pain pathways.

Finally, laboratory examinations are performed. If the site of disease appears to be in bones or joints, x-rays of those structures or radioisotope scans may localize it. First attention should be paid to the local site of pain but the physician should acquaint himself with the common referred patterns of pain (e.g., hip disease commonly causes knee pain, cardiac pain is frequently referred to the ulnar aspect of the arm and forearm, the pain of renal colic may be felt primarily in the groin and testicle, and pain resulting from disease of the throat may be referred to the ear).

Referred pain is pain perceived at a site remote from the source of the disturbance. Usually, referred pain is cutaneous and evoked by disease of deep structures innervated by the same dermatome. Referred pain may be associated with cutaneous hyperalgesia and even relieved by procaine injection into the area of referral. When pain is referred to the same dermatome or myotome as innervates the diseased structure (e.g., pain down the medial aspect of the arm [T1-T2] produced by myocardial infarction or angina pectoris), it is often helpful in diagnosis. However, pain is sometimes referred at a great distance from the primary site to segments not similarly innervated, and there the mechanism is perplexing (e.g., anginal pain referred to the jaw). Various theories have been suggested to account for referred pain. Such theories as division of the same nerve into deep and superficial branches, release of chemical mediators in the nervous system, and convergence of cutaneous and visceral nerves into common synaptic pools at the spinal cord all explain the dermatomal referral of pain but fail to explain pain at remote sites.

MANAGEMENT OF CHRONIC PAIN

In some patients, pain is best managed by treating the underlying disorder (e.g., steroids for giant cell arteritis relieve headache and muscle pain promptly; radiation therapy for bone pain caused by cancer is often helpful). In others, a particular kind of pain has a particular treatment (see Specific Pain Syndromes, below), but in many patients the pain is chronic and the physician is able neither to treat the underlying disturbances nor to offer specific therapy for that type of pain. In treating this type of chronic and severe pain, certain general principles should be followed:

1. The pain should be treated by the simplest means which will relieve it, but all efforts should be made to relieve it. Chronic pain is both physically debilitating and psychologically demoralizing. It should be treated by the physician as a serious symptom and all efforts made to relieve it to the extent that the patient is comfortable.

2. Pain should be treated early. There is both clinical and experimental evidence that if chronic pain goes untreated for an extended period of time, abnormal excitatory states arise in the central nervous system so that treatment directed toward peripheral structures which initially would have relieved the pain are no longer effective. In general, the earlier one undertakes to treat chronic pain, the more successful one is.

3. Pain should be treated promptly. Clinical evidence suggests that if analgesic drug doses are spaced so far apart that severe pain recurs, the analgesic becomes less effective. Thus patients should be encouraged to take analgesic agents when the pain first reappears rather than wait until it becomes unbearable.

4. Various treatments of pain are additive and should be used together rather than separately.

5. Narcotic drugs should be used with discrimination, but they should not be withheld if there is no alternative effective therapy. Long-term use of narcotics produces tolerance and physical dependence. These effects should not be confused with "addiction," which implies both a psychologic dependence and drug abuse for effects other than analgesia. The percentage of patients who actually become "addicted" to narcotics given for pain is unclear. Many physicians are impressed that narcotic "addiction" is unusual in patients treated for pain if the pain is later relieved by other means. The side effects of narcotic drugs include *tolerance*, which requires gradually increasing doses to maintain analgesia; *physical dependence*, which means that narcotics must be withdrawn gradually if they are to be discontinued after prolonged use; *constipation*, which requires careful attention to bowel function, including the use of stool softeners, laxatives and enemas; and at times *somnolence*. All narcotic drugs produce some degree of somnolence; in individual patients, if somnolence is a problem, lower doses should be given more frequently, amphetamines added, or several different narcotics tried, because the patient may tolerate a particular drug better than another in comparable doses. Other than those mentioned, the side effects of narcotic drugs are few. Methadone maintenance programs as well as other long-term studies have proved that patients can take narcotics in large doses over long periods of time without physical damage and continue to function usefully in society. Rarely, multifocal myoclonus and seizures may occur following repetitive doses of meperidine from accumulation of the metabolite normeperidine. Substitution of an alternative narcotic alleviates the seizures.

6. Psychogenic factors always play a role in chronic pain — the pain is more severe when the patient is anxious and stressed and less severe when he is relaxed. The physician must assess the psychologic factors in any patient with pain. However, no patient should be diagnosed as having psychogenic pain until an exhaustive examination has ruled out structural disease. Depression, whether endogenous or reactive, should be treated with antidepressant drugs. These may be effective in relieving pain by themselves, but more frequently are effective as analgesic adjuvants. Psychiatric consultation is necessary if psychogenic factors are causing the pain.

7. Placebo effects are important. In most clinical studies, about one third of patients report relief of pain when given a placebo, although the extent of relief is rarely equal to that achieved by analgesic drugs. The physician can utilize a patient's desire to be free of pain by approaching the therapy in an enthusiastic and reassuring manner. It is less important whether it is the placebo or the drug which was effective than that the patient be relieved of his pain.

8. Multidisciplinary pain clinics which diagnose and treat intractable pain exist in many centers and should be utilized to evaluate and treat severe problems.

Analgesic Agents

Analgesics are drugs which decrease pain without causing loss of consciousness. Analgesics (see accompanying table) can be divided clinically into those which are suitable for mild pain, generally non-narcotic agents; those suitable for moderate pain, usually narcotics or narcotic antagonists with low addiction potential; and those which are suitable for severe pain, generally narcotic agents except for methotrimeprazine. The mild analgesics appear to act peripherally by blocking the pain chemoreceptors and perhaps by relieving inflammation. There is also evidence for a central effect of some of these drugs as well.

The physician's strategy in treating chronic pain should begin with the mildest agents and add stronger agents or analgesic adjuvants only when mild agents fail to work. Drugs should always be given in sufficient amounts and at sufficiently short intervals to achieve relief of pain. Treatment should begin with aspirin or acetaminophen, 600 mg every three to four hours. If the pain is due to musculoskeletal spasm or if anxiety is prominent, one of the mild tranquilizers (diazepam or meprobamate) can be added. If the pain fails to respond to this mild regimen, one adds drugs used for the treatment of moderate pain (e.g., codeine or pentazocine). If the pain is still unrelieved and the physician satisfies himself that psychogenic factors are not responsible, the agents used for moderate pain should be discontinued, and agents used for severe pain should be added to the mild analgesic. Levorphanol, 2 mg, or methadone, 10 mg, every three to four hours is probably the agent of choice if oral drugs are to be used, and morphine, 10 mg every three to four hours, if a subcutaneous or intramuscular agent is necessary. If the pain continues as a chronic and unremitting problem not relieved by these drugs, or if anxiety and depression appear to be a major contributor to the pain, a major tranquilizer (phenothiazine) or antidepressant agent, or both, may be added to the mild analgesics and narcotic agents. At times a satisfactory resolution of an intractable problem may be achieved by the combined use of a narcotic and non-narcotic analgesic and a tranquilizer or an antidepressant. The physician must be careful to adjust the doses of each so as to produce maximal pain relief with minimal sedation and unpleasant side effects. The physician should be prepared to increase the dose of those particular drugs

Analgesic Agents

Type	Generic Name (Proprietary)	Usual Dose*		Comment
		Oral (mg)	Subcutaneous or Intramuscular (mg)	
Some agents used for mild to moderate pain	Aspirin	600 q 3–4 h		Side effects of dyspepsia and GI bleeding
	Acetaminophen (Tylenol)	650 q 3–4 h		Equal to aspirin but without GI side effects; less anti-inflammatory effect
	Phenacetin (aceto-phenetidin)	600 q 3–4 h		Probable renal toxicity with chronic use
	Dextropropoxyphene (Darvon)	65 q 3–4 h		Weak narcotic related to methadone, probably not superior to aspirin
	Indomethacin (Indocin)	25 qid		Useful only for pain associated with inflammation, probably not superior to aspirin
Some agents used for moderate to severe pain	Codeine	1 tab q 4–6 h	130 q 4–6 h	Narcotic with low addiction potential; additive effect if used with mild analgesics
	Oxycodone (with acetaminophen = Percocet)	5 q 4–6 h		Preferred over codeine by many patients
	Pentazocine (Talwin)	30–50 q 4–6 h	60 q 4 h	Narcotic antagonist (produces withdrawal in patients physically dependent on narcotics); low addiction potential; hallucinations and dysphoria in doses >80 mg IM or 200 mg PO
Some agents used for severe pain: narcotics and antagonists	Levorphanol (Levo-dromoran)	2 q 3–4 h	2 q 3–4 h	Long-acting oral narcotic
	Morphine		10 q 3–4 h	The standard narcotic agent for treatment of pain
	Meperidine (Demerol)	50–100 q 3–4 h	75 q 2–4 h	More rapid onset and shorter duration of action than morphine; possibly less spasmogenic and better for pain of biliary tree
	Methadone (Dolophine)	10–20 q 4 h	10–15 q 3–4 h	Long-acting oral narcotic; possibly less sedative effect than morphine
Non-narcotic	Methotrimeprazine (Levoprome)		20 q 4–6 h	Phenothiazine; no tolerance; produces sedation and postural hypotension
	Dextroamphetamine	10 q 6 h		Doubles narcotic effects and decreases somnolence in postoperative pain
Some agents used as analgesic adjuvants (probably little or no analgesic properties per se but used to relieve anxiety and/or depression)	Minor tranquilizers—muscle relaxants: Diazepam (Valium)	5 qid		Useful with mild analgesics for acute or subacute pain associated with muscle spasm and/or anxiety
	Meprobamate (Miltown)	200–400 qid		
	Antidepressants: Amitriptyline (Elavil)	75–100 hs		Reported useful in pain associated with depressive symptoms (esp. atypical facial pain); may be useful when combined with analgesic agents for chronic pain of many kinds; may cause oversedation or anticholinergic symptoms
	Phenelzine (Nardil)	15 tid		
	Imipramine (Tofranil)	25 qid		
	Phenothiazines: Chlorpromazine (Thorazine)	25–50 qid		Reported useful in pain associated with anxiety or depression and in some specific pain syndromes (e.g., thalamic pain, postherpetic pain); these drugs may have analgesic properties or potentiate analgesics; fluphenazine and amitriptyline have been reported to relieve postherpetic pain; may cause oversedation, depression, Parkinson-like syndrome, hypotension, or urinary retention
	Promazine (Sparine)	50–100 qid		
	Promethazine (Phenergan)	25–50 hs		
	Fluphenazine (Prolixin)	1–3 qd		

*Intramuscular dose of narcotics is equivalent to 10 mg of morphine. Since tolerance develops to these drugs, doses must be increased with continued use. Oral doses are not equivalent to intramuscular doses but represent usual starting doses.

to which tolerance develops as is necessary to control pain. No tolerance develops to non-narcotic analgesics.

NON-NARCOTIC MILD ANALGESICS. Aspirin and acetaminophen (Tylenol, Tempra) are the most useful of the mild analgesics. Either aspirin or acetaminophen may be given in doses of 600 mg every three to four hours, either alone for relief of mild pain or in conjunction with more potent drugs for relief of severe pain. The degree of pain relief is linearly related to the logarithm of the dose of the drug, higher doses being not significantly more effective until doses are reached which produce unpleasant side effects. The side effects of aspirin (clotting disorders, dyspepsia, and gastrointestinal bleeding) make acetaminophen a safer drug and probably the drug of choice. There is no evidence that aspi-

rin and acetaminophen together are more effective than either one alone, but either aspirin or acetaminophen plus codeine is more effective than codeine alone. There is no evidence that the other mild, non-narcotic analgesics are superior in any way to the two most commonly used drugs.

NARCOTIC ANALGESICS. Tolerance develops to all narcotics. Thus there is no set dose of the drug, and with continued usage the dose must increase. *The physician is wise to learn to handle two or three of these drugs and use those consistently rather than using all the drugs occasionally.* He must be prepared to use more than one, because some patients find that side effects of the drugs make one preferable to another. Morphine, 10 mg intramuscularly, is the standard by which other narcotic analgesics are judged. Intramuscular morphine has its maximal effect in 60 to 90 minutes and lasts between three and six hours. It requires 60 mg or more of morphine orally to give the same analgesic effect as 10 mg intramuscularly. Levorphanol has a relatively high oral/parenteral ratio for analgesia; 2 mg given intramuscularly is equal to 10 mg of morphine intramuscularly, and 4 mg given orally is equal in total effect to 10 mg of morphine given intramuscularly. Methadone also has a relatively high oral/intramuscular potency ratio; 10 mg intramuscularly or 20 mg orally equals 10 mg of morphine intramuscularly. Codeine and dihydrocodeine are also effective orally and are generally used in doses of 50 to 60 mg as a mild analgesic. They often cannot be used to relieve severe pain, because side effects preclude high doses. Pentazocine can be used as a mild analgesic when given in doses of 30 mg and is equal to morphine if given in intramuscular doses of 60 mg. It is a weak narcotic antagonist with a high analgesic potential and has a dependence potential substantially less than that of morphine or meperidine (Demerol). Pentazocine is not included in the Federal Controlled Substances Act. However, hallucinatory effects and toxic psychoses have been noted in its users, and like the other narcotics it can produce respiratory depression. Dextropropoxyphene (Darvon) is structurally related to methadone and is a prescription drug not subject to the Controlled Substances Act of 1970. It is a weak narcotic with a low analgesic potential.

OTHER AGENTS. The phenothiazine methotrimeprazine (Levoprome) is a potent analgesic agent. Given intramuscularly in doses of 20 mg, it is equivalent to 10 mg of morphine intramuscularly. The drug is an effective antiemetic, and does not suppress cough or respiration but does produce sedation and postural hypotension, making it useful only for hospitalized patients.

Sedative and anticonvulsant drugs as well as other phenothiazines have been utilized by some physicians in the treatment of chronic pain, particularly that associated with depression or other psychologic symptoms. The antidepressant amitriptyline (Elavil), given orally in a single dose of 75 mg at night (when it helps counter insomnia) or orally in divided doses of 25 mg three to four times a day, has been effective in relieving some chronic pain or in decreasing the narcotic dose required. In conjunction with the phenothiazine, fluphenazine, the drug has been reported useful in the treatment of postherpetic neuralgia (see below).

Dextroamphetamine has been reported to enhance the effectiveness of narcotic agents in postoperative patients while counteracting the undesirable side effects of sedation and possibly respiratory depression. Whether the drug is also an effective adjuvant for chronic pain remains to be established.

Physical Methods of Pain Relief

There are a bewildering array of physical methods designed to relieve pain. These vary from simply rubbing a partially denervated area with a soft towel to placing radiofrequency lesions stereotactically in the thalamic and hypothalamic reticular formations. The simpler procedures can be carried out by the general physician or even by the patient; the more complicated ones, depending on their nature, demand the expertise of a skilled anesthesiologist or neurosurgeon.

The physician's approach to the use of physical methods for intractable pain should embody certain general principles:

1. Nondestructive procedures should be tried first. Cutaneous stimulation, either by hand or by battery-driven electrodes, or local anesthetic blocks in conjunction with analgesic drugs may be effective in relieving pain. If these simple procedures fail, the services of an anesthesiologist or neurosurgeon should be procured and a treatment plan embodying the use of analgesics and physical procedures outlined.

2. The least destructive procedure should be tried first. In general, the procedure should be directed first at the peripheral nervous system, and only if this fails, at the spinal cord, brainstem, or cerebrum. Quantitative data on the incidence of pain relief and its duration are sketchy for most of these procedures and seem to vary from center to center, depending on the skill and enthusiasm of the investigator reporting.

3. Thus the choice of a particular procedure often depends not only on the nature of the patient's disease but on the particular skills, experience, and bias of the physician.

4. If and only if a full trial of analgesic drugs has failed should destructive procedures for relieving pain be tried. These destructive procedures can and should be used in conjunction with analgesic drugs, because, even if the drugs have failed to relieve pain on their own, they may act synergistically with physical methods. Nerve blocks and surgical procedures often yield only temporary relief in patients with chronic pain. Thus many of the enthusiastic reports in the literature refer to patients followed for only a short period of time. When the patients are followed over months or years, the pain which was relieved shortly after the procedure often returns and is as bad as or worse than it was prior to the operation. For this reason, patients with cancer who are not expected to live a long time are often better candidates for surgical destructive procedures than are patients with pain originating from more benign conditions.

5. Patients with chronic pain being considered for destructive procedures must be thoroughly evaluated psychiatrically. If psychogenic factors play a major role in the genesis of pain, surgical procedures will not help, and often the pain will be exacerbated after surgical intervention.

CUTANEOUS STIMULATION. Cutaneous stimulation of a painful area, particularly one which has been partly denervated, is often effective in relieving pain. This procedure, which probably has its greatest use in the treatment of postherpetic neuralgia, consists of rubbing the painful area with a soft cloth or terrycloth towel, almost constantly at first but then with gradually lengthening intervals of rest between rubbing periods. Often a period of rubbing will yield relief which long outlasts the stimulus, and continued intermittent rubbings may totally relieve the pain. The "gate theory" offers an explanation of the rubbing phenomenon, i.e., rubbing stimulates large fiber afferents which may close the gate against incoming pain fibers. Whatever the explanation, the procedure is often useful in the treatment of painful phantom limbs and in chronic cutaneous or extremity pain after surgery. Recently, battery-powered electrical stimulators which give one control over the frequency and intensity of the cutaneous stimulation have become available. The electrodes of the stimulator may be placed over the painful area or over the peripheral nerve supplying the painful area, and stimulation using an intensity and frequency which produces a vibratory sensation is applied.

ACUPUNCTURE ANALGESIA. Acupuncture analgesia has become increasingly popular in the past few years, but no carefully controlled studies have reported on its usefulness. A needle is placed under the skin, often in a place remote from the painful site but at times into the painful site, and the area is stimulated either by twirling the needle or by electrically vibrating it. Recent experiments in animals and man suggest that the analgesic effect of acupuncture is reversed by naloxone, leading to the hypothesis that the mechanism of acupuncture analgesia is through enkephalin release. The usefulness of acupuncture in Western medicine is still not clear.

NERVE BLOCKS. Direct block of peripheral nerves, using either anesthetic agents (lidocaine) or neurolytic agents (phenol), has been popular in the treatment of thoracic and abdominal pain, particularly that pain which follows surgery. Blocks may be dangerous if used in the extremities, because they may paralyze as well as anesthetize; but in areas where they can be used, relief of pain sometimes long outlasts the period of anesthesia. The procedure is a simple one when performed by a skilled anesthesiologist.

Subarachnoid injection of anesthetics or neurolytics directed at nerve roots has been utilized in patients with widespread and intractable pain. Phenol can likewise be injected into the subarachnoid space and directed at particular nerve roots by positioning the patient. The mechanism of action is destruction of nerve fibers; if material spills into the cauda equina, bladder and bowel dysfunction are common. The relief of pain may only be transient.

OTHER PROCEDURES. Several nondestructive procedures directed at the affective component of pain are currently in use. These include not only psychotherapy and hypnotism but also more recently developed techniques of biofeedback and operant conditioning. The latter two methods have been gaining in popularity, but their role in the treatment of chronic pain is not yet certain. Neither psychotherapy nor hypnotism has been particularly useful in patients with chronic pain due to organic disease.

Each nonsurgical procedure directed at the *peripheral nervous system* has its surgical counterpart. In patients with chronic pain such as that which follows herpes zoster, the skin has been undercut in an attempt to totally denervate it. Postoperative infection is a complication at times and the pain relief is transient, thus contraindicating this procedure. Peripheral nerves can be cut, particularly in the thorax and abdomen, but this should not be done unless prior nerve blocks have indicated that it will be effective and sustained. The peripheral nerves regenerate after a time, and often the pain returns. Dorsal root ganglia in the thorax and abdomen can be removed for chronic pain or the dorsal roots themselves cut. This procedure also should not be done unless nerve blocks have indicated that it will be effective. Several roots must be cut off either side of the painful area if one is to achieve long-term pain relief.

SURGERY OF THE CENTRAL NERVOUS SYSTEM. There are three kinds of surgical procedures directed at the central nervous system for the relief of pain. *The first type,* a direct outgrowth of the gate control theory, involves the placement of electrodes to stimulate large fiber pathways, thus "closing the gate" against pain fibers. Electrodes have been placed on the skin, along peripheral nerves, and along spinal cord pathways. A few years ago there was some enthusiasm about electrodes surgically placed on the dorsal columns with a subcutaneous power pack which would allow the patient to control frequency and intensity of stimulation. Failure of this method to give prolonged relief and the morbidity of the procedure have led neurosurgeons to abandon it. More recently, electrodes have been placed stereotactically in the periventricular gray matter, again using a power source controlled by the patient. Total body analgesia with increase in pain threshold has been observed for three to eight hours following stimulation, but tolerance develops to the analgesic effect. This procedure is still an experimental one, and its effectiveness requires further evaluation.

The second type of procedure destroys pain pathways in the spinal cord, brainstem, or brain. Spinothalamic tracts can be destroyed either surgically, after a laminectomy (open cordotomy), or by the placement of a radiofrequency lesion through a needle (percutaneous cordotomy). These procedures are particularly effective in relieving pain in the lower extremities and have the advantage that, although pain and temperature sensations are lost, cutaneous sensation and motor power remain intact. At times the level of anesthesia approaches within one or two cord segments of the level at which the destruction lesion is placed, but often there is a drop to about five segments below the placement of the lesion. Thus the lesion must be placed considerably higher than the site of pain. If the lesion is placed unilaterally, pain often reappears on the other side of the body, necessitating another lesion. Bilateral lesions considerably enhance the risk of motor weakness and bladder and bowel dysfunction, but in skilled hands these risks are low. Occasional patients with bilateral percutaneous lesions in cervical cord suffer loss of automatic respiratory function (Ondine's curse). Percutaneous spinothalamic tract cordotomy, when done by a skilled technician, produces satisfactory pain relief in 70 to 90 per cent of patients, with a small mortality (1 to 5 per cent) and morbidity. The procedure is particularly useful in patients with terminal cancer, because the pain relief is usually sustained until death and the procedure does not require a major operation. An analogous lesion in the low brainstem placed in the descending tract of the trigeminal nerve has been reported useful in relieving facial pain. Pain and temperature sensation are lost, but cutaneous sensation remains intact. Lesions have been placed in the spinothalamic tract of the midbrain, so-called mesencephalic tractotomies. The dangers of this lesion are considerably greater than those of spinal cord lesions, and most centers have abandoned the procedure. Several neurosurgeons have placed lesions in the thalamus, both in the ventral-basal complex and in the interlaminar nuclei. Although good results are occasionally reported for both, the ventral-basal lesions appear only to produce transient relief of pain, whereas those placed in the intralaminar nuclei at the end-point of the paleospinothalamic tract appear to be more successful. There are rare reports of removal of sensory portions of the parietal lobe in relieving chronic pain, but the rarity of the reports implies the ineffectiveness of the treatment.

The third surgical method directed at pain relief is to place lesions in the frontal lobe, particularly the limbic projection to the frontal areas, in an attempt to alter the patient's psychologic response to pain rather than alter the pain pathways themselves. Several different surgical procedures, including frontal lobotomy, frontal leukotomy, and cingulotomy, have been tried with varied success. These procedures, which alter the patient's personality as well as his suffering, probably deserve trial only when all other procedures have failed.

Good statistical data comparing the various surgical procedures for pain are difficult to come by. The best extant data indicate that initial relief of pain occurs with almost all procedures in 50 to 80 per cent of patients, with spinothalamic tract cordotomies yielding the best results. Longer-term follow-up suggests that considerably less than 50 per cent of patients achieve lasting relief, in many series the figure being as low as 20 per cent. Patients with malignant disease seem to have greater pain relief even initially than those with more benign conditions, probably because selection of patients with benign conditions often includes many with psychogenic pain.

SOME SPECIFIC PAIN SYNDROMES

TRIGEMINAL NEURALGIA. Trigeminal neuralgia (tic douloureux) is a disease characterized by sudden, lightning-like paroxysms of pain in the distribution of one or more divisions of the trigeminal nerve. The pain is usually unassociated with identifiable structural disease of the nervous system (idiopathic trigeminal neuralgia) but occasionally may be a symptom of a gasserian ganglion tumor, of multiple sclerosis, or of a brainstem infarct involving the descending root of the trigeminal nerve (symptomatic trigeminal neuralgia).

The history is diagnostic. The pain occurs as brief, lightning-like stabs, frequently precipitated by touching a trigger zone around the lips or the buccal cavity. At times, talking, eating, or brushing the teeth serves as a trigger. The pains rarely last longer than seconds, and each burst is followed by a refractory period of several seconds to a minute in which no further pain can be precipitated. The pains, however, often occur in clusters so that the patient may report that each pain lasts for hours. The pain is limited to the distribution of the trigeminal nerve, usually affecting the second and third division or both. Spontaneous remissions and exacerbations are common, the exacerbations tending to occur in spring and fall. Between paroxysms of pain, the patient is asymptomatic. Tic pain rarely occurs at night. In idiopathic trigeminal neuralgia, the neurologic examination is entirely normal. In symptomatic trigeminal neuralgia, there may be sensory changes in the distribution of the trigeminal nerve, and such a finding should prompt a careful search for structural disease of the nervous system.

Carbamazepine is the drug of choice for the treatment of trigeminal neuralgia. This anticonvulsant drug is given in doses varying from 400 to 800 mg a day, but because of its sedative properties the initial dose is 100 mg twice daily, gradually increased to the required maintenance dose. No more than 1200 mg should be taken daily. The drug is not an analgesic and is only effective for specific kinds of pain such as trigeminal neuralgia, glossopharyngeal neuralgia, and the light-ning pains of tabes dorsalis. Rarely, aplastic anemia has been reported, and complete blood counts are procured prior to the initiation of therapy and at intervals thereafter. Other side effects include dizziness and sedation. Phenytoin in doses of 400 mg a day is also effective in trigeminal neuralgia but less so than carbamazepine. There is no evidence that the two drugs are synergistic. If medical treatment fails, section of the nerve root proximal to the ganglion affords permanent relief. Local anesthesia of the ganglion or the peripheral branches of the nerve at some time prior to surgery is desirable because some patients find the anesthesia produced by nerve section less tolerable than the pain itself.

GLOSSOPHARYNGEAL NEURALGIA. Glossopharyngeal neuralgia is characterized by pain similar to that of trigeminal neuralgia but in the distribution of the glossopharyngeal and vagus nerves. The trigger zone is usually in the tonsil or posterior pharynx, and the pain spreads toward the angle of the jaw and the ear. Occasional patients suffer cardiac slowing or arrest during these attacks as a result of the intense afferent discharge over the glossopharyngeal nerve. Carbamazepine is often effective, but if it fails, glossopharyngeal nerve roots are sectioned in the posterior fossa. Symptomatic glossopharyngeal neuralgia is occasionally the presenting complaint in a patient with a tonsillar tumor, and careful examination of the pharynx and tonsillar fossa for mass lesions must be carried out.

LIGHTNING PAINS OF TABES. The lightning pains of tabes are acute, short-lived pains in the trunk or lower extremities which occur with structural lesions of the dorsal roots and particularly with tabes dorsalis. Lightning pains are analogous to trigeminal and glossopharyngeal neuralgia. Like those two disorders, the pain usually responds to carbamazepine. There is no surgical therapy. (See Ch. 171.)

"REFLEX SYMPATHETIC DYSTROPHIES." This is a term which applies to pain, hyperalgesia, hyperesthesia, and autonomic changes, usually after injury to an extremity. If the injury has involved a peripheral nerve, particularly the sciatic or median nerve, the syndrome is called *causalgia* (hot pain). If the injury has not involved a peripheral nerve, such terms as post-traumatic painful osteoporosis, Sudeck's atrophy, post-traumatic spreading neuralgia, minor causalgia, shoulder-hand syndrome, and reflex dystrophy have been applied, the particular term depending on the outstanding symptom. Whatever the term, the pathophysiology of all these disorders appears to be the same, as do their clinical manifestations and response to therapy.

The disorder may follow either a major or minor injury to an extremity, after which severe pain, usually of a burning quality, develops in the extremity. The pain is continuous but exacerbated by emotional stress and is associated with severe hyperpathia, so that moving or touching the limb is often intolerable. At first the pain is localized to the site of the injury or the distribution of the nerve injured, but with time it spreads, often to involve the entire extremity. Along with the pain there are vasomotor changes, first of vasodilatation (warm and dry skin) but later a change to vasoconstriction (edema, cyanosis, cool skin). Other autonomic disturbances include either hyperhidrosis or hypohidrosis; trophic changes in the skin, subcutaneous tissue, and muscles; and osteoporosis. The entire symptom complex is rarely present in any one patient, and one sign or symptom usually predominates. Untreated, severe reflex sympathetic dystrophy leads to muscle atrophy, fixation of joints, osteoporosis, and a useless extremity. The exact mechanism of the pain and sympathetic changes is not understood.

Treatment should be undertaken as early as possible, because there is evidence that the earlier the treatment, the more effective it will be. Treatment begins with local anesthetic infiltration of the painful site, using 2 to 5 ml of 0.5 per cent lidocaine, repeated frequently enough to maintain relief of pain. When local measures fail, most patients are relieved by sympathetic block with lidocaine. This procedure often gives permanent relief, but if repeated local anesthetics produce only transient benefit, surgical sympathectomy should be performed.

POSTHERPETIC NEURALGIA. Postherpetic neuralgia refers to severe and prolonged burning pain with occasional lightning-like stabs in the involved dermatome after an attack of herpes zoster. Severe postherpetic neuralgia is usually a disease of elderly patients and, like most chronic pain, is exacerbated by emotional upset and relieved to some degree by distraction. Touching the involved area usually exacerbates the pain. Treatment of postherpetic neuralgia is not entirely satisfactory, but the initial treatment should be directed toward stimulating the painful area. Brisk rubbing for many hours a day with a terrycloth towel or stimulation of the dermatome with a cutaneous electrical stimulator often brings relief which long outlasts the stimulus. Initially, when therapy is undertaken, the hyperpathia may be so severe that the patient is unwilling to have the area stimulated. One can then spray the area with a local anesthetic (e.g., ethyl chloride) before stimulation is undertaken. During the first 48 to 72 hours, stimulation should be done as often as possible while the patient is awake and then decreased gradually. Care must be taken to keep the rubbing light so as not to excoriate friable skin. Relief of pain may take several weeks. Analgesic drugs are sometimes beneficial, and psychotropic drugs (amitriptyline, 75 mg daily, and fluphenazine, 1 to 3 mg daily) have been reported to be useful. The results of surgical therapy are usually poor. In many patients the disease runs its course, and after a year or two the pain disappears spontaneously. Thus mutilating surgical procedures are probably not indicated.

PHANTOM LIMB PAIN. Phantom limb pain is a chronic and severe pain appearing to be localized in an amputated or totally denervated limb. All patients suffer phantom sensations after amputation, but in only about 10 per cent is it painful, usually when there has been severe pain prior to operation. The pain is frequently similar to that suffered before amputation, or at times it may resemble muscle pain with the phantom seeming to be in a cramped or uncomfortable position. In most instances, the pain lessens and disappears with time, but in occasional patients it is a chronic and severe problem. Therapy is difficult. A search should be made for painful neuromas, but these are an uncommon cause of phantom pain, and even if small neuromas are found and removed, the pain is not usually relieved. Surgical procedures directed at the central nervous system are often not helpful. The pain may be triggered by touching the amputation stump, but over the passage of time healthy areas of the body when touched may also trigger pain in the phantom. Phantom pain is sometimes permanently abolished by cutaneous stimulation, either rubbing or electrical stimulation, or by repeated anesthetic blocks of peripheral nerves proximal to the stump. Narcotic analgesics may be helpful; other analgesic agents are usually not helpful. Sympathetic blocks have been reported to relieve pain in some patients for prolonged periods, but sympathectomy rarely produces relief as lasting as with causalgia. The mechanism of phantom pain is unknown.

MYOFASCIAL PAIN SYNDROMES. Pain arising from skeletal muscle is common. Unaccustomed exercise causes soreness and tenderness in the involved muscles but is rarely a source of patient complaint. Prolonged tonic contraction of skeletal muscles, however, has an underlying pathogenesis of psychologic tension, resentment, and anxiety, and may produce pain in which the cause is not immediately apparent to the patient. Examples are tension headache arising from chronic contraction of paraspinous muscles at the base of the skull, anterior chest pain from contraction of pectoralis major, posterior thoracic or lumbar pain from paraspinous muscle contraction, and abdominal pain from rectus muscle retraction. The pain is initially localized over the area of muscle contraction but may spread widely into a distribution characteristic for the muscles involved. The muscles are usually tender to palpation, and there is often a particular tender area somewhere in the muscle, called a trigger area, which, when palpated, reproduces the entire distribution of the spontaneous pain. When the pain is acute, it may be treated with rest, local heat, and mild analgesic drugs, along with muscle relaxant drugs such as diazepam or meprobamate. When the pain is chronic or severe, particularly when a trigger area is found, local anesthesia with ethyl chloride spray or local injection of 0.5 per cent lidocaine sometimes affords relief. At times, a single injection breaks the pain–muscle tension–pain cycle and permanent relief is achieved. At other times, repetitive injections with the addition of analgesic agents and muscle relaxants are required.

Bonica, J. J. (ed.): Symposium on pain. Arch. Surg., 112:749, 861, 1971.
Bonica, J. J.: Management of Pain. 2nd ed. Philadelphia, Lea & Febiger, 1974.
Bonica, J. J., and Albe-Fessard, D. (eds.): Advances in Pain Research and Therapy. New York, Raven Press, 1976.
Guillemin, R., Bloom, F., Rossier, J., Minick, S., Henriksen, S., Burgus, R., and Ling, N.: Recent physiological studies with the endorphins. In Goodman, M., and Meinhofer, J. (eds.): Peptides 1977, Proceedings 5th American Peptide Symposium. New York, John Wiley & Sons, 1977.
Mayer, D., and Price, D. D.: Central nervous system mechanisms of analgesia. Pain, 2:379, 1976.
Sternbach, R.: Pain Patients: Traits and Treatment. New York, Academic Press, 1974.

261. HEADACHE

Fred Plum

INTRODUCTION

Headache is man's most common pain, and in one form or another it affects some 90 per cent of the population. In any consideration of headache, two major points stand out: one is that *most* headaches come from structures *outside* the skull, and the other is that increased intracranial pressure, as such, does not necessarily cause headache. The following is an outline of the principal types:

A. Extracranial headaches have several causes and are listed roughly in declining order of frequency.

1. Vascular headaches. These are recurrent and vary widely in intensity, duration, and frequency. The following subtypes are recognized:

a. *Classic migraine,* with sharply defined, transient visual, other sensory and/or motor prodromes.

b. *Hemiplegic or ophthalmoplegic migraine,* featured by sensory and motor phenomena that persist during and after the headache.

c. *Common migraine,* without striking prodromes and less often unilateral than (a) and (d). Synonyms are "atypical migraine" and "sick headache."

d. *Cluster headache,* predominantly unilateral, associated with flushing, sweating, rhinorrhea, increased lacrimation and, often, Horner's syndrome. The headaches are usually brief in duration and occur in close-packed groups separated by long remissions.

e. *Lower half headache,* of possible vascular mechanism, centered primarily in the lower face. In this group are some instances of atypical facial neuralgia, sphenopalatine ganglion neuralgia (Sluder), and vidian neuralgia (Vail).

2. *Muscle-contraction headaches.* These present as occipitofrontal pains or sensations of tightness, pressure, or constriction associated with sustained skeletal muscle contraction and no permanent structural change. The ambiguous terms "tension," "psychogenic," and "nervous" headache refer largely to this group.

3. Combination of vascular headache of the migraine type and muscle contraction headache.

4. Anterior headache and nasal discomfort (nasal obstruction, rhinorrhea, tightness, or burning) can result from congestion, edema, and inflammation of nasal and paranasal mucous membranes. This is "sinus" headache.

5. Nonmigrainous vascular headaches associated with generally nonrecurrent dilatation of extracranial arteries. The category includes post-traumatic and hypertensive headaches.

6. Ocular headache due to increased intraocular pressure, excessive contraction of ocular muscles, trauma, new growth, or inflammation.

7. Aural headache due to trauma, new growth, or inflammation.

8. Dental headache.

9. Headache due to spread of pain from noxious stimulation of other structures of the cranium and neck (periosteum, joints, ligaments, and muscles or cervical nerve roots).

10. Cranial neuritides (caused by trauma, new growth, or infection).

11. Extracranial arteritis.

B. Intracranial headache:

1. Traction headache. Headache resulting from traction on intracranial structures, mainly vascular, by masses:

a. Primary or metastatic tumors of meninges, vessels, or brain.

b. Hematomas (epidural, subdural, or parenchymal).

c. Abscesses (epidural, subdural, or parenchymal).

d. Headache following puncture ("leakage" headache).

e. Pseudotumor cerebri and various causes of brain swelling.

2. Headache due to inflammation of cranial structures resulting from usually nonrecurrent inflammation, sterile or infectious. Examples include infectious, chemical, or allergic meningitis, subarachnoid hemorrhage, postpneumoencephalographic reaction, arteritis, and phlebitis.

C. Cranial neuralgias: trigeminal (tic douloureux) and glossopharyngeal (see Ch. 260).

D. Headaches of a delusional or conversion reaction, in which a somatic pain mechanism is nonexistent. The diagnosis is rare and must be made cautiously. Closely allied are hypochondriacal and depressive reactions in which tissue abnormalities relevant to headache are minimal.

PATHOGENESIS OF HEADACHE. Wolff and his colleagues identified the principal intracranial and extracranial pain-sensitive structures. Almost all the *extracranial* tissues are pain sensitive, the arteries especially so. Among intracranial structures, only a limited group of tissues can cause pain. These include the great venous sinuses and their venous tributaries from the surface of the brain, parts of the dura at the base, the dural arteries and the cerebral arteries at the base of the brain, the fifth, seventh, ninth, and tenth cranial nerves, and the upper three cervical nerves.

The cranium (including the diploic and emissary veins), the parenchyma of the brain, most of the dura, most of the pia-arachnoid, and the ependymal lining of the ventricles and the choroid plexuses are not sensitive to pain.

The fifth cranial nerve contains the pathways for pain from sensitive intracranial structures located on or above the superior surface of the tentorium cerebelli. Pain from these structures is experienced in various regions in front of a line drawn coronally joining the ears across the top of the head.

The ninth and tenth cranial nerves and the upper two or possibly three cervical nerves contain the pathways for pain from pain-sensitive structures on or below the inferior surface of the tentorium cerebelli. Pain from these structures is experienced in various parietooccipital and upper cervical regions behind the line just described.

HEADACHE FROM INTRACRANIAL SOURCES

Headache from intracranial sources can result from the following mechanisms: (1) traction on and displacement of the great venous sinuses or of the veins that pass to them from the surface of the brain; (2) traction on and displacement of the middle meningeal arteries; (3) traction on and displacement of the large arteries at the base of the brain and their main branches; (4) dilatation and distention of intracranial arteries; (5) inflammation in or about any of the pain-sensitive structures of the head and portions of the pia and dura at the base of the skull; and (6) direct pressure by tumors on pain-sensitive cranial and cervical nerves. Intracranial diseases commonly cause headaches through more than one mechanism and may also cause secondary extracranial muscle-contraction headache, usually at the occiput, but often elsewhere.

The head pain associated with fever, bacteremia, sepsis, nitrite and foreign protein administration, carbon monoxide inhalation, hypoxia, and asphyxia is due principally to dilatation and distention of intracranial arterial structures. A similar mechanism probably causes the headaches that follow epileptic seizures (with or without convulsions) and certain "hangover headaches." Painful distention of intracranial arteries is responsible for the headaches that accompany sudden brisk rises in the arterial blood pressure, such as occurs with distention of the rectum or urinary bladder in paraplegics, rapid intravenous infusion of epinephrine, and the hypertensive crises occurring with pheochromocytoma or acute hypertensive encephalopathy.

The headache of meningitis is primarily related to the lowered pain threshold of inflamed tissues. The changes are usually most marked at the base of the brain. Under these circumstances, even the slight, usually painless arterial dilatation and distention during each cardiac systole become painful; hence, the characteristic throbbing headache.

Lumbar Puncture Headache

Dull, usually pulsating occipital headache develops in about one fifth of patients having lumbar puncture, particularly for the first time. For unexplained reasons, such headaches are less likely after repeated lumbar punctures. The headache usually begins 12 to 24 hours after the puncture, comes on in the erect position, and subsides if the subject lies flat. The headache usually disappears spontaneously in a day or so, and in most patients is made tolerable by routine analgesics. Occasionally, patients develop more prostrating symptoms that sometimes last as long as 10 to 14 days, accompanied by secondary muscle-contraction headache as well as nausea and vomiting.

The cause of postlumbar puncture headache is probably leakage of cerebrospinal fluid through the torn dural sac. The consequent loss of buoyance results in downward traction on unsupported, pain-sensitive posterior fossa tissues, particularly the veins. The headaches can often be avoided by accurate punctures, using No. 20 caliber sharp spinal needles, which minimize drainage through the dural needle wound.

Headache With Brain Tumor: With or Without Increased Intracranial Pressure

The headache with space-occupying lesions is deep, aching, steady, dull, and seldom rhythmic or throbbing. The pain is continuous in one tenth of the patients and is generally more intense in the morning. Aspirin, 0.3 gram, and local application of cold packs usually diminish the pain, and coughing or straining at stool may aggravate it. Some patients prefer the recumbent to the erect position. The headache is rarely as intense as that associated with migraine, ruptured cerebral aneurysm, or meningitis, and seldom interferes with sleep. Even when the tumor directly compresses and displaces pain-sensitive cranial nerves, headache may be absent or slight, and rarely is it as intense as the pain of tic douloureux, unless the tumor intermittently obstructs the cerebral ventricular system. In this instance, pain is excruciating and generalized, and may last 30 seconds to a half hour and then disappear as quickly as it commenced. During such an attack the sudden increases of intracranial pressure can be fatal.

Severe brain tumor headache is associated with nausea and vomiting. Vomiting caused by new growth also may occur with neither nausea nor headache, and is then usually the result of medullary compression. Being unexpected, such vomiting may be projectile.

When the headache is occipital or suboccipital, it is often associated with "stiffness" or aching of the muscles of the neck and tilting of the head toward the side of the lesion.

PATHOGENESIS. The initial headaches of brain tumor result from displacement of adjacent large arteries, veins, venous sinuses, and the cranial and somatic nerves, as mentioned. When the brain begins to shift away from the tumor, pain also can emanate form traction and displacement of structures remote from the space-occupying lesion. Increased intracranial pressure

per se need not cause headache, however. Indeed, in conditions such as benign intracranial hypertension, jugular venous obstruction or chronic communicating hydrocephalus, substantial elevations of intracranial pressure can occur with no headache.

(1) About one third of all headaches approximately overlie the tumor. (2) In the absence of increased intracranial pressure, two thirds of headaches are near or immediately over the tumor, and when unilateral are on the same side. (3) Occipital headache is almost always present and is the first symptom of posterior fossa tumors, except cerebellopontine angle tumors. When headache occurs with cerebellopontine angle tumors, it is frequently and sometimes solely postauricular. (4) Frontal headache is a first symptom in about one third of supratentorial tumors. Occipital headache rarely occurs with such growths unless associated with increased intracranial pressure or early tonsillar herniation. (5) A generalized headache with brain tumor signifies extensive displacement of the brain, usually with increased intracranial pressure, and has little localizing value.

MANAGEMENT. The most effective treatment for brain tumor headache is surgical removal of the mass. Transient decompression can be achieved by the intravenous infusion of either 500 ml of a 20 per cent sodium mannitol solution or 250 ml or a solution containing 30 per cent urea in 10 per cent invert sugar. Adrenal corticosteroids in high doses can also be employed to reduce brain edema and transiently decompress the mass. Lumbar drainage is contraindicated, nor does it predictably reduce headache of meningitis or subarachnoid hemorrhage.

If an inoperable tumor causes headache, ventricular drainage or shunting is sometimes employed.

Sometimes x-radiation or surgical procedures are justified in attempts to reduce headache caused by clearly defined metastatic disease. Headache resulting from craniopharyngioma or pituitary tumors does not in itself constitute an indication for surgical procedures, because removal provides no assurance that headache will be diminished or eliminated.

HEADACHES FROM EXTRACRANIAL STRUCTURES

Six main categories of head and face pain arise from extracranial tissues and related structures: (1) headaches due to painful dilatation and distention of cranial arteries; (2) headaches due to sustained contraction of skeletal muscle about the face, scalp, and neck; (3) headache from disease of the nose, paranasal spaces, eyes, ears, and teeth; (4) craniofacial pain of the major neuralgias and the postinfectious neuralgias and postinfectious neuritides; (5) headache due to nonspecific inflammation of cranial arteries ("cranial arteritis," "temporal arteritis"); and (6) head pain due to trauma, infection, or new growth involving extracranial tissues.

More than 90 per cent of all headaches are in the first two of these categories and occur or are intensified in a life setting that engenders frustration, resentment, anxiety, or depression.

Vascular Headaches

Vascular headaches are common; about 25 per cent of the population report having "migraine" or sick headaches, with about half this number suffering from unilateral headache. Such headaches are principally due to painful dilatation and distention of one or more of the extracranial and, probably, intracranial, i.e., dural, branches of the external carotid artery, with associated edema of adjacent tissues. The most common site of vascular headaches of the migraine type is the temple or the forehead, and one or both frontal, supraorbital, and superficial temporal arteries are most frequently involved, however. Many headaches at the back of the head and neck are associated with painful dilatation and distention of the postauricular and/or occipital arteries.

The lower half of the head and face and the upper jaw in the vicinity of the back teeth may all be the site of pain of vascular origin, with spread to the neck and even the shoulder. Such headaches may be accompanied by the awareness of unusually forceful throbbing in the neck. "Atypical facial neuralgia" is but one of the many designations applied to such headaches, which very probably result in good part from dilatation and distention of the extracranial portion of the middle meningeal artery, of the internal maxillary artery, and of the other branches and the trunks of the external and the common carotid arteries.

Migraine Syndrome

CLINICAL FEATURES. The migraine syndrome is a pattern of dysfunction integrated within the central nervous system and manifested as widespread bodily disturbances, both nonpainful and painful. The outstanding feature is periodic headache, usually unilateral in onset but at times becoming bilateral or generalized. The attacks may vary in duration from a few minutes to several days and, in severity, from trifling symptoms to prolonged disabling illness. The headaches are associated with "irritability," nausea, and often photophobia, vomiting, constipation, or diarrhea. Although most common in the temple, headaches may be experienced anywhere in the head, face, and neck. About 50 per cent of patients with classic migraine report a similar syndrome in a parent or grandparent.

Some patients experience vague symptoms for as much as several days before a migraine attack. These include a facial flushing or pallor and other transient cranial vasomotor phenomena such as vertigo. In the hour preceding the headache, a variety of visual and other neurologic abnormalities caused by transient local constriction of cerebral or retinal arteries occur in about 10 to 15 per cent of the instances. These prodromes may take the form of scintillating scotomas, visual field defects such as unilateral or homonymous hemianopsia, and, occasionally, hemiplegia. Rarely, more sustained neurologic defects and even cerebral infarction can occur. The risk of these cerebrovascular complications is higher in women than in men. The incidence of stroke reaches a fourfold increase over the control population in women with migraine who both smoke and take contraceptive pills. As the vasoconstriction phenomena recede, vasodilator headache commences, sometimes overlapping, sometimes beginning after a short symptom-free interval. The pain is throbbing and aching, is appreciably reduced by pressure on the common carotid and the affected superficial artery, and is characteristically eliminated or reduced by vasoconstrictor agents, particularly ergotamine tartrate. The walls of the dilated cranial arteries and the adjacent tissues become edematous and tender. With sustained vasodilata-

tion for several hours, the easily compressible arteries become rigid and relatively noncompressible, and the pulsatile pain becomes a steady ache. Redness and swelling of the eye with excessive tearing, and redness and swelling of the nasal mucosa with or without epistaxis, may occur. A secondary muscle contraction component of the headache may outlast the vascular pain and will not be modified by vasoconstrictor agents.

A variety of headache closely related to migraine is the *cluster headache*. This head pain is almost always unilateral, affects men more than women, and usually begins between the third and sixth decades. Attacks come on abruptly with intense throbbing pain arising high in the nostril and spreading to involve the region behind the homolateral eye and sometimes the forehead as well. During the attacks, which last up to two hours, the nose and eyes water. The skin reddens and a homolateral Horner's syndrome with pupillary constriction and ptosis may develop. The attacks tend to occur from once to several times daily, in clusters lasting weeks or, less often, months. Without apparent reason, the cluster subsides as suddenly as it began, and the patient commonly remains free of headache for weeks or months until another cluster begins. During a cluster period, but not between, alcohol is likely to induce attacks. When headaches recur in close succession, the Horner's syndrome may outlast the headache.

PATHOGENESIS. There is evidence of a general abnormality of vascular behavior in many migraine subjects, and the extracranial vessels of such subjects show more variability in their contractile patterns than those of normal subjects even during headache-free periods. Studies in man of the cerebral blood flow show that during the prodromal stages of the migraine attack the intracranial arteries are constricted, whereas during the headache itself the arteries become dilated. Humoral agents have long been sought as the basis of the migraine syndrome. Local fluid collected from sites of swelling at the point of maximal headache and tenderness during an attack contains a vasodilator polypeptide of the bradykinin type that lowers pain thresholds and may be a factor in a local sterile inflammation. However, kinins, histamine, or substances such as acetylcholine do not satisfactorily explain the generalized manifestations of the disorder. Several lines of evidence suggest that abnormalities in the metabolism of serotonin may play a role in the migraine syndrome. Reserpine, which induces a drop in serum serotonin levels, will often induce a migraine attack, and serum levels of serotonin have been found to drop spontaneously just before migraine attacks. During migraine attacks, an increased quantity of serotonin metabolites has been found in the urine. Evidence also indicates that a platelet abnormality may be connected with migraine. Transitory decreases in platelet monoamine oxidase activity have been recorded during migraine attacks. Increased platelet aggregability also has been noted; the full significance of these findings remains to be elucidated, however.

MANAGEMENT OF ACUTE HEADACHE. Traditionally, the vasoconstrictor effect of ergotamine tartrate taken orally, rectally, or by injection has provided the mainstay of treatment. Orally, two to eight Cafergot tablets (ergotamine tartrate, 1 mg; caffeine, 100 mg) may be given safely for any one headache attack. The intramuscular dose of ergotamine tartrate is 0.25 to 0.5 mg, and the rectal dose, by suppository, is 1 to 2 mg. Not more than 10 mg of ergotamine orally or 5 mg parenterally should be given in any week because of the hazards of arterial vasoconstriction. Recent evidence suggests that the combination of analgesics plus antiemetics sometimes may be superior to the use of ergotamine. Wilkinson reports that at the London Migraine Clinic most patients require for relief only an analgesic (aspirin, 0.6 to 0.9 gram, or acetaminophen, 0.5 to 1.0 gram) and an antiemetic (prochlorperazine, 5 mg). Codeine may be used judiciously, but using stronger narcotics threatens to produce addiction.

Cluster headaches are treated as above except that indomethacin almost specifically relieves some patients. Adrenocorticosteroids sometimes abort the clusters, but the effect is inconsistent. Methysergide has effects similar to its use in migraine.

PREVENTION. Prophylaxis against migraine is effective in perhaps 75 per cent of instances, and requires attention to both the medications and the personal problems of the patient.

Some patients relate recurrent headaches to the ingestion of chocolate, alcoholic beverages, or tyramine-containing foods such as cheese and wine. Such association deserves inquiry and appropriate restrictions. The most effective prophylactic drug is the serotonin antagonist methysergide, given as 2 mg three to four times daily. Methysergide must be used with caution, because it can cause a number of side effects, the serious ones including vascular insufficiency, retroperitoneal or pleural fibrosis, or fibrotic thickening of the heart valves. Side effects are minimized by enforcing drug-free periods of three to eight weeks' duration after every three-month treatment period. Less effective but sometimes successful agents used in prophylaxis include clonidine, cyproheptadine, and, occasionally, propranolol.

Patients with migraine often require considerable psychologic support and reassurance. Many such patients report becoming progressively more tense, resentful, and fatigued during periods of threat or conflict. Such feelings, along with a sense of anger or depression, often form the backdrop for a recurrence of headache. Treatment is best if it allows the patient free and repeated expression of his conflicts, resentments, and dissatisfactions; enables him to recognize the nature of his dilemma and its relationship to the physiologic basis of his pain; and guides him toward a more flexible attitude and personal adjustment.

Muscle-Contraction Headaches

The pain of a muscle-contraction headache is a steady, nonpulsatile, unilateral or bilateral ache located in the temporal, occipital, parietal, or frontal regions. Additional descriptive terms include tightness, bandlike or caplike sensations about the head, or sensations of weight, pressure, drawing, or soreness. Pain may be fleeting, with frequent changes in the site and intensity of recurrences, or localized in one region. The headache may last for weeks, months, or years.

PATHOGENESIS. The cause lies in long-sustained contraction of skeletal muscle about the face, scalp, and neck. Concurrent vasodilatation of the associated cranial arteries frequently contributes to the irritability of the involved muscles and the pain.

With prolonged sustained contraction, the muscles of the head, jaws, neck, and upper back become tender, causing the patient to limit their motion. Palpation may reveal sharply localized painful areas or nodules. Commonly, it hurts to comb or brush the hair or to don a hat. Exposure to cold, with shivering, may precipitate or aggravate the headache. Pressure on the contracted, tender muscles may augment the intensity and may elicit tinnitus, dizziness, and lacrimation — features that also occur spontaneously.

Sustained muscle contraction giving rise to headache is often secondary to other head pains, including migraine or disease in the eye, ear, nose, paranasal spaces, teeth, or scalp, and to brain tumor. Painful, sustained muscle contraction is also the primary source of many headaches associated with emotional tension states, especially during periods of tension, anger, or depression.

MANAGEMENT. Reassurance, massage, manipulation, and manual stretching of the nuchal and occipital muscles, aspirin, and phenobarbital (30 mg three times a day) reduce or eliminate most such headaches. Diazepam is often used but enhances feelings of depression. Heat, warm baths, and the passage of time are important adjuvants. Particularly among patients susceptible to recurrent headache of this type, the antidepressant amitriptyline in doses of 25 to 75 mg daily may bring considerable relief.

Other Types of Extracranial Headache

RECURRENT ("CHRONIC") POST-TRAUMATIC HEADACHE. Head injury may rarely be followed by headaches that stem from intracranial sources such as subdural hematomas or subarachnoid hemorrhages. However, most post-traumatic headaches stem from nonintracranial sources, four types being most common: (1) pain or tenderness resulting from local tissue damage in a scar or at a site of impact, (2) muscle-contraction headache, (3) attacks of throbbing and aching vascular headache, and (4) infrequently, delusional headaches for which no tissue abnormality exists. The first two varieties are most common and are sometimes accompanied by fleeting vertigo with sudden movement or rotation of the head, nausea, irritability, and insomnia.

Many injured patients harbor resentment related to the circumstances of their accident or fear that they have sustained permanent brain injury. These reactions and attitudes are intimately related to the pathophysiology and "chronicity" of post-traumatic headaches, and the headache often fails to subside as long as compensation claims remain unsettled.

HEADACHES ASSOCIATED WITH ARTERIAL HYPERTENSION. When otherwise symptom-free and in the absence of hypertensive encephalopathy or pheochromocytoma, about 10 per cent of persons with arterial hypertension may experience severe, even disabling, headaches, particularly during the morning hours. Fluctuations in blood pressure correlate only poorly with the headaches, nor is the extent of the elevation directly related to the severity of the attacks. However, headache attacks tend to be less frequent when the blood pressure is least elevated.

The headache associated with arterial hypertension resembles the vascular headaches of migraine and muscle tension and often regresses spontaneously with reassurance and the effective treatment of the hypertension.

NASAL AND PARANASAL STRUCTURES AS SOURCES OF HEADACHE. Sinus headache is predominantly a short-lived problem, always associated with objective evidence of acute sinusitis. Most of the discomfort comes from the ostia, which are many times more sensitive than the relatively insensitive walls of the sinuses. Typically, "sinus" headache commences in the morning (frontal) or early afternoon (maxillary) and subsides in the early or late evening. The pain is dull and aching, is made worse by changing head position, and is seldom associated with nausea and vomiting. It is due to mucosal inflammation, so that engorged turbinates, ostia, nasofrontal ducts and superior nasal spaces should be visible. Most patients have sinus tenderness. Headache not associated with turbinate engorgement and inflammation is probably not due to sinus or nose disease. Sinus headache is best treated with decongestants and analgesics. Persistent purulent discharges should be cultured and appropriate antimicrobial drugs employed. Chronic suppurative disease in the frontal, ethmoid, and sphenoid sinuses, or in the mastoid air cells, may result in osteomyelitis and inflammation of adjacent cranial tissues. Headache persisting after surgical drainage of the diseased sinus is evidence for extradural and possibly subdural infection.

HEAD PAIN AND DISEASE OF THE TEETH. Noxious stimuli in a tooth usually evoke local toothache, but when severe, such pain can be extremely difficult to localize. Afferent fibers for sensation in the teeth are contained in the second and third divisions of the fifth cranial nerve. Headache in the areas supplied by the latter is, in rare instances, associated with prolonged, intense toothache, or follows a tooth extraction. More commonly, in association with toothache, tooth extraction or a tender, diseased tooth, distant tissues exhibit surface hyperalgesia, tenderness, and vasomotor reactions, such as tender eyeballs, reddening of the conjunctivae, and tenderness of the auricular and temporal tissues. Because of secondary muscle contraction, other sites of tenderness and pain may be noted behind the ears, behind the lower border of the mastoid process, and in the muscles of the occiput, neck, and shoulders.

The upper teeth frequently hurt in association with disease of the nasal and paranasal structures. Occasionally, in coronary insufficiency, pain is experienced in the lower jaw because of the close approximation of the fifth cranial and upper cervical neural segments in the cord. The teeth rarely cause craniofacial pains or "neuralgias" in the absence of toothache. Headache may not be attributed to a diseased tooth unless the injection of procaine into the tissues about the suspected tooth greatly reduces the intensity of, or eliminates, such headache.

HEAD PAIN AND DISEASE OF THE EAR. The fifth, seventh, ninth, and tenth cranial nerves contribute to the sensory innervation of the ear, and branches from the upper cervical roots supply the immediately adjacent scalp and muscles. Severe pain in the vicinity of the ear can be caused by disease of the teeth, acute tonsillitis, inflammatory and neoplastic disease of the larynx and nasopharynx, temporomandibular joint disorders, tumors, and inflammation in the posterior fossa and disease of the cervical spine and its soft tissues. Pain in the ear is also associated with vascular headaches and atypical facial neuralgias as well as herpes zoster of the fifth and seventh cranial nerves and, rarely, the glossopharyngeal nerve. True glossopharyngeal neuralgia causes severe pain radiating from the tonsil into the ear. It has the usual timing feature of "tic."

Primary ear disease is relatively infrequent — but important — as a source of headache, because it almost always indicates inflammation or destructive disease. Acute otitis media (purulent or nonpurulent), furunculosis of the ear canal, traumatic rupture of the tympanum, and fracture of the anterior wall of the bony canal all cause pain in the ear associated with sustained tender contraction of adjacent skeletal muscles. Osteomyelitis of the mastoid bone may be associated with inflammation of the nearby periosteum as well as dura and adjacent tissues (epidural abscess) — both sources of pain in or behind the ear. Pain in this region also accompanies tumors of the acoustic nerve and inflammation and thrombosis of the lateral sinus.

THE EYE AS A SOURCE OF HEADACHE. Errors of refraction (hypermetropia, astigmatism, anomalies of accommodation), disturbances of ocular muscle equilibrium, and glaucoma are universally described as causing headache. Refractive errors are also said to give origin to such other symptoms as aching of the eyes, "sandy" feeling in the eyes, pulling sensations in and about the orbit, and conjunctival congestion. Headache usually starts around and over the eyes and subsequently radiates to the occiput and back of the head.

The pain of increased intraocular pressure at first remains localized in the eyeball, then extends along the rim of the orbit and, finally, throughout most of the area supplied by the ophthalmic division of the trigeminal nerve. Nausea and vomiting sometimes accompany such headaches.

Headache accompanying various ocular disturbances is regarded as secondary to (1) sustained contraction of the intraocular muscles, which is associated with excessive accommodation effort, or (2) sustained contraction of the extraocular muscles, resulting from the effort to produced distinct retinal images, and single binocular vision with fusion. Simple myopia does not evoke headache because the myope, in attempting to improve his vision by the contraction of his eye muscles, actually makes his vision worse and soon abandons the attempt.

With inflammation of the iris and ciliary body, light may cause intense pain in the eye and adjacent areas when the light stimulus is accompanied by movement of the inflamed iris. When the iris is immobilized, pain is allayed.

Dalessio, D. J.: Wolff's Headache and Other Head Pain. 3rd ed. New York, Oxford University Press, 1972.

Harper, A. M., MacKenzie, E. T., McCulloch, J., and Pickard, J. D.: Migraine and the blood brain barrier. Lancet, 1:1034, 1977.

Norris, J. W., Hachinski, V. C., and Cooper, P. W.: Changes in cerebral blood flow during a migraine attack. Brit. Med. J., 3:676, 1975.

Vinken, P. J., and Bruyn, G. W. (eds.): Headaches and Cranial Neuralgias. Vol. 5. Handbook of Clinical Neurology. Amsterdam, North-Holland, 1968.

Waters, W. E., and O'Connor, P. J.: Prevalence of migraine. J. Neurol. Neurosurg. Psychiatry, 38:613, 1975.

Wilkinson, M.: The treatment of acute migraine attacks. Headache, 16:291, 1976.

262. HEARING LOSS

Robert W. Baloh

INTRODUCTION

Hearing loss is usually expressed in terms of the ability to hear pure tones which are defined by their frequency and intensity. In order to quantify the magnitude of hearing loss, normal hearing levels are defined by an international standard. These levels approximate the intensity of the faintest sound that can be heard by normal ears. A patient's hearing level is the difference in decibels (db) between the faintest pure tone that he can hear and the normal reference level given by the standard. The range of audible frequencies is approximately 20 to 20,000 Hz in young normal ears. The ear is most sensitive between 500 and 4000 Hz, which roughly corresponds to the frequency range most important for understanding speech. The hearing level in this range has several practical implications in terms of the degree of handicap and the potential for useful correction with amplification. A 30 to 40 db hearing level in the speech range would impair normal conversation, whereas an 80 db hearing level would make everyday auditory communication almost impossible (the social definition of deafness).

TYPES OF HEARING LOSS

Hearing disorders can be classified as conductive, sensorineural, and central, based on the anatomic site of pathology. *Conductive hearing loss* results from lesions involving the external or middle ear. The tympanic membrane and ossicles act as a transformer, amplifying airborne sound and efficiently transferring it to the inner ear fluid. If this normal pathway is obstructed, transmission can occur across the skin and through the bones of the skull (bone conduction) but at the cost of significant energy loss. For example, simple interruption of the ossicles results in a hearing level of approximately 25 db, whereas complete absence of the conduction system on a congenital basis results in a hearing level of about 60 db, i.e., the level of bone conduction. Patients with conductive hearing loss can hear speech in a noisy background better than in a quiet background because they can understand loud speech as well as anyone.

Sensorineural hearing loss results from lesions of the cochlea and/or the auditory division of the eighth cranial nerve. The sensory cells of the cochlea are force transducers converting sound energy in the inner ear fluid to action potentials in the auditory nerve. The spiral cochlea mechanically analyzes the frequency content of sound. For high frequency tones only sensory cells in the basilar turn are activated, whereas for low frequency tones all or nearly all sensory cells are activated. Therefore with lesions of the cochlea and its afferent nerve, the hearing levels for different frequencies are usually unequal and the phase relationship (timing) between different frequencies may be altered. Patients with sensorineural hearing loss often have difficulty hearing speech that is mixed with background noise and may be annoyed by loud speech.

Three important manifestations of sensorineural le-

sions are diplacusis, recruitment, and tone decay. Diplacusis and recruitment are commonly seen with cochlear lesions; tone decay is usually seen with eighth nerve involvement. With diplacusis the tonal quality of a pure tone is distorted so that it may sound like a complex mixture of tones. Binaural diplacusis occurs when the two ears are affected unequally so that the same frequency has a different pitch in each ear, i.e., the patient hears double. Monaural diplacusis occurs when two tones or a tone and noise are heard simultaneously in one ear. With recruitment there is an abnormally rapid growth in the sensation of loudness as the intensity of a sound is increased so that faint or moderate sounds cannot be heard, whereas there is little or no change in the loudness of loud sounds. The inability to maintain perception of a continuous tone presented above auditory threshold is called tone decay. Patients with conductive or cochlear lesions can usually hear a continuous tone for at least 60 seconds, whereas the tone rapidly decays in patients with eighth nerve lesions.

Central hearing disorders result from lesions of the central auditory pathways. These consist of the cochlear and dorsal olivary nuclear complexes, inferior colliculi, medial geniculate bodies, auditory cortex in the temporal lobes, and interconnecting afferent and efferent fiber tracts. As a rule, patients with central lesions do not have impaired hearing levels for pure tones and they can understand speech as long as it is clearly spoken in a quiet environment. If the listener's task is made more difficult with the introduction of background noise or competing messages, performance deteriorates more markedly in patients with central lesions than in normal subjects. Lesions involving the eighth nerve root entry zone or cochlear nucleus, however, can result in unilateral hearing loss for pure tones. Since approximately 50 per cent of afferent nerve fibers cross central to the cochlear nucleus, this is the most central structure in which a lesion can result in a unilateral hearing loss.

EXAMINATION OF HEARING

BEDSIDE TESTS. A quick test for hearing loss in the speech range is to observe the response to spoken commands at different intensities (whisper, conversation, shouting). The examiner must be careful to prevent the patient from reading his lip movement. A high frequency stimulus such as a watch tick or coin click (approximately 4000 cps) should also be used, because sensorineural disorders often involve only the higher frequencies. Tuning fork tests permit a rough assessment of the hearing level for pure tones of known frequency. The clinician can use his own hearing level as a reference standard. The *Rinne test* compares the patient's hearing by air conduction with that by bone conduction. The fork (preferably 512 cps) is first held against the mastoid process until the sound fades. It is then placed one inch from the ear. Normal subjects can hear the fork about twice as long by air as by bone conduction. If bone conduction is greater than air conduction, a conductive hearing loss is suggested. The *Weber test* compares the patient's hearing by bone conduction in the two ears. The fork is placed at the center of the forehead or on a central incisor, and the patient is asked where he hears the tone. Normal subjects hear it in the center of the head, patients with unilateral conductive loss hear it on the affected side, and patients with unilateral sensorineural loss hear it on the side opposite the loss.

AUDIOMETRY. Tests Requiring Subjective Responses. *Pure tone* testing is the nucleus of most auditory examinations. Pure tones at selected frequencies are presented via either earphones (air conduction) or a vibrator pressed against the mastoid portion of the temporal bone (bone conduction). The minimal level that the subject can hear is determined for each frequency. Two *speech* tests are routinely used. The speech reception threshold (SRT) is the intensity at which the patient can correctly repeat 50 per cent of the words presented. The SRT is a test of hearing sensitivity for speech and should reflect the hearing level for pure tones in the speech range. The speech discrimination test is a measure of the patient's ability to understand speech when it is presented at a level that is easily heard. In patients with eighth nerve lesions, speech discrimination can be severely reduced even when pure tone thresholds are normal or nearly normal, whereas in patients with cochlear lesions discrimination tends to be proportional to the magnitude of hearing loss.

Recruitment is usually measured by the alternate binaural loudness balance (ABLB) test (if the hearing loss is unilateral). This test compares the loudness for tones of varying intensity as perceived by the pathologic ear and the normal ear. Recruitment is present if smaller increases in stimulus intensity are required in the poorer ear than in the better ear to maintain equal loudness. *Tone decay* is usually tested by presenting a tone at a prescribed suprathreshold level and asking the patient to respond as long as he hears the tone. Special tests for central auditory lesions assess the patient's ability to understand *distorted speech* or speech that is presented to one ear with a *competing message* in the other ear.

Tests Using Objective Measurements. By inserting a probe in the external canal that both presents and measures the sound pressure level of a tone, the acoustic impedance of the middle ear can be assessed. Two types of impedance measurements are routinely used: *tympanometry* and *stapedius reflex measurement*. Tympanometry, the measurement of impedance as a function of ear canal air pressure, is primarily useful for detection of middle ear disorders; stapedius reflex measurements are particularly useful for identifying lesions of the eighth nerve and/or brainstem. The stapedius muscle contracts and tightens the ossicular chain to protect the inner ear from excessively loud noises. The magnitude of the acoustic impedance change is an indirect measure of the strength of contraction of the stapedius muscle. The reflex arc consists of (1) auditory nerve, (2) brainstem interneurons, and (3) facial nerve. If the middle ear structures are intact, loss of the stapedius reflex suggests a lesion in this reflex arc.

Electrocochleography, a method for direct measurement of cochlear neural responses, and measurement of auditory evoked responses are two other promising objective tests of auditory function.

CAUSES OF HEARING LOSS

CONDUCTIVE HEARING LOSS. The most common cause of conductive hearing loss is *impacted cerumen* in the external canal. This benign condition is usually first noticed after bathing or swimming when a droplet of water closes the remaining tiny passageway. The most common serious cause of conductive hearing loss is inflammation of the middle ear, *otitis media*. Either infected (suppurative otitis) or noninfected (serous otitis) fluid accumulates in the middle ear, impairing the conduction of airborne sound. Since the air cavity of the middle ear is in direct connection with the mastoid air cells, infection can spread through the mastoid bone and occasionally into the intracranial cavity. Chronic otitis media with perforation of the tympanic membrane can result in an invasion of the middle ear and other pneumatized areas of the temporal bone by keratinizing squamous epithelium (cholesteatoma). Cholesteatomas can produce erosion of the ossicles and bony labyrinth, resulting in a mixed conductive-sensorineural hearing loss.

Otosclerosis commonly produces progressive conductive hearing loss by immobilizing the stapes with new bone growth in front of and below the oval window. Seventy per cent of patients with clinical otosclerosis notice hearing loss between the ages of 11 and 30, and there is a positive family history in approximately 50 per cent of cases. Initially, the hearing loss is purely conductive; but as the disease progresses, the cochlea may be invaded by foci of otosclerotic bone, producing an additional high frequency sensorineural hearing loss. Otosclerosis usually stabilizes when the hearing level reaches 50 to 60 db and rarely progresses to deafness. Other common causes of conductive hearing loss include trauma, congenital malformations of the external and middle ear, and glomus body tumors.

SENSORINEURAL HEARING LOSS. Congenital. Malformations of the inner ear can result from either abnormal genes or abnormal intrauterine factors. Genetically determined deafness may be present at birth, or it may become manifest years after birth as the normally developed inner ear structures deteriorate. In approximately one third of cases, there is a clearly defined syndrome, but in the majority of cases the diagnosis of *hereditary deafness* rests on the finding of a positive family history. In many instances the inheritance is through a recessive gene or a dominant gene with low penetrance, making it difficult to determine the genetic nature of the disorder.

Intrauterine factors resulting in congenital hearing loss include infection, toxic, metabolic, and endocrine disorders, and anoxia associated with Rh incompatibility and difficult deliveries. As many as 70 per cent of mothers who acquire *rubella* during the first trimester of pregnancy will produce a child with some degree of hearing loss. After conclusion of the first trimester, the risk is significantly less, but the infant's formed inner ear can still become infected from a maternal rubella infection. If the maternal infection occurs in the first six weeks of gestation, malformations of the eyes, cardiovascular system, and brain are also common. Since rubella rarely causes complete deafness, children with this type of congenital deafness may be helped with amplification. It is particularly important that children with congenital hearing loss of any variety be recognized, because they may be misdiagnosed as mentally retarded or brain damaged and appropriate educational opportunities not provided.

Acute. Infection of the inner ear (*labyrinthitis*) is the most common cause of sudden unilateral hearing loss.

Bacteria can enter the inner ear directly from the middle ear or from the cerebrospinal fluid via the cochlear aqueduct and internal auditory canal. In the former case, there is a history of recurrent or chronic otitis media; in the latter case, the patient has bacterial meningitis. In addition to the sudden hearing loss, the patient develops vertigo, nausea, and vomiting from involvement of the vestibular labyrinth. The end result is usually an irreversible unilateral deafness. In some instances there is not a direct bacterial invasion but rather an irritation of the labyrinth by bacterial toxins and endotoxins, producing biochemical damage to the membranes. This so-called toxic or serous labyrinthitis is associated with milder degrees of reversible hearing loss.

Viral labyrinthitis may be part of a systemic viral illness such as measles, mumps, and infectious mononucleosis or an isolated infection of the labyrinth without systemic symptoms. Mumps is a common cause of unilateral hearing loss in preschool and school-aged children, and there is serologic evidence that subclinical mumps infection may produce sudden unilateral hearing loss in adults. An infecting agent is rarely identified in adults with sudden unilateral hearing loss, but pathologic studies when obtained have suggested a viral cause in such patients.

Other common causes of sudden unilateral hearing loss include *head trauma* and *vascular occlusive disease*. Temporal bone fractures, particularly transverse fractures, are often associated with hearing loss. Sudden deafness that is either partially or completely reversible may also follow a blow to the head without skull fracture. This type of deafness is called inner ear concussion and is felt to be due to intense acoustic stimulation from pressure waves created by the blow. The role of vascular occlusion in the production of isolated sudden unilateral hearing loss is controversial, but this should be considered in patients with known vascular disease. Since the labyrinth is usually supplied by a branch of the anterior inferior cerebellar artery, transient hearing loss may be part of the basilar-vertebral insufficiency syndrome.

Subacute and Relapsing. *Meniere's syndrome* is characterized by fluctuating hearing loss and tinnitus, episodic vertigo, and a sensation of fullness or pressure in the ear. In the early stages the hearing loss is completely reversible, but eventually severe permanent loss develops. In approximately 20 per cent of patients bilateral involvement will occur. The principal pathologic finding is an increase in the volume of endolymph associated with distention of the entire endolymphatic sac (endolymphatic hydrops). Viral and bacterial, including presumed syphilitic, labyrinthitis can lead to endolymphatic hydrops and must be considered in the differential diagnosis; but in the majority of cases, the cause is unknown. Multiple causes have been proposed for idiopathic Meniere's syndrome, including allergy, endocrine disturbance, focal infection, sympathetic vasomotor disturbance, and psychophysiologic reaction.

Ototoxic drugs are an important cause of bilateral subacute hearing loss. Salicylates in high doses, ethacrynic acid, and furosemide often cause a reversible hearing loss, whereas aminoglycoside antimicrobials usually produce a permanent hearing loss. The primary pathologic change with each of these drugs is loss of hair cells in the cochlea and vestibular end-organs. Commonly used aminoglycosides that cause hearing loss include neomycin, kanamycin, and gentamicin. Neomycin has the undesirable effect of producing hearing loss weeks to months after administration of the drug. Each of these drugs must be used cautiously in patients with impaired renal function, as small doses can create high blood levels and an increased incidence of ototoxic effects.

Chronic Progressive. The bilateral hearing loss commonly associated with advancing age is called *presbycusis*. Presbycusis is not a distinct disease entity but rather represents multiple effects of aging on the auditory system. Presbycusis may include conductive and central dysfunction, although the most consistent effect of aging is on the sensory cells and neurons of the cochlea. The typical audiogram of presbycusis is a symmetrical hearing loss gradually sloping downward with increasing frequency. The most consistent pathology associated with presbycusis is degeneration of sensory cells and nerve fibers at the base of the cochlea. *Noise-induced hearing loss* is extremely common in industrialized societies. The loss almost always begins at 4000 cps and does not affect speech discrimination until late in the disease process. With only a brief exposure to loud noise (hours to days) there may be only a temporary threshold shift, but with continued exposure permanent injury begins. The duration and intensity of exposure determine the degree of permanent injury. Damage to sensory cells is often confined to a small area at the base of the cochlea, centering around the area sensing 4000 cps.

Slowly progressive unilateral sensorineural hearing loss can be caused by a small benign tumor arising from the sheath of the vestibular division of the eighth nerve *(acoustic neuroma, neurilemmoma, vestibular schwannoma)*. Acoustic neuromas initially compress the eighth nerve in the narrow confines of the internal auditory canal. As the tumor slowly enlarges, it protrudes through the internal auditory meatus, producing a funnel-shaped erosion of the bone surrounding the canal, stretching adjacent nerve roots over the surface of the mass and deforming the brainstem and cerebellum. The initial symptom is slowly progressive hearing loss in most cases, although rarely an acute hearing loss occurs from compression of the labyrinthine vasculature.

CENTRAL HEARING LOSS. Acute unilateral hearing loss is occasionally seen in patients with *multiple sclerosis* when a plaque involves the cochlear nerve root entry or cochlear nucleus. The hearing usually recovers in a period of days to weeks. *Infarction* in the lateral pontomedullary region can result in acute ipsilateral hearing loss along with multiple focal neurologic signs.

TREATMENT

Surgical treatment of hearing loss is limited to correcting abnormalities of the conduction system. *Hearing aids* amplify sound, usually with the goal of making speech intelligible. They are ideally suited for conductive hearing loss, but can also help sensorineural hearing loss if the inner ear is still able to discriminate speech. The most successful *medical treatment* of hearing loss is the use of appropriate drugs for microbial disease of the ear. The use of a low salt diet and diuretics may be effective in selected cases of Meniere's syndrome, particularly if episodes are precipitated by premenstrual water retention. There is little proof that vasodilator or anticoagulant drugs are effective in reversing sudden unilateral hearing loss of any cause. *Monitoring audiograms* in patients with noise or ototoxic drug exposure are critical for prevention of permanent hearing loss.

Davis, H., and Silverman, S. R. (eds.): Hearing and Deafness. 3rd ed. New York, Holt, Rinehart and Winston, 1970.

Dublin, W. B.: Fundamentals of Sensorineural Auditory Pathology. Springfield, Ill., Charles C Thomas, 1976.

Jerger, J. (ed.): Modern Developments in Audiology. New York, Academic Press, 1973.

Johnson, E. W.: Auditory test results in 500 cases of acoustic neuroma. Arch. Otolaryngol., 103:152, 1977.

Konigsmark, B. W.: Hereditary deafness in man. N. Engl. J. Med., 281:713, 1969.

Morrison, A. W.: Management of Sensorineural Deafness. Reading, Mass., Butterworth, 1975.

Schuknecht, H. E.: Pathology of the Ear. Boston, Harvard University Press, 1975.

263. DIZZINESS AND VERTIGO

David A. Drachman

THE COMPLAINT OF DIZZINESS

As a *complaint* rather than a *disease*, the term "dizziness" appropriately includes almost any sensation that a patient chooses to call by that name. By usage the term is applied to a number of uncommon sensations that are *not* part of daily experience. It is the thread of unfamiliar spatial disorientation that appears to bind these complaints together. When one listens carefully to a large number of "dizzy" patients, it is possible to sort their complaints into four types: a *rotational sensation, impending faint, dysequilibrium,* and *vague lightheadedness.*

Type I dizziness is a *definite rotational sensation* (vertigo) in which the patient feels that either he or the environment is spinning. Violent vertigo is often accompanied by nausea, vomiting, and a staggering gait. Oscillopsia — a visual hallucination of to-and-fro movement of the environment — may occur. The onset of vertigo is often instantaneous, and patients sometimes describe a sensation of being hurled to the ground. Although full-blown vertigo is unmistakable, with milder forms the patient may describe only a rocking sensation or vague lightheadedness. Recognition of mild vertiginous episodes is often aided by testing with the dizziness simulation battery described below.

Whenever the patient's dizziness is exclusively rotational, it is due to a disorder of the vestibular system: either the peripheral labyrinth or its central connections. Because of this close relationship, it is important to separate definite rotational vertigo accurately from other types of dizziness.

Type II dizziness is a *sensation of impending faint or loss of consciousness.* Pallor, dimness of vision, roaring in the ears, and diaphoresis, with recovery upon assuming the recumbent position, are common. Type II dizziness of cardiovascular origin is of abrupt onset and short duration. When faintness is gradual in onset or persists despite lying down, the relationship of the epi-

sodes to hypoglycemia or other disorders of cerebral metabolism should be sought.

The complaint of impending faint usually implies an inadequate supply of blood or nutrients to the entire brain, such as occurs in postural hypotension. It is not a feature of *focal* cerebral ischemia, although this mistaken impression is widely subscribed to by physicians. Other complaints of sudden alteration in the state of consciousness ("dreamy states") may be due to temporal lobe seizures, occurring in the absence of other, more obvious seizure phenomena.

Type III dizziness is *dysequilibrium:* the loss of balance *without* an abnormal sensation in the head. This experience occurs only when the patient is walking; it disappears as soon as he sits down. It is due to a disorder of motor system control.

Type IV dizziness is *vague lightheadedness* other than vertigo, faintness, or dysequilibrium. This designation includes dizziness that cannot be identified with certainty as any of the other types. When patients complain of lightheadedness, *fractional* or *poorly described* symptoms of vertigo, faintness, or dysequilibrium must first be looked for, e.g., a rocking sensation instead of spinning. Evidence of *hyperventilation* symptoms should next be sought, as well as symptoms pointing to a *psychiatric disorder,* particularly depression or anxiety. Finally, the evidence for *multiple sensory impairment* should be examined, especially a history of peripheral neuropathy, cervical spondylosis, or cataract surgery in an elderly or diabetic patient.

EVALUATING THE DIZZY PATIENT

The *history* must explore four major questions that critically distinguish the disorders producing dizziness: (1) the type of dizziness (I to IV) experienced by the patient; (2) the *abruptness* of attacks or *continuity* of symptoms; (3) the relation or independence of dizziness to *position or motion* (standing/sitting/lying; sudden change in position; walking); and (4) the *age* of the patient. The relation of these data to differential diagnosis will be discussed with specific entities.

A neurologic examination allows the distinction between central and peripheral causes of dizziness, and may reveal certain *patterns* of involvement that point to the diagnosis: e.g., brainstem syndrome (hemiplegia alternans), cerebellopontine angle syndrome, multiple sensory impairment.

The dizziness simulation battery is a series of eight bedside maneuvers that have proved valuable in distinguishing the various types of dizziness. Some produce dizziness in all patients, whereas others induce it only in patients with underlying disorders. After each maneuver the patient is questioned as to the similarity of the test-evoked sensation to his own dizziness. Identification of a provoked sensation as identical to the patient's dizziness is often more reliable than a verbal description, particularly if a single maneuver exclusively reproduces his symptoms.

1. *Orthostatic hypotension:* Blood pressure is measured supine, immediately on standing, and after three minutes.

2. *Potentiated Valsalva maneuver:* The patient squats for 30 seconds, then stands and blows into a mercury sphygmomanometer, raising the column to 40 mm Hg for 15 seconds.

3. *Carotid sinus stimulation:* The carotid sinus is unilaterally massaged for 15 seconds without continuous compression of the artery. ECG monitoring is required in the elderly, and the test should be omitted in patients with known cardiac disease.

TABLE 1. Positional Vertigo and Nystagmus

Benign	Central or Malignant
1. Latency of onset of vertigo and nystagmus	1. Immediate onset of vertigo and nystagmus
2. Adaptation and fatigue of vertigo and nystagmus	2. Persistence of nystagmus
3. Direction-fixed nystagmus	3. Direction-changing nystagmus
4. Severe vertigo and systemic symptoms	4. Mild vertigo; few systemic symptoms

4. *Neck-twist:* The patient rotates his head in each direction for 15 seconds as if watching an airplane fly past. Dizziness may result from "kinking" of a vertebral artery, cervicogenic dizziness, or a vestibular disorder.

5. *Walking and turning:* The patient walks in one direction and then quickly turns, reversing direction. This test reproduces dizziness occurring with multisensory deficits, gait apraxia, and disorders of balance.

6. *Hyperventilation:* The patient breathes deeply for three minutes.

7. *Nylen-Bárány maneuver:* The examiner carries the patient's head backward from a seated position, so that it is hanging 45 degrees below the horizontal and turned 45 degrees to one side. Vertigo *accompanied by nystagmus* indicates positional vertigo. The characteristics distinguishing a "benign" from a "malignant" form of this condition are listed in Table 1.

8. *Bárány rotation:* The patient is seated in a rotating chair, head tilted 30 degrees forward from the vertical. The examiner spins the patient in one direction ten times within 20 seconds, then abruptly stops the rotation.

LABORATORY TESTS (Table 2). *Electronystagmography* (ENG) may help to identify and distinguish disorders of the peripheral (labyrinth, eighth nerve) and central vestibular systems. Recording of the amplitude, speed, and duration of ocular movements is first made during a series of eye and head position maneuvers. In the *caloric test* the patient is positioned so that the horizontal semicircular canals are exactly vertical, and each ear is irrigated with cool and warm water (or air) to produce a convection flow of endolymph, which mimics rotational stimulation of each canal. Observations on the speed and duration of the nystagmus generated by this test provide information on the function of the vestibular apparatus.

Audiometric studies are used to evaluate lesions of the middle ear, labyrinth, and cochlear nerve, particularly in Menière's disorder and cerebellopontine angle tumors. Routine pure tone audiometry indicates the presence or absence of a hearing loss and may also distinguish banal causes (acoustic trauma, aging, otosclerosis) from specific cochlear and nerve disorders. More elaborate studies, such as the speech discrimination, alternate binaural loudness balance (ABLB), Békésy, threshold tone decay, and acoustic reflex tests, improve the accuracy of diagnosis. Recently, evoked re-

TABLE 2. Laboratory Tests in Dizziness

1. Electronystagmography (ENG) with caloric testing	6. Electrocardiogram with rhythm strip
2. Audiometry, ERA	7. Serum protein electrophoresis
3. Psychometric testing (MMPI)	8. Thyroid function studies
4. Skull x-rays with Stenvers' views	9. Electroencephalography
5. Cervical spine x-rays	10. Five-hour glucose tolerance test
	Optional: Petrous polytomography 24-hour cardiac monitoring

sponse audiometry (ERA), a signal averaging technique, has become a useful adjunct for distinguishing between brainstem and peripheral disorders.

SPECIFIC CONDITIONS PRODUCING DIZZINESS

It is not always simple to assemble the clinical and laboratory findings obtained from a dizzy patient into a specific diagnostic entity. A classification is provided here of the causes of dizziness, designed to parallel the four major complaints described earlier.

Vertigo and Other Vestibular Disorders

Vertigo accounts for only about a third of complaints of dizzy patients. When patients present with vestibular disorders, it is most important to distinguish between *peripheral* (labyrinthine) abnormalities and those involving *central* vestibular connections. The key to this distinction is the evidence for or against involvement of neighboring brainstem structures.

PERIPHERAL CAUSES OF VERTIGO. **Benign Positional Vertigo.** Benign positional vertigo is probably the most frequent cause of vertigo, accounting for about 25 per cent of patients with this complaint. The patient experiences a sensation of spinning when he rolls over in bed or makes other sudden head movements. Symptoms are greatest when he lies on his side with the affected ear underneath. The vertigo, sometimes accompanied by nausea and vomiting, lasts for less than five minutes, and between episodes the patient is free of symptoms. This condition, brought about *only* on change of position, differs from other vestibular disorders in which vertigo is increased by head motion but is present at other times as well. Benign positional vertigo occurs at any time during adult years; the cause is usually obscure, although it occasionally follows head trauma. The diagnosis is based on the typical history and on finding the "benign" type of vertigo and nystagmus on performing the Nylen-Bárány maneuver (Table 1). Caloric testing reveals depressed labyrinthine function in one ear in about half the patients. In the majority of cases symptoms persist for several weeks, although bouts may recur over a span of years with prolonged symptom-free intervals. This condition must be distinguished from so-called "central" or "malignant" positional vertigo and nystagmus (Table 1), which may occur with lesions (tumors, infarcts) involving posterior fossa structures; acute positional vertigo is uncommonly associated with such conditions.

Acute Peripheral Vestibulopathy ("Acute Labyrinthitis"; "Vestibular Neuronitis"). This condition is defined as a single bout of spontaneous vertigo, lasting for hours or days. Attacks occasionally follow a trivial respiratory or other infection, but the relation is not clear. Symptoms of vertigo, nausea, and vomiting usually improve within 48 hours, but may persist for 7 to 14 days. On examination the patient appears acutely ill, often pale and diaphoretic, resisting motion of the head. Nystagmus invariably accompanies the vertigo. As the patient recovers, he may feel "off balance" for weeks or months owing to unilateral impairment of vestibular function, present in about 50 per cent of patients. Hearing is not impaired in this condition.

Acute and Recurrent Peripheral Vestibulo-

pathy. Acute and recurrent peripheral vestibulopathy is clinically similar to the entity described above, but consists of *repeated* bouts of vertigo occurring over a period of months or years. This condition occurs in an older age group than acute peripheral vestibulopathy, and is associated with *less* severe vestibular impairment on caloric testing. Approximately half the patients presenting with a single attack of peripheral vestibulopathy experience a recurrence, linking this with the previous condition. The absence of auditory impairment distinguishes this condition from Menière's disorder.

Menière's Disorder. Menière's disorder is widely considered to be one of the most frequent causes of dizziness, but it actually accounts for only about 5 per cent of all dizziness and 10 to 15 per cent of vertigo. It usually occurs in adults and consists of recurring bouts of vertigo associated with *hearing loss* and *tinnitus* which may precede or follow the first bout of vertigo. Patients often complain of "fullness" in the ears, and are sometimes aware of *recruitment* as a sensation of auditory discomfort produced by loud noises. Bouts of vertigo last from hours to days, recurring as often as every week or as infrequently as every ten years. Hearing loss is unilateral in 80 to 90 per cent of patients, with a severe deficit in half the patients. Most patients develop chronic impairment of vestibular function, resulting in the syndrome of vestibular imbalance. In many patients the recurrent episodes of vertigo may "burn out" over the years.

Diagnosis depends on the characteristic history and the audiometric findings (low frequency pure tone impairment, poor speech discrimination comparable to the pure tone hearing loss, and recruitment). Caloric testing demonstrates abnormal vestibular function in 80 per cent of patients.

Pathologic studies have identified distention of the membranous labyrinth with endolymph as the immediate cause of this condition, but the explanation for the excess of endolymph remains obscure.

Toxic Damage to the Labyrinths. Drugs of the aminoglycoside groups (e.g., streptomycin, gentamicin) may produce toxic damage to the labyrinths. Although toxicity is generally dose related, some patients develop labyrinthine damage after brief treatment with ordinary doses of these drugs, particularly if renal function is impaired. Tinnitus, hearing loss, or vertigo may be the presenting symptom, along with severe impairment of balance, nausea, and vomiting. Vertigo continues for days or weeks. If the ototoxic drug is immediately discontinued, damage to the labyrinth is usually arrested. A characteristic loss of balance follows the acute stage of vertigo and may include blurring of vision on motion owing to loss of the vestibulo-ocular reflexes. With the loss of vestibular sensation, these patients are dependent on visual cues to maintain balance, and are unable to walk in the dark. After several months, adaptation to the loss of vestibular sensation develops, and many can lead fairly normal lives.

Diagnosis is based on the history of treatment with one of the ototoxic drugs, followed by the sequence described above. On examination the Romberg test is abnormal. Caloric tests demonstrate bilateral severe hypoactivity of the labyrinths. Bárány rotation may fail to elicit vertigo or nystagmus.

Other Peripheral Causes of Vertigo. Head trauma may be followed by persistent or positional vertigo. Dislocation of the otoliths from the macula of the utricle has been proposed as a cause of this condition. When vertigo immediately follows trauma, the etiologic relationship is clear, but in cases with medicolegal implications vertigo (and other forms of dizziness) may follow head trauma after a lengthy delay. It is often stated that the termination of pending litigation resolves such cases. *Cervicogenic vertigo,* although not vestibular in origin, may present with similar manifestations. Since the articulations and musculature of the cervical region provide extensive input to the brainstem vestibular system, cervical spondylosis or even painful muscular contraction may result in vertigo, nausea, and vomiting. *Dysproteinemias, hypothyroidism,* and *otitis media* are other occasional causes of vertigo.

TREATMENT. Management of vertigo resulting from most peripheral vestibular disorders is similar. When vertigo is severely disabling, the patient should be placed at bed rest or, in persistent cases, hospitalized. Meclizine, 25 mg four times daily, is of value in suppressing labyrinthine hyperactivity. Diazepam effectively suppresses central vestibular responses, and helps control the anxiety that often accompanies vertigo. Atropine tablets, 0.4 mg sublingually at the onset of attacks of vertigo, may abort the development of symptoms. Nausea and vomiting are controlled by trimethobenzamide hydrochloride (Tigan) suppositories, 200 mg every six hours, or in resistant cases by parenteral phenothiazines such as chlorpromazine (Thorazine), 25 mg every six hours.

Patients with benign positional vertigo may benefit from a soft foam rubber collar that limits cervical motion, thus preventing the stimulus for attacks.

Many patients with peripheral vestibular disorders have residual labyrinthine deficits after the acute vertiginous phase, and benefit from measures to improve their balance. A foam rubber collar is useful to limit neck motion, and methylphenidate (Ritalin) may enable them to react more quickly to the remaining sensory modalities. Balancing exercises help patients adapt to ambulation in the absence of normal vestibular function.

The treatment of acute attacks of Menière's disorder is similar to that for other vestibular disorders. A variety of medical and surgical treatments to prevent recurrences of vertigo and/or deterioration of hearing have been proposed; a discussion of their application and merits is beyond the scope of this chapter.

CENTRAL CAUSES OF VERTIGO. Cerebrovascular Disease. Cerebrovascular disease produces vertigo when basilar-vertebral artery ischemia damages the vestibular nuclei or their connections. In virtually all cases injury to adjacent brainstem structures occurs, and vertigo is unlikely to be due to a stroke when other neurologic symptoms or signs are absent. As with other patterns of cerebrovascular disease, elderly hypertensive patients with diabetes, heart disease, or hyperlipidemia are the most likely candidates. Caloric testing and evoked response audiometry (ERA) may help in the diagnosis by providing evidence of brainstem involvement of central vestibular and auditory pathways.

Transient ischemic attacks may be particularly difficult to diagnose, because at the time of examination the patient may have recovered completely. A reliable history of additional brainstem symptoms is necessary to establish the diagnosis. The treatment of cerebrovascular disease is discussed in Ch. 293 to 295.

Multiple Sclerosis. Multiple sclerosis may produce

vertigo in young patients, although this condition accounts for no more than 5 to 10 per cent of acute vertigo in those below age 40. Further, although multiple sclerosis may begin with vertigo, this is far less common than onset with optic neuritis or paresthesias. The diagnosis is discussed elsewhere; one must be aware that vertigo associated with ocular motor disorders that cannot be caused by purely peripheral vestibular disease (e.g., persistent diplopia, median longitudinal fasciculus syndrome, ophthalmoplegia) is strongly suggestive of this condition.

Treatment of the vertigo is similar to that for peripheral vestibulopathies; meclizine, diazepam, atropine, and Tigan are of value in controlling the vertigo and its associated nausea and vomiting.

Cerebellopontine Angle Tumors. Cerebellopontine angle tumors are a *rare* cause of vertigo, but must not be overlooked early in their growth when they are readily removable. The large majority are benign acoustic neuromas arising in the internal auditory meatus. These tumors develop in middle-aged patients who experience vague unsteadiness that progresses over a period of years. Vertigo when present may be of the "malignant" positional type (Table 1), and only rarely does acute spontaneous vertigo occur. Hearing loss, tinnitus, facial numbness or weakness, cerebellar ataxia, and occasional dementia complete the picture. Unilateral or bilateral acoustic neuromas are especially common in von Recklinghausen's disease (neurofibromatosis).

On caloric testing there is a markedly diminished response on the affected side. Audiometry demonstrates the findings of a "retrocochlear" lesion, including rapid tone decay, a diminished or absent acoustic reflex, and a Type III or IV curve on Békésy audiometry. Roentgenograms of the petrous bones are diagnostic and show erosion of the affected internal auditory meatus, a finding that is seen even earlier on polycyclic tomography.

Vertiginous Migraine. Vertiginous migraine may occur preceding the headache, during the headache phase, or as a "migraine equivalent" in place of the headache. Since both migraine and vertigo are common conditions, the occurrence of vertigo without a constant time relation to headache may represent only a coincidence in some unfortunate patients. Treatment is directed at prevention of the migraine attacks and control of the symptoms of vertigo, nausea, and vomiting as outlined above.

Viral Infections. Viral infections rarely cause vertigo except when herpes zoster affects the eighth nerve, often in conjunction with the Ramsay Hunt syndrome or geniculate herpes. Facial paralysis, vertigo, and hearing loss occur with herpetic vesicular lesions in the external auditory canal. Lymphocytes and polymorphonuclear leukocytes may be found in the cerebrospinal fluid. The diagnosis is established by demonstrating a rise of antibody titers to herpes zoster. Pathologically, lymphocytic infiltration of the sensory ganglia and nerve roots is seen. Treatment consists of the use of prednisone during the acute phase of the illness and the management of the vertigo, nausea, and vomiting as outlined above.

Cogan's syndrome is an uncommon vasculitis presenting in young adults with vertigo, deafness, and interstitial keratitis, as well as other systemic manifestations. Early in its course it may be mistaken for a minor vestibulopathy, although it may ultimately cause disability or death. Treatment with prednisone is of value and should be instituted promptly.

Deep-sea diving accidents may produce vertigo by a variety of mechanisms, including decompression sickness, air embolism, and rupture of the oval window. Investigation and treatment of these conditions should be carried out by physicians especially equipped to handle the problems of undersea medicine.

VESTIBULAR DISORDERS NOT PRODUCING VERTIGO. In some patients *hypoactivity* of the labyrinths may occur without antecedent episodes of vertigo. These patients describe lightheadedness on walking, turning, or changing position. The exact cause of the conditions producing these disorders is obscure. With *hyperactive* labyrinths, most often seen in anxious patients, instantaneous vertigo or loss of balance occurs on rapid turning. Caloric testing confirms the abnormal responsiveness of the labyrinths in either case. Patients with hypoactive or asymmetrical labyrinthine function benefit from methylphenidate (Ritalin), head restraint with a foam rubber collar, and a course of balancing exercises. Patients with hyperactive labyrinths are treated with meclizine, 25 mg three or four times daily, and diazepam, 5 mg three times daily.

Faintness: Syncopal and Seizure Disorders

SYNCOPAL DISORDERS (see also Ch. 264). **Orthostatic Hypotension.** In orthostatic hypotension the patient experiences faintness upon standing, resulting from a fall in blood pressure (at least 25/15 mm Hg). Acquired and idiopathic varieties are described. In the closely related Shy-Drager syndrome (see Ch. 278.6), manifestations of parkinsonism, peripheral neuropathy, dementia, and cerebellar abnormalities contribute to a multifactorial problem of dizziness. Recently, treatment with indomethacin, 50 mg three times daily, has been found to be effective in this condition.

Cardiac Arrhythmias. Patients with brief dizziness caused by episodic cardiac arrhythmias are often unaware of palpitations and complain only of faintness. When the arrhythmia is constantly present, it is easily recognized by observation of the jugular venous pulse, auscultation or electrocardiography. With infrequent runs of abnormal heart rhythm, the use of 12- or 24-hour ambulatory electrocardiographic monitoring is necessary. In young adults — especially women — mitral valve prolapse should be suspected as a cause of arrhythmia if a midsystolic click or late systolic murmur is heard on auscultation. Diagnosis and treatment are discussed in Ch. 364.

Carotid Sinus Hypersensitivity. Carotid sinus hypersensitivity resulting in bradycardia or temporary asystole may also present with Type II dizziness. The dizziness occurs abruptly and disappears rapidly, lasting no more than 15 seconds. The diagnosis is established by reproduction of symptoms with cautious carotid massage.

Vasovagal Syncope. Vasovagal syncope causes confusion with other forms of dizziness when the patient experiences faintness rather than actual loss of consciousness. The tendency to occur in young adults, the relation to precipitating emotional factors, the appearance of pallor at the onset, and the short duration are characteristic.

Cough, Micturition Syncope. Some patients experience faintness upon coughing or, with males, upon micturating while standing. The exact temporal relationship of faintness (or loss of consciousness) to these acts is diagnostic; the reproduction of symptoms by a potentiated Valsalva maneuver confirms the mechanism.

SEIZURE DISORDERS. Patients with temporal lobe seizures may describe feelings of "remoteness," "unreality," or, rarely, vertigo. When these events precede a typical psychomotor or generalized seizure, the cause is clearly *epileptic dizziness*. When the dizziness occurs as an isolated seizure phenomenon, it presents a diagnostic problem. Such patients *rarely* complain primarily of dizziness, however, because the epileptic phenomena dominate the picture.

Very rarely labyrinthine-induced vertigo may trigger "vestibulogenic epilepsy," a form of reflex seizure akin to reading epilepsy. If caloric testing is carried out while an electroencephalogram is taken, the observation of induced seizure activity establishes the diagnosis.

The reader is cautioned against diagnosing seizure disorders in patients whose dizziness is accompanied by mild abnormalities on electroencephalography without the other criteria mentioned.

Dysequilibrium: Impaired Balance

APRAXIA OF GAIT. This is a little-recognized but common disorder of the elderly. The patient walks with a broad-based gait, taking short steps and placing his feet flat on the ground, suggesting a person walking on ice. A tendency to retropulsion increases the danger of falling. On examination, motor power, coordination, and sensation are normal in the legs, although the gait is impaired and hopping on one foot is impossible. The finding of "frontal lobe" deficits, including dementia and grasp and suck reflexes, is confirmatory. Most cases of gait apraxia result from a degenerative process similar to Alzheimer's disease. Other causes include such conditions as subdural hematomas, tumors, normal pressure hydrocephalus, or a lacunar state.

When a specific disorder (e.g., a subdural hematoma) is found, treatment is directed appropriately. In the more common degenerative conditions treatment must be symptomatic. In some patients improvement may result from small doses of L-dopa (1.5 to 3.0 grams per day in divided doses). Mild stimulants (methylphenidate), balancing exercises, and a cane are of benefit, and patients should be encouraged to walk some distance *every day* to avoid total dependence.

PARKINSONISM. Patients with parkinsonism and a balance disturbance often complain of dysequilibrium. When tremor is minimal and impaired balance is prominent, it is difficult to distinguish between parkinsonism and gait apraxia. These patients often have a pronounced increase in axial tone, as well as frontal lobe signs and dementia.

CEREBELLAR LESIONS. Impairment of balance without other cerebellar signs may be seen in certain cerebellar lesions such as alcoholic cerebellar degeneration or tumors of the vermis. In addition some patients may develop "malignant" positional vertigo. Since a staggering gait and nystagmus are seen in peripheral vestibular disorders, the clinical distinction presents difficulties. Neurodiagnostic studies (radioisotope scan, computerized axial tomography, angiography) may be required to establish the diagnosis.

ASTASIA-ABASIA. Astasia-abasia is impairment of stance and gait on a psychogenic basis. In some patients the gait is quite bizarre, but in others it may resemble apraxia. The distinction depends on the absence of other frontal lobe signs and on the ability of the patient to walk *normally* under some circumstances, such as only indoors. Other evidence of a phobic or conversion reaction is often present.

Lightheadedness

Vague "lightheadedness" accounts for over 50 per cent of patients' complaints, and includes the largest spectrum of disorders.

Inevitably, some patients provide a *poor description of other types of dizziness* which more introspective or articulate patients would recognize as vertigo, faintness, or dysequilibrium. In addition, *fractional forms of other types of dizziness* are often described as "lightheadedness" even by observant patients. Almost half the patients who initially experience vertigo later complain of lightheadedness as their symptoms subside. The dizziness simulation battery helps to *identify* a sensation which the patient cannot easily *describe* verbally.

HYPERVENTILATION. This is the second most common cause of dizziness after vestibular disorders, and the most common under the age of 40. The disorder is discussed in detail in Ch. 265. In the acute form, young anxious patients present with brief episodes of shortness of breath, lightheadedness, paresthesias in the fingers and around the mouth, and feelings of panic. More difficult to identify is chronic hyperventilation, seen in patients who periodically sigh deeply.

The mechanism of hyperventilation-induced dizziness is presumed to be hypocapnia with secondary cerebral arterial contriction and diminished cerebral blood flow. Treatment of acute attacks with diazepam, 5 to 10 mg intramuscularly, is often effective. Rebreathing into a paper bag may abort the attack.

MULTISENSORY DIZZINESS. When several sensory modalities are impaired, perception of the environment becomes inadequate to maintain orientation, and the patient experiences dizziness when attempting to walk. The most common combinations of sensory impairment are peripheral neuropathy (with diminished touch, pressure, and proprioceptive sensation), visual loss from cataracts, and cervical spondylosis (with distortion of proprioception from cervical joints). Impaired vestibular and auditory function often add to the sensory disorientation. The aged and diabetic are especially prone to this condition. Patients with multisensory dizziness adopt a broad-based tentative gait, which may superficially resemble apraxia of gait, but the "frontal lobe" features are absent. Examination reveals the underlying neurosensory deficit — peripheral neuropathy, visual impairment, cervical arthritis, and hearing loss. Caloric testing may provide evidence of additional sensory impairment. When all five sensory modalities are severely impaired, patients may be unable to walk without assistance.

An important example of this condition is seen in the post-cataract-extraction patient who complains of disabling dizziness despite perfect restoration of visual acuity. Dizziness results from the distortion produced by the corrective lenses used after surgery. Patients who have no other sensory deficits are able to compensate for the visual distortions, but those with peripheral neuropathy cannot. Contact lenses eliminate these distortions, but unfortunately many elderly patients cannot manage them. Surgical replacement of opaque lenses wtih inert plastic implants promises to avoid this problem in suitable patients.

Treatment of multisensory dizziness includes balancing exercises and use of a foam rubber collar to eliminate extraneous head motion. A light cane should be used for balance. Methylphenidate (Ritalin) improves the speed of the patient's response to his perceived environment.

PSYCHIATRIC DISORDERS. In addition to patients with astasia-abasia or hyperventilation, some patients experience subjective dizziness on the basis of purely psychiatric disease. Some indicate that their dizziness consists of "difficulty concentrating"; others experience panic states when in crowded places; whereas some frankly psychotic patients describe the bizarre confusion of their perceived environments as "dizziness" for lack of a more explicit term.

In these patients, the diagnosis hinges on elimination of other causes of dizziness combined with evidence of significant psychiatric disease on interview or psychometric testing. It is often useful to demonstrate to such patients the negative findings on extensive tests for organic causes of dizziness, and to assure them that no cause has been overlooked.

Anxious patients complaining of lightheadedness may also manifest somatic symptoms, including tachycardia, palpitations, flushing, and tremulousness. In some cases the symptoms can be reproduced by the intravenous infusion of isoproterenol at a low rate (1 to 3 μg per minute), and have been attributed to "beta-adrenergic hyperactivity." Although the pathophysiology is obscure, such patients may derive benefit from treatment with propranolol hydrochloride, 10 to 40 mg four times daily.

Drachman, D. A.: Episodic vertigo. In Conn, H. (ed.): Current Therapy 1974. Philadelphia, W. B. Saunders Company, 1974, p. 684.

Drachman, D. A., and Hart, C. W.: An approach to the dizzy patient. Neurology, 22:323, 1972.

Fisher, C. M.: Vertigo in cerebrovascular disease. Arch. Otolaryngol. 85:529, 1967.

Harrison, M. S., and Ozsahinoglu, C.: Positional vertigo. Arch. Otolaryngol., 101:675, 1975.

Hart, C. W.: The evaluation of vestibular function in health and disease. In Otolaryngology. Vol. 1, Chap. 10. Hagerstown, Md., Harper & Row, 1972.

Naunton, R. F. (ed.): The Vestibular System. New York, Academic Press, 1975.

264. SYNCOPE

Albert Heyman

DEFINITION. Syncope is the cutting off or transient loss of consciousness. Although the term is usually applied to unconsciousness caused by a temporary decrease in cerebral blood flow, in this discussion a broader definition is employed that includes the brief disturbances in consciousness caused by changes in the chemical composition of the blood as in hyperventilation or hypoglycemia. Syncope has been found to occur in as many as 25 to 30 per cent of young, healthy adult males. It should be carefully differentiated from such disorders as epilepsy, vertigo, cataplexy, and strokes, all of which may produce transient disturbances in consciousness, generalized weakness, or inability to stand erect. The loss of consciousness in syncope may not be complete, but may consist of varying degrees of impaired sensorium with transient blurring of vision, weakness, and loss of postural tone. Such attacks may be described by the patient as dizziness, faintness, lightheadedness, or a "drunk feeling." These partial manifestations have the rapid onset, brief duration, and complete recovery characteristic of the fully developed faint.

PATHOGENESIS. Syncope is most frequently caused by a reduction in cerebral blood flow below a critical level and is usually associated with a sharp fall in blood pressure. This, in turn, is the result of either a loss of peripheral resistance, as seen in vasodepressor faint and in orthostatic hypotension, or a decrease in cardiac output, as in Adams-Stokes attacks. In many patients, however, loss of consciousness is not caused by reduction of blood pressure but by a decrease in such essential blood components as glucose, carbon dioxide, or oxygen. In other instances, as in micturition syncope and cough syncope, the faint seems to result from cerebral ischemia caused by extracardiac disturbances.

There are several features common to almost all types of syncope. Electroencephalographic changes usually appear, and consist of high voltage, 2- to 4-cycle per second slow waves that promptly return to normal after consciousness is regained. Brief convulsive movements, such as tonic or clonic contractions of the arms or turning of the head, can occur in all types of fainting, depending on the degree and duration of the cerebral ischemia. Fully developed seizures with tongue biting and urinary incontinence, however, are unusual. Recovery is usually hastened in the recumbent posture, which helps restore the normal cerebral circulation. The critical level of cerebral blood flow necessary to maintain consciousness has been estimated to be about 30 ml per 100 grams of brain per minute (normal value is 50 to 55 ml). The duration of asystole or the degree of hypotension necessary to produce critical levels of cerebral ischemia varies, depending upon the posture of the patient, the ability of the cerebral vessels to dilate, and other factors. In normal subjects in the erect posture, a mean arterial blood pressure as low as 20 to 30 mm of mercury or an asystole of four or five seconds' duration can produce syncope. In the recumbent position, longer periods of asystole may occur before loss of consciousness develops.

CLINICAL MANIFESTATIONS. Orthostatic Hypotension. Chronic orthostatic hypotension is a disorder of the autonomic nervous system in which syncope occurs when the patient assumes the upright posture. The condition is sometimes seen in diabetic neuropathy and in tabes dorsalis, but in many patients the site of the neurologic lesion is unknown. These people have an abnormality in the baroreceptor reflexes that ordinarily compensates for the pooling of blood in the lower extremities and viscera. When an attempt is made to stand upright, there is an inadequate degree of reflex arteriolar constriction, with a subsequent reduction in venous return. This is associated with an immediate and sharp fall in arterial blood pressure, followed by syncope. The pulse rate remains unchanged during the episode, and there are none of the usual prodromal symptoms of pallor, sweating, and nausea seen in vasodepressor faint. Orthostatic hypotension has also been associated with a Parkinson-like disorder sometimes referred to as the Shy-Drager syndrome (see Ch. 278.6).

A new syndrome of orthostatic hypotension known as hyperbradykininism has been reported, in which standing produces a fall in systolic blood pressure, an increase in diastolic pressure and heart rate, and purplish discoloration and ecchymoses over the legs. The disorder is characterized by high plasma levels of bradykinin, which may account for dilatation of the cutaneous venules and capillaries in the legs and reduction in venous return.

Failure of postural adaptation may appear after surgical sympathectomy for hypertension or the administration of vasodilating agents and antihypertensive drugs, especially the sodium-depleting diuretics and ganglionic blocking agents. Iatrogenic forms of syncope have also been noted in patients treated with tranquilizing agents such as phenothiazine derivatives or with L-dopa for Parkinson's disease. Commonly prescribed medications such as digitalis and quinidine may cause cardiac conduction disturbances resulting in arrhythmia and syncope. Patients recovering from chronic wasting illnesses associated with prolonged bed rest may experience syncope when they attempt to assume the upright position. Shorter periods of bed rest, particularly when associated with dehydration or electrolyte deficits, may also be associated with orthostatic hypotension.

Vasodepressor Syncope (the Common Faint). Vasodepressor syncope is by far the most frequent cause of transient loss of consciousness. The condition is characterized by a fall in blood pressure associated with the development of a variety of autonomic manifestations. In the early presyncopal period, there may be pallor, nausea, and sweating; in later stages pupillary dilatation, yawning, hyperpnea, and bradycardia appear. When the mean arterial pressure falls below critical levels, loss of consciousness and characteristic electroencephalographic changes occur. Bradycardia is often severe at the onset of unconsciousness, and pulse rates of 50 to 60 per minute may be observed even after recovery. The duration of syncope is brief, ranging from a few seconds to several minutes. In the postsyncopal period the patient may complain of headaches, weakness, nervousness, and slight confusion. Vasodepressor faint is most often evoked by sudden emotional stress associated with fear, anxiety, or pain. Hypodermic injections, trauma, minor surgery, and the sight of or withdrawal of blood are common precipitating events. Attacks usually occur in the standing or upright posture, and consciousness returns quickly once the patient is recumbent.

The initial event in this complex vascular and neurogenic reaction is dilatation of the vascular bed throughout the body, particularly in peripheral muscles. Vasodilatation in the limb muscles is a normal response to emotional stimuli, and is thought to represent preparation for "fight or flight." The absence of immediate muscle activity, however, and the fall in peripheral resistance are not compensated for by an increase in cardiac output, and as a result there is a reduction in cerebral blood flow.

Adams-Stokes Syndrome. In the early nineteenth century Morgagni, Adams, and Stokes separately observed and described fainting associated with a persistently slow pulse in the range of 40 per minute. Patients with this syndrome usually have a disordered atrioventricular conduction system. Syncope also occurs in patients with bilateral bundle branch disease, a condition which may precede complete heart block. The decision to insert a permanent pacemaker in such cases should be made only in patients with documented heart block or those with a clear-cut history of cardiac syncope. A rare form of syncope caused by ventricular fibrillation has been reported in children with hereditary prolonged Q-T intervals in the electrocardiogram, sometimes accompanied by congenital deaf mutism. Ventricular dysrhythmia and syncope caused by prolongation of Q-T intervals also has been described following drug intoxication and electrolyte imbalance. The clinical picture of syncope caused by cardiac arrhythmias is often characteristic. Loss of consciousness is abrupt; prodromal signs are not usually present. On regaining consciousness, the patient usually shows little confusion or postsyncopal residua. The attacks may occur several times a day and have no relation to posture or activity. Only a brief period of asystole of four or five seconds' duration will produce loss of consciousness in the erect position, but longer periods of asystole are not uncommon. In such instances, neurologic manifestations such as convulsive movements, pupillary dilatation, and prolonged confusion may be observed. Occasionally sudden death results from cardiac standstill. Syncope occurring for the first time in elderly patients should be suspected as being caused by heart block. Since these patients often have sinus rhythm with normal heart rate when seen by the physician, continuous tape-recorded electrocardiographic monitoring is often needed for diagnosis. Such monitoring can be carried out during the patient's routine activities; and by correlating the patient's symptoms with the appearance of an arrhythmia, a firm basis can be established for definitive treatment such as implantation of an intracardiac pacemaker.

Reflex Cardiac Standstill. Syncopal attacks may result from vagal reflex–induced cardiac standstill in persons without heart disease. A few authenticated cases of swallowing or deglutition syncope have been reported. Most such patients have been found to have diverticula or other disorders of the esophagus or underlying cardiac disease. Experimental distention of the esophagus with balloons can sometimes induce complete atrioventricular block and syncope. The alterations in consciousness and the electrocardiographic changes disappear when the pressure within the esophagus is relieved or after administration of atropine. The syncopal episode occasionally seen after drinking ice cold fizzy fluids, during digital prostatic examination (so-called prostatic prostration), or during thoracentesis or bronchoscopic examination may also be due to such reflex vagal mechanisms. Syncope caused by cardiac arrest has been observed in patients with paroxysmal pain in the throat due to glossopharyngeal neuralgia.

Carotid Sinus Syncope. In few patients is this the mechanism of actual syncope. Many persons, particularly those more than 60 years of age, show reflex slowing of the heart and fall of blood pressure during massage of one or both carotid sinuses. Such responses are frequent in patients with cardiac disorders, hypertension, or diseases of the carotid vessels such as atherosclerotic thrombosis or stenosis. The most common response to carotid sinus massage is either sinus bradycardia or sinoatrial block, both of which may be abolished by administration of atropine. Much less frequently, there may be a pure vasodepressor response without slowing of the heart. In a third but rare type of carotid response, fainting may appear in a few seconds without significant changes in either blood pressure or pulse; such instances probably occur only with vigorous pressure and when the opposite carotid is already thrombosed. Carotid sinus syncope is not accompanied by the prodromal symptoms seen in the common faint. It is more frequent in men, and usually occurs in the erect posture. It sometimes follows sudden head turning or pressure of a tight collar.

Very few of the patients who exhibit bradycardia or a reduction in blood pressure on carotid massage experience loss of consciousness. In eliciting carotid sinus responses, care should be taken to avoid obstructing blood flow to the brain by compression of the carotid vessels. Cerebral infarction and even death have been reported after carotid compression and massage. Massage of both carotid sinuses simultaneously may be hazardous. An increasing number of reports describe the use of a permanent demand pacemaker for relief of carotid sinus syncope. The rarity with which true syncope occurs with carotid sinus hypersensitivity, however, requires that such radical treatment be carefully evaluated.

Organic Heart Disease. Patients with myocardial infarction or valvular lesions may also have transient periods of unconsciousness. The mechanism of syncope in these disorders is not altogether clear, but may be related to a reduction in cardiac output with inadequate cerebral blood flow. In acute myocardial infarction, fainting probably results from decrease in stroke volume owing to a weakened myocardium. Transient arrhythmias, such as ventricular tachycardia, fibrillation, or heart block, may contribute to the syncopal reaction. Transient loss of consciousness may occur during attacks of angina pectoris, and is probably caused by ventricular fibrillation or various types of heart block associated with temporary periods of myocardial ischemia. Syncope also appears during paroxysmal tachycardia even in the absence of structural heart disease. In such cases the loss of consciousness usually occurs at the onset or at the end of the attack, at which time there may be a brief period of cardiac standstill.

Patients with aortic valvular or subvalvular stenosis often have syncope associated with physical exertion (effort syncope). The loss of consciousness in the early phases of such syncopal episodes may be due to shunting of blood to the peripheral muscles, but the later phases have been shown to be associated with transient ventricular asystole, tachycardia, or fibrillation, presumably caused by diminished coronary arterial blood flow. Sudden death may occur during these attacks. Effort syncope is also seen in patients with congenital heart disease such as patent ductus arteriosus or tetralogy of Fallot, as well as in those with pulmonary hypertension. Patients with atrial myxoma, on the right or left side, although rare, often present with recurrent syncope. In such cases, a pedunculated tumor intermittently obstructs the mitral or tricuspid valves.

Cough Syncope. Cough syncope usually follows a paroxysm of explosive and vigorous coughing. It is commonly observed in men but rarely in women. In adults, the condition is often seen in stocky, barrel-chested men with chronic lung disease or bronchitis; in children, it may occur during severe *pertussis*. The syncope is brief and there are no residua. The condition may recur in the recumbent patient or following hearty laughter. The loss of consciousness has been attributed to an increase in the intrathoracic and intra-abdominal

pressure caused by vigorous coughing. This, in turn, is thought to produce a sudden sharp elevation in cerebrospinal fluid pressure, thereby "squeezing" blood from the intracranial and cerebral vessels. Other theories maintain that the condition is due to a Valsalva effect with reduction in cardiac output or to cerebral "concussive effect" caused by rapid rise in the cerebrospinal fluid pressure. There is clinical evidence to suggest that the presence of an intracerebral lesion such as brain tumor or stenosis of a major cerebral artery may produce increased susceptibility to syncope after paroxysms of cough. Such patients may have focal neurologic symptoms such as paresthesias or clonic movements of one limb prior to loss of consciousness. Therapy consists of the relief of the force, frequency, and duration of the cough by clearing of the bronchial secretions and suppression of cough reflex. In refractory cases, tracheostomy may be beneficial by reducing intrathoracic pressure during the paroxysms of cough.

Micturition Syncope. This form of syncope is most often seen during or immediately after micturition in men who rise in the middle of the night to urinate. The loss of consciousness is brief and there is no postsyncopal confusion or weakness. Many such people give a history of drinking large quantities of beer before retiring, and considerable bladder deflation may take place during micturition. A similar fainting may be observed after drainage of a distended bladder in urinary retention or after removal of a large quantity of ascitic fluid by abdominal paracentesis. It has been suggested that the loss of consciousness may be due to a reflex vasodilatation of the peripheral vascular system, a situation thought to be the converse of the paroxysmal hypertension seen in paraplegics during bladder distention. It is not likely to be due to a Valsalva maneuver during micturition but may be related to peripheral vasodilation associated with a warm bed and perhaps the recent consumption of alcohol.

Hysterical Fainting. Hysterical fainting is seen almost entirely in young women with emotional illness. It differs from the vasodepressor faint and the hyperventilation syndrome in that the patient is relatively free of anxiety and shows little concern regarding the fainting episodes. The attack usually occurs in the presence of others. The patient generally slumps to the floor gracefully, sometimes dramatically, without injury or awkwardness. It thus resembles the mid-Victorian drawing room swoon. A few decades ago, hysterical fainting often occurred in groups of young women during mass excitement, particularly that caused by the presence of screen or television idols. Although excited behavior is now often observed among young women attending "rock" concerts, swooning is seldom seen.

During the attack the patient may be motionless or may show bizarre resisting movements. The attack may last from several minutes to as long as an hour or more, with fluctuations of responsiveness. There are no abnormalities in pulse, blood pressure, or skin color. The electroencephalogram is normal during the attack, indicating that there may be no actual loss of consciousness. The diagnosis can usually be made without difficulty on the basis of the setting of the episode, the patient's underlying emotional disturbance, and the absence of physical abnormalities.

Cerebral Arterial Occlusive Disease. Patients with generalized atherosclerosis may have frequent episodes of loss of consciousness over a period of days or weeks.

In most instances the attack is accompanied by signs of focal neurologic deficits such as motor weakness, sensory loss, or cranial nerve disorders. In such cases the diagnosis of transient focal ischemia can be made without difficulty. Syncopal episodes in older persons, however, are often not associated with focal neurologic symptoms but consist only of transient giddiness and visual blurring and occur particularly on arising from bed in the morning or standing upright after stooping or bending over. Such patients with "blind staggers" frequently have evidence of hypertension, cardiac disease, or obstructive lesions in the extracranial cerebral vessels, but these conditions may not be responsible for their disturbing postural symptoms. It appears that the reflexes that normally compensate for sudden changes in posture are impaired in these individuals. Attempts to relieve such symptoms by surgical correction of extracranial arterial occlusive disease or by administration of various medications are often unsuccessful.

Hypoglycemia. Low levels of blood sugar often produce symptoms of weakness, trembling, sweating, tachycardia, hunger sensation, and confused behavior. Syncope is not a common occurrence, but prolonged hypoglycemia may result in seizures, coma, and serious brain damage. The majority of patients with these symptoms have anxiety reaction rather than hypoglycemia. The diagnosis of hypoglycemia must therefore be based on documented low levels of blood sugar at the time of the clinical manifestations which, in turn, can be relieved by ingestion of food or sugar. It is also important that the type of hypoglycemia be established. Reactive hypoglycemia is the most common type and may appear in thin, emotionally tense persons a few hours after ingestion of a high carbohydrate meal. It sometimes follows extensive gastric resection in association with the dumping syndrome and occurs in some people with mild diabetes. Hypoglycemia may also be due to islet cell adenoma of the pancreas. In this condition, nervousness, weakness, trembling, and sometimes convulsions occur after fasting and exercise. The fasting morning blood sugar level may be low, in contrast to that of patients with reactive hypoglycemia, in whom this determination is usually normal. Other conditions such as pituitary insufficiency, Addison's disease, hepatic failure, and large sarcomas may also produce hypoglycemia.

DIAGNOSIS. The diagnosis of syncope depends almost entirely upon a careful history of the attack and the setting in which it occurs. Differentiation of syncope from an akinetic epileptic seizure, such as petit mal or psychomotor attack, may be difficult. Careful evaluation of the electroencephalographic findings, the onset and duration of the attack, and the postsyncopal manifestations can usually distinguish these conditions. These factors are also helpful in differentiating the various types of syncope. In vasodepressor faint, the patient usually has prodromal signs of autonomic hyperactivity such as pallor, sweating, salivation, and bradycardia. In cardiac arrest, orthostatic hypotension, and carotid sinus syncope, loss of consciousness occurs abruptly, and prodromal symptoms are not usually present. Postsyncopal confusion, headache, and weakness often follow vasodepressor faint and the hyperventilation syndrome. In chronic orthostatic hypotension and Adams-Stokes attacks, recovery of consciousness is rapid and complete without postsyncopal symptoms.

Most types of fainting occur in the erect or upright position, but in cardiac arrest, syncope may appear while the patient is recumbent. The duration of syncope is brief in postural hypotension but prolonged in hyperventilation and hypoglycemia. Most of these differentiating manifestations can be determined by careful history, but specific procedures should be carried out during the physical examination. These consist of voluntary hyperventilation for approximately two minutes, careful massage of the carotid sinuses (preferably with electrocardiographic and electroencephalographic monitoring), auscultation for murmurs over the cervical vessels and base of the heart to exclude possible obstruction of blood flow through the extracranial cerebral vessels and aortic valves, and, finally, observations of pulse and blood pressure during change in posture from recumbency to erect position. If the blood pressure falls appreciably but the heart rate fails to accelerate, dysfunction of the autonomic nervous system should be suspected. If the patient with syncope has orthostatic hypotension with an appropriate rise in heart rate, hypovolemia caused by salt and water depletion or diuretic therapy may be present. An electroencephalogram is indicated whenever convulsive movements develop during the syncopal episode, or when focal neurologic manifestations are noted. In older persons, long strips of the electrocardiogram should be searched for episodes of arrhythmia, and prolonged ambulatory cardiac (Holter) monitoring should also be carried out whenever recurrent syncope is not otherwise explained. A glucose tolerance test should be made if there appears to be a relationship of syncope to meals, prolonged duration of altered consciousness, or recovery following ingestion of carbohydrates.

TREATMENT. Therapy in syncope consists primarily of treatment of the underlying disorder. In all types of fainting, recovery is usually aided by maintaining the patient in a recumbent position with elevation of the lower extremities. Application of cold water to the face and head and inhalation of spirits of ammonia or other pungent aromatics are time-honored and certainly do no harm.

Ad Hoc Committee on Hypoglycemia: Statement on hypoglycemia. Arch. Intern. Med., 131:591, 1973.

Dhingra, R. C., Denes, P., Wu, D., et al.: Syncope in patients with chronic bifascicular block. Ann. Intern. Med., 81:302, 1974.

Noble, R. J.: The patient with syncope. JAMA, 237:1372, 1977.

Shillingford, J. P.: Syncope. Am. J. Cardiol., 26:609, 1970.

Thomas, J. E.: Hyperactive carotid sinus reflex and carotid sinus syncope. Mayo Clin. Proc., 44:127, 1969.

Walter, P. F., Reid, S. D., and Wenger, N. K.: Transient cerebral ischemia due to arrhythmias. Ann. Intern. Med., 72:471, 1970.

Wright, K. E., Jr., and McIntosh, H. D.: Syncope: A review of pathophysiological mechanisms. Prog. Cardiovasc. Dis., 13:580, 1971.

265. HYPERVENTILATION

Albert Heyman

HYPERVENTILATION SYNDROME. The hyperventilation syndrome is one of the most frequent causes of impaired consciousness, usually producing "faintness" and "lightheadedness" without actual syncope. It is almost always a manifestation of acute anxiety. At the onset of an attack, the patient may complain of tightness of the chest and a feeling of suffocation. He may not be aware of overbreathing but usually recalls excessive deep sighing. Later, a sense of unreality develops, accompanied by feelings of apprehension and sometimes panic. Symptoms related to the heart and gastrointestinal tract consist of palpitations or pounding of the heart, precordial oppression, fullness in the throat, and epigastric discomfort. The syndrome may last for as long as a half hour or more and may recur several times a day. Sensations of "numbness" and "coldness" of the hands, feet, and perioral areas often develop. In prolonged attacks, tetany has been noted with the appearance of carpopedal spasm and Chvostek's sign, i.e., unilateral facial spasm following finger tapping of the facial musculature. Some patients develop chest pain.

The pathogenesis of the individual symptoms of this disorder is not altogether clear. With normal subjects, hyperventilation in the recumbent posture for as long as an hour will not produce loss of consciousness. They may, however, have sensations of decreased awareness, lightheadedness, and blurring of vision, but do not have the trembling, sweating, palpitations, or precordial distress frequently seen in patients with spontaneous overventilation. The serum calcium level remains normal, but there is often a decrease in serum phosphate. Within 15 minutes after onset of hyperventilation in voluntary subjects, arterial P_{CO_2} falls to levels of 20 to 30 mm Hg, where it may remain with only an occasional sighing respiration. The hypocapnia caused by overventilation results in cerebral vasoconstriction, which decreases oxygen delivery to the brain. Studies in laboratory animals have shown that prolonged hyperventilation produces an increase in lactic acid in the cerebrospinal fluid and brain due probably to ischemic cerebral hypoxia. A slight fall in blood pressure also occurs during hyperventilation caused by muscular vasodilatation. These factors alone are usually insufficient to produce syncope, and the occasional loss of consciousness with this syndrome is probably due to vasodepressor mechanisms as in the common faint.

The hyperventilation syndrome is often precipitated by acute emotional stress and is most common in nervous, anxious women who have other functional disturbances related to tension. The syndrome can often be reproduced by having the patient hyperventilate voluntarily for two or three minutes. Although the patient is often reassured by the fact that he can control the attack somewhat by breath-holding or breathing in a paper bag, therapy directed at the underlying emotional disturbance is usually necessary.

HYPERVENTILATION COMBINED WITH VALSALVA MANEUVER. The physiologic alterations produced by a combination of hyperventilation and increased intrathoracic pressure (secondary to variants of the Valsalva maneuver) account for several unique types of syncope. The "mess trick," a prank often indulged in by schoolboys, consists of sudden manual compression of the chest of the victim after he has been hyperventilating for about a minute. Loss of consciousness may also occur in the "fainting lark," in which the victim is instructed to hyperventilate in the squatting position, stand quickly, and immediately perform the Valsalva maneuver. The loss of consciousness observed in athletes lifting weights ("weightlifter's blackout") is due to similar mechanisms. During competition, these individuals often hyperventilate vigorously and then squat before grasping the weight. Lifting of the weight produces high levels of intrathoracic pressure which reduces venous return and causes decrease in cardiac output, stroke volume, and pulse pressure. These alterations, combined with the peripheral vasodilation caused by squatting and cerebral vasoconstriction caused by hyperventilation, result in a reduction in cerebral blood flow and loss of consciousness. Voluntary syncope has also been observed in muscular teenage boys who can maintain a prolonged Valsalva maneuver by vigorous stretching of the trunk and back muscles. Such instances of "stretch syncope" are often self-induced to provide a curiously satisfying experience.

Klein, L. J., Saltzman, H., and Heyman, A.: Syncope induced by the Valsalva maneuver: A study of the effects of arterial blood gas tensions, glucose concentration and blood pressure. Am. J. Med., 37:263, 1964.

Saltzman, H. A., Heyman, A., and Sieker, H. O.: Correlations of clinical and physiologic manifestations of sustained hyperventilation. N. Engl. J. Med., 268:1431, 1963.

Section Ten NEUROLOGIC DIAGNOSTIC PROCEDURES

Kathleen M. Foley

266. INTRODUCTION

Neurologic diagnostic tests supplement but do not substitute for a meticulous neurologic history and examination. The yield from diagnostic tests is directly related to the skill of the physician who must order the appropriate test suggested by the neurologic history and examination, and who must interpret the test based on the clinical findings.

The most valuable and commonly used of the neurologic diagnostic tests are described in the following chapters. Special attention is directed at those procedures which the general physician is likely to use in evaluating a patient with neurologic symptoms. These include the lumbar puncture, skull and spine x-rays, the electroencephalogram (EEG), the radionuclide brain scan, and computerized tomography (CT or CAT scan). It is imperative for the physician to familiarize himself with the indications and limitations of these studies to ensure appropriate interpretation. There is also a series of more selective neurodiagnostic procedures (i.e., arteriography, pneumoencephalography, myelography, cisternography, electromyography) which the physician may find useful and which are usually performed after consultation with a neurologist or neurosurgeon. In this presentation these procedures are considered in less detail. Many of the procedures are also discussed elsewhere in this text in the context of neurologic illnesses, and, when applicable, reference will be made to those chapters.

Certain general principles should govern the physician in his choice of any neurologic diagnostic procedure: (1) *No procedure should be considered routine.* The physician should order only those tests appropriate to answer specific questions posed by the neurologic history and examination. (2) *The procedure which yields the most information with the least risk to the patient should be performed first.* For example, if a brain tumor is suspected, computerized tomography is superior to either plain x-rays or radionuclide brain scans because it is much more informative, and is superior to arteriography and pneumoencephalography because it is much less of a risk and is less costly. (3) *The responsible physician should discuss the diagnostic problem with the specialist performing the procedure before it is done* to assure that the maximal information related to the patient's problem will be procured. The responsible physician should also review the completed study with the specialist to ensure an interpretation based on the clinical findings. (4) *The patient should be properly instructed in the nature of the procedure and in its potential risks, complications, and benefits.* Since patient cooperation is essential in these studies, adequate sedation should be employed when necessary.

267. COMPUTERIZED TRANSAXIAL TOMOGRAPHY

(CT Scan, CAT)

Computerized tomography has had a profound impact on the diagnostic evaluation of the patient with neurologic symptoms. It provides a simple, rapid x-ray procedure, applicable on an ambulatory basis, with diagnostic accuracy comparable to that of arteriography and pneumoencephalography. The procedure is unique in that it provides a direct two-dimensional view of the head with adequate visualization of bone, brain parenchyma, and cerebrospinal fluid spaces. The method computes differences in x-ray density of the many cranial and intracranial structures and draws a tomographic picture of the brain (usually 0.8 to 1.3 cm in thickness) such that the calvarium appears white, whereas less dense brain tissue is depicted in varying shades of gray. Cortical gray matter is more dense than central gray or white matter, and cerebrospinal fluid has an unusually low density and appears black against the brain parenchyma, allowing for delineation of cerebral and cerebellar sulci and fissures. Contrast enhancement by the intravenous administration of an iodinated x-ray contrast agent increases the absorption coefficient (density) of some normal and a number of abnormal intracranial structures, allowing for identification of lesions not seen on the unenhanced scan. The radiation exposure is approximately equal to that for a skull series (below 2 rads) and is well below the exposure of either the arteriogram or pneumoencephalogram.

The CT scan is the initial diagnostic procedure to assess and localize intracranial pathology. As an emergency procedure, it is particularly valuable in patients with head trauma to identify abnormal collections of blood, shifts in the ventricular system, or parenchymal injury, including cerebral edema and infarction. In the comatose patient with focal neurologic signs, it allows for rapid localization of a mass lesion and gives information as to its cause with characteristic appearances for hematoma, tumor, infarction, and abscess. In the patient with transient ischemic attacks and focal neurologic signs, it allows one to differentiate between infarction and hemorrhage before using anticoagulants. In the patient with metabolic encephalopathy and focal neurologic signs, it is used to exclude a focal cerebral lesion. As an elective procedure, it can be performed on an ambulatory basis to diagnose mass lesions, to evaluate ventricular size, and, in the patient with dementia, to diagnose cerebral atrophy or normal pressure hydrocephalus. Demyelinating disease can also be assessed. It is an important follow-up procedure in patients who have had treatment for intracranial tumors, either radiation therapy or neurosurgical intervention, to assess any remaining tumor or the reappearance of new tumor, as well as in patients who have had shunt procedures to evaluate ventricular size. The usefulness of the CT scan as an elective procedure eliminates the need of hospital admission for diagnostic work-up in numerous patients and facilitates the care of the patient with a neurologic emergency. The limitations include the fact that abnormalities must be greater than 5 mm in diameter to be visualized. There are certain areas, specifically the suprasellar region and the posterior fossa, which are not well visualized and may require other tests. Cerebral vessels are not well visualized, and although aneurysms and vascular malformations have been diagnosed by CT scan, it is not the procedure of choice to assess cerebral vessels and their abnormalities. Subdural hematomas, even of a clinically important size, may not show up well. The only major contraindication to CT scanning is allergy to iodinated contrast materials. In such cases, a no-contrast CT scan in conjunction with a brain scan may provide the necessary information.

NEWER TECHNIQUES. The use of coronal and sagittal slices as well as cisternal enhancement with radiopaque iodinated contrast agents will further increase the applicability of CT scanning by providing increased definition of the brain and cerebrospinal fluid spaces.

268. LUMBAR PUNCTURE

Cerebrospinal fluid (CSF) is sampled through a needle inserted between the lumbar vertebrae into the lumbar subarachnoid space. The procedure is simple and may be performed at the bedside or in the emergency room. Because it is so simple and commonly performed, special attention is required to consider both its indications and the amount of CSF required for complete assessment before starting the procedure. The indications are specific, nonspecific, or therapeutic. Lumbar puncture is the specific procedure to evaluate meningeal infection, subarachnoid bleeding, and meningeal carcinomatosis, and to directly measure intracranial pressure. In multiple sclerosis, the characteristic gamma globulin profile confirms the diagnosis. In the differential diagnosis of brain tumor, spinal cord block, and cerebrovascular disease, the lumbar puncture provides information about changes in the content of the CSF which are neither specific nor diagnostic. Therapeutically, it provides the route of administration for anesthetic agents in spinal anesthesia and for the treatment of central nervous system infection or malignancy by the administration of antimicrobial drugs. The major contraindications include clinical evidence of increased intracranial pressure caused by mass lesions (see Ch. 316) and infection at the lumbar puncture site. Other important contraindications include bleeding diathesis, thrombocytopenia with platelet counts below 30,000, and congenital malformations of the lumbar cord.

PROCEDURE. Patient cooperation and proper positioning greatly facilitate the procedure. The patient should be placed in the lateral decubitus position with the knees flexed to allow for full extension of the space between the spinous processes. Under sterile conditions, local anesthesia should be administered. A 20-gauge stylet needle is then introduced slowly between the interspaces, most commonly L4-L5 or L3-L4 until it pierces the dura. The bevel should always be directed cephalad in order to pierce the dura in a vertical fashion. If the needle is advanced too far into the subarachnoid space, trauma to the ventrally located epidural venous plexus side will yield bloody fluid. Once the subarachnoid space is entered, a manometer should be attached to the lumbar needle and the opening pressure measured, with the patient as relaxed as possible, knees extended, and neck in a normal position. CSF should then be removed for study, and drugs or anesthetic agents administered. Lumbar puncture may also be performed in the sitting position but does not give reliable CSF pressure measurements. It does, however, allow for collection of CSF. In an unusually difficult situation, the procedure can be done under fluoroscopy to facilitate visualization of the normal bony landmarks. In special instances in which the lumbar route is not possible, CSF may be sampled from the cisterna magna. Although this is considered a routine method in other countries, the procedure should be done under fluoroscopy by a physician experienced in this technique. In patients with basilar meningitis from fungal or metastatic disease, a higher yield of positive cultures or of malignant cells may be found by this approach. The cisterna magna can also be the route of administration of radiopaque substances to outline the posterior fossa and the spinal cord above a spinal block. Once obtained, CSF samples are usually evaluated for cell count, glucose and protein content, and, if infection is suspected, Gram stain. Cell count and Gram stain are the responsibility of the physician performing the lumbar puncture (see Ch. 297). The sugar and protein content, bacterial, viral, and fungal cultures, and serologic and cytologic evaluation are customarily performed in hospital laboratories. More specialized studies to assess cerebrospinal fluid include viral cultures and titers, cryptococcal antigen, protein electrophoresis, and enzyme analysis. The normal values for CSF are found in Ch. 593. *Postspinal tap headache* is the most common complication of lumbar puncture and may be associated with bifrontal or occipital headache, neck stiffness, dizziness, and nausea. It resolves if the patient is placed in the prone or slightly head-down position, but may last up to ten days when the patient assumes the upright position. Although this is distressing for the patient, it does not produce any significant long-term effects. In rare instances transtentorial or cerebellar herniation may follow lumbar puncture, but if care is taken in the selection of patients, this complication should never occur.

269. CONVENTIONAL ROENTGENOGRAPHY

SKULL X-RAYS. Plain films of the skull identify developmental anomalies (such as basilar impression), in-

tracranial calcifications, fractures of the skull vault, and longstanding increased intracranial pressure. In patients with head trauma, medicolegal considerations mandate skull x-rays unless CT scan is done. In fact, for serious head trauma, the CT scan provides much more direct information about the effects on brain parenchyma. Skull x-rays play a minor role in the evaluation of patients with brain tumors (see Ch. 316) and cerebrovascular disease (see Ch. 293 to 295). Specific radiographic projections are required to answer specific clinical questions. The anteroposterior and lateral views provide the general information about bony configuration and structure. Towne's view best identifies a calcified pineal, the base view shows the jugular foramen and other foramina of the base of skull, the inclined frontal view assesses superior orbital fissures and frontal sinuses, and Stenver's view assesses the mastoid and petrous pyramids.

SPINE X-RAYS. Spine x-rays are the initial diagnostic procedure in patients with neck or back pain or dysfunction of the spinal cord. The spine films detect congenital anomalies, fracture or collapse of a vertebral body, inflammatory and degenerative diseases of the joint spaces, and spondylosis and spondylolisthesis of the spine. Prior to myelography they are required to assess the status of the lumbar spine. Three radiographic views provide the necessary information. These include the anteroposterior view, which provides information about the width of the spinal canal and integrity of the pedicles; the lateral view, which provides information about the status of the vertebral bodies, the disc spaces, and the size, shape, and alignment of the spinal canal; and the oblique view, which assesses the integrity of the joint and disc spaces, as well as the neural foramina. When necessary, specialized and coned-down views of the specific areas in question should be performed, particularly when one is concerned about areas which are poorly visualized on routine films, such as the C7-T1 region or the sacrum.

Plain radiographs of the skull and spine are limited by the fact that there must be 40 to 60 per cent change in bone density to detect changes on plain films. Alternative procedures include *the bone scan*, which provides a more sensitive method using specific radioisotopes, and which can demonstrate abnormalities three to four months before observable changes in plain x-rays; however, this procedure is nonspecific and cannot differentiate inflammatory diseases of bone from tumor. *Tomography* provides a more specialized radiographic technique to discern bony changes and is particularly useful in assessing areas of bony overlap such as the base of skull.

270. THE RADIONUCLIDE BRAIN SCAN

Radioisotope scans identify alterations of the blood-brain barrier and thus localize areas of intracranial pathology, especially tumor. Following intravenous injection of the radioisotope, most commonly technetium[99] pertechnetate, standard views of the brain are recorded on x-ray film, using a specialized scintillation camera, most commonly the gamma camera. This is a useful screening procedure to assess possible intracerebral mass lesions, infarction, subacute subdural hematomas, and abscess, because it provides a simple minimal-risk ambulatory procedure with a fair diagnostic accuracy. With the availability of the CT scan, however, its usefulness has diminished. At this time, radionuclide scanning is a second line procedure to futher clarify a normal or abnormal CT scan in the patient allergic to the contrast substances. The limitations of the procedure are significant: abnormalities must be 2 cm or greater to be visualized; changes in the skull vault may produce artifacts on the scan; and the diagnostic scope is restricted. Radionuclide scanning is not useful in assessing cerebral atrophy or ventricular enlargement, or in providing rapid diagnostic information in emergencies. Dynamic radionuclide brain scanning, available in some centers, employs a special camera attached to the scintillation camera which begins photographing the brain simultaneously with the injection of radioisotope. Cerebral blood flow, and particularly patency of the venous sinuses, can be estimated rapidly by this relatively low risk technique. In cerebrovascular disease, its diagnostic accuracy is less than that of arteriography. It is the initial procedure of choice to assess occlusion of the venous sinuses.

271. ELECTRO-ENCEPHALOGRAPHY

Electroencephalography (EEG) measures the electrical activity of the cortex, providing information about the functional status of the brain; it is considered in detail in Ch. 315. Because it is a simple and commonly available noninvasive procedure, it is often used by the general physician, but it provides limited diagnostic information except in certain types of epilepsy (petit mal), in patients with confusional states or unusual behavior who may display seizure activity on the EEG without motor or sensory component, and in patients with narcolepsy. The procedure provides nonspecific but, at times, important differential information in patients with metabolic encephalopathy (see Ch. 220). The EEG can help localize supratentorial brain tumors (see Ch. 316), but is not useful in the evaluation of posterior fossa tumors.

SPECIALIZED EEG TECHNIQUES. Specialized EEG techniques, used in some centers, include direct measurement of cortical activity with superficial and deep electrodes during ablative neurosurgical procedures for intractable epilepsy. Other techniques include computer analogues to assess sensory evoked responses of the visual, auditory, and sensory cortex in the evaluation of central visual and hearing loss, particularly in infants and children.

272. SELECTED NEURODIAGNOSTIC PROCEDURES

CEREBRAL ARTERIOGRAPHY. Cerebral arteriograms are performed by direct catheterization of the carotid artery in the neck or by catheterization of either the brachial or femoral artery and selective injection of the aortic arch and carotid and vertebral arteries, using a radiopaque contrast agent. Arteriography is the diagnostic procedure for assessing cervical or cerebrovascular occlusion, arteriosclerotic plaques, vasculitis, aneurysms, and other vascular malformations. Although it was formerly used as a diagnostic study in evaluating focal neurologic symptoms suggestive of brain tumor, the CT scan has replaced the arteriogram as the initial procedure.

PNEUMOENCEPHALOGRAPHY. This technique allows for visualization of the cerebrospinal fluid–filled ventricles, cisterns, and subarachnoid pathways, using air as the contrast agent. Special views and tomography are employed and selected by the radiologist during the examination. It is the specific diagnostic tool to assess the patency of the subarachnoid pathways, such as in patients with negative CT scans whose focal neurologic symptoms suggest pathology involving the parasellar area, the deep midline structures, or the posterior fossa. The major contraindications are those for lumbar puncture. The complications include transient fever, headache, and meningeal irritation, which usually clear within three to five days. In contrast to CT scans, this procedure is distressing for the patient, and in patients with normal pressure hydrocephalus it may produce transient worsening in their neurologic symptoms and signs.

MYELOGRAPHY. Myelography assesses abnormalities of the spinal cord, nerve roots, and meninges and is performed by the injection of a radiopaque contrast agent into the subarachnoid space, most commonly by the lumbar route. Although limited myelography is performed in some institutions, a full myelogram should be performed on every patient having the procedure. If a spinal block is suspected, a small amount of contrast is initially injected to assess the patency of the subarachnoid spaces. In cases of block, cisternal injection of contrast should also be performed to delineate the upper borders of the block and to assess the patency of the subarachnoid spaces above the block. This is particularly important prior to radiation treatment of patients with extradural metastatic disease and spinal cord compression who may have multiple blocks (see Ch. 332).

RADIOISOTOPE CISTERNOGRAPHY. Radioisotope cisternography involves the administration of a radioisotope into the subarachnoid space to study the dynamics of cerebrospinal fluid flow. Several radioisotope materials are currently used, and the basic principles of their dispersion involve both bulk flow and diffusion. The specific indications include the evaluation of patients with communicating hydrocephalus and cerebrospinal leaks, specifically CSF rhinorrhea.

ELECTROMYOGRAPHY. Electromyography is the investigative procedure which uses electrical activity of nerve and muscle to assess and localize disease involving the motor unit. Specifically, it provides the methods to differentiate lesions involving spinal motor neurons, roots, plexuses, entire nerves, branches of nerve, or muscle fibers. Its applicability is discussed in Ch. 338.

ECHOENCEPHALOGRAPHY. Echoencephalography uses pulses of ultrasound to detect shifts or alterations of structures within the cranial cavity, using the third ventricle as the reliable midline position. Although it is a simple, widely available procedure, it is nonspecific, and the patient requires further studies for a definitive diagnosis.

OTHER DIAGNOSTIC TESTS. The procedures outlined above, in conjunction with the neurologic history and examination, provide valuable information about the nature, site, and most likely pathologic process, but direct visualization of brain, nerve, and muscle provides the final diagnosis. *Brain biopsy* provides available tissue for neuropathologic evaluation and currently can be performed with minimal risk and discomfort to the patient. The specific indications are as follows: when the differential diagnosis is in question, e.g., benign vs. malignant disease; when knowledge of the pa-

thology will change or direct the therapy, e.g., brain abscess vs. tumor, toxoplasmosis encephalitis vs. herpes encephalitis; or when the pathology alone can provide the diagnosis and is necessary for genetic counseling, e.g., lipid storage diseases. *Muscle biopsy* is considered in Ch. 338.

Cohen, H. L., and Brumlik, J.: Manual of Electroneuromyography. New York, Harper & Row, 1976.
Gonzalez, C. F., Grossman, C. B., and Palacios, E.: Computed Brain and Orbital Tomography. New York, John Wiley & Sons, 1976.
Newton, T. H., and Potts, D. G. (eds.): Radiology of The Skull and Brain. St. Louis, C. V. Mosby Co., 1974.
Taveras, J. M., and Wood, E. H.: Diagnostic Neuroradiology. Baltimore, Williams & Wilkins Co., 1964.

Section Eleven THE EXTRAPYRAMIDAL DISORDERS

273. INTRODUCTION

Melvin D. Yahr

The basal ganglia or extrapyramidal diseases comprise a complex group of clinical disorders characterized by abnormal involuntary movements (dyskinesias), alterations in muscle tone, and disturbances in bodily posture. The major clinical states include parkinsonism, chorea, athetosis, dystonia, and hemiballism. These terms not only denote particular disease entities, but in a descriptive sense refer to a constellation of symptoms that may occur in a variety of central nervous system disorders involving the basal ganglia and/or their connections. They are recognizable, one from the other, by the degree, form, and combination of the triad of symptoms noted above and are distinguishable as disease entities by the age and mode of onset, the identification of particular etiologic and genetic factors, and the rate and manner of progression of symptoms.

The conventional anatomic concept of the basal ganglia as a group of nuclear masses in the forebrain has not proved adequate in explaining the clinical manifestations or what is known about the physiologic or pathologic aspects of these conditions. In consequence, neurologists have devised a functional anatomic approach that includes not only the basal ganglia nuclei, but also related structures in the brainstem as well as a neural network of connections with other parts of the nervous system. The structures of importance in this system are the caudate nucleus and putamen, which, because of their similarities in appearance, cellular structure, and phylogenetic development, are collectively known as the striatum; the globus pallidus or pallidum, an older structure but one in which many nonpyramidal pathways converge; the thalamus, another important way station and integrative region; and the subthalamic nucleus, red nucleus and substantia nigra, all brainstem centers with important connections to the basal ganglia. These nuclear masses, along with their connections with each other and with certain parts of the reticular formation, cerebellum, and cerebrum, make up an anatomic-physiologic unit that collectively has been

termed "the extrapyramidal system." The role of this system in maintaining normal motor activity in man is not definitely known, and has only been inferred from studies of animals, in which it is more highly developed and not dominated by the cerebral cortex. In submammalian forms, this system appears essential for maintaining normal locomotion, feeding, etc. In higher animals, except man, its integrity is necessary for the production of automatic movements and postural adjustments. Some believe that this same function is carried over to man and that coarse, gross automatic movements are mediated by the extrapyramidal system. Others have implied a more secondary role in which this system is incapable of initiating movements but provides a reinforcing and modulating influence on movements of cortical origin. The latter thesis seems more in keeping with present knowledge; hence it is best to view the pyramidal and extrapyramidal systems as operating in unison and constant balance. Movements having their origin in the cerebral cortex are mediated through the pyramidal tract but are influenced by reflex regulating mechanisms from various components of the extrapyramidal system. In this context, the prime role of the extrapyramidal system is automatic sensorimotor integration, which can be explained in terms of inhibition and facilitation of motor responses to appropriate stimuli. Hence dysfunction within this system results in motor responses that are delayed, slow, and incomplete and especially affect automatic or involuntary movements.

The manifestations of basal ganglia disorders fall into two general categories: those of a *positive* nature, such as abnormal movements, tremor, and chorea, and those of a *negative* nature, such as postural changes and loss of associated movements. Unfortunately, because of the nature of the disease processes affecting this region it has not been possible to correlate intimately the clinical symptoms with structural changes. Even the magnitude of the demonstrable morphologic changes often bears little relationship to the severity of the condition. During the past decade a growing body of evidence has related the underlying disturbance in these disorders to biochemical changes in the basal ganglia rather than to morphologic abnormalities.

The most prominent biochemical feature of the basal ganglia is their high content of putative neurotransmitter agents, notably acetylcholine (ACH), dopamine (DA), and gamma-aminobutyric acid (GABA). The substrates and enzymes necessary for their production and degradation are found within the cellular components of the basal ganglia. In some instances they are produced within the segment where they have their action, whereas in others cellular elements in one area produce the transmitters whence they are transported via connecting axons to another, where they are stored and then released to produce their effects. Experimental evidence is available indicating that dopamine, for example, is produced in the pars compacta of the substantia nigra and is transported via the nigrostriatal pathway to the caudate nucleus and putamen to exert its action. Normal function in the basal ganglia appears to depend on a balance among these various neurotransmitters. Neurophysiologically this balance may be viewed as existing between those whose action is inhibitory in nature (DA and GABA) versus those with excitatory properties (ACH). Disturbances of this balance result in symptoms. In general, dopamine deficiency allows for cholinergic hyperactivity and can be correlated with the akinetic rigid disorders such as parkinsonism. Dopamine hyperactivity and/or cholinergic hypoactivity results in the hyperkinetic phenomena encountered in Huntington's chorea. To a considerable extent present approaches to the etiogenesis and treatment of basal ganglia disorders are directed to a better understanding of the role of and re-establishing balance among these neurotransmitter agents.

In the clinical evaluation of extrapyramidal disorders it is essential to have a clear understanding of the many and varied symptoms encountered. Those of major significance are abnormal involuntary movements, alterations in muscle tone, and disturbances in bodily posture.

ABNORMAL INVOLUNTARY MOVEMENTS. *Tremor* is a rhythmic involuntary alternating contraction of opposing muscle groups, fairly uniform in frequency and amplitude. It may involve a limited segment such as fingers or lips, or may be widespread. Characteristically, tremor of extrapyramidal origin is augmented when the part is at rest and diminished or abolished during voluntary movements and sleep. It differs from that of anxiety, thyrotoxicosis, and those due to intoxications by being slower, of greater amplitude, and more rhythmic. Its occurrence at rest and suppression during voluntary movements and sleep distinguish it from the "action" tremor of cerebellar involvement. The anatomic and physiologic substrate of this type of tremor has not been defined with certainty. In Parkinson's disease in which such tremor is prominent, the substantia nigra invariably undergoes degeneration. However, not all such patients have tremor, and it remains controversial whether the pathologic changes are entirely limited to this structure. Discharges synchronous with the tremor have been recorded in certain thalamic nuclei, particularly lateralis posterior. These findings suggest derangement of a complex sensorimotor mechanism with possible multiple pathologic sites.

Athetosis denotes an involuntary movement that results from instability of posture combined with voluntary movement. The result is a slow, writhing, wormlike movement usually most prominent in the fingers and hand, but the face, neck, and feet may also be involved. Multiple areas of the extrapyramidal system, particularly the globus pallidus and striatum as well as the cerebral cortex, have shown pathologic changes.

Chorea refers to brief, distal, rapid, explosive movements which at first glance appear to be purposeful and coordinated but on closer inspection are aimless and uncoordinated. They involve upper and lower limbs, face, trunk, and head, and may occur with such rapidity that the individual appears in constant motion. Choreiform movements are accentuated by movement and environmental stimulation, and interfere with normal voluntary function. They are differentiated from tics by being unpatterned, unpredictable, and nonreproducible. Athetosis and chorea may coexist in such a pattern that they are indistinguishable from one another. Pathologic changes accompanying chorea have been found in many areas of the nervous system but especially in the striatum.

Dystonia is a term applied to an abnormally maintained posture resulting from a twisting, turning movement that usually involves the limbs, neck, or trunk. Although there is no specific pattern or posture that describes this disorder, the usual appearance is one of marked distortion of the affected part. The movements appear readily induced by ordinary stimuli, such as walking, talking, or light touch to the skin. The involved muscles appear to be alternately in a state of increased and decreased tone and, usually as the movement starts, the muscles involved appear to gradually build up tone. Patients with this type of movement cannot inhibit, modify, or terminate the posture, and voluntary movements become seriously impaired. In some instances the movements clear, but the abnormal postures become fixed with resultant torticollis, tortipelvis, and deformities of the limbs. Neither the pathologic nor physiologic substrate for this movement disorder has been defined.

Ballism is a violent dyskinesia consisting of forceful, flinging movements of the limbs. The muscles involved are in the shoulder and pelvic girdle, and usually only one side of the body or even one limb is affected. Ballism appears to be due to a discrete lesion, usually in the subthalamic nucleus of Luys or its immediate connections.

ALTERATIONS IN MUSCLE TONE. Although it is common to associate heightened muscle tonus (rigidity) with extrapyramidal disorders, some, such as chorea and athetosis, may show normal tone or hypotonus of the musculature. Rigidity, which is most commonly encountered in parkinsonism, must be differentiated from spasticity. The former is identifiable by passively flexing and extending the muscles of an extremity or rotating the hand on the wrist. The movement obtained is one of a series of interrupted jerks at regular intervals, the so called cog-wheel effect. Terms such as "plastic" or "lead pipe" are utilized to describe the homogeneous degree of rigidity. Rigidity may be limited to groups of muscles and may be evident only at some joints, or it may be generalized, affecting the entire musculature. The mechanism underlying the rigidity appears to be impairment of reciprocal inhibition of agonist and antagonistic muscle groups. Electromyographic analysis of these muscles shows continuing activity in both groups throughout a movement such as flexion of the forearm. Rigidity reduces muscle power and velocity of movement and also contributes to the production of deformities.

DISTURBANCES IN BODILY POSTURE. Patients with extrapyramidal disease, especially those with parkinsonism, have difficulty in preserving their equilibrium in the erect as well as the sitting position. They also have difficulty in changing from the horizontal to the upright position or in rolling over from back to front. Profound difficulties are noted in walking, when tendencies to propulsive or retropulsive gait are evident as well as shuffling and festination. Careful analysis of these defects has indicated that the subjects have loss of control of their center of gravity in both sagittal and coronal planes. These abnormalities are thought to be due to disturbances in righting reflexes, impairment of vestibular reflexes, and release of proprioceptor mechanisms subsequent to degeneration in the pallidum.

Carpenter, M. B.: Extrapyramidal pathways and interconnections. Pharmacol. Therap., 1:1, 1975.
Costa, E., Cote, L., and Yahr, M. D. (eds.): Biochemistry and Pharmacology of the Basal Ganglia. Hewlett, N. Y., Raven Press, 1966.
Duvoisin, R.: Clinical diagnosis of the dyskinesias. Med. Clin. North Am., 56:1321, 1972.
Lloyd, K. G.: Special chemistry of the basal ganglia 1. Monoamines. Pharmacol. Therap., 1:49, 1975.
Purpura, D. P.: Physiological organization of the basal ganglia. In Yahr, M. D. (ed.): The Basal Ganglia. New York, Raven Press, 1976, pp. 91–114.
Yahr, M. D.: Involuntary movements. In Scientific Foundations of Neurology. London, Heinemann, 1972, pp. 83–88.

274. THE PARKINSONIAN SYNDROME

(Paralysis Agitans, Shaking Palsy)

Melvin D. Yahr

274.1. INTRODUCTION

James Parkinson in 1817 first described the major manifestations of this syndrome, which is characterized by tremor, muscular rigidity, and loss of postural reflexes. Not only is it the most frequently encountered of the basal ganglia disorders, but parkinsonism is a prominent cause of disability. Its prevalence has been placed at close to one million patients in the United States, with the addition of 50,000 new cases each year. As a symptom complex its occurrence has been noted in a number of disease processes either as the sole manifestation or in association with other symptoms. However, in most cases no definable cause has yet been found; since the latter seem to have many features in common, particularly in regard to evolution, they have been designated as Parkinson's disease, paralysis agitans, or primary parkinsonism. The cases in which definable processes are found are best classified as secondary or symptomatic parkinsonism. This separation into clinical groups cannot be construed as indicative of a difference in pathophysiology or even pathogenic mechanisms for the production of symptoms, for all parkinsonism may well have a common origin. Indeed, from the standpoint of what is presently known about its chemical pathology, a deficiency of striatal dopamine is common to all types of parkinsonism. In most

instances of parkinsonism, regardless of cause, loss of pigmented neurons is found in the substantia nigra, locus ceruleus, and pigmented brainstem nuclei in association with other nonspecific changes diffusely distributed in the corpus striatum and cortex.

274.2. PARALYSIS AGITANS
(Parkinson's Disease)

The largest number of cases of parkinsonism fall into this category. The disease most frequently begins between the ages of 50 and 65 years. A rarely encountered juvenile form has been described. The disease affects both sexes and all races. There is no evidence to indicate a hereditary factor. Although the cause of Parkinson's disease is unknown, its appearance in the later years of life has suggested that it may relate to mechanisms involved in the aging process of neuronal cells, particularly in individuals in whom the nigral cells are highly vulnerable to such effects. One of the factors that has been given consideration and for which some evidence exists relates to the enzymes necessary for removing the oxidative products of catecholamine metabolism. Hydrogen peroxide is such a byproduct, and its removal depends on the enzymes peroxidase and catalase, both normally in high concentration in the substantia nigra and reduced with aging but more so in parkinsonian brains. Their reduction may allow for the accumulation of hydrogen peroxide and other toxic products which then leads to the destruction of nigral cells and the loss of tyrosine hydroxylase, the enzyme responsible for dopamine production.

The disease begins insidiously with any of its three cardinal manifestations either alone or in combination. Tremor usually in one or both hands, involving the fingers in a pill-rolling motion, is the most common initial symptom. This is often followed by stiffness in the limbs, general slowing of movements, and inability to carry out normal and routine daily functions with ease. As the disease progresses the face becomes "masklike," with a loss of eye blinking and failure to express emotional feeling; the body becomes stooped, and the gait becomes shuffling with loss of arm swing; and the patient is unable to readily gain and maintain an erect posture. Speech becomes slow and monotonous. There is a tendency to drool. The skin takes on an oily quality, and there is a tendency to seborrheic dermatitis. Although paralysis agitans is invariably progressive, the rate at which symptoms develop and disability ensues is extremely variable. Only rarely is the disease so rapidly progressive that the patient becomes disabled within five years of onset. In the majority, intervals of 10 to 20 years elapse before symptoms cause incapacity.

The major neurologic findings are as follows: (1) *Lack of facial expression*, with diminished eye blinking but ready induction of blepharospasm when the frontalis muscle is tapped (Myerson's sign). (2) *Tremor* of the distal segments of the limbs at rest, accentuated by suspension but decreased during active movements and eliminated in sleep. The tremor is rhythmical, alternatively affecting flexor and extensor muscles, and may involve upper or lower limbs, mouth, or head. (3) *Muscular rigidity*, readily evident on passive movement of a joint, and manifested by a series of interrupted jerks (cog-wheel phenomenon) rather than a smooth flowing, easy motion. (4) *Akinesia,* the tendency to slowness in the initiation of movement and sudden unexpected arrests of volitional movements while carrying out purposeful acts. The parkinsonian patient appears disinclined to move, and in the midst of performing a routine function suddenly finds himself "frozen" and unable to move through the sequence of motion necessary to complete the action. This is especially evident in writing or feeding and can be striking when, in attempting to walk, the patient finds that his feet are suddenly "frozen to the ground." (5) *Postural abnormalities,* most evident in the erect and sitting positions. The patient has a tendency to let his head fall forward on the trunk, and his body tends to fall forward or backward when seated on a stool unless supported; when pushed either from in front or behind in the erect position he falls, making no effort to catch himself either with a step or by movement of his arms. There is a tendency to deformities of the trunk, hands, and feet. Kyphotic deformity of the spine, causing a stooped posture, is a hallmark. There are ulnar deviations of the hand, flexion contractures of the fingers, and an equino-varus posture of the foot.

274.3. SECONDARY OR SYMPTOMATIC PARKINSONISM

In a long list of diseases and conditions of the nervous system parkinsonism has occurred as the predominant manifestation. Included are poisoning with carbon monoxide, manganese, and other heavy metals; brain tumors in the region of the basal ganglia; cerebral trauma; intoxication with neuroleptic agents; infectious processes such as encephalitis; multineuronal degenerative disorders of unknown cause; and association with cerebral arteriosclerosis as well as with endocrine dysfunction such as hypoparathyroidism. In most instances the presence of associated neurologic deficits, atypical features of the parkinsonian symptoms, and/or other systemic manifestations of the related disease process arouse suspicion that one is not dealing with primary parkinsonism. Of all the conditions noted, those most frequently encountered are postencephalitic and drug-induced parkinsonism and so-called arteriosclerotic pseudoparkinsonism.

POSTENCEPHALITIC PARKINSONISM

One of the most prominent sequelae of the epidemic of encephalitis lethargica (von Economo's disease) that occurred between 1919 and 1926 was the parkinsonian syndrome. The syndrome developed after mild as well as severe encephalitis lethargica, and, although in most instances it immediately followed the acute infectious process, in some patients prominent symptoms were not evident for intervals of up to ten years. The causative agent of encephalitis lethargica was never established. However, recent studies suggest that it was produced by a virus of the influenza A variety. Parkinsonism appears to have been a unique sequela of this form of encephalitis because it had rarely followed any other known viral encephalitides. There are still a significant number of survivors of encephalitis lethargica, and the evolution and consequences of this form of

parkinsonism differ from others, so its clinical recognition is of importance.

Postencephalitic parkinsonism has a number of distinctive features, including the following: (1) A history of encephalitis lethargica during the epidemic period 1918–1919. Since the pandemic of influenza occurred concurrently with encephalitis, it is essential that careful documentation be undertaken in differentiating these two infectious processes. (2) In addition to any or all of the parkinsonian symptoms indicated above, one or more of the following neurologic deficits may be found: hemiplegia, bulbar or ocular palsies, dystonic phenomena, tics, or behavioral disorders. (3) The parkinsonism itself is as a rule incompletely developed and has been static or slowly progressive over a period of years. (4) Episodes that have been termed oculogyric crises. These consist of attacks in which spasms of conjugate eye muscles occur so that the eyes are deviated upward, downward, or to one side for minutes or hours at a time.

DRUG-INDUCED PARKINSONISM

The use of neuroleptics as psychotherapeutic or antiemetic agents has resulted in the occurrence of a number of extrapyramidal syndromes. Parkinsonism indistinguishable from that previously described, dystonic movements involving the tongue and face, and akathisia, a restless fidgety state with a desire to be in constant motion, are those frequently encountered. Adults are more likely to develop parkinsonism and akathisia, whereas dystonic movements predominate in children. In some instances these reactions are dose dependent; in others they are related to individual susceptibility. The symptoms usually disappear within a few days when the drugs are withdrawn, but occasionally persist for months. In some subjects permanent remnants of parkinsonian symptoms have been found years after elimination of the drugs. Paradoxically, involuntary movements may make their initial appearance after withdrawal of neuroleptic agents. This condition, termed *tardive dyskinesia,* tends to occur in older patients who have been on phenothiazine drugs for extended periods of time, during which they have shown signs of parkinsonism. Stereotyped, repetitious movements of lips, tongue, and mouth and choreiform movements of limbs and trunk characterize this disorder. It may diminish in intensity or disappear spontaneously after weeks or months, but in some patients it has persisted indefinitely. Recently it has been shown that these abnormal movements may be controlled by the administration of large doses of choline chloride. In contrast, parkinsonism can be minimized by the simultaneous administration of one of the centrally active anticholinergic agents, such as benztropine (Cogentin) or trihexyphenidyl (Artane). In view of these potentially devastating side effects, physicians should employ neuroleptics cautiously with restricted doses. Drug holidays in those requiring long-term treatment should be routinely practiced and may be the best preventive measure.

ARTERIOSCLEROTIC PSEUDOPARKINSONISM

Atherosclerotic involvement of the cerebral vessels has been implicated by some as a cause of parkinsonism. Others have suggested that the nature of the symptoms warrants abandoning the term. Indeed, Critchley, who first proposed the term arteriosclerotic parkinsonism in 1929, has more recently re-emphasized the differing nature of the two disorders, and has recommended that when there is an underlying substrate of cerebrovascular disease, it be referred to as pseudoparkinsonism. Although the disorders superficially appear to resemble each other, there are distinctive differences as well as therapeutic implications. As a rule, the onset of symptoms is insidious, with most cases beginning in the seventh decade of life, although on occasion the occurrence has been noted in younger individuals as early as the fourth decade. Only rarely is there a history of a major stroke preceding onset, although symptoms referable to so-called minor strokes may be elicited. Early symptoms usually center around impaired mobility, with gait disturbance the most frequent complaint. Other presenting complaints may refer to pseudobulbar phenomena with dysarthria, some degree of dysphasia, and emotional incontinence. Some patients will present with progressive intellectual defects in association with poverty of movement. Tremor is rare, but alteration in muscle tone is common. It differs from the cog-wheel type, characteristic of Parkinson's disease, in that there is a stiffening of the limb in response to contact and a sense of resistance with attempted change of position. This type of alteration in muscle tone is known as gegenhalten. Hyperactive reflexes, abnormal plantar responses, and palmomental and snouting reflexes are all usually found. Pathologically, multiple small cerebral infarctions (lacunae) secondary to small vessel occlusion are found throughout the brain in these patients. The course of the disease is progressive, usually stepwise, and more rapid than that of Parkinson's disease. The usual antiparkinson drugs have little benefit.

274.4. MANAGEMENT OF THE PARKINSONIAN SYNDROME

GENERAL PRINCIPLES. Most patients will require lifelong treatment, consisting of the administration of specific medications, supportive psychotherapeutic measures, physical therapy, and, in rare instances, surgical intervention.

SUPPORTIVE PSYCHOTHERAPY. The major symptoms of parkinsonism are markedly influenced by psychic factors, and a patient's outlook and motivation will affect the extent to which he can overcome disability. It is important for the physician to provide reassurance, encouragement, and sympathetic understanding to the patient and family so that they may meet the numerous difficulties to be encountered at various stages of the illness. To allay anxieties both should be counseled regarding the meaning of various symptoms, the nature of the disease in terms of its long and variable course, and the potential that most patients can lead active and productive lives for long periods after symptoms begin.

PHYSICAL THERAPY. Simple measures such as heat and massage will alleviate painful muscle cramps and the muscle contraction headache that often accompanies pronounced rigidity of the cervical musculature. Exercises help in preventing flexion contractures. Gait training, walking exercises, and minor rehabilitative measures may enable the patient to maintain his independence with regard to personal hygiene and daily living activities for many more years than his disabilities might allow. Physical therapy in parkinsonism need not be elaborate, but when indicated should be done frequently and for an indefinite period. The patient should be instructed in simple home exercises and encouraged to develop a program of physical activity. Most patients in the earlier stages like to take long walks and should be encouraged to continue this habit as long as reasonably possible. Every effort should be made to keep them gainfully employed and to adjust their occupations as indicated by their symptoms.

DRUG THERAPY. The drugs now employed in the treatment of parkinsonism are theoretically capable of restoring normal activity to the striatum. Thus any agent that crosses the blood-brain barrier and enhances the brain's dopaminergic function or that reduces cholinergic activity may be expected to influence parkinsonism favorably. As a general rule a combination of agents with such properties works best.

The dopaminergic system may be functionally enhanced by agents that increase the synthesis of dopamine (this is presumably the modus operandi of levodopa), delay the catabolism of dopamine (monoamine oxidase inhibitors), promote its release from presynaptic storage sites (amphetamine), simulate its action at receptors (apomorphine, bromocriptine), and block the reuptake of monoamines at the synaptic cleft (anticholinergics). Of the numerous means for improving dopaminergic function that have been tried to date, the most effective has been the administration of levodopa (3,4-dihydroxyphenyl-L-alanine). Given alone or in combination with a peripheral dopa decarboxylase inhibitor (benserazide, carbidopa), it is appreciably more effective and less toxic than any therapeutic agent previously available for the treatment of Parkinson's disease.

In the selection of patients for treatment with levodopa, the over-all severity of parkinsonism and the degree of functional impairment, as well as the existence of concomitant diseases of other organs, must be carefully considered. Patients with minimal signs and symptoms who are able to meet the demands of daily living need not involve themselves in a treatment program that may be rigorous and demanding and carries an implicit risk. The presence of occlusive vascular disease involving the heart or brain warrants careful assessment. Severe angina pectoris or transient cerebral ischemic attacks contraindicate the use of levodopa. A history of episodic cardiac arrhythmia presents an additional hazard. When the arrhythmia is associated with myocardial disease, the use of levodopa must be undertaken with extreme caution. Evidence of prior mental illness, particularly affective disorders or major "psychotic breaks," contravenes the use of levodopa. Although requiring careful monitoring, levodopa has been administered without adverse effects to patients with hepatic, renal, gastrointestinal, and hematopoietic disorders. The presence of hemolytic anemia and glucose-6-phosphate dehydrogenase (G-6-DP) deficiency contraindicates its use.

Clinical treatment with levodopa comprises two phases. The first or "introduction phase" extends over a period of weeks or months in which the dosage is slowly built up to the therapeutic range. During this phase, tolerance develops to many of the side effects of levodopa; and although improvement of symptoms occurs in most patients, the optimal therapeutic response may not be evident. A "maintenance phase" follows, in which the full benefits of treatment most often occur, and careful patient monitoring with readjustment of dosage and ancillary therapeutic measures may be required to maintain a stable therapeutic response. Each of these phases requires cooperation on the part of the patient and careful management by the physician to achieve the best therapeutic response.

Levodopa is an aromatic amino acid that is a relatively inert compound by itself, but several of its metabolites have profound pharmacologic effects. Levodopa is available in two main forms in the United States. One is as tablets or capsules of 100, 250, and 500 mg of levodopa alone. The other combines levodopa with an extracerebral decarboxylate inhibitor, carbidopa, in tablets marketed as Sinemet, containing 10 or 25 mg of carbidopa plus 100 or 250 mg of levodopa. Available in most countries in the world but not in the United States is a similar combination utilizing benserazide, 20 or 50 mg, as a peripheral decarboxylase inhibitor with levodopa, 100 or 200 mg (Madopar).

Levodopa can be given in slowly increasing dosages, starting with 250 mg three or four times daily after meals and slowly increasing by 125 to 250 mg every few days until maximal therapeutic effect or side reactions are encountered. The optimal dose for adults is 5.0 grams or even more. At this dose level, however, many patients experience side effects, including anorexia, nausea, feelings of nervous tension, or hypotension. Occasional transitory alterations in blood chemistry, including elevations of serum glutamic oxaloacetic transaminase (SGOT), alkaline phosphatase, and blood urea nitrogen (BUN), as well as depression of white blood cell count and development of a positive Coombs test, have occurred. To date, these have not been associated with symptoms of dysfunction in organ systems, nor has autopsy material shown structural alterations.

Many of the aforementioned side effects of levodopa may be avoided by the simultaneous administration of carbidopa or benserazide. These agents prevent the peripheral utilization of levodopa, making it more readily and rapidly available to brain and avoiding extracerebral dopaminergic action. Consequently, the induction phase is considerably shortened and one may obtain optimal therapeutic responses within a matter of days. Sinemet, the carbidopa-levodopa combination, is effective when administered in total daily doses of 50 to 100 mg of carbidopa with 500 to 1000 mg of levodopa. In general one starts with modest doses of Sinemet 10/100 (carbidopa 10 mg, levodopa 100 mg) given four times a day with increases at two-day intervals as required. Not available in the United States but in most other countries of the world is Madopar, a combination of benserazide, 25 or 50 mg, and levodopa, 100 or 200 mg. The average required daily dose of this combination has been benserazide, 200 mg, and levodopa, 800 mg, in four equally divided doses. Sinemet and Madopar appear to have an equivalent therapeutic effect.

Most patients on long-term or high-dose levodopa therapy sooner or later develop side effects attributable to the central nervous system action of the drug. Adventitious movements consist of choreiform movements of hands or feet. Grimacing may affect the face. Variability in therapeutic response may lead to a loss of

dopa effect lasting for hours or even days. For all these reasons patients with parkinsonism need long-term supervision and drug adjustments to accomplish maximal benefits.

A number of other antiparkinsonian agents are useful as adjunctive drugs with levodopa; they are also indicated for those in whom levodopa is contraindicated and are preferred for patients with very mild symptoms in the very early stages of the disorder. Some are also the drug of choice in drug-induced parkinsonism. Most of these compounds possess central nervous system anticholinergic properties or augment striatal dopaminergic activity. Those most frequently used are trihexyphenidyl (Artane), available in 2 and 5 mg tablets; benztropine (Cogentin), as 1 and 2 mg tablets; cycrimine (Pagitane), as 1.25 and 2.5 mg tablets; and procyclidine (Kemadrin), 2 and 5 mg tablets. Treatment should be initiated with small doses such as trihexyphenidyl, 2 mg three times daily, and gradually increased until further increases yield no additional benefit or side effects reach an unacceptable degree of severity.

To obtain optimal results with anticholinergic drugs, careful titration of dosage against side effects is required. The goal is to find the dose that yields an optimal compromise between the limited symptomatic improvement of the parkinsonism and the disagreeable symptoms of cholinergic blockade of the central and peripheral nervous systems. Among the latter are blurring of vision, dryness of mouth and throat, anhidrosis, constipation, and urinary urgency or, sometimes, retention. The major symptoms of central anticholinergic intoxication are ataxia, dysarthria, hyperthermia, and a characteristic pattern of mental disturbances, including impairment of recent memory, confusion, delusional thinking, hallucinations, somnolence, and rarely coma.

A number of other agents, not primarily anticholinergics but with mild central anticholinergic properties, are useful. Diphenhydramine (Benadryl), orphenadrine (Disipal), and chlorphenoxamine (Phenoxene) are similar in pharmacologic action. In general, diphenhydramine has enjoyed the widest use and can be given in divided dosage up to 150 mg a day. It is particularly useful as an adjunct to levodopa, for in addition to benefiting symptoms of parkinsonism, it allays anxiety and tempers insomnia.

The antidepressants imipramine (Tofranil) and amitriptyline (Elavil) are minimally effective when used alone, but in combination with anticholinergic agents or levodopa they may be beneficial in relieving the depressive symptoms that so often accompany parkinsonism. With administration in limited dosage, one may avoid their adverse effects, which may resemble parkinsonism. Imipramine 10 to 15 mg given four times a day, or amitriptyline, 25 mg twice a day, can be safely administered for extended periods.

Introduced as an antiviral agent, amantadine HCl (Symmetrel) was accidentally found to have activity against parkinsonism. When used alone in doses of 100 mg twice a day, its therapeutic effects are evident within 48 to 72 hours, consisting of a mild reversal of symptoms of parkinsonism. More effective action can be achieved when it is added to an existing regimen of treatment consisting of anticholinergic agents or levodopa (or both). Its effects are short lived, tending to diminish after a month and rarely lasting for more than three months. Many of its side effects are similar to those of the anticholinergic agents, particularly the induction of confusional and delusional states. In some patients after long-term use, edema and a form of livedo reticularis develop over the limbs.

Recently clinical trials with a number of new agents designed to overcome the shortcomings of levodopa have been tried. In the main, they are directed toward patients who are unresponsive to levodopa, experience "on-off" response, or have an excessive degree of abnormal involuntary movements as a result of its use. Agents that have shown some promise are those having the property of directly activating postsynaptic dopamine receptors in brain — so-called dopaminergic receptor agonists. Some that have received particular attention are piribedil (Trivastal) and bromocriptine. Although piribedil has shown antiparkinson action, it has offered little advantage over levodopa administered with carbidopa (Sinemet). Indeed, its comparative efficacy is below that achieved with the latter combination. Bromocriptine in rather large doses, 100 to 200 mg a day, has produced beneficial effects in some patients who have been resistant to treatment. However, when added to an existing therapeutic regimen, in modest doses, it may add additional therapeutic benefit. Although the usual monoamine oxidase inhibitors have been avoided because of their potential for inducing hypertensive crises, when given with precursors of dopamine such reactions have not been encountered with the monoamine oxidase inhibitor deprenyl. Given in small doses, 10 mg a day, it has been possible to reduce the required dose of levodopa and produce a more efficacious therapeutic response. At the time of this writing, piribedil, bromocriptine, and deprenyl have not been approved by the Food and Drug Administration for general use in the United States.

At the time of this writing there is no doubt that levodopa given in combination with a decarboxylase inhibitor is the best available treatment for the large majority of parkinsonian patients. It is far from ideal, but its judicious use benefits a large proportion of those suffering from Parkinson's disease over an extended period of time.

SURGICAL MEASURES. Stereotaxic neurosurgical procedures, directed to the interruption of neural pathways in the brain responsible for producing symptoms of parkinsonism, were in considerable vogue before the advent of levodopa therapy. They have been almost entirely discontinued with the advent of the more successful medical therapy.

COURSE OF THE PARKINSON SYNDROME. All forms of parkinsonism reflect progressive disorders of the nervous system, leading over variable periods of time to a considerable degree of motor disability. The most progressive is the symptomatic form, in which, as part of a generalized disorder of the nervous system, marked disability and a fatal outcome can be expected within five years. Postencephalitic parkinsonism is unique in this regard, in that its evolution has been relatively slow and patients have remained functional for extended periods of time, in some instances for 30 years or more. Parkinson's disease, or what is now referred to as primary parkinsonism, prior to its treatment with levodopa, could be expected to produce severe disability or death in 25 per cent of patients within five years of onset, 65 per cent in the succeeding five years, and 80 per cent in those surviving for 15 years. Further, it had been estimated that those suffering from Parkinson's

disease had a mortality rate three times that of the general population matched for age, sex, and racial origin. Although there is no evidence to indicate that levodopa or any other therapeutic agent now in use alters the underlying pathologic process or stems the progressive nature of the disease, there are indications of a major impact on survival time and functional capacity. Recent studies show that the added risk of mortality from Parkinson's disease has been reduced by half and that longevity is extended by a number of years. More important, since the introduction of these newer therapeutic agents, the quality of life has been improved for parkinsonians in that they do not suffer the degree of incapacity and dependence which previously characterized this disease.

It must be emphasized, however, that the treatment of parkinsonism is still far from ideal. Long-term follow-up studies covering periods of up to eight years during which levodopa has been administered reveal a gradual loss of therapeutic efficacy. Optimal responses are obtained during the first three years of instituting treatment with levodopa regardless of duration of the disease, and then diminish. It is not known at this time whether this relates to intrinsic factors of the disease process itself or the loss of therapeutic efficacy of the drug.

Barbeau, A.: Parkinson's disease: Etiological considerations. *In* Yahr, M. D. (ed.): The Basal Ganglia. New York, Raven Press, 1976, pp. 281–289.

Cotzias, G. C., Papavasilou, P. S., and Gellene, R.: Modification of parkinsonism — chronic treatment with L-dopa. N. Engl. J. Med., 280:337, 1969.

Crane, G. E.: Persistence of neurological symptoms due to neuroleptic drugs. Am. J. Psychiatry, 127:1407, 1971.

Critchley, M.: Arteriosclerotic parkinsonism. Brain, 52:23, 1929.

Duvoisin, R. C., and Yahr, M. D.: Encephalitis and parkinsonism. Arch. Neurol., 12:227, 1965.

Gamboa, E. T., Wolf, A., Yahr, M. D., et al.: Influenza virus antigen in postencephalitic parkinsonism brain. Arch. Neurol., 31:228, 1974.

Hoehn, M. M., and Yahr, M. D.: Parkinsonism: Onset, progression and mortality. Neurology, 17:427, 1967.

Yahr, M. D. (ed.): Treatment of parkinsonism — the role of dopa decarboxylase inhibitors. Adv. Neurol., 2, 1973.

Yahr, M. D.: Evaluation of long-term therapy in Parkinson's disease: Mortality and therapeutic efficacy. *In* Birkmayer, W., and Hornykiewicz, O. (eds.): Advances in Parkinsonism. Basle, Editiones Roche, 1976, p. 435.

275.   ESSENTIAL TREMOR

(Familial Tremor)

Melvin D. Yahr

This is a monosymptomatic condition in which tremor involves the hands and/or head and face. The tremor is usually more rapid than that encountered in parkinsonism, is accentuated by emotional factors, may be worsened by volitional movement, and is usually suppressed by the use of alcohol. The age of onset is variable, but in most cases the disorder begins prior to the age of 25 years and tends to persist throughout life. Some progression of the intensity of tremor and spread to other bodily parts usually occur over the years, which may result in significant physical and social disability. There is a strong familial incidence, with occurrence in several successive generations and members of the same family, but the genetic pattern of inheritance has not been determined. Some have suggested its transmission as an autosomal dominant trait. To date no specific pathologic lesion has been reported in the nervous system of people with this condition. It has been suggested that the condition is an abortive form of parkinsonism, but this concept does not appear justifiable at present. There is no specific effective therapy for controlling the tremor, although beta-adrenergic blocking agents, such as propranolol in dosage of 120 to 180 mg a day divided equally into three or four doses, have been useful in some patients. Responses, however, are variable and unpredictable, and cardiovascular alterations may limit the use of optimal dosage. Sedatives such as phenobarbital, in dosage of 15 mg three times a day, may reduce the intensity of the tremor. It is of utmost importance to differentiate essential tremor from parkinsonism. By and large, the distinguishing characteristics are earlier age of onset; lack of severe progression, akinesia, rigidity, or postural abnormalities; and the strong family history of tremor.

Baughman, F. A., Jr., Higgins, J. V., and Mann, J. D.: Sex chromosome anomalies and essential tremor. Neurology, 23:623, 1973.

Marshall, J.: Observations on essential tremor. J. Neurol. Neurosurg. Psychiatry, 25:122, 1962.

McAllister, R. G., Markesbery, W. R., Ware, R. W., and Howell, S. M.: Suppression of essential tremor by propranolol: Correlation of effect with drug plasma levels and intensity of beta-adrenergic blockade. Ann. Neurol., 1:160, 1977.

Scopa, J., Longley, B. P., and Foster, J. B.: Beta-adrenergic blockers in benign essential tremor. Curr. Ther. Res., 15:48, 1973.

276. SENILE TREMOR

Melvin D. Yahr

Tremor is a frequent finding in the elderly, most often involving the upper limbs and head. It differs from parkinsonian tremor in that it is finer and more rapid and at first occurs only with voluntary movements. As time goes on it becomes more constant and is also present while the limbs are at rest. There is no associated weakness or alteration in muscle tone. These features differentiate this form of tremor from parkinsonism. The cause is unknown. Since senile tremor has both cerebellar and extrapyramidal features, in that it occurs at rest and with movement, the assumption is that some critical pathway linking these systems has undergone degeneration. There is no effective treatment, although mild benefit may be derived from sedatives or the use of diphenhydramine (Benadryl) given in 25 mg doses three times a day. Most patients accept it as another of the many changes that come with advancing years. Occasional patients have to be reassured that they do not have parkinsonism or some other progressive neurologic disorder.

277. THE CHOREAS

Melvin D. Yahr

277.1. INTRODUCTION

There are a number of disease entities that, though wholly unrelated etiologically, have choreiform movements as their major manifestation. In some, intimate relationships with infectious processes have been found, whereas in others familial tendencies have pointed to a strong genetic component. In the light of newer concepts of inheritance, a common pathogenesis for all may be found. Although controversy exists as to the exact anatomic site from which movements of this type may derive, pathologic changes are commonly found in the striatum, particularly in the small cell components of the caudate nucleus and putamen. The classification of chorea into separate entities is at present somewhat arbitrary and is based on age of onset, association with identifiable disease processes or familial tendency, and occurrence of other neurologic abnormalities.

277.2. ACUTE CHOREA
(Sydenham's or Infectious Chorea, St. Vitus' Dance)

Acute chorea is a movement disorder encountered primarily during childhood and having its greatest incidence between the ages of 5 and 15 years. Occurrence beyond this age is uncommon, and then is usually in association with pregnancy or in persons who have had symptoms earlier in life. Females manifest these symptoms at least twice as often as males. Acute chorea has been reported in people of all races.

Considered as a symptom complex rather than as a specific disease entity, acute choreiform movements have been encountered as initial manifestations of a variety of conditions. They have been reported in epidemic encephalitis, in the encephalopathies occurring with exanthema, with pertussis and diphtheria, in idiopathic hypocalcemia, hyperthyroidism, systemic lupus erythematosus, carbon monoxide poisoning, vascular disease, tumors, and degenerative processes of the basal ganglia. These instances, however, account for only a small percentage of cases. The closest relationship appears to be with rheumatic fever. In more than half of the cases, rheumatic manifestations consisting of carditis, valvular heart disease, or arthritis occur prior to, coincident with, or following an attack of chorea.

There are no specific pathologic changes or anatomic sites of involvement that can be correlated with acute chorea. In fact, because acute uncomplicated chorea is rarely fatal, there has been a paucity of detailed pathologic studies. Cases that have come to autopsy have shown scattered changes in the cortex, basal ganglia, cerebellum, and brainstem. These have consisted of varying degrees of arteritis combined with cellular degeneration.

The outstanding clinical features of chorea are involuntary movements, incoordination, muscle weakness, and emotional lability. Although the onset of symptoms may be abrupt and obvious, it is more often insidious and subtle. The most frequent initial complaints include clumsiness of the limbs, evidenced by dropping objects from the hands or an awkward gait, particularly during emotionally tense situations. When these are coupled with irritability, poor performance in school, and generally fidgety behavior, frequently a hasty conclusion is reached, blaming the child or implying a psychiatric disorder. The typical choreatic movements may be noted in any part of the body, limbs, face, hands, tongue, or trunk. They may at first appear to be a part of the natural pattern of coordinated movements but are soon noted to be completely random, jerking, aimless, and purposeless. They occur at rest, are accentuated by any attempt at volitional movement, and disappear in sleep. They may be very mild and may minimally affect normal function or may be so forceful and frequent as to be totally disabling. Facial grimacing and difficulty in speech, chewing, and swallowing occur when the muscles subserving these functions are involved. Interruption of voluntary movements by involuntary ones leads to incoordination so that the person drops objects, walks in an awkward, ungainly fashion, and, in general, appears uncoordinated. Attempts to maintain forceful muscular contraction are similarly interrupted, and the resultant "waxing and waning" of motor power results in a relative degree of motor weakness. Although actual paralysis is rare, there is a disinclination to use a part of the body that is severely affected by involuntary movements of this type. Generalized reduction of muscle tone is an invariable feature of chorea and is readily demonstrable by hyperextensibility at finger, wrist, and ankle joints. In almost all choreatic children some degree of emotional lability is evident. It varies from total apathy to irritability, restlessness, and, infrequently, wild, inappropriate behavior.

Certain cardinal features can be found in almost all patients. These include (1) pronation of the forearm when the upper limbs are raised and extended; (2) inability to sustain muscle contraction when the examiner grasps the patient's hand or when the patient protrudes his tongue so that it darts rapidly in and out of the mouth; and (3) abnormal posturing of hands in which the wrist is noted to be sharply flexed and the fingers hyperextended at the metacarpal pharyngeal joints.

There are no specific laboratory tests for chorea. The cerebrospinal fluid is normal. The electroencephalogram may or may not show diffuse abnormalities correlated with the severity of the disease. Unless there are associated disease processes that manifest themselves in abnormalities of blood count, chemistry, or sedimentation rate, these studies are normal.

The age of onset and the distinctive involuntary movements readily differentiate acute chorea from other disorders of the basal ganglia. Tics and habit spasms may be confused with mild cases, but their movements are quite different, being stereotyped repetitive patterns localized to a single group of muscles. Huntington's chorea rarely begins in childhood and, in addition, there is a strong familial tendency with associated dementia. Movement disorders associated with cerebral palsy occur in infancy but have an athetoid element. The use of phenothiazines may induce abnormal movements, but the history of drug ingestion will differentiate these.

Acute chorea is a self-limited disease, recovery occurring in two to six months. Recurrence, with as many as two or three attacks over a period of years, appears in almost one third of the cases. There is no specific therapy. Bed rest and reduction of external stimuli to a minimum, combined with sedative drugs such as phenobarbital or chloral hydrate, are beneficial in controlling the severity of the movements. Paradoxically, the phenothiazines, such as thorazine and chlorpromazine, as well as reserpine in doses commensurate with individual tolerance, although capable of inducing chorea, have also been shown to be effective in its control. Because

of the high incidence of rheumatic valvular heart disease complicating acute chorea, prophylaxis with antimicrobial drugs over a long interval of time similar to that utilized in acute rheumatic fever is now recommended. If emotional symptoms are intense, psychotherapy may be in order. When specific abnormalities of calcium metabolism or thyroid dysfunction are found, their correction may completely ameliorate the symptoms. With recovery most patients show few or no neurologic sequelae.

Aron, A., Freeman, J., and Carter, S.: The natural history of Sydenham's chorea. Am. J. Med., 38:83, 1965.
Schwartzman, J.: Chorea minor. Review of 175 cases with reference to etiology, treatment and sequelae. Rheumatism, 6:89, 1950.

277.3.   HEREDITARY CHOREA
(Chronic Progressive Chorea, Huntington's Disease)

Hereditary chorea is a progressive degenerative disease of the basal ganglia and cerebral cortex, beginning in adult life and characterized by choreiform movements and mental deterioration. The disease affects both sexes in equal numbers and is transmitted from parent to offspring in autosomal dominant fashion with full penetrance. Hence 50 per cent of children of sufferers will inevitably be affected. The disease is relatively rare, although its incidence may be high in geographic regions where affected families have resided for many generations.

Pathologically, widespread degenerative changes with cell loss and reactive gliosis are found, primarily in the cerebral cortex and caudate nucleus. Recently it has been demonstrated that glutamic acid decarboxylase and choline acetylase activity are reduced in the basal ganglia of patients with Huntington's chorea. This results in a deficiency of γ-aminobutyric acid, an inhibitory transmitter substance in brain, as well as depressed function of the excitatory transmitter acetylcholine. Disruption of the homeostatic relationship of these agents may underlie the choreatic manifestations of this disorder.

The clinical manifestations consist of choreatic movements, emotional disturbance, and intellectual deterioration in varying degrees, rate of appearance, and progression. The disease usually makes its appearance between the ages of 35 and 50 years, rather insidiously with any of the aforementioned symptoms, but as a rule with abnormal movements. The movements, though similar to acute chorea, are usually more jerky though less lightning-like and primarily involve the trunk and shoulder girdle and more often the lower limbs than the upper. This pattern of involvement tends to produce a dancing sort of gait, which is a prominent feature of the disease. In rare instances a Parkinson-like rigidity is encountered as the major manifestation rather than involuntary movements. The mental deterioration is similar to that of any organic dementia, with progressive impairment of memory and of intellectual capacity, and inattention to personal hygiene. Emotional disturbances include heightened irritability, bouts of depression, and fits of violent behavior.

With the typical triad of choreiform movements, dementia in adult life, and documentation of similar symptoms in family members, the diagnosis is readily evident. However, there is a tendency for families to deny the existence of mental disease, and it is sometimes difficult to obtain corroborative data even when the diagnosis is strongly suspected. Little difficulty occurs in differentiating hereditary chorea from acute chorea, but senile chorea may raise a problem. The latter, which comes on late in life, involves few mental changes, if any, lacks a familial history, and is usually benign in comparison. Other diseases such as the presenile psychoses, Alzheimer's and Pick's, because of their dementia and similarity in age of onset, may offer some difficulty, especially in instances in which choreiform movements are inconspicuous. Computerized axial tomography or pneumoencephalography demonstrating selective atrophy of the caudate nucleus may help to establish the correct diagnosis in such instances. There is a tendency to overdiagnose hereditary chorea, applying it to diverse neurologic disorders such as cerebellar degenerations and familial tremors. The dire implications of this form of chorea require strict adherence to the diagnostic criteria.

There is at present no known means of altering the underlying disease process or its progressive fatal outcome. Attempts to replace the defect in gamma-aminobutyric acid (GABA) metabolism by utilizing some of its precursors such as glutamic acid or to elevate its level by utilizing inhibitors of GABA catabolism such as dipropylacetic acid have been unsuccessful. Symptomatic control of the choreiform movements can be accomplished by the use of neuroleptic agents such as haloperidol and chlorpromazine. Recently it has been demonstrated that choline chloride given in dosages of up to 20 grams a day can ameliorate the choreiform movements to a considerable extent without the attendant rigidity occurring with the use of neuroleptic agents. Utilizing these drugs combined with supervision of the patient's daily activities allows for management at home during the early stages of the disorder. However, as the disease advances, confinement to a psychiatric facility becomes necessary. Of equal importance to treatment of the patient is appropriate genetic counseling of family members. They should be given a comprehensive understanding of the disease, their own risks as to inheritance as well as those of their children, and the value of predictive tests. In regard to such tests, none have been fully validated which permit detection of the disorder prior to development of symptoms.

Barbeau, A., Chase, T. N., and Paulson, G. W. (eds.): Huntington's chorea 1872–1972. Adv. Neurol., 1, 1973.
Bird, E. D., and Iversen, L. L.: Huntington's chorea: Post-mortem measurement of glutamic acid decarboxylase, choline acetyl transferase and dopamine in basal ganglia. Brain, 97:457, 1974.
Growdon, J. H., Cohen, E. L., and Wurtman, R. J.: Huntington's disease: Clinical and chemical effects of choline administration. Ann. Neurol., 1:418, 1977.
Paulson, G. W.: Predictive tests in Huntington's disease. In Yahr, M. D. (ed.): The Basal Ganglia. New York, Raven Press, 1976, pp. 317–329.

277.4. SENILE CHOREA

Infrequently, choreiform movements are encountered as an isolated symptom in persons above 60 years of age. As a rule, the movements are mild and may involve the limbs on one side of the body or bilaterally.

Involuntary complex movements of the face, mouth, and tongue may occur, in association with limb movements or as the only manifestation of this disorder. No associated mental disturbance occurs in such patients, and no family history indicative of Huntington's chorea can be obtained. In many instances the symptoms come on abruptly, are unilateral, and show little or no progression. This has suggested an underlying vascular lesion, which may be found in an exceptional case. More often than not the pathologic findings are similar to those of Huntington's chorea insofar as involvement of the caudate nucleus is concerned, but the cerebral cortex is spared. This has led to the contrary consideration that these cases are a variant of Huntington's chorea occurring sporadically. Probably this form of chorea has several causes. As a rule, the symptoms are mild and the course benign so that therapeutic considerations are unimportant.

Martin, J. P.: Hemichorea resulting from local lesions of the brain. Brain, 50:637, 1927.
Weiner, W. J., and Klawans, H. L., Jr.: Lingual-facial-buccal movements in the elderly. II. Pathogenesis and relationship to senile chorea. J. Am. Geriat. Soc., 21:318, 1973.

278. OTHER EXTRAPYRAMIDAL DISORDERS

278.1. TICS
(Habit Spasms)
Melvin D. Yahr

A tic is a sudden, abrupt, rapid, purposeless, involuntary contraction of a muscle or group of functionally related muscles. Usually an irregular sequence of such contractions occurs that may result in eye blinking, head shaking, shrugging of the shoulder, or any sudden gesture of limbs or face. Tics may be voluntarily controlled for brief intervals, but such a conscious effort is usually followed by more intense and frequent contractions. Many persons experience minor transitory tic phenomena under periods of stress that are of no consequence. More persistent, sustained, and gross movements may be related to particular personality disturbances, and may be amenable to psychotherapy. In some instances tics have occurred during the acute phase of encephalitis; these are thought to be an expression of extrapyramidal dysfunction. Tics in younger patients must be differentiated from chorea. Their patterned, predictable, and stereotyped character makes this distinction.

An unusual form of generalized tic (*maladie des tics, Gilles de la Tourette's disease*) involving facial twitching, continuous gestures associated with echolalia, foul language, and obsessional ideas is occasionally encountered in childhood. Although at onset it may be difficult to differentiate simple tic phenomena from Tourette's disease, the progressive nature and development of associated symptoms make the diagnosis of the latter apparent. A number of reports have appeared indicating that haloperidol (Haldol) in divided dosage of 6 to 20 mg a day is effective both in reducing the movement disorder and in overcoming the unfortunate verbal outbursts.

Bruun, R. D., Shapiro, A. K., Shapiro, E., Sweet, R., Wayne, H., and Solomon, G. E.: A follow-up of 78 patients with Gilles de la Tourette's syndrome. Am. J. Psychiatry, 133:8, 1976.

Sweet, R. D., Solomon, G. E., Wayne, H., Shapiro, E., and Shapiro, A. K.: Neurological features of Gilles de la Tourette's syndrome. J. Neurol. Neurosurg. Psychiatry, 36:1, 1973.

278.2.   ATHETOSIS
(Mobile Spasms)
Melvin D. Yahr

This involuntary movement disorder is most frequently encountered in early infancy. Although in some respects it resembles chorea and although there are, in fact, transitional forms (so-called choreoathetosis), the athetotic movements are distinguishable by being slower, coarser, and more writhing. They occur when pathologic conditions involve the basal ganglia, primarily the pallidum, as well as additional motor pathways such as the corticospinal tract. Athetosis is most often found in the heterogeneous group of conditions now lumped together under the term "cerebral palsy" (CP). More often than not, patients with cerebral palsy have marked alteration in muscle tone consisting of a combination of spasticity and rigidity. Their extrapyramidal movements may be widespread or limited and encompass a wide variety of dyskinetic phenomena. Congenital defects, anoxia or trauma at birth, and other degenerative conditions have all been implicated. Some attempt has been made to identify specific entities based on clinicopathologic correlations. One such is athetosis simplex or status marmoratus. Cases of this disorder, which exemplifies all of the features of athetosis, show at autopsy a distinctive marbled appearance of the basal ganglia, the result of an abnormal overgrowth of myelin sheaths and increased numbers of glial cells. The cause of this morphologic abnormality is unknown. Other cases have been grouped together in which the prime pathologic change is cell loss and failure of myelin sheath formation in the region of the basal ganglia — so-called status dysmyelination. Still other cases have been encountered in which abnormal deposits of pigments occur or one of the lipoidoses or other storage diseases is found with the predominant clinical picture of athetotic movements. Athetosis is infrequently encountered in adult life, but when it is, tumors, vascular insufficiency, or malformations and the effects of toxic agents have been found in the region of the basal ganglia.

Typical athetosis possesses the following features in varying degrees. One or both sides of the body are involved. The movements involve the upper limbs to a greater extent than the lower and primarily in their distal segments. The muscles innervated by the cranial nerves are invariably involved so that facial grimacing, writhing movements of the tongue, and disturbances in articulation and swallowing are encountered. Abnormal postures of the limbs are assumed. In the upper extremities, these consist of adduction and internal rotation at the shoulder, semiflexion at the elbow, flexion of wrist and metacarpal phalangeal joints, and extension at interphalangeal joints. In the lower limbs the foot is maintained in internal rotation and plantar flexion with

dorsiflexion of the toes. Superimposed on these abnormal postures are the athetotic movements described above. Muscle tone is increased during movement but is hypotonic during relaxation, and some degree of weakness is usually found. The reflexes may be hyperactive, with abnormal toe responses. In many instances some degree of intellectual impairment may be found.

The abnormal movements and postural abnormalities are distinctive enough to make this condition readily recognizable. The age at onset, the admixture of other neurologic abnormalities, and the manner in which the symptoms progress identify the disease. Since most instances of athetosis appear in early infancy, before one year of age, diseases of the perinatal period are considered primarily. Athetosis occurring in later childhood or adult life may be a part of other extrapyramidal disorders, such as dystonia, chorea, or hepatolenticular degeneration. Less frequently athetosis is a manifestation of a wide spectrum of neurologic disorders already mentioned in which the pallidum is coincidentally involved.

There is no specific therapy for the relief of athetosis. The use of anticholinergic agents as indicated in Ch. 274.4 may decrease the intensity of the movements. Thalamotomy has on occasion afforded some degree of relief, but one is hesitant to advocate this surgical procedure on a nervous system already extensively damaged by a variety of pathologic processes.

Courville, C. B.: Structural basis of athetosis in cerebral palsied children. Arch. Pediat., 78:461, 1961.

Mettler, F. A., and Stern, G.: On the patho-physiology of athetosis. J. Nerv. Ment. Dis., 135:138, 1962.

Narabayashi, H., and Nakamura, R.: Clinical picture of cerebral palsy in neurological understanding. Confin. Neurol., 34:7, 1972.

278.3.   DYSTONIA MUSCULORUM DEFORMANS
(Torsion Dystonia)
Melvin D. Yahr

The torsion dystonias comprise a group of movement disorders characterized by intense, irregular, sustained torsion spasms of the musculature, with resultant marked abnormalities of bodily posture. The dystonic movements may involve any or all of the musculature, but have a predilection for the trunk and shoulder and pelvic girdles. Although the site and underlying mechanisms by which symptoms are produced are unknown, sufficient evidence exists to indicate that they arise from dysfunction within the basal ganglia complex. In this regard a biochemical abnormality is suspected, because dystonic reactions may be induced by pharmacologic agents such as the phenothiazines and levodopa which affect striatal amine functions.

Based on genetic, clinical, and presumed causative factors, several forms may be recognized. In general, they fall into two categories: the symptomatic or acquired and the idiopathic or hereditary. The latter has a varied type of inheritance, being either autosomal recessive or autosomal dominant. Symptomatic dystonic movements occur with hepatolenticular degeneration, postencephalitic parkinsonism, tumors, or other diseases involving the basal ganglia. Morphologic changes indicative of these disease processes are found within one or another of the basal ganglia structures. In the idiopathic form no consistent morphologic abnormalities have been defined.

The autosomal recessive form is found most often in Ashkenazic Jews, beginning between the ages of 5 and 15 years. Its onset is variable but most frequently begins with intermittent spasmodic inversion of the foot, so that on walking the child finds difficulty in placing the heel on the ground. Bizarre stepping or a bowing gait may be noted when the dystonic movements affect the more proximal muscles of the leg or the spine. As the movements become more intense and the proximal musculature is more prominently involved, lordosis and tortipelvis appear. If the muscles of the neck and shoulder girdle are involved, torticollis is an early finding. Facial grimacing and difficulties in speech become evident as the muscles subserving these functions become involved. The continuous spasms over a period of time result in marked distortions of the body of a degree rarely seen in any other disease process. Although muscle tone and power appear to be normal, the involuntary movements interfere with function to such a degree as to make them useless. No changes in the deep tendon reflexes occur, and mentation remains normal.

The autosomal dominant form has its onset in early adult life and generally involves the axial musculature, with torticollis a frequent presenting symptom. In contrast to the recessive form, it remains more restricted in the regions of the body involved and is more slowly progressive. Recently it has been demonstrated that plasma dopamine beta hydroxylase activity is markedly elevated in the dominant form. This finding is strictly empiric, and although it is helpful in classification of the disease, neither the physiologic nor the biochemical significance of this finding has been elucidated.

In its early stages dystonia musculorum deformans must be differentiated from other movement disorders in which dystonic phenomena may occur. The history and physical findings exclude hepatolenticular degeneration and epidemic encephalitis. The age at onset and the involvement of proximal musculature in the movements are enough to differentiate it from athetosis. Chorea is characterized by movements more rapid and of shorter duration than those of dystonia. Hysteria is often a consideration; if it is not positively established by the personality characteristics of the patient, the course of the disease will soon suggest the correct diagnosis.

There is extreme variability in the rate of progression and eventual disability of both forms of the genetically determined disorder. In their early phases there may be complete remission of symptoms or lack of progression of initial symptoms for intervals of up to five years. Because the natural history is subject to wide variations, evaluation of the effects of treatment is difficult. Dystonic movements have been effectively controlled for varying periods of time by drugs and surgical intervention. Drugs which have proved useful are those which produce a degree of muscle relaxation, such as the benzodiazepines (diazepam [Valium], 15 to 30 mg per day, and clonazepam [Clonopin], 1.5 to 3 mg per day); and agents capable of inducing a degree of pseudoparkinsonism, such as the phenothiazines (chlorpromazine, 25 to 100 mg per day), butyrophenones (haloperidol, 6 to 10 mg per day), and carbamazepine (Tegretol,

800 to 1200 mg per day), which reputedly depresses neuronal activity in the thalamic nuclei. In mild cases a combination of these drugs with general supportive psychotherapeutic measures may be enough to control the patients' symptoms for years. Stereotactic thalamotomy has been reported to benefit patients for extended periods of time; however, it does require rather extensive bilateral lesions of the ventral lateral nuclei of the thalamus, which carries the risk of additional neurologic deficit, particularly speech disturbance. Attempts to utilize biofeedback mechanisms are of too recent origin to be assessed for value in this disorder.

Denny-Brown, D. E.: The nature of dystonia. Bull. N.Y. Acad. Med., 41:858, 1965.
Eldridge, R.: The torsion dystonias: Literature review and genetic and clinical studies. Neurology, 20(Part 2):1, 1970.
Marsden, C. D.: Dystonia: The spectrum of the disease. Res. Publ. Assoc. Res. Nerv. Ment. Dis., 55:351, 1976.

278.4. SPASMODIC TORTICOLLIS

Melvin D. Yahr

The restriction of dyskinetic movements to neck muscles so that abnormal postures of the head result is the distinguishing characteristic of this symptom complex. Involuntary activity involves the sternocleidomastoids, trapezius, and scalenus muscles in sustained contractions that result in slow, twisting, turning movements of the head (torticollis) or less often forward flexion (anterocollis) or forceful extension (retrocollis). In most instances there is bilateral involvement, and the resultant postural deformity is maintained for varying lengths of time. The muscles of the neck appear under tension, and the continual muscular activity may lead to some degree of hypertrophy, especially evident in the sternocleidomastoid. Similar activity may spread to facial and brachial musculature. The amount of active motion or static postural deformity is extremely variable.

Spasmodic torticollis has variably been described as a psychogenic disorder, a fragment of dystonia musculorum deformans, or a compensatory postural defect in persons with congenital ocular muscle imbalance or defects of the cervical spine or musculature. In some instances it has occurred as part of a wide spectrum of extrapyramidal disorders that follow encephalitis lethargica. There is no information at present regarding either its pathophysiology or pathology.

The disorder has been encountered at all ages, but most frequently makes its appearance during the third to sixth decades of life. The course is extremely variable, being transitory and remitting after a few months in some patients and relentlessly progressive and leading to incapacity in others. Some cases reach a static phase in which movements cease or are minimal, and a minor postural deformity of the head persists.

The evaluation of this condition includes a search for ocular and vertebral signs, major psychiatric disturbances, and other neurologic conditions with which it may be associated. Definable conditions account for only a small percentage of cases. In most, no known cause is uncovered.

There is no specific therapy for torticollis except when an underlying correctable disease process is found. Many measures have been recommended to ameliorate the symptoms. Sensory biofeedback techniques have been utilized with some success. Of the number of pharmacologic agents used, the benzodiazepines, including diazepam (Valium), 15 to 30 mg per day, and clonazepam (Clonopin), 1.5 to 3 mg per day, as well as haloperidol (Haldol), 6 to 10 mg per day, have been reported effective in some patients. In those more severely affected, a variety of surgical measures have been attempted with inconsistent results. Denervation of the affected muscles by section of the anterior cervical root and/or the spinal accessory nerve has been utilized. Although the movements decrease on the operated side, they frequently recur in the contralateral group of muscles. Bilateral procedures may result in extensive disability. Although bilateral thalamotomy has been performed with reported improvement, one is hesitant to recommend a procedure of this magnitude except in extreme situations. A procedure involving iontophoresis of saline into the middle ear, which presumably suppresses labyrinthine function unilaterally, has produced encouraging results in one series.

Gilbert, G. J.: The medical treatment of spasmodic torticollis. Arch. Neurol., 27:503, 1972.

Herz, E., and Glaser, G. H.: Spasmodic torticollis. Clinical evaluation. Arch. Neurol. Psychiatry, 61:227, 1949.

Korein, J., and Brudny, J.: Integrated EMG feedback in the management of spasmodic torticollis and focal dystonia: A prospective study of 80 patients. In Yahr, M. D. (ed.): The Basal Ganglia. New York, Raven Press, 1976, pp. 385–426.

278.5.   HEMIBALLISM

Melvin D. Yahr

This rather violent involuntary movement occurs when lesions involve the contralateral subthalamic nucleus, the corpus Luysii. Although a variety of pathologic processes such as tumor and infectious diseases have been found as underlying causes, most are a result of vascular lesions, either hemorrhagic or occlusive. In consequence, they are encountered in older patients, sometimes after a transitory hemiparesis. The event leading to the onset of this movement disorder often is an acute cerebrovascular accident with weakness and/or sensory deficit. As the neurologic signs clear or at a variable interval afterward, the ballistic movements begin. The movements do not occur during sleep, are localized to one side of the body, and involve the limbs in a forceful throwing movement, a result of almost continuous activity of the proximal musculature. Initially, their violence may exhaust and incapacitate the patient to such an extent that death may ensue. However, in most instances, the initial intensity decreases gradually so that they become tolerable, and in approximately six to eight weeks the movements stop spontaneously. Surgical measures, such as thalamotomy, are rarely needed for control. In this regard, it is interesting to note that hemiballism has followed attempted thalamotomy for other extrapyramidal disorders when poor localization for lesion placement has occurred. In such instances, the surgeon has inadvertently placed a lesion in the region of the corpus Luysii.

Carpenter, M. B.: Ballism associated with partial destruction of the subthalamic nucleus of Luys. Neurology, 5:479, 1955.

Hyland, H. H., and Forman, D. M.: Progress in hemiballismus. Neurology, 7:381, 1957.

Martin, P. J., and McCaul, I. R.: Acute hemiballism treated by ventrolateral thalamolysis. Brain, 82:104, 1959.

278.6.   IDIOPATHIC AUTONOMIC INSUFFICIENCY

(Idiopathic Orthostatic Hypotension, Shy-Drager Syndrome)

Ira B. Black

DEFINITION.   Idiopathic autonomic insufficiency is a rare degenerative disorder of unknown etiology which strikes during middle age, causing progressive autonomic dysfunction; severe debility or death may occur within 5 to 15 years of onset. Associated extrapyramidal abnormalities and lesions of pigmented brain nuclei may play a prominent role in the genesis of symptoms.

PATHOGENESIS AND PATHOLOGY.   Histologic examination at autopsy has disclosed degenerative changes in autonomic ganglia in the periphery, and in the preganglionic, intermediolateral cell column in the spinal cord. In the brain, virtually all cranial nerve nuclei may undergo degeneration, and similar changes may occur in the hypothalamus, nigrostriatal system, pontine nuclei, and globus pallidus. Postmortem biochemical studies have revealed marked depression of catecholamine biosynthetic enzyme activities in sympathetic ganglia and in central noradrenergic neurons of the nucleus locus ceruleus; the substantia nigra may be similarly affected in patients with extrapyramidal symptoms. More specifically, dopamine-β-hydroxylase, which converts dopamine to norepinephrine, is decreased in sympathetic ganglia, whereas tyrosine hydroxylase, the rate-limiting enzyme in catecholamine biosynthesis, is decreased in locus ceruleus. In parkinsonian patients, tyrosine hydroxylase may be depressed in substantia nigra.

The pathogenesis of the disease is unclear. A number of observations suggest that preganglionic neuronal dysfunction may be an early, perhaps primary, event. First, degeneration of preganglionic neurons may be prominent in many patients. Second, although basal levels of plasma norepinephrine may be normal in some patients, suggesting that postsynaptic adrenergic neurons are functional, stress fails to cause the normal elevation of plasma norepinephrine, suggesting dysfunction of central autonomic pathways. Lastly, indirect-acting drugs such as tyramine, which cause sympathetic activation by releasing endogenous norepinephrine, may exert normal effects in patients with obvious sympathetic abnormalities. However, more recent studies indicate that preganglionic disease may not be *the* primary phenomenon in all cases. Thus the preganglionic intermediolateral column neurons may be histologically normal in the disease. The preganglionic cholinergic terminals in sympathetic ganglia may be biochemically normal with demonstrable postganglionic histologic and biochemical lesions. Finally, the pattern of enzyme deficits in adrenergic neurons of sympathetic ganglia is not entirely consistent with trans-synaptic dysfunction. It is possible that several different subpopulations are now included in this disease category, and that the respective pathogeneses differ.

Indeed, several observers have suggested that at least two entities may comprise idiopathic autonomic insufficiency. The first may consist of autonomic insufficiency alone, whereas the second may be characterized by autonomic insufficiency in association with a variety of neurologic signs, including movement disorders resembling Parkinson's disease. The great degree of clinical overlap between these groups, however, is also consistent with the existence of a broad continuum rather than distinct entities.

CLINICAL MANIFESTATIONS. Symptoms of autonomic dysfunction predominate early in the course. Characteristically, initial difficulties consist of sexual impotence, urinary hesitancy, urgency, or incontinence, and/or anhidrosis. These early symptoms are frequently unrecognized and undiagnosed. Within months to years, the hallmark of the disorder, postural hypotension, appears. This may be manifested as dizziness, giddiness, or frank syncope upon standing. Less frequently, patients complain of generalized weakness, cervico-occipital discomfort, or leg weakness upon standing. Attendant autonomic symptoms, including intermittent diplopia, dysphagia, and diarrhea, fecal incontinence, or constipation, may also occur. As the disease progresses, a variety of movement disorders may appear. A parkinsonian disorder, consisting of bradykinesia, coarse tremor, and rigidity, is common, and tends to progress inexorably. Myoclonus, gait disturbance, and signs of olivopontocerebellar dysfunction may also occur.

Physical signs parallel the aforementioned symptoms and include evidence of autonomic dysfunction. Orthostatic hypotension, greater than a 30/20 mm Hg fall in blood pressure upon assumption of the erect position, constitutes the hallmark sign. Other signs of possible autonomic-cardiovascular dysfunction include absence of sinus arrhythmia, absence of increased heart rate upon standing, and absence of the normal overshoot in diastolic pressure during phase IV of the Valsalva maneuver. In addition, autonomic dysfunction may manifest as Horner's syndrome or as anhidrosis even with elevated ambient temperature, as well as the bladder and bowel dysfunction described above. Neurologic examination may reveal signs indistinguishable from those of Parkinson's disease. Cerebellar ataxia, dysmetria, and dysdiadochokinesia may also be elicited. Muscle wasting, fasciculation, and extensor plantar responses have been observed.

A variety of clinical laboratory tests may be employed to evaluate autonomic function, and only the simplest will be delineated here. In addition to the bedside examinations described above, other observations may be helpful. *Miosis* in response to ocular administration of dilute solutions of methacholine, or *mydriasis* after instillation of dilute epinephrine, suggests respective parasympathetic or sympathetic denervation supersensitivity. On the other hand, absence of mydriasis after ocular instillation of cocaine or hydroxyamphetamine suggests that endogenous norepinephrine stores are defective. Absence of sweating with elevation of the ambient temperature and absence of the axon reflex after intradermal histamine suggest denervation of cutaneous structures. The presence of an abnormally accentuated blood pressure response to the intravenous infusion of norepinephrine is consistent with widespread denervation supersensitivity. Vagal dysfunction may be manifested by absence of sinus arrhythmia, absence of bradycardia after carotid sinus massage, absence of increased gastric acidity after insulin hypoglycemia, and altered gastrointestinal motility with retention of barium in the small bowel during x-ray studies.

DIFFERENTIAL DIAGNOSIS. Orthostatic hypotension itself may accompany intravascular hypovolemia (as with massive hemorrhage or adrenal insufficiency), vasodepressor syncope, acute cardiac failure from a variety of causes, familial hyperbradykininism, and intracranial posterior fossa mass or vascular lesions. However, in these conditions other signs of autonomic dysfunction are absent. On the other hand, autonomic insufficiency, including orthostatic hypotension, may occur with any disease that alters peripheral or central autonomic pathways. Many disorders conform to this description. A variety of peripheral neuropathies may be accompanied by dysautonomia, including the acute Guillain-Barré syndrome, the chronic neuropathies of diabetes mellitus, amyloidosis, Wernicke's disease and porphyria, and the congenital Riley-Day syndrome. Ganglion dysfunction may result from ingestion of ganglioplegic agents. Tabes dorsalis is commonly accompanied by autonomic signs. Autonomic dysfunction may result from interruption of descending pathways in the spinal cord, as observed with syringomyelia, trauma, or spinal tumor. Pontine hemorrhage may interrupt descending sympathetic pathways in the brainstem, thereby causing sympathetic dysfunction. However, differentiation from these diseases is easily accomplished with suitable history, examination, and laboratory tests. For example, peripheral neuropathies characteristically produce distal sensory, and often motor, impairment.

COURSE AND TREATMENT. Although treatment does not alter the underlying pathologic process, it may allow an otherwise bedridden invalid to lead a virtually normal life. Orthostatic hypotension may be treated with a variety of measures, dictated by the severity of the problem. The first line of defense consists of antigravity stockings, which prevent pooling of blood in the lower extremities upon standing. In moderately severe cases, intravascular volume expansion may be achieved by using the mineralocorticoid 9-α-fluorocortisone and sodium chloride, with potassium supplementation. In severe cases, oral sympathomimetic agents, including ephedrine or hydroxyamphetamine, may be added. Such combination therapy is effective in virtually all cases. Recent work suggests that indomethacin may be effective in selected patients for the treatment of orthostatic hypotension. The use of monoamine oxidase inhibitors may be potentially hazardous in those patients who are subject to denervation supersensitivity. Although the diet may be rigorously regulated in the hospital setting, this is rarely possible on an outpatient basis. For example, such foods as cheese, broad beans, Chianti, raisins, bananas, and aged or smoked meat contain significant quantities of vasoactive amines. Inadvertent ingestion of microgram quantities of vasoactive amines in the diet may result in alarming elevation of blood pressure in patients being treated with monoamine oxidase for widespread sympathetic denervation.

Parkinsonian signs and symptoms may be successfully treated with L-dopa and the customary anticholinergic agents.

Bannister, R., and Oppenheimer, D. R.: Degenerative diseases of the nervous system associated with autonomic failure. Brain, 95:457, 1972.

Black, I. B., and Petito, C. K.: Catecholamine enzymes in the degenerative neurological disease idiopathic orthostatic hypotension. Science, 192:910, 1976.

Bradbury, S., and Eggleston, C.: Postural hypotension: A report of three cases. Am. Heart J., 1:73, 1925.

Shy, G. M., and Drager, G. A.: A neurological syndrome associated with orthostatic hypotension. Arch. Neurol., 2:511, 1960.

Ziegler, M. G., Lake, C. R., and Kopin, I. J.: The sympathetic-nervous-system defect in primary orthostatic hypotension. N. Engl. J. Med., 296:293, 1977.

Section Twelve INHERITED DEGENERATIVE DISEASES OF THE NERVOUS SYSTEM

Roger N. Rosenberg

279. INTRODUCTION

The classic eponymic neurologic diseases discussed in this section produce characteristic pathologic changes in specific nuclei and fiber tracts in brain, spinal cord, and peripheral nerve. The disorders are usually progressive and symmetrical in their pathologic and clinical expression and often have a clear genetic basis of inheritance or suggestion of familial involvement. The disorders involve specific regions or systems of the nervous system such as cerebellar nuclei and fiber tracts or the corticospinal or extrapyramidal motor system, resulting in specific neurologic symptoms and signs referred to as system degenerations.

Gowers in 1902 referred to these inherited degenerative diseases as abiotrophies. This term implies the occurrence of neurologic disease resulting from an impairment in the metabolic state of the brain, spinal cord, or peripheral nerve. Recently, as discussed below, enzyme deficiencies, chromosomal breaks, specific immunologic defects, abnormalities in nerve growth factor, and slow latent viral-like infections of the brain have been identified as specific etiologic bases for some of these abiotrophies.

It is of great interest and importance that in most of the inherited degenerative disorders to be discussed the primary impact of disease involves the neuron, changes produced in astrocytes and oligodendrocytes being presumably of a reactive and secondary nature. Intensive research is currently underway in many laboratories concerning most of the disorders mentioned here. The past decade has witnessed an exponential increase in our knowledge concerning the basic enzyme defects and metabolic consequences of many autosomal recessive disorders in the categories of the gangliosidoses, leukodystrophies, mucopolysaccharidoses, glycogenoses, and heavy metal storage disorders; these will be discussed in greater detail in other chapters. Using these autosomal recessive diseases as models, it is hoped that the basic molecular defect in several autosomal dominant system degenerations discussed in the following chapters, such as Huntington's disease, olivopontocerebellar atrophy, striatonigral degeneration, nigrospinodentatal degeneration, tuberous sclerosis, and neurofibromatosis, will be clarified.

280. STRIATONIGRAL DEGENERATION

Striatonigral degeneration (Joseph's disease) is a rare disease of the nervous system inherited as an autosomal dominant disorder in persons of Portuguese or Azorian ancestry. A nongenetic form of striatonigral degeneration also has been described by van der Eecken, Adams, and van Bogart. Patients with this form are diagnosed clinically as having Parkinson's disease, but the disease is different neuropathologically in that there is bilateral degeneration of the corpus striatum and substantia nigra, particularly the zona compacta portion. No cause has been found in any of the cases. Rosenberg, Nyhan, Bay, and Shore described a family of Portuguese ancestry with autosomal dominant striatonigral degeneration numbering 329 persons in eight generations, and Romanul et al. reported in another family of Portuguese-Azorian ancestry the presence of a striatonigral degeneration in a clinical setting of autosomal dominant disease with parkinsonism and polyneuropathy. No genetic link is present between these two families, who in fact come from separate and distant Azorian islands.

PATHOLOGY.   The major pathologic findings in one deceased family member are a severe loss of neurons and glial replacement in the corpus striatum and a severe loss of neurons in the zona compacta portion of the substantia nigra. There is also a moderate loss of neurons in the dentate nucleus of the cerebellum and in the nucleus ruber of the midbrain. The cerebellum, cerebellar peduncles, inferior olives, corticospinal tracts in the brainstem, and basis pontis do not show gross atrophy. The cerebellar and frontal cerebral cortex appears normal histologically. There is no evidence of demyelination in the cerebellum, its peduncles, or the brainstem. Although the putamen shows significant neuronal loss, there is no increased pigmentation characteristic of the nongenetic forms of the striatonigral degenerations.

CLINICAL MANIFESTATIONS.   The main neurologic findings include extremity weakness and spasticity of all extremities, especially the legs, often with associated dystonia of the face, neck, trunk, and extremities. Patellar and ankle clonus are common, as are extensor plantar responses. The gait is slow and stiff, with a slight increase in base and lurching from side to side due to spasticity. Affected persons have no truncal titubation. Pharyngeal weakness and spasticity cause difficulty with speech and swallowing. Of note are prominent horizontal and vertical nystagmus, the loss of the fast saccadic eye movements, hypermetric and hypometric saccades, and impairment of vertical gaze. Facial fasciculations, facial myokymia, and lingual fasciculations without atrophy are common and early manifestations.

The disorder is inherited as an autosomal dominant trait, the mean age of onset of symptoms in affected members examined being 25 years. Neurologic deficits increase progressively and result in death from debilitation within 15 years of onset. Patients retain full intellectual function, and the only significant involuntary movements are dystonia and tremor at rest in some affected members.

DIAGNOSIS. Autosomal dominant striatonigral degeneration should be considered in persons with an appropriate family history developing progressive dystonia, rigidity and spasticity of pharynx, trunk, and extremities, and associated hyperreflexia, clonus, and extensor plantar responses during the first or second decade. The entity is distinguished from Huntington's disease by the preservation of intellect and the absence of choreoathetosis. Dystonia musculorum deformans can be distinguished by the prominence of spasticity and the characteristic eye findings present in the striatonigral degenerations. The entity may be related to the nigrospinodentatal degeneration described by Woods and Schaumburg, which is also expressed as an autosomal dominant disorder producing rigidity and spasticity. However, the major pathology in their patients was in the dentate nuclei, the spinocerebellar tracts, and the middle cerebellar peduncle. Recent clinical and epidemiologic evidence indicates that this genetic disease can have a wide spectrum, and some patients in large families develop distal extremity atrophy, areflexia, distal sensory loss, hypotonia, and cerebellar truncal and extremity ataxia. Assays of the cerebrospinal fluid (CSF) for homovanillic acid are of value, as the mean concentration of this metabolite of dopamine in the CSF of five affected persons was 15.3 ng per milliliter as compared to a control value of 43.4 ng per milliliter.

281. MOTOR NEURON DISEASES

281.1. INTRODUCTION

The term motor neuron disease refers to a group of chronic neurologic disorders that selectively affect with varying combination and rapidity the anterior horn cells of the spinal cord and lower brainstem, plus, in some cases, those large motor neurons of the cerebral cortex that give rise to the corticospinal tract. Clinically significant sensory change or cerebellar dysfunction is absent in all instances. Cases in which upper motor neuron changes are prominent in addition to muscle fasciculation, atrophy, and weakness are called *amyotrophic lateral sclerosis* (ALS). *Progressive bulbar palsy* is a variant of ALS that produces relatively rapidly advancing upper and lower motor neuron involvement of the muscles of the jaw, pharynx, and tongue. Cases lacking signs of upper motor neuron disease and producing only a slow, progressive muscle wasting and weakness often are termed *progressive muscular atrophy* (PMA). A variety of clinical subtypes of PMA occur, some of which can produce restricted motor involvement that progresses extremely slowly over a period of many years. *Werdnig-Hoffmann disease* of infancy and young children and the *Wohlfart-Kugelberg-Welander disease* of older children and adolescents represent other variants of motor neuron disease. "Primary lateral sclerosis" is a nondisease. The ostensible condition included progressive spasticity but no lower motor neuron changes, and was at one time linked to the motor neuron diseases.

Subsequent studies have shown that such signs in fact always are attributable to other causes such as disseminated sclerosis, spinal cord compression, other degenerative disorders, or high spinal neoplasms.

281.2. AMYOTROPHIC LATERAL SCLEROSIS

Amyotrophic lateral sclerosis (ALS) can first affect bulbar muscles, a single limb, the extremities on one side of the body, the lower or upper extremities symmetrically, or all four limbs simultaneously, depending upon the individual case. The disorder occurs mainly in the fifth, sixth, and seventh decades of life and runs a progressive course lasting from as short as 18 to 24 months to as long as about seven years. The bulbar form runs a more malignant course. ALS usually occurs sporadically, but familial groupings of amyotrophic lateral sclerosis syndromes have occurred, indicating either a genetic predisposition for disease or common exposure to an unknown causative agent. Familial cases tend to come on younger and progress more rapidly than do cases in older adults. Recently Oldstone and associates have reported finding immune complexes associated with the mesangium of the renal glomerulus and basement membrane in patients with rapidly progressive but otherwise typical motor neuron disease. The implication in this instance is that motor neuron disease may be an autoimmune disorder. It also has been suggested that the disorder may be due to a slow latent viral infection such as a mutated poliovirus. Several reports cite the subsequent occurrence of motor neuron disease during late adulthood in patients having poliomyelitis in childhood. Despite these clues, the precise mechanism and cause of the motor neuron disorders is currently not known.

PATHOLOGY. The neuropathologic findings in ALS consist of degenerative changes and loss of the Betz cells in layers 3 and 5 of the precentral cerebral cortex, Brodmann's areas 4 and 6. These are absent in the more benign cases of progressive muscular atrophy. Neuronal loss also occurs in the motor cranial nuclei and the motor neurons in the anterior horns of the spinal cord. There are no characteristic features associated with the neuronal loss, and the musculature innervated by the affected motor cranial nuclei and anterior horn cells undergoes neurogenic atrophy as a result of denervation.

CLINICAL MANIFESTATIONS. ALS produces a variety of clinical patterns, all of which show muscle weakness and wasting but which vary in their rate of progression, the distribution of the major weakness, and the rapidity with which signs of upper motor neuron dysfunction occur. Patients develop a slowly progressive impairment of motor function affecting distal more than proximal structures, as evidenced by muscle atrophy involving the intrinsic muscles of the hand. Over a period of six months to a year, the process results in symmetrical muscle atrophy involving the hands, forearms, and shoulder girdle muscles. The disease may develop quite asymmetrically in some patients. Prominent and early in most patients is the occurrence of fasciculations due to acute and widespread denervation of entire motor units. The patient may have muscle cramps, as well as, rarely, mild distal paresthesias. The deep tendon reflexes are usually preserved in the upper extremities in the early phase of disease. Signs of upper motor neuron involvement may develop at any time but almost always by the time muscle involvement has lasted as long as a year. These include spasticity, particularly in the lower extremities with associated hyperreflexia, clonus, and extensor plantar responses on one or both sides. Characteristically, the superficial abdominal reflexes and the cremasteric reflexes as well as the bladder and anal sphincters remain normal. Generalized fasciculations and muscle atrophy in most instances involve the lower extremities later than the upper. These combinations of upper and lower motor neuron deficits are characteristic of ALS. Occasionally, spasticity predominantly involves the pharynx, larynx, and extremities, and signs of muscular atrophy and fasciculations are hard to detect; but they are always there, at least by electrical testing. The loss of the gag reflex, pharyngeal paralysis, lingual atrophy and fasciculations, and diffuse extremity atrophy and fasciculations with reduced myotatic reflexes would indicate a severe bulbospinal variant of ALS (progressive muscular atrophy almost always spares the cranial nerves). Musculature innervated by the fifth, seventh, tenth, eleventh, and twelfth cranial motor nuclei is involved in the bulbar form of ALS, but the disease spares the extraocular muscles. Patients may show signs of emotional lability, but intellectual functions are preserved, even in the terminal phases of the disorder. The cerebrospinal fluid is normal. The presence of fasciculations and other changes of acute muscle denervation can be confirmed by electromyography (EMG). The motor nerve conduction velocities remain normal, however, even in the presence of severe atrophy, a finding that separates this disorder from the peripheral motor neuropathies, in which conduction velocities are reduced.

DIFFERENTIAL DIAGNOSIS. Primary muscle disease, peripheral nerve disorders, spinal cord compression, or tumors and conditions damaging the corticospinal tracts so as to produce spasticity all can at least superficially resemble ALS. None of these conditions, however, are able to imitate the characteristic combination of painless, diffuse neurogenic muscle impairment plus spasticity and absent sensory change that marks severe motor neuron disease. Muscle disease can be separated by changes in serum enzymes, EMG, and biopsy. Peripheral nerve disorders mostly produce sensory impairment. They do not cause fasciculation, and they do cause slowing of nerve electrical conduction velocity. Cervical spinal cord compression from spondylosis or tumor often causes pain, and usually produces a destructive combination of weakness and atrophy restricted to the arms, plus spasticity and sensory changes in the legs.

Multiple sclerosis can result in spasticity, but not muscular atrophy or fasciculation, and sensory changes are usual. Intracranial disorders can produce bilateral spasticity, but other signs of brain involvement usually easily distinguish the condition.

TREATMENT. This must be symptomatic and supportive, as there is no specific therapy.

281.3. WERDNIG-HOFFMANN DISEASE

Werdnig-Hoffmann disease, occurring in infancy and early childhood, presents as a progressive impairment of the motor system. The lower motor neuron is exclusively involved, including musculature innervated by motor cranial nuclei and anterior horn cells of the spinal cord. Infants and young children may present with this syndrome at birth or in the first few months of life with diffuse flaccidity, muscular atrophy, muscle fasciculations, and reduced to absent myotatic reflexes with associated respiratory and swallowing difficulties. There may be prominent lingual fasciculations and atrophy in the first few months of life. A muscle biopsy indicates neurogenic atrophy, and the cerebrospinal fluid is entirely normal. Electromyography shows acute denervation with normal peripheral nerve conduction velocities. The disorder usually appears either sporadically or as an autosomal recessive genetic disorder. The cause is not known.

281.4. WOHLFART-KUGELBERG-WELANDER DISEASE

Wohlfart-Kugelberg-Welander disease is an autosomal recessive disorder in which symptoms begin during late childhood, adolescence, or early adulthood and include progressive proximal muscle atrophy, weakness, and fasciculations. It is very slowly progressive and is usually compatible with a life span into the third or fourth decade. Typical examples have been described in families in which other children have Werdnig-Hoffmann disease. Thus varying penetrance of a single gene mutation inherited in an autosomal recessive manner may produce either an aggressive form of motor neuron disease in childhood (Werdnig-Hoffmann disease) or a more benign form of motor neuron disease in later childhood and early adulthood (Wohlfart-Kugelberg-Welander disease). The onset in the first and second decades of life of proximal weakness and atrophy with fasciculations but with a very slow progression without evidence of upper motor neuron involvement separates this disorder from amyotrophic lateral sclerosis. The presence of denervation without the insertional irritability characteristic of polymyositis can be determined by electromyography. Both Wohlfart-Kugelberg-Welander disease and polymyositis may present with progressive proximal weakness and atrophy; if fasciculations are not prominent, electromyography and muscle biopsy are of important differentiating value. Neurogenic denervation can be identified in biopsied muscle, thus separating it from the acquired or inherited myopathies. The cause of the disorder is unknown, and specific therapy is not available.

282. SPINOCEREBELLAR DEGENERATIONS

282.1. INTRODUCTION

This term applies to a group of progressive degenerative disorders in which ataxia and dysmetria resulting from predominant involvement of the cerebellum and its pathways are combined to greater or lesser degrees, with impairment of other sensory and motor systems. All represent system degenerations, and many of the specific entities have a well established genetic basis. Although clinical signs of cerebellar involvement predominate, the extension of the disorders to involve other regions of the nervous system can produce more complex neurologic symptoms. The important and common inherited spinocerebellar degenerations include (1) Friedreich's ataxia; (2) Roussey-Lévy syndrome; (3) Bassen-Kornzweig syndrome, (4) Refsum's syndrome; (5) olivopontocerebellar degeneration; (6) Marie's ataxia; and (7) dyssynergia cerebellaris myoclonica.

As classified by Greenfield, the spinocerebellar degenerations can be grouped into predominant spinal forms, spinocerebellar forms, and cerebellar forms. Further subclassification exists in the olivopontocerebellar degenerations, with at least five subtypes identified by Konigsmark and Weiner with both autosomal dominant and autosomal recessive forms of inheritance. The spinocerebellar degenerations have common neuropathologic features from the peripheral nerve through the spinal cord and up to the cerebellum with its attendant connections. Although these disorders are well described both clinically and pathologically, only in Friedreich's syndrome, Refsum's disease, and the Bassen-Kornzweig syndrome do molecular insights exist into the cause. The similarity of neuropathologic findings in the Bassen-Kornzweig syndrome and Friedreich's syndrome despite very different molecular defects indicates the vulnerability of the spinocerebellar system to different chemical abnormalities as well as its limited neuropathologic response.

282.2. FRIEDREICH'S ATAXIA

This form of spinocerebellar degeneration begins in childhood and is mainly inherited as an autosomal recessive or dominant disorder. Sporadic cases presumably represent spontaneous mutations. Friedreich's ataxia comprises a syndrome including several subtypes with common clinical features and pathologic changes. Causes of Friedreich's syndrome include several inborn errors of metabolism, including disorders of lipids (phytanic acid storage disease, abetalipoproteinemia, moderate beta-galactosidase deficiencies, and juvenile arylsulfatase deficiency), diseases of oxidative metabolism (neuromuscular disorders with "ragged red" fibers and abnormalities of cytochrome B or of NADH oxidation), aminoacidurias (intermittent maple syrup urine disease, gamma-glutamylcysteinyl transferase deficiencies, and Hartnup disease) and the partial deficiency of hypoxanthineguanine phosphoribosyltransferase (HGPRT).

Recently Blass et al. have described children in whom pyruvate oxidation was low in muscles from 4 of 7 patients with Friedreich's syndrome, in 4 of 12 patients with other ataxias, and in 8 of 19 patients with familial or idiopathic neuropathies. In those studies the degree of pyruvate dehydrogenase complex activity correlated with the severity and rapidity of the spinocerebellar disease process. For example, patients with less than 15 per cent of normal pyruvate dehydrogenase activity but with normal oxoglutarate dehydrogenase generally had severe neurologic disease and lactic acidosis beginning in infancy. Severe deficiencies of both complexes have been described in one infant with severe disease. Several patients with 20 to 30 per cent of normal pyruvate

dehydrogenase activity had a milder illness in which ataxia was the most prominent sign. The patients with Friedreich's syndrome had the mildest defect, with 40 to 50 per cent of normal pyruvate dehydrogenase activity together with 50 per cent of normal oxoglutarate dehydrogenase activity. Thus a defect in pyruvate oxidation must be considered as a biochemical basis for one form of Friedreich's syndrome, and the evaluation of appropriate patients should include measurement of pyruvate oxidation.

PATHOLOGY. Demyelination with secondary gliosis affects the spinocerebellar tracts, the lateral corticospinal tracts, the posterior columns, and the peripheral nerves. Neuronal loss involves the primary sensory neurons in dorsal root ganglia as well as the cells of Clarke's column which give rise to the spinocerebellar tracts. Less often, neuronal loss affects the anterior horns of the spinal cord and cell layers in the cerebellar cortex and deep cerebellar nuclei. A diffuse and major loss of myocardial fibers with subsequent replacement by fibrosis may occur in some patients.

CLINICAL MANIFESTATIONS. Truncal ataxia appears first with impairment of gait, poor coordination, and frequent falling. Gait problems may be the only sign of disease for many years, but eventually dysarthria and ataxia of arm and hand emerge. By the midpart to end of the second decade of life most patients require assistance in walking. Nystagmus is an early and prominent feature, as is the loss of fast saccadic eye movements. A few patients develop optic atrophy during the later stages of the disease. Progressive skeletal deformities include kyphoscoliosis, pes cavus, and, less consistently, a deformed and high arched palate. Distal sensory deficits, especially in the legs, develop after several years and include impairment in position sense and vibratory sensation as well as, less prominently, a reduction in pain and temperature perceptions. Additional expressions of motor dysfunction include extensor plantar responses with normal or reduced tone in trunk and extremities and absent deep tendon reflexes. Moderate weakness and the occurrence of atrophy of the extremities and occasional fasciculations are late developments. About half the patients develop cardiomegaly, murmurs, bundle branch block, T wave inversions, and complete heart block on electrocardiograms. Cardiopulmonary arrest and congestive heart failure may occur. A small percentage of patients are mentally retarded.

DIAGNOSIS. The presence in childhood or young adolescence of insidiously beginning and slowly progressing truncal and extremity ataxia, with dysarthria and subsequent nystagmus, extensor plantar responses, and areflexia, is typical. When one adds the findings of scoliosis, pes cavus, and proprioceptive and vibratory loss in the lower extremities, hardly any other diagnosis is possible. Motor nerve conduction velocities are normal in the common neurogenic form of the disorder, but electromyography may detect denervation potentials, especially in the legs. In the hypertrophic neuropathic form of Friedreich's syndrome, the motor nerve conduction velocities are slowed and the peripheral nerves may be palpably enlarged with demyelination noted in peripheral nerve biopsies. The cerebrospinal fluid protein is normal. Muscle biopsies often show neurogenic atrophy but are unnecessary for diagnosis. The electrocardiogram may contain abnormalities as recorded above and the chest roentgenogram may show cardiomegaly.

DIFFERENTIAL DIAGNOSIS. Diagnosis of Friedreich's syndrome is not difficult if the case meets the aforementioned criteria. Multiple sclerosis and subacute combined degeneration of the spinal cord caused by vitamin B_{12} deficiency differ in both age of onset and clinical characteristics. Cerebellar or spinal tumors produce a more rapid course and, usually, pain. The *Roussy-Lévy syndrome* is inherited as an autosomal recessive trait characterized by onset in childhood of ataxia, areflexia, pes cavus–clubfoot deformity, and kyphoscoliosis. It differs from Friedreich's ataxia in sparing position and vibratory sensation and by the absence of extensor plantar responses as well as of nystagmus and dysarthria. The Roussy-Lévy syndrome may be an intermediate disorder between Friedreich's ataxia and Charcot-Marie-Tooth disease. Patients with *Refsum's disease* caused by elevated serum phytanate as a result of a defect in lipid alpha-oxidase can have a Friedreich-like ataxia but suffer the additional defects of optic atrophy, pigmentary retinal degeneration, ichthyosis, and deafness. Patients with the *Bassen-Kornzweig syndrome* have spinocerebellar signs but also prominent steatorrhea, abetalipoproteinemia, and acanthocytosis.

Hereditary spastic paraplegia expresses an autosomal dominant, recessive, or sex-linked recessive trait by the occurrence of peroneal muscular atrophy, skeletal deformities, nystagmus, and prominent spastic paraplegia. The syndrome overlaps with other forms of spinocerebellar degeneration in some families.

282.3. OLIVOPONTOCEREBELLAR DEGENERATIONS

The olivopontocerebellar atrophies represent a group of disorders manifested clinically by progressive involvement of cerebellar functions and pathologically by a reduction in neurons in the inferior olivary nuclei of the medulla, the basis pontis, the cerebellar cortex, and the deep cerebellar nuclei.

PATHOLOGY. Grossly, atrophy involves the cerebellum, cerebellar peduncles, and basis pontis. Microscopically, Purkinje cells, granule cells of the cerebellar cortex, and neurons from the dentate nucleus and other deep cerebellar nuclei all are severely reduced. Ultrastructurally, biopsies from the cerebellar cortex of patients at various stages of disease disclose a variety of nonspecific abnormalities but also reveal crystalloid inclusions resembling paramyxovirus-like tubular structures. These latter imply that infectious agents may participate in the pathogenesis of some autosomal dominant olivopontocerebellar degenerations.

CLINICAL MANIFESTATIONS. Olivopontocerebellar atrophy has several variants whose principal clinical manifestations vary with the phenotype. Sporadically arising cases outnumber those with clinically evident familial histories, but the pathologic changes are similar. Clinically, essential features include the development in mid-adult life of progressive ataxia, dysarthria, dysmetria, dysdiadochokinesia, nystagmus, and loss of fast saccadic eye movements. Subsequently, patients develop spasticity, optic nerve atrophy, distal sensory involvement, and late intellectual dysfunction.

In general, truncal ataxia develops initially in the second or third decades of life, and extremity ataxia and dysmetria and prominent dysarthria follow within a decade. After several years, perhaps a third of affected patients show spasticity with associated hyperreflexia, clonus, and extensor plantar responses. Nystagmus, optic nerve atrophy, and loss of fast saccadic eye movements occur frequently. A fraction of the patients display the late occurrence of muscle atrophy with fasciculations, including the facial muscles, muscles of mastication, and lingual musculature. Palatal myoclonus is an uncommon but almost pathognomonic accompaniment when it occurs. Variations in the illness include sensory deficits in a distal distribution, intellectual deterioration, signs of extrapyramidal dysfunction, external ophthalmoplegia, and early visual loss.

The olivopontocerebellar degenerations described by Holmes, Sanger-Brown, and Marie represent phenotypic variants of this general class of disease. The syndrome of *Ramsay Hunt's dyssynergia cerebellaris myoclonica* is another rare variant beginning in childhood and includes prominent, progressive ataxia and myoclonic seizures inherited as an autosomal dominant trait.

DIAGNOSIS. The olivopontocerebellar atrophies are readily characterized by the development early in adult life of progressive symmetrical involvement of cerebellar functions, followed in many instances by progressive and symmetrical development of spasticity in the legs. Abnormalities of eye movement, intellectual impairment, and muscle atrophy with sensory distal loss complete the clinical picture, sometimes with the addition of palatal myoclonus. Computerized tomography demonstrates cerebellar atrophy, pontine atrophy, and, late in the disease, cerebral atrophy and large lateral ventricles. Motor nerve conduction velocities may be slow, and muscle denervation may be detected by electromyography. The cerebrospinal fluid is normal. Neither specific diagnostic laboratory tests nor specific treatments exist. Progressive cerebellar deficits, which include truncal ataxia, nystagmus, and dysarthria, are also produced as a result of chronic malnutrition and as a remote effect of cancer, and these possibilities must be considered when a family history of cerebellar disease is lacking.

283.   SYRINGOMYELIA

Syringomyelia is derived from the Greek word syrinx, which means tube, and refers to the occurrence of a cavity within the spinal cord. Such cavities usually are located in the central region of the spinal cord at the cervical level; they often extend to higher levels in the medulla (syringobulbia) and may extend inferiorly into the thoracic and lumbosacral regions of the spinal cord. Acquired syringomyelia arises in association with approximately 25 per cent of intraspinal tumors. Syringomyelia in combination with spina bifida has been reported as a familial disorder.

PATHOLOGY. The syringomyelic cavity is usually associated with the central canal of the spinal cord but may be independent of it as well. The cavity may extend over many segments of the cervical cord and may be in direct anatomic communication with the fourth ventricle. The term hydromyelia is often used to describe those cavitary lesions of the spinal cord which do communicate with the fourth ventricle. The syringomyelic cavity dissects into and progressively replaces the gray matter of the posterior and anterior horns of the spinal cord, as well as disturbing the decussating fibers in the anterior commissure. The cavity wall is maintained by astrocytic glial and fibroblastic membranes and blood vessels. Most often, syringomyelia is associated with other congenital malformations at the cranial cervical junction, including the Arnold-Chiari malformation with herniation of the cerebellar tonsils, fusion of the cervical vertebrae (Klippel-Feil syndrome), or malformations at the lumbosacral region, including spina bifida and associated meningomyelocele. Hydrocephalus resulting from cranial cervical malformations or stenosis of the aqueduct of Sylvius occurs in some patients.

CLINICAL MANIFESTATIONS. Symptoms of syringomyelia most often begin in the second or third decade with a selective impairment in pain and temperature sensation with the preservation of the sense of touch. Earliest detected sensory changes are usually in the hands, but examination commonly discloses a similar dissociated sensory loss in the neck, shoulders, and upper chest and back. Sensory loss is accompanied by progressive atrophy of the musculature in the upper extremities with other skeletal malformations, principally kyphoscoliosis. These clinical manifestations are produced by the syrinx directly destroying the pain and temperature fibers in the anterior spinal commissure as well as the anterior horns to produce denervation of muscle. Progressive analgesia results in severe painless ulcers, burns, and Charcot joints. Atrophy of arm, forearm, and intrinsic hand musculature, fasciculations, and areflexia develop progressively. Later in the disease upper motor neuron signs arise in the legs owing to encroachment of the syringomyelic cavity into the lateral columns of the cord. Late involvement of vibratory and position sensations in the lower extremities and an associated Romberg sign indicate that the syrinx is extending into the posterior columns of the spinal cord. A preganglionic Horner syndrome may also develop due to dissection of the syrinx into the intermediolateral cell column of the lower cervical and first thoracic segment of the spinal cord containing sympathetic neurons. The kyphoscoliosis that sometimes heralds the disease results from the asymmetrical denervation and atrophy of paravertebral muscles. The disease process is progressive, usually symmetrical, and clearly evident in adult life.

Syringobulbia refers to the development of the syringomyelic cavity into the medulla with resultant destruction of the medullary structures in the lateral tegmentum. Dissociated impairment of pain and temperature over the face, nystagmus, pharyngeal and vocal cord paralysis, and lingual atrophy are most typical. Syringobulbia is always associated with syringomyelia and is not a separate process.

DIAGNOSIS. Lepromatous neuropathy, certain rare congenital and acquired peripheral neuropathies, and intramedullary destructive lesions of the spinal cord and brainstem are the only conditions causing insidiously developing and progressive, widespread, dissociated loss of pain and temperature sensation. Leprosy can be considered if the subject has grown up in an endemic area, but neither it nor other peripheral neuropathies produce signs of spinal cord involvement. When the dissociated sensory loss is coupled with signs of long tract disease in the lower extremities or is decidedly asymmetrical in distribution and dermatomal

in pattern, the principal differential consideration lies between congenital syrinx and intramedullary neoplasm. Pain is more frequent with tumors. Air or contrast myelography usually makes the necessary distinction, but even this may be difficult, especially when a secondary syrinx arises in association with a neoplasm. In such instances, surgical exploration may be necessary.

TREATMENT. Treatment generally is unsatisfactory. Surgical decompression of the distended syrinx by a laminectomy sometimes helps slow the disease progression. It has been claimed that dissection of the syringomyelic cavity also can be useful, but published results are few. Some surgeons claim that the placement of muscle tissue at the junction of the fourth ventricle and the upper cervical canal with or without a ventriculocardiac shunt has stabilized the neurologic status of patients. Syrinx associated with spinal tumor is treated by treating the tumor appropriately.

284. THE PHAKOMATOSES OR NEUROCUTANEOUS SYNDROMES

284.1. NEUROFIBROMATOSIS
(Von Recklinghausen's Disease)

Von Recklinghausen's disease or neurofibromatosis is a genetic disorder inherited as an autosomal dominant trait and characterized by the occurrence of pigmented skin lesions, multiple tumors of spinal or cranial nerves, tumors of the skin, and the associated occurrence of gliomas and intracranial meningiomas. There is an increased association with pheochromocytomas, cystic lung disease, renal vascular lesions causing hypertension, fibrous dysplasia of bone, gastrointestinal neurofibromas with chronic blood loss, and medullary thyroid carcinoma and other tumors of endocrine glands.

PATHOLOGY. The characteristic feature of the disease is the occurrence of multiple "neurofibromas" associated with nerves in their peripheral, intraspinal, or intracranial segments. Electron microscopic studies indicate that these tumors represent proliferation of fibroblasts or neurilemmal sheath cells (Schwann cells) in peripheral nerve. The tumors may become confluent in the region of the brachial or sacral plexus and produce large plexiform neuromas which can evolve into malignant sarcomas. Intracranial astrocytomas, ependymomas, glioblastomas, and meningiomas are also encountered with increased frequency, as are optic nerve gliomas in childhood. Stenosis of the aqueduct of Sylvius with noncommunicating hydrocephalus is also observed in this disease. The skin manifestations include pedunculated polyps, lightly colored pigmented lesions with sharp edges (referred to as café au lait spots), and depigmented lesions. Neoplasms of endocrine organs, including medullary thyroid carcinomas and pheochromocytoma with associated hypertension, have been reported in a number of patients.

Metabolic bone disease in some patients results in overgrowth of bone with the occluding of cranial foramina and rarefaction and cyst formation of bone due to replacement of normal bone with fibroblasts and fibrocytes in a pattern similar to that of fibrous dysplasia. The congenital absence of a portion of the sphenoid bone resulting in pulsating exophthalmos, congenital vertebral anomalies, bone cysts, pseudoarthrosis of the tibia, local gigantism of an extremity, and scoliosis are encountered in some patients. Histologic abnormalities of the cerebral cortex, ectopic islands of gray matter, and focal gliosis are described and may be the basis for the increased incidence of mental retardation.

Recently Schenkein et al. reported increases in nerve growth hormone–stimulating activity in serum from patients with neurofibromatosis. Nerve growth hormone or factor (NGF) is a protein which stimulates the proliferation and differentiation of spinal and sympathetic ganglia in vivo and induces differentiation of neurites from embryonic ganglion cells of the chick, mouse, and human neuroblastoma cells in culture. One can speculate that the high titer of the nerve growth factor during fetal life, when neurilemma sheath cells are most sensitive, induces a proliferation and transformation of sheath cells into benign tumor cells. Clinical manifestations of disease then result from the continued stimulation of these transformed tumor cells by the elevated levels of NGF. Possibly elevated NGF may serve as a useful marker in the future for individuals at risk for neurofibromatosis. Fialkow et al. studied tumor tissue from women with neurofibromatosis who also were heterozygous for the A and B genes at the X-linked glucose-6-phosphate dehydrogenase locus. The tissue contained both type A and type B isozymes. The implication is that hereditary neurofibromas have a multiple rather than a single cell origin.

CLINICAL MANIFESTATIONS. Neurofibromatosis, as is typical of diseases of dominant inheritance, can present in a variety of ways, but the presence of multiple cutaneous neurofibromas and café au lait pigmented skin lesions represent the hallmarks. The pigmented lesions are smooth with sharp, regular borders and occur most commonly over the trunk and in the axilla. Skin lesions greater than 3 cm in diameter and more than six in number are indicative of neurofibromatosis; smaller and fewer lesions can occur in persons who do not have this disorder. Nerve involvement can be solitary, involving individual nerves of the extremities, or multiple and diffuse. Multiple cranial nerves are affected as well, resulting in facial weakness, facial numbness, deafness, and visual loss with optic nerve atrophy. Multiple confluent tumors and fibrosis of the affected parts result in elephantiasis neuromatosa. A marked increase in the proliferation and overgrowth of skin and subcutaneous tissues of the skull, neck, and trunk can result in gross asymmetrical hypertrophy. Neurofibromas associated with the nerve root can invade the intervertebral foramen and result in compression of spinal cord or brainstem. Large neurofibromas of a cranial nerve can produce increased intracranial pressure due to hydrocephalus. Some such lesions present as a cerebellopontine angle mass lesion with ipsilateral cerebellar signs. The fifth, seventh, eighth, and tenth cranial nerves are commonly involved with neurofibromas, producing facial muscle weakness, facial numbness, weakness and atrophy of the muscles of mastication, deafness, and vertigo. Rarely, spontaneous fractures of vertebrae or long bones result because of fibrodysplasia or cystic bone formation.

The cerebrospinal fluid protein is elevated in patients having large tumors which result in cord compression. Roentgenograms of the skull and internal auditory meatus show erosion caused by adjacent tumors.

DIAGNOSIS. Neurofibromatosis is diagnosed readily by the occurrence of the characteristic neurofibromas and skin pigmented lesions. The tumors are often multiple and vary considerably in size. Most tumors are smooth, soft, and multilobulated, and can be palpated along the course of a peripheral nerve. Hypertensive patients must be evaluated for the possibility of renal artery stenosis as well as for pheochromocytoma with urinary determinations of catecholamines. Cranial nerve palsies and hydrocephalus signal the presence of an intracranial neoplasm and the need for computerized tomographic brain scans or angiography for precise definition. Cerebellopontine angle meningiomas and cranial nerve or spinal nerve tumors are usually resectable and must be considered in patients manifesting progressive brainstem or spinal cord deficits. There is no treatment for neurofibromatosis other than resection of symptomatic tumors and decompression of hydrocephalus.

284.2.   TUBEROUS SCLEROSIS
(Bourneville's Disease)

Tuberous sclerosis (Bourneville's disease or epiloia) is a neurocutaneous disorder inherited as an autosomal dominant trait. Its triad of findings include facial nevi (adenoma sebaceum), epilepsy, and mental retardation. Although the clinical and neuropathologic features are well described, the basic biochemical defect remains unknown.

PATHOLOGY. The gross brain has many firm nodules which are apparent on the surface. These firm nodules are also present in the deep layers of the cortex, the underlying white matter, and the basal ganglia, and they also line the lateral ventricles as projections referred to as "candle gutterings." In addition these nodules are also encountered in the substance of the spinal cord, the brainstem, and the cerebellum. The histologic appearance of the nodules shows a proliferation of primitive glia with multinucleated giant cells. Vascular malformations, meningiomas, gliomas, and hamartomas of the brain also occur.

The cutaneous lesions include characteristic facial nevi and areas of fibrosis. These nevi are not true adenomas of the sebaceous glands but take their origin from terminal nerves in the subcutaneous region of the skin and include a hyperplasia of connective tissue and blood vessels. Funduscopic examination can disclose similar nodules or phakomas consisting of glial elements, fibroblasts, and ganglion cells arising from the retina. Rarely an optic nerve glioma develops. Rhabdomyomas of the heart can occur, as can renal tumors and neoplasms of endocrine organs, including testis, pancreas, ovary, and thyroid.

CLINICAL MANIFESTATIONS. The clinical appearance is characteristic. Patients develop mental retardation and epilepsy during the first decade of life. The first manifestation of disease is usually focal or generalized major motor seizures without other focal neurologic deficits. The occurrence of mental retardation is not evident until six years of age. Several years after the development of seizures the characteristic cutaneous facial lesions first develop. The facial nevi occur in a symmetrical distribution on the malar and nasal regions and appear to be yellow or orange-red, varying in size from several millimeters to 1 cm. The occurrence of areas of roughening of the skin (shagreen patches) in the shape of small spheres caused by fibrous hyperplasia, café au lait spots, areas of depigmented nevi, and, rarely, subungual neurofibromas are characteristic of tuberous sclerosis and link it genetically to von Recklinghausen's neurofibromatosis. The concurrent neoplasms in other organs rarely cause clinical complications. Papilledema and other focal neurologic deficits signal the occurrence of a large intracranial tumor.

DIAGNOSIS. The triad of facial nevi, epilepsy, and mental retardation is diagnostic. Examination of other family members may help make the diagnosis in an infant or child who presents with generalized seizures but may not yet have the characteristic cutaneous lesions. The characteristic periventricular phakomas are demonstrable by pneumoencephalography. Large periventricular calcifications seen on skull roentgenograms are diagnostic as well. There is no specific treatment. Seizures should be managed by appropriate anticonvulsant medication and development of brain tumors or increased intracranial pressure by surgical intervention and shunting procedures. Since a few affected patients may have normal intelligence, educational programs should be individualized accordingly.

284.3. STURGE-WEBER DISEASE

Sturge-Weber disease produces a port wine–colored capillary hemangioma on the face, accompanied by a similar vascular malformation of the underlying meninges and cerebral cortex. The cause is unknown, although the defect has been reported in more than one family member, indicating a genetic predisposition.

PATHOLOGY. The cutaneous hemangioma follows the distribution of one or more divisions of the trigeminal nerve. The underlying meninges contain a similar vascular lesion, and the capillaries of the cortex may show thickening and calcification, especially in the second and third cortical layers. The cerebral cortex may undergo atrophy with loss of nerve cells and a proliferation of glia. Cerebral calcification clearly outlines the cortical mantle in an undulating manner.

CLINICAL MANIFESTATIONS. The presence of a port wine facial nevus following the sensory dermatomal distribution of the first, second, or third portions of the trigeminal nerve is diagnostic. Generalized or focal motor seizures may occur with or without associated mental retardation. The patient can develop hemiplegic atrophy with shortening of the extremities contralateral to the calcified atrophic hemisphere. Exophthalmos, glaucoma, buphthalmos, optic atrophy, and other cutaneous port wine nevi and retinal angiomas can be present. There is no specific treatment; seizures are managed with anticonvulsant drugs.

284.4. HIPPEL-LINDAU DISEASE

Hippel-Lindau disease is a familial disorder inherited without a clear mendelian pattern, producing heman-

gioblastomas of the cerebellar hemispheres with associated angiomas of the retina and cystic change in the kidney and pancreas. It presents in the fourth to sixth decades of life, usually not associated with cutaneous vascular lesions. The disorder can present with signs of cerebellar mass lesion, cerebellar hemorrhage, brainstem vascular malformations, or hemangioma of the retina. A clinical association with pheochromocytomas and polycythemia has been noted, especially in the patients with cerebellar hemangioblastomas. The diagnosis should be suspected in any patient with cerebellar brain tumor or cerebellar hemorrhage, especially in association with an elevated hematocrit. Diagnosis and treatment are as for other such mass lesions.

284.5. ATAXIA TELANGIECTASIA

Ataxia telangiectasia is a neurocutaneous disorder that begins in the first decade of life with prominent telangiectatic lesions involving the bulbar conjunctivae, malar eminences, ear lobes, and occasionally upper neck regions, associated with cerebellar ataxia and nystagmus. The condition is usually sporadic in occurrence but occasionally presents in a pattern consistent with an autosomal recessive disorder. A chromosome translocation involving chromosome 14, increased chromosome breakage, and reduced lymphocyte response to phytohemagglutinin have been described and represent the only molecular clues to pathogenesis.

PATHOLOGY. The most prominent neuropathologic changes include loss of Purkinje, granule, and basket cells in the cerebellar cortex as well as of neurons in the deep nuclei of the cerebellum. Neuronal loss is also present in the inferior olives of the medulla. The posterior columns of the spinal cord undergo demyelination, and there is a loss of anterior horn cells in the spinal cord and ganglion cells of the spinal ganglia. The most consistent defect of the lymphoid system is a poorly developed or absent thymus.

CLINICAL MANIFESTATIONS. The onset of the telangiectatic lesions occurs in the first decade of life and is associated with progressive deficits in cerebellar functions with early onset nystagmus. Truncal ataxia, extremity ataxia, dysarthria, extensor plantar responses, myoclonic jerks, areflexia, and distal sensory deficits occur in a pattern somewhat resembling that of Friedreich's syndrome. The patients have a high incidence of recurrent pulmonary infections and neoplasms of the lymphoreticuloendothelial system.

DIAGNOSIS. Ataxia telangiectasia is diagnosed by the characteristic telangiectatic lesions in association with a truncal ataxia, other cerebellar deficits, and apractic eye movements. Serum protein electrophoresis documents the common occurrence of a deficiency of gamma globulins, especially IgA and IgE. Cellular immune abnormalities include lymphocytopenia, a reduced response to skin test antigens, and lack of sensitization to dinitrochlorobenzene (DNCB).

Barnett, H. J. M., Foster, J. B., and Hudgson, P.: Syringomyelia. London, W. B. Saunders Company, 1974.

Blass, J. P., Kark, R. A. P., and Menon, N. K.: Low activities of the pyruvate and oxoglutarate dehydrogenase complexes in five patients with Friedreich's ataxia. N. Engl. J. Med., 295:62, 1976.

Brady, R. O.: Inherited metabolic diseases of the nervous system. Science, 193:733, 1976.

Crowe, F. W., Schull, W. J., and Neel, J. V.: A Clinical Pathological and Genetic Study of Multiple Neurofibromatosis. Springfield, Ill., Charles C Thomas, 1956.

Fialkow, P., Sagebiel, R., Gartler, S., and Rimoin, D.: Multiple cell origin of hereditary neurofibromas. N. Engl. J. Med., 284:298, 1971.

Hecht, F., McCaw, B., and Koler, R. D.: Ataxia-telangiectasia—clonal growth of translocation lymphocytes. N. Engl. J. Med., 289:286, 1973.

Horton, W. A., Eldridge, R., and Brody, J.: Familial motor neuron disease. Neurology, 26:460, 1976.

Konigsmark, B. W., and Weiner, L. P.: The olivopontocerebellar atrophies. Medicine, 49:227, 1970.

Kugelberg, E., and Welander, L.: Heredofamilial juvenile muscular atrophy simulating muscular dystrophy. Arch. Neurol. Psychiat., 75:500, 1956.

McFarlin, P. E., Strober, W., and Waldmann, T. A.: Ataxia-telangiectasia. Medicine, 51:281, 1972.

Meister, A.: The gamma-glutamyl cycle. Ann. Intern. Med., 81:247, 1974.

Oldstone, M. B. A., Perrin, L. H., Wilson, C. B., and Norris, F. H., Jr.:

Evidence for immune-complex formation in patients with amyotrophic lateral sclerosis. Lancet, 2:169, 1976.

Refsum, S.: Heredopathia atactica polyneuritiformis: Phytanic acid storage disease (Refsum's disease). In Vinken, P. J., and Bruyn, G. W. (eds.): Handbook of Clinical Neurology, Chap. 10, Vol. 21, Part I. Amsterdam, North Holland Publishing Company, 1975, pp. 181, 229.

Rosenberg, R. N., Nyhan, W. L., Coutinho, P., and Bay, C.: Joseph's disease in California, Massachusetts, and the Azores. In Kark, P., Rosenberg, R., and Schut, L. (eds.): The Inherited Ataxias. Proceedings of an International Symposium, Nov. 1977, Los Angeles. New York, Raven Press, 1978.

Schenkein, I., Bueker, E., Helson, L., Axelrod, R., and Dancis, J.: Increased nerve-growth stimulating activity in disseminated neurofibromatosis. N. Engl. J. Med., 290:613, 1974.

Schwartz, J. F., Rowland, L. P., Eder, H., Marks, P. A., Osserman, E. F., Hirschberg, E., and Anderson, H.: Bassen-Kornzweig syndrome. Deficiency of serum beta-lipoprotein. Arch. Neurol., 8:438, 1963.

Section Thirteen   NUTRITIONAL DISORDERS OF THE NERVOUS SYSTEM

Pierre M. Dreyfus

285.   INTRODUCTION

Malnutrition, undernutrition, and the deficiency of specific nutrients such as vitamins are known to affect normal function of some parts of the central and/or the peripheral nervous system. It is well established that an isolated or combined deficiency of vitamins B_1, B_6, B_{12}, niacin, pantothenic acid, and perhaps riboflavin can be associated with a variety of neurologic disorders. However, despite increasing knowledge regarding the role of these vitamins in general metabolism, the specific mechanisms by which a deficiency state affects the normal development and function of the nervous system remain essentially unknown.

Most of the neurologic disorders discussed in this section, although commonly associated with chronic alcoholism, have also been described in malnourished, chronically debilitated, nonalcoholic patients. The inveterate drinker is frequently the victim of a primary nutritional deficiency which alters the normal metabolic activity of the nervous system. During periods of heavy drinking, the chronic alcoholic patient may change the composition of his diet, sharply decreasing vitamin and other essential nutrient intake, because of decreased appetite. Vitamin absorption, intestinal transport, tissue storage, utilization, and conversion to metabolically active forms may be curtailed while the need for many vitamins and essential nutrients increases. In addition to causing abnormal vitamin metabolism, the prolonged and abusive intake of alcohol leads to a somewhat unusual and extreme state of nutritional imbalance characterized by an excess of carbohydrate, fatty acid, cholesterol, glycerol, glycogen, and calories combined with a severe deficiency of B vitamins and other essential nutrients. The chronic alcoholic patient may also suffer from a secondary nutritional deficiency which may be the result of a chronic illness, such as

infection, anemia, or blood loss, which increases his over-all metabolic demands.

The various nutritional syndromes described in this section may present separately in relatively pure form, but more frequently they occur together in varying combinations, some more prevalent than others. It is not known why, under seemingly identical circumstances, one nutritionally depleted patient develops one or several neurologic syndromes whereas another emerges essentially unscathed. Basic constitutional and genetic factors, such as aberrations in specific enzyme proteins, may underlie the individual response of patients to malnutrition and the chronic ingestion of alcohol.

Nutritional disorders of the nervous system are associated with one or more biochemical lesions which invariably antedate the appearance of symptoms and signs and histopathologic changes. These diseases all share the common neuropathologic attributes of other metabolic disorders of the nervous system by virtue of their predilection for specific areas or parts of the nervous system and because of the bilateral symmetry of the lesions.

286.   NUTRITIONAL POLYNEUROPATHY

(Dry Beriberi, Alcoholic Neuropathy)

CLINICAL MANIFESTATIONS.   Nutritional polyneuropathy, the most common of all the nutritional diseases of the nervous system, is characterized by progressive weakness and muscle wasting of varying degrees, involving, symmetrically, the legs more than the arms and the distal muscles more than the proximal ones. Weakness may be almost imperceptible or so severe that the legs are virtually paralyzed and the hands useless. Motor signs and sensory manifestations most frequently occur concomitantly. Abnormalities of sensation are usually striking. Patients complain of aching, coldness, hotness, deadness, numbness, prickliness, and tenderness, most commonly in the calves, on the plantar surfaces of the feet, and in the fingers. Deep pressure or light touch may be extremely unpleasant. In the most severe cases, the muscles become wasted, atrophic, flabby, and tender, and the skin may be dry, red, and shiny. Excessive perspiration of feet and hands is occasionally noted. The deep tendon reflexes, which may be exaggerated in some patients at the onset of the illness, are usually greatly diminished or totally abolished. The sensory loss is symmetrical, is most severe distally, and diminishes gradually over more proximal parts; all modalities are involved, some more than others. On rare occasions, severe burning, shooting, lightning, or "electric" types of pain can occur in the absence of clear-cut signs of neuropathy. The term "burning feet syndrome" has been applied to this variety of neuropathic disorder. This syndrome has been encountered in inmates of prison camps, chronic alcoholics, and patients undergoing dialysis for chronic renal failure. In rare instances, nutritional polyneuropathy may be accompanied by vertigo, deafness, hoarseness, dysphagia, and amblyopia.

The mode of evolution and the severity of nutritional polyneuropathy can be quite variable. Usually the onset is insidious, and the progression is slow. Sometimes the course is rapid and abrupt, crippling the patient in a matter of weeks. Recovery requires months and is sometimes incomplete. A temporary worsening of paresthesias and of weakness may follow the start of therapy. In early or mild cases, a prolonged nerve conduction velocity may be the only objective manifestation of the disease. Examination of the cerebrospinal fluid reveals a normal level or a very slight elevation of the protein content.

PATHOLOGY. The salient pathologic changes consist of demyelination and axonal destruction of peripheral nerves, involving distal parts to a greater degree than proximal ones. Occasionally dorsal root ganglia reveal a loss of nerve cells, and axonal reaction may be seen in some of the anterior horn cells of the spinal cord. In patients afflicted with hoarseness and dysphagia, degeneration of the vagus nerve and of the paravertebral sympathetic chain has been observed. It has been speculated that in nutritional polyneuropathy, primary axonal degeneration or a process of "dying back" results in destruction of both the axon and myelin sheaths in the periphery of the largest and longest nerve fibers.

PATHOGENESIS AND TREATMENT. Nutritional depletion probably alters the normal metabolism of peripheral nerves in several different ways. Both experimental and clinical studies support the view that a deficiency of several of the B vitamins can result in neuropathy. Certain neuropathies respond to the administration of thiamin alone. Recent studies have shown decreased levels of thiamin in the blood, urine, and muscles of patients afflicted with alcoholic neuropathy. Prior to nutritional replenishment, the activity of blood transketolase is usually reduced, and blood pyruvate levels,

measured before and after the administration of glucose, may be elevated. The fact that biochemical evidence of thiamin deficiency in nutritional polyneuropathy cannot always be obtained is explained by the slow evolution of this disorder. Whereas the biochemical lesion antedates all clinical manifestations of neuropathy, the latter linger on for many months after the metabolic insult has been removed. A deficiency of pyridoxine has also been blamed for nutritional polyneuropathy. A neuropathic disorder has been observed in patients who were given desoxypyridoxine, a metabolic antagonist of vitamin B_6. The neuropathy that develops in the course of isoniazid (INH) therapy can be reversed by pyridoxine alone. Isoniazid causes a deficiency of the essential cofactor pyridoxal phosphate by interfering with phosphorylation of the vitamin. Pyridoxal phosphate is an essential cofactor for a number of enzymatic reactions known to participate in protein metabolism. The specific role of these enzymatic reactions in the metabolism of peripheral nerves remains to be defined. A deficiency of pyridoxal phosphate results in the inadequate synthesis of nicotinic acid from tryptophan. Reduced blood levels of nicotinic acid and nicotinamide have been measured in some patients with nutritional polyneuropathy. Pantothenic acid deficiency may also be involved in the production of some forms of nutritional polyneuropathy. It has been claimed that the administration of pantothenic acid relieves the burning feet syndrome, regardless of its cause.

287. WERNICKE-KORSAKOFF SYNDROME

Of all the disorders of the central nervous system associated with the protracted and abusive intake of alcohol and nutritional depletion, Wernicke's disease and Korsakoff's psychosis are the most frequent. The term "cerebral beriberi" has sometimes been applied to these conditions.

CLINICAL MANIFESTATIONS. *Wernicke's disease* is characterized by disturbed ocular motility, ataxia, impaired mentation, and, occasionally, polyneuropathy. The patient may complain of diplopia and unsteadiness of gait, but is usually unaware of his deficit. On examination, bilateral weakness or paralysis of the external recti muscles and paralysis of lateral conjugate gaze are common. Horizontal nystagmus is almost always present, although it sometimes cannot be elicited until abducens function has improved. Vertical nystagmus, particularly on upward gaze, is frequently present. Occasionally there are ptosis, complete paralysis of eye movements, miosis, and, very rarely, unreactive pupils. The ataxia, which is almost always present, affects stance and gait primarily. It may be so slight that only special tests for cerebellar function betray its existence. When it is severe, the patient cannot stand or walk without help. Advanced polyneuropathy usually masks cerebellar ataxia. Intention tremor is less common and tends to affect the legs more than the arms. Scanning speech is a rarity. A mild to severe mixed sensory-motor polyneuropathy exists in at least 50 per cent of cases. When first seen, the patient with Wernicke's disease may display symptoms and signs attributable to alcohol withdrawal: i.e., delirium, tremulousness, confusion, agitation, hallucinosis, altered sense perception, and autonomic overactivity. More often, he lacks spontaneity, is apathetic, listless, indifferent, and disoriented in time and place, and tends to misidentify objects and people around him. Dull mentation, impaired retentive memory, and general lack of grasp are more common than drowsiness or unconsciousness. With improved nutrition and supplemental thiamin the patient becomes more alert, more attentive, and more readily testable. He may then display a characteristic amnestic syndrome known as *Korsakoff's psychosis.* In addition, the patient with Korsakoff's psychosis reveals a number of abnormalities of cognitive function. He may have a great deal of difficulty in forming visual and verbal abstractions. His capacity to shift from one mental set to another and his ability to learn are defective. Perceptual function and concept formation are affected. The most prominent and serious mental abnormality seen in Korsakoff's psychosis is the disordered memory function that renders some patients incapable of performing any but the simplest tasks. Recent retentive memory and the ability to learn newly presented material are strikingly impaired. An extensive retrograde amnesia covering a variable period of time is also common. Such patients may confabulate, i.e., fabricate fictitious or improperly sequenced stories. Confabulation is by no means unique to Korsakoff's psychosis and tends to disappear in the chronic stages of the illness.

Features of Wernicke's disease and Korsakoff's psychosis often coexist in the same patient. In many instances of Korsakoff's psychosis, slight, residual nystagmus and ataxia may be detected years later. The Wernicke-Korsakoff syndrome may be complicated by other stigmata of chronic malnutrition, including cirrhosis of the liver, anemia, and mucocutaneous lesions of various types. Many patients suffer from postural hypotension, dyspnea, and tachycardia, but full-blown beriberi heart disease is rare. The Wernicke-Korsakoff syndrome usually begins abruptly. Some degree of recovery is the rule, except in the most advanced cases and in those complicated by other illnesses. During the acute stage of the disease the mortality may be as high as 17 per cent. The ocular manifestations, except for nystagmus, respond promptly and dramatically to vitamin therapy. Ataxia improves more slowly, and incomplete recovery occurs in over half the patients; complete recovery from Korsakoff's psychosis occurs in less than one third of patients. The recovered patient usually shows permanent amnesia for the acute phase of the illness.

PATHOLOGY. The pathologic alterations that affect the cerebrum and the brainstem are remarkably constant. They almost always involve structures in a bilaterally symmetrical manner. Lesions are invariably seen in the mamillary bodies and the terminal fornices. Lesions in the periaqueductal region of the midbrain, in the floor of the fourth ventricle, in the vicinity of the dorsal motor nucleus of the vagus, and in the anterior superior parts of the cerebellar vermis probably account for the paralysis of gaze, nystagmus, and ataxia. The lesions involving thalamic nuclei (anteromedial, lateral dorsal, and pulvinar) and the hypothalamus and those seen in the mamillary bodies and fornices may underlie some of the psychologic abnormalities, particularly the amnestic syndrome. Microscopically, the lesions consist of necrosis of both nerve cells and myelinated structures. A striking glial reaction involves the center of the

lesion. Both endothelial proliferation and hemorrhages are found, but the latter are usually fresh and may represent a nonspecific, terminal change. In the vermis of the cerebellum the principal changes consist of a loss of Purkinje cells and gliosis of the molecular layer of the cortex.

PATHOGENESIS. There is now an overwhelming body of evidence that favors a specific lack of vitamin B_1 as the main nutritional factor in the Wernicke-Korsakoff syndrome. Most patients give a history of inadequate nutrition and weight loss. Other stigmata of malnutrition, such as loss of subcutaneous fat and skin turgor, mucocutaneous manifestations, and an enlarged liver, are frequent. Clinical studies have shown that the continued intake of alcohol is not followed by aggravation of symptoms, provided adequate nutritional repletion is undertaken promptly. Thiamin alone, given orally or parenterally, can dramatically reverse some of the symptoms and signs. Victor and Adams maintained patients with Wernicke's disease on either glucose or a boiled rice diet containing no vitamins for brief periods, then gave them B vitamins selectively. Ophthalmoplegia, apathy, listlessness, and inattentiveness began to improve within a few hours and cleared completely within a few days after thiamin had been added to the regimen. Nystagmus and ataxia diminished, but Korsakoff's psychosis did not improve significantly. Other B vitamins were ineffective. The improvement of neurologic signs can be closely correlated with levels of blood transketolase activity, which are reduced prior to thiamin administration and increase toward normal with clinical improvement, sometimes within four to five hours after the injection of 25 to 50 mg of thiamin.

A recent study has suggested the existence of a genetic abnormality of transketolase (a thiamin-dependent enzyme) in serially cultured fibroblasts and red blood cells of some patients who have recovered from the disease. The aberrant enzyme binds the active cofactor of thiamin less tightly than does the normal enzyme. It is postulated that the presence of the aberrant enzyme predisposes the individual to clinically significant thiamin deficiency.

Although most commonly associated with chronic alcoholism, Wernicke-Korsakoff syndrome has been observed in clinical settings totally unrelated to abusive drinking. It has been described as a complication of chronic hemodialysis, pernicious vomiting of pregnancy, thyrotoxicosis, and gastric carcinoma, as well as after prolonged intravenous therapy.

288. NUTRITIONAL AMBLYOPIA

(Tobacco-Alcohol Amblyopia, Nutritional Retrobulbar Neuropathy)

CLINICAL MANIFESTATIONS. A remarkably uniform and stereotyped disorder of vision sometimes appears in chronically undernourished persons. Characteristically it evolves slowly and subacutely, the mode of onset of symptoms being much the same from patient to patient. Visual impairment usually starts insidiously and reaches a maximum in several weeks to months. Blurred or dim vision, difficulty in reading, photophobia, and retrobulbar discomfort on moving the eyes are the common presenting complaints. On examination, the patient has bilaterally symmetrical central, centrocecal, or paracentral scotomata. Ophthalmoscopic changes are restricted at first to slight redness of the temporal margins of the optic discs; minimal pallor is observed at a later stage. Often, no abnormality is visible. The peripheral visual fields are usually intact. The visual disorder is, to a large extent, reversible with improvement of nutrition.

PATHOLOGY. The pathologic change in nutritional amblyopia consists of bilaterally symmetrical loss of myelinated fibers in the central parts of the optic nerves, chiasm, and optic tracts, corresponding in location to the papillomacular bundle. In severe cases, the retina loses macular ganglion cells, probably secondary to the "zonal" destruction of medullated fibers in the retrobulbar parts of the optic nerve.

PATHOGENESIS. Nutritional ambylopia has been encountered in undernourished populations all over the world. It is commonly seen during famine, and among civilian and military prisoners of war. It is endemic in certain parts of Africa, Asia, and South America. Among the more privileged populations in the western world, the syndrome is seen in persons chronically addicted to alcohol or, occasionally, to tobacco, who neglect their nutrition. A similar syndrome also occurs as a complication of vitamin B_{12} deficiency and of diabetes mellitus. This visual disorder accompanies other neurologic syndromes believed to have a nutritional cause, such as *Strachan's syndrome*, in which amblyopia is combined with paresthesias of the feet, hands, trunk, and, occasionally, face, loss of reflexes, dizziness, deafness, hoarseness, spasticity, ataxia, and a variety of mucocutaneous lesions (genital dermatitis, corneal degeneration, glossitis, and stomatitis). In the chronic alcoholic patient, amblyopia may occur in conjunction with Wernicke's disease, cerebellar degeneration, Marchiafava-Bignami's disease, and peripheral neuropathy. The nutritional basis is well established, for if such patients are renourished their vision improves even if they smoke or drink alcohol. As yet, the metabolic aberration or specific vitamin deficiency responsible for the development of amblyopia has not been defined. A lack of vitamin B_{12}, thiamin, riboflavin, and pyridoxine or a failure in the detoxification of cyanide present in tobacco smoke has been implicated in the genesis of the syndrome. Except for isolated findings of reduced serum vitamin B_{12} levels, the abnormal urinary excretion of methylmalonic acid, and low levels of blood transketolase activity, no specific biochemical abnormalities have been reported.

TREATMENT. Treatment with oral or parenteral B vitamins and improved nutrition are usually followed by improvement, depending upon the severity of the amblyopia and its duration before therapy is instituted.

289. CEREBELLAR CORTICAL DEGENERATION

Cerebellar cortical degeneration, or parenchymatous cerebellar degeneration, has often been referred to as alcoholic cerebellar degeneration, although well documented instances of cerebellar cortical degeneration have occurred as a result of chronic nutritional depletion not attributable to alcohol. This disorder can be set apart from all other known forms of acquired or familial cerebellar degeneration because of the uniformity of the clinical and pathologic manifestations. The clinical and pathologic findings are discussed in Ch. 282.

A substantial body of evidence favors the contention that cerebellar degeneration is due to nutritional factors. The history of chronic alcoholic patients is admittedly unreliable, yet most admit improper eating habits. Many patients with cortical cerebellar degeneration give a history of progressive weight loss before the onset of their symptoms. Signs of malnutrition are common, and the cerebellar syndrome frequently occurs in conjunction with cirrhosis and other nutritional complications of alcoholism. Furthermore, a number of nonalcoholic patients develop cortical cerebellar degeneration in the setting of other diseases associated with nutritional depletion, such as pellagra, amebiasis, and protracted vomiting. In general, improved nutrition and supplementary B vitamins result in some degree of improvement of ataxia.

290. CENTRAL PONTINE MYELINOLYSIS

Central pontine myelinolysis is a relatively rare disease characterized by demyelination of the central portion of the pons. It was described originally in patients afflicted with chronic alcoholism and malnutrition but has since been encountered in nonalcoholic patients who were nutritionally deprived. The illness affects adults mainly, but has been reported in children; males and females are equally afflicted. Although the precise clinical course has not yet been defined, the principal neurologic abnormalities are progressive weakness of facial muscles and tongue, causing severe impairment of speech and deglutition. In a number of cases, pseudobulbar phenomena such as emotional lability and pathologic crying have been noted. Quadriparesis at the onset of the illness usually leads to a flaccid and areflexic quadriplegia with Babinski signs. Lack of response to painful stimuli and absence of corneal reflexes are said to be common. Urinary incontinence, decerebrate posture, and respiratory paralysis have been reported in isolated cases.

The illness evolves rapidly over a period of two to three weeks, usually ending in stupor, coma, and eventual death. Most patients succumb to medical complications, such as pneumonia, sepsis, or uremia. In rare instances, slow, gradual, and sometimes complete recovery occurs.

The clinical diagnosis of the disease is difficult to establish, but brainstem auditory evoked potential studies may help demonstrate impaired function of pontine pathways. Examination of the cerebrospinal fluid is unremarkable.

Pathologic examination reveals demyelination, variable in size and extent, involving the center of the basal portion of the mid and upper pons. In some cases the demyelination may also involve the midbrain, basal ganglia, and cerebral white matter. Axis cylinders, nerve cells, and blood vessels are relatively well preserved. An appropriate glial and phagocytic reaction is seen within the lesions. Vascular or inflammatory changes are absent. The clinical symptoms and signs depend upon the size and location of the lesions.

The pathogenesis is in some way related to malnutrition and its treatment. The lesion has been found at postmortem examination in patients suffering from alcoholism, other forms of chronic malnutrition, neoplasia, renal disease, hepatic insufficiency, and a variety of infectious processes. It has been suggested that the disease may be related to the treatment of dehydration and electrolyte imbalance rather than to malnutrition or alcoholism per se; in most instances, patients die after a period of intensive treatment. To date no biochemical data have been obtained.

291. MARCHIAFAVA-BIGNAMI DISEASE

Marchiafava-Bignami disease is a rare disorder occurring in the setting of severe malnutrition, usually with alcoholism. The disease affects males of middle age predominantly. The course is variable; it may evolve over a period of a few days or several months. Complete recovery is rare. The patients are agitated and confused, and have hallucinations (visual, auditory, and gustatory), disturbance of memory, negativism, impaired judgment, and progressive dementia. Neurologic symptoms and signs suggest bilateral involvement of frontal lobes and include disturbance of language, gait and motor skills, seizures, incontinence, rooting, grasping, sucking, and delayed initiation of action. Tremulousness of the hands and dysarthria have been reported.

Pathologically, symmetrical zones of demyelination affect the central parts of the corpus callosum, beginning in the most anterior parts and extending caudally. Similar changes affect the central parts of the anterior commissure, the optic chiasm and tracts, and, in severe cases, the central white matter of the frontal lobes. In zones of demyelination, axis cylinders tend to be preserved. Occasionally, there is extensive tissue destruction and cavitation. The degree of glial reaction in these areas depends on the chronicity of the process.

The disease originally was reported in males of Italian descent who consumed excessive amounts of crude red wine. The illness has since been encountered in patients of varied ancestry and with other alcoholic preferences. The characteristic pathologic changes of Marchiafava-Bignami disease have been encountered in conjunction with Wernicke's disease and nutritional amblyopia as well as in malnourished, nonalcoholic patients.

292. VITAMIN B$_{12}$ DEFICIENCY

DEFINITION. Insufficient absorption of vitamin B$_{12}$ from the gastrointestinal tract can result in a subacute degeneration of the spinal cord, optic nerves, cerebral white matter, and peripheral nerves. Although the neurologic manifestations of vitamin B$_{12}$ deficiency are frequently associated with a macrocytic anemia (pernicious anemia), the latter is not always present. Neurologic symptoms develop in approximately 80 per cent of patients between the ages of 25 and 75 years afflicted with pernicious anemia. They rarely occur as a result of secondary vitamin B$_{12}$ deficiency complicating fish tapeworm (*Diphyllobothrium latum*) infestation, sprue, vegetarianism, or gastrointestinal surgery. (This subject is also dealt with in Ch. 479.)

CLINICAL MANIFESTATIONS. Symptoms and signs of spinal cord involvement (*combined system disease*) constitute the most common neurologic manifestations, and their mode of onset and progression is remarkably uniform. Symmetrical progressive paresthesias of the feet or hands in the form of numbness, tingling, burning, tightness and stiffness, and a feeling of generalized weakness constitute the most frequent initial symptoms. Vague asthenia and lameness progress to a measurable weakness and stiffness of the legs and an unsteadiness of gait that tends to be worse in the dark. The lower limbs may give way unexpectedly. The hands may be stiff and clumsy. When untreated, the illness progresses slowly and relentlessly. Spasticity, ataxia, and paraplegia ensue, often followed by bowel and bladder dysfunction. In the early stages of the disease, examination of the patient often reveals a few objective changes, but eventually signs of disturbed peripheral nerve and posterior and lateral column function become readily apparent. Diminution or loss of position and vibratory sense involves the legs, the hands, and, occasionally, the trunk, and tends to be pronounced. Pain, temperature, and tactile sensation are sometimes blunted over the distal parts of the legs in a pattern suggestive of peripheral nerve involvement. The motor examination reveals weak and, later, spastic legs and extensor plantar responses. The activity of the deep tendon reflexes is variable and appears to depend upon the severity of the illness. The knee jerks are often hyperactive and the ankle jerks absent. In advanced cases, all stretch reflexes may be diminished or absent, but may return when vitamin therapy has been promptly instituted. Psychologic symptoms range from apathy, irritability, and suspiciousness to confusion and dementia, and at times are the presenting neurologic abnormality. On rare occasions, failing vision caused by symmetrical centrocecal scotomata may be the presenting neurologic symptom of vitamin B$_{12}$ deficiency.

PATHOLOGY. The lesions associated with subacute combined degeneration involve in sequence the posterior columns, the lateral columns, and the cerebral white matter. The earliest visible change consists of swelling of individual myelinated nerve fibers in small foci. These lesions subsequently coalesce into large, irregular, spongy, honeycomb-like zones of demyelination. Fibers with the largest diameter are predominantly affected. Axis cylinders tend to be spared. Myelin destruction frequently begins in the cervical and upper thoracic segments of the cord, spreading axially to involve other segments. The cerebral white matter is affected last. The large fibers of the peripheral nerves may show minimal loss of myelin.

DIAGNOSIS. A number of diseases other than vitamin B$_{12}$ deficiency affect the posterior and lateral columns of the spinal cord, the most important being multiple sclerosis, tumors, cervical spondylosis, syphilitic meningomyelitis, and familial spastic paraplegia. These entities can usually be differentiated from one another clinically, but ancillary examinations such as myelography and special tests involving the cerebrospinal fluid may be necessary to establish a correct diagnosis. In B_{12} deficiency of the nervous system, the cerebrospinal fluid is usually normal. The electroencephalogram is often abnormal. The serum vitamin B_{12} content correlates well with the severity of the neurologic impairment and is invariably low in untreated cases. The Schilling test, using radioactive cyanocobalamin, is always positive, and gastric achlorhydria can be demonstrated in almost every instance. Blood and bone marrow examinations are of limited value, particularly when the patient has been treated with folic acid, which corrects the anemia but not the neurologic manifestations. The urinary excretion of methylmalonic acid, an intermediary metabolite in the conversion of propionic acid to succinic acid, is a sensitive indicator of vitamin B_{12} deficiency, but its relation to the lesions in the nervous system is as yet unknown.

PATHOGENESIS. The pathogenesis of the neurologic manifestations of vitamin B_{12} deficiency is unknown, although it probably differs from the biochemical lesion affecting the hematopoietic system, because the neurologic manifestations are independent of the anemia and may appear when folic acid corrects the anemia. The specific biochemical role of vitamin B_{12} in the nervous system has not yet been elucidated. It is an essential cofactor for at least two enzyme systems which exist in mammalian tissue, including brain: (1) methylmalonyl-CoA isomerase, which converts methylmalonyl-CoA to succinyl-CoA, a step in the utilization of propionic acid, and (2) N_5-methyltetrahydrofolate homocysteine methyltransferase, which is responsible for the synthesis of methionine from homocysteine. In experimentally induced vitamin B_{12} deficiency, the activity of both of these enzyme systems is reduced in brain. These enzymes may be essential to the maintenance of the myelin sheath. It has been shown that sural nerve specimens obtained from patients with pernicious anemia incorporate radioactively labeled propionate into abnormal fatty acids that have been identified as C_{15} branched-chain and C_{17} odd-chain acids. The presence of these abnormal fatty acids may explain, in part, the structural changes observed in central and peripheral myelin. An experimental approach to the study of the pathogenesis of the neurologic manifestations of vitamin B_{12} deficiency in animals has been greatly facilitated by the discovery of optic nerve and white matter lesions in monkeys maintained on a B_{12}-deficient diet for several years.

TREATMENT. Prompt initiation of therapy is of the utmost importance, because the early neurologic manifestations can be rapidly and completely reversed. The greatest degree of improvement is achieved in patients treated within three months of onset of symptoms, although variable degrees of amelioration can be attained after longer untreated periods (six to twelve months). In the first two weeks, daily intramuscular injections of 50 μg of cyanocobalamin, or an equivalent amount of liver USP, should be administered. During the next two months, 100 μg of cyanocobalamin should be injected twice a week. For the remainder of his life, the patient should receive a minimum of 100 μg intramuscularly every month to prevent a relapse. The administration of oral vitamin preparations containing folic acid must be avoided for patients with pernicious anemia, because folic acid may actually precipitate neurologic complications.

Agamanolis, D. P., Chester, E. M., Victor, M., Kark, J. A., Hines, J., and Harris, J. W.: Neuropathology of experimental vitamin B_{12} deficiency in monkeys. Neurology, 26:905, 1976.

Dreyfus, P. M., and Geel, S. E.: Vitamin and nutritional deficiencies. In Albers, R. W., Siegel, G. J., Katzman, R., and Agranoff, B. W. (eds.): Basic Neurochemistry. Boston, Little, Brown & Company, 1976, Chap. 29.

Gubler, C. J., Fujiwara, M., and Dreyfus, P. M.: Thiamine. New York, John Wiley & Sons, 1976.

Gyorgy, P., and Pearson, W. N.: The Vitamins. New York, Academic Press, 1967.

Kissin, B., and Begleiter, H.: The Biology of Alcoholism, Vol. 3, Clinical Pathology. New York, Plenum Press, 1974, Chaps. 7, 16.

Pant, S. S., Asbury, A. K., and Richardson, E. P., Jr.: The myelopathy of pernicious anemia — a neuropathological reappraisal. Acta Neurol. Scand., 44 (Suppl. 35), 1968.

Victor, M.: Polyneuropathy due to nutritional deficiency and alcoholism. In Dyck, P., Thomas, P. K., and Lambert, E. H. (eds.): Peripheral Neuropathy. Philadelphia, W. B. Saunders Company, 1975.

Victor, M., Adams, R. D., and Collins, G. H.: The Wernicke-Korsakoff Syndrome. Philadelphia, F. A. Davis Company, 1971.

Vinken, P. J., and Bruyn, G. W.: Handbook of Clinical Neurology. Vol. 28, Metabolic and Deficiency Diseases of the Nervous System. Amsterdam, North Holland Publishing Company, 1976, Chaps. 1–14.

Section Fourteen
CEREBROVASCULAR DISEASES

Fletcher H. McDowell

293.   INTRODUCTION

It is estimated that there are 2 million persons alive today who have neurologic manifestations of cerebrovascular disease and that cerebrovascular disease of all varieties is annually responsible for approximately 200,000 deaths in the United States. Fully a half million Americans each year suffer a new, acute cerebrovascular attack. The over-all problem is even more imposing than the annual incidence and mortality figures. Recurrent vascular accidents are common in nearly all forms of cerebrovascular disease, each recurrence carrying a high risk of mortality. For the survivors, disability and dependency are the usual result. The need for medical care and hospital facilities for these patients is enormous and is an imposing challenge to medical and social service agencies alike.

In the following chapters, the cerebral vascular diseases are divided into two general groups, those producing ischemic *cerebral infarction* and those producing *intracranial hemorrhage*. Much of the material is derived from observations on 966 patients with clinically diagnosed cerebral vascular disease undergoing long-term study at the Cornell Division of Bellevue Hospital in New York City. As a rough index of the frequency of the different types of cerebral vascular accident or "stroke," 88 per cent of these patients had acute infarction or less severe cerebral ischemic attacks, and 12 per cent had intracranial hemorrhage. Of the infarctions, about one in eight was attributed to cerebral embolism.

294. CEREBRAL ISCHEMIA AND INFARCTION

DEFINITION AND ETIOLOGY

Cerebral thrombosis and cerebral emboli produce clinical symptoms by causing cerebral infarction, which means neural death from ischemia. Cerebral ischemia is the result of either a generalized or a localized prolonged reduction of blood flow to the brain. If ischemia is transient, less than 10 to 15 minutes, usually no discernible neurologic deficit remains. If it lasts longer than that, neural damage results, producing neurologic dysfunction, disability, and death.

The causes of cerebral infarction are numerous. The following are the most common ones:

1. Atherosclerotic disease of the intra- and extracranial arteries.
2. Cerebral emboli with (a) rheumatic heart disease, (b) myocardial infarction, (c) cardiac disease and atrial fibrillation, (d) subacute bacterial endocarditis, (e) nonbacterial thrombotic endocarditis.
3. Reduced cerebral blood flow from severe hypotension or dysrhythmia of cardiac disease.
4. Cerebral arterial spasm following subarachnoid hemorrhage.
5. Generalized cerebral hypoxia from (a) cardiopulmonary insufficiency, (b) pulmonary emboli, (c) carbon monoxide poisoning.
6. Cerebral thrombosis due to arteritis: (a) collagen vascular disease, (b) giant cell arteritis, (c) bacterial arteritis, including syphilis.
7. Cerebral thrombosis due to polycythemia or ischemia caused by severe anemia.
8. Cerebral thrombosis adjacent to intracerebral hemorrhage.
9. Cerebral arterial vasoconstriction associated with migraine.
10. Dissecting aneurysm of the aorta or great vessels in the neck.

INCIDENCE AND EPIDEMIOLOGY

Cerebral infarction is most commonly the result of cerebral atherosclerosis and cerebral emboli. In the Cornell-Bellevue series of 873 cases with nonhemorrhagic stroke, 92 per cent were clinically related to cerebral atherosclerosis and 8 per cent to cerebral emboli. In the group with cerebral emboli 20 per cent occurred in association with myocardial infarction, 26 per cent with rheumatic heart disease, most commonly with mitral stenosis, and atrial fibrillation, and the remainder in patients with atrial fibrillation associated with other varieties of heart disease.

Cerebral infarction is almost twice as frequent in males as in females. The peak age period is 60 to 69 years, but the incidence of stroke rises linearly with increasing age. In the Cornell-Bellevue study, stroke occurred earlier than the age of 50 in only 8 per cent of the patients.

NEUROPATHOLOGY

The brain is exquisitely dependent on its oxygen supply. There is no reserve of oxygen in cerebral tissue to sustain cerebral metabolism during periods of reduced or absent cerebral blood flow. When the brain is acutely and completely deprived of oxygen generally or locally, the electroencephalogram changes within 10 to 20 seconds, and irreversible and extensive neural damage occurs in the cerebral hemispheres after three to ten minutes. The determinants of brain ischemia are hypoxia and reduced general or local cerebral perfusion. The more important of the two is a decrease in perfusion. When ischemia is prolonged, the ischemic tissue softens, and the usually distinct margins between gray and white matter become unclear and occasionally hemorrhagic. Under the microscope, neurons are seen to be necrotic and shrunken, i.e., infarcted.

Cerebral infarctions that follow ischemia may be "pale" (nonhemorrhagic) or hemorrhagic. The extravasation of blood into tissues more commonly follows an embolic arterial obstruction, and pale infarcts more frequently follow atherosclerotic or thrombotic arterial obstruction. Often the two varieties of infarction blend together, and there is little advantage in extensively weighing the difference of causation.

A variable amount of *cerebral edema* accompanies cerebral infarction. With large infarctions the edema may be so extensive that portions of the swollen hemisphere shift under the falx or down through the tentorium cerebelli. This change in intracranial space relationships further impairs the flow of blood and cerebrospinal fluid, thus increasing the ischemia and neurologic deficit. This is often followed by secondary congestion and ischemia of the upper brainstem, which is almost invariably fatal.

It is common to find numerous old, small cerebral infarctions in patients dying from other causes, indicating that cerebral infarctions need not always give rise to symptoms. Old infarctions that have been hemorrhagic are identified at postmortem examination by the presence of hemosiderin in the wall of the infarct. As the infarct ages, the necrotic area breaks down, is absorbed, and eventually may be replaced by a fluid-filled cavity lined with glial and fibrovascular tissue.

MECHANISMS

Cerebral infarction is usually accompanied by abnormalities in the state of the arterial conducting system from the heart to the brain or the venous system draining the brain; the efficiency of the heart as a pump in producing a constant blood flow at a sufficient arterial

Posterior commu-
nicating artery

Basilar artery

Anterior spinal artery

Anterior cerebral artery

Middle cerebral artery

Posterior cerebral artery

Internal carotid artery

Vertebral artery

External carotid artery

Common carotid artery

Subclavian artery

Arch of the aorta

Figure 1. The darkened areas on the arterial diagram show the common sites of atherosclerosis and obstruction in the cerebral vessels.

pressure; and the character of the circulating medium (blood), its viscosity, its oxygen-carrying capacity, and its capacity to change from a colloidal suspension to a gel. Most cerebral infarctions are due to simultaneous changes in several of these factors.

The arterial conducting system is most often altered by atherosclerotic disease. In the third decade of life atherosclerosis is usually evident in the arteries leading to the brain, particularly in the larger cerebral arteries. Sites of predilection for plaques (Fig. 1) are the origins of the common carotid artery; just above the common carotid bifurcation; the internal carotid in its siphonous portion; the origin of the middle cerebral artery; and the vertebral arteries just after they enter the skull and the basilar artery. The atheromatous process in cerebral arteries is the same as that found elsewhere in the body, with lipid deposition in the intima, fibrous tissue overgrowth, hemorrhage into the plaques, ulceration of the plaques, and vessel obstruction.

Although atheromatous vascular disease begins early, it is a silent process for most of the life of the patient, and rarely produces symptoms until the middle years, when myocardial infarction, cerebral infarction, and lower extremity infarction occur. Most postmortem studies show that 80 to 90 per cent of all adult patients examined at autopsy have significant atheromatous disease. Since by no means all of these had experienced adverse clinical effects, the factors determining symptomatic complications assume major importance.

The first factor of importance is the degree and extent of atheromatous vascular disase, both in the arteries in the neck leading to the head and in the intracranial cerebral arteries. In general, persons who have cerebral infarctions have the most extensive cerebrovascular dis-

ease in the arteries in the neck and in the head. However, the pathogenesis of infarction depends on several mechanisms, and patients with only small or moderate amounts of vascular disease sometimes suffer serious cerebral infarcts. Conversely, extensive atheromatous disease can be found in large and small intracranial and extracranial cerebral arteries in patients without cerebral infarction.

Diabetes or *hypertension* can be detected in over two thirds of patients who have had cerebrovascular accidents. Patients with either diabetes or hypertension develop atherosclerosis at an earlier age, and the process develops more rapidly than in patients without these complicating illnesses. The atherosclerotic disease is extensive and is found in the smaller intracranial arteries.

The condition of the *cerebral collateral circulation* influences the development of cerebral infarction in persons with atherosclerosis. Most collateral circulation from one major intracerebral arterial system to another is through the circle of Willis via the posterior communicating arteries or the anterior communicating artery. Other sites of collateral circulation include the interconnections of the pial arteries on the cerebral surface between the anterior, middle, and posterior cerebral arteries. Sites of collateral circulation that become functional only when circulation through other routes is impaired are also found between the external and the internal carotid artery system, via the ophthalmic artery, and through muscular branches between the vertebral arteries and the external carotid artery in the neck.

Anomalies of the circle of Willis occur in nearly half the population. The most common is atresia of the posterior communicating artery, which tends to isolate the anterior (carotid system) circulation from the posterior (vertebral basilar) circulation. Anomalies in the circle of Willis are even more common in patients with cerebral infarction, and thus are believed to increase the chances of stroke in patients with cerebral atherosclerosis.

Inflammatory states involving the cerebral arteries are another cause of cerebral infarction. Inflammation produces edema and fibrosis of the vascular wall, which reduces the carrying capacity of the vessel and causes a decrease in cerebral blood flow distally. Collagenvascular disease is the most common vascular inflammation causing cerebral infarction. Syphilis was formerly the most common inflammation of the cerebral arteries and a frequent cause of cerebral infarction, especially in young persons. Rarely, acute bacterial infections of the pharynx have been followed by vasculitis of the carotid arteries and cerebral infarction. Another uncommon illness is Takayasu's disease, which affects the origin of the cerebral arteries from the aortic arch and its branches, and often results in cerebral infarction, especially in young to middle-aged women.

Cerebral Emboli

Cerebral infarction can occur without intrinsic arterial disease when emboli block arteries and impair blood flow. The most common cause of cerebral emboli in patients under 50 is rheumatic heart disease with mitral stenosis and atrial fibrillation. Other conditions associated with embolus formation are myocardial infarction with mural thrombi, atrial fibrillation of unknown cause, subacute bacterial endocarditis, thyrotoxicosis with atrial fibrillation, and nonbacterial thrombotic endocarditis. Fat emboli are rare. Paradoxical emboli have been reported as a cause of cerebral infarction. These arise in distal veins, and are shunted through the heart to the brain through a patent foramen ovale.

The neuropathologic changes in the brain that follow embolic infarction are not different from those found with infarction from other causes except that hemorrhage into the infarct is found more often with emboli than with vascular occlusion from atherosclerotic disease. The actual embolic material is often not retrieved from the cerebral vessels at autopsy unless the embolus is large, presumably because most small emboli are lysed. This evanescence means that many instances of embolic cerebral infarction must be inferred by finding a source of emboli in other sites. Mutiple small areas of cerebral infarction are commonly found at autopsy in patients with embolic disease.

Cerebral emboli that originate from infected material with bacterial endocarditis or pulmonary infections may cause local inflammation as well as infarction. Infected emboli may produce cerebral abscess, local encephalitis, or mycotic aneurysm.

Recurrent emboli have been postulated as a cause for the transient attacks of neurologic dysfunction often seen in patients with cerebrovascular disease (see below). The surface of atheromatous plaques in the internal carotid artery is frequently ulcerated. A granular lipid debris is present on the ulcer, and the surface of some plaques has been noted to be covered with collections of platelets or organizing blood clot. It is believed that some of the granular or thrombotic material on the surface breaks off, is carried into and obstructs small cerebral vessels, and produces small areas of ischemia. Because only minute vessels are occluded, infarction usually does not occur. In support of this concept is the observation in the optic fundi of some patients having transient ischemic attacks of small white or yellow refractile bodies moving through or blocking the retinal arteries. These emboli have been identified as platelet collections or cholesterol crystals; it is believed that they represent atherosclerotic debris from plaques in proximal vessels and that similar emboli go to brain vessels, causing transient occlusions without necrosis. Embolic material from ulcerated atherosclerotic plaques can cause transient ischemic attacks in the absence of significant vascular obstruction.

Cerebral Venous Inflammation and Thrombosis

Cerebral infarction can result from thrombosis of one of the major venous sinuses, i.e., the superior sagittal sinus, the lateral sinus, or the cavernous sinus, or it can follow extensive thrombotic occlusion of cortical veins. The causes of cerebral venous thrombosis include dehydration, head injury, intracerebral hemorrhage, polycythemia vera, leukemia, infection, and the puerperal state. The most common cause is infection of the mastoid, the frontal sinus, or the subdural space. If the superior sagittal sinus is thrombosed anteriorly, both cerebral hemispheres become markedly congested, swollen, and hemorrhagic. The cerebral white matter may be involved, with small hemorrhages and edema. The surface veins become distended and filled with clot.

Thrombosis of surface veins is usually associated with cerebral or subdural abscess. The histologic picture is that of an acute inflammatory reaction with vascular congestion, edema, and neuronal loss.

Cavenous sinus thrombosis usually follows infection of the eye, face, or nose, and in many instances the thrombus extends through the perihypophyseal veins to involve the opposite cavernous sinus as well. Meningitis may follow spread of the infectious process through the sinus to the subarachnoid space.

Cardiac Disease

Hypotension and Hypertension

Cardiac disease contributes to infarction in patients with cerebral atherosclerosis as the result of periods of hypotension after myocardial infarction, congestive failure, and cardiac arrhythmia. In the Cornell-Bellevue series, clinical heart disease not only preceded cerebral infarction in half the patients, but was the actual cause of at least half the deaths after cerebral infarction.

HYPOTENSION. Both hypotension and hypertension have been implicated in the production of cerebral ischemia and infarction. Although cerebral blood flow in the normal person is relatively independent of the systemic blood pressure down to levels of 50 to 60 mm of mercury, it has been suggested that a lesser drop in blood pressure may produce cerebral ischemia when a significant obstruction is present in a vessel leading to the brain. A localized obstruction must reduce the vessel lumen by nearly 80 per cent to produce a significant distal drop in pressure, but luminal encroachment that extends over long distances theoretically could significantly decrease the distal arterial pressure with less severe grades of obstruction. However, the contribution to cerebral infarction of obstruction and distal decreases in blood pressure and flow is still an unsettled matter. Thus Marshall has reported that when patients with transient ischemic attacks were made briefly hypotensive with hexamethonium and tilting, nearly one half showed evidence of generalized cerebral ischemia only, and another one fourth developed evidence of generalized cerebral ischemia before any focal ischemia.

Failure to maintain the blood pressure may occur with cardiac arrhythmias and after myocardial infarction. The asystole that occurs in Stokes-Adams attacks, if prolonged, can reduce the cerebral blood flow so markedly that cerebral ischemia or infarction results.

HYPERTENSION. Longstanding hypertensive cardiovascular disease is probably the single biggest risk factor in stroke; the place of hypertension in the production of acute cerebral ischemia and infarction is less clear. Rapid elevations of blood pressure evoke an increase in cerebrovascular resistance, and model experiments have demonstrated that stenosis coupled with this increased resistance significantly reduces blood flow. In animal experiments, marked hypertension causes constriction in small cerebral vessels, leading, in turn, to areas of cerebral infarction. Transient marked increases in blood pressure may contribute to cerebral infarction.

Other physiologic changes in cerebral hemodynamics may contribute to cerebral ischemia. Osteoarthritis in the cervical spine may compress the vertebral arteries so that extension, flexion, or rotation of the head can reduce vertebral artery blood flow to the point that ischemic symptoms occur. Cerebral ischemia will be augmented in these instances if anomalies or extensive atherosclerotic deposits compromise the circle of Willis.

Changes in Blood: Clotting, Viscosity, and Anemia

A variety of blood changes have been linked to cerebral infarction. The most frequent is *thrombus formation*, although in many instances it is unclear whether this is primary or secondary to the ischemic process. Thus infarction is not invariably associated with clot-filled vessels, and when thrombi do occur, they arise most commonly in association with ulcerated atherosclerotic lesions or atherosclerotic plaques, which by themselves produce a marked degree of vessel obstruction. In vessels with greatly reduced or absent flow, clots form readily, and long, wormlike clots have been removed from the distal segment of a partially or completely obstructed internal carotid artery shortly after the development of symptoms and signs of cerebral ischemia. A plausible reconstruction of this sequence suggests that marked stenosis was present first and was suddenly increased by hemorrhage into the atherosclerotic plaque, after which clotting occurred distally to the occlusion.

Alterations in blood clotting suggesting hypercoagulability have been described in patients with cerebral infarctions. However, a state of altered clotting has not been observed before an infarction, and some evidence suggests that hypercoagulability is an epiphenomenon that follows, rather than precedes, infarction.

Other potentially deleterious changes in blood include *increased viscosity* with polycythemia and *decreased oxygen-carrying capacity* with anemia. About 15 per cent of patients with polycythemia die from thromboembolism in the brain. Transient ischemic attacks that occur in patients with polycythemia are believed to result from the increase in blood viscosity that occurs when the hematocrit rises above 55.

Severe *anemia* sometimes precipitates cerebral ischemia, particularly if the hematocrit falls below 20, i.e., if the oxygen-carrying capacity drops more than half. Any degree of anemia may supplement severe atherosclerosis, cardiac disease, or hypotension in causing cerebral ischemia.

Cerebral Infarction and Medication

Stroke occurring in young women of childbearing age is related to the use of oral contraceptive agents. The absolute risk of developing stroke in women of this age group is small (1 in 10,000), but with oral contraceptive agents it is increased five to six-fold. The risk is further increased in those women who have migraine or hypertension and who smoke. There is evidence relating the increased risk to the estrogen content of the medication, which is now known to alter blood clotting and intima of vessels. In patients with migraine and hypertension, when contraception is needed other means should be used.

THE PATHOGENESIS OF SYMPTOMS AND SIGNS IN CEREBROVASCULAR DISEASE

To make accurate clinical diagnoses in patients suspected of having cerebrovascular disease, the clinician requires an effective working knowledge of the structural and vascular anatomy of the brain. This is presented in the following paragraphs and diagrams, reference to which will explain why patterns of neurologic dysfunction after infarction or ischemia are related more to arterial territories than to specific neuroanatomic systems.

The brain is supplied by four large arteries, the two common carotids and the two vertebrals. One common carotid artery arises from the aortic arch and the other from the innominate artery in the upper thorax. The two vertebral arteries originate from the right and left subclavian artery. The common carotid artery bifurcates in the neck, forming the internal and external carotid arteries. Each internal carotid artery enters the skull through the homolateral foramen lacerum, passes through the cavernous sinus, and gives off branches in the following order: ophthalmic, anterior choroidal, and posterior communicating. It then bifurcates into the anterior and middle cerebral arteries.

The Anterior Cerebral Artery

As may be seen in Figures 2 and 3, the anterior cerebral artery supplies the medial and superior surfaces of the cerebral hemisphere and the whole of the most anterior portion of the frontal lobes. This area contains the motor and sensory cortex for the foot and leg and the supplementary motor cortex. The anterior cerebral artery also supplies several deep structures of impor-

Figure 2. The medial surface of the cerebral hemisphere, showing the course of the anterior and posterior cerebral arteries and the area of brain supplied by each.

Anterior cerebral artery

Areas of brain supplied by:
▨ Anterior cerebral artery
▧ Middle cerebral artery
▩ Posterior cerebral artery

Posterior cerebral artery

Figure 3. The cerebral hemispheres and the vascular supply, in coronal section.

tance, including the anterior nucleus of the thalamus and a portion of the anterior limb of the internal capsule.

The Middle Cerebral Artery

The middle cerebral artery (Figs. 3 and 4) supplies the lateral surface of the cerebral hemisphere with the exception of the occipital and frontal poles. The cortex supplied includes the primary motor and sensory area for the face, hand, and arm, the optic radiations, and, in the dominant hemisphere, the cortical areas for speech. The perforating branches of the middle cerebral artery reach the center of the cerebral hemisphere supplying the internal capsule and basal ganglia.

The Posterior Cerebral Artery

As shown in Figures 2 and 3, the posterior cerebral artery supplies the posterior pole of the lateral surface of the cerebral hemisphere and the posterior portion of the medial and inferior surfaces of the hemispheres. This area contains the calcarine cortex or the primary

visual receptive area. The short perforating branches of the posterior cerebral artery supply the thalamus, part of the optic pathways, and other diencephalic structures including the midbrain.

The Vertebral and Basilar Arteries

The vertebral arteries reach the head via a bony canal in the transverse processes of the sixth through the second cervical vertebrae and enter the skull through the foramen magnum. Immediately after entering the skull each vertebral artery gives off a medial branch (these unite to form the anterior spinal artery) and, just distal to this, the posterior inferior cerebellar artery. At all levels along the brainstem, the ventral medial portion is supplied by short paramedian vessels. The ventrolateral portion of the brainstem is supplied by short circumferential branches from the vertebrals or basilar artery. The dorsal lateral portion and cerebellum are supplied by long circumferential branches: the posterior inferior, the anterior inferior, and the superior cerebellar arteries.

The vertebral artery lies on the ventral lateral surface

Figure 4. The lateral surface of the cerebral hemisphere and the course of the middle cerebral artery. The sylvian fissure has been opened to better illustrate the course of the vessel.

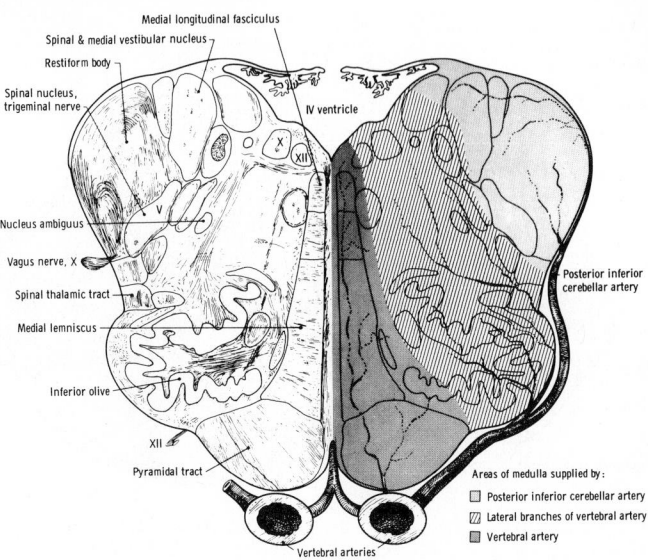

Figure 5. Cross section of the medulla oblongata seen from above at the level of the hypoglossal nuclei. The medial structures are supplied by short branches arising from the vertebral arteries and anterior spinal arteries. The lateral portions are supplied by longer branches and the dorsal and lateral areas by long circumferential branches, at this level called the posterior inferior cerebellar artery.

of the medulla oblongata, and from it and the anterior spinal artery short paramedian branches supply the pyramids, the inferior olives and medial lemniscus, the medial longitudinal fasciculus, and the emerging fibers of the hypoglossal nerve as shown in Figure 5.

The more dorsal portion of the medulla includes the spinothalamic tract, the vestibular nuclei, the sensory nucleus of the fifth cranial nerve, the restiform body, and the emerging fibers of the vagus and glossopharyngeal nerves, and is supplied by longer branches from the vertebral artery and branches from the posterior inferior cerebellar artery. The most cephalad and dorsal segment of the medulla includes the vestibular and cochlear nuceli, and it and the posterior portion of the cerebellum are supplied by the posterior inferior cerebellar artery.

At the lower border of the pons, the two vertebral arteries unite to form the basilar artery. From this artery in the pons, short perpendicular branches enter the brainstem to supply paramedian structures, including

the corticospinal tracts, the pontine nuclei, the medial lemniscus, the medial longitudinal fasciculus, and the pontine reticular nuclei (Fig. 6). Circumferential branches supply the lateral portion of the pons, which includes the emerging seventh and eighth cranial nerves, the trigeminal nerve root, the vestibular and cochlear nuclei, and the spinothalamic tracts. The anterior inferior cerebellar artery, the long circumferential branch at this level, also gives branches to the most dorsal and lateral of these structures as it runs dorsally to the cerebellum.

At the level of the midbrain the basilar artery lies in the interpeduncular fossa (Fig. 7). Short branches pass laterally and dorsally to both sides to supply the cerebral peduncles, the emerging third nerve roots, the medial portions of the red nuclei, the medial longitudinal fasciculus, the oculomotor nuclei, and the midbrain reticulum. Branches of the posterior cerebral artery supply the lateral portions of the peduncles, the red nuclei, and the medial lemnisci. The superior cerebellar arte-

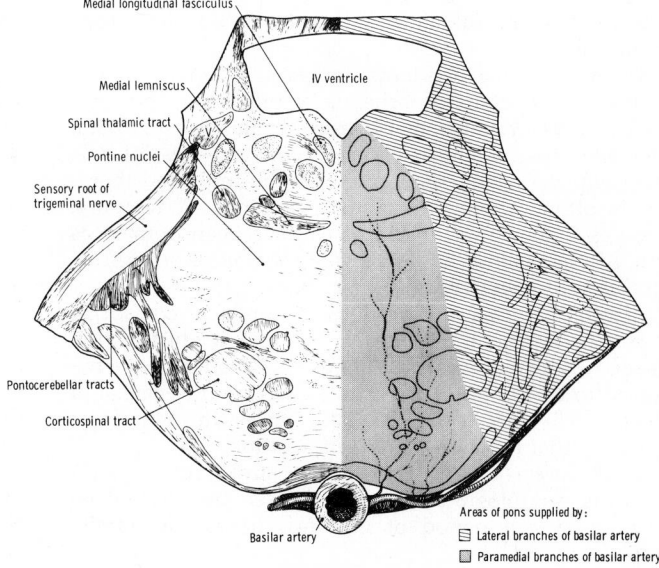

Figure 6. Cross section of the midpons. The most medial regions are supplied by short perforating branches from the basilar artery. The more lateral regions are supplied by lateral branches of the basilar artery. At this level, the more dorsal structures are supplied by the long circumferential branch, the anterior inferior cerebellar artery.

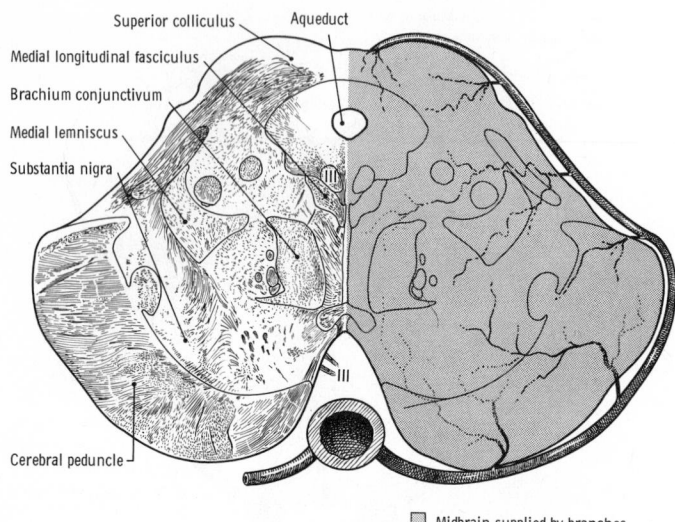

Superior colliculus
Aqueduct
Medial longitudinal fasciculus
Brachium conjunctivum
Medial lemniscus
Substantia nigra
III
III
Cerebral peduncle

Midbrain supplied by branches of the posterior cerebral artery

Figure 7. Cross section of the midbrain seen from below. The medial, lateral, and dorsal regions are supplied by short branches from the posterior cerebral artery as it passes around the midbrain.

ries supply some of the dorsal portions of the midbrain, including the colliculi and the anterior portion of the cerebellum on each side.

It will be clear from this review of neurologic and vascular anatomy that infarction can produce a large variety of clinical pictures, depending on the vessels involved. The pattern of most syndromes is helpful in localizing the area of the nervous system damaged by infarction, but only a few reliably indicate exactly which portion of the vascular tree is involved. As an example, diagnoses are often made of middle cerebral artery occlusion, but a review of the vascular anatomy of the brain quickly reveals why, with both anterior cerebral arteries filling from either side, an identical clinical picture can be associated with occlusion of the internal carotid artery at any point along its course.

SIGNS AND SYMPTOMS IN CEREBROVASCULAR DISEASE: STROKE SYNDROMES

An adequate exposition of the symptoms and signs of cerebrovascular disease requires a classification of the various clinical entities that make up the stroke syndrome.

Cerebrovascular accidents are classified on the basis of the anatomic site of ischemia or infarction, the cerebral vessels occluded or obstructed, and the temporal character of the entire clinical episode. The latter is clinically the most valuable in that the indicated therapy is often different for the three kinds of temporal profiles found. The three profiles have been defined as *transient ischemic attack, stroke-in-evolution* or *progressive stroke,* and *completed stroke.*

The term *transient ischemic attack* or incipient stroke refers to transient episodes of neurologic dysfunction caused by cerebrovascular disease. The attacks are believed to be caused by cerebral ischemia, and consist of fleeting, 5- to 30-minute disturbances in neurologic function that leave no permanent residue.

Stroke-in-evolution or progressive stroke refers to increasing neurologic dysfunction caused by cerebral ischemia over a period of minutes, hours, or, rarely, days.

Completed stroke refers to the clinical picture seen in patients who have ceased to show further progression in neurologic deficit or in those who have developed a slight to calamitous neurologic deficit earlier that is now stable or improving. *Cerebral embolism* is one cause of completed stroke in which the onset is an abrupt monophasic event, and there is clinically a demonstrable source of emboli.

Cerebral Transient Ischemic Attacks

The symptoms vary, depending upon which area of the brain is ischemic, but there are two main types: those associated with ischemia of parts or the whole of a cerebral hemisphere, and those associated with ischemia of the brainstem. The symptoms most often include transient contralateral weakness of the lower face, fingers, hand, arm, or leg, but such patients may also experience fleeting sensory symptoms such as tingling, "pin and needles," or numbness in parts of the body contralateral to the ischemia. Ischemia in the dominant hemisphere may cause dysphasia, with impairment in the context of speech and, at times, a transient lack of understanding.

Patients with ischemia in the portion of the brain supplied by the posterior cerebral artery may suffer blurred vision, or may notice transient hemianopic or altitudinal visual field defects or impairment of visual acuity.

Ischemia or insufficiency caused by internal carotid artery stenosis often produces transient retinal ischemia, resulting in monocular blindness or reduced acuity on the side of the stenosis, combined with contralateral weakness of the face, arm, or leg.

Ischemic attacks which result from involvement of the brain supplied by the vertebral and basilar arteries have an extremely wide range of symptoms. Common symptoms include vertigo, tinnitus, diplopia, dysarthria, dysphagia, and dysphonia. Patients may complain of unilateral or bilateral face, arm, and leg weakness and unilateral or bilateral sensations of numbness and tingling in the face, arms, or leg. There may be tinnitus, hearing loss, and ataxia. In addition, patients with brainstem ischemia may experience "drop attacks," in which they suddenly lose postural tone and fall to the ground without losing consciousness, then immediately regain postural control and rise quickly. The most common complaint with transient ischemic attacks from vertebrobasilar insufficiency is dizziness. However, dizziness is commonly associated with other physiologic disturbances and is rarely the only symptom of brainstem ischemia. When patients describe intermittent neurologic episodes with symptoms suggesting a generalized decrease in cerebral blood flow such as dizziness, lightheadedness, and generalized weakness, they should be carefully examined for cardiac dysrhythmia before being studied for the presence of extracranial arterial disease. Cardiac dysrhythmia, with a drop in cardiac output and subsequently in general cerebral blood flow, is a common cause of nonfocal transient ischemic attacks.

Symptoms of vertebral basilar artery ischemia, although variable, tend to occur in combinations that aid in their diagnosis. Vertigo, ataxia, dysarthria, paresthesia, diplopia, tinnitus, dysphagia, and focal weakness in the face, jaw, or pharynx tend to coexist, although not always in the same sequence or combination. Another grouping of symptoms is that of unilateral or bilateral weakness of the extremities with drop attacks and diplopia. The reason for these differences in symptom combinations can be found by referring to the diagrams of the blood supply to the brainstem. Ischemia of the dorsal and lateral portions of the brainstem supplied by the circumferential arteries produces the first group of symptoms. Ischemia of the more ventral portions supplied by the medial perforating arteries causes the second group.

Symptomatic vertebral basilar artery ischemia may occur with stenosis of the subclavian artery proximal to the origin of the vertebral artery. The arm on the side of the stenosis may be supplied by retrograde flow in the ipsilateral vertebral, and, during exercise, enough blood can be diverted from the vertebral system to the arm to cause symptoms of brainstem ischemia. This mechanism of producing brainstem ischemia has been called the *subclavian steal syndrome*. However, most instances of reversed vertebral artery flow with subclavian artery stenosis or occlusion are asymptomatic.

Ischemic attacks may occur many times a day or at weekly or monthly intervals. They may be intermittently present over several months or several years. Some patients with internal carotid artery occlusion have transient ischemic attacks for as long as two years before cerebral infarction occurs. Others have clusters of attacks lasting only a few hours or days before carotid occlusion becomes complete and causes infarction. *The major importance of transient ischemic attacks is that they signal the existence of significant cerebrovascular disease and clearly indicate the potential danger of cerebral infarction.* Studies of the natural history of transient ischemic attacks indicate that about one fourth to one third of patients afflicted will suffer a cerebral infarction within two to five years of onset of the attacks. It cannot always be predicted which patients with cerebral ischemia will develop cerebral infarction or even when it will occur. Transient ischemic attacks become more significant predictors of cerebral infarction if accompanied by extensive atherosclerosis as evidenced by abnormalities in the neurovascular examination, such as arterial bruit in the neck, absent temporal pulse, retinal embolization, and reduction of retinal artery pressure on the appropriate side. Some varieties of cerebral ischemic attacks carry a better prognosis than others. Attacks suggesting ventral brainstem involvement, such as bilateral paresis or unilateral transient paresis or drop attacks, connote a poor prognosis. Carotid ischemic attacks that occur close together in clusters carry a poor prognosis, for in a large percentage of such patients cerebral infarction rapidly follows.

In the interval between transient ischemic attacks, the neurologic examination is usually entirely normal. During a transient ischemic attack, patients commonly have neurologic deficits corresponding to their symptoms. Thus with ischemia of a cerebral hemisphere, there may be a hemiparesis with reflex asymmetry and an extensor plantar response, or a mild hemisensory or visual field deficit. If the dominant hemisphere is affected, dysphasia may be noted: the patient has difficulty in naming and recognizing objects. Patients examined during a brainstem ischemic attack often exhibit nystagmus, complete facial weakness, palate and tongue weakness, and deviation, dysconjugate eye movements, sensory defects, and weakness on one side or on both sides of the body. The evaluation of patients with transient ischemic attacks must always include careful examination of the optic fundus through a dilated pupil, searching for cholesterol (bronze debris) or platelet emboli (white or invisible plugs) in the arterial tree. *The presence of such emboli in one eye is important evidence of an embolic source in the carotid artery.* Patients with such emboli should have cerebral angiography, and the presence of ulcerated atherosclerotic plaques should be determined.

Consciousness is usually unimpaired during transient ischemic attacks, although thinking is sometimes slowed. This lack of alteration of consciousness coupled with the absence of either aura or convulsive movements helps to distinguish these attacks from convulsive seizures. Other conditions that must be considered in the differential diagnosis are Menière's syndrome (which is rare in the elderly), migraine headache, cerebral emboli, or the progressive neurologic deficits caused by cerebral neoplasm.

Stroke-in-Evolution
(Progressive Stroke)

The evolving stroke is characterized by the gradual development of paralysis and sensory impairment over a period of several hours and, at times, one to two days. The symptoms and signs may develop as a series of steplike changes or as an unbroken continuum of worsening. When first examined, a patient may have mild weakness which, as the hours pass, is found to be more and more marked and to involve more and more of the body. The symptoms and signs found are identical to those of completed stroke; only the time course of onset is different. This course also occurs with subdural hematoma and brain tumor, but, for these disorders, the duration usually extends over several days or weeks.

Cerebral Infarction
(Completed Stroke)

Cerebral infarctions resulting from cerebral emboli or from cerebral atherosclerosis and thrombosis, respectively, cannot be distinguished by the neurologic disorders they produce. Differences between these two causes of infarction do exist, however, in the mode of onset of symptoms and in the general physical evaluation.

The pattern of onset of neurologic symptoms and signs in cerebral infarction often suggests the cause. Cerebral embolism causes an abrupt onset of symptoms, and headache often precedes other neurologic symptoms by several hours. Cerebral infarction caused by atherosclerotic vascular obstruction or occlusion often has a less sudden onset. There may be a distinct series of steplike increases in neurologic symptoms and signs, or infarction may be preceded by a series of transient ischemic attacks. A gradual onset with increasing neurologic deficit over several (one to five) hours is characteristic of the progressing stroke. A gradual onset of symptoms and signs over two days or, occasionally, one week, does occur but is uncommon. The frequency of these different patterns can be inferred from the experience of one large series of patients with ischemic infarction; about one third had a sudden onset of symptoms, about one fifth had symptoms that progressively increased over one to 12 hours, and only about one in 20 had symptoms that progressed for as long as 12 to 24 hours. One fifth of the patients with occlusive vascular disease and cerebral embolism had the onset of neurologic signs during sleep.

Headache is present in many patients with embolic or atherosclerotic infarction. The headache is usually mild and localized to the side of the infarction. Headache is believed to be caused by vasodilation of unoccluded vessels near the infarcted area, and is most common when vessels near the base of the brain are occluded.

Consciousness is usually not lost at the onset of infarction of the cerebral hemispheres, but may be reduced, particularly when large infarcts involve the dominant hemisphere. When unconsciousness is present from the onset or is the initial symptom, brainstem infarction is the most likely cause. When large hemispheric infarctions are complicated by rapidly developing and severe brain edema, loss of consciousness caused by diencephalic and upper brainstem compression may occur shortly after the onset of symptoms. This may give the false impression of loss of consciousness from the onset unless a careful history documents a lucid period at the very beginning of symptoms. Convulsive seizures are rare at the onset of cerebral infarction, but they occur in about 8 per cent of patients at some time in the course of the acute or convalescent phase of the illness. They are usually focal, but may be generalized.

When infarction is limited to the cerebral hemisphere, there is weakness or paralysis in the extremities contralateral to the infarction. Patients may also be aware that sensory perception on the side of weakness is impaired and may complain of heaviness or numbness in the arm or leg. They rarely have other sensory symptoms such as pain or paresthesias. Defects in visual fields are common but often escape the patient's notice. The defect is suspected when patients pay little attention to visual stimuli on one side of the body. At times, the eyes may be constantly deviated to the side away from the neurologic deficits.

The most serious consequence of infarction in the dominant hemisphere is dysphasia, which can range from a mild deficit of expression to aphonic mutism. The dysphasia is almost invariably a mixture of difficulty with expression (expressive dysphasia) and difficulty in understanding what is said, written, or indicated by gesture (receptive dysphasia); one or the other may predominate. In patients who have infarction in the nondominant hemisphere, lack of awareness or concern about paralysis of the contralateral side is often evident. Such subjects may, at times, be so completely unaware of their neurologic disabilities that they are hospitalized only after family or friends notice their disabilities. This phenomenon, *anosognosia*, is most common when a patient is obtunded and when there is a significant sensory deficit on the paretic side as a result of infarction of the parietal lobe. It accompanies nearly one fourth of all large strokes, but usually persists only if the patient remains obtunded or confused or has little return of sensation.

Infarctions in the brainstem produce a wide variety of symptoms. Among the most conspicuous are vertigo, diplopia, dysarthria, dysphagia, and ataxia. In addition, the patient may note unilateral or bilateral sensory impairment or weakness. Often patients note clumsiness and difficulty in performing skilled acts without paresis.

Specific Vascular Syndromes

Internal Carotid Artery Occlusion

Occlusion of the internal carotid artery at its origin from the common carotid or intracranially is the site of the major vascular lesion in nearly 20 per cent of strokes. The usual lesion is atherosclerotic with, at first, partial obstruction and, finally, occlusion with a thrombus. Occasionally the internal carotid artery is obstructed by a large embolus.

Symptoms and signs specific for internal carotid artery occlusion in the neck are intermittent visual impairment or blindness in the eye on the side of the occlusion (retinal artery insufficiency) combined with a contralateral hemiparesis and sensory loss (middle cerebral artery insufficiency). This clinical picture often begins with a series of transient ischemic attacks and only later causes permanent weakness and sensory loss. *Unless the history of intermittent blindness can be obtained*, it is difficult, on clinical grounds alone, to distinguish occlusion of the internal carotid artery from middle cerebral artery occlusion.

On neurologic examination, patients with cerebral infarction caused by internal carotid artery occlusion have paresis of voluntary movement, with weakness most noticeable in the contralateral face and upper extremity. Infarcts produce motility defects as their main manifestations, but there is usually some impairment of sensory perception and, at times, visual field impairment as well.

In the paretic extremities, deep tendon reflexes are hyperactive, and pathologic reflexes such as the Babinski sign (extensor plantar response) are found. Muscle tone becomes increased on the weakened side, and spasticity may be so marked that early contracture is evident. Sensory impairment is most evident in modalities such as position sense, vibration sense, two-point discrimination, and tactile perception of shape and texture. Touch and pain perception may be moderately impaired, and extinction of stimuli on the involved side may be evident on double simultaneous stimulation. The size of the cerebral infarction produced by internal carotid occlusion is extremely variable. When there is no collateral circulation through the anterior communicating, posterior communicating, ophthalmic, or surface collateral arteries, the infarct can involve nearly the whole cerebral hemisphere, both lateral and medial surfaces. With a richer collateral circulation, smaller infarcts and proportionately fewer neurologic defects result. Occasionally occlusion of the internal carotid is asymptomatic, and is discovered only as an incidental finding at autopsy or when cerebral angiograms are done.

Internal carotid artery occlusion or stenosis sometimes causes partial Horner's syndrome (slight ptosis and miosis) on the side opposite the paresis. The eye changes have been attributed to ischemia of the sympathetic fibers that lie in the adventitia of the arterial wall adjacent to the occlusion, but are more probably due to direct hypothalamic damage, for they can also be observed in patients with similar infarcts who do not have occlusion of the carotid arteries. An audible bruit in the neck at the angle of the mandible is a helpful indicator of stenosis of the internal carotid artery at that site. Occlusion of the internal carotid artery is also suggested when the retinal artery pressure on the affected side, as measured with an ophthalmodynamometer, decreases 25 per cent or more below the arterial pressure in the other eye. Study of blood flow in the supratrochlear artery, using a directional Doppler flowmeter, may show reversal of the usual direction of flow, which can be stopped by compression of the temporal artery. This finding is highly indicative of carotid artery occlusion with collateral circulation from the extracranial to the intracranial circulation via the ophthalmic artery.

Middle Cerebral Artery Occlusion

The cerebral tissue supplied by the middle cerebral artery is the most common area for infarction from emboli or vascular insufficiency, and the neurologic picture produced by either is the same.

When a middle cerebral artery is occluded, infarction occurs in the lateral portion of the hemisphere and produces varying degrees of contralateral paresis and sensory loss, mainly in the face, the upper extremities, and the hand, and often blindness in the contralateral, homonymous visual field. Occlusions at the origin of the middle cerebral artery produce extensive neurologic disturbance with profound contralateral hemiplegia and sensory loss. Occlusions in branches of the middle cerebral artery may produce a variable clinical picture. At times, only paresis is evident in the arm and face. In some patients, sensory impairment is the dominant and occasionally the only neurologic abnormality, and some patients have only dysphasia.

Anterior Cerebral Artery Occlusion

Anterior cerebral artery occlusion causes infarction in the cortical areas that control motor and sensory functions of the contralateral lower extremity, and impairs voluntary movement and sensory perception of that leg. The upper extremity and face are spared. Cerebral infaction caused by occlusion of the proximal portion of the anterior cerebral artery is uncommon because collateral circulation through the anterior communicating artery is usually adequate to supply both hemispheres.

Posterior Cerebral Artery Occlusion

Posterior cerebral artery occlusion causes infarction of the posterior lateral and posterior medial surfaces of the cerebral hemisphere, including the calcarine cortex. Proximal occlusions of the artery result in infarction of the thalamus and upper brainstem as well. Extensive infarctions in the occipital cortex cause homonymous hemianopic field defects, and those involving the dominant hemisphere may produce disturbances in reading, visual learning, visual recognition, and visual spatial orientation.

Infarction of both occipital poles can follow basilar artery stenosis or occlusion. The result is a double hemianopia and cortical blindness, a striking feature of which is that the patient is usually unaware that he is blind and may vigorously deny it (Anton's syndrome).

Brainstem Infarction

Brainstem infarction, although not as common as hemisphere infarction, produces several distinct clinical syndromes, best categorized by noting whether the clinical picture suggests involvement of ventral paramedian, ventrolateral, or dorsal brainstem structures. As noted in the discussion of neurovascular anatomy, these three areas receive blood supply through different groups of arteries.

Many of the particular groupings of symptoms and signs associated with various brainstem infarctions that have been given eponyms are believed to be common occurrences with brainstem infarction. However, in an analysis of 50 patients with brainstem infarction from the Cornell-Bellevue series, only two clearly fitted into these syndromes as originally described. The remaining 48 had an extensive mixture of symptoms and signs indicating an overlap in the areas believed to be infarcted with occlusions in specific arteries.

Midbrain Infarctions

Occlusion of the paramedian branches from the apex of the basilar artery or of the proximal posterior cerebral arteries causes infarction of portions of one or both cerebral peduncles, the oculomotor nerves, the oculomotor nuclei, the brachia conjunctivae, the red nuclei, and the midbrain reticular formation. The resulting symptoms and signs may be unilateral or bilateral, depending on the extent of the infarction. Unilateral signs include (1) ipsilateral oculomotor palsy and contralateral hemiparesis (Weber's syndrome), (2) ipsilateral oculomotor palsy, ipsilateral ataxia of gait, and poorly coordinated arm and hand movements (Nothnagel's syndrome). Bilateral signs include impaired consciousness, quadriparesis, divergent gaze, impaired vertical eye movements and midposition, or dilated pupils unresponsive to light. Purposeless, flail-like, involuntary movements (hemiballismus) may occur, and usually involve the upper extremity more than the lower. Patients in coma caused by infarction of the midbrain often have an unusual appearance, seeming to be almost awake although unable to communicate in any manner. This state has been called *coma vigil* or *akinetic mutism*. Such patients, although unresponsive, may exhibit a sleepwalking cycle.

When the dorsal area, supplied by the posterior cerebral artery, is ischemic or infarcted, the spinothalamic tract, the red nucleus, the descending sympathetic tracts, and the medial lemniscus are involved. The clinical picture consists of slight ptosis and miosis (Horner's syndrome), ipsilateral ataxia, and choreiform adventitious movements and contralateral impairment of all modalities of sensory perception of the entire body, including the face. This clinical picture is often called the superior cerebellar artery syndrome.

Pontine Infarction

Infarction in the pons is usually associated with basilar artery obstruction. Occlusion of the paramedian branches of the basilar artery causes necrosis of the corticospinal tracts, the pontine nuclei, the medial lemniscus, the medial longitudinal fasciculus, the abducens nucleus, the pontocerebellar tracts, and the pontine reticulum. Ipsilateral abducens palsy, facial weakness, and contralateral corticospinal tract dysfunction (Millard-Gubler syndrome) and the same findings with lateral conjugate gaze palsy (Foville's syndrome) are two unilateral syndromes that occur with occlusion in the paramedian arteries to the pons. Bilateral signs include quadriparesis, reduced reaction to noxious stimuli, and abducens paresis. Other signs include coma, hyperventilation, apneustic or ataxic breathing, small pupils, and internuclear ophthalmoplegia. If only the most ventral portion of the pons is damaged, awareness may be maintained even though the patient is quadriparetic.

With occlusion of arteries to the lateral pons, the signs and symptoms are unilateral and include tinnitus, deafness, nausea, vertigo, impairment of facial sensation, complete ipsilateral facial paralysis, nystagmus, miosis and ptosis (partial Horner's syndrome), and impaired conjugate gaze toward the side of the lesion. Impaired pain and temperature perception of half the contralateral body below the face is usually found. This clinical picture is often referred to as the syndrome of anterior inferior cerebellar artery occlusion.

Medullary Infarction

Occlusion of the paramedian branches of the vertebral artery in the medulla causes contralateral paresis of the arm and leg, contralateral impaired sensory perception to touch, position sense and vibration sense in the arm, trunk, and leg, and ipsilateral tongue paralysis. With occlusion of arterial branches to the lateral medulla, the clinical picture includes vertigo, nausea, vomiting, dysarthria, dysphagia, nystagmus, ipsilateral Horner's syndrome, ipsilateral vocal cord paralysis, and impaired ipsilateral facial sensory perception to pain with impairment of pain sensation on the contralateral half of the body below the face. This clinical picture is referred to as the syndrome of posterior inferior cerebellar artery occlusion or Wallenberg's syndrome. It results from occlusion of the vertebral artery itself as frequently as or more frequently than it does from occlusion of its branches.

Basilar Artery Occlusion

When the basilar artery is completely occluded, infarction is found mainly in the ventral pons, midbrain, and occipital lobes. The clinical picture is like that seen with occlusion of the paramedian midbrain or pontine branches, but may include various defects in the visual fields and, at times, cortical blindness in addition. The brainstem tegmentum is almost invariably involved, causing major disturbances in consciousness.

Cerebral Embolism

The diagnosis of cerebral embolization is usually not difficult when it is remembered that the onset of neurologic symptoms and signs is abrupt, that they are often preceded by headache for a few hours before paresis is evident, and that a potential source for emboli is usually found on physical examination. Convulsive seizures occur at the onset, but they are uncommon. They are at first focal and later generalized in most patients. Loss of consciousness may occur and usually lasts for only a few minutes; but after onset, patients may be confused. The neurologic signs depend upon which artery is occluded; the most common clinical picture is that of middle cerebral artery occlusion. Cerebral emboli can lodge in any major cerebral artery, and emboli commonly recur often to the same artery. The cerebrospinal fluid is usually clear and without cells. When protein elevation and cells are found, subacute bacterial endocarditis should be suspected. Mitral stenosis with atrial fibrillation, myocardial infarction with mural thrombus, and subacute bacterial endocarditis are the cardiac disorders most commonly found. Normal sinus rhythm does not exclude the diagnosis of cerebral emboli, for it may be found in more than one third of such patients, particularly with a "tight" mitral stenosis or with past myocardial infarcts, respectively. Evidence of embolization to other sites strengthens the supposition that the cause of cerebral infarction is embolic.

Cerebral Venous Thrombosis

The symptoms of local cerebral venous thrombosis are headache, delirium, drowsiness, diplopia, and convulsions. The signs are usually those of increased intracranial pressure with papilledema and focal neurologic abnormalities. Focal fits are common, as are paresis and hemisensory loss. Such patients are restless, confused, and obtunded.

Superior sagittal sinus occlusion produces a somewhat similar clinical picture. At the New York Hospital, 21 patients with noninfective sagittal sinus thrombosis have been studied. Nine had terminal disease and marasmus, six had cyanotic congenital heart disease, and four had other, unexplained episodes of venous or arterial thromboses. Eleven of the 21 patients were children. Below the age of ten, cerebral infarction is more often due to venous than to arterial occlusion. Nearly all patients had fever, and their cerebrospinal fluids were under increased pressure, averaging 260 mm of fluid, and contained more than ten red blood cells. Neurologic symptoms appeared abruptly or progressed rapidly to a maximum, usually within 36 hours. Most patients were obtunded or confused and had headache. The white blood count was elevated in ten patients; in seven it was over 20,000. Nuchal rigidity was common, and papilledema, hemiparesis, and focal epileptic seizures occurred in about half the cases. Two patients presented later with signs of pseudotumor cerebri. The occurrence of hemiparesis or focal epilepsy was usually associated with cortical venous thromboses in addition to the sinus occlusion.

Cavernous sinus occlusion, usually a complication of sinus or paranasal skin infection, is characterized by proptosis, orbital chemosis, and edema, pain around the eye, papilledema, retinal hemorrhages, and fever. Extraocular palsy may be present. The disease carries a high risk of spread to the opposite cavernous sinus. Complications include meningitis and brain abscess.

Transverse or lateral sinus thrombosis, ususally secondary to mastoiditis, is now uncommon with the decline in the incidence of that disease. When it does occur, it is usually manifested by headache, tenderness over the mastoid process, and, occasionally, paresis of the structures supplied by the glossopharyngeal and accessory nerve, with dysphagia, dysphonia, and weakness of the ipsilateral sternomastoid and trapezius muscles.

In all varieties of cerebral venous thrombosis, there is usually some evidence of sepsis with fever, malaise, headache, and leukocytosis.

Although the condition is uncommon, a diagnosis of cerebral venous thrombosis should be kept in mind for patients with evidence of cerebral infarction who have focal seizures, increased intracranial pressure, or evidence of infection. Cerebral venous thrombosis is particularly likely as a cause of postpartum cerebral infarction.

PHYSICAL AND LABORATORY FINDINGS

The general evaluation of the patient with cerebral infarction usually reveals evidence of vascular disease at other sites as well as a variety of associated diseases. About one fifth of patients with atherosclerotic cerebral infarction in the Cornell-Bellevue series had had previous strokes, half of which had occurred in the preceding year. Another fifth had had myocardial infarction, usually within the previous year. Over one half of the patients were hypertensive, but the diastolic pressure was above 100 mm of mercury in only one third of the patients. Nearly one fifth of the patients had diabetes mellitus, and one in ten gave a history of peripheral vascular occlusive disease.

PHYSICAL EXAMINATION. The physical examination of most patients with cerebral infarction discloses a normal or slightly elevated body temperature. Careful examination of the heart should never be overlooked because the presence of cardiac enlargement, atrial fibrillation, and cardiac murmurs, suggesting rheumatic heart disease with mitral stenosis, aids in detecting the presence of cerebral emboli. Patients with cerebral infarction often have atherosclerotic cornary heart disease, and perhaps one fifth have had recent or associated myocardial infarcts.

Palpation may reveal absence of pulsation in easily felt peripheral arteries. In the lower extremities, this is indicative of atherosclerotic vascular disease in the aorta, iliac, femoral or popliteal arteries. In the upper extremities, it may indicate occlusions in the major branches of the aorta, such as the innominate or subclavian arteries. Absence of pulses in one or both upper extremities should alert the physician to such diagnoses as "pulseless disease" (Takayasu's syndrome) or the "subclavian steal syndrome."

Auscultation for bruit over the neck is helpful in identifying sites of extracranial stenosis. A bruit heard in the neck under the angle of the mandible suggests atherosclerotic disease of the carotid artery, and bruit heard just above the clavicles is associated with vertebral or subclavian artery stenosis. Bruit, when loud and localized, is associated with atherosclerotic obstruction at that site in more than three fourths of patients.

LABORATORY EXAMINATIONS. Laboratory tests are aimed at both confirming the diagnosis and identifying complications. Every patient suspected of stroke should have a lumbar puncture and skull roentgenograms, and, if there are any unusual features at all about the illness, computerized axial tomography (CAT scan) should be employed (see below).

The cerebrospinal fluid should be examined promptly to determine the presence of intracranial bleeding or an unsuspected infection. The lumbar puncture must be approached cautiously, however, when patients are in stupor or coma or when it is uncertain whether the illness is caused by stroke or by brain tumor, with increased intracranial pressure. In such instances, it is preferable to proceed with computerized axial tomography or an arteriogram, because lumbar puncture can inadvertently precipitate tentorial or foraminal herniation when there is an expanding intracranial mass.

The cerebrospinal fluid pressure is rarely over 200 mm of CSF in cerebral infarction. The fluid is usually clear and colorless, but bleeding and xanthochromia from hemorrhagic infarction may be found. The CSF protein level is usually normal, although slight elevations to 60 to 75 mg per 100 ml are found in perhaps one fifth of the patients. Elevations to 80 mg per 100 ml or above are found in less than 10 per cent, but particularly in those with basilar artery disease. With massive cerebral infarction, the protein may be raised to values of nearly 100 mg per 100 ml. Diabetes occasionally accounts for pronounced CSF protein elevations with stroke, probably by a leak of protein through damaged small vessels. Patients with high values should always be carefully reviewed for the possibility of brain tumor.

Skull roentgenograms should be examined for evidence of fracture, erosion of the posterior clinoids (suggesting chronically increased intracranial pressure), abnormal calcification, and pineal shift.

The general evaluation of patients with cerebral infarction should include an electrocardiogram (EKG) and a chest roentgenogram. The EKG may confirm the presence of an arrhythmia or may disclose a silent myocardial infarction. (A potentially confusing point is that the EKG may show minor T wave and S-T segment changes caused by cerebral infarction and not by primary cardiac disease.)

The development of computerized axial tomography (CAT scan) has added a major new dimension to the diagnosis and management of stroke and has replaced pneumoencephalography, electroencephalography, and echoencephalography in diagnosis. Its major use in cerebral infarction is in differential diagnosis, in which it is highly accurate in identifying or eliminating intracerebral hemorrhage and brain tumor as causes of neurologic deficit. It is the diagnostic means of choice to establish cerebral infarction as a cause of acute neurologic disability. It is further useful in defining the exact site and extent of an infarct. As the technique is based on the differential radiation absorption of tissue, during the first few days after infarction the CAT scan may not differentiate normal from infarcted brain, and small infarctions which are cystic may not alway be detected. On average the CAT scan will accurately detect cerebral infarction of 1 cm in diameter or larger in about 50 to 60 per cent of instances. Use of iodinated contrast media intravenously is useful in determining the degree of hemorrhage in an infarction. Computerized scans are helpful in delineating the degree of cerebral edema around an infarct and in following an infarct as it resolves.

Special Investigations

Arteriography

The technical quality and safety of arteriography has improved to the point that complications develop only in about 1 to 2 per cent of patients with cerebrovascular disease, and permanent worsening and death follow arteriography in less than 1 per cent of patients.

Cerebral angiography is indicated only for certain patients with cerebrovascular disease and has two main values. The first is in differential diagnosis for the patient with an atypical history and findings, or who is unable to give an accurate history because of dysphasia or depressed consciousness.

The second and more important value of cerebral angiograms is the accurate demonstration of the site, extent, and incidence of arterial obstructions and ulcerated atherosclerotic plaques that might be susceptible to surgical correction. Patients who need study include predominantly those who suffer transient ischemic attacks, very mild strokes, or strokes from which recovery has been substantial. In such cases, it is necessary to outline both the neck vessels and the nature and extent of the intracranial collateral circulation and the collateral channels from extracranial to intracranial vessels.

Rapid roentgenographic exposures have clarified some aspects of the physiology of cerebral blood flow in patients with cerebrovascular disease. Cerebral angiography may identify unusual patterns of blood flow in cerebral vessels, such as retrograde flow down one vertebral artery with proximal subclavian artery stenosis (subclavian steal). Ulceration of plaques can be demonstrated in about 41 per cent of patients with transient ischemic attacks coming to operation. The accuracy of the angiographic diagnosis when compared to findings at surgery is 90 per cent.

Brain scanning, using radiomercury-chlormerodrin or Tc^{99m} Pertechnetate, shows a high uptake of radioactive material in the area of a cerebral infarction. This technique may aid in accurate localization of the infarcted area, but an identical picture can result from brain tumor, thereby limiting its usefulness in differential diagnosis. A normal brain scan during the first few days after the onset of symptoms suggesting a stroke, followed by a positive brain scan, is highly suggestive of cerebral infarction.

DIFFERENTIAL DIAGNOSIS

The most common sources of error in the diagnosis of cerebral infarction are brain tumors, subdural hematomas, intracerebral hemorrhages, cerebral traumatic lesions, and cerebral infections.

When a clear history of the onset is available, cerebral infarction is seldom confused with other disorders. Stroke caused by cerebral emboli or cerebral thrombosis characteristically produces a maximal neurological deficit initially, with gradual improvement in function over days, weeks, or months. The first symptoms of brain tumor and subdural hematoma occasionally are mistaken for stroke, but the general tendency is for these two disorders to cause gradually progressive worsening, even though the first symptoms may seem to begin suddenly. In addition, both brain tumor and hematoma tend to produce disturbances in consciousness that are as prominent as or more prominent than focal neurologic defects, which helps in their differentiation from cerebrovascular disease. Often the problem in differential diagnosis is reversed in that the onset of stroke may include a gradual steady progression of symptoms and signs of focal neurologic defects, making the physician think first of tumor and only later of cerebral infarction. When doubt occurs about the diagnosis of infarction, subdural hematoma and neoplasm should be suspected, and cerebral angiograms and computerized axial tomography (CAT scanning) should be done.

Clinically, it is easier to confuse cerebral infarction with intracranial hemorrhage, for the onset is often similar. The cerebrospinal fluid examination usually helps, but blood can be found in both states —although considerably less often in cerebral infarction. Large amounts of blood in CSF under increased pressure is always caused by intracranial hemorrhage. Angiography or CAT scanning helps to settle the problem by demonstrating aneurysm, A-V anomaly, or intracerebral hematoma.

When it is not known where the patient could have suffered head trauma, it is often impossible to eliminate this as a cause of clinical states resembling cerebral infarction. Careful inspection for scalp lacerations and localized scalp edema and good quality skull roentgenograms identify most instances of trauma if it has been severe enough to cause neurologic injury. If trauma cannot be eliminated and the patient becomes progressively worse, CAT scanning or angiography must be done to eliminate consideration of subdural or epidural hematomas. CAT scanning is preferable, for it will not only indicate a hematoma but will also define other causes of illness such as tumor, or intracerebral hemorrhage.

Among the forms of intracranial sepsis only brain abscess is likely to be confused with cerebral infarction. The points that should alert the physician to the possibility of an abscess are a source of infection elsewhere in the body such as an ear, sinus, or chest infection; persistent headache; persistent low-grade fever; white cells, especially polymorphonuclear leukocytes, that persist more than 24 hours in the cerebrospinal fluid; a focal, highly abnormal EEG; and worsening of the clinical state. If abscess is suspected, angiograms performed on the side opposite the paresis will demonstrate the presence or absence of an intracerebral mass, which, if present, then must be surgically explored and drained to prove the diagnosis.

COURSE

Some improvement in function after the initial neurologic deficit can be expected after almost every cerebral infarction. During the first 72 hours, however, gradual worsening of neurologic deficits and increasing or beginning impairment of consciousness are frequent. This change may indicate extension of the cerebral infarction, but usually is associated with cerebral edema in and around the necrotic area. *Some degree of cerebral edema complicates every infarct.* It appears almost immediately, and with large infarctions may be so extensive as to shift the brain laterally and downward to produce herniation through the tentorium cerebelli and subsequent brainstem compression. This course of events, with its associated impairment of consciousness and other vital functions, is a common cause of death in patients with extensive infarction. The diagnosis of cerebral edema is especially likely when a patient shows a decline in awareness without a significant increase in focal neurologic deficits. Other causes of lethargy and stupor in patients with cerebral infarction are fever, electrolyte imbalance, the injudicious use of sedatives, tranquilizers or narcotics, and malnutrition.

In patients whose course is not complicated by severe cerebral edema, there is usually an early improvement in neurologic function. If some voluntary movement is preserved, there is a good chance for return of more. When function improves rapidly after the onset, the outlook for a good recovery is excellent. A slow return of function over weeks or months is associated with a less complete recovery. If flaccid paralysis is present from the onset with no return of voluntary movement over 30 to 60 days, the outlook for recovery is poor. Significant sensory loss impairs the chances of recovery of motor function. With brainstem infarction, the course is usually one of gradual improvement if the infarct is localized in the lateral medullary area. Symptoms of nausea, diplopia, and ataxia lessen and eventually disappear. Although some residual impairment of eye and extremity movement may be detected on examination, such patients often have little physical limitation. It is important to realize that recovery from cerebral infarction may continue for as long as one to two years.

PROGNOSIS

About one fourth to one fifth of patients with either thrombotic or embolic cerebral infarction die with their first attack. This figure varies somewhat with the cause of the infarction and especially with other factors such as age, cardiac status, and the degree of neurologic disability. The mortality rises sharply with increasing age; for patients over the age of 70 with cerebral infarction from atherosclerotic thrombosis or emboli the initial mortality is nearer 50 per cent. Patients with marked neurologic defects, coma, or extensive vascular disease elsewhere have an initial mortality of nearly 50 per cent. Infarction of the ventral portions of the brainstem after basilar artery occlusion, especially with quadriplegia, carries a poor outlook, although good medical and good nursing care may preserve a vegetative existence for long periods.

The prognosis for cerebral infarction is better in younger patients, in those with the least evidence of vascular disease at other sites, especially cardiovascular disease, and in those who do not have hypertension, diabetes, or severe neurologic defects.

About one fifth of patients who survive a cerebral infarction from atherosclerotic vascular disease suffer another cerebrovascular accident within the next 12 to 24 months. However, the most significant limiting factor on survival is not recurrent stroke but cardiovascular disease. *Thus in the Cornell-Bellevue series, fully half of the patients who survived the initial cerebral infarction died at a later date from myocardial infarction or cardiac failure.*

Recurrence of cerebral infarction is common with cerebral emboli. In the New York Hospital series about 22 per cent of patients with cerebral emboli suffered recurrences, and nearly all the patients had more than one embolus if extracerebral sites were included. There is a strong chance that each cerebral recurrence will cause death or further neurologic disability.

TREATMENT

GENERAL. Treatment of cerebral infarction has four goals: to preserve life, to limit the amount of brain damage, to lessen disability and deformity, and to prevent recurrences.

The treatment program designed to preserve life is similar to that outlined for all seriously ill patients with neurologic illness. Efforts are directed toward maintaining a clear airway, an adequate fluid, electrolyte, and caloric intake, and an adequate urine output. Constant care is required to protect the skin from ischemia and necrosis resulting from pressure. Such a program is necessary for the obtunded or comatose patient, and must often be continued for the remainder of his life.

In patients with hemispheric infarction *cerebral edema* can impair consciousness and vital function early in the course of the illness. When cerebral edema subsides, the patient may again be able to cough, swallow, and voluntarily move paretic parts. A variety of measures can often temporarily reduce the brain swelling and carry the patient through a period of severe difficulty. Hypertonic urea solution, 1 to 1.5 grams per kilogram of body weight given intravenously, dehydrates normal brain, giving more space for edematous brain. The effect is transient, and a rebound effect has been reported. Hypertonic invert sugar, mannitol, has been used with similar results except that less rebound has been reported. One and one half to 2 grams per kilogram of body weight is given intravenously in a 20 per cent solution. In patients with cerebral infarction and brain edema this therapy is reserved until there is a serious threat to life with declining brainstem function, for the benefits are transient, and most patients can be carried through periods of depressed consciousness with careful nursing care alone. Although glucocorticoids such as methylprednisolone are often dramatically effective in improving patients with brain edema from primary and metastatic brain tumor, they have been found in carefully controlled studies to be ineffective in reducing cerebral edema after infarction.

Several agents have been utilized to increase cerebral blood flow in an effort to decrease the amount of ischemic tissue and limit the extent of cerebral infarction. Nearly all known agents that produce vasodilatation, including aminophylline, papaverine, tolazoline hydrochloride, nicotinic acid, and histamine, have been used without clear evidence of success in cerebrovascular disease. The only agent that produces effective vasodilatation in cerebral vessels is carbon dioxide. Although it has been used to treat acute stroke, there is no evidence that it reduces the neurologic defects.

Treatment for the late acute and convalescent phase of a

stroke is directed toward lessening deformity and disability, a goal that requires daily passive exercise of paretic parts to prevent joint fixation and to maintain normal muscle and tendon length. Some increase in muscle tone with spasticity invariably accompanies hemiplegia and tends to be most marked in the flexor muscles in the upper extremities and in the extensor muscles in the lower extremities. If this increase in tone in one muscle group over another persists and cannot be overcome by voluntary movement, daily passive movement of weakened or paralyzed parts through the full range of motion must be carried out by a nurse, physician, physiotherapist, or member of the family to prevent muscle and tendon contracture that may be nearly impossible to correct later on.

REHABILITATION. After cerebral infarction, *programs of retraining and rehabilitation should begin as soon as there is no longer evidence of increasing infarction.* Stabilization of the neurologic findings for 12 to 24 hours with some evidence of improvement is usually sufficient evidence to permit a start. Rehabilitation programs have as their goal the retraining of the remaining functions for maximal effectiveness. Although a few patients do require and benefit from special hospital facilities for rehabilitation, most such programs can be carried out on medical services without the aid of extensive equipment. An internist or general physician who is interested in rehabilitation can direct programs of activity and exercise, and can achieve results in rehabilitating hemiplegic patients that are nearly as effective as those of specialized centers.

An active program of rehabilitation begins by increasing the patient's tolerance to sitting and standing, which is impaired both by weakness and by changes in the sense of balance. Patients are allowed to sit up and then stand for increasingly long periods, beginning with five to ten minutes. During this period daily active and passive exercises of weakened extremities are carried out. When patients begin standing they need firm support and often splinting or bracing of the knee on the weakened side; marked quadriceps weakness may even demand a long leg brace. Ambulation is one of the main goals of rehabilitation. Gait training should begin when the patient can comfortably stand for 15 to 20 minutes without fatigue, and the support of parallel bars or a walker should be depended upon at first. After ambulation has started, it may be necessary to brace the foot to avoid the foot drop and supination that commonly occur after hemiplegia. At the same time that the patient is relearning to walk he should be trained in developing new skills with his unaffected arm and improving the strength and function in the paretic arm. This is done by an active program of exercise and by observing and retraining the patient in the activities of daily living such as eating, dressing and undressing, and personal hygiene. More complete details of programs of rehabilitation are outlined in other sources such as Covalt (1965) and can be followed by patients and their families under the direction of the physician. Usually, the maximal effect is gained in six to eight months, but some patients continue to show improvement over periods lasting as long as two years. Passive exercise must be continued indefinitely for severely paralyzed patients if contractures are to be avoided.

For patients with cerebral infarction who have mild to moderate dysphasia, speech therapy may be helpful. With severe dysphasia, therapy is rarely able to restore usable speech.

PREVENTION

The probability of an asymptomatic individual developing an atherosclerotic cerebral infarction has been analyzed by the Framingham study. The risk of developing stroke is increased in either sex and at any age by hypertension, diabetes, electrocardiographic evidence of heart enlargement, hypercholesterolemia, and cigarette smoking. The risk is higher with more than one of these factors operant and increases with the age of the individual. At the moment, the only factor which, if altered, is clearly related to a reduced risk of cerebral infarction is hypertension. In view of this, careful control of blood pressure in hypertensive individuals emerges as an important factor in prevention of signs and symptoms of cerebral ischemia. For management of hypertension, see Ch. 361.

Prevention of recurrent attacks and of cerebral infarction in patients with transient ischemic attacks and prevention of recurrent infarction in patients with cerebral atherosclerosis and cerebral emboli are the goals of much of the currently recommended treatment for stroke. Four methods to achieve this have been extensively evaluated: anticoagulation, drugs which alter platelet adherence, surgical correction of arterial obstructions, and removal of ulcerated atherosclerotic plaques.

ANTICOAGULANT DRUGS OR SURGERY IN TRANSIENT ISCHEMIC ATTACKS. *Anticoagulant therapy* was introduced to treat transient ischemic attacks after its use in myocardial infarction suggested a beneficial action. Reported studies of anticoagulants in transient ischemic attacks indicate that as long as patients receive anticoagulants and their prothrombin times are kept at two to two and a half times the normal value, they have fewer ischemic attacks and less chance of having a cerebral infarction. As a result, anticoagulants are accepted as effective in treating patients with transient ischemic attacks. The question is, which patients should receive the anticoagulants and for how long? The natural history of attacks is variable; attacks often stop spontaneously; some varieties carry a better prognosis than others. Even admitting these differences, anticoagulants should be given to the patients with transient ischemic attacks who do not have contraindications to their use. They should be continued for three to six months and then gradually discontinued. If transient ischemic attacks recur, they should be given again. The management of patients on anticoagulants is discussed in Ch. 357.

Drugs which inhibit platelet aggregation have been used to reduce platelet emboli as a cause of transient ischemic attacks. These agents include aspirin, dipyridamole, sulfinpyrazone, and cyproheptadine. Use of aspirin has been shown to reduce the frequency of transient ischemic attacks and to significantly reduce the occurrence of stroke in males with transient ischemic attacks. The required dose of aspirin is 0.3 gram four times a day.

Surgical correction of extracranial arterial obstruction with removal of ulcerated atherosclerotic plaques has been successfully used in the treatment of patients with transient ischemic attacks. Most carefully evaluated studies show that transient ischemic attacks stop after surgery and that the chances of future cerebral infarction are reduced. Arteriography of all precerebral vessels in the neck and the intracranial vessels should precede consideration of surgery, as the number and extent of sites of atherosclerosis are related to the success of operation. Isolated single obstruction or atherosclerotic plaques in accessible sites carry the best chance of successful treatment. Patients with multiple sites of extensive atherosclerosis, extra- and intracranially, should not be treated surgically and are best managed with anticoagulants or platelet aggregation inhibitors. If skillful, experienced surgeons are unavailable or referral to such surgeons is impossible for other reasons, anticoagulants or platelet aggregation inhibitors are the treatments of choice.

ANTICOAGULANT DRUGS OR SURGERY IN PROGRESSING STROKE OR STROKE-IN-EVOLUTION. Anticoagulants have been shown to significantly reduce mortality and morbidity among patients with stroke-in-evolution. Such situations are emergencies, and unless specifically contraindicated, anticoagulation must begin with heparin and must be continued with coumarin derivatives. Anticoagulants are usually given for four to six weeks. Surgical correction of an arterial obstruction for the patient with progressing stroke has sometimes been attempted as a means of reducing neurologic disability, but with poor results. Those patients in whom it can be demonstrated that showers of emboli from an ulcerated atherosclerotic plaque in the carotid artery are the cause of the progression, and who do not respond to anticoagulation or platelet antiaggregation agents, should have immediate surgical removal of the ulcerated plaque.

ANTICOAGULANT DRUGS OR SURGERY IN COMPLETED STROKE. For the patient with an already completed stroke, there is no clear treatment for preventing recurrences. Most series of patients with completed stroke studied by angiograms illustrate the widespread nature of atherosclerotic obstructive vascular disease. Intra- and extracranial vessels are commonly affected simultaneously and impose limiting factors on the successful outcome of surgical correction of extracranial arterial defects. A controlled evaluation of surgical therapy in this group of patients has been carried out and shows that surgical correction of an isolated carotid stenosis in patients with a mild neurologic defect is effective in reducing future mortality and morbidity. Surgical correction of arterial obstruction in patients with severe neurologic defects or with evidence of extensive atherosclerotic disease and occlusion does not change future mortality or morbidity.

Anticoagulants, given for one to four months, are useful during the acute and early convalescent period after a cerebrovascular accident to prevent pulmonary emboli in paralyzed, bedridden patients. The use of anticoagulants has also been recommended on a long-term basis for prevention of recurrent stroke. However, most studies of this problem indicate that there is no benefit from this form of treatment and that the complication rate is too high to warrant its use. Anticoagulation, therefore, can be recommended only for highly selected patients after cerebral infarction.

ANTICOAGULANT DRUGS IN CEREBRAL EMBOLIZATION. Anticoagulants greatly reduce the mortality and morbidity associated with recurrent embolization, and patients with a well established diagnosis of cerebral embolus should be placed on these drugs if there are no contraindications. If the source of emboli is rheumatic heart disease, anticoagulants are given continuously. When emboli follow myocardial infarction, treatment is usually given for one year. Coumarin anticoagulants are used and should be started immediately after the diagnosis has been made and the lumbar puncture has revealed bloodless cerebrospinal fluid.

Patients with cerebral emboli who have atrial fibrillation are often considered for conversion to normal sinus rhythm. This may be valuable in increasing cardiac output, but does not clearly reduce the chance of recurrent cerebral emboli.

General management of anticoagulant therapy is outlined in Ch. 357.

Hemorrhagic complications from anticoagulants are serious in about 2 to 4 per cent of patients and fatal in 2 per cent. Minor bleeding does not require that the medication be discontinued, but with serious bleeding it should be. Minor surgical procedures can be undertaken safely in most patients on anticoagulants if the prothrombin time is slightly lowered. Head injury, even of a minor nature, in patients on anticoagulants must be carefully evaluated and followed, as the chance of subdural hematoma in this group is high.

Heparin is the anticoagulant of choice for the initial treatment of patients with progressing stroke.

Patients with transient ischemic attacks, progressing strokes, or established strokes who also have hypertension should be treated with antihypertensive medication. Studies of patients with atherosclerotic cerebrovascular disease and hypertension show that when the blood pressure is returned to normal or nearly normal levels, the recurrence rate and mortality rate of stroke are reduced. Hypertension, depending on its severity, should be continuously treated with reserpine, chlorothiazide, or hexamethonium, and the blood pressure should be maintained as nearly normal as possible (see Ch. 361).

To sum up the prophylaxis of strokes: Patients with transient ischemic attacks should be treated with anticoagulants or platelet antiaggregation agents. If arteriography indicates significant extracranial vascular disease, especially ulceration of an atherosclerotic plaque, and experienced surgical care is available, the patient should be offered this form of treatment. Patients with completed strokes are not likely to benefit from any prophylactic treatment. If they are to remain bedridden for long periods, anticoagulants help to reduce the chances of pulmonary embolism.

HYPERTENSIVE ENCEPHALOPATHY

Hypertensive encephalopathy is an uncommon, acute neurologic syndrome characterized by headache, nausea and vomiting, convulsive seizures, transient focal neurologic defects, retinal artery spasm, papilledema, stupor, and coma. The cerebrospinal fluid pressure and protein content are commonly elevated. The syndrome is encountered in patients with longstanding hypertension. Its occurrence is associated with sudden marked increases in blood pressure from various causes, including malignant hypertension, eclampsia, and glomerulonephritis.

The mechanism by which hypertension causes neurologic dysfunction is believed to be acute cerebral vasospasm causing cerebral ischemia and edema.

Mild transient focal neurologic defects can be encountered in this syndrome. When neurologic defects are severe and sustained, the correct diagnosis is more likely to be cerebral ischemia or cerebral hemorrhage. When the blood urea nitrogen is above 100 mg per 100 ml, hypertensive encephalopathy can be difficult to distinguish from uremia, or can blend into that state.

The outlook for patients with hypertensive encephalopathy has been greatly improved with the use of antihypertensive medication, and temporary recovery is now frequent. The appearance of the syndrome, however, is usually associated with the end-state phases of advanced hypertensive vascular disease.

Hypertensive encephalopathy is a medical emergency, and treatment should be given to rapidly lower the blood pressure, for this is the only effective way to eliminate the symptoms. Initial treatment should be intramuscular reserpine, 2 to 5 mg per day. Blood pressure will begin to fall in two to three hours after administration of reserpine, and it can be maintained at desired levels with daily injections. Care must be exercised to avoid cerebral ischemia from hypotension. Permanent medical therapy must be instituted to maintain the blood pressure at more nearly normal levels, utilizing hydrochlorothiazide, reserpine, or alpha methyldopa (see Ch. 361).

PROGRESSIVE SUBCORTICAL ENCEPHALOPATHY

Progressive subcortical encephalopathy, described by Binswanger, is a rare disorder that occurs in patients with hypertension and atherosclerotic vascular disease. Progressive dementia, seizures, and focal neurologic signs characterize the clinical picture. The diagnosis is usually made at necropsy; the brain shows atrophy mainly in the temporal and occipital regions and patchy demyelination in the white matter of the hemispheres.

Barnett, H. J. M., et al.: The Canadian Cooperative Stroke Study Group: A randomized trial of aspirin and sulfinpyrazone in treatment of stroke. N. Engl. J. Med., 299:253, 1978.

Genton, E., Barnett, H. J. M., Fields, W. S., Gent, M., and Hoak, J. C.: Cerebral ischemia: The role of thrombosis and antithrombotic therapy. Stroke, 8:150, 1977.

Kannel, W. B., et al.: Risk factors in stroke due to cerebral infarction. Stroke, 2:423, 1971.

Katzman, R., Clasen, R., Klatzo, I., Meyer, J. S., Pappius, H. M., and Waltz, A. G.: Brain edema in stroke. Stroke, 8:512, 1977.

McDowell, F. H., and Brennen, R. W. (eds.): Cerebral Vascular Disease. Transactions of the Eighth Princeton Conference, 1972. New York, Grune & Stratton, 1973.

Millikan, C. H.: Reassessment of anticoagulant therapy in various types of occlusive cerebrovascular disease. Stroke, 2:201, 1971.

Scheinberg, P.: Cerebrovascular Diseases. Tenth Princeton Conference. New York, Grune & Stratton, 1976.

Vinken, P. J., and Bruyn, G. W.: Handbook of Clinical Neurology. Vols. 11 and 12: Vascular Diseases of the Nervous System. New York, American Elsevier Publishing Company, 1972.

Whisnant, J. P., and Sandok, B. A.: Cerebrovascular Diseases. Ninth Princeton Conference. New York, Grune & Stratton, 1975.

295.   INTRACRANIAL HEMORRHAGE

DEFINITION

Intracranial hemorrhage, or apoplexy, comprises about one tenth of all acute cerebral vascular illness. Regardless of cause, intracranial hemorrhage is a serious illness with a high rate of mortality. At the bedside the physician can only suspect the diagnosis, which must be confirmed by finding blood in the cerebrospinal fluid or by the demonstration of a hematoma by computerized axial tomography, or angiography, or at surgery. The causes of intracranial hemorrhage are numerous, and the clinical pictures are similar regardless of the cause. It helps to understand the clinical problem better if one remembers that nontraumatic

bleeding within the cranium takes one of four separate anatomic courses and that these produce three relatively distinct clinical pictures:

1. Bleeding emanating from vessels on the surface of the brain and limited to the cerebrospinal fluid–filled space between the pial and arachnoid membranes is called *subarachnoid hemorrhage.*

2. *Subarachnoid hemorrhage with intracerebral extension* occurs when the sudden force of bleeding from a surface vessel also penetrates into the brain itself; signs and symptoms of both the subarachnoid and the parenchymal lesions result.

3. Bleeding from ruptured vessels within the substance of the brain is called *intracerebral hemorrhage.* This may remain isolated therein as a *cerebral hematoma.*

4. Intracerebral hemorrhage may extend through brain tissue to the ventricles or subarachnoid space, causing signs and symptoms of both the parenchymal and the subarachnoid lesions.

ETIOLOGY

Bleeding from ruptured arteries is the usual source of intracranial hemorrhage, although veins also may bleed. The accompanying table lists the common causes.

Arterial Aneurysms

BERRY ANEURYSMS. These are small, round, or saccular berry-shaped dilatations that form characteristically at arterial bifurcations at or near the circle of Willis. Their cause is uncertain, for aneurysms are not familial and they are rarely found in infants. They arise, however, from what are thought to be congenital defects in the media of cerebral vessels. The wall of an aneurysm is thin, composed usually only of intima and subintimal connective tissue. Muscle or elastic tissues may be evident at the origin of the aneurysmal sac from its parent vessel, but these tissues thin out and disappear as the sac enlarges. Most aneurysms are less than 1 cm in diameter; a few, however, dilate to as much as 2 to 5 cm. As the aneurysm enlarges, it may develop a narrow neck or may remain broadly attached to the vessel wall.

Most berry aneurysms, approximately 85 per cent, develop around the anterior portion of the circle of Willis, arising from the internal carotid, the posterior communicating, the middle cerebral, the anterior communicating, or the anterior cerebral artery, as shown in Figure 8. The most common site is the point of junction of the posterior communicating artery and the internal carotid. About 15 per cent of aneurysms arise from the vertebral-basilar artery system. Multiple aneurysms are found in about one of every six patients. Not all an-

---

Causes of Intracranial Hemorrhage

1. Arterial aneurysms
   a. *"Congenital" berry aneurysms*
   b. *Acquired arterial aneurysms*
      (1) Fusiform aneurysms
      (2) Mycotic aneurysms
2. Arteriovenous (A-V) anomalies
3. Hypertensive vascular disease
4. Vascular lesions associated with primary or metastatic brain tumors
5. Systemic bleeding diatheses
6. Undetermined and miscellaneous causes

- Internal carotid artery
- Anterior communicating artery
- Anterior cerebral artery
- Middle cerebral artery
- Posterior communicating artery
- Posterior cerebral artery
- Superior cerebellar artery
- Paramedian arteries
- Circumferential artery
- Anterior inferior cerebellar artery
- Basilar artery
- Vertebral artery
- Posterior inferior cerebellar artery
- Anterior spinal artery

Figure 8. The more common sites of berry aneurysm. The size of the aneurysm at the various sites is directly proportional to the frequency at that site.

eurysms bleed, and some are found incidentally at postmortem examination. Occasionally, they become so large that they compress adjacent cerebral tissue or cranial nerves, and, rarely, they enlarge sufficiently to cause a clinical state that simulates brain tumor.

What makes an aneurysm rupture at any given instant is not clear, although several factors seem important. These lesions gradually enlarge with time under the stress of the arterial blood pressure. They are more frequent in patients who are hypertensive, and their incidence is high in subjects with coarctation of the aorta and polycystic renal disease, both of which cause early hypertension. Atheromatous plaques form in their walls, and clots line the aneurysms, but whether either of these conditions increases the chance of rupture is problematic. Probably a change in the blood pressure is the single final event that precipitates perforation of the sac.

FUSIFORM ANEURYSMS. These spindle-shaped dilatations along the course of an artery, usually the basilar, sometimes the carotid artery in the cavernous sinus, are due to atherosclerosis. The resulting elongated and tortuous dilatation may be large enough to compress adjacent cranial nerves or the brain itself. Hemorrhage from such an aneurysm is unusual, but characteristically damages the brain fatally when it does occur.

MYCOTIC ANEURYSMS. Mycotic aneurysms are produced by septic emboli associated with bacterial endocarditis. A local necrotic vasculitis occurs at the site where the embolus lodges and results in thinning and dilatation of the vessel wall, which may eventually rupture. Such lesions tend to be multiple, and they are the only aneurysms found distally in the smaller branches of the middle cerebral artery.

Arteriovenous Anomalies or Cavernous Angiomas

Arteriovenous (A-V) anomalies or cavernous angiomas are tangled, interconnected networks of vessels in which arterial blood passes directly to venous drainage without intervening capillaries. These lesions tend to be supplied by more than one parent cerebral artery, and they range in size from the microscopic to a huge cavernous network large enough to cover most of one cerebral hemisphere or to occupy an entire lobe of the cerebellum. The vessels in an A-V anomaly are themselves malformed so that some structurally resemble arteries, others veins. Since these vessels are usually thin walled, circulating blood at arterial pressure distends and often eventually ruptures them, with a resultant subarachnoid hemorrhage, intracerebral hemorrhage, or both. Even without hemorrhage, large A-V malformations expand, and the neural tissue adjacent to the anomaly characteristically suffers an uneven pressure necrosis, causing progressively more abnormal neurologic signs and epilepsy. Hemorrhage can destroy all clinical evidence of a malformation of microscopic size and make postmortem diagnosis impossible.

Hypertensive Vascular Disease

Hypertension causes thickening and fibrinoid degeneration of the cerebral arterioles. Red cells can be found free in the perivascular spaces around many of the vessels, and microaneurysms have been described along the arteries since the time of Bouchard and Charcot in the nineteenth century. What part each of these abnormalities contributes to the eventual necrosis and rupture is still debated, although most contemporary pathologists view the fibrinoid degeneration as most important.

When hemorrhage occurs, it usually results from rupture of small arteries in the substance of the brain. This may occur anywhere; it is most common in the cerebrum and least common in the cerebellum and brainstem. In the cerebral hemispheres, small branches of the middle cerebral artery penetrating the region of the basal ganglia are most susceptible, and the lenticulostriate artery has even been termed "the artery of cerebral hemorrhage." In the brainstem, hemorrhages arise from paramedian perforating branches of the basilar more often than they do from the long circumferential branches of either the basilar or the vertebral arteries.

Hemorrhage in Brain Tumors

Hemorrhage may occur in either primary or metastatic lesions, usually in rapidly growing tumors with a large amount of vascular overgrowth. This complication is perhaps most common in glioblastoma multiforme and metastatic neoplasms from the lung. Among the more benign tumors pituitary adenomas have a tendency to cause apoplexy. Of the total number of cerebral hemorrhages, however, those from tumor contribute but a small fraction.

Bleeding Diatheses and Miscellaneous Causes

Leukemia, thrombocytopenia, and the ingestion of excessive amounts of anticoagulants all predispose to cerebral hemorrhage. In some patients it is difficult or impossible to establish what caused a cerebral hemorrhage. As mentioned, in some cases the hemorrhage may have erased the malformation. A hemorrhagic cerebral infarct can be so liquefied that it resembles a primary hemorrhage. However, with the increasing use of cerebral angiography and computerized axial tomography, more and more intracranial aneurysms and malformations are being demonstrated in all age groups as the cause of intracranial hemorrhage, and more strokes have been found to be small hemorrhages.

PATHOLOGY AND PATHOGENESIS

SUBARACHNOID HEMORRHAGE. Subarachnoid hemorrhage most commonly comes from rupture of a berry aneurysm, less commonly from an A-V anomaly or a mycotic or fusiform aneurysm. Blood suddenly released in this manner has several deleterious effects, each contributing to the seriousness of the disease. The sudden high pressure jet raises the intracranial pressure and sometimes acts like an acute concussion, causing sudden unconsciousness or, occasionally, rapid brain displacement and death. Blood is also a noxious agent, particularly as it hemolyzes and breaks down into its pigments. It irritates blood vessels, meninges, and the brain itself. Meningeal irritation causes the characteristic headache of subarachnoid hemorrhage, and later, within hours or days, the blood produces a sterile meningitis. This hemogenic meningitis itself becomes a source of considerable disability, for it not only causes subjective discomfort and systemic toxicity but leads to meningeal exudation, thickening, and scarring that can impair cerebrospinal fluid absorption and cause subacute or chronic communicating hydrocephalus. Moreover, the blood may irritate the underlying brain so as to evoke adverse descending autonomic discharges, causing hypertension and cardiac arrhythmias.

In addition to the brain destruction caused by the physical action of the hemorrhage, ischemic changes and infarction of brain tissue are found in as many as two thirds of patients dying from subarachnoid hemorrhage. The ischemia and infarction have been attributed to vascular spasm or vessel wall edema, and they are encountered most commonly in the area of the brain supplied by the artery with the ruptured aneurysm. Evidence for arterial spasm in subarachnoid hemorrhage comes from angiographic studies showing segmental vessel narrowing that correlates with a high incidence of clinical and pathologic evidence of cerebral infarction. The causative mechanism is believed to be a combination of the irritating effect of free blood and the production in the subarachnoid space of vasoactive substances, and of vessel injury. During surgery, mechanical stimulation of cerebral arteries causes significant and sustained vessel narrowing. Presumably, vascular spasm has a potentially protective action in reducing the amount of bleeding from a ruptured artery. Why in some instances it lasts long enough and is severe enough to reduce distal cerebral blood flow to the point of ischemia and neural death is unknown.

Extension of bleeding into the brain occurs in about half of all surface aneurysms and in nearly all A-V anomalies. The complication is particularly likely when the bleeding site lies close to cerebral tissue, as is true with aneurysms of the anterior communicating or anterior cerebral arteries, which are interposed between the frontal lobes, or of branches of the middle cerebral artery, which are buried within the sylvian fissure. Rupture from the anterior communicating vessel tends to damage one or both frontal lobes, and rupture of middle cerebral artery aneurysms tends to lacerate the temporoparietal or posterior frontal lobes.

INTRACEREBRAL HEMORRHAGE. Intracerebral hemorrhage is most often caused by hypertensive vascular disease or ruptured aneurysm, less often by a bleeding A-V malformation. The path that the blood takes with these lesions and the amount of bleeding are somewhat unpredictable. Some hemorrhages dissect the brain along fiber tracts, destroying relatively little brain tissue along the way. Others damage considerable amounts of neural tissue in the region of bleeding. All hemorrhages enlarge the brain and evoke cerebral edema. When the enlargement occurs rapidly, it displaces cerebral structures laterally across the midline under the falx and downward through the tentorium cerebelli, with resulting brainstem compression. Such a course of events is often fatal; at postmortem examination smaller areas of bleeding are found in the midbrain and pons in addition to the massive intracerebral hemorrhage. These secondary brainstem lesions have been attributed to venous obstruction and ischemia from transtentorial herniation.

Small intracerebral hemorrhages can remain entirely confined within the brain substance. Occasionally, the hematoma absorbs fluid, and this plus the surrounding edema can create the clinical picture of an expanding new growth. More often, however, the fluid is resorbed, and the remaining cavity shrinks almost to the point of disappearance.

Most large cerebral hemorrhages rupture into the subarachnoid space, the ventricular system, or both. Although serious consequences have been attributed to this course of events, it is likely that the large size of the hemorrhage causes the disastrous clinical effects rather than the fact that bleeding penetrated into the cerebrospinal fluid spaces.

CLINICAL MANIFESTATIONS OF INTRACRANIAL BLEEDING

SUBARACHNOID HEMORRHAGE. Subarachnoid hemorrhage has as its most common initial symptom a sudden violent headache. Initially the headache is usually described as an excruciating, intense, aching pain. Later it becomes dull and throbbing but remains severe, and most patients describe it as the most intense headache they have ever experienced. Even if it is at first localized, it soon becomes generalized, and frequently patients complain of severe neck and back pain. The initial localized headache is due to vascular distortion and injury. The later generalized headache is due to meningeal irritation from blood in the subarachnoid space.

Localization of headache at the onset is helpful in determining the site of the bleeding. Headache that begins in the back of the head suggests a posterior fossa origin of bleeding, and headache that begins in the anterior part of the head suggests a supratentorial bleeding source. If the initial headache is localized to one side, bleeding usually has occurred from a vessel on that side.

Other symptoms include dizziness, vertigo, vomiting, drowsiness, sweating and chills, stupor, and loss of consciousness.

Shortly after the onset of symptoms, the patient may lose consciousness for a few moments. With massive subarachnoid hemorrhage and intracerebral extension, the patient may lapse into and remain in coma until death. In some instances of subarachnoid hemorrhage death may be sudden and is related to intraventricular hemorrhage and sudden intense transtentorial herniation and brainstem compression. When hemorrhage is confined to the subarachnoid space or when intracerebral extension of bleeding is minor, consciousness is regained in a few minutes to a few hours. Delirium and lethargy often follow and may persist for as long as two weeks; severe mental clouding, delirium or coma usually indicates severe bleeding and brain damage.

Patients with subarachnoid hemorrhage usually complain of neck stiffness; this does not appear immediately in most patients but begins with the onset of the meningeal inflammatory reaction 6 to 12 hours later. When neck stiffness is evident shortly after the onset of symptoms, it is ominous and suggests that the meninges in the posterior fossa are stretched by beginning herniation of the cerebellar tonsils into the foramen magnum.

Although subarachnoid hemorrhage does occur during sleep, it most commonly occurs when patients are engaged in their usual activities. Many patients have reported that headache began during activity such as straining at stool, heavy lifting, or coitus.

Convulsions may occur, usually at onset, but sometimes during the acute phase of the illness. When present, they almost invariably indicate that the site of bleeding is in the anterior or middle fossa.

On examination the most conspicuous sign is marked neck rigidity and pain on attempting head movement. The most common localizing neurologic abnormality is pupillary inequality or paresis of vertical and medial movements of one eye that follows oculomotor nerve compression by aneurysms of the internal carotid artery.

Lateralizing neurologic signs, such as hemiparesis or hemiplegia, hemisensory defects or hemianopia, indicate either an intracerebral extension of bleeding or vascular spasm. The distribution of signs of neurologic dysfunction, particularly at onset, may be helpful in localizing the site of bleeding. Marked hemiparesis and severe hemisensory defects suggest bleeding from an aneurysm on the middle cerebral artery in the sylvian fissure. Unilateral oculomotor paresis with ptosis, diplopia, and mydriasis suggests that the bleeding source is from the region of the posterior communicating artery where it joins the internal carotid artery. This junction lies in close approximation to the oculomotor nerve as it passes from the posterior to the middle fossa. Bilateral paresis of the extremities suggests that the bleeding site is near the anterior cerebral–anterior communicating artery junction and suggests extension of bleeding into both frontal lobes. Paresis or sensory impairment present from onset is most likely to be caused by intracerebral extension of bleeding, whereas neurologic signs developing later are more often due to arterial spasm.

Examination of the optic fundi in patients with subarachnoid hemorrhage may reveal smooth rounded hemorrhages near the optic nerve head, "subhyaloid hemorrhages." They are often unilateral and, when present on one side, indicate the side of the bleeding. They are venous in origin and result from sudden increase in intracranial venous pressure at the time of the intracranial bleeding.

Fever caused by the hemogenic aseptic meningitis is common in patients with subarachnoid hemorrhage, appearing usually one to three days after onset and reaching 38 to 39° C. Greater elevations of body temperature usually suggest intraventricular or intracerebral extension of bleeding. Subsequent elevations of temperature during the course of the illness may suggest recurrent bleeding, but they are more often related to intercurrent infections.

RUPTURE OF AN ARTERIOVENOUS ANOMALY. The symptoms and signs of a subarachnoid hemorrhage from a ruptured A-V anomaly are identical to those from a ruptured aneurysm, because both bleed into the subarachnoid space or into the brain tissues. Bleeding into surrounding brain is common for a ruptured A-V anomaly, and symptoms and signs are like those of intracerebral hemorrhage from other causes. Seizures may occur at the onset of bleeding and are nearly always focal in pattern. The diagnosis of A-V anomaly is suggested by a history of pre-existing focal seizures or focal neurologic signs and of recurrent, always unilateral, vascular headache, each of which occurs in about a third of the patients. Rupture of A-V is more frequent at a younger age than is rupture of aneurysms, so that a history of focal seizures in a young patient with subarachnoid hemorrhage makes the diagnosis of arteriovenous anomaly particularly likely.

When the patient with an A-V malformation is examined, in addition to signs of meningeal irritation and focal neurologic defects, careful auscultation may disclose an audible bruit over the eyes or skull. Although bruits may be present with either A-V anomalies or aneurysms, they are more common with the former.

INTRACEREBRAL HEMORRHAGE. When intracranial hemorrhage occurs directly into the substance of the brain, the onset of symptoms is usually abrupt. Severe headache, nausea, and vomiting occur and sometimes precede other signs of a neurologic deficit or loss of consciousness by several hours. These early symptoms are the result of an acute increase in intracranial pressure. Focal neurologic dysfunction follows, with hemiplegia or hemisensory defects; this results from disruption or distortion of the main motor and sensory pathways in the cerebrum. Loss of consciousness within minutes after the onset occurs in more than one third of patients and indicates a large hemorrhage, intraventricular bleeding, or both. Among patients who are not initially in coma, half deteriorate with decline of awareness and eventually lapse into coma. With the progressive decline in consciousness, patients may show neurologic signs at first, indicating functional decortication and later indicating decerebration. This sequence follows herniation of the brain through the tentorial space with secondary brainstem compression.

In patients who retain consciousness but have motor or sensory deficits, it can be difficult to differentiate intracerebral hemorrhage from cerebral infarction until the cerebrospinal fluid is examined and found to be bloody. In about 20 per cent of patients, the intracerebral hemorrhage is circumscribed, and the fluid never becomes bloody. In these instances, except for the higher incidence of headache with intracerebral hemorrhage, it may be impossible to differentiate intracerebral hemorrhage from cerebral infarction.

The clinical picture produced by intracerebral hemorrhages at various sites is often characteristic and may enable an accurate localization of bleeding.

Capsular or Putamen Hemorrhage. Intracerebral bleeding into the region of the internal capsule causes abrupt flaccid hemiplegia, loss of sensory perception, and homonymous hemianopia. Capsular hemorrhages in the dominant hemisphere produce aphasia. When the hemorrhage is large, loss of consciousness promptly follows. With small hemorrhages changes are less severe. Paralysis is usually more prominent than sensory impairment, and paralysis of gaze to the side opposite the hemorrhage may be found.

Thalamic Hemorrhage. Hemorrhage into the thalamus also produces abrupt motor deficits, but in addition an impairment of all modalities of sensory perception is common and more prominent than deficits in motility or the visual fields. Consciousness is less likely to be lost with a thalamic than with a capsular hemorrhage. Thalamic hemorrhages are associated with distinct disturbances in eye movements. Patients commonly show paralysis of upward gaze. At rest, their eyes deviate downward and laterally and they are unable to look up on command or reflex. The pupils may be unequal and react poorly to light. There may be partial oculomotor palsy with ptosis and loss of convergence. The mechanism that causes the gaze palsy is compression of the region of the posterior commissure and the adjacent upper brainstem nuclei. Because the disturbances in gaze gradually clear, actual tissue destruction from extension of the hemorrhage into this area is probably not the cause of the defect.

Cerebellar and Brainstem Hemorrhage. Parenchymal hemorrhage in the posterior fossa can occur either in the cerebellar hemispheres or in the brainstem (usually pons). With intracerebellar hemorrhage, the patient may experience sudden severe occipital headache, diplopia, nystagmus, and ataxia. Examination reveals miosis, conjugate gaze palsy, and irregular respiration. In some subjects, these symptoms and signs may be present for several hours before any loss of consciousness; in others, loss of consciousness is immediate. When warning symptoms occur, the diagnosis can often be made from the clinical examination alone, and prompt evacuation of the hematoma can be lifesaving. Hemorrhage into the brainstem causes immediate impairment of consciousness, irregular breathing, pinpoint pupils, and quadriplegia followed by a rapid decline to death.

LABORATORY FINDINGS IN INTRACRANIAL BLEEDING

COMPUTERIZED TRANSAXIAL TOMOGRAPHY. Blood is more dense than brain tissue, and CAT scanning yields the diagnosis of most parenchymal hemorrhages greater than approximately 1 cm in diameter. Contrast enhancement with iodine accentuates the demarcation of such lesions.

CEREBROSPINAL FLUID EXAMINATION. Lumbar puncture can be safely carried out on most patients suspected of having intracranial hemorrhage, but should be done with caution when there is evidence of impaired consciousness or a progressive decline in awareness and focal neurologic defects. These signs indicate both extensive brain damage and the possibility of brainstem compression. With suspected intracerebral hemorrhages and hematoma, there is always the possibility of tentorial herniation, which may be precipitated or accentuated by changes in cerebrospinal fluid pressure

after puncture. In such instances lumbar puncture is best postponed until after CAT scanning has been carried out.

Examination of the cerebrospinal fluid shortly after the onset of intracranial bleeding (1 to 24 hours) reveals red cells with a constant red cell count in sequential samples. The supernatant fluid of a centrifuged specimen will have a pink color owing to the presence of oxyhemoglobin. The fluid reacts positively with benzidine. Cerebrospinal fluid examined after 24 hours will begin to show, in addition, a yellowish coloration (xanthochromia) caused by the degradation of oxyhemoglobin to bilirubin. This intensifies over a period of several days and usually reaches peak intensity at 36 to 48 hours after the onset of bleeding.

Bloody fluid caused by a traumatic lumbar puncture is indicated by the absence of pink or yellow discoloration of the centrifuged supernatant cerebrospinal fluid, i.e., not xanthochromic, by failure to obtain a positive benzidine test for hemoglobin in the supernatant fluid, and by a decreasing red cell count in sequential samples of the fluid. When there is still doubt about whether a traumatic lumbar puncture is the cause of bleeding, examination of the supernatant cerebrospinal fluid by spectrophotometry is helpful in proving that invisible amounts of hematin or bilirubin are not present and thus confirming the traumatic nature of the lumbar puncture.

The white cell count in the CSF, when determined shortly after bleeding, will be commensurate with the amount of bleeding — usually one white cell for every 1000 red cells. When the white cell count is made on specimens collected 12 hours or more after the onset of bleeding, it may be elevated. This increase in white cells is caused by the inflammatory reaction in the meninges and may reach levels as high as 500 per cubic millimeter. Early in the course of the inflammatory reaction, the cells may be polymorphonuclear leukocytes and lymphocytes; later, the cells are all lymphocytes.

An exudative reaction accompanies intracranial hemorrhage, and the cerebrospinal fluid protein is usually elevated to levels around 100 mg per 100 ml or more. During fresh bleeding, for each 10,000 red cells in the fluid, the protein is said to rise 15 mg per 100 ml. Protein elevations are maximal eight to ten days after bleeding and decline thereafter. The cerebrospinal fluid pressure is often elevated to levels of 200 to 300 mm (of CSF) with subarachnoid hemorrhage. Elevations may be much higher, 300 to 500 mm with large intracerebral hemorrhages. The white count in the peripheral blood can be elevated to levels up to 15,000, and some patients have a transient albuminuria and glycosuria.

ARTERIOGRAPHY. It is often impossible on clinical grounds alone to distinguish between a bleeding aneurysm, a bleeding A-V anomaly, or intracerebral bleeding of unknown cause. Cerebral arteriography is necessary to demonstrate the cause. Thus if the patient is a satisfactory operative risk, arteriography should be performed as soon as possible with the hope that specific treatment can be instituted.

Arteriography is most useful in demonstrating aneurysms and A-V anomalies. In patients with suspected ruptured aneurysm, cerebral angiograms will demonstrate the aneurysm in over 80 per cent of instances. They may also indicate whether the aneurysm can be approached surgically. In addition to the aneurysm, the angiogram may reveal distortion of the usual vessel patterns near the aneurysm, indicating a hematoma, and frequently there will be arterial narrowing. The technical details of arteriography are discussed elsewhere; however, the physician should see to it that the intracranial branches of both the right and left carotid arteries are visualized to determine whether more than one aneurysm is present. When more than one aneurysm is present, it is often difficult to determine which one ruptured. Points that are helpful are that the bleeding aneurysm is often irregular in outline and, in the surrounding area, there may be distortion of other vessels, suggesting a local hematoma, or the nearby vessels may show narrowing. Local hematoma is the most reliable evidence of bleeding. If an aneurysm is not seen in the carotid arterial tree, the vertebral and basilar arteries and their branches should be visualized. The demonstration of an aneurysm on the distal branches of the middle or anterior cerebral arteries is almost diagnostic of mycotic aneurysm.

A-V anomalies are readily demonstrated in cerebral angiograms, as the usually large flow of blood through these structures produces a characteristic picture of early arterial filling and venous drainage of the anomalous vessels.

Intracerebral hemorrhage often can be visualized on cerebral angiograms. Shift of midline vessels, widening of the space between the anterior and middle cerebral arteries, and downward or upward displacement of the middle cerebral branches are helpful evidence. However, roughly a quarter of small hematomas (20 to 30 per cent) escape detection by angiograms.

When hemorrhage has occurred into a cerebral neoplasm, angiograms help in demonstrating vascular changes suggestive of tumor. In addition to vessel distortion and shift of midline vessels, abnormal vessels in the tumor may fill with contrast media and produce a so-called "tumor stain."

PROGNOSIS

RUPTURED ANEURYSM. Subarachnoid bleeding from a ruptured aneurysm is extremely serious; the mortality rate is 45 per cent for each major attack, and there is a high risk of recurrence. Among those who succumb to bleeding, about one third do so within the first 48 hours, another one third within the next month, and the remainder from later major recurrences. Recurrence strikes about one patient in three, with the maximal danger during the first two weeks after the initial bleeding, when about 60 per cent of all rebleeding occurs. However, some patients bleed during the third and fourth weeks and about 20 per cent have late recurrences, most of which are within the first six months after leaving the hospital. Fatal recurrences have been reported as long as 20 years after the initial bleeding, and there is no way to predict which patient will have a recurrence of bleeding or when he or she is likely to have it. The high mortality and the frequency of recurrence make accurate statements of prognosis impossible for individual patients. In general, the longer a patient survives after the initial bleeding, the less are the chances of recurrence. Data submitted to the National Co-operative Study of Subarachnoid Hemorrhage indi-

cate that if a patient with subarachnoid hemorrhage is alive one week after onset, the chance of surviving five more weeks is 65 per cent. Patients living two weeks without recurrence have a 76 per cent chance of living four more weeks. Patients 20 to 50 years of age have a better chance of survival than those over 60. As might be expected, patients with the least neural damage and the least impairment of consciousness have the best chance of survival. Long-term prognosis studied during a ten-year period of follow-up indicates that for patients with aneurysm who are alive six months after subarachnoid hemorrhage, rebleeding occurs at a rate of 3.5 per cent per year, with mortality from rebleeding of about two thirds.

RUPTURED ARTERIOVENOUS ANOMALY. The prognosis for bleeding from A-V anomalies is better than for aneurysm. The initial mortality is about 25 per cent and the possibility of recurrence less than that. Because of their location and the tendency to bleed into brain tissue, the neurologic disability among survivors of bleeding A-V anomalies tends to be high. Seizures with A-V anomalies are common before bleeding, and patients who do not have seizures often develop them after bleeding.

HYPERTENSIVE VASCULAR DISEASE. The prognosis for intracerebral hemorrhage from hypertensive vascular disease is poor; the over-all mortality is more than 50 per cent. Mortality is highest with hemorrhage into the ventricle or when severe brain edema causes temporal lobe herniation with resultant compression of the midbrain. The initial mortality rises with the age of the patient. It is about 40 per cent for patients in the 40 to 60 age range, 50 per cent in patients over 60 and 80 per cent in patients over 70. Patients who are in coma when first seen have a mortality rate of 70 to 100 per cent. Recurrence of intracerebral hemorrhage is uncommon, but tissue destruction and displacement at the time of bleeding cause serious neural damage and residual neurologic dysfunction. Patients with small intracerebral hemorrhages usually are left with only slight disability.

TREATMENT

The treatment of intracranial hemorrhage has three goals: preserving life, reducing disability, and preventing recurrence. Treatment directed toward preservation of life is similar for all causes of intracranial hemorrhage and for most other life-threatening neurologic illnesses. During the acute phase of intracranial hemorrhage, the patient should be in bed for as long as the symptoms of headache, stiff neck, and prostration require. Rebleeding is unlikely with ruptured A-V anomaly and hypertensive vascular disease, and a patient with one of these disorders need not be kept in bed for a long period once he feels well enough to get up. Just when to mobilize the patient with subarachnoid hemorrhage from intracranial aneurysm is a question more difficult to answer. Four to six weeks of bed rest is usually recommended, because this is the period of maximal danger from rebleeding. Recurrent hemorrhage has been noted to occur with straining at stool and with other activity, and rest in bed is believed to lessen the chances for potentially dangerous activity.

When the patient is in coma or has impaired consciousness after intracranial hemorrhage, meticulous care must be taken to maintain an adequate airway, blood pressure, and fluid and electrolyte balance. The skin and eyes must be protected from pressure and irritation. The urinary bladder should not be allowed to become distended from urinary retention. These are common problems for all patients with neurologic illness and depressed consciousness; they are discussed more fully elsewhere.

Patients with intracranial hemorrhage who are conscious usually complain of severe headache and stiff neck. They also frequently are restless and delirious. Analgesics such as codeine sulfate by mouth or codeine phosphate intramuscularly in doses of 60 mg may be needed as often as every two hours to relieve headache; in most instances this also relieves restlessness. Other narcotics for analgesia should be avoided because they depress respiration. *Delirium may persist for as long as two weeks.* No specific treatment is indicated, but having a member of the family present at all times and reducing examinations and procedures to a minimum greatly reduce the patient's anxiety and restlessness.

Protracted stupor or depression of consciousness following subarachnoid hemorrhage sometimes can be attributed to progressive communicating hydrocephalus. CAT scans demonstrating progressive cerebral ventricular enlargement in such instances can be a useful guide to instituting appropriate decompression measures.

Initially, patients with intracranial hemorrhage should not take fluid or food by mouth for 24 to 48 hours because of the danger of vomiting and aspiration. Subsequently, it is best to give clear fluids for another 24 to 48 hours and then a soft diet. During the period of restricted fluid and food intake, intravenous fluids should be given in the usual physiologic quantities.

Constipation must be avoided. When patients require codeine for relief of pain, mild laxatives or stool softeners should be given if the patient is able to take medication by mouth. Otherwise, small enemas should be given every other day.

When the blood pressure is elevated, it should be returned to nearly normal levels, particularly in patients with bleeding from intracranial aneurysms. This should not be done rapidly, however, because of the risk of precipitating a hypotension-induced cerebral ischemic infarct. Methyldopa or reserpine orally or parenterally is usually an effective antihypertensive.

RUPTURED ANEURYSM. Prevention of recurrent bleeding from aneurysms is the primary goal of treatment and, in view of the close approximation of recurrent bleeding to the initial hemorrhage, should be attempted as soon as possible. Thus angiograms to identify the source and site of bleeding should be made as soon as practicable, once the diagnosis of intracranial hemorrhage has been made. Similarly, if the aneurysm is believed to be amenable to surgical therapy, this is performed as soon as the patient's condition allows. Patients with no depression of consciousness, who are under 60 and normotensive, who have no evidence of arterial spasm on angiograms, and who have minimal neurologic deficits are considered good surgical risks and can be treated surgically immediately if this form of therapy is indicated for the particular aneurysm. Patients with depressed levels of consciousness or coma or with major neurologic deficits are very poor candidates for surgery; operative mortality in this group is extremely high; operation, if indicated, should be postponed until improvement occurs. Patients over the age of 60 who are hypertensive and who have arterial spasm on angiograms also are poor operative risks, and surgery should be delayed until their condition improves.

The possibility that rebleeding is related to lysis of a clot plugging the aneurysmal sac has been suggested. Agents which inhibit the enhanced intrathecal fibrinolytic state that often follows subarachnoid hemorrhage have been evaluated to see if they decrease the chances of rebleeding. These agents include epsilon-aminocaproic acid and p-aminomethylbenzoic acid. Epsilon-aminocaproic acid must be given in large quantities, 20 to 30 grams per day intravenously, to be effective. Studies indicate that use of these agents reduces the chances of rebleeding and mortality. Complications related to altered blood clotting systemically are uncommon.

Surgical therapy is directed toward removal of the aneurysm or control of the bleeding by a direct surgical attack or toward decreasing the blood pressure in the feeding arterial tree by ligation of a proximal artery. Not all aneurysms can be treated surgically.

Some forms of surgical therapy are more suitable than others. In the past six years, several clinics and hospitals have worked together in a cooperative study to determine the type of surgery most suitable for a particular bleeding lesion. In the national cooperative study of ruptured aneurysm, surgical therapy has been found to reduce six-year mortality as compared to mortality in patients who did not have surgery. The reported mortality for patients with carotid artery aneurysm was 47 per cent; for middle cerebral artery aneurysm, 35 per cent; and for anterior cerebral artery aneurysm, 34 per cent. For those not surgically treated, mortality was 80 per cent. Carefully controlled studies in the United States and Britain have concluded that aneurysms arising from the internal carotid artery at the junction with the posterior communicating artery should be treated surgically, the procedure of choice being ligation of the common carotid artery in the neck or direct surgical attack on the aneurysm in good-risk patients.

The British controlled studies indicate that patients with anterior cerebral artery aneurysms probably do not benefit from surgery and may actually do worse. However, in properly selected patients, surgical correction of an aneurysm of the anterior cerebral or anterior communicating artery is beneficial.

The outcome of surgical treatment of middle cerebral artery aneurysms is more uncertain. In the British controlled treatment series, direct surgical attack provided better results in male patients, whereas women with middle cerebral aneurysms fared less well with surgery than when treated conservatively. The explanation of this difference appears to be that women are more prone to cerebral infarction after surgery than men. In addition, women have smaller, more fragile aneurysms that make surgery more difficult.

Aneurysms on the vertebral basilar vascular tree are difficult to reach surgically. The most successful surgery reported has been for aneurysms arising from the vertebral artery near the branching of the posterior inferior cerebellar artery.

Surgical treatment of ruptured intracranial aneurysm

is demanding, and should be performed using a surgical microscope. Surgical skill in this field is best maintained by frequent use. When physicians are considering surgery for their patients with aneurysm, these facts should be considered when selecting the surgeon.

If the patient is not suitable for surgical treatment or if surgery must be delayed, a program of medical treatment should be instituted as outlined above.

ARTERIOVENOUS ANOMALY. Surgery for A-V anomalies requires the tying of feeding vessels or the amputation of a portion of the brain containing the anomaly. The latter treatment is curative if the whole A-V malformation can be removed, but it is limited to those instances in which the anomaly lies entirely in or on the occipital pole or the frontal pole. The chance of neurologic disability associated with removal of A-V anomalies in other sites is usually too great to justify surgical therapy unless major disability had been present before bleeding.

Ligation of vessels feeding the anomaly has been recommended, but no carefully controlled evaluation of this form of surgical therapy has been done. Carotid ligation to reduce the blood pressure in the anomaly is also believed to reduce the chance of recurrent bleeding. Recently, artificial embolization with plastic spheres introduced into the feeding arteries has been reported to be successful in obliterating the anomaly.

Fortunately, the chance of recurrent bleeding with arteriovenous anomalies is less than with aneurysm. Also, bleeding carries a relatively low mortality, so that for most patients with A-V anomaly and intracranial hemorrhage, medical management identical to that described for ruptured aneurysm is the treatment of choice. The frequency of disability and mortality associated with surgical treatment is too high to justify its use except in highly special instances. Convulsive seizures are common with A-V anomalies and should be treated with anticonvulsants as outlined in Ch. 315.

INTRACEREBRAL HEMORRHAGE. Cerebral hemorrhage is a severe disease and one for which there is no satisfactory form of treatment. The immediate medical treatment was outlined earlier. It must include meticulous attention to the problems imposed by impaired consciousness and abrupt neurologic disability.

Whether and when to operate on cerebral hemorrhage is a recurrent question, and efforts have been made in this direction for years, although generally with poor results. Recently, McKissock and his colleagues in England carried out a carefully controlled evaluation of surgical treatment of acute cerebral hemorrhage caused by hypertensive disease, in which they showed that patients treated surgically fared less well than those treated conservatively. No matter what the treatment, patients in deep stupor or coma from intra-

cerebral hemorrhage rarely survive. For patients who survive the initial cerebral insult and become stable clinically, removal of a persistent encapsulated hematoma may lessen neurologic disability and hasten improvement.

Surgical removal of an intracerebral hematoma caused by bleeding from a ruptured aneurysm has been no more encouraging than when hypertensive vascular disease causes the hemorrhage. Patients with intracerebral hematoma from ruptured aneurysm are usually in coma and have severe neurologic dysfunction; survival in these circumstances is unlikely.

Removal of an intracerebral hematoma caused by bleeding from a ruptured A-V anomaly has been recommended for patients with neurologic disability. The results are difficult to appraise objectively, but surgical treatment has its best chance of offering relief if the patients have become stable clinically and have a well localized, encapsulated hematoma causing symptoms and signs of a mass lesion.

Patients who recover from intracerebral hemorrhage should begin programs of rehabilitation as soon as the effects of acute brain damage have subsided. Such a program begins with passive exercise of the paretic extremities to help avoid contractures and progresses to active exercises as voluntary movement returns. The program is as outlined under Treatment in Ch. 294.

Dinsdale, H. B.: Spontaneous hemorrhage in the posterior fossa. Arch. Neurol., 10:200, 1964.
Graf, C. J., and Nibbelink, D. W.: Cooperative study of intracranial aneurysms and subarachnoid hemorrhage. Report on a randomized treatment study, intracranial surgery. Stroke, 5:559, 1974.
McDowell, F. H., and Brennan, R. W.: Cerebral Vascular Diseases. Eighth Princeton Conference, 1972. New York, Grune & Stratton, 1973.
McKissock, W., Richardson, A., and Taylor, J.: Primary intracerebral hemorrhage. A controlled trial of surgical and conservative treatment in 180 selected cases. Lancet, 2:221, 1961.
McKissock, W., Richardson, A., and Walsh, L.: Anterior communicating aneurysms. A trial of conservative and surgical treatment. Lancet, 1:873, 1965.
McKissock, W., Richardson, A., and Walsh, L.: Middle-cerebral aneurysms. Further results in the controlled trial of conservative and surgical treatment of ruptured intracranial aneurysms. Lancet, 2:417, 1962.
Nibbelink, D. W., Torner, J. C., and Henderson, W. G.: Intracranial aneurysm and subarachnoid hemorrhage; antifibrinolytic therapy in recent onset subarachnoid hemorrhage. Stroke, 6:622, 1975.
Pool, J. L., and Potts, D. G.: Aneurysms and Arteriovenous Anomalies of the Brain: Diagnosis and Treatment. New York, Hoeber Medical Division, Harper & Row, 1965.
Sahs, A. L., Perret, G. E., Locksley, H. B., and Nishiotia, H.: Intracranial Aneurysms and Subarachnoid Hemorrhage. Philadelphia, J. B. Lippincott Company, 1969.
Whisnant, J. P., and Sandok, B. A.: Cerebrovascular Diseases. Ninth Princeton Conference, 1974. New York, Grune & Stratton, 1975.
Winn, H. R., Richardson, A. E. and Jane, J. A.: The long-term prognosis in untreated cerebral aneurysms: I. The incidence of late hemorrhage in cerebral aneurysm: A 10-year evaluation of 364 patients. Ann. Neurol., 1:358, 1977.

Section Fifteen INFECTIONS AND INFLAMMATORY DISEASES OF THE CENTRAL NERVOUS SYSTEM AND ITS COVERINGS

296. INTRODUCTION

Philip R. Dodge

The seriously ill patient with symptoms and signs of disease of the central nervous system and evidence of leptomeningeal inflammation presents a challenging diagnostic and therapeutic problem. Of crucial clinical significance is the determination of whether the involvement of meninges is primary, as in bacterial meningitis, or secondary, as in a variety of parenchymatous and parameningeal infections (e.g., encephalitis, brain abscess, subdural empyema). Central to this clinical problem is some degree of pleocytosis. Various bacteria, fungi, rickettsiae, viruses, and parasites may excite such a cerebrospinal fluid response. In addition, a similar reaction may be produced by a variety of noninfectious processes, including chemical irritation, hypersensitivity responses, and, occasionally, tumors. Elsewhere in this text many of the specific diseases that evoke an inflammatory response in the central nervous system and meninges are discussed. In this section emphasis will be placed on a systematic clinical approach to differential diagnosis and on the manner in which functions of the nervous system are deranged by such inflammatory processes.

297. AIDS TO DIAGNOSIS IN INTRACRANIAL AND INTRASPINAL INFLAMMATORY DISEASE

Philip R. Dodge

CEREBROSPINAL FLUID EXAMINATION

Because diagnosis rests in many instances on the cerebrospinal fluid (CSF) findings, the importance of a carefully performed lumbar puncture and of meticulous study of the CSF cannot be overstressed. The CSF findings characteristic of various inflammatory diseases of the central nervous system and meninges are outlined in Tables 1 and 2. Measurement of the initial pressure should be part of every CSF examination. In the presence of high pressure, just enough fluid should be removed slowly to allow for an adequate examination. Jugular compression (Queckenstedt's test) should be

avoided except in cases of suspected spinal cord compression. Deeply yellow (xanthochromic) fluid derives its color primarily from bilirubin pigment. In the absence of prior hemorrhage, this is most frequently associated with high concentrations of protein, and is often seen with impaired CSF circulation. Intense bilirubin staining of the CSF may also occur in jaundiced patients with meningitis (as in Weil's disease).

As few as 200 to 300 leukocytes per cubic millimeter will impart an opalescence to the fluid, and fluid containing thousands of cells will be turbid. The fluid should be examined promptly for cells in a counting chamber, and an accurate differential count should be performed on a stained smear of the sediment after centrifugation. In the event of a traumatic lumbar puncture, care must be exercised to ensure that an underlying pleocytosis is not missed. A gram-stained smear for bacteria should be studied. Recently, measurement of the concentration of bacterial antigens in CSF by countercurrent immunoelectrophoresis has proved highly reliable in the diagnosis of meningitis caused by *S. pneumoniae*, *N. meningitidis*, or *H. influenzae*. The test results can be provided within an hour. Whenever tuberculous meningitis is a consideration, a Ziehl-Neelsen or Kenyon stain should be performed on the sediment and on the protein coagulum or pellicle that frequently forms on standing. The India ink technique may outline *C. neoformans* in cases of cryptococcal meningitis (torulosis). The finding of budding forms of the yeast in CSF will help distinguish cryptococci from lymphocytes, with which they may be confused even by experienced observers; however, confirmation by culture is always necessary.

The CSF should be cultured whenever leukocytes are found or when an inflammatory process is suspected. A variety of media (blood agar, chocolate agar, thioglycollate broth) and various environmental conditions (reduced oxygen tension, increased CO_2 tension) are used routinely. Special media should be employed for the recovery of fungi or *M. tuberculosis*. The latter may also be injected into guinea pigs. Tissue culture techniques and inoculation of mice and embryonated eggs are used for virus isolation.

The concentration of protein in the CSF increases whenever there is interference with the blood-CSF barrier, as occurs with inflammation. In bacterial, tuberculous, mycotic, and carcinomatous meningitis the glucose concentration in the CSF is commonly reduced (hypoglycorrhachia). Although the mechanism of hypoglycorrhachia is incompletely understood, the high metabolic activity of rapidly growing cells, phagocyto-

TABLE 1. Initial Cerebrospinal Fluid Findings in Suppurative Diseases of the Central Nervous System and Meninges

	Pressure (mm H$_2$O)	Leukocytes per cu mm	Protein (mg per 100 ml)	Sugar (mg per 100 ml)	Specific Findings
Acute bacterial meningitis	Usually elevated; average, 300	Several hundred to more than 60,000; usually few thousand; occasionally less than 100 (especially meningococcal or early in disease); polymorphonuclears predominate	Usually 100 to 500, occasionally more than 1000	Less than 40 in more than half the cases	Organism seen on smear usually; recovered on culture in more than 90% of cases
Subdural empyema	Usually elevated; average 300	Less than 100 to few thousand; polymorphonuclears predominate	Usually 100 to 500	Normal	No organisms on smear or by culture unless concurrent meningitis
Brain abscess	Usually elevated	Usually 10 to 200; rarely fluid is acellular; lymphocytes predominate	Usually 75 to 400	Normal	No organisms on smear or by culture
Ventricular empyema (rupture of brain abscess)	Considerably elevated	Several thousand to 100,000; usually more than 90% polymorphonuclears	Usually several hundred	Usually less than 40	Organism may be cultured or seen on smear
Cerebral epidural abscess	Slight to modest elevation	Few to several hundred or more cells; lymphocytes predominate	Usually 50 to 200	Normal	No organisms on smear or by culture
Spinal epidural abscess	Usually reduced with spinal block	Usually 10 to 100; lymphocytes predominate	Usually several hundred	Normal	No organisms on smear or by culture; may enter abscess on L.P. and get pus
Thrombophlebitis (often associated with subdural empyema)	Often elevated	Few to several hundred; polymorphonuclears and lymphocytes	Slightly to moderately elevated	Normal	No organisms on smear or by culture
Bacterial endocarditis (with embolism)	Normal or slightly elevated	Few to less than 100; lymphocytes and polymorphonuclears	Slightly elevated	Normal	No organisms on smear or by culture
Acute hemorrhagic encephalitis	Usually elevated	Few to more than 1000; polymorphonuclears predominate	Moderately elevated	Normal	No organisms on smear or by culture

TABLE 2. Comparative Cerebrospinal Fluid Findings in Nonsuppurative Meningitis

	Pressure (mm H$_2$O)	Leukocytes per cu mm	Protein (mg per 100 ml)	Sugar (mg per 100 ml)	Specific Findings
Tuberculous	Usually elevated; may be low with dynamic block in advanced stages	Usually 25 to 100, rarely more than 500; lymphoyctes predominate except in early stages when polymorphonuclears may account for 80% of cells	Nearly always elevated, usually 100 to 200; may be much higher if dynamic block	Usually reduced; less than 50 in ³/₄ of the cases	Acid-fast organisms may be seen on smear of protein coagulum (pellicle) or recovered from inoculated guinea pig or by culture
Cryptococcal	Usually elevated; average, 225	0 to 800; average, 50; lymphocytes predominate	Usually 20 to 500; average, 100	Reduced in more than half of cases; average, 30; often higher in patients with concomitant diabetes mellitus	Organisms may be seen in India ink preparation or on culture (Sabouraud's medium); will usually grow on blood agar; positive skin test
Syphilitic (acute)	Usually elevated	Average, 500; usually lymphocytes; rarely polymorphonuclears	Average, 100; gamma globulin often high	Normal (reduced rarely)	Positive reagin test for syphilis; spirochete not demonstrable by usual techniques of smear or by culture; positive countercurrent immunoelectrophoresis
Sarcoid	Normal to considerably elevated	0 to less than 100 mononuclear cells	Slight to moderate elevation	Normal	No specific findings
Tumor	Usually elevated; may be considerably so	0 to several hundred mononuclears	Elevated often to high levels	Normal or greatly reduced; (low in ³/₄ of carcinomatous meningitis cases)	Neoplastic cells may be identified on smear, by Millipore filter technique or by tissue block
Viral	Normal to moderately elevated	5 to few hundred; but may be more than 1000, particularly with mumps or echovirus 9; lymphocytes predominate but may be more than 80% polymorphonuclears in first few days	Frequently normal or slightly elevated; less than 100; may show greater elevation in recovering stages (particularly poliomyelitis)	Normal (reduced rarely)	Viral agent may be recovered in tissue culture, embryonated egg or animal inoculation

sis, and impaired glucose transport may all be involved. The gamma globulin concentration may be disproportionately increased in certain inflammatory disorders such as syphilis, subacute inclusion body encephalitis, and certain demyelinating disorders (postinfectious encephalomyelitis, multiple sclerosis). In addition to the time-honored tests for syphilis reagin, countercurrent immunoelectrophoresis is also useful here.

RELATIONSHIP OF CEREBROSPINAL FLUID FINDINGS TO ANCILLARY CLINICAL AND LABORATORY DATA

An immediate etiologic diagnosis is possible only when the responsible agent is identified. However, the clinical and CSF data can help to exclude certain clinical entities early in the diagnostic study. For example, when the symptoms and signs reflect involvement of the meninges and there is no evidence of cerebral or spinal cord disease, primary meningitis is probable. If, in addition, the CSF contains about 100 or so lymphocytes, a normal quantity of sugar, and an only slightly elevated protein concentration, then bacterial, including tuberculous, and cryptococcal meningitis are less likely, and some form of aseptic meningitis should be suspected. (However, it should be emphasized that the CSF sugar may be normal on initial examination of patients with tuberculous meningitis and may be reduced in samples obtained subsequently. It should also be appreciated that on occasion the CSF glucose may be reduced in aseptic meningitis.) A history of exposure to mumps and manifest parotitis make a diagnosis of mumps meningitis probable. On the other hand, the same findings in the CSF in a patient recovering from varicella, especially if there are symptoms and signs of cerebellar ataxia, suggest a diagnosis of postinfectious (varicella) encephalitis. In addition to primary meningeal disease, parameningeal infections can produce CSF abnormalities similar to those just described. The coexistence of a progressive dysphasia, superior quadrantanopsia, and hemiparesis on the right side and a history of a chronic draining left ear should immediately direct the physician's attention to the diagnosis of a left temporal lobe abscess. Unfortunately, however, a definite diagnosis cannot be made from either the initial clinical or CSF findings in many cases. Every attempt should be made to amplify the immediate and remote history, including epidemiologic data. One should search for foci of infection adjacent to or remote from the meninges. The extent of the dysfunction of the nervous system should be defined by repeated neurologic examinations and by laboratory studies. In addition to culturing the CSF, blood cultures should be obtained, because bacteremia is present in about half the cases of primary bacterial meningitis, and similar CSF changes may occur in bacterial endocarditis. Secretions of the upper and lower respiratory tracts also should be cultured for bacteria and fungi. Enteroviruses cause aseptic meningitis and encephalitis, and recovery of these agents from the stools of patients may aid in establishing the diagnosis. The development of specific neutralizing and complement-fixing antibodies will help confirm the diagnosis. Acute phase sera should be obtained on admission, and a convalescent serum sample obtained two to three weeks later. A four-fold rise in complement-fixing or neutralizing antibody titer is usually evidence of a recent infection with that agent.

Roentgenograms of the skull, sinuses, chest, or spine may be helpful in establishing a diagnosis by disclosng a related focus of disease. An electroencephalogram or isotope scan may direct attention to a region of the brain that clinically is relatively silent. Computerized axial tomography (CAT), a noninvasive technique, is now established in the diagnosis of intracranial lesions and should be employed before resorting to invasive roentgenographic studies. Whether CAT will be equally reliable in the diagnosis of spinal lesions is now receiving study. Specialized contrast studies (myelography, pneumoencephalography, ventriculography, and angiography) are reserved for cases in which noninvasive studies are ambiguous or leave diagnosis in doubt. Occasionally the clinician must resort to a tissue biopsy; for example, the granulomatous lesions of sarcoidosis may be demonstrated in a lymph node or liver biopsy, and trichina, toxoplasma, or an unusual arteritis may be identified in microscopic sections of muscle tissue. Biopsy of the meninges or brain should be resorted to only rarely, but will at times help to establish the diagnosis in an obscure case. The pathologic findings in herpes, subacute sclerosing panencephalitis, and acute necrotizing hemorrhagic encephalitis are histologically specific enough to permit an exact diagnosis. Whenever tissue is obtained for routine histologic study, appropriate methods for the recovery of an infective agent should also be employed.

298. PARAMENINGEAL INFECTIONS

Morton N. Swartz

The three major localized intracranial suppurative lesions are *brain abscess, subdural empyema,* and *cerebral extradural abscess.* Of paramount importance in their early recognition and subsequent management is an understanding of the nature of the predisposing suppurative conditions and of the portals by which infection has spread intracranially. Not only must these conditions be distinguished from one another but they must also, from a therapeutic viewpoint, be clearly distinguished from meningitis caused by bacteria or other infective agents.

BRAIN ABSCESS

DEFINITION. Brain abscess represents a poorly or sharply delineated suppurative process of brain substance, resulting from extension from adjacent foci or from hematogenous spread.

INCIDENCE. Despite the introduction of effective antimicrobial therapy, the over-all incidence of brain abscess has not changed significantly over the past two decades (about 7 per 1000 neurosurgical operations). It is seen approximately one sixth as frequently as bacterial meningitis in a large general hospital.

PREDISPOSING FACTORS. More than one third of intracerebral infections are a consequence of an adjacent primary focus of infection: middle ear, mastoid, paranasal sinuses, face or scalp and skull (osteomyelitis, compound fracture with wound contamination, or craniotomy wound infection). Another one third or so are a consequence of bronchiectasis, lung abscess, empyema, skin infections, acute bacterial endocarditis, or congenital heart disease with right-to-left shunt. In the remainder of brain abscesses an underlying cause cannot be determined.

Subacute and Chronic Middle Ear Infection and Mastoiditis. Over one third of all brain abscesses stem from ear and sinus infection. Infection usually spreads from the ear by either of two routes: direct extension to the roof of the tympanic cavity or mastoid bone (osteomyelitis) and then through the meningeal covering of the brain, or by extension along veins of the inner ear through diploic vessels of the skull and through intracranial venous channels into the substance of the brain. Thrombophlebitis of the pial vessels and dural sinuses, by impairing cerebral circulation, may cause infarction of brain tissue and facilitate development of local infection. The temporal lobe and cerebellum adjacent to the ear and mastoid are the most common sites of otogenic abscess.

Infections of the Paranasal Sinuses. Frontal and sphenoid sinuses are most frequently implicated in "rhinogenic" brain abscess of the frontal and temporal lobes, respectively. Infection may erode the sinus wall and invade the brain directly or, as with otogenic infection, may spread by way of veins communicating with the cavernous sinus and brain.

Infections of the Face and Skull. Intracranial spread of infection from the face or nose to the frontal lobe occurs by way of a septic thrombophlebitis. Compound fractures of the skull may result in brain abscess, particularly when dura and brain are lacerated, leaving a nidus of bone or foreign body in the devitalized tissue. Such abscesses may develop directly after the injury, or as long as 20 to 30 years later. Occasionally, the original trauma has seemed trivial and been overlooked. Brain abscess caused by a pencil point introduced through the orbit has occurred. Brain abscess may complicate stereotactic surgery and ventriculovascular shunts.

ETIOLOGY. A wide variety of microorganisms cause brain abscesses, and a careful attempt to establish a bacteriologic diagnosis should be made in every case. A gram-stained smear of purulent material should be studied at the time of surgery, and aerobic and anaerobic cultures, as well as cultures for fungi, should be obtained. In about 20 per cent of brain abscesses cultures are sterile. In about 25 per cent, most often when there is a contiguous extracerebral focus, two or more microbial species are isolated.

Various streptococci (either anaerobic or non-group A strains) and *Staphylococcus aureus* are the most frequently isolated organisms. *Streptococcus pneumoniae,* formerly a leading cause of brain abscess, is rarely incriminated today. Enterobacteriaceae (*E. coli, Proteus, Klebsiella*) are sometimes isolated. Anaerobic bacteria (streptococci, *Bacteroides* species, *Fusobacterium, Veillonella*) are isolated from 40 to 80 per cent of brain abscesses, particularly those of otogenic or rhinogenic origin. Rarely *Actinomyces* and *Nocardia* species may be recovered from an abscess cavity. Of interest is the frequent association of pulmonary alveolar proteinosis with pulmonary and occasionally cerebral nocardiosis. *Hemophilus aphrophilus* and the fungus *Cladosporium trichoides* rarely infect human beings, but when they do they show a curious affinity for the central nervous system.

When *Entamoeba histolytica* causes brain abscess, there are associated lesions of the liver or lung in virtually every case. In Central and South America and parts of Europe and Asia cerebral cysticercosis (usually solitary cysts containing the larval form of the pork tapeworm *Taenia solium*) should be considered in patients presenting with symptoms of brain tumor. In the racemose form of disease, obstructive hydrocephalus results from the growth of cysts in the third or fourth ventricle. The clinical picture may suggest a diagnosis of pseudotumor cerebri. Very rarely the brain is the site of echinococcal cysts and granulomas of schistosomiasis.

PATHOLOGY. Abscesses resulting from direct spread of infection are found in the brain adjacent to the primary extracerebral site; those resulting from retrograde venous propagation are often located at some distance from the primary focus in the distribution of the nearest venous sinus. Thus, for example, cerebellar abscess from otitis media is the result of spread of infection from the middle ear to its deep venous drainage into the transverse sinus, and thence medially into the veins draining the anterior superior portion of the ipsilateral cerebellar hemisphere. Metastatic abscesses are usually found in the distribution of the middle cerebral artery.

Initially, the site is edematous and infiltrated with polymorphonuclear leukocytes. The lesion is poorly demarcated at this stage and represents a local suppurative encephalitis. Usually within two weeks of onset the center undergoes liquefaction necrosis. The surrounding zone of fibroblasts becomes progressively thicker and contains more collagen; this constitutes the wall of the abscess, and astrocytes proliferate in the adjacent cerebral tissue. Multiple satellite abscesses may develop and frequently communicate with the principal cavity. Since abscess cavities usually spread through the central white matter, they often extend to and through the ventricular wall, producing the dire complications of ventricular empyema and meningitis. Brain abscess seldom or never results from primary bacterial meningitis. Coincidental occurrence of brain abscess and meningitis is usually related to intraventricular leakage of the abscess. In support of this view, the three most common organisms in primary pyogenic meningitis (*S. pneumoniae, H. influenzae,* and *N. meningitidis*) occur only rarely as the cause of brain abscess.

CLINICAL MANIFESTATIONS. Age Incidence. Brain abscesses are most common in the second to fifth decades, but may occur at any age. They are rare in infancy, even in patients with congenital heart disease.

General Features. The natural history of brain abscess consists either of a subacute to acute febrile illness with headache accompanied or followed by localizing neurologic symptoms, or of a "stroke-like" or tumor-like development of focal signs and symptoms in which evidence of infection is lacking. A history of fever at the time of invasion of the brain by the infective agent may be elicited; but a third of patients will lack a history of fever and remain afebrile under observation. Blood cultures are usually sterile except in those with an underlying acute bacterial endocarditis.

Headache, the most frequent initial symptom of brain abscess, may develop suddenly or insidiously while the attention of the patient and physician is directed toward the primary infection of ear, sinus, or lung. The development of unexplained headaches in a child with congenital cyanotic heart disease should be regarded as due to abscess until proved otherwise. The headache may be localized to the side of the abscess, but it is often generalized and increases in severity as the infection progresses. Heightened intracranial pressure, manifested by nausea, vomiting, drowsiness, bradycardia, confusion, and stupor, is common. Papilledema is a relatively late finding that is recognized in a minority of cases. The increased intracranial pressure may result in signs of sixth- and, less often, in those of third-nerve palsy. They are often false localizing signs, because the abscess may be remote from the cranial nerves. Although, pathologically, brain abscess progresses through several phases, there is no clear correlation with the clinical course of most patients. In some patients, usually those with metastatic brain abscesses, the illness runs a fulminating course, ending fatally in 5 to 15 days. In most, however, the course is considerably prolonged, and a diagnosis of cerebral neoplasm is often suspected.

Specific Neurologic Syndromes. TEMPORAL LOBE ABSCESS. The temporal lobes are the site of 30 per cent of brain abscesses; most are secondary to ear infection. Involvement of the dominant temporal lobe may produce a nominal (inability to name objects) or Wernicke's (inability to read, write, or understand spoken words) aphasia. Homonymous upper quadrantic or hemianopic field defects may occur. The only motor deficit may be a slight contralateral faciobrachial monoparesis. Herniation of the temporal lobe through the tentorium may develop precipitously and cause a homolateral third-nerve paralysis, coma, and bilateral pyramidal tract signs.

The presence of a second abscess should not be overlooked in a patient whose clinical state fails to improve or worsens after surgical treatment of a brain abscess. This is especially true in cases of temporal lobe abscess secondary to mastoiditis, in which cerebellar abscess may coexist.

CEREBELLAR ABSCESS. Cerebellar abscesses are almost exclusively otogenic and comprise 15 to 20 per cent of all brain abscesses. Increased intracranial pressure, suboccipital headache, and stiff neck may be the only manifestations. The patient may stagger and veer to the side of the lesion. Impaired coordination of extremities on the same side, with poor performance of rapid, alternating movements and with intention tremor, may be present. Nystagmus is frequent and usually coarser when the gaze is directed to the side of the abscess. Associated diseases of the inner ear may contribute to the unsteady gait and nystagmus, and may produce vertigo. Seizures do not occur with abscesses restricted to the cerebellum.

FRONTAL LOBE ABSCESS. Frontal lobe abscesses (30 per cent of brain abscesses) are most commonly associated with disease of the frontal or, less frequently, the ethmoid sinuses. Drowsiness, inattention, disturbed judgment, and impaired intellectual functions are common; the findings may suggest a psychiatric diagnosis. Mutism and increased grasp, suck, and snout reflexes are often present. In about a fourth of cases focal or generalized convulsions occur; deviation of the head and eyes to the side opposite the lesion is a common pattern of seizure. When the abscess is large or in the posterior frontal region, a contralateral hemiparesis usually develops. Rarely, dysphasia results from a lesion on the dominant side.

PARIETAL LOBE ABSCESS. Parietal lobe abscesses are usually hematogenous, but large otogenic temporal lobe abscesses may extend to the parietal lobe. Impaired position sense, two-point discrimination, and stereognosis are characteristic signs of an anterior parietal lobe abscess. Focal sensory and motor seizures occur. Homonymous hemianopia, visual inattention (often demonstrated by bilateral simultaneous stimulation of visual fields), and impaired opticokinetic nystagmus are encountered with more posterior and deep lesions. Dysphasia is a feature of inferior parietal lobe abscess on the dominant side. When the posterior parieto-temporo-occipital region is affected, there may be impaired recognition of fingers, difficulty in differentiating left from right, acalculia, and agraphia (Gerstmann's syndrome).

BRAIN ABSCESS PRESENTING AS "ACUTE MENINGITIS." Occasionally patients with brain abscess present signs of meningitis, including fever, headache, stiff neck, and pleocytosis; focal neurologic signs are usually in evidence also. The syndrome is most often due to leaking of the abscess into the lateral ventricle. Massive rupture into the ventricle is a catastrophic event, with high fever, shock, and coma, and should be easily recognized. Pleocytosis with cell counts of more than 30,000 per cubic millimeter and reduced sugar concentrations are usual. Bacteria can often be seen on Gram stain and can be grown on culture.

In some patients with a similar clinical picture organisms are not found, and the syndrome may represent the phase of "bacterial encephalitis." The important point to be stressed is that one should be alert to the possibility of a brain abscess in any patients with chronic ear or sinus disease who develop "meningitis." These patients often improve on treatment of the meningitis only to develop evidence of an intracranial mass lesion one or two weeks later as encapsulation of the abscess progresses.

LABORATORY DIAGNOSIS. Modern neuroradiologic techniques presently provide the preferred and safest first step in laboratory diagnosis. When the diagnosis is suspected on clinical grounds, then skull films, supplemented as needed by x-rays of paranasal sinuses and mastoids, should be obtained. Brain scanning is the next step. The radionuclide scan will show increased uptake in almost all cases. Plain computerized tomography (CT) affords a similar high rate of detection of abnormality in cases of brain abscess and, in addition, provides much more detailed anatomic information, as well as increased accuracy in definition of multiple small lesions and loculi. Contrast enhancement may reveal an abscess capsule surrounding a central area of low absorption. (It should be recognized, however, that similar findings can be observed with cystic tumors, hematomas, or cerebral infarcts.) Angiography is generally less informative than the CT scan, but may provide further needed data (capsular staining, anatomic localization) when only the radionuclide scan is available. The EEG in brain abscess is localizing in the majority of cases, showing high voltage slow waves and, occasionally, sharp discharges over the margins of the abscess. However, it has little or no place if the CT scan is available.

The cerebrospinal fluid may require examination when meningitis is suspected, but lumbar puncture should be approached cautiously when clinical signs point to a mass lesion already being present. If the CT scan reveals no marked mass effect and that herniation is not occurring, lumbar puncture may be performed with less hazard. Cerebrospinal fluid pressure is commonly 200 to 300 mm H$_2$O, but may be considerably higher, particularly in the presence of intraventricular rupture. The cell count varies from a few to several hundred, with lymphocytes predominating. In cases of intraventricular rupture of the abscess, cell counts may be in excess of 50,000 (mainly neutrophils). Also, cell counts of several hundred to several thousand, with neutrophils predominating, may occur during the early phase of brain abscess ("bacterial encephalitis"). The glucose level is not reduced unless there is a simultaneous suppurative meningitis. The protein may be increased up to several hundred milligrams per 100 ml.

TREATMENT. Early diagnosis and prompt antimicrobial treatment are crucial. Intravenous mannitol is often employed to reduce brain edema. Parenteral corticosteroids have also been used for the same purpose during the perioperative period. Surgery is usually required once acute cerebral inflammation and edema are brought under control, and consists of initial aspiration of the abscess cavity, followed in some cases by excision at a later time, or primary total excision of the abscess. The method employed depends, to some extent, on the site of the lesion and the state of the patient, but whenever feasible, primary excision is probably preferable. The CT scan does provide a noninvasive means of following brain abscesses that have been drained rather than excised with an accuracy not previously possible.

Since in brain abscesses penicillin-susceptible organisms predominate, 10 million to 20 million units of penicillin per day intravenously should be started prior to operation. If there is reason to suspect an organism not susceptible to penicillin, e.g., gram-negative bacilli from a chronic ear infection, then chloramphenicol or similar drugs should be given concurrently. One of the semisynthetic penicillins, e.g., oxacillin, should be used if a penicillin-resistant *Staphylococcus* is suspected. The antimicrobial therapy should be modified as necessary at the time of operation, based on examination of a Gram-stained smear and culture of the abscess.

In selected cases it is possible that serial (plain or enhanced) CT scans will allow the delineation of the preabscess stage of acute bacterial encephalitis or cerebritis (previously not susceptible to definition except by invasive procedures), and the observation of its resolution or its evolution to abscess. However, it must be recognized that corticosteroid administration may significantly reduce contrast enhancement and obscure demonstration of an abscess capsule.

Mortality from brain abscess remains high despite antimicrobial and surgical treatment. Residual neurologic damage is frequent, and seizures are a significant sequela (up to 70 per cent) so that all patients should receive anticonvulsants for 24 months.

SUBDURAL EMPYEMA

DEFINITION. Subdural empyema refers to a collection of pus in the potential space between dura and arachnoid. It usually results from extension of infection from primary foci in the ears or sinuses. It is an infrequent complication of intracranial surgery, and may rarely represent a metastatic infection from a remote focus.

INCIDENCE. Subdural empyema is about one fifth as common as brain abscess. Its prevalence has not changed in the past two decades.

PREDISPOSING FACTORS AND PATHOLOGIC FEATURES. More than half the cases of subdural empyema develop in patients with chronic paranasal sinus infection, usually frontal. An acute exacerbation of the sinusitis just prior to the development of the subdural infection is common. Osteomyelitis of the frontal bone and an epidural abscess often accompany subdural empyema. Chronic otitis media and mastoiditis result in subdural empyema less often than formerly. Postoperative infection, penetrating wounds, infection in subdural hematomas, bacteremia, pulmonary infection, and (very rarely) bacterial meningitis are other sources of subdural empyema.

Infection spreads from the sinuses or mastoid by direct erosion of bone and dura or through infected veins. Thrombosis of cortical veins is observed in 90 per cent of fatal cases. Once pus forms in the subdural space it spreads widely over the convexity of the hemisphere and mesially along the falx. Rarely, the exudate extends beneath the falx to the opposite side. Purulent subarachnoid exudate is usually present immediately subjacent to the subdural exudate.

ETIOLOGY. Streptococci, often non-group A or anaerobic strains, are implicated most commonly, but a wide variety of gram-negative organisms are also found. Postoperative infections are usually due to *S. aureus*.

CLINICAL MANIFESTATIONS. The symptoms and signs of antecedent sinusitis, otitis, or osteomyelitis often blend into those of subdural empyema. Swelling and erythema of the tissues overlying the primary infection may be prominent, and percussion of the underlying bone may evoke considerable pain. In the early stages, pain or headache is mild and is limited to the area over the subdural infection. As the illness progresses, headache becomes generalized and severe; concomitantly high fever, chills, vomiting, and nuchal rigidity develop. Progressive obtundation, culminating in coma within 48 to 72 hours, occurs in untreated cases. Focal or generalized seizures and hemiparesis are common. Sensory deficits and visual field defects and dysphasia also occur. Although these signs are in part attributable to the compressive effects of a mass lesion, the associated thrombophlebitis of cortical veins and the consequent infarction of cerebral tissue are probably of equal importance. In the late stages, intracranial pressure is severely increased, but papilledema is rare except in chronic cases in which the clinical course has been modified by antimicrobial therapy. Without treatment, death usually occurs within a few days of onset of focal neurologic signs.

LABORATORY DIAGNOSIS. The cerebrospinal fluid pressure is elevated, and the fluid characteristically contains a few hundred to a thousand or more cells (either neutrophils or lymphocytes predominating), a normal glucose level, and no organisms. Roentgenograms of the skull may show destructive changes in the frontal or mastoid bones. In the past, carotid arteriography and/or burr hole examination have been diagnostic and distinguished subdural empyema from brain abscess. Although experience is as yet limited with the CT scan, it appears it can show up extracerebral collections of decreased density associated with a mass effect.

TREATMENT. The patient with a subdural empyema requires prompt and adequate surgical drainage by multiple burr holes or craniotomy. Surgical treatment of the accompanying sinusitis, frontal osteomyelitis, or mastoiditis is a secondary consideration and is usually postponed until the acute intracranial infection has subsided. Vigorous systemic therapy with penicillin (10 to 20 million units daily) and/or other antimicrobials, depending on the background of the case, is begun before surgery and continued until the infection has been completely controlled. The results of smear and culture of pus obtained at the time of operation may dictate changes in the antimicrobial regimen. Bacitracin or other antimicrobial drugs are commonly instilled into the subdural space at the time of operation and for a variable period thereafter.

CEREBRAL EPIDURAL ABSCESS

Epidural abscess is usually secondary to mastoiditis, sinus infection, osteomyelitis of the skull, skull fracture, or infection of an operative wound. Etiologic and pathogenetic considerations are identical to those described for subdural empyema. The close adherence of the dura to bone limits the size of the epidural abscess. It often represents granulations rather than a frankly purulent collection. Rarely, an extensive destructive osteomyelitis of the frontal bone ("Pott's puffy tumor") may be associated with an epidural abscess.

Diagnosis may be difficult. The patient is not as ill as with a subdural empyema, and the size of the collection is rarely sufficient to produce focal neurologic signs or increased intracranial pressure. Fever, pain, and tenderness over the affected area are the common manifestations. In most cases the cerebrospinal fluid is sterile, and contains few cells (lymphocytes predominating) and a normal concentration of glucose. Many times the diagnosis is made incidentally at the time of sinus or mastoid surgery or when intracranial surgery is performed for an associated subdural empyema or brain abscess. Some cases of epidural abscess are probably cured by antimicrobial therapy alone. Spread of infection from the mastoid along the ridge of the petrous bone may result in a small epidural granuloma or abscess that gives rise to a homolateral sixth-nerve palsy and temporoparietal pain from involvement of the sensory fibers of the fifth nerve (Gradenigo's syndrome).

THROMBOPHLEBITIS AND THROMBOSIS OF MAJOR VENOUS SINUSES

CORTICAL THROMBOPHLEBITIS. The syndrome of cortical thrombophlebitis characteristically appears some three to ten days after the onset of bacterial meningitis. The signs include a secondary rise in temperature, focal or generalized seizures, and focal neurologic deficits, such as a hemiparesis. In some instances at least, the underlying phlebitis has its inception earlier and is the basis for many of the seizures and signs of focal cortical disease encountered in the early stages of meningitis. Treatment includes continuation of the antimicrobial therapy and anticonvulsants. Anticoagulant drugs have no established place in therapy. In most cases the process is limited in extent and the patient recovers, but,

when the process is widespread, substantial neurologic deficits and death may result.

MAJOR DURAL SINUS THROMBOSIS

Thrombosis of the large dural sinuses may occur in meningitis, may complicate epidural or subdural abscesses, or may develop during the intracranial spread of infection from extracerebral veins. (For spontaneous sinus thrombosis, see Ch. 294.) The thrombotic process may spread to connecting sinuses and cortical veins. Abscess formation within the thrombosed vessel may result in septicemia and infected emboli that travel to distant sites. The cavernous, lateral, and superior sagittal sinuses are most frequently involved.

CAVERNOUS SINUS THROMBOSIS. Infection can spread to the cavernous sinus through venous channels by three routes: (1) from lesions of the upper half of the face through the facial veins communicating with the angular and superior ophthalmic veins, (2) from infections of the sphenoid and posterior ethmoid sinuses, inferiorly, and (3) from the ear, posteriorly. The initiating infection is usually a furuncle, acute sinusitis, or an ear infection. The use of antimicrobial drugs in the treatment of superficial infections has markedly reduced the incidence of this disease. The majority of infections are due to *S. aureus*.

Clinical Manifestations. The general clinical features are those of severe systemic infection: chills, fever, headache, nausea, lethargy, marked polymorphonuclear leukocytosis, and bacteremia. The specific findings are unilateral initially but become bilateral as the process extends to the opposite cavernous sinus via the connecting circular sinus. They include, in the case of infections about the face, unilateral edema of the forehead, eyelids, and base of the nose, as well as proptosis and chemosis — all caused by obstruction of the ophthalmic vein as it enters the cavernous sinus. The superficial veins over the forehead may be distended. The retinal veins become engorged or even thrombosed. Retinal hemorrhages and papilledema occur but may be late manifestations. Involvement of the ophthalmic branch of the fifth nerve produces pain in the eye, photophobia, and hyperesthesia of the forehead. Partial or even complete paralysis of the ocular muscles develops as a result of involvement of the third, fourth, and sixth cranial nerves as they pass through the sinus. The pupils are usually dilated but may be small; the pupillary reactions are often lost.

In infection spreading by the inferior route (e.g., sphenoid sinusitis) the process may be less acute initially. A meningeal reaction commonly occurs, usually without organisms in the cerebrospinal fluid, but pyogenic meningitis sometimes occurs. Rarely, infarction and abscess of the pituitary complicate septic cavernous sinus thrombosis.

Differential diagnosis includes other causes of proptosis, especially orbital cellulitis, abscess, or acute carotid-cavernous fistula. Retinal hemorrhages, papilledema, and palsies of cranial nerves innervating extraocular muscles rather than general restriction of ocular movement from the mechanical effects of orbital swelling are useful differential points.

LATERAL SINUS THROMBOSIS. Thrombosis of the lateral sinus is almost always a complication of acute or chronic otitis media, of mastoiditis, or of cholesteatoma formation. Rarely, infection may spread in a retrograde fashion from a focus in the neck or from a tonsillar abscess. Streptococci, predominantly group A, and staphylococci have been implicated most frequently. The clinical manifestations include chills, fever, and signs of increased intracranial pressure. Pain, venous engorgement, and edema behind the ear may result from associated involvement of the mastoid emissary vein and may extend into the neck over the jugular vein. Papilledema is common; it may be unilateral as a consequence of extension to the cavernous sinus on that side. A generalized increase in intracranial pressure is more frequent with occlusions of the right lateral sinus, which is commonly larger and more important for venous drainage than the left. Convulsive seizures and obtundation occur, but focal neurologic findings are rare except when the thrombophlebitis extends into cortical veins over the convexity of the hemisphere. Rarely, ninth-, tenth- and eleventh-nerve palsies develop, presumably owing to involvement of the jugular bulb and related venous channels.

Cerebrospinal fluid pressure is elevated, and the fluid contains several to many hundred leukocytes (lymphocytes predominating) but no bacteria.

SUPERIOR SAGITTAL SINUS THROMBOSIS. The superior sagittal sinus is less commonly involved in septic thrombosis than are the lateral and cavernous sinuses. Infection may spread from the lateral or cavernous sinuses, from the pelvis by way of the vertebral veins, from a primary meningitis, or from a contiguous osteomyelitis and peridural infection. If thrombosis is restricted to that portion of the sinus anterior to the rolandic veins, and there is no associated involvement of cortical veins, then the process is usually asymptomatic. Thrombosis of the posterior portion of the sinus results in increased intracranial pressure; at times there are engorgement of scalp veins and edema of the forehead. Extension of the inflammatory process into the cortical veins results in infarction of the underlying cortex. Focal seizures, which alternately involve one and then the other side of the body, are characteristic. Because the superior and mesial surfaces of the cerebral hemispheres are particularly liable to infarction, weakness and sensory changes are frequently more prominent in the legs. However, hemiparesis, homonymous hemianopia, aphasia, and paresis, or conjugate deviation of the eyes may occur.

The cerebrospinal fluid findings are similar to those in lateral sinus thrombosis. A suspected diagnosis of major venous sinus thrombosis can often be confirmed by angiographic study.

Treatment of Dural Sinus Thrombophlebitis. Appropriate antimicrobial drugs in high dosage and surgical drainage, with removal of infected bone and extradural or intrasinus abscess, constitute proper treatment for major sinus thromboses. Ligation of the jugular vein in lateral sinus thrombosis to prevent spread of infected emboli is usually not necessary. Because of the frequent involvement of penicillinase-producing staphylococci, the use of semisynthetic penicillins (nafcillin, oxacillin) is warranted until cultures are reported. Since infarction of cerebral tissue from venous thromboses tends to be hemorrhagic, anticoagulants are not employed. The prognosis for recovery is reasonably good when optimal treatment is given, although there are frequently residual neurologic symptoms and signs.

CEREBRAL MANIFESTATIONS OF BACTERIAL ENDOCARDITIS

Neurologic symptoms or signs occur in about 30 per cent of patients with bacterial endocarditis, and represent the major complaints in one half of these patients. The neuropathologic findings of subacute bacterial endocarditis (usually due to viridans streptococci) are distinct from those of acute bacterial endocarditis (see Ch. 131). Diffuse embolic infarctions, with a variable and usually limited inflammatory response about involved blood vessels and adjacent meninges, constitute the major neurologic findings in subacute bacterial endocarditis. Pyogenic brain abscess and purulent meningitis do not occur. The clinical picture can resemble that of diffuse encephalitis or toxic encephalopathy, or there may be focal signs such as hemiplegia and hemianopia. The cerebrospinal fluid contains modest numbers of polymorphonuclear leukocytes (sometimes red cells as well) and a normal concentration of glucose; bacteria are absent. Mycotic aneurysms, occurring in 2 to 10 per cent of patients with endocarditis, are generally small and located at the bifurcation of peripheral arteries. They are usually asymptomatic unless rupture occurs into brain or subarachnoid space. Clipping of superficial aneurysms may be possible; occasional mycotic aneurysms, demonstrated on angiogram, have been observed to disappear on subsequent study and following antimicrobial therapy.

In acute bacterial endocarditis caused by invasive pyogenic organisms (usually *Staphylococcus aureus*), brain abscess (usually small and multiple), acute purulent meningitis, and embolic infarction of cerebral tissue may occur.

Brain Abscess

Ballantine, H. T., Jr., and Shealy, C. N.: The role of radical surgery in the treatment of abscess of the brain. Surg. Gynecol. Obstet., 109:370, 1959.

Garfield, J.: Management of supratentorial intracranial abscess: A review of 200 cases. Br. Med. J., 2:7, 1969.

Gates, E. M., Kernohan, J. W., and Craig, W. M.: Metastatic brain abscess. Medicine, 29:71, 1950.

Heineman, H. S., and Braude, A. I.: Anaerobic infection of the brain. Am. J. Med., 35:682, 1963.

Matson, D. D., and Salam, M.: Brain abscess in congenital heart disease. Pediatrics, 27:772, 1961.

Samson, D. S., and Clark, K.: A current review of brain abscess. Am. J. Med., 54:201, 1973.

Swartz, M. N., and Karchmer, A. W.: Infections of the central nervous system. *In* Ballows, A., et al. (eds.): Anaerobic Bacteria. Role in Disease. Springfield, Ill., Charles C Thomas, 1974.

Zimmerman, R. A., Patel, S., and Bilaniuk, L. T.: Demonstration of purulent bacterial intracranial infections by computed tomography. Am. J. Roentgenol., 127:155, 1976.

Subdural Empyema

Conrood, D., and Dans, P. E.: Subdural empyema. Am. J. Med., 53:85, 1972.

Hitchcock, E., and Andreadis, A.: Subdural empyema: A review of 29 cases. J. Neurol. Neurosurg. Psychiatry, 27:422, 1964.

Kaufman, D. M., Miller, M. H., and Steigbigel, N. H.: Subdural empyema: Analysis of 17 recent cases and review of the literature. Medicine, 54:485, 1975.

Thrombophlebitis and Thrombosis of Major Venous Sinuses

Brown, P.: Septic cavernous sinus thrombosis. Bull. Hopkins Hosp., 109:68, 1961.

Kalbag, R. K., and Woolf, A. L.: Cerebral Venous Thrombosis. London, Oxford University Press, 1967.

Krayenbuhl, H.: Cerebral venous and sinus thrombosis. Clin. Neurosurg., 14:1, 1967.

Ray, B. S., and Dunbar, H. S.: Thrombosis of the superior sagittal sinus as a cause of pseudotumor cerebri: Methods of diagnosis and treatment. Trans. Am. Neurol. Assoc., 75:12, 1950.

Cerebral Manifestations of Bacterial Endocarditis

Jones, H. R., Siekert, R. E., and Geraci, J. E.: Neurologic manifestations of bacterial endocarditis. Ann. Intern. Med., 71:21, 1969.
Kerr, A., Jr.: Subacute Bacterial Endocarditis. Springfield, Ill., Charles C Thomas, 1955, Chap. V, p. 92.
Ziment, I.: Nervous system complications in bacterial endocarditis. Am. J. Med., 47:593, 1969.

299. SPINAL EPIDURAL INFECTIONS

Philip R. Dodge

DEFINITION. Spinal epidural infections consist of purulent or granulomatous collections contained within the spinal epidural space and overlying or encircling the spinal cord, roots, and nerves. Infection may be localized or may extend widely, at times involving the length of the spinal canal. In one large series an average extent of 4.3 bony segments was reported.

INCIDENCE. This is a rare type of infection in adults, being less than one twentieth — and in children one hundredth — as common as bacterial meningitis.

ETIOLOGY AND PATHOGENESIS. *Staphylococcus aureus* is involved in more than 90 per cent of cases, but group A streptococci, other streptococci, pneumococci, *Brucella*, *Salmonella*, and various other gram-negative organisms may be responsible. *M. tuberculosis* is an important cause of chronic epidural infections in areas where tuberculosis is prevalent; occasionally fungi and parasites may be recovered from epidural granulomas. There is a primary infective site remote from the spine in most cases. This usually involves the skin, and furuncles, boils, and cellulitis are the common underlying infections. Less often infections of the upper respiratory tract, genitourinary system, or bone may be responsible. Hematogenous or lymphatic spread of infection to the highly vascular epidural space is postulated. Occasionally the responsible organism may be cultured from the blood. Minor injury to the back frequently antedates the symptoms of epidural abscess, and trauma may in some way determine the site of infection. The lack of restraining fibrous tissue in the epidural fat allows the infection to spread caudally and rostrally, and epidural abscesses may extend into the extraspinal tissues; in contrast, the dura is rarely penetrated. In less than half the cases the spine and adjacent soft tissues are primarily affected, and the infection spreads secondarily to the epidural space. Only in tuberculous infections is primary osteomyelitis the rule. Epidural abscess may rarely complicate a lumbar puncture, myelogram, or spinal operation.

PATHOLOGY. The purulent material or granulomatous tissue is usually most abundant over the posterior aspect of the spinal cord. When the primary lesion is in a vertebral body, intervertebral disc, or some other anterior structure, the abscess may be predominantly ventral. Epidural abscess occurs most commonly in the thoracic region, but may develop at any level of the spinal axis. The lesion may be purulent or granulomatous.

The mechanism of neural dysfunction in spinal epidural abscess is uncertain. Since the lesion occupies space, direct compression of spinal cord, roots, and nerves is a prime consideration, but the small size of many epidural abscesses, in association with severe impairment of neural function, demands consideration of other possibilities. The most plausible of these and the one for which there are some supporting facts is a vasculitis with secondary venous and arterial occlusions resulting in infarction of neural tissues.

CLINICAL MANIFESTATIONS. Heusner has divided the clinical picture into four phases: spinal ache, root pain, weaknesses (voluntary muscles, sphincters, sensibilities), and paralyses.

Spinal Ache. The spinal ache, characteristically maximal at the level of the major pathologic process, soon spreads axially and may also include the paravertebral regions. Restricted movement of the spine, especially in the anteroposterior plane, is common. A functional or even a structural scoliosis may develop. The spines overlying the disease process are tender to percussion; pain so induced may be exquisite, particularly when there is vertebral caries. Signs of sepsis (fever, leukocytosis) are prominent, except in the more chronic cases. The diagnosis is rarely made at this stage.

Root Pain. Within two or three days (acute cases) nerve roots inevitably become encased by the purulent material, and radicular pains develop. Meningeal signs are present in most cases, and headache is a common symptom. At times reflex activity at the level of the involved segment may be depressed. An erroneous diagnosis of "neuritis" or "shingles" is frequently made, but at this stage of illness the combination of clinical symptoms and signs should permit an accurate diagnosis.

Weaknesses. The characteristic feature of this phase of the illness is progressive impairment of neural functions below the level of the lesion, the exact syndrome depending upon the site of maximal damage. If the abscess overlies the spinal cord, spastic weakness, heightened reflexes, and a sensory loss below the lesion are to be expected. There may be urinary urgency and incontinence. Abscesses in the lumbosacral region exert their effects on spinal roots and nerves, giving rise to dysesthesias in dermatomes supplied by the implicated nerves, along with appropriate pareses and depressed stretch reflexes. Pain is usually excruciating and nuchal rigidity extreme. The skin and soft tissues overlying the abscess may be swollen, warm, and red. High fever and signs of systemic toxicity are often present.

The diagnosis may be made as late as this with reasonable anticipation that prompt laminectomy and drainage of pus or removal of granulomatous tissue will effect considerable if not total recovery.

Paralyses. Within hours or at most a few days, severe or even total paralysis of nervous functions below the site of the lesion supervenes. Immediate surgical treatment is mandatory at this stage. Procrastination may vitiate the effect of any subsequent therapeutic measures, for *most patients who are paralyzed for more than a few hours remain so permanently*. When an epidural abscess remains unrecognized and untreated, death occurs in 25 to 33 per cent of cases.

It is axiomatic that the foregoing analysis of the clinical features of subdural abscess is arbitrary and somewhat artificial, because the various stages may merge one into the other. Yet, considered in this way the early stages are stressed and the importance of prompt diagnosis and treatment is underscored.

DIFFERENTIAL DIAGNOSIS. Spinal epidural abscess demands consideration in the patient with sepsis, back pain, and even minimal neurologic symptoms and signs. Confirmatory evidence may be obtained by tapping the epidural space with an ordinary spinal needle. This is most safely done in the lumbar area. Gentle suction is applied with a small (2 ml) syringe while slowly advancing the needle. If no purulent material is obtained, the stylet should be replaced in the needle and the subarachnoid space entered. The cerebrospinal fluid (CSF) is characteristically clear and xanthochromic. It may be acellular, but more often a few cells or a moderate pleocytosis (lymphocytes predominating) will be found. Normal sugar content and elevated CSF protein are the rule (several hundred to more than 2000 mg per 100 ml). A partial or complete manometric block below the lesion is found in most cases.

An acute viral, postinfectious, syphilitic, or necrotizing myelitis may produce a neurologic syndrome similar to that seen in stage 4 of a spinal epidural abscess, and may be associated with symptoms and signs of infection and CSF pleocytosis. There may be back pain in acute myelitis, but the duration of illness is compressed in time. Furthermore, xanthochromic CSF and manometric block are unusual in myelitis. They are seen, however, in progressive adhesive arachnoiditis, which may be confused with subacute or chronic epidural infections. Spinal caries, demonstrable by roentgenography in less than 20 per cent of cases of spinal epidural abscess, suggests the correct diagnosis. In questionable cases a myelographic study will confirm the presence of a space-occupying intraspinal lesion. Rarely, malignant tumors, especially lymphomas that lodge in the epidural space, may present with fever, backache, neurologic signs, and spinal block. Chronic epidural abscess in which evidence of an inflammatory disease is meager or wanting will, on occasion, be confused with the more benign intraspinal tumors.

TREATMENT. Prompt laminectomy with drainage of purulent material or removal of granulomatous tissue and the administration of appropriate antimicrobial drugs constitute proper therapy. The antimicrobials must be continued in high doses for a minimum of six weeks when pyogenic osteomyelitis is present.

Baker, A. S., Ojemann, R. G., Swartz, M. N., and Richardson, E. P., Jr.: Spinal epidural abscess. N. Engl. J. Med., 293:463, 1975.

Heusner, A. P: Nontuberculous spinal epidural infections. N. Engl. J. Med., 239:845, 1948.

Hulme, A., and Dott, N. M.: Spinal epidural abscess. Br. Med. J., 1:64, 1954.

300. TRANSVERSE MYELITIS OR MYELOPATHY

Philip R. Dodge

Transverse myelitis refers to a clinical syndrome in which there is evidence of complete or partial loss of neurologic functions below a lesion which pathologically usually has a limited longitudinal dimension in the spinal cord. Thoracic and cervical segments are most frequently involved. Although inflammation is implied, it should be appreciated that evidence for this is frequently lacking, and thus the term transverse myelopathy is preferred by many neurologists.

ETIOLOGY. As a syndrome rather than a disease, the spectrum of specific causes is broad (see accompanying table). However, the cause remains unknown in the majority of patients presenting with the typical clinical findings.

PREVALENCE. No precise epidemiologic data are available. Although rare in general medical practice, the syndrome is not uncommonly encountered in a neurologic setting. Sixty-seven cases (44 adults and 23 children) were encountered over a 25-year period at the Columbia Presbyterian Medical Center in New York. Males and females are affected about equally. Altrocchi, who reported on this experience, excluded compressive lesions, serious trauma, radiation myelopathy, those with evidence of concomitant cerebral involvement, and those thought to have multiple sclerosis.

PATHOLOGY. The pathology of myelitis or myelopathy includes varying degrees of destruction affecting either white or gray matter or often both, usually in an asymmetrical fashion with this irregular pattern of involvement present over the longitudinal extent of the lesion. Patchy destruction frequently involves several segments of the spinal cord but may be even more extensive. Demyelination, neuronal injury, and incomplete or complete necrosis of neural tissue have been described and may at times be associated with inflammatory cells, macrophages, or proliferation of astroglia. The form of the reaction is probably related to the du-

---

Diseases Which May Present as an Acute or Subacute Transverse Myelitis or Myelopathy

---

 I. Myelitis due to viruses
   A. Poliomyelitis
   B. Coxsackievirus
   C. Herpes zoster
   D. Rabies
   E. B virus myelitis
   F. EB virus
 II. Myelitis of unknown etiology
   A. Demyelination myelitis (acute multiple sclerosis)
   B. Postinfectious or postvaccinal myelitis
   C. Necrotizing myelitis (? myelopathy)
III. Myelitis secondary to inflammatory diseases of the meninges
   A. Syphilitic myelitis
     1. Acute meningitis
     2. Meningovascular spinal syphilis
     3. Tabes dorsalis
     4. Gummatous meningitis, including chronic spinal pachymeningitis
   B. Pyogenic or suppurative myelitis
     1. Subacute or chronic meningomyelitis
     2. Abscess of the spinal cord
     3. Subdural abscess
     4. Acute epidural spinal abscess or granuloma
   C. Tuberculous myelitis
     1. Pott's disease with spinal cord compression
     2. Tuberculous meningomyelitis
     3. Tuberculoma of the spinal cord
   D. Miscellaneous
     1. Parasitic and fungal infections producing an epidural granuloma, localized meningitis, or meningomyelitis
     2. Idiopathic meningomyelitis (chronic adhesive arachnoiditis)
IV. Myelopathies
   A. Vascular
     1. Anterior spinal artery occlusion
     2. Dissecting aneurysm with occlusion of major radicular arteries
     3. Arteritis, e.g., polyarteritis nodosa, lupus erythematosus
     4. Malformations
   B. Nutritional deficiencies

---

ration of the disease and its cause. Thickening of small arteries and veins within or adjacent to the parenchyma of spinal cord has been prominent in only a few of the recorded cases. Because death rarely occurs in the acute stage of the illness today, recent reports characteristically lack postmortem studies employing modern histochemical and cytologic techniques.

CLINICAL MANIFESTATIONS. The onset is usually abrupt, with the neurologic deficit evolving from the initial symptoms to maximal disability within hours to a few days or occasionally a few weeks. A premonitory history of an upper respiratory or other infection or minor trauma is reported in about 25 per cent of cases. The earliest symptoms are (1) muscle weakness, usually involving the lower limbs, (2) sensory aberrations, (3) back discomfort, or (4) root pain, all occurring with about equal frequency. Signs may be asymmetrical, but bilateral involvement of the spinal cord is invariable at some time in the course of disease. Bladder and bowel dysfunction are nearly universal as paresis of the limbs and sensory disturbances progress.

The degree of paraparesis is variable, but moderate to severe weakness of the legs obtains in about two thirds of patients. Weakness may affect the arms in as many as one quarter of patients. Sensory loss also is seen in approximately two thirds of reported cases, pain and temperature being more often affected than position and vibratory sensation. Segmental paresthesias and dysesthesias may occur. Stretch reflexes are often lost in the acute stage of the disease but become exaggerated later. Babinski signs are usual. Meningeal signs are encountered in up to one third of patients. There is fever in about one half of patients, although this may be referable to complicating infections of lung or urinary tract.

The cerebrospinal fluid (CSF) findings are extremely variable even during the acute stage of the disease. In some patients the CSF may be acellular with only a slight rise in the protein concentration, but there may be several hundred or a thousand or more leukocytes, often with a predominant polymorphonuclear reaction in the acute state. The protein concentration may be elevated to several hundred milligrams per 100 ml, and the percentage of gamma globulin can be increased significantly. The sugar content is typically normal. Spine radiographs are unrevealing, as is myelography, except in rare instances when spinal cord swelling is extreme, impeding the flow of dye. In such instances there also can be a manometric block.

DIAGNOSIS. Although the diagnosis of transverse myelitis or myelopathy can be suspected on clinical grounds, it is incumbent upon the physician to consider first those diseases which demand specific and prompt treatment. Spinal epidural abscess can mimic closely transverse myelitis, although the course of the latter condition is usually more rapid. Contrast myelography should be performed if there is any question about the diagnosis. (Spinal CAT myelography may eventually replace contrast myelograms, but this is not yet the case.) The risk of the myelography is minimal, and the danger of missing a compressive suppurative lesion which should be treated by surgery is of overriding concern. Intraspinal neoplasms and other compressive tumors will also be excluded by myelography except in those rare instances in which an acutely inflamed, swollen cord may mimic an intra-axial mass. Syphilis, especially the meningovascular form, may mimic nonspecific myelitis and deserves immediate treatment. The treatable nutritional myelopathies evolve more slowly and have a pattern of spinal cord involvement which is more diffuse. Other evidence of vitamin B_{12} deficiency or of pellagra should make exclusion of these disorders relatively easy. A vascular nevus at the segmental level of the spinal cord lesion should signal the possibility of an intraspinal vascular malformation which can be defined by selective spinal cord angiography. Every effort should be made to establish the diagnosis of specific viral infections by appropriate cultural and serologic means. A diagnosis of multiple sclerosis may become obvious only when lesions of the central nervous system disseminated in time and space appear.

TREATMENT. There is no specific treatment for transverse myelitis or myelopathy of unknown cause. The efficacy of pharmacologic doses of the glucocorticoids is unproved but might be considered, particularly if there is evidence of swelling of the spinal cord. Prevention or appropriate treatment for the complications of paraplegia is critical.

PROGNOSIS. Proper supportive care, including therapy for complicating infection, prevention of pressure sores, and attention to urinary tract function, renders the prognosis for survival excellent. According to Altrocchi, one third of patients make a good or complete recovery, one third do moderately well, and a poor recovery characterizes the course in the other third. Lipton and Teasdall found similar results. Recurrent neurologic problems are rare among the survivors.

Altrocchi, P. H.: Acute transverse myelopathy. Arch. Neurol., 9:112, 1963.

Greenfield, J. G., and Turner, J. W. A.: Acute and subacute necrotic myelitis. Brain, 62:227, 1939.

Hoffman, H. L.: Acute necrotic myelopathy. Brain, 78:377, 1955.

Lipton, H. L., and Teasdall, R. D.: Acute transverse myelopathy in adults. Arch. Neurol., 28:252, 1973.

301. SYPHILITIC INFECTIONS OF THE CENTRAL NERVOUS SYSTEM

Philip R. Dodge

A general exposition of *T. pallidum* infection is presented in Ch. 171. The following presentation is restricted to a discussion of neurosyphilis.

Although the spirochete invades the nervous system and its coverings during the early weeks of infection in nearly every case, neurosyphilis develops in less than 10 per cent of untreated cases.

PATHOLOGY. Involvement of the leptomeninges is an essential feature of all forms of neurosyphilis. A meningitis of varying severity and extent is present in every case of active neurosyphilis regardless of the neurologic syndrome. The cerebrospinal fluid (CSF) reflects this involvement. Even in cases of *asymptomatic neurosyphilis*, in which the presence of syphilis reagin constitutes the sole abnormality, rare postmortem examinations have disclosed definite meningeal inflammation and ependymal granulations. Similarly, in chronic tabes dorsalis with negative CSF examination, evidence of prior active meningeal disease will be revealed by pathologic study.

Postmortem study of a few cases of acute *syphilitic meningitis* has shown a meningeal inflammatory reaction in which lymphocytes and plasma cells predominate. Cellular aggregates collect about blood vessels, and evidence of early arteritis may be found, although cerebrovascular accidents are rare in this stage of the disease. Reactive fibrosis of the leptomeninges, especially about the base of the brain, is also seen. This accounts for the cranial nerve palsies and for impaired CSF circulation that can result in increased intracranial pressure. A granular ependymitis is commonly present, and, rarely, this may obstruct CSF flow through the aqueduct.

In so-called *meningovascular syphilis*, which is typically a more chronic disorder occurring months or a few years after the primary lesion, the inflammatory response is usually less acute and meningeal fibrosis more prominent. As the name suggests, there is an associated arteritis (usually small vessels) that predisposes to arterial occlusion and consequent infarction of neural tissue. When larger arteries become occluded, infarction of brain or spinal cord may be extensive. In some cases damage to regions of neural tissue adjacent to meninges occurs without obvious vascular occlusions.

In general paresis there is direct invasion of neural tissue by the spirochete, accompanied by meningeal involvement. In tabes dorsalis and primary optic atrophy, the pathogenesis is unclear. There is no convincing evidence that direct invasion by the spirochete plays a significant role; whether a reaction in the meningitis is important is uncertain. On gross inspection the dorsal roots appear gray and atrophic, and the dorsal aspect of the spinal cord appears wasted. Myelin sheaths are damaged as well, and demyelination of dorsal columns is easily demonstrated by appropriate stains. Involvement of anterior roots with resultant amyotrophy occurs also but is exceedingly rare. Why the syphilitic process shows a predilection for dorsal roots is unknown.

In general paresis one finds on gross examination meningeal thickening, atrophy of cerebral tissue (especially of frontal and temporal lobes), and enlargement of ventricles; a granularity of the ependymal surface is consistently present. Microscopically, diffuse destruction and loss of neurons, especially in the cortex, are found, and special stains may demonstrate a heavy infestation with *Treponema pallidum*. Reactive gliosis is often extreme, pleomorphic microglia being characteristically abundant. Inflammation of the meninges is prominent, and varying degrees of arteritis can be anticipated. Collections of subependymal astroglia account for the granularity noted grossly.

Focal *granulomatous accumulations* (gummas) are rare, but may occur in the meninges and extend into the parenchyma of the central nervous system. More diffuse granulomas of the dura (hypertrophic pachymeningitis) assume significance when they compress neural structures, especially the spinal cord.

CLINICAL SYNDROMES IN NEUROSYPHILIS

Asymptomatic Neurosyphilis

As the term suggests, the patient lacks symptoms or signs of neurologic disease, although pathologic involvement of the meninges and possibly of the nervous system parenchyma is implied. The diagnosis rests on the finding of cellular, chemical, or immunologic abnormalities of the CSF. This is the most common form of neurosyphilis and constituted about 30 per cent of cases in one large neurosyphilis clinic. With adequate treatment (see Treatment) the development of neurologic symptoms can be prevented in most cases.

Symptomatic Neurosyphilis

Meningitis

Symptoms and signs of an acute meningitis are encountered only rarely by physicians, an incidence of less than 2 per cent among syphilitic patients being reported from one general hospital series. It seems likely that some patients with mild or even moderate symptoms go unnoticed. Symptomatic syphilitic meningitis usually occurs during the early weeks or months of infection, often during the period of the secondary rash or concurrently with a mucocutaneous relapse in a patient previously but inadequately treated. The illness is usually of less than a month's duration, but symptoms may persist for longer periods. Headache, vomiting, malaise, and irritability are prominent symptoms. Kernig and Brudzinski signs develop. Occasionally, confusion, delirium, seizures, and cranial nerve palsies (seventh and eighth nerves most common) occur. Argyll Robertson pupils are not part of the constellation of findings in acute syphilitic meningitis. Acute syphilitic hydrocephalus with evidence of increased intracranial pressure, including papilledema, may lead to confusion with other inflammatory and neoplastic conditions. But the diagnosis should not be difficult if the physician considers the possibility of syphilis. The CSF will always contain an increased number of white blood cells (average about 500 per cubic millimeter — usually mononuclear, rarely polymorphonuclear), elevated total protein (average, about 100 mg per 100 ml), normal sugar concentrations (reduced rarely), and syphilitic reagins. An elevated gamma globulin concentration will be found in 70 per cent of cases. The serologic tests for syphilis are usually but not always positive.

The response to therapy is generally prompt and gratifying, although an occasional patient will subsequently develop some other form of neurosyphilis.

Meningovascular Syphilis

Although the incidence of this form of neurosyphilis is difficult to ascertain, a figure of 3 per cent of syphilitic patients has been recorded. As with the other forms of neurosyphilis, men are more often affected than women (3:1) Patients with meningovascular syphilis present most commonly from two to ten years after the primary lesion. Symptoms and signs of meningitis are lacking, although headache is a frequent complaint. The major neurologic abnormalities result from the arteritis and consequent arterial thromboses. The neurologic deficits may develop slowly as the circulation through small vessels becomes compromised, or there may be an abrupt loss of function consequent upon occlusion of a major vessel. The specific syndromes depend upon the distribution of infarction within the brain or spinal cord. The patient may develop hemiplegia, hemisensory defect, dysphasia, or homonymous hemianopia. Involvement of the cortex accounts for seizures in a small percentage of cases. Various spinal cord syndromes have been described. A transverse myelopathy can be expected to to produce varying degress of paraparesis, sensory loss, and impaired function of bladder and bowel. Infarction of the anterior two thirds of the cord, with resultant paraplegia and loss of pain sensation below the lesion, follows occlusion of the anterior spinal artery. Sensory functions subserved by the posterior columns are usually preserved. Asymmetric infarction of one half of the spinal cord will result in weakness and impairment of light touch and position sense on that side and diminished pain and temperature sensation on the opposite side below the anatomic lesion (Brown-Séquard's syndrome).

Some abnormality of the CSF is always found in meningovascular syphilis. A lymphocytic pleocytosis (few to 100 cells per cubic millimeter) and/or an elevated protein concentration is characteristic. The gamma globulin content is often elevated. Syphilitic reagins are nearly always present in the CSF as well as in the blood.

The progress of meningovascular syphilis can usually be halted by specific treatment, but the degree of functional recovery depends upon the extent and location of the infarcts and upon the many complex physiologic factors that condition recovery in cerebrovascular disease of any type.

General Paresis

(Dementia Paralytica, General Paralysis of the Insane)

This dread complication of syphilis makes its appearance from 2 to 30 (usually 10 to 25) years after the primary lesion. It occurs more often in men than in women (3:1) , and 89 per cent of cases occur between the ages of 30 and 60 years. In one large series about 60 per cent of patients presented with simple dementia, and less than 20 per cent displayed manic symptoms and megalomania. Often faulty judgment, impaired memory (recent memory affected first), disturbed affect (depression or euphoria), or paranoia suggests the presence of a serious mental disturbance. This behavioral change will be especially noticeable when the afflicted individual has been a competitive member of society. Delusions and hallucinations occur less often but, when present, prompt a quick referral to the physician. The patient himself may complain of "nervousness," but characteristically lacks insight into the nature of his difficulty. Fine or coarse tremors, often affecting facial muscles and tongue, are present in about two thirds of the patients with fully developed general paresis. Abnormal pupillary responses, including Argyll Robertson pupil (see Tabes Dorsalis, below), impassive facies, slurred or dysarthric speech, exaggerated stretch reflexes, and extensor plantar responses are additional neurologic signs. Convulsions occur in 10 per cent of patients, and strokes secondary to vasculitis are also seen. When symptoms and signs of tabes dorsalis accompany those of paresis, the designation taboparesis is used.

The CSF is always abnormal, containing in excess of 5 white blood cells per cubic millimeter (mononuclear) in 85 per cent of untreated cases, and more than 30 cells per cubic millimeter in about a fourth of cases. An ele-

vated total protein concentration (greater than 50 mg per 100 ml) of CSF can be anticipated in 75 per cent, and a level of 100 mg per 100 ml or higher in about 20 per cent of cases. An elevated gamma globulin level accounts for the first zone colloidal gold (Lange) curve, e.g., 5554433211, which is frequently found in general paresis. Nearly every patient will have a positive reagin test for syphilis in the CSF, and in more than 90 per cent of cases the blood serologic test will also be positive. Incomplete, prior treatment may modify but will not restore to normal the CSF.

General paresis, once established, evolves rapidly, and patients soon become disabled mentally, socially, and, in the late stage, physically. The term general paralysis of the insane derived from observations of patients helpless and bedridden in the terminal stages of the disease. Untreated general paresis is universally fatal, usually within three years.

If the disease is recognized early and treated vigorously, about 80 per cent of patients will return to some form of work, but only in about one half will complete recovery be achieved. There is little hope of a satisfactory result when treatment is delayed until the patient is demented, incontinent, and bedridden.

Tabes Dorsalis

(Locomotor Ataxia)

Tabes dorsalis develops in less than 5 per cent of patients with untreated syphilis, and symptoms usually become manifest 10 to 20 years after the primary infection. Rarely, there is a latent period of 30 or more years. Men are more often affected than women.

Dysfunction of affected posterior roots accrues slowly, and symptoms develop insidiously. Impaired joint position sense frequently results in stumbling and difficulty in walking, especially in the dark when visual compensation is imperfect. As the disease progresses, this sensory ataxia worsens, and a broad-based gait is assumed. Profound hypotonia, secondary to a lack of modulation of muscle tension by afferent fibers, is expressed frequently in a slapping gait. Paresthesias usually appear early in the disease but may be ignored by the patient until the appearance of lightning pains. These pains are characteristic of tabes dorsalis but are in no way specific, because they occur in other diseases affecting dorsal roots, e.g., diabetic neuropathy. Lightning pains develop in at least 75 per cent of patients and may appear in any area of the body, although they are most common in the lower extremities. Some patients insist that they are more troublesome when the barometric pressure is low. They may be described as sharp, burning, or aching. However, sharp jabs of pain are characteristic. These may be mild or excruciating, and frequently flit from one region to another. At times they are so transitory that by the time the patient has made the natural move to rub or massage the involved part, pain has disappeared. For a period of hours or days one spot will seem particularly vulnerable, but then the site of attack shifts to another place. Involvement of thoracoabdominal nerve roots gives rise to visceral pains (gastric or visceral crises), which may simulate intrinsic visceral disease and may lead to unnecessary surgery; in one series an estimated 25 per cent of tabetic patients had undergone operation for tabetic pain. The converse is also true: on rare occasions visceral pain has been ascribed to tabes dorsalis and suppurative appendicitis, or a ruptured peptic ulcer has gone undiagnosed. As the disease advances, pain sensation may be so dulled that recurrent trauma is unnoticed by the patient and indolent ulcers of the skin develop; the toes and balls of the feet are especially vulnerable. Weight-bearing joints and adjacent bone, deprived of pain sensation, are destroyed by the constant trauma of use in 5 to 10 per cent of tabetic patients (Charcot joints).

Unless general paresis coexists, as it does in a small percentage of cases *(taboparesis),* tabetic patients are mentally normal. Optic atrophy complicates tabes dorsalis in about 10 per cent of cases or occurs as an isolated disorder. Pupillary abnormalities, including meiosis, irregularity, poor responsiveness to light and mydriatics, but retained reaction in accommodation (Argyll Robertson pupils), are present in most cases of tabes dorsalis. Involvement of other oculomotor functions is occasionally seen. Hypotonia, ataxia, and broad-based gait can usually be demonstrated. Affection of the sensory arc of the myotatic reflexes accounts for the greatly diminished or absent stretch reflexes. The Achilles reflex is affected more constantly. The plantar responses are normal in most cases of uncomplicated tabes dorsalis. Loss or diminution of position and vibratory sensation is found in every case. Increased swaying when the eyes are closed and the patient is standing with feet together (Romberg's sign) results from the impaired position sense. Variable degrees of hypesthesia and hypalgesia in a root distribution can be anticipated but may be difficult to plot. Isolated areas of hypalgesia (Hitzig zones) are sometimes found. Delayed perception of a pain stimulus (from one to several seconds) often can be demonstrated. Impaired deep pain sensation may account for a dramatic lack of responsiveness to squeezing of the Achilles tendon or testicles. Because of involvement of sacral nerve roots, functions of the urinary bladder and bowel are impaired in up to one third of cases; overflow incontinence and constipation develop. Impotence is a major complaint in the male. Characteristically a csytometrogram shows an absence of, or reduction in, the normal muscular contractions of the bladder in response to filling; the patient may be unaware of a volume in excess of 500 ml. Hydronephrosis and pyogenic infection are common complications of a hypotonic bladder.

Early in the course of tabes dorsalis, the serologic tests for syphilis are, as a rule, strongly positive. The CSF may reflect the meningeal inflammatory process with pleocytosis, an elevated total protein, and a positive reagin test. Late in the disease, especially after some antisyphilitic treatment, the serologic tests may be negative (in 25 to 50 per cent of cases), and even the CSF is negative in up to 20 per cent of cases.

The course of tabes dorsalis is unpredictable, and the response to antisyphilitic therapy is variable. In general, patients who have had symptoms for a few months or at the most a few years, with significant CSF abnormalities and no prior therapy, are most likely to improve with treatment. Patients with far-advanced disease and severe degeneration of dorsal roots and who suffer from the painful complications will not benefit significantly from antisyphilitic therapy. At least partial relief of pain may be achieved by analgesics, but when narcotics are used the risk of addiction is significant.

Recently, some benefit has been reported with diphenylhydantoin (Dilantin) treatment (200 mg per square meter per day). Recourse to spinal cordotomy and other surgical measures to relieve pain should be deferred until all medical measures have failed. Urologic assistance may be required to deal effectively with the tabetic uropathies, and surgery may be required for management of penetrating ulcers of the skin and Charcot joints.

Optic Atrophy

Visual impairment in syphilis may result from iritis, choreoretinitis, increased intracranial pressure (consecutive optic atrophy), or primary optic atrophy. Optic atrophy occurs in 1 per cent of patients with untreated syphilis and is five times more common in males than in females. It is stated that blacks are more prone than whites to optic atrophy, whereas the reverse is reported in other forms of neurosyphilis.

Because the outer portions of the optic nerve are first affected, the visual impairment tends to be peripheral in the early stages. Ultimately, however, the papillomacular bundle lying in the center of the nerve becomes involved, and impaired visual acuity and central and paracentral scotomas develop. It has been estimated that, without treatment, 50 per cent of patients will be blind in two years and 90 per cent in ten years. One eye is typically affected before the other. Optic pallor is usually present by the time symptoms appear, but in the early stages it is recognizable only by the reduced vascularity. A chalk-white disc with sharp margins and prominent lamina cribrosa constitute the fully developed appearance of optic atrophy. The optic atrophy of syphilis is indistinguishable from that caused by other diseases of the optic nerve in which there has been no antecedent papillitis or papilledema. The CSF is abnormal in most patients with active disease of the optic nerve. Intensive antisyphilitic therapy may arrest the disease process and preserve what vision remains, but return of vision already lost should not be anticipated.

Gumma

This rare complication of syphilis usually declares itself as an intracranial or intraspinal mass lesion and behaves in every way as a slowly growing neoplasm. The correct diagnosis may be suspected from a positive serologic test for syphilis or from CSF abnormalities. Frequently, however, the diagnosis is not made until the patient is operated upon, and histopathologic studies are made. Removal of the tumor mass, supplemented by antimicrobial therapy (see Treatment), should alleviate symptoms and prevent spread of the disease.

Congenital Neurosyphilis

Syphilis acquired by the fetus from an infected mother after the first trimester of pregnancy tends to be a fulminant disease. Miscarriages and stillbirths are common, and a wide spectrum of clinical manifestations may be recognized in the infant or child who survives. *Neurosyphilis* develops in an estimated 10 to 20 per cent of infants and children with congenital syphilis. *Asymptomatic neurosyphilis* may be diagnosed in the early months or years of life by doing routine CSF examinations on children of syphilitic mothers. But, as with acquired neurosyphilis, symptoms and signs develop only after a latent period that, in the case of *juvenile paresis*, may be as long as 20 years. More often symptoms first appear late in the first decade or during adolescence. Clinical syndromes and CSF findings mirror those found with the acquired disease except that *tabes dorsalis* is exceedingly rare and *choreoretinitis* more common. Hydrocephalus, cranial nerve palsies (eighth cranial nerve especially), and seizures may complicate congenital syphilitic meningitis, and syphilis should be remembered as a cause of cerebrovascular accidents in children. Previous studies emphasize that more than a third of all children presenting with juvenile paresis have been retarded mentally since early life. Although mental retardation is very likely due to other factors in some cases, such statistics emphasize the vulnerability of the developing nervous system to syphilitic infection.

Other non-neurologic stigmata of congenital syphilis include dental deformities (Hutchinson's teeth), saddle nose, frontal bossing of the skull, saber shins, and interstitial keratitis (usually developing during the second decade). These signs are not seen in acquired syphilis. Fortunately, the current practice of doing routine serologic tests on all pregnant women and on infants of syphilitic mothers has all but eliminated congenital neurosyphilis in many areas of the world. In this regard it should be remembered that the mother can acquire syphilis at any time during pregnancy and that negative serologic studies obtained early do not exclude the possibility that they might become positive later in the course of pregnancy. In some institutions blood from the umbilical cord is routinely tested for the reagin of syphilis.

Early and intensive treatment of infants with congenital syphilis materially reduces the morbidity (see Treatment) from neurologic complications. Unhappily, results from even optimal treatment of patients with juvenile paresis remain poor.

TREATMENT

Penicillin is the preferred drug for treating neurosyphilis. Reasonable therapy for adults with all forms of neurosyphilis, except general paresis, is a total dose of procaine penicillin G of 6 to 12 million units given over two to three weeks. A total dose if 18 to 24 million units administered over the same period of time is used to treat patients with general paresis. For children, approximately one half of the adult dose is employed, and one quarter of the adult dose is given to infants. We prefer to treat patients with active neurosyphilis in hospital (mandatory in general paresis), but this is not always feasible. When outpatient treatment is necessary, an initial dose of 3 million units of long-acting penicillin (benzathine penicillin G, Bicillin) should be given. The sole use of benzathine penicillin G at weekly intervals in doses equivalent to those presented above has been advocated by some in the treatment of neurosyphilis. It must be stressed that these therapeutic regimens are empirical. Nevertheless, they are reasonable and have stood the test of time. The author suspects that early diagnosis of syphilitic infection is far more critical than the precise dosage and the time course of therapy.

For a further discussion of treatment, the reader is referred to Ch. 171.

Clarke, E. G., and Danbolt, N.: The Oslo study of the natural history of untreated syphilis. J. Chronic Dis., 2:311, 1955.

Green, J. B.: Dilantin in the treatment of lightning pains. Neurology. 11:257, 1961.

Hahn, R. D., et al.: Penicillin treatment of general paresis (dementia paralytica) — Results of treatment in 1086 patients, the majority of whom were followed for more than 5 years. Arch. Neurol. Psychiat., 81:557, 1959.

Hooshmand, H., Escobar, M. R., and Kopf, S. W.: Neurosyphilis. A study of 241 patients. JAMA, 219:726, 1972.

Idsøe, O., Guthe, T., and Willcox, R. R.: Penicillin in the treatment of syphilis. Geneva, Bull. WHO, Supplement to Vol. 47, 1972.

Merritt, H. H., Adams, R. D., and Solomon, H.: Neurosyphilis. New York, Oxford University Press, 1946.

Montgomery, C. H., and Knox, J. M.: Antibiotics other than penicillin in the treatment of syphilis. N. Engl. J. Med., 261:277, 1961.

Section Sixteen   VIRAL INFECTIONS OF THE NERVOUS SYSTEM

302.   INTRODUCTION

Richard T. Johnson

Viral infections of the nervous system, in general, represent uncommon but important complications of systemic infections. With a few exceptions such as rabies or B virus (*herpes simiae*), nervous system infections are caused by agents which often infect man. Some of these viruses, such as polioviruses and arthropod-borne encephalitis viruses, cause clinically significant disease only on the rare occasion when the nervous system is involved. Others, such as herpes simplex and mumps virus, are frequent causes of mild disease that assumes a more serious form when the central nervous system is infected.

Experimentally, viruses have been shown to invade the nervous system by centripetal growth or movement in peripheral nerves, by penetration across the olfactory mucosa, or by a viremia. In man most viruses which infect the nervous system spread to the brain and meninges from blood, although neural spread appears to be important in rabies, B virus, and varicella-zoster virus infections. The infrequency of nervous system involvement can be attributed to a variety of host defense mechanisms, including cellular and humoral responses, interferon production, anatomic barriers of nonsusceptible cells, and the activity of the reticuloendothelial system which clears viruses from the blood. Youth, severe nutritional deficiency, and defects of cellular immunity have been shown to increase the risk of nervous system infection with some viruses, but in the majority of patients the factors which have permitted central nervous system invasion are not evident.

Viral infections of the nervous system can lead to diverse clinical signs and symptoms, varied clinical courses, and protean pathologic changes. This diversity can be explained by the following two principles: (1) the varied cell populations of the nervous system have different susceptibilities to different viruses; and (2) viral infections can have varied effects on susceptible cells. If infection is limited to the meninges covering the nervous system, then signs of headache, fever, stiff neck, and pleocytosis (i.e., meningitis) may be the only clinical manifestations. If the infection spreads to the parenchymal cells of the brain, in addition to signs of meningeal irritation, there may develop a depression of the state of consciousness, seizures, focal neurologic deficits, or increased intracranial pressure (i.e., encephalitis). Some viruses cause even more selective involvement of specific cell populations in the brain and spinal cord and thus evoke characteristic clinical symptoms and signs. For example, in poliovirus infections the selective vulnerability of anterior horn cells leads to a characteristic clinical finding of acute meningitis with lower motor neuron paralysis. On the other hand, rabies virus infections in animals tend to spare the cortical neurons involved in most types of encephalitis and infect neurons of the limbic system. Therefore, instead of obtundation, seizures, and motor or sensory deficits, the infected animal shows alertness, loss of timidity, aberrant sexual behavior, and aggressive activity. This selective infection of cells of the limbic system appears to be a diabolic adaptation of the rabies virus to specific cell populations, so that the clinical disease in animals can drive the host to transmit the virus to another host by biting. Glial cell populations may also be selectively involved, such as in progressive multifocal leukoencephalopathy in which virus infection and cell lysis appear limited to the oligodendrocytes, causing a slowly progressive demyelinating disease.

The virus-cell interaction may be quite varied. There may be *acute lysis* of the infected cell, transformation of the cell with production of neoplasm, or *chronic infection* causing cellular dysfunction, cellular degeneration, or no abnormality. In acute viral infections the clinical and pathologic abnormalities may result either from an acute viral destruction of cells, as in acute viral meningitis or encephalitis, or from the host's immunologic response to the infection, as has been postulated in postinfectious encephalomyelitis. A *latent infection* is a virus-host relationship in which the virus remains present in some form in the host without giving rise to any signs of infection, but which can, when some trigger mechanism comes into play, emerge as an acute infectious process. This appears to occur in herpes zoster and possibly in some cases of herpes simplex encephalitis. *Chronic viral infections* are those in which there is an ongoing active infection, which may give rise to a somewhat irregular or unpredictable course extending over many months or years. Chronic inflammatory disease of the central nervous system is seen with fetal infections by rubella and cytomegaloviruses. In these indolent infections virus can be recovered for long periods of time postnatally and may or may not cause continuing or evolving clinical signs of disease. *Slow infections* have a more predictable course than chronic infections. They are defined as infections with an incubation period lasting for months to years, followed by a protracted but predictable clinical course ending in death. Slow viral infections of the nervous system in man include kuru, Creutzfeldt-Jakob disease, subacute sclerosing panencephalitis, and progressive multifocal leukoencephalopathy (see Ch. 310).

303. VIRAL MENINGITIS AND ENCEPHALITIS

Richard T. Johnson

Viral meningitis is a benign, self-limited illness with clinical signs of headache, fever, and meningeal inflammation. *Viral encephalitis* is a more severe illness in which fever, headache, and meningeal inflammation are complicated by depression of the state of consciousness, seizures, and/or focal neurologic deficits suggesting inflammation within the parenchyma of the brain.

The clinical syndrome of viral meningitis is also called *aseptic meningitis* or *serous meningitis*, since some bacterial infections and chemical irritants can cause identical clinical symptoms and cerebrospinal fluid changes. Encephalitis is also called *meningoencephalitis* or *encephalomyelitis*, the latter indicating concurrent signs of spinal cord involvement.

ETIOLOGY. A variety of viruses have been associated with meningitis and encephalitis (Table 1). The two syndromes represent a clinical continuum and are caused by the same spectrum of viral agents. However, some viruses tend to cause predominantly benign disease such as the coxsackie- and echoviruses, which cause about half of all cases of viral meningitis but are only rarely associated with encephalitis. Other viruses tend to cause more severe disease such as arthropod-

TABLE 1. Viruses Associated with Acute Central Nervous System Infections in the United States

Enteroviruses
  Polioviruses
  Coxsackieviruses, groups A and B
  Echoviruses
Togaviruses (arboviruses)
  Eastern equine
  Western equine
  Venezuelan equine
  St. Louis
  Powassan
  California
Herpesviruses
  Herpes simplex, type 1 and type 2
  Varicella-zoster
  Epstein-Barr
  Cytomegalovirus
Myxoviruses and paramyxoviruses
  Influenza
  Parainfluenza
  Mumps
  Measles (rubeola)
Adenoviruses
Lymphocytic choriomeningitis virus
Rabies virus

*Data from Neutropic Viral Diseases Surveillance Reports, Center for Disease Control.

TABLE 2.   Frequency of Association of Agents with Aseptic Meningitis and Encephalitis*

Etiologic Agent	Percentage of Cases of:	
	Aseptic Meningitis	Encephalitis†
Enteroviruses	30	8
Mumps	16	16
Lympocytic choriomeningitis	9	14
Leptospira	4	2
Herpes simplex	1	10
Arboviruses	1	14
Other‡	2	2

*Data from Meyer et al., 1960.

†Fatal cases in this study (eight of 139) associated only with herpes simplex and arbovirus infections.

‡Includes infectious mononucleosis, *Mycoplasma pneumoniae*, Rocky Mountain spotted fever, and fungal infections.

borne togaviruses (arboviruses) and herpes simplex virus, which are the major causes of fatal encephalitis (Table 2).

Enteroviruses are small, nonenveloped RNA viruses of the picornavirus family, and include polioviruses, group A and B coxsackieviruses, and echoviruses. The three serotypes of poliovirus are now largely controlled by immunization programs (see Ch. 307). Over 40 coxsackie- and echovirus serotypes have been associated with meningitis and encephalitis; the serotypes most frequently recovered from patients with viral meningitis are echoviruses 3, 4, 6, 9, 11, 18, and 30, coxsackievirus A9, and coxsackieviruses B1 through 5. Echovirus 9 has been associated with the largest epidemics.

Mumps virus is a large, enveloped RNA virus of the paramyxovirus group. Mumps is the single most common cause of viral meningitis and mild encephalitis. Lymphocytic choriomeningitis virus is a small, enveloped RNA virus of the arenavirus group, which also causes both meningitis and mild encephalitis.

Herpesvirus are large, structurally complex, enveloped DNA viruses which cause a variety of neurologic diseases. Type 1 herpes simplex virus is associated with severe encephalitis in adults and represents the most common cause of endemic fatal encephalitis. Type 2 herpes simplex virus, a major cause of fatal neonatal encephalitis, seldom causes severe encephalitis in adults but has been associated with cases of meningitis. Headache and pleocytosis often accompany herpes zoster infections, but it is not known whether meningitis without radicular pain or cutaneous eruptions can be a manifestation of recrudescences of latent varicella-zoster virus infections (see Ch. 305). The Epstein-Barr virus has been related to meningitis and encephalitis, complicating approximately 1 per cent of cases of infectious mononucleosis. Cytomegalovirus, like rubella virus, is associated primarily with chronic congenital infections. However, cytomegalovirus also causes encephalitis in immunocompromised adults, but such infections are usually asymptomatic and found incidentally at autopsy.

The acute neurologic disease associated with measles, vaccinia, and primary varicella (chickenpox) infections, in most cases, represents postinfectious encephalomyelitis (see Ch. 309.2). This may also be true of the encephalitis which has occasionally been reported with influenza and parainfluenza virus infections.

The arboviruses are small, enveloped RNA viruses of the togavirus family. Over 20 different arboviruses have been associated with encephalitis in varied geographic areas of the world; six cause encephalitis in the United States (Table 1). Over 100 cases of California virus encephalitis are reported annually over a wide geographic area. Eastern, Western, St. Louis, and Venezuelan equine encephalitis viruses cause localized epidemics; St. Louis virus has been the predominant cause of major epidemics in recent years.

Adenoviruses are respiratory viruses which only rarely cause meningitis or severe childhood encephalitis. Nonviral agents which cause clinical syndromes indistinguishable from viral meningitis or mild encephalitis include *Leptospira, Treponema pallidum, Mycoplasma pneumoniae,* and *Rickettsia.*

EPIDEMIOLOGY. Over 5000 cases of aseptic meningitis and over 2000 cases of encephalitis are reported to the Center for Disease Control annually, but this represents only a small fraction of the total number of cases per year in the United States. Both viral meningitis and encephalitis are reported with greater frequency during the later summer and early fall, and this increase results, in large part, from the seasonal dissemination of enteroviruses and arboviruses.

Epidemiologically the viruses causing meningitis and encephalitis in man fall into three categories: (1) Viruses that spread from man to man; these agents generally cause disease during a particular season of the year and often in epidemics. (2) Viruses acquired from infected animals (zoonoses); these agents may have distinct geographic distributions, and a history of animal contact in patients is often obtained. (3) Viruses spread by hematophagous arthropods and necessitating a cycle in the arthropod host; these viruses have very specific seasonal and geographic limitations.

The enteroviruses are spread from man to man by hand-to-mouth contact and to a lesser extent by respiratory spread or by fecal contamination of fomites or vectors. Virus growth is primarily in the intestinal tract. Although enteroviral infections occur throughout the year, the incidence of these infections increases dramatically in summer and early fall, often reaching epidemic proportions. Because of the mode of spread, family outbreaks are common, and the spread of virus is facilitated in families or communities with preschool children.

Mumps virus is spread by the respiratory route. Mumps occurs throughout the year, but there is a marked increase in incidence during the spring. Although the incidence of infection with mumps virus is equal between the sexes, males develop meningitis three times more frequently than females.

Lymphocytic choriomeningitis virus is the major zoonotic virus causing meningitis and encephalitis. The natural host of this virus is *Mus musculus*, the common house mouse, and the virus is present in its excreta. Man acquires the infection by contact with contaminated dust or food. Human disease is more common in winter, when the natural host tends to move indoors, increasing human exposure. Recently, lymphocytic choriomeningitis virus has also been found in hamsters, and human infections have been traced to laboratory and pet hamsters. Leptospiral infections are also acquired from both domestic and wild animals. These spirochetes are excreted in urine and contracted by man through contact with animal tissue, contaminated soil, or water polluted by animal urine.

Each of the arboviruses has a different epidemiologic cycle (see Ch. 101). In the United States, Eastern, Western, St. Louis, California, and Venezuelan equine encephalitis viruses are transmitted by mosquitoes. Powassan virus is transmitted by ticks. The seasonal occurrence of these infections is limited exclusively to seasons when the vectors are feeding. Eastern encephalitis virus is limited to the Atlantic and Gulf coasts and normally circulates between birds and salt marsh mosquitoes, which do not bite man. When ecologic changes alter the bird-mosquito balance, the virus can overflow into other arthropod vectors which feed on mammals. Regional deaths of horses or pheasants usually herald the rare human outbreaks. Western encephalitis virus is limited to the western two thirds of the country and normally circulates between mosquitoes and birds; horses and man become inadvertent hosts when bitten by infected mosquitoes. This virus causes many more human infections than does Eastern encephalitis virus, but only 1 in 100 of those infected develop encephalitis. St. Louis encephalitis virus causes both rural and urban disease over a large area of the United States. In the rural areas the virus has the same pattern as Western encephalitis virus, but in urban areas more explosive outbreaks can occur when the virus is introduced into urban breeding mosquitoes and urban birds and humans become the intermediate hosts. California virus has a different cycle involving woodland mosquitoes and small animals; birds are not involved. In recent years the virus has been related to encephalitis every year over a wide geographic area of the United States. Disease is confined almost entirely to children. Venezuelan equine encephalitis is transmitted from mosquitoes to animals, and the virus has recently spread into Florida and the southwestern states. Most people infected with the virus have an influenza-like illness, but about 3 per cent develop acute meningitis or encephalitis. Powassan virus has been found in ticks in Canada and along the northern border of the United States; it is a rare cause of encephalitis in man.

PATHOGENESIS AND PATHOLOGY. Viruses usually replicate in cells at the site of entry. For example, after oral ingestion enteroviruses grow in the gastrointestinal tract; after respiratory spread viruses grow in the respiratory tract; or after subcutaneous or intravenous inoculation arboviruses grow in local subcutaneous, vascular endothelial, or muscle cells. Following local replication, dissemination of virus usually occurs via the blood. Despite the longstanding belief that the blood-brain barrier was impervious to viruses, it is now evident that the majority of viruses invade the central nervous system from the blood. The cerebral capillary endothelium is nonfenestrated, has tight junctions, and is surrounded by a dense basement membrane with astrocytic processes apposed to the outer surface. These structures do constitute a relative barrier to virus invasion, but experimentally viruses are found to invade the nervous system both by infection of the vascular endothelial cells with subsequent infection of surrounding glia and neurons and by passage of virus through endothelial cells. Experimentally viruses have also been found to grow in the choroid plexus and to seed virus into the cerebrospinal fluid.

Since viral meningitis by definition is a benign disease, its histopathologic correlates are unknown. In fatal encephalitis an inflammatory reaction is usually prominent in the meninges and in a perivascular distribution within the brain. Although the perivascular inflammatory reaction is composed predominantly of mononuclear cells, polymorphonuclear cells may be evident. Neural cells may show degenerative changes, and apparent phagocytosis of neurons by macrophages or microglial cells (neuronophagia) is often found.

Pathologic changes in encephalitis cannot unequivocally distinguish the agent involved. Topographic localization of lesions is of little value except in distinguishing poliomyelitis, rabies, and herpes simplex virus infections. Intranuclear inclusions are seen in herpesvirus infections and in measles virus infections, and in the latter cytoplasmic inclusions may also be found. Cytomegalovirus infections produce a characteristic pathology with the induction of cytomegalic cells containing inclusion bodies. Although fatal cases of mumps virus encephalitis are rare, pathologic studies have shown both the acute inflammatory lesions usually seen in virus encephalitis and perivenular demyelination characteristic of postinfectious encephalomyelitis.

CLINICAL MANIFESTATIONS. Viral Meningitis. The major clinical manifestations of viral meningitis are headache, fever, and nuchal rigidity. Signs and symptoms are often abrupt in onset and may persist from three days to two weeks. Other symptoms may include general malaise, sore throat, nausea and vomiting, drowsiness, abdominal pain, and chills and fever. The headache is often frontal or retro-orbital and may be associated with photophobia. Fever is seldom elevated above 40° C. Nuchal rigidity may not be as severe as that seen in bacterial meningitis and may be detectable only with extreme flexion. Kernig and Brudzinski signs may or may not be positive.

Viral meningitis caused by several of the enteroviruses is often associated with rashes. The eruption usually appears at the same time as the fever and persists for four to ten days. In coxsackievirus A9 and 16 and echovirus 4, 6, 9, 16, and 30 infections the rash is typically maculopapular and nonpruritic, and may be confined to the face and trunk or may involve extremities, including the palms and soles. In echovirus 9 infections the rash may be petechial, causing confusion with meningococcal infections. In group A coxsackievirus infections herpangina may develop, characterized by grayish vesicular lesions on the tonsillar fossae, soft palate, and uvula. In coxsackievirus A5 and 16 infections a vesicular rash may involve hands, feet, and oropharynx (hand, foot, and mouth disease; see Ch. 95).

Mumps virus meningitis and encephalitis are associated with parotitis in approximately half the cases. However, the parotitis may precede or follow the meningitis by as much as a week. Oophoritis and pancreatitis may also be seen. Evidence of parotitis associated with meningitis is not diagnostic of mumps virus infection, because parotitis has also been reported with group B coxsackievirus and lymphocytic choriomeningitis virus infections.

Aseptic meningitis caused by the type 2 herpes simplex virus may coincide with the eruption of genital lesions. In some cases this meningitis has been associated with radicular pain simulating lumbar or sacral root compression.

Viral Encephalitis. In addition to headache, fever, and nuchal rigidity, alterations of consciousness characterize encephalitis; mild lethargy may progress to confusion, stupor, and coma. Focal neurologic signs usually develop, and seizures are common. Motor weakness, accentuated deep tendon reflexes, and extensor plantar responses may be observed. Abnormal movements are seen in some cases of encephalitis, and rarely a tremor characteristic of Parkinson's disease may develop. The hypothalamic-pituitary area may be involved, causing severe hyperthermia or poikilothermia, diabetes insipidus, and inappropriate antidiuretic hormone secretion. Involvement of the spinal cord can lead to flaccid paralysis, depression of tendon reflexes, and paralysis of bowel and bladder. Increased intracranial pressure can cause third and sixth cranial nerve palsies.

In herpes simplex virus encephalitis, signs often include bizarre behavior, hallucinations, and aphasia, suggesting the temporal lobe localization typical of that infection (see Ch. 304).

LABORATORY FINDINGS. Blood count may be normal, show moderate leukopenia, or show a moderate leukocytosis. Epstein-Barr virus infections are suggested by large numbers of atypical mononuclear cells, as well as by positive heterophil reactions. Serum amylase may be elevated with mumps virus infections. Lymphocyte choriomeningitis virus infections are frequently associated with pulmonary infiltrates.

Cerebrospinal fluid examination is essential to establish the diagnosis of aseptic meningitis and encephalitis, even though it is of little help in determining the specific virus involved. The cerebrospinal fluid may be under normal or moderately elevated pressure. The fluid is usually clear but may show xanthochromia if the protein content is over 100 mg per 100 milliliters. Cell counts are variable, but 10 to 1000 cells are usual with a predominance of mononuclear cells. If the fluid is examined early in the course of disease, there may be no cells or a preponderance of polymorphonuclear cells. Repeat examination in 24 hours will usually show the characteristic presence of mononuclear cells. Significant numbers of red cells are often present in herpes simplex virus encephalitis, but this finding is not a dependable point of differential diagnosis. The protein content is usually elevated. The glucose content in the cerebrospinal fluid is generally normal, although mild depressions are seen, particularly with mumps and lymphocytic choriomeningitis virus infections.

The electroencephalogram usually shows diffuse slowing, but shifting foci, marked asymmetry, and seizure activity may be evident in encephalitis. Diffuse slowing is not a grave sign in viral meningitis, because this abnormality can persist briefly even after the patient is asymptomatic.

Cerebral angiography, radioisotopic scans, and computerized axial tomography of the brain may show localization of lesions of the temporal lobes in herpes simplex virus encephalitis, but these studies are usually of no value in differentiating other forms of encephalitis.

DIAGNOSIS AND DIFFERENTIAL DIAGNOSIS. The most important aspect of differential diagnosis is to exclude those treatable diseases which may masquerade as viral infections. These include tuberculous and fungal meningitis, parameningeal infections, brain abscess, partially treated bacterial meningitis, subacute bacterial endocarditis, amebic encephalitis, and other illnesses which may present headache, fever, and nuchal rigidity. The differential diagnosis of encephalitis is important, as specific therapy is now recommended for herpes simplex virus encephalitis (see Ch. 304).

A definitive etiologic diagnosis can be determined only by appropriate virologic laboratory studies. However, an educated clinical guess regarding the cause can be based on public health information concerning agents currently being disseminated in the area; on knowledge of the agents endemic to the area and the season of the year; and on the patient's history, including past immunizations and illnesses, possible insect bites, place of residence, travel in areas where particular infections are prevalent, health of the family, and type of dwelling place.

The coxsackievirus and echovirus infections occur sporadically throughout the year but reach epidemic proportions in the late summer and fall. Furthermore, they cause family outbreaks and protean manifestations. Thus the patient with aseptic meningitis occurring in late summer or fall who gives a history of other family members with nonspecific illness, rash, pleurodynia, or other enterovirus-associated disease probably has meningitis due to a coxsackie- or echovirus. Transient lower motor paralysis reminiscent of poliomyelitis is also occasionally seen with these infections.

Mumps virus infections tend to occur in the spring, and a history of exposure is commonly obtained. Since there is no evidence that reinfection with mumps virus can occur, a clear-cut past history of parotitis during a mumps virus epidemic is good evidence against the patient's having mumps meningitis.

Patients with lymphocytic choriomeningitis virus infections often provide a history of living in mouse-infected houses or working in barns or other places frequented by mice. Alternatively, a history of exposure to or recent acquisition of a pet hamster should be sought. Lymphocytic choriomeningitis virus often causes a biphasic illness, with rather severe respiratory symptoms or pneumonitis preceding the abrupt onset of meningitis or encephalitis.

The mosquito-borne virus infections characteristically occur only in late summer and early fall before the frost. They vary in prevalence from year to year, depending on rainfall or other factors influencing mosquito, bird, and wildlife populations. Public health data regarding the dissemination of Eastern, Western, and St. Louis viruses in the population may be helpful in suggesting the diagnosis. California encephalitis virus shows little variation in frequency from year to year. Since this infection is usually acquired by children after exposure to woodland mosquitoes, a history of preceding recreational woodland exposure may be obtained.

Herpesvirus infections show no seasonal distribution. In type 1 herpes simplex virus infection, a past history of cold sores, exposure to herpes labialis, or presence of labial lesions at the time of encephalitis is of little help in ruling out or suggesting the diagnosis. The diagnosis is suggested by the severity of the encephalitis and signs of localization to the temporal lobes. In contrast, onset of type 2 herpes simplex virus meningitis may coincide with the appearance of genital lesions.

Obtaining a specific etiologic diagnosis in the laboratory necessitates obtaining acute and convalescent phase serum specimens. It is also useful to obtain specimens for isolation of virus (cerebrospinal fluid, stool, blood, and throat washings). Convalescent serum alone is of little value, as antibodies to most of the agents causing meningitis or encephalitis are widespread. Disease can be associated with a specific agent serologically only if a four-fold or greater increase in antibody is demonstrated between the early phase of disease and convalescence. Therefore blood should be drawn in the first few days of disease, and a subsequent serum specimen should be obtained two to six weeks later. The optimal specimens for viral isolation are dependent on the virus being sought. Arboviruses and enteroviruses can be isolated from the blood but are seldom recoverable at the time of clinical meningitis or encephalitis. During the acute disease coxsackie- and echoviruses are most readily isolated from stool or cerebrospinal fluid and, in some cases, throat washings. Lymphocytic choriomeningitis virus is most readily isolated from blood or cerebrospinal fluid. Mumps virus may be isolated from saliva, throat washings, or cerebrospinal fluid. Type 2 herpes simplex virus may also be isolated from the cerebrospinal fluid or blood. Unfortunately, type 1 herpes simplex virus can seldom be isolated from blood or cerebrospinal fluid, and serologic studies can be misleading. A definitive diagnosis of type 1 herpes simplex virus encephalitis at present still requires a brain biopsy.

TREATMENT. With the exception of adenine arabinoside, now recommended in treatment of herpes simplex encephalitis, specific antiviral therapy is not available for viral meningitis or other forms of encephalitis. Treatment consists of supportive therapy and the management of the complications of encephalitis, including coma, seizures, and increased intracranial pressure.

In both viral meningitis and encephalitis bed rest is indicated. Strict isolation procedures are not essential, as most of the viruses causing meningitis and encephalitis are common in our environment. If an enteroviral infection is suspected, precautions in handling of stools and handwashing should be instituted. If measles, chickenpox, rubella, or mumps virus infections are evident, the usual isolation from susceptibles is recommended.

The headache and fever of aseptic meningitis can usually be managed with judicious doses of aspirin. Severe hyperthermia may develop in encephalitis, necessitating use of more vigorous therapy, but it should be remembered that viruses are thermolabile. Therefore modest temperature elevations may serve as a natural defense mechanism, and attempts to reduce mild temperature elevations to normal or subnormal levels may be ill advised.

Patients with severe encephalitis are often in coma. Since these patients may make remarkable recoveries even after prolonged periods of coma, vigorous supportive therapy and avoidance of complications are essential. The airway must often be maintained by intubation or tracheostomy, and mechanical respiration may be necessary. Although intravenous fluids may suffice for brief periods, prolonged coma necessitates feeding with a nasogastric tube. Blood glucose and electrolytes should be checked frequently, because water, glucose, and salt control are not infrequently compromised during encephalitis. The respiratory tract, urinary tract, intravenous site, and skin are common sites of infection in comatose patients, and infections should be sought assiduously, treated vigorously, and avoided by skillful nursing, maintenance of bronchial drainage, frequent turning to avoid decubitus ulcers, and meticulous catheter care.

Although seizures frequently complicate encephalitis, prophylactic anticonvulsants are not usually recommended. If seizures develop, they can usually be managed with diphenylhydantoin and phenobarbital. If status epilepticus develops, more vigorous therapy should be instituted, remembering to treat the hypoxia and hyperthermia which complicate and aggravate status epilepticus.

Modest increases in intracranial pressure can be treated with glycerol given orally or by rectal tube. This osmotic agent is probably preferable to the use of urea or mannitol, because it can be given over a longer period of time. Steroids should generally be avoided in the treatment of encephalitis because of their inhibitory effects on host-immune responses and the potential of enhancement of viral invasion. However, when increased intracranial pressure is severe, the use of dexamethasone is probably indicated.

PROGNOSIS. Viral meningitis is a benign disease, and full recovery usually occurs within 5 to 14 days of onset, although some patients describe persistent fatigue, lightheadedness, and general asthenia which may persist for months.

The prognosis of encephalitis is dependent on the etiologic agent. The mortality rate of herpes simplex virus encephalitis is estimated at 50 per cent, with a high rate of sequelae in survivors. Encephalitis associated with arbovirus infections has variable mortality rates; the mortality rate with Eastern encephalitis is approximately 50 per cent; with St. Louis, 10 per cent; with Western, 10 per cent; with Venezuelan equine, 1 per cent; and with California, less than 0.5 per cent. The mortality rates for Western encephalitis are greater in children under one year of age, and for St. Louis encephalitis they are greater in the elderly. Nonfatal encephalitis caused by Eastern, Western, and St. Louis viruses leaves a relatively high rate of neurologic sequelae.

Encephalitis associated with mumps or lymphocytic choriomeningitis viruses is very rarely associated with death, and sequelae are infrequent. Recently, however, hydrocephalus has been reported as a late sequela of mumps meningitis and encephalitis in children.

Balfour, H. H., Siem, R. A., Bauer, H., and Quie, P. G.: California arbovirus (La Crosse) infections. I. Clinical and laboratory findings in 66 children with meningo-encephalitis. Pediatrics, 52:580, 1973.

Biggar, R. J., Woodall, J. P., Walter, P. D., and Haughie, G. E.: Lymphocytic choriomeningitis outbreak associated with pet hamsters. JAMA, 232:494, 1975.

Johnson, R. T., and Mims, C. A.: Pathogenesis of viral infection of the nervous system. N. Engl. J. Med., 278:23, 84, 1968.

Johnstone, J. A., Ross, C. A. C., and Dunn, M.: Meningitis and encephalitis associated with mumps infection. A 10-year survey. Arch. Dis. Child., 47:647, 1972.

McLean, D. M.: Arboviruses. In Rhodes, A. J., and Van Rooyen, C. E. (eds.): Textbook of Virology. 5th ed. Baltimore, Williams & Wilkins Company, 1968, p. 633.

Meyer, H. M., Jr., Johnson, R. T., Crawford, I. P., Dascomb, H. E., and Rogers, N. G.: Central nervous system syndromes of "viral" etiology. A study of 713 cases. Am. J. Med., 29:334, 1960.

304. HERPES SIMPLEX ENCEPHALITIS

J. Richard Baringer

DEFINITION. Adult encephalitis caused by herpes simplex virus is usually encountered as a sporadic illness, the consequence of infection by the antigenically distinct type 1 herpes simplex virus. Recently it has become apparent that most if not all of the cases previously designated as acute necrotizing encephalitis are related to infection by this virus. Electron microscopic examination of tissues from a number of these cases has revealed characteristic herpes simplex virus particles.

In newborn infants, herpes simplex virus encephalitis is seen as a result of maternal genital herpes infection. Usually the infection is due to type 2 herpes simplex virus, but some cases are related to infection by type 1 virus. The type 1 adult infection remains confined to the central nervous system, whereas in newborns the process is commonly disseminated in a variety of other organs, and the virus may be recovered from blood and cerebrospinal fluid. Type 2 virus may also occasionally produce a meningitis or polyradiculitis in adults, frequently in association with genital infection by the same strain.

Rarely the related B virus of monkeys has been incriminated as a cause of encephalitis in humans, usually as a result of accidental transmission of the virus to laboratory workers or attendants. This condition in humans is notable for its high mortality.

INCIDENCE. Because of the difficulty in establishing the diagnosis of herpes simplex encephalitis by currently available means, the precise incidence of the condition is unknown. It has been estimated that 4000 cases may occur in the United States each year. Herpes simplex virus probably causes fewer cases than either mumps or the arthropod-borne viruses. However, the considerable mortality and morbidity resulting from herpes simplex virus infection rank it as the most common cause of sporadic viral encephalitis with severe sequelae. In view of the tendency for some infections to undergo spontaneous resolution and the difficulty in establishing the virologic diagnosis, it is possible that herpes simplex virus may be a more frequent cause of mild encephalitic illness than is currently recognized.

ETIOLOGY. Herpes simplex virus is a large, 180 mμ diameter, enveloped, deoxyribonucleic acid–containing virus which is antigenically related to B virus of monkeys but antigenically distinct from the other herpesviruses. Herpes simplex virus has man as its natural host. It is known for its ability to cause recurrent cutaneous and oral or genital mucosal lesions. The virus commonly remains latent in trigeminal and sacral ganglion tissue of humans.

Early observations in man and laboratory animals suggested that various strains of herpes simplex virus behaved differently in regard to their ability to produce disease. Subsequent work has demonstrated that there are at least two distinct serotypes of herpes simplex virus (types 1 and 2) which differ not only antigenically but also in distribution. Type 1 is commonly isolated from oral and cutaneous lesions above the waist and from sporadic adult cases of herpes simplex encephalitis, whereas type 2 strains are commonly associated with genital infections and cutaneous lesions below the waist. Exceptions to these general rules are common. The two strains differ in several other respects. Type 1 has a slightly lower DNA density, produces smaller pocks on chick chorioallantoic membrane, produces a higher yield of virus in most tissue culture systems, possesses slightly less neurovirulence for mice and rabbits, and is slightly more sensitive to idoxuridine in tissue culture systems.

PATHOGENESIS. Many aspects of the pathogenesis of herpes simplex encephalitis in adults caused by type 1

virus are poorly or incompletely understood. Although most such infections appear to have resulted from a primary infection with the virus, in a few cases a previous history of recurrent cutaneous or oral herpes simplex lesions has been obtained. Rare cases have been reported in patients whose immune systems were compromised by disease or immunosuppressive drugs, but most cases are encountered in previously normal adults.

In adults, there is usually no evidence of involvement of other viscera. Within the cerebrum the pathologic process has a characteristic bilateral distribution, necrotic and hemorrhagic lesions being most prominent in the hippocampus, amygdala and medial temporal lobe, orbital surface of the frontal lobe, insular cortex, and cingulum. The distribution is usually asymmetric. The posterior portions of the cerebrum, the cerebellum, the brainstem, and the spinal cord are usually spared. Histologically, the lesions are characterized by severe necrosis of all elements of the tissue. The presence of eosinophilic intranuclear inclusions in neurons, oligodendrocytes, and astrocytes is suggestive but not diagnostic of herpes simplex encephalitis. There is a brisk inflammatory reaction, consisting of mononuclear cells and lymphocytes and usually a mild to moderate meningeal exudate. Small hemorrhages within the lesions and on the pial surface are common.

The route by which the virus produces nervous system involvement has been the subject of much speculation. The consistent involvement of portions of the brain subserving olfactory functions has suggested that the virus may enter the nervous system by way of olfactory mucosa whence it may travel along the olfactory tract to reach the brain. The ability of herpes simplex virus to travel within nerves has long been recognized, but there is little evidence from human studies to indicate that the olfactory bulb or tract is uniformly or even commonly involved in cases of herpes simplex encephalitis. The possibility that the nervous system involvement might be the consequence of a viremia and a special affinity or susceptibility of neurons in the limbic system to hematogenous virus has also been considered, but there is little evidence from clinical or experimental data to support this hypothesis. Further information concerning the pathogenesis of the disease awaits careful studies of the distribution of lesions and virus in human cases of herpes simplex encephalitis.

CLINICAL MANIFESTATIONS. Encephalitis caused by type I herpes simplex virus is a sporadic disease of the nervous system which often has devastating effects and a highly variable clinical course. It is uncertain whether or not the virus also causes a mild form of encephalitis, because the laboratory tests necessary to provide a definitive diagnosis are seldom feasible in patients with benign illness.

In contrast to other viral encephalitides in the United States, herpes simplex encephalitis is nonepidemic. In its severe form, the disease produces a combination of nonspecific signs and symptoms of an acute encephalitis plus focal manifestations of damage to the limbic system and frontal lobes. The onset in some patients is abrupt, with headache, fever, delirium, and, often, generalized or focal convulsions. Few illnesses can produce so much neurologic devastation in so short a time; within hours of the onset some patients may lose consciousness or undergo progressive dysphasia and/or unilateral or bilateral motor weaknesses.

Alternatively, the disease may have a subacute course. Behavioral changes are common early signs of disease and at times have prompted admission to psychiatric facilities. Some patients experience olfactory or gustatory hallucinations, presumably as a consequence of the focal involvement of temporal lobe structures. In others memory is impaired out of proportion to other cognitive functions, reflecting the bilateral involvement of the hippocampal system. Seizures may take the form of generalized, focal motor, temporal lobe, or occasionally myoclonic phenomena. Involvement of larger or deeper portions of the cerebrum is signaled by the appearance of hemiparesis, conjugate deviation of the eyes, or aphasia. The illness characteristically undergoes fluctuation in its intensity, and such fluctuation may help in distinguishing herpes simplex encephalitis from involvement of the cerebrum by tumor or abscess.

The type 2 herpes virus, which is the major cause of fatal disseminated herpes infections in the newborn, usually causes less severe neurologic disease in adults. This virus in adults has been associated with aseptic meningitis and with radicular pain, often over lower lumbar and sacral dermatomes. The pain may mimic symptoms of a herniated intravertebral disc but is often temporally associated with the eruptions of genital herpes.

DIAGNOSIS. The diagnosis of herpes simplex encephalitis rests upon clinical suspicion confirmed by laboratory data.

The cerebrospinal fluid (CSF) in most cases contains up to 500 cells per cubic millimeter, with lymphocytes or mononuclear cells predominating. Occasional cases, confirmed by isolation of the virus from the brain, have lacked cells in the CSF. Red cells in the CSF and/or xanthochromia frequently reflect the hemorrhagic nature of the lesions. The CSF protein concentration is commonly elevated, but this does not distinguish the process from a number of other affections. The CSF sugar is usually within the normal range, but occasionally is low.

Recent reports of the identification of herpesvirus antigen by fluorescent antibody study of cells in the CSF suggested a specific and convenient way of establishing the diagnosis, but further confirmatory experience is necessary. Attempts to isolate virus from the CSF have only rarely been successful.

Serologic tests for confirmation of the diagnosis have several inherent disadvantages. Comparison of acute and convalescent titers is of little practical value in the management of the acutely ill patient. Furthermore, fluctuations in the titer of antibody to herpes simplex virus are commonly encountered as a reaction to a variety of stimuli. Less than fourfold increases in titer do not necessarily signify recent herpes simplex virus infection; conversely in some confirmed cases of herpes simplex virus encephalitis, the titers have failed to rise. The utility of tests of complement requiring neutralizing antibody in serum or passive hemagglutinating antibodies in the CSF must await further experience from a variety of laboratories.

The electroencephalogram is virtually always abnormal, although the abnormality may not be specific. Diffuse slowing accentuated in one or both temporal lobes and the appearance of sharp waves or spikes in temporal areas are findings consistent with the diagnosis. Several cases have been associated with relatively specific, periodic sharp and slow wave complexes; such findings are highly suggestive of the disease, but their absence does not exclude it.

Brain scans reveal unilateral or bilateral uptake of the tracer substance, a reflection of the increased permeability of vessels in the lesions. Cerebral arteriography usually demonstrates an avascular mass in the temporal lobe with or without shift of midline structures. Computerized axial tomographic scans have frequently revealed bilateral low density temporal lobe lesions with positive uptake of contrast material.

A certain diagnosis of herpes simplex encephalitis requires the use of cerebral biopsy. This technique has several limitations and also some hazard, and it should be performed only in major medical centers possessing the necessary facilities for proper processing of the tissue. The limitations arise from the fact that the encephalitic process is often confined to the medial and undersurfaces of the temporal and frontal lobes, so that biopsy of the lateral or superior portions of temporal or frontal lobes or other portions of the brain may fail to demonstrate the process or identify the agent. The time at which the biopsy is performed is of additional importance. Herpes simplex virus disappears from neural tissue within a short time and cannot be recovered thereafter by ordinary techniques. Thus the biopsy should be performed as early as possible in the course of the illness, and the tissue should be subjected to histologic study, fluorescent antibody study, electron microscopy and viral culture. If the tissue is fixed in Bouin's solution for histology, intranuclear inclusions are stained to better advantage and can be more easily recognized than with formalin-fixed tissue. Fluorescent antibody study has the advantages of relatively great sensitivity for detection of viral antigen, and specificity for the virus when appropriate controls are included. The test may be completed within a few hours after the tissue is removed. Electron microscopy is less sensitive because of the inherent sampling problems. Viral culture offers the most sensitive method for demonstrating virus in nervous system tissue. The technique of inoculating trypsinized cells from the biopsy tissue onto indicator cultures may offer a better opportunity for recovery of virus than does inoculation of clarified suspension of homogenized brain.

Among conditions which must be distinguished from herpes simplex encephalitis, cerebral abscess presents the most difficult problem. Fever, headache, and seizures occur with cerebral abscess, and these features do not serve to differentiate abscess from herpes encephalitis. The presence of another site of pyogenic infection, especially in sinus or mastoid, should alert the clinician to the possibility of abscess. However, unusual psychiatric changes or an isolated disorder of memory are less common in cerebral abscess than in herpes, and abscesses usually produce more focal and fewer diffuse signs than herpes. CSF changes may be similar; there is some tendency for the protein to be higher and the cell count lower in cases of abscess than in encephalitis. In doubtful cases, the computerized axial tomographic scan, arteriogram, electroencephalogram, and brain scan are more apt to reflect the bilateral lesions in encephalitis, and periodic high voltage sharp waves which appear and disappear over a few days are characteristic of encephalitis but are not a feature of abscess. Rarely, proper diagnosis is not reached until craniotomy, but this is usually in patients in whom the diagnosis of encephalitis has not been given sufficient preoperative consideration.

The distinction between herpes encephalitis and a pyogenic or tuberculous meningitis is somewhat easier because of the prominence of meningeal signs, the more regular lowering of the CSF glucose, the presence of organisms, and the lesser frequency of focal signs in the latter conditions. Distinction between herpes simplex encephalitis and the postinfectious or other acute viral encephalitides may be difficult and rests with the history of one of the common viral exanthems or mumps in the weeks preceding the onset of the cerebral disorder. Cerebral neoplasm can usually be distinguished by its more slowly progressive course, by the absence of fever and of CSF findings suggestive of encephalitis, and by the appearance on scan and arteriographic studies.

TREATMENT. The difficulties in establishing the diagnosis of herpes simplex encephalitis, the infrequency with which cases are seen at any one medical center, and the great variation in course from one case to another have thwarted attempts to arrive at a reasonable evaluation of treatment. In any given case there is considerable uncertainty concerning the stage in the evolution of the disease at which treatment is instituted. In addition, recent improvements in supportive treatment may tend to invalidate comparisons between series of cases.

Individual reports involving single or small numbers of patients have appeared in which idoxuridine (IUDR) has been used to treat human encephalitis caused by herpes simplex virus. IUDR, a thymidine analogue, presumably exerts its antiviral effect by becoming incorporated into the viral DNA, thus producing a fraudulent molecule which cannot be replicated. However, controlled studies have shown it to lack effectiveness and to possess unacceptable toxicity.

Cytosine arabinoside (Ara-C), a pyrimidine nucleoside, has been shown to possess activity against herpes simplex virus both in tissue culture and with herpes simplex virus keratitis in animals. Although the drug has the practical advantages of being readily available and easily solubilized and there is more experience with its use, it retains some of the toxic effects of IUDR, including granulocytopenia and thrombocytopenia. Experience with Ara-C in treatment of herpes simplex encephalitis is limited to a few largely favorable reports. A controlled study of Ara-C in disseminated varicella-zoster infections revealed no therapeutic efficacy.

The purine nucleoside, adenine arabinoside (Ara-A), has been used in a small, placebo-controlled series of patients with biopsy-proved herpes simplex encephalitis. A reduction of mortality from 70 to 28 per cent was achieved with a daily dosage level of 15 mg per kilogram for 10 days. Toxicity appeared minimal. The material was effective only if given before loss of consciousness occurred. Further careful use of this compound in established cases of herpes encephalitis seems warranted on the basis of this information.

Some authors have recommended that corticosteroids be used in herpes simplex encephalitis to treat brain swelling and impending tentorial herniation. This effect must be weighed against the potential for corticosteroids to enhance the spread and delay the clearing of herpes and virus from lesions. Further data bearing upon this topic are necessary; in the meantime it would seem reasonable to use steroids only in situations in which brain swelling seems to be a critical factor threatening the patient's life, discontinuing their use as soon as possible.

PROGNOSIS. Because of the very great difficulty in establishing the diagnosis of herpes simplex encephalitis with certainty, as well as the tendencies for biopsy to be performed in more seriously ill patients and for cases to be reported only if they are confirmed by biopsy or autopsy, the outcome of herpes simplex encephalitis is quite difficult to predict. Published reports from many sources suggest that an over-all mortality of between 30 and 70 per cent is to be expected and that among survivors severe sequelae are common, including prominent impairment of memory. A few reports, however, emphasize that nearly complete recovery is possible even without any specific treatment.

Adams, H., and Miller, D.: Herpes simplex encephalitis: A clinical and pathological analysis of twenty-two cases. Postgrad. Med. J., 49:393, 1973.

Baringer, J. R.: Herpes simplex virus infection of nervous tissue in animals and man. Prog. Med. Virol., 20:1, 1975.

Boston Interhospital Virus Study Group and the NIAID-sponsored Cooperative Antiviral Clinical Study: Failure of high dose 5-iodo-2'-deoxyuridine in the therapy of herpes simplex virus encephalitis: Evidence of unacceptable toxicity. N. Engl. J. Med., 292:599, 1975.

Dayan, A. D., and Stokes, M. I.: Rapid diagnosis of encephalitis by immunofluorescent examination of cerebrospinal fluid cells. Lancet, 1:177, 1973.

Johnson, K. P., Rosenthal, M. S., and Lerner, P. I.: Herpes simplex encephalitis: The course of five virologically proven cases. Arch. Neurol., 27:103, 1972.

Sarubbi, F. A., Sparling, P. F., and Glezen, W. P.: Herpesvirus hominis encephalitis: Virus isolation from brain biopsy in seven patients and results of therapy. Arch. Neurol., 29:268, 1973.

Shope, T. C., Klein-Robbenhaar, J., and Miller, G.: Fatal encephalitis due to herpesvirus hominis: Use of intact brain cells for isolation of virus. J. Infect. Dis., 125:542, 1972.

Stevens, D. A., Jordan, G. W., Waddell, T. F., and Merigan, T. C.: Adverse effect of cytosine arabinoside on disseminated zoster in a controlled trial. N. Engl. J. Med., 289:873, 1973.

Thomson, J. L. G.: The computed axial tomography in acute herpes simplex encephalitis. Br. J. Radiol., 49:86, 1976.

Whitley, R. J., Soong, S., Dolin, R., Galasso, G. J., Ch'ien, L. T., Alford, C. A., and the Collaborative Study Group: Adenine arabinoside therapy of biopsy proved herpes simplex encephalitis: NIAID Collaborative Antiviral Study Group. N. Engl. J. Med., 297:289, 1977.

305. HERPES ZOSTER

Richard T. Johnson

Herpes zoster is an acute viral infection of sensory ganglia and the corresponding cutaneous areas of innervation. The disease is characterized by localized pain along the distribution of the nerve and a vesicular skin eruption over a single or adjacent dermatomes. The disease is due to the same virus that causes chickenpox (varicella) and is thought to represent an acute localized recrudescent infection by the varicella virus that has remained latent in the sensory ganglia since the primary attack of chickenpox. (For a description of chickenpox, see Ch. 85.) Herpes zoster is also called shingles or zona.

ETIOLOGY. The varicella or varicella-zoster virus is a herpesvirus. The virus core measures 45 to 50 mμ and contains deoxyribonucleic acid. This is surrounded by a capsid with a diameter of 50 to 100 mμ and an outer envelope, giving a total diameter of the virion of 150 to 250 mμ. The virus is naturally pathogenic only for man, although chickenpox has been seen in anthropoid apes in zoos. There is some evidence of experimental transmission of the virus to several species of monkeys. The virus can be grown in a variety of cell cultures of human and primate origin but not in nonprimate cells. The virus is avidly cell-associated and can usually be transmitted in the laboratory only by the inoculation of infected cells, although the virus is stable in a cell-free form in the vesicular fluid. Morphologically, varicella virus resembles herpes simplex virus, with which it shares some common antigens, but it is markedly different from herpes simplex virus in its inability to infect nonprimates and nonprimate cell cultures and in its loss of infectivity in most cell-free preparations.

INCIDENCE. Herpes zoster occurs at a rate of three to five cases per thousand persons per year. The attack rate increases with age. The disease is rare in childhood and is most frequently seen in persons over the age of 50 years. It is estimated that half the people reaching 85 years of age have suffered from at least one attack of herpes zoster. Rates are higher in persons with malignancies or diabetes mellitus and in patients receiving immunosuppressant drugs or radiation therapy.

EPIDEMIOLOGY, PATHOGENESIS, AND PATHOLOGY. It has long been recognized that chickenpox may develop after exposure to a patient with herpes zoster, although this is less likely than development of chickenpox after exposure to chickenpox. In contrast, zoster rarely develops after exposure to chickenpox or other cases of zoster. These observations are supported by the epidemiologic findings that chickenpox is a seasonal disease occurring mainly in the winter and spring and occurs in epidemic proportions every two to four years. In contrast, zoster is not a seasonal disease, and there is no increase in incidence during the years of chickenpox epidemics. There is, in fact, some evidence that the incidence of zoster decreases slightly during years when there are large numbers of cases of chickenpox.

The precise pathogenesis of herpes zoster is unknown, but the following hypothesis is widely accepted. Chickenpox is transmitted from man to man by respiratory spread, and in the susceptible person the virus is probably disseminated throughout the body by a viremia. Infection of the skin occurs through the blood, and vesicles develop most prominently over the face and trunk. It is postulated that virus then spreads centripetally via sensory nerve fibers to the sensory ganglia, where it becomes latent in some form within the neurons or stellate cells. This latency of varicella virus in ganglia has not been documented in man or laboratory animals, but the recent demonstration of latency of herpes simplex virus in sensory ganglia has added credence to this hypothesis for varicella virus. Virus replication is later activated. In some cases activation is associated with the development of malignancy, local x-irradiation, immunosuppressive therapy, trauma, treatment with arsenicals, neurosyphilis, or tumor entrapment of the dorsal root ganglia or nerve root. Nevertheless, in most patients, there is no obvious exciting cause, and it is thought that the decline of immunity with age and the lack of exposure to children with chickenpox may promote reactivation. When virus multiplies in the ganglia, an active ganglionitis develops, causing pain along its sensory distribution. Virus is then thought to pass down the nerve and multiply again in the skin, causing characteristic clusters of vesicles. The localized zoster lesions are most common over

trigeminal or thoracic dermatomes corresponding to the areas of major eruption during the antecedent chickenpox infection. The more rapid secondary immune response may prevent hematogenous dissemination. Resolution and limitation of the rash of herpes zoster do not correlate well, however, with the development of antibody but appear to correlate with the collection of inflammatory cells and the presence of interferon in the vesicular fluid. This theory of pathogenesis is consistent with the occurrence of the disease with increasing age or development of malignancy, the lack of seasonal association with chickenpox, the observation that pain usually precedes the skin eruption, the dermatomal localization of the lesions of herpes zoster, and the pathology and patterns of distribution of herpes zoster.

Pathologic studies of herpes zoster have shown an acute ganglionitis with an intense inflammatory response, cell necrosis, and occasionally hemorrhages within the ganglia. In addition, there is inflammation in the adjacent segments of the cord or brainstem which is predominantly unilateral, more prominent in gray matter, and involves the posterior more than the anterior horns. A mild leptomeningitis is generally found which is most intense over the segments of involvement. Inflammation in the roots distal to the ganglia is also present, representing a true peripheral mononeuritis.

In the skin innervated by the nerve there is degeneration of the basal and deep prickle cell layers of the epidermis. Ballooning degeneration of these cells causes the formation of the intradermal vesicles. Giant cells and eosinophilic intranuclear inclusions are found in the base of the vesicles.

CLINICAL MANIFESTATIONS. The eruption of herpes zoster is often preceded by malaise and fever for two to four days. Pain or dysesthesia along the segmental dermatome also precedes the rash usually for four to five days. The pain is often a superficial tingling or burning sensation, but may vary from severe deep pain, suggesting appendicitis, cholecystitis, or pleurisy, to very mild itching. The pain may be intermittent or constant. Tenderness or hypesthesia may be detected along the dermatome on examination during this pre-eruptive stage. The cutaneous lesions present first as small, red macules which rapidly vesiculate, becoming tense, clear vesicles on an erythematous base. On about the third day, the vesicular fluid becomes turbid as inflammatory cells collect within the vesicles. Within five to ten days, the vesicles dry and crusts develop. However, in severe cases the vesicles may become confluent with a gangrenous appearance, and healing may be delayed for many weeks. During the course of the rash, there is usually enlargement of the regional lymph nodes, and there is often spread of a few vesicles to adjacent dermatomes but seldom to the other side of the body. The pain or dysesthesia usually persists for one to four weeks, but approximately 30 per cent of the patients over the age of 40 have pain that persists for months to years. This postherpetic neuralgia is more common in the elderly when there has been a prolonged period of pain prior to cutaneous eruption and a more severe rash.

Although herpes zoster may occur over any sensory nerve distribution, the thoracic dermatomes are the sites in over two thirds of cases. Cranial nerve involvement is next in frequency, and this tends to be more severe, with greater pain, frequent signs of meningeal irritation, paralysis, and sometimes involvement of the mucous membranes. The ophthalmic division of the trigeminal nerve is the most common site of cranial involvement, accounting for 10 to 15 per cent of all cases of herpes zoster. Fortunately, the eye is usually spared, but occasionally a keratoconjunctivitis develops. With ophthalmic zoster it is not uncommon to have involvement of oculomotor function, with extraocular muscle weakness, ptosis, and paralytic mydriasis. The fourth and sixth cranial nerves may also be involved, indicating that the infection is not confined to the trigeminal ganglia and its ophthalmic fibers, but may involve the brainstem and other nerve roots. The association of vesicles in the external ear and ipsilateral facial palsy (Ramsay Hunt's syndrome) was originally ascribed to infection of the geniculate ganglia. This localization of zoster may be accompanied by hearing loss, vertigo, loss of taste, or vesicles on the tongue, and probably represents involvement of multiple cranial ganglia and the associated localized encephalitis and neuronitis.

Since the primary lesion of herpes zoster is in the nervous system, the cerebrospinal fluid commonly shows a pleocytosis and elevation of protein, even when clinical signs of meningeal irritation or encephalomyelitis are absent. Not infrequently, the peripheral mononeuritis or local encephalomyelitis may cause muscle paralysis and atrophy in the area of the segmental rash. Acute urinary retention, urinary or fecal incontinence, and hemidiaphragmatic paralysis have also been seen. Signs of major central nervous system infections with herpes zoster are rare, but cases of acute transverse or ascending myelitis, disseminated encephalitis, and acute cerebellar ataxia have been described.

Zoster sine herpete is typical pain in an appropriate sensory area which is not followed by the development of the characteristic vesicles. Whether some of the common transient intercostal pains represent activation of varicella virus in ganglia without spread to the skin is a matter of speculation. An antibody response to varicella virus has been demonstrated in the absence of a rash in patients with transient facial pain resembling trigeminal neuralgia and in patients with facial palsy (Bell's palsy). However, these are rare occurrences, and the vast majority of cases of trigeminal neuralgia and Bell's palsy are not associated with serologic evidence of activation of the varicella or any other known viral infection.

Cutaneous dissemination is rare, occurring in less than 2 per cent of the cases. Dissemination is more common in patients with underlying malignancies, and about one quarter of the patients with Hodgkin's disease show a progressive spread of vesicles beyond the original one or two dermatomes of involvement. Such cutaneous dissemination, however, generally does not progress for more than six days, and spontaneous recovery occurs in most patients.

DIAGNOSIS. Characteristic development of pain and vesicular eruptions over single or adjacent dermatomes served by a segmental or cranial nerve branch usually presents no problem in differential diagnosis. However, similar zosteriform lesions can be caused by herpes simplex virus in infants.

Diagnosis can be confirmed by the demonstration of multinucleated giant epithelial cells with intranuclear inclusions in Giemsa-stained scrapings from the base of an early vesicle. Virions can also readily be found in vesicular fluid by electron microscopic examination. However, neither of these tests differentiates zoster from herpes simplex virus infections, although they can be helpful in differentiating zoster or chickenpox from smallpox infections. Varicella and herpes simplex virus infections can be differentiated by fluorescent antibody staining of cells in scrapings from vesicles.

Virus can be isolated from vesicular fluid and, in some cases, from cerebrospinal fluid by inoculation of fluid onto cultures of human or primate cells. Serologic diagnosis can also be made, but in human sera some cross-reactions are found with herpes simplex virus, so that simultaneous serologic tests should be carried out against both viruses.

TREATMENT. Little can be done to treat the acute eruption of herpes zoster other than symptomatic application of powder or calamine lotion to the rash and the use of analgesics for the pain. A variety of previously advocated treatments such as protamide, vitamins, x-irradiation, vasodilators, antimicrobials, and gamma globulin have proved to be useless. In a controlled study corticosteroids have been shown not to affect the rate of healing of skin lesions but to shorten the period of the acute pain. This benefit must be weighed against the potential hazard that corticosteroids may promote dissemination.

Systemic cytosine arabinoside, a drug inhibitory against DNA virus replication in vitro, has been advocated for the control of severe and disseminated herpes zoster infections. However, in a placebo-controlled study, cytosine arabinoside was found to actually prolong the duration of dissemination in some patients compared to the placebo group. This adverse effect of cytosine arabinoside appeared to be related to its depression of antibody response, delay in vesicle interferon appearance, and possibly its effect on the cellular immune response. Preliminary results with adenine arabinoside and interferon have been encouraging, and definitive controlled studies are in progress to assess their value.

Postherpetic Neuralgia. The development of prolonged postherpetic neuralgia after recovery from herpes zoster presents a difficult problem in management. Although this pain usually abates over a period of months to years, it is very refractory to the usual analgesics. Application of cold to the area by use of an ethyl chloride spray may give some transient relief. Tranquilizers or sedatives can sometimes be of help, and tricyclic antidepressants (amitriptyline) in combination with substituted phenothiazines have been effective in relieving pain in some cases. Local injection or section of the nerve root is of no value, and narcotics should be avoided because of the problem of addiction. In the most severe cases when pain persists over long periods, the use of transcutaneous peripheral nerve stimulation or even cordotomy may be considered (see Ch. 260).

PROGNOSIS. There is a popular misconception that herpes zoster does not recur. However, zoster does not give immunity to further attacks, and the likelihood of a second attack is about the same as, if not slightly greater than, that of having suffered the first. Most patients recover uneventfully, although severe vesiculation may lead to permanent scarring. Scarring of the cornea after ophthalmic involvement may result in permanent visual impairment. Motor paralysis of the local nerves recovers to adequate function levels in over 75 per cent of cases. Even in patients with severe encephalomyelitis, the mortality rate appears to be less than 10 per cent, and permanent sequelae are rare. The prognosis, however, must be more guarded in those patients who have underlying neoplastic disease, in which both the disease and the chemotherapeutic agents used in the treatment of neoplasms may increase the possibility of cutaneous and visceral dissemination.

PREVENTION. No vaccine is available for varicella virus. Chickenpox can be modified if gamma globulin is given after exposure, and sera obtained from patients recuperating from herpes zoster can totally prevent chickenpox in children if given within 72 hours of the time of exposure. This zoster immune globulin is recommended for children on immunosuppressive therapy or with leukemia who have been exposed to chickenpox or herpes zoster. Similar measures are not recommended for disabled adults exposed to chickenpox or to zoster, although contact should be avoided in the adult patient with a compromised immune system, because it is in this group that occasional cases of zoster have been thought to be related to exposure to chickenpox or zoster.

Ch'ien, L. T., Whitley, R. J., Alford, C. A., Jr., Galasso, G. J., and the Collaborative Study Group: Adenine arabinoside for therapy of herpes zoster in immunosuppressed patients: Preliminary results of a collaborative study. J. Infect. Dis., 133 (Suppl):A184, 1976.

Hope-Simpson, R. E.: The nature of herpes zoster: A long-term study and a new hypothesis. Proc. R. Soc. Med., 58.9, 1965.

Jellinek, E. H., and Tulloch, W. S.: Herpes zoster with dysfunction of bladder and anus. Lancet, 2:1219, 1976.

Luby, J. P.: Varicella-zoster virus. J. Invest. Dermatol. 61:212, 1973.

McCormick, W. F., Rodnitzsky, R. L., Schochet, S. S., and McKee, A. P.: Varicella-zoster encephalomyelitis. Arch. Neurol., 21:559, 1969.

Stevens, D. A., Jordan, G. W., Waddell, T. F., and Merigan, T. C.: Adverse effect of cytosine arabinoside on disseminated zoster in a controlled trial. N. Engl. J. Med., 289:873, 1973.

Taub, A.: Relief of postherpetic neuralgia with psychotropic drugs. J. Neurosurg., 39:235, 1973.

Thomas, J. E., and Howard, F. M., Jr.: Segmental zoster paresis — a disease profile. Neurology, 22:459, 1972.

306. CYTOMEGALOVIRUS INFECTIONS

James B. Hanshaw

DEFINITION. Cytomegalic inclusion disease (CID), generalized salivary gland virus disease, cytomegaly, and inclusion disease are synonyms for an illness caused by cytomegalovirus infection. Although frequently an inapparent infection, it is a cause of fetal encephalitis with irreversible damage to the central nervous system. Disease also occurs in patients on immunosuppressive therapy and others subject to opportunistic infections. The virus has been associated with a mononucleosis-like illness in previously well patients and in individuals receiving transfusions of blood.

ETIOLOGY. Cytomegalovirus (CMV) infection is caused by a species-specific agent with the physiochemical and electron microscopic characteristics of a herpesvirus. It was isolated in human fibroblastic tissue culture in the mid-1950's from infants with CID as well as from the adenoid tissue of schoolage children. A cytopathic effect was noted in tissue culture which was characterized by large intranuclear inclusions. The propagation of the virus provided the basis for the development of specific serologic tests.

EPIDEMIOLOGY. Cytomegalovirus infection is worldwide in distribution. The prevalence of complement-fixing antibodies is especially high in communities where crowding and poor living conditions are extant. Although approximately 50 per cent of women in the child-bearing age group are seropositive, this may vary from 20 to 90 per cent. Approximately 4 per cent of pregnant women excrete the virus in the urine. In the several studies that have been done in this country and in the United Kingdom, 0.5 to 1.5 per cent of newborns are virus positive. Thus cytomegalovirus is the most common known fetal infection. In some countries infection occurs in the majority of infants at some time during the first year of life. In the United States complement-fixing antibody is present in approximately 5 to 15 per cent of infants from 6 to 24 months of age.

PATHOGENESIS AND PATHOLOGY. Cytomegalovirus does not induce a highly communicable infection. Thus a substantial number of individuals remain susceptible to the infection in adult life. The virus has been isolated from saliva, the upper respiratory tract, urine, milk, cervical secretions, semen, feces, and circulating leukocytes. Virus is probably transferred by intimate contact with an infected individual or by infusion of blood from an asymptomatic blood donor. Nursing personnel working on infant wards and newborn nurseries do not have a higher prevalence of complement-fixing antibody than women in the general population. There is evidence that the placenta itself is infected with the virus prior to transmission to the fetus.

The symptomatic newborn is rarely without neutralizing, complement-fixing, and immunofluorescent IgM antibodies in the cord serum. The presence of specific IgM antibody is of value in differentiating maternal from fetal antibody because of the failure of maternal macroglobulin to pass the placental barrier. Antibody in the serum of the congenitally infected infant does not prevent the persistence of virus excretion for years after birth. The precise mechanism of this remarkable persistence is not known.

Among adults undergoing immunosuppressive therapy after renal homotransplantation, over 90 per cent develop an active cytomegalovirus infection if they have cytomegalovirus antibody prior to surgery. Approximately half of the seronegative patients subsequently become infected on immunosuppressive therapy. Seronegative recipients receiving a kidney from a seropositive donor almost always develop a postoperative infection and are likely to develop symptoms.

CLINICAL MANIFESTATIONS. Congenital Infection. The most frequently encountered signs of the infection in symptomatic newborns are hepatosplenomegaly, jaundice, purpura, microcephaly, cerebral calcifications, and chorioretinitis—in approximate order of decreasing frequency. Any one of these signs may occur alone. A petechial rash on the first day of life is suggestive of CID. Occasionally there are no physical findings other than increased irritability or a general failure to thrive. Some infants have repeated respiratory infections. The incidence of various congenital abnormalities in infants with CID is increased. These include clubfoot, inguinal hernia, strabismus, high-arched palate, microcephaly, and deafness. There have been reports of associated congenital heart disease, but this coexistence may be coincidental.

The major complications of congenital cytomegalovirus infection relate to central nervous system sequelae. There is little evidence that extraneural involvement of viscera such as the liver, spleen, kidney, or lungs results in any permanent damage to these organs. Blindness is associated with macular chorioretinitis or optic atrophy. Deafness may be complete or limited to the higher frequencies. Spastic quadriplegia or hypotonia are common manifestations in severely affected infants. Psychomotor function may range from the vegetative state with no meaningful communication to milder abnormalities with minimal effect on speech, behavior, and motor coordination.

Acquired Infection. Cytomegalovirus acquired after birth is often inapparent but may also produce respiratory symptoms with pneumonia, paroxysmal cough, petechial rash, hepatomegaly, and splenomegaly. Central nervous system disease caused by infection acquired after birth has not been frequently demonstrated, although there are reports of associated myoclonic seizures in infants and infectious polyneuritis. Chorioretinitis has been documented after acquired infection.

Hepatomegaly and mildly abnormal liver function tests are found in well individuals excreting CMV in the urine as well as in patients with cytomegalovirus mononucleosis. The latter patients may experience malaise, fever, chills, myalgia, sore throat, headache, anorexia, and abdominal pain. On physical examination, pharyngeal edema without exudate, lymphadenopathy, and splenomegaly may be present. Atypical lymphocytosis is common. Some patients have maculopapular rashes, especially if ampicillin is administered, and abnormal serologic reactions, including cold agglutinins, antinuclear antibody, and cryoimmunoglobulins, have been described. An illness similar to cytomegalovirus infection has been described in patients who have received blood transfusions. This condition, referred to as post-transfusion mononucleosis, occurs two to four weeks after the administration of blood.

Acquired cytomegalovirus infection has also been associated with autoimmune hemolytic disease, ulcerative lesions of the gastrointestinal tract, posttransplantation pneumonia, and thrombocytopenic purpura.

There is equivocal evidence that the mild liver dysfunction associated with acquired CMV infection is capable of progressing to chronic hepatitis, granulomatous hepatitis, or cirrhosis of the liver. Children with chronic hepatitis or chronic liver disease may have a higher prevalence of active infection, but the relationship of this infection to the pathogenesis of chronic liver disease is uncertain. For the majority of CMV infections acquired *after* birth, recovery is without significant complications. Patients with CMV mononucleosis may experience recurrent or protracted periods of malaise, pharyngitis, and cervical adenopathy.

DIAGNOSIS. Congenital Infection. The diagnosis of congenital infection is usually not suspected at birth, because 90 per cent of infected infants are asymptomatic. The presence of infection (not necessarily disease) can be established by (1) virus isolation in human fibroblastic tissue culture from the urine, blood, upper respiratory tract, or biopsy material; (2) demonstration of cytomegalovirus IgM antibody in the cord or neonatal serum; (3) persistent cytomegalovirus complement-fixing or immunofluorescent antibody beyond the sixth month of life; or (4) demonstration of large nuclear inclusion-bearing cells in the urine sediment at birth.

Differential Diagnosis of Congenital Infec-

tion. TOXOPLASMOSIS. Cytomegalovirus infection resembles toxoplasmosis in striking detail. Toxoplasmosis, however, is more likely to be associated with microphthalmia, *scattered* cerebral calcifications, hydrocephalus, and chorioretinitis. The demonstration of specific toxoplasma antibody titers persisting beyond six months of age or the presence of toxoplasma IgM antibody is tantamount to isolation of the organism.

RUBELLA. Congenital CMV and congenital rubella may be difficult to distinguish in the neonatal period. Both can be associated with a purpuric rash, jaundice, microcephaly, and deafness. The presence of central cataracts, however, is strong presumptive evidence for rubella. If these are associated with a congenital heart lesion, the probability of rubella is high. Specific laboratory tests for rubella virus or rubella IgM antibody or serial hemagglutination-inhibition antibody tests are required for a definitive diagnosis.

HERPES SIMPLEX. Herpes simplex infection is usually transmitted to the infant during labor and has its onset in the second week of life. The disease is often fulminant in character and may present as a meningoencephalitis, pneumonitis, or undiagnosed vesicular rash. The virus is readily isolated from vesicular lesions (see Ch. 304).

BACTERIAL SEPSIS. Infants with bacterial sepsis usually are more lethargic than infants with CID and rarely have a petechial rash. Although the diagnosis rests on a positive blood culture, the decision to treat with antimicrobial drugs must be made on the basis of the early clinical findings.

Acquired Infection. The diagnosis of cytomegalovirus infection in a patient with mononucleosis-like symptoms can be established by virus isolation as described above. Serologic determinations, such as the presence of specific immunofluorescent IgM antibody or a fourfold rise or decline in complement-fixing antibody, must be interpreted with more caution than in the newborn period because of cross-reactions with other cell-associated herpesviruses, and a tendency for CF antibody to fluctuate widely in normal subjects. Patients with cytomegalovirus mononucleosis are always heterophil antibody negative.

Cytomegalovirus mononucleosis may be difficult to distinguish from heterophil antibody-negative *infectious mononucleosis,* because both conditions occur in young adults and both have atypical lymphocytosis, pharyngeal symptoms, abnormal liver function tests, splenomegaly, and fever. In addition, the cytomegalovirus IgM (FA) test is positive in cytomegalovirus and infectious mononucleosis, presumably because Epstein-Barr virus (EB virus) and cytomegalovirus share common antigens. A patient with cytomegalovirus mononucleosis usually has virus in the urine, upper respiratory tract, and peripheral leukocytes. EB virus antibody can be measured by an indirect immunofluorescence technique. The complement-fixation tests for EB virus and CMV are specific for each agent.

A jaundiced patient with CMV mononucleosis may clinically resemble one with *hepatitis A or B* infection. A serum glutamic oxaloacetic transaminase level above 800 units is unusual for CMV infections at any age and common in icteric A and B hepatitis. Both conditions may be associated with mild atypical lymphocytosis. Jaundice in an adult is far more unusual in CMV infections than in infections with the hepatitis viruses. A history of recent contact with a jaundiced person is strong evidence in favor of hepatitis A. Hepatitis B antigen may be detected in the serum of many patients with serum hepatitis.

PROGNOSIS. Congenital. The prognosis is guarded for completely normal psychomotor development in an infant with symptoms of CID at birth. Approximately 75 per cent or more usually have some central nervous system sequelae. Although asymptomatic infants discovered on routine surveys have a more favorable outlook, there is evidence that approximately 50 per cent of infants with cytomegalovirus IgM in the cord serum have detectable CNS sequelae five years after birth. Bilateral deafness may become apparent after the second year of life. The absence of cytomegalovirus IgM antibody in the cord serum and a birth weight above 3000 grams are favorable prognostic signs.

Acquired. Although acquired cytomegalovirus infections are usually benign, they may be life-threatening in a patient subject to opportunistic infection. This usually is manifest as a progressive pneumonitis but may take the form of a hemolytic anemia, purpura, gastrointestinal ulceration, hepatitis, pericarditis, and rarely encephalitis.

TREATMENT. There is no satisfactory treatment for cytomegalovirus infections. The use of corticosteroids, gamma globulin, and antiviral drugs such as deoxyuridine, floxuridine, cytosine arabinoside, and adenine arabinoside have been reported with equivocal, beneficial, or no effect on the clinical course. These reports are difficult to evaluate because of the small numbers of individuals treated, the multiple factors operating simultaneously, and the variability of virus excretion in individuals tested at different times.

PREVENTION. It is not possible to prevent cytomegalovirus infection at present. Handwashing and gown technique should be used in working with patients with cytomegalovirus infection in a hospital setting. Usually this is ineffectual because of the difficulty the physician has in recognizing the infection. Almost everyone in a given population will acquire CMV at some decade in life. The infection cannot be prevented by a live or killed vaccine, although this approach is under active investigation.

Benyesh-Melnick, M.: Cytomegaloviruses. *In* Lennette, E. H., and Schmidt, N. J. (eds.): Diagnostic Procedures for Viral and Rickettsial Infections, 4th ed. New York, American Public Health Association, Inc., 1969, pp. 701–732.

Hanshaw, J. B., Scheiner, A. P., Moxley, A. W., Abel, V., and Scheiner, B.: School failure and deafness after "silent" congenital cytomegalovirus infection. N. Engl. J. Med., 295:468, 1976.

Jordan, M. C., Rousseau, W. E., Stewart, J. A., Nobel, G. R., and Chin, T. D. Y.: Spontaneous cytomegalovirus mononucleosis: Clinical and laboratory observations in nine cases. Ann. Intern. Med., 79:153, 1973.

Plummer, G.: Cytomegaloviruses in man and animals. *In* Melnick, J. L. (ed.): Progress in Medical Virology. Basel, S. Karger, 1973, pp. 92–125.

Weller, T. H.: The cytomegaloviruses: Ubiquitous agents with protean clinical manifestations. N. Engl. J. Med., 285:203, 267, 1971.

307. ACUTE ANTERIOR POLIOMYELITIS

Fred Plum

DEFINITION. Acute poliomyelitis is a highly contagious viral disease which ranges widely in severity. An *inapparent infection* consists of an invasion by polio-

virus that produces an antibody response but no systemic symptoms. An *abortive infection* produces transient nonspecific symptoms of a minor illness without central nervous system involvement with a rise in antibody. In *nonparalytic poliomyelitis*, the major illness develops with signs and symptoms of central nervous system invasion and meningitis but no paralysis. *Paralytic poliomyelitis* consists of the major illness, often with a biphasic pattern, associated with flaccid weakness in one or more muscle groups, the result of the attack by the virus on the somatic motor and autonomic neurons of the spinal cord and lower brainstem.

Initially endemic in character, poliomyelitis became epidemic during the first half of this century in the highly developed countries of Western Europe and North America. Since the advent of effective vaccines in the 1950's, major epidemics have disappeared, but minor outbreaks have reappeared in groups of nonimmunized children and in specific areas such as the American-Mexican border.

ETIOLOGY. The polioviruses are small enteric viruses of the picornavirus group. The virus is naturally infectious only for selected primates, particularly man, and has no other known natural reservoir. Poliovirus can be classified immunologically into three distinct types. Infection with type 1, 2, or 3 confers immunity against subsequent infection with the same type, but cross-immunity from type to type is minimal, a fact reflected by well documented cases of second attacks of poliomyelitis. Occasionally cases of an acute paralytic illness clinically are caused by coxsackie- and echoviruses (see Ch. 90 to 98).

EPIDEMIOLOGY. The virus of poliomyelitis is worldwide, and the infection is spread largely if not entirely by human contact. In nonepidemic areas with poor sanitation and largely unvaccinated populations, the illness is mainly confined to infants and children who come in contact with fecal-borne virus during the early months of life. Such children have a high infection rate with all three types of virus. Presumably they get some protection from maternal antibody; there is little serious illness but an incidence of paralytic lameness in schoolchildren which is almost as high as the attack rate formerly reported from epidemics in the developed countries. Under the circumstances, a large percentage of the population develop antibodies early in life and, despite repeated exposures, become immune from epidemic spread. Once sanitation improves and infant mortality falls in a region, the average age incidence progressively rises, with a concomitant increase in the number of paralytic cases. Prior to the extensive use of preventive vaccines, as many as 35 per cent of affected patients in the northeastern United States were over 14 years old.

Individual epidemics are predominantly the result of a single virus type, although different types of virus may attack the same community in successive years. During epidemics, poliovirus can be recovered readily from the pharynx, nasopharyngeal secretions, and stools of both patients with clinical cases and those with inapparent infection. The ratio of inapparent infection to disease ranges from 50 to 1 to 500 to 1. Thus inapparent infections are by far the largest reservoir for transmission.

PATHOGENESIS AND PATHOLOGY. Naturally occurring poliomyelitis infection is transmitted by human contact. Poliovirus enters the body through the alimentary tract and multiplies in the oropharynx and lower intestinal tract. No symptoms accompany this early proliferative stage. From the alimentary canal, the virus disseminates to regional lymph nodes with subsequent viremia which corresponds to the early, nonspecific phase of the abortive illness. With inapparent and abortive attacks, although viremia occurs, the virus apparently fails to penetrate the barriers of the central nervous system.

Both virus and host factors influence whether poliomyelitis virus invades the central nervous system and the severity of CNS involvement. Different strains of the virus vary widely in virulence. Host factors are perhaps even more important. Both epidemiologic and tissue culture studies suggest that poliomyelitis in man is genetically determined. Age and excessive physical activity during the prodromal illness unfavorably influence the severity of paralysis. Pregnancy increases the risk of contracting paralytic poliomyelitis. Local injections received during the preceding six weeks appear to increase the risk of paralysis in the injected extremity, and previous tonsillectomy enhances the risk of bulbar poliomyelitis. Inapparent and abortive poliomyelitis infections presumably never invade the nervous system at all. In nonparalytic and paralytic cases, the distribution of lesions in the neural parenchyma is roughly similar, although the intensity of the changes increases proportionately to the degree of paralysis. No one knows just what factors govern the special susceptibility of the motor gray matter and the distribution of the virus along the neuraxis in any given patient. In paralytic cases, the spinal cord gray matter is diffusely reddened, swollen, and congested, particularly in the anterior horns; the involvement in fatal cases commonly extends rostrally to the hypothalamus and thalamus. Lesions in the cerebral cortex are confined to mild alterations of the motor area. Microscopically in regions of maximal damage there are marked perivascular cuffing and diffuse infiltrates of mononuclear cells. The anterior horn cells of the spinal cord and the motor nuclei of the lower brainstem show abnormalities ranging in severity from mild chromatolysis and pericellular infiltration to total destruction. Small areas of necrosis commonly dot regions of intense inflammation. Outside the anterior horns, the inflammatory reaction sometimes spreads into the intermediate horn of the spinal cord; posterior column demyelination and neuronolysis of dorsal root (sensory) ganglia are rare but well documented. In the brainstem, abnormalities can be found in the vestibular nuclei, the roof nuclei of the cerebellum, and that part of the reticular formation which regulates autonomic, respiratory, and circulatory functions.

Chronically active neural lesions do not follow poliomyelitis. In patients dying of motor neuron disease several years after poliomyelitis (see below), the pathologic changes have a degenerative rather than inflammatory character.

Outside the nervous system, pathologic changes of myocarditis may be found. Complications and secondary effects of the illness produce abnormalities in the lungs, gastrointestinal tract, urinary tract, bones, and muscles.

Cerebrospinal Fluid.   The cerebrospinal fluid (CSF) in poliomyelitis is characterized by pleocytosis, a moderate increase in protein content, and normal values for sugar and electrolytes. The pressure is not significantly elevated. As many as 10 per cent of patients may have an initially normal fluid, but persistently negative findings are rare.

The white cell counts range from 5 to 10 to as many as 3000 per milliliter in acutely ill patients. Polymorphonuclear cells predominate at first but give way to a lymphocytosis within 72 hours. The initial protein content ranges between 30 and 100 mg per 100 ml, values over 150 mg per 100 ml being unusual. After the first week of the disease, however, the CSF protein rises to 100 to 150 mg per 100 ml or more, and by this time the cell count often has returned to normal.

CLINICAL FEATURES.   One would not suspect that a systemic infection was caused by poliovirus unless the virus invaded the nervous system. Furthermore, once central nervous system invasion has taken place, the severity of the naturally occurring disease still has wide limits. Poliovirus can cause a relatively mild attack of aseptic meningitis in one patient but the most fulminating acute paralytic and encephalitic processes in another, all in the same epidemic. The illness often pursues a biphasic course. The early stage is the time of viremia and dissemination of virus in the tissues. The later phase reflects the effects of later damage to the cells of the nervous system. Nothing specific characterizes the early illness of poliomyelitis; vague malaise, low-grade fever, muscular aching, and sometimes headache are accompanied by coryza or moderate gastrointestinal difficulties with anorexia, sometimes nausea, and often diarrhea. This prodromal phase may subside in one to three days or can progress directly into the major illness. If it subsides, three to ten or more days of health may pass before the patient falls ill again.

Nonparalytic Poliomyelitis.   The major illness progresses with more severity and intensity. Moderate nonspecific malaise develops first, often with a sense of muscular aching or stiffness that leads to unwise exercise to "work off" the discomfort. Generalized headache appears early. Children may have coryzal symptoms. Anorexia, nausea, diarrhea, constipation, and sometimes vomiting are frequent in adolescents and adults. Chilliness is frequent, but shaking chills are rare. Other visceral symptoms are also prominent; many patients have insomnia as well as excessive and localized sweating. Some report urinary hesitancy or retention even before paralysis develops elsewhere.

As the illness progresses, *muscle pain* becomes prominent, usually antedating paralysis. Patients also complain of a deep-seated low back discomfort that repeated changes in position fail to alleviate. Occasionally, frank muscle twitching and cramping develop in the early stages of the illness, and diffuse fasciculations can be seen.

Fever ranges between 38.5 and 40° C. The pulse is elevated commensurately, usually between 100 and 120 per minute. Most patients have mild hypertension. Patients with poliomyelitis usually look acutely ill. Their skin is flushed, and the lips of those with severe illness may show a dark cherry hue, bssociated with circumoral pallor. There is usually some facial sweating, and localized sweating in dermatomes or restricted bodily parts. Many patients are restless and anxious, even at a stage when paralysis has not set in. Along with the diffuse autonomic changes of the early stages of the illness, the psychologic symptoms may reflect the widespread involvement of the brainstem reticular formation or hypothalamus.

A stiff neck and back along with tight hamstring

muscles are usually prominent in the early stages of nonparalytic or preparalytic disease. The muscles may be tender, and cutaneous hyperesthesia is often a complaint. Early in the illness, muscle stretch reflexes are often hyperactive.

Paralytic Poliomyelitis. Paralysis in poliomyelitis may develop with overwhelming rapidity, proceeding from barely detectable weakness to tetraplegia in but a few hours, or it may pursue a more indolent course in which additional weaknesses appear over a four- or five-day period. Rarely this indolent progression may last for as long as 10 to 12 days. In general, the more rapid the early progression, the more severe the eventual involvement.

The virus has a predilection for large motor neurons, with weakness about large joints usually being noted first. Spread of the disease shows no consistent pattern; although there is a tendency for adjacent spinal and brainstem segments to be involved together paralysis is nearly always asymmetric and at times widely scattered in its distribution. The lower extremities and lower trunk are involved most frequently, whereas upper extremities and cranial nerves are seriously paralyzed less often. These general incidences are of no help in predicting how the individual case will progress.

Poliomyelitis causes flaccid paralysis with the involved part becoming toneless and inert. The stretch reflexes become reduced, and then disappear. Fasciculations are inconstant and transient, and the paralyzed part is initially painless. Sensory loss does occur in acute poliomyelitis, but it is extremely rare, and in most instances the finding of reduced sensation indicates some other illness.

Bulbar Poliomyelitis. Cranial nerve paralysis may develop at any time. When bulbar palsy initiates the paralytic disease, it is a dangerous sign, for the progress of paralysis seldom halts in less than four to five days. With bulbar poliomyelitis certain signs herald trouble. During the early hours, agitation and fear may become pronounced. Delirium is prone to occur at night. Fulminating bulbar polioencephalitis can produce stupor, acute excitement, or myoclonic twitches. Nystagmus on the extremes of gaze is frequent and carries no serious significance. More severe forms of ophthalmoplegia with opsoclonia or even total external ophthalmoplegia are usually limited to fulminating cases. The pupils, if they show any abnormality at all, tend to be constricted. Funduscopic abnormalities are absent during the acute stage of the disease.

Abnormalities in the rest of the motor cranial nerves are more common than those in the oculomotor nerves. Trismus may precede paralysis of the jaw. Facial paralysis is usually restricted to one or more muscles and rarely produces a total facial diplegia. Paralysis of swallowing is the most frequent abnormality in cranial nerve function. Many such patients later show little or no residual pharyngeal weakness, implying that the acute dysfunction results from involvement of the integrating center for swallowing in the reticular formation of the medulla.

In addition to impaired swallowing, involvement of other somatic motor functions of the vagus is frequent. Muscle paralysis of the larynx creates the danger of respiratory obstruction. Total aphonia is rare, but laryngeal involvement may be so severe that the voice sounds are limited to hoarse cries. Vagal autonomic disturbances occur commonly and include anorexia, vomiting, and constipation.

Autonomic Abnormalities. Many autonomic abnormalities complicate acute poliomyelitis. Hypertension and excessive sweating have already been mentioned. Over 50 per cent of adults suffer at least transient acute urinary retention. Sialorrhea and bronchorrhea are usually profuse in patients with severe bulbar disease. The autonomic involvement in such patients sometimes progresses into fulminating elevations of blood pressure, tachycardia, and fatal pulmonary edema. Cardiac arrhythmias are frequent with bulbar poliomyelitis and consist of partial heart blocks, wandering cardiac pacemakers, supraventricular tachycardias, or auricular flutter. Electrocardiographic tracings show abnormalities in the configuration of the T waves.

DIFFERENTIAL DIAGNOSIS. Poliomyelitis is singular in producing an acute febrile illness with headache, stiff neck, and asymmetric, flaccid, multifocal, and progressive muscle paralysis. However, unless poliomyelitis invades the nervous system, it cannot be differentiated clinically from many other viral diseases producing myalgia or influenza-like symptoms. Similarly, aseptic meningitis can be caused by mumps, coxsackieviruses and echoviruses that can be identified only by tissue culture or serologic studies. Bacterial or fungal meningitides can usually be separated from nonparalytic poliomyelitis by their characteristic cerebrospinal fluid alterations, including the reduction of glucose.

Diseases in which muscle pain is combined with weakness and fever provide the greatest difficulty in diagnosis. *Acute polyneuritis* can be differentiated by the presence of sensory changes in approximately 80 per cent of cases. Furthermore, patients with polyneuritis are seldom systemically ill or febrile, and the CSF rarely shows a persistent or significant pleocytosis. Protein elevations in the CSF above 100 mg per 100 ml are frequent in polyneuritis but unusual in polio. Paralysis in poliomyelitis usually lacks the symmetry which characterizes polyneuritis. *Epidemic neuromyasthenia* (benign myalgic encephalomyelitis, Iceland disease) has many clinical similarities to early poliomyelitis. It is characterized by insidious onset, headache, fever, diffusely aching and tender muscles, and the development of muscular weakness in approximatly one quarter of the cases. The disease comes in epidemics, predominantly affects adolescents and young adults, and produces emotional instability and lassitude. However, the cerebrospinal fluid is normal, and paresthesias as well as mild sensory loss are often prominent. Paresis fails to progress to severe paralysis, and stretch reflexes are preserved. Viral, bacterial, and serologic studies have thus far failed to identify a cause for this obscure illness.

The course of *acute viral encephalitis* usually differs from poliomyelitis. Although headache and some stiff neck are present in encephalitis, such patients usually have drowsiness, lethargy, convulsions, or mental changes. There may be pupillary changes, ophthalmoplegia, or spastic pareses, but lower motor neuron involvement is absent. The cerebrospinal fluid often is normal in acute encephalitis. Specific neutralizing antibodies can be detected in the blood within seven to nine days after attacks of equine or St. Louis encephalitis.

Less frequent diagnostic problems include acute porphyria, in which fever is lacking and the cerebrospinal fluid normal, and hysteria, which commonly arises during poliomyelitis epidemics.

TREATMENT. There is no specific treatment for the poliomyelitis viral infection. Patients with known or suspected acute poliomyelitis are best kept at bed rest and should be hospitalized if signs of nervous system involvement are detected. Patients with paralytic and nonparalytic poliomyelitis are most comfortable if placed on a firm bed with the back and head supported. A low head pillow helps relieve neck pain, and a thin pad placed beneath the small of the back minimizes lumbar discomfort. Footboards to support the weight of bedclothes help to prevent foot drop.

During the acute illness, aspirin and other nonnarcotic analgesics should be used for pain relief. Narcotics and sedatives, with the exception of small doses of codeine, are dangerous and should be avoided. Hot packs provide comfort to painful muscles and should be gently laid on with minimal manipulations. More vigorous physical therapy should be deferred to the convalescent phase.

Patients should be on liquid or minimal diets until their appetite returns. If necessary, parenteral fluids totaling 2000 to 2500 ml should be given in order to maintain a high fluid intake and counteract the risks of immobilization. Either indwelling or intermittent catheterization can be employed to deal with urinary retention, parasympathomimetic drugs being of little help at this stage.

COMPLICATIONS. The acute complications of poliomyelitis result mainly from damage to motor neurons and autonomic centers in the upper spinal cord and the brainstem. *Swallowing paralysis* is common in bulbar poliomyelitis and is treated by a combination of withholding oral intake and postural drainage. If respiratory failure coexists, tracheostomy should be performed. *Respiratory failure* can result from either paralysis of the muscles of breathing (peripheral failure) or damage to the respiratory centers in the medulla oblongata (central failure). The treatment in either instance is the early and effective use of artificial respiration. The management of circulatory problems in poliomyelitis is similar to their management in other diseases.

During convalescence from acute poliomyelitis, almost all catheterized patients develop infections and many subsequently develop urinary calcium phosphate stones caused by the combination of skeletal demineralization and the alkaline, infected urine. Treatment should include effective antimicrobial therapy, and stones should be prevented by a high fluid intake and turning severely paralyzed subjects. Papilledema occurs in 5 to 10 per cent of patients during convalescence and has no serious significance. A few patients develop an unexplained but usually reversible increase in various muscle weakness as late as three to four weeks after the acute disease. A more severe complication is *late motor neuron disease after poliomyelitis.* This is the uncommon but well documented occurrence of clinically typical progressive muscular atrophy or amyotrophic lateral sclerosis developing 30 to 40 years after acute paralytic poliomyelitis. The frequency of the occurrence is several times that of spontaneous motor neuron disease and strongly suggests an association between the two illnesses. The pathogenesis is unknown.

PROGNOSIS. At the peak of the acute illness it is impossible to predict accurately how much recovery will take place. Less than 10 per cent of patients with paralytic poliomyelitis die when treated with modern methods. Only a few fail to recover significant strength during convalescence. It can generally be estimated that muscle groups which function partially at the end of the acute illness will recover considerably. Recovery or improvement in areas of total paralysis is less certain. Significant improvement in strength is unusual after the end of the first year, and improvement after this time is largely a matter of learning greater skill. Muscles that show no voluntary motion by three months after the illness rarely later develop functional usefulness.

Increased neuromuscular excitability with cramping on exercise or night cramps is sometimes a more or less permanent residuum of poliomyelitis. Many patients have fasciculations at least intermittently. These are sometimes so prominent and enduring as to suggest active motor neuron disease. In most instances such fascicular activity is benign and unaccompanied by any progression of weakness.

PREVENTION. Natural infection with any of the three types of poliovirus induces lifelong immunity to the specific infecting immunotype. Proper vaccination with either the inactivated poliovirus vaccine (IVP) or the live, attenuated oral poliovirus vaccine (OPV) appears to achieve a similar result and has largely eliminated epidemic poliomyelitis from the developed countries of the world. Nevertheless public apathy and failures of vaccine delivery in the United States have combined to produce a steady decline in immunization rates in both socioeconomically advantaged and disadvantaged groups as the menace of poliomyelitis has receded from public view. These unimmunized populations remain at risk of paralytic disease.

Although full courses of immunization with both IPV and OPV provide protective levels of serum antibodies in over 90 per cent of recipients, only OPV gives substantial immunity following a single dose. Moreover, OPV elicits secretory immunity of the alimentary tract, which prevents subsequent implantation of "wild" strains of poliovirus, thereby breaking the cycle of transmission. For these reasons OPV has almost completely replaced IPV in the United States. The chief disadvantage of OPV is the rare occurrence of vaccine-associated paralytic disease, estimated to be a risk of one case in a vaccine recipient for every 11.5 million persons vaccinated and one case in a household contact for every 3.9 million persons vaccinated. Two groups are at special risk: (1) young adult household contacts with normal immune status, and (2) immunodeficient children.

Immunization against poliomyelitis should be initiated in infancy, when a three-dose series of trivalent OPV should start at approximately two months of age. The second and third doses are given at eight-week intervals thereafter. A fourth dose should be given at 12 to 18 months of age. Additional doses are desirable on entrance to the first grade of school and the seventh grade. This last dose of OPV is designed to protect these young people in later years when they become parents, because it is then that they are at greater risk of paralytic poliomyelitis. Routine immunization is no longer recommended for adults residing in the United

States. If vaccination is required because of special occupational risk or travel to areas of high endemicity, the initial immunization of adults should be with IPV. IPV is also preferred for immunodeficient children and their siblings. In the event of an outbreak of poliomyelitis, the epidemic is best aborted by the use of either trivalent or homotypic monovalent OPV.

Grist, N. R., and Bell, E. J.: Enteroviral etiology of the paralytic polio-myelitis syndrome. Arch. Environ. Health, 21:382, 1972.

Horstmann, D. M.: Lagging immunity of our children. N. Engl. J. Med., 285:1432, 1971.

Mulder, D. W., Rosenbaum, R. A., and Layton, D. P.: Late progression of poliomyelitis or forme fruste amyotrophic lateral sclerosis? Mayo Clin. Proc., 47:756, 1972.

Nightingale, E. O.: Recommendations for a national policy on poliomyelitis vaccine. N. Engl. J. Med., 297:249, 1977.

Paul, J. R.: A History of Poliomyelitis. New Haven, Yale University Press, 1971.

Price, R. W., and Plum, F.: Poliomyelitis. In Vinken, P. J., and Bruyn, G. W. (eds.): Infections of the Nervous System. Part I, Vol. 000, Handbook of Clinical Neurology. Amsterdam, North Holland Publishing Company (in press).

308. RABIES

(Hydrophobia, Lyssa)

Hilary Koprowski

DEFINITION. Rabies is an acute infectious disease of the central nervous system to which all warm-blooded animals and man are susceptible. The virus, frequently present in the saliva of an infected host, is usually transmitted by bites, by licks, and occasionally by the respiratory route. The disease is characterized by a profound dysfunction of the central nervous system and ends usually in death.

HISTORY. Rabies is one of the oldest diseases of man. First mention of it dates to the twenty-third century B.C., when it was referred to in the pre-Mosaic Eshunna Code. In the Americas, rabies as a bat-transmitted disease fatal to man was probably first described in the sixteenth century. Since 1753, when it was first recorded, its presence has been evidenced throughout the North and South American continents.

In 1975, 64 countries in the world reported rabies (26 countries reported the absence of rabies). In most countries, dogs were the main source of bite wounds or other human contact that required treatment. Cats were the second most frequent source of exposure to rabies, with rats, squirrels, foxes, jackals, cattle, and bats a main source in several countries. On the basis of species, the total number of rabid animals reported was as follows: dogs, 18,026; cats, 1529; foxes, wolves and jackals, 10,686; bats, 73; mongooses, 234; farm animals, 33,559; and others, 2180.

The total number of human deaths from rabies reported in 1975 was 352, as compared with 294 in 1974. Of these human deaths, 68 had received antirabies treatment and 284 were untreated. However, 288,333 were reported to have received antirabies treatment in 1975. In 1975, antirabies treatment resulted in 27 paralytic reactions.

ETIOLOGY, HOST RANGE, AND EXPERIMENTAL INFECTION. Virus recovered in nature, the so-called *street virus*, is characterized by extremely variable, usually long incubation periods and by its ability to invade salivary glands as well as central nervous tissue. The term *fixed virus* is used for strains of rabies that have been adapted to laboratory animals by means of serial intracerebral passages and are characterized by their neurotropism and by causing disease after a shorter incubation period. Prolonged cultivation of some strains of rabies virus in the developing chick embryo or in tissue culture has resulted in modification to the point of complete loss of pathogenicity for animals injected extraneurally.

The physicochemical properties of the virus are shown in Table 1. In addition, the virus is readily inactivated by sunlight, ultraviolet irradiation, formalin, 50 to 70 per cent alcohol, and 0.1 to 1.0 per cent quaternary ammonium compounds, bichloride of mercury, and strong acids. It is relatively resistant to phenol. In aqueous solutions, its thermal death point is reached at $56°$ C after an exposure of one hour. It survives desiccation from the frozen state, and rabies-infected tissue may be stored successfully at $4°$ C in 50 per cent glycerol saline or kept frozen at temperatures below $-20°$ C.

All warm-blooded animals are susceptible to rabies. It is principally a disease of mammals, including bats. The virus is also pathogenic for birds, but to a lesser degree than for mammals. As far as we know, the disease is not transmissible by insects or arthropods. It has been found in all parts of the world, in all climates and seasons. The virus apparently cannot invade the body through intact skin, but infection through unabraded mucosa seems possible. An airborne transmission of infection in caves inhabited by rabid bats, as well as by inhalation of aerosolized virus in a laboratory, has been described in several human cases.

Rabbits, guinea pigs, mice, and hamsters are most commonly employed for experimental infection. Hamsters are remarkably susceptible to intramuscular infection with street virus, but intracerebral injection of mice is usually employed for diagnostic purposes.

Epizootics of rabies occur in any climate during any

TABLE 1. Specific Biologic Activities, Gross Chemical Composition, and Some Physical Properties of Purified Rabies Virus

Property	Observation
Specific infectivity	1×10^{10}–5×10^{10} PFU/mg protein
Specific hemagglutinating activity	10^4 HAU/mg protein
Specific complement-fixing activity	5×10^3 CFU/mg protein
Gross chemical composition	22% lipids 3% carbohydrates 1% RNA 74% protein
Virus structural proteins	Four major proteins, one of which is a glycoprotein and the other a phosphoprotein
Sedimentation coefficient	600 S
Buoyant density in sucrose solution	1.17 grams per cm³
Genome	Single-stranded RNA, 4.6×10^6 daltons molecular weight

PFU = Plaque-forming unit.
HAU = Hemagglutinating unit.
CFU = Complement-fixing unit.

season of the year. Wars and mass movements of men and animals favor the geographic spread of the disease. Man becomes an accidental host upon exposure to the infected saliva of the biting animal, and wild animals are often sources of human rabies. The attack rate in man, after exposure, depends to a certain extent on the location and on the severity of the inflicted wounds. Head and neck bites lead to a higher incidence of infection than bites on other parts of the body. The bites of rabid wolves are apparently very dangerous; an attack rate of 47 per cent was observed in 32 persons who were bitten by the same animal and did not receive antirabies treatment in time to be of any protective value.

PATHOLOGY. At autopsy, the brain is friable, edematous, and congested; the convolutions are broad and flattened. Severe vascular congestion of the white and gray matter may extend to the medulla and the spinal cord. Virus-infected salivary glands are usually soft and swollen. On microscopic examination of the central nervous system, the nonspecific findings consist of hyperemia, perivascular and perineuronal infiltration with mononuclear cells, and considerable neuronal degeneration. Mononuclear cell infiltration of periacinal interstitial tissue accompanied by degeneration of acinar cells may be observed in the parotid and sublingual and submaxillary salivary glands.

In the absence of Negri bodies (see below), the lesions are indistinguishable from those observed in some of the other viral encephalitides. The exact nature of the virus-host relationship is unknown.

INCUBATION. The incubation period in man varies from ten days to over twelve months. As minor and seemingly insignificant contacts with rabies virus in the saliva of an animal not obviously sick at the time of exposure are sometimes forgotten, claims of extended incubation periods (one to two years) have to be critically evaluated. In dogs, signs of rabies may appear after an incubation period of ten days to several months.

The length of the incubation period is related to the amount of virus introduced at the time of exposure and to the severity of the laceration. The *site* of the original exposure does not seem to affect the duration of the incubation period.

CLINICAL MANIFESTATIONS. Dogs. In dogs the prodromal phase of the disease lasts two to three days and consists of fever, anorexia, and, very frequently, a change in the tone of the bark. However, these signs are often so slight that only a trained observer may note them. The animal's disposition is altered, and symptoms give way to the excitation phase, usually lasting three to seven days, during which time the animal grows unnaturally restless and agitated. General tremor owing to stimulation of the muscular system appears frequently. In the furious type of the disease, agitation intensifies as the illness progresses. The animal, erratic and aggressive, growls and barks constantly. It will grab viciously at any object or animal encountered. At this stage, an unrestrained animal sometimes leaves home and travels great distances, inflicting damage on other animals and humans along the way. Convulsive seizures are often observed, and the animal may become completely paralyzed. In many cases, however, the excitation phase predominates until the time of death.

In the paralytic type of rabies, the excitation phase may be slight or totally absent, and the disease is characterized only by the paralytic syndrome. Paralysis of

the lower jaw, accompanied by excessive salivation, appears as an early symptom, and the animal acts as though it were choking on a foreign body. Paralysis of the muscles of phonation may lead to loss of the bark. As the disease progresses, paralysis of the posterior extremities sets in, followed by general paralysis and death. The time from the onset of the disease to the death of the animal ranges from one to eleven days. On the other hand, dogs may die suddenly without noticeable signs of illness.

Man. In man, the prodromal phase is marked by fever, anorexia, headache, malaise, nausea, and sore throat. *Abnormal sensations around the site of infection,* such as intermittent pain, tingling, or burning, are of diagnostic significance. Extreme stimulation of the general sensory system is manifested by hyperesthesia of the skin to temperature changes and to drafts, and by acute sensitiveness to sound and light. Other symptoms include increased muscular tonus, prompt gag and corneal reflexes, dilation of pupils, and increased salivation.

As the disease progresses, spasmodic contractions of the muscles of the mouth, pharynx, and larynx on drinking — and later at the mere sight of fluid — are observed in the majority of cases. This dysfunction of deglutition gave the disease its common name, *hydrophobia*, or fear of water. Spasms of respiratory muscles and convulsive seizures leading to opisthotonos also may occur. The pulse is very rapid. Periods of irrational and often maniacal behavior are interspersed with those of alertness and responsiveness. Paralysis of the muscles of phonation may lead to hoarseness or loss of voice.

The excitation phase may remain predominant until the time of death. However, in many cases it gives way shortly before death to cessation of muscle spasms, to hyporeflexia or areflexia, and to general paralysis of the flaccid type.

In rabies in man *resulting from vampire bat infection,* the excitation phase is almost totally absent, and the disease is characterized by ascending paralysis without hydrophobia. Without an adequate history of exposure, clinical diagnosis of this type of infection may be difficult.

DIAGNOSIS. Profound dysfunction of the central nervous system, accompanied by impairment in deglutition, in persons who either were exposed to a bite or lick of any animal or may have recently visited caves harboring bats, facilitates the clinical diagnosis. Isolation of virus from saliva obtained in the course of the disease and from brain tissue obtained at autopsy, followed by proper identification of the agent by means of neutralization test, will confirm the diagnosis. Syrian hamsters, rabbits, guinea pigs, and, preferably, suckling mice are used for diagnostic purposes. Demonstration of rabies virus antigen in smears of brain tissue obtained from either patient or animal (preferably brainstem, cerebellum, or Ammon's horn) by means of specific staining with antibody coupled with fluorescein isothiocyanate is of diagnostic significance. The presence of intracytoplasmic inclusion bodies in the neuron (Negri bodies) is pathognomonic, but their absence does not exclude the diagnosis of rabies, as the presence of virus may be demonstrated by other means.

PROGNOSIS. Although inapparent infection with

street virus may be induced artificially in laboratory animals, and although animals have recovered completely after exhibiting signs of the disease, there are only two cases reported of the recovery of a human from rabies after showing signs of disease. In all other reported cases, the disease proved fatal to humans.

TREATMENT. General Considerations. Confinement and observation of the biting animal, preferably under the supervision of a veterinarian, for a period of not less than ten days for dogs and cats, is one of the most important steps in deciding whether an individual has been exposed to rabies. Biting wild animals should be sacrificed and their brain tissue examined properly by immunofluorescent staining. Treatment of severely exposed persons should be started without awaiting results of the laboratory diagnosis. If the absence of rabies infection in the biting animal is reported, treatment may be stopped.

Local Treatment of Wounds. Since the most effective available mechanism of protection against rabies is the elimination of the virus at the site of infection, all bite wounds, as well as scratches and other abrasions exposed to licks of animals, should be treated immediately by thorough cleansing and adequate mechanical flushing of the wound with soap solution followed by treatment with substances such as 40 to 70 per cent alcohol, tincture or aqueous solutions of iodine, or 0.1 per cent quaternary ammonium compounds, which are lethal to rabies virus. If debridement is necessary, infiltration with local anesthetics is not contraindicated. Bite wounds should *not* be sutured immediately. After determination of sensitivity to antirabies serum, the serum should be used in local application upon the wound.

Preliminary application of antimicrobial drugs is of no value as a prophylactic measure. However, antitetanus treatment and local application of antiseptics and antimicrobials should be instituted if indicated.

Indications for Specific Treatment. These are summarized in Table 2, prepared by the Expert Committee on Rabies of the World Health Organization. Emphasis is placed on the condition of the biting animal at the time of exposure and during the ensuing ten days. It is assumed that the saliva of an animal that is not obviously ill at the time of exposure may be infectious during a maximal period of five days preceding the appearance of clinical signs of the disease.

New Human Vaccine. Plans have been well under way to have a new human rabies vaccine licensed in the United States. This human diploid cell vaccine, licensed in Europe and other countries, was used successfully in postexposure treatment of 45 Iranians who all survived after exposure to severe wolf and dog bites. This vaccine should be used preferentially for post- and pre-exposure immunization because it is more immunogenic than the currently available avian embryo vaccines and shows no side effects in contrast to the nervous tissue vaccines. The vaccine is administered either subcutaneously or intramuscularly in the upper arm. A single dose consists of 1 ml.

Administration of Postexposure Treatment. Passive-active immunization by the administration of antirabies serum of animal or human origin and immunogenically potent vaccine in repeated doses is the most effective protective specific treatment of the exposed persons. Experience indicates that vaccine alone is sufficient for minor exposures (see Table 2). Serum should be given in a single dose — 40 IU per kilogram of body weight for heterologous serum, and 20 IU for human antirabies gamma globulin; the first dose of vaccine is inoculated at the same time as the serum but at another site. Sensitivity to heterologous serum must be determined before its administration.

The human diploid cell vaccine (see above) is at present recommended to be given on days 0 (the day treatment begins), 3, 7, 14, 30, and 90. *All* other vaccines should be given daily for 14 consecutive days, with a booster inoculation given 10, 20, and 90 days after the regular course of vaccine. Treatments should be started as early as possible after exposure, but in no case should it be denied to exposed persons arriving late. In areas in which antirabies serum is not available, full

TABLE 2. Specific Systemic Treatment

| Nature of Exposure | Status of Biting Animal Irrespective of Previous Vaccination | | Recommended Treatment† |
	At Time of Exposure	During 10 Days*	
I. Contact, but no lesions; Indirect contact; no contact	Rabid	—	None
II. Licks of the skin; scratches or abrasions; minor bites (covered areas of arms, trunk, and legs)	(a) Suspected as rabid†	Healthy	Start vaccine; stop treatment if animal remains healthy for five days*‡
		Rabid	Start vaccine; administer serum upon positive diagnosis and complete the course of vaccine
	(b) Rabid; wild animal§ or animal unavailable for observation		Serum + vaccine
III. Licks of mucosa; major bites (multiple or on face, head, finger, or neck)	Suspect† or rabid domestic or wild animal,§ or animal unavailable for observation		Serum + vaccine; stop treatment if animal remains healthy for five days*‡

*Observation period in this chart applies only to dogs and cats.
†All unprovoked bites in endemic areas should be considered suspect unless proved negative by laboratory examination (brain FA).
‡Or if its brain is found negative by FA examination.
§In general, exposure to rodents and rabbits seldom if ever requires specific antirabies treatment.
FA = Fluorescent antigen.

vaccine therapy, including three booster inoculations, should be administered.

The administration of preventive treatment may give rise to local allergic reactions, to serum sickness (if combined serum-vaccine therapy is used), and to nervous system reactions (if vaccines containing nervous tissue are used). Treatment should then be either interrupted or continued with vaccines of non-nervous tissue origin. Many problems can be avoided if treatment is given only when specifically indicated (Table 2).

Treatment Once Clinical Signs Are Apparent. Although no specific therapeutic measures are available to save the life of a person exhibiting symptoms of the disease, the survival of two patients with human rabies indicates that all the tools of modern medicine should be used in the attempt to save the patient's life. These therapeutic measures should consist of (1) starting treatment immediately after signs of rabies appear; (2) placing the patient in the intensive medical care unit in a quiet environment, with constant monitoring to prevent cardiac failure; (3) using sedatives for the relief of anxiety and pain; (4) performing a tracheostomy and applying artificial breathing to maintain respiratory function; (5) using curare-like drugs to alleviate spastic muscular contractions if they occur; and (6) instituting intravenous perfusions and administering diuretics to assure proper hydration and diuresis. *Note:* Since rabies virus may be present in the saliva of the patient exhibiting signs of the disease, all attending personnel should be protected against contamination through the use of goggles, masks, and rubber gloves.

PRE-EXPOSURE IMMUNIZATION. Preferably, human diploid cell vaccine or, if that is not available, any other patent vaccine free from paralytic factors is recommended to be given at 1, 7, and 21 days to persons engaged in veterinary practice, experimental surgery involving handling of dogs and cats, spelunking, dog catching, or any other activity involving unusually high risk of exposure. The vaccinated person should be bled one month after the last vaccination to check the sera for the presence of antirabies antibodies. Such persons upon exposure may be given one booster dose of a *potent* vaccine. Persons without antibody should receive full treatment if re-exposed to rabies.

CONTROL MEASURES. Although the presence of rabies-infected bats in the Northern Hemisphere presents a difficult problem for rabies control, most human exposure can be prevented by the use of control measures that will rid an area of enzootics or epizootics of rabies.

The following measures should be applied in an efficiently organized rabies control program conducted by public health authorities: control of the canine population (registration, restraint, elimination of stray dogs), reduction in number of susceptible dogs by mass vaccination, reduction in number of wildlife species that are a reservoir of the virus, and continuous educational campaigns for the general public.

Baer, G. M. (ed.): The natural history of rabies, Vols. I and II. New York, Academic Press, 1973.

Bahmanyar, M., Fayaz, A., Nour-Salehi, S., Mohammadi, M., and Koprowski, H.: Successful protection of humans exposed to rabies infection. JAMA, 236:2751, 1976.

Expert Committee on Rabies: Sixth Report. WHO Techn. Rep. Ser., No. 523, 1973.

Hattwick, M. A. W., Weis, T. T., Stechschulte, C. J., Baer, G. M., and Gregg, M. B.: Recovery from rabies. A case report. Ann. Intern. Med., 76:931, 1972.

Hummeler, K., and Koprowski, H.: Investigating the rabies virus. Nature, 221:418, 1969.

Johnson, H. N.: Rabies. *In* Horsfall, F. L., Jr., and Tamm, I. (eds.): Viral and Rickettsial Infections of Man. 4th ed. Philadelphia, J. B. Lippincott Company, 1965.

Kaplan, M., and Koprowski, H. (eds.): Laboratory Techniques in Rabies. 3rd ed. Geneva, World Health Organization, 1973.

309. ENCEPHALITIC COMPLICATIONS OF VIRAL INFECTIONS AND VACCINES

Donald Silberberg

309.1. INTRODUCTION

Acute disseminated encephalomyelitis may be associated with banal viral diseases or may follow immunization. Neuroparalytic accidents following antirabies vaccination resemble acute disseminated encephalomyelitis, but specifically follow immunization against rabies. Reye's syndrome seems to be related to banal viral infections, but has distinctive features. Despite some points in common, these entities are best considered separately.

309.2. ACUTE DISSEMINATED ENCEPHALOMYELITIS

DEFINITION. Acute disseminated encephalomyelitis (postinfectious encephalomyelitis, postvaccinal encephalomyelitis, acute perivascular myelinoclasis, acute hemorrhagic leukoencephalitis) is an acute or subacute disease of the central nervous system which most commonly occurs after viral infections that do not normally affect the nervous system, or as a complication of immunization. Involvement of the brain and spinal cord may be widespread, or may be limited to discrete areas, such as optic nerves (optic neuritis, papillitis) or a single spinal cord level (transverse myelitis). Acute disseminated encephalomyelitis is characterized by varying degrees of perivenous mononuclear cellular infiltration and demyelination.

ETIOLOGY AND PATHOGENESIS. Predisposing factors include exposure to measles, mumps, varicella, rubella, influenza, infectious mononucleosis, smallpox, and banal upper respiratory infections. Similar disease has been associated with pertussis, tetanus, streptococcal infections, and mycoplasma pneumonia. Acute disseminated encephalomyelitis also follows immunization against smallpox, rabies, influenza, and tetanus. Disease occurring after immunization is often termed *postvaccination encephalomyelitis*, and the central nervous system disease which may follow immunization against smallpox with attenuated vaccinia virus is termed *postvaccinal encephalomyelitis*.

The neurologic complications of childhood viral diseases usually occur 4 to 18 days after the appearance of a skin rash or other systemic signs. However, encephalomyelitis can occur before, concomitant with, and even in the absence of systemic signs of viral infection.

The pathogenesis of acute disseminated encephalomyelitis may be viewed as the direct consequence of viral infection, as an immune disorder, or as the result of interaction of these two mechanisms. Historically an immune pathogenesis was considered first because of the histopathologic resemblance of acute disseminated encephalomyelitis to neuroparalytic accidents following antirabies vaccination and to experimental allergic encephalomyelitis (see Ch. 309.3).

There have been few attempts to recover an infectious agent from the central nervous system of patients with acute disseminated encephalomyelitis, using modern virologic techniques. Measles virus was isolated from the brain of a patient with postmeasles acute disseminated encephalomyelitis, using co-cultivation techniques. The patient's brain contained the typical histologic features of acute disseminated encephalomyelitis. Long after vaccination, vaccinia virus was isolated from the cerebrospinal fluid of a number of patients without neurologic symptoms, suggesting that persistent virus may play a role in postvaccinal encephalomyelitis. Mumps virus may be isolated from cerebrospinal fluid during the first few days of systemic illness in over half the patients.

At present no definite direct evidence exists for primary immune pathogenesis of human acute disseminated encephalomyelitis, except for the form that follows rabies immunization (see Ch. 308 and 309.3). However, several observations demonstrate that immune alterations occur in the course of the disorder. In the acute stages of disease, peripheral blood lymphocytes from patients show positive transformation on stimulation with homologous myelin basic protein. This may correlate with observations of lymphoblasts in the peripheral blood of similar patients. Cerebrospinal fluid lymphocytes from patients with acute disseminated encephalomyelitis also show an enhanced response to myelin basic protein, as do cerebrospinal fluid lymphocytes from patients with acute and progressive multiple sclerosis. These observations may relate to the liberation of myelin basic protein into cerebrospinal fluid, as has been shown in patients with multiple sclerosis.

INCIDENCE. Approximately 30 per cent of the reported cases of encephalitis in the United States are associated with childhood diseases. The incidence of neurologic complications may vary from epidemic to epidemic, but is approximately 1:1000 cases in measles, 1:5000 in rubella, and 1:8000 in scarlet fever, and probably exceeds these figures in pertussis. The fact that abnormalities in the electroencephalogram occur in approximately 50 per cent of neurologically uncomplicated cases of measles suggests that asymptomatic involvement of the nervous system is common. A variety of neurologic complications occur in approximately 1 per cent of patients with infectious mononucleosis, but acute disseminated encephalomyelitis is rare. In general, males are affected more frequently than females, approximating a ratio of 2:1 in some series. Infants younger than two years of age and the elderly are rarely affected; the age incidence reflects the age incidence of the precipitating disease.

Mumps resembles lymphocytic choriomeningitis in its central nervous system involvement. An increase of cells in cerebrospinal fluid is common in neurologically asymptomatic children with mumps. As many as 18 per cent of patients with mumps have convulsions, and signs of meningeal irritation are frequent. Despite this, the incidence of acute disseminated encephalomyelitis associated with mumps remains low.

Postvaccinal encephalomyelitis, which is practically unknown in infants under two years of age, occurred in 17 of 800,000 people who were vaccinated during the 1962 epidemic of smallpox in South Wales, suggesting an over-all incidence of approximately 1 in 50,000 vaccinations. Several other series report similar figures. There is a greater incidence of postvaccinal complications after primary vaccination than after revaccination, with the highest incidence among children of school age (3 per 100,000). A long interval between primary vaccination and revaccination increases the incidence.

PATHOLOGY. The basic lesion in acute disseminated encephalomyelitis is the presence of mononuclear cells around small veins, chiefly in white matter, but to a lesser extent in gray matter as well. This is accompanied by varying degrees of perivenous demyelination. Individual lesions are scattered and rarely coalesce to give large lesions. Severe cases may include destruction of axons and nerve cell bodies, serous exudate, fibrin impregnation of vessel walls, polymorphonuclear infiltration, and hemorrhages. The inclusion of hemorrhages as well describes acute hemorrhagic leukoencephalitis.

CLINICAL MANIFESTATIONS AND COURSE. Acute disseminated encephalomyelitis usually begins with fever, headache, vomiting, and drowsiness. This is quickly followed by depressed consciousness and often coma. Irritability, behavior disturbances, and convulsions are common. Multifocal signs, including ataxia, involuntary movements, paralyses of one or more extremities, visual impairment, or other focal neurologic signs occur, often accompanied by signs of meningeal irritation. Lesions restricted to the optic nerves producing optic papillitis or retrobulbar neuritis occur. The duration of symptoms varies from a few days to weeks and sometimes months.

Myelitis predominates in approximately 10 per cent of instances. The lesion may affect only one cord level (transverse myelitis), or may progress to involve the entire spinal cord, producing successive backache, urinary retention, paraparesis, paraplegia, quadriplegia, and bulbar signs.

The cerebrospinal fluid may be normal or may show increased pressure and pleocytosis up to 1000 cells per cubic millimeter. The cell counts usually range from 15 to 250. Most cells are mononuclear, although polymorphonuclear cells may predominate during the first several days of illness. Approximately 60 to 70 per cent of patients with neurologic complications have pleocytosis, but over 10 per cent of patients with neurologically uncomplicated exanthemata also have pleocytosis. Cerebrospinal fluid protein may be normal and rarely exceeds 100 mg per 100 ml. The cerebrospinal fluid changes have no prognostic significance and no relation to the type or severity of neurologic disorder. The electroencephalogram is almost always diffusely abnormally slow.

Neurologic manifestations may precede signs of systemic infection by up to ten days or follow signs of systemic infection by up to 24 days. The average latent period is about five days. The occurrence and severity of neurologic symptoms appear to bear no relation to the severity of the systemic disease.

The immediate and long-term prognosis varies somewhat with the individual virus. Encephalitis associated with rubella, measles, and mumps has a higher mortality (20 to 50 per cent) than in scarlet fever (13 per cent) or varicella (10 per cent). Sequelae are most common in scarlet fever (45 per cent) and measles (35 per cent), and less so in varicella (20 per cent) and rubella (2 to 5 per cent). The clinical sign which correlates best with prognosis is the level of consciousness.

DIAGNOSIS. Identification of acute disseminated encephalomyelitis is not difficult when neurologic symptoms are preceded by a recognizable viral illness. Differential diagnosis includes acute infectious encephalitis and acute multiple sclerosis. Encephalitis caused by neurotropic viruses is almost always accompanied by increased cells and protein in the cerebrospinal fluid which are often lacking in acute disseminated encephalomyelitis. Fever and meningeal signs are rare in multiple sclerosis. Correct diagnosis in the absence of precipitating illness may depend entirely on direct virus isolation from all possible sites and by serum antibody determinations during the course of the illness in an attempt to detect evidence of a virus infection. Fatal cases provide the opportunity for attempts at direct recovery of virus.

TREATMENT. Corticosteroid therapy appears to produce improvement in some patients with acute disseminated encephalomyelitis. However, no controlled studies have been feasible because of the low frequency of cases, and there is no convincing evidence to support the use of steroids in the absence of increased intracranial pressure. Appropriate measures to reduce increased intracranial pressure, including intravenous mannitol, high doses of corticosteroids, and hyperventilation, may be required to sustain life during severe acute illness. Appropriate symptomatic support include reduction of fever with aspirin, the use of anticonvulsants and antimicrobial drugs when indicated (such as for pneumonia), and management of fluid and electrolyte balance.

PREVENTION. Initial smallpox vaccination during infancy reduces the danger of postvaccinal disease. The use of measles, mumps, and pertussis vaccines to induce active immunity to these diseases will reduce the frequency of acute disseminated encephalomyelitis.

Alvord, E. C.: Acute disseminated encephalomyelitis and "allergic" neuroencephalopathies. In Vinken, P. J., and Bruyn, G. W. (Eds.): Handbook of Clinical Neurology. New York, American Elsevier Publishing Company, 1970, Vol. 9, pp. 500–571.

Cohen, S. R., Herndon, R. M., and McKhann, G. M.: Radioimmunoassay of myelin basic protein in spinal fluid. N. Engl. J. Med., 295:1455, 1976.

Lisak, R. P., Behan, P. O., Zweiman, B., and Shetty, T.: Cell-mediated immunity to myelin basic protein in acute disseminated encephalomyelitis. Neurology, 24:560, 1974.

Lisak, R. P., and Zweiman, B.: In vitro cell-mediated immunity of cerebrospinal fluid lymphocytes to myelin basic protein in primary demyelinating diseases. N. Engl. J. Med. 297:1207, 1977.

ter Mullen, V., Kackell, Y., Muller, D., Katz, M., and Meyermann, R.: Isolation of infectious measles virus in measles encephalitis. Lancet, 2:1172, 1972.

309.3. NEUROPARALYTIC ACCIDENTS FOLLOWING ANTIRABIES VACCINATION

The production of neurologic disease is a dreaded complication of immunization against rabies. Neuro-paralytic accidents following antirabies vaccination include a disease which resembles acute disseminated encephalomyelitis in its clinical manifestations and histology, and, less commonly, the Guillain-Barré syndrome. These complications are clearly related to the presence of brain tissue or other neural antigens in the vaccines. As vaccines produced in tissue cultures of human diploid cells replace the nervous tissue vaccines, the neurologic complications of antirabies vaccination described in this chapter should disappear (see Ch. 308).

The over-all incidence of postvaccinal encephalomyelitis varies from 1 in 2000 to 1 in 9000 of those receiving brain-containing vaccines. Practically no cases occur in young chidren, but as many as 1 per cent of young adults (20 to 40 years) developed encephalomyelitis after immunization with neural vaccines. The incidence after immunization against rabies with vaccines prepared in avian embryos is low, approximating 1 in 50,000.

With rare exceptions in which live rabies virus was accidentally introduced with vaccines, the pathogenesis of encephalomyelitis following antirabies vaccination seems to be immunologic. The low incidence and the age-related incidence strongly suggest that immune responsiveness plays a role in disease production. In addition, an experimental disease which is very similar histologically, experimental allergic encephalomyelitis (EAE), can be induced in a variety of animals by injection of homologous or heterologous brain tissue or myelin basic protein.

Encephalomyelitis following antirabies vaccination may be divided into encephalitic and myelitic forms. Both are distinguished by widely spread foci of demyelination and cellular infiltration throughout white and gray matter, but more pronounced in white matter. Brain lesions (encephalitic form) tend to be larger, and many are periventricular as well as perivenous. These lesions closely resemble plaques of multiple sclerosis. More acute lesions are distinguished by perivenous mononuclear cell invasion. Axis cylinders are spared in most instances. The myelitis form resembles acute disseminated encephalomyelitis, with smaller scattered areas of perivenous demyelination and cellular infiltration.

The interval from the last injection to the onset of symptoms averages 15 days with the myelitis form, and about 35 days with the encephalitic form. Headache, fatigue, and changes in mental function commonly precede the appearance of such focal neurologic signs as visual disturbance, hemiplegia, or paraplegia. Progression of neurologic signs and symptoms may proceed for days or weeks. Mortality is approximately 20 per cent, but most cases were reported before the availability of corticosteroids which may increase survival. Permanent sequelae occur, including changes in mentation or behavior.

If any signs of the possible development of encephalomyelitis develop during a course of immunization against rabies with a nervous tissue vaccine, immunization should be stopped. High doses of corticosteroids may be effective in reducing the morbidity of the acute process.

Immunization against rabies should be undertaken only when it is reasonably certain that there has been a bite by a rabid animal. Vaccines prepared in human diploid cells are unlikely to produce postvaccinal encephalomyelitis (see Ch. 308).

Shiraki, H.: The comparative study of rabies post-vaccinal encephalomyelitis and demyelinating encephalomyelinitis of unknown origin with special reference to the Japanese cases. *In* Bailey, O. T., and Smith D. E. (eds.): The Central Nervous System: Some Experimental Models of Neurological Diseases. Baltimore, Williams & Wilkins Company, 1968, pp. 87–123.

309.4. REYE'S SYNDROME

DEFINITION. Reye's syndrome describes an acute and often fatal encephalopathy of childhood that is characterized by acute brain swelling associated with fatty infiltration and dysfunction of the liver. Reye's syndrome may follow a variety of common viral infections.

ETIOLOGY AND PATHOGENESIS. Reye's syndrome has been reported after infections with influenza B, varicella, adenovirus type 3, coxsackievirus A and B, reovirus, echovirus, herpes simplex, and parainfluenza. Viral infection is suggested as the initiating factor by recovery of virus from a few patients, by the frequency of varicella as the prodromal illness in sporadic cases, and by the reported increased incidence concurrently with outbreaks of influenza B infection in two epidemiologic studies. The pathogenic relationship between virus infection and the encephalopathy and hepatic injury is unknown.

It is possible that the encephalopathy is secondary to metabolic effects of the hepatic lesion. The combination of hypoglycemia and ammonia retention, together with other abnormalities of intermediary metabolism, may be sufficient to produce the coma and cerebral edema which occur. The early occurrence of mitochondrial abnormalities in liver and brain suggests that induction of a partially reversible mitochondrial injury may be instrumental.

INCIDENCE. Reye's syndrome occurs in children 6 months to 15 years of age. Approximatley 1000 cases have been reported. Large series have been described from Australia, Canada, Thailand, and the United States. It occurs both as a sporadic, rare disease, and in minor outbreaks in a particular area. It is a leading cause of death in children one to six years old in Thailand, where it is associated with ingestion of the fungal toxin, aflatoxin.

PATHOLOGY. Marked cerebral edema occurs, with astrocyte swelling, myelin bleb formation, and injury of neuronal mitochondria which resembles the concurrent mitochondrial changes seen in the liver. The liver is swollen and orange to pale yellow. Fatty infiltration occurs initially as diffuse small vacuoles in the periportal areas, and spreads to cause massive involvement in fatal cases. Electron microscopic examination of liver biopsy specimens shows swollen pleomorphic mitochondria and small droplets of triglycerides in hepatocytes. Fat deposition also occurs in the renal tubules and in the myocardium.

CLINICAL MANIFESTATIONS AND COURSE. Typically, Reye's syndrome starts with an upper respiratory infection or mild gastrointestinal disturbance. A symptom-free interval of hours to several days is followed by persistent vomiting and then by delirium and coma. Convulsions are common. Hyperpnea or irregular deep respiration is common. There are no meningeal or focal neurologic signs. Decerebrate posturing may occur as increased intracranial pressure supervenes. Mild to moderate hepatomegaly is the only clinical suggestion of hepatic involvement, and even this is lacking in 50 per cent of cases.

Hypoglycemia is found less frequently now (5 per cent) than when the syndrome was first described. Cerebrospinal fluid protein is normal. Elevation of serum transaminases, hyperammonemia, and prolongation of the prothrombin time reflect hepatic damage. Bilirubin levels rise in a minority of patients. Hypocapnia, hyponatremia, and hypokalemia are common. Elevation of plasma free fatty acid levels reflects an initial impairment of fatty acid oxidation.

Deepening coma leading to death occurs in 25 to 50 per cent of patients. More recent reports indicate the lower mortality rates, both because of improved management and because milder cases are being diagnosed. Severe neurologic sequelae, such as mental impairment, seizures, or hemiplegia, occur in some survivors.

DIAGNOSIS. The diagnosis of Reye's syndrome is suggested by the clinical manifestations described above. Biopsy or autopsy demonstration of fatty infiltration of the liver is confirmatory but usually unnecessary.

TREATMENT. Treatment is empirical. Hypoglycemia and electrolyte disturbances should be corrected. Enemas, neomycin and low protein intake as employed in hepatic encephalopathy are commonly used. Peritoneal dialysis and exchange transfusions have been used to correct refractory metabolic abnormalities and to correct clotting factor deficiencies. Corticosteroids, mannitol, hyperventilation, and exchange transfusion may be used to reduce intracranial pressure.

Partin, J. C., Partin, J. S., Schubert, W. K., and McLaurin, W.: Brain ultrastructure in Reye's syndrome. J. Neuropathol. Exp. Neurol., 34:425, 1975.

Reye, R. D. K., Morgan, G., and Baral, J.: Encephalopathy and fatty degeneration of the viscera: A disease entity of childhood. Lancet, 2:749, 1963.

Schiff, G. M.: Reye's syndrome. Ann. Rev. Med., 27:447, 1976.

310. SLOW INFECTIONS OF THE NERVOUS SYSTEM

Richard T. Johnson

310.1. INTRODUCTION

Recently, slow viral infections have been related to several chronic and subacute neurologic diseases in which clinical signs of infection are lacking and in which the pathologic changes are those of degenerative or demyelinative processes. The term slow infection was originally coined in the veterinary literature to describe several transmissible diseases of sheep. Two of these sheep diseases, *scrapie* and *visna*, are the prototypes of slow infections of the nervous system. Both these diseases are transmissible. After inoculation of sheep with tissue from an affected sheep, there is a latent period of one to four years during which the sheep appear well. This is followed by the insidious onset of neurologic signs which progress without fever from one to six months and lead inevitably to death. Scrapie is clinically characterized primarily by ataxia and visna by progressive paralysis. Pathologically the diseases are very different. The lesions of scrapie are confined to the nervous system, where there is marked proliferation of astrocytes and the degeneration of neurons with vacuolization of their cytoplasms. By contrast, central nervous system lesions of visna are characterized by marked inflammation and demyelination. The agents responsible for these two slow infections of sheep are also very different. The scrapie agent has been transmitted to a variety of other animals, but the agent does not cause cytopathic changes in cell culture, and no virus-like particles have been found in infectious tissue by electron microscopy. The infectivity of this tissue remains remarkably stable on exposure to physicochemical treatments which inactivate classic viruses. Furthermore, animals naturally or experimentally infected with scrapie fail to develop any evidence of an immune response against the agent. In contrast, the visna virus is an enveloped RNA retrovirus. Although transmissible from sheep to sheep, it has not been transmitted to other animals but can be grown in a variety of tissue cultures. Of the four slow infections of the human central nervous system described below, kuru and Creutzfeldt-Jakob disease resemble scrapie pathologically, and the agents responsible for these diseases have properties similar to those described for the scrapie agent. Therefore scrapie, kuru, and Creutzfeldt-Jakob disease have been classified together as the subacute spongiform encephalopathies. Subacute sclerosing panencephalitis and progressive multifocal leukoencephalopathy, like visna, are due to classic viruses. These viruses have been visualized by electron microscopy, are antigenic in natural and experimental hosts, and can produce rapid cytolytic infection in some cell cultures even though they are capable of causing slow infections in man.

310.2.   KURU

Kuru is an endemic disease of Melanesian tribal people inhabiting a remote area of the Eastern Highlands of central New Guinea. The disease has been seen only among the Fore linguistic group and several neighboring groups with whom the Fore have intermarried. However, within this limited area, kuru, until recently, was the most common cause of death. The disease predominantly affected adult women, but children over age five were also affected but without sexual predilection. Adult males were least involved. The disease begins insidiously with unsteadiness of stance and gait. A progressive symmetrical cerebellar ataxia develops over a period of months and follows a relentless, afebrile course until the patient is unable to make the slightest movement without violent ataxic tremors. Late in the course of the disease, abnormalities of extraocular movement and mental changes develop. The disease invariably leads to death in three to six months. Extensive laboratory examinations have failed to show any abnormalities, and the cerebrospinal fluid remains normal. Pathologic changes are confined to the brain where there is a marked increase of astrocytes and degeneration of neurons with cytoplasmic vacuolization. The brain is diffusely affected, but the findings are most prominent in the cerebellum and pons and, to a

lesser degree, in the hypothalamus and basal ganglia. Inflammation is not found.

Because of the similarities between kuru and scrapie in terms of epidemiology, clinical progression, and pathologic changes, brain tissue from patients dying of kuru was inoculated into a variety of primates for long-term observations. After incubation periods of 18 months to 4 years, a similar disease developed in chimpanzees, and this disease has subsequently been transmitted from chimpanzee to chimpanzee and to several other species of primates. The agent can be transmitted with serial dilutions, proving that it replicates within the primate host. However, like scrapie, the agent of kuru has not been seen by electron microscopy, does not induce cytopathic changes in cell culture, is resistant to physical and chemical treatments that usually inactivate viruses, and fails to evoke a demonstrable immune response in man or experimentally infected primates.

In recent years, there has been a striking decline in the incidence of kuru, particularly among children, in whom the disease has disappeared. This decreasing incidence has coincided with the suppression of cannibalism is this primitive culture, and there is considerable circumstantial evidence indicating that kuru was transmitted during the practice of ritual cannibalism.

310.3.   CREUTZFELDT-JAKOB DISEASE

Creutzfeldt-Jakob disease is an uncommon form of rapidly progressive dementia accompanied by myoclonus and other neurologic signs. The disease usually develops between ages 40 and 65, is worldwide in distribution, and usually occurs sporadically, although a few familial cases have been reported. The dementia develops rapidly, so that deterioration from day to day or week to week is evident. Myoclonic jerks usually develop early in the disease, and often massive symmetrical myoclonic jerks of the limbs occur when the patient is startled by unexpected light or sounds. Pyramidal tract signs, cerebellar ataxia, visual disturbances, and muscle wasting with fasciculations are common but inconstant features. The disease is inexorably progressive, usually reducing the patient from good health to total helplessness or death in less than a year. The cerebrospinal fluid shows no abnormality; but the electroencephalogram becomes abnormal early in the disease, showing diffuse slowing with superimposed bursts of sharp waves.

Neuropathologic findings include diffuse loss of cortical neurons with a remarkable increase in fibrous astrocytes. Vacuoles are present in neurons and astrocytes, and this may give a spongiform appearance to the cerebral cortex. Inflammatory reactions and inclusion bodies are absent. Thus, despite clinical and epidemiologic differences, the pathologic findings in Creutzfeldt-Jakob disease are very similar to those of kuru and scrapie.

A similar disease develops in chimpanzees inoculated with brain tissue of most patients with Creutzfeldt-Jakob disease after an incubation period of 11 to 71 months. The chimpanzees developed somnolence, ataxia, tremor, fasciculations, and intermittent jerking of the extremities. The pathologic changes in the brains resembled those of Creutzfeldt-Jakob disease. The disease has also been transmitted from chimpanzee to chimpanzee, to Old and New World monkeys, to domestic cat, to guinea pig, and possibly to mouse. Little information is available on the agent of Creutzfeldt-Jakob disease, but the absence of virus-like particles on electron microscopic examination of infectious tissues, the failure to demonstrate cytopathic changes in cell cultures, and the absence of a demonstrable immune response suggest that the agent is similar to those causing kuru and scrapie.

The mode of spread is unknown, but the ability to transmit disease with tissues from familial cases suggests the importance of genetic factors or the possible vertical transmission of the agent. The failure to find increased incidences in medical personnel, laboratory investigations, or spouses of patients suggests a lack of significant communicability by respiratory, enteric, or sexual contact. Furthermore, the agent has not been detected in blood, sputum, or urine of patients, although it is present in extraneural tissue. On the other hand, apparent person-to-person transmission has been documented with the development of Creutzfeldt-Jakob disease in a patient 18 months after receiving a corneal transplant from another patient who proved to have the disease; by the occurrence of the disease in two young patients less than two years after cerebral corticography using the same implanted electrodes previously used in a patient with Creutzfeldt-Jakob disease; and by the occurrence of the disease in a number of patients within two years after undergoing intracranial surgery. In view of these observations, isolation of patients with Creutzfeldt-Jakob disease does not appear indicated, but careful disposal of needles and special sterilization of surgical instruments used on these patients appear mandatory. Medical personnel should avoid contamination of open sores or the conjuctiva with tissue, and no organs or corneas from patients with ill-defined neurologic diseases should be used for transplantation purposes.

No known treatment alters the relentless course of Creutzfeldt-Jakob disease.

310.4. SUBACUTE SCLEROSING PANENCEPHALITIS
(Dawson's Encephalitis, Subacute Inclusion Body Encephalitis)

This is an uncommon, subacute encephalitis that usually occurs in children or young adults between the ages of 4 and 20 years. The onset is usually insidious and is characterized by deterioration in school work and behavioral disorders. This is followed in weeks or months by overt mental deterioration and neurologic signs, the most characteristic of which is myoclonus. The disease usually terminates after a third stage of stupor, blindness, dementia, and decorticate rigidity, which may last months to several years. Characteristically, the cerebrospinal fluid is under normal pressure and shows no pleocytosis but an increased concentration in gamma globulin, corresponding in large part to antibodies against measles virus. During the stage of active myoclonus, the electroencephalogram usually shows a typical pattern of general suppression of activity, with periodic (8 to 15 seconds) synchronous bursts

of high-voltage slow and sharp waves. The clinical course is usually characterized by progressive deterioration, but occasionally an apparent arrest of the disease process or even transient clinical improvement is seen.

Although the disease follows a protracted afebrile course, a viral cause has long been suspected because of the pathologic changes. Perivascular infiltrates of mononuclear cells are characteristic, and eosinophilic intranuclear inclusion bodies are found in neurons and glial cells. Because of these inclusions, a herpesvirus was long suspected of being the etiologic agent. However, electron microscope studies of cerebral biopsies show virus-like particles resembling the nucleocapsids of paramyxoviruses. Astonishingly high levels of antibodies against measles virus can be demonstrated in the serums of most patients, and measles virus antigen is present in the brain. Nevertheless, the isolation of measles-like viruses from brains of patients with subacute sclerosing panencephalitis is difficult, requiring the establishment of cell cultures from brains of patients with the disease and subsequent cocultivation of these cultures with other cells. The measles virus associated with the disease is apparently defective.

The pathogenesis of subacute sclerosing panencephalitis is obscure. This disease bears little resemblance clinically or pathologically to the fulminating forms of measles virus infections, in which virus dissemination may lead to giant-cell pneumonia. Furthermore, it is quite distinct from parainfectious encephalomyelitis that occasionally complicates measles virus infections, in which acute neurologic disease occurs and perivascular demyelination is found in the brain and spinal cord. Epidemiologic studies have shown that subacute sclerosing panencephalitis is more common in males than females, in children of rural than of urban origin, and in patients with a history of measles during the first two years of life. These findings suggest that environmental factors and presence of residual transplacental passive immunity may play roles in inducing defective infection or precipitating disease.

Empirical treatments of patients with antiviral agents, interferon inducers, and immunosuppression and immunoenhancement therapies have provided no convincing evidence of beneficial effects. An apparent recent decline in numbers of cases suggests that the widespread use of measles vaccine may have some preventive effect.

In a small number of preadolescents with stigmata of congenital rubella virus infections, a progressive neurologic disease has developed which clinically resembles subacute sclerosing panencephalitis. In these patients antibodies to rubella virus have been elevated in serum and cerebrospinal fluid. Pathologic changes are similar to those of subacute sclerosing panencephalitis except that inclusion bodies are absent and mineralization, as seen in infantile congenital rubella encephalitis, is present. Rubella virus has been recovered from brain.

310.5. PROGRESSIVE MULTIFOCAL LEUKOENCEPHALOPATHY

This is a rare demyelinating disease of the central nervous system. It usually develops in patients having preexisting disorders of the reticuloendothelial system such as leukemia, lymphoma, or sarcoidosis, but has also developed in patients immunosuppressed thera-peutically or after organ transplantation. Although the underlying systemic disorder may be of long standing, the neurologic abnormalities develop rather suddenly and follow a subacute progressive course until death. The findings usually suggest multifocal disease. Abnor-malities of motor function, sensation, vision, or speech are common, and dementia frequently develops. The cerebrospinal fluid shows little if any abnormality, and the electroencephalogram shows only nonspecific slow-ing. Pathologic lesions in the brain consist of multiple foci of demyelination in various stages of evolution. Oligodendrocytes are depleted within the foci, but sur-rounding the foci they are enlarged and contain eosino-philic intranuclear inclusions. The astrocytes within the demyelinated areas are often bizarre and contain mi-totic figures. Inflammatory cells are usually not promi-nent.

The presence of the inclusion bodies and the occur-rence against a background of disorders associated with impaired immunologic responses led to speculation that the disease might be caused by a viral infection. Elec-tron microscopic examination in almost all cases has shown particles in the oligodendrocyte inclusions re-sembling small papovaviruses. Two small deoxyribonu-cleic acid viruses related to simian-virus 40 have been isolated from brain tissue of patients dying from pro-gressive multifocal leukoencephalopathy. The JC virus, a new human papovavirus to which the majority of peo-ple have antibody since childhood, appears to be the causative agent in most cases. Viruses antigenically in-distinguishable from simian-virus 40 have been related to two cases. Neither of these viruses has been asso-ciated with any disease in man except progressive mul-tifocal leukoencephalopathy. Therefore progressive mul-tifocal leukoencephalopathy apparently results from opportunistic infection of the brain by normally non-pathogenic agents. The viruses appear to selectively in-fect and lyse oligodendrocytes, the glial cells which maintain the myelin sheaths, and cause demyelination. The disease occurs in patients with impaired cellular immune responses, but it is not known whether this disease represents a primary infection of an immunolog-ically incompetent patient or whether it represents a reactivation of a latent or persistent papovirus infec-tion.

Evaluation of possible therapeutic agents has not been possible because of the rarity of cases and the in-frequency of diagnosis during life.

310.6.   OTHER NEUROLOGIC DISEASES

Since viruses can cause disease after a long incuba-tion period, can produce disease with a subacute or re-lapsing course, and can give rise to noninflammatory pathologic changes, the possible role of slow or latent virus infection in a variety of neurologic diseases has been entertained.

In several chronic or relapsing inflammatory diseases of the nervous system, a viral cause has been suspect-ed. *Chronic focal epilepsy* (epilepsia partialis continua, Kozhevnikov's epilepsy) is, in some cases, associated with a chronic focal inflammatory process in the brain. In the Soviet Union, this has been thought to represent

a persistent focal infection with tick-borne viruses after acute encephalitis; and in several Soviet laboratories, tick-borne encephalitis virus has been isolated from surgically removed cerebral epileptogenic foci. No viruses have been isolated from similar cases in other countries. Chronic focal epilepsy can be a manifestation of focal disease processes such as neoplastic, vascular, or traumatic lesions, but chronic infection may play a role in some cases.

Recurrent acute meningitis or encephalitis occurs in three clinical syndromes of unknown cause in which la-tent viral infection has been suspected. *Mollaret's men-ingitis* is a rare, recurrent meningitis characterized by repeated attacks of headache, fever, and nuchal rigidity. Each attack is abrupt in onset and lasts for two to three days; the patient is entirely well between episodes. During attacks, the cerebrospinal fluid may contain large numbers of both polymorphonuclear and mono-nuclear cells and also large, poorly staining "epithelial cells," characteristic but not pathognomonic of this dis-ease. More severe recurrent neurologic involvement can occur in *Behçet's syndrome* and in the *Vogt-Koyanagi-Harada syndrome*. Behçet's syndrome is a chronic dis-ease characterized by recurrent oral and genital ulcers and inflammatory ocular lesions, usually taking the form of acute recurrent iritis. In about one quarter of the patients neurologic signs develop, consisting either of cranial nerve palsies, focal seizures, hemiparesis, or other focal signs or of severe depression of conscious-ness, coma, or meningeal signs, suggesting more dif-fuse neurologic involvement. Neurologic deficits usual-ly remit and relapse but may be progressive. Neuropathologic findings include meningeal inflamma-tory reactions, perivascular inflammation, and focal areas of necrosis. The Vogt-Koyanagi-Harada or uveoencephalitic syndrome is characterized by depig-mentation of skin and hair, inflammatory ocular lesions (usually consisting of iridocyclitis or exudative retinal detachment), and meningitis. Unlike Behçet's syn-drome, neurologic involvement occurs in all cases, often precedes the ocular inflammation, and usually consists only of headache, nuchal rigidity, and a mono-nuclear cell pleocytosis. However, transient decrease in hearing and tinnitus may accompany the meningitis, or a severe encephalitis may develop, leaving permanent neurologic deficits. Neuropathologic findings have con-sisted only of a chronic arachnoiditis. Reports have been made of isolations of unidentified viruses from patients with Mollaret's, Behçet's, and Vogt-Koyanagi-Harada syndrome; but none of these claims have been entirely convincing. An allergic cause has also been postulated in each of these disorders, and consequently treatment with corticosteroids has been advocated.

Considerable interest in a possible viral cause of *mul-tiple sclerosis* has been stimulated by epidemiologic data that indicate the role of a common exposure factor, se-rologic studies showing higher antibody levels against measles virus in patients with multiple sclerosis, obser-vation of viral-like particles in brains, and unconfirmed claims of virus isolations. These data are still inconclu-sive. A notion that Parkinson's disease might have a viral cause has been entertained ever since the observa-tion was made that a form of parkinsonism was a fre-quent sequela of encephalitis lethargica (von Economo's disease). Similarly, the possible role of a slow infection in amyotrophic lateral sclerosis and in a variety of other demyelinating and degenerative diseases has also been postulated. Although the spectrum of neurologic disease that can be potentially attributed to slow, latent, or chronic viral infections has greatly broadened in recent years, evidence is still scant for incriminating a transmissible agent in these chronic neurologic diseases.

Bernoulli, C., Siegfried, J., Baumgartner, G., Regli, F., Rabinowicz, T., Gajdusek, D. C., and Gibbs, C. J., Jr.: Danger of accidental person-to-person transmission of Creutzfeldt-Jakob disease by surgery. Lancet, 1:478, 1977.

Gajdusek, D. C.: Unconventional viruses and the origin and disappearance of kuru. Science, 197:943, 1977.

Johnson, R. T., and Herndon, R. M.: Virologic studies of multiple sclerosis and other chronic and relapsing neurological diseases. Prog. Med Virol., 18:229, 1974.

Johnson, R. T., and ter Meulen, V.: Slow infections of the nervous system. Adv. Intern. Med., 23:353, 1978.

Lampert, P. W., Gajdusek, D. C., and Gibbs, C. J., Jr.: Subacute spongiform virus encephalopathies. Scrapie, kuru, and Creutzfeldt-Jakob disease: A review. Am. J. Pathol., 68:626, 1972.

Narayan, O., Penney, J. B., Jr., Johnson, R. T., Herndon, R. M., and Weiner, L. P.: Etiology of progressive multifocal leukoencephalopathy: Identification of papovavirus. N. Engl. J. Med., 289:1278, 1973.

Padgett, B. L., Walker, D. L., ZuRhein, G. M., Hodach, A. E., and Chou, S. M.: JC papovavirus in progressive multifocal leukoencephalopathy. J. Infect. Dis., 133:686, 1976.

Roos, R., Gajdusek, D. C., and Gibbs, C. J., Jr.: The clinical characteristics of transmissible Creutzfeldt-Jakob disease. Brain, 96:1, 1973.

Section Seventeen THE DEMYELINATING DISEASES

Labe C. Scheinberg

311. INTRODUCTION

The term *demyelinating diseases* is applied to disorders that selectively damage or destroy central nervous system myelin but relatively spare the axis cylinders of the nerve cells. Traditionally, the term has been applied principally to multiple sclerosis and its variants. Several other inherited and acquired disorders also can affect central myelin rather selectively, however. Accordingly, Poser, in 1957, suggested assigning the term "demyelinating" to those relatively common disorders in which myelin is apparently normally formed but from some cause breaks down later in life. Multiple sclerosis is the most frequent of these diseases. The term "dysmyelinating" was employed, on the other hand, to designate a group of relatively rare disorders in which a known or presumed genetically determined enzyme deficiency results in defective myelin early in life. The term includes the leukodystrophies, other lipodystrophies, and some of the aminoacidurias. Table 1 lists these disorders of myelin.

BIOLOGY OF MYELIN. Myelin in the central nervous system appears to be formed mainly, if not entirely, by the oligodendrocytes. Astrocytes, in turn, may contribute to maintaining the nutrition and the ionic-metabolic homeostasis of the central tissue once it is formed. As the central nervous system develops, oligodendrocytes wrap their external plasma membrane concentrically around the axons of the larger nerve cells, producing a lamellar proteolipid sheet (myelin) that insulates the axon and guarantees its proper conduction of impulses. One oligodendrocyte may, by multiple extensions, form the myelin of many axons; as a result, destruction or disease of only a few oligodendrocytes may lead to a relatively large lesion of myelinated tracts. As the unit membrane of the oligodendrocyte forms myelin, the internal surfaces become apposed to form what one sees by electron microscopy as the dark major period line. The external surfaces give rise to the lighter intraperiod line, and the entire wrapping produces a structure composed of layers of concentric, tightly packed membranes of uniform thickness. The results of studies employing x-ray diffraction, electron microscopy, and lipid analyses suggest that each layered unit membrane of myelin consists of a bimolecular lipid leaflet sandwiched between parallel layers of hydrated protein, in close contact with the polar groups of the lipids. The lipids that make up this leaflet appear to be interdigitated molecules of cerebroside, phospholipid, and cholesterol. Detailed chemical analyses of myelin indicate that protein (primarily proteolipid protein) makes up approximately 22 per cent of dry

TABLE 1. Disorders Selectively Affecting Myelin

I. Demyelinating diseases (acquired breakdown of preformed normal myelin)
  A. Known or suspected disorders of the host's immune response to a foreign protein
    1. Postimmunization encephalomyelitis (smallpox, rabies, etc.)
    2. Parainfectious encephalomyelitis (postexanthematous, postinfectious, etc.)
    3. Acute disseminated encephalomyelitis without antecedent cause
  B. Multiple sclerosis and its presumed variants
    1. Optic and retrobulbar neuritis
    2. Neuromyelitis optica (Devic)
    3. Transverse myelitis
    4. Acute disseminated encephalomyelitis
  C. Disorders of known viral cause
    1. Progressive multifocal leukoencephalopathy
    2. Subacute sclerosing panencephalitis
  D. Disorders of presumed nutritional origin
    1. Combined systems disease (cyanocobalamin deficiency)
    2. Demyelination of the corpus callosum (Marchiafava-Bignami)
    3. Central pontine myelinolysis
  E. Disorders of anoxic-ischemic origin
    1. Delayed postanoxic cerebral demyelination
    2. Progressive subcortical ischemic encephalopathy (Binswanger)
II. Dysmyelinating disorders (genetic or developmental failure to form or maintain normally constituted myelin)
  A. The leukodystrophies
    1. Simple storage type; metachromatic leukodystrophy, glial insufficiency type of sulfatidosis
    2. Sudanophilic (Pelizaeus-Merzbacher)
    3. Globoid cell (Krabbe)
    4. Adrenoleukodystrophy (Schilder)
    5. Miscellaneous and mixed types (Seitelberger, Lowenberg-Hill, Alexander, Canavan, etc.)
    6. Lipidoses (Tay-Sachs, Gaucher, etc.)
  B. Aminoacidurias and developmental disorders
    1. Phenylketonuria, maple syrup urine disease, etc.
    2. Congenital thyroid deficiency, etc.

weight. The lipids contain approximately equal molar ratios of cholesterol and phospholipids with about one half as much galactolipid. These lipids in the myelin sheath are remarkably inert; once deposited at the time of myelin formation, they undergo little subsequent turnover. The biologic half-life of cholesterol in myelin is about one year, for example, compared to about ten days in other biologic membranes. Myelin should not be considered as metabolically inactive, however, because the components of white matter, and particularly the glial cells, account for about 30 per cent of the brain's total oxygen consumption.

The central myelin sheath is a compact, highly organized membrane extension of the oligodendrocyte which, though metabolically active, must be regarded as one of the more permanent tissue elements of the body.

The foregoing considerations indicate that primary central demyelination must be considered not just as a problem of myelin breakdown or dysgenesis but as the result of a basic disorder of the oligodendrocyte. In most primary demyelinating disorders, the precise cause remains unknown. The pathogenic agent may attack either the perikaryon (cell body) or the plasma membrane of the oligodendrocyte to produce demyelination.

PATHOGENESIS OF MULTIPLE SCLEROSIS. Multiple sclerosis is by far the most prevalent and clinically significant myelin disorder, affecting as many as 500,000 persons in the United States. Until a valid biochemical or immunologic test exists or until the etiologic agent is identified with certainty, we cannot say that the various symptoms and signs collected under the rubric multiple sclerosis are more than a syndrome. Clinical experience has shown, however, that if certain diagnostic criteria are met (see below), a group of central nervous system disorders in adults may be defined which are accompanied by consistent neuropathologic changes. Developments in the past few years suggest that multiple sclerosis results when an exogenous agent, presumably a viral infection, precipitates in the body an autoimmune response which, in turn, destroys central nervous system myelin.

The strongest stimulus for suspecting allergic factors in the pathogenesis of demyelinating diseases lies in the similarity of the neuropathologic abnormalities in multiple sclerosis to those of rabies postvaccinal encephalomyelitis. Rivers and coworkers in 1933 showed that multiple intramuscular injections of normal rabbit brain into monkey resulted in an encephalomyelitis with neuropathologic lesions similar to those of rabies postvaccinal encephalomyelitis. This line of investigation was accelerated by the extensive work of Kabat, Wolf, and coworkers in the 1940's, who showed that experimental allergic encephalomyelitis (EAE) could be produced by a single injection of adult autologous, homologous, or heterologous central myelin mixed with Freund's adjuvant (paraffin oil and killed mycobacteria).

The critical antigenic material in white matter to produce EAE appears to be a protein known as myelin basic protein (BP). This BP with Freund's complete adjuvant can initiate EAE, but if injected into animals with paraffin oil alone, later challenge of the animals with the usual encephalitogenic agent fails to produce EAE. Unfortunately, subsequent investigations in animals have shown variable and sometimes contradictory results in the role of BP as a therapeutic agent. BP has no current role in the treatment of prophylaxis of multiple sclerosis.

Other studies have shown that EAE is a delayed hypersensitivity reaction mediated by thymus-dependent lymphocytes (T cells) and may be transferred from one guinea pig to another by sensitized lymphocytes. Serum from EAE animals and from patients with multiple sclerosis can destroy myelin in tissue culture.

The strongest direct evidence for immunologic abnormalities in patients with multiple sclerosis is the presence of increased levels of gamma globulin (IgG) both in the cerebrospinal fluid (CSF) and surrounding the demyelinating lesions in the brain of most patients with multiple sclerosis. The highest incidence of the CSF abnormality is detected by visualizing specific "oligoclonal" bands in the gamma globulin region, and this abnormality may be detected even when the percentage of IgG is normal.

Widespread acceptance of multiple sclerosis as a disease incorporating abnormalities of cellular and humoral immunity has led to several efforts at using these changes to provide laboratory tests of diagnosis or disease activity. Thus far none of these measures have achieved a sufficient consistency or specificity to be clinically useful. Among these studies, one has demonstrated that leukocytes from patients with multiple sclerosis adhere to measles-infected epithelial cells to form rosettes. Such responses are much less pronounced with normal leukocytes or with those from patients with other neurologic disorders. Also, patients with multiple sclerosis often have elevated levels of measles antibody in blood and CSF, but the response is inconsistent and often includes other increased antibody levels as well. Other efforts to determine the activity of multiple sclerosis employ BP in a radioimmunoassay of myelin fragments present in the CSF. The test has correlated a high concentration of BP in the CSF during supposed active myelin destruction or exacerbation, but is not specific to multiple sclerosis.

The hypothesis that a viral agent could cause the chronic relapsing and remitting lesions of multiple sclerosis is based on three principal pieces of indirect evidence. One is the recently acquired knowledge that slow or chronic viral infections can produce chronic neurologic disorders in animals and man (see Ch. 310). The second is the evidence suggesting an excessive immunologic response to an exogenous agent in the tissues and CSF of patients with multiple sclerosis. The third is epidemiologic evidence that multiple sclerosis arises predominantly in individuals who have been exposed prior to a certain age to a (possibly infectious) environmental agent.

Multiple sclerosis (MS) is from three to over thirty times more prevalent in northern than in southern latitudes. Several epidemiologic investigations have shown that individuals who move from areas of higher to areas of lower MS prevalence after the age of about 15 years retain a risk of developing MS that is the same as in their original environment. Those who move before 15 years of age, however, develop the risk engendered by the new environment. A virus (e.g., measles) that differently affected adults and children and that infected individuals at an earlier age in southern than in northern latitudes could explain these observations. Poliomyelitis, for example, when it attacks at an early age, may cause mild illness yet afford lifelong immunity, but at a later age often produces paralytic disease. Factors of geography, economics, climate, and hygiene all seem to play significant roles in the prevalence of MS and are consistent with the theory of viral etiology.

Inconclusive or inconsistent results have attended efforts to identify a virus in the tissues of patients with MS. Reports of visualizing viral particles in the tissues by electron microscopy have not been confirmed. Parainfluenza viruses have reportedly been recovered from affected brains by co-cultivation techniques by some laboratories, but not others. Other laboratories have claimed that agents in the tissues of patients with MS will induce specific abnormalities in animals or cells in tissue culture, but this finding also stands as unconfirmed. Even the oligoclonal band in the CSF of patients with multiple sclerosis has thus far not been demonstrated to contain predominantly antibody to any specific virus.

Even if it turns out that MS results from infection by a virus, the epidemiologic data indicate that most of those infected do not get the disease. This implies a possible genetically determined susceptibility, and evidence supporting this speculation is gained from the fact that certain patterns of histocompatibility antigens are found more frequently in patients with MS than in normals. According to theory, an MS susceptibility gene occurs in close association with genes determining the body's immune response to viruses and modifies the response to such infection.

Since the HLA patterns associated with MS show differences in different parts of the world, however, the full significance of the association remains to be determined.

312. MULTIPLE SCLEROSIS

DEFINITION. Multiple or disseminated sclerosis (MS) is the most common demyelinating disorder. The disease characteristically is marked by recurrent attacks of demyelination (dissemination in time) distributed widely in the brain and spinal cord (dissemination in space). The disease includes a number of well recognized and readily diagnosed syndromes, but borderline cases may be difficult to categorize clinically and pathologically. The lack of comprehensive diagnostic laboratory tests adds to this difficulty. Generally, MS is chronic and relapsing, but fulminating attacks occur and as many as 30 per cent of the patients progress steadily from the onset. Most of the symptoms and signs reflect involvement of central myelin, but occasionally symptoms of neuronal or gray-matter involvement occur when the plaques extend into such areas.

PREVALENCE. The prevalence of MS in the United States varies from about 10 per 100,000 in the South to 60 per 100,000 in the North, with similar prevalence and distribution in Europe. The disease affects males and females about equally. About 67 per cent of cases begin between the ages of 20 and 40 years and 95 per cent between 10 and 50 years.

Populations residing between latitudes 40° N and 40° S (tropical and subtropical zones) have a low risk of MS, whereas populations residing north of this latitude in North America and Europe are at higher risk. Exceptions to these generalizations are found in other parts of the world; e.g., a low incidence is reported in the Union of South Africa and in Japan. Racial factors seem to play little part in the United States, because the incidence in blacks is almost the same as in whites. Reports of a greater family incidence than could be expected by chance fail to exclude the common effects of environmental factors. A purely hereditary basis seems to be excluded by a lack of concordance in identical twins.

PATHOLOGY. The external surface of the brain and cord generally shows no abnormality. Occasionally there is atrophy of the optic nerves, and rarely there is focal or generalized atrophy of the cerebral hemispheres. Acute large lesions may cause swelling of the cord. Rarely there may be sufficient focal swelling of the cerebrum to give the appearance of a neoplasm in roentgenologic contrast studies.

Cut sections of the brain or spinal cord reveal numerous scattered, grayish, well defined lesions that are slightly depressed and vary in diameter from a few millimeters to a few centimeters. These are found throughout the white matter of the brain, optic nerves, and spinal cord and occasionally extend into gray matter. The number of lesions is usually greater than would be expected from the clinical picture.

Microscopic abnormalities depend on the age of the lesion. Acute lesions show an infiltration of microglial phagocytes and mononuclear cells about vessels, as well as scattered in the lesion itself. The myelin sheaths are affected to varying degrees, from partial to complete destruction, with relative sparing of axons, glia, and other structures. In more severe lesions there may be total destruction of tissue and cyst formation. As the lesions become chronic, there is a proliferation of glial cells and fibers to give the typical "sclerotic plaque." The axons in these areas may be preserved or destroyed.

AGGRAVATING FACTORS. An *infective process* (upper respiratory infection, "influenza," urinary tract infection, gastroenteritis, etc.) is said to precede the initial attack or a relapse of MS in 10 to 40 per cent. *Immunizations* are without apparent effect on the course of the disease, and any exacerbations seen following these are probably coincidental.

Many workers have stated that *pregnancy* aggravates the disease, but this is open to question. The disease and pregnancy occur in the same age group, and although some studies show a higher incidence in married childbearing women, more attacks occur during the puerperium than during pregnancy itself. The physician must consider many nonmedical factors when advising on this problem. Pregnancy is generally considered nondeleterious to the course of MS in any patient who has had no attack in two years.

There seems to be no clear-cut association of attack or relapse with surgical procedures, and indications for *surgery* in patients with MS should be judged solely on their merit.

There is no statistical evidence to support a relationship between peripheral *trauma* and the onset or relapses of MS. There is a tendency for patients to associate trauma with the onset of an attack or relapse, but in many cases it is more likely that the trauma resulted from the disability of MS. *Emotional stress* has been incriminated as a precipitant of attacks or relapses of MS. This is difficult to substantiate, but it is reasonable to assume that cerebral changes in MS make it difficult for the patient to cope with emotional stress.

TABLE 2.   Frequency of Occurrence of First Symptom of Multiple Sclerosis in Cases Proved by Clinical Study and Autopsy

Symptom	Autopsy (Carter et al.) (46 Cases)	Autopsy (Poser) (111 Cases)	Clinical Diagnosis (Carter et al.) (539 Cases)
	per cent	per cent	per cent
Weakness	42	39	54
Diplopia, impaired vision	35	32	21
Tremor, ataxia, incoordination	20	6	19
Paresthesias	13	16	32
Pain	11	1	—
Sphincter impairment	11	1	7
Dizziness or vertigo	7	1	8
Changes in muscle tone	7	—	—
Facial pain	2	—	—
Mental changes	2	2	—
Seizures	—	—	3

Certain diagnostic procedures such as lumbar puncture, pneumoencephalography, cerebral angiography, and myelography have been implicated in the worsening of symptoms in MS. However, these procedures are performed usually in patients whose disease is progressing or soon after an attack or relapse. They should be reserved for patients in whom one has serious questions whether a neoplasm exists in the nervous system, and not performed simply because "there's nothing else to be done."

CLINICAL MANIFESTATIONS. The clinical picture of MS is pleomorphic, but there are usually sufficient typical features to enable one to diagnose the disorder in the absence of a specific diagnostic test or without extensive "excluding" diagnostic procedures. The disease is chronic, often characterized by exacerbations and remissions, with evidence of multiple lesions in central white matter occurring in young adults without other systemic disorders. The symptoms of central white matter involvement are usually those of supranuclear weakness, incoordination, paresthesias, and visual complaints. Other symptoms and signs that are more characteristic of lesions in gray matter, e.g., aphasia, seizures, fasciculations, and neurogenic atrophy, are rare. Mental changes have an intermediate incidence and affect perhaps 30 per cent of patients.

The onset may be acute, with symptoms appearing within minutes to hours, or it may be insidious, with gradual, slow progression of symptoms over a period of months.

The frequency of occurrence of the first symptom of MS is given in Table 2.

The weakness usually begins or is most prominent in the lower extremities, but the upper extremities may be involved. When both lower extremities are involved, there are usually accompanying urinary complaints such as urgency or frequency. The weakness may be minimal, or there may be a total paralysis. There are usually upper motor neuron signs such as spasticity, hyperreflexia, and pathologic reflexes.

Visual complaints include blurring of vision with a central scotoma and decreased visual acuity or diplopia with extraocular paresis and nystagmus.

The incoordination is seen as ataxia or clumsiness and intention tremor of the upper extremities. Often a combination of spastic-ataxic gait is seen.

The paresthesias may involve any or all of the extremities. Usually there is impairment of vibratory sense and position sense in the lower extremities, whereas cutaneous sensation is relatively spared.

The typical clinical course of MS is one of exacerbations and remissions over a period of years, with increasing neurologic deficits caused by an increasing number of disseminated lesions. Less frequent are (1) an acute, severe course progressing to death in a few days or weeks; (2) a chronic, progressive course over a period of years; and (3) a benign form with relatively few presenting symptoms and signs and long-lasting remissions. In middle age the insidious onset of a progressive spastic paraparesis is often seen as the major clinical manifestation, particularly in women.

MS is sometimes divided into clinical types, depending upon which portion of the neuraxis is most involved, e.g., spinal, cerebral, brainstem-cerebellar, or mixed. The most common form is spinal with prominent features of spastic paraparesis, lower extremity paresthesias, and urinary complaints. The brainstem-cerebellar variety with prominent visual complaints, cranial nerve signs, nystagmus, vertigo, and incoordination is also common, but the cerebral form with mental changes and hemiparesis and hemisensory changes is uncommon.

Although most cases may be classified as one of these forms early in the course, almost all patients appear to have a mixed type of involvement after about 15 years.

In Table 3 may be noted the frequency of various symptoms and signs of MS in clinical and autopsy series reported by Carter et al. and by Poser.

Certain uncommon symptoms and signs such as nausea, vomiting, facial pain, seizures, dysphagia, atrophy, hearing loss, tinnitus, and changes in states of consciousness occur in 2 to 10 per cent of cases. Signs such as internuclear ophthalmoplegia are highly characteristic of multiple sclerosis; headache and aphasia are rare.

LABORATORY DATA. Abnormal findings in MS are usually confined to the cerebrospinal fluid (CSF). In the acute disease, there may be a mild mononuclear pleocytosis of as much as 200 to 300 cells per cubic millimeter, but usually less than 40. The protein content is usually normal or slightly elevated (50 to 100 mg per 100 ml); values higher than this are rare. The gamma globulin content is elevated in about two thirds of the cases and, correspondingly, there is often an abnormal colloidal gold curve (first or second zone), accompanied by a negative serologic test for syphilis. Closer examination of the gamma globulin region of the CSF by starch-gel or agar-gel electrophoresis shows specific oligoclonal bands of immunoglobulin in a majority of cases. These may be detected even when the percentage of gamma

TABLE 3. Frequency of Occurrence of Symptoms and Signs in Course of Multiple Sclerosis

	Carter et al. (46 Cases)	Poser (111 Cases)
	per cent	per cent
Weakness (symptom or sign)	89	96
Abnormal movements	67	
Abnormal reflexes (absent superficials, Babinski signs, or hyperreflexia)	99	95
Sphincter and genital difficulties	78	82
Visual disturbance (symptom or sign)	100	85
Nystagmus (any type)	85	70
Disc pallor, atrophy, decreased acuity	75	85
Third nerve impairment (and internuclear ophthalmoplegia)	67	
Tremor, ataxia	93	79
Impaired vibration and position sense	81	58
Impaired touch, pain, temperature sense	35	35
Mental changes (symptom or sign)	61	45
Paresthesias	44	65
Pain	42	19
Vertigo or dizziness	18	15

globulin is normal. Such oligoclonal bands also occur occasionally in neurosyphilis, subacute sclerosing panencephalitis, Guillain-Barré syndrome, brain tumor, and cerebrovascular disease, and are not of themselves diagnostic.

The electroencephalogram may be mildly abnormal in about two thirds of cases, but is not useful in diagnosis. Computerized tomography (CT) scans detect large confluent areas of cerebral demyelination but are not useful for diagnosis in most cases. Recently described blood immunologic tests require independent confirmation before they can be relied upon for diagnosis.

Visual evoked responses can extend the diagnostic examination in patients with suspected MS. The test involves the presentation of a patterned stimulus to the retina and recording the response at the occipital cortex by scalp electrodes. Abnormalities of the latency and/or configuration of the computer-averaged cortical response are readily detected and identify subclinical involvement of the visual pathways.

DIAGNOSIS. Because of the pleomorphic nature of the disease, it is often necessary to exclude many other neurologic disorders. Most often one must consider spinal cord, brainstem or cerebellar tumors, degenerative diseases such as the spinocerebellar degenerations, and combined system disease.

The fact that MS has a remitting nature in many instances and the dissemination of symptoms and signs should indicate that one is not dealing with an expanding lesion involving the nervous system. If all the symptoms and signs can be explained by a single lesion, then one should assume that the condition is not MS. If the patient complains of headache, seizures, or progressive focal neurologic signs, which are uncommon in MS, and if these are accompanied by abnormalities such as increased CSF pressure, roentgenographic changes in the skull or spine, and marked elevation of CSF protein, then one must proceed further to exclude a neoplasm. This can be done in most cases by a neuroroentgenologic procedure such as myelography, pneumoencephalography, cerebral angiography, or CT scan. Vascular disease, particularly that involving the brainstem, can be confused with MS in middle-aged patients. In some of these cases only prolonged follow-up reveals the true diagnosis.

Certain degenerative disorders of the nervous system can be confused with MS. However, the former tend to have a family history, to be slowly progressive without remission, and to confine themselves to systems, e.g., cerebellar, extrapyramidal, or motor system. In the differential diagnosis of spastic paraparesis of middle age, one should consider, respectively, motor neuron disease (amyotrophic lateral sclerosis), cervical spondylosis, or spinal cord tumor. The first has no sensory abnormalities, and the latter two both have characteristic roentgenologic abnormalities. Combined system disease can be excluded in most cases by hematologic studies and gastric analysis.

TREATMENT. There are several aspects to the management of MS. The first is to attempt to treat or affect the course of the disease itself. The second is to attempt to manage the painful and disabling complications of the disease, e.g., spasticity, tremor, decubiti, and urinary problems. The third aspect is the management of the patient with a chronic, unpredictable, and occasionally disabling disease.

Many authorities believe that adrenocorticosteroids favorably influence the onset or acute exacerbations of MS, and recommend the administration of ACTH, 40 to 80 units per day, or prednisone, 40 to 80 mg per day, over a period of three to four weeks, taking suitable precautions against complications. Controlled studies have suggested that such measures induce the more rapid clearing of acute symptoms and signs but leave the long-term outcome of the disease unaffected. Because of potential complications, long-term maintenance therapy with ACTH or corticosteroids is contraindicated. No evidence indicates that immunosuppressant agents have long-term benefit.

The greater gain in treatment lies in the management of some of the painful or disabling complications of the disease. Some are specifically neurologic and related to MS, whereas others are seen in any chronic disease. Three neurologic symptoms are responsible for most of the disability seen in MS: spasticity, incoordination, and urinary bladder problems. Spasticity with flexor spasms seems best controlled by use of baclofen, a substituted gamma-aminobutyric acid compound which inhibits central synaptic transmission. In doses of 30 to 100 mg per day* it is effective in most patients and causes few side effects or complications. Gait incoordination or truncal ataxia responds poorly to most measures, although intention tremor of the arm seems to respond to contralateral cryothalamotomy. Bilateral

---

*See p. vi, Dosage Notice, immediately following Preface.

thalamic surgery is not advised because of the occurrence of pseudobulbar symptoms. Pharmacologic agents such as propanolol, 40 to 320 mg per day, have been reported sometimes to relieve tremor. The management of the urinary bladder is of extreme importance regarding both the life expectancy of the patient and his or her self-esteem. Primarily the effort must be made to avoid a large residual urine with eventual infection of the bladder. Intermittent daily catheterization probably carries a lower risk of infection than prolonged use of an indwelling catheter, and many women can be taught self-catheterization. The prevention and management of decubiti, nutritional deficiency, contractures, infections, and psychologic problems are similar to those in other diseases. In MS, because of its often undeserved grim reputation, there is a frequent attempt to keep the diagnosis from the patients. This often results in unnecessary distress for the patients and family and loss of confidence in the physician. Usually, it is advisable to inform the patient when the diagnosis is established and to be supportive and optimistic. Statistics indicate an average survival of 35 years from onset of MS, with about two thirds of the patients remaining productive if not in physically demanding occupations.

The third aspect of the management of the patient with chronic, unpredictable, and occasionally disabling disease is the most important, rewarding, and neglected aspect. These patients are told often that there is no treatment — and indeed there is none for the MS itself — but this does not imply that one can do nothing for its complications. Medical neglect combines with disease progression in taking physical and psychologic toll on patient and family. In addition to disclosure and open discussion of the disease with the patient and family, one must be continuously supportive and even optimistic. Sexual problems, financial insecurity, and physical disability are reflected in a higher divorce and unemployment rate and should be met with counseling and judicious planning. Occupational therapy, with emphasis on activities of daily living, probably contributes more than physical therapy. Exhausting physical exertion and even exhausting physiotherapy may cause greater distress in patients already suffering lassitude. An increased body temperature may aggravate the symptoms of MS, and consequently swimming in a cool pool is a much advised form of therapy and general conditioning exercise. Splinting, tenotomy, and neurectomy may be necessary in the final stages to manage contractures and decubiti.

Pregnancy generally is best avoided within two years of an acute attack because of the associated fatigue and weakness. Pregnancy probably does not adversely influence the course of the disease over the years. The timing of elective surgery and other unnecessary stresses should be carefully weighed by patient and physician.

PROGNOSIS.   In the early stages of the disease it is not possible accurately to predict the course, although certain symptoms seem to indicate a better prognosis. Monosymptomatic and acute symptoms lasting hours to weeks tend to give a better prognosis than polysymptomatic or slowly progressive manifestations. Cranial nerve, visual, and sensory symptoms carry a better prognosis for remission or a benign course than do motor or cerebellar symptoms. More than half the cases remit after an initial attack, but one cannot predict the next attack. The remission of certain symptoms, e.g.,

retrobulbar neuritis, may be so complete as to make the clinician doubt the history.

Within the first five years after onset, about 70 per cent of patients are able to be employed, although with occasional interruptions in some cases. By the end of ten years this drops off to 50 per cent. At the end of 20 years 35 per cent are still employed, with minor interruptions, and about 20 per cent of patients succumb to complications of the disease by this time. The major disabilities are spasticity, disturbances of coordination, and disturbance in bladder and bowel function.

Life expectancy varies considerably, ranging from a few weeks to over 50 years after the initial attack regardless of whether one considers hospitalized severe cases or the more benign forms. The average life expectancy in all patients is about 35 years after onset. This represents an increase of about 10 years in the last generation and is due to better management of intercurrent genitourinary or respiratory infections, the usual causes of death.

313.   POSSIBLE MULTIPLE SCLEROSIS VARIANTS

OPTIC AND RETROBULBAR NEURITIS

Optic neuritis is a term used to describe involvement of the optic nerve as a result of inflammation, demyelination, or degeneration. When the site of the lesion is intraocular, ophthalmoscopy reveals papilledema and the terms *papillitis* or intraocular neuritis are employed. *Retrobulbar neuritis* indicates involvement of the orbital or intracranial optic nerve behind the eye. There is often a predilection for the papillomacular bundle, producing a characteristic central scotoma but usually with minimal or absent ophthalmoscopic abnormalities in the acute stage.

Optic neuritis has many known causes, such as nutritional deficiency, intoxications (tobacco, alcohol), local inflammatory conditions (sinusitis, meningitis, orbital infections), and metabolic diseases (diabetes mellitus, pernicious anemia, other vitamin deficiencies). Once these have been excluded, demyelinating disease must be considered as a likely cause. In several large series of patients who presented with retrobulbar neuritis and were followed for many years, 15 to 30 per cent later developed other manifestations of MS. Conversely, about 50 per cent of patients with MS exhibit symptoms of optic neuritis at some time during the course of the disease.

Both optic and retrobulbar neuritis are characterized by an abrupt or progressive loss of vision that is rarely total and is usually unilateral. Associated with the visual loss may be pain in and around the eye that is accentuated by ocular movement. There may be tenderness on palpation of the eyeball. Visual testing reveals decreased acuity and central or paracentral scotomas. In *intraocular neuritis* or *papillitis,* the optic disc appears inflamed, and there may be hyperemia, blurred margins, and even elevation. A few hemorrhages may be seen in the retina adjacent to the disc. In *retrobulbar neuritis* the ophthalmoscopic picture is normal, but the features are otherwise similar to those of optic neuritis.

It is essential to differentiate optic neuritis from papilledema associated with increased intracranial pressure or other conditions. Papilledema is almost always bilateral, and vision is usually well preserved until late in the course. The disc elevation is usually greater in papilledema, and the only visual field defect is an enlarged blind spot. In optic neuritis the cerebrospinal fluid pressure is almost always normal, and there may be other findings indicative of MS.

Optic and retrobulbar neuritis may be treated with ACTH or corticosteroids. However, almost complete spontaneous recovery often occurs, and the benefits of therapy are difficult to assess.

The prognosis in a single attack of optic or retrobulbar neuritis is usually good. There may be complete recovery, or there may be residual visual field defects, temporal pallor of the discs, or optic atrophy. The visual acuity may be further impaired with subsequent attacks, but complete visual loss is rare.

ACUTE TRANSVERSE MYELITIS

Acute transverse myelitis may appear as the initial event in a subsequently typical form of MS, or it may develop during the course of the disease. The findings include complete or partial paralysis of both legs or of all four limbs, variable sensory loss, and bladder and bowel involvement. The condition is described in detail in Ch. 300.

Subacute necrotizing myelopathy is often associated with vascular malformations of the spinal cord or thrombophlebitis (Foix-Alajouanine syndrome). In acute necrotizing myelopathy there is hemorrhagic necrosis of the spinal cord without any associated vascular malformation. Such cases, which are rare, show a rapidly ascending motor and sensory paralysis with polymorphonuclear cells in the cerebrospinal fluid, and death may occur in weeks or months.

NEUROMYELITIS OPTICA (DEVIC'S DISEASE)

This clinical syndrome is characterized by acute transverse myelitis and optic neuritis. It may be considered to be a variant of MS and may occur as the initial illness or later during the course of the disease. There may be sudden loss of vision in both eyes, with central scotoma or sudden onset of paraplegia with sensory loss. The ocular involvement may be due to optic or retrobulbar neuritis, and the transverse myelitis may be partial or complete. Days or weeks may elapse between the onsets of the two symptom complexes. In severe cases the motor symptoms tend to be permanent, but otherwise the course, laboratory data, and treatment are similar to those of MS.

TRANSITIONAL SCLEROSIS

Transitional sclerosis is probably a pathologic variant of MS in which the disseminated plaques tend to become confluent, creating large areas of myelin loss. Clinically these cases are indistinguishable from cases of typical MS. Transitional sclerosis probably represents an intermediate pathologic form between MS and Schilder's cerebral sclerosis.

ACUTE NECROTIZING HEMORRHAGIC ENCEPHALOMYELITIS

This is a rare and fulminant variant of demyelinating disease that often progresses to death in days or weeks. The disease is characterized by a rapid course, fever, headache, convulsions, progressive change in state of consciousness from drowsiness to coma, nuchal rigidity, and hemiplegia or quadriplegia. The cerebrospinal fluid examination reveals a pleocytosis up to several thousand white blood cells that are predominantly polymorphonuclear leukocytes, and an elevated protein content. On pathologic examination, there are large foci of hemorrhagic necrosis of white matter. Although most patients succumb within a few weeks, there are rare alleged reports of recovery. There appears to be an experimental allergic model of this disorder with similarities on histologic examination. The only therapy that can be offered is supportive, though ACTH and corticosteroids should be tried.

ACUTE DISSEMINATED ENCEPHALOMYELITIS

Occasionally acute neurologic symptoms may occur without apparent preceding infection. The clinical picture is dependent on the location of the lesions and may include the symptoms and signs of meningitis, encephalitis, myelitis, or any combination of the preceding. Some cases blend indistinguishably into chronic, typical MS and so may represent the initial acute attack of that disease. Other cases may be uniphasic, and the patient may recover with or without neurologic residua and have no further attacks. Only prolonged follow-up with a recurrence or progression of neurologic symptoms can enable one to diagnose acute MS and exclude acute disseminated encephalomyelitis.

DIFFUSE SCLEROSIS

There is a group of progressive neurologic disorders of young patients who manifest severe neurologic deficits of various types and progressive visual and mental deterioration. In three publications from 1912 to 1924, Schilder described three cases of diffuse disease of white matter that he proposed grouping under the name encephalitis periaxialis diffusa (called Schilder's disease). Additional publications by Schilder and others followed. It now seems likely that three separate conditions have been included under the rubric of Schilder's disease and that the eponymic designation should be discarded. Some of these cases represent the result of severe, confluent extensions of the myelinoclastic lesions of MS. Some represent leukoencephalitides of known viral origin, such as subacute sclerosing panencephalitis and progressive multifocal leukoencephalitis. A third group undoubtedly includes the leukodystrophies listed in Table 1. Among these, it is probable that adrenoleukodystrophy was the disorder that Schilder identified in one of his early cases. This condition only recently has been delineated fully. It is genetically transmitted, probably as a sex-linked recessive trait, and affects young boys, usually before the age of ten years.

The onset of adrenoleukodystrophy is usually insidious but may be acute. It is usually slowly progressive, but there may be successive bursts to simulate the course of MS. A typical presenting picture is of insidious mental deterioration with loss of recently acquired intellectual achievements, and this progresses slowly to dementia. Many patients develop aphasia, apraxia, and dysarthria. Visual loss with cortical blindness is characteristic, and auditory complaints with cortical deafness may follow involvement of the cortical radiations. Clinical signs of adrenal insufficiency occur in only a minority of the patients, but tests of adrenal function are almost always abnormal. Pathologic examination of the adrenal gland shows abnormalities predominantly in the zona fascicularis and zona reticularis. Neuropathologically, the changes in brain myelin resemble many of the abnormalities of MS, yet contain abnormal cytoplasmic inclusions. Since these ultrastructural abnormalities also occur in other tissues, adrenoleukodystrophy presently is regarded as an inherited metabolic disorder.

314. LEUKODYSTROPHIES

This group includes heredofamilial diseases in which normal myelin is probably not formed because of some genetically determined enzymatic defect. The classsification is not completely satisfactory; the group tends to merge with the lipidoses of the nervous system, so that authorities differ in their classifications. Only further elucidation of the enzymatic defects of myelin metabolism in these disorders will lead to a satisfactory classification.

METACHROMATIC LEUKOENCEPHALOPATHY

These are otherwise known as the glial insufficiency forms or the sulfatide lipidoses. This group includes those cases in which large amounts of metachromatic material accumulate in the central nervous system. The disease is inherited as an autosomal recessive and begins in the first ten years of life, usually with gait disturbances, convulsions of various types, hypotonia, ocular palsies, and dysarthria. There are coarse tremors of the extremities and, terminally, severe mental deterioration and spasticity or rigidity.

The cerebrospinal fluid protein is usually elevated (100 to 200 mg per 100 ml), and metachromatic material (staining red with toluidine blue) can be found in the urinary sediment. The metachromatic material also collects in the kidney, liver, gallbladder, spleen, or peripheral nerves, and biopsy confirms the diagnosis. Gallbladder function studies may be abnormal. The course is one of progressive neurologic deterioration leading to death in one to four years, although some patients have survived 10 to 20 years. Some cases may begin later in childhood and run a more protracted course. The disorder is one of the more common leukodystrophies and can often be diagnosed in life. There is no therapy.

SUDANOPHILIC LEUKODYSTROPHY
(Pelizaeus-Merzbacher Disease)

This is a very rare, familial leukodystrophy, predominantly of males. The pathologic changes consist of extensive diffuse demyelination in the cerebral hemispheres and cerebellum. The disease appears to be transmitted as a sex-linked recessive and begins in early life with a slowly progressive course. Disturbances of coordination such as intention tremor, gait disturbances, dysarthria, spasticity, abnormal movements, and mental deterioration occur. The illness lacks pathognomonic features, but the predominant progressive cerebellar symptoms in a male with a positive family history should make one suspect the entity. It runs a course of several years or more before fatal termination. There is no therapy.

GLOBOID CELL LEUKODYSTROPHY
(Krabbe's Disease)

This rare familial type of leukodystrophy begins in infancy and rapidly progresses to death. The typical pathologic feature is the deposition of cerebrosides in globoid cells of the brain. These may be glial or another type of macrophage. The cases described by Krabbe began at about four months of age with seizures, spastic quadriplegia, abnormal startle responses, cortical blindness, and optic atrophy, and progressed rapidly to death in one or two years. The protein in the cerebrospinal fluid is usually elevated. There is no therapy.

SPONGY DEGENERATION OF WHITE MATTER
(Canavan's Disease)

In this rare familial leukodystrophy there is widespread demyelination accompanied by microscopic vacuolation that gives rise to a spongy appearance. It appears to be transmitted as an autosomal recessive and seems to be most common among Jews. Usually it begins early in infancy with atonia of the neck muscles, spastic paraplegia, severe mental retardation, optic atrophy, abnormal reflexes, and enlargement of the head. Laboratory studies, except for skull roentgenograms showing enlargement, are usually normal. Death usually occurs at about 18 months of age. There is no therapy.

LIPIDOSES OF THE CENTRAL NERVOUS SYSTEM

These comprise disturbances of metabolism that result in an increase of lipids in the brain. Included are amaurotic idiocy, or Tay-Sachs disease (gangliosidoses) (see below); Niemann-Pick disease (sphingomyelin) (see Ch. 533.3); Gaucher's disease (cerebrosides) (see Ch. 533.2); and Hurler's disease (mucopolysaccharides) (see Ch. 538.1).

The dividing line is by no means sharp between the dysmyelinating diseases, characterized by faulty myelin formation, and the lipid storage diseases, characterized by the accumulation of lipid-staining materials within nerve cell bodies. The distinction is further blurred by the fact that demyelination also occurs in many of the lipidoses, particularly amaurotic idiocy.

Amaurotic idiocy, or cerebromacular degeneration, can have an infantile (Tay-Sachs), late infantile (Bielschowsky), or juvenile (Batten-Spielmeyer-Vogt) onset. The Tay-Sachs variety is found chiefly among children of Jewish descent and has a recessive genetic pattern. The incidence of the other forms is genetic recessive and nonracial. All three are characterized by a progressive decrease in vision leading to complete blindness within one to two years. Concomitantly, there is a progressive and usually severe dementia combined with convulsions and advancing weakness, leading eventually to the patient's being bedridden with paralysis. Diagnosis in all three forms depends upon the characteristic clinical combination of dementia and blindness plus, in the Tay-Sachs and Batten-Spielmeyer-Vogt varieties, either a cherry-red or red-purple discoloration, respectively, marking the area of macular degeneration in the retina. An adult form (Kufs') has also been recognized. This group of late onset neuronal storage disorders without organomegaly is characterized by seizures, pigmentary degeneration or cherry-red spot changes in the retina, pyramidal signs, basal ganglia signs, cerebellar signs, and dementia. The problem remains whether these disorders are examples of identical or different genetically determined enzymatic defects of the nervous system. Clinicopathologic changes are not diagnostic. Rectal biopsy disclosing fat-packed ganglion cells in Meissner's plexus provides morphologic confirmation of the diagnosis.

Carter, S., Sciarra, D., and Merritt, H. H.: The course of multiple sclerosis as determined by autopsy proven cases. Am. Res. Nerv. Ment. Dis. Proc., 28:471, 1950.

Davison, A. N., Humphrey, J. H., Liversedge, L. A., McDonald, W. I., and Porterfield, J. S. (eds.): Multiple Sclerosis Research. London, Her Majesty's Stationery Office, 1975.

McAlpine, D., Lumsden, C. E., and Acheson, E. D.: Multiple Sclerosis. A Reappraisal. London, E. & S. Livingstone Ltd., 1965.

Porterfield, J. S. (ed.): Multiple sclerosis. Br. Med. Bull., 33:1, 1977.

Poser, C. M.: Recent advances in multiple sclerosis. Med. Clin. North Am., 56:1343, 1972.

Prineas, J. W.: Paramyxovirus-like particles associated with acute demyelination in chronic relapsing multiple sclerosis. Science, 178:760, 1972.

Raine, C. S., Powers, J. M., and Suzuki, K.: Acute multiple sclerosis. Confirmation of "paramyxovirus-like" intranuclear inclusions. Arch. Neurol., 30:39, 1974.

Schaumberg, H. H., Powers, J. M., Raine, C. S., Suzuki, K., and Richardson, E. P.: Adrenoleukodystrophy. A clinical and pathological study of 17 cases. Arch. Neurol., 32:577, 1975.

Shein, H. M. (ed.): Interaction of brain cells and viruses. In Schmitt, F. O., and Worden, F. G. (eds. in chief): The Neurosciences: Third Study Program. Cambridge, Mass., M.I.T. Press, 1975.

Vinken, P. J., and Bruyn, G. W. (eds.): Multiple Sclerosis and Other Demyelinating Diseases. Handbook of Clinical Neurology, Vol. 9, Amsterdam, North-Holland Publishing Company, 1970.

Section Eighteen   THE EPILEPSIES

315.   THE EPILEPSIES

Gilbert H. Glaser

DEFINITION AND PREVALENCE. Epilepsy is derived from the Greek *epilepsia,* meaning a "taking hold of" or "a seizing." It refers to the many types of recurrent seizures produced by paroxysmal excessive neuronal discharges in different parts of the brain that can be due to a variety of cerebral and general bodily disorders. Designation of "the epilepsies" as symptom complexes, therefore, is more appropriate, and the term encompasses convulsions or convulsive disorders with loss of consciousness as well as nonconvulsive seizures with only slight changes in conscious awareness.

An accurate epidemiology of the epilepsies is difficult, but various studies indicate an over-all incidence of between 0.5 and 1.0 per cent in general populations involving all age groups. The experience of a single seizure is more common, especially in early childhood, but recurrence is necessary for the diagnosis of an epilepsy.

PATHOGENESIS.   Basic Mechanisms of Epileptic Discharge.   Given the sufficient and proper electrical and chemical stimuli, abnormal discharges and seizures can arise in even the normal brain. Certain regions of the brain are particularly sensitive to seizures, having a low threshold and a high susceptibility. These include particularly the motor cortex and the structures within the limbic system. The temporal lobe and its deeper nuclear aggregates, the amygdala and hippocampus, are especially susceptible; their vascularity is vulnerable to compression, and the tissues themselves are especially sensitive to biochemical disturbances. It sometimes is difficult to separate cause from effect in temporal lobe lesions, because morphologic abnormalities in these regions may result when a severe seizure produces secondary vascular insufficiency and hypoxia.

Factors related to age and development are important in the genesis of the epilepsies, and brain lesions acquired during the perinatal period often require many years to mature and produce clinical epileptic phenomena. Certain seizure types such as massive spasms are more common in infants; petit mal seizures appear in childhood rather than later in life. This is reflected by different electroencephalographic patterns associated with seizures in infancy and childhood, compared with those in older age groups. The immature brain also is more susceptible than that of the adult to biochemical disturbances such as hypoxia, hypocalcemia, hypoglycemia, and hyponatremia. The occurrence of seizures with high fever is almost confined to early childhood. The periodicity of epilepsy correlates with sleep or menstrual cycles in some patients.

Seizures may be *focal,* arising from an abnormal focus or a number of foci, or *generalized from the onset,* seemingly without focal origin. However, generalization throughout the brain of an initially focal paroxysmal discharge sometimes occurs so rapidly that the focal origin can be obscured. The attacks of many patients with fixed cerebral lesions and *secondary or symptomatic seizures* are in this category. It is still uncertain whether generalized seizures, such as idiopathic grand mal convulsions and the brief seizures of petit mal absence (see below), develop immediately as generalized cerebral discharges involving specific pathways or whether they are initiated by a localized discharge. Convulsions caused by metabolic disturbances such as water intoxication, hypocalcemia, or hypoglycemia may be considered examples of those generalized from the onset. In these instances, the initial detonation starting the seizure is believed to be in the subcortical mesodiencephalic nonspecific reticular systems with diffuse propagation bilaterally into the cerebral cortex. The rapid loss of consciousness that first occurs and the marked memory disturbance after the seizure can be related to this spread.

Hughlings Jackson concluded many years ago from clinical observations that most seizures develop from a focus or aggregate of abnormally excitable neurons, and many studies since his time have supported this hypothesis. It is postulated that the nerve cells of patients with epilepsy contain intrinsic intra- and extracellular metabolic disturbances which produce excessive and prolonged depolarization of the membrane, producing a defect in the recovery process after excitation. The cortical regions containing such cells generate shifts in slow or standing wave potentials as a result of abnormal electrical activity arising in the region of neuronal dendrites. The neurons in the abnormal, epileptic focus are a hyperexcitable aggregate, and they tend to discharge paroxysmally. Clinical seizures develop if the discharge propagates along neural pathways or if sufficient local recruitment occurs. The abnormal discharges, once initiated, spread through essentially normal brain; the manifestations of the particular seizure then depend upon both the focus of origin and the region of the brain subsequently involved in the propagated discharge. In certain cases, seizures may be provoked by various sensory stimuli ("reflex" or sensory-induced epilepsy), especially flickering light or visual patterns and sound. At other times, peripheral sensory stimulation can arrest the development of a seizure.

The metabolic environment of epileptogenic neurons is most important in the genesis of attacks, and many metabolic disturbances may be associated with seizures. For example, a balance of electrolytes is required to maintain the resting potential of the neuronal membrane. An alteration in membrane permeability with an increased, intraneuronal sodium content could be a significant change preceding seizure discharge. Initiation and maintenance of neuronal hyperexcitability have been related to increases in extraneuronal potassium. Depletion of available calcium ions upsets membrane stability and causes oscillations; conversely, an increase in calcium has a depressant, anticonvulsive effect. Both hypoxia and hypoglycemia deprive neurons of basic substrates, allowing insufficient energy for the maintenance of appropriate ionic gradients. However, if effects of excessive muscle metabolism and apnea during generalized convulsive seizure activity are eliminated, such seizures do not induce cerebral hypoxia; actually, cerebral blood flow increases to meet cerebral oxygen demands in this state.

The coenzyme function of pyridoxal phosphate is directly involved in the metabolic pathway of gamma-aminobutyric acid, which has neuronal inhibitory activity. Experimental alterations of this system can be produced by such substances as the antimetabolite methoxypyridoxine and the hydrazides, but pyridoxine deficiency seizures occur only rarely and in infants. The toxicity of isoniazid in high doses operates by this mechanism.

ETIOLOGY. It is customary to divide epilepsy into two categories, *idiopathic* and *symptomatic or acquired*. A diagnosis of idiopathic epilepsy is made when no specific cause is found; in acquired epilepsy the cause can be determined by available diagnostic procedures. Present techniques fail to uncover a specific structural or biochemical cause of epilepsy in up to 75 per cent of patients.

Idiopathic Epilepsy. Idiopathic epilepsy undoubtedly stems from a number of cryptic causes, in many instances accompanying a genetic predisposition to seizures. A family history of seizures exists in high incidence for some groups of seizures, particularly those beginning in early life. The relatives of patients with idiopathic epilepsy have a 3 to 5 per cent incidence of epilepsy, six to ten times that in the ordinary population. There is also an increased incidence of electroencephalographic abnormality in the relatives of seizure patients, particularly in monozygotic twins, in whom the incidence of concordant abnormalities may exceed 20 per cent. Since epilepsy may be but a symptom associated with other neurologic abnormalities, an inheritance pattern for a specific cerebral disease must be considered in some cases. There are also a number of indirect factors, such as cerebral birth trauma resulting from a narrow maternal pelvis, that tend to produce seizures in families.

Acquired Epilepsy. Most diseases or structural abnormalities of the brain may be associated with seizures. *Congenital malformations* induced chromosomally or otherwise, such as microgyria, porencephaly, and hemangiomas, have a varying incidence of associated epilepsy, depending upon the intensity of the abnormality and possibly on more general genetic factors. Maternal infection, as by rubella, can produce multiple cerebral abnormalities, and severe toxemia of pregnancy also can affect the fetus. Perinatal difficulties causing *birth trauma* and *asphyxia* are relatively common causes of cerebral damage and later epilepsy.

Acute, subacute, and chronic infections of the brain and its coverings, such as meningitis, encephalitis, and abscess, cause seizures, both during the active process and later as healing leaves cerebral scars. Acute viral encephalitis often causes seizures, and convulsions caused by cerebral tuberculomas (more often by tuberculous meningitis) remain common in certain countries such as India. Cysticercosis and schistosomiasis have specific geographic distributions and are frequent causes of seizures in highly endemic areas.

Febrile convulsions commonly accompany nonspecific infections in infants and young children and are to be distinguished from direct infection of the nervous system. The seizure usually accompanies a high rise in fever in an otherwise neurologically normal child. About 30 per cent of these children develop epilepsy later without fever. Sometimes febrile convulsions precipitate status epilepticus, which, in turn, causes permanent cerebral damage. The deep temporal lobe structures are particularly sensitive to the ill effects of prolonged seizures; the resulting lesions may later result in psychomotor seizures.

Head injury is a major cause of acquired epilepsy, the seizures occurring both in the acute phase and as a chronic residual. The incidence of late epilepsy after head injury is given differently in different accounts, but in Jennett's comprehensive series it was 5 per cent. Acute hematoma, seizures occurring immediately after the trauma, and depressed skull fracture all raise the risk. With severe head and depressed skull fracture or open penetration of brain in the sensorimotor area, the incidence of late epilepsy can rise to 50 per cent.

Brain tumors are an important cause of seizures, particularly in adults, but it has been difficult to ascertain the relative incidence of brain tumor with the large population of epileptics. Between 30 and 40 per cent of all patients with cerebral tumors have seizures especially if the tumor is supratentorial. The seizure is apt to be focal and, in 15 to 20 per cent of cases, is the first symptom. The brain tumors most likely to cause seizure are astrocytomas, meningiomas, and metastatic neoplasms, especially those from the lung.

Cerebral vascular disease is a relatively common cause of seizures, particularly in the older age groups. The attacks may result either from localized vascular insufficiency and secondary ischemic hypoxia or from a chronic residual scar, left after thrombosis, embolism, or hemorrhage. Episodes of loss of consciousness owing to diminished cerebral blood flow may progress into seizures, as in severe states of carotid sinus sensitivity and Adams-Stokes syndrome caused by heart block. Seizures appear in up to 20 per cent of patients with the various collagen disorders, e.g., systemic lupus erythematosus and periarteritis nodosa, and are the result of small vascular lesions involving the brain.

Various *allergic reactions* may be related to single seizures, but usually not recurrent epilepsy. Convulsions have been reported after immunizations in drug sensitivity reactions, and after insect bites.

Certain generalized *cerebral degenerative and demyelinating diseases* carry a significant incidence of seizures; in multiple sclerosis this is 5 per cent, and patients with Alzheimer-Pick dementia may experience generalized and myoclonic seizures. The complex cerebral lesions of tuberous sclerosis often produce seizures, including infantile massive spasms. The cerebral lipidoses, such as Tay-Sachs disease, may cause generalized and myoclonic seizures.

Toxic and metabolic disorders are an important cause of seizures since treatment may be directed quite specifically. Seizures are prominent during withdrawal from chronic drug intoxications, particularly from barbiturates (and other sedatives and tranquilizers), and from alcohol. Seizures developing in association with alcoholism usually appear within 48 hours after cessation of drinking and may precede delirium tremens. Carbon monoxide intoxication and other forms of hypoxia may cause seizures. Lead poisoning has been a common cause of convulsions in young children. Water intoxication or excessive hydration, with hemodilution, can produce seizures, again especially in the young. Other pertinent metabolic causes are pyridoxine deficiency, phenylketonuria, hypocalcemia (with or without hypoparathyroidism), porphyria, and hypoglycemia. Hypoglycemia may be a complication of the treatment of diabetes or may accompany islet cell tumors of the pancreas and other endocrine disturbances such as hypopituitarism. Seizures, especially myoclonic, are common in acute and chronic renal insufficiency but are relatively unusual in hepatic failure. Secondarily induced magnesium deficiency, such as follows severe gastrointestinal fluid loss, has been implicated in the production of seizures.

It is likely that, in many patients, several factors combine to produce attacks: a genetically determined predisposition, an increased cerebral excitability related to a general metabolic disturbance, the presence of a focal brain lesion or a tendency to vascular insufficiency, and a triggering disturbance such as emotional crisis or an excessively flickering light. Each patient, therefore, must be evaluated from many different aspects in order to establish full cause and develop appropriate total therapy.

CLINICAL MANIFESTATIONS. The classification of seizures employed here is based mainly on a combination of clinical manifestations and electroencephalographic correlates. Table 1 gives a recently adopted, more detailed international classification of the epilepsies.

Generalized Seizures (Grand Mal or Major Convulsions). The major tonic-clonic seizures have many causes and arise in all age groups. These seizures usually start with a *prodromal phase* that lasts minutes or even hours, with a change in emotional reactivity or affective responses, such as increasing anxiety or depression, often difficult to recognize. More commonly, the specific onset of the seizure is the *aura*, a brief experience directly related to the locus of origin of the seizure. Frequently experienced auras are a sense of fear, a peculiar epigastric sensation welling up into the throat, an unpleasant odor, various visual and auditory hallucinations, and strange sensations in an arm or leg. At times, localized movements of an extremity or portions of the face precede the onset of the general convulsion. The *convulsion* itself occurs with sudden vocalization (the "epileptic cry"), loss of consciousness, tonic extensor rigidity of the trunk and extremities, then clonic movements, a brief cessation of respiration, cyanosis, and then heavy, stertorous breathing. Incontinence of urine and feces can occur; subjects often bite the tongue and cheeks in the clonic phase. After some minutes, the excessive motor activity ceases, breathing becomes more normal, and consciousness gradually returns. Frequently a *postictal state* appears, characterized by confusion, general fatigue, headache, and, some-

---

TABLE 1. A Classification of Seizures

I. Generalized seizures (bilaterally symmetrical and without local onset)
1. Tonic-clonic seizures (grand mal)
2. Tonic seizures
3. Clonic seizures
4. Absence seizures (petit mal); may be simple or complex (i.e., with brief automations)
5. Bilateral epileptic myoclonus (myoclonic jerks)
6. Infantile spasms
7. Atonic seizures (often with myoclonic jerks)
8. Akinetic seizures (loss of movement)
II. Partial seizures or seizures beginning locally (focal seizures)
A. Elementary or simple (generally without impairment of consciousness)
1. Motor (with march, as in jacksonian; or without; adversive, aphasic)
2. Sensory (somatosensory, visual, auditory, vertiginous, olfactory, gustatory)
3. Autonomic
B. Complex (generally with some impairment of consciousness; may begin as simple)
Includes symptoms of cognitive, affective, psychosensory, and psychomotor disturbance, i.e., the psychomotor–temporal lobe–limbic seizure complex
C. Partial seizures with secondary generalization
III. Unilateral or predominantly unilateral seizures (mostly in childhood); these are mainly unilateral tonic, clonic, or tonic-clonic seizures
IV. Unclassifiable epileptic seizures (usually because of incomplete data)

times residual neurologic signs such as hemiparesis or monoparesis, sensory disturbances, and dysphasia. Automatic behavior may be present. As with the aura, these postictal phenomena can imply focal origins of the generalized seizure. The postictal paralysis, sometimes called "Todd's paralysis," ordinarily lasts for several minutes to hours after the seizure. In general, there is amnesia for a generalized seizure with the exception of possible recollections of the prodromal phase or the aura.

The designation *fragmentary seizure* is given to the occurrence of brief components of the generalized complex. For example, only auras may appear and may or may not be followed by abortive tonic movements or loss of consciousness. Such fragments occur particularly during therapy with anticonvulsant drugs and reflect incomplete control.

Grand mal seizures vary in their frequency from once or twice yearly to many times daily; 20 per cent of patients may have only nocturnal seizures. In women the seizures may appear cyclically with or immediately before the menstrual periods, and the incidence may increase or decrease with pregnancy, being increased by toxemia and water retention.

The *electroencephalographic (EEG) patterns associated with generalized seizures* are difficult to distinguish during the attack from movement artifact. Between attacks, the EEG often contains paroxysms of bilateral, synchronous, 4- to 7-cycle-per-second discharges from all areas, interspersed with nonspecific patterns of high amplitude spikes and slow waves. A paroxysmal or slow wave discharge localized to one region of the scalp suggests a focal cerebral lesion. Between seizures up to 25 per cent of patients have an electroencephalogram within the normal range.

Petit Mal (Absence Attack).   The petit mal seizure is a specific form of minor epilepsy, consisting of a sudden brief lapse of consciousness, usually lasting no longer than 30 seconds, more commonly 5 to 10 seconds. Petit mal almost always appears in childhood, with onset usually between the ages of three and ten. The attacks diminish during postpuberty, and rarely persist into adult life after the age of 30. Usually, no specific cause is found. In rare instances a specific brain lesion such as a vascular calcified tumor of the frontal lobe or diffuse cerebral lipidosis has been reported with petit mal seizures, but the EEG was seldom entirely characteristic.

Clinically, the patient with petit mal has a sudden cessation of activity and stares blankly, making no movements, except at times a 3-per-second blinking of the eyelids, a slight deviation of the eyes and head, or brief minor movements of the lips and hands. The end of the spell is equally abrupt. More complex behavioral disturbances or postictal confusion or drowsiness suggest another type of minor seizure such as psychomotor automatism rather than petit mal. The attacks of petit mal can be as few as a flurry every several days to as many as 100 or more per day. As the frequency increases, the repeated absences sometimes produce difficulties in continuing motor tasks and in learning. The designation *petit mal status* or absence state refers to many attacks occurring close together for minutes to hours and producing confusion and disorientation.

The electroencephalographic correlate of the petit mal or absence seizure is a rhythmic 3-cycle-per-second spike and wave discharge appearing synchronously from all scalp regions both during and between seizures. Usually a discharge of more than a few seconds' duration is associated with a clinical absence. The characteristics of the seizure and the typical electroencephalographic discharge have led to these seizures being designated as "centrencephalic," implying an origin in the centrally placed, "integrating," mesodiencephalic regions of the brain. Experimentally, there is evidence to support this hypothesis, although direct confirmation in the human is inconclusive.

Akinetic Seizure.   The term akinetic attack is applied to a generalized seizure associated with loss of consciousness and simple falling. It may be accompanied by an absence and minor movements, but generally there is a marked diminution of postural tone with falling and, often, self-injury. Afterward, the appearance of normal posture and mental clarity is common, although there may be a brief period of confusion. Electroencephalographically, there is a diffuse abnormality with slow wave discharges or atypical spike waves, often slower than 3 per second.

Myoclonic Seizures.   These are characterized by sudden involuntary contractions involving an integrated response of a single muscle or several muscle groups, producing relatively simple arrhythmic jerking movements about a single joint or several joints, or of a segment of the body. The jerks may exist as an independent entity, as a phenomenon preceding and building up to a generalized grand mal convulsion, or as an accompaniment to petit mal absences in children. Myoclonic attacks are often sensitive to sensory stimulation and may be precipitated or accentuated by sound or light, by change in posture, by movement of an extremity, by drowsiness, or by an emotional upset. Myoclonic jerks occur as a normal phenomenon in normal subjects during drowsiness.

Myoclonus Epilepsy.   The myoclonus epilepsy of Unverricht refers to generalized myoclonus and mental deterioration secondary to a diffuse degenerative metabolic disorder of undetermined origin. Other forms of myclonus appear in diseases of cerebral lipid metabolism, in subacute encephalitis, and with rare forms of cerebellar disease. A severe myoclonus appearing in the first 18 months of life and associated with general cerebral deterioration is called *infantile massive spasms* or jackknife seizures. In this condition, the infant develops severe flexion spasms of the head, neck, and trunk and extension of the legs and arms. Some known causes of this disorder are phenylketonuria, tuberous sclerosis, and Down's syndrome, but in most instances neither a biochemical nor an anatomic abnormality can be found.

The *electroencephalographic correlates of the myoclonic seizure* are variable depending on the severity of the seizure state; in mild instances, generalized, synchronous slow spike and wave complexes or sharp and slow wave elements occur intermittently, with relatively normal electroencephalographic patterns between. Infantile massive spasms are commonly associated with *hypsarrhythmia*, which consists of more or less continuous, nonsynchronous, asymmetric discharges of spike and sharp wave elements along with slow waves from all regions.

Focal or Partial Seizures.   Involvement by a lesion of a specific region of the brain may be manifested by characteristic seizures. They are typical of acquired epilepsy, although occasionally no anatomic abnormality is found. As indicated above, a focal onset seizure can occasionally spread extremely rapidly to become generalized, but in seizure states specifically classified as focal or partial, the attack usually remains limited. There often is a disturbance of consciousness or awareness with varying degrees of amnesia, but total loss of consciousness occurs only with general spread.

Lesions involving any of the motor regions of the brain, but particularly the so-called motor cortex, produce focal motor seizures. The classic *jacksonian motor seizure*, caused by a lesion sharply localized in a specific region of the motor cortex, begins as a repetitive movement of a distal portion of an extremity, such as the fingers or toes, and then spreads by a march of the clonic contractions up the extremity toward the trunk. Such a seizure usually remains limited to the extremity, but it may spread to the rest of the ipsilateral side, the face, and the contralateral side. Occasionally, these seizures begin at the corner of the mouth and are associated with masticatory movements and speech disturbances. Other focal motor seizures involve gross movements of the arms or legs without the classic jacksonian march. *Adversive seizures* produce turning movements of the head, eyes, and trunk toward the side opposite the cerebral lesion, which is usually in the profrontal cortex.

Focal seizures originating from the *supplementary motor area* of the mesial frontal supracingulate cortex are not common; they are characterized by gross body movements, especially raising of the contralateral arm with the head turning toward that arm, rhythmic bilateral arm and leg movements, and repetitive speech, usually of syllables, not words. Occasionally, speech is slowed or totally inhibited during such a seizure. Other experiences are peculiar sensations in the abdomen, generalized flushing, and palpitations.

Focal sensory seizures caused by a lesion involving the sensory cortex may be jacksonian with a march of abnormal sensations such as numbness and tingling spreading up an extremity. Other sensory areas of the cerebral cortex produce more complex seizures with paroxysmal visual, auditory, olfactory, gustatory, and vertiginous components in varying degrees of organization. As with other types of focal attacks, the pattern of onset is often the most accurate guide to the locus of an abnormal cerebral lesion.

Autonomic seizures are produced by focal lesions in the regions of the brain associated with autonomic representation, namely, the deep temporal, limbic, and diencephalic (hypothalamic) areas. Many autonomic symptoms are associated with other focal or generalized seizures, but they also appear in attacks more or less by themselves, as paroxysms of abdominal pain, sweating, piloerection, incontinence, salivation, and, rarely, fever.

Psychomotor (temporal lobe, limbic system) epilepsy is due to seizure activity involving the temporal lobe, its deeper nuclear masses (the amygdala and hippocampus), and their associated limbic system structures. Psychomotor epilepsy is common in both children and adults and occasionally coexists with grand mal seizures. Such patients often give a history of febrile seizures and status epilepticus in infancy. Evidence of an acquired lesion is found in more than half the patients, with a frequent history of trauma at birth or, later, encephalitis or neoplasm. Some patients with psychomotor seizures are found to have focal frontal or occipital

lobe lesions, but even with these there is evidence that the discharges produce their eventual manifestations by propagation through temporal-limbic lobe structures.

Psychomotor-temporal-limbic seizures can take a number of forms, and several combinations can occur of the symptoms given in the following description. Many such attacks are manifested by an initial aura of anxiety and visceral symptoms, especially by a peculiar epigastric sensation welling up into the throat. An alteration in consciousness follows, associated with complex feeling and thinking states, as well as automatic somatic and autonomic motor behavior. Memory loss, disorientation, or a sense of re-experiencing the environment (déjà vu) may be prominent. Motor activity is first arrested or suspended, then simple movements can ensue, such as chewing, swallowing, sucking, lip smacking, and aimless twistings of the arms and legs. Automatisms of varying complexity can involve either partially purposeful or inappropriate and bizarre behavior. Usually, such automatisms are stereotyped, but, despite this, the movements usually interplay with the environment, and occasionally they appear to be determined in part by psychologic factors. The activities in this phase of the seizure may merge into normal behavior. The complex attack beginning with unpleasant olfactory hallucinations caused by lesions of the mesial portions of the temporal lobe, the uncus, was specifically called an uncinate seizure by Jackson, who also described the "dreamy" and confused state of the patient. Visceral manifestations are common in young patients, who experience hunger, nausea, vomiting, and abdominal pain as well as urinary incontinence. Destructive aggressive behavior occasionally occurs but usually is not goal-directed unless patients are forcibly restrained. Affective disturbances may include expressions of fear, anger, and depression. Occasionally, prolonged fuguelike states with running or wandering may last many minutes or even hours. During some psychomotor–temporal lobe seizures, patients experience hallucinations, visual or auditory as well as interpretive illusions involving their own bodies or the immediate environment. These symptoms frequently are associated with ideational blocking and forced thinking as well as peculiar feelings of familiarity called "déjà vu" and "déjà pensée." Amnesia is usually present.

ELECTROENCEPHALOGRAPHIC CONCOMITANTS OF FOCAL SEIZURES. These are represented by discharges of slow waves, spikes, and sharp and slow complexes localized over the particular cerebral region involved. Frequently, the abnormalities are bilateral but asynchronous, representing transmission and diffusion of the abnormal discharge from one hemisphere to its mirror point on the other. At times, deeply situated lesions produce only minimal or no significant alteration in the ordinary electroencephalogram recorded from the scalp.

Status Epilepticus. The rapid repetitive recurrence of any type of seizure without recovery between attacks is called status epilepticus. The term is usually applied to attacks of generalized epilepsy in which the patient remains unconscious and in continuous seizures, with tonic and clonic fluctuations, incontinence, severely disturbed breathing, high fever, excessive sweating, and elevation of blood pressure. Such status may last for hours, even days, and requires emergency medical treatment because of the possible dangers of cerebral damage, thought to be due to ischemic anoxia (or "consumptive" hypoxia) and cardiac and renal failure. Careful attention to ventilation and oxygen demands during such severe seizure activity reduces the associated risk of brain damage, but only stopping the seizures guarantees that no more damaging consequences will occur. Although status epilepticus sometimes begins spontaneously, most attacks follow sudden withdrawal from anticonvulsant medication or a too rapid shift of medication.

Focal motor seizures may recur in continuous fashion, lasting many hours; this state has been called *epilepsia partialis continua*.

Petit mal status is associated with sustained 3-cycle-per-second spike-wave discharges in the electroencephalogram. The patient is in a state of confusion, has a continuously dazed expression, and has minor movements around the lips or in the arms and legs. *Psychomotor* or *temporal lobe status* also occurs, but less frequently. Such patients are found in a confused state with persistent, inappropriate, bizarre complex behavior patterns lasting over many hours, occasionally associated with fluctuating visceral symptoms.

The Interseizure State. A patient with a progressive cerebral degenerative disease, an extensive cerebral malformation, a severe encephalitis, or an expanding brain tumor may develop changes in behavior and intellectual functioning, primarily because of the underlying structural lesions and not directly because of any seizures that might be present. In the past much attention has been paid to the possibility of a specific personality distortion in epileptic patients. Most patients subject to seizures have normal behavior and intellectual functions between attacks and adjust appropriately to society, often excelling. In some instances, however, severe emotional problems do develop, usually in response to environmental restrictions. *Neurotic, maladjusted behavior* occurs with obsessional, particularly religious, preoccupations. Often, under these circumstances, the seizures increase and become more difficult to control.

An undetermined number of patients with frequent recurrent generalized seizures, especially status epilepticus, or with recurrent psychomotor temporal-limbic seizures, develop continuing defects in intellectual functions. Psychologic tests reveal persistent impairments of concentration and attention, memory lapses, word-finding distortions, subtle losses in the ability to associate, and perceptual difficulties. It is possible that prolonged subclinical seizure activity contributes to these disturbances.

More severe personality disturbances, ranging all the way to psychosis with schizophrenic manifestations, complicate the interseizure course of a few patients with either psychomotor or severe grand mal epilepsy. The psychotic reactions often have psychologic precipitating factors; occasionally, they follow control of the actual seizures by medication, and these instances may be related, in part, to a reaction to the drug. The symptoms include paranoid, depressive, and hallucinatory reactions, catatonic disorders, flattening of the affect, and severe obsessional states. The patients suffer marked difficulty in concentration and disorientation of time sequences. Defects in memory are present and are accompanied by abnormalities in perception as well as difficulties in word finding, in calculating, and in analyzing the thought content of written material. However, the patients usually attempt to maintain contacts

with reality, and major withdrawal is not present, in contrast to most examples of spontaneous schizophrenic illness. Diffuse electroencephalographic abnormality, with either bilateral temporal lobe involvement or diffuse spike wave paroxysms, accompanies some of these clinical phases, but with others the electroencephalogram remains normal.

DIAGNOSIS IN EPILEPSY. The patient with epilepsy should receive a thorough diagnostic evaluation to determine causative factors and precipitating circumstances. This requires a thorough history, a detailed medical and neurologic physical examination, and selected laboratory investigations, with particular reference to blood chemistry tests, cerebrospinal fluid analysis, electroencephalography, and special roentgenologic studies. Every effort should be made to identify a specific medical illness or a focal cerebral lesion.

History. The history must contain a detailed description of the attacks to help establish the fact of recurrent seizures. As much recollection as possible should be obtained from the patient, particularly of experiences of the aura and the onset of the seizure. The patterning or course of events during and after the seizure should be documented, especially by eyewitness accounts, with special attention to any phenomena that might possess localizing significance. Information should be sought as to the various circumstances under which seizures occur, such as the time of day or night, the frequency of attacks and how medication influences them, their relationship to the menstrual cycle, pregnancy, food intake, sound or light stimulation, intake of alcoholic drinks, or psychologic stresses. All symptoms of neurologic disturbances should be described, such as headache, hemiparesis, hemisensory disturbances, dysphasia, visual difficulties, or vertigo.

The *past medical and developmental history* is of great aid in establishing the cause. Information should be obtained concerning pregnancy, delivery, the neonatal period, the developmental neurologic milestones, head injuries, and reactions to immunizations and the various childhood illnesses such as measles, mumps, and chickenpox. The occurrence of any severe illness with delirium or coma that might be considered an encephalitis should be inquired about, as well as any exposure to toxic substances. Drug intake needs particular investigation, particularly with adults suspected of taking barbiturates or tranquilizer drugs. One must inquire into the patient's social development and behavior in and out of the family setting, his intellectual performance at school, and his vocational adjustments and performance. Any alteration in these phases of existence should be related to seizure occurrence, to the interseizure state, and to the possible effects of medication.

A *family history* of susceptibility to seizures may delineate a significant number with a history of febrile seizures in early childhood as well as of generalized and focal seizures extending into later life. The family history may reveal not only genetically determined cerebral disorders associated with seizures but also other neurologic abnormalities.

The *general medical history* can reveal evidence of pertinent cardiovascular disease, blood dyscrasias, and metabolic and endocrine disorders; a seizure may be the first manifestation of a cerebral metastasis or of a generalized vascular disease.

Clinical Examination. In most patients with seizures, physical examination fails to disclose significant physical or neurologic abnormalities. Nevertheless, a thorough general examination is warranted; careful examination of the skin, for example, may produce the diagnosis in cases of tuberous sclerosis, neurofibromatosis, or cerebral hemangioma. Examination of the lungs provides evidence for consideration of metastatic tumor or abscess; evaluation of the peripheral circulation and blood pressure gives an indication of the possibility of the various types of cerebral vascular lesions or aids in differentiating between syncope and seizure.

The *neurologic examination* serves two purposes: to elicit signs of any general neurologic disorder and to determine whether or not focal signs of a localized cerebral lesion are present. A neurologic examination is particularly valuable at the time of, or shortly after, a seizure if it reveals a transitory hemiparesis or related signs.

A battery of *psychologic tests* can aid the evaluation of both intellectual capabilities and psychologic adjustments. Simple tests of memory and perception are part of the regular neurologic examination. For more complete studies, the most useful tests include the Wechsler Intelligence Scale (especially the Kohs block test), the memory scales, the Bender-Gestalt, the Rorschach, and the Thematic Apperception tests. Attention should be paid to the patient's performance during these tests as well as to the actual scores.

Laboratory Investigations. Each patient with recurrent seizures, no matter the age, should be examined with certain laboratory investigations at least once and more often if changes develop in seizure patterns or neurologic signs. At different ages certain tests are more apt to produce results leading to specific etiologic diagnosis. Additional studies are necessary to evaluate the general health of the patient and follow the potentially toxic effects of medications.

There are no abnormal laboratory findings consistently associated directly with seizure activity except electroencephalographic discharges. Urinalysis is necessary to determine the state of kidney function; if abnormal, a specific renal disorder may be present, and certain drugs cannot be administered. Similarly, a complete blood count is necessary. Severe seizure states such as status epilepticus may be associated with proteinuria, leukocytosis, and fever as secondary manifestations. In certain instances, special blood chemistry studies are warranted, such as the blood sugar for the diagnosis of suspected hypoglycemia and in the evaluation of a diabetic with epilepsy, and the serum calcium determination for infants and young children with seizure states. Evaluation of fluctuations in serum electrolytes and acid-base balance is necessary to study both children and adults with disorders of the kidney, liver, heart, and lungs, or those suspected of water intoxication. Serologic tests help to diagnose past infections.

The *cerebrospinal fluid* is apt to be normal in all constituents and pressures, except in the minority of patients who have specific neurologic disease. After severe seizures, there may be a slight increase in the cerebrospinal fluid protein and white cell count. In structural neurologic disorders with seizures, the protein and/or pressure may be elevated persistently, and the specific diagnosis then depends on other tests, such as contrast roentgenologic studies. Chronic nervous system infection can be associated with an increase in the white cell count of the cerebrospinal fluid; occasionally, a cerebral tumor may be revealed by neoplastic cells in the fluid.

Roentgenograms of the skull and chest may be taken of all patients. The film of the skull may reveal asymmetry caused by early injury or maldevelopment, abnormal calcifications, shift of the calcified pineal, or signs of increased intracranial pressure. The chest film potentially detects pulmonary infection or tumor and aids in evaluating the cardiac status. Roentgenologic studies of the intracranial contents employing contrast media are extremely useful diagnostic procedures if employed at the proper time, but must be selected with care because of their morbid potential. Such procedures are considered when a focal intracranial lesion is suspected. In many countries, *computerized axial tomography* (CT scanning) of the brain has largely replaced ventriculography and pneumoencephalography in the diagnosis of suspected brain tumors or atrophic lesions. CT scanning with contrast material certainly is indicated in any epileptic in whom the least suspicion of a focal abnormality exists or in adults with seizures of recent onset. *Cerebral arteriography* is useful to demonstrate localized abnormal vascular patterns in neoplasms as well as intracranial hematomas, vascular malformations, and the location of vascular occlusions.

Radioactive isotopic brain scanning has largely been supplemented by CT scanning as a diagnostic tool in epilepsy.

Electroencephalography. The various electroencephalographic correlates of the different types of seizures have been described. The electroencephalogram is an indicator of a certain kind of cerebral activity determined by recording electrodes upon the scalp. This is important to realize, because electroencephalograms from up to 25 per cent of patients with seizures are normal; yet, abnormal discharges are disclosed in many of these same patients by depth electrodes recording from deeper cerebral structures such as the amygdala and hippocampus. The electroencephalogram, therefore, has limited diagnostic applications and must be correlated with other information from the various physical and neurologic examinations. It can be utilized to confirm the presence of a seizure disturbance, particularly if paroxysmal discharges are recorded during and correlated with a seizure. The use of television monitoring during electroencephalographic recording sometimes aids in establishing the specificity of the electroencephalographic pattern. An example of this specificity is that up to 85 per cent of children with petit mal will have the typical 3-cycle-per-second spike and wave discharges both during and between seizures, and in many instances these discharges can be precipitated during the recording by overventilation and light stimulation.

In other instances of epilepsy, the electroencephalogram contains generalized, nonspecific slow wave discharges that merely indicate the presence of cerebral dysfunction, but not a definite seizure disorder. Focal slow wave abnormalities in the electroencephalogram suggest a localized structural lesion and ordinarily lead to further investigations. In certain forms of focal epilepsy, the electroencephalogram may show focal discharges of spikes, sharp waves, and complex components indicative of the epileptogenic nature of the focus. Yet, in some of these instances, such an abnormality might be transmitted, the basic discharging focus being elsewhere.

In most laboratories of electroencephalography the test procedure involves recording in the waking state and during voluntary overventilation. Additional attempts are usually made to provoke generalized and focal paroxysmal discharges by means of sleep, sensory stimulation with light and occasionally sound, and sometimes by utilizing certain metabolic and pharmacologic adjuvants.

The recording of the electroencephalogram during sleep is useful in the attempt to demonstrate focal temporal lobe discharges in patients with psychomotor–temporal lobe epilepsy. In adults, such discharges are increased during sleep in up to 75 per cent of patients, but in children the increase occurs in only 30 per cent. In many patients, sleep produces increased bilateral appearance of abnormal temporal discharges. The use of sleep deprivation prior to a recording, then followed by sleep, may produce more abnormal discharges. The use of sphenoidal electrodes is occasionally of some help in lateralizing temporal lobe discharge, particularly when patients are being evaluated for surgical therapy. At times, barbiturate-induced fast wave activity is found to be diminished on the side of the involved temporal lobe. Photic stimulation identifies patients with light-sensitive epilepsy and, occasionally, produces lateralized discharges in patients with a sensitive focus. There have been many attempts to alter the electrical activity of the brain in susceptible patients by inducing metabolic changes, such as hydration after an injection of Pitressin. Various stimulant drugs have been used, such as pentylenetetrazole (Metrazol) and bemegride (Megimide). All these methods, particularly the use of the drugs, may produce paroxysmal discharges as well as clinical seizures, usually generalized. However many normal subjects respond with seizures to these procedures. Accordingly, these methods are not recommended for general use in the diagnosis of epilepsy. Occasionally, it may be important in the evaluation of a specific patient to study in detail the phenomena of the seizure and to determine focal components either in the electroencephalogram or clinically. In selected cases, this can be accomplished by the administration of a controlled dose of a seizure-producing drug, under very careful monitoring.

The use of the electroencephalogram in following patients with epilepsy is limited, because in many instances some degree of electroencephalographic abnormality persists even though seizures are controlled. This is most often the case in patients with psychomotor–temporal lobe epilepsy and least often in children with petit mal and myoclonic seizures.

DIFFERENTIAL DIAGNOSIS. The diagnosis of epilepsy has profound medical and psychologic implications as it affects the total life situation of the patient and his family. Consequently, careful attention must be given to make this diagnosis positively and specifically, and to differentiate it from nonepileptic disturbances that produce somewhat similar abnormalities of neurologic function.

Consciousness may be disturbed episodically by inadequate cerebral blood flow in attacks of *cerebrovascular insufficiency* or of *syncope* of various types, particularly the vasodepressor form. Disturbances of cerebral circulation affect older persons especially, and such pa-

tients generally suffer other evidence of hypertension and cerebral arteriosclerosis. Periodic blackouts and recurrent confusional states are manifestations of basilar artery insufficiency, as are other episodic signs of brainstem and cerebellar dysfunction. Patients with carotid arterial insufficiency characteristically experience transitory hemiparesis and hemisensory disturbances along with dysphasia, but the clonic movements of a paroxysmal disorder usually are absent. The electroencephalographic findings of paroxysmal discharge do not occur with cerebrovascular disease although, at times, bilateral rhythmic discharges are observed related to vascular lesions of the upper brainstem. The differential diagnosis is sometimes difficult and may require arteriographic confirmation of a vascular lesion as well as the usual evaluation of the history and general medical state of the patient.

Syncopal episodes may resemble akinetic or brief motor seizures; prolonged syncope can progress into a convulsion resulting from the persistence of cerebral ischemia and hypoxia. Girls and young women are more prone than boys to such severe syncopal attacks. The patient with syncope usually has indications of disturbed vasomotor reactivity with excessive sweating, pallor, and tachycardia. Specific precipitating factors often are present such as fear or other psychologic upset. The confusion, headache, and drowsiness that occur after a generalized seizure usually do not appear in syncope. The electroencephalogram during simple syncope consists of diffuse asynchronous slow waves without paroxysmal or focal discharges.

Certain *psychogenic disorders* resemble epileptic states and can be difficult to differentiate. Hysterical "seizures" not only occur as independent problems, but also complicate the course of a limited number of patients with known seizures, the combination being called "hysteroepilepsy." The clinical problem is difficult to unravel because of the interrelationships between the actual seizure and the reactive psychologic disturbance. The hysterical seizure is not associated with neurologic signs of reflex abnormality and, during it, the electroencephalogram contains no paroxysmal discharges. The pattern of hysterical seizures is often bizarre and not a stereotyped tonic-clonic movement sequence. During true seizures the pupils are fixed, and following grand mal convulsions caloric responses are briefly lost; neither change occurs with hysteria. Self-injury is an unusual result of hysterical seizures, and the postictal states of confusion, headache, and drowsiness are absent. Hysterical or psychotic fugue disturbances and dissociative reactions must be distinguished from psychomotor–temporal lobe seizures. The diagnosis of an hysterical seizure state requires careful psychiatric evaluation because of the severe neurotic process involved.

TREATMENT. Treatment of the epilepsies must take into account not only the patient and his disorder, but his family and general life situation. Much depends on the diagnostic evaluation and the finding of specific causes whenever possible that can be treated directly. This is clearly defined in instances in which metabolic disturbance is obvious, such as hypoglycemia and hypocalcemia, or when an operable cerebral tumor is found. However, in many cases of acquired epilepsy, the basic cause of the seizure cannot be treated directly. Seizures may continue in patients even after removal of a brain tumor because of scarring, or when the tumor

TABLE 2.   Most Frequently Used Anticonvulsant Drugs: Dosage, Indications, and Toxic Effects

Acetazolamide (Diamox)

Dose: 250 mg tablets

Daily dosage: Children: 0.75 to 1.0 gram; adults: 1.0 to 1.5 grams. Use intermittently; tolerance occurs

Indications: As an adjuvant in all types of seizures, especially those in females related to menstrual cycles

Toxic effects: Anorexia, acidosis, drowsiness, numbness of extremities; rarely, blood dyscrasias

Carbamazepine (Tegretol)

Dose: 0.2 gram tablets

Daily dosage: Children: 20 mg per kg; adults: 0.2 to 0.8 gram

Indications: Complex partial (psychomotor–temporal lobe) and other focal seizures, grand mal

Toxic effects: Leukopenia, anorexia, "dizziness," drowsiness, rash

Clonazepam (Clonopin)

Dose: 0.5 mg, 1.0 mg, 2.0 mg tablets

Daily dosage: Children: 1.5 to 4 mg; adults: 3 to 12 mg

Indications: Myoclonic, minor motor, akinetic, petit mal, some complex partial seizures

Toxic effects: Drowsiness, ataxia, behavioral problems, anorexia, hematologic (anemia, leukopenia)

Diphenylhydantoin (phenytoin, Dilantin)

Dose: 0.03 gram and 0.1 gram capsules; 0.05 gram tablets; 0.1 gram delayed action capsules; 0.025 gram per ml suspension; 0.1 gram in oil, capsules; 0.25 gram ampules for parenteral use

Daily dosage: Children: 0.15 to 0.3 gram; adults: 0.3 to 0.6 gram. Effective blood level 10 to 20 μg/ml

Indications: Grand mal, psychomotor and focal seizures; most useful in combination with phenobarbital or primidone

Toxic effects: Rash, fever, gum hypertrophy, gastric distress, diplopia, ataxia, hirsutism (young females); drowsiness, uncommon; megaloblastic anemia (due to secondary folic acid deficiency); lymphadenopathy

Ethosuximide (Zarontin)

Dose: 0.25 gram capsules

Daily dosage: Children: 0.75 to 1.0 gram; adults: 1.5 grams. Effective blood level range 40 to 80 μg/ml

Indications: Petit mal seizures (now the drug of choice); used with Dilantin in mixed seizure states

Toxic effects: Blood dyscrasias (pancytopenia, leukopenia) unusual; dermatitis, anorexia, nausea, drowsiness, dizziness

Ethylphenylhydantoin (Peganone)

Dose: 0.25 gram, 0.5 gram tablets

Daily dosage: Children: 0.5 gram to 1.5 grams; adults: 2.0 to 3.0 grams

Indications: Grand mal, psychomotor and focal seizures

Toxic effects: Similar to those of Dilantin but less frequent; may be substituted for Dilantin, but is generally less effective

Methylphenylethylhydantoin (Mesantoin)

Dose: 0.1 gram tablets

Daily dosage: Children: 0.1 to 0.4 gram; adults: 0.4 to 0.8 gram

Indications: Grand mal, psychomotor, and focal seizures

Toxic effects: Rash, fever, drowsiness, ataxia, gum hypertrophy (less than Dilantin), neutropenia, agranulocytosis

Paramethadione (Paradione)

Dose: 0.15 gram, 0.3 gram capsules; 0.3 gram per ml solution

Daily dosage: Children: up to six years of age, 0.3 to 0.9 gram; over six years of age, 0.6 to 1.8 grams; adults: 1.2 to 2.4 grams

Indications: Peti mal, myoclonic, and akinetic seizures, massive spasms, occasionally psychomotor seizures (in children); often useful in combination with Dilantin and phenobarbital; somewhat less effective and less toxic than Tridione

Toxic effects: Rash, gastric distress, visual symptoms (glare, photophobia), neutropenia, agranulocytosis

Phenacemide (Phenurone)

Dose: 0.5 gram tablets; 0.3 gram enteric-coated tablets

Daily dosage: Children over five years of age, 0.5 gram to 2.0 grams; adults: 1.5 grams to 3.0 grams

Indications: May be effective in all types of seizures, especially psychomotor-temporal lobe seizures; should be used only in very resistant cases

Toxic effects: A highly toxic drug, producing liver damage, agranulocytosis, psychotic reactions, and rashes

Phenobarbital

Dose: 0.015 gram, 0.030 gram, 0.060 gram, 0.1 gram tablets; 4 mg per ml elixir

Daily dosage: Children: 0.045 gram to 0.1 gram; adults: 0.1 gram to 0.3 gram. Effective blood level range 15 to 30 μg/ml

Indications: All seizure states: grand mal, petit mal, psychomotor and other focal; most useful in limited dosage in combination with other drugs such as Dilantin

Toxic effects: Drowsiness, dulling, rash, fever; irritability, and hyperactivity in some children

Primidone (Mysoline)

Dose: 0.05 gram, 0.25 gram tablets; 250 mg per 5 ml suspension

Daily dosage: Children: 0.25 gram; adults: 0.75 to 2.0 grams. The daily dosage should be built up very slowly. Effective blood level range 5 to 15 μg/ml

Indications: Grand mal, psychomotor and focal seizures; occasionally, petit mal; useful in combination with Dilantin

Toxic effects: Drowsiness, ataxia, dizziness, rash, nausea, leukopenia (rare)

Trimethadione (Tridione)

Dose: 0.15 gram tablets; 0.3 gram capsules; 0.15 gram per 4 ml solution

Daily dosage: Same as paramethadione, above. Effective blood level range 10 to 30 μg/ml

Indications: Petit mal, myoclonic and akinetic seizures, massive spasms; often useful in combination with Dilantin and phenobarbital

Toxic effects: Rash, gastric distress, visual symptoms (glare, photophobia) neutropenia, agranulocytosis, nephrosis

Valproic Acid (Depakene)

Dose: 0.25 gram capsules, 0.25 gram per ml syrup

Daily dosage: 15 mg/kg/day, increasing at one-week intervals by 5 to 10 mg/kg/day until seizures controlled or side effects preclude further increase; maximum daily dosage is 30 mg/kg/day; if daily dose exceeds 250 mg, it should be given in a divided regimen

Indications: Petit mal (simple and complex absence seizures); adjunctive therapy in multiple seizure types

Toxic effects: Nausea, vomiting, diarrhea, anorexia, sedation, ataxia, hair loss (rare, transient), rash, emotional reactions, altered bleeding time, leukopenia, hepatotoxicity (rare); may cause an increase in serum phenobarbital levels, and decrease or increase in serum phenytoin (diphenylhydantoin)

The following drugs may be used in the emergency treatment of status epilepticus:[*]

Diazepam (Valium): 2.5 to 10 mg intravenously

Sodium phenobarbital: 0.25 to 0.50 gram intravenously

Sodium amytal: 0.25 to 0.50 gram intravenously

Dilantin sodium (parenteral): 0.25 gram intravenously in patients previously receiving this drug or as much as 1.0 to 1.5 in previously untreated patients). *Caution:* Dilantin intravenously must be given slowly in 0.05 gram increments to avoid vasodepression

*General anesthetics such as ether, Avertin, and xylocaine have a limited usefulness in the treatment of status epilepticus. Careful nursing and attention to fluid and electrolyte balance, airway, cardiac and renal functions, and temperature control are essential in the over-all management of status epilepticus.

is found to be inoperable or incompletely removable. The diagnosis of an acquired epilepsy after head injury or encephalitis usually does not lead to specific therapy. Only a limited number of patients with post-traumatic epilepsy are satisfactory candidates for surgical removal of a localized meningocerebral scar. The administration of anticonvulsant drugs is necessary, therefore, for the majority of patients.

Medical Therapy. There are many available anticonvulsant drugs, but those listed in Table 2 are the main ones used by the general physician. No drug will achieve total seizure control in all patients, but careful selection and utilization in each case often leads to optimal results. Each physician should learn to use a number of these drugs well and to recognize disturbing side effects as early as possible. Periodic blood counts, urinalyses, and liver function tests are necessary with certain drugs.

The basic mechanisms of anticonvulsant drugs are not definitely known. Most of the drugs are neuronal depressants with certain variations in action. The hydantoin drugs reduce the synaptic activity of post-tetanic potentiation; the oxazolidine (methadione) drugs decrease nerve transmission during repetitive stimulation. The drugs are believed to increase the stability of excitable neuronal membranes by acting upon electrochemical characteristics involved in ion permeability and membrane polarization. Such stabilizing effects would decrease the activity of the hyperexcitable neuronal aggregates in an epileptogenic focus and prevent the spread of discharge through normal neuronal circuits.

The anticonvulsant drugs are administered to achieve the desired effect of seizure control and must be built up in dosage while not producing untoward toxic reactions. It is best to start with one drug of choice, but usually a single drug is not totally effective, and a second is necessary. Two drugs might be needed initially for patients with two different types of seizure such as grand mal and petit mal. This occurs in from 25 to 50 per cent of children with petit mal. The process may require weeks of adjustment, and during this time the patient's or parent's cooperation in reporting effects on seizure frequency or side reactions is most important. Determination of anticonvulsant blood levels, i.e., diphenylhydantoin, phenobarbital, primidone, may be helpful in identifying patients who are obtaining unsatisfactory control because they either fail to take the drug or metabolize it abnormally. Drugs should be started slowly and their doses changed gradually. Frequent and rapid shifting or replacement of drugs produces side effects and can precipitate seizures. Following blood levels in each individual patient and using the blood level to adjust medication dosage into the therapeutic range improves seizure control and reduces the risk of inducing toxicity.

Diphenylhydantoin metabolism is impaired in patients with acute and chronic liver disease, resulting in elevations of blood levels when standard doses of the drug are taken. By contrast, in the presence of uremia, the blood level of diphenylhydantoin is reduced; however, apparently adequate amounts of the drug unbound to plasma protein may be achieved with administered low dosage.

Other drugs can alter the rate of diphenylhydantoin metabolism induced in liver microsomal enzymes so as to lead to an increase in diphenylhydantoin blood levels even to toxicity. These drugs include isoniazid, bishydroxycoumarin, phenyramidol, disulfiram, methylphenidate, diazepam, chlordiazepoxide, phenylbutazone, chlorpromazine, prochlorperazine, and some estrogens. Carbamazepine and ethanol have been reported to lower diphenylhydantoin blood levels. On the other hand, diphenylhydantoin has been reported to lower blood levels of digitoxin, bishydroxycoumarin, metyrapone, and DDT. Diphenylhydantoin also has been found to stimulate enzymes which rapidly turn over endogenous or exogenously administered adrenocorticosteroids; this has resulted, in some instances, in increased adrenocorticotropic and cortisol production by negative feedback effects.

A specific anticonvulsant drug for each type of seizure is not available. However, there is one major therapeutic division; petit mal absences respond best to either succinimide or oxazolidines (methadiones). These drugs are not effective in the treatment of major generalized (grand mal) or focal cerebral seizures, nor are the hydantoins (used in grand mal and other seizures) effective in petit mal. It is stated that the drugs used in the therapy of petit mal may worsen a generalized seizure state, but this has not been proved.

Generalized grand mal and focal motor seizures are best treated by diphenylhydantoin sodium and phenobarbital. Initially, either drug may be administered to patients who have infrequent attacks, but generally the combination of diphenylhydantoin and phenobarbital produces the most effective seizure control. The average dose of diphenylhydantoin is 0.3 to 0.4 gram per day usually administered as 0.2 gram in the morning after breakfast and 0.2 gram after dinner. The dosage of phenobarbital is initially 60 mg at bedtime, with 30 mg increments over the day, up to three times daily, if necessary, limited by the unwanted sedative effect.

Patients with psychomotor–temporal lobe epilepsy are often more difficult to control. Many trials of different agents and different doses may be necessary in these cases; the best results are to be expected with diphenylhydantoin and either phenobarbital or primidone. Although in some clinics the two latter drugs are used together, primidone is partially converted to phenobarbital, and their sedative effects combine to make such administration difficult. It is most important with primidone to start therapy with small doses, such as 125 mg, increased at weekly intervals to reach a maximal dosage of 0.75 gram for children or 1.0 to 2.0 grams per day for adults.

Carbamazepine (Tegretol) is being administered more frequently to patients with psychomotor–temporal lobe seizures, often in combination with diphenylhydantoin, rather than the barbiturate-related drugs, as it is less sedative. The tendency for carbamazepine to produce leukopenia must be monitored carefully.

Acetazolamide is an adjuvant to the treatment of any type of seizure. It seems to have a general effect upon hyperexcitable cerebral neurons because of its properties of inhibition of carbonic anhydrase and production of acidosis. Because tolerance develops, the drug should be administered intermittently. It is occasionally useful, for example, in helping to control seizures appearing periodically in females at the time of menstruation. Under these circumstances, acetazolamide is administered for a week prior to and during menses.

Status epilepticus with major motor seizures is a medical emergency and requires immediately effective treatment to minimize the risk of brain damage. The first step is to establish an adequate airway and oxygenation. This requires insertion of an endotracheal tube if the subject remains unresponsive for more than 30 minutes or so. Anticonvulsants should be given intravenously, diazepam, 10 mg, being the initial drug of choice to stop convulsions. This can be repeated up to three times with 20-minute intervals, as it has a short duration of action. Maintenance anticonvulsants should follow immediately, injecting diphenylhydantoin slowly intravenously, 0.05 gram every one to two minutes to a total of 0.5 gram in patients previously receiving the drug and up to 1.0 or 1.2 grams in previously untreated patients. With the higher dosage, one should monitor pulse and blood pressure closely after each successive dose and stop the administration if any sign of bradycardia or hypotension develops. Additional anticonvulsants, including phenobarbital or diphenylhydantoin, can be given intramuscularly, as indicated.

The *results of drug therapy* are difficult to predict. With careful attention to individual details and general management, most patients with occasional generalized and psychomotor seizures achieve either complete or nearly complete reduction of seizures. Satisfactory or complete control can be achieved in most children with petit mal absences. However, each group of patients, especially those with grand mal and psychomotor epilepsy, contains a refractory number who suffer from troublesome side effects of drugs and from increasing psychologic and sociologic difficulties as the years go by.

In a relatively small number of patients under treatment with diphenylhydantoin and occasionally phenobarbital-related drugs, a paradoxical increase in seizures occurs, along with depressed mentation and increased electroencephalographic abnormalities. The blood levels of the drugs are usually in a "toxic" range, but not always, and other signs of "toxicity," such as nystagmus and ataxia, may not be present. Reduction of anticonvulsant drug dosage, in these instances, leads to a diminution of seizure activity and clearing of mental functions.

When to stop drugs for a patient whose seizures are completely controlled is a recurrent question. Some authorities recommend cautiously withdrawing anticonvulsants if patients have been free of attacks for two years. In relatively few cases, however, can drugs be withdrawn without seizures recurring even after symptom-free periods of three to five years. Thus continued treatment is indicated for most adults with grand mal and psychomotor epilepsy. The electroencephalogram may remain abnormal in clinically seizure-free patients, indicating persistent seizure potentiality, but even in patients with normal electroencephalograms drug withdrawal may be unsuccessful. Yet, in the management of some patients, it is understandable that a calculated risk of drug withdrawal be considered if this represents a psychologic achievement of great magnitude. Under these circumstances, the drug should be withdrawn carefully with some decrements over many weeks. Drug elimination may be carried out more successfully in children with controlled petit mal, particularly because there is a natural tendency for the absences to diminish with age and maturity.

Adrenocorticotropic hormone (ACTH) and adrenocortical steroids are now used in the treatment of massive spasms in infancy associated with the "hypsarrhyth-mic" electroencephalogram. Such therapy is administered after primary causes of massive spasms, such as phenylketonuria, have been excluded. Although initial improvements in the spasms and the electroencephalogram may occur, the prognosis is poor, particularly with regard to the mental deterioration accompanying this condition. Nothing is known about the mechanism of action of the hormones in this disorder; this is somewhat paradoxical because these hormones are known to raise cerebral excitability and precipitate seizures in older persons and in experimental situations.

Dietary Treatment. There are no dietary restrictions for the patient with epilepsy, nor is there a specific diet capable of aiding most patients. A diet high in fat content, the *ketogenic diet,* occasionally helps in treating young children with intractable petit mal and generalized motor seizures. Anticonvulsant drugs usually have to be continued, and the diet is difficult to maintain because it is unpleasant.

Psychologic Therapy and Sociologic Management. Many problems in the life adjustments of the patient need management even though drugs can achieve control of seizures. In many cases, the coexistence of seizures and personality problems requires a combination of medical therapy and psychologic management.

The sedative properties of anticonvulsant drugs usually are not used directly. The so-called tranquilizing drugs have limited usefulness in the management of seizure patients; chlordiazepoxide (Librium) and diazepam (Valium) may reduce disturbed behavior, particularly in children. The phenothiazine drugs have variable effects; an alerting phenothiazine, fluphenazine, is of some use in controlling abnormal behavior in certain patients with psychomotor seizures. However, other drugs in the chlorpromazine group are known to provoke seizures and paroxysmal discharges in the electroencephalogram.

Some patients in a state of psychologic turmoil experience increased seizures and require greater amounts of anticonvulsant drugs. The subsequent achievement of psychologic adjustment decreases the frequency of seizures and lessens the drug requirement. This needs to be developed in various ways, depending on the patient's age and his family and social circumstances. Family understanding is of primary importance, because the child with seizures has to live, insofar as possible, as a normal person within home and school settings. A great problem, still to be overcome, is the stigma attached by society to the diagnosis of epilepsy, and the lack of understanding that not only exists among people in general but is reflected by various restrictive legal practices. Most children with seizures are able to attend schools and vocational programs successfully; most adults with controlled seizures are capable of developing productive careers and engaging in the activities that are so much a part of our culture, such as marriage, childbearing, obtaining an education, driving an automobile, traveling from country to country, and working with appropriate safeguards, protected by insurance and worker's compensation programs. Only a relatively small number of patients require a protected environment, such as that in schools or colonies specifically developed for epileptic patients. Even these no longer should be institutions where many hundreds of epileptic patients are kept in essentially custodial care. "Colonies" with schools, homelike units, and small villages exist in Great Britain, Holland, and Denmark and take care of relatively small numbers of patients (up to a few hundred at most in each), involved in intensive programs of medical therapy, psychologic management, education, and vocational training. From these places increasing numbers of adequately controlled patients are sent out into the general community, where they live well adjusted and productive lives.

Only a few occupations are contraindicated for patients with seizures. These include activities of potential danger to either the patient or others, such as work requiring unprotected climbing to great heights and work utilizing heavy power equipment or dangerous chemical substances.

Informal and formal psychotherapeutic measures can be undertaken in order to reduce emotional disturbances. The role of the family physician is all-important in these considerations. Often he alone can judge the problems that exist in a family, school, or social setting. His understanding and guidance help both the patient and his family to overcome the feelings of despair, anxiety, fear, and self-consciousness that otherwise interfere with the normal adjustments of everyone involved. It is only when anxieties and depressive tendencies develop into more severe reactions, associated with paranoid states, increased withdrawal, and excessive obsessional tendencies, that more intensive psychiatric treatment becomes necessary. Occasionally, brief periods of hospitalization help in the evaluation of the intensity of the psychologic disturbance and any associated intellectual difficulties that may interefere with the patient's performance. Drug schedules may be revised at the same time, under controlled conditions.

Even the child with epilepsy and behavioral disorder can be cared for best if he attends a regular school in an understanding environment and is associated with a clinical outpatient service in which the physician and social service department work together with both the child and the family. It is becoming less necessary to arrange for either home tutoring or the placement of such children into schools or other facilities for the maladjusted.

Surgical Therapy. The patient with a potentially remediable lesion, such as a brain tumor, usually is considered for operation, whatever the state of the seizures. Surgical intervention for the removal of a focus of abnormal discharge is appropriate only for selected patients who have focal epilepsy that remains intractable after intensive medical therapy. A constant focally discharging area should be confirmed by serial electroencephalographic studies, and the region of brain considered for excision must be such that the patient will not be left afterward with a severe speech, memory, or other disabling neurologic deficit.

Patients so evaluated usually do not have gross space-occupying lesions, but the epileptogenic region eventually excised may contain an area of scarring (secondary to previous seizures, i.e., mesial temporal scle-

rosis), a hematoma, a small tumor, a vascular lesion, or a scar secondary to trauma or previous encephalitis. The surgical approach has been utilized particularly for patients with focal motor and psychomotor–temporal lobe seizures. Even though many patients are considered for surgical therapy, relatively few are chosen, and the numbers of patients so treated are still only in the hundreds the world over. In carefully selected series, about half the patients enjoy significantly improved control of seizures postoperatively, although this sometimes merely represents less anticonvulsant drug requirement. In some patients, generalized seizures appear instead of previous psychomotor–temporal lobe attacks. A small number experience relief from severe personality disturbances, particularly aggressive psychotic behavior, but this is an uncertain effect, and surgical intervention usually is not primarily directed toward this. Bilateral operations on the temporal lobe have been of limited success and have produced severe memory disturbances.

Cerebral hemispherectomy has been accomplished in a small number of carefully selected children with severe infantile hemiplegia, intractable convulsions, and behavior disturbances. Improvement in the seizures and behavior has occurred despite the persistence of motor and sensory neurologic disability.

Much more must be learned about the natural history of the epilepsies in order to evaluate thoroughly the different therapies. Adequate seizure control can be achieved now for most patients. The drugs involved are increasingly less toxic, but anticonvulsant medication remains essentially nonspecific and is directed against mechanisms of neuronal hyperexcitability that are little understood. A relatively small number of cases not responding to other management can be selected for surgical intervention. It is hoped that combined physiologic and biochemical studies of disturbed cerebral and bodily functions in the epilepsies will lead eventually to more rational and effective therapy.

Brazier, M. A. B. (ed.): Epilepsy. Its Phenomena in Man. New York, Academic Press, 1973.

Gastaut, H.: Clinical and electroencephalographic classification of epileptic seizures. Epilepsia, 11:102, 1970.

Glaser, G. H.: Limbic epilepsy in childhood. J. Nerv. Ment. Dis., 144:394, 1967.

Jasper, H. H., Ward, A. A., and Pope, A.: Basic Mechanisms of the Epilepsies. Boston, Little, Brown & Company, 1969.

Jennett, B.: Epilepsy After Non-missile Head Injuries. 2nd ed. Chicago, Heinemann–Year Book, 1975.

Laidlaw, J., and Richens, A.: A Textbook of Epilepsy. London, Churchill Livingstone, 1976.

Lennox-Buchthal, M. A.: Febrile Convulsions. A Reappraisal. Amsterdam, Elsevier Scientific Publishing Company, 1973.

Ounsted, C., Lindsay, J., and Norman, R.: Biological Factors in Temporal Lobe Epilepsy. London, Heinemann Medical Books Ltd., 1966.

Penfield, W. G., and Jasper, H. H.: Epilepsy and the Functional Anatomy of the Human Brain. Boston, Little, Brown & Company, 1954.

Solomon, G., and Plum, F.: Clinical Management of Seizures. Philadelphia, W. B. Saunders Company, 1976.

Woodbury, D. M., Penry, J. K., and Schmidt, R. P. (eds.): Antiepileptic Drugs. New York, Raven Press, 1972.

Section Nineteen INTRACRANIAL TUMORS AND STATES CAUSING INCREASED INTRACRANIAL PRESSURE

Robert A. Fishman

316. INTRACRANIAL TUMORS

Intracranial tumors include neoplasms, both benign and malignant, and other space-taking lesions of chronic inflammatory origin that develop in brain, meninges, or skull. Their clinical manifestations are diverse and vary according to tumor type and location. Errors in diagnosis are relatively common because the clinical manifestations of tumor may simulate a variety of neurologic disorders. Brain tumors occur at any age; they are common in children under ten, but have their peak incidence in the fifth and sixth decades of life. Race, occupation, and history of trauma have not been established as predisposing factors. Genetic factors are relevant to the occurrence of a few tumor types, e.g., hemangioblastomas, neurofibromas, and certain gliomas.

CLASSIFICATION AND PATHOLOGY. Most classifications include (1) primary tumors originating in brain, (2) meningeal tumors, (3) vascular tumors, (4) pituitary tumors, (5) congenital tumors, (6) adnexal tumors, (7) metastatic tumors, and (8) granulomas and parasitic cysts.

Primary Brain Tumors. The largest group of primary brain tumors are the gliomas, composed of malignant glial cells. These include the following:

GLIOBLASTOMA MULTIFORME. These most malignant gliomas are composed of very undifferentiated cells. Complete surgical removal is impossible. The average life expectancy varies from 6 to 36 months or so, according to location and treatment. They have a very rapid growth rate and are characterized by tissue necrosis and brain edema.

ASTROCYTOMA. Astrocytomas are composed of astrocytes that infiltrate the brain and are often associated with cysts of varying size. They are generally slow growing and may run a course of many years or even decades. They may infiltrate normal brain widely but with relatively little effect on brain function early in the illness. Complete surgical excision of cystic astrocytomas of the cerebellum may be possible, particularly in children, but in most other instances their invasiveness of brain prevents complete removal. Astrocytomas may undergo malignant change, and a highly malignant glioblastoma may develop within a relatively benign astrocytoma.

OLIGODENDROGLIOMA. Oligodendrogliomas, composed of oligodendroglial cells, are similar in behavior to astrocytomas and are distinguishable only on histologic study.

EPENDYMOMA. Ependymomas are derived from ependymal cells. They arise from the walls of the ventricular system, filling or obstructing the ventricles and invading adjacent tissues. They are malignant and cause death in about three years.

MEDULLOBLASTOMA. Medulloblastomas develop from a primitive cell within the cerebellum. They are chiefly tumors of childhood but can occur in older patients. They are highly malignant and frequently metastasize throughout the subarachnoid space to involve the cerebrum or spinal cord.

Meningeal Tumors. The most important tumor arising in the meninges is the *meningioma*, which may invade the adjacent bone as well as compressing and distorting the brain. It is slow growing, well circumscribed, often highly vascular, and may be calcified. It is benign, and complete removal is often possible unless the tumor involves critical structures.

Vascular Tumors. Tumors composed of vascular elements include the arteriovenous malformations (angiomas) and hemangioblastomas. The angiomas are congenital malformations composed of an abnormal collection of blood vessels of adult structure. They are present from birth but slowly enlarge and may not cause symptoms for many years. They may compress normal brain, may bleed intracerebrally or into the subarachnoid space, may be manifest only as a source of seizures, or may be an incidental finding at autopsy. Hemangioblastomas are true neoplasms composed of primitive vascular elements that may be quiescent for many years or may enlarge very slowly. They are most commonly found in the cerebellum but occur also in the cerebrum. Cerebellar hemangioblastoma may be associated with angiomatosis of the retina and cysts of the kidney and pancreas (the von Hippel–Lindau syndrome).

Pituitary Tumors. Pituitary tumors may arise from chromophobe, eosinophil, or basophil cells of the anterior pituitary. Of these, chromophobe adenomas are the most common. Chromophobe adenomas are nonfunctioning tumors that give symptoms by compression of the normal pituitary gland as well as the optic chiasm, the hypothalamus, and the adjacent brain with their suprasellar growth. Eosinophilic adenomas give rise to hyperpituitarism, acromegaly in adults, and gigantism in children, but do not generally compress suprasellar structures unless the tumor is mixed with chromophobe elements. Basophil adenomas are small and, although associated with Cushing's syndrome, are not responsible for symptoms by compression of adjacent tissues. *Craniopharyngiomas* derived from Rathke's pouch may be intrasellar or suprasellar in location, may compress the pituitary and optic chiasm, and are similar in effect to the chromophobe adenoma. They are frequently calcified and often contain cysts filled with thick, lipid-laden fluid. Endocrine aspects of pituitary tumors are discussed in Ch. 543.5.

Congenital Tumors. These tumors develop from congenital rests and include craniopharyngiomas of the pituitary, chordomas, dermoids, and teratomas. Chordomas are composed of cells derived from the embryonic notochord. They are midline and usually arise on the clivus, posterior to the sella. They grow slowly, but are highly invasive, and their total extirpation can seldom be accomplished. Dermoids and teratomas may occur anywhere in the central nervous system, particularly near the midline, adjacent to the ventricular system, or at the distal end of the cord. They tend to become symptomatic during the first decade of life, but may be silent for many years.

Adnexal Tumors. These tumors include those originating within the pineal body and those derived from the choroid plexus, the choroid papilloma. Pinealomas are rare tumors that cause symptoms by compressing the aqueduct, resulting in obstructive hydrocephalus and giving paralysis of vertical gaze by involvement of the pretectum of the midbrain. They may compress the hypothalamus and give rise to precocious puberty or diabetes insipidus. Choroid plexus papillomas are benign lesions that may cause intraventricular bleeding. They may cause increased intracranial pressure by obstructing the ventricular system or by excessive formation of cerebrospinal fluid.

Metastatic Tumors. Metastatic tumors constitute 10 to 25 per cent of brain tumors. They may originate from almost any primary tumor, most commonly those of breast and lung, but also from neoplasms of the gastrointestinal and genitourinary tracts, bone, thyroid, or nasal sinuses. They may be single or multiple, well encapsulated or diffuse, spread by extension from adjacent tissues or hematogenously. They may occur as a late manifestation in widespread carcinomatosis or as the first manifestation of an unrecognized primary visceral malignancy.

Granulomas and Parasitic Cysts. Granulomas affecting the nervous system include those associated with tuberculosis, mycotic infection, sarcoidosis, parasitic infestation, and syphilis. *Tuberculoma* may present as a solitary mass lesion within the brain; although rare in the United States, it is more common in Central and South America and in India. Tuberculoma usually develops without evidence of tuberculous meningitis, although evidence of pulmonary tuberculosis is common. Favorable results with surgical excision and antituberculosis therapy have been reported. *Toruloma* is the most common mycotic granuloma affecting brain. This is usually associated with evidence of meningeal involvement. The *granulomas of sarcoidosis* occur in the brain; there is usually evidence of meningeal or posterior pituitary involvement, although the evidence for systemic sarcoid may be minimal. *Cysticercosis*, caused by the larvae of *Taenia solium* or *Taenia saginata*, may be responsible for single or multiple cerebral masses. This is seen chiefly in South America and in the Middle East and India. *Syphilitic gummas* are extremely rare, presenting like slow-growing cerebral gliomas.

PATHOPHYSIOLOGY. Intracranial tumors give rise to focal disturbances in brain function and to increased intracranial pressure. Focal manifestations occur because brain is compressed or infiltrated by tumor, because the blood supply of the region is compromised, resulting in tissue necrosis, and because of cerebral edema. Tumors may be located either within or outside brain parenchyma, i.e., intra-axial or extra-axial in location. Brain dysfunction is generally greatest with rapidly growing, infiltrative intra-axial tumors, e.g., glioblastoma, because of marked infiltration, compression, and necrosis of brain. Cyst formation within tumors also compresses adjacent normal brain. Cerebral edema about tumors may greatly increase the neurologic deficit. It has the features of *vasogenic brain edema* with increased brain water and sodium and an expanded extracellular fluid volume. Extra-axial tumors, e.g., meningioma, which slowly compress brain, may reach great size with few, if any, clinical signs.

Tumors cause a generalized increase in intracranial pressure when they reach sufficient mass, because of the fixed volume of the intracranial cavity. Obstruction of the ventricular system also increases intracranial pressure and causes hydrocephalic dilatation of the proximal ventricles and thinning of the cerebral hemispheres. Tumors that obstruct the intracranial venous sinuses also cause increased intracranial pressure. Complete compensation with very little or even no rise in pressure can occur with slowly growing neoplasms, but with rapidly growing malignant tumors, increased intracranial pressure is an early sign. Increased intracranial pressure becomes life threatening when there is sufficient displacement of brain to cause herniation of the uncus or cerebellum. In *uncal herniation*, the most medial gyrus of the temporal lobe, the uncus, is displaced inferiorly by a hemispheric mass through the tentorial notch, thus causing compression of the midbrain. This results in depression of consciousness and ipsilateral or bilateral dilated and fixed pupils owing to compression of the third nerve. In *cerebellar herniation*, the tonsils are displaced downward through the foramen magnum by a posterior fossa mass, causing compression of the medulla and respiratory arrest. Characteristic vasomotor changes ensue with increased intracranial pressure when rapid or severe. These include *progressive bradycardia* caused by vagal slowing of the heart; *systemic hypertension*, which occurs as the intracranial pressure begins to approach arterial diastolic pressure, inducing medullary ischemia and compensatory systemic vasoconstriction; and, finally, *central respiratory failure*. Carbon dioxide retention will further increase intracranial pressure because of its cerebrovasodilator effects, and therefore adequate ventilation with maintenance of a clear airway is essential for the patient with increased intracranial pressure. (Drugs such as morphine, which depress respiration sufficiently to raise arterial carbon dioxide levels, are therefore contraindicated.)

CLINICAL MANIFESTATIONS. The natural history of intracranial tumor is characterized by insidious onset and progression of focal or general neurologic deficits, or both. Many tumors have rather characteristic manifestations that point to the diagnosis (see below). There is great variation, depending upon location and rate of growth. Occasionally symptoms may be explosive in onset, suggesting a vascular lesion, and there may also be variations in course, suggestive of a remission. The symptoms and signs of intracranial tumor are discussed below.

Headache. Headache is a major but not invariable symptom of intracranial tumor. Patients with extensive tumors may not complain of headache, particularly if they have slowly growing infiltrative tumors (astrocytoma) or slowly growing extra-axial tumors (such as meningiomas, acoustic neuromas, or pituitary tumors). Similarly, when tumors interfere with the higher intellectual functions, headache may not be reported. Tumors give rise to headache by displacing the pain-sensitive structures within the cranial cavity (see Ch. 261).

Mental Changes. Mental changes may occur either early or late in the history of brain tumor, depending upon tumor location. Subtle evidence of personality change may be the first manifestation of a mass in the cerebral hemispheres, particularly involving the frontal lobes. This may take several forms. The symptoms may be chiefly affective, simulating an involutional depression. Some patients develop confusional states, at times associated with episodes of bizarre behavior. The most common mental changes are progressive impairment of abstraction, recent memory and judgment, and a shortened attention span (see Ch. 226 to 231). However, some patients, particularly those with slowly growing neoplasms in the right (nondominant) hemisphere, may harbor huge tumors with only minimal impairment of intellect. Drowsiness progressing to stupor and coma accompanies severely increased intracranial pressure.

Disturbances of Speech. Various forms of aphasia occur with neoplastic involvement of the dominant hemisphere. The aphasic disorders are insidious in their development, and minor disturbances may be overlooked or erroneously attributed to psychologic factors. The various discrete forms of apraxia and agnosia may occur in evolution of the tumor syndrome, and may be the initial symptom in otherwise well persons.

Papilledema and Vision. The presence of the characteristic ophthalmoscopic appearance of papilledema suggests increased intracranial pressure; however, the funduscopic findings may be indistinguishable from those of optic neuritis or pseudopapilledema. Pseudopapilledema is a congenital change in the funduscopic appearance of the disc that simulates the swelling associated with increased intracranial pressure. Differential points include the late loss of visual acuity in increased intracranial pressure as opposed to early and more severe visual loss in optic neuritis. Visual acuity is generally unaffected in pseudopapilledema. Episodes of *amaurosis fugax*, fleeting moments of dimming vision, may be associated with a marked degree of papilledema and are a dangerous warning sign of potential loss of vision. The visual fields in true papilledema or pseudopapilledema may show enlargement of the blind spots. Disturbance of vision in patients with intracranial tumor also can be caused by extra-ocular muscle palsies, disturbances of the central visual pathways (see below), and disorders of visual interpretation, as in the alexias and visual agnosias. Uniocular papilledema with contralateral optic atrophy occurs characteristically, with subfrontal tumors that cause optic atrophy by direct involvement of the nerve and papilledema in the opposite eye owing to increased intracranial pressure. The fundi may not reveal papilledema despite very elevated intracranial pressure; this may be attributable to glaucoma when present, but may also occur for unexplained reasons.

Diplopia and Hemianopia. Diplopia with brain tumors is due to involvement of one or both sixth cranial nerves, either directly by the tumor or, more commonly, indirectly because of generalized increase in intracranial pressure (see False Localizing Signs, below). Third-nerve palsy may be due to involvement of the superior orbital fissure by meningioma, although the nerve may be involved by a variety of other lesions anywhere along its course. Hemianopias result from involvement of the visual pathways. Lesions affecting the optic chiasm, notably originating in or near the pituitary, give rise to bitemporal hemianopia. Lesions of the optic tract, optic radiation, or occipital cortex give rise to contralateral homonymous hemianopias. Lesions of the anterior temporal pole characteristically cause a contralateral homonymous, superior quadrantopsia.

Ataxia and Hemiplegia. Unsteadiness in walking may occur with tumor in various intracranial sites. Lesions affecting the midline cerebellum cause a characteristic truncal ataxia with lateralized ataxia of the extremities if the cerebellar hemispheres are also involved. Disease in the frontal lobes may give rise to unsteadiness in walking, an apraxia of gait, which may simulate cerebellar truncal ataxia. Drug intoxication caused by diphenylhydantoin or barbiturates may potentiate ataxia. Tumors of the hemisphere characteristically cause contralateral spastic hemiparesis; initially the signs may be so minimal as to be easily overlooked.

Sensory Disturbances. Hemisensory defects occur with intracranial tumors affecting the contralateral sensory pathways. The primary sensory modalities of touch, pain, temperature, and proprioception are impaired when the thalamus or the ascending spinothalamic pathways are involved. Tumors of the parietal sensory cortex cause loss of cortical sensory functions that results in impairment of sensory localization, two-point discrimination, graphesthesia, stereognosis, and position sense. Tumors of the thalamus may be manifested by episodes of pain affecting the contralateral side of the face or body. Tumors of the cortex may cause focal sensory seizures with a jacksonian march; these may be reported as an aura before a grand mal seizure. Pain in the face occurs with tumors affecting the base of the skull, particularly those arising in the nasopharynx and paranasal sinuses. Tumors affecting the trigeminal nerve may give rise to paroxysms of pain in the face simulating trigeminal neuralgia (tic douloureux), but unlike the latter there is also some loss of facial sensation.

Seizures. Seizures may serve as the first clinical manifestation of brain tumor, or may occur at any time in the course of the illness. The types include classic grand mal seizures and various forms of focal seizures. Typical petit mal is probably never due to neoplasm; minor seizures that at first may resemble petit mal generally are, in fact, either fragmentary grand mal seizures or a variety of psychomotor attack. With any cerebral seizure, it is extremely important to note its aura or the pattern of its onset, for this often provides a reliable indicator of the location of the neoplasm. Focal motor and sensory seizures may be limited to one region of the body or may progress (jacksonian seizures) to involve the entire body. Lesions in the temporal lobe characteristically give rise to psychomotor seizures. These may be associated with olfactory hallucinations (uncinate fits), disorders of visual or auditory perception, experiential attacks such as déjà vu, and various types of automatic behavior, for which the patient is generally amnesic (see Ch. 315). The onset of convulsions in an otherwise healthy subject over the age of 20 without history of convulsions raises the possibility of an expanding lesion.

Nausea and Vomiting. Nausea and vomiting occur as a result of direct or reflex stimulation of the emetic center of the medulla. This is most likely to occur in association with increased intracranial pressure, particularly with displacement of the brainstem owing to herniation or the presence of bleeding into the cerebrospinal fluid. The vomiting may occur without preceding nausea and may be projectile. Brain tumor is not suggested by the occurrence of nausea and vomiting alone, i.e., there are invariably other clinical manifestations of the tumor. Antiemetic drugs, e.g., the phenothiazines, inhibit this type of centrally induced vomiting.

Stiff Neck. Signs of meningeal irritation may occur in brain tumor, as a manifestation of cerebellar herniation through the foramen magnum, because of the effects of bleeding into the subarachnoid space, or with meningeal involvement. Cervical rigidity may be striking, but Kernig's sign is generally absent (see Tumors of the Cerebellum, below).

Vasomotor and Autonomic Changes. These occur as ominous late signs. They include bradycardia and hypertension, as described above. Apnea generally precedes cardiac arrest in fatal cases. Autonomic manifestations of brain tumor include gastric ulceration (Cushing's ulcer), which may present as a massive gastrointestinal hemorrhage. This may occur with mass lesions anywhere in the intracranial cavity. (The use of adrenocortical steroids in the management of patients with brain tumor may further increase this hazard.) Fever may also occur in patients with mass lesions in the absence of pulmonary, urinary, or other infection, because of a central disturbance, presumably of hypothalamic origin. Hyperthermia is not uncommon just prior to death, but hypothermia may also occur. Fever commonly accompanies the presence of blood in the subarachnoid space. This may occur with rapidly growing neoplasms or as a result of surgery. Disturbances of sweating may occur, lesions of hypothalamus and brainstem giving rise to contralateral signs of sympathectomy.

Metabolic Manifestations. The complex interrelationships between the hypothalamus and the anterior and posterior pituitary may be deranged with intracranial tumors, giving rise to various systemic metabolic disorders. These include diabetes insipidus, inappropriate secretion of antidiuretic hormone, hypopituitarism, and precocious puberty (see Ch. 544.2, 530, 543.6, and 548.3, respectively).

False Localizing Signs. These may occur with increased intracranial pressure or with shift of intracranial structures. The most common such sign is unilateral or bilateral lateral rectus palsy due to sixth-nerve compression. This need not imply neoplastic involvement of the nerve, for it frequently occurs as a pressure palsy of the nerve resulting from increased intracranial pressure itself. Signs of hemiplegia can occur ipsilateral to the tumor owing to compression of the opposite cerebral peduncle on the tentorium; i.e., hemiplegia need not be contralateral to the mass. There are relatively silent areas in brain, wherein tumors reach large size with relatively little clinical deficit; these are the right frontal and temporal lobes. This must be considered in evaluating patients with the syndrome of increased intracranial pressure without localizing signs (see below).

DIAGNOSIS. Patients suspected of having an intracranial tumor require complete medical evaluation to establish the relationship of the neurologic findings to possible coexisting systemic disease. Appropriate laboratory studies should be obtained to search for a primary systemic neoplasm, e.g., lung, breast, gastrointestinal, genitourinary, or thyroid malignancies. The major neurologic diagnostic techniques are described below.

Skull Roentgenograms. The films should be examined for the following: (1) changes suggestive of increased intracranial pressure, (2) bone destruction, (3) bony thickening or hyperostosis, (4) abnormal vascular channels, (5) abnormal calcifications, (6) the shape of the sella turcica, (7) the position of the pineal if calcified, and (8) the relationship of the skull to the cervical spine in suspected platybasia, basilar impression, and related disorders (see Ch. 321).

Characteristic roentgenographic changes may occur with chronically increased intracranial pressure as a result of pressure atrophy of bone, which produces a beaten-silver appearance in the cranial vault, decalcification of the clinoid processes, and separation of the sutures in children. Bone destruction is characteristic of metastatic neoplasms arising from distant organs and of directly invasive tumors that arise in the paranasal sinuses and nasopharynx. Focal hyperostosis of the skull, i.e., thickening of the inner or outer tables of the skull, or both, with increased calcification, is characteristic of meningioma. Generalized thickening of the skull occurs with Paget's disease. Hyperostosis frontalis interna, localized bilateral thickenings of the inner table of the skull, is generally considered an incidental finding without clinical significance. The vascular markings of the skull, which accompany arterial and venous channels, vary greatly in the normal subject. Focal enlargements of the markings occur characteristically with meningioma involving adjacent meninges and skull. Abnormal calcifications characteristically occur in very slowly growing primary neoplasms (astrocytoma, oligodendroglioma, craniopharyngioma, meningioma), in arteriovenous malformations, in aneurysmal walls, and in the glial nodules associated with tuberous sclerosis. Calcifications may also occur in the gliotic walls of old abscesses, in hemorrhagic cavities, and in granulomas of cerebral toxoplasmosis. Displacement of the pineal laterally more than 2 mm is pathologic, and this or a shift superiorly or inferiorly suggests the presence of a space-taking lesion.

Electroencephalography. The electroencephalogram can be used in screening for possible brain tumor when computerized tomography is not available. Focal changes, particularly slowing in frequency of the record, are common with tumors in the cerebral hemispheres. Rapidly growing tumors are more likely to evoke focal changes than are slowly progressive tumors with only minimal clinical manifestations, and with the latter the record may be normal. The electroencephalogram is often normal with posterior fossa neoplasms.

Cerebrospinal Fluid. Examination of the cerebrospinal fluid (CSF) for pressure, protein, sugar, cell count, cultures, serologic tests, and cytologic analysis is often helpful in the diagnosis of intracranial tumor. The incidence of abnormalities varies with the stage of the illness and the site and nature of the neoplasm. The fluid is crystal clear unless the protein exceeds about 150 mg per 100 ml or unless bleeding has occurred. With slowly growing neoplasms the intracranial pressure will remain normal, less than 200 mm, until late in the illness, whereas in rapidly growing tumors increased pressure may be an early manifestation. Jugular compression for the Queckenstedt test is contraindicated in patients who are suspected of having brain tumor. A protein content greater than 100 mg per 100 ml is frequently associated with rapidly growing tumors near the ventricles or subarachnoid space. With slowly growing tumors, the protein may be normal despite the presence of a huge mass. Of the posterior fossa neoplasms, acoustic neuroma commonly results in marked elevation of the protein, 100 to 500 mg per 100 ml. The fluid is normal in most patients with brainstem gliomas. The cell count is elevated from 5 to 100 white cells per cubic millimeter in about one third of the cases, and may exceed 1000 white cells, particularly when the tumor involves the ventricular wall and has undergone necrosis. Malignant cells may be detected with suitable techniques. The glucose content is normal with brain tumor, apart from patients with diffuse neoplastic involvement of the meninges, when it is characteristically reduced to levels below 40 mg per 100 ml; in some cases this may be the sole abnormality, although commonly 10 to 100 mononuclear cells are seen, and with special cytologic techniques malignant cells may be detected.

Lumbar puncture may be hazardous; it is *contraindicated* in critically ill patients with clinical signs of incipient herniation because the removal of fluid from the lumbar sac may increase the degree of *pre-existing* herniation of the temporal lobe or of the cerebellar tonsils.

Computerized Tomography. The increasing availability of computerized tomography has provided a great advance in diagnostic evaluation (see Ch. 267). As a relatively noninvasive test, and especially when used with contrast enhancement, it is very useful in screening patients suspected of having single or multiple brain tumors. Its excellent visualization of the ventricular system has reduced the need for pneumoencephalography or ventriculography as well as the frequency of hospitalization.

Roentgenographic Contrast Studies. *Pneumoencephalography* by the lumbar route, *ventriculography*, and *arteriography* are used in the diagnosis and localization of brain tumor. Lumbar pneumography delineates the ventricular system and the subarachnoid space and thus may reveal the presence of a mass lesion. In ventriculography, air is injected via burr holes in the skull directly into the lateral cerebral ventricles; this may prove necessary for patients with increased intracranial pressure, in whom the lumbar route is deemed hazardous, and for patients in whom there is nonfilling of the ventricular system by the lumbar route. Cerebral angiography may yield much information concerning the location and size of a tumor. The vascular patterns of the tumor, arterial, capillary, and venous, may give indications of its histology. The decision as to which contrast technique is most likely to give maximal information in any patient depends upon the specific circumstances of the diagnostic problem in question and must be resolved individually.

Isotope Encephalography. Various scanning techniques permit the recording of the radioactivity present over regions of the skull after intravenous administration of radioiodinated human serum albumin, technetium, and other gamma emitters. The isotope may enter more rapidly and in greater concentration into the tumor and its adjacent area of edema because of the greater permeability of the capillaries and adjacent cellular membranes. The isotope scan does not readily differentiate between focal changes caused by neoplasm,

sepsis, or infarction, and is often negative with slowly growing tumors.

Ancillary Laboratory Tests. Audiometry and vestibular tests are necessary in evaluating patients with suspected tumor of the eighth nerve, and visual fields are valuable in assessing lesions of the visual system.

TUMOR SYNDROMES. Tumors of the Skull. Benign osteomas rarely reach a size sufficient to compress underlying brain; generally these can be extirpated. Malignant tumors arising in the paranasal sinuses or nasopharynx directly invade the base of the skull and cause chronic facial pain and multiple cranial nerve involvement. Tumors of the glomus jugulare (nonchromaffin paraganglioma) arise near the jugular bulb and often lead to progressive deafness and a bloody discharge in the external auditory canal. Other lesions that give roentgenographic evidence of bone destruction and that must be differentiated include Paget's disease, Hand-Schüller-Christian disease, eosinophilic granuloma, and cholesteatoma (epidermoids).

Diffuse Meningeal Neoplasia (Carcinomatous Meningitis). Carcinomas, gliomas, sarcomas, melanomas, and lymphomas may diffusely infiltrate the leptomeninges and subarachnoid space to produce a syndrome of chronic meningitis, which may simulate chronic meningitis caused by fungi, tuberculosis, sarcoidosis, and meningovascular syphilis. Common manifestations include headache, mental changes, cranial nerve palsies, areflexia, and minimal if any signs of meningeal irritation. The cerebrospinal fluid findings generally will establish the diagnosis. The pressure is usually normal; sugar content may be below 45 mg per 100 ml and as low as 10 mg per 100 ml; protein content is normal or elevated; cell count reveals from 5 to several hundred mononuclear cells; cultures are negative; cytologic studies usually reveal malignant cells. The diagnosis may not be apparent at autopsy because gross lesions are not seen, and microscopic sections are needed to verify the diagnosis.

Tumors of the Cerebral Hemispheres. Tumors affecting the cerebral hemispheres are characterized by progressive focal neurologic deficits and, commonly, by generalized or focal convulsive seizures. Hemispheric tumors involving any lobe may be associated with contralateral hemiplegia; when located in the parasagittal region the paralysis is greater in the leg than in the arm. Tumors of the frontal lobes are also characterized by early impairment of intellectual function. Tumors in the parietal region cause contralateral cortical (interpretive) sensory deficits, impairment of primary sensation, and homonymous hemianopia. Tumors in the occipital region also cause contralateral homonymous hemianopia plus disorders of visual interpretation. Tumors in the temporal lobe, in the nondominant hemisphere, are relatively silent apart from contralateral superior quadrantopsia. Tumors of regions adjacent to the sylvian fissure of the dominant hemisphere give rise to aphasic disorders; anterior lesions in the frontal lobe cause expressive aphasia, posterior lesions in the parietal region cause the receptive aphasias, and lesions in the superior temporal gyrus cause anomic aphasia.

Tumors of the Cerebellum. The common tumors of the cerebellum include medulloblastomas, which affect the midline vermis most commonly in childhood, and tumors of the cerebellar hemisphere, chiefly gliomas and metastatic tumors. Early manifestations of tumor of the midline vermis include truncal ataxia on tandem walking and symptoms of increased intracranial pressure. Tumors of the cerebellar hemisphere cause ipsilateral limb ataxia as an early manifestation. Tilting of the head to one side may be an early sign as well. Stiffness of the neck is often seen in posterior fossa neoplasms as an early sign of herniation.

Brainstem Tumors. These intrinsic tumors of midbrain, pons, and medulla are most commonly gliomas. The initial symptoms are those of cranial nerve dysfunction, most commonly affecting the extraocular muscles (nuclear or internuclear ophthalmoplegia), chewing and swallowing, as well as the long tracts, ascending and descending. Headache and other manifestations of increased intracranial pressure occur late in the course. The cerebrospinal fluid is often normal.

Pituitary Tumors. The earliest symptoms may be those of endocrine disturbances (see above) or may be due to effects on the visual system. Frontal headache may be an early symptom. Pituitary tumors may invade the sphenoid sinus and thus permit the development of bacterial meningitis. The cysts associated with craniopharyngioma may release lipid-laden fluid into the subarachnoid space, thus causing bouts of sterile meningitis.

Optic Nerve Glioma. Gliomas may develop in the intraorbital, retro-orbital, or chiasmatic region of the optic nerve, the first of these being the most common location. These tumors usually occur in early childhood with uniocular loss of vision as the most common presenting symptom. Proptosis is seen in about one third of cases. Uniocular optic atrophy or papilledema may be noted. Roentgenographic evidence of enlargement of the optic foramen is common. The tumor is most often a slowly growing astrocytoma and may be associated with neurofibromatosis.

Acoustic Neuroma (Cerebellopontine Angle Tumor). These neurofibromas (schwannomas) of the eighth nerve begin within the auditory canal or in the subarachnoid space. They are slowly growing and characteristically cause progressive tinnitus and nerve deafness. The vestibular portion is more seriously involved than the acoustic portion, and in patients who do not have a dead labyrinth on caloric testing, the diagnosis is suspect. There are few symptoms referable to loss of vestibular function. A mild sensation of giddiness or unsteadiness is common, but recurrent episodes of vertigo are very rare in acoustic tumors. Adjacent cranial nerves are also commonly involved, particularly the fifth, sixth, and seventh nerves. Large tumors cause ipsilateral cerebellar signs and manifestations of increased intracranial pressure. Meningiomas of the cerebellopontine angle may give a similar clinical picture without, however, enlargement of the auditory canal on roentgenograms of the skull.

Metastatic Tumors. The clinical pictures that result from metastatic neoplasms are very variable, depending on the site and number of metastases and their rate of growth. The diagnosis is readily made in patients with evidence of widespread metastatic disease who then develop focal neurologic signs. Frequently the metastatic tumor becomes symptomatic in brain with few if any manifestations of the primary tumor. Therefore patients with an apparently single intracranial mass lesion should be studied for a hidden neoplasm.

DIFFERENTIAL DIAGNOSIS. A wide variety of neurologic diseases may simulate brain tumor because they are also characterized by progressive focal neurologic signs or signs of increased intracranial pressure. Some of the more common problems in differential diagnosis are considered in the following paragraphs.

Syndrome of Increased Intracranial Pressure Without Localizing Signs. A major diagnostic problem is seen in the patient who presents with increased intracranial pressure manifested by headache and papilledema and who is otherwise apparently normal. The many diagnostic possibilities (see Ch. 318) include extra-axial neoplasms that obstruct the ventricular system, such as tentorial meningioma and pinealoma, and intraventricular tumors like ependymoma and glioma. Some patients have the syndrome of aqueduct stenosis, hydrocephalus, or chronic meningitis. Tumors of relatively silent areas like the right frontal and temporal lobes must be excluded. The diagnosis of idiopathic benign intracranial hypertension is made by exclusion of the many specific causes of the syndrome (see Ch. 318).

Tumor vs. Vascular Disease. The differential diagnosis between tumor and vascular disease is generally made on the basis of history; most tumors have an insidious onset and progress slowly, but most vascular lesions characteristically have an abrupt onset. However, some neoplasms such as glioblastoma or metastatic tumors may have a very abrupt onset, most often caused by bleeding into the tumor. Also, the stepwise progression ("stuttering onset") of hemiplegia in some patients with vascular disease of the extracranial portions of the internal carotid and vertebral arteries and, at times, of the intracranial arteries, may pose diagnostic uncertainty.

Tumor vs. Subdural Hematoma. The clinical picture in these patients simulates an expanding hemispheric mass: e.g., headache, drowsiness, papilledema, hemiparesis. About one third of patients with chronic subdural hematoma provide no significant history of head injury. The diagnosis can be made almost always with computerized tomography or arteriography.

Tumor vs. Demyelinating Diseases, Multifocal Leukoencephalopathy. The more common forms of multiple sclerosis do not usually simulate expanding intracranial lesions. Diagnostic difficulty may be encountered in patients with another disorder of white matter, multifocal leukoencephalopathy, which occurs in association with the lymphomas and malignant disease arising in lung and other organs. In this disorder, multiple foci of demyelination are associated with electron microscopic evidence of viral infection. Clinically, there are signs of multiple lesions in the brain that can simulate metastatic disease. However, despite clinical evidence of multiple lesions and rapid progression, signs of increased intracranial pressure are absent. Characteristic, confluent low density lesions in the white matter seen with computerized tomography assist the premortem diagnosis.

Tumor vs. Presenile Dementia. Progressive development of an organic dementia in middle age may be caused by many diseases, including frontal or bifrontal neoplasms. Tumors most likely to present with dementia include frontal and subfrontal tumors (olfactory groove meningioma and tumors of the corpus callosum, "butterfly glioma"). Roentgenographic contrast studies may be necessary to establish the diagnosis. A CSF protein greater than 100 mg per 100 ml favors tumor over the degenerative dementias.

Tumor vs. Abscess, Granuloma. Encapsulated brain abscess and the granulomas associated with cysticercosis may simulate brain tumor. Cysticercosis must be considered in any patient in an endemic area having signs of a cerebral mass lesion. An eosinophilic pleocytosis in the cerebrospinal fluid favors cysticercosis. Differentiation between tumor and abscess may be particularly difficult because patients with encapsulated brain abscess generally do not have systemic manifestations of infection (fever, leukocytosis), and the primary source of infection may be obscure. The cerebrospinal fluid may show little or no inflammatory change. The correct diagnosis of abscess or granuloma may not be made until surgery is performed.

Tumor vs. Epilepsy. The common occurrence of convulsive seizures with intracranial tumors requires consideration of this diagnosis when patients develop seizures (apart from true petit mal, which is never due to brain tumor). This is particularly true of patients in whom seizures first develop after the age of 20. The occurrence of transient focal neurologic signs in the postictal state (Todd's paralysis) favors the presence of a structural lesion as basis for the attacks. It is estimated that about 20 per cent of patients who develop seizures after the age of 20, who do not have post-traumatic seizures, will in time be shown to have intracranial tumors. The likelihood of a brain tumor diminishes with the passage of years if focal signs do not appear.

TREATMENT. Surgical Therapy. Total surgical removal without sacrifice of normal cerebral tissue is possible only with tumors that are extra-axial in location, such as some meningiomas, osteomas, neurofibromas, and pituitary tumors. Total surgical extirpation of the primary tumors of brain, glioblastomas, and the less malignant gliomas, is not possible, although there are rare exceptions, e.g., cystic astrocytomas of the cerebellar hemisphere. Complete surgical removal of angiomas may be possible. Therefore it is essential to establish the precise location and tumor type to allow optimal therapy. Surgical attack on primary brain tumors may be helpful as palliative therapy, e.g., internal decompression or partial removal of tumor and edematous brain may relieve headaches and prolong useful life, particularly if the tumor is cystic and in the nondominant frontal or temporal lobes. There is no absolute rule for the surgical treatment of metastatic tumors. In some patients with major symptoms caused by an apparent single brain tumor without widespread systemic disease, surgical excision may offer useful palliation.

Radiotherapy. The gliomas may have a high degree of sensitivity, and x-ray therapy is generally indicated for palliation. Although biopsy and tissue diagnosis are highly desirable prior to instituting radiotherapy, a specimen is not always obtainable, particularly when the tumor is located in an inaccessible area like the brainstem. In such cases, diagnosis must be made on clinical and roentgenographic grounds. Unfortunately, the response of the gliomas to radiation is often brief, and recurrent growth supervenes.

Supportive Measures. Anticonvulsant drugs are indicated for patients with a history of convulsive seizures and for patients who have had intracranial surgery. Diphenylhydantoin, 300 to 500 mg per day, and phenobarbital, 30 to 60 mg three times a day, are common dosages. Higher dosages of these and other anticonvulsant drugs may be necessary for seizure control (see Ch. 315). The use of hypertonic intravenous solutions such as 25 per cent mannitol to lower intracranial pressure has a limited place in management of patients with increased intracranial pressure. This is chiefly for very acute situations while the patient awaits neurosurgical intervention. Adrenal corticosteriods, such as dexamethasone, in high dosages help to reduce cerebral edema associated with brain tumors, particularly in the postoperative period and during radiotherapy; gastrointestinal bleeding, however, is a potential complication. Dosages of dexamethasone of 22 mg in the first 24 hours and 16 mg per day thereafter have been recommended. The toxic effects of such high doses make such long-term use hazardous. The administration of parenteral fluids must be planned carefully when hydrating patients with increased intracranial pressure, because intravenous infusion of 5 per cent glucose in water can result in a significant increase in intracranial pressure. This danger can be avoided by use of normal saline, 5 per cent glucose in saline, or 5 per cent glucose in 0.42 per cent saline. The phenothiazines may be used as antiemetic agents for patients with severe vomiting. These drugs are depressants and must be used cautiously. A variety of chemotherapeutic agents for the treatment of brain tumor are under active study, but their value has not yet been established.

Dastur, H. M., and Desai, A. D.: A comparative study of brain tuberculomas and gliomas based upon 107 case records of each. Brain, 88:375, 1965.

Dixon, H. B. F., and Lipscomb, F. M.: Cysticercosis: An Analysis and Follow-up of 450 Cases. Medical Research Council Special Report, Series No. 299. London, Her Majesty's Stationery Office, 1961.

Fishman, R. A.: Brain edema. N. Engl. J. Med., 293:706, 1975.

Samson, D. S., and Clark, K.: A current review of brain abscess. Am. J. Med., 54:201, 1973.

Vinken, P. J., and Bruyn, G. W. (eds.): Tumors of the brain and skull. In Handbook of Clinical Neurology, Vols. 16, 17, and 18. New York, American Elsevier Publishing Company, 1974.

Walker, M. D., and Weiss, H. D.: Chemotherapy in the treatment of malignant brain tumors. In Friedlander, W. J. (ed.): Advances in Neurology, Vol. 13. New York, Raven Press, 1975.

317. RADIATION INJURY OF THE NERVOUS SYSTEM

Radiation injury of the nervous system occurs as a complication of x-ray therapy when tissue dosage has been excessive. Signs of injury may appear within hours or days of high-dosage irradiation in laboratory animals; in man, with the doses used therapeutically, the onset is delayed. Characteristically, a progressive neurologic deficit develops after a latent period of many months or years after the termination of radiotherapy. This complication occurs when irradiation has been directed at neoplasms of the brain or at other tumors in the head and neck. The spinal cord is also subject to injury from excessive radiation, whether directed at a primary cord tumor or at tumors overlying the spine and paraspinal regions, e.g., tumors of the thyroid or mediastinum. Peripheral nerves are relatively radioresistant but are injured also by high doses.

PATHOLOGY. The response of the central nervous system to ionizing radiation can be recognized in three phases: an acute phase of meningoencephalitis, a period of apparent normalcy, and a period of late nerve cell damage, demyelination, and vascular change. The lesions in the nervous system attributed to irradiation are extensive in both white and gray matter. There are hyaline thickenings in the walls of blood vessels that may partially or completely occlude the lumen. There is a variable degree of cellular necrosis and degeneration of myelin. Astrocytosis and thickening of the leptomeninges are common. The long latent period between the time of irradiation and the onset of progressive signs is poorly understood; it has been attributed to progressive ischemia caused by gradual narrowing of the vascular lumen. Latent radiation effects in skin are readily attributable to vascular and connective tissue damage; this lends weight to the primary importance of the vascular injury in the brain, although it is likely that neuronal degeneration is not due to progressive ischemia alone. It has been suggested that autoimmune mechanisms play a role in the tissue damage that develops after a latent period.

DOSAGES. The precise tissue dosage that will induce radiation injury is uncertain. The minimal dose in Lindgren's series of 71 cases that produced pathologic evidence of brain necrosis was 4500 to 5000 roentgens, with delivery through medium-sized fields over a period of 30 days. The spinal cord is vulnerable to somewhat lower doses; radiation myelopathy has been reported after 4000 r in 28 days directed toward the mediastinum. Boden has defined the tolerance of the brainstem and spinal cord from a review of his own material. With small treatment fields of 10 by 7 cm or less, tissue doses up to 4500 r in 17 days or their biologic equivalent seem to be tolerated by the cord and brainstem. With large fields, a tissue dose of 3500 r is considered as the maximal tolerance dose to the brainstem and cord. There is considerable biologic variation in susceptibility of normal tissue to radiation damage, and precise definition of the effects of various dosages on normal tissue is difficult.

CLINICAL MANIFESTATIONS. When radiotherapy has been administered to tumors close to, but sparing, the brain and spinal cord, the development of a focal neurologic deficit after a latent period raises the possibility of radiation injury. After radiotherapy to brain or spinal cord tumors, clinical improvement that persists for one to five years with subsequent regression suggests the possibility of late radiation damage to normal nervous tissue. A transient form of radiation myelopathy is not uncommon; its major manifestation is the occurrence of Lhermitte's sign 2 to 37 weeks after radiation. Symptoms most often appear about a year after irradiation. The onset is insidious, and the rate of subsequent progress is unpredictable. The process may become arrested or may progress to cause a major cerebral hemispheric deficit or complete functional spinal cord transection. The clinical differentiation between radiation injury and recurrent tumor growth may be very difficult and uncertain pending pathologic confirmation at autopsy, and both may be coexistent. A repeated roentgenographic contrast study may help in differentiation. There is no specific therapy for radiation injury of the nervous system.

Goodwin-Austen, R. R., Howell, D. A., and Worthington, B.: Observations on radiation myelopathy. Brain, 98:557, 1975.

Holdorff, B.: Radiation damage to the brain. *In* Vinken, P. J., and Bruyn, G. W. (eds.): Handbook of Clinical Neurology, Vol. 23. New York, American Elsevier Publishing Company, 1975, p. 639.

Lindgren, M.: On tolerance of brain tissue and sensitivity of brain tumours to irradiation. Acta Radiol. (Stockholm), (Suppl. 170):1, 1958.

Samaan, N. A., Bardash, M. M., Caderao, J. B., Cangir, A., Jesse, R. H., and Ballantyne, A. J.: Hypopituitarism after external irradiation. Evidence for both hypothalamic and pituitary origin. Ann. Intern. Med., 83:771, 1975.

318. BENIGN INTRACRANIAL HYPERTENSION

(Pseudotumor Cerebri)

DEFINITION. Benign intracranial hypertension (BIH) describes the syndrome of increased intracranial pressure in which intracranial mass lesions, obstruction of the cerebral ventricles, intracranial infection, and hypertensive encephalopathy have been *excluded*. It has also been termed pseudotumor cerebri, serous meningitis, and otitic hydrocephalus. BIH includes a heterogenous group of disorders in which a number of different etiologic factors have been identified, although in most cases the cause and pathogenesis of these syndromes are poorly understood. They are termed "benign" because spontaneous recovery generally occurs; however, serious threats to vision may occur.

CLINICAL MANIFESTATIONS. The presenting symptoms are headache and disturbance of vision. The headache is often worse on awakening and is aggravated by coughing and straining. It is often relatively mild and may be entirely absent. The most common ocular complaint is visual blurring, a manifestation of papilledema. Some patients complain of brief, fleeting movements of dimming or complete loss of vision, occurring many times during the day (amaurosis fugax), at times accentuated or precipitated by coughing and straining. This ominous symptom indicates that the patient's vision is in serious jeopardy. Visual loss may be minimal despite severe chronic papilledema, including retinal hemorrhages; however, blindness rarely may develop very rapidly — in less than 24 hours. Visual fields characteristically show enlargement of the blind spots, and may show constriction of the peripheral fields and central or paracentral scotoma. Diplopia caused by unilateral or bilateral sixth nerve palsy may develop as a result of increased intracranial pressure. The neurologic examination is otherwise normal. A major clinical point is that patients with BIH commonly look well; that is, their appearance and apparent well-being belie the ominous appearance of the papilledema. Although the disorder may last for months or perhaps even years, no serious sequels usually follow. In some patients, however, BIH may be responsible for the development of the *"empty sella syndrome,"* in which there is enlargement of the sella turcica on x-ray simulating a pituitary tumor. The enlarged sella is filled with CSF due to a defect of its diaphragm.

PATHOPHYSIOLOGY. The signs and symptoms of BIH are due to the effects of increased intracranial pressure; pressures between 300 and 600 mm are frequent. The intracranial pressure is normally between 50 and 180 to 200 mm of water as measured in the lumbar sac or ventricles with the patient in the lateral recumbent position. This pressure is dependent upon the pressure-volume relationships within the intracranial and spinal cavities. The intracranial cavity contains about 1400 ml of brain, 75 ml of blood, and 75 ml of CSF, and an additional 75 ml in the spinal subarachnoid space. The CSF pressure is directly dependent upon the intracranial venous pressure; changes in the latter pressure are readily transmitted to the CSF, and thus a sustained increase in intracranial venous pressure may result in the syndrome of chronically increased intracranial pressure. The intracranial pressure is largely independent of the systemic arterial pressure, and it is normal in essential hypertension; however, it falls with acute systemic hypotension and rises acutely with very acute increases in systemic blood pressure, e.g., with the administration of vasopressor drugs or in the syndrome of acute hypertensive encephalopathy. Increased intracranial pressure also accompanies increased cerebral blood flow resulting from CO_2 retention, as in acute asphyxia or with chronic pulmonary insufficiency. In patients with BIH apart from those with obstruction of the intracranial venous system and chronic pulmonary insufficiency, the mechanism of the increase in intracranial pressure is unknown.

The occurrence of a special form of "interstitial" brain edema has been suggested to occur in some forms of BIH associated with decreased CSF absorption at the arachnoid villi. This hypothetical mechanism has been invoked to explain the occurrence of BIH in patients with polyneuritis and spinal tumors; a similar defect in CSF absorption may occur in the more common forms of BIH in which there is no apparent explanation for the intracranial hypertension.

ETIOLOGIC FACTORS AND ASSOCIATED DISORDERS (Table). **Intracranial Venous Sinus Thrombosis.** Increased intracranial pressure as a result of occlusion of the intracranial venous sinuses occurs as a consequence of otitis media with extension of the infection into the petrous bone and to the wall of the lateral sinus. This syndrome has been termed otitic hydrocephalus. It occurs as a complication of both acute and chronic infection; at times the evidence for otitis media is minimal and readily overlooked. The sixth cranial nerve may also be involved, giving rise to diplopia on lateral gaze. Thrombosis of the superior longitudinal sinus may occur as a consequence of relatively mild closed head injury and may give rise to a pseudotumor syndrome. (Occlusion of this sinus that drains both cerebral hemispheres is more likely to result in hemorrhagic infarction in the cerebrum as the thrombosis extends into the cerebral veins, giving rise to bilateral signs. In such cases, the course is frequently fulminant and the prognosis guarded, although occasionally complete recovery may occur.) Aseptic or primary thrombosis of the superior longitudinal sinus may also be responsible for a pseudotumor syndrome. This develops as a complication of pregnancy and has been reported to occur during the first two to three weeks post partum, at the end of the first trimester of pregnancy, and with the use of oral progestational drugs. A disorder of the blood clotting mechanism has been suggested as basis for these events during the postpartum period, although this has not been substantiated. Sinus thrombosis occurs as a complication of cachexia ("marantic" thrombosis), and in association with cryofibrinogenemia.

Endocrine and Metabolic Disorders. The most common association is the occurrence of BIH in women with a history of menstrual dysfunction. The women are frequently moderately to markedly overweight (without evidence of alveolar hypoventilation). Menstrual irregularity is common, often with amenorrhea.

Benign Intracranial Hypertension: Etiologic Factors and Associated Disorders

1. Intracranial venous sinus thrombosis
   a. Mastoiditis and lateral sinus thrombosis
   b. After head trauma
   c. Pregnancy and postpartum
   d. Oral progestational drugs
   e. "Marantic" sinus thrombosis
   f. Cryofibrinogenemia
2. Endocrine and metabolic disorders
   a. Obesity and menstrual irregularities
   b. Pregnancy and postpartum (without sinus thrombosis)
   c. Menarche
   d. Addison's disease
   e. Hypoparathyroidism
   f. Diabetic ketoacidosis
   g. Dialysis dysequilibrium syndrome
3. Drugs and toxins
   a. Adrenal steroids and steroid withdrawal
   b. Female sex hormone
   c. Vitamin A
   d. Tetracycline and nalidixic acid
4. Hematologic disorders
   a. Iron deficiency anemia
   b. Infectious mononucleosis
   c. Wiskott-Aldrich syndrome
   d. Polycythemia
5. Pulmonary encephalopathy
   a. Paralytic hypoventilation
   b. Pulmonary emphysema
   c. Pickwickian syndrome
6. High cerebrospinal fluid protein
   a. Spinal cord and cauda equina tumors
   b. Polyneuritis
7. Miscellaneous
   a. Roseola infantum
   b. Sydenham's chorea
   c. Familial
   d. Lupus erythematosus
   e. Empty sella syndrome
8. Idiopathic

Galactorrhea is a rare associated symptom. The histories usually emphasize excessive premenstrual weight gain. Endocrine studies thus far have not revealed any abnormalities of urinary gonadotropins or estrogens, and the pathogenesis is unknown. BIH has been reported as a complication of Addison's disease, improvement occurring with replacement therapy. The mechanism is obscure. Hypoparathyroidism may present with evidence of increased intracranial pressure. The presence of hypocalcemic seizures or cerebral calcifications roentgenographically may further complicate the clinical picture. Increased intracranial pressure disappears with replacement therapy.

Drugs and Toxins. BIH has been reported in patients treated with adrenal corticosteroids for prolonged periods. Many of the patients have been children with allergic skin disorders or asthma. The syndrome is more likely to occur when the steroid dosage is reduced, suggesting that relative adrenal insufficiency might have been present, but this has not been substantiated. BIH has been reported in women taking oral progestational drugs when angiography has excluded sinus thrombosis. BIH has been reported in otherwise healthy adolescents taking huge doses of vitamin A for the treatment of acne. Doses as low as 25,000 units per day orally have been noted to cause headache and papilledema; there is rapid improvement after cessation of the therapy. The syndrome is said to have occurred in Arctic explorers who consumed polar bear liver, a great source of the vitamin. A few cases of BIH, manifested by bulging fontanelle and papilledema, have been reported in children after the administration of tetracycline or nalidixic acid. The mechanisms involved are obscure. Spontaneous rapid recovery occurs when the drugs are stopped.

Hematologic Disorders. Papilledema and increased intracranial pressure have been attributed to severe iron deficiency anemia, with striking improvement after treatment of the anemia. The mechanism presumably is dependent upon the marked increase in cerebral blood flow that accompanies profound anemia. BIH occurs with infectious mononucleosis and the Wiskott-Aldrich syndrome, but its mechanism is not known.

Pulmonary Encephalopathy. BIH can be a major complication of chronic hypoxic hypercapnia caused by paralytic states such as muscular dystrophy and cervical myelopathy, as well as of obstructive pulmonary disease and the pickwickian syndrome. The mechanism is dependent upon the chronic increase in cerebral blood flow resulting from the anoxemia and carbon dioxide retention (see Ch. 344).

High Cerebrospinal Fluid Protein. BIH occurs rarely with tumors of the spinal cord or cauda equina as well as with polyneuritis. Papilledema and headache have disappeared with treatment of the spinal lesion or regression of the polyneuropathy. The mechanism may involve the effects of a very high CSF protein upon CSF absorption at the arachnoid villi, both in the cranial and spinal subarachnoid spaces.

Idiopathic. One of the more common forms of BIH is its occurrence in otherwise healthy subjects in the absence of any of the etiologic factors described above. Both sexes are involved, and the occurrence is most often between the ages of 10 and 50 years. These cases represent the idiopathic form of BIH; its pathogenesis is a mystery. There are rare case reports of BIH with roseola infantum, Sydenham's chorea, and lupus erythematosus in which the mechanism is unknown.

DIAGNOSIS. The patient with headache and papilledema without other neurologic signs must be considered to have an intracranial mass, ventricular obstruction, or intracranial infection until proved otherwise. Although the diagnosis of BIH may be suspected by the appearance of apparent well-being and by the history of some of the associated features listed above, the diagnosis is essentially one of exclusion dependent upon ruling out the more common causes of increased intracranial pressure. Brain tumor, particularly when located in relatively silent areas such as the frontal lobes or right temporal lobe or when obstructing the ventricular system, may be manifest only by headache and papilledema. Patients with chronic subdural hematoma, without history of significant trauma, may present in the same way. Diagnostic evaluation requires skull films, electroencephalography, and arteriography and/or air studies. Computerized tomography, when available, has negated the need for angiography or air studies in many cases. Lumbar puncture is necessary in these patients, but is generally deferred until arteriography or computerized tomography has revealed that the ventricular system is normal in size and location. Laboratory studies regarding possible hypoadrenalism or hypoparathyroidism may be rewarding in rare cases of these disorders that present with the pseudotumor syndrome. The cerebrospinal fluid pressure is elevated, between 250 and 600 mm, but the fluid is otherwise normal. The protein content is generally low normal, and lumbar CSF protein levels below 15 mg per 100 ml are common. The

electroencephalogram is normal in BIH. Pseudopapilledema may be a source of diagnostic confusion. It is a developmental anomaly of the fundus wherein the ophthalmologic appearance may be indistinguishable from that of the true papilledema; there is elevation of the optic disc, but exudates or hemorrhages are absent. The visual acuity is normal, although visual fields may show some enlargement of the blind spots. The unchanging appearance of the fundus in subsequent examinations favors the diagnosis of pseudopapilledema, as does the finding of normal CSF pressure on lumbar puncture.

TREATMENT. In patients with lateral sinus thrombosis caused by chronic infection in the petrous bone, surgical decompression is often indicated. When the pseudotumor syndrome is a manifestation of hypoadrenalism of hypoparathyroidism, replacement therapy is indicated. Vitamin A intoxication disappears when administration of the vitamin is stopped. Anticoagulation therapy has been recommended for patients with dural sinus thrombosis; however, for patients with extension of the clot into cerebral veins with infarction of tissue, anticoagulation is hazardous because it increases the likelihood of hemorrhagic infarction.

The idiopathic form of BIH and its occurrence in patients with menstrual disorders and obesity require individualized management. This syndrome is self-limited in most cases, and after some weeks or months spontaneous remissions occur, making evaluation of therapy difficult. Recurrent episodes have been noted in about 5 per cent of cases. In rare instances, the illness may last for years. In the very obese, weight reduction is recommended. The use of daily lumbar punctures has been advocated to lower pressure to normal levels by removing sufficient fluid; 15 to 50 ml of fluid may be required, but its value is dubious. Subtemporal decompression has been widely used in the past. This procedure may be necessary for patients with serious threat to vision caused by pressure, although its efficacy has been questioned in a number of reports. A CSF shunting procedure, such as a lumbar-peritoneal shunt, is probably the surgical procedure of choice in such cases. The use of dexamethasone has been advocated because it minimizes cerebral edema of diverse causes. Acetazolamide has been used because this carbonic anhydrase inhibitor has been shown to reduce CSF formation. Furosemide also reduces CSF formation and may be useful. Hypertonic intravenous solutions (25 per cent mannitol) to lower intracranial pressure can be used in acute situations when there is rapidly failing vision, while one awaits neurosurgical intervention; however, prolonged dehydration therapy is impossible because of its deleterious systemic effects. The use of oral glycerol has the disadvantage of high caloric intake for obese patients. Management of these patients is difficult and requires the attention of neurologists and neurosurgeons experienced in these problems.

Boddie, H. G., Banna, M., and Bradley W. G.: Benign intracranial hypertension: A survey of clinical and radiological features, and long-term prognosis. Brain, 97:313, 1974.

Johnston, I., and Patterson, A.: Benign intracranial hypertension: I. Diagnosis and prognosis, II. CSF pressure and circulation. Brain, 97:289, 1974.

Jordan, R. M., Kendall, J. W., and Kerber, C. W.: The primary empty sella syndrome. Am. J. Med., 62:569, 1977.

Lombaert, A., and Carton, H.: Benign intracranial hypertension due to A-hypervitaminosis in adults and adolescents. Eur. Neurol., 14:340, 1976.

Weisberg, L. A.: Benign intracranial hypertension. Medicine, 54:197, 1975.

319. INTRACRANIAL HYPOTENSION

The normal intracranial pressure is 70 to 200 mm water (or 5 to 15 mm Hg). Symptoms of intracranial hypotension occur with pressures of about 70 mm water or less; at times the CSF pressure is not measurable and the fluid can be obtained only by aspiration with a syringe. The symptoms of intracranial hypotension include severe headache precipitated by the erect position and relieved by the supine position. Symptoms are aggravated by cough or strain. There also may be nausea and vomiting precipitated by similar postural changes. A unilateral or bilateral sixth nerve palsy may accompany low pressure syndromes. The most common cause is previous lumbar puncture with persistent CSF leakage into the subdural or epidural spaces. Low pressure syndromes also occur owing to spontaneous or post-traumatic cerebrospinal fluid rhinorrhea, and with pituitary tumors. Bacterial meningitis may complicate such cases. Traumatic avulsions of spinal roots may also result in a CSF leak. Severe dehydration also results in intracranial hypotension. An erroneously low CSF pressure may be recorded in the presence of spinal block.

The management of post–lumbar puncture headache includes bed rest, preferably in the prone position, adequate hydration, and analgesics (see Ch. 261). In patients with persistent symptoms, the use of the "blood patch," in which 10 ml of the patient's blood is carefully injected into the *subdural* space, has proved valuable. Major CSF leaks, e.g., CSF rhinorrhea, require surgical closure.

Bell, W. E., Joynt, R. J., and Sahs, A. L.: Low spinal fluid pressure syndromes. Neurology, 10:512, 1960.

MacGee, E. E.: Cerebrospinal fluid fistula. *In* Vinken, P. J., and Bruyn, G. W. (eds.): Handbook of Clinical Neurology, Vol. 24. New York, American Elsevier Publishing Company, 1976.

Ostheimer, G. W., Palahniuk, R. J., and Shnider, S. M.: Epidural blood patch for post-lumbar-puncture headache. Anesthesiology, 41:307, 1974.

320. HYDROCEPHALUS

DEFINITIONS. Hydrocephalus is a pathologic state characterized by dilatation of the cerebral ventricles with an increase in volume of cerebrospinal fluid (CSF), almost always caused by an obstruction in the circulation of this fluid. In children, prior to fusion of the cranial sutures, there is enlargement of the skull. Hydrocephalus must be distinguished from other causes of macrocephaly in infancy, including subdural hematoma. In older subjects, cranial enlargement cannot occur. Hydrocephalus is termed "active," i.e., progressive and associated with increased intraventricular pressure, or "arrested," i.e., when the intraventricular pressure has returned to normal and is no longer a stimulus for ventricular enlargement. These forms of hydrocephalus are distinguished from hydrocephalus ex vacuo, which is characterized by an increase in the volume of CSF under normal pressure that is compensatory to a primary atrophy of the brain. Normal pressure occult hydrocephalus refers to the syndrome of ventricular dilatation associated with inadequacy of the subarachnoid spaces without evidence of increased intracranial pressure (see below).

ETIOLOGY AND PATHOPHYSIOLOGY. There are three possible mechanisms for the development of hydrocephalus: overproduction of CSF, defective absorption of CSF, and obstruction of the CSF pathways. *Overproduction* of the fluid has been documented to occur only with the rare papilloma of the choroid plexus. *Defective absorption* of the CSF at the arachnoid villi, where the fluid passes through these membranous structures to enter the venous sinuses, may occur with subarachnoid hemorrhage, with meningitis, and with a very high CSF protein. *Obstruction* of the CSF pathways, which results in dilatation of the channels proximal to the site of obstruction, is the most common underlying mechanism in both the hydrocephalus of infancy and of adults. When the block is within the ventricular system, the process is termed *noncommunicating hydrocephalus,* whereas *communicating hydrocephalus* describes ventricular dilatation in which there is free flow of fluid and air between the ventricular system and the spinal subarachnoid space. Communicating hydrocephalus is characterized by extraventricular obstruction of the CSF pathways, most commonly in the subarachnoid spaces about the brainstem at the incisura of the tentorium or in the subarachnoid spaces about the cerebral hemispheres, or both. Ventricular dilatation develops in hydrocephalus because the intraventricular pressures (both the mean pressure and the pulsatile pressures, synchronous with cardiac systole) are pathologically increased; these give rise to a transmural pressure gradient across the cerebral mantle sufficient to cause compression of the adjacent white matter that has a loss of protein and lipid but an increase in water and sodium content. The magnitude and duration of the transmural pressure gradient necessary to induce ventricular dilatation have not been well defined. These changes may be reversible if surgical therapy can successfully relieve the increased intraventricular pressure (see below).

The major causes of obstruction in the CSF pathways that produce hydrocephalus are neoplasms, congenital malformations, and post-traumatic and postinflammatory lesions.

Neoplasms most likely to give rise to hydrocephalus are those that arise within or adjacent to the ventricular system and obstruct the flow of CSF. These include gliomas and ependymomas of the third and fourth ventricles and of the aqueduct (see Ch. 316). Congenital stenosis of the aqueduct may give rise to symptoms early in life, or manifestations may be absent until adulthood. Congenital malformations of the craniovertebral junction also may be associated with hydrocephalus (see Arnold-Chiari Malformation in Ch. 321). Most frequently, hydrocephalus is related to postinflammatory or post-traumatic obstruction of the basilar cisterns, particularly in the region of the tentorium. In infancy, this follows intracranial bleeding at the time of birth, at times unrecognized, or episodes of bacterial meningitis or toxoplasmosis. These processes lead to progressive fibrosis of the subarachnoid pathways at the base of the brain, with subsequent obstruction. In adults, postinflammatory hydrocephalus may develop with or after purulent, tuberculous and mycotic meningitis or with cysticercosis, and also may follow subarachnoid hemorrhage caused by trauma or ruptured congenital aneurysm.

CLINICAL MANIFESTATIONS. The major signs and symptoms of hydrocephalus are those of increased intracranial pressure (see Ch. 316). In infancy, this is manifest by a greater than normal growth rate and size of the head and by distended scalp veins; in severe cases there is downward displacement of the eyes and mental retardation. Although the head size (occipitobregmatic circumference) in comparison with the chest circumference is of importance, repeated observations of the *rate* of head growth are more significant. Additional information can be obtained from measurements of the anterior fontanelle, as active hydrocephalus does not occur in conjunction with a closing fontanelle. On the other hand, a fontanelle enlarging from month to month is evidence for increased intracranial pressure, and further investigations are warranted.

In older children and adults, the major manifestations include headache, diplopia caused by sixth nerve palsy, papilledema, visual blurring, nausea, and vomiting. Thus occult hydrocephalus that is due to a benign process must be differentiated from intracranial mass lesions, including tumor without localizing signs and chronic subdural hematoma, as well as from the various forms of benign intracranial hypertension and the chronic meningitides, including fungal meningitis, sarcoidosis, and diffuse meningeal neoplasia (carcinomatous meningitis).

Occult "Normal Pressure" Hydrocephalus. In recent years, a new syndrome has been delineated as occult "normal pressure" hydrocephalus. Typically, there is a gradual development over weeks or months of a mild impairment of memory with mental and physical slowness which progresses insidiously to a severe dementia with unsteady gait and urinary incontinence. The patients are usually headache-free and have no signs of increased intracranial pressure e.g., they have normal fundi and normal CSF pressure at lumbar puncture. Computerized tomography reveals ventricular enlargement without cortical atrophy. Pneumoencephalography reveals enlarged ventricles and a lack of filling of the subarachnoid space over the hemispheres. Isotope cisternography (intraspinal injection of isotope with serial scanning of the skull) has revealed a pathologic reflux of the isotope into the ventricular system with delayed and inadequate visualization of the cortical subarachnoid space. Some patients have a previous history of head injury or subarachnoid bleeding; in others, the cause is obscure. Striking improvement in the mental state and gait has been noted to follow shunting procedures. Patients with short histories are more likely to respond to surgery. This treatable syndrome is uncommon but must be differentiated from the more frequent forms of organic dementia as discussed in Ch. 226 to 231.

DIAGNOSIS. Detailed neurologic study is necessary to determine the cause of increased intracranial pressure and ventricular dilatation. Skull films show characteristic signs of increased intracranial pressure in young children; the signs in adults are generally less striking and may be absent. Computerized tomography is valuable in demonstrating ventricular enlargement and the presence of obstructive lesions. Electroencephalograms may be normal or may demonstrate bilateral slowing of nonspecific nature. Carotid angiography will show displacement of the arteries and veins characteristic of ventricular enlargement. Air contrast studies will reveal the degree of ventricular enlargement, the presence of obstructive lesions in the cerebrospinal fluid pathways, and the adequacy of the subarachnoid spaces about the brainstem, base, and cerebrum. Precise neuroradiologic analysis is essential to establish the diagnosis. The cerebrospinal fluid pressure is characteristically, but not invariably, increased in the cerebral ventricles and lumbar sac. The protein content is generally normal; elevated protein levels favor an underlying neoplastic process in the absence of bleeding or chronic meningitis.

TREATMENT. The treatment of hydrocephalus is surgical; it is directed toward reducing the volume and pressure of cerebrospinal fluid by bypassing obstruction. A wide variety of shunting procedures have been used. The choice of procedure will depend upon technical factors and the skill and experience of the operating surgeon. If the block exists in the third ventricle, aqueduct, or fourth ventricle (as with intraventricular tumors or with "aqueduct stenosis"), the Torkildsen procedure is often employed (ventriculocisternal shunt), wherein a catheter is placed from one or both lateral ventricles over the occiput into the cisterna magna to enable normal CSF reabsorption into the intracranial venous sinuses. In patients with communicating hydrocephalus, direct shunting of the ventricular fluid into the venous system is generally used, particularly the ventriculoatrial shunt wherein the fluid exits from the ventricle through a valved tube, which extends into the superior vena cava and right atrium of the heart. There are many variations of these procedures in use, including shunting to other body cavities, e.g., ventriculopleural, ventriculoabdominal, and lumbar peritoneal shunts. Infections and recurrent obstruction of the shunt are common complications of the various shunting procedures, and the results of treatment particularly in young children are frequently discouraging. Acetazolamide, a carbonic anhydrase inhibitor, reduces the rate of formation of CSF; but there is no convincing evidence that it is useful in the management of the various forms of hydrocephalus. Some hydrocephalic children will have spontaneous arrest and may function within the normal range with only a prominent forehead and large hat size as residual defects. Shunting procedures have established occult "normal pressure" hydrocephalus as a treatable dementia.

Fisher, C. M.: The clinical picture in occult hydrocephalus. Clin. Neurosurg., 24:270, 1977.

Mathew, N. T., Meyer, J. S., Hartmann, A., and Ott, E. D.: Abnormal cerebrospinal fluid-blood flow dynamics. Implications in diagnosis, treatment and prognosis in normal pressure hydrocephalus. Arch. Neurol., 32:657, 1975.

Messert, B., and Wannamaker, B. B.: Reappraisal of the occult hydrocephalus syndrome. Neurology, 24:224, 1974.

Milhorat, T. H.: Hydrocephalus and Cerebrospinal Fluid. Baltimore, Williams & Wilkins Company, 1972.

321. ANOMALIES OF THE CRANIOVERTEBRAL JUNCTION, SPINE, AND MENINGES

A wide variety of neurologic syndromes are associated with morphologic anomalies in the region of the foramen magnum of the skull that are due to distortion of the brainstem, cervical cord, and cerebellum. The most common of these are (1) Arnold-Chiari malformation, (2) fusion of the cervical vertebrae (Klippel-Feil syndrome), (3) basilar impression and platybasia, and (4) spina bifida and meningocele. These defects may occur singly or together, with or without clinical symptoms. Symptoms result from compression, distortion, or malformation of adjacent neural structures. These are most often congenital lesions, but acquired defects caused by bone disease or neoplasms of this region may give rise to similar syndromes.

ARNOLD-CHIARI MALFORMATION

This congenital anomaly is characterized by downward displacement of the cerebellum through the foramen magnum of the skull and by similar caudal elongation of the medulla. These cases can be divided into two major types, the infantile and the adult.

INFANTILE FORM. The infantile form is commonly associated with other midline defects such as spina bifida and meningocele, hydrocephalus caused by aqueductal or fourth ventricular obstruction, and other congenital malformations of the brain and cord. The infantile form of the Arnold-Chiari malformation usually presents itself because of hydrocephalus in the early months of life, with evidence of spina bifida or frank paraparesis resulting from myelomeningocele. Therapy is directed toward surgical relief of the hydrocephalus with a ventricular shunting procedure and repair of the meningomyelocele. Prognosis is poor for patients with extensive defects.

ADULT FORM. The malformation may be asymptomatic until adult life, when there is the onset of symptoms and signs of damage to the cerebellum, lower cranial nerves, pyramidal tracts, and posterior columns. The presenting signs may be due to hydrocephalus secondary to obstruction of the cerebrospinal fluid pathways or to coexisting syringomyelia of the cervical spinal cord and medulla (see Ch. 320 and 334.3). Commonly, there is evidence, clinical or roentgenographic, of fusion of the cervical vertebrae, platybasia, or basilar impression. The Arnold-Chiari malformation in adults may simulate syndromes produced by tumors near the foramen magnum and by multiple sclerosis. Surgical enlargement of the foramen magnum and decompression of the cervicomedullary junction are beneficial in selected cases.

CONGENITAL FUSION OF CERVICAL VERTEBRAE
(Klippel-Feil Syndrome)

Fusion of one or more of the cervical vertebrae is a congenital malformation that may be an asymptomatic finding, detected only with roentgenograms of the cervical spine; malformation of the atlas and axis may coexist. Multiple fusions and condensaton of vertebrae result in shortening of the cervical spine, which produces a characteristic appearance of a short, thick neck, head set low on the shoulders, and limitation of neck movements.

Coexisting abnormalities are common, including undescended scapula (Sprengel's deformity), platybasia, basilar impression, Arnold-Chiari malformation, and other "dysrhaphic" disorders such as syringomyelia and meningomyelocele. Clinical evidence of spinal cord involvement is most likely to be due to coexisting syringomyelia. "Mirror movements" may occur with the Klippel-Feil syndrome and other anomalies of the craniovertebral junction and high cervical cord, in which voluntary movements of one upper extremity are involuntarily imitated by the other upper extremity. Surgical decompression may be indicated if there is evidence of spinal cord compression.

BASILAR IMPRESSION AND PLATYBASIA

Basilar impression refers to abnormal invagination of the cervical spine into the base of the posterior fossa of the skull. The diagnosis is made from lateral roentgenograms of the skull when there is excessive protrusion of the tip of the odontoid process of the axis above Chamberlain's line, that is, a line drawn from the back of the hard palate to the posterior margin of the foramen magnum. Other radiologic criteria are also useful. *Platybasia* refers to flattening of the base of the skull, wherein lateral roentgenograms of the skull reveal flattening of the angle between the orbital plates of the anterior fossa and the clivus, the sloping anterior floor of the posterior fossa. The angle is normally 135 degrees and becomes 145 degrees or more in platybasia. Platybasia alone is asymptomatic.

These malformations, which commonly coexist or may exist alone, are usually developmental in origin, and there may be hereditary transmission. Occasionally, these deformations of the base of the skull may result from metabolic bone diseases such as rickets, osteitis deformans, osteomalacia, or osteogenesis imperfecta. The congenital form may be associated with the Klippel-Feil syndrome, Arnold-Chiari malformation, and other congenital malformations of the atlas and axis, such as fusion of the atlas to the base of the skull, malpositioning of the odontoid process, or atlantoaxial subluxation. Minor degrees of deformity of the base of the skull give rise to no symptoms. The neck appears shortened, and its movements may be limited. With more severe invagination, there may be signs of impaired function of the cerebellum, lower cranial nerves, pyramidal tracts, and posterior columns. Syringomyelia and syringobulbia may also be present. Increased intracranial pressure may develop owing to obstruction of the foramina of the fourth ventricle and the basal cisterns. The clinical manifestations must be differentiated from those caused by neoplasms in the region of the foramen magnum and multiple sclerosis. When neurologic signs are progressive, surgical decompression of the posterior fossa and upper cervical cord may be indicated.

SPINA BIFIDA AND MENINGOCELE

Various malformations of the meninges and spinal cord result from developmental defects in the closure of the bony canal. Although many of these are obvious at birth, some may not be symptomatic until adult life. The classification of these defects would include the following: (1) *Complete rachischisis*, in which the bony vertebral arches are missing in the lumbar region, the cord is undeveloped or aplastic, and the nerve elements have no covering. (2) *Meningomyelocele*, an obvious soft tissue saccular mass which extends over the lumbosacral spine. The cerebrospinal fluid may leak from a defect which may be responsible for bacterial meningitis. (3) *Meningocele*, a bony defect in the spine associated with a meningeal diverticulum covered by atrophic skin. The spinal cord and roots are generally not involved and there may be no associated neurologic defect. (4) *Spina bifida occulta*, a defect in the bony arches in the lumbar region often discovered incidentally on roentgenographic examination. In most cases, neither cord nor roots are involved. The overlying skin may be the site of a tuft of hair, a pilonidal dimple, or a dermal sinus, which is continuous with the subarachnoid space. The latter may serve as a portal of entry for recurrent bouts of meningitis. It should be sought in all patients presenting with bacterial meningitis. These malformations may be associated with Arnold-Chiari malformation and with hydrocephalus. There may also be evidence of syringomyelia. The neurologic deficit varies with the degree of involvement of the spinal cord, conus medullaris, and cauda equina. In adults the chief manifestation may be a neurogenic bladder and defective anal sphincter. Asymptomatic spina bifida requires no therapy. Dermal sinuses, when responsible for bacterial meningitis, require surgical excision. In patients with neurologic deficits, attempts at surgical correction may be indicated.

Appleby, A., Foster, J. B., Hankinson, J., and Hudgson, P.: The diagnosis and management of the Chiari malformations in adult life. Brain, 91:131, 1968.
Embry, J. L., and MacKenzie, N.: Medullo-cervical dislocation deformity (Chiari II deformity) related to neurospinal dysraphism (meningomyelocele). Brain, 96:155, 1973.
Greenberg, A. D.: Atlanto-axial dislocations. Brain, 91:655, 1968.
Schmidt, H., Sartor, K., and Heckl, R. W.: Bone malformations of the craniocervical region. In Vinken, P. J., and Bruyn, G. W. (eds.): Handbook of Clinical Neurology, Vol. 32. New York, American Elsevier Publishing Company, 1978, p. 1.
Wilkinson, M.: The Klippel-Feil syndrome. In Vinken, P. J., and Bruyn, G. W. (eds.): Handbook of Clinical Neurology, Vol. 32. New York, American Elsevier Publishing Company, 1978, p. 111.

Section Twenty NONMETASTATIC EFFECTS OF CANCER ON THE NERVOUS SYSTEM

Jerome B. Posner

322. INTRODUCTION

When patients with systemic cancer develop nervous system dysfunction, metastasis is usually the cause. However, cancer also exerts deleterious effects on the nervous system in the absence of direct metastatic involvement. Recognition of these nonmetastatic neurologic complications can prevent inappropriate and perhaps harmful therapy directed at a nonexistent metastasis. Since at times the nervous system symptoms precede the discovery of the cancer, they can also lead the physician to the diagnosis of an otherwise occult neoplasm.

An almost bewildering variety of neurologic disorders have been ascribed to effects of systemic cancer, as shown in the accompanying table. Many of these bear only an indirect nutritional or metabolic (e.g., hepatic coma) relationship to cancer and are discussed elsewhere in this book. The term "remote effects of cancer on the nervous system" as used in this section applies to nervous system dysfunction of unknown cause occurring in association with cancer (see accompanying table). The classification is similar to that of Brain and Adams (see Brain and Norris), but progressive multifocal leukoencephalopathy is not included in the text, because its cause (a viral infection by a papovavirus) is known.

Remote effects of cancer on the nervous system are uncommon. Croft and Wilkinson found remote effects in 96 of 1465 patients, an incidence of 6.6. per cent, but a rather ill-defined weakness and wasting of proximal muscles associated with diminished deep tendon reflexes accounted for two thirds of their patients. The incidence varied according to the type of cancer, with ovary (16.4 per cent) and lung (14.2 per cent) leading the list. Rectal (0.5 per cent) and uterine (1.3 per cent) cancer rarely caused remote effects. Since carcinoma of the lung is much more common than ovarian carcinoma, about half of all their patients with remote effects had lung cancer, usually of the oat cell type. My experience is that "remote effects" are less common than the aforementioned series suggests, and the diagnosis should never be accepted until a thorough evaluation has excluded metastatic or other nonmetastatic (e.g., infection, vascular disease) causes of neurologic dysfunction. In particular, infiltration of nerve roots by tumor in the leptomeninges (meningeal carcinomatosis) may mimic a "remote" peripheral neuropathy.

The etiology and pathogenesis of these "remote effects" are unknown; suggestions for their cause have included autoimmune reactions, viral infections, toxins secreted by the tumor, and nutritional deprivation. It is possible that different mechanisms are responsible for the several types of remote effects. Although the neurologic disorders described below are separated into anatomic categories, there is often an overlap. This is particularly true of the dementias, which are often lumped together with brainstem, cerebellar, and spinal cord lesions as "carcinomatous encephalomyelitis," and of myopathy and peripheral neuropathy associated with cancer, often called "carcinomatous neuromyopathy." The latter term was also applied by Brain to all the remote effects of cancer on the nervous system.

323. BRAIN AND CRANIAL NERVES

CEREBRUM. About 40 per cent of patients suffering from remote effects of cancer on the nervous system are demented. The dementia may be the only neurologic abnormality or may be associated with other neurologic findings. The dementia is insidious in onset and progressive. There is usually a striking loss of recent memory and an alteration of the affect, either anxiety or depression. Generalized seizures are prominent in some patients, and others have a fluctuating confusional state mimicking metabolic encephalopathy. When other abnormal neurologic signs are present, they usually point

Nonmetastatic Effects of Systemic Cancer on the Nervous System

I. "Remote effects," cause unknown
  A. Brain and cranial nerves
    1. Dementia
    2. Bulbar encephalitis
    3. Subacute cerebellar degeneration–opsoclonus*
    4. Optic neuritis – retinal degeneration
  B. Spinal cord
    1. Gray matter myelopathy
      a. "Amyotrophic lateral sclerosis"
      b. Subacute motor neuropathy
      c. "Autonomic insufficiency"
    2. Subacute necrotic myelopathy
  C. Peripheral nerves and roots
    1. Dorsal root ganglionitis*
    2. Sensorimotor peripheral neuropathy
    3. Acute polyneuropathy, "Guillain-Barré" type
    4. Autonomic neuropathy
  D. Neuromuscular junction and muscle
    1. Polymyositis and dermatomyositis (dermatomyositis in older men*)
    2. "Myasthenic" syndrome*
    3. Myasthenia gravis (thymoma)
    4. Neuromyotonia
II. Metabolic encephalopathy
  A. Destruction of vital organs
    1. Liver (hepatic coma)
    2. Lung (pulmonary encephalopathy)
    3. Kidney (uremia)
    4. Bone (hypercalcemia)
  B. Elaboration of hormonal substances by tumor
    1. "Parathormone" (hypercalcemia)
    2. "Corticotropin" (Cushing's syndrome)
    3. Antidiuretic hormone (water intoxication)
  C. Competition between tumor and brain for essential substrates
    1. Hypoglycemia (large retroperitoneal tumors)
    2. Tryptophan (carcinoid)
  D. Malnutrition
III. Infections (usually associated with lymphomas)
  A. Parasites
    1. Toxoplasma cerebral abscess
  B. Fungi
    1. Meningitis (cryptococcosis)
    2. Encephalitis (aspergillus, mucormycosis)
  C. Bacteria
    1. Meningitis (*Listeria monocytogenes*)
  D. Viruses
    1. Herpes zoster (radiculitis, myelitis, encephalitis)
    2. Progressive multifocal leukoencephalopathy
IV. Vascular disease
  A. Intracranial hemorrhage (secondary to bleeding disorders)
    1. Subdural hematoma
    2. Subarachnoid hemorrhage
    3. Intracerebral hemorrhage
  B. Cerebral infarction
    1. Thrombotic (due to "disseminated intravascular coagulation")
    2. Embolic (tumor emboli, marantic endocarditis)
V. Effects of therapy
  A. Steroids
    1. Myopathy
    2. Psychosis
  B. Chemotherapy
    1. Central effects (asparaginase encephalopathy)
    2. Peripheral effects (vinca alkaloid neuropathy)
  C. Radiation
    1. Encephalopathy
    2. Myelopathy
    3. Neuropathy
    4. Radiation-induced neoplasms

*Neurologic disorders which may precede diagnosis of cancer but strongly suggest its presence.

to brainstem, cerebellar, or peripheral nerve involvement (see below). The electroencephalogram in the demented patients is diffusely slow, and there are sometimes 10 to 40 lymphocytes per cubic milliliter in the cerebrospinal fluid and a slight elevation of the protein content.

Pathologically, there are two main groups. In some patients, particularly those who also have subacute cerebellar degeneration, bulbar encephalitis, or carcinomatous neuropathy (q.v.), no significant pathologic changes can be found in the cerebrum despite clinical dementia. Other patients demonstrate widespread cerebral neuronal loss with perivascular collections of lymphocytes, particularly in the temporal lobes (limbic encephalitis) or the thalamus.

The etiology of the dementing illness is unknown, but the inflammatory changes have led some to propose that a virus is responsible. The differential diagnosis includes metastatic disease of the brain or meninges, fungal or parasitic infections of the brain, a metabolic encephalopathy, and multifocal leukoencephalopathy. In the first three, focal cerebral signs other than dementia are present, and appropriate contrast and cerebrospinal fluid studies support the diagnosis of infectious or metastatic disease of the brain. Metabolic encephalopathy can usually be diagnosed by appropriate laboratory tests, as indicated in Ch. 220. The presence of a progressive dementia in middle age accompanied by cerebellar, brainstem, or peripheral nerve dysfunction but no other focal cerebral signs suggests carcinomatous dementia. There is no treatment for the dementias associated with carcinoma.

BULBAR ENCEPHALITIS. Henson et al. have reported a few patients with brainstem dysfunction and usually dementia, which develops insidiously or subacutely and is progressive. The brainstem signs include vertigo, nystagmus, dysphagia, ophthalmoplegia, and at times ataxia and extensor plantar reflexes. The pathologic changes, predominantly in the lower pons and medulla, are those of neuronal loss and perivascular lymphocytic cuffing. The lymphocytic infiltration is responsible for the term encephalitis. The cause is unknown, and there is no effective treatment.

CEREBELLUM. Subacute cerebellar degeneration due to cancer has a clinical picture sufficiently characteristic to suggest strongly that cancer is present even if the neurologic symptoms predate the appearance of the tumor. There is a subacute onset of bilateral and symmetrical cerebellar dysfunction, the patient being equally ataxic in arms and legs. Severe dysarthria is usually present, but nystagmus is generally absent or mild. Many patients have neurologic signs pointing to disease outside the cerebellum: extensor plantar responses are common; tendon reflexes may be either diminished or exaggerated; and dementia occurs in about half. The cerebrospinal fluid is usually normal, but there may be as many as 40 lymphocytes per cubic milliliter and an elevated protein content. The disease, which is usually associated with either carcinoma of the lung or of the ovary, precedes the discovery of the neoplasm by periods of from weeks to three years in more than half the patients, and it tends to run a progressive course over six to eight weeks, rendering the patient severely disabled. Characteristic pathologic changes consist of diffuse loss of Purkinje cells in all areas of the cerebellum with lymphocytic cuffs around blood vessels. There is often additional neuronal degeneration of brainstem nuclei and subthalamic structures as well. This illness can be distinguished from cerebellar metastases by the symmetry of its signs and the absence of increased intracranial pressure, and from alcoholic-nutritional cerebellar degeneration because dysarthria and ataxia in the upper extremities are prominent in the carcinomatous cerebellar degenerations, and are usually mild or absent in the alcoholic variety. The hereditary cerebellar degenerations rarely run so rapid a course. There is no treatment for this disorder, and its cause is unknown. There is no evidence that treatment of the tumor reverses the neurologic disability.

Another, less common, cerebellar syndrome is that of opsoclonus (spontaneous, conjugate, chaotic eye movements most severe when voluntary eye movements are attempted). Opsoclonus is frequently associated with cerebellar ataxia and myoclonus of the trunk and extremities. It has been reported in adults as a remote effect of cancer, but is more common in children as a remote effect of neuroblastoma. In children, the neurologic symptoms respond to adrenocorticosteroid therapy and to removal of the tumor.

OPTIC NERVES. Acute optic neuritis is a rare remote effect of cancer which may precede the discovery of the cancer by months or years. The disease is bilateral, acute or subacute in its onset, and associated with decreased vision, central scotomas, and papilledema. The cerebrospinal fluid is normal, and vision usually does not improve. Pathologically, there is widespread demyelination of the optic nerves with relative preservation of the axis cylinders and occasional perivascular cuffings with lymphocytes. The illness cannot be distinguished from the optic involvement which is a common accompaniment of meningeal carcinomatosis except by examination of the cerebrospinal fluid, which in meningeal tumor usually reveals increased protein and decreased glucose concentrations and the presence of malignant cells. Blindness from optic nerve or chiasm involvement has also been reported as an untoward effect of radiation therapy and chemotherapy in patients with leukemia, but in these instances the history is diagnostic. Treatment of the acute optic neuritis with corticosteroids is not helpful. Blinding caused by degeneration of retinal photoreceptors has recently been described as a remote effect of oat cell carcinoma.

324. SPINAL CORD

Two rare but distinct myelopathies complicate cancer. The first, which involves spinal gray matter (particularly anterior horn cells), has clinical and pathologic findings at times indistinguishable from amyotrophic lateral sclerosis, except that the patients with cancer are usually older and suffer a more indolent course. Alternatively, the course may be subacute, more like poliomyelitis, but sometimes with sensory changes. In these patients, there are inflammatory changes in the spinal gray matter as well as neuronal loss. Rarely, gray matter myelopathies with clinical courses resembling syringomyelia or autonomic insufficiency (q.v.) complicate systemic cancer. The second myelopathy is that of a subacute necrotic destruction of the spinal cord in which both gray and white matter are affected to an equal degree. Clinically, there is a rapidly ascending sensory and motor loss, usually to midthoracic levels, the patient becoming paraplegic and incontinent within hours or days of the onset of symptoms. The neurologic symptoms often precede the discovery of the neoplasm, and the illness is clinically and pathologically indistinguishable from idiopathic subacute necrotic myelop-

athy. Since epidural spinal cord compression from metastatic tumor or arteriovenous spinal cord anomalies may present similar clinical signs, a myelogram is essential to the diagnosis. In addition to the two aforementioned entities, many patients with carcinomatous cerebellar degeneration develop extensor plantar responses, mild sensory changes, and reflex asymmetries and weakness associated with degenerations of long tracts and anterior horn cells of the spinal cord. However, spinal cord symptoms do not predominate in these patients.

325. PERIPHERAL NERVES

Four types of peripheral nerve disorders occur in association with cancer. Characteristic of carcinoma is a subacute sensory neuropathy (dorsal root ganglionitis) marked by loss of proprioception and cutaneous sensory modalities with relative preservation of motor power. The illness sometimes precedes the appearance of the carcinoma and progresses over a few months, leaving the patient with a moderate or severe disability. The cerebrospinal fluid protein is usually elevated. Pathologically, there is destruction of posterior root ganglia with perivascular lymphocytic cuffing. There is wallerian degeneration of sensory nerves. Many of the patients have inflammatory and degenerative changes in brain and spinal cord as well. The entity is rare; in one series no examples were found on examination of 1476 patients with cancer. The illness is of interest, however, because it is almost pathognomonic of cancer. The pathogenesis is unknown. There is no treatment.

More common than sensory neuropathy is a distal sensorimotor polyneuropathy characterized by motor weakness, sensory loss, and reflex absence distally in the extremities. Croft et al. subdivided their 33 patients with cancer and sensorimotor polyneuropathy into three groups: (1) a mild neuropathy often occurring in terminal patients (10 patients), (2) a more severe subacute or acute neuropathy at times preceding discovery of the cancer (15 patients), and (3) a remitting or relapsing neuropathy (8 patients). The illness is pathologically characterized by both segmental demyelination and wallerian degeneration of sensory and motor peripheral nerves. Dorsal root ganglia are never involved to the same degree that they are in the purely sensory neuropathy. Pathologically and clinically, the sensorimotor neuropathy is indistinguishable from nutritional polyneuropathies as well as those associated with uremia and other metabolic defects. Indeed, some have suggested that the late or terminal polyneuropathy may be due to nutritional deprivation associated with cancer. Its etiology, however, is not clear, and it does not respond to treatment with vitamins and other nutritional supplements.

A polyneuritis clinically and pathologically indistinguishable from acute postinfectious polyneuropathy (Guillain-Barré syndrome) also complicates cancer, particularly Hodgkin's disease, in which it is probably related to impaired immunity. A few patients with neuropathy limited to the autonomic nervous system as a remote effect of cancer, usually oat cell carcinoma, have been reported.

326. NEUROMUSCULAR JUNCTION AND MUSCLES

NEUROMUSCULAR JUNCTION. *Myasthenia gravis* is associated with thymomas but not other systemic tumors. However, Lambert and Eaton described a *"myasthenic syndrome"* occurring predominantly in men over 40 and associated with intrathoracic tumors in 70 per cent of the patients (see Brain and Norris). The patients complain of weakness and fatigability of proximal muscles, particularly of the pelvic girdle and thighs. The cranial nerves and respiratory muscles are involved less. In addition, patients complain of dryness of the mouth, impotence, pain in the thighs, and peripheral paresthesias. On examination there is weakness of the proximal muscles, but strength increases over several seconds of a sustained contraction. The deep tendon reflexes are diminished or absent. The diagnosis is made by electromyographic studies in which repeated nerve stimulations at rates above ten per second cause a progressive increase in the size of the muscle action potential (exactly the opposite of the effect of myasthenia gravis). The neuromuscular defect in this illness is believed to be deficient release of acetylcholine. The illness responds poorly to anticholinesterase drugs, but does respond to guanidine hydrochloride given in doses of 15 to 40 mg per kilogram per day. There is no direct relationship between treatment of the tumor and change in the myasthenic syndrome.

MUSCLE. Typical *dermatomyositis* or *polymyositis* may appear as a remote effect of cancer. About 10 per cent of patients with this disorder have cancer, but this figure is higher in patients with dermatomyositis, particularly in men over 40. In at least 60 per cent of males over 40 with dermatomyositis, a cancer either can be found when the disease develops or will appear within a few months or years. The clinical picture is indistinguishable from that of dermatomyositis or polymyositis. Pathologically there may be two groups: one with the typical inflammatory lesions of polymyositis, and one with little inflammation but severe muscle necrosis. The latter group may suffer an explosive clinical course. The patients respond somewhat less well to corticosteroid therapy than do those with dermatomyositis unaccompanied by cancer, although improvement with steroid treatment does occur in some.

327. MUSCLE WEAKNESS

Some patients with cancer complain of weakness and fatigability which seems worse than can be accounted for by their cancer alone. Cachexia and weight loss alone do not usually cause measurable muscle weakness. The weakness is usually proximal and produces particular difficulty climbing stairs and getting out of low chairs. Ankle reflexes may be diminished or absent. Further neurologic evaluation does not yield findings diagnostic of one of the remote effects of cancer described above. Brain and his colleagues have labeled this entity a "neuromyopathy" because its exact anatomic locus is unclear, but Hildebrand and Coers have suggested that it is a nonspecific accompaniment of cachexia and systemic illness. Engle has demonstrated that specific (type II) muscle fiber atrophy develops early in patients with systemic cancer. The cause and treatment of the weakness are unknown, but Sloane and Truong suggest that some of the patients have mild neuromuscular transmission disorders of the "myasthenic syndrome" type and respond to guanidine HCl.

Brain, R., and Norris, F. H., Jr.: The Remote Effects of Cancer on the Nervous System. New York, Grune & Stratton, 1965.

Croft, P. B., and Wilkinson, M.: The course and prognosis in some types of carcinomatous neuromyopathy. Brain, 92:1, 1969.

Curries, S., Henson, R. A., Morgan, H. G., and Poole, A. J.: The incidence of the nonmetastatic neurological syndromes of obscure origin in the reticuloses. Brain, 93:629, 1970.

Thompson, R. A., and Green, J. R. (eds.): Neoplasia in the Central Nervous System. Advances in Neurology, Vol. 15. New York, Raven Press, 1976.

Section Twenty-One   INJURIES OF THE HEAD AND SPINE

Russel H. Patterson, Jr.

328. INJURIES OF THE HEAD

Trauma claims over 110,000 lives each year in the United States and ranks in frequency as a cause of death after heart disease, cancer, and stroke. Head injury accounts for death in 70 per cent of cases and surpasses all other causes in persons between the ages of 1 and 35. Good management can benefit many of these patients, but often responsibility for their care falls first on someone who lacks formal training in the field of cerebral trauma. This need not be a disadvantage if the physician follows a few simple principles of management based on an understanding of the pathophysiology of the injury. Properly prepared, he can recognize the indications for specialized diagnostic procedures and possible surgery.

PATHOPHYSIOLOGY. The scalp, hair, skull, and bones of the face protect the brain from trauma by absorbing energy from blows to the head. When struck by a blow of moderate velocity, the calvaria bends inward, but a few centimeters away the skull bends outward, and linear fractures radiate toward and away from the point of impact. A blow of higher kinetic energy may comminute or penetrate the skull to cause a depressed fracture.

Beneath the point of impact intracranial pressure may increase for a few milliseconds to as much as 5000 mm Hg, and low or even negative pressure can be recorded simultaneously in the brain at the opposite side of the skull. Cavitation occurs in the brain in regions of low pressure, which accounts for many contrecoup injuries. The pressure gradients distort the brain, which attempts to flow toward the foramen magnum, inducing shear stresses in the brainstem and upper cervical spinal cord. Other shearing forces, induced by rapid acceleration and deceleration of the head, tear axonal processes; this is manifest pathologically by chromatolysis in the cell body of the neuron and microglial proliferation in the white matter associated with abnormalities of the myelin sheath. These changes may not be visible macroscopically at autopsy but account for widespread dysfunction in the cerebral hemispheres, basal ganglia, and brainstem.

The brain and skull respond at different rates to forces of acceleration and deceleration produced by a blow which results in mass movements of the brain. Sharp and irregular surfaces inside the cranial cavity such as the orbital surface of the frontal fossa, the sphenoid ridge, the falx, and the tentorium lacerate and contuse the moving brain. Rotational forces shear nervous tissue around arterioles and result in parenchymal hemorrhages; fragile cerebral veins draining into the dural venous sinuses may tear and fill the subdural space with blood. Fractures that divide meningeal arteries or major venous sinuses commonly cause bleeding in the epidural space.

After brain injury cerebral blood flow may decrease in some areas owing to vasospasm, whereas in other areas the arterioles dilate and lose their capacity to regulate flow in response to change in arterial blood pressure. Loss of the normal autoregulatory mechanism accompanies many, but by no means all, severe head injuries. The resulting dilation of the vascular bed combines with cerebral edema and any hematoma that might be present to increase the intracranial pressure. The elevated intracranial pressure fluctuates rhythmically and, in cases of severe injury, periodically may rise further to levels of 25 to 100 mm Hg for several minutes at a time. These additional pressure elevations, known as *plateau waves*, are often associated with a transient deterioration in neurologic status.

Cerebral contusions and lacerations accompany 90 per cent of severe nonpenetrating injuries. Blood stains the cortical surface and subarachnoid space over both cerebral hemispheres, areas of hemorrhage are found in the brain parenchyma, and clots form in the subdural and epidural spaces. Edema further crowds the contents of an unyielding cranium. The swollen cerebrum displaces the uncus of the temporal lobe through the tentorial notch to compress the oculomotor nerve and the midbrain. Continued pressure obstructs the posterior cerebral artery and basilar vein, inducing ischemia and augmenting edema.

The supratentorial structures generally are most susceptible to damage from head trauma because a heavy layer of muscle protects the contents of the posterior fossa. But should the effects of an injury swell the cerebellum, the tonsils herniate downward through the foramen magnum to compress the medulla while the vermis pushes upward through the apex of the tentorial notch to squeeze the vein of Galen against the corpus callosum, which is backed by the rigid falx.

Increased intracranial pressure causes constriction of the peripheral vascular bed, bradycardia, and increased return of venous blood to the heart. The left ventricle of the heart may be unable to increase cardiac output suf-ficiently to prevent the development of high pressure in the left atrium and pulmonary edema. Even in the absence of pulmonary edema, pulmonary arteriovenous shunts may open in response to both the increased blood flow in the pulmonary artery and increased sympathetic tone in the pulmonary vascular bed. The consequence is frequently arterial hypoxemia even if the patient's ventilation is adequate to maintain normocapnia or hypocapnia. If the tongue or secretions obstruct the airway, hypoxia develops in association with hypercapnia. Hypercapnia augments cerebrovasodilatation and causes a further increase in intracranial pressure with the grave consequences outlined above. In addition, blood flow may be shunted to one area of the brain through a portion of the vascular bed that is dilated and of low resistance, thereby reducing circulation to other areas that become relatively ischemic.

Hemorrhages are found about the pituitary gland and hypophyseal stalk in about two thirds of patients dying of craniocerebral trauma. Necrosis of the anterior lobe is present in more than a fifth of cases and has been attributed to shock, swelling of the gland, and obstruction of the portal vessels. The consequence may be some combination of diabetes insipidus, absence of thirst, and hypoadrenalism producing a varied picture of abnormal fluid and electrolyte metabolism which can range from hypernatremia to water intoxication.

CONCUSSION

Concussion is a clinical term that may be defined as loss of consciousness after an injury to the head without macroscopic damage to nervous tissue. Recovery is usually prompt after less severe injuries, but long periods of unconsciousness or death may occur, and amnesia for events before and after the accident is common. Concussion implies that contusions and lacerations of the brain have not accounted for the symptoms, but the diagnosis must be presumptive except in occasional fatal cases studied at autopsy. Information about the pathophysiology of concussion therefore is derived largely from experiments with laboratory animals.

How an injury to the head causes unconsciousness is not entirely clear. Transmitted pressure gradients and rotational forces distort the brainstem, but bilateral injury to the cerebral hemispheres may be equally important. Changes in the brainstem probably account for the apnea and bradycardia that immediately follow the blow as well as for the unsteadiness and giddiness with change in position of which patients often complain for a time. Amnesia, forgetfulness, irritability, fatigue, and impaired memory are attributed to neuronal damage in the cerebrum, although long persistence of these vague symptoms after cerebral trauma may be hard to evaluate, particularly if a lawsuit is unsettled.

Microscopic changes in the brain after a concussive blow are observed in the neurons and glia within a few hours. Some cells may recover, but others do not, and thus permanent damage to the nervous system occurs. Psychologic tests and neurologic examination may not reveal evidence for the loss of a relatively few neurons, but the effects of repeated small injuries are cumulative as the dull, querulous behavior of the punchdrunk fighter testifies.

EVALUATION OF THE ACUTE HEAD INJURY

The initial examination of the head-injured patient is particularly important not only because it will guide immediate management but also because it serves as a baseline for subsequent observations. The physician must be able to assess neurologic improvement or deterioration in order to make decisions about the need for special diagnostic and therapeutic procedures.

Details of the accident suggest what parts of the brain may be injured, and the physician should remember that drugs, alcohol abuse, or underlying disease may contribute to the clinical picture. The duration of unconsciousness is a rough index to the severity of the injury; even brief unconsciousness is evidence of enough damage to merit hospitalization and careful observation. The neurologic examination is repeated at intervals to detect any change in consciousness, breathing, pupillary diameter, motor strength, speech, or vision, which may signal the presence of an expanding intracranial mass.

The blood pressure, pulse, respirations, and temperature should be recorded frequently after an injury to the head. However, the classic response to increasing intracranial pressure of bradycardia and arterial hypertension may not occur, and any instability of vital signs implies a change in intracranial homeostasis.

The head should be inspected carefully for evidence of trauma, remembering that a scalp laceration can be overlooked easily under a heavy growth of hair. If a scalp laceration is present, the underlying skull should be palpated under sterile precautions because sometimes a fracture will be discovered that is not obvious on subsequent roentgenograms. Likewise, ecchymosis around the mastoid or the leakage of blood or cerebrospinal fluid from the auditory canal may be the only evidence of a basilar skull fracture. If the patient is unconscious, the neck should be stabilized until roentgenograms and the clinical course show that the cervical spine is not fractured or dislocated.

As death after trauma is usually due to failure of the respiratory and circulatory centers, the physician must be particularly alert to the early signs of damage to the brainstem. Coma may result from extensive injury to both cerebral hemispheres, but stupor that progressively deepens usually results from distortion of the brainstem caused by an enlarging clot or progressively edematous brain. The evolution of these signs of dangerous rostral-caudal deterioration is emphasized later in this discussion. Grave signs, however, are fixed pupils, impaired oculovestibular responses, and decerebrate posturing.

If edema or a clot herniates the temporal lobe through the tentorial notch, the uncus compresses the ipsilateral third cranial nerve, and the pupil first dilates, then fixes to light. Occasionally the contralateral third nerve is first affected, but eventually both nerves are paralyzed, and both pupils dilate. Later, when sympathetic centers in the midbrain are damaged, the pupils may contract to become fixed in midposition. Treatment, to be fully effective, must reverse the process before this advanced stage.

Sometimes retinal hemorrhages follow intracranial bleeding, or an occluded venous sinus causes papilledema, but mydriatics alter pupillary responses and for this reason should not be used to obtain a better view of the ocular fundus.

DIAGNOSTIC PROCEDURES. Roentgenograms. Roentgenographic examination of the skull should be performed without undue delay in all cases of injury to the head. Fractures of the calvaria are generally visible, but most basilar fractures are obscured in the bony detail. The presence of skull fracture is reason enough to admit a patient to the hospital after an injury even if he appears to have sustained no brain damage. Roentgenograms perhaps will reveal an indriven fragment of bone, a displaced pineal gland, or intracranial air if a fracture through a paranasal sinus tears the dura and arachnoid. The patient is a likely candidate for an intracranial blood clot if fracture is found which crosses a venous sinus or meningeal artery.

Lumbar Puncture. Lumbar puncture is helpful in the differential diagnosis of coma because the cerebrospinal fluid is commonly xanthochromic after being centrifuged in cases of trauma. However, if a good history is available, lumbar puncture is better avoided because in a patient with an edematous brain or an intracranial clot the withdrawal of fluid can precipitate transtentorial or foramen magnum herniation.

Echoencephalography. A shift of the midline structures of the brain caused by edema or hematoma can be identified by a displaced pineal gland on roentgenograms of the skull or by echoencephalography if the gland is uncalcified. After evacuation of a clot, the displaced midline structures return to their normal position unless the clot reaccumulates. The absence of a shift does not necessarily mean that an intracranial clot is not present; bilateral subdural hematomas are common and may cause transtentorial herniation of the temporal lobes without shift of the midline structures.

Electroencephalography. The electroencephalogram is rarely helpful in the management of acute injury to the head. An abnormal tracing is common immediately after the trauma and tends to improve as recovery takes place. In cases of chronic subdural hematoma the electroencephalogram may be of value if low voltages and abnormal wave forms are recorded from the scalp overlying the hematoma.

Radioactive Scan. Chronic subdural hematomas are often well demonstrated by the radioactive scan technique. In acute injuries a scan is less helpful because the study does not differentiate space-occupying lesions from contused areas of brain.

Cerebral Angiography. Angiography is widely used in evaluating trauma to the head, and in some cases, such as subdural hematoma, the films are almost diagnostic. The procedure is not without danger, particularly when the circulation to a region of the brain is already impaired by an injury. Consequently, angiography is best reserved for patients in whom progressive deterioration or focal signs such as hemiparesis raise suspicion that a blood clot may be present.

Burr Holes. Burr holes placed in the skull can be used to diagnose and treat subdural and epidural hematoma. The advantages of the procedure lie in the speed with which the clot can be evacuated if the patient's condition is rapidly worsening. However, computed tomography (CT scanning) and angiography have many advantages over burr holes as diagnostic procedures. Consequently, burr holes are reserved for emergencies or occasions when the more complex studies are not available.

Air Encephalography. Air encephalography provides less information than angiography or CT scanning in patients with trauma and carries more risk because of the possibility that a change in pressure relationships in the head may precipitate an unfavorable shift in the brain with serious consequences. As a result, air studies are employed infrequently in the management of head injury.

Computed Tomography.   CT scanning has proved of great value in the management of head injury. Acute intracranial hematomas are well identified and localized because of the high absorption of x-rays by freshly shed blood. In addition, the CT scan often can demonstrate areas of contused and edematous brain, displacement or hydrocephalic enlargement of the ventricles, the presence of pneumocephalus, and skull fractures.

Obtaining a CT scan in a restless patient may be difficult and require sedation with drugs such as diazepam. The airway must be preserved during the scanning procedure, so many patients will require tracheal intubation and perhaps supplemental oxygen. Roentgenograms of the cervical spine prior to the scan are also desirable to rule out a spine fracture, particularly in unconscious patients.

In managing acute head injury, enhancement with intravenous contrast agent is rarely necessary. However, contrast enhancement is appropriate in evaluating some of the subacute and chronic effects of injury, since the membranes and walls of hematomas and of abscesses may be made visible.

MANAGEMENT OF ACUTE HEAD INJURY

Although it sometimes accompanies a severe head injury, hypovolemic shock is rarely the consequence of moderate head trauma or a scalp laceration. Consequently, a patient with a head injury who is in shock deserves investigation for a source of an occult hemorrhage, such as a pelvic fracture with retroperitoneal bleeding. Scalp lacerations are best repaired in the emergency room before roentgenograms are obtained in order to control bleeding and to prevent infection. This is the time to initiate baseline observations of vital signs and neurologic status and to examine the patient for associated injuries of the skeleton, viscera, and soft tissues. Prophylaxis against tetanus is administered, as are antimicrobial agents if open fractures are present.

RESPIRATION.   A number of steps may be taken to reduce edema in the brain after an injury. The most important is the establishment of an adequate airway. Hypoxia and hypocarbia have grave consequences on cerebral homeostasis as outlined earlier. If a stuporous patient is unable to clear his own airway, the trachea should be intubated.

Blood gases should be monitored even in patients who appear to be respiring adequately, because pulmonary edema and shunting in the lung, described above, may result in low values of arterial Po_2 that the administration of oxygen can correct. When spontaneous respirations cease, even if cardiac action continues, death is inevitable, and mechanical ventilation is unavailing.

Opiates and sedatives are avoided for patients with injuries to the head. These drugs further depress an already damaged nervous system, impair respirations, and increase stupor. Urinary retention often accounts for restlessness in drowsy patients and is readily treated by catheterization.

BLOOD AND FLUID REPLACEMENT.   Motor vehicle accidents commonly result in multiple injuries. Hypovolemic shock occurs and is best treated by the ordinary measures except that the head-low position is avoided if the brain is damaged. Elevation of the extremities increases the return of blood to the heart without contributing to cerebral edema.

Cerebral swelling is increased when hypotonic fluids are administered. Five per cent dextrose in water becomes hypotonic as the sugar is metabolized, and therefore should not be given in large quantities. Isotonic saline or 5 per cent dextrose in one half isotonic saline is less hazardous, because sodium chloride passes the blood-brain barrier poorly. Consequently, fluids are mildly restricted for patients with brain injury, and more saline is employed than in ordinary practice.

Patients with head injury sometimes develop inappropriate secretions of antidiuretic hormone with consequent water intoxication, even if fluids are replaced with care. The resulting symptoms of stupor and seizures are often mistakenly attributed to extensive parenchymal damage. Water intoxication is confirmed by demonstrating a serum sodium of less than 120 mEq per liter associated with a serum osmolality of less than 280 mOsm per kilogram and a urinary sodium greater than 25 mEq per liter. The primary treatment consists of restricting water and perhaps giving small amounts of intravenous 5 per cent saline.

Occasionally trauma damages homeostatic centers in the hypothalamus so that diabetes insipidus results. A patient who is alert will ordinarily drink enough to prevent dehydration. However, if osmoreceptor mechanisms are also disturbed or the subject is in stupor with a lack of thirst, serum hyperosmolarity with high electrolyte levels occurs if adequate fluids are not administered. Replacement of water, restriction of salt, and administration of Pitressin (usually as Pitressin tannate in oil) are indicated until the condition corrects itself, as it usually does.

Severe injuries to the brain are sometimes associated with impaired renal function despite the absence of shock, or a reaction to blood transfusion, or other common causes of damage to the renal tubules. Characteristically the ouput of urine remains good, but the specific gravity is fixed at 1.010, albuminuria is present, and the sediment contains red cells, white cells, and casts. Death from renal failure may occur in spite of treatment. The mechanism of the renal damage is not entirely clear, but stimulation of certain cortical areas and destructive lesions in the hypothalamus cause similar renal lesions in laboratory animals.

OSMOTIC DIURETICS.   By administering a hypertonic solution it is possible to establish an osmotic gradient across the blood-brain barrier that removes water from the brain and reduces cerebral edema. Drugs that penetrate the brain slowly are employed, such as a 30 per cent solution of urea in 10 per cent invert sugar or 20 per cent mannitol given intravenously or glycerin given by mouth.

The administration of an osmotic diuretic often stabilizes or improves the neurologic status of a patient who is deteriorating rapidly after a head injury. The beneficial effects, if observed, are only temporary, but respite even for an hour or two may be enough to obtain diagnostic studies. If the patient is sufficiently ill to warrant the use of osmotic diuretics, his state is serious enough to deserve prompt and vigorous management. Any temporary improvement that might follow their use should not lull the physician, because the patient's neurologic status once again may worsen rapidly when the drug effect wears off.

INTRACRANIAL PRESSURE MONITORING. In most cases of severe head injury the physician is faced with treating diffuse brain damage complicated by cerebral swelling and edema rather than intracranial hematomas that need surgical drainage. Changes in brain swelling are reflected by changes in intracranial pressure, which can be measured continuously by a variety of methods that employ an intraventricular cannula or devices positioned in the subdural or epidural space. As described earlier in this chapter, periodic elevations in intracranial pressure to greater than 25 mm Hg may be associated with neurologic deterioration. These increases in pressure can be aborted by the administration of an osmotic agent or perhaps a diuretic such as furosemide (Lasix). Sometimes the drugs must be given as often as every two to four hours, in which case the serum electrolytes need close monitoring.

The aggressive use of dehydrating agents to treat brain swelling is presently under study not only in cases of head injury but also in other conditions such as Reye's syndrome. Their ultimate value in head injury remains to be established. Possibly their use may improve the rate and quality of survival in certain cases, or they may prove unrewarding, as have surgical attempts at controlling brain swelling through extensive cranial decompression.

STEROIDS. The administration of steroids, which has been of great value in managing the edema associated with brain tumor, has proved disappointing in treating post-traumatic cerebral edema. Although steroids are widely used, various prospective studies have failed to show any benefit in patients treated with doses of up to 40 mg per day of dexamethasone. Some preliminary reports have suggested that higher doses (in the range of 100 mg per day) may be helpful, but this remains to be proved. The fact that the pituitary gland becomes necrotic in as many as 25 per cent of patients with severe head injury suggests that at least replacement doses of steroids may sometimes be necessary.

COMPLICATIONS OF HEAD INJURY

CRANIAL NERVE INJURY. Damage may occur to the cranial nerves as they exit from the skull. Among the more common complications, anosmia and blindness are often permanent in contrast to extraocular palsies and facial paralysis, which usually improve.

DEPRESSED FRACTURES. The incidence of epilepsy is 30 per cent or more after depressed fractures and penetrating wounds, but the risk is reduced if the fracture is elevated and fragments of bone and other foreign bodies are promptly removed. As seizures may occur even if the site of fracture is remote from the motor areas of the cerebral cortex, all depressed fractures should be elevated except possibly a small depression over a major venous sinus. If a laceration of the scalp overlies a depressed fracture, antimicrobial agents are administered to prevent the occurrence of osteomyelitis and intracranial infection.

Debridement of a depressed fracture or penetrating missile wound often leaves an unsightly cranial defect that a properly executed cranioplasty will correct. The current use of synthetic material such as tantalum, acrylic plastic, and stainless steel has simplified this operation and improved its cosmetic results. Some have thought that cranioplasty both ameliorates such subjective symptoms as headache and giddiness and reduces the frequency of convulsive seizures, but properly controlled studies do not bear this out.

BASILAR SKULL FRACTURE AND CEREBROSPINAL FLUID FISTULA. Because they are often not visible on skull roentgenograms, basilar fractures are usually diagnosed by clinical signs such as anosmia, Battle's sign, bilateral periorbital ecchymoses, and the drainage of blood or cerebrospinal fluid from the nose or ears. Cerebrospinal fluid can be distinguished from a mucoid nasal discharge by testing for sugar, which is best done by analysis rather than the use of paper test strips. Patients with cerebrospinal fluid fistulas should be treated prophylactically with antimicrobial agents to prevent meningitis until the leak stops, as it does in 75 per cent of cases of rhinorrhea and almost all cases of otorrhea. The ear or nose should not be probed or packed, and sealing of the leak may be hastened by repeated lumbar punctures in which 30 ml or more of cerebrospinal fluid is withdrawn. A fistula which persists more than 10 to 14 days demands surgical repair.

EPILEPSY. The incidence of epilepsy after head injury varies with the severity of the injury to the brain. Seizures occur in 40 per cent of patients who sustain penetrating missile wounds, but follow only 10 per cent of the blunt injuries characteristic of civilian life. Depressed skull fracture is associated with an increased incidence of epilepsy, which reaches 40 per cent if accompanied by evidence of severe brain damage such as traumatic amnesia lasting more than 24 hours. Elevation of the depressed fracture, debridement of the wound, prevention of infection, and the prophylactic use of anticonvulsant agents can reduce this toll.

The first convulsive seizure occurs within the first week after injury in 95 per cent of cases. These early seizures are typically focal motor in type and many do not recur. Late epilepsy, meaning seizures which occur after the first week, has a more ominous prognosis. It is treated by anticonvulsants. Fortunately in many patients the attacks decrease in frequency as the years pass and ultimately stop in half the cases. A persistent, debilitating convulsive disorder can sometimes be improved by surgical excision of the epileptogenic focus.

INTRACRANIAL HEMATOMAS. Both increasing edema and an enlarging hematoma cause neurologic signs that progress. As the two are difficult to distinguish, progressive signs are a justifiable reason in any patient to search for a clot by the diagnostic procedures outlined earlier in this chapter.

Epidural Hematoma. Although small amounts of blood are often found in extradural space after fracture of the skull, large hematomas are uncommon, occurring in only 1 or 2 per cent of injuries to the head. Despite their rarity, epidural hematomas are important because they are potentially fatal, yet proper treatment is followed by recovery with little or no neurologic deficit if the brain has not sustained other injuries.

Epidural hematomas most frequently occur in the temporal region from a tear in the middle meningeal artery but are sometimes found in the frontal parietal, occipital, and suboccipital areas. Typically, a patient receives a blow on the temple that results in transitory unconsciousness. After a lucid interval of a few minutes or hours the expanding clot causes headache, drowsiness, contralateral hemiparesis, and paralysis of the ipsilateral third cranial nerve. Signs of decompensation of the brainstem soon follow, and death results.

The classic case is easily recognized but not often encountered. The patient may relate that the blow was light and unconsciousness brief. His prompt recovery and normal roentgenograms apparently substantiate the unimportance of the injury. Yet an epidural hematoma may be present and may reach a critical size some hours later, and death may ensue if the patient has been sent home with inadequate observation.

Variations from the typical pattern are common. An associated serious brain injury may cause the patient to remain stuporous without the lucid interval, or symptoms may be delayed several days if the bleeding is slow or intermittent. Progressive coma without localizing signs is the rule with clots over the cerebellum, and occasionally occurs with supratentorial clots. At times a hematoma is missed at operation, especially in children in whom the dura adheres to the suture lines of the skull and restricts the spread of blood over the convexity.

About 40 per cent of patients with epidural hematoma die or are permanently incapacitated. Because the hematoma often occurs in patients with other severe injuries to the brain, some morbidity doubtless is inevitable. But the gratifying recovery that may follow surgery justifies a meticulous evaluation of every patient with severe head injury in a search for this infrequently occurring intracranial clot.

Subdural Hematoma. Subdural hematomas are conveniently divided into categories of acute, subacute, and chronic, which differ in both symptomatology and prognosis. A subdural hematoma is called acute when a rapid progression of symptoms leads to its discovery within hours or a day or two after the injury. Prospects for recovery depend on the severity of the associated brain damage. The fatality rate is 90 per cent in patients whose symptoms warrant operation within 12 hours of injury, but the outlook is much improved if the need for surgery is evident only after several days have passed.

Chronic Subdural Hematoma. Chronic subdural hematoma in adults usually occurs after the age of 50 and often in alcoholics because of their unsteadiness and frequent falls. With age the brain shrinks away from the dural lining of the skull and leaves a space that can fill with blood if a fragile vein should tear. The trauma that initiates the bleeding is often trivial and even forgotten when symptoms commence several weeks later. The clinical importance of such hematomas depends on their size, and many hematomas of 60 ml or less probably cause no symptoms. With larger clots, headache occurs in 90 per cent of cases. Even if a confused patient denies it, the family may testify to his earlier complaints of pain or to his increased consumption of aspirin. Fatigue and irritability are followed insidiously by drowsiness, urinary incontinence, and stupor, which may be attributed erroneously to a natural deterioration in senescence. Hemianopsia, hemiparesis, or pupillary abnormality is observed in less than half the cases. Lumbar puncture usually reveals normal pressure, but in 50 per cent of cases the fluid is xanthochromic. Bruises about the head are frequently present, but a fracture of the skull is identified in only one third of

cases, and a calcified pineal is displaced in only one fifth.

The patient usually deteriorates at an irregular rate. Intervals of substantial improvement interrupt the gradual decline and give hope of recovery, but sudden decompensation and unexpected death may occur.

Small clots may be tolerated or occasionally resorbed, especially when treated with a course of corticosteroid agents. Persistent mass lesions cause edema and irreversible anoxic-ischemic demyelination of the underlying brain. Most subdural hematomas are therefore best treated by surgical drainage. The diagnosis is confirmed readily by angiography or trephination. CT scanning, even with contrast enhancement, may not demonstrate a hematoma when it is between two and six weeks of age because the hematoma is in an "isodense" stage. At this time, shift of the ventricles, if present, may provide the only evidence of hematoma. The results of treatment are good except that irreversible effects of pressure on the brain may leave a noticeable defect in mentation after recovery, particularly in elderly patients. If treatment is delayed until stupor signals dysfunction of the brainstem, evacuation of the clot and the administration of steroids and osmotic diuretics may be unable to reverse progressive transtentorial herniation that results in death.

Intracerebral Hematoma. Scattered petechial hemorrhages are commonly observed in fatal injuries to the brain, but large parenchymal hematomas occur in only 1 to 2 per cent of cases and are usually located in the frontal or temporal lobes or, less frequently, in the occipitoparietal region or cerebellum. The diagnosis is difficult because stupor from associated concussion or contusions may mask the focal neurologic signs produced by the hematoma. The mass is best demonstrated by CT scanning or angiography. The results of surgery are often disappointing because the hemorrhage has destroyed sufficient cerebral tissue to leave a substantial neurologic deficit.

VASCULAR COMPLICATIONS. A blow to the head may rupture the carotid artery within the cavernous sinus and establish a *carotid–cavernous sinus fistula*. The arterial pressure dilates the tributaries of the sinus such as the orbital veins, with the result that the eye protrudes and pulsates, a bruit is usually heard, and chemosis and extraocular palsies occur. Altered arterial circulation to the eye causes loss of vision and, eventually, blindness. If the fistula is small, the symptoms may progress slowly, but spontaneous cure is uncommon. Repair by a direct approach to the fistula through the cavernous sinus is possible but requires the complicated technique of profound hypothermia and circulatory arrest. Ligation of the carotid artery in the neck or trapping the fistula by ligating in addition the intracranial carotid artery is sometimes successful. Better results have been achieved by embolizing the fistula with bits of muscle, often after intracranial ligation of the carotid artery. A recent development is to pack the cavernous sinus with fine copper wire, which precipitates an asymptomatic thrombosis of the cavernous sinus, thereby eliminating the fistula.

Trauma about the head occasionally leads to *thrombosis of the internal carotid artery* in the neck, resulting in hemiplegia. Less frequently, *thrombosis of the middle cerebral artery* by a dissecting aneurysm accounts for an unexpected paralysis several days after the injury.

Depressed fractures may cause *occlusion of the superi-*

or longitudinal sinus, blocking venous drainage from the cerebral hemispheres and thereby raising intracranial pressure and causing the rapid appearance of papilledema and hemorrhages in the ocular fundus. Patients display paralysis of both lower limbs and often of one or both upper limbs.

INFECTION. Osteomyelitis of the skull, meningitis, and abscesses of the brain occasionally complicate open injuries of the head, and may recur for years after the injury. Antimicrobial therapy and proper debridement of the wound greatly reduce the incidence of these infectious complications.

CEREBRAL SWELLING. Enthusiasm for aggressive surgery to cope with cerebral edema in patients with serious head injury waxes and wanes. Experience has shown that extensive cranial decompression is rarely rewarded by survival with an acceptable degree of neurologic function.

CEREBRAL FAT EMBOLISM. Fat embolism is an infrequent complication observed after severe trauma in which a long bone is fractured, or occurs occasionally with just extensive soft tissue injury. Symptoms start between 12 and 48 hours after the accident; a frequent history is that a patient has remained comatose after general anesthesia to reduce a fractured extremity. Cerebral symptoms and signs consist of rapidly progressive stupor often associated with extensor plantar responses and decerebrate posturing but with preservation of pupillary responses. Petechiae may appear on the chest and in the conjunctivae; dyspnea, tachypnea, and cyanosis are evidence that the lungs are affected. The diagnosis is best made by bedside examination, but the finding of fat globules in urine and sputum can lend laboratory support to the clinical impression.

Although cerebral fat embolism has an ominous prognosis, some patients recover even after long periods of coma. Treatment consists of taking measures to prevent shock and hypovolemia, providing ventilatory support, and perhaps administering steroids to reduce cerebral edema. The value of intravenous ethanol or of anticoagulation with heparin, which have been suggested, remains to be seen.

PROGNOSIS IN SEVERE HEAD INJURIES. About 45 per cent of patients with severe head injury die of their illness. Among survivors, the young are more likely to make a good recovery than older patients. Signs indicating a relatively poor outcome include abnormal pupillary responses, abnormal oculovestibular responses, and extensor posturing of the extremities, either spontaneous or in response to noxious stimulation. Patients between 20 and 50 years old who remain in coma for as long as two weeks rarely make a good recovery, whereas patients less than age 20 sometimes recover from coma lasting several weeks. In patients over age 30, the combination of abnormal motor responses and coma makes recovery unlikely.

After head injury some patients remain in a *vegetative state;* in such a case the patient awakens but is unresponsive to his environment. At autopsy, multiple lesions are likely to be present throughout the brain, with the most consistent pathologic changes to be found in the periaqueductal gray matter of the rostral brainstem. Less severely damaged patients profit from intensive care in a rehabilitation center where their physical, emotional, and social disabilities receive appropriate attention. Recovery from the injury continues

for a long time, even several years. Ultimately 80 per cent can be returned to work, but others remain handicapped by permanent neurologic defects. Even some who appear to make a good recovery have subtle defects in memory, concentration, and comprehension which prevent their achieving their expected potential at work. Others manifest distressing psychopathology, ranging from mildly asocial behavior through psychosis or dementia.

329. INJURIES OF THE SPINE

GENERAL CONSIDERATIONS. The first morphologic changes in laboratory animals suffering experimental spinal cord injury appear in the microvasculature. Within minutes small hemorrhages appear in the gray matter, and in severe injuries the hemorrhages coalesce and blood flow to the region ceases for a long interval. Although blood flow is maintained for a few minutes in the white matter, axonal transmission is lost immediately, which suggests that mechanical trauma rather than hemorrhage or ischemia accounts for the acute loss of function following injury. In animals that recover from experimental trauma, blood flow in the white fiber tracts decreases transiently but tends to return toward normal by one hour. In contrast, impaired blood flow in the white matter lasts many hours if the paraplegia is to be permanent. Late changes seen in paraplegic animals include edema in the white fiber tracts and hemorrhagic necrosis in the central gray matter. The mechanism of these changes remains unclear. Experimental efforts at treatment have been attempted with reserpine, regional hypothermia, splitting of the cord to decompress swelling, and the administration of glucocorticoids and epsilon-aminocaproic acid. All have appeared helpful in certain circumstances, but their usefulness in the management of the spinal cord–injured patient remains to be established.

THE ATLAS AND AXIS. Most fractures of the atlas result from blows to the vertex. They are of two types: those of the posterior arch, and the less frequent burst fractures of the lateral masses (Jefferson's fracture). The former can be treated with a cervical collar, whereas the latter generally require traction with skull tongs.

One common fracture of the axis is known as the "hangman's fracture." It consists of a fracture through the lateral arch of the axis and may be associated with a dislocation between the axis and C3. These fractures are inherently stable and heal in traction. In contrast, fractures across the base of the odontoid process cause instability of the atlantoaxial joint that may lead to dislocation. For this reason they are often treated by spinal fusion.

THE MIDCERVICAL SPINE. Patients with hyperextension injuries of the cervical spine often can be identified clinically because of the presence of abrasions on the forehead. They may have cervical spine roentgenograms which are normal or show only a chip fracture of the anterior inferior corner of the vertebral body. However, the forced neck extension buckles the ligamentum flavum forward and pinches the spinal cord, especially in elderly patients, who often have arthritic spurs present anteriorly. A central cord syndrome is a common result.

The upper limbs are weaker than the lower, and a variable sensory loss occurs with relative sparing of touch, position, and vibration sense.

Flexion injuries may lead to unilateral or bilateral locking of the articular facet joints and a variety of vertebral body fractures. They have a propensity for blocking the circulation in the anterior spinal artery or for injuring the radicular arteries or the vertebral arteries in the intervertebral foramina. The resulting ischemic injury is most severe in the anterior portion of the spinal cord and often causes motor paralysis with relative preservation of position sense. Actual thrombosis of the anterior spinal artery is rare.

Patients with injury to the cervical spine must be handled carefully to prevent an unfavorable shift of the fracture-dislocation from further damaging the spinal cord. A conscious patient usually gives warning of his plight, but the possibility of an unstable spine is easily overlooked if the patient is unconscious. A gentle pull on the head in line with the spine is advisable to keep traction on the neck whenever the patient is moved. Spine boards to which the head and trunk can be strapped commonly are used to protect the spinal cord when removing a patient from a wrecked automobile. If one is not available, a bulky wrapping about the neck which supports the chin and occiput will help reduce motion that might be dangerous. A firm board or a door makes a better litter than a sagging canvas stretcher that flexes the neck. Roentgenograms are best obtained on the litter to avoid the manipulation of a transfer to the x-ray table.

The primary treatment of fracture-dislocation of the cervical spine is traction with tongs or wires inserted in the skull to achieve and maintain the reduction. The pull should be in the line of the spine, and weights exceeding 30 pounds should be used with care to prevent a sudden shift from causing further damage.

After reduction is obtained, traction can be continued for six weeks, after which the patient is ambulated in a collar that is worn for three months. An acceptable alternative that shortens the period of immobilization is to perform an operation at which loose fragments of bone and disc are removed and the vertebral bodies fused anteriorly. Atlantoaxial dislocations are characteristically unstable and are appropriately treated by early fusion of the first three cervical vertebrae.

THE THORACOLUMBAR SPINE. Fractures of the upper and mid-thoracic spine may range from the wedge fracture of the elderly to an injury in which a strong force applied to the dorsal surface of the spine shears the upper portion of the spine from the lower. The result of the latter injury is usually a stable fracture but accompanied by complete spinal paralysis. Injuries at the thoracolumbar junction result from a variable combination of flexion, rotation, and compression. This produces wedging of the vertebral body or sometimes a horizontal fracture through the vertebral body associated with facet fracture and vertebral dislocation.

Thoracolumbar fractures in the past have been treated by hyperextension in bed, plaster jackets, and decompression laminectomy. More recently it has proved possible to restore normal alignment to the spine in severe injuries by inserting metal rods at operation. Whether or not this will improve the final outcome remains to be established. Certainly, in most cases, the position of a stable fracture can be accepted and the patient treated by bed rest until the pain subsides, at which time progressive ambulation is begun.

SURGICAL DECOMPRESSION. Whether surgical decompression restores function to a traumatized spinal cord is a matter of controversy. Here the initial neurologic examination assumes importance because almost no patient with complete loss of motor power and sensation that persists more than 24 hours ever regains much useful function regardless of treatment. Examination should include the testing of perianal sensation, and current clinical research includes efforts to record electrical activity in the cerebral cortex when sensory nerves below the level of the lesion are stimulated. If either a trace of motor activity or persistent sensation confirms that the cord has been only partially interrupted, surprising improvement may take place and may continue as long as two years, even without surgery.

All agree that the rare patient who shows progression of the neurologic defect after an injury should have a decompressive operation. Surgical debridement and closure prevent a spinal fluid fistula in open fractures, and possibly damaged nerve roots of the cauda equina benefit from decompression. At present many patients with fracture-dislocation of the cervical spine are operated upon by the anterior approach to achieve decompression of the cord and fusion of the vertebral bodies. The results are difficult to assess because of the relatively good prognosis without surgery when the damage to the cord is incomplete, and a conservative approach is usually justified.

Babcock, J. L.: Cervical spine injuries. Diagnosis and classification. Arch. Surg., 111:646, 1976.

Becker, D. P., Miller, J. D., Ward, J. D., Greenberg, R. P., Young, H. F., and Sakalas, R.: The outcome from severe head injury with early diagnosis and intensive management. J. Neurosurg., 47:491, 1977.

Fell, D. A., Fitzgerald, S., Moiel, R. H., and Caram, P.: Acute subdural hematoma. Review of 144 cases. J. Neurosurg., 42:37, 1975.

Fuld, P. A., and Fisher, P.: Recovery of intellectual ability after closed head-injury. Dev. Med. Child Neurol., 19:495, 1977.

Gronwall, D., and Wrightson, P.: Cumulative effect of concussion. Lancet, 2:995, 1975.

Jennett, B., Teasdale, G., Braakman, R., Minderhoud, J., and Knill-Jones, R.: Predicting outcome in individual patients after severe head injury. Lancet,:1031, 1976.

Lepistö, P., and Alho, A.: Diagnostic features of the fat embolism syndrome. Acta Chir. Scand., 141:245, 1975.

Marar, B. C.: The pattern of neurological damage as an aid to the diagnosis of the mechanism in spinal cord injuries. J. Bone Joint Surg., 56-A:1648, 1974.

Miller, J. D., Becker, D. P., Ward, J. D., et al.: Significance of intracranial hypertension in severe head injury. J. Neurosurg., 47:503, 1977.

Norrell, H. A.: Fractures and dislocations of the spine. In Rothman, R. H., and Simeone, F. A. (eds.): The Spine. Philadelphia, W. B. Saunders Company, 1975, p. 922.

Rish, B. L., and Caveness, W. F.: Relation of prophylactic medication to the occurrence of early seizures following craniocerebral trauma. J. Neurosurg., 38:155, 1973.

Rutherford, W. H., Merrett, J. D., and McDonald, J. R.: Sequelae of concussion caused by minor head injuries. Lancet,:1, 1977.

330. SEVERE SPINAL CORD DYSFUNCTION AND PARAPLEGIA

Many disorders, including spinal trauma, neoplasms, acute myelitis, poliomyelitis, and multiple sclerosis, can result in extensive spinal paralysis and cause similar problems in care and in the management of complications.

Antimicrobial agents and improved medical care have greatly reduced the mortality among patients with paraplegia or other forms of extensive spinal paralysis. Life expectancy is related to the severity of the neurologic deficit. Patients who are partially paraplegic or tetraplegic have a mortality about twice that of the normal population, whereas complete paraplegia carries a mortality four times the normal, and complete tetraplegia twelve times the normal. The mortality stems from an increased incidence of renal disease, cardiovascular disease, and cancer, in that order.

PROGNOSIS. The degree of independence that a paraplegic achieves largely depends on how many muscle groups escape paralysis. The lower the spinal level of the injury or disease, the more skills a well motivated patient can develop if good care prevents the complications of muscle spasm, decubitus ulcers, and infection of the urinary tract.

An understanding of how much recovery is possible sets goals and supplies a yardstick with which to measure progress during rehabilitation. The patient with a complete or extensive lesion of the spinal cord just below C5 retains innervation of the neck musculature and some of the shoulder girdle. He is unable to move in bed, and becomes easily fatigued because of poor respiratory reserve, but he may be able to feed himself with special equipment. With lesions of the lower cervical cord, function of more muscles of the upper limb is preserved; thus the patient is able to roll over, sit up, propel a wheelchair, and possibly learn a job at home that does not require strength and dexterity of the hands. He depends upon an attendant for most of his needs.

High levels of thoracic spinal cord injury leave a functional upper limb, but the trunk is unstable, and intercostal breathing is not possible. The patient can transfer to and from a wheelchair, but even with bracing cannot develop a useful gait. Lower thoracic injuries, which leave a strong pectoral girdle and good respiratory reserve, permit the patient to be independent in all his daily activities. Bracing is still cumbersome, and ambulation is generally not practical.

Patients with lesions at T12 to L3 can usually walk in long leg braces and even negotiate stairs, but depend heavily on wheelchairs. Even with an injury below L3 a patient may sometimes use a wheelchair because such acts as arising from the sitting position, climbing steps, and standing for prolonged periods are difficult.

EMOTIONAL ASPECTS. Severe depression may accompany the realization that paralysis and partial dependency are permanent. Progress in rehabilitation is slowed, and recently learned skills may be temporarily lost, but emotional support from the hospital staff does much to reduce the depth and length of the depression. The environment of a center where others face and overcome similar hurdles also bolsters the morale of the paraplegic.

CARDIORESPIRATORY SYSTEM. Injuries in the cervical region paralyze the intercostal muscles and leave only diaphragmatic respiration. Exercise quickly results in dyspnea, so that the usefulness of a hand-driven wheelchair or braces for walking is limited.

Interruption of motor pathways in the cervical spinal cord isolates the thoracic sympathetic centers from higher control. Consequently, the patient cannot constrict peripheral arteries when he sits or stands. Blood pools in the limbs and viscera, thus reducing venous return to the heart, and even elastic supports cannot adequately compensate. Venostasis in the lower limbs also accounts for a higher incidence of pulmonary embolus in paraplegics who are confined to bed.

GASTROINTESTINAL SYSTEM AND NUTRITION. Paralytic ileus commonly follows spinal injury or acute poliomyelitis for a few days. In treatment oral feedings should be omitted until bowel activity returns. If abdominal distention occurs, a nasogastric tube is advisable to decompress the intestinal tract.

Most paraplegics eventually begin to defecate without an enema. However, fecal impactions are frequent in patients with acute spinal paralysis, so that stool softeners, gentle laxatives, or low enemas may be needed at first. As recovery progresses, a regular dietary schedule and adequate fluids are important to achieve spontaneous evacuation. Some patients initiate reflex evacuation by abdominal massage or digital stimulation of the rectum.

Adequate nutrition is imperative for recovery but is difficult to attain, particularly for patients confined to bed. A diet high in protein and calories helps repair injured tissue and prevent bedsores. A reasonable goal at first is 2000 to 2500 calories daily, although this may have to be lowered later to avoid obesity. During the early months the daily calcium intake should be kept below 0.5 gram to minimize the likelihood of urinary calculus. Transfusions to correct anemia and low blood volume in poorly nourished patients are often beneficial.

SKIN. Decubitus ulcers are a serious problem for paraplegics and can occur in any paralyzed, immobilized patient who is neglected. The danger of an anesthetic region is that it tolerates continuous pressure without the pain that ordinarily prompts a shift in position. After about two hours of immobility, ischemic changes begin in the subcutaneous tissue and are manifested by erythema of the overlying skin. Repeated ischemic insults are followed by ulceration.

Bedsores can be prevented by turning the patient at least every two hours, protecting reddened skin from further pressure, and maintaining adequate nutrition. Alternating air mattresses and rotating frame beds help to vary pressure points but are not by themselves guarantees against ulcers forming over the occiput, heels, trochanters, and sacrum. The weight of bedding is sometimes sufficient to erode the tips of the toes. Plaster casts over anesthetic areas may ulcerate the skin, and even supporting braces are dangerous.

Bedsores that heal with scar tissue remain particularly vulnerable to pressure. Therefore the most satisfactory coverage of a sizable decubitus ulcer is obtained by rotating pedicle tissue into the defect after trimming off any underlying bony prominence.

MUSCULOSKELETAL SYSTEM. Many operations and mechanical devices have been used to compensate for paralyzed muscles. Crutches, braces, or wheelchairs restore mobility. An automatic lift enables anyone to transfer a patient from bed to chair. Bracing or surgery can reconstruct the loss of pinch between the thumb and index finger and thus allow the patient to feed and shave himself.

Kyphosis or lordosis is a grave consequence of the unequal pull of partially paralyzed muscles that distorts the growing spine of a child. Spinal fusion halts progression of such deformity, and often can correct a moderate curvature. Good results have been reported with internal fixation of the spine to avoid the complications of plaster immobilization.

Although a certain amount of muscle spasm may help a paraplegic to support the trunk or to position an extremity, painful or recurrent spasms that forcibly flex or adduct the lower limbs interfere with sitting and ambulation and thus prevent rehabilitation. As flexor spasms are reflex responses, the first step is to remove sources of noxious, afferent stimuli such as infection of the bladder and bedsores. If these measures plus physical therapy fail, more drastic procedures may be required, such as myelotomy, excision of the distal end of the spinal cord, anterior rhizotomy, subthecal injections, peripheral neurotomy, or division of muscles and tendons. Any procedure that increases the neurologic deficit of an already paralyzed subject is undesirable. Accordingly, division of spastic muscles and tendons or a myelotomy that disconnects the afferent sensory input from the efferent limb of the spinal reflex is appropriate if motor or sensory function is present. Subthecal alcohol, anterior rhizotomy, or excision of the cord is suitable only for those who have no useful spinal cord function.

URINARY TRACT. Renal calculi, pyelonephritis, and hydronephrosis are the major causes of death in paraplegics and are sources of considerable disability in patients with lesser paralysis. These renal complications follow incomplete emptying of the bladder, which initially necessitates catheterization. Secondary infection and vesicoureteral reflux follow. These complications can be minimized by providing a low calcium diet, intermittently turning patients soon after the onset of paralysis, forcing fluids to achieve 1500 to 2000 ml of daily urine output, and treating culturally proved urinary tract infections promptly — but not prophylactically — with antimicrobial drugs. During recovery, nearly all patients with poliomyelitis and about 80 per cent of paraplegics become able to void without catheterization. Patients with poliomyelitis regain essentially normal bladder function. In paraplegics with high lesions of the spinal cord, reflex micturition occurs, mediated through the distal spinal segments. If an injury has destroyed sacral roots, suprapubic pressure may be necessary to empty the bladder.

Regaining spontaneous voiding after spinal injury is always difficult. In many patients a fluid intake of 3000 to 4000 ml daily and either intermittent catheterization or intermittent clamping of an indwelling catheter may establish spontaneous, automatic voiding. Intermittent catheterization using aseptic technique has given the best results as the urine remains sterile in three quarters of patients; if a catheter is left indwelling, one of the Gibbon type is preferred to the more irritating Foley. Some may need a transurethral resection of obstructing tissue at the bladder neck. If there is spastic hypertrophy of the bladder, especially with vesicoureteral reflux, satisfactory voiding usually cannot be obtained without partially interrupting the reflex arc. If there are no undesirable muscle spasms of the lower limbs, graded sacral rhizotomy is the most satisfactory procedure for enabling some patients to master bladder training. Myelotomy, as described earlier, is useful in managing patients with disabling spasticity of both the bladder and lower limbs. The more extensive procedures will also relieve autonomic hyperreflexia manifested by unpleasant episodes of sweating, hypertension, and headache triggered by contraction of bladder, bowel, or skeletal muscle. Recently, electrical stimulation of the conus medullaris to induce micturition has shown some promise, although the stimulus may also induce unwanted motion of lower limbs and penile erection.

Even patients who have apparently established satisfactory micturition may have slowly progressive hydronephrosis that, if unrecognized, will eventually cause death. Consequently, all patients should be evaluated periodically by intravenous pyelography. Progressive renal damage is an indication for urinary diversion, usually by implantation of the ureters into an ilial conduit.

Geisler, W. O., Jousse, A. T., and Wynne-Jones, M.: Survival in traumatic transverse myelitis. Paraplegia, 14:262, 1977.

Grimes, J. H., Nashold, B. S., and Currie, D. P.: Chronic electrical stimulation of the paraplegic bladder. J. Urol., 109:242, 1973.

Guttman, L.: Spinal Cord Injuries, Comprehensive Management and Research. Oxford, Blackwell Scientific Publications, 1976, p. 731.

Ivan, L. P., and Wiley, J. J.: Myelotomy in the management of spasticity. Clin. Orthop., 108:52, 1975.

Long, C., II, and Lawton, E. B.: Functional significance of spinal cord lesion level. Arch. Phys. Med. Rehabil., 6:249, 1965.

Wilcox, N. E., and Stauffer, E. S.: Follow-up of 423 consecutive patients admitted to the spinal cord centre, Rancho Los Amigos Hospital, 1st January to 31st December, 1967. Paraplegia, 10:115, 1972.

Section Twenty-Two
MECHANICAL LESIONS OF THE NERVE ROOTS AND SPINAL CORD

Albert J. Aguayo

331. SYMPTOMS OF NERVE ROOT AND SPINAL CORD COMPRESSION

Certain diseases result in compression of the nerve roots or spinal cord within the spinal canal. In general the symptoms and signs that accompany such intraspinal lesions may be classified into two groups: radicular syndromes due to spinal root injury, and myelopathy caused by compression of the spinal cord; but a combination of both syndromes is common.

RADICULAR SYNDROMES

Compression of nerve roots causes pain, paresthesia, sensory loss, weakness, atrophy, and reflex changes which are confined to a radicular anatomic distribution. A single nerve root can be compressed, as in most cases of intervertebral disc protrusion, but several roots are often involved in arachnoiditis or when there is neoplastic invasion of the spinal canal.

The pain caused by root compression is experienced in the overlying spine, deep in certain muscles, or along the cutaneous distribution of the injured root (*dermatome*). This pain is often influenced by movement and increases with strain. Radicular pain is usually unilateral, but some intraspinal lesions, by compressing roots bilaterally, can give rise to pain in both limbs or on both sides of the thorax or abdomen. The most common sensory symptoms are hypesthesia and paresthesia, both of which may be described by patients as numbness. These sensory symptoms are usually accompanied by sensory impairment in the distribution of the compressed root or roots. Because of the more extensive overlapping of adjacent innervation for touch, this sensory loss is better outlined by testing responses to pinprick than to light touch.

Muscles supplied by roots that originate from the same spinal cord segment constitute a *myotome*. Because most muscles are supplied from more than one segmental level, compression of a single root causes different degrees of weakness and atrophy in different muscles. The effects of a root lesion on a muscle ultimately depend on the importance of the innervation provided by the injured root; weakness of certain muscles within a particular myotome may be difficult to elicit, whereas other muscles may be severely affected. For example, although fibers from the L5 root innverate approximately 30 different muscles in the lower limb, severe changes after compression of this root may be clearly apparent in only two: the extensor hallucis longus and extensor digitorum brevis muscles.

Muscle stretch reflexes are diminished or absent when reflex arcs are interrupted by root compression. At the level at which they can be clinically tested, reflex changes have an important localizing value (Table 1).

Differentiation between symptoms caused by nerve root and peripheral nerve lesions must follow anatomic guides (see figure and Table 2). In radiculopathy, as mentioned above, weakness and atrophy of muscles occur within a myotome. In a neuropathy weakness and reflex changes are confined to the anatomic distribution of the nerve, and sensory deficits do not fully

TABLE 1. Clinical Findings in the Four Most Common Radicular Syndromes

Root	Usual Distribution of Pain	Principally Affected Muscles	Sensory Loss	Muscle Stretch Reflexes Affected
C6	Neck, parascapular, lateral aspect of arm and forearm	Biceps, brachioradialis, wrist extensors and flexors	Radial border of forearm, thumb	Biceps and/or brachioradialis may be diminished
C7	Neck, parascapular, posterolateral arm, dorsum of forearm	Triceps, wrist, finger flexors and extensors	Dorsum of forearm; index and middle fingers	Triceps
L5	Low back, buttock, lateral thigh, dorsum of foot	Dorsiflexors of foot and toes	Anterolateral aspect of lower leg, dorsum of foot	Usually none, but ankle jerk may be diminished
S1	Low back, buttock, posterior thigh	Calf muscles, plantar flexors	Outer edge of foot and sole	Ankle jerk

TABLE 2. Peripheral Nerve and Radicular
Innervation of Muscles

Upper Limb:

Nerves	Radicular Innervation					
	C-4	C-5	C-6	C-7	C-8	T-1
Suprascapular	– –Supraspinatus– –					
Axillary		– –Deltoid– – – –				
Musculocutaneous		– – Biceps– – – – – – –				
Median			– –Flexor carpi radialis– –			
				– – – –Flexor pollicis longus– –		
				– –Flexor digitorum– –		
				– –Abductor pollicis longus– –		
					– –Opponens pollicis– – – –	
Ulnar				– –Flexor carpi ulnaris– – – –		
				– –Opponens digiti quinti– –		
					– –Abductor digiti quinti– – – –	
					– –Interossei– – – – –	
Radial				– –Triceps brachialis– – – – – – – – –		
		– –Brachioradialis– –				
			– –Extensor carpi radialis– –			
			– –Extensor carpi ulnaris– –			
			– –Extensor digitorum longus– –			

Lower Limb:

Nerves	Radicular Innervation						
	L-1	L-2	L-3	L-4	L-5	S-1	S-2
	– –Iliopsoas– – – –						
Gluteal				– –Gluteus maximus– – – – –			
Femoral			– –Quadriceps femoris– –				
Obturator		– –Adductors– – – –					
Sciatic					– – – –Hamstrings– – – – –		
C. Peroneal			– –Tibialis anterior– –				
			– – Extensor digitorum brevis– –				
Tibial					– – – – –Gastrocnemius– –		
			– –Abductor hallucis				
				– –Abductor digiti quinti– –			

correspond to individual dermatomes. Differentiation is made easier when the affected muscles are supplied by different nerves (e.g., the deltoid and biceps may be weak in lesions of the C5 root; these muscles are supplied by different nerves: axillary and musculocutaneous nerves, respectively). Because of the proximity of roots and spinal cord within the spinal canal, both structures may be compressed together. Associated signs of spinal cord compression are not a feature in peripheral neuropathies except in rare disorders such as familial hypertrophic neuropathy, in which pathologically enlarged roots may encroach upon the spinal cord (Symonds and Blackwood).

SPINAL CORD COMPRESSION

The clinical symptomatology depends on the speed of compression, the transverse and longitudinal extent of the lesion, the functional role of the compressed level of the spinal cord, and the cause of compression.

The spinal cord accommodates to slow forms of compression such as occur with meningiomas and neurofibromas. As a result these tumors in their early stages may cause few symptoms and signs. However, an acute intervertebral disc protrusion or an epidural hematoma will result in rapid impairment of function with severe paralysis, sensory loss, and loss of bladder and bowel control.

The effects of compression may be limited to only a portion of the transverse area of the cord. When one half of the spinal cord is injured at levels higher than the tenth thoracic, the symptoms and signs that follow may be those of *Brown-Séquard's syndrome*. Such patients have spastic weakness, exaggerated muscle stretch reflexes, and an extensor plantar response (Babinski sign) all on the same side as the lesion. Joint position and vibration sense are decreased ipsilaterally, but pain and temperature are impaired on the opposite half of the body. The contralateral loss of pain and temperature sensation is due to crossing of spinothalamic fibers subserving these modalities. Spinothalamic fibers are somatotopically arranged within the ventrolateral columns of the spinal cord, with fibers originating at lower levels lying most laterally. Because of this anatomic organization, extrinsic compression tends to first produce symptoms below the site of the lesion, the level of sensory impairment gradually ascending as the compression affects deeper parts of the spinal cord. Conversely, because deep-seated lesions may spare superficially arranged fibers, sensation may be normal in the lower dermatomes in patients with intramedullary lesions (sacral sparing).

In addition, intramedullary lesions may give rise to sensory dissociation with loss of pain and temperature sensation and relative preservation of touch. This occurs when mainly crossed fibers are interrupted by a central cord lesion (*commissural or syringomyelia-like syndrome*). In addition, by predominantly disturbing postural sensibility, cord compression may cause ataxia.

Schematic representation of dermatomes and peripheral nerve sensory areas:

1. Trigeminal 1st division
2. Trigeminal 2nd division
3. Trigeminal 3rd division
4. Greater auricular nerve
5. Branches from cervical plexus
6. Axillary nerve
7. Radial nerve
8. Medial brachial cutaneous nerve
9. Musculocutaneous nerve
10. Median nerve
11. Ulnar nerve
12. Lateral femoral cutaneous nerve
13. Femoral nerve
14. Saphenous nerve
15. Peroneal nerve
16. Sural nerve

LEVELS OF INTRASPINAL COMPRESSION

FORAMEN MAGNUM AND UPPER CERVICAL SPINE. Compression at this level may cause symptoms resulting from spinal cord, nerve root, or intracranial involvement. Pain in the neck and back of the head is the most common and earliest sign. The pain is made worse by head movement, particularly nodding. There may be weakness and atrophy of muscles of the neck and shoulder girdle with spasticity in the lower limbs. Paresthesia and sensory deficits may also occur in the occipital head region (C2 dermatome) and the neck (C3 dermatome). Motor and sensory signs may even extend to involve the hands (C6 to C8 segmental level); this extension to the mid- and lower cervical cord has been thought to be due to impaired circulation from compression of spinal vessels. Tumors of the formen magnum may also extend intracranially and cause increased intracranial pressure, cerebellar dysfunction, nystagmus, trigeminal sensory loss, and atrophy of the tongue.

The most common causes of compression at the craniocervical junction are bony abnormalities which result in basilar invagination, dislocation of the atlantoaxial and atlanto-occipital joints, and neoplasms, meningiomas in particular.

CERVICAL REGION. Compression at this level characteristically produces spinal and radicular signs in the upper limbs combined with long tract signs in the lower extremities.

There is loss of power and bulk in muscles of the shoulder girdle and arms. The biceps, brachioradialis, or triceps jerks mainly depend on the integrity of the C5, C6, or C7 reflex arcs, respectively, and may be diminished or absent. In addition, there can be "inversion" of the brachioradialis reflex; tapping the tendon of this muscle elicits a brisk reflex contraction of the hand and finger flexor muscles and not the usual flexion and supination of the forearm. This unusual response is due to efferent interruption of the segmental reflex arc; the spread of the response and hyperreflexia at lower spinal levels results from pyramidal tract involvement.

When sensory symptoms extend along the radial border of the forearm and thumb ("numb thumb"), they suggest involvement of the C6 cord segment or nerve root. Symptoms in the index and middle fingers point to C7, and sensory impairment in the ring and little fingers suggest C8. Lesions at the cervicothoracic junction can cause unilateral Horner's syndrome which can be associated with wasting of the small muscles of the hand and a sensory deficit on the ulnar border of the hand and forearm (C8, T1).

The most common causes of compression at this level are cervical spondylosis and protrusion of an intervertebral disc, but intramedullary and extramedullary tumors also occur.

THORACIC REGION. Compression is suggested by the finding of normal upper limbs and spasticity in the legs. When thoracic radicular symptoms are present, a more precise localization is possible. It is useful to remember that the projection of the thoracic segments coincides with that of the intercostal spaces. Important landmarks are the level of the nipples for the fourth thoracic, the xiphoid process for T7, and the umbilicus and groin for T10 and T12, respectively. Patients will often complain of a tight, bound feeling which usually coincides with the compressed root or segment. In addition, intercostal muscles may be wasted. In low thoracic lesions the umbilicus may elevate when the patient, in the supine position, raises his head against resistance (Beevor's sign).

Common causes of compression at the thoracic spine level are metastatic tumors, meningiomas, and neurofibromas. Intervertebral disc protusions are comparatively rare at this level.

LUMBOSACRAL REGION. Lower Spinal Cord. There is a close relation between the segments in the lower cord and the roots that form the cauda equina. As a result, pain, sensorimotor signs in the lower limbs, and loss of sphincter control can result from the involvement of either cord or roots. It is seldom that a discrete spinal cord segmental lesion can be clinically identified at this level.

Cauda Equina. In cauda equina compression, dull, aching pain may be experienced in the sacrum or perineum or can radiate to the legs in a sciatic distribution.

Symptoms depend on the level of compression and number of motor and sensory roots affected. Often there is atrophic, areflexic paralysis combined with asymmetrical bilateral radicular sensory impairment. Sensory dissociation does not occur. Progression of signs is usually slow, and loss of bladder and bowel control may occur late.

Presumably because of interference with blood supply to the roots of the cauda equina by compression, some patients with a narrowed lumbar spinal canal experience transient, radicular signs or pain in the calf muscles when walking or after prolonged standing. This syndrome has been named intermittent claudication of the cauda equina.

The most important cause of single or multiple root compression at the lower lumbar and sacral level is an intervertebral disc protrusion. Cauda equina compression occurs in congenital spinal stenosis and lumbar spondylosis, Paget's disease, and achondroplasia. Ependymomas, teratomas, and lipomas may constrict the lower segments of the cord and cauda equina. Tabes dorsalis, diabetic neuropathy, and other lesions affecting peripheral nerves to the lower limbs must be differentiated from lesions compressing the lumbosacral roots.

Aids to the Investigation of Peripheral Nerve Injuries. London, Her Majesty's Stationery Office, 1960.

Haymaker, W.: Bing's Local Diagnosis in Neurologic Diseases. 15th ed. St. Louis, C. V. Mosby Company, 1969.

Keegan, J. J., and Garett, F. D.: The segmental distribution of the cutaneous nerves in the limbs of man. Anat. Rec., 102:409, 1948.

Klenerman, L.: Cauda equina and spinal cord compression in Paget's disease. J. Bone Joint Surg., 48B:365, 1966.

Rewcastle, N. B., and Berry, K.: Neoplasms of the lower spinal canal. Neurology (Minneap.), 14:608, 1964.

Symonds, C. P., and Blackwood, W.: Spinal cord compression in hypertrophic neuritis. Brain, 85:251, 1962.

332. LABORATORY AIDS TO INVESTIGATION

To localize and establish the nature of lesions causing intraspinal compression, several diagnostic tests may be used. Roentgenographic investigations are the most important, but electrophysiologic techniques, radioisotope scanning, and cerebrospinal fluid examination are also helpful.

ROENTGENOGRAPHIC METHODS

Roentgenographic investigation should begin with plain films of the suspected site of spinal cord or root compression. Frontal, lateral, and oblique views are required for examination of the cervical spine; frontal and lateral views are generally satisfactory for visualization of the thoracic and lumbosacral spine. Lateral films of the cervical spine in flexion and extension are needed if recurrent subluxation is suspected. In certain situations, tomography may be necessary to define a bone lesion more precisely.

Plain films of the spine should be systematically examined, noting the number, shape, density, and alignment of the vertebrae and the contour of the pedicles, the size of the intervertebral foramen, the size and shape of the spinal canal, the width of the disc spaces,

and the presence of abnormal soft tissue shadows or calcifications. The anteroposterior depth of the spinal canal is a particularly important measurement. Sagittal diameters of less than 10 mm at any level of the cervical spine usually indicate spinal cord compression; bony compression of the cord is also possible with canals measuring 10 to 13 mm but improbable if measurements are greater than 13 mm. Increases in the transverse diameter of the spinal canal may be associated with thinning of the pedicles and are seen with syringomyelia or intramedullary tumors. Narrowing of the spinal canal with compression of the spinal cord or roots may occur in spondylosis, achondroplasia, and Paget's disease.

Plain x-rays of the vertebral column may suggest certain specific conditions. Dumbbell-shaped neurofibromas which enlarge the intervertebral foramen will become readily apparent in such x-rays. Congenital anomalies of the vertebral bodies are at times associated with intraspinal teratomas or lipomas. Bone caries suggests an infectious process such as tuberculosis, typhoidal infection, or brucellosis. Vertebral bone destruction by infection often involves the intervertebral discs; conversely, tumor metastases to the vertebral column spare the discs.

When surgical treatment is contemplated, radiopaque *oil myelography* by lumbar or cisternal injection is required for precise localization. In expert hands, *air myelography* is also a useful tool for the assessment of spinal cord size and for a diagnosis of small tumors. *Spinal angiography* is a specialized technique necessary for the detailed investigation of tumors and vascular malformations.

Computerized tomography using a body scanner is a new, yet to be fully evaluated tool for the investigation of lesions in the spinal canal and surrounding tissues.

SCANNING AND ELECTROMYOGRAPHY

Bone scanning after radioisotope injection may be helpful if metastases are suspected as cause of bone destruction. However, fractures, infection, and ankylosing spondylitis may also cause increased radioisotope uptake.

Electromyography is useful for the localization of intraspinal lesions affecting the motor unit at the anterior horn cell or the nerve root levels, as noted in Ch. 272.

CEREBROSPINAL FLUID EXAMINATION

Cerebrospinal fluid examination rarely provides specific diagnostic information about compressive spinal cord or root lesions. Therefore because satisfactory myelograms are difficult to obtain in patients who have had lumbar puncture in the preceding week, cerebrospinal fluid examinations are usually best performed at the time of myelography. In general, the examination of cerebrospinal fluid may suggest certain diagnostic possibilities. Xanthochromic fluid is seen with intraspinal hemorrhage or block of cerebrospinal fluid circulation. Intraspinal bleeding may originate from vascular malformations, ependymomas, or melanomas. Inflammatory cells indicate an infectious process or chemical meningitis caused by a ruptured teratoma or dermoid cyst. Tumor cells may be identified in the cerebrospinal fluid of patients with carcinomatous infiltration of the meninges.

In the absence of a block in the circulation of cerebrospinal fluid, elevations of CSF protein over 60 mg per 100 ml suggest other intraspinal lesions than an intervertebral disc protrusion or spondylosis. Spinal fluid blocks are best established by myelography; because irreparable damage to the spinal cord may result from displacement of an intraspinal mass after pressure changes resulting from jugular compression (Queckenstedt test), this procedure should not be done if spinal cord compression is suspected.

Aguilar, J. A., and Elvidge, A. R.: Intervertebral disc disease caused by the Brucella Organism. J. Neurosurg., 18:27, 1961.

Ambrose, G. B., Alpert, M., and Neer, C. S.: Vertebral osteomyelitis. A diagnostic problem. JAMA, 97:101, 1966.

Charkes, N. D., Sklaroff, D. M., and Young, I.: A critical analysis of strontium bone scanning for detection of metastatic cancer. Am. J. Roentgenol. Radium Ther. Nucl. Med., 96:647, 1966.

DiChiro, G., and Doppman, J. L.: Differential angiographic features of hemangioblastomas and arteriovenous malformations of the spinal cord. Radiology, 93:25, 1969.

Elsberg, C. A., and Dyke, C. G.: Diagnosis and localization of tumors of the spinal cord by means of measurements made on x-ray films of vertebrae and the correlation of clinical and x-ray findings. Bull. Neurol. Inst., 3:359, 1934.

Hammerschlag, S., Wolpert, S., and Carter, B.: Computer Tomography of the spinal canal. Radiology, 121:361, 1976.

333. MANAGEMENT OF PATIENTS WITH SUSPECTED NERVE ROOT OR SPINAL CORD COMPRESSION

The specific management of intraspinal compression of nerve roots or cord depends on the suspected diagnosis, the severity of the symptoms, and the extent of the neurologic signs.

CONSERVATIVE MANAGEMENT AIMED AT REDUCING PAIN AND PREVENTING FUTURE RECURRENCES. Patients in this category have acute localized pain in the spinal or paraspinal region with or without peripheral radicular radiation; they do not have neurologic deficits indicative of spinal cord or severe root compression. The most likely diagnosis is an acute intervertebral disc protrusion, and with time complete recovery can usually be anticipated. This approach is particularly justified when there is no history of similar previous episodes and when the pain follows minor trauma, effort, or strain.

Patients may stay at home and should rest on a firm bed and make no physical effort. Analgesics and muscle relaxants are given for symptomatic relief. When pain subsides, exercises aimed at strengthening the muscular support of the spinal column may help prevent recurrences.

Plain x-rays of the involved segment of the spine help ascertain changes in the vertebral bodies or discs. Initially, however, these investigations can be deferred if the patient is in considerable pain.

CONSERVATIVE MANAGEMENT AIMED AT DECIDING IF THE COURSE OF INTRASPINAL ROOT COMPRESSION IS PROGRESSIVE. Acute pain may be accompanied by signs of moderate sensory or motor deficit in a root distribution. Such signs are represented by some loss of strength, paresthesia, and mild sensory impairment or a loss of muscle stretch reflexes. If these signs worsen or do not subside after a trial of conservative treatment, admission to hospital should be arranged to assure immobilization and rest and to arrange further investigations.

MANAGEMENT AIMED AT POSSIBLE SURGICAL DECOMPRESSION. This approach is indicated for patients showing signs of spinal cord compression. It is also advisable for patients with nerve root compression if there is intractable or severe recurrent pain or if there are signs of severe neurologic deficit, particularly marked weakness and muscle atrophy. These patients should be admitted to hospital for investigation. If there are no contraindications to surgery, myelography should be performed to establish a diagnosis and determine the site and extent of compression. If indicated, operative treatment should soon follow.

PROMPT INVESTIGATION AND SURGICAL DECOMPRESSION. This approach is required for patients who rapidly develop spinal cord or cauda equina compression. A particular emergency is represented by impaired bladder or rectal control. Patients should be immediately admitted to hospital to undergo only those investigations which enable a localization of the lesion. Such investigations usually include plain films of the spine and an emergency myelogram. In the course of these investigations, patients should be kept fasting to allow for immediate anesthesia if surgical intervention is decided upon.

334. SPECIFIC DISORDERS THAT CAUSE NERVE ROOT OR SPINAL CORD COMPRESSION

334.1. INTERVERTEBRAL DISC PROTRUSION

Each intervertebral disc consists of fibrocartilage and has a soft center, the nucleus pulposus, surrounded by thicker fibrous tissue, the anulus fibrosus. The nucleus pulposus constitutes most of the disc substance in the young, but with age it loses volume and resilience. When, during effort or trauma, the disc is suddenly compressed and the nucleus pulposus is caused to protrude through the anulus, fragments of disc may be extruded into the spinal canal. The herniated disc is usually directed toward the spinal canal because the anulus and longitudinal ligament are thinner posteriorly. Disc disease is more common in the cervical and lumbar spine, where there is greater mobility; in the thoracic spine, where movement is limited, disc herniations are rare.

The signs and symptoms of disc herniation result from compression of pain-sensitive structures within the spinal canal, including nerve roots or the spinal cord itself. Posterolateral disc herniations tend to involve individual nerve roots at the intervertebral foramina, whereas central protrusions may compress the spinal cord or cauda equina. Commonly the compressed root approximately corresponds to the level of the protruded disc, but this may not be the case in the lumbosacral region where several roots can be compressed by a single disc. Furthermore, extruded disc material may move several centimeters along the dural sac and compress roots situated below the site of disc rupture.

CLINICAL MANIFESTATIONS. Pain is the main symptom of an intervertebral disc protrusion. It is usually severe and accompanied by local reflex contraction of paraspinal muscles. Other symptoms and signs depend upon the localization of the protruded disc.

Herniated Cervical Discs. Cervical disc herniations occur most frequently at the fifth and sixth interspaces with fewer protrusions at C4 and C7 interspaces. Symptoms are often precipitated by sudden twisting, hyperextension, or hyperflexion of the neck. The pain may radiate to the shoulder and parascapular region and usually has a boring, aching quality. If nerve roots are compressed below the midcervical level, pain may extend into the upper extremity. Movements of the neck, but particularly hyperextension and tilting toward the affected side, are limited by pain. Symptoms caused by compression of the C6 and C7 roots are summarized in Table 1, Ch. 331. More rarely cervical disc protrusion results in cord compression. In such patients, long tract signs which develop below the level of the lesion are mainly due to involvement of the corticospinal tract.

Herniated Lumbar Discs. The most common disc protrusions are in the lower lumbar region and affect the L5 and S1 roots (Table 1). There is often a poorly localized low backache (lumbago), and pain may radiate into the buttocks, thigh, and lower leg (sciatica). The pain is generally severe and follows effort, such as lifting. In some patients, however, the pain may be spontaneous; occasionally sensory and motor deficits caused by disc herniation occur in the absence of pain. In most patients, the radiation of pain is unilateral; when there is a central disc protrusion, however, pain may occur in both lower extremities.

On examination patients show straightening of the normal lumbar curvature, and the pelvis may be tilted away from the side of the protrusion. Paraspinal muscles and vertebral spinous processes are tender to palpation. Straight leg raising (Lasègue's maneuver) on the side of compression is limited by pain. In addition, the pain can occur with raising of the opposite leg ("crossover pain"). There may be tenderness on palpation of the sciatic notch.

Compression of several of the roots of the cauda equina may give rise to pain, asymmetric bilateral sensory and motor changes, and even to loss of sphincter control. Occasionally, bladder control may be lost in the absence of other symptoms.

DIAGNOSIS. The symptoms of an intervertebral disc protrusion must be differentiated from those caused by arthritis of the spine and other bone and joint diseases. Neuropathies caused by entrapment, neuralgic amyotrophy, and diabetic neuropathy may enter the differential diagnosis because they may present with localized pain, and with sensory and motor deficits.

Plain x-rays of the spine reveal narrowing of disc spaces in less than half the patients. In the cervical spine, oblique views are necessary to establish whether there is a reduction in the size of intervertebral foramina. *Myelography should be performed only when the cause of compression is doubtful or when surgical treatment is contemplated.* Disc protrusions are evidenced by myelography as a filling defect at the level of the interspace. Obliteration of the root sleeve by a protruded disc may also be demonstrated by this procedure. The cerebrospinal fluid protein may be normal or increased; in the absence of complete block of cerebrospinal fluid circulation, protein values are usually below 60 mg per 100 ml.

TREATMENT. Patients presenting with acute pain should be treated with analgesics, muscle relaxants, rest, and immobility. A cervical collar or a lumbar brace may reduce mobility, and rest in bed on a hard mattress is often helpful. If improvement follows such measures, usually no investigations other than plain x-rays of the spine are necessary. If pain and other symptoms persist after a period of rest, hospitalization must be considered to ensure immobilization. Intractable pain, persistent disability, or development of progressive sensory or motor signs of radicular compression requires consideration of surgical treatment. Prompt operative treatment is mandatory when signs of progressive cord involvement or impairment of bladder or rectal sphincter control develop.

Recurrent symptoms after discoidectomy may be due to an incomplete removal of the disc, to disc herniation at an adjacent level, or to arachnoiditis. In addition the possibility that a herniated disc may have been associated with another type of intraspinal disease must be considered.

Fisher, R. G.: Protrusions of thoracic disc. The factor of herniation through the dura mater. J. Neurosurg., 22:591:1965.
Kessler, L. A., and Stein, W. Z.: Posterior migration of a herniated disc. Radiology, 76:104, 1961.
Love, J. G., and Schorn, V. G.: Thoracic disc protrusions. JAMA, 191:627, 1965.
Scott, P. J.: Bladder paralysis in cauda equina lesions from disc prolapse. J. Bone Joint Surg., 47B:224, 1965.
Spanos, N. C., and Andrew, J.: Intermittent claudication and lateral lumbar disc protrusions. J. Neurol. Neurosurg. Psychiatry, 29:273, 1966.
Spurling, R. G.: Lesions of the Lumbar Intervertebral Disc. Springfield, Ill., Charles C Thomas, 1953.
Spurling, R. G.: Lesions of the Cervical Invertebral Disc. Springfield, Ill., Charles C Thomas, 1956.

334.2. MYELOPATHY AND NERVE ROOT COMPRESSION DUE TO SPONDYLOSIS

Spondylosis refers to degenerative changes in the spine which may be neurologically asymptomatic or may cause symptoms by compression of nerve roots or spinal cord.

Spondylotic changes consist of intervertebral disc narrowing, osteophyte formation, and thickening of spinal ligaments. These changes most frequently involve the cervical or lumbar spine and are rare in the thoracic region. The term spondylosis is not generally used to describe acute protrusion of intervertebral discs, although the two conditions may be associated.

PATHOGENESIS. Spondylosis presumably results from the "wear and tear" of repeated spinal movement. Although more than one half of people older than 50 years of age have cervical spine osteophytes, associated neurologic symptoms and signs are much less frequent.

The single most important factor in the development of clinical manifestations caused by spondylosis is the size of the spinal canal. If the canal is congenitally narrow, the spinal cord may be compressed by relatively small osteophytes or ligamentous hypertrophy; on the other hand, a wide spinal canal may accommodate extensive spondylotic changes without causing appreciable neurologic signs of compression.

When the cervical spinal cord is compressed by osteophytes from the vertebral bodies or by thickening of the posterior longitudinal ligament and ligamentum flavum, symptoms and signs may follow trauma caused by neck movement or from impairment of spinal cord circulation. The cauda equina may also be injured in lumbar spondylosis. At both the cervical and lumbar levels, nerve roots are compressed by degenerative changes in bone and soft tissues adjacent to the intervertebral foramina.

CERVICAL SPONDYLOSIS

The most important symptoms and signs of cervical spondylosis are due to spinal cord (cervical myelopathy) and root (cervical radiculopathy) compression.

CERVICAL MYELOPATHY. Cervical myelopathy commonly develops insidiously, but symptoms may be precipitated by minor trauma. Sensory abnormalities are usually less striking than signs of disturbed motor function. Spastic paresis, clonus, and hyperreflexia in the legs as well as extensor plantar responses are the most common neurologic signs of this myelopathy.

In the upper limbs, there may be segmental muscle weakness and atrophy, as well as loss of muscle stretch reflexes, particularly if there is an associated radiculopathy. Vibration sense may be diminished in the lower limbs, but loss of joint position sense or pain and temperature sensation is uncommon. As a rule, bladder and bowel control are normal in patients with cervical myelopathy.

CERVICAL RADICULOPATHY. Cervical radiculopathy may occur in the absence of cervical myelopathy. Various radicular syndromes may develop, depending on the particular root affected. In the cervical spine the most common radiculopathies are those of the C6 and C7 root (Table 1, Ch. 331).

Pain and limitation of neck movements are common in cervical spondylosis, and some patients may present with occipital headaches.

DIAGNOSIS. X-rays of the cervical spine confirm the presence of cervical spondylosis. However, there is a high incidence of asymptomatic spondylotic changes, and careful clinical correlation is required for interpretation of such radiologic findings. To prove the diagnosis of cervical spondylotic myelopathy, the anteroposterior diameter of the cervical canal must be measured. If this measurement is less than 10 mm, there is almost certain cord compression. The extent of compression can best be determined by myelography which also shows soft tissue changes in spondylosis. Oblique x-ray views demonstrate narrowing of the intervertebral foramina.

PROGNOSIS AND TREATMENT. Because of wide variations in the natural course of cervical spondylotic myelopathy, it is difficult to assess the relative merits of conservative and surgical management. By and large, surgical treatment rarely is indicated for radiculopathy, but should be undertaken when clear evidence indicates progressive myelopathy. Most patients can usually be managed effectively with analgesics, muscle relaxants, and cervical immobilization.

LUMBAR SPONDYLOSIS AND SPINAL STENOSIS

In addition to compression of individual nerve roots by osteophytes encroaching upon intervertebral foramina, spondylosis of the lumbosacral spine may significantly reduce the size of the spinal canal. In such circumstances, spinal canal stenosis may cause injury to the cauda equina.

The pathogenesis of neurologic symptoms in patients with lumbar stenosis is similar to that in other bone diseases resulting in shallow lumbar canals, namely, congenital spinal stenosis, achondroplasia, and Paget's disease. In all these disorders, further narrowing by osteophytes, disc herniation, or ligamentous hypertrophy may give rise to compression of the cauda equina.

CLINICAL MANIFESTATIONS. The only symptom in patients with lumbar spinal stenosis may be backache after prolonged standing or effort. Signs of single or multiple root compression may develop gradually or have a sudden onset. These radicular symptoms are similar to those of intervertebral disc herniation and other causes of lumbosacral nerve root compression. Patients with lumbar spinal stenosis may suffer acute compression of the cauda equina after minor trauma or when subjected to prolonged hyperextension as during anesthesia for certain surgical procedures.

Intermittent Claudication of the Cauda Equina. Intermittent claudication of the cauda equina is a rare syndrome which may present in association with narrowing of the spinal canal. Typically, symptoms and signs are evoked or accentuated by walking and disappear soon after stopping. In other patients symptoms follow prolonged standing. In both varieties of intermittent claudication of the cauda equina, roots are compressed within a narrow spinal canal. The onset of symptoms has been explained by postulating that transient additional spinal narrowing is caused by the lordotic posture adopted during walking and standing. Patients usually present with pain in the low back and legs and may show weakness and sensory symptoms. During examination signs of motor and sensory deficit, as well as diminished reflexes, may be temporarily elicited by asking the patient to walk until symptoms reappear.

The absence of signs of vascular insufficiency in the iliofemoral and other arteries to the lower extremities helps differentiate claudication caused by compression from that which results from primary vascular disease.

DIAGNOSIS. The diagnosis of lumbar spinal stenosis requires radiologic demonstration of a narrow lumbar canal and myelographic confirmation of cauda equina compression.

TREATMENT. In advanced lumbar spinal stenosis, progressive signs of individual root or cauda equina compression can be relieved by surgical decompression.

Ehni, G., et al.: Significance of the small lumbar spinal canal: Cauda equina compression syndromes due to spondylosis: (Parts I to V). J. Neurosurg., 31:490, 1969.

Naylor, A.: Surgery in the treatment of cervical and thoracic disc protrusions. Br. Med. J., 1:821, 1977.

Stoltmann, H. F., and Blackwood, W.: The role of the ligamenta flava in the pathogenesis of myelopathy in cervical spondylosis. Brain, 87:45, 1964.

Turnbull, I. M. Microvasculature of the human spinal cord. J. Neurosurg., 35:141, 1971.

Waltz, T. A.: Physical factors in the myelopathy of cervical spondylosis. Brain, 90:395, 1967.

Wilkinson, M. (ed.): Cervical Spondylosis. Its Early Diagnosis and Treatment. Philadelphia, W. B. Saunders Company, 1971.

334.3. SPINAL CORD TUMORS

Depending upon their anatomic relation to the dura mater, tumors affecting the spinal cord may be classified as *extradural tumors*, which usually arise in the bone of the spinal column or within the extradural space; *intradural extramedullary tumors*, which lie between the dura mater and the spinal cord; and *intramedullary tumors*, which arise within the substance of the cord itself. The relative incidence in a general hospital population is approximately 50, 40, and 10 per cent, respectively.

EXTRADURAL TUMORS

Such tumors are usually manifested by symptoms and signs of spinal cord compression and are most often caused by extradural bone metastases. Common primary sources are carcinomas of the lung, breast, kidney, and prostate; less frequent sources are the gastrointestinal tract and thyroid gland. Spinal extradural compression may also occur in multiple myeloma, sarcomas, or lymphomas. Most metastases give rise to localized compression, but a few, particularly lymphomas and sarcomas, may extensively infiltrate the epidural space.

Pain resulting from bone destruction or root compression is the first symptom in the majority of patients with extradural tumors. It is usually dull, constant, and localized, is made worse by movements of the spine or pressure over the vertebral spinal processes, and is often exacerbated by bed rest. Radicular symptoms usually follow the local pain and are often bilateral. Pain alone is usually present for weeks or months before signs of spinal cord dysfunction develop; but once spinal cord signs appear, they usually progress rapidly over a few days or weeks to produce, if untreated, complete paralysis. More rarely, compression develops acutely, because of pathologic collapse of an infiltrated vertebral body or from hemorrhage within the metastasis. In either event, spastic weakness and loss of vibration and joint position sense below the level of the lesion are the first spinal cord signs to develop, whereas disturbances of bladder and/or bowel control generally occur late.

Radiologic changes are present on the plain x-ray films of most patients with malignant extradural metastases. Signs vary from osteoporosis to frank destruction of bone. When ordinary x-ray films of the spine are normal, evidence of bone involvement may be provided by radioisotope scanning. A definitive diagnosis of malignant extradural metastasis, however, can be made only by myelography, which must be carried out promptly if there is clinical suspicion of spinal cord compression, no matter what the plain radiograms reveal.

As a rule the cerebrospinal fluid protein is elevated, but there are no malignant cells. The CSF glucose is normal, in contrast to the decreased levels often seen in patients with carcinomatous invasion of the subarachnoid space.

Because metastatic tumors are a frequent cause of spinal cord compression in adults, this possibility should always be considered in patients with signs or symptoms of compression. In particular, the lungs and breasts should be carefully examined as sources of a possible primary malignancy. Anemia, bone pain, mediastinal enlargement, hepatomegaly, or splenomegaly all suggest metastatic disease or lymphomas. Bone x-rays, serum electrophoresis, testing for Bence Jones protein in the urine, and bone marrow examinations are all of help in diagnosing multiple myeloma.

Hormones, radiotherapy, and/or chemotherapy are used in the treatment of most of the extradural tumors involving the spine. The best results of medical therapy are usually obtained in patients with myeloma and lymphomas. Surgical decompression may be indicated when such therapy is ineffective, when there are signs of rapidly progressing compression of the cord, and when the etiologic diagnosis is unknown. Whatever form of treatment is chosen, it must be begun promptly and be vigorous, because if neurologic signs are mild, the chances of maintaining or improving neurologic function are better.

INTRADURAL EXTRAMEDULLARY TUMORS

The two most important tumors in this category are meningiomas and neurofibromas, which together account for almost two thirds of all primary intraspinal neoplasms. Less common tumors are teratomas, arachnoid cysts, some lipomas, and meningeal invasion by carcinoma.

Meningiomas show a high incidence among middle-aged women. They are usually single, relatively small, and located posterior or lateral to the spinal cord. Excluding those that occur in the region of the foramen magnum, approximately 90 per cent are found in the thoracic region. Signs of spinal cord compression develop insidiously so that an ataxic, spastic syndrome, which superficially resembles subacute combined degeneration of the spinal cord, may result. Moderate localized or segmental pain is presented in only 50 per cent of patients and is the central symptom in only 20 per cent. Tenderness on percussion of the vertebral spinous processes may be present. Tumors of the foramen magnum are particularly difficult to diagnose. Spastic ataxia and nystagmus can be early symptoms and may suggest multiple sclerosis rather than such a tumor. With foramen magnum tumor there may be pain or sensory loss in the C2 distribution, and the CSF protein is elevated.

X-ray may show bone erosion or calcification within a meningioma (4 per cent). Myelography is required for a precise localization of intraspinal meningiomas. In tumors of the foramen magnum a routine myelogram may be negative; therefore if such a tumor is suspected, myelography must be done in the supine as well as in the prone position to localize high, posteriorly placed tumors.

Neurofibromas arise from dorsal nerve roots, affect both sexes equally, occur at all ages, and may be present at any level of the spinal canal. Neurofibromas may extend extradurally but may also grow within the substance of the spinal cord. In some cases the tumors are part of a generalized neurofibromatosis. A small percentage of neurofibromas undergo sarcomatous changes and become invasive or metastasize.

Patients with intraspinal neurofibromas often give a history of longstanding radicular pain, and this symptom usually long precedes any sign of cord compression. When neurofibromas extend on either side of an intervertebral foramen, they may adopt a dumbbell or hourglass shape. X-rays, including oblique views of the spine, may show enlargement of a foramen and thinning of the adjacent pedicle. The degree of radiographic change may be out of proportion to the presenting symptoms. When the intraspinal portion of the tumor is small in comparison to the extraspinal, the latter may grow to such a large size that it is palpable externally even when there are few signs of cord compression.

As with meningiomas, the cerebrospinal fluid protein is almost always elevated. Myelography is essential for precise localization. A complete recovery usually follows the early surgical removal of both meningiomas and neurofibromas.

INTRAMEDULLARY TUMORS

Most of these tumors arise from constituent cells of the spinal cord. Ependymomas are the most common, followed by astrocytomas, glioblastomas, and oligodendrogliomas. In addition, vascular tumors (hemangioblastomas), lipomas, and even metastases may occur as intramedullary tumors.

Ependymomas arise at all levels of the spinal cord but have a preference for the caudal region. They represent more than two thirds of the tumors of the conus medullaris and are common causes of tumors of the filum terminale. Ependymomas may extend through several segments of the spinal cord; in rare instances the entire length of the cord is involved. Syringomyelia may develop in association with these and other intramedullary tumors. Spontaneous hemorrhages into ependymomas and hemangioblastomas occur and may give rise to sudden pain and neurologic deficit. Excluding glioblastomas and metastases, most intramedullary tumors have a slow progression. Dull, localized aching pain, muscle weakness or atrophy, impotence in males, and sphincter disturbances in both sexes are common early symptoms. Intramedullary tumors affecting the cervical or thoracic cord may cause sensory dissociation with predominant pain and temperature impairment. In such cases the sacral dermatomes are usually spared. In some patients, however, signs and symptoms may resemble Brown-Séquard's syndrome.

Longstanding intramedullary tumors may cause radiologically visible widening of the spinal canal and erosion of the pedicles. Contrast myelography usually demonstrates an enlarged spinal cord. In the lumbosacral region tumors may present as a pedunculated mass involving the cauda equina. Tumors of the filum terminale may be mobile and be a source of confusion for myelographic localization.

Successful surgical removal of intramedullary tumors is sometimes possible. Operative success is particularly high with ependymomas and hemangioblastomas, but recurrences may occur; gliomas respond poorly to any form of treatment, and lipomas are technically difficult to remove.

Davis, R. A., and Washburn, P. L.: Spinal cord meningiomas. Surg. Gynecol. Obstet., 131:15, 1970.
Harries, B.: Spinal cord compression. Br. Med. J., 1:611, 673, 1970.
Posner, J. B.: Neurological complications of systemic cancer. Med. Clin. North Am., 55:625, 1971.
Posner, J. B.: Management of central nervous system metastases. Semin. Oncol., 4:81, 1977.
Thomas, J. E., and Miller, R. E.: Lipomatous tumors of the spinal canal. Mayo Clin. Proc., 48:393, 1973.
White, W. A., Patterson, R. H., Jr., and Bergland, R. M.: Role of surgery in the treatment of spinal cord compression by metastatic neoplasm. Cancer, 27:558, 1971.

334.4. SPINAL ARACHNOIDITIS

Spinal arachnoiditis results from a low grade inflammation of the spinal meninges with formation of fibrous adhesions and loculation of cerebrospinal fluid. The changes extend throughout the length of the subarachnoid space or may be confined to a few segments. The adhesions may compress roots or the spinal cord itself.

Arachnoiditis may result from spinal surgery or spinal anesthesia and, more rarely, from myelography. It can be a late complication of subarachnoid hemorrhage, syphilis, tuberculosis, or other bacterial or parasitic spinal meningitides. In some cases no cause is found.

The development of symptoms and signs is insidious, the earliest symptoms usually reflecting multiple root involvement. This is particularly true if the adhesions extend into the lumbosacral spinal region, thereby involving the cauda equina. Pain is common and may be unrelated to movement; sensory symptoms usually exceed motor deficit. Signs of cord compression gradually develop and may progress to paraplegia; in other cases the disease process spontaneously arrests.

The diagnosis of spinal arachnoiditis depends upon the clinical course, as well as on examination of the cerebrospinal fluid and myelography. The CSF protein is elevated, and there may be pleocytosis. On myelography there are spotty, irregular collections of oil and an impairment of the flow of contrast material in the subarachnoid space.

When a specific infectious agent is identified, appropriate chemotherapy is indicated. Surgical exploration may provide histologic evidence as to the diagnosis, but laminectomy and removal of adhesions are not always beneficial for the relief of spinal and root compression.

Davidson, S.: Cryptococcal spinal arachnoiditis. J. Neurol. Neurosurg. Psychiatry, 31:76, 1968.
Guidetti, B., and LaTorre, E.: Hypertrophic spinal pachymeningitis. J. Neurosurg., 26:496, 1967.
Seaman, W. B., Marder, S. N., and Rosenbaum, H. E.: The myelographic appearance of adhesive spinal arachnoiditis. J. Neurosurg., 10:145, 1953.
Weiss, R. M., Sweeney, L., and Dreyfuss, M.: Circumscribed adhesive spinal arachnoiditis. J. Neurosurg., 19:435, 1962.
Wise, B. L., and Smith, M.: Spinal arachnoiditis ossificans. Arch. Neurol., 13:391, 1965.

334.5. ARTERIOVENOUS MALFORMATIONS AND OTHER VASCULAR LESIONS OF THE SPINAL CORD

Vascular malformations may be present on the surface of the spinal cord or within its substance. They may thus give rise to subarachnoid hemorrhage, intramedullary hemorrhage (hematomyelia), or both. Rarely, a spinal epidural hematoma results from such bleeding. The sudden development of partial or complete transverse myelopathy is the most common form of onset. This is manifested by paralysis, sensory impairment, and loss of sphincter control. If there is bleeding into the subarachnoid space, pain in the neck and back and other signs of meningeal irritation occur. Sudden headache, neck stiffness, and blood in the cerebrospinal fluid may be mistakenly attributed to hemorrhage of intracranial rather than intraspinal origin.

Arteriovenous malformations may also compress the spinal cord or give rise to hemodynamic changes that result in spinal ischemia. Distortion and compression of the cord by enlarged, abnormal vessels occur only gradually, and patients present with slowly progressive symptoms of spinal cord dysfunction. Transient exacerbation of symptoms may occur in association with menstrual periods or pregnancy.

Complete or partial recovery of function can follow episodes of spinal cord ischemia or even small hemorrhages. The unchanging localization of the attacks and the prominence of pain help to differentiate those symptoms caused by arteriovenous malformations from other recurrent neurologic disorders such as multiple sclerosis. In some patients a spinal bruit may be heard by auscultation over the site of the malformation.

Cavernous angiomas of the spinal cord are vascular hamartomas which may be associated with cysts and tumors in the organs or with hemangioblastomas of the cerebellum. Retinal vascular changes (von Hippel–Lindau syndrome) and cutaneous vascular nevi may be associated with spinal vascular malformations. The presence of these associated signs lends support to the assumption that, in a patient who presents them, spinal symptoms may be due to a vascular malformation.

Intraspinal bleeding caused by vascular malformation must be differentiated from bleeding that occurs as a complication of hemorrhagic diathesis, anticoagulant therapy, or collagen disease such as polyarteritis nodosa. In these conditions, however, there are usually signs of a more general disorder, cutaneous hematomas or other skin lesions, hematuria, or abnormal laboratory investigations.

In most patients with vascular malformations presenting with acute symptoms, examination of the cerebrospinal fluid reveals bloody or xanthochromic fluid, but, when there has been no recent bleeding, the only finding may be an elevated protein. Plain x-rays of the spine may show erosion, coexistent vertebral hemangiomas, or calcification within the spinal canal. On myelography, serpentine streaks within the column of oil

may reveal the site of the vascular malformation. Angiography with regional catheterization of radicular vessels is a necessary preliminary to surgical treatment. Advances in microsurgery have increased considerably the chances for a satisfactory removal of spinal vascular malformations.

Antoni, N.: Spinal vascular malformations (angiomas) and myelomalacia, Neurology, 12:795, 1962.

Fine, R. D.: Angioma racemosum venosum of spinal cord with segmentally related angiomatous lesions of skin and forearm. J. Neurosurg., 18:546, 1961.

Henson, R. A., and Parsons, M.: Ischaemic lesions of the spinal cord: An illustrated review. Quart. J. Med., 36:205, 1967.

Houdart, R., Djindjian, R., Hurth, M., and Rey, A.: Treatment of angiomas of the spinal cord. Surg. Neurol., 2:186, 1974.

Matthews, W. B.: The spinal bruit. Lancet, 2:1117, 1959.

Taylor, J. R., and Van Allen M. W.: Vascular malformation of the cord with transient ischaemic attacks. J. Neurosurg., 31:576, 1969.

334.6. SPINAL EPIDURAL HEMATOMA

Bleeding into the spinal epidural space may occur spontaneously but is more commonly associated with trauma, bleeding diathesis, or vascular malformations. It is a particular risk in patients receiving anticoagulants. The hemorrhage usually originates in the epidural venous plexus, and the hematomas tend to collect over the dorsum of the thoracic dura mater. Epidural hematomas vary in size, but the larger ones cause spinal cord compression. The clinical picture is characterized by the sudden onset of severe, localized back pain. Cord compression, when it occurs, results in the rapid development of flaccid paralysis, sensory loss, and impaired bladder and bowel control. The sudden onset of signs of cord compression in a patient on anticoagulants should allow few doubts as to the likelihood of a spinal epidural hematoma.

In epidural hematomas the cerebrospinal fluid may be clear or very slightly hemorrhagic.

Emergency surgical evacuation of the hematoma is essential. Although myelography is of great help in diagnosis and localization of epidural hematomas, this and other investigations should not take the place of prompt surgical intervention in order to avoid irreversible spinal cord damage.

Bidzinski, J.: Spontaneous spinal epidural hematoma during pregnancy. Case report. J. Neurosurg., 24:1017, 1966.

Jacobson, I., McCabe, J. J., Harris, P., and Dott, N. M.: Spontaneous spinal epidural hemorrhage during anticoagulant therapy. Br. Med. J., 1:522, 1966.

Markham, J. W., Lynge, H. N., and Stahlman, G. E. B.: The syndrome of spontaneous spinal epidural hematoma. Report of three cases. J. Neurosurg., 26:334, 1967.

Section Twenty-Three DISEASES OF THE PERIPHERAL NERVOUS SYSTEM

Peter James Dyck

335. DEFINITION OF PERIPHERAL NEUROPATHY

The term peripheral neuropathy includes any primary disorder of peripheral motor, sensory, and autonomic neurons. The clinical hallmarks are muscle weakness, with or without atrophy, sensory change, autonomic manifestations, or admixtures of these, from disease of peripheral neurons. The various clinical involvement patterns are of help in differential diagnosis and will be discussed in subsequent chapters.

The precise cause for many neuropathies is unknown, and the diagnosis of many neuropathies depends on their association with other diseases such as diabetes mellitus, carcinoma, or uremia.

Pathologic classifications are based on the nature of the fiber degeneration (wallerian, axonal degeneration, segmental demyelination) or the site of the pathologic changes, as well as on the specific histologic pattern (vasculitis, granulomatous reaction, hypertrophic repair, amyloidosis, and specific infective organism).

336. MONONEUROPATHIES AND PLEXUS NEUROPATHIES

336.1. CRANIAL NERVES

OLFACTORY NERVE. Anosmia is often the result of local disease of the nose, skull fracture, or brain tumor and may be reported by the patient as altered taste. Brief occurrences of stereotyped bad odors (or taste) not experienced by associates are from uncinate seizures — a condition not due to disease of the olfactory nerve but due to disease of the temporal lobe.

OPTIC NERVE. Altered vision is a symptom which may be due to refractive error, extra- and intraocular disease, developing diplopia or ptosis, optic nerve, optic tract, and optic radiation disease, and altered states of consciousness. Because of its serious implications and because treatment is available for many of its causes, this symptom should be investigated promptly by the appropriate medical specialist.

Disease of the optic nerve presents with loss of vision and a visual field defect. Temporary loss of visual activity followed by a pulsatile or sick headache is typical of migraine but may occasionally indicate cerebrovascular disease. Unilateral loss of vision accompanied by a central scotoma and an elevated optic disc is typical of papillitis. The appearance of the disc through the ophthalmoscope in papilledema may be no different from that of papillitis. Vision is not impaired in papilledema unless it is of long duration. In retrobulbar neuritis which not infrequently develops as a harbinger of more widespread multiple sclerosis, the patient has loss of vision (from a central scotoma) but no accompanying ophthalmoscopic abnormality. Intrinsic lesions of the optic nerve tend to produce scotomas, whereas untreated compressive lesions tend to produce monocular and binasal or bitemporal visual field defects. Such lesions include meningiomas, craniopharyngiomas, cholesteatomas, and chromophilic adenomas. Homonymous visual defects are usually the result of lesions of the optic pathways posterior to the chiasm from intrinsic brain disease.

OCULOMOTOR, TROCHLEAR, AND ABDUCENS. The motor nerves to the eyes may be damaged by a variety of diseases located anywhere in their long course from brainstem to orbit. In order of frequency the broad categories causing neurogenic extraocular palsies and pupillary disturbances are vascular disease (especially brainstem ischemia, hemorrhage and infarction, and aneurysm), neoplasm (both primary and secondary tumors), trauma, infections and postinfectious states, and congenital causes. The latter two causes are particularly common in the pediatric age group, whereas the vascular cause is especially common in old age, in hypertension, and in diabetes. The predominant symptom of dysfunction of these nerves is diplopia. Persons with a congenital palsy and those with disturbances of consciousness (especially in diseases affecting midbrain and pons) may be unaware of diplopia. Fluctuating diplopia, especially if improved with rest, suggests the diagnosis of myasthenia gravis.

The differential diagnosis of patients with an extraocular palsy and/or of a pupillary disturbance may not be easy. Congenital and traumatic causes are usually readily identified. In the former the deficit has been present since birth and is usually without symptoms. Trivial trauma does not as a rule produce extraocular palsy, and the maximal deficit is related in time to the trauma with usually slow improvement thereafter. An important cause of bilateral sixth cranial nerve palsy is increased intracranial pressure. Third cranial nerve palsy with pupillary enlargement and lid ptosis accompanying an ipsilateral cerebral hemisphere tumor is a sign of impending uncal herniation through the tentorium. Pontine gliomas, pituitary tumors, and nasopharyngeal and other tumors may directly displace the brainstem and cause damage of these cranial nerves. Episodic diplopia and pupillary disturbances may occur in transient cerebral ischemia (basilar artery), infrequently in migraine, and in berry aneurysm. Infectious and postinfectious states cause many of the transitory ocular palsies that affect children and young people. Extraocular palsies are especially common in chronic meningitis such as from tuberculosis, sarcoid, and cancer. They also may accompany presumptive viral meningitis and occur after trivial infections and exanthems. Short-lived extraocular palsy is not uncommon in acute inflammatory polyradiculoneuropathies. Third nerve palsy with sparing of pupillomotor function is associated with diabetes mellitus.

Abnormalities of pupillary size, shape, and reaction are not confined to third nerve injuries. The Argyll Robertson pupil is small, irregular, and usually bilateral, constricts to convergence accommodation but not to light, and responds poorly to mydriatics; it is common with neurosyphilis and rare with diabetes. The pupils of diabetics are often unequal, however, and may be nonreactive to light. Adie's myotonic pupil may cause confusion. It reacts only slowly to light or accommodation-convergence, but constricts to fresh 2.5 per cent methylcholine instilled into the conjunctival sac; a normal pupil lacks the latter reaction.

Bilateral external ophthalmoplegia of rapid or sudden onset occurs with four diseases, all of which are potentially serious and demand prompt treatment: acute myasthenia gravis, acute thiamin deficiency with Wernicke's encephalopathy, botulism, and acute inflammatory cranial polyneuropathy.

TRIGEMINAL. Generally speaking, disturbances of sensation of the face and anterior scalp are more likely to be due to brainstem lesions than to involvement of the gasserian ganglion, its roots, or its divisions. When they do occur, peripheral lesions are caused by tumor, infection, collagen disease, immunologic states, and intoxications. Herpes zoster and herpes simplex infections are discussed in Ch. 304 and 305. Painful states in the distribution of the trigeminal nerve include herpes zoster, trigeminal neuralgia (discussed in Ch. 260), and atypical face pain. Disturbed sensation in the face may accompany scleroderma. A hyperalgesic trigeminal neuropathy may be caused by stilbamidine and trichloroethylene.

FACIAL. Brain injury above the facial nucleus usually spares the innervation of the brow and forehead muscles because they are bilaterally represented at higher nervous levels; injury to the facial nerve at or peripheral to its nucleus paralyzes all the ipsilateral facial muscles. An intrapontine lesion causing facial weakness usually also affects abducens nerve function. As the facial nerve leaves the pons and enters the internal auditory meatus along with the acoustic nerve, it also carries fibers for lacrimation, salivation, and taste. As the nerve descends through the petrous bone, fibers to the lacrimal glands branch off first, and then salivary and taste fibers depart in the chorda tympani and cross the middle ear. Only motor fibers to the face emerge from the stylomastoid foramen. Thus the syndrome of seventh nerve damage varies according to the site of the injury. Acoustic neurinomas and other tumors of the cerebellopontine angle often involve the facial nerves, as do infections and neoplasms of the meninges.

Bell's palsy is a peripheral facial weakness of unknown cause and rapid onset, occasionally attended by aching pain about the angle of the jaw or behind the ear. Recent work has shown that the point of nerve conduction block is usually in the vicinity of the internal auditory meatus. Retraction of the angle of the mouth and eye closure are impaired, and the forehead is smooth on the affected side. Taste perception on the anterior part of the involved half of the tongue may be distorted. Rarely, hyperacusis results from paralysis of the stapedius muscle. Recovery usually begins within a week, and three of four patients fully recover over a period of several weeks. Occasionally, some permanent deficit remains after a protracted course. In such patients, asynchronous facial spasms may accompany voluntary facial movement. The use of adrenal corticosteroids begun near the onset of the illness and continued for seven to ten days is thought to speed recovery.

Herpes zoster affecting the geniculate ganglion produces a severe facial paralysis that is associated with a painful eruption within the external ear canal. This affection, often referred to as the Ramsay Hunt syndrome, may also involve the auditory nerve.

Chronic facial hemispasm affects middle-aged or older women somewhat more commonly than men, with spontaneous, unilateral, frequent, sudden, strong, brief contractions of part or all of the facial musculature. The condition usually begins in the orbicularis oculi muscle and, over many years, spreads to involve more of the face. In a few instances the disorder follows Bell's palsy. More often the cause is not known, but a slowly progressive, degenerative condition of the facial nucleus in the pons has been postulated, as has compression of the facial nerve by adjacent structures in the posterior fossa. Relief can be obtained by alcohol injection or section of the facial nerve, but it must be weighed against the facial paralysis necessarily produced. Relief has also been reported following intracranial surgical freeing of the facial nerve from adjacent structures.

Facial myokymia describes a condition of constant wormlike contractions of facial muscles. Such undulating, writhing, continuous movement is quite different from fasciculations, which are brief, synchronized contractions of muscle fibers. Myokymia is caused by intrapontine lesions such as tumors and multiple sclerosis.

AUDITORY. Disturbances of eighth nerve function are discussed in Ch. 262 and 263.

GLOSSOPHARYNGEAL. Glossopharyngeal neuralgia is described in Ch. 260.

HYPOGLOSSAL. This motor nerve to the tongue is uncommonly involved in its peripheral course, usually by neoplasms. Atrophy and fasciculation of the ipsilateral half of the tongue are seen, and the tongue deviates toward the affected side upon protrusion.

336.2. MONONEUROPATHY

PHYSICAL INJURY

Spinal nerves, plexuses, and peripheral nerve trunks may be injured by traction, compression, contusion, and laceration. Nerves may be damaged by electricity and radiation. Fractured bones may lacerate or compress nerves. Excessively tight casts or tourniquets may damage nerves by direct compression or by ischemia. Injection of penicillin or other medications into the sciatic nerve can cause serious injury, particularly if the vehicle for the medications is oil.

Recovery of nerve function is usually complete following acute compressive lesions and incomplete, faulty, or lacking in transected nerves. Recovery after contusion or section is greater in the young than in the old and in good than in poor fascicular apposition.

COMPRESSION AND ENTRAPMENT

The peripheral nerve trunks of the limbs are particularly prone to compression and entrapment, although any nerve passing over a rigid promontory or through a bony canal or tight fascial plane is vulnerable. The degree of compressive damage to nerves depends on the magnitude and duration of the force, on whether the force is repeated, on whether the nerve is anatomically situated next to soft or hard structures, on the physical habitus of the person, and on disease susceptibility. Malnutrition, diabetes mellitus, renal disease, and inflammatory neuropathy all are thought to predispose to compression damage. The tendency to compression damage is inherited in some families. For many years, investigators have differed as to whether ischemia or mechanical compression was the factor that produced nerve damage from compression. At an earlier time, the evidence favored ischemia; now it favors mechanical compression. Contusion and hemorrhage and later scarring may complicate some of the compressive lesions in man.

The term *entrapment* is given to the process by which nerves are damaged by repeated compression as they pass over a rigid structure or through a tight bony or fascial canal. Such injury occurs more readily when swelling, inflammation, or degeneration develops in adjacent joints and tendons (as may happen in pregnancy, rheumatoid arthritis, myxedema, and acromegaly). Suggestive evidence that multiple minor episodes of bruising of the nerve may contribute to the development of signs of entrapment comes from the common experience that excessive use of the wrist, in knitting or in gardening in the patient with the carpal tunnel syndrome, or in prolonged walking in patients with Morton's neuroma, will worsen symptoms. Sites of compression for the median nerve include the pronator teres muscle and the carpal tunnel ligament; for the ulnar nerve, the elbow wrist, pisohamate tunnel, palm, and metacarpal heads; for the radial nerve, the axilla, posterior aspect of the humerus, the supinator muscle, and radial aspect of distal forearm; for the lateral femoral cutaneous nerve, the pelvic brim; for the femoral nerve, the groin; for the saphenous nerve, the medial side of the knee; for the obturator nerve, the obturator canal; for the common peroneal nerve, the lateral aspect of the knee; for the superficial and deep peroneal nerves, muscle and fascial sheaths near their origin; for the posterior tibial nerve, the tarsal tunnel; and for plantar nerves, the sole of the feet.

The three most common entrapment neuropathies are the carpal tunnel syndrome, tardy ulnar palsy, and tardy peroneal nerve palsy.

CARPAL TUNNEL SYNDROME. In the carpal tunnel syndrome the median nerve is compressed as it passes through the canal made by the carpal bones and ligament. Some cases are idiopathic, and, in these, surgeons report a flattening of the median nerve just distal to the crease of the wrist and either thickening of the ligament or, more commonly, noninflammatory thickening of the synovia of the flexor tendons. The median nerve may be compressed within the carpal tunnel by a ganglion or by degenerative joint and synovial changes from rheumatoid arthritis, myxedema, and acromegaly.

This common disorder especially affects women. Pricking numbness and pain in the fingers and hands, coming on especially during the night and relieved by changing the position of the hands (shaking them), are characteristic. It is uncommon for patients to localize the numbness to the exact cutaneous distribution of the median nerve. Furthermore, the aching discomfort that may accompany the numbness may extend up the arm. Atrophy of the muscles innervated by the median nerve (for example, the thenar muscles) is not an early sign. In many cases it is possible to reproduce the painful numbness by holding the wrist in extreme flexion (Phalen's sign). Also, a burst of tingling may occur when the skin over the nerve at the wrist is percussed (Tinel's sign). There may be sensory loss in the distribution of the median nerve, although more frequently none is detected.

Measurement of Nerve Conduction. This provides an important confirmatory test and consists in determining the time from stimulation of the median nerve at a point above the carpal ligament to the appearance of the thenar muscle action potential. Similarly, one can determine the time from stimulation of digital fibers to the obtaining of an action potential in electrodes overlying the median nerve above the carpal ligament. In the carpal tunnel syndrome, the latency of both responses is usually prolonged.

Since the carpal tunnel syndrome may be brought on by an excess of gardening, ironing, sewing, crocheting, or similar activity, relief may follow the discontinuation of these activities. Immobilization of the wrist during the hours of sleep with a posterior splint of forearm and hand may give relief. Injections of corticosteroid preparations beneath the carpal ligament sometimes help. Treatment for an associated disease (myxedema, rheumatoid arthritis, acromegaly) may effect an improvement. However, in most instances the treatment of choice is surgical section of the carpal ligament, which usually provides almost immediate relief.

TARDY ULNAR NERVE PALSY. The ulnar nerve may be injured at the elbow, especially in persons with a shallow ulnar groove, those who rest their weight on their elbows excessively, and those who are cachectic and lie in bed.

Contrary to the findings in the carpal tunnel syndrome, muscle weakness and atrophy characteristically predominate over sensory symptoms and signs, possibly because the ulnar nerve at the elbow has relatively fewer sensory fibers than the median nerve at the wrist. Characteristically, the patient notices atrophy of the first dorsal interosseous muscle or difficulty in performing fine manipulations. There may be numbness of the small finger and contiguous half of the proximal and middle phalanges of the ring finger and ulnar border of the hand. Treatment consists of prevention of further injury. A doughnut cushion for the elbow may be helpful. Mobilizing and transplanting the nerve to a position in front of the medial epicondyle may prevent further progression of the disorder.

ACUTE RADIAL NERVE PALSY. The radial nerve may be compressed against a hard edge or surface in persons insensitized by an excess of alcohol or sedatives (Saturday night palsy) or may be compressed for excessive periods by the weight of a bed partner's head (bridegroom's palsy). Time usually provides complete recovery.

ACUTE AND TARDY PERONEAL NERVE PALSY. The common peroneal nerve is vulnerable where it crosses the head of the fibula, and can be injured when a person falls asleep in the sitting position with the knees crossed. A more chronic form occurs in cachectic patients who lie for prolonged periods with the legs externally rotated. In this disorder, dorsiflexion of the foot at the ankle and extension of the toes are weak, but usually little or no sensory loss is found over the lateral surface of the leg and on the dorsum of the foot.

TARSAL TUNNEL SYNDROME. Fractures of the ankle may compress the posterior tibial nerve, resulting in pain and numbness of the sole of the foot.

MERALGIA PARESTHETICA. Fat people wearing tight corsets, people wearing gun belts, and people with pendulous abdomens may develop superficial paresthesia and burning discomfort in the distribution of the lateral cutaneous nerve of the thigh. Presumably the trouble results from compression of this nerve as it passes beneath the inguinal ligament, but the condition sometimes arises without evident cause.

THORACIC OUTLET SYNDROME. Formerly, paresthesias of the fingers were frequently attributed to compression of the brachial plexus by a cervical rib or a tight scalene anterior muscle. Most such patients, however, prove to have either nerve root compression from a cervical disc or carpal tunnel syndrome.

336.3. MULTIPLE MONONEUROPATHY

Multiple mononeuropathy replaces the old term mononeuropathy multiplex. The term implies dysfunction that develops in the distribution of several individual nerve trunks at different times. At one time it was thought erroneously that this clinical pattern arose predominantly in association with vasculitis. It is now realized that the pattern may occur in leprosy (see Ch. 170), in necrotizing angiopathy, in inflammatory-immunologic disorders, in some metabolic diseases (some cases of uremia and diabetes mellitus), in familial disposition to pressure palsies, and in rare conditions involving blood and foreign body emboli to nerves and with iatrogenic nerve lesions.

A *necrotizing angiopathy* affects small arteries and arterioles within the epineurium of nerve trunks in periarteritis nodosa (see Ch. 53), in rheumatoid arthritis (see Ch. 56), and in other vasculitides. Such patients often have evidence of a multisystem disease affecting joints, skin, skeletal muscles, kidney, and other parenchymatous organs as well as evidence of a systemic illness with fever, cachexia, weight loss, and elevation of the sedimentation rate, and laboratory evidence suggesting a collagen-vascular involvement. Characteristically, the disorder begins with pain, paresthesias, or weakness in the distribution of a peripheral nerve which progresses to a maximal deficit within a few hours to several days. Other nerves become affected within days. The nerves of the lower extremities are affected more often than those of the upper, and neurologic signs are usually asymmetrical. After the initial involvement the disorder may improve,

relapse, or deteriorate. This type of neuropathy is a common manifestation of polyarteritis nodosa; it occurs less commonly with rheumatoid arthritis, Wegener's granulomatosis, Sjögren's syndrome, and Churg-Strauss syndrome.

The pathologic changes in most instances of necrotizing angiopathy affect the epineurial arteries of nerves. These may show degeneration of the media, fragmentation of the internal elastic lamina, thickening of the intima, and infiltration of the media and adventitia by mononuclear and polymorphonuclear cells (especially eosinophils). At necropsy segments of arterioles with occluded lumens may be widespread along the length of the nerve. Regions of nerve fiber degeneration do not coincide with these occluded vessels, but begin in isolated central regions of fascicles at watershed levels of poor blood perfusion. For the ulnar and median nerves this level is thought to be at mid-upper arm; for the peroneal and tibial nerves it is at midthigh. Because of separation and recombination of fascicles along the length of nerve, degenerating fibers arising from the focal areas of damage may be more randomly mixed with intact fibers in distal nerve.

336.4. PLEXUS NEUROPATHIES

BRACHIAL PLEXUS INJURY AND NEUROPATHY

The brachial plexus can be injured by traction, penetrating wounds, or compression. *Acute nontraumatic brachial plexus neuropathy* is a disorder of unknown cause. Antecedent needle injections into shoulder muscles, intercurrent infections, and an allergic basis have been suggested as possible etiologic factors. Factors causing it are also discussed in Ch. 337.3. Typically this disorder begins with aching pain in the lateral aspect of the shoulder or, less often, in the region of the elbow or arm. Muscle weakness develops within a few hours or days, and atrophy follows; sensory loss is usually minimal and is restricted to a small patch in the cutaneous distribution of the axillary nerve. The upper brachial plexus is affected more commonly than the lower, and therefore the weakness and atrophy are more often located in the region of the shoulder. In mild cases, improvement begins in a few weeks, and clinical recovery is complete within months. More characteristically, improvement does not begin for several months and may not be complete for years. Nevertheless, eventual complete or almost complete recovery is likely. Rarely, as one side improves, the other brachial plexus becomes affected. Careful examination by electromyography may reveal more extensive involvement of nerves than expected from the clinical examination. The cerebrospinal fluid is usually normal. There is no known treatment.

LUMBAR AND SACRAL PLEXUS AND ROOTS

Under the term *femoral neuropathy* (also called diabetic amyotrophy), a disorder has been described which in many cases involves lumbar roots and plexus. Many such cases occur in association with diabetes as described in Ch. 337.8, but sometimes no associated illness is found. Pain centered in the thigh and extending to the medial side of the leg may herald the onset of muscle weakness and atrophy, which usually develops rapidly over the next week. If the onset is abrupt and the neurologic signs are restricted to the distribution of the femoral nerve, an infarction of that nerve is a possibility. Careful examination and electromyography, however, often indicate that branches of multiple lumbar and sacral roots are affected with or without involvement of lumbar and sacral plexuses (in reality a lumbosacral radiculoplexus neuropathy). The cerebrospinal fluid protein may be elevated. Recovery may require months or years.

Occasionally, patients with lumbosacral plexus neuropathy present with the symptoms of sciatica, which differs from that caused by disc disease in the lack of a history of injury, the lack (usually) of marked back symptoms, and the clinical and electromyographic evidence of involvement of multiple roots and a negative myelogram. Although marked muscle weakness and wasting may occur, the outlook is usually favorable. The cause, pathology, and treatment are unknown.

337. POLYNEUROPATHY

337.1. DIFFERENTIAL DIAGNOSIS OF PERIPHERAL NEUROPATHY

SYMPTOMATOLOGY. Muscle weakness and atrophy are common in neuropathy. The first thing to decide is whether the weakness is myelopathic, neuropathic, neuromuscular, or myopathic. Spasticity, hyperreflexia, the Babinski sign, and a sensory level indicate a myelopathy. Muscle weakness associated with sensory symptoms, a reduction of tendon reflexes of a greater degree than accounted for by muscle atrophy, fasciculations, and a distal distribution of involvement favors neuropathy. In the absence of sensory changes, reliable differentiation of neuropathic from myopathic and from neuromuscular weakness depends heavily on the characteristics of nerve conduction and electromyographic examination. Reduction or absence of sensory nerve fiber action potentials, low nerve conduction of motor fibers, and the finding of fibrillation potentials with or without an increase in the size of motor unit potential favor a neuropathy. In myopathy motor unit potentials are small in amplitude and often polyphasic. Abnormalities of neuromuscular transmission in myasthenia gravis are recognized by a fall in amplitude of the muscle action potential when 3 per second supramaximal stimuli are given to the nerve. The abnormalities of neuromuscular transmission are different between the myasthenic syndrome, botulism, and drug-induced defects of neuromuscular transmission.

If it has been decided that the muscle weakness is neurogenic, one needs to know whether it is focal or diffuse and from what level along the length of the peripheral nerve it arises — roots, plexus, or nerve trunks. Proximal limb and axial involvement suggests proximal nerve involvement, raised cerebrospinal fluid protein suggests leptomeningeal (or root) involvement, and paraspinal denervation confirms this locus.

Sensory symptoms are typical of neuropathy and include two kinds. The first type occurs spontaneously and consists of symptoms of an "asleep feeling," "tightness," "coolness," "burning," "tingling," "aching," "tenderness," or other so-called "positive symptoms." These may be particularly bothersome during inactivity, as at night when they are characteristic of the "restless leg syndrome." In other patients "positive symptoms" of the feet are accentuated by walking and of the hands by their use in work or play. The second type of sensory symptom expresses the functional deficit from abnormal sensation, the so-called "negative symptoms." Unsteadiness, clumsiness, inability to recognize objects by feel, and mutilation without pain are examples of this group of symptoms.

Autonomic abnormalities are characteristic of some neuropathies. Postural hypotension is the most striking and usually implies involvement of the greater splanchnic nerves to the viscera. Impotence, incontinence of bladder and bowel, and anhidrosis are other important autonomic symptoms.

Peripheral neuropathy does not always present with the characteristic triad of distal limb muscle weakness and atrophy, absent tendon reflexes, and sensation loss. To illustrate, early in the course of neuropathy, loss of muscle stretch reflexes or reliable evidence of sensation loss may not be present. Several patterns of neuropathic symptomatology are useful in differential diagnosis.

PATTERNS OF NEUROPATHIC SYMPTOMS

HIGH ARCHES; CURLED UP TOES; AND PAINFUL CORNS AND CALLUSES. The recognition that a patient has a pes cavus foot deformity or other skeletal abnormality suggests an inherited neuromuscular disorder. If lower motor neurons are predominantly affected, such patients have a progressive muscular atrophy (hereditary motor neuropathy); if primary sensory neurons are predominantly affected, probably a hereditary sensory neuropathy; and if both lower motor and primary sensory neurons are affected, a hereditary motor and sensory neuropathy. Pes cavus is also common (probably because of the associated involvement of lower motor neurons) in spastic paraplegia and in spinocerebellar degenerations such as Friedreich's ataxia. Rarely, high arches are observed in longstanding myopathy.

CLAW HAND. This is the counterpart in the hand of pes cavus in the foot. Unlike pes cavus, however, which is usually due to neuromuscular disorders which begin in infancy or childhood, claw hand may come on at any age. If it occurs asymmetrically and without sensory abnormality, it may signal the onset of motor neuron disease or an unusual lower brachial plexus neuropathy. An associated sensory loss suggests the diagnosis of tardy ulnar palsy, cervical spondylosis, syringomyelia, intramedullary cervical tumor, or adult onset Tangier disease.

MUSCLE WEAKNESS OF LOWER LIMBS WITHOUT SENSORY SYMPTOMS. The absence of sensory signs is the important characteristic to look for. To confirm the lack of sensory involvement, recording of the latency and amplitude of afferent potentials over median, ulnar, and sural nerves should be obtained. Muscle weakness of lower limb muscles results in difficulties described as "unsteadiness," "stumbling," and "awkwardness in walking." Patients with bilateral foot drop tend to trip or stumble, and to walk with a steppage gait. Patients with weakness of plantar and dorsiflexion are unable to "stand still without holding onto something," or they may need to "brace their knees" against the cabinet of the sink when washing the face or shaving. Patients with quadriceps weakness may experience "collapsing" or "buckling" of the lower limb, to the point of falling down. They may not be able to arise from a seated position without the use of the hands or to climb stairs without a rail. A waddling gait reflects gluteal weakness.

The aforementioned symptoms suggest the possibility of a myopathy, a disorder of motoneurons, or, less often, a disorder of neuromuscular transmission. Reliable methods to distinguish myopathy and defects of neuromuscular transmission from neurogenic involvement are provided by the specialized techniques of electromyographic laboratories. Among neurogenic causes of weakness, poliomyelitis and motor neuron disease have mainly an asymmetrical distribution, whereas inflammatory polyradiculoneuropathy, porphyria, and hereditary motor neuropathy are mostly symmetrical.

BILATERAL DISTAL WEAKNESS OF THE HANDS, AND PROXIMAL WEAKNESS OF THE UPPER LIMBS WITHOUT SENSORY SYMPTOMS OR SIGNS. The list of conditions to be considered resembles that of the preceding category. Hyperreflexia, the Babinski sign, and long-tract sensory signs in the lower limb suggest possible cervical cord disease.

MUSCLE WEAKNESS OF LOWER LIMBS WITHOUT "POSITIVE" SENSORY SYMPTOMS BUT WITH SENSORY SIGNS. With a few exceptions, the lack of "positive" sensory symptoms in the presence of a testable abnormality of cutaneous sensation implies longstanding disease to which the patient has accommodated. The differential diagnosis includes inherited motor and sensory neuropathy, acute and chronic inflammatory polyradiculoneuropathy, and other rare conditions.

MUSCLE WEAKNESS OF LOWER LIMBS WITHOUT "POSITIVE" SENSORY SYMPTOMS. Sensory symptoms may be roughly divided into those found in patients with acute and subacute degeneration of large fibers, those associated with degeneration of small fibers, and those with mixtures of both.

Selective degeneration of large fibers of limb nerves results in abnormalities of touch-pressure, of vibration, and of joint position and motion sensations. Patients may describe their toes or feet as "asleep" or feeling as if a local anesthetic has been injected. The term pseudotabes has been applied when impairment of joint position is sufficient to result in locomotor ataxia. A similar involvement in the upper limbs may produce a disability to recognize the shape of objects by the sense of feel.

Selective degeneration of small myelinated and unmyelinated fibers often produces symptoms of hyperalgesia, described as "burning," "stinging," "prickling," or "aching." Tenderness and hypersensitivity are characteristic. The feet may have a raised threshold of sensation yet be hypersensitive once the threshold is exceeded, producing painfulness in walking.

Disorders which tend to affect large fibers selectively include inflammatory polyradiculoneuropathy, neuropathy associated with multiple myeloma, leukemia, and dysproteinemias, and neuropathy associated with hy-

pothyroidism. Disorders which tend to involve predominantly small fibers include amyloidosis, inherited sensory neuropathy, Fabry's disease, and Tangier disease. A variety of toxins, drugs, and vitamin deficiencies (particularly thiamin deficiency associated with alcoholism and vitamin B_{12} deficiency in pernicious anemia), as well as less clear insults associated with uremia, amyloidosis, peripheral vascular disease, and malabsorption, may affect both large and small fibers. Diabetic neuropathy can affect large fibers, small fibers, or both.

SENSORY LOSS OF DISTAL LOWER LIMBS WITHOUT MUSCLE WEAKNESS. The differential diagnosis depends on whether large or small fibers are predominantly affected and on the chronicity of the disorder. Large fiber involvement is particularly seen in posterior inflammatory polyradiculoneuropathy and in spinocerebellar degeneration. Small fiber involvement with or without large fiber involvement occurs with herpes zoster, in hereditary sensory neuropathies, in carcinomatous sensory neuropathy, and in some cases of inflammatory sensory polyradiculoneuropathy. Mild neurogenic weakness in affected segments is common.

Patients with neuropathy involving small fibers often have autonomic symptoms, including postural hypotension, anhidrosis, impotence, and disturbances of gut motility. Whether these symptoms reflect preganglionic or postganglionic involvement or degeneration, or both, is not known for most disorders. The symptoms are characteristic of amyloidosis, hyperalgesic diabetic neuropathy, malabsorption syndromes, the Riley-Day syndrome, and the Shy-Drager syndrome.

DIFFERENTIAL DIAGNOSIS BY CHARACTERISTICS OF NERVE CONDUCTION AND ELECTROMYOGRAPHY

The determination of nerve conduction velocity and electromyography have assumed an increasingly important role in establishing the presence and type of neuropathic involvement. As described below, involvement of large, alpha motoneurons may be of at least three types: (1) rapid degeneration of the entire neuron (neuronal degeneration), (2) axonal degeneration of the distal axon (dying-back) with or without atrophy and with or without secondary segmental demyelination, and (3) primary segmental demyelination. In neuronal degeneration, nerve conduction velocity tends to remain within normal limits until marked muscle weakness occurs. Needle electromyography shows denervation and an increased size of motor unit potentials. In axonal degeneration, low conduction velocity occurs only when the majority of fibers show the features of axonal atrophy and secondary segmental demyelination and remyelination. The features of the electromyogram will be similar to those of anterior horn cell disorders. In primary segmental demyelination, Schwann cell function is altered because of an inborn error of metabolism, by toxin, or by immunologic mechanism. Nerve conduction velocity is reduced and muscle action potentials are reduced in size and dispersed. Special techniques can determine low conduction in both proximal and distal segments of nerve. Denervation, which often accompanies segmental demyelination, implies concomitant axonal degeneration.

The evaluation of abnormality of A alpha primary afferent neurons by clinical neurophysiologic techniques is less complete than for alpha motoneurons. A decrease in amplitude and increase in latency of ulnar, median, and sural nerve action potentials provide evidence of such an abnormality. Adequate clinical neurophysiologic evaluation of gamma motoneuron fibers, of A delta and somatic C fibers, and of sympathetic C fibers is not possible at this time. This lack is often not a serious limitation, as most neuropathic conditions also involve A alpha fibers.

DIFFERENTIAL DIAGNOSIS OF PERIPHERAL NEUROPATHY BY PATHOLOGY

Pathologic changes in peripheral nerve tissue can be divided broadly into interstitial and parenchymatous. Interstitial pathologic changes arise outside the nerve and Schwann cells and may damage these cells secondarily. Usually in interstitial neuropathies the initial change is in the supporting tissue of the nerve or in its blood vessels. Examples include amyloidosis, necrotizing angiopathy, and acute, chronic, and relapsing inflammatory polyradiculoneuropathy. In parenchymatous neuropathies, the nerve and Schwann cells are primarily affected from various causes such as inherited metabolic diseases, toxic substances, deficiency states, and other metabolic diseases. Examples of parenchymatous neuropathies are those caused by alcohol, lead, arsenic, diphtheria, and metachromatic leukodystrophy.

To help characterize the pathologic involvement it is helpful to ask the following questions: Which populations of neurons are affected? What is the level of damage within neurons? What is the type of fiber degeneration? How extensive? What kind of repair or regeneration has occurred?

A highly selective involvement by population of neurons may occur in neuropathic disease, e.g., in hereditary motor neuropathy, lower motor neurons; in Fabry's disease, A delta and somatic C neurons; and in Friedreich's ataxia, A alpha neurons.

The level of involvement within neurons may be characteristic for various neuropathies. To illustrate, in some neuropathies the entire neuron degenerates. This is seen in so-called anterior horn cell diseases, e.g., in poliomyelitis and in motor neuron disease. Such generalized neuronal degeneration may also affect primary afferent neurons, e.g., in herpes zoster and in Friedreich's ataxia. The degeneration of entire neurons is in contrast to diseases in which distal axons degenerate — dying-back neuropathies, e.g., in uremic neuropathy.

Several types of nerve fiber degeneration are recognized. In both wallerian and axonal degeneration, involvement of the axon is primary. In wallerian degeneration from crush or section of nerve, the distal axon inevitably degenerates by a series of rapid stereotyped histologic changes. In man wallerian degeneration occurs from compression, crush, or traction and from transection of fibers as, for example, in necrotizing angiopathic neuropathy. In axonal degeneration the course may be less rapid than in wallerian degeneration, axonal atrophy may precede degeneration, and electron microscopic abnormalities of axis cylinders may be present prior to dissolution of the myelinated fiber. Also, focal axonal abnormalities in some disorders may lead secondarily to wallerian degeneration of the distal axon.

At least two types of segmental demyelination are recognized. In primary segmental demyelination, the Schwann cells are affected first and predominantly. For example, in inflammatory polyradiculoneuropathy, involvement of interstitial mononuclear cells results in myelin damage, whereas in lead neuropathy a metabolic poisoning of Schwann cells probably is involved. A secondary segmental demyelination (secondary to axonal atrophy or disease) seems to characterize those neuropathies with axonal atrophy, e.g., in Friedreich's ataxia and in uremia.

The neurologic deficits from demyelinating lesions tend to be less severe and shorter lived than those from axonal degeneration. Nerve repair following a crush lesion is rapid and more complete than when the nerve trunk is transected. Nerve regeneration tends to be better in the young than in the old.

NERVE BIOPSY

Nerve biopsy can usually provide specific answers to the following questions: Is neuropathy present? What populations of fibers are affected? What type of fiber degeneration is occurring? How severe and how fast is it? Is regeneration or fiber repair occurring? Can specific diagnostic features be recognized? Cutaneous nerve biopsy (usually of the sural nerve) may provide diagnostic information in amyloidosis, in necrotizing angiopathic neuropathy, in leprosy, in sarcoidosis, and in various lipidoses such as metachromatic leukodystrophy and Fabry's disease. A presumptive diagnosis from nerve biopsy may be possible in inflammatory neuropathies, in lymphoproliferative disorders, and in myxedema. Despite its usefulness in diagnosis, however, nerve biopsy should be used sparingly because it may leave a longlasting, disagreeable, and sometimes painful numbness. Nerve biopsies should probably be performed only in centers which have specialized laboratories expert in dealing with this tissue.

337.2. NEUROPATHY ASSOCIATED WITH INFECTION

Diphtheria is commonly complicated by paralysis of the nasopharynx and oculomotor and ciliary muscles. More widespread cranial polyneuropathy is uncommon. A more generalized peripheral neuropathy may occur several weeks after the pharyngeal infection has subsided. The disease is discussed fully in Ch. 145.

Herpes zoster, with infection of the gasserian or spinal ganglia, produces a characteristic cutaneous lesion followed by a persistent hyperalgesic, anesthetic monoradiculopathy in the affected dermatome. The first division of the gasserian ganglion and intercostal dermatomes are most frequently affected. Although the painful state may persist for prolonged periods, it eventually remits in almost all instances (see Ch. 305).

Leprosy is one of the most common neuropathies on a worldwide scale. Diagnosis depends on recognizing the distinctive sites of predilection and the associated cutaneous involvement, and on histologic studies. New forms of treatment are completely changing the way these patients are being handled and their prognosis. This subject is discussed in Ch. 170.

337.3. NEUROPATHY ASSOCIATED WITH INFLAMMATION AND PRESUMED ALTERED IMMUNITY

Serum sickness neuropathy typically begins within seven to ten days of the injection of a foreign protein. The condition was more frequent when bacterial infections were treated with foreign antisera. A brachial plexus neuropathy occurs more frequently than does more diffuse peripheral neuropathy. One should consider serum sickness when the neuropathy is superimposed on a history of arthralgia, skin eruption, fever, albuminuria, and possible cerebral symptoms. Episodes of neuropathic involvement may recur over the course of several weeks. The pathogenesis is as follows: The introduction of foreign protein elicits an immune response. Initially because of an excess of antigen, the immune complexes are small and circulate freely. As antibodies build up, immune complexes become large and less soluble and are deposited between endothelial cells and basement membranes of blood vessels. Serum complement is bound and activated, and polymorphonuclear leukocytes release hydrolases which damage vessel walls. An acute inflammatory necrotizing vasculitis ensues.

337.4. ACUTE INFLAMMATORY POLYRADICULONEUROPATHIES

Acute inflammatory polyradiculoneuropathies are a group of disorders which probably have a similar pathologic and etiologic basis but can differ in their anatomic sites of predilection and their temporal profile. Understanding of etiologic and pathologic factors is incomplete, but investigators generally believe that infection, particularly by viruses, plays a role. Because a diverse group of viruses, bacterial agents, and foreign proteins may produce similar disorders, it seems unlikely that direct infection of nerve cells by these organisms is involved. Most likely, viruses produce an indirect effect through immunologic mechanisms. The pathologic hallmarks of the disorder are infiltrates of mononuclear cells around capillaries within nerve tissue, edema of the endoneurial compartment, and segmental demyelination and remyelination. Sensitized lymphocytes are thought to be involved in the myelin damage. The disorder may recur in some patients. Since the disorder may affect more than one family member, genetic factors may influence susceptibility. The pathologic lesions are patchy and tend to be widely distributed along the length of the nerves. In the motor variety, the predominant pathologic changes lie in the ventral spinal roots; in the sensory variety, in the posterior spinal roots; and in the autonomic variety, possibly in the sympathetic and autonomic ganglia of the abdomen. Four clinical syndromes are recognized: motor polyradiculoneuropathy, sensory polyradiculoneuropathy, autonomic neuropathy, and polyneuritis

cranialis. The clinical and pathogic features, at least of the motor and sensory syndromes, are sufficiently alike to seem to be explained by different anatomic sites of involvement rather than by different mechanisms. Pure syndromes of motor and of sensory involvement are uncommon. In mixed syndromes motor symptomatology predominates.

ACUTE INFLAMMATORY MOTOR POLYRADICULONEUROPATHY
(Landry-Guillain-Barré-Strohl Syndrome)

Approximately one half of patients give a history of a mild upper respiratory infection one to two weeks before the onset of muscle weakness. For the most part the specific virus or bacterial infection remains unknown, but the syndrome has been known to follow infection with measles, mumps, rubella, influenza A, influenza B, varicella-zoster, cytomegalovirus, infectious mononucleosis, vaccinia, variola, infectious hepatitis, coxsackievirus, and echoviruses. Cases have been described to follow the injection of a foreign protein, cat scratch, dog bite, blood transfusion or immunization, as was seen in the widespread influenza vaccine program of 1976 (see Ch. 82).

All the polyneuropathies tend to begin subacutely with relatively mild initiating symptoms and few or no systemic symptoms and signs. A small percentage of patients have unspecific malaise and headache, but chills, fever, stiff neck, and severe headaches are generally absent. Signs and symptoms of neurologic dysfunction usually appear first in a restricted part of the body, and are often relatively mild at onset. The rate of further progression varies widely. Some patients become severely paralyzed within no more than a few days, whereas in others the neuropathy worsens insidiously and slowly over a period of several days or even weeks.

In the syndrome originally described by Landry, there is an ascending paralysis which develops over the course of approximately one week, reaches a plateau for several weeks, and then improves. Most often, symptoms of acute polyneuropathy begin with some abnormality of walking, climbing stairs, or rising from a seated position. Muscle weakness tends to involve both proximal and distal limb muscles. The extent of paralysis varies widely from patient to patient. In the more severe cases, most of the cranial nerves except for the first, second, and eighth may be affected. Facial weakness and weakness of chewing and swallowing occur most frequently. Muscle weakness can affect all skeletal muscles of the limb and trunk.

Although muscle weakness and atrophy predominate in most patients, few fail to develop evidence of sensory involvement at some time during the course. Patients may report feelings of prickling numbness, bandlike tightness, altered sensation when the skin is touched, thermal sensations, and painful sensations. Typically these involve the feet but may extend upward to other parts of the lower limbs or the body. Sensory symptoms may accompany the onset of muscle weakness and then disappear, or may persist throughout the entire illness and be a major component of the disease. Some patients may have symptoms of unsteadiness in walking and severe loss of tactile sensation.

Involvement of the autonomic nervous system may

occur even in these predominantly motor polyradiculoneuropathies. Most commonly this is reflected by postural hypotension in the sitting or standing position after prolonged recumbency. Cramping abdominal pain may result from an atonic bowel. Bladder or bowel incontinence is rare.

The diagnosis is confirmed by the characteristic clinical course, the cerebrospinal fluid findings, the typical characteristics of the nerve conduction and electromyographic examination, and the lack of laboratory evidence of other disease. Characteristically the cerebrospinal fluid pressure is normal and the fluid is clear, contains less than 5 lymphocytes per cubic millimeter, and contains an elevated protein content. On occasion, however, either an increased number of lymphocytes or a normal protein level is found in otherwise typical cases. In approximately two thirds of cases, conduction velocity of motor fibers of distal limb nerves is less than 60 per cent of normal values. In such cases, the amplitude of the muscle action potential may be reasonably well preserved. When more proximal sites along the length of the limb nerves are stimulated, a reduction in muscle action potential may occur, implying a proximal block of motor fibers. In one third of cases, motor nerve conduction may be normal. In such instances, a proximal block or slowing of nerve fiber conduction would provide evidence of a segmentally demyelinating lesion in the proximal portion of nerves.

The differential diagnosis of acute inflammatory polyneuropathy includes acute intermittent porphyria and the neuropathy associated with leukemia, lymphoma, and multiple myeloma. Acute intermittent porphyria is recognized by the additional features of a delirium and by laboratory evidence of porphobilinogen excretion. The polyradiculoneuropathies associated with carcinoma and with lymphoma usually develop more insidiously and may be recognized by their radiographic and systemic alterations.

The first concern in the treatment of acute inflammatory motor polyradiculoneuropathy is to maintain an adequate airway and to provide ventilatory assistance as necessary. Fluid and food intake must be monitored so that supplementation may be begun either by tube feeding or by intravenous feeding. Corticosteroid hormones are reported to provide a small but significant improvement in the rate of recovery. The risk of complications is reduced by restricting such treatment to short periods of time. Convalescence may last for months or several years and should include physical therapy. Initially this should consist of passive exercises and later of active exercises. If at all possible the education of students should continue during this illness. Most patients make an almost complete improvement from this neuropathic disease.

ACUTE INFLAMMATORY SENSORY POLYRADICULONEUROPATHY

Involvement predominantly of the posterior root and spinal ganglion results in a sensory polyradiculoneuropathy which is probably the counterpart of the ventral spinal root involvement described above. As in the motor variety, a preceding infection may antedate the neurologic syndrome by several weeks. Typically the onset is marked by combinations of sensory dysfunction and pain. The sensory dysfunction is most commonly described as unsteadiness in gait or clumsiness in the use of the hands. Even more incapacitating are the painful dysesthesias which develop in some patients. Varying combinations of lancinating pain, prickling hyperesthesia, constricting band-like sensations, and burning or coldness of skin may be described. Most patients appreciate that the hyperesthetic skin is insensitive but that when the threshold for sensation is exceeded the discomfort is excessive. Any region of the body may be affected, and the disorder involves proximal as well as distal dermatomes. On clinical examination the lower extremities tend to be affected more than the upper, and the various modalities of sensation may be affected to different degrees. The patients often exhibit sensory ataxia, and, because of the severe impairment of joint position, the limbs may be held in distorted positions. Tendon reflexes are often diminished or absent.

Minor degrees of involvement of motor and autonomic neurons are not uncommon. In addition, patients have difficulty is sustaining muscle contraction in the presence of severe involvement of their afferent peripheral nervous system. The cerebrospinal fluid changes are similar to those in the motor variety. The motor nerve conduction velocity, the amplitude of the muscle action potential, and the distal latency may be within normal limits. By contrast, nerve action potentials cannot be elicited from stimulation of afferent nerve fibers either because the afferent fibers have degenerated or because the action potential is so dispersed.

Prognosis for recovery in sensory polyneuropathy is less good than in the motor variety, and symptoms of cutaneous hyperpathia often persist or recur for many years. The sensory ataxia usually improves but likewise often does not recover completely. This persistence of the neurologic deficit probably is explained by irreversible damage of spinal ganglion neurons. Affected craftsmen and professionals whose work depends on manual dexterity often require retraining in less skilled work.

ACUTE INFLAMMATORY AUTONOMIC NEUROPATHY
(Pandysautonomia)

Acute inflammatory autonomic neuropathy is a poorly understood, rare condition which may be the autonomic counterpart of the motor and sensory varieties described above. The onset and time course are similar to the motor and sensory neuropathies, but to date pathologic studies are unavailable. The principal symptoms include postural hypotension, cramping abdominal pain, and varying amounts of diarrhea and constipation. The hypotension may be so severe that the patient cannot sit up without losing consciousness. The cramping abdominal pain presumably is caused by regions of atonic bowel. Affected subjects reportedly improve with time, but few long-term follow-up studies are available. The use of fitted elastic stockings and oral fludrocortisone may hasten resumption of the erect position. The cramping abdominal pain may be modified by the use of frequent small bland feedings and antispasmodic agents.

337.5. CHRONIC INFLAMMATORY POLYRADICULONEUROPATHY

(Including Recurrent Polyradiculoneuropathy)

In chronic inflammatory polyradiculoneuropathy the neurologic deficit tends to develop slowly over months or years and persists for years. Some patients have a monophasic course over many years. Others have a stepwise progression to their maximal deficit and then slowly improve. Still others have a recurrent course with ultimate worsening or ultimate improvement. A few patients progress slowly to death several years later. As in the acute inflammatory polyradiculoneuropathies, the process tends to involve symmetrical proximal body structures and to affect motor, autonomic, and sensory peripheral neurons in varying proportions. The cerebrospinal fluid protein is usually elevated. The pathologic alterations initially resemble those of the acute variety, but with time hypertrophic neuropathy develops. Sural nerve biopsy may show features of the disease without cellular infiltrates. The characteristics of the nerve conduction and electromyographic examination are not unlike those of the acute variety, except that there probably are fewer cases with preserved normal nerve conduction. Over a period of years most patients eventually improve beyond their maximal deficit but continue to have a significant neurologic problem.

The use of prednisone often indicates a dramatic improvement. Regrettably, such effects soon wear off in most instances, and long-term steroid therapy should be avoided because of its complications.

337.6. SARCOID NEUROPATHY

Sarcoid neuropathy most commonly affects the facial nerve, and when it does it is indistinguishable from Bell's palsy. Occasionally other cranial nerves may be affected, or a more generalized neuropathy may be found (see Ch. 65).

337.7. NEUROPATHY ASSOCIATED WITH MESENCHYMAL DISEASE AND NECROTIZING ANGIOPATHY

Neuropathy is a relatively common complication of periarteritis nodosa, of Wegener's and other granulomas, and of rheumatoid arthritis. It is less commonly associated with Sjögren's syndrome and with cranial arteritis. Mononeuropathy may develop in any of these patients when nerves are compressed by immobilization, recumbency, or inflamed tissue within tight compartments. More often, these patients develop a characteristic and distinctive multiple mononeuropathy as a result of a necrotizing angiopathy. Usually such patients first develop a neurologic deficit in the distribution of a major limb nerve such as the peroneal or the ulnar. Characteristically, with peroneal nerve involvement, the patient becomes aware of his inability to dorsiflex the foot at the ankle. This is followed within hours or days by burning discomfort of the top of the

foot and lateral side of the leg. In short succession other limb nerves may sequentially become affected. Pathologically, nerve fibers in regions of poor blood perfusion (usually at midthigh and mid-upper arm levels) become damaged only after occlusion of multiple epineurial arteries so that clinically one is seeing a late stage of the pathologic process. Corticosteroids are commonly used for treatment, usually with at least symptomatic improvement.

337.8. NEUROPATHY ASSOCIATED WITH DIABETES MELLITUS

FREQUENCY AND EPIDEMIOLOGY. The reported frequency of neuropathy among diabetic patients ranges widely, from 5 to 60 per cent. The difference is mainly due to differences of definition of what constitutes neuropathy and of the criteria and techniques used to diagnose it. If a mild reduction of nerve conduction velocity is used, neuropathy occurs in approximately 60 per cent of diabetics. The frequency of neuropathy increases with age and with the duration of diabetes.

ETIOLOGY. It seems unlikely that a single mechanism underlies the various types of diabetic neuropathy. Nerve damage from ischemia to distal lower limbs represents one variety, and compression may be another. The mechanism of nerve fiber damage in the more diffuse types of neuropathy is less well understood. A diffuse microangiopathy of endoneurial capillaries with alteration of blood nerve barrier seems a reasonable possibility. Alternative explanations include immunologic or biochemical derangements, insulin deficiency, or phospholipid deficiency. No explanation stands fully proved.

CLINICAL SYMPTOMATOLOGY AND CLASSIFICATION. The various types of diabetic neuropathy overlap each other, but the following classification illustrates the diverse types.

Asymptomatic Neuropathy. Although incompletely studied, asymptomatic low nerve conduction velocity is associated with morphologic abnormality of nerve fibers.

Neuropathy with Peripheral Vascular Disease. Diabetic patients with severe peripheral vascular disease affecting the distal lower limb may develop a distal, stocking-like ischemic neuropathy. Sensory and autonomic symptoms predominate. Only nerves in the territory of the ischemia are affected.

Ataxic Neuropathy (Pseudotabes Diabetica). A diffuse symmetrical distal neuropathy especially affecting the lower limbs is common in diabetics, particularly in longstanding disease and even in patients with mild diabetes mellitus. In most cases the neuropathy involves both large and small afferent fibers, as well as autonomic fibers and motor fibers. Mild cases produce nonpainful numbness of the toes and the front part of the foot. Varying degrees of sensory ataxia are found with more severe cases. The Achilles and, less frequently, the quadriceps reflex disappear. Touch-pressure, joint position, and vibration sensations are variably abnormal in the distal lower limb, less so in the upper. Pain and thermal discriminations tend to be spared.

Hyperalgesic Neuropathy. With hyperalgesic neuropathy the patients have burning painfulness of the skin of the toes, feet, and legs. In addition lancinating pain, tightness, hypersensitivity of the feet, and deep aching in the limbs may be present. Night pain in the legs, with the features of restless legs, can be improved only by movement such as getting out of bed and moving about. Autonomic involvement resulting in postural hypotension, anhidrosis, and impotence is more common in hyperalgesic than in ataxic neuropathy.

Autonomic Neuropathy. Autonomic symptoms of mild degree are common in diabetes, especially with neuropathy. In the variety called *autonomic neuropathy,* postural hypotension, impotence in the male, and bladder and bowel incontinence in both sexes are particularly troublesome. These patients tend to have hyperalgesic symptoms as well.

Diabetic Lumbosacral Plexus Neuropathy (Diabetic Amyotrophy and Femoral Neuropathy). The terms used to describe this type of diabetic neuropathy draw attention to different clinical presentations. So-called *femoral neuropathy* often begins suddenly with pain in the anterior aspect of the thigh, followed within a few days by marked weakness, and later atrophy, of the quadriceps muscle. The pattern of electromyographic denervation reveals that the disorder extends beyond the femoral nerve and involves either the lumbosacral plexus or the roots, or both. A rapid improvement in some cases speaks against the disorder's being due to vascular occlusion. If muscle weakness and atrophy predominate and the disorder affects both legs, the term *diabetic amyotrophy* has been applied.

TREATMENT. Only weak evidence indicates that close diabetic control prevents or ameliorates diabetic neuropathy. The pain in hyperalgesic diabetic neuropathy must be approached in several ways. One must allay anxiety and depression, encourage a normal sleep pattern, and find ways of dealing with the pain without addicting the patient. Cool soaks of the feet given for 15 minutes twice a day may help. Some patients find relief with phenytoin or carbamazepine. Aspirin with codeine may help others. Sedation should be reserved for night sleep. In the well adjusted male with impotence, an inflatable prosthesis may allow sexual function. Patients with insensitive feet should be instructed according to the direction given in Ch. 337.17.

337.9. NEUROPATHY ASSOCIATED WITH UREMIA

ETIOLOGY. The cause of uremic neuropathy is unknown. The lesion appears to be occurring less frequently than in the early days of hemodialysis, suggesting an effect from improved technique. Neuropathy generally disappears after renal transplantation.

PATHOLOGY. Abnormal nerve conduction is frequent in chronic uremics on hemodialysis. Pathologic studies in the diffuse symmetrical polyneuropathies show an axonal atrophy with secondary segmental demyelination that appears to precede a distal degeneration of nerve fibers.

CLASSIFICATION AND SYMPTOMATOLOGY. Subclinical neuropathies are common in patients with end-stage uremia on hemodialysis. Such patients may have slight

weakness or dorsiflexion of the foot, absent ankle reflexes, and mild abnormalities of touch-pressure and vibration sensations. Patients with uremia are cachectic and prone to both compression and traumatic mononeuropathy. They also appear to be abnormally susceptible to acute inflammatory polyradiculoneuropathy. The most typical neuropathy seen in uremics, however, is a symmetrical, distal process in which variable severe sensory symptoms predominate, accompanied by mild motor and autonomic symptoms. Older men especially are predisposed. Uremic neuropathy develops earlier in patients with creatinine clearances below 5 ml per minute and more frequently when diabetes mellitus or polycystic kidneys are present. Treatment is difficult, and the benefit of hemodialysis in preventing or in improving the neuropathy is uncertain.

337.10. NEUROPATHY ASSOCIATED WITH HEPATIC DISEASE

Several kinds of peripheral neuropathy can accompany liver disease. These include those of nutritional deficiency as well as those associated with infectious mononucleosis, acute intermittent porphyria, various vasculitides, amyloidosis, celiac disease, and various intoxications. Acute inflammatory polyneuropathy can follow viral hepatitis. A sensory neuropathy may be associated with primary biliary cirrhosis.

337.11. NEUROPATHY ASSOCIATED WITH ENDOCRINE DISEASES

Hypothyroidism is associated with both a mononeuropathy and a diffuse peripheral neuropathy. Myxedematous changes of the connective tissues of the carpal tunnel often result in compression of the median nerve. Thyroid replacement may be curative. Diffuse peripheral neuropathy associated with myxedema tends to affect predominantly the lower limb. A sensory ataxia with or without hyperesthesia or hyperalgesia is characteristic. Motor and sensory nerve fiber conduction velocity is reduced, and the muscle action potential is dispersed. Thyroid replacement therapy results in clinical and electrophysiologic improvement.

Hyperthyroidism may also be associated with a neuropathy, but this may be a chance association.

Acromegaly commonly produces entrapment neuropathies at wrist and elbow. A diffuse and sometimes severe hypertrophic neuropathy may also occur. The neuropathy of acromegaly seldom improves with hormone replacement. The effects of hypophysectomy have not been well studied.

Inherited multiple endocrine neoplasia, commonly associated with thyroid and medullary adrenal carcinoma, is usually associated also with a peroneal muscular atrophy. The patients have pes cavus, peroneal muscular weakness, and sensory loss of the feet and legs. The facial features are distinctive, consisting of thickened lips and adenomas of the tongue, lips, and conjunctiva. Such patients and their relatives should be studied for the presence of endocrine neoplasms.

337.12. AMYLOIDOSIS

Inherited amyloidosis is frequent only in endemic regions such as Portugal and Japan. In the Portuguese variety, which is inherited as an autosomal dominant trait, the disorder usually begins in the third, fourth, and fifth decades and affects predominantly small sensory and autonomic fibers. Lumbosacral dermatomes show a syringomyelia-like loss of nociception and thermal discrimination with preservation of touch-pressure sensation. Loss of potency in the male, postural hypotension, and bladder and bowel incontinence are common in advanced stages. The disorder tends to progress over a decade or so. Biopsied sural nerves show a reduction in unmyelinated and small myelinated fibers with nodular deposits of amyloid along the nerve trunks.

In the Indiana type of inherited amyloidosis symptoms begin in the hands. Numbness of the thumb and first three fingers from compression of the median nerve at the carpal tunnel ligament is characteristic.

Noninherited amyloidosis may be divided into primary and secondary varieties. The peripheral neuropathy of primary amyloidosis also affects the distal aspects of the lower extremities more than the upper extremities and includes small fibers as much as or more than larger fibers. When typical symptoms of neuropathy are associated with heart enlargement, nephropathy, and enlargement of the tongue, the diagnosis of amyloidosis should be strongly suspected and can be confirmed by histologic examination of rectal mucosa, kidney, carpal ligament, muscle, gingivae, nerve, or bone marrow. No effective treatment for the neuropathy is available.

Some patients with multiple myeloma develop a symmetrical predominantly motor neuropathy with many of the clinical features of chronic inflammatory polyradiculoneuropathy. It is sometimes assumed that neuropathies associated with multiple myeloma are due to amyloidosis. Although amyloid deposition has sometimes been found in the nerves in myeloma, it is not clear that this causes the neuropathy. Multiple myeloma should be considered in chronic neuropathy of unknown cause.

Recently a new syndrome with peripheral neuropathy associated with solitary osteosclerotic myeloma has been reported from Japan. The patients had the additional features of skin hyperpigmentation and gynecomastia.

337.13. NEUROPATHY ASSOCIATED WITH CARCINOMA AND OTHER MALIGNANCY

Direct compression of nerves by metastatic tumors occurs within the spinal canal, within intervertebral foramina, and behind tight fascial sheaths, as in the retroperitoneal space of the pelvis. Bronchogenic, renal, prostatic, and breast carcinomas are especially prone to such metastases. The nonmetastatic neurologic effects of cancer are described in Ch. 322 to 327.

NEUROPATHY ASSOCIATED WITH NUTRITIONAL DEFICIENCY

See Ch. 286.

337.14. NEUROPATHY ASSOCIATED WITH THE USE OF DRUGS

Many drugs produce a peripheral neuropathy, some more frequently than others. When prescribing such agents, the risk-benefit ratio must always be considered.

The vinca alkaloids, particularly vincristine and vinblastine, are employed in the treatment of leukemias, lymphomas, and Hodgkin's disease. The drugs predictably produce a sensory neuropathy with sometimes painful paresthesias of the feet and a severity proportional to the dosage.

The use of clioquinol has been associated with a severe neurologic disorder, reported especially in Japan, called subacute myeloptical neuropathy (SMON). This disorder is characterized by loss of vision, ascending numbness, motor weakness, and autonomic involvement.

Nitrofurantoin commonly produces neuropathy when used for urologic infections in patients with impaired renal function who then develop high blood levels of the drug. Most common are paresthesias, but an ascending paralysis can occur.

Isoniazid used as an antituberculous agent interferes with pyridoxine metabolism. Paresthesias of the toes and feet associated with lower limb weakness can be prevented by pyridoxine supplementation.

Hydralazine occasionally produces a neuropathy, probably by producing pyridoxine deficiency.

The anticonvulsant phenytoin can produce a mild asymptomatic neuropathy with hyporeflexia.

Chloramphenicol occasionally produces mild peripheral neuropathy or optic neuritis.

Gold, used as sodium aurothiomalate for rheumatoid arthritis, can produce a peripheral neuropathy and cranial neuropathy as well as a confusional state.

Sodium cyanate is potentially useful in the management of sickle cell anemia but produces a distressing polyneuropathy in both man and laboratory animals.

Ethambutol, an otherwise promising antituberculous drug, produces optic neuritis and occasionally a peripheral neuropathy.

337.15. NEUROPATHY ASSOCIATED WITH HOUSEHOLD AND INDUSTRIAL POISONS

Large outbreaks of polyneuropathy can occur from inhalation of toxic substances in factories and from adulteration of food and drinking water. A variety of chemicals used as euphoriants or for suicidal purposes produce neuropathy.

Arsenic continues to cause a few cases of peripheral neuropathy each year in the United States. Often it is difficult even with intensive investigation to determine whether the intent of ingestion was homicidal or suicidal. A typical hyperalgesic neuropathy affects the feet and lower legs, and is accompanied by distal muscle weakness and a gastrointestinal upset. Cerebral and hepatic symptoms may occur. The skin may darken. Diagnosis depends on finding elevated arsenic levels in blood, in urine, in nail clippings, and in hair. Several months are required before one can reliably detect the diagnostic Mees lines on the fingernails.

Lead neuropathy is now rare. Abdominal colic, anemia, and wrist drop suggest the diagnosis.

Thallium neuropathy resembles arsenical neuropathy but with superimposed alopecia.

Methyl mercury, an industrial toxin, produces an encephalopathy with delirium and may be associated with loss of vision and a peripheral neuropathy. *Organophosphorus compounds* may produce an initial cholinergic block resulting in respiratory paralysis and at a later time a peripheral neuropathy. Of the organophosphorus compounds, tri-ortho-cresyl phosphate has resulted in the greatest number of cases of neuropathy in man owing to contamination of medicines and cooking oils.

Acrylamide, used for the waterproofing of underground tunnels and for various scientific purposes, when ingested results in a severe distal neuropathy.

Pesticides such as DDT and kepone (an ant insecticide) may be associated with a peripheral neuropathy.

A variety of organic solvents and plasticizers are associated with neuropathy. n-Hexane, used industrially in shoe factories and misused as a euphoriant agent, is known to produce neuropathy. Other toxic industrial chemicals producing neuropathy include methyl n-butyl ketone, hexachlorophene, carbon disulfide, and trichloroethylene.

337.16. INHERITED DISORDERS OF PERIPHERAL NEURONS

These represent a group of nonremitting, slowly progressive disorders probably caused by inborn errors of metabolism. Pathologically they are system atrophies which affect selective populations of neurons by type and size. In those with primary neuronal involvement, distal axonal atrophy and secondary segmental demyelination are characteristic.

The disorders are characterized by the type of inheritance, by their natural history by which population of neurons is involved, and by the nature of the pathologic involvement. Predominant involvement of lower motor neurons is called progressive muscular atrophy (inherited motor neuropathy); of sensory neurons, inherited sensory neuropathy; of both motor and sensory neurons, inherited motor and sensory neuropathy; and of autonomic neurons, dysautonomia. Predominant involvement of large sensory fibers and of corticospinal and spinocerebellar tracts constitutes spinocerebellar degeneration. Predominantly cerebellar involvement constitutes cerebellar ataxia. Predominant involvement of corticospinal tracts plus, as a rule, lower motor and sensory neurons constitutes spastic paraplegia.

The expression of clinical symptoms in inherited neuronal disorders varies widely from patient to patient and generation to generation. Usually functional disability is less than might be expected from the chronic neurologic signs. To confirm the presence of an inherited neuronal degeneration the patient's relatives often must be examined neurologically and by nerve conduction and electromyography.

DISORDERS OF PERIPHERAL MOTOR NEURONS
(Progressive Muscular Atrophies)

These are discussed fully in Ch. 281.

337.17. DISORDERS OF PERIPHERAL SENSORY NEURONS

Patients with disorders of peripheral sensory neurons characteristically suffer from pain, cutaneous injury from lack of sensation, unsteady movement from kinesthetic sensory loss, or combinations of these. Frequently they also have autonomic dysfunction. The nature of these symptoms and the associated sensory loss correspond reasonably well with the populations of fibers affected. Thus patients with loss of pain and temperature sensation and with autonomic impairment have degeneration, mostly of unmyelinated and small myelinated fibers, whereas patients with loss of touch-pressure sensation have degeneration of large myelinated fibers of cutaneous nerves. In advanced disease this selectivity of involvement by fiber size tends to be lost.

HEREDITARY SENSORY NEUROPATHY, TYPE I

Hereditary sensory neuropathy, Type I, is a dominantly inherited sensory radicular neuropathy. It has been variously described as perforating ulcers of the feet, mutilating acropathy, acrodystrophic neuropathy, and hereditary sensory radicular neuropathy. Variability in severity is commonplace. Sensory loss is usually much more severe over the feet and legs than in the hands and forearms, and some patients have lancinating pains. Pain and temperature sensation are affected more than touch-pressure sensation, and sensory ataxia is absent. Loss or decrease of sweating usually corresponds to the region of sensory loss. Nerve conduction of motor fibers is usually normal. Denervation may affect foot and leg muscles. The ankle tendon reflex may be absent. Life expectancy is normal in most cases. Late in the disorder, perforating ulcers of the foot may develop, especially when there has been poor foot care. In kinships, signs such as pes cavus, hammer toes, plantar calluses, inability to walk on heels, and sensation loss of acral parts of lower limbs point to an incomplete expression of the affliction.

HEREDITARY SENSORY NEUROPATHY, TYPE II

This is a recessively inherited disorder, also called congenital sensory neuropathy, which usually manifests itself in infancy or childhood with a mutilating acropathy characterized by paronychia, whitlows, ulcers of the fingers and plantar surfaces of the feet, and, frequently, unrecognized fractures of the extremities. Sensory loss affects all types of cutaneous and sometimes kinesthetic sensation and is most marked distally in all four limbs. Tendon reflexes are usually absent. Sweating loss usually occurs over the distal limbs. Nerve action potentials of afferent fibers of cutaneous and limb nerves cannot be detected. Pathologically, there is an almost complete absence of myelinated fibers from the cutaneous nerves of the distal lower limb with preservation of decreased numbers of unmyelinated fibers.

HEREDITARY SENSORY NEOROPATHY, TYPE III
(Dysautonomia of Riley-Day)

Familial dysautonomia is a recessively inherited disorder of Jewish infants and children. It affects peripheral autonomic neurons, peripheral sensory neurons, peripheral motor neurons, and probably other central nervous system neurons. Characteristic are an onset in infancy, a history of poor feeding, repeated episodes of vomiting and pulmonary infections, autonomic disturbances, and premature death. Autonomic abnormalities include defective lacrimation, defective temperature control, skin blotching, excessive perspiration, hypertension, and postural hypotension. There are also insensitivity to pain, areflexia, corneal insensitivity, and absence of the fungiform papillae of the tongue. An abnormality of catecholamine metabolism has been demonstrated.

HEREDITARY SENSORY NEUROPATHY, TYPE IV

In this recessively inherited sensory neuropathy, insensitivity to pain, anhidrosis, and mental retardation are found. This disorder has been attributed to an abnormality of differentiation of the neural crest.

ANGIOKERATOMA CORPORIS DIFFUSUM
(Fabry's Syndrome)

This rare disorder is characterized by angiokeratomas, impaired renal function, and small purple to black spots distributed especially over the lower trunk and buttocks along segmental lines. Typically, patients have pain and numbness in the limbs but no motor symptoms. A deposition of glycolipids in the cell bodies of peripheral sensory neurons and a decrease in the number of small neurons of spinal ganglia and of unmyelinated and small myelinated fibers have been observed and may be important in explaining the painfulness of the disorder.

TREATMENT OF INSENSITIVE HANDS AND FEET

Persons with pain and temperature insensitivity of hands and feet are vulnerable to many injuries which potentially can cascade into ulceration, cellulitis, lymphangitis, osteomyelitis, and osteolysis. These events are seen particularly in the disorders of leprosy, inherited amyloidosis, and other inherited and acquired neuropathies with the aforementioned sensory loss. Congenital neuropathies with such sensory loss are particularly difficult to manage, because they occur at an age when it is difficult to obtain the cooperation of the patient. The goal in treatment is to prevent the onset of tissue damage or, when it has occurred, to promote healing and prevent further damage. Persons with loss of pain and temperature sensation should not engage in most forms of manual labor or perform repetitive tasks with hands and feet which can cause bruising. Repeated inspection of the feet and hands is necessary. Any bruise or ulcer on the foot should lead one to stop weight bearing until healing has occurred. Shoes should be wide and well constructed. The inside of the shoes must be inspected to remove retained objects or nails. The feet of such patients should be soaked in lukewarm water for 15 minutes twice a day and lightly covered with petrolatum lotion to retain moisture in the softened skin.

337.18. INHERITED DISORDERS OF PERIPHERAL MOTOR, SENSORY, AND AUTONOMIC NEURONS

The disorders are usually inherited and progressive and have symmetrical signs. The pathologic features are nonfocal, and the nerve fibers show axonal atrophy and degeneration. The molecular cause is unknown.

HEREDITARY MOTOR AND SENSORY NEUROPATHY, TYPE I
(Dominantly Inherited Hypertrophic Neuropathy Type of Peroneal Muscular Atrophy)

This is a fairly common, mild, dominantly inherited variant of peroneal muscular atrophy. Affected persons may have no symptoms or signs, but may be identified by their position in a kinship and by low conduction velocities of all nerves.

Pathologically the disorder affects mainly myelinated fibers, producing segmental demyelination and remyelination and varying degrees of onion-bulb formation (the hallmark of hypertrophic neuropathy).

In involved kinships affected persons can be recognized by higher plantar arches, hammer toes (curled-up toes with convexity upward), frequent corns or calluses, and a high-stepping, awkward gait caused by paresis of the dorsiflexor muscles of the ankle and instability of the ankle joint. Persons with greater weakness may have weakness and wasting of the intrinsic hand muscles and weakness of the plantar flexor muscles. Ankle joint instability makes it difficult to stand still. The amount of muscle atrophy is usually not great. Typically, the tendon reflexes are reduced or absent, disappearing successively from the Achilles tendon, the quadriceps, and the upper extremity. Sensory loss is mild, affecting the modalities of touch-pressure, two-point discrimination, and joint position and motion in the distal parts of the extremities. Clinical enlargement of peripheral nerves may be detected in about one fourth of the cases. Some members of kinships have, in addition to the clinical features mentioned, a tremor of the head and outstretched hands which is indistinguishable from essential tremor (Roussy-Lévy syndrome). Foot ulcers occasionally occur. Corrective surgery should be reserved for patients who develop ulcers at pressure points owing to excessively high arches and for those with excessive inversion of the foot. Footdrop springs or braces may be used to elevate the toes in walking and to stabilize the ankle.

HEREDITARY MOTOR AND SENSORY NEUROPATHY, TYPE II
(Neuronal Type of Peroneal Muscular Atrophy; Charcot-Marie-Tooth Disease)

This dominantly inherited disorder usually begins in the second decade of life, occasionally as late as the fifth or sixth decade. Symmetrical muscle weakness with atrophy begins in small foot muscles, peroneal, long toe extensor, and ankle dorsiflexor muscles. Pes cavus and hammer toes may or may not be associated with the weakness. Initial symptoms include inability to pick up the toes in walking, instability of the ankle, difficulty in standing immobile, and visible atrophy of muscles. Later, weakness of small hand muscles develops. The muscle atrophy of the lower limbs may be typical of peroneal muscular atrophy, with a greater degree of atrophy in the distal aspect of thigh muscles and with much atrophy of leg muscles. Tendon reflexes are usually diminished or absent in the lower limbs. Touch-pressure, joint position, and vibration sensation are mildly decreased distally in lower limbs. Conduction velocities of motor fibers are normal in upper limbs and only slightly reduced in lower limbs. Sporadic cases occur. Leg braces that stabilize the ankle joint often permit these patients to stand still without losing balance.

HEREDITARY MOTOR AND SENSORY NEUROPATHY, TYPE III
(Recessively Inherited Hypertrophic Neuropathy)

This is a rare disorder transmitted as an autosomal recessive trait and beginning in infancy. Affected children learn to walk late, have great difficulty in walking even at their best point of neuromuscular development (ages 8 to 12), and are usually in wheelchairs by the age of 20 years. The patients are usually short, and most have a severe, symmetrical sensory motor neuropathy affecting predominantly the distal extremities with enlarged peripheral nerves. Some weakness of proximal muscles of the extremities usually is present also. Sometimes there are associated miosis and nystagmus. The conduction velocities of motor and sensory fibers of peripheral nerves are among the lowest determined in electromyographic laboratories. Pathologically, marked segmental demyelination and remyelination are found in myelinated fibers; unmyelinated fibers are not decreased in number but are probably affected also. A systemic biochemical abnormality involving ceramide hexoses and their sulfates has been found. No specific treatment is available.

HEREDITARY MOTOR AND SENSORY NEUROPATHY, TYPE IV
(Recessively Inherited Hypertrophic Neuropathy with Excess of Phytanic Acid; Refsum's Disease)

This rare progressive or relapsing disorder is inherited as an autosomal recessive trait and is due to the inability of affected subjects to alpha-oxidize ingested phytanic acid. Clinical manifestations usually begin in the second decade with night blindness and constriction of the visual fields owing to an atypical retinitis pigmentosa. Additionally, symptoms caused by a distal sensorimotor neuropathy develop, as well as an ataxia which is thought to be greater than that accounted for by kinesthetic loss. Ichthyosis, skeletal abnormalities, and death in the third or fourth decade from involvement of the heart all provide evidence of systemic extraneural involvement. The cerebrospinal fluid protein is usually markedly elevated. Pathologically, the peripheral nerves contain evidence of segmental demyelination and remyelination and onion-bulb formation. Pathognomonic is the occurrence of elevated levels of 3, 7,11,15-tetramethylhexadecenoic acid (phytanic acid) in the serum, red blood cells, liver, heart, kidneys, and skeletal muscles. Treatment consists of withholding dietary phytols (chlorophyll-free diet); if begun early, it can result in great improvement.

HEREDITARY MOTOR AND SENSORY NEUROPATHY WITH OPTIC ATROPHY, TYPE VI

In this very rare dominantly inherited disorder, there is optic atrophy in addition to peroneal muscular atrophy.

HEREDITARY MOTOR AND SENSORY NEUROPATHY WITH RETINITIS PIGMENTOSA, TYPE VII

This disorder has many of the features of Refsum's syndrome but without elevated plasma phytanic acid levels.

Asbury, A., Victor, M., and Adams, R.: Uremic polyneuropathy. Arch. Neurol., 8:413, 1963.

Austin, J.: Recurrent polyneuropathies and their corticosteroid treatment. Brain, 81:157, 1958.

Cooke, W., and Smith, W.: Neurological disorders associated with coeliac disease. Brain, 89:683, 1966.

Croft, P., Urich, H., and Wilkinson, M.: Peripheral neuropathy of sensorimotor type associated with malignant disease. Brain, 90:31, 1967.

Dyck, P. J., Lais, A. C., Ohta, M., Bastron, J. A., Okazaki, H., and Groover, R. V.: Chronic inflammatory polyradiculoneuropathy. Mayo Clin. Proc., 50:621, 1975.

Dyck, P., and Lambert, E.: Dissociated sensation in amyloidosis. Compound action potential, quantitative histologic and teased-fiber, and electron microscopic studies of sural nerve biopsies. Arch. Neurol., 20:490, 1969.

Dyck, P. J., Thomas, P. K., and Lambert, E. H.: Peripheral Neuropathy. Philadelphia, W. B. Saunders Company, 1975.

Iwashita, H., Ohnishi, A., Asada, M., Kanazawa, Y., and Kuroiwa, Y.: Polyneuropathy, skin hyperpigmentation, edema and hypertrichosis in localized osteosclerotic myeloma. Neurology, 27:675, 1977.

Raff, M., Sangalang, V., and Asbury, A.: Ischemic mononeuropathy multiplex associated with diabetes mellitus. Arch. Neurol., 18:497, 1968.

Sunderland, S.: Nerves and Nerve Injuries. Edinburgh and London, E. and S. Livingstone Ltd., 1968.

Thomas, P. K., and Lascelles, R.: The pathology of diabetic neuropathy. Quart. J. Med., 35:489, 1966.

Tyler, H.: Neurological complications of dialysis, transplantation and other forms of treatment in chronic uremia. Neurology, 15:1081, 1965.

Wiederholt, W., Mulder, D., and Lambert, E.: The Landry-Guillain-Barré-Strohl syndrome or polyradiculoneuropathy. Historical review, report on 97 patients, and present concepts. Mayo Clin. Proc., 39:427, 1964.

Section Twenty-Four   DISEASES OF MUSCLE AND NEUROMUSCULAR JUNCTION

Lewis P. Rowland

338.   INTRODUCTION

DEFINITIONS. Muscles can be weakened by many different disorders. When muscles become weak, they may waste away. Until recently it has been conventional to ascribe the varied causes of weakness and wasting to neurogenic and myopathic disorders, a fundamental pathologic distinction originally made a century ago. In the neurogenic disorders, the brunt of pathologic change was seen in the motor neuron or peripheral nerve; changes in muscle were less pronounced or could be attributed to secondary effects of denervation. In the myopathic disorders, the histopathologic changes in muscle were of different type and there was little abnormality in nerve cell or peripheral nerve.

Pathologic criteria, however, have limitations when one is dealing with living people. Muscle biopsy is possible, but there is no way of obtaining a sample of the spinal cord. Other criteria were therefore introduced to separate neurogenic and myopathic disorders: clinical and genetic characteristics, electromyography, nerve conduction velocity, and assay of serum activity of sarcoplasmic enzymes. Together, these criteria have provided a reasonably consistent basis for continued separation of those syndromes characterized by weakness into neurogenic and myopathic groups.

The concept, however, has been shaken in recent years. Denervation and cross-innervation studies of fast and slow muscles have shown that physiologic and biochemical characteristics of muscle are under neural control. A new kind of electrophysiologic evidence has been adduced to indicate a neurogenic cause for the muscular dystrophies, long held to be the prototype of myopathy. Unsurprisingly, there is confusion, perhaps more than necessary. Under the circumstances, the traditional separation of neurogenic and myopathic disease will be perpetuated in this section.

An air of vagueness pervades some of the language used to describe neuromuscular diseases, and the same words have different meanings to different authorities. Since the ideas are important, it is appropriate to define some of the more prevalent words.

The word *atrophy* means, literally, "lack of nourishment." It has come to mean wasting of muscle, or loss of muscle bulk from any cause, and it is also used to denote single muscle fibers that are smaller than normal when viewed microscopically. But when used in the name of a disease, it always implies that the muscle wasting is secondary to a neural disorder, e.g., infantile spinal muscular atrophy, progressive spinal muscular atrophy, or peroneal muscular atrophy. To avoid ambiguity, it is therefore appropriate in examining patients to use "wasting" rather than "atrophy" to describe diminution in muscle bulk unless the cause is known to be neurogenic. *Myopathies* include disorders characterized by weakness or some other symptom of muscle dysfunction that is not due to emotional or neurogenic cause. Some authors speak of "primary" or "secondary" myopathies but there is little evidence that any muscle disease is really "primary," in the sense that there is an abnormality in muscle and nowhere else. In some myopathies, as in thyrotoxic myopathy, the fundamental disorder is elsewhere, and this could be true even in genetically determined diseases. The *dystrophies* are a subgroup of myopathy with three special characteristics: heritable transmission, progressive weakness, and histologic evidence of degeneration of muscle with no evidence of abnormally stored material or structural abnormality of the fibers. There are other genetic disorders of muscle in which the weakness seems to be stationary, and some in which progressive weakness is not the dominant symptom (transient attacks of weakness in periodic paralysis, cramps, and myoglobinuria in some glycogen diseases, or myotonia); other names are given to these conditions individually.

DIFFERENTIATION OF NEUROGENIC AND MYOPATHIC DISEASE

Sick muscles are usually weak. Few other symptoms result; sometimes muscles ache (myalgia); sometimes they relax with difficulty (myotonia); sometimes they shorten abruptly and painfully (cramp or contracture). Weakness is also the symptom that results from neurogenic diseases affecting corticospinal pathways, motor neurons, or peripheral nerves. The differential diagnosis of muscle disease is therefore a problem in distinguishing myopathic from neurogenic causes. Corticospinal disorders have characteristic signs that immediately identify them, and therefore they do not often enter into this differential diagnosis. Disorders of the lower motor neuron or peripheral nerve may be difficult and sometimes impossible to separate from muscle disease. In this kind of neurogenic disorder and in myopathies, weakness, wasting, and depression of myotatic reflexes are common to both groups. Neurogenic disorders are apt to affect distal muscles primarily, whereas myopathic disorders are more likely to affect proximal muscle, but there are so many exceptions that this is an unreliable guide. (Distal myopathy is rare but does occur; proximal weakness is not so rare in motor neuron disease or peripheral neuropathy.) Twitching of muscle is probably a reliable guide to motor neuron disease, but it is not yet definitely excluded as a myopathic sign. The combination of active reflexes in a limb with weak, wasted, and twitching muscles is almost pathognomonic of amyotrophic lateral sclerosis, especially if there are also Babinski signs. Sensory loss and an increased protein content of the cerebrospinal fluid are reliable guides to peripheral neuropathy, but once it is established that there is a peripheral neuropathy, it may be difficult or impossible to state whether there is also a concomitant myopathy. Because of these ambiguities in clinical diagnosis, increasing attention has been directed to three laboratory aids: serum enzymes, electromyography and nerve conduction velocities, and muscle biopsy. Some syndromes are virtually defined by electromyography: distal myopathy and "juvenile muscular atrophy simulating muscular dystrophy."

SERUM ENZYMES. Several different enzyme activities are increased in the serum of patients with X-linked dystrophies and polymyositis, whereas they are not increased in neurogenic diseases. It is often stated that determination of creatine phosphokinase (CPK) activity is the most sensitive. This enzyme is significantly increased in almost all muscle diseases, but it is, if anything, too sensitive; it picks up all the myopathic cases, but it is sometimes also increased in neurogenic disease. Other serum enzyme levels, e.g., SGOT or lactate dehydrogenase (LDH) and others, do not rise so much in myopathies, but neither do they give falsely positive reactions in neurogenic disorders. For this reason, it is useful to couple determinations of CPK with SGOT or LDH in evaluating individual cases. CPK has one other considerable advantage: it is not present in erythrocytes or liver and is therefore normal in serum contaminated by hemolysis or in patients with liver disease. Isoenzyme analysis has not improved diagnosis.

ELECTROMYOGRAPHY. Needle electromyography has been refined to a very useful technique. Normal muscle is electrically silent at rest, and patterns of potentials evoked by voluntary contraction have been analyzed in terms of frequency, duration, and amplitude of individual motor unit potentials. In denervated muscle, there is spontaneous activity (fibrillations from single muscle fibers or fasciculations from motor units), the number of potentials during a voluntary contraction is reduced, and the duration of potentials is increased. In myopathic disorders, there is usually no spontaneous activity, there is no reduction in the number of potentials under voluntary control, and the potentials are reduced in duration. These signs are usually reliable, but in some cases the results are equivocal, and there may be features of both a neurogenic and myopathic disorder.

NERVE CONDUCTION VELOCITIES. The speed of conduction along motor nerves can be recorded accurately, and slowing of conduction is a reliable guide to neuropathy. A normal conduction velocity, however, does not exclude a nerve lesion.

MUSCLE BIOPSY. The features of neurogenic and myopathic diseases can usually be differentiated in a muscle biopsy, especially with the new techniques of the rapid examination of frozen tissue and the application of histochemical methods. The electron microscope has opened new approaches that are still in the process of refinement. Only a few diseases can be definitively identified by muscle biopsy: periarteritis nodosa, trichinosis, sarcoidosis, and most (but not all) cases of lipid or glycogen storage disease. The congenital myopathies are best identified by histochemical and other special procedures.

In most cases, the results of all these special studies are consistent, one with the other. In some cases, however, the results are conflicting, and problems of classification remain.

Black, J. T., Bhatt, G. P., DeJesus, P. V., et al.: Diagnostic accuracy of clinical data, quantitative electromyography and histochemistry in neuromuscular disease. J. Neurol. Sci., 21:59, 1974.
Buchthal, F.: Electrophysiological signs of myopathy as related with muscle biopsy. Acta Neurol. Scand., 32:1, 1977.
Dubowitz, V., and Brooke, M. H.: Muscle Biopsy: A Modern Approach. Philadelphia, W. B. Saunders Company, 1973.
Lenman, J. A. P., and Ritchie, A. E.: Clinical Electromyography. Philadelphia, J. B. Lippincott Company, 1970.
McComas, A. J., Sica, A. E. P., and Campbell, M. J.: "Sick" motoneurones. A unifying concept of muscle disease. Lancet, 1:321, 1971.
Rowland, L. P.: Are the muscular dystrophies neurogenic? Ann. N. Y. Acad. Sci., 228:244, 1974.

339. INHERITED DISEASES

339.1. MUSCULAR DYSTROPHIES

DEFINITION. Muscular dystrophies are inherited myopathies, characterized primarily by progressively severe weakness. In the absence of known biochemical abnormality, they are distinguished from similar diseases by lack of histologic evidence of any metabolic storage material, or by changes other than those of degeneration and regeneration of muscle or tissue reactions to these processes.

ETIOLOGY. Although it is generally believed that inherited diseases must be due to a missing or structurally abnormal protein (either an enzyme or a structural protein), this abnormality has not been identified in any form of dystrophy. Increasing biochemical and ultrastructural evidence implicates the muscle surface membrane as the site of fundamental disorder. There is evidence of dysfunction of enzymes which are an integral part of the membrane, and there are gaps in the plasma membrane that permit the entry of large molecules such as horseradish peroxidase, a protein, or procion yellow, a dye. Membranes of erythrocytes from patients with Duchenne or myotonic dystrophy also exhibit biochemical and functional deviations from normal, although this is not reflected in any symptomatic disorder of red blood cells or anemia. Pathologic and biochemical abnormalities can be detected in muscle, and there is no clear evidence of neural abnormality in traditional terms. It is conceivable, however, that the fundamental abnormality is in another organ (such as the liver or bowel) and that the muscular abnormalities are secondary. There is still debate about the possible role of altered motor neurons, and some writers postulate a debatable vascular cause, functional ischemia of muscle.

CLASSIFICATION. No classification of the muscular dystrophies is entirely satisfactory, but clinical and genetic analysis provides the best approach at present. The classification in the accompanying table is based upon the clearly identifiable features of Duchenne dystrophy, facioscapulohumeral dystrophy, and myotonic muscular dystrophy. Limb-girdle dystrophy is probably not a single disease, but encompasses cases that do not fall into the other categories.

INCIDENCE. None of the muscular dystrophies are common. Incidence rates vary from 5 per million births for facioscapulohumeral dystrophy to about 250 per million births for Duchenne dystrophy. Many cases

Classification of Human Muscular Dystrophies

	Duchenne Dystrophy	Facioscapulohumeral Dystrophy	Limb-Girdle Dystrophy	Myotonic Dystrophy
Genetic pattern	X-linked, recessive	Autosomal, dominant	Autosomal, recessive	Autosomal, dominant
Age at onset	Before age 5	Adolescence	Adolescence	Early or late
First symptoms	Pelvic	Shoulders	Pelvic	Distal; hands or feet
Pseudohypertrophy	+	0	0	0
Predominant weakness, early	Proximal	Proximal	Proximal	Distal
Progression	Relatively rapid; incapacitated in adolescence	Slow	Variable	Slow
Facial weakness	0	+	0	Occasional
Ocular, oropharyngeal weakness	0	0	0	Occasional
Myotonia	0	0	0	+
Cardiomyopathy	0 or late	0	0	Arrhythmia, conduction block
Associated disorders	None (?mental retardation)	None	None	Cataracts; testicular atrophy and baldness in men
Serum enzymes	Very high	Slight or no increase	Slight or no increase	Slight or no increase
Prevalence (per million population)	38	5	20	25
Incidence (per million births)	251	5	47	—
Mutation rate	9×10^{-5}	5×10^{-7}	3×10^{-5}	10×10^{-6}

seen to be sporadic; the mutation rate of Duchenne dystrophy is high, 7×10^{-5}, and about two thirds of the cases appear sporadically, with no other affected individual in the family.

PATHOLOGY. Pathologic abnormalities are restricted to skeletal muscle, sometimes involving cardiac muscle. The brain, spinal cord, and peripheral nerves are devoid of histologic change, although some authors have implicated the brain because of a seemingly high incidence of mental retardation in children with Duchenne dystrophy. Terminal pneumonia may cause changes in the lungs, and there may be a variety of associated diseases not directly linked to the dystrophy. In myotonic muscular dystrophy, baldness and testicular atrophy are integral parts of the disease in men, and corneal opacities affect both sexes.

The abnormalities in muscle seem to involve all fibers in random fashion. Early, there is scattered evidence of necrosis and regeneration, with prominent variation in fiber size, including many fibers much larger than normal and many fibers that appear hyalinized. Later, fibers disappear, to be replaced by fibrous connective tissue and fat. "Pseudohypertrophy" is probably due to both "true" hypertrophy (large fibers) and increased accumulation of fat and connective tissue. In myotonic dystrophy, unusual figures form "ring fibers" (with one fiber running at right angles, encircling the other fibers in the same bundle) and "sarcoplasmic masses," or accumulations of sarcoplasm that are free of myofilaments. However, these abnormalities

occur occasionally in other diseases and are not pathognomonic of myotonic dystrophy. In Duchenne dystrophy, the myocardium may be affected by similar changes, but cardiac symptoms are rarely evident in life, a discrepancy that has been attributed to the sedentary life imposed upon the patients by advanced muscular weakness. Myopathic changes in the heart are common in myotonic dystrophy. There is no good evidence that smooth muscle is affected in any form of dystrophy. Ultrastructural investigations suggest an early, and perhaps primary, abnormality of the muscle surface membrane, but it is not clear how this might be related to the progressive degeneration of muscle. Disruption of myofibrillar structure, alterations of mitochondria, and degeneration of tubules and sarcoplasmic reticulum all seem to proceed together.

CLINICAL MANIFESTATIONS. The symptoms and signs of all forms of the muscular dystrophies are related to weakness alone, except that additional systems are involved in myotonic dystrophy. In other forms, the symptoms depend upon the distribution of weakness and the age at onset. In *Duchenne dystrophy* weakness is primarily proximal at onset, and symptoms begin early. By definition, girls are not affected. There are no symptoms in the first year of life, but walking may be somewhat delayed beyond 18 months. Once the child walks, some abnormality is usually evident to an experienced observer (either a parent with a previously affected child or a skilled physician). The boys tend to waddle when they walk, or walk on their toes, or fall frequently and have difficulty rising. They are probably never able to run, because they have difficulty raising their knees. These symptoms become more evident as the children grow older, and even the most unsuspecting parent becomes aware of some abnormality by age five. Teachers sometimes may detect the difficulty when the child starts school. Some cases are averred to start between ages five and ten, but these must be exceptional. It is difficult to examine individual muscles of a young child, but the waddling gait, the typical method of rising from the ground by "climbing up" himself (Gowers' sign), enlargement of calf or other muscles, and inability to run are characteristic. Myotatic reflexes may be normal at first, but by three years the knee jerks are usually lost, and later the ankle jerks disappear. As the child grows, increased growth and coordination may compensate temporarily for the concurrent progressive weakness and wasting, but the disease always prevails. There is increased difficulty walking. Going up grades or stairs first requires aid, then becomes impossible. Weakness of the trunk muscles leads to increased lordosis and a protuberant abdomen. Then the arms become weak. Finally, in early adolescence, the child becomes unable to walk. This may be accelerated by a period of inactivity after an injury or an orthopedic operation. Contractures appear, at first in the feet, as the gastrocnemius muscles tighten. When the child stops walking, flexion contractures limit motion of the knees, and scoliosis becomes more a problem with prolonged sitting. Ultimately respiration becomes shallow and the child is increasingly subject to pulmonary infection. Sooner or later, one of these infections is fatal, usually in the third decade. Although muscles are ravaged from the neck down, the cranial muscles are entirely spared. Congestive heart failure and abnormalities of cardiac rhythm are rare.

Becker dystrophy has manifestations similar to those of Duchenne dystrophy, but the onset is later in childhood or in adolescence, and the tempo is slower and more variable. This form may also be devastating, but some patients are able to function, albeit with limitations, well into adult life. The clinical similarities include pseudohypertrophy of calf muscles and increased serum content of creatine phosphokinase and other sarcoplasmic enzymes. However, although the two forms are similar, they are genetically separate; there are no mildly affected individuals in typical Duchenne families, nor are children affected severely in Becker families. In some families it is admittedly difficult to decide whether the disorder is Duchenne dystrophy of relatively late appearance or Becker dystrophy of relatively early appearance. The distinction awaits recognition of the biochemical abnormalities in the two or more forms.

The manifestations of *limb-girdle dystrophy* are also similar because weakness of muscles of the pelvic girdle usually initiates the syndrome, but symptoms start in late childhood or adolescence. Girls are affected as often as boys, and pseudohypertrophy is rare. Waddling gait, difficulty in walking and climbing, and frequent falls are common. Occasionally, symptoms begin in the shoulder girdle. In either case, there is usually weakness in all four limbs by the time the patient seeks medical attention. The severity, age at onset, and rate of progression vary considerably, suggesting that this category contains more than one disease.

Facioscapulohumeral dystrophy is distinct. Symptoms vary in severity so that some affected individuals never have any disability (but can be recognized by the signs), whereas others become incapacitated early; there are all grades in between. The first symptoms are apt to be related to difficulty in raising the arms or to prominence of the scapulae. Weakness of the legs may affect pelvic girdle muscles, or equally prominent weakness of the anterior tibial muscles may lead to a steppage gait. Truncal weakness may lead to prominent scoliosis. The face is always involved on examination; the perioral muscles may be more affected than those of the upper face, but ultimately patients develop difficulty in closing the eyes. The sternal head of the pectoral muscle is affected earlier than the clavicular head, a selectivity that can be detected on testing the individual muscles, and leads to a peculiar appearance of the axillary folds when the arms are dependent, because the anterior axillary fold of normal people is formed by the sternal portion of the pectoral muscle. Winging of the scapulae can be seen when the patient leans against a wall with the arms extended, and the weakness of shoulder girdle muscles leads to an unusual appearance because, viewed from the front, the superior margin of the scapula is higher than the clavicle.

Myotonic muscular dystrophy diverges from the preceding types in several respects. (1) The distribution of weakness differs in that cranial muscles are often affected and limb weakness is initially more marked in distal muscles. Thus weakness of the hands (as in twisting bottle caps or using tools) precedes shoulder weakness, and footdrop or steppage gait precedes symptoms of pelvic muscle weakness. *Ptosis, facial weakness,* and *dysarthria* are signs not seen in the other forms of dystrophy. Moreover, there is almost always selective weakness and smallness of the sternomastoids. The masticatory muscles either are poorly developed or waste early (even when not symptomatically weak), causing a characteristic long, lean facial facial appearance. (2) Myotonia, or difficulty in relaxation, may be symptomatic, and after a firm grip the patient may have difficulty letting go. Myotonia may cause other symptoms in patients with myotonia congenita (see below), but in the dystrophy only the hands are affected by this kind of stiffness. Myotonia of grip may be evident on examination, and can also be elicited by percussing the thenar eminence. In normal persons this evokes a rapid twitch, whereas in patients with myotonia, a sustained contraction of the adductor pollicis muscle persists for several seconds, only gradually relaxing. Similar responses to percussion may be elicited uncommonly in other limb muscles, but can often be seen in the tongue. Although myotonia is a dramatic sign and a symptom that can be relieved by drugs, it is not the symptom that causes the major disability in myotonic dystrophy; weakness is the problem. (3) Other systems are involved in this pleomorphic disorder; cataracts appear sooner or later in all patients, and are sometimes the only sign of the disease; most of the men (but not the women) have frontal baldness; testicular atrophy affects most of the men, but often after they have already sired children to perpetuate the disease (there is no definite evidence of gonadal insufficiency in affected women); the basal metabolic rate is often low, but other tests of thyroid function are normal (extrathyroidal hypometabolism). The incidence of diabetes mellitus may be increased. (4) Conduction defects are common in the electrocardiogram, and may lead to clinically significant arrhythmia or congestive heart failure.

Certain rare forms of muscular dystrophy are named after the prominent manifestations. *Ocular dystrophy* is a slowly progressive disorder in which ptosis of the eyelids and progressive immobility of the eyes are the cardinal features. The pupils are spared, and both eyes are usually affected symmetrically so that diplopia is uncommon. Other muscles of the head, neck, and limbs may also be affected, varying from family to family. This syndrome raises problems of definition; some cases probably are myopathic in origin, but this kind of ophthalmoplegia is often associated with other manifestations that are clearly neurogenic (such as spinocerebellar degeneration or peripheral neuropathy). The final distinction is often difficult or impossible to make because in the ocular muscles signs of myopathy in muscle biopsy or electromyography are not valid. In some patients with myopathic ophthalmoplegia, structural and biochemical abnormalities may be found in limb muscles. Abnormally large mitochondria are present in increased numbers; this can be seen dramatically in electron microscopy, and the numbers are sufficient to stain fibers red in the trichrome stain for light microscopy, leading to the appellation "ragged red fibers." In these cases there is apt to be an accumulation of glycogen, but the biochemical cause of this has not been ascertained.

Distal myopathy, as the name implies, affects distal leg and hand muscles first. It is probably the rarest form of dystrophy, and can be identified only by characteristic signs of myopathy in electromyography and muscle biopsy.

In the *scapuloperoneal syndrome* distal weakness in the legs resembles that of neurogenic peroneal muscular atrophy, but sensory loss is lacking, and there is proximal weakness in the shoulder girdle similar to that of facioscapulohumeral dystrophy. Some of these cases are myopathic and some neurogenic as distinguished by electromyography, muscle biopsy, and serum enzymes. In either case, autosomal dominant inheritance and a relatively slow progression seem characteristic.

DIAGNOSIS. The clinical picture of Duchenne dystrophy entails little diagnostic confusion. In its first stages, some children are merely regarded as clumsy, and some receive orthopedic care because of toe-walking; otherwise the diagnosis becomes obvious. As noted, the trait is transmitted as a sex-linked recessive, and once a case is recognized, members of the family rapidly detect the signs in subsequently affected youngsters. Once a family is known, affected individuals can be identified in the neonatal period because the serum enzymes are already markedly abnormal. Limb-girdle and facioscapulohumeral dystrophy must be differentiated from neurogenic diseases, from congenital myopathies, and from polymyositis, as will be discussed below. Myotonic dystrophy may be confused with endocrine disorders or, because of the distal weakness, with neuropathy or amyotrophy, or with hypothyroidism or gonadal disorders. Ocular myopathy must be differentiated from myasthenia gravis; there is no fluctuation of symptoms in the myopathy, and the weakness does not respond to cholinergic drugs.

These familial cases of progressive ophthalmoplegia (ocular muscular dystrophy) also have to be distinguished from an unusual syndrome that seems to be sporadic, not yet reported in more than one person in a family. This form is identified by progressive ophthalmoplegia, pigmentary degeneration of the retina, and onset before age 15. When these three features are identified, almost all the patients will be found to have evidence of heart block on the electrocardiogram and cerebrospinal fluid protein content of more than 100 mg per deciliter. More than half of these patients also have short stature, hearing loss, and evidence of corticospinal tract or cerebellar disease. The constellation is sufficiently consistent to warrant designation as the Kearns-Sayre syndrome.

The differential diagnosis of the myopathies depends also upon the age of the patient. In childhood and adolescence, the major problems involve peroneal muscular atrophy (Charcot-Marie-Tooth) and "muscular atrophy simulating muscular dystrophy" (Wohlfart-Kugelberg-Welander). In adults, amyotrophic lateral sclerosis is the major problem. At all ages, polyneuritis must be considered.

TREATMENT. There is no specific treatment for the weakness of any form of dystrophy. Physical therapy exercises, splints, braces, and corrective orthopedic surgery are applied in different centers with varying degrees of enthusiasm. Some claim that walking can be prolonged into late adolescence in Duchenne dystrophy. The most poignant decisions concern the use of antimicrobial drugs or supported respiration for young men paralyzed from the neck down and with no hope of ultimate recovery. The myotonia of myotonic dystrophy can be relieved by diphenylhydantoin (0.3 to 0.6 gram daily), quinine (0.3 to 1.5 grams daily), or procainamide (4 to 6 grams daily), but this is rarely the problem, and nothing can be done for the weakness. Cataracts are treated surgically upon appropriate indication, and cardiac arrhythmias or congestive heart failure are managed accordingly.

PROPHYLAXIS. Genetic counseling offers the only possibility to control muscular dystrophy at present. Carriers of Duchenne dystrophy may often but not always be identified by abnormally increased serum enzyme activity (higher than normal, but not as high as in affected boys). In some centers, antenatal detection of sex allows selective prophylactic abortion. There is presently no way to determine whether a male fetus is affected, however. The development of methods to sample fetal blood has led to attempts to measure creatine phosphokinase. This technique may ultimately provide the way to identify the true biochemical abnormality in the fetus, assuming that it will be the same in both muscle and erythrocytes, an assumption that is not proved. Birth control ought to be effective in dominantly inherited diseases such as facioscapulohumeral and myotonic dystrophy, but since many cases are mild, few will accept continence. The high rates of mutation do not encourage optimism that genetic restriction can be the ultimate goal.

Berenberg, R. A., Pellock, J. M., DiMauro, S., et al.: Lumping or splitting? "Ophthalmoplegia plus" or Kearns-Sayre syndrome? Ann. Neurol., 1:37, 1977.

Mokri, B., and Engel, A. G.: Duchenne dystrophy: Electron microscopic findings pointing to a basic or early abnormality in the plasma membrane of the muscle fiber. Neurology, 25:1111, 1975.

Panayiotopoulos, C. P., and Scarpalezos, S.: Muscular dystrophies and motoneuron diseases. Neurology, 26:721, 1976.

Roses, A. D., Herbstreith, M., Metcalf, B., and Appell, S. H.: Increased phosphorylated components of erythrocyte membrane spectrin band II with reference to Duchenne dystrophy. J. Neurol. Sci., 30:167, 1976.

Rowland, L. P. (ed.): Pathogenesis of Human Muscular Dystrophies. Amsterdam, Excerpta Medica, 1977.

Walton, J. N.: Disorders of Voluntary Muscle. 3rd ed. Edinburgh, Churchill Livingstone, 1974.

Cornelio, F., DiDonato, S., Pelúchetti, D., et al.: Fatal cases of lipid storage myopathy with carnitine deficiency. J. Neurol. Neurosurg. Psychiat. 40:170, 1977.

DiMauro, S., and Eastwood, A. B.: Disorders of glycogen and lipid metabolism. Adv. Neurol., 17:123, 1977.

339.2. OTHER INHERITED BIOCHEMICAL DISORDERS

Although the glycogen storage diseases are discussed in more detail in Ch. 531.4, it is necessary to mention them here, because they enter into differential diagnosis and because they were the first inherited muscle diseases in which the biochemical defect was discerned. Of the several forms, the only ones that do not affect muscle are type 1 (lack of glucose-6-phosphate dehydrogenase) and type 6 (lack of liver phosphorylase).

Pompe's disease, the infantile form of glycogen storage disease Type 2, is associated with lack of acid maltase. It affects motor neurons and muscle, causing a clinical disorder that resembles Werdnig-Hoffmann disease, from which it is distinguished by glossomegaly and cardiomegaly with congestive heart failure. It is uniformly fatal by one year of age. In another group of disorders, the same enzyme is missing, but the disease starts later in childhood, or even in adult years. The syndrome is one of proximal limb weakness that resembles either limb-girdle dystrophy or polymyositis, and the only clinical clues to the nature of the disease are the prominence of respiratory failure and the presence of myotonic discharges in the electromyogram. Histologically, there is a vacuolar myopathy, which can be shown to be due to deposition of glycogen. Lack of acid maltase is demonstrated by biochemical assay of muscle homogenates or in the urine. Ketogenic diet and other dietary manipulations have been attempted, with little therapeutic effect.

Type 3 glycogen storage disease, caused by lack of the debrancher enzyme system, is usually manifest by hepatomegaly and hypoglycemia, but skeletal muscle may be involved with the liver, or even alone. This disorder may also resemble limb-girdle dystrophy or polymyositis. Again, diagnosis is suspected on the basis of histochemical study of muscle and proved by biochemical analysis. Types 5 and 7, resulting from lack of phosphorylase or phosphofructokinase, are causes of recurrent myoglobinuria.

Another group of diseases sometimes involves storage of glycogen, but the dominant biochemical abnormalities are lipid storage in muscle, sometimes with lactic acidosis, and often with proliferation of malformed mitochondria. These disorders may be manifest by a proximal myopathy alone, or in combination with mental retardation and seizures. One form of lipid storage disease is associated with abnormally low content of carnitine in muscle with no systemic abnormalities. Oral carnitine therapy may be beneficial. In another form, the liver is affected as well, with low tissue concentrations of carnitine in that organ and also in blood plasma, and the clinical disorder is punctuated by episodes of hepatic encephalopathy that may be fatal.

339.3. CONGENITAL MYOPATHIES

DEFINITION. These are rare diseases characterized by weakness that is usually mild but persists throughout life, either progressing slowly or remaining stationary.

ETIOLOGY. The cause is not known. A few of these disorders are familial and suspected of having a genetic basis, but so many cases are sporadic that other causes are not excluded, and there are no clear clues.

PATHOLOGY. These diseases are defined in terms of pathology, and most of them have been delineated within the past 15 years since the introduction of histochemical techniques to study muscle biopsy. The names of the diseases reflect the predominant anatomic disorder.

In *central core disease*, the central portion of the muscle fiber appears rather amorphous, in contrast to the fibrillar appearance of the surrounding normal portion. In cross-section, the central portion appears blue when stained with Gomori's trichrome, in striking contrast to the red periphery. The central areas lack all oxidative enzyme activity, and there are no mitochondria in this region. In *nemaline myopathy or rod myopathy*, small threadlike or rod bodies are scattered throughout the fiber. The rods are barely visible in conventional hematoxylin and eosin stains, but can be seen readily in phase contrast or with the trichrome stain. In electron microscopy the structures seem to originate in the Z-band, and circumstantial evidence suggests that they are composed of tropomyosin. *Myotubular myopathy* designates the appearance of myofibers that resemble a stage in the early development of fetal muscle, with nuclei located centrally rather than at the periphery and surrounded by a halo of apparently empty space. Because the pathogenesis of this appearance is uncertain, some investigators prefer the name *centronuclear myopathy*. In other disorders mitochondria have appeared abnormal, either in number (too many) or size (too large), often associated with accumulations of lipid droplets.

CLINICAL MANIFESTATIONS. Although designated "congenital," these disorders are only exceptionally symptomatic in the first year of life, except that the onset of walking may be delayed. Later, the symptoms of proximal limb weakness become evident: waddling gait, difficulty in climbing stairs, frequent falls, and scoliosis. Later, there may be weakness of the arms. There are few clinical clues to each specific histologic abnormality. Among the nemaline cases there have been skeletal abnormalities (kyphoscoliosis, pigeon breast, pes cavus, high palate, and an unusually elongated face). In two families with myotubular disease, ophthalmoplegia was present as well as limb weakness. Central core and mitochondrial disorders have not been associated with distinctive clinical signs other than proximal limb weakness. Abnormal mitochondria have been found in a variety of different clinical syndromes: euthyroid hypermetabolism (Luft's syndrome), proximal limb weakness with or without lactic acidosis or lipid storage, ocular myopathies, the Kearns-Sayre form of progressive ophthalmoplegia, variable limb weakness, cramps, and fatigue syndromes, among others. In none of the structurally defined congenital myopathies, therefore, is it possible to link the morphologic abnormality to a biochemical or physiologic cause of the weakness.

DIAGNOSIS. Proximal limb weakness in a young child is usually myopathic in origin, but must be distinguished from the neurogenic Wohlfart-Kugelberg-Welander syndrome and from polyneuritis. Myopathic abnormalities in the electromyogram, an abnormal family history, an incidence in girls, and especially the histologic abnormalities define the individual entities. The serum enzymes may be normal or slightly increased. In some clinics most cases of apparently congenital myopathy fail to meet the specific histologic criteria, showing only nonspecific myopathic changes in biopsy. There is no better designation for these cases than "congenital myopathy," but it is likely that there is more than one cause.

In infancy, the major cause of weakness is a form of motor neuron disease (Werdnig-Hoffmann disease). Among infants with multiple congenitally fixed joints (arthrogryposis multiplex), some prove to have myopathic disease as defined by muscle biopsy and electromyography. In some cases, neonatal difficulty in swallowing is followed by delayed onset of walking, possibly persistent weakness, obesity, childhood diabetes, mental retardation, and a characteristic facial appearance (Prader-Willi syndrome), but there is no abnormality on muscle biopsy or electromyogram.

TREATMENT AND PROGNOSIS. There is no specific treatment for any of these disorders. Physical therapy and orthopedic corrective measures are of value. There are too few cases to generalize about the course of these illnesses; most seem to be mild and nonprogressive, but occasional cases are more severe.

Afifi, A. K., Ibrahim, M. Z. M., Bergman, R. A., Haydar, N. A., Mire, J., Bahuth, N., and Kaylani, F.: Morphologic features of hypermetabolic mitochondrial disease. J. Neurol. Sci., 15:271, 1972.

Bharucha, E. P., Pandya, S. S., and Dastur, D. K.: Arthrogryposis multiplex congenita. J. Neurol. Neurosurg. Psychiatry, 35:425, 1972.

DiMauro, S., Schotland, D. L., Bonilla, E., et al: Mitochondrial myopathies. Which and how many? In Milhorat, A. T. (ed.): Exploratory Concepts in Muscular Dystrophy II. Amsterdam, Excerpta Medica, 1974, pp. 506–516.

Dubowitz, V.: The Floppy Infant. London, Spastics International Medical Publications, 1969.

Gordon, A. S., Rewcastle, N. B., Humphrey, J. G., and Stewart, B. M.: Chronic benign congenital myopathy; fingerprint body type. Can. J. Neurol. Sci., 1:106, 1974.

Hall, B. D., and Smith, D. W.: Prader-Willi syndrome: A résumé of 32 cases, J. Pediat., 81:286, 1972.

Kinoshita, M., Satoyashi, E., and Matsuo, N.: Myotubular myopathy and type 1 fiber atrophy in a family. J. Neurol. Sci., 26:575, 1975.

Kinoshita, M., Satoyashi, E., and Suzuki, Y.: Atypical myopathy with myofibrillar aggregates. Arch. Neurol., 32:417, 1975.

339.4. MYOTONIA CONGENITA

(Thomsen's Disease)

DEFINITION. Myotonia congenita is a rare disorder characterized by difficulty in relaxation of skeletal muscle after forceful contraction, present from early childhood.

ETIOLOGY. There are occasional sporadic cases, but most are inherited in a pattern corresponding to an autosomal dominant trait. In a few families, the disease seems to be autosomal recessive. The biochemical fault is not known, but the muscle membrane is electrically unstable and tends to fire repetitively. The abnormality must be inherent within the muscle, because myotonic

phenomena may be elicited after all neural influences are abolished by spinal anesthesia, block of motor nerves by local anesthesia, or blockade of the neuromuscular junction by intra-arterial injection of d-tubocurarine. Myotonia is abolished, however, by the intramuscular administration of procaine. In human myotonia congenita, as in a genetic myotonia of goats, there seems to be an abnormality of chloride conductance in muscle, and this could account for the tendency to discharge repetitively. The disorder in myotonic muscular dystrophy seems to differ, and it is possible that the biochemical abnormality is different in each of the several forms of inherited human myotonia.

CLINICAL MANIFESTATIONS. The difficulty in relaxation is widespread. Difficulty in relaxing the grip may lead to prominent and sometimes embarrassing symptoms. Ocular muscles may be affected, so that the eyes seem momentarily "stuck" in one position, or the eyelids may remain closed after forceful closure. Sometimes oropharyngeal muscles are affected, with difficulty in speaking or swallowing. Startle reactions may induce stiffness of the legs, thwarting sudden attempts to catch a bus or run from home plate. There is no weakness, and one unexplained characteristic is the unusual muscular development of many patients, causing a Herculean appearance, perhaps related to involuntary and repeated isometric exercise. The myotonia can be elicited by tapping any muscle in severely affected cases. Reflexes are unaltered.

DIAGNOSIS. The major problem is in distinguishing the disorder from myotonic muscular dystrophy. Here the only symptoms and signs are related to myotonia. There is no weakness, cataract, baldness, or gonadal atrophy. So-called "transitional cases" are probably patients in families with myotonic muscular dystrophy who are only mildly affected and show only myotonia before the other manifestations. There may be some weakness in families with the rare autosomal recessive form of myotonia congenita. In general, families with myotonia congenita breed true.

TREATMENT. For many years, quinine was the staple treatment in doses of 0.3 to 1.5 grams daily. Recently, phenytoin has proved equally effective and less apt to cause disagreeable side effects in therapeutic doses of 0.3 to 0.6 gram daily. Should this fail, procainamide may also be used, in doses of 4 to 6 grams daily, but this drug is prone to induce lupus erythematosus.

Barchi, R. L.: Myotonia. An evaluation of the chloride hypothesis. Arch. Neurol., 32:1575, 1975.

Becker, F.: Myotonic syndromes. In Rowland, L. P. (ed.): Pathogenesis of Human Muscular Dystrophies. Amsterdam, Excerpta Medica, 1977.

339.5. FAMILIAL MYOGLOBINURIA

Most cases of myoglobinuria are sporadic, and they will be described in Ch. 340.3. Some persons, however, have repeated attacks from early childhood, suggesting some genetic fault, and sometimes more than one individual in a family is affected. Some of these familial cases are due to lack of muscle phosphorylase or phosphofructokinase. They can be recognized by the ischemic work test in which contracture is induced and venous lactate fails to rise. (See Ch. 531.4.) In several families, recurrent myoglobinuria has been associated with lack of carnitine palmityl transferase, the enzyme necessary for the oxidation of long-chain fatty acids. In other cases, however, no abnormality has been found of either glycogen or lipid metabolism.

Bank, W. J., DiMauro, S., Bonilla, E., Capuzzi, D. M., and Rowland, L. P.: A disorder of lipid metabolism and myoglobinuria. Absence of carnitine palmityl transferase. N. Engl. J. Med., 292:443, 1975.

339.6. FAMILIAL PERIODIC PARALYSIS

DEFINITION. Periodic paralysis is characterized by recurrent attacks of flaccid weakness usually associated with abnormally high or low serum potassium concentrations. Many cases are familial. In sporadic cases the abnormality may be secondary to aberrations of potassium metabolism.

ETIOLOGY AND PATHOGENESIS. Familial cases are distributed in a pattern consistent with autosomal dominant inheritance. Hypokalemia during attacks was the first metabolic abnormality to be recognized, with no loss of potassium in urine. It was presumed that potassium shifted from extracellular to intracellular compartments, especially muscle. This has been difficult to prove, and the anticipated hyperpolarization of the muscle membrane potential has not been substantiated by direct measurement with intracellular electrodes. Abnormalities of glucose metabolism have been suspected, because attacks can be precipitated by infusions of glucose and insulin, by eating a large meal, or by administration of epinephrine. However, biochemical studies have failed to pinpoint the abnormality.

During the past two decades it has been recognized that the serum potassium tends to rise in some patients, and attacks in these individuals are induced by the ingestion of potassium. This variety is therefore called "hyperkalemic periodic paralysis," and is generally considered to be the mirror image of the hypokalemic type, with potassium presumably shifting out of muscle and into blood during attacks. Why this should happen is not clear, but at least in the hyperkalemic type there are alterations of the intracellular potential in the direction required by theory. There are clinical differences between the two forms of periodic paralysis, but there are so many areas of overlap and so many common features that it is difficult to decide just how many genetically distinct forms there really are.

PATHOLOGY. In both forms of periodic paralysis there may be vacuoles within muscle fibers. These may be numerous or scanty, and it is not clear whether they are more frequent in paralyzed muscle. Most electron microscopists believe that the vacuoles are derived from the sarcoplasmic reticulum, but others think they originate in the T-system in areas of necrotic muscle. Glycogen seems to be increased in amount in ultrastructural studies, but the results of biochemical analysis have been inconsistent. There is no evidence that other organs are affected in either form of the disease. The heart is usually spared pathologically.

CLINICAL MANIFESTATIONS. There are clinical differences between the two forms. In the hypokalemic variety, attacks tend to start in late childhood or adolescence, frequently occur at night, are apt to be severe, and last for a day or more. In the hyperkalemic variety, attacks start at an early age, occur much more frequently, tend to be milder, and may last minutes or hours.

Moreover, patients with hyperkalemic periodic paralysis usually have some evidence of myotonia, often limited to percussion myotonia of the tongue. Lid-lag and Chvostek's sign are identified with the hyperkalemic type. These clinical distinctions may break down in application to individual cases and are only crude guides. Moreover, many features are common to both types: a dominant pattern of inheritance, a susceptibility to attacks during periods of rest after vigorous exercise, the ability to ward off attacks by mild exercise after a mild attack has begun, persistent weakness between attacks, vacuoles in muscle, a lack of clear relation between the serum potassium concentration and the severity of paresis, the induction of local weakness by cooling, and protection against attacks by acetazolamide. Some patients are affected by attacks in which the serum potassium may be either high or low.

Typical attacks start with weakness of the legs that ascends to the arms. Cranial muscles are affected in severe attacks only, and respiratory insufficiency is exceptional. The attacks may be mild and brief, or severe and prolonged, with all gradations in between. During severe attacks, the myotatic reflexes are lost, and the muscles are electrically inexcitable. Attacks are rarely apoplectic in onset and usually take an hour or more to develop, except that attacks beginning in sleep may be fully developed when the patient awakes. Paresthesias and myalgia may be prominent at the onset, or may be completely lacking. Some patients are aware of oliguria during the attack and of diuresis afterward.

The serum potassium is in the range of 2.5 to 3.5 mEq per liter in hypokalemic attacks, and 5.0 to 7.0 mEq per liter in the hyperkalemic type. Between attacks serum potassium values may be normal. The electrocardiogram is altered as would be predicted from the serum values, with low T waves in hypokalemia and peaked T waves in hyperkalemia.

Patients with hyperkalemic periodic paralysis may have mild myotonia, especially of the hands. When individuals in a family are studied, some may be found to have myotonia without any history of periodic paralysis.

In both types of the disease, there may be persistent weakness between attacks, most often proximal, sometimes distal. In the past this has been attributed to a permanent "myopathy," but experience with acetazolamide therapy indicates that even longlasting weakness may be reversible, regardless of pathologic changes in muscle. A few patients with intermittent normokalemic or hyperkalemic paralysis have had persistent cardiac arrhythmia, especially bigeminy, and bouts of ventricular tachycardia. The cardiac disorder is neither temporally related to attacks of limb weakness nor related to serum potassium content.

DIAGNOSIS. Periodic paralysis can be recognized by the history of typical attacks; no other disease causes this pattern of recurrent weakness. In myasthenia gravis, weakness may come and go, but less abruptly and with a duration of weeks rather than hours or days; remissions are less frequent so that it is less "periodic." Polymyositis may be transient, but episodes are rarely shorter than several weeks or months. Attacks of myoglobinuric weakness could conceivably be confusing if the pigmenturia were not recognized, but myalgia and malaise are so prominent that it is rarely mistaken for periodic paralysis. Hysterical attacks might be confusing.

If the patient is seen during the attack and the serum potassium is abnormal, other causes of hypo- or hyperkalemia must be considered. Low serum potassium concentrations with paralysis are also encountered in hyperaldosteronism; potassium-losing nephritis; potassium depletion caused by laxative abuse, diuretics, or diarrhea; and thyrotoxicosis. *Thiazide* and *thalidone diuretics* are in such widespread use nowadays that these drugs are likely to be an increasingly frequent cause of hypokalemic weakness; in one series, about 25 per cent of randomly chosen patients receiving these drugs had serum potassium contents below normal. Hyperkalemia is most often due to renal insufficiency, but may also occur in adrenal insufficiency, after administration of spironolactone, or as a manifestation of aldosterone deficiency.

Thyrotoxicosis can produce a variant of periodic hypokalemic paralysis closely resembling the familial variety. The condition especially occurs in young Chinese and Japanese men in their third or fourth decade, although other Asians and even women have occasionally been affected. The clinical manifestations of hyperthyroidism usually are not prominent, although tachycardia and even cardiac arrhythmias are frequent. Attacks commonly are precipitated by exercises or heavy carbohydrate meals. Serum potassium is low. Effective treatment of the thyrotoxicosis is curative.

A family history of periodic paralysis is useful in diagnosis, but sporadic cases may be indistinguishable from the familial disorder. If the patient is not having a spontaneous attack when studied, the only way to distinguish the two forms is to provoke an attack. The techniques to be described have been used in numerous centers with many patients, without serious complications. But induced attacks may be frightening to patient and physician, and should be left to experienced investigators. Facilities for supported respiration should be immediately available. Appropriately informed consent is mandatory. Because of the uncertainty of clinical distinction, it is advisable to start with glucose (100 grams) given intravenously in one hour with 20 units of regular insulin either in the infusion or given subcutaneously. Hypoglycemic symptoms should be anticipated, and the electrocardiogram should be monitored. Hypokalemia is induced as the blood sugar falls, usually within one hour after the infusion is completed. If an attack is induced, it can be terminated with administration of 7 to 10 grams of potassium chloride (KCl) by mouth. Whether or not an attack is induced by glucose and insulin, but especially if it is not, the patient should then be challenged with potassium. This poses problems because it is not clear how much potassium constitutes an adequate challenge. The writer starts with 3 grams of KCl by mouth. If this fails the dose is gradually increased on successive days to a maximum of 8 or 10 grams. Patients with hyperkalemic paralysis have attacks with serum potassium levels between 5 and 8 mEq per liter.

Other members of the family should be investigated clinically and electromyographically for evidence of myotonia.

TREATMENT. Acute attacks of hypokalemic paralysis are best treated with oral KCl, 5 to 10 grams. Relief of weakness usually commences within 30 minutes but may take several hours, and some attacks are peculiarly refractory. Hyperkalemia may be relieved by infusions of glucose and insulin. Chlorothiazide and calcium gluconate have also been reported to be effective. In severe attacks, weakness may persist even after the serum potassium has returned to normal concentrations.

The traditional method used to protect patients against hypokalemic paralysis was, until recently, a low-sodium diet supplemented by oral KCl, or perhaps by spironolactone or dexamethasone. Then, acetazolamide in small doses, sometimes only 250 per mg daily, sometimes more, was found to be effective prophylaxis in the hyperkalemic type. Subsequently, it was found that similar doses of acetazolamide were equally effective in the hypokalemic variety, so a single drug is beneficial in both forms. How it exerts this effect is not known. The best-known effects of this compound relate to its ability to inhibit carbonic anhydrase, but muscle lacks this enzyme, and no definite systemic effects of the drug have been recognized in the doses used, but respiratory acidosis may be responsible.

Gordon, R. M., Green, J. R., and Lagunoff, D.: Studies on a patient with hypokalemic familial periodic paralysis. Am. J. Med., 48:185, 1970.

Griggs, R. C., Engel, W. K., and Resnick, J. S.: Acetazolamide treatment of hypokalemic periodic paralysis: Prevention of attacks and improvement of persistent weakness. Ann. Intern. Med., 73:39, 1970.

Pearson, C. M., and Kalyanaraman, R.: Periodic paralyses. *In* Stanbury, J. B., Wyngaarden, J. B., and Fredrickson, D. S. (eds.): The Metabolic Basis of Inherited Disease. 3rd ed. New York, McGraw-Hill Book Company, 1972, pp. 1180–1203.

Ramsay, I.: Thyroid Disease and Muscle Dysfunction. Chicago, Year Book Medical Publishers, 1974.

Vroom F. Q., Jarrell, M. S., and Maren, T. H.: Acetazolamide treatment of hypokalemic periodic paralysis. Probable mechanism of action. Arch. Neurol., 32:385, 1975.

Zierler, K. L.: Speculations on hypokalemic periodic paralysis. Am. J. Med. Sci., 266:131, 1973.

339.7. MYOSITIS OSSIFICANS

This rare disorder is most dramatic in its consequences, producing the "stone man" of circus sideshows. Symptoms usually begin in early childhood, with transient and localized swellings of the neck and back. Ultimately there is progressive rigidity of the neck, trunk, and limbs. Palpable plates are discernible beneath the rigid parts. Severely affected patients may be able to stand and walk, and yet unable to bend so that they must be raised from bed with assistance. The bars beneath the skin are visible roentgenographically. Microscopically, muscle is replaced by bone and connective tissue. Whether the primary disorder is in the fibroblasts (leading to abnormal ossification) or in the muscle itself is not resolved. Muscle biopsy early in the disease may show widespread necrosis and inflammation, but serum enzymes are not always elevated, nor is the electromyogram always myopathic. Few cases are familial, but the disorder is believed to be inherited because digital abnormalities are almost always present in both the patients and other members of the family in a pattern suggesting an autosomal dominant inheritance. Microdactyly commonly affects the great toe, and clinodactyly (curved digits) may affect the hands. There is no detectable systemic abnormality of calcium and phosphate metabolism, and there has been no effective therapy, but recent reports suggest that administration of disphosphonates may prevent the deposition of bone. Once bone is formed, however, these drugs are ineffective.

Bassett, C. A. L., Donath, A., Macagno, F., Preisig, R., Fleisch, H., and Francis, M. D.: Diphosphonates in the treatment of myositis ossificans. Lancet, 2:845, 1969.

Lutwak, L.: Myositis ossificans progressiva. Am. J. Med., 37:269, 1964.

340. SPORADIC DISORDERS

340.1. THE PROBLEM PRESENTED BY DERMATOMYOSITIS AND POLYMYOSITIS

The main discussion of these conditions is found in Ch. 51. However, the concept of polymyositis is central to the analysis and concepts of acquired myopathies of adult life, and thus it is appropriate to review some of the problems here.

These conditions are usually considered together, but this practice may prove imprudent. *Dermatomyositis* is a recognizable syndrome, characterized by a rash and myopathy, both with distinctive features. The name is derived from the inflammatory cellular response that is usually found in skeletal muscle, but lymphocytic reaction is not present in all cases. This lack causes problems in defining *polymyositis,* a disorder presumably identical with dermatomyositis but without the rash.

There probably is such a disease as true dermatomyositis with scarcely detectable skin lesions. The rash of dermatomyositis may be so mild that it could be overlooked by parents or inexperienced clinicians, and there are patients with no history of rash who develop subcutaneous calcinosis, implying that the skin had been involved without visible dermatitis. But once the rash is taken away, an essential sign of dermatomyositis is withdrawn, and it becomes impossible to define polymyositis as the same condition. Polymyositis, therefore, is a syndrome, probably of diverse causes, and is identifiable by the following set of diagnostic criteria.

DIAGNOSIS. The diagnosis of dermatomyositis is a clinical diagnosis, depending upon the characteristic rash and limb weakness. In some patients, features of scleroderma may also be present, warranting the name "sclerodermatomyositis." However, there is no overlap with lupus erythematosus or periarteritis nodosa, and the visceral lesions of these conditions do not occur in dermatomyositis.

When there is no rash, the syndrome must be differentiated from the dystrophies by lack of family history, onset after age 35 (because no familial limb-girdle dystrophy starts so late), rapidity of onset in weeks or months rather than years, spontaneous improvement (which does not occur in dystrophy, by definition), distribution of weakness affecting cervical and cranial muscles, or systemic symptoms such as arthralgia or Raynaud's syndrome. Severe inflammation, when present, supports the diagnosis of polymyositis, but lack of leukocytic infiltration does not exclude the diagnosis. The electromyogram is helpful, but, again, not distinctive; there are the usual features of myopathy with the additional evidence of irritable muscle (increased insertional activity and some spontaneous activity). Serum enzymes tend to be high. There may also be an increased erythrocyte sedimentation rate, increased serum gamma globulin concentration, or a positive latex fixation test for rheumatoid factor. Evidence of lymphocytes sensitized to muscle may be demonstrable, but this has not yet attained diagnostic reliability.

The problem of diagnosis is best exemplified by a patient with limb weakness commencing at age 40 and evidence of myopathic disease in muscle biopsy and electromyogram. Search must be made for the known causes of muscle disease, to be discussed below. If none is found, the diagnosis of exclusion is polymyositis, no matter what the laboratory data show or do not show. That this residual group is all due to one disease seems unlikely, not only because there is clinical heterogeneity, but also because if there are so many known causes of the syndrome, others still remain to be recognized. Because inflammatory cells are not always seen in the muscle biopsy, some authorities eschew the word "polymyositis" and prefer "myopathy of unknown cause." This, at least, identifies the problem, but for the present "polymyositis" seems to be entrenched. Clinicians should recognize, however, that "polymyositis" is no more a specific diagnosis than "headache," "polyneuritis," or "convulsive disorder," terms that also imply inadequately defined syndromes of diverse etiology.

340.2. OTHER ACQUIRED MYOPATHIES

Proximal limb weakness in patients with no rash, with or without inflammatory lesions in muscle, and with or without increased serum enzyme activity, occurs in several disorders. These may be considered diseases associated with polymyositis, causing poliomyositis or simulating poliomyositis. To identify these disorders, appropriate diagnostic tools must be utilized.

CARCINOMATOUS MYOPATHY. Muscle weakness without rash may occur in patients with carcinoma of the lung or of any other primary site. Myeloma, macroglobulinemia, and other gammopathies may also be associated with myopathy. The tumor itself may or may not be symptomatic, and treatment of the tumor may or may not affect the muscular symptoms.

COLLAGEN DISEASES. Proximal limb weakness may occur in the course of systemic lupus erythematosus, progressive systemic sclerosis, rheumatoid arthritis, and, rarely, periarteritis nodosa or giant cell arteritis. In these circumstances, the myopathy is treated as part of the general disorder.

ENDOCRINE DISEASE. Thyrotoxic myopathy is a well-recognized syndrome. Usually there is clinical evidence of hyperthyroidism, but not always ("apathetic hyperthyroidism"). Signs of hypermetabolism are especially apt to be lacking in elderly patients. This myopathy inevitably disappears when the patient is rendered euthyroid by treatment. Similarly, weakness may complicate hypothyroidism. Another muscle syndrome of hypothyroidism is Hoffmann's syndrome, a peculiar difficulty in relaxing muscles that lack the characteristic electromyographic abnormalities of myotonia and is therefore called "pseudomyotonia," but may appear similar clinically. This, too, disappears with appropriate replacement therapy. Infants with cretinism may have unusually well developed muscles but not the disorder of relaxation.

Hyperparathyroidism and hyperadrenocorticism may also be responsible for weakness that looks like any other proximal myopathy. Surprisingly, because asthenia has so long been regarded as prominent, Addison's disease seems not to be a cause of this syndrome. Weakness may be part of hyperpituitarism, but acromegalic features always overshadow the myopathy. Myalgia, with or without weakness, may be a prominent symptom in patients with osteomalacia, and the muscular disorder may respond dramatically to administration of vitamin D.

INFECTIONS. Structures resembling viral particles have been seen with the electron microscope with polymyositis, and sometimes there are acute myopathic disorders in individuals with serologically proved influenza or other viral infections, or with encephalomyelitis assumed to be viral in origin. In one special form, children with congenital agammaglobulinemia develop dermatomyositis, and echovirus can be isolated from cerebrospinal fluid. Other infections or infestations that can be associated with clinical polymyositis are trichinosis, toxoplasmosis, cysticercosis, schistosomiasis, and trypanosomiasis.

SARCOIDOSIS. In muscle clinics, sarcoidosis is recognized as a significant cause of polymyositis. Usually there is other evidence of the disease, but sometimes the first symptoms are due to weakness, and in a few cases only muscle seems to be involved. Myalgia may be severe in these patients.

DRUGS. A variety of drugs used to treat more common disorders may themselves cause muscular weakness, especially triamcinolone and other fluorinated adrenal steroids (but probably all steroids), vincristine, chloroquine, bretylium, and guanethidine. Repeated injections of narcotics and other drugs may lead to fibrosis of muscle that simulates a diffuse myopathy.

ALCOHOLIC MYOPATHY. The clearest myopathic disorder in alcoholic persons is acute myoglobinuria. Some of these individuals, and some who never have an attack of pigmenturia, also suffer from proximal limb weakness, especially affecting the legs. The serum creatine phosphokinase is often elevated. The problem in some of these patients, however, is that they also suffer from the typical polyneuritis of alcoholism, and it then becomes difficult to prove that the muscular weakness is not also secondary to a neurogenic disorder. Too few patients have been evaluated to know whether abstinence and a good diet will reverse the persistent weakness. Chronic hypokalemia from any cause may be associated with the syndrome of polymyositis: weakness of relatively abrupt onset, muscle necrosis in biopsy, and high serum enzymes. This is most commonly seen in patients taking thiazide diuretics, but may also occur in hypokalemic states caused by chronic diarrhea. Hypokalemia may also contribute to some cases of alcoholic myopathy. (Other acquired disorders of potassium metabolism are discussed under Diagnosis in Ch. 339.6.)

Dietzman, D. E., Schaller, J. G., Ray, C. G., and Reed, M. E.: Acute myositis associated with influenza B infection. Pediatrics, 57:255, 1976.

Floyd, M., Ayar, D. R., Barwick, D. D., Hudgson, P., and Weightman, D.: Myopathy in chronic renal failure. Quart. J. Med., 43:509, 1974.

Frame, B., Heize, E. G., Block, M. A., and Manson, G. A.: Myopathy in primary hyperparathyroidism. Ann. Intern. Med., 68:1022, 1968.

Mastaglia, F. L., Gardner-Medwin, D., and Hudgson, P.: Muscle fibrosis and contractures in a pethidine addict. Br. Med. J., 4:532, 1971.

Perkoff, G. T.: Alocholic myopathy. Ann. Rev. Med., 22:125, 1971.

Rowland, L. P., Clark, C., and Olarte, M.: Therapy for dermatomyositis and polymyositis. Adv. Neurol., 17:63, 1977.

Scarpalezos, S., et al.: Neural and muscular manifestations of hypothyroidism. Arch. Neurol., 29:140, 1973.

Schott, G. D., and Wills, M. R.: Muscle weakness in osteomalacia. Lancet, 1:626, 1976.

Sharp, G. C., Irvin, W. S., Tan, E. S., Gould, R. G., and Holman, H. R.: Mixed connective tissue disease; an apparently distinct rheumatic disease syndrome associated with an antibody to extractable nuclear antigen. Am. J. Med., 52:148, 1972.

Silverstein, A., and Siltzbach, L. E.: Muscle involvement in sarcoidosis. Arch. Neurol., 21:235, 1969.

340.3.   SPORADIC MYOGLOBINURIA

DEFINITION. Sporadic myoglobinuria comprises a group of disorders characterized by injury of muscle and excretion of myoglobin in the urine. *Rhabdomyolysis* has been proposed as a more precise term, but it is never used except when there is myoglobinuria and is therefore of dubious value.

PATHOGENESIS. Myoglobin may be released from muscle whenever there is extensive and rapid destruction. Sometimes the cause is evident, as in the *crush injuries* of World War II. Similar pressure injuries may occur in comatose persons who lie on one side without moving for prolonged periods. This kind of injury is perhaps more apt to occur when there are other causes of *metabolic depression;* for instance, in coma after suicidal ingestion of barbiturates or carbon monoxide intoxication, or prolonged unconsciousness in the snow. A similar effect may be induced by *arterial occlusion* by tourniquet or embolism, or even by prolonged knee-chest posture under anesthesia.

In other patients, the cause is less discernible. In every series of patients with myoglobinuria, a disproportionate number are *alcoholics*, but why this should occur is not known. Sometimes there has been exposure to a known *membrane toxin*, such as the bite of the Malayan sea snake. In some addicts, heroin itself seems to cause myoglobinuria. Or there may be *metabolic alterations* that do not ordinarily cause this kind of trouble, such as diarrhea with hypokalemia; potassium depletion caused by diuretics, amphotericin, or licorice; diabetic acidosis; or systemic infection with fever. In many attacks, however, not even these clues prevail.

The most common cause of myoglobinuria is probably unusually *vigorous exercise* by an otherwise normal person. Most cases have been reported by military physicians, and local designations include such titles as the "squat-jump syndrome." Some cases are attributed to "march hemoglobinuria." When large numbers of recruits endure these tortures, a certain number will have attacks of myalgia followed by pigmenturia. Why these individuals have attacks and others are spared is not clear, but this seems to be a "normal" variation. In civilians, cases have been caused by the excess muscular activity of an initiation rite into a club or fraternity, and isolated attacks have occurred after the vigorous muscular activity induced by succinylcholine before it achieves relaxation. In *malignant hyperthermia*, there is a rapid rise in temperature, widespread muscular rigidity, hyperkalemia, and metabolic acidosis, with a fatal outcome in about 75 per cent. The offending agents are usually halothane and succinylcholine. Increased serum activities of sarcoplasmic enzymes are the rule, and often there is myoglobinuria. The intense muscular contraction may be the proximate cause of myoglobinuria in this syndrome, but the widespread metabolic disorder probably contributes. Spontaneous convulsions and electroconvulsive therapy have also been followed by myoglobinuria. If an individual is subject to repeated attacks, it may be suspected that there is some kind of undiscovered genetic defect, although the only ones recognized now are deficiencies of phosphorylase, phosphofructokinase, or carnitine palmityl transferase.

CLINICAL MANIFESTATIONS. In attacks other than those caused by local crushing or arterial occlusion, the clinical picture is similar. Affected muscles are apt to be the ones subject to greatest physical strain (the legs in squat-thrusts, the arms after chinning or push-ups, the arms and legs after wrestling matches). The muscles ache, may be swollen, and are weak. Sometimes there is so much edema that local vascular abnormalities are suspected. There may be fever and considerable malaise. Symptoms persist for several days even though pigmenturia rarely lasts more than 48 hours. Recovery may be gradual. Cranial muscles are rarely involved, and although respiratory failure is uncommon it is a hazard. The most important threat to life is renal injury secondary to excretion of heme. There may be red cells or myoglobin in the urine as well as casts. Oliguria is followed by azotemia and hyperkalemia. This may be treated by appropriate measures.

DIAGNOSIS. The diagnosis of myoglobinuria can be made on clinical grounds and with relatively simple tests, but precise identification of the pigment depends upon biochemical analysis. The urine may appear red-brown because of hemoglobin, myoglobin, or porphyrins. The latter would not give a positive test with benzidine (or other heme-reacting reagents), and would give a positive Watson-Schwartz test for porphobilinogen. Besides, the neurologic disorder of porphyria is neuropathy, not an acute myopathy. If the urine gives a positive test for heme and contains no or few erythrocytes, the pigment is either myoglobin or hemoglobin. If it is hemoglobin, the serum would be pink (after a hemolytic reaction), whereas the color of the serum in myglobinuria is normal. (This distinction depends upon the affinity of serum haptoglobin for hemoglobin and not for myoglobin. Hemoglobin is not excreted until haptoglobin is saturated by visible amounts of the pigment, whereas myoglobin is excreted at much lower concentrations.) Furthermore, in attacks of myoglobinuria, the muscular weakness and myalgia are distinctive, and serum enzymes are greatly increased, whereas they are not in hemolysis. Positive identification of myoglobin can be achieved by several tests: absorption spectrophotometry is direct and simple, but in many laboratories the most convenient method is electrophoresis on starch gel or cellulose acetate. Immunochemical methods are gaining in favor.

Myoglobinuria should be considered a possible cause in cases of acute renal failure of uncertain etiology. If the serum content of sarcoplasmic enzymes is very high (e.g., creatine phosphokinase values to 10,000 to 50,000 units, with a method giving normal maximal values of 50 units), myoglobinuria is the likely cause.

TREATMENT. If there is no renal injury, myoglobinu-ria is not threatening. The hazards of renal injury are not directly correlated to the amount of pigment excreted, and other factors are probably involved. Once an attack starts, it is useful to encourage excretion of dilute urine, and some authorities favor alkalinizing agents although it has not been clearly demonstrated that these treatments protect the kidneys. Few patients are left with residual weakness, but in some the syndrome is characterized by prolonged weakness punctuated by attacks of myoglobinuria.

Demos, M. A., Gitlin, E. L., and Kagen, L. G.: Exercise myoglobinuria and acute exertional rhabdomyolysis. Arch. Intern. Med., 134:669, 1974.

Grossman, R. A., Hamilton, R. W., Morse, B. M., Penn, A. S., and Goldberg, M.: Nontraumatic rhabdomyolysis and acute renal failure. N. Engl. J. Med., 291:807, 1974.

Knochel, J. P.: Environmental heat illness. An eclectic review. Arch. Intern. Med., 133:841, 1974.

Moulds, R. G. W.: Biochemical basis of malignant hyperthermia. Br. Med. J., 2:241, 1974.

Rowland, L. P., and Penn, A. S.: Myoglobinuria. Med. Clin. North Am., 56:1233, 1972.

Ryan, J. F.: Procaine for malignant hyperthermia. N. Engl. J. Med., 291:210, 1974.

340.4. MYASTHENIA GRAVIS

DEFINITION. Myasthenia gravis is a disease of unknown cause, due to circulating antibodies to acetylcholine receptors, and manifest by weakness that has special characteristics: predilection for ocular and other cranial muscles, tendency to fluctuate in severity, no signs of neural lesion, and amelioration of weakness by cholinergic drugs.

ETIOLOGY. Although the initiating event is not known, it seems clear that myasthenic weakness results from the presence of circulating antibodies to acetylcholine receptor (AChR). It has been found that rabbits and other species can be immunized with purified AChR. When antibodies appear in the blood, weakness results, and this weakness has all the essential physiologic and pharmacologic properties found in the human disease. Also, as in human myasthenia, there are morphologic changes at the neuromuscular junction, especially simplification of the postjunctional folds, and antibody can be demonstrated on the postjunctional membrane by immunocytochemical methods. As a result, the postjunctional membrane becomes less sensitive to the application of acetylcholine or other agonists.

When this experimental autoimmune myasthenia gravis was demonstrated and confirmed in other laboratories, similar antibodies to AChR were soon demonstrated in the blood of patients with myasthenia gravis. In a transient syndrome of infants born to myasthenic mothers, the symptoms disappeared when the antibodies disappeared. When purified IgG from patients was injected into mice, characteristics of myasthenia were induced in the animals, and if the plasma of patients was removed by plasmapheresis or thoracic duct drainage, the symptoms were ameliorated.

Some questions remain. Foremost is the nature of the events that initiate the formation of the antibodies. Also, it is not clear what role sensitized lymphocytes play, for there is evidence of altered cellular immunity, too. There are questions about the antibodies themselves, for they seem to be directed to antigenic sites on the AChR other than the combining site for acetylcholine. Simple blockade of AChR by steric hindrance is one possible mechanism, but the antibodies also seem to accelerate the loss of AChR, and other mechanisms of interference are possible. In intercostal muscle from patients with the disease, miniature end-plate potentials are reduced in amplitude and there is decreased sensitivity to cholinergic agonists.

Other evidence of an autoimmune disorder include abnormalities of the thymus gland in most patients, either germinal centers or thymoma; accumulation of lymphocytes in muscle and other organs; increased coincidence with other presumed autoimmune diseases; and increased frequency of nonspecific autoantibodies against nuclear antigens (ANA), striation-binding muscle antigens, and thyroid antigens.

NEUROMUSCULAR DISORDER. The symptoms of myasthenia gravis resemble those of curare intoxication. This observation led to the use of curare antagonists in the treatment of myasthenia gravis. All effective therapies have been derived from this initial observation, and all drugs currently in use are inhibitors of the enzyme cholinesterase. These drugs also partially repair a physiologic defect that can be detected in patients by relatively simple techniques. When the ulnar nerve of normal individuals is stimulated at rates of 15 per second or less, the action potential of the hypothenar muscles is sustained at a constant amplitude. In patients with myasthenia, however, there is a rapid decline in the height of the evoked potentials. If the patient is then given neostigmine, the amplitude of the evoked potentials is restored to normal. This abnormality has been regarded as characteristic and is consistent with the reduced amplitude of miniature end-plate potentials found in intercostal muscle. The use of repetitive stimulation for diagnostic purposes has disadvantages because it causes some discomfort to the patient and because decrementing responses can be encountered in diseases other than myasthenia gravis. Attention has therefore been given to single-fiber electromyography (SFEMG), which is less painful but has not yet been validated for specificity. In SFEMG, the intervals are measured between discharges of different fibers within the same motor unit. These intervals vary normally, a variation called "jitter," and the temporal limits have been defined. In myasthenia, jitter increases; when the intervals are very long, expected potentials do not appear, a phenomenon called "blocking," and the number of blockings increases in myasthenia. These abnormalities are attributed to slowing of and uncertainty of neuromuscular transmission.

INCIDENCE AND PREVALENCE. The prevalence of myasthenia gravis is about 33 per million population and the annual incidence about 2 to 5 million. Cases occur in all decades of life, most frequently at about age 40. Among young adults, the disease affects women about three times more frequently than men. Among children and older persons, however, men and women are affected equally. There are few familial cases, perhaps somewhat more than would be expected by chance, and there may be increased incidence of thyroid or other autoimmune disease in relatives of patients with myasthenia. Some genetic predisposition is suggested by a disproportionate frequency of particular transplantation antigen haplotypes in affected individuals, and these may differ in those with thymoma and in younger patients with no tumor.

PATHOLOGY. Pathologic changes in myasthenia gravis are limited to muscle and thymus. Skeletal muscles may appear completely normal, but there are often collections of lymphocytes around blood vessels. In some cases there is evidence of degeneration of muscle fibers, and the inflammatory cellular response may be more extensive. Rarely, similar lesions are encountered in the myocardium. The thymus gland is often abnormal. Encapsulated tumors (thymoma) occur in about 15 per cent of the cases, almost all after age 30. In about 25 per cent of these tumors there is evidence of local invasion, but distant metastases are virtually unknown and the local invasiveness is not a cause of symptoms. Lymphocytic proliferation, in the form of germinal centers, is seen in the thymus glands of almost all other patients, but sometimes the gland appears normal, and in some older individuals the gland is so involuted that it cannot be found. Patients dying of this disease usually have some pulmonary disorder (edema, atelectasis, infection) secondary to the terminal events. It has not been shown that myasthenia occurs more frequently in patients with cancer than might be expected on the basis of chance.

CLINICAL MANIFESTATIONS. The most common presenting symptoms relate to weakness of eye muscles, ptosis or diplopia. At the onset these symptoms may last only a few days, then disappear, only to return weeks or months later. Ptosis frequently varies even in the course of a single day. Diplopia may be noted in particular directions of gaze. Difficulty in chewing, dysarthria, and dysphagia are common. Limb weakness is more often proximal in accentuation, so that patients have difficulty climbing stairs or rising from chairs, or have difficulty lifting heavy objects or raising the arms overhead. However, distal weakness is not uncommon, and the initial symptoms may be related to the strength of the hands or fingers. Selective respiratory weakness is unusual. There is no alteration of consciousness, no pain, and, in untreated patients, no cramps or muscular twitching. Difficulty in chewing and swallowing may lead to considerable loss of weight, but there is no specific wasting of muscle except in patients with severe chronic weakness.

On examination, evidence of weakness of the appropriate muscle groups is found. If any sensory abnormality is found, there must be some other disorder, alone or in combination with myasthenia. Similarly, hyperactive reflexes and Babinski signs imply some other disorder, as does the complete loss of reflexes. Weakness is responsible for all the signs of myasthenia. Ptosis may be unilateral or bilateral. Most often, there is asymmetrical weakness of several ocular muscles in a pattern that cannot be explained by disorder of a particular ocular motor nerve. In addition, there is frequently weakness of eye closure because of paresis of the orbicularis oculi. Muscles of the lower face are involved later. Lingual and palatal weakness are evident in patients with dysarthria, producing a nasal twang and indistinct speech. In advanced cases, patients support the chin with one hand to help them talk, a maneuver almost pathognomonic of myasthenia. Neck weakness may be mild or severe enough to cause difficulty in holding the head erect. Limb weakness may be mild or so severe that the patient cannot walk or even turn in bed. Ventilatory insufficiency occurs only in severely affected patients and usually in generalized disease, but some patients with oropharyngeal weakness may be unable to breathe unassisted even though limb muscles are strong. Even though weakness fluctuates, a normal neurologic examination is inconsistent with the diagnosis of myasthenia gravis if the patient is symptomatic at the time.

COURSE. It is the experience of most clinicians that the nature of the disease in a given patient is established within weeks or months of onset, with fluctuations afterward. If after one year, or certainly after two years, myasthenia is still restricted to ocular muscles, it is most unlikely to become generalized; purely ocular myasthenia may account for 20 per cent of all cases.

SPECIAL FORMS OF MYASTHENIA. Neonatal Myasthenia. Infants born to myasthenic women may have a transient syndrome of weakness. The most prominent symptom is difficulty in sucking and swallowing. This may be the sole manifestation, or there may also be noticeable reduction in spontaneous movement and in the vigor of the baby's cry. Only rarely is there respiratory difficulty, but unrecognized neonatal myasthenia has been fatal in exceptional cases. The condition can be identified by the intramuscular injection of neostigmine (0.1 to 0.25 mg), followed by improved sucking, a louder cry, better response to the Moro reflex, and stronger spontaneous movements. Small doses of cholinergic drugs may be administered therapeutically, but more often all that is needed is a nasogastric tube to ensure adequate nutrition. Symptoms subside within a week or, at most, a month.

Congenital Myasthenia. Myasthenia gravis may commence at any age. But there are some children who seem to have had ophthalmoplegia from birth, with or without other signs of myasthenia. Although presumably congenital, this disorder rarely causes concern in the first year of life. It is only later, when the ophthalmoplegia is recognized, that the parents state the child's eyes have always been that way. There may be a disproportionate number of familial cases among children with congenital myasthenia; ophthalmoplegia occurs in almost all of them, and there may be somewhat less tendency for crisis and remission. Otherwise, there are no characteristics that distinguish this syndrome from myasthenia at any other age.

Thyrotoxicosis. About 5 per cent of patients with myasthenia have thyrotoxicosis at some time. Usually the two disorders occur simultaneously, but sometimes hyperthyroidism is evident for weeks or months before there are myasthenic symptoms. Only rarely does myasthenia come long before the thyrotoxicosis, and patients who appear euthyroid do not ordinarily have laboratory evidence of thyroid overactivity. Treatment of the two disorders is directed according to the usual indications for each.

DIAGNOSIS. In almost all cases the diagnosis of myasthenia is obvious from the history and examination. The diagnosis is immediately confirmed by the response to cholinergic drugs. For adults, 1 ml of edrophonium (10 mg) is given by vein intermittently; after injection of 2 to 3 mg, specific muscle groups are evaluated. If there is no response within 30 seconds, a second dose of 3.0 mg is given and the patient is evaluated once again. If there is still no response, the remainder is given, a total of 10 mg. This drug is preferred when cranial muscles are being tested because the response is prompt and dramatic. Cranial weakness cannot be simulated voluntarily, and placebo injections are therefore not necessary.

If it is desired to evaluate limb strength, the injection of neostigmine has advantages because the effect lasts longer, permitting more leisurely testing. The adult dose is 1.5 mg intramuscularly, and it is usually combined with atropine, 0.5 mg, to avoid the muscarinic symptoms of abdominal cramps and sweating. When limb strength is evaluated, it is sometimes advisable to evaluate placebo responses by giving the atropine 30 minutes before the neostigmine. In all cases of myasthenia gravis there is some response to these drugs, but the response is sometimes slight, and the test may have to be repeated on several occasions to provide convincing evidence.

To provide confirmatory evidence, the electromyographic response to ulnar nerve stimulation may be studied. The characteristic decline in amplitude of the evoked potential is usually seen in affected muscles, but the response may be normal when the disease is restricted to the eyes. As noted above, SFEMG is finding increasing use in diagnosis. Rarely, it is desirable to administer d-tubocurarine, a drug to which myasthenics are unusually sensitive. There are hazards in the administration of this drug, however, and its use should probably be left to research centers; d-tubocurarine should never be given without appropriate precautions to support respiration.

The most important diagnostic laboratory test is likely to be the demonstration of antibodies to AChR, as this seems to be present in virtually all these patients but not in the other diseases. The most sensitive and most specific assay system reported so far involves use of human AChR as antigen, and this is difficult to obtain. AChR from denervated rat muscle or from the electric organs of torpedo or eel may substitute, but seem less sensitive.

It is useful to perform a standard series of studies. Thymomas can almost always be identified in standard roentgenograms of the chest, supplemented by oblique views. Laminagrams may provide more information, but there is little need for thymic venography or mediastinal pneumography. Thyroid function should be tested, and it is useful to evaluate immunologic disorders by serum protein electrophoresis, LE cell preparation, latex fixation test for rheumatoid factor, and antinuclear antibodies. Tests for muscle antibodies or lymphocyte sensitivity are performed in special centers.

The differential diagnosis requires special consideration. Probably the most frequent error in diagnosis concerns patients with emotional fatigue states and hysterical weakness. There are no cranial muscle symptoms in these patients (except globus hystericus), whereas cranial muscles are involved in virtually all myasthenics. Their symptoms are not those of weakness but of exhaustion, and in tests of strength against resistance there is apt to be marked variation in effort, or dramatic giving way. The diagnosis of acute myasthenia may be mistakenly made in a patient with botulism. As the discovery of botulism calls for urgent action, for both patient and eating companions, the physician should be aware of this diagnostic pitfall (see Ch. 22.3). Amyotrophic lateral sclerosis and peripheral neuropathy may be confused with myasthenia when these disorders affect cranial muscles, but signs indicative of a neurogenic disorder distinguish them from myasthenia. Polymyositis may be confusing, but ocular muscle paresis is not found. There is some debate about the specificity of the therapeutic effect of cholinergic drugs, but for practical purposes it may be taken that an authentic (not placebo), convincing (not equivocal), and reproducible (not seen by one examiner only) effect is found only in myasthenia gravis.

TREATMENT. Therapeutic efforts fall into two categories: those which affect symptoms without influencing the course of the disease (cholinergic drugs), and those designed to induce remission of the disease itself (thymectomy, steroids, immunosuppressive drugs). Management starts as soon as the diagnosis is made, using cholinergic drugs. Then decisions are made regarding other forms of treatment.

Cholinergic Drug Therapy. The major drugs used to treat myasthenia gravis are inhibitors of cholinesterase, neostigmine and pyridostigmine. Another drug, ambenonium, is also used in some clinics, but has no special advantages. It is best to use only one drug; there is no benefit from combinations of two or more. Neostigmine is provided in 15 mg tablets, and pyridostigmine in 60 mg tablets; these are essentially interchangeable. The choice of drugs is arbitrary because there is no evidence that the maximal benefit achieved by one is more than that of the other. Most patients, but not all, prefer pyridostigmine because it is less apt to cause abdominal cramps and diarrhea, and it is less apt to cause noticeable peaks and valleys of strength. But these advantages have never been proved objectively, and some patients do very well with neostigmine. Pyridostigmine is also provided in a slow-release capsule (Timespan) of 180 mg, said to provide 60 mg immediately and the remainder in 8 to 12 hours. Some clinicians use the prolonged-action preparation throughout the day, but because of uncertainties of release, it seems advisable to use this only at bedtime for patients who would otherwise have to awaken at night or who are very weak on waking in the morning. (For patients who cannot swallow pills, both drugs may be administered parenterally, and pyridostigmine may be given as a syrup. The intramuscular dose is about one tenth of the oral dose, and the intravenous dose is one thirtieth of the oral dose.) Decisions about optimal dosage are sometimes difficult. Some authorities advocate the use of edrophonium to evaluate oral drug therapy; a test dose of 2 mg is given intravenously. If the patient improves, oral therapy has been too little. If there is aggravation of weakness, oral therapy has been too much. But other authorities find this an unreliable guide, and we do not use this technique. If edrophonium is not used, there is nothing but clinical observation to guide the therapist. For mild cases, two tablets of either neostigmine or pyridostigmine three times daily, with meals, is useful. If there is inadequate response, the dose may be increased, first by shortening the interval between doses, then by increasing the quantity of drug with each dose. Problems arise because these drugs never completely reverse symptoms. Therefore the dose should be increased only so long as there is clear-cut response, and it should not be increased beyond the amount giving some perceptible benefit.

Overtreatment itself can cause weakness; cholinesterase inhibitors may cause a depolarizing block at the neuromuscular junction. This probably does not occur often.

Drugs advocated as "adjuvants" include potassium chloride, ephedrine, and guanidine; they may have some effect in individual patients, but their true value is unproved.

Steroids and Immunosuppressive Drugs. Prednisone now enjoys widespread popularity in the treatment of myasthenia, but it has never been put to an adequately controlled prospective therapeutic trial. Some investigators report improvement in as many as 80 per cent of patients treated, with virtually no side effects. Others are less enthusiastic about beneficial effects and are more concerned about deleterious effects. Some treat virtually all patients; others restrict therapy to those with incapacitating disease. It is agreed that the minimal dose should be about 50 mg daily for an adult, often given as 100 mg on alternate days. For patients who are seriously ill, larger doses have been used. Alternatively, because worsening of myasthenia may attend initiation of therapy, some start with 25 mg on alternate days and gradually increase to the full dose. Some use prednisone in preparation for thymectomy; others reserve steroids until some interval after thymectomy. If there is no beneficial response, it is not clear how long prednisone should be continued before deeming the trial a failure; a minimum of three months at full dosage seems reasonable. No matter how used, steroid drugs should be initiated with close supervision and probably in hospital because of the danger of their temporarily increasing the weakness.

The mechanism of action of steroids in myasthenia is not known, but current theories favor an immunosuppressive role. More specific immunosuppressive drugs such as azathioprine, methotrexate, or cyclophosphamide have also been used. There is no indication that these drugs are any better than prednisone, and evaluation of them is probably best performed in research centers.

Surgical Treatment. A reasonable program for patients with myasthenia starts with thymectomy for those still disabled after cholinergic drug treatment. Thymectomy is followed by significant improvement in about two thirds of patients with myasthenia and no tumor. Patients with thymoma fare worse whether the tumor is excised or not. Chest surgeons, anesthesiologists, and respirator units for postoperative care are now so skillful that the risks of operation are almost negligible. Because it is difficult to predict which patients will benefit, however, there is still some uncertainty in the selection of patients. Some recommend the operation for all patients who are incapacitated in daily living for more than six months despite adequate drug therapy. In preparing patients for operation, their usual oral dosage is continued until the day of operation, then stopped. Endotracheal intubation is used for all patients with oropharyngeal weakness, and intermittent positive pressure breathing is used in the postoperative period. The endotracheal tube may have to be replaced by tracheostomy after a few days, but endotracheal intubation alone suffices in most cases. Specific cholinergic drug therapy is withheld for several days, until fever subsides, and then started again at a level of one half or less of the preoperative dose.

Crisis. Patients with myasthenia gravis may suddenly develop difficulty breathing, severe enough to require artificial ventilation. This may be induced by systemic infection or major surgical procedures, but often there is no apparent cause. Patients with oropharyngeal weakness are especially liable to this threat, perhaps because of aspiration. Whenever there is doubt about the adequacy of ventilation or the state of the airway, endotracheal intubation should be used for short periods of respiratory support, obviating the need for tracheostomy. The insertion of a cuffed tube makes intermittent positive pressure breathing feasible, and also reduces the hazard of aspiration. Patients are best transferred to a respiratory intensive care unit. Cholinergic drugs are stopped. After several days, usually after fever (an almost inevitable concomitant of crisis and tracheostomy) has started to subside, drugs may be started once again, at half the precrisis dosage. The cause of crisis is not clear, but it is usually transient, and will subside if the patient can be kept alive. The mortality rate of crisis was formerly about 50 per cent, but since the advent of intensive care units, only about 10 per cent die, and these are mostly elderly patients with complicating cardiac and renal disease.

Some patients require assisted ventilation for prolonged periods, some longer than one year. For these patients, trial programs of prednisone seem advisable.

PROGNOSIS. The course of myasthenia is variable. The disease may be restricted to ocular muscles for many years, with no threat of life. Other patients are disabled to a variable degree by oropharyngeal or limb weakness, and a few are crippled. Crisis occurs in about 25 per cent of the cases. The over-all mortality is probably about 15 per cent, and although myasthenia itself was formerly the main hazard, intercurrent and unrelated disease is now more often the cause of death.

Drachman, D. B.: Medical progress: Myasthenia gravis. N. Engl. J. Med., 298:136, 186, 1978.

Genkins, G., Papatestas, A. E., Horowitz, S. H., and Kornfeld, P.: Studies in myasthenia gravis. Early thymectomy. Am. J. Med., 58:517, 1975.

Harvey, A. M.: Myasthenia gravis: The first 100 years in perspective. Trans. Am. Clin. Climatol., 82:149, 1970.

Jaretski, A., III, Wolff, M., Olarte, M., et al.: A rational approach to total thymectomy in the treatment of myasthenia gravis. Ann. Thorac. Surg., 24:120, 1977.

Johns, T. R.: Treatment of myasthenia gravis. Long-term administration of corticosteroids with remarks on thymectomy. Adv. Neurol., 17:99, 1977.

Lindstrom, J. M., Einarson, B. L., Lennon, V. A., et al.: Antibody to acetylcholine receptor in myasthenia gravis; prevalence, clinical correlates, and diagnostic value. Neurology, 26:1054, 1976.

Lindstrom, J. M., and Lambert, E. H.: Content of acetylcholine receptor and antibodies bound to receptor in myasthenia gravis, experimental autoimmune myasthenia gravis and Eaton-Lambert syndrome. Neurology, 26:130, 1978.

Pinching, A. J., Peters, D. K., and Davis, J. N.: Remission of myasthenia gravis following plasma exchange. Lancet, 2:1373, 1976.

340.5. EATON-LAMBERT SYNDROME
(Myasthenic Syndrome)

DEFINITION. The Eaton-Lambert syndrome is defined essentially in terms of electromyography. It is a disorder with muscular weakness in which the amplitude of the first muscle action potential evoked by stimulation of the nerve is reduced, and with repetitive stimulation the amplitude of the action potential increases to more than three times the original height.

PATHOGENESIS. The first cases were associated with oat-cell carcinoma of the lung, but cases have been found with other tumors, other diseases, and sometimes with no complicating disorder. Microelectrode studies indicate that the defect is due to impaired release of acetylcholine at the nerve terminals.

CLINICAL MANIFESTATIONS. The first evidence of the Eaton-Lambert syndrome may be prolonged apnea after curarization for surgery. Formal testing with d-tubocurarine also indicates that patients are unduly sensitive. Other patients may have symptoms of limb weakness, but cranial muscle weakness is never prominent. The response to cholinergic drugs is usually equivocal at best. Pain in the limbs may be prominent. Movements may be peculiarly slow. In tests of strength it may seem as though the patient gets stronger with continued effort. Myotatic reflexes are frequently depressed.

DIAGNOSIS. The signs listed above diverge sufficiently from myasthenia to avoid confusion; only limb weakness and curare sensitivity are similar. The remainder of the syndrome resembles polymyositis, and polyneuritis would also have to be considered. The diagnosis is made by the response to repetitive stimulation. Antibodies to AChR have not been found in typical cases.

TREATMENT. Guanidine promotes the release of acetylcholine, and the drug is effective in daily doses of 35 mg per kilogram of body weight, given orally. This drug may suppress bone marrow in many patients, however, and great caution must be taken. This effect limits treatment seriously, and the drug should probably not be used unless the neuromuscular disorder is disabling.

Eaton, L. M., and Lambert, E. H.: Electromyography and electric stimulation of nerves in diseases of motor unit: Observations in myasthenic syndrome associated with malignant tumors. JAMA, 163:1117, 1957.

Elmqvist, D., and Lambert, E. H.: Detailed analysis of neuromuscular transmission in a patient with myasthenic syndrome sometimes associated with brochogenic carcinoma. Mayo Clin. Proc., 43:689, 1968.

Oh, S. J., and Kim, K. W.: Guanidine hydrochloride in the Eaton-Lambert syndrome. Neurology, 23:1084, 1973.

340.6. UNUSUAL CAUSES OF NEUROMUSCULAR BLOCK

Botulism and *tick paralysis* are described in Ch. 22.3 and 33.12. Both cause a syndrome of flaccid quadriplegia with paresis of cranial muscles, and must be differentiated from polyneuritis, myasthenia gravis, and periodic paralysis. In neither is there a sensory disorder, but autonomic fibers may be affected in botulism, especially pupilloconstrictor fibers (resulting in a dilated, fixed pupil). The physiologic disorder in both syndromes is impaired release of acetylcholine from motor nerve terminals. The electromyogram in botulism may resemble that in the Eaton-Lambert syndrome, an observation that may be diagnostically important. Guanidine has been used with benefit to treat botulism and might also be effective in tick paralysis. Supportive therapy (tracheostomy and assisted respiration) is mandatory in severe cases. Tick paralysis is reversed by removal of the organism.

Several *aminoglycoside antimicrobial drugs* interfere with the release of acetylcholine, and may cause clinical syndromes in man. The offending drugs include neomycin, streptomycin, colistin, polymyxin, and kanamycin. The most common manifestation is postoperative apnea without other evidence of paralysis. This is most apt to occur in patients with renal failure, presumably with unusually high blood levels of the antimicrobial drug. In occasional cases, however, there may be flaccid quadriplegia. Administration of calcium and guanidine may be helpful, but the essence of management is supportive treatment and use of a safer antimicrobial.

Cherington, M., and Ryan, D. W.: Botulism and guanidine. N. Engl. J. Med., 278:931, 1968.

de Jesus, P. V., Slater, R., Spitz, L. K., and Penn, A. S.: Neuromuscular physiology of wound botulism. Arch. Neurol., 29:425, 1973.

McQuillen, M. P., Cantor, H. E., and O'Rourke, J. R.: Myasthenic syndrome associated with antibiotics. Arch. Neurol., 18:402, 1968.

Swift, T. R., and Ignacio, F. J.: Tick paralysis: Electrophysiologic studies. Neurology, 25:1130, 1975.

340.7. SYNDROMES OF MUSCULAR OVERACTIVITY: CRAMPS AND RELATED DISORDERS

Cramps, caused by painful, abrupt shortening of muscle, affect almost everyone at some time or other, Electromyographic investigation indicates that motor units fire at a rate of about 300 per second, much higher than the most vigorous voluntary contraction. It is presumably the high rate of discharge that causes the palpable muscle tautness and the pain. The pain can be relieved by stretching the affected muscle, or by massage. The stimulus responsible for cramps is not known; relief by stretching suggests that some central mechanism is involved, since this is the stimulus for receptors in muscle that inhibit discharge of the motor neuron to the same muscle. Certain conditions are associated with a propensity to cramps: denervation (especially amyotrophic lateral sclerosis), pregnancy, and electrolyte disorders (especially water intoxication and hyponatremia). Some people are more susceptible than others for unknown reasons. Sometimes cramps occur only at night, and can be prevented by quinine sulfate, 0.3 gram orally at bedtime. Sometimes cramps occur frequently during the day, occasionally so often that the individual is effectively crippled. Diphenylhydantoin, 0.3 to 0.6 gram daily, may be helpful to these patients, but some are resistant to this and to other drugs that may be tried, including diazepam and procainamide.

Tetany is a special form of cramp, identified by its predilection for flexor muscles of the hand and fingers, its association with laryngospasm, and its relationship to hypocalcemia. Tetany can be painful. It differs from other cramps electromyographically because of the characteristic rhythmic grouping of discharging potentials.

Contracture is the term reserved for the painful shortening of muscles in glycogen storage diseases, in which the muscles are electrically silent although maximally shortened.

Myokymia has been used to describe a variety of apparently different disorders characterized by cramps in association with spontaneous twitching of muscle. In some cases there are prolonged trains of spontaneous potentials, whereas in others there is grouping of potentials. Some of these patients have difficulty in relaxing grip, but, unlike myotonia, the muscular activity is abolished by neuromuscular blocking agents, indicating a neural rather than a muscular origin. Hyperhidrosis is prominent in some patients and is secondary to the increased muscular activity.

Continuous shortening of the muscle would lead to abnormal postures and abnormally increased resistance to passive movement. These abnormalities, of course, are often due to central neurologic disorders. In recent years, however, an increasing number of patients have been described because of fluctuating rigidity of axial and limb muscles. For want of a better name, and lacking understanding of the pathogenesis, this has been called the *stiff man syndrome*. The diagnosis requires that there be no signs of cerebral or spinal cord disease, and there must be continuous electromyographic activity despite authentic attempts to relax. Ordinary cramps may be superimposed upon the persistent stiffness. Diazepam, 30 to 60 mg daily, may bring dramatic relief.

A variety of other names have been applied to these syndromes, including *quantal squander, armadillo diease, neuromyotonia,* and *continuous muscle fiber activity.* Some cases of brief duration may be related to mild cases of tetanus. It will take some time to sort out the variety of causes. If these unusual forms can be analyzed, we may yet understand why an otherwise normal individual occasionally has a cramp.

Editorial: Writer's cramp. Br. Med. J., 1:67, 1972.

Garner-Medwin, D., and Walton, J. N.: Myokymia with impaired muscular relaxation. Lancet, 1:127, 1969.

Gordon, E. E., Januszko, D. M., and Kaufman, L.: A critical survey of stiff man syndrome, Am. J. Med. 42:582, 1967.

Isgreen, W. P.: Normocalcemic tetany. Neurology, 26:825, 1976.

Layzer, R. B., and Rowland, L. P.: Cramps. N. Engl. J. Med., 285:31, 1971.

Wallis, W. E., Van Poznak, A., and Plum, F.: Generalized muscular stiffness, fasciculations and myokymia of peripheral nerve origin. Arch. Neurol., 22:430, 1970.

PART XII
RESPIRATORY DISEASE

341. INTRODUCTION

John F. Murray

Normal respiration includes all of the processes concerned with O_2 uptake and CO_2 elimination. The lungs are the major organs of gas exchange, but the nose, oropharynx, extrapulmonary airways, brain, spinal cord, nerves, thoracic cage, respiratory muscles, and cardiovascular system are also involved. Thus respiratory diseases, literally interpreted, incorporate a large variety of abnormalities arising in all the different structures that contribute to gas exchange. In general, however, a more limited definition applies, and respiratory diseases are considered to include disturbances of the air passages, lungs, pleura, chest wall, muscles of respiration, and mediastinum (excluding the heart, systemic vessels, and esophagus).

Acute respiratory diseases are probably the most common affliction of mankind and are responsible for more absences from school and work than any other illness. Chronic respiratory diseases, particularly emphysema and bronchitis, are second only to cardiovascular diseases as causes of disability payments. Cancer of the lung kills more persons each year than any other kind of malignancy. Because of the remarkable incidence of these and other respiratory diseases, it is important that all physicians, not just internists and chest specialists, be well versed in the clinical manifestations and methods of diagnosis, treatment, and prevention of the most common disorders. The material concerned with respiratory diseases here and elsewhere in the book is intended as a primer of necessary knowledge with which to recognize and to treat the major respiratory diseases; additional information is available in the references cited at the end of each chapter.

Acute infections of the upper and lower respiratory tract caused by viruses, bacteria, fungi, protozoa, and helminths are discussed in appropriate chapters in Parts IX and X of the text. Although most infectious diseases of the air passages and lungs are viral in origin and prove to be relatively benign and self-limiting, the importance of other infections in the differential diagnosis of patients with respiratory disease cannot be overemphasized. These remain a major cause of morbidity and mortality that can largely be prevented by early diagnosis and use of appropriate chemotherapy. For example, tuberculosis, an eminently curable disease, is too often forgotten and tragically identified only at postmortem examination.

In view of their systemic manifestations, diseases that commonly involve the lungs such as sarcoidosis (see Ch. 65), Wegener's granulomatosis (see Ch. 68), eosinophilic syndromes (see Ch. 72), and the "collagen diseases" (see Ch. 49 to 53) are also discussed elsewhere. Another group of diseases that frequently involve the lungs both primarily and secondarily are disorders of the pulmonary circulation. Of these, pulmonary embolism and infarction (see Ch. 357.3) are by far the most important, but patients with primary pulmonary hypertension (see Ch. 358) and other vasculitic disorders are occasionally encountered. A major feature of many respiratory diseases, but not a disease itself, is pulmonary edema; this is discussed in part in Ch. 351 and in part in Ch. 355.

Part XII begins with a review of basic respiratory physiology (Ch. 342). Knowledge of physiologic principles provides the background for understanding how respiratory diseases affect the function of the lungs and for ordering and interpreting various pulmonary function tests. Next, Ch. 343 deals with the work-up of the patient with respiratory disease, including discussion of the indications for selecting particular diagnostic procedures among those traditional and newly available methods that have improved and often simplified the diagnosis of many diseases. These chapters are followed by those on categories of respiratory diseases: diseases associated with airways obstruction (Ch. 344); abnormalities of lung aeration (Ch. 345); diffuse infiltrative diseases (Ch. 346); lung abscess and bronchiectasis (Ch. 347); physical and chemical irritants (Ch. 348); neoplasms of the lung (Ch. 349); and diseases of the pleura, diaphragm, chest wall, and mediastinum (Ch. 350). Finally, because virtually all respiratory disorders can lead to disturbances of gas exchange, Ch. 351 discusses the diagnosis and treatment of respiratory failure. In this context the term respiratory is used in its broadest meaning to include abnormalities anywhere in the body that cause decreases in arterial Po_2 and increases in Pco_2.

342. RESPIRATORY STRUCTURE AND FUNCTION

John F. Murray

342.1. INTRODUCTION

Knowledge of normal pulmonary physiology is a necessary background for understanding how abnormalities affect the function of the lungs. This information enables practicing physicians to order and to interpret results of the pulmonary function tests that have proved of considerable value in the diagnosis and management of patients with many types of lung disease.

Respiration can be defined as "those processes concerned with gas exchange between an organism and its environment." This definition, which emphasizes that the chief function of the respiratory system is *gas exchange*, is sufficiently comprehensive to apply to all animals, ranging from simple one-celled protozoa to infinitely more complex mammals. In human beings, the basic processes leading to gas exchange, or the uptake of O_2 and the elimination of CO_2, are usually separated into four functional subdivisions:

(1) *Ventilation* — the movement of air from outside to inside the body and the distribution of air within the tracheobronchial system to the gas exchange units of the lungs.

(2) *Diffusion* — the movement of O_2 and CO_2 across the alveolar-capillary membrane between the gas in alveolar spaces and the blood in pulmonary capillaries.

(3) *Perfusion* — the flow of mixed venous blood through the pulmonary arterial circulation, distribution of the blood to the capillaries of the gas exchange units, and removal of the blood from the lungs through pulmonary veins.

(4) *Control of breathing* — the regulation of ventilation, usually in accordance with changing metabolic demands.

342.2. VENTILATION

Air moves from outside the body into the gas exchange units of the lung because contraction of the muscles of respiration normally generates sufficient force to expand the lungs and chest wall and to overcome the resistance and inertia in the system. Accordingly, the volume of gas that reaches the individual gas exchange units is determined by the mechanical properties of the lung parenchyma, airways, and chest wall, and by the force provided by the muscles of respiration (or by a mechanical ventilator).

The amount of air that enters the lung with each breath is called the *tidal volume*. When the lungs are fully expanded, the amount of gas they contain is called the *total lung capacity*. The maximal volume of gas that a person can exhale from total lung capacity is called the *vital capacity*, and the amount of gas remaining in the lungs at the end of maximal expiration is called the *residual volume*. Another important static lung volume is the *functional residual capacity*, which is the volume of gas in the lungs at the end of a normal breath. The relationships among these different lung volumes, which vary in different disorders and which will be frequently referred to, are shown in Figure 1.

STATIC PROPERTIES

Both the lungs and chest wall are elastic structures. This means that they can distend and, when the distending force is removed, recoil back to their resting volumes. Although the lungs and chest wall are similar in this respect, they differ considerably in their respective resting volumes when there is no expanding force.

The elastic properties of isolated lungs are shown by the dashed line in Figure 1. The slope of the line, or the change in volume (ΔV) for a given change in pressure (ΔP), is known as the compliance of the lung. This curve demonstrates that (1) the lungs collapse almost completely when there is no distending pressure, (2) the slope of the volume-pressure curve is relatively steep at low lung volumes (i.e., as the lungs are beginning to inflate, their compliance is high), and (3) at high lung volumes, the curve flattens (compliance decreases) so that little increase in volume results from a large increase in pressure. The elastic forces of the lungs originate within the tissues that are being stretched, particularly those containing elastin and collagen, and from the surface tension of the film of *sur-*

Figure 1. Schematic representation of the volume-pressure relationships of the chest wall (dotted line), lungs (dashed line), and chest wall and lungs combined (solid line). Total lung capacity (TLC) occurs when the lungs are fully expanded, and residual volume (RV) is the amount of gas remaining in the lungs at the end of a maximal expiration. Functional residual capacity (FRC) occurs at that volume at which the recoil pressures of the chest wall and lung are equal and opposite (i.e., the distending pressure = 0 cm H_2O). The bar graph on the right shows the vital capacity (VC) and RV subdivisions of TLC.

factant that lines the air-liquid interface of alveolar spaces. The static properties of the isolated chest wall (including the diaphragm and abdominal contents that must be displaced during breathing) are shown by the dotted line in Figure 1. The chest wall is a compressible and distensible structure that contains an appreciable volume in its resting state. To decrease the volume of the thorax, a force must be applied to overcome the tendency of the chest wall to resist compression and recoil back to its resting position. Conversely, to increase the volume of the thorax, the applied force must overcome the elastic forces in the chest wall that also cause it to recoil back to its resting position.

It is useful conceptually to consider the behavior of the lung and chest wall separately, but obviously they function together. Because their action is coupled by the pleural pressure that keeps the lung expanded against the chest wall, the lungs and chest wall ordinarily change their volumes by exactly the same amount. Thus the pressures required to inflate and deflate the respiratory system (or lung and chest wall combined) are obtained by simply adding the pressures necessary to achieve a given volume. The solid line in Figure 1 indicates the pressure that must be produced by contraction of the respiratory muscles, or by a mechanical ventilator, to inflate or deflate both the lungs and chest wall. Figure 1 also shows that functional residual capacity is the volume at which the inward recoil force of the lung is equal and opposite to the outward recoil force of the chest wall; in other words, functional residual capacity is that volume at which the net force of the respiratory system is zero.

During inspiration, the force developed by the contracting muscles of inspiration meets progressively increasing (inward) recoil forces from the combined expansion of the lung and chest wall. Furthermore, because shortening muscle fibers generate progressively less force, inspiration finally ceases at that volume (total lung capacity) at which the weakening inspiratory muscle forces can no longer overcome the increasing forces required to expand the lungs and chest wall. Similarly, during expiration, the net force developed by the contracting muscles of expiration meets progressively increasing (outward) recoil forces from the chest wall. In children and young adults, expiration ceases at that volume (residual volume) at which the decreasing expiratory muscle forces can no longer overcome the increasing forces required to compress the chest wall. In older persons, residual volume is governed mainly by factors that regulate the caliber and patency of peripheral airways; thus even though the expiratory muscles are capable of further compression, emptying is prevented by airway closure and trapping of gas in the lungs.

Vital capacity, or the volume between total lung capacity and residual volume, is determined by the factors that influence maximum inspiration and expiration, i.e., the balance of forces generated by the muscles of respiration and by the mechanical properties of the lungs and chest wall combined. Changes in these variables explain the characteristic changes in lung volumes that occur in patients with the respiratory disorders discussed in subsequent chapters.

Lung volumes also vary among healthy persons according to their age, sex, and physical structure (especially height). Because body build varies slightly from one ethnic group to another, it is important to have normal data that pertain to the population being studied. Measured volumes are usually expressed as both the observed value and the percentage of the predicted value for a normal subject of the same age, sex, and height.

$$\text{Per cent predicted} = \frac{\text{observed value}}{\text{predicted value}} \times 100$$

Measured values should not be considered abnormal unless thay are clearly outside the range of values likely to be found in normal persons (100 per cent ± 20 per cent for vital capacity and 100 per cent ± 25 per cent for total lung capacity, residual volume, and functional residual capacity).

Vital capacity is easily measured with a spirometer or one of a variety of commercially available recording systems. Most spirometers can also be used to determine airflow rates (see Dynamic Properties, below) but they do not measure total lung capacity, functional residual capacity, or residual volume.

To measure *all* the gas in the lungs at any of these volumes, one of two basically different methods must be used: either dilution or washout of an inert gas or whole body plethysmography. Functional residual capacity is usually determined because it is the normal end-expiratory lung volume and an easy volume for subjects to maintain during the breathing test. After measuring functional residual capacity, residual volume is derived by subtracting expiratory reserve volume, and total lung capacity is obtained by adding vital capacity to the residual volume.

Gas dilution or washout involves measurement of the volume and concentration of an inert gas such as nitrogen (N_2), neon (Ne), or helium (He). These methods measure the amount of gas that communicates freely with the airways during the breathing maneuver; dilution or washout techniques do not detect gas trapped beyond closed (or very narrowed) airways and in poorly communicating regions, like bullae.

Body plethysmography involves placing the subject in the plethysmograph, a large airtight box resembling a telephone booth, and having him breathe through a mouthpiece in which a shutter can be closed to stop the flow of air. When the subject attempts to pant against the closed shutter, the volume of the thorax and gas in the lungs expands and contracts, which changes the pressure measured inside the mouthpiece. Movement of the thorax also changes the pressure in the box by compressing and expanding the gas surrounding the subject. From application of Boyle's law, which states that the pressure times the volume of a gas is constant if temperature remains the same, the volume of gas in the thorax can be calculated. The body plethysmograph measures all the gas present during the breathing maneuver, including that in freely communicating airspaces and any that may be trapped behind poorly communicating airways or in closed spaces (pneumothorax).

In normal subjects, measurements of functional residual capacity by dilution (or washout) and plethysmographic techniques are virtually identical. In contrast, in patients with airways obstruction or bullous disease, the communicating volume may be considerably less than the plethysmographic volume and the difference is a measure of the noncommunicating (sometimes called trapped) volume.

DYNAMIC PROPERTIES

To cause air to flow from outside the body into the gas exchange units, a muscular (or other mechanical) force must be exerted to overcome not only the elastic recoil properties of the lungs and chest wall but also their resistive and inertial properties. In contrast to distensibility, which is not affected by the rate of movement, the forces required to offset resistance and inertia are markedly influenced by the velocity of airflow. Except in a few patients (e.g., those with severe obesity), inertial forces are normally small and usually ignored; thus only those factors affecting airways resistance need be considered in detail.

Resistance to airflow is affected chiefly by the caliber of the airways. Although the diameter of each successive generation of airways decreases, their combined total cross-sectional area increases steadily throughout the tracheobronchial tree from the main bronchi to the peripheral airways. This means that airways resistance progressively decreases and that most of the resistance of the human tracheobronchial tree resides in large airways: direct measurements reveal that about 80 per cent of total airway resistance originates in airways *greater than* 2 mm in diameter. A corollary of this observation is that changes can occur in the caliber of the small peripheral airways without having much effect on total airways resistance. Hence, small airways have been called the lung's "quiet zone," and because they are frequently involved early in the evolution of clinically important lung disease, new tests have been devised to examine their functional behavior.

Changes in the cross-sectional area of airways can also result from changes in lung volume and diseases of the lung parenchyma and airways. During inflation of the lungs from functional residual capacity, airways are

Figure 2. Schematic representation of a normal forced vital capacity (FVC) maneuver (expired volume against time, heavy line) and the derivation of several variables commonly used to evaluate airways obstruction. $MEFR_{200-1200}$ = maximal expiratory flow rate, measured between expired volumes of 200 and 1200 ml; $MMER_{25-75}$ = maximal mid-expiratory flow rate, measured between 25 and 75 per cent of the total FVC; FEV_1 = forced expiratory volume in one second, expressed as percentage of total FVC; FEV_3 = forced expiratory volume in three seconds, expressed as percentage of total FVC.

pulled open so that resistance to airflow decreases; during deflation, airways narrow and their resistance increases. Airway caliber changes during inflation and deflation because of the combined effects of the tethering action of the attachments between the lung parenchyma and small airways and the distending effect of pleural pressure on large airways. Elastic recoil of the lung, which governs the pull of the attachments and the magnitude of pleural pressure, affects the size of all airways. It follows that when elastic recoil is decreased, as in patients with emphysema, airways are narrowed and resistance is increased; this mechanism accounts for much of the airflow obstruction found in patients with emphysema.

Airway narrowing can also result from bronchospasm, edema of the mucosal lining, and secretions within the lumen. Also, changes in the viscosity and density of the inspired gas affect airways resistance, and gas mixtures of different densities are sometimes used to study the dynamic properties of the tracheobronchial system.

Airways resistance can be measured in a body plethysmograph; however, this procedure has limited clinical usefulness. Fortunately, the important dynamic properties of the respiratory system can be assessed by several readily available tests of airways function. The simplest and most widely used of these is the forced expiratory volume in one second (FEV_1), expressed as a ratio of the forced vital capacity (FVC), or FEV_1/FVC (Fig. 2). To perform the FVC maneuver, the subject inhales fully and then exhales as rapidly and completely as possible. In normal persons, the FVC equals the vital capacity from a slow or nonexpulsive maneuver, but in patients with airways obstruction, vigorous expiration may cause airways to narrow or close so that the FVC may be less than the vital capacity; the magnitude of

the difference between the two values is an indication of the amount of air trapped behind compressed airways. The FEV_1/FVC decreases with age in normal persons after reaching adulthood and is usually higher in women than in men at all ages.

Additional measurements of airways behavior besides the FEV_1 can be obtained from the tracing obtained during the FVC maneuver (Fig. 2): several derivatives of time such as the $FEV_{0.5}$ and FEV_3 (the subscript denoting the number of seconds after beginning expiration at which the expired volume is measured), the maximal expiratory flow rate (MEFR or often $MEFR_{200-1200 \; ml}$, indicating that the flow rate was measured between expired volumes of 200 and 1200 ml), and the maximal mid-expiratory flow rate (MMFR or often $MMFR_{25-75\%}$, indicating that the rate was measured between expired volumes of 25 and 75 per cent of the FVC). None of these has any particular advantage over the FEV_1 except that the MMFR is less dependent on the effort exerted by the subject than the other variables and reflects the flow properties of small as well as large airways.

Another way of examining the events during an FVC maneuver is by recording flow against volume instead of volume against time, which provides a maximal expiratory flow–volume curve. From these records, maximal flow rates at any given fraction of the vital capacity, usually 50 per cent ($\dot{V}max_{50}$) or 25 per cent ($\dot{V}max_{25}$), can be determined and reported as the percentage of the predicted values for a subject of the same age, sex, and body size. The early portion of the maximal expiratory flow–volume curve, which includes peak flow, is determined by the effort exerted by the subject and is thus called the effort-*dependent* segment; the later portion is less influenced by effort and is called the effort-*independent* segment. Failure of increasing expiratory effort to augment the velocity of airflow (during the effort-independent portion of the curve) is explained by a fortuitous combination of circumstances through which increasing effort narrows airways by the phenomenon of dynamic compression, and increases airways resistance by just the right amount to offset the effect of the extra effort. Dynamic compression occurs mainly in large airways, from the trachea out to about the segmental bronchi. Compression is important during coughing because the increased lateral velocity of airflow in the narrowed airways produces a shearing effect that removes particles and other material deposited on the luminal surface.

Because events recorded in the effort-independent portion of the flow-volume curve require less cooperation and understanding by the subject, they are more reproducible than those in the effort-dependent portion. Once the effort-independent portion of the maximal expiratory flow–volume curve is reached, maximal flow is determined by only two factors: the elastic recoil of the lungs and the geometry (i.e., cross-sectional area) of the airways between the alveoli and the airways in which dynamic compression occurs. This concept means that tests of peak flow, MEFR, and even FEV_1 reflect mainly resistance to airflow offered by central "large" airways, whereas tests of MMFR and $\dot{V}max_{50}$ and $\dot{V}max_{25}$ reflect chiefly the characteristics of airflow in peripheral or "small" airways. Maximal expiratory flow-volume curves can also be recorded after a few breaths of 79 per cent He and 21 per cent O_2 (He-O_2) as well as after breathing room air (79 per cent N_2 and 21 per cent O_2). In normal persons, the two curves differ from each other because He is a less dense but more viscous gas than N_2. Thus higher flow rates are achieved with He-O_2 during the early and mid portions of expiration in which turbulence and convective acceleration (both density-dependent phenomena) occur; later, when slow laminar flow develops, viscous effects prevail and the He-O_2 curve is identical with or even lower than the room air curve. In general, in normal subjects, flow rates are higher with He-O_2 than with room air throughout most of expiration; appreciable differences in flows are evident at 50 per cent ($\Delta\dot{V}max_{50}$) and 25 per cent ($\Delta\dot{V}max_{25}$) of the vital capacity, and the volume at which the two curves intersect ($Viso_{\dot{V}}$) is close to residual volume.

In the presence of narrowing of peripheral airways, turbulence and convective acceleration are less prominent, so the He-O_2 curve is nearer to the room air curve than it should be; this means that $\Delta\dot{V}max_{50}$ and $\Delta\dot{V}max_{25}$ decrease and $Viso_{\dot{V}}$ increases. Comparison of maximal expiratory flow–volume curves obtained while breathing room air and He-O_2 may prove to be one of the most sensitive tests for demonstrating abnormalities that are presumably located in the small airways of the lungs; however, the value of these tests in detecting early bronchitis and emphysema remains to be proved.

DISTRIBUTION OF VENTILATION

During the movement of air from outside the body into the lungs during inhalation, the airstream is partitioned as it flows through the tracheobronchial to the terminal respiratory units where gas exchange takes place. Even in healthy persons ventilation is not distributed uniformly, and marked derangements may develop in patients with lung disease.

The unevenness of ventilation found in normal subjects results from the vertical gradient of pleural pressure between the uppermost and lowermost parts of the lungs. The origins of the vertical gradient are complex and include the weight of the lungs, their attachments at the hilum, and the shape and effects of the chest wall and abdominal contents. Because of the gradient in the pressure surrounding the lungs, alveoli are larger at the top than at the bottom, and the distribution of inspired ventilation differs from top to bottom.

When breathing normally from functional residual capacity, more inspired air is distributed to the dependent regions of the lungs than to the superior regions because the differences in pleural pressure cause the two regions to function on different segments of the same volume-pressure curve. Because the *change* in intrapleural pressure during quiet breathing is the same throughout the pleural space, the lower regions inflate more than the upper regions because they are operating on a steeper part of the curve and thus receive more volume for the same pressure change. When inspiration continues to total lung capacity, alveoli at the top and bottom of the lung inflate to nearly the same size because both regions are functioning on the flat portion of the volume-pressure curve even though the pleural pressure difference persists. During exhalation, the pleural pressure surrounding the most dependent portion of the lung becomes positive; this causes airways in that region to close. As expiration continues, airway closure progresses from the lowermost regions up the lungs involving more and more airways.

Regional differences in the distribution of ventilation can be examined by the test of closing volume, which is carried out by labeling alveolar gas during inspiration from residual volume to total lung capacity by one of two methods (bolus or resident gas techniques); in either case, the uppermost regions contain a higher concentration of the label than the lowermost regions. The gas concentration measured at the mouth during the subsequent exhalation varies according to the sequence of regional emptying and demonstrates that the first gas inhaled is the last gas exhaled. Phase 1 reflects the composition of gas from the tracheobronchial system and contains none of the label; the concentration rapidly rises during Phase 2 as alveoli containing the label begin to empty; a near-plateau is evident in Phase 3 as alveoli throughout the entire lung deflate; finally, the plateau terminates abruptly with a steep rise in concentration during Phase 4. Closing volume is the junction between Phases 3 and 4 and is that volume at which airways in the dependent regions of the lung begin to close; accordingly, the rising concentration of the label in the subsequent expirate indicates the progressively increasing contributions from the preferentially labeled alveoli in the upper regions of the lung.

Because an increase in closing volume reflects premature closure or narrowing of airways, an increase in closing volume occurs in patients with lung disorders in which the caliber of peripheral airways is decreased from either decreased elastic recoil (e.g., in emphysema) or abnormalities of the airways themselves (e.g., in bronchitis or asthma). Furthermore, increases in closing volume have been detected in asymptomatic patients, usually smokers, and may be an early manifestation of lung disease. In addition, the slope of Phase 3 is useful because it provides a sensitive measure of the adequacy of the distribution of ventilation. Well ventilated units fill and empty more completely and rapidly than poorly ventilated units; this means that the concentration of the label will be lower in the better ventilated regions that empty early during exhalation than in the poorly ventilated regions. Thus the more uneven the distribution of ventilation within the lung, the steeper the slope of Phase 3. The physiologic principles that govern the slope of Phase 3 in the closing volume test are the same as those in the single breath O_2 test for the distribution of ventilation designed by Comroe and Fowler many years ago.

Other tests of the distribution of ventilation utilize the gamma ray–emitting properties of certain radioactive gases, chiefly ^{133}Xe, which are nontoxic and can be detected after inhalation in low concentrations by external counters. The distribution of ventilation can be assessed during a breath hold at end-inspiration after a single breath of ^{133}Xe or at intervals during its elimination by normal breathing after the lung has been labeled uniformly by rebreathing ^{133}Xe from a closed system.

ABNORMALITIES OF VENTILATION

Lung diseases that cause abnormalities of ventilation are usually divided into two different categories: restrictive and obstructive ventilatory disorders. This classificaton is not completely satisfactory because it ignores the fact that disturbances of the distribution of ventilation are the earliest and by far the most common

TABLE 1. Characteristic Changes in Lung Volumes and Tests of Airways Resistance in Patients with Restrictive and Obstructive Ventilatory Disorders*

Test	Restrictive	Obstructive
Vital capacity	Decreased	Decreased or normal
Residual volume	Decreased	Increased
Total lung capacity	Decreased	Normal or increased
RV/TLC	Normal or slightly increased	Markedly increased
FEV$_1$/FVC	Normal or increased	Decreased
MMFR	Normal or decreased	Decreased
Single-breath O$_2$	Normal or increased	Increased

*Abbreviations: RV/TLC = residual volume to total lung capacity ratio; FEV$_1$/FVC = forced expiratory volume in one second to forced vital capacity ratio; MMFR = maximum mid-expiratory flow rate.

abnormality of ventilation and can occur in the absence of manifestations of coexisting obstructive or restrictive disorders.

DISTURBANCES OF DISTRIBUTION. Whenever a disease process involves the lung parenchyma or airways unevenly, abnormalities in the distribution of ventilation are likely to occur because more inspired gas will reach the normal regions of the lung compared with the regions distal to the site of bronchial narrowing, or the regions in which the distensibility is impaired. Whether these functional changes can be detected depends on the extent and severity of the disease and the sensitivity of the test being used. The single breath O$_2$ test, the slope of Phase 3 of the closing volume maneuver, and the washout of radioactive gases are all sensitive methods of detecting early abnormalities in the distribution of ventilation. Frequency dependence of compliance is also a sensitive test for distribution of ventilation but is seldom used owing to its technical complexities.

RESTRICTIVE VENTILATORY DISORDERS. The term *restrictive ventilatory disorder* denotes a pattern of abnormalities in lung function. The word "restrictive" is employed to indicate a restriction of or limitation to the amount of gas within the lungs. Thus restrictive ventilatory disorders are characterized by reductions in lung volumes (Table 1). The hallmark of restriction is a decreased vital capacity, but because this change also occurs in obstructive ventilatory disorders, it is important to exclude the presence of airways obstruction (see Obstructive Ventilatory Disorders, below) or demonstrate the presence of reductions in other lung volumes, particularly total lung capacity.

Many components of the lung, chest wall, and respiratory control system determine the amount of gas that can be breathed into the lungs. Accordingly, restrictive ventilatory disorders can develop in diseases that (1) affect the chest wall or respiratory muscles (pectus excavatum, myasthenia gravis), (2) cause infiltrations in the lung parenchyma or air spaces (diffuse interstitial fibrosis, pulmonary edema), (3) involve the pleura (pleural thickening), (4) occupy space within the thorax (tumors, effusions, cardiac enlargement), and (5) occur after lung resection (pneumonectomy).

OBSTRUCTIVE VENTILATORY DISORDERS. The term *obstructive ventilatory disorder* denotes the constellation of abnormalities that results from airways obstruction, regardless of its cause. Because the functional disturbances depend on the presence of increased resistance to

airflow, obstructive ventilatory disorders are detected mainly by tests of the behavior of the respiratory system under dynamic conditions (Table 1). The FEV$_1$/FVC test is the most widely used, but tests of maximal flow-volume relationships are being used increasingly and may prove superior to the FEV$_1$/FVC in the *early* diagnosis of airways obstruction, especially when the obstruction is situated in peripheral airways.

Obstructive ventilatory disorders are found in patients with asthma, bronchitis, emphysema, advanced bronchiectasis, or other diseases that cause narrowing of the tracheobronchial system. When the term "obstructive" was originally employed, it was not possible to differentiate among these various entities, so they were lumped together in the nonspecific category of chronic obstructive pulmonary disease. Now, however, it is possible by means of specialized tests of lung function to sort out the various diseases that cause airways obstruction, even when they coexist; the characteristic features of asthma, chronic bronchitis, and emphysema are described in subsequent chapters.

342.3. DIFFUSION

Diffusion can be defined as the movement of molecules from a region of higher to one of lower concentration; accordingly, diffusion tends to eliminate differences in concentration within the various regions accessible to the molecules. Diffusion is a passive process that results from the kinetic motion of the molecules and no extra energy is required. In the lung, O$_2$ moves by diffusion from alveolar gas into pulmonary capillary blood; similarly, in the tissues, O$_2$ moves by diffusion from capillary blood in peripheral tissues into neighboring cells. Carbon dioxide also moves by diffusion but usually in the direction opposite to that of O$_2$. Both O$_2$ and CO$_2$ undergo chemical reactions in the bloodstream at the start and finish of their journeys between the lungs and the peripheral tissues; O$_2$ reacts solely with hemoglobin, and CO$_2$ reacts in part with hemoglobin and in part to form bicarbonate.

DIFFUSING CAPACITY

The diffusing capacity of the lung for any gas (G) indicates the quantity of that gas that diffuses across the alveolar-capillary membrane per unit time ($\dot{V}_G$) in response to the difference in mean pressures of the gas within the alveolus (P_{A_G}) and pulmonary capillary ($P\bar{c}_G$). The diffusing capacity of the lung for any gas (D_{L_G}) is expressed by the following general equation:

$$D_{L_G} = \dot{V}_G / P_{\bar{A}_G} - P\bar{c}_G$$

Most inert gases (e.g., N$_2$) diffuse across the air-blood barrier so rapidly that the amount taken up by the lung is not detectably limited by the diffusibility of the gas and the properties of the lung and blood but is determined solely by the solubility of the gas and the volume of tissue and blood into which it can dissolve. This phenomenon enables use of highly soluble gases like acetylene, dimethyl ether, or nitrous oxide to measure lung tissue volume and pulmonary capillary blood flow.

The only two gases that measure the diffusing capacity of the lungs are O_2 and CO. Because of their unique ability to combine with hemoglobin, both have to diffuse across the alveolar-capillary membrane in large quantities to saturate the available hemoglobin at the gas pressure prevailing in the alveoli. Thus it may not be possible for complete equilibrium to occur before the hemoglobin-containing red blood cells leave the pulmonary capillaries and gas transfer ceases. Of the two gases, CO is much more widely used for the measurement of diffusing capacity than O_2 because of the ease and convenience of applying the various CO tests and because CO uptake is always diffusion limited. In contrast, O_2 uptake is not limited by diffusion (i.e., is not a test of diffusing capacity) in normal subjects except during heavy exercise or while breathing low concentrations of O_2.

The physical definition of the diffusing capacity of the lung and its mathematic definition are simple and straightforward. However, despite technical improvements in testing procedures, the interpretation of the results in normal subjects and especially in patients with lung disease is open to question. The chief problem lies in the difficulty of obtaining a true "mean" alveolar Pco. None of the several available methods of measuring diffusing capacity with CO yields a value for Pco that summarizes accurately the events taking place in the 100,000 gas exchange units of the lung, in each of which Pco varies according to the ventilation and blood flow to the unit. Despite this shortcoming, measurements of the diffusing capacity of the lung have provided useful empirical information concerning the function of the lung in healthy persons and patients with lung diseases.

Two general types of tests are available that involve either a breath-holding maneuver (single breath method) or continuous rebreathing (steady state methods). (1) The single breath test for the measurement of pulmonary diffusing capacity is noninvasive, easy for the subject to perform, rapid, and safe. Accordingly, it is widely used not only in pulmonary function laboratories but also in screening clinics for early detection of lung disease. However, some patients with severe dyspnea cannot hold their breath for ten seconds; similarly, the breath-holding requirement limits use of the single breath tests for CO-diffusing capacity during exercise. (2) All six steady state methods involve the continuous breathing or rebreathing of a gas mixture containing a small amount of CO, but each has a different approach to the derivation of mean alveolar CO pressure. Although steady state methods take longer to apply than the single breath method and nonuniformity of ventilation and blood flow probably affect the results of steady state methods more than those of the single breath technique, steady state methods are easier to use during exercise.

The quantity of CO that will diffuse in a known period of time from alveolar gas into capillary blood and combine with hemoglobin in response to a given pressure difference between gas and blood depends on (1) the solubility and diffusibility of CO in each layer of the air-blood barrier, (2) the surface area and thickness of the barrier, and (3) the rate of the chemical reaction between CO and hemoglobin within red blood cells. Because the solubility and diffusibility of CO are physical characteristics that presumably do not change under ordinary circumstances, the two chief components of diffusing capacity are the area and thickness of the alveolar-capillary membrane available for diffusion (DM) and the pulmonary capillary blood volume (Vc) (i.e., the reservoir of hemoglobin) with which the CO combines at a finite rate (θ).

It is now possible to derive the two components of overall diffusing capacity by performing several measurements of DL_{CO} with the subject breathing gas mixtures of different concentrations of CO and O_2. Because CO and O_2 compete with each other for available positions on the hemoglobin molecule, changing the O_2 concentration changes the rate with which CO reacts with hemoglobin, in other words θ, and thus affects DL_{CO}. The values from a series of tests can be plotted and solved graphically for DM and Vc according to the equation developed by Roughton and Forster that expresses the interrelationships among the various factors:

$$1/DL = 1/DM + 1/\theta Vc$$

Approximately half the total resistance to diffusion of CO from alveolar gas to capillary blood resides in the membrane compartment and the other half in the chemical reaction that takes place in the pulmonary capillary blood volume. Accordingly, changes in the hemoglobin concentration have a calculable effect on total CO diffusion that should be taken into account when establishing the predicted "normal" value for a patient with anemia or polycythemia.

Normal values for CO-diffusing capacity depend chiefly on the person's lung volume and therefore closely correlate with body size, especially height. Because single breath and steady state methods yield different results in the same subject, appropriate regression equations must be solved to obtain predicted normal values according to the test being used.

Diffusing capacity is normally higher in the supine than erect posture because position changes Vc. When blood flow to the lung increases, as in muscular exercise, Vc also increases owing to recruitment of previously nonperfused capillaries and dilatation of others; these phenomena account for the progressive increase in DL_{CO} during increasingly strenuous levels of exercise. Similarly, the elevated pulmonary arterial pressures encountered in persons who live at high altitudes also recruit capillaries, increase Vc, and cause an increase in "normal" DL_{CO}. For unexplained reasons (possibly genetic), natives of high altitudes have higher DL_{CO} values than sojourners fully acclimatized to the same altitude.

ABNORMALITIES OF CO-DIFFUSING CAPACITY

Based on the physiologic principles that govern the diffusion of CO, it can be inferred that DL_{CO} may increase or decrease in patients with various cardiopulmonary disorders that affect Vc, DM, or both. When tests of diffusing capacity were first used to study patients with various forms of lung disease, it was assumed that abnormalities of gas transfer would result from thickening of the air-blood barrier by a pathologic process that lengthened the pathway for diffusion of gases; this concept led to the formulation of what became widely known as the *alveolar-capillary block syndrome*. The "block" meant that the distance CO molecules had to travel from gas to blood was increased and, in turn, that extra time was required for diffusion to reach equilibrium across the air-blood barrier. This means that alveolar–end-capillary O_2 differences might occur during the period of time red blood cells normally spend in the pulmonary capillary. Now it is known that the importance of alveolar-capillary block has been greatly exaggerated because (1) arterial hypoxia in patients at rest with decreased diffusing capacities has been shown to be caused mainly by ventilation-perfusion inequalities and not by diffusion abnormalities and (2) decreases in D_L from changes in D_M, such as would occur with a "block," are rare, whereas decreases in D_L from changes in V_C are common.

Pulmonary vascular disorders, such as pulmonary emboli and pulmonary vasculitis, that affect (directly or indirectly) the pulmonary capillary bed decrease D_L through a decrease in V_C. Similarly, $D_{L_{CO}}$ is reduced because of decreases in V_C in patients with infiltrative disorders of the interalveolar septum that obliterate or destroy capillaries. This is the usual mechanism underlying reduction of $D_{L_{CO}}$ in patients with sarcoidosis, diffuse interstitial fibrosis, berylliosis, or collagen diseases of the lung.

Changes in D_M account for a decreased $D_{L_{CO}}$ in patients with diseases in which some form of intra-alveolar filling process has occurred and the air-to-blood diffusion pathway is actually lengthened: pneumonia, pulmonary edema, alveolar proteinosis. A decrease in both D_M and V_C produces a low $D_{L_{CO}}$ in patients with disorders associated with removal or destruction of lung tissue, such as resectional surgery and emphysema.

An increase in $D_{L_{CO}}$ results occasionally from an increase in V_C secondary to hemodynamic changes in the pulmonary circulation: an increase in pulmonary arterial or left atrial pressures or an increase in pulmonary blood flow. The $D_{L_{CO}}$ is sometimes increased in patients with bronchial asthma during an attack, but the cause of this change is not known.

342.4.   PERFUSION

The pulmonary circulation delivers blood in a thin film to the gas exchange units so that O_2 uptake and CO_2 elimination can occur. The physiologic determinants of pulmonary blood flow are analogous to those of ventilation in that the total volumes of ventilation and blood flow must be adequate to meet metabolic needs, and the distribution of both must be such that proportionate amounts of inspired fresh air and incoming mixed venous blood are delivered to individual gas exchange units. Ventilatory volume is controlled by the factors that regulate breathing (see Ch. 342.5), whereas the volume of blood flowing through the lungs is determined mainly by the extrapulmonary mechanisms that govern cardiac output.

DISTRIBUTION OF PULMONARY BLOOD FLOW

Pulmonary blood flow is not distributed uniformly throughout the lung but is normally greatest in the dependent regions where pulmonary arterial pressure is highest and, conversely, is least in the superior regions where pulmonary arterial pressure is lowest. In the upright subject under resting conditions, the apices of the lungs are barely perfused and considerably more blood flows, even allowing for differences in the amount of lung tissue, to the basilar regions. The presence of nonuniform blood flow, which is not matched by comparable changes in ventilation, leads to important differences between regions of the lung in their defense capabilities and efficiency of gas exchange.

Distribution of pulmonary blood flow can readily be measured by injecting radioactive substances, such as ^{125}I-albumin aggregates or ^{133}Xe dissolved in saline, and then detecting their location in the lung with an external counter system. Abnormalities in the volume and distribution of pulmonary blood flow may result from diseases that involve the blood vessels themselves (emboli, vasculitis, emphysema), from compression of blood vessels (tumors, cysts), or from reactivity of blood vessels (vasoconstriction secondary to alveolar hypoxia).

OTHER FUNCTIONS

The pulmonary circulation has important functions besides providing blood flow for continuous gas exchange: (1) it acts as a filter of virtually the entire venous drainage; (2) it supplies substrates for the nutrition and metabolic needs of the lung, including the synthesis of surfactant; (3) it serves as a reservoir of blood for the left ventricle; (4) it affects endocrine function by modifying the pharmacologic properties of a variety of circulating substances; and (5) it provides a large surface area for the absorption and filtration of liquids and solutes.

342.5.   CONTROL OF BREATHING

The respiratory system must maintain gas exchange during periods of stress, such as exercise and other forms of increased metabolic needs. The O_2 consumption may increase more than tenfold from rest to strenuous exercise; over this range, arterial P_{O_2} remains remarkably constant. The correspondence between the volume of ventilation and the demands for O_2 uptake and CO_2 elimination results from the responsiveness of three reasonably well characterized receptor systems that interact to regulate breathing in normal subjects and patients with a variety of disease states: (1) receptors in the airways and lung parenchyma, (2) peripheral chemoreceptors, and (3) central chemoreceptors. Nerve impulse traffic from these receptors is integrated and modulated in the medulla with impulses arising from higher centers in the brain. The medulla can be viewed as the main headquarters for initiating, processing, and relaying messages concerning breathing to other parts of the body via nervous pathways. Some of the resulting medullary neural activity may reach the cerebral cortex and evoke conscious perception of breathing (i.e., the symptom of dyspnea); other impulses may travel through efferent pathways in the autonomic nervous system to the lungs and other organs; still other impulses may descend in the spinal cord to be processed with afferent impulses from peripheral nerves at different cord segments before finally being transmitted to the muscles of respiration and other effectors.

ABNORMALITIES OF CONTROL OF BREATHING

Variations, usually increases, in the rate and depth of breathing occur in patients with many common clinical disturbances such as fever, metabolic diseases, or psychiatric disorders. Several frequently used drugs (e.g., aspirin, antidepressants, and alcohol) also affect ventilation. *Hyperventilation* occurs when ventilation increases out of proportion to CO_2 production and arterial Pco_2 decreases; *hypoventilation* is the converse. *Hyperpnea* signifies an increase in the rate and depth of breathing, such as occurs during exercise, but carries no implication concerning arterial Pco_2 values. It should be emphasized that a decrease in the O_2 pressure (Po_2) of arterial blood has several causes. In contrast, the pressure of CO_2 (Pco_2) is governed simply by the relationship between CO_2 production ($\dot{V}co_2$) and CO_2 elimination by alveolar ventilation ($\dot{V}alv$):

$$Pco_2 = k\dot{V}co_2 / \dot{V}alv$$

Because alveolar ventilation normally changes to keep pace with CO_2 production, for practical purposes abnormal arterial Pco_2 values can always be interpreted as indicating hyper- or hypoventilation.

Abnormalities of the control of breathing can result from excitation of intrapulmonary receptors (pulmonary embolism, pneumonia, asthma), depression of peripheral chemoreceptors (natives of high altitudes, sedative drugs, severe chronic bronchitis), stimulation of peripheral chemoreceptors (drugs such as doxapram), depression of central chemoreceptors (sedative drugs, obesity, myxedema, neurologic disorders), and stimulation of central chemoreceptors (drugs such as aspirin, irritative neurologic lesions). Special tests of the ventilatory response to breathing gas mixtures with increased CO_2 or decreased O_2 help in defining the physiologic derangements among these disorders.

342.6. GAS EXCHANGE

The end product of respiration is gas exchange, which in human beings consists of maintaining the values for Po_2 and Pco_2 in arterial blood within normal limits. As stated previously, respiration consists of ventilation, including the distribution of inspired air throughout the tracheobronchial system, diffusion, blood flow, including the distribution of mixed venous blood throughout pulmonary capillaries, and the control of breathing. Each of these contributes in a unique way to gas exchange such that an impairment in one process cannot be compensated for by improvement in another.

Normal values for the pressures of O_2, CO_2, N_2, and H_2O at sea level (barometric pressure 760 mm Hg) in ambient air, conducting airways (i.e., the dead space), gas exchange units, and arterial and mixed venous blood are given in Table 2. Ambient air consists primarily of N_2 and O_2 with varying amounts of water vapor. As air is inhaled, it is warmed to the subject's body temperature and fully saturated with water vapor (PH_2O 37° C = 47 mm Hg); the addition of water vapor has the effect of diluting the inspired mixture of N_2 and O_2 and reduces their respective pressures proportionately. During gas exchange in the alveoli, more O_2 is removed than CO_2 is added; this causes the volume of each respiratory unit to decrease slightly and raises the concentration and pressure of N_2 slightly.

The values given in Table 2 indicate that gas exchange in the healthy lung is not perfect because there is a small (5 mm Hg) difference between the Po_2 values in (mean) alveolar gas and arterial blood. The difference, known as the alveolar-arterial Po_2 difference, occurs because of the normal presence of a slight nonuniformity in the distribution of ventilation with respect to perfusion and a small right-to-left shunt. Note that the sum of the pressures of the individual gases in mixed venous blood is less than the total atmospheric pressure. Because the tissues and spaces of the body are in approximate equilibrium with venous blood, these structures are also subatmospheric. The "suction" serves to keep the lung expanded against the chest wall and to cause the reabsorption of gas from tissue spaces (e.g., a pneumothorax).

ABNORMAL GAS EXCHANGE

Measurements of arterial Po_2 and Pco_2 and calculations of the alveolar-arterial Po_2 difference are reliable guides to the over-all adequacy of respiration. In determining whether or not an abnormality is present, it must be remembered that normal values for Po_2, but not Pco_2, vary with age and that both Po_2 and Pco_2 are influenced by the altitude at which the subject is living. There are five physiologic mechanisms known to cause arterial hypoxia, defined as a decrease below normal of arterial Po_2: (1) hypoventilation, (2) decreased diffusion, (3) ventilation-perfusion imbalance, (4) right-to-left shunting of blood, and (5) breathing air (or a gas mixture) with a low Po_2. Except for a few uncommon clinical examples, such as breathing air with its Po_2 reduced by combustion of O_2 and addition of smoke or suffocation, item 5 can be ignored. Items 1 to 4 can be separated, at least for practical clinical purposes, by analyzing the values from a given blood specimen and a few easy tests.

TABLE 2. Normal Gas Pressures (in mm Hg) During Inspiration in Ambient Air, Conducting Airways, Terminal Respiratory Units (Alveoli), and Arterial and Mixed Venous Blood

Gas Pressure	Ambient Air	Conducting Airways	Terminal Respiratory Units	Arterial Blood	Mixed Venous Blood
Po_2	156	149	100	95	40
Pco_2	0	0	40	40	46
PH_2O	15*	47	47	47	47
PN_2	589	564	573	573	573
P_{TOTAL}	760	760	760	755	706

*PH_2O varies according to humidity and has a proportionate effect on Po_2 and PN_2.

HYPOVENTILATION. The simplest disturbance of gas exchange occurs when not enough fresh air is breathed into alveolar spaces to raise pulmonary capillary Po_2 to normal levels and to allow CO_2 to leave the bloodstream. Although arterial Pco_2 may theoretically increase in patients with other disturbances of gas exchange (ventilation-perfusion abnormalities and right-to-left shunts), for clinical purposes an elevated value should be interpreted as indicating alveolar hypoventilation.

Pure hypoventilation is a relatively uncommon clinical event. When it is found, depression of the central nervous system resulting from anesthetic agents or other sedative drugs is the usual cause. More commonly, hypoventilation occurs in association with other disturbances of oxygenation. When these coexist, they can be recognized by the fact that the decrease in arterial Po_2 is more than can be accounted for by the increase in arterial Pco_2.

IMPAIRED DIFFUSION. Decreased diffusion, from either loss of pulmonary capillaries or thickening of the air-blood barrier, does not usually cause important alveolar-arterial Po_2 difficulties *at rest*. Thus abnormalities of diffusion can be ignored in patients with arterial hypoxia whose blood specimens are obtained while they are resting. In contrast, impaired diffusion is one of the two major causes of severely worsening hypoxia during exercise (right-to-left shunting of blood is the other). Regardless of the cause of the diffusing impairment, under resting conditions there is sufficient time to allow gas transfer to reach equilibrium between gas and blood. However, during exercise, cardiac output and the velocity of blood flow through pulmonary capillaries increase; thus the time for gas transfer is reduced and marked alveolar–end-capillary Po_2 differences occur.

VENTILATION-PERFUSION MISMATCHING. Because the distributions of inspired air and pulmonary blood flow in normal subjects are neither uniform nor proportionate to each other, a slight ventilation-perfusion imbalance exists in healthy persons. Moreover, increased (above normal) mismatching of ventilation and perfusion is by far the most common cause of arterial hypoxia encountered clinically. Virtually all forms of lung disease are associated with a detectable ventilation-perfusion abnormality.

When a unit is underventilated relative to its perfusion (i.e., has a low ventilation-perfusion ratio), O_2 uptake by that unit must decrease so that the Po_2 of its end-capillary blood is lower than normal; Pco_2 tends to increase but cannot rise above the value in mixed venous blood. Thus the process affects values for Po_2 more than Pco_2. Furthermore, in those units that are overventilated owing to a redistribution of inspired air, the high ventilation-perfusion ratio causes Po_2 to increase and Pco_2 to decrease. But there is an important difference in the effects of these changes in pressures on the actual quantities (contents) of O_2 and CO_2 in the capillary blood leaving units with high ventilation-perfusion ratios. Given the shapes of the respective dissociation curves, O_2 content is not appreciably increased but CO_2 content is decreased. Thus increasing ventilation with respect to perfusion in some regions corrects the tendency to CO_2 retention that would otherwise exist but does not correct the hypoxia caused by low ventilation-perfusion relationships in other units. Another invariable consequence of a ventilation-perfusion abnormality is an increase in the alveolar-arterial Po_2 difference.

RIGHT-TO-LEFT SHUNTING. A small right-to-left shunt of blood is found in normal persons, and shunts of considerable magnitude may occur in patients with pulmonary disease. A right-to-left shunt may be visualized as a pathway(s) through which mixed venous blood flows from the right to the left side of the heart without having contacted functioning gas exchange units along the way. Thus there is a continuous admixture of venous blood with arterialized blood that has come from normal pathways in the lungs. Arterial hypoxia and an increased alveolar-arterial Po_2 difference occur that vary in severity with the magnitude of the shunt and its O_2 content. Right-to-left shunts occur through intracardiac communications in patients with congenital heart disease. In patients with lung disease, although shunts may be extremely large, they seldom occur through abnormal vascular channels such as pulmonary arteriovenous fistulas; instead, they are caused by blood perfusing normal vessels in regions of lung that are atelectatic or in which alveoli are filled with edema fluid, pus, or blood; in either case, because gas transfer is impossible, a shunt occurs.

The consequences of a right-to-left shunt are similar to those of a ventilation-perfusion imbalance owing to basic similarities between the two disturbances. A shunt can be viewed as an extreme ventilation-perfusion abnormality in which there is perfusion but *no* ventilation at all. It is impossible to differentiate between a ventilation-perfusion disturbance and a right-to-left shunt while the subject is breathing ambient air; therefore the effects of both are combined and designated as venous admixture or a "shunt-like" effect. The two causes of hypoxia can be separated by giving the patient 100 per cent O_2 to breathe and measuring arterial Po_2 after all the N_2 has been washed out of the lungs. When a ventilation-perfusion abnormality exists, the N_2 is replaced by O_2 and all the blood perfusing the lungs equilibrates at a high Po_2 (approximately 600 mm Hg); in this way 100 per cent O_2 is said to "correct" a ventilation-perfusion disturbance. In contrast, in the presence of a right-to-left shunt, the admixture of mixed venous blood continues despite breathing 100 per cent O_2 and arterial hypoxia persists. In fact, the alveolar-arterial Po_2 difference in patients with a right-to-left shunt is higher during breathing of 100 per cent O_2 compared with room air, whereas the opposite occurs in patients with ventilation-perfusion inequalities.

SIGNIFICANCE OF ARTERIAL BLOOD GAS VALUES

The availability of accurate rapid analyzers for measuring Po_2, Pco_2, and pH has been one of the major clinical advances of the last 25 years. Virtually the entire therapeutic approach to patients with acute and chronic respiratory failure is dictated by the presence and magnitude of blood gas and pH abnormalities (see Ch. 351). Every physician should know the mechanisms of arterial hypoxia and how to differentiate them because it is important clinically whether a patient's hypoxia results from hypoventilation, impaired diffusion, ventilation-perfusion mismatching, or right-to-left shunting. Evaluating the course and prognosis of the lung disease, determining the need for and outcome of therapy, and assessing disability, operability, and the limits of resection in patients considered for pulmonary surgery all depend to some extent on the findings of blood gas analysis. Thus all physicians who care for patients must become familiar with the technique of arterial puncture and must know how to interpret the results of blood gas analysis.

Bates, D. V., Macklem, P. T., and Christie, R. V.: Respiratory Function in Disease; An Introduction to the Integrated Study of the Lung. 2nd ed. Philadelphia, W. B. Saunders Company, 1971.

Campbell, E. J. M., Agostoni, E., and Davis, J. N.: The Respiratory Muscles; Mechanics and Neural Control. 2nd ed. Philadelphia, W. B. Saunders Company, 1970.

Comroe, J. H., Jr., Forster, R. E., II, DuBois, A. B., Briscoe, W. A., and Carlsen, E.: The Lung; Clinical Physiology and Pulmonary Function Tests, 2nd ed. Chicago, Year Book Medical Publishers, 1962.

Comroe, J. H., Jr., and Nadel, J.: Screening tests of pulmonary function. N. Engl. J. Med., 282:1249, 1970.

Cotes, J. E.: Lung Function, 3rd ed. Philadelphia, J. B. Lippincott Company, 1975.

Jones, N. L. Campbell, E. J. M., Edward, R. H. T., and Robertson, D. G.: Clinical Exercise Testing. Philadelphia, W. B. Saunders Company, 1975.

Murray, J. F.: The Normal Lung: The Basis for Diagnosis and Treatment of Pulmonary Disease. Philadelphia, W. B. Saunders Company, 1976.

343. SPECIAL DIAGNOSTIC PROCEDURES IN PULMONARY DISEASE

Gordon L. Snider

Pulmonary disease comes to light because the patient has respiratory symptoms, because the physician finds abnormalities on physical examination, or because a chest roentgenogram has disclosed an abnormal shadow. With the data in hand from the history and physical examination, chest film (see below), and basic blood and urine laboratory tests, the physician must choose among a broad array of special procedures in order to establish a diagnosis and develop a plan of management. Clinical pulmonary function testing is discussed in Ch. 342. In the following chapters the special diagnostic procedures applicable to pulmonary disease will be reviewed, with comments on when they are to be used and on their limitations.

343.1. THE CHEST ROENTGENOGRAM

STANDARD VIEWS. As already noted, the chest roentgenogram can detect abnormalities in the asymptomatic patient with a normal physical examination of the chest. Even in the presence of respiratory symptoms, the chest roentgenogram may be abnormal when the physical examination is nonrevealing. On the other hand, the full inspiration chest roentgenogram provides no dynamic information, and rales denoting parenchymal disease or rhonchi indicating bronchial disease may be present when the lung fields appear normal in the roentgenogram. It follows that complete evaluation of the respiratory system in the individual who is symptomatic, or who is suspected on other grounds of having pulmonary disease, must include both a physical examination and a chest roentgenogram.

The standard projections are the posteroanterior (PA) and lateral views of the chest. The PA view is taken in full inspiration with the patient's anterior chest wall against the film and the scapulae rotated anterolaterally; the x-ray tube is about 2 meters from the patient so that divergence of the x-ray beam is minimal and the images of the heart and any pulmonary lesions are not magnified. The lower neck and upper abdomen should be included in the field of view. The lateral chest film is an essential part of the roentgenographic examination because it exposes to view portions of the lungs obscured in the PA view by the heart, the mediastinal structures, and the leaflets of the diaphragm. Precise localization of a lesion usually requires display in both the PA and lateral projections.

The normal chest roentgenogram is formed from images of the soft tissues, the bones, the air columns of the trachea and main bronchi, the heart and great vessels, pleural planes observed on end, and the pulmonary parenchyma. The last-named has two major components: (1) the respiratory tissues are strikingly radiolucent because they are more than 90 per cent air at total lung capacity; and (2) the pulmonary vessels present as a branching pattern of denser shadows gradually tapering from the hilum to the periphery but normally seen in a film of good quality to within 1 cm of the edge of the lung. The air columns in lobar and smaller bronchi are not usually seen except adjacent to the lung roots. Variations in density of the lung fields are caused not just by disease processes but also by differences in the depth of respiration and the technical factors of positioning the patient, x-ray exposure, and processing of the film.

Parenchymal abnormalities may be manifest by either an increase or a decrease in roentgenographic density. Diseases which cause an increase in density may be classified into predominant air-space disease, predominant interstitial disease, or shadows due to atelectasis. Air-space consolidation is characterized by poorly marginated densities, often patchy in distribution, and with a tendency to coalesce. Shadows of the air-filled bronchi may become visible in contrast to the consolidated lung tissue surrounding them, an appearance known as an air bronchogram. Densities abutting pleural surfaces are sharply marginated, a property which aids in their localization. The volume of affected lung is normal or even increased. Bacterial pneumonia and pulmonary edema are examples of air-space consolidation.

Processes which predominantly affect the parenchymal interstitium such as viral pneumonia and chemical injury of the lung tend to give rise to linear or lacy patterns of abnormal shadows. The processes are widespread but often uneven in intensity and may be accompanied by some degree of alveolar exudation. Fibrosis with incorporation of alveoli into the interstitium and loss of lung volume may occur.

Atelectasis is a state in which lung tissue is shrunken and airless. The process may be due to bronchial obstruction, to compression of lung by air or fluid in the pleural space, to pulmonary fibrosis, or to alveolar collapse from impaired surfactant activity. The volume of lung affected may vary from less than a segment to an entire lung. The shadows of atelectasis may be nonhomogeneous, but air bronchograms tend to be absent. Loss of volume is evidenced by shifts toward the lesions of the interlobar fissures, the chest wall, or mediastinal structures.

Dense, circumscribed shadows may result from neoplasms, inflammatory processes, or fluid-filled cysts. These shadows may be well or poorly marginated and single or multiple, and may range in size from less than 1 cm to densities which almost fill a hemithorax. It is common to refer to large solitary circumscribed shadows as mass lesions. Central radiolucencies representing necrosis and cavitation may be seen in circumscribed lesions.

There are a number of parenchymal processes which give rise to a decrease in roentgen density. In emphysema (see Ch. 344), the destruction of lung parenchyma results in increased transradiancy and attenuation of the vascular pattern. When the process is very severe locally, bullae may be evident as localized radiolucent zones partially or completely surrounded by arcuate hairline shadows. Increased transradiancy of lung parenchyma is also observed in conditions in which there is high-grade obstruction of the distal airways with pulmonary overdistention, as in severe asthma (see Ch. 344.1) and obliterative bronchiolitis (see Ch. 344.1). A decrease in the amount of blood in relation to tissue is also noted in congenital or acquired narrowing or obstruction of the pulmonary arteries. All the processes referred to above may be widespread or they may be confined to one lung, one lobe, or an even smaller moiety of lung tissue.

Some disease processes show predilections for particular zones of the lung. For example, postprimary tuberculosis occurs most frequently in the apical-posterior segments of the upper lobes; pulmonary embolism and infarction favor the lower lobes. These preferential localizations, although not always rationally explained, are often helpful in differential diagnosis.

Pleural fluid, whether serous, bloody, purulent, or chylous, causes an increase in roentgenographic density; the different types of fluid are not roentgenographically distinguishable. The fluid when free in the subcostal pleural space and small in amount presents as obliteration of the costophrenic angle; larger amounts of fluid present as homogeneous basilar densities with an upper border which is concave. Pleural fluid may occasionally present atypically with a border which is convex upward, mimicking an elevated hemidiaphragm — a so-called infrapulmonary effusion. Fluid may also be loculated in the interlobar fissures, in the subcostal pleura, or paramediastinally. Such shadows usually present as sharply marginated, homogeneous, ovoid densities. The pleura may also be the site of fibrous thickening, calcification, or neoplastic processes.

Pneumothorax is identified by the presence of a radiolucent zone without vascular markings which subtends part or all of the subcostal parietal pleura. In massive pneumothorax, the underlying lung may be completely collapsed and the mediastinum is shifted to the contralateral side. With lesser degrees of pneumothorax, the lung will be variably aerated and the sharp margin of the visceral pleural can be identified, separating the pneumothorax on one side and the slightly denser lung on the other. If fluid accompanies the pneumothorax, its upper border is horizontal, presenting as an air-fluid level.

FLUOROSCOPY. Fluoroscopy permits inspection of the chest during motion and is useful for establishing the diagnosis of diaphragmatic paralysis, for localizing circumscribed dense shadows in preparation for further roentgenographic study, or for guiding placement of a needle, a bronchial brush, or a biopsy forceps. The extent of diaphragmatic excursion during deep breathing is readily determined; paradoxical upward movement of the hemidiaphragm during an inspiratory sniff or downward movement during cough helps confirm the suspicion of paralysis. The anteroposterior placement of a shadow can be located by observing the lesion while the patient rotates on the vertical axis. The degree of motion is related to a structure of known anterior or posterior location such as a rib. The less relative motion there is between the lesion and the reference point, the closer they are together. Attempts to differentiate transmitted from intrinsic pulsation in studying a mediastinal or a paramediastinal mass are usually not helpful.

INSPIRATION-EXPIRATION VIEWS. Films taken a few moments apart in full inspiration and full expiration provide a record of the respiratory system at total lung capacity and at residual volume. The technique is useful for confirming the presence of a small pneumothorax. The air in the pleural space shows an apparent increase in size without change in radiographic density but air leaves the underlying lung, making it more dense and enhancing contrast with the pneumothorax. Inspiration-expiration films are also useful for the demonstration of unilateral or focal obstruction of airways, whether by foreign body or tumor in the large airways or by generalized disease of the small airways. In the expiratory film, the parenchyma beyond the involved airways will empty poorly and the mediastinum will shift away from the involved lung.

SPECIAL VIEWS AND TECHNIQUES. The lordotic projection throws the images of the clavicles and anterior ends of the first ribs upward, thus bringing the structures in the apical-posterior segments of the upper lobes into clear view. This projection demonstrates small nodular shadows due to granulomatous disease and may occasionally show a cavity which is not seen in the plain PA film; however, the lordotic view may conceal a lesion in the anterior segment of the upper lobe.

Overpenetrated PA and lateral views may be taken to more clearly see lesions which are concealed by overlapping structures such as the heart or thickened pleura. Portable films are views taken at the bedside in seriously ill patients using a portable x-ray machine. The views are anteroposterior (AP) in projection with the patient "upright" at an angle of 45 to 80 degrees. The tube-film distance is about 4 feet, resulting in magnification of the heart shadow. These films have more limitations in diagnostic potential than standard PA films but are frequently necessary. Some of these limitations may be overcome by ordering supine or upright AP films done with the patient lying or sitting on a litter in the x-ray department, but such films require the transporting of a seriously ill patient.

Lateral decubitus views are made with the patient lying on one side with the x-ray beam oriented in a horizontal plane. This technique is of great value in the identification of pleural effusions which are free in the major pleural space. Comparison of the lateral decubitus and PA films reveals the appearance in the former of a dense shadow along the lateral chest wall due to fluid which has flowed from above the diaphragm in response to the effects of gravity. Less than 100 ml of fluid may be identified, and the presence of fluid with an atypical presentation may be readily shown. The technique may also be used to confirm the presence of air-fluid levels in the thorax and for demonstrating whether a structure which appears within a cavity is really an intracavitary, freely moving body such as a mycetoma (fungus ball).

Comparison of current PA and lateral views with old films often yields information of signal importance. A solitary pulmonary nodule may be shown to have been present and unchanging for years or alternatively to have appeared in the recent past. The nature of a shadow may be made clear as with no other procedure, e.g., it may become obvious that an air-fluid level in the lung represents an infected bulla rather than a lung abscess. Few diagnostic procedures will as richly repay the physician's efforts as an assiduous search for old chest roentgenograms.

Special views for study of the bones are often helpful. Rib films in suspected fracture and spine films in the evaluation of chest pain are examples. Contrast studies of the esophagus and stomach are valuable in studying mediastinal masses and diaphragmatic hernias as well as in the detection of disorders of esophageal function such as achalasia or intrinsic disorders of these organs.

TOMOGRAPHY. Tomography is a technique in which films are exposed while the x-ray tube and the film move proportionally in opposite directions. The effect is to allow selective visualization of a predetermined layer of tissue to the exclusion of structures lying superficial or deep to this layer. In essence, the image is that of a thin "slice" of lung. The level of the slice which is in focus may be varied at will and is usually recorded as the number of centimeters from the roentgenograph table on which the patient is positioned.

The main indications for the procedure are providing more precise delineation of the morphology of lesions visible on plain films but obscured by overlying densities. Accurate diagnosis of the presence of cavitation within the lung is a good example of this application. Tomography is also capable of clearly demonstrating the presence of calcification within lesions, which is not readily seen in the plain films. The large airways are well shown, and pulmonary arteries and veins may also be more clearly delineated with this method, at times permitting their separation from other shadows such as lymph nodes or demonstrating the decrease in caliber characteristic of pulmonary emphysema. Tomograms may reveal shadows within the lung which are beyond the resolving power of the plain film. For example, small nodules of metastatic neoplasm not seen in the PA or lateral films may be detected tomographically.

BRONCHOGRAPHY. Bronchograms are made by taking a roentgenogram of the chest after the surface of the bronchial mucosa is coated by a contrast medium. The procedure is most often carried out after topical anesthesia of the bronchial tree but may be performed under general anesthesia. The contrast medium is usually oily propyliodone, although other contrast media have been used. Excellent films have been obtained with powdered tantalum, but this material has not yet been released for general use.

Bronchography is most useful for the diagnosis of bronchiectasis, although it is sometimes of value in investigating segmental bronchial obstruction when the nature of the obstructing process is not readily apparent from bronchoscopy or tomography. The procedure

is used on occasion for the study of air-filled or solid densities within the thorax such as giant bullae or intralobar sequestration. The bronchogram also reveals dilation of submucosal mucous gland ducts in chronic bronchitis as well as impairment of filling of the smallest radicles of the bronchial tree in conditions such as chronic bronchitis, asthma, and obliterative bronchiolitis; filling of the microbullae of centrilobular emphysema presents a characteristic pattern known as the mimosa or lily-of-the-valley pattern; bronchography is virtually never justified for the sole purpose of displaying these abnormalities.

The performance of a bronchogram causes transient impairment of ventilatory and gas exchange function, with the amount of function loss dependent upon the amount of bronchographic medium used and the presence of a bronchoconstrictor response to the local anesthetic or bronchographic medium, as in asthma. Needless to say, in patients with pulmonary insufficiency, a bronchogram can precipitate acute respiratory failure. As with any diagnostic procedure, the risks must be weighed against the benefits, and in general the procedure should not be carried out unless its outcome is going to directly influence action taken by the physician.

ANGIOGRAPHY. **Pulmonary Angiography.** Pulmonary angiography is the making of a sequential series of chest roentgenograms, following the rapid injection of a contrast medium into the pulmonary arterial circulation. Although the bolus of contrast medium is sometimes injected into the inferior vena cava, better visualization is obtained if the injection is made through a catheter positioned in the pulmonary artery. More selective pulmonary angiograms may be made by injection into the right or left main pulmonary arteries or even into smaller branches. Although most information is obtained from a study of the opacified pulmonary arteries, the contrast medium is also usually followed as it passes through the capillary circulation of the lung into the pulmonary veins; the pulmonary angiogram also gives information about vascular transit times and the presence of anomalous vascular communications.

Pulmonary angiography is most frequently used for the diagnosis of pulmonary embolism and is the most accurate test for that entity. The presence of pulmonary emboli is revealed by the demonstration of areas of decreased perfusion or intravascular filling defects.

A less frequent but nevertheless important use of pulmonary angiography is the demonstration of oligemic areas in patients with unilateral hyperlucent lungs or in patients with giant bullous emphysema who are being considered for surgical therapy. In the latter group, pulmonary angiography usefully identifies lung which is being compressed by the giant bullae; the procedure is of less risk to the patient than bronchography. Pulmonary angiography is also useful for demonstrating congenital anomalies of the pulmonary vascular tree such as agenesis or hypoplasia of a pulmonary artery, stenosis of peripheral pulmonary vessels, idiopathic dilation of the pulmonary artery, and arteriovenous malformation of the lungs, including pulmonary venous varix. Rarely, pulmonary angiography may be the only way of settling whether an enlarged hilum is due to a dilated pulmonary artery or to lymphadenopathy.

In general, the procedure is well tolerated even by seriously ill patients. However, there is a decidedly increased risk of cardiopulmonary arrest when this test is performed in patients with severe pulmonary hypertension. If, in this circumstance, the physician decides that the procedure still must be done, the amount of contrast medium injected should be sharply decreased and consideration given to carrying out several small, selective injections.

Aortography. Aortography, best carried out by direct catheterization of the aorta by a percutaneously inserted catheter, is useful for the diagnosis of aneurysm of the aorta and the differentiation of dilations and distortions of the great vessels from other mediastinal masses. The procedure should also be performed prior to exploratory thoracotomy in a patient who may have intralobar sequestration of the lung in order to identify the anomalous aortic vessel which often supplies such a sequestration.

Superior Vena Cava Angiography. The superior vena cava is opacified by the injection of contrast medium into a catheter which has been passed into the vessel or into one of its large tributaries. The technique is useful in the investigation of obstruction of the superior vena cava, especially with incomplete manifestations of the superior vena cava syndrome. It is also used occasionally in preoperative staging of patients with carcinoma of the bronchus, especially when the primary lesion is in the right upper lobe, adjacent to the mediastinum.

Azygography. The azygos and hemiazygos veins can be outlined by injecting contrast medium directly into the intraosseous space of a lower rib or into a catheter which has been introduced percutaneously into the azygos vein. This technique has been used for evaluating the presence of mediastinal metastases in carcinoma of the lung and for studying enlargement of the azygos vein in obstruction of the superior vena cava, congestive heart failure, and severe cirrhosis of the liver. However, the technique has added little to other methods of study and is rarely used.

Bronchial Arteriography. The bronchial arterial circulation can be opacified by the injection of contrast medium through a catheter which has been passed through the aorta directly into one of the bronchial arteries. Bronchial arteriography carries the risk of spinal cord injury if contrast medium is injected into a vessel communicating with the anterior spinal artery. This technique has been useful in elucidating the hyperplasia of the bronchial circulation which occurs in such conditions as pulmonic stenosis and bronchiectasis, but has no proved value as a diagnostic tool. Bronchial arterial embolization is currently being explored as a means of controlling life-threatening hemoptysis.

COMPUTERIZED TOMOGRAPHIC SCANNING. Computerized tomographic (CT) scanning provides a 180 degree transverse image of a thin "slice" of the thorax. A thin beam or beams of x-rays passes through the thorax, and the change in the attenuation of the x-rays is measured by a series of detectors. A computer reconstructs a pictorial image which represents the differential absorption of the x-ray beam through the chest. Newer equipment performs two adjacent levels of scanning in approximately two to ten seconds, a time which permits breath-holding. The examination is usually performed in the supine position, but prone and lateral recumbent projections can also be utilized.

Experience with the method is still limited in the thorax, but preliminary studies show the equipment to be more accurate than conventional tomography in the evaluation of mediastinal mass lesions, especially those due to fat deposition, cystic lesions, and vascular enlargements. The method appears to be more sensitive than tomography in screening for the small nodular shadows of suspected metastatic neoplasm and is of unique value in differentiating pleural from peripheral pulmonary lesions. CT scanning is also extremely sensitive in detecting calcification and is therefore of value in studying solitary pulmonary nodules. The technique is also used for identifying pulmonary lesions in areas which are ordinarily poorly seen in conventional roentgenograms or laminograms such as the lung adjacent to mediastinal structures, including the paravertebral areas (especially at the thoracoabdominal junction) and the posterior costophrenic sulci. Lesions in the parenchyma which are obscured by complex pleural or parenchymal shadows are well shown.

Felson, B.: Chest Roentgenology. Philadelphia, W. B. Saunders Company, 1973.

Fraser, R. G., and Paré, J. A. P.: Diagnosis of Diseases of the Chest. Philadelphia, W. B. Saunders Company, 1970.

Heitzman, R. E.: The Lung; Radiologic-Pathologic Correlations. St. Louis, C. V. Mosby Company, 1973.

343.2. RADIONUCLIDE IMAGING

In a relatively few years, radionuclide lung scanning has come into widespread use. The procedure is most often carried out with the gamma scintillation camera coupled to a digital computer system and cathode ray display; photographs of the display are made for permanent records. Lung scanning is most often used for the diagnosis of pulmonary embolism; however, the technique is also used clinically for the evaluation of regional lung function.

We will first consider the lung perfusion scan, which is based on the following considerations. There are billions of arterioles and capillaries in the lung which are less than 30 μm in diameter. Following the injection of about 50,000 microspheres of radioactive human serum albumin of 30 μm diameter, a small proportion of these vessels will be blocked temporarily by the particles. Because the density of the microspheres is comparable to that of red blood cells, their distribution throughout the lungs will be determined by the distribution of pulmonary arterial blood flow. External imaging of the radioactivity within the lung can be carried out in four projections: the anterior, posterior, and both lateral projections. Foci of the lung with impaired arteriolar and capillary perfusion will be disclosed as areas partially or completely devoid of radioactivity. Vessels occluded by emboli will thus be revealed as fairly sharply defined segmental or lobar defects. However, areas of parenchymal pulmonary infiltration caused by pneumonia, fibrosis, or tumor will also show as impaired zones of perfusion; the presence of such areas can, of course, be detected by a study of the plain chest roentgenogram. Emphysematous lung or areas where there is impaired perfusion due to focal increase in intra-alveolar pressure, as in asthma, will also appear as areas of impaired perfusion. Such perfusion defects are usually nonsegmental in nature and are vague in outline. It is apparent that this latter class of perfusion defects is not readily detectable from a study of the plain chest roentgenogram.

Regional ventilation can be determined by imaging with a scintillation camera the initial distribution and subsequent washout of air mixed with a radioactive gas, [133]xenon. Imaging after an initial period of breathing the gas to equilibration reveals "cold" areas of lung which may be aerated (as seen in the chest films) but not communicating with the bronchial tree. Study of images done at regular intervals during washout of the ^{133}Xe permits estimation of total and regional rates of ventilation. The normal lung is cleared of xenon at the end of about three minutes of breathing air. The perfusion scan, of course, gives information regarding regional perfusion. Regional ventilation and perfusion relations may be assessed visually or by processing of the information with the computer. The two lungs may be studied separately to give information comparable to that obtained by differential bronchospirometry but without the need for using an invasive technique. The computer may also be programmed to provide the ventilation-perfusion relationships of more limited zones of the lung such as the upper, middle, and lower lung zones of each of the lungs separately.

A negative perfusion lung scintigram of good technical quality excludes the diagnosis of angiographically detectable pulmonary embolism. In pulmonary embolism without infarction, perfusion of the embolized area is profoundly impaired, with minimal impairment of ventilation; in emphysema both regional perfusion and ventilation are impaired. Consequently, the combination of impaired perfusion with maintained ventilation permits improved accuracy in the diagnosis of pulmonary embolism.

Regional ventilation and perfusion relationships are also useful in preoperative evaluation of the risk of pulmonary surgery, in the evaluation of unilateral hyperlucent lung, and in more precise evaluation of the localized severity of emphysema than is possible in the plain chest roentgenogram. Impairment of perfusion with maintenance of ventilation has been demonstrated in patients with bronchogenic carcinoma who have involvement of their pulmonary arteries by tumor. Such patients have been shown to have a decreased rate of operability and of survival when resectional surgery is carried out.

[67]Gallium citrate, a radioisotope with a half-life of 78 hours which emits gamma rays, concentrates in rapidly dividing cells. Thus the radioisotope will appear in rapidly growing tumors and in inflammatory lesions. Although this technique is largely of research interest in pulmonary disease, it has been used to detect occult mediastinal metastases in patients with known bronchogenic carcinoma. Its use in establishing the activity of such diseases as idiopathic interstitial pulmonary fibrosis and sarcoidosis of the lungs is presently being explored.

Anderson, P. O., Rujanavech, N., Secker-Walker, R. H., and McNight, R. C.: Role of ^{133}Xe ventilation studies in scintigraphic detection of pulmonary embolism. Radiology, 120:633, 1976.

Bell, W. R., and Simon, T. L.: A comparative analysis of pulmonary perfusion scans with pulmonary angiograms. Am. Heart J., 92:700, 1976.

Gilday, D. L., and James, E., Jr.: Lung scan patterns in pulmonary embolism versus those in congestive heart failure and emphysema. Am. J. Roentgenol., 115:739, 1972.

Siemsen, J. K., Grebe, S. F., Sargent, E. N., and Wentz, D.: Gallium-67 scintigraphy of pulmonary diseases as a complement to radiography. Radiology, 118:371, 1976.

Wagner, H. N., Jr.: The use of radioisotope techniques for evaluation of patients with pulmonary disease. State of the art. Am. Rev. Respir. Dis., 113:203, 1976.

343.3. ULTRASONOGRAPHY

Ultrasound is the term applied to a class of mechanical pressure waves that can be propagated through liquids and solids and which, for medical use, have a frequency of oscillation between 1 and 20 MHz. A high frequency sound wave is emitted from a transducer which is applied to the patient's skin. A portion of the wave is reflected back to the transducer as it passes through the tissues being scanned. An image is produced on a cathode ray tube for immediate viewing or is photographed for producing permanent records. Ultrasonography can be applied in a variety of different modes which permit localization of the depth of visualized structures, show the rate of motion of structures such as the diaphragm and heart valves, or generate cross-sectional images which can show outlines of solid viscera such as the liver, large blood vessels, and solid or cystic masses.

Ultrasound waves do not penetrate far into the aerated lung, and the technique is therefore applicable only in pleural or juxtamediastinal disease. Ultrasonography has proved to be helpful in the evaluation of pleural opacities, especially in the localization and identification of loculated pleural effusions. Pleural effusion, whether serous, sanguineous, or purulent, presents as an echo-free space. Consolidated lung conducts sound but, unlike pleural fluid, produces numerous echoes. Pleural fibrosis behaves similarly to consolidated lung. Ultrasonography is useful for determining the site of thoracentesis and may be used to determine the depth to which the needle or a chest tube must be inserted in order to drain a pleural loculation. In most circumstances, ultrasonography is superior to fluoroscopy or chest roentgenography in assisting in the diagnosis and management of loculated pleural effusion. Its use is unnecessary in uncomplicated pleural effusion.

Doust, B. D., Baum, J. K., Maklid, N. F., and Doust, V. L.: Ultrasonic evaluation of pleural opacities. Radiology, 114:135, 1975.

Sandweis, D. A., Hanson, J. C., Gosink, B. B., and Moser, K. M.: Ultrasound in diagnosis, localization and treatment of loculated pleural empyema. Ann. Intern. Med., 82:50, 1975.

343.4. SKIN AND SEROLOGIC TESTS

Skin and serologic tests are of value in the investigation of many viral, bacterial, and fungal diseases of the lungs as well as in the investigation of hypersensitivity lung diseases. Skin tests may be divided into three broad categories: immediate or wheal-and-flare reactions, immune complex or Arthus-type reactions, and delayed or tuberculin-type reactions.

IMMEDIATE SKIN REACTIONS. Immediate, wheal-and-flare or Type I skin reactions result from the release of chemical mediators from IgE-sensitized basophils and mast cells which have contacted a specific antigen. Solutions for skin testing are made from extracts of material which are inhaled or ingested, and which may be causing symptoms, such as the pollens of trees, grasses and weeds, house dust, animal danders, mold spores, or foods. Dilutions may also be made from insect venoms and animal serums. These tests are most safely performed by applying the test solutions to scratches or pricks and demonstrating a wheal-and-flare reaction, which is usually obvious within 15 to 20 minutes after the test is performed and which is greater than the reaction produced by a simultaneously applied test diluent. Intradermal tests may be done with 0.02 ml amounts of solution when scratch tests have been negative. As with any laboratory test the results of skin tests must be interpreted in their clinical context.

The presence of antigen-specific serum IgE may also be detected by the radioallergosorbent test. In this test an insoluble polymer-antigen conjugate is mixed with the serum to be tested. IgE specific for the antigen present in the serum will attach to the conjugate. The quantity of antigen-specific IgE in the serum is quantified by adding[125] I-labeled anti-IgE antibody and measuring the amount of radioactivity taken up by the conjugate.

Bronchial inhalational challenge may be carried out by using graded doses of a highly dilute extract of the allergen to be tested. Development of airways obstruction is demonstrated by serial measurements of airways resistance or indices derived from the forced expiratory spirogram or flow volume loop. This method remains largely a research procedure.

IMMUNE COMPLEX SKIN REACTIONS. Skin test reactions manifest by an erythematous, edematous area developing about six hours after the intradermal injection of the test solution are known as Type III or immune complex reactions. They are believed to result from the deposition of a soluble circulating antigen-antibody (immune) complex in the vessels or tissues. Both wheal-and-flare and immune complex reactions may occur following the same skin test material, as with aspergillus antigen solutions. Except for aspergillosis, this type of skin test reaction has limited clinical use.

DELAYED SKIN REACTIONS. Delayed, tuberculin-type hypersensitivity or Type IV reactions are believed to be caused by activation of sensitized lymphocytes after contact with antigen. An inflammatory reaction results from direct cytotoxicity or from the release of lymphokines. A positive reaction is manifest by an area of induration occurring 48 hours or more after the injection of an appropriate test solution.

The intracutaneous or Mantoux test is the "gold standard" of delayed-type hypersensitivity testing in tuberculosis; 0.1 ml of stabilized solution of PPD-tuberculin containing 5 tuberculin units in injected intradermally into the skin of the forearm. The test is read on the second or third day after injection: 10 mm or more of induration is interpreted as a positive reaction indicating infection with *Mycobacterium tuberculosis*, with or without associated disease; induration of 5 to 9 mm diameter is interpreted as doubtful (such reactions can result from either infection with *M. tuberculosis* or one of the atypical mycobacteria), and the test must be interpreted in clinical context and may have to be repeated; 0 to 4 mm induration is interpreted as a negative reaction, representing either no evidence of infection with *M. tuberculosis* or low grade sensitivity caused by atypical mycobacterial infection.

Multiple puncture tests, such as the tine test, should be used only for screening, and positive reactions should be confirmed by an intradermal test. Skin tests with antigens produced from atypical mycobacteria may give larger reactions in patients with such infections than the tuberculin test done with standard PPD-tuberculin. Although these tests have proved useful in epidemiologic studies, they are rarely useful in establishing a diagnosis in the individual case, and skin testing materials are not available for general use.

Skin testing materials are available for studying patients who may have coccidioidomycosis (coccidioidin, spherulin) and histoplasmosis (histoplasmin); 0.1 ml of a 1:100 dilution is given intradermally, and induration of 5 mm or greater is interpreted as a positive reaction. As with the tuberculin reaction, the test may take several weeks after infection to become positive, is often negative in severe or disseminated disease, and may be falsely negative when there is cutaneous anergy as in advanced age or severe febrile illnesses, especially those due to viruses. The state of skin reactivity may be established by testing with a common antigen such as mumps or *Trichophyton*. Skin tests for blastomycosis, cryptococcosis, nocardiosis, and actinomycosis are not clinically useful. Many physicians believe that since, as noted below, the histoplasmin skin test often causes a rise in histoplasmin complement-fixing titer and is often negative in early or disseminated disease, this skin test is also of very limited clinical usefulness.

THE KVEIM TEST. The Kveim test for sarcoidosis is performed by intradermally injecting 0.1 to 0.2 ml of a crude saline suspension of tissue prepared from spleen or lymph node of a patient with active sarcoidosis. A positive reaction consists in the development of a sarcoid granuloma in tissue biopsied four to six weeks after the injection. The reaction is said to be positive in up to 80 per cent of patients; false-positive reactions are low with most but not all batches of the test material. Kveim antigen is not commercially available in the United States, and the test remains a research procedure.

SEROLOGIC TESTS. Serologic tests, which demonstrate the presence of specific antibodies in the patient's serum and which depend on agglutination, precipitating, complement-fixation, or other reactions, are useful in a variety of bacterial, viral, and mycotic infections. The specificity and sensitivity of these tests varies, and the experience of a particular laboratory with a particular test must generally be known to permit the most useful interpretation. The tests must always be interpreted in the light of the full clinical picture, and the results must often be considered confirmatory or supportive rather than diagnostic.

In acute viral, mycoplasmal, and rickettsial infections, the occurrence of recent infection must generally be documented by showing a rise in titer to the antigen occurring over time (10 to 21 days). A single positive test may indicate nothing more than infection in the distant past. Thus these tests are often of most value in identifying the nature of an epidemic in a community rather than being of help in the diagnosis and treatment of the acutely ill patient.

Nonspecific cold agglutination antibodies are found in about half the patients with *Mycoplasma pneumoniae* infections, and a rising titer of cold agglutinins in an appropriate clinical setting is strong evidence for the presence of this disease.

Precipitin reactions are positive during the early weeks of histoplasmosis and coccidioidomycosis and then wane. Complement-fixation (CF) tests then become positive. In coccidioidomycosis a rising CF titer, especially above 1:64, presages dissemination. In histoplasmosis, complement-fixing antibodies tend to disappear with dissemination. The coccidioidin skin test does not affect the coccidioidin CF test, but the histoplasmin skin test tends to cause a rise in histoplasmin CF titer. Serologic tests for blastomycosis are not useful.

Precipitin and CF tests for aspergillosis tend to be positive in patients with invasive aspergillosis and aspergilloma and in many patients with allergic bronchopulmonary aspergillosis. However, these tests are not highly specific and must be regarded as confirmatory rather than diagnostic.

Cryptococcal antigen in blood, or especially spinal fluid, is helpful in establishing the diagnosis of infection with *Cryptococcus neoformans* and in following the course of treatment; as the patient improves, antigen levels tend to fall and antibodies to the cryptococcus are detectable in increasing titer. These tests have had little application in uncomplicated pulmonary cryptococcosis.

In autoimmune disorders, antibodies may develop to various components of the individual's own cells (see Ch. 38). These antibodies may be specific for components of the nucleus or of the cytoplasm of the cells. One of the most widely used of these is the antinuclear antibody test. The demonstration of the lupus erythematosus cell is also dependent upon this type of immune disorder.

Serologic tests have proved to be disappointing in the diagnosis of hypersensitivity lung disease. Although precipitin antibodies to the agent in question are often demonstrated in patients with these diseases, they are also frequently found in persons who have had inhalational exposure to the causative organic dusts but who have not developed any illness. The tests thus have a confirmatory rather than a pathognomonic role in diagnosis.

Emmons, C. W., Binford, C. H., and Utz, J. P.: Medical Mycology. Philadelphia, Lea & Febiger, 1970.

The Tuberculin Skin Test. Supplement to Diagnostic Standards and Classification of Tuberculosis and Other Mycobacterial Diseases. New York, American Lung Association, 1974.

343.5. EXAMINATION OF THE SPUTUM

COLLECTION OF THE SPECIMEN. It is estimated that the tracheobronchial glands and goblet cells produce about 100 ml of secretion per day. Virtually all this material is swallowed after being carried to the oropharynx by the mucociliary elevator. Expectoration of bronchial secretions represents an abnormal state, and much information can be garnered by a study of sputum using microscopic and cultural methods. In patients with acute or chronic pulmonary disease who are not expectorating sputum, a specimen may be obtained by passing a suction catheter through the nose into the trachea (the nasotracheal specimen), or sputum production may be induced by having the patient inhale an ultrasonically generated aerosol of physiologic saline for 15 minutes. An aerosol of a 10 to 15 per cent sodium chloride solution heated to near body temperature may also be used for this purpose. When cultural studies are to be carried out for organisms such as *M. tuberculosis* or pathogenic fungi, which can withstand an acid milieu, a specimen of lower respiratory secretions can generally be obtained by early morning aspiration of gastric contents. However, specimens obtained in this way do not have a higher yield than induced sputa.

Since expectorated sputum is always contaminated by mouth flora, anaerobic cultures can be performed only on specimens obtained by transtracheal aspiration. Transtracheal aspiration is performed under local anesthesia by inserting a thin-walled needle through the cricothyroid membrane into the lumen of the trachea. A sterile plastic catheter is threaded through the needle into the trachea, and secretions are aspirated after a few milliliters of sterile saline are instilled to provoke cough. Routinely obtained bronchoscopic specimens are invariably contaminated with mouth organisms.

INSPECTION. Inspection of sputum with the naked eye serves to distinguish mucoid from mucopurulent sputum and discloses the presence of blood, black pigment as in anthracosis, or stones and gravel as in broncholithiasis. The viscosity of the sputum and the presence of plugs or casts of the bronchi can be ascertained.

MICROSCOPIC EXAMINATION. A fleck of sputum, carefully chosen because it is opaque, is placed on a microscope slide. This is spread out under a coverslip and, after scanning with the low power lens, is examined with the oil-immersion lens with the condenser racked down and the diaphragm adjusted to give a quasi-darkfield effect. In such a preparation eosinophils can be recognized by their large, brightly refractile granules and a bilobed nucleus. The granules of neutrophils are smaller and often display brownian motion; these cells have multilobed nuclei. The numbers of cells present indicate whether grossly observed purulence of the sputum is due to eosinophils or neutrophils. The presence of more than 20 per cent eosinophils suggests the presence of atopic disease. Macrophages are larger, are rounded, and often contain granular and pigmented inclusions. These cells come only from the lower respiratory tract and are observed in large numbers in the quiescent phases of chronic bronchitis. In lipoid pneumonia, clear lipid droplets abound in their cytoplasm. Hemosiderin-laden macrophages are observed in chronic left ventricular failure and in idiopathic hemosiderosis.

Charcot-Leyden crystals, which are elongated, rhomboid, needle-like shapes varying from 10 to 400 μm in length, are derived from the granules of eosinophils and have the same significance. Fungi such as the budding forms of candida, sometimes with their pseudohyphae, the septate hyphae characteristic of aspergillus, and the endospore-filled spherules of coccidioidomycosis can be recognized. Detection of fungi may be improved by clearing the specimen with potassium hydroxide.

Epithelial cells are often seen. The presence of squamous epithelial cells identifies contamination with oral secretions, indicating that further microscopic and cultural examination should not be carried out on that portion of the specimen. Study of the morphologic variants of bronchial-epithelial cells by this method is of little clinical value.

The coverslip can be removed from the wet preparation and the smear may be stained with Gram's stain for evaluation of bacterial flora. Eosinophils and neutrophils cannot be distinguished in this preparation, but squamous epithelial cells are easily identified, and areas near such cells should be avoided or another smear made. The morphology and Gram-staining characteristics of organisms can be identified. The morphology of bacteria often permits tentative identification such as the flame-shaped, gram-positive diplococci that denote the pneumococcus or the clumped, rounded, gram-positive cocci of the staphylococcus; the fine gram-negative rod of *Hemophilus influenzae* can usually be differentiated from the plump, sometimes encapsulated gram-negative rod that is *Klebsiella pneumoniae*.

The predominance of large numbers of one organism suggests infection of the respiratory tract rather than colonization. Sheets of gram-negative rods, to the virtual exclusion of other organisms, suggest a gram-negative bacillary infection; a large number of gram-negative and gram-positive organisms of great morphologic variability suggests the possibility of a mixed anaerobic infection. Needless to say, the Gram stain is of little value by itself, but is often helpful in establishing a clinical diagnosis when its results are carefully integrated with all other clinical information. Although cultures of sputum provide the most accurate qualitative information, integration of the sputum Gram stain with cultural data provides the best easily available estimate of quantitative bacteriology of the respiratory tract.

Examination of a sputum smear stained by the acid-fast or Ziehl-Neelsen method (direct smear technique) provides the possibility of rapid discovery of acid-fast bacilli in the sputum and the diagnosis of a mycobacterial infection in the appropriate clinical setting. Concentration of sputum with low bacillary counts by smear of the sediment after solubilization of mucus by adding agents such as N-acetyl-cysteine increases the sensitivity of both the smear and cultural techniques and, when sputum is scanty, may be applied to sputum collected over a period of several days. Mycobacteria may be seen with even more sensitivity but somewhat less specificity in sputum smears stained with fluorochrome dyes and examined by ultraviolet microscopy.

SPUTUM CULTURES. Cultures of sputum may be made for pyogenic organisms, mycobacteria, and fungi; drug susceptibility testing can be carried out on the pyogens and mycobacteria. Reports on pyogens are usually available within 24 to 72 hours, but mycobacterial cultures take from three to eight weeks from time of planting and fungal cultures take about three weeks. As noted previously, mouth flora contaminates all expectorated sputum, and cultural studies must be interpreted in the context of a Gram stain and the clinical findings. Positive blood cultures in the appropriate clinical setting provide the most powerful evidence of the etiology of bacterial pneumonia.

When dealing with an exacerbation of a chronic bronchopulmonary process, it is appropriate to start antibiotic therapy for the most commonly found organisms (*D. pneumoniae* or *H. influenzae*) without doing a culture, provided that the Gram stain does not show predominance of some other organism.

Cultures for mycobacteria done on concentrated specimens are much more sensitive diagnostically than microscopic examination, and accuracy improves as multiple cultures, up to five in number, are performed. Cultures are also required for precise identification of mycobacteria.

SPUTUM CYTOLOGY. Smears are prepared for cytologic examination either by ethanol-ether fixation of a freshly expectorated specimen or by homogenization and concentration of a specimen previously expectorated into a fixative solution. Staining is carried out by the Papanicolaou method. Tumor cells can be identified in as high a proportion as 90 per cent of central tumors and a lower proportion of midzonal tumors. Cytologic study is of little value in diagnosing peripheral tumors. Diagnostic yield increases with the examination of multiple specimens, but there is little increase in the rate of return after five specimens have been examined. In many instances, the cytologist can accurately identify the histologic type of the tumor. It should be remembered that positive sputum cytology can result from neoplasms in the nasopharynx, larynx, mouth, and esophagus, a fact that is of special importance when the chest roentgenogram is negative.

Chodosh, S.: Examination of sputum cells. N. Engl. J. Med., 282:854, 1970.

Davies, D. F.: A review of detection methods for the early diagnosis of lung cancer. J. Chron. Dis., 19:819, 1966.

Epstein, R. L.: Constituents of sputum: A simple method. Ann. Intern. Med., 77:259, 1972.

343.6.   EXAMINATION OF PLEURAL FLUID

Inspection of pleural fluid, an inevitable part of every thoracentesis, provides useful information. The diagnosis of empyema is evident if pus is obtained. Hemorrhagic effusions are more frequent in carcinoma and pulmonary infarction than in infectious processes. The obtaining of milky white fluid establishes the diagnosis of chylous effusion, and the presence of shimmering reflections from the top of a test tube of pleural fluid suggests the presence of a cholesterol-containing pleural effusion.

Laboratory examinations of pleural fluid are definitive only if tumor cells are seen in cytologic examination of the specimen or when a specific agent is recovered which proves the etiology of an infectious process. However, the integration of relatively inexpensively obtained laboratory data with the clinical information often provides important clues to the diagnosis. Thus pleural fluid transudates, often a part of systemic edematous states, generally have a specific gravity of less than 1.015, total protein of less than 2.5 grams per 100 ml or a pleural fluid to serum protein ratio of less than 0.5, lactic dehydrogenase (LDH) levels of less than 200 IU, and pleural fluid to serum LDH ratios of less than 0.6. Pleural exudates, reflecting an inflammatory process, have a specific gravity greater than 1.018 and total protein of greater than 3 grams per 100 ml or a pleural fluid to serum protein ratio of greater than 0.5; the pleural fluid to serum LDH ratio is greater than 0.6.

In infectious effusions, glucose is often decreased to values of about half the serum value, but in rheumatoid pleural effusion, glucose is characteristically less than 10 mg per 100 ml.

Total and differential cell counts are helpful except when the pleural fluid is grossly purulent. A predominance of polymorphonuclear leukocytes (PMN's) suggests that bacterial infection is the cause, e.g., the pleural effusion accompanying a pneumonia. Such a fluid may be sterile, or microscopic examination of a pleural fluid smear stained with Gram's stain may reveal bacteria. A predominance of small lymphocytes, particularly with few mesothelial cells and total cell counts above 1000 per cubic millimeter, strongly suggests tuberculosis. Tubercle bacilli are rarely observed in acid-fast stains and are not commonly recovered on cultures. Lymphoma of the pleura is much less readily diagnosed on cytologic preparations than carcinoma. With pulmonary infarction, a mixture of PMN's, lymphocytes, and numerous mesothelial cells is often observed. Lupus erythematosus cells may be seen in the pleural fluid in systemic lupus erythematosus. Eosinophils in the pleural fluid have no diagnostic significance except to indicate chronicity of the process.

The pleural fluid complicating pancreatitis usually demonstrates an amylase concentration several times higher than that in serum. Pleural fluid pH of 7.2 or below tends to be associated with empyema or loculated effusions requiring drainage. In the cholesterol or pseudochylous effusion, cholesterol concentration is high but neutral and fatty acid concentrations are low. Such effusions are the result of longstanding chronic pleural disease, most commonly tuberculosis or rheumatoid disease. In chylothorax, the lipid content of the fluid is high as manifest by sudanophilic fatty droplets and a high concentration of neutral fat and fatty acids; the cholesterol content is low.

Black, L. F.: The pleural space and pleural fluid. Mayo Clin. Proc., 47:493, 1972.

Light, R. W., MacGregor, M. I., Luchsinger, P. C., and Ball, W. C.: Pleural effusions: The diagnostic separations of transudates and exudates. Ann. Intern. Med., 77:507, 1972.

343.7. BRONCHOSCOPY

Bronchoscopy is the inspection of the lumen of the tracheobronchial tree with a lighted optical system or endoscope. Prior to 1967, all bronchoscopies were performed with the rigid bronchoscope, a hollow metal tube with a blunted tip, and a system for providing light at the end of the bronchoscope, either a minature electric light bulb or a fiberoptic light carrier. This instrument may be passed under either local or general anesthesia. The neck must be hyperextended and flexed to the right or left side to permit entry into the left or right bronchial trees, respectively. Visualization of the lobar and segmental orifices of both lower and the right middle lobes is readily possible. Visualization of the upper lobe bronchi bilaterally is usually possible but more difficult; segmental orifices can sometimes be seen using telescopes fitted with prisms which permit visualization at 45- or 90-degree angles to the axis of the telescope. These instruments permit ready appreciation of fixation of the bronchial tree owing to lymph node involvement by tumor; biopsy or surgical treatment of bronchoscopically visualized lesions and the removal of foreign bodies can be carried out.

During the last ten years the use of the rigid bronchoscope has been rapidly superseded by the flexible fiberoptic bronchoscope. In these instruments, light is carried to the tip of the device by fiberoptic light carrying bundles and the image is returned to the eye through an objective lens and fiberoptic bundle. Bronchoscopes for use in adults have a 5 to 5.2 mm tip and an aspiration channel which is approximately 2 mm in diameter. Aspiration may be carried out directly through this channel, or suction catheters, bronchial brushes, and various types of biopsy and grasping forceps can be passed through the channel. The distal end of the bronchoscope can be angulated to facilitate visualization and entry of various portions of the bronchial tree by moving a lever at the proximal end of the instrument.

The flexible fiberoptic bronchoscope can be passed through either the nose or the mouth with the neck in its normal position. Inspection of the tracheobronchial tree down to subsegmental bronchi or beyond is readily possible. Cytologic specimens can be collected on the bronchial brush, and fragments of bronchial wall can be readily removed with the biopsy forceps for histologic examination. Brush or biopsy forceps can be passed directly into solid lesions under fluoroscopic control. Small fragments of pulmonary parenchyma can be obtained with the biopsy forceps by grasping the walls of distal, thin-walled bronchi, a procedure known as transbronchoscopic lung biopsy. The small diameter of the bronchoscope permits ready bronchoscopy of patients who are receiving mechanically assisted ventilation. The instrument is passed through either the endotracheal or tracheostomy tube, and special adapters are used to maintain assisted ventilation during the procedure.

Bronchoscopy is a major tool in evaluating the patient with suspect bronchogenic carcinoma. Such patients present with hemoptysis or a shadow in the chest film which suggests bronchial obstruction or a mass lesion; the method is of greatest value in central and mid-zonal lesions. Although the flexible bronchoscope can be used for foreign body removal, the rigid bronchoscope is much more versatile for this purpose. Bronchoscopy can be used therapeutically for aspirating secretions, but since the method cannot be applied at frequent intervals, it is of limited value; the rigid bronchoscope accepts larger suction devices than can be passed through the flexible bronchoscope.

Although flexible fiberoptic bronchoscopy is much more widely applicable than rigid tube bronchoscopy, the procedure is not innocuous. Asthmatic patients may have an adverse reaction to the local anesthetic agent; mild hypoxemia is a regular accompaniment of the procedure and, although not troublesome in individuals with normal lung function, may be hazardous in patients with underlying lung disease. Life-threatening hemorrhage may complicate bronchial wall or transbronchoscopic lung biopsy. Fever may occur without a parenchymal pulmonary infiltration, and pneumonia may be a complication of bronchoscopy, especially in elderly individuals with obstructing bronchial lesions.

As with any diagnostic procedure, the risks of the procedure should be weighed against the benefits, and alternative methods for diagnosis should be considered. Thus, if precise anatomic information regarding the presence of an endobronchial tumor is not necessary, sputum cytology should be considered first for tumor diagnosis. In the elderly, seriously ill individual with a large peripheral tumor, cytologic examination of a specimen obtained by percutaneous fine-needle aspiration may entail a lower risk than bronchoscopy.

Khan, M. A., Whitcomb, M. E., and Snider, G. L.: Flexible fiberoptic bronchoscopy. Am. J. Med., 61:151, 1976.

Sackner, M. A.: Bronchofiberscopy. State of the art. Am. Rev. Respir. Dis., 111:62, 1975.

343.8. BIOPSY TECHNIQUES

LYMPH NODE BIOPSY. Biopsy of palpable superficial lymph nodes is generally helpful in evaluating pulmonary disease that is part of a systemic process or when primary tumor of the lung has spread outside the confines of the thorax. When lymph nodes are not palpable, the scalene lymph node, situated on the anterior scalene muscle, may be biopsied through a small supraclavicular incision. Scalene lymph node involvement is much more likely when there is involvement of the paratracheal lymph nodes as observed in the chest roentgenogram. This procedure has a high yield in granulomatous disease such as sarcoidosis but a much lower yield in neoplastic disease.

MEDIASTINOSCOPY. Mediastinoscopy is performed under general anesthesia, using an endotracheal tube. An incision is made in the suprasternal notch, and the mediastinoscope, a metal tube with light carried to its beveled end, is inserted via the tissue planes adjacent to the trachea as far as the carina. Anterior mediastinal, right paratracheal, and even subcarinal lymph nodes may be seen and biopsied. The left paratracheal area is more difficult to approach because of the presence of the aortic arch. This procedure has almost 100 per cent yield in granulomatous disease such as sarcoidosis. The method is being widely used for staging patients with bronchogenic carcinoma, but the exact indications remain controversial.

PLEURAL BIOPSY. Biopsy of the parietal pleura using the side-cutting Cope or Abrams needles is of major importance in the diagnosis of pleural effusion. In patients who do not have an obvious explanation for pleural effusion, biopsy should be considered at the time of the initial thoracentesis. The Abrams needle has the advantage that large pieces of tissue can be obtained with a very low risk of inducing a pneumothorax, and several biopsies tangential to the needle puncture can be obtained with a single insertion of the needle. The Cope needle produces smaller pieces of tissue than the Abrams needle. An end-cutting core-biopsy needle, such as the Silverman needle, can be used when the pleura is very thick and adherent to the lung.

The major risk of pleural biopsy is bleeding due to injury of the intercostal artery, and biopsy should never be performed on the cephalad side of the intercostal puncture wound. The procedure should obviously not be performed on patients with a coagulopathy. Because of the focal nature of pleural disease, a second or third biopsy is often performed if the first biopsy has failed to yield diagnostic information. Consideration should always be given to culturing a piece of tissue as well as to histologic examination, because the yield of positive cultures for *M. tuberculosis* is much higher from tissue than from pleural fluid. Surgical or open pleural biopsy adds little to twice or thrice repeated needle biopsy of the pleura and is rarely used.

LUNG BIOPSY. In instances in which simpler diagnostic studies have not been fruitful, consideration should be given to obtaining lung tissue for laboratory diagnosis. The approach to sampling lung tissue for cytologic, histologic, or bacteriologic diagnosis varies, depending on whether the patient has a diffuse pulmonary lesion or has a circumscribed and presumably solid lesion.

The endoscopic approach to solid lesions by the means of the fluoroscopically guided biopsy forceps or brush has been referred to above. Material for cytologic examination can often be obtained by fine needle aspiration of the mass lesion carried out under fluoroscopic control. If the lesion is not adherent to the pleura, pneumothorax may result, requiring the insertion of a chest tube. When the lesion is adherent to the chest wall, core biopsy with a cutting needle, obtaining material for both cytologic and histologic examination, is probably a preferable procedure. Percutaneous methods

should be considered only when surgical therapy is contraindicated or the risk is so high that this form of treatment would not be undertaken without proof of diagnosis.

Diffuse pulmonary lesions may be approached by transbronchoscopic lung biopsy. This method should be particularly considered when the differential diagnosis includes lesions which can be readily diagnosed by the pathologist on small amounts of tissue. Included in this category are granulomatous and neoplastic lesions and the suspected presence of infectious agents readily identified histologically such as *Pneumocystis carinii*, aspergillus, or one of the obligatory pathogenic fungi. The procedure is less helpful in diagnosing lymphoma than carcinoma and is of limited value in the diagnosis of chronic interstitial fibrosis in which the histology of small amounts of tissue is nonspecific and there is a serious sampling problem. In the latter circumstance, open lung biopsy performed through a short intercostal incision permits biopsy of a larger portion of lung, often from two sites, and provides enough tissue for a variety of histologic, cultural, and immunopathologic examinations. Core biopsy, using the high speed air-powered biopsy drill or one of the core biopsy needles, has been applied to diffuse pulmonary lesions; but except in the hands of the most highly skilled and experienced operators, it carries more hazard than either transbronchoscopic or open lung biopsy.

Carr, D. T., Soule, E. H., and Ellis, F. H., Jr.: Management of pleural effusions. Med. Clin. N. Am., 48:961, 1964.

Gaensler, E. A., Moister, V. B., and Hamm, J.: Open lung biopsy in diffuse pulmonary disease. N. Engl. J. Med., 270:1319, 1964.

Gunstensen, J., and Wade, J. D.: Mediastinoscopy. An analysis of 320 consecutive cases. Br. J. Surg., 59:209, 1972.

Levine, H., and Cugell, D. W.: Blunt-end needle biopsy of pleura and rib. Arch. Intern. Med., 109:516, 1962.

Lillington, G. A., and Jamplis, R. W.: Scalene node biopsy. Ann. Intern. Med., 59:101, 1963.

Manfredi, F., and Krumholz, R.: Percutaneous needle biopsy of the lung in evaluation of pulmonary disorders. JAMA, 198:1198, 1966.

Niden, A. K., Burrows, B., Kasik, J. E., and Barclay, W. R.: Percutaneous pleural biopsy with a curetting needle. Special reference to biopsy without effusion. Am. Rev. Respir. Dis., 84:37, 1961.

Nordenstrom, B.: Transthoracic needle biopsy. N. Engl. J. Med., 276:1081, 1967.

Skinner, D. B.: Scalene-lymph node biopsy: Reappraisal of risks and indications. N. Engl. J. Med., 268:1324, 1963.

Steel, S. J., and Winstanley, D. P.: Lung biopsy with a high speed air drill. Thorax, 22:286, 1967.

Zavala, D. C.: Diagnostic fiberoptic bronchoscopy techniques and result of biopsy in 600 patients. Chest, 68:12, 1975.

343.9. MISCELLANEOUS PROCEDURES

THE ELECTROCARDIOGRAM. Electrocardiographic changes occur in only a small proportion of patients with pulmonary embolism, but the procedure is noninvasive and inexpensive and should therefore be regularly used when this diagnosis is suspected. The changes are transient so that serial examination is helpful; P pulmonale, right bundle branch block, right axis deviation, and supraventricular arrhythmias are most frequently seen (see Ch. 364). Electrocardiographic evidence of right ventricular hypertrophy correlates quite well with the degree of pulmonary hypertension and cor pulmonale in patients with disorders causing restriction of the vascular bed of the lung. The electrocardiogram is a less sensitive indicator of right ventricular enlargement in patients whose cor pulmonale is due to chronic bronchitis and emphysema (see Ch. 344). The changes of myocardial ischemia may be helpful in discerning the etiology of chest pain, and those of ischemia and left ventricular hypertrophy may be helpful in patients with acute cardiogenic pulmonary edema, especially when the presentation is atypical (see Ch. 356).

EXTRAPULMONARY RADIONUCLIDE IMAGING. Scintiscanning of the neck and mediastinum after administration of radioiodine is useful in the evaluation of an upper mediastinal mass which may be substernal goiter (see Ch. 546). Liver scans are useful in detecting bacterial or amebic abscess of the liver but are neither very sensitive nor specific in detecting metastatic bronchogenic carcinoma, and the technique should not be routinely used in the preoperative evaluation of patients with this neoplasm (see Ch. 349.2). Bone scans after ^{99m}technetium-labeled polyphosphate often can detect metastatic carcinoma before lesions are roentgenographically visible; however, focal injury to bone from any cause may cause increased concentration of radionuclide, and some highly lytic lesions may not be revealed by this method (see Part XXII).

TESTS OF MUSCLE FUNCTION. Disorders of the muscular system may involve the muscles of the respiratory system and be suspected because of loss of vital and total lung capacities. Brief reversal of the impaired vital capacity after administration of the short-acting anticholinesterase edrophonium supports the diagnosis of myasthenia gravis (see Ch. 340.4). Electromyography may be helpful in establishing this diagnosis as well as that of other neurologic or muscular disorders (see Ch. 272). Elevation of serum creatine phosphokinase and aldolase levels is helpful in the diagnosis of polymyositis or dermatomyositis (see Ch. 51).

SPECIAL TESTS. Sweat chloride concentrations above 60 mEq per liter in the absence of adrenal insufficiency or nephrogenic diabetes insipidus support the diagnosis of cystic fibrosis of the pancreas; 95 per cent of adult males with this disorder have azoospermia (see Ch. 412). Patients with Kartagener's syndrome (situs inversus, sinusitis, and bronchiectasis) have ultrastructurally identifiable abnormalities of their cilia which can be detected in nasal or bronchial mucosal biopsies. In homozygous alpha$_1$ antitrypsin deficiency, serum alpha$_1$ globulin and serum trypsin inhibitory capacity levels are markedly decreased.

344. DISEASES ASSOCIATED WITH AIRWAYS OBSTRUCTION

Benjamin Burrows

344.1. GENERALIZED AIRWAY DISEASES

The present discussion deals with chronic or recurrent generalized airways disorders which are not the direct result of an underlying "specific" bronchopulmonary disease. It includes asthma, the chronic bronchitis syndromes, emphysema, and chronic obstructive pulmonary disease.

INTRODUCTION

DEFINITIONS OF TERMS AND INTERRELATIONSHIPS OF DIAGNOSTIC ENTITIES. The bronchopulmonary system may respond in different ways when exposed to irritants or allergens. The type of response depends on the nature and severity of the exposure and on host susceptibility.

In subjects with hyperreactive or "twitchy" airways, exposure to a variety of provocative factors can lead to bronchospasm (i.e., constriction of bronchial smooth muscles, often accompanied by edema of bronchial walls and abnormal mucus production). Recurrent episodes of bronchospasm of sufficient severity to lead to symptoms are called *asthma*. Asthma is especially likely to develop in allergic individuals in whom exposure to inhaled allergens provokes recurrent Type I allergic bronchospasm. But it also occurs in nonallergic individuals who have hyperreactive airways, and, as used in this discussion, the term "asthma" has no specific etiologic implications.

The response is different when there is chronic, relatively low-grade exposure to bronchial irritants in a subject without hyperreactive airways. This results in stimulation of the mucus-secreting elements of the airway, reduction in bronchial ciliary activity, and impaired resistance to bronchial infection. In the present discussion, the resulting syndrome, characterized primarily by chronic productive cough, is called *simple chronic bronchitis*.

In a relatively small proportion of subjects, chronic exposure to bronchial irritants results in severe irreversible narrowing of airways, a condition called *chronic obstructive bronchitis*. Much of the obstruction is in airways less than 2 mm in diameter, including bronchioles as well as bronchi, and the term *"small airways disease"* has been introduced to emphasize this point. There would seem little use, however, in delineating this as a separate disease.

Finally, the lung may respond to noxious stimuli by developing *emphysema*, a condition characterized by dilatation of air spaces distal to the terminal bronchiole with destruction of their walls. As with chronic obstructive bronchitis, there appears to be considerable variability in susceptibility to the disorder. Emphysematous changes reduce the elastic recoil of the lung, allowing excessive airways collapse on expiration and leading to an irreversible obstructive problem.

The definitions of the aforementioned terms are in no way mutually exclusive. Indeed, in view of their common dependence on exposure to inhaled irritants, one would expect them to coexist frequently. Patients with chronic obstructive bronchitis may show superimposed recurrent bronchospasm, thereby fulfilling the criteria for asthma. Most patients with emphysema have a chronic productive cough at some stage of their illness, allowing a secondary diagnosis of simple chronic bronchitis. Some obliteration of small airways generally accompanies emphysema, and without elaborate tests it may be difficult to determine the relative importance of chronic obstructive bronchitis and emphysema in a severe irreversible airways obstructive disorder. This has led to the use of general terms such as *chronic obstruc-*

Figure 1. A schematic model of the respiratory system during forced expiration. The pleural pressure (Ppl) is applied to both alveoli and intrathoracic airways. The pressure driving air out of the system is the alveolar pressure (Palv), which is the sum of Ppl and the elastic recoil of the lung (Pst(l)). The pressure within the airway falls as one proceeds mouthward. At the equal pressure point (EPP), pressure within the airway just equals Ppl. In airways upstream (US) of this point, intraluminal pressure exceeds Ppl and airways remain dilated. Mouthward or downstream (DS) of this point, compression of intrathoracic airways occurs, and this acts as a governor on flow, causing a maximal flow (Vmax) to be achieved which is essentially independent of the Ppl generated by the expiratory muscles. (From Burrows, B., Knudson, R. J., and Kettel, L. J.: Respiratory Insufficiency. Copyright © 1975 by Year Book Medical Publishers, Inc., Chicago. Used by permission.)

tive pulmonary (or lung) disease (abbreviated COPD) to describe this clinical syndrome.

In practice, one generally applies the single diagnostic term which best describes the patient's major problem. But this must not limit one's therapeutic efforts. For example, a diagnosis of emphysema should not imply that measures directed at amelioration of bronchitis or prevention of bronchospasm are inappropriate. Therapy should be directed at all features of the patient's disease, not simply at those which determine the primary diagnosis.

The term *chronic bronchitis,* unqualified, has been used in various ways by different authors, sometimes referring to a simple smoker's cough and at other times (especially in the British literature) to severe COPD. In view of its ambiguity, it will be used in the present discussion only when qualified as "simple" or "obstructive."

PATHOPHYSIOLOGY OF AIRWAYS OBSTRUCTION. In clinical practice, airways obstruction is synonymous with slowing of forced expiration. To understand the determinants of the speed of forced expiration, one must consider the pressures which develop within the thorax during a maximum expiratory effort. These are depicted in Figure 1. The high intrapleural pressure (Ppl) developed by the expiratory muscles tends to drive air from the alveoli, but its effect on flow is limited by its tendency to compress intrathoracic airways. This "dynamic compression of airways" is resisted by the recoil of the lung (Pst) which causes the pressure within the alveoli and peripheral airways to exceed Ppl. Owing to flow resistance, however, the high pressure within the alveoli and peripheral airways is dissipated as air progresses mouthward, and during a forced exhalation there will be a point within the thorax where the pressure inside the airway just equals Ppl. Mouthward of this "equal pressure point," the pressure outside the airways exceeds that within, and airways compression occurs. This airways compression

acts as a governor on flow, and a maximum expiratory flow (Vmax) occurs which is essentially independent of the effort exerted by the subject. It depends only on the intrinsic resistance of the airways, the recoil of the lungs, and the compressibility of the airways mouthward of the equal pressure point. A high airways resistance, low lung recoil, or excessive collapsibility of airways will lead to a reduction in Vmax.

In determining whether Vmax is normal, its relationship to lung volume must be taken into account. When the lung volume is large, airways are maximally dilated and have a low resistance. Also, lung recoil is high. Thus Vmax is high when the lung is near full inflation. As lung volume decreases, airways resistance rises and lung recoil falls, leading to a reduction in Vmax. The relationship between lung volume and Vmax is readily seen in a maximum expiratory flow volume (MEFV) curve, depicted in Figure 2A. The same information is contained in a standard spirogram (Fig. 2B) in which volume is displayed against time; in this case, the rapidity of change in volume (the slope of the curve) reflects Vmax. The total volume exhaled during the test is called the "forced vital capacity" (FVC). Values for the volume exhaled during the first second of a forced exhalation (the FEV_1) or for the average flow during the middle half of the FVC (the MMEF or $FEF_{25-75\%}$) are readily determined from standard spirograms and are commonly used indicators of the speed of forced expiration. Instantaneous Vmax values are more readily measured from MEFV curves. They are most commonly

Figure 2. Solid lines are used to show a normal maximum expiratory flow-volume (MEFV) in *A* and a normal spirogram in *B*. Broken lines indicate typical curves for a patient with mild airways obstruction. Measurements of the forced vital capacity (FVC), the forced expiratory volume at one second (FEV_1), and forced flow rates at 50 per cent and 75 per cent of the FVC ($Vmax_{50\%}$ and $Vmax_{75\%}$) are depicted as vertical lines.

determined at 50 per cent or 75 per cent of the forced expired volume ($\dot{V}max_{50\%}$ or $\dot{V}max_{75\%}$, respectively*).

The $Vmax_{75\%}$ appears more sensitive than the FEV_1 for detecting subclinical airways dysfunction and has become popular in epidemiologic studies. However, since it is easily measured, is highly reproducible, has a relatively narrow normal range, and tends to reflect the clinical severity of disease, the FEV_1 is more widely used in clinical practice.

In order to determine that a low FEV_1 results from slowing of expiration rather than from a marked restriction in the total volume exhaled, the FEV_1/FVC ratio is examined. This ratio is regularly below 65 per cent in clinically significant airways obstructive diseases. Once the presence of airways obstruction has been confirmed by the presence of a low FEV_1/FVC ratio, the severity of the abnormality is best assessed from the degree of reduction in the FEV_1 itself.

Airways obstruction leads to an increased work of breathing. It also causes a diminished response to a ventilatory stimulus. The latter may lead to underventilation and hypercapnia if the disease is severe, if ventilatory drive is reduced (as with sedatives or narcotics), or if there is respiratory muscle weakness or fatigue.

Since the airways abnormalities and any accompanying parenchymal lesions are nonuniformly distributed throughout the lung, ventilation becomes uneven and may be poorly matched to blood flow. The nonuniformity of alveolar ventilation can be demonstrated by an increased "slope of phase III" on the single breath nitrogen test, by an abnormality in the nitrogen washout curve, or by prolongation of the helium equilibration time.

Continued perfusion of poorly ventilated regions of lung causes some alveoli to have very low ventilation/perfusion ($\dot{V}/\dot{Q}$) ratios. The blood traversing such areas does not become well oxygenated, an effect called "venous admixture," "physiologic shunting," or "relative shunt." This is the major cause of hypoxemia in airways obstructive diseases.

As a result of the mismatched ventilation and perfusion, other alveoli show very high $\dot{V}/\dot{Q}$ ratios. The ventilation which reaches these alveoli is largely wasted, resulting in an increased "physiologic dead space." This reduces the effective alveolar ventilation and necessitates an increase in overall ventilation if hypercapnia is to be avoided.

Obstructed airways tend to close prematurely during a maximum exhalation, leading to trapping of air and an increase in residual volume. In emphysema and during attacks of asthma, the total lung capacity is also increased. As might be expected, the pulmonary diffusing capacity measurement is almost always reduced in emphysema. It is usually within normal limits in asthma and gives variable results in chronic obstructive bronchitis.

The small airways have a very large total cross-sectional diameter, and extensive changes in this "quiet zone" of the lung are required to produce a discernible effect on measurements such as the FEV_1. More sensitive tests are needed to detect mild small airways ab-

normalities. Many new tests have been proposed, including measurements of $\dot{V}max$ late in forced expiration, "closing volume," and "frequency dependence of compliance." Although these tests may prove useful for detecting subclinical disease and in research studies, their specificity for small airways abnormalities is doubtful, and they have no proved clinical application. Recently, there has also been much interest in the helium responsiveness of the MEFV curve. In normal subjects, $\dot{V}max_{50\%}$ shows a marked increase after helium breathing. A smaller than normal increase in $\dot{V}max_{50\%}$ is considered evidence for small airways obstruction. The role of this test in clinical practice remains uncertain.

A report of the ACCP/ATS Joint Committee on Pulmonary Nomenclature: Pulmonary terms and symbols. Chest, 67:583, 1975.

Burrows, B., and Hasan, F. M.: Abnormalities in small airways. Disease-a-Month, Vol. 23, No. 10, July 1977, pp. 2–34.

Despas, P. J., Leroux, M., and Macklem, P. T.: Site of airway obstruction in asthma as determined by measuring maximal expiratory flow breathing air and a helium-oxygen mixture. J. Clin. Invest., 51:3235, 1972.

Knudson, R. J., and Burrows, B.: Early detection of obstructive lung diseases. Med. Clin. North Am., 57:681, 1973.

Macklem, P. T.: The pathophysiology of chronic bronchitis and emphysema. Med. Clin. North Am., 57:669, 1973.

Macklem, P. T., Thurlbeck, W. M., and Fraser, R. G.: Chronic obstructive disease of small airways. Ann. Intern. Med., 74:167, 1971.

Mead, J., Turner, J. M., Macklem, P. T., and Little, J. B.: Significance of the relationship between lung recoil and maximum expiratory flow. J. Appl. Physiol., 22:95, 1967.

Thurlbeck, W. M.: Chronic bronchitis and emphysema. Med. Clin. North Am., 57:651, 1973.

SIMPLE CHRONIC BRONCHITIS

PREVALENCE AND PATHOGENESIS. In epidemiologic studies, simple chronic bronchitis is diagnosed when productive cough is present on most days for at least three months of the year. Using this criterion, the diagnosis may be applied to a large proportion of heavy cigarette smokers, especially after age 45. Exposure to occupational or environmental air pollutants adds to the effects of smoking. Only a small fraction of subjects with this syndrome consult a physician. Most accept their "smoker's cough" as a penalty for their cigarette habit. Those who do see a physician are likely to have recurrent respiratory infections or some type of wheezing problem in addition to their cough.

The disorder results from three apparently direct effects of inhaling bronchial irritants: (1) stimulation of the mucus-secreting elements of the airway; (2) interference with ciliary activity with impaired mucus clearance; and (3) disturbance of alveolar macrophage function with reduced resistance to bronchopulmonary infection. Accumulation of secretions leads to cough. Bacterial colonization is common, the normally sterile bronchi now harboring organisms similar to those found in the nasopharynx.

PATHOLOGY. The most characteristic finding is hypertrophy of mucous glands and goblet cells. The "Reid index," representing the ratio of mucous gland to total bronchial wall thickness, exceeds its normal limit of 0.4. In addition, one finds retained bronchial secretions and variable degrees of inflammatory change in the bronchial walls. Even in the absence of clinically significant obstruction, careful studies may show narrowing or obliteration of some small airways and scattered centrilobular emphysema. Similar small airways and em-

---

*There is considerable confusion in use of these symbols. It has been recommended that $\dot{V}max_{50\%}$ and $\dot{V}max_{75\%}$ be expressed as $FEF_{50\%}$ and $FEF_{75\%}$, respectively. Also, the $\dot{V}max_{75\%}$ as defined herein is sometimes reported as $\dot{V}max_{25\%}$, the 25% then referring to the portion of the FVC remaining when the flow measurement is made.

physematous changes are noted in asymptomatic smokers, however, and it is uncertain that they are related to simple chronic bronchitis except through their common association with cigarette use.

CLINICAL MANIFESTATIONS. In mild disease, cough is noted primarily on arising or after smoking the first cigarette of the day, is productive of a small quantity of mucoid sputum, and is present most regularly during the winter months. As the disorder becomes more severe, cough tends to recur throughout the day, symptoms persist throughout the year, larger volumes of sputum are raised, and increasingly severe paroxysms of cough are noted. Wheezing is common at the end of a severe coughing spell, probably representing cough-induced bronchospasm. Wheezing may also occur on reclining; this may first be noted by the patient's spouse. This type of wheeze is probably a direct result of retained secretions, as it is often relieved by cough.

Periodic exacerbations of symptoms occur, often accompanied by purulence of the sputum. Most such episodes appear to follow viral respiratory infections, and purulence of the sputum is regarded as evidence of bacterial overgrowth. Cultures generally show the normal nasopharyngeal flora, although *H. influenzae* and *S. pneumoniae* are often present as well. These organisms probably represent secondary invaders rather than primary causes of the exacerbations. Varying degrees of bronchospasm may occur during exacerbations, and there is no clear distinction between such episodes and asthma. Blood-streaked sputum occurs occasionally, but repeated or severe hemoptysis should lead one to suspect a more serious disease than simple chronic bronchitis.

With further progression of the disorder, the sputum may become chronically purulent. The term *mucopurulent bronchitis* is sometimes applied to this stage of illness. Sputum cultures may now reveal drug-resistant organisms such as *P. aeruginosa;* this is especially likely to occur if the patient has received a variety of antibiotics.

Physical examination may be entirely normal in mild disease. Later, scattered rhonchi and variable coarse rales are heard. These may clear or change location after cough. A wheeze or paroxysm of coughing is often induced by a forced expiratory effort.

LABORATORY FINDINGS. In uncomplicated cases, blood counts and differential smear are normal, as is the chest radiograph. Sputum examination shows variable numbers of leukocytes and a mixed flora of organisms, as already noted. Bronchograms reveal the enlarged ducts of hypertrophied mucous glands, mucus plugs which prevent filling of some medium-sized bronchi, and often mild diffuse dilatation of bronchi on inspiratory films. Bronchoscopy reveals retained secretions, diffuse hyperemia, and some mucosal edema. Spirometry may be within normal limits but often shows slight slowing of forced expiration.

COURSE AND PROGNOSIS. Patients with simple chronic bronchitis often show considerable fluctuation in symptoms. Cough and sputum production worsen with increased cigarette use, during inclement weather, and following acute respiratory infections. In mild cases, symptoms usually disappear completely with cessation of smoking. Although simple chronic bronchitis is often associated with slight reduction in ventilatory function, at least one prospective study has failed to show that smokers with chronic productive cough have a significantly greater rate of decline in lung function than asymptomatic smokers. This suggests that the effect of cigarette smoke on airways function is essentially independent of its effect on mucus secretion. It is clear, at least, that a diagnosis of simple chronic bronchitis does not imply that the patient will inevitably develop progressive disabling respiratory insufficiency.

DIFFERENTIAL DIAGNOSIS. The diagnosis is basically one of exclusion. It is justified when there is persistent cough which cannot be ascribed to a parenchymal lung disease, a disorder of the upper respiratory tract, a specific endobronchial disease, or an allergic reaction of the airway. Thus a chest radiograph is required to exclude a parenchymal lesion. A careful examination of the upper airway is indicated, and one must exclude physical findings which might indicate a localized airways disorder (such as a persistent localized wheeze). In children or in young adults with severe symptoms, mucoviscidosis also must be excluded.

One should be cautious in diagnosing simple chronic bronchitis in the absence of an obvious source of chronic bronchial irritation. In a nonsmoker, in a patient whose history suggests an association between symptoms and exposure to allergens, or in a patient with episodes of wheezing dyspnea, one should check for eosinophilia in the sputum and blood. High eosinophil levels suggest that the disorder is a variant of asthma. In any case, a secondary diagnosis of asthma is justified when recurrent reversible airways obstruction is an important feature of the disease.

Repeated or severe hemoptysis, or physical findings suggesting localized disease may call for bronchoscopy and even bronchography to rule out an endobronchial lesion or localized bronchiectasis, but these procedures are not indicated in the routine case. Some authorities recommend sputum cytology on all subjects with chronic bronchitis, especially over age 40. Spirometry should be carried out to determine the degree of associated ventilatory impairment.

There may be a problem in distinguishing severe mucopurulent bronchitis from bronchiectasis. Mild diffuse cylindrical dilatation of bronchi is noted in many severe bronchitics. Recurrent hemoptysis, repeated pneumonias in the same lung region, or areas of honeycombing on chest radiograph suggest that there may be areas of frank saccular bronchiectasis. Bronchography is required for accurate diagnosis but is usually indicated only if resection of the bronchiectatic areas would be considered. Otherwise, there is little difference in the therapy of mucopurulent bronchitis and bronchiectasis.

TREATMENT. Removal of the provocative factors (usually cigarettes) is of primary importance and may totally relieve the condition. When symptoms persist despite maximal efforts to avoid bronchial irritants or are severe enough to require more immediate relief, the following measures are employed:

Antibiotic Therapy. Noneosinophilic purulent sputum is regarded as evidence of infection and is treated with a seven- to ten-day course of tetracycline or ampicillin, 1 gram daily in divided doses. If the sputum fails to clear, further antibiotic therapy should be determined by sputum culture and sensitivity. Successive doses of different antibiotics should be avoided, however, because they tend to lead to a resistant flora. Failure of therapy is more often related to poor drainage of bronchial secretions than to inadequate antibacterial agents.

Recurrent infections may be treated with prophylactic tetracycline, prescribing 0.5 to 1.0 gram daily either continuously or for three weeks out of each month. Alternatively, the patient may be given a supply of tetracycline and advised to begin a seven- to ten-day course promptly if the sputum becomes purulent or if there are other signs of a lower respiratory tract infection. Prophylactic therapy appears to reduce the severity and duration of exacerbations but does not reduce their frequency.

Very severe exacerbations of disease generally respond better to ampicillin or cephalothin than to tetracycline, and it is reasonable to use these agents as initial therapy when the specific infecting organism is unknown. (Penicillin has proved inappropriate therapy for severe purulent exacerbations of bronchitis.) When resistant organisms are cultured from the sputum, the antibiotic regimen may have to be adjusted in accord with drug susceptibility studies.

Bronchodilator Agents. These are indicated on a regular basis for patients with mild reversible airways obstruction and for patients with prominent posttussic wheezing. Doses may have to be increased or medications first prescribed during exacerbations of disease. Inhaled bronchodilators are also useful adjuncts to bronchial hygiene treatments, as described below. Some degree of bronchospasm is generally present in patients with severe paroxysmal cough, and in them a trial of bronchodilators is justified even when frank expiratory slowing cannot be demonstrated. Bronchodilator therapy is discussed in more detail under the treatment of asthma.

Bronchial Hygiene Measures. The objective of these measures is to clear retained bronchial secretions. The most important steps are deep breathing followed by deliberate coughing. This may be made more effective by positioning the patient so that the most affected lung regions are in a superior position (postural drainage). In some subjects, chest percussion and vibration further increase sputum production.

Premedication with an inhaled bronchodilator may greatly improve the patient's tolerance of bronchial hygiene measures and increase their effectiveness. This may be followed by inhalation of bland mist in an attempt to loosen secretions. It has been difficult to show objective effects from bland mist therapy, but some patients are convinced of its beneficial effects. There is no evidence that use of complicated apparatus such as IPPB machines improves the effectiveness of therapy.

Thus for patients with troublesome cough or retained secretions, a bronchial hygiene treatment might consist of inhaling a bronchodilator medication followed by breathing of a bland mist, postural drainage, deep breathing with deliberate cough, and even chest percussion and vibration. Treatments are usually prescribed twice daily for ambulant patients and more often during exacerbations. It should be appreciated, however, that patients vary in their reactions to such therapy. Only those measures which prove effective for the individual patient should be continued, as the full program is time consuming, uncomfortable, and costly.

All patients should be encouraged to keep well hydrated to avoid inspissation of secretions. In acute exacerbations, this may require intravenous fluids. The usefulness of expectorant medications is questionable. Some authorities recommend 10 to 12 drops of a saturated solution of potassium iodide three times a day. This does seem to be effective in some patients, but it is associated with a high rate of side effects, some of which can be severe. Cough syrups and lozenges may help relieve a "tickle" in the throat but have little effect on the viscosity of bronchial secretions. Cough sedatives are generally contraindicated. They should be used only for acute episodes of severe nonproductive cough.

Burrows, B., and Lebowitz, M. D.: Characteristics of chronic bronchitis in a warm, dry region. Am. Rev. Respir. Dis., 112:365, 1975.
Burrows, B., and Nevin, W.: Antibiotic management in patients with chronic bronchitis and emphysema (editorial). Ann. Intern. Med., 77:993, 1972.
Ferris, B., Jr.: Chronic bronchitis and emphysema. Classification and epidemiology. Med. Clin. North Am., 57:637, 1973.
Fletcher, C. M., Elmes, P. C., Fairbairn, A. S., and Wood, C. H.: The significance of respiratory symptoms and the diagnosis of chronic bronchitis in a working population. Br. Med. J., 2:257, 1959.
Fletcher, C. M., and Peto, R.: The natural history of chronic airflow obstruction. Br. Med. J., 1:1645, 1977.
Proceedings of the Conference on Scientific Basis of Respiratory Therapy. Aerosol therapy. Physical therapy. Intermittent positive pressure breathing. Am. Rev. Respir. Dis., 110:85, 129, 169, 1974.

ASTHMA

PREVALENCE AND PATHOGENESIS. Approximately 3 per cent of the United States population are known to have asthma. In addition, there are many subjects in the population who have symptoms suggesting a subclinical form of the disease or who have features of asthma associated with a primary diagnosis of chronic bronchitis or chronic obstructive pulmonary disease. The disease often begins in childhood but may have its onset quite late in life. Childhood asthma is more common in boys.

The basic problem in asthma is hyperreactivity or "twitchiness" of the airways, causing the subject to develop bronchospasm in response to a variety of stimuli. Provocative factors include allergens; bronchial infections; irritant particles, fumes, and gases; mechanical irritation of the airways; certain pharmacologic agents; vigorous exercise; psychologic stresses; and irritation of the nasopharynx.

Bronchial Reactivity. The factors which lead to bronchial hyperreactivity are uncertain. They may include (1) the quantity, anatomic arrangement, or inherent contractility of bronchial smooth muscles; (2) the number of bronchial mast cells or their ability to produce and release mediators of bronchoconstriction; (3) the sensitivity of airways receptors and of vagally mediated bronchoconstrictor reflexes; and (4) the sensitivity of bronchial beta$_2$-adrenergic receptors. To some extent, bronchial reactivity is an inherited characteristic, but it is also susceptible to environmental influences. For example, increased reactivity may be noted for a prolonged period following an acute viral bronchitis. Also, postexercise bronchospasm is much more marked in young asthmatics who are still having attacks than after a prolonged remission. It appears that recurrent bronchospasm may cause the bronchi to become more irritable, hence the adage, "Asthma begets asthma."

Provocative Factors and Mechanisms of Their Effect. In children and young adults, inhaled allergens are usually important provocative factors. Typically, they produce immediate, "Type I," IgE-mediated, allergic reactions in the airway, although "Type III," IgG-mediated reactions may also occur in some individuals. The Type I reaction depends on release of chemical mediators of bronchoconstriction by bronchial mast cells. An inhaled allergen which traverses the bronchial mucosa bridges two antigen-specific IgE antibodies which are bound to a mast cell wall, leading to the formation of active mediators. Mediators include histamine, slow-reacting substance of anaphylaxis (SRS-A), eosinophilic chemotactic factor of anaphylaxis (ECF-A), prostaglandins, and a variety of other substances. The importance of each of these mediators remains to be determined, but histamine appears to be relatively less important in asthma than in some other allergic disorders. The ability of the mast cell to form mediators is moderated by intracellular levels of 3'5' cyclic AMP. Agents which increase 3'5' cyclic AMP, such as beta-adrenergic agonists and methylxanthines, tend to inhibit mediator production.

The parasympathetic nervous system also plays an important role in the asthmatic response. Cooling or cutting of the vagus nerve ameliorates experimental allergic bronchoconstriction. Cholinergic stimulation induces mediator production in the mast cell and causes contraction of bronchial smooth muscle. Parasympathetic reflexes apparently augment mucus secretion and may be responsible for the cough and hyperventilation associated with bronchospastic attacks. "Nasobronchial" reflexes are involved in the bronchoconstriction induced in some subjects by stimulating the upper airway with cold air or certain chemicals. The parasympathetic system also appears important in the bronchoconstriction induced by direct irritation or infection of the bronchial mucosa, and such reactions can be blocked with anticholinergic agents.

Vigorous exercise produces bronchoconstriction in some asthmatic subjects. The precise mechanism is uncertain, but release of mast cell mediators appears to be involved in many cases.

Asthmatic subjects are also unusually susceptible to bronchoconstrictor drugs, and responses to graded doses of inhaled histamine or methacholine have been used to assess the degree of bronchial reactivity. Therapeutically employed beta-adrenergic blockers (such as propranolol) may induce bronchospasm in asthmatic patients. By mechanisms which are less clear, aspirin, indomethacin, and certain yellow coloring agents used in foods and medications may also induce asthmatic attacks. This reaction to aspirin does not have an immunologic basis and usually occurs in nonatopic subjects.

Asthma-like reactions to inorganic chemicals and to organic dusts are described in Ch. 348.14.

The role of psychogenic factors is difficult to assess. Attacks can be precipitated by suggestion in some subjects, and many patients appear to have exacerbations of disease when subjected to emotional stress.

PATHOLOGY. In fatal cases, the lungs are hyperinflated and there is hypertrophy of bronchial smooth muscle. The bronchial walls are edematous and show eosinophilic infiltration as well as variable numbers of neutrophils, lymphocytes, and plasma cells. Extensive mucous plugging is noted in small and medium-sized bronchi.

CLINICAL MANIFESTATIONS. Several types of asthma have been described. There are atopic patients in whom most attacks appear to be related to inhalation of allergens. These are generally younger subjects, and their disease is designated as "extrinsic," "atopic," or "allergic" in type. Hay fever is common in such subjects and often precedes the onset of asthma. Some patients give a past history of infantile eczema, and a family history of allergies is common. Attacks are likely to occur when environmental pollen counts are high (spring or fall) or in relationship to exposure to an obvious specific allergen, such as an animal dander. These subjects show other evidences of atopy, including multiple allergy skin test reactions and high levels of circulating IgE. Approximately 70 per cent of subjects with an onset of asthma before age 30 have this form of illness. Even in typical extrinsic asthma, attacks may be precipitated by nonallergic factors, including exercise, infections, nonspecific irritants, and even emotional factors.

A special form of allergic asthma is associated with *Aspergillus* organisms which grow in bronchial mucus plugs. The resulting syndrome, *allergic aspergillosis*, is characterized by relatively persistent asthma; recurrent pulmonary infiltrates, which may lead to lung fibrosis; localized bronchiectasis of relatively large airways; marked immediate hypersensitivity to *Aspergillus* (noted both by RAST and allergy skin tests); and very high circulating IgE. Findings suggesting a Type III allergy (modest levels of serum precipitins to *Aspergillus* and an Arthus reaction at the site of an intradermal allergy skin test) are common, and in some cases *Aspergillus* can be cultured from the sputum.

A second type of asthma, called "intrinsic" or "nonallergic," is characteristic of adult onset disease and is not associated with evidences of atopy. Attacks are generally precipitated by infections, exposure to nonspecific irritants, or emotional factors. Most patients deny a relationship to season, but some claim worsening during the winter months. Vasomotor rhinitis and nasal polyps are common. Many patients have some degree of chronic productive cough and are prone to recurrent respiratory infections. Approximately 70 per cent of asthma beginning after age 30 is of the "intrinsic" or "nonatopic" type. Aspirin intolerance is noted in some subjects, and the combination of persistent asthma, nasal polyps, and aspirin sensitivity has been called the "aspirin triad."

Another form of asthma is that which occurs in some patients with chronic obstructive lung disease. Even mild superimposed bronchospasm in such subjects may lead to a life-threatening exacerbation.

Regardless of the type of disease, the history is usually characteristic. After a period of relative well being, a sense of tightness or congestion is noted in the chest, usually accompanied by wheezing and slight cough. Over a period varying from minutes to days, symptoms increased in severity. Severe episodes culminate in an attack of incapacitating dyspnea. Although the attacks of dyspnea are often described as sudden in onset, the disease is usually more chronic than is appreciated by the patient. Serial spirometric measurements may show a gradual decline in FEV_1 long before the patient is aware of an attack. Symptoms then seem to develop suddenly when the airways obstruction reaches a level intolerable to the patient. Patients vary in the diurnal pattern of their attacks. In some, episodes are primarily nocturnal.

During a frank attack, physical examination reveals

obvious respiratory distress, hyperinflated chest, marked prolongation of forced expiration, frank wheezing, and, in severe cases, cyanosis. With increasing severity of the attack and marked diminution in expiratory flow rates, wheezing may become less pronounced, an ominous sign. As the episode is relieved, thick mucoid sputum may be raised. It often contains bronchial casts which illustrate the mucous plugging characteristic of the disease.

When symptoms persist despite bronchodilator therapy, *status asthmaticus* is said to exist. After many hours in "status," especially if the patient has been unable to sleep, respiratory muscle fatigue may develop, leading to hypoventilation and hypercapnia.

LABORATORY FINDINGS. During an attack, forced expiratory flow rates and the forced vital capacity are markedly reduced. Physiologic studies suggest that the obstruction is likely to involve the small airways to a greater extent in intrinsic than in extrinsic asthma. The residual volume and total lung capacity are increased, and the chest radiograph reveals hyperinflation. In some patients, recurrent pulmonary infiltrates accompany asthmatic episodes. These may result from subsegmental atelectasis behind a mucus plug. They may also result from an eosinophilic infiltrate in the lung, a characteristic finding in allergic aspergillosis.

During an acute episode, blood gases reveal variable degrees of hypoxemia. This may worsen temporarily after bronchodilator administration. Early in the episode, the arterial carbon dioxide tension is generally low, reflecting hyperventilation. With prolonged status asthmaticus the arterial carbon dioxide may return to normal or even become elevated, a grave prognostic sign.

In mild disease, spirometric tests generally return to normal between acute episodes, but more sensitive lung function studies often show subtle persisting abnormalities. In more severe disease, some slowing of forced expiration is likely to persist between attacks. This generally improves transiently following inhalation of a bronchodilator.

Sputum and blood eosinophilia are common and tend to reflect the activity of the disease. Eosinophilia occurs in both intrinsic and extrinsic forms of the disease.

In atopic subjects, serum IgE levels are elevated. The presence of IgE's specific for suspected antigens may be demonstrated directly by the RAST or indirectly by allergy skin tests.

COURSE AND PROGNOSIS. Asthma having an onset in childhood usually diminishes in severity during adolescence, and only 5 to 10 per cent of asthmatic children continue to have severe symptoms as adults. A history of infantile eczema is associated with a poorer prognosis. The prognosis is also less favorable for adult onset asthmatics. In them, symptoms tend to fluctuate in severity, but complete remission occurs in less than 25 per cent of cases. Persistence of frank spirometric abnormalities between symptomatic episodes and the presence of nasal polyps are poor prognostic signs.

Considering the high prevalence of the disease, death from asthma is relatively uncommon. Occasional sudden unexpected deaths do occur, however, even in young patients. Some of these may be the result of overuse of sympathomimetic drugs, leading to cardiac arrhythmias. Occasional deaths also occur in patients with status asthmaticus despite apparently optimal medical management.

A small number of subjects, especially those with late onset intrinsic asthma, appear to progress from typical paroxysmal asthma to persistent irreversible airways obstruction, but the actual relationship between asthma and COPD remains uncertain.

DIFFERENTIAL DIAGNOSIS. There is usually little difficulty in diagnosis. The recurrent episodes of wheezing dyspnea, often associated with known provocative factors, are quite characteristic. In patients with nocturnal episodes or with symptoms provoked by exertion, one must exclude congestive heart failure. Episodic dyspnea in the latter condition is almost always accompanied by cardiomegaly and other evidence of primary cardiac disease. Occasionally, however, a trial of diuretic therapy may be needed to distinguish nocturnal asthma from paroxysmal nocturnal dyspnea of cardiac origin.

It is also possible to mistake the hyperventilation syndrome for asthma on the basis of a casual history. In the hyperventilation syndrome, dyspnea is usually described as an inability to fill the chest sufficiently and is accompanied by a sighing rather than labored type of breathing. The conditions are readily distinguished if the patient is seen during an attack, because the hyperventilation syndrome is not associated with slowing of forced expiration.

Bronchospasm may be precipitated by aspiration, it may occur as part of the carcinoid syndrome, or it may represent a feature of a generalized immunologic disorder, particularly periarteritis nodosa.

In older subjects, it is sometimes difficult to distinguish asthma from COPD, and many patients show features of both disorders. In fact, the degree of reversibility of COPD (its "asthmatic component") can only be determined by a therepeutic trial. This is discussed further in the therapy of COPD.

THERAPY. Treatment of the Ambulent Patient. Asthma is a chronic disease characterized by hyperreactive airways. Regular management in an attempt to normalize function and prevent episodes of bronchospasm is essential, especially because the tendency to recurrent attacks appears to be reduced following a prolonged induced remission. The following measures are employed in the ambulant asthmatic patient:

AVOIDANCE OF PROVOCATIVE FACTORS. A careful history is required to identify factors which tend to aggravate symptoms. Nonspecific irritants, including smoking, should be eliminated or avoided. Dust suppression measures should be implemented in the home and work environment. Respiratory infections should be treated promptly and antibiotics prescribed if recurrent infections are a problem, as outlined in the treatment of simple chronic bronchitis. Aspirin and related compounds and beta-blocking agents should be used cautiously if at all in asthmatic subjects.

Allergens clearly related to attacks should be avoided. Unfortunately, identification of allergens responsible for attacks is often difficult. Atopic individuals usually have specific IgE's and positive skin tests to a wide variety of foreign proteins. Only a few are likely to be important in producing bronchospasm. Bronchial challenge tests with suspected allergens may be more specific, but these tests are difficult and time consuming, and their reliability in identifying clinically significant allergens remains uncertain. Immunologic tests are helpful in determining the general atopic predisposition of the patient, but they must be evaluated in conjunction with the clinical history in identifying agents of etiologic significance in the disease.

Severe asthmatics are often tempted to change their place of residence in order to avoid local allergens. For many, this does result in symptomatic improvement. Frequently, however they soon develop reactions to the aeroallergens in the new locale.

ANTIALLERGIC THERAPY. When it is clear that a few specific allergens cause a large fraction of the patient's symptoms, immunotherapy ("hyposensitization") is sometimes recommended. Such therapy, consisting of injections of increasing doses of antigen, induces the formation of IgG antibodies which block antigen binding with IgE. It may also lead to a reduction in specific IgE. Unfortunately, hyposensitization is prolonged, expensive, and only partially effective.

Antihistamines are generally ineffective except for controlling nasal symptoms. In fact, they should be used with caution in asthma, as they tend to lead to inspissation of secretions.

Immunosuppressive therapy of the type used in transplant patients has been attempted in very severe asthmatic subjects. Results are equivocal, and such therapy is rarely justified except in a research environment.

BRONCHODILATOR AGENTS. These are the mainstays of therapy for asthma, for control of any reversible component in COPD, and for management of bronchospasm associated with simple chronic bronchitis. Both the main classes of bronchodilators, beta-adrenergic agonists and methylxanthines, raise the level of 3'5' cyclic AMP in mast cells and bronchial smooth muscles, thereby inhibiting mediator production and reducing bronchial muscle contractility. Beta-adrenergic agents cause a conversion of ATP to 3'5' cyclic AMP by increasing adenylcyclase activity. Methylxanthines inhibit degradation of 3'5' cyclic AMP by interfering with phosphodiesterase activity. These agents may have additive or even synergistic effects. They are useful both to relieve existing bronchospasm and to prevent recurrent attacks.

Doses of beta-adrenergic drugs are limited by their side effects, and new drugs are continuously being introduced which have less alpha and beta$_1$ (cardiac) adrenergic effects while retaining beta$_2$ activity on bronchial mast cells and smooth muscles. Thus ephedrine, for many years the standard oral medication for asthma in doses of 25 mg three to four times daily, is being replaced by drugs such as metaproterenol, terbutaline, and salbutamol. (Salbutamol is not yet available in the United States but is considered the drug of choice in many other countries.) Oral medications are begun in small doses and gradually increased, depending on the patient's tolerance (e.g., terbutaline, 2.5 mg three times a day, increasing to 5 mg four times a day). The major side effects are tachycardia and tremulousness. Ephedrine may still have a role in some subjects, but it must be used with caution in older persons and should be not used in hypertensives or in men with prostatic disease, in whom it tends to cause urinary retention.

The newer beta-adrenergic drugs may also be used by aerosol and are replacing isoproterenol, long the standard inhaled bronchodilator. Metaproterenol, terbutaline, and salbutamol have longer durations of action as well as more specific beta$_2$ activity. Individual patients differ in their responses to these agents, however, and some still prefer isoproterenol (0.1 mg per inhalation) to newer aerosolized medications. Inhaled bronchodilators may be used regularly as preventive medication. They are especially useful as premedication for bronchial hygiene treatments, as described in the treatment of simple chronic bronchitis. In subjects with infrequent attacks, the aerosols may be used prior to exposure to known provocative factors or as therapy for episodes of dyspnea.

Inhaled bronchodilators are most conveniently administered from a pressurized container, but some authorities prefer a hand or powered nebulizer. One must limit use of aerosol medications to four or five times per day. Abuse of these is common and can lead to refractoriness or side effects such as cardiac arrhythmias. There is no evidence that complicated apparatus such as IPPB machines add significantly to the effectiveness of inhaled bronchodilator medications.

Methylxanthines are frequently given instead of, or in combination with, adrenergic agents. Oral therapy is begun with 100 to 200 mg of aminophylline three to four times daily and the dose increased gradually (up to 400 mg four times daily) until a satisfactory therapeutic effect is obtained or adverse side effects such as nausea occur. Aminophylline may also be administered rectally, using 250 to 500 mg of the drug in a suppository or rectal solution. Rectal aminophylline can be used at bedtime to prevent nocturnal attacks, but offers no real advantage over long-acting oral preparations.

Atropine and related drugs are effective in reversing bronchospasm in some subjects, but the place of anticholinergic agents in the management of asthma remains unclear.

DISODIUM CROMOGLYCATE (CROMOLYN). This unique type of therapy consists of inhalation of a powder containing 20 mg of cromolyn four times daily, using a special spinhaler. The only known effect of cromolyn is to stabilize mast cells, preventing mediator release. It is relatively effective preventive therapy for allergen- or exercise-induced attacks but is of no value for treatment of established bronchospasm as it is not a bronchodilator and must be used regularly to be effective prophylaxis. It has to be given for at least four weeks to determine its usefulness. It is generally ineffective, even as prophylaxis, in older intrinsic asthmatics. Cromolyn is irritating for some subjects, and the agent may be better tolerated if an aerosolized bronchodilator is used shortly before each cromolyn treatment. Cromolyn has no known side effects.

ADRENOCORTICAL HORMONES. The exact mechanism of action of adrenocortical steroids, the most potent antiasthmatic medications, remains unclear. They probably minimize inflammation by stabilizing lysosomes. Their use in asthma is justified when significant airways obstruction persists or recurs frequently despite maximal bronchodilator and cromolyn therapy. In the ambulant patient, drugs are given in moderate doses (e.g., 20 to 40 mg of prednisone per day) for a few days and rapidly tapered to the lowest level compatible with sustained improvement. In many cases, improvement is rapid and the medication may be discontinued totally within five to seven days. Occasional relapses are then treated by repeated short "bursts" of steroids. In some patients, however, symptoms recur when the steroid dose falls below a certain level. One must then taper slowly to the lowest dose compatible with patient comfort and reasonably normal ventilatory function. If possible, maintenance steroids should be administered as a single dose given on alternate days.

Once a maintenance dose has been reached, an attempt should be made to replace some or all of the oral corticosteroid with an inhaled nonabsorbed preparation such as beclomethasone. This agent is supplied in a pressurized container, and the standard dose is two inhalations (100 μg) four times a day. This generally replaces 7.5 to 10 mg per day of oral prednisone and produces no discernible systemic side effects. Some patients require premedication with an inhaled bronchodilator to ameliorate irritation from the beclomethasone aerosol.

Several problems may occur when inhaled steroids are substituted for oral medications. In the steroid-dependent patient who has received oral medication for many months or years, systemic medication must be discontinued very slowly (over several months) to avoid adrenal insufficiency. Nasal symptoms, previously suppressed with oral medications, may exacerbate, requiring reinstitution of oral medications. In some subjects (up to 30 per cent in some series) oropharyngeal candidiasis occurs. Fortunately, this responds promptly to specific therapy and rarely requires discontinuation of inhaled steroids.

OTHER MEASURES. There are some asthmatic subjects in whom cough and sputum production are significant persistent problems. Such patients may be helped by the bronchial hygiene measures described in the therapy of simple chronic bronchitis.

Much has been written about a possible psychogenic basis for asthma. More often than not, however, emotional problems prove to be a result rather than a cause of the disease. Regardless, one must cope sympathetically with anxiety in both the patient and the family. Patients should be encouraged to lead as normal a life as possible. A full program of medications should be used to prevent attacks rather than severely limiting the patient's activities in an attempt to avoid provocative factors.

One must provide medications to use at home (e.g., an aerosol bronchodilator, rectal theophylline, or epinephrine for subcutaneous use) should a mild attack occur. One must also assure that the patient has emergency medical care readily available should home remedies fail to terminate an attack. Most importantly, one should encourage the patient to make regular office visits to be sure his disease remains in good control and to seek medical attention promptly if symptoms worsen.

Treatment of the Acute Attack. Mild attacks in subjects not receiving regular bronchodilator management may respond promptly to an aerosol bronchodilator, rectal aminophylline, or even oral bronchodilator agents. In young subjects not already receiving adrenergic drugs, 0.1 to 0.2 ml of 1:1000 epinephrine subcutaneously is traditional therapy. In older subjects, 5.6 mg of aminophylline per kilogram of body weight given intravenously over 20 minutes may terminate an acute attack. (In patients already receiving aminophylline, the intravenous dose is lower and generally should not exceed 250 mg.) Since episodes tend to recur when effects of medications wear off, maintenance therapy should be prescribed until the patient returns for a regular office visit.

When patients fail to respond promptly to the aforementioned measures, *status asthmaticus* is said to exist and admission to hospital is generally required. Following the loading dose of intravenous aminophylline noted above, this medication is given as a continuous intravenous infusion in an attempt to maintain a therapeutic blood level, generally considered to lie between 10 and 20 mg per liter. A dose of 0.9 mg per kilogram of body weight per hour is commonly recommended, but patients vary in their aminophylline requirements, and the dose may have to be adjusted, depending on the patient's clinical response. Blood theophylline measurements can be helpful in regulating therapy.

In addition, patients should inhale beta-adrenergic agents, followed by bronchial hygiene measures, every four to six hours.

Supplemental oxygen is given in a dose sufficient to maintain the arterial oxygen tension in the range of 60 to 70 torr. Large doses of corticosteroids are indicated and should be begun early because their effect is delayed for several hours. An initial dose of 200 mg of hydrocortisone intravenously, followed by 100 mg every hour or two until symptomatic relief occurs, is conventional therapy. Even larger doses, up to 5 grams per day, have been used in refractory cases. When these measures fail to produce significant improvement over the first 12 to 24 hours, one should consider intravenous isoproterenol. Sedatives and narcotics should be avoided, as they may lead to underventilation. Should this occur, as evidenced by a rising arterial CO_2 tension, endotracheal intubation and mechanical ventilation are indicated. At this stage, sedatives and muscle relaxant agents may be used; they are sometimes required to allow the patient to coordinate with the ventilator.

Once bronchospasm is controlled, oral therapy is substituted for intravenous, and steroids are reduced slowly. Patients should remain in hospital until they have returned to their baseline state and should always be discharged on a full program of maintenance bronchodilators and steroids. Otherwise, return of severe symptoms is likely within 72 hours.

Antic, R., and Macklem, P. T.: The influence of clinical factors on site of airway obstruction in asthma. Am. Rev. Respir. Dis., 114:851, 1976.

Austen, K. F., and Orange, R. P.: Bronchial asthma: The possible role of the chemical mediators of immediate hypersensitivity in the pathogenesis of subacute chronic disease. Am. Rev. Respir. Dis., 112:423, 1975.

Brogden, R. N., Speight, T. M., and Avery, G. S.: Sodium cromoglycate (Cromolyn sodium): A review of its mode of action, pharmacology, therapeutic efficacy and use. Part I: Asthma. Drugs, 7:164, 1974.

Burrows, B., Lebowitz, M. D., and Barbee, R. A.: Respiratory disorders and allergy skin-test reactions. Ann. Intern. Med., 84:134, 1976.

Davies, G., Thomas, P., Broder, I., Mintz, S., Silverman, F., Leznoff, A., and Trotman, C.: Steroid-dependent asthma treated with inhaled beclomethasone dipropionate. Ann. Intern. Med., 86:549, 1977.

Godfrey, S., and König, P.: Exercise-induced bronchial lability in atopic children and their families. Ann. Allergy, 33:199, 1974.

Gold, W. M., Kessler, G.-F., and Yu, D. Y. C.: Role of vagus nerves in experimental asthma in allergic dogs. J. Appl. Physiol., 33:719, 1972.

Kaufman, J., and Wright, G. W.: The effect of nasal and nasopharyngeal irritation on airway resistance in man. Am. Rev. Respir. Dis., 100:626, 1969.

Klaustermeyer, W. B., DiBernardo, R. L., and Hale, F. C.: Intravenous isoproterenol: Rationale for bronchial asthma. J. Allerg. Clin. Immunol., 55:325, 1975.

Mitenko, P. A., and Ogilvie, R. I.: Rational intravenous doses of theophylline. N. Engl. J. Med., 289:600, 1973.

Pepys, J., and Hutchcroft, B. J.: Bronchial provocation tests in etiologic diagnosis and analysis of asthma. Am. Rev. Respir. Dis., 112:829, 1975.

Pepys, J., and Simon, G.: Asthma, pulmonary eosinophilia, and allergic alveolitis. Med. Clin. North Am., 57:573, 1973.

Woolcock, A. J.: Inhaled drugs in the prevention of asthma (editorial). Am. Rev. Respir. Dis., 115:191, 1977.

CHRONIC OBSTRUCTIVE PULMONARY DISEASE

PREVALENCE AND PATHOGENESIS. Chronic obstructive pulmonary disease (COPD) is a major cause of disability in older subjects, ranking behind heart diseases and schizophrenia in United States Social Security statistics. It is also an increasingly important cause of mortality. Reported United States mortality rates, which are almost certainly underestimates, have increased several-fold over the last few decades, and the true mortality from COPD probably approaches that from lung cancer. The disease is usually first diagnosed between ages 55 and 65. It is much more common in men than in women, most series reporting a male:female ratio close to 9:1, but this may reflect only the different smoking habits of the sexes earlier in the century.

As already noted, COPD results from some combination of chronic obstructive bronchitis and pulmonary emphysema. Both disorders are closely related to cigarette smoking. The intrinsic airways disease is generally considered a direct consequence of bronchial irritation in a susceptible individual, but a possible role of chronic infection cannot be excluded. It is now generally believed that emphysema results from the effect of proteolytic enzymes on lung tissue. When there is a very severe congenital deficiency of serum antiproteolytic activity, emphysema is likely to develop by middle age even if the subject does not smoke. Without such a severe deficiency (which accounts for only 0.5 to 2 per cent of COPD), the development of emphysema depends on prolonged exposure to noxious irritants, usually cigarette smoke. Presumably, such exposure leads to reduction in lung defense mechanisms, low grade inflammatory changes in the lung parenchyma, and release of sufficient leukocytic proteases to overwhelm the body's antiproteolytic mechanisms.

Epidemiologic studies reveal a close relationship between cigarette smoking and slowing of forced exhalation. Whereas the average nonsmoking adult shows a rate of decline in FEV_1 of 20 to 25 ml per year of age, the average heavy smoker shows a decline of 40 to 45 ml per year. Thus an FEV_1 of 4.0 liters in a 25 year old would be expected to decline to approximately 3.1 liters by age 65 if he did not smoke but, on the average, would be close to 2.2 liters if he smoked one to two packs of cigarettes per day throughout adult life. The excess rate of decline appears to cease if smoking is discontinued. But this average effect of cigarettes is not sufficient to explain the much more severe impairment of FEV_1 noted in clinically significant COPD. Presumably, there are subjects who are especially susceptible to the effects of smoking.

There is great interest in identifying factors which cause a minority of smokers to develop clinically significant COPD. Respiratory disorders in childhood and intercurrent respiratory infections may be contributory factors. Genetic factors may also play a role. Certainly there are a few families in whom a deficiency of serum antiproteolytic activity is associated with a susceptibility to COPD. The serum's trypsin inhibitory capacity is determined by the *p*rotease *i*nhibitor or "Pi" phenotype of the subject. A normal individual has two M genes (Pi phenotype MM). Severe deficiency of alpha$_1$ globulin, which contains most of the serum's antiproteolytic (antitrypsin) activity, occurs with a ZZ phenotype. This is found in approximately 1:4000 of the population. It is associated with hepatitis in infancy as well as emphysema in middle age. A heterozygotic state (phenotype MZ) is much more common, occurring in 3 to 5 per cent of the population. It is associated with moderate reduction in serum antiproteolytic activity. In some families, such an MZ phenotype appears to be associated with an increased tendency to COPD. On the other hand, general population studies have failed to show any over-all tendency for MZ subjects to develop an excess of respiratory disease or for respiratory disorders to be related to the level of serum trypsin inhibitory capacity except in ZZ subjects. A variety of other Pi genes have been identified (of which S is the most common), but only the Z gene is clearly associated with COPD.

The generally accepted concept of the early, preclinical history of COPD is that susceptible subjects who smoke show a very excessive rate of decline in lung function throughout adult life, a decline approximating 75 ml per year. According to this concept, the subject who will later develop COPD should be recognizable by age 40 because he will already show a mild ventilatory abnormality. This has led to some enthusiasm for screening of young to middle-aged adults in order to detect early COPD. There is no direct evidence, however, that the individual who will later develop severe disabling disease can be identified reliably by any physiologic test applied early in life. Indeed, it remains possible that the usual subject who develops COPD is indistinguishable from the average smoker until a relatively few years prior to the onset of symptoms when ventilatory function declines extremely rapidly.

PATHOLOGY. The basic defect in emphysema is destruction of alveolar walls, leading to a reduced number of enlarged air spaces. This is often most severe in the central portion of the lobule (centrilobular emphysema) but it may occur uniformly throughout the acinus (panacinar emphysema). Both types of change may occur in the same lung, and severe centrilobular changes may progress to a point at which the process appears to involve the entire acinus. Centrilobular changes are closely related to chronic obstructive bronchitis, whereas panacinar changes, especially severe at the lung bases, are characteristic of homozygotic (ZZ) alpha$_1$-antitrypsin deficiency states.

Changes in the large airways characteristic of simple chronic bronchitis vary considerably in severity. But there are usually widespread abnormalities in small bronchi and bronchioles, including inflammation in and around air passages with narrowing of their lumens, mucous impaction, and obliterative changes. The extent of the abnormalities in small airways is not obvious on casual examination of the lung and can be quantified only by morphometric studies.

Small airways changes and emphysema may not be totally unrelated. Indeed, it is likely that one may induce the other. However, there is wide variability in the relative importance of intrinsic airways disease and emphysema among subjects with COPD, and these differences are reflected in the clinical and physiologic manifestations of the disease.

CLINICAL MANIFESTATIONS. Dyspnea is the most common chief complaint, but some patients first see a physician because of cough, wheezing, recurrent respiratory infections, or even weakness or weight loss. The dyspnea is usually described as insidious in onset and progressive. Some patients, however, are aware of shortness of breath only during exacerbations of disease and give a history more suggestive of asthma than COPD. Others date their chronic symptoms from an acute respiratory infection.

Most patients admit to some cough and expectoration, but often this consists only of clearing a small quantity of mucus from the chest shortly after awakening. Other patients complain of more severe cough and more copious, sometimes purulent sputum.

Physical findings are extremely variable and depend to some extent on the stage of the disease. In relatively early illness (FEV_1 above 1.0 liter), the examination is often normal except for slowing of forced expiration. Rhonchi may be present or the chest may be unusually quiet on auscultation. Other physical findings occur with increasing frequency as the disease progresses. There may be gross overinflation with low diaphragms and a decreased area of cardiac dullness. Labored breathing, sometimes through pursed lips, may be present after slight exertion or even at rest. The patient may assume a stooped posture, tend to lean on his elbows when sitting, and use accessory muscles of respiration. Cyanosis may be present, and slight dependent edema is common.

Evidences of cor pulmonale generally appear only in advanced stages of illness when the FEV_1 is below 1 liter, but the severity of cardiac complications is quite variable. Pulmonary hypertension and cor pulmonale in COPD are more closely related to the severity of hypoxemia than to the degree of ventilatory impairment and are generally noted only when the resting arterial Po_2 is below 45 torr. Occasionally, patients first seek medical attention at this stage of illness, their major presenting features being those of heart failure secondary to cor pulmonale.

The variability in findings in patients with COPD is explained, at least in part, by differences in the severity of their emphysema and their intrinsic airway disease. Occasionally, relatively distinctive syndromes can be distinguished which relate to the underlying pathology. These have been called the emphysematous (Type A) and bronchial (Type B) types of COPD. Their features are summarized in the accompanying table. Since typical Type A

patients often hyperventilate, thereby maintaining reasonably normal arterial oxygen tensions, they have been described as "pink puffers." Cyanosis and congestive heart failure are more common in Type B disease, and patients with these features have been called "blue bloaters." It should be recognized, however, that these clinical types represent extremes of a spectrum of presentations. Most patients display a mixture of findings, especially if followed over a period of time.

LABORATORY FINDINGS. Except for some erythrocytosis in severely hypoxemic patients, the routine blood count and differential are normal. The finding of eosinophilia should lead one to suspect that there is a reversible (asthmatic) component to the disease.

The chest radiograph may be entirely normal early in the disease, or it may reveal only the residua of previous inflammatory changes. With severe emphysema, marked overinflation is noted with flattening of the diaphragms, increased retrosternal space, and regional attenuation of vessels. In some cases, there are frank bullae demarcated by hairline margins. In homozygotic alpha$_1$-antitrypsin deficiency, emphysematous changes are usually most marked at the bases of the lungs.

The most characteristic feature of COPD is persistent reduction in forced expiratory flow rates. The residual volume is increased, as is the residual volume : total lung capacity ratio. Nonuniformity of ventilation and some mismatch of ventilation and perfusion are generally noted, but the severity of physiologic shunting and hypoxemia varies greatly from case to case. Most other pulmonary function abnormalities are also variable and depend to some extent on the relative severity of the emphysema and intrinsic airways disease, as indicated in the table.

Isotopic lung scans show the uneven ventilation and perfusion. Areas of diminished perfusion may even be mistaken for pulmonary emboli, and lung scans must be interpreted cautiously in patients with any chronic pulmonary disease.

The electrocardiogram is often normal, especially early

Features of the Bronchial and Emphysematous Types of COPD

	Emphysematous (Type A)	Bronchial (Type B)
Clinical features		
Dyspnea	Insidious onset, slowly progressive	Often noted first only during chest infections
Sputum	Usually scant and mucoid	Often copious and purulent
Weight loss	Often marked	Usually slight or absent
Chronic cor pulmonale with heart failure	Infrequent until terminal stages of the disease	Common
Chest examination	Quiet chest (except slight wheeze at end expiration), marked hyperinflation	Noisy chest, slight hyperinflation
Chest radiograph	Hyperlucent, overinflated lung; often regional attenuation of vessels	Often evidence of old inflammatory disease
Physiologic tests		
Total lung capacity	Increased	Normal or slightly decreased
Residual volume	Markedly increased	Moderately increased
Lung compliance, static	Increased	Near normal
Lung compliance, dynamic	Normal or slightly low	Very low
Lung recoil	Markedly reduced	Variable
Inspiratory airways resistance	Normal	Increased
Diffusing capacity	Markedly reduced	Variable
Arterial Po_2	Slight reduction at rest; usually falls with exertion	Often very low at rest; variable change with exertion
Arterial Pco_2	Usually normal or low	Often chronically elevated
Resting pulmonary artery pressure	Normal or slightly elevated at rest; increases with exertion	Often markedly elevated at rest
Cardiac output	Often low	Usually near normal

in the disease. Later, one may find some right axis shift and a delayed transition of the QRS complexes across the precordial leads. Peaked P waves ("P pulmonale") may be noted, especially during exacerbations of disease. These changes, although characteristic of severe COPD, are not well correlated with pulmonary hypertension or cor pulmonale. The most reliable indication of the latter condition is the presence of R waves over the right precordium.

COURSE AND PROGNOSIS. The initial response to therapy is variable and depends on the degree of bronchospasm associated with the disease. Some patients show considerable initial symptomatic and physiologic improvement. After this, the disease tends to progress slowly, with an average decline in FEV_1 between 50 and 75 ml per year. The rate of loss of function can be assessed only after several years of follow-up, however, because the variability in FEV_1 may exceed its true annual decline. Almost all symptoms also tend to worsen slowly. Cough and sputum production are exceptions. These often improve, especially if the patient stops smoking.

As a rule, patients note dyspnea on moderate exertion when the FEV_1 is between 1.2 and 1.5 liters, become limited to relatively sedentary activity when the FEV_1 is near 1 liter, and become invalided as the FEV_1 approaches 500 ml. Chronic hypercapnia, severe hypoxemia, and cor pulmonale are usually noted only when the FEV_1 is below 1 liter. Median survival is approximately ten years when the FEV_1 exceeds 1.2 liters, is near five years when the FEV_1 is 1.0, and approaches 2.0 years when the FEV_1 is less than 700 ml, but there is considerable variability around these median survivals, some patients living 12 to 15 years despite a very low initial FEV_1. Rapid heart rate at rest, severe blood gas abnormalities, or evidences of cor pulmonale are poor prognostic signs. Longevity is reduced in patients residing at altitudes in excess of 3500 feet.

Many patients show periodic exacerbations of their disease characterized by increased cough and dyspnea. These exacerbations often follow acute respiratory infections and are associated with variable degrees of bronchospasm. In patients with severe COPD, such exacerbations are life threatening, leading to acute respiratory failure and to heart failure secondary to cor pulmonale.

DIFFERENTIAL DIAGNOSIS. There are three criteria for the diagnosis of COPD: (1) there must be slowing of forced expiration, and the reduction of FEV_1 must be disproportionate to any reduction in FVC (i.e., both the per cent predicted FEV_1 and the FEV_1/FVC ratio must be reduced); (2) the expiratory slowing must persist despite prolonged and intensive medical therapy; and (3) specific bronchopulmonary diseases which might explain the physiologic abnormalities must be excluded. Failure to demonstrate extensive parenchymal disease on chest radiograph and an absence of any signs of upper airway obstruction (e.g., stridor, neck mass, or narrowing of the upper airway on chest radiogram) are generally considered sufficient for the last criterion. It is more difficult to exclude reversibility of the disease. This is discussed further under Treatment.

Determining the relative importance of intrinsic airways changes and emphysema may also present a challenge, but attenuation of vascular markings and increased transradiancy of the lung are usually noted on the chest radiograph if the emphysema is severe. A well-preserved diffusing capacity suggests that extensive emphysema is not present, whereas a relatively normal airways resistance measurement suggests that intrinsic airways abnor-

malities are limited in extent. The esophageal balloon measurements required to measure the elastic properties of the lung (the best guide to the severity of emphysema) are rarely justified for clinical evaluation.

In children and young adults, any syndrome resembling the bronchial type of COPD should suggest mucoviscidosis.

A homozygotic alpha$_1$-antitrypsin deficiency should be suspected when there is a family history of emphysema or when there is an early age of onset of an emphysematous type of COPD, especially if the patient is a nonsmoker or is female, or when the radiograph reveals a bilateral basilar distribution of the emphysematous changes. The diagnosis is confirmed by almost complete absence of alpha$_1$ globulin, by very low serum trypsin inhibitory capacity, and, most definitively, by demonstration of the pattern of a ZZ phenotype on crossed immunoelectrophoresis of the serum.

TREATMENT. The goals of therapy of COPD are as follows: (1) relief of any reversible component of the airways obstruction; (2) control of cough and bronchial secretions; (3) elimination and prevention of bronchopulmonary infection; (4) increase in exercise tolerance to the limits imposed by the patient's permanent physiologic impairment; (5) control of remediable complications of the disease, including cardiovascular problems and excessive hypoxemia; (6) avoidance of factors which may aggravate the disease such as inhaled irritants, sedatives and narcotics, or unnecessary surgery; and (7) relief of depression and anxiety which often accompany the disorder.

A comprehensive therapeutic program can ameliorate symptoms, reduce the frequency of hospital admission, prevent premature death, and allow patients to lead more active and more satisfying lives. Although it is true that most patients with severe COPD show a slow progression of ventilatory impairment despite treatment, this should not lead to therapeutic nihilism.

The usefulness of a team approach to therapy of COPD has been well demonstrated. There is no evidence, however, that equally satisfactory results cannot be obtained by a dedicated individual physician, perhaps assisted by an office nurse to help patients with bronchial hygiene and physical therapy measures.

Initial Treatment. One cannot predict accurately the degree of reversibility of the airways obstruction when the patient is first seen, and all patients should be regarded as having potentially reversible disease. Bronchodilators should be given to tolerance, as described in the therapy of asthma. Smoking should be eliminated or minimized and other sources of bronchial irritants avoided. Bronchial hygiene measures and, when appropriate, antibiotics should be used, as outlined in the therapy of simple chronic bronchitis. If signs of congestive heart failure are present, diuretics should be prescribed.

The appropriateness of this regimen should be evaluated after its effects on symptoms and ventilatory tests have been observed. Therapy may have to be adjusted to minimize side effects, and apparently useless measures (such as postural drainage which leads to no sputum production or symptomatic relief) should be discontinued. The physician must then decide if the possibility of further reversibility of the disease is sufficiently great to justify a three- to four-week trial of corticosteroids.

Although there are no hard and fast rules, the following features suggest potential reversibility of the disease and indicate that a trial of steroids is worthwhile in a patient with apparent COPD: (1) improvement in FEV_1 of greater than 20 per cent after inhalation of a bronchodilator; (2) similar degree of improvement in FEV_1 over several weeks of intensive bronchodilator therapy; (3) history of considerable fluctuation in severity of symptoms or of acute attacks of wheezing dyspnea not precipitated by exertion; (4) prominent wheeze or noisy chest on physical examination; (5) chest radiograph which appears normal except for hyperinflation; (6) eosinophilia of the blood or sputum; (7) evidences of atopy, such as a history of hay fever, positive allergy skin tests, or high serum IgE level; (8) associated vasomotor rhinitis or nasal polyps; or (9) normal pulmonary diffusing capacity measurement.

Corticosteroids are given in moderate doses (e.g., 20 to 40 mg per day of prednisone) for three to four weeks, and their effectiveness is assessed by changes in spirometric tests. Full doses of bronchodilators are maintained during this trial period. If significant improvement in FEV_1 is not observed, steroids should be discontinued gradually over one to two weeks. If improvement does occur, medications should be tapered to the smallest possible maintenance dose, as described in the therapy of asthma.

Maintenance Therapy. Even if no objective improvement is obtained with bronchodilator drugs, maintenance doses of theophyllines, perhaps in conjunction with beta-adrenergic drugs, are usually advised to prevent episodes of superimposed bronchospasm. Adrenergic aerosols may also be used prior to exposure to known bronchial irritants, for treatment of acute attacks of dyspnea, or as part of a bronchial hygiene program. In patients who show significant improvement with bronchodilators or with adrenocortical hormones, these drugs should be maintained as described in the therapy of asthma. Those measures described for the treatment of simple chronic bronchitis are fully applicable to patients with COPD who suffer from productive cough, recurrent bronchopulmonary infection, or retained secretions. Certain other types of treatment are more uniquely applicable to COPD.

PHYSICAL THERAPY. Unless contraindicated by a cardiac disorder, a program of gradually increasing exercise should be prescribed. This should have a specific goal which is important to the patient, such as walking a greater distance so the patient can go to a neighborhood store. Exercise does not improve lung function but it does train skeletal muscles to function more efficiently, thereby increasing exercise tolerance. For very severely disabled patients, exercise therapy may have to be initiated by a trained physical therapist, but in the usual case an appropriate program can be recommended directly to the patient by his physician. Patients with severe exertional hypoxemia may need supplemental oxygen during exercise, and it is advisable to obtain arterial blood gas at rest and after exercise before embarking on a vigorous exercise program in patients with an FEV_1 below 1 liter.

"Breathing exercises" are sometimes recommended. These generally consist of attempts to train the patient to breathe abdominally, in the hope of encouraging diaphragmatic activity. It is doubtful, however, that one can alter the patient's usual breathing pattern. More realistically, one can teach the patient that dyspnea per se is not harmful, that slow deep breathing relieves dyspnea more quickly than rapid shallow "panic breathing," and that breath holding during exertion is to be avoided. Mechanical devices, such as emphysema belts and IPPB machines, are of no proved value.

OXYGEN THERAPY. There are clear indications for home oxygen therapy in some patients with COPD. Low flow oxygen by nasal cannula may be employed during exercise in patients with severe exertional hypoxemia. Other patients require regular oxygen therapy to control severe pulmonary hypertension which has led to cor pulmonale and recurrent episodes of heart failure. In the latter instance, oxygen is generally administered during sleep, and there is a suggestion that it should be given for at least 15 hours per day to achieve maximum effects. The proper oxygen dose is one which achieves an arterial oxygen tension between 55 and 65 torr (usually 1 to 2 liters per minute by nasal prongs). In patients with resting arterial oxygen tensions consistently below 40 torr, continuous oxygen therapy may be needed to maintain ambulation and prevent congestive failure.

Oxygen should not be used to treat episodes of dyspnea. Patients become habituated to this form of therapy, adding to their invalidism.

ENVIRONMENTAL CONTROL. The possibility of a change in climate or locale is often considered for severely impaired patients. A move to a lower altitude is certainly justified for patients living at altitudes above 4000 feet. (All patients with severe COPD should be advised to avoid high altitudes, and those with severe hypoxemia may require supplemental oxygen when traveling by air.) A change in residence may also be indicated for patients residing in areas of very heavy air pollution.

Many patients consider moving to escape a cold winter climate. Some find relief in warm humid regions, whereas others prefer dry warm desert climates. There is no evidence that the overall course of the disease is altered by a move to either type of area. A decision to relocate in a more salubrious climate should be made only after weighing the possible symptomatic relief against the social and economic hardships of the move. The specific area is best chosen on the basis of a trial period to assess both symptomatic relief and the patient's fondness for the locale.

TREATMENT OF EDEMA AND COR PULMONALE. Pedal edema is common even in the absence of other evidences of congestive heart failure and is usually readily controlled with small doses of diuretics. Recurrent or chronic congestive failure secondary to cor pulmonale is a more difficult problem. In addition to the usual therapy for heart failure (using digitalis with great care), phlebotomies may be needed to maintain the hematocrit below 56, and all treatments may fail unless hypoxemia is controlled with oxygen therapy.

TREATMENT OF HYPERCAPNIA. Chronic hypercapnia is common in late stages of the disease. It requires no specific therapy but does indicate the need to monitor blood gases closely during exacerbations of the disease and to avoid totally the use of sedatives, tranquilizers, or narcotics. There is no justification for respiratory stimulants or mechanical assistance to ventilation in patients with chronic stable hypercapnia.

SURGICAL THERAPY. A few patients with very large bullae which compress relatively normal lung may be benefited by bullectomy. However, the selection of suitable operative candidates requires careful and detailed preoperative evaluation.

SUPPORTIVE MEASURES. It is essential that patients understand the nature of their disease, the significance of symptoms which may develop (e.g., purulent sputum), the possible side effects of medications, and the goals of therapy. Provision must be made for prompt treatment of exacerbations. Most importantly, patients must be encouraged to live active and interesting lives within the limits imposed by their respiratory impairment and within the constraints imposed by any therapeutic measures which are employed. Occupational therapy and vocational rehabilitation are useful for some patients.

Treatment of Exacerbations. Mild symptomatic exacerbations, often associated with infection, are treated with more vigorous application of the measures mentioned above. Antibiotics, increased bronchodilators, and even a course of steroids are often indicated. Blood gases should be monitored and cardiovascular status assessed. Severe hypoxemia, increasing arterial carbon dioxide tension, or evidence of congestive heart failure dictates immediate hospitalization. The management of acute respiratory failure and heart failure from cor pulmonale are discussed in Ch. 351.5 and 355. Patients with refractory bronchospasm superimposed on their COPD should receive the same type of management as patients with status asthmaticus, as described in the therapy of asthma.

Burrows, B., and Earle, R. H.: Course and prognosis of chronic obstructive lung disease. N. Engl. J. Med., 280:397, 1969.

Burrows, B., Fletcher, C. M., Heard, B. E., Jones, N. L., and Wootliff, J. S.: The emphysematous and bronchial types of chronic airways obstruction. Lancet, 1:830, 1966.

Burrows, B., Knudson, R. J., Cline, M. G., and Lebowitz, M. D.: Quantitative relationships between cigarette smoking and ventilatory function. Am. Rev. Respir. Dis., 115:195, 1977.

Burrows, B., Knudson, R. J., and Lebowitz, M. D.: The relationship of childhood respiratory illness to adult obstructive airway disease. Am. Rev. Respir. Dis., 115:751, 1977.

Filley, G. F., Beckwitt, H. J., Reeves, J. T., and Mitchell, R. S.: Chronic obstructive bronchopulmonary disease. II. Oxygen transport in two clinical types. Am. J. Med., 44:26, 1968.

Fletcher, C. M., and Peto, R.: The natural history of chronic airflow obstruction. Br. Med. J., 1:1645, 1977.

Hogg, J. C., Macklem, P. T., and Thurlbeck, W. M.: Site and nature of airway obstruction in chronic obstructive lung disease. N. Engl. J. Med., 278:1355, 1968.

Lertzman, M. M., and Cherniack, R. M.: Rehabilitation of patients with chronic obstructive pulmonary disease. Am. Rev. Respir. Dis., 114:1145, 1976.

Lieberman, J.: Alpha₁-antitrypsin deficiency. Med. Clin. North Am., 57:691, 1973.

Morse, J. O., Lebowitz, M. D., Knudson, R. J., and Burrows, B.: Relation of protease inhibitor phenotypes to obstructive lung diseases in a community. N. Engl. J. Med., 296:1190, 1977.

Proceedings of the Conference on the Scientific Basis of Respiratory Therapy: Oxygen therapy. Am. Rev. Respir. Dis., suppl. to Vol. 110, Dec. 1974, pp. 25–84.

344.2. LOCALIZED AIRWAY OBSTRUCTION

Localized obstruction to airflow may result from extrinsic compression of airways, from diseases of the airways themselves, or from intraluminal obstructions. Signs and symptoms depend on whether the lesion is above or below the tracheal bifurcation, on whether the obstruction is complete or partial, and on the cause of the obstruction.

OBSTRUCTION ABOVE THE TRACHEAL BIFURCATION

PARTIAL OBSTRUCTION. The characteristic finding in partial obstruction above the tracheal carina is stridor, often accompanied by inspiratory retraction of the intercostal spaces. Slowing the air flow is noted on both forced inspiration and forced expiration, and the MEFV curve may have a characteristic appearance, showing a plateau which reflects a relatively constant forced expiratory flow over a large portion of the FVC. With severe obstruction,

adequate over-all ventilation may not be maintained, resulting in hypercapnia and hypoxemia.

Diseases intrinsic to the airways which may lead to partial obstruction include enlarged tonsils and adenoids (especially in young children); neoplasms of the hypopharynx, larynx, vocal cords, or trachea; stenosing lesions secondary to trauma; bilateral vocal cord paralysis; laryngeal edema or spasm; and inflammatory lesions of the pharynx (as in peritonsillar abscess), larynx (as in croup), or trachea (as in diphtheria). Extrinsic compression of the larynx or trachea may occur secondary to enlarged thyroid, paratracheal neoplasm, or, rarely, mediastinal infection. If the primary cause of the obstruction cannot be eliminated, an artificial airway, tracheostomy, or surgical repair is indicated.

COMPLETE OBSTRUCTION. Unless promptly relieved, complete obstruction above the tracheal carina leads to rapid asphyxiation. The presentation is pathognomonic with lack of air flow at the mouth despite inspiratory efforts and inspiratory retraction of the intercostal spaces. Acute obstruction is most commonly caused by aspiration of poorly chewed food. This emergency is treated by applying forceful pressure to the epigastrium, using the *Heimlich maneuver*.

Episodic complete obstruction of the upper airway occurs during sleep in a few very obese individuals owing to falling back of the glossopharyngeal structures. This form of sleep apnea causes frequent awakening, troubled sleep, and somnolence. The resulting clinical picture can be confused with the pickwickian syndrome.

Complete obstruction secondary to trauma, intractable laryngospasm, or chronic disease must be bypassed with an artificial airway or tracheostomy.

OBSTRUCTION BELOW THE TRACHEAL BIFURCATION

PARTIAL OBSTRUCTION. Characteristically, this results in a localized expiratory wheeze over the site of obstruction and hyperinflation of the distal lung. It is most commonly caused by a primary neoplasm which grows into or compresses an airway, but it may result from acute or chronic inflammatory lesions of the bronchi, aspiration of foreign bodies, compression of bronchi from enlarged hilar lymph nodes, or mucus plugs. Since airflow from the remaining lung is unimpaired, spirometry may be relatively normal, but other tests will reveal evidence of nonuniformity of ventilation. The area of diminished airflow may be detected by ventilation scans. Definitive diagnosis generally depends on bronchoscopy, and treatment is directed at the underlying disease.

Partial bronchial obstruction impairs clearance of secretions from the distal lung, leading to infection and even abscess formation. Recurrent infections in the same area of lung, slow clearing of pneumonia, or lung abscess should make one suspect partial obstruction of the bronchus leading to the affected region.

COMPLETE OBSTRUCTION. Air in the lung distal to a complete obstruction is absorbed into the bloodstream, leading to collapse of the affected region, a condition called "obstructive atelectasis." Its features are discussed under Atelectasis in Ch. 345. Any of the disorders mentioned above as causes of partial obstruction may progress to the point of complete occlusion of a bronchus and lead to obstructive atelectasis.

Ainger, L. E.: Large tonsils and adenoids in small children with cor pulmonale. Br. Heart J., 30:356, 1968.

Heimlich, H. J.: A life-saving maneuver to prevent food-choking. JAMA, 234:398, 1975.

Sackner, M. A., Landa, J., Forrest, T., and Greeneltch, D.: Periodic sleep apnea: Chronic sleep deprivation related to intermittent upper airway obstruction and central nervous system disturbance. Chest, 67:164, 1975.

Shim, C., Corro, P., Park, S. S., and Williams, M. H., Jr.: Pulmonary function studies in patients with upper airway obstruction. Am. Rev. Respir. Dis., 106:233, 1972.

345. ABNORMALITIES OF LUNG AERATION

Benjamin Burrows

LOCALIZED HYPOAERATION (ATELECTASIS)

Atelectasis refers to diminished aeration of the lung. It is a feature of many bronchopulmonary diseases, and several types of atelectasis have been described. When total airlessness of a portion of the lung occurs, blood traversing the region fails to participate in gas exchange and behaves as if it were being shunted directly from the right to the left side of the heart. Thus total atelectasis leads to an "anatomic-like" or "absolute" shunt. Unlike the "physiologic" or "relative" shunt noted in most bronchopulmonary diseases, the "absolute shunt" produced by atelectasis is not fully corrected by inhalation of 100 per cent oxygen.

TYPES OF ATELECTASIS AND THEIR PATHOGENESIS. When there is complete obstruction of an airway distal to the tracheal bifurcation, air in the lung behind the obstruction is gradually absorbed into the bloodstream, leading to complete collapse over a period of a few hours, a condition called *obstructive atelectasis*. The rate of collapse is limited by the poor solubility of nitrogen and is much more rapid in an oxygen-filled than in an air-filled lung. Thus high inspired oxygen tensions encourage the development of atelectasis behind obstructing mucus plugs.

Atelectasis may also occur when the recoil of a local area of the lung is greatly increased by fibrotic changes. This results in shrinkage of the involved region rather than total airlessness and is called *contraction atelectasis*.

When widespread alveolar instability occurs in the respiratory distress syndromes (in newborns owing to a surfactant abnormality), *patchy atelectasis* may develop throughout the lung.

A portion of the lung may be allowed to decrease in volume when the intrapleural pressure is elevated as a result of a large pneumothorax, pleural effusion, or other space-occupying lesion in the thorax. This has been called "compression atelectasis" but is more properly termed *relaxation atelectasis*, because it occurs as a result of the lungs' own tendency to recoil when distending forces are relaxed. With marked relaxation atelectasis, small airways in the affected region collapse, and any air remaining distally is removed by the bloodstream.

Finally, a condition called *plate-like atelectasis* may be noted on a chest radiograph. Its pathologic significance is uncertain. The horizontal radiopaque streaks which characterize the condition occur most often at the bases of the lung. They are associated with poor aeration of the lung and are commonly seen when the diaphragm is elevated or when the patient has been unable to breathe deeply for a prolonged period.

CLINICAL MANIFESTATIONS. The clinical and physiologic consequences of atelectasis depend on the extent and chronicity of the process. Sudden collapse of a large portion of the lung may cause severe dyspnea and profound hypoxemia. Over a period of hours, blood flow through the nonventilated lung diminishes, and both symptoms and hypoxemia become less severe. The acute picture is apt to be noted when obstructive atelectasis develops rapidly from retained secretions (as occurs occasionally in the postoperative period) or from aspiration of a foreign body. When the obstruction develops slowly, as is usually the case with bronchial neoplasms, there may be few or no symptoms and only minimal hypoxemia.

Physical findings depend on the type of atelectasis. With relaxation atelectasis, the findings are those of the underlying condition (e.g., pneumothorax or pleural effusion). In patchy atelectasis, findings are those of the respiratory distress syndrome, which is discussed in Ch. 351. Plate-like atelectasis is not associated with any distinctive physical findings and is basically a radiographic interpretation. With contraction or obstructive atelectasis, physical findings depend on the amount of lung involved. If the atelectatic area is sufficiently large, the trachea and mediastinum are deviated to the affected side, the diaphragm is raised, and the entire hemithorax may be smaller and show less respiratory motion than the unaffected side.

DIAGNOSIS AND TREATMENT. The presence of atelectasis is confirmed radiographically. If the appearance suggests an obstructive type of disease, bronchoscopy is needed to determine its specific etiology. Occasionally, it is possible to remove the occluding material through the bronchoscope. Obstructive atelectasis in a patient who is not severely ill always should raise the question of a bronchogenic neoplasm.

In nonobstructive types of atelectasis, treatment is directed at the underlying cause of the disorder.

THE RIGHT MIDDLE LOBE SYNDROME. In relaxation atelectasis, the lung is usually restored to normal when it is allowed to re-expand (as with relief of a large pneumothorax). With obstructive atelectasis, however, secondary infection is common, leading to fibrosis, abscess formation, and localized bronchiectasis. Thus after prolonged collapse, the affected lung may fail to re-expand normally when the obstruction is relieved. This is commonly noted when the right middle lobe bronchus has been compressed by large hilar lymph nodes in primary tuberculosis or other granulomatous lung diseases. When the lymph nodes finally decrease in size, the affected lung may fail to re-expand fully. It often shows bronchiectatic changes and becomes the site of recurrent or chronic infection. This has been called the *right middle lobe syndrome*. Less commonly, the same sequence of events occurs in other lung regions. When recurrent pneumonia, chronic suppuration, or hemoptysis occurs, the involved lung may have to be resected.

Albo, R. J., and Grimes, O. F.: The middle lobe syndrome; A clinical study. Dis. Chest, 50:509, 1966.

Wanner, A., Landa, J. F., Nieman, R. E., Jr., Vevaina, J., and Delgado, I.: Bedside bronchofiberscopy for atelectasis and lung abscess. JAMA, 224:1281, 1973.

LOCALIZED HYPERAERATION

A partial bronchial obstruction may lead to overinflation of the affected lung. Increased aeration is also seen in emphysematous lung regions, and pockets of air may be noted within cysts, abscesses, or cavities. Lung bullae and the so-called "unilateral hyperlucent lung" are discussed in Ch. 349.1.

346. INFILTRATIVE DISEASES OF THE LUNG

Gareth M. Green

346.1. INTRODUCTION

DEFINITION. Pulmonary infiltration is a radiologic term which connotes a variable but rather characteristic reticulonodular pattern on the chest radiograph. This radiographic pattern is nonspecific with regard to etiologic agent, pathologic entity, or mechanistic process, or as a guide to treatment or prognosis. It is seen as a terminal stage in lymphoma, leukemia, or carcinomatosis, in advanced metabolic derangement such as uremia, in acute viral infections, and in congestive failure, either acute or chronic; it can be found as the only manifestation of a chronic low level exposure to an occupational or environmental agent, such as silica dust or metals or exposure to an air pollutant or to a drug. However, since the radiograph is commonly the first point of recognition of an underlying disorder, these diverse diseases have been grouped by their generally similar radiographic appearance, a somewhat characteristic clinical presentation, and a set of common physiologic abnormalities.

In the past, the infiltrative diseases of the lungs have been classified chiefly according to pathologic reactions, and therefore diagnosis has depended either on examination of pulmonary tissue by lung biopsy or on strong historical evidence of exposure to an occupational or environmental agent known to be associated with the infiltrative or fibrotic process in the lung. Recent and current research has directed much more attention to biologic mechanisms in these diseases. As this new knowledge develops, a more organized and fruitful approach to diagnosis becomes possible and new classifications are introduced.

This chapter will commence with a discussion of features of the syndrome that are common to most of the group. Rather than explain each separate disease as a distinctive clinical entity — an unwarranted practice because of the great variation between and among the disorders — the different diseases will be distinguished by etiology, pathogenesis, or histopathology. Clinical features particularly characteristic of one specific disorder will be mentioned in the discussion of that disease, although it should be remembered that differentiation and diagnosis depend more on the meticulous collection and analysis of historical and laboratory data than on any clustering of clinical, physiologic, or radiologic findings.

The clinical presentation of diffuse infiltrative lung diseases (DILD) varies from asymptomatic to acute or chronically progressive dyspnea, tachypnea, and cyanosis. Commonly, an environmental or occupational exposure is not recognized, although it is the responsibility of the physician to ferret out this information from the history and recognize when an individual has been exposed to an agent that might account for the symptoms and pulmonary abnormalities. The chest film characteristically shows reticulonodular infiltrations diffusely throughout the lung, or localized to upper and lower lung fields or to one region, lobe, or segment. The syndrome, however, includes radiographs with a characteristic ground glass appearance and areas with localized consolidations and even cavitations. Although not characteristic, pleural effusions occur and enlargement of the hilar nodes is seen, particularly in infectious disorders, mineral dust exposures, and sarcoidosis. Cardiac enlargement of the right ventricular type reflects cor pulmonale in either acute or chronic form.

Abnormalities of respiratory physiology are variable, depending upon the chronicity and duration of the process. However, as a general statement, this group of diseases contrasts with obstructive pulmonary disorders by showing relatively little change in air flow dynamics, but, rather, reduction in pulmonary volumes, including vital capacity, functional residual capacity, and residual volume, and in pulmonary compliance and diffusing capacity. Minute ventilation is frequently elevated, distribution of ventilation is well maintained, and perfusion may be reduced and ventilation-perfusion ratios deranged by disease of the small airways. Reductions in both arterial P_{O_2} and P_{CO_2} are characteristic, with either a normal or elevated arterial pH. The symptoms of tachypnea and dyspnea are generally attributed to the changes in compliance and in the efficiency of gas transfer. The relatively stiffer lungs require greater respiratory effort, particularly on inspiration, a finding frequently reflected in augmented work of inspiration, the increased audibility of respiratory effort, and perceptible intercostal retractions. Additional findings on physical examination include tachypnea, increased tactile and vocal fremitus, coarsening of breath sounds with a tendency toward bronchovesicular and bronchial breathing, fine or crackling rales, particularly in the lower lung fields, normal percussion note unless there is consolidation or pleural effusion, accentuated S-2, prominent subxiphoid cardiac impulse, and peripheral cyanosis and clubbing of the digits in more severe cases.

ETIOLOGY. The infiltrative lung diseases are associated particularly with the inhalation of a wide variety of particulate agents, including minerals, metals, radioactive dusts, fungal spores and other allergenic substances, bacteria, viruses, and other microbial organisms. Infiltrative reactions also occur in response to the inhalation of irritant gases, such as nitrogen dioxide, ozone, and components of cigarette smoke; radioactive gases, such as radon; and a variety of other fumes produced principally as occupational exposures. Infiltrative reactions occur as the pulmonary component of disseminated vasculitis, systemic collagen vascular diseases, lymphatic carcinomatosis of the lung, or chronic congestive cardiac failure, particularly mitral stenosis; as a manifestation of pulmonary thromboembolic and veno-occlusive disease; and as epithelial cell proliferation associated with certain drug reactions. The medical challenge is to discover by historical, epidemiologic, or laboratory analysis the specific agent producing the infiltrative response, to eliminate further exposure to that agent, and to suppress or control the infectious or inflammatory process by appropriate drug therapy. Since environmental and occupational agents loom large in the list of agents producing infiltrative responses in the lung, a detailed knowledge of such agents found both in the environment and as hazards of occupations is required for an astute diagnostic evaluation.

EPIDEMIOLOGY. As a group, the infiltrative lung diseases have not received the attention of the research and practicing medical profession warranted by the probable importance of this type of reaction in the lung. When studies have been made, it has become apparent that diffuse pulmonary infiltration and fibrosis are far more widespread than was previously suspected. The reason is that the medical profession has tended to rely on the chest radiograph for detection and diagnosis of these diseases. It is becoming increasingly apparent that the chest radiograph is considerably less sensitive to low-level chronic infiltrative and fibrotic processes in the lung than to the acute inflammatory variety. Thus an acute viral infection shows up well on the radiograph, whereas the diffuse early fibrosis associated with cigarette smoking and other environmental exposures can lead to considerable functional derangement before radiographic changes are apparent. Likewise, recent studies in the granite industry indicate that functional impairment may occur in advance of radiographic signs.

Thus epidemiologic studies relying principally on the chest radiograph do not indicate reliably the true prevalence of infiltrative lung disease in an exposed population. Recent advances in pulmonary physiologic and other laboratory techniques available for epidemiologic surveillance mandate extensive new studies of working and other populations before the true extent and significance of environmental and occupational exposure can be known.

PATHOGENESIS. As the name implies, infiltrative lung disease results from the infiltration of fluid, cells, fibrous tissue, inhaled particulates, or lipid substances into the interalveolar septa, the alveolar spaces, and the peribronchial and perivascular lymphatics. The pathology is widely variable, even with a fairly constant radiographic picture. Inhaled particles are phagocytized by alveolar macrophages and other alveolar phagocytic cells, which eradicate the inhaled particle in situ, exit up the bronchial ciliary escalator carrying the phagocytized burden, become immobilized in the interstitium of the lung with long-term retention of the particle, or trigger by release of chemotactic and other factors acute and/or chronic inflammatory processes.

Exposure to inert dust, such as coal, results in long-term passive accumulation of dust-laden cells which degenerate in time to leave coal dust deposits in the perivascular and peribronchial lymphatics. Exposure to highly irritant dusts such as silica or asbestos causes intracellular damage to phagolysosomal structures with release of proteolytic enzymes and stimulation of inflammatory processes and fibrosis. Inhalation of immunogenic particles leads to the influx of thymus-derived and/or bursa-equivalent lymphocytes which respond to the antigen by the synthesis of immune globulins or the transformation of sensitized lymphocytes. These cells in turn liberate additional mediators, with exacerbation or evolution of the inflammatory

process frequently associated with granuloma production, vasculitis, and fibrosis. The process seems to depend both on the physical, chemical, or immunogenic properties of the inhaled particle and gas and on poorly defined qualities in host defense mechanisms. In low grade fibrogenic exposures, such as to cigarette smoke, the response to exposure may not be associated with any inflammatory process. There appears to be a direct fibrinogenic relationship between the injured phagocytic cell on the one hand and the infiltrating fibroblast on the other. Although less dramatic than the more acute inflammatory processes, this form of silent fibrosis may be the most common cause of idiopathic progressive impairment and disability.

DIFFERENTIAL DIAGNOSIS. The differential diagnosis of infiltrative lung diseases is encyclopedic in terms of the specific agents which can produce a limited variety of histopathologic response in the lung. The classification used in this chapter is somewhat empiric but of clinical utility; it is based on the clustering of disease entities related by clinical or laboratory manifestations, association with systemic disorders, exposure to external agents such as drugs or occupational or environmental agents, or a variety of different agents producing disease by a common and defined pathogenic mechanism. Even with this type of classification, there is still a group of disorders simply classified as "other," without common agent, disease mechanism, histopathologic picture, or diagnostic or therapeutic approach.

Diseases associated with diverse immunologic mechanisms are the pulmonary infiltrates with eosinophilia, the pulmonary manifestations of systemic collagen vascular diseases, hypersensitivity pneumonitis or alveolitis, Wegener's granulomatosis and allergic granulomatosis, drug-induced infiltrative reactions in the lung, and Goodpasture's syndrome. Diseases caused by the inhalation of physically or chemically active agents include the pneumoconioses, pulmonary fibroses (caused by a variety of metallic fume and oxidant gas exposures), and fibrosis associated with exposure to ionizing radiation.

A group of diseases of unknown cause, but of rather characteristic clinical, radiologic, or pathologic presentation, includes sarcoidosis, eosinophilic granuloma, hemosiderosis, alveolar proteinosis, diffuse interstitial pneumonitis, desquamative interstitial pneumonitis, lymphoid interstitial pneumonitis, and usual interstitial pneumonitis (UIP) with fibrosis. Finally, diseases associated with lymphatic stasis include chronic passive congestion associated with mitral stenosis, lymphatic carcinomatosis, and thromboembolic disease of the lungs. A word should be said here about the *Hamman-Rich syndrome*, which is perhaps associated more with a characteristic tempo and intensity of inflammatory process in the lung than with any specific etiologic agent. It is a virulent form of infiltrative lung disease with active inflammatory and epithelial proliferative processes associated with acute shortness of breath and cyanosis, and an unrelenting course with death in three to six months. It is not yet clear that this is a specific etiologic entity or simply one end of a spectrum that is common to a variety of diffuse infiltrative lung disorders.

The diagnosis in this heterogeneous group of disorders is made by systematic analysis of the history for detection of etiologic or associated disease factors; by a study of respiratory tract cells and secretions for detection of characteristic cellular elements, such as eosinophils; by a detailed and specific immunologic evaluation of both the respiratory tract and the systemic immunologic system for evidence of immunization against specific environmental antigens; and by tissue biopsies of draining lymph nodes, of distant organs such as liver and bone marrow, or, most usually, of lung parenchymal tissue obtained by transbronchial or transthoracic needle.

TREATMENT. The selection of therapeutic agents to combat this group of pulmonary disorders is limited largely to the anti-inflammatory agents such as corticosteroids; immunosuppressive agents such as cyclophosphamide; specific antibiotics when appropriate; treatment of underlying diseases such as the collagen vascular diseases, neoplasias, and cardiovascular abnormalities; and removal and avoidance of any identified environmental or ingested causative agents (such as drugs). When the history fails to reveal a specific environmental agent known to produce a characteristic clinical picture, when the immunologic work-up is negative for the identification of a specific antigenic agent, and when examination of pulmonary secretions fails to reveal an etiologic agent, it is best to proceed to the analysis of a tissue specimen obtained either by transbronchial or transthoracic needle biopsy or by open lung biopsy. Although the needle biopsy procedures are capable of providing a diagnosis in more than 80 per cent of cases, the heterogeneity of the pulmonary reactions and the limited size of the biopsy obtained by the needle frequently do not provide a representative assessment of what is going on in the lungs. Under such circumstances, an open lung biopsy is required to fix the diagnosis.

There is growing research interest in the role of subsegmental bronchoalveolar lavage to obtain pulmonary cells and secretions for diagnostic purposes. This technique has become well established in the diagnosis of pulmonary alveolar proteinosis, has recently been found to be effective in the diagnosis of occult infectious processes, and is showing promise of giving useful information in the assessment of the nature of the inflammatory process in the lungs and possibly the state of activity of the disease in the lungs. It is too soon to know the full value of this procedure; but as more becomes known about the etiology and pathogenesis of diffuse infiltrative lung diseases, and as new technology, such as fiberoptic bronchoscopy and subsegmental lavage, becomes available, there will be less need to resort to invasive procedures such as open lung biopsy. Perhaps the two best examples of how developments in scientific knowledge and technology have virtually eliminated the role of open lung biopsy in diagnosis are in hypersensitivity alveolitis, in which diagnosis can frequently be made by immunologic assessment; and in occult infections of the lung in the immunosuppressed host, specifically *Pneumocystis carinii*, in which bronchopulmonary lavage may substitute for needle or open lung biopsy in identifying the causative agent.

PROGNOSIS. The prognosis in infiltrative lung disease is highly variable and difficult. In general, the acute actively inflammatory diseases respond more favorably to agents such as corticosteroids than do diseases of a chronic and slowly progressive variety that are discovered only late in their course. Acute inflammatory disorders more often give rise to symptoms

which bring the patient to the doctor, whereas chronic asymptomatic but progressive disorders are unlikely to do so until the late onset of symptoms of dyspnea and fatigue, when the pathologic process is well advanced and difficult to alter. When a specific agent can be identified and removed from the patient's surroundings, or from the therapeutic regimen, the disease process may subside completely. This is particularly true of diseases associated with drug ingestion and the immunologically produced diseases associated with inhalation of fungal spores or other antigenic material that can be identified and removed from the environment. On the other hand, when no agent can be identified and the pathologic process is obscure, as in the case of pulmonary manifestations of collagen vascular diseases or pulmonary fibrosis of unknown cause, the response to treatment may be minimal.

PREVENTION. A significant portion of the infiltrative lung diseases provides one of the best opportunities in medicine for prevention of disease. Infiltrative diseases associated with environmental exposures in the form of air pollutants, occupational exposures, or avocational exposures to materials around the home can be completely prevented if the disease process is recognized, if the susceptibility of the individual to the agent is identified, and if the offending agent is effectively removed. However, since many of these agents produce asymptomatic disease, it is not possible to rely on the symptomatic patient in order to control the disease. Instead, efforts must be developed to systematically and continuously monitor working and other populations exposed to a wide variety of environmental materials. This will require greatly increased skills and professional capability, but it is here that epidemiology and preventive medicine offer the greatest hope of long-term control of respiratory disease.

American College of Radiology Committee on Audio-visuals: Radiologic Diagnosis of Interstitial Disease of the Lung (videorecording). Chevy Chase, Md., 3M Company, 1975.

Baum, G. L.: Textbook of Pulmonary Diseases. 2nd ed. Boston, Little, Brown & Company, 1974.

Fraser, R. G., and Paré, J. A. P.: Diagnosis of Diseases of the Chest. Philadelphia, W. B. Saunders Company, 1977, p. 342.

Green, G. M., et al.: State of the art: Defense mechanisms of the respiratory membrane. Am. Rev. Respir. Dis., 115:479, 1977.

Petty, T. L.: Pulmonary Diagnostic Techniques. Philadelphia, Lea & Febiger, 1975, pp. 51, 171, 203, 243.

Schofield, N. C., et al.: Small airways in fibrosing alveolitis. Am. Rev. Respir. Dis., 113:729, 1976.

Spencer, H.: Pathology of the Lung: Excluding Tuberculosis. 3rd ed. Oxford and New York, Pergamon Press, 1976.

346.2.   PULMONARY INFILTRATE WITH EOSINOPHILIA

(PIE)

Pulmonary infiltrate with eosinophilia (PIE) includes a variety of disease entities which have in common pulmonary infiltrations with local and/or systemic eosinophilia (Table 1). Although the diseases included under this term have little else in common, the grouping is useful as an easily recognized point of departure along the diagnostic pathway or for the identification of a specific entity. This clustering is also of interest because it illustrates that diseases of diverse etiology and clinical presentations have in common the attraction of a specific blood leukocyte, the eosinophil. This cell has

TABLE 1. Pulmonary Eosinophilia*

Classification	Clinical Data	Radiologic Features	Pathologic Findings
Simple pulmonary eosinophilia (Löffler's syndrome)	Minimal symptoms; peripheral blood eosinophilia; spontaneous resolution within one month	Migratory, patchy "infiltrates" with a predominantly peripheral distribution	Not well characterized
Prolonged pulmonary eosinophilia	Symptoms may be severe: fever, weight loss, cough, dyspnea; duration greater than one month or may be fatal; diminished pulmonary function; response to steroids, but relapse possible	Dense, progressive infiltrates primarily at periphery and nonsegmental	Variable, but may include eosinophilic and mononuclear cell collections in alveoli and interstitium; occasional granuloma formation and even microangiitis
Tropical eosinophilia	Persistent pulmonary symptoms, including cough, dyspnea, asthma; malaise, fever, weight loss; marked blood eosinophilia; high levels of antifilarial antibody and very high levels of serum IgE; improvement after antifilarial chemotherapy (e.g., diethylcarbamazine)	Diffuse finely nodular infiltrates; increased interstitial markings	Granulomatous nodules often surrounding degenerate microfilaria or with necrotic centers; alveolar and interstitial infiltrates composed of eosinophils and mononuclear cells
Pulmonary eosinophilia with asthma	Most commonly allergic bronchopulmonary aspergillosis, either as complication of longstanding asthma or as a cause of adult-onset asthma; elevations of both specific reaginic and precipitating antibodies	Nodular opacities of varying size; recurrent pneumonia; atelectasis; occasional bronchiectasis	Eosinophilic and mononuclear cell infiltrates of alveoli and interstitium; increased numbers of mast cells in walls of the air spaces
Pulmonary eosinophilia with periarteritis nodosa, and variants	Severe symptoms: pulmonary, systemic, and multisystem	Variable: interstitial markings, peripheral infiltrates, consolidations, nodules, and sometimes cavitations	Variable, but characterized by vasculitis and granuloma formation, both sometimes associated with eosinophils

*From Ottesen, E. A.: In Kirkpatrick, C. H., and Reynolds, H. Y. (eds.): Immunologic and Infectious Reactions in the Lung, Volume 1. New York, Marcel Dekker, Inc., 1976, p. 289.

long interested both clinicians and researchers, and it is only recently that significant information has accumulated to determine why it responds in such a wide variety of disease processes.

The eosinophil has long been associated with allergic and immunologic processes. Recently, a link between the eosinophil response and the lymphoid immune system has been determined through the identification of at least four distinct eosinophilotactic substances: eosinophil chemotactic factor of anaphylaxis (ECF-A), a product of the mast cell; eosinophil chemotactic factor produced by complement activation (ECF-C); eosinophil stimulation promoter (ESP); and a lymphocyte-derived eosinophil chemotactic factor (ECFP) requiring the presence of specific antigen-antibody complexes. These chemoatactic factors have been attributed to specific types (Type I through IV) of immunologic responses of the Coombs-Gell system, and this linkage has provided a rationale for the appearance of eosinophilia in immune responses of widely different pathogeneses. Individual rationales will be discussed further under the headings that follow.

SIMPLE PULMONARY EOSINOPHILIA
(Löffler's Syndrome)

Simple pulmonary eosinophilia is asymptomatic or minimally symptomatic in individuals who present with migratory pulmonary infiltrates which are generally patchy and peripheral or pleural based, most often in the upper lung fields, unilateral or bilateral, transient and migratory, and associated with peripheral blood eosinophilia. The condition is self-limited, with spontaneous resolution occurring usually within a month. These manifestations are attributed to an allergic response to a variety of causative agents, and the features of this response are compatible with a Type I allergic reaction in which the allergen interacting with mast cell bound antibody, the reaginic (IgE) antibody, elicits the release of biologically active mediator substances, including SRS-A (slow reacting substance of anaphylaxis), histamine, and ECF-A (eosinophil chemotactic factor of anaphylaxis). These mediators act at local vessels to increase the concentration of cells and fluid giving rise to the characteristic pulmonary infiltrates. The most notable agents to elicit such responses are the tissue-invading parasitic helminths, including *Ascaris lumbricoides,* Strongyloides stercoralis, the dog and cat ascarids, *Toxocara canis* and *Toxocara cati,* and *Ancylostoma braziliense,* the dog hookworm. In addition, drugs, such as p-aminosalicylic acid, sulfonamides, and chlorpropamide, and chemicals, such as nickel carbonyl, also produce Löffler's pneumonia. There are, in addition, other unknown causes of this syndrome.

As the disease is self-limited and ordinarily results in no tissue damage, the importance of this syndrome is to differentiate it from infectious or other causes of pulmonary infiltration of more serious import. No specific treatment is indicated, except for the underlying parasite infestation if identified and for the removal of any offending drug that might be the cause of the reaction.

PROLONGED PULMONARY EOSINOPHILIA

This group of diseases is distinguished from simple pulmonary eosinophilia by the prolonged duration and more severe character of the clinical symptoms of fever, night sweats, weight loss, cough, and dyspnea. The specific causes for this syndrome are diverse, including parasitic, bacterial, and fungal infections, hypersensitivity pneumonitides, and drug allergies. The tissue reaction is more severe with accumulation of eosinophils, mononuclear cells, and occasionally multinucleate giant cells; with an edematous interstitium infiltrated with eosinophils and mononuclear and plasma cells; and with granulomas often showing necrosis and, on occasion, minimal microangiitis. The mechanism of disease appears to be a combination of immune complex (Type III) and cell-mediated immune (Type IV) responses, and responds dramatically to corticosteroid treatment. Recognition is important for this reason and to distinguish this form of pulmonary infiltration from pulmonary infections and other forms of pulmonary infiltration and fibrosis.

TROPICAL EOSINOPHILIA

Tropical eosinophilia bears a relationship to filarial infection and is characterized by persistent pulmonary symptoms of cough, paroxysmal nocturnal asthma, dyspnea, malaise, weight loss, fatigue, low-grade fever, peripheral blood eosinophilia greater than 2000 to 4000 cells per cubic millimeter, and high levels of antibody in all classes to filarial organisms. Duration is a few weeks to months, and clinical improvement occurs by treatment with antifilarial chemotherapy. For reasons that are not clear, the syndrome appears under certain circumstances in infection with the human filarial parasites *Wuchereria bancrofti* and *Brugia malayi*. In particular circumstances, it appears that the host localizes the larval infections to the pulmonary parenchyma, as there is no generalized microfilaremia and the pathologic lesions show microfilaria surrounded by necrotic tissue or eosinophilic leukocytes with granulomatous responses composed of epithelioid histiocytes, fibroblasts, and multinucleate giant cells. This granulomatous response is associated with interstitial infiltrates composed of eosinophils, lymphocytes, macrophages, and plasma cells. This pathologic response may represent immune injury from Type I and Type IV allergic responses mediated by ECF-A and ECF-C (the complement derived eosinophilic chemotactic factor) associated with antigen-antibody complex. Treatment is for the underlying filarial infection.

PULMONARY EOSINOPHILIA WITH ASTHMA

Eosinophilia may occur as a complication of longstanding asthma or in association with adult onset asthma. The disease is characterized by persistent wheezing, cough, fever, and tenacious sputum with rusty brown bronchial plugs. In addition to the pulmonary infiltrates, the syndrome is characterized by recurrent pneumonia, atelectasis, and proximal bronchiectasis. The finding of dilated proximal bronchi associated with pulmonary infiltrates, rubbery brownish bronchial casts, and eosinophilia is strong evidence for the diagnosis. The disease is most commonly caused by allergy to a noninvasive colonization of the bronchial airways by species of *Aspergillus* organisms. The fungal spores serve as potent immunogens, giving rise to both reaginic (IgE) and precipitating (IgG and IgM) antibodies in the patients. Stains of bronchial casts show masses of fungal filaments, and cultures yield the offending organism.

The Type I reaginic response appears to pave the way for the Type III antigen-antibody–mediated reaction, with asthma characterized by gradual onset, prolonged

duration, greater severity, poor reversibility, fever, and leukocytosis. These responses are probably mediated by the activation of complement, with eosinophils responding to the complement-derived eosinophil chemotactic factor (ECF-C). Treatment with corticosteroids will interrupt this immunologic reaction, suppress the inflammatory response and lead to a reduction of secretions, fever, leukocytosis, and symptoms. Recurrence of the syndrome, however, is common, and control can be difficult.

PULMONARY EOSINOPHILIA WITH PERIARTERITIS NODOSA

This entity is included for completeness to distinguish the eosinophilias associated with vasculitis from those described above. However, it more logically belongs in the discussion of the collagen vascular diseases below. Pulmonary eosinophilia may also occur with a wide variety of other conditions, including infection, pulmonary infarction, neoplasia, and cardiac myopathies. However, in these conditions other aspects of the disease predominate and are likely to distinguish them from the aforementioned groupings of pulmonary infiltrates with eosinophilia. In all these disorders, the eosinophilia most likely results as a response to one of several eosinophil chemotactic factors, reflecting the immunologic mechanisms of the underlying disease.

Adickman, M., et al.: Pulmonary infiltrates and eosinophilia associated with drug reactions and parasitic infections. Postgrad. Med., 60:143, 1976.

Ottesen, E. A.: Eosinophilia and the lung. *In* Kirkpatrick, C. H., and Reynolds, H. Y. (eds.): Immunologic and Infectious Reactions in the Lung. Volume 1. New York, Marcel Dekker, Inc., 1976, p. 289.

Turner-Warwick, M., et al.: Cryptogenic pulmonary eosinophilia. Clin. Allergy, 6:135, 1976.

346.3.   HYPERSENSITIVITY PNEUMONITIS
(Extrinsic Allergic Alveolitis)

DEFINITION. Hypersensitivity pneumonitis, also known as extrinsic allergic alveolitis, is perhaps the most important immunologically mediated pulmonary disease to recognize because of the ubiquity of etiologic agents, the severity of acute symptoms, and the potential for permanent fibrotic damage to the lung, but, most importantly, because this disease is entirely preventable by removal of the etiologic environmental agent. Hypersensitivity pneumonitis is an inflammatory interstitial pneumonia that results from an Arthustype immunologic reaction in response to a variety of inhaled organic dusts (Table 2). The reaction also involves the terminal and small airways and may present with an asthmatic component in addition to the symptoms and signs of pneumonitis. Precipitating antibody of the IgG class is generated in response to the inhalation of fungal spores of a variety of species frequently, although not always, associated with an occupational exposure. Recognition of the disease depends on knowledge of its clinical presentation, its timing with an environmental exposure, and the ability to identify one of the many possible etiologic agents.

ETIOLOGY. Hypersensitivity pneumonitis may result from the inhalation of small particle antigenic material

TABLE 2. Etiologic Agents in Hypersensitivity Pneumonitis*

Disease	Exposure	Antigen
Farmer's lung	Moldy vegetable compost	
Mushroom worker's lung	Moldy vegetable compost	*Micropolyspora faeni*
Bagassosis	Moldy vegetable compost	*Thermoactinomyces vulgaris*
Humidifier or air conditioner lung	Contaminated forced air system	*Thermoactinomyces saccharii*
Maple bark stripper's lung	Moldy bark	*Cryptostroma corticale*
	Moldy malt	*Aspergillus clavatus*
Sequoiosis	Moldy redwood dust	*Aureobasidium pullulans*
Paprika splitter's lung	Paprika dust	*Mucor stolonifer*
Wheat weevil disease	Wheat flour weevils	*Sitophilus granarius*
Cheese worker's lung	Cheese mold	*Penicillium caseii*
Suberosis	Moldy cork	*Penicillium sp.*
Bird breeder's lung	Pigeons, parakeets, etc.	Avian proteins
Pituitary snuff lung	Porcine, bovine pituitary	Porcine, bovine proteins

*From Fink, J. N.: *In* Kirkpatrick, C. N., and Reynolds, H. Y. (eds.): Immunologic and Infectious Reactions in the Lung, Volume 1. New York, Marcel Dekker, Inc., 1976, p. 229.

of biologic origin from animal or plant sources. The most common forms result from the inhalation of fungal spores, dried and fragmented fungal or insect particles, or particulate animal proteins, such as are found in pigeon or parakeet droppings or in pituitary powder originating from beef or pig serum proteins and used as snuff. The responsible fungal species are varied, but most belong to the thermophilic actinomycetes identified as *Micropolyspora faeni* or *Thermoactinomyces vulgaris* and *saccharii*. These fungi grow best at 45 to 60°C, usually in decaying vegetation as in molding hay, sugar cane, or other vegetable products. Fungi may also grow in heated water associated with air conditioning and may be disseminated to a rather large population through air conditioning or air heating systems in residential or commercial buildings. Other fungal materials, such as are found in wood dust or in association with tree bark, molding cheese, or brewery materials, may also be responsible agents. A partial list is shown in Table 2. The alert physician may discover new agents by careful study of the patient's environmental exposure, and by microbiologic characterization of discovered fungal species.

EPIDEMIOLOGY. Hypersensitivity pneumonitis most commonly occurs with an occupational exposure as in farmers, sugar cane workers, and bird handlers, or in the general population exposed to contaminated forced air systems, but the physician must be alert to the potential for this type of exposure in a wide variety of circumstances, e.g., snuff taking, moldy cellars, or molding wallpaper. Physicians who specialize in this area have patients with unique and unusual kinds of exposures that have been identified only after repeated hospitalizations and treatments for infectious or other pneumonias. In studies of air conditioning or forced air heating system exposure, it has been found that approximately 15 per cent of the individuals exposed to these particles will develop symptoms of hypersensitivity pneumonitis, and this may be taken as an index of the magnitude of the susceptible population in any given exposure. The development of hypersensitivity pneumonitis in housewives after inhalation of small particles of proteolytic enzymes in laundry detergents is perhaps the best example of how the right combination of susceptible population and conditions of exposure can lead to the disease in any epidemiologic setting.

PATHOGENESIS. The pathogenesis of hypersensitivity pneumonitis involves factors both in the environment and in the host. Vegetation decaying under conditions which give rise to temperatures between 45 and 60° C, such as in composting or when hay is baled wet, is favorable to the development of vast numbers of fungal spores of a particle size appropriate to reach the terminal airways of the lungs when the dust is released by breaking open the hay bale, turning the compost heap, starting up a forced air system in the fall, stripping off maple bark, or other such suitable conditions for exposure. The small respirable particles (between 2 and 5 microns) reach the depths of the lung where they are phagocytized by macrophages and other phagocytic cells of the alveolar surface. An immunologic response is characterized by development of precipitating IgG antibody to the antigen.

Only a fraction of those who develop antibodies exhibit symptoms and signs either acutely or chronically, depending on the nature of the exposure and other factors that are poorly understood. The precipitating antibody interacts with freshly inhaled or deposited antigen with the deposition of immune complexes. Their rephagocytosis by inflammatory cells and the release of inflammatory mediators, chemotactic agents, and lymphokines set up an acute or chronic inflammation. Although the disease is largely thought to be mediated by a Type III immune complex reaction in the pulmonary tissues, there is also evidence of granuloma production and the probable involvement of the Type IV cell-mediated immune response. Evidence of alveolar phagocyte involvement can be seen in histopathologic sections in which histiocytes contain foamy cytoplasm and are surrounded by large numbers of lymphocytes in the interstitium and in the alveolar space. Sarcoid-like granulomas may develop, and some may show foci of central necrosis. More severe cases, and particularly the chronic variety of disease, develop fibrosis in the interalveolar tissues with thickening of the walls of bronchioles and luminal obstruction by granulation tissue.

CLINICAL MANIFESTATIONS. Hypersensitivity pneumonitis is unified as a disease more by the character of the immunologic response than by etiology or by clinical manifestations. A wide variety of clinical presentations may occur, but in general the disease presents in either acute or chronic form. The *acute form* follows inhalation of the antigenic dust in patients previously sensitized to the agent at work or at home. Symptoms include dyspnea, fever, cough, chills, malaise, and myalgia, characteristically four to six hours after exposure. Symptoms persist for up to 12 hours, but spontaneous recovery is the rule. Patients may be treated repetitively for a mistaken diagnosis of acute respiratory infection until the immunologic nature is recognized and the etiologic agent identified.

On physical examination, patients may appear dyspneic, toxic, and acutely ill with bibasilar end-inspiratory moist rales. The chest x-ray most often shows diffuse and nodular reticulations throughout the lung fields, most marked in the lower lung fields, looking very much like an interstitial pneumonia. Pleural effusion is not part of the syndrome. A leukocytosis up to 25,000 cells may occur with a marked shift to the left and occasionally eosinophilia. Pulmonary function studies usually show an acute restrictive defect with a decrease in forced vital capacity and one second forced expiratory volume, but with little air flow obstruction. These signs appear four to six hours after exposure and may be accompanied by mild hypoxemia, hypocapnia, and decrease in pulmonary compliance.

Another type of response follows a two-stage course, with an immediate asthmatic type reaction with decrease in forced vital capacity and forced expiratory volume as well as expiratory flow rates. This pattern is then followed in four to six hours by the restrictive response described above.

The *chronic form* of disease is not accompanied by acute respiratory symptoms and presents with signs of respiratory failure, including dyspnea and cyanosis, fixed restrictive ventilatory impairment with decrease in total lung capacity and vital capacity, marked decline in diffusing capacity, and noncompliant lungs. However, in some of the chronic advanced forms of hypersensitivity pneumonitis, elevated residual volume and diminished respiratory flow rates with loss of pulmonary elasticity suggestive of emphysema are found.

DIAGNOSIS. The diagnosis of hypersensitivity pneumonitis used to depend on pathologic examination of lung tissue obtained by biopsy. However, recent advances in understanding the immunologic pathogenesis of the disease now make it possible to achieve the diagnosis in most cases on the basis of historical, radiographic, and immunologic features. A careful history reveals the relationship of the symptoms to the suspect exposure as part of an occupational or home environment. The radiograph reveals the characteristic reticulonodular interstitial infiltrations of either acute inflammatory disease or advanced fibrosis. Careful culture for environmental agents found in the suspect moldy vegetation, such as hay, or in dusts or contaminated liquids, such as in humidifiers, reveals the antigen. Subsequent exposure of the antigen to the serum from the patient may reveal the diagnostic precipitin lines. The diagnostic loop is completed on occasion by careful inhalation challenge of the patient with the suspect antigen in a laboratory setting, or to the suspect work or home environment such as barnyard or coop. After exposure the patient is carefully observed for 12 to 24 hours with blood pressure, temperature, white blood count, and pulmonary function studies. A characteristic decline in vital capacity and forced expiratory volume and sometimes an elevated temperature and leukocyte count occur at four to six hours following the exposure. These laboratory abnormalities, even in the absence of acute symptoms, in response to exposure to the agent and the finding of precipitins in the blood are considered diagnostic.

TREATMENT. Treatment with corticosteroids is indicated when acute symptoms fail to respond within 12

to 24 hours of observation, when symptoms are extreme and there is hypoxemia, or when an extensive exposure has occurred over a fairly long period of time. Corticosteroid treatment is provided to determine whether the fibrotic reaction is reversible. Steroid treatment should be followed with repeat studies of radiographic appearance and pulmonary function changes to determine the extent of response to treatment.

PREVENTION. Hypersensitivity pneumonitis is completely preventable by avoidance of exposure to the etiologic antigen. The principal deficiency in clinical management of this disease is failure to recognize the nature of the hypersensitivity process or to discern the etiologic antigen by careful historical assessment and by environmental analysis. The diagnosis made in the clinic or hospital should be the beginning of a systematic search of the patient's environment with either elimination of the offending agent, such as by the burning of moldy hay, or by engineering the work environment so that the patient no longer becomes exposed to an antigen, even when it is almost impossible to remove it from the work environment. For example, great advances have been made in the dairy industry in the designing of barns and the feeding process such that minimal or no exposure to the offending antigen takes place. At the very least, a person who is not sensitive to the antigen should substitute at the work step where exposure occurs. Careful attention to these aspects of the work environment rather than callously ordering the patient to give up his occupation will usually permit the patient to maintain his livelihood without undue hazard to his health.

PROGNOSIS. The prognosis for the acute disease is excellent provided that repetitive exposure to the offending antigen is avoided. Prognosis in the chronic fibrotic form is poor as far as reversal of pulmonary dysfunction is concerned, but good in terms of progression of the disease if further exposure is avoided. Corticosteroid treatment is generally not effective in improving pulmonary function in the chronic and fibrotic form of the disorder. Thus long-term prevention depends principally on alertness to the acute immunologic cause of diffuse infiltrative lung disease which might otherwise be mistaken for an acute pulmonary infection or, in a chronic form, for idiopathic pulmonary fibrosis.

Fink, J. N.: Hypersensitivity pneumonitis. *In* Kirkpatrick, C. H., and Reynolds, H. Y. (eds.): Immunologic and Infectious Reactions in the Lung, Volume 1. New York, Marcel Dekker, Inc., 1976, p. 229.
Kilburn, K. (ed.): International conference on pulmonary reactions to organic materials. Ann. N. Y. Acad. Sci., Vol. 221, 1972.
Richardson, H. B.: Allergic alveolar diseases. Problems in diagnosis and management. Postgrad. Med., 60:121, 1976.

346.4. PULMONARY VASCULITIS AND GRANULOMATOUS VASCULITIS (INCLUDING WEGENER'S GRANULOMATOSIS)

DEFINITION AND CLINICAL MANIFESTATIONS. Pulmonary vasculitis and granulomatous vasculitis are characteristic tissue reactions common to a broad group of systemic diseases that may also affect the lung and to a few diseases which primarily involve the lung. The pathologic entities usually require tissue diagnosis either by biopsy of the parenchymal lung tissue or by presumptive diagnosis through biopsy of other tissues, such as skin, muscle, or kidney, in the case of systemic disorders. Pulmonary vasculitis is associated with disseminated vasculitis in systemic lupus erythematosus and other collagen vascular diseases, in some of the drug-induced hypersensitivity states, in rheumatoid arthritis with vasculitis, in serum sickness, and potentially in any disorder in which disseminated vasculitis occurs. The pulmonary reaction may be an incidental or prominent part of this systemic disorder.

Pulmonary granulomatous vasculitis is characterized by granuloma formation in addition to the vascular inflammation. Diseases with this pathology primarily involve the lung, although reactions in other tissues, particularly the kidney, may be found. *Wegener's granulomatosis* is perhaps the best known of these diseases and is characterized by the triad of necrotizing granulomatous vasculitis of the upper and lower respiratory tracts, focal glomerulitis and glomerulonephritis, and a greater or lesser degree of disseminated vasculitis. Involvement of the upper respiratory tract may be manifested by mucosal ulcerations of the nose and by chronic and recurrent infections of the sinuses and middle ear. The renal involvement, when present, represents the most serious threat to life because of progressive renal failure (see Ch. 68 and 374.4). For this reason, the renal tract should always be carefully assessed and treatment modified accordingly. Carrington and Liebow have described a limited form of Wegener's granulomatosis which spares the kidney.

The pulmonary lesions may be asymptomatic, but more usually involve cough, hemoptysis, pleuritic pain, and sometimes neurologic symptoms associated with central nervous system involvement. The radiographs are frequently characteristic, showing solitary or multiple nodular densities resembling localized areas of pneumonia, with secondary cavitation in necrotic centers a common sequel. The nodules may be solitary or multiple, varying in size from 1 to several centimeters and may be unilateral or bilateral. The lack of mediastinal lymph node enlargement as well as the cavitation helps distinguish these lesions from acute sarcoidosis, although definitive diagnosis usually requires obtaining tissue by biopsy of the lung or, in the case of upper respiratory tract or renal involvement, tissue from those organs, respectively.

Less common forms of pulmonary granulomatous vasculitis are allergic granulomatosis with vascular necrosis involving the lungs, heart, skin, and nervous system in patients with an allergic background, and lymphomatoid granulomatosis in which a proliferative lymphoreticular disease is associated with necrotizing granulomatous vasculitis involving predominantly the lungs.

PATHOGENESIS. The mechanism of the vasculitis is thought to involve the deposition of circulating immune complexes (Type III allergic reaction) or the Type IV reaction caused by antigen reacting with sensitized lymphocytes, with the release of lymphokines and other mediators of inflammation in and around the blood vessels. Deposition of immune complex has been demonstrated in systemic lupus erythematosus, serum sickness, and rheumatoid arthritis, as well as in periarteritis nodosa. In these diseases, the predominant manifestations are those of the systemic disorder. Granulomatous arteritis and tissue and blood eosinophilia may follow a respiratory illness and lead to periarteritis nodosa, presumably because of a hypersensitivity state to

some agent initiating the respiratory illness. Asthma is usually not found in this type of periarteritis nodosa. Drugs such as sulfonamides, penicillin, busulfan, and others may induce vasculitis as part of a serum sickness–like syndrome, whereas the prolonged administration of hydralazine and procainamide has been associated with a lupus-like syndrome with small vessel periarteritis and vasculitis.

TREATMENT. Corticosteroid therapy is the treatment of choice for pulmonary vasculitis other than in Wegener's granulomatosis. When pulmonary vasculitis is associated with systemic disease, as in lupus erythematosus or rheumatoid arthritis, the treatment is generally governed by the systemic factors. In serum sickness and drug-induced hypersensitivity states, discontinuation of exposure to the agent will usually result in a clearing of the signs of the disease. However, a brief course of corticosteroid therapy is probably effective in reducing the inflammatory responses to the mediators released by the immunologic reactions and also in diminishing the release of proteolytic lysosomal enzymes by the stabilization of lysosomal membranes. Corticosteroids may also affect the immunologic process by suppressing the blastogenic lymphocyte response to mitogens.

Wegener's granulomatosis is the one disease in this group that has been determined to show an excellent response to the cytotoxic agents, particularly cyclophosphamide or azathioprine. Presumably these agents are effective through suppression of the production and proliferation of the lymphocytes which mediate the disease. Treatment with these agents is associated with lymphocytopenia, with a greater suppression of bursa-equivalent than of thymus-derived lymphocytes, a decrease of elevated serum immunoglobulin levels to normal, suppression of primary induction of delayed hypersensitivity in antibody responses to new foreign antigens, and decreased in vitro lymphocyte blastogenic response to certain antigens, but with intact mitogen-induced in vitro lymphocyte blastogenic response.

Fauci, A. S.: Pulmonary vasculitis. *In* Kirkpatrick, C. H., and Reynolds, H. Y. (eds.): Immunologic and Infectious Reactions in the Lung, Volume 1. New York, Marcel Dekker, Inc., 1976, p. 243.

346.5. THE CONNECTIVE TISSUE DISORDERS

Although recognized and characterized primarily by their systemic manifestations, connective tissue diseases frequently show significant and often serious manifestations in the lungs. Indeed, pulmonary infiltration, pleuritis, and pleural effusion may be the earliest sign of the systemic connective tissue disorders. In addition to direct involvement in the connective tissue disease process, the lungs show increased susceptibility to pulmonary infection, so that a significant proportion of the pulmonary infiltrates call for treatment with antibiotic agents. Although the systemic connective tissue disorders may show nonspecific (or noncharacteristic) pathologic change such as vasculitis, the major diseases — systemic lupus erythematosus, rheumatoid arthritis, polymyositis-dermatomyositis, and scleroderma — can be recognized as distinct entities through their pulmonary manifestations. More general descriptions of these diseases are found in Ch. 50, 51, 52, and 56.

SYSTEMIC LUPUS ERYTHEMATOSUS

Pulmonary involvement in systemic lupus erythematosus (SLE) occurs in more than 50 per cent of patients. It is characterized radiographically by serosal as well as parenchymal changes. Serositis is manifested by cardiac enlargement, pericardial effusion, and pleuritis with or without effusion. The effusions are usually small, are frequently bilateral, are exudative in character, and may show LE cells. Pulmonary infiltrates most frequently involve the lung bases, are patchy, interstitial and migratory in nature, and are caused by infection, vasculitis, or interstitial pneumonitis. These parenchymal abnormalities produce the characteristic pulmonary functional abnormalities of volume restriction, impairment of diffusing capacity, and arterial hypoxemia, with the usual symptoms of cough and dyspnea.

Treatment should be governed by the systemic manifestations of the disease, and usually includes corticosteroids.

RHEUMATOID ARTHRITIS

Pulmonary involvement is a frequent and often unsuspected manifestation of rheumatoid arthritis, giving rise to pleuritis with or without effusion, diffuse interstitial pneumonitis, rheumatoid nodules often associated with dust exposure or pneumoconiosis as in *Caplan's syndrome,* and vasculitis with pulmonary hypertension. Pleural disease is probably the most common pulmonary manifestation of rheumatoid arthritis, occurs primarily in males, may precede or follow the onset of joint involvement, and may result in empyema and fibrothorax. The pleural fluid is an exudate, but its characteristically low glucose level (less than 30 mg per cent) is virtually diagnostic if tuberculous and malignant effusion can be excluded. This finding is useful in distinguishing rheumatoid from other causes of effusion and in indicating the likely cause of associated infiltrative or nodular disease in the lungs.

The fibrosing alveolitis found in rheumatoid arthritis is nondistinctive but may be diagnosed by the associated findings indicated above and by the serologic finding of rheumatoid factor. The pulmonary disease may precede or complicate joint manifestations. Whereas overt radiologic interstitial fibrosis is relatively uncommon in rheumatoid arthritis, evidence of parenchymal disease is more commonly found by pulmonary function studies, the characteristic findings being restrictive ventilatory impairment, reduced diffusing capacity, and hypoxemia.

The nodular form of rheumatoid pulmonary disease is more characteristic than the interstitial form. These nodules occur more frequently in men than in women and may be associated with occupational exposures such as coal mining, sandblasting, asbestos work, pottery, boiler scaling, and brass and iron work. Radiographically, the lesions are single or multiple, may develop rapidly, are characteristically rounded and sharply circumscribed, and may undergo cavitation. These radiographic changes may appear prior to the onset of joint disease and may be diagnosed clinically by lung biopsy and by association with high titers of rheumatoid factor. Patients with rheumatoid lung disease may show enhanced susceptibility to infection,

which should systematically be excluded when new symptoms and infiltrates appear.

DIFFUSE SYSTEMIC SCLEROSIS
(Scleroderma)

Scleroderma is a connective tissue disease primarily of females in the middle years, and is characterized by atrophic sclerosis of the skin, musculoskeletal system, heart, lungs, kidneys, and gastrointestinal tract. Involvement of the skin, esophagus, and lungs often presents a triad, and the presence of pulmonary fibrosis, vascular disease, or pleuritis occurs in over 80 per cent of the patients. Manifestations include cough and dyspnea, signs of hypoxemia, interstitial fibrosis, and, later, cor pulmonale. Progressive fibrosis with cystic changes, pulmonary calcifications, pleural effusion and pleural thickening, and enhanced pulmonary vascular markings and hypertension are other evidences of the progressive pulmonary disorder. Pulmonary function studies show reduction of pulmonary volumes, diffusing capacity, and lung compliance. Pathologic study of lung biopsy and postmortem material has shown the abnormality much more frequently than expected, with histopathologic findings focused principally in the blood vessels, which show marked intimal thickening with loose myxomatous connective tissue in the small pulmonary arteries and arterioles.

POLYMYOSITIS AND DERMATOMYOSITIS

Polymyositis and dermatomyositis, which are systemic diseases primarily affecting striated muscle, also affect the lungs, with interstitial pneumonitis and pneumonia. The pneumonia is a secondary complication of aspiration and hypostasis related to atrophy and weakening of chest wall muscles, with impairment of ventilation and cough. However, primary interstitial pneumonitis does occur in a small percentage of patients with these diseases, either in acute form or with gradual onset of dyspnea, cough, and diffuse pulmonary infiltrate. The histopathology is noncharacteristic, showing the changes of idiopathic fibrosing alveolitis with arteriolitis. There may be some improvement with corticosteroid therapy.

Matthay, R. A., et al.: Pulmonary manifestations of systemic lupus erythematosus: Review of twelve cases of acute lupus pneumonitis. Medicine, 54:397, 1975.

Matthay, R. A., Schwarz, M. I., and Petty, T. L.: Pleuro-pulmonary manifestations of connective tissue diseases. Clin. Notes Respir. Dis., 16:3, 1977.

346.6.   DRUG-INDUCED REACTIONS

DEFINITION. Among the many adverse reactions to drugs is allergy or hypersensitivity. This is thought to account for only 25 per cent of all drug-induced disease, and therefore other types of adverse reactions should be ruled out. Specific evidence of allergy or hypersensitivity, such as that established by laboratory immunologic investigation, should be obtained whenever possible to implicate that mechanism as responsible for the pathogenesis of the observed disease.

PATHOGENESIS.   In order to induce immune response

TABLE 3. Drugs that Produce Pulmonary Disease Possibly Through a Hypersensitivity Mechanism

Antibiotics
  Nitrofurantoin
  Sulfonamides
  Penicillin
Chemotherapeutic agents
  Busulfan, cyclophosphamide
  Methotrexate
  Bleomycin
  Procarbazine
  Melphalan
Analgesics, neuroactive and vasoactive agents
  Heroin
  Hexamethonium
  Methadone
  Methysergide
  Propoxyphene
Miscellaneous
  Blood
  Chlordiazepoxide
  Drugs that induce systemic lupus erythematosus
  Hydrochlorothiazide
  Pituitary snuff

and hypersensitivity reactions, a drug must first bind irreversibly to tissue macromolecules by covalent bonding. It thus serves as a hapten against which the antigenic determination is made. Hypersensitivity to drug reactions may occur as anaphylactic, cytotoxic, Arthus, or delayed hypersensitivity reactions. At least the last three, and probably all types, can be associated with acute or chronic diffuse pulmonary infiltration.

ETIOLOGY. A vast number of drugs are potentially associated with pulmonary hypersensitivity reactions, as listed in Table 3.

Nitrofurantoin. Probably the most commonly reported drug associated with diffuse infiltrative pulmonary disease is nitrofurantoin, a drug used over long periods of time as an antibacterial agent in the urine. The disease can occur in acute form with fever, cough, and pulmonary infiltrates, and it may be associated with pulmonary infiltration with eosinophilia; it is presumably of the Type II or Type III immune reaction. The reaction can begin within hours or days of beginning treatment, and a chest roentgenogram may have the appearance of noncardiac pulmonary edema. Eosinophilia and bronchospasm can occur, or even anaphylactic reaction, but remission occurs within 24 to 48 hours after the drug is discontinued. A positive response can be elicited by a small rechallenge dose.

Chronic disease associated with nitrofurantoin ingestion develops insidiously as cough and dyspnea over months to years after initiation of nitrofurantoin therapy. The disease is much like other forms of pulmonary fibrosis radiographically, functionally, and histopathologically. Diagnosis is made by history of drug ingestion and compatible histopathology by lung biopsy. Therapy is discontinuation of the drug and use of corticosteroids.

Busulfan, Cyclophosphamide, Methotrexate, and Methysergide. A very different histopathology is seen in the interstitial pneumonitis and fibrosis associated with busulfan and cyclophosphamide ingestion. Cough, dyspnea, and fever develop subacutely three to four years after starting the treatment. The pulmonary infiltrate may be interpreted as an opportunistic infection or a neoplastic infiltration. Lung biopsy shows a bizarre hyperplastic reaction of Type II alveolar cells

that appear almost neoplastic. Corticosteroids are of little benefit, and the patient usually dies even though the drug is discontinued. A similar disease without the atypical Type II cells can be produced by methotrexate. Methysergide, on the other hand, produces a fibrotic lung and pleural fibrosis.

Drug-Induced Systemic Lupus Erythematosus (SLE). A variety of drugs may be followed by diffuse pulmonary infiltration with pleuropulmonary reactions and laboratory findings of systemic lupus erythematosus. These drugs are listed in Table 4. Drug-induced SLE shows less renal and cutaneous reaction and more pleuropulmonary disease than spontaneous SLE. The reaction appears to be dose related and may simply represent an unmasking of a pre-existing propensity to SLE.

DIAGNOSIS. The x-ray and the laboratory offer little help in the diagnosis of diffuse infiltrative diseases of the lung induced by drug ingestion. In vitro detection of drug-induced antibodies is possible through physical, chemical, serologic, and in vitro live cell tests, but these are not generally available or useful clinically. The diagnosis depends almost entirely on physician awareness of the possibility of drug-induced diffuse infiltrative disease, careful elicitation of history, or, on occasion, the contribution of an alert pharmacist. Specific inquiry must be made into the drugs that may account for the clinical picture, for many individuals fail to recognize that a drug which they have taken routinely and for years, such as nitrofurantoin, is in fact a drug at all. Of course, all patients should be carefully questioned as to previous drug reactions, because the predisposition to drug reactions and hypersensitivity may indicate the possibility of cross-reactions, and such a patient is at a greater risk than one with no prior history. Rechallenge or provocative test is the most definitive method of diagnosing the drug-related nature of the patient's disease. This procedure, however, should be reserved for situations in which the drug is required as a therapeutic agent, because it is dangerous and may give rise to serious anaphylactic, inflammatory, or pancytopenic hypersensitivity reactions.

TREATMENT AND PREVENTION. Treatment consists of withdrawal of the drug, suppression of inflammatory or

TABLE 4. Drugs Thought to Induce Systemic Lupus Erythematosus*

Definite	Reported
Chlorpromazine	Aminosalicylic acid
Diphenylhydantoin	Digitalis
Ethosuximide	Gold
Hydralazine	Griseofulvin
Isoniazid	Guanoxan
Mephenytoin	Isoquinazepon
Phenobarbital	Methyldopa
Primidone	Methylthiouracil
Procainamide	Oral contraceptives
Trimethadione	Penicillamine
	Penicillin
	Phenylbutazone
	Practolol
	Propylthiouracil
	Reserpine
	Streptomycin
	Sulfonamides
	Tetracycline
	Thiazides

*Adapted from Schwarz, J. A. Von: Arzneim-Forsch./Drug Res., 27:1856, 1977.

anaphylactic reactions with corticosteroids or sympathomimetic amines, and other supportive measures as indicated. Preventive measures are most important, for legal as well as for medical reasons. Patient education as to the cause of illness and risks of re-exposure to the same or related drug and potential for cross-reactions with other drugs should be assiduously carried out. As always, thorough record keeping is mandatory, along with a mechanism available to alert others in the health care system to the risks of a patient's drug hypersensitivity. The use of Medic-Alert tags or bracelet or wallet cards and the availability of integrated computerized records, are recent and valuable approaches to prevention of recurrent episodes.

Bone, R. C., et al.: Desquamative interstitial pneumonia following chronic nitrofurantoin therapy. Chest, 69(2 Suppl.):286, 1976.

Gould, V. E., et al.: Sclerosing alveolitis induced by cyclophosphamide. Ultrastructural observations on alveolar injury and repair. Am. J. Pathol., 81:513, 1975.

Lundgren, R., et al.: Pulmonary lesions and autoimmune reactions after long-term nitrofurantoin treatment. Scand. J. Respir. Dis., 56:208, 1975.

Petty, T. L.: Editorial: What else can injure the lungs? N. Engl. J. Med., 294:954, 1976.

Rosenow, E. C., III: Drug-induced hypersensitivity disease of the lung. In Kirkpatrick, C. H., and Reynolds, H. Y. (eds.): Immunologic and Infectious Reactions in the Lung, Volume 1. New York, Marcel Dekker, Inc., 1976, p. 261.

346.7. INFILTRATIVE DISEASES ASSOCIATED WITH CAPILLARY BLEEDING

GOODPASTURE'S SYNDROME

Goodpasture's syndrome can now be considered a distinctive disease entity, characterized clinically by hemoptysis, pulmonary infiltrates, and hematuria. The glomerulonephritis and pulmonary hemorrhage are caused by complement-mediated damage to pulmonary and renal tissue produced when autoantibodies react with glomerular and alveolar basement membranes. Although the etiologic agent (or agents) is unknown, the immune reactions are probably triggered by an inhaled antigen or infectious agent. Progressive glomerulonephritis with proteinuria, hematuria, and renal insufficiency is punctuated with frequent episodes of hemoptysis, bilateral pulmonary infiltrates, and dyspnea. The clinical course is one of progressive renal failure, although cases of spontaneous resolution have been reported. Approaches to treatment have included corticosteroids, immunosuppressive therapy, and nephrectomy. The diagnosis is suspected by the clinical and laboratory findings, and substantiated by kidney or lung biopsies showing antglomerular or pulmonary capillary basement membrane antibody. This syndrome is also described in Ch. 374.4.

From the renal standpoint, the disease must be distinguished from Wegener's granulomatosis, acute glomerulonephritis, or other forms of glomerulonephritis or renal vein thrombosis. From the pulmonary standpoint, the disease must be distinguished from viral or bacterial pneumonia, allergic alveolitis, pulmonary edema, and other forms of pulmonary vasculitis. Goodpasture's disease is distinguished by the episodic nature of hemoptysis and dyspnea, the rapid resolution of the pulmonary infiltrates, the appearance of hemosiderin-laden macrophages in the sputum, hypochromic anemia and iron deficiency responding to iron therapy, the circulating anti-glomerular basement membrane antibody, the evidence of glomerulonephritis with microhematuria and red blood cell casts, and positive tissue immunofluorescence tests for anti-basement membrane IgG. Episodes of hemoptysis may vary from microscopic evidence only to massive hemoptysis with death from exsanguination or asphyxia. Treatment with prednisone is indicated because of the anti-inflammatory effect of this agent, with immunosuppressive agents such as cyclophosphamide to suppress immunoglobulin and cell-mediated immune reactions, and, in rare instances, with nephrectomy, presumably to remove the offending antigen.

IDIOPATHIC PULMONARY HEMOSIDEROSIS

Idiopathic pulmonary hemosiderosis is a disease entity of children and young adults characterized by cough, dyspnea, fatigue, pulmonary infiltrates, and microcytic hypochromic anemia with iron deficiency, progressing to pulmonary fibrosis. Although hemoptysis is occasionally manifested, the disease is characterized more by the symptoms of the anemia and the associated acute or chronic pulmonary infiltrates. Pathologic examination shows pulmonary inflammation and fibrosis with large numbers of hemosiderin-filled pulmonary macrophages with associated hematologic findings of hypochromia and deficiency of iron stores in the bone marrow. It appears that the cause of the disease is unknown. The pathogenesis is characterized by chronic and recurrent extravasation of blood into the pulmonary tissues, with subsequent low-grade inflammation and fibrosis and phagocytosis of blood elements, with permanent storage of the hemosiderin pigment isolated in the macrophages. The clinical characteristics, the nonspecificity of the pathology, and the absence of immunologic involvement are the keys to diagnosis.

The disease is distinguished from other forms of pulmonary interstitial disease by the evidence of the anemia and the large amounts of iron stored in the tissues. It is distinguished from Goodpasture's syndrome by absence of glomerulonephritis and anti-basement membrane autoantibodies. Suspicion of the disease should prompt examination of sputum with iron stains for hemosiderin; this finding indicates only that bleeding has occurred in the lung, but does not indicate the cause. The chronicity of the condition, the degree of pulmonary fibrosis, and the anemia without other apparent cause for blood loss should lead to a pulmonary biopsy to confirm the diagnosis. Also in the differential diagnosis is the chronic hemorrhage and pulmonary fibrosis associated with mitral stenosis, which may be similar pathologically to idiopathic pulmonary hemosiderosis. Other forms of chronic cardiac failure may produce a similar pathologic picture, although generally less severe, with clinical attention more appropriately focused on the cardiac disease. The disease must also be distinguished from other forms of pulmonary vasculitis and pulmonary manifestations of systemic connective tissue disease; again, these are more likely to show extrapulmonary manifestations with less predominance of blood loss anemia.

Benoit, F. L., et al.: Goodpasture's syndrome: A clinicopathologic entity. Am. J. Med., 37:424, 1964.

Dolan, C. J., Jr., et al.: Idiopathic pulmonary hemosiderosis. Electron microscopic, immunofluorescent, and iron kinetic studies. Chest, 68:577, 1975.

Donald, K. J., et al.: Alveolar capillary basement membrane lesions in Goodpasture's syndrome and idiopathic pulmonary hemosiderosis. Am. J. Med., 59:642, 1975.

Everett, D. E., et al.: Goodpasture's syndrome: Response to mercaptopurine and prednisone. JAMA, 214:1849, 1970.

Gonzalez-Crussi, F., et al.: Idiopathic pulmonary hemosiderosis: Evidence of capillary basement membrane abnormality. Am. Rev. Respir. Dis., 114:689, 1976.

Nowakowski, A., et al.: Goodpasture's syndrome: Recovery from severe pulmonary hemorrhage after bilateral nephrectomy. Ann. Intern. Med., 75:243, 1971.

Poskitt, T. R.: Immunologic and electron microscopic studies in Goodpasture's syndrome. Am. J. Med., 49:250, 1970.

Soergel, K. H., and Sommers, S. C.: Idiopathic pulmonary hemosiderosis and related syndromes. Am. J. Med., 32:499, 1962.

Wilson, C. B., and Smith, R. C.: Goodpasture's syndrome associated with influenza A2 virus infection. Ann. Intern. Med., 76:91, 1972.

346.8. SARCOIDOSIS

Sarcoidosis is "a disease characterized by the presence in all of several affected organs and tissues of non-caseating epithelioid cell granulomas proceeding either to resolution or to conversion into featureless hyaline connective tissue." The disease is usually systemic, affecting lungs, liver, spleen, eye, skin, and even heart. The systemic aspects of the disease are presented in Ch. 65; the disease is included here because it is commonly recognized first as a pulmonary disorder, characterized clinically by dyspnea, shortness of breath, and hypoxemia, and radiologically as a localized or diffuse pulmonary interstitial infiltration and/or characteristically enlarged "potato nodes" in the hilar regions.

DIAGNOSIS. The diagnosis of sarcoidosis depends on the accumulation of evidence that the symptoms and signs presented by the patient are related to a widespread noncaseating epithelioid cell granulomatosis with the clinical, immunologic, and pathologic characteristics associated with sarcoid. Diagnosis is strongly influenced by clinical and radiographic signs; by the age, sex, and race of the patient; by immunologic characteristics, including depressed cell-mediated immunity and reactivity to the Kveim antigen; and by characteristic histopathology. Lung biopsy is rarely needed, as histopathologic confirmation can be obtained by biopsy of lymph nodes, particularly of the mediastinum. Biopsy at the site of injection of the Kveim antigen in the presence of characteristic or concordant symptoms and signs and radiographic presentation is sufficient for diagnostic purposes.

In patients with pulmonary sarcoid, diagnostic work-up should include stains and cultures of respiratory tract secretions or washings and biopsy material for acid-fast bacilli, mycobacterial organisms, and fungi. There will occasionally be some confusion between mycobacterial disease and sarcoid when characteristics of both are present, particularly when acid-fast bacilli may be seen on smear in a case that is otherwise characteristic of sarcoid. It is more appropriate to refer to both possibilities in the diagnostic categorization than to eliminate either one prematurely. Particular difficulty arises if the evidence of sarcoidosis is limited only to the lung without evidence of granulomas in other organs, and if the Kveim test is negative or inconclusive. In such cases, greater reliance must be placed on clinical analysis and observation and on the biopsy of lymph nodes or lung tissue. Diagnosis should also consider other findings associated with systemic sarcoidosis such as erythema nodosum, bilateral hilar adenopathy, uveitis, or other signs of systemic sarcoidosis, such as hypercalcemia and hypercalciuria.

TREATMENT. Treatment of sarcoidosis is nonspecific, as no etiologic agent has been identified against which therapy may be directed. The use of corticosteroids in pulmonary sarcoidosis is governed by evidence of active and progressive deterioration of pulmonary function rather than by the appearance of the chest x-ray. Indeed, the chest radiograph may look severely abnormal in acute inflammatory sarcoidosis, which may turn out to be self-limited with spontaneous resolution. Although clinical signs such as breathlessness may be used as guides, the best index is a measure of gas transfer such as the single breath diffusing capacity. Although measurements of arterial blood oxygen tension or pulmonary vital capacity will similarly reflect interference of pulmonary function, the single breath diffusing capacity, when measured serially, is a more useful guide to the activity of the disease and the response to corticosteroid therapy.

Initial treatment is with relatively large doses of corticosteroids (e.g., 40 to 60 mg of prednisone), continued until maximal improvement of pulmonary function is observed on sequential studies. At this point, the dose can be reduced slowly to the smallest dose that maintains the level of improvement. Treatment should be continued for six to twelve months, at which time there should be further gradual reduction of the dose, accompanied by careful observation of symptoms, radiographic appearance, and tests of pulmonary function. It is not uncommon for the inflammatory process to recur, even six to twelve months after initiation of corticosteroids, and indeed the flare-up may be more difficult to control than the original process. In the event of recrudescence, the steroid dose should be increased once again as in the original treatment schedule. It should be remembered that the majority of sarcoid cases require no treatment, even though radiographic findings may be substantial in the early phases. The tendency of the disease to recur when steroids are withdrawn, the limited evidence that steroid therapy of even long-term duration affects the fibrotic course of disease, the common finding that steroid treatment may require continuation for years, and the serious complications of long-term steroid therapy should temper the physician's decision to treat acute sarcoidosis automatically at the time of diagnosis. Indeed, it is better to follow the patient for several weeks or months to determine the natural course of the disease, whether self-limited or progressive, before commencing a long and potentially hazardous course of corticosteroid therapy.

Baum, G. L., Schwarz, J., and Barlow, P. B.: Sarcoidosis and specific etiologic agents: A continuing enigma. Chest, 63:488, 1973.

Editorial: Diagnosis of pulmonary sarcoidosis. Br. Med. J., 4:540, 1975.

Hirsch, J. G., Nelson, C. J., and Siltzbach, L. E.: The Kveim test. N. Engl. J. Med., 284:1327, 1971.

Israel, H. L.: Sarcoidosis. Postgrad. Med. J., 46:524, 1970.

Israel, H. L., Fouts, D. W., and Beggs, R. A.: A controlled trial of prednisone treatment of sarcoidosis. Am. Rev. Respir. Dis., 107:609, 1973.

Mitchell, D. N., and Scadding, J. G.: Sarcoidosis. In Murray, J. F. (ed.): Lung Diseases: State of the Art, 1974-75. New York, American Lung Association, 1976.

Siltzbach, L. E. (ed.): Seventh international conference on sarcoidosis. Ann. N. Y. Acad. Sci., Vol. 278, 1976.

346.9. MISCELLANEOUS INFILTRATIVE DISEASES

PULMONARY ALVEOLAR PROTEINOSIS

DEFINITION, ETIOLOGY, AND PATHOGENESIS. Pulmonary alveolar proteinosis, a disease of unknown cause and pathogenesis, is characterized by chronic and progressive filling of the alveoli with a proteinaceous, lipid-rich, granular material thought to represent surfactant and cellular debris. The disease is often found on a background of acute or chronic exposure to inhaled dusts or chemicals, and some have thought there to be an immunologic abnormality. Because of the diversity of preceding history, pulmonary alveolar proteinosis is thought to be a pattern of pulmonary response to a variety of environmental agents.

CLINICAL MANIFESTATIONS. The diagnosis may be suspected when there are progressive dyspnea and hypoxemia, with scanty sputum, x-ray infiltrates of a characteristic ground-glass appearance involving first the lower lung fields and later the upper lung fields, and pulmonary function tests showing ventilatory restriction, reduction in lung volumes, and hypoxemia. Arterial oxygen desaturation may be severe, with arterial blood oxygen tensions as low as 28 to 33 mm Hg in ambulatory patients with this disorder. Nevertheless, definitive diagnosis is usually made by lung biopsy. The histopathology shows essentially normal alveolar septal structure, with the alveolar spaces packed with eosinophilic, PAS-positive, proteinaceous, granular material rich in lipids. In the active phases of the disease, numerous macrophages may be seen, but few leukocytes or inflammatory cells are found. Recent electron microscopic studies of biopsies and bronchial washings in pulmonary alveolar proteinosis have demonstrated abundant annular inclusions in pulmonary alveolar macrophages, showing concentric layering of the bilamellar material characteristic of surfactant. The disease is thought to represent an accumulation of surfactant material due either to overproduction or decreased clearance, with secondary phagocytosis of the material by alveolar macrophages. Complicating infections may be a problem; for example, several cases have been reported in which nocardiosis developed.

DIAGNOSIS AND TREATMENT. Definitive diagnosis of the disease is important for two reasons: first, because blind steroid treatment renders the patient susceptible to secondary bacterial infection and produces no effect on the disease process; and second, because effective therapy can be rendered by the *technique of whole lung lavage* with massive volumes of balanced salt solution. The technique of large-volume lavage has been developed specifically for treatment of pulmonary alveolar proteinosis and involves careful volume-controlled inflow of fluid to minimize adverse effects on pulmonary blood flow. The course of the disease is highly variable; some patients show spontaneous resolution and some show resolution after lavage, but most patients will have a recurring accumulation of the material and a repeated need for lung lavage. Patients with an associated interstitial inflammatory process have in general a poorer prognosis than those in whom the alveolar septal structure is essentially normal. No preventive measures are known, except general measures to avoid inhaled dusts and chemical irritants.

EOSINOPHILIC GRANULOMA

Eosinophilic granuloma is a disease of unknown cause, found typically in young, adult, white males, either localized to the lung or presenting as a multifocal disease involving bone, brain, and endocrine organs as well as spleen, bone marrow, and lymph nodes. The pathologic lesion is one of granulomatous fibrosis, infiltration of histiocytes, macrophages, and eosinophils, and occasionally extensive endarteritis of the small blood vessels. The disease, when localized to the lung, presents with nonspecific symptoms of cough, shortness of breath, and weight loss, and x-ray findings of diffuse pulmonary infiltration or, in more severe cases, honeycomb lung. In multifocal disease symptoms of adrenal insufficiency, hypothyroidism, neurologic abnormalities, and diabetes insipidus may be found. The pulmonary disease is complicated by pneumothorax in about a quarter of the patients, and indeed some patients present with this complication.

The course is variable. In localized disease, it tends to be benign and may show spontaneous remission. Mortality is associated with extensive soft tissue involvement. In the progressive disease, treatment is not satisfactory and focuses on corticosteroids and immunosuppressive agents. Because of the granulomatous pathology and the response to corticosteroids and immunosuppressive agents, as well as abnormalities of delayed hypersensitivity and immunoglobulin levels, the disease is thought to have an immunologic mechanism and perhaps to reflect an immunologic response to an exogenous inhaled agent.

DESQUAMATIVE INTERSTITIAL PNEUMONITIS (DIP)

Desquamative interstitial pneumonitis, or DIP, is a disease of unknown cause but characteristic histopathology, consisting of the proliferation and desquamation into the alveolar spaces of Type II epithelial cells. The disease may be associated with a variety of environmental exposures to chemicals and dusts, and may be preceded by a history of respiratory infection, suggesting the possibility of viral involvement. Clinical, functional, and radiographic features do not distinguish it from other forms of diffuse infiltrative diseases of the lung, but diagnosis is important because the appropriate treatment is corticosteroids, to which this disease responds reasonably well. No other known therapy is available. Histopathology suggestive of DIP may be found simultaneously with areas that resemble pulmonary alveolar proteinosis and pulmonary fibrosis. These processes may be successive steps in the low grade inflammatory and fibrotic response of the lung to environmental agents. The factors that govern the appearance of one form or another are not understood.

USUAL INTERSTITIAL PNEUMONITIS (UIP)

Usual interstitial pneumonitis is a term coined to designate a fairly common and characteristic histopathologic picture in patients with clinical, functional, and radiographic evidence of diffuse infiltrative disease of the lung who have no identifiable environmental exposure, associated connective tissue disease, identifiable immunologic reaction, or other etiologic agent. Response to treatment with corticosteroids is variable.

LYMPHOID INTERSTITIAL PNEUMONITIS
(LIP)

This disorder is similar to UIP, except that the histopathology is characterized by an extensive infiltration with lymphocytic cells and a tendency to be associated with the later appearance of diffuse lymphoma.

INFILTRATIVE DISEASE CAUSED BY PHYSICAL AND CHEMICAL AGENTS

Diffuse infiltrative and fibrotic diseases of the lung that are caused by identifiable physical or chemical agents such as inorganic dusts, industrial chemicals, or exposure to ionizing radiation are covered more extensively in Ch. 348, but are included here because of the importance of the differential diagnosis in considering the preceding diseases. Although some of these exposures produce a rather characteristic radiographic picture and histopathology, more frequently the x-ray is indistinguishable from those of other diseases in this group and the diagnosis is made by the historical association with an environmental or occupational exposure, or by a previous history of radiotherapy for lung cancer or pulmonary lymphoma. Diseases in this category do not usually call for lung biopsy when an adequate explanation for the changes can be found by historical evidence of exposure. For this reason, a careful and exhaustive occupational and environmental history is extremely important in all cases of diffuse infiltrative lung disease so that an agent can be implicated when present, the patient removed from exposure, and unnecessary lung biopsy avoided.

OTHER CAUSES OF INFILTRATIVE LUNG DISEASE

Diffuse infiltrative pulmonary disease can be a manifestation of a variety of other disorders: viral and bacterial infections; mycotic pneumonitis; rickettsial infection (psittacosis); gastric acid aspiration; cardiogenic pulmonary congestion and edema related to mitral stenosis or left ventricular failure, or to fluid overload; parasitic infestations; pneumonia caused by *Pneumocystis carinii*; diffuse pulmonary calcifications known as pulmonary alveolar microlithiasis; blood-borne anaerobic infection; septic emboli; the early stages of adult respiratory distress syndrome, occurring postoperatively or related to trauma and pulmonary contusion; kerosene or gasoline ingestion; and metabolic infiltrates associated with uremia, myxedema, and acute hypervolemia. This list is included to alert the physician to the wide range of agents and conditions which can induce diffuse interstitial pulmonary infiltrations and to encourage the student of disease to look more intensively to the lungs not only to recognize and resolve diseases of that organ, but to gain clues and insight into systemic disorders and diseases of other organs as well.

Costello, J. F., et al.: Diagnosis and management of pulmonary alveolar proteinosis: The role of electron microscopy. Thorax, 30:121, 1975.

Rogers, R. M., et al.: Hemodynamic response of the pulmonary circulation to bronchopulmonary lavage in man. N. Engl. J. Med., 286:1230, 1972.
Villar, T. G., Avila, R., and Marques, R. A.: Eosinophilic granuloma of the lung and the extrinsic pulmonary granulomatoses. Ann. N.Y. Acad. Sci., 278:612, 1976.
Zinkham, W. H.: Multifocal eosinophilic granuloma: Natural history, etiology, and management. Am. J. Med., 60:457, 1976.

347. LUNG ABSCESS AND BRONCHIECTASIS

Sydney M. Finegold

347.1. LUNG ABSCESS

DEFINITION. Lung abscess is a suppurative pulmonary infection producing destruction of lung parenchyma with the formation of a cavity with an air-fluid level. Some workers describe a similar process with multiple cavitations each less than 2 cm in diameter as necrotizing pneumonia. The distinction is arbitrary; they are different expressions of the same pathologic process.

ETIOLOGY. By far the most important background factor for abscess of the lung or necrotizing pneumonia is aspiration, usually related to altered consciousness. Common causes of altered consciousness in such patients are alcoholism, cerebral vascular accident, general anesthesia, drug overdose or addiction, seizure disorder, diabetic coma, shock, and other serious illness. Other factors in aspiration include dysphagia caused by either esophageal disease or neurologic disease, intestinal obstruction, and tonsillectomy or tooth extraction. Next to aspiration, the most important factor predisposing to lung abscess or necrotizing pneumonia is periodontal disease or gingivitis. Lung abscess is rare in an edentulous person and suggests the possibility of an associated bronchogenic carcinoma. Other underlying processes include bronchiectasis and secondary infection of a bland pulmonary embolus with infarction. Anaerobic bacteria are the primary organisms recovered. About 60 per cent of cases have only anaerobic bacteria as etiologic agents, with the majority of the balance having both anaerobes and facultative or aerobic forms recovered concurrently. There is generally an average of three organisms per case. The predominant anaerobes recovered are *Fusobacterium nucleatum*, *Bacteroides melaninogenicus*, *Peptostreptococcus*, *Peptococcus*, and microaerophilic streptococci. *Bacteroides fragilis* and *Fusobacterium necrophorum* may also be found. The predominant nonanaerobes recovered are streptococci of various types. Actually, the microaerophilic streptococci produce lactic acid as the major end-product of fermentation and therefore officially belong in the genus *Streptococcus*. However, anaerobic techniques are usually required for their isolation and characterization so that most workers continue to consider them along with the anaerobes.

Pneumonia, particularly that caused by *Staphylococcus aureus*, *Klebsiella pneumoniae*, and *Streptococcus pyogenes*, may be complicated by abscess formation. Pneumococcal pneumonia is rarely or never associated with abscess formation unless other organisms are involved in the infectious process with the pneumococci. *Pseudomonas aeruginosa* may cause necrotizing pneumonia but seldom causes lung abscess per se. Uncommon causes of lung abscess are actinomycosis, glanders, and melioidosis. Patients with impaired host defense mechanisms, particularly patients receiving high doses of corticosteroids or chemotherapy for malignancy, are predisposed to necrotizing pneumonia and lung abscess. An important cause in this group, although it may occur in the absence of such background factors as well, is *Nocardia asteroides.*

Bronchial obstruction may lead to lung abscess. Most often the obstructing lesion is a bronchogenic carcinoma, but it may be a foreign body or an enlarged mediastinal lymph node. Carcinoma of the esophagus may also be complicated by lung abscess, most often on an aspiration basis.

Metastatic lung abscess may occur, usually as a result of septic emboli from right-sided bacterial endocarditis (*Staphylococcus aureus* is the major pathogen in this setting) or from pelvic or other deep vein thrombophlebitis. Septicemia may result in lung abscess.

Occasionally, subphrenic abscess or other intra-abdominal infection will extend directly or indirectly to involve the lung. In this situation and with intestinal obstruction, *Bacteroides fragilis* is much more common than in the usual aspiration type of lung abscess.

Tuberculosis must always be a consideration in necrotizing pneumonia, and fungal infection (particularly histoplasmosis, coccidioidomycosis, and aspergillosis) may also produce this type of pathology. Bronchogenic cysts, which are lined with an epithelium containing secretory elements, commonly contain fluid which may constitute a good culture medium for various microorganisms. Factors which favor aspiration of oropharyngeal flora or which interfere with drainage may lead to infection of lung cysts. The bacteriology of these infected lung cysts is not unlike that of lung abscess.

Lung abscess is the primary manifestation of pleuropulmonary amebiasis, but pleural complications may occur as well.

INCIDENCE AND PREVALENCE. Although lung abscess was more common prior to the introduction of antimicrobial agents, large general hospitals still see at least ten cases each year; if necrotizing pneumonias are included, the figures are considerably higher.

EPIDEMIOLOGY. Lung abscess and necrotizing pneumonia are primarily of endogenous origin. Most of the bacteria involved are elements of the normal flora of the upper respiratory tract. Infections involving *Staphylococcus aureus*, *Klebsiella*, and occasionally other organisms may be of hospital origin.

PATHOGENESIS AND PATHOLOGY. The primary site of lung abscess is the posterior segment of the right upper lobe, with the same segment on the left less commonly affected. Next in frequency of involvement are the apical segments of the lower lobes. These segments are dependent, and the distribution relates to the fact that aspiration or inhalation is the primary background factor. Normally, aspirated material is handled effectively by ciliary action, cough, and alveolar macrophages; but if the protective mechanisms are not effective, infection may result. Thick or particulate matter and foreign bodies are not easily removed and thus may lead to bronchial obstruction and atelectasis. With aspiration, gastric acid and enzymes may be primary offending agents.

Subdiaphragmatic infection may extend to the lung or pleural space by way of lymphatics, directly through the diaphragm or defects in it, or by way of the bloodstream. Most amebic lung abscesses are located in the right lower lobe adjacent to the diaphragm, since they typically arise by direct extension of hepatic abscesses through the diaphragm. Infection may arise in or behind an obstructing neoplasm.

Although the virulence of the infecting organism(s) may be a factor determining the nature and extent of the infectious process, this is not usually important in the case of the anaerobes except for *Fusobacterium necrophorum*. However, the number of organisms aspirated may well be an important factor. With certain of the nonanaerobes, such as *Klebsiella*, *Staphylococcus*, and Group A streptococci, virulence may play an important role.

In the early stages of infection the pathology is that of an ordinary pneumonia. Later, necrosis supervenes upon the inflammation, and cavitation or abscess formation takes place. Subsequently, the abscess cavity may become partially lined with regenerated epithelium, and localized bronchiectasis and emphysema may develop. There is usually no significant vascular involvement in either necrotizing pneumonia or lung abscess. However, septic or bland pulmonary embolus may be the initial event. Once underway, the infection itself may give rise to pulmonary arteritis as in infection caused by *Pseudomonas aeruginosa.*

CLINICAL MANIFESTATIONS. The illness often begins as an acute pneumonic process with fever, malaise, cough, and often pleuritic pain. As a frank abscess is produced, the cough becomes productive of copious amounts of purulent sputum that is usually foul smelling. There may be hemoptysis. Symptoms have usually been present for two weeks or longer at the time of admission, and weight loss and anemia are common. When lung abscess complicates pneumonia caused by *Staphylococcus aureus* or *Klebsiella pneumoniae*, the symptoms are those of a severe pneumonia. There may be a history of unconsciousness, evidence of alcoholism, diseased gums, absence of the gag reflex, or other indications of the predisposing condition.

The physical findings are those of pneumonia, with or without pleural effusion, early in the course of the illness. Later there may be amphoric or cavernous breath sounds. Clubbing of the fingers is noted on occasion. In addition to the usual findings on roentgenograms (see Diagnosis, below), mediastinal lymphadenopathy may be seen on occasion. This may make the differential diagnosis more difficult.

The onset not uncommonly is more insidious than with acute pneumonia. There may be weeks or even months of malaise, low grade fever, productive cough, and significant weight loss before the patient seeks medical attention.

Approximately one third of lung abscesses are complicated by empyema. This may be seen with or without bronchopleural fistula. Brain abscess may also be a complication in patients not receiving appropriate therapy early.

In patients with amebic lung abscess, the symptoms of the associated liver abscess often have been present prior to the rupture through the diaphragm. Following perforation of the liver abscess into the lung, there is gradual development of cough and expectoration of a peculiar chocolate or anchovy sauce–like sputum. There is no odor to the sputum. The development of pulmonary amebic abscess varies from a very insidious phenomenon to a dramatic disease with sudden attack of severe cough productive of a large amount of brownish red sputum. There may be a history of diarrhea and appropriate travel. Complications of amebic abscess include spontaneous perforation to create a cutaneous sinus, hepatobronchial fistula, empyema, secondary bacterial infection, and amebic abscess of the brain.

In cases of secondary lung abscess, the basic process (bacteremia, endocarditis, or septic phlebitis) is usually evident in addition to the pulmonary process.

DIAGNOSIS. A typical lung abscess can be suspected on clinical grounds. Most diagnoses are made from the chest roentgenogram, specifically from the presence of a cavity with an air-fluid level. As indicated earlier, the majority of lung abscesses are located in dependent segments, most often the posterior segment of the right upper lobe, the posteroapical segment of the left upper lobe, and the superior segments of the lower lobes. The basilar segments of the lower lobes may also be involved. Diagnosis of the specific cause, as well as differentiation from similar lesions, depends on bacteriologic studies. Because of the universal presence of large numbers of anaerobes as indigenous flora in the mouth and the common presence, particularly in hospitalized individuals, of potential pathogens such as *Staphylococcus aureus* and *Klebsiella pneumoniae* as colonizers in the mouth and upper respiratory tract, it is necessary to obtain a specimen other than expectorated sputum for bacteriologic diagnosis. When empyema fluid is available, this provides an excellent source. On occasion, particularly in metastatic lung abscess, blood cultures may be positive and provide the specific etiologic diagnosis. However, in most cases of primary lung abscess or necrotizing pneumonia there is no accompanying bacteremia. In the absence of the aforementioned sources, percutaneous transtracheal aspiration is the easiest, safest, and most dependable way of establishing the specific etiology of lung abscess or necrotizing pneumonia. The procedure should not be used in individuals with a significant bleeding tendency or in those in whom it is difficult to provide adequate oxygenation. Percutaneous transthoracic aspiration has been used on occasion in adults but is more hazardous and, in the case of necrotizing pneumonia, provides a much smaller specimen than can be obtained by transtracheal aspiration. It is possible that specimens obtained through a fiberoptic bronchoscope, using special precautions to minimize contamination from normal upper airway flora, may be suitable when quantitative aerobic and anaerobic culture is employed. However, this remains to be established. The antibacterial activity of the topical anesthetic employed with bronchoscopy presents another problem with regard to that type of specimen. It is essential that material obtained for culture be placed under anaerobic conditions promptly before transport to the laboratory. It is usually desirable to aspirate the material to be cultured into a syringe, to expel all bubbles of air or gas from the syringe and needle, and to then transfer the specimen to a tube which has been gassed out with oxygen-free gas for transport to the laboratory.

Amebic lung abscess often provides distinctive clues, i.e., evidence of the disease in the liver. Although demonstration of underlying liver abscess is basic to the diagnosis of amebic involvement of the lung, one may be able to demonstrate motile trophozoites of *Entamoeba histolytica* in the patient's sputum. Presence of Charcot-Leyden crystals in the sputum is very suggestive of amebic infection. The usual procedures for diagnosis of intestinal or hepatic amebiasis should be undertaken. This would include stool examination, sigmoidoscopy, barium enema, and serologic tests. The vast majority of patients with extraintestinal amebiasis have high titers in hemagglutination or complement fixation tests.

Bronchogenic carcinoma can simulate lung abscess when a large tumor undergoes necrosis and cavitation. In addition, the two diseases may coexist. A true lung abscess may develop peripheral to a bronchus obstructed by tumor. In the case of a peripheral cavitating carcinoma, bronchoscopy may not provide the diagnosis. Factors which suggest a cavitating carcinoma rather than lung abscess include absence of predisposing factors for an aspiration abscess (including edentulous state), location of an abscess in a nondependent segment, irregular abscess wall, and failure to respond to antibacterial therapy. Tuberculosis may also simulate lung abscess or necrotizing pneumonia and should always be excluded in cases in which these diagnoses are considered. Cavitating fungal infection may also be confused with lung abscess but is usually distinguished without difficulty. Patients with infected lung cysts typically lack the systemic symptoms which may be seen in lung abscess, the cavity wall is thin, and there is no surrounding pneumonitis. Films taken prior to the illness may have shown an air-containing cyst. Other lesions which may occasionally simulate lung abscess include a cavitating bland pulmonary infarct, cystic bronchiectasis, and cavitating lesions of Wegener's granulomatosis.

TREATMENT. The primary therapy is administration of antimicrobial agents for prolonged periods of time. Treatment may have to be continued for two to four months in order to achieve cure without likelihood of relapse.

With the exception of the *Bacteroides fragilis* group and occasional strains of other anaerobes, the anaerobes involved in lung abscess or necrotizing pneumonia are susceptible to penicillin G. Penicillin V, ampicillin, and amoxicillin are roughly comparable in activity against the anaerobes. Carbenicillin and ticarcillin, in the high dosage usually employed, are active against 95 per cent of strains of the *Bacteroides fragilis* group. However, these agents would not ordinarily be the drugs of choice for this type of infection unless there was another indication for their use. Since some of the anaerobic cocci may require 8 units per milliliter or more of penicillin G for inhibition, one should use large doses of this agent (10 to 20 million units intravenously daily) in patients who are quite ill. The usual adult with anaerobic lung abscess is not seriously ill and usually responds satisfactorily to doses of 2 to 6 million units of penicillin G daily. After there has been a good clinical response, the regimen can usually be changed to 600,000 units of procaine penicillin G intramuscularly every 12 hours. Patients not very ill may be treated satisfactorily with one of the oral penicillins. It should be noted that penicillins other than those mentioned above are typically less active than penicillin G and often considerably less active.

Cephalosporins not uncommonly are less active against anaerobic bacteria than are the penicillins.

However, respiratory tract anaerobes are usually susceptible to cephalosporins (*Bacteroides fragilis* is a major exception), and oral cephalosporins such as cephalexin or cephradine may be used with good effect. Cefoxitin, an investigational beta-lactamase–resistant cephamycin, is much more active than the cephalosporins; 90 per cent of strains of the *Bacteroides fragilis* group are susceptible to this compound and virtually all other anaerobes, with the exception of some clostridia, are as well. Doxycycline and minocycline are more active than other tetracyclines against anaerobes, but a significant percentage of strains of most species are resistant. Accordingly, these compounds should be used only when susceptibility data are available or when the patient's illness is minor so that a therapeutic trial in the patient can be undertaken safely. Clindamycin is active against most anaerobes with the exception of some strains of *Peptococcus* and some strains of clostridia other than *C. perfringens*. It is almost always active against *Bacteroides fragilis*. Accordingly, it represents a good choice in individuals who have significant allergy to penicillins or cephalosporins and in seriously ill patients in whom the *Bacteroides fragilis* group may be present. It may be given intravenously or orally in a dose of 15 to 30 mg per kilogram of body weight per day in four equal doses every six hours. Chloramphenicol is active against nearly all anaerobes and represents another option in a seriously ill patient with necrotizing pneumonia or lung abscess in whom the *Bacteroides fragilis* group may be present. The succinate derivative may be given intravenously in a dosage of 30 to 60 mg per kilogram of body weight per day in adults, using four equal portions every six hours and giving the drug slowly, over a period of 30 minutes. Metronidazole, still investigational for treatment of anaerobic infections, has a broad spectrum of activity and is consistently bactericidal. All strains of *Bacteroides fragilis* are susceptible. However, some of the cocci, particularly those not obligately anaerobic, and *Actinomyces* are resistant.

For staphylococcal infections a penicillinase-resistant penicillin is preferable, but one of the parenteral cephalosporins or vancomycin may be used in the event of significant allergy. Penicillin G is the drug of choice for group A streptococcal infection. For infections caused by *Klebsiella pneumoniae* or other facultative or aerobic gram-negative bacilli which may be involved in the type of pulmonary infection under discussion, one of the aminoglycosides would represent the drug of choice. Gentamicin is ordinarily suitable, but in certain settings significant numbers of gram-negative bacilli are resistant to gentamicin, and then amikacin is the next choice. In seriously ill patients, particularly those who may be immunosuppressed, the use of carbenicillin or ticarcillin along with the aminoglycoside is desirable.

For nocardiosis, sulfonamides or co-trimoxazole, minocycline, and ampicillin all have significant activity. In seriously ill patients, a sulfonamide plus one of the antibiotics should be used. In amebiasis, drugs used for treatment of amebic liver abscess (in particular, metronidazole or emetine) constitute effective therapy, along with appropriate drainage. Treatment for the primary intestinal amebiasis should also be included.

Postural drainage is an important aspect of therapy of lung abscess. Bronchoscopy may be helpful in effecting good drainage at times and also permits removal of foreign bodies and biopsy diagnosis of tumors. Surgical resection of lung abscess is rarely required unless there is a coexisting malignant process. Indeed, surgery is contraindicated because of the hazard of uncontrollable spread of infection or asphyxiation from spillage of abscess contents during positioning of the patient on the table. Surgical drainage of lung abscess through the chest wall is almost never indicated. In the case of accompanying empyema, drainage is crucial and usually requires an open procedure with rib resection.

PROGNOSIS.   The prognosis varies with the type of underlying or predisposing pathologic process, if any, and, in the case of acute severe necrotizing pneumonias, the speed with which appropriate therapy is instituted. The mortality in anaerobic lung abscess is 15 per cent or less. In anaerobic necrotizing pneumonia it is 25 per cent. The mortality may be significantly higher in acute pneumonias caused by *Staphylococcus aureus*, *Klebsiella pneumoniae*, and other facultative or aerobic gram-negative bacilli. Prognosis in amebic lung abscess is good when diagnosis and treatment are prompt. Nocardiosis often has a relatively poor prognosis, especially when it complicates a serious underlying disease.

PREVENTION.   When possible, care should be taken to minimize the likelihood of aspiration. Thus nasogastric tube feedings should be employed with care. The head of the bed should be elevated for patients with achalasia or similar problems. If aspiration does occur, particulate material should be removed promptly. Proper treatment of periodontal disease and gingivitis will minimize pulmonary complications. Acute pneumonias and bacteremias should be treated promptly with appropriate drugs.

347.2.   BRONCHIECTASIS

DEFINITION.   Bronchiectasis refers to abnormal dilatation of the bronchial tree. The distribution of the disease is patchy. There are usually no signs or symptoms directly related to the bronchial dilatation. The clinical picture is due to chronic or recurrent infection and hypersecretion of mucus.

ETIOLOGY.   Various infections may cause peripheral bronchial obstruction and stasis which may then lead to bronchiectasis. At present, bronchopneumonia is the most common causative factor. Obstruction related to a foreign body or to tumor may also lead to chronic infection and development of bronchiectasis distal to the obstruction.

True congenital bronchiectasis may be seen in Kartagener's syndrome. This syndrome consists of dextrocardia, sinusitis, and bronchiectasis. In cystic fibrosis of the pancreas or mucoviscidosis, the thick secretions obstruct the lumen of the bronchi, resulting in distal atelectasis. Bronchiectasis commonly results from infection superimposed on the aforementioned process. Recurrent infection in individuals with congenital agammaglobulinemia also leads to bronchiectasis. Tuberculosis may cause it by distortion of bronchi in association with healing disease, obstructing lymph nodes, or destruction due to endobronchial disease.

PATHOGENESIS AND PATHOLOGY.   Irreversible dilatation of the bronchi results from prolonged bronchial obstruction and infection. The infection may extend into the bronchial wall, disrupting smooth muscle and elastic tissue and, at times, invading adjacent peribronchial tissue. Ciliated columnar epithelium is replaced by nonciliated cuboidal epithelium and sometimes fibrous tissue, resulting in the formation of localized areas of dilatation or saccules. These anatomic changes lead to further stasis of infected secretions, and there may be traction as a result of peribronchial scarring. The posterior basal segments of the lower lobes are the areas most commonly affected by bronchiectasis. When the left lower lobe is involved, the lingular segment of the left upper lobe is also commonly involved. Upper lobe bronchiectasis tends to be in the posterior or apical segments and is commonly secondary to healed tuberculosis.

CLINICAL MANIFESTATIONS. As noted earlier, bronchiectasis is asymptomatic in the absence of superimposed infection. Some individuals with bronchiectasis may be asymptomatic for extended periods of time. The classic symptoms of bronchiectasis are cough productive of mucopurulent sputum, hemoptysis, and recurrent pneumonitis. The cough may be particularly bothersome when the patient lies down, thus emptying secretions from the dilated saccules of the dependent lower lobes into the larger bronchi. Large amounts of mucopurulent sputum are produced each morning. Classically, such sputum, when collected in a jar, will show three layers: a bottom layer consisting of pus cells and elastic tissue, a central watery layer, and a frothy top layer. The sputum is not uncommonly foul or putrid smelling but may have a sickening sweet odor. The hemoptysis may be massive on occasion. Recurrent pneumonitis involving the same segment or lobe repeatedly should raise suspicion of the possibility of underlying bronchiectasis, as well as of tumor or foreign body.

Many patients with bronchiectasis also have sinusitis and gingival or periodontal disease, but the relationship of the latter processes to bronchiectasis does not seem to be one of cause and effect.

Exertional dyspnea may be noted by patients with extensive disease. There may be pleuritic pain, usually mild in nature. Fatigue and malaise are common. Patients appear chronically ill. A significant number exhibit clubbing of the fingers and toes. The most characteristic finding is persistent moist, coarse rales over the area of involvement.

DIAGNOSIS. In overt cases the diagnosis is readily established clinically. Such cases are not nearly so common as in the preantimicrobial era. Roentgenograms of the chest may show increased coarse lung markings and even honeycombing. In extreme cases of saccular bronchiectasis there may be ring shadows and fluid levels. Ordinarily, bronchography is the most effective means of establishing the diagnosis. In the case of suspected endobronchial obstruction underlying the bronchiectasis, bronchoscopy is important.

TREATMENT. The treatment of choice, when it is feasible because of localized disease, is resection of the involved areas. Aside from this, treatment consists of use of antimicrobial agents in limited courses for complications such as pneumonitis or acute exacerbations of the disease. There is a paucity of good bacteriologic data as to cause of the infection in these patients, but what is known suggests that it is comparable to that observed in lung abscess and necrotizing pneumonia. Accordingly, penicillin G is ordinarily the drug of choice. Individuals who have had repeated and extended courses of antimicrobial therapy, patients with cystic fibrosis in

particular, may have infection with more resistant organisms such as *Staphylococcus aureus* or *Pseudomonas aeruginosa*. For them, a penicillinase-resistant penicillin or aminoglycoside such as gentamicin or amikacin represents the drug of choice. A major aspect of therapy is postural drainage.

Before contemplating surgery for localized disease in a newly diagnosed case, the clinician should undertake conservative management and observation of the patient. It is important to realize that spontaneous reversion of the process may take place. Reversible bronchiectasis may follow pneumonia or expansion of a collapsed lobe. In some cases, it may take many months for the process to revert to normal.

PROGNOSIS. The disease is usually not progressive, and with judicious use of antimicrobial therapy the life expectancy can be normal.

Bartlett, J. G., and Finegold, S. M.: Anaerobic infections of the lung and pleural space. Am. Rev. Respir. Dis., 110:56, 1974.

Bartlett, J. G., Gorbach, S. L., Tally, F. P., and Finegold, S. M.: Bacteriology and treatment of primary lung abscess. Am. Rev. Respir. Dis., 109:510, 1974.

Brock, R. C.: Lung Abscess. Springfield, Ill., Charles C Thomas, 1952.

Finegold, S. M.: Anaerobic Bacteria in Human Disease. New York, Academic Press, 1977.

Ochsner, A., and DeBakey, M. E.: Pleuropulmonary complications of amebiasis: An analysis of 153 collected and 15 personal cases. J. Thorac. Surg., 5:225, 1936.

Wynn-Williaus, N.: Bronchiectasis: A study centered on Bedford and its environs. Br. Med. J., 1:1194, 1953.

348. PHYSICAL AND CHEMICAL IRRITANTS

Margaret R. Becklake

348.1. INTRODUCTION

Man, in taming his environment, in developing his complex industrial society, and, more recently, in pursuit of his hobbies, has become increasingly exposed to a wide variety of *inhaled agents, including particles, fumes, or vapors,* which are capable of affecting his lungs to the point of producing disease. Apart from community air pollution, most *such exposures occur in relation to occupations.* Although the title of this chapter implies that the harmful effects of all such agents can be attributed to *physical or chemical irritation,* it is in reality often difficult to characterize the mechanisms whereby they produce biologic effects, even though the physical and chemical properties of the environmental agents concerned can be precisely measured. Often when the precise nature of the agent is not known, the practical solution may be to *link the disease with the occupation concerned.*

The physician usually makes this link through *the occupational history.* An industrial physician is sensitized to the need for a detailed occupational history and the environmental hazards associated with different occupations. However, in many communities working men and women first seek medical advice from their personal physician who may easily fail to recognize an occupational exposure because it occurs in a small plant, using experimental materials, or in the processing as a secondary user of dangerous products whose hazards are neither recognized nor appreciated. Thus *a work history should always be exhaustive* and should cover every job ever held, even part-time or vacation jobs, together with the materials handled directly or indirectly, as well as safety measures recommended on the job and information about the health of co-workers. Furthermore in the past, the role of women in the workplace was often forgotten; thus the listing of a middle-aged or elderly woman's occupation as that of housewife may result in failure to recognize, for example, a link between pleural calcification and work in a talc factory when she was younger. In addition, place of residence is also important, as well as the occupation of other family members, because *neighborhood* and *"take-home"* risks are increasingly being identified, e.g., mesothelioma developing years later in someone whose childhood home was beside an asbestos plant, or in the wife or child of a previous asbestos worker.

Thus today *occupational lung disease* covers the reaction of the lung to *a variety of physical and chemical agents.* It includes those conditions originally described by the term *pneumoconioses,* which refers to lung disease consequent to the inhalation of dust, in keeping with its Greek derivation. The term has recently been redefined by the International Labor Organization (ILO) to mean *the accumulation of dust in the lungs and the tissue reactions to its presence.* For the purpose of this definition, "dust" means an aerosol of solid inanimate particles. The tissue reaction may be *noncollagenous,* i.e., alveolar architecture remains intact, stromal reaction is minimal and consists mainly of reticulin fibers, and the reaction is potentially reversible. By contrast, *collagenous* pneumoconioses are associated with permanent scarring of the lung. Although the term was originally applied only to inorganic (mineral) dusts, it has subsequently been extended to cover organic (biologic) "dusts" as well, because exposure to the latter is also frequently occupational. However, besides any nonspecific reaction these biologic "dusts" may evoke, especially if exposure is heavy, they may act as stimulants to the subject's immune mechanisms (see Ch. 346). In this chapter the ILO definition will be followed. A large number of variants of the term pneumoconiosis

Physical and Chemical Irritants: Working Classification of their Pulmonary Effects

Category of Agents	Effect on Lung	Agent	Circumstances of Exposure, Including Occupation(s) or Industry at Risk
Inorganic dusts	1. Pneumoconiosis (noncollagenous)	Carbon, tin, iron, coal, graphite	Mining, welding
	2. Acute silicolipoproteinosis	Free silica (uncombined SiO_2)	Tunnelling, sandblasting: exposure to high doses of fine particles
	3. Pneumoconiosis (collagenous)		
	a. Nodular	Free silica	Hardrock mining of any sort; quarrying, stonecutting and dressing; foundry, pottery, and enamel workers
	b. Diffuse	Asbestos (all fiber types)	Asbestos mining, milling and manufacturing; insulating
		Fume and other fine silica	Sandblasting
		Beryllium	Fluorescent light and space industry
	c. Complicated	An altered response to usually nonfibrogenic dust	Coal miners (progressive massive fibrosis)
	4. Neoplasia (lung) (see Ch. 349.2)	Asbestos (all fiber types)	Mining and industrial exposures
		Radioactive dusts	Mining operations
		Metal mining	Hematite, chrome
		Metal refining	Nickel, chrome
	5. Neoplasia (pleura) (see Ch. 350.1)	Asbestos (excluding anthophyllite)	Industrial exposure more at risk than mining exposures
	6. Chronic bronchitis	All dusts, given a high enough dose	Probably all types of exposure
Organic dusts	1. Asthma-like reactions (see Ch. 344.1)	Enzymes of *B. subtilis*	Manufacture of detergents
		Western red cedar dust	Wood workers
	2. Late onset airflow obstruction (eventually irreversible)	Cotton, hemp, flax, and jute	Processing of vegetable fiber, especially carding of cotton
	3. Hypersensitivity pneumonitis (see Ch. 346.3)	Fungal spores, especially *M. faeni*	Haymaking, grain handling, mushroom cultivating, sugar cane picking or processing the residue
	4. Chronic bronchitis	Organic material (nonspecific)	Grain handling
	5. Chronic interstitial pneumonia	Vaporized mineral oil	Smoking blackfat tobacco (Guyana); certain industrial exposures
Chemicals, including fumes and vapors	1. Acute pulmonary edema	Oxides of nitrogen	Silo filling, fire fighting
		Phosgene	Fire fighting
		Certain insecticides, e.g., paraquat	Accidental ingestion
	2. Asthma-like reactions (see Ch. 344.1)	Complex platinum salts	Platinum refining
		Aluminum solder flux	
		Toluene di-isocyanate (TDI)	Manufacture of polyurethane plastic
	3. Acute bronchitis	TDI (in heavier doses)	Manufacture of polyurethane plastic
		SO_2	Pulp and paper mills
		NH_3	Refrigeration industry
		Vanadium	
	4. Chronic bronchitis	All the aforementioned agents in lower dose	As above
	5. Pneumonitis	Cadmium, Hg, Mn	
Radiation	1. Pneumonitis	X-radiation	Medical treatment
	2. Neoplasia (see Ch. 349.2)	Radioactive dusts	Uranium and other mining

have been coined to describe specific occupations at risk or specific dust diseases, and these will be referred to where appropriate.

The accompanying table, although it implies more precise understanding of the mechanisms of lung response to the different agents than is justified by current knowledge, does, however, provide a working and essentially practical approach for diagnosis. Included also is reference to the recognized associations between these agents and neoplasia, although of course the mechanism of action is probably more complex than physical and/or chemical "irritation."

Pneumoconiosis redefined. Br. Med. J., 2:552, 1972.

348.2. INORGANIC DUSTS: DOSAGE, CLEARANCE, AND CELLULAR REACTION

The main biologic effects of inorganic dusts depend on their retention in the lungs of man for long periods of time, measured usually in years, not months. It has been suggested that any mineral dust, if relatively insoluble and not immediately toxic, can produce a pneumoconiosis when inhaled in sufficient quantities. The physician is probably better advised to adopt this over-suspicious attitude to mineral dusts than to fail in recognizing old as well as new pneumoconioses. In addition to effects attributable to retention of dust in lung tissue, less specific effects on airway function are being increasingly recognized, and will be discussed under the heading of occupational bronchitis (see Ch. 348.10).

Human lungs have been aptly called "size-selective dust samplers." Airborne dust, when inspired into the lung, undergoes a process of separation based on its aerodynamic behavior or falling rate, a function mainly of diameter, but also of size, shape, and density. Once particles make contact with any part of the airways or airspaces, they are not resuspended in the expiratory airstream. Other factors which influence penetration and deposition include breathing patterns, including the amount of time spent mouth breathing, as well as tidal volume and minute ventilation. There is also evidence to suggest that the state of the airways in smokers is such as to favor central deposition rather than deeper penetration of particles. Over 80 per cent of larger particles (6 μ and over) impact on the mucous lining of the larger airways to be removed, usually quite rapidly (i.e., within hours), by ciliary escalation; however, some particles of considerable length, e.g., asbestos fibers up to as much as 100 μ in length, may penetrate as far as terminal respiratory units. Small dust particles penetrate more deeply, fine particles (below 2 μ) constituting the majority of those which reach the alveolar spaces. The retention rate is about 40 per cent in the 2 to 1 μ size, and higher for those below 0.2 μ (see Fig. 1). It is ironic that in many industrial situations mechanization has resulted in an increase in the environmental risks, increasing not only the overall dust levels but in particular the fine particles with a higher retention rate.

Particles deposited in the major airways are removed rapidly (within hours) by the mucociliary escalator. However, since the respiratory bronchioles and alveoli are lined with surfactant, not mucus, dust particles set-

Figure 1. Deposition rate of particles in the human lung in the nose and supraglottic structures (URT) and in the tracheobronchial tree and lung parenchyma (LRT) in relation to aerodynamic diameter, a measurement which refers to the actual diameter in the presence of water vapor which may exceed the particle size in dry air. (Courtesy of Professor Paul Morrow, University of Rochester, N.Y. Reproduced from Lee, D. H. K. [ed.]: Environmental Factors in Respiratory Disease. New York, Academic Press, 1972.)

tling here are handled by other clearance mechanisms, which are slower, with half-clearance times of between 24 hours and 100 days. Important to them all is the process of alveolar phagocytosis; dust-laden phagocytes migrate toward the alveolar ducts and terminal bronchioles; if not extruded into the airways they may penetrate into lung interstitium and lymphatics. Furthermore, clearance mechanisms may be provoked, i.e., mucus and surfactant production, ciliary activity, and endocytosis may all increase, in response to the inhalation of irritants, particularly if exposure is intermittent. Heavy doses, on the other hand, tend to overwhelm the removal mechanisms, and their efficiency may also be reduced by associated pollutants, either industrial or personal (tobacco smoke).

The *lung tissue response to inorganic dust* has been likened to the color spectrum to emphasize the variety in the type of response and its intensity, ranging from noncollagenous tissue reactions in the presence of large amounts of retained dust, e.g., cotton and coal, to intense collagen fibrosis in association with relatively small amounts of retained dust. The nature of the tissue response is thought to depend on the physicochemical properties of the dust as well as on its antigenic properties. It is almost certainly dose related to *the amount of dust retained* (not to the exposure dose), which in turn is the consequence of the integrated personal exposure less the integrated clearance over the years, and probably also relates to how long the dust has been resident in the lung. Other factors which may influence the response are the presence or absence of infection, and possible synergistic or antagonistic effects of other respirable materials in the environment. Finally, although dust dose is probably the most important factor determining the lung response, there appear to be between-individual differences in susceptibility; it is not clear, however, whether this is a reflection of between-individual differences in clearance and therefore retention, or between-individual differences in tissue response.

The nodular pneumoconioses, either noncollagenous or collagenous, are caused by the relatively insoluble dusts, and the diffuse pneumoconioses by relatively soluble dusts.

Brain, J. D., and Valberg, P. A.: Models of lung retention based on the ICRP Task Group Report. Arch. Environ. Health, 28:1, 1974.

Seal, R. M. E., and Wagner, J. C.: Pathologic reactions of the lung to dust. *In* Morgan, W. K. C., and Seaton, A. (eds.): Occupational Lung Diseases. Philadelphia, W. B. Saunders Company, 1975, p. 39.

348.3. INORGANIC DUST PNEUMOCONIOSES: DIAGNOSIS, LUNG FUNCTION, AND DISABILITY

The criteria for *diagnosis* of an inorganic dust pneumoconiosis depend on the purpose for which the diagnosis is to be used (e.g., working diagnosis, screening, or attributability for compensation), as well as the degree of certainty required. In general, it will be based on the characteristic changes in the chest roentgenogram, *provided that the subject in question has an appropriate exposure history*. Furthermore it is not unusual for there to be no physical signs and no impairment of physical performance, even in the presence of marked radiographic changes. In no other field therefore is the quality of the chest radiograph more important, and the technique used should be appropriate; e.g., low kv to define pleural calcification, high kv to define the pulmonary parenchyma and noncalcified pleural changes, oblique views often being necessary to demonstrate the latter. In addition, use of standard films in conjunction with the UICC/Cincinnati Classification of Radiographic Appearances of the Pneumoconioses (1970) will improve the accuracy of film interpretation. In this classification, which is descriptive rather than etiologic, parenchymal changes are classified according to *type* (round or irregular); *size* (p, q, and r for rounded opacities of <1.5, 1.5 to 3.0, and >3.00 mm diameter, respectively; s, t, and u for fine, medium, and coarse irregular opacities; A, B, and C for large opacities of <1.0, 1 to 5, and >5 cm in diameter, respectively); and *profusion* (from 0/- to 3/4 on a 12-point scale, with provision for indicating the zones involved). Provision is also made for recording pleural thickening (according to site, width, and extent, and whether the costophrenic angle is involved), ill-defined diaphragm and cardiac outline, and pleural calcification (according to its site, thickening and extent), as well as other changes in the hila, mediastinum, and heart. In the absence of an exposure history, or if the exposure is considered to be too short to account for the amount of radiologic change seen, it may be necessary to establish a *tissue diagnosis* by *mediastinal node biopsy or transbronchial* or *open lung biopsy*. However, the pathologic findings may also be inconclusive, because lung tissue has only a limited number of response patterns and a given response may be evoked by several stimuli, e.g., irritants and infections, and every attempt should therefore be made to identify the agent. This may require examination under the electron microscope, e.g., for asbestos fibers, as well as chemical analysis and mineralogic study with x-ray diffraction of adequate tissue samples (for which open biopsy is usually necessary). The electron microprobe may ultimately allow precise characterization of mineral in very small tissue samples, or even in the single ferruginous (asbestos) body. Since most pneumoconioses develop as a consequence of occupational exposure, *precise evaluation of disability* is frequently called for, with a view to establishing compensation; hence, the many studies of pulmonary function in pneumoconiosis. However, the relationships between *organ malfunction* (as reflected in what might be called descriptive measurements of the lung, e.g., its size or volumes, and measurements reflecting its mechanical properties, including gas mixing and airway caliber), *organ failure* (generally considered to be present only when gas exchange function is impaired), and *disability* (diminution of performance as perceived by the subject himself) are not straightforward. Thus considerable organ malfunction (i.e., abnormality of lung function tests) can be present without organ failure (i.e., abnormal arterial blood gases) even under the stress of effort. It is generally believed that *dyspnea* is felt when the respiratory effort (either minute volume or muscular effort) for a given task is greater than the subject habitually experiences. In health there exists a tremendous reserve of cardiopulmonary function, indicated by the capacity to increase O_2 consumption (going from rest to maximal exercise) by a factor varying from 20 in the young athlete to perhaps 10 in the middle-aged man. In its early stages pneumoconiosis may produce only very minor measurable changes in organ function, affecting performance at high levels of exercise only, and this may well be interpreted by the subject as the natural consequence of aging. As the condition progresses, dyspnea may be more easily related to demonstrable changes in the lung function. In the following chapters, an attempt is made to describe the usual clinical picture and lung function findings in the different pneumoconioses in their different stages of development, and, because of the universal nature of the smoking habit, the effect that smoking will have in further modifying function. *In evaluating the individual case*, however, *there is no substitute for the detailed study of pulmonary function at rest and on effort*, with a view to determining performance at an average aerobic workload (such as many jobs demand) and possibly to determine maximal aerobic work capacity. This information can then be interpreted in the light of industrial history, the physical demands of the individual's job, dust exposure (quality and quantity), medical history (in particular, previous and present heart and lung disease), and appropriate laboratory investigations.

In a case of industrial lung disease, the physician's responsibility to his patient does not cease until he has assured himself that the case has been referred to the correct local authority in charge of industrial safety. This referral has social implications at two levels. In the first place, there is the question of attributability and compensation for the individual and for his dependents. In the second place, it is evident that the occurrence of a case of occupational disease represents failure of control measures, and it is essential that this point of failure be identified so that appropriate action can be taken to protect the future health of a new generation of workers, the younger colleagues and children of today's cases. The physician must ensure that these steps have been taken.

Bates, D. V. B., Macklem, P. T., and Christie, R. V.: Response to chemical and physical irritants. *In* Respiratory Function in Disease. Philadelphia, W. B. Saunders Company, 1971, p. 361.

Becklake, M. R.: Pneumoconioses. *In* Handbook of Physiology. Respiration. II. Baltimore, Williams & Wilkins Company, 1965, p. 1601.

ILO U/C International Classification of Radiographs of Pneumoconiosis. Geneva, International Labour Office, 1972.

348.4. NONCOLLAGENOUS PNEUMOCONIOSES

EXAMPLES. Examples include *coal workers' pneumoconiosis; siderosis* in welders; *pneumoconiosis* in hematite and magnetite miners; *stannosis* in tin miners; *baritosis* in barium miners; *pneumoconiosis* in *chromite* and *china clay* miners, and in *Fuller's earth* and *mica* workers. It should be noted that information on the noncollagenous pneumoconiosis is derived largely from coal workers' pneumoconiosis, which, because of the large numbers of men at risk in many countries and the resurgence of coal as a source of energy, has been under extensive study in recent years.

PATHOGENESIS AND MECHANISMS. The dusts mentioned above elicit a virtually noncollagenous response in the lung; hence the diseases associated with such exposure have been called the *"benign" pneumoconioses.* Thus particles which are phagocytosed by macrophages accumulate in these cells without killing them. Dustladen macrophages then move toward the respiratory bronchioles, where they aggregate. Similar aggregations develop in pulmonary lymphoid tissue and round small vessels. As the bronchiolar aggregations enlarge, dustladen macrophages collect upstream, resulting in the development of dust macules located in a centrilobular position, and visible to the naked eye on whole lung sections. At first the macules are little more than dust collections (see Fig. 2), but later reticulin fibers appear, with some collagen, usually distributed in a radial rather than a concentric fashion. Thus even in the presence of as much as 30 grams of coal dust per lung (autopsy measurements) the stromal reaction tends to remain for the most part noncollagenous; however, it is influenced by the other constituents of the dust, in particular mineral and silica content. This probably explains such regional differences as exist, for example, among the dust macule of the Welsh soft coal miner, the more fibrous macule of his counterpart in Belgium, and the *stellate "mixed dust" nodule* of the foundry worker. Indeed, if the silica content of lung dust exceeds 18 per cent, the associated lung lesions will almost certainly be collagenous, resembling those of classic silicosis. In addition, the radiodensity of the

Figure 2. *A,* Coal macule located next to a distal airway; note the lack of collagenous response (× 30). *B,* Asbestos bodies in alveolar macrophages in an alveolus (× 500). *C,* Classic silicotic nodule showing a central core of dense hyalinized collagen fibers surrounded by loose fibers, arranged in a concentric manner; normal alveolar walls to one side (× 125). *D,* Classic silicotic nodule showing doubly refractile dust particles (× 300). (Courtesy of Dr. Nai-San Wang, Department of Pathology, McGill University, Montreal, Canada.)

nodules appears to be related to their iron content, endogenous iron accumulating around dust as it does around other foreign bodies. In time the respiratory bronchioles around the dust foci dilate, perhaps because of the local traction of the dust-encased bronchioles on the surrounding lung parenchyma, with bronchiolar dilatation and the development of *focal emphysema,* believed to be distinguishable from the more common centrilobular emphysema by the absence of an associated bronchiolitis. Indeed, it has been suggested that the dust sheathing accounts for this being a distention rather than a destruction emphysema.

The pathologic changes of generalized emphysema may also be seen in lungs which are affected by these nodular pneumoconioses, particularly when the nodulation is of the smaller variety (pinhead rather than micronodular). Such changes occur more frequently and to a more disabling degree (leading to pulmonary hypertension and right heart failure) in certain geographic areas, e.g., the iron mines of Lorraine and the coal mines of Belgium. Finally, pulmonary emphysema has been shown to occur more frequently in the lungs of miners than in the lungs of the nonmining population, even in the absence of pneumoconiosis, thus strengthening the evidence that dust exposure, particularly in the cigarette smoker, is a factor contributing to the development of chronic obstructive lung disease.

CLINICAL MANIFESTATIONS. The term "tattooing" of the chest roentgenogram has been applied to this group of *"benign" noncollagenous nodular pneumoconioses,* because even in the presence of diffuse radiologic nodular densities symptoms and signs of chest disease are rarely present. Thus the diagnosis is made on the basis of the presence of small rounded opacities on the chest roentgenogram characteristically distributed in the mid and upper zones; indeed, because of the close relationship between radiologic category and lung dust content, it has been suggested that the chest film remains "the only feasible method of determining and quantifying dust exposure in life." Likewise, most tests routinely used to evaluate pulmonary function, such as measurements of lung volume, flow rates, diffusing capacity at rest, and even the pulmonary mechanics, have been found to be within the normal limits in keeping with the histology of the dust macules. However, as the profusion of dust macules (reflected by advancing radiologic category) increases, detectable changes include an increase in residual volume, and a decrease in expiratory flow rates at the end of a forced expiration and in diffusing capacity (possibly related to the smaller type of nodulation), as well as abnormalities of gas distribution (reflected in dead space ventilation) and in gas exchange (reflected in A-a O_2 differences). Such changes, demonstrable at rest and exaggerated during effort, presumably reflect regional inequalities in ventilation vis-à-vis perfusion. However, they do not appear to affect function enough to cause symptoms or cause disability affecting performance; the latter, if present, is usually attributable to chronic obstructive airway disease.

EPIDEMIOLOGY AND PROGNOSIS. The prevalence rate of simple pneumoconiosis varies very much from operation to operation, even within the same industry; for example, in the 1970–71 National Coal Board survey in Britain, rates varied from 3.3 to 15.9 per cent of working miners, whereas in the 1969 Interagency study in the United States coal pits, rates varied from 4.6 to 46.0 per cent. In small uncontrolled operations prevalence may well be higher. These differences are thought to be related to the dust exposure levels, although differences in the reading of the chest roentgenogram, particularly for the lower categories of change, cannot be ignored. Prevalence usually falls dramatically as dust control becomes effective, e.g., in the Dutch coal miners rates fell from 270 to 160 per 1000 working miners over a seven-year period, but rates have leveled off in some countries, e.g., Britain — a trend attributed to increased mechanization and longer running times for coal machinery. An unfavorable influence of mechanization on prevalence has also been observed elsewhere, e.g., in the coal mines of central India. In addition, the British Coal Board study has shown that radiologic progression is related to mean mass concentration of airborne dust (not to particle counts), and occurs more rapidly in those men who develop radiologic change sooner.

In addition to the pathologic evidence quoted above, there is also epidemiologic evidence that the prevalence of symptoms of chronic bronchitis (e.g., sputum production) is increased in coal miners and that this is related to their occupation since dose relationships have been shown. However, other factors which influence its prevalence include environment (e.g., in some areas bronchitis appears to be as common among miners' wives as among the miners themselves) and cigarette smoking, since miners are frequently heavy smokers. Thus attributability is a taxing and difficult problem for compensation commissions, especially as the noncollagenous nodular pneumoconioses do not usually per se produce significant disability.

It is *unusual* for these noncollagenous pneumoconioses *to develop for the first time or to progress after exposure has ceased,* but this does occur. Likewise, the disappearance of radiologic changes after removal from exposure, though unusual, has been described, and is in keeping with animal experiments showing that dust nodules are not static structures but are the site of continuing phagocytic activity. Life expectancy does not appear to be affected by the presence of the noncollagenous pneumoconioses, provided that complicated pneumoconiosis, e.g., progressive massive fibrosis in coal miners, does not develop. This complication, by contrast, is associated with disability and premature death (see below).

Doig, A. T.: Baritosis: A benign pneumoconiosis. Thorax, 31:30, 1976.
Morgan, W. K. C., and Lapp, N. L.: Respiratory disease in coal miners. Am. Rev. Respir. Dis., 113:531, 1976.
Ryder, R., Lyons, J. P., Campbell, H., and Gough, J.: Emphysema of coal workers' pneumoconiosis. Br. Med. J., 3:481, 1970.

348.5. COLLAGENOUS PNEUMOCONIOSES (NODULAR)

EXAMPLES. Examples of these disorders include *classic silicosis of hardrock miners* (e.g., gold, tin, copper, uranium, chromite) and of *granite workers* and *cutters;* and silicosis in *iron and steel workers* and *sandblasters,* in the *pottery industry,* in industries using *silica flour,* and in those processing *bentonite* clays.

PATHOGENESIS AND MECHANISMS. If the dusts of carbon and coal represent those at the low end of the response spectrum, free crystalline silica dust represents the opposite end, with its almost unique biologic capacity to evoke a powerful fibrogenic tissue response. Silica particles are rapidly ingested by macrophages, but are only briefly retained within the phagosomes created by the invaginated cell wall before these rupture, owing to the action of lysosomal enzymes, thus freeing the particles now apparently in activated form, since cell death follows rapidly. This contrasts with the fate of the less fibrogenic dusts, which may be retained for long periods within the phagosomes of the macrophages without cell death. Other macrophages are recruited, perhaps by an autoimmune reaction, to reingest the particles with the same result. Released particles may penetrate lung tissue, with lymphatic clearance to the hilar lymph nodes, and preferential clearance from the lower lobes may explain why the subsequent tissue reaction appears more frequently in the mid and upper zones. Collagen formation follows, resulting from stimulation of fibroblasts, and finally hyalinization of the collagen to form the *characteristic fibrous silicotic nodule,* made up of whorled fibrous connective tissue like an onion. These appear first in the hilar nodes, and then in peribronchial, perilymphatic, or perivascular locations, presumably at the sites of accumulation of the activated dust particles, which, however, tend to remain on the periphery of the nodule and thus are capable of enlarging it or stimulating the formation of new nodules (see Fig. 2). Autoimmunity may play a role in recruiting macrophages to sustain the reaction and in altering the development of already established lesions, since diseases such as systemic sclerosis, which are thought also to be mediated through autoimmune mechanisms, occur with increased frequency in subjects with established silicosis and in some instances even in miners with dust exposure but no evident dust disease. An *unusual form of silicotic lung lesion* has recently been described in *Elliot Lake* (Ontario) *uranium miners,* in which the granulomas resemble those of sarcoid more than the classic silicotic nodule; the presence of radioactivity may account for this modified type of lung reaction. Extensive and marked fibrosis may be present in the lungs at autopsy with only relatively small amounts of dust (up to 10 grams, of which perhaps half is silica). Involvement of the hilar and mediastinal lymph nodes is common, occasionally with *egg-shell calcification,* but abdominal nodes are only occasionally affected. *Acute silicotic reactions* occur with heavy exposures to fine particles and may be associated with alveolar wall thickening and the accumulation of proteinaceous fluid in the alveolar spaces *(alveolar lipoproteinosis),* thought to be due in part to overloading of the clearance mechanisms and accumulation of surfactant. Sarcoid-like granulomas may also be seen, and complicating infection, particularly by mycobacteria, including atypical forms, is frequent. In nature, free crystalline silica occurs almost exclusively as quartz; however, other free crystalline silicas, e.g., crystobalite, tridymite, though rare in natural geologic formation, may be formed from quartz in steel-making and in other high-heat smelting processes, and probably have a more powerful silicosis-producing action than quartz.

Conglomerate silicosis is the result of the matting together by fibrosis of silicotic nodules, often with obliteration of bronchi and blood vessels, and frequently associated with caseous areas and cavitation, which often but by no means always show conclusive histologic evidence of tuberculosis. These changes account for the right heart strain, hypertrophy, and failure which may

develop subsequently, perhaps as a consequence of the pulmonary vascular bed's being reduced by the fibrosis and tissue loss and associated emphysematous changes in the adjacent lung. A reversible element in the pulmonary hypertension may also be present, related perhaps to hypoxia or hypercapnia or both.

CLINICAL MANIFESTATIONS. Nodular silicosis is essentially a chronic disease, and radiologic changes rarely appear before 20 years of exposure. However, even in this disease in which the radiologic lesions are fibrous nodules, not noncollagenous dust macules, there may be no clinical manifestations and no apparent impairment in pulmonary function, particularly for Category 1 radiologic disease. However, the proportion of cases without signs and symptoms is probably only about 20 per cent, in contrast to about 90 per cent in the noncollagenous pneumoconioses of equivalent radiologic category.

The first complaint in nodular silicosis is commonly *shortness of breath,* brought on by moderate, and then progressively less, exercise until it is present at rest. This symptom is probably due to the increased muscular work required to ventilate incompliant lungs and is aggravated by increased minute ventilation to offset impaired gas exchange. Lung volumes are reduced as the nodular disease becomes more widespread. Other changes may follow, including a reduction of diffusing capacity commensurate with the volume reduction, a further fall in compliance, impaired mixing, and disturbances of gas exchange (attributed to impairment of regional ventilation-perfusion balance), eventually with hypoxemia, first on exercise and then at rest. However, the over-all function profile is by no means always restrictive; in particular, miners who smoke may present with the symptoms, signs, and classic lung function pattern of chronic obstructive lung disease, even though the radiologic pattern is primarily that of diffuse nodular pneumoconiosis. Additional symptoms include *cough* and *sputum* (usually the consequence of cigarette smoking), *hemoptysis* and *chest pain* (usually associated with intercurrent infection), and, rarely, pressure effects of calcified hilar nodes on neighboring structures (superior vena cava, esophagus, phrenic nerves, and bronchus).

When *complicated pneumoconiosis* develops *on a background of classic silicosis,* the symptoms, signs, and clinical presentation usually represent a progression from an already symptomatic state, and the diagnosis is made from the chest radiograph which shows a conglomeration of existing lesions, usually in the upper mid-zones, often bilateral, with eventual progression to the characteristic bilateral "angels' wings" shadows. The lung function pattern may suggest restrictive disease but frequently shows a pattern characteristic of obstructive disease, or there may be a mixed picture. Infection with *M. tuberculosis* is more likely to be demonstrable in conglomerate silicosis than in the progressive massive fibrosis of coal workers, and is more likely to behave and progress as in the nonsilicotic lung with constitutional symptoms (see below). Right heart strain and failure may complicate the picture, particularly if chronic bronchitis and emphysema are present. *An accelerated form of silicosis* may develop with a shorter incubation period after first exposure (e.g., four to eight years) if exposure has been heavy. Its clinical features are similar to those of the chronic form, but the over-all course to death is rapid (approximately ten years), and complicating infection by mycobacteria is common (about 25 per cent of cases).

Acute silicolipoproteinosis, a variant of accelerated silicosis with characteristic histopathologic changes, runs an even more rapid course. Clinical features include weight loss, weakness, diffuse rales, and hypoxemia. Infection with mycobacteria (often atypical) is invariable, and the clinical course to death is usually only a matter of months.

In addition, the presence of silicosis appears to be associated with an *increased prevalence of autoimmune diseases,* such as rheumatoid arthritis, systemic sclerosis, and diffuse lupus erythematosus, which occurred, for example, in 10 per cent of New Orleans sandblasters who had developed an accelerated form of silicosis. An increased incidence of systemic sclerosis has also been reported in Witwatersrand gold miners.

EPIDEMIOLOGY AND PROGNOSIS. Prevalence rates vary between as well as within mines or other operations, the variations reflecting differences in airborne dust levels and, most important, its free silica content. Thus in the Witwatersrand gold mining industry, rates fell from 40 per 1000 underground miners in the 1920's to less than 10 per 1000 in the 1950's, and the average period of mining service prior to diagnosis rose from 10 to 23 years over this period. Comparable over-all prevalence figures for the United States metal mining industry for 1958 to 1961 were 34 per 1000. Complacency about exposures to dusts thought to be low in silica content, e.g., in bentonite mining in the United States or granite quarrying in the West country of the United Kingdom, has accounted for recent outbreaks and should alert the physician to exploring in full the occupational history even in industries not recognized to have a health risk. In addition, epidemiologic studies have now shown that *occupational exposure to most mining environments* is a risk factor in the *development of bronchitis,* the prevalence of which is dose related to estimated exposure (see Ch. 344.1) when the greater effect of cigarette smoking has been taken into account. This is not linked to the presence of pneumoconiosis. Thus it appears that exposure to the mining environment is associated with two types of tissue response: one specific (the fibrosis of pneumoconiosis), and one nonspecific (chronic mucus hypersecretion or chronic bronchitis)—both dose related to exposure, but not apparently related to each other. The simple silicosis of hardrock miners is undoubtedly a less benign disease than the simple pneumoconiosis of coal miners, despite the fact that it does not appear to affect life expectancy, and figures for Sweden indicate that, after withdrawal from exposure, x-ray changes never regress but progress in the majority of cases (Fig. 3).

Ziskind, M., Jones, R. N., and Weill, H.: Silicosis. Am. Rev. Respir. Dis., 113:643, 1976.

348.6. COLLAGENOUS PNEUMOCONIOSES (DIFFUSE)

EXAMPLES. These pneumoconioses include *asbestosis* in mining, milling, manufacturing, and all the secondary industrial uses of asbestos, including insulation workers, particularly those pulling out old insulation in ships and buildings; *aluminosis,* as in Shaver's disease; *talcosis* in miners and millers of talc in some industrial

Figure 3. Rate of progression of different pneumoconioses after removal from dust exposure. The figures are based on five occupational groups of Swedish workers (each containing a minimum of ten cases) followed for 15 years after dust exposure ceased. (From Bruce, T., Nystrom, A., and Ahlmark, A. L.: Scand. J. Resp. Diseases, Supp. 63, 1968.)

processes, and also in its intravenous administration by drug users who inject solutions of talc-containing tablets; and *chronic beryllium disease of the lung.*

PATHOGENESIS AND MECHANISMS. Asbestos, the most important mineral in this group, occurs in several forms: *chrysotile* (a magnesium silicate, occurring as long, white, flexible fibers), the chief asbestos of commerce, mined primarily in Canada and the U.S.S.R. as well as in Italy and in Southern Africa; and the *amphiboles,* iron silicates (occurring as brittle fibers such as amosite, anthophyllite, and blue crocidolite) mined in South Africa, Australia, and Finland. Exposure occurs in mining and milling, and in the manufacture of a wide variety of the commodities used by modern man. *Asbestos cement products,* such as tiles and pipes, account for 70 per cent of production, and *insulation materials,* including floor tiles, for another 10 per cent; the rest is used in *paper, friction materials* (car brake and clutch linings), and *textiles* for use as protection against heat in industry and in homes.

The extent to which asbestos fibers penetrate the lung in all likelihood depends on their physical properties, the curly fibers of chrysotile being more likely to impinge on the mucus blanket than the short straight amphibole fibers. Some fibers appear to penetrate the interstitium directly and remain there, perhaps undergoing chemical and physical degeneration but nevertheless visible in much greater profusion than was ever suspected before the use of electron microscopy in their detection. Other fibers become engulfed by macrophages, and still others, but probably only a very small proportion of the longer fibers, become coated by a smooth protein film which becomes iron-impregnated, giving rise to the typical drumhead, golden-brown *asbestos bodies* (see Fig. 2), a process also attributed at least in part to macrophage action. There is some evidence that the coating of a fiber renders it nonfibrogenic. The pleura also appears to be a target organ, although it is not clear how the fibers gain access to the pleura, for pleural reactions may occur even in the absence of demonstrable fibers in the lung, and coated fibers are rarely seen in the pleura. It is possible that small fibers may be cleared to subpleural lymphatics and for some reason undergo dissolution here more readily than in other parts of the lung. *Pleural reactions* include *effusion* (often bloody); dense, fibrous, *adhesive pleurisy; plaques* and *calcification* involving parietal rather than visceral pleura; and malignancy in the form of *mesothelioma* (see below).

It is not known which fibers are, or become, fibrogenic; nor is their precise mode of action known. However, observed cytogenic effects include an interaction with the cell membrane, increasing permeability, and an interreaction of already ingested particles with the lysosomal membrane. Target cells include the macrophage, mesothelial cells, alveolar epithelial cells, and fibroblasts. Fibers deposited in alveolar structures elicit a cellular reaction similar to *desquamative alveolitis;* others at the level of the respiratory bronchiole produce an appearance of *bronchiolitis obliterans;* a third reaction is characterized by *interstitial edema* going on to *collagenization.* Nonspecific antinuclear antibodies may accelerate the fibrosis once it has started, and it eventually becomes confluent, obliterating air spaces and replacing them with cystic spaces lined by flattened epithelium ("honeycomb" lung). Other mineral dusts which produce this pattern of diffuse fibrosis are talc and diatomaceous earth.

Generalized pulmonary fibrosis may also be found in *chronic beryllium disease* of the lung, now thought to be the end result of a Type IV immune reaction to the inhalation of beryllium salts. The granulomas which characterize the earlier stage of the process are indistinguishable histologically from those of sarcoidosis, and may vary from loose collections of histiocytes to large circumscribed granulomas, often containing giant cells with various inclusion bodies. Although the lung is the organ most seriously affected, presumably because it is the portal of entry, granulomas are found throughout the body, involving hilar, mediastinal, and abdominal lymph nodes, liver, spleen, skin, and in fact all organs involved in sarcoidosis except the eye, parotid, and tonsil. Beryllium has been isolated, in varying amounts, from all these tissues (about 0.5 gram of tissue is necessary for this analysis), and the diagnosis can be made with certainty only by isolation of the element beryllium in tissues or body fluids. There is often a very long period of latency, up to 30 years, and initial exposure may have been only indirect, e.g., neighborhood exposure (residence close to a plant using beryllium), so that cases related to the manufacture of fluorescent light in the United States during World War II continue to be reported today, even though the use of beryllium in the fluorescent lamp industry ceased in 1949. Although its modern uses, particularly those concerned with space exploration, appear to be better controlled, physicians should remain vigilant because new cases continue to be added to the U.S. Beryllium Registry at the Massachusetts General Hospital.

CLINICAL MANIFESTATIONS. These are no different from those of diffuse pulmonary fibrosis, whatever the underlying cause. In some subjects *dyspnea* is the first symptom, brought on at first by considerable exertion and then by progressively less effort, until it is eventually present at rest. In other subjects, an *irritating dry cough* precedes the awareness of shortness of breath, often by many years. With the progress of the disease, the cough may become productive, and *spells of chest pain* may be associated with the coughing. When the condition is advanced, there are usually diffuse basal rales, but these may also occur early before radiologic evidence of lung changes. The lung signs may be modified by the presence of pleural thickening or calcification. Respiratory failure may only appear late in the course of the disease, with pulmonary hypertension, right heart strain, and right heart failure. Nor is the victim of these diffuse pneumoconioses immune from the attack by general atmospheric pollutants — in particular, cigarette smoking — which may encourage the development of chronic bronchitis and bronchiectasis and increase the risk of bronchial neoplasm.

The *radiologic changes* are also no different from those seen in all other forms of diffuse interstitial fibrosis except for the *prominence of the associated pleural changes;* in particular, calcification should direct attention to the possibility of exposure to asbestos or talc. Thus for the purpose of diagnosis of the individual case, the features to be evaluated are, in particular, prevalence, extent and character of *small irregular opacities in the parenchyma,* and the site, width, and extent of *pleural thickening or calcification,* as outlined in the ILO classification. Rounded opacities are more frequent when the exposure includes silica.

In certain parts of the world, e.g., Finland, *pleural calcification* may appear as the only manifestation of exposure to anthophyllite, asbestos, and less commonly talc and mica. It is rarely seen under 20 years of industrial exposure, and neighborhood cases are seen with diminishing frequency as the circumferential distance of the place of residence from the industry increases.

The *established case of asbestosis* is associated with changes in pulmonary function characteristic of restrictive lung disease, i.e., small volumes, reduced compliance, impaired gas exchange with reduced diffusing capacity, and hyperventilation on effort and eventually at rest. The earliest function changes in response to asbestos dust exposure appear to be reduced vital capacity and increased exercise ventilation, tests which may eventually prove useful in the longitudinal surveillance of exposed workers. In addition, the function changes of chronic obstructive lung disease are not infrequently seen, particularly in workers who smoke.

In addition, changes in lung function may be detected in the healthy worker before symptoms and sometimes before radiographic changes occur, changes which are thought to reflect the effects of asbestos exposure in the lung and which vary from subject to subject, presumably according to the particular location of the tissue responses in his lung, i.e., peribronchiolar, pleural, or interstitial. These include changes in tests thought to represent small airway status, as well as in vital capacity, exercise ventilation, and possibly diffusing capacity. Small changes in tests of this sort, particularly the vital capacity, although not likely to be useful in the diagnosis of the individual case, may, however, eventually prove useful in the *long-term surveillance of exposed workers,* particularly if followed over time from their recruitment into the industry.

EPIDEMIOLOGY AND PROGNOSIS. The *attack rate of asbestosis* varies in different industries from under 10 per cent of miners working in open pits, as in Quebec, up to over 70 per cent in men with long exposure in the insulation and construction industries. These differences are thought to reflect primarily differences in exposure levels to respirable dust, which is often higher in industrial operations with the progressive manipulation of the fiber and its fractionation into small particles, which penetrate the lung further with higher retention rates.

The epidemiology of *population exposure* to *asbestos* has been established from the search for asbestos bodies in lung scrapings or extruded lung fluid in routine autopsies. Positive results are reported in many parts of the world, ranging from 1 per cent in rural Italy to over 50 per cent in Finland, the site of the world's oldest known asbestos deposits; prevalence is also consistently higher in men than in women, increases with age, and shows within-city variation in relation to proximity of residence to industrial areas. Insofar as the lung is an accumulator over time, and the world's use of asbestos is increasing dramatically, it is not surprising that this percentage is increasing in adults in London; New York studies by contrast report between 50 and 60 per cent both in recent and in 1934 autopsy material. It must be emphasized that the presence of *ferruginous bodies* (as experts now urge that they be called) indicates exposure, not disease. Nor are they specific for asbestos, because other types of fibers, e.g., glass, wool, cotton, talc, may constitute their core, and the lung probably uses this method to "inactivate" a large variety of inhaled particles. However, their presence in the sputum or other biologic material should alert the physician to the strong possibility of an occupational exposure, past, even remote past, or present, which he should explore with vigor for its relationship to any current pulmonary disease.

Becklake, M. R.: Asbestos-related diseases of the lung and other organs: Their epidemiology and implications for clinical practice. Am. Rev. Respir. Dis., 114:187, 1976.

Hamilton, A., and Hardy, H. L.: Industrial Toxicology. 3rd ed. Acton, Mass., Publishing Sciences Group, Inc., 1974, p. 43.

348.7. COMPLICATED PNEUMOCONIOSIS

EXAMPLES. Examples of the complicated pneumoconioses include *progressive massive fibrosis of coal workers* and *Caplan's syndrome*.

PATHOGENESIS AND MECHANISMS. Progressive massive fibrosis (defined as a radiologic lesion greater than 1 cm in diameter) may develop as a complication of most inorganic dust pneumoconioses, including those which are noncollagenous, usually on the background of Category 2 or 3 disease, and this complication may occur even after exposure has ceased. Thus, although initially the response to dust exposure may be a macrophage reaction producing a noncollagenous response with little effect on the lung architecture, years later the same lung tissue may react to the same dust with severe fibrosis which obliterates and destroys all anatomic structure. On macroscopic examination the lesions of *progressive massive fibrosis in coal workers* (PMF) are amorphous, irregular, rubbery, and relatively homogeneous. Microscopic examination shows the central core of the lesion to be made up of an insoluble protein complex; its capsule consists of dust irregularly mixed with bundles of coarse, hyaline collagen fibers. Few blood vessels and air passages are seen, but the persistence of internal elastic lamellae suggests that they have been obliterated by invading fibrous tissue. In addition, there is sclerosis of the vessel walls, often with invasion by dust-laden cells and evidence of endarteritis at the periphery of the lesion; *emphysema,* usually of an *irregular* nature, frequently develops in association with the lesions of PMF which often distort the major and medium-sized airways, and histologic or bacteriologic evidence of *Mycobacterium tuberculosis* is found in a high proportion of cases.

Several mechanisms may be operative in the development of complicated pneumoconiosis, of which infection by *M. tuberculosis* and/or atypical mycobacteria is probably the most frequent (the recovery rate of organisms both in life and at autopsy increases with increasing effort and has exceeded 50 per cent in some autopsy series). Clinical evidence includes the observation of an increased attack rate of PMF in miners who developed active tuberculosis after gastrectomy for peptic ulcer. However, the disease has been shown to develop in a substantial number of subjects with negative tuberculin skin tests (particularly in the United States), whereas in the Rhonda Fach in Wales a decline in attack rate of tuberculosis was not accompanied by a concomitant decline in the attack rate of PMF. Thus in some cases, other mechanisms may be important; these include the overwhelming of clearance mechanisms by lung dust; aseptic necrosis owing to interference with blood supply; significant silica contamination of the coal dust; and, finally, reaction on an immunologic basis, in which the coal dust acts as an absorptive surface for proteins. Immune mechanisms are also thought to play a role in the development of *Caplan's syndrome*. Caplan observed an association between rheumatoid arthritis and a particular radiologic picture in miners, characterized by well-defined opacities 0.5 to 5 cm in diameter, widely distributed and developing rather more suddenly than progressive massive fibrosis, often on a background of slight or no pneumoconiosis. Some lesions eventually cavitate, then shrink, perhaps with calcifications, and may later become incorporated into a mass radiologically indistinguishable from progressive massive fibrosis. Histologically, the rheumatoid nodule contains a central core of necrotic collagen separated by bands of dust, with a peripheral zone of active inflammation and a well-marked arteritis in the adjacent vessels. Caplan's syndrome, though first recognized and most frequently seen in coal miners, has been described in workers in foundries, asbestos, potteries, sandblasting, and boiler scaling. Most of the evidence supports the view that the lung lesions in Caplan's syndrome are a manifestation of *rheumatoid disease facilitated by the presence of dust*. Thus in Wales there is no evidence that coal mining predisposes to the development of rheumatoid arthritis, but the prevalence of PMF (and incidentally of tuberculosis) was increased in miners with this disease. Furthermore rheumatoid factor was positive with greater frequency in miners with Caplan's syndrome (approximately 70 per cent) than in those with PMF (30 to 40 per cent), whereas lower figures were observed in men with simple pneumoconiosis. By contrast in Appalachian coal miners, the prevalence of rheumatoid factor appeared to relate not to radiologic lesions suggesting Caplan's syndrome but to the type of coal mined, being highest in anthracite miners with PMF (74 per cent). Thus there remain aspects of the interrelationships of simple pneumoconiosis, PMF, and Caplan's syndrome which require clarification.

CLINICAL MANIFESTATIONS. In coal workers, the appearance of progressive massive fibrosis usually marks the onset of symptoms and signs of lung disease. The first symptom is commonly *dyspnea* on heavy effort, and subsequently at lesser work loads until it becomes evident at rest. The changes in function initially suggest loss of functioning volume, followed by a generalized restrictive lung disease. The symptom of cough does not appear to be more common in the earlier stages of complicated pneumoconiosis than in simple pneumoconiosis. *Melanoptysis* (sudden coughing up of a moderate amount of jet black fluid) is not uncommon, and frequently relates to cavitation. *Chest pain*, dull and aching, and diffusely located, is common, and there is an increasing tendency to *acute purulent bronchitis*. Pulmonary hypertension and right heart hypertrophy, leading ultimately to *right heart failure*, is present in many instances, with the usual symptoms and signs. When infection with *M. tuberculosis* appears to be the factor precipitating the development of the complicated pneumoconiosis, it is seldom accompanied by the usual systemic symptoms, i.e., fever, weight loss, and hemoptysis.

When the chest roentgenogram suggests Caplan's syndrome (see above), serum tests for rheumatoid factor are positive in over 70 per cent of cases, whereas arthritis, already present in about 50 per cent of cases, may develop in others only after a delay of several years.

EPIDEMIOLOGY AND PROGNOSIS. *Attack rates of PMF vary* within a region, chiefly in relation to the *background of radiologic category* (e.g., 0.7 and 4.3 per cent per year for Category 1 and 3, respectively, in South Wales), but they also decline steeply in relation to *age.* They tend to be higher in those whose chest radiographs show the *more rapid progression of disease*, but are apparently uninfluenced by smoking, energy expenditure, tuberculous infection, and even continued exposure. Considerable between-region differences (e.g., high in France and eastern Pennsylvania, low in Utah) may well be due to variations in some of the factors mentioned above. Rheumatoid pneumoconiosis occurs in 2 to 6 per cent of United Kingdom coal miners affected by pneumoconiosis, and should be suspected when PMF develops suddenly in an individual with minimal or no pneumoconiosis. By contrast with simple coal workers' pneumoconiosis, PMF does affect mortality, but it is of interest that this does not apply to lesions less than 20 sq cm in size on the chest radiograph.

Benedek, T.: Rheumatoid pneumoconiosis: Documentation of onset and pathogenic considerations. Am. J. Med., 55:515, 1973.
Morgan, W. K. C.: Coal workers' pneumoconiosis. *In* Morgan, W. K. C., and Seaton, A. (eds.): Occupational Lung Diseases. Philadelphia, W. B. Saunders Company, 1975, p. 149.

348.8.   INORGANIC DUST PNEUMOCONIOSES: TREATMENT AND PREVENTION

TREATMENT. There is *no specific treatment for the simple nodular or diffuse inorganic dust pneumoconioses* once the diagnosis is established. Nor does it seem likely that any of the materials mentioned under Prophylactic Substances, below, will be effective, although so far aluminum is the only one to have received a careful clinical trial. Despite this, the physician has an extremely important role to play in management, both in support of and advice to an individual faced with a threat to his livelihood due to diagnosis of a disease related to the source of his livelihood. Advice depends primarily on evaluating *factors which influence outcome*, most important of which is diagnosis of whether the *pneumoconiosis is noncollagenous (and likely to affect health, function, or longevity)* or *collagenous (carrying threats to all of the above)*. Other factors include the *immune status* and *skin reactivity* to mycobacteria, *age*, and an *evaluation of the current as opposed to past risks* (including dust levels) in the *particular working environment* concerned. The physician must attempt to answer the following questions as accurately as he can: (1) *What is the likely outcome* in this particular case? (2) *Should he advise the patient to seek other employment?* These questions are easier to answer when the subject is a "patient" with complaints for which he seeks the physician's help, but much harder when the individual is working and believes himself to be in good health, but has an abnormality on the chest roentgenogram and/or a small loss of lung function. For the noncollagenous pneumoconioses, most physicians will permit continued employment given regular health surveillance measures. For the collagenous pneumoconioses, progression to complicated disease appears to depend as much on past as on subsequent exposure (see Fig. 2), and the decision is much more difficult. Although animal studies do suggest that withdrawal from exposure slows progression, extrapolation of these results to man must be done with caution, despite the intuitive reaction to act on them.

In *complicated pneumoconiosis*, the medical management of associated chronic obstructive lung disease and right heart failure and pulmonary heart disease is the same whether or not it coexists with pneumoconiosis (see Ch. 351). When active tuberculous infection with mycobacteria, including atypical types, can be demonstrated, and probably even when the only evidence is a positive skin test to PPD, appropriate chemotherapy should be instituted (see Ch. 167). The addition of rifampin to the treatment regimen has received favorable comment. Nevertheless, although treatment is usually successful in respect of sputum conversion, radiologic clearing is less impressive; and controlled clinical trials do not support the routine use of tuberculosis chemoprophylaxis in all cases of PMF irrespective of whether active tuberculous infection can be demonstrated. Neither antituberculous treatment nor steroids appear to influence the evolution of Caplan's syndrome. Since complicated pneumoconiosis is invariably accompanied by disability, often associated with right heart failure, most patients with complicated pneumoconiosis will have already left the industry concerned. Opinion is divided on the advisability of withdrawal from exposure if the patient is still so occupied.

In *acute silicosis*, progression to death is rapid and does not appear to be halted by any treatment measures, including steroids. Lung transplant has been carried out in two cases, one with survival up to ten months. The management of *alveolar lipoproteinosis* associated with silica exposure is no different on this account; however, if bronchial lavage is considered, the addition of PVNO (see below) to the lavage fluid might be considered on purely theoretical grounds, without as yet any published practical report.

DUST CONTROL. Inorganic dust pneumoconioses cannot be treated effectively, but they can be prevented, and *prevention* means, essentially, *dust control.* Attack rate increases with exposure, and there is a dust dose–disease relationship. Thus *control should be at an epidemiologic level,* aiming at controlling the exposure of the community at risk, not at a personal level with the use of masks or respirators, which should preferably be regarded as a measure for temporary use when circumstances force the suspension of other control measures. Indeed their use, often incorrectly, in the past has led to a false sense of security on the part of the worker and his employer; for instance, *inside* the hoods used, though not consistently, by Gulf sandblasters, respirable dust of high silica content reached average levels of three times, ranging up to 50 times, in excess of recommended standards. Dust can seldom be completely eliminated from industrial operations. However, disease could be controlled if the minimal exposure which produces health effects in a given industry were known, and increasing efforts are being made to translate available scientific information, in particular epidemiologic studies, into estimates of health risk. For instance, it has been estimated that the probability of a British coal worker developing Category 2 (or higher) pneumoconiosis is 3.4 per cent given a 35-year working exposure at an average dust concentration of 4.3 mg per cubic meter. Similarly, the risk of developing asbestosis has been estimated at under 1 per cent for a 50-year working exposure at an average fiber level of 2 per cubic centimeter. It is possible to envisage a future in which, using cumulative ongoing records of each worker's exposure, operations could be planned so that no worker would be likely to exceed the exposure known to produce disease within his working life. Such an ambitious scheme, already under way in the West German coal mining industry, is likely to be set up only in large industries able to mount extensive research programs. However, for smaller industries, it is quite valid to assert that *less dust means less disease.* Equally important aspects of environmental control are work practices, often best controlled not by directive but by worker education and worker participation in environmental monitoring with posting of information. Provision of laundry facilities at work to avoid the "take-home" hazards of the past—e.g., asbestos, beryllium—is equally important. *Threshold limit values* are annually revised by bodies such as the American Conference of Governmental Industrial Hygienists and provide general reference standards. However, it should be clear to the physician that these are only estimates of safe levels, based on the information presently available, and he should not be deterred from making the diagnosis of pneumoconiosis because the individual has worked in a controlled environment only; controls may fail and estimates may be inaccurate, and the physician must not automatically assume that his patient is "protected."

TUBERCULOSIS CONTROL IN WORKING POPULATIONS. Medical attention should be directed toward reducing the attack rates of complicated pneumoconiosis and silicotuberculosis. All subjects with pneumoconiosis are at a higher risk in terms of tuberculosis

than the general population; in addition the circumstances of employment may favor infection, e.g., recruitment of workers from populations in which infection with tubercle bacilli occurs relatively late in life. Case finding and control of tuberculosis should thus be of a particularly high standard in populations exposed to an inorganic dust hazard; at the very least this should include a pre-employment tuberculin skin test and chest roentgenogram, the latter to be repeated subsequently at appropriate intervals. Finally, gastrectomy for peptic ulcer should be avoided in subjects with pneumoconiosis (see above).

PROPHYLACTIC SUBSTANCES. Studies in laboratory animals have indicated that certain substances (ferric oxide, iron, coal, aluminum, and, more recently, poly-2-vinyl-pyridine-N-oxide or PVNO) depress or inhibit the biologic effects of silica dust. Of these materials only aluminum has received a trial in man as a prophylactic or preventive measure when it was introduced into the gold mines of Ontario in 1943; however, no conclusive evidence on its effectiveness has come out of this experience, and this type of prophylaxis is a sorry substitute for proper environmental dust control. PVNO has also received a limited trial in Europe.

Becklake, M. R.: Asbestos-related diseases of the lung and other organs: Their epidemiology and implications for clinical practice. Am. Rev. Respir. Dis., 114:187, 1976.

Dubois, P., Gyselen, A., and Prignot, J.: Rifampin-combined chemotherapy in coalworker's pneumoconiotuberculosis. Am. Rev. Respir. Dis., 115:221, 1977.

Kennedy, M. C. S.: Aluminum powder inhalations in the treatment of silicosis of pottery workers and pneumoconiosis of coalminers. Br. J. Industr. Med., 13:85, 1956.

Morgan, W. K. C., and Seaton, A.: Occupational Lung Diseases. Philadelphia, W. B. Saunders Company, 1975, pp. 108, 203.

348.9. NEOPLASIA ASSOCIATED WITH DUST EXPOSURE

ASBESTOS. The carcinogenic potential of asbestos has been amply confirmed by animal experiments, and human exposure should also be regarded as always potentially carcinogenic. Thus in man it has been shown that exposure increases the attack rate (probably in a dose-related fashion) of *bronchial carcinoma,* and also of *laryngeal cancer,* particularly in smokers, suggesting a synergism between these carcinogens. It has been estimated that if smoking and asbestos exposure separately increase the risk of developing bronchogenic cancer about ten-fold, the two factors together increase the risk about 80-fold. In addition, the risk is increased by the presence of asbestosis, and some reports indicate that neoplasia will develop in 50 per cent of patients with already established asbestosis. However, the belief that all excess lung tumors are "scar cancers" (i.e., adenocarcinomas) is supported by only some of the studies examining cell types of cancer in asbestos-exposed victims of this disease. Exposure to asbestos dust is also associated with increased risk of *gastrointestinal neoplasia,* presumably because of dust swallowing. An unusual feature is the occurrence of multiple cancers, e.g., in lung and gut. Thus far, however, no link between nonoccupational exposure (e.g., to asbestos fibers in drinking water) and gastrointestinal neoplasia has been shown. Finally a rare tumor, *mesothelioma of the pleura and/or peritoneum,* occurs with greater frequency not only in industrially exposed populations, but also in association with indirect exposure, often after a long latent period, e.g., neighborhood exposure as a child 40 years before. This led to the supposition that this type of cancer was not dose related to exposure. However, careful fiber counts in affected lungs suggest that for this cancer, too, there is a dose relationship to fibers retained in the lung.

Although all types of asbestos fiber are implicated in the increased incidence of neoplasia, the order of increase varies, being on the whole higher for those engaged in processing and using than for those engaged in mining or milling. To what extent these differences are attributable to dust dose, fiber type, changes in physical and chemical properties with processing, and/or contamination by co-carcinogens remains to be determined. For mesothelioma, however, the evidence to date suggests that fiber type is important, the risk being greatest with exposure to crocidolite, less with amosite, and possibly even less with chrysotile.

AIRBORNE RADIOACTIVE PARTICLES. Knowledge of an excess mortality in the Schneeberg metal miners dates back to the sixteenth century, and is likely to have been due to lung cancer associated with the radioactivity of these mines. This risk has persisted into the twentieth century. In North America, an increased number of deaths from lung cancer have been observed in Colorado as well as Ontario uranium miners, the risk being related to the estimated radiation dose with a preponderance of small cell cancers. In these men also, smoking considerably increased the risk. Furthermore, regular sputum cytology examinations in this occupational group have shown progression from mild through moderate to marked atypia, over a time span of, on the average, up to ten years before the identification of a carcinoma in situ, information which permits a realistic evaluation of sputum cytology as a screening procedure. Increased deaths from lung cancer have also been observed in miners handling other materials, thought to be noncarcinogenic, in whom exposure has occurred to mine air contaminated by radon decay products from the ore-bearing rock or mine water, e.g., fluorspar miners of St. Lawrence, Newfoundland, and hematite miners in Cumberland, England.

OTHER OCCUPATIONS AT RISK. Increases in mortality from lung cancer have been reported in a number of other occupations which involve exposure to dusts and/or fumes and chemicals, without identification of the specific agent implicated. These include *chromate workers, workers in nickel refineries and in copper smelters, coke oven workers* in the United States, *gas workers* in the United Kingdom, and workers exposed to chlormethyl-ether. Indeed Doll has estimated that up to 50 per cent of cigarette-caused lung cancer may be dependent on the synergistic effect of an atmospheric pollutant, and the ever expanding number of occupations for which an increased risk has been demonstrated is in keeping with this belief.

Whether or not a neoplasm is occupation associated makes no difference to the outcome as far as the individual patient is concerned; *recognition of this association* on the part of the attending physician may, however, be important both from the patient's point of view (because of the question of compensation) and from the point of view of the patient's working colleagues, since index cases serve to direct attention to as yet unrecognized occupational hazards. It has been suggested as a rule of thumb that *for a working population of 1000 men, diagnosis of the second case of cancer of the lung* should arouse suspicion in the mind of the occupational physician that there is an excess lung cancer risk requiring investigation.

Becklake, M. R.: Asbestos-related diseases of the lung and other organs: Their epidemiology and implications for clinical practice. Am. Rev. Respir. Dis., 114:187, 1976.

Seaton, A.: Occupational pulmonary neoplasms. *In* Morgan, W. K. C., and Seaton, A. (eds.): Occupational Lung Diseases. Philadelphia, W. B. Saunders Company, 1975, p. 357.

348.10. OCCUPATIONAL BRONCHITIS

Chronic bronchitis may be defined as a *clinical syndrome* characterized by *sputum production*, often with a *cough*, and frequently associated with *airflow obstruction*. A *relationship with exposure to cigarette smoke* was strongly suspected by clinicians, but was difficult to confirm by clinical observation alone for a number of reasons: a persistent cough is so frequently accepted as a "normal" phenomenon in a smoker, smoking is such a widespread habit, and few individuals consult a doctor for just a cough. It was through the study of its manifestations in the population at large, using the techniques of epidemiology, that the strength and importance of this relationship were revealed, a relationship which is now accepted as causal. By this the epidemiologist means that the relationship is consistent (i.e., has been found in almost all populations studied, in almost all circumstances, and in almost all countries), and is dose-related, including the influence of withdrawal (i.e., the manifestations occur more frequently in those who smoke more heavily, and tend to diminish in those who quit), as well as having a consistent time relationship (i.e., manifestations develop *after*, not *before*, the smoking habit is taken up). Additional *environmental risk factors* shown to be important are urban (as opposed to rural) living and social class (at least in Britain); *host factors* which influence its prevalence include sex, age, race, childhood health, and probably some genetic factors. In passing, it should be pointed out to the clinician who generally regards with scorn the epidemiologist's definition of bronchitis (positive answers to a standardized questionnaire indicating the presence of "cough with production of sputum occurring on most days for at least three months of the year during at least two years") that this definition, never intended for clinical diagnosis, was developed for use in population studies as an indicator of the presence of a clinical condition, and as such has proved a powerful tool in discerning the risk factors listed above.

Occupations which result in individuals being exposed to the *inhalation of dusts* (see above), *fumes, and vapors* (see below) have also been suspected by clinicians of contributing to the development of chronic bronchitis, but a problem has been to disentangle the relative importance of smoking (usually practiced by over 60 per cent of any particular occupation group). In addition, *in studies* in which the *population* has also been *at risk for developing other dust-related diseases*, in particular pneumoconiosis, *the two diseases (chronic bronchitis and pneumoconiosis) do not appear to be directly linked*. A likely explanation is that each represents the response to a different size range of dust particles, pneumoconiosis representing the lung tissue response to the smaller particles which penetrate deeply and are more likely to be retained, whereas chronic bronchitis is the consequence of the deposition of larger particles in major airways with perhaps irritation and stimulation of mucus glands and probably also goblet cells. When the possible responses to dust inhalation are considered separately in this way, and when smoking has been taken into account, an *increased prevalence of chronic bronchitis has been consistently found in mining populations*, and has invariably been shown to be dose related to estimated dust exposure. Occupations in which the prevalence of bronchitis appears to be increased include coal mining (in the United States, United Kingdom, Belgium, and Germany), gold mining (in South Africa), asbestos mining (in Canada), chemical workers (in the United Kingdom and Canada), and coke oven workers (in the United Kingdom), as well as cement workers, rubber workers, cotton workers, wool workers, and grain handlers. This list is not exhaustive.

A consistent finding, however, has been the *predominant influence of cigarette smoking compared to that of occupations* on the prevalence of bronchitis. Furthermore, some studies have shown the excess prevalence to be present in smokers only; others suggest synergism between the two factors, and yet others suggest the opposite. Nor is the association with airflow obstruction (reflected in pulmonary function tests) always clear. A next step is to re-evaluate the influence of dust exposure on symptoms (i.e., mucus hypersecretion) and airflow obstruction separately; it may be that these, too, are separate responses to dust exposure, in the same ways as they have recently been shown by Fletcher to be separate responses to cigarette exposure. Other unanswered questions include the relative importance of withdrawal from dust exposure and quitting smoking on symptoms and on airflow obstruction thought to be dust related, and the influence, if any, of both on morbidity and mortality.

There can be little doubt that *chronic bronchitis (either as diagnosed by the clinician or as detected by the epidemiologist) is a disease of multifactorial etiology, with risk factors attributable to both the host and the environment*, one of which is *exposure to different industrial environments in the pursuit of different occupations*. As in other conditions of multifactorial etiology, not only are difficulties encountered by the scientist attempting to study these factors and elucidate their relative importance in populations, but difficulties are also encountered by the physician attempting to translate this information into clinical practice, both in management of the individual case and in evaluation for compensation purposes. Society, through legislative action, is equally at a loss to know how to act, because it is as yet impossible to apportion relative importance of the different risk factors in an individual case. Should occupation be considered the only risk factor, and so compensated? Or should it be relegated to second place in the presence of the most important other risk factor, the cigarette? Neither seems just, and for the moment and until further evidence becomes available, a preferable way to proceed seems to be by clinical diagnosis, a procedure which, in scientific parlance, proposes the "best available hypothesis" to explain the known facts about the individual and all the occupations he has ever pursued, past and present.

Fletcher, C., and Peto, R.: The natural history of chronic airflow obstruction. Br. Med. J., 1:1645, 1977.

Higgins, I. T.: Epidemiology of Chronic Respiratory Disease: A Literature Review. Publication No. EPA-650/1–74–007. Washington, D.C., Office of Research and Development, Environmental Protection Agency, 1974.

Lapp, N. L.: Industrial bronchitis. *In* Morgan, W. K. C., and Seaton, A. (eds.): Occupational Lung Diseases. Philadelphia, W. B. Saunders Company, 1975, p. 265.

348.11. ACUTE AIRWAY REACTIONS TO ORGANIC PARTICLES

EXAMPLES. Examples include "asthma" in workers exposed to the enzymes of *B. subtilis* in the manufacture of detergents and asthma in workers with Western red cedar (*Thuja plicata*) and in grainhandlers.

PATHOGENESIS AND MECHANISMS. Inhalation of organic materials may provoke *airway reaction on a nonimmunologic basis*, the result of *stimulation of cough and irritant receptors* which cause *reflex constriction of the airways via vagal pathways*. These receptors are believed to be located in the complex network of nerve endings beneath and between the cells of the alveolar epithelium, cough receptors occurring in the major airways (especially in the larynx and carina), whereas irritant receptors, stimulation of which also results in hyperpnea, occur in the more peripheral airways. The trigger mechanism is likely to be *mechanical irritation* due to the deposition of inhaled particles. Of interest is the fact that *receptor reactivity may be enhanced in the presence of pathologic changes in the airways*, e.g., inflammation, and may account for epidemics of *acute febrile episodes associated with asthma* reported, for instance, by grain handlers, in association with the contamination of grain by bacterial toxins. Similar episodes have been described in cotton weavers.

In addition, inhaled organic materials may evoke *airway reactions on an immunologic basis*, and reactions may be immediate (within minutes), late (within the hour), delayed (within hours), nocturnal (following exposure), and even recurrent nocturnal (on subsequent nights without subsequent exposure) (see Ch. 344). *In the individual subject the mechanism underlying an airway response* will be determined not only by his *immunologic reactivity* (atopic status and probably also nonspecific airway reactivity), and *nature of the exposure* (in particular, whether there has been a previous sensitizing contact with the offending material), but also by the *dose of inhaled material* (heavy doses appear to be capable of provoking immune reaction in nonatopic individuals), as well as the *particle size distribution* (which will influence the site of deposition). More than one type of reaction may occur in the same individual so that it is not always possible clinically to determine the mechanism(s) responsible in a particular patient.

For a detailed discussion of the mechanisms, as well as the diagnosis, treatment, and management of the patient with airways reactions (asthma) of an immunologic nature attributed to the inhalation of organic material, the reader is referred to Ch. 344. Indeed, the list of respirable organic particles capable of producing asthma in the atopic individual is virtually limitless and includes not only those generated in daily living but also the wide variety of others generated by industrial and commercial enterprises. It is the relatively *heavy exposure* to the latter of *large numbers of individuals together in a workplace* that has directed attention to the often widespread occurrence of *asthma-like reactions in nonatopic individuals* and resulted in clarification of the nonimmunologic nature of their response, the subject for consideration here.

Two such exposures, recognized and studied over the last decade, are mentioned above under Examples. Reactions to these occupational exposures occur usually within months of first exposure in the case of the enzymes, but often only after years in the case of *Thuja plicata*. The nonatopic individual is as much at risk as the atopic individual, with up to 50 per cent of workers in some plants being affected. In the case of *detergent workers who are atopic*, bronchial provocation tests invariably elicit a dual response, i.e., immediate and late (within hours), attributed to Type I (IgE-mediated) and Type III (precipitin-mediated) hypersensitivity, respectively. In *nonatopic workers* (usually the majority of the factory personnel), the immediate effects appear to be on a nonimmunologic basis, but there is some evidence that the late effects are precipitin mediated and may involve the alveoli as well (see Ch. 344). Skin reactions are positive in about half the workers, but do not distinguish the symptomatic from the nonsymptomatic.

CLINICAL MANIFESTATIONS.   In sensitized workers, symptoms follow exposure within minutes and include chest tightness, cough, and wheezing, with audible rhonchi. Without bronchodilators, the symptoms subside slowly over about four hours, to be followed by the development of *dyspnea, wheezing,* and *rhonchi,* and the general symptoms of headache, malaise, and muscle pains at about six hours. *Nocturnal exacerbations of wheezing* are also characteristic and have been attributed to inhibition of endogenous regulatory mechanisms, and their association with a daytime occupational exposure can easily be missed. There is no present evidence of serious and permanent lung damage, but the manufacture of these detergents is too recent to be certain that such effects may not occur, particularly because animal exposures, admittedly to much higher doses, have produced diffuse emphysema. The use (as opposed to the manufacture) of enzyme detergents may on occasion pose a risk, but probably only in the atopic individual, and the risk is probably less when the enzyme component is added in granular rather than powder form to the washing powder. A case of chronic granulomatous lung disease attributed to the inhalation of cedar sawdust has been reported.

TREATMENT AND PREVENTION.   Sensitized individuals should be removed from exposure promptly once the diagnosis of an immunologically mediated airways reaction is established, but it may take several weeks for symptoms to disappear completely. However, since some 50 per cent of exposed workers appear to become reactive in many instances, control *must* be environmental. Improvements in plant housekeeping, including changes in production techniques and dust control measures, have successfully reduced the frequency of acute effects in a number of plants. In addition, coating the enzyme particles to increase their size (from 0.5 to 1.0 mm) reduces the chance that they will be inhaled into smaller airways. However, complacency is not justified in the detergent industry until more is known about long-term outcome of exposure, even to low levels.

Biological effects of proteolytic enzyme detergents (report of a symposium). Thorax, 31:621, 1977.

Nadel, J. A.: Parasympathetic nervous control of airway smooth muscle. Ann. N.Y. Acad. Sci., 221:99, 1974.

Seaton, A.: Occupational asthma. *In* Morgan, W. K. C., and Seaton, A. (eds.): Occupational Lung Diseases. Philadelphia, W. B. Saunders Company, 1975, p. 251.

348.12. AIRWAY OBSTRUCTION (EVENTUALLY CHRONIC) DUE TO ORGANIC PARTICLES

EXAMPLES.   Examples include *byssinosis* in association with the processing of *cotton* (particularly spinning), *flax,*

and *soft hemp dusts; jute* may be implicated; sisal probably is not.

CLINICAL MANIFESTATIONS.   An acute response to cotton dust may occur at first exposure. This type of response appears to occur in the atopic subject only, is almost certainly mediated through the subject's immune system, and may be very severe. However, this is not what is meant by *byssinosis,* a term reserved for the symptom complex described below which usually develops only after a number of years' exposure, and its appearance is unrelated to the subject's atopic status, with the nonatopic individual as much at risk as the atopic one. The diagnosis is made on the basis of a characteristic symptom pattern in a subject with *cough, tightness in the chest,* and *breathlessness,* occurring at first only occasionally on the first day of the working week (Grade 1/2), then regularly on Monday morning (Grade 1), then persisting beyond Monday (Grade 2), and finally, after several years, persisting throughout the week (Grade 3), when it is indistinguishable from nonindustrial chronic obstructive lung disease. There are no specific radiologic changes. Attack rates may reach over 90 per cent of exposed populations; a family history of atopy, with hypersensitivity to inhaled histamine, is unusual, and immediate skin reactions to cotton dust are infrequent — all observations in favor of a nonimmunologic mechanism to explain the airway reactions. The only host factor which appears important is cigarette smoking, which increases the risk and severity of the disease. The nonsymptomatic worker generally has normal pulmonary function; he may react to exposure with small shift decreases in tests reflecting major airway status such as FEV_1 and forced expiratory flow rates, or he may not (see Fig. 4). By contrast, the worker with the *Monday morning dyspnea of byssinosis* is likely to have lower spirometric values than his nonsymptomatic counterpart, and exposure usually results in more marked effects on FEV_1 and on the forced expiratory flow rates, particularly toward the end of expiration, as well as effects on residual volume and (less consistently) closing volumes, with, on occasion, arterial hypoxemia suggesting a response in peripheral as well as central airways. The airway effects can be improved by

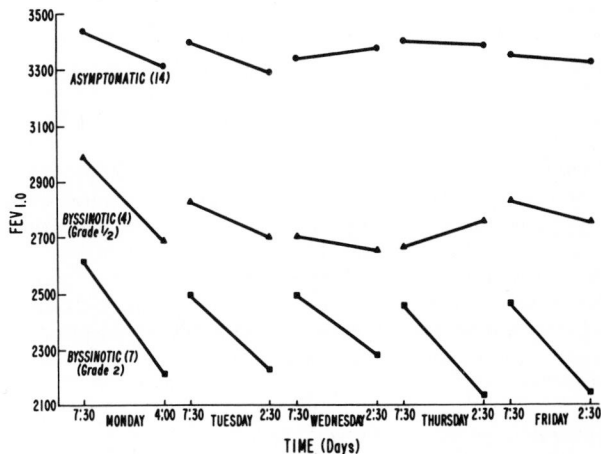

Figure 4.   The pattern of physiologic response of exposure to cotton dust; $FEV_{1.0}$ during a five-day working week in 25 carders in a textile plant. (Courtesy of Dr. J. A. Merchant, Director, Appalachian Laboratory for Occupational Safety and Health, NIOSH, Morgantown, W. Va. Reproduced from Ann. N.Y. Acad. Sci., 221:39, 1974.)

isoproterenol inhalation. Antihistaminic drugs may also improve the flow rates in byssinosis without necessarily affording subjective relief, a finding pointing to the probable importance of small airway involvement. Pretreatment with orciprenaline, antihistamines, and ascorbic acid appears to diminish the biologic response to cotton dust.

PATHOGENESIS AND MECHANISMS. Despite the many studies and the variety of approaches used, the mechanism underlying the airway reactions in byssinosis is not fully understood. The hypothesis that the reactions are nonspecific, the result of stimulation of cough and/or irritant receptors, is no longer tenable. There is evidence to support the view that some fraction of the offending dusts (probably the protein fraction) causes the nonantigenic release of histamine and perhaps of other pharmacologically active substances; these reduce the caliber of large and/or small airways, the site of action perhaps being related to dust size and site of maximal deposition. Whether the histamine release is entirely nonantigenic, as originally proposed, or whether there is an antigenic component to the reaction (e.g., a Type III or Arthus reaction to a condensed polyphenol derived from the cotton plant), as recently proposed, has not been determined. Information on the long-term effects comes from published autopsy reports, the largest series being 43 patients compensated for byssinosis in the United Kingdom, in over half of whom no emphysema was noted. All lungs showed heavy dust pigmentation, but there was no excess fibrosis, granulomas were not noted, and vasculature was not remarkable. Mucous gland hyperplasia in the lobar bronchi suggests this as the site of major involvement rather than the smaller ones. In addition, occasional "ferruginous" bodies, more rounded than the usual asbestos body, were noted, containing what was assumed to be cotton fibers. There is a single report of extensive fibrosis with plasma cell infiltration, suggesting an immunologic background for the disease in that particular case, but this does not appear to be the rule.

EPIDEMIOLOGY AND PROGNOSIS. Attack rates of byssinosis vary widely, and are thought to relate to the *quality of the cotton* (being very low when high quality cotton is processed), to the *care with which it is picked* (there is some evidence that the active component is in the bracts), and usually, though not invariably, to the *environmental levels of cotton dust*. In addition, the jobs of carding and stripping carry a higher risk. In some instances plant modernization and air conditioning have even led to increased environmental dust. Reported rates for Egyptian workers vary from 0 to 90 per cent; for Swedish, Dutch, and British workers, about 50 per cent; and for American workers, up to 30 per cent (it has been estimated that at present there are 20,000 American workers with byssinosis, and this does not take into account those already retired). A study of retired rural Spanish workers shows a high prevalence of chronic disease. There are no data on the rate and inevitability of progression from Grade I (essentially reversible) to Grade III (essentially irreversible) disease. However, it is not insignificant and annual decrements of FEV_1 up to over 100 ml have been reported. Indeed, the recognition of byssinosis resulted from the observation of increased mortality and morbidity rates for cardiovascular and respiratory disease in certain Lancashire cotton workers.

PREVENTION. Present efforts to control byssinosis are directed toward dust control by means of environmental engineering, and its success depends on the accuracy with which it is possible to estimate the dust levels which constitute risk. *Reprocessing the cotton* by autoclaving has been found to diminish by ten-fold the incidence of the biologic response. Thus dust control of the future may well be a source intervention as envisaged many years ago by Schilling. Medical aspects of prevention include a *pre-employment examination* (to eliminate those with pre-existing lung disease and those who show a marked response to dust) and *regular medical surveillance* to detect reactors and, if feasible, relocate them in a nonexposed job. Indeed, this may be one of the few industrial exposures in which progression to chronic disease may be halted by removal from exposure at any early clinical stage of the disease.

Bouhuys, A., Gilson, J. C., and Schilling, R. S. F.: Byssinosis in the textile industry. Arch. Environ. Health, 21:475, 1970.

Edwards, C., McCartney, J., Rooke, G., and Ward, F.: The pathology of the lungs in byssinotics. Thorax, 30:612, 1975.

Merchant, J. A., Lumsden, J. C., Kilburn, K. H., O'Fallon, W. M., Copeland, K., Germino, V. H., McKenzie, W. N., Baucom, D., Currin, P., and Stilman, J.: Intervention studies of cotton steaming to reduce biological effects of cotton dust. Br. J. Industr. Med., 31:261, 1974.

Morgan, W. K. C.: Byssinosis and related conditions. *In* Morgan, W. K. C., and Seaton, A. (eds.): Occupational Lung Diseases. Philadelphia, W. B. Saunders Company, 1975, p. 251.

348.13. INTERSTITIAL (LIPOID) PNEUMONIA

EXAMPLES. Those affected have *inhaled vaporized mineral oil*, e.g., while oilspraying (usually *occupational exposures)*, or while smoking tobacco (blackfat tobacco smokers' lung).

PATHOGENESIS AND MECHANISM. *Aspiration of oil in liquid form* into the lungs is associated with *acute reactions* such as hemorrhagic bronchopneumonia if the *oil is irritant* (usually the case if it contains animal fats), and with more *insidious reactions leading to chronic disease* in the case of the more *bland mineral oils*. Localization of such chronic disease to a zone or lobe is usual, and is attributed to the influence of gravity at the time of the aspiration. When chronic reactions result from *aspiration of mineral oil in vaporized form*, e.g., in association with its industrial use in cleaning aircraft parts, they tend to be more generalized in distribution, and may pose a much more series threat to health, as revealed by a recent investigation in Guyana. Here an unusually high prevalence of diffuse interstitial pulmonary fibrosis in older individuals, recognized for at least 25 to 30 years, has now been shown to be due to a chronic interstitial lipoid pneumonia, the consequence of many years of smoking blackfat tobacco. Blackfat tobacco is unusual in that certain oils are added to the leaf during processing, and smoking causes these to distil over into the lungs. The pathology (based on three postmortem lung biopsies) is in keeping with published reports on aspiration lipoid pneumonia. Thus in the early stages the lipid is present in the alveolar phagocytes, lying free in alveoli or in collections in the interstitium in a peribronchiolar or subpleural location where they evoke first a cellular and eventually (if the dose is large) a collagenous response, with lesions resembling those of liquid paraffin granulomas. The end result is a diffuse interstitial fibrosis and vasculitis, with deposits of lipid and black material in the walls of blood vessels and in the interstitium. The absence of any marked inflammatory reaction was in keeping with previous evidence that mineral oil is comparatively bland in its effect on lung tissue. It was possible to exclude hypersensitivity to the suspected agent, teichoic acid, and extrinsic allergic alveolitis as the background of the chronic interstitial fibrosis in the Guyana study.

CLINICAL MANIFESTATIONS. Localized disease may be asymptomatic and discovered by chance on a routine chest roentgenogram. When disease is diffuse, as in the Guyana series, symptoms include cough, dyspnea, and rather striking weight loss, with eventually pulmonary heart disease. Basal crepitations are characteristic, and wheezing is unusual except during superimposed infection. Radiologic and functional changes are those of diffuse interstitial fibrosis, except in the Guyana series, in which the function profile was obstructive rather than restrictive, perhaps because of the association with another inhaled pollutant, tobacco smoke. The finding of fat droplets in macrophages in the sputum is evidence of exposure, not disease.

TREATMENT, EPIDEMIOLOGY, AND PREVENTION. There is some evidence that x-ray changes associated with the aspiration of mineral oil of short duration (months, not years), are reversible on steroids. Presumably this occurs when the tissue reaction is primarily cellular rather than collagenous. Thus this form of treatment certainly merits consideration in the patient with recent occupational exposure to vaporized mineral oil. Once diffuse fibrosis has developed, however, treatment is essentially palliative, no different from that of other chronic interstitial lung diseases. In the Guyana series, giving up the smoking of blackfat tobacco was no guarantee that symptoms would not develop in the future. The steady decline in blackfat tobacco smoking in Guyana suggests that this local health problem is also on the decline. However, *recognition that inhaled additives to tobacco* can produce *long-term effects* of a *low-grade inflammatory type* on the lungs is of great importance to physicians the world over who are concerned with the health effects of tobacco smoking.

Fraser, R. G., and Paré, J. A. P.: Diagnosis of Diseases of the Chest, Vol. II. Philadelphia, W. B. Saunders Company, 1970, p. 964.

Miller, G. I., Ashcraft, M. T., Beadrell, H. M. S., Wagner, J. C., and Pepys, J.: The lipoid pneumonia of black fat tobacco smokers in Guyana. Quart. J. Med., 160:457, 1971.

348.14. ASTHMA-LIKE REACTIONS TO CHEMICAL AGENTS

EXAMPLES. Those affected include workers with *toluene di-isocyanate* (TDI) and *other isocyanates* (e.g., di-isocyanato diphenyl methane, [MDI]) used in the application of certain lacquers and resins and in the manufacture of polyurethane foams for cushioning, insulation, and soft toys; consumers using do-it-yourself polyurethane; and *cable jointers* using certain aluminum soldering flux. *Platinosis* (describing rhinorrhea, asthma, and urticaria) results from exposure to complex platinum salts in refineries.

PATHOGENESIS AND MECHANISMS. From carefully controlled occupational-type provocation tests monitored by measurements of forced expiratory volumes, it has been shown that immediate, late, and dual asthmatic reactions occur in workers sensitized to the chemical vapors, fumes, and dusts listed above. These reactions may be mechanically (due to irritation) or, less commonly, immunologically mediated. The presence of reaginic and precipitating antibodies against *platinum salts* and against *soldering flux* in symptomatic subjects suggests an immunologic basis (Types I and III allergy) for reactions to these materials, and others may well come to light in the future. However, it has not been possible to date to show an allergic mechanism for *TDI sensitivity*, in keeping with the clinical observations that large numbers of those exposed have symptoms but are not atopic. Nor is skin reactivity to TDI correlated with respiratory responsiveness, which appears to be dose related. An alternative possibility is TDI interaction with specific IgE antibodies localized to the respiratory tract, with release of pharmacologic mediators. In addition, there is some evidence that TDI may increase bronchial reactivity. These reactions, which may follow exposure to very low doses, should be distinguished from the well recognized *irritant effects of the same chemicals in higher doses* and other chemicals discussed subsequently. Thus sensitization to isocyanate vapors may occur at very low exposure levels (0.002 parts per million) which is well below the present threshold limit value of 0.02 ppm, which is again below the level at which the irritant effects of isocyanates are seen. Even when measured environmental levels do not exceed 0.02 ppm, an excess fall in expiratory flow rates in the long term, linked to the occurrence of acute effects, has been shown in one study; however, this may be related to factors peculiar to that exposure and has not been shown in other studies.

CLINICAL MANIFESTATIONS. Symptoms (cough, chest pain, and tightness suggesting asthma which may be immediate and/or late and often nocturnal) develop after periods varying from one week to several months after first exposure and, if possible, should be distinguished from those of high dose irritation, of which eye, nose, and throat irritation are the most common. Decreases in forced expiratory volumes and flow rates, immediate, late, or delayed, accompany the symptoms. Symptoms subside after removal from exposure, and function may return to normal within days or weeks. However, re-exposure regularly results in recurrence, often more violent. Most exposed persons show some reduction in expiratory flow rates during working hours, a change eliminated by the oral administration of an aminophylline compound.

DIAGNOSIS, TREATMENT, AND PREVENTION. Diagnosis depends on a high degree of suspicion, particularly when symptoms occur predominantly at night, and can be confirmed using carefully controlled occupational-type provocation tests as suggested by Pepys. These should be carried out only under hospital supervision with monitoring of forced expiratory flow tests, together with observation of the effects of isoproterenol and disodium cromoglycate on the reactions. Objective demonstration of sensitization is important, particularly for platinum salts and solder flux where an immunologic mechanism is likely, because it may be necessary to advise removal from exposure with potential financial and other hardships for the worker.

Since TDI sensitivity is rarely immunologically mediated, diagnosis in an individual exposed in a plant with other workers must be brought to the attention of the appropriate authority, because control should clearly be at the environmental and not the personal level. Thus the variation in the number of sensitized workers, ranging from 4 to 100 per cent, is most likely a reflection of plant housekeeping. Nor can satisfactory environmental control be assumed on the basis of area monitoring, which does not necessarily correlate directly with monitoring by personal sampler, and it should be supplemented by vigilant health surveillance of the working population with prompt action when cases are detected.

Butcher, B. T., Jones, R. N., O'Neil, C. E., Glindmeyer, H. W., Diem, J. E., Venkatram, D., Weill, H., and Salvaggio, J.: Longitudinal study of workers employed in the manufacture of toluene-diisocyanate. Am. Rev. Respir. Dis., 116:411, 1977.

Pepys, J., and Hutchcroft, B. J.: Bronchial provocation tests in etiologic diagnosis and analysis of asthma. Am. Rev. Respir. Dis., 112:829, 1975.

Peters, J. M., and Murphy, R. L. H.: Pulmonary toxicity of isocyanates. Ann. Intern. Med., 73:654, 1970.

348.15. ACUTE CHEMICAL BRONCHITIS AND/OR PNEUMONITIS

EXAMPLES. *Chemical agents with principal effects on airways,* with industries or occupations at risk for exposure, *include sulfur dioxide,* SO_2 (in the manufacture of pulp and refrigerators); *ammonia,* NH_3 (in the production of fertilizers, refrigerators, explosives, and plastics); *chlorine,* Cl_2 (in the production of alkalis, bleaches, and disinfectants); *phosgene,* Cl_2CO (in the chemical industry and in fire-fighting); and *hydrogen fluoride,* HF (in etching and metal refining).

Chemical agents with principal effects on both airways and pulmonary parenchyma, with occupations or industries at risk for exposure, *include osmium tetroxide,* OsO_4 (in alloy production); *vanadium pentoxide,* V_2O_5 (in the chemical industry); *cadmium oxide* (welding and ore smelting); *chromates* (in electroplating); *zinc chloride* (dry cell manufacture); and *trimellitic anhydride* (used to harden epoxy resins).

Neither of these lists is exhaustive, and they should be supplemented by consulting specialized texts.

PATHOGENESIS AND MECHANISMS. Reaction to chemical agents, usually inhaled in the form of fumes and/or vapors, tends to be primarily at the level of the airways for agents with a high solubility in biologic fluids, and further down the bronchial tree involving the parenchyma for agents with lower solubility. Thus when compared to CO_2, the most soluble of the physiologic gases (56.7 vols per cent in water at 37°C at 1 atmosphere), those whose effects are primarily on airways have a much greater solubility: equivalent values for SO_2, Cl_2 and NH_3 being 280, 257, and 139 vols per cent, respectively. Accidental inhalation of high concentrations results in rapid solution in the mucous membranes of the upper airways with the formation of irritant compounds, e.g., H_2SO_3 from SO_2, NH_4OH from NH_3, HCl from Cl_2. The initial irritation causing *bronchorrhea* is rapidly followed by sloughing and a *frank necrotizing bronchitis.* In fatal cases, the bronchial mucosa may be stripped down to the cartilage. If exposure is prolonged or unduly heavy, the lower respiratory tract becomes exposed, with the development of an *acute chemical pulmonary edema.* Recovery may be complete. However, residual mucosal scars and submucosal thickening are not uncommon, particularly if the mucosal sloughs were deep and secondary infection prominent. Acute chemical irritation may also result from the *aspiration of vomited or regurgitated material high in HCl content,* an event more common in the frail and elderly than is generally supposed, or in relation to blunting of the gag reflex as in anesthesia, head injuries, and alcohol-

ic or other intoxications. If the aspirate is chiefly water or saline in small amounts, absorption is quick and the consequences usually slight.

CLINICAL MANIFESTATIONS. When exposure to a chemical irritant is heavy, clinical manifestations are invariably immediate, the patient is alerted to his exposure, and he makes every effort to remove himself therefrom. *Conjunctivitis, irritation* and *burning* in the *mucosa* of the mouth and throat, *laryngitis, laryngospasm,* and *difficulty in breathing* are in keeping with the usual site of damage, i.e., upper respiratory tract, and coarse *rhonchi* are a characteristic physical finding, often with profound *mucorrhea,* which may be bloodstained. *Cough* is usually also a prominent symptom, although it is believed that the cough receptors are less responsive to chemical stimuli than are the irritant receptors. More profound *dyspnea* usually implies alveolar involvement resulting from either chemical edema or aspiration of bronchial sloughs. These complications can frequently be suspected from chest roentgenograms and may result in profound impairment of pulmonary blood-gas exchange with *severe arterial hypoxemia* and a low arterial CO_2 tension. Nausea, vomiting, and stupor may complicate the picture.

If the patient survives the acute event, complete recovery is usual. However, some patients may be left with chronic bronchitis or saccular bronchiectasis or both, sometimes of considerable severity, with residual effects on pulmonary function.

Chronic irritation from long-term exposure to low doses, e.g., SO_2, as in city air pollution, Cl_2, as in chlorine plants, may perhaps be more important in terms of community health, particularly in relation to the etiology of chronic obstructive lung disease.

TREATMENT. Recognition, the most important aspect of treatment, poses no difficulty for the acute accidental heavy exposure, but it seems likely that many exposures producing less dramatic effects go unrecognized in the complex modern industrial processes. These are more likely to be identified if a substantial number of individuals are affected, e.g., the outbreak of upper and lower respiratory tract disease in a Wisconsin rubber tire plant when a new thermosetting resin, containing resorcinol and a trimere of methylene aminoacetonitrile, was introduced into the tire formulation. Over 200 workers in all were affected, and lung biopsy revealed evidence of interstitial fibrosis as well as chronic peribronchiolar and perivascular inflammation. This shows that an exhaustive occupational history is an essential part of the investigation of all cases of idiopathic pulmonary fibrosis.

Acute chemical bronchitis and *acute chemical pulmonary edema* are *medical emergencies.* In the acute phase, survival depends on maintaining airway patency and adequate oxygenation. To aspirate sloughs, it may be necessary to employ intubation, lavage with saline, using modest amounts only (10 ml at a single flush), and even bronchoscopy. Controlled oxygen administration is usually necessary, and frequently must be supplemented with positive pressure respiration, assisted in mild cases, controlled in the severe ones. Corticosteroids, thought to modify the acute inflammatory reaction at the gas-exchange surface, should always be given in the presence of pulmonary edema and indeed are recommended by some in all cases of exposure on a prophylactic basis. Heavy initial doses should be reduced as the clinical picture improves. Infection should be controlled by the use of antimicrobial drugs.

DoPico, G. A., Rankin, R., Chosy, L. W., Reddan, W. O., Barbee, R. A., Gee, B., and Dickie, H. A.: Respiratory tract disease from thermosetting resins. Ann. Intern. Med., 83:177, 1975.

Fraser, R. F., and Paré, J. A. P.: Diagnosis of Diseases of the Chest, Vol. II. Philadelphia, W. B. Saunders Company, 1970, p. 948.

Hamilton, A., and Hardy, H. L.: Industrial Toxicology. Section Three: Chemical Compounds. Acton, Mass., Publishing Sciences Group, 1974, p. 203.

Walton, M.: Industrial ammonia gassing. Br. J. Industr. Med., 30:78, 1973.

348.16. CHEMICAL PULMONARY EDEMA

EXAMPLES. Chemical pulmonary edema can result from exposure to *oxides of nitrogen* in freshly filled silos *(silo-filler's disease)*; welding in poorly ventilated spaces; misfires in blasting operations carried out in closed spaces (e.g., mines); burning of N_2-containing materials in closed spaces; *exposure to phosgene* after its liberation from many chlorinated substances, e.g., carbon tetrachloride in fire extinguishers; or *accidental ingestion of the herbicide paraquat*.

PATHOGENESIS AND MECHANISMS. The immediate clinical effects of exposure to the oxides of nitrogen and phosgene may be mild, but a severe, chemical pulmonary edema, often fatal, may develop after a *delay of several hours to several days*. The physicochemical processes underlying this delay are not fully understood, but changes in permeability and liquid transport appear to follow the direct injury to pulmonary alveolar and capillary cells by the inhaled agents, and the edema fluid is high in protein content. If the acute event is not immediately fatal, healing by fibrosis may lead to the development of *bronchiolitis fibrosa obliterans*, usually four to eight weeks after initial exposure, often with a fatal result. Autopsy studies show widespread organization of exudates, primarily located in the terminal bronchioles; atelectasis is not seen, however, presumably because of the collateral ventilation now recognized to be extensive in man.

Acute chemical pulmonary edema of delayed onset (one to three days) may also follow the *accidental ingestion of the herbicide paraquat* (1,1'-dimethyl-4,4'-dipyridilium), a common constituent of commercial weed-killers. Thus the acute effects of this poison, which also include acute oral, esophageal, hepatic, and renal damage, become evident only after a delay of several days, i.e., after the peak blood levels and at a time when most of the material has been excreted. These characteristics have earned it the name of the "hit and run" poison, and once the pulmonary damage starts, it invariably runs a relentless course to death within weeks from respiratory failure caused by a *diffuse progressive pulmonary fibrosis* and replacement of gas-exchanging tissue by cystic changes. Its mechanism of action is unknown, but it has been suggested that the primary action is to inactivate or depress formation of surfactant.

CLINICAL MANIFESTATIONS. Immediate effects of exposure to the oxides of nitrogen and phosgene, which may include cough, chest irritation, and sputum, are often so mild that the victim may even fail to report to the first-aid post, only to return from hours to several days later with the symptoms, signs, and chest roentgenogram of *acute, severe, pulmonary edema*. Hence it is reasonable to suggest observation in hospital for 48 hours after possible exposures (e.g., for firefighters who have been inside burning buildings), perhaps even giving steroid

therapy if suspicion of exposure is strong. In the mild case of edema, symptoms may escape attention, changes on the chest film at the most may be equivocal, and the diagnosis depends on the finding of coarse rales, sometimes lasting over a short period only, with a transient hypoxemia. Clinical management has been discussed above; in cases of frank, severe edema, steroid therapy should probably be prolonged for six to eight weeks to cover the period when the subacute complication of bronchiolitis obliterans is likely to develop. This complication, probably avoidable if steroid therapy is given early, should be suspected when symptoms recur or appear at three to six weeks, and generally responds to steroid therapy.

Management of a patient known to have ingested paraquat should include heroic measures to prevent absorption. In laboratory animals bentylol and/or Fuller's earth by mouth has been shown to inactivate the material more effectively than charcoal. Forced diuresis and hemodialysis are recommended once blood levels have risen. There is some evidence that corticosteroids may be effective in the treatment of the pulmonary edema, and that O_2 therapy should be used with the utmost caution, experimental work indicating that it potentiates the action of the poison.

EPIDEMIOLOGY. Large-scale heavy exposure to, for instance, oxides of nitrogen occurs only in relation to mass disasters, e.g., in the Cleveland clinic fire in 1929 owing to the burning of stored x-ray film, and in the Cocoanut Grove fire in Boston in 1943 owing to the burning of nitrogen-containing plastics. Many modern plastics no longer contain nitrogen. However, in most fires involving domestic buildings in which wood is used, circumstances exist in which these fumes could be evolved, and three or four cases are seen annually in most city hospitals.

Fraser, R. F., and Paré, J. A. P.: Diagnosis of Diseases of the Chest, Vol. II. Philadelphia, W. B. Saunders Company, 1970, p. 948.

348.17. RADIATION

Increased use of x-irradiation in the treatment of cancer of the breast and of various intrathoracic organs led to the recognition that the lungs themselves may be affected by this procedure. *Acute changes* may come on within weeks of the onset of treatment up to six months after its cessation and possibly much longer, but rarely manifest themselves clinically while treatment is in progress. The initial damage is believed to occur in the capillary endothelium, which becomes necrotic and eventually collagenized; this is associated with an alveolar cellular reaction, followed by desquamation and exudation of protein-rich material, which itself is followed in some instances by hyaline membrane formation. Focal necrosis of the bronchial mucosa may develop as a result of damage to capillary endothelium with subsequent necrosis and vascular occlusion. These changes may resolve or go on to loss of lung volume, sometimes of marked degree, occurring rather suddenly, and usually ascribed to fibrosis, shrinkage, and hyalinization, particularly if there has been infection. Studies in animals, however, suggest that the loss of volume may, on occasion, be due to atrophy and that the hyalinization may be in part due to autohypersensitivity, the consequence of new cell antigens formed as a result of the ionizing radiation.

There may be no clinical manifestations of *radiation pneumonitis* even in the face of definite radiologic changes. Likewise, lung damage detectable by pulmonary function tests may occur in the absence of roentgenographic changes. The most common symptom is a persistent, hacking dry cough. Fever, some dyspnea, and weakness may be seen, and the symptoms of radiation esophagitis are common. On physical examination the effects of radiation on the skin of the thorax are usually evident; rales and a friction rub may be found. The chest film characteristically reveals regional or diffuse haziness usually corresponding to the area irradiated, and pulmonary function tests indicate a restrictive pattern. Spontaneous remission over weeks is frequent. Recommended therapy includes steroids (to lessen the chances of healing by fibrosis) and, less commonly, anticoagulants (which may lessen the ischemic effects of small-vessel thrombosis commonly seen at autopsy). When *radiation fibrosis* supervenes, clinical presentation will depend on how much functioning lung tissue is lost and on the function in the remaining lung. In severe cases the loss of lung volume is striking, with obliteration of all lung architecture and evidence of traction on the hilum and mediastinum. Respiratory failure, pulmonary hypertension, and right heart failure may all follow.

Some authors suggest that there is a parenchymal reaction to ionizing radiation of the thorax in 100 per cent of cases so exposed, that some degree of pneumonitis is common if not invariable, though symptoms occur in a smaller number (estimated at 10 per cent), and that progression to radiation fibrosis is rare. Factors thought to affect the attack rate include total dose (broadly speaking, there is a dose relationship but with considerable individual variation), the *time over which it is given* (the longer the time, the less likely an unfavorable reaction), and the technique of application. Clinically important reactions are unusual at total doses below 2000 rads and invariable above 6000 rads. The age of the patient, the chest wall thickness, the condition of the lung before treatment, and the presence of complicating disease may also be important. Individual factors remain to be identified, however, since identical doses can be harmless to one person and cause a severe reaction in another.

Gross, N. J.: Review: Pulmonary effect of radiation therapy. Ann. Intern. Med., 86:81, 1977.

349. CYSTS AND NEOPLASMS OF THE LUNG

Leo F. Black

349.1. CYSTIC LESIONS OF THE LUNG, BULLOUS DISEASE OF THE LUNG, AND UNILATERAL HYPERLUCENT LUNG

Classification of different types of cysts in the lungs is confusing because there is considerable variation in the definition of the terms cysts, blebs, bullae, and pneumatoceles. For this presentation, cysts will be considered to be abnormal air-containing spaces lined with bronchial epithelium. Blebs are collections of air within the layers of the visceral pleura. Blebs are formed by air that ruptures out of alveoli along the lobular septa and bronchovascular sheaths and dissects toward the pleura within the connective tissue framework. Bullae are emphysematous spaces at the pleural surface or within the lung parenchyma. Pneumatocele is a term sometimes used to describe a bullous lesion. At other times, this term is used more specifically to describe an intraparenchymal air collection caused by obstruction of small airways by an inflammatory process. This most commonly occurs with staphylococcal pneumonia in children. Infections in the lung parenchyma due to many bacteria, fungi, and parasites may be associated with abnormal air spaces, which are generally referred to as cavities rather than cysts, although they may have a similar appearance on the thoracic roentgenogram.

BRONCHOGENIC CYSTS

Bronchopulmonary foregut malformations are a group of developmental abnormalities that include bronchogenic cysts, enterogenous cysts, and bronchopulmonary sequestrations. Bronchogenic cysts may be located in the mediastinum or within the lung parenchyma. The cysts are thin walled, are lined with ciliated columnar epithelium, and usually are filled with mucus. They may contain all the elements normally found in the tracheobronchial tree such as cartilage, mucous glands, fibrous tissue, and smooth muscle. The respiratory epithelial lining may be destroyed when a cyst is infected, and in this instance it may be difficult to distinguish a congenital cyst from an acquired air-containing space.

In infants and young children, some authors describe congenital alveolar cysts that are considered to develop at the embryologic stage of alveolar formation. These cysts are usually peripheral and multiloculated. Both these and bronchogenic cysts may be asymptomatic, or they may produce coughing, wheezing, and respiratory distress by expanding and compressing the tracheobronchial tree and the surrounding lung parenchyma. They also may be associated with recurrent pulmonary infections. Treatment is surgical resection with conservation of as much normal pulmonary tissue as possible.

In adults, bronchogenic cysts are frequently asymptomatic and are discovered incidentally on the thoracic roentgenogram. They may, however, produce chest discomfort and be associated with recurrent pulmonary infections. The diagnosis of a bronchogenic cyst may be suspected on the basis of clinical findings and the findings on the thoracic roentgenogram. These cysts, when intrapulmonary, are most often in the lower lobes and present as solitary masses. If they have been infected and a bronchial communication has developed, then an air-fluid level may be visible. Bronchogenic cysts in the mediastinum may present as masses in the paratracheal, carinal, hilar, or paraesophageal regions on the thoracic roentgenogram. Definite diagnosis frequently cannot be made until thoracotomy. Treatment is surgical resection, with preservation of as much functioning lung tissue as possible.

Hutchin, P.: Congenital cystic disease of the lung. Rev. Surg., 28:79, 1971.

BRONCHOPULMONARY SEQUESTRATION

Bronchopulmonary sequestration is a congenital malformation that arises from accessory budding of the tracheobronchial tree early in its development. Sequestrations may present as masses separate from the lung (extralobar) or may occur within the visceral pleura of a lobe (intralobar).

Extralobar sequestrations represent maldeveloped pulmonary tissue that is enclosed in its own visceral pleura. The arterial supply is from the aorta or one of its branches. Venous drainage is into the systemic circulation. Approximately 90 per cent are on the left side and present as a mass between the lung and the diaphragm; the lesion may also be within the diaphragm or below it. It is frequently associated with an ipsilateral congenital diaphragmatic hernia. Because this type of sequestration has its own pleural covering, infection is unusual. This lesion is usually detected in infancy, and surgical excision is the treatment of choice.

Intralobar sequestration consists of a nonfunctioning portion of lung within the visceral pleura of a lobe. It has poorly developed respiratory structures and may be filled with mucus. The epithelium may be flat or ciliated columnar. The arterial supply is from the aorta or one of its branches, and the venous drainage is into the pulmonary veins. These sequestrations most commonly develop in the lower lobes, especially in the posterior basal segments. If infection has occurred and a bronchial communication has developed, cystic changes with air-fluid levels may be visible on the thoracic roentgenogram. Intralobar sequestrations are frequently not diagnosed until adulthood. They may be detected in asymptomatic patients when a routine thoracic roentgenogram reveals a solid or cystic lesion in the posterior portion of the lower lobes. In some patients, recurrent pulmonary infections are associated with the sequestration. Aortography may aid in diagnosis by demonstrating the abnormal arterial blood supply to the lesion. Treatment is surgical excision.

Heithoff, K. B., Sane, S. M., Williams, H. J., Jarvis, C. J., Carter, J., Kane, P., and Brennom, W.: Bronchopulmonary foregut malformations: A unifying etiological concept. Am. J. Roentgenol., 126:46, 1976.

HONEYCOMB LUNG

This term refers to the presence of multiple small cysts in the lung and is the end result of pulmonary involvement by many diseases, such as interstitial pneumonitis and fibrosis, histiocytosis X, rheumatoid lung, and scleroderma. The fibrotic lungs contain multiple cysts that are formed from dilated bronchi and bronchioles and are lined by columnar or cuboidal epithelium. They are associated with a grossly distorted pulmonary architecture. The cysts may have thickened fibrous walls. Occasionally, rupture into the pleural space produces pneumothorax. Treatment is directed at the underlying disease process responsible for the diffuse pulmonary changes.

BULLOUS DISEASE OF THE LUNG

DEFINITION. Bullous disease of the lung refers to the presence of bullae in the lung, and they may or may not be associated with obstructive airway disease.

PATHOLOGY. Bullae may result from any form of emphysema, including the panacinar, paraseptal, and irregular types. Reid has described several different types of bullae, based on their anatomic characteristics. Type 1 bullae are subpleural, are more common in the upper lobes, have a narrow neck, and represent small units of lung tissue that have become greatly expanded. These tend to occur independent of widespread emphysema and may represent examples of paraseptal or irregular emphysema. Type 2 bullae are subpleural, have a broad neck, and may be associated with panacinar or centrilobular emphysema as well as paraseptal and irregular emphysema. Type 3 bullae represent overdistention of relatively large areas of lung, may affect any lobe, and are located within the lung parenchyma.

CLINICAL MANIFESTATIONS. The symptoms produced by bullae vary greatly. In general, the presence of dyspnea depends on the size of the bullae and the functional status of the remainder of the lung. Bullae also may become infected and produce symptoms related to this. Pneumothorax is another possible complication.

Some patients have bullae in the apical areas of the lung and have no chronic symptoms. These may be discovered incidentally on a thoracic roentgenogram, or they may produce a pneumothorax, which results in acute pain and dyspnea. Another group of patients may have single or multiple bullae in one area of the lung and also have no symptoms unless pneumothorax develops.

Patients with multiple bullae may present with symptoms of chronic obstructive airway disease, such as cough and dyspnea. In them, it is not always easy to determine the relative contribution of the chronic airway disease and the bullae to the dyspnea. In many, the bullae represent emphysematous areas of the lung that are part of the basic problem of chronic obstructive airway disease. Some patients, however, have bilateral bullae demonstrable on the thoracic roentgenogram years before symptoms of chronic bronchitis develop. In such cases, bronchial obstruction secondary to bronchial compression by the bullae may have a role in the development of chronic bronchitis.

DIAGNOSIS. The diagnosis of bullae is usually established on the basis of the thoracic roentgenogram, which reveals single or multiple hyperlucent areas with a decreased vascular pattern. The hyperlucent areas may be bordered by hairline-curved densities representing the walls of the bullae and surrounding compressed lung. When bullae are infected, an air-fluid level may be detected.

Physical examination of the lungs may reveal suppression of breath sounds over the bullous areas if the bullae are large. If the patient has chronic obstructive airway disease, physical findings may include slowing of a forced expiration and generalized suppression of breath sounds.

Angiography and perfusion lung scanning may offer the best indications of the condition of the remaining lung in patients with obvious bullae. Pulmonary function tests reveal variable findings, depending on the size of the bullae and the presence or absence of chronic obstructive airway disease. In general, patients with bullae but no obstructive airway disease have relatively normal pulmonary function until the bullae become very large. The vital capacity may be reduced. The total lung capacity, measured by a gas dilution method, may be increased, normal, or decreased, depending on the degree to which the bullae communicate with the airways. Total lung capacity measured with the body plethysmograph will be increased in patients with large bullae. Expiratory flow rates, such as the one-second forced expiratory volume and the maximal midexpiratory flow rate, are mildly reduced in the presence of large bullae. The diffusing capacity for carbon monoxide will be normal or decreased, depending on the extent of compression of the surrounding lung.

When chronic obstructive airway disease is present in addition to the bullae, pulmonary function tests may reveal a decreased vital capacity, increased total lung capacity, decreased expiratory flow rates, and a decreased diffusing capacity for carbon monoxide. Arterial blood gases may be abnormal depending on the extent of the disease.

TREATMENT. Treatment depends on the symptoms of the patient. Asymptomatic patients with bullae and no accompanying chronic obstructive airway disease require no specific therapy other than periodic follow-up to determine any progressive enlargement of the bullae. When the bullae are large (greater than one third the volume of one lung), resection may be considered when the patient is symptomatic. In the presence of chronic obstructive airway disease, the decision to resect the bullae is often very difficult. Occasionally, a patient will experience considerable benefit from resection of large bullae. Decisions regarding resection should be made only after the patient has been on a medical program for the airway disease and when the course of the disease has been determined by regular follow-up examinations.

When recurrent pneumothorax occurs owing to bullae, abrasion of the pleural space and resection of the bullae are indicated to prevent further recurrences.

Boushy, S. F., Kohen, R., Billig, D. M., and Heiman, M. J.: Bullous emphysema: Clinical, roentgenologic and physiologic study of 49 patients. Dis. Chest. 54:327, 1968.
Pride, N. B., Barter, C. E., and Hugh-Jones, P.: The ventilation of bullae and the effect of their removal on thoracic gas volumes and tests of over-all pulmonary function. Am. Rev. Respir. Dis., 107:83, 1973.
Reid, L.: The Pathology of Emphysema. Chicago, Year Book Medical Publishers, 1967, p. 211.
Thurlbeck, W. M.: Chronic Airflow Obstruction in Lung Disease. Philadelphia, W. B. Saunders Company, 1976.

UNILATERAL HYPERLUCENT LUNG

DEFINITION. Unilateral hyperlucent lung (Swyer-James syndrome, Macleod's syndrome) is characterized by the presence of a hyperlucent lung on the thoracic roentgenogram with a normal or smaller than normal lung volume.

PATHOLOGY AND PATHOGENESIS. The entire lung is characteristically abnormal, although not uniformly involved by the pathologic process. At times, only one lobe may be involved. Morphologically, there is evidence of bronchitis, bronchiolitis, and bronchiolitis obliterans. The patchy involvement allows some ventilation of the involved lung, and pathways of collateral ventilation prevent alveolar collapse. The lung parenchyma frequently shows panacinar emphysema, although sometimes there is minimal parenchymal destruction. The number of alveoli and finer branches of the pulmonary artery are reduced, thus suggesting that hypoplasia of these structures may be secondary to air

way obstruction early in life, preventing the normal growth of these structures. Lower respiratory infections, especially viral, may be the cause of the widespread bronchial and bronchiolar disease. The pulmonary artery on the affected side, when examined at surgery, is larger than it appears on angiography but may be smaller than normal.

CLINICAL MANIFESTATIONS. Patients with this condition may be asymptomatic, and the abnormality is discovered on a routine thoracic roentgenogram. Some of them complain of cough and dyspnea on exertion, whereas others have histories of repeated lower respiratory tract infections.

DIAGNOSIS. Generally, the diagnosis can be established on the basis of the clinical findings and inspiratory and expiratory thoracic roentgenograms. Physical examination reveals decreased excursion of the affected hemithorax. Breath sounds are diminished over the involved lung, and occasionally scattered rales are heard.

The inspiratory thoracic roentgenogram reveals a hyperlucent lung of normal or smaller than normal overall lung volume. The hyperlucency is due to decreased vascular perfusion of the affected lung. The pulmonary artery to the involved lung may appear to be smaller than normal. The vascular markings of the contralateral lung may appear more prominent than normal because most of the pulmonary blood flow goes through the contralateral lung. The expiratory thoracic roentgenogram reveals air trapping in the involved lung and shifting of the mediastinum to the opposite side.

Bronchoscopy reveals the absence of an obstructing lesion in major airways on the affected side. Bronchograms show irregular dilated segmental bronchi that end abruptly or may terminate in small pools or dilations. The peripheral bronchi do not fill with the contrast material.

Radioisotope lung scans reveal decreased ventilation to the involved lung and delayed clearance of the isotope. Perfusion scans reveal reduced to absent pulmonary blood flow to the affected lung. Pulmonary angiograms reveal a small pulmonary artery on the affected side, the peripheral arterial tree is smaller than normal, and the vessels appear to be narrow and attenuated.

Pulmonary function studies reveal variable findings. The vital capacity may be reduced, as may be the expiratory flow rates. The diffusing capacity for carbon monoxide may be normal or reduced. Arterial blood gases may be normal or may reveal hypoxemia at rest or with exercise. Bronchospirometric measurements have shown decreased ventilation and oxygen uptake in the involved lung.

The presence of expiratory air trapping documented by expiratory thoracic roentgenograms differentiates this condition from agenesis of a pulmonary artery and embolic or thrombotic obstruction of a pulmonary artery. Hyperlucency of one lung secondary to partial bronchial obstruction generally is associated with increased lung volume on the affected side. Bronchoscopy is of diagnostic aid in ruling out a bronchial-obstructing lesion.

TREATMENT. Treatment of this condition consists of prompt therapy for respiratory infections. The prognosis is good.

Gottlieb, L. S., and Turner, A. F.: Swyer-James (Macleod's) syndrome: Variations in pulmonary-bronchial arterial blood flow. Chest, 69:62, 1976.

Macleod, W. M.: Abnormal transradiancy of one lung. Thorax, 9:147, 1954.

Swyer, P. R., and James, G. C. W.: A case of unilateral pulmonary emphysema. Thorax, 8:133, 1953.

Weg, J. G., Krumholz, R. A., and Hackleroad, L. E.: Unilateral hyperlucent lung: A physiologic syndrome. Ann. Intern. Med:, 62:675, 1965.

349.2. NEOPLASMS OF THE LUNG

The lung may be the site of many types of neoplasms. Benign tumors such as hamartomas, lipomas, and papillomas occur infrequently compared with malignant tumors. Primary and metastatic malignancies involving the lung are common clinical problems. The classification of primary lung neoplasms by the World Health Organization is shown in Table 1. Groups I through V constitute approximately 90 per cent of the primary lung neoplasms and are commonly designated bronchogenic carcinomas.

BRONCHOGENIC CARCINOMA

DEFINITION. The frequency distribution of the different histologic types of bronchogenic carcinoma varies in several reported series, but in general the incidence is epidermoid carcinoma, 40 to 50 per cent; adenocarcinoma (bronchogenic and bronchiolo-alveolar), 15 to 20 per cent; large cell carcinoma, 15 to 20 per cent; and small cell anaplastic carcinoma, 15 to 20 per cent. Lung cancer is now the leading cause of cancer deaths in men and is the third leading cause of cancer deaths in women, after cancer of the breast and colon. Bronchogenic carcinoma occurs most frequently between the ages of 45 and 75 years, and there is a male-to-female preponderance of about 7:1. However, in the United States, mortality rates from lung cancer are now increasing more rapidly for women than for men, and the sex ratio has started to decline.

ETIOLOGY AND PATHOGENESIS. The major factor in the development of bronchogenic carcinoma is the inhalation of carcinogenic pollutants, especially tobacco smoke, by susceptible hosts. Epidermoid and small cell anaplastic carcinomas have been most closely associated with cigarette smoking. The evolution of changes in the respiratory epithelium related to smoking has received detailed study. Three principal types of changes related to smoking have been described: a loss of cilia, an increase in the number of cell rows, and the presence of atypical cells. Each of these three changes increases with increased amounts of cigarette smoking. Epithelial lesions are much more frequent in cigarette smokers than in pipe and cigar smokers. Eventually, the columnar epithelial lining is replaced by metaplastic squamous epithelium. Subsequently, atypical proliferation, dysplasia, and carcinoma develop. When carcinomatous change is present and located above the basement membrane, the lesion is referred to as carcinoma in situ. Invasive epidermoid carcinoma is the end result of this progression. Studies have shown that ex-smokers have fewer hyperplastic epithelial cells than do current smokers. Ex-smokers also have fewer cells with atypical nuclei than do current smokers, and the number of such cells decreases progressively as the number of years of nonsmoking increases, although they do not reach the level seen in never-smokers. In agreement with these observations is the finding that the incidence of bronchogenic carcinoma decreases in ex-smokers compared with current smokers, although not reaching the incidence level in never-smokers.

Because many smokers do not develop lung cancer, host factors may be important in the development of this disease. Indeed, there is a significant excess mortality from lung cancer among relatives of lung cancer patients that cannot be accounted for by smoking. There appears to be a synergistic interaction between the familial and smoking factors. The nature of this familial influence has not been determined.

An increased incidence of lung cancer has been recognized in association with certain other environmental exposures. Higher mortality rates from lung cancer have been noted in heavily industrialized areas, where air pollution is characterized by elevated concentrations of benzo(a)pyrene and other polynuclear aromatic hydrocarbons. The increased incidence of lung cancer in asbestos workers is well documented. The frequency of lung cancer has been reported to be eight times the expected value in insulation workers employed in that industry for more than 20 years. It is of interest that lung cancer develops rarely in nonsmoking asbestos workers. The effects of smoking and asbestos exposure appear to be multiplicative rather than additive, thus resulting in the increased frequency of lung cancer in this group. The relative risk for the development of cancer also depends on the type of exposure and the type of asbestos fiber involved. Most, but not all, patients in whom lung cancer develops relative to asbestos exposure also have evidence of pulmonary fibrosis due to exposure to asbestos fibers.

Workers in uranium mines have an increased incidence of lung cancer which cannot be explained solely

TABLE 1. World Health Organization Classification of Primary Lung Neoplasms

I. Epidermoid carcinomas
II. Small cell anaplastic carcinomas
  1. Fusiform cell type
  2. Polygonal cell type
  3. Lymphocyte-like ("oat-cell") type
  4. Others
III. Adenocarcinomas
  1. Bronchogenic
    a. Acinar ⎤
    b. Papillary ⎦ with or without mucin formation
  2. Bronchiolo-alveolar
IV. Large cell carcinomas
  1. Solid tumors with mucin-like content
  2. Solid tumors without mucin-like content
  3. Giant cell carcinomas
  4. "Clear" cell carcinomas
V. Combined epidermoid and adenocarcinomas
VI. Carcinoid tumors
VII. Bronchial gland tumors
  1. Cylindromas
  2. Mucoepidermoid tumors
  3. Others
VIII. Papillary tumors of the surface epithelium
  1. Epidermoid
  2. Epidermoid with goblet cells
  3. Others
IX. "Mixed" tumors and carcinosarcomas
X. Sarcomas
XI. Unclassified
XII. Mesotheliomas
  1. Localized
  2. Diffuse
XIII. Melanomas

by smoking. The histologic types of these cancers are mainly epidermoid and small cell anaplastic carcinomas. The incidence of the lung cancers is related to cumulative radiation dosage. More recently, an increased incidence of lung cancer was reported in workers exposed to chloromethyl methyl ether. All these patients were males, and their ages ranged from 33 to 55 years. Most were smokers, but some had never smoked. The duration of exposure to this chemical varied from 3 to 14 years. These tumors were predominantly small cell anaplastic carcinomas. Other occupations in which an increased incidence of lung cancer has been reported include those in which workers are exposed to chromium, arsenic, nickel, and mustard gas.

Several reports have suggested that lung cancer, especially adenocarcinoma, may develop in areas of pulmonary fibrosis or scars. Such lesions may result from proliferating epithelial changes that are sometimes associated with chronic inflammation in the pulmonary parenchyma.

CLINICAL MANIFESTATIONS. The clinical manifestations of bronchogenic carcinoma depend on several factors related to the type and anatomic extent of the tumor. Symptoms may be related to the primary lesion, extension of the tumor beyond the lung parenchyma, distant metastasis, and syndromes produced by systemic nonmetastatic effects of the neoplasm. Many patients with lung cancer are asymptomatic when the pulmonary lesion is discovered.

Cough is a common symptom of lung cancer, and it may be a particularly troublesome symptom when the lesion is located near the carina. Because many lung cancers develop in smokers, a change in the character of a chronic cough may signal the development of the new lesion. *Sputum production* commonly accompanies the cough. The amount is generally small. Profuse expectoration may at times result from the presence of a diffuse bronchiolo-alveolar cell carcinoma, but even with this tumor large amounts of sputum are unusual. *Hemoptysis* occurs frequently owing to ulceration of the primary bronchial lesion. Usually, this is in the form of blood streaking of the sputum. Occasionally, the bleeding is more vigorous, as small blood vessels are eroded by the tumor. Massive hemoptysis leading to death occasionally occurs in advanced disease when the neoplasm erodes into a large blood vessel. *Dyspnea* is a frequent complaint. This may result from the primary tumor, an associated disease, or a combination of both. When lung function is otherwise normal, dyspnea may develop when the neoplasm involves a main bronchus and compromises ventilation to one lung or when it has spread extensively within the thorax.

Frequently, patients have associated chronic obstructive pulmonary disease, and this process is a factor in the development or worsening of dyspnea. The onset of dyspnea may be associated with the development of a pleural effusion due to the neoplasm, and at times, this occurs when the primary neoplasm is small but has spread extensively to the pleural space. Rarely, a primary lung neoplasm may be associated with the development of a pneumothorax, leading to an acute episode of dyspnea. *Fever and chills* resulting from pneumonitis may occur secondary to a bronchogenic carcinoma. The tumor may produce partial or complete bronchial obstruction, leading to an obstructive pneumonitis or atelectasis. Any patient with recurrent pneumonitis or an unresolved pneumonitis should be evaluated for the

possibility of a bronchial neoplasm. *Loss of weight* is a frequent symptom of bronchogenic carcinoma but generally occurs with more extensive disease beyond the time when the neoplasm is limited to the lung parenchyma. *Wheezing* occasionally may be the primary complaint of the patient when the primary bronchial lesion has narrowed a major airway to the degree that impaired air flow and secretion removal lead to the production of this symptom.

When the primary neoplasm has extended beyond the confines of the lung parenchyma, numerous additional symptoms may be present. *Chest pain* may be due to pleural involvement by the tumor or to direct involvement of the ribs and chest wall. The pain may have pleuritic qualities or may be dull and boring in character. *Dysphagia* may result from invasion or compression of the esophagus by a tumor that has spread into the mediastinum. *Hoarseness* is usually due to involvement of the recurrent laryngeal nerve owing to extension of a tumor from the left lung. *Superior vena caval compression or obstruction* results from mediastinal extension of a tumor. This produces edema of the face, neck, and upper extremities, along with a dilated superficial venous pattern in these areas. Some of these patients complain of headache and dizziness or vertigo. Neoplasms at the extreme apex of the lung may invade contiguous structures, producing the *Pancoast syndrome*. In this condition, pain is the most common initial complaint. This pain may be felt in the shoulder, scapular or interscapular area, upper anterior chest, arm, neck, or axilla. Other components of the syndrome include Horner's syndrome, muscle weakness of the upper extremity, and sensory disturbances in the upper extremity. The pain is due to neoplastic involvement of the pleura, ribs, spinal column, and brachial plexus. Horner's syndrome results from tumor extension into the inferior cervical sympathetic ganglion. The upper extremity weakness and sensory disturbances result from involvement of the inferior trunk of the brachial plexus or the eighth cervical and first and second thoracic nerves. Occasionally, such patients complain of hoarseness, which is due to tumor invasion of the right laryngeal nerve, which normally passes around the right subclavian artery in this area.

Distant metastasis is common with bronchogenic carcinoma and may result in a wide variety of symptoms. *Bone pain* may result from osseous metastasis, especially to the ribs, spinal column, and pelvis. *Headache, cranial nerve palsy, monoparalysis, hemiplegia*, and various other neurologic symptoms may result from metastasis to the central nervous system. *Lymphadenopathy*, especially in the supraclavicular and cervical areas, is common, and occasionally this finding is the first abnormality noted by the patient. *Anorexia, epigastric distress, and jaundice* may result from hepatic metastasis.

In recent years, a wide variety of syndromes have been noted in patients with lung cancer from the systemic effects of the neoplasm but not from metastasis. In some of these conditions, hormone or hormone-like secretion by the primary neoplasm has been demonstrated (see Ch. 525). In lung cancer the most commonly encountered endocrine syndromes are *inappropriate antidiuretic hormone secretion, Cushing's syndrome*, and *gynecomastia*. Small cell anaplastic carcinoma especially is associated with the development of these syndromes, suggesting hormone overproduction. Small cell anaplastic carcinoma may be derived from malignant change in the Kulchitsky or K-type cell in the basal layer of the bronchial epithelium. These cells may be of neural crest derivation and may have the potential for secreting many different chemical mediators.

Hypercalcemia associated with lung cancer may be due to metastatic destruction of bone, ectopic formation of parathyroid hormone, or formation by the tumor of an osteolytic substance other than parathyroid hormone. Hypercalcemia may be accompanied by such symptoms as nausea, vomiting, lethargy, polydipsia, polyuria, and mental confusion. The most common cell type of lung cancer associated with this finding is epidermoid carcinoma. Depending on the type of radioimmunoassay utilized, 20 to 70 per cent of tumors that cause hypercalcemia do so by producing ectopic parathyroid hormone. The serum phosphorus level varies, depending on the presence or absence of azotemia, but generally in nonazotemic patients the level is decreased. Removal of the primary lung tumor may lead to prompt return of the serum calcium and phosphorus levels to normal. Recurrence of the tumor may return the electrolyte abnormalities.

Hypertrophic pulmonary osteoarthropathy may be associated with various neoplasms, but it is most commonly associated with bronchogenic carcinoma. In one series, 41 per cent were epidermoid carcinomas, 22 per cent were adenocarcinomas, 16 per cent were large cell carcinomas, and 8 per cent were small cell carcinomas; the remainder included lymphomas, bronchial carcinoids, and other more infrequent tumors. This syndrome occurs frequently with large localized fibrous mesotheliomas of the pleura and may occur with metastatic tumors to the lung from the breast, uterus, and prostate. The syndrome consists of a symmetric proliferating subperiosteal osteitis with subperiosteal new bone formation. This process most commonly involves the distal long bones of the arms and legs. The ankles, knees, and wrists may show chronic synovitis, effusion, pannus formation, and cartilage erosion. This produces arthralgias, limitation of motion, and tenderness on palpation. The circumference of the limbs may be increased, and at times severe edema of the legs may be noted. Hypertrophic pulmonary osteoarthropathy is almost always associated with *digital clubbing*, but the latter frequently occurs alone. On pathologic examination, the subperiosteal new bone formation that takes place around the distal ends of the long bones of the extremities is characterized by a vascular, edematous osteoid matrix. The connective tissue overlying the periosteum undergoes proliferative changes and contains numerous thick-walled vascular channels, which appear to be arteriovenous anastomoses. Increased blood flow to the involved extremities has been demonstrated. In some way, a neural reflex appears to be involved also, because vagotomy decreases the abnormal blood flow in the extremities of patients with this syndrome. In animals with this syndrome, atropine does not produce the same effects as vagotomy, thus suggesting that the vagus may have a role as the afferent limb in a neurovascular reflex. The symptoms from this syndrome may precede, occur simultaneously with, or follow the development of symptoms related to the lung tumor. Removal of the lung tumor produces relief of symptoms, and in some cases vagotomy alone relieves symptoms. Bone changes may gradually revert to normal after resection of the tumor.

A number of *neurologic syndromes* that are not due to metastasis have been associated with lung cancer. The cause of these syndromes is unknown. These may be due to immunologic reaction, infection due to altered immunity, toxin production by the tumor, or utilization of an essential metabolite by the tumor. The neurologic symptoms may antedate discovery of the tumor by several years, may occur at the same time as symptoms from the tumor, or may develop after resection of the tumor. There is no correlation between the neurologic symptoms, the size of the tumor, and the presence or absence of metastasis. The neurologic symptoms may occur when the lung tumor is curable, but the neurologic manifestations generally do not change after resection of the tumor. The lung cancer is frequently of small cell anaplastic type, but the syndromes have been associated with all types of bronchogenic carcinoma. The neural and neuromuscular syndromes include *corticocerebellar degeneration, spinocerebellar degeneration, peripheral neuropathy, myasthenia,* and *myopathy* (see Ch. 322 to 327).

Thrombophlebitis, when it is recurrent or migratory and without apparent cause and when it is resistant to treatment with anticoagulants and involves unusual sites, suggests the possibility of an underlying lung neoplasm.

Nonbacterial thrombotic endocarditis may occur with lung neoplasms, especially with bronchiolo-alveolar cell carcinomas and adenocarcinomas. Vegetations occur most frequently on the mitral valve, but they may occur on the aortic valve alone or on both the aortic and mitral valves. These lesions may result in cerebral and myocardial embolization.

DIAGNOSIS. The diagnosis of bronchogenic carcinoma is generally established by some combination of clinical history, physical examination, thoracic roentgenogram, sputum cytologic examination, bronchoscopic examination, biopsy of involved structures, and thoracotomy. The many symptoms that bronchogenic carcinoma may produce have been described, and most of them are not specific for carcinoma. Physical examination of the chest may reveal a localized wheeze due to bronchial obstruction, dullness to percussion and decreased breath sounds due to presence of a pleural effusion, or other abnormalities such as rhonchi and expiratory slowing. However, in many patients, examination of the chest reveals no abnormalities. A complete physical examination is very important because it may reveal, for example, evidence of mediastinal spread of the tumor producing the signs of superior vena caval obstruction, as well as evidence of distant metastasis to supraclavicular or cervical lymph nodes or to the liver, with resultant hepatomegaly. Such findings are important in guiding the subsequent workup and evaluation of the patient.

The *thoracic roentgenogram* may reveal the presence of the neoplasm, give clues as to the histologic cell type of the neoplasm, and provide information on the extent of the neoplasm within the thorax. Epidermoid carcinomas most frequently present as hilar or perihilar masses, although they also may present as peripheral nodules. At times, the thoracic roentgenogram reveals obstructive hyperlucency, obstructive pneumonitis, or atelectasis that is secondary to the intrabronchial tumor. Cavitation has been reported to occur in about 7 per cent of patients with epidermoid carcinomas. The cavity may be thick walled and contain an air-fluid level, thereby resembling a lung abscess. The cavitation may be central or eccentric. Small cell anaplastic carcinoma generally presents as a hilar or perihilar mass, frequently with mediastinal widening. There may be associated obstructive pneumonitis or loss of lung volume. Large cell carcinoma appears most commonly as a peripheral mass. Cavitation may occur with this tumor, and the cavity usually appears to have a thick wall. Adenocarcinoma usually appears as a peripheral mass, and rarely it may also undergo cavity formation. Bronchiolo-alveolar cell carcinoma may present as single or multiple nodules or as diffuse lobar infiltrates. At times, one can recognize radiolucent spaces within the nodules. The margins of the nodules in alveolar cell carcinoma may be less sharply defined and less dense than nodules of metastatic tumor, and this may aid in the differential diagnosis of multiple pulmonary nodules.

In addition to these findings concerning the primary lung neoplasm, the thoracic roentgenogram also may demonstrate hilar and mediastinal lymph node involvement, pleural effusion due to the tumor, rib metastasis, elevation of a hemidiaphragm, tracheal compression or distortion, and pericardial effusion. Special roentgenographic studies may be helpful. Bilateral decubitus thoracic roentgenograms will demonstrate free pleural fluid and may demonstrate small amounts of pleural fluid that are not apparent on routine films. Tomograms of pulmonary nodules are helpful if they demonstrate central calcification suggestive of a granuloma or stippled calcification suggestive of a hamartoma. Eccentric calcification does not necessarily indicate a benign process because the calcium may have been engulfed by an enlarging neoplasm. Whole-lung tomograms may be helpful in differentiating a primary lung cancer and a metastatic lesion from a previously resected cancer elsewhere in the body. If these tomograms reveal multiple lesions, which may not be apparent on routine films, the diagnosis of metastatic disease is favored. Pulmonary nodules must be at least 1 cm in diameter before they can be detected on the routine thoracic roentgenogram. Lesions even larger than this may be hidden by overlying bone structures, the diaphragm, and the heart and great vessels.

Cytologic studies of the sputum are very helpful in establishing the diagnosis of bronchogenic carcinoma. The frequency of positive results in patients with lung cancer depends on the number and types of specimens examined and the location of the neoplasms. Centrally located lesions may be positive in about two thirds of cases, whereas peripheral lesions are positive in about one third of cases or less. Epidermoid and small cell anaplastic carcinomas that are central in location are most frequently associated with positive cytologic examinations. Bronchiolo-alveolar carcinoma, when present as a diffuse lesion rather than as a discrete nodule, can also be identified frequently by this means. Sputum for examination may be collected as a one-day spontaneous specimen, a three-day pooled spontaneous specimen, or an induced sputum specimen. Studies have shown that the three-day pooled specimen is superior to the one-day spontaneous specimen and has a similar percentage of positivity to induced sputum specimens. The induced sputum technique is of greatest value in patients who cannot expectorate spontaneously. Experienced cytologists can be very accurate in providing information regarding the cell type in epidermoid and small cell carcinomas and adenocarcinomas.

The sputum cytologic examination and the thoracic roentgenogram have been shown to be complementary in several studies. The thoracic roentgenogram is especially valuable in detecting early peripheral lesions, whereas sputum cytologic examination is more helpful in detecting early central lesions. False-positive sputum cytologic examinations are unusual, but can occur with such illnesses as acute pulmonary infections and pulmonary infarctions.

Bronchoscopic examination is an important technique in the diagnosis and localization of bronchogenic carcinoma. The recent introduction of the bronchofiberscope has increased the ability of this technique to establish a diagnosis, largely because this instrument enables close examination of the segmental and subsegmental bronchi in the upper lobes, which was not possible with previous instruments. A definitive diagnosis frequently can be established by direct visualization and biopsy of the lesion. Bronchial washings also may be obtained for cytologic examination. In addition, brushing of a peripheral lesion under fluoroscopic guidance may yield the diagnosis when direct biopsy is not possible.

Lung cancer may spread extensively within the thorax and metastasize widely throughout the body. The extent of local spread and distant metastases must be documented to determine prognosis and to plan therapy. *Biopsy of enlarged cervical and supraclavicular nodes* will establish the presence of extrathoracic metastasis. Liver metastasis is common, and when clinically suspected it may be detected by *liver function tests* and *isotope scans. Liver biopsy* may be indicated. *Bone roentgenograms* and *bone isotope scans* in patients with bone pain may demonstrate bone metastasis. Most metastatic lesions from lung cancer are osteolytic. The brain is a frequent site of metastatic disease, and when neurologic symptoms are present, this involvement can be documented by *neurologic examination, skull roentgenography, computerized tomographic studies*, and *angiography. Mediastinoscopy* may be needed to demonstrate metastasis to the mediastinal nodes and may preclude the need for thoracotomy. Some authorities employ this procedure almost routinely before deciding on surgery. Pleural effusion may be due either to direct tumor involvement of the pleura or to lymphatic obstruction by the tumor, or may be secondary to obstructive pneumonitis. Generally, the effusion is an exudate with a protein concentration that is greater than 3 grams per deciliter. Frequently, it is bloody or serosanguineous. *Cytologic examination of the pleural fluid or pathologic examination of material obtained by needle biopsy of the pleura* usually will establish the cause for the effusion. Some patients present with single nodules in the lung, and for various reasons they may not be suitable candidates for thoracotomy. The diagnosis of lung cancer in these patients frequently can be made by *cytologic examination of transthoracic needle aspirates.* The procedure is carried out under fluoroscopic guidance.

STAGING OF BRONCHOGENIC CARCINOMA. A method for staging lung cancer has been proposed that is helpful in determining prognosis and aids in the selection of proper therapy. This method, proposed by the American Joint Committee for Cancer Staging and End-Results Reporting (Table 2), is based on an estimate of the anatomic extent of the disease. In this system, the letter T describes the extent of the primary tumor, the letter N describes the presence or absence of regional lymph node involvement, and the letter M describes

TABLE 2. Staging of Bronchogenic Carcinoma Proposed by the American Joint Committee for Cancer Staging and End-Results Reporting

TNM Classification

Primary tumor (T)

TO: No evidence of primary tumor

TX: Tumor proved by the presence of malignant cells in broncho-pulmonary secretions but not visualized roentgenographically or bronchoscopically, or any tumor that cannot be assessed

TIS: Carcinoma in situ

T1: A tumor that is 3.0 cm or less in greatest diameter, surrounded by lung or visceral pleura, and without evidence of invasion proximal to a lobar bronchus at bronchoscopy

T2: A tumor more than 3.0 cm in greatest diameter, or a tumor of any size that either invades the visceral pleura or has associated atelectasis or obstructive pneumonitis extending to the hilar region; at bronchoscopy, the proximal extent of demonstrable tumor must be within a lobar bronchus or at least 2.0 cm distal to the carina; any associated atelectasis or obstructive pneumonitis must involve less than an entire lung, and there must be no pleural effusion

T3: A tumor of any size with direct extension into an adjacent structure as the parietal pleura or chest wall, the diaphragm, or the mediastinum and its contents; or a tumor demonstrable bronchoscopically to involve a main bronchus less than 2.0 cm distal to the carina; or any tumor associated with atelactasis or obstructive pneumonitis of an entire lung or pleural effusion

Regional lymph node involvement (N)

N0: No demonstrable metastasis to regional lymph node

N1: Metastasis to lymph nodes in the peribronchial or the ipsilateral hilar region, or both, including direct extension

N2: Metastasis to lymph nodes in the mediastinum

Distant metastasis (M)

MX: Not assessed

M0: No (known) distant metastasis

M1: Distant metastasis present in lymph nodes, brain, bones, liver, contralateral lung, bone marrow, pleura, skin, eye, or other areas

Stage Grouping

Occult carcinoma

TX N0 M0 — An occult carcinoma with bronchopulmonary secretions containing malignant cells but without other evidence of the primary tumor or evidence of metastasis to the regional lymph nodes or distant metastasis

Stage I

TIS N0 M0 — Carcinoma in situ

T1 N0 M0 / T1 N1 M0 / T2 N0 M0 — A tumor that can be classified T1 without any metastasis or with metastasis to the lymph nodes in the peribronchial and/or ipsilateral hilar region only, or a tumor that can be classified T2 without any metastasis to nodes or distant metastasis

NOTE: TX N1 M0 and T0 N1 M0 are also theoretically possible, but such a clinical diagnosis would be difficult if not impossible to make; if such a diagnosis is made, it would be included in stage I

Stage II

T2 N1 M0 — A tumor classified as T2 with metastasis to the lymph nodes in the peribronchial and/or ipsilateral hilar region only

Stage III

T3 with any N or M / N2 with any T or M / M1 with any T or N — Any tumor more extensive than T2, or any tumor with metastasis to the lymph nodes in the mediastinum, or any tumor with distant metastasis

the demonstrable extent of the disease that staging of it is not very helpful.

TREATMENT AND PROGNOSIS. *Surgery* remains the most effective therapy for bronchogenic carcinoma. One exception is in the patients with small cell anaplastic carcinoma. This tumor has an extremely poor prognosis, and for limited disease radiation therapy is superior to surgery. Many clinical trials utilizing polychemotherapy are now under way for this neoplasm. For stages I and II bronchogenic carcinomas, surgical resection is recommended. Some stage III carcinomas are resectable if the extent of the disease is such that all the cancer can be excised. This may be true for some peripheral lesions that directly involve the chest wall in which the entire disease can be removed en bloc. Overall, the prognosis for all patients with lung cancer is poor. The five-year survival rate for all stages of bronchogenic carcinoma has been about 9 per cent for the last 20 years. However, it is well recognized that the size and extent of the primary lesion are important determinants of survival. Relatively high five-year survival rates of about 70 per cent have been reported for patients with carcinoma in situ or minimally invasive carcinoma. Patients with peripheral lesions 4 cm or less in diameter also have been shown to have improved survival rates. In one study of 193 patients with peripheral lesions of this type, resection for cure was carried out in 182 patients or 94 per cent of the group. The operative mortality was 7 per cent. Of patients who survived surgery, the five-year survival rate was 51 per cent. The five-year survival rate for patients with lesions 2 cm or less in diameter was 68 per cent; for patients with lesions 2.1 to 3 cm in diameter, it was 46 per cent; and for patients with lesions 3.1 to 4 cm in diameter, it was 42 per cent. In this study, 49 per cent of the lesions were adenocarcinomas, 21 per cent were large cell carcinomas, 18 per cent were epidermoid carcinomas, 10 per cent were bronchiolo-alveolar cell carcinomas, and 2 per cent were small cell anaplastic carcinomas. The survival rates for patients with adenocarcinoma, epidermoid carcinoma, and large cell carcinoma were similar. The survival rate for those with bronchiolo-alveolar carcinoma was higher. Other studies have reported five-year survival rates of 50 to 80 per cent for patients with localized bronchiolo-alveolar cell carcinomas. Patients with the diffuse variety of bronchiolo-alveolar cell carcinoma have a uniformly poor prognosis. Further evidence of the importance of the extent of disease on survival can be noted in Table 3, in which two-year survival rates for various types of lung cancer are shown, based on the stage of the disease determined by the method previously discussed. Thus improvement in survival of patients with lung

the presence or absence of distant metastases. Utilizing this system, a clinical-diagnostic stage for all patients can be determined after the initial examination. If the patient undergoes thoracotomy, a surgical-evaluative stage or a postsurgical treatment–pathologic stage may be determined. A re-treatment stage may be assigned if the cancer recurs after treatment. Small cell anaplastic carcinoma has such a poor clinical course regardless of

TABLE 3. Percentage of Two-Year Survivals in Carcinoma of the Lung*

Cell type	Stage of Disease		
	I	*II*	*III*
Epidermoid	46.6	39.8	11.5
Adenocarcinoma	45.9	14.3	7.9
Large cell	42.8	12.9	12.9
Small cell	6.0	5.0	3.8

*Adapted from Mountain, C. F., Carr, D. T., and Anderson, W. A. D.: Am. J. Roentgenol., 120:130, 1974.

cancer probably will come from earlier diagnosis of the neoplasm, at least until chemotherapy or other forms of treatment become more effective.

When a patient presents with a lesion that is compatible with a bronchogenic carcinoma, it is important to determine whether the patient is a surgical candidate. Surgery may not be feasible because of spread of the primary tumor or because of associated diseases. The patient is generally considered to be inoperable if there is widespread mediastinal lymph node metastasis, superior vena caval obstruction, neoplastic pleural involvement, or evidence of distant metastasis. Evaluation of general health is important, especially in relation to the presence of chronic obstructive pulmonary disease. When such disease is present, one must estimate the pulmonary function that the patient will have after the operation. In evaluating this, it is important to consider the extent of the contemplated surgery — lobectomy or pneumonectomy — and whether the tumor is significantly impairing pulmonary function preoperatively. For example, in a patient with a tumor occluding a mainstem bronchus, the results of pulmonary function tests before operation probably closely reflect what the patient will be able to do after the operation. However, a patient with a small peripheral lesion will undoubtedly lose functioning lung in the course of the operation. Patients with reduction of 50 per cent in the forced vital capacity, the one-second forced expiratory volume (expressed as a percentage of the forced vital capacity), maximal voluntary ventilation, and diffusing capacity for carbon monoxide are high-risk patients, but many can successfully undergo surgery. Additional studies, such as isotope perfusion scans, to evaluate the pulmonary capillary bed may help the clinician determine whether a patient can tolerate surgery in selected instances. With modern methods of intensive respiratory care, it is often surprising how well resectional surgery is tolerated.

Radiation therapy is recommended for stages I and II bronchogenic carcinoma only when surgical treatment is contraindicated. This form of therapy is indicated for stage III neoplasms when the disease is limited to the involved hemithorax and ipsilateral supraclavicular lymph nodes and when surgical treatment is not possible. Such therapy can eliminate evidence of cancer in as many as 30 per cent of such patients. Failure to cure such patients results from presence of metastatic lesions outside the field of therapy. Preoperative radiation to lung cancers has not increased survival rates in general. Preoperative radiotherapy to superior sulcus tumors has been advocated in some studies. Patients with advanced lung cancer frequently may receive palliation with radiotherapy. Bone pain, superior vena caval obstruction, pleural effusion, brachial plexus involvement, and hemoptysis may be controlled in as many as 75 per cent of the patients. When radiation therapy is considered for limited disease in patients with pulmonary insufficiency, it is important to realize that the radiation therapy will damage the adjacent lung tissue and thereby further impair lung function.

The poor over-all prognosis for lung cancer is related to the early and widespread dissemination of the cancer. *Chemotherapy* would seem to be a reasonable approach to this problem. At this time, many clinical trials are under way using chemotherapeutic agents, such as nitrogen mustard, cyclophosphamide, methotrexate, 5-fluorouracil, Adriamycin, and bleomycin. The responses to single drugs have been disappointing, but some combination-drug programs have produced encouraging results, particularly in patients with small cell anaplastic carcinoma.

Immunotherapy is currently being considered for bronchogenic carcinoma. This approach has been based on studies that suggest an impaired cellular immunity in patients with carcinoma. The cellular immune response has been evaluated by quantifying the number of circulating T cells and B cells, by skin testing with antigens such as purified protein derivative, mumps, *Candida*, and 2,4-dinitrochlorobenzene (DNCB), and by testing the ability of lymphocytes to undergo blast transformation in response to mitogens. At present, there is considerable uncertainty in regard to how and when the impaired cellular immunity develops in a patient with lung cancer and what the effect of this impaired immunity is on prognosis and survival. Animal experiments suggest that immunotherapy may be most effective when only a limited amount of tumor is present. Because immunotherapy is likely to be most effective when the tumor burden is minimal, clinical trials using nonspecific immunostimulating agents such as BCG vaccine as surgical adjuvants are under way. It is too early to know what the benefits will be.

In spite of the poor prognosis for most patients with advanced lung cancer, much can be done to alleviate their distress. Judicious use of analgesics and narcotics, together with appropriate radiotherapy, will control pain in many patients. Occasionally, neurosurgical procedures are necessary for symptomatic relief. Antibiotics for symptoms of obstructive pneumonitis, and bronchodilator therapy for dyspnea due to or aggravated by accompanying chronic obstructive pulmonary disease, are helpful. Occasionally, oxygen therapy at home aids in relieving dyspnea. Recurrent pleural effusion may be benefited by intercostal tube drainage with the instillation of sclerosing agents, such as nitrogen mustard or tetracycline.

Auerbach, O., Stout, A. P., Hammond, E. C., and Garfinkel, L.: Changes in bronchial epithelium in relation to cigarette smoking and in relation to lung cancer. N. Engl. J. Med., 265:253, 1961.

Auerbach, O., Stout, A. P., Hammond, E. C., and Garfinkel, L.: Changes in bronchial epithelium in relation to sex, age, residence, smoking and pneumonia. N. Engl. J. Med., 267:111, 1962.

Byrd, R. B., Carr, D. T., Miller, W. E., Payne, W. S., and Woolner, L. B.: Radiographic abnormalities in carcinoma of the lung as related to histological cell type. Thorax, 24:573, 1969.

Carbone, P. P., Frost, J. K., Feinstein, A. R., Higgins, G. A., Jr., and Selawry, O. S.: Lung cancer: Perspectives and prospects. Ann. Intern. Med., 73:1003, 1970.

Fontana, R. S., Sanderson, D. R., Woolner, L. B., Miller, W. E., Bernatz, P. E., Payne, W. S., and Taylor, W. F.: The Mayo Lung Project for early detection and localization of bronchogenic carcinoma: A status report. Chest, 67:511, 1975.

Holmes, E. C.: Immunology and lung cancer. Ann. Thorac. Surg., 21:250, 1976.

Jackman, R. J., Good, C. A., Clagett, O. T., and Woolner, L. B.: Survival rates in peripheral bronchogenic carcinomas up to four centimeters in diameter presenting as solitary pulmonary nodules. J. Thorac. Cardiovasc. Surg., 57:1, 1969.

Mountain, C. F., Carr, D. T., and Anderson, W. A. D.: A system for the clinical staging of lung cancer. Am. J. Roentgenol., 120:130, 1974.

Nathanson, L., and Hall, T. C.: Lung tumors: How they produce their syndromes. Ann. N.Y. Acad. Sci., 230:367, 1974.

Selawry, O. S.: The role of chemotherapy in the treatment of lung cancer. Semin. Oncol., 1:259, 1974.

Stenseth, J. H., Clagett, O. T., and Woolner, L. B.: Hypertrophic pulmonary osteoarthropathy. Dis. Chest, 52:62, 1967.

Tokuhata, G. K., and Lilienfeld, A. M.: Familial aggregation of lung cancer in humans. J. Natl. Cancer Inst., 30:289, 1963.

CARCINOID TUMORS

DEFINITION. The term "bronchial adenoma" has been used in the past to describe slow-growing intrabronchial lesions that subsequently have been subdivided into three distinct pathologic entities: bronchial carcinoids, cylindromas, and mucoepidermoid tumors. Because these tumors have different biologic courses, as well as different histologic features, they should be considered as separate entities rather than under the broad category of bronchial adenoma. True bronchial adenomas of bronchial gland origin are extremely rare. Carcinoid tumors arising elsewhere in the body are discussed in Ch. 551.

PATHOLOGY. Carcinoid tumors may develop from Kulchitsky's cells, which are found in the bronchial epithelium and in bronchial glands. These are of neural crest origin and contain neurosecretory granules. Also, small cell anaplastic carcinoma may be derived from them. At times, the pathologist may have difficulty in distinguishing, on a small biopsy specimen, a carcinoid tumor from a small cell anaplastic carcinoma. Carcinoids tend to grow into the bronchial lumen, but there is frequently considerable extension below the mucosa. Carcinoids may metastasize to the regional lymph nodes, liver, and bones. The bone metastatic lesions may be osteoblastic or osteolytic. About 10 per cent of these tumors may be pathologically classified as "atypical carcinoids." These have increased mitotic activity, pleomorphism, and irregularity of nuclei with prominent nucleoli, areas of increased cellularity with disorganization of the architecture, and areas of tumor necrosis. These tumors have a more aggressive clinical course.

CLINICAL MANIFESTATIONS. Carcinoid tumors have an equal sex distribution. The average age of the patient at diagnosis is about 48 years, with a range reported in one series to be from 15 to 73 years. As expected from this intrabronchial lesion, the most common symptoms are cough, hemoptysis, and recurrent pneumonitis.

Bronchial carcinoids may produce the carcinoid syndrome, with cutaneous flushes, diarrhea, bronchoconstriction, and cardiac valvular lesions (see Ch. 551).

DIAGNOSIS. The diagnosis may be suspected on the basis of the history, particularly if the clinical course has been prolonged, because the tumor is slow growing and many patients have cough or recurrent hemoptysis for several years. The findings on physical examination depend on the degree of bronchial obstruction produced by the tumor. There may be decreased breath sounds and dullness to percussion owing to atelectasis, or a localized wheeze may be audible because of partial bronchial obstruction.

The thoracic roentgenogram may reveal a peripheral nodule, a hilar mass, or secondary manifestations of the intrabronchial lesion such as loss of volume, atelectasis, obstructive hyperinflation, or obstructive pneumonitis. Results of sputum cytologic examination are generally negative. Bronchoscopic examination is the best procedure for diagnosis of lesions within the range of the bronchoscope. Care should be taken while these tumors are being biopsied, because excessive bleeding may ensue.

TREATMENT AND PROGNOSIS. The treatment of choice is surgical excision. The extent of the surgery depends on the findings at operation. Sleeve resection of a part of a bronchus, segmental resection, lobectomy, or pneumonectomy may be required. The over-all five-year survival rate for patients with typical bronchial carcinoids has been reported to be 94 per cent; if regional nodes are involved with metastasis, the five-year survival rate decreases to 71 per cent. Patients with "atypical" carcinoids, based on a more aggressive pathologic appearance of the tumor, have a poorer prognosis; metastasis develops in 70 per cent compared with 5 per cent for patients with typical carcinoids, and 57 per cent of patients with "atypical" carcinoids survive five years. Corticosteroids and the phenothiazine drugs have been reported useful in patients with the carcinoid syndrome due to bronchial carcinoids.

Melmon, K. L., Sjoerdsma, A., and Mason, D. T.: Distinctive clinical and therapeutic aspects of the syndrome associated with bronchial carcinoid tumors. Am. J. Med., 39:568, 1965.

Okike, N., Bernatz, P. E., and Woolner, L. B.: Carcinoid tumors of the lung. Ann. Thorac. Surg., 22:270, 1976.

PRIMARY LYMPHOMA OF THE LUNG

The major discussions of lymphomas are to be found in Ch. 500 to 503. The lung and intrathoracic lymph nodes may be the primary sites of Hodgkin's disease and non-Hodgkin's lymphoma. Pseudolymphoma and lymphocytic interstitial pneumonitis are additional entities that may lead to difficulties in establishing a diagnosis.

The clinical manifestations produced by Hodgkin's disease and non-Hodgkin's lymphoma are variable, depending on the extent of the disease. Fever, cough, dyspnea, pleuritic pain, and loss of weight are frequent.

With Hodgkin's disease, the thoracic roentgenogram may reveal a solitary mass that may cavitate, an area of parenchymal consolidation, pleural effusion, or obstructive pneumonitis or atelectasis due to bronchial occlusion. Mediastinal lymph node enlargement is common. The anterior mediastinal nodes are often involved, a finding that is rare in sarcoidosis, and may be helpful in the differential diagnosis of mediastinal adenopathy. Direct parenchymal invasion via the lymphatic vessels may occur and produce a pattern of diffuse linear infiltration on the thoracic roentgenogram. Non-Hodgkin's lymphoma may produce similar roentgenographic patterns. When this disease is primary in the lung, the most common pattern is that of a homogeneous mass within the lung parenchyma with or without hilar and mediastinal lymph node enlargement. Bronchial obstruction rarely occurs, and cavitation in the parenchymal mass is uncommon. Lesions caused by non-Hodgkin's lymphoma may seem to progress very slowly on serial thoracic roentgenograms.

Pseudolymphoma and lymphocytic interstitial pneumonitis are lymphoproliferative disorders that are incompletely understood at present. The pathologic changes are similar in both, with the pseudolymphoma presenting as a nodular lesion and lymphocytic interstitial pneumonitis presenting as a diffuse infiltrate. Pathologically, these lesions may be very difficult to distinguish from a well-differentiated malignant lymphoma of the lymphocytic type. In fact, some patients who were considered to have pseudolymphoma or lymphocytic interstitial pneumonitis initially have developed true malignant lymphoma. Involvement of the hilar or mediastinal lymph nodes in a patient in whom the differentiation is difficult points strongly toward the diagnosis of a malignant lymphoma.

Diagnosis of intrathoracic lymphoproliferative disease depends on obtaining tissue for pathologic examination. Bronchoscopy and cytologic studies of the sputum and bronchial washings are generally not helpful. Occasionally, bronchoscopic biopsy of an endobronchial lesion will be diagnostic in Hodgkin's disease. Transbronchoscopic lung biopsy, mediastinoscopy, mediastinotomy, and thoracotomy are employed to establish the diagnosis when the disease is limited to the thorax.

Hodgkin's disease and non-Hodgkin's lymphoma are treated with radiation therapy and chemotherapy. Surgical resection of non-Hodgkin's lymphoma localized to the lung parenchyma has been carried out at the time of thoracotomy for diagnosis, with radiotherapy given postoperatively in many patients. These studies report a five-year survival of about 45 per cent. Pseudolymphoma of the lung is generally resected when surgical exploration is carried out to obtain the diagnosis. The proper therapy for lymphocytic interstitial pneumonitis has not been established. Some clinicians have treated these patients with immunosuppressive drugs.

Greenberg, S. D., Heisler, J. G., Gyorkey, F., and Jenkins, D. E.: Pulmonary lymphoma versus pseudolymphoma: A perplexing problem. South. Med. J., 65:775, 1972.

Thiessen, P. N., and Couves, C. M.: Primary lymphosarcoma of the lung: A case report and review of the literature. Can. J. Surg., 17:117, 1974.

UNCOMMON PRIMARY LUNG MALIGNANCIES

Cylindromas or adenoid cystic carcinomas derive from the mucous glands of the bronchial epithelium. Most are located in the trachea or main bronchi. There is an equal sex incidence, and the age range at the time of diagnosis has been reported to be between 30 and 65 years. Cylindroma is the second most common tumor of the trachea (the most common being epidermoid carcinoma). It produces its symptoms by bronchial irritation and obstruction. Bronchoscopic examination reveals a polypoid infiltrative tumor that partially or completely obstructs the airway and may bleed easily. Treatment is surgical resection. The prognosis must be guarded because of the tendency for distant metastasis to develop ultimately.

Mucoepidermoid tumors are rare structures of mucous gland origin, occurring in the age range of 40 to 55 years. On bronchoscopic examination, they present as polypoid masses with a smooth surface. Treatment is surgical resection, and the prognosis is better with these than with adenoid cystic carcinomas.

Carcinosarcoma is a rare entity that has both malignant epithelial and sarcomatous elements. It may present as a peripheral parenchymal mass or as an endobronchial lesion with bronchial obstruction. Treatment is surgical resection.

Pulmonary blastoma probably is a malignancy of primitive mesodermal cells capable of producing both epithelial and stromal components. It tends to arise in the peripheral portion of the lung. Treatment is surgical resection, and the prognosis is poor.

Payne, W. S., Ellis, F. H., Jr., Woolner, L. B., and Moersch, H. J.: The surgical treatment of cylindroma (adenoid cystic carcinoma) and muco-epidermoid tumors of the bronchus. J. Thorac. Cardiovasc. Surg., 38:709, 1959.

METASTATIC NEOPLASMS OF THE LUNG

The lung is a frequent location of metastases from carcinomas and sarcomas. These lesions may have several different patterns on the thoracic roentgenogram, patterns which may provide clues to aid in the search for the primary lesion if it is not apparent. *Solitary metastatic lesions to the lung* commonly originate from carcinomas of the colon, rectum, breast, kidney, testis, and cervix and from melanomas. Osteogenic and synovial cell sarcomas may produce this pattern. *Diffuse hematogenous metastasis* may appear as multiple micronodular shadows or large masses on the thoracic roentgenogram. Nodules may be of one size, suggesting one shower of tumor emboli, or may vary in size, suggesting tumor embolization at different times. A fine micronodular pattern is suggestive of metastasis from thyroid, renal, or trophoblastic tumors or from bone sarcomas. Rarely, diffuse hematogenous metastasis may produce a clinical pattern of cor pulmonale, with the thoracic roentgenogram revealing large hilar vessels but no parenchymal infiltration or nodules. *Diffuse lymphatic metastasis* may develop owing to involvement of the bronchomediastinal lymph nodes, with retrograde spread through the pulmonary lymphatics, or to vascular metastasis, with invasion of the peripheral lymphatic vessel and spread toward the hilar regions. Tumors that frequently present these findings are carcinomas from the breast, stomach, pancreas, thyroid, larynx, and lung. The roentgenographic pattern is one of increased linear and reticulonodular markings throughout the lung. *Cavitation* in metastatic lesions is suggestive of an epidermoid carcinoma from the head and neck regions and female reproductive organs, of a carcinoma of the colon, or of a metastatic sarcoma. *Calcification* in metastatic lesions is suggestive of an osteogenic sarcoma or a chondrosarcoma. *Pleural effusions* may be produced by metastasis from almost any primary neoplasm. *Pneumothorax* may be due to metastatic lesions, especially from bone, or to synovial cell sarcomas.

Cytologic examination of the sputum may be positive in as many as 50 per cent of patients with lung metastasis, depending on the extent of the disease. Bronchoscopy with biopsy of endobronchial lesions due to metastasis is occasionally helpful in renal, pancreatic, and adrenal carcinomas and malignant melanoma.

Surgical resection should be considered for solitary metastases to the lung. Five-year survival rates of 30 per cent have been reported, with the rate for carcinomas being 32 per cent and for sarcomas, 23 per cent. The resection should be conservative, and the primary neoplasm should be controlled. There should be no other evidence of metastatic disease. It has been suggested that a patient with a presumed solitary metastasis should be observed three months to see if additional lesions develop before proceeding with surgery. In some situations (patients with metastatic osteogenic sarcomas), multiple lung resections have been performed, with good results. It is important to remember that a solitary nodule in a patient with a previous malignancy may be a new primary lung malignancy.

Thomford, N. R., Woolner, L. B., and Clagett, O. T.: The surgical treatment of metastatic tumors in the lungs. J. Thorac. Cardiovasc. Surg., 49:357, 1965.

BENIGN TUMORS OF THE LUNG

In comparison with malignant neoplasms of the lung, benign tumors are uncommon. They present as solitary nodules in asymptomatic persons or as endobronchial lesions. In the latter instance, they may produce cough, hemoptysis, dyspnea, and recurrent pneumonitis, depending on size and location. The *hamartoma*, the most common benign lung neoplasm, is composed of tissues normally present in the lung, but these elements are unorganized, and include fat, epithelial tissue, fibrous tissue, and cartilage. These tumors are usually not diagnosed until adulthood, and there is a 2:1 or 3:1 male predominance. Most of them are peripheral and present as a solitary lung nodule. There may be calcification in the lesion, and sometimes this has the characteristic stippled or "popcorn" appearance. About 10 per cent of hamartomas are endobronchial. Treatment is surgical excision, and the prognosis is excellent.

Papillomas are most often encountered as laryngeal tumors in children. They may involve the trachea and bronchi. Histologically, they are composed of vascular connective tissue covered by stratified squamous epithelium. They may be of viral cause. In an unusual situation in which multiple papillomas extend throughout many bronchi, the clinical course may be characterized by repeated pneumonitis, atelectasis, bronchiectasis, and chronic pulmonary infection. Management is difficult and includes repeated bronchoscopic removal of the tumors if possible. Malignant change has been reported.

Granular cell myoblastomas are rare benign tumors usually found in the walls of the large bronchi. They may present as a mass lesion on the thoracic roentgenogram or with symptoms suggestive of a bronchial obstructing lesion. Treatment is surgical resection. Other uncommon benign lung tumors include *lipomas, fibromas, leiomyomas, chondromas,* and *hemangiomas.*

Arrigoni, M. G., Woolner, L. B., Bernatz, P. E., Miller, W. E., and Fontana, R. S.: Benign tumors of the lung: A ten-year surgical experience. J. Thorac. Cardiovasc. Surg., 60:589, 1970.

350. DISEASES OF THE PLEURA, MEDIASTINUM, DIAPHRAGM, AND CHEST WALL

John H. McClement

350.1. THE PLEURA

INTRODUCTION

The pleura, a serous membrane of mesodermal origin, covers the lung, the chest wall, the diaphragm, and the mediastinum. It is a closed sac which encloses the pleural space and separates the lung from adjacent structures. The visceral pleura designates that portion of it which covers the lung; the remainder is the parietal pleura. The parietal pleura receives its blood supply from the systemic circulation, whereas the visceral is supplied by the pulmonary circulation. The normal pleural space contains no gas and only a small amount of serous fluid. During quiet breathing, the elastic recoil of the lung produces a subatmospheric pressure (-4 to-10 cm H_2O) in the pleural space.

Pleural pain and signs and symptoms secondary to collections of fluid and gas in the pleural space are principal indicators of pleural disease.

Pleural pain originates in the parietal pleura; stimulation of the visceral pleura does not cause pain. Typically, pleural pain is sharp, aggravated by respiration and thoracic motion, and relieved by splinting of the involved area. When it arises from the pleura of the chest wall, the pain is referred to the chest wall overlying the involved area; pain arising from the pleura of the central portion of the diaphragm is referred to the posterior part of the shoulder area; pain from the costal portions of the diaphragm is referred to adjacent parts of the chest wall and abdomen.

The formation and removal of pleural fluid are dependent on those forces which regulate the exchange of fluid into and out of capillary beds, and on lymphatic drainage. The hydrostatic pressure in the pleural capillaries (Pc), the hydrostatic pressure in the pleural space (Ppl), the oncotic pressures of the plasma (OPp) and the pleural fluid (OPpf), and the permeability of the pleural capillaries (K) are the factors which regulate the transport of fluid (F) into and out of the pleural capillaries. According to Starling's law of transcapillary exchange, this can be expressed as follows:

$$F = K(Pc - OPp) - (Ppl - OPpf)$$

The visceral pleura is supplied by arterioles from the low pressure pulmonary arterial system, whereas the parietal pleura is supplied by the higher pressure systemic arteries. There is evidence that the permeability (K) of the visceral capillaries is less than that of the parietal pleura. Normally a balance of these forces favors absorption of fluid by the visceral pleura at about the same rate it is formed. However, all these forces may be altered by disease, and the removal of fluid may be slowed or its formation increased. An increase in capillary permeability (K) from inflammation, a decrease in the oncotic pressure of the plasma proteins (OPp) from hypoalbuminemia, and an increase in the hydrostatic pressure in the pulmonary capillaries (Pc) are the common alterations that lead to pleural fluid collections. Uncommonly a decrease in the hydrostatic pressure in the pleura (Ppl) from a collapsed and nonexpandable lung will cause effusion. Protein, red blood cells, and particulate matter are removed from the pleural space by the pleural lymphatics. The absorption and transport of pleural fluid by way of the lymphatics is increased by diaphragmatic and intercostal activity. Decrease in this activity or obstruction of local or distant lymphatic channels may prolong or prevent reabsorption of pleural fluid.

METHODS OF EXAMINATION IN PLEURAL DISEASE

HISTORY AND PHYSICAL EXAMINATION. Pleural pain and shortness of breath are the symptoms which most often call attention to pleural disease. A dry, irritating, nonproductive cough may sometimes accompany the pleural pain. Shortness of breath may sometimes be caused by severe pleural pain, but usually indicates the presence of fairly large amounts of intrapleural fluid or gas. Early in the course of pleural inflammation a friction rub may be heard over the involved area. As fluid forms, the friction rub and the pain disappear, and dullness to percussion and diminished breath sounds on auscultation appear. At the upper limits of pleural fluid, egophony is sometimes elicited. Pleural disorders for the most part arise from derangements in cardiac, hepatic, or renal function which lead to increased collections of fluid, or by extension of disease from adjacent structures such as the lung, mediastinum, chest wall, esophagus, or the upper abdomen. Evidence of disease in these structures must be searched for in the history and physical examination.

RADIOLOGIC EXAMINATION. Up to 300 ml of fluid may be present in a pleural space and not be apparent on the usual upright chest x-ray film. Small amounts of fluid may sometimes be suspected, especially on the left side, from the presence of a density or apparent widening of the diaphragmatic shadow as it is seen between the gas-containing stomach and the lower limits of the lung. Decubitus films taken with the involved side dependent may also sometimes make small amounts of fluid apparent on the x-ray film. With larger amounts of fluid the characteristic density of pleural fluid with its curvilinear upper border appears. However, if pleural fluid occurs in a pleural space in which previous inflammatory disease has produced adhesions, the distribution of the fluid may produce varied shadows. The x-ray shadows of pleural fluid are characteristically adjacent to the chest wall; rarely fluid will collect in or become encapsulated in one of the interlobar fissures and produce a pattern similar to a parenchymal pulmonary tumor.

EXAMINATION OF PLEURAL FLUID. A detailed chemical, bacteriologic, and cytologic analysis of all pleural fluids aspirated is essential in patients in whom the diagnosis is not completely clear. Analysis for total protein and lactic acid dehydrogenase (LDH), a complete blood count with a differential count, cultures for bacteria including mycobacteria, a Gram-stained smear, and a search for malignant cells should be carried out initially on virtually all pleural fluids. Glucose, pH, amylase, fat, and cholesterol measurements may also sometimes be indicated. The specific gravity of pleural fluid was once recommended as a measurement that would help differentiate between exudates and transudates. Because the specific gravity depends almost entirely on the protein content of the pleural fluid, and because it is a measurement that is frequently inaccurate, it can usually be omitted if an accurate measure of protein content is available.

The differentiation of pleural transudates and exudates is most helpful diagnostically and can usually be accomplished from examination of pleural fluid. Transudates are those fluids which occur in response to a decrease in the oncotic pressure of plasma, an increase in hydrostatic pressures in the pleural capillaries, or a decrease in intrapleural pressure. Exudates result from infections or from inflammatory or neoplastic processes which alter the permeability of pleural capillaries. Characteristically, transudates have a low protein content, a low specific gravity, and few white blood cells, whereas exudates have a high protein, high specific gravity, and increased numbers of white blood cells. Arbitrary limits have been chosen to separate transudates and exudates (e.g., total protein more than 3.0 ml per 100 ml and specific gravity greater than 1.015). Unfortunately, when these arbitrary limits are tested in patients who have pleural fluid in which the cause is certain, both transudates and exudates are sometimes misclassified. Light and his associates have examined the cellular and chemical characteristics of pleural fluid from patients in whom a definite diagnosis could be established. On this basis they were classified as transudates or exudates. The three measurements which they found most reliable in differentiating transudates and exudates were the pleural fluid to serum protein ratio (greater than 0.5 in exudates), the level of LDH (greater than 200 IU in exudates) and the ratio of pleural fluid to serum LDH (greater than 0.6 in exudates). Although white blood counts greater than 10,000 per cubic millimeter are usually found only in exudates and counts of greater than 2500 per cubic millimeter suggest that the fluid is an exudate, counts below 2500 per cubic millimeter do not distinguish transudates from exudates.

Chylothorax refers to the presence of chyle in the pleural space and results from trauma to or obstruction (most often by a neoplastic process) of the thoracic duct or some other major intrathoracic lymphatic. Chylous pleural effusions are characteristically milky in appearance and have a high fat content which can be identified both microscopically and chemically. The protein content is usually about half that of plasma.

Milky-appearing pleural collections may also occur late in the course of tuberculous pleural effusion, in the pleural effusions of rheumatoid lung disease, and in other chronic effusions from the accumulation of cholesterol and cholesterol crystals in these fluids. Chemical analysis of such fluids will show a high cholesterol content and a low fat content and distinguish them from chylous effusions.

PLEURAL BIOPSY. Biopsy of the pleura with a Cope or Abrams needle is indicated in nearly every patient in whom the diagnosis is not clear, and who has sufficient pleural fluid to make this a safe procedure. Material from the biopsy should be submitted not only for histologic examination, but also for culture for tubercle bacilli. Pleural biopsy has been particularly useful in establishing the diagnosis of tuberculous pleurisy and malignant neoplastic implants in the pleura.

SIMPLE HYDROTHORAX

Pleural fluid collections occur more often as a result of cardiac, hepatic, or renal disease than from inflammatory or malignant disease of the pleura. These fluid collections most often result either from increases in hydrostatic pressures in the pleural capillaries, from a decrease in the oncotic pressure of the plasma, or from a combination of these factors. There is some exchange of fluid between the peritoneum and the pleura through the diaphragmatic lymphatics, and in patients with ascites this mechanism may result in pleural collections. Clinically these fluid collections are usually identified by physical examination, from x-rays of the chest, or, if they are large, from the appearance of dyspnea. They occur much more frequently on the right side than on the left. Pleural fluid in patients with simple hydrothorax will have those characteristics of a transudate which have been described. Because the parietal pleura is thin and uninvolved, pleural biopsy often fails to yield any identifiable pleural tissue. The treatment of these pleural collections is the treatment of the underlying disease, and pleural aspiration should be used therapeutically only if these measures fail and dyspnea requires relief.

PULMONARY EMBOLISM AND PULMONARY INFARCTION

Pulmonary embolism frequently produces pleural manifestations. In patients with pulmonary embolism, confirmed by pulmonary angiography, more than half will have a clinically detectable pleural effusion. The pleural effusion does not appear immediately and is usually identified more than 24 hours after the embolic event. The pleural effusion is an exudate and sometimes has moderate numbers of red blood cells; however, it is usually a clear amber fluid. Unless repeated embolization occurs, the pleural fluid disappears as the pulmonary infarction resolves.

PLEURAL EFFUSIONS WITH PNEUMONIA: EMPYEMA

Inflammation of the adjacent pleura occurs in most patients with pneumonia whatever the cause. Bacterial pneumonia frequently has clinically significant pleural involvement; in most pneumonias caused by viruses and mycoplasma, pleural disease is not clinically prominent.

The extent of pleural inflammation in bacterial pneumonia varies widely from case to case. There may be minor inflammation which produces pleural pain with clinically undetectable amounts of fluid, and which leaves no clinical residue; or large collections of grossly purulent fluid containing large numbers of bacteria (empyema) resulting in marked pleural fibrosis and fibrothorax. In practice one encounters patients who produce a continuum between these two extremes. Treatment of these effusions depends largely on the severity and intensity of the pleural inflammation, but is primarily the treatment of the associated pneumonia with appropriate antimicrobial drugs. The less intense small serous effusions with relatively small numbers of white blood cells and few organisms will usually respond to drug treatment alone. With larger collections of fluid and more white blood cells, aspiration by means of closed drainage through an intercostal tube may speed resolution and lead to smaller pleural residues. The finding of a pH of lower than 7.30 in the pleural exudate correlates with a more protracted and complicated course and may be an indication for earlier surgical drainage. With grossly purulent fluid and larger numbers of bacteria, surgical rib resection and open dependent drainage may be necessary. Infrequently pleural inflammatory disease leads to persistent massive fibrous entrapment of the underlying lung even after the infection has been controlled. A so-called fibrothorax results; the affected lung has its volume greatly decreased; ventilation and perfusion are reduced; there is a shift in the mediastinum toward the entrapped lung, and overdistention of the contralateral

lung occurs. In such cases surgical decortication may free the entrapped lung and restore pulmonary function.

TUBERCULOSIS OF THE PLEURA

DEFINITION. Localized tuberculosis of the pleura probably occurs in most patients with pulmonary tuberculosis. It is usually clinically inapparent, but does result in pleural adhesions over the involved area.

Tuberculosis of the pleura with pleural effusion and without apparent pulmonary tuberculosis is the principal or first clinical manifestation of tuberculous disease in a few patients. Characteristically it is a febrile illness, accompanied by a serous pleural effusion. Although the acute illness, even if untreated, usually subsides in a few weeks with resorption of the fluid, it is very frequently followed by pulmonary tuberculosis or some other form of tuberculosis. Roper and Waring found that 65 per cent of patients with serofibrinous pleurisy who did not receive antituberculous chemotherapy developed tuberculosis during the next five years. Thus recognition of the tuberculous cause is of great importance. Infrequently pleural effusions that are grossly purulent and contain large numbers of tubercle bacilli are encountered; such cases are designated as tuberculous empyema.

EPIDEMIOLOGY. Tuberculous pleurisy with effusion can occur at any age but occurs most often in older children and young adults. It usually occurs soon after tuberculous infection, and is uncommon in patients who are known to have had tuberculous infection for a long time.

PATHOLOGY AND PATHOGENESIS. Tuberculosis of the pleura in nearly all cases results from extension of disease from the lung. Extension from tuberculosis of adjacent bones or lymph nodes is rare. Usually this extension from the lungs results only in localized pleural disease, and pleural effusion is not significant. In an occasional patient there is a massive outpouring of pleural fluid, and tuberculous infection is generalized over the visceral and parietal pleura. Myriads of typical tubercles stud the pleural surfaces. The immunologic reasons why some patients have this acute, widespread disease whereas others have only insignificant localized disease are not known. In a few weeks the acute reaction subsides, the pleural fluid decreases and then disappears, and fibrous adhesions between the visceral and parietal pleura form. Infrequently the fluid persists, becomes more purulent, and has increased numbers of tubercle bacilli; a chronic tuberculous empyema is established, which may persist for many years. Perhaps because the adjacent subpleural area is richly supplied with lymphatics, there is easy access for the dissemination of tubercle bacilli. In any case the subsequent development of tuberculosis in the lung and in other organs is a common event after untreated tuberculous pleurisy with effusion.

CLINICAL MANIFESTATIONS. The onset of tuberculous pleurisy with effusion is usually fairly sudden and acute. Sharp, fairly severe pleural pain is the most common first symptom. It is usually unilateral, made worse by breathing, and relieved by splinting the affected area. It is sharpest and most painful for the first few days, and then with the outpouring of pleural fluid it becomes duller and gradually subsides. Shortness of breath which is sometimes severe results from large collections of pleural fluid. Fever, which is sometimes as high as 39 to 40° C, is usually present in the first two or three weeks, and gradually subsides. Physical examination and x-ray examinations will identify the presence of variable amounts of fluid. In the typical case the parenchymal focus in the lung from which the disease originated is not apparent radiologically.

DIAGNOSIS. The diagnosis of tuberculous pleurisy should be considered in every patient with a pleural effusion; should be strongly suspected if this is accompanied by skin reactivity to 0.0001 mg of PPD; and should be presumptively diagnosed if, in addition, the fluid has the characteristics of an exudate and another diagnosis cannot be firmly made. Fortunately, methods for making the diagnosis of pleural tuberculosis have improved to such an extent that, if they are all used in a concerted fashion before treatment is started, the number of cases in which only a presumptive diagnosis must be made is small. Tubercle bacilli can be cultured from pleural fluid in up to 20 per cent of cases, from the sputum in a similar number, and from pleural biopsy material in over 60 per cent of cases. Typical tuberculous granulation tissue is seen in over 60 per cent of pleural biopsies from cases of tuberculous pleurisy. Although none of these methods are diagnostic in all cases, if they are used together, bacteriologic or histologic evidence of tuberculosis will be found in most cases.

Congestive heart failure, metastatic carcinoma involving the pleura, pulmonary infarction, and the effusions of bacterial pneumonia are the most commonly encountered conditions from which tuberculous pleurisy with effusions must be differentiated. Pleural mesothelioma, subdiaphragmatic abscess with an associated pleural effusion, rheumatoid pleural disease, and disseminated lupus erythematosus are less common conditions that may resemble tuberculous pleurisy.

TREATMENT. The treatment of tuberculous pleurisy is the prolonged administration of isoniazid and at least one other antituberculous drug and is the same as that for pulmonary tuberculosis (see Ch. 167). Surgical decortication to free a lung trapped by pleural adhesions (fibrothorax) after chemotherapy has controlled the infection is rarely necessary. With prompt and adequate chemotherapy, pleural residues are usually minor and do not benefit from surgical correction.

NEOPLASMS OF THE PLEURA

METASTATIC CARCINOMA. Implants of metastatic carcinoma of the pleura are, especially in older age groups, a common cause of pleural effusions. Carcinomas of the lung and breast are the tumors that most commonly extend to the pleura, but almost any carcinoma can have this complication. If the primary tumor has already been identified, the diagnosis is usually quickly made. If the pleural effusion is the first indication of the tumor, the diagnosis may not be so apparent. Characteristically the pleural effusions of malignant implants in the pleura are not accompanied by fever, the fluid is an exudate and often contains a large number of red blood cells, and the course is marked by the continued outpouring of fluid. The diagnosis can be established by finding malignant cells in the pleural fluid, by the presence of tumor in the parietal pleura on

pleural biopsy, or by open surgical biopsy of the pleura.

Treatment is aimed at preventing the accumulation of fluid in the pleural space and eliminating the need for repeated thoracenteses for the relief of dyspnea. Obliteration of the pleural space may be produced by the instillation of various irritating substances (e.g., atabrine, nitrogen mustard, cyclophosphamide, tetracycline, radioactive gold), followed by aspiration of the fluid to assure that the visceral and parietal layers are opposed. The insertion of an intercostal tube attached to suction is sometimes used for continuous aspiration after the irritating material has stimulated an inflammatory response.

MESOTHELIOMA. Pleural mesotheliomas may be either localized or diffuse. The localized tumor, the so-called fibrous mesothelioma, is relatively benign, may grow to a very large size, is sometimes cured by surgical resection, but does have a tendency to recur. The diffuse mesothelioma is a highly malignant tumor which involves the pleura widely and produces massive encroachment on the pleural space with fluid and tumor. Formerly this was believed to be a very rare tumor. It is now being seen with increased frequency, and its association with exposure to asbestos has been established (see Ch. 348.9).

OTHER PLEURAL TUMORS. Benign tumors of the pleura include lipomas, fibromas, vascular tumors, and pleural cysts. Primary malignant tumors of the pleura other than mesotheliomas include various sarcomas. They are all very uncommon.

Pleural effusions from intrathoracic lymphoma are not uncommon and apparently can result either from direct involvement of the pleura or from intrathoracic lymphatic obstruction. Chylothorax is sometimes seen when there is lymphatic obstruction.

SPONTANEOUS PNEUMOTHORAX

The pleural space normally does not contain gas, and if gas is instilled into the pleural space, it is absorbed. The total pressure of dissolved gases in venous blood is 54 mm Hg less than the atmospheric pressure which is transmitted to the pleura. This negative gradient keeps the intact pleural space gas free. Air may enter the pleural space through either the chest wall or the lung. Trauma to the chest wall or lung, medical procedures that permit the entry of air through the chest wall or that puncture the lung, and the spontaneous entry of gas from a ruptured emphysematous bleb are the most common causes of pneumothorax. The rupture of lung abscesses and tuberculous cavities into the pleura are less common causes. Spontaneous pneumothorax occurs in at least two distinct populations: the young, tall, otherwise healthy male, and the older person with underlying and usually clinically apparent chronic obstructive pulmonary disease or some other disease that has produced pulmonary fibrosis and localized emphysema.

CLINICAL MANIFESTATIONS. Pleural pain and shortness of breath are the principal symptoms of spontaneous pneumothorax. The severity of the shortness of breath may vary from insignificant to very severe and depends on the amount of gas in the pleural space and the amount of underlying pulmonary disease which is present. Physical examination of the chest will sometimes show increased resonance to percussion over the affected side, but a decrease in the intensity of the breath sounds is a more definite and discernible sign. If the pneumothorax is large and there is a marked increase in intrapleural pressure, a shift in mediastinal structures away from the affected side may be detected. The chest x-ray will show air in the pleural space and the amount of collapse of the lung which has occurred.

DIAGNOSIS. The possibility of spontaneous pneumothorax should be considered whenever there is the sudden onset of shortness of breath and particularly when it is accompanied by chest pain. It is a diagnosis which is usually made easily when it occurs in an otherwise healthy person and when the clinical findings which have been enumerated are present. The diagnosis is occasionally missed when it occurs in an asthmatic, a patient with obstructive pulmonary disease, or in other patients who have some other disease that seems to explain their shortness of breath. Because it can be lethal in such patients if untreated, the possibility of its occurrence should be kept prominent.

If a vessel in the lung or chest wall is torn when a pneumothorax occurs, a hemopneumothorax may result. When the chest x-ray shows the presence of fluid as well as air, this possibility should be considered, and a thoracentesis should be performed. Massive intrapleural bleeding is uncommon, but if present it requires surgical correction.

TREATMENT. The treatment of pneumothorax is concerned with its immediate and acute management, and with the prevention of recurrences.

The methods used in the early management of spontaneous pneumothorax will depend on the size and cause of the pneumothorax, the presence or absence of complicating pulmonary disease, and whether the leak between the lung and the pleura is closed or continuing. If the pneumothorax has occurred in a young healthy person, is small (e.g., 10 to 15 per cent), is causing few or minimal symptoms, and does not increase during the first 12 hours of observation, it requires no treatment. However, the fact that it has indeed resorbed should be confirmed by chest x-ray about two weeks later. In a similar patient with a larger pneumothorax, and especially if there is significant shortness of breath, the gas may be removed by inserting a small venous catheter through a thoracentesis needle and aspirating the intrapleural gas. This simple method will usually succeed in patients who do not have underlying pulmonary disease and who do not have a continuing leak. If there is significant pulmonary disease, pleural adhesions, or evidence of a continuing bronchopleural fistula, a larger intercostal tube should be inserted and attached to an underwater seal. The relief of an increasing and positive pressure — a *tension pneumothorax* — by prompt decompression is occasionally lifesaving. If there is a significant continuing leakage of air or evidence of respiratory insufficiency, continuous suction is required. If the lung cannot be re-expanded or there is continued leakage for more than a few days, an open thoracotomy with resection and closure of the bronchopleural fistula may be required.

Recurrence. Spontaneous pneumothorax may recur once or many times over several years after the first episode. Recurrences may be on the same side or the opposite side. The possibility of recurrence can be greatly reduced or eliminated by surgical treatment. Surgical treatment includes the resection of blebs and bullae if they are sufficiently localized to permit this and the obliteration of the pleural space. The removal of the parietal pleura, the application of irritating substances to the pleura, and the scarification of the pleura followed by intrapleural suction are methods which are used to obliterate the pleural space.

MISCELLANEOUS PLEURAL DISEASES

The pleura is involved in a great variety of systemic diseases and in diseases of the lung and adjacent structures.

COLLAGEN VASCULAR DISEASES. Systemic lupus erythematosus and rheumatoid arthritis are the collagen vascular diseases in which pleural effusions are most often encountered. In rheumatoid arthritis pleural effusions are usually seen in older men in whom the arthritis is of long duration. The fluid is an exudate and characteristically has a very low glucose content.

PANCREATITIS. Pleural effusions secondary to acute and chronic pancreatitis are occasionally encountered. They may occur in either pleural space, but are more common on the left. There is often an associated pancreatic pseudocyst. The fluid is an exudate, may have extremely high amylase content (500 to 50,000 units per milliliter), and characteristically has a higher level of amylase than the serum.

ASBESTOSIS. Inhalation of asbestos dust commonly leads to pleural disease. Serous pleural effusion, pleural fibrosis, pleural calcification, and pleural mesothelioma are all complications of asbestos dust exposure.

The pleural effusion of asbestos exposure is commonly bilateral and frequently recurrent; the fluid is usually an exudate and is often serosanguineous. Pleural effusion is often accompanied by clinically apparent parenchymal fibrosis, but can occur in the absence of obvious asbestosis. Duration and intensity of exposure to asbestos can vary widely.

Pleural fibrosis is a common accompaniment of pulmonary asbestosis and has been identified in up to 14 per cent of cases of asbestosis. Like pleural effusion it may be seen in patients who do not have evident parenchymal fibrosis.

Pleural calcification is common among asbestos workers and has been found in more than 10 per cent of workers with prolonged exposure. It is often bilateral, predominantly involves the basilar portions, is primarily in the parietal pleura, and usually occurs only after lengthy exposures to asbestos.

Although pleural mesothelioma has been reported to follow these more benign forms of pleural disease from asbestos, it is an uncommon complication.

MEIGS' SYNDROME. Ascites, pleural effusion, a benign fibroma, or fibroma-like ovarian tumor, with cure of the ascites and pleural effusion by removal of the tumor, is a syndrome that Meigs called attention to in 1934. It is an uncommon cause of pleural effusion, but many cases of the syndrome have been reported. Most often the fluid is found in the right pleural space, but it can be present in either or both pleural spaces. The fluid is usually a clear transudate, but exudative fluids and serosanguineous collections have been reported. The amount of fluid in both the pleural and peritoneal spaces is variable, and in some cases the amount of ascites has been quite small. The mechanism for the formation of the pleural and peritoneal fluid has not been completely explained, but it is suggested that somehow the fibroma causes the ascites which is then transported to the pleural space by diaphragmatic lymphatics. Because this uncommon condition can be cured by pelvic surgery, it should be considered in women with pleural effusion of obscure origin, especially if there is evidence of concurrent ascites and pelvic disease.

SUBDIAPHRAGMATIC ABSCESS. Pleural effusion and pleurodiaphragmatic pain, particularly on the right side, are common manifestations of a subdiaphragmatic abscess, and are frequently the first indicators of the location of the infection. The pleural effusion is most often a serous exudate, and the organism in the subdiaphragmatic abscess is often not found in the pleural fluid. Amebic infection from the liver may also extend through the diaphragm and cause a pleural exudate, which is characteristically purulent and chocolate-colored and may contain amebae.

Berger, H. W., Rammohan, G., Neff, M. S., and Buhain, W. J.: Uremic pleural effusion. Ann. Intern. Med., 82:362, 1975.

Besson, L. N., Ferguson, T. B., and Burford, T. H.: Chylothorax. Ann. Thorac. Surg., 12:527, 1971.

Black, L. F.: The pleural space and pleural fluid. Mayo Clin. Proc., 47:493, 1972.

Gaensler, E. A., and Kaplan, A. I.: Asbestos pleural effusions. Ann. Intern. Med., 74:178, 1971.

Killen, D. A., and Gobbel, W. G., Jr.: Spontaneous Pneumothorax. Boston, Little, Brown & Company, 1968.

Light, R. W.: Management of parapneumonic effusions (editorial). Chest, 70:324, 1976.

Light, R. W., MacGregor, M. I., Luchsinger, P. C., and Ball, W. C., Jr.: Pleural effusions: The diagnostic separation of transudates and exudates. Ann. Intern. Med., 77:507, 1972.

Meigs, J. V.: Fibroma of the ovary with ascites and hydrothorax — Meigs' syndrome. Am. J. Obstet. Gynecol., 67:962, 1954.

Mellins, R. B., Levine, O. R., and Fishman, A. P.: Effects of systemic and pulmonary venous hypertension on pleural and pericardial fluid accumulation. J. Appl. Physiol., 29:564, 1970.

Potts, D. E., Levin, D. C., and Sahn, S. A.: Pleural fluid pH in parapneumonic effusions. Chest, 70:328, 1976.

Scharer, L., and McClement, J. H.: The isolation of tubercle bacilli from needle biopsy specimens of parietal pleura. Am. Rev. Respir. Dis., 97:466, 1968.

Szucs, M. M., Brooks, H. L., Grossman, W., Banas, J. S., Meister, S. G., Dexter, L., and Dalen, J. E.: Diagnostic sensitivity of laboratory findings in acute pulmonary embolism. Ann. Intern. Med., 74:161, 1971.

Wallach, H. W.: Intrapleural tetracycline for malignant pleural effusions. Chest, 68:510, 1975.

Yeoh, C. B., Hubaytar, R. T., Conklin, E. F., Simpson, D. G., and Ford, J. M.: Spontaneous pneumothorax: Treatment with small lumen polyethylene tube. New York State J. Med., 70:779, 1970.

350.2.   THE MEDIASTINUM

The mediastinum is that anatomic space which lies in the mid-thorax, separates the two pleural cavities, and is delineated by the diaphragm below and the suprasternal thoracic outlet above. It contains the heart, pericardium, esophagus, various great vessels, nerves, lymph nodes, and numerous other structures. Diseases of the mediastinum arise for the most part from infections, tumors, and other disorders of these contained structures. Because defining the principal anatomic locus of mediastinal disease may be helpful, the mediastinum has been arbitrarily divided into three or more zones: a superior area, above the heart, which contains the great vessels, thymus, and substernal extensions of the thyroid; a lower anterior area, which contains the heart, pericardium, and lymph nodes; and

a posterior area, which contains the esophagus, the descending aorta, and many different nerves.

INFECTIONS.   Acute mediastinitis is fortunately rare and most often results from endoscopy, surgery, or trauma to the esophagus. Fever, widening of the mediastinal shadow by x-ray, and a history of surgery, perforation, trauma, or manipulation of the esophagus may suggest the diagnosis. X-ray studies with suitable contrast material may demonstrate esophageal perforation, or the development of a complicating pleural effusion may be observed. Repair of the esophageal perforation, if it is identified early, surgical drainage of mediastinal abscesses, and microbial treatment are the usual therapies.

Chronic mediastinitis from extension of tuberculosis or histoplasmosis of mediastinal lymph nodes is extremely rare but may cause organizing mediastinal fibrosis with venous obstruction (see Ch. 71).

MEDIASTINAL EMPHYSEMA.   Mediastinal emphysema occurs when air enters the mediastinum from some adjacent air-containing organ. Although it may result from trauma to or rupture of the eosphagus or a large bronchus, in which case it has serious impact, it most often results from a dissection of air from the peripheral airways into the pulmonary interstitium either from a spontaneous tear or as a complication of positive pressure artificial ventilation. There then occurs a dissection of air along the peribronchial and perivascular structures into the mediastinum. Precordial pain or discomfort may be present, and on physical examination there may be a loud crunching sound over the precordium which is related to the heartbeat and not to respiration (*Hamman's sign*). Dissection of air out of the mediastinum and into the neck or even very extensively over much of the body may occur. The air in the mediastinum sometimes can be seen on the x-ray of the chest as x-ray translucencies that outline the pericardium, the heart, and other mediastinal structures. Mediastinal emphysema is usually a benign, self-limited condition that resolves without treatment and does not interfere with venous return or other mediastinal organ function. Surgical relief of intramediastinal pressure is rarely helpful or necessary.

TUMORS.   Tumors of the mediastinum are the most common major disorder of this region. In young adults they are often primary in the mediastinum and benign; in older adults they are more often malignant and metastatic. Symptoms of mediastinal tumors may arise from pressure on or invasion of adjacent structures, and result in cough, shortness of breath, dysphagia, venous congestion, substernal pain, or phrenic or recurrent laryngeal nerve paralysis. Malignant tumors may cause constitutional symptoms. Many mediastinal tumors come to medical attention only because an asymptomatic mass is identified on an x-ray of the chest.

Tumors of the superior mediastinum are often of thymic origin and may be benign or malignant. Intrathoracic extensions of thyroid adenomas are also common causes of upper mediastinal tumors. Metastatic carcinoma from the lung or breast may involve the lymph nodes of the upper mediastinum. If there is extension to the superior vena cava, the so-called *superior vena caval syndrome* may result, with edema and swelling of the head, eyes, and upper extremity. Involvement of the various nerves in the upper mediastinum may result in vocal cord paralysis (especially on the left) or diaphragmatic paralysis.

Lymphoma may be a cause of upper anterior mediastinal tumor, but most often tumors of the anterior mediastinum are teratodermoids, usually benign. They may vary from a simple cyst to complex mixed tumors of ectodermal origin. Pericardial cysts arise from and are attached to the pericardium and must be differentiated from other tumors of this region. Congenital cysts that arise from the bronchi, bronchogenic cysts, usually are attached to the trachea or the large central bronchi and radiologically are seen as tumors of the central mediastinum. They are usually fluid filled and by x-ray present as solid spherical masses. Occasionally a bronchial communication is established, they contain air, and by x-ray they appear as cystic air-containing spaces.

In the posterior mediastinum the most common tumors are of neural origin; these, too, are usually benign. Neurofibromas may arise from the dorsal roots and the sympathetic chain.

Although many mediastinal tumors are benign and do not cause symptoms, the inability to establish a certain diagnosis, together with the possibility that they will undergo malignant degeneration, has usually resulted in their treatment by surgical removal.

Hamman, L.: Spontaneous mediastinal emphysema. Bull. Johns Hopkins Hosp., 64:1, 1939.
Sabiston, D. C., Jr., and Oldham, H. N., Jr.: The mediastinum. *In* Sabiston, D. C., Jr., and Spencer, F. C. (eds.): Gibbons' Surgery of the Chest. 3rd ed. Philadelphia, W. B. Saunders Company, 1976, pp. 406–424.

350.3. THE DIAPHRAGM

The diaphragm is the principal muscle of respiration. It separates the thorax and the abdomen, and it confines to the thorax the negative pressure of the pleura during inspiration. It arises from and is attached to the sternum, the lower ribs, the upper lumbar vertebrae, and from the fascia of the quadratus lumborum and the psoas muscles. It inserts into the central tendon of the diaphragm. Motor and sensory fibers reach the diaphragm by the phrenic nerves; some sensory fibers come from the lower intercostal nerves.

HERNIAS.   Hernias of the diaphragm may be congenital, developmental, or traumatic.

Herniation of abdominal organs through the congenital and persistent foramina of Bochdalek and Morgagni is quite uncommon. Hernias of Bochdalek are more common than hernias of Morgagni; they occur in the posterolateral chest on either side, are predominantly a disease of infants and children, may result in massive herniation of small intestine or other abdominal viscera into the chest with collapse of the lung and intestinal obstruction, and often require emergent surgical correction.

Hernias of Morgagni are located anteriorly, in or close to the midline, and on either side, but more often on the right. Part of the liver or the omentum is the structure that most often protrudes through them; other abdominal viscera, e.g., colon, stomach, or small intestine, may be in the hernia. These hernias are often asymptomatic, found on a routine x-ray, and they present the diagnostic problem of an anterior mass connected to or adjacent to the diaphragm. Radioisotopic scans of the liver and x-rays of the gastrointestinal tract will often make the diagnosis. Diagnostic pneumoperitoneum with abdominal x-ray has sometimes been used.

Surgical exploration for diagnosis and repair is usually carried out.

The much more common herniation of the stomach through the esophageal hiatus is considered in Ch. 396.

Traumatic hernia of the diaphragm may result from direct injury to the diaphragm, e.g., knife or bullet wounds, or indirectly from severe abdominal trauma with compression. Because this complication may not be appreciated at the time the trauma occurs, it may come to attention later when abdominal viscera are found located in the thorax. Unfortunately the cause of the abnormalities is not always recognized, and the chest x-ray findings may be confused with a paralyzed diaphragm or a pneumothorax. These usually require surgical correction.

PARALYSIS.   Paralysis of the diaphragm may result from interruption of the phrenic nerve anywhere in its course. It may be caused by trauma, infection (e.g., diphtheria), surgical interruption, or tumor, or it may be of unknown cause. Invasion of the phrenic nerve by a malignant tumor in the mediastinum is the most common cause. The paralyzed diaphragm is elevated and may move paradoxically in inspiration. If inspiration is performed swiftly, as with an inspiratory sniff, this paradoxical motion is accentuated and usually is very apparent.

Most of the physiologic studies in diaphragmatic paralysis were done on patients who had tuberculosis at a time when unilateral interruption of the phrenic nerve was a form of therapy. The physiologic changes were minor and consisted of some changes in the lung volumes.

EVENTRATION.   Rarely, one of the diaphragms or part of one of the diaphragms is atrophic, and is replaced by a thin nonmuscular membranous structure. The cause is unknown, but is probably congenital. The involved portion of the diaphragm is high and moves paradoxically. It is often confused with a paralyzed diaphragm. The patient with an eventration is often asymptomatic, and the defect may be found on a routine x-ray examination. If it produces either thoracic or abdominal symptoms, surgical correction may be necessary.

HICCUP.   Hiccup is an involuntary quick inspiration interrupted by a quick closure of the vocal cords. It is usually of unknown and benign cause and of short duration, and stops spontaneously or as a result of various self-administered respiratory maneuvers. Occasionally it is a symptom of serious disease, e.g., uremia. It occurs in various pulmonary, cardiac, pleural, and abdominal processes that irritate the diaphragm. In a rare case of persistent hiccup, if exhaustion becomes a problem, local anesthesia of a phrenic nerve has sometimes been successful. Fluoroscopy to determine if the process is unilateral should precede this therapy.

Agostoni, E., and Sant'Ambrogio, S.: The diaphragm. *In* Campbell, E. J. M., Agostoni, E., and Davis, J. N. (eds.): The Respiratory Muscles. Philadelphia, W. B. Saunders Company, 1970.
McCredie, M., Lovejoy, F. W., Jr., and Kaltreider, N. L.: Pulmonary function in diaphragmatic paralysis. Thorax, 17:213, 1962.
Paris, F., Tarazona, V., Casillas, M., Blosco, E., Conto, A., Pastor, J., and Acosta, A.: Hernia of Morgagni. Thorax, 28:631, 1973.

350.4. THE CHEST WALL

The chest wall may be disturbed in its structure and function by a variety of congenital, inflammatory, neuromuscular, pulmonary, pleural, and idiopathic diseases. The most common disturbances are from diseases of the spine that result in gross bony disarrangement (kyphoscoliosis), various congenital defects of the anterior thorax (pectus excavatum, pectus carinatum), and those that are secondary to pulmonary or pleural disease or its surgical treatment.

KYPHOSIS AND SCOLIOSIS

DEFINITION. Scoliosis is lateral curvature of the spine. It is almost always accompanied by some posterior curvature (kyphosis). It may occur in any part of the spine, but produces its greatest disturbance when it is in the thoracic region. In scoliosis there is usually a compensatory curve in the opposite direction in the spine below the primary curvature. Scoliosis is categorized as to the right or left according to the direction of the convexity of the primary curvature, and its degree is expressed as the angle which the converging limbs of the curvature form when measured on an x-ray of the spine. Kyphosis is described by the angle which the upper limb of the deformity forms with the vertical plane.

ETIOLOGY AND MECHANISMS. Most cases (70 to 80 per cent) of kyphoscoliosis are of *unknown cause* and are first recognized in childhood. A smaller and decreasing number are due to neuromuscular disease, especially poliomyelitis. Another relatively uncommon cause of kyphoscoliosis and scoliosis is intrinsic disease of the spine. Pulmonary and pleural disease, as well as chest surgical procedures, e.g., extensive thoracoplasty, may cause kyphoscoliosis.

CLINICAL MANIFESTATIONS. The most common disturbance which kyphoscoliosis or kyphosis causes is the psychologic effect of the skeletal deformity. Unless the scoliosis or kyphosis is severe, cardiorespiratory insufficiency usually does not appear. In the carefully studied group of patients observed by Bergofsky and his associates, this complication was seen only in those patients whose scoliosis exceeded 100 degrees or whose kyphosis exceeded 20 degrees. The effect of the kyphosis and scoliosis seemed to be additive.

Probably most patients with kyphoscoliosis have no pulmonary complaints. If their pulmonary function is measured, they will be found to have only minor decreases in lung volumes and ventilatory capacity without disturbances in gas exchange.

With more advanced skeletal deformity and especially with advancing age, some patients have first shortness of breath on exertion, hypoxia, and hypercapnia. Others will have extreme dyspnea on exertion, severe hypoxia and hypercapnia, even at rest, and cor pulmonale with profound right ventricular failure.

The mechanism for this cardiorespiratory failure was long thought to be due to complicating bronchitis and emphysema. It is now clear that this is usually not the case and that the skeletal and chest wall deformity leads to an increased work of breathing and eventually to decreased alveolar ventilation, hypoxia, hypercapnia, polycythemia, decreased carbon dioxide responsiveness, and increased pulmonary vascular resistance.

PROGNOSIS. Although it is known that cardiorespiratory failure occurs only with severe degrees of kyphoscoliosis, it is not certain how many individuals with severe deformities develop this complication.

Once cor pulmonale develops, the prognosis is poor; but vigorous treatment sometimes reverses many of the derangements, and with good care and medical supervision some patients have done well for many years after an episode of cardiorespiratory failure.

TREATMENT. Early prophylactic treatment of the skeletal deformity is primarily an orthopedic problem, but aggressive surgical treatment aimed at correcting and stabilizing the deformed spine in children and adolescents seems warranted and promising.

In older adults who are deformed but stable and asymptomatic, all measures which may prevent the development of complicating bronchitis should be taken, e.g., removal of bronchial irritants, prompt treatment of bronchial infection.

The treatment of severe cardiorespiratory insufficiency requires a multifactorial approach like that used in other forms of cardiopulmonary failure, in which one strives to identify reversible physiologic defects and correct them. Decreased alveolar ventilation may require assisted ventilation, although the chest deformity may make this difficult. Marked hypoxia may indicate the need for supplemental oxygen if ventilation can be maintained. Congestive failure should be treated with diuretics and digitalis. Sometimes with vigorous treatment, patients with severe cardiorespiratory failure recover, improve, and maintain this improvement for long periods. Nocturnal assisted ventilation with a Drinker respirator has been used chronically in some patients with decreased alveolar ventilation.

ANKYLOSING SPONDYLITIS

Ankylosing spondylitis of the thoracic spine produces a characteristic deformity of the chest with marked flexion of the thoracic spine, and rigidity from vertebral fusion (see Ch. 58.1). This disorder most commonly causes limitation in thoracic mobility and reduced vital capacity but little pulmonary disability. Recently it has been recognized that a small group of patients with ankylosing spondylitis also have pulmonary or pleural disease. Most commonly there is fibrobullous disease of the upper lobes; infrequently it is complicated by *Aspergillus* colonization or severe respiratory insufficiency. Pleural effusions or pleural fibrosis are also rare complications.

DEFORMITIES OF ANTERIOR CHEST WALL

PECTUS EXCAVATUM. This congenital defect is sometimes also called funnel chest. It consists of a shortening of the distance between the xiphoid and the vertebral bodies, backward displacement of the body of the sternum, and deformity of the costal cartilages to accommodate this displacement.

For most patients the only disability arises from the cosmetic effects and the psychologic symptoms it engenders. Extremely rarely the defect may be so severe that it causes cardiorespiratory symptoms. Surgical correction is possible but rarely necessary.

PECTUS CARINATUM. This defect has also been called pigeon breast. It is less common than pectus excavatum and consists of a swinging forward of the xiphoid and lower portion of the sternum and a lengthening of the costal cartilages. It causes cardiorespiratory symptoms even less frequently than pectus excavatum, and correction of the cosmetic defect is a rare indication for surgical correction.

Bergofsky, E. H., Turino, M., and Fishman, A. P.: Cardiorespiratory failure in kyphoscoliosis. Medicine, 38:263, 1959.

Gacad, G., and Hamosh, P.: The lung in ankylosing spondylitis. Am. Rev. Respir. Dis., 107:286, 1973.

Rosenow, E. C., Strimlam, C. V., Muhm, J. R., and Ferguson, R. H.: Pleuropulmonary manifestations of ankylosing spondylitis. Mayo Clin. Proc., 52:641, 1977.

Sinha, R. and Bergofsky, E. H.: Prolonged alteration of lung mechanics in kyphoscoliosis by positive pressure inflation. Am. Rev. Respir. Dis., 106:47, 1972.

351. RESPIRATORY FAILURE

John F. Murray

351.1. INTRODUCTION

Adequate respiration consists of the uptake of sufficient amounts of O_2 and the elimination of sufficient amounts of CO_2 to maintain Po_2 and Pco_2 in arterial blood at their respective normal values. It follows that *respiratory failure* is associated with disturbances in the exchange of O_2 and CO_2 between gas in alveoli and blood in pulmonary capillaries and that these abnormalities must be reflected by changes in the Po_2 and Pco_2 in arterial blood. Thus respiratory failure is defined as a condition in which arterial Po_2 is below the normal range (excluding hypoxemia from intracardiac right-to-left shunting of blood), or arterial Pco_2 is above the normal range (excluding respiratory compensation for metabolic alkalosis). This definition, which is physiologically precise as well as clinically applicable, implies that the diagnosis of respiratory failure depends chiefly on laboratory analysis of arterial blood and not on clinical findings.

Respiratory failure is not a disease but a disorder of function that can be caused by a variety of conditions that affect the lungs; in some instances, the lungs are completely normal (e.g., overdose of sedative drugs). Respiratory failure is analogous to heart failure and renal failure, both of which represent the consequences of impaired normal function resulting from numerous disparate diseases.

Respiratory failure is traditionally divided into acute and chronic varieties, depending on the time it takes for the abnormalities in gas exchange to occur. This arbitrary classification does not take into account the common clinical occurrence of an acute worsening of arterial Po_2 and Pco_2 in a patient who already has chronic respiratory failure as a result of some underlying disorder. However, the distinction between acute and chronic respiratory failure has important etiologic and therapeutic connotations and will be referred to frequently.

351.2. PATHOPHYSIOLOGY OF RESPIRATORY FAILURE

In human beings, respiration has been subdivided into four functional processes: ventilation, diffusion, perfusion, and control of breathing. Each of these contributes uniquely to the maintenance of normal values of Po_2 and Pco_2 in arterial blood. Therefore, abnormalities in any one of the four processes, if sufficiently severe, will cause respiratory failure; furthermore, in many common respiratory disorders, multiple abnormalities coexist.

NORMAL GAS EXCHANGE

The physiology of normal gas exchange is described in Ch. 342.6 and will not be reviewed here. However, understanding what is meant by normal is important, because arterial Po_2 varies with age and both arterial Po_2 and Pco_2 vary according to the altitude (i.e., the prevailing barometric pressure) at which the person happens to be when the blood specimen is obtained and to the extent of acclimatization. The normal range includes the biologic variabilities among individuals and the analytic variations inherent in the measurements. Because the diagnosis of respiratory failure should be made in the laboratory and not at the bedside, the physician's ability to establish the diagnosis depends on the accuracy of the laboratory tests used to measure Po_2 and Pco_2. Normal mean arterial Po_2 (Pa_{O_2}) values in subjects 20 years of age or older can be calculated from the regression equation $Pa_{O_2} = 100.1 - 0.323$ (age in years). The normal range of variation is ± 5 mm Hg from the mean value. Arterial Pco_2 does not vary with age and is normally within the range of 40 ± 5 mm Hg in healthy persons at sea level. Values of Po_2 *below* or Pco_2 *above* normal limits indicate the presence of respiratory failure.

ABNORMAL GAS EXCHANGE

The pathophsiology of abnormal gas exchange is also discussed in Ch. 342.6. Hypoventilation, impaired diffusion, ventilation-perfusion mismatching, right-to-left shunting of blood, and breathing air with a low Po_2 all cause arterial hypoxia (a decrease below normal of Po_2); in contrast, for practical purposes only hypoventilation causes arterial hypercapnia (an increase above normal of Pco_2). In view of the therapeutic importance of recognizing the abnormal mechanism(s) leading to a patient's respiratory failure, each will be reviewed briefly.

HYPOVENTILATION. As just mentioned, alveolar hypoventilation is present when the arterial Pco_2 is increased. Furthermore, as arterial Pco_2 increases, Po_2 decreases *except* when the patient is breathing gas with an enriched concentration of O_2. Because arterial Po_2 and Pco_2 change in opposite directions by nearly the same amount during hypoventilation, the contribution of hypoventilation to the patient's arterial hypoxia can be readily assessed. (In a 60-year-old person, for example, if $Po_2 = 50$ mm Hg and $Pco_2 = 70$ mm Hg, both have changed from their normal values by the same amount [30 mm Hg] and "pure" hypoventilation is present; in contrast, if $Po_2 = 30$ mm Hg and $Pco_2 = 70$ mm Hg, the change from normal of Pco_2 does not account for the entire change in Po_2; some other cause in addition to hypoxia from hypoventilation must be present.) Arterial hypoxia from alveolar hypoventilation is not associated with an increased alveolar-arterial Po_2 difference and is "corrected" by breathing 100 per cent O_2.

IMPAIRED DIFFUSION. Abnormalities of diffusion do not cause arterial hypoxia in persons at rest unless they are extremely severe. Although these occur in occasional patients with respiratory failure, for practical purposes the possible contribution of an abnormality of diffusion to a given patient's arterial hypoxia can be ignored except during exercise. This practice is permissible because diffusion disturbances can cause only relatively small increases in the patient's alveolar-arterial Po_2 difference, and this abnormality, if it exists, is readily corrected by adding small amounts of O_2 to the inspired air.

VENTILATION-PERFUSION IMBALANCE. When gas exchange units receive more blood flow than ventilation, arterial hypoxia results. Mismatching of ventilation-perfusion is by far the most common cause of arterial hypoxia and can be recognized by giving the patient 100 per cent O_2 to breathe; this causes the alveolar-arterial Po_2 difference from pure mismatching that is present while the patient breathes room air to decrease and arterial Po_2 to increase to normal values (>550 mm Hg). Although a "pure" ventilation-perfusion inequality can lead to CO_2 retention, this is an uncommon cause of hypercapnia because as arterial Pco_2 tends to increase, it stimulates peripheral and central chemoreceptors and increases ventilation; this, in turn, reduces Pco_2 back to normal values but, owing to the shape of the oxyhemoglobin dissociation curve, does not correct the hypoxia.

RIGHT-TO-LEFT SHUNTS. Shunts of blood from right to left may occur through abnormal anatomic communications in the lung (e.g., a pulmonary arteriovenous fistula) and frequently by perfusion of lung units that are completely unventilated because they are either collapsed (atelectasis) or filled with fluid (pulmonary edema, pneumonia, alveolar proteinosis). Regardless of the cause, an alveolar-arterial Po_2 difference results that increases when the patient breathes 100 per cent O_2 compared with the value obtained while breathing room air. For reasons similar to those occurring in patients with ventilation-perfusion imbalances, CO_2 retention seldom occurs in patients with right-to-left shunts.

HYPERCAPNIA. In contrast to arterial hypoxia, which may result from five different pathophysiologic derangements, arterial hypercapnia can always be interpreted as signifying alveolar hypoventilation. This is true because arterial Pco_2 (Pa_{CO_2}) is governed by the relationship between CO_2 production ($\dot{V}co_2$) and alveolar ventilation ($\dot{V}A$); $Pa_{CO_2} = k\dot{V}co_2/\dot{V}A$. Normally, however, even when CO_2 production increases markedly, alveolar ventilation increases proportionately and arterial Pco_2 is maintained within narrow limits. Thus an increase in arterial Pco_2 can always be viewed as respiratory failure in the sense that alveolar ventilation is inadequate to eliminate all the CO_2 being produced at that time. Severe ventilation-perfusion imbalances and right-to-left shunts can produce CO_2 retention, but this is uncommon because, as already emphasized, alveolar ventilation increases and corrects the disturbance.

An increase or decrease in Pco_2 in the blood has a direct effect on the amount of carbonic acid in the blood and a reciprocal effect on pH. Acute changes in Pco_2 have a more profound effect on pH than chronic changes owing to differences in plasma bicarbonate. With acute increases or decreases in Pco_2, there is little change in bicarbonate level and a considerable change in pH; after three to five days of sustained changes in Pco_2, renal compensation has increased plasma bicarbonate in hypercapnia and decreased it in hypocapnia, both tending to restore pH toward normal. Many patients with respiratory failure have mixed respiratory and nonrespiratory acid-base disturbances. Knowledge of the time course of a patient's problem as well as the magnitude of changes in plasma bicarbonate is extremely useful in providing the necessary understanding for appropriate treatment of all components of the disorder.

RIGHT HEART FAILURE

Acute respiratory failure can cause acute right heart failure (acute cor pulmonale). The right ventricle cannot sustain sudden pressure loads over 40 to 50 mm Hg and fails. Thus acute right heart failure may develop in any condition in which pulmonary vascular resistance increases abruptly; this happens most commonly in patients with multiple pulmonary emboli with obstruction of much of the pulmonary vascular bed (usually >60 per cent). At times, acute cor pulmonale complicates the course of patients with severe bronchial asthma or other forms or marked airways obstruction.

Acute right heart failure may also occur in patients with chronic lung disease during an episode of acute respiratory failure. Most of these patients have right ventricular hypertrophy (chronic cor pulmonale) to begin with, and a subclinical or stable condition is worsened by the added effects of the superimposed acute lung disease (usually bronchitis or pneumonia). In these patients, resistance to blood flow through the lungs increases above its previous value for several reasons: (1) alveolar hypoxia and acidemia cause pulmonary arterial vasoconstriction; (2) certain lung diseases reduce the cross-sectional area available for perfusion; (3) hyperinflation of the lung increases pulmonary vascular resistance; and (4) arterial hypoxia may depress myocardial contractility. These factors are important to recognize because they are reversible and usually respond well to appropriate treatment of the intercurrent acute disorder.

351.3. CAUSES OF RESPIRATORY FAILURE

Because respiratory failure is defined as the presence of arterial hypoxia with or without hypercapnia, it is obvious that a large variety of disorders are capable of producing these abnormalities. For convenience, the multiple causes of respiratory failure can be classified (Table 1), depending on which component of the respiratory system is involved. Because most of these disorders characteristically cause either acute or chronic respiratory failure, they can be subdivided further into these categories.

DISEASES CAUSING AIRWAYS OBSTRUCTION

ACUTE. Obstruction may result from acute diseases that involve any portion of the upper and lower airways. The presence of respiratory failure depends on the magnitude and extent of the narrowing. Obstruc-

TABLE 1. Classification of Common Disorders Associated
with Respiratory Failure

**TABLE 1. Classification of Common Disorders Associated
with Respiratory Failure**

Diseases causing airways obstruction
  Acute
    Epiglottitis
    Laryngeal edema (croup)
    Foreign body
    Bronchiolitis
    Bronchial asthma
  Chronic
    Bronchitis
    Emphysema
    Bronchiectasis
Diseases causing parenchymal infiltration
  Acute
    Pneumonia
    Immunologic reactions
  Chronic
    Sarcoidosis
    Pneumoconioses
    Diffuse interstitial fibrosis
Diseases causing pulmonary edema
  Cardiogenic
    Myocardial infarction
    Mitral or aortic valve disease
    Left ventricular failure
  Noncardiogenic
    High altitude
    Shock from any cause
    Heroin
    Inhalation of chemical substances
    Sepsis
    Neurologic disorders
Pulmonary vascular diseases
  Acute
    Pulmonary emboli (blood clots)
    Fat emboli
  Chronic
    Pulmonary vasculitis
    Recurrent thromboembolism
Diseases of the chest wall and pleura
  Acute
    Flail chest
    Pneumothorax
  Chronic
    Kyphoscoliosis
    Obesity
    Massive pleural effusion(s)
Disorders of the neuromuscular system
  Brain disorders
    Sedative drugs, anesthesia
    Vascular diseases
    Infections
    Tumors
  Muscular disorders
    Muscular dystrophy
    Myasthenia gravis
  Peripheral nerve disorders
    Polyneuritis
    Poliomyelitis

op in infants and young children who have smaller and hence more vulnerable upper passages than older children and adults.

Acute obstruction of the lower airways is usually caused by swelling of the mucosa, secretions in the lumen, or bronchospasm. Accordingly, bronchial asthma, infections, bronchiolitis, and the inhalation of chemicals (such as nitrogen dioxide in silo-filler's disease) are important causes of acute respiratory failure.

CHRONIC. Diffuse obstruction may result from disorders originating in large bronchi (bronchiectasis), small bronchi (bronchitis), or the lung parenchyma (emphysema). These abnormalities characteristically progress gradually and lead to chronic respiratory failure. Of considerable importance are the intercurrent episodes of acute disease, usually pneumonia or bronchitis, that complicate the underlying disorder and often worsen the severity of existing respiratory failure.

DISEASES CAUSING PARENCHYMAL INFILTRATION

ACUTE. The most common cause of acute infiltration of the parenchyma is pneumonia, which may have a viral, bacterial, or occasionally chemical origin. Whether acute respiratory failure develops depends on the extent and severity of the disease. Immunologic reactions from drugs, migrating parasites, or leukoagglutinins are uncommon causes of acute respiratory failure but are important because of their special therapeutic requirements.

CHRONIC. There are over 100 different conditions that can cause chronic diffuse parenchymal infiltration. When severe, any of these can cause chronic respiratory failure. As in patients with chronic airways obstruction, patients with chronic infiltrative diseases may have intercurrent episodes of bronchopulmonary infection that cause acute worsening of their underlying respiratory status.

DISEASES CAUSING PULMONARY EDEMA

CARDIOGENIC. Pulmonary edema in patients with heart disease may be acute or chronic in onset; both varieties are caused by an increase in the hydrostatic pressure within pulmonary capillaries. Pulmonary edema may follow an acute myocardial infarction and acute left ventricular failure of any cause (hypertensive crisis, arrhythmias), or it may be precipitated in patients with valvular or other forms of chronic heart disease by sudden changes in their circulatory status (from arrhythmias, pulmonary emboli, or increased systemic blood pressure). Chronic pulmonary edema is found in patients with chronic, usually refractory, heart failure, but even in these patients the amount of edema increases and decreases according to changing hemodynamics and therapy.

NONCARDIOGENIC. It has long been recognized that acute pulmonary edema can accompany certain conditions that do not involve the heart. The basic pathophysiologic abnormality in most of these disorders appears to be an increased permeability of the pulmonary capillary endothelium, but other forms of pulmonary edema (high altitude pulmonary edema, re-expansion pulmonary edema) also occur. Pulmonary edema result-

tion of the *extra*thoracic airway (nasopharynx, larynx, extrathoracic portion of the trachea) usually causes stridor, a characteristic alteration of breathing that is associated with harsh, high-pitched respiratory noises that are louder and more pronounced during inspiration than expiration. In contrast, obstruction of the *intra*thoracic airways causes wheezing, an abnormality of breathing in which expiration is louder and longer than inspiration.

Obstruction of the upper airways can result from (1) inflammation-induced swelling of the mucosa secondary to infections, allergic reactions, and, less commonly, thermal or mechanical injuries, and (2) impaction of foreign bodies or, occasionally, tumors. Acute obstruction of the upper airways is particularly likely to devel-

TABLE 2. Partial List of Conditions That Have Been Associated with the Adult Respiratory Distress Syndrome

Shock of any etiology	Inhaled toxins
Infections	O_2 (high concentrations)
Gram-negative sepsis	Smoke
Viral pneumonia	Corrosive chemicals (NO_2, Cl_2,
Bacterial pneumonia	NH_3, phosgene, cadmium)
Trauma	Hematologic disorders
Fat emboli	Intravascular coagulation
Lung contusion	Massive blood transfusion
Nonthoracic trauma (including	Metabolic disorders
head injury)	Pancreatitis
Liquid aspiration	Uremia
Gastric juice	Paraquat ingestion
Fresh and salt water (drowning)	Miscellaneous
Hydrocarbon fluids	Increased intracranial pressure
Drug overdose	(including seizures)
Heroin	Eclampsia
Methadone	Postcardioversion
Propoxyphene	Radiation pneumonitis
Barbiturates	Postcardiopulmonary bypass
Colchicine	

ing from increased permeability is an important and apparently steadily increasing cause of acute respiratory failure, especially in patients who are hospitalized with serious medical or surgical illnesses that initially do not involve the lungs. After a latent period of 6 to 24 hours, these patients develop progressive arterial hypoxia, decreased compliance, and extensive roentgenographic infiltrations; in fatal cases, the lungs are found to be nearly airless, intensely congested, and filled with a proteinaceous edema fluid that also contains large numbers of red blood cells; occasionally, hyaline membranes are found. This constellation of clinical, physiologic, and pathologic events is now known as the *adult respiratory distress syndrome* and has been reported as a complication of many apparently unrelated conditions (Table 2). The feature common to all these disorders is the presence of diffuse injury to the alveolar-capillary membrane. Once damage has occurred, probably by many different pathways, and the permeability of the membrane is increased, pulmonary edema follows; thus the clinical, physiologic, and pathologic manifestations are similar, regardless of the cause of the injury.

PULMONARY VASCULAR DISEASES

ACUTE. Pulmonary embolism is usually accompanied by a decreased arterial Po_2 and Pco_2, the latter reflecting the hyperventilation that nearly always occurs. Pulmonary embolism is also an important cause of worsening respiratory failure in patients with underlying chronic lung disease. Fat emboli and emboli from platelet-fibrin aggregates can cause marked hypoxia by increasing the permeability of the alveolar-capillary membrane and producing severe pulmonary edema.

CHRONIC. Pulmonary vasculitis and recurrent thromboembolism are not common conditions and, when present, usually do not cause respiratory failure until the late stages of the disease. Recurrent thromboembolism occurs in intravenous drug abusers and in patients with chronic peripheral venous thrombi, sickle cell anemia, and schistosomiasis. Pulmonary vasculitis occurs in patients with scleroderma, other collagen diseases, and primary pulmonary hypertension.

DISEASES OF THE CHEST WALL AND PLEURA

ACUTE. The most important cause of sudden respiratory failure from acute disorders involving the thoracic cage is injury to the chest wall. Segmental fractures of several ribs or fractures of ribs on both sides of the sternum can result in a flail chest. Besides the impairment of ventilatory function that results from the unstable chest wall, gas exchange abnormalities are often compounded by contusion of the lung underneath the site of injury. Spontaneous or traumatic pneumothorax is an important cause of acute respiratory failure, which may be severe and which often afflicts otherwise healthy persons.

CHRONIC. Severe idiopathic or acquired kyphoscoliosis can cause chronic respiratory failure, which is often associated with cor pulmonale. Similarly, massive obesity is a well known cause of chronic respiratory failure. Patients with massive pleural effusion(s) or with thickened, constrictive pleural layer(s) may also have chronic respiratory failure.

DISORDERS OF THE NEUROMUSCULAR SYSTEM

Disorders of the neuromuscular system are classified into which part of the effector system is involved, i.e., the brain, neuronal pathways, or muscles of respiration, rather than into acute and chronic varieties. Patients with these disorders often have normal lungs; respiratory failure occurs from lack of ventilation.

BRAIN DISORDERS. Probably the most common cause of respiratory failure from impaired function of the central nervous system comes from the use of sedative drugs or anesthetic agents. Suppression of ventilatory drive from opiates, barbiturates, psychic depressants, alcohol, and a variety of sedative drugs results in hypoxia and hypercapnia that may be life threatening. Ventilatory stimuli can also be depressed by many diseases of the central nervous system, including vascular diseases, tumors, and infections.

SPINAL CORD AND PERIPHERAL NERVE DISORDERS. Injuries to the cervical or high thoracic spinal cord may produce immediate respiratory failure from paralysis of the muscles of respiration. Loss of anterior horn cell function in patients with poliomyelitis was an important cause of acute and chronic respiratory failure but is seldom encountered now because of the widespread use of vaccination. Polyneuritis, whether postinfectious (Guillain-Barré syndrome) or toxic, is an uncommon but important cause of respiratory failure in view of its inherent reversibility.

MUSCULAR DISORDERS. The final effectors in the system that controls breathing are the skeletal muscles of respiration. When these muscles are involved by generalized myopathies, such as muscular dystrophy or myasthenia gravis, respiratory failure results. Respiratory failure in patients with myasthenia gravis occurs during myasthenic or cholinergic crises. In contrast, respiratory failure in patients with muscular dystrophy is nearly always chronic and related to an advanced stage in the progression of the disease.

351.4. CLINICAL MANIFESTATIONS

Given the great variety of disorders that can cause respiratory failure (Table 1), it is obvious that the clinical manifestations in a given patient depend in large part on which underlying disease he has; these are dealt with elsewhere in this book. When respiratory failure ensues and if the blood gas disturbances are sufficiently severe, the signs and symptoms of hypoxia, and possible hypercapnia, become superimposed upon the signs and symptoms of the underlying disease. It should be emphasized that the clinical manifestations of hypoxia and hypercapnia are nonspecific and usually occur late in the evolution of the clinical problem. This statement underscores the earlier axiom that respiratory failure is a laboratory diagnosis and not a clinical diagnosis.

HYPOXIA

The signs and symptoms of acute hypoxia are chiefly caused by abnormalities in central nervous system and cardiovascular function. Characteristic features are impaired judgment and motor instability, a clinical picture closely resembling acute alcoholism. As hypoxia worsens, the brainstem is affected and death results from depression of the medullary respiratory centers. The initial cardiovascular effects of acute hypoxia are tachycardia and increased blood pressure; when hypoxia is very severe, bradycardia, myocardial depression, and shock ensue. Recognizable cyanosis of the lips, mucous membranes, and nail beds usually occurs when the concentration of reduced hemoglobin in the capillaries is >5 grams per 100 ml. Accordingly, cyanosis can result from decreases in either arterial Po_2 or blood flow. In patients with lung disease, cyanosis cannot be detected by most physicians until arterial Po_2 is <50 mm Hg; some observers cannot recognize cyanosis unless arterial Po_2 is <40 mm Hg!

In patients with chronic hypoxia, the central nervous system manifestations are drowsiness, inattentiveness, apathy, fatigue, and delayed reaction time. The chronic cardiovascular effects are often minimal, but pulmonary hypertension or even cor pulmonale with signs of right heart failure may be detected on clinical examination. One of the hallmarks of chronic hypoxia is erythrocytosis, which may cause noticeable plethora and changes in the hemoglobin concentration, hematocrit ratio, or red blood cell count. However, the increase in red blood cell mass in many patients with chronic hypoxia is masked by an almost proportionate increase in plasma volume; in these patients, the usual peripheral blood indexes of the red blood cell production (hemoglobin, hematocrit) do not reveal the full extent of the erythropoietic response.

HYPERCAPNIA

The physiologic consequences of hypercapnia depend not only on the amount of excess CO_2 in the body but also on the rate at which retention develops. Increases in Pco_2 from acute respiratory failure lead to a constellation of progressive disturbances of central nervous system function: apprehension, confusion, drowsiness, coma, and death. The vascular responses represent a mixture of vasoconstriction, from generalized sympathetic activity, and vasodilation, from local accumulation of CO_2; thus the cardiovascular abnormalities are variable and depend on whether vasoconstrictor or vasodilator influences predominate. There is usually tachycardia and sweating, but blood pressure may be high, low, or normal.

In contrast, if Pco_2 increases slowly, compensation takes place and the clinical consequences may be minimal at values of arterial Pco_2 that would cause death if reached suddenly. There are numerous patients with arterial Pco_2 values over 100 mm Hg who are ambulatory and at times living active lives, although most breathe supplementary O_2 to prevent life-threatening hypoxia. Patients with hypercapnia from chronic respiratory failure frequently complain of headaches and drowsiness; these symptoms are probably attributable to the potent cerebral vasodilating effect of excess CO_2. In addition, patients with chronic hypercapnia may have papilledema, muscular twitching, coarse myoclonic jerky motions, and asterixis. At times, the neurologic findings simulate those of a brain tumor.

351.5. TREATMENT OF ACUTE RESPIRATORY FAILURE

The time course of worsening abnormalities varies in patients with acute respiratory failure from almost instantaneous (flail chest, pulmonary embolism) to a gradual crescendo during a period of several hours or even days (respiratory tract infections, bronchial asthma). The demands for treatment and the speed with which it must be provided obviously differ from one patient to another. It is difficult to generalize about such an extremely variable clinical condition, but the principles of treatment of acute respiratory failure are as follows: *first,* establish an airway, administer O_2, and maintain adequate alveolar ventilation; *second,* identify and treat the underlying condition and monitor the patient's progress carefully.

ESTABLISH AN AIRWAY

The upper airway tends to be occluded in unconscious patients because of relaxation of the oropharyngeal muscles and tongue and the presence of saliva, vomitus, and other secretions. When respiratory arrest occurs away from medical facilities, clear all material from the oropharynx and place the victim on his or her back with the head tilted backward as far as possible and extend the jaw forward. Sometimes these simple maneuvers are all that is required to enable breathing to resume spontaneously. If it does not, start mouth-to-mouth breathing; after three or four quick full breaths without allowing time for deflation to occur, maintain deep breaths once every five seconds until the emergency is over.

An airway can be established by three different methods: an oropharyngeal tube, an endotracheal tube passed via the nose or mouth, and a tracheostomy. Selection of the procedure depends on available facilities and personnel and on the site and severity of the obstruction.

OROPHARYNGEAL AIRWAY. An oropharyngeal airway is valuable in unconscious patients who are breathing spontaneously (e.g., during recovery from general anesthesia, after a cerebrovascular accident). An oropharyngeal airway is also useful in patients who are apneic during emergency resuscitation but who are receiving some form of assisted ventilation (mouth-to-mouth respiration, bag-mask system) Although an oropharyngeal tube is commonly used in these clinical circumstances, its role must be viewed as temporary, either while the patient is waking up or until an endotracheal tube can be inserted.

ENDOTRACHEAL TUBE. The preferred method of establishing an airway in most emergencies is with an endotracheal tube. Once inserted, the tube is used to remove secretions and to provide ventilation. Endotracheal tubes can usually be passed quickly through the nose or, at times, through the mouth into the trachea by an experienced person; the airway is then sealed by inflating a balloon near the tip of the tube. Endotracheal tubes should be used in nearly all patients with acute respiratory failure severe enough to require control of their airways.

TRACHEOSTOMY. Emergency tracheostomy was formerly the only way of quickly establishing an airway in patients with acute respiratory failure. Now, emergency tracheostomy is contraindicated except in one clinical situation: acute obstruction of upper airways (e.g., from foreign bodies, trauma, or inflammation). Otherwise, intubation with an endotracheal tube is the treatment of choice for acute respiratory failure. Tracheostomy, if needed, can be performed at a later time in the operating room under ideal conditions. There is virtually no mortality and very little morbidity with an elective tracheostomy, in contrast to the high incidence of complications associated with emergency tracheostomy performed at the bedside.

The decision to convert a satisfactory endotracheal intubation to a tracheostomy is not an easy one and must be individualized in each case. The availability of tubes of inert plastic with low pressure cuffs permits endotracheal tubes to be used for weeks rather than days without prohibitive injury; the main mechanical difference between endotracheal and tracheostomy tubes is the trauma to the vocal cords from the former. The usual reasons for performing a tracheostomy in a patient with a satisfactory endotracheal tube are (1) failure to control secretions (sometimes it is difficult to suction the lungs adequately, especially the left side, through a long endotracheal tube) and (2) the need for prolonged (i.e., several weeks) intubation for assisted ventilation and/or removal of secretions (these circumstances are uncommon but occur particularly in patients with neuromuscular disease and chest wall injuries).

The presence of a tube and its cuff in the airway can cause necrosis of the mucosa of the trachea; at times the entire airway wall may be eroded with penetration of the esophagus (tracheoesophageal fistula) or a neighboring blood vessel (innominate artery), causing severe hemorrhage. Delayed complications after extubation are caused by damage to the trachea or larynx from the tube or cuff; injury to the vocal cords merely impairs phonation, but serious and life-threatening obstruction can result from stenosis or malacia of the tracheal wall. These complications should be considered and evaluated in any patient who complains of persisting hoarseness or who develops breathlessness or stridor at any time after endotracheal intubation.

HUMIDIFICATION. Insertion of an endotracheal or tracheostomy tube bypasses the normal source of humidification of the inspired air. When this occurs and unhumidified air or gas mixture is breathed, the result is drying of the mucosa and impairment of mucociliary clearance. Thus as long as the upper airway is bypassed, patients must receive air or a mixture of O_2 that is fully saturated with water vapor at their body temperature. This is easily accomplished if the patient is being ventilated with most commercial ventilators that have heated humidifiers in the circuit. If the patient is breathing spontaneously, humidifed gas can be delivered through a T-piece connected to the endotracheal or tracheostomy tube. When proper humidification is carried out, remember that there is *no* insensible water loss through the respiratory tract when evaluating the patient's daily fluid balance.

ADMINISTER OXYGEN

Acute respiratory failure, by definition, includes decreased arterial Po_2. When respiratory failure is severe, death results from the central nervous system or cardiovascular consequences of hypoxia. During emergencies, supplementary O_2 is given without worrying about the concentration being used; in general, the higher the concentration of O_2, the better. After the patient's emergency condition has stabilized, attention is directed to administering O_2 in the lowest possible concentration required to correct the hypoxia. Any more O_2 than required to raise arterial Po_2 to a safe level exposes the patient to the direct toxicity of O_2 on the lung parenchyma and other undesirable effects: suppression of alveolar macrophage function and mucociliary clearance. Another possible complication of O_2 therapy that should be kept in mind is suppression of ventilatory drive; hypoventilation develops in patients with chronic CO_2 retention who are insensitive to hypercapnia and whose chief stimulus to breathe comes from the effect of hypoxia on the peripheral chemoreceptors. When these patients are given high concentrations of O_2, correction of their hypoxia removes the stimulus to breathe and further hypoventilation results. Deaths from severe hypercapnia and respiratory acidosis have resulted from this iatrogenic complication. However, the sequence occurs only in patients with chronic lung diseases, particularly airways obstruction, who are hypercapnic to begin with, and is one of the reasons for using "low-flow" O_2 therapy as in Ch. 351.6.

The usual goal of O_2 therapy in acute respiratory failure is to raise arterial Po_2 to between 60 and 80 mm Hg. Because these values lie on the flat portion of the oxyhemoglobin dissociation curve, most of the available hemoglobin is saturated with O_2; raising arterial Po_2 values even higher adds very little additional O_2 to the blood and may require increases in alveolar Po_2 concentrations to toxic levels. At times, especially when the mechanism of arterial hypoxia is right-to-left shunting of blood, arterial Po_2 may be considerably less than 60 mm Hg even with the patient breathing 100 per cent O_2. When this occurs, other maneuvers such as addition of end-expiratory pressure are required to raise arterial Po_2 and to allow a reduction in inspired O_2 concentration.

There are several ways of giving supplementary O_2 to a patient. Which method is chosen depends on the cause and severity of the arterial hypoxia and convenience to the patient. It is important to emphasize that no method can be relied upon to produce a certain increase in arterial Po_2; the response depends on which physiologic mechanism(s) is responsible for the hypoxia. Thus it is always advisable to monitor the effects of O_2 administration by serial analyses of arterial blood.

NASAL CANNULAS OR PRONGS.   The concentration of O_2 in the inspired air can be enriched by nasal cannulas, catheters, or prongs. These devices work well even when patients breathe through their mouths. However, because of the drying effects of unhumidified O_2 on the nasal mucous membranes, if >3 to 5 liters per minute is needed to achieve satisfactory arterial oxygenation, other methods of administration are advisable.

VENTURI MASKS.   These masks work on the principle of entrainment of a fixed proportion of air that mixes with the O_2 being supplied, and results in a constant inspired concentration: 24, 28, 35, or 40 per cent O_2. Although a properly used Venturi mask ensures that the inspired O_2 concentration is constant, the effects on arterial Po_2 vary considerably from one patient to another. The mask is somewhat uncomfortable and must be removed for eating and drinking. Because of these disadvantages and high cost, other simpler and cheaper methods usually suffice to deliver relatively low (21 to 41 per cent) concentrations of O_2.

RESERVOIR MASKS.   When high concentrations of O_2 (40 to 80 per cent) are needed in patients who are not intubated, reservoir masks are used. To ensure optimal efficiency of operation, the masks must be tight fitting to avoid leaks; because this often causes discomfort, it is difficult to deliver high concentrations of O_2 by reservoir masks for long periods.

OTHER METHODS.   Most of the recently developed mechanical ventilators have regulators that can be set to deliver an inspired O_2 concentration that ranges from 21 to 100 per cent. One of the best ways of ensuring that patients actually receive high concentrations of O_2 (60 to 100 per cent) is to use a mechanical ventilator connected to an endotracheal or tracheostomy tube.

MAINTAIN ALVEOLAR VENTILATION

Emergency resuscitation after respiratory arrest requires ventilation by mouth-to-mouth respiration or a bag and mask device. As soon as possible thereafter, if the patient does not resume spontaneous breathing, intubation and ventilation by a mechanical ventilator are required. Similar considerations apply to patients with acute respiratory failure whose breathing is insufficient to maintain adequate gas exchange. Because these patients are often receiving supplementary O_2, arterial Po_2 is not a good guide to the adequacy of their alveolar ventilation and reliance is placed on arterial Pco_2. Intubation and mechanical ventilation are indicated in most patients with acute respiratory failure whose arterial blood gas studies reveal substantially elevated or increasing Pco_2 values.

MECHANICAL VENTILATION.   Two types of mechanical ventilation can be used to provide assisted ventilation: pressure ventilators, in which a certain (adjustable) airway pressure is reached by the machine during each breathing cycle, or volume ventilators, in which a constant (adjustable) tidal volume is delivered to the patient with each breath. Most commercially available ventilators of both types can be set either to cycle automatically or to assist breathing once it is initiated by the patient. Most instruments also provide means of controlling inspiratory and expiratory flow rates. Pres-

sure ventilators were widely used for many years, but emphasis is now shifting from pressure to volume ventilators, which are more versatile and more reliable.

In general, pressure ventilators work best when the pressure required to deliver a satisfactory tidal volume does not exceed 30 to 40 cm H_2O — in other words, when the compliances of the lung and chest wall are normal or only slightly decreased and airways resistance is normal or only slightly increased. In contrast, volume ventilators deliver a preset tidal volume regardless of any respiratory mechanical abnormalities that might be present; these machines are particularly useful in patients with flail chests, massive obesity, or adult respiratory distress syndrome.

END-EXPIRATORY PRESSURE.   Mechanical ventilators ordinarily raise airway pressure during inspiration and allow it to fall to zero (atmospheric) during expiration; this pattern of assisted ventilation is known as intermittent positive pressure ventilation, or IPPV. At times, it is desirable to add positive pressure to the airway during expiration as well as inspiration to hold the lung at a higher end-expiratory lung volume (functional residual capacity) than it would reach at zero end-expiratory pressure; this pattern of assisted ventilation is known as continuous positive pressure ventilation, or CPPV. Keeping the lung at a high functional residual capacity prevents closure of alveoli and airways during expiration and often improves arterial Po_2 considerably. Positive end-expiratory pressure (or PEEP) is most useful in patients with the conditions that cause the adult respiratory distress syndrome (Table 2).

Although end-expiratory pressure usually results in an improvement in arterial Po_2 and O_2 content, it may also decrease cardiac output by impairing myocardial contractility and increasing pulmonary vascular resistance. Accordingly, the actual delivery of O_2 to the tissues of the body may decrease. Thus it is important to monitor both the respiratory and circulatory responses to end-expiratory pressure to determine the optimal amount of pressure and the need for additional therapeutic interventions. Another common and serious hazard of end-expiratory pressure is its tendency to cause spontaneous pneumothorax and pneumomediastinum.

IDENTIFY AND TREAT THE UNDERLYING CONDITION

Acute respiratory failure always has a precipitating cause. Consequently, the cause of the condition should be identified as soon as possible after emergency measures have been started and the patient's condition has stabilized. Usually, the diagnosis can be established easily by a thorough history and physical examination, analysis of the blood and urine, and chest roentgenogram. Helpful auxiliary tests include those that evaluate central nervous system or cardiac function, those that determine the presence of drugs or poisons in the body, and bacteriologic study of secretions and blood.

Treatment obviously depends on the underlying cause, and the reader is referred to the appropriate chapters of this book for information about the therapy of specific pulmonary and other disorders that lead to acute respiratory failure. In all patients with acute respiratory failure, careful attention should be paid to fluid balance. Overhydration is a frequent and serious complication that can usually be avoided by careful attention to fluid replacement and monitoring of pulmonary capillary (wedge) pressure.

MONITOR THE PATIENT'S PROGRESS

The need for monitoring varies from patient to patient according to the response to initial treatment. If the disorder is readily reversible (e.g., bronchial asthma), the patient may respond sufficiently to go home shortly after being seen and treated. Other less rapidly responding conditions causing acute respiratory failure often require hospital care, and seriously ill patients are best treated in special acute care facilities (intensive care units) when available. Intensive care units provide an institutional focus of trained personnel and special equipment for the care of critically ill patients.

All seriously ill patients should have frequent measurements of blood pressure, constant monitoring of heart rate, careful recording of fluid intake and output, and determination of weight daily. Arterial blood gas analysis should be performed as often as needed but usually at least once daily. Special studies include measurement of cardiac output and placement of a Swan-Ganz catheter in the pulmonary artery for determination of pulmonary arterial and wedge pressures and sampling of mixed venous blood; this information is very helpful in guiding fluid replacement and ventilator adjustments, including levels of end-expiratory pressure. In general, wedge pressure values should be maintained in the normal range (5 to 10 mm Hg) and not allowed to increase above 10 mm Hg, especially in patients with the adult respiratory distress syndrome. Values of mixed venous O_2 saturation provide a rough guide, but the best presently available, to the balance between O_2 delivery to and utilization by all the organs of the body. Although satisfactory levels probably vary from one patient to another, saturations greater than 60 per cent or Po_2 values above 30 mm Hg should be maintained in mixed venous blood by various maneuvers that increase O_2 delivery: breathing supplementary O_2, increasing cardiac output, and increasing hemoglobin concentration. Per cent O_2 saturation of mixed venous blood is probably a better guide to the adequacy of O_2 transport than Po_2 because the affinity between O_2 and hemoglobin (i.e., the position of the oxyhemoglobin dissociation curve) may vary markedly in critically ill patients.

351.6.   TREATMENT OF CHRONIC RESPIRATORY FAILURE

Patients with chronic lung disease often have sufficient alterations in their arterial Po_2 and Pco_2 values that they are said to be in chronic respiratory failure. Therapeutic regimens for these patients, whose disease is relatively stable, are delivered mainly on an outpatient basis and are designed to meet two objectives: (1) preventing or minimizing the number and severity of the intercurrent complications that would otherwise occur, and (2) treating maximally all reversible elements of the underlying disorder. Many of the specific remedies are used for both purposes, and the approaches to preventive and maintenance therapy for patients with the most common chronic lung diseases, asthma, bronchitis, and emphysema, are discussed in Ch. 344.

Despite emphasis on preventing intercurrent complications, these attacks continue to plague the lives of patients with chronic lung disease. Acute episodes of bronchopulmonary infection, pneumothorax, pulmonary embolism, surgical procedures, and misuse of sedatives all add their effects to those of the underlying lung disease and frequently produce serious disturbances of blood gases. These episodes are potentially life threatening, are usually associated with prolonged morbidity, and frequently require hospitalization. The principles of therapy are to maintain oxygenation while treating all new, presumably reversible, elements of the disease in an effort to restore the patient to his or her former state of health.

OXYGEN

Patients with chronic obstructive lung disease and superimposed episodes of acute respiratory failure nearly always have severe hypoxia from a combination of hypoventilation and ventilation-perfusion mismatching. Typical arterial blood values are Po_2 of approximately 30 mm Hg, Pco_2 of 70 mm Hg, and pH of 7.30. Neither the hypercapnia nor the acidemia is life threatening, but the hypoxia is potentially fatal. Thus treatment is directed mainly at alleviating the disturbance in oxygenation; the changes in Pco_2 and pH will return to baseline values as the acute condition improves. In view of the possibility that O_2 therapy may depress ventilation further by withdrawing the hypoxic stimulus to breathe, O_2 is given initially in low concentrations (1 to 3 liters per minute). The goal is to raise Po_2 to satisfactory levels (50 to 60 mm Hg) without depressing ventilation to the extent that unacceptable increases in Pco_2 and decreases in pH (particularly) occur.

The O_2 is usually started at 2 liters per minute, and an arterial blood specimen is analyzed 15 to 30 minutes later to determine the patient's response. Depending on the Po_2 value, the flow of O_2 can be adjusted. If hypoventilation and acidemia result from too much O_2 (e.g., Po_2 80 mm Hg, Pco_2 80 mm Hg, and pH 7.25), the supplementary O_2 should *not* be discontinued but the flow rate should be decreased. The Po_2 decreases much faster than the stimulus to breathe returns, and cardiac arrest or other serious complications of hypoxia may result.

INTUBATION-ASSISTED VENTILATION

Low-flow O_2 given in the manner described provides satisfactory relief of hypoxia in nearly all instances. Although the goal of low-flow O_2 is an arterial Po_2 of 50 to 60 mm Hg, at times one has to be satisfied with 40 to 50 mm Hg. When oxygenation cannot be achieved without intolerable hypercapnia and acidemia, the decision whether to intubate and ventilate the patient must be made. Experience with intubation and mechanical ventilation in this group of patients has been extremely unrewarding, particularly because of the prolonged need for assisted ventilation once intubation is performed and the poor prognosis for prolonged survival and return to useful life after recovery from the acute episode. Although each case must be considered individually, in general, patients with chronic obstructive pulmonary disease who develop superimposed acute respiratory failure should not be intubated. The major exception to this axiom is the need for ventilator support during the postoperative period. Doxapram (see Respiratory Stimulants, below) often allows administration of "extra" O_2 without depressing ventilatory drive.

BRONCHODILATORS

Most intercurrent episodes of acute respiratory failure in patients with chronic obstructive pulmonary disease are associated with increased airways resistance from the presence of secretions, edema of the mucosa, and bronchospasm. Because it is impossible to discriminate among these, bronchodilator drugs are always included in the treatment regimen to take advantage of the reversibility of whatever element of bronchospasm is present.

When patients seek medical attention for intercurrent attacks, they frequently have already tried — and failed to respond to — oral and aerosolized bronchodilators. In this circumstance, intravenous aminophylline is the initial drug of choice. Aminophylline can be injected slowly in 250-mg or 500-mg boluses, or, if the patient has been hospitalized and prolonged treatment is envisioned, by a loading dose (5.6 mg per kilogram of body weight) and constant sustaining infusion (0.9 mg per kilogram of body weight per hour). These dosages should be reduced in patients who have been receiving aminophylline, who are elderly, or, especially, who have liver disease or heart failure. It is advisable to determine the aminophylline plasma level 24 to 36 hours after the constant infusion regimen has been started to ensure that values are in the therapeutic range (10 to 20 mg per 100 ml) and to avoid toxicity.

Selective β-2 sympathomimetic drugs, administered either parenterally or by aerosol, are begun or continued at appropriate intervals. Aerosolized drugs that work topically should not be relied upon solely, because they fail to penetrate effectively throughout the tracheobronchial system in the presence of airways secretions and severe narrowing.

The indications for and dosage of corticosteroids in this clinical setting are controversial. Most patients who have typical attacks of intercurrent infectious bronchitis can be managed satisfactorily without corticosteroids. These drugs should be used in patients with either status asthmaticus or severe episodes of superimposed acute respiratory failure in which an important component of bronchospasm and airways inflammation is presumed to exist. Hydrocortisone, 100 mg intravenously every four hours or the equivalent dose by constant infusion, is indicated. Much higher doses of corticosteroids (e.g., methylprednisolone, 15 mg per kilogram of body weight per day in divided doses) have been recommended, but there is no evidence to suggest that these are more efficacious than the suggested dose of hydrocortisone.

ANTIMICROBIALS

Infections are the most frequent and important cause of acute respiratory failure in patients with chronic underlying lung disease. Intercurrent attacks usually begin as a typical cold, with rhinitis, pharyngitis, and headaches. Shortly afterward, lower respiratory involvement appears with increasing cough, sputum production, purulence, wheezing, and breathlessness. These episodes occur several times a year in most patients with chronic obstructive pulmonary disease. (It should be noted that fever, leukocytosis, and new roentgenographic infiltrations are uncommon in this setting.) When airway infection is present, the sputum is not only purulent but usually contains numerous microorganisms detectable by Gram stain of the secretions. Sputum cultures, however, often fail to reveal pathogenic bacteria, although at times *Diplococcus pneumoniae* and/or *Hemophilus influenzae* may be grown. Regardless of the presence or absence of identifiable pathogens, oral treatment with ampicillin (250 to 500 mg every six hours) or tetracycline (250 to 500 every six hours) frequently results in decreased volume of sputum, thinning of the secretions, change in sputum appearance from purulent to mucoid, and improvement in blood gases.

When pneumonia is present, signified by the presence of new infiltration(s) on the chest roentgenogram, Gram stain of the sputum is likely to show one bacterial species predominating, and the initial selection of antimicrobials should cover this organism. Therapy can be revised, if necessary, when the results of the sputum cultures are available.

CONTROL OF SECRETIONS

Many patients complain of thick tenacious sputum that is troublesome to clear. Although it seems desirable to attempt to alter the character of these secretions to facilitate their removal, there is no clear evidence that it is possible to do so by pharmacologic means. Iodides, enzymes, detergents, and acetylcysteine, administered orally or by aerosol, have been tried extensively, but none has been shown convincingly to be effective. Moreover, each has potential toxic side effects. Similarly, mist tents and ultrasonic nebulizers, once widely used, are seldom employed today. The best way to control secretions is to control infection with antimicrobials and to ensure adequate (but not excessive) hydration by the administration of intravenous fluids.

Patients with troublesome sputum retention may require intermittent nasotracheal suction to control the volume of secretions. Manual or mechanical percussion serves to loosen secretions and enhances their removal. Respiratory physical therapy, especially when carried out by a skilled therapist, often results in increase in arterial Po_2 related to the improvement in the distribution of ventilation from clearance of sputum.

TREATMENT OF HEART FAILURE

Cor pulmonale is an inevitable complication of severe chronic lung disease. Right-sided heart failure occurs secondary to the increased work load imposed on the right ventricle by the changes in the pulmonary circulation from the effects of lung disease. Resistance to blood flow through the lungs increases when pulmonary blood vessels are destroyed (as in emphysema), obstructed (as in pulmonary thromboembolism), narrowed (from vasoconstriction), or compressed (breathing at high lung volumes), or the blood is unusually viscous (polycythemia). Patients whose cor pulmonale is well compensated or even inapparent while their chronic lung disease is stable often develop acute right heart failure during intercurrent attacks of acute respiratory failure. Peripheral edema, increased venous pressure, and enlarged, painful liver are important clues to the presence of acute cardiac decompensation.

Most patients with right heart failure from cor pulmonale, even if severe, have a satisfactory diuresis when put to bed, given O_2, and treated appropriately for their underlying lung disease. Diuretics may make patients feel more comfortable by diminishing peripheral edema and hepatic and gastrointestinal congestion faster than spontaneous diuresis; but if used, the drugs should be administered orally in low doses. Intravenous ethacrynic acid or furosemide can cause excessive renal loss of Cl^- that worsens existing acid-base disturbances and depletes intravascular volume sufficiently to decrease cardiac output and blood pressure. A particularly dangerous situation occurs in patients who already have coexisting nonrespiratory (metabolic) alkalosis, often from Cl^--losing diuretics, in addition to their hypercapnia from chronic respiratory failure; when the measures designed to improve ventilation lower arterial Pco_2, the nonrespiratory alkalosis becomes "unmasked" and arterial pH becomes markedly alkaline. When this occurs, the patients can develop cardiac arrhythmias, become comatose, or manifest convulsive seizures or other focal neurologic abnormalities.

If an element of pulmonary edema or pulmonary vascular congestion is present from left heart failure, this may also respond to diuretics. Whether left heart failure can occur secondary to purely right-sided disease is controversial, but there is probably little or no relationship. Of greater importance are coexisting causes of left-sided involvement (e.g., valvular disease, coronary atherosclerosis); furthermore, chronic hypoxia and severe polycythemia may impair left ventricular as well as right ventricular function.

There is no clear evidence that digitalis or its derivatives are beneficial in patients with cor pulmonale; in fact, most of the recent evidence is to the contrary. Also, the use of digitalis is hazardous in patients with chronic respiratory failure owing to the sudden shifts in acid-base balance and electrolyte concentrations that may occur in these patients. Therefore digitalis should be used only in patients with digitalis-responsive arrhythmias or coexisting left heart failure.

RESPIRATORY STIMULANTS

With few exceptions, respiratory stimulants are obsolete. Nikethamide, picrotoxin, and ethamivan have been replaced by other less hazardous and more efficient methods of maintaining ventilation. Doxapram, a drug that works by stimulating carotid chemoreceptors rather than neurons in the brain, appears to be much safer than centrally acting stimulants. The chief use of doxapram is to minimize or prevent the depression of ventilation, with consequent increase in Pco_2 and decrease in pH, that occurs in some hypoxic patients with hypercapnia who are given O_2 to breathe.

SEDATION

All sedative drugs should be avoided in patients with chronic lung disease and intercurrent acute respiratory failure, including diazepam (Valium) and chlordiazepoxide (Librium), which can suppress ventilation. Exceptions to this cardinal rule are made from time to time, but usually only when the patient is being mechanically ventilated and sedation is required to enable breathing synchronous with the machine.

POSTOPERATIVE COMPLICATIONS

Patients with chronic respiratory failure are high risk operative candidates. Moreover, the closer the surgical incision to the thorax, the higher the incidence of postoperative complications. Despite this caveat, it is safe to say that virtually *all* patients who have respiratory failure can safely undergo *non*thoracic surgery. Postoperative complications can be anticipated and often prevented by attention to the general principles of care outlined in this chapter. Close observation and monitoring are usually required, and these can best be carried out in an intensive care unit.

Abraham, A. S., Cole, R. B., Green, I. D., Hedworth-Whitty, R. B., Clarke, S. W., and Bishop, J. M.: Factors contributing to the reversible pulmonary hypertension of patients with acute respiratory failure studied by serial observations during recovery. Circ. Res., 24:51, 1969.

Campbell, E. J. M.: The J. Burns Amberson Lecture. The management of acute respiratory failure in chronic bronchitis and emphysema. Am. Rev. Respir. Dis., 96:626, 1967.

Hopewell, P. C., and Murray, J. F.: The adult respiratory distress syndrome. Ann. Rev. Med., 27:343, 1976.

Moser, K. M., Shibel, E. M., and Beamon, A. J.: Acute respiratory failure in obstructive lung disease. Long-term survival after treatment in an intensive care unit. JAMA, 225:705, 1973.

Pontoppidan, H., Geffin, B., and Lowenstein, E.: Acute Respiratory Failure in the Adult. Boston, Little, Brown, & Company, 1973.

Sykes, M. K., McNicol, M. W., and Campbell, E. J. M.: Respiratory Failure. Oxford, Blackwell Scientific Publications, 1976.

Zwillich, C. W., Pierson, D. J., Creagh, C. E., Sutton, F. D., Schatz, E., and Petty, T. L.: Complications of assisted ventilation. A prospective study of 354 consecutive episodes. Am. J. Med., 57:161, 1974.

PART XIII
CRITICAL CARE MEDICINE

Byron D. McLees

352. THE MEDICAL INTENSIVE CARE UNIT

352.1. INTRODUCTION

Critical care medicine may be defined as the observation, diagnosis, treatment, and rehabilitation of patients with overt or potential failure of vital functions. Morbidity and mortality can be reduced by the concentration of these patients in special units where staff and equipment are oriented to special methods of care. In the following pages attention is focused on common problems of critically ill patients. Emphasis is placed on the distortions of physiology in patients hospitalized on intensive care units and the techniques and concepts of care integral to their treatment. Problems encountered in the critically ill are unique not only in their impact on all the vital systems but also in their time course of development and in the types of data required for adequate evaluation and treatment.

The most important requirement of an intensive care unit (ICU) is that there be an organization. The essential aspects for the organization of an ICU include the following points:

1. Formal educational programs for the nursing, technical, and medical staff.

2. Protocols for the management of commonly encountered problems to aid in the consistent application of a therapeutic approach to patient care by all members of the team.

3. Staffing patterns for nursing and technical personnel which are designed to meet the needs of each specific unit and not calculated from empirical formulas based on fixed ratios of patients to staff.

4. Patient selection criteria which are carefully developed and implemented.

5. Appropriate record-keeping to attempt to establish the effectiveness of the ICU.

Recognition, treatment, and rehabilitation are well recognized phases in the care of the critically ill patient. We must now emphasize *anticipation* as a critical stage in patient care, because early, appropriate management of the critically ill patient can frequently alter the natural history of the illness and perhaps obviate the need for major life support systems. The fact that intensive care units frequently treat patients presenting in extremis should not be interpreted as license to allow an illness to reach catastrophic proportions before transfer to an ICU.

GOALS AND LIMITATIONS OF INTENSIVE CARE: MEDICO-LEGAL ASPECTS. Definition of therapeutic goals is an important requirement in the total care of a critically ill patient. Failure to define goals can lead to the application of maximal life support measures for the sake of appearances long after hope for survival has been abandoned. A prognostic classification system has been developed to aid in the assessment of patients, particularly with respect to deciding when a specific intervention (including cardiopulmonary resuscitation) is no longer advisable (Tagge et al.). This system establishes a process regularly exercised by the ICU staff to address the question of what is best for the whole patient and promises open communication regarding the elements of life and death decisions in the critical care setting.

Both the termination of life-supporting interventions and the failure to initiate therapy have substantial legal implications. The legal aspect of discontinuing life support is a controversial subject at present. Courts throughout the United States are concerned with this problem. Neurologic criteria are now frequently used as the basis for pronouncing the patient dead. The Harvard criteria for brain death have gained considerable medical acceptance: (1) absence of responsivity or receptiveness; (2) absence of spontaneous movement, breathing, or reflex activity; (3) presence of isoelectric EEG; and (4) all examinations repeated at two intervals 24 hours apart in the absence of hypothermia or drug ingestion.

These criteria provide the physician with a concrete means for determining clinical death and have been used to determine the time at which organs may be removed from transplantation donors. However, even these widely used criteria are not recognized by civil law in all states. The legal status of the termination of life-supporting therapy in patients who do not meet the criteria for brain death is not defined, and the medicolegal aspects of such action are far from clear. Both civil and criminal litigation could be involved. The law regarding failure to initiate therapy, thus permitting natural death from a fatal illness, is ambivalent; however, the practice has been upheld by the courts in cases in which the choice has been made by competent adults. There is no record of criminal action against a physician for neglecting to engage in the active treatment of a dying patient. The physician has the responsibility for the life of his patient but must also have an intelligent and sympathetic concern for the patient's death. It is incumbent upon the physician to formulate his ethical and medical decisions in the best interests of the patient and in recognition of the status of the law surrounding such action.

352.2. INSTRUMENTATION FOR THE INTENSIVE CARE UNIT

The purpose of this chapter is to discuss the instrumentation commonly used to facilitate care of the critically ill patient. The details of data collection and interpretation will be discussed in the chapters devoted to specific clinical problems.

AUTOMATED DATA MANAGEMENT. An intensive care unit has the potential to generate large amounts of data, and much effort is directed toward obtaining appropriate measurements to guide patient therapy. Unfortunately, less effort and thought may be given to the manner in which the data will be displayed and stored. It may be impossible to interpret very accurate cardiac output data because changes in fluid balance and medications relevant to the regulation of cardiac output were not recorded appropriately. Intelligent care of the patient frequently depends upon a knowledge of the patient's response to previous therapy. The most accurate and sophisticated data may become useless without detailed and accurate flow sheets, which should be tailored to each intensive care unit and to the individual patient.

The development of dedicated mini-computers designed specifically for critical care medicine permits the use of a computer-generated flow sheet. Some of the commercially available systems collect data directly from electronic transducers and conduct on-line processing and computation of the data. Data which cannot be collected directly, such as intake and output, body weight, and appearance, can be entered at a small bedside keyboard by the nursing staff. Computing systems complete with software (programs) are now commercially available; as the cost of these devices decreases, they may become more readily available to all intensive care units.

CARDIAC OUTPUT DEVICES. Contemporary care of the critically ill patient requires knowledge of the cardiac output. Serial determinations of cardiac output provide information essential to the cardiorespiratory and pharmacologic management of the patient. The development of bedside pulmonary artery catheterization permits the use of indicator dilution techniques for determination of cardiac output. Many substances have been used as indicators, but the two most commonly used are indocyanine green and cold saline or water. More recent thermodilution computers can use room temperature solutions.

Dye dilution is more cumbersome than the thermodilution technique, but will produce a more reliable value for cardiac output in the critically ill patient. A small volume of dye is injected into the pulmonary artery, and its appearance is measured spectrophotometrically at the arterial side of the circulation (brachial or femoral artery). Blood is withdrawn from the artery at a fixed rate by a mechanically powered syringe and passed through a densitometer, which records the dilution of dye with respect to time. Commercially available devices are available to calculate and digitally display the cardiac output in liters per minute immediately following injection of the indicator.

The thermodilution technique employs a bolus of cold indicator (10 ml of 5 per cent dextrose in water or normal saline) which is injected through a special purpose catheter. The bolus passes through a side hole located approximately 30 cm proximal to a thermistor, which is positioned near the tip of the catheter and senses the change in temperature as the indicator flows into the pulmonary artery. The thermodilution system does not require an arterial puncture; hence serial determinations may be performed without withdrawing blood samples. In some hands the thermodilution technique has been as reliable as the dye dilution technique, even in the critically ill patient.

FLUOROSCOPIC IMAGE INTENSIFIER. Intensive care medicine has been greatly facilitated by the availability of small, inexpensive image intensifiers which can be used at the bedside without special wiring or lead shielding. These devices can be used by the ICU staff, thus obviating the need to move critically ill patients for simple roentgenographic studies. Hydraulic, radiolucent beds simplify fluoroscopic interpretation but are not absolutely necessary. The effective and accurate use of vascular catheters and endotracheal and nasogastric tubes is greatly simplified by safe, rapid, and convenient fluoroscopy.

MASS SPECTROMETER. Stable low cost mass spectrometers have been developed to provide automated systems for monitoring respiratory gases on a practical clinical basis. These commercially available systems provide for the real time, simultaneous noninvasive measurement of inspired and expired gas concentrations on up to 12 patients. The partial pressures of oxygen, carbon dioxide, and nitrogen can be displayed and printed at preselected time intervals ranging from 10 to 60 minutes. Respiratory gas monitoring permits earlier detection of changes in respiratory function than blood gas determinations. Audible and visual alarms are activated if end-tidal gases exceed preset limits.

TRANSDUCERS. Pressure is quantified by strain gauges or transducers. Hydrodynamic pressure is transmitted to a diaphragm through a fluid-filled tube system attached to the catheter and is converted to an electrical signal. This signal is detected and amplified by an amplifier which displays the pressure on an oscilloscope or other suitable display device. The fluid-filled manometer has no role in the measurement of systemic or pulmonary artery pressures, and it is clearly a second choice even for measurement of venous pressures.

VENTILATORS. The function of a mechanical ventilator is to deliver an adequate volume of gas to the patient's airway. Many devices are available which fulfill this function; selection of a ventilator is principally a matter of preference, provided that the desired volume can be delivered at the desired rate. A mechanical ventilator should be simple and provide for the control of pressure, volume, flow rate, expiratory time, and oxygen concentration. The parameter used to regulate the quantity of gas delivered is frequently used to classify ventilators into pressure-, volume-, or time-cycled devices. *Pressure-cycled devices* terminate the inspiratory phase of ventilation when the airway pressure reaches a predetermined level regardless of the volume of gas delivered, and initiate the expiratory phase. These devices may be used for uncomplicated ventilation problems and are frequently successful in ventilating patients with respiratory failure accompanying chronic obstructive pulmonary disease. The tidal volume delivered is a function of chest wall and lung compliance (stiffness) and airway resistance; consequently, the expired volume must be measured frequently to ensure that the desired gas volume is being delivered. Patients with the syndrome of acute respiratory failure require large tidal volumes and may suffer frequent and rapid changes in pulmonary mechanics. Pressure-cycled devices are frequently inadequate and always inconvenient to use in this setting.

Volume-cycled ventilators deliver a predetermined gas volume regardless of the airway pressure. The simplicity, reliability, and reproducibility of the volume-cycled devices have made them popular ventilators for the management of patients with acute respiratory failure.

Time-cycled devices are also reliable and acceptable ventilators for the management of patients with acute respiratory failure; however, they have not been widely used in the United States, perhaps because of their expense and foreign manufacture. The cycling pattern in the time-cycled ventilators is determined by regulation of the length of the inspiratory and expiratory phases of the respiratory cycle. The tidal volume is determined by adjustment of the flow rate so that an appropriate volume is delivered during the time scheduled for inspiration.

Fluidic and pneumatic ventilators are commercially available as gas-powered, volume-cycled, and time-cycled devices. They require no electrical power and are especially useful for the transportation of critically ill patients requiring large tidal volumes, high oxygen concentrations, and end-expiratory pressures — conditions in which use of resuscitation bags is at best a tenuous means of respiratory support.

The performance of a ventilator is no better than its operator. If a machine is capable of delivering the required tidal volume at the desired rate and is appropriately adjusted, there is little to suggest any special therapeutic advantage for a particular ventilator over any other device capable of delivering the desired volumes and rates.

352.3. ACUTE RESPIRATORY FAILURE

The term acute respiratory failure includes pathologic states frequently labeled adult respiratory distress syndrome, post-traumatic pulmonary insufficiency, shock lung, or wet lung. Respiratory failure associated with decompensation of chronic lung disease is discussed separately in Ch. 351 because it is a different disease process in terms of etiology, pathophysiology, and therapy. It must be emphasized that the discussion to follow does not apply to decompensated obstructive bronchopulmonary disease, and the treatment outlined here for acute respiratory failure may result in substantial morbidity and possible mortality if applied to the patient with chronic obstructive lung disease as the *primary* illness.

Acute respiratory failure occurs in many clinical settings; Table 1 lists the etiologic factors frequently associated with this syndrome. The inclusion of so many diverse entities under the guise of a single syndrome is obviously unsatisfactory and should not be interpreted to suggest that etiology is irrelevant or unimportant. As our understanding of this syndrome increases, it may become unnecessary to lump undoubtedly separate entities into a single category termed acute respiratory failure. Unfortunately, the patient frequently presents to the intensive care unit with severe, progressive respiratory failure under conditions in which single etiolo-

TABLE 1. Etiologic Factors in Acute Respiratory Failure

Fat emboli
Fluid overload
Shock
Aspiration
Pulmonary infarction
Oxygen toxicity
Multiple transfusions
Disseminated intravascular coagulation
Sepsis
Pancreatitis
Septic abortion
Massive trauma and burns

gic factors cannot be defined. In each instance a detailed and diligent investigation should be conducted to define the etiologic factors which alone or in combination could be responsible for respiratory insufficiency. Frequently a number of factors, taken singly, seem insufficient to account for the onset of progressive respiratory failure; however, taken together they become sufficient to cause acute respiratory failure. If the search for an etiology is unrewarding, a pragmatic approach should be taken to management of the acute respiratory failure syndrome. Appropriate and effective therapy can usually be designed despite the inability to define an etiology, because the distortions of lung pathology and physiology are similar regardless of the initial insult.

CLINICAL FEATURES. Moore et al. have described the clinical features of acute respiratory failure and have outlined four phases which characterize progression of the syndrome.

Phase I: Injury and Resuscitation. This is the period immediately following the initial injury, hemorrhage, or infection. During this period the patient has almost invariably been resuscitated from a low flow state by infusion of large volumes of crystalloid or colloid and, perhaps, by cardiopulmonary resuscitation. Alkalosis is frequently present, but there is no evidence of respiratory distress and the chest x-ray is clear. It is important to recognize this setting as the milieu in which the syndrome of acute respiratory failure may appear so that appropriate plans can be made for careful observation of the patient.

Phase II: Circulatory Stabilization. Tissue perfusion, as reflected by mental status, renal function, and blood pressure, has returned to normal. This phase may last for five to seven days before the onset of pulmonary insufficiency becomes clinically apparent. The signs of acute respiratory failure frequently occur in an otherwise stable patient. *The most important* and frequently the earliest sign of incipient respiratory failure is hyperventilation, which may persist long after the initial injury and at a time when the chest x-ray and auscultatory findings are normal. The hyperventilation is frequently and erroneously attributed to anxiety, pain, or subclinical pulmonary congestion. The arterial oxygen tension is slightly decreased (60 to 70 mm Hg) on room air. However, measurement of the arterial oxygen tension following a 20-minute trial on 100 per cent oxygen will reveal a large alveolar-arterial oxygen tension difference (Aa_{DO_2}) consistent with a large intrapulmonic shunt. These findings are frequently overlooked or dismissed because the patient looks and feels well and all are pleased with the results of a successful resuscitation; however, the presence of a large Aa_{DO_2} points strongly to the incipient development of the acute respiratory failure syndrome. The intrapulmonic shunt (Qs/Qt) may be as high as 15 to 30 per cent at this phase of the patient's course. Aggressive therapeutic intervention promptly initiated may alter the natural course of the illness.

Phase III: Progressive Pulmonary Insufficiency. This phase is characterized by increasing respiratory difficulty manifested by tachypnea, progressive hypoxemia, and hypocarbia. Auscultation reveals scattered rales and rhonchi; the x-ray film shows spotty, diffuse infiltrates compatible with bronchopneumonia. Entities such as congestive heart failure, pulmonary emboli, bronchopneumonia, atelectasis, and aspiration pneumonitis are frequently invoked to explain this constellation of signs and symptoms. The assistance of a mechanical ventilator will frequently be required to support the patient's respiration. Sputum cultures may show growth of nosocomial organisms such as *Klebsiella, Pseudomonas,* or *Serratia* species. As time passes, the roentgenogram begins to show large areas of consolidation and the powerful respiratory drive begins to disappear; the patient becomes less alert. Hypoxemia is progressive, requiring increased oxygen concentrations to maintain satisfactory arterial oxygen tensions. The hypocapnia associated with the initial hyperventilation gradually disappears and may be replaced by hypercapnia in spite of mechanical ventilation with large minute volumes. Progressive hypercapnia precedes the terminal phase of illness; the mixed venous oxygen tension begins to fall, and the patient becomes comatose.

Phase IV: Terminal Hypoxia and Hemodynamic Decompensation. This phase of illness is usually brief, but with advanced life support techniques it may last several days. It is characterized by progressive coma, increasing intrapulmonary shunt, hypercapnia, and metabolic acidosis. The cardiac output finally begins to fall and requires pharmacologic support. Atrial and ventricular arrhythmias appear. Tissue perfusion deteriorates in spite of increasing hemodynamic support, and bradycardia and terminal asystole frequently mark the death of the patient.

The four phases of acute respiratory failure may be telescoped into a very short course of seven to ten days or may last up to several weeks. Unfortunately, the diagnosis of acute respiratory failure is frequently not entertained until the patient has progressed to the second phase of the illness; it is even more unfortunate when transfer to critical care facilities is delayed until the patient has progressed to the third or fourth phase of the syndrome. The importance of early recognition of the illness is again emphasized because early intervention with institution of appropriate therapy may be capable of modifying the natural history of the disease.

PATHOLOGIC CHANGES. Many types of injurious conditions which affect lung architecture produce similar reactions at the cellular level and cause a series of uniform morphologic responses to injury. The pulmonary capillaries are lined with endothelial cells which may be important in active transport and metabolism. The alveolar side of the capillary is lined with epithelial cells, termed Type I pneumocytes. Large, distinct cells, termed Type II or granular pneumocytes, are frequently located at junctions of the interalveolar septa. The Type II pneumocytes are progenitor cells and are thought to be capable of replacing the Type I pneumocytes. The capillary endothelial cells and the alveolar epithelial cells are separated by basement membrane and connective tissue components which compose the interstitium of the lung. The pulmonary capillaries course from arteriole to venule through the interstitial space of the interalveolar septum.

The pulmonary lymphatics represent a third circulating system for the lung and are of particular importance in the prevention of extravascular fluid accumulation. They are well designed to participate in the removal of fluid from the interstitial space and serve to protect the lung against increases in interstitial fluid.

The response of the lung to acute injury is characterized by the accumulation of fluid in the interstitial space; transudated fluid forms during oxygen toxicity, shock, and other acute injuries. A consideration of the determinants of capillary permeability in the absence of heart failure provides a convenient framework for the construction of a picture of acute respiratory failure. Swelling and disruption of the mitochondria in the endothelial cells of the pulmonary capillary are produced by many types of injuries. This process eventually leads to swelling of the capillary endothelial cells and causes the tight junctions between these cells to open, permitting the escape of fluid into the interstitial space. These junctions may become so distorted that cellular elements escape into the interstitium, followed ultimately by their deposition into the alveolus.

Extensive cellular damage involving the Type I and Type II pneumocytes is also observed. The Type I cells become detached from the basement membrane, leaving a completely denuded surface; Type II cells then line the alveoli as regeneration begins to take place. The Type II cells become vacuolated because of the destruction of the lamellar bodies. This may be an anatomic representation of the decrease in surfactant content found in the lungs of patients with acute respiratory failure. Many investigators feel that the common pathway for pulmonary injury is mediated through a decrease in surfactant production. The loss of surfactant tends to favor transudation of fluid from the vascular bed into the air spaces. The precise magnitude of the physical forces producing fluid movement at the alveolar-capillary junction is unknown, but it is likely that the sum of the Starling forces is normally slightly positive, producing a liquid layer which coats the air-tissue interface and is responsible, in part, for the normal pulmonary lymph flow. This normal flux of fluid into the lung may explain the genesis of severe pulmonary edema following capillary injury. Mechanical occlusion of the pulmonary capillary bed decreases its volume and may also produce pulmonary capillary hypertension with subsequent fluid transudation. Microaggregates containing erythrocytes, platelets, leukocytes and fibrin-containing thrombi are frequently found occluding the pulmonary arterioles and capillaries of patients dying from acute respiratory failure, but the extent of this microaggregation is generally thought to be insufficient to explain capillary hypertension on a purely mechanical basis. There is evidence, however, that these aggregates of cellular material may release intracellular substances which are capable of inducing capillary hypertension and directly altering capillary permeability. Prostaglandins, ADP, serotonin, and histamine all have the potential to produce pulmonary vasoconstriction and may play a role in the induction of pulmonary hypertension and pulmonary edema seen in acute respiratory failure. Thrombin produced by intravascular coag-

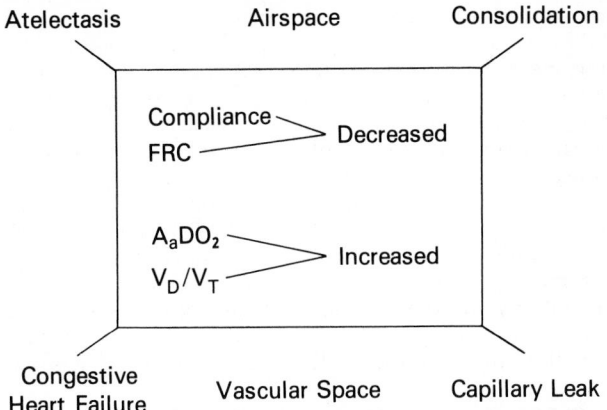

Figure 1. Interrelationship between primary pathologic changes in acute respiratory failure and alterations in pulmonary physiology. (From Wilson, R. F., and Pontoppidon, H.: Crit. Care Med., 2:293, 1974.)

ulation may directly cause an increase in pulmonary vascular resistance, in addition to its role in platelet aggregation and fibrin formation. The histologic features of pneumonitis may be produced in experimental animals following the release of vasoactive peptides, mediated perhaps through the action of lysosomal enzymes. When blood from septic dogs is perfused through an isolated canine pulmonary lobe, the pulmonary resistance is increased. A histologic picture of pneumonitis is produced only in the perfused lobe, and pretreatment of the septic animal with a protease inhibitor (Trasylol) prior to the perfusion will prevent the appearance of these lesions. In advanced stages of pulmonary injury the alveoli are filled with a hemorrhagic fibrinous exudate containing leukocytes, macrophages, and cellular debris. Fibrin covers many of the alveolar surfaces, alveolar ducts, and distal airways and may contribute to the formation of hyaline membranes.

In summary, the common morphologic and pathologic features of acute respiratory failure are (1) microaggregation of platelets and leukocytes within the pulmonary capillaries; (2) swelling and degeneration of the pulmonary capillary endothelium; (3) interstitial edema and hemorrhage; (4) marked reduction in capillary bed integrity; (5) extensive proliferation of granular pneumocytes, with the production of a cuboidal epithelial lining in the air spaces; (6) alveolar hemorrhage and edema; (7) hyaline membrane formation; (8) atelectasis; and (9) bronchopneumonia.

PHYSIOLOGY OF ACUTE RESPIRATORY FAILURE. The anatomic and morphologic changes discussed above produce the distortions of physiology seen in the clinical management of acute respiratory failure (Fig. 1). The functional residual capacity (FRC) equals the volume of gas in the lung at the end of tidal respiration; it is the equilibrium lung volume when the tendency of the lung to collapse is balanced by the tendency of the chest wall to "spring outward." The FRC serves two physiologic functions: (1) it buffers inspired gases to prevent large tidal swings in alveolar gas tension, and (2) it acts to keep airways open.

Reductions in the FRC may occur as a consequence of interstitial edema, hemorrhage, and pneumonitis; however, abdominal distention, pain, and body position also decrease FRC. Changes in lung volume affect pulmonary function primarily through changes in the distribution of ventilation. In large measure, the distribution of ventilation to the basilar or apical regions of the lungs depends upon the region of the pressure-volume curve over which ventilation is occurring. The effect of inspiration on the pressure-volume curve of the lung is illustrated in Figure 2. The degree of expansion manifested by any region of the lung depends upon its position on the pressure-volume curve. The base of the lung will undergo a larger change in volume than the apex because of its location on the steep part of the curve; it will, consequently, receive better ventilation than the apex in spite of the small resting volume.

Figure 2. Change in pressure-volume relationships in the lung with acute respiratory failure. In the normal upright lung (*A*), the transpulmonary pressure is less at the base than apex. During inspiration the change in transpulmonary pressure will be of equal magnitude at the base and apex of the lung; however, the alveoli at the base will expand more than those at the apex because of their position on a steeper portion of the curve. The slope of the curve for basal alveoli (compliance = volume/pressure) is greater for the basal alveoli; thus inspired air will preferentially move to the basal lung regions. If the lung volume is decreased by edema or atelectasis, as seen in acute respiratory failure (*B*), the alveoli at the base will remain closed with the initial change in transpulmonary pressure, causing the inspired gas to preferentially move to the apex. Once the critical opening pressure of the alveoli has been overcome, their volume will increase and proceed to move up the inspiratory limb of the curve. (From West, J. B.: Respiratory Physiology: The Essentials. Baltimore, Williams & Wilkins Company, 1974.)

Ventilation at low lung volumes can result in better ventilation of the apices because of airway closure in the poorly expanded basal portion of the lungs. The closing volume is operationally defined as the lung volume at which airway closure is detected. During expiration to very low lung volumes, the small airways, probably in the region of the respiratory bronchioles, functionally close or collapse. As long as the volume at which closure occurs is below the FRC, gas exchange will probably not be adversely affected; however, the reduction in FRC seen in acute respiratory failure may produce circumstances in which airways close prior to the end-expiratory position (FRC), resulting in impairment of gas exchange. If the volume required to open the airways (critical opening volume) is not achieved, the gas entrapped distal to the airway closure will be absorbed, resulting in atelectasis.

Compliance is defined as the change in volume per unit change in pressure and is determined by the slope of the pressure-volume curve (Fig. 2). A reduction in compliance signifies that the lungs are becoming stiffer and more difficult to ventilate, and reflects the decrease in FRC and the presence of edema, hemorrhage, and pneumonitis commonly seen in patients with acute respiratory failure. As the FRC decreases, more alveoli approach closing volume, producing atelectasis, impaired gas exchange, and further decrease in compliance. The fall in compliance, perhaps coupled with an increase in airway resistance secondary to airway edema and congestion, causes an increase in the work of breathing. The total work of breathing can be approximated by the following equation:

$$W = \frac{(V_T)^2}{2C} + 2R(V_T)^2 \, f \qquad \text{(Eq. 1)}$$

W = Work of breathing
R   = Resistance to flow
V_T = Tidal volume
f   = Respiratory frequency
C   = Compliance

It can be seen that ventilation at small tidal volumes will minimize the work required for ventilation; the shallow, rapid respiration of the patient with acute respiratory failure typifies this pattern of breathing.

The volume of each breath which fails to reach functioning terminal respiratory units is termed wasted ventilation or physiologic dead space. Wasted ventilation may be calculated from a modification of the Bohr equation:

$$V_D = \frac{(Pa_{CO_2} - Pe_{CO_2})}{Pa_{CO_2}} \cdot V_T \qquad \text{(Eq. 2)}$$

V_D = Wasted ventilation (dead space)
Pa_{CO_2} = Partial pressure CO_2 in arterial blood
Pe_{CO_2} = Partial pressure CO_2 in mixed expired gas
V_T = Tidal volume

For bedside measurement a 10-liter Douglas bag may be used to collect the mixed expired gas sample over several breaths; a simultaneous sample of arterial blood should be obtained to permit calculation of the ratio of wasted ventilation, V_D, to tidal volume, V_T (V_D/V_T ratio). The $V_D V_T$ ratio is normally 0.3. An increase in the ratio implies that the efficiency of the lung for CO_2

removal is impaired and an increase in tidal volume will be required if the Pa_{CO_2} is to remain constant. During mechanical ventilation corrections should be made for mechanical dead space and gas volume compressed within the ventilator system (Caldwell and Moya). The most important factors influencing the V_D/V_T ratio are processes which deprive alveoli of perfusion, causing an increase in the ratio of ventilation to perfusion. In moderate respiratory failure the V_D/V_T ratio may assume values of 0.5 to 0.6, and occasionally values up to 0.8 may be present. Changes in the V_D/V_T ratio parallel alterations in compliance, FRC, and x-ray appearance and provide a simple means for evaluating pulmonary function in addition to the measurement of gas exchange.

BLOOD GAS EXCHANGE. The effectiveness of blood gas exchange is assessed by comparison of the gas tension in the arterial blood with that present in the alveoli. The mean alveolar gas tension can be calculated from a modification of the alveolar gas equation:

$$PA_{O_2} = FI_{O_2}(PB - 47) - \frac{Pa_{CO_2}}{RQ} \qquad \text{(Eq. 3)}$$

PA_{O_2} = Mean alveolar oxygen tension (mm Hg)
FI_{O_2} = Fractional concentration of O_2 in inspired gas
PB   = Barometric pressure (mm Hg)
47   = Vapor pressure of water (mm Hg, 37° C)
Pa_{CO_2} = Arterial carbon dioxide tension (mm Hg)
RQ   = Respiratory quotient (usually assumed to be 0.8)

This equation can be simplified for use at the bedside to:

$$PA_{O_2} = 713 \cdot FI_{O2} - 1.25 \cdot Pa_{CO2} \text{ (assume PB} = 760 \text{ mm Hg)} \quad \text{(Eq. 4)}$$

An example is given for a patient with the following data:

$$FI_{O_2} = 0.40 \; Pa_{O_2} = 150 \text{ mm Hg } Pa_{CO_2} = 35 \text{ mm Hg}$$

The mean alveolar oxygen tension can be calculated as shown:

$$PA_{O_2} = (713)(0.40) - (1.25)(35) = 241 \text{ mm Hg}$$

The normal difference between the alveolar and arterial oxygen tensions is approximately 10 mm Hg; hence the predicted Pa_{O_2} would be 231 mm Hg. The alveolar-arterial oxygen tension difference (Aa_{DO_2}) in this patient is 91 mm Hg and denotes a severe disorder of gas exchange in spite of what, superficially, appears to be an acceptable arterial oxygen tension (150 mm Hg).

The Aa_{DO_2} may be used to evaluate the etiology of arterial hypoxia (Table 2). It is characteristically increased in parenchymal pulmonary disease through one or more of the following mechanisms:

1. Impaired diffusion resulting principally from thickening of the alveolar capillary membrane, a reduction in pulmonary capillary blood volume, or both.

2. Nonuniform distribution of alveolar ventilation and blood flow to the gas exchange units, producing a ventilation-perfusion imbalance. A mismatch in ventilation and perfusion causes the ventilation-perfusion (Va/Q) ratio to deviate from the normal value of 0.8 and results in an abnormally wide Aa_{DO_2}.

3. Physiologic or intrapulmonary (right to left) shunt

TABLE 2. Causes of Arterial Hypoxia (a Reduction in Po_2) and Their Effect on Alveolar-Arterial Po_2 Differences (Aa_{DO_2})

Cause	Effect on Arterial Po_2	Effect on Aa_{DO_2}
Hypoventilation	Decreased	No change
Diffusion abnormality*	No change	No change
Ventilation-perfusion imbalance	Decreased	Increased
Right to left shunt	Decreased	Increased
Reduction in inspired Po_2	Decreased	No change

*Effects of diffusion abnormalities are infrequently encountered at rest and are more likely to be evident during exercise.

of blood past nonventilated alveoli to return mixed venous blood to the left atrium.

Intrapulmonary shunts are believed to be a major cause of arterial hypoxia in acute respiratory failure. The normal or physiologic shunt represents 3 to 5 per cent of the cardiac output and arises from bronchial and mediastinal veins, which anastomose with the pulmonary veins, and from the thebesian veins of the myocardium, which empty directly into the left ventricle. These physiologic shunts are responsible for an Aa_{DO_2} of approximately 8 mm Hg or less in normal subjects breathing room air; an Aa_{DO_2} of 20 to 40 mm Hg is found in normal subjects following exposure to 100 per cent oxygen. The pathologic changes of atelectasis, edema consolidation, and hemorrhage, discussed earlier, are associated with a decrease in FRC and compliance and result in the perfusion of nonventilated respiratory units. Shunting of blood past nonventilated alveoli provides a source of mixed venous blood which dramatically lowers the oxygen tension of normally arterialized blood at the level of the left atrium. This fall in oxygen tension is produced by the addition of blood containing unsaturated hemoglobin to fully oxygenated blood and explains why the arterial blood oxygen tension in patients with large intrapulmonic shunts (Qs/Qt) is refractory to the inhalation of increased oxygen concentrations. The Qs/Qt term represents the degree of venous admixture expressed as per cent of the total cardiac output and can be calculated from the following expression:

$$\frac{Qs}{Qt} = \frac{Cc_{O_2} - Ca_{O_2}}{Cc_{O_2} - Cv_{O_2}} \qquad \text{(Eq. 5)}$$

Where Cc_{O_2} = end-capillary blood oxygen content
Ca_{O_2} = arterial blood oxygen content
Cv_{O_2} = mixed venous oxygen content

The pulmonary-capillary oxygen tension cannot be measured but is assumed to be equal to that of the blood if it were allowed to equilibrate at mean alveolar oxygen tension. The value of the capillary oxygen content may be calculated from the following expression:

$$Cc_{O_2} = So_2 \times Hb \times 1.34 + (Pa_{O_2} \cdot 0.0031) \text{(Eq. 6)}$$

Where: Cc_{O_2} = end capillary blood oxygen content (vol per cent)

Hb = hemoglobin concentration (grams per 100 ml)

1.34 = ml oxygen combined with 1 gram hemoglobin

0.0031 = factor used to convert oxygen tension (mm Hg) to oxygen content (ml per 100 ml) in solution

So_2 = per cent saturation of hemoglobin

A similar expression can be applied to calculate the arterial oxygen content. Substitution of the expressions for arterial and end-capillary oxygen contents into Equation 5 gives the following expression in terms of oxygen tensions and is valid under conditions when the hemoglobin is *fully* saturated:

$$\frac{Qs}{Qt} = \frac{(0.0031)\,(Aa_{DO_2})}{(0.0031)\,(Aa_{DO_2}) + (Ca_{O_2} - Cv_{O_2})} \qquad \text{(Eq. 7)}$$

By assuming a value for the ($Ca_{O_2} - Cv_{O_2}$) term, this equation can be used to approximate the intrapulmonic shunt when only arterial blood gas data are available. This equation provides justification for using the Aa_{DO_2} as an index to the size of the right to left shunt during ventilation with 100 per cent oxygen. The Aa_{DO_2} is a practical, useful bedside tool for evaluation of a patient's status, but it is important to be aware of factors other than the shunt fraction which may affect the value of the Aa_{DO_2} (Table 3). The theoretical relationship between Qs/Qt, Pa_{O_2}, Pa_{O_2}, and mixed venous oxygen content is shown in Figure 3. At moderate values of Qs/Qt it is apparent (Fig. 3B) that small changes in the mixed venous oxygen content are reflected by large changes in the Pa_{O_2}. Failure to estimate the Aa_{DO_2} in a patient suspected of early acute respiratory failure may delay the initiation of therapy. The arterial Pa_{O_2} on room air may be abnormal, but this does not necessarily indicate that the patient is critically ill. However, if the Pa_{O_2} increases to only 100 mm Hg following ventilation with 100 per cent oxygen (Aa_{DO_2} = 560 mm Hg), then the presence of a large shunt is likely, and the patient should be considered to have acute respiratory failure and to be in the high risk category until proved otherwise. As a rule of thumb an approximation of an Aa_{DO_2} of 15 mm Hg (on 100 per cent oxygen) reflects a right to left shunt of approximately 1 per cent of the cardiac output, *provided that the cardiac output is close to normal*. In the example cited above, the Aa_{DO_2} of 560 mm Hg could be used to estimate the shunt to be 37 per cent. The development of balloon flotation catheters has permitted the safe and convenient sampling of pulmonary arterial blood for determination of the mixed venous oxygen content (Cv_{O_2}) and direct calculation of Qs/Qt (Eq. 5) to eliminate many of the uncertainties inherent in the use of the Aa_{DO_2} for estimation of the shunt fraction. The Cc_{O_2} term is calculated from Equation 6; the arterial and venous oxygen contents can be calculated from knowledge of the per cent saturation, hemoglobin concentration, and oxygen tension of the appropriate blood samples. A sample calculation of Qs/Qt, using the shunt equation (Eq. 5), is given on the following page.

TABLE 3. Factors Affecting the Aa_{DO_2}

FI_{O_2}
Impaired pulmonary function
Cardiac output
Oxygen consumption
Position of the oxyhemoglobin dissociation curve
Mixed venous oxygen content

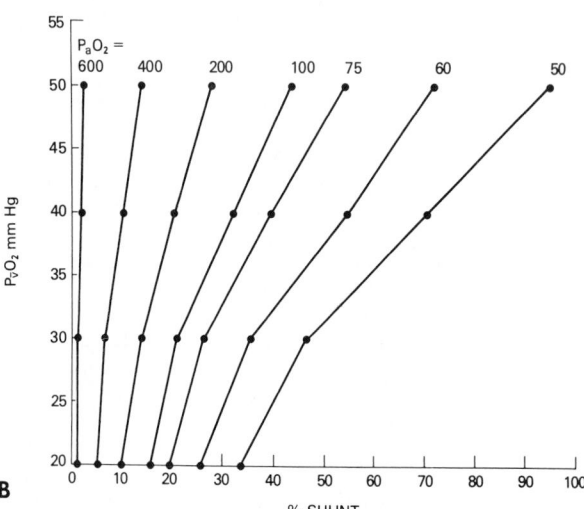

Figure 3. *A,* Relationship between arterial oxygen tension (PO_2) and intrapulmonary right to left shunt at various levels of alveolar PO_2 (PA_{O_2}). The PA_{O_2} varies with the inspired oxygen concentration. Note that the arterial PO_2 changes relatively slowly at shunt fractions exceeding 30 per cent. (From Pontoppidon, H., Laver, M. B., and Geffin, B., *In* Welch C. E. [ed.]: Advances in Surgery, Vol. 4. Chicago, Year Book Medical Publishers, 1970.) *B,* Effect of mixed venous oxygen tension (Pv_{O_2}) on shunt fractions Qs/Qt at constant arterial oxygen tensions (Pa_{O_2}) during inhalations of 100 per cent oxygen. For a given shunt fraction, the Pa_{O_2} becomes dependent upon the mixed venous oxygen tension; this relationship becomes more marked at the higher shunt fractions. (From Moore, F. D., et al.: Post-Traumatic Pulmonary Insufficiency. Philadelphia, W. B. Saunders Company, 1969.)

T	$= 38°$ C	pH $= 7.20$	$Sa_{O_2} = 98$ per cent
Pa_{O_2}	$= 163$ mm Hg	$FI_{O_2} = 1.0$	$Sv_{O_2} = 35$ per cent
Pa_{CO_2}	$= 40$ mm Hg		
Pv_{O_2}	$= 25$ mm Hg		
Hb	$= 13$ grams per 100 ml		

$PA_{O_2} = (760-47) (1.0) - (1.25) (40) = 663$ mm Hg
$Ca_{O_2} = (0.98) (13.0) (1.34) + (163) (0.0031) = 17.58$ vol per cent
(Continued at top of next column)

$Cc_{O_2} = (1.0) (13.0) (1.34) + (663) (0.0031) = 19.47$ vol per cent
$Cv_{O_2} = (0.35) (13.0) (1.34) + (25) (0.0031) = 6.17$ vol per cent

$$Qs/Qt = \frac{(19.47 - 17.58)}{(19.47 - 6.17)}$$

$$= 14 \text{ per cent}$$

The patient has only a 14 per cent shunt; the large $Aa_{D_{O_2}}$ measured on 100 per cent oxygen is a consequence of the wide arterial-venous oxygen content difference (11.4 vol per cent), associated with a low cardiac output. In spite of the superficial appearance of a large Qs/Qt based on the $Aa_{D_{O_2}}$, direct calculation of the shunt fraction shows only a modest venous admixture and, in fact, represents the situation in a patient virtually moribund with septic shock and low cardiac output. Therapeutic efforts must be directed toward improvement of the cardiac output and decreasing the arterial-venous oxygen content difference.

HEMODYNAMIC RESPONSES. Myocardial function must be understood if the results of therapeutic interventions in acute respiratory failure are to be properly interpreted. In experienced hands it is relatively uncommon for death to occur because of failure of parenchymal lung function; survival in acute respiratory failure is frequently critically dependent upon myocardial function and pharmacologic support for a compromised circulation.

In the absence of tricuspid disease central venous or right atrial pressure measurements have frequently been used to evaluate ventricular function. Numerous studies have shown that the central venous pressure does not correlate with left ventricular function as determined by direct measurement of left atrial pressure. In view of this evidence, it is disturbing that central venous pressure is still widely used as a monitor of left ventricular function. Furthermore, disparate function of the right and left ventricles in the critically ill patient is now well recognized. This imbalance between right and left ventricular functions requires separate determination of both right and left ventricular filling pressures if myocardial function is to be critically evaluated.

The development of balloon-tipped flotation catheters now permits direct measurement of pulmonary artery and pulmonary capillary wedge pressures. The pulmonary capillary wedge pressure is the pressure value obtained when the tip of a catheter is wedged into a small, distal branch of the pulmonary vascular tree. This maneuver interrupts blood flow, and the value measured under these circumstances is an equilibrium pressure transmitted retrogradely from the left atrium through the pulmonary veins and capillaries to the catheter tip. The wedge pressure may also be obtained through the use of a balloon-tipped flotation catheter; use of this device is described in detail later in this chapter.

The pulmonary capillary wedge pressure is of major importance in the care of patients with acute respiratory failure. It is closely related to the left atrial pressure (± 1 mm Hg), which (in the absence of mitral valve disease) parallels the left ventricular end-diastolic pressure; hence the mean pulmonary capillary wedge pressure is of major importance in the assessment of left ventricular function. In the absence of pulmonary disease the pulmonary artery diastolic pressure is nearly identical to the pulmonary capillary wedge pressure; however, conditions which increase the vascular resis-

Figure 4. Relationship between CVP and pulmonary capillary wedge pressure (PCWP) in hemorrhagic shock. Prior to transfusion, the patient was severely hypotensive with an elevated CVP and low wedge pressure. Following successful volume replacement, CVP gradually fell to normal range and (PCWP) was increased to an acceptable level.

tance, such as hypoxemia, acidosis, or pulmonary fibrosis, convert the high capacitance pulmonary vascular bed to a low capacitance circuit, causing the diastolic pulmonary artery pressure to increase and exceed the capillary wedge pressure. Under these conditions the pulmonary artery diastolic pressure may be much higher than the capillary wedge pressure, and consequently the wedge pressure becomes a relatively useless guide to filling pressure and left ventricular function. The left atrial pressure is fundamentally related to pulmonary congestion; hence the capillary wedge pressure may be extremely useful in the evaluation of pulmonary congestion and establishing safe limits for volume expansion. Figure 4 illustrates the value of the capillary wedge pressure in patient care.

Measurement of the central venous pressure alone may have prompted therapeutic decisions to withhold the administration of plasma expanders and, perhaps, to administer a diuretic agent. Since the evaluation of ventricular function based on the measurement of filling pressures may be of limited value, it is frequently advisable to assess function of the myocardium through determination of ventricular function curves at the bedside. The effect of a carefully controlled volume challenge on the right atrial and capillary wedge pressures and cardiac output is determined over a 15- to 20-minute interval. If the cardiac output increases with only a small (2 to 3 mm Hg) increase in atrial or wedge pressure, the preload is again increased by rapid infusion of volume to obtain an optimal position on the function curve. The effects of pharmacologic support for the vascular system can be evaluated by the determination of function curves in a similar manner.

The importance of these measurements in the patient with acute respiratory failure cannot be overemphasized. The diagnosis of noncardiogenic pulmonary edema should not be considered unless left ventricular failure can be excluded unequivocally. Precise therapeutic manipulation of the cardiovascular system can

be accomplished only through measuring right and left atrial pressures and cardiac output and observing their response to volume expansion.

TREATMENT. The first problem in the management of acute respiratory failure centers on early recognition of the syndrome. It is important to be aware of the clinical settings which predispose the patient to the development of acute respiratory failure. Patients recovering from severe trauma, hemorrhage, or shock are, of course, at high risk; however, a number of other clinical settings have been recognized to contribute to the development of the syndrome (Table 1). If a trial on 100 per cent oxygen demonstrates the presence of a large Aa_{DO_2}, further studies should be conducted to help formulate the therapeutic plan.

Evaluation of Need for Mechanical Ventilation. The decision to institute mechanical ventilation requires clinical experience and judgment. A serious error frequently results when mechanical ventilation is postponed until the patient is in extremis. Such errors in judgment occasionally occur because of failure to appreciate the difference between the physiology of a patient with acute respiratory failure and that of a patient with decompensation of chronic obstructive bronchopulmonary disease. The patient with acute respiratory failure will be moribund if allowed to reach the stage of decompensation permitted in chronic obstructive bronchopulmonary disease prior to institution of mechanical ventilation. Pontoppidan and coworkers have formulated several useful guidelines in assessment of the need for mechanical ventilation (Table 4). These are only guidelines and should not be viewed as absolute criteria. Many patients who appear well but meet the criteria for mechanical ventilation will only deteriorate further if respiratory support is deferred on the basis of subjective clinical observations. In borderline or questionable situations the serial, frequent determination of the parameters listed in Table 4 will usually resolve the uncertainty.

Airway Control. Once the decision has been made to begin mechanical ventilation, attention must be directed toward airway control and endotracheal intubation. The choice between oral endotracheal or nasotracheal intubation is largely a matter of personal preference and skill of the intubationist, but patient comfort and maintenance of tube position and patency are frequently more satisfactory with nasotracheal tubes. Oral endotracheal intubation is the method of choice in emergency situations. It may frequently be necessary to paralyze the combative or disoriented patient with neuromuscular blocking agents prior to laryngoscopy and intubation when this route is utilized. The use of a fiberoptic bronchoscope as a guide to introduce either the oral endotracheal or nasotracheal

TABLE 4. Indications for Mechanical Ventilation

Pa_{O_2} (mm Hg)	<60 (on mask O_2)
Aa_{DO_2} ($FI_{O_2} = 1.0$)	>400
Qs/Qt	30–40%
Respiratory rate	>35
Tidal volume (ml/kg)	<4
Vital capacity (ml/kg)	<15

These values suggest that mechanical ventilation should be considered; a downward trend from these values would make mechanical ventilation mandatory in the majority of patients.

tube decreases patient discomfort and increases the speed and safety of the procedure. The tube is passed over the tip of the bronchoscope, which is placed into the trachea under direct visualization. Supplemental oxygen can be administered through the suction channel of the bronchoscope during the procedure. This technique is especially valuable for intubation of the patient with cervical traction or limited neck motion. The recent introduction of low pressure, "floppy," large residual volume, highly compliant cuffs has resulted in the mechanical ventilation of patients for weeks without tracheal damage; however, inappropriate or careless management of even the best, most modern endotracheal tube for only a few hours can result in severe tracheal damage. The risk of cuff-induced tracheal damage is the same with either endotracheal or tracheostomy tubes. The use of endotracheal tubes subjects the patient to the uncommon complication of laryngeal destruction, with the resulting possibility of aphonia. The placement of a tracheostomy tube eliminates this complication and also improves patient comfort during long-term mechanical ventilation. Overinflation of the cuff by only 1 ml can result in unacceptable and dangerous pressures against the wall of the trachea and cause tracheal damage. Some general guidelines for the management of endotracheal tubes should be considered:

1. The minimal leak technique of ventilation should be utilized; the cuff should be inflated to allow an audible air leak at the end of inspiration. Such a leak will not be sufficient to affect the delivery of the desired volume or to interfere with the use of end-expiratory pressure. This technique will decrease the likelihood of cuff overinflation.

2. The volume of air necessary to achieve the minimal leak condition is recorded on a flow sheet for each nursing shift. If the volume of air begins to increase, a careful evaluation of the trachea should be conducted. Increasing cuff diameters may reflect the onset of tracheomalacia as the cuff begins to accommodate to a dilating tracheal wall.

The care of a tracheostomy tube should follow the same guidelines outlined for the endotracheal tube. It is important that the tracheostomy tube be connected to the respirator through a swivel connector and flexible tubing to minimize motion of the tip, which can produce trauma to the tracheal stoma and mucosa. The tracheostomy tube should be changed 72 hours after tracheostomy if the patient's condition is stable. The first postoperative tube change should be performed by a physician experienced in airway management. A tracheostomy tray should be immediately available, and the tube should be removed over a small catheter or guide wire placed into the trachea to facilitate placement of the new tube into position. Accidental extubation prior to maturation of the stoma is a potential emergency; it may be impossible to rapidly replace the tube because of the inability to identify the tracheostomy tract or stoma. If this situation should occur and the tube fails to be repositioned in a single try, the stoma should be sealed with a dressing and the patient ventilated by mask until an endotracheal tube can be positioned from above. Surgical assistance should be immediately obtained.

An uncommon complication of tracheostomy is massive hemorrhage from a tracheal innominate artery fistula, which may occur at any time following surgery. Hemorrhage occurring at the tracheostomy site which is not obviously superficial in origin should prompt immediate surgical consultation. The cuff should be tightly inflated and left in this position until surgical help arrives. If massive hemorrhage occurs following maximal cuff inflation, digital pressure should be applied against the anterior tracheal wall by insertion of a finger through the tracheal stoma. It is the physician's responsibility to see that appropriate equipment and personnel are always at hand for maintenance of airway control. Deaths have occurred because suction devices failed to function or because adapters needed to couple the endotracheal tube to a bag or ventilator could not be located. Such catastrophes reflect directly on the physician assuming responsibility for care of the patient and maintenance of airway control. These details cannot be delegated to the nursing staff, central supply, or other personnel.

Mechanical Ventilation. A description of ventilators suitable for use with the critically ill patient is presented in Ch. 352.2. A general approach to the selection of an optimal ventilation pattern is described below; the details of each pattern will of course vary, depending on the specific clinical condition. The optimal pattern is achieved through the use of large tidal volume ventilation. An initial tidal volume of 15 ml per kilogram should be selected; if the airway pressure at this volume exceeds 50 to 55 cm H_2O, the use of a smaller tidal volume should be considered in order to minimize the possibility of barotrauma (the airway pressure should be measured under no flow conditions). This can be easily achieved on the MA-I ventilator by reading the plateau pressure when the expiratory resistance knob is turned fully clockwise. (On other machines it may be necessary to occlude the expiration line momentarily at peak inspiration.) The use of periodic sighs or hyperinflations is superfluous with the large tidal volume ventilation, because each breath approaches a sigh in volume. A respiratory rate between 10 and 20 breaths per minute is desirable, and most patients will spontaneously assist at these rates as they become accustomed to the large tidal volume pattern. When the tidal volume and rate have been established, the ratio of inspired to expired time (I:E ratio) should be adjusted to provide a value between 1:2 and 1:3. On volume-cycled machines the ratio is adjusted by determining the length of the inspiratory phase with the flow control.

The ventilation pattern is selected and established without regard for the value of the Pa_{CO_2}. The pattern described above may be associated with a minute ventilation of 15 to 20 liters per minute (normal = 6 liters per minute) producing hypocapnia, frequently with Pa_{CO_2} values less than 30 mm Hg. Hypocapnia below 30 mm Hg should be corrected because it is deleterious and may be dangerous; it may cause an important decrease in oxygen delivery by changing the parameters listed in Table 5. Correction of severe hypocapnia can

TABLE 5. Effects of Hypocapnia

Decreased cardiac output
Decreased cerebral blood flow
Decreased seizure threshold
Sensitization of heart to arrhythmia
Hypoxemia secondary to ventilation-perfusion
Perfusion imbalance

frequently produce a substantial increase in the Pa_{O_2}. The Pa_{CO_2} should not be corrected through reductions in either tidal volume or respiratory rate. Normocapnia is best achieved by the addition of carbon dioxide to the inspired line of the ventilator or by the addition of dead space tubing to the breathing circuit. When possible, the ventilator should be operated in the assist mode, which allows the patient to receive a breath in response to a small inspiratory effort to trigger the machine. This mode of ventilation is often more acceptable to the patient, because a breath is delivered with each inspiratory effort. Occasionally the tachypneic, restless patient will trigger the machine at unacceptably high rates of respiration. In these circumstances the frequent use of reassurance and encouragement, coupled with the administration of morphine for relief of pain and diazepam to make the patient more comfortable, will usually result in the production of a more satisfactory respiratory rate. The rate should never be controlled by decreasing the ventilator sensitivity to a point at which the machine fails to respond to a few initial inspiratory efforts, but finally triggers in response to a desperate inspiratory gasp. This technique will undoubtedly decrease the respiratory rate, but it is antithetical to the primary goals of mechanical ventilation, which include the elimination of respiratory distress and a reduction in the work of breathing.

If the respiratory rate cannot be satisfactorily controlled by reassurance, sedation, and adequate oxygenation, it may rarely be necessary to eliminate the respiratory drive through muscular paralysis with a neuromuscular blocking agent such as pancuronium bromide or curare. The former has been especially safe and effective when used in the critically ill patient because of its lack of effect (except for tachycardia) on the cardiovascular system. Paralytic therapy not only represents another level of control from which the patient must be weaned, but also precludes neurologic evaluation of the patient, renders communication with the patient impossible, and totally obliterates the cough reflex with an attendant increase in the risk of infection. These agents greatly increase the danger associated with accidental disconnection of the electrical power and must not be used simply because the patient requires frequent emotional and pharmacologic support to synchronize respiration with the machine. The benefits of paralysis must be carefully weighed against these risks. If the patient is paralyzed, every attempt must be made to limit the duration of such treatment to the briefest possible period.

The syndrome of oxygen toxicity in the critically ill patient is poorly understood and does not develop in a predictable fashion. Prolonged exposure to high concentrations of oxygen can produce oxygen toxicity with pathologic changes similar to those described in acute respiratory failure, i.e., edema, hemorrhage, and hyaline membrane formation. The development of oxygen toxicity is considered to be both time and concentration dependent; oxygen concentrations of less than 40 per cent can be tolerated over long periods of time without apparent risks; concentrations of 60 per cent can certainly be tolerated in many patients for sustained periods of time without apparent damage, but this is generally considered to be an unsafe concentration for long-term ventilation. Attempts to avoid oxygen toxicity at the expense of hypoxemia will almost certainly result in unsatisfactory clinical results.

The patient should be ventilated at the lowest oxygen concentration capable of maintaining an arterial hemoglobin saturation of 90 per cent. If 100 per cent oxygen is required to maintain adequate oxygenation, it should be used until it is safe to reduce the inspired oxygen concentration. Patients ventilated on 100 per cent oxygen for two to three days or longer have survived. It must be remembered that most patients requiring oxygen concentrations greater than 60 per cent will have intrapulmonic shunts, with Qs/Qt exceeding 30 per cent, a range at which the Pa_{O_2} is not a sensitive function of the inspired oxygen concentration (Fig. 3A). Clinically, this means that a reduction in the $F_{I_{O_2}}$ from 1.0 to 0.7 will be associated with only a very small decrease in the Pa_{O_2}. However, a large fall in the Pa_{O_2} will occasionally accompany a modest decrease in the inspired gas concentration, so such trials should be conducted with caution.

Positive End-Expiratory Pressure. During conventional mechanical ventilation the airway pressure is returned to 0 at the end of expiration. If the expiratory limb of the breathing circuit is submerged under a column of water, the end-expiratory pressure will be positive and the magnitude of the pressure will depend upon the length of tubing below the water surface. The same effect has been more conveniently achieved by the design of the expiration valve so that a desired level of end-expiratory pressure can be obtained from a simple adjustment on the control panel. The reduction in lung volume and interstitial edema described in acute respiratory failure combine to produce airway closure during tidal breathing. These changes, collectively, are responsible for the physiologic intrapulmonic shunt and the increased $Aa_{D_{O_2}}$ difference described earlier. The goal of therapy with end-expiratory pressure is to increase the number of alveoli remaining open by raising the pressure at end-expiration above the critical opening pressure. The patient with acute respiratory failure usually has a marked reduction in FRC and may be expected to benefit from the application of end-expiratory pressure because the potential exists to "recruit" these collapsed alveoli. As more alveoli are recruited, the FRC increases and the shunt and $Aa_{D_{O_2}}$ decrease. Patients with a high or normal FRC are unlikely to respond to the application of end-expiratory pressure, because alveolar collapse is unlikely to be significant in the presence of a normal FRC. Excessive amounts of end-expiratory pressure may overdistend normal alveoli, decreasing perfusion to these units as the intra-alveolar pressure increases. This overdistention increases the dead space and may be associated with a rise in the Pa_{CO_2} and a decrease in the Pa_{O_2}; ultimately, overdistention may cause alveolar rupture and pneumothorax.

End-expiratory pressure will, of course, increase the mean airway pressure and may have a profound effect on the cardiac output because of the impedance to venous return reflected by changes in ventricular filling pressures. The importance of the increased airway pressure in producing changes in the circulation depends principally on the extent to which it is transmitted through the lung parenchyma to the pleural space. In the severely diseased noncompliant lung of acute respiratory failure the airway pressure may not be transmitted to the pleural space and, consequently, may have little effect on the filling pressures and cardiac output. In the more common situation in which airway pressure is transmitted to the pleural space, the pleural pressure will rise (become less negative) during inspiration, and the measured atrial and wedge pres-

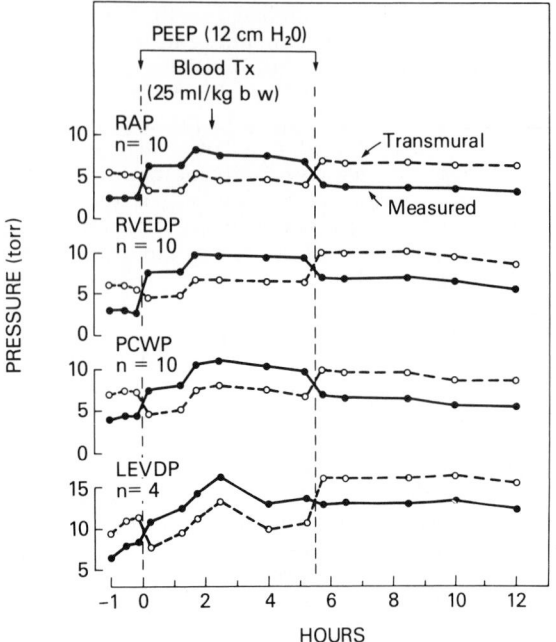

Figure 5. Pattern of response of right atrial pressure (RAP), right ventricular end-diastolic pressure (RVEDP), pulmonary capillary wedge pressure (PCWP), and left ventricular end-diastolic pressure (LVEDP) during 12 hours of positive end-expiratory pressure (PEEP). Note that the measured pressure (relative to the atmosphere) rose while the transmural pressures (measured pressure − pleural pressure) actually fell with application of PEEP. This pattern was reversed when PEEP was removed. (From Quist, J., et al.: Anesthesiology, 42:45, 1975.)

sures will increase secondary to the changes in pleural pressure. These pleural pressure changes will cause the measured values of the pulmonary artery, central venous, and capillary wedge pressures to increase as the end-expiratory pressure is increased. The measured pressure values, however, are determined with respect to atmospheric pressure and are not the correct values to be used in assessment of cardiovascular performance. The pressure across the vessel wall is the transmural pressure:

$$\text{Transmural pressure} = \text{measured pressure} - \text{pleural pressure}$$

The relationship between measured and transmural atrial pressure is shown in Figure 5. The transmural filling pressure actually decreases while the measured pressure increases following the application of end-expiratory pressure. Volume augmentation increases the ventricular preload and returns the transmural filling pressure and cardiac output to normal. Ventricular function curves have shown that these changes in cardiac output can be related solely to changes in filling pressure and not to changes in myocardial contractility. The sudden increase in venous return which occurs when end-expiratory pressure is suddenly discontinued may result in the appearance of pulmonary congestion. This paradoxical deterioration in cardiovascular function is most likely to occur in patients with underlying myocardial disease and physiologically may be considered analogous to the results of rapid volume expansion in the patient with pre-existing congestive heart failure. The appropriate use of end-expiratory pressure requires considerable thought. An increase in the

Pa_{O_2} may be negated by the decrease in cardiac output associated with the inappropriate use of end-expiratory pressure. The application of end-expiratory pressure solely to maximize the arterial oxygen tension is a potentially lethal maneuver; the cardiac output may be decreased by as much as 30 per cent with very little change in blood pressure. The enthusiasm associated with a dramatic initial increase in the Pa_{O_2} will subsequently be replaced by disappointment and frustration as the patient develops metabolic acidosis and hypotension and deteriorates in iatrogenic shock. Because pleural pressures are not routinely measured at the bedside and pulmonary capillary wedge pressures are probably unreliable at values of end-expiratory pressure exceeding 10 cm H_2O, it is advisable to examine other ways to assess the response of the cardiovascular system to the application of end-expiratory pressure. The mixed venous oxygen content and the arterial-venous oxygen content difference may be used along with cardiac output to measure the responses of the vascular system to the application of end-expiratory pressure. Careful examination of all parameters of cardiovascular function will usually provide sufficient data to resolve any doubts about the vascular response to end-expiratory pressure. If the response to volume augmentation is equivocal or uncertain, the fluid administration should be continued only with extreme caution. The administration of an inotropic agent will frequently provide sufficient hemodynamic support to permit the use of end-expiratory pressure under conditions in which its use would otherwise be impossible because of ventricular failure.

Suter and coworkers have shown that the end-expiratory pressure value associated with maximal oxygen transport (defined as cardiac output × the arterial oxygen content) is associated with maximal values of effective compliance as estimated from the tidal volume and plateau pressure registered by the airway pressure dial on the ventilator. The end-expiratory pressure corresponding to the maximal effective compliance has been termed the "best PEEP" value, because increases in the Pa_{O_2} obtained at end-expiratory pressures exceeding this value were negated by decreases in oxygen transport. It should be noted that the "best PEEP" values were determined in normovolemic patients who did not require changes in volume status during therapy. As a general rule the end-expiratory pressure should be increased by a maximum of 5 cm H_2O every 30 to 40 minutes. The response of the Pa_{O_2} is time dependent and may not reach the maximal value until 30 to 40 minutes after application of the end-expiratory pressure; when it is discontinued, the Pa_{O_2} may return to baseline values within three to five minutes. Concern is frequently expressed about the use of positive end-expiratory pressure during ventilation in the assist mode, because the inspiratory efforts may cause the airway pressure gauge to deflect in a negative direction, indicating that such efforts have caused a reduction of the positive end-expiratory pressure. The gradient of pressure across the lung (airway pressure to pleural pressure) will not be changed by the inspiratory efforts, and the effectiveness of the end-expiratory pressure is not lost under these conditions. The effectiveness of positive end-expiratory pressure depends upon this pressure gradient and not upon the absolute value of pressure indicated by the airway pressure gauge. Most important, there is no reason to sedate or paralyze the patient receiving end-expiratory pressure simply to eliminate the effects of respiratory efforts.

Use of the Swan-Ganz Catheter. Precise measurements of cardiac output, pulmonary capillary wedge pressure, and right atrial pressure are required to evaluate the nature and severity of pulmonary congestion and to direct therapeutic manipulations. These data also permit the need for hemodynamic support with inotropic agents to be assessed objectively. The development of the balloon-tipped flow-directed catheter has greatly facilitated bedside measurement of these parameters. A particularly useful version of the flow-directed catheter is a triple lumen device, which also contains a small thermistor for thermal dilution cardiac output determinations (see Ch. 352.2). One lumen is used to inflate the balloon with air or CO_2 (not saline or water). When the balloon is inflated to the volume denoted on the body of the catheter, it is carried by the blood flow through the right atrium and right ventricle into the pulmonary artery. A second lumen opens at the tip of the catheter and is used for recording pressures and for withdrawing pulmonary arterial blood samples for determining mixed venous oxygen content. A third lumen is positioned to open into the right atrium when the tip of the catheter is placed within the pulmonary artery. This permits the simultaneous determination of atrial and pulmonary capillary wedge pressure. A thermistor is located approximately 4 cm from the catheter tip and senses the temperature of the pulmonary artery blood to permit determination of the cardiac output, as described previously.

Catheterization of the pulmonary artery can be conducted at bedside with only pressure and electrocardiographic monitoring. A portable image intensifier (see Ch. 352.2) can greatly facilitate placement of the catheter but is not usually necessary. The catheter can be inserted percutaneously or through a small cutdown site at the antecubital fossa. Following insertion, the catheter is advanced into the thorax, denoted by the superimposition of respiratory variations upon the pressure tracing. The balloon is inflated and the catheter is rapidly advanced under continuous pressure monitoring (Fig. 6). The catheter is advanced until the wedge tracing is obtained. The balloon is deflated, and the pulmonary artery pressure waveform should immediately reappear. The validity of the wedge pressure tracing should be confirmed by the following points:

1. Balloon inflation should change the contour of the pulmonary artery pressure, and deflation of the balloon should cause immediate reappearance of the pulmonary artery waveform.

2. The wedge pressure should be less than or equal to the diastolic pulmonary artery pressure.

3. The trace should vary with respiration.

Figure 6. The change in pulmonary artery pressure to pulmonary capillary wedge pressure occurs when the balloon is inflated and the pulmonary artery is occluded proximal to the catheter tip.

4. A pressure trace which drifts up or down following balloon inflation is unsatisfactory.

5. The catheter tip is in the appropriate position if arterialized blood can be drawn through the distal lumen while the balloon is inflated.

The tip of the catheter should be positioned in a major branch of the pulmonary artery. After passage of the catheter into a wedge position, it is important to allow the catheter to assume a position independent of balloon inflation. The balloon should be reinflated to the volume at which the pulmonary artery trace changes to that of the wedge pattern. If this volume is significantly less than the balloon capacity, the catheter position should be readjusted so that balloon volumes approaching the capacity of the balloon are required to produce the wedge pressure trace.

The catheter frequently tends to migrate distally after insertion, causing the production of a continuous wedge pressure pattern with the balloon deflated. The pressure must be continually monitored so that the catheter may be repositioned immediately if such a fixed wedge tracing appears. Pulmonary infarction can result from such catheter migration. A digital display of the arterial pressure does not allow changes in the pressure waveform to be easily detected and, by itself, is not an adequate monitoring system for a Swan-Ganz catheter. The use of the Swan-Ganz catheter is not associated with a high risk to the patient; however, the complications of pulmonary infarction, pulmonary artery rupture, and air embolism are real, and the guidelines described above (Swan-Ganz) should be carefully followed if the values are to be reliable and disasters are to be avoided. Blood for the determination of mixed venous oxygen content can be aspirated from the distal lumen of the catheter with the balloon deflated. If the catheter is positioned as described above, the sample obtained should be representative of the mixed venous blood, provided that the withdrawal rate is 3 ml per minute or less. Large errors may occur if the blood is withdrawn rapidly or if the catheter is positioned peripherally within the pulmonary artery. These errors result from contamination of the mixed venous pulmonary blood with arterialized blood drawn from the pulmonary capillaries and veins.

General Considerations in the Treatment of Acute Respiratory Failure. Every attempt should be made to diagnose and treat the syndrome of acute respiratory failure as soon as possible after the onset of symptoms. Tachypnea, hypocapnia, and hypoxemia associated with intrapulmonary shunts have been discussed as early warning signs. Treatment must be initiated before the patient has developed obvious signs of respiratory distress.

Initial therapy should consist of administration of methylprednisolone sodium succinate (30 mg per kilogram intravenously every six hours for 48 hours). Corticosteroid therapy should be started as soon as the diagnosis of acute respiratory failure is entertained; following the appearance of overt respiratory failure, it is fruitless. The action of corticosteroids in this syndrome will undoubtedly depend upon the etiology and precise physiologic profile at the time therapy is started. There is impressive experimental evidence and suggestive clinical evidence for the efficacy of methylprednisolone in the prevention of the progressive pathologic features of pulmonary insufficiency. Pharmacologic doses of methylprednisolone have been reported to reduce the mortality from acute respiratory failure following shock and hypotension; however, there are no convincing clinical data to justify the use of corticosteroids in this syndrome. Wilson and colleagues have shown that the microcirculatory changes seen in the dog lung during shock can be almost totally prevented by the prior administration of corticosteroids. There are ample data to support the safety of pharmacologic doses of corticosteroids administered over a 48- to 72-hour period. Hyperglycemia is the only systemic side effect likely to be seen following the use of corticosteroids as outlined above. The fact that corticosteroids may alter the progression of respiratory failure while subjecting the patient to only a minimal risk suggests that their use may be prudent in a disorder associated with such a high mortality rate.

Intensive nursing care in the early phases of respiratory failure may do much to obviate the eventual need for mechanical ventilation. Frequent coughing and deep breathing should be coupled with position changes every 30 minutes without fail. Oxygen should be administered by mask to maintain an arterial hemoglobin saturation of 90 per cent. Ultrasonic nebulization may also be used to deliver medications to the airway and to augment humidification of the tracheobronchial tree. The incentive spirometer may be particularly useful for encouraging the cooperative patient to take deep breaths; the routine use of intermittent positive pressure breathing will probably be of little value unless carefully and expertly administered. The routine of mucolytic agents should be avoided; good nursing care and humidification should obviate the use of these agents, which may cause bronchoconstriction and bronchial irritation. Abdominal distention should be relieved and restlessness eased with gentle sedation. The use of salicylates to reduce fever may decrease the over-all energy expenditure of the patient. The over-all goals of therapy at this stage should be to obtain a well oxygenated, relaxed, comfortable patient and to encourage postural drainage, deep breathing, coughing, and frequent position changes.

Fluid Balance. The roentgenographic features of acute respiratory failure are frequently indistinguishable from those of acute pulmonary edema. Any questions regarding the presence or absence of congestive heart failure must be resolved, and it will frequently be necessary to measure vascular pressures to decide this question. Volume overload may cause profound hypoxemia and greatly prolong the course of the disease because of the inability to mobilize the extravascular lung water in this syndrome. Diuretic therapy and dehydration may be ineffective, perhaps because of changes in capillary permeability coupled with damage to the pulmonary lymphatics. As a first step the vascular volume should be adjusted to be as close to normal as possible; baseline values establishing the state of fluid and electrolyte balance should be collected. Perhaps because of the resemblance of the syndrome of acute respiratory failure to pulmonary edema, attempts are frequently initiated to dehydrate the patient by fluid restriction and diuretic therapy. Such therapy is potentially very dangerous; rapid diuresis can lead to reductions in cardiac output, with subsequent reductions in tissue perfusion leading to renal failure. There is no direct evidence that reduction of venous pressure improves pulmonary function; however, excessive lung water is present in acute respiratory failure, and it is probably desirable to initiate a carefully controlled, gradual reduction in the vascular volume. This reduction in volume should not

proceed unless it is unequivocally demonstrated that tissue perfusion is not compromised by this maneuver. A urine output of 1 ml per kilogram per hour will usually be sufficient to reflect adequate renal perfusion. The administration of furosemide (20 mg intravenously) once or twice daily will prevent the gradual accumulation of fluid frequently associated with mechanical ventilation. Failure to maintain adequate urine flow or to administer small amounts of a diuretic agent will almost invariably lead to the gradual accumulation of excess fluid. A critically ill patient receiving conventional intravenous fluid therapy can be expected to lose 0.5 kg per day; a stable body weight indicates that the patient is retaining fluid.

Patients receiving high levels of positive end-expiratory pressure may retain large quantities of fluid manifested as daily weight gain, but still require administration of fluid to maintain hemodynamic stability. Decisions regarding volume status should integrate all the clinical data, including input, output, osmolality, weight, and electrolyte concentrations. If uncertainty remains or if the patient fails to improve, the collection of hemodynamic data becomes essential. Pulmonary capillary wedge pressures greater than 16 mm Hg may contribute to pulmonary congestion, and, in general, myocardial performance should be optimized without exceeding this value of filling pressure. The use of colloids to increase the plasma oncotic pressure and assist in the mobilization of fluid from the interstitial space is controversial. Colloid may pass through the damaged capillary endothelium into the interstitial space and there act to potentiate interstitial edema. The administration of albumin should probably be limited to those patients with frank hypoalbuminemia (<2.0 grams per 100 ml). Hyperalimentation should be considered in all patients likely to require long-term mechanical ventilation. Parenteral hyperalimentation can be safely instituted as soon as hemodynamic stability has been achieved.

Hemodynamic Support. Signs of hemodynamic instability or deterioration are particularly ominous in the patient with acute respiratory failure. Deterioration of cardiopulmonary function is more frequently the immediate cause of death than failure to achieve adequate gas exchange. The use of inotropic agents should be considered for patients requiring high filling pressures (>16 mm Hg) to maintain an adequate cardiac output. A low cardiac output in the critically ill patient may represent a serious degree of hemodynamic decompensation, because the stress in these patients is virtually always associated with at least a high normal cardiac output in patients with normal cardiovascular responses. Isoproterenol and dopamine are useful inotropic agents; they can be easily titrated to the desired level and rapidly discontinued if necessary. They should not be reserved for the terminal, hypotensive patient, but should be used at the first sign of decreased perfusion to provide hemodynamic stability and to prevent further decompensation. The administration of these agents is discussed in more detail in Ch. 352.4.

Infection Control. Infection is a major cause of death in respiratory failure. The presence of infection may be particularly hard to establish in the critically ill patient with acute respiratory failure. The chest x-ray is frequently difficult or impossible to interpret; a leukocytosis may be present for other reasons or conversely may fail to appear in the seriously ill patient. Most patients have preexisting, intermittent low grade temperature elevations and may not become overtly febrile when infection develops. Cultures from the airway systems are always positive due to colonization of organisms. The physician is frequently presented with a picture of gradual deterioration in gas exchange coupled with slight changes in the chest x-ray. There is no simple answer to the management of this situation, but every attempt should be made to identify the presence of infection and the type of organism responsible prior to committing the patient to antimicrobial therapy. A positive sputum culture is not of itself sufficient indication for the initiation of antimicrobial therapy; however, if bacterial invasion occurs, it will frequently be caused by organisms colonizing the respiratory system. Daily Gram stains and sputum cultures are useful to monitor the changes and nature of the respiratory flora. If the patient fails to show a definite response to antimicrobial therapy, a more aggressive approach to the diagnosis of the problem should be entertained. Open lung biopsy can be performed on patients requiring mechanical ventilation with acceptable risks. Antimicrobial therapy for presumed infections will almost always give unacceptable clinical results if no signs of improvement are seen within 72 hours. This situation frequently leads to superinfection with resistant organisms, and the concern about infection turns into a self-fulfilling prophecy. Reactivation of tuberculosis can and does occur in the catabolic, critically ill patient, and this possibility should be considered in any patient developing a pneumonia on the intensive care unit.

Monitoring the Results of Therapy. Arterial blood gas tensions are frequently used to follow the progress of a patient with acute respiratory failure; unfortunately, they provide little information about oxygen delivery. There is no satisfactory measurement of oxygen delivery at the tissue level, but the mixed venous oxygen tension (Pv_{O_2}) can provide additional insight into the delivery of oxygen throughout the body and is a valuable guide to the over-all changes in oxygen delivery. A mixed venous $Pv_{O_2} > 40$ mm Hg is normal and reflects good oxygenation, whereas values between 30 and 40 mm Hg reflect modest disturbances in oxygenation. Values of Pv_{O_2} between 20 and 30 mm Hg reflect severe disturbances in oxygen delivery and call for some intervention to improve the situation; values < 20 mm Hg are seldom compatible with life. In sepsis the Pv_{O_2} will occasionally be misleadingly high because of poor oxygen extraction by the peripheral tissues; the interpretation of this (and all) physiologic measurement must be considered in the total clinical context of the patient. Sequential changes are much more important than any single measurement. Metabolic acidosis caused by the accumulation of lactic acid is a late sign of circulatory failure. Any degree of acidosis in the critically ill patient should be assumed to be a consequence of hypoperfusion until proved otherwise. If the acidosis appears to be a consequence of poor oxygen delivery, every attempt should be made to improve the patient's status because of the very poor prognosis associated with metabolic acidosis, regardless of its severity. Cardiac output and arterial venous oxygen content difference can also be used to evaluate the hemodynamic status of the patient. These measurements are particularly valuable when it is necessary to optimize the hemodynamic status through the construction of ventricular function curves. They should also be obtained when changes in pH or mixed venous oxygen tensions suggest a deterioration in oxygen delivery. The delivery of oxygen is a function of the hemoglobin content, the cardiac output, and the level of hemoglobin

saturation. Each factor can be measured separately, and attempts can be made to improve oxygenation through the optimization of each value. In general, patients receiving adequate therapy with less than 40 per cent inspired oxygen concentration and less than 10 cm H_2O end-expiratory pressure will not require hemodynamic monitoring in the absence of other complicating factors. As long as the patient is hemodynamically stable, has normal renal function, and shows no evidence of hypoperfusion, careful sequential monitoring of the conventional clinical parameters will suffice. As treatment progresses, the patient should show a progressive improvement in effective compliance, Aa_{DO_2}, and V_D/V_T.

Intermittent Mandatory Ventilation. A system of mechanical ventilation has been developed which allows the patient to breathe spontaneously (Downs et al.) and still permits a mechanical ventilator to inflate the lungs at a predetermined rate. Figure 7 shows a schematic diagram of such a system (IMV). This technique of ventilation has been used primarily to facilitate weaning of patients from mechanical ventilators following long-term ventilation. It has also been reported to be effective in reducing the impedance to venous return caused by high levels of positive end-expiratory pressure. Used in these circumstances intermittent mandatory ventilation permits the use of levels of end-expiratory pressure which otherwise would be prohibited because of the deleterious effect on cardiac output related to decreased venous return.

352.4. SHOCK

The definition, classification, and general features of the shock syndrome are discussed in Ch. 356. The purpose of this chapter is to discuss the problems of diagnosis and treatment of this syndrome as frequently encountered in the intensive care unit. Cardiogenic shock is discussed in Ch. 356.

DIAGNOSIS OF SHOCK. The classic description of shock is well known: cold, clammy skin, restlessness, oliguria, diaphoresis, systolic hypotension (less than 90 mm Hg), and tachycardia associated with a metabolic acidosis. The patient with all or most of these signs would be dangerously, perhaps even irretrievably ill with irreversible

IMV CIRCUIT
(Respirator Off)

Figure 7. Schematic diagram of intermittent mandatory ventilation (IMV) circuit. The patient's inspiratory effort opens the one-way valve, which permits delivery of fresh humidified gas. During ventilator-generated mandatory breath the one-way valve is closed.

shock. It should be remembered that hypotension is a relatively late sign in shock and appears only after the initial compensatory mechanisms are no longer able to conserve vascular volume. The diagnosis of frank overt shock should present little or no difficulty; however, the recognition of incipient, early shock presents a more challenging problem. Blood pressure is an important indicator of hemodynamic status but does not necessarily parallel cardiac output or blood flow.

The earliest manifestation of shock, particularly septic shock, is frequently hyperventilation, and the appearance of this sign should prompt immediate attention. Arterial blood gas analysis will show a respiratory alkalosis characterized by a low Pco_2, an elevated pH, and a normal bicarbonate value. Determination of the Aa_{DO_2} following the administration of 100 per cent oxygen at this stage will generally fail to disclose a significant intrapulmonic shunt. If a shunt does exist, the situation is even more urgent. Restlessness, apprehension, and changes in mental status are particularly frequent manifestations of early shock, and their appearance should be assumed to represent an early stage of abnormal perfusion until further investigation can clearly resolve the problem. A cold, clammy skin frequently reflects the presence of increased systemic vascular resistance developed in compensation for a decrease in vascular volume. Inadequate renal perfusion may be indicated by a progressive decline in urine flow coupled with an increase in urine osmolality.

Metabolic acidosis can be considered an early sign of shock only in the sense that it may present prior to the onset of hypotension or oliguria; however, the presence of a metabolic acidosis resulting from abnormal perfusion always signifies a major derangement in the circulatory status and calls for immediate therapy.

ACID-BASE DISTURBANCES IN SHOCK. The metabolic (lactic) acidosis associated with shock is well recognized, but it is less well appreciated that the acid-base disturbances frequently progress as follows: normal → respiratory alkalosis → metabolic acidosis. The major significance of the respiratory alkalosis is to alert the physician to the incipient development of shock or respiratory failure. The recognition of metabolic acidosis is frequently delayed because of the presence of a mixed acid-base disturbance. A pH of 7.50 associated with a Pco_2 of 20 mm Hg will usually represent a mixed respiratory alkalosis and metabolic acidosis in spite of a pH value which indicates an alkalemia. This point is important, because an underlying acidosis suggests a serious and potentially catastrophic defect in perfusion. Nothing would be gained by delaying therapy until the development of frank acidemia. Valuable time will be lost if the situation is allowed to progress further, because the acidosis becomes more difficult to correct with the passage of time and will require the administration of very large amounts of sodium bicarbonate.

Lactate acidosis causes deleterious effects on myocardial contractility, cardiac rhythm, and serum electrolytes. Correction of the underlying circulatory or perfusion disturbance is the cornerstone of therapy for the metabolic acidosis of shock. If the acidosis is not corrected by aggressive therapy of the perfusion disturbance or if the pH falls below 7.30, the administration of bicarbonate should be instituted. Maintenance of the arterial pH above 7.30 may avoid the necessity for the rapid administration of large quantities of base. Sodium bicarbonate is the most convenient agent for the correction of acidosis. The amount of bicarbonate to be administered can be approximated from the following relationship: mEq HCO_3 = (base deficit) × 0.30 body weight (kilograms). The base deficit is approximated by subtraction of the carbon dioxide content from the normal bicarbonate value of 25 mEq per liter. The rapid administration of large quantities of base may cause severe disturbances in fluid and electrolyte balance. One half the calculated amount of bicarbonate should be administered at a rate not to exceed 5 mEq per minute. The remainder should be administered as indicated by pH determinations. In the presence of severe acidosis the volume of distribution of bicarbonate can be assumed to be 100 per cent of body weight. The approach to correction of metabolic (lactic) acidosis is considerably different from that applied in the management of diabetic ketoacidosis, in which treatment with bicarbonate is generally reserved for pH values of 7.1 or lower. The metabolic acidosis associated with shock may progress very rapidly and can be extremely difficult to correct under any conditions. It is prudent to correct the acidosis as early as possible, because lethal acidemia may develop even in the face of heavy bicarbonate therapy. The administration of base for the correction of acidosis substantially changes the serum potassium and ionized calcium levels; the consequences of these changes should be considered when treating metabolic acidosis.

Metabolic alkalosis is frequently encountered in the critically ill patient and is most often a consequence of diuretic administration or nasogastric suction; it may occur rarely as a consequence of poorly understood metabolic responses to shock. The first line of therapy for metabolic alkalosis is, naturally, to discontinue the administration of all alkalinizing agents. Antacids, bicarbonate, and diuretic agents are the most common offenders. Nasogastric suction should be discontinued and the serum potassium concentration maintained within normal limits. The administration of potassium chloride in addition to the measures above is frequently sufficient to correct the alkalosis. In severe alkalosis or in the face of hyperkalemia, the intravenous administration of hydrochloric acid (0.10 M) can safely correct the problem. This reagent should be administered into a central vein and the rate of flow adjusted by careful sequential measurements of the arterial pH.

In summary, acid-base disturbances should be diagnosed by frequent analysis of the appropriate electrolyte and blood gas data. Abnormalities should be corrected slowly after the perfusion and volume deficits have been treated. The correction of acid-base disturbances requires a knowledge of the interrelationship of pH, potassium, calcium, and magnesium levels.

ASSESSMENT OF THE PATIENT IN SHOCK. The patient in shock must be assessed and followed very carefully. Therapy will sometimes be necessary without the comfort of laboratory data and before vascular monitoring catheters can be placed for baseline values. All patients can be followed by observation and by recording the items listed in Table 6. The sequential measurement of these parameters will be sufficient to guide therapy when shock has been diagnosed early and the patient responds rapidly to initial treatment. This will frequently be the case for the younger patient without multisystem failure, but if the patient fails to respond to the initial administration of 1.5 to 2.0 liters of crystalloid for volume replacement or if multisystem failure is present, more sophisticated monitoring and treatment will generally be required.

TABLE 6. Critical Measurements for Patients in Shock

Arterial blood pressure
Pulse rate
Respiratory rate
Arterial pH
Arterial blood gases
Mental status
Urine flow and osmolality
Chest roentgenogram

The blood pressure can frequently be followed by sphygmomanometry, but this procedure may give falsely depressed values in the presence of severe vasoconstriction. In patients without obtainable blood pressures or with mean pressures calculated to be below 60 mm Hg, an arterial catheter should be placed for measurement of intravascular pressure. In the seriously ill or unstable patient the intravascular pressures provide a continually visible indication of vascular stability and allow the nursing personnel to spend time more profitably than by measuring cuff pressures. The radial artery pressure can be conveniently monitored by percutaneous insertion of a 20 gauge arterial cannula. The brachial artery should be avoided if possible because of the lack of collateral circulation around the elbow. In patients with severe vasoconstriction there may be substantial differences between the peripheral arterial pressure and that measured centrally in the aorta. In these circumstances a special catheter can be advanced from the brachial artery to the proximal aorta; alternatively a femoral cannula may be inserted to record pressures from the distal aorta. The use of these sites may be associated with substantial complications, and they should not be used without defined, specific reasons and unless the operator has previous experience in the placement of such devices.

The blood pressure should be monitored and maintained at a level sufficient to produce (1) a urine flow of at least 0.5 ml per kilogram per hour, (2) a normal mental status, and (3) a normal electrocardiogram. A mean systemic pressure of 55 to 60 mm Hg is usually sufficient to achieve these goals. It should be remembered that there is no obligatory relationship between blood flow and blood pressure, and that blood pressure values alone are not acceptable parameters in the management of a patient in shock. Urine flow is frequently correlated with renal blood flow and may also be used to reflect perfusion of other organs; however, urine flow alone may not be a valid reflection of renal function. The urine volume and specific gravity should be recorded systematically every 15 to 30 minutes. The use of simple laboratory tests can be of considerable value in the assessment of oliguria. The measurement of central venous pressure may be of some value as a guide to the replacement of volume in the patient with *simple* shock caused by hypovolemia; however, it is usually much more important to follow the urine flow, blood pressure, mental status, and indicators of peripheral perfusion. As with all clinical measurements, the change or trend of these values is worth more than any single measurement.

Careful chest auscultation is important during the rapid administration of large volumes of fluid. Pulmonary congestion may develop with surprising speed during volume replacement and may be a prelude to acute respiratory failure. The appearance of rales or an increase in the Aa_{DO_2} requires careful assessment of the clinical situation.

The use of the Swan-Ganz flotation catheter has been fully discussed in Ch. 352.3. Changes in the pulmonary capillary wedge pressure should also be interpreted very carefully in response to volume expansion. Extreme caution should be exercised at wedge pressures exceeding 18 mm Hg. The blind use of any physiologic measurement to the exclusion of careful clinical assessment of the patient, including auscultation and recording of urine flow, is a certain invitation to disaster.

Cardiac activity should be monitored to detect trends in the pulse rate and to identify arrhythmias. Tachycardia is the rule in shock; however, bradycardia may present in elderly patients with coronary artery disease and may contribute further to the abnormal perfusion state. Arrhythmias are important both in terms of electrical malfunction of the heart and because they may contribute substantially to deterioration in hemodynamic performance. Careful observation of the arterial blood gases will be rewarded by the detection of metabolic acidosis and deteriorating pulmonary function at a time when they may still be responsive to treatment.

Serum chemical concentrations should be followed frequently; the blood urea nitrogen, glucose, and serum electrolytes may have to be followed twice daily or even more frequently. The serum albumin, calcium, phosphorus, SGOT, LDH, bilirubin, and uric acid values should be followed at least every two to three days unless specific circumstances dictate the necessity for more frequent determinations. It is also important to follow daily determinations of the hemogram, including, during the acute phase of illness, prothrombin and partial thromboplastin times and platelet counts. The examination of each stool for occult blood is important, along with daily examination of the gastric aspirate for occult blood if a nasogastric tube is in place. Wound, tracheal, and urine cultures should be monitored frequently as long as endotracheal tubes and catheters are in position. Collection and analysis of data in a systematic manner will maximize the chance for early therapeutic intervention and recovery of critically ill patients.

FLUID REPLACEMENT. The appropriate replacement fluid for the patient in shock is controversial. Crystalloid solutions contain isotonic sodium chloride as the principal constituent. Colloid solutions contain osmotically active particles as the principal constituent. There is little objective evidence to dictate the selection of one crystalloid preparation over another. Comparison of patients resuscitated with either saline or Ringer's lactate solution showed no difference in survival or in electrolyte or acid-base balance. Comparison of resuscitation programs using blood plus colloid and blood plus saline suggested that the latter is a better combination for the resuscitation of combat casualties. The critically ill patient may sequester large amounts of fluid in areas of trauma or other third spaces such as the peritoneum or intestine. Alterations in cellular membrane potential may result in the movement of fluid from the extracellular to the intracellular space in addition to third space accumulation. The infusion of colloid contributes to expansion of the vascular space, but crystalloid infusion contributes expansion of the entire extracellular space and perhaps results in an improved chance for recovery. Blood is the only replacement fluid which can restore oxygen-carrying capacity; it also contains protein, which contributes to the maintenance of osmotic pressure. The principal disadvantage to the use of blood is its potential to transmit hepatitis; it can also cause serious transfusion reactions and is an expensive replacement fluid. Albumin is occasionally used in resuscitation from shock but principally to restore serum osmolality.

Resuscitation of the patient from shock may begin with the administration of 2 to 3 liters of crystalloid. If this results in hemodynamic stabilization with hematocrit above 30 per cent, the crystalloid administration should be continued at a maintenance level. If the patient is still unstable after the crystalloid administration and the hemoglobin concentration is adequate, at least one third to one half of the administered fluid should be in the form of colloid solution such as plasma or plasmanate. If the hematocrit falls below 30 per cent, the administration of packed red cells should be initiated. Sufficient albumin should be administered to maintain an albumin concentration greater than 2.0 to 2.5 grams per deciliter to maintain the serum colloid osmotic pressure.

The appropriate use of crystalloid has reduced the amount of blood required for the resuscitation of the patient from shock. Blood should not be considered to be the only replacement fluid for the patient in shock but one of the components which may be chosen for the individual patient. The replacement program described above permits the loss of 2 to 3 units of blood before replacement by transfusion is indicated. The use of blood for situations requiring massive blood transfusions is discussed in Ch. 352.6.

THE USE OF VASOACTIVE DRUGS IN SHOCK. Pharmacologic support of the vascular system is frequently required in the treatment of resistant or refractory shock. Replacement of volume deficits is the first priority in all forms of shock; patients failing to respond to volume augmentation have a poor prognosis and will frequently require the addition of a vasoactive drug to support their hemodynamic status. The use of such agents in hypovolemic shock has been popular because of their ability to produce an elevation in systemic blood pressure. The increase in blood pressure is usually produced through an increase in the systemic vascular resistance, which results in decreased tissue perfusion and serves to potentiate the abnormal perfusion pattern. The objective of treatment is to improve blood flow to the tissues, and the use of agents to raise the blood pressure by elevation of systemic resistance through vasoconstriction can be dangerous and should be undertaken only on good indication. For example, the elderly patient with clinical evidence of myocardial, cerebral, or renal ischemia is particularly susceptible to the effects of hypotension and may benefit from the judicious use of agents that increase peripheral vascular resistance to maintain a perfusion pressure to these vital organs.

The general use of specific vasoactive drugs and their combinations are discussed in Ch. 356. The use of dopamine, isoproterenol, and calcium in the critically ill patient deserves special consideration.

Dopamine produces vasodilation of the coronary, cerebral, renal, and mesenteric vascular beds. The administration of 1 to 5 μg per kilogram per minute (low dose) will frequently produce a dramatic increase in urine flow in the oliguric patient and cause little detectable change in cardiac output or blood pressure. The administration of dopamine at this dosage level may have value in the preservation of renal function in the critically ill patient, and its use for this purpose requires further investigation. Improvement in cardiac output and tissue perfusion is generally obtained by increasing the rate of administration to the

range of 5 to 20 μg per kilogram per minute. Alpha-adrenergic stimulation begins to occur as the rate of administration is increased beyond this range and the function of the drug becomes similar to that of the conventional alpha agonists.

Isoproterenol is predominantly a beta stimulator. It decreases peripheral resistance as well as renal and coronary resistance to produce an increase in cardiac output and tissue perfusion. Isoproterenol frequently produces tachycardia and myocardial irritability; but if appropriate concentrations are used and the rate of administration is carefully controlled, these complications can be minimized. A concentration of 2.0 mg in 250 ml of diluent will facilitate the safe and convenient administration of this drug. The rate of administration should begin at 0.80 μg per minute and be increased slowly to obtain the desired hemodynamic response.

The use of alpha agonists such as norepinephrine is usually associated with a dramatic improvement in systemic blood pressure, but, unfortunately, the increase in blood pressure is frequently associated with a decrease in cardiac output, manifested by cold, cyanotic extremities and a decreased urine flow. These changes may also be accompanied by substantial increases in central venous and left atrial pressures. The use of alpha agonists alone will seldom contribute to improvement in the hemodynamic status of the patient. Their use when combined with vasodilators is discussed in Ch. 356.

Severe abnormalities in *calcium* metabolism occur in the critically ill patient. The administration of calcium is recommended following the transfusion of every 4 units of blood; however, there is little evidence that decreases in ionized calcium sufficient to cause coagulation abnormalities occur in association with blood transfusion. Patients receiving pharmacologic support of the circulation may undergo a marked depression of the serum ionized calcium levels. This depression of ionized calcium may occur in the absence of transfusions and while the total calcium level is normal. If facilities for the determination of ionized calcium are not available, every patient with persistent hypotension should receive a trial of intravenous calcium chloride. This may result in surprising improvement in cardiac output and tissue perfusion.

Many patients with refractory shock have impairment of myocardial function, but the use of digitalis preparations in patients with variable renal function and labile electrolyte and acid-base disorders can be particularly difficult. The safety, ease of administration, and ability to regulate the minute to minute dosage of agents such as dopamine and isoproterenol have led to the widespread use of these agents in place of digitalis in the unstable, critically ill patient. If digitalis is selected for use, digoxin is the agent of choice because of its relatively short half-life and rapid onset of action.

SEPTIC SHOCK. The terms sepsis and septicemia refer to a number of ill-defined clinical conditions in addition to bacteremia. The shock syndrome in sepsis is presumed to result from the effects of endotoxin. Organisms which are considered normal flora as well as highly virulent bacteria are capable of causing sepsis. Viruses, fungi, protozoa, and rickettsiae have all been implicated as etiologic agents in septic shock.

Gram-negative bacteria are a ready source of infection because of their prevalence in the hospital environment and their contribution to the patient's normal oropharyngeal, gastrointestinal, and dermal flora. The organisms are frequently resistant to all drying and chemical disinfectants; these properties are largely responsible for their role in the transmission of infection by contaminated medical devices.

Underlying host factors not only influence susceptibility of the patient to infection but also determine the likelihood of survival. The severity of the underlying disease is a more important determinant of survival than either the administration of an appropriate antimicrobial agent or the species of bacteria. In one study (Freid and Vosti), the mortality rate in patients with gram-negative bacteremia who were in otherwise good health was 16 per cent. If the underlying disease was anticipated to prove fatal in four to five years, the mortality was 46 per cent; the mortality rate was 90 per cent if the underlying disease was anticipated to prove fatal in less than one year.

Pathophysiology. The pathophysiology of septic shock is poorly understood and largely speculative, but the hemodynamic changes may result from a series of interactions occurring through activation of the complement system, which results in the production of chemotactic factors, histamine and bradykinin. The hemodynamic changes characteristic of gram-negative sepsis are illustrated in Table 7.

Diagnosis. Resuscitation from shock depends upon prompt recognition and treatment of sepsis. The classic description of shock, including tachycardia, cold, clammy skin, weak pulse, and hypotension, is discussed under Diagnosis of Shock, above, and applies in part to septic shock; however, some patients with sepsis present with a different clinical picture. The hallmark of this pattern is arterial vasodilation associated with an increased cardiac index and a hyperdynamic circulation. The blood pressure is usually lower than the patient's baseline pressure but not so low as the values associated with the classic picture of frank shock. The extremities may be warm and pink; occasionally the vasodilation may produce striking erythema. The mental status, electrocardiogram, and urine flow may be normal or may show only slight deterioraton. Hyperventilation is frequently present. In spite of the clinical appearance of apparently excellent perfusion, a metabolic acidosis may document the presence of an abnormal microcirculation. A mild hypoxemia may be present in spite of the hyperventilation. These hemodynamic findings reflect an increased blood flow associated with peripheral vasodilation and arteriovenous shunting. If this hyperdynamic circulatory state progresses or is unresponsive to therapy, the high output state gradually merges into the low output syndrome classically associated with shock.

Treatment. The best treatment of septic shock is prevention, especially because many patients develop this syndrome during hospitalization. Meticulous attention must be directed toward sterile techniques for the managagement of all catheters and cannulas placed into the patient. The use of prophylactic antimicrobials should be sharply curtailed and proper attention directed to nutritional support of the chronically ill, debilitated patient. These steps, coupled with restraint in the use of immunosuppressive drugs and an effective infectious disease committee, can do much to reduce the incidence of bacteremia and septic shock.

Shock associated with sepsis progresses rapidly. If sepsis is suspected on clinical grounds, a rapid examination of the patient for a source of infection should be conducted. Cultures and Gram stains should be performed on all appropriate specimens; at least three separate blood cultures should be obtained. All indwelling catheters should be removed and cultured; antimicrobials must be started as soon as cultures and smears are obtained. Definitive therapy for sepsis depends upon control of the infection with antimicrobials and surgical debridement and drainage when indicated. The institution of these steps should be considered an emergency and must not be postponed until supportive measures such as monitoring systems, fluid administration, and hemodynamic support can be established.

Surgical therapy, if indicated, should be performed as soon as the patient's condition is stabilized and may be required before the patient responds to therapy. If the infection cannot be controlled, the situation is hopeless and even the best supportive therapy will fail.

Antimicrobial selection and administration will be required before culture and sensitivity data are available. The choice of antimicrobial agent should be based on the most likely etiologic agent and the susceptibility pattern of bacteria applicable for each institution. Occasionally, in the presence of life-threatening infection, particularly in the compromised host, shotgun therapy with broad-spectrum antimicrobials may be appropriate, but the routine use of this practice is to be condemned because of the risk of superinfection with resistant organisms. Treatment of bacteremia with an appropriate antimicrobial will decrease the frequency of shock and subsequent fatal outcome; however, there is no difference in survival rates related to use of bactericidal or bacteriostatic antimicrobial agents.

The basic principles underlying fluid therapy have been discussed under Fluid Replacement, above. Patients with hypodynamic shock will have inadequate filling pressures and will respond to appropriate volume augmentation. If the hemoglobin concentration is adequate, the initial volume replacement should consist of a crystalloid solution. If hemodynamic stability has not been achieved following administration of 1000 to 1500 ml of fluid, a pulmonary artery catheter should be inserted to guide further therapy. The central venous pressure will frequently be high, but the pulmonary capillary wedge pressure will almost always be low (Fig. 4). The failure to initiate adequate volume augmentation is a serious error; however, it is

TABLE 7. Hemodynamic Changes in Sepsis

	Blood Pressure	Pulse	Cardiac Output	AVO$_2$D	Central Venous Pressure	Total Peripheral Resistance
Hypodynamic	↓	↑	↓	↑	↕	↑
Hyperdynamic	N ↓	↑	↑	↓	↕	↓ N

AVO$_2$D = Arterial-venous oxygen content difference.

equally important to avoid fluid overload and its disastrous pulmonary consequences.

The hemoglobin concentration should not be allowed to fall below 13 grams per 100 ml; blood transfusions will frequently be required to maintain the hemoglobin concentration in this range. Therapy for the hyperdynamic pattern of shock is not well established. One approach has been to optimize ventricular function through determination of wedge pressure and cardiac output values. It is important to ensure that these patients do not become volume depleted with resulting sudden deterioration manifested by the appearance of atypical hypodynamic shock. The hyperdynamic pattern of shock is frequently refractory to vasoactive drugs. The general principles underlying the use of these drugs in hypovolemic shock apply equally well to the treatment of septic shock. The administration of pharmacologic doses of steroids should be initiated as soon as sepsis is suspected and continued for 48 hours.

REFRACTORY SHOCK.   Resuscitation from shock can fail for a number of reasons, but failure is frequently related to myocardial, renal, pulmonary, or hepatic insufficiency. Myocardial dysfunction is an important element in refractory shock and may even be seen in young patients with no pre-existing heart disease. Subclinical coronary artery disease and the direct action of endotoxin have been suggested as causes of myocardial depression. A myocardial depressant factor (MDF) has been described in the plasma of animals following many forms of shock. If further studies document the authenticity of this factor, believed to be a small peptide, many episodes of myocardial failure associated with shock may be explained.

Renal failure accompanying shock is associated with a very high mortality. Dialysis does not alter the mortality associated with renal failure in this setting, and every therapeutic effort should be expended to prevent this catastrophic complication in the critically ill patient.

The pulmonary lesion in shock is discussed in detail in Ch. 352.3. Early and appropriate therapy of shock can do much to reduce the mortality associated with this disorder. Disseminated intravascular coagulation may be detected, but is not often a clinically important problem. When pathologic bleeding occurs in association with disseminated intravascular coagulation, the prognosis is extremely poor. The patient in shock with underlying hepatic disease has a particularly grave prognosis, perhaps attesting to the central role of the liver in maintaining metabolic homeostasis. Unless the patient responds rapidly to initial therapy, the mortality has been greater than 90 per cent. Advanced life support systems can maintain such patients for very long time periods but seldom with satisfactory results.

A number of reversible factors can be responsible for the lack of response to appropriate therapy: (1) inadequate or inappropriate fluid therapy; (2) sepsis, unrecognized or refractory to treatment; (3) pulmonary emboli; (4) pneumothorax; (5) occult adrenal insufficiency; or (6) malnutrition. A careful and systematic search for one or more of these factors should be conducted in every patient refractory to therapy for shock.

352.5. RENAL FUNCTION IN THE CRITICALLY ILL PATIENT

Acute renal failure is discussed in Ch. 372. The present discussion is limited to those aspects of renal failure relevant to the critically ill patient. Oliguria is defined as a urine flow less than 400 ml per day for a 70-kg patient and is the most common renal problem encountered in the seriously ill. The volume of urine excreted depends upon (1) the ability of the kidney to concentrate and (2) the solute load. A normal subject is capable of maximal urinary concentration to 1300 to 4000 mOsm per kilogram of water. This solute load will require a urine volume of 1 liter for excretion. A catabolic patient may require excretion of 1200 mOsm of solute per 24 hours; however, the seriously ill patient may be unable to concentrate urine to greater than 600 mOsm per liter. This set of conditions requires a large urine volume for the excretion of increased osmolar loads. The septic, catabolic patient may, in fact, be oliguric, with urine flows approaching 800 ml per day. A *minimal* output of 0.5 ml per kilogram per hour will usually provide a sufficient margin of safety to permit excretion of the increased solute loads in the presence of a decreased concentrating ability without the appearance of azotemia; however, urine flows of 0.8 to 1.0 ml per kilogram per hour provide a more acceptable margin of safety. Oliguria may be present if the hourly urine flow decreases below this level.

Oliguria is associated with a high incidence of renal failure. The need for immediate therapy requires oliguria to be characterized as prerenal, renal, or postrenal in origin. A rapid, thorough search must define the cause of oliguria in each case. Prerenal azotemia is caused by a decreased renal blood flow which is insufficient to cause intrinsic renal damage. Peripheral vasodilation, myocardial failure, and hypovolemia are all causes of prerenal oliguria. The kidney responds to minimize volume loss through secretion of aldosterone, antidiuretic hormone, and increased proximal tubular reabsorption of sodium. The increased reabsorption of sodium and water results in the production of urine characterized by a high solute concentration. The urine volume is decreased, whereas the concentration of sodium is low (<20 mEq per liter) and the potassium concentration is high. Tubular concentrating mechanisms function effectively in prerenal oliguria; the urine to plasma osmolality ratio is greater than 2:1, and the urine to plasma creatinine ratio is usually greater than 50. The use of the simple laboratory measurements in assessing the cause of oliguria is more fully discussed in Ch. 372. Postrenal failure must be considered if the patient remains oliguric following bladder drainage. Considerable judgment must be used in assessment of a patient for postrenal failure. Diagnostic aids include KUB films, intravenous pyelography, and retrograde pyelography. The hazard of infection associated with urinary tract instrumentation is real, and these procedures should be undertaken only in patients with specific indications pointing to bilateral ureteral obstruction.

If renal and postrenal uropathy are eliminated as causes of oliguria, the adequacy of vascular volume must be established. Oxygen delivery should be optimized through appropriate attention to cardiac output and hemoglobin concentration. If optimization of perfusion fails to produce an adequate urine flow, a trial of diuretics should be administered. The administration of large initial doses of furosemide to the hemodynamically unstable patient can produce severe hypotension unrelated to the diuretic effect of the drug. Large doses of loop diuretics are unlikely to alter the course of renal failure, and their use for this purpose is controversial; however, the administration of diuretics may convert oliguric renal failure to non-oliguric failure, which greatly simplifies the convenience and ease of patient management. The initial dose of furosemide should be 20 to 40 mg given intravenously, and this may be doubled every hour until a maximum single dose of 500 to 600 mg or a maximum cumulative dose of 1 gram in 24 hours has been administered. Dialysis should be instituted as soon as the diagnosis of acute renal failure is established. The patient should not be allowed to become uremic; frequent dialysis will also facilitate the administration of a high caloric intake. The hemodynamically unstable patient usually tolerates peritoneal dialysis well.

The preceding discussion has emphasized the importance of oliguria in assessment of the renal status. It is equally important to realize that a normal or high urine flow does not guarantee that renal function is normal. It may be used as an indicator of change in renal function, but other parameters such as BUN and creatinine should be used to monitor the renal status.

Patients with sepsis may have abnormally high urine flows; if these losses are not carefully replaced, oliguria may develop. The erroneous use of diuretics under these circumstances can be particularly hazardous because of the likelihood of volume depletion. The urine sodium concentration can be particularly useful in following such patients.

Polyuric syndromes have been described (1) following resuscitation from shock, (2) associated with sepsis, and (3) accompanying nonoliguric renal failure. The syndrome of acute nonoliguric renal failure is characterized by azotemia and a high urine flow. The urine sodium is less than 20 mEq per liter, and isosthenuria is usually present. Hyperkalemia is found less frequently than in the oliguric form of renal failure. The management of nonoliguric renal failure may be simplified because fluid restriction is not required, but the condition is by no means benign. The mortality is only slightly less than that reported for oliguric renal failure.

352.6. MASSIVE BLOOD TRANSFUSIONS

The principles underlying blood replacement are discussed in Ch. 352.4; however, special problems are encountered in massive blood transfusions. Massive blood loss requires replacement by typed, cross-matched blood. Blood should be transfused within 60 minutes of its removal from the blood bank unless proper storage facilities are available at the bedside. Patients requiring multiple blood transfusions over several days should have their serum tested for compatibility each day, because antibodies may develop to the transfused blood and react with future transfusions. Type-specific, cross-matched blood is always the first choice for replacement therapy, but under emergency circumstances blood may have to be administered under less than ideal conditions. The second choice is partially cross-matched, type-specific blood. Such blood should be available after a 15- to 20-minute delay; this blood is provided after the conventional cross-match procedure has been performed but before the Coombs test is completed. Type-specific ABO and Rh (D) noncross-matched blood may be administered if a five- to ten-minute delay is acceptable. In truly exsanguinating hemorrhage, type O Rh-negative blood may be administered while a cross-match is performed. Transfused antibodies may accumulate when a nongroup O patient receives type O blood. A substantial risk may be involved in returning the patient to type-specific blood, and it may be necessary to continue administration of type O blood until this antibody titer decreases. Blood transfusions are frequently administered to improve the recipient's oxygen delivery. The hemoglobin-oxygen dissociation curve is shifted to the left during the first few days of blood storage, and this shift may remain for up to 24 hours following the transfusion of banked blood. Storage of blood in citrate-phosphate-dextrose (CPD) anticoagulant maintains the 2,3-diphosphoglycerate level, which increases the potential of transfused blood to deliver oxygen. Many blood banks are changing from the conventional acid-citrate-dextrose (ACD) solutions for this reason.

COMPLICATIONS OF MASSIVE BLOOD TRANSFUSIONS. The complications from transfusion of more than 5 units of blood are (1) pulmonary insufficiency, (2) leukocyte sensitization, (3) hypothermia, (4) acidosis, (5) hypocalcemia, (6) hyperkalemia, and (7) hemorrhage.

Banked blood stored in either acid-citrate-dextrose or citrate-phosphate-dextrose solution contains significant quantities of debris composed of platelets, leukocytes, and fibrin. This debris has been shown to produce changes in pulmonary hemodynamics; there is a substantial body of experimental evidence to implicate a contributory role for microaggregates of this debris in the pathogenesis of respiratory failure. Ultrafiltration of banked blood with small pore filters will remove the microaggregates. These filters are now commercially available and are capable of removing over 500 mg of microaggregated material per unit of stored blood. Most of these filters are manufactured of woven Dacron and can be used without causing substantial damage to the blood components or decreasing the flow rate. Failure to use these devices for administration of over 3 units of blood may place the patient at increased risk for the development of acute respiratory failure.

Sensitization of the recipient to leukocytes or platelets of the donor has been proposed as a cause of noncardiogenic pulmonary edema. The sudden appearance of pulmonary edema without evidence of circulatory overload following the administration of only 2 to 3 units of blood may be the only presenting sign of this phenomenon. Therapy for this rare syndrome has not been established, but the use of dextran and antihistaminic agents has been suggested.

The rapid administration of banked blood can quickly lower core temperature. A temperature decrease of only 0.5° C can induce shivering, which greatly increases oxygen consumption and cardiac output. These effects may be extremely deleterious in the patient with a marginal hemodynamic status. The incidence of cardiac arrest and ventricular arrhythmias during massive blood transfusion has been decreased by warming the blood prior to or during transfusion. A number of safe, inexpensive heat exchangers or blood warmers are now available and should be used for transfusions of more than 2 units.

The individual acid-base responses to blood transfusion are extremely variable; pH should be monitored during massive transfusion therapy to assess to need for bicarbonate administration. The rapid administration of large quantities of ACD blood may contribute to the development of metabolic acidosis, in part because the pH of ACD blood may approach 6.5 following 14 days of storage.

Citrate intoxication may produce circulatory depression secondary to the binding of ionized calcium by citrate; there is little evidence to establish the clinical importance of hypocalcemia said to be associated with blood transfusions.

Hyperkalemia is frequently listed as a major complication of multiple blood transfusion; however, significant hyperkalemia does not frequenlty accompany administration of banked blood to patients with normal renal function. The patient with compromised renal function, hypovolemia, and massive trauma, however, is predisposed to hyperkalemia on other grounds unrelated to blood transfusion. It should be appreciated that the patient with normal renal function and not in frank shock may, in fact, become hypokalemic following massive transfusion and may actually require the administration of potassium to prevent the development of hypokalemia.

A hemorrhagic diathesis, manifested by bleeding from venipuncture sites, hematuria, or petechiae, may be seen following the administration of large amounts of stored blood. This bleeding tendency may be the result of dilutional thrombocytopenia, deficiency of factors V and VIII, or disseminated intravascular coagulation (DIC). Blood storage at 4° C may be capable of altering platelets sufficiently to cause their removal by the reticuloendothelial system soon after infusion. Infusion of ACD blood stored for more than 24 hours can produce dilution of the available platelet pool in patients losing large amounts of blood. This phenomenon is perhaps the most important cause of bleeding tendencies following massive blood transfusion. Factors V and VIII may decrease to values as low as 20 per cent of normal following three weeks of blood storage. This deficiency is rarely the cause of post-transfusion bleeding, but may act to intensify bleeding from other causes. The administration of fresh frozen plasma can correct this deficiency.

352.7. COAGULATION DISORDERS IN THE CRITICALLY ILL PATIENT

The most important coagulation disorders identified in the critically ill patient are those related to activation of the coagulation or fibrinolytic processes following shock or trauma and those related to therapy.

DISSEMINATED INTRAVASCULAR COAGULATION. The most important coagulopathy is termed disseminated intravascular coagulation. This syndrome is characterized by intravascular coagulation occurring within the peripheral vessels. This extensive coagulation process consumes normal clotting factors in the plasma to the point at which normal hemostasis is impossible and uncontrollable hemorrhage begins. Conditions frequently associated with intravascular coagulation are hypotension, shock, sepsis, burns, anaphylactoid reactions, hepatic disease, massive trauma, and cancer. Plasma factors I, II, V, and VIII and platelets are consumed through activation of both the intrinsic and extrinsic clotting systems. Activation proceeds through a final common pathway to the formation of thrombin which cleaves fibrinogen to form a fibrin clot. Thrombin also promotes the conversion of plasminogen to plasmin, which acts on fibrin to form fibrin split products. The hemorrhagic process is perpetuated by the split products which inhibit the action of thrombin on fibrinogen. The clinical manifestations of disseminated intravascular coagulation classically involve the skin. The petechiae, purpura, and hemorrhage at venipuncture sites are common clinical presentations of disseminated intravascular coagulation. Oral cyanosis and gangrene are also manifestations of disseminated intravascular coagulation. The diagnosis of this syndrome must be made from serial coagulation studies which include the partial thromboplastin time and prothrombin time, both of which are prolonged by consumption of clotting factors. The fibrinogen level and platelet count also decrease because of their consumption in the clotting process. The thrombin time is also frequenlty prolonged, but this may result from hypofibrinogenemia or the presence of even minute quantities of heparin. The use of these tests to diagnose disseminated intravascular coagulation and the special problems of their interpretation in the presence of hepatic disease are discussed more fully in Ch. 521.5.

The basic treatment of disseminated intravascular coagulation lies in the correction of the underlying disease process. In life-threatening hemorrhage the appearance of disseminated intravascular coagulation in the critically ill patient is associated with a grave prognosis, perhaps because of its frequent relationship to irreversible shock. In life-threatening hemorrhage a trial of heparin therapy may be initiated in an attempt to control the widespread coagulation process. The use of heparin in this condition is not established and is controversial, but in the face of life-threatening hemorrhage associated with disseminated intravascular coagulation its use can perhaps be justified. In any case, its use can, at best, only provide additional time for correction of the underlying disorder. The course of heparin therapy is best followed by its regulation to prolong the whole blood clotting time between two and three times normal. The partial thromboplastin time cannot be used, because depletion of the clotting factors and the presence of fibrin split products interfere with interpretation of the test. The administration of heparin should begin at 15 units per kilogram per hour. Several days may be required before the effects of heparin become apparent, and it may require even longer before improvement in the thrombocytopenia is noted. Heparin excretion depends both on renal and hepatic function; the dosage may require reduction in the presence of either hepatic or renal compromise. After the intitution of heparin therapy, the replacement of consumed factors may be considered. Fresh frozen plasma may be used to replace factors V and VIII; platelets may be given if necessary, and plasma may be administered if the fibrinogen level fails to respond to appropriate therapy. The role of fibrinolysis in disseminated intravascular coagulation is unclear, but primary fibrinolysis unrelated to disseminated intravascular coagulation is rare. The use of drugs to treat primary fibrinolysis can precipitate thrombotic complications if disseminated intravascular coagulation is present.

THROMBOCYTOPENIA. Thrombocytopenia is probably the most frequently encountered hematologic disorder in the critically ill patient. Its presence probably reflects increased platelet utilization caused by immune antibodies, drugs, or infections. Generalized marrow suppression may occur as a consequence of inanition or drug therapy. As a general rule platelet counts greater than 50,000 per cubic millimeter are not associated with an increased incidence of hemorrhage; however, if large numbers of inadequately functioning platelets are present, substantial hemorrhage may occur even in the presence of adequate numbers of platelets. A number of drugs interfere with platelet function, including aspirin, dipyridamole, phenylbutazone, indomethacin, glyceryl, guaiacolate, chlorpromazine, and diphenhydramine. Platelet dysfunction is also seen as part of the uremic syndrome and may be corrected by dialysis.

VITAMIN K DEPLETION. Factors II, VII, IX, and X are vitamin K dependent clotting factors. The prothrombin time and partial thromboplastin time are both prolonged by deficiencies of these factors. Biliary tract obstruction and malnutrition produce clotting disorders which are corrected by the administration of vitamin K. Unfortunately, malnutrition is still a problem in patients receiving long-term life support. It is hoped that the use of hyperalimentation techniques will reduce the incidence of this cause of clotting disorder. The vitamin K dependent clotting factors may be replaced by either infusion of fresh frozen plasma or a concentrate of factor IX.

Civetta, J. M.: The daily problems in the intensive care unit. Adv. Surg., 8:221, 1974.
Collins, J. A., and Ballinger, W. F.: The treatment of shock. In Ballinger, W. F., Rutherford, R. B., and Zuidema, G. D. (eds.): The Management of Trauma. 2nd ed. Philadelphia, W. B. Saunders Company, 1973.
Downs, J. B., Klein, E. F., Desautels, D., et al.: Intermittent mandatory ventilation, a new approach to weaning patients from mechanical ventilators. Chest, 64:331, 1973.
Freid, M. S., and Vosti, K. L.: The importance of underlying disease in patients with gram negative bacteremia. Arch. Intern. Med., 121:418, 1968.
Moore, F. D.: Post-traumatic pulmonary insufficiency. In Hardy, J. D. (ed.): Critical Surgical Illness. Philadelphia, W. B. Saunders Company, 1971.
Murray, J. F.: The Normal Lung. The Basis for Diagnosis and Treatment of Pulmonary Disease. Philadelphia, W. B. Saunders Company, 1976.
Pontoppidan, H.: Bedside pulmonary tools and their interpretation. In Caldwell, T. B., and Moya, F. (eds.): Advances in Respiratory Care and Physiology. Springfield, Ill., Charles C Thomas, 1973.
Pontoppidan, H., Geffin, B., and Lowenstein, E.: Acute Respiratory Failure in the Adult. Boston, Little, Brown & Company, 1973.
Rutherford, R. B.: The pathophysiology of trauma and shock. In Ballinger, W. F., Rutherford, R. B., and Zuidema, G. D. (eds.): The Management of Trauma. 2nd ed. Philadelphia, W. B. Saunders Company, 1973.
Suter, P. M., Fairley, H. B., and Isenberg, M. D.: Optimum end expiratory airway pressure in patients with acute pulmonary failure. N. Engl. J. Med., 292:284, 1975.
Tagge, G. F., Adler, D., Bryan-Brown, C., et al.: Relationship of therapy to prognosis in critically ill patients. Crit. Care Med., 2:61, 1974.
West, J. B.: Ventilation/Blood Flow and Gas Exchange. Oxford, Blackwell, 1970.
Wilson, R. F., Leblane, L. P., and Walt, A. J.: Shock due to trauma. In Walt, A. J., and Wilson, R. F. (eds.): Management of Trauma; Pitfalls and Practice. Philadelphia, Lea & Febiger, 1975.

353. CARDIOPULMONARY RESUSCITATION

DEFINITION. Cardiopulmonary arrest is a clinical syndrome characterized by apnea, pulselessness, unconsciousness, and a death-like appearance in a person not otherwise expected to die. Physiologically this syndrome is characterized by a sudden cessation of sufficient oxygen to maintain viability of the heart and brain.

SCOPE OF THE PROBLEM. In this chapter we will discuss the recognition of cardiopulmonary arrest and the application of resuscitation techniques necessary to maintain life until the patient recovers or until advanced life support measures become available. The causes of cardiopulmonary arrest in the hospital are legion. Virtually every diagnostic and therapeutic procedure performed has been complicated by cardiopulmonary arrest, which emphasizes the importance of a knowledge of the hazards and side effects of all medications and procedures administered by the hospital staff. The long-term survival following resuscitation from cardiopulmonary arrest occurring inside the hospital depends upon the environment in which the arrest occurs. Survival rates as high as 70 to 80 per cent have been reported for patients experiencing cardiopulmonary arrest following acute myocardial infarction. By contrast, survival rates of only 10 to 20 per cent have been reported for patients with chronic underlying disease who arrest on hospital wards. The survival of persons who arrest outside the hospital is even less, but is improved when there is widespread training in basic life support techniques, and when mobile coronary care units are available.

The most effective treatment for cardiopulmonary arrest is prevention; the identification of patients with specific risk factors at the time of hospitalization should permit the application of appropriate monitoring and treatment to decrease the over-all incidence of cardiopulmonary arrest. The relationship between etiology, prevention, and treatment of cardiopulmonary arrest can best be appreciated through an understanding of the underlying pathophysiology. Jude has defined four vectors which may interact to cause cardiac arrest: (1) decreased cardiac output, (2) decreased coronary perfusion, (3) decreased myocardial function, and (4) cardiac arrhythmias. These vectors may be considered to be the proximate cause(s) of cardiopulmonary arrest, producing a decreased delivery of oxygen and substrate to the tissues and resulting in cellular hypoxia. Each vector can be associated with anatomic, physiologic, or biochemical situations representing the etiologic factors leading to the arrest. The cardiac arrest circle (Fig. 8) facilitates treatment directed toward each vector and thus provides a logical basis for management of the appropriate pathophysiologic factor.

DEFINITION OF BASIC AND ADVANCED LIFE SUPPORT. The classic mechanistic approach toward cardiopulmonary arrest is a basic life support system designed to maintain the circulation of oxygenated blood to the tissue. This approach facilitates a reflex response by both medical and nonmedical personnel which suffices for all causes of cardiopulmonary arrest. It is a pragmatic approach of proven effectiveness, but it will not lead to an understanding of cause; nor will it direct attention to prevention of recurrence. Basic life support

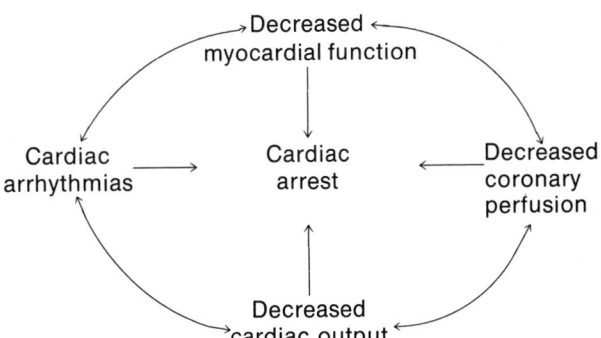

Figure 8. Cardiac arrest circle. The interaction of these four vectors may lead to the loss of effective circulation and cardiac arrest. Identification of factors giving rise to each vector facilitates a systematic approach to the causative factor(s). This permits a plan of treatment to be developed on a logical basis. (Modified from Jude.)

is emergency first aid designed for the management of cardiopulmonary arrest. It includes steps frequently recalled by the mnemonic *ABC*, which stands for *A*irway, *B*reathing, *C*irculation. These measures may be applied by medical or nonmedical personnel and do not require specialized equipment or the administration of drugs. Advanced life support includes monitoring, defibrillation, drug administration, and other therapies and equipment required to stabilize the patient; it requires the presence of highly trained personnel and the supervision of a physician (Fig. 9).

RECOGNITION OF CARDIOPULMONARY ARREST. Patients with unexpected collapse or loss of consciousness should be considered to have sustained cardiopulmonary arrest. Gasping respiration and absence of the cardiac impulse and major arterial pulses are important clinical criteria for recognition of cardiopulmonary arrest. The cessation of respirations may not occur for one to two minutes following circulatory failure, and dilatation of the pupils may take two to three minutes; hence these signs should not be required for the initiation of cardiopulmonary resuscitation. There must be a sense of emergency about initiating the basic life support steps in cardiopulmonary resuscitation. The initial seconds are critical. Chances of survival decrease rapidly with each minute of delay. The differential diagnosis can be considered after the institution of basic life support; the situation usually clarifies itself after beginning of the initial resuscitative efforts. Cardiopulmonary resuscitation should commence as soon as a cardiopulmonary arrest is suspected, and assistance should be summoned. All hospitals should have a well rehearsed plan for bringing personnel and equipment to the bedside in the shortest possible time.

ESTABLISHMENT OF AIRWAY. The first aspect of basic life support is the establishment and maintenance of airway control. The most frequent mistake is failure to open the airway prior to artificial ventilation. The airway is easily opened by placing the patient on his back and tilting his head backward as far as possible (unless there is a neck injury; see below). The rescuer places one hand beneath the patient's neck and the other hand on the forehead in order to tilt the head backward. This procedure (1) extends the neck and (2) moves the tongue from the posterior oropharynx. This decreases the possibility of airway obstruction by the tongue, opens the airway, and may even allow breathing to resume spontaneously. The head should be maintained in this position throughout resuscitation without fail.

If a neck injury is suspected, e.g., following an automobile or diving accident, the neck must not be hyperextended. In this case, the airway should be opened by using a modified jaw thrust, keeping the victim's head in a fixed, neutral position.

ASSISTED BREATHING. If the patient does not begin spontaneous respirations when the airway is opened, artificial ventilation must be started. The methods available for artificial ventilation are as follows: (1) expired air ventilation — mouth to mouth or mouth to nose; (2) bag-valve-mask system; (3) endotracheal intubation; and (4) esophageal obturator airway.

Mouth to Mouth. To perform mouth-to-mouth ventilation the patient's head is maintained in a position of maximal backward tilt while debris is removed from the patient's mouth. The patient's nostrils are closed; the resuscitator takes several deep breaths, makes a tight mouth-to-mouth seal, and exhales slowly into the patient's mouth. He then removes his mouth and allows the patient to exhale passively, while watching the chest fall. This cycle is repeated every five seconds (12 breaths per minute). The adequacy of ventilation can

Figure 9. An approach to the management of cardiopulmonary arrest, incorporating elements of basic and advanced life support systems. (Modified from Jude.)

be assured by seeing the chest rise and fall with each breath and feeling the compliance and resistance of the patient's lungs as they expand. If difficulty is encountered in securing a tight seal about the patient's mouth, mouth-to-nose resuscitation can be used; with this technique the patient's lips are sealed by lifting the mandible during ventilation; subsequently it may be necessary to open the mouth slightly during expiration to allow the air to escape.

Bag-Valve-Mask Devices. The principal advantage of the manually operated, self-inflating bag-valve-mask units lies in their ability to deliver supplemental oxygen. With mouth-to-mouth or mouth-to-nose resuscitation the concentration of exhaled oxygen is approximately 18 per cent, which, under ideal conditions, will correspond to an alveolar tension of 80 mm Hg. This may result in marked hypoxemia because of substantial physiologic shunting and ventilation-perfusion imbalance which frequently accompany an arrest. The resuscitator bag devices usually provide tidal volumes less than are delivered by mouth-to-mouth ventilation, and it is very difficult to maintain a leakproof seal between the mask and face while assuring an adequate open airway. Considerable training and practice are required to ventilate a patient successfully with a resuscitator bag assembly; it is frequently more effective for the resuscitator to hold the mask and effect a seal to the patient's face while an assistant squeezes the bag. The resuscitator bag assembly should always be used with supplemental oxygen and should ideally have a reservoir assembly to permit administration of 100 per cent oxygen. Care must be taken to ensure that oxygen flows are not so high as to jam the valve system, rendering the bag useless and giving the impression that the valve malfunctions. Gas flow in the range of 8 to 10 liters per minute should be tolerated by a high quality bag assembly. If supplemental oxygen is not available, mouth-to-mouth resuscitation will provide more effective ventilation than use of the mask-bag-valve resuscitator bag assemblies.

Endotracheal Intubation. Cuffed endotracheal tubes undoubtedly provide ventilation superior to the methods discussed above. Mouth-to-mouth and bag-valve-mask ventilation promote gastric distention, posing the hazard of regurgitation and aspiration of gastric contents into the lungs. With a cuffed endotracheal tube the airway is patent, aspiration is prevented, and delivery of high concentrations of supplemental oxygen is ensured. In spite of these advantages, valuable time should not be wasted in attempts to intubate the patient during the first few minutes of resuscitation. This should be attempted only after the patient has been well oxygenated by mouth-to-mouth or bag-valve-mask ventilation. No more than ten seconds should be allowed for intubation. If the airway cannot be secured within this period of time, the patient should be ventilated with 100 per cent oxygen for a few minutes before the next attempt. Any interruption of ventilation and assisted circulation for longer periods of time will contribute to the irreversibility of the process. It is far better to use mouth-to-mouth resuscitation than to waste time while inexperienced personnel attempt to intubate the patient. If the airway cannot be established, an emergency cricothyroidotomy should be performed. The cricothyroid membrane should be incised and a 6 mm (OD) tube inserted into the tracheal lumen.

There is probably no role for a tracheostomy during cardiopulmonary resuscitation.

Esophageal Obturator Airway. Oxygenation of the lungs by exhaled air methods or by simple airway adjuncts often results in gastric distention, which may interfere with breathing or result in regurgitation. This can be avoided by endotracheal intubation; however, this technique requires special training, is often difficult in emergency situations, may cause delays and interruptions in administration of cardiopulmonary resuscitation, and may have serious complications. The esophageal obturator airway may be a useful alternative to endotracheal intubation. The airway may be introduced more easily and quickly than an endotracheal tube, and direct visualization is not required. Gastric distention and regurgitation are prevented by the soft plastic obturator, which blocks the distal orifice of the tube, and by the inflatable cuff, which completes the total occlusion of the esophagus. Multiple openings in the tube at the level of the pharynx provide adequate air flow in the trachea and ventilation of the lungs. This airway should be used only in patients who are not breathing or who are unconscious. Precautions must be taken to minimize or prevent regurgitation and aspiration of stomach contents during insertion and removal of the tube.

EXTERNAL CARDIAC COMPRESSION. The absence or questionable presence of a pulse is indication for starting artificial circulation by means of external cardiac compression. When cardiopulmonary arrest occurs, the airway must be controlled, artificial ventilation initiated, and external cardiac compression commenced in very rapid succession. The rescuer must (1) establish unresponsiveness of the patient and maintain the airway, (2) quickly ventilate the lungs four times, demonstrating good chest expansion, and (3) while maintaining an open airway, check for presence of the carotid pulse. The following procedure should be used in the application of external cardiac compression:

1. The patient remains supine in bed, or on the floor or ground, but is positioned on a firm surface such as a board or tray placed under the back.

2. Effective cardiac compression requires sufficient pressure to depress the lower sternum from 1½ to 2 inches. The heel of the hand should be palced on the lower portion of the sternum approximately 1 to 1½ inches from the xiphoid process toward the patient's head. The rescuer's fingers should not rest on the patient's ribs during compression, because lateral pressure increases the possibility of rib fractures. The heel of the hand should remain in constant contact with the chest wall during relaxation, but pressure on the sternum should be *completely* released so that it returns to its normal resting position between compressions. The compression should be smooth and regular, with the cycle equally divided between compression and relaxation time.

3. It is always preferable to have two rescuers, because artificial ventilation must be combined with artificial circulation. Under these conditions one rescuer positions himself at the patient's head *to maintain the airway* and to perform rescue breathing, while the other rescuer positions himself at the side of the patient to perform external cardiac compression. With two rescuers the compression rate is 60 per minute. This rate facilitates timing at 1 compression per second and per-

mits optimal coordination of ventilation and circulation by the rapid interposition on one breath after each five chest compressions *without* interruption of the mechanical compression (5:1 ratio). It is important to deliver the breath without a pause in external compression, because any interruption in cardiac compression results in a decrease in blood flow and blood pressure to zero. When there is only one rescuer, the compression rate is increased to 80 per minute, and two *quick* full lung inflations are delivered after each 15 compressions. This procedure produces a 15:2 ratio of compression to ventilation and results in an actual compression rate of 60 per minute. The two breaths must be delivered in rapid succession without allowing full exhalation to occur in order to maintain an adequate number of breaths and compressions per minute.

4. Palpation of the femoral and carotid pulses may be used to assess the effectiveness of circulatory support; however, there is often poor correlation between recorded intra-arterial pressures and the strength of the pulse to palpation.

It must be remembered that even under the best of conditions the cardiac output is less than 50 per cent of normal when external cardiac compression is applied. It is possible to achieve systolic pressures approaching 100 mm Hg (mean arterial pressure of 30 to 50 mm Hg); however, the average pressure obtained during resuscitation is frequently 40 to 60 mm Hg. External cardiac compressions must not be interrupted for longer than five seconds, even for insertion of intravenous lines or monitoring of cardiac rhythm, if a resuscitation is to be successful. Any interruption in cardiac compression results in a drop in blood flow and blood pressure to zero. The use of a stopwatch to time the interruptions of external massage is frequently useful to prevent additional hypoxic damage related to cessation of cardiac compression. Occasionally external cardiac compression will not provide adequate tissue perfusion. Progressive metabolic acidosis results, and the resuscitation is unsuccessful. Certain conditions preclude effective external massage; these include massive obesity and thoracic deformities such as kyphoscoliosis, pectus excavatum, and severe emphysema. In addition, hypovolemia, pneumothorax, and cardiac tamponade may produce poor ventricular filling and result in ineffective resuscitation. These three conditions are easily correctable and should come to mind when resuscitative efforts appear to be unsuccessful. Since the cardiac output during cardiopulmonary resuscitation is so dependent upon ventricular filling, it is frequently efficacious to elevate the legs during external cardiac compression to increase venous return and augment the cardiac output. If external cardiac massage is ineffective, open chest massage should be considered. This procedure is rarely performed outside the operating room and requires trained personnel, adequate equipment, and the presence of a thoracic surgeon. During prolonged resuscitation the efficiency of mechanical external compression decreases because of fatigue; rotation of individuals performing external compression should be considered at least every ten minutes. Mechanical devices are available to perform external cardiac compression, and they may be of great value in cases in which massage must be continued for more than an hour or the patient must be transported in a vehicle. They should not be used ini-

tially because of the time consumed at such a critical stage in the resuscitation.

FAILURE AND COMPLICATIONS. The most common causes for failure in cardiopulmonary resuscitation are excessive delay in initiating the resuscitative efforts, improper management of assisted ventilation and circulation, and extensive myocardial damage. Especially important in contributing to the failure of resuscitation efforts is the detrimental effect of discontinuing cardiac compression during endotracheal tube insertion or placement of intravenous lines.

Complications arising from cardiopulmonary resuscitation do occur and may be potentially lethal. The most frequent are fractures of the rib and sternum, which may be associated with laceration of the liver, esophagus, spleen, or kidney. Hemopericardium and pneumothorax may be related to rib fracture or intracardiac administration of drugs.

If the airway is patent and appropriate ventilation and perfusion are provided through basic cardiopulmonary resuscitation, definitive therapy can be formulated, based on an accurate diagnosis.

VENTRICULAR FIBRILLATION. Ventricular fibrillation is the most common cause of cardiac arrest and is treated by electrical defibrillation with a direct current defibrillator. If a defibrillator is not available and the patient is pulseless, a single thump should be delivered to the immediate mid-sternum–precordial area; if successful, this maneuver may restore the patient's circulation and obviate the need for cardiopulmonary resuscitation. If the single thump is unsuccessful, no harm will have resulted, provided that resuscitation has not been delayed unduly. If a defibrillator is available, the electrode paddles are placed at the cardiac apex and at the base of the heart at the right upper sternal portal. If electrocardiographic monitoring is not immediately available, a single 400 watt-second shock should be delivered prior to cardiopulmonary resuscitation. An unmonitored attempt at defibrillation will not adversely affect the patient with asystole or heart block. If a single countershock is unsuccessful, no further defibrillabion should be attempted until electrocardiographic monitoring is available; basic cardiopulmonary resuscitation must be continued. If ventricular fibrillation or asystole is shown to be present, basic resuscitation should be continued while an intravenous infusion route is established. A peripheral vein should be used if possible; the femoral or jugular veins provide acceptable alternative routes if a peripheral vein cannot be easily cannulated. The insertion of a subclavian intravenous cannula can be extremely difficult in the presence of *uninterrupted* cardiopulmonary resuscitation. Drug therapy with sodium bicarbonate (1 mEq per kilogram administered as a bolus) and epinephrine (0.5 mg, i.e., 5 ml of a 1:10,000 solution) should be initiated after the intravenous route is established. These drugs should not be mixed together, because epinephrine may be inactivated by the alkaline bicarbonate solution. External cardiac compression must be continued following injection to circulate the drugs. The cardiac rhythm may than be reassessed, and, if ventricular fibrillation is still present or rapidly returns after a brief episode of sinus rhythm, further administration of sodium bicarbonate and perhaps lidocaine is indicated. If the ventricular fibrillation presents a fine fibrillatory electrocardiographic pattern, epinephrine (5 ml of 1:10,000 solution) should be administered intravenously to produce a course pattern prior to further attempts at defibrillation. Continued failure to defibrillate the patient demands a reassessment of the perfusion, oxygenation, and pharmacologic management of the patient. Hypoxemia and acidosis are frequently responsible for the presence of ventricular fibrillation refractory to electrical conversion.

If reassessment of the cardiac rhythm shows the return of normal sinus rhythm, a bolus of lidocaine (1 mg per kilogram) should be administered, followed by a continuous infusion of 1 to 4 mg per minute. It may be necessary to repeat the bolus administration at three- to five-minute intervals, but extreme caution should be used in the administration of doses exceeding 300 mg because of the possibility of drug toxicity. Lidocaine toxicity is especially likely to occur in the presence of acute reductions in cardiac output, and this should be kept in mind with respect to individualizing the dosage for each patient.

If normal sinus rhythm returns, the pulse is checked and basic resuscitation discontinued if appropriate. If bradycardia is present *and associated with hypotension*, atropine (0.5 mg) may be administered intravenously and repeated every five minutes up to a total dose of 2.0 mg.

The presence of asystole or electromechanical dissociation (electrical myocardial activity without palpable pulse) indicates the need for further pharmacologic intervention and perhaps the use of a pacemaker.

Epinephrine (5 ml of 1:10,000 solution) given *intravenously* should be administered for the presence of asystole or electromechanical dissociation. This drug should not be administered by intracardiac injection if an intravenous route is present. The hazards of intracardiac administration include interruption of cardiac compression and ventilation, coronary artery laceration, pneumothorax, and intramyocardial injection, which may produce intractable ventricular fibrillation. If there is a delay in establishing the intravenous route, epinephrine may be given by intracardiac injection in the same dose. Calcium chloride (5 ml of a 10 per cent solution) may be especially useful in the presence of electromechanical dissociation and also in the restoration of an electrical rhythm during asystole. Isoproterenol (1 to 20 μg per minute) may be useful in the management of profound cardiovascular collapse associated with asystole or electromechanical dissociation; however, it must be used cautiously because it may result in the production of serious dysrhythmias.

DRUG THERAPY. The most important pharmacologic maneuvers in cardiopulmonary resuscitation are the administration of oxygen to combat hypoxemia and sodium bicarbonate to treat acidosis. All drugs are preferably administered through an intravenous line, followed by one to two minutes of external cardiac compression to ensure circulation of the agent. There is no indication for the intracardiac injection of any pharmacologic agent during cardiopulmonary resuscitation, provided that an intravenous route is present.

Ineffective perfusion and ventilation result in the appearance of metabolic and respiratory acidosis within minutes of the onset of cardiopulmonary arrest. Effective resuscitation critically depends upon the proper maintenance of acid-base balance. After the initial injection of sodium bicarbonate (discussed above), further administration should be titrated on the basis of pH and arterial blood gas measurements determined every five to ten minutes during resuscitation. If laboratory facilities are not available, repeated doses of 1.0 mg per kilogram should be given every ten minutes until spontaneous circulation is restored.

If laboratory facilities are available, the dose of bicarbonate can be approximated as follows:

$$mEq\ bicarbonate = \frac{base\ deficit\ (mEq\ per\ liter) \times patient\ weight\ (kg)}{4}$$

The base deficit may be approximated as follows:

$$pH\ change\ of\ 0.15 = base\ change\ of\ 10\ mEq\ per\ liter\ per\ liter$$

The use of these two expressions allows one to approximate the amount of bicarbonate required from pH data alone. The respiratory component of acid-base balance can be assessed by correcting the measured pH appropriately for deviations of the P_{CO_2} from 40 mm Hg. Every 10 mm Hg change in P_{CO_2} is associated with a 0.08 unit change in pH. Using these guidelines, the measured pH can be corrected for the respiratory contribution; the corrected value can then be used to calculate the base deficit, which is then used in conjunction with the patient's weight to estimate the dose of bicarbonate. The full calculated dose of sodium bicarbonate should be administered during cardiopulmonary resuscitation. Correction of the acidemia will improve myocardial contractility and render the heart more sensitive to cardiovascular drugs; however, frank alkalemia is deleterious, because it sensitizes the myocardium to arrhythmias and results in a decreased release of oxygen because of the pH dependency of the oxyhemoglobin dissociation curve.

Vasopressor agents such as norepinephrine and epinephrine are frequently useful after the return of a regular cardiac rhythm to increase the peripheral vascular resistance, elevate central venous pressure, and improve coronary and cerebral blood flow. Their use should be limited to very brief time periods and discontinued as soon as the patient's status can be evaluated and adequate manipulations of the vascular volume and inotropic agents can be instituted to maintain cardiac output and peripheral perfusion. These powerful vasoconstrictor agents should not be needed for longer than a few minutes under most conditions.

PACEMAKERS. Persistent asystole or bradycardia resistant to therapy may require insertion of a pacemaker. Percutaneous insertion of a pacemaker into the left ventricle will usually provide sufficient myocardial contact to permit satisfactory pacing. Insertion of a transvenous pacemaker via the internal jugular vein will also usually provide for satisfactory pacing. Balloon-tipped flotation-directed catheters are difficult to place in emergency situations, because the blood flow is insufficient to provide a guiding force for the catheter. Electrical depolarization of the myocardium will be ineffective in the presence of acidemia and hypoxemia.

POSTARREST TREATMENT. After successful resuscitation, attention must be directed toward maintenance of the appropriate life support systems until the patient's primary disorder can be corrected. The maintenance of life support systems has been discussed in detail in Ch. 352.

Many patients experience recurrent cardiopulmonary arrest within minutes to hours of the initial episode. It is essential to provide continuous monitoring and evaluation of the patient during the first 24 to 48 hours following such an episode.

If central nervous system dysfunction persists following resuscitation, treatment should be administered to minimize adverse effects of the hypoxia-induced cerebral edema. Cerebral edema should be managed by (1) elevation of the head and chest, (2) mild hyperventilation (Pco_2 maintained between 25 and 35 mm Hg), (3) dexamethasone (6 mg every four hours), (4) diuretic administration (mannitol), and (5) mild hypothermia (temperature no lower than 32° C). If clinical absence of central nervous system function persists beyond 72 hours, an electroencephalogram should be obtained for further evaluation.

CONCLUSION. There is need for training in emergency cardiopulmonary resuscitation for all health professionals, especially physicians.

Committee on Emergency Cardiac Care, American Heart Association: Advanced Cardiac Life Support. Dallas, American Heart Association, 1975.

Committee on Emergency Medical Services, National Academy of Sciences, National Research Council: Standards for cardiopulmonary resuscitation and emergency cardiac care. J.A.M.A., 277:837, 1974.

Jude, J. R.: Classification of etiology, prevention and treatment of cardiac arrest. In Safar, P. (ed.): Advances in Cardiopulmonary Resuscitation. New York, Springer-Verlag, 1975.

PART XIV
CARDIOVASCULAR DISEASES

354. INTRODUCTION

354.1. PREVALENCE AND EPIDEMIOLOGY OF CARDIOVASCULAR DISEASE

Robert I. Levy

It is difficult to overemphasize the magnitude of the medical, social, and economic burden of cardiovascular diseases. An estimated 30 million Americans have some form of cardiovascular disease. Each year about 25,000 children are born with congenital heart disease, and of the 6000 of these children who die annually approximately half are less than one year of age. Over 100,000 children and 1.6 million adults have rheumatic heart disease, of whom almost 15,000 die each year. More than 4 million Americans have overt clinical signs of atherosclerosis, primarily of the coronary, cerebral, and peripheral blood vessels. Over 23 million adult Americans (15 per cent of the adult population of the United States) have hypertension as defined by a blood pressure of 160/95 or higher. Furthermore, the latter two major etiologic processes, atherosclerosis and hypertension, are interactive and result in an estimated 1.25 million heart attacks (of which 750,000 are first events) each year — a rate of 3400 per day or two per minute — and 500,000 strokes (of which 400,000 are first events) each year. In 1975, cardiovascular diseases accounted for 994,513 deaths or 52.5 per cent of all deaths in the United States, of which almost 650,000 were due to coronary artery disease (heart attack and sudden death) and 194,000 to cerebrovascular disease (stroke).

The age-adjusted death rate from rheumatic heart disease in the United States declined from 20.5 to 6.3 per 100,000 population between 1940 and 1970 and from 6.3 to 4.8 per 100,000 population between 1970 and 1975 (a 25.4 per cent decline). Although there are few reliable studies of the incidence of rheumatic fever, the data that are available indicate that a significant decrease in both severity and incidence of the disease has occurred in this country since 1940. It has been estimated that approximately 12,000 new cases of rheumatic fever occur at present in subjects between 5 and 14 years of age, based on a mean incidence rate of 11.0 per 100,000 population. Data on the prevalence of rheumatic heart disease are usually based on surveys of school children, with rates ranging between 0.5 and 3.7 per 1000.

The major risk factor for the development of rheumatic fever is the existence of a prior group A beta-hemolytic streptococcal throat infection; from 0.3 to 3.0 per cent of individuals so infected develop the disease. Environmental factors have been identified as significant additional risk factors, the most important being overcrowded living conditions. Other risk factors include low socioeconomic status, ethnic status, malnutrition, climate, and geography.

The onset of the downward trend in morbidity and mortality preceded the introduction of antibiotics, although the trend declined more precipitously following the introduction of effective treatment of streptococcal infections. Recurrent attacks of the disease have decreased dramatically following the institution of secondary prevention programs, in which effective drug therapy was utilized to prevent streptococcal infections in subjects who had previously experienced an episode of rheumatic fever. The additional impact of altered environmental factors, such as overcrowding, must be significant. Despite this decrease in morbidity and mortality, rheumatic fever and rheumatic heart disease continue to be the leading cause of death from heart disease in subjects between 5 and 24 years of age and second only to coronary heart disease as a reason for adults undergoing cardiovascular surgery.

The prevalence of coronary, cerebrovascular, and hypertensive diseases rises sharply with age. Although 8 per cent of adults under age 45 have hypertension, few have other manifestations of cardiovascular disease. Overt coronary heart disease is present in 6 per cent of males ages 45 to 64 and 11 per cent of males age 65 and over. For females the corresponding rates are 3 per cent and 7 per cent. Cerebrovascular disease, present in 1 per cent of persons ages 45 to 64, is present in 5 per cent age 65 and over. Hypertension is present in 44 per cent of women age 65 and over — compared to 37 per cent for men in that age group. In terms of mortality from these diseases, it is from coronary heart disease that mortality is highest. As in prevalence statistics, death rates rise steeply with age, especially after age 35, and for ages under 65 rates for coronary heart disease in men are more than double the rates in women. Death rates for cerebrovascular and hypertensive disease are large in number only after age 65.

Cardiovascular diseases rank second only to respiratory diseases in terms of days of bed disability. They rank first in terms of limitation of activity, Social Security disability, hospital discharges, and total hospital bed days (48 million per year). In terms of economic costs, cardiovascular diseases also rank first among all medical disorders. The estimated economic cost of cardiovascular diseases to the nation in 1976 totaled over $47 billion. Of this amount, $17 billion was related to the direct costs of illness and over $30 billion was due to indirect costs secondary to lost wages and productivity.

In America in 1900, infectious processes, such as pneumonia, influenza, and tuberculosis, reigned as our major health problems. As these disorders were brought under control, cardiovascular disease (especial-

TABLE 1. Age-Adjusted Death Rates* for Major Cardiovascular-Renal Diseases and All Other Causes of Death Combined—United States, Decades 1900–1970 and 1975†

Year	All Causes	All Causes Except Cardiovascular-Renal Diseases	Cardiovascular-Renal Disease				
			Total	Heart Disease	Cerebro-vascular	Renal	All Other
1900	1778.5	1356.5	422.0	167.3	134.4	97.0	23.3
1910	1578.8	1101.6	477.2	201.7	126.4	107.0	42.1
1920	1423.6	952.2	471.4	203.6	122.6	105.9	39.3
1930	1246.1	754.9	491.2	252.7	106.5	102.5	29.5
1940	1076.1	590.3	485.8	292.7	91.0	79.0	23.1
1950	841.5	401.4	440.1	307.6	88.8	14.5	29.2
1960	760.9	361.6	399.3	286.2	79.7	5.7	27.7
1970	714.3	364.5	349.8	253.6	66.3	3.5	26.4
1975	638.3	338.4	299.9	220.5	54.5	2.8	22.1

*Rate per 100,000 population, age-adjusted to the United States population, 1940.
†Source: Vital Statistics of the United States, National Center for Health Statistics.

TABLE 2. Age-Adjusted Death Rates* for Four Subgroups of Cardiovascular Disease—United States, 1940–1975†

Year	Coronary Heart Disease	Hypertensive Disease	Rheumatic Fever and Rheumatic Heart Disease	Congenital Heart Disease
1940	207.2	69.3	20.5	4.8
1945	208.2	59.7	17.1	4.9
1950	226.4	56.0	14.0	4.6
1955	226.0	41.2	11.2	4.3
1960	238.5	29.6	9.7	4.7
1965	237.7	22.4	7.5	4.3
1970‡	228.1	7.9	6.3	3.7
1975‡	196.1	5.1	4.8	3.1

*Rate per 100,000 population; age-adjusted to the United States population, 1940.
†Source: Vital Statistics of the United States, National Center for Health Statistics.
‡Rates since 1968 are not totally comparable with rates for previous years due to the change in the International Classification of Diseases.

TABLE 3. Recent Mortality from Cardiovascular Diseases—United States, 1970–1976*

Year	Total	Cardiovascular Diseases					Noncardiovascular Causes of Death
		Coronary Heart Disease	Stroke	Hypertension	Rheumatic Heart Disease	Other Cardiovascular Disease†	
				Numbers of Deaths			
1970	1,032,500	666,500	207,000	23,500	15,000	120,500	888,500
1971	1,041,500	674,000	209,000	22,000	14,500	122,000	886,000
1972	1,060,000	684,500	213,500	21,500	14,000	126,500	904,000
1973	1,062,000	684,000	214,000	20,000	13,500	130,000	911,000
1974	1,035,000	665,000	207,500	19,000	13,500	130,000	899,000
1975	994,500§	642,500	194,000	17,500	13,000	127,500	898,500
1976‡	996,500	647,000	188,500	16,500	13,000	131,500	907,500
				Death Rate Per 100,000 Population (age-adjusted)¶			
1970	350.0	228.1	66.3	7.9	6.3	41.4	364.3
1971	344.4	225.1	65.2	7.2	6.0	40.9	355.5
1972	343.7	223.9	65.0	6.8	5.7	42.3	358.1
1973	336.6	218.9	63.7	6.3	5.4	42.3	356.3
1974	320.1	207.7	59.9	5.7	5.1	41.7	346.1
1975	300.3	196.1	54.5	5.1	4.8	39.8	338.0
1976	298.3	195.1	52.8	4.9	5.1	40.4	336.1

*Source: Vital Statistics of the United States, National Center for Health Statistics.
†Includes congenital heart disease.
‡Provisional.
§Below 1,000,000 for the first time since 1964.
¶Adjusted by age to the United States population, 1940.

TABLE 4. Percentage of All Deaths Due to Cardiovascular Diseases* by Age—United States, 1962, 1975†

Age	1962	1975
Total	55.1	52.5
Under 25	7.6	7.4
25–44	27.7	20.1
45–64	50.2	44.2
65–74	61.3	54.9
Over 74	71.3	67.5

*Includes congenital heart disease.
†Source: Vital Statistics of the United States, National Center for Health Statistics.

ly that of the coronary arteries) became more prevalent and virulent, raising the specter in the late 1940's and 1950's of an "epidemic" of cardiovascular disease and accounting for 55.1 per cent of all deaths in 1962. Over the last 30 years, however, this tide has gradually turned; age-adjusted cardiovascular death rates have been declining slowly since 1950 and then more sharply since 1963. In total, since 1950 age-adjusted cardiovascular death rates have decreased by more than 31 per cent. Most significantly, the decline in coronary and cerebrovascular disease mortality rates has been even more precipitous since 1970 (stroke deaths down 18 per cent and coronary deaths down 14 per cent between 1970 and 1975) and has continued through 1977. This decline in cardiovascular mortality rates has been observed in both sexes and all age decades from ages 20 to 29 to 70+ and has been so sharp that, despite a growing and aging United States population, cardiovascular disease accounted for fewer than 1 million deaths in 1975 and again in 1976 for the first time in a decade. This trend is generally not paralleled in the rest of the world, however. Between 1969 and 1973 the mortality from cardiovascular disease increased sharply in Sweden, Denmark, Norway, England, Scotland, and Hungary, with lesser increases documented in other countries. In spite of the encouraging trends in the United States, cardiovascular disease remains a problem of staggering proportions, causing over 50 per cent of all deaths in 1976. The gaps in our knowledge and management of cardiovascular disease thus continue to pose a formidable challenge.

It is hard to attribute the ebb and flow in cardiovascular morbidity and mortality to specific events. Clearly, the two major etiologic processes damaging both the heart and the blood vessels are hypertension and atherosclerosis. Both processes are silent but incessant. We now know that hypertension may be present for long periods, as measured by simple blood pressure measurement, without producing signs or symptoms and, similarly, that atherosclerosis develops secretly in focal areas in blood vessels beginning in the first and second decades of life. This secret process may then proceed for two to six decades with no overt signs or symptoms until after two thirds of a vessel's lumen is occluded or the lesion breaks off or hemorrhage occurs. Symptoms appear suddenly in the form of heart attack, sudden death, angina, claudication, or stroke. It is because of their silent nature that these processes did not receive more attention earlier. Because of their ultimately devastating effects on the cardiovascular system, they are now the major subject of cardiovascular disease investigation. As basic researchers seek the cause(s) of arteri-

osclerosis and hypertension, as well as a better understanding of their basic pathophysiologic effects on the heart and blood vessels, cardiovascular physiologists have sought to develop better invasive (angiography) and noninvasive methods (e.g., echocardiography, nuclear imagery, x-ray densitometry) to diagnose abnormalities of the blood vessels, heart muscle, and heart valves long before signs or symptoms appear. During the past 30 years, cardiovascular epidemiologists have also made important contributions by detecting risk factor traits or habits in individuals to identify those who are at increased risk for specific cardiovascular diseases.

Much of the epidemiologic evidence regarding the role of certain personal characteristics ("risk factors") in the occurrence of coronary heart disease derives from several long-term prospective studies of fairly large population samples. The Framingham Heart Study, conducted by the National Heart, Lung, and Blood Institute, is a prototype study in which a general population sample of 5209 residents of the town of Framingham, Massachusetts, has been followed. At their first examination in 1948–1950, these men and women were 30 to 62 years old. Every two years they are reexamined to assess their medical status and to measure the characteristics to be described below. In 1977–1979 the fifteenth biennial cycle of examinations is being conducted, yielding 28 years of follow-up experience on this group. The Tecumseh Study followed a similar design, using all the residents of Tecumseh, Michigan, of whom 8624 participated in the initial examination in 1959. Three subsequent examinations have been completed.

Similar epidemiologic studies included studies in Albany, using male civil servants aged 39 to 54 years; in Chicago, using male employees of the Chicago Peoples Gas Company aged 40 to 59 years, and another using male employees of Western Electric Company aged 40 to 55 years; and in Evans County, Georgia, using a total community in which one third of the population was black. The Tecumseh, Framingham, and Evans County studies included women as well as men.

A long list of major and minor cardiovascular risk factors have now been enumerated by these studies. They include as major factors *age, male sex, hypertension, cigarette smoking, plasma LDL and HDL cholesterol,* and *blood glucose,* and as lesser factors *overweight, sedentary way of life, hardness of water, family history of heart disease before age 65, personality type,* and *stress.*

Prospective epidemiologic studies in other areas have tended to confirm the findings of the aforementioned studies. Most of the other studies have used populations with lower over-all rates of heart disease such as Japanese men in Japan, Hawaii, and California, Puerto Rican men, urban and rural men in Yugoslavia, and male civil servants in Israel. The essential features of each of these studies were (1) an effort to obtain a large representative sample of the population, (2) careful assessment of a variety of measurements prior to the onset of clinically overt coronary disease, and (3) complete ascertainment of all cardiac events occurring during the subsequent years of follow-up.

As a result of studies such as those mentioned above, there is little doubt of the predictive power of the major cardiovascular risk factors (see accompanying figure). Estimates based on the Framingham Heart Study and

	Low Risk	High Risk
Sys. BP	105	150
Chol	185	285
Smoke	No	Yes
Glu. Intol.	No	Yes

Probability of developing coronary heart disease (CHD) in eight years by age, sex, and risk category. (From Feinleib, M.: Am. J. Epidemiol., 104:457, 1976.)

national vital statistics indicate that two out of every three coronary events (myocardial infarction, coronary death, or coronary insufficiency) occur in high risk subjects. As detailed in the basic prevalence figures, older age and male sex both are associated with increasing cardiovascular disease. Females seem to have a 15- to 20-year protective buffer before cardiovascular events begin to manifest themselves increasingly in the seventh and eighth decades of life.

Cigarette smoking has clearly been shown to be an independent, potent risk factor for coronary, cerebral, and peripheral vascular disease. Sudden cardiac death, heart attack, angina, claudication, and stroke incidence and prevalence can be related to the number of cigarettes one smokes. The heavier the cigarette smoking history, the higher the risk. Both the nicotine and carbon monoxide inhaled with cigarette smoking have been incriminated as causative factors, but definite understanding of cause and effect still eludes us. Cigar and pipe smoking are not associated with this heightened degree of cardiovascular risk. Furthermore, in contrast to the apparently cumulative relationship of cigarette smoking to lung cancer, a series of prospective and retrospective studies now indicates that if one stops smoking cigarettes, over 90 per cent of the increased cardiovascular risk disappears within 18 months.

Hypertension is not only a major direct cause of cardiovascular disease but also appears to greatly accelerate the atherosclerotic process, especially that of the coronary and cerebral vessels. Although we define blood pressures above 160/95 as hypertension, cardiovascular risk begins to increase at considerably lower levels. For example, in a 35-year-old man with a normal blood pressure of 120/80, the risk of mortality over the

next 20 years would increase almost two-fold if his pressure were 142/90. That risk increases 2.2 times with a pressure of 142/95, whereas a level of 152/95 raises the 20-year mortality risk 2.5 times.

An elevation of plasma cholesterol levels has long been associated with increased cardiovascular risk. Through second and third generation epidemiologic studies, our focus has become more specific. It is now clear that the cholesterol-rich low density lipoproteins (LDL), the major carriers of cholesterol in our blood, are directly and independently associated with cardiovascular risk. It has been observed recently that another plasma carrier of cholesterol, high density lipoprotein (HDL) (usually accounting for less than 25 per cent of the total plasma cholesterol) is independently but *inversely* related to cardiovascular risk. The higher the level of HDL, the lower the cardiovascular event rate. Although the biochemical basis of the apparently protective effect of HDL is still speculative, it is clear that the measurement of the plasma levels of HDL and LDL gives more information than the determination of total plasma cholesterol alone. LDL levels are in part genetically determined, although environmental factors, especially diet, appear to have major effects on the plasma levels of this lipoprotein. Diets high in cholesterol and saturated fats increase plasma LDL levels, whereas diets low in cholesterol and saturated fat and/or high in unsaturated fat decrease LDL levels. Plasma levels of HDL are much more stable in any given individual and appear to be under stronger genetic control. Exercise and modest ingestion of alcohol do appear to raise HDL levels, however. From the time of adolescence, males have levels of HDL that are 10 to 20 per cent lower than those of females, whereas LDL levels are 10 per cent higher. This sex difference may be explained by the direct inverse effects of estrogen and testosterone on plasma HDL and LDL levels.

Blood glucose is another independent cardiovascular risk factor, with higher levels directly related to the extent of vascular disease. This relationship is true for both the juvenile and adult onset diabetic, and in both groups premature macrovascular disease is the major cause of death. Of special interest is the observation that the female diabetic appears to lose all the protective cardiovascular effect usually attributed to the female sex.

Overweight, although associated with increased cardiovascular risk, does not appear to be an independent risk factor for cardiovascular disease. When other associated variables are factored out through multivariate analysis, obesity loses all its predictive risk power. It appears, rather, to exert its cardiovascular effect through other risk factors. Thus weight gain raises blood pressure, LDL cholesterol, and blood glucose levels and increases sedentary behavior, whereas weight loss has the opposite effect, lowering each of these variables.

The association of sedentary behavior, family history of premature heart disease, water hardness, and personality type with vascular disease risk seems clear cut. However, whether they represent primary or independent risk factors still must be clarified.

Although the existence of the risk factors enumerated above and their predictive value in assessing cardiovascular risk in an individual or group is now firmly established, evidence that modification of risk factors will alter cardiovascular risk is incomplete. Prospective and retrospective analysis leaves little doubt that cessation of cigarette smoking will decrease cardiovascular risk; in fact, it has been suggested that if all Americans stopped smoking, cardiovascular deaths would be reduced by 150,000 per year. Little doubt exists of the beneficial effects on many body functions of weight control and regular modest exercise. Therefore, although it has not been firmly established that weight reduction or exercise conditioning will decrease cardiovascular events, these measures are usually recommended. In the case of high blood pressure, there is little doubt that treatment of moderate and severe hypertension will decrease stroke, renal failure, and heart failure; hence we treat hypertension aggressively. However, whether treatment of high blood pressure will prevent heart attack has not been definitely proved in man. Similarly, it remains unclear whether treatment of mildly elevated blood pressure or elevated blood pressure in the elderly is efficacious. Furthermore, the potential preventive benefit of salt restriction and weight control in those at risk for hypertension remains to be definitely proved.

There is little doubt that dietary modifications in cholesterol and saturated fats will reduce levels of LDL cholesterol, and nonhuman primate studies suggest that cholesterol lowering through diet will actually lead to regression of existent atherosclerosis. However, we await the results of ongoing clinical trials in man to prove conclusively the benefit of lowering LDL. Similarly, the beneficial effect of lowering blood sugar levels is still being debated.

Conclusive demonstration of the benefit of risk factor modification is of central importance to our current approach to cardiovascular disease. It is increasingly apparent that the first clinical signs of cardiovascular disease may also be the last, because one fourth of first heart attacks manifest as sudden death. Epidemiologic evidence shows clearly that after a coronary event, the state of the heart and the degree of damage are more crucial than any of the aforementioned risk factors. There is little doubt therefore that the primary prevention of cardiovascular disease is important. If it can be demonstrated that the basic process of arteriosclerosis and hypertension can be delayed or prevented, either through risk factor modification or by other means, we will clearly have a very cost-effective remedy.

The striking association of the current waning cardiovascular "epidemic" with clear evidence of changing American life styles and habits is very hopeful. Since 1966, the number of cigarette smokers has declined in men by 25 per cent, in women by 10 per cent, and in physicians of both sexes by 33 per cent. Between 1963 and 1975, there has been a 22.4 per cent decline in per capita tobacco consumption, a 19.2 per cent decline in the consumption of fluid milk and cream, a 31.9 per cent decline in butter consumption, a 12.6 per cent decline in egg consumption, a 56.7 per cent decline in the ingestion of animal fats and oils, and a 44.1 per cent increase in the ingestion of vegetable fats and oils. These concomitant changes have been associated with evidence of a 4 to 8 per cent decline in plasma LDL cholesterol levels in the United States in the past ten years. Americans are more conscious of the need for exercise. Since 1972, a government-sponsored National High Blood Pressure Education Program has increased by over 8 million the number of adult Americans aware of having hypertension, increased patient visits for hypertension by 50 per cent, and increased by an estimated 4 to 6 million the number of Americans under effective blood pressure control. These life style and habit changes coincide with a declining United States cardiovascular death rate (reinforced by the lack of evidence for a decline in either cardiovascular rates or risk factor status in Europe) and augur a potentially bright future for preventive cardiology.

Dawber, T. R.: Risk factors in young adults: The lessons from epidemiologic studies of cardiovascular disease — Framingham, Tecumseh, and Evans County. J. Am. College Health Assoc., 22:84, 1973.

Gordon, T., Garcia-Palmieri, M. R., Kagan, A., Kannel, W. B., and Schiffman, J.: Differences in coronary heart disease in Framingham, Honolulu and Puerto Rico. J. Chron. Dis., 27:329, 1974.

Kannel, W. B.: Prevention of cardiovascular disease. Cur. Prob. Cardiol., 1:1, July 1976.

National Center for Health Statistics, National Health Survey, 1972.

Stamler, J., and Epstein, F. H.: Coronary heart disease: Risk factors as guidelines to preventive action. Prev. Med., 1:27, 1972.

World Health Statistics Annual, 1972–1976. World Health Organization.

354.2. CIRCULATORY FUNCTION AND CONTROL

William W. Parmley

The normal cardiovascular system has a remarkable capacity to alter its performance. Such adjustments can increase cardiac output three to five times and heart rate two and a half times above basal values. The mechanisms responsible for this reserve capacity have been carefully studied over the years, resulting in a plethora of information about the circulatory system. The purpose of this chapter is not to detail these studies, but to provide a general overview of cardiovascular function. In particular, clinically important concepts will be stressed more than the details of data. Following a brief discussion of functional anatomy, the balance of the chapter will discuss the factors determining cardiac pump performance and overall circulatory function, and then discuss selected aspects of the response of the circulatory system to stress and heart failure.

FUNCTIONAL ANATOMY

The normal adult heart (weight approximately 300 grams) is about the size of a person's clenched fist — a gesture, interestingly enough, that the patient with angina pectoris frequently uses to describe the character of his cardiac discomfort. The atria are thin-walled shallow cups whose functional role is three-fold. When the atrioventricular (AV) valves are closed during ventricular systole, the atria serve a reservoir function by collecting blood from the systemic or pulmonary veins. In early diastole therefore there is rapid ventricular filling following opening of the AV valves. In mid-diastole, the AV valves remain open so that the atria serve as a conduit for the continuous flow of blood from the veins to the ventricles. Toward the end of diastole active atrial contraction ejects another increment of blood into the ventricle just prior to ventricular systole (about 20 per cent of stroke volume). The normal atria are thin walled, because they pump into the ventricles during diastole at low pressure.

The right ventricle is a thin-walled volume pump which has a low filling pressure (about 5 mm Hg) and ejects blood into the low pressure pulmonary artery (about 20 mm Hg). The right ventricle is formed by a concave free wall which opposes the convex septal wall, thus creating a crescent-shaped slit between them. Ejection of blood occurs by both shortening of the free wall and movement toward the interventricular septum, which compresses the chamber by a bellows action. This latter mechanism is extremely efficient in ejecting a large volume of blood with a minimum of muscle shortening, but can only function effectively at the low pressures normally found in the right-sided circulation.

The left ventricle is somewhat conical in shape, with its apex forming the apex of the heart. It can be considered as a thick-walled pressure pump whose medial wall is the thick interventricular septum. Ejection of blood from the left ventricle is primarily accomplished by a constriction of the muscular wall, although there is some shortening of the chamber.

The thickness of the ventricular wall is dependent on the relationship between wall stress, intraventricular pressure, and the radius of wall curvature as defined by the Laplace relation:

$$\sigma = \frac{PR}{2h}$$

(σ = wall stress [force/cross-sectional area], P = intraventricular pressure, R = radius of curvature of the wall, and h = wall thickness.) In general, wall stress is relatively constant throughout the heart. Thus the radius of curvature and wall thickness tend to be related. At the apex of the heart where the radius of curvature is short, the wall is thin. By contrast, the free wall of the left ventricle has a longer radius of curvature and a proportionally thicker wall.

Although emphasis is usually placed on a description of the systolic function of the heart, a greater appreciation of the importance of the diastolic properties of the heart has occurred over the past few years (Fig. 1). A thick hypertrophied ventricle with decreased compliance causes increased resistance to filling. This frequently leads to atrial dilatation and hypertrophy in order to maintain the atrial contribution to ventricular filling. The importance of this contribution is apparent in patients with severe hypertrophy due, for example, to aortic stenosis or idiopathic hypertrophic subaortic stenosis. Loss of an appropriately timed atrial contraction (as with atrial fibrillation) often results in marked exacerbation of left heart failure. In these patients during sinus rhythm, the left ventricular end-diastolic pressure is markedly elevated due to a large A wave, whereas mean diastolic pressure, which is reflected back through the pulmonary veins into the lungs, is maintained at a lower level. When atrial contribution and the A wave kick are lost, however, there is an increase in mean left atrial and pulmonary venous pressures in an attempt to maintain the same level of end-diastolic pressure and cardiac output. This frequently leads to disabling dyspnea.

Recent observations have also pointed out how the apparent compliance of the ventricles can be acutely altered by hemodynamic factors, such as raising and lowering arterial or right-sided pressures. Since the two ventricles are enclosed in a common pericardial sac,

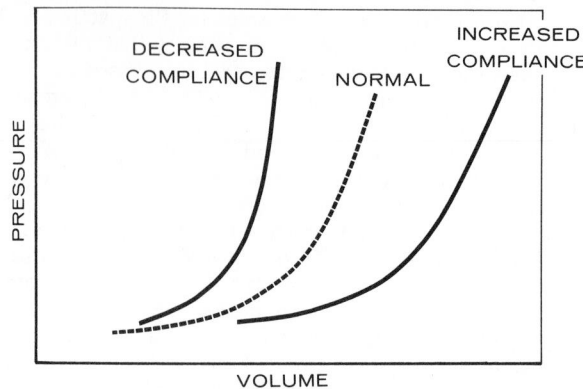

Figure 1. Representative passive pressure-volume relations of the left ventricle. The general exponential relationship between left ventricular diastolic pressure and volume is shown. At low pressures a small increase in pressure results in a large volume increment, whereas at higher pressures lesser volume increments occur with a rise in pressure. Chronic shifts in the passive pressure-volume relation can occur with various disease states. For example, with aortic stenosis and concentric hypertrophy, the left ventricular volume may be reduced at a given end-diastolic pressure (decreased compliance curve). On the other hand, with volume overload (e.g., mitral or aortic insufficiency) the curve may shift to the right with a larger volume at each end-diastolic pressure. In addition, recent evidence suggests that acute shifts in the left ventricular pressure volume relation may occur with changes in hemodynamics or ischemia. Vasodilator drugs which lower arterial pressure may produce a slight shift of the curve to the right (increased compliance).

which is quite stiff at high filling pressures, pressure or volume influences on one side of the ventricle can be transmitted to the other side of the heart. For example, administration of vasodilator drugs, such as nitroprusside or nitroglycerin, which reduce arterial and right-sided pressures in patients with heart failure, will tend to reduce left ventricular end-diastolic pressure at the same left ventricular end-diastolic volume. The presumed mechanism is a reduction in right ventricular volume (the more compliant chamber) and a reduction in the transpericardial pressure gradient, both of which result in an apparent increase in compliance of the left ventricle. Appreciation of the interaction of the right and left ventricles in a common intrapericardial space is important in any patient undergoing therapeutic maneuvers which rapidly alter right- and left-sided filling pressures.

CARDIAC PERFORMANCE

We will first consider the factors which alter the performance of the heart and then integrate these factors into the over-all function of the intact cardiovascular system. The four most important factors in determining the pump performance of the heart are preload, afterload, contractility, and heart rate.

Preload refers to the initial loading conditions of the heart. In isolated heart muscle, it is defined as the initial resting force stretching the muscle prior to contraction. In the intact heart, it is less easily defined. Estimates of preload include measurements of end-diastolic volume or end-diastolic pressure of the ventricle. In patients, it is often convenient to measure the filling pres-

INTERACTION OF PRELOAD (LVFP) AND AFTERLOAD ON STROKE VOLUME

Figure 2. Representative ventricular function curves following changes in afterload (impedance). Stroke volume is plotted as a function of left ventricular filling pressure (left atrial pressure). A vasodilator drug such as sodium nitroprusside, which decreases impedance, will shift the ventricular function curve up and to the left. Beginning at a high filling pressure, there will be a decrease in filling pressure and an increase in stroke volume (line A). Beginning at a low filling pressure, nitroprusside will also shift the patient to a new curve, but there may be a reduction in stroke volume (line B) because the patient moves down the ascending limb of the function curve. (From Chatterjee, K., and Parmley, W. W.: Prog. Cardiovasc. Dis., 29:305, 1977.)

sures (atrial pressures) of the ventricles as an index of preload. Within limits, as one increases the preload (end-diastolic pressure or volume of the heart), there is an increase in cardiac performance, manifested by an increase in the pressure developed or in the volume of blood ejected. This represents the ascending limb of the familiar Frank-Starling relationship (Fig. 2). The classic explanation of this phenomenon has been related on an ultrastructural basis to the degree of overlap of cross-bridges between the thick myosin filaments and the thin actin filaments of each sarcomere. Newer evidence suggests that initial muscle length also has an effect on the amount of calcium available for contraction (length-dependent activation).

This over-all relationship is often referred to as a ventricular function curve (Fig. 2). Some measure of cardiac performance, such as stroke volume or stroke work (stroke volume × arterial pressure), is plotted as a function of some measure of preload, such as atrial filling pressure or end-diastolic pressure. The concept of the ventricular function curve is important for several reasons. First of all, it allows for a comparison between subjective signs and symptoms and objective measurements. Thus as the level of left atrial pressure rises, the symptoms and signs of pulmonary congestion and edema appear. The ensuing dyspnea is the most common symptom associated with heart failure. The second major symptom complex in heart failure is fatigue due to reduced cardiac output. This is related to the vertical axis of the ventricular function curve, because cardiac output is the product of stroke volume and heart rate. This correlation between subjective symptoms and objective measurements is an important conceptual one in evaluating patients with cardiovascular disease.

An important application of preload alteration is exemplified by the therapy of patients with severe acute power failure. In such hypotensive patients, optimization of left ventricular filling pressure will maximize stroke volume or stroke work. The normal left atrial pressure is about 10 mm Hg. The optimal left atrial pressure in critically ill patients appears to be approximately 15 to 20 mm Hg. At higher pressures, there is no further improvement or, in some cases, an actual decline in cardiac performance, whereas the symptoms of pulmonary congestion will increase. In patients who are hypotensive with a very low left ventricular filling pressure, volume administration is appropriate therapy to raise the filling pressure up to 15 to 20 mm Hg. This therapy is often sufficient to reverse the hypotension and low cardiac output state. An appreciation of preload therefore is of great practical importance in the characterization and management of patients with heart failure.

An important distinction must be made between the right atrial pressure, which represents the filling pressure of the right ventricle, and the left atrial pressure, which is the filling pressure of the left ventricle. Each atrial pressure is related to the functional status of its respective ventricle. In manipulating the volume status of the patients, however, it is far preferable to measure left ventricular filling pressure, because the left ventricle has a more important role in determining arterial pressure and forward cardiac output.

The term *afterload* refers to the load against which the heart must contract. In isolated heart muscle studies, it can be carefully defined as the load resisting shortening as the muscle is stimulated. In the intact heart, it is loosely approximated as the arterial pressure or impedance against which the heart has to work. The effect that afterload has on performance is relatively straightforward. As one increases arterial pressure, the stroke volume will go down because the ventricle has greater difficulty in ejecting blood against a higher load. Conversely, if one can reduce systemic vascular resistance and arterial pressure with vasodilator drugs, one can increase forward stroke volume and cardiac output. One must avoid severe hypotension, however, which will compromise coronary blood flow and therefore reduce cardiac performance. The principle of afterload manipulation is one of the most important new concepts in cardiac therapy within the past several years. Vasodilator therapy for both acute and chronic heart failure is emerging as one of the most important adjuncts to more standard forms of therapy.

It should also be pointed out that there is a close relationship between changes in preload and afterload. Thus as the arterial pressure is increased, the ventricle has greater difficulty in ejecting blood and tends to retain more end-diastolic volume, thus increasing its preload. The opposite sequence of events occurs when the afterload is reduced. Therefore when one monitors arterial pressure and left atrial pressures simultaneously, particularly in patients with heart failure, the two frequently undergo directionally similar changes.

In terms of a ventricular function curve, vasodilator drugs which reduce both preload and afterload may affect function differently, depending on the initial level of left ventricular filling pressure. As illustrated in Figure 2, a vasodilator drug such as sodium nitroprusside, which reduces the resistance (impedance) to aortic ejec-

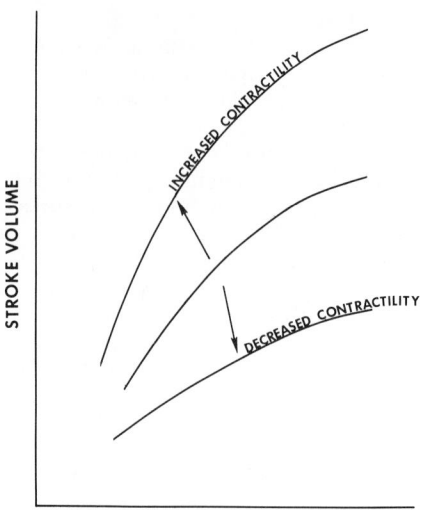

Figure 3. Representative shifts in ventricular function curves following changes in contractility. Left ventricular stroke volume is plotted as a function of left ventricular end-diastolic pressure. If the middle curve represents a baseline, drugs which increase contractility shift this curve upwards and to the left, while interventions which decrease contractility shift the curve down and to the right.

tion, will shift the ventricular function curve upward. Beginning at a high filling pressure (20 mm Hg), there will be both a reduction in filling pressure and an increase in stroke volume (line A, Fig. 2). At a normal filling pressure (10 mm Hg), however, the reduction in filling pressure will move the patient down the ascending limb of the ventricular function curve, and may reduce stroke volume (line B), even though the patient is on a higher curve.

Contractility refers to the vigor of contraction of heart muscle and is best defined in isolated heart muscle as an increased velocity of shortening at a given load. Drugs such as digitalis or the catecholamines increase contractility, whereas hypoxia, ischemia, acidosis, and certain antiarrhythmic drugs or beta-adrenergic blocking agents may reduce contractility. In terms of a ventricular function curve, drugs which increase contractility tend to increase stroke volume or stroke work at a given end-diastolic pressure. With a depression of contractility, the ventricular function curve shifts down and to the right with a reduction in stroke volume at a given left ventricular end-diastolic pressure (Fig. 3). Alterations of contractility may not always be beneficial. For example, in patients with coronary artery disease and limited coronary flow, a positive inotropic agent such as a catecholamine will markedly increase contractility and the need for myocardial oxygen. The partially obstructed coronary circulation may not be able to deliver the necessary increase in coronary blood flow. Under these circumstances, myocardial oxygen demand may outstrip supply and produce further ischemia and deleterious effects on the myocardium.

Heart rate is an obvious determinant of cardiac performance, and is one of the most important mechanisms available to the heart to increase cardiac output (cardiac output = stroke volume × heart rate). The magnitude of the heart rate may be an important indicator of the cardiovascular status of an individual patient. For example, in a patient with acute failure who

has a sinus tachycardia of 140, it is evident that the reduction in stroke volume (downward shift in ventricular function curve) is so great that a marked elevation of heart rate has resulted in an effort to maintain cardiac output at an acceptable level. Of course, stroke volume may be reduced because of low preload (hypovolemia) or because of severe failure with a high preload. It may be necessary to measure the preload to resolve this dilemma. Other factors which raise heart rate must also be considered, including fever, anemia, thyrotoxicosis, and others.

The effects of changes in heart rate on cardiac contractility are related to the interval strength relation. If one has a premature ventricular depolarization, that contraction is reduced, whereas the contraction following the pause is augmented (post-extrasystolic potentiation). This augmented contractility is apparently related to an increased availability of calcium during the subsequent beat. Although an increase in heart rate in and of itself causes a slight increase in the contractility of heart muscle, this is not a major effect when compared to interventions such as the catecholamines.

Although the importance of the ascending limb of the Frank-Starling curve is established, there is some question regarding the importance of a descending limb as preload is increased to extremely high levels. In general, studies in isolated heart muscle and whole heart preparations have shown that there is *not* a prominent descending limb. However, in patients with reduced cardiovascular reserve, it is possible to demonstrate a "descending limb" (reduction in cardiac performance and marked increase in preload) by provoking an exercise or afterload stress. For example, arterial pressure can be increased with drugs such as angiotensin or during isometric exercise, a potent mechanism for increasing arterial pressure. Under these circumstances, patients with reduced ventricular reserve may have a marked increase in left ventricular filling pressure and a decrease in stroke volume or stroke work index.

In response to an afterload stress, the heart utilizes the Frank-Starling mechanism and increased contractility to maintain compensation. When the limits of these compensatory factors are exceeded, a descending limb of the ventricular function curve will appear, predominantly related to the increase in afterload and not specifically to a descending limb of muscle function.

As quantitative indices of cardiac performance, cardiac pressures and volumes can be measured in the cardiac catheterization laboratory, or in patients in critical care units. For reference, normal pressures, volumes, cardiac output, and vascular resistance are listed in the accompanying table. Volume measurements are normalized for interpatient comparison by dividing by the body surface area (square meters). This latter value is obtained from a standard table, based on height and weight. One useful index of left ventricular function is the ejection fraction, which is defined as stroke volume per end-diastolic volume. A normal ejection fraction is 0.55 or greater. In severe heart failure, ejection fraction may be reduced to less than 0.20.

PERIPHERAL CIRCULATION

The arterial system represents the conduit system for delivery of blood to all parts of the body. Blood pressure remains relatively constant in this system until one

Pressures and Volumes in the Normal Heart

Pressures
  Left-sided
    1. Left atrial pressure (normal mean pressure $\leq$ 12 mm Hg)
    2. Left ventricular pressure
      a. Peak systolic pressure (wide normal range, usually 100–150 mm Hg in adults)
      b. Left ventricular end-diastolic pressure (normal $\leq$ 12 mm Hg)
    3. Aorta
      a. Systolic pressure (wide normal range, usually 100–150 mm Hg in adults)
      b. Diastolic pressure (wide normal range, usually 60–100 mm Hg in adults)
  Right-sided
    1. Right atrial pressure (normal mean pressure $\leq$ 6 mm Hg)
    2. Right ventricular pressure
      a. Peak systolic pressure (normal 15–30 mm Hg)
      b. Right ventricular end-diastolic pressure (normal $\leq$ 6 mm Hg)
    3. Pulmonary artery
      a. Systolic pressure (normal 15–30 mm Hg)
      b. Diastolic pressure (normal 4–12 mm Hg)
Volumes
  Left-sided (at rest)
    1. Left ventricular end-diastolic volume (normal 70–100 ml/m^2)
    2. Left ventricular end-systolic volume (normal 25–35 ml/m^2)
    3. Stroke volume (wide normal range, usually 40–70 ml/m^2)
    4. Ejection fraction (stroke volume divided by end-diastolic volume (normal 0.55–0.80)
Time-related measurements
    1. Heart rate (wide normal range, usually 60–100 beats/minute)
    2. Cardiac index (2.8–4.2 liters/minute/m^2)
Resistances
    1. Systemic vascular resistance (770–1500 dynes sec cm^{-5})
    2. Pulmonary vascular resistance (20–120 dynes sec cm^{-5})

reaches the level of the terminal arteries and arterioles. There is about an 80 per cent drop in pressure across this latter network, which is primarily responsible for regulating the peripheral vascular resistance. The subsequent cross-sectional area of the capillaries is enormous so that the relatively large velocity of blood in the aorta (40 to 50 cm per second) is reduced to about 0.07 cm per second in the capillaries.

The venous system is not only responsible for return of blood to the heart, but at one time contains about 75 to 80 per cent of the total blood volume. These larger thin-walled vessels therefore are extremely important in regulating shifts in blood volume between the central and peripheral circulation, depending on their relative constriction or dilatation. Various therapeutic agents can produce important volume shifts. For example, in patients with heart failure, a potent diuretic such as furosemide and sublingual nitroglycerin both produce prompt dilatation of systemic veins, resulting in a redistribution of blood away from the central circulation into the peripheral circulation. This is effective in reducing pulmonary venous and left atrial pressures, thus improving the symptoms of pulmonary congestion.

Cardiac output has an important regional distribution, which may be altered in various pathologic states. For example, the kidney accepts a high proportion of cardiac output (approximately 20 per cent), which is necessary for appropriate renal function. Abrupt reductions in cardiac output can compromise renal flow and markedly reduce urine output. Regional circulations, such as the cerebral and coronary circulations, have powerful autoregulatory capabilities so that blood flow can be maintained despite reductions in arterial pressure. Other regional circulations, including the skin and splanchnic bed, are often "sacrificed" during hypotension so that blood may be preferentially shunted to more vital organs.

The primary function of the heart is to pump nutrients and oxygen to all parts of the body. The amount of oxygen delivered to the body is the product of the cardiac output and the arterial-venous oxygen difference. During periods of reduced cardiac output, increased oxygen extraction by peripheral tissues can increase oxygen delivery to the body, although this is a minor compensatory mechanism. The kidneys receive a large share of cardiac output, but have relatively less demand for oxygen so that the arterial-venous oxygen difference across the kidneys is less than the rest of the body. At the other end of the spectrum, the heart itself tends to extract oxygen nearly maximally from the blood delivered through the coronary arteries. Thus an increase in oxygen delivery to the myocardium is accomplished primarily by an increase in coronary flow, rather than by an increase in oxygen extraction.

The capillary system has an enormous total surface area, which facilitates passage of substances into and out of the circulation. Lipid-soluble substances such as O_2 and CO_2 diffuse directly across the capillary walls. Blood flow in capillaries is not uniform and is dependent on the contractile state of the precapillary sphincters. True capillaries have no smooth muscle cells and therefore cannot actively change their cross-sectional area. Ions and small molecules move across the capillary walls at surprising rates, through pore sizes of 40 Å. The primary factor which restrains fluid from leaving the capillaries is the osmotic pressure of the plasma proteins, the most important of which is albumin. The Starling hypothesis states that hydrostatic forces are primarily responsible for fluid movement out of the capillaries, whereas oncotic pressure is primarily responsible for fluid movement back into capillaries. An example of imbalance between these forces is seen in pulmonary edema secondary to an increase in pulmonary venous pressure. Under these circumstances hydrostatic pressure exceeds oncotic pressure, resulting in movement of fluid into the interstitial space and eventually into the alveoli.

Figure 4. Schematic representation of the circulatory system. See text for details.

INTEGRATED CARDIOVASCULAR FUNCTION

A simplified overview of the circulatory system is diagrammatically illustrated in Figure 4. The four factors directly affecting cardiac muscle performance have already been discussed in relation to left ventricular performance. Similar factors would apply to right ventricular performance and the pulmonary circulation, although they are not separately shown in Figure 4. The discussion to follow will summarize information related to these and other major factors listed in the diagram.

HEART RATE. The heart rate is determined by the frequency of the sinoatrial node impulses, which are related to the rate of depolarization of phase four of their action potential. Heart rate is also markedly affected by the autonomic nervous system. Branches of the sympathetic nerves increase heart rate via norepinephrine release, whereas branches of the vagus nerve decrease heart rate by release of acetylcholine. It appears that the parasympathetic system is the dominant factor in the normal control of heart rate. In individuals who have undergone exercise conditioning and have slow resting heart rates, the initial increase in heart rate during exercise is mediated by a gradual reduction in vagal tone. Only at higher levels of exercise are the sympathetic nerves active in increasing heart rate. On the other hand, in individuals who are not physically conditioned, the sympathetic influence is utilized much sooner in increasing heart rate. Emotional factors have an important influence on heart rate, as is evident during anxiety, fear, or anger. An increase in heart rate also occurs in anticipation of physical exertion before the exercise has been initiated.

Stretch receptors in both the carotid body and aortic arch exert important effects on heart rate. A change in arterial blood pressure alters the frequency of impulses from the baroreceptors to the central nervous system. In general, a drop in arterial pressure induces an acceleration of the heart, whereas an increase in arterial pressure tends to slow the heart. Similarly, externally applied digital pressure on a sensitive carotid body can promptly reduce heart rate. There are a number of other reflex effects mediated through the vagus nerve which may slow heart rate. These include stimulation of the respiratory tract as with intubation, nausea and vomiting, or painful stimuli of various kinds. On the other hand, an increase in heart rate accompanies any activity in which there is an increase in sympathetic tone or in circulating catecholamines.

CARDIAC OUTPUT AND VENOUS RETURN. In general, the cardiac output is normally determined by the peripheral needs of the body. Thus the heart is a relatively passive organ in the circulatory system. It merely pumps out all the blood that is returned to it, and cardiac output is determined by the venous return to the heart.

Changes in venous return and cardiac output are largely produced by the altered capacity of the peripheral vascular bed. Either an augmentation of blood volume or a reduction of venous capacitance will tend to augment venous return and thus raise cardiac output.

Any venoconstriction will improve cardiac filling by slightly elevating the pressure gradient for venous return, thereby displacing blood from the peripheral circulation toward the cardiopulmonary circulation. Since only about 20 per cent of the blood volume is in the arterial system, it is clear that there can be little or no displacement of blood by constriction of arteries or arterioles.

If one alters heart rate substantially under normal resting conditions, there is usually no change in cardiac output. As the heart rate goes up (as for example by artificial pacing), the stroke volume goes down in a reciprocal manner, and cardiac output remains constant. This further emphasizes the importance of peripheral factors in determining the normal cardiac output. The heart becomes the limiting factor in regulating cardiac output only when it begins to fail. When the diseased heart is unable to pump out all the blood that has returned to it and is unable to supply blood sufficient for the metabolic needs of the body, then a state of heart failure can be said to exist. Under these circumstances, the changes in cardiac output are extremely dependent on myocardial function, which then becomes the limiting factor. Under normal circumstances, however, the heart basically responds to the increased needs of the body and supplies the blood required by the organism at that particular time. Variations in venous return as produced by alteration in posture, activity, or intrathoracic pressure transiently influence cardiac output considerably. When one assumes the upright posture, gravitational forces tend to pool blood in the dependent parts of the body, which may transiently reduce venous return, central blood volume, and diastolic volumes of the heart. The normal changes in intrathoracic pressure which occur with breathing also influence the return of blood to the heart. During inspiration, the negative intrathoracic pressure enhances cardiac filling and stroke volume, whereas the reverse occurs during expiration. Changes in intrapericardial pressure may also markedly affect venous return to the heart in pathologic states. Pericardial effusion with tamponade, restrictive pericarditis, or endocardial fibrosis all markedly limit venous return and thereby limit forward cardiac output.

The most important factor in determining venous return and cardiac output is a change in peripheral metabolic needs such as might occur with exercise, fever, or thyrotoxicosis. The most common example of this increased need occurs during exercise in which the arterioles of the exercising muscle are dilated, resulting in a marked increase of blood flow to the exercising muscles. As catecholamine influence increases during exercise, there is also a constriction of the venous bed which markedly enhances the return of blood to the heart. Thus any activities associated with sympathetic stimulation would be expected to constrict the venous bed and augment venous return. Although elevation of venous pressure has some role in returning peripheral blood to the heart, the pressure difference between small veins and right atrium is too small to be an important factor. Furthermore, the venous bed is quite compliant so that even marked venoconstriction or venodilatation may result in only small changes of venous pressure relative to arteriolar pressure. Even though the pressure changes that occur may be relatively small, the displacement of volume and change in venous return may be quite substantial. Exercising leg muscles which compress veins with a one-way valve system are also quite important in returning venous blood to the heart during exercise.

ARTERIAL PRESSURE. In order for an individual to carry out a wide range of activities with a reasonably constant arterial pressure, it is clear that a stabilizing and regulatory system of some magnitude must exist. In this regard it is useful to consider the relation between blood pressure, cardiac output, and systemic vascular resistance. The formula relating them states that blood pressure = cardiac output × systemic vascular resistance. This equation assumes that central venous or right atrial pressure is small. Although a marked increase in cardiac output can lead to some elevation of blood pressure, the principal factor which regulates blood pressure is the peripheral vascular resistance, as primarily influenced by reflex neurogenic control.

Both extrinsic and intrinsic mechanisms influence systemic vascular resistance. Most important among the extrinsic mechanisms are neurogenic stimuli, although circulating hormones, including catecholamines and prostaglandins, have some minor role. The intrinsic mechanism for altering active tension of smooth muscle in arterioles has been termed autoregulation. Both the kidney and the heart have extraordinary abilities to autoregulate their arterioles and thus maintain blood flow at a needed level over a fairly wide range of perfusion pressures. This autoregulation is produced by two opposing mechanisms. Stretching of the vascular tissues increases the spontaneous activity of the smooth muscle and thus initiates progressive vasoconstriction. On the other hand, accumulation of tissue metabolites exerts a local vasodilator influence so that the opposing effects of pressure-induced vasoconstriction and metabolite-induced vasodilation tend to maintain flow at a level appropriate to the needs of the tissue. It is also possible that a decrease in oxygen in and of itself may be responsible for vasodilation. One clinically important vascular bed, however, that responds to hypoxia with vasoconstriction is the pulmonary bed, where pulmonary hypertension and pulmonary edema may occur at high altitudes with reduced oxygen content.

Although there are several pressure-sensitive receptors, the best studied baroreceptor involved in blood pressure control is the carotid body, which is located at the junction of the common carotid artery with its internal and external branches. Pressure-sensitive nerve endings in the wall of the receptor alter their discharge rate according to the pressure that is applied. At extremely high pressures the discharge rate is increased, whereas at low pressures the discharge rate from the carotid body is reduced. These impulses pass through the cardiovascular regulatory centers in the medulla, which then alter the relative magnitude of vagal and sympathetic tone. For example, as arterial pressure is increased, the impulses from the carotid body to the cardioregulatory center are also increased. These (1) stimulate the motor nucleus via the vagus to slow heart rate, and (2) inhibit the cardioaccelerator center, which reduces sympathetic tone and peripheral vascular resistance. This latter effect returns blood pressure toward the previous level. Alterations in the sympathetic vasoconstrictor outflow appear to be the most important mechanism for altering or producing changes in peripheral vascular resistance.

Chemoreceptors lying near the carotid bifurcation and in the aortic arch also respond to changes in pH, Pco_2 and Po_2. Reduced oxygen, increased CO_2, or lowered pH stimulates the chemoreceptors and leads to an elevation of systemic arterial pressure. A marked reduction in arterial pressure can also make the brainstem ischemic and result in severe peripheral vasoconstriction mediated through the sympathetic nerves. This is presumably an attempt to raise arterial pressure up to levels that would relieve the central nervous system ischemia. In general, these latter mechanisms are operative only under extreme conditions and probably are not involved in the normal regulation of arterial pressure.

There is considerable fluctuation in blood pressure around the clock, as influenced by all the factors of everyday life, including posture, emotion, exercise, stress, and sleep. For example, exercise generally causes an increase in both systolic and diastolic pressure which persists for some time after the termination of exercise. Sleep, on the other hand, usually results in a reduction in blood pressure, although intense dreaming may produce an elevation of both heart rate and blood pressure.

CARDIOVASCULAR RESPONSE TO STRESS. A major principle related to the evaluation of the cardiovascular system is the importance of its response to an imposed stress. Under certain circumstances, resting function may be normal, whereas the response to an imposed stress may be grossly abnormal, thus detecting the individual with reduced cardiovascular reserve. This principle is implicit in history taking when one inquires about shortness of breath, fatigue, chest pain, or other symptoms provoked by exercise and other activities.

The cardiac response to exercise involves the interrelated effect of increased heart rate, catecholamine stimulation, and the utilization of the Frank-Starling mechanism. A treadmill exercise test or other specialized tests are useful in quantitating cardiovascular reserve. Two different stresses which have been used are isotonic and isometric exercise, which represent the two major types of exercise conditioning. Isometric exercise implies little change in the length of exercising skeletal muscles. This would occur during weight lifting or any exertion in which there is little movement of muscles. The usual response to isometric exercise is some degree of peripheral vasoconstriction with an increase in arterial pressure. There is an increase in sympathetic outflow which increases the contractility of the heart and may result in a slight increase in cardiac output. There is also an increase in heart rate in response to the increased sympathetic tone. In patients with normal cardiovascular reserve, the ventricular function curve therefore shifts generally upward with little change in pulmonary capillary wedge pressure (Fig. 5). Patients with poor ventricular reserve, however, may

have an adverse response to the increased afterload produced by vasoconstriction. This is characterized by a substantial reduction in stroke volume or stroke work index, and a marked rise in left ventricular filling pressure (Fig. 5). The response to isometric exercise therefore can be useful in quantitating the cardiovascular reserve of individual patients.

Isotonic exercise implies considerable muscle movement against a constant but low load. This is characteristic of walking, jogging, or running. Those who engage regularly in isotonic exercise programs will "train" their cardiovascular system. This results in a lower resting heart rate with a far greater capacity to increase cardiac output during subsequent exercise. With isotonic exercise, there is a marked reduction in systemic vascular resistance, primarily in the exercising muscles. This improves forward flow and markedly increases cardiac output.

The normal distribution of cardiac output at rest is indicated in Figure 4. With exercise, there is a substantial increase in relative and absolute blood flow to the skeletal muscles and skin. There is also an increase in flow through the coronary circulation, but little absolute change in flow to the splanchnic, cerebral, or renal beds.

With the onset of heart failure and a reduced resting cardiac output, there is a reduction in the percentage flow to the renal bed and skin. Exercise during heart failure produces a marked reduction in relative flow to the renal and splanchnic beds, with a greater proportion of flow going to exercising muscles. The absolute increase of flow to skeletal muscle, however, is far less than that found in a normal person during exercise.

Initially, it was assumed that changes in preload (Frank-Starling mechanism) were responsible for the increased cardiac output during exercise. It is apparent, however, that most of the changes in cardiac output are mediated by an increase in heart rate. The adrenergic nervous system increases both heart rate and contractility, and leads to peripheral vasodilation. The tachycardia which occurs due to the increase in sympathetic tone tends to reduce the cardiac dimensions, and thus to counteract the changes which might occur if the heart were allowed to dilate via the Frank-Starling mechanism. During light or initial exercise, there may be a slight reduction in end-diastolic volume. Because of the increase in contractility of the heart, however, stroke volume tends to remain relatively constant, and the increase in cardiac output is produced primarily by the increase in heart rate. At more profound levels there may be a slight increase in heart size as the Frank-Starling mechanism is utilized.

BLOOD VOLUME. The magnitude of blood volume is another important factor affecting cardiovascular function. Some of the factors involved in the maintenance of extracellular fluid and blood volume are listed on the right-hand side of Figure 4.

An increase in blood volume as might occur by an increased intake of salt and water would increase cardiac output. This, in turn, would tend to increase arterial pressure and renal perfusion and thus increase urine output, which would decrease blood volume back toward normal. Atrial receptors sensitive to dilatation are also responsible for vasodilating reflexes to the kidneys, and reflexes to the central nervous system to diminish the secretion of ADH. Both these factors would tend to

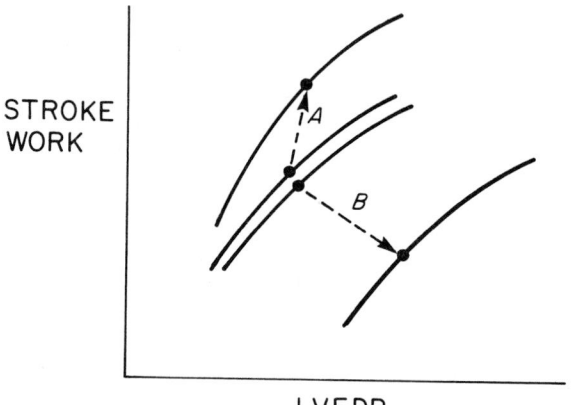

Figure 5. Altered ventricular function due to an elevation of arterial pressure produced by handgrip isometric exercise. A normal integrated response (patient A) shows an increase in stroke work with little change in left ventricular end-diastolic pressure (LVEDP). In this case, the increased contractile reserve has overcome the effects of the increased afterload (aortic pressure). The response of patient B indicates a substantial reduction in cardiovascular reserve. Under these circumstances, the marked increase in afterload has reduced the cardiovascular performance and produced a large rise in end-diastolic pressure.

increase the output of urine. These volume receptors, however, appear to have only transient effects and are not operative during heart failure with high atrial pressures.

Loss of fluid volume occurs primarily through the kidneys. Sweating, respiratory, and gastrointestinal losses are usually less important, except during extreme conditions. Since approximately 20 per cent of the resting cardiac output passes through the kidneys, they provide an ideal location for regulating salt and water balance. Since this subject is discussed in detail elsewhere, only some of the pertinent factors will be mentioned here.

Reduction in renal perfusion (reduced pressure and flow) is sensed by the juxtaglomerular apparatus, which releases renin. Other factors, such as ischemia and sodium depletion, have also been suggested as stimuli that affect renin release. Over-all, the phrase "effective blood volume" is a useful concept to keep in mind. Thus, decreased effective blood volume results in increased renin release, whereas increased effective blood volume turns off the stimulus for renin release. This concept forms the basis for alterations in sodium intake and volume as provocative tests for altering renin levels. Renin promotes the formation of angiotensin I from its precursor in the bloodstream. Angiotensin I is then converted to angiotensin II. Although angiotensin II is a powerful vasoconstrictor substance, this may not be its most important effect on blood pressure. Small subpressor doses of angiotensin II may increase aldosterone secretion, which may be one of its most important roles in regulating blood pressure. Angiotensin is also a potent stimulus for catecholamine release via the central nervous system vasomotor center and from the adrenal medulla.

Aldosterone promotes retention of salt and water. Under normal circumstances, salt and water intake are carefully balanced by their excretion. With congestive heart failure, there is an increased retention of salt and water which leads to edema formation and increased blood volume. There are usually increased aldosterone levels in severe heart failure secondary to reduced renal perfusion, and probably also due to decreased metabolism of aldosterone in the liver. It should be recalled that splanchnic flow is often reduced in heart failure, particularly during exercise.

In some patients with severe heart failure, free water excretion may also be severely impaired, and patients may be hyponatremic despite excess body sodium. Under such circumstances, restriction of fluid intake may be necessary to reduce fluid accumulation and reverse the hyponatremia. The potent diuretics available today are usually extremely effective in reversing the excess salt and water retention associated with heart failure. In some cases, excessive diuresis can lead to relative volume depletion and hypovolemia. Although uncommon, it is important to recognize this syndrome, because the associated hypotension and low cardiac output are effectively treated by liberalization of salt and water intake.

CIRCULATORY FAILURE. Heart failure is due to a number of causes, including mechanical or valvular defects, failure of the myocardium (cardiomyopathy), or loss of myocardium (myocardial infarction). In general, as myocardial failure occurs, there is reduction in heart muscle contractility, and the heart becomes the limiting factor in maintaining an appropriate level of cardiac output. In terms of the factors we have discussed, several characteristic alterations occur. First of all, cardiac output is decreased, and the preload of the heart is generally increased due to the reduced ability of the heart to eject blood (reduced ejection fraction) and to an increase in circulating blood volume. This may lead to elevated filling pressures on *both* the right and left sides of the heart. Second, there is evidence that the reduction in cardiac output which accompanies heart failure leads to a reflex increase in peripheral vascular resistance in an attempt to maintain arterial blood pressure. This increase in peripheral vascular resistance increases the resistance to ejection and may therefore further reduce cardiac output, resulting in a vicious cycle. The presumed existence of this cycle is supported by the fact that arteriolar dilating drugs such as hydralazine are extremely effective in increasing forward cardiac output in patients with severe heart failure, with no essential change in arterial pressure, heart rate, or pulmonary capillary wedge pressure. This suggests that systemic vascular resistance may be inappropriately high in heart failure for the level of cardiac output required. It should also be noted that the baroreceptor reflex mechanisms are markedly blunted in congestive heart failure. Thus interventions which reduce arterial pressure do not produce the same reflex increase in heart rate as in the normal individual.

In heart failure, there is a generally heightened sympathetic tone to the peripheral vasculature and to the myocardium, in an attempt to maintain cardiovascular compensation. This increased sympathetic tone causes more venoconstriction than in the normal individual, presumably in an attempt to maintain venous return and cardiac output. Heart rate may also be chronically elevated in heart failure in an attempt to maintain cardiac output. Arterial pressure often tends to be somewhat lower in heart failure as the ventricle loses the capacity to generate a normal or high blood pressure. In patients with hypertensive heart failure, however, blood pressure may remain at elevated levels for some time.

A consideration of the aforementioned factors suggests a rationale for the usual interventions employed in the treatment of chronic heart failure. Thus salt restriction and diuretics tend to reduce intravascular volume and therefore reduce preload below the level responsible for dyspnea. Digitalis stimulates the failing myocardium to increase its contractile state and thus improves the ability of the heart to eject blood. An inappropriately high systemic vascular resistance can be treated with arteriolar dilators to reduce the resistance to ejection and thus increase forward cardiac output. Venodilators, such as nitroglycerin, which predominantly dilate veins can redistribute blood away from the central circulation and also reduce pulmonary capillary wedge pressure.

In general, one does not attempt to control the sinus heart rate during heart failure, as this is the result of cardiac decompensation rather than a cause which has to be corrected. Of the four factors which affect cardiac performance therefore, therapy can be directed toward a correction of three of them (preload, afterload, and contractile state), and improved compensation will be reflected by a reduction in an elevated heart rate.

In summary, the cardiovascular system is a complex,

carefully regulated system which has extraordinary capabilities for altering its performance over wide ranges in response to the needs of the body. Usually the cardiac output is determined by the peripheral needs of the body as regulated by changes in venous return. Only when the heart is unable to meet these peripheral needs does a state of "heart failure" occur. At this point, the four factors affecting cardiac muscle performance become important considerations, and their regulation forms the basis of most of our therapeutic interventions in chronic heart failure.

Braunwald, E.: Control of cardiac performance. In Berne, R. (ed): Handbook on Circulation. Baltimore, Waverly Press, 1978, in press.

Chatterjee, K., and Parmley, W. W.: The role of vasodilator therapy in heart failure. Prog. Cardiovasc. Dis., 19:301, 1977.

Crexells, C., Chatterjee, K., Forrester, J. S., Dikshit, K., and Swan, H. J. C.: Optimal left heart filling pressure in acute myocardial infarction. N. Engl. J. Med., 289:1263, 1973.

Guyton, A. C.: Circulatory Physiology: Cardiac Output and Its Regulation. Philadelphia, W. B. Saunders Company, 1963.

Kivowitz, C., Parmley, W. W., Donoso, R., Marcus, H., Ganz, W., and Swan, H. J. C.: Effects of isometric exercise on cardiac performance: The grip test. Circulation, 44:994, 1971.

Parmley, W. W., and Talbot, L.: Heart as a pump. In Berne, R. (ed.): Handbook of Circulation. Baltimore, Waverly Press, 1978, in press.

Parmley, W. W., Tyberg, J. V., and Glantz, S. A.: Cardiac dynamics. Ann. Rev. Physiol., 39:277, 1977.

Rushmer, R. F.: Structure and Function of the Cardiovascular System. Philadelphia, W. B. Saunders Company, 1976, Chapters 3-7.

354.3. APPROACH TO THE PATIENT WITH CARDIOVASCULAR DISEASE

Andrew G. Wallace

This chapter describes an approach to the collection of cardiovascular data, the principles behind certain laboratory tests used to obtain data, and strategies about data acquisition. The objective is to complement the following chapters, which emphasize the data in specific conditions and their use in management decisions.

A textbook of medicine is customarily organized by system. Diseases are presented for each system according to diagnostic categories, and for each category topics such as etiology, pathophysiology, symptoms, physical signs, laboratory data, and treatment are discussed. This approach provides the reader with an integrated picture of diseases that affect the system. The merits of the approach are numerous and outweigh shortcomings; however, there are shortcomings. One is that patients usually do not present to the doctor with an established diagnosis. Another is that textbooks frequently describe a composite of the manifestations of a disease; often patients fail to match this description, either because the description conveys inadequately the continuum of symptoms and signs produced by variable amounts of disease or because the evolution of symptoms and signs over time receives less than optimal attention. Establishing whether or not cardiovascular disease is present is the first objective of a complete evaluation. When disease is present, the diagnosis includes not only a definition of the structural abnormality it produces, but also its etiology and severity. The approach to the patient is at least as important as a knowledge of the clinical and laboratory characteristics which are expected in any given disease.

In an effort to exclude cardiovascular disease or to define more precisely structural changes and severity of

diseases that are evident from clinical examination, the physician relies on laboratory methods. There are many laboratory methods available which give information about cardiovascular structure and function. Each method has particular conditions for which it is best suited, each has a predictable sensitivity and specificity with respect to particular questions, and among various methods there is an element of redundancy so that essentially the same information can be obtained in more than one way. Laboratory studies vary in cost and risk to the patient. They may give false or misleading information about a condition, especially if it is interpreted out of context with clinical data or other laboratory studies. The optimal approach to the patient requires a knowledge of changes in laboratory results produced by a disease, and also a strategy regarding which test and what sequence of studies will help in making the diagnosis and appropriately directing management of the patient.

Making a diagnosis is an important step in defining a clinical problem, but the diagnosis is not an end in itself. Patients within a given diagnostic category typically do not come to common end points within a predictable time. This is especially true in common chronic cardiovascular diagnoses such as hypertension, angina pectoris, and mitral stenosis. Prognosis is important to the patient because he or she wants to know what the future holds. Prognosis is important to the doctor because he or she needs to prescribe therapy and to select a therapeutic program. The number of descriptors which enable a physician to predict outcomes accurately is generally greater than the number needed to make a diagnosis. Large numbers of patients within a diagnostic category are needed to define which descriptors discriminate against certain outcomes. Finally, estimating prognosis is essentially an exercise in the application of probability statistics. The optimal approach to management decisions involves accurate collection of data which contribute to a definition of outcomes, the availability of information on many patients similar to the one being evaluated, and valid systems for assessing the impact of management choices.

COMPONENTS OF THE CARDIOVASCULAR DATA BASE

There are five components of the cardiovascular data base: the history, physical examination, electrocardiogram, chest x-rays, and laboratory studies. Patients with heart disease may or may not have symptoms, and they may be referred by one physician to another because of an abnormality or a suspected abnormality in any of the components of the data base. In practice, therefore, the starting point may be anywhere in this scheme. The sequence of acquiring data is less important than a thorough approach to each component. Indeed, it is instructive and useful to start purposefully with a different component of the scheme on different occasions, because it increases the likelihood of a thorough approach and skillful interpretation of each component.

THE HISTORY. The cardinal symptoms of cardiovascular disease include chest pain, shortness of breath, hemoptysis, palpitations, swelling, faintness or syncope, and cyanosis. Chest pain is usually characterized by its location, quality, severity, duration, radiation, and factors which cause, aggravate, or alleviate the symptoms.

These features are sought in the history in an effort to distinguish between the common causes of chest pain: ischemic heart disease, pericardial disease, pulmonary infarction, aortic aneurysm, chest wall pain, and pain related to gastrointestinal disease. Shortness of breath may occur at rest, only with exertion, or only in certain positions. The history is designed to help distinguish between shortness of breath related to heart failure, pulmonary emboli, intrinsic lung disease, and anxiety. Hemoptysis is the production of bloody sputum during coughing. The quantity of blood, its color, and how it is mixed within the sputum (i.e., streaks, clumps, evenly mixed, or pure blood) all are important in distinguishing bronchitis, pulmonary infarction, pulmonary edema, and hemorrhage from a ruptured bronchial vein such as in mitral stenosis. Palpitation is an awareness of the heart beating in the chest. This sensation is not unusual in normal subjects when lying in bed or after vigorous exercise. On the other hand, when the sensation has an abrupt onset and termination, or is described as irregular or a skipping sensation, it usually signifies an arrhythmia. Swelling is edema in any part of the body. Edema implies retention of salt and water and is a common manifestation of heart failure. Local factors may cause or contribute to the site of edema formation. For example, edema of only one leg suggests venous disease. Dizziness or syncope may be a consequence of one of several mechanisms: arrhythmias, obstruction to blood flow, an orthostatic drop in blood pressure, loss of blood volume, or drugs. The history is particularly important in syncope, because abnormal signs are frequently absent. The relation to preceding incidents, associated symptoms such as pain and palpitations, and a history of blood loss or drug use are important to elicit. Other important causes of syncope include cerebrovascular disease, seizures, and hyperventilation.

To obtain a good cardiovascular history, remember these two principles: First, let the patient tell the story. Patients will frequently include information that would not come forth in response to a series of directed questions. Gestures used by the patient to describe symptoms and the situations in which they appear are often significant in subsequent management decisions. Second, after hearing the patient's story, ask direct questions to fill in any missing information and to determine the presence or absence of the cardinal symptoms of cardiovascular disease. Pursue each positive response in appropriate detail. Establish the chronology of the history, the severity of present symptoms, and whether the course is stable, progressive, or cyclic. Whenever possible, use the patient's words, not your own.

THE PHYSICAL EXAMINATION. There are five parts to the cardiovascular physical examination: physical appearance, venous pressure and pulse, arterial pressure and pulse, precordial movements, and auscultation.

Physical Appearance. The physical appearance of a patient is important for two reasons: it may give clues to a systemic disease that also affects the heart, and it may provide data relevant to the nature and severity of heart disease. Marfan's syndrome involves a typical body habitus and is sometimes associated with mitral and aortic insufficiency and aneurysms of the aorta. Mongolism (trisomy 21) is associated with endocardial cushion defects. Bony abnormalities of the upper extremity (especially a fingerized thumb) are associated with atrial septal defect and together constitute the Holt-Oram syndrome. Dis-

turbances of gait may suggest Friedreich's ataxia with associated cardiomyopathy. Acromegaly, disturbances of thyroid function, and rheumatoid arthritis are frequently associated with myocardial, pericardial, or valvular disease. Cyanosis and clubbing are clues to reversal of a shunt in congenital heart disease. A head bob and exaggerated arterial pulsations in the neck suggest increased diastolic run-off, as in aortic insufficiency. Edema and ascites suggest heart failure; when combined with obvious cachexia, they indicate longstanding and severe heart disease.

Venous Pressure and Pulse. There are two objectives to examination of the neck veins. The first is to estimate central venous pressure, and the second is to evaluate the wave form of the venous pressure pulse (Fig. 1). The examination is a visual one seeking a volume change in the veins. Because the venous system is a low pressure system, neck veins are nearly empty when the patient is sitting up, and they are distended when lying flat without a pillow. In either position a change in volume synchronous with the heartbeat is usually absent. To examine neck veins ideally, elevate the patient's head to an angle which maximizes the volume change in the veins throughout the cardiac cycle. The external jugular vein is a more reliable source to estimate venous pressure, but the internal jugular vein is a more reliable source to evaluate venous pulsations. Venous pressure is estimated by identifying the undulating meniscus in the jugular vein, measuring its height in centimeters above the sternal angle of Louis and adding 5 cm. The "A" wave results from atrial contraction and is exaggerated with right ventricular hypertrophy (reduced compliance), tricuspid stenosis, arrhythmias in which atrial contraction occurs against a closed tricuspid valve (i.e., cannon waves), and constrictive pericarditis. Obliteration of the "X" descent and a prominent "CV" wave are characteristic of tricuspid insufficiency. Elevated venous pressure with exaggerated "X" and "Y" descents is typical of pericardial constriction.

Figure 1. Normal jugular venous pulse.

Figure 2. Bifid or bisferious carotid pulse in asymmetric septal hypertrophy with obstruction.

Arterial Pressure and Pulses. Arterial pulses are examined by palpation with the fingertips. The artery is compressed until it is displaced by the force of the arterial pressure pulse. This sensation of force on the fingertips is related to the amplitude of the pressure pulse, i.e., the difference between systolic and diastolic pressure, and not to pressure or flow per se. The carotid arteries are generally the most valid reflection of cardiac activity because they are centrally located and not influenced importantly by local factors which will affect the amplitude of the radial artery pulse independent of changes in cardiac activity. The amplitude of the carotid pulse is increased with anemia, thyrotoxicosis, and aortic insufficiency. In these conditions stroke volume and the rate of left ventricular ejection are enhanced. The carotid pulse is attenuated in myocardial failure, with rapid heart rates such as atrial fibrillation, and in aortic stenosis. These conditions are characterized by either a reduced stroke volume or a decreased rate of left ventricular ejection, or both. The arterial pulse becomes bifid in certain conditions in which left ventricular ejection is initially very rapid, producing a percussion wave, which is then followed by tidal wave which represents a reflected pulsation from the periphery (Fig. 2). A bifid or bisferious pulse is typically seen in asymmetric septal hypertrophy with obstruction (i.e., hypertrophic subaortic stenosis) and sometimes in aortic valve disease with predominate aortic insufficiency. In addition to examination of the carotid pulse, peripheral arterial pulses should be felt and compared. A diminished or delayed pulse at one site compared to another suggests arterial occlusion. If such a discrepancy is noted, it can be exaggerated by exercising the extremity supplied by the obstructed artery. In patients with claudication arterial pulses are frequently normal at rest, but they become reduced in the affected leg or foot with walking. This happens because at rest the distal arterial bed is constricted, flow in the leg is low, and as a consequence there is little or no gradient across the stenosis. With exercise the distal arterial bed opens up, flow into the leg is limited by the stenosis, and a gradient develops with a marked drop in pressure distal to the stenosis.

Arterial blood pressure should be measured with a cuff of appropriate size. If an elevated blood pressure is obtained in the arm, pressure in one leg should also be recorded. This procedure is used to exclude coarctation of the aorta in hypertensive patients. The arterial blood pressure should be recorded in both the supine and the standing positions. If the patient's blood pressure is elevated on the first measurement, several recordings should be obtained. Blood pressure is recorded to establish the presence or absence of hypertension. Discrepancies between pressure at two sites suggest obstruction or an arterial anomaly. A marked postural drop in arterial pressure suggests either hypovolemia or an inadequate sympathetic vasoconstrictor response. A change of systolic arterial pressure on alternate beats in sinus rhythm is referred to as pulsus alternans (observed in severe myocardial failure), and a change of systolic blood pressure of greater than 10 mm Hg with respiration is referred to as pulsus paradoxus (observed in pericardial tamponade).

Precordial Movements. Precordial movements should be evaluated by inspection and by palpation at the apex, in the left parasternal region, and in the right and left second intercostal spaces. The normal apical impulse is ascribed to left ventricular activity and is seen and felt as a tap of brief duration localized in the fourth or fifth interspace at the midclavicular line. Its distance from the midsternal line should be measured in centimeters and recorded. When the left ventricle is dilated, the impulse is displaced to the left and downward and occupies a larger area. With systolic overloads such as hypertension or aortic stenosis, the impulse is not displaced (in the absence of dilation) but is more forceful and sustained than normal (Fig. 3). Right ventricular enlargement typically produces an exaggerated left parasternal early systolic lift or thrust. A soft late systolic lift may be produced by mitral insufficiency. Dilation of the pulmonary artery or aorta (aneurysm) may produce a systolic pulse or tap in the second left or right intercostal spaces, respectively. In regional myocardial disease or in coronary disease with regional infarction, there is a paradoxical outward systolic movement felt in the third or fourth left intercostal space between the sternum and the nipple. Accentuated heart sounds are often palpable. Gallop sounds are usually palpable when they can be heard and reflect altered ventricular compliance. Palpation of the precordium is directed primarily at assessing ventricular size, ascertaining whether an increase in chamber size is due to dilation or concentric hypertrophy, assessing

Figure 3. Apex cardiogram showing an exaggerated and prolonged outward systolic plateau (SP) due to left ventricular hypertrophy in a patient with aortic stenosis.

changes in compliance, and detecting asynchronous contraction of a region of the ventricle due to a regional disease process. For the experienced observer many cardiac diagnoses can be anticipated even before listening with a stethoscope.

Auscultation. The first principle of cardiac auscultation is to choose a stethoscope which fits the ears comfortably and which has tubing as short as possible. The second important principle is to carry out the examination in a room where the ambient noise level is as low as possible. Clinical experience and studies in hearing laboratories have shown that acoustic phenomena of diagnostic importance can be missed even by experienced observers if either of these principles is compromised.

The next important step in auscultation is to remember that you only hear what you listen for. A systematic approach in which you listen at specific locations and focus on specific sounds and parts of the cardiac cycle is essential. Devise a *mental check list* which you move through in stepwise fashion. For example, starting at the apex, ask yourself the following questions: (1) Which is the first and which the second heart sound? (2) What are their relative intensities, and is either accentuated? (3) Is there more than one component to either sound? (4) If there are two components to the first sound, is the extra component an S_4, an ejection click, or splitting? (5) Are there midsystolic or diastolic sounds? (6) Can a murmur be heard in either systole or diastole? Remember that high frequency sounds are best heard with the diaphragm, whereas low frequency sounds are best heard with the bell. Make it a standard part of your examination to listen with the patient supine, in the left lateral position, standing, and after exercise.

In chapters that follow this introduction, details of the physical examination in each of the major cardiac disorders will be presented. The point stressed here is the approach to the patient. The examination should be systematic. Abnormal physical findings may be so striking that they cannot be missed; more often, however, they are subtle. Therefore the most reliable approach is a mental check list. Progress through the list in an orderly fashion, and at each step optimize the conditions for eliciting the phenomenon which is sought.

It is rare for a cardiac condition to have only one manifestation on the physical examination. For example, when you see cyanosis you can anticipate certain findings on palpation or auscultation which will help explain it. When you feel an enlarged right ventricle, a palpable first heart sound, and a systolic pulse over the pulmonary artery in a middle-aged female, you can anticipate that auscultation may elicit an opening snap and diastolic rumble. Anticipating the next step is useful in examining a patient. For one thing, it is likely to increase the precision of the next step in the examination so that less will be missed. Absence of an anticipated finding may redirect tentative conclusions about the diagnosis. Finally, an anticipatory approach encourages synthesis of data as the examiner progresses through the check list. A diagnosis results from a synthesis of data; whether the history and physical examination yield a diagnosis or a definition of the problem which falls short of a diagnosis, synthesis helps to define what the next step should be and whether or not that step is necessary.

Laboratory studies play a central role in the diagnosis of cardiovascular diseases and, even more importantly, in quantifying the severity of these disorders. The paragraphs below are designed to highlight the role of commonly employed laboratory tests in cardiovascular diagnosis. It seems appropriate to discuss briefly the physical or physiologic principles behind these tests, because in some instances these techniques have been applied to cardiovascular studies only in the recent past, or because these principles help to clarify the uses and limitations of a particular test.

THE ELECTROCARDIOGRAM. Cardiac muscle is an excitable tissue. On each beat excitation begins at some site in the heart (normally the sinoatrial node), spreads from cell to cell initially over the atrium, then through the atrioventricular node, and finally to the ventricles. The form of the electrocardiogram at any point in time is determined by the location, size, and geometry of boundaries between excited and unexcited regions.

Whenever a boundary exists, the voltage difference across the boundary produces an electrical field at any point in the body. The positive side of this boundary can be viewed as a source of current, and the negative side of the boundary can be viewed as a sink. Regions on the body surface that face the current source will be on the positive side of the field, whereas those that face the current sink will be on the negative side of field. Because the location, spatial orientation, and size of the boundary change throughout excitation and recovery, the field changes in strength and orientation. On the body surface the amplitude and sign of the potential change with time. An electrocardiogram is a record of the voltage difference between two points on the body surface with respect to time.

The electrocardiogram is the most widely used and useful noninvasive cardiac diagnostic technique. Its diagnostic value has developed over the years of use through (1) correlations with clinical states and pathologic material, (2) physiologic studies designed to establish the relation between the electrocardiogram and normal and abnormal states, and (3) simulation. Analyses of the P wave and the QRS complex, their rate, and their temporal relation to each other provide a definitive approach for recognizing most disturbances of cardiac rhythm. The electrocardiogram gives diagnostic and localizing information about most myocardial infarctions. Criteria have been established for recognizing hypertrophy of the right or left atrium and the right or left ventricle. The electrocardiogram is an important diagnostic aid also in various forms of congenital heart disease. Because it can be obtained repeatedly in the same individual or monitored continuously over days, it is of particular value in assessing pathophysiologic phenomena that change over the interval between records (rhythm, hypertrophy, infarction or ischemia, electrolytes, and drug effects). The electrocardiogram is easily recorded during exercise.

THE X-RAY. Chest roentgenography is the oldest and one of the most useful techniques for imaging the heart. Radiographic examination utilizes x-rays which are a form of electromagnetic energy. X-rays are created by an energy conversion that occurs when rapidly moving electrons strike a metal target and atoms which comprise the target are converted from one energy state to another. This conversion is produced in an x-ray tube which is a modified vacuum diode tube. The cathode of an x-ray tube consists of a filament which is heated by electrical current. Electrons emitted from the cathode are accelerated by the voltage potential across the tube. These electrons strike the anode or target, which is usually made up of tungsten, and x-rays are emitted from the target. Useful x-rays emerge through a diaphragm at the base of the tube to form a beam which is directed at the patient. This beam consists of x-ray photons which are packets of electromagnetic energy. In passing through the chest a variable fraction of photons is absorbed by body tissues where absorption is determined by the composition of the tissues, their thickness, and the quality of the beam. The photons that emerge from the subject are used to expose a film. The picture created on the film is a superimposition of structures within the chest that absorb x-rays to a variable extent. The cardiovascular structures form silhouettes because of the marked difference between their x-ray absorptive characteristics and those of bone and lung.

The standard radiographic examination of the heart involves a posteroanterior view and a lateral view, usually supplemented by left and right oblique views with barium in the esophagus. Each view is designed to optimize conditions for visualizing various cardiac structures. With appropriate views one can assess the size of individual cardiac chambers, the size of the superior vena cava, the aorta, and the pulmonary artery. The pulmonary vessels can be seen on conventional x-rays, and typical patterns are produced by pulmonary venous engorgement, by increased or decreased pulmonary blood flow, and by pulmonary hypertension. Calcification of valves, the anuli of valves, coronary arteries, and pericardium can be observed, although conventional x-rays are less sensitive than fluoroscopy in detecting calcium. With fluoroscopy one also can visualize the motion of cardiovascular structures.

In many forms of congenital and acquired heart disease, a diagnosis can be made or strongly suspected on the basis of chest x-rays. In practice, however, x-rays are interpreted together with the history, physical examination, and electrocardiogram. In this context, the most useful role of the x-ray is to confirm structural changes suspected by physical examination, to identify structural changes not suspected by physical examination, and to assess on a semiquantitative basis the severity of anatomic and physiologic consequences of heart disease. One of the greatest values of the x-ray is to provide a method for determining the size of cardiovascular structures over time.

THE ECHOCARDIOGRAM. Echocardiography is a noninvasive technique in which high frequency sound waves are directed into the thoracic cavity and echoes reflected from moving cardiac structures are recorded (Fig. 4A). Echoes are produced at the interface between tissues of different acoustic impedance (i.e., at the epicardial surface, at the interface of endocardium and blood, and at the interface of structures such as septa and valves and the blood). The echoes produced by these structures vary in distance from the transducer throughout the heart cycle, and they vary in distance from each other with respect to time (Fig. 4B). With appropriate instrumentation and technique high quality echocardiograms can be obtained in approximately 75 per cent of individuals.

A complete examination should include visualization of the mitral, aortic, tricuspid, and pulmonary valves, and the left atrium, left ventricle, and right ventricle; a sweep from the left ventricle into the aortic root; and assessment of the presence or absence of pericardial fluid.

The importance of echocardiography can be inferred from several observations about its use and diagnostic valve. An echocardiogram is completely noninvasive, is without risk, and requires approximately 30 minutes. Mitral stenosis can be easily recognized, and the orifice of the stenotic valve can be measured. Aortic stenosis can be easily recognized, and although the orifice size is difficult to measure precisely, a demonstration of cusps which open to the periphery of the aortic root rules out significant aortic stenosis. A pulmonary artery diastolic pressure above 20 mm Hg produces a typical change in the diastolic contour of the pulmonary valve. Echocardiography is probably the most sensitive technique available for recognizing left atrial myxoma, mitral valve prolapse, and asymmetric septal hypertrophy with or without subaortic obstruction. It is the only available technique for visualizing vegetations on the valves in infectious endocarditis. The presence of small amounts of pericardial fluid can be detected, and the volume of fluid can be closely estimated. Although there are serious limitations to quantitation of ventricular volume and function from echo studies, chamber dimensions and a qualitative assessment of wall motion have proved to be reliable estimates of chamber size and left ventricular function. Images which are diagnostic of certain forms of congenital heart disease have also been reported. From this brief survey it can be concluded that echocardiography is capable of establishing the diagnosis in several important types of cardiac disease, and it provides important information about structure and function that is otherwise not available short of cardiac catheterization.

RADIONUCLIDE STUDIES. Radionuclide studies of the cardiovascular system involve the injection of an isotope into the circulation and subsequent detection of the energy emitted from the isotope by an appropriate external instrument. Isotopes vary in their mode of decay (for example, emission of electrons or positrons), in their half-life, and in the energy of photons that are liberated as a consequence of decay of the isotope. After variable absorption in body tissues, photons exit from the body and are available for detection. Most detection instruments rely on a thallium-activated sodium iodide crystal which has the property of giving off electrons (a photoelectric event) when struck by photons. The current generated by this event is then amplified many times by a photomultiplier tube and used to expose film or to modulate an oscilloscope beam, or, after conversion to a voltage, is stored in a computer. Imaging devices are of several types. The rectilinear scanner is a single small collimated probe that is moved over the area of interest. The Anger camera is a much larger crystal coupled to an array of 19 to 91 separate photomultiplier tubes which view a very large field. Multicrystal cameras consist of as many as 294 separate crystals. With appropriate collimation, scintillation cameras can be focused to produce tomographic images.

Decay of the positron-emitting isotope results in the emission of two photons per event, and the photons are directed at 180 degrees relative to each other. By placing detectors on opposite sides of the source and operating the detectors in a coincidence mode, events are recorded only if both detectors sense the annihilation photons simultaneously. This amounts to electronic collimation. By rotating the crystal array around the patient, positron cameras can be used to provide tomographic images; and

Figure 4. *A,* The ultrasound beam of an echocardiograph and its intersection with various cardiac structures. *B,* The echocardiogram, which shows the motion of various cardiac structures with respect to time and each other.

by an array of 48 crystals surrounding the patient, three-dimensional reconstruction or cross-sectional images can be produced.

Radionuclides can be used to label the blood pool and thus produce images of the cardiac chambers throughout the cardiac cycle to estimate chamber volume, ejection fraction, and wall motion (Fig. 5). A special application is the construction of time-activity plots over specific regions and the application of indicator dilution principles to locate and quantitate intracardiac shunts. Radionuclides such as potassium-43 and thallium-201 are extracted by normal muscle in proportion to blood flow and can be used to evaluate relative regional myocardial perfusion at rest and during exercise. Technetium-99m phos-

phate is localized to acutely necrotic myocardium and gives images that are diagnostic of acute infarction (positive images from 12 hours to three to five days after infarction). Theoretically, positron-emitting isotopes can be used for any of the aforementioned applications. A unique application of positron images results from the availability of isotopes of carbon, oxygen, and nitrogen which can be used to label natural metabolites and thus study regional metabolism of ischemic zones noninvasively and sequentially. It can be projected that noninvasive nuclear cardiology will replace the need for cardiac catheterization in some instances, complement catheterization in other situations, and provide unique data about cardiovascular function unattainable by other methods.

Figure 5. Radionuclide angiogram. Diastolic and systolic images at rest and during exercise are shown for three subjects: (a) a normal, (b) a patient with two vessel coronary artery disease, and (c) a patient with disease of the left main coronary artery. In the normal sujbect ejection fraction improves with exercise. In the patients with coronary artery disease, ejection fraction deteriorates with exercise.

CARDIAC CATHETERIZATION. Cardiac catheterization provides a method by which the pressure in any or all of the cardiac chambers can be measured with considerable accuracy. Gradients across stenotic valves can be measured, cardiac output and pulmonary blood flow can be estimated, and shunts between the systemic and pulmonary circulation can be localized and quantitated. Contrast agents can be injected to define radiographically the dimensions of the cardiac chambers, to estimate the volume of regurgitation through insufficient valves, and to visualize the anatomy of simple and complex congenital malformations. The aorta and most of its branches, including the coronary arteries, can be selectively catheterized, and deviations from normal anatomy can be defined. The contractile performance of heart muscle can be evaluated, and the adequacy of cardiac output and flow to many individual organs, including the heart, can be deduced from measurement of flow and the arteriovenous difference of several metabolites, including oxygen. Electrode catheters can be used to define the location of conduction delays within the heart, the sequence of excitation, and the mechanism of certain alterations of cardiac rhythm. Catheterization is a powerful diagnostic technique which provides definitive data about many cardiovascular disorders.

There are many cardiac conditions in which the diagnosis can be established by history, physical examination, and noninvasive tests. The severity of the condition can also be assessed with sufficient clarity to judge that the patient is a surgical candidate. Catheterization in these circumstances is performed primarily to provide the surgeon with anatomic and physiologic detail which will help direct his approach to the patient (e.g., an open or closed approach to mitral stenosis, or which coronary arteries should be bypassed in a patient with angina pectoris). Catheterization may also reveal conditions that are unsuspected on clinical grounds or that cannot be judged quantitatively with the accuracy needed to guide the surgical approach (e.g., the presence of associated anomalous pulmonary venous return in a patient with atrial septal defect or aortic insufficiency which was underestimated on clinical grounds in a patient with pre-

dominant mitral regurgitation). Catheterization provides information about myocardial function which may not be adequately assessed on clinical grounds and hence contributes to the evaluation of surgical risk and the likelihood that correction of a valvular, congenital, or coronary lesion will prolong survival and reduce symptoms.

Another role of cardiac catheterization in patients with known heart disease is to enhance our knowledge of the severity of the condition when there is a discrepancy between symptoms and data obtained from physical examination and noninvasive techniques. One of the most noteworthy examples of this situation is the question of whether or not significant mitral stenosis has persisted or recurred in a patient who had mitral commissurotomy with an initially favorable response. On the other hand, patients with hydraulically significant stenosis of the aortic or pulmonary valve or with atrial septal defect may present with clinical signs and EKG and x-ray findings which indicate the need for surgical correction, and yet there may be few symptoms or none at all.

In certain situations cardiac catheterization is performed as a diagnostic procedure in patients in whom a diagnosis can only be suspected on clinical grounds or to clarify the basis of symptoms or signs of unknown significance. Probably the most frequent example is the adult patient with recurrent chest pain compatible with angina in whom the electrocardiogram at rest and during exercise fails to provide evidence of myocardial ischemia. When other noncardiac causes of angina-like chest pain have been searched for and excluded, coronary artery disease cannot be confirmed or excluded as a basis for the symptoms without coronary arteriography. In this situation a normal arteriogram may be very useful in directing attention away from the heart. Similarly, the finding of significant coronary artery disease may lead to a course of therapy (medical or surgical) which is successful in relieving a symptom which was causing significant incapacity.

Despite the usefulness and necessity of cardiac catheterization for situations of the type described above and many others, most cardiac conditions can be recognized and their severity adequately assessed without resorting to catheterization. Catheterization requires hospitalization, it is an expensive test, it causes some discomfort to the patient, and there are risks of arterial injury, embolization, myocardial infarction, reactions to contrast agents, and even death. Fortunately, these occurrences are extremely rare. Cost and the incidence of untoward events are not sufficient reasons to defer or refrain from catheterization when a significant condition is present or suspected and the probability of obtaining data which will be useful to management of the patient is high. Conversely, catheterization should not be undertaken if significant heart disease can be reasonably excluded on the basis of history and physical examination with or without the use of noninvasive laboratory tests. Similarly, cardiac catheterization is not indicated even in the presence of heart disease if the data obtained will not contribute substantially to decisions about management. Furthermore, even when cardiac catheterization can contribute data which would be useful to management, it is not needed if the same or more definitive data can be acquired by a less invasive, less expensive, and lower risk procedure.

STRATEGIES

When the physician has obtained a thorough history and performed a complete physical examination of the cardiovascular system, the next question frequently is whether or not laboratory studies are indicated and, if so, what tests and in what sequence. The answer to this question is not as straightforward as it might seem. What is important is to have a general strategy and a willingness to adapt that strategy in a manner which is appropriate to the problem which led the patient to the doctor, or to the findings obtained from the clinical examination. In any situation it is appropriate to pursue studies until a potential problem has been reasonably excluded or until an actual problem has been defined at the level which is necessary to make a decision about the need for further tests or treatment.

The role of laboratory studies is influenced in part by the age of the patient and the reason for seeking the advice of a doctor. For example, when a teenager is evaluated prior to participating on a high school athletic team and the history and physical examination are normal, most doctors would agree that no laboratory studies are indicated. If the same individual is referred to a cardiologist because of a systolic murmur at the base which radiates to the carotid arteries, and the physical examination, x-ray, and electrocardiogram are otherwise normal, an echocardiogram may show a bicuspid aortic valve without evidence of stenosis. This additional information would provide a basis for encouraging athletic participation, and also advice about prophylactic antibiotics and follow-up over the years ahead.

Is there an age at which certain laboratory tests become routine even in the absence of a history of cardiovascular disease or abnormalities on the physical examination? Many physicians would respond to this question in the affirmative. One example is the physician who is oriented toward preventive cardiology and is interested not only in detecting the presence or absence of disease, but also in detecting conditions which may substantially increase the risk of disease in later life. This strategy is invoked by those who advocate measuring serum cholesterol and its distribution between high and low density lipoproteins at least once in early adult life, particularly if there is a family history of premature atherosclerotic disease or hyperlipidemia.

There is another justification for obtaining selected tests on a routine basis in young adults. As patients grow older there is an increased probability that they will develop cardiovascular disease. There is also an increased probability that they will develop conditions which may require surgery (e.g., hernia repair, hip replacement). At that stage the consultation of an internist is frequently sought, particularly if the patient is over age 50, and an electrocardiogram and chest x-ray are obtained. If an abnormality is observed on one or both of these tests, it is useful to have a prior x-ray or electrocardiogram. It can be argued that the yield of abnormal electrocardiograms or chest x-rays does not justify obtaining them on a routine basis annually, especially prior to the age of 45 or 50. On the other hand, for the physician who is seeing patients over the age of 45, the availability of one electrocardiogram and chest x-ray at an earlier age when no disease was suspected can be of enormous value in evaluating later records.

When patients present with a history that indicates heart disease or with abnormal physical findings, laboratory tests take on a different role. At one level, certain tests are used to confirm or help interpret an abnormal physical finding. For example, the phonocardiogram can be used to confirm and document the presence and timing of abnormal sounds or murmurs, the apex cardiogram can confirm and document abnormal precordial movements, and external pulse recordings can confirm and document abnormal venous or arterial pulsations. These techniques are useful in teaching and they can be very important when a patient moves from the care of one doctor to another. Echocardiography is a new and exciting noninvasive cardiovascular diagnostic technique. It is probably the most sensitive available method to detect mitral valve prolapse, mitral stenosis, pericardial fluid, left atrial myxoma, and asymmetric septal hypertrophy. Not only is the method sensitive in these conditions, but it is probable that modern two-dimensional echocardiography will eliminate the need for cardiac catheterization to diagnose these conditions.

The most important point is that laboratory studies should be selected and pursued until the nature and severity of the disease can be established with reasonable certainty. If that can be accomplished with noninvasive methods, then tests of greater expense and potential risk are not necessary. On the other hand, when symptoms or signs suggest a severe disease potentially amenable to surgery, or if significant disease is suspected but cannot be clarified by noninvasive techniques, then catheterization is clearly indicated.

Most forms of heart disease are chronic. The approach of a physician whose focus is on prognosis, management, and follow-up requires more information than is required to make a diagnosis. Furthermore, accurate assessments of severity of disease and the response to management require quantifiable and reproducible descriptors. These considerations never justify the performance of costly unnecessary tests which subject the patient to a risk of complications. They emphasize, however, that a complete cardiac evaluation very often includes the use of laboratory procedures which exceed the minimal data base required to make a diagnosis.

355. HEART FAILURE

Alfred P. Fishman

The heart is part of an elaborate circulatory apparatus that is designed to serve two major functions: (1) to provide the tissues with sufficient blood (carrying oxygen, substrates, and nutrients) for their metabolic needs, both at rest and during activity; and (2) to reapportion the cardiac output according to the physiologic priorities of the moment, e.g., muscular exercise, heat loss, digestion. The same regulatory mechanisms that satisfy physiologic priorities in health also serve to protect vital organs, e.g., the heart and brain, when cardiac output is seriously compromised.

As a pump, the heart is remarkable not only for its capacity to adjust rapidly to metabolic need and to varying loads, but also for its durability. Unfortunately, it is also vulnerable to a wide array of congenital, metabolic, inflammatory, and degenerative disorders that affect its muscular walls, its linings, its valves, and particularly its nutrient vessels, i.e., the coronary arteries. Some cardiac disorders, such as arteriosclerosis of the small coronary arteries, progress slowly and insidiously, and their disease takes a lifetime to become clinically evident. Others, such as bacterial infection of the aortic valve, are often dramatic in onset and catastrophic in their consequences.

In general, signs and symptoms of heart disease are of two different kinds: those referable to the heart itself, such as pain and palpitation, and others that are extracardiac and originate in congested circulatory beds and hypoperfused organs. Considered out of context, each extracardiac manifestation may be disappointingly nonspecific. For example, breathlessness is a common symptom that is shared by disorders of the heart, the lungs, and the brain. Nonetheless, when breathlessness develops in a patient with left heart disease in association with other evidence of congested and edematous lungs, and grows worse when the patient lies flat, there is little question that the patient is suffering from left heart failure.

Subsequent chapters in Part XIV will deal with individual cardiac disorders. The present chapter will be concerned with heart failure, a final common pathway for many of the diverse etiologies and pathogenic mechanisms that will be discussed subsequently.

GENERAL ASPECTS

Heart failure may be considered in clinical, physiologic, or biochemical terms. *Clinically,* "heart failure" refers to a distinctive constellation of symptoms and physical signs that has emerged in a patient with an underlying cardiac disorder. *Physiologically,* heart failure is defined as the inability of the heart to match its output to the metabolic needs of the body (determined as O_2 consumption) even though filling pressures of the heart are adequate. The biochemical features are not as certain as the hemodynamic, but appear to involve defective conversion by the heart muscle of chemical energy to mechanical work.

No definition of heart failure is universally acceptable. However, experts generally use the term in one of two ways: (1) to indicate that inadequate performance of some part of the heart, i.e., valves or myocardium, has evoked the florid clinical picture of pulmonary and systemic venous congestion, or (2) as a synonym for inadequacy of heart muscle secondary either to overloading or to intrinsic disease. In this chapter, the second alternative is chosen, and *heart failure* is used as a synonym for *myocardial failure.* This approach has some distinct advantages: the inept performance of the heart, and the clinical picture that ensues, can be related to physiologic and biochemical events in heart muscle and to the pathogenesis of the heart failure; it avoids confusion with nonmyocardial disorders, which often evoke the same clinical picture but which have different origins and require different therapeutic measures, e.g., valve replacement for aortic stenosis; and it requires that distinction always be maintained between left and right ventricular failure in tracing pathogenesis and with respect to applying therapeutic measures. This stipulation automatically excludes syndromes in which the seat of the difficulty is in abnormalities of the heart valves or pericardium or excessive heart rates — each of which can compromise the circulation even though the cardiac muscle is normal.

Disproportion between hemodynamic load and myocardial capacity to cope with it initiates the sequence that culminates in heart failure. In general, the heart tolerates volume overloads better than pressure overloads. For example, *volume* overload of the left ventricle produced by aortic insufficiency may exist for years without causing distress; in contrast, *pressure* overload from aortic stenosis generally elicits signs and symptoms of heart failure much earlier. Sustained overloads are also accommodated better than acute overloads. Thus chronic mitral regurgitation caused by rheumatic heart disease often lasts for years without signs of heart failure, whereas the acute mitral regurgitation produced by a ruptured chorda tendinea is apt to precipitate a disastrous syndrome of heart failure.

The myocardium responds differently to volume and pressure loads. Volume overloads generally elicit dilatation followed by hypertrophy; conversely, pressure overloads characteristically elicit hypertrophy until late in the natural history when dilatation supervenes. Primary myocardial disease generally elicits both dilatation and hypertrophy.

Categories of Heart Failure

In the clinic, the type of heart failure is generally identified by its duration (acute or chronic), initiating mechanisms, the ventricle that is primarily affected, the characteristic clinical syndrome, and the underlying physiologic derangements.

ACUTE VS. CHRONIC HEART FAILURE. The manifestations of heart failure usually begin insidiously, blurring at the outset with those of the underlying cardiac disorder and continuing gradually into a chronic state. However, the syndrome may also begin acutely, as after myocardial infarction. Between these extremes of acute and chronic heart failure are many instances of subclinical heart failure in which a successful cardiotonic program, coupled with self-restriction of activity by the patient, minimizes signs and symptoms even though cardiac performance remains seriously compromised. On the other hand, it is not uncommon for the course of chronic heart failure that is nicely controlled to be punctuated by bouts of acute heart failure that stem either from lapses in therapy or from progression of the underlying heart disease.

Both acute and chronic heart failure elicit compensatory adjustments. These include increase in peripheral vascular resistance, redistribution of blood flow, and increase in erythropoietic activity. But the adaptive mechanisms differ strikingly in type, degree, and intensity, and even in direction. For example, *acute* distention of the left atrium generally promotes a sodium-poor diuresis, whereas *chronic* distention of the left atrium elicits salt and water retention. This distinction between acute and chronic heart failure must be borne in mind when attempting to relate observations on experimental heart failure in animals to the clinical syndrome of chronic heart failure in man, because experimental heart failure is generally acute in onset, is fulminating in course, and is generally ended abruptly by the death of the animal.

INITIATING MECHANISMS. Each initiating mechanism generally imposes its own distinctive stamp upon the clinical syndrome. Thus rheumatic heart disease leads to a different constellation of symptoms and signs from that of hypertensive heart disease; in turn, both have a different natural history from cor pulmonale. Indeed, even a single etiology, arteriosclerosis, may have distinctly different consequences; progressive narrowing and gradual occlusion of *peripheral* branches of the coronary arteries may be so covert that the characteristic shortness of breath and undue fatigue of left ventricular failure may be misinterpreted as evidence of the general physical decline of advancing age. Conversely, abrupt closure of a major coronary artery, as a consequence of thrombosis superimposed on an arteriosclerotic plaque, may elicit massive myocardial necrosis, followed by extensive myocardial scarring and unremitting heart failure.

LEFT VS. RIGHT HEART FAILURE. With rare exception, one ventricle fails before the other. Because of the prevalence of cardiac disorders which overload or damage the left ventricle, e.g., coronary arteriosclerosis and hypertension, heart failure usually begins with the left ventricle. Breathlessness, the key clinical expression of pulmonary congestion and edema, is the most common initial complaint. Conversely, when the right ventricle fails, systemic venous congestion and peripheral edema generally predominate. Left ventricular failure is the most common cause of right ventricular failure, and breathlessness often improves as right ventricular output falls and pulmonary congestion diminishes.

The mechanism by which left ventricular failure causes the right ventricle to fail is not clear. The conventional explanation puts the blame on pulmonary hypertension secondary to left ventricular failure. But the degree of pulmonary hypertension in this circumstance is rarely enough to constitute a formidable burden on the right ventricle. Much more likely as a predominant mechanism is the continuity of heart muscle that envelops both ventricles. In contrast to the fact that left ventricular failure is the most common cause of right ventricular failure, how often right ventricular failure causes left ventricular failure is still a matter of debate. Resolution of this problem is difficult because of the frequency with which independent and unrelated left ventricular disease coexists with right ventricular failure.

The combination of left and right ventricular failure, in which evidences of systemic and pulmonary venous hypertension predominate, is traditionally referred to as "congestive heart failure." This is a colloquialism that conveys the image of severe physical incapacity, breathlessness, distended neck veins, hepatic engorgement, and troublesome peripheral edema. But it also highlights clinical features that can be measured at the bedside: a high venous pressure, a prolonged circulation time, and a diminished vital capacity, all of which improve as the patient gets better.

BACKWARD VS. FORWARD HEART FAILURE. Somewhat reminiscent of the fable about the blind men and the elephant is the vintage controversy about "backward" versus "forward" heart failure. "Backward failure" calls attention to the damming up of blood in the veins proximal to the failing ventricle and attributes to this venous congestion a critical role in the evolution of the syndrome of heart failure; "forward failure" assigns the same pivotal role to a decrease in cardiac output and underfilling of the arterial tree. In reality this distinction is meaningless, because it is inevitable in a closed circuit that the inability of the heart to sustain its output (forward failure) and the pooling of blood on the venous inflow side (backward failure) must go hand in hand.

LOW VS. HIGH OUTPUT FAILURE. Cardiac catheterization in man has made it possible to sort myocardial failure according to the level of the cardiac output. This practice has served at least three purposes: (1) to separate, on clinical and physiologic grounds, a type of myocardial failure ("high output failure") in which the circulation remains vigorous and the extremities remain warm despite venous congestion, edema, and a lower cardiac output than existed prior to the heart failure; (2) to emphasize that the level of the cardiac output and the circulatory adjustments during myocardial failure are, to large extent, a consequence of the cardiac output that existed prior to heart failure; and (3) to relate etiology and clinical evidences of heart failure to the state of the circulation: the more common causes of heart failure — arteriosclerosis, hypertension, myocardial disease, valvular disease, and pericardial disease — tend to be low output states; less common causes, such as hyperthyroidism, Paget's disease, anemia, beriberi, and arteriovenous fistula, tend to be high output states. But the hemodynamic hallmark of cardiac failure remains the same regardless of the level of cardiac output at rest: an inability of the heart to increase its output (or stroke volume or stroke work) as end-diastolic volume (as well as pressure) is increased (see Preload, below).

The separation into "high" and "low" output failure is concerned with the clinical manifestations, rather than the causes, of myocardial failure. But it is also a hemodynamic frame of reference to which the anatomist and the biochemist can relate the myocardial origins of heart failure. For example, "high output" failure probably has different biochemical bases from "low output" failure. Nor are all types of "low output" or "high output" failure apt to have the same biochemical origins. For example, it is unlikely that the "high output" failure of a peripheral arteriovenous fistula has the same anatomic or biochemical beginnings and evolution as the "high output" failure of severe anemia or malnutrition.

CONGESTIVE FAILURE VS. CONGESTED STATE. Overfilling of the circulation, without myocardial failure, is the hallmark of the "congested state." It may be induced by rapid infusions; it is common in severe anemia and in chronic renal insufficiency. Similar but less dramatic venous congestion may also complicate Paget's disease or beriberi. In each of these situations, venous hypertension arises from a combination of an expanded venous volume and heightened venomotor tone, rather than from heart failure.

It is true that persistence of a "hyperkinetic" congested state may, in time, cause the heart muscle to fail from overwork. The onset of myocardial failure may then be difficult to detect on clinical grounds, because the hyperkinetic circulation persists and the congestion may be only slightly increased during myocardial failure. Accordingly, the transition from the congested state to congestive heart failure may be difficult to detect on clinical grounds alone. But when heart failure does supervene, cardiac catheterization will disclose an inadequate increase in cardiac output during exercise as well as a considerable increase in cardiac output after digitalis. Fortunately, identification of the transition from a "congested state" to "congestive heart failure" is of greater theoretical than practical importance, because therapeutic measures, such as the administration of diuretics and the replacement of particular nutrients, e.g., thiamin in beriberi, are effective in both situations. However, digitalis will exert an important therapeutic effect once the myocardium has failed, whereas it is clinically useless when administered to a heart that is coping well with an overfilled circulation.

Subcellular Bases for Contraction

With each beat, the heart develops force and expends energy. Electrical activity at the cell surface activates the contractile machinery. Connecting the electrical activity at the surface and the contractile machinery within the muscle cell is the sarcoplasmic reticulum which plays a critical role in the release and uptake of calcium during contraction and relaxation.

For the development of the contractile force, heart muscle depends on interactions among contractile proteins, the hypothetical "elastic components" with which they are connected in series, and the constraining bounds within which the contractile elements function. The contractile proteins are contained within sarcomeres, repeating units that comprise the individual muscle fibers (myofibrils). Within the sarcomere, the contractile proteins are arranged in two orderly groups of myofilaments, one consisting of myosin, the other predominantly of actin. Holding the contractile apparatus at bay are two modulator proteins, troponin and tropomyosin. Delivery of calcium to troponin from the sarcoplasmic reticulum and sarcolemma sets the contractile process into motion.

To account for changes in the length of heart muscle during contraction and relaxation, the sliding filament hypothesis of Huxley is generally invoked: during contraction, the thin actin filaments slide past the thicker myosin filaments to shorten the sarcomere; the entire muscle cell follows suit. Conversely, during relaxation, the sarcomeres and the muscle cell resume their initial lengths as the original actin-myosin relationships are restored. Nearby mitochondria generate energy for the contractile machinery by oxidative phosphorylation of free fatty acids and glucose supplied by the circulation.

The tension that is developed in cardiac muscle during contraction depends on actin-myosin relationships. Projecting from the myosin filaments are cross-bridges. Before activation, these bridges are not attached to actin filaments. Upon activation, the cross-bridges on the myosin filaments lock into receptor sites on the actin filaments, thereby developing the force that leads to contraction. As the muscle shortens, the cross-bridges disengage and slide along the actin filament, like a pawl on a ratchet, to engage other sites. Depending on the number of cross-bridges that are interlocked at the same time, different tensions will be developed.

In addition to these subcellular elements that are directly involved in the contractile process, there appears to be a subcellular beta sympathomimetic system that can enhance the inotropic state. Although an increase in intracellular calcium is involved, the precise mechanism is unclear.

Evidence exists that for the sarcomere, as for the whole heart (see Preload, below), the tension developed during contraction is directly related to its initial length. This correspondence implies that, for the whole heart, stretching increases the ability of its individual contractile elements to develop force. Also, since stretching does not affect the rate of interaction of active sites, elongation of cardiac muscle fibers before contraction should not affect the velocity of the subsequent contraction. These considerations underlie many current notions about cardiac contractility. But it is still unclear whether the ultrastructural-physiologic correlations are real or simply models for eliciting a new kind of reflection about an exceedingly complicated problem.

PATHOPHYSIOLOGIC INTERPLAY

Each ventricle functions as a separate muscular pump supplied by its own booster pump (atrium). The two ventricles empty in unison, simultaneously dispatching their respective contents: the right ventricle sending blood to the lungs for arterialization, the left ventricle sending arterialized blood to the rest of the body for metabolic purposes. In the normal heart, at least 50 per cent of the end-diastolic volume is ejected with each beat. Much of the ejection force is the result of the inherent properties (fiber-length and inotropism) of the myocardium. But a wide range of adaptability to the ever-changing metabolic needs of daily life is provided by a superimposed series of extrinsic neurohumoral adjustments which, in daily life, modify and obscure the intrinsic inherent properties of the heart muscle.

Each ventricle, as with any man-made machine, is endowed with a finite capacity for stress, strain, and repair. The two ventricles also have somewhat different designs in keeping with their different long-range functions as pumps. The rate of obsolescence of each ventricle depends on the wear and tear to which it is subjected, its supply of nutriments and substrates, and its continuing state of good health. Before birth, both ventricles are taxed equally, because they bear the same pressure loads. After birth, as pulmonary arterial pressure falls, the right ventricular burden decreases and its walls thin. Consequently, other influences remaining equal, the durability of right ventricular performance is destined from birth to exceed that of the left ventricle. The brighter prospects of the right ventricle for longevity in performance are intensified by the greater vulnerability of the left side of the heart to disease and to disorders in its blood supply.

Assessment of Cardiac Performance

With respect to evaluating cardiac performance, the heart may be regarded from three points of view: as a pump; as a muscle; and as a component of the circulation. Hemodynamic measurements are used to characterize its behavior as a pump: cardiac output, stroke output, stroke work, stroke power, ventricular end-diastolic pressure, ejection fraction, and ventricular end-diastolic volume. To ascertain its behavior as a muscle, principles of muscle mechanics are applied. Its adequacy as a component of the circulation is reflected in the derangements that result from the low cardiac output, the redistribution of blood flow among tissues and organs, organ hypoperfusion, and venous congestion.

Heart as a Pump: Hemodynamics

By the time the heart fails, a variety of mechanisms are operating to bolster its flagging performance. In contrast to the inappropriately low cardiac output, the blood pressure generally remains normal or even increases.

CARDIAC OUTPUT. At each level of activity, in health and disease, a complicated interplay automatically adjusts the extent of shortening of myocardial fibers and, consequently, the stroke volume and the cardiac output. Four principal determinants set the stroke volume: preload (Table 1), afterload (ventricular emptying during

systole), the inotropic characteristics of the heart, and the coordinated pattern of contraction. A fifth determinant, the heart rate, sets the cardiac output (stroke volume times heart rate). For practical purposes, three of these five principal determinants of cardiac output — preload, afterload, heart rate — are quantifiable. Attempts are currently under way to depict quantitatively the fourth, i.e., the contribution of different regions of the ventricular myocardium to the ejection of blood from the heart. But the fifth, i.e., the inotropic state, remains difficult to assess (Fig. 1) except in the extreme, i.e., when the heart is large and evidence exists of venous congestion and organ hypoperfusion.

Relationships among these determinants are not fixed; they play greater or lesser roles, depending on the state of the heart. Thus when the inherent contractility (inotropic state) is impaired, stroke output and cardiac output may be maintained by ventricular dilatation (Frank-Starling mechanism). This flexible arrangement limits the value of cardiac output as a measure of cardiac contractility (inotropic state) to situations in which preload, afterload, and heart rate can be held constant. Unfortunately, this degree of control of loading conditions and heart rate is easier to achieve in the experimental laboratory than in clinical situations.

Indicator-dilution techniques are now widely used for the bedside determination of cardiac output. The normal range in adults at rest is between 2.5 and 3.6 liters per minute per square meter. A decrease in cardiac output at rest represents a late stage in abnormal cardiac performance. Failure to increase cardiac output during exercise occurs much earlier. Thus in normal subjects exercising in a supine position, the increase in cardiac output exceeds 600 ml per minute for each 100 ml increase in oxygen consumption. Lower values indicate abnormal cardiac performance. In heart failure, the arteriovenous difference for oxygen is abnormally wide,

TABLE 1. Terms Used to Describe Mechanical Performance of the Heart

Term	Relation to Cardiac Function
Inotropic state	A measure of contractility.
Preload	Stretch of myocardial fibers at end-diastole.
Afterload (during ejection)	Force that the ventricle must develop during systole in order to eject the stroke volume. The two major determinants are aortic impedance and left ventricular volume. Afterload is usually expressed as wall stress or wall tension; also, as instantaneous force at some point during ventricular ejection or as mean wall force throughout systole.
Wall tension (during ejection)	Total force per unit of ventricular circumferential length. Determined as product of systolic pressure and radius of ventricle in accord with Laplace equation. Independent of wall thickness.
Wall stress (during ejection)	Force per unit of cross-sectional wall area. Determined as product of pressure and radius divided by wall thickness. Reduced by thickening of wall in ventricular hypertrophy.
Impedance (during ejection)	Instantaneous relationship between rate of change in aortic pressure and aortic blood flow. The aortic input impedance reflects the forces external to the heart that impose a load on the left ventricle, including stiffness of aortic wall. Determined primarily, but not exclusively, by total peripheral vascular resistance to run off from the arterial tree. Normal peripheral resistance is approximately 1500 dynes sec/cm^{-5} or 15 peripheral resistance units.
Energetics	Generally determined as myocardial oxygen consumption. For any contractile state, the force developed and maintained during contraction represents the major mechanical determinant of oxygen consumption. An increase in myocardial wall force (tension or stress) that accompanies an increase in filling pressure and radius (Laplace equation) in heart failure increases the energy cost of contraction.

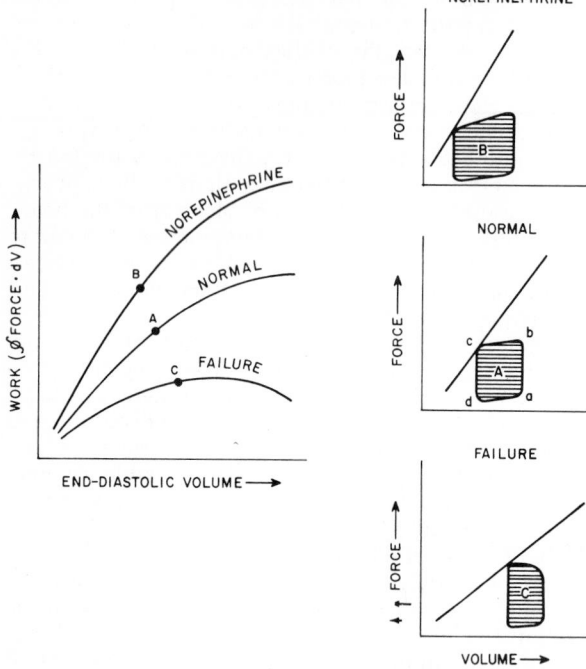

Figure 1. Schematic ventricular function (Frank-Starling) curves (left). By using work (instead of stroke output) on the ordinate, the work done per beat can be analyzed using force-volume curves (right). The three curves correspond to the normal (A), failing (C), and highly contractile (B) hearts on the Frank-Starling curves.

Left, The effects of preload and contractility on ventricular function curves. The normal left ventricle (A) increases its stroke output as preload (measured clinically as pulmonary wedge pressure) increases, moving up the ascending limb of the curve until preload reserve is exhausted. In severe heart failure, the ventricular function curve is displaced downward and to the right. The preload reserve is gone, and the heart is operating chronically on the descending limb of curve (C). An increase in contractility, as after administering norepinephrine, displaces the curve to the left, i.e., a large stroke output is accomplished at lower filling pressures (B).

Right, Work loops per beat corresponding to points B, A, and C on the ventricular function curves. The sloping line in each curve defines the contractility of the particular heart under consideration. On the perimeter of the work loop in the cardiac cycle are indicated the following landmarks: a = end diastole; b = opening of aortic valve; c = closure of aortic valve; d = start of filling of heart.

In comparison with the normal heart (center), the failing heart (lower) does just about as much work (total area under curve), at a high filling pressure, but ejects less per beat (d-a). Norepinephrine improves the contractility, so that the end-diastolic volume and pressure decrease whereas the stroke output (d-a) improves greatly. (Based on Weber and Janicki.)

resulting almost entirely from the low oxygen content of venous blood returning to the heart rather than from impaired oxygenation in the lungs.

During exercise, heart rate and cardiac output increase as linear functions of oxygen consumption. This is true during both supine and upright exercise, but for any level of exercise the cardiac output is appreciably lower in the upright position. These increases in cardiac output are accomplished principally by acceleration of the heart rate rather than by increase in the stroke volume. In heart failure, cardiac output is even more

dependent on heart rate, both at rest and during exercise.

VENTRICULAR END-DIASTOLIC PRESSURE. Inadequate ventricular emptying during systole leads to an increase in the residual volume of blood in the ventricle after systole, and thereby to an increase in end-diastolic ventricular volume. Since end-diastolic ventricular volumes are difficult to measure, end-diastolic ventricular pressures are generally substituted. This practice depends on the premise that a change in pressure is effected by a change in ventricular volume. However, exceptions to this rule do occur: structural changes in the myocardium (fibrosis, edema, hypertrophy, hemorrhage) and pericardial restriction cause end-diastolic pressure to increase without increment in volume, i.e., compliance is decreased. Conversely, in some states of chronic volume overloading of the ventricle, compliance decreases so that large volumes are accommodated at end-diastole without increasing pressure to abnormal levels.

An end-diastolic pressure in the *left* ventricle greater than 12 to 15 mm Hg is abnormal; for the right ventricle, the corresponding upper limit of normal is 10 mm Hg. It is rather simple to estimate the right ventricular end-diastolic pressure by measuring the central venous pressure; the left ventricular end-diastolic pressure is more difficult to estimate because of its inaccessibility. However, in the absence of mitral obstruction or of an increase in pulmonary vascular resistance, pulmonary arterial diastolic pressure provides a useful estimate of left ventricular end-diastolic pressure. Pulmonary wedge pressure is now widely used as a measure of left ventricular end-diastolic pressure.

The performance of the heart depends on two essential components: fiber length (Frank-Starling mechanism) and the inherent contractility (inotropic state) of the muscle. The normal heart is keyed to respond automatically to maintain the cardiac output. The factors that are involved are preload, afterload, contractility, and heart rate. In response to chronic overloading, the heart undergoes dilatation or hypertrophy or a combination of the two.

PRELOAD (THE FRANK-STARLING MECHANISM). According to this mechanism, an increase in end-diastolic volume (preload) is followed by a more forceful contraction that improves ventricular emptying. To assess the Frank-Starling mechanism, only preload should vary, i.e., afterload and heart rate are kept constant for each level of contractility. A distinctive "ventricular performance" curve exists for each state of contractility (Fig. 1). Thus the curve for a failing ventricle is depressed and flat so that small stroke volumes are delivered at abnormally high end-diastolic volumes. The high filling pressures are responsible for congestion and edema in the venous beds that lead to the ventricle that has failed.

In the normal heart, the Frank-Starling mechanism operates chiefly to match the stroke outputs of the two ventricles. But in heart failure, this mechanism plays an important part in sustaining the cardiac output.

AFTERLOAD. Afterload refers to the force that the ventricle must develop during systole in order to eject the stroke volume. In principle, it provides a measure of all factors that oppose active shortening of the ventricular fibers. In practice, because of the difficulties of estimating all these factors, impedance is estimated either from the arterial blood pressure or from a calculation of systemic vascular resistance (ratio of blood pressure to flow, expressed in dynes sec/cm^{-5} or in peripheral resistance units).

For clinical purposes, the relationship of blood pressure to cardiac output and peripheral resistance (P/Flow = R) is quite useful. For example, any intervention that causes a large increase in cardiac output without changing systemic blood pressure presumably causes vasodilation, thereby decreasing calculated peripheral vascular resistance, impedance, and afterload (wall force). Accompanying the improved emptying of the left ventricle is a decrease in its filling pressure (measured by pulmonary wedge pressure).

Increasing the afterload on the normal heart (while preload and contractility remain constant) decreases both the degree and speed of wall shortening; reduction in afterload has the opposite effect.

CONTRACTILITY. Increase in sympathetic nervous activity provides the major inotropic effect for the normal heart (in conjunction with increase in heart rate and venous tone). In contrast to the Frank-Starling mechanism, the increase in force and velocity of contraction is accomplished without corresponding increase in fiber length (end-diastolic ventricular volume). Contractility does not limit the performance of the normal heart. In contrast, the failing heart is limited in its myocardial performance as indicated by displacement of the ventricular function curve downward and to the right. An increase in afterload in severe heart failure moves the heart to the descending limb; conversely, improvement in contractility displaces the heart toward the normal curve.

Inotropic State. Clinicians would welcome an objective index of myocardial contractility in which the inotropic state (intrinsic contractility of the muscle) could be measured independent of change in the length of myocardial fibers (Frank-Starling relationship). This would be useful in three different ways: (1) to examine the effects on the myocardium of an acute intervention, such as the administration of digitalis, (2) to determine consecutive changes in the inotropic state of the myocardium in the same individual during the evolution of heart failure and in response to treatment; and (3) to compare the inotropic state in different individuals.

Unfortunately, distinction between the effects of fiber length and of intrinsic contractility is difficult to accomplish for the heart. The main obstacle stems from the strong influence of mechanical loading conditions on hemodynamic measurements. Thus a change in either the preload (length of ventricular fibers at end-diastole) or the afterload (force developed in ventricular muscle during systole) can modify ventricular performance greatly without affecting its intrinsic inotropic state. Another complication is the inability of conventional hemodynamic measurements to take heart size into account so that comparisons of contractility in hearts of different size are generally unreliable.

Because changes in mechanical loading conditions confuse determinations of inotropic state, attempts are being made (1) to make these determinations under constant conditions of mechanical loading (constant diastolic volume, aortic pressure) and heart rate, (2) to devise methods for determining inotropic state that are insensitive to loading conditions, or (3) to interpret hemodynamic values in terms of a change in inotropic state when loading conditions can be adequately dis-

counted. But when determinants of mechanical performance other than inotropic state cannot be discounted — which is usually the case — more independent indices of contractility have been sought, particularly the rate of rise in ventricular pressure in the pre-ejection phase of ventricular contraction and force-velocity relationships.

Rate of Increase in Intraventricular Pressure (dp/dt). Several indices of dp/dt are being used. In practice dp/dt is determined electronically as the first derivative of the ventricular pressure. For comparative purposes, measurements are generally made at some preselected point(s) in the cardiac cycle, e.g., at 40 mm Hg. Often the value for dp/dt is further standardized by reference to some common denominator; e.g., peak dp/dt may be divided by total pressure instead of being used as dp/dt, per se. At present, application in man of the dp/dt determinations is handicapped by the need for extraordinarily high fidelity recording systems and by the difficulty in reproducing loading conditions. Although it holds considerable promise for comparisons of contractile performance in a single patient before and after intervention, it has little prospect for comparing different hearts.

As in the case of pressure, the rate of development of wall tension is also decidedly abnormal in heart failure. Moreover, in contrast to the normal heart in which wall tension decreases during systole, wall tension in heart failure remains high throughout systole so that both the velocity and the degree of shortening are abnormal.

Velocity of Contraction. The use of the velocity of contraction as a measure of contractility became popular a few years ago. In principle, it was based on force-velocity relationships developed by A. V. Hill for skeletal muscle. However, the great promise that was envisaged for this approach has not materialized.

EJECTION FRACTION. The fraction of the end-diastolic volume that is ejected per beat is termed the "ejection fraction." It is widely used as a measure of contractility and is estimated angiographically or by echocardiography. The normal systolic ejection fraction ranges from 0.56 to 0.78. A reduction in ejection fraction suggests that the ventricle is excessively dilated as a result of a depressed inotropic state.

SYSTOLIC TIME INTERVALS. Simultaneous recording of the electrocardiogram, phonocardiogram, and carotid arterial pulse allows indirect bedside appraisal of cardiac function. By this combination of recordings, total electromechanical systole is subdivided into left ventricular ejection time and the pre-ejection period. In patients with abnormalities of myocardial contractility — even before overt congestive heart failure — pre-ejection time usually lengthens, whereas ejection time shortens (the normal ratio of pre-ejection time to left ventricular ejection time is 0.35 ± 0.04 SD). This noninvasive technique is most useful in chronic coronary artery disease, arterial hypertension, and the cardiomyopathies. It does not distinguish between inotropic state and other mechanical determinants of contractility, particularly loading of the ventricle. Disturbances in conduction, valvular disease, and other unanticipated disorders may invalidate the determinations.

Chronic Compensatory Mechanisms

In principle, the heart that is chronically in a state of failure has recourse to four compensatory mechanisms:

Figure 2. Laplace relationship applied to the dilated heart. The tension developed in the wall of the heart during systole (T) is a directional force that is proportional to the product of the mean pressure that the wall is supporting (P) and the mean radius (r). Dilatation of the heart ($r_2 > r_1$) at the same pressure ($P_1 = P_2$) increases wall tension ($T_2 > T_1$). Should the wall become thinner during dilatation, the wall stress would increase as the cross-sectional area of myocardium (h) decreased (equation 2). The use of wall force (equation 3) which is proportional to the pressure and volume of the chamber eliminates considerations of chamber size and shape and of the thickness of the myocardial wall.

$$\begin{aligned} \textit{Wall tension} &= \text{Force per circumferential length of myocardium} \\ &= \frac{P \cdot \pi r^2}{2\pi r} \\ &= \frac{P \cdot r}{2} \end{aligned} \tag{1}$$

$$\begin{aligned} \textit{Wall stress} &= \text{Force per cross-sectional area of myocardium} \\ &= \frac{P \cdot \pi r^2}{2\pi rh} \\ &= \frac{P \cdot r}{2h} \end{aligned} \tag{2}$$

$$\begin{aligned} \textit{Wall force} &= \text{Pressure} \cdot \text{cross-sectional area of chamber} \\ &= P \cdot \pi r^2 \end{aligned} \tag{3}$$

increased contractility due to sympathetic nervous activity, tachycardia, hypertrophy, and dilatation. Of the four, the increase in sympathetic activity is more of a burden than a blessing, since it increases peripheral vascular resistance without contributing appreciably to the inotropic state of the faltering heart. Sympathetic activity does, however, contribute indirectly to support the cardiac output by reflexly increasing the heart rate.

HEART RATE. Chronic tachycardia is a feature of heart failure. Much of the increase in heart rate stems from cardiac reflexes that are stimulated by distention of the great veins at their junctions with the atria (Bainbridge reflex). However, in terms of energetics, tachycardia is a costly way to run the heart. Indeed, it is possible to produce, or to precipitate, heart failure by inducing tachycardia.

DILATATION. Progressive and persistent dilatation marks the transition between ventricular hypertrophy and failure. For a long while, dilatation may serve as a compensatory mechanism, increasing the contractile force of the heart by way of the Frank-Starling relationship. But dilatation gradually becomes inadequate to maintain stroke output.

Several different mechanisms seem to be involved in the ultimate inability of the dilated heart to maintain its output: (1) slippage and rearrangement of sarcomeres during progressive dilatation; as a result, they neither produce a coordinated contraction nor are properly stretched to enhance contractility as the heart dilates further; (2) high wall tension in accord with the law of Laplace (Fig. 2); as the volume of the ventricle increases so that its wall tension for a given pressure in the ventricular cavity during contraction is greater than normal, the myocardial oxygen consumption increases accordingly; (3) protracted maintenance of high wall tension during contraction; in contrast to the normal heart, in which the wall tension decreases in the course of systole, wall tension remains high in the dilated heart; (4) high energy requirements coupled with an inefficient conversion of chemical to mechanical energy; despite the decrease in stroke output, the dilated heart does more internal work and has a higher myocardial oxygen consumption than does the normal heart. Because of these limitations, chronic enlargement is an inefficient and ill-fated mechanism for achieving sustained improvement in cardiac performance.

HYPERTROPHY. Chronic exposure to abnormal pressure and volume loads leads to hypertrophy, i.e., an increase in ventricular mass. This increase in muscle mass takes time to develop. It involves increased protein synthesis in response to mechanical overload or dilatation. The stimulus for hypertrophy may be an increase either in wall force (tension) in accord with the Laplace relationship (Fig. 2) or in the energy requirements of a heart that is chronically dilated or operating at high filling pressures.

The pattern of hypertrophy depends on the load. In response to chronic volume overloading, e.g., arteriovenous fistula, the total mass increases as the chamber size enlarges but thickness does not change. This pattern is known as "eccentric" hypertrophy. In contrast, in chronic exposure to increased afterload, e.g., systemic hypertension, the end-diastolic volume remains unchanged, whereas the wall thickens. This pattern is known as "concentric" hypertrophy.

Normal ventricular contraction is a smoothly coordinated process by which the ventricular wall moves inward during systole to eject its contents. Abnormal electrical conduction interferes with this smooth performance and with ventricular function. The coordinated mechanism is further disrupted by local disease that causes zones of fibrosis to alternate with normal zones. This disposition of normal and abnormal areas leads to hypertrophy of functioning muscle not only because the geometry of the abnormal ventricle causes it to operate at a mechanical disadvantage but also because normal muscle is obliged to do work, and to expend energy, in moving and stretching damaged muscle or scar upon which it abuts.

Early in hypertrophy, muscle mass and capillary vessels increase proportionately and the contractile properties of the myocardium are preserved. But later, the inotropic behavior becomes abnormal and the capacity of the myocardium to synthesize adrenergic transmitter decreases. Indeed, once hypertrophy begins, the myocardium has been eased on the road to failure.

In the depressed inotropic state associated with hypertrophy, circulatory function is maintained for a long while by the combination of the increase in muscle mass, the Frank-Starling mechanism (Fig. 2), and augmented sympathetic stimulation by way of circulating catecholamines. But as the myocardial inotropic state continues to deteriorate, perhaps after intrinsic catecholamine stores have been depleted, circulatory compensation can no longer be maintained. Resting cardiac output then fails and filling pressures increase, leading to the clinical and hemodynamic manifestations of congestive heart failure.

Heart As A Muscle

Most studies of ventricular performance during heart failure have centered around the contraction phase. Before embarking upon these considerations, it is pertinent to consider how events during diastole influence the subsequent contraction and how the energy for cardiac contraction is derived.

RELAXATION AND DISTENSIBILITY. Filling of the ventricle during diastole depends not only on the time available but also on the pattern of relaxation. Relaxation consists of two components: an active one, which promotes relaxation by way of intrinsic mechanisms; and a passive one, arising from extension of the fibers by the inflowing blood. Incomplete relaxation would be expected not only to increase the filling pressure of the heart but also to dissipate energy. In the normal heart, the active and passive components appear to work synergistically to minimize losses in chemical energy. But in heart failure the viscous and elastic properties of the heart muscle seem to change so that there is a diminished resistance to filling (decreased "impedance") and an increased extent of ventricular expansion on filling (increased "compliance"). Thus not only the velocity and duration of relaxation but also changes in the physical properties of the muscle seem involved in heart failure.

ENERGETICS. The heart does work and expends energy during each contraction. For its supply of energy, it depends on aerobic metabolism. Some energy is expended to satisfy its basic oxygen requirements and those of activation. But the bulk of the energy is spent during contraction.

Attempts have been made over the years to dissect physiologically the major determinants of oxygen consumption of the heart. The variables that have been examined are ventricular pressure, volume, work, wall force, and contractile state. The major determinant for any given contractile state has proved to be the force (calculated as the product of ventricular volume and pressure) that is developed in the myocardium at the start of ejection and that continues to the end of systole. At each instant during ejection this wall force is changing. It is the integral of systolic force that relates closely to myocardial oxygen consumption. Other important influences in addition to wall force are heart rate and contractility. In contrast, fiber shortening has negligible effect on myocardial oxygen consumption.

For its contraction, the heart depends on the conversion of the chemical energy of oxidizable substrates into the mechanical energy of muscular contraction. ATP participates in this process as the principal store of energy released by oxidation; its breakdown by myosin ATPase is the principal way by which chemical energy is transformed into mechanical energy. ATP resynthesis in the myocardium is accomplished chiefly through oxidative phosphorylation. The rate of ATP breakdown and the quantity of energy used by the myocardium depend chiefly on the tension that is developed in the myocardial fibers rather than on the degree of shortening or the work done; this developed tension causes the ventricular walls to contract and the blood to be ejected. From a biochemical point of view, the muscle of a ventricle has failed when its generation of free energy, or its utilization of that energy in the process of contraction, is insufficient for the circulatory load which it has to handle.

Unfortunately, the biochemical basis for heart failure is not yet settled. But it is now clear that there are no consistent defects in energy metabolism or in protein synthesis. The investigative focus at present is on excitation-coupling and the role of calcium in the contractile process.

Any physiologic change or pharmacologic intervention will increase myocardial oxygen requirements if it increases either preload or afterload, increases the contractile state of the myocardium, or increases the heart rate. The usual compensatory mechanisms in severe heart failure tend to increase myocardial oxygen requirements by increasing all these parameters: fluid retention increases preload; sympathetic mechanisms increase afterload, contractility, and heart rate. Similarly, the usual interventions employed in heart failure may or may not increase myocardial oxygen requirements further, depending on the balance of changes in the aforementioned determinants in each individual case.

Heart as Component of Circulation

As the overburdened ventricle fails, it elicits venous hypertension and slowed circulation, and sets into motion peripheral mechanisms to sustain blood pressure and cardiac output.

VENOUS HYPERTENSION. With the onset of failure, the ventricle fails to empty properly during systole so that the volume of blood left in the ventricle after contraction increases, i.e., ejection fraction decreases. An increase in diastolic pressure in the ventricles and in the atrium and veins that lead to the ventricle accompanies the increase in ventricular volume. Several other elements contribute to the venous hypertension: (1) heightened venomotor tone; (2) expansion of the blood volume as a consequence of sodium retention by the kidney; and, on occasion, (3) regurgitation of blood from ventricle to atrium as the atrioventricular valve becomes incompetent either from ventricular dilatation or from improper closure during an arrhythmia.

SLOWED CIRCULATION. The circulation time depends on the cardiac output and the volume of blood interposed between the sites of sampling and injection. Should either ventricle fail, the time for a tracer substance to pass from the site of intravenous injection to the site of detection will be prolonged. For example, in left heart failure, the arm-to-tongue circulation time, measured by using Decholin as a tracer, will be prolonged beyond the normal limits of 10 to 15 seconds; delay of the tracer in traversing the pulmonary circulation and dilated left heart, as well as excessive dilution of the tracer by the enlarged intervening blood volume, contributes to the delay. Similarly, the arm-to-breath circulation time measured after the intravenous injection of ether will be prolonged in right heart failure. By relating the circulation times to the central venous pressure, it may be possible to establish at the bedside which ventricle has failed. For example, in left heart failure, central venous pressure and ether circulation time will be normal, whereas Decholin time will be prolonged.

PERIPHERAL MECHANISMS TO SUSTAIN CARDIAC OUTPUT AND BLOOD PRESSURE. In order to sustain the cardiac output, to apportion it selectively, and to maintain the systemic arterial blood pressure, a variety of peripheral mechanisms are activated.

Autonomic Nervous System. Normally, a four- or fivefold increase in oxygen consumption elicits a doubling of the cardiac output. When the increase in cardiac output cannot keep pace with the level of activity, distribution of blood flow is altered to defend vital areas, e.g., brain and heart. The autonomic nervous system is deeply involved in this rearrangement of the circulation. It also contributes to activation of the mechanisms for retaining sodium and water.

Peripheral vasoconstriction and tachycardia are the hallmarks of the usual forms of heart failure. Paradoxically, despite a generalized increase in sympathetic nervous activity, norepinephrine stores in the heart muscle are depleted because of defective local synthesis. Consequently, the failing heart, denied local adrenergic support for its inotropic and chronotropic responses, is obliged to rely on norepinephrine delivered to it by the blood from the adrenal medulla and the peripheral vasculature. Pharmacologic agents, such as guanethidine, which further deplete the heart of its catecholamines, aggravate heart failure. In many respects, the performance of the human heart that has failed resembles that of both the "denervated" heart and the isolated heart-lung preparation that Starling used. The role that the parasympathetic nervous system plays in heart failure is ill defined, but evidence does exist to indicate that its contribution to the control of heart rate and baroreceptor activity is impaired.

PERIPHERAL VASOCONSTRICTION. Peripheral arteriolar and venoconstriction, mediated by heightened sympathetic nervous activity, are essential compensatory mechanisms in heart failure. The extent to which accumulation of sodium and water in the arteriolar wall contributes to increased arteriolar resistance is as yet unclear. Selective arteriolar vasoconstriction helps not only to sustain the blood pressure but also to preserve function in critical organs. The pattern of selective vasoconstriction, in turn, influences the cardiac output by determining the total peripheral resistance to cardiac emptying.

Selective venoconstriction promotes venous return by transfer of returning blood to the central veins. Although peripheral venoconstriction may contribute importantly to the increase in central venous pressure, the major determinant is myocardial incompetence in coping with the venous return.

REDISTRIBUTION. In order to maintain oxygen delivery to vital organs (brain and myocardium) during heart failure, blood flow is diverted by heightened sympathetic nervous activity from skin, kidneys, splanchnic viscera, and muscle. At first the redistribution of blood flow among organs occurs during activity or stress, i.e., as cardiac output fails to increase appropriately for the increment in metabolism; later it operates also at rest. The mechanism for diversion is the balance between sympathetic innervation and local metabolism: the circulations to skin, kidney, splanchnic organs, and skeletal muscle are richly innervated, and these viscera have low metabolic rates; sympathetic nervous vasoconstriction easily overrides local metabolites. In contrast, the circulations to brain and myocardium are poor in alpha-adrenergic receptors; these organs, with high oxygen consumption, produce ample metabolic dilators to counterbalance heightened sympathetic activity.

In the normal subject during exercise, as need for heat dissipation increases, cutaneous hyperemia develops. In contrast, the patient in heart failure fails to develop cutaneous hyperemia despite increasing need for heat dissipation. The net effect is that the patient in heart failure, suffering from a low cardiac output during exercise, preserves blood pressure and blood flow to vital organs by paying the penalty of impaired heat loss as well as inadequate blood flow to exercising muscles.

VALSALVA MANEUVER. An abnormal response to the Valsalva maneuver, in which intrathoracic pressure is maintained at approximately 40 mm Hg for 10 to 12 seconds, is a useful test for left heart failure. The autonomic nervous system, operating in conjunction with the expanded volume of blood in the left side of the heart and pulmonary venous system, contributes to the abnormal response. During strain, the normal subject manifests a characteristic decrease in blood pressure and pulse pressure and increase in heart rate; when straining stops, the blood pressure, pulse pressure, and bradycardia "overshoot." In contrast, the patient in left heart failure demonstrates a "square wave response" of blood pressure: at the start of straining, blood pressure increases abruptly, stays high during the maneuver, and drops precipitously to baseline after the maneuver, without overshoot. Throughout the procedure there is little or no change in pulse pressure and no tachycardia. The lack of reflex changes stems from the failure of stroke output or arterial pulse pressure to change during the straining phase, so that no reflex changes are elicited in peripheral vessels.

Salt and Water Retention. As the patient slips into heart failure, the reduction in cardiac output is associated with a decrease in renal blood flow and glomerular filtration rate, and with a redistribution of blood flow within the kidneys. These hemodynamic changes undoubtedly contribute to the sodium and water retention of heart failure, but in different ways and to different degrees according to the stage of heart failure. Early in heart failure, when filtration rate is decreased, much of the sodium retention is attributable to the decrease in the filtered load of sodium presented to the tubules for reabsorption. Later on, humoral factors, predominantly hyperaldosteronism and a group of extra-adrenal, sodium-retaining influences ("factor III") predominate.

There is little doubt that disturbed hemodynamics are importantly involved in the release of the humoral factors. Thus a large role is currently envisaged for diminished baroreceptor stimulation in the renal afferent arterioles or a decrease in the sodium load passing the macula densa, or both, in activating the renin-angiotensin-aldosterone mechanism. In addition, baroreceptor effects arising in the distended left atrium or underfilled arterial tree may affect renal hemodynamics and the renin-angiotensin-aldosterone system. Other reflexes engaged in the intense sympathetic activity of heart failure may also be involved. Clearly, the hemodynamic-neurohumoral interplay that results in sodium and water retention is complex and incompletely understood. On the other hand, awareness of the important role of hyperaldosteronism in the genesis of sodium and water retention has provided new approaches to the therapy of heart failure using aldosterone antagonists.

Not only urine but also sweat and saliva are sodium poor. But the underlying mechanisms are different. Antidiuretic hormone is not directly involved in the genesis of the edema of heart failure.

The expansion of the circulating blood volume contributes to sustaining the cardiac output and the perfusion of vital organs. Rarely is the expansion in blood volume marked, usually ranging from 10 to 20 per cent in moderately severe heart failure to 30 to 50 per cent in severe, refractory heart failure. But even modest expansion helps to augment the ventricular-end-diastolic volume, thereby improving ventricular performance by way of the Frank-Starling principle. Unfortunately, the high end-diastolic volume and pressures promote the formation of edema by raising capillary pressures in the circulation behind the failing ventricle. At a time when circulation blood volume may be increased by 20 per cent, the extravascular fluid volume may have doubled.

CLINICAL MANIFESTATIONS OF HEART FAILURE

The signs and symptoms of heart failure depend on the ventricle that has failed and the duration of the failure. The clinical syndrome of left ventricular failure is dominated by *symptoms* of pulmonary congestion and edema. In contrast, right ventricular failure is dominated by *signs* of systemic venous congestion and peripheral edema. Fatigue and weakness are common in both types of heart failure.

Left Ventricular Failure

Symptoms

Complaints of respiratory discomfort or distress dominate the symptoms of left ventricular failure. They vary with position, stress, and activity. They are often associated with physical signs of disturbances in the lungs or in respiratory control mechanisms.

DYSPNEA. Like pain or anxiety, dyspnea is subjective and difficult to quantify. Because breathing is ordinarily automatic and effortless except after strenuous exertion, the complaint of breathlessness may signify anything from awareness to distress. Dyspnea during modest exertion is usually the first symptom of left heart failure. Usually dyspnea is associated with increased rate of breathing (tachypnea).

The physiologic basis for the sensation of dyspnea remains unclear. Both lungs and the chest muscles may contribute. Thus interstitial edema in the vicinity of the pulmonary capillaries stimulates juxtacapillary receptors ("J-receptors"), thereby reflexly setting a pattern of rapid, shallow breathing; associated with this abnormal pattern is an increase in the work and oxygen cost of moving the stiff lungs. However, this increased amount of work on the lungs is done in the face of diminished blood flow to the respiratory muscles, a consequence of the diminished cardiac output and redistribution of blood flow. Consequently, the disproportion between work done by the respiratory muscles and the supply of blood delivered to them may contribute to fatigue of the respiratory muscles and to the sensation of dyspnea. Sensory elements within the respiratory muscles may also contribute to respiratory discomfort by registering the disproportion between the inordinate amount of energy that is being spent by muscles and the amount of ventilation that they produce.

Although precise mechanisms for dyspnea remain uncertain, its occurrence in left heart failure clearly depends on the increase in the blood and water content of the lungs at the expense of the air volume. Ventilation increases as the air volume is progressively encroached upon, and, as the minute ventilation approaches the maximal ventilatory capacity, the likelihood of dyspnea increases.

ORTHOPNEA. Progressive, and often urgent, dyspnea that occurs soon after lying flat is designated as orthopnea; it is relieved by sitting up. The physiologic basis for orthopnea is the augmented venous return from the lower extremities and splanchnic bed to the lungs that results from redistribution of gravitational forces in the supine position and the reabsorption of diurnal edema. In the patient with heart disease, orthopnea is reliable evidence of left ventricular failure. In contrast, the dyspnea of chronic lung disease or musculoskeletal disorders is rarely aggravated by lying flat.

The patient learns to avoid respiratory distress at night by supporting head and thorax by two or more pillows. In severe heart failure, orthopnea may force the patient to sleep upright in a chair rather than in bed. In some patients with extensive coronary artery disease and left ventricular failure, orthopnea occurs only in the left lateral position; the mechanism for this is unclear.

Cough and expectoration are common in left heart failure, presumably a consequence of reflexes from the congested lungs and bronchi. The patient may also manifest an orthopneic cough which has the same significance as orthopnea, and is presumably the consequence of venous congestion and edema of the tracheobronchial walls. In some patients, precordial distress may substitute for breathlessness in the supine position. This "nocturnal angina" is also somehow related to the mobilization of water from the tissues to the circulation when the patient goes to bed.

PAROXYSMAL NOCTURNAL DYSPNEA. A bout of urgent respiratory distress, verging on suffocation, may rouse the patient unexpectedly from sleep and cause him to seek relief desperately, either by sitting up or by rushing to the open window to breathe "fresh air." Respiration may be labored and wheezing, hence the designation "cardiac asthma." The episodes represent intolerable aggravation of pulmonary congestion and edema during sleep in the supine position. A combination of dulling of the respiratory center to sensory input from the lungs during sleep and increase in venous return to the lungs makes it possible for pulmonary venous congestion and edema to accumulate to the point of precipitating the frightening episode of breathlessness.

ACUTE PULMONARY EDEMA. In an acute episode of left ventricular failure, such as that which follows myocardial infarction, the inability of the left ventricular myocardium to handle the blood that the competent right ventricle is delivering to it may result in an abrupt increase in pulmonary venous and capillary pressure, followed by flooding of the interstitial spaces and alveoli. If the edema is confined to the interstitial spaces of the lungs, an increase in respiratory frequency because of stiff lungs would be expected to produce alveolar hyperventilation and respiratory alkalosis; conversely, once free fluid enters the terminal bronchioles and mounts the respiratory tree, respiratory acidosis may occur because of imbalances between alveolar ventilation and alveolar blood flow (ventilation-perfusion inhomogeneities).

Pulmonary edema may begin with a cough, with wheezing, or with breathlessness. Often there is a sense of oppression in the chest. At first, except for the abnormal breathing pattern and the evidences of heart disease, there may be few physical signs. In time, as free fluid enters the distal airways, rales become audible, most marked in the dependent parts of the lungs, but extending upward as the attack worsens. In a severe attack, the patient is pale, sweating, cyanotic, obviously gasping for breath, and usually producing frothy sputum which may be blood tinged.

HEMOPTYSIS. Rusty sputum, laden with heart failure cells (alveolar macrophages containing hemosiderin), occurs frequently in severe left heart failure. Frankly bloody sputum is generally a sign of pulmonary infarction. In severe pulmonary edema caused by left ventricular failure, the frothy fluid that pours from the bronchial tree is often pink, i.e., blood tinged, owing to the escape of red cells into the alveoli from the congested minute vessels of the lungs.

CHEYNE-STOKES RESPIRATION. Some patients with severe heart failure display periodic breathing characterized by alternate periods of apnea and hyperventilation. Cyclic changes in arterial blood gas tensions accompany this waxing and waning of the ventilation: during apnea, the arterial P_{O_2} reaches its peak, whereas the arterial P_{CO_2} reaches its nadir. At the same time, alveolar gas tensions are exactly opposite: the alveolar P_{O_2} reaches its peak during hyperpnea; the alveolar P_{CO_2} reaches its nadir during hyperpnea. This discrepancy between arterial and alveolar gas tensions has been attributed to the fact that changes in arterial blood gases *cause* the swings in ventilation, whereas the changes in alveolar gas tension are the *consequences* of the changes in ventilation. The critical role of the arterial blood gases stems from the prolonged circulation time between the lungs and the respiratory centers in the brain. This slowing of the circulation exposes the central respiratory control mechanisms to arterial blood that differs in gaseous composition from that in pulmonary venous blood. In essence, because of slowing of the circulation, negative feedback is delayed. As expected, the longer the circulation time, the longer the cycles of hyperventilation and apnea. The neurologic and cerebrovascular changes of old age predispose to Cheyne-Stokes breathing.

Physical Signs

In addition to being breathless, the patient is generally pale, a bit dusky, and sweaty. His handshake is cold because of peripheral vasoconstriction. The heart rate is rapid and the pulse pressure is narrow, with a modest increase in diastolic blood pressure. If only the left ventricle has failed, the neck veins are not distended.

THE HEART. Enlargement of the heart is usually evident to inspection and palpation of the apical impulse and is confirmed by roentgenologic and radiographic examination. Angina pectoris is not a manifestation of heart failure, nor is palpitation common unless overzealous administration of digitalis and diuretics has occasioned digitalis toxicity. As the left ventricle fails and pulmonary venous pressure increases, pulmonary arterial pressure also increases, and the heart sound attributable to pulmonary valve closure increases in intensity. Also, as the left ventricle dilates, the mitral valve leaflets fail to appose properly, resulting in mild mitral incompetence.

Gallop Rhythm. The advent of a third heart sound during diastole in an adult with heart disease signifies the advent of heart failure. The fixed sequence of the two normal sounds and the abnormal third sound, in conjunction with an increase in heart rate, is responsible for the characteristic cadence of a gallop rhythm. The third heart sound ("S-3 gallop") occurs early in diastole during the state of rapid ventricular filling. This ventricular gallop presumably originates in the vibrations of the ventricular walls as the rapidly inflowing blood is abruptly arrested; this extra sound, normal in young children and in young adults, is generally a reliable sign of ventricular failure in the middle-aged or elderly patient with heart disease.

A gallop rhythm may also originate in the atrial contribution to ventricular filling. This atrial or "S-4 gallop" is not unique for heart failure, because it may reflect diminished ventricular compliance resulting from hypertrophy or ischemia rather than myocardial failure. If a patient with a fourth heart sound develops heart failure, a third sound appears to cause a quadruple rhythm. If the heart rate is rapid or the P-R interval is prolonged, the atrial and ventricular gallop sounds summate ("summation gallop"). In the candidate for heart failure, summation gallop has the same implication as other diastolic gallop rhythms, particularly if it persists as the heart is slowed.

Pulsus Alternans. In patients with heart disease, particularly if the cause is hypertension, cardiomyopathy, or coronary arteriosclerosis, the appearance of alternating strong and weak beats, even though the fundamental rhythm remains regular, heralds the onset of heart failure. This pulsus alternans may be detected by palpation or by sphygmomanometry. It often follows an extrasystole. Rarely is this mechanical alternans associated with electrical alternans. The mechanism for pulsus alternans has been attributed to alternations in fiber length (ventricular end-diastolic volume) or to alternating increase and decrease in the number of contractile units, or to both.

THE LUNGS. A characteristic consequence of interstitial edema and pulmonary venous congestion is tachypnea. As left heart failure progresses, interstitial edema is succeeded by alveolar edema and fluid in the terminal bronchioles, particularly at the lung bases. Accordingly, bilateral basal rales are common in moderate failure of the left ventricle.

Electrocardiogram

Abnormalities in the electrocardiogram arise from the underlying cardiac disorder and from therapeutic agents, e.g., digitalis and diuretics, rather than from heart failure per se.

Radiologic Aspects

The x-ray can be exceedingly helpful in the diagnosis of left ventricular failure. Typically, the cardiac silhouette is enlarged, often assuming telltale configurations that are determined by the underlying disorder. In contrast to the normal, in which pulmonary *arteries* are prominent in the lower lung fields, pulmonary vasculature is prominent at the apices, reflecting pulmonary *venous* hypertension and redistribution of blood flow because of edema and fibrosis at the bases. Enlarged hilar shadows accompany the prominent pulmonary veins in the upper lung fields.

Prominent septal lines, particularly near the costophrenic angles (Kerley's lines), indicate the presence of interstitial edema. The advent of alveolar edema is signaled by a generalized clouding of the lung fields. Pleural effusion may occasionally occur in left heart failure, but is much more apt to occur in biventricular heart failure. Evidence of interstitial and alveolar edema often lessens or disappears when right ventricular failure supervenes. However, hydrothorax generally persists. A widened shadow of the superior vena cava may provide reliable evidence of right ventricular failure and systemic venous congestion.

Pulmonary Function Tests

Traditionally, the course of overt failure of the left ventricle, particularly the response to treatment, has been followed by consecutive determinations of vital capacity. This is an insensitive measure, usually associated with decrease in compliance and occasionally with increase in airway resistance. Recently it has been shown that earlier in the course of pulmonary edema — presumably when the excess fluid is still confined to the interstitial space around alveoli and terminal airways (less than 2 mm in diameter) — expiratory flow rates at *low lung volumes* are reduced and peripheral airways tend to close prematurely during expiration, trapping gas within the lungs and disturbing the distribution of alveolar gas with respect to pulmonary capillary blood. This has led to a variety of tests (e.g., "closing volumes") which are designed to detect premature closure and resultant maldistribution of air — presumably by interstitial edema — long before compliance falls and total resistance of airways increases. During recovery there is usually a delay before expiratory flow rates and closing volumes return to normal, even though left atrial pressure is again within normal limits. The basis for the persistent abnormalities is presumably the gradual removal of interstitial edema from the vicinity of the small airways and blood vessels.

Associated with the high closing volume is evidence of ventilation-perfusion abnormalities manifested by widening of the alveolar-arterial ΔPo_2 and a decrease in arterial Po_2 caused by "venous admixture." Nonetheless, arterial oxygen saturation is generally near normal unless independent lung disease is present. Along with the decrease in arterial Po_2 is a widening of the arterial venous difference in O_2 content owing to the increased extraction of oxygen in the tissues. Arterial CO_2 tension remains normal or low unless free fluid enters the terminal airways in the course of pulmonary edema. Abnormally high values for CO_2 tension indicate that considerable free fluid has made its way into the airways.

Right Ventricular Failure

Clinical Manifestations

Isolated failure of the right ventricle is uncommon, generally a consequence of cor pulmonale secondary to intrinsic lung disease. More often, right ventricular failure is a sequel to left ventricular failure. In right ventricular failure, neck veins are distended and fill from below; the engorged liver may be tender to gentle pressure, and compression causes a surge of blood into the neck veins (hepatojugular reflux). In time, when both ventricles have failed, evidence of right ventricular failure may dominate the scene; but continuing dyspnea and rales attest to the persistence of left ventricular failure, and the continuing low cardiac output is manifested by signs of increased sympathetic nervous activity and of organ hypoperfusion.

Weakness may be marked and is occasionally associated with anorexia, weight loss, and malnutrition ("cardiac cachexia"). Not only severe heart failure but also digitalis, diuretics, and electrolyte disturbances are generally involved in the genesis of this cachectic state.

CYANOSIS. Bluish discoloration of the skin and mucous membranes is designated as cyanosis. It is due to an abnormal concentration of reduced hemoglobin (more than 5 grams per 100 ml) in the subpapillary venous plexus of the skin. In right heart failure, the congested venules, containing blood from which considerable oxygen has been extracted because of the slow flow, account for the cyanosis. In left heart failure, cyanosis is usually caused by a complication, e.g., pneumonia, unless overt pulmonary edema is present.

ABNORMAL HEART AND LUNGS. Although the breathlessness of the left ventricular failure may be somewhat relieved by right heart failure, usually some dyspnea persists along with tachypnea and basal rales. Severe right heart failure (and dilatation) may produce tricuspid valvular insufficiency, thereby contributing to systemic venous engorgement. The murmur of tricuspid insufficiency is distinguished from that of mitral insufficiency by its location (lower left border of sternum) and by its tendency to increase during inspiration. Hydrothorax, generally unilateral, is more common than in isolated left ventricular failure.

SYSTEMIC VENOUS CONGESTION. Distention of systemic veins is a hallmark of right heart failure. Several different mechanisms contribute to its genesis: (1) the inability of the failing right ventricle to cope adequately with the venous return; (2) the increase in the quantity of blood contained in the large systemic veins; and (3) increased venomotor tone, resulting from heightened sympathetic nervous activity. The increase in systemic venous pressure underlies the hepatomegaly, splenomegaly, and peripheral edema that characterize right heart failure. Less apparent are the congestion and edema of the gastrointestinal tract that the systemic venous hypertension produces.

Pressure in the superficial jugular vein is a useful index of right atrial pressure and, with experience, may be reliably estimated from the height of the fluid column distending the cervical vein. Normally, the cervical veins are flat in the erect position, whereas in right heart failure they are prominent and distended, usually with a level that pulsates. Functional tricuspid insufficiency, complicating dilatation of the right heart, distorts the normal venous pulse by increasing its v wave. Usually superficial venous distention precedes the onset of hepatomegaly and peripheral edema. Occasionally, compression of the abdomen over the liver (hepatojugular reflux) is necessary to display the increased blood volume in the venous system.

LIVER. The liver is usually enlarged and palpable in right heart failure, often in association with mild abdominal discomfort, and generally somewhat tender to compression. In severe right heart failure, particularly if the onset is acute, constraint of the swollen liver by its tight capsule may cause right upper quadrant pain. Tricuspid insufficiency accompanying right ventricular dilatation may cause synchronous pulsations in neck veins and liver. Splenomegaly is uncommon except in prolonged congestion of the liver. Rarely is the enlarged spleen tender from congestion per se.

Early in hepatic congestion, sensitive liver function tests, such as the handling of Bromsulphalein, are apt to be abnormal, and modest increases in the concentrations of cellular enzymes in serum, such as glutamic oxaloacetic transaminase (SGOT) increases in serum bilirubin, are not uncommon. The hyperbilirubinemia consists of a combination of quick- and slow-reacting bilirubin, presumably a consequence of decreased oxygen delivery to the liver arising from hypoperfusion and venous hypertension. But jaundice is uncommon unless hepatic congestion is associated with longstanding pulmonary congestion and, often, with pulmonary infarction.

If cardiac output is severely curtailed and liver congestion is marked and protracted, hypoglycemia may occur, presumably owing to depletion of glycogen stores in the liver and increased formation of lactic acid from glucose because of hypoxia. During physical activity, hepatic blood flow in heart failure decreases further, resulting in a marked decrease in aldosterone breakdown, thereby furthering sodium retention.

Repeated bouts of right heart failure elicit atrophy and necrosis of liver cells in the vicinity of the central veins and stimulate extensive fibrosis ("cardiac cirrhosis"). Many months of reduced hepatic blood flow and high venous pressures are required for this reaction, which may result in a shrunken, fibrotic liver difficult to distinguish from posthepatitic cirrhosis. Hepatic coma is a rare, preterminal complication of severe hepatic congestion and fibrosis.

EXTRACELLULAR FLUID COMPARTMENTS. In normal subjects, the fluid compartments of the body are held remarkably constant as the result of an automatic interplay among *intake* (governed by thirst and appetite), *transcellular exchanges* of fluid and electrolytes (governed by passive and active mechanisms), and *excretion* (regulated mainly by the kidneys). In heart failure, this automatic balance tends to be upset mainly because of inordinate retention of salt and water by the kidneys. The result is an isosmotic expansion of the extracellular fluid in which the circulating blood volume shares. It is conceivable that early in heart failure the conservation of salt and water may serve a useful purpose by expanding the blood volume either to sustain venous return to the failing heart or to relieve the arterial baroreceptors from undue stimulation as the cardiac output fails. But this teleologic explanation does not apply when the myocardium can no longer respond to increased filling pressures and volumes, and the retention of salt and water only aggravates congestion and edema.

The distribution of the excess extracellular fluid varies from patient to patient. In the patient who is up and about, edema accumulates in the feet and ankles under the influence of gravity; in the bedridden patient, the fluid shifts to the sacral region. Low tissue pressure, as around the back of the ankle, predisposes to localization. The level of colloid osmotic pressure and the integrity of the lymphatic system also influence the distribution of the excess fluid.

Subcutaneous Edema. Dependent edema, manifested as swelling of feet or ankles, developing gradually during the day and subsiding by morning, is a characteristic feature of right heart failure. Invariably, it is anteceded by systemic venous congestion, but after diuresis subcutaneous edema may linger even though systemic venous hypertension has been relieved by the reduction in venous blood volume. Usually a gain in weight precedes clinical evidence of edema. If edema is allowed to persist, complications such as low-grade cellulitis may occur. The combination of edema and slowed venous flow predisposes to thrombosis and to pulmonary embolism. The massive pitting edema of the lower extremities that was commonly seen before the advent of potent diuretics is now rarely encountered except in instances of gross neglect.

Hydrothorax. It is so uncommon for hydrothorax to complicate isolated failure of the right ventricle, that the association of pleural effusion and cor pulmonale should lead to search for an independent mechanism for the pleural effusion, e.g., pulmonary infarction. On the other hand, as indicated previously, it is quite common in combined heart failure (right and left). The pathogenesis of hydrothorax involves impaired removal of water from the pleural space because of high venous pressures in both the pulmonary and systemic circulations, thereby not only compromising transcapillary exchange of water in the pleura but also impeding lymphatic drainage. Hydrothorax contributes to dyspnea not only by encroaching on the air volume but also reflexly, probably by stimuli from lungs and chest wall. Pulmonary infarction may cause pleural effusion in two ways: by direct contiguity of the infarcted area of the lung and the pleural space, or by aggravation of heart failure.

Ascites. Clinically evident excess of free fluid in the abdominal cavity is designated as ascites. It is a late manifestation of right heart failure, generally associated with marked systemic venous hypertension, severe peripheral edema, and hydrothorax. It occurs most frequently in patients with tricuspid valvular disease (or with constrictive pericarditis). Portal and hepatic venous hypertension, coupled with high pressure in the systemic veins draining the peritoneum, seem to be involved in the etiology of ascites; but retention of salt and water is a fundamental prerequisite for ascites to occur. Usually ascites is first noticed by the patient as a gradual increase in abdominal girth. But in severe right heart failure, it may cause anorexia, abdominal discomfort, or pain.

Pericardial Effusion. In severe and persistent heart failure, abnormal quantities of transudate may accumulate in the pericardial sac. Rarely does fluid accumulate to the level of tamponade.

Anasarca. Massive right heart failure may cause excess fluid to accumulate everywhere in the body, most conspicuously in subcutaneous tissues and abdominal and thoracic cavities. Because of the influence of gravity, face and arms are spared until preterminally.

GASTROINTESTINAL TRACT. The bowel wall shares in the systemic venous congestion and edema. These changes rarely interfere with absorption of drugs or foods unless heart failure is extreme. In severe congestive heart failure, anorexia, nausea, and vomiting may occur from reflex, central, or local causes. Occasionally, when right heart failure is severe, a protein-losing enteropathy may develop.

BRAIN. Neurasthenia, headache, and insomnia are common in heart failure. Usually these manifestations are attributed to a combination of a modest diminution of cerebral blood flow and triggering mechanisms, e.g., dyspnea contributing to insomnia. Cerebral manifestations are more frequent when the reduction in cerebral blood flow is superimposed on antecedent cerebrovascular disease, e.g., arteriosclerosis, or personality disorder. Severe heart failure is often associated with irritability, restlessness, and difficulty in fixing attention, particularly in older persons. Preterminally, stupor and coma may develop. The possibility exists that central nervous abnormalities may be enhanced by the delivery to the brain of abnormal products elaborated by remote organs (liver, endocrines, gastrointestinal tract) that suffer deranged metabolism during heart failure as a result of congestion and hypoperfusion.

KIDNEY. Oliguria occurs in both right and left heart failure but is much more striking in the latter. As the heart improves, urinary output increases. The urine is poor in sodium but has a high specific gravity (1.020 to 1.030). Azotemia is common but generally moderate except when intrinsic renal disease is present or after vigorous diuresis. The combination of azotemia and high specific gravity is distinctive for heart failure (and dehydration) and contrasts with the low specific gravity of intrinsic renal disease. Proteinuria is common but rarely severe — usually less than 1 gram per day. A variety of casts accompany the proteinuria. Renal function, as determined by clearance techniques, is only slightly depressed except in severe right failure of long standing.

OTHER MANIFESTATIONS. In severe congestive heart failure, the accumulation of edema may obscure the gradual loss of tissue mass. Often this tissue wasting is associated with *weakness*. In extreme instances, *cachexia* may

develop. At this late stage, the patient is usually suffering from anorexia, gastrointestinal upsets, anemia, and electrolyte upsets. Part of the picture undoubtedly stems from organ hypoperfusion and congestion, but often a large contribution has been made by overvigorous use of diuretics and digitalis.

Anxiety. It is not surprising that patients with organic heart disease become anxious. Indeed, anxiety is a regular feature by the time the heart fails. But not always is it an easy matter to distinguish between cardiac complaints as manifestations of anxiety or of the cardiac disorder. Part of the difficulty stems from the nonspecific nature of complaints, such as breathlessness, especially if the patient does have organic heart disease. The difficulty is compounded if the patient misinterprets or exaggerates his symptoms unconsciously. For example, the severely anxious patient may hyperventilate to the point of alkalosis, producing the characteristic lightheadedness, cold hands, and tingling fingers of hypocapnia, reduced cerebral blood flow, and peripheral vasoconstriction, thereby reinforcing his view of the organic nature of his breathlessness. Palpitation is also commonly misinterpreted by the patient suffering from anxiety as a telltale sign of organic heart disease.

The standard approach for the physician is the separate assessment of the organic versus the psychosomatic aspects of the heart disease. Particularly helpful in this regard are excessive or inconsistent complaints for the role of the cardiac disease. Not infrequently, hemodynamic measurements may be required to settle the role of organic heart disease in producing the clinical symptoms.

CLINICAL MANAGEMENT

General Measures

The aim of treatment in heart failure is to arrest and reverse the pathogenic sequence that led to the clinical signs and symptoms. The response to treatment of the more common types of heart failure, i.e., hypertensive and arteriosclerotic, is often dramatic. But each relapse marks another milestone on the road to refractory heart failure, not only by signaling progressive deterioration of the myocardium, but also because intensified and protracted treatment enhances the prospect for eliciting the toxic manifestations of the therapeutic agents.

INCREASING CARDIAC OUTPUT. In most forms of chronic heart failure, the cardiac output can be made to increase by decreasing the cardiac load, by improving myocardial contractility, or by a combination of the two. In the patient with severe bradycardia associated with heart failure, acceleration of the heart rate by cardiac pacing may cure heart failure that would otherwise be refractory. Conversely, severe tachycardia must be arrested if filling times of the ventricles are too greatly curtailed by the abbreviated diastole.

DECREASING THE WORK OF THE HEART. Lightening the cardiac load is prerequisite for the successful treatment of heart failure. The load is always assessed with respect to the state of the myocardium, i.e., a damaged heart may not be able to cope with a blood pressure or volume load that a normal heart handles easily. The aim of treatment is to promote ventricular emptying so that the stroke output of the heart will increase. If successful, the improved cardiac performance reverses the train of clinical manifestations that the low cardiac output had initiated.

The traditional mainstays of cardiotonic therapy are rest, digitalis to improve the inotropic state of the myocardium, and diuretics to reduce the filling pressure of the failing ventricle. Rest is sometimes overlooked as an effective instrument for decreasing the cardiac burden. It must be both physical and mental. For the patient in left ventricular failure, simply sitting upright and breathing more easily is conducive to mental ease. Reassurance is essential to decrease metabolic activity and tachycardia and to relax peripheral vasoconstriction. No amount of reassurance will suffice to relieve a patient experiencing the pangs of severe constipation or urinary retention. Oxygen by nasal catheter (4 to 6 liters per minute) often makes the patient more comfortable even though the degree of arterial hypoxemia is exceedingly modest, possibly by increasing oxygen delivery to the brain. After recovery from an acute bout of heart failure, a new life style of lessened activity may be required as part of the cardiotonic program. Should reassurance prove inadequate, sedatives or tranquilizers (such as chloral hydrate, 0.5 to 1.0 gram, phenobarbital, 15 to 30 mg, or diazepam, 2 to 10 mg, taken orally three times per day and at bedtime) may be needed to promote mental ease, particularly as the patient improves and grows restless. Narcotics are rarely needed in heart failure unless pulmonary edema has generated intolerable anxiety. Excessive sedation, to the point of immobilizing the patient, enhances the risk of venous thrombosis and embolism, particularly in the elderly.

It is remarkable how often the proper use of rest as the initial step in treatment will promote a vigorous diuresis, slow the heart rate, and relieve dyspnea, thereby allowing a more leisurely use of other cardiotonic agents, such as digitalis and diuretics. On the other hand, if metabolic demands remain high, as during undetected thyrotoxicosis or fever, heart failure may prove refractory to the conventional cardiotonic program until the thyroid overactivity is curtailed.

Acute Pulmonary Edema

Treatment of the acute pulmonary edema of left ventricular failure is begun with the patient in the sitting position, thereby draining the upper portions of his lungs of excess fluid. Meperidine, 50 mg, or morphine, 10 to 15 mg, is administered intravenously for restlessness or dyspnea. These agents seem to act primarily by relieving anxiety and agitation. Morphine is the traditional agent. How it works is still a matter of debate. Most clinicians credit its effectiveness to its role in relaxing the patient and in decreasing tachycardia. Evidence for a direct venodilating effect that would withhold blood from the overloaded ventricle is more convincing under experimental conditions than in human heart failure. Unfortunately, distressing side effects, such as nausea, vomiting, and urinary retention, are sometimes troublesome and force recourse to other sedatives. A rapid-acting diuretic, ethacrynic acid or furosemide, is administered intravenously. Even though arterial oxygenation may be near normal, high concentrations of humidified oxygen, 50 to 100 per cent, are frequently used empirically to relieve dyspnea, restlessness, and confusion.

Most initial or mild episodes of pulmonary edema respond quickly to the aforementioned program of rest,

reassurance, morphine, and diuretic. When the prospect of severe and progressive pulmonary edema is likely, attempts are generally instituted to reduce preload or afterload, or both. The drugs that are used are considered subsequently under Unloading Agents. In addition to drugs, several other interventions are in common practice: rotating tourniquets on the extremities, phlebotomy (of the order of 200 to 300 ml of blood), or positive pressure breathing which impedes venous return. All three of these interventions have become less popular since the advent of vasodilator therapy. Systemic hypotension is a contraindication to phlebotomy or to positive pressure ventilation.

Digitalis is more essential for supporting the myocardium after the loads on the heart have been lessened than during the acute bout of pulmonary edema. However, a digitalis preparation is usually part of the first wave of therapy in the emergency room. Digitalis (digoxin or lanatoside C, 1.0 mg) may be administered intravenously if the patient has had none during the preceding two weeks. However, the urgency for intravenous injection of digitalis has decreased considerably since the advent of potent, rapid-acting diuretics. An exception to this generalization is the attack of pulmonary edema precipitated by a bout of tachycardia which can be slowed by digitalis, e.g., paroxysmal atrial fibrillation. In this instance, digitalis relieves the heart failure primarily because of its effect on slowing atrioventricular conduction and consequently the ventricular rate, rather than because of its inotropic effect on the heart. In ectopic tachycardias, it may be necessary to resort to DC electroshock in order to restore normal heart action and tolerable heart rates.

Face to face with a patient in pulmonary edema, the physician often feels compelled to apply a battery of strenuous measures in rapid succession or simultaneously. Especially for patients in poor condition, this treatment may be worse than the disorder, which is usually self-limited once the upright position has been assumed, mental rest accomplished, and a potent diuretic administered. As soon as the crisis is over, a more conventional cardiotonic program is begun, and a search is made for the cause of the left heart failure as well as for the mechanism that precipitated the episode.

The role of left heart failure in producing high-altitude pulmonary edema is not clear. Prompt recovery usually follows bed rest, descent to lower altitude, and the administration of oxygen.

Inotropic Agents: Digitalis

Although immediate therapeutic agents for coping with the acute episode of heart failure may not include digitalis, once the crisis is over, lasting improvement almost invariably requires the use of digitalis glycosides. Unfortunately, establishing the proper dose of digitalis is not always straightforward, because optimal doses vary somewhat from patient to patient and with associated clinical disorders. Moreover, unless standard brands of predictable potency are prescribed, tablets may vary considerably in effectiveness. Finally, the concomitant administration of other, apparently unrelated, medications may lead to drug interactions which interfere with the effect of the digitalis.

DRUG INTERACTIONS. Multiplicity of drugs is the rule in modern therapy. Some drugs are deliberately prescribed in combinations, either to reinforce a desirable therapeutic effect or to avoid an untoward side effect. A familiar example of this practice is the combination of digitalis, a potassium-losing diuretic, and potassium supplements for the treatment of heart failure; the dosage of each is individualized to achieve maximal inotropic effect on the heart and to relieve circulatory congestion. But other drugs, such as sleeping pills and anticoagulants that are administered concomitantly for subsidiary or unrelated purposes, may interact and decrease the effectiveness of the cardiotonic program.

There are several ways by which one therapeutic agent can influence the effects of another. Among these are (1) chemical interaction (cholestyramine, a cholesterol-lowering, ion-exchange resin, impedes absorption of digitoxin [and, to a much lesser extent, of digoxin] by binding in the intestine); (2) competition for binding sites on plasma proteins (digitoxin and ethacrynic acid compete for albumin); (3) induction of drug-metabolizing enzymes (phenobarbital and phenylbutazone enhance the metabolism of digitoxin by hepatic microsomal enzymes); and (4) enhanced excretion (polar metabolites of digitoxin are eliminated more rapidly in urine and bile than is digitoxin per se). In conventional dosages, few of these interactions seem to be clinically significant even though cholestyramine has been advocated in treating digitoxin intoxication. But they do introduce an element of unpredictability into standard therapeutic programs, and they do urge caution whenever medications are either added to or deleted from a stable therapeutic regimen.

Related to the concept of drug interaction is the broader concept of drug-biologic interaction which determines how drugs act. This broader concept includes reactions between the pharmacologic agent and some biologic aspect of the living subject. For example, digitalis effects depend heavily on ion fluxes at ultrastructural membranes; changes in ionic composition and behavior are known to modify the clinical influence of digitalis. Or the physiologic state of the patient may shape the response: acidosis blunts the effectiveness of norepinephrine; the administration of a conventional dose of a ganglionic blocking agent, when sympathetic vasomotor tone is high because of vigorous diuresis and depletion of blood volume, may precipitate circulatory collapse.

The concept of drug-biologic interaction is complicated by individual variability in responsiveness to drugs. Part of this variability is undoubtedly inherited; part is immunologic; most remains to be explained.

DIGITALIS: GENERAL ASPECTS. Digitalis improves the contractility of the failing myocardium regardless of the type of heart failure, the rate, or the rhythm. After digitalis has been given in effective doses and myocardial contractility has increased, the heart shrinks in size, cardiac output increases, end-diastolic volume and pressure decrease, venous pressure normalizes, and evidences of peripheral vasoconstriction, circulatory congestion, and organ hypoperfusion disappear. In the reordering of the circulation that follows relief of congestive heart failure, blood that had been sequestered in the splanchnic venous bed is redirected to the systemic veins by appropriate adjustments in vascular tone, thereby helping to sustain the improved cardiac output.

Molecular Bases. Although the full picture of how the digitalis glycosides improve cardiac contractility is not yet clear, they do seem to act by altering surface and intracellular (sarcoplasmic reticulum and mitochondria)

membranes so that they release calcium ions more readily. Another manifestation of a change in cellular membrane characteristics caused by the glycosides is inhibition of the Na^+-K^+-ATPase activity. However, it is unsettled whether this interference with ATPase, as well as the associated decrease of sodium pumping into the cell, is directly related to the inotropic effect of the glycosides.

Effect on Inotropic State. In low output heart failure, digitalis increases the cardiac output and restores the end-diastolic pressure in the left ventricle to normal. This is a consequence of increased myocardial contractility. A similar effect on contractility occurs in the normal myocardium, but the cardiac output does not increase because of a direct vasoconstricting effect of digitalis on the peripheral resistance vessels. But in low output heart failure in which sympathetic nervous activity is consistently high, restoration of the cardiac output by digitalis reflexly diminishes sympathetic tone, thereby overriding the direct vasoconstricting effects of digitalis on the vessels. These distinctions underscore the unique property of digitalis glycosides as inotropic agents because of their ability to improve myocardial contractility in heart failure without simultaneously eliciting antagonistic effects, such as peripheral vasoconstriction (or tachycardia).

Myocardial Oxygen Consumption. The increase in the strength of contraction produced by the digitalis glycosides increases the oxygen consumption of the myocardium in the normal heart. But this tendency is neutralized in the failing heart which responds to glycosides by shrinking in volume, thereby reducing wall tension and its associated oxygen consumption. Accordingly, the increase in contractility produced in the dilated failing heart is generally accomplished with no increase in myocardial oxygen consumption.

Catecholamine Depletion. Although reduction in cardiac catecholamines is a feature of chronic heart failure, this depletion leaves unaffected the positive inotropic effects of the digitalis glycosides.

Coronary Circulation. In the normal unanesthetized animal, ouabain elicits coronary vasoconstriction. Unfortunately, nothing is known about the behavior of the coronary circulation in response to digitalis during heart failure.

Systemic Circulation. Digitalis elicits an increase in cardiac output, thereby reducing the reflex vasoconstriction of the low output state. But because of the direct constrictor action of cardiac glycosides on vascular smooth muscle, there is apt to be a brief period of increase in systemic arterial pressure, particularly if large doses of cardiac glycosides are administered intravenously.

CHOICE OF DIGITALIS PREPARATION. Five digitalis preparations are in common use today in the United States: digitalis leaf, digoxin, digitoxin, deslanoside (Cedilanid-D), and ouabain. Their basic pharmacologic actions on the heart and their toxic-therapeutic ratios are quite similar. But they do differ considerably with respect to the rate and degree of absorption from the intestine and both the onset and duration of action.

Digoxin and digitoxin have replaced digitalis leaf for chronic oral administration; ouabain and deslanoside, as well as digoxin, are administered intravenously. Digitoxin is not as satisfactory an intravenous agent, because it is relatively slow in reaching its peak effect. Digitalis leaf is gradually disappearing from use, because it varies

TABLE 2. Administration of Common Cardiac Glycosides

| Preparation | Digitalization | | | Cardiotonic Effects | | Blood Levels | |
	Loading Dose* (mg/24 hrs)	Initial Dose† (mg)	Maintenance Dose (mg)	Onset of Activity (min)	Peak Effect (hrs)	Steady State Therapeutic Level¶ (mg/ml)	Half-Life (hrs)
Digoxin (oral)	2.5	1.0	0.25	60–120	1–3	1.5	36
Digitoxin (oral)	1.2	0.75‡	0.1	30–120	4–6	17	96–144
Deslanoside (IV)	1.6	0.8§	–	10–30	1–2	–	33
Ouabain (IV)	0.25	0.25§	–	3–10	0.5–2	0.5	21

(These values are examples to illustrate orders of magnitude.)

*Total quantity to be administered in 24 hours for therapeutic effect.
†Assuming no prior digitalis during previous two weeks.
‡The same dose may be administered intravenously if urgent digitalization is required.
§When feasible, switch to oral maintenance doses of digoxin or digitoxin.
¶On conventional maintenance doses.

in potency, requires bioassay for standardization, and has no therapeutic advantage over digitoxin which is its principal constituent.

Traditional practice in digitalization has relied on a preliminary loading phase to achieve a therapeutic level, followed by maintenance dosage to sustain a balance between intake and elimination. Accordingly, the preset loading dose is administered over a period of one to three days (Table 2), providing enough digitalis to load body stores and to compensate for daily elimination. Unless a desperate situation — such as a life-threatening cardiac arrhythmia — calls for acute digitalization, slow digitalization is preferable. Indeed, if there is no hurry, continued administration of the maintenance dose, without a loading dose, has proved to be a practical way to achieve digitalization.

Dosages listed in Table 2 are intended to indicate orders of magnitude rather than precise schedules. Dosage is determined individually according to the nature and severity of the heart disease, the clinical setting, the use of other drugs such as potassium-losing diuretics, and continued observation of the patient's response.

Oral Preparations. Digoxin and digitoxin have replaced digitalis leaf for chronic oral administration.

DIGOXIN. The maintenance dosage of digoxin is determined by a balance between renal excretion, dose, and absorption. Ordinarily, between 75 and 90 per cent of an oral dose is absorbed. Digoxin is lipid soluble and absorbed from the small intestine by diffusion. Some variation in absorption may occur, depending on the solubility of digoxin molecules in the intestinal fluids. Variability in absorption may also result from different preparations of digoxin. Consequently, once a digoxin

preparation from one manufacturer has proved effective, changes should be avoided.

Digoxin is excreted primarily by the kidney, and most of the drug appears unchanged in the urine. When fully digitalized, the concentration of digoxin in serum is approximately 1 per cent or less of total body stores of digoxin. If renal function is normal, approximately one third of the body stores is eliminated per day; the maintenance dose replenishes this daily loss. The half-life of digoxin in serum is approximately the same in normal subjects and in patients with heart failure, averaging one and one half days. However, the half-life is prolonged in renal failure. The serum level of digoxin in renal insufficiency is directly related to the creatinine clearance and inversely to the concentration of urea nitrogen in the blood (BUN). Formulas have been devised to take these relationships into account, recognizing that, in contrast to the normal daily elimination of one third of body stores of digoxin, the anuric patient eliminates about one seventh. Accordingly, the anuric patient will require one half or less of the usual maintenance dose.

Only 5 per cent of digoxin in serum is bound to protein. Its polar structure accounts for the difference between its concentration and that of digitoxin (nonpolar) in the serum (Table 3).

Without an initial loading dose, patients receiving digoxin orally reach a steady state in the serum, reflecting equilibrium between body stores, intake, and elimination in about one week. The steady state level in serum is approximately 1 per cent or less of total body stores of digoxin. Body stores are related to lean body weight, because digoxin does not accumulate in fat or interstitial fluid. In an adult patient, body stores are generally of the

TABLE 3. Features of Cardiac Glycoside Preparations in Common Use

Preparation	Source	Usual Route of Administration*	Gastrointestinal Absorption	Protein Binding†	Principal Route of Elimination
Digoxin	*Digitalis lanata*	Oral	75–90%‡	23%‡	Kidneys
Digitoxin	*Digitalis purpurea*	Oral	90–100%	97%	Liver; kidney for metabolites
Deslanoside	*Digitalis lanata*	Intravenous	Erratic	–	Kidneys
Ouabain	*Strophanthus gratus*	Intravenous	Erratic	0	Kidneys

(These values are examples to illustrate orders of magnitude.)

*All can be administered intravenously.
†Affinity for protein (albumin) determines rate of urinary excretion and persistence in body.
‡Varies according to preparation. Different tablets differ in bioavailability of digoxin.

order of 0.01 mg per kilogram of body weight. Rarely are body stores required greater than 0.02 mg per kilogram of body weight. Therefore for a 70-kg patient, digitalization usually requires a minimal dose of approximately 0.7 mg. Should this digitalizing dose be exceeded in order to achieve better control of the clinical state, the prospects for toxicity will increase accordingly.

The essential features in using digoxin therapeutically are summarized in Table 2. Because of its short half-life, a single dose per day will cause a wide swing in serum concentration (and in body stores, including the heart) before the next dose is administered. In practice this swing is often unimportant; but, if desirable, its magnitude may be reduced (and therapeutic control improved) by administering one half the daily dose at 12-hour intervals. Many clinicians use digoxin for intravenous as well as oral administration, because its hemodynamic and biologic properties are comparatively well understood, and dosages are relatively easy to adjust.

DIGITOXIN. This agent is widely used for chronic administration. It differs importantly from digoxin in its metabolism and its slow rate of elimination; the main route of elimination is by metabolism in the liver, only a small fraction being eliminated by the kidney.

Digitoxin is completely absorbed after oral administration so that oral and intravenous dosages are identical. Body stores and digitalizing doses are approximately the same, but maintenance doses are quite different because of different rates of elimination. Approximately 12 per cent of body stores of digitoxin is eliminated per day in patients with normal renal function. The usual body store is estimated to be of the order of 0.8 mg in a 70-kg adult. Therefore the daily maintenance dose is generally 0.1 mg per day (0.12×0.8 mg). Because of its slow dissipation and elimination, serum levels of digitoxin vary less from hour to hour than do digoxin levels. But the drug accumulates insidiously so that maintenance doses established at the onset often prove to be toxic in time.

In contrast to digoxin, digitoxin has a strong avidity for albumin so that 97 per cent in plasma is nondialyzable. This combination is a critical factor in limiting glomerular filtration and excretion of digitoxin by the kidneys. After an oral dose of 1.0 mg, 50 per cent of the inotropic effect is reached in one hour; 85 to 100 per cent is achieved in four hours and sustained for the rest of the day. The average half-life is approximately five days. Digitoxin enters into an enterohepatic cycle. Between 30 and 60 per cent of the 1.0 mg dose is eliminated in the feces and urine, the larger fraction generally in the urine. The remainder is metabolized, primarily to digoxin, which is eliminated in the urine. Digoxin is preferable to digitoxin in renal or hepatic insufficiency.

Intravenous Preparations. As a rule, these are reserved for life-threatening situations. These include acute heart failure complicating a bout of atrial fibrillation with rapid ventricular rate, fulminating pulmonary edema as a complication of left ventricular failure, and the onset of heart failure or a serious arrhythmia during surgery. As a rule, the larger the dose of the glycoside, the more apt it is to create problems, particularly arrhythmias, of its own.

An intravenous bolus of a digitalis preparation may elicit a bout of hypertension, particularly if the dose is large, e.g., 1.0 mg of digoxin. The increase is generally of the order of 20/10, and the effect is generally short lived. But it may suffice to overburden the failing heart and to aggravate the situation until it subsides and is succeeded by the inotropic effect. Hypertension is rarely a problem if the intravenous dose is modest and administered slowly.

OUABAIN. This is the traditional digitalis preparation for intravenous use. It is a pure crystalline substance that is unsuitable for oral use because of erratic absorption from the gastrointestinal tract. Its latency after intravenous injection is exceedingly brief (less than five minutes); it is rapidly eliminated so that it is not suitable for maintenance of digitalization. The initial intravenous dose is 0.25 to 0.3 mg, administered slowly. An additional 0.15 or 0.3 mg may be repeated after 24 hours.

DESLANOSIDE. This preparation is identical with digoxin except for the addition of a glucose residue. It is gradually replacing ouabain in popularity for intravenous use. Its digitalizing effect appears in 10 to 30 minutes after intravenous injection, reaches peak effect in one to two hours, and regresses in 24 hours. For rapid intravenous digitalization, the full 1.6 mg may be given at once, or, preferably, 0.8 mg may be followed by another 0.8 mg, either in four hours or in divided doses, at two- to four-hour intervals for two or three additional doses. Maintenance of digitalization is preferably done by oral digoxin or digitoxin. But, if necessary, 0.4 mg may be given intravenously or intramuscularly at 8- to 12-hour intervals.

DIGOXIN. For rapid digitalization, 0.5 mg is given initially, followed by 0.25 mg every two to four hours as needed, but taking care to avoid exceeding a total dose of 2 mg in 12 hours. As soon as practical, the oral route is substituted for the intravenous route.

Diagnostic Preparations. ACETYLSTROPHANTHIDIN. This is a partial synthetic which, because of its exceedingly rapid onset of action and dissipation, has been advocated more as a diagnostic test for adequacy of digitalization than as a therapeutic agent for heart failure. In practice, repeated injections of the substance (0.25 mg in 5 ml of glucose and water) are made until toxic or therapeutic effects are observed. Because it is potentially dangerous, other diagnostic tests are being investigated.

GUIDES TO PROPER DOSAGE OF DIGITALIS. A major problem in using digitalis for its inotropic effect is the threat of inducing arrhythmias by virtue of its other effects on the heart (Fig. 3). On the other hand, if rapid atrial fibrillation coexists with heart failure, slowing of the ventricular rate, a consequence of slowed atrioventricular conduction, has proved to be a practical guide to digitalis dosage. Fortunately, slowing of the heart rate when atrial fibrillation coexists with heart failure also provides a rough measure of the inotropic effect (and of serum levels of the glycoside). On the other hand, when heart failure coexists with a normal sinus rhythm, slowing of the heart is a treacherous index of inotropic effect. Digitalis toxicity is common if large doses are administered in the attempt to slow the sinus tachycardia, particularly if a mechanism such as pulmonary emboli, infection, or hyperthyroidism is operating to sustain the rapid heart action.

The clinician now has available several different and effective digitalis preparations. Although none of these has any intrinsic advantage over the others with respect to myocardial contractility, they vary considerably with respect to speed of action, time course of effectiveness, and rates of elimination. Because of the ever-present prospect of digitalis toxicity, before starting to administer digitalis it is important to know whether digitalis, in any form, has been taken during the preceding week or two.

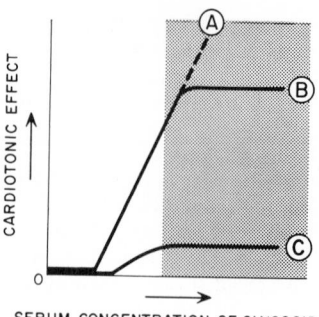

Figure 3. Hypothetical effects on contractility elicited by increasing doses (and serum concentrations) of digitalis. Once the inotropic effect of the digitalis preparation begins, it is unlikely that it will continue indefinitely as in A. Instead, it is likely that beyond a certain point the inotropic effects will taper to a plateau despite increasing serum concentration. When this plateau will occur depends on the capability of the heart to respond; a left ventricle that is suffering its first bout of failure is apt to manifest an excellent inotropic response for small increments in serum concentration before the plateau is reached (B). On the other hand, a spent heart that has suffered multiple myocardial infarctions may only manifest a sluggish inotropic response from the start and plateau early despite enormous increments in serum levels of glycoside (C). The shaded area is intended as a reminder of the increasing likelihood of serious arrhythmias as serum glycoside levels continue to increase.

Longer may be required if renal failure is present, particularly if digoxin was used. It cannot be overemphasized that the intravenous administration of a bolus of a digitalis preparation to a patient who has recently taken digitalis may precipitate ventricular tachycardia or fibrillation.

Clinical manifestations and the electrocardiogram are the key guides to dosage. As the circulation improves and signs and symptoms of heart failure abate, conventional dosage schedules are tailored to individual needs. The usual changes in the S-T segment and in the T waves produced by digitalis merely indicate that appreciable quantities of digitalis have been taken but provide no measure of dosage or efficacy. On the other hand, digitalis toxicity may first be manifested by electrocardiographic changes of abnormal conduction and of ectopic pacemakers.

Prophylactic. The perennial question of administering digitalis prophylactically, especially before surgical procedures, is again being discussed. This practice requires the administration of a preset dose without conventional criteria for distinguishing between adequacy and toxicity. Therefore uncertain guidelines for safe administration are coupled with questionable therapeutic benefits. Compounding this uncertainty is the prospect of hypoxia and electrolyte imbalance during surgery. Because of the availability of digitalis preparations that do act rapidly and effectively, there seems to be little basis at present for prophylactic digitalization.

DIGITALIS TOXICITY. Digitalis preparations are among the most dangerous, as well as the most useful, of current medications. The incidence of cardiotoxicity is staggering — of the order of 10 to 20 per cent in hospitalized patients receiving conventional doses of digitalis — and mortality from digitalis cardiotoxicity is estimated to run into the thousands per year.

Several different reasons account for much of this morbidity and mortality. (1) The narrow margin between therapeutic and toxic doses; this predisposes to digitalis toxicity during ordinary use but enhances its prospects when dosages are increased in the attempt to deal with increasing congestive heart failure. (2) The heavy reliance on slowing of heart rate and clearance of circulatory congestion as indices of improved contractility; this practice works well in atrial fibrillation but may be disastrous in normal sinus rhythm. (3) The ease with which changes in the clinical situation can derange stability of control; among the more common upsetting influences are electrolyte disturbances (particularly hypopotassemia), acute myocardial ischemia, upset acid-base balance, hypoxemia, renal impairment, autonomic nervous imbalances, other drugs, and infection. (4) Incomplete understanding by the physician of the distinctions in the clinical pharmacology of the various digitalis preparations; for example, differences in the renal handling of digoxin and digitoxin must be taken into account when choosing the proper glycoside in patients with renal insufficiency.

Recognition. The electrocardiogram is generally the final arbiter of digitalis cardiotoxicity. But three categories of clinical clues direct attention to the electrocardiogram: (1) the appearance of central nervous system evidence of digitalis toxicity, particularly anorexia and aversion to food; (2) a change in the arrhythmia, including unusual slowing or acceleration of the heart rate; and (3) regularization of the heart rate in the patient with atrial fibrillation while taking maintenance doses of digitalis.

Although serum levels are now quite popular as indices of digitalis toxicity, the lack of close correspondence between serum levels of glycosides and moderate cardiotoxicity in individual patients has kept alive interest in other tests to evaluate myocardial sensitivity to digitalis. These include the acetylstrophanthidin tolerance test, which is dangerous and should be reserved for experts. Among the more recent and innocuous is the salivary electrolyte test which relies on increases in the concentration of calcium and potassium in the saliva as an index of digitalis toxicity. This test is as yet empirical, because the mechanism for the increase in the concentration of these electrolytes is unknown. The practical value of this test remains to be established.

Digitalis cardiotoxicity is primarily a matter of arrhythmias. As might be expected from the diverse effects of digitalis on the heart, the arrhythmias are generally nonspecific. However, the coincidence of depressed atrioventricular conduction and stimulation of ectopic pacemakers is virtually unique for digitalis toxicity. This combination accounts for arrhythmias characterized by simultaneous rapid atrial rates and slow ventricular responses, for escape beats, and for nonparoxysmal junctional tachycardia. For example, atrial tachycardia with atrioventricular block, generally precipitated by overzealous administration of potassium-losing diuretics, is characteristic, although not specific, for digitalis toxicity. Even more distinctive is atrioventricular dissociation with junctional rhythm, in which two pacemakers operate independently above and below the intervening area of atrioventricular block. In atrial fibrillation, the advent of serious digitalis toxicity may be signaled by regularization of the ventricular rate because of acceleration of an ectopic focus below a high degree of atrioventricular block.

The usual cause of death in digitalis toxicity is ventricular fibrillation. Rarely does it appear unexpectedly. More often, it is presaged by multifocal premature contractions and runs of ventricular tachycardia. Consequently, premature ventricular beats that appear after digitalis has been started or during maintenance therapy have to be regarded as serious warnings of toxicity, particularly if they are multifocal in origin and if there is bigeminy involving premature beats that are bizarre in appearance. Rarely do ventricular arrhythmias occur without other evidence of digitalis intake, including the characteristic ST-T deformations, disturbances in atrial ventricular conduction, and atrial arrhythmias.

Treatment. The mainstay for treating digitalis cardiotoxicity is to stop the digitalis and to discontinue diuretics that contributed to hypokalemia. There is no specific antidote. Fortunately, most digitalis-induced arrhythmias are arrested by stopping digitalis. Thus junctional rhythms without excessive ventricular rates or evidence of ventricular irritability are generally treated without specific medication or intervention. But if the arrhythmia is characteristic of ventricular irritability or if it has caused hemodynamic upset in the form of hypotension, heart failure, and pulmonary edema, medical intervention is mandatory.

Potassium is the agent of choice for suppressing digitalis-induced automaticity. But because it slows conduction through the myocardium and specialized conduction tissues, thereby potentiating the depression produced by digitalis, it must be used with extreme caution when atrioventricular block is severe. In the latter case, the introduction of a temporary perivenous cardiac pacemaker may prove useful in tiding the patient over the period needed to eliminate the excess digitalis, particularly if antiarrhythmic drugs are to be used to suppress ectopic atrial or ventricular beats.

If the arrhythmia has produced no crisis, if renal function is adequate, and if there is no hyperkalemia, potassium salts (4 to 6 grams of potassium chloride per day) may be administered orally. On the other hand, if the situation is deteriorating rapidly because of ectopic beats or uncontrollable tachycardia, potassium salts may be administered intravenously. Continuous electrocardiographic monitoring is mandatory during intravenous administration. The combination of continuous monitoring and careful intravenous titration of the arrhythmia is generally safer than is oral administration. The usual preparation for intravenous use contains 40 mEq of potassium in a 500 ml solution of 5 per cent glucose in water; this is administered slowly, e.g., at a rate of 40 mEq per hour. This may be repeated, if necessary, for up to three doses. Hypotension may limit the amount of potassium that can be given by vein. The electrocardiogram is monitored throughout, recognizing that high plasma concentrations of potassium may per se cause death through cardiac depression, arrhythmias, or arrest. The characteristic changes in the EKG are disappearance of the P wave, widening of the QRS complexes, changes in the S-T segments, and tall, peaked T waves.

Antiarrhythmic drugs which decrease ventricular automaticity by slowing diastolic depolarization, such as procainamide, lidocaine, propranolol, and diphenylhydantoin, are effective but must be used cautiously. Procainamide is useful when potassium fails to control the arrhythmia or if potassium is contraindicated because of uremia or hyperkalemia. It also has the advantage of sustained action if digitalis toxicity should persist. But it runs the risk of hypotension, depression of contractility, and producing AV block.

Lidocaine (1 to 2 mg per kilogram in one to two minutes by intravenous injection or as continuous infusion) has been used to control premature ventricular beats and ventricular tachycardia resulting from digitalis. It produces an effect within 45 to 90 seconds which is dissipated within 20 minutes. It has the advantage over procainamide of not causing hypotension. Doses less than 750 mg per hour are rarely associated with significant toxic effects, i.e., neurologic disorders and convulsions.

Diphenylhydantoin has been advocated for the treatment of digitalis-induced arrhythmias because it does not depress atrioventricular conduction. It is administered intravenously at a rate of 5 to 10 mg per kilogram over a 5- to 15-minute period. Propranolol, quinidine, and chelating agents are also being used. Electroconversion by DC shock, which has proved to be remarkably effective in controlling many arrhythmias, is a desperate measure of last resort in digitalis-toxic arrhythmias because of the likelihood of producing uncontrollable paroxysmal ventricular arrhythmias.

BLOOD LEVELS. The pharmacologic effectiveness of most drugs depends on concentration at the site of action. Dosage may be a poor guide to this effective concentration because of biologic unpredictability with respect to absorption from the gastrointestinal tract, patterns of distribution throughout the body, and rates of metabolism and excretion. In general, it is anticipated that concentration of a drug in the blood (serum or plasma) will relate better to therapeutic consequences, including toxicity, than will dosage.

In recent years, as a result of advances in radioimmunoassay technology, determination of serum concentrations of some cardiac glycosides became practical and available as well as reliable, accurate, and specific. The application of these tests to patients taking digitalis preparations (digoxin, digitoxin) has shown that the frequency and severity of toxic effects increase progressively as serum concentrations exceed therapeutic levels.

But some overlap in concentrations does occur, particularly in the zone between toxic and therapeutic levels. Moreover, occasionally there is a complete disparity between serum concentration and clinical consequences. These divergences are not unexpected because of the multiplicity of physiologic, pathologic, and biochemical influences that can modify the response to a given concentration of glycoside in the serum (and at the site of action): e.g., hypokalemia, acid-base disturbances, hypoxemia, interaction with other drugs, hypoproteinemia, acquisition of tolerance. But the exceptions do emphasize that serum concentrations must be interpreted critically in the light of the clinical setting.

Currently, determination of serum concentration of a digitalis glycoside is most useful in patients who are suspected of digitalis toxicity but are unable to provide an accurate account of digitalis dosage. It also has a place in guiding dosage in candidates for digitalis toxicity, e.g., heart failure complicated by renal insufficiency or by violent biochemical and physiologic perturbations, as after cardiac surgery. At the other extreme, determination of serum concentration may indicate that refractory heart failure may simply be a consequence of inadequate dosage.

DIGITALIS IN ACUTE MYOCARDIAL INFARCTION. As a general rule, digitalis is the drug of choice for myocardial failure. Since some degree of left ventricular failure is characteristic of acute myocardial infarction, it might seem reasonable to afford high priority to digitalis in the therapeutic program. Although this generalization still applies to *severe* heart failure during acute myocardial infarction, particularly if the heart is enlarged, the value of digitalis in less urgent degrees of left ventricular failure during acute myocardial infarction is much less certain.

The dilemma stems from the noninfarcted myocardium. If the noninfarcted ventricle has failed, considerable improvement is to be expected from the inotropic effects of digitalis; conversely, if the noninfarcted ventricle is normal, the inotropic effect will be of little consequence, particularly when compared with the inotropic effects of circulating catecholamines that the acute crisis has promoted. The possibility also exists that, even if digitalis does enhance contractility of the noninfarcted area, the net effect on cardiac performance may not be impressive because of the paradoxical motion of the infarcted area during cardiac contraction.

In addition to these uncertainties concerning enhanced contractility, the threat exists that digitalis may promote ventricular irritability in the peri-infarcted, ischemic zone of the myocardium, thereby predisposing to ectopic foci and uncontrollable ventricular arrhythmias. This likelihood is accentuated by a variety of other concomitant influences that predispose to ventricular arrhythmias: increased sympathetic activity, hypokalemia, and hypoxemia (to which excess sedation may contribute).

These reservations, plus the availability of effective diuretics to clear pulmonary congestion and edema during the first few days of an acute myocardial infarction, encourage extraordinary circumspection in using digitalis during the acute episode. On the other hand, if heart failure persists after the acute crisis — because of either extensive scarring or unremitting hemodynamic overload — digitalis is clearly required because the myocardium has failed globally. Moreover, should atrial fibrillation with a rapid ventricular response complicate acute myocardial infarction early or late in its course, digitalis may be lifesaving. For other supraventricular arrhythmias, which generally require larger doses of digitalis and may even prove refractory, antiarrhythmic agents or electrical conversion are preferable during the phase of increased ventricular irritability.

OTHER INOTROPIC AGENTS: SYMPATHOMIMETIC AMINES. Although fashions in diuretics continue to change, no inotropic agent has as yet been found to compete with digitalis. Substitutes have been sought among the sympathomimetic amines which also stimulate the myocardium but differently from digitalis. The qualifications that have been sought include effectiveness after oral administration, improved contractility in conjunction with peripheral vasodilation, increased renal excretion of sodium, and a greater increase in coronary blood flow than in myocardial oxygen consumption. Three catecholamines have been singled out for close scrutiny because of their ability to stimulate the heart and to decrease peripheral resistance: epinephrine, isoproterenol, and dopamine. Unfortunately, none of these is on a clinical par with digitalis: all three provoke tachycardia; epinephrine decreases the elimination of sodium by the kidney, whereas isoproterenol usually has no effect on sodium excretion; dopamine has to be given intravenously, acts briefly, and causes undesirable increments in systemic arterial pressure.

Glucagon, a polypeptide hormone produced chiefly by the α cells of the pancreas, attracted considerable attention for a while as a possible adjunct for the patient in refracto-

ry heart failure who can tolerate no more digitalis. Like the catecholamines, glucagon presumably exerts its cardiotonic effects by activating adenyl cyclase. It has been given by continuous intravenous infusion (2 to 4 mg per hour for 10 to 13 days) and by injections of large single doses (10 to 25 mg). In these doses, the major side effect was nausea; abnormalities in blood sugar levels were uncommon. Unfortunately, enthusiasm for this agent has begun to wane because of recent evidence that the effects of glucagon on myocardial contractility are far less consistent in chronic heart failure than in the normal heart.

UNLOADING AGENTS (VASODILATOR THERAPY). The use of vasodilator agents began with refractory heart failure. Some patients with severe heart failure become unresponsive to increasing dosages of digitalis and diuretics and manifest toxicity. Because of their bleak outlook, the idea of improving the performance of the heart by administering vasodilators immediately caught hold. Its popularity was ensured by the availability of a wide assortment of agents for trial. At present, criteria have been liberalized so that the use of vasodilators is no longer restricted to refractory heart failure (Table 4). Indeed, questions are being raised about the feasibility of using these agents prophylactically.

Principles. The normal ventricle usually adjusts automatically to a change in afterload so that cardiac output and stroke volume remain virtually unchanged; if cardiac output does increase, it is because of an increase in heart rate. In contrast, the failing ventricle improves its emptying when afterload is reduced (Fig. 4), thereby increasing stroke volume and cardiac output without increasing heart rate. By this tactic, the failing heart responds to a decrease in afterload by shifting its ventricular function curve toward normal even though the inotropic state of the myocardium is unchanged. Thus by reducing afterload the failing heart can increase its output without increasing either preload or contractility. Since contractility, preload, and heart rate are major determinants of myocardial oxygen consumption, the use of agents that reduce afterload in heart failure includes the attractive prospect that better emptying of the ventricle will be achieved while decreasing myocardial oxygen requirements.

An early attempt at reducing afterload in severe heart failure was the use of arterial counterpulsation. This approach is still being used to treat patients who experience shock after myocardial infarction and involves the placement of an intra-aortic balloon device to reduce afterload and to raise diastolic aortic blood pressure. More recently, reduction in afterload has been approached using pharmacologic agents that induce systemic vasodilatation.

TABLE 4. Current Clinical Uses of Reduction in Afterload

Chronic myocardial failure
  Refractory heart failure in ambulatory patients
  Acute heart failure unresponsive to standard cardiotonic and
    diuretic program
Acute myocardial infarction
  Particularly with hypertension
  With severe heart failure
  With cardiogenic shock
Acute left ventricular failure due to cardiac overload
  Hypertensive crisis
  Acute aortic insufficiency
  Complications of acute myocardial infarction
    Ruptured chordae tendineae leading to mitral regurgitation
    Ventricular septal defect

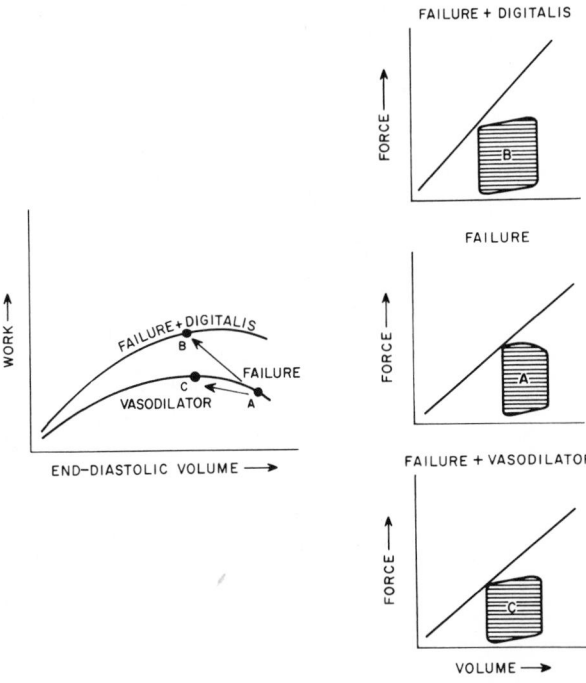

FAILURE + DIGITALIS

FAILURE

FAILURE + VASODILATOR

Figure 4. Schematic ventricular function curves comparing effects of vasodilator (reduction in afterload, per se) and vasodilator plus digitalis (inotropic effect) in heart failure. *Left,* The administration of a vasodilator in severe heart failure (A) moves the heart to an improved position on the lower curve of impaired contractility (B). Digitalis shifts the heart to a curve of improved contractility (C). *Right,* Analysis of work done per beat for points B, A, C shown on left. The landmarks on the work loops are the same as in Figure 2.

Three broad categories of vasodilators have been tried: arteriolar, venous, and a combination of the two (Table 5). The prototype is nitroprusside, which exerts its vasodilator effects directly on systemic arterioles and veins. Venodilation operates by pooling blood in peripheral veins, thereby decreasing venous return to the heart and decreas-

ing left ventricular end-diastolic volume and pressure (preload). Arteriolar dilatation decreases the impedance to left ventricular ejection (afterload). The over-all unloading effect of nitroprusside depends on the hemodynamic state of the heart. If the heart is not in failure so that output and filling pressures are normal, nitroprusside has little or no effect on stroke output; left ventricular end-diastolic pressure falls. The unchanged output and the concomitant decrease in filling pressure presumably reflect an equivalent reduction in preload and afterload by the nitroprusside. In contrast, if myocardial function is severely impaired, stroke output increases as left ventricular end-diastolic pressure falls because nitroprusside causes a greater decrease in afterload than in preload. In practical terms, the unloading effect of nitroprusside is most apt to be helpful when the left ventricular end-diastolic pressure is greater than 12 to 15 mm Hg and the cardiac output is low. Unloading of the heart by nitroprusside is not accompanied by a change in heart rate or in contractility. However, as systemic arterial pressure and end-diastolic volume fall, ventricular wall tension decreases and consequently the myocardial oxygen requirement falls. Thus in severe heart failure nitroprusside affords the prospect of achieving better emptying of the ventricle while decreasing myocardial oxygen requirements.

Phentolamine accomplishes vasodilation somewhat differently from nitroprusside. It is an alpha-adrenergic blocking agent as well as a direct dilator of systemic arterial and venous blood vessels. As in the case of nitroprusside, the effects of phentolamine on stroke output depend on the level of left ventricular filling pressure. However, phentolamine is less of a venodilator than an arteriolar dilator, so that it exerts a greater effect on impedance to ventricular emptying than on preload.

Nitroglycerin exerts its greatest effect directly by relaxing venous smooth muscle. As a result, venous return to the heart decreases. Therefore the predominant therapeutic effect of nitroglycerin is accomplished by reducing ventricular preload. Although nitroglycerin does have a vasodilator effect on systemic arterioles, the venodilator effect predominates.

Other vasodilator agents that are currently being tried are indicated in Table 5. Undoubtedly new agents will

TABLE 5.   Representative Vasodilators Used to Reduce Afterload in Heart Failure

Agent	Route of Administration	Usual Dosage	Predominant Sites of Action	Blood Pressure	Cardiac Output	PA Wedge	Heart Rate	Comment
				Predominant Hemodynamic Effects				
Sodium nitroprusside	IV	Start with 15 μg/min and increase gradually;* maximum of 400 μg/min: usual, 65 μg/min	A, V†	+	++	++	0 or +	Hazard of thiocyanate or cyanide toxicity during prolonged therapy or high doses
Phentolamine	IV	Start with 0.1 mg/min;* maximum of 2 mg/min	A, V	+	++	++	+	Chief effect on arterioles; causes tachycardia
Nitroglycerin	IV Sublingual		V	+	+	+++	0	Transient (15-30 min); negligible effect on arterioles
Isosorbide dinitrate	Oral Sublingual	20-40 mg 2.5-10 mg	V	+	+	+++	0	Same as nitroglycerin but longer (1-4 hrs)
Hydralazine	Oral	50-75 mg q 6 hrs	A	0 or +	+++	0 or +	0	Sometimes used in conjunction with venodilator
Trimethaphan	IV	Start with 2-4 mg/min; decrease, maximum of 6 mg/min	A, V	+	++	++	0	No reflex increase in heart rate; adjust dose carefully to avoid marked hypotension

*Increase every 10 to 15 minutes, using arterial blood pressure and pulmonary wedge pressures as guides. Avoid large fall in systemic blood pressure while pulmonary wedge pressure is returning to about 15 mm Hg.

†A = Arterial bed. V = Venous bed.

continue to appear during the next few years. In applying any of these it is important to relate their predominant and side effects to the hemodynamic state of the patient.

Clinical application of agents that reduce afterload is not yet standardized. Vasodilators, such as hydralazine, trimethaphan, and diazoxide, have been successfully used to manage acute heart failure as a complication of hypertensive heart disease. This practice has been logically extended to the management of acute myocardial infarction and impaired ventricular performance in a patient with hypertensive heart disease. Vasodilators have also proved useful in managing heart failure that complicates acute myocardial infarction even though blood pressure is normal. At present, trials are being made of vasodilator agents in the management of chronic congestive heart failure in patients with chronic coronary heart disease.

Dramatic clinical improvement has followed the use of vasodilators in mitral regurgitation that follows papillary muscle dysfunction in acute or chronic coronary heart disease and in cardiomyopathies. Infusion of nitroprusside has increased the stroke output into the aorta while the regurgitant fraction decreases. Accompanying these changes is a decrease in left ventricular filling pressure and in systemic vascular resistance. In a similar fashion, nitroprusside decreases left-to-right shunting across a ventricular septal defect that occurs in the course of acute myocardial infarction; the drop in systemic arterial resistance that nitroprusside produces results in an increase in stroke output that decreases the left-to-right shunting and pulmonary congestion. Nitroprusside has also been of great value in improving cardiac function in the patient with severe aortic valvular insufficiency.

Diuretics

Inordinate retention of salt and water, followed by expansion of the plasma and the interstitial tissue compartments of the extracellular fluid volume, is a hallmark of congestive heart failure and is responsible for many of its symptoms. Consequently, elimination of the excess salt and water and contraction of the extravascular fluid volume by diuresis are essential for the successful treatment of heart failure.

"DRY" WEIGHT. The use of diuretics entails two separate problems: elimination of excess fluid, and the maintenance of edema-free ("dry") weight. In the hospital, where the patient is at rest and salt intake is precisely controlled, low dosages of diuretics may suffice to maintain dry weight. Out of the hospital, where the patient engages in various degrees of exercise, and salt intake is neither readily monitored nor controlled, larger doses may be needed. However, continued use of large doses of diuretics inevitably leads to serious derangements in electrolyte balance, often predisposing to digitalis toxicity by way of hypokalemia. Consequently, once the urgent need for brisk diuresis has passed — as during an episode of acute pulmonary edema — the optimal cardiotonic program relies heavily on digitalis and salt restriction and depends on diuretics as an ancillary measure.

SALT AND WATER RESTRICTION. Restriction of sodium intake should be directed not only at sodium chloride per se but also at sodium-containing medications, e.g., antacids. Restriction of water intake is rarely necessary except after the use of potent diuretics which predispose to hyponatremia and water intoxication. In mild heart failure, sodium intake is generally restricted to less than 3

grams per day; in severe congestive heart failure, intake of less than 0.5 gram per day is often needed to promote diuresis and to reduce the blood volume and venous pressure. Overzealous sodium restriction in conjunction with potent sodium-losing diuretics, particularly in the elderly or in others with impaired renal function, may lead to weakness, oliguria, and azotemia.

THE SODIUM CONTROL SYSTEM. The major diuretics increase the rate of sodium excretion by the renal tubule. As indicated previously, the tubule is the end organ of an elaborate control system that is influenced by hemodynamic and neurohumoral mechanisms. For some mysterious reason, the control system seems to be reset in heart failure so that an expanded extracellular fluid volume, usually a stimulus to diuresis, coexists with antidiuresis. Nonetheless, despite this reset, it is possible to modify the handling of sodium by intervening at several different sites in the control system.

The diuretics that will be considered interfere with the control system by modifying the reabsorption of sodium, with its accompanying anions and water, by the end organ, the renal tubule (Fig. 5). Five distinct categories of diuretics are in common use (Table 6). Each affects tubular reabsorption somewhat differently, and each produces its own characteristic abnormalities in electrolyte pattern, hydration, and acid-base balance. These abnormalities represent the pharmacologic consequences of effective drug action. When carried to extremes, or when effects interact, they are responsible for the toxicity of these different diuretics.

Figure 5. Schematic representation of a nephron, indicating predominant sites of action of the five groups of diuretics. Carbonic anhydrase inhibitors exert predominant effects on the proximal tubule. The potassium-retaining diuretics affect the distal nephron. The major diuretic effect of the thiazides is at a site of urine dilution in the cortical portion of the ascending limb of the loop of Henle. Ethacrynic acid, furosemide, and the organomercurials act chiefly on the loop of Henle, affecting both the diluting and concentrating segments to achieve potent diuretic effects.

TABLE 6. Diuretic Agents in Heart Failure

Type of Diuretic	Effect on Kidney		Effect on Electrolytes		Toxic Manifestations	Special Features
	Principal Site of Action	Mechanism	In Urine	In Blood		
Thiazides (chloruretic sulfonamides)	Ascending limb of loop of Henle; distal tubule	Interference with dilution of urine	Increased excretion of Na, Cl, K	Hypochloremic alkalosis; hypokalemia	Nausea; vomiting; skin rashes; hyperuricemia; hypercalcemia; hyperglycemia; azotemia	Loss of effectiveness and hypokalemia are common on continued administration
Ethacrynic acid*	Ascending limb of loop of Henle; distal tubule; probably proximal tubule	Interference with dilution and concentration of urine	Increased excretion of Na, Cl, HCO_3, K, H	Hypochloremic alkalosis; hypokalemia; hyponatremia	Hypotension; contraction alkalosis; hyperuricemia; hypercalcemia; azotemia; hyperglycemia; hearing loss	Causes renal vasodilatation; effective in renal insufficiency, systemic acidosis or alkalosis; potent diuresis often followed by rebound
Organomercurials	Proximal and/or distal tubule	Decrease of isosmotic reabsorption	Increased excretion of Na, Cl, H	Hypochloremic alkalosis	Mercury intoxication; sudden death (after IV injection); occasional agranulocytosis	Inactivated by hypochloremic alkalosis; hazardous in oliguria
Potassium-sparing†	Distal tubule	Aldosterone antagonism for Na-K exchange	Decreased excretion of K and H; slight increase in Na, Cl, HCO_3	Hyperkalemia	Generally nontoxic; GI upset; gynecomastia; rare agranulocytosis	Synergistic with thiazides and ethacrynic acid; avoid in renal insufficiency and in hyperkalemia
Carbonic anhydrase inhibitors	Proximal tubule	Inhibition of enzyme involved in acidification of urine	Increased excretion of Na, K, HCO_3; decrease in H	Hyperchloremic acidosis; hypokalemia	Generally nontoxic; mild GI and mental upsets; occasional sulfonamide idiosyncrasy	Not very potent and loses effectiveness in a few days

*Furosemide (Lasix), a nonthiazide sulfonamide, has practically the same indications and effects despite its different chemical structure.
†Spironolactone (Aldactone) operates as a competitive inhibitor of endogenous aldosterone; triamterene and amiloride are noncompetitive inhibitors and produce the characteristic effects on the urine even though aldosterone is absent.

THIAZIDES. Because of their effectiveness by mouth, their reliability, and their relative freedom from toxicity if administered circumspectly, the benzothiadiazine drugs are usually the diuretics of choice in cardiac edema. The prototypes of this group are chlorothiazide and hydrochlorothiazide (Table 7). *Acute* administration promotes the urinary excretion of sodium, chloride, and potassium without consistent change in urinary pH or bicarbonate excretion. The predominant diuretic effect (natriuresis and chloruresis) has been localized to inhibition of sodium absorption at a diluting site in the distal nephron (Fig. 5). Although there is also a carbonic anhydrase–inhibiting effect, it is generally insignificant until large daily doses are reached (of the order of 2000 mg per day). Kaliuresis depends on an increase in the quantity of sodium delivered to the distal nephron. Intravenous administration of chlorothiazide is uricosuric, whereas chronic administration results in hyperuricemia. The mechanisms responsible for the paradoxical uric acid effects are still unclear.

Hypokalemia is particularly apt to arise after intensive diuresis with thiazides or after prolonged thiazide therapy. Supplementary doses of potassium may then be required. Several generalizations have proved useful as practical guides to therapy. Acute hypokalemia that is modest in degree is managed by diet; if diet fails to correct the hypokalemia, supplementary doses of potassium may be required. Potassium chloride is generally the agent of choice for oral supplementation, because hypochloremic metabolic alkalosis usually accompanies diuretic-induced hypokalemia. For severe hypokalemia, intravenous infusions are used. To prevent hypokalemia during chronic administration of potassium-losing diuretics, aldosterone inhibitors are useful.

Certain precautions merit attention in applying these guides to therapy. Potassium salts administered orally in any form cause gastric irritation. This side effect is generally tolerable, especially in the hospital, where potassium chloride can be safely given in liquid form after meals.

Prolonged administration of potassium salts, particularly if enteric coated, is particularly hazardous because of the high incidence of intestinal ulceration, perforation, and peritonitis, often followed by intestinal stenosis and obstruction. No matter how administered, excessive doses of potassium are apt to lead to hyperkalemia. This likelihood is enhanced in older persons who often have slight renal impairment, especially if an aldosterone inhibitor is given concomitantly.

ETHACRYNIC ACID AND FUROSEMIDE. These are the most potent natriuretic agents currently available. Both are organic acids but otherwise are quite different chemically. Furosemide is a sulfonamide–anthranilic acid derivative related to the thiazide diuretics, whereas ethacrynic acid is a ketone derivative of aryloxyacetic acid (Table 7). Like the thiazides, they are effective orally and are rapid acting. They exert powerful diuretic effects by inhibiting both the renal diluting and concentrating mechanisms in the ascending limb of the loop of Henle (Fig. 5). Ethacrynic acid is without appreciable effect on carbonic anhydrase, whereas furosemide does elicit modest anti-carbonic anhydrase activity. Ethacrynic acid appears to relax vascular smooth muscle by a direct effect. Although this effect could contribute importantly to unloading the failing heart, it is exceedingly difficult to dissociate from the diuretic effect per se.

Ethacrynic acid, administered orally, exerts its effects in 30 minutes and continues to act for six to eight hours; administered intravenously, it acts within a few minutes, reaching its peak activity in one hour. Both agents elicit a marked increase in urine flow containing large quantities of sodium and chloride (of the order of 20 to 30 per cent of the filtered load). Kaliuresis is consistent and appreciable. In conventional doses, neither drug consistently increases bicarbonate secretion or modifies urine pH. But chronic administration of ethacrynic acid promotes hydrogen loss in a bicarbonate-free urine, i.e., produces metabolic alkalosis.

A cardinal virtue of these agents (in contrast with thia-

TABLE 7. Administration of Diuretics

	Example	Relevant Chemical Structure	Preferred Route of Administration	Usual Range of Daily Dosage	Suggested Pattern of Administration
Thiazides	Chlorothiazide (Diuril)	Benzothiadiazine derivative	Oral	500 mg × 2–4	Standard type of diuretic to start treatment; few days on, few days off to avoid refractoriness and serious electrolyte disturbances
Ethacrynic acid*	Ethacrynic acid (Edecrin)	Ketone derivative of aryloxyacetic acid	Oral or IV*	50 mg × 2–3	Reserve for serious or refractory edema
Organomercurials	Mersalyl and theophylline	Theophylline plus organic mercurial	IM	2 ml	Adjunct diuretic or for moderately rapid response in hospital
Potassium-sparing†	Triamterene (Dyrenium)	Pteridine derivative	Oral	200 mg	Continuous administration in conjunction with more potent potassium-losing diuretics; do not use with potassium supplements
Carbonic anhydrase inhibitors	Acetazolamide (Diamox)	Sulfanilamide derivative	Oral	250 mg × 4–6	Episodic as booster diuretic; useful before injection of organomercurial for chloride-retaining effect

*Furosemide and ethacrynic acid may be given intravenously as well as by mouth. For ordinary use, however, furosemide is administered as a single oral dose in the morning. In an urgent situation (pulmonary edema), furosemide, as well as ethacrynic acid, may be administered intravenously (50 mg). Intravenous administration should not be administered at less than six-hour intervals.

†Spironolactone (Aldactone), 75 to 100 mg per day, is commonly used as a potassium-sparing diuretic. In refractory heart failure doses of 100 to 600 mg per day have proved helpful.

zides and carbonic anhydrase inhibitors) is their lack of effect on filtration rate or renal plasma flow unless sodium depletion occurs. This lack of direct hemodynamic effect is fortunate, because a decrease in filtration rate interferes with their action; conversely, increase in filtration rate, as by intravenous administration of mannitol or albumin, enhances their effects. At peak effect, both agents decrease renal vascular resistance.

Ethacrynic acid and furosemide remain effective despite gross electrolyte disturbances and hypoalbuminemia. If pushed, either may cause hyponatremia, volume depletion, fall in blood pressure, fall in urine volume, azotemia, and water retention. Because of the upsets in the electrolyte concentrations which they induce, other diuretics are preferred for maintenance treatment. They are most valuable in three situations: in acute pulmonary edema (25 to 50 mg intravenously), in severe or refractory heart failure, or when renal function is impaired (because they increase renal blood flow). Both agents produce "contraction alkalosis," i.e., an increase in plasma bicarbonate consequent to the decrease in extracellular fluid volume that follows excretion of a large volume of bicarbonate-poor urine. The metabolic alkalosis that follows hydrogen depletion and "contraction" predisposes to alveolar hypoventilation through its depressant effects on respiratory control mechanisms.

ORGANOMERCURIAL DIURETICS. Until the advent of potent oral diuretics, the organomercurials, generally a combination of an organic mercurial and theophylline, were the diuretic agents of choice in heart failure. Now they are generally reserved for parenteral administration in hospital. After administration of a maximally effective dose intravenously, large (and approximately equal) amounts of sodium and chloride are eliminated in the urine. The normal subject is apt to eliminate 10 per cent of the filtered load, whereas the individual who has been primed to the stage of hyperchloremic acidosis by prior administration of ammonium chloride may eliminate up to 20 per cent of the filtered load. Bicarbonate excretion does not increase, and urinary acidity persists during the diuresis. The effect on potassium excretion is variable and generally small, depending on prior rates of excretion. Generally they tend to decrease potassium.

Like ethacrynic acid and furosemide, the organomercurials exert an important inhibitory effect on sodium reabsorption in the loop of Henle, impairing both the diluting and concentrating mechanisms. In Figure 5, the organomercurials are shown as acting predominantly on the distal tubule, beyond the predominant sites of action of the thiazides, ethacrynic acid, and furosemide. However, these distinctions are far from absolute. Theophylline-containing mercurials usually elicit transient increases in filtration rate, but this effect is generally neutralized by volume concentration if diuresis is effective.

The organomercurials are almost invariably administered intramuscularly. After intramuscular injection, the onset of action is in one to two hours, reaching a peak in six hours, and lasting for 12 to 24 hours. Early in treatment, a brisk diuresis and natriuresis occur. But with continued use, refractoriness may result, generally for one of two reasons: (1) the onset of a hypochloremic hypokalemic alkalosis (with fairly normal sodium levels); responsiveness may then be restored by administering ammonium chloride; or (2) the advent of a low-salt syndrome in which sodium as well as chloride levels in the serum are severely depressed; this state responds to water restriction.

ALDOSTERONE ANTAGONISTS. A characteristic feature of chronic heart failure is high circulating levels of renin and aldosterone. Aldosterone, either by providing energy for active transport or by increasing permeability, enhances the movement of sodium through the distal tubular cell, from lumen to interstitium. Water follows passively. In addition to promoting sodium reabsorption, aldosterone also increases potassium excretion by a mechanism that is not entirely clear but is more than an ion-exchange mechanism. In heart failure the hyperaldosteronism causes continuing sodium retention, whereas potassium excretion remains normal, i.e., no hypokalemia. Aldosterone antagonists interfere with these actions, causing potassium retention and sodium excretion.

Three agents are available: spironolactone, triamterene, and amiloride (MK-870). Spironolactone is most popular; amiloride is not yet available for general use. Although all three act by competing for receptor sites in the distal tubule, the intimate mechanisms involved in electrolyte secretion may be quite different. The major site of action of spironolactone is in the distal tubule, in the region of the aldosterone-stimulated secretion of hydrogen and potassium. It is a specific competitive inhibitor of aldosterone and has no action if aldosterone is absent. It promotes natriuresis, water loss, and potassium retention by depressing aldosterone-dependent sodium-potassium exchange in the distal tubule. It is only effective in the presence of high levels of mineralocorticoid activity; it is devoid of effect after adrenalectomy. Conversely, triamterene (Table 7) and amiloride are noncompetitive inhibitors that inhibit potassium and hydrogen ion excretion even if aldosterone is absent. Their mechanism of action is unclear. Although these natriuretic agents are far less potent than the thiazides, ethacrynic acid, furosemides, and the organomercurials, they have the extraordinary advantage for prolonged use of continuing effectiveness, minor electrolyte derangements, and the virtual absence of toxicity as long as hyperkalemia is avoided. These agents are unique in that they are given without interruption, because, in contrast to the thiazides, ethacrynic acid, and furosemide, they do not lose effectiveness in a few days nor do they cause violent electrolyte upheavals.

Spironolactone is expensive but effective. Oral doses, ranging from 100 to 400 mg per day, are well tolerated for months. A few days may elapse before its action becomes apparent. It is currently being used primarily to potentiate the effects of the more powerful diuretics, particularly if potassium depletion is a serious consideration.

CARBONIC ANHYDRASE INHIBITORS. These agents are effective by mouth. They elicit an increase in excretion of bicarbonate, sodium, and potassium and an increase in urine pH. The most striking increments are in bicarbonate and potassium. By interfering with carbonic anhydrase activity in the kidney, they inhibit hydrogen ion secretion primarily in the proximal and distal portions of the nephron, exerting lesser effects on the loop of Henle, i.e., little effect on urinary diluting or concentrating mechanisms.

The prototype of this group is acetazolamide (Table 7). It is a weak diuretic and loses its effectiveness as hyperchloremic metabolic acidosis develops because of diminished hydrogen ion excretion (usually in 48 hours). Like ammonium chloride, this class of diuretics is particularly valuable in patients with high serum bicarbonate, as occurs in cor pulmonale or metabolic alkalosis. They are valuable in preparing for a mercurial diuresis because of the hyperchloremic acidosis that they produce. This group also enhances natriuresis produced by thiazides, ethacrynic acid, and furosemide. A contraindication for its use is severe acidosis, as from renal failure or hepatic insufficiency.

SPECIAL DIURETICS. This is a miscellaneous group of agents that are used with extreme caution and under special conditions. For example, osmotic diuretics such as mannitol and albumin, which expand the circulating blood volume, have the potential for increasing the renal blood flow and for blocking the reabsorption of sodium and water at the proximal tubule. However, in heart failure they entail the risk of circulatory overload and pulmonary edema.

COMBINATIONS. There are two main reasons for introducing a combination of diuretics into a cardiotonic program: to avoid serious electrolyte upsets that are bound to occur if the powerful primary diuretics are administered without pause, in large dosage, for long periods; and to stimulate diuresis when the prevailing cardiotonic program no longer suffices to prevent edema. In either case, the net diuretic effect of the combination will be determined by a wide variety of influences: the respective sites of action on the renal tubule of each agent, the extent of competitive inhibition at common receptor sites, the dose-response curves of the individual drugs, strategic timing of the administration of one agent with respect to the other, and the acid-base and electrolyte balances at the time that the agents are given.

A currently popular duo of diuretics is a potassium-sparing agent (triamterene or spironolactone) that is taken daily and a thiazide that is taken intermittently (e.g., for four days of each week). In time, the thiazide may be succeeded by ethacrynic acid or ethacrynic acid may be given sporadically as needed to sustain the edema-free state. On occasion, particularly in the hospital, a mercurial diuretic (after prior acidification) may prove helpful in overcoming a resistant state of edema. In contrast to the foregoing, other combinations hold little promise for success. Thus the combined use of acetazolamide and a mercurial diuretic is not apt to be exceedingly effective, because, by preventing acidification of the urine, the carbonic anhydrase inhibitor is apt to block, rather than to enhance, the diuretic effect of the mercurial.

The same general principles govern the use of combinations of diuretics in the treatment of refractory edema. This troublesome state is now relatively uncommon because of the advent of powerful primary diuretics, particularly furosemide and ethacrynic acid, coupled with a better understanding of the sites of action of the auxiliary diuretics. On the other hand, refractory edema may again become tractable by reversing electrolyte and acid-base imbalances that have been produced by unremitting administration of the primary diuretics for long periods. As a working principle, resistance to diuresis is overcome by deliberate selection of agents that act on different parts of the tubule. This approach presupposes that digitalis dosage is optimal. On occasion, aminophylline, by its inotropic effect, may reinforce the diuretic action of a thiazide or ethacrynic acid. Clearly, many opportunities exist for the physician to devise original sequences and combinations of diuretics. However, a restraining influence is imposed by the complicated interplay that is to be expected, not only between the diuretic agents per se, but also within the broad context of a deranged internal environment that generally is a feature of the state of refractory edema.

REFRACTORY EDEMA. This is a state of edema that resists conventional cardiotonic and diuretic measures. Before embarking on an endless train of drug combinations, the patient should be carefully re-evaluated for either a complication or an underlying disorder that has been overlooked: a surgically correctable disorder, such as mitral stenosis or constrictive pericarditis; a medical disorder, including hyperthyroidism, anemia, pulmonary emboli, bacterial endocarditis, persistent infection, and arrhythmias; inappropriate or excessive diuretic therapy that elicits serious disturbances in blood volume and electrolyte composition, digitalis toxicity, and water intoxication; physical overactivity; excessive salt intake and renal disease; sodium-containing medicaments, such as antacids, or agents such as reserpine, propranolol, and guanethidine which depress the myocardium to the point of failure.

COMPLICATIONS. A variety of disturbances may complicate effective diuretic therapy. These include hypotension and vascular collapse from rapid, massive diuresis; sodium depletion, usually the consequence of prolonged and effective diuretic therapy in conjunction with excessive water intake; hypokalemia from uninterrupted use of diuretics, predisposing to digitalis toxicity; hyperkalemia from injudicious administration of aldosterone antagonists and potassium supplements; metabolic alkalosis, either from a massive excretion of a bicarbonate-poor urine or from a combination of increased hydrogen ion excretion in the urine and alveolar hypoventilation as produced by ethacrynic acid or potassium depletion; and hyperuricemia after prolonged administration of small doses of the thiazides, ethacrynic acid, and furosemide, which share an inhibiting effect on uric acid excretion. In predisposed individuals, the hyperuricemia of prolonged diuretic therapy may precipitate an episode of gout. The thiazides, and occasionally furosemide, may precipitate diabetes which is rarely severe.

GENERAL COMMENTS. In treating heart failure, rarely is there a desperate need to restore everything to normal at once by vigorous diuresis. The temptation to restore the patient immediately to dry weight and to free him of breathlessness and congestion must be tempered by the penalty of dehydration and severe electrolyte disturbances. The more leisurely the diuretic therapy, the more durable and tolerable the relief.

The ability of these potent diuretics to elicit dramatic diuresis has led to their abuse. Thus without direct inotropic effect on the heart, a single injection of ethacrynic acid can effect a decrease in blood volume, a decrease in intracardiac filling pressures, an increase in cardiac output, and clear edema. But ethacrynic acid is rarely advisable as the mainstay of therapy unless edema is refractory and less drastic measures have proved ineffective. Only when coupled with a full cardiotonic program can judicious control of heart failure be maintained, particularly if the underlying heart disease is progressive and severe complications of diuretic therapy are to be avoided.

SURGICAL THERAPY OF REFRACTORY HEART FAILURE. Attempts are under way in several medical centers to provide temporary respite for the heart in acute refractory failure that is judged to be reversible, e.g., after myocardial infarction. The common feature of the different approaches is to unload the heart for hours to days while it is recuperating. The most popular devices are (1) venoarterial bypass, which assists the heart by diverting blood to a pump that returns it to the arterial tree, and (2) counterpulsation, which operates in synchrony with the heartbeat to adjust the aortic blood pressure by rhythmically changing either the volume of blood in the aorta (using an external pump) or the capacity of the aorta (using an internal balloon). All methods aim to reduce the external work of the heart and the tension that it develops during systole and to decrease myocardial oxygen consumption at the same time as coronary arterial perfusion is improved. Technical problems have restricted the use of these appliances in man to biding time in desperate situations, e.g., in cardiogenic shock. As yet, there are very few long-term survivors.

Cardiac replacement and the development of an artificial heart to assist or replace the failing heart are also being pursued as last measures for refractory heart failure. Experience with cardiac replacement began ten years ago, and approximately one fifth of the 346 heart transplant patients are still alive, the oldest nine years after transplantation. Because of great skill in surgery and in related techniques, expectations for one-year survival have improved to two out of three who undergo transplantation. However, the procedure is limited in applicability because of shortage of donor hearts and the burden of long-term immunosuppression and its complications.

The artificial heart program currently has the greatest promise as an assist device for the left ventricle. This modality is still experimental, has no long-term survivors, and is handicapped by incompatibilities between blood and artificial materials that comprise the synthetic heart.

Braunwald, E., Ross, J., Jr., and Sonnenblick, E. H.: Mechanisms of Contraction of the Normal and Failing Heart. Boston, Little, Brown & Company, 1976.
Cohn, J. N., and Franciosa, J. A.: Vasodilator therapy of heart failure. N. Engl. J. Med., 297:27, 254, 1977.
Dollery, C. T., George, C. F., and Orme, M. L. E.: Drug interaction in cardiovascular disease. Prog. Cardiol. 1:31, 1972.
Fishman, A. P. (ed.): Heart Failure. Washington, D.C., Hemisphere, 1978.
Fishman, A. P.: Pulmonary edema. The water-exchanging function of the lung. Circulation, 46:390, 1972.
Goldberg, M.: The renal physiology of diuretics. In Berliner, R. W., and Orloff, J. (eds.): Handbook of Physiology — Renal Physiology. Washington, D.C., American Physiological Society, 1973.
Mason, D. T.: Congestive Heart Failure. New York, Dun-Donnelley Publishing, 1977.
Weber, K. T., and Janicki, J. S.: Instantaneous force-velocity-length relations: Experimental findings and clinical correlates. Am. J. Cardiol., 40:740, 1977.

356. SHOCK

Francois M. Abboud

Shock is a complex clinical state which demands immediate care to avoid a fatal outcome. Few other clinical situations require such vigilant medical attention, careful hemodynamic monitoring, and thorough understanding of the basic principles of circulatory control and of the pharmacology of cardiac and vasoactive drugs. This chapter covers the basic principles of *circulatory control* as they relate to the shock syndrome, the *cellular mechanisms* involved in the pathogenesis of shock, and the *therapy* of shock.

DEFINITION. The common denominator in shock, regardless of cause, is a failure of the circulatory system to deliver the chemical substances necessary for cellular survival and to remove the waste products of cellular metabolism. In other words, the perfusion of tissues and cells with blood is restricted despite compensatory adjustments. This leads to cellular membrane dysfunc-

tion, abnormal cellular metabolism, and eventually cellular death. The goal is to recognize this state early and attempt to restore tissue perfusion.

The clinical picture is usually that of a patient who is hypotensive (with a systolic arterial pressure of 90 mm Hg or less); is hyperventilating; has cold, clammy, and cyanotic skin, constricted peripheral veins, a thready rapid pulse, and a dulled sensorium; may be confused or combative; and is oliguric, with a urinary output of less than 20 ml per hour. This basic clinical picture is present in addition to the signs and symptoms of the underlying precipitating disease, e.g., severe chest pain of acute myocardial infarction or dissecting aneurysm, visible bleeding, burn, peritonitis, sepsis.

STAGES OF SHOCK. The progress of this syndrome and its pathogenesis may be described in *three stages* which reflect the severity of the decline in tissue perfusion and intensity of cellular membrane damage. The basic elements in the pathogenesis of shock as they relate to the stages of the syndrome and the types of shock are portrayed in the accompanying figure. The causes and initiating mechanisms are listed in Table 1.

Stage I: Compensated Hypotension. Hypotension may be caused either by a fall in cardiac output or by vasodilatation. The initial event in a great majority of cases of shock is a fall in cardiac output rather than vasodilatation, except in septic shock in which peripheral vascular resistance is decreased significantly and cardiac output may be increased initially. The fall in cardiac output and hypotension trigger effective compensatory mechanisms mediated through the symptho-adrenal and renin-angiotensin systems and other hormonal and local metabolic factors. These restore arterial pressure, and tend to restore blood flow to the more vital organs such as brain and heart. During this early stage the patients may not present with sufficient symptoms and signs to allow the clinician to suspect the possibility of impending shock. It is during this phase that intervention might be most effective in preventing further deterioration of the circulation and cellular death.

Stage II: Decreased Tissue Perfusion. Here the compensatory mechanisms to maintain perfusion of vital organs are maximal but insufficient. The evidence of decreased cerebral perfusion may be apparent from the mental status of the patient; decreased renal perfusion may reduce urinary output, and patients with coronary artery disease may begin to suffer from myocardial ischemia. The external appearance of the patient also reflects the excessive sympathetic discharge, with cyanosis and coldness and clamminess of the skin. The majority of patients are seen in this phase, and rapid aggressive intervention to restore cardiac output and perfusion of the tissues may reverse the shock syndrome.

Stage III: Microcirculatory Failure and Cellular Membrane Injury. Excessive and prolonged reduction of tissue perfusion leads to significant alterations in cellular membrane function, aggregation of blood corpuscles, and "sludging" in the capillaries. The vasoconstriction which has taken place in the less vital organs in order to maintain blood pressure is now excessive and has reduced flow to such an extent that cellular damage occurs.

Arterial pressure continues to fall progressively to a critical level at which even the perfusion of vital organs such as brain and heart is limited. Critical impairment

Pathophysiology of shock.

of renal perfusion leads to acute tubular necrosis as a result of ischemia of the cortical regions of the kidney. Ischemia of the gastrointestinal tract may lead to serious necrotic damage of the mucosa and the absorption into the circulation of bacteria and toxic bacterial products, which could have significant detrimental effects on other organs and might lead to a state of generalized endothelial damage with disseminated intravascular coagulation. Bacterial toxins react with neutrophils and cause the release of vasodilator poly-peptides, which contribute to the fall in arterial pressure despite the excessive sympathoadrenal discharge and other vasoconstricting compensatory mechanisms. The severe acidosis resulting from anaerobic metabolism also contributes to vasodilatation. The decreased perfusion pressure of the coronary vessels, particularly in patients with coronary disease, results in reduction of myocardial perfusion, which in turn decreases myocardial contractility and creates a vicious cycle situation as the decreased contractility causes further decrements in arterial blood pressure. Similarly, reduction in perfusion pressure and ischemia of the central nervous system impair reflex neurogenic circulatory adjustments which help in maintaining arterial pressure. The loss of integrity of the capillary membranes leads to loss of fluid and proteins through the capillaries, with exacerbation of hypovolemia and hypotension. Damage to cellular membranes from ischemia leads to the leak of lysosomal enzymes and intracellular ions, to the progressive reduction in high energy phosphate reserves, and to cellular destruction.

CIRCULATORY CONTROL IN SHOCK

Major Determinants of Tissue Perfusion

The major determinants of hemodynamics and tissue perfusion are listed in Table 2. The perfusion of any organ is dependent upon the systemic arterial pressure (which is the driving force for blood to flow through all organs), the resistance offered by the vasculature of that organ, and the patency of nutritional capillaries. Systemic arterial pressure is in turn determined by the vigor of contraction of the heart (cardiac output) as well as the resistance of the total vascular tree. Vascular resistance is predominantly a function of the radius or caliber of blood vessels. Vascular caliber is influenced by neurogenic, humoral, and myogenic factors that regulate the tone of vascular smooth muscle. Thus blood flow to any one organ is dependent on cardiac function and on muscle tone and caliber of vessels in all the arterial tree as well as in the organ itself. The determin-

---

TABLE 1.   Causes of Shock and Initiating Mechanisms

I. Blood loss and decreased intravascular volume
   A. Acute hemorrhage: gastrointestinal bleeding, hemoptysis, hemoperitoneum, retroperitoneal bleeding, ruptured aneurysm
   B. Excessive fluid loss
      1. Vomiting (intestinal or pyloric obstruction)
      2. Severe diarrhea and dehydration
      3. Peritonitis, pancreatitis, splanchnic ischemia, intestinal obstruction and gangrene
      4. Fractures and extensive muscle injury
      5. Burns
   C. Relative hypovolemia
      1. Neurogenic vasodilatation: anesthesia (spinal), ganglionic and adrenergic blockers, spinal cord injury
      2. Metabolic, toxic, or humoral vasodilatation: septicemia (gram-negative endotoxemia or gram-positive bacteremia)
II. Cardiac
   A. Myocardial infarction, cardiac rupture
   B. Myocarditis and myocardial depression (hypoxia, acidosis, septic shock, myocardial depressant factors [MDF], drugs)
   C. Arrhythmias: severe bradycardia, tachycardia, and fibrillation
   D. Mechanical compression or obstruction
      1. Pericardial effusion or tamponade
      2. Positive pressure ventilation
      3. Pulmonary embolism
      4. Ball-valve thrombus or atrial myxoma
III. Microcirculatory endothelial injury and aggregation
   A. Anaphylaxis
   B. Disseminated intravascular coagulation
   C. Burns, septic shock, trauma
IV. Cellular membrane injury
   A. Septic shock
   B. Anaphylaxis
   C. Ischemia, prolonged hypoxia, pancreatitis, tissue injury

TABLE 2. **Major Determinants of Hemodynamics and Tissue Perfusion**

I. Systemic arterial pressure
  A. Total vascular resistance
    1. Total arteriolar resistance, vascular muscle tone
      a. Tissue metabolism
      b. Neurohumoral factors, toxins
    2. Viscosity of blood
  B. Cardiac output
    1. Heart rate
    2. Stroke volume
      a. Cardiac filling pressure
        i. Venous (vascular) tone
        ii. Blood volume
          Capillary hydrostatic pressure: post-precapillary resistance
          Capillary permeability
          Oncotic pressure, plasma proteins
      b. Myocardial contractility
        i. Arterial blood pH, Po₂
        ii. Myocardial O₂ supply
          Increase supply:
            ↑ Diastolic arterial pressure (norepinephrine, dopamine)
            Capillary diffusion
            Coronary dilatation (nitroglycerin, dopamine, metabolites)
          Decrease supply:
            ↓ Diastolic arterial pressure (isoproterenol, vasodilators)
            Coronary artery disease, myocardial infarction
            Hypoxia, anemia
        iii. Myocardial O₂ demand
          Increase demand:
            ↑ Cardiac size (pulmonary wedge pressure)
            ↑ Afterload (systolic arterial pressure, impedance)
            ↑ Contractility (norepinephrine, dopamine, isoproterenol) and heart rate
          Decrease demand:
            ↓ Cardiac size
            ⎰ Digitalis, ↑ ejection fraction
            ⎱ Venodilatation (nitroprusside, nitroglycerin, phentolamine)
            ⎱ Diuretics
            ↓ Afterload, impedance (vasodilators)
            ↓ Contractility and heart rate
        iv. Humoral factors
          Catecholamines
          Myocardial depressant factors
        v. Drugs
          Increase norepinephrine, dopamine, isoproterenol, digitalis
          Decrease propranolol, anesthetics
II. Organ vascular resistance
  A. Occlusive arterial disease
  B. Local arteriolar resistance
  C. Local venular resistance
  D. Viscosity of blood
III. Patency of nutritional capillaries
  A. Precapillary sphincter tone
  B. Intracapillary aggregation of corpuscles
  C. Capillary endothelial integrity

ant of exchange of substrates and metabolites with the tissues is the microcirculation. A patent nutritional capillary network is the critical interface between the circulation and the cell.

This discussion deals with cardiac, vascular, and microcirculatory factors.

CARDIAC FACTORS. Cardiac output is the product of heart rate and stroke volume. A rate of 70 beats per minute and a stroke volume of 70 ml per beat give a cardiac output of approximately 5 liters per minute, an amount more than sufficient to deliver 250 ml of oxygen per minute to all the tissues. This consumption of oxygen reflects metabolic needs at rest. A drop in cardiac output below 2 liters per minute per square meter is an indication of severe shock.

Heart Rate. Tachycardia usually increases cardiac output, but a marked increase in heart rate may limit cardiac filling time and result in a low cardiac output and arterial blood pressure. For example, ventricular tachycardia or rapid atrial fibrillation in a patient with recent myocardial infarction causes a reduction in cardiac output and arterial pressure which, if uncorrected, could result in cardiogenic shock. Immediate treatment to restore heart rate is essential. In considering the treatment of tachycardia in shock, one has to be cautious in avoiding treatment of a "compensatory tachycardia" often seen in patients with fever, anemia, sepsis, hemorrhage, or severe hypovolemia. Tachycardia is often an appropriate reflex circulatory adjustment to maintain cardiac output.

Extreme bradycardia may also cause a low output and hypotension. Sinus bradycardia and atrioventricular block are often seen immediately following myocardial infarction and should be reversed if they contribute to hypotension. Severe bradycardia is also seen in the "common faint" syndrome or vasovagal syncope; the patient usually falls to the horizontal position and recovers spontaneously. Rarely is it necessary to treat such patients with atropine.

Stroke Volume. A decrease in stroke volume may be caused by (1) a decrease in filling pressure, (2) a decrease in myocardial contractility, or (3) a mechanical obstruction to blood flow.

DECREASE IN FILLING PRESSURE. The amount of blood filling the ventricles at the end of diastole regulates the subsequent contraction and stroke volume (Starling's law of the heart). Although there are many factors that determine filling pressure such as the rate and duration of filling, ventricular compliance, and venous tone, a most important determinant is total blood volume. Reduction in blood volume may be either absolute or relative to the capacity of the vascular tree. Absolute reductions in blood volume are apparent when blood or fluids are lost, causing a hypovolemic state leading to hypovolemic shock. This is seen in hemorrhage (either external or internal bleeding), excessive vomiting, diarrhea, burns, renal loss of fluids such as in diabetes mellitus or diabetes insipidus, excessive diuresis, and excessive perspiration without fluid replacement. Internal losses of fluid occur in peritonitis, intestinal obstruction with extravasation of fluid, splanchnic ischemia with bowel necrosis and gangrene, fractures with extensive muscle trauma, hemothorax, and hemoperitoneum.

Relative decreases in blood volume occur when there is loss of vascular tone because of the administration of anesthetics or ganglion blockers, after spinal cord injury, and in patients with neuropathy or autonomic insufficiency. Pooling of blood thus results in a decrease in filling pressure. Compression of the heart may also prevent its filling, as is seen during pericardial tamponade, in tension pneumothorax, or in the superior vena caval syndrome.

DECREASE IN MYOCARDIAL CONTRACTILITY. Reduced contractility of the heart is the primary cause of shock after myocardial infarction, and it is a complicating factor in the late phases of any shock. There are many factors that contribute to it.

Hypoxia. Hypoxia resulting from ventilation-perfusion abnormalities of the lung occurs in the early phases of shock. In late shock malignant hypoxia accompanies the pathologic entity of shock lung. Hypoxia has several effects on the circulation. A direct, vascular effect tends to decrease vascular resistance and cause vasodilatation in organs such as the heart, brain, or contracting skeletal muscle, thus permitting the redistribution of blood to the organs with higher oxygen demand. Hypoxia also activates chemoreceptors, causing a sympathetic vasoconstrictor response in vessels of skeletal muscle, skin, and splanchnic bed, allowing for a redistribution of flow to the more vital organs. When the central nervous system is hypoxic and ischemic, a significant sympathetic discharge also takes place. Despite these and other compensatory adjustments, myocardial performance is impaired in the presence of decreased arterial Po_2. The severity of arterial hypoxia is often a reflection of the extent of myocardial damage following myocardial infarction. It is an important, potentially reversible cause of depression of myocardial contractility.

Acidosis. Acidosis results from anaerobic metabolism with release of lactate, from decreased renal perfusion with accumulation of organic acids, and possibly from hypoventilation of certain pulmonary segments, leading to respiratory acidosis. Acidosis reduces myocardial contractility and the vasoconstrictor response to various neurohumoral factors involved in the circulatory adjustment to the shock syndrome. This is another cause of myocardial depression which should be treated.

Myocardial Ischemia and Perfusion Pressure. Myocardial performance depends on perfusion of the ischemic myocardium, which is determined to a great extent by the level of arterial diastolic pressure. The fall in arterial pressure during hemorrhagic or hypovolemic shock in patients with coronary artery disease may complicate the syndrome by causing myocardial ischemia. Thus restoration of arterial pressure in any shock situation is critical to preservation of myocardial function. As stated above, the perfusion of any organ is dependent on arterial pressure and on the resistance to flow created by the vessels supplying that organ. In the presence of coronary artery disease, the resistance to flow is due to structural changes in the vessel wall, and the degree of reversible increase in vasomotor tone is minimal because of the excessive accumulation of metabolites downstream from the site of coronary narrowing and in the region of ischemia. Thus arterial pressure becomes the determinant of perfusion of the ischemic segment through collateral vessels or across a narrowing or a plaque.

Increased Myocardial Oxygen Demand Relative to Supply. Although oxygen supply to the ischemic myocardium is increased by increasing arterial pressure, hypertension is detrimental, as it increases myocardial work and oxygen demand. Conversely, hypotension decreases myocardial work and oxygen needs, but it also reduces myocardial perfusion as mentioned earlier. Thus judicious restoration of arterial pressure is necessary.

Increased cardiac size is associated with greater myocardial oxygen consumption as myocardial wall tension increases. Reductions in preload, cardiac size, and oxygen demand may be achieved with appropriate venodilator and diuretic therapy. Drugs such as isoproterenol might increase myocardial oxygen demand out of proportion to the associated increase in coronary flow and

would have a net detrimental effect. Conversely, propranolol decreases myocardial oxygen demand and could be protective, but its myocardial depressant action in patients with cardiogenic shock would be a hazardous complication.

Other Factors That Depress Contractility. Drugs may depress cardiac output by a direct effect on the myocardium such as might occur with the barbiturates or, more frequently, by suppression of the adrenergic drive to the myocardium such as is seen following the administration of propranolol, the administration of a ganglion-blocking drug, the use of catecholamine depleters such as reserpine or guanethidine, a high spinal anesthetic, spinal cord injury, or an intracranial lesion involving the medullary centers. These interventions not only depress myocardial contraction but also decrease peripheral tone and create a state of "relative hypovolemia" and a reduction in "effective blood volume."

Myocardial depressant factors (MDF) may be released from damaged cells in various organs during shock from burns, septicemia, or hemorrhage, and add an element of myocardial depression which compounds the syndrome.

MECHANICAL OBSTRUCTION TO BLOOD FLOW. Cardiac output may rapidly decline in situations in which there is a major obstruction to blood flow either in the heart or in the pulmonary circulation. In the heart, a ball-valve thrombus in the left atrium or an atrial myxoma might contribute to progressive hypotension and possibly shock. Similarly, extensive pulmonary embolism or acute occlusion of the large pulmonary vessels will result in severe shock. In these situations, early recognition and removal of the obstruction can be lifesaving.

VASCULAR FACTORS. These determine the resistance to blood flow and transcapillary exchange.

Arterial blood pressure is determined by cardiac output and total vascular resistance. The resistance to flow of blood to any organ is determined by the viscosity of blood and by the length and the cross-sectional area of the vessels. The cross-sectional area is the most important component, because the calculated resistance is inversely proportional to the fourth power of the radius of the vessels. The caliber of the vessels is in turn determined by the tone of vascular smooth muscle in the wall of the vessels. The vascular smooth muscle tone is modulated by neurogenic influences mediated primarily through the sympathoadrenal system and by circulating humoral and local metabolic factors.

Neurogenic Control. The sympathoadrenal discharge to the circulatory system is regulated by medullary neurons in the vasomotor center. The activity of these neurons is modulated by afferent neural impulses originating in various receptors located in strategic areas around the body. Some of these receptors trigger impulses which suppress the sympathoadrenal drive to the circulatory system, and others increase the activity of the sympathoadrenal system. Important among these receptors are the arterial and cardiac baroreceptors, the chemoreceptors, the somatic receptors in skeletal muscle, and the thermal receptors. Activity originating in various parts of the central nervous system (cerebellum, fastigial and vestibular nuclei, and hypothalamus) also impinges upon the vasomotor center to modulate its output. Activation of cardiac sensory afferent receptors, particularly those in the left ventricle during stretch of the myocardium, inhibits sympathoadrenal activity, causing hypotension and bradycardia. The severe bradycardia and hypotension often seen following myocardial infarction, especially the inferior-posterior wall infarction, could be ascribed to dyskinesis of the infarcted ventricle. Conversely, reduction in the stretch of these ventricular receptors during hypovolemia and hemorrhage releases the sympathoadrenal efferent activity to cause reflex tachycardia and vasoconstriction, to restore arterial blood pressure, and to release renin. The arterial baroreceptors, activated by a rise in blood pressure, suppress sympathoadrenal tone; conversely, during hypotension they increase sympathoadrenal drive and restore arterial pressure.

Severe hypoxia, often associated with shock from any cause, activates the chemoreceptor reflex and causes an increase in sympathoadrenal drive. Afferent impulses from baro- and chemoreceptors may be activated simultaneously during shock, and their interaction results in the ultimate response in the clinical situation. The reduction of central or cardiopulmonary blood volume and arterial pressure during hemorrhage activates the cardiopulmonary reflex and the arterial baroreceptor reflex simultaneously, and the two reflexes are synergistic with respect to the final sympathetic efferent activity. Similarly, the combined activation of the arterial baroreceptor reflex by hypotension and the chemoreceptor reflex by hypoxia results in a significant synergistic effect on the ventilatory response as well as the circulatory sympathetic drive. On the other hand, there may be situations in which the reflex responses have opposite effects. This may occur, for example, when cardiac receptors are activated following acute myocardial infarction by the dyskinetic bulge of the left ventricle, while the arterial baroreceptors are unloaded because of hypotension.

In the experimental preparation the inhibitory influence of the bulging left ventricular wall on the sympathetic outflow predominates and overrides the arterial baroreflex, preventing vasoconstriction and thus causing a decrease in cardiac afterload for the damaged left ventricle. Teleologically, this effect may be beneficial, as it will tend to decrease left ventricular work following its acute insult. There have been few studies of the effects of endotoxin on neurocirculatory reflexes. An increase in baroreceptor activity for any level of arterial blood pressure has been reported in endotoxemia, a situation which would tend to inhibit sympathoadrenal tone, and might explain in part, if confirmed, the decreased vascular resistance often seen in septic shock.

Humoral Factors. The release of hormones such as renin, vasopressin, steroids, prostaglandins, and kinins is partly mediated through the sympathoadrenal system and cardiovascular mechanoreceptors. In addition to their direct cardiovascular and renal effects these hormones have significant indirect effects by modulating central or peripheral adrenergic transmission and the release of the neurotransmitter (norepinephrine) at the adrenergic terminal.

RENIN-ANGIOTENSIN. Circulating levels of renin or angiotensin are too small to cause significant circulatory effects in physiologic states. However, angiotensin and renin may traverse the blood-brain barrier in the area postrema, where they influence medullary cardiovascular centers. A fall in arterial blood pressure or an increase in sympathoadrenal sympathetic discharge to the kidney causes the release of renin. The resulting formation of angiotensin causes peripheral vasoconstriction,

maintains arterial pressure, stimulates the release of aldosterone to retain sodium and water, and has an intrarenal effect on tubular sodium reabsorption which permits greater sodium and water absorption and preservation of blood volume during hypotensive states.

VASOPRESSIN. This important constrictor hormone is released from the posterior pituitary primarily in response to changes in osmolality, and may also play a role in the circulatory control in shock. Its release may be significantly reduced by stretch of the left atrial receptors during hypervolemia or by stretch of the arterial baroreceptor during hypertension; conversely, during hemorrhage and systemic hypotension, or when patients are on cardiopulmonary bypass, the blood levels of vasopressin increase significantly. Recent observations suggest that thirst and the release of vasopressin may be induced by a central nervous system action of angiotensin.

KININS. A variety of potent vasodilator polypeptides are formed by the action of certain proteolytic enzymes on plasma protein precursors. The substance bradykinin serves as the prototype for this class of endogenous peptides. Their major physiologic role may be the local regulation of blood flow and function of such organs as the salivary gland and pancreas. In pathophysiologic states, kinins are believed to play a part in the hyperemia associated with inflammation and as vasodilators in hypotension produced by anaphylactic reactions and anaphylactic shock.

SEROTONIN AND HISTAMINE. Serotonin released from platelets and histamine released from mast cells during anaphylaxis or during complement activation in shock may play an important role in regulating local vascular tone and capillary permeability.

PROSTACYCLIN AND THROMBOXANE A$_2$. Prostaglandins are a family of endogenous acidic lipid-soluble materials with widespread distribution in the body and with diverse cardiovascular effects. They may be released in various organs during periods of ischemia and may therefore contribute to the reactive hyperemia and vasodilatation. The prostaglandin endoperoxides formed in platelets and in blood vessels from arachidonate are pivotal in the synthesis of two potent substances with opposing effects on the formation of thrombi. Prostacyclin, a powerful vasodilator and inhibitor of platelet aggregation, is synthesized in the vascular wall, mostly in the endothelial layers, from endoperoxides. In the platelets, however, endoperoxides are converted to thromboxane A$_2$, which causes vasoconstriction and platelet aggregation. In shock, damage to endothelial cells may inhibit synthesis of prostacyclin; in addition, platelets may release thromboxane A$_2$, causing intravascular platelet aggregation, clumping, and vasoconstriction.

Local Autoregulatory Adjustment of Blood Vessels. Blood vessels have an intrinsic ability to regulate vascular tone and thereby maintain blood flow to the organ over a wide range of perfusion pressures. This property has been referred to as the autoregulatory capacity for blood flow and is independent of systemic neurogenic influences or humoral factors. Different vascular beds vary with respect to their ability to maintain blood flow. The cerebral, coronary, and renal circulations are most potent. Thus during a fall in arterial pressure, vasodilatation of the cerebral, coronary, and renal vasculatures maintains blood flow and oxygen delivery to the brain and heart as well as sodium and water balance. Although a myogenic response intrinsic to the smooth muscle may explain the phenomenon, accumulation of tissue metabolites following a transient period of ischemia may also cause vasodilatation and restore blood flow. The specific mediator of metabolic vasodilatation is not known, but it is likely that a combination óf changes in oxygen, carbon dioxide, hydrogen ion, and other cations, in osmolality, in the amount of adenosine compounds, and in Krebs cycle intermediates and other metabolites released in the immediate environment of blood vessels contributes to adjustments in vascular tone.

MICROCIRCULATION AND TRANSCAPILLARY EXCHANGE. Perhaps the most critical aspect of the pathogenesis of the shock syndrome takes place at the level of the microcirculation. The delivery of a significant amount of blood to an organ does not ascertain that all the segments of that organ and all capillaries are perfused appropriately.

Intraorgan Blood Flow Distribution. Adequate tissue perfusion depends on blood flow through vascular channels in which diffusion between the blood and tissues may occur. These are referred to as nutritional capillaries, as contrasted with non-nutritional vessels which do not permit capillary exchange. The latter are also referred to as arteriovenous shunts, although there may be little anatomic evidence for the existence of such shunts. An example of the importance of the intraorgan redistribution of blood flow is observed in myocardial infarction, in which an increase in coronary blood flow may not increase perfusion to the infarcted segment. Under some circumstances a coronary vasodilator might redistribute flow away from the ischemic into the nonischemic regions.

Similarly, intraorgan blood flow distribution may be critical in the kidney. Acute tubular necrosis associated with shock may reflect a reduction in glomerular filtration in the outer cortex because of a localized increase in vascular resistance in this region and a selective reduction in blood flow. Interventions that alter total renal blood flow can produce significant redistribution of flow within the kidney; for example, renal vasoconstriction following adrenergic discharge tends to shunt blood away from the outer cortex, whereas renal vasodilators such as furosemide shunt blood toward the outer cortical nephrons.

Pre- and Postcapillary Resistance. The *precapillary sphincters* regulate the patency of nutritional or "exchange" capillaries. The tone of those sphincters may be modulated by neurohumoral factors which contribute to the circulatory adjustments in shock. The metabolic products at the local tissue level are important determinants of the patency of these sphincters, which regulate the total capillary surface area and in turn determine the intravascular-extracellular fluid and solute exchange. The capillary hydrostatic force driving fluid out of the capillaries into the extracellular space is dependent on the ratio of the post- to the precapillary resistances. In hypovolemic or hemorrhagic shock, the fall in arterial pressure causes activation of the sympathoadrenal system, constriction of the precapillary resistance vessels, and a fall in capillary hydrostatic pressure, facilitating the movement of fluids from the extracellular into the intravascular space. This partially restores intravascular volume. Hematocrit and viscosity of blood and plasma oncotic pressure fall. The decline in plasma oncotic pressure may be partially corrected

by rapid synthesis of new proteins; but as the hypotension persists and ischemia is prolonged, the vasoconstrictor response of the precapillary resistance vessels becomes less pronounced because of tissue acidosis but the resistance of *postcapillary* vessels (venules) increases, a situation in which more fluid is lost from the vascular to the interstitial space. Thus *venular resistance* and the reactivity of venules to the various vasoactive agents involved in the shock syndrome become important. The venules may even be *relatively* more reactive than the precapillary resistance vessels to catecholamines which activate constrictor alpha receptors. This differential effect in favor of postcapillary vasoconstriction also increases further hydrostatic pressure and intravascular fluid loss. The administration of alpha blockers in this situation might reverse this detrimental imbalance between post- and precapillary resistance. The ratio of post- to precapillary resistance and the consequent hydrostatic pressure may vary significantly from organ to organ as well as during the various stages of shock, and it is difficult to propose a specific uniform course of management directed at a reversal of that particular state, although one might consider the administration of a vasodilating drug in late stages of shock, in which the failure of the microcirculation is a predominant factor.

Capillary Permeability and Oncotic Pressure. The colloidal osmotic pressure (COP) is a major determinant of the intravascular volume. Albumin (molecular weight, 69,000) is the main osmotically active protein in plasma. The balance between the colloidal osmotic pressure and the capillary hydrostatic pressure determines the balance between the intravascular and extracellular fluid spaces. A significant degree of hypovolemia and hemoconcentration may take place either because of excessive capillary hydrostatic pressure from an increase in the ratio of post- to precapillary resistance or because of a reduction in plasma protein and consequently reduction of plasma oncotic pressure. Reduction of plasma protein and oncotic pressure might come about as the result of increased capillary permeability and loss of plasma protein from the intravascular to the extracellular space. The balance between oncotic and hydrostatic pressures is also an important determinant of the level of pulmonary edema and is critical in the management of shock and particularly of the shock lung syndrome with fluid replacement. Plasma oncotic pressure should be restored through careful selection of the type of fluid to be used in volume replacement. Fluids containing crystalloids may be undesirable, as these further decrease the oncotic pressure. On the other hand, administration of blood or colloids would be more appropriate, particularly to reduce pulmonary edema and accumulation of interstitial pulmonary fluid if pulmonary venous (or wedge) pressure is low.

Shock resulting from increased vascular permeability, such as anaphylactic shock or snake venom poisoning, is characterized by a dramatic reduction of plasma volume. Hematocrit rises sharply and oncotic pressure drops. This increase in capillary permeability may be partly related to the release of histamine from macrophages or the release of other metabolites or humoral factors which alter endothelial permeability.

Intravascular Hemagglutination and "Blood Sludging." The erythrocytes, leukocytes, and platelets undergo agglutination to a variable degree in association with the shock syndromes of thermal burn, sepsis, trauma, and perhaps even hemorrhagic shock. These aggregates may cause obstruction of capillaries as well as arterioles. The precipitating events are numerous. They may include platelet aggregation by catecholamines; damage to endothelial lining of small blood vessels and capillaries with subsequent fibrin deposition and accumulation of microthrombi; hypoxia increasing the rigidity of red cells; and release of vasoactive peptides and anaphylatoxins as a result of complement activation, which may in turn have an effect on permeability of endothelial cells and tone of precapillary sphincters, leading to further reduction in tissue perfusion and tissue damage.

Disseminated intravascular coagulation is a syndrome often seen in shock, particularly from gram-negative septicemia. The syndrome causes predominantly renal cortical necrosis and may contribute also to the pathogenesis of the shock lung.

Shock Lung. Pathologic studies of the lungs in patients dying from the shock syndrome may reveal marked capillary dilatation, pulmonary edema, alveolar hemorrhages, massive pulmonary vascular congestion and hyaline membrane formation, atelectasis, superimposed bronchial pneumonia, and, if the patient survives for weeks or months after the initial injury, pulmonary fibrosis. Shock affects the lung by producing endothelial damage in the vast capillary bed or precapillary arterioles. Microaggregates of platelets, polymorphonuclear leukocytes, and red cells block capillaries, destroy capillary endothelial cells by releasing hydrolytic enzymes, and eventually cause the increased capillary permeability that is responsible for the pulmonary interstitial edema seen in shock. In the balance of forces responsible for interstitial fluid in the lung, one must keep in mind the role of lymphatic drainage. Lymph flow is greatly increased in the very early stages of shock, and patients dying in hemorrhagic shock may have a widely distended pulmonary lymphatic system filled with proteinaceous material.

The decrease in pulmonary blood flow may also interfere with the production of surfactant. Lack of surfactant reduces the patency of alveoli and perpetuates leakage of fluid across pulmonary arterioles. Pulmonary venular constriction in response to tissue hypoxia may also contribute to pulmonary capillary congestion. It is also possible that with cerebral ischemia and hypoxia, neurogenic influences on the lung may cause a differential increase in venular resistance and increase capillary hydrostatic pressure and permeability. During *Pseudomonas* infusions in animals, there may be a direct effect of the endotoxin on capillary permeability, although sometimes a delayed response suggests an immune reaction with release of serotonin, contributing to the pulmonary edema. Regardless of its cause, the damage to the pulmonary capillary endothelium in shock perpetuates the resistance to blood flow, systemic hypoxia, and accelerates cellular death.

CELLULAR AND BIOCHEMICAL FACTORS IN SHOCK

OXYGEN-HB AFFINITY. Arterial blood with normal hemoglobin and oxygen saturation of 90 per cent at a P_{O_2} of 100 mm Hg carries close to 20 ml of O_2 per deciliter to the tissues. The mixed venous blood has an oxygen saturation of 75 per cent at a P_{O_2} of 40 mm Hg and contains 15 ml of O_2 per deciliter. The normal arteriovenous oxygen difference is 5 ml per deciliter. The extraction of oxygen from Hb by the tissues is not complete and depends to a large extent on the affinity of O_2 to Hb, i.e., the shape of the oxygen dissociation curve. Hydrogen ion (Bohr effect), carbon dioxide, and 2,3-diphosphoglyceric acid (2,3-DPG) cause greater dissociation of O_2 from Hb because of their preferential affinity for reduced hemoglobin. 2,3-DPG concentration in red cells results from a side reaction of glycolysis and increases during anemia, hypoxia, and acidosis. A drop in hemoglobin, hypoxia, and acidosis may thus be partly compensated for by a shift of the O_2 dissociation curve to the right, favoring greater delivery of O_2 to the tissues at the same P_{O_2}. This compensatory mechanism, in addition to the increase in cardiac output, provides for better oxygenation as extraction of O_2 from the O_2 reserve in venous blood increases. In certain tissues, however, such as the myocardium, extraction of O_2 at rest is already large, and any additional oxygen demand or a decrease in oxygen-Hb dissociation such as in alkalosis requires greater delivery of O_2, i.e., higher coronary blood flow.

In shock, the pH, carbon dioxide, and 2,3-DPG levels are changing, and one cannot calculate oxygen extraction from values of P_{O_2} because the shape of the O_2 dissociation curve cannot be predicted accurately. It is preferable to measure O_2 content or saturation of venous and arterial blood; if saturation is lower than predicted from values of P_{O_2}, one can deduce that there is a shift of the dissociation curve to the right, and vice versa. Overzealous correction of acidosis with bicarbonate may, through the Bohr effect on Hb affinity for O_2, actually reduce O_2 delivery to the tissues. Hypophosphatemia reported during hyperalimentation may decrease 2,3-DPG and O_2 delivery.

MITOCHONDRIAL FUNCTION. Survival of aerobic cells depends on the availability of substrates and oxygen to the mitochondria, which provide most of the high energy phosphate needs of the cell and utilize most of the available oxygen in the process. During oxidative phosphorylation, 36 moles of adenosine triphosphate (ATP) is produced per mole of glucose, whereas in the anaerobic state, glycolysis provides only two ATP molecules during the breakdown of one glucose molecule. Synthesis of the ATP from adenosine diphosphate (ADP) is associated with the most active state of respiration in mitochondria (state 3 respiration) and is determined by the cell energy demands. In addition to oxidative phosphorylation and ATP synthesis, the mitochondria bind and accumulate calcium. This function determines calcium availability for other intracellular organelles and thereby regulates biochemical processes or contractile events, as in cardiac or vascular muscle. Hypoxia may reduce the rate of ATP synthesis by mitochondria, but it does not cause significant damage to mitochondrial membrane functions unless it is severe, sustained, or associated with ischemia, which also reduces the availability of other substrates. In fact, an adaptation to hypoxia appears to take place such that when mitochondria are isolated from animal tissues after the animals have been exposed to brief periods of hypoxia (at P_{O_2} of 30 to 40 mm Hg), their capacity to respire and synthesize ATP in vitro is even enhanced. One of the earliest effects of hemorrhagic and endotoxin shock on mitochondrial function is the reduction in calcium transport by mitochondrial membranes, particularly in the organs that become ischemic. Effects on respiratory activity and ATP synthesis appear later, and finally mitochondrial damage ensues. The mechanism by which ischemia induces mitochondrial damage is not known. Whether such mitochondrial changes are the direct effects of deprivation of vital substrates during ischemia or are secondary to the release of lysosomal enzymes, changes in intracellular pH, or other changes in cellular ionic environment with accumulation of metabolites is not apparent.

Glucocorticoids may exert a protective effect on mitochondrial function in endotoxemia in rats. Very large doses of glucocorticoids completely protected the mitochondria when rats were given an LD 60 dose of endotoxin. The protective effect was not apparent, however, when a dose of LD 90 was given. One may summarize the mitochondrial effects by saying that hypoxia by itself triggers some adaptive mechanisms which tend to increase respiratory activity if oxygen and ADP become available, but ischemia during shock can induce significant mitochondrial damage which heralds cellular death.

CELLULAR STRUCTURE AND FUNCTION IN SHOCK. Several structural changes take place in cellular membranes in shock, and reversibility may occur at various stages. The earliest manifestation consists of swelling of the cell associated with an increase in intracellular sodium and clumping of nuclear chromatin, followed by dilatation of the endoplasmic reticulum. In this phase the cell membrane is unstable, and "blebs" may appear at the surface. The mitochondria will then begin to swell, and electron-dense clumps of flocculent material will appear within them. As the swelling of the mitochondria continues, Ca^{++} may or may not accumulate in them, depending on the type of cellular damage. The process of cell death becomes irreversible, lysosomes begin to disappear from the cell, and finally the cell is converted to a mass of debris, with large inclusions resembling myelin.

Two processes may lead to cellular death. One is a marked inhibition of the electron transport system caused by severe ischemia or anoxia or by the administration of cyanide or actinomycin A. This process leads to depletion of ATP, and the electron microscopic appearance of the cells undergoing that type of death does not show any calcium phosphate accumulation in the mitochondria. The other type of cell death is initiated by an injury to the cell membrane caused by activation of complement, by an antigen-antibody reaction, or by the administration of certain polyenes, such as amphotericin B, or certain bacterial or microbiologic products, such as the phospholipases or antitoxin. This type of cellular membrane damage is generally characterized by the precipitation of calcium phosphate in the mitochondria, presumably because active processes requiring ATP are preserved until late stages and calcium can be transported into the mitochondria.

One can relate the sequence of structural changes in the cellular membranes to specific biochemical changes. Initially there is probably an increase in cellular permeability for sodium and water causing cellular swelling, followed by increased sodium-potassium ATPase activity in an attempt to drive sodium out of the cell. Increased ATPase activity might eventually lead to the depletion of ATP and cyclic AMP, the latter leading to alteration of the cellular response to insulin, glucagon,

catecholamines, and other hormones. For example, the effect of insulin on glucose uptake in muscle of animals that have been subjected to hemorrhagic shock is reduced. The unresponsiveness to insulin in the peripheral tissues may be one of the reasons for hyperglycemia of injured individuals. There is also a marked decrease in ATP, particularly in the liver in early shock and in most other organs in late shock. It is difficult to determine the critical level of ATP that is necessary for cellular function, but it is believed that as long as there is ADP and oxygen, and substrate is provided, ATP generation can be resumed within minutes. The organs that are most seriously affected in the process of shock include, in descending order, the liver, kidneys, muscle, and lung.

THE LYSOSOMAL THEORY. Lysosomes are cytoplasmic granules which contain a variety of potent hydrolytic enzymes bound in a latent form in a relatively impermeable membrane. These enzymes are capable of hydrolyzing a wide variety of both natural and synthetic substances and can digest all intra- and extracellular macromolecules if they are released from their membranes. When released from the organelles, either inside or outside the cell, as a consequence of certain forms of cellular injury, they may contribute to the pathogenesis or the propagation and perpetuation of shock. They are most active at an acid pH, which would make them potentially more destructive in the setting of hypoxia and shock.

Numerous morphologic and biochemical observations implicate the lysosomal enzymes in the perpetuation of shock, but at this time the evidence for their primary involvement is not convincing. In organs such as liver, spleen, and intestine, the lysosomes enlarge and lose their granules during the early phases of shock. This is associated with a decrease in the total activity of lysosomal hydrolases in tissues and a corresponding increase in activity in the soluble fraction of the tissue homogenate. This has been interpreted to indicate a loss of lysosomal membrane integrity in vivo. When examined in vitro, the lysosomes obtained from animals in shock demonstrate an enhanced release of enzymes. A reduction in lysosomal membrane integrity has also been observed in animals after the administration of endotoxin. In several animal studies the levels of hydrolases found in blood, lymph, or serum seem to correlate with severity of shock.

The appearance of a *myocardial depressant factor* or factors (MDF) in shock, although still controversial, may be an indirect manifestation of the effect of lysosomal enzymes. In experimentally induced pancreatitis and in a variety of other shock states, plasma MDF activity closely parallels lysosomal hydrolases in the plasma. It has been suggested that pancreatic ischemia associated with shock results in the release of lysosomal and other enzymes within the pancreas, which act on an endogenous substrate to yield a peptide with low molecular weight and MDF activity, which is then released into the circulation. The resulting myocardial depression maintains the state of low cardiac output and sustains shock.

Another indication of the involvement of MDF has been the reproducibility of the shock syndrome with infusion of lysosomal hydrolases in animals. These animals demonstrate the hypotension, circulatory collapse, and pathologic changes in the tissues that are seen in experimental forms of shock.

Other suggestive evidence of the involvement of MDF has been the responsiveness of certain animals in shock to large amounts of corticosteroids. In vitro corticosteroids stabilize the lysosomal membranes and prevent their lysis. Treatment with steroids has been shown to suppress circulating serum levels of lysosomal hydrolases in a variety of shock states.

Endotoxemia is associated with increased levels of serum hydrolases, but in vitro the endotoxins do not increase the lysis of lysosome. It has been suggested that endotoxins may cause the formation of a lysosomal releasing factor, LRF, through activation of the alternative as well as the classic complement pathways. Activation of complement in fresh human serum has been found to generate a factor (LRF) which stimulates human polymorphonuclear leukocytes to release their lysosomal enzymes. This factor has many of the properties of human C5a, a complement component known to have chemotactic and anaphylatoxin activities.

COMPLEMENT ACTIVATION IN SHOCK. The complement system consists of a series of discrete plasma proteins which are present as inactive precursors until they are activated by highly specific biochemical reactions, some of which involve limited proteolytic cleavage. Nineteen components have been isolated and characterized. The activity of the immune system may depend on "complements" which may be the primary humoral mediators of antigen-antibody reactions. Not all antigen-antibody reactions depend on "complements." For example, the anaphylactic shock seen after penicillin or pollen antigens involving the IgE antibodies does not include complement. IgE immunoglobulins may act directly on cells to release histamine, slow reactive substance, and eosinophil chemotactic factor. In contrast, many other antigen-antibody reactions, particularly those involving the IgG and IgM immunoglobulins, which can also evoke an acute anaphylactic reaction, depend on complement as the primary humoral mediator of that reaction. The complement, when activated, can promote certain specialized functions by the cell, but could also eventually impair membrane function and cause cellular death. The various types of complements are designated numerically, and from a functional standpoint one could think of these various proteins as having a *recognition*, an *activation*, or a *cellular attack* function. The recognition function is carried out by three proteins forming a macromolecular complex in the plasma, which attaches itself to the membrane surface of a target cell with the appropriate antibody. The activation mechanism is triggered primarily by the antigen-antibody complex (classic pathway), but it may also be triggered by bacterial or fungal mucopolysaccharides without the participation of any immunoglobulins (alternative pathway). Regardless of pathways of activation, the results in terms of generation of various effectors, anaphylatoxins, or direct cellular damage are the same. Activation of complement causes the release of several low molecular weight vasoactive peptides from the complement molecules by cleavage, and these in turn have significant biologic effects. For example, during the activation of C2, a cleavage product occurs which has kinin-like activity, which then can significantly influence capillary permeability. Two other activation peptides, C3a and 5a, release histamine from mast cells, have chemotactic activity, and constrict vascular smooth muscle. Another fragment, C3b, acts as an opsonin and facilitates phagocytosis. Polymorphonuclear leukocytes may be attracted chemotactically through activation of esterases on their surface and may release their lysosomal enzymes if the concentration of the complement reaction product C5a is large enough. Platelets may have an increase in their procoagulant activity, and endothelial cells may contract. In addition to the direct and indirect effects of the fragments of activated complement on cells, their aggregation as decamolecular complexes on the surface of the cell membranes causes cellular destruction. The expressions of all these effects are increased capillary permeability; increased leukocyte accumulation and infiltration, such as is sometimes observed in glomerulitis; release of lysosomal enzymes, which could cause necrotizing vasculitis; and intravascular coagulation factors, which would induce the Shwartzman reaction, thrombocytopenia, and other manifestations of microcirculatory collapse and intravascular plugging seen in prolonged shock and in endotoxemia.

Although the side effects of complement activation in shock are detrimental, leading to cellular death, the fundamental biologic activities of the complement components are beneficial in enhancing phagocytosis and mediating the inflammatory response to local infection or irritation, in the vital neutralizing of viruses, and, finally, in modulating the immune response.

TREATMENT OF SHOCK

There are three main goals in the management of shock: (1) to restore or increase cardiac output to meet the demands of the tissues, (2) to distribute blood flow to vital organs if cardiac output cannot be increased effectively, and (3) to maintain arterial blood pressure in order to assure perfusion of the brain and of the ischemic myocardial segments in myocardial infarction, and to maintain glomerular filtration.

MYTHS IN THE TREATMENT OF SHOCK. *Myth 1: "All patients in shock die."* It is true that patients with extensive myocardial infarction, extensive burns, or overwhelming sepsis have a very meager chance for survival. On the other hand, a large number of patients with hypotension who are in the early phases of shock can be saved if an aggressive management is carried out to restore cardiac output and arterial blood pressure, particularly in situations in which reversible factors are contributing to the myocardial depression and hypotension.

Myth 2: "Norepinephrine (Levophed) is a lethal drug that should not be used in shock." This is another misconception which has emerged over the years from the assumption that all patients in shock have intense generalized vasoconstriction. Such is not the case in many shock syndromes, even after myocardial infarction, and particularly in septic shock. Furthermore, norepinephrine has a cardiotonic effect in addition to its vasoconstricting action, which will increase cardiac output and improve perfusion. Finally, it has a selective vasoconstrictor effect which spares the coronary and cerebral circulations and thus maintains perfusion of these vital organs and elevates arterial pressure for the perfusion of ischemic myocardial segments and glomerular filtration.

Myth 3: "Patients in cardiogenic shock should not receive intravenous fluid." This concern reflects the fact that patients in cardiogenic shock may have left ventricular failure and are bordering on pulmonary edema.

With careful monitoring of the pulmonary capillary wedge pressure (with a Swan-Ganz catheter), one can avoid fluid overload and yet administer sufficient fluid to compensate for hypovolemia and maintain a high left ventricular end-diastolic pressure necessary for an optimal stroke volume. It is also true that sometimes the shock lung syndrome associated with excessive transcapillary fluid loss into the lung may be reduced not by restricting fluid, but by giving fluids with high molecular weight colloids to increase oncotic pressure and reduce pulmonary edema.

Myth 4: "All patients in shock should be given a vasodilator." The assumption here is that the only way to improve tissue perfusion is to dilate blood vessels and decrease cardiac afterload. Drugs which produce vasodilatation may reduce arterial pressure, and thereby decrease perfusion of critically ischemic regions of the myocardium. For example, a vasodilator such as isoproterenol may increase blood flow to skeletal muscle, and a greater proportion of the cardiac output is diverted to that particular vascular bed, but the associated hypotension may reduce perfusion of the ischemic myocardium. Furthermore, unless vasodilatation includes the microcirculation, it might not necessarily be beneficial. This can be assessed by evaluating the metabolic changes in organs following the administration of a vasodilator. Isoproterenol, for instance, increases total myocardial blood flow; however, the distribution of flow within the microcirculation is such that perfusion of "exchange capillaries" is not increased and thereby the anaerobic state of that organ is not improved. In patients with myocardial infarction the intravenous administration of isoproterenol increases lactate production by the myocardium.

MONITORING PATIENTS IN SHOCK. Monitoring should include the following measures:

1. *The electrocardiogram.* Electrocardiographic monitoring promptly detects any premature ventricular contraction which could herald ventricular tachycardia and fibrillation or complete heart block, severe sinus bradycardia, or atrial arrhythmias, all of which should be treated if hypotension and low output are to be corrected.

2. *Arterial blood gases and pH.* These should also be monitored routinely. Correction of acidosis and hypoxia are essential elements in the management of the early phases of shock.

3. *Central venous and Swan-Ganz catheters.* The monitoring of central venous pressure provides an index of the status of absolute and relative blood volume and of the need for fluid replacement. The catheter should be inserted through the antecubital or external jugular vein; only if the physician is experienced should it be introduced through the subclavian or the internal jugular vein. Central venous pressure obtained with the catheter advanced to the superior vena cava is normally between 5 and 8 mm Hg, but it should be elevated to 10 mm Hg if one is to expect an adequate cardiac output in patients in shock. Central venous pressure reflects the filling pressure of the right ventricle.

The filling pressure of the left ventricle can be estimated from measurement of the "pulmonary capillary wedge" pressure with a Swan-Ganz balloon-tip catheter. A double lumen No. 7 F. catheter is introduced intravenously with or without fluoroscopy but with electrocardiographic monitoring. Its tip is advanced to the pulmonary artery; the balloon is inflated with air

and it can be floated to a wedge position in one of the pulmonary arteries. The recorded pressure downstream from the inflated balloon is the "pulmonary capillary wedge" pressure, and the appearance of the left atrial pressure wave form on the oscilloscope confirms the position of the catheter tip. The wedge pressure reflects left ventricular end-diastolic pressure, but a discrepancy between the two may occur if there is severe mitral stenosis or left atrial tumors. If for some reason one is unable to get the wedge pressure, the pulmonary artery diastolic pressure might be a useful index of the wedge pressure.

The double lumen Swan-Ganz catheter has been modified to include an extra lumen that allows measurement of right ventricular end-diastolic pressure simultaneously with the wedge pressure. Another modification includes a temperature sensor device at the tip that allows the detection of changes in temperature following injection of cold dextrose in the right atrium, and the temperature dilution curve obtained with the temperature sensor provides an estimate of cardiac output. A further modification of the Swan-Ganz catheter includes an electrical lead to allow the continuous monitoring of intracardiac electrocardiogram.

The Swan-Ganz catheter is expensive, and complications may accompany its use, such as arrhythmias, sepsis, or pulmonary infarction; nevertheless, it is a very important tool for monitoring patients with severe shock and for providing an important data base for judicious administration of fluids and sympathomimetic amines. One can suspect pulmonary infarction as a complication of Swan-Ganz catheterization if the pulmonary artery pressure rises, so occasional monitoring of the pulmonary artery pressure would be useful. The catheter should probably be removed within 48 hours after its insertion to avoid sepsis or pulmonary infarction, and should not be left continuously in the "wedged" position. The normal wedge pressure is 12 mm Hg, but it should be raised to 15 to 20 mm Hg in shock.

A discrepancy between right atrial and left atrial pressures may occur in patients with acute myocardial infarction, sepsis, or trauma when a high left atrial or pulmonary capillary wedge pressure may be accompanied by a low right atrial pressure, and under those circumstances monitoring right atrial pressure alone might lead to a dangerously aggressive replacement of blood volume. Conversely, patients with pulmonary disease, pulmonary embolism, pulmonary hypertension, and right ventricular infarction have relatively high levels of right atrial pressure compared to the pulmonary capillary wedge pressure, and the avoidance of fluids under those circumstances might deprive the patient of important therapy.

4. *Urinary catheter.* This allows the routine hourly measurement of urinary output. A decline in urinary output to less than 20 ml per hour is an indication of the inadequacy of arterial pressure and renal perfusion. It is a sensitive index of the progress of the shock syndrome and reflects the effectiveness of management. The most frequent cause of oliguria in shock is hypovolemia. Fluid deficits are often underestimated, particularly in the presence of sepsis. If oliguria persists despite adequate administration of fluid, diuretic therapy may be necessary to avoid acute renal tubular necrosis which complicates prolonged hypotension.

5. *Arterial catheterization for arterial pressure monitoring.* Patients with severe or persistent hypotension and

shock in whom it is difficult to measure blood pressure with the sphygmomanometer are candidates for intra-arterial pressure monitoring. There is often a discrepancy between the intra-arterial pressure measurements and the cuff pressure. There may be a low or even no recordable arterial pressure by the cuff technique when intra-arterial pressure by cannulation is normal or even at times slightly elevated. This discrepancy may result from severe peripheral vasoconstriction and low output and pulse pressure. Since the sphygmomanometric measurement of arterial pressure in shock may be erroneously low, it is advisable to palpate the femoral artery in the groin to get a better index of the strength of the pulse pressure in this more proximal large artery and to introduce an arterial cannula for monitoring arterial pressure before administration of vasopressors or resorting to counterpulsation. An arterial cannula also allows the frequent determination of blood gases and pH. The radial, brachial, or femoral arteries may be cannulated. We prefer to cannulate the femoral artery because of its size and the greater ease in identifying the pulse pressure in patients who are in shock.

6. *Cardiac output.* Measurement of cardiac output by thermal or dye dilution techniques is used for management of selected patients or for the evaluation of new therapeutic regimens. The mixed venous blood oxygen content may be used as an index of total body perfusion. Within certain limitations, one can estimate the effectiveness of total body perfusion and delivery of oxygen to the tissues by monitoring the oxygen content of mixed venous or pulmonary arterial blood. The assumptions are that the total body oxygen consumption is constant or does not change drastically and that the arterial oxygen content is high and does not vary significantly. An arteriovenous oxygen difference of 6 ml per deciliter or more indicates poor tissue perfusion.

MANAGEMENT. General Measures. Patients in shock may be in pain, apprehensive, and frightened. They should be reassured and put in a horizontal position with the legs slightly elevated, unless this position is uncomfortable or causes shortness of breath. In that case, they should be allowed to be in the most comfortable position. Pain should be relieved with morphine sulfate intravenously, preferably in small repeated doses of 2 to 5 mg; if side effects occur, such as hypotension, cold clammy skin, bradycardia, nausea, and vomiting, atropine may cause some relief. Another analgesic, meperidine, 50 to 100 mg, may be given intravenously. Intravenous fluid and monitoring of various functions should begin promptly to guide further therapy. Oxygen, norepinephrine, or dopamine may be initiated while the cause of shock is determined. Reversible factors which decrease cardiac output and cause hypotension should be corrected promptly.

CORRECTION OF HYPOVOLEMIA. Hypovolemia may occur in any type of shock whether or not it is associated with external signs of blood or fluid loss. If there is no evidence of actual fluid or blood loss, there may be a significant shift of fluid from the intravascular to the extracellular space because of increased capillary permeability and endothelial damage. This may occur in any vascular bed, but more specifically in the splanchnic and the pulmonary vasculature. Fluid may also shift intracellularly because of changes in cellular membrane permeability with increased intracellular sodium and water in any shock syndrome associated with decreased tissue perfusion. Fluid replacement is essential for the

restoration of cardiac output. Without an adequate filling pressure, there will not be an adequate cardiac output. The administration of potent cardiotonic drugs in the presence of hypovolemia and low cardiac filling pressure may be ineffective. On the other hand, these drugs increase cardiac output significantly if left ventricular end-diastolic pressure and volume are adequate.

If the patient has cardiogenic shock or if there are signs of pulmonary congestion or edema, one should insert a Swan-Ganz balloon catheter into the pulmonary artery or pulmonary arterial wedge position for measurements of the pulmonary artery diastolic pressure or the pulmonary capillary wedge pressure. If the pulmonary artery diastolic or pulmonary artery wedge pressure is less than 15 mm Hg, one should give 100 ml of Ringer's lactate, saline, or dextran every 10 to 15 minutes. If perfusion improves and wedge pressure remains less than 15 mm Hg, one should continue infusion at the same rate, trying to achieve a pressure between 15 and 20 mm Hg. If perfusion of the tissues is unchanged or worse, if wedge pressure increases above 20 mm Hg, or if there are signs of pulmonary congestion, one should stop volume expansion. Improvement in tissue perfusion is evaluated by examining the degree of cyanosis, clamminess of the skin, the level of arterial blood pressure, and urinary output, as well as the sensorium and alertness of the patient, blood gases, and pH.

In other types of shock, or if wedge pressure cannot be obtained, the insertion of a central venous catheter is a helpful guide for administration of fluids. If the central venous pressure is less than 10 mm Hg, one should expand volume until arterial pressure and tissue perfusion return to satisfactory levels, central venous pressure is between 10 and 15 mm Hg, or pulmonary congestion develops. The central venous or pulmonary capillary wedge pressures should be measured with careful reference to a constant point marked on the chest at the level of the right atrium or the phlebostatic axis. Patients who are on respirators or are receiving positive pressure assistance or positive pressure ventilation will have an abnormally elevated pressure. Under those circumstances, the filling pressure should be recorded at the time the respirator is transiently disconnected.

Treatment for hemorrhagic hypotension is with blood replacement; but while waiting for typing and cross-matching, the patient should be given isotonic glucose or Ringer's lactate. The effects of these fluids are transient, because the crystalloids will rapidly leave the intravascular space. A more effective treatment might include colloids that stay longer in the circulation and increase oncotic pressure. This is particularly important when patients have manifestations of the shock lung syndrome, when extensive endothelial damage and interstitial edema are suspected, or when patients are chronically ill or malnourished and have hypoalbuminemia. Under those circumstances, dextran or mannitol, albumin or plasma would expand blood volume. The excretion of dextran or mannitol by the kidney will increase oncotic pressure in Bowman's capsule and create a favorable hydrostatic-oncotic pressure gradient across the glomerulus, facilitating filtration even at low arterial pressure. If arterial pressure is not rapidly restored or oliguria persists despite the administration of diuretics such as furosemide in conjunction with fluid replacement, then there might be danger of overexpansion of plasma volume and accentuation of the pulmonary edema. Dextran might not be indicated in the presence of hypofibrinogenemia and bleeding dyscrasias. The development of pulmonary edema is closely correlated with the gradient between plasma oncotic and pulmonary artery wedge pressure, which reflects the capillary hydrostatic pressure in the lung. Plasma oncotic pressure of normal adults is approximately 25 mm Hg, whereas pulmonary wedge pressure is 10 to 12 mm Hg. Capillary filtration takes place normally in the lung despite a low hydrostatic and a relatively high oncotic pressure, because of the equally high interstitial oncotic pressure in the lung. Plasma oncotic pressure may fluctuate. After 12 hours of bed rest, for example, it declines markedly. If oncotic pressure remains significantly higher (>8 mm Hg) than pulmonary capillary hydrostatic pressure, the risk of pulmonary edema is negligible; but if oncotic pressure is only 1 to 3 mm Hg higher than pulmonary wedge pressure, the patient is at high risk for pulmonary edema.

Types of Fluid. The isotonic saline solution contains 140 mEq of sodium and 140 mEq of chloride, whereas Ringer's lactate solution has 130 mEq of sodium, 4 mEq of potassium, 108 mEq of chloride, and 28 mEq of lactate. Lactate and acetate are converted to bicarbonate and maintain the alkalinity of the blood when large volumes of fluid are necessary. When large volumes of fluid are administered, isotonic saline causes a dilution acidosis, which can be avoided if Ringer's lactate is used.

Human serum albumin comes in two concentrations, 5 grams per deciliter, which is the usual dose used, or 25 grams per deciliter salt-poor albumin. The 25 grams per deciliter will be necessary only in the presence of severe hypoalbuminemia. An alternative is purified plasma protein, which is free of hepatitis virus contamination but has some contamination with vasoactive substances, causing the Food and Drug Administration to express concern about its use. Both albumin and purified plasma protein are expensive. They cost between $50 and $100 per 500 ml and represent a significant strain on blood donor programs. They should not be used indiscriminately.

There are two types of dextran: dextran 40 with 40,000 molecular weight, and dextran 70 with approximately 70,000 molecular weight. Dextran 70 comes in a 6 per cent solution, and dextran 40 comes in a 10 per cent solution. The dextran solutions maintain intravascular volume for several hours; but if given in amounts exceeding 1 liter, they may cause serious side effects, including platelet dysfunction and abnormalities in bleeding and coagulation, the nature of which is not clearly defined, and occasional anaphylactoid reactions. Approximately 5 per cent of patients receiving dextran have had such reactions, but very few of these are fatal.

With dextran 40 there is an incidence of acute renal failure, presumably because the rapid filtration of the low molecular weight dextran into the urine is accompanied by maximal reabsorption of the filtered salt and water, leading to a high intratubular concentration with an increase in intratubular viscosity and possibly physical occlusion of the renal tubule by dextran 40 precipitates. This does not seem to occur with dextran 70 because it is filtered at a much slower rate owing to its molecular size.

Another colloid is hydroxyethyl starch or hetastarch, which maintains volume expansion almost twice as long as dextran and has few of the side effects of dextran. It interferes minimally with coagulation, it has a very mild anaphylactoid effect, and its cost is one fifth that of albumin.

CORRECTION OF HYPOXIA. Often administration of 100 per cent oxygen by intranasal catheter may be sufficient to correct the hypoxia, although occasionally the use of positive pressure respirators to improve gas exchange has been necessary. Positive pressure ventilation may simultaneously decrease the venous return by increasing intrathoracic pressure, and thereby perpetuate and aggravate a low output state. Also, 100 per cent oxygen by mask may lead to toxic changes in the lung if continued more than a few hours. Thus when a respirator is required, the preferred approach is to select an F_{IO_2} of 50 per cent, and to increase the F_{IO_2} and employ positive pressure only if needed to achieve a P_{O_2} of about 70 mm Hg.

CORRECTION OF ACIDOSIS. If the arterial blood pH is less than 7.3 and respiratory acidosis has been ruled out, it is advisable to give 1 vial of sodium bicarbonate intravenously (44.6 mEq). On the other hand, if the arterial blood pH is less than 7.2, 2 vials intravenously may be administered and values repeated for further therapy in 15 to 30 minutes. Overcorrection of acidosis to alkalosis may decrease oxygen delivery to tissues by shifting the oxyhemoglobin dissociation curve.

TREATMENT OF ARRHYTHMIAS. Arrhythmias, particularly after myocardial infarction, may limit cardiac output and perpetuate shock.

Sustained ventricular tachycardia may be treated first with intravenous lidocaine in doses of 50 to 100 mg; if there is associated hypotension or any evidence of hemodynamic deterioration, electroshock should be used immediately. Ventricular fibrillation should be treated immediately with electroshock. If the first or second shock is unsuccessful, the patient must receive closed chest massage, mouth-to-mouth respiration, and possibly intravenous sodium bicarbonate before again attempting electrocardioversion.

Accelerated idioventricular rhythm is seen frequently in patients with myocardial infarction, particularly in those with diaphragmatic infarction. The rate is slightly faster than sinus rhythm, and a period of sinus bradycardia seems to favor the development of this arrhythmia. This benign condition can occasionally deteriorate into a fatal ventricular arrhythmia and should be treated with lidocaine or with atropine to increase the sinus rate.

Supraventricular arrhythmias (atrial tachycardias, flutter, fibrillation, or junctional rhythms) should generally be treated with digoxin; but if the rhythm persists or there is an associated hypotension or hemodynamic deterioration, electroshock therapy should be utilized immediately. Sinus bradycardia, if severe (less than 40 beats per minute), can contribute to hypotension. It is more commonly associated with inferior diaphragmatic infarction, and, if accompanied by frequent premature ventricular beats, restoration of a more rapid sinus rhythm can eliminate them. Atropine is most effective intravenously in doses of 0.4 mg up to 1 or even 2 mg. If bradycardia persists and hypotension or other signs of hypoperfusion are evident, electrical pacing should be instituted.

Conduction disturbances such as atrioventricular block carry a variable prognosis. The conduction disturbance which occurs with inferior diaphragmatic infarction has a better prognosis. It generally occurs early, is associated with sinus bradycardia, and may be caused by a temporary reflex increase in vagal tone to the conduction system or by atrioventricular nodal ischemia with only localized necrosis of this discrete structure. In anterior wall infarction, on the other hand, heart block is related to ischemic damage of the three fascicles of the conduction system, which results from a more extensive degree of necrosis and is associated with higher mortality. Patients with inferior infarction benefit from temporary electrical pacing if they do not respond to atropine, whereas those with anteroseptal infarction generally require a permanent pacemaker.

Treatment of Sepsis. Both gram-negative and gram-positive organisms have been associated with septic shock. In gram-negative septicemia, *E. coli* is the predominant organism, and infections with *Klebsiella-Aerobacter* (enterobacter) groups are not uncommon; endotoxin is an important factor in the pathogenesis of this syndrome. Gram-positive infections without endotoxemia, such as in pneumococcal pneumonia, *Staphylococcus aureus,* or streptococcal bacteremia, may cause shock. Chronic alcoholism is a common associated illness among these patients.

The characteristic hemodynamic abnormality in septic shock (whether gram-positive or gram-negative) is a marked decrease in peripheral vascular resistance; cardiac output may be increased, normal, or decreased. In contrast, in cardiogenic shock cardiac output is low and peripheral resistance is normal, increased, or occasionally decreased, and in hypovolemic shock cardiac output is low and peripheral resistance is increased. The treatment of septic shock includes the aggressive treatment of the infection with antibiotics and drainage of any abscesses. Although cardiac output may be normal or high, it may be insufficient to meet metabolic needs of the tissues, and an absolute or relative decrease in intravascular volume requires fluid administration. Therefore volume replacement with crystalloids or colloids is necessary to restore and raise central venous pressure to levels of 10 to 15 mm Hg or pulmonary wedge pressure to 20 mm Hg.

Use of Steroids. The use of corticosteroids in septic shock has been adopted by most physicians and is used in very large doses early in the treatment of shock. Their beneficial effect appears to be related primarily to their action on cellular membranes. Steroids interact with biomembranes and probably become incorporated within their bilayer structures. The stabilizing effect of corticosteroids on biomembranes has been demonstrated in vitro in studies of lysosomes isolated from animals that have been treated with these agents. These lysosomes have a markedly increased resistance to lysis in vitro. Apparently this beneficial action of corticosteroids is not limited to their glucocorticoid properties. For example, testosterone is another potent membrane stabilizing agent. The reason for the continued question concerning the effectiveness of corticosteroids is that the consequences of membrane stabilization by corticosteroids in vivo are not really known. Experimental studies in animals subjected to septic, endotoxin, or hemorrhagic shock indicate improved survival with administration of corticosteroids. In shock, considerable damage to the microcirculation may be attributed to membrane interactions between platelets, polymorphonuclear leukocytes, and endothelium. Activation by the bacteria of the alternative complement pathway with the release of various peptides may favor platelet aggregation with endothelium and leukocytes, clot formation, and obstruction of the microcirculation. Corticosteroids may prevent these membrane interactions in vivo. Animals pretreated with cortisone exhibit an impressive resistance to endotoxin-mediated shock. On the other hand, it is not apparent whether corticosteroids are effective in the advanced shock state in which the physician often finds the patient. The use of corticosteroids in doses of 30 mg per kilogram of methylprednisolone as early as possible in patients with septicemia and hypotension might be justifiable, based on extensive work in vitro. The extension of the use of corticosteroids to patients with cardiogenic shock is unwise. There is evidence of malignant arrhythmias developing after the administration of corticosteroids to such patients, and the incidence of ventricular aneurysms may be increased because of interference with the inflammatory and healing processes of the myocardium.

It is claimed that corticosteroids have significant cardiovascular effects with possibly alpha receptor blocking activities, but pharmacologic studies indicate that the steroids have little if any significant direct cardiovascular action; they may augment the action of catecholamines, but they do not block alpha receptors.

Use of Sympathomimetic Amines. These drugs are used to increase cardiac output through their cardiotonic effect, and to redistribute blood flow to vital organs by their selective vasoconstricting action; by virtue of these two effects, they raise arterial pressure and allow the perfusion of ischemic regions, particularly in the myocardium, through collateral vessels. There are two potential problems with their use. If arterial pressure is elevated significantly, the hypertension may be detrimental, as it increases myocardial work and oxygen demand. Thus judicious elevation of arterial pressure to levels between 110 and 120 mm Hg systolic pressure would be reasonable. One cannot predict the optimal arterial pressure necessary to perfuse the coronaries in any particular patient because one does not know the severity of coronary disease and its extent, or the extent of myocardial reserves that would allow the heart to cope with a slight increase in afterload induced by the rising arterial pressure. Nevertheless, hypotension, particularly following myocardial infarction, should be corrected and arterial pressure maintained. The second potential problem with use of these drugs is their vasoconstricting effect; however, some vasoconstriction can be beneficial if it occurs in nonvital organs and if it is associated with increased cardiac output. This combination of effects raises arterial pressure and improves perfusion of vital organs. Therefore the proper use of sympathomimetic amines in shock requires a thorough knowledge of their cardiovascular effects. They have a structure similar to that of the natural adrenergic neurotransmitter norepinephrine and activate adrenergic receptors in various cells. Their action depends upon their affinity for various types of adrenergic receptors.

Adrenergic Receptors. The adrenergic receptors may be classified as alpha or beta receptors with respect to their cardiovascular action. The alpha receptors are predominantly in blood vessels and mediate vasoconstriction. The beta receptors are present in the blood vessels as well as the myocardium. Activation of the beta-1 receptors in the myocardium causes an increase in myocardial contractility and in heart rate, whereas activation of beta-2 receptors in blood vessels causes vasodilatation. The same catecholamine may activate both alpha and beta receptors, depending on the dose and the organ in which it is acting.

Norepinephrine. Norepinephrine increases myocardial contractility by activating beta-1 receptors and thus may increase cardiac output. On the other hand, in blood vessels it activates primarily alpha or vasoconstricting receptors. The magnitude of its effect on alpha receptors varies from one organ to another. It is a very potent vasoconstrictor in skin, muscle, and splanchnic beds, whereas in the coronary vessels it activates the beta-2 receptors as well as the alpha receptors; and because there is a paucity of alpha receptors in the coronary vessels in contrast to other vascular beds, the drug causes vasodilatation of the coronaries.

It offers several distinct advantages in the treatment of shock. It increases cardiac output and redistributes blood flow away from the extremities and toward the heart and brain and increases arterial pressure, which in turn increases coronary flow to ischemic myocardium. It should be administered intravenously through an indwelling catheter to avoid the risk of extravasation, which results in necrosis of subcutaneous tissues. Two ampules of Levophed (4 mg base per ampule) may be dissolved in 500 ml glucose and water and an infusion rate started at a very low level to determine the smallest necessary dose to maintain arterial pressure between 100 and 120 mm Hg, which should provide adequate perfusion to the heart, brain, and kidney (unless the patient was hypertensive or has extensive arteriosclerotic disease). A dose of 4 μg per minute may occasionally be adequate; however, many patients require up to 40 μg per minute; and in general if such doses are necessary to maintain pressure, prognosis is poor. An average dose would be between 10 and 15 μg per minute. The lack of response to norepinephrine is probably an indication of significant myocardial damage if hypoxia, hypovolemia, and acidosis have been considered and corrected.

DOPAMINE. This is a naturally occurring catecholamine which is the precursor of norepinephrine. It has a different cardiovascular effect, depending on its dose level. When given in low concentrations, approximately 200 μg per minute, it has a vasodilator action in the renal and mesenteric vessels, with only slight dilatation of cerebral and coronary vessels. The dilator effect is mediated through beta-2 receptors and through specific dopaminergic receptors. In doses of 500 to 1000 μg per minute, it increases myocardial contractility and cardiac output through the activation of beta-1 receptors. In larger doses of 1500 to 3000 μg per minute, it causes vasoconstriction through activation of alpha-adrenergic receptors of arteries and veins in most vascular beds. Thus this drug may redistribute blood flow away from the extremities and toward the kidney, gut, heart, and brain; however, it may be necessary to give large doses to maintain arterial pressure and coronary blood flow, particularly following myocardial infarction, and these large doses will then tend to oppose to some degree the beneficial vasodilator effects seen in some vascular beds.

EPINEPHRINE. Epinephrine is released from the adrenal gland; it activates myocardial beta-1 receptors and vasoconstrictor alpha receptors in most vessels except in skeletal muscle and coronary vessels, where it activates beta-2 receptors when administered in low doses. It increases cardiac output, but redistributes flow away from the kidney and splanchnic circulations toward skeletal muscle. Given in a dose range from 2 to 30 μg per minute intravenously, its effect on the redistribution flow is not optimal, and its effect on arterial pressure is only modest because of its vasodilator effect in skeletal muscle.

ISOPROTERENOL. Isoproterenol is a synthetic sympathomimetic amine which activates primarily vascular beta-2 receptors, causing vasodilatation, and myocardial beta-1 receptors, increasing cardiac output. The magnitude of the vasodilator effect of isoproterenol varies in different vascular beds, depending on the density of beta-2 receptors and the affinity of the drug for them. The major vasodilator action of isoproterenol is in skeletal muscle beds.

This drug is not recommended in either cardiogenic or septic shock. In hemorrhagic shock, burns, or trauma the major line of treatment should be blood or fluid replacement. In cardiogenic shock, isoproterenol significantly increases myocardial oxygen requirement, and, despite the increase in coronary flow, there is evidence that the ischemic region of the myocardium may be hypoperfused as indicated by increased lactate production. In contrast, the administration of norepinephrine tends to decrease lactate production by the heart. Dopamine is also beneficial if arterial pressure is maintained. The use of isoproterenol should probably be limited to the treatment of complete heart block in an attempt to maintain an idioventricular rhythm until more definitive therapy can be carried out. The usual dose of isoproterenol is 0.5 to 4 μg per minute.

One can summarize the use of sympathomimetic amines by saying that the goal is to attain an arterial pressure sufficiently adequate to perfuse the kidney, the ischemic myocardial segment, and the brain without overloading the left ventricle. The drug should redistribute blood flow toward the more vital organs and away from skin and muscle for the optimal utilization of the limited cardiac output in shock. Finally, the drug should also have an inotropic action, and drugs such as methoxamine and phenylephrine, which only cause arterial vasoconstriction by activating alpha receptors without stimulating the heart, should be avoided. With these goals in mind, norepinephrine and dopamine should be chosen in the management of shock, regardless of the initiating cause.

Vasodilator Therapy. The beneficial effects of vasodilator therapy are (1) to decrease myocardial oxygen demands by decreasing preload or cardiac filling pressure and cardiac size and decreasing afterload by decreasing arterial pressure and arterial impedance, and (2) to dilate microcirculatory vessels.

The effectiveness of vasodilators (nitroprusside, nitroglycerin, phentolamine, or hydralazine) is impressive in the acutely failing heart following myocardial infarction without shock and with an elevated left ventricular end-diastolic pressure or capillary wedge pressure above 20 or 25 mm Hg; but the presence of *hypotension* should be a contraindication to the use of this therapy alone. Under those circumstances one may have to use a vasodilator drug along with norepinephrine or dopamine.

REDUCTION IN PRELOAD. One can reduce oxygen demand of the myocardium by decreasing cardiac volume in patients who have a high filling pressure. Reduction in cardiac size decreases myocardial wall tension, which is a major determinant of myocardial oxygen requirements. It may be achieved by administration of diuretics or venodilator drugs, which reduce filling pressure by pooling blood in the peripheral veins. The goal of "venodilator therapy" is to decrease preload and cardiac size and not to decrease arterial blood pressure. This effect is desirable as long as cardiac filling pressure does not drop excessively, causing a drop in cardiac output. In some patients with severe pulmonary congestion and high cardiac filling pressure with systemic arterial hypotension, it might be necessary to combine the vasodilator therapy with another drug that will cause selective arteriolar vasoconstriction in certain organs and will increase peripheral vascular resistance and raise and maintain arterial pressure, such as dopamine or norepinephrine.

REDUCTION IN AFTERLOAD. This is a beneficial effect of the vasodilators, because it will decrease the arterial impedance against which the left ventricle ejects its blood; thus ejection fraction may improve. This is desirable as long as it is not associated with a significant reduction in systemic arterial diastolic pressure, particularly in patients who are normotensive or have borderline hypotension. The dose of the vasodilator drug may be adjusted so that it would not cause a significant reduction in diastolic arterial pressure. Any drop in arterial pressure by more than 10 mm Hg should be avoided, and the diastolic pressure should certainly not be allowed to decrease below 65 mm Hg. Reduction in afterload is ideal in patients with chronic severe congestive failure with high filling pressure, pulmonary congestion, and low cardiac output, but without a significant reduction in arterial pressure. Patients with cardiomyopathy without coronary artery disease may be the best candidates for this therapy.

Neither a vasodilator alone nor propranolol, which also reduces myocardial oxygen demand, has a place in the management of cardiogenic hypotension following myocardial infarction. The elimination of the cardiotonic effect of the normal sympathetic drive by propranolol may significantly impair cardiac output and precipitate failure. If the patient has continuing pain and *a normal or elevated blood pressure,* despite the administration of narcotics, morphine or meperidine, and nitroglycerin, the administration of propranolol might then be considered.

MICROCIRCULATORY VASOCONSTRICTION AND ALPHA RECEPTOR BLOCKERS. In some patients, despite prolonged administration of dopamine or norepinephrine, tissue perfusion is not improved. The reasons may be that the myocardial infarction or the cellular damage is extensive. It is also possible that constriction of microcirculatory vessels may be preventing the perfusion of exchange capillaries. The alpha receptor blocker phentolamine has a specific effect on the vasoconstricting α-receptors and does not block the beta receptors in the myocardium. Thus the cardiotonic effect of sympathomimetic amines would not be prevented, yet vasoconstricting effects at the microcirculatory level would be antagonized. Phentolamine has a preferential inhibitory effect on alpha receptors in venules and veins as opposed to arterioles, and its dilator action may therefore be greater in veins than in arterioles. This effect calls for a note of caution, because rapid relaxation of large veins may abruptly lower cardiac filling pressure if the patient is hypovolemic. For this reason, it is essential to ascertain that the patient has received adequate amounts of fluid before giving phentolamine.

In this setting of shock with high circulating catecholamines and after prolonged infusions of high concentrations of norepinephrine and dopamine and with persisting evidence of decreased tissue perfusion, the use of the alpha receptor blocker phentolamine offers several theoretical advantages over other vasodilators based on animal work. It dilates venules to decrease capillary hydrostatic pressure and opens up precapillary sphincters, which allow perfusion of nutritional capillaries. Other vasodilators may have a negligible effect on veins and venules, and although they increase blood flow, they do not necessarily increase perfusion of the microcirculation. Unfortunately there are no clinical studies which would confirm the

beneficial effects of phentolamine* in that stage of shock, which in general carries a poor prognosis. An initial dose of 2 mg given intravenously, followed by 5 mg, should be attempted, with careful monitoring of the intra-arterial and central venous pressures to ascertain that the patient is not hypovolemic and does not have a decreased effective blood volume. If hypotension results from this small dose, more rapid fluid replacement will be necessary before adding phentolamine. Generally phentolamine may be added to the intravenous fluid containing norepinephrine. One or 2 ampules of phentolamine (5 mg per ampule) may be added for each ampule of norepinephrine in the intravenous fluid. If given alone, 4 ampules in 500 ml or 40 μg per milliliter is a reasonable concentration, and the usual dose is between 20 and 80 μg per minute.

NITROPRUSSIDE. This is a very effective vasodilator drug that causes relaxation of veins to decrease preload and some relaxation of arterioles to decrease arterial impedance. It may be started intravenously at a dose of 16 μg per minute and increased to 200 μg per minute with constant monitoring of arterial pressure. Occasionally larger doses have been necessary.

Other vasodilator drugs, such as hydralazine, which primarily exert an action on the arterioles, would not be very effective in reducing cardiac size and myocardial oxygen demand, and may be detrimental in causing a significant reduction in arterial blood pressure.

Digitalis. One should consider the administration of digoxin to patients with cardiogenic shock only if there is evidence of pulmonary congestion and an elevated pulmonary artery wedge pressure. The initial loading dose of digoxin may be reduced because in the setting of myocardial infarction hypoxia may predispose to myocardial irritability, and the renal excretion of digoxin may be impaired because of decreased renal perfusion and arterial blood pressure.

Surgical Treatment in Cardiogenic Shock. In cardiogenic shock, experience has been obtained with the use of intra-aortic balloon counterpulsation. The balloon is introduced into the aorta at the end of a catheter inserted through the femoral artery. It is inflated during early diastole and is collapsed during systole. This sequence increases the pressure during diastole and reduces it during systole, thus decreasing afterload during ejection and increasing diastolic coronary perfusion pressure and coronary flow during diastole. Improvement of the hemodymic status has been observed, but because a large number of patients with myocardial infarction and shock have extensive coronary artery disease, the long-term survival is still disappointing. The balloon counterpulsation appears to be of greatest potential benefit in the support of patients who have seriously compromised hemodynamics after myocardial infarction and who are candidates for a surgical procedure. This mechanical assistance sustains the hemodynamics during cardiac catheterization and coronary arteriography in preparation for surgery. Emergency revascularization surgery or infarctectomy, which has been carried out on occasion, has not been encouraging. Two complications of myocardial infarction require surgical intervention and carry a reasonable prognosis; these are ruptured papillary muscle and interventricular septal perforation. In both, there is decreased ejection from the left ventricle and a fall in arterial pressure. Attempts to increase systemic arterial pressure with drugs exaggerate the regurgitation or the left to right shunt. In these circumstances, the selective

---

*Experimental drug for this purpose.

lowering of arterial systolic pressure with intra-aortic balloon counterpulsation is ideal, as it will facilitate ejection and reduce mitral regurgitation or left to right shunt. A significant reduction in afterload and vasodilatation may also be achieved with drugs such as nitroprusside or nitroglycerin, but the associated fall in diastolic pressure may extend the myocardial ischemia. Surgical management, as soon as it is feasible and safe, should be the course to pursue. Severe papillary muscle dysfunction or papillary muscle rupture (the posterior more frequently than the anterior) may cause significant left ventricular failure, and the surgical replacement of the mitral valve has been satisfactory, particularly in patients with good myocardial function. Patients with a perforation of the ventricular septum have congestive failure in association with the sudden appearance of a pansystolic murmur, often accompanied by a thrill. Clinically, it is often impossible to differentiate this condition from a ruptured papillary muscle. The demonstration of a left to right shunt by cardiac catheterization confirms the diagnosis. Rupture of the septum should be treated surgically, preferably six to eight weeks after infarction, so that the margins of the defect can have sufficient scar tissue to permit surgical closure with relative ease.

Abboud, F. M., et al: Reflex control of the peripheral circulation. Prog. Cardiovasc. Dis., 18:371, 1976.

Braunwald, E.: Protection of the ischemic myocardium. Circulation, 53 (Suppl. 1):1, 1976.

Braunwald, E.: The Myocardium: Failure and Infarction. New York, H. P. Publishing Company, 1975.

Goldberg, L. I.: Dopamine — clinical uses of an endogenous catecholamine. N. Engl. J. Med., 291:707, 1974.

The Cell in Shock. Proceedings of a Symposium on Recent Research Developments and Current Clinical Practice in Shock. The Upjohn Company, April 1976, pp. 16–29, 30–34, 35–38.

The Organ in Shock. Proceedings of the Second Symposium on Recent Research Developments and Current Clinical Practice in Shock. The Upjohn Company, April 1977, pp. 8–15, 24–31, 38–49.

Weil, M. H., et al.: Treatment of circulatory shock. JAMA, 231:1280, 1975.

Winslow, E. J., et al.: Hemodynamic studies and results of therapy in 50 patients with bacteremic shock. Am. J. Med., 54:421, 1973.

357. THROMBOEMBOLIC DISEASES

357.1. THROMBOSIS

Patrick A. McKee

A *thrombus,* as defined by Welch in 1899, is "a solid mass or plug, formed in the living heart or vessels from constituents of the blood." This definition remains valid, and thrombosis, which is the formation of a thrombus, can be contrasted with the term blood clotting or blood coagulation, which refers to the conversion of blood from a liquid to a solid outside the circulatory system. The primary difference between the two terms has to do with the mode of initiation and the in vivo contribution of flowing blood to the microanatomy of the thrombus. The term *embolus* refers to the dislodgment, in total or in part, of a thrombus from its site of origin and its movement by the flow of blood to a more distant site within the circulatory system. The general topic of *thromboembolism* refers to all those diseases which have as part of their pathogenesis, course, or outcome the occlusion of some part of the vascular system by a mass formed from blood constituents. Al-

though the exact mortality and morbidity attributable to thromboembolic diseases are not known precisely, it is known that the incidence of thromboembolic diseases has increased appreciably in proportion to man's longevity. As an index of the over-all importance of this condition, it is estimated that diseases either complicated or caused by thromboembolism occur approximately three times more frequently than cancer in general. Despite extensive research, the precise mechanisms involved in the pathogenesis of thrombosis have not been defined, and the general circumstances which predispose to thrombi remain the sharpest features of our understanding about their pathogenesis. These situations are defined by the presence of one or more features of Virchow's triad of abnormalities of blood flow, the vessel lining surface, and the blood constituents. To date our ability to measure meaningful changes in any one of these three descriptors remains elusive.

The consensus is that all thrombi, whether developing in arteries or veins, are initiated by platelets adhering to the endothelial surface of the vessel. For many years it has been known that venous thrombi are mostly influenced by marked slowing in the flow of blood, i.e., "stasis," and that this somehow leads to the activation of certain serine protease clotting factors with the formation of thrombin and then the conversion of fibrinogen to fibrin. This type of thrombus has been termed a "red thrombus" because it contains a fairly even distribution of red and white blood cells and platelets in a network of fibrin. More recent data, however, strongly suggest that, even in veins, platelets comprise the initial nidus of thrombi and that such an aggregate of platelets is analogous to the head of an arterial thrombus, which is referred to classically as a "white thrombus." The latter has long been recognized as being initiated and attached to the arterial endothelium by a large mass of platelets that grossly has a whitish appearance in contrast to the rest of the thrombus. Pathologic examinations have shown that deep venous thrombi usually begin in the concavity formed by the juncture of a venous valve leaflet with the vein wall. At this site, layers or aggregates of platelets can be seen, and it is believed by many that these platelet clumps trigger the events which culminate in the conversion of fibrinogen to fibrin and hence the formation of a thrombus. In the arterial vasculature overt stasis is not very important as a predisposing factor to thrombosis; however, relative stasis, such as might occur in areas of nonlaminar blood flow, may contribute significantly to the development and progression of a thrombus. Since arterial thrombi occur mostly in diseases characterized by atherosclerotic lesions, and on or in close proximity to such lesions, it is commonly believed that this attests to the importance of both disrupted laminar flow and an abnormal endothelial surface predisposing to thrombosis. The mechanism by which platelets adhere to a damaged endothelial surface is presumably due to the exposure of collagen fibrils in the subendothelial area. Although this can be shown to occur in vitro, it is not unequivocally established that the same phenomenon occurs in life. As platelets adhere to a surface, adenosine diphosphate (ADP) is released, which causes additional platelet aggregation. Other substances are also recognized as important in platelet-surface and platelet-platelet interactions; for example, the soluble plasma protein, von Willebrand factor, is known to be required for certain platelet adhesion and aggregation reactions. In addition, arachidonic acid, precursor to prostaglandin synthesis, and prostaglandin G_2 and thromboxane A_2, which are formed and released by the metabolically active platelet during platelet aggregation, promote further platelet aggregation. As platelets aggregate, other important components are also released which participate in reactions occurring at the blood-platelet membrane interface. This leads to the activation of certain plasma clotting factors, particularly those of the intrinsic system, thereby initiating a cascade of reactions which generates thrombin and culminates in the conversion of fibrinogen into fibrin (see Ch. 519 for blood clotting scheme).

Despite numerous studies, it is still unknown whether measurable changes in the levels of various blood clotting factor activities predispose to thrombosis. There are a number of nonspecific and not very sensitive differences in the levels of various clotting factors which have been found statistically significant when large populations of patients with certain thromboembolic disorders have been compared to those without such problems. For example, a shortened whole blood clotting time, a shortened partial thromboplastin time, increased levels of fibrinogen, circulating fibrin multimers, excess levels of activity of factors V, VII, and VIII, the presence of fibrin degradation products, increased platelet number or stickiness, decrease in the concentration of normal plasma serine protease inhibitors (antithrombins and antiplasmins), and reduction of the normal fibrinolytic activity have each been taken to signify a tendency to form thrombi. The results of such tests, however, have been ambiguous, and in general they are not very useful measurements for the diagnosis or management of thromboembolic disorders. In actuality, the presence of certain risk factors or the presence of certain diseases correlates better with the ability to predict or suspect thromboembolic disease than any laboratory assessment currently in use. Although in most instances local atherosclerotic changes are a prerequisite for arterial thrombosis, and venous stasis is recognized as the major predisposing factor to deep vein thrombosis, the question of whether "hypercoagulable" blood changes are also required in either situation remains debatable. Clearly, many of the reports that indicate such changes are necessary may have quantitated the result rather than the cause of thrombosis. The most important evidence to suggest that blood constituents may themselves trigger thrombosis is derived from observations that show thrombi do form in situations in which no obvious disturbance of flow has occurred and on endothelial surfaces which, as closely as one can detect, appear normal.

Recently it has become apparent that there are normally occurring plasma proteins which inhibit certain of the blood clotting factor enzymes, particularly those which are serine proteases. Since their inhibitory effects are relative with respect to specificity, rate, and completeness, these inhibitors can be viewed as modulators of the over-all activity of the blood clotting system. The more important inhibitors are thought to be antithrombin III, α_2-macroglobulin, and antiplasmin. The best evidence of their biologic importance is the well established observation that congenital deficiencies of antithrombin III predispose to venous thromboses in otherwise normal, healthy young people. Whether transient, acquired deficiencies of these inhibitors truly predispose to thromboses remains unknown. Of interest, however, is the fact that probably the most frequently reported and reproducible abnormality of the blood clotting system in women taking oral contraceptives is a decrease in antithrombin III concentration. Lastly, diminished fibrinolytic activity has also been offered as an explanation for the propensity to develop and sustain a thrombus. Most data supporting this notion are derived from epidemiologic studies, particularly those conducted in Africa, which show an increased fibrinolytic state to be associated with an absence of vascular disease. Studies in other countries have frequently not confirmed this. Isolated reports of patients who have reduced fibrinolytic activity and a predisposition to thromboses have also been used to marshal support for this theory.

Included among the more common thromboembolic diseases are deep venous thrombosis, pulmonary embolism, ischemic heart disease, cerebral vascular disease, thromboembolism as a complication of prosthetic heart valves, and thromboses confined to the microcirculatory system (e.g., diffuse intravascular coagulation, thrombotic thrombocytopenic purpura). Thromboembolism causes a reduction or cessation of blood flow to an organ or area of the body with attendant impairment or loss of function. When such blockage occurs in the microcirculation, microangiopathic hemolytic anemia may develop if red cell damage occurs when blood is forced through a vessel lumen partially obstructed by fibrin strands; paradoxically, a bleeding disorder due to utilization of coagulation factors and platelets in the microthrombi may also develop. Thromboembolism frequently complicates the course of malignancies, possibly by the release into the circulation of thromboplastin, which then interacts with certain of the clotting factors. Similarly, thromboplastin or analogous substances may enter the circulatory system, which becomes open during certain complications of pregnancy. Finally, in women receiving oral contraceptive agents, the problems of spontaneously occurring thromboses, particularly in the deep leg veins with subsequent pulmonary embolism or cerebral arterial thrombosis, have also received considerable attention.

Besides the more or less acute type of thromboembolic disorders, it has also been postulated that the blood coagulation system is involved in the pathogenesis of the initial atherosclerotic lesion. The initial stimulus is thought to be endothelial damage, probably due to shear stresses exerted on its surface by hypertensive blood pressure levels. This is believed to be followed by the formation of a nonocclusive, platelet-rich thrombus that becomes adherent to the arterial endothelial surface and then over time becomes organized, infiltrated with lipid, and partially endothelialized. During the attachment of platelets to subendothelial structures, the platelets are believed to release substances which stimulate smooth muscle cells to proliferate and migrate toward the lumen. Gradually a multiple-layered lesion composed of smooth muscle cells develops and protrudes into the lumen of the vessel; this lesion is thought eventually to become infiltrated with lipid and, ultimately, to become an atherosclerotic plaque. It is important to emphasize that, although currently very popular, this is only one theory of atherogenesis.

The therapy of thromboembolism continues to be aimed at altering the coagulability of the blood or the ability of platelets to stick to surfaces or each other. Because some epidemiologic studies have indicated that acetylsalicylic acid may be useful in preventing the development of thrombosis, it has received considerable attention; however, it is still not clear whether it prevents thromboses associated with any disease or predisposing situation. Biochemical data indicate that aspirin acetylates, and thereby inhibits, cyclo-oxygenase, which is an enzyme important in forming prostaglandin G_2 from arachidonic acid; as a consequence, the stimulant effect on platelet aggregation of prostaglandin G_2 and the subsequent metabolite, thromboxane A_2, is greatly diminished. Very low levels of aspirin are required to do this, and the effect seems to be irreversible during the life span of the platelet. *Coumarin* derivatives continue to be the mainstays in the long-term management of thromboembolism, particularly in situations such as deep vein thrombosis or recurrent pulmonary embolism. Recent analyses of older studies and results of new studies suggest that their use may decrease both morbidity and mortality in the acute and chronic stages of myocardial infarction. Coumarins serve as vitamin K antagonists in reactions which, although poorly understood, lead to the attachment of an additional carboxyl group on certain glutamic acid residues to form the dicarboxylic amino acid, γ-carboxyglutamic acid, in the vitamin K dependent clotting factors. It is thought that the dicarboxylic acid groups are important in binding calcium and lipid during the conversion of the zymogen forms of these clotting factors to active serine proteases. When a coumarin is administered, the clotting factor is synthesized without the addition of the extra carboxyl group to the specific glutamic acids, and as a result the conversion of the precursive form of the clotting factor to the active enzyme is greatly impaired. The levels of the zymogen protein, however, are normal. The other commonly used anticoagulant, *heparin,* is usually employed in a hospital setting where it is given subcutaneously or intravenously. The introduction of low-dose heparin therapy, i.e., doses administered subcutaneously in the range of 5000 units two or three times daily, has effected a dramatic reduction in the incidence of fatal thromboembolism following major thoracoabdominal surgery. This level of heparin does not ordinarily prolong the whole glass clotting time or the partial thromboplastin time. It is to be emphasized that low-dose heparin has only been found effective for the prevention of thromboses; much higher heparin levels are recommended for the treatment of established thromboembolism. To date no oral form of heparin has been found useful. For heparin to be effective as an anticoagulant, it requires a protein cofactor in plasma, antithrombin III. Evidence suggests that heparin temporarily binds and alters the shape of antithrombin III, thereby greatly accelerating the rate of covalent bond formation between an amino acid in its sequence and the active site serine amino acid residue in several of the clotting factor proteases. This mode of inhibition occurs rapidly at fairly low levels of heparin and is believed to be permanent.

Obviously advances have occurred in our understanding of the diseases and situations which predispose to thromboses, the biochemistry of blood clotting, and the therapy of thromboembolic disorders. Of concern, however, is our lack of knowledge about the precise mechanisms which trigger and perpetuate thromboses. It is probable that these must be defined if thromboembolism is to be prevented.

Chalmers, T. C., Matta, R. J., Smith, H. J., and Kunzler, A-M.: Evidence favoring the use of anticoagulants in the hospital phase of acute myocardial infarction. N. Engl. J. Med., 297:1091, 1977.

Davie, E. W., and Hanahan, D. J.: Blood coagulation proteins. *In* Putnam, F. W. (ed.): The Plasma Proteins. 2nd ed. New York, Academic Press, 1977, pp. 422–544.

Majerus, P. W.: Why aspirin? Circulation, 54:375, 1976.

Rosenberg, R. D.: Actions and interactions of antithrombin and heparin. N. Engl. J. Med., 292:146, 1975.

Ross, R., and Glomset, J. A.: The pathogenesis of arteriosclerosis. N. Engl. J. Med., 295:369, 420, 1976.

Salzman, E. W., Deykin, D., Shapiro, R. M., and Rosenberg, R.: Management of heparin therapy. N. Engl. J. Med., 292:1046, 1975.

Sherry, S.: Low-dose heparin prophylaxis for post-operative venous thromboembolism. N. Engl. J. Med., 293:300, 1975.

Sherry, S., Brinkhous, K. M., Genton, E., and Stengle, J. M. (eds.): Thrombosis. Washington, D.C., National Academy of Sciences, 1969.

357.2.   THROMBOPHLEBITIS AND PHLEBOTHROMBOSIS

Sol Sherry

The presence of a thrombus in a vein is referred to clinically as thrombophlebitis or phlebothrombosis. Adherence to the vein wall incites an inflammatory reaction with local symptoms, and because of the associated phlebitis the process is referred to as thrombophlebitis. When the thrombus is poorly adherent and extends primarily into the free-flowing circulation, local symptoms of phlebitis may be minimal or absent, and the process may be referred to as phlebothrombosis. Since the two states are, for the most part, identical and subject to the same complications, little virtue attaches to such a clinical differentiation; hereafter only the term thrombophlebitis will be used.

ETIOLOGY, RISK FACTORS, PATHOGENESIS, AND PREVALENCE. Multiple causes probably initiate venous thrombosis. Injury to the vessel wall by mechanical trauma, infection, chemical irritants, or the process of thromboangiitis obliterans is responsible for some cases, particularly the superficial variety.

In most instances, stasis with slowing of blood flow and venous distention appears to be the major predisposing factor, e.g., in the venous thrombi which frequently complicate the use of constricting garments, and in such clinical conditions or states as the hyperviscosity syndromes (including polycythemia vera), severe obesity, varicose veins, postoperative and postpartum states, trauma (particularly when extensive or involving fractures of the pelvis or femur), acute myocardial infarction, heart failure, hemiplegia, debility, and cachexia. Long periods of cramped sitting, e.g., in travel or watching television, or in fact any state involving partial or complete immobilization, particularly in the older age group, because of the loss of the normal pumping action of the leg muscles, is subject to an increased incidence of venous thrombosis. The risk of stasis-mediated as well as other forms of venous thrombosis is increased when there has been a previous episode of thrombophlebitis or pulmonary embolism.

Alterations in blood components have received much attention, but a "hypercoagulable state," i.e., one predisposing to thrombus formation, has defied simple description. Rather, it is recognized that many disorders of the blood may be associated with predisposition to venous thrombosis. These include thrombocythemia as well as certain thrombocytopathies, particularly those involving shortened survival and increased platelet functional activities (adhesion, aggregation, and coagulant properties), dysfibrinogenemias, accelerated thromboplastin generation, constitutionally elevated levels of plasma factors V and VIII, heightened antifibrinolytic activity, and decreased antithrombin III activity.

Finally, many other clinical conditions are associated with an increased incidence of thrombophlebitis, but the responsible factors have not been adequately elucidated. These include ulcerative colitis, malignancies of all types (possibly more so of the pancreas), homocystinuria, and prolonged administration of large doses of estrogens or estrogen-containing oral contraceptive agents. The presence of a "migratory thrombophlebitis" should cause suspicion of an underlying malignancy, collagen disease, thromboangiitis obliterans, or polycythemia vera. When thrombosis occurs without evidence of a known predisposing factor or associated clinical condition, the term *idiopathic* thrombophlebitis may be used.

Thrombosis in veins occurs most commonly in the deep and superficial veins of the lower extremities. Deep leg vein thrombi usually begin in the soleal arcade of the calf muscles where they may resolve, organize, extend, or trigger additional thrombi at independent sites. As long as the thrombus remains limited to the soleal veins, no significant clinical problem is posed. However, once extension into the major deep vessels of the leg occurs, or additional thrombi appear at other sites in the major deep veins, the patient is at significant risk for one or more complications (circulatory obstruction, valve damage, postphlebitic insufficiency syndrome, pulmonary embolism). When extension occurs from the soleal vessels, the thrombus extends proximally into larger vessels, frequently progressing to involve the popliteal, superficial femoral, common femoral, and iliac veins. More rarely the inferior vena cava is also affected. Thrombi originating in the major deep veins usually begin at the base of valve pockets and then extend either up along the vein wall or into the flowing circulation, or they may completely obstruct the entire vascular lumen. When the latter occurs, retrograde thrombosis as well as continued proximal growth is likely.

Next in frequency to thrombi in the deep leg veins are thrombi in the pelvic venous network, the right cardiac chambers, and the veins of the upper extremities. However, thrombi may occur in any veins (retinal, cerebral, renal, hepatic, portal, mesenteric) and contribute significantly to disease of the organ system involved.

Until recently, data on the incidence and frequency of leg vein thrombi were inadequate, because most of these are inapparent clinically. In studies in which leg vein dissections were carried out post mortem, the incidence was shown to be very high, varying from 27 to 80 per cent, depending on the nature of the series and the extent of the dissection; in most, the incidence ranged from 44 to 65 per cent. This incidence did not appear to depend on sex or clinical diagnosis, for the likelihood of thrombosis was similar in patients dying of medical, surgical, and traumatic causes. The most important factors influencing the frequency of leg vein thrombosis appeared to be the duration of bed rest and advancing age, although other factors undoubtedly contributed to those incidence figures.

With the advent of the ^{125}I-labeled fibrinogen leg-scanning technique, important epidemiologic and prevalence data are being obtained on leg vein thrombi appearing during life and in nonfatal situations. For example, in Kakkar's study of 469 consecutive patients aged 40 or over, undergoing elective surgery, 28 per cent developed deep vein thrombosis; older patients undergoing major operations had an incidence of over 50 per cent. Half the thrombi developed within the first 24 hours postoperatively, and the remainder occurred three to seven days after surgery; in one third of the patients, the thrombi were bilateral. The incidence in other conditions was as follows: fractured hips, 75 per cent of pertrochanteric and 34 per cent of subcapital femoral neck fractures; retropubic prostatectomy, 50 per cent; acute myocardial infarction, 38 per cent; stroke, 60 per cent in the hemiplegic lower extremity; gynecologic patients over 30 years of age and undergoing major abdominal or vaginal surgery, 18 per cent; and obstetric patients during the puerperium, 4 per cent. Probably the highest risk is in patients undergoing reconstructive or total hip replacement.

In over 90 per cent of the patients undergoing thrombosis, leg vein thrombi appear first in the veins of the calf; one fifth of these soleal thrombi extend proximally into the major deep vessels of the leg and thigh; of the latter, half embolize. In acute myocardial infarction, in which the over-all incidence of leg vein thrombosis is approximatley 20 to 25 per cent, 5 per cent of patients may be expected to develop thrombi in the major deep vessels of the leg or thigh, and in 2 to 3 per cent the illness will be complicated by an acute pulmonary embolism; the risk of leg vein thrombosis, extension, and embolization, however, is doubled in patients in the older age group who develop shock or congestive heart failure with their infarction.

CLINICAL MANIFESTATIONS AND DIAGNOSIS. Thrombophlebitis occurs suddenly or gradually. Superficial thrombophlebitis is not difficult to diagnose, because the thrombosed vessel can usually be felt beneath the skin as a tender cord, and the lesion may be accompanied by a surrounding area of localized inflammation. With more extensive use of the venous route for both therapy and drug abuse, the incidence of this form of thrombophlebitis has increased sharply. Although it is usually benign, a significant number of patients may become infected, e.g., after the use of contaminated equipment or when intravenous catheters have been left in situ for periods of more than 48 hours, and this may lead to a serious septic state.

Deep vein thrombophlebitis is much more difficult to diagnose, because it may or may not be accompanied by local (pain and tenderness) and systemic (fever) symptoms; these occur in only 20 to 30 per cent of patients. In the absence of local findings, the diagnosis should be suspected when there is a "doughy" feeling or an unexplained increase in the circumference of the limb and the presence of *Homan's sign* (pain in the calf and/or popliteal space on dorsiflexion of the foot). The *sphygmomanometer cuff pain test of Lowenberg* may also prove useful, particularly when carried out during ambulation. A blood pressure cuff around the involved part of the extremity is slowly inflated to 200 mm Hg and then deflated. During inflation, discomfort is normally experienced at or above 160 mm Hg. In venous obstructive disease, discomfort or tenderness is evident at a lower level (60 to 150 mm Hg). The test may often be positive when other symptoms and signs are absent, but it is not sufficiently specific to be considered diagnostic. The most useful noninvasive diagnostic techniques are the *augmented Doppler ultrasound examination* and *electrical impedance phlebography* with a thigh cuff; with experience, the results of these latter tests will correlate well with venography. However, these tests are positive only when the major deep veins are obstructed; they do not detect thrombi limited to the soleal veins. *Venography* is the most specific for diagnostic purposes, but it has limitations; it is expensive, may require a cut-down, and cannot be interpreted properly unless all the deep veins, including the soleal vessels, are filled adequately; there is also the possibility (still unresolved) that the large amounts of dye used in the procedure will aggravate an underlying thrombophlebitis.

Unless the patient has local complaints, the signs of venous thrombosis are often overlooked until the occurrence of pulmonary embolism calls attention to the limbs. Therefore special attention should be paid to the possibility of venous thrombi in all patients who are predisposed, and frequent observations should be made in older patients immobilized for any period of time.

Local tenderness in the calf and pain on forced dorsiflexion of the foot should suggest involvement of the deeper branches of the popliteal vein. Edema and mottled cyanosis will be present when the superficial femoral vein is affected; these findings are absent when adequate collateral channels exist. When the disease extends to involve the common femoral and iliac veins, edema and cyanosis of the leg may develop rapidly, often with diminished pulsation of the femoral artery. When associated perivenous inflammation and pelvic lymphatic involvement accompany thrombosis of the iliac vein, the swelling can be massive and result in a "milk leg" or *phlegmasia alba dolens*. In a particularly serious from of deep vein thrombosis called *phlegmasia cerulea dolens*, cyanosis and swelling of the extremity are associated with a disappearance of the arterial pulses; the leg becomes cold; gangrene appears imminent and may follow. This is associated with massive venous occlusion involving the deep, superficial, and intercommunicating veins so that there is almost total outflow obstruction; the rapid rise in tissue pressure compromises the arterial inflow and produces the picture of combined arterial and venous occlusive disease.

Damage to the venous valves resulting from an extensive episode or repeated attacks of deep vein thrombophlebitis may cause venous stasis and insufficiency; this leads to chronic edema, fibrosis, pigmentation, and trophic ulceration in the limb. The eventual deformity in this *postphlebitic syndrome* may be extreme and disabling. However, the most frequent and serious complication of thrombophlebitis is pulmonary embolism, a subject discussed in Ch. 357.3.

PROPHYLAXIS. Stasis should be eliminated whenever possible, particularly in the older patient. This includes the wearing of elastic or supportive hose in the presence of varicose veins; avoidance of long periods of cramped sitting and of constricting garments about the abdomen and lower extremities; and the use of appropriate measures during periods of immobilization or illness or after surgery, trauma, or fracture. The value of elastic hose during periods of immobilization is very limited, as are foot and leg exercises, even when carried out frequently and in the elevated position. More effective are physical devices which ensure repeated calf muscle contraction or intermittent pulsation of the leg veins. Early but active ambulation is to be encouraged after illness, surgery, or trauma.

Iatrogenic thrombophlebitis can be minimized by avoiding prolonged use of intravenous catheters or administration of hypertonic or chemically irritating solutions.

Prophylactic therapy with anticoagulants is to be considered in high risk groups, i.e., those most likely to develop venous thrombi and pulmonary embolism. Included in this category are patients over the age of 50 who will be bedridden or immobilized for long periods of time as a result of extensive fractures, particularly of the femur, or other forms of trauma, debilitating disease, cardiac failure, myocardial infarction, or surgery, particularly hip arthroplasty. The pharmacologic basis for the use of anticoagulation in the prevention of venous thrombotic disease is sound, and its effectiveness in reducing thromboembolic complications after fractured hips or extensive trauma, during the postoperative state, and after acute myocardial infarction has been established in several series of observations. When indicated, anticoagulant therapy should be instituted immediately; it can be carried out solely with *oral agents (coumarin or indandione compounds),* for although these agents take several days to induce an appropriate antithrombotic state, the danger period for pulmonary embolism usually begins somewhat later. Anticoagulation should be continued until full mobilization is completed, because the risk of thrombosis remains as long as stasis exists. Such anticoagulation is not a contraindication to surgery or other procedures. Surgery can be performed without much danger either before or shortly after the institution of anticoagulant treatment, because hemostasis is not impaired for several days; later, in the more chronically anticoagulated patient, surgery can be undertaken after reduction of the level of anticoagulation with careful attention to wound hemostasis. Nevertheless, despite its proved value, physicians have been reluctant to use such prophylactic anticoagulant therapy except in cases of recurrent thrombophlebitis or pulmonary embolism; cited are the hazard of bleeding and the difficulties in maintaining adequate anticoagulation in older patients. Some of these difficulties can be avoided by elimination of a loading dose and recognition of the various factors which influence drug responsiveness (see below).

Infusion of *dextran* 40 or 75 (500 to 1000 ml on day of surgery, 500 ml daily for next five days)* can also be used to prevent postoperative thrombophlebitis, presumably by increasing blood flow and preventing surface interactions. However, although effective, it provides little advantage over anticoagulants, because it also enhances the risk of bleeding and is tolerated poorly in individuals with impaired cardiac reserve.

The most important advance in the prevention of deep vein thrombi in immobilized patients is administration of small doses of *heparin,* i.e., 5000 units twice a day subcutaneously into the abdominal wall during periods of high risk. This regimen maintains circulating heparin blood levels at a fraction of that ordinarily achieved with conventional therapeutic doses as used in the treatment of established thrombosis (see below), and does not significantly affect the Lee-White clotting time and activated partial thromboplastin time; nor

---

*Experimental drug for this purpose.

does it enhance the risk of bleeding. However, there is sufficient circulating heparin to activate enough heparin cofactor (antithrombin III) to block the action of earlier activated enzymes of the clotting reaction (notably Xa and IXa). In several trials, prophylactic therapy with low dose heparin has strikingly reduced the incidence of venous thrombosis occurring postoperatively (except after femoral fractures and hip arthroplasty) and after acute myocardial infarction as measured by ^{125}I-labeled fibrinogen scanning. A large multicenter, multinational study also has revealed that this mode of prophylaxis results in a significant reduction in pulmonary embolism in older patients following major abdominothoracic surgery.

The use of *platelet function inhibitors*, e.g., *aspirin, dipyridamole*, and *sulfinpyrazone*, for the prevention of deep vein thrombosis remains unclear; aspirin (600 mg twice daily) has been claimed to be effective in preventing deep vein thrombosis following reconstructive hip surgery, and sulfinpyrazone (600 to 800 mg daily) has been found useful in reducing the incidence of arteriovenous shunt thrombosis in patients undergoing chronic renal dialysis, and in decreasing the frequency of attacks in patients with recurrent thrombophlebitis who are refractory to coumarin therapy. When sulfinpyrazone is used with coumarin, the dose of the latter should be lowered because of occupation by sulfinpyrazone of coumarin-binding sites.

TREATMENT. General Measures. Acute superficial thrombophlebitis is most often self-limited, unless infected, and usually responds promptly to analgesics, bed rest, warm moist packs, and elevation of the affected limb. Pulmonary embolism is a rare complication unless there is also involvement of the deep venous system. Antimicrobial drugs are not indicated except in septic phlebitis, in which the choice of agent depends on the organism responsible for the infection.

Acute deep vein thrombophlebitis must be managed more aggressively because of the tendency of these thrombi to extend, embolize, and produce serious venous obstruction and damage to venous valves (a postphlebitic insufficiency syndrome occurs in about 5 per cent of those with an ascending thrombophlebitis). In addition to the local measures described above, the objectives of treatment are to prevent further disease and, if indicated, to remove the obstructing thrombus.

Anticoagulants. Currently the principal therapeutic agents for the prevention of further extension and embolization are the anticoagulants, and with their use alone most cases can be managed successfully and without complication. In the absence of contraindications (bleeding diathesis, hemorrhagic lesions, malignant hypertension, known allergy to heparin) anticoagulation should be instituted immediately with heparin, for it is the most effective of the agents available and induces an immediate antithrombotic state.

Heparin can be administered intravenously or by the intramuscular and subcutaneous routes. Based on control of antithrombotic effects, the intravenous route is most often recommended, particularly for the first several days of therapy. Because of local pain and frequent hematomas, intramuscular injections are the least desirable. Even with the intravenous route, dosages and regimens vary. Continuous intravenous infusions of heparin, although requiring special care in administration, are becoming the preferred mode of therapy; control of dosage is easier and, more important, evidence

is accumulating that bleeding complications can be reduced significantly. A suggested procedure is to begin with a loading dose of 75 IU per pound of body weight, followed by a sustaining infusion of 10 IU per pound per hour through an indwelling plastic catheter placed above the antecubital fossa. Subsequent dosage is adjusted to maintain the activated partial thromboplastin time at twice normal (range 1½ to 2½); with Lee-White clotting times, the range is 2 to 2½ times normal. If the intermittent injection technique is employed, it is suggested that 60,000 IU be given during the first day (e.g., 10,000 units every four hours) and that, beginning on the second day, dosage be regulated by coagulation determinations; one hour before the next injection, the activated partial thromboplastin time or Lee-White clotting time should be at the level recommended above for sustaining infusions.

Once the dose requirement has been established, the clotting time may be checked once daily at an appropriate time to exclude possible increase or decrease in the anticoagulant effect and to allow for variations in heparin requirement during the course of therapy. Not infrequently, patients in whom thrombosis is occurring require more heparin in the first 24 to 48 hours of treatment than several days after the institution of therapy. Heparin therapy is recommended for periods of seven to ten days before relying solely on oral anticoagulation with coumarin drugs; this will ensure the most potent antithrombotic state and allow the underlying thrombus to become firmly fixed to the vessel wall.

"Burning fingers" and an occasional allergic reaction may be seen with heparin (osteoporosis and alopecia are additional adverse effects associated with long-term administration), but the primary risk in heparin therapy is bleeding. In one series it was as high as 50 per cent in women over the age of 60; usually the incidence is of the order of 5 to 8 per cent. This risk can be reduced by better control of the anticoagulant state, eliminating aspirin and aspirin-containing compounds, and avoiding intramuscular injections and invasive procedures. It should be remembered that patients whose hemostatic mechanism is impaired before heparin is instituted are predisposed to bleed. When significant bleeding occurs, heparin in the circulation can be immediately neutralized with protamine sulfate; the latter reacts with heparin stoichiometrically and on a milligram per milligram basis. Protamine is administered slowly intravenously after dilution in physiologic saline in an amount equivalent to half the last dose of heparin but not in excess of 100 mg.* For this calculation 100 units of heparin can be taken to represent 1 mg.

Oral anticoagulation with *coumarin* (or, less popularly, *indandione*) compounds should be instituted several days before the discontinuation of heparin therapy. It should be continued for six weeks to six months, unless the phlebitis is associated with immobilization, in which case the drug should be continued until full physical activity is resumed. If thrombi recur when anticoagulants are discontinued, the treatment should be resumed, and long-term therapy may be necessary. Patients with known recurrent episodes of phlebitis may require prophylactic anticoagulant therapy extending over years.

The action of coumarin compounds is indirect, i.e., the induction of a hypocoagulable state, in contrast to

---

*See p. vi, Dosage Notice, immediately following Preface.

the action of heparin as an immediate activator of antithrombin III. At present, the aim of therapy is to reduce the level of the prothrombin complex factors (factors II, VII, IX, and X) to approximately 20 per cent of normal and sustain it there. (Antithrombin III levels are increased during coumarin administration and may contribute to the antithrombotic effect.) This is achieved by regulating dosage so as to prolong the one-stage prothrombin time test to one and a half to two times the control time by the Quick test. Levels of two and a half times or greater are associated with an increased incidence of bleeding, and levels of less than one and a half times the control may not be effective.

There is little difference in the onset of effect or smoothness of control among the various coumarin derivatives, and vitamin K_1 is equally effective in counteracting their action. Because factor VII of the various vitamin K dependent factors (II, VII, IX, and X) has the shortest half-life, it is depressed most quickly by coumarin therapy. However, the rapid depression of factor VII does not provide good antithrombotic protection but does enhance the risk of bleeding. Accordingly, previous regimens involving the use of a loading dose are being employed less frequently. A suggested regimen is to give warfarin, 10 to 15 mg daily, until the desired effect on the prothrombin time is achieved and the dose adjusted to maintain that level. Individualization of dosage is essential, because a variety of drug interactions, other pharmacologic considerations, and metabolic factors influence the sensitivity and response to the coumarin compounds. *Drugs to be avoided during warfarin therapy* include aspirin, phenylbutazone, oxyphenbutazone, and indomethacin, and the following have been shown to potentiate its effect: anabolic steroids, certain antimicrobials (particularly chloramphenicol and those which affect the intestinal bacterial flora), chloral hydrate, clofibrate, disulfiram, ethacrynic acid, glucagon, mefenamic acid, methylphenidate, quinidine, quinine, and sulfinpyrazone. Those agents which inhibit the prothrombinopenic effect of warfarin include barbiturates, corticosteroids, cholestyramine, ethchlorvynol, glutethimide, griseofulvin, haloperidol, meprobamate, and oral contraceptives. Also, older patients, particularly women, are more sensitive to warfarin, as are individuals suffering from febrile illnesses, malnutrition, steatorrhea, and hepatic or pancreatic disease, as well as those in the immediate postoperative state. Increased resistance to warfarin is associated with hyperlipidemia and hyperuricemia. Warfarin also interferes with the metabolism of other drugs; it enhances the action of diphenylhydantoin, chlorpropamide, and tolbutamide.

In patients being switched from heparin to warfarin therapy, a period of overlap is necessary because of the delay in the antithrombotic effect of the coumarin. A suggested procedure is to give warfarin, 10 to 15 mg daily for two to three days, until the desired therapeutic range for the prothrombin time is achieved; then, while continuing maintenance warfarin therapy, heparin dosage is progressively reduced over another three- to four-day period before discontinuation. Since prothrombin times are influenced by the presence of heparin, such assays should be carried out on blood specimens with a normal or near normal activated partial thromboplastin time; otherwise, the in vitro addition of protamine may be necessary.

Bleeding is a significant hazard with oral anticoagula-

tion, occurring in 3 per cent or more of patients on long-term therapy; vitamin K_1 in doses of 5 to 10 mg is usually corrective. Long-term therapy should not be undertaken unless a reliable laboratory is available and the patient's cooperation can be assured. Individuals on such therapy should avoid contact exercise, aspirin, and aspirin-containing compounds, and should be observed carefully even after slight trauma (subdural hematoma in the aged is often an unsuspected complication of coumarin therapy). Invasive procedures, including needle biopsies and spinal taps, are to be avoided unless the prothrombin time is first restored to or near the normal range. Other adverse effects are minimal; probably of most interest is the occasional appearance of skin necrosis and the rare "purple toe syndrome." Contraindications to coumarin therapy are similar to those previously mentioned for heparin and, in addition, pregnancy. Not only has coumarin administration been shown to increase teratogenicity in animals during the first trimester but, unlike heparin, it crosses the placental barrier and can produce fetal hemorrhage. The use of coumarins also should be avoided, when possible, for patients with severe liver disease or advanced renal insufficiency.

Other Antithrombotic Agents. Low molecular weight *dextran* infusions, based on their ability to improve flow rates by expanding plasma volume and to inhibit platelet adherence and aggregation, have been recommended by some as a useful adjunct in the management of acute thrombophlebitis. In contrast to its proved value in prevention, the efficacy of such therapy for thrombophlebitis remains to be established; at present there is little justification to have dextran infusions replace anticoagulant therapy. Also, there is considerable interest in the use of defibrinating agents; the most promising agents in this respect are the highly purified fraction *(Arvin)* obtained from the venom of the Malayan pit viper, and *Defibrase*. It remains to be established whether these agents will have advantages over heparin.

Surgical Therapy. Surgical procedures may be helpful in the management of some cases of thrombophlebitis; *proximal interruption of venous flow* can be employed to prevent embolization, and thrombectomy to relieve obstruction. The surgical procedures of choice to protect adequately against pulmonary embolization from the lower extremities and pelvis are inferior vena caval ligation, plication, or the insertion of an appropriate filter or umbrella. The last-named can be accomplished transvenously and does not require abdominal surgery. Each procedure has its adherents, and all but the first obviate the difficulty of sudden acute fluid sequestration with hypovolemia and impaired venous return, an event which may be tolerated poorly by people with underlying heart disease. Since all these procedures are usually followed by retrograde thrombosis, and consequently carry a significant incidence of distressing sequelae, both immediate and late, and do not permanently protect (large collaterals develop in several months and may provide a new route for embolization), they are not given consideration except in the presence of pulmonary embolism, or when pulmonary embolism has been known to occur in the past and there is a contraindication to the use of anticoagulant therapy.

Thrombectomy, including the use of Fogarty and similar types of catheters, has been employed successfully in the management of occasional cases of phlegmasia cerulea dolens. However, since this procedure is often followed by venous rethrombosis as well as complicating the subsequent use of anticoagulation, it is currently indicated only for those patients in whom acute fluid sequestration and high tissue tension sufficiently jeopardize the arterial circulation as to threaten the survival of the limb.

Thrombolytic Therapy. Clot-dissolving agents are useful in selected cases as adjuncts in the management of deep vein thrombophlebitis, for they provide the only medical means for directly lysing a thrombus already formed. The most useful agents for thrombolytic therapy are *streptokinase* and *urokinase*, activators of the naturally occurring human fibrinolytic enzyme system. Streptokinase is a secretory product of the hemolytic *Streptococcus* and can be produced readily in large quantities and relatively inexpensively for therapeutic purposes. Its major disadvantage is its antigenicity; this poses problems in dosage and, more important, in retreatment should thrombosis recur. Urokinase, a normal constituent of human urine, is nonantigenic and simpler to use therapeutically, but more expensive. Although originally prepared from urine, currently it is being processed from the culture medium of fetal kidney tissue cells. Both agents are given intravenously; for thrombophlebitis, a suggested procedure for streptokinase is to give 250,000 units as a loading dose over a 20- to 30-minute period, followed by a sustaining infusion of 100,000 units per hour for 48 to 72 hours; with urokinase, 2000 units per pound of body weight is given as a loading dose, followed by a sustaining infusion of the same amount per hour for 24 to 48 hours. Heparin therapy is instituted at the termination of the fibrinolytic therapy so as to prevent rethrombosis. Although both agents when used in appropriate dosage age capable of lysing large thrombi in the deep leg veins, the intense fibrinolytic state has a propensity to induce bleeding. Consequently, current recommendations are to limit their use to those patients with extensive occlusions of the major deep veins of the extremity or with a rapidly ascending thrombophlebitis or pulmonary embolism.

Follow-up Therapy. When the systemic symptoms and signs of thrombophlebitis have subsided and the involved limb is pain free and nontender, the patient can begin walking with the leg supported by elastic stockings, unless such activity is followed by return of symptoms. After walking has been resumed, the patient should be advised to elevate the extremity above heart level for several half-hour periods a day. Elastic stockings should be worn until measurement of the extremity reveals no accumulation of edema fluid. Early and persistent therapy is important to prevent development of the postphlebitic syndrome. Once the brawny swelling and induration of the postphlebitic limb have occurred, they may be relieved somewhat by long periods of elevation, elastic compressions, vigorous massage, special exercises and mechanical devices, providing that there has been no recent recurrence of phlebitis. Gross deformities, ulcerations, and persistent or repeated infections may ultimately require one or more surgical procedures.

Basu, D., Gallus, A., Hirsh, J., and Cade, J.: A prospective study of the value of monitoring heparin treatment with the activated partial thromboplastin time. N. Engl. J. Med., 287:324, 1972.

Coon, W. W., Willis, P. W., III, and Keller, J. B.: Venous thromboembolism and other venous disease in the Tecumseh Community Health Study. Circulation, 48:239, 1973.

Foster, C. S., Genton, E., Henderson, M., Sherry, S., and Wessler, S. (eds.): The epidemiology of venous thrombosis. Milbank Memorial Fund Quarterly, 50(1), Part 2:9, 1972.

Gallus, A. S., Hirsh, J., Tuttle, R. J., et al.: Small subcutaneous doses of heparin in prevention of venous thrombosis. N. Engl. J. Med., 288:545, 1973.

Genton, E.: Guidelines for heparin therapy. Ann. Intern. Med., 80:77, 1974.

Harris, W. H. Salzman, E. W., Athanasoulis, C. A., et al.: Aspirin prophylaxis of venous thromboembolism after total hip replacement. N. Engl. J. Med., 297:1246, 1977.

Koch-Weser, J., and Sellers, E. M.: Drug interaction with coumarin anticoagulants. N. Engl. J. Med., 285:547, 1971.

O'Reilly, R. A., and Aggeler, P. M.: Studies on coumarin anticoagulant drugs. Institution of warfarin therapy without a loading dose. Circulation, 38:169, 1968.

357.3. PULMONARY EMBOLISM AND INFARCTION

Sol Sherry

DEFINITION. Pulmonary embolism is the impaction in the pulmonary vascular bed of a previously detached thrombus or foreign matter. Its major complication, pulmonary infarction, is the necrosis of lung parenchyma resulting from interference with blood supply. Since pulmonary embolism is the more common event, is not invariably accompanied by infarction, and has distinguishing features of its own, this chapter will be devoted primarily to pulmonary embolism; however, discussion of pulmonary infarction will be included as indicated.

ETIOLOGY. Pulmonary embolism is a complication, not a primary disease; therefore its etiology is considered in terms of the nature and source of the offending embolus. Almost all pulmonary emboli originate as thrombi; on occasion nonthrombotic materials such as amniotic fluid, fat, air, bone marrow, or tumor may embolize to the lung.

Venous thrombi in the deep veins of the lower extremities are the most common source for pulmonary emboli, accounting for 80 to 90 per cent. Another important source for pulmonary embolization is thrombi in the pelvic veins and prostatic plexus. Prostatic vein thrombosis may accompany malignant disease of the prostate but more frequently follows prostatic surgery. In the female, thrombosis in the pelvic veins may follow parturition or surgery; a particularly severe form, with frequent and protracted embolization, may complicate septic abortion. Pulmonary emboli may also arise from the right heart and are seen in association with cardiac failure, atrial fibrillation, myocardial infarction, the primary cardiomyopathies, and bacterial endocarditis (involving the tricuspid or pulmonic valves). Thrombi in the right heart frequently embolize and are said to account for approximately 25 per cent of pulmonary emboli among cardiac patients.

The factors controlling detachment of the whole or part of a venous thrombus into the general circulation are even less well understood than thrombus formation itself; frequently such thrombi will break away without apparent cause. It was formerly believed that embolization occurred more frequently with phlebothrombosis, but evidence to support this concept is lacking, and symptomatic thrombophlebitis is often complicated by embolization. Of more importance are the location of the vessel (embolism is rare from a superficial vein but very frequent from the iliofemoral vein), the presence of a free floating tail, and factors which acutely change pressure relationships in veins or suddenly increase venous blood flow; these include straining at stool, exertion, and ambulation after a long period of immobilization.

Once a thrombus is released into the venous circulation, it is usually carried rapidly through the great veins and right heart into the pulmonary arteries, except under those circumstances in which the embolus is shunted, through a patent foramen ovale or other defect, into the heart and systemic circulation (*paradoxical embolization*). However, even this latter condition tends to occur most frequently after a bout of pulmonary embolism, for the associated pulmonary hypertension predisposes to paradoxical embolization.

INCIDENCE AND PREVALENCE. Pulmonary embolism with or without infarction is a common disorder and a most important cause of morbidity and mortality. It is frequently misdiagnosed. Next to pneumonia, it is the most common acute pulmonary lesion seen in hospitalized patients today. Thirty per cent of pulmonary emboli occur in cardiac patients, another 30 per cent occur among medical noncardiac patients (particularly among the aged), and most of the remainder occur postoperatively. Immobilization, venous disease, and prior cardiopulmonary disease are the factors most frequently predisposing to pulmonary embolism. The over-all incidence of pulmonary embolism in general autopsy series ranges from 5 to 14 per cent, but the incidence is considerably higher (25 per cent) in institutions for the care of the aged, and highest (30 to 45 per cent) among cardiac patients. The incidence of pulmonary embolism appears to have increased progressively over the past several decades.

Embolism to the main pulmonary artery or its primary branches so as to occlude acutely the major portion of the circulation through the lungs, although less frequent than embolism of smaller vessels, is the third most common cause of sudden death (5 per cent) among hospitalized patients. It occurs in about 3 per cent of general autopsy series, but with antemortem diagnosis of only one in eight.

Embolism to medium-sized vessels, i.e., lobar and segmental vessels, is observed approximately three to five times more frequently in autopsy series than is embolism of the major vessels; but since the former is commonly not fatal and is often recurrent, the actual incidence of acute episodes is relatively much greater. Furthermore, in contrast to embolism of the major vessels, the presence of medium-sized emboli at autopsy can be considered only incidental in two thirds of the cases; in the other third, the clinical features are such as to suggest some relation to the fatal termination. Pulmonary infarction complicates embolism of medium-sized arteries in less than 25 per cent of cases. In cardiac patients, the incidence of infarction after such embolism is considerably increased; in one autopsy series, more than 90 per cent of the lungs of cardiac patients with emboli were found to have areas of infarction.

Embolism to small-sized vessels, i.e., subsegmental arteries and their branches, probably occurs with great frequency, but the incidence is difficult to assess. As an isolated and focal lesion, such embolization has little clinical significance, for it usually is not large enough to produce a macroinfarction, and in routine autopsies the

lesion is likely to be overlooked unless there are associated emboli in the larger vessels. However, multiple small emboli scattered throughout the lungs are frequently observed in association with embolic occlusions of larger vessels; under these circumstances they contribute significantly to the impairment of pulmonary circulation and associated morbidity. Miliary small vessel occlusion is also the major cause of morbidity when nonthrombotic emboli, such as fat, amniotic fluid, air, or nitrogen, are involved.

PATHOLOGY. Pulmonary emboli may be single or multiple and vary in size from microscopic particles to large saddle emboli that completely occlude the pulmonary artery and its major branches. In addition a large embolus may break up during passage through the heart or upon impaction and not only obstruct a major vessel but further embolize into one or more smaller branches in both lung fields. Also, there is evidence that, subsequent to impaction, emboli may shift or further fragment into previously unobstructed pulmonary vessels.

With occlusion of the main pulmonary artery or of both its primary branches, or when there is extensive involvement of medium-sized vessels so as to cut off the major portion of the pulmonary arterial circulation, there is acute mechanical obstruction to pulmonary blood flow; the pulmonary artery is distended by the presence of both clot and blood, the right ventricle is acutely dilated, the peripheral veins are engorged, and the liver is congested. Acute infarction rarely occurs; either the lung parenchyma is fairly normal or there is moderate atelectasis, usually explained by the loss of surfactant, and edema. Although the low incidence of acute infarction is possibly attributable to the rapidity with which death occurs (90 per cent of the deaths from acute pulmonary embolism occur within the first two hours), other factors are probably responsible for this phenomenon. In 40 per cent of the cases there is evidence of previous embolization and infarction.

Emboli which pass beyond the pulmonary artery and its major branches tend to impact the arteries of the lower lobes, more often the right than the left. Embolism to other lobes is much less frequent; combined, they account for only 25 per cent of cases. The more frequent involvement of the lower lobes is believed to be due to the fact that these areas lie in the more direct stream of the pulmonary arteries.

When *infarction* occurs, its spreads to involve a pleural surface, either peripheral or interlobar. The infarcted area is airless and hemorrhagic; the hemorrhage is both interstitial and alveolar. Because of the associated pleuritis, hypoventilation, and pre-existing disease, there may be surrounding atelectasis and edema as well. Although occlusion of the larger medium vessels, e.g., interlobar arteries, tends to be associated with infarcts of larger size, the relation between size of vessel occlusion and infarction is a poor one; other factors appear to be more critical in determining the presence and size of the infarct. By roentgenography, infarcts are poorly visualized on the first day. Thereafter they usually appear as humped, wedge-shaped, or, less commonly, rounded shadows. When they occur near the bases, considerable diaphragmatic elevation and restriction of motion may be observed. In 30 to 40 per cent of cases, infarcts are associated with a variable amount of *pleural effusion* that may be serous, serosanguineous, or frankly hemorrhagic; usually the specific gravity is in the range of 1.014 to 1.017 (protein, 3 to 3.5 grams per 100 ml) and there is mild to moderate increase in cell content.

Some shadows clear rapidly (two to three days) on roentgenographic examination and have been referred to as "incomplete" infarcts; however, it is likely that this clearing represents reventilation of an atelectatic or congested area occasioned by the embolic occlusion rather than true resolution of an infarct. "Complete" infarcts clear slowly over a two- to three-week period, ending as an area of linear fibrosis.

MECHANISMS OF DISEASE, INCLUDING PULMONARY INFARCTION. Emboli lodging in the pulmonary arterial tree acutely reduce the circulation distal to the site of obstruction. Potentially, the effects are four-fold: (1) less blood proceeds through the pulmonary circuit to the left heart and systemic circulation; (2) there is a damming back of blood behind the mechanical obstruction; (3) hemorrhagic necrosis of the ischemic area may occur; and (4) pulmonary function is impaired (pulmonary capillary perfusion and diffusion; later, ventilation may be compromised as well).

Except for the occurrence of infarction, which must be considered as a localized or focal disorder, the average person is believed capable of withstanding considerable obstruction of the pulmonary arterial bed without serious consequences to the vascular dynamics; in normal animals, a 60 to 70 per cent obstruction is usually well tolerated. Nevertheless, exceptions occur, particularly in the presence of underlying heart disease, when less extensive occlusions may elevate pulmonary arterial pressure or significantly reduce pulmonary venous outflow and when pulmonary circulation has been previously impaired by disease or prior embolization.

With a large occlusion of the main pulmonary artery or its primary branches, the effects are acute and primarily mechanical: rapidly rising pulmonary artery pressure, failure of the right ventricle, cyanosis, venous engorgement, and hepatic congestion. The consequences of impaired pulmonary venous return are sharp reduction in left ventricular filling, diminished cardiac output, reduced coronary and cerebral blood flow, hypoxia (also caused by pulmonary blood shunting), dyspnea, pallor, tachycardia, and hypotension, often progressing quickly to shock and death. Sudden dyspnea and retrosternal pain are frequently the most prominent initial complaints; the dyspnea is believed to be due to anoxia, apprehension, and stimulation of Hering-Breuer and other reflexes; the angina is usually attributed to acute coronary insufficiency, but direct stimulation of sensory nerves in the wall of a rapidly distending pulmonary artery may also play a significant role.

The effects of embolization to medium-sized vessels depend on the number, size, and distribution of the emboli and the prior state of the lung and circulation. Several patterns may be observed. (1) There may be no observable effects; a transient episode of dyspnea may be the only clue to its occurrence. (2) The picture may be predominantly one of pulmonary infarction with hemoptysis, pleuritic chest pain, friction rub, and abnormal roentgenographic shadows. Often, however, some elements of this pattern may be absent, notably the hemoptysis or the evidence of pleural involvement. (3) There may be an acute picture similar to, but frequently not as severe as, that seen with embolization of the main pulmonary artery or its primary branches, in which pattern the primary difficulty is one of extensive and sudden compromise of the pulmonary arterial circulation but here by multiple emboli or recurrent embolization; it may or may not be complicated by infarction. (4) There may be a chronic and insidiously developing syndrome of cor pulmonale from progressive pulmonary hypertension that has evolved slowly after repeated episodes of embolization with or without infarction. This is often superimposed and obscured by the presence of other underlying chronic disease.

Controversy exists concerning the factors that acutely compromise the pulmonary circulation when emboli impact in medium-sized or smaller vessels. Some hold that vasoconstriction (pulmonary and perhaps coronary), mediated through reflexes from occluded arterioles or by the local release of serotonin, prostaglandins, or other vasoactive substances, plays an important role. It seems probable, however, that the continuing effects of most pulmonary emboli are primarily mechanical; when a major segment of the circulation is organically occluded, pulmonary hypertension and decreased venous outflow result. The suggestion has been made, and experimental studies have been cited to support the concept, that idiopathic pulmonary hypertension and pulmonary arteriosclerosis may result from repeated small pulmonary emboli.

The mechanism of pulmonary infarction is poorly understood. It does not result from ligation of pulmonary vessels and is unusual after embolization in animals with normal lungs; however, it does occur with great frequency in the congested, infected, or hypoventilated lung. Currently the best working hypothesis is that when medium-sized embolization occurs, enhancement of the circulation through the bronchial artery collaterals and bronchopulmonary vascular anastomoses distal to the embolus ordinarily serves to sustain the lung. However, in the presence of congestion or other conditions that predispose to local intrapulmonic circulatory stasis, augmentation of the collateral circulation is delayed or its benefits voided, and infarction occurs.

Hemorrhagic necrosis of the lung tissue and the overlying pleural inflammation are responsible for the characteristic clinical features of pulmonary infarction. The former accounts for the hemoptysis, cough, and fever; the latter for the pleural friction rub and pain. Since both lung tissue and the visceral pleura are devoid of sensory nerves, infarcts that do not extend to the outer surface of the lung to involve the parietal pleura do not cause pleural pain. When pain is present, it usually occurs over the ribs in the axillary region, but occasionally it may appear in the abdomen along the costal margin, or, when there is involvement of the parietal diaphragmatic pleura, in the shoulder or neck. The mechanism of the pain has usually been attributed to friction over an inflamed pleura, but an alternative explanation that may better explain its features (accentuation only on inspiration) is tension exerted during inspiration on those sensitized nerve ends of the parietal pleura that are attached to the intercostal muscles.

CLINICAL MANIFESTATIONS. The manifestations of *massive pulmonary embolism* (defined for clinical purposes as occlusion of 50 per cent or more of the pulmonary arterial circulation and representing approximately one third to one half of the suspected cases) may include sudden dyspnea; tachypnea; cyanosis; precordial or substernal oppressive pain, occasionally with radiation to shoulders and neck; evidence of right-sided cardiac dilatation and failure; tachycardia; restlessness; anxiety; syncope, occasionally with convulsions; and hypotension.

With massive embolism, death may be sudden or may occur over a period of several hours. In the latter instance, shock with vascular collapse becomes prominent. In an additional 2 to 3 per cent of patients, death may be delayed from one to several days; but when blood pressure spontaneously returns to normal, recovery is likely (unless the course is complicated by recurrence or an underlying disease). The physical signs noted include pulsation in the second left interspace, accentuation of P_2, a pseudo- or pleuropericardial friction rub, systolic or diastolic murmurs in the second left interspace, an interscapular bruit, S_3 or S_4 gallop rhythm, increased cardiac dullness to the right, distended neck veins, increased venous pressure with an hepatojugular reflex, and enlarged liver. Dislodgment of a large obstructing embolus may be associated with the dramatic transient appearance of a "red arterial wave" suddenly passing over a pallid cyanotic face.

Serial *electrocardiograms* reveal transient changes in most patients (85 per cent), but the pattern is extremely variable. The most frequent initial finding is T wave inversion (40 per cent). The electrocardiographic signs of acute cor pulmonale ($S_1Q_3T_3$, complete right bundle branch block, P pulmonale, or right axis deviation) are present in only 25 per cent of patients; left axis deviation is observed more frequently than right axis deviation. Rhythm disturbances (most commonly, premature ventricular beats) are observed in 10 per cent, as is a pseudoinfarction pattern. Patients with prior cardiopulmonary disease have a greater frequency of arrhythmias, conduction disturbances, and QRS changes; patients with extensive embolization demonstrate more QRS, RST, and T wave changes. In general, little change occurs during the first 24 hours, but after five to six days the QRS, primary RST segment, and T wave abnormalities begin to disappear. Roentgenographically, massive pulmonary embolism may result in the appearance of a large pulmonary arterial shadow that terminates abruptly; in some cases the ischemia may produce radiolucency of portions of the lung field (Westermark's sign).

With *submassive embolism*, i.e., occlusion of less than 50 per cent of the pulmonary circulation and usually involving the medium-sized or smaller vessels, the clinical manifestations may vary from a transient episode of dyspnea or the sudden or insidious worsening of an underlying pulmonary or cardiac disease, to the full-blown picture described for massive embolism (submassive embolism in patients with prior embolism or severe underlying cardiopulmonary disease frequently presents with the findings usually attributable to massive embolism); however, when pulmonary infarction occurs, its manifestations may also be superimposed.

The manifestations of *pulmonary infarction* are usually less dramatic. They vary in intensity from silent to those characterized by pleuritic chest pain, hemoptysis, cough, moderate dyspnea, fever, tachycardia, pleural friction rub, areas of dullness or flatness on percussion, and diminished breath sounds, occasionally with tubular breathing and rales. The leukocyte count is usually elevated, the sedimentation rate is accelerated, and, subsequently, the serum bilirubin and serum lactic dehydrogenase levels rise. Roentgenographic examination may show typical humped or wedge-shaped shadows; on occasions the lesions are rounded or indistinguishable from pneumonic infiltrates. At other times, a pleural effusion may be the only clue to an underlying infarct. The average patient with pulmonary infarction runs a moderately febrile course for a few days, which is followed by clearing of roentgenographic and physical signs in one to three weeks.

DIAGNOSIS.   Despite the introduction of such diagnostic aids as pulmonary isotopic and ventilation photoscanning and selective pulmonary angiography, the diagnosis of pulmonary embolism with or without infarction is accurately made in no more than 50 per cent of cases when compared to autopsy findings. Frequently the diagnosis is overlooked because the disorder appears in the guise of congestive heart failure or pneumonia rather than as a distinctive syndrome; furthermore, the cardinal features do not occur with any great regularity. In half the patients subsequently proved to have recurrent infarction, no evidence of phlebitis, pleural pain, pleural friction rub, or hemoptysis is present, and in any one episode the incidence of each of these is less than 20 per cent. Thus in the absence of classic features, the diagnosis must be made on the basis of a high index of suspicion followed by confirmatory laboratory findings.

Pulmonary embolism with or without infarction should be suspected in all cases of chest pain of unknown cause, atypical pleural effusion, or bronchopneumonia. The possibility of this complication should also be considered in any patient who has a proved or suggestive history of a previous episode (present in 25 per cent of cases), in groups at high risk for deep vein thrombosis, and, most carefully, in critically ill patients with congestive heart failure; the incidence among the last-named group approaches 50 per cent and is much higher among those who exhibit unexplained fever or the *triad of tachycardia, digitalis toxicity, and edema unresponsive to diuretic therapy.*

Actually, the presence of one or more of the following symptoms, signs, or laboratory findings should raise the possibility of pulmonary embolism for consideration: sudden or increased dyspnea, tachypnea, cough, or cyanosis; substernal or pleuritic chest pain; hemoptysis; phlebitis; acute right-sided failure or sudden worsening of congestive heart failure; shock; pulmonary consolidation; pleural friction rub; roentgenographic evidence of pulmonary infiltration, elevated diaphragm, large areas of increased radiolucency, or pleural effusion; unexplained arrhythmias or electrocardiographic changes, particularly when the latter is indicative of acute right heart strain or dilatation; pulmonary function studies indicating an increased ventilatory dead space, i.e., reduction in the mean alveolar carbon dioxide tension in the presence of a normal or nearly normal arterial carbon dioxide tension; or unexplained fever, leukocytosis, elevated erythrocyte sedimentation rate, serum bilirubin, lactic dehydrogenase, and fibrinogen/fibrin split products (normal levels of fibrinogen/fibrin split products and fibrin monomer are rare in pulmonary embolism).

The most reliable *screening procedures* for excluding an acute pulmonary embolism are pulmonary isotopic photoscanning with technetium-labeled microspheres or macroaggregates of human serum albumin, and an arterial Po_2 determination; a negative four-positional (anterior, posterior, and both laterals) lung scan virtually eliminates acute embolism, and it is rare when the arterial Po_2 is 90 mm Hg or above.

Confirmation of the diagnosis can often be achieved through the use of either selective pulmonary angiography or pulmonary isotopic photoscanning; on occasion, both techniques will be necessary. Since selective *pulmonary angiography* provides direct visualization of the vascular tree, it is the more definitive of the two procedures, and is the choice for establishing the diagnosis of pulmonary embolism. However, there are limitations to its usefulness. It is expensive and requires a skilled team; catheterization of the pulmonary artery is associated with some morbidity; the technique does not distinguish between new and old emboli; the subsegmental and smaller vessels are not visualized adequately; and there may be errors in interpretation unless the angiographer is experienced and strict criteria are used.

Pulmonary isotopic photoscanning has the advantages of convenience and lack of significant morbidity, and allows for repeated observation in following the course of the patient. However, unlike pulmonary arteriography, photoscanning does not visualize the pulmonary arterial tree; rather, it is a measure of the distribution of blood flow or pulmonary capillary perfusion, and defects in perfusion may be misinterpreted as to cause, especially in the presence of any underlying pulmonary lesion, e.g., infiltrates, blebs, cysts, emphysema, an acute asthmatic attack, or alterations in perfusion as a result of previous or associated disease. Since the scan is not specific for pulmonary embolism, perfusion defects should be characterized as to whether they are segmental or not and only interpreted as having a high, medium, or low probability of being due to an embolism. Although emphysema may also be responsible for high probability perfusion defects, the differential diagnosis can usually be resolved by a radioactively labeled xenon ventilation scan, because such a scan is unaffected by pulmonary embolism, at least for a period of five days. Pulmonary isotopic photoscanning is most useful for demonstration and quantitating the perfusion defect of a pulmonary embolism when the chest roentgenogram is normal; it may also be diagnostic by revealing multiple perfusion defects (indicative of multiple pulmonary embolism) when only an isolated infiltrate or lesion is present roentgenographically. Resolution of the perfusion defect after an embolism occurs progressively (50 per cent in two weeks), and this, too, may be useful diagnostically. It is noteworthy that patients with underlying cardiac disease have an impaired resolution rate.

Acute pulmonary embolism may be most readily confused with acute myocardial infarction, pulmonary edema, acute asthma, atelectasis, pericarditis, spontaneous pneumothorax, ball-valve thrombus in the left atrium, dissecting aneurysm, and pulmonary artery thrombosis. The last-named condition occurs rarely as a primary form of obscure cause or as a complication of a partially obstructing embolus, invading tumor, narrowed vascular lumen, or atherosclerotic plaque; it is also seen in sickle cell disease and the mixed sickle cell hemoglobinopathies.

The differential diagnosis of pulmonary infarction includes pneumonia, pleurisy, other forms of pleural effusion, neoplasm, acute upper abdominal conditions, and the various causes of pulmonary hemorrhage. During resolution, an occasional infarct may slough out, leaving a thin-walled cavity which may be confused with an abscess.

To distinguish between an infarct and pneumonia may be difficult, yet this question arises frequently. Findings that are helpful in pointing to the diagnosis of infarct are a history or the presence of one of the preconditions of infarct, e.g., recent surgery, trauma, cardiac disease, previous venous disease, or pulmonary embolism; an extremely rapid appearance of roentgenographic abnormalities from the time of the first respiratory symptom; illness that seems disproportionately mild in relation to the extent of the pulmonary involvement or leukocytosis; and relative lack of cough or lack of preceding respiratory disease.

A spontaneous form of pulmonary infarction occurs in sickle cell disease, in the mixed sickle cell hemoglobinopathies, or in persons with sickle cell trait who are exposed to high altitude.

TREATMENT. General Measures. Supportive treatment for the usual acute embolism should include bed rest, an analgesic or narcotic (preferably meperidine hydrochloride [Demerol]) for pain and apprehension, and oxygen as indicated. The administration of antimicrobial drugs to prevent bacterial disease of the lungs is not indicated unless a septic infarct is suspected. All sudden effort should be avoided, especially straining at stool. Stool softeners and colonic lavages may prove useful. Pleural effusions may require aspiration, particularly if dyspnea is progressive. Digitalization is indicated if cardiac failure appears or worsens, but usually is of little benefit.

In more severe cases, continuous oxygen therapy should be employed, and positive pressure oxygen may prove particularly useful when pulmonary edema is present. Cardiac arrhythmias, which occur in 10 per cent of cases, should be treated appropriately. If shock occurs, fluids and isoproterenol should be given. Intravenous fluids should be monitored by central venous pressure measurements but maintained below 150 mm saline to prevent pulmonary edema. For hypotension, isoproterenol, because of its inotropic effect on the heart, is the agent of choice. It should be given intravenously slowly, usually at a rate of 2 μg per minute to sustain the systolic blood pressure at about 100 mm Hg (preferably at 120 mm Hg in previously hypertensive patients). Aminophylline, 250 to 500 mg (by suppository, intramuscularly, or by slow intravenous administration), may prove useful, particularly when dyspnea is prominent or pulmonary edema is present. Venesection may be dangerous, however, because of impaired left ventricular filling. The value of pulmonary vasodilators, e.g., papaverine, and bronchodilators, e.g., atropine, is still highly controversial.

Anticoagulants. In the absence of contraindications, heparin therapy should be instituted immediately in all patients with pulmonary embolism to lessen the danger of a recurrent and frequently fatal embolic accident (when heparin allergy is present, anticoagulation should be instituted immediately with coumarin compounds). Hemoptysis from pulmonary infarction is not a contraindication to anticoagulant therapy. The regimen for heparin therapy and subsequent oral coumarin anticoagulation is as described under the treatment of thrombophlebitis (Ch. 357.2). Aspirin and aspirin-containing compounds should be avoided because of the increased risk of bleeding. Coumarin therapy is continued for six weeks unless there is a chronic disease, e.g., cardiac failure, that predisposes to repeated venous thrombus formation; under these circumstances anticoagulant therapy should be continued for prolonged periods.

Thrombolytic Agents. These provide an important adjunct to the management of the more seriously ill patient with pulmonary embolism. Clinical trials have demonstrated that urokinase and streptokinase lyse pulmonary emboli extensively, reduce the hemodynamic abnormalities, improve pulmonary capillary perfusion, and increase gas exchange. These effects are observed fairly rapidly and are most striking in patients with massive embolism. Regimens as described previously for thrombophlebitis also will reduce significantly the need for surgical embolectomy, particularly when the therapy is combined with temporary cardiac bypass to tide the patient over the most critical period. Whether local perfusion of the agent directly into the pulmonary artery has any advantage over intravenous administration remains to be established. At present, thrombolytic agents are not indicated for the treatment of submassive embolism when stable vital signs are present; in the absence of complications, the patient is destined to recover and there is little need to increase the risk of bleeding; however, they are indicated in massive embolism with or without shock and in submassive embolism with shock. *Arvin*, the defibrinating agent, may also prove to be of benefit in the management of acute pulmonary embolism, but its advantage over heparin remains to be established.

Surgical Therapy. Inferior vena caval ligation, plication, or the insertion of a filter or umbrella should be reserved for those patients in whom anticoagulants are contraindicated, must be discontinued, or whose disease for one reason or another cannot be successfully managed with this form of therapy. Since these procedures carry a significant incidence of sequelae, they are not indicated unless there has been massive embolism or there is evidence of recurrent embolization (a minor recurrence of symptoms, due either to further small emboli or a shift in the position of a previous embolus, is observed in about 10 per cent of patients during the first few days of heparin therapy, and should not be considered as a failure of anticoagulant therapy unless the episode is significant clinically or continues to recur during adequate levels of anticoagulation).

Surgical embolectomy may be lifesaving in critically ill patients. However, this procedure requires cardiac bypass, and because of the condition of the patients, the mortality in patients treated with surgical embolectomy is still very high. At present, the indication for embolectomy is limited to patients who are in extremis or are deteriorating with angiographic evidence of massive embolism of the main pulmonary artery or its primary branches and with sustained peripheral hypotension despite the use of appropriate supportive measures, including thrombolytic therapy. Pulmonary embolectomy may also be considered for patients who have survived a massive embolism but in whom pulmonary hypertension resulting from the presence of an accessible embolus is leading to the development of cor pulmonale.

PROGNOSIS. The prognosis of pulmonary embolism is difficult to establish because the clinical diagnosis is frequently obscure. Of those who succumb, approximately 90 per cent die immediately or within the first two hours. Another 2 to 3 per cent die of protracted shock during the next 48 hours. Once stable vital signs are established, subsequent mortality approximates 7 per cent and is usually attributable to recurrent embolism or adverse effects on an underlying cardiopulmonary disease. The likelihood of a fatal episode is increased with succeeding embolic attacks and, most important, in the presence of a significant impairment of cardiopulmonary reserve. The greatest hope for the management of this problem is prevention.

Unfortunately, such measures as the use of elastic stockings or bandages, leg exercises for immobilized patients, and early ambulation postoperatively have not greatly affected the high incidence of pulmonary embolism; nevertheless, the intelligent use of such measures, and particularly of the more recently developed mechanical devices which enhance blood flow, is to be encouraged. In addition, serious consideration should be given to the use of anticoagulants for all patients predisposed to thrombus formation. When used carefully, anticoagulants have significantly reduced the incidence of pulmonary embolism after fracture of the femur and in cases of congestive heart failure. This form of therapy should not be undertaken lightly, because the hazards, in any specific case, may outweigh the benefits to be derived. Low-dose heparin should obviate this problem.

Anticoagulation also has an important role to play in the *prevention of arterial embolism.* Coumarin therapy is useful in avoiding systemic embolization from endocardial mural thrombi in the left ventricle, e.g., after acute transmural infarction, and in the left atrium, e.g., in rheumatic mitral disease or during an electrical conversion of an arrhythmia. For acute myocardial infarction, coumarin therapy should be administered to those at high risk for such embolic episodes; the high risk factors include age over 60, previous myocardial infarction, shock, congestive heart failure, and evidence of large transmural infarction as judged by the levels of serum enzymes, fever, leukocytosis, sedimentation rate, and the extent of the electrocardiographic abnormalities. Therapy should be initiated at the onset of the illness and continued for a period of four weeks. Patients with rheumatic mitral disease with a nonseptic embolus (anticoagulants are contraindicated in subacute bacterial endocarditis) should be maintained on long-term anticoagulation or until surgical correction of the lesion. For individuals undergoing electrical conversion of an arrhythmia, coumarin therapy should be initiated two to three weeks prior to attempting reversion to a sinus rhythm in all patients with previous emboli or evidence of mitral stenosis; in other situations the need for anticoagulation should be considered and evaluated on an individual basis.

Coumarin anticoagulation is less effective for the prevention of platelet emboli such as may occur from prosthetic heart valves and in the transient ischemic attack syndrome. Better results are being obtained for the former condition when coumarin anticoagulation is combined with antiplatelet agents, e.g., sulfinpyrazone* (800 mg daily) or dipyridamole* (400 mg daily). For the transient ischemic attack syndrome, aspirin (1.2 grams daily) appears to be the antiplatelet agent of choice.

Medical therapy of an acute embolic event with antithrombotic agents is as described under the management of thrombophlebitis and pulmonary embolism.

Anticoagulants in acute myocardial infarction. Results of a cooperative clinical trial. JAMA, 225:724, 1973.

Kakkar, V. V., Corrigan, T. P., and Fossard, D. P.: Prevention of fatal postoperative pulmonary embolism by low doses of heparin: An international multicentre trial. Lancet, 1:45, 1975.

Kakkar, V. V., Howe, C. T., Flanc, C., and Clarke, M. B.: Natural history of postoperative deep vein thrombosis. Lancet, 2:230, 1969.

McIntyre, K. M., and Sasahara, A. A.: The hemodynamic response to pulmonary embolism in patients without prior cardiopulmonary disease. Am. J. Cardiol., 28:288, 1971.

Miller, G. A. H., Hall, R. J. C., and Paneth, M.: Pulmonary embolectomy, heparin and streptokinase: Their place in the treatment of acute massive pulmonary embolism. Am. Heart J., 93:568, 1977.

Paraskos, J. A., Adelstein, S. J., Smith, R. E., et al.: Late prognosis of acute pulmonary embolism. N. Engl. J. Med., 289:55, 1973.

Sasahara, A., Hyers, T. M., Cole, C., et al. (eds.): The urokinase pulmonary embolism trial. Circulation, 47 (Suppl. II):II-5, 1973.

Stein, M., and Moser, K. M. (eds.): Pulmonary Thromboembolism. Chicago, Year Book Medical Publishers, 1973.

---

*Experimental drug for this purpose.

358. PULMONARY HYPERTENSION

Daniel S. Lukas

358.1. INTRODUCTION

Morphologically and physiologically, the circulation of the lungs differs from that of all other organs. Although the entire cardiac output passes through the lungs, a mean pressure in the pulmonary artery only one ninth of the pressure in the aorta is needed to sustain this flow. Under a wide variety of physiologic circumstances, simple adjustments of the pulmonary vascular bed minimize increases of pulmonary arterial pressure. Because many diseases of the heart and lungs can seriously compromise this regulatory capacity, pulmonary hypertension is a common clinical phenomenon. In some disorders elevations of pulmonary arterial pressure are acute and episodic, whereas in others the pulmonary hypertension is chronic and progressive.

The mechanisms producing pulmonary arterial hypertension in the major categories of disease are sufficiently different to warrant separate consideration and are best appreciated in the context of the normal structure and funciton of the pulmonary circulation.

THE NORMAL PULMONARY CIRCULATION

STRUCTURE. The pulmonary arterial tree consists of three distinct types of arteries that differ from each other in the composition of their walls and in size. The elastic arteries include the main pulmonary artery, its major branches, and arteries with external diameters greater than 1.0 mm. The muscular pulmonary arteries range in diameter from 0.1 to 1.0 mm. The smallest pulmonary arteries, the arterioles, have diameters less than 0.1 mm. The walls of all three types of arteries are much thinner than those of systemic arteries, and aside from the main pulmonary artery and its branches, these vessels have no strict anatomic counterparts in the systemic vascular bed.

The media of the main pulmonary artery and the elastic arteries contains a small amount of smooth muscle, collagen, and elastic fibers that are short, irregularly branching, and fragmented in appearance. The media of the aorta, in contrast, is 1.5 to more than 2 times thicker, and its elastic fibers are long, unbranching, and distributed in parallel fashion.

The muscular pulmonary arteries are closely apposed to the bronchioles and alveolar ducts. They have a large lumen and a thin wall that is composed of an intima and a thin media of concentrically oriented smooth muscle fibers bounded by internal and external elastic laminae.

The arterioles differ vastly from those of the systemic circuit, because they contain no muscle except at their point of origin. They consist of an endothelium, a single elastic lamina, and a scanty adventitia.

The pulmonary capillaries are the most prominent structural component of the alveolar walls, in which they form an extensive, interlacing network that is separated from the alveolar air by the lining cells of the alveoli and their basement membrane. The total surface of the capillaries that is available for gas exchange in adults has been estimated to comprise 60 to 70 square meters.

The pulmonary venules are thin-walled structures histologically indistinguishable from the arterioles. The structure of the veins is less ordered than that of the muscular arteries. The media, which is not bounded by well-defined elastic laminae, blends indistinguishably with the adventitia, and both contain smooth muscle and fragmented elastic fibers. The main venous trunks acquire a layer of cardiac muscle before they enter the left atrium. The venules and veins, unlike the arteries, do not course with the bronchial tree but are lodged in the septa that separate lobules and segments of the lung.

The bronchial arteries wind in spiral fashion around the bronchi and anastomose extensively with each other in and around the walls of the airways. They also form vasa vasorum in the adventitia of the elastic and larger muscular pulmonary arteries. Evidence that the two arterial systems intercommunicate in the normal lung is inconclusive. The bronchial veins, however, normally form numerous, small anastomotic channels with the pulmonary veins.

It is of considerable significance that the pulmonary arteries in the fetus and newborn differ structurally from those of the adult and do not attain their final form until the sixth to twelfth month of postnatal life. In the newborn, the media of the main pulmonary artery is as thick as that of the aorta and contains numerous, tightly packed, long, elastic fibers that are fairly uniform in thickness and are arranged in parallel fashion as in the aorta. Progressively after birth, the media diminishes in thickness, and the elastic fibers become fragmented, irregularly shaped, randomly distributed, and less densely packed, until they assume the full adult appearance. The muscular pulmonary arteries in the newborn resemble small systemic arteries. Typically, the wall contains a wide media composed of circularly oriented smooth muscle, and its thickness exceeds the diameter of the lumen. Rapid increase in luminal and external diameters and thinning of the media occur during the first sixth months of life. The arterioles at birth are surrounded by dense connective tissue and their lumina are barely patent. Their wall:lumen ratio likewise rapidly diminishes in the first few months of life.

During the early days of the postnatal period, the mean pulmonary arterial pressure is two or more times greater than that of the adult and may be high enough to reverse flow through the ductus arteriosus. The pulmonary arterial pressure declines to normal adult values within the first month, well before the metamorphosis of the pulmonary vasculature has been completed.

HEMODYNAMICS. The average normal pressure in the pulmonary artery at rest is 19/6 mm Hg (systolic/diastolic) with a mean pressure of 11 mm Hg. Normally at rest, the systolic pressure does not exceed 25 mm Hg, and the mean pressure is not greater than 15 mm Hg. Mean pressures in the large pulmonary veins and left atrium are essentially identical, ranging from 3 to 8 mm Hg, with an average of 5 mm Hg. Thus a pressure gradient from the pulmonary artery to the large pulmonary veins of only 6 mm Hg is sufficient to sustain a blood flow in the normal adult at rest of approximately 6.0 liter per minute. These values are eloquent testimony to the low resistance offered to the flow of blood by the thin-walled and capacious pulmonary vessels. Calculated in the conventional manner as the mean pressure gradient divided by flow, the normal pulmonary vascular resistance is 1.0 mm Hg per liter per minute, or 80 dyne sec cm^{-5}, a value only 7 per cent of the normal systemic vascular resistance. The linear distribution of resistance in the pulmonary vascular bed is uncertain, but measurements in dogs indicate that the pulmonary arteries are responsible for approximately half the total resistance, the pulmonary capillaries for 30 per cent, and the veins for 20 per cent.

Several observations testify to the capacity of the pulmonary vascular bed to accommodate increases in blood flow with disproportionately small increases in pressure. During exercise, two- to three-fold increases in cardiac output are associated with increments of only 25 to 50 per cent in mean pulmonary arterial pressure, but the pressure doubles when the output rises to four to five times the resting value. Large left-right shunts through an atrial septal defect that commonly triple the pulmonary blood flow are tolerated for many years with no more than slight elevations of pulmonary arterial pressure. After pneumonectomy or occlusion of either main branch of the pulmonary artery by a balloon catheter and in patients with congenital absence of a main branch of the pulmonary artery, the pulmonary arterial pressures remain within the normal range at rest if the perfused lung is normal.

Augmentation of pulmonary blood flow is facilitated and concomitant changes in pressure are minimized by several mechanisms that combine to expand the net cross-sectional area of the pulmonary vessels and thereby decrease the resistance they offer to the flow of blood. One of these mechanisms relates to the effect of changes in intravascular pressures on the caliber of the vessels. It has been demonstrated that increases in pulmonary arterial pressure well within the normal operational range are associated with large decreases in pulmonary vascular resistance and that the resistance declines further with the addition of a 2 to 3 mm Hg rise in left atrial pressure. The vessels are also subjected to the deforming effects of the pressures that surround them. The total pressure that acts on the vascular wall is the transmural pressure, or the difference between the intravascular and perivascular pressures. Some uncertainties exist regarding perivascular pressures in the lungs, but for vessels that are not intrinsic components of the alveolar structure, perivascular pressure is considered to approximate pleural pressure; for intraalveolar vessels, the alveolar pressure has been regarded as the extravascular pressure. Since the vessels that account for the major fraction of the pulmonary vascular resistance are exposed to the normally negative pleural pressure, their transmural pressures exceed the hydrostatic pressures within them.

During exercise, the more negative pleural pressures generated to augment tidal volume increase the transmural pressure gradients acting on the extra-alveolar vessels, thereby stretching them open further and decreasing their resistance to flow. Pressure changes within the pleura and the lungs can profoundly affect the pulmonary vasculature. For example, when intrapleural and alveolar pressures are greatly increased, as during a Valsalva maneuver, pulmonary vascular transmural pressures fall, some vessels collapse, and the resistance rises markedly.

Primarily because of gravitational effects on regional intravascular pressures, the lungs are not evenly perfused. In the erect position, the height of the blood column from the apices of the lungs to the midpoint of the left atrium is sufficient to reduce pressures within the pulmonary arteries at the apices almost to zero and to decrease the transmural pressures of the pulmonary capillaries and veins in these regions to less than zero. Consequently, the vascular bed in the apices is not open, whereas at the bases of the lungs the vessels are subjected to the distending effects of the overlying column of blood and all are patent. These regional differences in vascular resistance produce a progressive decrease in regional blood flow within the lungs from base to apex, and in the upright position blood flow per unit volume of lung is eight times greater at the base than at the apex. At some point below the apices of the lungs, the transmural pressures of the arteries and the arterial limbs of the alveolar capillaries are high enough to maintain patency of the vessels, but the pressure within the venous segment of the capillaries or the venules is less than or just equals the perivascular pressure. The collapsible vascular segments in this region behave like sluices; they are either barely open or closed, and flow of blood through them no longer depends on the pressure gradient between the arterial and venous limbs but varies directly with the pressure difference between the arterial end of the segment and the pressure surrounding the collapsed segment. These hemodynamic conditions have been compared to those of a waterfall.

With increases in pulmonary flow, small changes in intravascular pressures open previously closed or partially collapsed vessels, thus expanding the size of the vascular bed and further lowering resistance to flow. This recruitment of small vessels and capillaries partly explains the increase of pulmonary diffusing capacity that occurs during exercise.

The volume of blood contained by the pulmonary vessels of an average size adult is approximately 400 to 500 ml, 70 to 100 ml of which is in the pulmonary capillaries. Because of its geometric complexity and the probably nonuniform dimensional rearrangements that the pulmonary vascular bed undergoes with changes in volume, the interrelationships among resistance, pressures, flow, and blood volume in the vessels of the lungs are far from simple. It is clear that the distensibility of the pulmonary arterial tree is much greater than that of the systemic arteries, and that this partially accounts for its lower resistance to flow. The large pulmonary veins, however, are less compliant than the major systemic venous segments. Also, the compliance of the small pulmonary vessels is not uniform; the capillaries are less distensible than the arteries and veins. In one study of normal subjects during an exercise that evoked an almost two-fold increase in cardiac output, the pulmonary blood volume increased by only 27 per cent, mean pulmonary arterial pressure increased slightly, and pulmonary vascular resistance fell. The pulmonary vasoconstriction produced by hypoxia is associated with a decrease in pulmonary blood volume, despite the increase of pressure in the elastic pulmonary arteries.

The compliance of the pulmonary vessels is finite, and changes in the volume of blood in the lungs do produce changes in vascular pressures. For example, the intense constriction of the systemic vessels that sometimes occurs after injury to the brain (*Cushing reflex*) results in systemic hypertension, displacement of blood from the systemic circuit into the lungs, and marked pulmonary venous and pulmonary arterial hypertension.

Whereas the systemic vessels are closely regulated by the autonomic nervous system and respond to a wide variety of endogenous compounds and drugs, adjustments of the pulmonary vascular bed appear to result almost entirely in response to physical forces. The pulmonary arteries are supplied with autonomic nerves, and there is experimental evidence in animals that the larger pulmonary arteries can be reflexly induced to stiffen, but reflex control of the pulmonary circulation has not been convincingly demonstrated in man. Similarly, many pharmacologic agents considered on the basis of experiments in animals to exert a vasoconstrictor action on the pulmonary arteries (norepinephrine, epinephrine, and serotonin) or a vasodilator effect (bradykinin, isoproterenol, and acetylcholine) have been shown to have either little or no direct action on the normal human pulmonary vascular bed. Because these compounds profoundly affect the systemic circulation and may alter pulmonary mechanics, the changes in pulmonary vascular pressures and resistance that are observed after they are administered are mainly secondary consequences of their actions elsewhere.

HYPOXIA. Ample evidence of several types indicates that hypoxia directly constricts the pulmonary bed and elevates the pulmonary vascular resistance by direct action on the muscular pulmonary arteries, which are separated from the inner surface of the small airways by only 0.1 mm. Extensive investigations in the past have failed to disclose the mechanism of this effect, but some studies have shown that in contrast to its action on systemic arterial smooth muscle, hypoxia may stimulate production of adenosine triphosphate and facilitate membrane depolarization in pulmonary arterial smooth muscle. Evidences that the actions of hypoxia on the pulmonary vessels are mediated by catecholamines, histamine, prostaglandins, angiotensin II, or serotonin generated or released by the lung either are inconclusive or have been convincingly refuted.

The vasoconstrictor response to hypoxia is greatly potentiated by increases in blood hydrogen ion and is almost abolished by alkalosis. The hypoxic reflex serves a useful local regulatory function by limiting blood flow to underventilated pulmonary segments and thereby restores the regional ventilation-perfusion ratio to normal, but when the hypoxia is generalized, the response is far from beneficial. Inhalation of 12 per cent oxygen at sea level (Po_2: 91 mm Hg) promptly results in twofold increases of pulmonary vascular resistance and pulmonary arterial mean pressure, with no increase in cardiac output or left atrial pressure.

PULMONARY ARTERIAL PRESSURE AT HIGH ALTITUDE. Chronic exposure to the hypoxia of high altitude produces a sustained increase in pulmonary arterial pressure. The average values of pulmonary arterial pressure in natives of Morococho, Peru, which is at 14,900 feet above sea level (Po_2: 80 mm Hg), are 41/15 mm Hg (systolic/diastolic), with a mean pressure of 28 mm Hg at rest and 77/40 (mean: 60 mm Hg) during exercise. Their right ventricles are hypertrophied, and their small pulmonary arteries are thicker and contain increased amounts of smooth muscle, which extends farther down into the smallest vessels than normally. After two years of residing at sea level, the pulmonary

arterial pressures of these people fall to normal values at rest but still rise to abnormal values with exercise.

Studies of the pulmonary circulation in residents of Leadville, Colorado (altitude: 10,200 feet; Po_2: 100 mm Hg), have emphasized the considerable individual variation in the reactivity of the pulmonary vasculature to chronic hypoxia. The average mean pulmonary arterial pressure at rest in one group of subjects was increased to 25 mm Hg, but it varied from 10 to 45 mm Hg, and in one 15-year-old woman the pressure rose to 105 mm Hg during exercise. This subject's pressure became normal after she had resided at sea level for 11 months.

The individuality of the response to hypoxia is further emphasized by the occurrence of acute pulmonary edema at high altitudes in susceptible persons who are otherwise normal. The pathogenesis of the pulmonary edema, which responds promptly to inhalation of oxygen, has not been fully elucidated, but it is not due to left ventricular failure, and pulmonary venous constriction has not been proved to be the cause. It occurs at altitudes greater than 9000 feet in persons who have not previously been exposed to altitude as well as in residents at high altitude within 12 to 36 hours after returning from even a brief sojourn at a lower level. Such persons are liable to recurrence of pulmonary edema with each transition from low to high altitude. Studies of susceptible subjects have revealed hyperreactivity of their pulmonary vessels to hypoxia. Their pulmonary hemodynamics and pulmonary function were normal at sea level, but at 10,000 feet after a day of exposure to the altitude and a period of vigorous activity at higher altitude, despite the maintenance of normal pulmonary wedge pressures and no evidence of pulmonary edema, their pulmonary arterial pressures were two to three times greater than those of normal subjects at the same altitude.

In many disease states affecting the pulmonary circulation, including those not producing alveolar hypoxia, individual variations in pulmonary vascular reactivity are common, and the spectrum of physiologic and structural abnormalities of the pulmonary vessels in each condition is usually wide.

358.2. PRIMARY PULMONARY HYPERTENSION

Primary pulmonary hypertension is a disease of unknown cause characterized by marked increase in the pulmonary vascular resistance and pulmonary arterial pressure. Despite exhaustive search while the patient is alive, or at autopsy, no evidence can be found of underlying diseases known to produce pulmonary arterial hypertension, such as congenital or acquired heart disease, pulmonary disease, disorders of respiration, and systemic diseases that affect the pulmonary vessels.

INCIDENCE. Primary pulmonary hypertension is uncommon. In one series of 10,000 patients with heart disease, it was found in only 17. Among reported cases, the patients ranged in age from 1 to 68 years, but most were 20 to 40 years old. There were three times as many women as men; most of the women were in their early thirties and had borne children. The disease is known to occur in a familial form. Among 20 families reported, the ratio of males to females in the 47 members with the disease was approximately 2 to 1. In six families, apparent parent-to-offspring transmission was documented, and in one kindred five members of three generations manifested the disease. The mode of genetic transmission is uncertain. In five families, the mother and either a daughter or a son were affected; in the other family, the father and his son and daughter died of the disease.

PATHOLOGY. In all patients, the pulmonary arteries show structural abnormalities characteristic of hypertensive pulmonary vascular disease usually of the most advanced degree (Grades 4 to 6 of Heath and Edwards). The walls of the muscular arteries and arterioles are greatly thickened, and their lumina are markedly narrowed and even obliterated. The smooth muscle in the media of the muscular arteries is hypertrophied and extends well down into the arterioles, which normally do not have a distinct media. In the arterioles and extending back to the smaller muscular pulmonary arteries less than 0.3 mm and occasionally those as large as 0.5 mm, marked cellular proliferation and fibrosis of the intima are seen. In some of the vessels, the intimal proliferation is concentric, shows an onion-layering appearance, and encroaches evenly on the lumen; in others, the masses of protruding fibrous tissue are unevenly distributed and create an eccentric, irregularly shaped lumen. The fibrous tissue contains elastic fibrils and eventually assumes a hyaline appearance.

Although the media attains a thickness equivalent to 30 per cent of the external diameter of the small arteries in some areas, in other areas the media is atrophied and the vessels dilated. Such generalized dilatations of the arterial wall are often found at and downstream from an occluded segment of a small muscular artery or arteriole and upstream from occlusions in the medium-sized arteries.

In addition to the generalized dilatations, localized dilatations that form morphologically complex, saccular structures develop from the walls of the smallest muscular arteries and arterioles. One of these structures, known as a plexiform lesion, is characterized by a thin-walled sac protruding from the wall of the vessel. The sac frequently contains a thrombus, over which an area of cellular intimal tissue has proliferated to form a complex, plexiform pattern. An overlying layer of fibrous tissue is continuous with the intimal proliferative layer of the artery. In other dilatation lesions, groups of thin-walled, cavernous vessels arise from thin-walled branches of muscular arteries, or occluded arteries give rise to veinlike branches that have been misinterpreted as arteriovenous anastomoses. Because of their thin walls, the vessels of dilatation lesions are subject to rupture and are associated with focal collections of hemosiderin-laden macrophages in the pulmonary tissue.

In the most advanced stage of hypertensive pulmonary vascular disease (Grade 6), fibrinoid necrosis occurs in the media of some of the muscular arteries. The necrotic muscle produces an inflammatory reaction consisting of polymorphonuclear leukocytes and some eosinophils that may invade all layers of the vessel. The necrotizing arteritis may destroy the entire vessel or only a segment of it, and thrombi are found in the lumina of some of the affected arteries.

The elastic pulmonary arteries, especially the main trunk and its branches, are greatly dilated, but the walls are thick. The media shows an increase in muscle mass that in the main pulmonary artery causes the thickness of the media to approximate or exceed that of the aortic media. The elastic fibers in the media are fragmented, irregularly shaped, and arranged in a loose network characteristic of the adult pulmonary artery. This configuration of the elastic tissue is evidence that the pulmonary hypertension was acquired rather than present at birth, because in patients with congenital heart diseases that produce pulmonary arterial hypertension from birth, the elastic fibers of the main pulmonary artery retain their fetal form and appear like those in the aorta. In a few reported cases of primary pulmonary hypertension, an orderly array of elastic fibers in the media signified that the hypertension existed in the neonatal period. In all cases, the media contains an excess of acid mucopolysaccharides that can accumulate in cystic fashion. A few atheromas are often found in the intima of the main pulmonary arteries; in occasional patients, they are numerous and scattered throughout the intima of all the elastic arteries.

The capillaries, veins, and parenchyma of the lungs are normal.

The right ventricle is extensively hypertrophied and dilated, and the ring of the tricuspid valve is often dilated. The right atrium is also dilated, and in a few patients, the foramen ovale is patent. The systemic arteries are usually free of significant abnormalities, although James has reported the occurrence of fibrous lesions in the intima of the small arteries of the sinus node in patients with primary pulmonary hypertension.

ETIOLOGY AND PATHOGENESIS. None of the several theories proposed for the pathogenesis of primary pulmonary hypertension has been verified. Amniotic fluid embolization of the pulmonary arteries has been suggested as a cause because of the preponderance of young women among patients with the disease, some of whom experienced their first symptoms after pregnancy. Congenital defects in the pulmonary arteries, such as medial aplasia or failure of the pulmonary arteries to undergo normal transformation from their fetal form, have been suggested; however, with only a few exceptions, the appearance of the elastic fibers in the media of the main pulmonary artery of patients with primary pulmonary hypertension indicates that the hypertension was not present from birth, as would be expected if the pulmonary arteries maintained their thick-walled, fetal form. The theory of medial aplasia holds that the areas of dilatation and thinning of the media observed in the muscular arteries represent congenital defects of the media and that the intima over these areas is subject to the development of intimal proliferation that then acts as the primary obstructive lesion. This explanation neglects the fact that all patients with primary pulmonary hypertension do not manifest dilatation lesions or defects of the media other than hypertrophy.

The occurrence of Raynaud's disease in some patients with primary pulmonary hypertension has prompted the speculation that the hypertension is due to vasospasm or to involvement of the pulmonary arteries by a systemic disease of a collagen, autoimmune, or allergic variety. Pulmonary vascular lesions and marked pulmonary hypertension are the predominant abnormalities in rare patients with lupus erythematosus, scleroderma, or sarcoidosis, but other stigmata of these diseases are evident during life or at autopsy. Neurogenically or humorally induced spasm of the pulmonary arteries is an attractive possibility, especially because these vessels in a few patients manifest medial hypertrophy with only slight abnormalities of the intima, but the hypothesis lacks support. Alveolar hypoxia, a potent pulmonary vasoconstrictor, is not present in these patients, and there is no history of residence at altitude, although an occasional patient may first experience symptoms during an excursion to a region several thousand feet above sea level.

The possibility that primary pulmonary hypertension is the consequence of multiple pulmonary emboli is most difficult to deny. Recurrent, small emboli to the lungs are often "silent" and can eventually produce marked increase in pulmonary arterial pressure and a clinical and physiologic syndrome identical to that of primary pulmonary hypertension. It is often difficult to distinguish between the two conditions by examination of the vasculature of the lungs, because the small pulmonary arteries in widespread pulmonary embolization often exhibit the medial hypertrophy and intimal proliferation of hypertensive pulmonary vascular disease, and recanalized, fibrotic emboli in the small arteries can resemble occlusive intimal lesions. Differentiation of the two conditions depends on identification in the embolic disease of intraluminal thrombi, recent or old, throughout the pulmonary arteries, especially in the larger elastic arteries, and absence of plexiform and dilatation lesions and necrotizing arteritis, which do not occur in the embolic disorder.

The practical difficulty in discriminating between pulmonary hypertension of the primary type and that caused by recurrent pulmonary embolization can be illustrated by the author's experience with 14 patients who after extensive study were considered to have primary pulmonary hypertension. Nine of these came to autopsy, and no cause for the hypertension other than the pulmonary vascular lesions of primary pulmonary hypertension was found in five. All five were women 32 to 33 years of age, except for one who was 44. In the other four patients, multiple thromboemboli were present in the pulmonary arteries. Two of these were men age 37 and 60 years, and two were women, 48 and 53 years of age. This and other reported experiences suggest the likelihood of an embolic cause of unexplained pulmonary hypertension in patients older than 40 years, especially if they are men. These data were collected before the widespread use of oral contraceptives, and it is conceivable that the proportion of young women with thromboembolism among patients with cryptic pulmonary hypertension may be modified in the future. Predisposition to pulmonary thromboembolism in one reported family with pulmonary hypertension was suggested by elevated plasma and serum antiplasmin activity in seven of its members.

An apparent increase in the frequency of pulmonary hypertension followed the introduction in a few countries of aminorex (2-amino-5-phenyl-2-oxazoline), an appetite depressant with pharmacologic actions similar to those of amphetamine. Although many of the patients had taken the drug, its role in the production of the "epidemic" of pulmonary hypertension was not established, and even after prolonged administration of large doses the compound does not cause pulmonary hypertension or pulmonary vascular lesions in laboratory animals. An association, probably also coincidental, of pulmonary hypertension with use of phentormin has been reported.

Whatever the cause, it appears that once pulmonary hypertension is established, the media of the pulmonary arteries reacts by progressive hypertrophy of its smooth muscle mass, probably as a consequence of increased arterial wall tension and work. The intima subsequently responds to the elevated pressure by proliferation, perhaps as the arterioles do in systemic hypertension. Thus each structural response of the pulmonary arterial tree leads to further compromise of its patency, further elevation of pressure, and the eventual development of the highest grades of hypertensive pulmonary vascular disease.

PATHOLOGIC PHYSIOLOGY. The cardinal hemodynamic abnormality is marked increase in the pulmonary vascular resistance with no evident physiologic cause. The resistance is usually 12 to 18 times normal and in the range of the systemic vascular resistance, and in an occasional patient it exceeds the systemic resistance. In one series, the average pulmonary arterial systolic pressure was approximately 110 mm Hg and the mean pressure approximately six times normal. During exercise the pulmonary vascular resistance remains fixed, and the pulmonary arterial pressures rise further. At rest and during exercise, the pulmonary wedge and left atrial pressures are normal. In contrast, the right ventricular end-diastolic and right atrial pressures are usually greatly increased. In some patients, the cardiac output is normal at rest, but more often it is only 50 to 60 per cent of normal and fails to increase appropriately with exercise. As the function of the right ventricle declines under its enormous afterload, cardiac output dwindles further, and evidences of tricuspid regurgitation may appear. Because of the small stroke volume, systemic arterial systolic and pulse pressures are frequently low.

The arterial oxyhemoglobin saturation is usually normal at rest and during exercise, but a few patients display mildly (91 to 92 per cent) and rarely substantially diminished (less than 90 per cent) saturation. Slight reduction in arterial carbon dioxide tension reflects the hyperventilation that commonly exists.

Infusion of tolazoline or acetylcholine into the pulmonary artery has been observed to produce slight to moderate decrease of pulmonary vascular resistance and pulmonary arterial pressure in some patients. Inhalation of oxygen has little effect.

CLINICAL MANIFESTATIONS. These are the direct result of the physiologic and anatomic disturbances produced by the disease. Dyspnea during exertion, closely intertwined with fatigue and weakness, is a universal symptom. An oppressive substernal sensation and even frank angina are commonly experienced during effort, although this symptom, which is most likely the result of right ventricular ischemia, can occur in some patients in the form of recurrent and exceedingly disturbing episodes at rest. Syncope on exertion is an ominous sign because patients with primary pulmonary hypertension are subject to sudden death. There is evidence that an abrupt fall in cardiac output secondary to acute right ventricular failure or arrhythmia is the essential mechanism producing the syncopal attacks. Rupture of the flimsy walls of localized arterial dilatation lesions probably accounts for the intermittent minor hemoptyses experienced by some patients. An occasional patient may experience hoarseness related to compression of the left recurrent laryngeal nerve by the enlarged left pulmonary artery.

Overt signs of right ventricular failure develop in many patients before death and initially respond to digitalis and diuretics, but within a short period of time become increasingly more difficult to control. Because of the marked and fixed obstruction to flow in the pulmonary vessels and severe impairment of right ventricular function, the cardiac output is not only low but does not increase on demand to meet peripheral needs. Consequently, systemic arterial pressure can fall precipitously and fatally during anesthesia; after vasodepressor drugs, such as barbiturates; with physiologic stresses, such as fever and hemorrhage; and during diagnostic procedures, such as cardiac catheterization and angiocardiography. Because of the enormous obstruction to blood flow in the lungs, resuscitation from cardiopulmonary arrest is usually unsuccessful.

The patient usually appears normally developed and in good nutritional state. Occasionally the nail beds are slightly cyanotic, but the peripheral origin of the cyanosis is demonstrated by its disappearance after rubbing the digits. Clubbing is absent. Its presence should promptly suggest other causes of the pulmonary hypertension. Depending on the state of right ventricular function, the jugular veins may be distended; almost invariably, they show a prominent and sustained atrial contraction wave ("a" wave). If right ventricular failure and dilatation are advanced, the systolic wave of tricuspid regurgitation can also appear. The carotid arterial pulse is usually small.

The heart may be of normal size or considerably enlarged to the left and right. In contrast to the localized and unimpressive apical impulse, the heave associated with vigorous contraction of the hypertrophied right ventricle can be seen and felt along the left sternal border. Especially in patients with thin-walled and long chests, the prominent systolic pulsation of the enlarged main pulmonary can be seen and palpated for several centimeters to the left of the sternal border in the second left intercostal space. In almost every patient, a loud, sharp, pulmonic ejection sound can be heard and often felt. The second sound is usually closely split (0.02 to 0.03 sec), but in some patients the splitting may be wider (0.04 to 0.05 sec) and may vary relatively little during the respiratory cycle. The sound of pulmonic valvular closure is invariably accentuated in intensity, sharp or ringing in quality, and often palpable. Murmurs may be absent, but in many patients a systolic ejection murmur that is rarely harsh is heard in the third left interspace and extends well up along the left sternal border over the pulmonary artery. The diminuendo, medium-high-pitched murmur of pulmonic valvular regurgitation is audible in the third and fourth left interspaces in patients whose main pulmonary artery is very large, and is most easily detected with the patient erect and his chest held in full expiration. Either an atrial gallop sound (fourth sound) or an early diastolic gallop sound (third sound) or both are often heard over the lower right ventricle; increase in their intensity with inspiration signifies that they are generated in the right heart. When both gallop sounds are present, they can create the auditory illusion of a mitral diastolic rumble, an illusion that is enhanced by the early ejection sound, which may be misidentified as the loud closure sound of a stenotic mitral valve. A systolic murmur of tricuspid regurgitation that increases with inspiration may be heard in the fourth and fifth intercostal spaces along the left sternal border; it occasionally radiates well toward the apex if the tricuspid valve has been displaced to the left by a very enlarged right atrium and right ventricle. The usual signs of right ventricular failure and systemic venous congestion may be present.

Early in the course of the disease, the only abnormality in radiograms of the chest is enlargement of the main pulmonary artery and its major branches. Hypertrophy of the right ventricle is first manifested by its encroachment on the retrosternal space in lateral films and by a globular appearance of the heart in the posteroanterior projection. The heart is seldom massively enlarged, but the right ventricle may be sufficiently hypertrophied and dilated to displace the heart posteriorly, thereby creating some difficulty in assessing the size of the left ventricle. The right atrium usually appears rounded in frontal view, and eventually it and the superior vena cava dilate well into the right chest. The lung fields appear normal or slightly avascular, and the normal size of the small pulmonary arteries contrasts sharply with the dilated central arteries, which can attain considerable size. The pulmonary veins and left atrium are normal in size.

The electrocardiogram invariably reveals evidences of right ventricular hypertrophy, usually of the type associated with a systemic arterial systolic pressure in the ventricle. The mean QRS axis is at 90 degrees or more to the right. Lead V_1 shows an R wave of 1.0 to 1.5 mV with a small S wave, and the T waves in leads V_1 and V_2 are inverted. The P waves are tall (greater than 0.25 mV) and peaked in leads II, III, and aV_f; in V_1 the P wave is upright, peaked, narrow, and associated with a long PR segment. Higher grades of right ventricular hypertrophy are reflected by increasing amplitude of the R wave in V_1 and V_2, prominent S waves in the left precordial leads, and depression of the S-T segment and increasingly negative and coved T waves in V_1 and V_2 and even V_3.

Polycythemia occurs in some patients late in the course of the disease despite a normal or only slightly decreased arterial oxyhemoglobin saturation.

DIAGNOSIS. Although the diagnosis of primary pulmonary hypertension can be made on the basis of the clinical, radiographic, and electrocardiographic manifestations, it is very difficult in some patients to be certain on these grounds alone that an underlying lesion of the heart, such as septal defect, cor triatriatum, or silent mitral stenosis, does not exist. It is especially difficult to exclude multiple pulmonary emboli or a systemic disease as the fundamental disorder.

In the rare patient with marked pulmonary arterial hypertension and auscultatorily silent mitral stenosis, enlargement of the left atrium and calcification of the mitral valve may be the only clinical clues to the presence of the valvular lesion and should be assiduously sought by radiographic and electrocardiographic means. Echocardiography is exceptionally effective in identifying stenosis and other abnormalities of the mitral valve (see Ch. 360.2 to 360.4) and in measuring the dimensions of the left atrium and ventricle. Since it can also detect a left atrial myxoma, cor triatriatum, and septal defects, all patients suspected of having primary pulmonary hypertension should be carefully studied by this noninvasive method before submitting them to cardiac catheterization.

Cardiac catheterization should be performed to establish the diagnosis, to assess the severity of the hemodynamic derangements, and to demonstrate conclusively that the pulmonary arterial hypertension is not secondary to a congenital defect, mitral stenosis, or other lesion that produces left atrial or pulmonary venous hypertension. In pulmonary angiograms, filling defects or occlusions of the larger elastic pulmonary arteries are certain signs of pulmonary thromboemboli that are not found in primary pulmonary hypertension. Large areas lacking radioactivity in the lung fields in radioisotopic perfusion scans of the lungs constitute further evidence of the presence of embolic obstruction of large pulmonary arteries.

Because death of patients with primary pulmonary hypertension has been reported to occur during or immediately after cardiac catheterization and angiocardiography, considerable judgment and care must be exercised in performing these studies and determining how extensive they should be. The general state of the patient, the blood pressure, and the electrocardiogram should be meticulously monitored throughout the procedure and for some time afterward. Arrhythmias and frequent ectopic beats should be promptly suppressed; significant falls in blood pressure should be immediately corrected with an infusion of norepinephrine to maintain perfusion of the right ventricular myocardium. Many patients with primary pulmonary hypertension have undergone these essential diagnostic studies without complication.

The appropriate laboratory tests, including skin biopsy to exclude scleroderma and lupus erythematosus, should be performed in all patients with primary pulmonary hypertension, especially those who manifest Raynaud's phenomenon. Sarcoidosis involving the pulmonary arteries almost exclusively and producing pulmonary hypertension is exceedingly rare and has only recently been reported. The author has also observed one such case in which the cause was uncovered only at autopsy. The possibility of reversing the pulmonary hypertension by the administration of corticosteroids should prompt a search for signs of this disease.

Lung biopsy should not be performed because of the great risk and because the vessels in the tissue obtained may not manifest representative lesions of the pulmonary hypertensive vascular disease, which typically vary widely in type and severity throughout the lungs. A small pneumothorax in a patient with primary pulmonary hypertension was reported to precipitate an alarming increase in pulmonary arterial pressure and death.

Pulmonary function studies in patients with primary pulmonary hypertension usually reveal no major abnormalities aside from slight arterial hypoxemia and hyperventilation. If the patient does not have a right-left shunt through a patent foramen ovale, substantial hypoxemia at rest or during exercise owing to intrapulmonary arteriovenous shunting greatly increases the probability that thromboemboli are the cause of the pulmonary hypertension.

TREATMENT. No effective method for producing a sustained decrease in the pulmonary arterial pressure has been found. Chronic treatment with tolazoline or prolonged infusions of this drug or acetylcholine into the pulmonary artery have proved to be ineffective. Nor is there evidence that long-term administration of oxygen decreases the pulmonary arterial pressure or in any way modifies the course of the disease. Transplantation of a single lung is an appealing therapeutic maneuver but is impractical because of the currently short viability of pulmonary homotransplants. Because of the difficulty in excluding recurrent pulmonary emboli and because in situ thrombosis can occur in pulmonary arteries affected by hypertensive pulmonary vascular disease, chronic anticoagulation therapy has been widely advocated. Such therapy should be closely monitored in view of the deleterious consequences of hemorrhage in these patients. The usual cardiac glycosides, diuretic agents, and restriction of sodium intake should be used to control cardiac failure. The patient should not travel to altitudes above sea level.

PROGNOSIS. The patient usually dies during a syncopal spell, or after an acute, short-lived, shock-like episode, or of intractable right heart failure within three to four years after the onset of symptoms. Rarely, dissection of the main pulmonary artery is the lethal event. An occasional patient may survive for 12 or more years, but with progressively disabling dyspnea, angina, and syncope with exertion.

358.3. OTHER CAUSES OF PULMONARY VASCULAR DISEASE

CONGENITAL HEART DISEASE

These remarks are intended to supplement the discussion of congenital heart disease in Ch. 359.

Pulmonary arterial hypertension is exceedingly common in patients with congenital defects that produce left-right shunting of blood within the heart or between the great vessels. The hypertension is usually the result of augmentation of pulmonary blood flow by the left-right shunt, structural abnormalities within the pulmonary arterial tree, or most commonly both. There are distinct differences in the frequency and severity of the pulmonary vascular abnormalities associated with these congenital lesions.

In patients with left-right shunts that traverse the left ventricle, such as those produced by ventricular septal defect, patent ductus arteriosus, aortic septal defect, and ostium atrioventricularis with a large ventricular septal defect, hypertensive pulmonary vascular disease is very frequent. The severity of the arterial lesions varies among patients, depending on the size of the defect, the magnitude of the left-right shunt it is capable of conducting, and individual susceptibility. If the communication is small and produces a pulmonary blood flow that exceeds systemic blood by 50 per cent or less, the pulmonary arteries are usually normal or show minimal changes and the pulmonary vascular resistance and pulmonary arterial pressure are also normal or only slightly elevated.

With larger defects, hypertensive pulmonary vascular disease of the type described in Ch. 358.2 is almost universally present. Most commonly, the small pulmonary arteries and arterioles simply manifest thickening of their walls owing to hypertrophy of the smooth muscle of the media (Grade 1 hypertensive pulmonary vascular disease, according to the classification of Heath and Edwards), but other obstructive lesions may be superimposed on this basic abnormality to produce increasingly advanced vascular disease. An early additional change is cellular proliferation of the intima of the arteries (Grade 2), which may subsequently undergo fibrosis and fibroelastic organization (Grade 3). The development of generalized and focal dilatations of the arterial wall with the formation of complex vascular structures occurs in Grade 4 disease, and in Grade 5 the dilatations are scattered throughout the lung and associated with hemosiderosis. Necrotizing arteritis occurs in the most severe form of the disease (Grade 6).

The development of the vascular disease is initiated shortly after birth by failure of the pulmonary arteries to undergo normal transformation from their fetal form. Instead of regressing, the increased mass of smooth muscle in the arterial walls persists, hypertrophies, and extends distally into the arterioles. The elastic fibers in the media of the main pulmonary artery and its major branches also fail to develop their adult form. They persist as dense, thick structures in parallel array, closely resembling their appearance in the media of the aorta. This important histologic sign indicates that the pulmonary vascular disease began in the neonatal period; it is not found in patients who acquired their pulmonary hypertension later in life.

The size of the communication determines the subsequent development of arterial lesions. Ventricular septal defects larger than 1 sq cm and patent ducti that approximate 1 cm in diameter are usually associated with more advanced grades of pulmonary vascular disease. Progression of the vascular lesions appears to occur early in life, but the most advanced abnormalities are found in patients older than 15 to 20 years. The pulmonary vascular resistance, however, in patients with only moderate pulmonary arterial hypertension (systolic pressure of 50 to 60 mm Hg) does not appear to increase significantly during the course of many years.

Why pulmonary vascular lesions develop in patients with post-tricuspid valvular shunts is uncertain. One possible factor is that these shunts early in life load the left ventricle and consequently produce higher left ventricular diastolic, left atrial, and pulmonary venous pressures than would normally exist, thus from the outset exhausting the distensibility of the pulmonary arteries and subjecting them thereby to higher pressures. Another theory holds that the transmission directly into the pulmonary arteries of part of the kinetic energy that is generated in the left ventricle is the responsible factor.

The height of the pulmonary arterial pressure in patients with ventricular septal defect or patent ductus arteriosus is determined by the pulmonary vascular resistance, the size of the left-right shunt, and consequently the magnitude of the pulmonary blood flow. If the resistance is only slightly increased, large shunts and pulmonary flows as large as twice the systemic blood flow can occur with pulmonary arterial mean pressures three times normal and systolic pressures of 60 to 70 mm Hg. With increasing resistance, the pulmonary arterial pressures rise and the left-right shunt diminishes. Evidence of right-left shunting at first appears only during exercise when pulmonary arterial and right ventricular

pressures increase further or under circumstances when the systemic vascular resistance falls. Eventually, the pulmonary arterial systolic pressure attains systemic arterial levels at rest and the right-left shunt becomes larger and more sustained. Despite persistence of bidirectional shunting, the pulmonary blood flow declines to values usually less than normal. As a consequence of the right-left shunt and the diminished pulmonary blood flow, chronic arterial hypoxemia that is accentuated by exertion appears. In patients with patent ductus arteriosus, because the right-left shunt is directed into the descending segment of the aortic arch, the arterial unsaturation is more pronounced or even confined to the lower body and, occasionally, may also appear in the left arm and left side of the head. It is possible that the polycythemia and consequent increase in blood viscosity contribute to the resistance to flow in the pulmonary vessels.

Aside from cyanosis, which is usually accompanied by clubbing of the fingers and toes, the clinical signs and symptoms of patients with marked pulmonary hypertension and right-left shunts are similar to those of patients with primary pulmonary hypertension, but the course is usually considerably longer, and survival to an age of 30 to 40 years occurs frequently. The cyanosis is especially striking when polycythemia is marked. In patent ductus arteriosus with bidirectional shunting, the toes are cyanotic and clubbed, whereas the fingers are not or are much less so. Some signs of the underlying cardiac lesion are often evident. A precordial bulge is usually present. In some patients, the characteristic murmurs are intermittently audible, but in most, the murmurs are greatly modified. A pulmonic ejection sound is almost always present; the sound of pulmonic valvular closure is loud and sharp in quality, and a diastolic murmur of pulmonic regurgitation is frequent. Persistent enlargement of the left ventricle may be manifested by a forceful, diffuse apical thrust. Suggestive evidences of left ventricular enlargement may also be present in radiograms of the heart and in the electrocardiogram, but these and the radiographic signs of increased pulmonary blood flow tend to disappear as the pulmonary vascular disease advances.

In patients with a left-right shunt that does not traverse the left ventricle, structural abnormalities in the pulmonary arteries are slight, and the pulmonary arterial pressure remains normal or only slightly increased until late in the course of the disease. An atrial septal defect of the secundum type is the most common lesion producing such a shunt; other causes are partial or complete anomalous drainage of the pulmonary veins into the right atrium or its main venous trunks. Only in occasional patients with enormous shunts, caused by complete anomalous pulmonary venous drainage or an atrial septal defect of such size that the atria are converted into a common chamber, are pulmonary vascular disease and significant pulmonary hypertension established early in life. In most patients, despite pulmonary blood flows consistently 2.5 to 3 times greater than normal, the pulmonary arterial pressure remains at the upper limits of normal for 20 to 30 years and even longer. Thereafter, however, pulmonary vascular lesions begin to appear and the pulmonary arterial pressure rises. The earliest structural abnormality is fibrosis of the pulmonary veins followed by cellular proliferation of the endothelium of the widely dilated arterioles and small muscular arteries. At this stage, the pulmonary vascular resistance may no longer be less than normal as it must be to maintain a normal pulmonary arterial pressure in the presence of the large blood flow. The resistance is also fixed, and even though its value is within the limits of normal, the persistently augmented flow produces a proportionate increase in pulmonary arterial pressure.

The pulmonary venous pressure remains normal in atrial septal defect until the onset of myocardial failure, manifested by elevation of the diastolic pressures of both ventricles. As a consequence of the increased left ventricular diastolic pressure, the pressures in the left atrium and pulmonary veins rise to three to four times their usual values. A substantial left-right shunt nevertheless persists, and pulmonary arterial systolic pressure commonly attains values of 60 to 70 mm Hg.

Episodes of pulmonary embolization, which are common in patients with atrial septal defect, and progression of the hypertensive pulmonary arterial lesions eventually produce seven-fold or greater increases of pulmonary vascular resistance that throttle the pulmonary flow and promote right-left shunting through the defect.

The classic clinical, radiographic, and electrocardiographic features of atrial septal defect (see Ch. 359.2) usually persist throughout the patient's course, and provide for ready recognition of the lesion. The diagnosis is less evident in the occasional patient who has developed high-grade pulmonary vascular disease and pulmonary hypertension early in life and shows little evidence of increased pulmonary blood flow and a hypertrophied but not very large right ventricle.

TREATMENT. The response of the pulmonary arterial pressure to closure of a septal defect or patent ductus arteriosus is governed by the relative roles of the left-right shunt and the pulmonary vascular resistance in elevating the pressure. If the pulmonary vascular resistance is normal preoperatively, the pulmonary arterial pressure declines to normal values postoperatively. When the shunt constitutes 50 per cent or more of the pulmonary blood flow and the resistance is only moderately increased, a substantial decrease can be expected. When the left-right shunt is small and the pulmonary vascular resistance and pressures approximate those in the systemic circuit, and especially if a significant right-left shunt exists, the pressure does not decrease and the risk of death during or shortly after the surgical procedure is great. Decision as to advisability of surgical correction of the lesion should be made on an individual basis after consideration of all physiologic and clinical data. Some have advocated preoperative measurements of the response of the pulmonary arterial pressure and pulmonary vascular resistance to infusion of tolazoline or inhalation of oxygen as a means of identifying a vasospastic component of an increased resistance.

Except in occasional infants with lower grades of hypertensive pulmonary vascular disease, the pulmonary vascular resistance does not usually fall after closure of an atrial or ventricular septal defect, and although the patient may be greatly benefited by the procedure, some degree of pulmonary hypertension persists.

STENOSIS OF PULMONARY ARTERIAL BRANCHES. Although multiple coarctation-like, congenital stenoses of the large branches of the pulmonary artery produce an increase in pressure only in the pulmonary arterial segments upstream from the stenotic regions, the malformation in some patients raises the systolic pressure in the main pulmonary artery and right ventricle to 70 to 80 mm Hg and can create difficulty in diagnosis. The lesions can occur in isolated form, but they often coexist with supravalvular aortic stenosis or an atrial septal defect. The total obstructive effect is usually slight, and the systolic pulmonary arterial pressure is increased to only 35 to 40 mm Hg at rest. The stenoses generate a continuous murmur or simply a systolic murmur that can be heard over the upper right or left precordial region. The diagnosis is conclusively established by an angiogram of the pulmonary arteries. An acquired form of pulmonary arterial branch stenosis can be produced by mediastinal fibrosis.

PULMONARY EMBOLI

Thrombi, globules of fat, and particulate matter of amniotic fluid can embolize the pulmonary arteries and produce acute pulmonary hypertension. The pathophysiologic basis for the hypertension is described in Ch. 357. Repeated embolization of the pulmonary arteries by thrombi (see Ch. 357 and 358.2), schistosomal ova (see Ch. 210), tumors, and cotton fibers and foreign matter contained in some drugs illicitly administered by vein cause chronic, progressive pulmonary hypertension by their primary obstructive effects and by the subsequent development of hypertensive pulmonary vascular lesions. In addition, schistosomal ova and particulate foreign matter evoke a granulomatous inflammatory reaction in the intima and walls of the arteries.

Although fragments of several types of cancer can embolize the pulmonary arteries after the tumor has invaded the liver or the inferior vena cava, the propensity of choriocarcinoma (chorioepithelioma) to metastasize in this manner deserves special consideration. Choriocarcinoma may remain undetected for several years after pregnancy, but soon after it originates it can invade the inferior vena cava and repeatedly discharge fragments of tissue into the pulmonary circulation. These emoblic episodes may give rise to symptoms and signs of acute pulmonary embolization, or they can be clinically silent. The consequent obstruction of the larger pulmonary arteries can be extensive and give rise to marked pulmonary hypertension before the tumor invades the walls of the pulmonary arteries and appears in the lung fields.

Choriocarcinoma should be suspected in a woman who has had a recent pregnancy or even one a few years previously and has repeated bouts of pulmonary embolization or unexplained pulmonary hypertension. An increased concentration of human chorionic gonadotropin in the urine and the demonstration of multiple occlusions of the pulmonary arteries by angiography confirm the diagnosis. The tumor is exquisitely sensitive to methotrexate, actinomycin D, and 6-mercaptopurine, and complete cure has been achieved in 50 per cent or more of patients by administration of these agents.

COLLAGEN AND MULTIPLE SYSTEM DISEASES

Pulmonary hypertension caused by the pulmonary arterial lesions of scleroderma, lupus erythematosus, and sarcoidosis has been discussed in Ch. 358.2. The clinical features and diagnosis of these diseases are presented in Ch. 50, 52, and 65, respectively. It is worth emphasizing that the pulmonary hypertension and its secondary effects may rarely be the only clinically apparent manifestations of these disorders. Hemodynamic studies of patients with scleroderma have demonstrated the high frequency of increases in pulmonary vascular resistance and slight pulmonary hypertension without involvement of the pulmonary parenchyma by the disease.

HEPATIC CIRRHOSIS AND PORTAL HYPERTENSION: THE PORTOPULMONARY HYPERTENSION SYNDROME

The development of marked pulmonary hypertension has been observed in a number of patients with portal hypertension secondary to longstanding hepatic cirrhosis or obstruction of the portal vein by a congenital malformation or thrombus. Collateral vessels joining the portal and systemic veins were present in all patients and were often extensive. In some patients, the manifestations of pulmonary hypertension appeared only after a portacaval or equivalent shunt had been surgically created to alleviate bleeding from esophageal varices.

Except for the presence of portal hypertension in all the patients and hepatic cirrhosis in most of them, the clinical features, course, and hemodynamic disturbances were identical with those of primary pulmonary hypertension and are readily distinguishable from those of the high cardiac output state, which is a far more common circulatory complication of alcoholic or postnecrotic cirrhosis. The hyperkinetic state affects both cardiac ventricles and can produce mild to moderate pulmonary arterial hypertension when the pulmonary venous pressure rises as the result of faltering left ventricular function. In the portopulmonary hypertension syndrome, the pulmonary arterial pressure and vascular resistance are usually strikingly elevated, the right ventricle reacts to this burden and often fails, pulmonary venous pressure is normal, and left ventricular function appears unimpaired.

Morphologic studies of the pulmonary vessels at autopsy of patients with the syndrome have revealed the typical lesions of advanced pulmonary hypertensive disease, including plexiform lesions in all and necrotizing arteritis in a few. In almost 75 per cent of the cases, thromboemboli in various stages of organization were widespread throughout the muscular pulmonary arteries. The portal veins of a few patients contained large thrombi, and clots were also present in the eosphageal and gastric varices of one patient.

Naeye attributed the pulmonary vascular disease to the effects of multiple small pulmonary emboli that originated in the portal venous bed and entered the right heart via the copious portal systemic venous collateral vessels, thereby escaping entrapment in the liver. He was the first to propose that thrombogenic materials which are released into or generated in the portal venous blood and normally inactivated in the liver could in similar fashion gain access to the pulmonary circulation and incite the formation of thrombi therein. Others have proposed that vasoconstrictive or vasculotoxic substances which arise from the gut and normally undergo hepatic transformation to inactive compounds might serve as the pathogenetic agents. In searching for models of the syndrome, attention has been focused on the capacity of *Crotalaria spectabilis* (a leguminous annual plant used as a cover-crop) and monocrotaline, a complex alkaloid contained by the plant, to produce hepatic damage, pulmonary vascular disease, and marked pulmonary hypertension in animals. In man, however, ingestion of the plant leads to liver injury without evidences of pulmonary hypertension.

In reconstructing the pathogenesis of the hypertensive pulmonary vascular disease, it is difficult to exclude a primary role for pre-existing hyperkinemia. In 50 per cent of patients with portal cirrhosis, the cardiac output at rest is increased and is generally higher in those with a surgically created portacaval shunt. Outputs that are twice and even three times normal have been measured, and augmentation of output during exercise is greater than normal. Such marked increases in pulmonary blood flow, especially when they are of long standing, may in some patients promote the development of structural abnormalities in the pulmonary arteries as they do in patients with intracardiac left-right shunts. The few available hemodynamic studies of the syndrome have shown that the cardiac output is usually low to normal, but in occasional patients the output exceeded normal values, thereby enhancing the severity of the pulmonary hypertension.

The frequency of the portopulmonary hypertension syndrome is unknown, but it appears to be rare. Nevertheless, patients with portal hypertension and naturally occurring or surgically produced portacaval anastomoses should be periodically and carefully monitored for signs of pulmonary hypertension. Treatment for the condition is like that for primary pulmonary hypertension. It is difficult to advance a blanket recommendation concerning anticoagulant therapy in the syndrome because of the enormous risks of such therapy in these patients.

358.4.   LEFT ATRIAL AND PULMONARY VENOUS HYPERTENSION

Elevation of pulmonary venous pressure is the most common cause of pulmonary arterial hypertension. Most frequently, left atrial and pulmonary venous hypertension are the result of dysfunction of the left ventricle characterized by impairment of its contractile state, decrease in its compliance, or both. Even in the absence of clinical signs of left ventricular failure, left ventricular end-diastolic pressure can be elevated, at first only with physical exertion or stress; later, as ventricular function becomes more impaired, it is chronically increased even at rest. Two-fold increases in left atrial, pulmonary venous, and pulmonary arterial pressures are common. During episodes of acute left ventricular failure, pressures in the pulmonary veins and capillaries rise to levels exceeding 25 mm Hg.

The state of left atrial function is a significant determinant of the degree of left atrial and pulmonary venous hypertension. A properly timed, vigorous atrial contraction will generate a considerably increased left ventricular end-diastolic pressure without the need for much increase in left atrial pressure during the rest of diastole, but when the pumping function of the left atrium is lost because of atrial arrhythmia or left atrial failure, its pressure throughout diastole becomes greater. Thus for a given level of ventricular end-diastolic pressure, mean pressures in the atrium and the entire pulmonary vascular circuit are higher in the presence of left atrial failure or arrhythmia, such as atrial fibrillation, than in the presence of normal atrial function.

Disorders of the mitral valvular apparatus are another frequent cause of left atrial hypertension. In general, stenosis of the mitral valve and stenosis combined with regurgitation produce more severe degrees of left atrial hypertension than does mitral regurgitation alone. Nevertheless, in certain patients with chronic, marked mitral regurgitation caused by rheumatic valvular disease or rupture of the chordae tendineae, high-grade hypertension can occur in the left atrium, pulmonary veins, and pulmonary artery.

Less common causes of obstruction at the mitral valve are left atrial myxoma and left atrial ball-valve thrombus. A ball-valve thrombus almost invariably occurs with pre-existing mitral stenosis. A myxoma which is tethered by a stalk attached to the atrial septum in the region of the fossa ovalis, produces left atrial hypertension by obstructing blood flow through the mitral orifice in diastole, but it can also pass through the mitral valve and obstruct left ventricular outflow. Other tumors of the left atrium can obstruct the mitral valve and may also grow into and obstruct the main pulmonary veins.

Cor triatriatum, a congenital anomaly in which an abnormal diaphragm with one or more small perforations partitions the pulmonary venous outflow region from the main left atrial chamber, mimics mitral stenosis in its effects on the pulmonary circulation. However, it is often not associated with a diastolic murmur and can thus escape clinical detection. Although cor triatriatum and left atrial myxoma are rare, their recognition is of great importance because they can be completely corrected by appropriate surgical procedures.

Mediastinal collagenosis with constriction of the extrapulmonary veins and diffuse pulmonary veno-occlusive disease are rare causes of pulmonary venous hypertension. The etiology of the latter disease, which occurs predominantly in women, is unknown. The small and medium-sized pulmonary veins are narrowed and occluded by thrombi and fibrous tissue without evidence of inflammation in the venous walls. The clinical picture resembles that of primary pulmonary arterial hypertension; however, because of increased pressure in the pulmonary capillaries, radiographic evidence of pulmonary congestion and edema is present. The disease leads relentlessly to death in a few weeks to five years after the onset of symptoms.

PULMONARY CIRCULATION IN MITRAL STENOSIS

The physiologic and anatomic modifications of the pulmonary circulation induced by various degrees of chronic pulmonary venous hypertension are well illustrated by the extensive observations that have been made in patients with mitral stenosis. When the mitral orifice is only slightly restricted, left atrial pressure and intravascular pressures throughout the pulmonary circuit may be normal when the patient is at rest, but they exceed normal values with exercise or during other states accompanied by augmentation of cardiac output, such as fever, anemia, pregnancy, thyrotoxicosis, and hypermetabolism of other causes. Tachycardia alone, by abbreviating diastole, requires the generation of a higher left atrial pressure to maintain cardiac output through the stenotic valve. At this stage, as in animals with acutely produced mitral stenosis not severe enough to cause pulmonary edema, the modest vascular hypertension dilates the small pulmonary vessels and produces a decrease in their resistance to flow. In these circumstances, the increase in pulmonary arterial pressure is less pronounced than the increase in pulmonary venous and left atrial pressures.

In moderate and severe mitral stenosis with valvular orifice areas less than 1.5 sq cm, left atrial mean pressure at rest is often in the range of 25 to 30 mm Hg and rises with slight exercise to values of 40 to 55 mm Hg, especially if cardiac output increases substantially. Even if the pulmonary vascular resistance is normal, the pronounced pulmonary venous hypertension causes the mean pressure in the pulmonary artery to exceed normal values by three- to six-fold. In most patients, however, pulmonary vascular resistance is greater than normal, resulting in an increase of pulmonary arterial pressure that is disproportionately greater than that caused by the left atrial hypertension alone.

The range of abnormality of pulmonary vascular resistance in mitral stenosis is wide. In a series of 180 patients studied by the author, the resistance was two or more times greater than normal in 67 per cent of the patients. In 11 per cent, the resistance and consequently the pulmonary arterial pressure equaled or exceeded systemic arterial values. Patients with such advanced disturbances usually have very severe mitral stenosis and appear also to have a predisposition to advanced alterations in the pulmonary arteries in response to hypertension in the pulmonary veins and arteries that is not shared by other patients whose mitral obstruction and left atrial hypertension are equally pronounced. The clinical features of such patients resemble in many respects those of patients with primary pulmonary hypertension. A mitral diastolic murmur may not be audible, mainly because the cardiac output is greatly diminished as the result of the pulmonary vascular restriction and marked right ventricular dysfunction. Normal sinus rhythm persists in many of them despite the advanced mitral stenosis. Unlike patients with primary pulmonary hypertension, however, they do not experience frequent syncope.

In mitral stenosis, structural lesions are present in all segments of the pulmonary vascular bed. The pulmonary veins are dilated, and their walls are greatly thickened by medial hypertrophy and proliferation of the intima. In some patients, numerous anastomoses develop between the pulmonary and bronchial veins. These anastomotic channels form submucosal varicosities in the bronchi that can rupture and produce brisk hemoptysis when the left atrial pressure rises acutely.

The basic anatomic expression of increased hydrostatic pressure in the pulmonary capillaries is dilatation and engorgement of these vessels with edema of the alveolar walls and leakage of edema fluid into the alveolar spaces. Measurements made by the simultaneous injection of isotopically labeled water and a nondiffusible indicator into the pulmonary artery of patients with mitral stenosis and with pulmonary venous hypertension of other causes have demonstrated expansion of the interstitial pulmonary water volume directly related to the increase in left atrial pressure. At left atrial pressures of 25 to 30 mm Hg, the extravascular water volume is three or more times normal. Increased transport by the lymphatics is reflected by dilatation of these vessels. When the pulmonary capillary pressure exceeds values of 20 mm Hg, which is on the threshold of plasma protein osmotic pressure, the lymphatic vessels and the edematous interlobular septa at the bases of the lungs become sufficiently radiopaque to appear as short lines extending horizontally to the pleura (Kerley B lines) in radiograms of the chest.

Rupture of alveolar capillaries and pulmonary venules leads to scattered microhemorrhages and subsequent hemosiderosis. When the edema is of long standing, it promotes the development of interstitial fibrosis in the alveolar walls and the surrounding parenchyma that is most marked in the bases of the lower lobes and the lower segments of all lobes. These regional differences attest to the gravitational augmentation of capillary pressure and the consequently greater and more persistent edema in the dependent regions of the lungs. In these regions, the alveolar septa are markedly thickened and the pulmonary capillaries are compressed or obliterated. Rarely, the fibrotic regions become ossified and appear as small calcified nodules scattered throughout the lower lung fields.

The small pulmonary arteries manifest the medial hypertrophy, proliferation and fibrosis of the intima, increased wall thickness, and diminished internal diameter characteristic of hypertensive pulmonary vascular disease; however, dilatation lesions and necrotizing arteritis that are the hallmarks of the most advanced grades of pulmonary vascular disease are very rarely found. Also, in contrast to the hypertensive pulmonary vascular disease associated with congenital heart disease and primary pulmonary hypertension, the distribution of the arterial lesions conforms to a regional pattern. The arteries in the lower lobes are most affected and show the greatest restriction of their lumina; even in the upper lobes, in which the larger arteries are dilated and the small arteries are relatively spared, the vascular lesions are more prominent in the lower segments. As a consequence of the pattern of distribution of the vascular abnormalities and probably because of the more pronounced interstitial fibrosis in the lower lobes, blood flow is preferentially directed to the upper zones of the lung and away from the lower zones, resulting in reversal of the normal ratio of perfusion between the two zones. The ratio of upper zone perfusion to lower zone perfusion can be as large as 4:1 in contrast to the normal ratio of 1:8. The degree to which perfusion of the upper zones exceeds that of the lower regions is directly related to the height of the pulmonary venous pressure. The ratio also increases directly with the pulmonary vascular resistance, but when the resistance attains values in the range of the systemic vessels, the ratio decreases toward normal, probably because of more widespread distribution of the vascular abnormalities.

Pulmonary embolization and infarction are exceedingly frequent in mitral stenosis and in one series were found at autopsy in approximately one third of the patients who had manifested moderate to severe pulmonary arterial hypertension during life. These occlusions and the secondary effects on the parenchyma of the lung undoubtedly contribute to the restriction of the pulmonary vascular bed.

The main pulmonary artery and its central branches are dilated, and their intima often contains atherosclerotic plaques. The cross-sectional diameter of these vessels increases directly with the pulmonary arterial pressure. When the internal diameter of the main pulmonary artery is 4.0 cm or more, the murmur of pulmonic regurgitation (Graham Steell murmur) commonly appears.

Some insight into the mechanisms producing the pulmonary arterial hypertension and the relative roles of the various vascular disturbances in the genesis of the increased pulmonary vascular resistance is offered by observations of the hemodynamic changes that occur after successful mitral valvotomy or replacement of the mitral valve by a prosthetic valve with a functionally adequate orifice. In almost all patients whose left atrial pressure is lowered by the surgical procedure, the pulmonary vascular resistance decreases and the decline in pulmonary arterial pressure is consequently even greater than that of the pulmonary venous pressure. Substantial decreases in pulmonary vascular resistance have been observed as early as two days after surgery and have been attributed to dilatation of muscular pulmonary arteries that had been reflexly induced to constrict by the left atrial and pulmonary venous hypertension. However, failure of the resistance to fall immediately after the surgical procedure despite the decrease in left atrial pressure has been interpreted as indicating that interstitial and perivascular edema exert a cardinal role in the pathogenesis of the increased resistance and that resolution of the edema lags behind the fall of pulmonary venous pressure. In the ensuing weeks and months, the pulmonary vascular resistance often decreases further; even in patients whose preoperative values exceeded systemic vascular resistance, the arterial pressure and vascular resistance in the lungs can eventually attain values only slightly in excess of normal. The most striking changes occur in patients whose left atrial pressures postoperatively at rest and during exercise are normal or only slightly greater than normal. Evidence is now available that regression of the medial hypertrophy and intimal proliferation in the small pulmonary arteries is responsible for the progressive decline of the vascular resistance, but the way in which the pulmonary venous hypertension initiated the development of the structural abnormalities in the pulmonary arteries remains uncertain.

358.5.   PULMONARY DISEASES AND DISORDERS OF RESPIRATION

Constriction of the pulmonary arteries by hypoxia and destruction or restriction of the pulmonary vascular bed are the two basic mechanisms that operate to increase the pulmonary arterial pressure in diseases of the lungs and disorders of the respiratory system. Primary alveolar hypoventilation is an example of a condition in which the disturbances in gas exchange alone initiate the pulmonary hypertension; but in most diseases of the lungs, anatomic restriction of the pulmonary vessels alone in the early stages of these diseases usually increases pulmonary arterial pressure only slightly because of the enormous reserve capacity of the pulmonary vasculature. By the time that the disease process has obliterated enough of the vessels to produce high-grade pulmonary hypertension, structural damage of the pulmonary parenchyma is sufficiently advanced to result in marked disturbances in gas exchange. In most pulmonary diseases therefore both mechanisms are operative.

Since diseases of the lungs and respiratory system are described in Part XII, only those features of significance in the production of pulmonary hypertension, its consequences, manifestations, and treatment are considered here.

PATHOLOGIC PHYSIOLOGY.   In *chronic obstructive pulmonary disease,* loss of pulmonary capillaries accompanies the loss of alveoli. Some muscular arteries adjacent to terminal bronchioles may show intimal fibroelastosis of sufficient extent to obliterate their lumina. The media of the muscular arteries is slightly thickened, but these vessels and the arterioles show few of the changes characteristic of hypertensive pulmonary vascular disease.

The loss of pulmonary vessels is tolerated with little or

no increase of pulmonary arterial pressure at rest, although the pressure does rise to abnormal levels when pulmonary blood flow is augmented by exercise. In such patients, defects in distribution of ventilation and perfusion within the lungs and reduction in diffusing capacity exist but are not severe enough to cause hypercapnia and more than slight hypoxemia. With increase in the extent of hypoventilated but perfused pulmonary segments, marked hypoxemia develops and the pulmonary arterial pressure rises in direct proportion to the degree of oxygen unsaturation of systemic arterial blood. The hypercapnia that accompanies more widespread alveolar hypoventilation does not appear to affect the pulmonary arteries directly, and its effect on blood pH is minimized by concomitant increase in plasma bicarbonate concentration. Acidosis, arising as the consequence of sudden increase in carbon dioxide tension or failure of the buffering capacity to keep pace with the hypercapnia, potentiates the pulmonary vasoconstrictor response to the hypoxia and further raises the pulmonary arterial pressure.

The greater afterload to ejection of blood created by the increased pulmonary vascular resistance and pulmonary hypertension is met by hypertrophy of the right ventricle. Since the pulmonary arterial mean pressure at this stage is usually no more than twice normal, the right ventricle does not fail until a bronchopulmonary infection or some other event aggravates the bronchial obstruction and the disturbances in gas exchange and produces marked, generalized alveolar hypoventilation. Under such circumstances, as much 80 per cent of the cardiac output perfuses underventilated alveoli, and the arterial oxyhemoglobin saturation falls to values of 40 to 80 per cent; the arterial carbon dioxide tension rises to 60 to 80 mm Hg, and the arterial pH falls to values as low as 7.20. Renal blood flow and glomerular filtration decrease; the excretion of sodium and water diminishes, and the extracellular volume expands. The consequent increase in blood volume is augmented by hypoxia-induced polycythemia of variable degree. The end-diastolic pressure of the right ventricle increases and raises the pressure in the right atrium and systemic veins. The contractile function of the right ventricular myocardium is progressively depressed, and the right ventricle dilates and fails. Several studies have demonstrated that left ventricular function, if it was previously normal, is not disturbed by these events, and that left atrial and pulmonary venous pressures remain within the range of normal.

The relative pathogenic role of each physiologic disturbance in producing the sudden increase in pulmonary arterial pressure in this complex state has been difficult to assess. Correction of the hypoxemia or the acidosis while the failure persists reduces the pulmonary arterial pressure, but it remains considerably elevated. Phlebotomy does not promptly lower the pulmonary arterial pressure. In some patients, because of infection and hypermetabolism, the cardiac output is higher than in the prefailure period, but in many patients the cardiac output is subnormal.

It is striking that as the manifestations of acute respiratory insufficiency and congestive right ventricular failure resolve with appropriate treatment, the pulmonary arterial pressure gradually falls and, together with the systemic arterial oxyhemoglobin saturation, finally returns to its prefailure values. It is difficult to avoid assigning a cardinal role to hypoxia in the pathogenesis of the marked pulmonary hypertension and the overt cor pulmonale.

During recurrent acute exacerbations of respiratory failure, and occasionally as the result of pulmonary thromboembolism to which these patients are prone, signs of increased pulmonary hypertension and right ventricular failure reappear. Eventually these manifestations and the disturbances in gas exchange do not respond fully to treatment, and the cor pulmonale becomes chronic.

In *fibroproliferative and chronic inflammatory diseases of the lungs,* the pulmonary vascular bed is compromised in many ways. In the diffuse interstitial disorders that affect the alveolar walls, such as *sarcoidosis* and other granulomatous diseases, the *Hamman-Rich syndrome, scleroderma, polymyositis, berylliosis, asbestosis, lymphangitic carcinomatosis, radiation fibrosis,* and *idiopathic pulmonary hemosiderosis,* the alveolar capillaries are compressed or obliterated. In massive pulmonary fibrosis caused by *silicosis* or coal miner's *pneumoconiosis,* the fibrotic nodules develop in proximity to muscular and small elastic arteries, and as they enlarge, they engulf and obliterate these vessels.

In all these disorders, increasing disruption of parenchymal structures and fibrosis cause progressive distortion, obstruction, and obliteration of pulmonary vessels. With the development of pulmonary hypertension, the medial hypertrophy and intimal proliferation of hypertensive pulmonary vascular disease are superimposed.

Early in the course of the pulmonary disease, as for example in the interstitial disorders of the lung, pulmonary hypertension may be only slight at rest despite marked restriction of lung volume, but the pressure usually rises steeply with exercise. Similarly, hypoxemia is only mild at rest, but the arterial oxygen saturation usually falls during exercise. With diminution of pulmonary diffusion capacity, the development of marked maldistribution of alveolar ventilation and perfusion, and increase in the extent of intrapulmonary arteriovenous shunting, oxygenation of arterial blood is progressively impaired, pulmonary arterial pressure rises further, and the right ventricle fails. Episodic exacerbations of failure are often precipitated by respiratory infections as in obstructive pulmonary disease, but reduction of pulmonary arterial pressure with treatment is less impressive, and once right ventricular failure occurs, it usually becomes chronic. The highest grades of chronic pulmonary hypertension secondary to pulmonary disease are found in fibrotic diseases of the lungs.

In bronchiectasis, tuberculosis, and other chronic inflammatory diseases of the lungs, extensive intercommunications can develop between the bronchial and pulmonary arteries; occasionally, the mammary and intercostal arteries participate in the formation of the anastomoses. The bronchial collateral flow through these channels is usually small, but in a rare patient it is large enough to constitute a significant left-right shunt that increases the pulmonary blood flow, further elevates the pulmonary arterial pressure, and taxes the left ventricle.

Alveolar hypoventilation pronounced enough to produce hypoxemia and hypercapnia, secondary constriction and hypertension in the pulmonary arteries, and right ventricular failure is encountered in a group of disorders characterized by a *defective ventilatory apparatus.* The fundamental defect exists in the chest bellows, as in *kyphoscoliosis, marked obesity* and *neuromuscular diseases* that affect the respiratory muscles, or in the respiratory control centers, as in hypoventilation of central nervous origin (*Ondine's curse*). The lungs and pulmonary vessels are intrinsically normal except in patients with severe kyphoscoliosis, whose pulmonary vascular bed is restricted by the inordinately small dimensions of the lungs and in whom concomitant bronchiectasis, areas of atelectasis, and bronchopulmonary infections are common.

Regardless of the nature of the basic defect in this group of diseases, alveolar ventilation not only is diminished at rest, but also fails to increase normally with exercise and increased metabolic demand, which consequently accentuates the hypoxemia and hypercapnia. In patients with these disorders, as well as in those with primary lung diseases who have had bouts of hypercapnia, the sensitivity of the chemoreceptors to both carbon dioxide and hypoxemia is progressively impaired, and the loss of ventilatory response to these stimuli enhances the propensity to the development of cor pulmonale. A respiratory infection commonly precipitates the development of marked pulmonary hypertension and right ventricular failure.

CLINICAL MANIFESTATIONS AND DIAGNOSIS. Pulmonary disease is usually readily identified by the history, the physical findings, and radiograms of the chest, but clues to the presence and severity of pulmonary hypertension may be masked by the pulmonary disease. In some patients, the classic signs of pulmonary hypertension described in Ch. 358.2 may be present, but in others, especially those with chronic obstructive disease, the cardiac sounds are barely audible or are obscured by adventitious pulmonary sounds, and enlargement of the right ventricle and main pulmonary artery cannot be detected with certainty. Despite considerable pulmonary hypertension, the sound of pulmonic valvular closure may not be audibly accentuated.

The patient with right ventricular failure typically presents a history of a recent respiratory infection followed by exacerbation of his usual respiratory symptoms and progressive dyspnea. He presents the appearance and physical signs of a patient with acute pulmonary insufficiency. Cyanosis is usually marked, especially in the presence of polycythemia, but often it is not impressive despite pronounced decrease in the arterial oxyhemoglobin saturation. If hypercapnia exists, drowsiness and the other central nervous system manifestations of hypercapnia may be evident. The jugular veins are distended and are further engorged by applying pressure over the enlarged, usually tender liver. Edema of the lower extremities may be present. The cardiac rate is rapid, and an early diastolic gallop sound may be audible over the mid-left precordium.

Radiograms usually reveal a prominent main pulmonary artery and enlargement of its main branches; but if the pulmonary hypertension is not marked or has not been sustained for a prolonged period of time, these vessels may appear normal in size. Especially in patients who have manifested chronic cardiac failure, the right ventricle and the right atrium are grossly enlarged. In other patients with obvious failure, the cardiac dimensions seem surprisingly normal, but serial films will often show diminution in the size of the right ventricle and right atrium with recovery from the failure.

The electrocardiographic manifestations of right ventricular hypertrophy are also modified by lung disease; even in patients with considerable pulmonary hypertension and right ventricular hypertrophy, the usual criteria considered diagnostic of hypertrophy and enlargement of the right ventricle are often not present. Large S waves in the precordial leads as far to the left as V_5 or V_6, a small rS or rSR' complex in V_1, negative T waves in the right precordial leads, a vertical or slight rightward displacement of the mean QRS axis in the frontal plane, and peaked P waves in the limb leads (P pulmonale) may be the only signs that the right ventricle is hypertrophied. These electrocardiographic alterations may not be present if the pulmonary arterial pressure is not two or more times greater than normal at rest. Regression of these electrocardiographic features in the course of recovery from an episode of respiratory failure often permits a retrospective appreciation of their significance. Atrial arrhythmias, especially flutter and fibrillation, and ventricular premature contractions are common in patients with acute respiratory insufficiency and cor pulmonale. Although it appears most commonly in such patients, chaotic atrial rhythm is an infrequent complication and bears a poor prognosis.

The findings of a reduced oxyhemoglobin saturation, diminished oxygen tension and pH and elevated carbon dioxide tension in the arterial blood, increase in plasma bicarbonate, and polycythemia support the diagnosis of pulmonary hypertension caused by pulmonary disease or respiratory disorder. Studies of pulmonary function are useful in defining the disorder, monitoring the effects of treatment, and assessing the probability that cor pulmonale will develop. Primary alveolar hypoventilation of central origin as the cause of pulmonary hypertension and congestive cardiac failure may go undetected without measurements of arterial blood gases and studies of the ventilatory response to carbon dioxide. In some patients with cardiac murmurs or evidence of left ventricular enlargement, the issue of whether the pulmonary hypertension is primarily due to the pulmonary disease or is secondary to an intracardiac lesion or left ventricular dysfunction may sometimes be resolved only by hemodynamic and angiographic studies. Pulmonary disease does not protect the patient from the development of coronary arteriosclerosis or systemic hypertension, which may compromise left ventricular function. The left ventricle may also be directly affected by scleroderma, polymyositis, sarcoidosis, certain forms of muscular dystrophy, and obesity. The features of the cardiopulmonary syndrome of obesity, in which marked pulmonary hypertension can occur, are described in Ch. 474.

TREATMENT. Treatment must be simultaneously directed at improving the function of both the lungs and the heart. The specific measures to be used are described in Part XII. When cardiac failure appears, a cardiac glycoside and a diuretic, such as hydrochlorothiazide or furosemide, should be administered. Losses of body potassium during diuresis should be replaced, but because of pre-existing disturbances in potassium balance and impairment of renal function, serum potassium should be closely monitored as a guide to such replacement. The hypoxemia, hypercapnia, acidosis, and electrolyte imbalances appear to predispose the heart of patients with cor pulmonale to arrhythmias and to the toxic effects of cardiac glycosides. Daily maintenance doses larger than 0.1 mg of digitoxin or 0.25 mg of digoxin should be used with caution, and manifestations of digitalis intoxication should be watched for. Correction of hypoxemia by inhalation of oxygen in concentrations that do not depress alveolar ventilation is a cardinal feature of therapy during an acute episode of failure, and chronic administration of oxygen may be indicated to control pulmonary hypertension in patients with marked chronic hypoxemia. Because polycythemia enhances the tendency to develop thromboemboli and increases viscosity of the blood and consequently the resistance to its flow, periodic phlebotomy is indicated to maintain the hematocrit at 50 per cent in patients with marked polycythemia.

PROGNOSIS. The development of pulmonary arterial hypertension and right ventricular failure in patients with pulmonary disease is a serious complication, but its prognostic significance depends on the underlying disorder. With appropriate treatment, the patient with chronic obstructive pulmonary disease may survive repeated bouts of cardiac and pulmonary failure over the course of many years. In patients with pulmonary fibrosis, the course after the onset of cardiac failure is variable but generally much shorter.

Blount, S. G., Jr., and Grover, R. F.: Pulmonary hypertension. *In* Hurst, J. W., and Logue, R. B. (eds.): The Heart, Arteries and Veins. 2nd ed. New York, McGraw-Hill Book Company, 1970, p. 1126.

Fishman, A. P.: Hypoxia on the pulmonary circulation. How and where it acts. Cir. Res., 38:221, 1977.

Harris, P., and Heath, D.: The Human Pulmonary Circulation. Its Form and Function in Health and Disease. Baltimore, Williams & Wilkins Company, 1962.

Heath, D., and Edwards, J. E.: The pathology of hypertensive pulmonary vascular disease. A description of structural changes in the pulmonary arteries with special reference to congenital cardiac septal defects. Circulation, 18:533, 1958.

Levine, O. R., Harris, R. C., Blanc, W. A., and Mellins, R. B.: Progressive pulmonary hypertension in children with portal hypertension. J. Pediat., 83:964, 1973.

Naeye, R. L.: "Primary" pulmonary hypertension with coexisting portal hypertension. A retrospective study of six cases. Circulation, 22:376, 1960.

Wagenvoort, C. A., and Wagenvoort, N.: Primary pulmonary hypertension. A pathologic study of the lung vessels in 156 clinically diagnosed cases. Circulation, 42:1163, 1970.

Yu, P. N.: Pulmonary Blood Volume in Health and Disease. Philadelphia, Lea & Febiger, 1969.

359. CONGENITAL HEART DISEASE

Joseph K. Perloff

359.1. INTRODUCTION

DEFINITION. "Congenital" is a Latin derivative from *con*, together, and *genitus*, born. However, the simple implication that congenital heart disease merely means "present at birth" requires qualification. The natural history begins before delivery, because most anomalies compatible with six months of intrauterine life permit live offspring at term. A congenital anomaly originating in the developing fetus is often considerably modified, at least physiologically, by the dramatic circulatory adjustments at birth. Weeks, months, or even years may elapse before the anomaly evolves into the "typical" clinical picture. Both physiologic and structural changes subsequently continue. The ductus in a premature infant sometimes remains widely patent for months, finally closing spontaneously, leaving the baby with a normal heart. A ventricular septal defect that delivers a large left to right shunt in infancy may gradually develop progressive infundibular pulmonic stenosis, so that years later the physiologic and the clinical picture resembles cyanotic Fallot's tetralogy. A congenital bicuspid aortic valve that is functionally normal at birth can take two, three, or more decades to stiffen, calcify, and

present as overt aortic stenosis. Accordingly, congenital heart disease should not be viewed narrowly as a fixed group of anatomic defects present at birth, but as dynamic anomalies that originate in fetal life and alter during postnatal development. Certain defects that are not "anatomic" in the gross morphologic sense are nevertheless considered congenital, such as congenital complete heart block, whereas others that are anatomic, such as the aortic root disease of Marfan's syndrome, are, by convention, not classified as congenital.

INCIDENCE, CHANGING POPULATION, AND ROLE OF THE INTERNIST AND MEDICAL CARDIOLOGIST. The prevalence of congenital heart disease has little meaning unless certain preconditions are met. An impression of over-all prevalence can be derived from population figures at the beginning of this decade when 3,718,000 live births were registered in the United States. An estimated 28,000 infants were born with congenital heart disease, i.e., 0.8 per cent. About half died within the first year, leaving 14,000 survivors. Both over-all incidence and incidence of specific defects vary according to patient age (neonate, infant, child, adolescent, young adult, older adult) and according to whether figures are derived from living subjects or necropsy material. A further distinction must be made between incidence based upon *natural* history and the incidence modified by *palliative* or *corrective surgery*. It is now possible to perform palliative or corrective surgery on almost all congenital cardiacs, even the most complex. Survival patterns are affected, often profoundly. We are therefore confronted with a changing population of congenital heart disease. Recent decades of intense diagnostic and therapeutic effort have resulted in survival of increasing numbers of adolescents, postadolescents, and adults with congenital defects of the heart or circulation. Accordingly, postpediatric congenital heart disease is represented not only by anomalies with a natural tendency for long survival, but also by those in which palliative or corrective surgery has been successfully employed. Operation not only increases life expectancy in anomalies with a natural tendency for long survival, but may also permit larger numbers of patients with disorders hiterto fatal in infancy or childhood to reach postadolescence or even adulthood. Appropriate long-term management requires an understanding of both the preoperative anomaly and the effects of surgical repair. *Thus congenital heart disease from the point of view of patient care should be considered not only in terms of age of onset, but also in terms of the age range that potential survival now permits.* Such patients require specialty care, be it by a pediatric cardiologist who extends an interest in older subjects or by a medical cardiologist who has a satisfactory comprehension of congenital cardiac disease. By the same token, just as it is necessary for the pediatrician to provide primary general pediatric care for the infant or child with congenital heart disease, the internist must provide primary general medical care for the late teenager and adult with these malformations.

ETIOLOGY. Congenital heart disease is etiologically multifactorial, the result of a complex interplay between genetic and environmental factors. These determinants in part include heredity, chromosomal defects, teratogens, prematurity, altitude at birth, sex, and maternal age.

Some tendency exists for congenital heart disease to

run in families. There is an increased incidence of defects in the offspring of propositi. Distribution and incidence are difficult to ascertain, because survival into the reproductive age is a requirement for transmission. Atrial septal defect commonly permits adult survival, and can be both familial and recurrent through a number of generations. Parents who in childhood experienced spontaneous closure of ventricular septal defects may live to adulthood and produce offspring with ventricular septal defects. There is also the prospect that increasing numbers of *operated* congenital cardiacs will reach childbearing age and produce a higher incidence of offspring with congenital defects of the heart or circulation. About 2 per cent of siblings of propositi have congenital heart disease. If one of a nonidentical twin pair has a congenital cardiac anomaly, the incidence in the co-twin is about the same as for sibs in general, but about 25 per cent of identical twins with congenital heart disease have affected co-twins with a high probability of identical defects.

Certain abnormal chromosome patterns are associated with predictable types of congenital cardiac disease, although chromosomal abnormalities per se are uncommon in the general population of congenital cardiacs. Down's syndrome (trisomy 21) has a high incidence of endocardial cushion defects, and about 50 per cent of patients with complete endocardial cushion defects have trisomy 21. Typical Turner's syndrome (phenotypic female with XO) occurs with coarctation of the aorta; trisomy 18 occurs with right ventricular origin of both great arteries; the Holt-Oram syndrome heightens suspicion of ostium secundum atrial septal defect, and the Ellis–van Creveld syndrome predicts common atrium.

The role of *teratogens* at critical times in fetal development is epitomized by the effects of thalidomide taken by the pregnant mother. Maternal rubella (German measles) during the first trimester increases the risk of offspring with patent ductus arteriosus and stenosis of the pulmonary artery and its branches.

Ventricular septal defect and patent ductus arteriosus are relatively common in *premature infants*. It has been postulated that the expected intrauterine time of ventricular septal closure is not limited to early fetal life but sometimes continues through gestation into the postpartum period. Delayed closure of the ductus arteriosus is more likely to occur in premature infants, and the duct may remain patent for as long as four to six months after birth. Incompletely developed cholinergic innervation and reduced constrictor response to oxygen of the premature ductus may in part account for this.

The *altitude at birth* is another factor that influences the occurrence of congenital heart disease. Patency of the ductus arteriosus is six times as frequent in people born at high altitudes as in those born at sea level. Reduced oxygen tension in ambient air at high altitudes may provide inadequate stimulus for ductal constriction even if cholinergic innervation of the ductal wall is well developed.

Parental age has been considered an etiologic factor. There is no evidence that paternal age plays a role, but *maternal age* has been called into question. Late maternal age (immediate premenopausal) seems to increase the risk of Fallot's tetralogy.

Sex distribution has been a point of interest in congenital diseases of the heart and circulation. The bicuspid aortic valve is predominantly a male disease. In fact, aortic valve disease in general has a strong male prevalence. The male-to-female ratio in ventricular septal defect with aortic regurgitation is twice as high as in uncomplicated ventricular septal defect. Aortic atresia is almost exclusively a disease of male infants. On the other hand, patent ductus arteriosus predominates in females (sex ratio of 2 or 3:1). Female predominance in ostium secundum atrial septal defect is estimated to be as high as 3.5:1, and females predominate in partial endocardial cushion defects. Congenital aneurysms of sinuses of Valsalva carry a male-to-female ratio of 4:1. A similar male-to-female ratio occurs in complete transposition of the great arteries, with a range of 2 to 4:1.

PHYSIOLOGIC ADAPTATION AFTER BIRTH. The concept has been underscored that congenital heart diseases are not static in time, but change anatomically and functionally during the course of their natural histories. A given congenital cardiac defect may exist in harmony with the fetal circulation, but is confronted with dramatic circulatory changes at birth that alter this harmony to widely varying degrees. It is therefore appropriate to examine briefly the principal immediate and delayed circulatory alterations at birth and in the neonatal period. The immediate changes consist of (1) a colossal fall in pulmonary vascular resistance associated with expansion of the lungs; (2) a pronounced rise in systemic vascular resistance associated with elimination of the low resistance placental circulation; (3) a fall in blood flow to the right atrium owing to abolition of umbilical venous return; (4) an abrupt rise — as much as tenfold — in pulmonary blood flow, which is promptly translated into a rise in left atrial volume and pressure; (5) functional closure of the valve of the foramen ovale caused by the rise in left atrial and the fall in right atrial pressure; and (6) constriction of the ductus arteriosus at about 12 hours after birth in response to an increase in systemic arterial Po_2. Several important delayed changes complete the picture. The thick-walled fetal pulmonary arterioles are designed to meet the full force of systemic right ventricular pressure the instant the lungs expand. After this need has been met, the fetal arterioles involute during the first few months of life. As respiration is established at birth, there is a marked rise in alveolar and systemic arterial oxygen tension to which pulmonary arterioles are exquisitely sensitive, setting the stage for dilatation and anatomic involution. In addition, the larger pulmonary arteries may also play a role — though much less — in determining the total drop in pressure across the lungs after birth. Maturational changes may affect the neonatal disparity in size between the main and branch pulmonary arteries as well as the angulation at the origins of the right and left branches; both these factors have been held responsible for a physiologic drop in pressure distal to the pulmonary trunk. The third important delayed change relates to the fetal right ventricle, which slowly loses its relative thickness during the first year of life. Adaptive hypertrophy is an expected feature of the fetal right ventricle, which ejects at systemic pressure via the ductus arteriosus. After birth, with the stimulus of right ventricular afterload eliminated, there is a gradual reduction in its thickness relative to septum and left ventricle. The thick neonatal right ventricular wall does not undergo regression; it merely does not increase its thickness as rapidly as the left in the growing infant.

These physiologic adaptations of the normal heart to the events at birth are remarkable in their own right. It is no surprise that congenital defects of the heart or circulation will, to varying degrees, interact with or be modified by adaptations to extrauterine life. A few examples suffice. At one end of the spectrum is the ductus arteriosus, which is a normal part of the fetal circulation. However, when the fetal ductus remains widely patent after birth, the neonatal fall in pulmonary vascular resistance establishes a left to right shunt; pulmonary blood flow increases; the left ventricle is volume overloaded and may fail under the burden. Thus a normal structure in the fetus becomes a potentially hazardous congenital defect after birth. At the other end of the spectrum, aortic atresia is an example. This anomaly is characterized by an atretic aortic valve, a rudimentary left ventricular cavity, and a rudimentary or atretic mitral valve. The left atrium has no effective exit, but in the fetus this is not a handicap, because flow into the left atrium via the lungs is negligible and right to left flow across the foramen ovale is not vital. Accordingly, survival to term is the rule, because systemic venous blood received by the fetal right heart is pumped into the systemic circulation via the ductus, bypassing the left heart. However, at birth, the lungs expand and pulmonary blood flow suddenly and dramatically increases, abruptly delivering a large volume into a left atrium that has no effective outlet because forward flow through the left ventricle is totally obstructed by the atretic mitral and/or aortic valves. Temporary survival depends upon decompression of the left atrium via a herniated valve of the foramen ovale. Death follows shortly. An intermediate case in point is large ventricular septal defect which, although abnormal, does not disturb the fetal circulation because it allows right ventricular blood to enter the aorta in a fashion analogous to the fetal ductus. However, after birth, a fall in pulmonary vascular resistance establishes a left to right shunt which may significantly disturb the postnatal circulation. Subsequently, the pulmonary vascular resistance may rise again and, in a decade or more, reverse the shunt (Eisenmenger's complex), re-establishing a circulatory state similar to the intrauterine presence of the ventricular septal defect.

The principle to be extracted from these examples is clear. The anatomy and physiology of the heart and circulation in congenital heart disease change with the passage of time from the fetus, to the dramatic changes at birth, to further changes in the infant, child, adolescent, and adult survivor. Some of these changes result in neonatal death; others express themselves gradually over weeks, months, years, or decades. A satisfactory comprehension of the clinical manifestations of congenital heart disease requires that these patterns be taken into account.

DIAGNOSIS. The clinical diagnosis of congenital heart disease can represent the epitome of applied medical logic. When sound inferences are drawn from accurate observations, correct diagnoses can be made with gratifying frequency. The clinical expressions of congenital cardiac disease are best dealt with in terms of the anatomic and physiologic mechanisms responsible for their production. Logical thought should be encouraged and memorization minimized. The pathologic anatomy must first be clarified in order to shed light on the resulting physiologic derangements. The question can then be asked: "What clinical manifestations result from these anatomic and physiologic derangements?" The stage is now set for the clinical diagnosis, which depends upon a synthesis of information derived from the history, the physical signs, the electrocardiogram, the x-ray, and the noninvasive and cardiac catheterization laboratories. Similarly, the physical diagnosis consists of a synthesis of information from its own five sources, namely, physical appearance, the arterial pulse, the jugular venous pulse, precordial movements and palpation, and auscultation. It is axiomatic that emphasis is placed on the *relationship of the parts to the whole*, a relationship that ideally results in a complete, harmonious picture devoid of internal contradictions, and *not* a loose confederation of unrelated observations. Maximum data should be extracted from each clinical source while relating information from one source to another. A simple principle emerges — on the one hand, depth; on the other, synthesis. Each step should advance our thinking and narrow the diagnostic possibilities. By the end of the clinical appraisal, untenable considerations should have been abandoned, diagnostic possibilities retained for due consideration, and high priority probabilities brought into sharp focus. Conclusions should become more and more refined as the clinical evaluation progresses step by step. The essence of this thesis stems from Herophilus' adage that the best physician is one who is able to distinguish between the possible and the impossible. A single additional word gives this comment modern relevance — distinguish between the *probable*, the possible, and the impossible.

Diagnostic thinking benefits from the devices of anticipation and supposition. Anticipate what the next step might reveal, and less will be missed. Having drawn tentative conclusions from the history, it is useful to pause momentarily and ask, "If these assumptions are correct, what can I expect the physical examination to reveal? What specific points might I anticipate in the electrocardiogram or x-ray in order to support or refute the conclusions based on the history?" The device of *anticipation* not only helps achieve a synthesis of each step with the next but also serves to heighten interest and suspense as the clinical assessment progresses. The device of *supposition* lends itself to the clinical classification of congenital heart disease in Table 1. Clinical information can be directly related to this classification so that orderly thinking begins apace. For example, we can ask, "*Suppose* this were a *congenital* cardiac defect in an *acyanotic* patient with a *left to right shunt*; which if any of the malformations in this category are appropriate to the information thus far at hand?" By simply asking, "Suppose this were so, what is likely to follow?" one is permitted the dual advantages of thoughtful consideration without inflexible commitment.

Diagnostic information is best handled within the framework of an orderly classification (Table 1) selected because it is practical, is clinical, and can be used effectively irrespective of which of the five sources of information one is dealing with. There are shortcomings in any classification, but these shortcomings, provided they are recognized and minimized, should not obscure the value of a practical, orderly grouping. *The fact that a number of defects are listed in more than one category simply emphasizes the variability of their clinical expressions.* The classification, first proposed by Paul Wood over two decades ago, is based upon the answers to the

TABLE 1. A Clinical Classification of Congenital Heart Disease*

General

Innocent or normal murmurs
Congenitally corrected transposition of the great arteries
Congenital positional anomalies of the heart—cardiac malpositions
Congenital complete heart block

Acyanotic without a Shunt

Malformations originating in the left heart
1. Aortic stenosis
   a. Valvular
   b. Discrete subvalvular
   c. Supravalvular
2. Congenital aortic regurgitation
3. Coarctation of the aorta
4. Congenital mitral regurgitation
   a. Endocardial cushion defect
   b. Congenitally corrected transposition of the great arteries
   c. Primary endocardial fibroelastosis (dilated)
   d. Anomalous origin of the left coronary artery from the pulmonary trunk
   e. Miscellaneous (e.g., double orifice mitral valve, congenital perforations, accessory commissures with anomalous chordal insertion, congenitally short or absent chordae, cleft posterior leaflet, parachute mitral valve)
5. Primary endocardial fibroelastosis
6. Congenital obstruction to left atrial flow
   a. Cor triatriatum
   b. Mitral stenosis
   c. Pulmonary vein stenosis

Malformations originating in the right heart
1. Pulmonic stenosis
   a. Valvular
   b. Infundibular
   c. Supravalvular (stenosis of the pulmonary artery and its branches)
   d. Subinfundibular
2. Idiopathic dilatation of the pulmonary trunk
3. Congenital pulmonary valve regurgitation
4. Primary pulmonary hypertension
5. Ebstein's anomaly of the tricuspid valve

Acyanotic with a Shunt (Left to Right)

Shunt at atrial level
1. Atrial septal defect (isolated)
   a. Ostium secundum
   b. Ostium primum
   c. Sinus venosus
2. Atrial septal defect with mild pulmonic stenosis
3. Total anomalous pulmonary venous connection with low pulmonary vascular resistance
4. Partial anomalous pulmonary venous connection with intact atrial septum
5. Atrial septal defect with mitral stenosis (Lutembacher's syndrome)

Shunt at ventricular level
1. Ventricular septal defect (isolated)
   a. Infracristal
   b. Supracristal
   c. Muscular
   d. Endocardial cushion location
2. Ventricular septal defect with mild pulmonic stenosis
3. Ventricular septal defect with right ventricular origin of both great arteries
4. Ventricular septal defect (infracristal) with congenitally corrected transposition of the great arteries
5. Ventricular septal defect with aortic regurgitation
6. Ventricular septal defect with left ventricular to right atrial shunt

Shunt between aortic root and right heart
1. Coronary arteriovenous fistula
2. Ruptured sinus of Valsalva aneurysm

3. Anomalous origin of the left coronary artery from the pulmonary trunk

Shunt at aorticopulmonary level
1. Patent ductus arteriosus
2. Aorticopulmonary septal defect
3. Truncus arteriosus with large pulmonary arteries and low pulmonary vascular resistance

Shunts at more than one level
1. Complete endocardial cushion defect (complete persistent common atrioventricular canal)
2. Ventricular septal defect with patent ductus arteriosus
3. Ventricular septal defect with atrial septal defect

Cyanotic

Increased pulmonary blood flow
1. Complete transposition of the great arteries
2. The Taussig-Bing anomaly (right ventricular origin of both great arteries with supracristal ventricular septal defect or right ventricular aorta with biventricular pulmonary trunk)
3. Truncus arteriosus with large pulmonary arteries
4. Total anomalous pulmonary venous connection
5. Single ventricle with low pulmonary resistance and absent or mild pulmonic stenosis
6. Common atrium
7. Fallot's tetralogy with pulmonary atresia and increased collateral arterial flow
8. Tricuspid atresia with large ventricular septal defect and no pulmonic stenosis
9. Atrial septal defect with caval connection to left atrium

Normal or decreased pulmonary blood flow
1. Dominant left ventricle
   a. Tricuspid atresia
   b. Ebstein's anomaly with right to left interatrial shunt (mechanical dominance)
   c. Pulmonary atresia with intact ventricular septum and diminutive right ventricle
   d. Congenital vena caval to left atrial communication
   e. Single ventricle with pulmonic stenosis and non-inversion of the infundibulum
   f. Large pulmonary arteriovenous fistula in infancy
2. Dominant right ventricle
   Normal or low pulmonary arterial pressure
   a. Pulmonic stenosis or atresia with ventricular septal defect and right to left shunt (cyanotic Fallot's tetralogy)
   b. Pulmonic stenosis with right to left interatrial shunt
   c. Complete transposition of the great arteries with severe pulmonic stenosis
   d. Pulmonic stenosis with right ventricular origin of both great arteries
   e. Pulmonic stenosis with single ventricle and inversion of the infundibulum (electrical dominance)
   f. Truncus arteriosus with hypoplastic or absent pulmonary arteries
   Elevated pulmonary arterial pressure (pulmonary hypertension)
   a. Atrial septal defect with reversed shunt
   b. Ventricular septal defect with reversed shunt (Eisenmenger's complex)
   c. Patent ductus arteriosus or aorticopulmonary septal defect with reversed shunt
   d. Right ventricular origin of both great arteries with high pulmonary vascular resistance
   e. Hypoplastic left heart (aortic atresia, mitral atresia, complete interruption of the aortic arch)
   f. Complete transposition of the great arteries with high pulmonary vascular resistance
   g. Single ventricle with high pulmonary vascular resistance
   h. Total anomalous pulmonary venous connection with high pulmonary vascular resistance
3. Normal or nearly normal ventricles
   a. Pulmonary arteriovenous fistula
   b. Congenital vena caval to left atrial communication

*From Perloff, J. K.: The Clinical Recognition of Congenital Heart Disease. 2nd ed. Philadelphia, W. B. Saunders Company, 1978.

TABLE 2. Five Basic Questions

1. Is the patient acyanotic or cyanotic?
2. Is pulmonary arterial flow increased or not?
3. Does the malformation originate in the left or right heart?
4. Which is the dominant ventricle?
5. Is pulmonary hypertension present or absent?

TABLE 6

Acyanotic with a shunt. Where is the left to right communication, i.e., where does it originate and what chamber or vessel receives the shunt? Start proximally and end distally:

1. Atrial level
2. Ventricular level
3. Great artery level (aortic root, aortic arch)

TABLE 3

TABLE 7

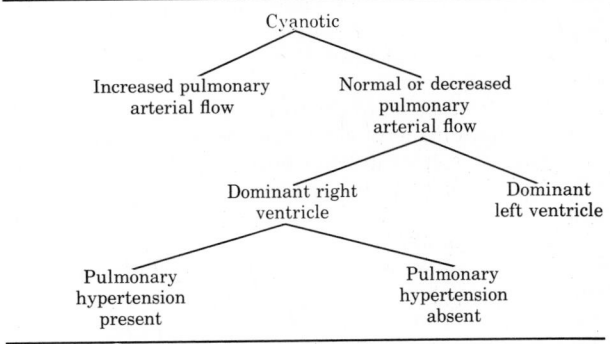

TABLE 4

Acyanotic without a shunt, malformation originating in the right heart. Start proximally (venae cavae) and end distally (pulmonary arteries):

1. Venae cavae
2. Right atrium
3. Tricuspid valve
4. Right ventricular inflow
5. Right ventricular outflow
6. Pulmonary artery and branches
7. Pulmonary arterioles

TABLE 8

Cyanotic with normal or decreased pulmonary arterial flow, dominant right ventricle, and pulmonary hypertension. Where is the right to left shunt? Start proximally and end distally.

1. Atrial level
2. Ventricular level
3. Great artery level

TABLE 5

Acyanotic without a shunt, malformation originating in the left heart. Start proximally (pulmonary veins) and end distally (aorta):

1. Pulmonary veins
2. Left atrium
3. Mitral valve
4. Left ventricular inflow
5. Left ventricular outflow
6. Thoracic aorta

TABLE 9

Cyanotic with normal or decreased pulmonary arterial flow, dominant right ventricle, and no pulmonary hypertension.

1. Pulmonic stenosis or atresia with right to left shunt at ventricular level.
2. Pulmonic stenosis or atresia with right to left shunt at atrial level.

five questions in Table 2. It is not even necessary to ask all five questions for each patient, although the first two questions are obligatory. If the answer to question 1 is "acyanotic," only two additional questions need be posed, first: "Is pulmonary arterial flow increased or not?" (i.e., is a shunt absent or present?), and second, if a shunt is absent: "Does the malformation originate in the left or right heart?"

Let us illustrate by dealing first with an acyanotic patient (Table 3). If the patient is *acyanotic* and the answer to question 2 is negative (acyanotic without shunt), we must then ask question 3: "Does the malformation originate in the left or right heart?" Now move step by step in the direction of blood flow. If the malformation originates in the right heart (Table 4), is it at the level of the venae cavae (persistent left superior vena cava) tricuspid valve—right ventricular inflow (Ebstein's anomaly), right ventricular outflow (stenosis or regurgitation, the former infundibular, valvular, or supravalvular), or the pulmonary arterioles (primary pulmonary hypertension)? Similarly, if the malformation originates in the left heart (Table 5), is it at the level of the pulmonary veins (congenital pulmonary vein stenosis), left atrium (cor triatriatum), mitral valve (stenosis or regurgitation), left ventricular inflow (endocardial fibroelastosis), left ventricular outflow (stenosis or regurgitation, the former subvalvular, valvular, or supravalvular), or the thoracic aorta (coarctation)? If the answer to question 2 (Table 2) is that pulmonary arterial blood flow is *increased* in an acyanotic patient, then the shunt by definition is left to right because cyanosis is absent. We can then consider methodically the origin of the shunt and the chamber or vessel that receives it. Again, move step by step through the heart in the direction of blood flow (Table 6), i.e., shunts at atrial level (atrial septal defect), ventricular level (ventricular septal defect), from the aortic root to right heart (e.g., coronary arteriovenous fistula), or from aortic arch to pulmonary artery (patent ductus).

Now, let us deal with *cyanotic* patients (Table 7; see accompanying figure). If pulmonary arterial blood flow is *increased*, there are, for all practical purposes, about eight or nine possibilities (Table 1, Cyanotic with Increased Pulmonary Blood Flow), only three of which are relatively common — namely, complete transposition of the great arteries, truncus arteriosus, and total anomalous pulmonary venous connection. If pulmonary arterial flow is *normal or decreased* (Table 7), and the *left* ventricle is dominant (question 4), there are six possibilities, only two of which are likely — namely, tricuspid atresia and Ebstein's anomaly of the tricuspid valve. If the *right* ventricle is dominant, question 5 must be asked: "Is pulmonary hypertension present or absent?" If pulmonary hypertension is *present*, again move step by step through the heart in the direction of blood flow (Table 8). Is one dealing with a pulmonary hypertensive right to left shunt at atrial, ventricular, or great artery level, i.e., reversed shunt through a pulmonary hypertensive atrial septal defect, ventricular septal defect, or patent ductus arteriosus? *Absence of pulmonary hypertension* (Table 9) necessarily implies obstruction to outflow into the pulmonary bed, i.e., normal or low pulmonary arterial pressure with high right ventricular pressure. In practical terms, the probabilities are two: pulmonic stenosis with right to left shunt at atrial or ventricular level, i.e., pulmonic stenosis with reversed flow through a foramen ovale or atrial septal defect, or through a ventricular septal defect (Fallot's tetralogy).

In dealing with the history, physical examination, electrocardiogram, x-ray, and diagnostic laboratories, it is worthwhile briefly to call attention to a few points especially appropriate to congenital heart disease. In the history, questions should include the pregnancy, for example, maternal exposure to teratogens such as rubella in the first trimester, or the altitude at which the patient was born. Maternal age may be important. Details of a cardiac murmur — the detection of which often heralds the diagnosis of congenital heart disease — should be precise regarding

A, Hand of a cyanotic adult, showing the change in skin color of the distal phalanges. *B*, Profile of the index finger of another cyanotic adult, showing both a change in skin color and dramatic clubbing. (From Perloff, J. K.: The Clinical Recognition of Congenital Heart Disease. 2nd ed. Philadelphia, W. B. Saunders Company, 1978.)

onset and intensity. Was the murmur present at birth (newborn nursery), or was it first detected in early infancy, adolescence, or young adulthood? Was the murmur consistently and readily heard irrespective of patient cooperation (conspicuous murmur), or was it absent at times, difficult to hear, or believed to be unimportant? Was a new murmur ever commented upon (ventricular septal defect with subsequent aortic regurgitation)? Cyanosis should similarly be defined precisely according to time of onset, degree, and distribution. A history of squatting in a cyanotic patient typically applies to Fallot's tetralogy. Patterns of growth and development should be established. It is worth recalling that the clinical manifestations of congestive heart failure differ in infants, older children, and adults. Family history of congenital cardiac disease may shed light on the defect in the patient, especially if kinship is close. Susceptibility to lower respiratory infections suggests large left to right shunts. Neck pulsations (arterial or venous) may provide useful clues. A history of infective endocarditis calls attention to a relatively limited number of susceptible defects.

Physical appearance should apply to the presence of certain *somatic* congenital defects that are associated with specific types of congenital *cardiac* anomalies, such as *mongolism* (endocardial cushion defect), *Turner's syndrome* (coarctation of the aorta), *peculiar facies and dentition* associated with supravalvular aortic stenosis and pulmonary artery stenosis, the *Holt-Oram syndrome* (defects in the atrial septum), the *Ellis–van Creveld syndrome* (common atrium), or trisomy 18 (double outlet right ventricle).

The arterial pulses should be compared in the upper and lower extremities (coarctation of the aorta), but the brachials should also be palpated (cyanotic male infant with absent brachials and present femorals may mean aortic atresia). Right and left systemic arterial pulses should be compared (increased pulse pressure in the right carotid and brachial arteries in supravalvular aortic stenosis). The jugular venous pulse deserves special attention as soon as the patient is old enough to permit such observation (the short neck of the infant usually makes examination difficult or impossible). Percussion is useful in establishing visceral positions (cardiac and hepatic dullness and gastric tympany) to avoid missing a congenital postitional anomaly. Palpation should carefully define each precordial movement according to chamber or great artery of origin, avoiding vague, meaningless terms such as "point of maximum impulse." During auscultation, designations such as "pulmonary area, aortic area, or mitral area" should be avoided, because they assume normal topographical anatomy of the heart, i.e., situs solitus without transposition of the great arteries and without ventricular inversion, assumptions which cannot be made, especially in the context of congenital heart disease. Simple descriptive terms should be used, such as apex, left or right lower, mid or upper sternal border, and the like. Murmurs should be precisely characterized, especially their timing in the cardiac cycle, with systolic murmurs classified as early, mid, late or holosystolic; diastolic murmurs as early diastolic, mid-diastolic or presystolic; and the continuous murmur defined as one that begins in systole and continues without interruption through the second heart sound into all or part of diastole.

The 12-lead surface electrocardiogram should be supplemented by leads V_3R and V_4R, and a vectorcardiogram is often necessary to clarify complex electrocardiograms. Technically satisfactory plain films of the chest in the posteroanterior, lateral, right and left oblique positions have for all practical purposes replaced intracardiac fluoroscopy except for the detection of intracardiac calcium. *Echocardiography* is a valuable source of diagnostic information and can be repeated without discomfort or risk. Cardiac catheterization and angiocardiography should be an extension of clinical judgment, a judgment which should decide not only when and which patients should be selected for study, but also which type of investigation is most appropriate for a given subject. Accurate diagnosis depends upon synthesis of the broad range of clinical data with the results of carefully planned and well-executed laboratory studies.

SCOPE OF THESE CHAPTERS. Survival in congenital heart disease results from natural selection or from surgical intervention. Ch. 359.2 to 359.5 will emphasize defects with a natural tendency to survive beyond the pediatric age group. Such emphasis is appropriate for a textbook of medicine. It must be stated, however, that congenital cardiac disease is a continuum from birth to adult life and that the only way to understand the patterns of postpediatric survival is to have dealt at some point with the same disorders in the infant and young child. The following categories will be considered: (1) *common* congenital cardiac defects in which postpediatric survival is expected; (2) *uncommon* congenital cardiac defects in which postpediatric survival is expected; (3) *common* congenital cardiac defects in which postpediatric survival is exceptional; and (4) *uncommon* congenital cardiac defects in which postpediatric survival is exceptional. Congenital cardiac anomalies (common or uncommon) in which postpediatric survival is unknown will not be considered. Chief emphasis will be placed on the common or uncommon anomalies with *expected* postpediatric survival. The common or uncommon defects with exceptional postpediatric survival will be touched upon more briefly to provide necessary perspective. It should be borne in mind, however, that as time goes on more and more congenital cardiacs beyond the pediatric age group will be postoperative; this is only as it should be.

359.2. COMMON CONGENITAL CARDIAC DEFECTS IN WHICH POSTPEDIATRIC SURVIVAL IS EXPECTED

FUNCTIONALLY NORMAL BICUSPID AORTIC VALVE

The frequency of congenitally bicuspid aortic valves — functionally normal, stenotic, and/or incompetent — may approach 2 per cent of the population. If this figure is correct, it means that the bicuspid aortic valve is not only the most frequent congenital anomaly of the heart or great vessels, but that the most common congenital cardiac defect in man manifests itself in the *postpediatric population*. The typical bicuspid aortic valve consists of two commissures and two cusps. One cusp, generally the larger, contains a low ridge or raphe ("false commissure"), adjacent to the aortic wall but not reaching the edge of the leaflet. If the free edges of a congenital bicuspid aortic valve are sufficiently redundant to permit unimpeded forward flow (no systolic gradient) yet not redundant enough to cause malapposition in diastole (little or no aortic regurgitation), then the bicuspid aortic valve is said to be "functionally normal." The natural history of such a valve is variable. A bicuspid aortic valve that functions normally at birth may continue to do so throughout life and be found incidentally at necropsy in late adult life. However, the same valve may take three unfavorable courses. The first is the tendency to become thickened, fibrotic, calcified, and stenotic during early or mid-adulthood. Second, infective endocarditis may convert a functionally benign lesion into the catastrophic mechanical fault of acute severe aortic regurgitation. Third, the larger of the two cusps may progressively evert or prolapse, causing progressive aortic regurgitation that ultimately can be severe. It is not yet known what determines which of these courses a given functionally normal congenitally bicuspid valve will take.

A functionally normal bicuspid aortic valve can be suspected clinically especially in teenagers and young adults. Innocent systolic murmurs in this age group, except for infraclavicular radiation of the innocent brachiocephalic systolic murmur, are not maximally heard at the right base. Accordingly, a short, somewhat impure Grade I to II midsystolic murmur loudest at the right base in a child, adolescent, or young adult is suspect. If that murmur is introduced by an ejection sound and if careful auscultation detects the soft murmur of aortic regurgitation, the clinical diagnosis reaches a high degree of probability. Physical interventions that increase aortic pressure (squatting, isometric exercise with clenched fists) increase audibility of faint murmurs of aortic regurgitation. Suspicion is always greater in males, because the congenital bicuspid aortic valve, whether functionally normal or not, is predominantly a male disease. If clinical suspicion is high, an argument can be made for verification by thoracic aortography, because the bicuspid aortic valve is highly susceptible to infective endocarditis and appropriate antimicrobial prophylaxis must be recommended. However, the simplest means of verification is echocardiography.

CONGENITAL VALVULAR AORTIC STENOSIS

Congenital obstruction to left ventricular outflow can be *valvular*, *subvalvular*, or *supravalvular*. The most common type is valvular and, in the adult, is usually characterized by narrowing of a bicuspid valve which can be intrinsically stenotic from birth or, more typically, becomes stenotic after progressive thickening and calcification (see above). Unicommissural unicuspid aortic valves are relatively frequent causes of intrinsically stenotic aortic valves at birth but, like the congenital bicuspid valve, sometimes exhibit delayed obstruction owing to thickening and rigidity.

Congenital valvular aortic stenosis is much more prevalent in males, with a sex ratio approximating 4 or 5:1. If the obstruction is present at birth, the murmur is likely to date from the newborn nursery. On the other hand, the functionally normal congenital bicuspid aortic valve is usually undetected in infancy or childhood, but may subsequently generate the prominent murmur of aortic stenosis in the second, third, or fourth decade. Angina and effort syncope arouse suspicion of aortic stenosis in acyanotic young patients with a history of

dyspnea, fatigue, and a prominent cardiac murmur dating from infancy or a murmur appearing in the second, third, or fourth decade. Cerebral symptoms can be subtle, consisting of nothing more than mild giddiness or lightheadedness, especially with effort. On the other hand, recurrent syncope is dangerous and heralds sudden death even in childhood or adolescence. Inappropriate sweating sometimes occurs and increases with the advent of cardiac failure. Infective endocarditis is a serious complication of congenital valvular aortic stenosis; all varieties are susceptible. The pulse pressure is small, and is accompanied by a slow rate of rise, a sustained peak, and a gentle collapse when obstruction is severe.

Precordial palpation reveals a left ventricular impulse that varies from normal (mild stenosis) to the strong, sustained heaving movement characterizing the hypertrophied left ventricle of severe obstruction. Presystolic distention of the left ventricle implies increased force of left atrial contraction, and is good evidence in young adults that the obstruction is significant. The thrill of aortic stenosis may be trivial or absent with mild obstruction, or with severe obstruction and advanced heart failure. The typical aortic stenotic thrill radiates upward and to the right, is maximal in the second right interspace, and is readily detected in the suprasternal notch and over both carotids. In some patients the thrill is confined to the apex or, if the heart is small, to the lower left sternal edge where the atypical location can be misleading. In addition to the thrill, the sharp impact of an ejection sound can often be palpated at the apex in congenital valvular aortic stenosis.

An ejection sound is a characteristic although not invariable feature. The sound is caused by abrupt upward movement of the dome-shaped or truncated congenitally stenotic valve and implies good valve motion. In adults calcification may impair valve mobility so that the ejection sound diminishes or vanishes. The aortic stenotic murmur begins after the first sound (or with the ejection sound), rises in a crescendo to a systolic peak, and declines in a decrescendo to end before the aortic component of the second sound. The quality at the right base is harsh, rough, and grunting, especially when loud. Although configuration, length, and loudness do not necessarily relate to the degree of stenosis, the longer and louder the murmur and the later its systolic peak, the greater the likelihood of severe obstruction. However, an unimpressive midsystolic murmur — or none at all — may occur in severe aortic stenosis with advanced heart failure or in adults with increased anteroposterior chest dimensions. The right basal location and radiation of the murmur of valvular aortic stenosis are related to the upward and rightward direction of the high velocity jet within the ascending aorta. The second heart sound should be judged with regard to the intensity of the aortic component and the presence, degree, and type of splitting. In congenital valvular aortic stenosis with mobile valve, the aortic component of the second sound is well preserved even in the presence of appreciable obstruction. Prominent inspiratory splitting usually (but not invariably) means mild obstruction, because the duration of left ventricular ejection is not prolonged. *Paradoxical* splitting is a sign of severe obstruction and generally indicates that the duration of left ventricular ejection is appreciably prolonged. However, the majority of patients with aortic stenosis exhibit a second sound that is single or closely split through a wide range of severity.

A soft murmur of aortic regurgitation may be heard with congenital valvular aortic stenosis but is more common with discrete subvalvular obstruction because of cusp distortion (see below). A fourth heart sound in aortic stenosis is the acoustic counterpart of presystolic distention of the left ventricle and is likely to mean appreciable obstruction. However, after age 40, the fourth heart sound is not a reliable sign of severity, because there is an age-related incidence.

Electrocardiographic estimates of severity should be made with caution; mild valvular aortic stenosis sometimes occurs with left ventricular hypertrophy, and severe obstruction occasionally exists with a normal electrocardiogram. Sudden death may occur in patients with severe congenital aortic stenosis and normal electrocardiograms. Although these points must be borne in mind, they should not obscure the value of the scalar tracing. The best electrocardiographic index of appreciable obstruction is the combination of both voltage and repolarization criteria for left ventricular hypertrophy, especially in preadolescent patients. In congenital valvular aortic stenosis the x-ray features are poststenotic dilatation of the aorta with a relatively convex, globular left ventricular contour. In adults, aortic calcification is presumptive evidence of valvular obstruction and must be sought with the aid of echocardiography and an image intensifier.

Despite considerable clinical sophistication, cardiac catheterization and angiocardiography are generally required to be precise about the morphologic type and severity of congenital valvular aortic stenosis. If clinical evidence strongly points to mild obstruction, diagnostic intervention may be deferred, the risk of postoperative endocarditis far exceeding the benefits of operation. When clinical findings point to severe obstruction, diagnostic investigation should precede selection for surgery. If valvular obstruction is severe and the patient is *asymptomatic*, surgical intervention depends in large part upon the morphologic type of obstruction. Direct repair may provide excellent results at low risk. Severe valvular aortic stenosis in the *symptomatic* patient — especially with angina or syncope but without significant congestive heart failure — requires surgical intervention even if this means valve replacement. In severe obstruction, the greater the left ventricular dysfunction, the smaller the gradient, the smaller the ejection fraction, the higher the surgical risk, and the poorer the results.

COARCTATION OF THE AORTA

The basic anatomic fault is a localized deformity of the media manifested by a curtain-like infolding that eccentrically narrows the aortic lumen. The zone of coarctation is characteristically located distal to the origin of the left subclavian artery at or just beyond the insertion of the ligamentum arteriosum. Occasionally coarctation is situated at or just proximal to the left subclavian artery so that the orifice of that vessel is in the low pressure zone.

Nearly 25 per cent of patients with coarctation of the aorta have bicuspid aortic valves which may be functionally normal or may take one of the courses described above. The most important noncardiac anomaly is an aneurysm of the circle of Willis which may remain clinically silent or may announce itself by rupture.

Aortic coarctation predominates in males. After early infancy, patients are usually asymptomatic when the malformation is diagnosed. Serious symptoms are relatively uncommon before age 15 years, but it is uncommon for symptoms to be absent after age 30. The majority of patients live to adult life, but only a minority reach age 40, and only 10 per cent live beyond age 50. The longest survival was recorded in 1828 by Reynaud in his account of coarctation in a 92-year-old man. Discovery of systemic hypertension provides the initial suspicion unless the brachial and femoral pulses are palpated. A number of minor symptoms such as headache, spontaneous epistaxes, and leg fatigue sometimes occur. Major symptoms are related to four complications: congestive heart failure, rupture of the aorta or dissecting aneurysm, infective endocarditis or endarteritis, and cerebral hemorrhage. The incidence of cardiac failure is highest in early infancy or after the third decade and can develop in adults previously devoid of symptoms related to the malformation. Rupture of the aorta or dissecting aneurysm occurs most frequently in the 20's and 30's. The rupture originates either in the proximal ascending aorta or in a postcoarctation aneurysm. Infective endocarditis or endarteritis is most frequently implanted on the peculiarly susceptible bicuspid aortic valve; endarteritis at the site of coarctation occurs less frequently. Cerebral hemorrhage, the fourth major complication, is usually due to rupture of an aneurysm of the circle of Willis. In the pregnant female with coarctation, blood pressure fluctuations are similar in direction to those of uncomplicated pregnancy. The incidence of toxemia is lower in women with coarctation than in pregnant women with other forms of hypertension; intracranial hemorrhage is not more likely to occur, and cardiac failure seldom develops. However, pregnancy does increase the risk of rupture of the aorta, especially at the end of the third trimester. Furthermore, the bacteremia that may accompany labor and delivery can cause endocarditis or endarteritis.

The physique in coarctation is at times impressive; an athletic appearance of the chest and shoulders contrasts with narrow hips and thin legs. Coarctation of the aorta is sometimes suspected because of the characteristic physical appearance of *Turner's syndrome*, namely, a female with short stature, webbing of the neck, absent or scanty pubic and axillary hair, wide-set nipples, low hairline, small chin, and wide carrying angle of the arms.

Abnormal differences in upper and lower extremity arterial pulses are the clinical hallmarks of coarctation of the aorta. Diagnostic differences in arm and leg blood pressures should be based upon systolic and not diastolic levels. These pressure differences between arm and leg are exaggerated by exercise, which can therefore be a useful adjunct in confirming mild coarctation. The level of upper extremity blood pressure must be interpreted according to the patient's age. A blood pressure that is normal in an adult may be hypertensive in a child. As patients with coarctation grow older, the systolic pressure rises relatively more than the diastolic, so the pulse pressure increases. Such patients exhibit conspicuous, forceful carotid and suprasternal pulsations resembling aortic regurgitation, which may coexist. In addition, the subclavian arteries can sometimes be seen pulsating below the clavicles. Collateral arteries, even when abundant, are seldom obvious and must be specifically sought by having the patient stand and bend forward with the arms hanging at the sides. The examiner inspects the back, particularly around and between the scapulae, using a tangential light source to expose the subcutaneous collaterals in shadowed relief. The retinal arteries may be tortuous and narrowed, but hypertensive retinopathy is rare.

The right and left brachial arteries should be simultaneously compared by palpation and blood pressure determination. An absent or relatively small left brachial pulse means that the coarctation is at or just proximal to the left subclavian artery. In aortic stenosis with coarctation, the brachial arterial pulse (and pressure) may be relatively normal rather than hypertensive, whereas the femoral pulses are diminished or absent. Conversely, aortic regurgitation increases the femoral pulse, especially in mild coarctation, so the clinical diagnosis of the combined defects may be obscured.

Precordial palpation detects a left ventricular impulse that varies from normal to the sustained heaving impulse of ventricular hypertrophy. A dilated ascending aorta can cause a visible and palpable systolic impulse at the right base. Suprasternal thrills are relatively frequent in uncomplicated coarctation, but precordial thrills are seldom present without coexisting aortic stenosis.

An aortic ejection sound increases suspicion of coexisting bicuspid aortic valve, although the sound may arise in the dilated aortic root. Coarctation of the aorta is associated with systolic, diastolic, or continuous murmurs. Systolic murmurs originate from arterial collaterals, the coarctation itself, and the bicuspid aortic valve. Collateral systolic murmurs are distributed widely over the thorax. There is a tendency for these murmurs to be especially conspicuous along the left sternal border (the left internal mammary artery). Collateral murmurs are crescendo-decrescendo in shape and delayed in onset because of origin in arteries distant from the heart. The coarctation itself is responsible for a localized midline posterior murmur, the level of which is related to the site of aortic constriction. With mild coarctation, the posterior systolic murmur is relatively short; as the degree of obstruction increases, the murmur gets longer and may extend well into diastole, becoming "continuous." The most common *diastolic* murmur is aortic regurgitation, a useful sign of bicuspid aortic valve.

Isolated *right* ventricular hypertrophy is for all practical purposes confined to infants in the first six months of life with heart failure and reactive pulmonary hypertension. In uncomplicated coarctation, left ventricular hypertrophy is manifested by both voltage and repolarization criteria. However, prominent S-T segment depressions with deeply inverted T waves seldom occur with uncomplicated coarctation and suggest coexisting aortic stenosis.

The x-ray provides considerable information regarding both the diagnosis and the anatomic variations of coarctation of the aorta. Notching of the ribs results from collateral flow through dilated, tortuous, pulsatile *posterior* intercostal arteries. The notches typically appear as irregular, scalloped areas on the undersurfaces of the posterior ribs. The *anterior* ribs are spared because the anterior intercostal arteries do not run in costal grooves. Notching seldom appears before six or seven years. When the coarctation is located *proximal* to the left subclavian artery, collateral circulation fails to develop on the left side; *unilateral* notching appears in the *right* posterior ribs. In older children or adults, the lateral x-ray may show *retrosternal* scalloping caused by dilated tortuous internal mammary arteries. In classic coarctation of the aortic isthmus, the hypertensive ascending aorta is dilated. Aortic dilatation *distal* to the zone of coarctation (poststenotic enlargement) produces a recognizable leftward convexity of the descending thoracic aorta. When this sign is accompanied by the convex shadow of a dilated left subclavian artery, the two convexities form a typical "figure 3" in the frontal projection.

Cardiac catheterization and angiocardiography define the anatomic features of coarctation, including the collateral circulation, but as a rule they are not necessary for a secure clinical diagnosis upon which a therapeutic decision can be based. If there is clinical suspicion of coexisting bicuspid aortic valve, the inclination to perform thoracic aortography is increased, because confirmation gives insight into the postoperative natural course and the need for continued prophylaxis for infective endocarditis. The presence of all but mild coarctation warrants consideration for surgical repair. It is still the consensus that optimal age for correction awaits the seventh year. On the other hand, selection of patients for elective repair at earlier ages has been liberalized, because subsequent recurrence of coarctation has been shown to be negligible even when correction is done in early childhood. In fact primary repair in small infants with persistent heart failure is now selectively and successfully accomplished. In older patients, risk of technical complications during surgery increases. Irrespective of the quality of the repair, the risk of infective endocarditis on a coexisting bicuspid aortic valve is not diminished, and we do not know whether the risk of intracranial hemorrhage (berry aneurysm) is affected. Although the incidence of heart failure continues to rise during the fourth decade in unoperated coarctation, after age 40 there appears to be an even chance of death from incidental causes. In those surviving to this age, the efficacy of correction becomes debatable. Furthermore, long-term analyses of patients after surgical correction of coarctation of the aorta have revealed a high incidence of premature cardiovascular disease despite adequate operation. Particularly disturbing in this regard are the data on unexplained late postoperative hypertension.

PULMONIC STENOSIS

Congenital obstruction to right ventricular outflow can be valvular, subvalvular, or supravalvular. *Valvular* pulmonic stenosis, the most common variety, is characterized by a conical or dome-shaped valve with a narrow outlet at its apex. Three raphes extend from the small central opening to the wall of the pulmonary artery, although separate leaflets cannot be identified. Males and females are equally affected. Rarely, valvular pulmonic stenosis is caused by myxomatous dysplasia of the valve.

The functional consequences of valvular pulmonic

stenosis are related to the resistance to right ventricular outflow. Early discovery of the murmur is the rule, because the anatomic and physiologic conditions necessary for its production are present at birth. Survival into adulthood is relatively common. The tendency for the valve to grow in proportion to body size may in part account for this. However, with advancing age fibrous thickening and even calcification may reduce valve mobility and increase the degree of obstruction.

Familial occurrence is not a feature of ordinary valvular pulmonic stenosis. However, in congenital pulmonic stenosis caused by dysplasia of the valve, some relatives may have pulmonary valve dysplasia and others typical dome-shaped valvular pulmonic stenosis.

Subjective complaints tend to increase with age, although equivalent degrees of stenosis may handicap one patient in childhood yet leave another relatively unlimited in the fourth decade. An appreciable number of patients with moderate to severe stenosis are virtually symptom free well into the postpediatric age group. Dyspnea and fatigue are the most common symptoms. These complaints tend to remain absent as long as the right ventricle can maintain a normal stroke volume at rest and augment its output with effort. Right ventricular failure is the single most common natural cause of death. Patients with valvular pulmonic stenosis sometimes experience giddiness, lightheadedness, or frank syncope, especially with effort. Children as well as adults occasionally have chest pain resembling myocardial ischemia. Some patients with severe pulmonic stenosis are subjectively aware of giant A waves in the jugular venous pulse, especially during effort or excitement. The stenotic valve is susceptible to infective endocarditis.

Infants with typical valvular pulmonic stenosis may appear remarkably healthy, with good fat deposits and chubby round faces. Even older patients may have faces that are wide, full, or even bloated, with highly colored cheeks. Males or females with many of the phenotypic features of Turner's syndrome but normal chromosomal complements (46XX or XY) tend to have valvular pulmonic stenosis. *Myxomatous dysplasia* of the pulmonic valve may be associated with slow body growth and abnormal facies (triangular face with hypertelorism, ptosis of the eyelids, and low-set ears).

The jugular venous pulse exhibits an A wave that gets progressively larger as the degree of obstruction increases. Exercise and excitement augment these A waves. In addition, powerful right atrial contraction may be associated with presystolic pulsation of the liver. An increase in the height of the V wave occurs with the advent of right ventricular failure and tricuspid regurgitation.

Thrills mirror the location and intensity of accompanying murmurs (see below). In valvular pulmonic stenosis, the thrill is maximal in the second or occasionally third left interspace, radiating upward and toward the left, because the intrapulmonary jet is directed toward the left pulmonary artery. A right ventricular systolic impulse is an important physical sign of pulmonic stenosis and, when absent, casts doubt on the diagnosis. The location of the parasternal right ventricular impulse can sometimes be related to the level of obstruction, because the transmitted systolic movements originate in the high-pressure zone proximal to the level of stenosis. Presystolic distention of the right ventricle is caused by forceful contraction of the right atrium and is typically accompanied by a large jugular venous A wave.

An ejection sound is a characteristic feature of valvular pulmonic stenosis and is important in identifying this form of obstruction. The pulmonic ejection sound is high pitched, sharp or clicking, and maximal in the second left interspace, often selectively decreasing during inspiration. An ejection sound is not present in valvular pulmonic stenosis caused by myxomatous dysplasia or in the rare adult with a calcified pulmonic valve.

The systolic murmur of typical valvular pulmonic stenosis is maximal in the second left interspace, although it may be just as loud in the third. The lower location may be related to secondary subvalvular hypertrophy. The murmur, like the thrill, radiates upward and to the left, and when loud may be heard in the suprasternal notch and at the base of the neck, especially on the left. Loudness per se is not necessarily an index of severity, although as a rule intensity tends to vary directly with the degree of obstruction. However, the magnitude of stenosis is the major determinant of the *duration* of right ventricular ejection which, in turn, determines the *length* of the systolic murmur. A soft, symmetrical murmur, peaking in midsystole, is a feature of mild pulmonic stenosis; whereas a loud murmur, peaking late in systole and extending well beyond aortic closure, is a feature of severe obstruction.

The intensity of the pulmonic component of the second sound varies from normal to inaudible as severity increases. However, the *timing* of the pulmonic component is more important than intensity in assessing severity. A relatively slight increase in expiratory splitting, with normal intensity of the pulmonic component, is evidence of mild stenosis, whereas a marked increase in splitting with a faint or absent pulmonic component is evidence of severe obstruction.

The electrocardiogram commonly shows tall, peaked P waves. The QRS axis in the frontal plane shifts to the right, the degree of right axis deviation tending to vary directly with right ventricular pressure. The severity of pulmonic stenosis corresponds fairly well to the R/S ratios in V_1 and V_6 and to the height of the R wave in V_1. In mild pulmonic stenosis an rSr' pattern in V_1 is sometimes difficult to distinguish from normal. In severe pulmonic stenosis, leads V_1 and V_3R exhibit tall monophasic R waves, and lead V_6 shows an rS pattern. Between these extremes all gradations exist. In severe pulmonic stenosis, deeply inverted T waves that curve upward on the downstroke and that extend beyond V_2 are typical and assume greater significance when accompanied by ST segment depressions. Upright T waves occur with increased right ventricular pressure in young children, and upright T waves in the right precordium are the only electrocardiographic signs of right ventricular hypertension in some children with mild pulmonic stenosis.

The x-ray evaluation of valvular pulmonic stenosis should concentrate on (1) the peripheral intrapulmonary) vascular pattern, (2) the main pulmonary artery and its branches, and (3) the size and contour of the right ventricle and right atrium. The peripheral pulmonary vascular pattern is normal even in severe valvular stenosis until the output of the right ventricle falls. Poststenotic dilatation of the pulmonary trunk is characteristic and is often accompanied by conspicuous enlargement of the left branch. Calcification of the congenitally stenosed pulmonary valve is rare and confined to adult survivors. The left anterior oblique view is best for defining the right ventricular contour, whereas a prominent right atrial sweep may be seen in the posteroanterior projection. A conspicuous increase in right heart size is almost always a sign of severity, especially at an early age. Cardiac catheterization and angiocardiography permit definitive diagnosis of the level, morphologic type, and severity of obstruction to right ventricular outflow. However, patients with mild valvular pulmonic stenosis can be identified with such clinical confidence that invasive diagnostic investigation is generally not required. But in this group, clinical distinction from idiopathic dilatation of the pulmonary trunk may be difficult or impossible.

In typical valvular pulmonic stenosis, surgical repair is probably indicated for patients with resting gradients of 50 mm Hg or more, although a single determination may be misleading, because gradients vary considerably with cardiac output (transvalvular flow). The risk of operative repair in valvular pulmonic stenosis is low, and results are excellent. Postoperative pulmonary regurgitation often occurs, but as a rule it is mild and functionally unimportant. In severe valvular pulmonic stenosis, secondary hypertrophic subpulmonic stenosis may require resection. This intervention should not be taken lightly, because right ventriculotomy is necessary, although repair via the tricuspid valve is feasible.

ATRIAL SEPTAL DEFECT

Atrial defects are designated according to their sites in the septum: (1) in the region of the fossa ovalis (ostium secundum), (2) between the fossa and the inferior vena cava, (3) in the upper part of the septum (sinus venosus), (4) in the lower part of the septum (ostium primum), and (5) in the position normally occupied by the coronary sinus. The most common variety that will be dealt with here is referred to as *ostium secundum defect.*

The physiologic consequences of an atrial septal defect depend chiefly upon the magnitude and duration of the shunt, the adaptive response of the volume-loaded right ventricle, and the behavior of the pulmonary vascular bed. Two mechanisms have been proposed to explain left to right shunting. First, in infancy the right and left ventricles have similar distensibility characteristics and hence should have similar end-diastolic volumes. As pulmonary vascular resistance falls in the neonatal period, the right ventricle ejects into a low resistance bed and would be expected to have a larger ejection fraction than the left. During the subsequent diastole the volume received by the right ventricle would increase, and a left to right shunt would therefore be established. Second, as the pulmonary arterioles involute, the relatively thick-walled neonatal right ventricle becomes thinner and offers less resistance to filling than the left. Conditions become appropriate for augmenting flow from left atrium across the defect. The left to right shunt occurs in the presence of low pulmonary vascular resistance *and* normal pulmonary arterial pressure. This may in part explain the relative infrequency of subsequent pulmonary hypertension in young people with atrial septal defect. Pulmonary hypertension is rare in infants and children with uncomplicated atrial septal defects and does not reach its peak incidence of about 14 per cent until early adult life.

In ostium secundum atrial septal defect the female-to-male ratio ranges from 2 to 3.5:1. Family history is important, because these defects not only can be familial, but also may recur through a number of generations.

Atrial septal defects often go unrecognized for years, because symptoms may be trivial or absent and physical signs subtle. The relatively soft pulmonic midsystolic murmur is easily overlooked in restless or crying children and may be mistaken for an innocent murmur in both children and young adults. In apparently healthy normal adults, atrial septal defect is often first suspected because of a routine chest x-ray. Life expectancy is shortened, although adult survival is the rule, and some patients live to an advanced age. Survival is more limited in young adults who develop pulmonary hypertension, but even in them the span of life generally averages more than 40 years. It is not rare to find atrial septal defects beyond age 70 years. Death may be unrelated to the defect, but when a relationship exists, cardiac failure is the most common natural cause. Since the natural history of uncomplicated ostium secundum atrial septal defect spans the childbearing age and since the majority of such patients are female, it is noteworthy that pregnancy is usually well tolerated. After the third or fouth decade, complications arise, and practically all patients who survive to the sixth decade are symptomatic. Effort dyspnea and fatigue are most frequent. Older patients with large left to right shunt atrial septal defects may experience not only effort dyspnea but also orthopnea. In the presence of decreased lung compliance caused by longstanding large left to right shunts, the work of breathing is greater in the supine than in the sitting position.

Infective endocarditis is rare in isolated ostium secundum atrial septal defect, a rarity attributed to the absence of jet lesions or turbulence because of the low velocity diastolic shunt.

Older patients with ostium secundum atrial septal defects deteriorate chiefly on three accounts. First, degenerative diseases such as coronary artery disease or systemic hypertension cause the left ventricle to become less distensible, so a larger volume of left atrial blood preferentially flows across the defect, adding to the work of an already overloaded right ventricle. The second problem is a rise in pulmonary arterial pressure in the face of a persistent large left to right shunt. The third concern is the advent of atrial arrhythmias — fibrillation, flutter, or paroxysmal atrial tachycardia. After the fourth decade atrial arrhythmias increase in frequency and represent one of the most serious complications.

Physical appearance of adults with ostium secundum atrial septal defect is generally normal, but children often exhibit a delicate, frail, or gracile habitus, with weight affected more than height. A left precordial bulge is common and is often associated with Harrison's grooves. A distinctive appearance that heightens suspicion of an ostium secundum atrial septal defect is the *Holt-Oram syndrome.* The thumb is hypoplastic, with an accessory phalanx that gives it a "crooked" appearance. Apposition of the thumb with other digits is difficult, and in some cases the thumb is rudimentary or absent.

The jugular venous pulse in ostium secundum atrial septal defect may show A and V waves of equal heights, because the two atria are in free communication. Pulmonary hypertension results in an increased force of right atrial contraction and a dominant A wave which may reach giant proportions.

Precordial movement and palpation characteristically detect a right ventricular impulse that is hyperdynamic, even tumultuous, and relatively brief in duration. This pattern occurs because the left to right shunt distends the right ventricle in diastole, and the chamber then contracts vigorously into a low resistance pulmonary bed. The dilated pulmonary trunk is often palpated in the second left interspace. A systolic thrill at that site indicates either a very large shunt or coexisting valvular pulmonic stenosis. In the presence of pulmonary hypertension, the right ventricular impulse becomes sustained and less dynamic, and presystolic distention may result from an increased force of right atrial contraction.

The "first heart sound" at the left sternal edge and apex may be split and the *second component* relatively loud. It has been variously proposed that the loud second component originates from the tricuspid valve or represents a pulmonic ejection sound. The location and lack of selective attenuation with inspiration favor the former, although the two mechanisms may coexist. The typical murmur accompanying atrial septal defect results from rapid ejection of a large right ventricular stroke volume into a dilated pulmonary trunk. The murmur is usually Grade 3 or less, maximal in the second left intercostal space, beginning after the first heart sound, crescendo-decrescendo in shape, peaking in early or midsystole, and ending well before both components of the second heart sound. The septal defect itself is, with rare exception, acoustically silent. A murmur exceeding Grade 3 is likely to mean an unusually large shunt or associated valvular pulmonic stenosis. In slightly built patients, widely distributed thoracic systolic murmurs can sometimes be heard in the right chest, axilla, and back because of rapid flow through peripheral pulmonary arteries in low resistance, high-flow atrial septal defects.

A hallmark of atrial septal defect is the behavior of the second heart sound. The aortic and pulmonic components are widely and persistently split and exhibit little or no change in the degree of splitting with respiration or Valsalva maneuver. The relative loudness of the two components is usually normal, although at times the second component is increased despite little or no pulmonary hypertension. Proximity of the dilated pulmonary trunk to the chest wall and the brisk elastic recoil of the distended pulmonary trunk may account for this.

Two types of diastolic murmurs occur in atrial septal defect with left to right shunt. One is mid-diastolic and is caused by torrential flow across the tricuspid valve, indicating a sizable left to right shunt. The second diastolic murmur is rare and is due to pulmonary regurgitation in the absence of pulmonary hypertension; a very large pulmonary trunk is probably responsible.

Auscultatory signs in atrial septal defect with pulmonary hypertension differ from the foregoing. The pulmonic midsystolic flow murmur is replaced by a softer, shorter midsystolic murmur caused by ejection of a normal stroke volume into a dilated pulmonary trunk. Tricuspid flow murmurs vanish. Typical pulmonic ejec-

tion sounds appear, especially in the second left interspace, and exhibit characteristic respiratory variation (selective decrease with inspiration). The pulmonic component of the second heart sound becomes progressively louder, although fixed splitting persists as long as a significant left to right shunt exists. With abolition or reversal of the shunt, the pulmonic component becomes very loud, and the wide fixed split disappears. A *Graham Steell murmur* may develop. The holosystolic murmur of tricuspid regurgitation appears when the pressure load of pulmonary hypertension results in right ventricular failure. Since the right ventricle occupies the cardiac apex in atrial septal defect, the tricuspid murmur is heard at that site and can be mistaken for the murmur of mitral regurgitation.

After the third decade *atrial arrhythmias* increase, especially atrial fibrillation, but atrial flutter and paroxysmal atrial tachycardia also occur. When right atrial P waves are present, they generally manifest themselves by peaking in lead II rather than by an increase in amplitude. The QRS duration is usually upper limits of normal with a tendency to prolong with age. As QRS duration increases, the pattern resembles complete right bundle branch block, but this rarely develops before the fourth decade. Depolarization is typically clockwise, with q waves in inferior leads and a vertical QRS axis. These electrical directions are important, because they distinguish ostium secundum from ostium primum defects in which the axis is directed upward and to the left and depolarization is counterclockwise (see below).

An electrocardiographic sign of atrial septal defect is the rSr' complex in right precordial leads. This feature is believed to stem from delayed activation of the crista supraventricularis, depolarization of which causes the terminal electrical forces to be directed superiorly, to the right, and anteriorly. These terminal force patterns do not result from interference of electrical impulses through the proximal right bundle branch. In fact, the sequence of ventricular activation is normal, so the term "incomplete right bundle branch block" is inappropriate. With the advent of pulmonary hypertension, the right ventricular free wall thickens and lead V_1 exhibits an increase in the amplitude of the R' wave together with a gradual decrease in the depth of the S wave.

The *chest x-ray*, especially in postadolescents and adults, is often distinctive. The lung fields show increased pulmonary arterial vascularity that generally extends to the periphery. The combination of a small aorta and a markedly dilated pulmonary trunk with disproportionate enlargement of the right branch can be striking. With the advent of pulmonary hypertension, peripheral pulmonary vascularity is replaced by relatively clear lung fields, the pulmonary trunk and its proximal branches get still larger, and the right branch presents as a huge inverted comma with an abrupt cut-off that makes the contrast between large central vessels and clear lung field stand out in bold relief. In an occasional older subject, the main pulmonary artery and its branches dilate aneurysmally and calcify.

Right atrial enlargement is ordinarily seen as a rightward convexity in the posteroanterior projection. Although radiographic signs of left atrial enlargement are occasionally found in adults, this is rarely so in children. Dilatation of the right ventricle is an expected feature, resulting in a convex lifted apex that usually forms an acute angle with the diaphragm. Dilatation of the outflow tract sometimes causes relatively smooth continuity or even a hump-shaped appearance below the enlarged pulmonary trunk. In the left oblique projection the right ventricle casts a rather typical convex anterior shadow.

Although uncomplicated ostium secundum atrial septal defect in the young is among the most easily diagnosed congenital malformations of the heart, the same anomaly may be misleading in some adults. Mitral stenosis with pulmonary hypertension comes under suspicion because of dyspnea, orthopnea, atrial fibrillation, an increased V wave in the jugular venous pulse, a right ventricular impulse, a loud first heart sound, a delayed pulmonic component of the second sound that is mistaken for an opening snap, a tricuspid flow murmur mistaken for a mitral diastolic murmur, vascular peripheral lung fields believed to represent pulmonary venous congestion, and a cardiac silhouette that exhibits dilatation of the pulmonary trunk and occasionally of both right and left atria. Similarly, mitral regurgitation may be suspected because the holosystolic murmur of tricuspid regurgitation is heard at the apex which is occupied by the right ventricle. A delayed pulmonic component of the second sound followed by a tricuspid flow murmur may be mistaken for the opening snap and the mid-diastolic murmur of coexisting mitral stenosis. In older subjects, coronary artery disease, systemic hypertension, atrial arrhythmias, or inverted left precordial T waves may cloud the issue. A catalogue of these misleading clinical points makes impressive reading, but it is rare to be confronted with all of them at once. However, even when the entire clinical picture is considered, the correct diagnosis may remain uncertain, although clues generally emerge to provide the background for an intelligently planned laboratory study.

Echocardiography has been a major step forward in the noninvasive diagnosis of atrial septal defect, defining not only the expected large right ventricular dimensions but also paradoxical motion of the interventricular septum. Normally, the interventricular septum moves *away* from the anterior chest wall during systole, behaving as part of the left ventricle. In ostium secundum atrial septal defect (volume overload of the right ventricle), the septum moves *toward* the anterior chest wall in systole.

Cardiac catheterization is generally employed even in patients in whom the clinical diagnosis is not in doubt. Such an intervention provides precise preoperative quantitative data that set the stage for comparative postoperative assessment. In addition to quantification of the shunt and confirmation of intracardiac pressures, there are a number of other reasons why cardiac catheterization is undertaken. An attempt should be made to separate ostium secundum from sinus venosus atrial septal defects which clinically can be indistinguishable. Patients with pure ostium secundum atrial septal defects sometimes exhibit mitral leaflet prolapse. This movement can be detected by left ventricular angiography and echocardiography and need not be accompanied by auscultatory signs.

Patients with high flow, low resistance uncomplicated ostium secundum atrial septal defects (pulmonary to systemic flow ratios of 2:1 or more) should be electively repaired, optimally in childhood. At this age, surgical risk is minimal, and delay gives rise to concern over postoperative residua, especially regression of dilatation and hypertrophy of the right ventricle. There has been debate regarding surgical correction in older patients (beyond age 40), but current experience has shown that patients in the fifth, sixth, or even seventh decades with relatively low resistance–high flow ostium secundum atrial septal defects benefit from surgical repair which can be undertaken at comparatively low risk. What is still more encouraging is that older patients can be operated upon at an acceptable risk despite moderate pulmonary hypertension and cardiac failure, provided there is still a sizable left to right shunt. In patients of any age in whom pulmonary resistance has reached or exceeded systemic so that the left to right shunt has been abolished, operative repair is contraindicated.

PATENT DUCTUS ARTERIOSUS

Patent ductus arteriosus represents persistence of a normal fetal vascular channel between the pulmonary artery and the aorta. The pulmonary orifice of the ductus is located immediately to the left of the bifurcation of the pulmonary trunk. The aortic end of the duct usually arises just beyond the origin of the left subclavian artery. A patent ductus is apt to be largest at its aortic insertion, exhibiting the shape of a truncated cone, because the tendency to close begins at the pulmonary arterial end. The ductus arteriosus in full-term infants normally undergoes an initial stage of *functional* closure, followed by a later stage of *anatomic* closure. At the end of a week the ductus is generally no more than probe patent, and by four to eight weeks anatomic closure is usually established.

The physiologic consequences of persistent patency of the ductus arteriosus depend upon the size of the communication and the level of pulmonary vascular resistance. When the ductus is small, the pulmonary arterial pressure remains normal; the left to right shunt and hemodynamic burden are negligible despite continuous aortic to pulmonary flow. When the duct is large, aortic pressure is transmitted directly into the pulmonary trunk, so pulmonary hypertension exists with pressure overload of the right ventricle. Under these circumstances the direction of flow through the ductus depends upon the relative resistances in the pulmonary and systemic beds. If pulmonary resistance is appreciably lower than systemic, a sizable left to right shunt exists, with volume overload of the left heart and pressure overload of the right. If pulmonary resistance is appreciably higher than systemic, left to right flow through the ductus is abolished, leaving a pure right to left shunt and pure pressure overload of the right ventricle. The vast majority of patients with isolated patent ductus arteriosus, literally 95 per cent, have left to right shunts with pulmonary arterial pressures considerably below systemic. Only 5 to 7 per cent have very high pulmonary vascular resistances with exclusive right to left shunts.

For all practical purposes the history in patent ductus arteriosus does not begin at birth, because the diagnosis is usually not entertained in the newborn. The mother is likely to report that her infant was examined and pronounced normal. As the neonatal pulmonary vascular resistance falls, a left to right shunt is established, the ductus murmur emerges, and the diagnosis becomes apparent. Patent ductus arteriosus predominates in females, with a sex ratio as high as 3:1. The female preponderance is even greater in older patients with this anomaly. Family history is important, because patent ductus tends to recur in siblings. The prenatal history also deserves comment, especially regarding maternal rubella in the first trimester. Patent ductus arteriosus (together with pulmonary artery stenosis) is the most common congenital cardiac defect in the offspring of mothers who have had rubella in the first trimester. Birth weight in uncomplicated patent ductus is normal but in the rubella syndrome low birth rate is the rule, and there is failure to thrive even when the shunt is small and cardiac failure absent. Another interesting point in the history is the *altitude* at which the patient is born. It has been estimated that persistence of the ductus arteriosus is six times as frequent in patients born at high altitudes as in those born at sea level, and there is a tendency for such patients to develop pulmonary hypertension. The physical appearance in patent ductus may be characterized by underdevelopment owing to a large shunt, cardiac failure, and recurrent respiratory infections. In addition, maternal rubella results not only in patent ductus and low birth weights, but also in poor growth irrespective of the size of the duct. Differential cyanosis and clubbing occur when pulmonary vascular resistance exceeds systemic so that unoxygenated pulmonary arterial blood flows through the ductus and enters the aorta distal to the left subclavian artery; this unoxygenated blood goes to the lower extremities so that the toes are cyanotic and often clubbed.

A wide pulse pressure is an important physical sign of patent ductus with large left to right shunt. Diastolic flow from aortic root into pulmonary artery lowers the aortic diastolic pressure, whereas the large left ventricular stroke volume caused by the left to right shunt results in elevation of aortic systolic pressure.

Precordial impulses are normal with small patent ductus. A moderately large ductus causes isolated volume overload of the left heart; the left ventricular impulse is somewhat dynamic, the right ventricular impulse is unimpressive, and a continuous thrill with systolic accentuation is present in the first or second left intercostal space. A large ductus with appreciable left to right shunt results in marked volume overload of the left ventricle with pulmonary hypertension; the left ventricular impulse is hyperdynamic, and a heaving right ventricular impulse appears. If a thrill is present, it is more likely to be systolic. When flow through the ductus is reversed, pulmonary hypertension exists without volume overload of the left ventricle. Palpation detects right ventricular and pulmonary arterial impulses and a loud pulmonic component of the second sound, but the ductus thrill is absent and a left ventricular impulse is trivial or absent.

Auscultation is virtually diagnostic when the classic murmur of uncomplicated patent ductus arteriosus rises to a peak in latter systole, continues without interruption through the second sound, and declines in intensity during the course of diastole. High velocity flow through a small duct results in a relatively soft high-frequency continuous murmur. The larger ductus is likely to cause a loud, noisy "machinery" murmur, accentuated in latter systole and punctuated with "eddy" sounds. The ductus

murmur is typically loudest in the first or second intercostal space or just beneath the left clavicle. With progressive elevations in pulmonary vascular resistance, the classic murmur is shortened, always beginning with the diastolic portion, and is finally abolished, to be replaced by auscultatory signs of pulmonary hypertension per se. Such patients present with pulmonic ejection sounds, short pulmonic midsystolic murmurs, a single or closely split second heart sound, and a loud pulmonic component of the second sound followed by the Graham Steell murmur of pulmonary regurgitation. Under these circumstances the diagnosis of patent ductus arteriosus cannot be made on auscultatory grounds. Differential cyanosis (cyanotic toes, acyanotic fingers) may be the key.

The electrocardiogram is normal when the ductus is small. Variations depend upon the degree and duration of volume overload of the left heart and pressure overload of the right.

In the x-ray, the ductus can sometimes be seen in the frontal projection as a separate convexity between the aortic knuckle and the pulmonary trunk. In older patients calcium is occasionally identified in the ductus; this should be sought in the frontal, left oblique, and lateral projections. A large left to right shunt *without* appreciable pulmonary hypertension results in varying degrees of pulmonary plethora while the pulmonary trunk and its branches increase in size. The ascending aorta is normal in infants but tends to enlarge in older children or adults because shunt flow traverses the aortic root. Volume overload of the left heart results in left ventricular dilatation and left atrial enlargement. The increase in left atrial size is usually mild to moderate but can occasionally be marked. In infants and young children, a sizable patent ductus arteriosus with left to right shunt and pulmonary hypertension is often associated with congestive heart failure and appreciable cardiomegaly; all four chambers contribute to the cardiac silhouette.

When flow through the ductus is reversed (suprasystemic pulmonary vascular resistance), a different radiologic picture emerges. The left ventricle and the left atrium are normal in size, and the right ventricle is hypertrophied but not conspicuously dilated. The pulmonary trunk and its main branches enlarge, but the ascending aorta tends to be normal, and the peripheral pulmonary vasculature is normal or reduced.

The typical patient with uncomplicated patent ductus in childhood, adolescence, or early adult life can be confidently diagnosed clinically. However, the sick infant with congestive heart failure and large left to right shunt should be investigated preoperatively, not only to confirm the clinical suspicion of patent ductus but also to determine the presence or absence of coexisting anomalies, especially ventricular septal defect. Also requiring diagnostic investigation are patients (generally postadolescent) with increased pulmonary vascular resistance, in whom the degree of left to right shunt must be firmly established before division of the ductus is recommended.

Typical patent ductus presenting in childhood is corrected by surgical division. A number of variations in therapeutic judgment are required, however. Since patency of the ductus with *delayed* spontaneous closure is frequent in premature infants, there is a tendency to delay surgery in such patients because of the prospect of spontaneous closure within months. On the other hand, large patent ductus is a relatively common cause of congestive heart failure in acyanotic infants, and generally requires operative intervention which may take the form of ligation rather than division. After the first year of life most patients with patent ductus are asymptomatic. Division of the ductus in such patients not only carries a low risk but also results in complete anatomic and physiologic correction. The adult poses a more complex problem. The simplest decision is in the adult with a large left to right shunt, relatively low resistance patent ductus, and no ductal calcification. Operation should be advised once the diagnosis is established. Calcification of the patent ductus increases the risk, but, if the shunt is large, operation is still advisable. When pulmonary resistance has exceeded systemic, abolishing the left to right shunt, patients are inoperable. A difficult decision occurs in the occasional adult with a small hemodynamically insignificant patent ductus. The answer hinges on a comparison of the risk of infective endocarditis as opposed to the risk of surgery. Each case requires individual judgment. If there has been a previous episode of infective endocarditis and the patient expresses concern regarding recurrence, surgical correction should be advised. If there has been no previous episode of infective endocarditis and the patient is reluctant to undergo thoracotomy, operation should be deferred.

VENTRICULAR SEPTAL DEFECT WITH PULMONIC STENOSIS

(Fallot's Tetralogy)

This combination encompasses a wide anatomic, physiologic, and clinical spectrum. Two elements of the tetralogy are of prime importance, namely, pulmonic stenosis and a nonrestrictive ventricular septal defect (right ventricular pressure at systemic levels). Large ventricular septal defect with mild to moderate pulmonic stenosis is looked upon as *acyanotic* Fallot's tetralogy; large ventricular septal defect with severe pulmonic stenosis and right to left shunt as *classic cyanotic Fallot's tetralogy;* and large ventricular septal defect with complete obstruction to right ventricular outflow as *Fallot's tetralogy with pulmonary atresia*. It is wise to remain flexible, however, and use appropriate *anatomic* designations instead of, or coupled with, the eponym, to serve the cause of clarity.

In classic cyanotic Fallot's tetralogy, the aorta may be left ventricular in origin, or biventricular to varying degrees, but the posterior aortic wall maintains anatomic continuity with the anterior mitral leaflet. Pulmonic stenosis can be located in the pulmonary trunk, pulmonary valve, infundibulum, or subinfundibular zone, although typically the obstruction is infundibular. Pulmonary atresia can be viewed as the ultimate expression of pulmonic stenosis and therefore the most severe form of Fallot's tetralogy. With pulmonary atresia, the pulmonary circulation is supplied chiefly by large collateral arteries, especially bronchial.

The degree of obstruction to right ventricular outflow may progress with the passage of time. When life expectancy is prolonged by an anastomotic operation, the patient may develop progressive narrowing of the zone of stenosis culminating in complete closure (atresia). Furthermore, infundibular stenosis in acyanotic patients with sizable left to right shunting can progress

sufficiently to reverse the interventricular shunt. Accordingly, a single patient may exhibit a broad spectrum of severity ranging from mild stenosis with large left to right shunt to marked obstruction with reversed shunt.

A number of *additional congenital cardiac malformations* have a tendency to occur with Fallot's tetralogy: (1) right aortic arch, (2) persistent left superior vena cava, (3) hypoplasia, stenosis, or absence of a pulmonary artery, (4) absence of the pulmonary valve, (5) incompetence of the aortic valve, and (6) a coronary arterial anomaly consisting of origin of the left anterior descending coronary artery from the right coronary artery.

The *physiologic consequences* depend upon three variables, namely, the degree of pulmonic stenosis, the size of the interventricular communication, and, to a lesser extent, the systemic vascular resistance. These variables can best be understood by beginning with a large ventricular septal defect upon which increasing degrees of pulmonic stenosis are imposed. When the stenosis is mild, the shunt is entirely left to right, and the condition closely resembles large isolated ventricular septal defect with increased pulmonary blood flow and volume overload of the left heart. As the degree of obstruction increases, the left to right shunt diminishes. When the resistance offered by the obstruction equals systemic resistance, the shunt is balanced. As the stenosis increases still further, a right to left shunt is established because it becomes easier for the right ventricle to eject into the aorta than into the pulmonary trunk. Since right ventricular blood under these circumstances preferentially enters the aorta, circulation to the lungs is reduced and the left heart is underfilled. When the stenosis is complete (pulmonary atresia), the entire right ventricular output is ejected through the ventricular septal defect into the aorta. No matter how severe the pulmonic stenosis, the right ventricle decompresses into the aorta via the large ventricular septal defect, so right ventricular systolic pressure does not exceed systemic. The magnitude of right ventricular systolic overload is then determined by *aortic* pressure.

The *history in typical Fallot's tetralogy* generally dates from the neonatal period because of detection of a murmur or cyanosis. Arterial unsaturation is usually obvious by three to six months. When an infant is born with very severe pulmonic stenosis or atresia, cyanosis dates from birth, and the murmur is relatively inconspicuous. A history of *squatting for relief of dyspnea* has long been a hallmark of Fallot's tetralogy. In addition, Taussig clearly described the preference for certain other postures, such as the knee-chest position, sitting with the legs drawn underneath, or lying down. A history of right ventricular failure is rare in classic Fallot's tetralogy. The neonatal right ventricle is well equipped to pump at systemic pressures, and is seldom called upon to do more, because the ventricular septal defect permits direct decompression into the aorta. A number of other complications occur in the natural history, such as recurrent cerebral hypoxia that can lead to brain damage and mental retardation, cerebral venous sinus thromboses, cerebral embolism, or brain abscess. Death from brain abscess is twice as frequent in cyanotic Fallot's tetralogy as in any other form of congenital cardiac disease. Infective endocarditis sometimes occurs on the zone of pulmonic stenosis. There are two chief determinants of long survival: a degree of pulmonic stenosis that permits adequate but not excessive pulmonary blood flow with little or no cyanosis, and pulmonary stenosis that evolves gradually enough to permit the formation of a well developed collateral circulation.

After age four, most cyanotic children with congenital heart disease have Fallot's tetralogy. This malformation is also present in the largest number of *cyanotic adults* with congenital heart disease.

The physical appearance of the majority of patients with cyanotic Fallot's tetralogy is characterized by small size and physical underdevelopment. When Fallot's tetralogy occurs with little or no cyanosis, the physical appearance is generally normal.

Knowledge of the brachial arterial systolic pressure allows an accurate bedside estimate of the gradient. Since right ventricular systolic pressure is the same as systemic, the gradient across the zone of stenosis is simply the difference between the brachial arterial systolic pressure and the estimated pulmonary arterial systolic pressure (15 to 25 mm Hg).

The jugular venous pulse in classic cyanotic Fallot's tetralogy is seldom elevated; the A wave is normal or nearly so, because the right ventricle maintains its neonatal capability of ejecting at systemic pressures without extra help from its atrium.

Precordial movement and palpation in classic Fallot's tetralogy detect a relatively inconspicuous right ventricular systolic impulse that is usually located inferior to the third left intercostal space because of the stenosed infundibulum. The right ventricle ejects at systemic pressures without an appreciable increase in the vigor of contraction and without dilating. In cyanotic Fallot's tetralogy, especially in the presence of pulmonary atresia, a right aortic arch is relatively frequent, and can sometimes be suspected because of movement imparted to the right sternoclavicular junction.

The auscultatory signs mirror the pathologic physiology. The incidence of aortic ejection sounds varies inversely with the degree of obstruction; the more hypoplastic the pulmonary trunk, the larger the aortic root, and the more likely an aortic ejection sound. The systolic murmur in cyanotic Fallot's tetralogy originates at the zone of stenosis and not across the ventricular septal defect. The murmur tends to be maximal in the third left interspace, because obstruction is usually infundibular. The length and loudness of the murmur (and accompanying thrill) are of considerable importance in estimating the severity of obstruction. A loud, long murmur extending up to the aortic component of the second sound means that an appreciable amount of blood is being ejected into the pulmonary trunk. As resistance at the zone of stenosis arises, there is an increase in the right to left shunt and reciprocal fall in pulmonary blood flow; the murmur gets shorter and softer. When obstruction is complete (pulmonary atresia), the pulmonic stenotic murmur vanishes altogether and is replaced by a soft midsystolic murmur caused by ejection into the dilated aorta. A continuous murmur is an auscultatory sign of pulmonary atresia because of flow through collateral arterial circulation. The pulmonic component of the second heart sound is inaudible in cyanotic Fallot's tetralogy and pulmonary atresia, but when cyanosis is mild or absent a soft delayed sound can sometimes be detected. When a large ventricular septal defect is associated with mild pulmonic stenosis, the auscultatory signs resemble those of uncomplicated ven-

tricular septal defect, although the murmur tends to have midsystolic accentuation (a combination of the ventricular septal defect and pulmonic stenotic murmurs) and there is likely to be moderately wide splitting of the second heart sound.

The *electrocardiogram* is another useful index of the physiologic spectrum encompassed by ventricular septal defect with pulmonic stenosis. Since the force of right atrial contraction is not appreciably increased, P waves of right atrial enlargement are absent about half the time. The mean QRS axis in the frontal plane is rarely to the right of 150 degrees so that right axis deviation takes the form of a dominant S wave in lead I but dominant R waves in leads II and III. In the precordial leads, a tall monophasic R wave is usually confined to lead V_1 with rS complexes in the remaining chest leads. In left precordial leads, q waves are conspicuous by their absence in cyanotic Fallot's tetralogy, because the left ventricle is underfilled. When the shunt is balanced, right ventricular pressure remains at systemic levels, so the electrocardiogram continues to exhibit right ventricular hypertrophy as described. However, the left heart is no longer underfilled, so left precordial leads exhibit well developed R waves and small q waves. When a large ventricular septal defect exists with mild pulmonic stenosis, the electrocardiogram resembles that of isolated ventricular septal defect with right ventricular hypertension.

The *x-ray* in ventricular septal defect with pulmonic stenosis shows vascular markings that are normal or increased when a large defect exists with a balanced or left to right shunt. Severe obstruction to right ventricular outflow diverts more right ventricular blood into the aorta, so that pulmonary blood flow falls and lung vascularity diminishes. In adults, these oligemic lungs may have an emphysematous appearance. In cyanotic Fallot's tetralogy the pulmonary artery segment is characteristically represented by a *concavity*. The aortic arch size varies inversely with the pulmonary trunk. In pulmonary atresia the aorta receives the entire output from both ventricles, so the rightward sweep and knuckle are especially prominent. A right aortic arch occurs in 20 to 30 per cent of patients with cyanotic Fallot's tetralogy, the incidence increasing with the severity of pulmonic stenosis, so that a right arch is most frequent with pulmonary atresia. In cyanotic Fallot's tetralogy the left atrium and left ventricle are normal or small because the left heart is underfilled; the right atrium and right ventricle cope with systemic pressure without dilating, so the cardiac size is normal or nearly so. In pulmonary atresia, however, the cardiac silhouette tends to be larger, especially in older subjects. The configuration of the heart has long been a subject of interest in cyanotic Fallot's tetralogy because of the distinctive boot-shaped appearance caused by a combination of concentric hypertrophy of the right ventricle, an abnormally small left ventricle, a relatively horizontal ventricular septum, and a concave pulmonary artery segment. In Fallot's tetralogy with little or no cyanosis (balanced or bidirectional shunt), the right ventricle remains concentrically hypertrophied, but the left ventricle is not underfilled. The cardiac apex is more likely to be smooth and rounded. When a large ventricular septal defect exists with mild pulmonic stenosis, the x-ray in many ways resembles that of large isolated ventricular septal defect except that the size of the pulmonary trunk may be comparatively small.

The *echocardiogram* serves a useful purpose in identifying biventricular origin of the aorta and continuity between posterior aortic wall and anterior mitral leaflet. Cardiac catheterization and angiocardiography are important in characterizing the morphology of the right ventricular outflow tract, in identifying the location of the ventricular septal defect, and in ruling out right ventricular origin of both great arteries. Intracardiac repair is technically a lesser problem in the patient with large ventricular septal defect, left ventricular aorta, and acquired pulmonic stenosis, even if the stenosis is severe enough to have reversed the shunt. Large ventricular septal defect with biventricular aorta and hypoplastic right ventricular outflow tract is far more difficult to repair (classic cyanotic Fallot's tetralogy). Primary intracardiac repair (total correction) is the treatment of choice and can be accomplished even in infancy. Nevertheless, shunt operations (Waterston or Blalock) are still applied in cyanotic symptomatic infants, especially those less than one year old. A previous shunt operation adds to the risk of complete repair. Postoperative "complete right bundle branch" is expected after right ventriculotomy. The long-term effects of ventriculotomy per se and of a patch for relief of outflow obstruction are still to be assessed.

359.3. UNCOMMON CONGENITAL CARDIAC DEFECTS IN WHICH POSTPEDIATRIC SURVIVAL IS EXPECTED

SITUS INVERSUS. The term "situs inversus" refers to an organ arrangement the reverse of normal (mirror image dextrocardia). Situs inversus is often accidentally discovered on a routine chest x-ray or physical examination, because the malposition is likely to occur with an otherwise normal heart. Such patients experience normal longevity and hence fall into age groups that are susceptible to acquired cardiac disease. Pain of myocardial infarction may be referred to the *right* chest and pain of acute appendicitis to the *left* lower quadrant. Palpation and percussion identify the cardiac apex and stomach on the right and the liver on the left; the left ventricular impulse forms the apex. The heart sounds are louder in the right chest, and splitting of the second sound is detected in the second right intercostal space. The electrocardiogram shows negative P, QRS, and T waves in lead I; the complexes in lead aVR and aVL are the reverse of normal, and right precordial leads resemble those normally recorded from the left chest. The x-rays are the exact mirror image of normal, so that the viewer must identify the symbols on the film that designate left and right. The aortic arch and stomach bubble are on the right, together with the cardiac apex.

DEXTROVERSION OF THE HEART. This term applies when thoracic and abdominal viscera are in normal position but the cardiac *apex* is on the *right* (right thoracic heart). In early fetal life the cardiac apex begins on the side opposite to that which it ultimately occupies. When the apex remains on the right while the aortic arch, left atrium, and stomach are in their normal left-sided positions, the term "dextroversion" is used. Dextroversion of the heart is likely to be detected because of other congenital cardiac anomalies which almost invariably coexist. The most common of these are congenitally corrected transposition of the great arteries (see below), pulmonic stenosis, and ventricular or atrial septal defect. Palpation and percussion identify the cardiac apex and liver on the right with the stomach on the left (normal abdominal situs with right

thoracic heart). Heart sounds and murmurs are louder on the right. The electrocardiogram shows upright P waves in lead I, because the atrial situs is normal. Prominent R waves or RS complexes are recorded from the right chest, whereas the left chest leads exhibit small septal q waves and small r waves. The x-ray shows the aortic arch and stomach bubble on the left but the apex on the right; the heart retains its peculiar silhouette whether or not the film is reversed.

CONGENITAL COMPLETE HEART BLOCK. This is a straightforward diagnosis by electrocardiogram. The AV block is identified as congenital if the slow heart rate existed from infancy (or in utero) and if the QRS configuration exhibits a "supraventricular configuration," i.e., a normal sequence of ventricular excitation. If liberal use were made of the electrocardiogram in infants and children with inappropriately slow heart rates, few cases of congenital heart block would be missed. The conduction defect is generally discovered accidentally in otherwise healthy asymptomatic children, or an alert obstetrician may detect a slow fetal heart rate. The arterial pulse is inappropriately slow for age, the upstroke brisk, the pulse pressure wide, and the rhythm regular. The jugular venous pulse shows intermittent "cannon waves" (right atrial contraction against a closed tricuspid valve), with independent A waves occurring at rates faster than the carotid pulse. The left ventricular impulse is dynamic (large stroke volume). The first heart sound varies in intensity from booming to soft, and there are short midsystolic basal flow murmurs, soft intermittent fourth heart sounds, and intermittent summation sounds. The x-ray may show mild cardiac enlargement related to increased diastolic filling (slow heart rate). The slow rate, regular rhythm, intermittent cannon waves, and variation in intensity in the first heart sound constitute a diagnostic combination.

CONGENITALLY CORRECTED TRANSPOSITION OF THE GREAT ARTERIES. In this anomaly there is a right to left interchange of the ventricles and their respective AV valves. Right atrial blood flows across an AV valve that is morphologically mitral into a venous ventricle that is morphologically left, and then into the pulmonary trunk. Left atrial blood flows across an AV valve that is morphologically tricuspid into an arterial ventricle that is morphologically right, and then into the aorta. Since the pulmonary trunk springs from an anatomic left ventricle and the aorta from an anatomic right ventricle (ventriculo–great artery discordance), the term "transposition of the great arteries" is appropriate. Since right atrial blood finds it way into the pulmonary trunk (albeit across a mitral valve and through an anatomic left ventricle) and since left atrial blood finds its way into the aorta (across an anatomic tricuspid valve and through an anatomic right ventricle), the "transposition" can be considered "congenitally corrected." Hemodynamic consequences of congenitally corrected transposition depend chiefly upon the presence of *associated defects*, the most common of which are (1) incompetence of the left AV valve which is tricuspid and deformed by Ebstein's anomaly (see below), (2) ventricular septal defect, and (3) disturbances in AV conduction. Theoretically, *uncomplicated* congenitally corrected transposition (a rarity) should cause little or no physiologic disturbance. However, even when the malformation is uncomplicated, "spontaneous" failure of the systemic ventricle tends to occur before the fourth decade, although some patients live longer. The unanswered question is the durability of an anatomic right ventricle as a systemic pump, i.e., whether a right ventricle subjected to systemic work loads will fail for that reason alone.

IDIOPATHIC DILATATION OF THE PULMONARY TRUNK. This malformation is characterized by congenital dilatation of the main pulmonary artery and occasionally its branches in the absence of anatomic or physiologic cause. Patients are asymptomatic, and physical appearance, arterial pulse, and jugular venous pulse are entirely normal. Palpation of the precordium may detect a pulmonary arterial impulse but no right ventricular impulse. Auscultation discloses a characteristic pulmonic ejection sound that introduces a soft, short pulmonic midsystolic murmur and normal or exaggerated splitting of the second heart sound. The electrocardiogram is normal. The chest x-ray is also normal except for a conspicuous convexity caused by the dilated pulmonary trunk.

DISCRETE SUBVALVULAR AORTIC STENOSIS. There are two relatively common forms of discrete congenital subaortic stenosis — the tunnel, tubular or fibromuscular, and the localized fibromembranous. "Tunnel" subaortic stenosis is represented by a long narrow fibromuscular channel; the lesion is typically severe at its onset, is usually associated with hypoplasia of the aortic ring, and is seldom seen beyond childhood. Somewhat more appropriate to this discussion is the fibromembranous variety, which is characterized by a thin (1 to 2 mm), crescent-shaped fibrous membrane 2 cm or less below the aortic valve. The membrane extends across the anterior portion of the left ventricular outflow tract, each end inserting onto the anterior mitral leaflet. Fibrous thickening and mild incompetence of the aortic valve commonly coexist and are believed to result from impact of the high velocity jet from the zone of subaortic obstruction. Accordingly, this anomaly is susceptible to infective endocarditis. Fibromembranous subaortic stenosis has a relatively high incidence in the young (11 per cent of left ventricular outflow obstruction below age 15 years), but survival into or beyond the fifth decade is a rarity. Progression in severity and perhaps later transformation into fibromuscular (tunnel) and/or asymmetric septal hypertrophy apparently conspire to shorten life span, accounting for the age-related difference in prevalence in children and adults. The arterial pulse is similar to that of valvular aortic stenosis. The systolic thrill is maximal in the first or second right interspace with radiation into the neck. The left ventricular impulse is sustained, and presystolic distention with an accompanying fourth heart sound may be present. *An aortic ejection sound is typically absent.* The midsystolic stenotic *murmur* is rough and noisy, and its location and radiation correspond to the thrill. The aortic component of the second heart sound is normal or reduced; a soft early diastolic murmur of aortic regurgitation is relatively common (see above). The electrocardiogram is indistinguishable from other forms of discrete aortic stenosis. In the x-ray, the ascending aorta is usually normal, although slight to moderate poststenotic dilatation may occur.

Precise characterization of the level and degree of obstruction requires cardiac catheterization and angiocardiography. The echocardiogram is characterized by abnormal echoes within the left ventricular outflow tract, abnormal systolic movement of the aortic valve (spike plateau contour caused by rapid opening followed almost immediately by partial closure for the rest of systole), and concentric hypertrophy of the left ventricle. Discrete fibromembranous subvalvular aortic stenosis is amenable to direct surgical repair, although it should be remembered that the aortic leaflets are often distorted and that care must be taken not to damage the anterior mitral leaflet to which the subvalvular fibrous collar is attached.

SUPRAVALVULAR AORTIC STENOSIS. This malformation is typically characterized by a segmental hourglass-shaped narrowing immediately above the aortic sinuses. Occasionally there is tubular hypoplasia of the ascending aorta. Associated mental retardation is presumptive evidence that the aortic stenosis is supravalvular. Under these circumstances stenosis of the pulmonary artery and its branches almost always coexists. Physical appearance is sometimes sufficiently typical to permit these diagnoses to be entertained at a glance: small chin, large mouth, malformed teeth, abnormal bite, and retarded growth. The brachial and carotid arterial pulses may be asymmetrical, with the pulse pressure and rate of rise conspicuously greater on the right. The left ventricular impulse is similar to other forms of discrete aortic stenosis. An aortic ejection sound is absent, and the midsystolic stenotic murmur tends to be more conspicuous in the *first* right intercostal space with disproportionate radiation to the right neck. The aortic component of the second sound is normal or soft, and the murmur of aortic regurgitation is rare. The electrocardiogram is similar to that of valvular or discrete subvalvular aortic stenosis. The x-rays are distinguished by one chief feature — not only is poststenotic dilatation of the aorta absent but the ascending aorta is usually undersized. Precise diagnosis of morphology and severity requires cardiac catheterization and angiocardiography. Surgical repair, although possible, is difficult and at times untenable, as with tubular hypoplasia of the ascending aorta.

SUBVALVULAR PULMONIC STENOSIS. The location can be either infundibular or, rarely, subinfundibular. Discrete infundibular stenosis generally results from localized narrowing of the entrance to the outflow tract, beyond which the infundibulum may be somewhat dilated. Subinfundibular stenosis, a rare variety of right ventricular outflow obstruction, may be caused by hypertrophy of either abnormal muscle groups or normal bulbar muscle. Subvalvular pulmonic stenosis is uncommon as an isolated anomaly and is generally associated with ventricular septal defect. Isolated infundibular pulmonic stenosis can be suspected if the right ventricular impulse does not reach the third left interspace, if the murmur and thrill are maximal in the fourth interspace, if an ejection sound is absent, and if the x-ray shows a nondilated pulmonary trunk, a right aortic arch, and a local indentation at the site of the ostium of the infundibulum. Cardiac catheterization and angiocardiography delineate the level of obstruction, its morphologic type, and the degree of severity. It must be borne in mind that surgical correction may require right ventriculotomy, so operative risk is greater than with valvular pulmonic stenosis.

SUPRAVALVULAR PULMONIC STENOSIS (STENOSIS OF THE PULMONARY ARTERY AND ITS BRANCHES). This defect results from narrowing of the pulmonary trunk, its bifurcation, or its primary or peripheral branches; it may be unilateral or bilateral, single or multiple. Stenosis of the pulmonary artery and its branches causes hypertension in the proximal pulmonary trunk, whereas the converse is true with valvular or subvalvular obstruction. Isolated stenosis of the pulmonary artery and its branches exhibits the following features: murmurs, which may be discovered in early life but are sometimes inconspicuous or even absent in infants and young children; an occasional history of maternal rubella with low birth weight, physical and mental underdevelopment, cataracts, and deafness; familial occurrence; rarely hemoptysis from rupture of thin-walled poststenotic aneurysms; or the distinctive appearance associated with supravalvular aortic stenosis (see above). Auscultatory signs include absence of an ejection sound, normal intensity and splitting of the second heart sound, and left basal midsystolic murmurs with peripheral murmurs of nearly equal intensity in the axillae and back. X-rays show little or no dilatation of the pulmonary trunk but may reveal clusters of poststenotic dilatation of intrapulmonary vessels. Cardiac catheterization and angiocardiography establish the severity and define the anatomic pattern and distribution. Stenosis of the pulmonary artery and its branches is not currently amenable to surgical repair except in the occasional patient with isolated segmental obstruction confined to a zone within the pulmonary trunk.

CONGENITAL PULMONARY VALVE REGURGITATION. Healthy, asymptomatic individuals may be found to have cardiac murmurs and dilatation of the pulmonary trunk on routine chest x-rays. When congenital pulmonary regurgitation accompanies *idiopathic dilatation of the pulmonary trunk*, the clinical features are those of idiopathic dilatation (see above) plus the characteristic diastolic murmur described below. Regurgitation caused by *structural abnormalities of the valve itself* results in the following picture. Palpation detects a right ventricular impulse that becomes progressively more dynamic as the degree of incompetence increases. Systolic expansion of the pulmonary trunk may cause an additional impulse in the second left intercostal space. Auscultation reveals a characteristic diastolic murmur maximal in the second or third left interspace, medium to low in frequency, crescendo-decrescendo in shape, delayed in onset, short in duration, and louder during inspiration. A midsystolic pulmonic flow murmur may also be heard; the second sound can be normal or widely split and the pulmonic component soft or inaudible. The electrocardiogram is generally normal or exhibits volume overload of the right ventricle with an rSr' pattern in lead V_1. The echocardiogram should display systolic anterior motion of the ventricular septum (paradoxic septal motion due to right ventricular volume overload). The x-ray shows moderate dilatation of the pulmonary trunk and occasionally of the right ventricle.

EBSTEIN'S ANOMALY OF THE TRICUSPID VALVE. Displaced, fused, malformed portions of tricuspid valvular tissue project into the right ventricular cavity. The portion of the right ventricle underlying adherent tricuspid valvular tissue is thin and functions as a receiving chamber analogous to the right atrium (*"atrialized right ventricle"*). Abnormal function of the right heart is related to three derangements: the malformed tricuspid valve, the "atrialized" portion of right ventricle, and the reduced capacity of the pumping portion of the right ventricle. Ineffective emptying of the right atrium may result in an appreciable increase in right atrial volume and a right to left shunt through a foramen ovale or an atrial septal defect, although most patients are acyanotic. Tricuspid regurgitation caused by the malformed leaflets adds to the hemodynamic burden. However, Ebstein's anomaly is compatible with a relatively long and active life, because there is a considerable range of severity. The majority of patients survive into the second, third, or fourth decade, but fewer than 5 per cent live beyond age 50.

Ebstein's anomaly can generally be diagnosed clinically. Bouts of paroxysmal rapid heart action — especially in cyanotic subjects — raise the index of suspicion. A key to the clinical recognition of Ebstein's malformation with right to left shunt is the combination of cyanosis with normal or diminished pulmonary blood flow and a functionally dominant *left* ventricle (see Table 1). A right ventricular impulse is conspicuously lacking, although the infundibulum may be palpable. A large jugular venous V wave is lacking despite tricuspid regurgitation because of decompression in the large right atrium. The murmur of tricuspid regurgitation is either absent or early systolic, because tricuspid regurgitation occurs with normal or low right ventricular systolic pressure. The murmur is of medium frequency, tending to be maximal over the region of the displaced tricuspid valve, i.e., further toward the cardiac apex. Third and fourth heart sounds commonly cause triple or quadruple rhythms. Short mid-diastolic or presystolic murmurs occur, especially when the P-R interval is prolonged, which is often the case. Type B Wolff-Parkinson-White electrocardiograms are noteworthy, and, in the context of cyanotic congenital heart disease, are likely to mean Ebstein's anomaly. The electrocardiogram otherwise shows prominent right atrial P waves and generally right bundle branch block but no right ventricular hypertrophy. The chest x-ray may have a relatively characteristic appearance with normal or clear lung fields, small vascular pedicle, and globular cardiac silhouette caused by rightward convexity of the enlarged right atrium and leftward convexity of the infundibulum. On echocardiography, recordings are readily obtained from the large mobile anterior tricuspid leaflet. These echoes are consistently abnormal, showing marked delay in tricuspid leaflet closure as well as increased amplitude of motion and an abnormally anterior position of the leaflet throughout diastole.

CONGENITAL PULMONARY ARTERIOVENOUS FISTULA. The fistula consists either of one or more relatively large vascular trunks or of a thin aneurysmal sac or a tangle of distended tortuous vascular channels. The arterial supply is derived from one or more abnormal branches of the pulmonary artery. Drainage is almost always through anatomically recognizable dilated pulmonary veins. Such connections are truly *pulmonary* arteriovenous. The physiologic consequences depend chiefly on the amount of unoxygenated blood delivered through the right to left shunt. As a rule the shunt is sufficient to cause cyanosis but not large enough to impose a hemodynamic burden. These fistulas are usually discovered in healthy young adults who are found to have abnormal densities in routine chest x-rays or who exhibit cyanosis or hereditary hemorrhagic telangiectasia. Dyspnea and fatigue are mild even in the presence of conspicuous cyanosis. Intermittent hemoptysis may punctuate the history. Recurrent bleeding also occurs from nose, mouth, or lips (telangiectasia), and members of the family may have similar complaints. Cerebral symptoms include dizziness, vertigo, paresthesias, faintness, visual aberrations, speech disturbances, headache, extremity weakness, mental confusion, and convulsions, although the mechanisms are unclear. Physical appearance is characterized by cyanosis and clubbing, together with small ruby patches (telangiectasia) on the face, tongue, lips, skin and nail beds, and nasal or oral mucous membranes. Thoracic auscultation detects delayed systolic murmurs (or none at all), or occasionally continuous murmurs with systolic accentuation, usually located over the lower lobes or the right middle lobe. The murmurs are generally less than Grade 3 and may get louder with inspiration or Müller's maneuver and softer with expiration or Valsalva's maneuver. The lung fields show densities that are single or multiple, unilateral or bilateral, small or large, typically located in the lower lobes or right middle lobe. The opacities are homogeneous, rounded or lobulated, fairly well demarcated, and attached to the hilus by bandlike shadows that represent dilated vessels entering and leaving the fistula. The size of a mass tends to decrease with Valsalva's maneuver and to increase with Müller's maneuver. In simple terms, pulmonary arteriovenous fistula is a cause of cyanosis with normal ventricles (see Table 1). The combination of cyanosis and telangiectasia with normal electrocardiogram and normal cardiac silhouette is distinctive in its own right, and conclusive when the fistulas cause shadows in the films.

LUTEMBACHER'S SYNDROME. The eponym generally refers to a congenital atrial septal defect upon which acquired mitral stenosis is superimposed. A large atrial septal defect has an ameliorating effect upon mitral stenosis, which in turn aggravates the hemodynamic effects of the interatrial communication. Left atrial pressure is relatively low, and symptoms of pulmonary venous congestion are attenuated. Atrial fibrillation is relatively common, and the systemic arterial pulse may be small owing to a decrease in left ventricular stroke volume. The jugular venous pulse can exhibit a prominent A wave in the absence of pulmonary hypertension, because the left atrial pressure pulse is transmitted into the right atrium. The right ventricular impulse tends to be especially dynamic. Auscultation does not readily detect the telltale signs of mitral stenosis which as a rule are incomplete or absent altogether. The pulmonary flow murmur is prominent, because an especially large right ventricular stroke volume is ejected into a dilated pulmonary trunk. The electrocardiogram shows P waves of combined atrial enlargement, although left atrial P waves need not be present; evidence of right ventricular hypertrophy is common. The x-ray exhibits pulmonary plethora without pulmonary venous congestion; the right atrium and right ventricle are conspicuously dilated, and the pulmonary trunk may reach a remarkable size. Lutembacher's syndrome is more common in females, because the sex predilection exists for both isolated atrial septal defect and isolated mitral stenosis. The echocardiogram is useful in identifying both volume overload of the right ventricle (systolic anterior motion of the ventricular septum) *and* mitral stenosis (slow EF slope and diastolic anterior motion of the posterior mitral leaflet). Lutembacher's syndrome is amenable to complete intracardiac repair.

COMMON ATRIUM. This relatively rare variety of interatrial communication is the result of complete or virtual absence of the atrial septum. The right-sided portion of the common chamber has anatomic features of a *right* atrium and receives both venae cavae and the coronary sinus. The left-sided portion has anatomic features of a *left* atrium and receives the pulmonary veins. Absence of the septum means that the septum primum is deficient, so that elements of the endocardial cushion malformation coexist, especially a cleft anterior mitral leaflet with or without regurgitation. The physical appearance of the Ellis–van Creveld syndrome heightens suspicion. The clinical picture resembles large atrial septal defect, with the following exceptions: (1) symptoms begin earlier and are generally

more severe; (2) cyanosis exists without sufficient pulmonary hypertension to account for its presence; (3) the physical signs are those of atrial septal defect in which a large left to right shunt persists despite the presence of cyanosis (cyanosis with shunt vascularity; see Table 1); (4) the P wave axis tends to shift leftward, because there is absence of the upper or sinus venosus portion of the atrial septum with absence of a right sinus node); the QRS shows left axis deviation resembling endocardial cushion defect; and (5) the chest x-ray resembles a large atrial septal defect in which pulmonary arterial blood flow is increased even though cyanosis is present. Common atrium can be surgically corrected, more readily if mitral regurgitation is trivial or absent.

CONGENITAL CORONARY ARTERIOVENOUS FISTULA. Both coronary arteries arise from the aorta, but a fistulous branch of one communicates directly with a cardiac chamber or the pulmonary trunk. The right coronary artery is more frequently involved than the left. However, the *drainage* site is of greater clinical importance than the vessel of origin. Ninety per cent of coronary arterial fistulas drain into the right heart (arteriovenous). Most of these enter the right atrium, coronary sinus, or right ventricle, whereas relatively few enter the pulmonary trunk. Congenital coronary arteriovenous fistula should be considered when an asymptomatic acyanotic child or young adult is found to have an atypically located precordial continuous murmur that is relatively soft and "superficial"; the suspicion is heightened when the murmur does not peak around the second heart sound but instead is louder in either systole or diastole. The precordial location is determined by the chamber or vessel that receives the fistula and not by the vessel of origin. In young patients with small fistulas, an "atypical" continuous murmur is likely to be the only clinical abnormality. Larger flows acting over longer periods of time can result in the following pictures. When the fistula enters the *right atrium* or *coronary sinus*, precordial palpation detects both left and right ventricular impulses; the continuous murmur tends to be louder in systole and maximal along the right sternal border, over the lower sternum, or close to the lower left sternal edge; volume overload of both ventricles may be seen in the electrocardiograms; the x-ray shows increased pulmonary arterial flow. When the communication drains into the body of the *right ventricle*, palpation detects right and left ventricular impulses; the continuous murmur is louder in either systole or diastole and is maximal along the mid to lower left sternal border or subxiphoid area; volume overload of both ventricles may be seen in the electrocardiogram; the x-rays exhibit increased pulmonary arterial flow. When the pulmonary artery receives the fistula, palpation detects only a left ventricular impulse; the continuous murmur is usually indistinguishable from patent ductus arteriosus in both configuration and location; volume overload of the left ventricle may appear in the electrocardiogram; the x-ray may show increased pulmonary arterial flow. Coronary AV fistulas should be surgically ablated to abolish the left to right shunt, to eliminate the risk of infective endocarditis, and to channel coronary blood flow into the capillary circulation.

CONGENITAL ANEURYSMS OF THE SINUSES OF VALSALVA. Sinuses of Valsalva are three small dilatations in the wall of the aorta immediately above the attachments of each aortic cusp. More than 90 per cent of congenital aneurysms originate in the right or noncoronary sinus and project into the right ventricle or right atrium. The typical aneurysm begins as a blind pouch or diverticulum; the entire sinus is not dilated, but instead the aneurysm projects as a finger-like or nipple-like extension with a perforation at its tip. Acute rupture of a large aneurysm creates a dramatic clinical picture; a previously healthy young adult, generally male, develops sudden chest pain, dyspnea, a loud continuous murmur, bounding arterial pulse, and relentless cardiac failure that follows a period of temporary improvement. The arterial pulse resembles that of aortic regurgitation; the jugular venous pulse is elevated, and dynamic biventricular impulses are palpable. The continuous murmur is maximal below the third intercostal space along the right or left sternal border or over the lower sternum. The murmur is usually louder in either systole or diastole and does not peak around the second heart sound as in patent ductus. The electrocardiogram is likely to show biatrial P waves and left ventricular or combined ventricular hypertrophy. The chest x-ray displays increased pulmonary arterial flow which may be obscured by pulmonary venous congestion, dilatation of both ventricles, and enlargement of the right and occasionally the left atrium. Small perforations sometimes progress slowly and at first go unnoticed. Such patients come to attention because continuous murmurs are detected. Occasionally, unruptured aneurysms announce themselves by to-and-fro or diastolic murmurs, or because of heart block or myocardial ischemia resulting from coronary arterial compression by the aneurysm.

Cardiac catheterization and angiocardiography are usually definitive. Ruptured congenital aneurysms of the sinuses of Valsalva are amenable to complete correction by relatively simple intracardiac repair.

VENA CAVAL TO LEFT ATRIAL CONNECTION. Isolated drainage of a vena cava into the left atrium is a rare anomaly, but its presence can be suspected with a high degree of accuracy. The malformation is a form of *cyanotic* congenital heart disease *without* right ventricular hypertrophy (see Table 1). Cyanosis dates from early life, but cardiac symptoms are absent or nearly so. A right ventricular impulse is absent, whereas the left ventricle is normal or slightly thrusting. There are no significant murmurs. The electrocardiogram is usually normal but occasionally exhibits left ventricular hypertrophy. The x-ray reveals a normal cardiac silhouette, normal or diminished pulmonary blood flow, and perhaps the shadow of a persistent left superior vena cava.

359.4. COMMON CONGENITAL CARDIAC DEFECTS IN WHICH POSTPEDIATRIC SURVIVAL IS EXCEPTIONAL

VENTRICULAR SEPTAL DEFECT. The most common variety of ventricular septal defect lies below and posterior to the crista supraventricularis in the region of the membranous septum. Variations in both location and size of ventricular septal defects deserve special comment. The normal growth of the heart is most rapid in the first two years of life, during which the defect remains about the same in size or enlarges less rapidly than the rest of the heart. Accordingly, there is a tendency for the *relative* size of the defect to diminish. This tendency ideally results in complete spontaneous closure. Ventricular septal defects are

seldom seen after the fourth decade, not because patients have succumbed but probably because their communications have spontaneously closed or diminished to the point that they are clinically unrecognizable. The physiologic consequences of an isolated ventricular septal defect depend chiefly upon its size and the pulmonary vascular resistance. Both variables may change with time, and the physiologic and clinical manifestations will vary accordingly. A small defect causes little or no functional disturbance, because the shunt is negligible and the pressures in the right heart are normal. With moderately large defects, the left to right shunt increases and, up to a point, occurs with little or no elevation in pulmonary arterial pressure. In such patients the physiologic derangements are essentially due to volume overload of the left heart. A large defect (nonrestrictive) results in equalization of systolic pressures in the two ventricles. The amount of flow into the pulmonary and systemic beds then depends upon their relative vascular resistances. Three regulatory mechanisms affect the volume and direction of the interventricular shunt and the level of pulmonary arterial pressure in infants born with large ventricular septal defects: first, the pattern taken by the pulmonary vascular resistance; second, the relative decrease in size that the defect undergoes, especially in the first two years of life; and third, the development of obstruction to right ventricular outflow, i.e., acquired infundibular pulmonic stenosis.

A *small ventricular septal defect* is ordinarily suspected because of a prominent holosystolic parasternal murmur in a patient in whom cardiac evaluation is otherwise normal. The murmur is generally absent at birth but is readily detected at the first well-baby examination. With passage of time, if the size of the defect decreases, the holosystolic murmur becomes shorter, softer, and higher pitched and is early systolic prior to complete closure. Similarly, *very small defects* are associated with soft, localized high frequency early systolic murmurs. *Large ventricular septal defects* with appreciable left to right shunts cause congestive heart failure in infancy, with retarded growth and development (failure to thrive), diaphoresis, poor feeding, and recurrent lower respiratory infections. Physical examination reveals hyperdynamic biventricular impulses, a harsh holosystolic left parasternal murmur accompanied by a thrill, an apical mid-diastolic flow murmur, and normal or wide splitting of the second heart sound with a relatively prominent pulmonic component. The electrocardiogram exhibits biatrial and biventricular hypertrophy with volume overload of the left ventricle. The x-ray shows pulmonary plethora, a large pulmonary trunk, a normal ascending aorta, dilatation of both ventricles, and often dilatation of the left and right atria as well. Spontaneous improvement is related to a reduction in left to right shunt caused by a decrease in the size of the defect, especially in the first year, by an increase in pulmonary vascular resistance, or by acquired infundibular stenosis (see above).

In *large ventricular septal defect with reversed shunt (Eisenmenger's complex)*, cyanosis ordinarily dates from childhood but not from birth. Effort dyspnea occurs without left ventricular failure. The jugular venous pulse is usually normal and the precordium quiet, with moderate right ventricular and pulmonary arterial impulses. There are auscultatory signs of pulmonary hypertension but *no murmur of ventricular septal defect*. The electrocardiogram shows right ventricular hypertrophy with little or no evidence of volume overload of the left heart. The x-ray exhibits normal or decreased pulmonary vasculature, a relatively normal cardiac silhouette, moderate dilatation of the pulmonary trunk, and normal aortic arch (see Table 1).

In patients with typical small ventricular septal defects, the clinical diagnosis is so evident and the physiologic consequences so benign that cardiac catheterization and angiocardiography are not necessary; such patients should be followed expectantly. They are, however, at risk of infective endocarditis. Patients with *large* ventricular septal defects and pulmonary hypertension (nonrestrictive defects) require investigation to establish the magnitude of left to right shunt and pulmonary vascular resistance, the location of the defect or defects, and the absence or presence of coexisting anomalies.

Large ventricular septal defect with congestive heart failure in infancy is a special problem that will not be dealt with here. Beyond infancy, patients with ventricular septal defects and pulmonary to systemic flow ratios in excess of 1.7:1 should have elective correction. If the pulmonary to systemic flow ratio is less than 1.5:1 because the defect is small, the benign functional consequences do not warrant the risk of operative repair. If a similar flow ratio is the result of *high pulmonary resistance* with *large* ventricular septal defect, operative risk is high and results are poor, because little or no beneficial effect on the pulmonary resistance follows elimination of such a small shunt.

VENTRICULAR SEPTAL DEFECT WITH AORTIC REGURGITATION. The murmur of the ventricular defect is usually known from infancy. Between the ages of three and eight years a *new* murmur appears, together with the gradual development of bounding arterial pulses and a dynamic left ventricular impulse. The combined murmurs are *not* continuous but are holosystolic and early diastolic. The electrocardiogram and x-ray show left ventricular hypertrophy and enlargement out of proportion to the estimated size of the left to right shunt. As time goes on, the ventricular septal defect may decrease in size while the aortic regurgitation progressively worsens. Survival to adult life occurs, although cardiac failure eventually develops because of the volume of regurgitation.

ENDOCARDIAL CUSHION DEFECT. The endocardial cushions of the embryo contribute to the development of the mitral and tricuspid valves and to the growth and convergence of the atrial and ventricular septa. Defects therefore include varying combinations of anomalies in these four contiguous parts of the heart. Three general categories are recognized, namely, complete endocardial cushion defect, partial or incomplete endocardial cushion defect, and transitional forms. In the complete variety, separate atrioventricular valves do not exist as such. There is a common AV valve lying in a canal formed by an atrial septal defect above and a ventricular septal defect below. The partial or incomplete form is represented by an ostium primum atrial septal defect and a cleft mitral valve. Transitional forms represent intermediates between complete and partial endocardial cushion defects. Less commonly, any one of the four component lesions occurs as a clinically isolated anomaly. The physiologic consequences depend upon the presence and degree of the various combinations of the four anatomic components. The following remarks will relate to partial endocardial cushion defects in which postpediatric survival is possible.

An ostium primum atrial septal defect with cleft mitral valve occurs more frequently in females than males. The physical signs resemble ostium secundum atrial septal defect except that the left ventricle occupies the apex and is accompanied by the holosystolic murmur of mitral regurgitation. Congestive heart failure may begin in childhood, especially when marked mitral regurgitation exists with a large left to right shunt. Growth and development are poor and lower respiratory infections frequent. If mitral regurgitation is relatively mild and the left to right shunt moderate, symptoms may be delayed for one or two decades. The incompetent left atrioventricular valve is susceptible to infective endocarditis. Mongolism occurs, but not so frequently as with transitional or complete endocardial cushion defects. The electrocardiogram is important, because the frontal plane exhibits counterclockwise depolarization with left axis deviation; precordial leads show the rSr' pattern of expected volume overload of the right ventricle. In persistent ostium primum with cleft but competent mitral valve, this electrocardiogram is the only distinguishing clinical feature from ostium secundum defect.

The most important laboratory study in identifying endocardial cushion defect is a left ventricular angiocardiogram in the frontal projection which shows a characteristic "goose neck" deformity of the outflow tract caused by the cleft anterior mitral cusp and its abnormal chordal arrangements. The echocardiogram is likely to show displacement of the anterior mitral leaflet into the left ventricular outflow tract with prolonged diastolic apposition to the left side of the ventricular septum. Surgical repair in partial endocardial cushion defect is complicated chiefly by the degree of mitral regurgitation rather than the presence of the atrial septal defect.

TRICUSPID ATRESIA. In this disorder tricuspid valvular tissue cannot be identified. A small imperforate dimple is found on the floor of the right atrium, but no direct connection exists between right atrium and right ventricle. The only outlet for the right atrium is an interatrial communication which can take the form of a fossa ovale or an atrial septal defect. Variations beyond the mitral valve form the basis of Edwards' anatomic classification from which physiologic inferences can be drawn and clinical manifestations of tricuspid atresia understood. According to this classification, tricuspid atresia occurs either with or without transposition of the great arteries and, in each of these two categories with no pulmonic stenosis, with pulmonic stenosis, or with pulmonary atresia. Given an adequate interatrial communication, pulmonary blood flow is the chief determinant of longevity. Life expectancy is greatest when pulmonic stenosis of just the right degree exists so that blood flow to the lungs is favorably regulated. When the great arteries are normally related, the subpulmonic obstruction is generally marked, and most patients die in the first year. Nevertheless, occasional examples of survival have been recorded from the second through the fifth decade, with one exceptional survival to age 57. When the great arteries are *transposed*, pulmonic stenosis is more likely to permit longer survival. Sporadic patients in this category have lived into the second, third, and fourth decades, and one died at age 56. The key to the clinical diagnosis of tricuspid atresia is the presence of cyanosis, normal or diminished pulmonary blood flow, and a dominant left ventricle (see Table 1). The electrocardiogram shows right atrial P waves with left axis deviation and adult progression of the QRS in the precordial leads. Definitive diagnosis is achieved by angiocardiography. Palliative surgery is possible through (1) creation of an atrial septal defect in those patients with a foramen ovale, or (2) a shunt operation to improve pulmonary blood flow.

In addition, blood from the right atrium has been directed through a conduit to the pulmonary artery, permitting the right atrium to act as a pumping chamber for the pulmonary circulation.

COMPLETE TRANSPOSITION OF THE GREAT ARTERIES. According to Elliott and Edwards: "In complete transposition, there are two ventricles. . . . The aorta, with the coronary arteries arising from it, takes origin from the right ventricle, while the pulmonary trunk takes origin exclusively from the left ventricle. Both atrioventricular valves are patent and have the corresponding structure of the right and left sided atrioventricular valves of the normal heart. The connections of the systemic, pulmonary and coronary veins are normal." Survival in complete transposition requires the presence of some means of blood exchange between the pulmonary and systemic circulations which exist in parallel rather than in series. The term "transposition" is best applied to hearts exhibiting ventriculo–great artery discordance, i.e., each great artery arises separately from an anatomically inappropriate ventricle (pulmonary artery–left ventricle; aorta–right ventricle). Connections between the greater and lesser circulations may take the form of an interatrial communication, ventricular septal defect, or patent ductus arteriosus. As a general rule, complete transposition of the great arteries is a congenital cardiac anomaly that exists with *cyanosis* and *increased* pulmonary blood flow (see Table 1). The large majority of patients die within the first year, often within the first months. Isolated examples of unusual longevity have been recorded into the second, third, or fourth decade; one patient aged 56 years at autopsy was believed to have complete transposition. Definitive diagnosis is by angiocardiography. Two physiologic corrective operations are currently applied. The Mustard operation redirects venous inflows, whereas the Rastelli operation achieves redirection of ventricular outflows.

359.5. UNCOMMON CONGENITAL CARDIAC DEFECTS IN WHICH POSTPEDIATRIC SURVIVAL IS EXCEPTIONAL

Anomalous origin of the left coronary artery from the pulmonary trunk is characterized by normal origin of the right coronary artery from the aorta and anomalous origin of the left coronary artery (LCA) from the pulmonary trunk. The aberrant left coronary artery is relatively small and thin walled, resembling a venous channel, whereas the right coronary artery is dilated and tortuous, especially in patients who survive childhood. Myocardial ischemia is a serious problem. The ischemic derangement is not due to the fact that only *one* coronary artery originates from the aorta, but is due instead to direct flow from the right coronary artery to the LCA through intercoronary anastomoses which bypass the capillary bed. Thus the anomalous left coronary artery distributes blood *into* the pulmonary trunk but does not receive blood from it.

In the natural history of this anomaly, three general patterns emerge: serious symptoms in early infancy with death before one year; early illness followed by improvement so that by childhood symptoms may be absent or nearly so; and absence or virtual absence of early symptoms with survival into adulthood. About 15 to 20 per cent of individuals with anomalous origin of the LCA reach adulthood; relatively few survive through the fourth decade, although one of the first known patients with this anomaly was a 50-year-old woman. The intercoronary anastomoses often result in a continuous murmur, and the myocardial ischemia results in papillary muscle dysfunction with mitral regurgitation. The electrocardiogram is important, because at a relatively early age deep Q waves appear in leads I and aVL. Definitive diagnosis is by cardiac catheterization and aortography or selective right coronary arteriography. A left to right shunt from right coronary through intercoronary anastomoses to anomalous LCA into the pulmonary trunk is identified. Selective coronary arteriography (injection into the right coronary) traces this pathway and provides specific anatomic diagnosis. Two surgical interventions have been applied. In infancy, ligation of the anomalous left coronary artery interrupts retrograde flow and improves capillary circulation. In older children or adults, the left subclavian artery or the internal mammary artery or a saphenous vein graft can be directly anastomosed to the left coronary artery, which is then ligated at its origin from the pulmonary trunk.

Cor triatriatum is characterized by drainage of the pulmonary veins into an accessory left atrial chamber that lies proximal to the true left atrium. The distal compartment communicates with the mitral valve and contains the left atrial appendage and the fossa ovalis. The fibrous or fibromuscular diaphragm that partitions the left atrium harbors one or more openings, the size of which determines the degree of left atrial obstruction. Cor triatriatum is therefore a congenital anomaly that is acyanotic without a shunt, with the malformation originating in the left heart (see Table 1). Severe cor triatriatum is ordinarily detected in infants or young children, but symptoms may not begin until adolescence or adulthood. Patients with mild obstruction may be entirely asymptomatic. The functional consequences are analogous to mitral stenosis with elevated pulmonary venous and pulmonary arterial pressures. However, the auscultatory signs of mitral stenosis are lacking, and enlargement of the left atrial appendage is absent, because that structure is in the distal low pressure compartment. It is wise to consider cor triatriatum in postadolescents with clinical signs of obstruction to left atrial flow but without signs of mitral stenosis. The diagnosis is materially assisted by echocardiography that detects a nonstenotic mitral valve, and by angiocardiography which, with pulmonary arterial injection of contrast material, defines the zone of obstruction as dye opacifies the left heart. Surgical intervention can completely remove the partition and relieve the left atrial obstruction.

Total anomalous pulmonary venous connection (TAPVC) is a condition in which all venous blood from both lungs enters the right atrium directly or through one of its tributary veins. The four anomalously connecting pulmonary veins emerge individually from the lungs and either enter the right atrium directly or, more often, unite in the mediastinum to form a confluence which joins the right atrium via (1) the coronary sinus, (2) an anomalous vertical vein or left superior vena cava, that connects the left innominate vein to the right superior vena cava, or (3) the right superior vena cava directly or via the azygos vein. In the right atrium, there is mixing of systemic and pulmonary venous blood, part of which enters the left heart via an atrial septal defect and most of which enters the right ventricle and low-resistance pulmonary bed. Accordingly,

TAPVC is classified as a cyanotic congenital anomaly with increased pulmonary arterial blood flow (see Table 1). The clinical picture in many ways resembles isolated atrial septal defect with large left to right shunt except for cyanosis which varies from subtle to marked. However, the patient is likely to be male, and symptoms generally begin in early childhood, although some individuals reach adult life with surprisingly little disability. The jugular venous pulse may exhibit a large A wave because of pulmonary hypertension. Palpation and auscultation are similar to atrial septal defect with large left to right shunt, but signs of pulmonary hypertension are more likely to coexist. Similarly, the electrocardiogram shows right atrial and right ventricular hypertrophy. The x-ray resembles atrial septal defect with large left to right shunt, but there is one distinctive picture. When the pulmonary veins communicate with the left innominate vein via a left vertical vein, the heart may exhibit a "figure of 8" appearance. The upper part of the figure of 8 is the left vertical vein on the left and the dilated right superior vena cava on the right. The lower part is the cardiac silhouette itself, i.e., dilated right atrium and right ventricle.

Diagnosis is established by cardiac catheterization and angiocardiography; the latter defines the specific connecting pathways. Echocardiography is similar to a large shunt ostium secundum atrial septal defect. Surgical correction is achieved, especially when the confluence of pulmonary veins can be anastomosed directly to the left atrium and the vascular channel to the systemic venous bed divided.

Right ventricular origin of both great arteries and "double outlet right ventricle" are synonymous terms for a congenital malformation in which the pulmonary artery arises in its normal position but the aorta arises wholly from the right ventricle. A ventricular septal defect provides the left ventricle with its only outlet. Pulmonary stenosis may or may not coexist. Right ventricular origin of both great arteries can exist with a ventricular septal defect above or below the crista supraventricularis. In double outlet right ventricle with infracristal ventricular septal defect and no pulmonic stenosis, two steps help in clinical diagnosis. The first step involves recognition of large ventricular septal defect with left to right shunt and pulmonary hypertension. Since both great arteries originate from the right ventricle, pulmonary arterial pressure is by definition systemic. It is a good rule to consider double outlet right ventricle in all patients who present with the picture of large left to right shunt pulmonary hypertensive ventricular septal defect. The second step in the clinical diagnosis consists of recognizing a QRS that exhibits left axis deviation and counterclockwise depolarization. The clinical diagnosis depends chiefly on left axis deviation in the presence of a pulmonary hypertensive ventricular septal defect with a large left to right shunt. Favorable adjustments in pulmonary vascular resistance sometimes regulate pulmonary blood flow so that, even though increased, it is not excessive. Under these circumstances longevity is improved; patients occasionally survive into young adulthood, and one underwent successful surgical correction at 53 years of age.

In right ventricular origin of both great arteries with supracristal ventricular septal defect, the defect lies just beneath the pulmonary valve (subpulmonic). This anomaly, called *Taussig-Bing complex,* is a diagnostic consideration in patients with *increased* pulmonary blood flow and *cyanosis* from birth or early infancy. Radiologic, electrocar-diographic, and physical signs of pulmonary hypertension are obligatory. In the presence of patent ductus arteriosus (which often coexists) and high pulmonary vascular resistance, a distinctive type of reversed differential cyanosis occurs in which the toes are less cyanotic than the fingers, because oxygenated blood from the left ventricle is ejected into the pulmonary trunk and then through the ductus into the descending aorta, whereas unsaturated right ventricular blood is ejected into the aortic root and brachiocephalic vessels. It is a good rule to consider the Taussig-Bing anomaly in patients who appear to have Eisenmenger's complex but in whom cyanosis dates from birth or early infancy.

Right ventricular origin of both great arteries occurs with all grades of pulmonic stenosis (mild to severe to complete, i.e., pulmonary atresia). The ventricular septal defect is usually infracristal if pulmonic stenosis coexists. Double outlet right ventricle with mild to moderate pulmonic stenosis resembles ordinary large ventricular septal defect with equivalent pulmonic stenosis except for the electrocardiogram, which may exhibit counterclockwise depolarization with left axis deviation (see above).

Right ventricular origin of both great arteries with severe pulmonic stenosis closely resembles cyanotic Fallot's tetralogy and should be considered whenever the clinical diagnosis of cyanotic Fallot's tetralogy is entertained. Clinical distinction between the two is difficult, although some points favor double outlet right ventricle: (1) auscultatory evidence of a holosystolic murmur at the lower left sternal edge despite the presence of cyanosis (obligatory left to right shunt through the ventricular septal defect); (2) palpable left ventricular impulse in this context; and (3) electrocardiogram showing small q waves in leads I and aVL and relatively broad slurred S waves in leads I, aVL, and V_{5-6}. The echocardiogram may assist by identifying lack of continuity between the posterior aortic wall and anterior mitral leaflet, because in double outlet right ventricle there is no continuity between the anterior mitral leaflet and the wall of *either* artery. Definitive diagnosis is angiographic. Corrective surgery is technically feasible, although complex.

Truncus arteriosus is a congenital anomaly in which a single great artery leaves the base of the heart through a single semilunar valve. The truncus is situated just above a ventricular septal defect, receives blood from both ventricles, and gives rise to the coronary arteries and to the pulmonary and systemic circulations. No remnant of a second semilunar valve is present. Truncus arteriosus with large pulmonary arteries occurs with cyanosis and pulmonary plethora (see Table 1). Both pulmonary branches may arise from a common short pulmonary artery that emerges from the truncus, or the two branches may arise directly from the truncus.

The outlook is better when the pulmonary arteries are moderately stenotic at their truncal origins, advantageously controlling pulmonary blood flow and delaying death from cardiac failure. Occasional patients with favorably regulated pulmonary circulations have survived into the third or fourth decade, and one died at the age of 43 years. However, postpediatric survival is rare, especially with truncus arteriosus and large unobstructed pulmonary arteries.

Definitive diagnosis of truncus arteriosus is by angiocardiography. Physiologic correction is feasible, employing an operation which joins the two pulmonary arteries to the outflow of the right ventricle with a conduit.

Single ventricle refers to a congenital anomaly in which there are two atria but only one anatomic ventricular chamber that receives both the mitral and tricuspid valves. The usual type is a morphologic left ventricle or primitive ventricle with a small outlet chamber that represents the infundibular portion of the right ventricle. The infundibulum is a subdivision of the single ventricle, not a separate ventricular chamber. The great arteries are almost always transposed. If the infundibulum is situated at the right basal aspect of the heart, this arrangement is called "noninversion"; if the infundibulum is situated at the left basal aspect of the heart (corresponding to its expected location with congenitally corrected transposition), this arrangement is termed "inversion." Pulmonic stenosis may or may not coexist. Single ventricle without pulmonic stenosis occurs with increased pulmonary blood flow, and hence is an anomaly exhibiting cyanosis with pulmonary plethora (see Table 1). In single ventricle with high pulmonary vascular resistance, cyanosis is conspicuous and pulmonary blood flow normal or diminished (see Table 1). Single ventricle with pulmonic stenosis is an anomaly exhibiting cyanosis with normal or diminished pulmonary blood flow (see Table 1).

Survival depends chiefly upon a favorable balance between resistances to flow into the pulmonary trunk and aorta. Although the average patient dies in childhood, survival into adolescence or early adult life is not rare. The natural history occasionally extends into the third, fourth, or even fifth decade, with one survival to age 56 years. Moderate pulmonic stenosis without aortic obstruction favors longevity. Definitive diagnosis depends upon cardiac catheterization and angiocardiography, although precatheterization diagnoses are accomplished with a high degree of accuracy. On echocardiography, separate AV valves (tricuspid and mitral) are simultaneously recorded *without* an intervening septal echo. On a base to apex scan, there is absence of the ventricular septal echo in any of its expected locations. Surgical intervention is palliative, and consists of either banding the pulmonary trunk to limit pulmonary plethora or providing a shunt operation to improve pulmonary blood flow in patients with critical pulmonic stenosis or atresia.

de la Cruz, M. Z., Anselmi, G., Romero, A., and Monroy, G.: A quantitative and qualitative study of the ventricles and great vessels of normal children. Am. Heart J., 60:675, 1960.

Edwards, J. E., Carey, L. S., Neufeld, H. N., and Lester, R. G.: Congenital Heart Disease. Philadelphia, W. B. Saunders Company, 1965.

Feigenbaum, H.: Echocardiography. 2nd ed. Philadelphia, Lea & Febiger, 1976.

Gault, J. H., Morrow, A. G., Gay, W. A., and Ross, J., Jr.: Atrial septal defect in patients over age 40 years. Clinical and hemodynamic studies and the effects of operation. Circulation, 37:261, 1968.

Higgins, C. B., and Mulder, D. G.: Tetralogy of Fallot in the adult. Am. J. Cardiol., 29:837, 1972.

Higgins, I. T.: The epidemiology of congenital heart disease. J. Chronic Dis., 18:699, 1965.

Maron, B. J., Humphries, J. O., Rowe, R. D., and Mellits, E. D.: Prognosis of surgically corrected coarctation of the aorta. A 20-year postoperative followup. Circulation, 47:119, 1973.

Mitchell, S. C., Korones, S. B., and Berends, H. W.: Congenital heart disease in 56,109 births. Circulation, 43:323, 1971.

Morganroth, J., Perloff, J. K., Zeldes, S. M., and Dunkman, W. B.: Acute severe aortic regurgitation. Ann. Intern. Med., 87:223, 1977.

Nadas, A. S., and Flyer, D. C.: Pediatric Cardiology. 3rd ed. Philadelphia, W. B. Saunders Company, 1972.

Nora, J. J.: Multifactorial inheritance hypothesis for the etiology of congenital heart disease. Circulation, 38:604, 1968.

Perloff, J. K.: Pediatric congenital cardiac becomes a postoperative adult. The changing population of congenital heart disease. Circulation, 47:606, 1973.

Perloff, J. K.: The Clinical Recognition of Congenital Heart Disease. 2nd ed. Philadelphia. W. B. Saunders Company, 1978.

Perloff, J. K.: Postpediatric congenital heart disease: Natural survival patterns. Cardiovasc. Clin., in press.

Polani, P. E., and Campbell, M.: An aetiological study of congenital heart disease. Ann. Hum. Genet., 19:209, 1955.

Roberts, W. C.: The congenitally bicuspid aortic valve. Am. J. Cardiol., 26:72, 1970.

Rudolph, A. B.: Changes in the circulation after birth. Their importance in congenital heart disease. Circulation, 41:343, 1970.

360. ACQUIRED VALVULAR HEART DISEASE

John Ross, Jr.

360.1. INTRODUCTION

Before considering the characteristic features and treatment of each acquired valvular heart lesion, it will be useful to consider broad differences in the physiologic effects of these lesions and to suggest a general diagnostic approach to the patient with valvular heart disease. It will also be worthwhile to discuss the indications for cardiac catheterization, as well as the general considerations that enter into a decision to recommend surgical treatment.

GENERAL PHYSIOLOGIC EFFECTS OF VALVULAR HEART DISEASE

The consequences of stenosis or regurgitation of the heart valves may be considered in relation to their direct effects on the cardiac chamber that must compensate for the valvular lesion by undergoing hypertrophy or dilatation, and their secondary effects on intravascular pressures and blood flow in the aorta, pulmonary vascular bed, and systemic veins. When a semilunar valve of the heart (aortic or pulmonic) is stenotic or regurgitant, or when an atrioventricular valve (mitral or tricuspid) is regurgitant, the primary burden is placed upon the adjacent *ventricle*. With aortic stenosis and regurgitation, important secondary effects occur in the aortic pressure pulses, and with mitral regurgitation there are major secondary effects on the pulmonary venous bed. When an atrioventricular valve is stenotic, the primary burden is placed on the *atrium*, and secondary effects are prominent on the adjacent venous bed; in tricuspid stenosis, for example, there are right atrial overload and secondary elevation of pressure in the systemic veins. These general consequences of stenotic and regurgitant valvular lesions are summarized in Figure 1.

Aortic stenosis places an overload on the left ventricle during systole, a pressure gradient being developed to overcome the obstruction at the aortic valve (see Fig. 1). This leads to progressive hypertrophy of the left ventricular wall without an increase in chamber volume. Aortic regurgitation, in contrast, places a volume overload on the left ventricle during diastole. This leads to an augmented forward stroke volume into the aorta which, in turn, causes a substantial increase in the systolic pressure in the aorta and left ventricle, an increase

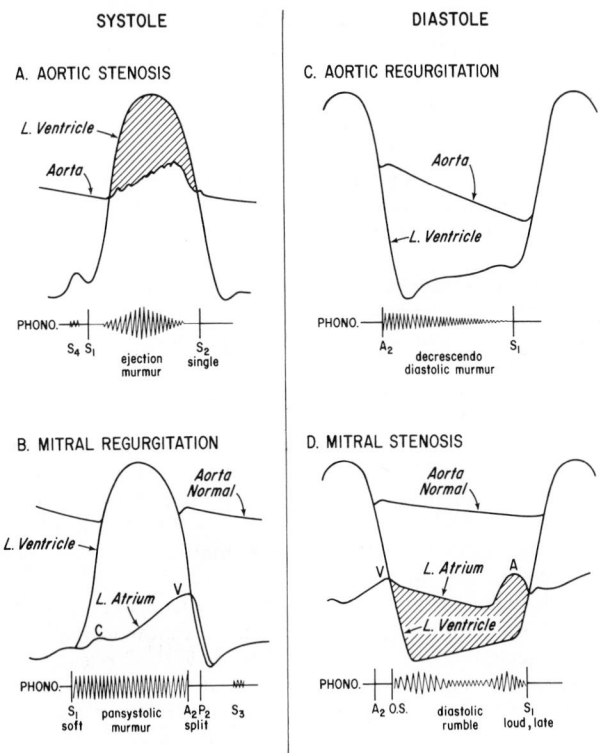

SYSTOLE | DIASTOLE

A. AORTIC STENOSIS

C. AORTIC REGURGITATION

B. MITRAL REGURGITATION

D. MITRAL STENOSIS

Figure 1. Diagrams of pressure tracings and phonocardiograms in valvular heart disease. The left-hand panels illustrate systole; the right-hand panels, diastole.

A, Pressure tracings in the aorta and left ventricle in aortic stenosis. The shaded area indicates the pressure gradient between left ventricle and aorta. The presystolic (A wave) in the left ventricle is shown, which correlates with the atrial diastolic gallop (S_4) on the phonocardiogram (Phono.). The murmur follows the time course of the pressure gradient during ventricular ejection, and the prolonged left ventricular ejection time results in a single second heart sound (S_2).

B, Pressure tracings in the aorta, left ventricle, and left atrium in mitral regurgitation. (Similar events occur in the right atrium, jugular venous pulse, and right ventricle in tricuspid regurgitation.) A prominent V wave is visible in the left atrium, and the pansystolic murmur on the phonocardiogram persists as long as there is a pressure gradient from left ventricle to left atrium across the leaking mitral valve. The A_2P_2 interval is more widely split than normal because of a shortened left ventricular ejection time in severe mitral regurgitation. The rapid filling wave in the left ventricle and left atrium is illustrated, which is often accompanied by a ventricular diastolic gallop (S_3).

C, Pressure tracings in the aorta and left ventricle in aortic regurgitation. There is a widened arterial pulse pressure with a rapidly falling aortic diastolic pressure. On the phonocardiogram the decrescendo diastolic murmur can be seen to follow the time course of the diminishing diastolic pressure gradient from the aorta to the left ventricle across the leaking aortic valve.

D, Pressure tracings in the aorta, left ventricle, and left atrium in mitral stenosis. (Similar events occur in the right atrium, jugular venous pulse, and right ventricle in tricuspid stenosis.) The left atrial pressure is elevated and the pressure gradient between left atrium and left ventricle during diastole is indicated by the shaded area. The slow fall in left atrial pressure after the V wave (slow Y descent) indicates obstruction to left atrial emptying, and the prominent A wave of left atrial contraction is not transmitted to the ventricle. The dumbbell-shaped diastolic rumble of mitral stenosis in the presence of normal sinus rhythm follows the time course of the pressure gradient, which is greatest early and again late in diastole. It can be seen how an increase or a decrease in the height of the left atrial pressure will move the mitral opening snap (O.S.) closer to or farther from, respectively, the aortic closure sound (A_2); similarly a higher left atrial pressure will result in a later and louder first heart sound (S_1).

in left ventricular volume, and moderate hypertrophy of the left ventricular wall. An excessive oxygen consumption by the left ventricle occurs in aortic stenosis because of the hypertrophy and increased pressure required to drive blood across the narrowed valve, and myocardial oxygen consumption also is increased to some degree in aortic regurgitation because of the large stroke volume and the increased systolic pressure in the aorta. In addition, there is a low diastolic aortic pressure available for coronary artery perfusion in aortic regurgitation and a low aortic pressure relative to left ventricular pressure in severe aortic stenosis (see Fig. 1), which can lead to imbalances between coronary

blood flow and myocardial oxygen demands. Angina pectoris is therefore common in both these conditions. Both aortic stenosis and regurgitation, in time, lead to left ventricular myocardial dysfunction.

Mitral regurgitation also places a diastolic volume overload on the left ventricle, but it differs importantly from aortic regurgitation in that the regurgitant leak occurs during ventricular systole and takes place into a relatively low pressure chamber, the left atrium (see Fig. 1). The ventricular chamber dilates to allow the increased total stoke volume (forward plus backward flow), but the ventricular systolic pressure is not elevated, wall hypertrophy is only moderate, oxygen demands are not greatly augmented, and coronary artery perfusion pressure is normal. Therefore this lesion, when it develops slowly, tends to be well tolerated, and left ventricular myocardial dysfunction develops late in the course of the disease. Mitral stenosis does not place an overload on the left ventricle; rather, obstruction at the mitral valve overwhelms the capacity of the atrial booster pump to maintain forward blood flow, and progressive elevation of left atrial pressure ensues (see Fig. 1).

The secondary effects of these valvular lesions on the arterial and venous beds are many. As mentioned above, the reduced aortic pulse in aortic stenosis and the wide aortic pulse pressure with low diastolic pressure in aortic regurgitation have important effects on coronary artery perfusion. In addition, when valvular lesions are sufficiently severe, or when left ventricular myocardial failure supervenes, the forward cardiac output becomes reduced, the arterial pulse weakens, and there is reflex systemic vasoconstriction with cool extremities and peripheral cyanosis. Such signs constitute evidence of *"forward" cardiac failure*. The effects of *"backward" cardiac failure* in the presence of left-sided valvular lesions are due to left atrial and pulmonary venous hypertension, and they are reflected in the lungs and the right heart. In mitral stenosis, obstruction to left atrial emptying leads to left atrial hypertension, distention of the pulmonary veins, interstitial edema of the lung, reactive pulmonary arteriolar constriction, and eventually pulmonary arterial hypertension. However, the same sequence of effects can also occur when aortic stenosis becomes extremely severe, or when left ventricular myocardial dysfunction becomes significant in the presence of aortic valve disease or mitral regurgitation. The common denominator under these conditions is marked elevation of the left ventricular diastolic pressure, and late in the course of each of these left-sided valvular lesions left atrial and pulmonary venous hypertension, lung congestion, and pulmonary arterial hypertension can also occur, as in mitral stenosis.

Once severe pulmonary hypertension develops, the resulting pressure overload on the right ventricle may then result in secondary right ventricular failure, tricuspid regurgitation, and right atrial hypertension. This, in turn, leads to congestion of the systemic venous bed and the peripheral tissues (liver, abdomen, and extremities). Tricuspid stenosis alone can produce such effects, the right atrial hypertension being caused by mechanical obstruction at the tricuspid valve.

APPROACH TO THE PATIENT WITH VALVULAR HEART DISEASE

Five basic steps in the evaluation of a patient with acquired valvular heart disease should be taken in a logical sequence: (1) the history, (2) the physical examination, (3) the chest roentgenogram (usually with multiple views and barium swallow), (4) the electrocardiogram, and (5) other special tests (phonocardiogram, echocardiogram, cardiac catheterization). The patient is often seen initially, of course, because of an abnormal finding in one of these areas (cardiac murmur, abnormal electrocardiogram, unusual chest x-ray).

HISTORY. The clinical course of patients with each major type of acquired valvular lesion tends to be

rather characteristic, and often the findings to be encountered on physical examination can be predicted on the basis of a careful history alone. Thus in mitral stenosis the earliest symptoms are those due to episodic left atrial hypertension and pulmonary congestion, occurring particularly when the heart rate is rapid during exercise, and during intermittent atrial fibrillation or tachycardia. Such symptoms often begin in early adult life, and the dyspnea increases as the mitral valve narrowing progresses and reaches a critical degree. In contrast, patients with aortic stenosis or regurgitation, or mitral regurgitation, tend to develop dyspnea in relation to the duration and severity of the overload on the left ventricle. In acquired isolated aortic stenosis, there is often a long period without symptoms while the stenosis progresses and left ventricular hypertrophy increases; this is followed by a rather abrupt downhill course over four or five years, beginning at age 55 or 60, as the compensatory mechanisms are exhausted. The average downhill course in patients with chronic rheumatic aortic regurgitation tends to be less precipitous than that of aortic stenosis after symptoms begin, taking place over seven or eight years, but it usually begins somewhat earlier in life. On the other hand, in chronic mitral regurgitation the onset of symptoms is gradual and deterioration tends to be slow owing to the relatively favorable loading conditions on the left ventricle, discussed above.

These average clinical courses represent those of patients who experienced rheumatic fever in childhood, or who develop progressive stenosis of a congenitally bicuspid aortic valve. Departures from the typical patterns occur when, for example, coronary artery disease leads to angina pectoris in the presence of mild aortic stenosis, or when mitral regurgitation occurs acutely as a consequence of chordal rupture or papillary muscle dysfunction associated with coronary heart disease. Such deviations from the usual history should arouse the suspicion of a nonrheumatic etiology of valve dysfunction, or of other associated disease.

PHYSICAL EXAMINATION. In examining the heart, it is well to develop an ordered approach, commencing with careful inspection of the neck veins, palpation of the carotid arteries, and inspection and palpation of the precordium. Palpation of the carotid arteries may be highly useful, for example, in differentiating aortic stenosis caused by valvular obstruction from that caused by hypertrophic subaortic stenosis. Estimation of the jugular venous pressure (which, with practice, can be done reliably within 1 or 2 cm H_2O) and examination of the contour of the jugular venous pulse waves carry great importance, because these veins provide direct clues to events occurring in the right atrium. The jugular veins therefore serve as an "external manometer," and the characteristically slow downslope of the jugular venous pulse (Y descent) associated with tricuspid stenosis (see Fig. 1) or the dominant V wave of tricuspid regurgitation, may suggest organic tricuspid valve involvement. The jugular venous pulse waves often disclose atrial arrhythmias, or provide a clue to the presence of pulmonary hypertension and right ventricular hypertrophy, evidenced by a prominent venous A wave.

Auscultation of the heart is of course the key to an accurate diagnosis in valvular heart disease. An orderly sequence for listening should be developed, each area being examined first for normal or abnormal heart sounds and then for cardiac murmurs. Simultaneous palpation of the carotid artery and observation of the neck veins should be used as aids in the proper timing of the heart sounds and murmurs. By listening first at the aortic area, the aortic component of the second heart sound can be readily identified; the intensity of the pulmonic closure sound and its movement with respiration can then be assessed at the pulmonic area. As one moves down the left sternal border with the diaphragm of the stethoscope, the opening snap of mitral stenosis may be revealed even before the murmur is heard at the apex, or the high-pitched blowing murmur of aortic regurgitation may be audible. The tricuspid and mitral areas should then be examined for the characteristics of the first heart sound. Sometimes a very loud first heart sound alerts the examiner to the possibility of mitral stenosis, whereas mitral regurgitation leads to a reduction in the intensity of the first heart sound at the apex (see Fig. 1).

The duration and intensity of the murmurs of valvular heart disease occur with, and tend to follow, the time course of the pressure gradients between two adjacent cardiac chambers or between a chamber and its great vessel. Thus the diamond-shaped systolic murmur ("ejection" murmur) of aortic stenosis increases and decreases with the pressure gradient, and the velocity at which blood is forced across the narrowed aortic orifice rises and falls (see Fig. 1); this type of murmur does not occur during isovolumetric ventricular contraction and relaxation, and therefore begins well after the first heart sound and ends before the second sound. The decrescendo murmur of aortic regurgitation occurs as the diastolic pressure gradient between the aorta and the left ventricle gradually falls during left ventricular filling (see Fig. 1). The holosystolic (pansystolic) murmur of mitral or tricuspid regurgitation begins with the first heart sound and persists as long as active ventricular contraction maintains a positive pressure gradient from the ventricle to the passively filling atrium (see Fig. 1). The duration and intensity of the diastolic rumbling murmurs of mitral or tricuspid stenosis closely follow the diastolic pressure gradient across the valve from atrium to ventricle (see Fig. 1). Presystolic accentuation of the murmur during the A wave of atrial systole tends to disappear when atrial fibrillation occurs; and if the stenosis is mild, the pressure gradient and the murmur may disappear midway during diastole. It also can be seen from Figure 1 why the first heart sound is both late and loud in mitral stenosis, the left ventricle contracting rapidly and forcefully by the time it has built up sufficient pressure to close the mitral valve, and why the interval between the aortic closure sound and the mitral opening snap becomes progressively shorter as left atrial pressure rises.

Finally, it is important that changes in body position and certain other maneuvers become a regular part of the complete physical examination in a patient with valvular heart disease. The murmur of mitral stenosis may not be heard until the patient is placed in the left lateral decubitus position; the same position may be required to move the left ventricle sufficiently close to the chest wall to allow a ventricular diastolic gallop to be appreciated. The diagnosis of mitral stenosis should also not be excluded until a brief period of muscular exercise, or an isometric handgrip, has been performed

to accentuate the murmur by increasing the heart rate and cardiac output, thereby augmenting the pressure gradient across the mitral valve. The handgrip maneuver tends to increase aortic pressure as well, and it is useful for augmenting a left ventricular gallop, or for accentuating the murmur of aortic regurgitation. The faint murmur of mild aortic regurgitation may also be detected only when the patient leans forward and breathes out completely. Sometimes the standing position is required to bring out the murmur of hypertrophic subaortic stenosis; the Valsalva maneuver is also useful for accentuating this murmur and for diminishing the murmur of valvular aortic stenosis. Other maneuvers, such as amyl nitrite inhalation, sometimes are used to produce characteristic changes in murmurs; for example, the murmur of rheumatic mitral regurgitation is diminished, whereas that of mitral valve prolapse is prolonged by this agent, and the murmur of aortic stenosis is increased.

CHEST ROENTGENOGRAM. As mentioned above, the jugular venous pulse provides a "direct access" route to the right atrium and allows estimation of the right atrial or systemic venous pressure. The pulmonary veins, of course, are inaccessible to physical examination, and therefore the chest roentgenogram is relied upon heavily to aid in detecting left atrial and pulmonary venous hypertension. Often, when there is left atrial hypertension, enlargement of the upper lobe pulmonary veins reflects redistribution of pulmonary blood flow, with reduced perfusion of the lung bases relative to the upper lobes (reversing the normal pattern in the upright posture), and there are signs of interstitial pulmonary edema (such as the Kerley B line) which usually precede the development of pulmonary (intra-alveolar) edema.

Oblique, overpenetrated views of the heart with barium swallow provide valuable information in evaluating valvular heart disease. Left atrial enlargement may be disclosed in the frontal view by a round "double density" or by elevation of the left mainstem bronchus in the frontal view, but it also may be detected only in the right anterior oblique view as a discrete, posterior displacement of the barium-filled esophagus. This view is also useful for identifying right ventricular enlargement in patients suspected of having pulmonary hypertension. The left anterior oblique projection is the most reliable for detecting enlargement of the left ventricle. Other clues to the location of valvular heart lesions include poststenotic dilatation of the aorta in valvular aortic stenosis or calcification in a heart valve. Sometimes the latter is detected only by image intensification fluoroscopy.

THE ELECTROCARDIOGRAM. In acquired valvular heart disease, the electrocardiogram should be carefully scrutinized for signs of chamber enlargement. Left atrial enlargement may be the only electrocardiographic sign of isolated mitral stenosis in the patient with sinus rhythm, and this single sign disappears when atrial fibrillation occurs. The presence or absence of left ventricular hypertrophy is of importance in considering the hemodynamic severity of aortic stenosis and in assessing the degree of mitral regurgitation; in the patient with mitral stenosis who has an apical systolic murmur, the presence of left ventricular hypertrophy may indicate that associated mitral regurgitation is of significance. The suspicion of associated coronary heart disease or myocardial disease may be raised by a bundle branch block pattern or by evidence of a previous myocardial infarction. Prominent (septal) Q waves associated with left ventricular hypertrophy can also occur with hypertrophic subaortic stenosis. Right axis deviation or right ventricular hypertrophy suggests significant pulmonary hypertension. Sometimes the vectorcardiogram is employed to confirm the presence or absence of myocardial infarction or ventricular hypertrophy.

SPECIAL LABORATORY TESTS. Short of cardiac catheterization (discussed below), two other noninvasive tests are highly useful in the precise diagnosis of acquired valvular heart disease: the *phonocardiogram* and the *echocardiogram*.

The *phonocardiogram* is of value particularly for ascertaining the timing of normal and abnormal heart sounds. Recorded with the heart sounds are the indirect carotid pulse wave, which substitutes for the arterial pressure tracing; the indirect jugular venous tracing, which resembles the atrial pressure pulse; and the apex cardiogram, which corresponds roughly to the diastolic left ventricular pressure pulse. For example, a mitral opening snap can be identified by its close relation to the onset of left ventricular filling on the apexcardiogram, and its precise timing in relation to the aortic closure sound can be determined from the carotid pulse wave (see Fig. 1). A prolonged left ventricular ejection time and a single second heart sound are often associated with the abnormal carotid pulse wave of severe aortic stenosis (see Fig. 1). The phonocardiogram is not particularly useful for detecting soft cardiac murmur; these are better identified by careful auscultation at various locations and by the several maneuvers described above.

The *echocardiogram* can aid considerably in reaching an accurate clinical diagnosis (Fig. 2). Thus the characteristically abnormal pattern of anterior mitral valve leaflet motion can be demonstrated in mitral stenosis (see Fig. 2), or the fluttering movement of this leaflet associated with a diastolic Austin-Flint murmur can be identified. The echocardiogram may show posterior mitral leaflet prolapse when mitral regurgitation is associated with the click-murmur syndrome or with papillary muscle dysfunction (see Fig. 2). The characteristic anterior movement of the mitral leaflet during systole (see Fig. 2) and echocardiographic identification of septal hypertrophy have simplified the diagnosis of hypertrophic subaortic stenosis (hypertrophic cardiomyopathy with obstruction). In this condition, there is also asymmetric septal hypertrophy (ASH) (see Ch. 366.2). The applications of echocardiography are many, and the technique is finding increasing application in the study of cardiac diseases of all types.

DECISIONS CONSIDERING CARDIAC CATHETERIZATION AND OPERATION

Cardiac catheterization is rarely necessary for the *diagnosis* of valvular heart disease. An accurate diagnosis can usually be accomplished by careful application of the approaches described above, including the use of special noninvasive techniques such as echocardiography when necessary. Therefore cardiac catheterization and angiography are generally reserved until the patient is considered a potential candidate for a corrective operation. Of course there are some occasions when

cardiac catheterization is used to make a definitive diagnosis, such as in differentiating angina pectoris caused by aortic stenosis from that resulting from associated coronary atherosclerosis, or in the differential diagnosis of pulmonary hypertension. In the latter situation, it is clearly important not to make a diagnosis of primary pulmonary hypertension until valve obstruction has been carefully excluded by hemodynamic studies.

Prior to considering a surgical procedure, cardiac catheterization is usually undertaken for several purposes: (1) To determine whether the valve lesion (stenosis or regurgitation) is sufficiently severe to make it likely that surgical correction will relieve symptoms. (2) To assess carefully the degree of left ventricular myocardial dysfunction or failure associated with aortic valve lesions and mitral regurgitation. (3) To detect significant associated lesions, such as unexpectedly severe mitral regurgitation or aortic stenosis in a patient with mitral stenosis. (4) To study the coronary circulation, particularly in older subjects or in patients with aortic valve disease in whom symptoms may be due primarily to coronary heart disease rather than the valvular lesion. (5) To assess the relative significance of myocardial and valvular disease in patients with recurrent symptoms after previous cardiac surgery.

Once appropriate information has been assembled concerning the mechanical severity of the valve defect, the degree of involvement of the left ventricular myocardium, the severity of any associated coronary artery disease, and possible complicating illnesses (such as diabetes mellitus, liver disease, anemia, or thyroid disease), a decision concerning the advisability of a cardiac operation can be undertaken. Such a decision must also be based upon knowledge in several other important areas:

1. The risk to the patient's life of the proposed operation versus the risk of medical management alone. Operative risk is related to the nature of the surgical intervention required. Must a valve prosthesis be inserted, or is a commissurotomy possible? Is more than one valve involved? Is there associated coronary artery disease that will require a myocardial revascularization procedure? The patient's age and the presence of associated noncardiac illness also influence the operative risk.

2. The usual natural course of the valve lesion and the long-range outlook after operation. Knowledge of the natural history as well as the likely course after operation is important. For example, once significant symptoms begin in patients with aortic stenosis, the downhill course is usually rapid and the risk of *not* operating outweighs that of the surgical procedure. The average downhill course is somewhat slower after the onset of symptoms in patients with aortic regurgitation, but the degree of secondary left ventricular myocardial dysfunction must be considered, and operation should be undertaken before myocardial disease becomes irreversible. A similar consideration applies in patients with chronic mitral regurgitation, but their more gradual downhill course allows a more leisurely decision concerning the proper time for surgical intervention. The probable finite limitations in the life span of the various valvular prostheses should be taken into account before recommending operation in a young patient who has only moderate limitation of activity.

3. The social setting. This must be considered care-

Figure 2.   Characteristic normal and abnormal motions of the mitral valve.

Upper panel, Simplified diagrammatic echocardiogram of the motions of normal mitral valve as obtained by M-mode echocardiography. AML = Anterior mitral leaflet; PML = posterior mitral leaflet. ECG = simultaneously recorded electrocardiogram. The scale is in centimeters from anterior (ANT) to posterior (POST). During left ventricular systole the two leaflets are normally closed and there is a gradual anterior motion, as the whole heart moves forward during ventricular ejection. With the onset of diastole (D) the leaflets open rapidly in opposite directions, and during early rapid ventricular filling the anterior leaflet rapidly reaches its most forward position (E). The anterior leaflet then moves back to a partially closed position as rapid filling diminishes (E to F slope), and a brief period of slow filling or diastasis is shown, followed by another rapid opening of both leaflets due to late rapid filling during atrial contraction which reaches a peak at point A. With atrial relaxation the leaflets again close. The onset of mechanical ventricular contraction sometimes causes a notch (not shown) at point B, and is then followed by closure of the mitral valve at point C.

Lower panel, Abnormal mitral valve motions indicated by dashed lines.

In the typical patient with severe mitral stenosis (MS), the abnormalities are represented by the dashed lines during diastole. *Both* the anterior and posterior mitral leaflets move anteriorly during diastole; the forward excursion of the anterior leaflet to the E point is much reduced, and its E to F slope is greatly diminished.

In the patient with hypertrophic subaortic stenosis, during systole (on the left) the dashed line illustrates marked systolic anterior movement (SAM) of the anterior mitral leaflet. In some instances this motion may cause the anterior leaflet to touch the hypertrophied interventricular septum during systole, thereby leading to obstruction in the left ventricular outflow tract.

Mitral valve prolapse (MP) occurs during left ventricular systole, as illustrated in the right-hand systolic period. Typically, the leaflets move posteriorly during the latter half of systole, the motion often being most marked in the posterior leaflet, as shown. Occasionally, the posterior movement is holosystolic.

fully, for in the final analysis the expected benefits of the operation must be judged in relation to the patient's age, occupational needs, family responsibilities, and expectation of substantially improved longevity and functional capacity.

360.2.   MITRAL STENOSIS

ETIOLOGY AND PATHOLOGY.   Mitral stenosis in the adult usually develops as a sequel to rheumatic fever;

only rarely is obstruction caused by such malformations as congenital cor triatriatum (see Ch. 359.5) or left atrial myxoma. It is the most common single valvular lesion to follow acute rheumatic fever, accounting for over half the patients with chronic rheumatic heart disease. About two thirds of the subjects are female.

The rheumatic mitral valve shows fibrosis and thickening of the cusps, with partial fusion of the commissures; in patients with longstanding disease, leaflet fusion may produce restriction of the mitral orifice to as little as 0.5 sq cm. There are thickening and shortening of the chordae tendineae, and there may be heavy calcium deposits in the valve. The left ventricle is generally normal in size and weight unless there is associated mitral regurgitation or disease of the aortic valve, but the left atrium is enlarged and thick walled. Microscopic examination of the myocardium often shows evidence of old rheumatic myocarditis (Aschoff bodies). In the lungs, there is thickening of the muscular walls of the pulmonary arterioles and venules with intimal proliferation, and in the late stages of mitral stenosis there is diffuse hemosiderosis (primarily disintegrated hemoglobin within alveoli), and there may be interstitial fibrosis and pulmonary infarction.

PATHOLOGIC PHYSIOLOGY. The primary physiologic abnormality in mitral stenosis is mechanical obstruction to emptying of the left atrium produced by the narrowed valve orifice. Left ventricular function is usually normal, and therefore the defect in mitral stenosis stands in marked contrast to that of mitral regurgitation, or of aortic valve disease, in each of which a chronic overload is placed in the left ventricle.

When the mitral valve orifice is only mildly reduced, the mean left atrial pressure and filling of the left ventricle remain normal at rest. However, the rate of blood flow across the mitral valve is dependent not only on the orifice area of the valve and the driving pressure gradient (from left atrium to left ventricle), but also on the *time* available for flow across the mitral valve during diastole. With an increase in heart rate, the duration of left ventricular systole shortens only slightly, and tachycardia therefore occurs mainly at the expense of diastolic filling time per minute. Hence patients with mild mitral stenosis generally experience their earliest symptoms only during severe exertion, or with the onset of rapid atrial fibrillation. With exertion, both the normal tachycardia of exercise and the increased cardiac output lead to an increased left atrial pressure, whereas with atrial fibrillation and an uncontrolled ventricular rate the increased rate alone leads to a left atrial pressure elevation because of compromised filling time per minute.

With increased narrowing of the mitral orifice, the mean left atrial pressure becomes somewhat elevated at rest (over 12 mm Hg), but as the mitral orifice is reduced to below 1 sq cm the resting cardiac output can be maintained only at the expense of a markedly elevated left atrial pressure (often in excess of 20 mm Hg), in which the high pressure gradient forces blood across the narrowed orifice at high velocity. In this stage of the disease, the increased left atrial pressure and critically narrowed mitral valve often lead to pulmonary edema. Although pulmonary edema theoretically should occur when the pulmonary venous pressure exceeds about 30 mm Hg, higher levels have occasionally been recorded without its occurrence. This may be related to thickening of the alveolar-capillary membrane, which has been noted in the lungs of patients with mitral stenosis.

As the disease progresses, the elevated pressure in the pulmonary veins leads to pulmonary artery hypertension (see also Ch. 358.4). When pulmonary hypertension becomes persistent at rest, it reflects two major factors: first, the elevated left atrial pressure is transmitted retrogradely and requires an increased pressure head in the pulmonary artery to drive blood forward; and second, pulmonary arteriolar vasoconstriction occurs. This vasoconstriction is accompanied in time by organic changes, mainly intimal proliferation and medial thickening in the walls of the small pulmonary arteries. At this stage, the pulmonary vascular resistance becomes elevated, which in turn leads to a reduction in the resting cardiac output. This sequence tends to limit any further increase in the left atrial pressure, which may even fall somewhat as the cardiac output becomes diminished. Symptoms of pulmonary venous congestion and pulmonary edema often diminish at this stage. In late mitral stenosis, pulmonary hypertension may become extreme, with the systolic pressure in the pulmonary artery equal to or exceeding that in the systemic arterial bed. Even with less marked elevations in pulmonary arterial pressure, the right ventricular end-diastolic volume and pressure become elevated, and this may lead to functional tricuspid regurgitation. Finally, signs of right ventricular failure appear with peripheral venous congestion.

CLINICAL MANIFESTATIONS. **Symptoms and Clinical Course.** After one or more attacks of rheumatic fever in childhood, there is a latent period averaging about 12 years before mitral stenosis becomes clinically manifest, symptoms and signs usually first becoming apparent in young adulthood. There is commonly then a relatively long period (five to eight years) of mild to moderate symptoms as the scarring and obstruction at the valve gradually progress.

The earliest manifestation of mild to moderate mitral stenosis is dyspnea caused primarily by the increased cardiac output and tachycardia of exercise, leading to transient elevation of left atrial pressure, as discussed above. Elevation of the left atrial pressure causes pulmonary venous hypertension, increasing lung stiffness and the work of breathing, and thereby leads to the subjective sensation of dyspnea. As the disease progresses, orthopnea at night commences as a result of redistribution of the peripheral blood volume into the central circulation and of peripheral resorption of fluid caused by the supine posture. Coughing, particularly at night, may also be a troublesome symptom. Dyspnea eventually becomes extreme with minimal activity, and hemoptysis may occur owing to rupture of dilated endobronchial vessels, which appear to form collateral channels between the pulmonary and bronchial venous systems. The hemoptysis, consisting of bright red blood which can accumulate in sufficient quantities to cause atelectasis, usually subsides with bed rest and sedation with opiates; most commonly it occurs in patients who do not have severe elevation of the pulmonary vascular resistance. An increased number of pulmonary infections may occur, perhaps related to the interstitial pulmonary edema present in this stage of the disease, and other factors such as severe emotional stress, sexual activity, and fever with tachycardia may acutely worsen the patient's symptoms.

Significant left atrial enlargement develops as the left atrial hypertension becomes persistent, and atrial premature beats, paroxysmal atrial tachycardia, or atrial fibrillation commonly occur. The sudden onset of atrial fibrillation with rapid ventricular rate may precipitate acute pulmonary edema when the obstruction at the mitral orifice is of sufficient severity. Eventually, sustained atrial fibrillation supervenes, requiring control of the ventricular response with digitalis. Intermittent atrial fibrillation, in particular, may be associated with peripheral embolic phenomena, and the incidence of emboli in patients with chronic atrial fibrillation is substantial. As the left atrium enlarges and stasis occurs, thrombus formation is most frequent within the left atrial appendage, and adherent clots have been found at operation in this location in about 30 per cent of patients. Small emboli may break loose to become lodged in the renal, splenic, or cerebral circulations, and the effects of such emboli, causing a convulsion or perhaps a renal infarction, sometimes provide the initial symptom in a patient with mitral stenosis. Coronary artery embolization with myocardial infarction has also been reported. Sometimes a large embolus to the brain results in serious and permanent sequelae, and saddle embolus in the aorta has been encountered on a number of occasions. Infrequently a thrombus within the left atrium may become sufficiently large to obstruct a pulmonary vein, leading to localized unilateral pulmonary edema, and rarely a pedunculated "ball-valve thrombus" can be formed which mimics the findings of left atrial myxoma (see below).

As mitral stenosis progresses further, the pulmonary vascular resistance rises, tending to limit flow across the pulmonary bed; with the associated diminution of pulmonary venous hypertension, hemoptysis and pulmonary interstitial edema diminish. Thus in patients with longstanding, severe mitral stenosis, dyspnea on exertion and orthopnea often become less prominent and fatigue now predominates. The development of functional tricuspid regurgitation may result in a further drop in the cardiac output and some reduction in the pulmonary artery pressure. In this stage of the disease weakness and signs of right heart failure become extreme, and abdominal discomfort with hepatomegaly, ascites, and peripheral edema dominate the clinical picture. Pulmonary embolus with pulmonary infarction is a common late complication.

Physical Findings. The patient (usually a female) with severe mitral stenosis may exhibit peripheral cyanosis and a "mitral facies" (blue-tinged with malar flush), and often there is some degree of emaciation. In such advanced cases, peripheral edema and ascites may also be evident.

The peripheral arterial pulses are typically small, and the blood pressure is normal or low. The jugular venous pulse is initially normal in the presence of moderate mitral stenosis, but as pulmonary hypertension develops, the mean venous pressure is increased and the A wave becomes prominent owing to right ventricular hypertrophy and elevation of the right ventricular end-diastolic pressure. In the presence of atrial fibrillation, there is a dominant V wave in the jugular veins.

In patients with mitral stenosis without pulmonary hypertension, palpation of the precordium may be unremarkable except for the presence of a diastolic thrill localized just inside the left ventricular apex. The accentuated first heart sound and sometimes an opening snap may be palpable. The apical impulse is otherwise normal, and the heart is not enlarged. In patients with pulmonary hypertension, there is a right ventricular lift in the left parasternal area, and the bulging pulmonary artery segment and pulmonic closure may be palpable at the upper left base if the mean pulmonary arterial pressure is in excess of 50 mm Hg.

On auscultation, the first heart sound is generally loud, snapping in quality, and somewhat delayed (see

Fig. 1, Ch. 360.1). These features occur because the left atrial pressure is elevated, and additional time is required for the left ventricle to build up sufficient pressure to close the mitral valve; the rate of change of left ventricular pressure (dP/dt) is rapid by that time, which results in the more forceful than normal mitral valve closure. The aortic closure sound is normal, but a mitral opening snap follows the second sound, the snap being audible at the lower left sternal border and the apex. A general correlation exists between the severity of mitral stenosis and the timing of the opening snap, necessitating careful evaluation of the interval between aortic closure and the opening snap on the phonocardiogram. As the left ventricular pressure declines during the isovolumetric relaxation period after aortic valve closure, eventually it falls below the left atrial pressure and the stenotic mitral valve then snaps open. The higher the left atrial pressure, the closer this event must occur in relation to aortic closure (A_2). This time interval (the so-called A_2-OS interval) tends to be long (0.10 second or more) in patients with mild mitral stenosis and mean left atrial pressures below 15 mm Hg, whereas in patients with severe mitral stenosis and mean left atrial pressures of 20 mm Hg or more, the interval is usually shorter (less than 0.09 second). As might be expected, however, the interval will vary considerably with the heart rate. If the heart rate is below 100 and the interval 0.07 second or less, the mitral stenosis is usually of significant degree.

The opening snap is followed immediately by a low-pitched *diastolic rumble* resulting from turbulent flow across the stenotic mitral orifice. The murmur is usually localized to an area about 2 cm in diameter near or just inside the left ventricular apex in the fourth or fifth left intercostal space, and it is best brought out by positioning the patient in the lateral decubitus position. The mitral rumble is loudest in early diastole; it diminishes somewhat as the pressure gradient between left atrium and left ventricle falls, and, in patients with sinus rhythm, it then becomes loud (presystolic accentuation) as the left atrium contracts to again raise the pressure gradient (see Fig. 1, Ch. 360.1). When the stenosis is mild, the diastolic murmur may not be audible until the patient is placed in the lateral decubitus position *after* performing mild exercise or during a handgrip maneuver, when the cardiac output and heart rate are increased, thereby augmenting the pressure gradient across the valve. In the presence of atrial fibrillation, presystolic accentuation disappears; when the ventricular rate is slow, the murmur may occur only in the early and middle phases of long diastolic periods, because given sufficient time the left atrial and left ventricular pressure will come into equilibrium. In patients with severe mitral stenosis and a very low cardiac output, the murmur may be unusually difficult to appreciate. It is most important therefore to position the patient properly and to listen carefully over a wide area of the left chest for the well localized murmur, as well as to carry out the aforementioned exercise maneuvers. When such precautions are taken, "silent" mitral stenosis will be encountered rarely. Occasionally the murmur is inaudible when massive right ventricular enlargement places the left ventricle far posteriorly from the chest wall.

Individuals with "pure" mitral stenosis have a small fixed orifice, and it is not uncommon to hear a soft systolic murmur at the cardiac apex, which presents a trivial mitral regurgitant leak. When a louder pansystolic murmur at the left ventricular apex is accompanied by a third heart sound, by left ventricular enlargement on physical examination, or by electrocardiographic signs of left ventricular hypertrophy, the associated mitral regurgitation is undoubtedly of significance. In the patient with severe pulmonary hypertension, when a very large right ventricle fills the anterior chest and displaces the left ventricle posteriorly, the murmur of tricuspid regurgitation can mimic that of mitral regurgitation. The systolic murmur of tricuspid regurgitation is ordinarily heard best at the lower left sternal border; it increases with inspiration, and is not heard in the axilla or over the spine posteriorly, features which serve to distinguish it from the murmur of mitral regurgitation. With severe pulmonary hypertension the high-pitched, early diastolic blowing murmur of pulmonic regurgitation (the Graham Steell murmur) may also be audible. This murmur, heard best at the left sternal border, is usually indistinguishable from that of mild aortic regurgitation.

DIAGNOSIS. Electrocardiogram. In patients with moderate mitral stenosis and sinus rhythm, the electrocardiogram may be normal, or it may show only left atrial enlargement, with a notched and prolonged P wave in the limb leads and an increased negative component of the P wave in lead V_1. When there is atrial fibrillation, patients with rheumatic heart disease tend to show coarse fibrillation waves, presumably owing to the thickened atrial wall and enlarged chamber volume, a finding which contrasts with the fine fibrillatory waves often found in patients with coronary heart disease.

The right ventricle is the next chamber to be affected as mitral stenosis progresses, and in severe mitral stenosis with pulmonary hypertension the electrocardiogram often shows right axis deviation. Usually, if the QRS axis is 100 degrees or more or the R/S ratio in V_1 exceeds unity, the mean pulmonary artery pressure is over 35 mm Hg. Evidence of left ventricular hypertrophy in a patient with mitral stenosis generally indicates accompanying aortic valve disease or significant associated mitral regurgitation.

Roentgenographic Features. Minimal enlargement of the left atrium may be the only radiographic abnormality in patients with moderate mitral stenosis. It may be apparent only with barium swallow, the right anterior oblique view showing best the localized, posterior displacement of the barium-filled esophagus. As the disease progresses, left atrial enlargement becomes distinct, and this chamber is visible as a large round "double density" in the center of the cardiac shadow on the frontal view. The left mainstem bronchus is elevated by the enlarged left atrium (the angle formed by the bronchus with a central, vertical line increasing to more than 45 degrees), and enlargement of the left atrial appendage results in straightening of the left heart border.

As left atrial and pulmonary venous hypertension develop, there is a redistribution of the pulmonary vascularity in the lung fields. Initially, in the upright posture the normal, relative avascularity of the upper lobes is lost, and the pulmonary vascular pattern appears equal in the upper and lower lungs. In later stages of the disease, vascularity in the upper lobe vessels is increased.

Redistribution of the pulmonary vascular pattern generally occurs when left atrial pressure exceeds 15 mm Hg, and evidence of interstitial pulmonary edema commonly appears when the mean left atrial pressure at rest exceeds 20 mm Hg. Interstitial edema may be evidenced by *Kerley's B lines*, transverse linear densities about 1 cm in length and located at the lung bases laterally above the diaphragm, representing engorged septal lymphatic vessels. Acute pulmonary edema is reflected by typical butterfly densities in the hilar regions.

As pulmonary hypertension develops, the pulmonary artery segment becomes enlarged, the peripheral pulmonary arteries become dilated, and enlargement of the right ventricle and right atrium is evident. With long-standing pulmonary hypertension a diffuse reticular pattern in the lung fields may result from pulmonary hemosiderosis. Calcification in the mitral valve should be searched for, using image intensification fluoroscopy. The presence of calcification makes it less likely that the valve will prove amenable to valvuloplasty.

Phonocardiography. The phonocardiogram is particularly useful for timing the A_2-OS interval (see Physical Findings). Also, the configuration of the apexcardiogram, as it reflects diastolic events in the left ventricle (see Fig. 1, Ch. 360.1), may show loss of a rapid early filling wave and absence of a presystolic (A) wave in patients with significant mitral stenosis.

Echocardiography. Reflected ultrasound to confirm the presence of mitral stenosis and to estimate its severity has found widespread application. The echo recorded from the mitral leaflets exhibits characteristic features in the presence of significant mitral stenosis, the degree of the abnormality correlating in general with the severity of stenosis. Thickening of the anterior and posterior leaflets can often be identified, and there is a reduced anterior excursion of the leaflet during diastole (see Fig. 2, Ch. 360.1). Also, the degree of separation of the anterior and posterior leaflets during diastole is reduced in the presence of mitral stenosis. Both the anterior and posterior leaflets move forward with diastole as the domed, stenotic valve opens (in a normal valve, the posterior leaflet opens in an opposite direction to the anterior leaflet). Because of the persistent pressure gradient from left atrium to left ventricle, the normal posterior floating motion of the anterior mitral leaflet during mid-diastole does not occur; the leaflet is held open in an anterior position and moves only slowly posteriorly (see Fig. 2, Ch. 360.1). This posterior motion (the so-called E to F slope) is reduced to less than 15 mm per second when mitral stenosis is severe and is usually less than 25 mm per second when it is moderate. Although a general relation exists between the hemodynamic severity of mitral stenosis and the degree of reduction of the E to F slope, the slope by itself has not proved to be a reliable measure of the severity of stenosis; thus other factors such as the cardiac output and the left ventricular diastolic compliance also affect this measurement. Cross-sectional echocardiography, as with a mechanical sector scanner, offers the promise of direct estimates of the mitral valve orifice area, but this approach remains to be further validated.

The detection of characteristic moving echoes from behind the mitral valve can indicate the presence of left atrial myxoma or a ball-valve thrombus.

Pulmonary Function Tests. Patients with longstanding mitral stenosis generally have a reduced pulmonary compliance owing to elevation of the left atrial pressure and interstitial pulmonary edema. The vital capacity, total lung capacity, maximal breathing capacity, and oxygen uptake per unit of ventilation may be reduced, and abnormalities of ventilation-perfusion relations are often seen as well.

Cardiac Catheterization. In the young patient with obvious features of pure mitral stenosis and marked symptoms, cardiac catheterization is not performed in some centers prior to operation. On the other hand, when there is uncertainty about the severity of the stenosis in relation to the level of symptoms, cardiac catheterization should be performed to document objectively the degree of valve narrowing, and to calculate the orifice area. At cardiac catheterization, the typical patient with significant mitral stenosis will exhibit an elevated mean pulmonary artery wedge pressure. If a satisfactory wedge pressure tracing cannot be obtained, transseptal left atrial puncture is often performed. If the patient is in sinus rhythm, the forceful left atrial contraction produces a dominant A wave in the tracing, and there is a slow fall in the pressure after the V wave (reduced rate of the Y descent), reflecting obstruction to left atrial emptying during diastole. The left ventricular end-diastolic pressure is usually normal (below 12 mm Hg). The pressure gradient from left atrium to left ventricle is high early in diastole, falling progressively as left ventricular filling occurs, but the gradient is again increased late in diastole by left atrial contraction (see Fig. 1, Ch. 360.1). In patients with atrial fibrillation, the V wave is dominant and left atrial pressure continues to fall throughout diastole until the onset of ventricular systole.

The *mitral valve orifice area* can be calculated if both the cardiac output and the pressure gradient are known. By the Gorlin formula, the valve orifice area is directly proportional to the flow across the valve per second of diastole and is inversely proportional to the square root of the pressure gradient. In simple terms, this means that if the flow doubles, the pressure gradient will quadruple. Because of this nonlinear relation, measurement of the left atrial or wedge pressure alone can be misleading in assessing the severity of the mitral stenosis. Thus if the cardiac output is unusually high, an elevated left atrial mean pressure may give a false picture of the severity of the stenotic lesion; if it is low, a moderate left atrial pressure elevation may belie the presence of severe stenosis. Also, if the heart rate is abnormally rapid or slow and a shorter or longer diastolic filling time is available, the left atrial mean pressure may not reflect accurately the size of the mitral orifice. The area of the normal mitral valve is about 4 sq cm. Mitral stenosis is generally considered mild when the calculated orifice area is over 1.2 sq cm, moderate when it is between 1.2 and 0.9 sq cm, and severe when it is below 0.8 sq cm. Thus an area of 1.1 sq cm or less is usually considered to represent stenosis of sufficient severity to warrant operation.

Left ventriculography usually shows the left ventricle to contract normally, with a normal end-diastolic volume. It also provides information concerning the degree of thickening and fusion of the chordal attachments of the mitral valve, the pliability of its leaflets, and the degree of associated mitral regurgitation. All

these factors, together with the presence or absence of valve calcification, weigh in the decision of whether to perform mitral valvuloplasty, or whether to recommend replacement of the valve with a prosthesis.

In older patients, selective coronary arteriography is indicated to search for significant coronary vascular disease. Cardiac catheterization will also document the severity of any associated aortic valvular disease; in patients with recurrent systemic emboli, a pulmonary angiogram may verify the presence of a left atrial thrombus.

DIFFERENTIAL DIAGNOSIS. Clinical findings of pulmonary hypertension should raise the suspicion of mitral stenosis. *Primary pulmonary hypertension* usually occurs in young females; it is associated with hyperventilation, chest pain, fatigue and dyspnea, and effort syncope, but with a relative paucity of objective physical findings. Whenever this diagnosis is considered, mitral stenosis and left atrial myxoma, treatable causes of left atrial and pulmonary hypertension, should be excluded by measurement of left atrial pressure directly or from an adequate pulmonary arterial wedge pressure. *Pulmonary hypertension caused by severe chronic lung disease* usually presents no diagnostic difficulty; but sometimes patients are given a diagnosis of ordinary bronchial asthma, when in fact their wheezing is due to mitral stenosis with left atrial hypertension ("cardiac asthma").

The murmur of rheumatic mitral stenosis may be mimicked by that resulting from a *left atrial myxoma*. However, with the latter lesion there may be other abnormal diastolic sounds, and the murmur may disappear when the patient's position is altered. In addition, symptoms can vary with changes in body position, syncope may occur, and there is usually an elevated sedimentation rate, anemia, fever, or other evidence of systemic disease. Echocardiography may detect the left atrial myxoma. In the young patient, *congenital cor triatriatum* (a rare malformation consisting of a fibrous partition within the left atrium above the mitral valve) may be considered.

The diastolic rumble which occurs in the presence of severe aortic regurgitation, the *Austin Flint murmur*, may be attributed to organic mitral stenosis. This murmur is typically ushered in by a ventricular diastolic gallop (S_3) rather than an opening snap, and it is loudest in mid-diastole. Amyl nitrite inhalation decreases this murmur by lowering diastolic aortic pressure, but the reflex tachycardia and increased cardiac output increase the murmur of mitral stenosis. Echocardiography is particularly helpful in differentiating the Austin Flint murmur from that of mitral stenosis by detecting a characteristic fluttering motion of the anterior leaflet during diastole as its motion is affected by the regurgitant jet.

In the older patient, *atrial septal defect* is occasionally mistaken for mitral stenosis. In atrial septal defect, the tricuspid closure sound is loud, the widely split second heart may mimic the opening snap of mitral stenosis, and the rumble of excessive flow across the tricuspid valve may be confused with the murmur of mitral stenosis. The murmur of mitral stenosis diminishes with inspiration, in contrast to this murmur and the murmur of tricuspid stenosis, which increase.

TREATMENT. Medical Management. In the patient with mild mitral stenosis and few symptoms, restriction of strenuous activity may result in many years of comfortable existence. If the patient is under 40 years of age, monthly Bicillin injections or oral penicillin (sulfonamides may be used in the allergic patient) are advisable to prevent infection with the beta-hemolytic *Streptococcus* and recurrence of acute rheumatic fever (see Ch. 130). In addition, antimicrobial drugs in therapeutic doses should be recommended prior to and after dental procedures or surgical manipulations, particularly those on the genitourinary tract, to prevent infective endocarditis (see Ch. 131).

In patients with moderate symptoms, limitation of activity should be combined with *sodium restriction* and/or administration of a *diuretic* agent. There is little rationale for the use of digitalis in patients with sinus rhythm, because left ventricular function is normal and this agent has no effect on exercise-induced tachycardia. *When atrial fibrillation occurs* for the first time, one or more attempts at *electrical reversion of the rhythm,* followed by maintenance with oral quinidine, are generally indicated. When mitral stenosis is significant, however, permanent atrial fibrillation will generally supervene in time, despite such therapy. In the presence of chronic atrial fibrillation, *digitalis* should be administered to maintain the ventricular rate at an acceptable level both at rest and during moderate exertion. In patients in whom the ventricular rate is difficult to control even with high doses of digitalis, the addition of a *beta-adrenergic blocking agent* (such as propranolol) in small doses may result in very effective control of the ventricular response. Moreover, during acute stress, such as a pneumonia, patients with atrial fibrillation may develop a rapid ventricular response caused by enhanced atrioventricular conduction consequent to excessive sympathetic nervous discharge; under these circumstances the addition of a beta-adrenergic blocking agent to digitalis may allow effective reduction of the ventricular rate in a safer manner than with high doses of digitalis alone. When the ventricular rate is refractory to digitalis in the absence of acute stress, or when signs of heart failure are out of proportion to the degree of mitral stenosis, hyperthyroidism should be suspected. Obvious signs of thyrotoxicosis may be masked in the presence of cardiac disease; but if such hyperthyroidism is detected and treated, symptoms caused by mild mitral stenosis may disappear.

In patients who have suffered a systemic embolus originating from the left atrium, long-term *anticoagulation* with Coumadin derivatives has been shown to be effective in preventing recurrence. The risk of recurrent embolization is greatly increased by atrial fibrillation and may occur even with mild mitral stenosis accompanied by atrial fibrillation. Minor neurologic episodes, or a frank convulsion, often provide the earliest sign of systemic embolization. Emboli also may occur to the legs, to the spleen, or to the mesenteric artery (causing abdominal pain and bowel necrosis), and prompt surgical treatment with embolectomy is required. Coronary artery embolization also occurs occasionally. If systemic embolization recurs while the patient is on adequate anticoagulant therapy, a mitral valve operation with removal of left atrial clot may be recommended for the patient with somewhat milder mitral stenosis, or with less marked symptoms than are usually required for an elective operation.

When pregnancy occurs in a patient with mitral stenosis, symptoms frequently develop for the first time or intensify. Such symptoms become most severe during the second trimester, when increased cardiac output and blood volume are maximal, and a substantial period of hospital treatment may be required. Generally, such symptoms diminish during the third trimester, and only rarely is a mitral commissurotomy necessary during pregnancy.

Once severe symptoms begin in the patient with tight mitral stenosis (New York Heart Association [N.Y.H.A.] Class III), the average mortality in patients treated medically approaches 30 per cent at five years. In severely limited patients (Class IV), the outlook without operation is extremely poor, less than 20 per cent of patients being alive after five years if data gathered prior to the cardiac surgical era are considered. Surgical treatment has greatly altered this outlook.

Surgical Treatment. In the typical younger patient with symptoms on normal activity (N.Y.H.A. Class II) and findings of pure mitral stenosis, the decision of whether to recommend operation is usually reached by considering the individual in his desired activity setting. In the patient with significant mitral stenosis who has had a complication such as a systemic embolus and who develops symptoms on ordinary exertion, operation is usually recommended. In the older patient in functional Class II who has evidence of mitral valve calcification on x-ray and physical findings suggesting a thickened and immobile mitral leaflet (soft first heart sound and reduced or absent opening snap), or in whom significant associated mitral regurgitation is suspected, a waiting period until symptoms are more severe is justified, because mitral valve replacement with a prosthesis will undoubtedly be necessary. Other features which indicate that valve replacement will probably be required are evidence of left ventricular hypertrophy, previous valvotomy, and a markedly thickened, immobile anterior leaflet on echocardiography. In patients with symptoms on less than normal activity (N.Y.H.A. Class III) or at rest (Class IV), the outlook without surgical treatment is poor and the indication for operation is clear.

The presence of severe pulmonary hypertension was considered at one time to represent a relative contraindication to operation, but more recent studies have indicated that even marked elevations of the pulmonary vascular resistance invariably regress postoperatively. Some reduction in the pulmonary vascular resistance occurs within a few hours postoperatively. In most patients studied by cardiac catheterization six months to one year after operation, the pulmonary artery pressure and pulmonary vascular resistance have returned to normal or near normal levels, provided the left atrial pressure is normal.

Surgical practices differ somewhat as to the type of procedure performed in the patient with mitral stenosis. Closed mitral valvulotomy by opening the valve commissures with the finger, inserted through the left atrial appendage, sometimes combined with the use of a mechanical dilator passed through the left ventricular apex, is still employed by some surgeons without the use of cardiopulmonary bypass (heart-lung machine). In many centers, open mitral commissurotomy is now carried out even in the uncomplicated patient, the left atrium being opened with the patient on cardiopulmonary bypass and the mitral stenosis relieved by blunt and sharp dissection under direct vision. The operative risk of such a mitral valvuloplasty is now about equal to that of cardiopulmonary bypass alone (under 2 per cent). This approach also allows removal of any clot that may be present within the left atrium. If significant mitral regurgitation is produced by the attempted valvuloplasty, it is then possible to proceed readily with replacement of the mitral valve by a ball-valve or other prosthesis.

The late results of valvuloplasty have been poor when there is significant mitral regurgitation, or if there is calcification with severe shortening and thickening of the chordae tendineae and immobilization of the mitral valve leaflets. When the valve exhibits such unfavorable anatomic signs, it is replaced with a prosthetic device, the caged ball-valve (Starr-Edwards) and, more recently, the glutaraldehyde-preserved porcine aortic valve xenograft being employed in many centers.

After a valvuloplasty, the average patient experiences 8 to 12 years of symptomatic relief, but a second operation is often necessary (usually mitral valve replacement). The average age at the time of mitral valve replacement is between 50 and 53 years, and about 30 per cent of patients have had a previous mitral commissurotomy. Most experience has been obtained with the caged ball-valve (Starr-Edwards) type of prosthesis. Operative mortality currently averages between 3 and 7 per cent, but it is higher in patients who are in N.Y.H.A. Class IV (average 20 per cent) and in patients who have objective findings of a very large left atrium and right ventricular hypertrophy. Mitral valve replacement usually results in marked alleviation of symptoms and appears to offer substantial prolongation of average life expectancy, when compared to earlier studies on the natural history of medically treated patients with mitral valve disease who were in Classes III and IV. At five years postoperatively, about 75 to 80 per cent of the patients who survive mitral valve replacement are alive, and about two thirds are still alive at the end of a ten-year follow-up. The long-term outlook is poorer for Class IV patients, however, with only about 50 per cent surviving at the end of six years. Thus results appear to support the desirability of operating on patients with mitral valve disease before Class IV symptoms appear, and before great left atrial enlargement with right ventricular overload are present. Thromboembolism is a significant complication with the ball-valve prosthesis, and continuous anticoagulation with sodium warfarin is customarily employed. Embolism occurs at rates of from 3 to 8 per cent per year, depending upon the adequacy of anticoagulation, the type of valve (cloth-covered versus non-cloth-covered), and the size of the left atrium. There also is some risk of a major complication, or death, from bleeding complications associated with the anticoagulation, and about one quarter of late deaths are related to the ball-valve prosthesis (e.g., thrombotic occlusion of the valve, bacterial endocarditis, embolism, or bleeding).

The follow-up after replacement of the mitral valve with the porcine xenograft valve is shorter and involves fewer patients. However, the incidence of thromboembolism has been lower (approximately 1 to 3 per cent per year), and generally patients have not been maintained on anticoagulants after the first three postoperative months. Anticoagulation may be continued, however, in those patients with left atrial enlargement and atrial fibrillation. Some centers have reported lower operative mortalities after xenograft mitral valve replacement than with the ball-valve prosthesis, and late deaths related to the xenograft so far have been rare. Long-term valve durability beyond five years is still an unresolved question with this type of valve substitute.

360.3.   MITRAL REGURGITATION

ETIOLOGY AND PATHOLOGY.   A wide spectrum of disease processes can result in mitral regurgitation, although rheumatic involvement is easily the most common cause. Rheumatic mitral regurgitation occurs more commonly in males, in contrast to mitral stenosis, and the murmur is commonly heard during or soon after the acute rheumatic episode, again in contrast to the relatively late development of the murmur of mitral stenosis. In chronic rheumatic disease, the left ventricle is generally dilated and the wall thickened, there is left atrial enlargement, and the mitral valve exhibits mild, diffuse scarring of the leaflets associated with some thickening of the chordae tendineae. The finding of associated aortic valve disease favors a rheumatic cause.

Other forms of mitral regurgitation include rupture of one or more chordae tendineae, most commonly resulting from bacterial endocarditis, but also sometimes attributed to rheumatic disease, trauma, or unknown causes. Papillary muscle dysfunction is usually secondary to necrosis or fibrosis of one or both papillary muscles owing to coronary artery disease, mitral regurgitation resulting from poor contraction of the muscles, and systolic eversion of the mitral leaflets. In acute myocardial infarction, rupture of a papillary muscle causes sudden, severe mitral regurgitation (see Ch. 363.3). Congenital mitral regurgitation can occur as an isolated condition, but more commonly it accompanies such lesions as ostium primum atrial septal defect or Marfan's syndrome in which the valve may resemble that found in the floppy valve syndrome, but is associated with other stigmata.

Mitral regurgitation also occurs as a secondary phenomenon in patients with obstructive hypertrophic cardiomyopathy, as discussed subsequently. In primary myocardial disease, mitral regurgitation may be secondary to massive dilatation of the left ventricle and the mitral anulus. Acquired, heavy calcification of the mitral anulus, which typically occurs in elderly women, is sometimes associated with significant mitral regurgitation. The mitral valve prolapse syndrome has been recognized with increased frequency and is considered in Ch. 360.4.

PATHOLOGIC PHYSIOLOGY.   With insufficiency of the mitral valve of the type found in chronic rheumatic heart disease, regurgitation of blood from the left ventricle into the left atrium commences as soon as the left ventricular pressure during early systole exceeds that in the left atrium, and persists until the left ventricular pressure falls below the left atrial pressure. Therefore the regurgitation is pansystolic, commencing with the first heart sound and often ending with or just after the second heart sound, and at the peak of the atrial V wave. The prominent V wave in the left atrial pressure pulse is due to the normal inflow of blood from the pulmonary veins (when the mitral valve is ordinarily closed) which is augmented by the regurgitant leak.

An important physiologic characteristic of mitral regurgitation relative to the function of the left ventricle is that this lesion provides a relatively low impedance pathway for blood to exit from the left ventricle, pressure in the left atrium being lower than that in the aorta. The pressure in the left ventricle tends to fall more abruptly than normal late in ventricular systole because of the leak, and the average afterload or active tension in the wall of the left ventricle is thereby reduced. This effect favors increased shortening of the myocardial wall because of the inverse relation between force and fiber shortening (and velocity), and the ratio of stroke volume to end-diastolic volume (ejection fraction) may therefore be normal or even high in mitral regurgitation. In addition, although myocardial oxygen consumption is greatly enhanced by lesions which cause increased systolic pressure work or augmented wall tension, it is little affected by the increased volume load imposed by mitral regurgitation. These favorable mechanical loading conditions and the minimal effect of this lesion on oxygen consumption help to explain the prolonged clinical course observed in many patients with chronic mitral regurgitation.

In chronic mitral regurgitation the diastolic volume of the left ventricular chamber becomes increased because of ventricular dilatation and increased muscle mass. The increased diastolic ventricular size allows delivery of a much larger than normal *total* stroke volume during systole (forward stroke volume plus the regurgitant volume), but with a normal extent of shortening of each unit of the enlarged left ventricular circumference. When left ventricular myocardial function is not impaired, the left ventricular end-diastolic pressure is normal or only slightly elevated, and the forward cardiac output is well maintained. Under these conditions, the *mean* left atrial pressure may be minimally elevated, because the exaggerated V wave occurs only briefly during the cardiac cycle. There is no impairment of left atrial emptying into the left ventricle and hence little or no rise in mean left atrial pressure during exercise.

With longstanding, severe mitral regurgitation, left ventricular myocardial contractility is eventually depressed. When this happens, the extent of shortening of the left ventricular wall becomes reduced, the residual volume in the left ventricle at the end of ejection increases, the ejection fraction falls, and the end-diastolic volume and left ventricular end-diastolic pressure rise. The latter, in turn, leads to elevation of the mean left atrial pressure and subsequently to pulmonary hypertension. Left atrial hypertension also occurs when there is some associated narrowing of the mitral valve. The mechanism of pulmonary hypertension in mitral regurgitation resembles that in mitral stenosis, and in later stages elevations of the pulmonary vascular resistance as severe as those seen with mitral stenosis have been encountered.

The aforementioned description encompasses most patients with chronic rheumatic mitral regurgitation, but there are unusual physiologic manifestations seen late in the course of chronic disease or with acute mitral regurgitation, such as that caused by ruptured chordae tendineae. In the former category is the finding of giant left atrium with low mean left atrial pressure and greatly reduced cardiac output. This syndrome appears to be due to a combination of poor left ventricular function with reduced forward cardiac output and diminished regurgitant volume, as well as to a capacious and compliant left atrium, which absorbs the regurgitant leak with little change in the pressure. At the other extreme is the situation in sudden, severe mitral regurgitation. In this setting, the left atrium is small, distended, and noncompliant, and the large regurgitant leak produces a giant V wave which can reach 70 to 80 mm Hg (so-called "ventricularization" of the left atrial pressure pulse). Severe pulmonary hypertension and reduced forward cardiac output accompany such marked, acute regurgitation.

CLINICAL MANIFESTATIONS. Symptoms and Clinical Course. As mentioned earlier, the mean left atrial pressure may not be significantly elevated at rest in patients with mitral regurgitation in whom the left ventricle is compensated, and, unlike mitral stenosis, there is little increase in left atrial pressure during exercise or with tachycardia. Therefore the earliest symptom in mitral re-

gurgitation is often exertional fatigue, which reflects inability to maintain a normal forward cardiac output to supply the exercising skeletal muscles. Mild symptoms of this type may persist for many years without significant dyspnea or pulmonary congestion.

Later in the course of severe chronic mitral regurgitation, with the onset of early left ventricular failure, the ventricular end-diastolic pressure increases, left atrial hypertension develops, and dyspnea on exertion and orthopnea occur. However, paroxysmal nocturnal dyspnea and acute pulmonary edema are distinctly unusual in this condition. With the onset of pulmonary hypertension, right heart failure accompanied by venous distention and peripheral edema may occur. Atrial fibrillation is a common complication, but left atrial thrombi are relatively unusual, and systemic emboli occur much less commonly than with mitral stenosis.

Chronic mitral regurgitation is the best tolerated of the lesions involving the left side of the heart. Frequently, patients remain relatively asymptomatic for 10 or 20 years, even in the presence of severe regurgitation, and it is not uncommon for patients to respond well to medical therapy for an additional 10 years or more before progressive left ventricular failure causes serious progressive difficulty and death. This long clinical course undoubtedly reflects in part the favorable loading conditions of this lesion on the left ventricle, as discussed earlier. It seems likely that a sizable number of patients with only moderate mitral regurgitation never experience serious difficulty and may have a normal life expectancy.

Physical Findings. When mitral regurgitation is severe, the peripheral pulse is sharp and abbreviated, owing to lack of sustained forward stroke volume in the face of the regurgitant leak. The jugular venous pulse is normal unless there is pulmonary hypertension or tricuspid valve disease. Atrial fibrillation is frequently present.

On palpation of the precordium, the left ventricle is enlarged, the apex beat is hyperactive and displaced laterally, and frequently there is a systolic thrill at the apex. In the lateral decubitus position, a rapid outward movement in early diastole (rapid filling wave) may be palpable. If pulmonary hypertension is present, there is a right ventricular lift. When the left atrium is markedly enlarged and the mitral regurgitation is severe, expansion of this chamber during systole may push the right ventricle and pulmonary artery out against the chest wall in the third and fourth left interspaces during late systole, a finding which may be confused with right ventricular enlargement.

The characteristic feature of mitral regurgitation in chronic rheumatic disease is a high-pitched *pansystolic murmur* at the cardiac apex which is transmitted to the left axilla (see Fig. 1, Ch. 360.1). If the lesion is severe, it is accompanied by four other findings: (1) soft first heart sound, (2) loud ventricular diastolic gallop (third heart sound), (3) short early diastolic rumble, which accompanies the rapid inflow of blood to the left ventricle, and (4) wide splitting of the second heart sound caused by early closure of the aortic valve. The last-named finding is caused by shortening of the left ventricular ejection time consequent to the regurgitant leak.

Although the murmur of mitral regurgitation is usually pansystolic, variations may be heard. When mitral regurgitation is due to papillary muscle dysfunction, the murmur begins well after the first heart sound and may have a crescendo-decrescendo quality. These characteristics result from posterior herniation of the mitral leaflet as the papillary muscles fail to contract normally late during ventricular systole. In the *click-murmur* or mitral valve prolapse syndrome, late ballooning of the mitral leaflets into the left atrium also occurs, but caused by intrinsic mitral valve disease. In this condition the late systolic murmur may be ushered in by one or more midsystolic clicks. In sudden, severe mitral regurgitation, sinus rhythm is often preserved and there may be a loud fourth heart sound, a most uncommon finding in chronic mitral regurgitation. When a giant left atrial V wave accompanies acute mitral regurgitation, the murmur may occur early in systole; but it is short and terminates before the end of systole, because the left ventricular pressure and massive left atrial V wave equalize near or even before the time of aortic valve closure.

DIAGNOSIS. Electrocardiogram. In patients with mild to moderate mitral regurgitation the electrocardiogram may be normal; but with longstanding moderate disease or with severe regurgitation the electrocardiogram usually shows left ventricular hypertrophy and atrial fibrillation. Typically, there is evidence of a so-called diastolic overload pattern, with upright T waves and voltage criteria for left ventricular hypertrophy. Right ventricular hypertrophy may develop in the late stages of the disease when there is pulmonary hypertension. If sinus rhythm is present, left atrial enlargement may be evident.

In the "click-murmur syndrome" S-T segment and T wave abnormalities may be observed and evidence of old or recent myocardial infarction may be seen with papillary muscle dysfunction caused by coronary heart disease.

Roentgenographic Features. The left ventricle and left atrium are usually enlarged. Occasionally, the left atrium is of giant size and can extend well into the right chest. The left ventricle is observed to contract vigorously on fluoroscopy, and systolic expansion of the left atrium may be striking. The presence of calcium in the mitral valve suggests some degree of associated mitral stenosis. If left atrial hypertension is marked, the findings in the lung fields resemble those of mitral stenosis.

Echocardiography. The echo from the mitral valve leaflets can be particularly useful in detecting abnormal posterior prolapse of one or both mitral leaflets into the left atrium during systole (see Ch. 360.4). A flail mitral leaflet may be identified in the presence of a ruptured chorda.

Cardiac Catheterization. Cardiac catheterization is indicated prior to considering cardiac surgery in order to confirm the presence of severe regurgitation, assess the degree of left ventricular myocardial dysfunction, exclude associated coronary artery disease, and assess the severity of any associated valvular lesions.

The severity of mitral regurgitation can be estimated by cineangiography, with injection of contrast medium into the left ventricle. The backward regurgitation of contrast medium into the left atrium during ventricular systole is readily apparent, and it is also possible to calculate the diastolic volume of the left ventricle, the total stroke volume, and the ejection fraction. If the forward cardiac output and forward stroke volume are calculated by the Fick method, when the regurgitation is severe the regurgitant volume per beat may be well in excess of the forward stroke volume.

An elevated V wave in the left atrium (peak of the V wave over 20 mm Hg) may be detected on the pulmonary artery wedge pressure tracing, or from direct measurement by transseptal puncture, with relatively normal mean left atrial pressure. The increased V wave is followed by a rapid pressure fall (the Y descent) as the ventricle

relaxes, the mitral valve opens, and an excessively rapid inflow of blood (forward plus regurgitant volume) crosses the mitral valve in early diastole (see Fig. 1, Ch. 360.1). Even with pure mitral regurgitation, there is often a pressure gradient across the mitral valve in early diastole, reflecting functional mitral stenosis in the presence of increased flow. A normal, simultaneous rise in left atrial and left ventricular pressures then ensues later in diastole, with no pressure gradient.

With the onset of left ventricular dysfunction, the ventricular end-diastolic pressure increases, the ratio of stroke volume to ventricular end-diastolic volume (ejection fraction) falls to less than 55 per cent, and the forward cardiac output diminishes. At this stage of the disease, pulmonary hypertension of moderate degree is generally present.

Mitral regurgitation due to ruptured chordae tendineae may result from bacterial endocarditis or may occur spontaneously with rheumatic or other types of degenerative valve disease, such as Marfan's syndrome or the click-murmur syndrome. In some patients the onset is insidious, but in others it is acute and characterized by a small left atrium, a murmur that is not prominent, sinus rhythm with S$_3$ and S$_4$ gallops, and severe congestive heart failure.

DIFFERENTIAL DIAGNOSIS. Several conditions may produce a systolic murmur resembling that of mitral regurgitation. The thrill and murmur of *ventricular septal defect* are pansystolic, but their location at the lower left sternal border is characteristic. The murmur of *tricuspid regurgitation* may be heard well to the left of the sternum whenever the right atrium and right ventricle are markedly enlarged, but the prominent V waves in the jugular venous pulse and the characteristic increase in intensity of the murmur with inspiration should help differentiate this lesion from mitral regurgitation.

When the jet of mitral regurgitation caused by a leak through the posterior mitral leaflet strikes the interatrial septum, the murmur is heard well in the aortic area, and it may be confused with the murmur of *aortic stenosis*. However, the murmur of mitral regurgitation increases when systemic arterial pressure is raised (as with the handgrip maneuver), and it decreases when the systemic arterial pressure is lowered (as with amyl nitrite inhalation), whereas opposite responses tend to occur in aortic stenosis.

The ejection type of murmur associated with *idiopathic hypertrophic subaortic stenosis* may be well heard at the apex, as well as at the left sternal border. The characteristic increase of this murmur with the Valsalva maneuver should provide a point of differentiation.

TREATMENT. Medical Management. In the absence of significant symptoms, the only therapeutic measures necessary are *antimicrobial prophylaxis* against streptococcal infections in the younger patient with a history of rheumatic fever and antimicrobial prophylaxis against bacterial endocarditis with dental or surgical procedures. With the onset of fatigue, dyspnea, or atrial fibrillation, the use of *digitalis* is indicated both to control the ventricular rate and to improve the contractile function of the left ventricle. Frequently, even in patients with severe mitral regurgitation, the use of an oral diuretic and digitalis, together with reduced sodium intake, will serve to maintain the patient in a comfortable status for a number of years.

In patients with sudden, severe mitral regurgitation, as with ruptured chordae tendineae, the use of a peripheral vasodilating agent such as sodium nitroprusside, to reduce the afterload on the left ventricle, often will improve the cardiac output and decrease left ventricular failure until replacement of the mitral valve can be carried out.

Surgical Treatment. Surgical treatment is generally indicated when symptoms of severe fatigue or dyspnea occur on less than normal activity (N.Y.H.A. Class III or IV), despite appropriate medical management. Such symptoms generally indicate the onset of significant left ventricular myocardial disease. Obviously, in reaching the decision to recommend operation, the prolonged natural course of this disease should be kept in mind, and the low incidence of serious complications such as acute pulmonary edema, systemic emboli, and sudden death should be considered. Nevertheless, it is desirable to recommend operation prior to the development of irreversible left ventricular myocardial disease, and the persistence of significant symptoms while the patient is maintained on adequate medical therapy is generally considered to presage the onset of this process.

Occasionally, the surgical repair of a ruptured chorda or of a deficient posterior leaflet is possible. Almost always, however, in rheumatic and other forms of mitral regurgitation, replacement of the valve with a prosthesis is necessary. Sudden, severe mitral regurgitation is not well tolerated and generally requires early surgical intervention. Different types of prostheses, complications, and late results of mitral valve replacement are discussed in Ch. 360.2.

360.4. THE MITRAL VALVE PROLAPSE SYNDROME

This syndrome, initially recognized by its auscultatory features, has received a variety of names, including the "floppy mitral valve" syndrome and the mid-systolic click–late systolic murmur or "click-murmur" syndrome. It has been recognized with increasing frequency in recent years as a result of the enhanced diagnostic accuracy available through echocardiography. It now seems likely that this common disorder, with some exceptions, is generally associated with a benign clinical course.

ETIOLOGY AND PATHOLOGY. Pathologic findings in the mitral valve prolapse syndrome include myxomatous degeneration of the mitral valve, often associated with redundant valve tissue and with elongation and other abnormalities of the chordae tendineae. Sometimes degenerative changes in the valve are associated with deposition of acid mucopolysaccharide material. The cause of these pathologic abnormalities is unknown, although the disorder has been associated with the Marfan syndrome (in its complete or incomplete forms), osteogenesis imperfecta, and other connective tissue diseases, as well as occasionally with coronary artery disease. It has been reported in up to 15 per cent of patients with ostium secundum atrial septal defect. The syndrome is seen more frequently in women than in men, and it occurs quite commonly in several members of the same family.

PATHOLOGIC PHYSIOLOGY. The abnormal mitral valve structure involves both the anterior and posterior leaflets, but effects often are most prominent on the posterior leaflet. With the onset of left ventricular contraction normal closure of the mitral valve initially takes place, but during ventricular ejection, as cardiac volume decreases, there is abrupt movement of the valve leaflets toward the left atrium; this rapid posterior motion is followed by

tensing of the chordae and other valve structures, leading to the mid-systolic click. The subsequent prolapse or herniation of the leaflets into the left atrium is associated with the late systolic murmur of mitral regurgitation. In some patients, the posterior prolapse of the leaflets starts more gradually early in systole and is not associated with a click. Mitral regurgitation can be absent, mild, or severe, and occasionally it is progressive over several years. Also, rupture of a mitral valve chorda with acute mitral regurgitation (sometimes associated with infectious endocarditis) occurs with increased frequency in patients with this syndrome.

Localized regional contraction disorders of the left ventricle have been described in many patients studied by angiocardiography, but whether or not they are causally related to the prolapse is not clear. In some patients, infusion of a pressor agent has reproduced their symptom of chest pain, suggesting the possibility of subendocardial ischemia, and it has also been suggested (without direct evidence) that small vessel coronary artery disease may play a role. Generally the major coronary arteries are normal, and there is no clear pathologic explanation for the chest pain or the frequent dysrhythmias that are observed in patients with this disorder.

CLINICAL MANIFESTATIONS. Symptoms and Clinical Course. The spectrum of symptoms is broad, but most commonly they include chest pain, weakness, fatigue, palpitations, lightheadedness, and dyspnea. The chest pain usually is not typical of angina pectoris; commonly it is nonexertional, and it may be prolonged. Sometimes symptoms are vague in nature, and there is an increased incidence of abnormal psychologic tests in patients with this disorder. Symptoms of lightheadedness or palpitations ordinarily are not associated with simultaneous cardiac rhythm abnormalities. Complaints of dyspnea usually are not progressive, nor are they accompanied by signs of cardiac failure.

The natural history of the mitral valve prolapse syndrome has not yet been defined clearly. However, its relatively high frequency in the general population (probably well over 1 per cent) suggests that symptoms never occur in many individuals. In one retrospective follow-up study of over 50 patients identified an average of 14 years earlier, there was an over-all incidence of serious complications of 15 per cent. These included progressive mitral regurgitation (9 per cent), bacterial endocarditis (6 per cent) (one patient died after rupture of a chorda), and nonfatal ventricular fibrillation (one patient); one patient died suddenly following institution of quinidine therapy for frequent ventricular premature beats. A late systolic murmur, rather than an isolated systolic click, was present in the patients with complications. Prospective studies are needed to define whether or not the few patients at risk of complications can be identified early in their course.

Physical Findings. The hallmark of this syndrome is the occurrence of one or more mid-systolic clicks, which generally occur 0.14 second or more after the first heart sound. Sometimes this finding is present alone, but more commonly the click is followed by a crescendo-decrescendo late systolic murmur; occasionally, patients with the echocardiographic features of mitral prolapse exhibit a holosystolic murmur without a click. Alterations in the characteristics of the click and murmur produced by certain maneuvers aid in the identification of the syndrome. Maneuvers which decrease cardiac volume tend to increase mitral valve prolapse, thereby causing the click and murmur to occur earlier during systole (prolonging the murmur), whereas those that increase cardiac volume tend to move the click and the murmur later in systole. The standing position and the Valsalva maneuver decrease the left ventricular volume, moving the click closer to the first heart sound and prolonging the murmur. Inhalation of amyl nitrite typically produces a biphasic response, initially only decreasing the intensity of the murmur, but later moving the click and murmur closer to the first heart sound. The squatting position (or production of bradycardia with agents such as propranolol) increases cardiac volume and moves the click later in systole while shortening the murmur. It is usually possible to document clearly the effects of these interventions by the use of phonocardiography.

DIAGNOSIS. Electrocardiogram. The electrocardiogram is abnormal in a relatively large proportion of patients, the most common finding being T wave inversions in leads II, III, and aVF and occasionally in leads V_5 and V_6; ST segment changes and Q waves are rather uncommon. Prominent U waves and prolongation of the QT interval have also been reported, particularly in patients with a positive family history. ST segment abnormalities are sometimes seen on the exercise ECG, but do not consistently correlate with the occurrence of chest pain. A variety of rhythm disturbances are common, and some surveys have shown frequent ventricular ectopic beats in 40 to 50 per cent of nonselected patients during 24-hour ECG monitoring; in a significant proportion of patients with frequent ventricular ectopic beats, brief or even prolonged bouts of ventricular tachycardia have been reported. Atrial premature contractions and supraventricular tachycardia also are quite common. As mentioned earlier, subjective complaints of palpitations and dizziness usually do not correlate well in time with dysrhythmias recorded on the ECG. In many patients, arrhythmias can be brought out by exercise stress testing, although 24-hour ECG monitoring appears to be the most sensitive method of detection.

Echocardiography. Two types of echocardiographic abnormalities have been described. In the more common variety, an initially normal closure of the anterior and posterior leaflets is followed by a horizontal or slightly posterior motion during early ventricular ejection and then by abrupt posterior motion of the valve during the latter half of left ventricular systole (a pattern said to resemble a "question mark placed on its side") (see Fig. 2, Ch. 360.1). Often, multiple echoes are recorded from the redundant valve tissue. The second type of abnormality consists of posterior motion of the mitral valve leaflets early after the onset of systole, reaching the most posterior position during mid-ejection, followed by a gradual motion anteriorly (yielding a "hammock" configuration). The first echocardiographic pattern tends to be associated with the click and late systolic murmur; the second, with a holosystolic murmur alone. These findings on the echocardiogram have also occasionally been reported to occur without associated physical findings, and rarely the echocardiogram is normal despite typical findings on physical examination.

Cardiac Catheterization. Left ventriculography has shown abnormalities in almost all patients studied. Usually, the intracardiac pressures and cardiac output are normal, except in those uncommon patients with associated hypertrophic cardiomyopathy or severe mitral regurgitation. The frontal and lateral plane angiocardiograms generally show markedly enlarged, scalloped mitral valve leaflets that prolapse into the left atrium during systole; often, scalloping and prolapse of the posterior leaflet are most prominent. Left ventricular contraction abnormalities, including hypokinesis of the posterior wall, systolic cavity obliteration, and the so-called "systolic contraction ring," are often observed. Some patients have been found to have angiographic evidence of associated prolapse of the tricuspid valve as well. An accompanying atrial septal defect may be detected in some patients.

DIFFERENTIAL DIAGNOSIS. The murmur closely resembles that associated with papillary muscle dysfunction and mitral regurgitation due to coronary heart disease. In its physical findings the mitral valve prolapse syndrome also closely resembles hypertrophic subaortic stenosis (hypertrophic cardiomyopathy, asymmetric septal hypertrophy), although many other features and the ECG differ (see Ch. 366.2). The murmur of hypertrophic subaortic stenosis has a crescendo-decrescendo character and responds in a qualitatively similar manner to that of mitral valve prolapse during the maneuvers described above, but it is greatly intensified during the Valsalva maneuver, whereas that of the prolapse syndrome tends instead to become more prolonged. Moreover, the murmur of hypertrophic subaortic stenosis is not initially decreased with amyl nitrite inhalation intensity, but is increased throughout the inhalation; if ectopic beats are present, the murmur of hypertrophic subaortic stenosis increases during the postextrasystolic beat, whereas that of mitral valve prolapse diminishes.

Systolic anterior motion of the anterior mitral leaflet in hypertrophic subaortic stenosis is followed by posterior motion ("SAM"; see Fig. 2, Ch. 360.1), but this event occurs anterior to the C point of the echocardiogram, whereas with mitral valve prolapse the posterior motion occurs posterior to the C point (see Fig. 2). Amyl nitrite administration during echocardiography enhances systolic anterior motion in hypertrophic subaortic stenosis but increases posterior motion in the mitral prolapse syndrome.

TREATMENT. In some patients with significant symptoms, beta-adrenergic blockade with propranolol (up to 320 mg per day in divided doses) has been found to relieve chest pain, whereas nitroglycerin often is ineffective. Propranolol may, however, increase symptoms of fatigue or dyspnea. Although dysrhythmias are common, treatment with antiarrhythmic drugs usually is reserved for patients with severe symptoms or life-threatening arrhythmias. In patients with significant symptoms, 24-hour ECG monitoring is recommended. Sudden death has been reported rarely, usually in association with a positive family history, and ventricular fibrillation has been reported in individuals with a prolonged Q-T interval. Therefore antiarrhythmic therapy appears warranted in patients with either of these features, as well as in patients with a history of ventricular fibrillation or syncope. In some patients, palpitations may respond to propranolol. Often, however, the control of arrhythmias with propranolol or other antiarrhythmic medications is difficult.

The true incidence of infectious endocarditis is not known, but there have been several reports of this complication, usually associated with viridans streptococci. Therefore prophylaxis against endocarditis at the time of dental or surgical procedures should be recommended in all patients with the mitral valve prolapse syndrome.

Rarely, mitral regurgitation appears to be progressive, and, if unresponsive to medical management, mitral valve replacement may be required. Also, following rupture of a chorda tendinea, some patients may require valve replacement for acute, severe mitral regurgitation.

It should be re-emphasized, however, that in most patients the clinical course of this disorder is benign. Thus reassurance of the patient usually is in order, and specific therapy should be reserved for patients with disabling symptoms or serious dysrhythmias.

360.5. AORTIC STENOSIS

ETIOLOGY AND PATHOLOGY. There is evidence that a congenitally bicuspid aortic valve is present in more than one half of adult patients with isolated aortic stenosis, most of the remainder being of rheumatic cause. Although the bicuspid valve is frequently not stenotic in early life, this malformation sets up abnormal stresses within the valve, leading to progressive fibrosis and thickening, with eventual immobility of the leaflets and calcification. This sequence may take many years, and the typical patient presents with findings of significant stenosis in the sixth decade of life. Three quarters of patients with isolated valvular aortic stenosis in adult life are male. The varieties of congenital aortic stenosis as they present in childhood and adolescence are discussed in Ch. 359.2. When aortic stenosis is due to rheumatic heart disease, the sex distribution is relatively equal, and frequently there is evidence of associated mitral valve involvement. With rheumatic disease, the aortic valve is tricuspid and shows fusion of one or more commissures and scarring and thickening of the leaflets; calcification may also be present. Acquired aortic stenosis may also occur in elderly subjects as a degenerative process without fusion of the commissures, stenosis resulting from heavy deposition of calcium within the valve leaflets. When calcification of the aortic valve is marked, the calcium may extend into the anulus and even into the upper portion of the ventricular septum, leading to involvement of the bundle of His or the left bundle branch.

When aortic stenosis is significant, the left ventricle shows concentric hypertrophy with marked thickening of the left ventricular wall, and there is poststenotic dilatation of the ascending aorta. The left atrium is usually normal unless there has been left ventricular failure.

PATHOLOGIC PHYSIOLOGY. The earliest physiologic response to obstruction at the aortic valve, as in acute experimental constriction of the ascending aorta, is an increased left ventricular diastolic volume and pressure and compensatory use of the Frank-Starling mechanism. Consequent to the more forceful contraction, the systolic left ventricular pressure is elevated and a pressure gradient is created across the aortic valve, forcing blood across the narrowed orifice at high velocity. The chronic effect of longstanding systolic pressure overload on the left ventricle is to induce hypertrophy of the ventricular wall, a compensatory process which tends to maintain the force or tension in the wall relatively normal, without substantial enlargement of the left ventricular cavity. (Wall tension, or stress, is directly related to systolic pressure but inversely proportional to wall thickness, and in concentric hypertrophy the increased pressure load is distributed over a larger number of muscle fibers.) The stroke volume is generally well maintained by these mechanisms until very late in the disease. Even when the pressure gradient across the aortic valve

is quite large, the compensatory left ventricular hypertrophy, coupled with a forceful left atrial contraction, serves to maintain the cardiac output at a normal level. This strong left atrial "booster pump" generates a prominent presystolic wave in the pressure tracings, leading to an elevated end-diastolic pressure in the hypertrophied and noncompliant ventricle (often near 20 mm Hg). However, elevation of the end-diastolic pressure by this mechanism does not indicate left ventricular failure, and the mean left atrial pressure is maintained relatively normal.

It should be recognized that a significant gradient is not produced across the aortic valve until the valve orifice is narrowed substantially, by more than 60 per cent of its normal area. A murmur may be created by turbulent flow in the absence of a pressure gradient; but as the stenosis progresses beyond this critical point, an increasing systolic pressure gradient develops between the left ventricle and aorta.

With the increased heart rate which accompanies muscular exercise, diastole is primarily abbreviated, and therefore more time is available per minute for systolic ejection. Hence the aortic valve gradient does *not* tend to increase during exercise, despite an augmented cardiac output, and the left ventricular end-diastolic pressure and mean left atrial pressure may also remain unchanged. This finding is in marked contrast to the situation in mitral stenosis, when filling occurs during diastole and less time is available for flow during exercise.

The arterial pulse pressure is usually narrow when there is significant aortic stenosis, and an important accompanying effect is a tendency toward reduction of the diastolic aortic pressure. The perfusion pressure available to the coronary circulation is therefore diminished. In addition, the oxygen demands of the left ventricle are increased because of the hypertrophy and the need to maintain an elevated systolic pressure in the ventricle (often well over 200 mm Hg in severe aortic stenosis). Heart rate, as well as pressure development, is an important determinant of myocardial oxygen consumption, and the increased heart rate during exertion, together with a limitation of coronary perfusion pressure, can lead to an imbalance between oxygen supply and demand in the left ventricle. Thus *angina pectoris* is common in aortic stenosis in the absence of coronary artery disease. Transient myocardial ischemia in the hypertrophied heart may also explain, at least in part, the tendency toward *sudden serious arrhythmia* which can lead to sudden death. Likewise, this mechanism, perhaps coupled with transient hypotension caused by momentary inability to maintain cardiac output (such as may occur with sudden assumption of the upright posture), may have a role in the *syncopal attacks* which sometimes mark the clinical course of patients with aortic stenosis.

Longstanding pressure overwork by the hypertrophied left ventricle in aortic stenosis eventually leads to evidence of myocardial disease with inability of the heart muscle to maintain normal basal contractile processes, often associated with some degree of myocardial fibrosis. With the onset of left ventricular dysfunction, the degree of emptying becomes reduced. This, in turn, leads to an increased residual ventricular volume and elevation of the end-diastolic volume, with a further increase in the end-diastolic pressure. Elevation of the left atrial mean pressure then ensues, with the onset of orthopnea and exertional dyspnea through the same mechanisms discussed in Ch. 360.2. In the late phases of myocardial failure, pulmonary hypertension develops and cardiac output falls.

CLINICAL MANIFESTATIONS. Symptoms and Clinical Course. Usually there is a latent period of many years, during which aortic stenosis is present and progressing in severity but symptoms are absent. When congenital aortic stenosis is severe, symptoms may occur in childhood, but typically they begin in middle or late life. If there is associated mitral valve disease in patients with rheumatic aortic stenosis, particularly mitral stenosis, the onset of symptoms may be much earlier and may lead to earlier detection of the associated aortic lesion. The three cardinal symptoms of aortic stenosis are (1) angina pectoris, (2) syncope, and (3) symptoms caused by left ventricular failure.

The pathophysiology of *angina pectoris* in aortic stenosis, an imbalance between oxygen supply and demand, is discussed above. It may mimic in every way the exertional chest pain which occurs in patients with coronary artery disease. In the older patient, the *coexistence* of coronary heart disease should be considered. Thus even when the aortic stenosis is moderate, or when stenotic lesions in the coronary vessels are moderate, increased oxygen utilization by the myocardium may lead to angina pectoris. Angina pectoris is often the first symptom in patients with aortic stenosis, and in the young patient it usually indicates severe obstruction to left ventricular ejection.

Syncope is sometimes the initial symptom in patients with aortic stenosis. This may be due to a transient arrhythmia such as atrial or ventricular tachycardia. The tendency of the hypertrophied ventricle to develop transient ischemia undoubtedly makes it more susceptible to ventricular fibrillation or ventricular tachycardia. Other mechanisms for syncope may consist of a transient fall in blood pressure during or immediately after exercise, or upon abruptly assuming the upright posture; such mechanisms are related to transient inability of the left ventricle to maintain a normal forward cardiac output, as discussed earlier, or are perhaps associated with metabolic or reflex peripheral vasodilatation. So-called presyncope may also occur, in which the patient experiences a transient graying out or loss of vision.

One of the major problems in the patient with hemodynamically significant aortic stenosis is the occurrence of *sudden death*, which is occasionally the first sign of the disease. In postmortem studies of patients who have died from aortic stenosis, death was sudden in about 15 per cent. It should be recognized, however, that most of these patients had significant symptoms, and that only 3 to 4 per cent of the patients who die do so without prior symptoms. The mechanism of sudden death is unclear, but it may be due to serious arrhythmia or mechanisms similar to those occurring with syncope.

With longstanding pressure overload, and increasing obstruction at the aortic valve, *left ventricular myocardial dysfunction* eventually develops. The earliest symptom of left ventricular dysfunction is usually orthopnea, caused by elevation of the left atrial mean pressure. Mild dyspnea on exertion may then ensue, which progresses to dyspnea on minimal exertion. In the late stages of aortic stenosis, pulmonary edema or evidence of pulmonary hypertension with right ventricular failure and peripheral edema may occur.

The onset of *atrial fibrillation* in patients with aortic stenosis is uncommon, but when it occurs in the absence of mitral valve disease it is ominous. Usually it indicates an elevated mean left atrial pressure with left atrial distention. Because of the loss of left atrial contribution to ventricular filling, further elevation of the mean left atrial pressure, fall in the cardiac output, and severe cardiac failure may ensue.

The onset of symptoms in a patient with significant aortic stenosis has real importance, because the subsequent course is generally downhill. Although earlier mortality figures based on retrospective clinical analyses of patients with aortic stenosis may be modified somewhat by the advent of modern diuretic, antiarrhythmic, and antimicrobial therapy, the typical course after symptoms begin remains relatively short. Thus the average life expectancy in an adult patient after the onset of congestive heart failure is 18 months to 2 years; after the onset of angina pectoris it is about 5 years; and when syncope begins it is about 6 years, although survivals as long as 18 to 20 years after onset of syncope have been reported. The natural history in the patient with severe stenosis who has few or no symptoms has not been clearly established.

Complications of aortic stenosis include *infective endocarditis*, which has been estimated to occur in as many as 25 per cent of patients during their lifetime. Rarely, hemolytic anemia has been seen in patients with severe calcific aortic stenosis, presumably owing to local blood trauma at the valve, and perhaps also to intrinsic red blood cell abnormalities. Systemic emboli have been reported as a result of calcium or fibrin particles breaking loose from the aortic valve.

Physical Findings. The primary findings on physical examination can be related to three features: abnormal ejection of blood into the arterial bed, turbulent flow and prolonged ejection across the stenotic aortic orifice, and left ventricular hypertrophy. Physical findings reflecting all three phenomena can generally be detected in hemodynamically significant aortic valve obstruction; but despite their helpfulness, such signs do not always predict accurately the degree of stenosis in the individual patient.

The patient with aortic stenosis is typically not debilitated or wasted, the cardiac output being well maintained until late in the course of the disease. The mean jugular venous pressure is generally normal, although the A wave may be prominent in patients with hemodynamically significant aortic stenosis, presumably because of septal hypertrophy with decreased right ventricular compliance. The carotid pulse is small, the upstroke is delayed, and a systolic thrill may be felt in the carotid vessels. The blood pressure is usually low-normal, with narrowing of the pulse pressure, but in elderly patients having reduced compliance (increased stiffness) of the aortic wall and arteries it is not unusual to find an elevated *systolic* blood pressure, even in the presence of significant aortic stenosis. However, marked systemic hypertension with a substantial diastolic pressure elevation is not encountered in the presence of severe aortic stenosis.

On palpation of the precordium, there is a systolic thrill at the aortic area, the apex beat is enlarged, and there is a sustained apical impulse. A presystolic atrial impulse may be palpable at the apex in the lateral decubitus position. The first heart sound is usually normal, and the aortic component of the second heart sound is diminished. Often, the second heart sound is single owing to a prolonged left ventricular ejection time; or aortic valve closure may even follow pulmonic valve closure, leading to paradoxical splitting of the second heart sound (decreased splitting during inspiration) (see Fig. 1, Ch. 360.1). The *systolic murmur* of aortic stenosis is crescendo-decrescendo in quality, is loudest at the aortic area, is transmitted to the carotid arteries, and is also audible at the apex. Being ejection in type, the murmur begins well after the first heart sound and ends before the second heart sound. In the presence of severe aortic stenosis, the murmur is long and peaks in mid- or late systole. Frequently there is an atrial diastolic gallop (fourth heart sound), which reflects both reduced compliance of the thickened left ventricular wall and forceful left atrial contraction. This gallop is best heard in the left lateral decubitus position.

When aortic stenosis is mild, there tends to be less delay of the carotid upstroke, the duration of ventricular ejection may be normal, and the second heart sound splits normally with respiration. The systolic murmur tends to be less intense and shorter, peaking early in systole. It should be appreciated, however, that in the late stages of aortic stenosis, when cardiac failure and low cardiac output supervene, the murmur of aortic stenosis may also become markedly diminished in intensity. Under these circumstances, the left ventricle is generally substantially enlarged, and there are symptoms and signs of cardiac failure.

It is not uncommon to hear a soft, early diastolic blowing murmur at the left sternal border caused by mild aortic regurgitation, even in patients with severe aortic stenosis. This small leak occurs because of the small, fixed orifice. The murmur of associated mitral stenosis should be searched for carefully, particularly in female patients with aortic stenosis, because the association of these two obstructive lesions serves to diminish the physical findings of each. When mitral and aortic stenosis coexist, the cardiac output tends to be reduced, the severity of aortic stenosis may be underestimated, and the murmur of mitral stenosis may be difficult to appreciate.

DIAGNOSIS (see table). **Electrocardiogram.** In both children and adults, a normal electrocardiogram is rarely found in the presence of significant aortic stenosis. In children under 10 or 12 years of age, the degree of left ventricular hypertrophy on the electrocardiogram tends to relate to the degree of obstruction, but in adults relatively marked degrees of left ventricular hypertrophy are sometimes seen in mild or moderate obstruction. Typically, the electrocardiogram shows voltage criteria for left ventricular hypertrophy, with associated S-T segment and T wave changes and left atrial enlargement. Occasionally, intraventricular conduction delay or left bundle branch block is seen, particularly late in the course of the disease, and atrial fibrillation is a late and relatively uncommon problem. Complete heart block has been reported in some patients resulting from extension of aortic calcification into the conduction system.

Roentgenographic Features. There may be little or no over-all cardiac enlargement, but when aortic stenosis is significant some degree of left ventricular enlargement is usually discernible, with straightening of the left heart border, downward displacement of the left ventricular apex, and overlapping of the spine by the left ventricular shadow at 60 degrees of rotation in the left anterior oblique view. In the presence of left ventricular failure, the chamber is enlarged and the left atrium is also usually dilated, causing posterior displacement of the barium-filled esophagus. When significant left atrial

Differential Diagnosis in Aortic Stenosis

	Valvular Aortic Stenosis	Idiopathic Hypertrophic Subaortic Stenosis
Carotid pulse	Delayed	Rapid and bifid
Systolic murmur, location	Second right ICS, neck and apex	LLSB and apex
Effect of Valsalva maneuver	Murmur decreased	Murmur increased
Aortic closure sound	Soft	Normal
Systolic ejection click	Common when valve not calcified	Rare
Diastolic murmur of aortic regurgitation	Common	Rare
Electrocardiogram	LVH	Marked LVH; deep Q waves (septal in origin); left atrial enlargement
Chest roentgenogram	Normal heart size	Cardiomegaly (left ventricular); left atrial enlargement
Poststenotic dilatation of aorta	Present	Absent
Calcium in aortic valve	Present	Absent

LLSB = Lower left sternal border; ICS = intercostal space; LVH = left ventricular hypertrophy.

enlargement is seen, however, it should always raise the suspicion of associated mitral stenosis. Poststenotic dilatation of the ascending aorta is common in the frontal view, and calcification of the aortic valve should be searched for on the plain roentgenogram. However, image intensification fluoroscopy may be necessary for detection of mild valve calcification. In the presence of left ventricular failure, there is evidence of pulmonary venous engorgement and interstitial pulmonary edema.

Phonocardiography. Recording of heart sounds and the external carotid pulse wave may help in assessing the severity of aortic stenosis by documenting the presence or absence of a single second heart sound, paradoxical splitting, or a prolonged ejection time. A slow rising carotid pulse wave and the characteristics of the ejection murmur can also be documented. Usually, the carotid wave has an anacrotic notch or shudder and continues to slowly rise throughout the duration of the murmur (see Fig. 1, Ch. 360.1).

Echocardiography. In the presence of valvular aortic stenosis the echocardiogram will usually detect thickening of the aortic leaflets; if the opening of the leaflets is less than 1.5 cm during left ventricular systole, the diagnosis of aortic stenosis may be suspected. However, because of multiple echoes and difficulty in assuring that the echocardiographic beam is precisely traversing the aortic orifice, this sign is difficult to quantify and often unreliable. Sometimes because of eccentric placement of the aortic orifice relative to the aortic wall, it is possible to ascertain that a bicuspid valve is present. Hypertrophy of the left ventricular wall (posterior wall thickness over 1.1 cm) may further support the diagnosis of aortic stenosis. Cross-sectional echocardiography of the aortic valve may allow, in the future, a more quantitative assessment of aortic valve orifice size.

Cardiac Catheterization. In patients who have symptoms, cardiac catheterization is carried out to determine whether the degree of mechanical obstruction at the aortic valve is sufficient to warrant surgical treatment. It is important to measure both the systolic pressure gradient between left ventricle and aorta (see Fig. 1, Ch. 360.1) and the cardiac output at the time of left heart catheterization because of the nonlinear relation between the pressure and flow across the stenotic orifice, the orifice area being directly related to flow and inversely proportional to the square root of the pressure gradient (see Ch. 360.2). Thus if the cardiac output is reduced by 30 per cent, the pressure gradient will fall by about 50 per cent and the severity of the stenosis will be underestimated if the pressure gradient alone is relied upon. For example, when myocardial failure is responsible for a reduced resting cardiac output, the peak gradient from left ventricle to aorta may be below 50 mm Hg, even in the presence of marked aortic valve narrowing.

When the cardiac output is normal, with relatively mild aortic stenosis the aortic valve orifice area is between 0.75 and 1.5 sq cm in the adult (normal area 2.5 sq cm), and the systolic pressure gradient across the aortic valve is small. When aortic stenosis is moderate, the orifice area is 0.5 to 0.75 sq cm and the peak pressure gradient usually exceeds 50 mm Hg. With very severe or "tight" aortic stenosis, the orifice area is 0.5 sq cm or less, there may be a left ventricular systolic pressure in excess of 250 mm Hg, and the transvalvular pressure gradient is often over 100 mm Hg. The right heart pressures are normal, unless there is left ventricular failure which can produce pulmonary hypertension. Simultaneous measurements should be made of the pulmonary artery wedge pressure and the left ventricular pressure to exclude associated mitral stenosis.

It is important that selective left ventricular angiography be carried out to document the functional status of the left ventricle. Such a study will indicate whether or not the left ventricular end-diastolic volume is elevated and the ejection fracton reduced to below 55 per cent, factors which bear on the operative risk in the individual patient. In older patients, it is also important that selective coronary arteriography be performed. Lack of appreciation of significant coronary artery lesions can lead to difficulty during surgical treatment, and coronary revascularization procedures are sometimes carried out at the time of the aortic valve replacement.

DIFFERENTIAL DIAGNOSIS. An ejection murmur at the aortic area and lower left sternal border can be heard in the patient with *hypertrophic subaortic stenosis* (hypertrophic cardiomyopathy, asymmetric septal hypertrophy), although the murmur is generally poorly transmitted to the carotid vessels and has other special features. The key differentiating points between this lesion and valvular aortic stenosis are shown in the table. The echocardiographic features of each are also distinctive (see Ch. 360.1).

In the younger patient who has a murmur suggesting congenital aortic stenosis, other locations for the lesion (supravalvular, subvalvular membrane) should be considered. Occasionally the murmur of papillary muscle dysfunction or ruptured chordae tendineae, caused by mitral regurgitation through the posterior leaflet, can mimic the murmur of aortic stenosis. The mitral regurgitant jet impinges on the interatrial septum, which is directly contiguous to the posterior wall of the aorta, leading to transmission of the murmur to the aortic area; however, this murmur tends to transmit poorly to the carotid arteries; it increases with isometric handgrip and diminishes with amyl nitrite inhalation, whereas the murmur of aortic stenosis will behave in an opposite manner with these two maneuvers.

TREATMENT. Medical Management. The adult patient with findings suggestive of moderate aortic stenosis and no symptoms may be followed carefully, although cardiac catheterization is sometimes done to be certain of the severity of obstruction. In such patients, very strenuous physical exertion, such as competitive athletics, should be prohibited in order to minimize risk of sudden death. Antimicrobial prophylaxis for dental or surgical procedures is advised to prevent the development of bacterial endocarditis. In children or adolescents with congenital aortic stenosis who are suspected of having obstruction, cardiac catheterization is generally advised even when they are without symptoms.

Early symptoms of orthopnea or mild dyspnea may respond temporarily to digitalis, sodium restriction, and diuresis. However, as soon as significant symptoms appear (angina, syncope, or symptoms of left ventricular failure), the adult patient should usually be sent for cardiac catheterization and coronary arteriography, and consideration should be given to early operation.

Surgical Treatment. In children or young adult patients with congenital aortic stenosis, surgical treatment is generally advocated even in the absence of significant symptoms if the obstruction is severe, because the risk of operation appears to be lower than the risk of sudden death. The bicuspid valve in the young patient is generally favorable for a valvuloplasty, and clinical improvement may be experienced for a number of years.

In the adult patient with symptoms and significant narrowing of the aortic orifice (less than 0.75 sq cm) or peak systolic pressure gradient over 50 mm Hg with normal cardiac output, aortic valve replacement, using a prosthesis or a graft, is carried out, using cardiopulmonary bypass. Without operation, the outlook for such patients is poor. The average age at which such operations are performed is about 56 to 58 years. Associated coronary artery disease is often found in older patients, and insertion of one or more coronary artery bypass grafts sometimes is combined with replacement of the aortic valve. Sometimes mitral valve replacement also is necessary if an associated mitral valve lesion is sufficiently severe. Most experience has been obtained with the caged ball-valve (Starr-Edwards) prosthesis. The average operative mortality currently is between 5 and 10 per cent, but patients who are in NYHA Class IV exhibit a higher risk (approximately 15 per cent). Great improvement in symptoms generally occurs after the operation. Also, life expectancy is prolonged in survivors of the operation, 75 to 80 per cent being alive at five years and about 60 per cent of patients surviving after ten years. These late survival figures appear to be modified by the size of the left ventricle; thus if the ventricle is small, five-year survival is 95 per cent; whereas if it is greatly enlarged, five-year survival is approximately 60 per cent. The incidence of thromboembolism is significant after ball-valve replacement, averaging 2 to 3 per cent per year if the patient is continuously anticoagulated with sodium warfarin, although the use of certain types of cloth-covered ball-valves may improve this figure somewhat. If anticoagulation is inadequately maintained, the embolic rate is up to 8 per cent per year. Also, with long-term anticoagulant therapy, the incidence of important complications from bleeding (such as intracranial hemorrhage) averages about 1.5 per cent per year. Figures are comparable for prostheses such as the tilting disc (Björk-Shiley) device.

There is relatively less experience with application of porcine xenograft valves for aortic valve replacement. Operative mortalities and survival rates appear to be comparable to those reported with ball-valve devices, but the rate of embolization appears to be significantly lower with the xenograft, and long-term anticoagulation has not been employed. However, unless a large valve size can be inserted, blood flow characteristics through xenograft valves in the aortic position have been less favorable than with ball-valves of comparable ring size, and significant pressure gradients across this valve have sometimes been found postoperatively. The question of the durability of xenograft valves beyond five years also remains to be settled, although early results have been promising.

The question of whether the adult patient with documented, hemodynamically severe aortic stenosis but with few symptoms should be operated upon is not settled at present. The risk of aortic valve replacement is now relatively low in many centers, but whether the risk of sudden death in asymptomatic patients over a period of several years approaches this figure is unknown. Therefore older patients are referred for operation only if they have significant symptoms.

360.6.   AORTIC REGURGITATION

ETIOLOGY AND PATHOLOGY. Aortic regurgitation is usually the result of rheumatic fever, but it has been described as a complication of an increasing number of systemic diseases (see below). A careful history may be of substantial help in ascertaining etiology. In chronic aortic regurgitation of rheumatic etiology, the aortic valve leaflets are scarred, thickened, and retracted and do not close during diastole. With longstanding disease, marked dilatation of the ascending aorta and the aortic anulus may add further to the insufficiency. Combined aortic stenosis and regurgitation are most frequently associated with rheumatic disease, but can also be seen in the late stages of a congenitally bicuspid valve. Aortic regurgitation may be associated with the most marked enlargement and hypertrophy of the left ventricle encountered in valvular heart disease. Approximately 70 per cent of patients with predominant aortic regurgitation are male.

Isolated congenital aortic regurgitation has rarely been reported as a consequence of a bicuspid aortic valve, but congenital aortic regurgitation can occur as a complication of discrete subvalvular stenosis which produces secondary thickening and insufficiency of the aortic leaflets. In younger children, ventricular septal defect may be complicated by prolapse of an aortic valve leaflet, thereby causing aortic regurgitation.

Acquired aortic regurgitation occurs in association with the following conditions: (1) *Syphilis,* which causes scarring and degeneration of the media and intima of the ascending aorta, resulting in part from disease of the vasa vasorum. There can be an aneurysm in the ascending aorta and dilatation of the aortic anulus, with thickening of the aortic leaflets, as well as narrowing of the coronary ostia caused by syphilitic involvement of the aortic intima. (2) *Ankylosing spondylitis,* in which associated medial disease of the aorta results in significant aortic regurgitation. (3) *Rheumatoid arthritis;* degeneration of the aortic valve leaflets and the ascending aorta have been described. (4) *Marfan's syndrome,* in which loss of elastic tissue and connective tissue degenerative changes can lead to marked dilatation of the aorta and aortic anulus with severe aortic regurgitation. (5) *Hurler's syndrome,* or mucopolysaccharidosis, which may be accompanied by significant aortic regurgitation. (6) *Relapsing polychondritis,* which can exhibit associated aortic root involvement with aortic regurgitation. (7) *Severe systemic hypertension,* which can be associated with aortic dilatation and relative aortic insufficiency; other complications associated with hypertension, such as ascending aortic aneurysm or dissecting aneurysm, may also cause aortic regurgitation. (8) *Infective endocarditis,* which usually occurs on a deformed valve, and can lead to rapid progression of aortic regurgitation or to fenestration of the leaflets.

PATHOLOGIC PHYSIOLOGY. The physiologic defect in aortic regurgitation is retrograde leakage of blood from the aorta into the left ventricle during diastole. This results in low diastolic aortic pressure and increase in the end-diastolic volume of the left ventricle. The amount of blood ejected during systole is abnormally large, because it consists of the normal stroke volume plus blood regurgitated during the previous diastolic period. In severe aortic regurgitation the amount of blood regurgitated per beat may equal or even exceed the forward stroke volume. The initial compensation to this volume overload on the left ventricle is by the Frank-Starling mechanism (increased end-diastolic volume), and in mild aortic regurgitation there is increased systolic emptying as well, with little chronic dilatation of the ventricle. As regurgitation becomes more severe, the left ventricle slowly dilates, and new sarcomeres are laid down both in parallel and in series in the left ventricular wall during the process of dilatation and hypertrophy. This compensatory mechanism allows the enlarged left ventricle to deliver a greater stroke volume, but with normal shortening of each unit of the enlarged circumference.

The pathophysiology of aortic regurgitation somewhat resembles the volume overload of mitral regurgitation, but there are two important differences. (1) The increased foward stroke volume is delivered into a high impedance system (the aorta), and because the total forward stroke volume is increased, the left ventricular and aortic systolic pressures are elevated (sometimes to 160 mm Hg or higher). This, together with the increased size of the left ventricular chamber, leads to pressure as well as volume overloading and a somewhat elevated myocardial oxygen consumption. (2) The lowered diastolic aortic pressure tends to impair coronary artery perfusion. Normally the coronary blood flow occurs during diastole; with the reduced diastolic pressure which accompanies aortic regurgitation, coronary blood flow may become inadequate either during exercise or when heart rate and hence the diastolic pressure become very low, as during sleep. The increased myocardial oxygen consumption coupled with relative underperfusion of the coronary bed may lead to an imbalance between oxygen supply and demand. Thus unlike patients with mitral regurgitation, patients with severe aortic regurgitation commonly develop *angina pectoris* in the absence of coronary artery disease.

With adequate left ventricular myocardial contractility the ejection fraction of the left ventricle (ratio of stroke volume to end-diastolic volume) is maintained at normal (over 55 per cent), the forward cardiac output is normal, and left ventricular end-diastolic pressure may remain nearly normal despite ventricular dilatation. However, because longstanding overload leads to myocardial damage and depression of contractility, the extent of wall shortening during ejection tends to diminish, the residual volume in the left ventricle rises, and the end-diastolic pressure in the left ventricle becomes elevated. Indeed, in the late stages of severe aortic regurgitation the diastolic pressure in the aorta and that in the left ventricle may reach equilibration near the end of diastole, leading to an abbreviation of the murmur. Occasionally, "preclosure" of the mitral valve even occurs, leading to a dissociation between the rising left ventricular pressure and the left atrial pressure, which remains at a lower level. This situation may occur in sudden severe aortic regurgitation, such as with bacterial endocarditis, when sufficient time has not elapsed for ventricular dilatation and hypertrophy to occur. Such mitral valve preclosure may be audible as a snapping sound in mid- to late diastole.

In the late stages of aortic regurgitation the cardiac output decreases, and the left ventricular end-diastolic pressure becomes further elevated because of myocardial failure. The mean left atrial pressure then rises, leading to decreased pulmonary compliance and interstitial edema, and acute pulmonary edema occasionally occurs.

CLINICAL MANIFESTATIONS. Symptoms and Clinical Course. The typical patient with rheumatic aortic regurgitation has experienced acute rheumatic fever in childhood, and a period of about ten years then follows during which the severity of the regurgitant lesion progresses. Marked aortic regurgitation may become apparent by age 18 or 20, and there often follows a period of compensation during which the patient is asymptomatic, despite the presence of severe regurgitation. Occasionally during this stage of the disease, palpitations caused by transient atrial arrhythmias, headache caused by the high systolic blood pressure during exercise, or subjective sensations resulting from cardiac hyperactivity may be noted. Studies in children followed for many years after developing severe aortic regurgitation indicate that even after 20 years about 25 per cent of the individuals with this lesion remained asymptomatic. However, the average duration of the latent or asymptomatic period in severe aortic regurgitation is about ten years.

The earliest symptoms are usually due to the onset of left ventricular dysfunction or to coronary insufficiency. Mild dyspnea on exertion is noted as a result of elevation of the left ventricular end-diastolic and mean left atrial pressures during exercise. The length of time between onset of this symptom and death of the patient averages seven to ten years, although it should be recognized that many of these data were derived before the advent of modern diuretic therapy and rheumatic fever prophylaxis. Angina pectoris usually begins somewhat later, postdating the onset of dyspnea by two to three years. It may occur during exertion, and may or may not respond to nitroglycerin. Angina pectoris can also be atypical and occur at rest or at night, presumably caused by low heart rate which can lead to very low diastolic aortic pressure and inadequate coronary perfusion during long diastolic periods. The onset of severe nocturnal angina associated with profuse sweating, particularly in young patients, can portend a poor prognosis. Also, in young patients with rheumatic aortic regurgitation without significant symptoms who were followed prospectively, it has been reported that a triad of findings portends the occurrence of angina, heart failure, or death within six years in nearly 90 per cent of patients; these included marked left ventricular hypertrophy in the electrocardiogram, roentgenographic evidence of moderate or marked left ventricular enlargement, and a systolic arterial pressure over 140 mm Hg and/or a diastolic pressure below 40 mm Hg.

Once left ventricular decompensation begins, patients with severe aortic regurgitation usually tolerate infections poorly. They may experience severe congestive heart failure, and they are also at some risk of unexpected death. There are no clear-cut figures on the incidence of sudden death in patients with severe aortic regurgitation; although not as common as in aortic stenosis, it is by no means rare and probably results from sudden ventricular arrhythmia. In the late stages of severe aortic regurgitation, orthopnea and paroxysmal nocturnal dyspnea occur, and eventually symptoms and signs of right ventricular failure may supervene.

The natural history in the other forms of aortic regurgitation depends largely on the rapidity with which the lesion develops and on its severity. Patients with aortic regurgitation caused by syphilis may exhibit a course resembling that of rheumatic disease, although it usually begins later in life. With acute regurgitation such as that in bacterial endocarditis, there is insufficient time for chronic compensation to occur, and the clinical course may be fulminating. Under these circumstances, severe intractable left ventricular failure may develop.

Physical Findings. The diastolic pressure determined by sphygmomanometry correlates generally with the severity of the regurgitant leak, although in some patients there is severe regurgitation with diastolic pressure as high as 60 mm Hg. A diastolic sound over the artery is usually audible down to 0 mm Hg when regurgitation is severe, but the level at which the diastolic sound muffles corresponds reasonably well to the directly measured aortic pressure at the end of diastole, determined by a needle within the artery. The systolic arterial pressure is elevated. Characteristic clinical features caused by the large stroke volume and rapid runoff of blood from the aorta consist of *head bobbing* (a nodding motion of the head with each systole, which may be visible from a considerable distance), *visible pulsations of the carotid arteries*, a *Corrigan or water-hammer pulse* (sharp upstroke with collapsing quality), *Quincke's sign* (on light compression of the fingernail, alternate blushing and blanching are visible in the nailbed with each cardiac cycle), *pistol shot sounds* on auscultation with a stethoscope over the femoral arteries, and *Duroziez' murmur* (a to-and-fro bruit over the femoral artery, using slight compression with stethoscope diaphragm). Palpation of the carotid arteries may reveal a bisferious or bifid pulse, particularly if there is some associated aortic stenosis.

On palpation of the precordium, a diastolic thrill may be felt at the lower left sternal border, and a systolic thrill is palpable at the aortic area, the jugular notch, and the carotid arteries. The left ventricle is enlarged, the apex is displaced laterally, and the apex beat is hyperkinetic with marked retraction during systole.

The first heart sound may be normal or slightly reduced; the aortic component of the second heart sound is diminished or inaudible in the presence of severe regurgitation. Frequently, a loud third heart sound is audible at the apex, and there may also be a fourth heart sound. The most characteristic feature of the lesion is a decrescendo, blowing *diastolic murmur* at the left sternal border in the third and fourth intercostal spaces (see Fig. 1, Ch. 360.1). In the presence of mild aortic regurgitation, this murmur is high pitched, soft, and heard only in early diastole; it may be appreciated only with the patient in an upright position, leaning forward, and with held expiration. With a more severe regurgitant leak, the murmur may have a somewhat rougher quality and may last throughout diastole. Late in the course of severe aortic regurgitation, or with acute aortic regurgitation, the diastolic murmur may be shortened by equilibration of aortic pressure with a markedly elevated left ventricular end-diastolic pressure before the end of diastole; occasionally, a snapping sound caused by mitral valve "preclosure" is audible (see above). In patients in whom the aortic regurgitation is due primarily to aneurysmal dilatation of the ascending aorta or to enlargement of the aortic anulus, as in Marfan's syndrome, the diastolic murmur may be loudest to the *right* of the sternum, thereby providing a clue to the cause.

Invariably, when aortic regurgitation is severe, there is a systolic ejection murmur at the aortic area which is transmitted to the jugular notch and carotid arteries. This may be very loud even in the presence of pure aortic regurgitation, reflecting the extremely large stroke volume delivered across a deformed aortic valve, but usually there is little or no pressure gradient from left ventricle to aorta during systole. Frequently in the presence of severe aortic regurgitation, an *Austin Flint diastolic rumble* is audible at the apex. Although true mitral stenosis may accompany aortic regurgitation of rheumatic origin, the Austin Flint rumble is characterized by its onset with a third heart sound; it is loudest in mid-diastole and often exhibits some presystolic accentuation. The Austin Fint murmur is probably due not only to interference with opening of the anterior mitral leaflet by the regurgitant jet, but also to a more rapid rise in the left ventricular than the left atrial diastolic pressure. The effect is to prevent full opening of the normal mitral leaflets during diastole, leading to turbulent flow across the mitral orifice (see Differential Diagnosis in Ch. 360.2).

Sometimes, in the late stages of aortic regurgitation when left ventricular dilatation and failure are present, a holosystolic murmur of relative mitral regurgitation may be audible at the cardiac apex. Signs of pulmonary hypertension and right ventricular enlargement may also be encountered in the late stages of the disease.

DIAGNOSIS. Electrocardiogram. The electrocardiogram usually shows left ventricular hypertrophy, sometimes of marked degree, with associated S-T segment and T wave changes. Left atrial enlargement may also be present, particularly when the left ventricular end-diastolic pressure becomes elevated. When myocardial disease develops, left axis deviation, intraventricular conduction defects, or left bundle branch block may occur. Atrial fibrillation is a late and relatively uncommon complication.

Roentgenographic Features. The major findings are enlargement of the left ventricle and aorta with vigorous pulsations of the ascending aorta on fluoroscopy. The left ventricular enlargment is characterized by a downward and lateral displacement of the left ventricular apex, the left ventricle being particularly prominent and overlying the spine in the left anterior oblique view. With severe aortic regurgitation, left atrial enlargement may be apparent on the right anterior oblique view with barium in the esophagus. When aortic regurgitation is associated with aortic root disease, the ascending aorta may be markedly dilated or aneurysmal, although sometimes the major dilatation takes place posteriorly and may not be visible on the plain chest films. Occasionally, calcium is seen in the aortic valve, and calcification in the ascending aortic wall is characteristic of syphilitic involvement.

Echocardiography. By the use of ultrasound, calculation of the diameter of the aortic root and of left ventricular chamber size may be feasible. In addition, in the presence of an Austin Flint rumble there is a characteristic fluttering motion of the anterior mitral leaflet during diastole caused by the impinging aortic regurgitant jet. This finding, together with absence of mitral valve thickening and normal excursion of the posterior leaflet, provides evidence against organic mitral stenosis. However, such diastolic fluttering has not proved to be a reliable sign of the severity of the leakage. Often the echocardiogram will reveal left ventricular dilatation or hypertrophy when aortic regurgitation is severe, and there may also be left atrial enlargement. In severe aortic regurgitation, particularly of the acute variety, the echocardiogram may detect early closure of the mitral valve in mid-diastole. Such premature mitral valve closure appears to be due to massive aortic regurgitation associated with rapid elevation of the left ventricular diastolic pressure until it exceeds the more slowly rising left atrial pressure, whereupon the mitral valve closes. Sometimes, a group of multiple eccentric echoes from the aortic valve will signify the presence of vegetations due to infectious endocarditis.

Cardiac Catheterization. It is generally desirable to perform cardiac catheterization prior to undertaking cardiac surgery in order to characterize the status of left ventricular myocardial function and to exclude associated lesions. Supravalvular injection of contrast medium into the aortic root often provides adequate radiographic visualization of the left ventricle and the anatomy of the ascending aorta, and also allows assessment of the severity of the aortic regurgitation. The systolic, left ventricular, and aortic pressures are moderately elevated; there may be a slight systolic pressure gradient across the aortic valve and a low diastolic aortic pressure (see Fig. 1, Ch. 360.1). A normal or moderately elevated left ventricular end-diastolic pressure (less than 20 mm Hg) is encountered when left ventricular myocardial function is maintained, and the forward cardiac output is normal. There may be an early diastolic gradient across the mitral valve from the pulmonary artery wedge or left atrial pressure tracing to the left ventricle; this is probably related to the rapid early rise of left ventricular diastolic pressure and impaired opening motion of the anterior mitral leaflet consequent to the aortic regurgitation. Simultaneous recordings of this nature should exclude the presence of associated organic mitral stenosis, in which there is usually a pressure gradient throughout diastole. In longstanding aortic regurgitation there is elevation of the calculated left ventricular end-diastolic volume (in excess of 90 ml per square meter), with or without an elevation of the left ventricular end-diastolic pressure.

A reduced ejection fraction, an impaired forward cardiac output, and marked elevation of the left ventricular end-diastolic pressure all indicate depressed left ventricular myocardial function, which may increase the operative risk. Under these conditions, the left ventricular and aortic diastolic pressures may become equal late in diastole at a pressure of 35 to 40 mm Hg, or even higher. It is under the latter circumstances that early closure of the mitral valve can occur (see above), leading to a higher pressure in the left ventricle than in the left atrium in the last portion of diastole. Finally, selective coronary arteriography should be carried out in older patients to search for significant coronary artery disease.

DIFFERENTIAL DIAGNOSIS. When mild aortic regurgitation is associated with mitral valve disease, the aortic pulse pressure may be normal and the early diastolic blowing murmur may be confused with that of pulmonic regurgitation (Graham Steell murmur). If severe mitral valve disease with pulmonary hypertension is present, it may not be possible to make this differentiation on physical examination; but when aortography is performed, such a murmur has been shown to be due most commonly to aortic regurgitation. Handgrip, which increases aortic pressure, augments the murmur of aortic regurgitation but usually does not affect that of pulmonic regurgitation.

TREATMENT. Medical Management. In marked aortic regurgitation, some restriction of physical exertion is advisable to reduce the likelihood of sudden arrhythmia. In the younger patient with a history of rheumatic fever, prophylaxis against streptococcal infection is indicated, and the use of antimicrobial drugs to prevent bacterial endocarditis during and after dental or surgical procedures is important at all ages. Patients with syphilitic aortic regurgitation should receive a full course of treatment with penicillin. When acute aortic regurgitation occurs, as in patients with infective endocarditis, the use of a vasodilator such as sodium nitroprusside can, by reducing the afterload, relieve acute left ventricular failure until operation can be undertaken.

In the patient with angina pectoris, nitroglycerin is not always effective, but it may be worth a cautious trial; it should be recalled, however, that nitroglycerin causes peripheral arterial vasodilatation and may lower the aortic diastolic pressure even further. With the onset of dyspnea or orthopnea (symptoms of early left ventricular failure), the use of digitalis, sodium restriction, and diuretics when necessary can result in substantial improvement, and consideration for operation can sometimes be postponed.

Surgical Treatment. Once signs of left ventricular failure become significant, the course of the disease tends to be downhill. Although the natural course is not as abrupt as that in aortic stenosis, the life expectancy averages only about seven years after onset of significant symptoms. When dyspnea or angina becomes troublesome on less than ordinary activity (N.Y.H.A. Class III) despite optimal medical management, surgical treatment should clearly be considered. In younger patients with the triad of severe left ventricular enlargement, marked electrocardiographic changes, and systolic arterial pressure over 140 mm Hg or diastolic arterial pressure below 40 mm Hg, it appears that a large percentage of such patients will develop symptoms or die within a few years, and operation may therefore be recommended even in the absence of significant symptoms.

An additional factor in selecting the appropriate time for operation is the finding that in some patients, despite hemodynamic improvement after aortic valve replacement, left ventricular dilatation and myocardial dysfunction may persist. Therefore it is desirable that surgical treatment be undertaken prior to the onset of such irreversible left ventricular disease. It may be hoped that improved noninvasive methods eventually allow detection of this potential problem before permanent changes occur.

Sudden, severe aortic regurgitation is poorly tolerated, and the average life expectancy is short. Therefore surgical treatment should usually be undertaken promptly.

In the great majority of patients, replacement of the diseased aortic valve with a prosthesis is necessary. The average age at the time of aortic valve replacement for aortic regurgitation is between 45 and 47 years. In some patients with marked dilatation of the aortic root and aneurysm formation, aortic valve replacement is combined with replacement of a portion of the ascending aorta. The various types of prosthetic aortic valves employed, the complications, and the results of operation are discussed in Ch. 360.5.

360.7.   TRICUSPID VALVE DISEASE

TRICUSPID STENOSIS

Tricuspid stenosis is rare as an isolated lesion. Almost always it accompanies rheumatic involvement of other cardiac valves, and it is of clinical significance in only about 5 per cent of patients with rheumatic heart disease. Seventy to 80 per cent of patients with tricuspid stenosis are female, and most often they have accompanying disease of both the mitral and aortic valves. *Rare causes* of tricuspid stenosis include *carcinoid heart disease, endomyocardial fibroelastosis, congenital malformations,* and obstruction from a *right atrial myxoma.*

The primary abnormality in tricuspid stenosis, like that in mitral stenosis, is mechanical obstruction to atrial emptying. This results in an elevated right atrial pressure and a pressure gradient across the tricuspid valve during diastole. It is important to measure simultaneous pressures in the right atrium and right ventricle at cardiac catheterization, because signs of peripheral venous congestion may occur with substantially lower pressure gradients (less than 10 mm Hg; often only 3 or 4 mm Hg) than are observed with mitral stenosis. Generally, the cardiac index is reduced substantially.

Tricuspid stenosis should be suspected particularly in the patient who has signs of multivalve disease and severe right-sided venous congestion but no evidence of marked pulmonary hypertension. The patient may also be relatively free of signs and symptoms of pulmonary venous congestion, despite the presence of mitral valve stenosis. This feature may be due to a limiting effect of this lesion on the cardiac output (a protective effect of the tricuspid stenosis) which may prevent sudden augmentation of blood flow into the pulmonary vascular bed. Such an effect would help explain the unusually prolonged clinical course seen in some patients with tricuspid stenosis.

On physical examination, the mean jugular venous pressure is elevated, and in patients with sinus rhythm there is a very sharp, prominent A wave which reflects right atrial contraction against the stenotic valve. There is a characteristic slow fall in the jugular V wave (delayed Y descent), caused by the obstruction to right atrial emptying and the resulting slow fall in right atrial pressure during diastole (see Fig. 1, Ch. 360.1).

On palpation of the precordium, the right ventricle is not enlarged, and a diastolic thrill may be palpable at the lower left sternal border. The diastolic murmur of tricuspid stenosis will often be missed unless specifically searched for at that location. It resembles that of mitral stenosis, having a low-pitched rumbling quality often beginning with a tricuspid valve opening snap (somewhat later than a mitral opening snap), and an early diastolic decrescendo murmur is followed by presystolic accentuation if sinus rhythm is present. A characteristic feature in differentiating the murmur from that of mitral stenosis is augmentation in the intensity of the tricuspid rumble during *inspiration,* or during the *Müller maneuver* (attempted inspiration against a closed glottis). This augmentation is due to the transitory increase in right atrial filling and tricuspid valve flow, which results from the negative intrathoracic pressure. Both these maneuvers diminish the murmur of mitral stenosis. There may be an associated abnormal increase in the venous pressure during such inspiration in tricuspid stenosis. When atrial fibrillation is present, the murmur is even more difficult to detect, because it may occur only in early diastole and can be confused with the murmur of pulmonic regurgitation.

The electrocardiogram, if sinus rhythm is present, exhibits peaked P waves in leads II and V_1, evidence of right atrial enlargement, but atrial fibrillation is often present. There is no evidence of right ventricular hypertrophy. On the chest roentgenogram, in addition to the findings caused by associated valvular lesions, there is enlargement of the right atrium. Echocardiography may detect a reduced posterior diastolic motion (low E to F slope) of the anterior leaflet of the tricuspid valve similar to that observed in mitral stenosis, although here also it should be recognized that this slope is influenced by tricuspid valve flow as well as by right ventricular diastolic compliance.

Surgical treatment is not indicated for mild tricuspid stenosis, but if it is severe or if the patient must undergo operation for a mitral valve lesion, surgical treatment may be undertaken. The tricuspid valve is usually not favorable for valvuloplasty, and most often a tricuspid valve prosthesis is inserted. Sometimes the tricuspid stenosis is not detected prior to a mitral valve operation, and is recognized only when unexpected signs of right-sided congestion develop postoperatively.

TRICUSPID REGURGITATION

Tricuspid regurgitation, like tricuspid stenosis, is usually associated with rheumatic disease of other cardiac valves, particularly the mitral. It may occur as an organic lesion, or more commonly it is a functional lesion secondary to right ventricular dilatation with severe pulmonary hypertension. Such functional tricuspid regurgitation usually occurs late in the course of mitral valve disease. Other forms of severe pulmonary hypertension, such as the Eisenmenger reaction in congenital heart disease or pulmonary hypertension caused by chronic lung disease, can also cause functional tricuspid regurgitation. Rheumatic involvement of the tricuspid valve can result in tricuspid regurgitation when the right ventricular systolic pressure is normal, although most frequently such organic lesions are of mixed variety, with both stenosis and regurgitation. Isolated tricuspid regurgitation can occur congenitally (as in Ebstein's malformation), and progressive tricuspid

regurgitation caused by traumatic damage to the valve has been reported after crush injuries of the chest. The normal tricuspid valve can serve as a focus for bacterial endocarditis, particularly in drug addicts.

Tricuspid regurgitation constitutes a leakage of blood retrograde into the right atrium during right ventricular systole, which places an augmented volume load on the right ventricle. The pathophysiology resembles that of mitral regurgitation but involves the right heart. In mild tricuspid regurgitation, when the right ventricular end-diastolic pressure is not elevated, the right atrial mean pressure is normal and the V wave may not be particularly prominent. As the right ventricular and mean right atrial pressures rise in the presence of more severe regurgitation, the V wave becomes increased. If the right ventricle fails, the right ventricular diastolic and mean right atrial pressure rise, and the V wave becomes markedly enlarged.

Examination in severe tricuspid regurgitation may show the V wave in the jugular venous pulse high in the neck, with the patient in the upright position. Sometimes the height of the venous pressure may be difficult to discern, because the mean pressure may exceed 20 cm of water, and the top of the column may not be visible even in the sitting position. Systolic hepatic pulsations may be present, and there may be marked hepatomegaly, ascites, and peripheral edema. In tricuspid regurgitation secondary to severe pulmonary hypertension, there is a palpable pulmonary artery segment in the second left interspace, and a markedly accentuated pulmonic closure sound is evident. With severe tricuspid regurgitation, there is a thrill over the lower left sternal border and lower sternum, and an enlarged right ventricle is palpable along the left sternal edge and in the subxiphoid region. A pansystolic murmur is heard near the lower left sternal border and lower sternum, transmitted to the right sternal edge or the subxiphoid region. An early diastolic rumble caused by increased blood flow across the tricuspid valve may be audible; when there is organic involvement of the tricuspid valve by rheumatic disease, a longer diastolic murmur caused by associated tricuspid stenosis may be present. A characteristic feature of the murmur of tricuspid regurgitation is its augmentation during inspiration (*Carvallo's sign*), and the murmur can also be increased by the Müller maneuver (see Tricuspid Stenosis, above). These maneuvers lead to decreased intensity of a mitral regurgitant murmur.

There is electrocardiographic evidence of right ventricular hypertrophy, and atrial fibrillation is usually present in severe tricuspid regurgitation. Enlargement of both the right atrium and the right ventricle is evident on the chest roentgenogram. Infectious vegetations on the tricuspid valve may be detected by echocardiography, particularly when there is infective endocarditis secondary to intravenous drug use.

The *treatment* of tricuspid regurgitation, if moderate and secondary to severe pulmonary hypertension, is conservative. Generally, the patient will respond to medical measures aimed at the left-sided valvular disease (sodium restriction, diuresis, digitalis). When aortic or mitral valve surgery is undertaken, such functional tricuspid regurgitation generally disappears gradually after relief of the left-sided lesion, as the pulmonary hypertension regresses. Occasionally, plication of the tricuspid valve anulus is done in patients with functional tricuspid regurgitation who are undergoing operation on other cardiac valves. If the functional tricuspid regurgitation is very severe, or if organic disease of the tricuspid valve is present in the absence of severe pulmonary hypertension, replacement with a prosthesis is necessary.

360.8. PULMONIC VALVE DISEASE

PULMONIC REGURGITATION

Regurgitation at the pulmonic valve most commonly accompanies severe pulmonary hypertension caused by left-sided valvular heart disease. The murmur is high pitched, decrescendo in quality, and best heard at the lower left sternal border. It may be indistinguishable from the murmur of mild aortic regurgitation; however, it should be noted that by far the most common cause of such a murmur in the patient with rheumatic valvular heart disease is aortic regurgitation. Isolated congenital pulmonic regurgitation with a normal pulmonary arterial pressure occurs rarely, and in this situation the murmur occurs later in diastole, is lower in pitch, and may be confused with the murmur of tricuspid stenosis. Pulmonic regurgitation with a normal pulmonary artery pressure can also occur in association with bacterial endocarditis on a normal pulmonic valve, particularly in drug users. Occasionally, if antimicrobial therapy is unsuccessful in this condition, excision of the pulmonic valve has been used to eradicate the source of infection, and this procedure does not appear to result in serious hemodynamic difficulties.

PULMONIC STENOSIS

Pulmonic stenosis usually occurs as a congenital malformation and is discussed in Ch. 359.2. Occasionally, acquired subpulmonic stenosis occurs in association with hypertrophic subaortic stenosis, owing to bulging of the interventricular septum into the right ventricular chamber. Rarely an intrapericardial tumor can compress the main pulmonary artery or right ventricular outflow tract, resulting in a pressure gradient between the right ventricle and the pulmonary artery.

Barnhorst, D. A., Oxman, H. A., Connolly, D. C., Pluth, J. R., Danielson, G. K., Wallace, R. B., and Mcgoon, D. C.: Long-term follow-up of isolated replacement of the aortic or mitral valve with the Starr-Edwards prosthesis. Am. J. Cardiol., 35:228, 1975.

Braunwald, E., Lambrew, C. T., Rockoff, S. D., Ross, J., Jr., and Morrow, A. G.: Idiopathic hypertrophic subaortic stenosis. I. A description of the disease based upon an analysis of 64 patients. Circulation (Suppl. 4), 30:3, 1964.

Cohen, L. S., Gault, J. H., and Ross, J., Jr.: Mitral regurgitation. In Barondess, J. A. (ed.): Diagnostic Approaches to Presenting Syndromes. Baltimore, Williams & Wilkins Company, 1971, p. 1.

Feigenbaum, H.: Echocardiography. 2nd ed. Philadelphia, Lea & Febiger, 1976.

Hancock, E. W., and Fleming, P. R.: Aortic stenosis. Quart. J. Med., 29:209, 1960.

Mills, P., Rose, J., Hollingsworth, J., Amara, I., and Craige, E.: Long-term prognosis of mitral valve prolapse. N. Engl. J. Med., 297:13, 1977.

O'Rourke, R. A., Crawford, M. H., Johnson, A. D., Davidson, R. M., LeWinter, M. M., and Karliner, J. S.: Prolapsing mitral valve leaflet syndrome. West. J. Med., 122:217, 1975.

Rees, J. R., Epstein, E. J., Criley, J. M., and Ross, R. S.: Haemodynamic effects of severe aortic regurgitation. Br. Heart J., 26:412, 1964.

Ross, J., Jr., and Braunwald, E.: Aortic stenosis. Circulation (Suppl. 5), 37:61, 1968.

Ross, J., Jr., Braunwald, E., Gault, J. H., Mason, D. T., and Morrow, A. G.: On the mechanism of the intraventricular pressure gradient in idiopathic hypertrophic subaortic stenosis. Circulation, 34:558, 1966.

Salazar, E., and Levine, H. D.: Rheumatic tricuspid regurgitation, the clinical spectrum. Am. J. Med., 33:111, 1962.

Salomon, N. W., Stinson, E. B., Griepp, R. B., and Shumway, N. E.: Mitral valve replacement: Long-term evaluation of prosthesis-related mortality and morbidity. Circulation (Suppl. 2), 56:11, 1977.

Sanders, C. A., Harthorne, J. W., DeSanctis, R. W., and Austen, W. G.: Tricuspid stenosis: A difficult diagnosis in the presence of atrial fibrillation. Circulation, 33:26, 1966.

Segal, J., Harvey, W. P., and Hufnagel, C.: A clinical study of one hundred cases of severe aortic insufficiency. Am. J. Med., 21:200, 1956.

Spagnuolo, M., Kloth, H., Taranta, A., Doyle, E., and Pasternack, B.: Natural history of rheumatic aortic regurgitation. Criteria predictive of death, congestive heart failure, and angina in young patients. Circulation, 44:368, 1971.

Wood, P.: An appreciation of mitral stenosis. Parts I and II. Br. Med. J., 1:1051, 1113, 1954.

361. ARTERIAL HYPERTENSION

C. T. Dollery

DEFINITION. A wide range of blood pressure values is found among human populations. The values are not normally distributed, and there is a skew toward higher ones. The distribution of blood pressure readings (Fig. 1) has no natural break separating normality from abnormality, so the definition of what constitutes hypertension is empirical. Much effort has been expended, probably needlessly, in trying to define hypertension. Several different operational definitions are possible. Very high values of blood pressure — say, above 230 systolic and 130 diastolic mm Hg — are associated with a high probability that the individual will develop left ventricular failure or accelerated hypertension and thus present with a clinical illness which can be termed hypertension. Below this level of pressure most patients are not ill, but there is an increasing incidence of some symptoms such as morning headache with pressure from approximately 170 systolic and 110 diastolic mm Hg upward. However, the real problem for the individual with a blood pressure in the upper part of the distribution range is not the development of

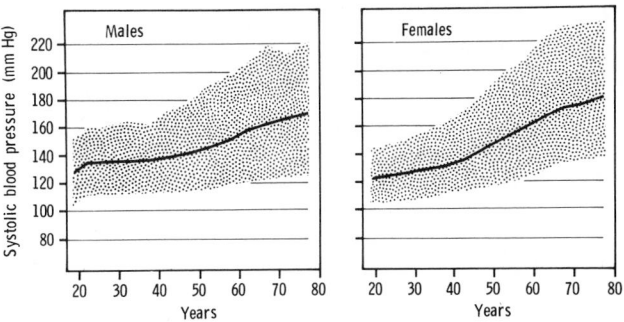

Figure 1. Median systolic blood pressure with 5 per cent and 95 per cent limits in male and female inhabitants of Bergen, Norway, over the whole span of age found in an adult population sample. (From Boe et al.: Acta Med. Scand., Suppl. 321, 157:1–252, 1957.)

symptoms due to the blood pressure but the sudden and apparently unpredictable catastrophe of a myocardial infarction or a cerebrovascular accident. Several prospective epidemiologic studies of human populations have shown that the risk of such a catastrophe is graded with the level of blood pressure throughout the range of pressures found. Normality in the sense of freedom from risk has no meaning in relation to blood pressure.

Thus the main clinical importance of hypertension is not that it is a disease in the usual sense but that it is the most important single factor that enables a physician to make a prediction about the future risk of vascular disease, and that furthermore it is a risk that can be controlled by lowering the blood pressure.

MEASUREMENT OF BLOOD PRESSURE. The sphygmomanometer column is calibrated in 10- and 2-mm divisions. Most physicians show a strong preference for numbers ending in zero and record the blood pressure only to the nearest 10 mm Hg. As decisions about patient management may be altered by differences in diastolic pressure of this magnitude, it is much preferable to read the instrument to the nearest 1 or 2 mm. It is also important to deflate the cuff slowly when taking blood pressure. Rapid deflation may bring about a considerable difference in the pressure in the cuff and that indicated by the column because of the inertia of the mercury. Furthermore, it is almost impossible to read the column accurately if the meniscus is rushing past the calibration points.

It is useful to make a rough check of the systolic pressure by palpation during inflation and to start deflation from 20 mm Hg above the systolic value. This avoids the problem of errors caused by "silent zones" during deflation which can cause the observer to fail to record the true (and much higher) level of systolic pressure. As the column falls, the silence is broken by a faint but distinctive tapping sound in time with the pulse. This is phase 1 of the sounds described by Korotkoff and corresponds with the systolic pressure. Less skilled observers usually record this value more accurately than the diastolic pressure, which has a less clear-cut endpoint. During further deflation the quality of the sound changes. At first it grows louder and has a roaring quality and then it becomes abruptly muffled. The point of muffling is the fourth phase, and the disappearance of sound, which usually occurs soon afterward, is the fifth phase. The true diastolic pressure lies between the fourth and fifth phase sounds, but as it is usually closer to the fifth, it is now official policy to record this as the diastolic blood pressure. Some individuals may have a diastolic pressure that is difficult or impossible to record precisely because the sound fades gradually without a clear point of muffling or disappearance. This is a particular problem if the peripheral circulation is dilated after exercise or under the action of a vasodilator drug. Under such circumstances the systolic pressure is much more reproducible.

The blood pressure varies widely with mood and activity. A patient seen for the first time is usually more anxious than on the second or third visit to the same doctor and clinic. It is common to find a fall of 10 mm Hg in systolic pressure from the first visit to the second, and about 4 mm Hg from the second to the third. A blood pressure taken at the beginning of a consultation is almost always higher than one taken near its end. There has been much debate as to which, if any,

of these is the most representative. The blood pressure taken on the first visit without any special preparation is often termed "casual" blood pressure. It probably corresponds most nearly to those used in epidemiologic surveys. The blood pressure recorded under conditions of rest, tranquillity, and even sedation is sometimes referred to as the "basal" blood pressure. As there is no generally agreed preparation for recording a "basal" reading, it cannot be precisely defined. There is evidence that a series of readings taken over the waking day provides a better prediction of prognosis than a single casual one, but portable equipment to provide such readings is expensive and not generally used.

Reading the mercury column of the sphygmomanometer is prone to systematic bias as well as digit preference and boundary avoidance. For exact work such as therapeutic trials and epidemiologic surveys, it is usual to employ an instrument that has provision for concealing the mercury columns, which are stopped by pressing a switch, or for incorporating a device to offset the zero by up to 80 mm Hg, so that the observer cannot anticipate any particular pressure level. The zero offset can only be read after the systolic and diastolic pressures have been recorded.

EPIDEMIOLOGY. Many factors affect the blood pressure of an individual within a population or may cause differences between two populations. Study of these factors may yield information about pathogenesis and suggest possible preventive measures.

Age and Sex. Blood pressure tends to rise throughout life, although the rate of rise varies at different ages. There is a relatively rapid rise from the low values of the neonate to the higher values of a child and young adult. The upward trend is slower between the ages of 20 and 45 years in both men and women; it then resumes an upward march, rising at an average rate of 0.5 to 1.0 mm Hg of systolic pressure each year until the seventh decade is reached. Values in older people are affected by differential mortality of those with higher pressures, and population means tend to level out or even fall in extreme old age. Women have slightly lower pressures than men in the third and fourth decades and slightly higher ones thereafter. The rate of rise of pressure is not uniform within a population, and the range of pressures found widens as age advances. There is some evidence that this occurs because those in the higher part of the range have a pressure that increases more rapidly than those in the lower part of the range. Recent work has suggested that individuals who ultimately develop pressure levels requiring treatment may lie in the upper part of the distribution as young as the age of one year.

Race and Environment. Studies of the distribution of blood pressure values have been carried out in many countries of the world, and almost all populations show a progressive rise in pressure with age and a distribution of values resembling in varying degrees that found in Western Europe and the United States. Although the pattern is similar, the proportion falling into higher pressure categories shows some interesting geographical and racial variations. Black people in West and East Africa, the West Indies, and the United States have a similar proportion of higher values to those found in whites, and in some samples significantly more. The proportion of individuals with higher values appears to be somewhat lower in population samples from the Indian subcontinent. Some communities have been found in which the blood pressure shows little increase with age and the distribution curve lacks the upward skew of higher values found in Caucasians. Such communities include nomads in East Africa, bushmen in Southern Africa, and the inhabitants of some Pacific islands such as Pukapuka in the Northern Cook Islands.

There is conclusive evidence that blood pressure is heritable, but wide divergencies of opinion exist concerning the proportion of the blood pressure variability in populations which is genetically controlled. Estimates of the genetic contribution to variation in systolic blood pressure range from as high as 82 per cent to as low as 30 per cent. The evidence of a major genetic contribution comes from several sources. Blood pressures of parents and their natural children are highly significantly correlated (r 0.3), whereas those of adopted children are not. There is a much lower correlation of spouse blood pressures than of family members who are genetically related. The correlation of blood pressures in monozygotic twins (0.55) is higher than that in dizygotic twins (0.25). It was once contended that blood pressure distribution in populations was bimodal and controlled by a single gene. The error arose because of digit preference for blood pressures ending in zero and boundary avoidance of pressures around 150 mm Hg systolic. It is now generally agreed that blood pressure is unimodally distributed and must be controlled by several genes. How many genes are important and what they control are still in doubt.

Extremes of body weight and salt intake can alter blood pressure, so that differences in body weight and salt intake found between races probably exercise some influence on the range of blood pressures that prevail among them. There is also the question of how much urban and social pressures may contribute to the elevation of arterial pressure. The evidence here is conflicting. Some studies of rural populations have demonstrated pressures as high as, or even higher than, those of genetically similar people living in crowded conditions in cities. A group with one of the highest proportions of high blood pressure values ever reported is black people living in rural Georgia in the United States. Yet studies of Pacific islanders have suggested that groups in closer contact with modern society have higher pressure values than those found in communities from which they migrated. The practical implication of these results is that, with the possible exception of obesity, no factor has yet been identified that can be utilized in a program to prevent high blood pressure.

Body Weight. Many epidemiologic studies have demonstrated a positive correlation between body weight and both systolic and diastolic blood pressure. The correlation is strongest among young and middle-aged adults. Prospective studies suggest that weight gain is associated with a significant rise in blood pressure in those initially normotensive, and, conversely, that weight loss lessens the chance of developing hypertension in those who were normotensive at the outset. There is also epidemiologic evidence that loss of weight among individuals who are hypertensive lowers blood pressure. Clinical studies have been conflicting in that loss of weight does not always lower blood pressure, and it has been argued that when it does so reduced sodium intake may be as important as reduced total calorie intake and body mass.

The improved nutrition of many countries that has resulted from improvements in agriculture and food distribution may increase the number of individuals who are both overweight and hypertensive as well as increasing the number with glucose intolerance. The prevention of obesity is a worthwhile objective in relation to several other health problems besides hypertension, but practical ways of reducing the food intake of whole populations, short of famine or war, have not been identified.

Salt Intake. One of the earliest effective methods of lowering the blood pressure was the rice diet introduced by Kempner which owed its efficacy to its very low content of sodium chloride. Unfortunately, few patients were willing to persist with this tasteless and monotonous regimen, and such an extreme reduction of salt intake would be impractical as a preventive measure. Even the word salary is a reminder that the Roman legionaries were partly paid in salt, and the craving for this substance is deep seated in man and animals. Several studies have been made both within and between communities to establish how far variability in blood pressure is due to salt intake. Variations between communities are difficult to interpret because of genetic differences, but it has been established that the range of salt intake found in western populations does not appear to be an important influence upon levels of blood pressure. It appears unlikely that any practical degree of reduction of salt intake would lower blood pressure. Interesting selective breeding experiments have been carried out in a rat colony at Brookhaven, in which it has proved possible to breed a strain of animal that readily develops severe hypertension when given a high salt intake. Another strain was bred from the same original stock that was highly resistant to the blood pressure–elevating effect of a high salt intake. If there is a human counterpart to this experiment, it would probably involve extremes of salt intake that are rarely encountered in the population.

RISK FACTORS FOR PREDICTING VASCULAR DISEASE. Physicians are accustomed to making predictions about the likely future course of an illness to recovery or death. The use of risk factors to predict the future likelihood of developing an illness is no more than an extension of the same principle. The first to make extensive use of this concept were the life insurance companies, who recognized that factors such as high blood pressure, overweight, and proteinuria increased the probability of their having to pay out the proceeds of a policy, and they learned to adjust their premiums accordingly. It is instructive to reflect that life insurance companies were loading premiums for individuals with moderately elevated blood pressures at a time when their physicians were still patting them on the back and telling them that there was nothing to worry about. As a result of prospective epidemiologic studies such as those carried out in Framingham, Massachusetts, by the National Institutes of Health, it has been possible to study whole populations and to calculate correlation coefficients for many factors that have predictive power in relation to the risk of developing vascular disease. The concept is a most important one to grasp, because it alters radically the clinical management of a patient with a given level of pressure, depending upon the burden of associated factors of risk. It is also important to grasp the difference between absolute risk and relative risk. A young man with a systolic blood pressure of 160 mm Hg has two and one half times the chance of dying compared with a stand-

TABLE 1. Effect of Associated Risk Factors upon Outcome in Hypertension*

	Case I	Case II
Age	45 years	45 years
Sex	Male	Male
Systolic blood pressure	170 mm Hg	170 mm Hg
Cigarette smoker	Yes	No
Serum cholesterol	260 mg/100 ml	185 mg/100 ml
Glucose intolerance	Yes	No
Left ventricular hypertrophy on the ECG	Yes	No
Relative risk compared with age/sex average	7.15	0.78
Patient's risk of developing cardiovascular disease over eight years	54.1	6.33
Average risk for this age and sex group over eight years	8.0	8.0

*Based upon data from the Framingham Survey (program by courtesy of Dr. R. H. Roberts, Ciba-Geigy, Summit, N.J.).

ard risk. In an older man, the ratio is slightly lower. But as older men who are not hypertensive have a much higher chance of suffering a stroke or myocardial infarction, the absolute risk for the older man is much greater than for the younger one.

The three most important risk factors for predicting the future risk of myocardial infarction are level of blood pressure, level of blood lipids, and cigarette smoking habit. Other important factors include the presence of both voltage and T wave signs of left ventricular hypertrophy, glucose intolerance, and obesity. In absolute terms age and sex are most important, because the incidence of morbidity and mortality from vascular disease increases sharply as age advances, but the incidence at younger ages is less in women than in men. Simple computer programs have been constructed that make it possible to calculate the relative risk by providing information about these risk factors, and their importance is illustrated by two case histories for a man of 45 years who has a systolic pressure of 170

mm Hg with and without a high risk category in other respects (Table 1).

A further illustration is given in Figure 2, which shows histograms of risk of developing coronary disease at various levels of systolic pressure from 105 to 195 mm Hg as the burden of other risk factors increases. It can be seen that the risk of the lower pressure category in someone with a full load of other factors is greater than that of someone in the highest pressure category who is free of other risk factors.

The concept of risk factors is very important, but it has certain limitations. The demonstration of a correlation with predictive power does not by any means prove that there is a cause-and-effect relationship. It cannot be assumed that reduction of a risk factor will automatically bring about a proportional, or indeed any, reduction in risk. However, if a risk factor can be diminished without any obvious countervailing disadvantage, it is a matter of common sense to try to reduce it while awaiting the scientific evidence. This argument

Figure 2. Risk of cardiovascular death according to systolic blood pressure at specified levels of other risk factors in 40-year-old men in Framingham, Mass. (By permission of Dr. W. B. Kannel.)

applies especially strongly to reduction of cigarette intake and body weight. The value of reducing lipids is a matter that has caused great controversy. There is evidence that lipid fractions such as the low and very low density lipoproteins may be more important than the total cholesterol or triglycerides. Measures that reduce blood lipids may not automatically reduce the amount of lipid in atheromatous lesions of the arterial wall. Drugs used for this purpose have not been entirely free of unwanted effects, and thus far there is no evidence of benefit in secondary prevention trials, i.e., when they have been used in individuals who have already suffered a myocardial infarction. The results of primary prevention trials are awaited.

CAUSES OF DEATH IN HYPERTENSION. The main causes of death in hypertensive individuals are from damage to blood vessels in vital organs causing myocardial infarction, stroke, peripheral vascular disease, and renal failure. The only causes of death that relate directly to the level of pressure at the time are accelerated hypertension, cerebral hemorrhage, heart failure, and (possibly) dissecting aneurysms. Myocardial infarction is by far the most important and accounts for over half the deaths.

A number of prospective studies, such as that carried out at Framingham, have demonstrated the steep gradient of risk with levels of blood pressure for each of these causes of death. Comparing normotensive individuals with those having a pressure exceeding 160 systolic and 95 diastolic mm Hg, the gradients were threefold for coronary disease and peripheral vascular disease, four-fold for congestive heart failure, and seven-fold for stroke. The increase in risk with level of blood pressure is most striking for stroke deaths. In the age group 40 to 49 years the risk of stroke is ten times higher in individuals with a diastolic pressure exceeding 104 mm Hg than in those in whom it is below 85 mm Hg.

These data also highlight a problem when the control of blood pressure is used as a public health measure to decrease the incidence of stroke and coronary disease. The risk is much greater at high pressure levels, but the number of individuals involved is relatively small. Individuals with modest elevations of blood pressure are so much more numerous that they account for a large fraction of the hypertension-related morbidity and mortality, although at present many of them would probably not be considered for treatment.

CLINICAL MANIFESTATIONS. The assessment of the patient with hypertension has three main objectives: to ascertain the extent of organ damage that has already resulted from the high pressure, to detect any treatable cause, and to define and, when possible, to reduce the factors that determine a high risk of cardiovascular disease. Information relevant to these three factors can be obtained from the history, physical examination, and laboratory investigations.

The Extent of Organ Damage. Patients with severe hypertension may present to the physician with symptoms, although most patients with mild to moderate hypertension have no symptoms directly referable to the disease. Common symptoms include headache, dyspnea, giddiness, and blurred vision. The relationship of headache to hypertension has caused much confusion. Most headaches, including those in the majority of patients with a high blood pressure, bear no rela-

tionship to the level of blood pressure. However, patients with diastolic pressures exceeding about 110 mm Hg, especially younger patients, often complain of morning headaches similar to those seen in patients with other causes of raised intracranial pressure. These headaches are related to the level of blood pressure. Breathlessness and/or a slow walking pace are also common symptoms at higher pressure levels, but many patients with these complaints also have ischemic heart disease. The complaint of giddiness or unsteadiness is common in patients with untreated hypertension, although rather similar complaints may arise as a result of reducing the pressure to a point where cerebral perfusion is impaired. Blurred vision usually indicates the presence of cotton wool spots and/or macular edema, but also arises as a result of a branch retinal vein occlusion, which is more common in hypertensives than in normotensive people. There is a change in the normal diurnal rhythm of urine flow in many patients with hypertension, and they may complain of nocturia even though there is little other evidence of impaired renal function. Hypertension also commonly presents as a result of local ischemia which has resulted from atheromatous narrowing or occlusion of an artery in the brain, heart, or lower limbs. Unfortunately, some patients with hypertension have already suffered such severe damage to the function of the brain or myocardium as to make the value of treatment debatable.

Clinical examination is mainly focused upon the cardiovascular system and the brain. Patients with severe hypertension usually have an apex beat which is displaced to the left and which has a forceful sustained character. They frequently also have an atrial sound. In some patients there may also be signs of left ventricular failure, basal crepitations in the lungs, a third heart sound, pulsus alternans, or congestive heart failure with a raised jugular venous pressure and peripheral edema. Patients with mild to moderate hypertension often have a normal heart on clinical examination. It is important to feel the main arterial pulses, including the femoral, posterior tibial, and dorsalis pedis, and to time the femoral against the brachial artery pulse. The carotid artery should be auscultated at the angle of the jaw, the renal artery just above and about 2 inches lateral to the umbilicus, and the femoral artery at the inguinal ligament.

Careful retinal examination is essential, and this should be done in a darkened room, if possible, with the pupils dilated. The disc margin and the disc color should be carefully inspected, and the presence of the normal optic cup confirmed. The four main vessel groups should be followed for at least three diameters from the disc, taking note of the caliber of the artery, the uniformity of its diameter, the color of the blood column, and the shape of the crossings. The blood vessel wall is not visualized in the normal retina. The red lines of the "vessels" are the column of red cells within them. The cells are surrounded by a shell of plasma and a transparent vessel wall, neither of which is visible with the ophthalmoscope. When the wall becomes thickened and fibrosed, it begins to obscure the red cells column and may ultimately become an opaque white sheath. Cotton wool spots usually occur within three diameters of the optic disc and close to the main vessel groups. Flame-shaped hemorrhages have a similar distribution. Hard exudates are usually best seen close to the macula as radial spokes.

The most important investigations designed to assess organ involvement are the ECG, the chest radiograph, and tests of renal function, particularly the serum creatinine concentration. The ECG should be carefully examined. Common findings are an increased voltage and flattening or inversion of the T waves in leads 1, aVL, and V_{4-6}. The chest radiograph may confirm the clinical assessment of left ventricular enlargement. There is frequently some evidence of aortic disease such as dilatation or tortuosity with unfolding of the thoracic aorta. The degree of renal impairment varies, but some reduction of glomerular filtration rate is present in most patients with severe hypertension, although usually only to about 65 ml per minute if the patient is not in the accelerated phase. Mild and moderate hypertension usually leave renal function unimpaired.

Detection of Treatable Causes. There has been much controversy about the extent to which it is desirable to investigate patients for etiologic factors which may be treatable by surgery. The three main classes of treatable causes are excess catecholamine production from a tumor of the chromaffin tissue; excess mineralocorticoid production from the adrenal, e.g., Cushing's syndrome or hyperaldosteronism; and vascular obstruction such as coarctation of the aorta or renal artery stenosis. Causes of renal disease other than arterial disease are less important, because they less commonly lead to cure of hypertension.

The basic screening investigation for pheochromocytoma is the urinary vanillylmandelic acid (VMA), which some clinics measure in all hypertensive patients. It should certainly be measured in patients with a suggestive history or severe hypertension. The simplest screen for mineralocorticoid excess is measurement of serum potassium and sodium concentrations. There is debate about the extent to which it is necessary to search for renal artery disease if there are no suggestive features such as resistance to treatment or rapid onset of a high pressure level.

Evaluation of Risk. Much of the basic data for evaluating risk will have been derived from the patient's history. This includes date of birth, sex, previous vascular episodes, family history of hypertension and vascular disease, and history of renal disease or diabetes. These findings will be reinforced by the clinical examination and in particular by the blood pressure, body weight and height, and urinalysis for protein and sugar. The only information of value in prediction of risk to be derived from investigations is the ECG for evidence of left ventricular hypertrophy and/or ischemia.

Case Finding. As most patients with elevated levels of blood pressure are symptomless, the only practical way of detecting them before a catastrophe occurs is to conduct an active case-finding program. This means that every physician ought to take the blood pressure of every patient he sees, whatever the primary reason for the consultation. Several attempts have been made to develop rules about the frequency of rescreening if the pressure has been taken in the past. Based upon epidemiologic data, it seems reasonable to rescreen after ten years if the initial diastolic pressure is less than 80 mm Hg, after five years if it lies in the range of 80 to 89 mm Hg, and every year if it is in the range of 90 to 104 mm Hg. Higher pressures than this would normally be treated as would some in the range of 90 to 104 mm Hg.

CLINICAL SYNDROMES OF HYPERTENSION. High blood pressure can present clinically in a wide variety of ways. Before treatment of mild to moderate hypertension became widespread, patients frequently presented with accelerated hypertension, left ventricular failure, or cerebral hemorrhage. A few patients still slip through the net of case-finding programs and suffer these catastrophes prior to initiation of antihypertensive therapy, but these are less common than they used to be. The clinical presentation of hypertension is now most commonly as part of the spectrum of risk factors in a patient who has suffered a stroke or a myocardial infarction, or as a chance finding during clinical examination for another purpose.

Malignant or Accelerated Hypertension. The patient with malignant hypertension is almost always ill with symptoms such as morning headaches, blurred vision, dyspnea, and/or symptoms of uremia. Such patients are commonly in their fourth, fifth, or sixth decade of life, and about half have underlying chronic renal disease. Their blood pressure is almost always above 110 mm Hg diastolic in adults and frequently much higher, with diastolic pressures in the range of 130 to 170 mm being commonplace. Clinical examination usually reveals an enlarged left ventricle and early signs of pulmonary edema such as persistent rales at the lung base. The retinal finding of cotton wool spots and papilledema is essential to make the diagnosis. Investigation usually shows some degree of renal impairment with raised blood urea and serum creatinine values. The serum potassium concentration is often reduced. The blood film may show evidence of intravascular coagulation of "microangiopathic hemolytic anemia" with circulating red cell fragments and fibrin degradation products. The platelet count may be reduced. Irrespective of whether the underlying cause is renal, there is likely to be proteinuria and microscopic hematuria. The characteristic pathologic change of accelerated hypertension is fibrinoid necrosis of small arterioles. Evidence will be presented later that the insudation of plasma and deposition of fibrin follow sudden dilatation of small arterioles whose smooth muscle cells have been unable to generate sufficient tension to withstand the intravascular pressure. This process can be termed high pressure autoregulatory failure, as it represents the upper limit of pressure at which tissue perfusion can be held approximately normal by progressive constriction of arterioles in the face of a rising systemic arterial pressure. High pressure autoregulatory failure is particularly likely to occur if the pressure has risen rapidly or if there are associated factors such as anemia which may impair autoregulation. If the rate of rise of pressure is slow, both smooth muscle hypertrophy and replacement of muscle by fibrous tissue increase the strength of the vessel wall and render it better able to stand the bursting strain of the high intravascular pressure. This probably explains the infrequency of accelerated hypertension in the elderly even though high pressure levels are very common among them. Conversely, younger patients, especially children, may develop the retinal features of accelerated hypertension at lower levels of pressure than is the case in older people.

Accelerated hypertension is a medical emergency because this condition is causing progressive damage to the blood vessels in vital organs, particularly the kidney. Such a patient is also in severe danger of suffering cerebral hemorrhage. When the diagnosis is made, a patient should be admitted to hospital at once for blood pressure reduction.

RETINOPATHY IN ACCELERATED HYPERTENSION. The diagnosis of malignant or accelerated hypertension is based clinically upon the retinal finding of cotton wool spots, linear hemorrhages, and papilledema, and its pathologic hallmark is the presence of fibrinoid necrosis in the arterioles of many organs, particularly the kidney. The retinal changes in accelerated hypertension are all direct consequences of the pressure elevation. As the pressure rises, the arterioles constrict and thus maintain an approximately normal pressure in the distal arterioles and the capillaries. If the pressure rises to a very high level, particularly if it does so quickly, the arterioles may not be able to withstand the high level pressure and begin to give way. The result is that a much higher pressure than usual is applied to the proximal ends of capillaries. In the retina the high pressure capillaries fed directly from the arterioles lie amid the nerve fibers; when hemorrhage takes place from these capillaries, its spread is confined by the nerve fibers so that it has a linear or flame-shaped appearance. A general transudation of fluid as a result of the disturbed Starling pressure equilibrium in the capillary leads to the formation of a grayish retinal edema. The walls of some arterioles which have given way in the face of the high pressure become disrupted, allowing the insudation of plasma through the endothelial cells into the wall. The plasma penetration is often accompanied by cellular elements such as platelets and red cells. This stage can be recognized on a fluorescence angiogram of the retina by the presence of multiple leaking points on small arterioles. The swelling and disruption of the arteriolar wall as a result of the penetration of plasma may obstruct the lumen and lead to a small retinal infarct downstream. This infarct is the cotton wool spot. Pathologic examination of the wall of the arteriole at this stage shows necrosis of myofibrillae in smooth muscle cells, penetration of plasma, and precipitation of fibrin. This is the appearance which pathologists term fibrinoid necrosis. The term is exactly descriptive of the appearances but misleading in the terms of the pathophysiology, because the deposition of fibrin has little or nothing to do with the causation of the lesion. Autoregulatory failure in the vessels of the nerve head causes swelling, engorgement of the capillaries, transudation of fluid, and sometimes also formation of cotton wool spots on the nerve head itself. Keith, Wagener, and Barker (1939) described the presence of hemorrhages and exudates as the third grade of retinopathy, and papilledema as the fourth. As they have the same basic pathogenetic mechanisms, it seems best to describe both as accelerated hypertension. Hard exudates are not present in the earlier stage of the development of hypertensive retinopathy, but they appear soon after cotton wool spots and papilledema are established and are often arranged in radial spokes from the macula, giving the appearance of a star or fan. Hard exudates are fine, punctate, shiny deposits of lipid in the deep layers of the retina and are readily distinguished with the ophthalmoscope from the larger, more diffuse white cotton wool spot with blurred edges which lies in the nerve fiber layer. The cotton wool spot is made up of swollen ischemic axons. The ischemia leads to an interruption of both anterograde and retrograde axoplasmic flow, so that organelles and other materials which are normally moving up and down the axon come to rest in the area of ischemia. These lead to swelling of the axon and its cloudy white appearance. Eventually some of these materials aggregate into dense masses within the neuron, where they have the superficial appearance of a cell nucleus. The swollen axon containing its pseudonucleus is sometimes referred to as a cytoid body. As cotton wool spots clear, they can take on a punctate appearance which may be confused with hard exudates. The punctate white areas are the cytoid bodies.

Hypertensive Encephalopathy. This term tends to be misused to describe any transient neurologic deficit in a patient with severe hypertension. True hypertensive encephalopathy is the cerebral counterpart of the retinal pathology of accelerated hypertension. It is caused by cerebral autoregulatory failure, which brings about generalized cerebral edema and patchy damage to arterioles with leakage of plasma constituents into their walls. Hypertensive encephalopathy often occurs in patients who also have the retinal features of accelerated hypertension, but these are not always present.

The patients usually present clinically with a very high level of pressure and increasingly severe headaches. These progress to general impairment of higher functions and eventually to stupor. Focal and usually transient neurologic signs may develop in the course of the illness. Investigation shows generalized swelling of the brain substance, and animal studies have demonstrated leakage of plasma from arterioles. The diagnosis is a most important one to make accurately, because the patient's condition will improve rapidly if the blood pressure is reduced to a level at which cerebrovascular autoregulation is once again possible.

There is a resemblance between hypertensive encephalopathy and other syndromes in brain autoregulatory failure such as high altitude cerebral edema or carbon dioxide narcosis, although these less commonly manifest focal neurologic signs.

Hypertension in Pregnancy. A raised arterial pressure during pregnancy usually leads to impaired placental function and a small baby. There is an increased risk of intrauterine death and increased neonatal mortality because of prematurity. Toxemia of pregnancy is characterized by a rise in blood pressure from 28 weeks' gestation onward, with edema and proteinuria. The most feared complication is progression to severe hypertension with fits and coma. Eclamptic convulsions are essentially hypertensive encephalopathic attacks occurring in a previously normotensive young woman who has suffered a rapid rise in blood pressure. They should never occur in women who have received proper antenatal care and control of blood pressure. Toxemia is hypertension provoked by pregnancy, but many women who have mild hypertension become pregnant or may be first found to be hypertensive when they consult a physician at about 8 to 12 weeks of pregnancy for antenatal care. Because of the separation that exists between medical specialties, there was in the past a different approach to treatment in a pregnant hypertensive than in the nonpregnant female with high blood pressure. This view is now changing, and most physicians and obstetricians use the same methods of management in pregnancy as at other times but aim to achieve particularly accurate control of pressure during the pregnancy. There is evidence that effective antihypertensive therapy reduces fetal loss during pregnancy, and the aim should be to keep the pressure below 140 systolic and 90 diastolic mm Hg if possible. The main drug used to control blood pressure is methyldopa. There has been concern that antihypertensive drugs might damage the development of the fetal nervous system by interfering with catecholamine pathways, but studies of babies whose mothers have been treated for hypertension with these drugs are reassuring. Some obstetricians are concerned about the use of beta-adrenergic blocking drugs because it obscures the interpretation of fetal bradycardia, an important clinical sign of both fetal and neonatal hypoxia.

Hitherto, pregnant hypertensives often had to spend many weeks resting in hospital to keep the blood pressure down. This is sometimes still necessary, but in many cases the blood pressure can be controlled with drugs and the patient can remain ambulatory.

Cerebral Hemorrhage. Abrupt onset of major neurologic signs, sometimes accompanied by severe headache and progressing rapidly to loss of consciousness, usually signifies the onset of intracranial bleeding in a hypertensive patient. The bleeding may occur into the subarachnoid space from a berry aneurysm, but the common source in hypertensive patients appears to be the minute arterial aneurysms on the striate arteries on the base of the brain, first described by Charcot and Bouchard in France over 100 years ago. These aneurysms are rare in individuals who have a normal blood pressure. Their pathogenesis has not been completely elucidated, but there may be areas of high pressure autoregulatory failure on the thin-walled cerebral vessels. The hemorrhage usually begins in the substance of the brain but may rupture into the ventricular system. Once intracranial bleeding has reached the subarachnoid space, the prognosis is very poor. Small hemorrhages have a better prognosis and can be difficult to differentiate clinically from the cerebral infarction caused by vascular occlusion. If there is any question of using anticoagulants, this differentiation can be important, and in such cases further investigation by lumbar puncture and computerized axial tomography is indicated. Carotid arteriography is indicated if there is clinical suspicion of a berry aneurysm and if the patient's condition improves sufficiently to warrant consideration of neurosurgical intervention.

Hypertensive Left Ventricular Failure. The presence of a high systemic arterial pressure increases the afterload of the left ventricle, and in consequence the ventricle hypertrophies. As the pressure rises to a very high level, the ventricles dilate and eventually fail, and the patient then presents with pulmonary edema. This may range in severity from a patient who is asphyxiating with airways full of white or pink froth to mild dyspnea on exertion or occasional attacks of nocturnal dyspnea. In older people with hypertension the clinical presentation of pulmonary edema is frequently precipitated by the onset of atrial fibrillation or by ischemic heart disease. If pulmonary edema is caused by high pressure, the clinical improvement as a result of pressure reduction can be almost miraculous in its rapidity.

"Benign Essential" Hypertension. Patients with an elevated pressure who are not in the accelerated phase are often described as having benign essential hypertension. The term benign is inappropriate, as an elevated blood pressure always carries some risk. Although no cause can be identified in most individuals with high pressure, the use of the word essential to describe it adds nothing, and it, too, is probably better avoided.

What then are the clinical features of hypertension which is not in the accelerated phase? They are rarely dramatic. The elevated level of pressure is often the only clinical finding of note. A mild degree of left ventricular hypertrophy may be identified clinically, or by means of the electrocardiogram or chest x-ray. Vascular damage may be evident either from its consequences on the heart or brain or by loss of pulses or arterial bruits.

RETINOPATHY IN "BENIGN" HYPERTENSION. Keith, Wagener, and Barker applied the terms grade I and grade II retinopathy to the retinal changes found in hypertensive patients who are not in the accelerated phase. The main features which they described included narrowing of the arterioles, often with caliber irregularity, and nicking of the veins at the crossing. The appearance of the arteriole wall changed so that it became shinier and more irregular, whereas the color of the underlying blood columns was partly concealed so that it took on a coppery or silvery hue. Narrowing of the retinal vessels is due to vasoconstriction. All the other changes represent thickening of the vessel wall as a result of muscle hypertrophy and fibrous replacement. The problem with these features is that none of them is by itself characteristic of hypertension. Elderly people who are normotensive may show all of them. They are still of clinical value if the patient is young but of little use in drawing conclusions about the severity of hypertension in the elderly. Recording of these features is very prone to observer error, and attempts to standardize the recording of the diameter of the arteries by comparing them with the nearby veins have foundered on the variability of the branching pattern of the retinal vessels. The presence of these features does not add much to knowledge of the patient in most cases.

MECHANISMS. The systemic arterial pressure must be maintained at a level which permits the brain and eye to function and allows pressure filtration in the kidneys and perfusion of the coronary arteries. It is not surprising that this most vital function is defended by several different control systems which prevent its falling too low. The blood pressure must also be prevented from rising too high, because vascular damage might result. Four control systems play the major part in maintaining the blood pressure between these limits. These are the arterial baroreflex, the regulation of body fluid volume, the renin-angiotensin system, and vascular autoregulation. All these mechanisms participate in blood pressure regulation in normotension and in hypertension. It is uncertain how far derangement of any one of them plays a role in the pathogenesis of hypertension.

The Arterial Baroreflex. The main concentration of pressure sensors lies in the carotid sinus, although there are others in the aorta and the wall of the left ventricle. These sensors continually monitor the level of arterial pressure, and their rate of firing changes between systole and diastole. They form the afferent limb of the fastest responding blood pressure regulating system. Sensory impulses from the baroreceptors are relayed and processed in the brainstem. Norepinephrine and epinephrine containing fibers around the nucleus of the solitary tract play an important part in regulating the gain of the baroreflex. The efferent fibers proceed through sympathetic adrenergic nerves to the heart and blood vessels and through vagal cholinergic fibers. A sudden rise in pressure causes baroreflex discharge, which results in vagally mediated cardiac slowing and vasodilatation with decreased sympathetic tone. The result is to lower the blood pressure, although not all the way to the prestimulus level. A sudden fall in pressure diminishes the rate of firing and causes sympathetic stimulation of the rate and force of cardiac contraction and constriction of peripheral arterioles and veins. The result is partly to restore the level of blood pressure. Denervation of the carotid sinus in animals causes extreme lability of blood pressure, which is sometimes termed neurogenic hypertension. However, the rise in arterial pressure is not usually very great except when the animal is stimulated, and the characteristic is more of extreme instability than sustained elevation of pressure.

It is important to realize that the baroreflex arc is not simply a fixed feedback loop such as might be found in an amplifier. Depending upon the physiologic circumstances, the response to the same level of blood pressure can be quite different. A blood pressure of 85 systolic and 55 diastolic mm Hg caused by bleeding would cause an intense sympathetic discharge and tachycardia. The same level of pressure during deep sleep would be accompanied by the normal bradycardia of the sleeping subject. A pressure of 200 systolic and 100 diastolic mm Hg is readily achieved during heavy exercise and is accompanied by tachycardia. The same pressure brought about by infusion of norepinephrine would cause severe cardiac slowing mediated by the baroreflex. The pressure is the same, but the interpretation at CNS level is completely different.

If the pressure remains elevated, the baroreflex begins to regulate at the new level within 24 to 48 hours. The ability of the baroreflex to reset so quickly argues against its playing an important role in long-term pressure regulation. Baroreflex function in patients with hypertension appears to be intact and not to differ qualitatively from that found in normotensives.

The effector side of the baroreflex is chiefly the sympathetic nervous system through its ability to constrict arteries and veins and to stimulate cardiac contractility and rate. The importance of this side of the reflex is seen in the postural hypotension suffered by many patients in whom it is inhibited by ganglion-blocking or adrenergic neuron–blocking drugs. The baroreflex is not the only control system that uses the adrenergic nerves to raise blood pressure. The rise in pressure that occurs with fear, anxiety, pain, or mental activity is also mediated by increasing cardiac output or peripheral resistance through these pathways. One possible mechanism for long-term elevation of blood pressure would be excessive central nervous system–mediated stimulation of adrenergic nerves. Evidence for this possibility has been sought by comparing the level of blood pressure at rest with the plasma concentration of the adrenergic neurotransmitter norepinephrine. Some research workers have found a very close relationship between blood pressure and plasma norepinephrine; others have not. It has not proved possible to devise any method of measuring the basic level of sympathetic impulses other than the plasma and urinary catecholamines that represent the totality of these processes and not just the vascular ones. There is evidence for a wider spread of norepinephrine levels in plasma in hypertensives, about 40 per cent of them lying above the normal range, but not yet sufficient to conclude that hypertension in some individuals is caused by the brain.

Fluid Volume. If the body is severely depleted of salt and water, the blood pressure falls; if it is overloaded, the pressure rises. The mechanisms involved are complex and have been discussed cogently by Guyton. Changes in fluid volume alter the distention of the venous system and change the venous return to the heart. If the cardiac filling pressure rises, so does the cardiac output; if it falls, the output also falls. The short-term effects of cardiac output changes upon blood pressure are buffered by the baroreflex, but in the longer term changes in tissue perfusion which are inappropriate to metabolic requirements lead to autoregulatory changes in the peripheral resistance and thus to changes in the blood pressure. If the kidneys are intact, a rise in pressure leads to a diuresis and a fall in pressure to conservation of salt and water. Thus the feedback loop is closed, and Guyton has claimed that this system, unlike the baroreflex, has infinite gain so that it can exactly restore the previous level of pressure.

Pathologic changes that alter the pressure threshold at which the kidneys excrete salt and water will alter the level of systemic arterial pressure. At one extreme a complete lack of kidneys should lead to a great sensitivity to changes in volume, and this has proved to be the case. Relatively small increases in salt and water intake in nephrectomized individuals cause a large increase in blood pressure. This type of hypertension is sometimes termed "renoprival." Other mechanisms such as the lack of a renal depressor substance may also play a part in the abnormal pressure regulation. If excretory function is diminished, the blood pressure will become responsive to an abnormally high sodium load. Mineralocorticoid excess will cause the kidney to retain salt at a pressure level at which it would normally be excreted and thereby raise the arterial pressure. Anything that increases the pressure gradient between the aorta and the glomeruli will tend to raise the systemic arterial pressure as renal retention of salt and water endeavors to restore the preobstruction renal perfusion pressure. This will apply to obstruction of the main renal arteries and of the arterial branches within the kidney. An experimental analogy is the one-kidney Goldblatt model. Here one kidney has been removed and the other has an arterial clip upon it. The renin levels are low, and the pressure gradient across the renal artery appears to be the important factor in causing the hypertension through the salt and water retention that results from diminished perfusion pressure applied to the clipped kidney.

Renin and Angiotensin. Renin is an enzyme released from the kidney which splits a decapeptide from a plasma globulin substrate. This decapeptide, angiotensin I, has little pharmacologic activity, but a dipeptide residue is removed by a converting enzyme in the lung to form an octapeptide, angiotensin II. Until the discovery of the thromboxanes, this was the most potent vasoconstrictor agent known. Angiotensin II has a direct action upon blood vessels, but it is also an important physiologic stimulant of aldosterone secretion from the adrenal gland.

Renin and angiotensin levels in the blood respond in the direction anticipated if they were participating in physiologic blood pressure regulation. Standing or salt depletion raises renin, and recumbency and salt loading reduce it. In conditions of primary mineralocorticoid excess the renin falls to a low value. Four control mechanisms have been identified that control the release of renin from the kidney. The first mechanism is the renal barostat, which senses changes in renal perfusion pressure and releases renin when the pressure falls; the second mechanism is the short feedback loop of plasma angiotensin II levels upon renin release. If angiotensin effects are blocked with its competitive antagonist saralasin, renin levels rise rapidly. The third mechanism is mediated by beta-adrenergic receptors in the kidney which release renin when they are stimulated, and the fourth mechanism depends upon sensing the tubular concentrations of sodium.

The importance of angiotensin II in maintaining blood pressure at any particular time depends upon the level of sodium intake. In a sodium replete individual inhibition of angiotensin II has little effect upon blood pressure; but if the same person is salt depleted, the result of inhibition may be a substantial fall. There is good evidence that angiotensin II is the cause of the blood pressure elevation in the experimental two-kidney Goldblatt hypertension and in human hypertension caused by renal artery stenosis. In the two-kidney Goldblatt model one kidney is clipped and the other is not. Thus the unclipped kidney should be able to prevent a rise in pressure due to salt and water retention resulting from the pressure gradient across the clipped artery. In the first phase of this form of hypertension the blood pressure rises and so do the plasma renin and angiotensin. Infusion of the competitive angiotensin II antagonist saralasin causes a prompt fall to a normal level of pressure. However, in experimental hypertension and probably also in human hypertension the pressure continues to rise in the second phase, whereas the renin subsides almost to normal. Short-term infusion of saralasin will not lower the blood pressure, which appears to be no longer angiotensin dependent. However, a 12-hour infusion of saralasin or a converting enzyme inhibitor gradually lowers the pressure to normal in animals and may do so in man. Thus the hypertension in phase II is still angiotensin dependent but apparently by a different mechanism.

The role of angiotensin II in other forms of human hypertension remains to be elucidated in full, but it seems very unlikely that it plays a central role in the majority of patients. In malignant hypertension the renin levels are usually high because of the multiple small areas of ischemia within the kidney. Angiotensin II plays some part in the maintenance of blood pressure and is undoubtedly responsible for the secondary hyperaldosteronism that frequently causes mild potassium depletion in these patients.

Vascular Autoregulation. In many tissues, of which the brain is the best example, a change in perfusion pressure does not cause a corresponding change in tissue perfusion. Instead, the vascular resistance is adjusted by local mechanisms to keep perfusion roughly constant over a wide range of arterial pressures. This phenomenon is known as "vascular autoregulation." If flow changes rather than pressure, autoregulation will diminish the vascular resistance in response to a reduction in flow and raise it in response to an increase. Thus changes in cardiac output which are inappropriate to metabolic demand should produce corresponding changes in blood pressure. It seems likely that this is an important mechanism in the causation of the hyper-

tension that accompanies salt and water overload, but it is uncertain how significant it is in other circumstances. It has been suggested that some patients with essential hypertension may go through a phase of increased cardiac output before hypertension becomes established, but this has not been proved beyond doubt. Reduction of cardiac output may be the main mode of action of beta-adrenergic blocking drugs in lowering the blood pressure, but this, too, remains to be established.

Circulatory Dynamics. In broad terms the level of the systemic arterial pressure is set by the match between cardiac output and peripheral vascular resistance. Elevation of blood pressure could result from either or both. In the early stages of hypertension some patients have a raised cardiac output and some a raised peripheral resistance, but in the majority of patients with established hypertension the cardiac output is normal and peripheral resistance is raised. In the later stages of severe hypertension the cardiac output is often less than normal and the peripheral resistance is greatly increased. Thus in looking for new factors that may cause hypertension, it seems most profitable to concentrate upon those which raise the peripheral resistance.

Elevation of the arterial pressure causes many other changes in the cardiovascular system. A high level of pressure stimulates hypertrophy of the vessel wall and increases the thickness of the smooth muscle coat. These changes probably account for the enhanced sensitivity to pressor stimuli in patients with established or early hypertension. Such stimuli include exposure to cold, fear, mental arithmetic, and so forth. A greater thickness of muscle means that the change in vessel caliber for a given degree of fiber shortening will be greater. Hypertrophy of the vessel wall also raises the minimum vascular resistance of tissues such as the human forearm under conditions of maximal vasodilatation.

Besides the hypertrophic changes, other structural changes take place in the arteries. Some of the muscle in the thickened wall is replaced by fibrous tissue. The most important vascular change is that the deposition of atheroma is increased by the presence of hypertension. The reason is not known, but it is a change manifest in pulmonary hypertension as well as systemic hypertension. As the predominant causes of death in hypertensive patients are stroke and myocardial infarction, the significance of accelerated formation of atheroma cannot be denied, but the mechanism is uncertain.

The cardiac muscle also hypertrophies, and, if pressure elevation is extreme, the cavity of the ventricle dilates. Local imbalance between metabolic demand and perfusion within the increased muscle mass may lead to relative ischemia and areas of fibrosis. These may lead to ineffective contraction which, combined with the dilated chamber and the afterload of the high pressure, will eventually bring about heart failure.

The regulation of plasma volume is altered in hypertension. Some patients have a relatively contracted plasma volume with a high hematocrit, probably because of the increased capillary pressure. There is a marked diurnal variation of plasma volume, with the value almost 10 per cent lower in the morning than in the evening in hypertensive subjects. An infused sodium load is excreted more rapidly by hypertensive patients than by normotensive controls.

ETIOLOGY. In most diseases the need to establish a diagnosis is paramount because the prognosis and the treatment given may be entirely different, depending upon which of the possible alternatives is the cause of the illness. The position with hypertension is somewhat different. There are very few causes of hypertension which are life threatening other than by their effect upon the blood pressure. The most important condition in this category is renal failure, but this is usually readily detected clinically, or by the use of a biochemical screen at presentation. Only coarctation of the aorta and a pheochromocytoma are sufficiently serious in themselves as well as through the pressure elevation they cause as to make it essential that they should be diagnosed at once. Although it is desirable to make a diagnosis of renal artery stenosis or primary hyperaldosteronism, if present, some delay will not usually cause harm to the patient if the pressure has been controlled with drugs in the meantime. Thus the diagnostic problem in a patient with hypertension is how to detect as large a proportion as possible of the rare treatable causes without exposing millions of patients without such factors to unnecessary and uncomfortable investigations. The answer is to use screening tests and to be willing to reconsider the diagnosis in treated patients if the clinical course is atypical.

Obstruction or Loss of Elasticity in the Large Arteries. Coarctation of Aorta (see Ch. 359.2). Routine palpation of the femoral pulses with simultaneous timing against the radial is part of the basic clinical examination of a patient with hypertension. Other clinical features, such as a wide pulse pressure in the arteries fed by the aorta proximal to the coarctation, palpable or visible collaterals, or tortuous retinal arteries, help to confirm the diagnosis that has been made. Occasionally the diagnosis is first made radiologically by direct visualization of the coarctation or of rib notching on a routine chest radiograph. Operative treatment is indicated if it is technically feasible.

Systolic Hypertension. Many elderly patients and some younger ones present with considerable elevation of the systolic pressure while having a relatively normal diastolic pressure. A typical pressure might be 200 systolic and 80 diastolic mm Hg in such an individual. The principal factors governing the magnitude of the pulse pressure are the stroke volume and acceleration of the blood from the left ventricle and the elasticity of the large arteries, particularly the aorta. Factors that increase the stroke volume such as bradycardia, aortic incompetence, anemia, and anxiety may all lead to an increase in systolic pressure with a normal or low diastolic pressure. In the elderly the most common cause is not an increase in stroke volume but a loss of elastic compliance of the large arteries. Epidemiologic studies have shown that such patients have an increased risk of cardiovascular morbidity and mortality even if their diastolic pressure is relatively low. However, it is not clear whether this cardiovascular disease is a cause or consequence of the systolic hypertension. It may be that the presence of a systolic hypertension is itself a marker of arterial disease and the level of systolic pressure has no other significance. There is no evidence as to whether reduction of systolic hypertension with a normal diastolic pressure conveys any advantage to the patient.

Hypertension Associated with Catecholamine Excess. Pheochromocytoma (see Ch. 550). Pheochromocytoma is a very rare cause of hypertension. It can be suspected clinically in half to two thirds of the patients. Pounding palpitations and/or headaches, paroxysmal skin color changes, tremor, sweating, agitation, glycosuria, and hypermetabolism may all point to the likelihood of this diagnosis.

Some patients are aware that pressure over the tumor area can provoke an attack. A very rare but striking example is the precipitation of a paroxysm by micturition in a patient with pheochromocytoma of the bladder. In some patients there are only occasional spikes of hypertension, or even of hypotension, whereas in others there may be a sustained elevation in the blood pressure. There is sometimes quite marked orthostatic hypotension in the absence of the use of drugs with a postural effect.

It is common practice to measure the urinary VMA as a screening test to detect pheochromocytoma in all hypertensive patients irrespective of clinical suspicions. A single estimate is about 80 per cent reliable in detecting a pheochromocytoma, but many slightly elevated values occur as false positives. Once firmly suspected, the diagnosis should be confirmed by further measurements of the urinary VMA and of metanephrines or catecholamines. Other causes of increased sympathetic activity such as left ventricular failure and myocardial infarction should be ruled out. Increasingly the measurements of plasma norepinephrine are being used to make and confirm the diagnosis of pheochromocytoma. These, combined with segmental venous sampling, may supplement radiologic methods of localizing the tumor.

Monoamine Oxidase Inhibitors: Interaction with Tyramine. Patients taking drugs which inhibit the monoamine oxidase in the gut wall and in the body at large may develop paroxysmal hypertension if they consume food or drink containing tyramine or medicines such as cold cures which contain indirectly pressor amines such as phenylpropanolamine. Tyramine and phenylpropanolamine are both capable of releasing norepinephrine from adrenergic nerve endings. Normally the amounts of these releasing agents that penetrate into the body are small because of metabolism by monoamine oxidase in the gut wall. If this enzyme is inhibited, larger amounts reach the systemic circulation where the adrenergic nerve endings contain an excessive amount of norepinephrine because of the local inhibition of monoamine oxidase. The result can be a catastrophic increase in circulating norepinephrine, causing a very high blood pressure with a risk of cerebral hemorrhage or paroxysmal cardiac arrhythmia.

Clonidine Withdrawal. The imidazoline clonidine is an effective antihypertensive agent. It acts centrally as an alpha-adrenoceptor agonist and causes a decrease in the sympathetic outflow. If treatment with the drug is suddenly withdrawn, patients may develop a syndrome of catecholamine excess 16 to 48 hours later which closely resembles a pheochromocytoma. Patients complain of anxiety, tremor, palpitations, and insomnia with severe headache. Both plasma and urinary catecholamines can reach levels found in patients with pheochromocytoma. The precise mechanism underlying this reaction has not yet been determined, but sympathetic efferent activity is greatly increased. The blood pressure can be controlled by restarting clonidine or by use of alpha-adrenergic blocking agents.

Catecholamine Excess in Essential Hypertension. A wide range of values of both plasma norepinephrine and urinary metabolites of catecholamines are found in both normotensive and hypertensive individuals. Some studies have found a fairly close correlation between the height of the blood pressure and the concentration of norepinephrine in the plasma, but this has been denied by others. The plasma norepinephrine rises slightly as age advances, and this may account for some of the reported differences between values in hypertensives and normotensive laboratory controls. It is still an open question whether prolonged chronic sympathetic overactivity is one of the causes of essential hypertension.

MANAGEMENT OF CATECHOLAMINE EXCESS HYPERTENSION. The long-term treatment of hypertension associated with gross excess of circulating catecholamines is to treat the cause. However, in the short term the blood pressure and cardiac rhythm disturbances, if present, must be controlled. Alpha-adrenergic blocking drugs such as injections of phentolamine should be used to control the immediate rise in pressure; oral agents such as phenoxybenzamine which alkylate the alpha receptor can be used in longer-term treatment. Tachycardia or tachyarrhythmias can be controlled by use of beta receptor blocking agents, such as propranolol. Patients with a pheochromocytoma should always be prepared for surgery by pharmacologic control of hypertension and cardiac arrhythmias.

Renal Hypertension. All forms of chronic renal disease may be associated with an increased incidence of hypertension. This is true of chronic glomerulonephritis due to immune complex deposition, chronic pyelonephritis due to infection, vascular lesions such as occur in polyarteritis nodosa and lupus erythematosus and in the main renal arteries due to congenital bands, intimal fibroplasia, and atheroma. Renal carcinoma can cause hypertension as can polycystic disease, although isolated renal cysts rarely do so. Obstructive uropathies, analgesic abuse, and renal calculi can also cause hypertension. Acute renal failure resulting from glomerulonephritis or tubular necrosis can cause rapid elevation of blood pressure, especially in fluid-overloaded patients.

There are two main reasons for making an accurate diagnosis of renal hypertension. The first is that the renal or urologic condition which has caused the hypertension may itself require treatment, e.g., infection, stone, obstruction, tumor. Of the conditions that fall into this category, infection is the most important. Pyelonephritis is an important cause of renal damage and hypertension, especially in children. Its numerical importance in relation to adult hypertension is difficult to establish because of the difficulty of proving a diagnosis of chronic pyelonephritis.

The relationship between bacilluria and hypertension is disputed, but there is an increased incidence of hypertension in patients whose urograms show "pyelonephritic scars." There are vascular lesions in the vicinity of these scars, and there seems little doubt that the scars are ischemic in origin. Such lesions can be caused by hypertensive changes in the vessels without any infection, and it is not clear how far infection of the renal parenchyma can cause vascular lesions and initiate the ischemia that leads to scar formation and hypertension in a previously normotensive individual. But in children with vesicoureteral reflux, urinary infection, renal scars, and hypertension, there seems little doubt that reflux and infection start the whole process.

If there are renal symptoms or a history of urinary infection, the urine should be cultured; if the culture is positive, an appropriate antimicrobial should be given.

There is no evidence that this will modify the course of the hypertension, but it may prevent further loss of renal parenchyma due to infection. Investigation of urologic causes of recurrent infection such as stone should proceed as it would in a normotensive patient.

The second reason for investigating a patient to determine if hypertension has a renal cause is the possibility of surgical cure of renovascular disease or unilateral renal disease. Cure of hypertension has resulted from nephrectomy in several types of unilateral renal disease, including pyelonephritis, hydro- and pyonephrosis, and tumor. One of the best pieces of direct evidence that pyelonephritis can cause hypertension is the cases of surgical cure when the disease was predominantly unilateral. Unfortunately, pyelonephritis is rarely completely unilateral; and as cure rates are only 30 to 40 per cent even in carefully selected patients, modern policy is to conserve functioning renal tissue when possible. Attempts at cure are focused on renovascular disease.

SALT AND WATER OVERLOAD HYPERTENSION. Patients without kidneys or those in terminal renal failure with very low values of glomerular filtration are extremely sensitive to changes in salt and water balance. The plasma renin and angiotensin II levels are usually low unless the patient has entered the accelerated phase of hypertension. This form of hypertension can usually be managed successfully by restriction of salt and water intake and elimination of excess by dialysis. The body weight is often a better guide to progress than the sphygmomanometer. The experimental counterpart to this form of hypertension is salt-loading animals that have had one kidney and part of another removed or else have had one kidney removed and an arterial clip applied to the other.

RENIN-DEPENDENT HYPERTENSION. The extent to which renin contributes to elevation of blood pressure in the majority of patients with hypertension is controversial, but most studies suggest that the proportion is quite small. The spread of renin values is wider among hypertensives than normotensives, and those above and below the normal range, related to sodium intake, are often called "high renin" and "low renin" hypertensives. It was suggested that renin might be itself a factor causing damage to blood vessels and that high renin hypertensives had a much increased incidence of stroke and myocardial infarction. That view has found little support from further studies. As plasma renin falls with age and the risk of vascular disease increases, a negative association has been proposed based upon epidemiologic studies. Renin contributes to the elevation of blood pressure in accelerated hypertension and causes it in renal disease associated with ischemia. Many types of renal disease can be associated with localized areas of ischemia, but the most important is renal artery obstruction caused by medial fibroplasia or atheromatous disease. The detection of these conditions has given rise to much controversy on the grounds of prevalence, costs, and results of surgery.

RENAL ARTERY STENOSIS. There are no reliable figures for the incidence of renal artery stenosis in the community. It may cause 3 to 5 per cent of severe hypertension treated in hospital but probably less than 1 per cent of the mild hypertension now being treated in the community.

There are few clinical features that help in making a diagnosis. Suspicion should be aroused by severe hypertension in a patient under 35 years old, or sudden increase in severity in an older patient. Rarely an attack of flank pain may point to a renal artery embolus, and a bruit above and radiating laterally from the umbilicus may be helpful. Unfortunately the majority of bruits heard over the abdominal aorta do not originate in the renal arteries. The most common means of diagnosis is an intravenous urogram. Typical features include one kidney more than 1.5 cm shorter than the other, delay in appearance of contrast on the ischemic side on a two-minute film, and delay in emptying on that side later in the urogram because of the low flow of concentrated urine. The most reliable means of confirming the diagnosis is an angiogram of the abdominal aorta and renal arteries. At one time a high proportion of patients with hypertension were subjected to abdominal aortography, but the yield of cases was low and appreciable discomfort and cost were involved. Routine aortography has now been abandoned almost everywhere. Some have argued against the value of the urogram in hypertension, especially when there is no indication other than the level of pressure itself. The cost of the investigative procedures per patient eventually cured of hypertension is rather high.

When the diagnosis of renal artery stenosis has been confirmed anatomically, it is still necessary to try to establish whether the elevation of blood pressure is due to it. The methods used currently include measurement of renin concentration in blood drawn from both renal veins. The difference should exceed 1.5 to 2 times, and the unprotected kidney has its production of renin suppressed. Antagonism of the effect of circulating renin is another promising method of establishing the diagnosis. This can be done by infusing the angiotensin II antagonist Sar-1-Ala-8-angiotensin II (saralasin) or a converting enzyme inhibitor such as the nonapeptide SQ 20881. The predictive power of these tests for results of surgery is good but not perfect.

At present the usual method of managing renin-dependent hypertension is to seek a treatable cause such as renal artery obstruction and to repair it by surgical means. Results depend upon the skill of the surgeon, but normotension has been achieved in half to two thirds of patients in some centers. In patients in whom operation is not technically feasible or whose general health does not permit, the blood pressure can be lowered by antihypertensive drugs, and the long-term survival of operated and medically managed patients is similar. Mortality tends to be high in both groups, because patients with atheromatous stenosis of the renal artery usually have extensive atheroma elsewhere. A special situation may arise in patients with renal failure and bilateral renal artery obstruction, in whom surgery can sometimes improve overall renal function. Drugs that reduce the sympathetically mediated release of renin are indicated if medical management is to be used, and a beta-adrenergic receptor blocking agent such as propranolol would be the first choice. As propranolol only inhibits sympathetically mediated renin release, it is not completely effective in reducing the plasma renin. Inhibitors of the converting enzyme active by the oral route hold out more promise but are still at an early stage of clinical trial.

MINERALOCORTICOID EXCESS HYPERTENSION. Mineralocorticoids, both natural and synthetic, can cause retention of salt and water and resultant hypertension. Thus hypertension is a common complication of Cushing's syndrome, both natural and iatrogenic. The contraceptive pill is capable of causing elevation of blood pressure, and there are worrying indications that this may be progressive over several years. The elevation each year is a trivial 1 or 1.5 mm rise in diastolic pressure, but the cumulative effect over several years can begin to be significant in epidemiologic terms in relation to the incidence of stroke and myocardial infarction. Blood pressure elevation may also result from the salt-retaining effects of carbenoxolone sodium given to treat gastric ulcer.

Among these factors the contraceptive pill gives rise to by far the greatest difficulty because of the extent of its use. Severe hypertension in users of the pill is very uncommon, although accelerated hypertension has been reported. More commonly a woman who has used the pill for several years develops a pressure level which is on the threshold of an indication for treatment. There is no certain method of establishing whether the pill is responsible short of stopping it for six weeks. Some women taking the pill are unwilling to stop taking it for fear of unwanted pregnancy, and it may be necessary to treat their hypertension without establishing beyond doubt that the contraceptive pill is its cause.

Endogenous mineralocorticoid excess can also pose difficult problems of detection and treatment. Cushing's syndrome or congenital adrenal hyperplasia as a cause of hypertension can usually be diagnosed clinically, although patients with an ACTH-producing malignant tumor may present with hypertension and severe hypokalemia without much other evidence of Cushing's syndrome. The main problem is the diagnosis of primary hyperaldosteronism. Some patients will give a history that suggests potassium depletion with muscle weakness and edema, but most do not. The presence of hypokalemia is a useful guide if the patient has not received a thiazide diuretic, but most patients have been treated with these agents before they get to a hospital clinic. If potassium depletion is severe and the serum sodium is high, the diagnosis is very likely to be hyperaldosteronism, and it can be confirmed by measuring plasma or urinary aldosterone and plasma renin. A patient with primary hyperaldosteronism has an increased production of aldosterone with a suppressed plasma renin. A trial of treatment with the aldosterone antagonist spironolactone predicts fairly accurately the eventual response of both blood pressure and serum potassium concentration to operative removal of an adrenal tumor. Primary hyperaldosteronism can be caused by an adrenal adenoma or by diffuse "micronodular" hyperplasia. A few patients have been described with hypertension due to primary hyperaldosteronism who had a normal serum potassium level some or all of the time. These patients are impossible to diagnose without full investigation of aldosterone and renin, and this does not appear justified as a routine procedure for the very low yield of treatable cases likely to result.

TREATMENT. The intellectual challenge of diagnosis often attracts more interest than the time-consuming persistent effort required for effective long-term drug treatment. The problem is evident in the management of hypertension, in which surgically treatable patients have tended to attract more attention than those requiring drug therapy. Although it is important for the patient with a surgically treatable cause to be detected, this must not be done at the expense of the great majority of patients who do not require elaborate clinical investigation but do need careful blood pressure control by use of drugs to diminish the risk of cardiovascular disease. The proportion of hypertensive patients in the community who might benefit from pressure reduction and who have a surgically remediable cause is very small, probably only 1 to 2 per cent of those requiring treatment.

Reduction of Risk. The aim of patient management in hypertension is to reduce the likelihood of cardiovascular complications, and the approach adopted depends upon the level of blood pressure and the burden of associated risk factors. If the blood pressure is very high, this is the dominant consideration, and other considerations can be deferred until the pressure has been reduced. However, in many patients with only moderate elevation of pressure, other factors such as cigarette smoking, serum lipids, glucose intolerance, and obesity may be of comparable significance to the blood pressure. Careful assessment is required to decide which factors should receive the most attention. A patient who is told to stop smoking, to lose 20 pounds in weight, and to take pills to lower blood pressure is likely to find the task so difficult that he will end up doing none of them. Failure to comply with the physician's advice is the most common cause of treatment failure, and strategies must be developed to try to improve it. A close relationship between the patient and a single physician is a significant factor. A patient who knows, likes, and trusts his physician is more likely to take his advice irrespective of its quality. That advice should be simple and unequivocal. A general advice to lose weight rarely has much impact, but a specific instruction to lose 1 pound per week for 20 weeks backed up by regular weighing and scrutiny of the results may succeed.

The drug regimen should consist of as few different drugs and tablets as possible, and regimens that require doses to be taken during the working day should be avoided. The patient should know the name and purpose of each tablet, and when and how many to take. The very fact that the doctor takes an interest in the drugs reinforces their importance in the eyes of a patient. A hastily written prescription handed over without an explanation may have the contrary effect. Patients often find it helpful to purchase a small metal pillbox and to count their tablets for the next day into it just before they go to bed. If the box is empty again by the next evening, the patient will know he has taken exactly the right amount. If the patient is elderly or confused, a family member can be enlisted to help count out the tablets and make sure they have been consumed. A wife or husband often seems more concerned about the outcome of therapy than the patient does.

Despite these measures to improve compliance with advice, some patients will drop out from treatment and attendance at follow-up. Few will do so by deliberate rejection of therapy, which is their right. In most cases it is more a matter of oversight. A well-run clinic should have a system to detect nonattendance and to issue reminders. A special register for hypertensive patients is the best arrangement.

Antihypertensive Drugs. In most countries there are many different antihypertensive drugs available, and the range of choice may seem bewildering. If the drugs are categorized in terms of their main pharmacologic action, much of this confusion disappears, and the choice of a particular drug within a group is of less importance than the correct choice of the main action. The main groups of drugs used to lower blood pressure are diuretics, beta receptor–blocking drugs, vasodilators, and centrally acting sympathetic inhibitors (Table 2). Drugs that blockade autonomic ganglia and adrenergic neurons are used less often than formerly. There has been increased interest in drugs that blockade alpha-adrenergic receptors, and in the combination of more than one property in a single molecule, e.g., alpha- and beta-adrenergic blockade.

DIURETICS. Most of the diuretics used to treat hypertension are based upon the molecular structure of chlorothiazide and, despite differences in activity per unit weight and duration of action, are of similar efficacy. It is more convenient for the patient to use a diuretic with a long duration of action for hypertension, because a sudden diuresis is an inconvenience. All diuretics of this type cause depletion of salt and water with a loss of extracellular and plasma fluid volume. During long-term treatment these changes in volume are less marked but the blood pressure reduction is maintained. There is a reduction of peripheral vascular resistance without alteration in the cardiac output. The dose response curve is relatively flat, which is an advantage, as it permits use of a single fixed dose in most patients. The precise mechanism of action in reducing peripheral resistance is not well defined, but probably depends upon changes in the fluid and ionic content of the blood vessel wall. The main advantage of the thiazides and related diuretics is that they cause few symptoms in most patients, and in this respect they approach the ideal more closely than any other antihypertensive drug. Serious toxicity is rare. The main long-term

TABLE 2. Drugs and Doses Used to Treat High Blood Pressure

Type of Action	Drug Name	Dose Range in General Use (mg per Day)
Diuretic	Bendrofluazide	5–10
	Hydrochlorothiazide	50–100
	Chlorthalidone	25–50
	Polythiazide	1–2
Beta-adrenergic blocker	Propranolol	40–640
	Oxprenolol	40–640
	Atenolol	50–100
	Metoprolol	200–600
Centrally acting alpha agonist	Methyldopa	500–3000
	Clonidine	0.3–1.0
Vasodilator	Hydralazine	50–300
	Minoxidil*	5–40
Alpha receptor antagonist	Prazosin†	0.5–15
Norepinephrine-depleting agents	Reserpine	0.1–0.25
Adrenergic neuron–blocking drug	Guanethidine†	10–100

*Investigational drug.
†Special care is needed to avoid postural hypotension. Start with a low dose.
See manufacturers' data sheets for full prescribing information and contraindications.

concern with thiazide diuretics has been in respect of their metabolic effects such as potassium depletion, hyperuricemia, glucose intolerance, and reduction of urinary calcium excretion. Some reduction of serum potassium value, averaging about 0.6 mEq per liter, almost always occurs, but this rarely causes any problem unless the patient is on a digitalis glycoside. The serum potassium concentration can be increased by eating a diet rich in high potassium foods (e.g., fruit, meat), and by taking oral potassium supplements or a potassium-retaining diuretic (amiloride, triamterene, or spironolactone). It is questionable whether routine use of potassium supplements or potassium-retaining diuretics is necessary.

Reduction of urate clearance and elevation of serum urate values are also almost invariable accompaniments of treatment with thiazide diuretics. Use of a diuretic occasionally precipitates an acute attack of gout, but it is not clear whether the mild hyperuricemia of prolonged diuretic therapy increases the incidence of acute gouty arthritis. Routine use of allopurinol or probenecid does not appear to be necessary.

A potentially more serious problem is a slow deterioration of glucose tolerance among patients treated with thiazides. Decreased glucose tolerance is much more likely if it is already abnormal, such as in patients with obesity. At present there is not sufficient evidence to seek to restrict the use of thiazides, but administration for very long periods should be accompanied by occasional urine testing for sugar. There is also a moderate increase in serum lipid concentrations during treatment with the thiazides, but the significance of this in relation to cardiovascular risk factors is still open.

Thiazide diuretics also reduce the urine calcium concentration and cause a small increase in the serum concentration, averaging about 0.15 mEq per liter. This is probably not of significance unless there is an additional cause of hypercalcemia such as sarcoidosis.

BETA-ADRENERGIC RECEPTOR BLOCKING DRUGS. Beta-adrenergic receptors are widely distributed in the heart, lungs, blood vessels, and metabolic and endocrine systems. Beta-adrenergic receptor blocking drugs cause competitive blockade of the action of norepinephrine and other beta receptor agonists. Their main cardiovascular action is to reduce the rate and force of cardiac contraction and thus lower the cardiac output. They also blockade bronchial beta receptors and may precipitate asthma in susceptible individuals. Among the many other consequences of beta receptor blockade are inhibition of sympathetically mediated renin release from the kidney and inhibition of sympathetically mediated mobilization of muscle glycogen. Some beta receptor–blocking drugs readily penetrate the central nervous system, and central sites of action have been postulated.

The mechanism of the hypotensive action of beta receptor–blocking drugs is still disputed among four main hypotheses. These are reduction of cardiac output, inhibition of renin release, a central action upon sympathetic receptors, and a peripheral action upon a beta receptor on the presynaptic surface of the adrenergic nerve endings. Reduction of cardiac output with loss of the full baroreflex-mediated compensatory increase in peripheral resistance seems the most likely of these explanations. Low concentrations of propranolol will cause maximal inhibition of renin release, but higher concentrations are required for an optimal effect upon blood pressure.

Beta-adrenergic blocking drugs do not cause a large and immediate fall in blood pressure such as can be seen with a drug that blocks sympathetic transmission elsewhere, at the alpha receptor or the sympathetic nerve ending, for example. However, the blood pressure begins to fall in two to four hours after a large dose, and most of the hypotensive effect is manifest within two or three days. In mild hypertension the fall in pressure achieved is comparable to that obtained with diuretics, but in more severe hypertension results comparable to those with methyldopa and guanethidine have been obtained. The reduction in pressure is similar in the lying and standing positions, and the normal rise in pressure on exercise is much reduced. A wide range of doses of propranolol has been used to treat hypertension, and the dose response curve appears to be steeper than it is for the diuretics. Other beta-blocking drugs such as atenolol have a flatter dose response curve.

The main contraindications to the use of beta-blocking drugs are a history of asthma or wheezing and the presence of cardiac conduction defects. The risk of precipitating an attack of asthma is greatest in patients with a history of this disease and is less in patients with a history of chronic bronchitis and emphysema. It is very rare for an asthmatic attack to be precipitated in a patient with no previous history of wheezing. The main concern about cardiac conduction defects has been that a patient who develops complete heart block while on beta-blocking drugs may have a dangerously slow ventricular rate. Opinions differ about the wisdom of using these drugs in patients with bundle branch or fascicular block, but they are probably best avoided in any situation in which a serious conduction disturbance is particularly likely to occur, such as the sick sinus syndrome and atrioventricular or intraventricular block. Less categorical contraindications include heart failure and diabetes requiring hypoglycemic agents. A failing heart depends upon sympathetic drive to maintain its contractility and beta receptor blockade may worsen heart failure. It would be most unwise to use beta receptor–blocking drugs in the early stages of treatment of a patient with severe heart failure, but once the blood pressure has been reduced these drugs can be used with little hazard. In patients with an enlarged left ventricle who are not in failure, the use of beta-blocking drugs in combination with diuretics is often effective and is rarely attended by evidence of impaired cardiac function. Recovery from hypoglycemia depends chiefly upon the mobilization of liver glycogen which is alpha-adrenergic receptor mediated in man. If the liver glycogen is depleted by starvation or ketosis, mobilization of muscle glycogen by beta-adrenergic receptor stimulation becomes important, and this cannot be achieved if the patient is beta blocked. Beta-blocking drugs should be used with great care, if at all, in unstable diabetics on insulin or sulfonylureas.

Beta-adrenergic blocking drugs cause many symptoms, but few of them are disabling. The reduction of cardiac output may cause cold extremities in cold weather and may worsen intermittent claudication in patients with obstructive disease of their leg arteries. Central nervous system side effects include a feeling of "muzziness," an exactly descriptive English word that appears to have no American equivalent, vivid dreams, and insomnia. Some patients may suffer daytime visual hallucinations. Serious toxicity has been very rare, but one beta-adrenergic blocking drug, practolol, had to be withdrawn from use because it caused a dry eye, progressing in some cases to perforation of the anterior chamber, a psoriasiform skin rash, and peritoneal fibrosis. It appears that this toxicity was unique to practolol, but some concern about the safety of new beta-adrenergic blocking drugs is bound to remain until much longer experience has accumulated.

Besides competitive beta receptor blockade, these drugs may possess in varying degree three other pharmacologic properties. These are cardioselectivity, membrane effects, and partial agonist activity. Cardioselective agents appear to be just as effective in lowering the blood pressure as nonselective ones. Their main advantage is a lesser degree of blockade of bronchial beta receptors and thus a lesser likelihood of precipitating asthma and a greater ease of treating it with beta receptor agonists if it occurs. Unfortunately the degree of selectivity for the cardiac, or beta-1, receptors is insufficient to avoid a substantial amount of bronchial beta blockade, especially at higher doses. Membrane activity such as is seen with the local anesthetic lidocaine is demonstrated by some beta-blocking drugs such as propranolol, but it is insignificant at the concentrations achieved by the usual dosage schedules in hypertension. Partial agonist activity means the ability to stimulate as well as blockade the beta receptors; it is sometimes referred to as "intrinsic sympathomimetic activity" or ISA. The consequence of partial agonist activity is less slowing of the resting heart rate. Claims have been made that drugs with partial agonist activity are less likely to precipitate heart failure of asthma and cause a lower incidence of cold extremities. The evidence to support these claims, particularly the first two, is slender, and it seems unlikely that the comparatively minor stimulation of beta receptors makes much difference to the therapeutic use of the drug.

Beta receptor–blocking drugs also vary in their lipid solubility and thus in the readiness with which they enter the central nervous system. The more hydrophilic drugs may have less tendency to cause vivid dreams and sleep disturbance than the lipid-soluble ones that enter the brain in high concentration.

CENTRALLY ACTING DRUGS. The level of efferent sympathetic activity is controlled by the brain. Drugs such as methyldopa and clonidine diminish the flow of impulses in peripheral sympathetic nerves as a result of a direct action upon alpha receptors in the brainstem. Methyldopa must be transformed into methylnorepinephrine to exert this effect, but clonidine is an alpha receptor agonist in its own right. Stimulation of alpha receptors in the brain potentiates the effect of the vasodepressor baroreflex, and this is one reason why the action of these drugs is accompanied by slowing of the heart rate. The reduction of sympathetic activity is manifest by a lowering of the plasma norepinephrine concentration and reduced amounts of catecholamine metabolites in the urine. As the baroreflex remains intact, postural adjustments of pressure can still be made, although there is sometimes a degree of fall in pressure on standing. The main problem of this type of action is that stimulation of brain alpha receptors also causes sedation and reduction in the flow of saliva. These are troublesome side effects for some patients, especially in the early days of therapy or after an increase in dose. In other respects, there are important differences between methyldopa and clonidine.

Methyldopa must be decarboxylated in the brain before it can exert its effect, and there is a delay of three to six hours after an oral dose before the full hypotensive effect is seen. In part the delay is caused by slow absorption from the gut, and in part by the need for metabolic transformation to the active form. Methyldopa modifies the rise in pressure on exercise but to a much lesser extent than beta receptor–blocking drugs. Apart from its central nervous system side effects, the main concern with methyldopa has been with its toxicity. Ten to 30 per cent of patients given the drug develop a direct antiglobulin test on their red cells, depending upon the dose used. A very small proportion of these will go on to develop an autoimmune hemolytic anemia. Mild diarrhea is a common symptom. A less common problem is the development of a maculopapular skin rash. Rarer forms of toxicity include a drug-induced fever, usually manifest in the first 14 days of therapy, and a hepatitic type of liver damage. However, the drug has been very widely used and is effective, and problems with toxicity have necessitated withdrawal in only a small proportion of patients.

Clonidine has a similar action to methyldopa, but the sedation and dry mouth it causes are marginally more prominent than with the equiactive doses of methyldopa. Clonidine causes constipation rather than diarrhea and is free of other types of toxicity. The main concern with the drug has been a syndrome of sympathetic hyperactivity with tachycardia, high blood pressure, tremor, sweating, and insomnia that occurs if the drug is stopped suddenly. Pressure begins to rise within 16 to 24 hours of cessation of therapy.

NOREPINEPHRINE-DEPLETING AGENTS. A number of hypotensive agents deplete neuronal stores of norepinephrine, but only the reserpine alkaloids appear to do this as their main pharmacologic action. The substances available include rauwolfia (whole root), reserpine, alseroxylon, deserpidine, rescinnamine, and syrosingopine. The differences among the action of these drugs are small, and reserpine itself is the most widely used. In high doses reserpine is an effective hypotensive agent and at one time injections of 1 to 5 mg parenterally were used to treat hypertensive crises. Chronic oral dosing at this level produces an unacceptable incidence of severe depression, and only low doses are now used. At these low doses reserpine is not of much use as single drug but is a valuable agent in combination with diuretics and vasodilators. Unfortunately, even in low doses reserpine increases the incidence of depression. There have also been several reports of increased incidence of breast cancer in middle-aged women treated with reserpine. Other studies have not supported this contention, although the argument has not been completely settled. Perhaps in consequence of these problems and also because of their greater efficacy, there has been a change to the use of beta-adrenergic blocking drugs in circumstances in which reserpine was used in the past. Reserpine has the virtue of cheapness, and it is worth recalling that the Veterans Administration trials, which still provide the best evidence of the efficacy of hypotensive therapy, used a triple combination of reserpine, hydralazine, and a diuretic.

VASODILATORS. As the main hemodynamic abnormality in hypertension is an increased peripheral vascular resistance, it would appear that use of a drug that directly dilates the blood vessels might be the most logical approach to treatment. Hydralazine is the most widely used drug of this class, although minoxidil and diazoxide are also important. Vasodilators share many properties in common. Acute administration leads to dilatation of arteriolar beds, with flushing of the skin, a fall in pressure, stimulation of the baroreflex, and a reflex increase in heart rate and force. If the patient has ischemic heart disease, the resultant increase in left ventricular work can precipitate angina or even myocardial infarction. Concurrent use of a beta-adrenergic blocking drug prevents most of the increase in heart rate caused by vasodilators, and as a result there has been a great increase in the use of this combination.

Hydralazine, the most widely used vasodilator, becomes tightly bound to the smooth muscle of blood vessel walls and in consequence has a much longer duration of action than its plasma half-life would suggest. The duration of action is such that twice or even once daily dosing will give effective control of pressure through the day and night. The main problem with hydralazine is its toxicity if the dose is increased above 200 mg daily. A proportion of patients develop a drug-induced lupus syndrome with arthralgia, muscle pains, fever, and skin rashes. As in other drug-induced lupus syndromes, the DNA binding is normal.

Hydralazine is a hydrazine, and like other hydrazines such as isoniazid it is metabolized by acetylation. In Caucasian populations there are roughly equal numbers of slow and fast acetylators, and it is the slow acetylators who develop the lupus syndrome. If the acetylator phenotype is known to be fast, it is possible to increase the hydralazine dose to 300 mg daily without undue risk of drug-induced lupus. Because of the limitation on dosage imposed by its toxicity, hydralazine is only a moderately effective hypotensive agent and is usually combined with both a beta-adrenergic blocking drug and a diuretic.

Several other vasodilators are under investigation, and two that have been studied extensively are diazoxide and minoxidil. Diazoxide is little used by the oral route because it causes diabetes in a high proportion of patients, but minoxidil is as effective as high doses of hydralazine but without the problems of lupus syndrome. The main problems associated with minoxidil therapy are fluid retention, which requires high doses of a loop diuretic in some cases, and increased growth of lanugo hair on the face, body, and limbs. The drug has shown considerable promise in controlling the pressure of patients with very severe hypertension otherwise difficult to control with existing drugs.

ADRENERGIC NEURON–BLOCKING DRUGS. These drugs — examples include guanethidine, bethanidine,* and debrisoquine* — are concentrated in adrenergic nerve endings by the amine pump and, once they achieve a high enough concentration, blockade transmission by preventing norepinephrine release. The result is to inhibit both alpha and beta adrenoceptor–mediated responses. The drugs are effective hypotensive agents, but interfere more severely than other agents with normal blood pressure regulation. There is often a substantial fall in blood pressure on standing and after exercise. Ejaculation during

sexual intercourse in the male may be inhibited. Because of these problems these drugs are less widely used, although they are still an effective alternative when other measures fail or are contraindicated. Tricyclic antidepressants, which blockade the amine pump in adrenergic nerve endings, interfere with the hypotensive effect of adrenergic neuron–blocking drugs.

ALPHA-ADRENERGIC RECEPTOR–BLOCKING DRUGS. The alpha-adrenergic receptor–blocking drugs phentolamine and phenoxybenzamine have been known for some years and are used to treat hypertension due to excess circulating catecholamines. They are not very effective hypotensive agents in patients without excess catecholamines in the circulation. This in itself is surprising, because drugs that prevent stimulation of alpha receptors by diminishing catecholamine release are effective. The explanation may be that there are alpha receptors on both sides of the synaptic cleft, on the innervated structure and on the neuron. Inhibition of the neuronal presynaptic receptors causes increased release of norepinephrine, which partly negates the effect of postsynaptic receptor blockade. Prazosin, a new hypotensive agent, has an alpha receptor–blocking action which is almost entirely upon the postjunctional alpha receptor. It is a powerful hypotensive agent, although prone to cause postural hypotension, especially with the first dose, unless this is very small. It appears that some degree of postural hypotension is an unavoidable consequence of alpha receptor blockade, although the extent varies, and only a minority of patients have sufficient fall in blood pressure on standing to cause symptoms of faintness and weakness.

COMBINED DRUG TREATMENT OF HYPERTENSION. The main groups of antihypertensive drugs lower the blood pressure by somewhat different mechanisms; if more than one type of action is used at the same time, the result is often an additive effect. As unwanted drug effects are often dose related, this opens the possibility that drug combinations could be used to achieve the same or greater fall in pressure without so many side effects. A second possibility is that the effect of the use of two drugs might be greater than the addition of the two individual actions because of a synergistic action of the combination. The most widely used combination is that of a vasodilator with a beta-adrenergic blocker with the aim of minimizing the reflex rise in cardiac output caused by the vasodilator and the fall in cardiac output caused by beta-adrenergic blockade. This appears to be because other reflex adjustments such as a sympathetically mediated vasoconstriction are not completely inhibited. However, even if there is no synergy, there may be a useful additive effect such as has been demonstrated with the components of the vasodilator–beta blocker–diuretic combination and for combinations of diuretics with all other types of hypotensive agents (Table 3).

EMERGENCY REDUCTION OF BLOOD PRESSURE. There are only a few circumstances in which it is necessary to reduce

*Investigational drug.

TABLE 3. Blood Pressure Response to Combined Drug Therapy*

Regimen	Fall in Pressure from Placebo (mm Hg)
Diuretic alone	21/11
Beta-adrenergic blocker alone	26/16
Diuretic + beta-adrenergic blocker	34/20
Diuretic + beta-adrenergic blocker + vasodilator	46/26

*Figures taken from Wilcox and Mitchell: Br. Med. J., 2:547, 1977.

the blood pressure rapidly. These include hypertensive left ventricular failure, hypertensive encephalopathy, including eclampsia, and accelerated hypertension. Other situations such as intracranial bleeding and dissecting aneurysm need careful evaluation before a decision is reached. Sudden reduction of blood pressure may be dangerous, and it is rarely necessary to reduce the level abruptly to 120 systolic and 80 diastolic mm Hg or below. Reduction to a level which relieves the immediate crisis is all that is necessary; fine adjustment can more safely be done later with oral therapy.

There are many methods of lowering the blood pressure quickly. If an immediate action is needed, an intravenous bolus injection of 300 mg of diazoxide or an infusion pump–controlled administration of sodium nitroprusside is effective in most cases. The patient must be carefully monitored with frequent readings of blood pressure, and baseline investigations such as an ECG and plasma electrolytes should be taken, if possible, before lowering the pressure. If reduction within a few hours is the objective, an oral loading dose of 1000 mg of methyldopa is effective, but the sedation that accompanies the fall in pressure may be diagnostically confusing in some circumstances. Diuretics and beta-adrenergic blocking drugs are not usually suitable for rapid reduction of pressure. Hydralazine is useful, but given alone it causes flushing and tachycardia and may precipitate angina. Pretreatment with a beta-adrenergic blocking agent will obviate this problem but may cause delay.

Stopping Hypotensive Therapy. Once drug treatment of hypertension has begun, it can rarely be stopped. Both patient and doctor should understand the long-term nature of the decision they have taken. If the drugs are stopped, the subsequent course of the blood pressure is highly variable. It may return to pretreatment levels within a few days, but more commonly it slowly rises over a few weeks or months. At one stage it was hoped that reversal of cardiovascular hypertrophy and a downward resetting of the pressure control mechanisms might make it possible to withdraw treatment after several years of blood pressure control. Results in the small number of patients in whom it was tried were disappointing, but the amount of hard data available on this point is small. Withdrawal of treatment is usually brought up in three circumstances: extreme old age, intercurrent illness, and surgery. If the main reason for treating hypertension is to prevent a late risk of myocardial infarction or stroke, there is little point in continuing it in a patient who is terminally ill. Old age of itself is not a reason for stopping therapy, but extreme senility would be. There is usually no need to interrupt therapy for a surgical operation, but it is essential that the anesthesiologist should be aware of current therapy.

Therapeutic Choices. Three main considerations govern the choice of antihypertensive drugs for a particular patient: simplicity, tolerability, and efficacy. Absent from this list is one important consideration, the prediction of individual drug response.

As some patients do not respond well to one drug but do to another, it would be advantageous if an accurate prediction could be made to avoid the delays of trial and error. Some progress has been made in making predictions. There is evidence that the small proportion of hypertensives who have a low plasma renin respond less well than other patients to beta-adrenergic blocking drugs such as propranolol. However, a response to propranolol can be

obtained even in low renin patients by using higher doses of propranolol (greater than 240 mg daily), although the response is never as great as in normal or high renin patients. There is also some evidence that patients with a urinary VMA in the higher part of the normal range respond better to a centrally acting hypotensive agent such as methyldopa than do patients with a urinary VMA in the lower part of the normal range. Patients with a low renin respond particularly well to diuretics, and, surprisingly, high VMA patients also respond well to diuretics. It has been suggested, largely on theoretical grounds, that patients with a raised cardiac output would respond particularly well to beta-adrenergic blocking agents, but this does not seem to be borne out in practice, and it is possible that the converse may be true.

It is too early to translate these findings into a flow chart to predict the optimal drug for a particular patient, although that stage may be reached in the medium-term future. One difficulty is that the unresponsive groups, low renin and low VMA, are a relatively small fraction of the total number of patients. A more substantial difficulty lies in the general use of drug combinations. There is no evidence about the predictability of response to drug combinations, and it may be that the "catch-all" philosophy of two- or three-drug combination therapy largely obviates the need to find the optimal single drug.

The ideal treatment for hypertension would be a once for all intervention that permanently lowered blood pressure. Surgical thoracolumbar sympathectomy at one time promised that this might be possible, but the effects waned as the nerves regenerated. In animals central administration of 6-hydroxydopamine, which destroys adrenergic nerve endings in the brain, seems to produce a long-lasting fall in blood pressure, but this agent is too damaging to contemplate using in man. Long-term daily administration of hypotensive agents — effective but inconvenient — is all that we have to offer at present.

Two measures are possible to simplify the patient's regimen. The first is to use drugs with a long duration of action to avoid the necessity of a midday drug dose, and, when possible, to give the drugs only once a day. The second is to be prepared to use combined drug preparations when the mutual efficacy of the components has been well proved. Thus combinations of diuretic, beta-adrenergic blocker, and vasodilator in a single tablet are useful, just as similar combinations in which reserpine replaced the beta blocker were in the past.

Making a regimen tolerable for a patient is chiefly the ability to predict the acceptability of drug side effects. Drugs which interfere with male sexual function, such as the adrenergic neuron–blocking drugs and, to a lesser extent, the centrally acting drugs, are unsuitable for younger men. Fatigue on exertion and cold extremities or a past history of Raynaud's phenomenon would be a contraindication to the use of beta blockade in a patient who had to do heavy muscular work and/or work out of doors in cold weather. Sedation and dry mouth are tiresome side effects for patients who have to do intellectual work or speak in public. Some patients who speak in public find a positive virtue in the lessening of palpitations and shaking hands brought about by beta-adrenergic blockade. Younger women do not relish the hirsute face and limbs brought about by minoxidil. A patient troubled by insomnia may find his problem worse while taking propranolol, but better on methyldopa. A depressed patient is always much more troubled by drug side effects than one with a normal mood, and drugs with prominent side effects should be avoided in such a patient.

It may seem a strange inversion to deal with efficacy last, but the truth is that there are a number of equally effective regimens available, and no drug is effective if the patient will not take it. A simple step care approach should prove adequate in all but the most severely hypertensive patients.

Because of freedom from side effects and a flat dose response curve, it is wise to use a thiazide diuretic as the first choice in patients with diastolic pressures up to 114 mm Hg. A fixed dose can be used. The second step is a beta-adrenergic blocking drug. In most cases the dose should be started low and titrated upward. If the patient has a diastolic pressure of 115 mm Hg or higher, it would be sensible to begin treatment with both a thiazide diuretic and a beta-adrenergic blocking agent. The alternative to the beta-blocking drug is to use a centrally acting drug or reserpine. The third step would be to add a vasodilator such as hydralazine to the existing two-drug combinations, beginning with a low dose and increasing quickly to the practical maximum. If these three steps are inadequate and minoxidil is available, this should be substituted for the hydralazine. Alternatively an adrenergic neuron–blocking drug or a combination of alpha- and beta-adrenergic blockade should be tried. Never accept poor pressure control too readily. It can always be improved, provided that sufficient time and care are spent. Depending upon the type of patient, it is reasonable to anticipate that about half the patients can be controlled with one drug, and another 30 per cent with two; the remaining 20 per cent will require three or more.

Blood pressure should be reduced as close to normal as symptoms will allow. The target of reducing the diastolic blood pressure below 100 mm Hg, which many clinics set when treating severe hypertension in the 1960's, is quite inadequate today. A diastolic of 90 mm Hg might be acceptable, but one of 80 to 85 mm Hg would be even better.

PROGNOSIS. In patients with accelerated hypertension and left ventricular failure the results of treatment are so dramatically beneficial that a controlled clinical trial was never considered necessary to establish them. Improvement in pulmonary edema is often evident within seconds of lowering the blood pressure, although full resolution may take much longer. The retinopathy of accelerated hypertension ceases to progress within two or three days of pressure reduction, and those lesions that appear after pressure reduction were probably already in process of formation at the time treatment began. All the features of accelerated hypertensive retinopathy will eventually regress in periods varying from 6 to 12 weeks for the cotton wool spots, linear hemorrhages, and papilledema, to up to a year or more for the macular star figure of hard exudate. Renal function ceases to deteriorate at a rapid rate, and in patients with an abrupt onset of accelerated hypertension there may be some improvement in glomerular filtration. The survival of patients with accelerated hypertension is greatly improved by treatment, although still dominated by the extent of deterioration of renal function at the time of diagnosis. Patients with severe impairment of renal function tend to continue to deteriorate despite pressure control. The availability of renal dialysis and transplant programs has become the main consideration in the long-term survival of these patients. However, the five-year survival of patients with accelerated hypertension under treatment is now 35 to 50 per cent without the help of renal support, which compares with only 1 to 5 per cent prior to the introduction of antihypertensive therapy. Accelerated hypertension should be looked upon as a preventable condition, and the widespread introduction of treatment for mild to moderate hypertension is leading to a progressive decrease in the number of patients with accelerated hypertension who are being diagnosed.

The great majority of patients with elevated blood pressure are not in the accelerated phase, and the benefits of treatment are less obvious in the short term. Some symptoms such as headache in the mornings are relieved by blood pressure reduction, but the loss of some symptoms is often roughly balanced by the gain of others which are due to the drugs. The only objective signs of improvement may be a reduction in the size of the heart and a reduction in the voltage and improvement in repolarization abnormalities in the electrocardiogram. Retinal vascular changes such as caliber irregularity and crossing changes rarely show much change when the pressure is lowered. However, if the rise in pressure has been recent and rapid and the retina shows a uniform narrowing of the retinal arteries, there may be some dilatation when the pressure is lowered.

The benefits of treatment of this type of hypertension had to be established by controlled clinical trials. Considering the very large numbers of patients who might potentially be treated, proof of the benefit of treatment rests upon a very small number of properly controlled trials. Of these the largest and best known are those conducted by the Veterans Administration in the United States. Only men were included in these trials, and the incidence of complications among the control groups was rather high, probably because the patients were drawn from those referred to hospitals rather than from a community sample. The pressure levels quoted in the trial are those after six weeks on placebo, a point to bear in mind when relating them to first visit casual pressures. In individuals with diastolic pressures of about 115 mm Hg, the benefits of treatment were so striking that the trial was stopped on ethical grounds. Deaths and major complications such as stroke, heart failure, and progression to accelerated hypertension appeared entirely in the placebo-treated group. For patients with diastolic pressures of between 105 and 114 mm Hg, there was a statistically significant benefit with treatment, with fewer deaths and many fewer hypertensive complications than in the control group, although the difference was less dramatic than in the patients with a diastolic of 115 mm Hg and higher. For the group with diastolic pressures of between 90 and 104 mm Hg there were fewer incidents in the treated group than in their controls, but this difference did not reach statistical significance. Based upon these results, most physicians have concluded that patients with diastolic pressures above 105 mm Hg on the first visit would benefit from treatment, and no further placebo-controlled trials among patients with this level of pressure are being undertaken. It should be noted that there is no direct proof that this is the case in women, as almost all of the clinical trial evidence was derived from men. Women with untreated hypertension have fewer complications over a given time than men.

Two major areas of doubt remain concerning the efficacy of hypotensive therapy. The first concerns the benefit of treatment in the great majority of hypertensive patients whose casual pressure lies in the range 90 to 104 mm Hg. Trials are in progress in the United Kingdom, the United

States, and Australia to try and answer this question. Until the results are available in the early to mid-1980's, it seems reasonable to treat those patients with a particularly high burden of risk factors but not to treat those who lie in a relatively low risk group. The second question concerns the effects of treatment upon different types of cardiovascular pathology. The vascular pathology of accelerated hypertension does not rise in patients whose blood pressure has been well controlled throughout. If a patient already has accelerated hypertension, the progression of the vascular changes is halted but tissue damage, had it already taken place, remains. The onion skin proliferative changes of the intima of renal arteries is still present in patients many years after their accelerated hypertension has been brought under control. The risk of death from cerebral hemorrhage is also very greatly reduced by lowering the blood pressure, and this probably indicates that the Charcot-Bouchard aneurysms are remodeled or obliterated after a period of pressure control. The effect of hypotensive therapy upon atheromatous disease and particularly myocardial infarction is much more difficult to answer, yet is of central importance. The majority of deaths in patients with mild to moderate hypertension occur as a result of myocardial infarction. None of the individual clinical trials thus far carried out has shown a significant reduction in morbidity or mortality from myocardial infarction, although the pooled results of several trials suggests that there may have been a reduction of as much as 50 per cent. There is room for modest optimism about the prospect of achieving a worthwhile reduction of the incidence of myocardial infarction by hypotensive therapy, but full proof is still necessary. The widespread use of beta-adrenergic blocking drugs may alter the picture, as two of these, alprenolol and practolol, have been shown to reduce the risk of sudden death in the first three years after a myocardial infarction.

Berglund, G., Hansson, L., and Werkoe, L. (eds.): Conference on Pathophysiology and Management of Arterial Hypertension. Moelndal, Sweden, Lindgren & Soner, 1975.
Dollery, C. T.: Adrenergic drugs in the treatment of hypertension. Br. Med. Bull., 29:158, 1973.
Genest, J., Koiw, E., and Kuchel, O. (eds.): Hypertension. New York, McGraw-Hill Book Company, 1977.
Pickering, G. W.: High Blood Pressure. 2nd ed. London, J. & A. Churchill, 1968.
Sackett, D. L., and Haynes, R. B. (eds.): Compliance with Therapeutic Regimens. Baltimore, Johns Hopkins University Press, 1976.
Stamler, R., and Pullman, T. N.: The Epidemiology of Hypertension. New York, Grune & Stratton, 1967.
Veterans Administration Cooperative Study Group on antihypertensive agents. JAMA, 202:1028, 1957, and 213:1143, 1970.

362.   ATHEROSCLEROSIS

Harvey Wolinsky

HISTORY. The antiquity of atherosclerosis has been established from studies of Egyptian mummies. Attempts to relate pathologic changes in the coronary vessels to clinical symptoms, particularly angina pectoris, followed upon early descriptions of sclerotic vessels by Leonardo da Vinci in the sixteenth century. The term *atheroma,* derived from the Greek word meaning porridge, was not used in the context of arterial disease until 1904, when Marchand coined the term *atherosclerosis.* This disease is lipid rich, as contrasted with *arteriosclerosis,* an older and more general term for thickening and stiffening of the vessel wall. Another important distinction still made today is that arteriosclerotic involvement of a blood vessel wall tends to be concentric and diffuse, whereas atherosclerotic lesions are more eccentric and focal. The interrelation among coronary disease, myocardial damage, and clinical syndromes was not appreciated before the emergence of pathology as a separate discipline in the latter part of the nineteenth century. It was not until 1918 that the proposal by Herrick of a connection between clinically detected nonlethal heart damage and atherosclerotic coronary disease gained acceptance.

OCCURRENCE AND EPIDEMIOLOGY. Atherosclerosis tends to involve large and medium-sized arteries. Most commonly affected are the aorta and the iliac, femoral, coronary, and cerebral arteries. Clinical symptoms occur because the mass of the atherosclerotic plaque reduces blood flow through the involved artery and thereby compromises tissue or organ function distal to it.

Ischemia or necrosis of the perfused tissue results in characteristic clinical syndromes, and myocardial infarction and sudden death are common fatal outcomes. In terms of public health, cardiovascular diseases, particularly myocardial infarction and stroke, are the most common lethal diseases in the United States and other industrialized societies, accounting for more than 50 per cent of all deaths. For example, well over 500,000 deaths per year in the United States are attributable to acute myocardial infarction. The risks of developing clinical evidence of a cardiovascular disease by age 65 are 37 per cent for a man and 18 per cent for a woman. A downward trend in death rates from myocardial infarction of approximately 20 per cent has been documented since 1970. The precise reasons for this are not yet clear.

PATHOLOGY. By the time it is large enough to cause clinical events, the atherosclerotic plaque is a complicated mixture of three components: (1) cells, mostly smooth muscle in origin, (2) connective tissue (elastin, collagen, glycosaminoglycans), often concentrated as a "cap" on the lesion, and (3) lipid deposits, both intra- and extracellular, representing complex aggregates of cholesteryl ester, cholesterol, triglyceride, and phospholipids. Cell necrosis is a prominent feature which contributes to the gruel-like nature of the lesion. Calcification is often present in advanced lesions, and hemorrhage from small ingrowing vessels frequently occurs. A slowly progressive increase in the plaque mass is usually responsible for its clinical sequelae. Other events in the blood vessel wall which can provoke acute symptoms include transient or progressive deposition of platelet clumps or thrombus on the irregular luminal surface, rupture of the plaque and release of its components, hemorrhage into a plaque, or dissection of blood into the wall.

Basic knowledge of the progressive stages of atherosclerosis is essential to the physician who cares for patients with vascular disease and who attempts to influence its progression. Clinical events in middle age which are associated with the advanced plaque represent the culmination of decades of slow growth of the lesion beginning in childhood. In the first decade of life, blood vessels undergo structural remodeling, which mainly involves the intima. This takes the form of concentric fibromuscular intimal thickening and development of intimal cushions at branch sites. In all human populations studied (even all mammals), this thickening develops progressively throughout life. However, in those populations which have a predilection for development of later atherosclerosis, this arteriosclerotic thickening is especially well developed long before lipid deposition is prominent. Enhanced intimal thickening of certain artery segments, especially in the male, also predicts patterns of subsequent atherosclerotic lesions. In those human societies not vulnerable to atherosclerosis, this concentric intimal thickening, even when prominent, does not in itself seem to seriously compromise blood flow.

Upon this matrix, lipid accumulates in the form of *fatty streaks* in all populations. These yellow, soft, raised lesions may be transient, but their prevalence increases with age to a peak in the third decade of life. Microscopically, these consist largely of smooth muscle cells in the intimal layer which are filled with lipid deposits, mainly cholesterol and cholesteryl ester. In populations prone to atherosclerotic vascular disease, *plaques,* as described above, begin to be seen in the third decade and become more numerous with time in common disease sites, such as the proximal coronary vessels. The *fibrous plaque* is grayish white, focal, and raised and microscopically consists of a prominent extracellular matrix, with less prominence of visible lipid (although by biochemical analysis the lipid content is high). It is thought that these lesions may arise de novo at times, but that they usually develop from fatty streaks. The forces required for this transformation in susceptible populations are not well understood, but hypertension seems to be one such stimulus. The further accumulation of cells, connective tissue, and fat over decades results in the severe or *complicated lesions* which are so often found at autopsy to provide the "explanation" for a clinical event.

LOCALIZATION. Although tending to occur in large elastic and muscular arteries, the distribution of atherosclerosis is far from uniform. The aorta is heavily involved, particularly its abdominal portion. The large caliber of this distributing vessel makes it an uncommon site for occlusive symptoms, although it may be a source of embolic clot or plaque material to peripheral branches. Atheromas are most common in the proximal coronary tree, although lesions occur peripherally as well. Curiously, lesions occur in the extramural portions of the coronary blood vessels and not in those segments which are intramural and surrounded by muscle. It is also of interest to those who stress the role of hemodynamic factors in localization that the renal arteries, arising from the heavily diseased abdominal aorta, are remarkably spared of disease despite having a caliber similar to that of the main coronary arteries.

Arteries of the lower extremities have much more atherosclerosis than those of the upper limbs. The distribution patterns may be focal and proximal or more diffuse. Clinical symptoms rarely arise from isolated lesions because of the rich collateral blood supply. The major hazard to those having peripheral vascular disease, even when symptomatic, stems from the likelihood of concurrent coronary artery disease in the same individuals.

The vertebral or carotid vessels may develop patchy lesions which present clinically with neurologic deficits. Particularly likely sites are the proximal portions of these arteries or the carotid bifurcation. Intracranial predisposed sites are the basilar artery, the middle cerebral artery, and the carotid artery as it angulates in the region of the carotid siphon.

Atherosclerosis of the smaller muscular arteries is especially common in individuals who use cigarettes or have glucose intolerance. Since basement membrane abnormalities also frequently occur in small blood vessels of diabetics, it is not certain that atherosclerotic involvement alone explains the notable symptoms of vascular insufficiency in these individuals.

Again of special interest to the proponents of hemodynamic factors in atherogenesis is the observation that the low-pressure venous system and pulmonary arteries are infrequent sites of atherosclerosis except under circumstances of increased intravascular pressure, as occurs in pulmonary hypertension.

RISK FACTORS. The concept of risk factors for atherosclerosis derives from epidemiologic studies. A profile of risk can be obtained from evaluation of the frequency with which specific characteristics and chemical measurements are associated with occurrence of certain clinical events in a given population. It should be stressed that the epidemiologist can only point out associations; he can neither determine mechanism nor even be certain of a direct interaction between a particular characteristic and the presence of disease. The value of these constructs, however, is that they identify high-risk populations in which "reduction" of risk factors can be attempted, and they suggest to the experimentalist potentially fruitful areas of investigation to elucidate mechanisms of pathogenesis. Possible links between known risk factors and aspects of cellular involvement in atherogenesis are summarized under Pathogenesis, below.

Finally, it is important to stress that for virtually every risk factor, the risk is a continuous gradient throughout the entire range of observed values, habits, or characteristics. For example, an increasing risk of occurrence of a cerebrovascular event is seen with increasing blood pressure, even within the "normotensive" range of blood pressures. It is only within the "hypertensive" range, however, that the growing gradient of risk is generally felt to justify intervention.

Age. The risk of myocardial infarction increases with age regardless of sex. Little is known about this factor, although it is assumed that it simply represents duration of exposure to other factors. For example, recent epidemiologic studies of children have shown the appearance of significant subgroups in the teenage years with blood pressures and serum lipids at levels of the general adult population.

Sex. A 10- to 15-year lag in extent of atherosclerosis of the coronary, cerebral, and peripheral vasculature and its sequelae is seen in women compared to men until approximately 50 years of age. After that point, which roughly corresponds to the menopause, the rates of disease in both sexes are more similar. This may represent increased risk in women or decreased risk in men due to early elimination of high-risk males. The acceleration of vascular disease in younger individuals with diabetes mellitus blurs the usual sex differences.

Blood Pressure. Experimental and clinical evidence has convincingly shown the importance of blood pressure as an accelerator of atherosclerosis. A systolic blood pressure of greater than 160 mm Hg or a diastolic of greater than 95 mm Hg carries a five-fold increased risk of coronary heart disease compared to normotensive individuals. Hypertension is the strongest risk factor over-all for clinical disease in individuals older than 45 years; it is especially predictive of atherosclerotic brain infarction. (In the absence of uniform autopsy reporting, this designation may include pure hemorrhagic stroke as well as atherosclerotic sequelae.) Recent studies have shown a clear-cut effect of blood pressure reduction on the incidence of stroke, when hypertension is defined as a diastolic pressure of 105 to 115 mm Hg, but, disappointingly, no reduction in myocardial infarction was found after a three-year period of treatment. This difference might reflect the major contribution of pressure to stroke, whereas the coronary lesion reflects the chronic, degenerative aspects of atherosclerosis which, once established, may be more difficult to reverse.

Hyperlipidemia. Another major risk factor is the presence of elevated circulating blood lipids — cholesterol and triglyceride. The problem may be broken down into two components: (1) the generally elevated lipid levels in industrialized populations compared to agricultural societies, and (2) identification of high-risk individuals with high lipid levels within a given population range. The increased levels found in entire populations seem largely due to diet, although genetic factors may play a role. The increased intake of saturated fat, refined sugar, and total calories by a sedentary population seems of major importance.

Using ultracentrifugal and electrophoretic techniques, four major lipoprotein classes have been identified as carriers of lipid in plasma (see Ch. 532.3). For the purposes here, it is necessary only to summarize briefly the major constituents of these lipoprotein classes. Chylomicrons are the largest particles, contain the most lipid (mainly triglyceride) and least protein (1 to 2 per cent by weight), and are normally found in the circulation only shortly after meals. In the fasting state, very low density lipoproteins (VLDL) carry most circulating triglycerides as well as lesser amounts of cholesterol and cholesteryl ester. Low-density lipoproteins (LDL) are derived from metabolism of VLDL and carry most of the serum cholesterol and cholesteryl ester. High density lipoproteins (HDL), the smallest particles, contain the most protein (50 per cent by weight); phospholipid and cholesterol account for about 45 per cent and 35 per cent, respectively, of the lipid. HDL are involved in the esterification of free cholesterol released into plasma from the tissues. It has been shown that whole plasma triglyceride accurately reflects VLDL levels and that total plasma cholesterol generally reflects LDL-cholesterol levels in man, although this latter relationship is not as consistent (see below).

The three most common electrophoretic patterns of serum lipoproteins in individuals with premature atherosclerotic vascular disease are increased LDL or Type IIa (elevated cholesterol, normal triglyceride), increased VLDL and LDL or Type IIb (elevated cholesterol, elevated triglyceride), and increased VLDL or Type IV (normal or slightly increased cholesterol, elevated triglyceride). These three patterns appear with about equal frequency in survivors of an acute myocardial infarction below age 60. Approximately one third of all such individuals will have one of these patterns, and familial distributions of each have been demonstrated. Whereas Types IIa and IV show autosomal dominant inheritance and are clearly monogenic, the inheritance of Type IIb is not yet completely defined. What is important, however, is that when Type IIb is found in a proband, familial expressions may include elevations mainly of

cholesterol or triglyceride or both. To screen for the most common disorders, therefore, measurement of total plasma cholesterol and triglyceride provides the same detection of risk as do the more complicated lipoprotein pattern analyses. In adults under age 55, a value of plasma cholesterol greater than 250 mg per deciliter or fasting triglyceride greater than 150 mg per deciliter indicates the need for further investigation (see Ch. 532.3).

Current knowledge about lipoprotein metabolism does not permit a clear-cut assessment of the precise roles of various lipoproteins in the clinical definition of risk for unselected populations. However, prospective epidemiologic studies do show a positive correlation between plasma cholesterol levels (particularly LDL) and risk of clinical atherosclerotic events. This relationship is evident under age 50, but is not detectable in older age groups. Increasing plasma VLDL (triglyceride) levels seem to add risk to a given plasma LDL (cholesterol) level. Triglyceride levels alone, however, are less strongly related to clinical atherosclerotic events. The risk associated with triglyceride, seen more clearly in women, is eliminated when obesity or glucose intolerance is taken into account and may therefore not be an independent variable. More recently, the emergence of HDL as an important protective factor has complicated the use of total plasma cholesterol to assess risk. That is, the risk of coronary heart disease is inversely related to the level of HDL cholesterol. Since this can only be detected by examining isolated HDL and LDL, the total cholesterol level alone is less informative. HDL levels are significantly higher in women than in men at all age levels, are reduced by the presence of diabetes mellitus, are increased by regular exercise (e.g., jogging), and are not predictably related to levels of LDL in the same individual. Therefore a plasma lipid profile of total cholesterol, HDL cholesterol, and fasting triglyceride may be the best predictor of coronary disease.

Cigarette Smoking. Increased risk of atherosclerotic vascular disease manifested by stroke, myocardial infarction, and intermittent claudication is seen in male smokers compared to nonsmokers; in female smokers, the occurrence of intermittent claudication is increased. By age 45, the excess risk in males approaches 70 per cent. The increased incidence of atherosclerosis found in smokers at autopsy correlates with the degree of previous smoking activity. In addition to atheromatous changes in larger coronary blood vessels, small intramyocardial arteries show increased diffuse fibromuscular intimal thickening. Not only are these changes related in degree to numbers of cigarettes smoked, but cigar and pipe smokers have impressive increases over nonsmokers as well.

Sudden death is the most frequent clinical event associated with cigarette smoking. Cessation of smoking promptly and sharply reduces the risk of this event. Levels of carboxyhemoglobin are significantly increased in smokers, of whom about 15 per cent regularly achieve levels of carboxyhemoglobin of 5 per cent or more. Men in the age group of 30 to 69 years who achieve this level of carboxyhemoglobin show a 20-fold increased prevalence of atherosclerotic vascular disease events (myocardial infarction, angina pectoris, intermittent claudication) compared to nonsmokers or smokers with levels of 3 per cent or less. A narrowed coronary artery may be unable to deliver the 20 per cent increase in blood flow required to offset the decreased availability of oxygen from blood containing 5 per cent carboxyhemoglobin and thereby prevent ischemia. Indeed, a lower threshold for angina pectoris occurs in cardiac patients in whom comparable levels of carboxyhemoglobin have been experimentally achieved. Nicotine, once considered a culprit, has not been implicated in recent studies. Glycoprotein components of tobacco leaf and tar, which contain rutin moieties, appear to promote thrombosis in normal animals and cardiac arrhythmias in sensitized experimental animals, and have also been shown to be allergenic in man.

Glucose Intolerance. Glucose intolerance, defined as a casual blood glucose of 120 mg per deciliter or more or the presence of glucose in the urine, acts independently of other commonly associated risk factors, namely, triglyceride elevation, obesity, and hypertension. It is somewhat more important in women than in men. The excess risk associated with glucose intolerance may be 100 per cent. Intermittent claudication is the cardiovascular symptom most associated with glucose intolerance. When present in combination with a fasting plasma triglyceride level of greater than 150 mg per deciliter, a marked synergistic effect of diabetes mellitus on development of angiographically demonstrable, diffuse coronary artery disease is found. The contribution to this process of basement membrane abnormalities found in the small coronary branches in diabetics is not known.

Obesity. Obesity, particularly at 20 per cent or more above ideal weight, carries significantly increased risk. However, when associated variables, including hypertension, hyperlipidemia, and diabetes mellitus, are removed, obesity per se makes no clear contribution. The salutary effect of weight reduction on the other variables, however, makes it a prime focus of intervention.

Physical Activity. It is difficult to separate the risk of this variable from other confounding factors. Sedentary individuals have many other risk factors operating as well. Epidemiologic studies show that only heavy physical work, of the type done in rural communities or by the most active dockworkers, is associated with decreased risk of myocardial infarction and sudden death. The remarkably striking decrease in sudden death in these groups suggests that exercised myocardium may be less vulnerable to a fatal ischemic event. Exercise tolerance can be improved in individuals with coronary artery disease through a program of regular, moderate exercise.

Personality Factors. A strong suspicion has long been held that angina pectoris and sudden death are strongly associated with emotional stress or anxiety. The Type A pattern of behavior (enhanced aggressiveness, ambitiousness, competitive drive, and chronic sense of time urgency) is frequently associated with many other risk factors, and the converse Type B is less closely associated. A prospective study by the Western Collaborative Group showed that even after removal of associated risk components, Type A behavior, determined from interviews, had a residual two-fold risk of clinical coronary heart disease over the Type B personality type. The possible metabolic, genetic, and other components of this behavior pattern have not been identified, nor has behavior modification been convincingly shown to be feasible or effective in modifying risk.

Genetic Factors. Familial inheritance patterns of hyperlipidemia, hypertension, and diabetes mellitus are well known. Segregation of behavioral factors within families, including tobacco smoking, obesity, and perhaps physical activity, is also seen. These associations may provide the physician his best opportunities to detect clusters of risk factors and to attempt preventive measures.

Other. A host of other variables associated with cardiac risk have been enumerated, but in sum they appear to contribute only a minor portion of risk. Included among many others are lung vital capacity, blood uric acid level, blood group type, and mineral salt content of local drinking water. Moderate alcohol consumption seems to be associated with decreased risk of myocardial infarction, perhaps through a positive effect on HDL:LDL ratios. Electrocardiographic evidence for left ventricular hypertrophy carries about a three-fold risk for new coronary artery disease, independent of other variables, including blood pressure.

Unknown. All known risk factors taken together account for approximately 50 per cent of the risk of an individual's developing coronary heart disease in the United States. It is clear that important risk determinants remain to be discovered. For example, little has been said about the contribution made by inherent properties of vascular tissue, genetic or otherwise, to cardiovascular disease. Each risk factor must ultimately be expressed at the tissue or cellular level if it is in fact related to the development of the manifest vascular disease we call atherosclerosis. Therefore further identification of specific cellular and tissue metabolic patterns under well defined conditions of risk may provide additional risk factors.

PATHOGENESIS. Atherosclerosis is undoubtedly multifactorial in origin and progression. The sharp contrast between the frequent suddenness of clinical events and the slow progressiveness of vascular lesions suggests that different factors are responsible for each and that different strategies might be needed for intervention. Pioneering studies of quite advanced lesions generated the classic theories which invoked processes such as vascular injury, lipid infiltration, thrombosis, and hemorrhage. Although still useful in a descriptive pathologic sense, these terms are being incorporated into concepts more consonant with newer knowledge of cell biology. Vascular tissue is increasingly appreciated to be a dynamic responsive organ system of great complexity, rather than a conduit arrangement with rather limited responses. The normal blood vessel is a tightly organized, highly regulated, and closely integrated fibrocellular system. The two major cell types found in blood vessel walls are smooth muscle cells and endothelial cells. Each has been shown experimentally to have characteristic, far-ranging metabolic capabilities. Endothelium seems to be important in determining the rate of entrance of circulating materials, including lipoproteins, into the blood vessel wall and in maintaining the nonthrombogenicity of the vascular surface. Smooth muscle cells elaborate the extensive connective tissue matrix of the arterial wall and metabolize those circulating plasma components which gain entrance to the vessel wall. When atherosclerosis occurs, the same basic wall components are present, but the picture is a distorted one of smooth muscle cell proliferation, connective tissue deposition, and lipid accumulation.

Alteration in the functional or structural barrier presented by the endothelial cell-lining layer is thought to be an early event in the pathogenesis of atherosclerosis. Local turbulence or shear force generated by blood flowing at high pressure could determine the special susceptibility of certain sites to disruption of the surface layer. Two major consequences of endothelial loss would be increased thrombogenicity of the denuded sites and increased entrance of circulating lipoproteins and other plasma components into the blood vessel wall. Platelet adhesion and aggregation quickly occur on the exposed region; platelets contain a mitogen which can stimulate smooth muscle cell proliferation in vitro. Other evidence obtained in vitro suggests that LDL itself might stimulate proliferation of these cells. The recent evidence that cells in each human atherosclerotic plaque tend to be monoclonal raises the possibility that selective growth advantage or even neoplastic transformation of certain cells could contribute to this aspect of plaque growth. Experimentally produced atherosclerotic lesions are polyclonal, so that this issue is far from resolved.

Increased connective tissue synthesis is closely linked to cell proliferation whether studied in the intact blood vessels or in isolated cell systems. Specific stimuli at the cellular level for increased synthesis of connective tissue proteins have not been identified, although hypertension in particular seems to promote fibrosis and estradiol given experimentally seems to retard it. Circulating lipoprotein, particularly LDL, can be immunologically detected in very low concentrations in normal human blood vessels. With loss of endothelial integrity, it is presumed that an increased influx of this lipoprotein occurs which may result in progressive accumulation of lipid by two mechanisms. First, binding to excessive extracellular matrix in more advanced lesions might occur. Perhaps a more important determinant in early lesions, however, is the metabolic capacity of the vascular smooth muscle cell to cope with the incoming lipid. The ability of the cell to maintain balance among internalization and catabolism of complex lipoproteins (including hydrolysis of cholesteryl ester to free cholesterol and fatty acid) and synthesis of lipid may determine its susceptibility to intracellular lipid accumulation. In the sense that ingress of substrate may exceed egress of product, the lipid accumulation can be thought of as a subtle form of storage disease in the muscle cell, which becomes a repository of slowly permeant cholesteryl ester and other lipids. Based on available information, it seems plausible that many "risk factors" exert an influence on this influx-efflux balance. For example, the relationships among LDL and HDL levels and risk of disease may derive at least in part from the putative role attributed to LDL of carrying cholesterol to the cell and to HDL of carrying cholesterol away from the cell. The influence of sex, age, and exercise as risk factors might stem, at least in part, from associated changes in levels of these lipoproteins. The increased vascular permeability seen with hypertension could lead to increased influx of lipoprotein into the cell, and, based on recent experimental evidence, diabetes mellitus might act to reduce efflux from the cell.

Plasma membrane receptors, endocytosis, lysosomal function and intracellular lipoprotein metabolism by this cell, and the nature of lipid transfer between isolated lipoprotein fractions and the cell are therefore active areas of inquiry in current research. Perhaps the best evidence for the appropriateness of the recent emphasis on the cellular biology of vascular tissue comes from the observation that a phenotypic hypercholesterolemia with monogenic inheritance is associated with a specific deficiency of surface receptors for LDL molecules in cultured cells obtained from afflicted individuals. Absence of the normal function of these receptors in regulating intracellular cholesterol synthesis results in hypercholesterolemia. The mechanisms by which this deficiency is translated into a marked predisposition to lipid accumulation by these cells and by which other "risk factors" exert their effects at the cellular level are yet to be identified.

TREATMENT, REGRESSION, AND PREVENTION. Current treatment of clinical atherosclerotic complications revolves around highly sophisticated coronary care units, replacement of diseased vascular segments with prosthetic or natural grafts, the use of antiarrhythmic agents, anticoagulants and plasma lipid lowering agents, and even heart transplantation. Although these approaches are remarkable accomplishments, they are addressed to the late stages of a disease process for which prevention is clearly the best goal. Significant regression of modest lesions in nonhuman primates follows extreme manipulation of diets from cholesterol-rich to cholesterol-poor content. However, the great reductions in serum lipid levels after this maneuver are not usually possible in man. Although an occasional study suggests that progression of atherosclerotic lesions may be slowed or arrested by stringent risk factor control in man, conclusions about real benefit are premature. Despite these uncertainties about the ultimate effects of available preventive measures on the atherosclerotic process, the clinician might adopt an approach which emphasizes a "prudent" course for his patients. Moderation of intake of total calories and saturated fat, reduction of elevated blood pressure and cigarette use, and control when possible of the other risk factors at the very least carry real benefits of improved general well-being and decreased likelihood of other serious diseases.

Benditt, E. P., and Benditt, J. M.: Evidence for a monoclonal origin of human atherosclerotic plaques. Proc. Natl. Acad. Sci. USA, 70:1753, 1973.

Fowler, S., and Wolinsky, H.: Lysosomes in vascular smooth muscle cells. In Bohr, D., Somlyo, A. P., and Sparks, H. V. (eds.): Vascular Smooth Muscle. Handbooks on Circulation. Washington, D.C., American Physiological Society, 1979.

Fry, D. L.: Responses of the arterial wall to certain physical factors. In Porter, R., and Knight, J. (eds.): Atherogenesis: Initiating Factors. Proceedings, Ciba Foundation Symposium No. 12. Amsterdam, Elsevier, 1973, pp. 93–120.

Geer, J. C., and Haust, M. D.: Smooth muscle cells in atherosclerosis. In Pollak, O. J., Simms, H. S., and Kirk, J. E. (eds.): Monographs on Atherosclerosis. New York, S. Karger, 1972, Volume 2.

Goldstein, J. L., and Brown, M. S.: The low-density lipoprotein pathway and its relation to atherosclerosis. Ann. Rev. Biochem., 46:897, 1977.

Goldstein, J. L., Hazzard, W. R., Schrott, H. G., Bierman, E. L., and Motulsky, A. G.: Hyperlipidemia in coronary heart disease. J. Clin. Invest., 52:1533, 1544, 1569, 1973.

Gordon, T., Castelli, W. P., Hjortland, M. C., Kannel, W. B., and Dawber, T. R.: High density lipoprotein as a protective factor against coronary heart disease. The Framingham Study. Am. J. Med., 62:707, 1977.

Kannel, W. B., Castelli, W. P., Gordon, T., and McNamara, P. M.: Serum cholesterol, lipoproteins, and the risk of coronary heart disease. The Framingham Study. Ann. Intern. Med., 74:1, 1971.

McGill, H. C., Jr. (ed.): The Geographic Pathology of Atherosclerosis.

Baltimore, Williams & Wilkins Company, 1968. (Reprinted from Lab. Invest., 18:463, 1968.)

Ross, R., and Glomset, J. A.: Atherosclerosis and the arterial smooth muscle cell. Science, 180:1332, 1973.

Wissler, R. W., Vesselinovitch, D., and Getz, G. S.: Abnormalities of the arterial wall and its metabolism in atherogenesis. Prog. Cardiovasc. Dis., 18:341, 1976.

363. DISORDERS OF THE CORONARY ARTERIES

363.1. INTRODUCTION

Desmond G. Julian

Disorders of the coronary arteries are the most common causes of death in developed countries and are responsible for much disability. The most frequent disease process involved is coronary atherosclerosis; other abnormalities include embolism, luetic aortitis, spasm, and, rarely, arteritis.

Coronary arterial disease usually exists for many years before it has any adverse effects upon the myocardium. Ischemic heart disease develops when the coronary circulation is insufficient to supply myocardial oxygen demands. The development of ischemia depends upon the location and severity of the stenosis or stenoses, the presence or absence of collateral vessels, and the demands of the myocardium.

Ischemic heart disease has three major manifestations: angina pectoris, myocardial infarction, and sudden death. Angina pectoris is a clinical syndrome resulting from transient and reversible myocardial hypoxia. Myocardial infarction is the term used to describe acute necrotic changes in the myocardium which are usually secondary to coronary occlusion.

It is important to recognize the differences in concept between the two syndromes. One — angina pectoris — is essentially a symptom complex; the other — myocardial infarction — by definition is a pathologic entity. The borderline between them is by no means always clinically distinct, and there are patients who exhibit features characteristic of both conditions. Some such patients, suffering from the "intermediate syndrome," may have symptoms suggesting myocardial infarction but no evidence of necrosis; others may have typical features of angina pectoris when, in fact, necrosis has taken place.

The initial presentation and course of ischemic heart disease vary strikingly from one patient to another. In about 25 per cent of cases, the first manifestation of ischemic heart disease is sudden death. In others, sudden death complicates acute myocardial infarction, whereas in still others it follows a prolonged period of angina pectoris. Myocardial infarction may be the first presentation, although it is frequently preceded by new or worsening attacks of angina pectoris. The patient who has recovered from myocardial infarction may be symptom free but often experiences angina pectoris and is liable to sudden death. The patient with angina pectoris may retain this symptom without any complications for years or decades. However, at any time other manifestations of ischemic heart disease may supervene.

The prognosis in ischemic heart disease is determined to a large extent by the location and severity of coronary arterial stenosis and the state of the myocardium, although other factors such as coexistent hypertension and cigarette smoking play a role.

363.2. ANGINA PECTORIS

Desmond G. Julian

DEFINITION. Angina pectoris describes a syndrome of discomfort in the chest and adjacent areas resulting from transient and reversible myocardial hypoxia.

The term was originally coined by William Heberden, whose description in 1768 has not been bettered:

"There is a disorder of the breast marked with strong and peculiar symptoms, considerable for the kind of danger belonging to it, and not extremely rare which deserves to be mentioned more at length. The seat of it, and the sense of strangling and anxiety with which it is attended, may make it not improperly be called angina pectoris.

"They who are afflicted with it, are seized while they are walking (more especially if it be uphill, and soon after eating) with a painful and most disagreeable sensation in the breast, which seems as if it were to extinguish life, if it were to increase or continue; but the moment they stand still, all this uneasiness vanishes.

"In all other respects the patients are, at the beginning of this disorder, perfectly well, and in particular have no shortness of breath, from which it is totally different. The pain is sometimes situated in the upper part, sometimes in the middle, sometimes at the bottom of the os sterni, and often more inclined to the left than to the right side. It likewise very frequently extends from the breast to the middle of the left arm."

ETIOLOGY. Coronary atherosclerosis is responsible for angina pectoris in about 90 per cent of cases. Coronary angiographic and postmortem studies have demonstrated that it is usual for at least one of the three major coronary arteries to be stenosed by 80 per cent or more before angina develops. In most cases, two or three of the major vessels are involved.

Another important cause of the syndrome is aortic stenosis; angina occurs less often in aortic regurgitation if this is isolated, but it is common in combined lesions. It is also a feature of syphilitic aortitis, although this is now a rare cause.

Coronary arterial spasm is being increasingly recognized as a mechanism of angina pectoris, but its frequency has not yet been established.

Rarer causes of angina pectoris include congenital anomalies of the coronary arteries, cardiomyopathies, mitral valve disease (particularly mitral valve prolapse), and diseases affecting small coronary arteries, including the connective tissue disorders such as systemic lupus erythematosus and polyarteritis nodosa.

Angina may also occur with marked right ventricular hypertrophy associated with pulmonary stenosis and pulmonary hypertension.

Conditions which may aggravate angina pectoris, although seldom responsible for it in the absence of other forms of disease, include hypotension, thyrotoxicosis, anemia, and polycythemia.

PATHOPHYSIOLOGY. Angina pectoris occurs when

there is an inadequate supply of oxygen for the needs of the myocardium. The quantity of oxygen available to the heart depends upon the coronary blood flow and the arteriovenous oxygen difference. In the normal heart under basal conditions, the heart extracts a very high percentage of the oxygen in the coronary arterial blood. The reserve available for increased demands is therefore very limited, and these can only be met by an increase in coronary blood flow. Coronary blood flow is determined by aortic pressure and coronary vascular resistance. Only a modest increase in coronary blood flow can be obtained by increasing arterial pressure; in the normal heart augmentation of flow in response to increased demands is mainly achieved by coronary vascular dilatation. Dilatation of the coronary vessels seems to be activated by oxygen lack, although the mechanism by which this occurs is not yet clearly identified.

The increase in coronary vascular resistance which is present in coronary arterial disease cannot be readily compensated for by an increase in arterial pressure or by increased oxygen extraction. However, as the disease process often affects only one or two of the major proximal vessels, the development of a collateral circulation may compensate. The degree of narrowing necessary to produce symptoms is variable, but in general a reduction in coronary blood flow in the basal state will be seen only when at least one vessel is obstructed 80 per cent or more, although there may be a limitation of coronary flow on exercise in the presence of only 50 per cent reduction. In patients with critically narrowed arteries, the coronary vessels beyond the obstructions are maximally dilated and are therefore unable to respond by further dilatation to increased demand.

The main determinants of myocardial oxygen demand are the contractile state of the myocardium, the heart rate, and the tension in the ventricular wall. Exercise, the chief provoking agent of angina, increases all three of these factors. In the presence of coronary arterial stenosis, it is usual for there to be segmental inadequacy of coronary blood flow, in spite of the presence of any collaterals. Furthermore, subendocardial blood flow suffers disproportionately.

During an attack of angina pectoris it is usual for there to be a moderate tachycardia, a rise in systemic blood pressure, and an increase in the end-diastolic pressure in the left ventricle. It seems probable that the last of these is due to decreased compliance (increased stiffness) in the ventricular wall. The contractility of the affected region of myocardium is impaired; contraction may cease completely and the ischemic area may move paradoxically.

Regional hypoxia also leads to metabolic changes, including loss of potassium and excessive lactate production as a result of anaerobic glycolysis. The actual cause of anginal pain is undetermined, although it seems probable that some as yet unidentified chemical stimulates the nerve endings. Many substances — acetylcholine, adenosine, histamine, and the kinins — have been thought to be possibly involved, but in no case has this been proved.

CLINICAL MANIFESTATIONS. Angina pectoris is by definition a symptom complex, and the diagnosis can usually be made readily from the patient's description. Sometimes, however, the features may be atypical or the individual's powers of expression inadequate. Observations which suggest or prove myocardial hypoxia at the time of the discomfort are of value, although they cannot prove the diagnosis.

Symptoms. There are four cardinal features of the angina syndrome: its site, its character, its relationship to exertion, and its duration. In the most typical case, all these features are present in their characteristic form, but one or more of them may be atypical.

Site. Angina pectoris is most commonly located in the region of the middle or upper third of the sternum. However, it is quite frequently most severe in other areas or radiates to or from them. Such areas include the lower sternal region, the xiphisternal region, one or both sides of the chest (particularly the left), the arms (particularly the left), and the neck or lower jaw. More rarely, the pain is epigastric, interscapular, or over one scapula.

In milder attacks the discomfort may be located at only one site, but as it becomes more severe it may spread to the other areas. Similarly, when angina first occurs it is often localized, but with advancing severity it becomes more diffuse.

In its most typical form, the discomfort starts in the sternal region and radiates to the left shoulder and upper arm. It frequently extends further down one or both arms to the elbow, wrists, or fingers. In many cases, areas are "skipped" so that some patients complain of pain in the left shoulder and hand with the rest of the arm being uninvolved. In a few patients, the discomfort arises first in a peripheral area such as the jaw or wrists, and only with increasing severity is the sternal region involved. It is important to emphasize that the left submammary region is seldom involved in angina, and only very rarely is it the only site.

Character. The discomfort of angina pectoris is usually of mild to moderate severity and can be controlled by slowing down or stopping. Many patients emphatically deny that the discomfort in their chest is a pain. The sensation may be described as one of oppression, heaviness, or tightness. Other descriptions include "bandlike" or "viselike"; it is not knifelike or stabbing.

The discomfort in the arms is usually described as a heaviness or sense of uselessness or ache, but in the fingers there is often the sensation of numbness or tingling. In the neck, the feeling is one of choking, whereas in the jaw it is an ache, sometimes similar to toothache.

Exercise, Emotion, and Other Provoking Factors. The most common provoking factor of angina pectoris is physical exercise, and it is usual for the subject to be first aware of discomfort when walking uphill or in a hurry. Many patients manage to continue at their occupations even if they involve physical labor but find travel to or from work difficult. The syndrome is more likely to occur in the cold or after a meal. There is a marked variation in the amount of exercise that may be required to provoke the pain from time to time, and symptoms may disappear in warm weather only to return in the winter. In general, there is a tendency to progressive worsening over a period of several years.

Although less common, anginal pain may be readily provoked by arm movements, and for a given amount of work, it would seem that arm movements are more likely to produce angina than is walking. In the most severe cases, such activities as rubbing oneself after a shower or shaving may provoke angina.

Emotion is almost as important as exercise as a precipitating factor. Anger and anxiety are obvious causes, and the watching of competitive sport is frequently responsible. Car driving and public speaking are other common provokers of angina. Angina on sexual intercourse is particularly common, but frequently is not spontaneously mentioned by the patient.

Many patients complain of angina when first getting into bed, and others are troubled by being awakened by it, sometimes being aware that the syndrome is preceded by dreams which may be exciting or involving physical exercise. Angina which occurs whenever a patient lies down — "angina decubitus" — is rare and usually indicates advanced disease.

In most cases of angina, there is a clear precipitating factor. However, in a proportion of patients attacks of angina occur quite unexpectedly and in relation to no evident cause. Such patients often exhibit S-T elevation in the ECG, in contrast with the usual S-T depression which is a feature of exercise- or emotion-induced angina pectoris. Such cases, often classed as "Prinzmetal's angina" or "variant angina," will be discussed at the end of this chapter.

The ways in which angina may be relieved are almost as specific as its provoking factors. When it is provoked by exertion, rest usually produces relief of symptoms within a short time. Similarly, the pain subsides with the relief of emotion. Carotid sinus pressure may abbreviate an attack, provided that bradycardia can be induced. This test should be carried out with the patient recumbent and should not be undertaken if there is any evidence of carotid artery stenosis. Nitroglycerin can usually terminate an attack of angina pectoris in less than three minutes; an inability to achieve this relief should then cause one to question the diagnosis. In particular, when pain is more prolonged and is unresponsive, myocardial infarction should be suspected.

DURATION. Most attacks of angina pectoris last for about two or three minutes. It is rare for them to last less than a minute or for more than 15 minutes, although, particularly in emotion-induced angina, longer attacks may occur. However, too much emphasis must not be placed on the patient's estimation of duration, as most people find it difficult to know precisely how long an attack has lasted.

"NONVERBAL" DESCRIPTIONS OF ANGINA. It is always difficult to describe a pain and to know how long it has lasted. This appears to be particularly so in the case of angina pectoris, but there are some "nonverbal" ways in which the patient conveys valuable information about his discomfort. Patients may lay their hands across the chest or sweep them from side to side, a gripping motion may be made in front of the sternum, one hand may be placed on each side of the chest with the fingers touching over the sternum, or both hands may be placed laterally in this way. All these gestures are suggestive of angina, whereas the diagnosis is exceedingly unlikely if the patient points to the location of the pain with the tip of a finger, particularly if he points to the left submammary region.

ACCOMPANYING SYMPTOMS. Although Heberden pointed out the difference between dyspnea and angina, the two symptoms commonly coexist. Specific questions may have to be asked to elicit a history of one in the presence of other.

Palpitation is uncommon, except in those cases in which paroxysmal arrhythmias are responsible for the syndrome. Nausea and sweating sometimes occur, and some patients experience "angor animi" — a sense of impending dissolution. Dizziness occurs occasionally, but loss of consciousness is very unusual except when bradycardia, resulting from either sinus slowing or atrioventricular block, is responsible for both the chest discomfort and syncope.

Physical Examination. Physical examination plays a relatively small role in the diagnosis of angina pectoris, except in those patients in whom such disorders as aortic stenosis or cardiomyopathy are responsible. On the other hand, it may reveal important abnormalities which must be taken into account in the assessment of the patient and which may require correction. Such factors include overweight, hypertension, and anemia.

Apart perhaps from detecting high blood pressure, examination of the cardiovascular system is relatively unhelpful in most patients between attacks. There may, however, be features of myocardial malfunction due to old myocardial infarction or hypertension. Thus there may be cardiomegaly or left ventricular hypertrophy; a fourth heart sound is not uncommon. A third heart sound is much rarer, as is the murmur of mitral regurgitation secondary to papillary muscle malfunction. Occasionally, the paradoxical pulsation of a ventricular aneurysm may be detected.

During an actual attack of angina pectoris, the pulse rate is usually moderately increased and the blood pressure higher than prior to the attack. Other features which are occasionally noted are a fourth heart sound, paradoxical splitting of the second heart sound, and pulsus alternans. More rarely, an apical systolic murmur resulting from transient mitral regurgitation can be heard.

DIAGNOSIS. As angina pectoris is a symptom complex, the diagnosis depends upon an accurately taken and interpreted history. Because it is essentially a subjective phenomenon, no test can prove or disprove the diagnosis, but investigations are valuable in confirming the presence of concomitant myocardial ischemia and for demonstrating the pathologic processes which are responsible for it or are the consequences of it.

Electrocardiography. The ECG is normal in some 50 to 75 per cent of patients with angina pectoris. Changes which may be found in the remainder include evidence of old myocardial infarction, particularly Q waves and, less often, persistent S-T segment elevation or T wave inversion. The changes of left ventricular hypertrophy secondary to hypertension may be present. In many patients there are minor ECG abnormalities, such as flattening or inversion of the T waves; in others there may be arrhythmias.

Attacks of angina pectoris at rest are seldom witnessed, and ECG recordings are therefore not often obtained in this situation. However, if such attacks are observed, particularly in the context of an intensive care unit or by Holter monitoring, it is most usual to see depression of the S-T segments. However, in cases of so-called Prinzmetal's angina, S-T segment elevation develops.

Because the ECG is so often normal at rest and because angina is characteristically a symptom evoked by exercise, stress tests provide valuable evidence in its diagnosis. The longest established method of doing this is the so-called Master two-step test, which involves the performance of 15 to 25 trips up and down two steps each 9 inches high in a period of 1½ minutes. The number of trips is varied, depending on the age, weight, and sex of the patient. The test is discontinued if the pain is experienced, but is repeated if the patient remains symptom free and the ECG remains normal. ECG records are recorded immediately and for up to ten minutes after the conclusion of the test. S-T segment depression of 0.5 mm is suggestive of myocardial ischemia, provided that it is horizontal or downward sloping, but more severe degrees of S-T depression provide more definite evidence of ischemia. This test is rather unsatisfactory, as few patients can exercise themselves sufficiently to produce chest pain or the tachycardia which usually precedes it. An additional major disadvantage of the Master two-step test is the inability to monitor the ECG during the exercise.

Most cardiac centers now carry out exercise tests using either a treadmill or bicycle ergometer. These may be either "submaximal" or "symptom-limited" tests. In submaximal tests, the patient is exercised to a target heart rate which is related to the maximum anticipated heart rate for an individual of a given age and sex. Increasingly, symptom-limited maximal exercise tests are being undertaken, because it is common for patients with heart disease to reach symptom-limited work capacity before they achieve the expected target heart rate. Several different techniques are used, but all should include the recording of at least three chest leads during exercise and the recording of leads I, II, and III and three chest leads immediately after exercise and several times over the succeeding ten minutes. During the test, the workload is progressively increased at three-minute intervals until fatigue, chest pain, dyspnea, or other symptoms limit it. Blood pressure is recorded each three minutes, and the ECG is continuously monitored. The test should be discontinued if marked S-T changes develop, if the blood pressure falls, or if there are any other untoward signs. It may be regarded as positive if there is a 1-mm depression of the S-T segment persisting until 0.08 second after the J point, and it is most diagnostic if this is downward sloping. The heart rate and blood pressure response is extremely important, and it is essential to note at what level angina or S-T segment changes develop and at what work load the test has to be discontinued. Failure to raise the blood pressure significantly during the test or discontinuance of the test at low heart rates is suggestive of severe disease of the proximal parts of the coronary arteries.

Exercise ECG stress tests must be interpreted with considerable caution, as there are many false-positive and false-negative results. These tests are of little value when the patient is receiving digitalis or has certain ECG abnormalities such as bundle branch block.

There is almost no risk in a carefully conducted exercise test, provided that the precautions mentioned are observed. Very rarely, ventricular tachycardia or fibrillation may ensue, and it is essential to have a defibrillator and other apparatus available for cardiopulmonary resuscitation.

An alternative method of stress testing is by pacing of the atrium during cardiac catheterization. The tachycardia so induced increases oxygen demand, although not to the same extent as an equivalent degree of tachy-

cardia produced by exercise. The heart rate is accelerated to 160 to 180 beats per minute or until chest pain or S-T changes develop. Although not as satisfactory a test of myocardial ischemia as the exercise test, it is valuable in assessing patients who are unable to perform satisfactorily on a bicycle or treadmill.

The demonstration of lactate production by coronary sinus sampling during stress testing provides further evidence of myocardial ischemia.

Chest Roentgenogram. This is of little value in the diagnosis of angina except when calcification of a coronary artery can be seen, but the demonstration of cardiomegaly or of a ventricular aneurysm may be important in assessing prognosis or planning treatment.

Coronary Arteriography. Coronary arteriography enables one to visualize the major coronary arteries and their branches and to demonstrate areas of narrowing in these vessels. It is the only method of proving the diagnosis of atherosclerotic disease, and is essential in patients being considered for coronary artery surgery. It also provides valuable information on prognosis. Notwithstanding the advantages of this technique, its dangers and its limitations must be borne in mind, and it should not be undertaken unless one or more of a number of indications are present.

The investigation is carried out either by means of a brachial arteriotomy (Sones technique) or by a percutaneous femoral approach, using special preformed catheters (Judkins technique). The method in experienced hands should have a mortality of less than 0.5 per cent. It should only be undertaken in laboratories in which at least 100 such investigations are undertaken annually and in which there is a highly trained team. Risks include ventricular fibrillation, bradycardia and hypotension, provocation of myocardial infarction, and dissection of a coronary artery, as well as local disorders in the intubated artery. All these complications are very unusual in competent hands. The risks are particularly low in those with little or no coronary arterial disease and are highest in patients with disease of the left main coronary artery. Measurement of the left ventricular pressure and left ventriculography are carried out at the same procedure. It has been shown that prognosis is closely related to the number of coronary vessels involved and to the nature and extent of ventricular malfunction.

Coronary arteriography is a quite sensitive test for coronary atherosclerosis, but one cannot assume that the presence of this pathologic process proves the presence of angina or ischemia, for such changes are common in symptom-free populations.

Coronary arteriography is indicated when the possibility of surgery on the coronary arteries is under consideration. The major group of patients is that for whom medical treatment has failed to control the symptoms. It is also of value in the diagnosis of coronary arterial disease and is particularly useful when it is desired to rule out coronary atherosclerosis in younger patients, in whom such a diagnosis would have adverse effects on their careers and future plans.

Nuclear Imaging. Imaging techniques are rapidly coming into widespread use in spite of their expense and the restricted availability of appropriate gamma cameras. The techniques used in angina are of two main kinds.

One of these is "cold spot scanning," in which an

isotope is injected which is taken up uniformly by well-perfused myocardium but poorly in ischemic areas. The most commonly used indicator at present is thallium-201. If this isotope is injected during exercise-induced angina, the isotope is not taken up in the ischemic area; when this area recovers, the "cold spot" disappears.

A different technique involves the use of gated blood pool scanning in the ventricles, using a label such as technetium-labeled albumin, to permit visualization of the ventricle in systole and diastole and, with more sophisticated techniques, throughout both periods. This allows an assessment both of over-all left ventricular function and of regional abnormalities.

DIFFERENTIAL DIAGNOSIS. A positive diagnosis of angina pectoris can usually be made on the basis of history, buttressed if necessary by the exercise ECG, but difficulties may arise when the pain is atypical.

Musculoskeletal pains are frequent in the chest wall, and often no cause can be found. Such pains may be aggravated by exertion, but the areas affected are often tender and seldom in the midline. The pain is most likely to be provoked by such factors as lifting, rotating the trunk, and pulling, which produce tension in the muscles attached to the ribs. Among more specific musculoskeletal conditions are Tietze's syndrome (in which there is inflammation of one or more costochondral junctions), metastatic lesions in the ribs, and fractured ribs. The pain of cervical spondylosis may be most severe in the upper chest region and is accompanied by discomfort in the shoulders and arms. However, such pains are not so clearly related to walking or emotion and are most likely to be provoked by movements of the neck.

Patients with anxiety neuroses are prone to chest pains and frequently think that these are due to cardiac disease. Most often they take the form of a persistent aching over the left breast region, but stabbing pains may also occur in the same area. If there is a relationship to exercise, this is usually after rather than during the effort. Chest pain in these patients forms a part of a group of symptoms which include breathlessness on little or no exertion, sweating, and faintness. On examination, the physical signs of anxiety are present, with cold moist hands and sighing respiration. Patients with these symptoms and signs have been designated in the past as suffering from "neurocirculatory asthenia," "effort syndrome," or "soldier's heart." Although it is possible to differentiate these features from those of angina pectoris, particularly if there is a clear-cut psychologic cause, angina and an anxiety state may coexist.

Rarely, the pains of pericarditis or pleurisy may be confused with that of angina, particularly as these may be aggravated by exercise. However, a carefully elicited history will show that the pain is aggravated on taking a deep breath or, perhaps, by lying flat.

One of the conditions most difficult to differentiate from angina pectoris is that of an esophageal reflux, which may be associated with hiatus hernia. The pain is usually central in the lower sternal region; it may radiate up toward the neck, but rarely to the shoulders or arms. It may be provoked by exercise, but is more commonly related to stooping or lying flat. It may be associated with flatulence or heartburn and be relieved by alkalis. The mere presence of a hiatus hernia does not prove the diagnosis, but the demonstration of esopha-gitis by esophagoscopy and the provocation of pain by an acid perfusion test are virtually diagnostic.

The pain of peptic ulceration may radiate from its usual site in the epigastric region to the chest. There is usually associated epigastric tenderness, and the pain is related to food rather than exertion. It is usually relieved by alkali or milk and not by nitroglycerin. Cholecystitis and cholelithiasis may also give rise to pain in the lower sternal region, but it is usual for there to be tenderness in the right hypochondrium.

The pain of angina pectoris has, of course, to be differentiated from that of myocardial infarction. The pain of infarction is usually more prolonged and severe but is not necessarily either. However, the lack of relationship to exercise, the greater systemic upset, and the eventual ECG and enzyme abnormalities permit the establishment of the diagnosis of myocardial infarction, although 24 to 48 hours may elapse before one can be certain.

PROGNOSIS. Although in the lay mind angina pectoris is a diagnosis with sinister connotations, the majority of patients with this condition live for many years, and perhaps one half survive at least ten years. However, the risk of sudden death and myocardial infarction exists even in those apparently doing well. The severity of symptoms is, indeed, a poor guide to prognosis, and those with severe symptoms may live for many years, whereas those with mild angina may die suddenly. Clinical features which carry a bad prognosis include cardiomegaly, a third heart sound, and electrocardiographic abnormalities at rest. Hypertension is an unfavorable feature, as is marked S-T depression on the exercise test. Cardiac failure is particularly sinister.

More accurate prognosis may be obtained from coronary angiography and left ventriculography. If only one of the main coronary arteries is involved, the annual mortality is 2 to 4 per cent; if two are involved, it is 6 to 8 per cent; and if three are involved, it is 10 to 12 per cent. If the left main coronary artery is involved, the mortality is even higher. Malfunction of the left ventricle is also important. Those with apparently normal left ventricular function have an excellent prognosis in contrast to those whose ventricles contrast very poorly, whose mortality is very high.

TREATMENT. The aims of treatment are (1) to alleviate the patient's symptoms, (2) to educate him to live as rewarding a life as possible within his limitations, and (3) to improve prognosis.

General Management. The general management of a patient with angina is of paramount importance. Whether or not his symptoms can be controlled with medical or surgical measures, the patient will have to reappraise his life style in the light of the disorder. First of all the physician must reassure him that the diagnosis of angina pectoris is not a sentence of death. The relatively good prognosis should be stressed, but the long-term benefits of general health measures such as the avoidance of overweight and the stopping of smoking must be emphasized.

Moderate exercise, provided that this does not provoke angina, should be encouraged, and, if possible, a program of increasing activity should be prescribed. On the other hand, the patient should be cautioned against strenuous exercise, particularly if it involves heavy lifting or walking uphill against a wind.

The known risk factors for coronary arterial disease

should be controlled, particularly in the younger patient. Hyperlipidemia should be corrected by appropriate dietetic and, if necessary, drug measures. Coexistent hypertension should be treated. Often the most appropriate therapy for this is a beta-adrenergic blocking drug, which is also of value in the management of the chest pain. Smoking must be stopped.

Drugs. Attention to such factors as obesity and modifications of life style can often completely abolish angina pectoris, if only for some months. If symptoms can be controlled in this way, there seems no special point in prescribing drugs, but many patients do indeed require pain relief.

For more than 100 years, nitrates have been used to control angina. Their mode of action is still not entirely understood. They can be shown to have a dilator effect on the coronary arteries, but this is probably not the reason for their effectiveness except in patients who have coronary arterial spasm. They also dilate the peripheral arteries and veins and thereby reduce both the afterload and the preload on the myocardium. This in turn leads not only to a reduction in oxygen demand but also to a fall in left ventricular end-diastolic pressure, which allows a relative increase in endocardial blood flow.

Glyceryl trinitrate (nitroglycerin) is the drug in most common use. It must be administered sublingually and acts within about two minutes, its duration of action lasting for about 45 minutes. Patients should be encouraged to use it both prophylactically and therapeutically. Long-acting nitrates are also in common use, but are probably best reserved for those whose angina is proving troublesome or for those who find unacceptable the headache which may be produced by nitroglycerin. Isosorbide dinitrate, 2.5 to 5 mg sublingually, may give relief for one to two hours.

The beta-adrenergic blocking drugs have achieved an importance almost equal to that of the nitrates in the management of angina. Several double-blind studies have proved their efficacy, provided that they are given in adequate doses. Beta-adrenergic blocking drugs reduce the oxygen demand on the myocardium. They slow the heart rate, reduce the rise of blood pressure that occurs on exercise, and diminish the velocity of cardiac contraction. Propranolol is the most commonly used drug in this group and the only one currently available in the United States. It is classified as a "nonselective" drug in that it blocks both the beta receptors in the heart (beta-1) and those in bronchial smooth muscle and in the peripheral arterioles (beta-2). As a consequence, it may lead to bronchoconstriction in patients with obstructive airways disease and may cause cold extremities, particularly in those with peripheral atherosclerosis or poor peripheral circulation. Selective beta blockers, such as metoprolol and atenolol, which are available in most other countries, effectively block only the cardiac receptors. They reduce the risks of bronchoconstriction and also seem less liable to produce cardiac failure, which may occur with propranolol therapy.

Because of the risks of provoking cardiac failure and bronchospasm, it is wise to start propranolol in a relatively small dose of 10 mg four times daily. If this is well tolerated, there is usually little problem with larger amounts, and the daily dose may be rapidly increased to 160 mg, 240 mg, or higher as necessary. Bradycardia at rest may be produced by quite small doses, but full beta blockade has not been achieved until the tachycardia of exercise has been largely abolished.

The major side effects of propranolol are cardiac failure and bronchospasm, but these are uncommon if patient selection is careful. Minor side effects are more common but are frequently overlooked. They include fatigue and depression, nightmares, cold extremities, and the aggravation of intermittent claudication. Propranolol should not be withdrawn abruptly, as this may lead to the sudden worsening of angina or even the precipitation of myocardial infarction.

Several new drugs, not yet available in the United States, are of value in patients who respond inadequately to beta-adrenergic blocking drugs.

Perhexilene, 100 to 200 mg twice daily, effectively relieves pain in many otherwise resistant patients. Its toxic effects include dizziness, ataxia, and, rarely, peripheral neuritis. Liver function test results are sometimes disturbed, but no untoward effects seem to ensue.

Prenylamine, 60 mg four times daily, is effective in a few patients but can cause repetitive ventricular arrhythmias.

Verapamil, 60 mg thrice daily, is particularly effective in coronary arterial spasm (Prinzmetal's angina). It has few side effects but may produce atrioventricular block.

Surgery. Surgery plays a major role in the management of angina pectoris (see Ch. 363.5). The discomfort can be relieved in nearly all subjects and abolished in most. The effect on mortality for coronary disease is still uncertain, except in the case of severe disease of the left main coronary artery, in which there appears to be undoubted benefit. The benefits and risks of coronary artery bypass operations should be considered when the patient with angina is first seen and should be regularly reappraised from time to time.

Surgery is clearly called for when anginal symptoms cannot be adequately controlled by medical measures. However, there is as yet insufficient evidence to recommend surgery for the improvement of prognosis.

UNSTABLE ANGINA. The term unstable angina is used to describe an increase in the severity of angina for which there is no obvious explanation. Although it has been applied to the first appearance of the symptom, it is better reserved for those patients in whom there is a progressive deterioration, with the pain becoming more prolonged or occurring on minimal exertion or at rest. It has been long recognized that patients with this condition are at a relatively high risk of proceeding to myocardial infarction, and the syndrome has been described as "impending infarction" or "preinfarction angina." This situation has also been described as "acute coronary insufficiency." It is likely that a variety of circumstances can be responsible. Thus in some cases a small myocardial infarction may have occurred, in others coronary arterial spasm may be responsible, and in yet others such factors as arrhythmias, anemia, or increased catecholamine drive following acute stress may be involved. Most commonly, however, it is likely that unstable angina develops because the natural progression of the disease has reached a critical stage.

During the attacks of pain, the S-T segments become depressed or the T waves inverted, although in a few cases the S-T segments may become elevated. By definition, no diagnostic enzyme changes occur, nor do the

Q waves of infarction appear. Some 10 to 20 per cent of affected patients proceed to myocardial infarction within the succeeding days or weeks; a small number die suddenly from ventricular fibrillation.

In the majority of patients, the situation can be stabilized by putting the patient to bed and treating with nitroglycerin, long-acting nitrates, and beta-adrenergic blocking drugs. In a few, symptoms continue to be severe in spite of these measures; coronary artery surgery should then be considered.

PRINZMETAL'S (VARIANT) ANGINA. A relatively uncommon but important variant of angina pectoris is characterized by recurrent attacks of angina, usually at rest, accompanied by S-T elevation and, sometimes, by ventricular arrhythmias. Coronary arteriography during the spells of pain has shown that there is usually spasm affecting one of the major coronary arteries. This may occur in an otherwise normal artery or in one affected by coronary atherosclerosis. The pain usually responds to nitroglycerin. Long-acting nitrates are helpful in prevention. Beta-adrenergic blocking drugs may either help or provoke the syndrome. Coronary arterial surgery is indicated only if there is severe concomitant coronary atherosclerotic disease.

Braunwald, E.: Control of myocardial oxygen consumption: Physiological and clinical considerations. Am. J. Cardiol., 27:416, 1971.

Bristow, J. D., Burchell, H. B., Campbell, R. W., Ebert, P. A., Hall, R. J., Leonard, J. J., and Reeves, T. J.: Report of the ad hoc committee on the indications for coronary arteriography. Circulation, 55:969a, 1977.

Dunkman, W. B., Perloff, J. K., Kastor, J. A., and Shelbourne, J. C.: Medical perspectives in coronary artery surgery — a caveat. Ann. Intern. Med., 81:817, 1974.

Gorlin, R.: Pathophysiology of cardiac pain. Circulation, 32:138, 1965.

Julian, D. G. (ed.): Angina Pectoris. Edinburgh, Churchill Livingstone, 1977.

Ross, R. S.: Ischemic heart disease: An overview. Am. J. Cardiol., 36:496, 1975.

Sheldon, W. C., Rincon, G., Pichard, A. D., Razavi, M., Cheanvechai, C., and Loop, F. D.: Surgical treatment of coronary artery disease — "pure" graft operation. Prog. Cardiovasc. Dis., 18:237, 1976.

Vlodaver, A., and Edwards, J. E.: Pathology of coronary atherosclerosis. Prog. Cardiovasc. Dis., 14:256, 1971.

363.3. MYOCARDIAL INFARCTION

Desmond G. Julian

DEFINITION. Myocardial infarction is the term used to describe acute necrotic changes in the myocardium due to a sudden and catastrophic diminution in coronary blood supply.

ETIOLOGY AND PATHOLOGY. Atherosclerosis of the major coronary arteries is responsible for nearly all cases of acute myocardial infarction. Infarction may also result from such conditions as coronary embolism complicating rheumatic heart disease or the use of prosthetic valves, or from the occlusion of a coronary artery from syphilitic aortitis.

Infarction usually follows acute coronary arterial occlusion from thrombosis, subintimal hemorrhage, or rupture of an atheromatous plaque. However, a coronary artery may occlude without causing infarction if collateral blood flow is adequate. Infarction can also occur without total occlusion and without thrombosis.

Many patients dying during acute heart attacks do so within two hours of the onset of acute symptoms. In such cases, it is unusual to be able to demonstrate the classic features of acute myocardial necrosis. This may be due to the fact that no such necrosis has taken place and death has been due to an arrhythmia. On the other hand, changes may not be found because currently available pathologic techniques are unable to detect the earliest changes of infarction. When a patient dies several hours or days after the onset of the attack, necrotic changes can nearly always be seen.

The role of thrombosis in infarction remains a controversial issue. Thrombosis appears to be relatively uncommon in those who die suddenly or with a subendocardial infarction. It is nearly always present in patients dying with full thickness infarctions, particularly if there has been left ventricular failure or shock.

PATHOPHYSIOLOGY. The most important factor determining the hemodynamic response to myocardial infarction is the amount of myocardium involved. The size of the infarct depends on the location of the coronary arterial lesion responsible for it and the state of the other coronary artery vessels, but it is important to appreciate that the area of myocardium which is eventually infarcted is affected by influences operating after the onset of the heart attack. These include factors which increase or decrease the preload and afterload on the heart.

In the early stages after infarction, particularly if it is located inferiorly, there may be a strong vagal discharge with sinus bradycardia and hypotension. Many patients have a sympathetic response which leads to vasoconstriction, hypertension, and tachycardia unless a coexistent vagal effect is more powerful. Inadequate preload resulting from hypovolemia may lead to a lowered arterial pressure, which, although it diminishes afterload, may reduce the coronary perfusion below a critical level. Drugs which increase myocardial oxygen demand by increasing either contractility or afterload may have deleterious effects. Such drugs include digitalis, isoproterenol, and norepinephrine. The arrhythmias also may impair myocardial function by causing excessive bradycardia or tachycardia. In severe cases, arterial acidosis and hypoxia develop, and these may further damage the myocardium.

Other complications include papillary muscle malfunction or rupture leading to mitral regurgitation, rupture of the ventricular septum, and asynergy caused by left ventricular aneurysm.

In patients with mild attacks, the cardiac output is maintained or slightly abnormal; in those who proceed to heart failure or shock, it is profoundly depressed. In such patients, there may be elevation of left ventricular end-diastolic, left atrial, and pulmonary arterial pressures. The right atrial pressure may rise, especially when the infarction affects the right ventricle, as it may in inferior infarction.

Generally speaking, the severity of the hemodynamic disturbance parallels the seriousness of the clinical condition; but when pump failure supervenes, it may be difficult to determine the mechanisms responsible. Careful monitoring of the patient with intracardiac pressure recordings may be necessary to delineate the factors involved.

CLINICAL FEATURES. Symptoms. The most common presentation is with the onset of pain which may either develop abruptly or build up gradually over a period of minutes or hours. Sometimes it occurs in a stuttering fashion with short episodes lasting ten minutes or more. Although often severe, there may be only a slight discomfort. The sensation may be described as "heavy," "tight," or "vise-like." It may also be choking, aching, or bursting. The pain usually persists for half an hour to several hours, but sometimes lasts for only a few minutes. It is usually located in the region of the middle or upper sternum but may be lower down. It frequently radiates to one or both sides of the chest, to the neck and lower jaw, and to one or both arms. In some patients, more particularly the elderly, chest pain is either absent or overshadowed by other symptoms such as dyspnea or syncope. Other common complaints include sweating, giddiness, nausea, and vomiting.

Some two thirds of the patients have experienced an exacerbation of pre-existing angina or the onset of new angina in the month prior to the attack itself.

Physical Examination. At the start of the attack, the patient who is experiencing severe pain appears distressed, sweating, pale, and cold. Either bradycardia or tachycardia may occur at this time; similarly, blood pressure may be either raised or abnormally low. The patient may look "shocked," but this appearance is usually related to the severity of the pain and disappears rapidly when this is relieved. These features may be the consequence of increased vagal tone or sympathetic activity. Many patients look surprisingly normal within an hour or two.

Hypotension may occur transiently with the pain in the initial stages but may in this case be quickly reversed. However, there is usually a gradual fall in the blood pressure over the next few hours or days, followed by a slow rise which may or may not reach the preinfarction level. In 10 to 20 per cent of patients, blood pressure falls progressively until cardiogenic shock develops; such patients frequently die.

The venous pressure is often slightly raised in the first hours after infarction but usually subsides toward normal again. Persistent venous engorgement caused by right-sided heart failure is a feature of severe myocardial damage and usually takes some days to develop.

The apex beat is often impalpable but may be displaced to the left and downward, particularly if there is left ventricular enlargement secondary to longstanding hypertension or previous myocardial infarction. If the infarction has affected the anterior wall of the heart, it is common for a systolic pulsation to be felt in an area internal to and above the apex beat.

On auscultation, first and second heart sounds are often abnormally soft. A fourth heart sound can frequently be heard; a third heart sound or gallop rhythm is less common and indicates left ventricular failure. A soft systolic murmur at or internal to the apex, resulting from functional mitral regurgitation, is common; rarely, a loud systolic murmur can be heard due to rupture of the ventricular septum or of a papillary muscle. A pericardial rub can be heard in about 10 to 20 per cent of patients; it usually lasts for only a few hours and occurs on the second or third day. Crepitations are frequently audible at the lung bases. If they are widespread and persist after coughing, they suggest the presence of left ventricular failure but can occur in its absence in the recumbent patient. Most patients with myocardial infarction sustain a mild pyrexia which develops within 12 to 24 hours, reaches its peak by the second day, and gradually subsides over the next few days.

Most of the abnormal physical signs disappear over the succeeding two or three days. In patients with left ventricular failure, sinus tachycardia and a third heart sound may persist.

CLINICAL COURSE. The mortality of acute coronary heart attacks in the first four weeks is about 40 per cent. About half of these deaths occur within the first two hours of the onset of symptoms. Patients who survive to reach hospital have, without special care, a 20 to 30 per cent risk of dying. The most common mechanism of death is ventricular fibrillation, which is responsible for the majority of early deaths. Shock and left ventricular failure are responsible for most of the deaths after the first day.

Some 50 to 70 per cent of patients have a relatively uncomplicated course and escape severe arrhythmias, hypotension, or pulmonary congestion.

Early Complications. ARRHYTHMIAS AND DEFECTS OF CONDUCTION. Some disorder of rate, rhythm, or conduction is almost invariable. In about half the patients, they are severe enough to be of clinical importance.

Sinus tachycardia is common. When encountered soon after the onset, it may be the result of apprehension or pain; but when it is persistent, it usually indicates severe myocardial damage and is a feature of cardiac failure and shock. Sinus bradycardia is common during the first three hours and is particularly associated with inferior infarction. It can also result from therapy with drugs such as morphine and digitalis. In the early stages it may be dangerous because of hypotension or may be responsible for ventricular ectopic rhythms, but when seen later on during the course it is usually a good prognostic feature.

Atrial tachycardia and flutter are rare, but atrial fibrillation occurs in about 10 to 15 per cent of patients, mostly developing on the second or third day. It is often brief and self-limiting; but if the ventricular rate is fast, cardiac failure may be induced or aggravated.

Ventricular ectopic beats can be detected in most patients. Although they have been regarded as harbingers of ventricular fibrillation, this is probably not the case except when they are of the R-on-T variety or in prolonged runs, constituting ventricular tachycardia. Ventricular tachycardia is dangerous not only because of its association with ventricular fibrillation but because it can lead to cardiac failure and hypotension. Ventricular fibrillation is seen in 5 to 10 per cent of patients with myocardial infarction treated in hospital. It is responsible for most of the many deaths that occur in the first two hours, usually developing at home or at work.

Minor degrees of heart block are common in the first few hours and are usually vagal in origin. More persistent and severe atrioventricular conduction disturbances usually complicate inferior myocardial infarction. This association is a result of the right coronary artery supplying both the atrioventricular nodal tissue and the diaphragmatic surface of the heart. This form of block may be well tolerated but can cause hypotension or episodes of asystole. It usually resolves spontaneously within hours or days. A less common but more sinister type of atrioventricular block occurs in anterior myocardial infarction; it results from interruption of conduction in the right bundle and both fascicles of the left bundle. Widespread myocardial damage is usually present, and the prognosis is poor.

THE SHOCK SYNDROME. Between 5 and 15 per cent of

patients admitted to hospital with myocardial infarction develop shock; in the majority of cases this leads to a fatal outcome. The features of the shock syndrome include hypotension associated with a cold and clammy skin, pallor, mental dulling, and oliguria. Characteristically, the systolic blood pressure is less than 90 mm Hg, but may be higher than this in patients who were previously hypertensive. The most important factor in shock is probably the amount of contracting myocardium that is lost. Apart from the initial pathologic cause of the myocardial infarction, during the early hours additional factors come into play which, if they are not corrected, may augment the size of the eventual infarct. These include arterial hypotension, excess catecholamine drive, arrhythmias, and hypovolemia. It is probable that severe pain may be a factor in the early stages, associated as it is with sinus tachycardia and hypotension.

LEFT VENTRICULAR FAILURE. In most patients, there is no evidence of left ventricular failure on admission to hospital, although in a few this is the presenting feature. However, the majority of patients develop some evidence of pulmonary congestion within the first 48 hours. Signs of left ventricular failure include tachycardia, a third heart sound, and widespread pulmonary rales. On the chest roentgenogram the features of pulmonary venous congestion or edema may be demonstrated.

THROMBOEMBOLISM. Thromboembolic episodes in myocardial infarction may be either pulmonary or systemic.

Pulmonary embolism was common in former years when patients were confined to bed for several weeks in the management of myocardial infarction. Anticoagulants were found beneficial in reducing the many deaths which used to occur from this cause. With earlier ambulation, pulmonary embolism is much less common and is largely confined to patients with severe complications such as cardiac failure, in which prolonged recumbency is the rule.

Massive pulmonary embolism may cause sudden breathlessness, hypotension, or syncope. Any of these features accompanied by raised venous pressure, cyanosis, and the ECG patterns of right heart strain or right bundle branch block suggest the diagnosis. More commonly, pulmonary embolism is manifested by pulmonary infarction, which may produce pleuritic pain or hemoptysis and which can be detected on a chest roentgenogram.

Systemic emboli usually arise from thrombus originating in the left ventricle on the endocardial surface of a myocardial infarction. In some cases, however, they can arise in the atrium, particularly when there is atrial fibrillation.

PERICARDITIS. Pericarditis develops in 15 to 20 per cent of patients, usually on the second or third day. It often produces the recurrence of chest pain, but one that is typically aggravated by deep breathing, lying flat, or swallowing. A pericardial rub may be heard, but it is frequently transient, lasting only for minutes or hours. Usually, the only treatment required is the relief of pain. If the patient is on anticoagulants, these should be discontinued unless there is a strong reason for their continuation, as hemorrhagic pericarditis leading to tamponade may occur.

CARDIAC RUPTURE. Rupture of the myocardium is most likely to occur several days after the onset of symptoms. Rupture through the free wall of the left ventricle usually causes sudden collapse with loss of blood pressure

and pulse but with the electrocardiogram demonstrating persistence of sinus rhythm. In a few cases, classic cardiac tamponade ensues over a period of minutes or hours; in such cases it may be possible to correct the defect surgically. Rupture through the interventricular septum occurs in approximately 0.5 per cent of patients with myocardial infarction, mainly those who have anteroseptal infarcts with bundle branch block. The usual clinical picture is of the sudden onset of severe heart failure, with a systolic thrill and loud murmur developing in the region of the left sternal edge. In most cases, the patient deteriorates rapidly and dies within a few days; in a small proportion of cases there may be survival for several weeks. The diagnosis may be confirmed by floating a Swan-Ganz catheter into the right side of the heart and demonstrating a left-to-right shunt at the ventricular level. If the patient is too ill to withstand corrective surgery at the time of the acute event, he may be kept alive by intra-aortic balloon counterpulsation for one or two weeks until surgery can be more safely undertaken.

PAPILLARY MUSCLE RUPTURE AND MALFUNCTION. Mitral systolic murmurs caused by papillary muscle malfunction are common during the first few days after myocardial infarction but usually disappear subsequently. In a small proportion of patients a papillary muscle ruptures and leads to severe cardiac failure, accompanied by a loud systolic murmur with thrill internal to the apex. Death may occur within the next few hours or days; as with interventricular septal rupture, the patient may be kept alive with intra-aortic balloon counterpulsation until mitral valve surgery can be undertaken.

DIAGNOSIS. In most cases, the presence of myocardial infarction is suspected because of the severe, prolonged nature of the chest pain with its typical heavy or gripping character and its radiation to the arms and throat. The patient's extreme distress and the changes in heart rate and blood pressure also help to suggest the diagnosis. However, this can never be regarded as proved unless there are ECG abnormalities, preferably supported by enzyme changes.

The Electrocardiogram (see also Ch. 364.2). The electrocardiogram in myocardial infarction is associated with changes in three different features of the ventricular complexes. The most specific of these is the appearance of Q waves, indicating myocardial necrosis. Highly suggestive, but less diagnostic, are elevation and alteration in configuration of the S-T segment, indicating myocardial injury. Least specific are the T wave changes of myocardial ischemia.

The earliest changes are usually those of the S-T segment, which develop within minutes or hours of the onset of the attack. The raised S-T segment may initially retain its normal upward concavity, but within a short time it usually becomes convex upward. The S-T elevation develops in relation to the area of the infarct; other leads may show "reciprocal" S-T depression. Usually, the S-T segment returns to the isoelectric line within a few days. Persistence of the S-T segment elevation suggests an aneurysmal or akinetic segment. The S-T changes described, although nearly always due to myocardial infarction, are not specific. Similar changes may be seen in Prinzmetal's angina. However, when the characteristic pattern develops over a period of days and is supported by enzyme abnormalities, a confident diagnosis of infarction may be made.

Q waves, which usually develop between the first and

sixth hour after the onset of symptoms, are much more specific. Indeed, the development of pathologic Q waves (i.e., 0.03 sec or more) in appropriate leads in association with a typical history can be regarded as diagnostic of infarction even though enzyme abnormalities have not been demonstrated. However, Q waves, because they indicate necrosis, may persist indefinitely. The mere presence of Q waves therefore does not prove recent infarction; the changes may be old. When Q waves are present, the infarction is often called transmural, although in such cases the whole ventricular wall is not necessarily involved. When no Q waves can be seen, the infarction may be described as subendocardial or nontransmural.

T wave changes usually occur late in the first day or subsequently and become more pronounced as the S-T segment returns to the isoelectric line. These changes are quite nonspecific and may be seen in a number of different conditions. One should therefore be hesitant to make the diagnosis of infarction when the only ECG abnormalities detected are those of T waves.

The electrocardiogram is of great value in demonstrating the location of the infarct. Anteroseptal infarctions lead to changes in leads V_2 to V_4; anterolateral infarctions, in V_3 to V_6. Inferior or diaphragmatic infarctions produce abnormalities in leads II, III, and aVF. The electrocardiogram is less satisfactory in demonstrating infarctions affecting the posterior surface of the left ventricle; in this situation, none of the conventional leads overlies the infarct, but the loss of posterior left ventricular forces leads to apparent right ventricular preponderance, with a tall R wave appearing in V_1 and V_2. Right bundle branch block does not obscure the changes of myocardial infarction, a common variety being the appearance of an initial Q wave in V_1 to V_4, as opposed to the initial R wave expected in right bundle branch block. On the other hand, left bundle branch block usually obscures the changes of myocardial infarction because of the abnormal initial QRS vector.

Serum Enzyme Concentrations. The myocardium contains many enzymes which are released into the circulation by necrosis. The different enzymes vary from one another in the rate at which they are released; the pattern of enzyme rises in the serum is of diagnostic importance.

Creatine phosphokinase (CPK) occurs in heart, skeletal muscle, and brain. The CPK activity in serum rises within six hours of the onset of infarction and reaches its peak in 18 to 24 hours. It may become normal by 72 hours. Apart form myocardial infarction, high levels of CPK are seen in muscle diseases and cerebrovascular damage. Unfortunately, intramuscular injections can give rise to high CPK levels; as these are often given in the early phases of infarction, they may reduce the value of the enzyme level as a diagnostic test. Three CPK isoenzymes can be identified by electrophoresis. These have been designated BB, characteristic of brain; MM, found in skeletal and heart muscle; and MB, found only in myocardium. Changes in MB isoenzyme activity are virtually specific for myocardium and highly suggestive of myocardial infarction. Unfortunately, the assay is relatively expensive and is not in universal use. Glutamic oxaloacetic transaminase (GOT) is found particularly in the heart, skeletal muscle, brain, liver, and kidney. Normal values vary somewhat from laboratory to laboratory, but in most normal serum activity is 20 to 40 Frank-Karmen units or 30 to 60 international units. After myocardial infarction, the serum activity rises in about 12 hours, reaching its peak in 36 to 72 hours and gradually falling to normal by about the fifth day. As with other enzymes, repeated estimation on a daily basis is desirable in establishing the diagnosis. Caution must be exercised in the presence of liver disease. In general, the height of the GOT reflects the severity of acute myocardial infarction. Sometimes, extremely high levels are encountered in myocardial infarction, e.g., 2000 or 3000 units; when this occurs, it suggests acute hepatic necrosis due to a severe reduction in the splanchnic blood flow associated with shock.

Lactate dehydrogenase (LDH) is also found in the heart. There are five LDH isoenzymes, of which the rapidly migrating isoenzyme LDH I predominates in the heart. The same isoenzyme is found in red cells. The rise in lactate dehydrogenase occurs later than the other enzymes mentioned, reaching its peak 48 hours or more after the onset of infarction; it may remain abnormal for one to three weeks. LDH is less specific than the other enzymes, but is valuable when it is suspected that the infarct has occurred some days prior to sampling or when concomitant diseases diminish the significance of CPK or GOT findings.

It has been shown that the release into the serum of enzymes from the myocardium reflects the severity of myocardial damage. This observation has been used to quantitate the severity of infarct by analyzing the area under the CPK curve. The validity of such estimates remains to be determined.

Nuclear Imaging. Certain chemical substances, such as pyrophosphate and diphosphonate, accumulate in the mitochondria of ischemic or infarcted myocardial cells. Technetium-labeled pyrophosphate and diphosphonate have been used for "hot-spot" scanning for the diagnosis of myocardial infarction. This has proved to be a quite sensitive method of detecting myocardial infarction, but its specificity remains undetermined.

Other Laboratory Abnormalities. A polymorphonuclear leukocytosis occurs in most cases, starting on the first day and persisting for five to seven days. The increase is usually to 12,000 to 15,000 leukocytes per cubic millimeter. In general, the extent of the leukocytosis reflects the severity of the infarction, but levels beyond 15,000 should suggest some other complication. The erythrocyte sedimentation rate rises more slowly and may remain elevated for several weeks.

DIFFERENTIAL DIAGNOSIS. The most common diagnostic problem is the differentiation of myocardial infarction from *angina*, particularly of the "unstable" type. The pain of myocardial infarction is usually more severe and prolonged and is more likely to be accompanied by breathlessness, syncope, nausea, and vomiting, as well as by evidence of hypotension and cardiac failure. None of these features is diagnostic, however, and the distinction between these disorders depends essentially on the finding of the characteristic ECG and enzyme abnormalities of myocardial infarction.

Massive pulmonary embolus may present great diagnostic difficulty, particularly in the patient recovering from surgery or trauma. Massive pulmonary embolism often presents with acute dyspnea, tachypnea, and cyanosis, rather than severe chest pain, although this can be present. Syncope is sometimes the only major manifestation. Additional diagnostic evidence is provided by the features of deep vein thrombosis. Many of the physical signs occur in both conditions, including tachycardia, hypotension, and gallop rhythm.

Many patients with pulmonary embolism have a persistently normal ECG, but Q waves and T wave inversion may appear in lead III; in these cases there is commonly an S wave in lead I. Other ECG abnormalities include P pulmonale, partial or complete right bundle branch block, and transient T wave inversion in the right chest leads. The S-T depression of myocardial ischemia is sometimes seen, but S-T elevation is not a feature. Enzyme abnormalities, including elevation of GOT, CPK, and LDH, may occur in pulmonary embolism, although not to the same extent as is found in myocardial infarction. The MB isoenzyme of CPK remains normal in pulmonary embolism. A lung scan may demonstrate unperfused areas of lung, which is highly suggestive, particularly if the chest roentgenogram is normal. The diagnosis may be established firmly by carrying out a pulmonary angiogram.

Acute pericarditis may produce a pain similar to that of an acute myocardial infarction, although it is usually made worse by lying flat, by breathing, or by swallowing. It is often sharper in character than the pain of myocardial infarction and seldom radiates to the arms, although it may reach the shoulders, neck, and upper abdomen. Acute pericarditis is commonly a complication of a viral infection, in which case pyrexia usually precedes rather than follows the onset of the pain, as in myocardial infarction. In pericarditis Q waves do not appear, but there is usually S-T elevation, which usually remains concave upward but is followed by T wave inversion. The ECG abnormalities tend to be more widespread than they are in myocardial infarction, and reciprocal S-T depression is not characteristically seen. Enzyme abnormalities are either absent or slight.

Dissecting aneurysm of the aorta may be difficult to diagnose. As with infarction, the pain is central and severe. However, it is often described as "tearing" in character and frequently starts in the back rather than in the front of the chest. Furthermore, it tends to move to the front of the chest and sometimes to the abdomen. The patient often has the appearance of shock with pallor and diaphoresis, but the blood pressure is frequently in the hypertensive or normal range, having previously been raised. Features which suggest the diagnosis of dissecting aneurysm include weakness or transient paralysis of the limbs, hemiplegia, hemothorax and aortic regurgitation, and differences in the pulses in the peripheral arteries. Roentgenographic features include a left pleural effusion and widening of the mediastinum. The ECG usually either is normal or shows the features of left ventricular hypertrophy. Transient elevations of serum enzyme activities may occur, although they are usually not great. Aortography can demonstrate the presence of the aneurysm, but is potentially hazardous.

Spontaneous pneumothorax may sometimes produce central chest pain, but usually it is pleural in character. The physical signs and roentgenographic features are diagnostic.

Perforation of a peptic ulcer is usually associated with severe abdominal pain accompanied by tenderness and rigidity. A roentgenogram taken in the upright position will usually demonstrate air under the diaphragm.

Rupture of the esophagus may simulate myocardial infarction, but is usually precipitated by violent vomiting. The chest roentgenogram may show air in the mediastinum.

Pancreatitis may also simulate myocardial infarction, although the pain is usually predominantly in the abdomen. It may radiate into the lower chest, and the picture is made more confusing by the quite frequent occurrence of S-T and T wave abnormalities in the electrocardiogram. Transaminase levels may be raised, but in pancreatitis the serum and urinary amylase levels are usually markedly elevated.

Biliary colic may mimic myocardial infarction, particularly when it is due to a gallstone wedged in the cystic duct. The pain may radiate to the chest and right shoulder region but not to the arms. Vomiting is frequent, and there is virtually always tenderness or rigidity in the right hypochondrium or epigastrium. The diagnosis may be established by appropriate roentgenographic examinations.

PROGNOSIS. The mortality of acute heart attacks is approximately 40 per cent within one month of the onset. A substantial proportion of these deaths are instantaneous or nearly so. The fatality rate in the remainder is in the order of 30 per cent, but this varies considerably with the age of the patient as well as other factors such as a previous history of coronary disease, the presence or absence of other diseases, and the complications of infarction. The mortality below 50 years of age is little more than 10 per cent, but it rises to more than 50 per cent in the elderly. Quite apart from the very early deaths, mortality is highest during the first day and progressively decreases thereafter. Death on the first day is usually due to ventricular fibrillation, although shock and failure may be fatal at this time. These latter complications are responsible for most of the deaths on the second and third days, but they become less common causes subsequently. Later, death may be due to cardiac rupture, pulmonary embolism, or recurrent myocardial infarction.

Unfavorable prognostic features include cardiogenic shock, persistent tachycardia, gallop rhythm, and the development of right-sided heart failure. Bundle branch block, high serum enzyme levels, and persistent arrhythmias are also sinister observations.

There is a high mortality in the first six months after myocardial infarction, but it progressively decreases over the first year and in succeeding years. Over-all, some 85 per cent of patients surviving one month after infarction live for one year, and about 70 per cent live for five years.

In those who survive an acute infarction, the most important correlate with early death is the severity of left ventricular malfunction. Indices of this include cardiomegaly, persistent tachycardia, a third heart sound, and signs of pulmonary congestion or edema. Ventricular arrhythmias are also associated with a bad prognosis, although this may be because they reflect the severity of left ventricular damage rather than being independent risk factors.

TREATMENT. The aims of treatment are (1) to relieve the patient's discomfort, (2) to minimize the oxygen demands of the myocardium in the hope of limiting the extent of the infarction, and (3) to prevent or correct complications.

Relief of Symptoms. The most urgent measure in most cases is the relief of pain. This usually requires the use of morphine sulfate in a dose of 5 to 15 mg given intravenously or intramuscularly. This may have to be repeated. Morphine may produce respiratory depression, hypotension, or bradycardia. It should not be given if possible in those with known obstructive airways disease. Bradycardia can be avoided by simultaneously administering atropine. Alternatively, morphine may be given with an antihistamine drug which diminishes the risk of vomiting and hypotension. It is probably unwise to use meperidine, as this may also cause hypotension and can increase the ventricular rate undesirably. In patients with less severe pain, pentazocine, 15 to 30 mg intravenously, may be helpful. When these powerful pain-relieving drugs are not available, the inhalation of nitrous oxide, 50 per cent, and oxygen, 50 per cent, is useful and can be administered by paramedical personnel.

Most patients respond well to these drugs and the pain is relieved within a short period of time. Furthermore, apprehension, a common feature of myocardial infarction, will usually be alleviated. If it is not, chlordiazepoxide (Librium) or diazepam (Valium) may be used.

General Management. PLACE OF CARE. The initial care of a patient with myocardial infarction will usually be in his home or at his place of work. Ideally, appropriately trained personnel will attend him where he develops the attack and treat his symptoms and complications immediately. This is best achieved by a mobile coronary care unit (see below). In most cases, and as soon as the patient has been made comfortable and any complications corrected, he should be transferred to hospital and admitted to a coronary care unit.

Although hospital admission is the almost invariable practice in the United States, the wisdom of transferring a patient from his home has been questioned in some European countries, notably the United Kingdom. Some controlled studies have suggested that patients do as well at home as they do in hospital, and it has been claimed that the physical and emotional stress of an ambulance journey and admission to an unfamiliar environment may evoke unfavorable responses, including dangerous arrhythmias. These studies are not scientifically satisfactory, and the high risk of unexpected sudden death within the first few hours suggests strongly that it is advisable for patients to be under intensive care during this period. This applies particularly to the younger patient, but it is not unreasonable to treat those patients at home who are seen there many hours after the onset of symptoms, particularly if they are in good general condition or if they are elderly.

BED REST. The obvious need to restrict demands on the myocardium has led many physicians in the past to insist on bed rest for a period of some weeks. The apparent advantages of such strict rest are outweighed, however, by the disadvantages that immobility imposes. The risks of deep vein thrombosis and subsequent pulmonary embolism are well known, but there is also a danger of "deconditioning" so that, when the patient becomes ambulatory, there is a tendency to orthostatic hypotension and undue increases in heart rate. Furthermore, the psychologic effects of the disorder are enhanced, and the patient is more liable to anxiety and depression.

It certainly seems wise to keep the patient in bed for at least 48 hours, although a bedside commode may be used except for those who have severe hypotension. If the patient's initial condition appears satisfactory, he may be allowed to feed himself and should be encouraged to exercise his legs gently. Within a few days, he may be allowed to sit out of bed although still resting in a comfortable armchair. Patients with mild cases may be permitted to walk a few steps after four to five days and be ready for hospital discharge in one to two weeks.

On the other hand, if the infarction has been more severe, being complicated by dangerous arrhythmias, cardiac failure, or shock, a more prolonged period of strict bed rest may be required until the complication has been brought under control. Affected patients need careful observation over the next two to three weeks and may require three to six weeks in hospital.

REASSURANCE. Rehabilitation is often impeded by undue anxiety on the part of the patient and his relatives. This anxiety is frequently engendered by inappropriate remarks made by doctors and nurses. By the time a patient is admitted to a coronary care unit, the most dangerous phase of the illness has already passed and the major complications which may yet develop can usually be controlled. The patient and his relatives can therefore be reassured that there is an excellent chance of survival and that there will be a probability of return to work within the subsequent two or three months. An optimistic attitude must be conveyed to the patient from the moment of his admission and constantly reinforced by his medical attendants. There is often a period of enhanced anxiety when the patient leaves the protective atmosphere of a coronary care unit for progressive care; it must be emphasized to the patient that he has done so well that careful monitoring is no longer necessary. Similarly, a sense of dependence on the hospital must be avoided so that at the time of discharge there is not another period of worry.

DIET. As the acutely ill patient usually has little appetite in the first few days, it is desirable to provide an attractively prepared, low calorie diet with moderate sodium restriction. When the acute phase is over, a normal diet may be given except for the overweight patient, for whom the calorie content should remain low.

SMOKING. Smoking should be absolutely prohibited during the phase of acute infarction and allowed subsequently only with the greatest reluctance.

BOWEL AND BLADDER FUNCTION. Patients are often constipated during the first few days in hospital, partly because of bed rest, partly because of inhibitions imposed by the unfamiliar surroundings, and partly because of the use of narcotics. Bedpans should be used only if they are essential, and in most cases patients should be allowed to use a bedside commode. Many will benefit from the use of a stool softener such as dioctyl sodium sulfosuccinate (Colace), 100 mg twice daily.

Some patients, particularly those with mild prostatic obstruction, develop urinary retention in the first few days. This may be aggravated by such drugs as atropine and disopyramide. If there is evidence of urinary retention, and particularly if there is hypotension, a knowledge of the urinary output is of great importance in management, and an indwelling catheter should be inserted with aseptic technique.

OXYGEN THERAPY. Nearly all patients with myocardial infarction have arterial hypoxemia; in many this is so mild that the additional discomfort of oxygen administration does not seem worthwhile. However, any patient who is breathless, or who has other features of cardiac failure or of shock, should receive oxygen, which is best given by nasal cannula or Venturi mask. High oxygen concentrations should be given except to patients suspected of having obstructive airways disease, in which case the concentration of oxygen should be limited to 28 per cent.

ANTICOAGULANT THERAPY. In the days when patients were confined to bed for long periods of time, it was shown that anticoagulant therapy reduced the risk of deep vein thrombosis and serious pulmonary embolism. With early ambulation and the encouragement of limb movements in bed, these risks have been substantially reduced and are largely confined to those with more severe reactions to the infarction. There is no evidence that anticoagulant therapy has any effect upon coronary thrombosis or the development of the myocardial infarction, although it may have a beneficial effect in reducing the risk of systemic embolism. It seems appropriate to confine anticoagulant treatment to those patients who have evidence of a severe course, including left- or right-sided cardiac failure, shock, and prolonged arrhythmias, particularly atrial fibrillation. They should be given to patients with a previous history of deep vein thrombosis or pulmonary embolism, but avoided if possible in those with known history of ulcer or hemorrhagic tendency, and in the presence of pericarditis.

Disorders of Rate and Rhythm. Sinus bradycardia is usually well tolerated and requires no treatment. However, particularly in the early stages, it may lead to hypotension, cardiac failure, or ventricular ectopic rhythms. The heart rate may be accelerated if the venous return is increased by raising the patient's legs. If this maneuver fails, atropine should be given, starting with not more than 0.5 mg but repeating it if necessary. The action of this drug usually lasts two to four hours. Larger doses may give rise to an undesirable degree of tachycardia, which may rarely lead to ventricular arrhythmias, including ventricular fibrillation. The drug should not be repeated many times, as it may provoke mental confusion and urinary retention and aggravate pre-existing glaucoma. Sinus bradycardia usually disappears after a few hours; but even if it persists, it seldom gives rise to serious hemodynamic disturbances. If it should do so, temporary pacing can be established with the electrode tip placed in the right ventricle. This procedure is particularly helpful when the "sick sinus syndrome" is present, as it permits the use of digitalis or other drugs required to control the concomitant atrial arrhythmias.

ATRIAL ARRHYTHMIAS. Frequent atrial premature beats require no treatment, although they may presage other atrial arrhythmias. Atrial tachycardia may respond to carotid sinus pressure. If it does not do so, therapy should depend upon the hemodynamic disturbance which it has caused. If the patient is in good condition, treatment with digoxin is adequate. However, if the patient is distressed and the blood pressure has fallen precipitately, synchronized direct current shock should be administered. If paroxysmal atrial tachycardia with block occurs, one should first check whether digitalis could have been responsible; if it has not, digitalis is called for if the heart rate is fast. Atrial flutter may be treated as atrial tachycardia.

When atrial fibrillation occurs, the ventricular rate may not be very fast. If this is the case, no treatment may be necessary. However, if the ventricular rate is sufficient to cause hemodynamic disturbance, it may be treated with digoxin in the first place. If this does not produce an adequate fall in heart rate, direct current shock may be necessary. Following a reversion to sinus rhythm, digitalis should be administered for several days because there is a risk of recurrence.

VENTRICULAR ECTOPIC BEATS. In recent years, ventricular ectopic beats and short runs of ventricular tachycardia have been regarded as harbingers of ventricular fibrillation, and therefore great efforts have been expended on detecting and treating them promptly. Certain types of ventricular ectopic beat have been regarded as particularly

sinister: those which occur in pairs or are multiform, or those of the R-on-T variety. The most effective drug in this situation is lidocaine. Therapy should be started with an intravenous injection of 50 to 100 mg given over a period of one to two minutes (*not* rapidly as a "push," as this may produce neurotoxic effects). Subsequently, an intravenous infusion of this drug should be given, starting with 3 to 4 mg a minute for the first half hour and then gradually reducing to 2 mg a minute and 1 mg a minute over the next 12 to 24 hours. Further injections of 75 to 100 mg may be required to suppress recurrences of ventricular ectopic beats.

There is increasing dissatisfaction with this method of trying to prevent ventricular fibrillation. In the first place, many episodes of ventricular fibrillation occur without "warning" arrhythmias. Secondly, conventional monitoring techniques often fail to detect "warning" ventricular arrhythmias. It seems more logical therefore to use lidocaine prophylactically in all cases in which it is not contraindicated. However, the drug has important side effects if given in excessive doses. Mild confusion is common; more serious effects include convulsions and coma. It is preferable to give the drug by an infusion pump.

Several alternative drugs are available if lidocaine fails. These include procainamide and quinidine sulfate. Diphenylhydantoin is less effective but occasionally of value when the other drugs are unsuccessful. The adrenergic blocking drug bretylium tosylate* may also be valuable in difficult cases. An alternative method of treatment is by overdrive suppression, using a temporary pacing electrode.

VENTRICULAR TACHYCARDIA. The management of ventricular tachycardia is similar to that of ventricular ectopic beats, except that the treatment is more urgent. If drug therapy is not immediately successful, consideration should be given to direct current shock therapy.

VENTRICULAR FIBRILLATION. This should be corrected immediately by direct current shock. Usually 200 watt-seconds is sufficient; but if this fails, larger shocks should be administered. If the first shock is not successful, the usual techniques of cardiopulmonary resuscitation, including ventilation and closed chest cardiac compression, should be undertaken (see Ch. 353). Acidosis usually ensues and should be corrected by intravenous sodium bicarbonate; recurrence of ventricular fibrillation should be prevented by intravenous lidocaine, or by other drugs used for suppressing ventricular ectopic beats.

Disorders of Conduction. First-degree heart block (prolonged P-R interval) requires no treatment, but monitoring for more advanced degrees of block should be undertaken. The Wenckebach type of second degree block is a common complication of inferior infarction, usually requires no treatment, and, in the first few hours, can often be corrected by atropine administration. It generally carries a good prognosis but may progress to complete heart block. Mobitz type II heart block, in which there are unexpected dropped beats or 2:1 heart block, occurs with a slow ventricular rate, is usually due to extensive myocardial damage to the bundle branches, and is liable to lead to an extremely slow heart rate or asystole. Such patients should have an electrode inserted with the tip in the right ventricle. Pacing should be instituted if the heart rate is slow enough to cause hypotension or if episodes of asystole have occurred. Therapy of complete heart block depends on the anatomic location of the block

---

*Investigational drug.

and the heart rate. When complete heart block is due to inferior myocardial infarction, the ventricular rate is often adequate and the hemodynamic status satisfactory. When heart block complicates anterior infarction, the block is usually in the bundle branches and the idioventricular rate is slow. Transvenous pacing is called for when the bradycardia leads to hypotension or cardiac failure or to episodes of asystole or ventricular fibrillation. If electrical pacing is not immediately available, isoproterenol may be administered as intravenous infusion of 2 to 5 mg in 500 ml dextrose. The rate of infusion should be adjusted to keep the heart rate between 70 and 100 per minute. Atrioventricular conduction defects in acute infarction nearly always resolve spontaneously within hours or days. Only very rarely is long-term pacemaking required, although there is a risk of late recurrence of heart block and sudden death in those with anterior infarction. Some physicians consider that long-term pacemaker therapy should be instituted in such patients even though normal conduction appears to have been restored.

BUNDLE BRANCH BLOCK. When infarction leads to block in two or more of the fascicles, such as the right bundle and the left anterior or left posterior fascicle, there is a risk of the sudden onset of complete heart block or asystole. Many physicians think it wise to insert a pacing electrode with its tip in the right ventricle as a prophylactic measure and to remove it when the danger of heart block appears to have passed.

Shock.   When the shock syndrome has developed, the mortality is high whatever treatment is given. Prevention is therefore of great importance, and this depends upon the avoidance of hypotension, if possible, in the early phase, the relief of pain, and the correction of such unfavorable factors as arrhythmias and hypovolemia.

Once the features of the shock syndrome have developed, it is desirable to monitor the patient's hemodynamic status carefully, preferably with a Swan-Ganz catheter positioned in the pulmonary artery. If there is severe hypotension and the other features of shock, but left ventricular filling pressure is in the normal range, one may infuse fluid provided that the pulmonary capillary wedge pressure does not exceed 20 mm Hg. It is important not to rely on the right atrial (central venous) pressure in this context, as this may be within normal limits when the pulmonary wedge pressure is high.

Controversy persists as to the value of vasopressors in the management of shock syndrome. Norepinephrine and isoproterenol have been used in the past in this context, but both these drugs potentially may increase the size of the myocardial infarction and, in the case of isoproterenol, may produce peripheral vasodilatation. Myocardial oxygen consumption may be increased, which leads to an increase in the size of myocardial infarction. Dopamine and dobutamine may be of greater value in this context.

The most effective way of counteracting shock is by the use of intra-aortic balloon counterpulsation (see Ch. 356). With this technique, aortic systolic pressure is lowered and diastolic pressure is augmented, thus increasing coronary perfusion and reducing the work of the left ventricle.

Cardiac Failure.   Mild degrees of pulmonary congestion may require no treatment; but when dyspnea or pulmonary edema is present, it is wise to give a diuretic such as furosemide intravenously or orally. The role of

digitalis remains controversial. There is evidence that it may, by increasing myocardial contractility, lead to a disproportionate myocardial oxygen demand and thus increase the size of the infarct. Furthermore, the drug is particularly likely to induce arrhythmias in the context of myocardial infarction. On the other hand, when there is cardiomegaly, the drug, by reducing cardiac size, may improve cardiac efficiency. It may be wise therefore to reserve cardiac glycosides for patients with cardiomegaly and, of course, for those with atrial arrhythmias.

Substances which reduce cardiac afterload, e.g., nitroglycerin and sodium nitroprusside, may be effective in improving left ventricular performance; the combination of one of these drugs with an inotropic drug such as dopamine may be particularly beneficial.

Coronary Care Unit.   The natural mortality in the first two or three days after the onset of myocardial infarction is very high. Some of the major causes of death, notably ventricular fibrillation, can be prevented if the patient is under close observation and if appropriate therapy, including cardiopulmonary resuscitation, can be applied without delay. In order for this to be done, the patient himself and his electrocardiographic and hemodynamic status must be under continuous observation. This can best be achieved by concentrating patients at maximal risk in specially designed areas, by ensuring that they are cared for by nurses and doctors with appropriate training, and by having apparatus for monitoring and resuscitation immediately available. The patients are best accommodated in a quiet environment, preferably in single rooms but under direct visual inspection by nurses at a central monitoring station. The nurses require training in the recognition of arrhythmias, in the administration of the main antiarrhythmic drugs, and in the techniques of cardiopulmonary resuscitation, including the application of direct current countershock. The patient's electrocardiograms are under continuous scrutiny so that any important arrhythmias are detected and treated without delay. In many coronary care units, not only are the electrocardiographic features observed but continuous hemodynamic monitoring is carried out in patients with suspected pump failure.

It is believed that coronary care units have substantially reduced mortality from acute myocardial infarction in hospitals, mainly by the prevention of death from ventricular fibrillation, but also by the more skillful care of the patient with pump failure. However, because many patients die before reaching the coronary care unit, the concept of mobile coronary care has been developed. The mobile coronary care unit is a facility for bringing the principles and practices of coronary care units to patients wherever they may be, at home, in the street, or in the factory. The patients who probably benefit most from this are those who "drop dead" away from hospital and are kept alive initially by cardiopulmonary resuscitation until the mobile unit can arrive and give appropriate therapy. These units are usually staffed by highly trained paramedical personnel, who are authorized to give antiarrhythmic drugs and to carry out defibrillation, as necessary.

PREVENTION OF RECURRENT HEART ATTACKS.   Several approaches have been made to the prevention of recurrent heart attacks. The earliest of these involved the use of anticoagulant drugs such as warfarin. Although in some studies, there appeared to be a reduction in recurrent infarction, the risks of this form of therapy and the difficulty of controlling treatment have meant that the earlier enthusiasm for long-term anticoagulant therapy has dissipated. Recently, the use of sulfinpyrazone as a form of antithrombotic therapy appears to have reduced the incidence of recurrent heart attacks in patients who have recovered from myocardial infarction. Further information is needed before this form of therapy can be widely recommended.

As discussed in Ch. 363.4, there is evidence that certain beta-adrenergic blocking drugs, e.g., alprenolol, may reduce the incidence of death and, particularly, of sudden death in the months following an acute myocardial infarction. Whether these observations are applicable to propranolol is not yet known.

LATE COMPLICATIONS. Ventricular Aneurysm. A ventricular aneurysm has been defined as a protrusion of a localized portion of the external aspect of the ventricle accompanied by a corresponding protrusion of a ventricular cavity. Such aneurysms occur in 10 to 20 per cent of patients following acute myocardial infarction. They occur when the infarction affects the full thickness of the ventricular wall, which becomes extremely thinned and replaced by fibrosis. The asynergy adds to the load on an already impaired ventricle and may lead to cardiac failure. It is rare for aneurysms to rupture, and although they almost invariably contain organized clot, embolism is not common. They may be suspected clinically in any patient who, following a myocardial infarction, has persistent cardiac failure, a systemic embolism, or persistent arrhythmias. The characteristic physical sign is the presence of a palpable and visible systolic expansion in the anterior chest wall, giving rise to a double apical impulse. Third and fourth heart sounds are often present. The ECG usually shows evidence of old myocardial infarction, and in many cases there are large Q waves associated with persistent S-T segment elevation in the affected leads. The S-T elevation may become more pronounced on exercise. An abnormal rounded bulge may be seen on chest roentgenogram, but this is often absent. The diagnosis is best established by left cineventriculography, which shows the paradoxical movement of the affected area. If symptoms are troublesome, it should be removed surgically.

Postmyocardial Infarction Syndrome (Dressler's Syndrome). This syndrome occurs in 1 to 5 per cent of patients and usually begins one to six weeks after the onset of myocardial infarction. It is thought to be due to an autoimmune reaction to cardiac muscle damage and affects particularly the pericardium, pleura, and lungs. Pleural or pericardial pain is accompanied by malaise and pyrexia. Large effusions and tamponade are unusual, but anticoagulants should be discontinued because of the risk of hemopericardium. Many minor cases resolve spontaneously; but if severe symptoms persist, they can be brought under control quickly by corticosteroids or indomethacin.

Shoulder-Hand Syndrome. A small number of patients develop limitation of movement in the shoulder joint, especially the left, associated with pain and stiffness in the arm. There may also be swelling of the associated hand, the skin of which may become tense and shiny. It is less common than it used to be and is probably a consequence of prolonged immobility. It usually responds to physiotherapy.

Bigger, J. T., Jr., Dresdale, R. J., Heissenbuttel, R. H., Weld, F. M., and Wit, A. L.: Ventricular arrhythmias in ischemic heart disease: Mechanism, prevalence, significance, and management. Prog. Cardiovasc. Dis., 19:255, 1977.

Chatterjee, K., and Swan, H. J. C.: Hemodynamic profile of acute myocardial infarction. *In* Corday, E., and Swan, H. J. C. (eds.): Myocardial Infarction. Baltimore, Williams & Wilkins Company, 1973, Chap. 6.

Coronary Drug Project Research Group: Factors influencing long-term prognosis after recovery from myocardial infarction: Three-year figures of the coronary drug project. J. Chron. Dis., 27:267, 1974.

Fowler, N. O. (ed.): Treatment of acute myocardial infarction. *In* Cardiac Diagnosis and Treatment. 2nd ed. New York, Harper and Row, 1976, Chap. 35.

Meltzer, L. E., and Dunning, A. J. (eds.): Textbook of Coronary Care. Amsterdam, Excerpta Medica, 1972.

Multicentre International Study: Improvement in prognosis of myocardial infarction by long-term beta-adrenoreceptor blockade using practolol. Br. Med. J., 3:735, 1975.

Pantridge, J. F., Adgey, A. A. J., Geddes, J. S., and Webb, S. W.: The Acute Coronary Attack. London, Pitman Medical, 1975.

363.4. SUDDEN DEATH

Desmond G. Julian

Death is often sudden and unexpected. Every year almost half a million inhabitants of the United States die instantaneously or within 24 hours of the onset of fresh signs or symptoms. A high proportion of these succumb within less than half an hour of the onset of the final disorder. Nearly all these very rapid deaths are due to cardiovascular causes, predominantly coronary atherosclerosis. Other cardiac causes include aortic stenosis, cardiomyopathies, and various rare types of rhythm disorder, including Wolff-Parkinson-White syndrome and the prolonged Q-T syndromes. Noncardiac causes include cerebral hemorrhage; drug overdose, toxicity, or idiosyncrasy; pulmonary thromboembolism; and chronic obstructive pulmonary disease. Patients with chronic alcoholism may also die within a few hours of the onset of an acute illness.

MECHANISM OF SUDDEN CARDIOVASCULAR DEATH. Most cases of sudden death take place in circumstances in which the determination of the mechanism is impossible. However, a sufficient number of cases have been observed to occur under close observation and electrocardiographic monitoring to assert that the majority of sudden deaths are due to ventricular fibrillation. It is particularly common in patients dying with severe coronary atherosclerosis, either with or without an accompanying acute myocardial infarction. Ventricular asystole or extreme bradycardia may be responsible for death in some cases. This is relatively rare as a consequence of atherosclerosis but is more common in those with chronic heart block or the sick sinus syndrome. Death may also occur from a sudden reduction in cardiac output, as in acute massive pulmonary embolism, or from cardiac tamponade from such causes as acute pericarditis and cardiac rupture. Death often occurs suddenly in cases of severe aortic stenosis; the mechanism is not known in many cases, although arrhythmias are responsible for some. In others, it would appear to be due to sudden ventricular failure, and this may also be the cause of death in some patients with acute myocardial infarction. Acute vasodepressor reflexes may be responsible for some deaths, including those of the so-called "voodoo" type. In such cases, there may be a sudden reduction in arterial pressure and heart rate. Organic causes include pulmonary thromboembolism, carotid sinus syndrome, and primary pulmonary hypertension.

PREDICTION OF SUDDEN DEATH. The identification of

the person liable to sudden death is clearly important, as it is only by instituting prophylactic therapy in such individuals that the mortality of acute coronary disease can be substantially reduced. In general, it is true that the risk factors for sudden death are essentially the same as those for myocardial infarction, although heavy cigarette smokers may be at particular risk. The situation is different in those who have already sustained a myocardial infarction. The risk of sudden death in the months after infarction is particularly high in those who have evidence of serious left ventricular malfunction, such as cardiomegaly and persistent sinus tachycardia, in the convalescent phase; those who additionally show ventricular arrhythmias are especially vulnerable.

PREVENTION OF SUDDEN DEATH. Many people can be saved from sudden death by the prompt treatment of ventricular fibrillation. This is relatively easy in the emergency room or in the coronary care unit, but most sudden deaths take place away from hospital. Success in such cases depends on the rapid initiation of artificial ventilation and closed chest cardiac massage by lay or paramedical personnel until a defibrillator can be made available. There are now many areas where mobile coronary care is provided so that a defibrillator can be brought to the patient wherever cardiac arrest takes place. The value of such a scheme has been demonstrated particularly clearly in Seattle, where more than 50 patients each year are resuscitated successfully from ventricular fibrillation. This has required the organization of a very rapid response system operated by fire department paramedical personnel and, importantly, the training of a quarter of the whole population of the area in the techniques of cardiopulmonary resuscitation. Notwithstanding the impressive results, the consequent reduction in mortality from acute coronary heart attacks is probably of the order of only 5 to 8 per cent. More substantial reduction in sudden death must depend on preventive measures, either of coronary atherosclerosis or, more particularly, of ventricular fibrillation.

There is good evidence that one important factor in sudden death is the habit of smoking cigarettes. Stopping smoking appears to lead to a reduction in the risk of sudden death, certainly in those who have recovered from an infarction. There is also highly suggestive evidence that certain beta-adrenergic blocking drugs, e.g., alprenolol, can prevent sudden death in postinfarction patients. Whether this also applies to patients who have not had an infarction and whether other beta blockers are so effective have yet to be established. As yet, there is no definite evidence that coronary arterial surgery or the long-term use of antiarrhythmic drugs prevents sudden death.

Cobb, L. A., Baum, R. S., Alvarez, H., and Schaffer, W. A.: Resuscitation from out-of-hospital ventricular fibrillation: Four years' follow-up. Circulation (Suppl. 3), 51–52:223, 1975.

Goldstein, S.: Sudden Death and Coronary Heart Disease. Mount Kisco, N.Y., Futura Publishing Company, 1974.

Kannel, W. B., Doyle, J. T., McNamara, P. M., Quickenton, P., and Gordon, T.: Precursors of sudden coronary death. Circulation, 51:606, 1975.

Kuller, L., Cooper, M., and Perper, J.: Epidemiology of sudden death. Arch. Intern. Med., 129:714, 1972.

363.5. SURGICAL TREATMENT OF CORONARY ARTERY DISEASE

David C. Sabiston, Jr.

Although a number of surgical procedures have been devised to revascularize the myocardium, the development of the aortocoronary bypass graft during the past decade has made a remarkable impact on the management of ischemic heart disease. For the first time, significant numbers of patients with symptomatic coronary disease have undergone a direct surgical attack, and this procedure is currently the most common operation performed in the field of cardiac surgery. Although aortocoronary bypass grafts (CABG) have been supported by both cardiologists and surgeons with encouraging results, a cautious attitude nevertheless remains appropriate until a final assessment based upon long-term evaluation is available. Controversy continues concerning the effect of the CABG procedure on extending the life span of patients with symptomatic coronary disease, but there is general agreement that complete relief of anginal pain is achieved in the majority of patients. For specific anatomic lesions, such as significant stenosis of the left main coronary artery, it is also clear that patients managed surgically survive longer than those treated by medical means, as demonstrated in randomized studies.

A knowledge of the natural history of coronary atherosclerosis is of considerable importance in selecting the appropriate therapeutic approach, and a number of factors are of significance in evaluating the prognosis of a patient with angina pectoris. These factors include the number of coronary arteries involved, the severity and extent of the atherosclerotic lesions, the status of left ventricular performance, and the presence of associated conditions such as a valvular lesion or ventricular aneurysm. The prognosis in these patients is known to be adversely affected by several other factors, including a familial history of coronary disease, hypertension, diabetes, and a history of cigarette smoking.

Studies of the natural history of angina pectoris indicate that significant stenosis (greater than 70 per cent) of a *single* coronary artery is associated with a relatively low threat to life, the mortality in this group being in the range of 2 to 4 per cent each year. As the extent of the disease increases, the risk of death becomes greater such that with significant lesions in *two* main vessels the death rate increases to 7 to 8 per cent annually. For *three*-vessel disease, the annual mortality is even greater, being 10 to 15 per cent. Finally, for patients with *left main* coronary lesions, the death rate is even higher, leading to the position that nearly all patients with this condition are candidates for surgery.

SELECTION OF PATIENTS FOR SURGICAL THERAPY. It is difficult to state precisely the number of patients who are appropriate candidates for myocardial revascularization. However, it is generally estimated that some 20 per cent of those with angina do not obtain satisfactory pain relief by pharmacologic means alone. In some patients, drug intolerance becomes a problem, whereas in others the anginal pain is refractory to medication, especially in those with severe and diffuse coronary lesions. The most common indication for CABG is *relief of anginal pain,* and the majority of patients obtain complete relief, and all but a few of the remainder are considerably improved. In appropriate circumstances, CABG is also indicated for other manifestations of myocardial ischemia, including refractory cardiac dysrhythmias, preinfarction angina, and congestive heart failure in the presence of a ventricular aneurysm.

In selection of patients for myocardial revascularization, selective coronary arteriography is essential. The diseased vessels which are to be potentially grafted should have a reasonable lumen, and whenever possible the distal runoff should indicate a patent peripheral coronary bed. A coronary artery suitable for anastomosis should have a diameter of at least 1 mm. If extensive intrinsic disease is present in the distal coronary arteries, the postoperative result is apt to be unsatisfactory. Experience has shown that in 80 to 90 per cent of patients with symptomatic coronary disease the anatomy *is* appropriate for direct aortocoronary grafts. The majority of surgical candidates have several significant lesions in the proximal portions of the major coronary arteries, which are potentially correctable by a graft. It should be emphasized that in patients with *complete* occlusion of a proximal coronary artery the collateral circulation at the time of arteriography may be inadequate to opacify the vessel distally despite the fact that a lumen is present, as studies have demonstrated that a significant number of distal vessels which do not opacify can be shown to be patent at the time of operation or autopsy.

In addition to selective coronary arteriography, cardiac catheterization frequently adds many data of importance for an understanding of the total hemodynamic status. Such studies are not only helpful but often essential in objectively documenting left ventricular function. Cardiac catheterization reveals the status of left ventricular wall motion and also provides an assessment of the aortic and mitral valves. Certain features are associated with an *increased* surgical risk; these include cardiomegaly, a low ejection fraction (below 25 per cent), an increased left ventricular volume, a large arteriovenous oxygen difference (greater than 6 volumes per cent), and, to a lesser extent, an elevated left ventricular end-diastolic pressure. It should be emphasized, however, that the presence of any of these abnormalities does not necessarily represent a contraindication to operation or to a successful result.

The use of noninvasive radionuclide angiography has simplified the diagnostic approach, and with this technique it is possible to obtain objective values for ventricular volume, ejection fraction, cardiac output, and left ventricular wall motion not only at rest but during exercise. Thallium injections, which demonstrate ischemia during exertion, and ventricular function studies, which demonstrate a deterioration of ejection fraction and local abnormalities of wall motion, enhance ability to recognize ischemia by noninvasive techniques and to assess the significance of coronary arterial lesions demonstrated by angiography. With the use of a bicycle ergometer, the cardiodynamic status can be assessed both at rest and — of more importance — during graded exercise. Such data provide very helpful information in the total assessment of myocardial function and of the potential role of myocardial revascularization.

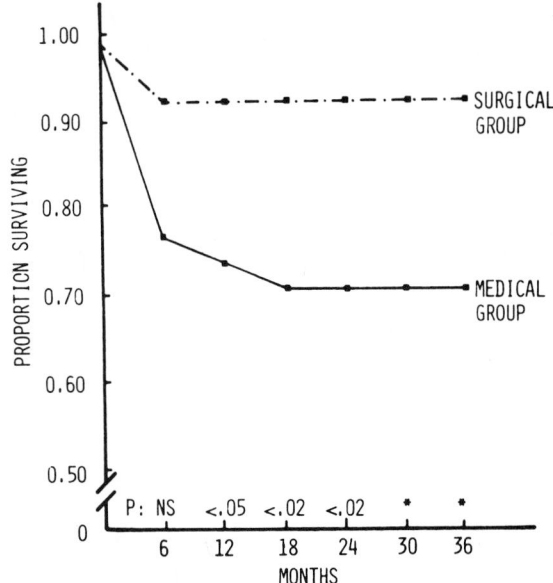

Accumulative survival rates of 83 patients with significant lesions of the left main coronary artery, who were randomly allocated into medical or surgical treatment groups in 1972, 1973, and 1974. There were 41 patients in the medical group and 42 patients in the surgical group. (From Takaro, T., Hultgren, H. N., Lipton, M. J., and Detre, K. M., and Participants in the Study Group: Circulation [Suppl. 3], 54:107, 1976.)

Significant stenosis of the *left main* coronary artery is known to be associated with considerable risk, and several studies have confirmed the fact that the death rate ranges up to 50 per cent in the two-year period following diagnosis by arteriography (Cohen et al.). In another study of 30 patients with left main arterial lesions, among those in whom operation was not performed the mortality was 33 per cent, with all deaths occurring within a month after arteriography. In an important and frequently cited cooperative study conducted by Veterans Administration Hospitals, 83 patients with critical stenosis of the left main coronary artery were randomized into surgical and medical groups for a three-year period. In the 41 patients in the medical group, 70 per cent survived, whereas among the 42 patients managed surgically, the survival was 93 per cent (see accompanying figure).

Left ventricular *aneurysms* may follow myocardial infarction and are hazardous both for the paradoxical dilatation which occurs during systole, producing cardiac inefficiency, and also as a source of systemic arterial embolism. These aneurysms may also be the site of electrical instability and cause refractory dysrhythmias.

Urgent or emergency aortocoronary bypass grafts have been recommended for patients with impending myocardial infarction (preinfarction or unstable angina) with good results. Nevertheless, others prefer to withhold operation for these patients until a procedure can be done electively.

Several groups have made an intensive effort to reduce the mortality of *acute* myocardial infarction associated with intractable *shock* with modest success. An immediate CABG procedure is performed, often combined with resection of ventricular wall for either dyskinesia or frank aneurysm formation. In this situation, the use of an intra-aortic balloon pump for diastolic augmentation has been extremely helpful. Despite the salvage made in some of these patients, the surgical mortality remains high and emergency operation in the immediate postinfarction period is generally not recommended. Most believe that myocardial revascularization is indicated for the survivors who have persistent refractory angina, with performance of the procedure three to six months following the infarct.

Another complication of myocardial infarction, which may require surgical intervention, is an acquired *ventricular septal defect*. These lesions develop in 1 to 2 per cent of patients following infarction, and the prognosis is quite poor unless operation is performed. In one series of 157 patients, 24 per cent died on the first day, 65 per cent by the end of two weeks, and 81 per cent at two months. Only 7 per cent survived a year after the development of the ventricular septal defect. Since the natural history is very poor, surgical closure is indicated in nearly all patients. When possible, it is preferable to allow the infarct to heal to permit the edges of the defect to become fibrotic and permit a better repair. Intractable heart failure often ensues following the development of these defects, and earlier or even urgent operation may be necessary. *Multiple* ventricular defects are present in approximately a third of patients and should be carefully sought at operation. The defect is generally closed with the use of a plastic prosthesis, and coronary bypass procedures may also be necessary in order to provide adequate ventricular function. If early operation is mandatory, the results are less favorable than for those who are able to survive for several weeks with elective scheduling of the operative procedures.

SURGICAL PROCEDURES. For most patients undergoing a CABG procedure, an *autologous vein* is anastomosed between the ascending aorta and the coronary artery distal to the obstruction. The saphenous vein is usually chosen, and the vessel is reversed to permit blood flow in the direction of open valves. Extracorporeal circulation is used to assure a quiet heart and to permit a careful coronary arterial anastomosis to be performed. It is well recognized that meticulous attention to detail is essential in making the anastomosis if a good postoperative result is to be obtained. The use of a very fine monofilament suture, often placed with the use of magnifying lenses, has been quite helpful in achieving long-term patency in these small vessels. It has also been shown that all major coronary arteries with significant stenoses should be grafted if the best results are to be obtained. Moderate total body hypothermia is usually employed, and the temperature of the heart may be further lowered by infusion of a potassium solution at 4° C to produce cardioplegia. During the procedure, the heart can also be continuously surrounded by cold saline or ice slush. The cardioplegia produces a flaccid heart, and the hypothermia simultaneously reduces the oxygen consumption to a very low level, preventing ischemic cellular changes within the myocardium. After placement of the coronary grafts, intraoperative electromagnetic flowmeter determinations have shown that significant volumes of blood flow through the anastomoses. Average flows for right coronary grafts are approximately 60 ml per minute (range of 28 to 150 ml), for the anterior descending coronary artery 80 ml per minute (range of 20 to 160 ml), and for the circumflex artery 75 ml per minute (range of 60 to

90 ml). In some patients with severe lesions and with borderline ventricular performance, the use of an intra-aortic balloon from the beginning of the operative procedure has been found helpful. This device is also of considerable importance in weaning difficult patients from cardiopulmonary bypass following the revascularization procedure. In those with extensive disease, the heart may be unable to assume a normal cardiac output immediately, and an intra-aortic balloon pump may be necessary for a period of several hours or days, during which time cardiac function improves sufficiently to maintain the circulation. Its use under these circumstances has clearly led to improved survival. In extenuating circumstances, this device has been used up to several weeks with successful results.

In the recent past there has been an increasing awareness of the association of severe coronary artery disease in patients who present primarily with disorders of the aortic and mitral valves. In these individuals, a surgical attack on the valve alone may be inadequate, and a simultaneous CABG for coronary lesions may be necessary. Similarly, patients with infarction of the papillary muscle and resulting mitral insufficiency often require a CABG procedure in addition to replacement of the mitral valve.

While autologous veins are chosen for the bypass graft in most patients, the internal mammary artery may be used in appropriate circumstances. In some reports, long-term patency has been greater in this vessel than with venous grafts.

POSTOPERATIVE MANAGEMENT. A number of postoperative problems may arise in patients following myocardial revascularization, and prompt diagnosis and immediate therapy are of prime importance. Adequate oxygenation is essential, and the endotracheal tube is generally left in place for the first day to assure adequate ventilation by a respirator. The effectiveness of the ventilatory support should be assessed by blood gas measurements, including Po_2, Pco_2, and pH. The cardiac output should be maintained at a normal level by continuous monitoring of central venous pressure, systemic arterial pressure, the electrocardiogram, and urinary output. Determinations of cardiac output are also important, especially if doubt exists concerning the circulatory status. Should a *low cardiac output syndrome* develop postoperatively, isoproterenol, dopamine, nitroprusside, and other agents should be employed as necessary with careful and continuous monitoring, including pulmonary artery diastolic and left atrial pressures. Cardiac dysrhythmias are common and may require the use of appropriate drugs or electrical cardioversion.

Myocardial infarction following CABG is usually reported in the range of 5 to 15 per cent, and in some series has been higher. The incidence of perioperative myocardial infarction is largely dependent upon the sensitivity of the diagnostic tests employed. For example, when CPK-MB isoenzyme activity is determined, the incidence of intraoperative and perioperative myocardial infarction is generally 30 per cent or more, as this determination is quite sensitive. This contrasts with an incidence of 15 per cent or less in studies in which new Q wave development is the primary criterion upon which the infarction is based. It is interesting that the presence of a perioperative myocardial infarction is generally not dependent upon whether or not the segment of myocardium involved received a graft or, indeed, if the graft was patent postoperatively. Moreover, in most patients in whom perioperative infarction occurs, the clinical manifestations are minimal and the diagnosis is made primarily upon electrocardiographic and enzymatic changes. It is relatively unusual for such patients to experience the signs and symptoms of a clinical myocardial infarction in the characteristic sense. In other words, in the majority of these patients, the infarction might well be unrecognized were it not for the electrocardiographic alterations and changes in serum enzymes.

RESULTS. Although the surgical *mortality* in early reports following CABG ranged up to 12 per cent or more, the figure has fallen considerably in the last several years and is currently in the range of 1 to 2 per cent for patients with *uncomplicated* angina pectoris. The mortality is correspondingly higher in those with severe left ventricular dysfunction, ventricular aneurysms, or associated valvular disease.

Relief of Pain. In nearly all series, an excellent symptomatic response is obtained. In approximately 65 per cent of patients the angina is *completely* relieved with no further medication being required, and much improvement occurs in an additional 25 per cent. With the passage of time pathologic changes may occur in some of the vessels, both in the native coronary arteries and in the inserted grafts. Such changes may be responsible for reappearance of symptoms. When these are present, further clinical evaluation, including coronary arteriography, is indicated.

Graft Patency. The patency rate of venous grafts during the first year following operation approximates 90 per cent. Later, intimal fibrosis may occur in the vein graft and reduce its caliber or produce complete obstruction. The graft may also thrombose, and this is generally the cause of *early* graft failure. In addition, technical features at the site of the anastomosis such as kinking of the graft can produce obstruction. Nevertheless, the distinctive fibrous proliferation which occurs in these grafts is the most common cause of failure and has been described in detail. Of additional interest is the continuation of the basic atherosclerotic process which progresses in the coronary arteries. In one series of patients followed one to four years postoperatively with repeat arteriography, 55 per cent of the original lesions *proximal* to the graft had progressed, whereas only 7 per cent of lesions *distal* to the anastomosis progressed. In this series, 14 per cent of the ungrafted vessels showed progression of atherosclerosis (McLaughlin et al.).

Reoperation. If symptoms recur following myocardial revascularization, reoperation may be indicated. However, the technical problems of the procedure are appreciable, due primarily to epicardial scarring and fibrosis, which make difficult the dissection and anastomosis of the coronary arteries. In one group of 21 patients undergoing reoperation, 33 per cent obtained complete relief of angina, 29 per cent obtained partial relief, and in 38 per cent there was no change. It is therefore apparent that the results following reoperation are less satisfactory than for the original procedure. For this reason, careful consideration should be given the indication when a second CABG procedure is planned.

RESULTS OF MEDICAL VERSUS SURGICAL MANAGEMENT IN RANDOMIZED STUDIES. The preferred method for resolving a problem concerning a controversial form of therapy is its evaluation by a double-blind, randomized study. For surgical forms of therapy, the double-blind feature is generally not feasible, but a randomized study of medical versus surgical treatment can be appropriately undertaken. With this objective, a group of cardiologists and surgeons in a group of Veterans Administration Hospitals combined to perform a cooperative study of patients with ischemic heart disease (Murphy et al.). The patients were randomized to medical and surgical management in an effort to determine the effect upon survival. In a series of 596 patients, 310 were managed by medical means and 286 were randomized to the surgical group. In the latter group a CABG procedure was performed, and the operative mortality at 30 days was 5.6 per cent. At an average of one year following operation, 69 per cent of the grafts were patent and 88 per cent had at least one patent graft. At 36 months, 87 per cent of the medical group and 88 per cent of the surgical group were alive.

This study has been the subject of much interest and considerable controversy, because the results suggest that the CABG procedure does not increase the life span when compared randomly with patients managed medically. Supporters and critics of this study have been numerous, and the principal points of view have been concisely summarized. Controversies of this type frequently arise when the goal of therapy is not *cure*, but rather *improved quality of life*. It has been difficult to define objective criteria to assess the results of either medical or surgical therapy for this group of patients as a whole. Critics of the VA study call attention to the high operative mortality in the series (5.6 per cent) and of the low rate of graft patency (69 per cent at one year), especially when these figures are compared to those which currently prevail. Another criticism is that selectivity was involved in the VA study, with exclusion of patients with unstable angina, left main coronary disease, ventricular aneurysms, and generalized poor ventricular contraction, as well as patients with markedly increased end-diastolic pressure and a large left ventricle with a poor ejection fraction. By exclusion of such patients, the series may have been artificially weighted.

In summary, for those patients who fail to achieve relief of anginal pain despite adequate medical therapy, myocardial revascularization is indicated and can be performed with expectation of very favorable clinical results and a low mortality. In addition, patients known to have a poor prognosis with medical management alone, such as those with significant lesions of the left main coronary artery, are also candidates for revascularization and have been shown in randomized studies to have an improved life expectancy when compared with similar patients managed medically. In a consideration of the total group of patients with symptomatic myocardial ischemia, questions remain concerning the ultimate effect of revascularization upon the life span, and further long-term evaluation will be required before this problem is finally clarified.

Cohen, M. V., Cohn, P. F., Herman, M. V., and Gorlin, R.: Diagnosis and prognosis of main left coronary obstruction. Circulation (Suppl. 1), 45–46:57, 1972.

Daggett, W. M., Guyton, R. A., Mundth, E. D., Buckley, M. J., McEnany, T., Gold, H. K., Leinbach, R. C., and Austen, W. G.: Surgery for postmyocardial infarct ventricular septal defect. Ann. Surg., 186:260, 1977.

Humphries, J. O.: Survival after myocardial infarction. Prognosis and management. Modern Concepts Cardiovasc. Dis., 46:51, 1977.

Kaiser, G. C., Marco, J. D., Barner, H. B., Codd, J. E., Laks, H., and Willman, V. L.: Intraaortic balloon assistance. Ann. Thorac. Surg., 21:487, 1976.

McLaughlin, P. R., Berman, N. D., Morton, B. C., McLoughlin, M. J., Aldridge, H. E., Adelman, A. G., Goldman, B. S., Trimble, A. S., and Morch, J. E.: Saphenous vein bypass grafting. Changes in native circulation and collaterals. Circulation (Suppl. 1), 51–52:66, 1975.

Murphy, M. L., Hultgren, H. N., Detre, K., Thomsen, J., Takaro, T., and participants of the Veterans Administration Cooperative Study: Treatment of chronic stable angina. A preliminary report of survival data of the randomized Veterans Administration Cooperative Study. N. Engl. J. Med., 297:621, 1977.

Rerych, S. K., Scholz, P. M., Newman, G. E., Sabiston, D. C., Jr., and Jones R. H.: Cardiac function at rest and during exercise in normals and in patients with coronary heart disease. Evaluation by radionuclide angiocardiography. Ann. Surg., 187:423, 1978.

Sabiston, D. C., Jr.: The coronary circulation. The William F. Rienhoff, Jr., Lecture. Johns Hopkins Med. J., 134:314, 1974.

364. CARDIAC ARRHYTHMIA

Anthony N. Damato

364.1. INTRODUCTION

Normally, the pacemaker of the heart is the sinoatrial (SA) node, which is an elongated structure (1.5 cm in length) located at the junction of the superior vena cava and the lateral border of the right atrium. In 55 per cent of cases the SA node receives its blood supply from the right coronary artery, and in 45 per cent of the cases, from the left circumflex artery. Cells of the SA node possess the property of automaticity which is responsible for the spontaneous rhythmicity of the heartbeat. Automatic or pacemaker cells undergo spontaneous diastolic depolarization (phase 4 depolarization) in contrast to nonautomatic or working myocardial cells which maintain a steady diastolic or resting potential. When an automatic cell achieves threshold potential, it undergoes depolarization and serves as the excitatory or depolarizing stimulus for adjacent cells. Increasing the rate of diastolic depolarization of sinoatrial nodal pacemaker cells increases the heart rate and vice versa. The property of spontaneous diastolic depolarization can also be found in certain cells of the atrium, atrioventricular (AV) junction, bundle branches, and Purkinje network, but not in ordinary working myocardial cells. These specialized cells serve as latent or potential pacemakers of the heart, and their rate of spontaneous diastolic depolarization is normally less than that of the sinoatrial node. However, if sinus node function is depressed, latent pacemaker activity can emerge and establish an escape rhythm. At other times, certain stimuli such as digitalis excess, ischemia, or hypoxia can enhance the rate of spontaneous diastolic depolarization of latent pacemakers beyond that of normal sinus node automaticity, which then results in an ectopic rhythm.

The transmission of impulses from the sinus node to the ventricles occurs along specialized conducting tissue which includes the AV node, the bundle of His (also called the common AV bundle), the right bundle branch, the left bundle branch, including its fascicular divisions, and the subendocardial Purkinje network. The bundle of His, bundle branches, and Purkinje network are commonly referred to as the His-Purkinje system or the ventricular specialized conducting system. In addition, three internodal connecting pathways (anterior, middle, and posterior internodal tracts) have been described which originate from the sinus node region and insert into different parts of the AV node.

Fibers from these internodal pathways also spread in various degrees from the right to the left atrium. It has been suggested by some investigators that transmission of the sinus node impulse to the AV node and between the atria is along these specialized and preferential pathways and not by radial spread alone. Internodal pathways have also been invoked to explain some cases of short P-R interval in which it is suspected that an atrial impulse either partially or completely bypasses the AV node during its conduction to the ventricles.

The AV node lies beneath the right atrial endocardium, anterior to the os of the coronary sinus, and above the insertion of the septal leaflet of the tricuspid valve. The human adult AV node measures between 5 and 7 mm in length, and its deep surface abuts the central fibrous body of the heart. Anteriorly, the AV node is directly continuous with the bundle of His. Most of the fibers of the internodal tracts, mentioned above, enter the superior and posterior margins of the AV node, and a smaller number of fibers enter along its lateral margin. Conduction velocity within the AV node is slow (0.05 meter per second), which accounts in part for the normal physiologic AV delay that is reflected in the P-R interval. In most human hearts, the AV node receives its blood supply from the right coronary artery, which explains the association of AV nodal conduction abnormalities seen in some cases of inferior or diaphragmatic myocardial infarctions.

The anterior and deep part of the AV node becomes the common AV bundle or bundle of His in which the muscle fibers are arranged in parallel. The bundle of His penetrates the collagenous central fibrous body and lies on the upper margin of the muscular interventricular septum. At the posterior margin of the membranous interventricular septum the common bundle gives off a relatively wide left bundle branch which courses over the left side of the interventricular septum. The left bundle branch divides into anterior and posterior fascicles which enter the anterior and posterior papillary muscles, respectively. In addition, fibers from the left bundle insert directly into the interventricular septum. On the right side of the heart, the common bundle continues as a slender right bundle branch which courses over the interventricular septum and enters the anterior papillary muscle. Peripheral arborization of the right and left bundle branches constitutes the Purkinje network. In contrast to the AV node, the velocity of conduction throughout the His-Purkinje system is more rapid, being within the order of 1.0 to 3.5 meters per second.

The AV node and the proximal portion of the bundle of HIs are in close anatomic relationship to the tricuspid and mitral valve rings. In addition, the distal part of the bundle of His and the proximal portions of the bundle branches lie in close proximity to the noncoronary artery aortic cusp. These anatomic relationships of the AV conducting system are important to bear in mind, because inflammation, fibrosis, or calcification of the valve rings or central fibrous body may cause different types of AV block.

The P-R interval represents a combination of intra-arterial, AV nodal, and His-Purkinje conduction times. Unfortunately, the electrical activities of the sinus node, AV node, bundle of His, bundle branches, and subendocardial Purkinje network are not recorded by the surface electrocardiogram. Figure 1 presents in a schematic way the electrical events occurring during the P-R in-

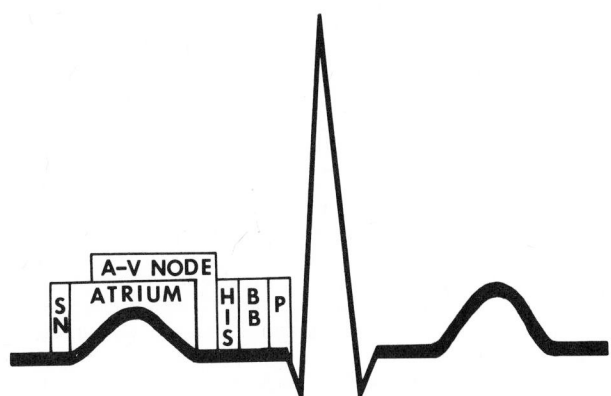

Figure 1. Schematic representation of the sequence of AV conduction in relationship to the P wave, P-R segment and QRS complex. SN = sinus node impulse; AV node = atrioventricular node; HIS = His bundle; BB = bundle branches; P = subendocardial Purkinje system. (Modified from Hoffman, B. F., and Singer, D. H.: Prog. Cardiovasc. Dis., 7:226, 1964.)

terval. The sinus node generates an impulse prior to the inscription of the P wave. As the atrial muscle is being depolarized (P wave), the sinus node impulse enters the AV node. Conduction within the bundle of His, bundle branches, and subendocardial Purkinje network occurs during the P-R segment. The QRS complex represents depolarization of the ventricular muscle.

It has become possible to record electrical activity of the bundle of His in man, using an electrode catheter which is fluoroscopically positioned in the region of the tricuspid valve. The electrode catheter records a low atrial electrogram (A), a His bundle deflection (H) which appears as a bi- or triphasic deflection within the P-R segment, and a ventricular electrogram (V) (Fig. 2). His bundle recordings permit division of the P-R interval into two subintervals, namely the A-H and H-V intervals. The A-H interval represents an approximation of AV nodal conduction time, and the H-V interval represents conduction time within the His-Purkinje system. Normal values for A-H and H-V inter-

Figure 2. Tracings from top to bottom are as follows: surface ECG; a recording from the high right atrium (HRA); His bundle electrogram recording (HBE); and time lines (T) at 10 and 100 msec. A = Low atrial electrogram; H = His bundle electrogram; V = ventricular electrogram. During sinus rhythm the sequence of activation is from the high to low atrium. During retrograde conduction across the AV node, the sequence of atrial activation is reversed; the low atrial electrogram precedes the high atrial electrogram.

vals have varied slightly as reported by different investigators, but in general are 60 to 140 msec and 30 to 55 msec, respectively. Bundle of His recordings provide a more precise method of localizing sites of AV conduction delay and block which may occur proximal to, within, or distal to the bundle of His. In addition, bundle of His recordings provide an accurate method for determining whether beats are of supraventricular or ventricular origin. Beats of supraventricular origin are preceded by His deflections with H-V intervals which are normal or greater than normal. In general, beats of ventricular origin are not preceded by His deflections.

364.2. ARRHYTHMIAS

SINUS ARRHYTHMIA

Sinus arrhythmia is characterized by irregular changes in the sinus rate which most often occur in relationship to the phases of respiration. The sinus rate increases at end inspiration and decreases at end expiration. The respiratory changes in sinus rate are believed to result from changes in vagal tone. Sinus arrhythmia is a normal phenomenon seen more frequently in children and young adults and tends to become less pronounced with increasing age. Electrocardiographically the P wave configuration is normal but may show slight changes in shape. The P-P intervals show cyclical increases and decreases in relation to the phase of respiration, whereas the P-R intervals remain fairly constant. Sinus arrhythmia requires no treatment.

SINUS BRADYCARDIA

Sinus bradycardia has been arbitrarily defined as a sinus rate of less than 60 per minute. It is a normal finding in a significant number of young healthy adults and is the expected finding in well trained athletes. Sinus bradycardia may result from administration of drugs such as digitalis, propranolol, morphine, reserpine, and prostigmine. Normal sinus rates return when these drugs are withdrawn. A temporary sinus bradycardia may occur during acute diaphragmatic myocardial infarction. Usually, sinus bradycardia is associated with normal AV conduction (1:1 AV response with a normal P-R interval). In older patients sinus bradycardia and AV block may coexist. Sinus bradycardia at rates of 40 per minute or less should raise the possibility of a 2:1 sinus node exit block, which is a rare phenomenon (see Fig. 4).

In general, sinus bradycardia requires no treatment. In most cases, the sinus rate shows a normal acceleration in response to exercise, atropine, or other appropriate stimuli. An inappropriate response to such stimuli raises the possibility of the sick sinus syndrome. If symptoms such as lightheadedness, syncope, congestive heart failure, or angina pectoris are the result of a low resting heart rate or inappropriate acceleration of the heart rate during stressful situations, a permanent ventricular pacemaker should be inserted.

SINUS TACHYCARDIA

For adults, sinus tachycardia is defined as a sinus rate in excess of 100 per minute. Most often, sinus tachycardia represents a normal physiologic response to stressful situations such as exercise, fright, emotional upset, fever, congestive heart failure, and hypotension. Under these conditions, the increase in sinus rate is generally associated with a normal or less than normal P-R interval, because the sympathetic stimuli causing sinus node acceleration also enhance AV nodal conduction. Vagolytic drugs, such as atropine, can also produce a sinus tachycardia. The treatment for sinus tachycardia is that of the underlying condition. Carotid sinus pressure will produce a temporary and incomplete slowing of the sinus rate which quickly returns to original levels. If sinus tachycardia is the result of congestive heart failure, digitalis will slow the sinus rate as the failure improves. However, digitalis will be ineffective in sinus tachycardia from other causes such as fever or thyrotoxicosis.

SICK SINUS SYNDROME

The sick sinus syndrome (SSS) refers to a variety of electrocardiographic abnormalities which result from dysfunction of the sinoatrial node. Included in SSS are the following:

1. Persistent, severe, or unexpected sinus bradycardia. At times, sinus bradycardia may alternate with episodes of supraventricular tachyarrhythmias, and this combination has been termed the bradycardia-tachycardia syndrome.

2. Sinoatrial block or exit block not related to drug therapy.

3. Sinus arrest (cessation of sinus rhythm) for short or long intervals, during which time either no escape rhythm arises or an atrial, junctional, or ventricular rhythm emerges.

These electrocardiographic abnormalities result because (1) the sinus node fails as an impulse generator, or (2) the sinus node impulse is delayed or blocked in its conduction out to the atrial muscle. Often, patients with SSS have an associated AV block or intraventricular conduction abnormality. The most commonly encountered symptoms in SSS are lightheadedness, dizziness, syncope, convulsions, dyspnea, fatigue, and angina pectoris.

Sinus Bradycardia

Sinus bradycardia may be the initial manifestation of SSS, and consequently not all sinus bradycardias are benign. SSS should be suspected when sinus bradycardia occurs in a symptomatic patient or is an inappropriate response to the clinical environs, such as during exercise, fever, pain, or congestive heart failure. Failure of the sinus rate to increase after atropine administration should raise the possibility of SSS, and further observations are indicated.

Bradycardia-Tachycardia Syndrome

The bradycardia-tachycardia syndrome is included in the spectrum of SSS and is characterized by sinus bradycardia alternating with episodes of atrial tachycardia, atrial fibrillation, or atrial flutter. The atrial tachycardia may be ectopic in origin or may result from AV nodal re-entry (Fig. 3). Symptoms may be related to either slow or rapid heart rates or both.

TREATMENT. Sinus bradycardia as a manifestation of SSS is generally, although not always, unresponsive to pharmacologic treatment. If belladonna alkaloids, atropine, or sympathomimetic amines are ineffectual in speeding up the sinus rate and the patient is symptomatic from the slow heart rate, a permanent ventricular pacemaker should be inserted. In the bradycardia-tachycardia syndrome the therapeutic problem is compounded by the fact that not only are agents such as procainamide and quinidine often ineffectual in controlling the atrial tachyarrhythmias, but these drugs may aggravate the sinus bradycardia. Likewise, digitalis, which can effectively slow the ventricular response during a period of supraventricular tachycardia, may also worsen the bradycardia. The most effective therapy to date has been the insertion of a permanent ventricular pacemaker by which the ventricular rate can be controlled and pharmacologic agents more safely administered to control the atrial arrhythmia.

SINOATRIAL BLOCK

The tissue surrounding the sinoatrial node normally imposes a conduction delay between the sinus node impulse and depolarization of the atrial myocardium. Disturbances in conduction of the sinus node impulse can take the form of first, second, or third degree SA block, all of which constitute uncommon manifestations of the clinical spectrum of SSS. Because of the inability to record the sinus node impulse in man, the diagnosis of SA block is an inferential one based primarily on the behavior of the P waves.

Figure 3. Bradycardia-tachycardia syndrome. After two sinus beats (rate, 45 per minute), two ectopic atrial beats occur, the second of which initiates an AV nodal re-entrant tachycardia. The initial part of the tachycardia shows aberrant ventricular conduction.

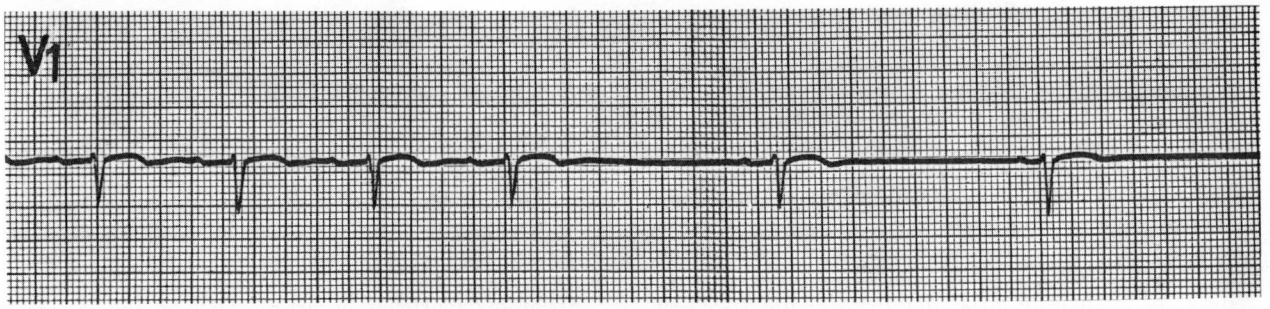

Figure 4. 2:1 SA exit block. The sinus rate is suddenly halved.

First Degree SA Block

In the first degree SA block the sinus node impulse is conducted more slowly out to the atrial myocardium. However, the clinical diagnosis of uncomplicated first-degree SA block cannot be made, because each sinus impulse elicits a P wave and the degree of delay is not reflected in the EKG recording.

Second Degree SA Block

Second degree SA block, like second degree AV block, has been classified into types I and II.

Type I Second Degree SA Block

In type I second degree SA block, sinoatrial conduction is of a Wenckebach type in which there is progressive conduction delay until a sinus node impulse fails to elicit a P wave. Like AV nodal Wenckebach cycles, the increment of SA conduction delay increases throughout the cycle so that the P-P intervals progressively shorten prior to the dropped wave. The P-P interval encompassing the dropped P wave is less than twice the P-P interval preceding the absent P wave.

Type II Second Degree SA Block

In type II second degree SA block, a sinus P wave is intermittently and unexpectedly dropped. The resultant pause is equal to twice the normal P-P interval. Atrial extrasystoles, which are hidden in the T wave and followed by a near compensatory pause, may simulate a type II SA block. In 2:1 SA block the normal sinus rate is halved. The resultant bradycardia is indistinguishable from the usual variety of sinus bradycardia unless an abrupt spontaneous doubling of the heart rate occurs (Fig. 4). Atrial bigeminy in which the ectopic P waves are masked by the T wave may simulate 2:1 SA block.

Third Degree SA Block

In third degree SA block, all the sinus impulses are blocked and there is absence of P waves. After a period of arrest, a subsidiary pacemaker located in the atrium, AV junction, or ventricles usually emerges as an escape rhythm. Third degree SA block is indistinguishable from sinus node arrest in which the pacemaker cells fail to generate impulses (Fig. 5).

Figure 5. Third degree SA block. After three sinus beats, the sinus node impulse either fails to be generated or to exit from the sinus node. An AV junctional pacemaker emerges, followed by resumption of sinus rhythm. During the AV junctional rhythm, the QRS complexes are similar to those of sinus origin.

ABERRATION

Ventricular aberration is defined as an alteration in the sequence of ventricular activation which results whenever an impulse of supraventricular origin is asynchronously conducted within the His-Purkinje system. Aberration results because a supraventricular impulse enters the His-Purkinje system during its refractory period. For atrial impulses the determinants of aberration include (1) the degree of prematurity of the atrial impulse; (2) the cycle length (R-R interval) preceding the premature atrial impulse; (3) the speed of AV nodal conduction; and (4) the state of recovery of excitability of the His-Purkinje system. In general, the more premature an atrial impulse, the greater the tendency for aberration to occur. Fast or relatively rapid AV nodal conduction enhances the possibility of aberration, because the premature atrial impulse can be delivered to the His-Purkinje system during its refractory period. However, at very close coupling intervals, aberrant ventricular activation may disappear if the premature atrial impulse encounters sufficient AV nodal delay that its arrival time within the His-Purkinje system is delayed and the latter is no longer refractory.

A direct relationship exists between cycle length (R-R interval) and refractoriness within the His-Purkinje system. Refractoriness of the His-Purkinje system increases with longer R-R intervals and decreases as the R-R interval shortens. A long R-R interval preceding a sufficiently premature atrial beat favors aberration, whereas decreasing the preceding cycle length may abolish aberration.

Aberrant conduction involving the right bundle branch is seen more commonly than aberration involving the left bundle branch. Given the right conditions, aberrant ventricular activation can occur in normal or abnormal hearts and therefore is not a sign of heart disease. Aberrant conduction of consecutive beats during a surpaventricular tachycardia can mimic a ventricular tachycardia. Examples of aberrant conduction of supraventricular impulses are shown in Figures 3, 6, and 8.

ATRIAL EXTRASYSTOLES

Atrial extrasystoles are premature depolarizations of the atria resulting from impulses which originate in ectopic foci located anywhere within the atria. Atrial extrasystoles are also referred to as premature atrial beats, premature atrial contractions, or premature atrial systoles.

Atrial extrasystoles result in P waves (P') which are different from sinus P waves. These differences, which may be marked or subtle, are due to an altered sequence of atrial activation resulting from an ectopic origin of the depolarizing impulse.

Atrial extrasystoles may have a constant or inconstant coupling interval to the preceding sinus beat and can occur in a bigeminal or trigeminal sequence. Three or more consecutive atrial extrasystoles occurring at a rate of 100 per minute or greater constitute an ectopic atrial tachycardia.

Atrial extrasystoles occurring late in the diastolic period may be associated with little or no AV conduction delay, in which case the P-R interval will be the same as or close to that of the sinus beats. Extrasystoles of greater prematurity are almost always associated with an increased P-R interval (relative to sinus beats), which may be due to conduction delay within the AV node, His-Purkinje system, or both.

Atrial extrasystoles may result in normal or aberrant ventricular activation, the determinants of which are discussed above. Aberrant ventricular activation may mimic premature ventricular extrasystoles if the premature atrial P' wave is not recognized or is obscured within the T wave of the preceding QRS complex (Fig. 6). Atrial extrasystoles which are not conducted to the ventricles may block within the AV node or His-Purkinje system. A nonconducted atrial extrasystole may result in prolongation of the P-R interval of one or more subsequent sinus beats — a phenomenon which is called concealed conduction.

Atrial extrasystoles generally invade and prematurely depolarize the sinus node pacemaker, causing a reset of the sinus cycle which is reflected in the pause that follows the atrial extrasystole. If the delay in the appearance of the postextrasystolic sinus beat equals the prematurity of the atrial extrasystole, the pause is said to be compensatory. In a fully compensatory pause, the sum of the pre- and postextrasystolic R-R intervals equals two sinus cycle lengths. Complete compensatory pauses are uncommonly associated with atrial extrasystoles. More often, one sees postextrasystolic pauses which are incompletely compensatory; that is, the sum of the pre- and postextrasystolic pauses is less than two sinus cycles. Occasionally, one may see significant suppression of sinus node automaticity after an extrasystole.

Atrial extrasystoles are common and may occur in completely normal individuals or may be associated with various types of organic heart disease. They may presage atrial fibrillation, atrial flutter, ectopic atrial ta-

Figure 6. The third, sixth, and ninth P waves (P') are atrial extrasystoles which occur with trigeminal regularity. The first and third atrial extrasystoles are aberrantly conducted to the ventricles. The second atrial extrasystole is blocked.

Figure 7. Untreated atrial fibrillation. There is absence of P waves with an irregular ventricular rate.

chycardias, or AV nodal re-entrant tachycardias. Very often, patients are unaware of the presence of infrequent atrial extrasystoles, and no special treatment is required. The patient may complain of "skipped beats" and "palpitations" which are the result of the pause and forceful ventricular contraction that follow the extrasystole. Mild sedation and abstinence from alcohol, tobacco, or caffeine may be all that is required to treat occasional extrasystoles which produce mild symptoms. Quinidine sulfate is used to treat atrial extrasystoles which cause disturbing symptoms, foreshadow other atrial arrhythmias, or are unabated by conservative measures.

ATRIAL FIBRILLATION

Atrial fibrillation is a frequently encountered cardiac arrhythmia which commonly occurs in association with some form of organic heart disease. Most cases of atrial fibrillation are associated with arteriosclerotic heart disease, followed in frequency by rheumatic and hypertensive heart disease. A high incidence of this rhythm disorder is seen in patients with thryotoxicosis. The greater tendency for enlarged atria to fibrillate may explain the frequent occurrence of atrial fibrillation in patients with congestive heart failure and mitral valvular disease. Atrial fibrillation, usually paroxysmal in nature, can occur in apparently healthy individuals who have no detectable evidence of associated heart disease.

The exact mechanism(s) underlying the development of atrial fibrillation is uncertain. Many of its characteristics are compatible with re-entry of multiple activation fronts. However, the fact that atrial fibrillation is frequently induced by premature atrial extrasystoles suggests that alterations in automaticity also play a role in the mechanism of this arrhythmia. Factors which favor the development and perpetuation of atrial fibrillation include frequent atrial extrasystoles, increased vagal tone, and an increase in atrial muscle mass wherein significant differences in conduction and refractoriness exist in adjacent fibers. Atrial fibrillation can be precipitated by a single atrial extrasystole which occurs in the so-called vulnerable period of the atrial cycle. At sinus cycle lengths the atrial vulnerable period has been estimated to be between 180 and 300 msec after a sinus P wave.

ELECTROCARDIOGRAPHIC FEATURES. Atrial fibrillation is characterized by absence of P waves and an irregular ventricular response. Normal sinus P waves are replaced by irregular chaotic and rapid atrial impulses occurring in excess of 400 per minute. The presence or absence of P waves is best observed in leads II and V_1. Atrial fibrillation has been described as "coarse" when the baseline of the electrocardiogram presents rapid, irregular fibrillatory (f) waves of varying amplitude, and "fine" when practically no atrial activity is detected. In untreated and uncomplicated atrial fibrillation, the irregular and rapid ventricular response is generally between 110 and 160 per minute, and most or all of the QRS complexes are of normal configuration for that patient (Fig. 7).

Concealed conduction within the AV node is the major determinant of the irregular R-R cycles during atrial fibrillation. The inherent capacity of the AV node to accept and transmit impulses to the ventricles is exceeded by the rapid, irregular atrial rate in atrial fibrillation. Consequently, many atrial impulses are blocked or concealed within the AV node, thereby altering its state of refractoriness which in turn affects the conduction of subsequent impulses. Impulses which exit from the AV node and enter the His-Purkinje system almost invariably result in a ventricular response. Uncommonly is the His-Purkinje system the site of concealment. Digitalis, propranolol, or increased vagal tone increases the degree of concealment or block within the AV node and thereby slows the ventricular response. The irregular R-R intervals during atrial fibrillation predispose to the occurrence of aberrant intraventricular conduction. In atrial fibrillation the distinction between aberrant conduction and ventricular ectopy is an important one which unfortunately is made more difficult because of the absence of P waves. The diagnosis of aberrant conduction is favored (80 per cent of the time) if the beat in question (1) has a right bundle branch block pattern, (2) terminates a short cycle which is preceded by a long cycle, and (3) has initial vector forces which are the same as known supraventricular beats. No single criterion or combination of criteria provides absolute evidence for the origin of any beat. The distinction can be made with bundle of His recordings. In atrial fibrillation with a rapid ventricular response, aberration may persist for many consecutive cycles and may simulate ventricular tachycardia. The occurrence of aberrant conduction during digitalis administration for atrial fibrillation is not a contraindication to continued use of the drug. In fact aberration usually disappears when the desired effect of ventricular slowing is achieved with digitalis. On the other hand, ventricular ectopy may signify digitalis toxicity or the presence of an additional dysrhythmic problem.

TREATMENT. Treatment of atrial fibrillation depends upon the urgency of the situation. If the irregular rapid ventricular response is causing severe dyspnea, hypotension, congestive heart failure, or severe anginal pain, conversion to normal sinus rhythm by DC countershock is the treatment of choice. DC countershock is contraindicated if it is suspected that digitalis intoxication is the cause of atrial fibrillation, which is uncommon. In less urgent situations, ventricular slowing is achieved with digitalis. Digoxin, 0.5 mg, is given intravenously and followed by a second dose in one half to one hour. If the ventricular rate is slowed (80 to 100 per minute), maintenance therapy of 0.25 mg digoxin per day is started. If the ventricular rate is not slowed within two hours of the initial dose, 0.25 mg digoxin is given every three to four hours until the desired effect is obtained. Infrequently, digitalis may convert atrial fibrillation to sinus rhythm. Propranolol may be used in conjunction with digitalis for those patients requiring excessive amounts of digitalis to slow the ventricular rate.

Once the ventricular rate is under control, consideration is given as to whether conversion to sinus rhythm is indicated. Conversion should not be attempted in those patients who have longstanding chronic atrial fibrillation, or in whom previous conversions have been unsuccessfully maintained. In some patients with severe heart disease, the loss of atrial contribution to the cardiac output may be significant, and conversion to sinus rhythm is necessary in order to avoid intractable heart failure. Patients with atrial fibrillation of recent onset should be converted to sinus rhythm, using either DC countershock or quinidine sulfate. The maintenance dose of digitalis should be withheld for one to two days prior to DC countershock.

ATRIAL FLUTTER

Atrial flutter is characterized by a rapid, regular atrial rate between 220 and 350 beats per minute. However, there is no universal agreement about which range of atrial rates specifically defines atrial flutter and separates it from an ectopic atrial tachycardia. There can be an overlap in the lower ranges of atrial rate; some ectopic atrial tachycardias may achieve trial rates of 220 beats per minute, whereas some cases of atrial flutter may be associated with rates of less than 220 beats per minute. Atrial flutter is almost always associated with some form of organic heart disease (coronary artery disease, cor pulmonale, rheumatic valvular disease), and rarely does it occur in normal healthy individuals. Digitalis is rarely a cause

of atrial flutter. Clinical symptoms associated with atrial flutter are related primarily to the ventricular response. Atrial flutter with a 3:1 or 4:1 AV conduction ratio may result in no symptoms, and the patient may be unaware of any dysrhythmia. On the other hand, during a 2:1 or a varying AV conduction ratio, the patient may experience palpitations, shortness of breath, anginal symptoms, or congestive heart failure.

ELECTROCARDIOGRAPHIC FEATURES. The following are the commonly found electrocardiographic features associated with atrial flutter: (1) the atrial rate is between 220 and 350 beats per minute; (2) the P waves are broad, bizarre atrial deflections which have been termed F waves; (3) leads II, III, and AVF show a "sawtooth effect with absence of an isoelectric period between flutter waves." One flutter wave appears to be merging directly with the next. The "sawtooth" effect may be absent in lead I and left-sided chest leads (v_5, V_6); (4) in most cases of atrial flutter, atrial activation is in a caudocranial direction; and (5) some degree of AV block exists which may be fixed, alternating, or variable. Many of the characteristic features associated with atrial flutter are presented in Figure 8.

A 1:1 AV response in atrial flutter is very uncommon, because atrial rates of 220 or greater generally exceed the inherent transmission capacity of the AV node. The presence of atrial flutter with a suspected 1:1 AV response should raise the possibility of an accessory or anomalous AV pathway such as exists in the Wolff-Parkinson-White syndrome. Conduction ratios of 2:1 or 4:1 are more commonly observed. Effective vagotonic maneuvers such as carotid sinus pressure temporarily increase the degree of AV block, permit a more positive identification of the atrial flutter waves, and do not significantly affect the atrial flutter rate. At times an increase in vagal tone which causes a shortening of atrial refractory period may convert atrial flutter to atrial fibrillation. By a similar mechanism, digitalis may convert atrial flutter to fibrillation.

TREATMENT. Direct current countershock is very effective in converting atrial flutter to sinus rhythm and is often the treatment of choice. Conversion can be achieved with low energy discharges. Direct current countershock is certainly the treatment of choice when the ventricular response is rapid and the patient is symptomatic.

Atrial pacing by means of an electrode catheter at rates slightly or greatly in excess of the inherent flutter rate has been used in the treatment of atrial flutter. Cessation of pacing may result in normal sinus rhythm or atrial fi-

Figure 8. Atrial flutter with varying degrees of AV block. In the middle of the tracing, a period of high degree AV block occurs, during which time the atrial flutter waves are more easily identified. The second to the sixth beats after the long pause are aberrantly conducted with a right bundle branch block pattern.

Figure 9. Re-entry within the AV node resulting in paroxysmal atrial tachycardia. In panels *A* and *B,* the tracings from top to bottom are electrocardiographic leads 1, 2, and V$_1$, a high right atrial electrogram (HRA), His bundle electrogram (HBE), and time lines (T) at 10 and 100 msec. In each panel, the first two beats are the last in a series of paced atrial beats at a constant cycle of 700 msec (A$_1$-A$_1$). The A-H and H-V intervals are 80 and 45 msec, respectively. Note that the sequence of atrial activation for paced atrial beats and sinus beats (fourth beat in Panel *A*) is from the high to low, right atrium. In Panel *A,* a premature atrial depolarization (A$_2$) is induced 390 msec after A$_1$. A$_2$ conducts with some AV nodal delay (A-H 110 msec), after which sinus rhythm resumes. In Panel *B,* A$_2$ is introduced 350 msec after A$_1$ and conducts more slowly through the AV node (A-H 250 msec). For this patient an AV nodal conduction time of 250 msec was apparently sufficient to induce an AV nodal re-entrant tachycardia at a cycle length of 345 msec. Note that during re-entry, atrial activation (Ae) occurs within the QRS complex and from the low to high right atrium.

brillation. Usually atrial fibrillation is not sustained and may convert to normal sinus rhythm in a matter of seconds or hours. The atrial pacing technique is useful when repeated DC shocks are required because of recurrent or persistent atrial flutter.

Digitalis and quinidine sulfate are the primary drugs used in the treatment of atrial flutter. Depending upon the urgency of the situation, digitalis may be given intravenously or orally. Its main function is to increase the degree of AV nodal block and to slow the ventricular rate. Rarely does digitalis convert atrial flutter directly to sinus rhythm; it may, however, convert flutter to atrial fibrillation, whereupon withdrawal of digitalis may re-establish sinus rhythm or atrial flutter may resume. Once the ventricular rate is controlled with digitalis, quinidine sulfate is given orally to convert the atrial flutter to sinus rhythm. It is preferred not to give quinidine initially without first digitalizing the patient, because quinidine may slow the atrial flutter rate, enhance AV nodal conduction, and precipitate dangerously rapid ventricular rates. If digitalis and quinidine are the primary therapies and prove to be unsuccessful, cardioversion by direct current countershock can be used but only after digitalis has been withheld for several days, because countershock and excessive amounts of digitalis may precipitate more serious ventricular dysrhythmias.

PAROXYSMAL ATRIAL TACHYCARDIA

Paroxysmal atrial tachycardia (PAT) is a relatively common arrhythmia. Several types of PAT are recognized which differ in etiology, underlying mechanism, and therapeutic approach. PAT may result from sustained re-entry within the AV junction or may be ectopic in origin. Three types of AV junctional re-entry have been reasonably well defined; these include AV nodal re-entry, re-entry utilizing a VA accessory pathway, and the Wolff-Parkinson-White syndrome (considered below). Undoubtedly, there are other types of junctional re-entries, but these appear less common and less well defined.

PAT Due to Sustained Reciprocation or Re-entry Within the AV Node

PAT that is due to AV nodal re-entry is seen in all age groups and frequently occurs in the absence of any clinically detectable heart disease. Characteristically, these tachycardias begin and terminate abruptly. During the tachycardia the patient may be keenly aware of a rapid heart rate and may complain of a fluttering within the chest or palpitations. Other associated symptoms include dyspnea, lightheadedness, or diaphoresis. Syncope may occur upon termination of the tachycardia if a sufficiently long pause follows prior to re-establishment of sinus rhythm or the occurrence of an escape beat. In patients with coronary artery disease, episodes of PAT may produce angina pectoris and significant S-T segment depression.

ELECTROCARDIOGRAPHIC FEATURES. Sustained re-entry within the AV node is almost always initiated by an atrial extrasystole. It is uncommon for this type of tachycardia to be precipitated by a ventricular extrasystole. If an atrial extrasystole encounters sufficient antegrade delay within the AV node (as indicated by a prolonged P-R or A-H interval), the impulse may at some point enter a nonrefractory pathway within the AV node and may be retrogradely transmitted back to the atria. If the retrogradely conducted impulse finds the antegrade pathway recovered, it may re-enter it, and the sequence is repeated, resulting in sustained reciprocation and a paroxysmal atrial tachycardia (Fig. 9).

During the reciprocating tachycardia, the atria are retrogradely activated. The P waves are inverted in leads II, III, and AVF and most often occur during the inscription of the QRS complex. The rate of these tachycardias is generally between 150 and 250 per minute. Aberrant conduction may occur for the first few beats or may persist for the entire episode of the tachycardia, thereby mimicking a ventricular tachycardia.

Perpetuation of a re-entrant tachycardia depends primarily upon a balance of refractoriness and conduction between the reciprocating limbs within the AV node. Consequently, any intervention which alters AV nodal conduction or refractoriness can terminate these tachycardias. Abrupt termination of these tachycardias can be achieved by increasing vagal tone with carotid sinus massage, gagging, Valsalva maneuvers, or raising the blood pressure. Propranolol and digitalis, both of which increase AV nodal conduction time and refractoriness, have been used successfully to treat AV nodal re-entrant tachycardias.

Prophylactic therapy could be directed toward eliminating atrial extrasystoles, which are the most frequent initiating cause, or toward altering refractoriness and conduction within the AV node. Quinidine can be used to eliminate atrial extrasystoles, whereas digitalis alone or in combination with propranolol can be used to affect the AV node.

PAT Due to Re-entry via a V-A Accessory Pathway

Evidence has accumulated supporting the idea that there exist within the AV junction accessory pathways which conduct unidirectionally, i.e., from ventricles to atria. These VA accessory pathways, located at the base of the heart, may be right or left sided; they differ (at least functionally) from the classic Kent bundles of the Wolff-Parkinson-White syndrome in that there is no antegrade conduction and hence no telltale sign of a delta wave. It is estimated that approximately 20 per cent of patients previously thought to have PAT due to AV nodal re-entry represent re-entry due to a V-A accessory pathway.

It is thought that during sinus rhythm, atrial impulses block at or within the atrial end of the accessory pathway, leaving it refractory even for retrograde conduction after the ventricles are activated. However, if a properly timed atrial extrasystole encounters sufficient AV delay, the accessory pathway may recover after the ventricles are activated and permit retrograde conduction back to the atria. Recovery of the AV node for anterograde conduction would then set the stage for a re-entrant tachycardia to occur. The AV conduction delay may be within the AV node (long P-R interval) or within the bundle branch (aberrant conduction) ipsilateral to the site of the accessory pathway. The basal location of these pathways means that the atria are retrogradely activated after the inscription of the QRS complex. Thus re-entry via a VA accessory pathway should be suspected in any patient in whom the inverted P waves (leads II, III, and AVF) during a PAT appear after the QRS complex (Fig. 10). In most cases of PAT due to AV nodal re-entry, the retrograde P waves are within the QRS complex (compare Figs. 9 and 10). Properly timed ventricular extrasystoles may also initiate re-entrant tachycardias if the impulse is retrogradely conducted to the atria via the VA accessory pathway and simultaneously blocked in the bundle branch AV nodal pathways.

Evidence that one is dealing with a VA accessory pathway can be obtained from electrophysiologic studies, using His bundle recordings and the ventricular extrastimulus technique. In patients with VA accessory pathways, a closely coupled premature ventricular extrasystole will result in atrial activation prior to the ventricular impulse depolarizing the bundle of His.

Therapy for re-entry via a VA accessory pathway is similar to that for AV nodal re-entry. Therapy may be directed toward abolishing atrial or ventricular extrasystoles (quinidine, procainamide) or altering the conducting characteristics of the AV node (digitalis, propranolol).

Ectopic Atrial Tachycardia

Areas within the atria but outside the sinus node can serve as the pacemaker of the heart. Depolarization of the atria by an ectopic atrial pacemaker in excess of 100 beats per minute constitutes an ectopic atrial tachycardia. The atrial rates of most ectopic tachycardias are between 150 and 220 per minute. The tachycardias may be sustained for long periods of time or occur in paroxysms lasting seconds to hours. Ectopic atrial tachycardias can occur in all forms of heart disease. They may occur in association with digitalis toxicity, chronic obstructive lung disease, or enlarged diseased atria, or may be associated with no apparent heart disease.

ELECTROCARDIOGRAPHIC FEATURES. In ectopic atrial tachycardias the configuration of the P waves is different from that of sinus beats. If all the ectopic P waves are of the same size and shape, it is called unifocal ectopic atrial tachycardia. A multifocal ectopic tachycardia is one in which the ectopic atrial impulses arise from different parts of the atria, and consequently the configuration of P waves varies.

Depending upon the atrial rate and the capacity of the AV node to transmit impulses to the ventricle, ectopic atrial tachycardias may be associated with 1:1 AV conduction with normal or prolonged AV conduction times, AV nodal Wenckebach cycles, or 2:1 AV block. Digitalis toxicity is a frequent cause of rapid unifocal ectopic atrial tachycardias with 2:1 AV block (Fig. 11). Multifocal ectopic atrial tachycardias are frequently associated with chronic obstructive lung disease or marked atrial disease and may precipitate atrial fibrillation.

The differentiation between paroxysmal atrial tachycardias caused by AV nodal re-entry from a unifocal ectopic tachycardia may at times be difficult. Tachycardias

Figure 10. PAT in a patient with a VA accessory pathway. In panels *A* and *B*, the tracings from top to bottom are as follows: electrocardiographic leads 2 and V₁, a high right atrial electrogram (HRA), His bundle electrogram (HBE), and time lines at 10 and 100 msec. In each panel the first two beats are of sinus node origin with upright P waves in lead 2, a high to low sequence of atrial activation, AV nodal conduction time of 165 msec, and His-Purkinje conduction time of 45 msec. In panel *A*, a premature atrial depolarization (P′ or A₂) introduced 300 msec after the sinus beat (A₁) is conducted with an AV nodal delay of 380 msec. After activation of the ventricles sinus rhythm resumes. In panel *B*, a slightly earlier atrial extrasystole (P′ or A₂) encounters greater AV nodal delay as indicated by an A-H interval of 440 msec, which for this patient was sufficient to initiate a re-entrant tachycardia at a cycle length of 520 msec. Note that atrial activation occurs after the inscription of the QRS complex and is from the low to high right atrium, and that the P waves are inverted in lead 2. Atrial activation during the tachycardia is indicated by a P* on the surface ECG and by Ae on the intracardiac recordings.

associated with inverted P waves in leads II, III, and AVF favor re-entry within the AV node as the mechanism but do not exclude a rhythm of ectopic origin. Upright P waves in these same leads strongly suggest an ectopic tachycardia. If the configuration of the P waves during the tachycardia is the same as the initiating atrial extrasystole, ectopy is favored, especially if the P waves are upright in leads II, III, and AVF. If the initiating atrial extrasystole is upright in II, III, and AVF and inverted in these same leads during the tachycardia, re-entry is likely. Abrupt termination of the atrial tachycardia by carotid sinus massage or an electrically induced atrial extrasystole favors a mechanism of AV nodal re-entry. These maneuvers generally produce a temporary slowing or pause in the ectopic atrial tachycardia, followed by resumption of its inherent firing rate.

TREATMENT. The treatment of digitalis-induced ectopic atrial tachycardias is withdrawal of the cardiac gly-coside and administration of potassium supplements. Treatment of ectopic tachycardias in patients with chronic obstructive lung disease should first be directed toward correcting hypoxemia, hypercapnia, acid-base imbalance, or other metabolic imbalances, which frequently are present and are the initiating cause of these rhythm disturbances. Ectopic atrial tachycardias or other causes should be treated with either quinidine or procainamide.

VENTRICULAR EXTRASYSTOLES

Ventricular extrasystoles (ventricular premature beats, contractions, or systoles) are a common occurrence in patients with and without heart disease. In young healthy individuals, the incidence varies between 0.5 and 2.0 per cent. They may be caused by emotional stress, tobacco, alcohol, caffeine, anoxia, sympathomimetic

Figure 11. Digitalis-induced atrial tachycardia with 2:1 AV block.

Figure 12. Ventricular bigeminy. A single premature ventricular extrasystole is coupled at a constant interval to each sinus beat.

drugs, or exercise. They are associated with all forms of heart disease and occur frequently (up to 80 per cent) in patients with acute myocardial infarction. Digitalis excess is a common cause of ventricular extrasystoles, especially if hypokalemia is present. Patients with occasional or even frequent ventricular extrasystoles may be completely unaware of their presence. On the other hand, some patients complain of "pauses," "palpitations," or "thumping" in the chest.

ELECTROCARDIOGRAPHIC FEATURES. Ventricular extrasystoles are characterized by wide QRS complexes (0.12 sec) with S-T and T wave changes. They may occur early or late in the cardiac cycle and very often have a constant coupling interval to the preceding sinus beat. The coupling interval is considered constant if the variation is within 0.08 sec (80 msec). A single ventricular extrasystole occurring after each sinus beat is referred to as ventricular bigeminy (Fig. 12). The term trigeminy refers to repeat cycles of either two sinus beats followed by a single extrasystole or one sinus beat followed by two consecutive ventricular extrasystoles.

Recurrent ventricular extrasystoles which always exhibit the same QRS morphology are referred to as unifocal in origin (arising from the same ectopic focus), whereas recurrent extrasystoles of different morphologies are termed multifocal in origin. Ventricular extrasystoles can arise anywhere within the bundle branch–Purkinje network. Extrasystoles arising from the left side of the conduction system result in QRS complexes which resemble right bundle branch block patterns, and those arising from the right side result in QRS complexes resembling a left bundle branch block pattern. Infrequently, extrasystolic impulses may arise high in one of the bundle branches, close to the bundle of His, and conduct with slight asynchrony down both bundle branches, resulting in narrow QRS complexes.

Most ventricular extrasystoles occur late in the cardiac cycle, i.e., after completion of the T wave of the preceding sinus beat, and are frequently coupled to the preceding sinus beat by a fairly constant interval. Less commonly, ventricular extrasystoles occur in early diastole, near the peak of the T wave or on its descending limb. This has been called the R on T phenomenon; it may reflect a very serious situation, because extrasystoles occurring near the so-called vulnerable period of the ventricle may lead to ventricular tachycardia or ventricular fibrillation.

Ventricular extrasystoles may be associated with various types of retrograde conduction patterns. The more common of these patterns include the following:

1. Complete retrograde conduction may occur across the AV conducting system, resulting in premature retrograde depolarization of the atria with inverted P waves in leads II, III, and AVF.

2. The extrasystolic impulse may retrogradely block within the AV node. This may result in the phenomenon of retrograde concealed conduction in which the next sinus impulse either is blocked or conducts with a P-R interval longer than sinus beats.

3. During prolonged retrograde AV nodal conduction delay, the extrasystolic impulse may reciprocate within the AV node and return to the ventricles, producing a ventricular echo beat.

4. Very premature extrasystolic impulses may retrogradely block within the His-Purkinje system. This type of retrograde conduction pattern cannot be determined from the electrocardiogram.

TREATMENT. The treatment of ventricular extrasystoles depends upon their cause, the underlying cardiac condition, severity of symptoms, their frequency, the coupling interval, and whether they are unifocal or multifocal in origin.

Ventricular extrasystoles which are related to emotional upsets, tobacco, alcohol, or sympathomimetic drugs may require only reassurance, mild sedation, or abstinence. Withholding of digitalis therapy for one or more days, in conjunction with oral potassium supplements, may be all that is necessary to treat extrasystoles caused by excess digitalis.

Ventricular extrasystoles occurring during an acute myocardial infarction require antiarrhythmic therapy. Therapy is urgently indicated if the extrasystoles have a close coupling interval, occur at a rate of five or more per minute, or are multifocal in origin. Irrespective of the underlying cardiac condition, antiarrhythmic therapy is indicated for ventricular extrasystoles which demonstrate the R on T phenomenon, are multifocal in origin, or occur consecutively in pairs.

VENTRICULAR TACHYCARDIA

Three or more consecutive beats occurring at rates greater than 100 per minute and arising from a focus located below the bundle of His constitute an episode of ventricular tachycardia. Most ventricular tachycardias occur at rates between 120 and 180 beats per minute; they may occur in paroxysms lasting a few seconds to several minutes or may persist for hours or days. Ventricular tachycardia is almost always associated with some form of organic heart disease, the most common being arteriosclerotic, rheumatic, and hypertensive heart diseases. As many as 50 per cent of patients with acute myocardial infarction may have one or more episodes of ventricular tachycardia of varying duration. Toxic doses of digitalis are a common cause of ventricular tachycardia. Other precipitating causes of paroxysmal ventricular tachycardia include hypoxia, hypokalemia, exercise, drugs (such as epinephrine, quinidine, and procainamide), cardiac catheterization of either the right or left heart, and anesthetic agents (cyclopropane, chloroform). Ventricular aneurysms may be the cause of recurrent or drug-resistant ventricular tachycardias.

Paroxysmal ventricular tachycardia has been reported to occur in young patients (less than 30 years old) in whom no evidence of heart disease could be detected. In this group, some attacks have been demonstrated to occur during exercise or emotional stress, implying a relationship between increased sympathetic tone and the ventricular dysrhythmia. In other patients, no precipitating factor could be demonstrated.

ELECTROCARDIOGRAPHIC FEATURES. In ventricular tachycardia, the QRS complexes are wide (0.12 sec or greater) and bizarre, recurring regularly at rates over 100 per minute (usually 120 to 180). Since the pacemaker is located below the bundle of His (i.e., within the bundle branches or Purkinje network), ventricular tachycardia is characterized electrophysiologically by the absence of a His bundle electrogram preceding the onset of ventricular activation. The bundle of His is retrogradely activated, and although in most cases it is not discernible, it is located within the ventricular electrogram. Initiation of the tachycardia may begin with a premature ventricular beat occurring close in time to the peak of the T wave of a preceding sinus beat; at other times, the initiating beat is located at the end of or after inscription of the T wave. Once initiated, ventricular tachycardia may be continuous for long periods of time or intermittent with one or more sinus beats interspersed (Fig. 13).

Often, it is extremely difficult to define the pattern of atrial activity during episodes of ventricular tachycardia from standard electrocardiographic tracings. Esophageal or intra-atrial recordings can be quite helpful in defining the frequency of atrial activity and its relationship to the QRS complexes.

During ventricular tachycardia, the atria may be dissociated from the ventricles, in which case independent P waves will be observed. At other times, various degrees of retrograde capture of the atria will occur (1:1, 2:1 retrograde Wenckebach cycles). If discernible, the P waves would be inverted in leads II, III, and AVF during retrograde activation of the atria.

An important and sometimes difficult clinical problem is the differentiation of supraventricular tachycardia with aberration from ventricular tachycardia. In aberrant conduction a His deflection with a normal or greater than normal H-V interval precedes ventricular activation, whereas in ventricular tachycardia there is absence of a His bundle electrogram preceding ventricular activation.

From the electrocardiographic point of view the presence of fusion beats during a sustained tachycardia provides strong supportive evidence that the rhythm in question is of ventricular origin. Fusion beats refer to partial activation of the ventricles by both supraventricular and ventricular impulses. During ventricular tachycardia, fusion beats may result because the atria are dissociated from the ventricles, and a sinus impulse occurring at an appropriate time in the cardiac cycle penetrates the AV conducting system and partially activates the ventricles; or during retrograde Wenckebach cycles, the impulse may reciprocate within the AV node and return to the ventricles, resulting in partial activation of that chamber. Complete activation or capture of the ventricles by either of the aforementioned mechanisms may terminate the tachycardia for one or more cycles, during which time sinus beats may appear, after which the tachycardia usually resumes.

A diagnosis of ventricular tachycardia is favored if one can discern independent atrial activity at a rate slower than the ventricular rate. On the other hand, supraventricular tachycardia with aberration is favored if carotid sinus pressure or other vagal maneuvers abruptly terminate the tachycardia.

TREATMENT. The choice and urgency of treatment for ventricular tachycardia depends on a number of factors, including its cause, the age and general condition of the patient, the severity and type of the underlying heart disease, blood pressure, and the state of consciousness. Causative factors such as hypoxia, hypokalemia, or other metabolic imbalances must be recognized and corrected.

DC countershock and drug therapy are the two commonly used methods for treating ventricular tachycardia. DC countershock is generally reserved for emergent situations in which the ventricular dysrhythmia is continuous or causes profound hemodynamic disturbances, or when drug therapy is ineffective. DC countershock is not the preferred treatment for ventricular tachycardias caused by digitalis toxicity.

Lidocaine is the most commonly used drug for the conversion of ventricular tachycardia to sinus rhythm. It is administered intravenously as a 50 to 100 mg bolus which can be repeated in two to three minutes if the initial injection is totally or partially ineffective. After suppression of the arrhythmia, lidocaine may be given as a continuous intravenous drip of 1 to 4 mg per minute. Ap-

Figure 13. A short episode of a unifocal ventricular tachycardia interspersed between periods of sinus rhythm.

Figure 14. Accelerated idioventricular rhythm which begins just prior to the fourth sinus P wave. The rates of the sinus node and idioventricular pacemakers are nearly identical, thereby resulting in a period of isorhythmic AV dissociation.

proximately 90 per cent of ventricular tachycardias can be suppressed at lidocaine blood levels of 2 to 4 μg per milliliter. The more common side effects of lidocaine include drowsiness, paresthesias, decrease in auditory acuity, agitation, and convulsions. Since lidocaine is metabolized by the liver, lower doses of the drug may cause side effects in patients with hepatic dysfunction.

Intravenous procainamide is also highly effective in the treatment of ventricular tachycardia. The drug can be administered at a rate of 25 to 50 mg per minute until either the tachycardia is terminated or 1000 mg has been administered. Most ventricular tachycardias are suppressed at blood concentrations of 4 to 8 μg per milliliter. Occasionally, higher concentrations are required. Continued suppression of the tachycardia can be achieved by a continuous intravenous drip at a rate of 2.5 mg per minute. Procainamide, like most antiarrhythmic drugs, may cause significant hypotension after intravenous administration, especially if the underlying myocardial dysfunction is severe. At other times the arrhythmia is the cause of a lowered blood pressure which improves when normal sinus rhythm is restored.

If lidocaine and procainamide are ineffective in controlling the arrhythmia, one can use diphenylhydantoin, propranolol, or quinidine sulfate. On occasion, a combination of drugs is required.

If ventricular tachycardia is associated with an underlying complete or high degree of AV block, an electrode catheter should be positioned within the right ventricular cavity and endocardial pacing initiated immediately upon terminating the ventricular tachycardia with drug therapy. This is required because effective drug therapy may suppress all idioventricular pacemaker activity and ventricular asystole may ensue.

ACCELERATED IDIOVENTRICULAR RHYTHMS

Accelerated idioventricular rhythms (AIVR) is a term applied to ectopic ventricular rhythms with rates intermediate between idioventricular escape rhythms (30 to 40 per minute) and ventricular tachycardia (120 to 180 per minute). Most frequently the rates are between 75 and 100 per minute. Accelerated idioventricular rhythms are commonly associated with myocardial infarction or digitalis toxicity. Current thinking holds that AIVR represents an enhancement of the normal escape rhythm of latent ventricular pacemakers. Like other ventricular rhythms, the QRS complexes are bizarre and wide (0.12 sec). The rate of the AIVR is usually close to that of the sinus rate, and consequently it becomes manifest when

sinus rhythm is slowed by an increasing vagal tone (carotid sinus massage) or premature atrial extrasystoles, or when some degree of AV block develops. AIVR usually begins late in the cardiac cycle, and it may start with a fusion beat (Fig. 14). AIVR may also begin early in the cardiac cycle. If dissociation between the atria and ventricles is present, fusion beats may occur frequently. If 1:1 retrograde conduction occurs, the AIVR may persist for long periods of time. Some patients manifest, at different times, episodes of AIVR and ventricular tachycardia in which the QRS morphology during both rhythm disturbances is the same. The AIVR may represent ventricular tachycardia with a degree of exit block from the ventricular focus. Acceleration of the sinus rate by atropine or atrial pacing usually suppresses the AIVR. AIVR can also be suppressed with lidocaine or procainamide. Treatment of AIVR is the same as that of ventricular tachycardia. Also, acceleration of the sinus rate by atropine or atrial pacing can and usually does suppress AIVR.

BIDIRECTIONAL TACHYCARDIA

Bidirectional tachycardia is an infrequently encountered arrhythmia which is characterized by (1) rapid regular rate of 140 to 180 beats per minute, (2) alternating rightward and leftward axis shifts in the frontal plane, and (3) a constant right bundle branch block pattern in lead V_1. Most bidirectional tachycardias occur in the presence of severe myocardial disease or digitalis toxicity and are associated with a poor prognosis. Hypokalemia has also been implicated as a cause of bidirectional ventricular tachycardia. Two different mechanisms have been proposed to explain the electrocardiographic pattern of bidirectional tachycardia. One suggested mechanism is that bidirectional tachycardia originates from a supraventricular tachycardia in which there is permanent aberrant conduction within the right bundle branch along with alternating aberrant conduction in the two divisions (anterior and posterior fascicles) of the left bundle branch. The other mechanism, confirmed by His bundle recordings, indicates that bidirectional tachycardia results from an ectopic focus located in the left ventricle, which would account for the permanent right bundle branch block pattern observed (Fig. 15). It is as yet unclear whether the alternating rightward and leftward axis shift is the result of alternating routes of ventricular activation by a single ectopic left ventricular focus of alternating discharge of two separate left ventricular foci. The treatment of bidirectional tachycardia is withdrawal of digitalis and administration of potassium and an antiarrhythmic agent such as lidocaine or diphenylhydantoin.

Figure 15. Bidirectional ventricular tachycardia. The first six QRS complexes show a persistent RBBB pattern in lead V_1 and alternating left and right axis deviation in lead 2. The ventricular origin of these beats is indicated by absence of a His deflection preceding the QRS complex. Ventricular activity is dissociated from atrial activity. The last beat shows a normally conducted atrial impulse with normal A-H and H-V intervals. (From Kastor, J. A., and Goldreyer, B. N.: Circulation, *48*:897, 1973. Copyright 1973, American Medical Association.)

VENTRICULAR FIBRILLATION

Ventricular fibrillation consists of rapid, disorganized, multifocal depolarizations of the ventricular myocardium. The absence of rhythmic coordinated muscular contractions produces a loss of the pumping action of the heart and causes a precipitous fall of the blood pressure to zero levels and unconsciousness. Ventricular fibrillation is most often seen in patients with significant underlying cardiac disease, especially ischemic heart disease. It may also occur in patients without clinical or pathologic evidence of heart disease. It may accompany digitalis toxicity, especially if hypokalemia or other metabolic imbalances are present. Quinidine sensitivity or toxicity may also be the cause of ventricular fibrillation. Ventricular extrasystoles occurring within the so-called vulnerable period of the ventricles (R on T phenomenon) may initiate ventricular fibrillation (Fig. 16).

The treatment of ventricular fibrillation must be prompt and decisive. The patient must be ventilated and defibrillated, using DC countershock at 400 watt-seconds.

AV DISSOCIATION

AV dissociation is a general term which describes any rhythm in which the atria and ventricles are independently activated by different pacemakers discharging at similar or dissimilar rates. The atria may be activated by either the sinus node or an ectopic atrial pacemaker, whereas the ventricles may be under the control of either a junctional or an idioventricular pacemaker. AV dissociation may occur with an essentially intact AV conduction system and may be of short duration, lasting for one or a few cardiac cycles, or it may persist for much longer periods. AV dissociation may be caused by (1) acceleration of a junctional or idioventricular pacemaker (Fig. 14), (2) slowing of an atrial pacemaker accompanied by an escape rhythm located in either the AV junction or ventricles, or (3) SA or AV block accompanied by an escape rhythm (Fig. 5).

Isorhythmic AV dissociation is one type of dissociated rhythm in which (1) the atria and ventricles are controlled by independent pacemakers discharging at equal or nearly equal rates, and (2) the P waves remain in close proximity to the QRS complexes; they may precede, occur simultaneously with, or follow the QRS complex. An example of isorhythmic AV dissociation in which the ventricles come under control of a junctional pacemaker is shown in Figure 17. As the atrial cycle length increases, the ventricles come under control of a junctional pacemaker, and the P waves which remain under control of the sinus node appear to be "marching" into the QRS complex and maintain a fixed R-P relationship, during which time the atria may remain under control of the sinus node or be retrogradely activated by the junctional pacemaker. After a variable period of time, acceleration of the sinus rate occurs, the P waves reappear in front of the QRS complex, and sinus rhythm is re-established. Sinus acceleration results from changes in baroreceptor activity, consequent to changes in arterial pressure or the

Figure 16. Ventricular fibrillation initiated by a rapid burst of ventricular activity (arrow).

Figure 17. Isorhythmic AV dissociation. After the first five sinus beats, the sinus rate slows and an AV junctional pacemaker emerges, starting with the sixth QRS complex. The atria continue to be activated by the sinus node, and the P waves are obscured within the QRS complex. In the bottom strip, accelerating forces cause an increase in the sinus node rate and sinus rhythm is reestablished.

effect of right atrial stretch, or both. Acceleration of the sinus rate is dependent upon the magnitude of these accelerating influences and the responsiveness of the sinus node.

JUNCTIONAL RHYTHMS

Traditionally, AV nodal rhythms have been described as arising from the upper, middle, or lower portions of the AV node. This classification has been based primarily on the relationship of inverted P waves (leads II, III, AVF) to the QRS complex. In upper AV nodal rhythms the inverted P wave precedes the QRS complex, whereas in middle or lower AV nodal rhythms the P wave occurs simultaneously with or follows the QRS complex, respectively. It has been recommended that the terms "junctional" or "AV junctional rhythms" replace that of "AV nodal rhythms," because (1) experimentally it has been difficult to consistently and convincingly demonstrate pacemaker activity (phase 4 depolarization) in all three regions of the AV node and (2) pacemaker activity in other areas of the heart (coronary sinus, left atrium, and bundle of His) can result in electrocardiographic patterns similar to those ascribed to AV nodal rhythms.

AV junctional rhythms are primarily escape rhythms with rates usually in the range 40 to 70 per minute. They become manifest if there is (1) significant sinus slowing, (2) AV block, or (3) SA block. If the discharge rate of the sinus node falls below that of a subsidiary junctional pacemaker, as may occur during sinus bradycardia or after premature discharge of the sinus node by an extrasystolic impulse, an area within the AV junction can take over as the pacemaker of the heart. In similar fashion, an escape junctional rhythm can emerge when sinus node impulses fail to conduct to surrounding atrial myocardium such as occurs in SA block (Fig. 5). Escape junctional rhythms also occur during AV block in which supraventricular impulses block in the AV node and proximal to the site of a junctional pacemaker (see Fig. 27). In complete AV block in which the nonconducted atrial impulses block below the bundle of His, the escape rhythms are located below the AV junction (idioventric-

ular pacemaker). AV junctional rhythms result in QRS complexes which are similar to those of sinus rhythm.

JUNCTIONAL EXTRASYSTOLES

Extrasystolic impulses arising from the AV node or bundle of His are referred to as junctional extrasystoles. Their occurrence late in the cardiac cycle results in normal QRS complexes which are not preceded by P waves. More premature extrasystolic impulses may result in aberrant ventricular conduction, producing a wide QRS complex which mimics a ventricular extrasystole. Closely coupled extrasystolic impulses may encounter anterograde refractoriness within the bundle branches (no QRS complex) and retrogradely block in the AV node. Retrograde concealment in the AV node may affect conduction of subsequent sinus impulses. A variety of AV conduction patterns may result, depending upon frequency, regularity, and coupling interval of these concealed junctional extrasystoles. These include (1) sudden and expected prolongation of a P-R interval, (2) type I second degree AV block, (3) type II second degree AV block, (4) 2:1 AV block, and (5) alternation of the P-R interval. Patients exhibiting type II second degree AV block produced by a concealed junctional extrasystolic impulse do not require pacemaker therapy. Concealed junctional extrasystoles may disappear spontaneously, or may be suppressed during exercise or administration of atropine. When they occur in patients receiving digitalis, withholding the glycoside for a few days may be all that is necessary. Lidocaine and procainamide are also effective treatment. Diagnosis of concealed junctional extrasystoles can be made when the aforementioned conduction abnormalities occur in ECG tracings along with junctional extrasystoles, which are conducted to the ventricles.

SYNDROME OF SHORT P-R INTERVAL, NORMAL QRS COMPLEXES, AND SUPRAVENTRICULAR TACHYCARDIAS
(Lown-Ganong-Levine Syndrome)

The syndrome of short P-R interval (0.12 sec or less), normal QRS complexes (0.10 sec), and paroxysmal supraventricular tachycardias is known as the Lown-Ganong-Levine syndrome. The mechanisms responsible for both the short P-R interval and the tachycardias have remained obscure. Several theories, based primarily on anatomic considerations, have been proposed to explain the short P-R interval. The most popular theory centers on the presence of specialized internodal pathways by which atrial impulses can partially or completely bypass the AV node. Recent electrophysiologic studies, using His bundle recordings and atrial pacing techniques, have shown that most cases of short P-R interval are associated with AV nodal conduction times which are at the lower range of normal values. The A-H intervals were 60 to 80 msec, whereas H-V intervals were between 30 and 55 msec. In addition, in most patients when the right atrium was stimulated at progressively increasing rates, the expected A-H interval increases were qualitatively similar to, but quantitatively less than, that observed for subjects with normal P-R intervals. In only an occasional patient with a short P-R interval was the A-H interval found to be less than 60 msec or did the A-H interval not increase as the paced atrial rate was increased. These limited data suggest that most cases of short P-R interval are due to an abbreviated AV nodal conduction time which could be due to (1) atrial impulses partially bypassing the AV node (? specialized internodal tracts), (2) an anatomically small AV node, (3) preferential intranodal pathways, or (4) a combination of these. In only occasional patients are the electrophysiologic data compatible with a complete bypass of the AV node, accounting for the short P-R interval. It should be pointed out that prolonged periods of isorhythmic AV dissociation can mimic a short P-R interval with normal QRS complexes. Studies to date have shown that AV nodal re-entry is a common mechanism for the paroxysmal supraventricular tachycardias in this syndrome.

WOLFF-PARKINSON-WHITE SYNDROME

The electrocardiographic pattern of the Wolff-Parkinson-White syndrome is characterized by a short P-R interval (less than 0.12 sec) and a widened QRS complex, starting with an initial delta wave. This abnormal electrocardiographic pattern occurs in approximately 0.1 to 0.4 per cent of routine tracings. A significant number of patients exhibiting this pattern have episodes of supraventricular tachycardia. The Wolff-Parkinson-White syndrome may be associated with Ebstein's anomaly of the tricuspid valve and idiopathic hypertrophic subaortic stenosis (IHSS). Other terms used to describe this phenomenon include anomalous AV excitation, ventricular pre-excitation, and accessory AV conduction.

Over the years, many hypotheses have been put forth to explain the electrocardiographic findings in this syndrome. Currently, there is anatomic as well as electrophysiologic evidence indicating that atrial impulses pre-excite the ventricles via accessory bypass tracts composed of myocardial fibers which connect the atria and ventricles. These bypass tracts are referred to as bundles of Kent. Atrial impulses are simultaneously conducted to the ventricles via the normal AV nodal His-Purkinje conducting system and the accessory pathway. AV conduction via the latter results in shortening of the P-R interval, and pre-excitation of the ventricle produces the delta wave. In most cases, the QRS complex in the Wolff-Parkinson-White syndrome represents fusion activation, the delta wave being an expression of ventricular excitation via the accessory pathway, and the remaining portion of the QRS the result of excitation via the normal AV nodal His-Purkinje conducting system. If significant delay or block exists within the AV nodal His-Purkinje pathway, the QRS complex may represent one of total pre-excitation. Alternatively,

Figure 18. Wolff-Parkinson-White syndrome, showing Type A QRS complexes. The delta wave can be seen in almost all leads. The precordial leads resemble a right bundle branch block pattern. In leads 2, 3, and AVF the delta wave produces a Q wave which mimics a diaphragmatic myocardial infarction.

Figure 19. The first two QRS complexes show a Wolff-Parkinson-White type of ventricular excitation in which the delta wave (d) in leads II and III mimics a diaphragmatic myocardial infarction. Atrial impulses are also conducted along the AV nodal His-Purkinje system; bundle of His activation occurs at about the time of the onset of the delta wave. The third P wave (A₂) is premature and finds the accessory pathway refractory. Exclusive conduction along the AV nodal His-Purkinje system results in normal ventricular activation, followed by a re-entrant supraventricular tachycardia. Note the absence of electrocardiographic evidence of myocardial infarction.

if AV nodal conduction time is shortened, as may occur with increased sympathetic tone or during an isoproterenol infusion, activation of the ventricles by the AV nodal His-Purkinje system is increased and the QRS tends toward normalization. Anomalous AV excitation may be always present during sinus rhythm, or it may intermittently alternate with periods of normal activation. At times, anomalous AV excitation may mimic the electrocardiographic pattern of a myocardial infarction (Fig. 18). Bundle of His recordings in conjunction with atrial pacing techniques can establish the correct diagnosis (Fig. 19).

For a long time, the Wolff-Parkinson-White syndrome was divided into types A and B. In type A the accessory bundle crosses the AV sulcus on the left side, causing pre-excitation of the base of the left ventricle. The vector of the delta wave is directed anteriorly in all precordial leads (upright in V₁ V₆), and the QRS pattern resembles right bundle branch block pattern (Fig. 18). In type B, the accessory bundle pre-excites the lateral margin of the right ventricle and the initial delta forces are directed leftward and posteriorly, producing a biphasic or negative delta wave in V₁ and QRS complexes resembling the left bundle branch block pattern.

It is now known from intraoperative epicardial mapping studies that accessory pathways may be located at a variety of sites within the tricuspid and mitral annuli. Accessory pathways have been located in the anterior,

Figure 20. Patient with known Wolff-Parkinson-White syndrome who develops atrial fibrillation with rapid conduction over the accessory pathway (wide, negative QRS complexes). Intermittently, activation of the ventricles occurs over the normal AV nodal His-Purkinje system, producing upright QRS complexes of normal duration.

lateral, posterior (paraseptal), and medial aspects of the tricuspid annulus, as well as the anterior, lateral, and posterior (paraseptal) regions of the mitral annulus. On standard ECG tracings, pre-excitation of the ventricles from these various sites produces different delta wave vector forces which can be used to approximate the earliest site of epicardial excitation.

Supraventricular Tachycardias in Wolff-Parkinson-White Syndrome

Between 25 and 70 per cent of patients with Wolff-Parkinson-White type QRS complexes have episodes of supraventricular tachycardia, and most of these appear to be re-entrant in nature. However, it should be noted that atrial tachycardias which are ectopic in origin may also occur in these patients. Most re-entrant tachycardias occurring in the patients with the Wolf-Parkinson-White syndrome have normal QRS complexes with long P-R intervals and are initiated by premature atrial beats. Less commonly are re-entrant tachycardias associated with pre-excitation type QRS complexes.

There are two possible mechanisms to explain re-entrant supraventricular tachycardias with normal QRS complexes in patients with the Wolff-Parkinson-White syndrome. If a closely coupled premature atrial beat finds the accessory pathway refractory to antegrade conduction, it may traverse the AV nodal His-Purkinje conducting system (usually with some delay) and activate the ventricles, producing a normal QRS complex. If sufficient time has elapsed to permit recovery of excitability of the accessory pathway, retrograde conduction back to the atria will occur via the accessory pathway. If, after atrial activation, the AV nodal His-Purkinje conducting system has recovered, activation of the ventricles will follow and a self-sustaining re-entrant tachycardia will result (Fig. 19). Alternatively, a re-entrant supraventricular tachycardia with normal QRS complexes could be initiated by a premature ventricular beat which was retrogradely blocked within the His-Purkinje AV nodal conducting system but which retrogradely activated the atria via the accessory pathway. Recovery of excitability of the AV nodal His-Purkinje conducting system would allow antegrade conduction to ventricles to follow retrograde activation of the atria; if the process is repetitive, a sustained tachycardia with normal QRS complexes will result.

The second mechanism involved in producing re-entrant supraventricular tachycardias with normal QRS complexes is one in which reciprocation or re-entry occurs only within the AV node; the accessory pathway, although present, is not utilized in the re-entrant process. This type of re-entry is the same as that occurring in patients who have paroxysmal atrial tachycardia without Wolff-Parkinson-White complexes.

Re-entrant supraventricular tachycardias with pre-excitation type QRS complexes result when antegrade conduction occurs via the accessory pathway and the impulse is retrogradely returned to the atria via the AV nodal His-Purkinje pathway.

A potentially life-threatening situation may occur in patients with the Wolff-Parkinson-White syndrome who develop atria fibrillation (Fig. 20). Rapid irregular activation of the ventricles via the accessory pathway exclusively or both pathways simultaneously may lead to ventricular fibrillation. DC countershock is the treatment of choice in this situation.

TREATMENT. Most re-entrant tachycardias associated with the Wolff-Parkinson-White syndrome respond to vagotonic maneuvers such as carotid sinus stimulation, the Valsalva maneuver, or elevation of blood pressure (Fig. 21). Increased parasympathetic tone alters the re-entrant pathway by increasing refractoriness and delaying conduction within the AV node. Similarly, digitalis and propranolol can terminate re-entrant tachycardias by the same mechanism. DC countershock is reserved (1) for those tachycardias which are resistant to vagotonic maneuvers and require excessive amounts of drug therapy, (2) for those associated with very rapid ventricular responses and hemodynamic compromise, and (3) for atrial fibrillation with anterograde conduction over the accessory pathway.

Prophylactic drug therapy can be directed at (1) suppressing the atrial extrasystoles which are a common initiating cause of re-entrant tachycardias in the Wolff-Parkinson-White syndrome; quinidine sulfate may be used for this purpose; (2) altering refractoriness and conduction in the AV node so that re-entry cannot be sustained; digitalis and propranolol alone, or in combination, have been successfully used; or (3) altering conduction and refractoriness of the accessory pathway; procainamide or quinidine may be tried to accomplish this end. We have found digitalis, given daily with or

Figure 21. Paroxysmal atrial tachycardia in a patient with type A Wolff-Parkinson-White syndrome. Top tracing shows PAT with normal QRS complexes. Retrograde P waves are buried within the S-T segment. Bottom tracing depicts termination of the tachycardia by carotid sinus pressure with the characteristic QRS complexes of pre-excitation during the subsequent sinus rhythm.

Figure 22. First degree heart block due to AV nodal delay.

without propranolol, an effective form of therapy for most of our patients. Arrhythmias are either not sustained or more easily terminated by carotid sinus massage or Valsalva maneuvers.

A small percentage of patients with the Wolff-Parkinson-White syndrome have frequent severe episodes of supraventricular tachycardia which, in addition to causing disabling and life-threatening symptoms, are resistant to control by drug therapy alone. An operative procedure has been devised for surgically interrupting the anomalous atrioventricular bypass tract which can effectively prevent or significantly modify recurrences of tachycardias. Surgical therapy in these selective patients requires that the region of the anomalous bypass tract be localized by epicardial mapping studies.

Preoperative evaluation in these patients should be directed toward (1) documenting that the patients' symptoms are related to arrhythmias caused by the presence of a bypass tract; (2) documenting that the arrhythmias are resistant to single and combination drugs (blood levels of drugs should be obtained and side effects noted); and (3) determining whether any associated cardiac anomalies exist, such as Ebstein's anomaly of the tricuspid valve or IHSS. A preoperative electrophysiologic study should be performed with the following goals in mind: (1) Confirming the presence of an accessory pathway and presumptively localizing its site. Some patients may have more than one accessory pathway. (2) Identifying the nature of the arrhythmias which the patient is experiencing and the participation of the accessory pathway in those arrhythmias. (3) Characterizing the functional characteristics of both the accessory pathway and the normal AV nodal–His–Purkinje systems. Examining the effect of drugs on both the normal and accessory pathways. A postoperative electrophysiologic study should also be performed to determine the effectiveness of surgical interruption of the accessory pathway.

DISORDERS OF AV CONDUCTION

First Degree Heart Block

In adults a P-R interval of more than 0.20 sec constitutes electrocardiographic evidence of first degree heart block which most commonly (90 per cent or more) is due to conduction delay occurring within the AV node. First degree heart block in the presence of normal QRS complexes is almost always due to AV nodal conduction delay, an example of which is presented in Figure 22. Bundle of His recordings reveal that the A-H interval was

prolonged at 310 msec and His-Purkinje conduction time was within normal limits at 39 msec.

Drugs such as digitalis and propranolol cause P-R prolongation by delaying conduction within the AV node. Neither drug affects conduction within the His-Purkinje system to any significant degree. The A-H interval returns to normal when these drugs are discontinued. At times, first degree AV nodal block may alternate with periods of type I second degree AV block or 2:1 AV block. In general, no specific treatment for first degree AV block is required. In most patients an increase in sympathetic tone, such as occurs during exercise or vagal blockade by atropine (0.5 to 1.0 mg intravenously), causes a decrease in the A-H interval concomitant with an increase in sinus rate so that 1:1 AV conduction is maintained.

His-Purkinje Delay

Less commonly, first degree heart block is due solely to conduction delay within the His-Purkinje system. Figure 23 is an example of P-R prolongation and right bundle branch block in which AV nodal conduction (A-H interval) is within normal limits and His-Purkinje conduction time (H-V interval) is markedly prolonged at 90 msec. The presence of a prolonged H-V interval is almost always associated with a bundle branch block pattern or widened QRS complex. However, not all patients with a bundle branch block pattern have prolonged H-V intervals. A prolonged H-V interval (greater than 60 msec) in the presence of a bundle branch block pattern usually indicates that there is conduction delay within the contralateral bundle. In asymptomatic patients, no specific treatment is required.

AV Nodal Plus His-Purkinje Conduction Delay

First degree AV block may be due to conduction delays in both the AV node and His-Purkinje system.

Intra-His Bundle Delay

Conduction delay occurring within the bundle of His itself can cause a prolongation of the P-R interval. However, this is an uncommon cause of first degree heart block.

Second Degree AV Block

Second degree heart block has been classified into two types. Type I second degree heart block (Wenckebach phenomenon, Mobitz type I AV block) is electrocardio-

Figure 23. First degree heart block due to a prolonged H-V interval (90 msec) in a patient with right bundle branch block.

graphically characterized by a progressive prolongation in the P-R interval preceding a nonconducted atrial beat. After the nonconducted P wave, the P-R interval is shorter. Type II second degree AV block (Mobitz II) is electrocardiographically characterized by a constant P-R interval preceding an unexpected nonconducted atrial impulse.

Type I Second Degree AV Block

The electrocardiographic pattern of type I second degree AV block can result from Wenckebach type conduction occurring within (1) the AV node, (2) the bundle of His itself, or (3) the bundle branch–Purkinje system. Delay in the AV node is by far the most common cause (more than 90 per cent) of type I AV block. The next most common site is the bundle branch–Purkinje system, and the least common is the bundle of His itself.

Classically the AV nodal Wenckebach phenomenon is depicted as one in which the greatest increment in P-R interval occurs with the second beat of the Wenckebach cycle and thereafter progressively diminishes. This results in a decreasing R-R interval in the presence of increasing P-R intervals. Some AV nodal Wenckebach cycles do not follow this classic pattern, and the greatest increment in P-R interval may occur with the last conducted beat. Also, one may observe little or no change in the P-R interval for several beats throughout the cycle.

Figure 24 is an example of type I second degree AV block resulting from progressive conduction delay and block within the AV node. Type I AV block in the presence of normal QRS complexes is almost always AV nodal in origin. At times, the second beat of the Wenckebach

cycle may be aberrantly conducted to the ventricles. Aberrant conduction is favored by the fact that the nonconducted atrial impulse of the preceding Wenckebach cycle results in a long R-R interval. In a 3:2 AV nodal Wenckebach cycle, aberrant conduction of every second beat may simulate a ventricular bigeminy, especially if the P wave of the aberrant beat is obscured by the T wave of the preceding QRS complex.

Type I AV block occurring within the AV node may be associated with inferior wall myocardial infarctions or excessive digitalis administration, and in both of these situations the block is generally reversible. Small doses of atropine, which enhances AV nodal conduction, usually re-establish 1:1 AV conduction. However, in some cases atropine may increase the sinus rate without appreciably affecting AV nodal conduction, and higher degrees of AV block (2:1, 3:1) may result. In type I AV block of AV nodal origin, the ventricular rate is seldom slow enough to warrant aggressive drug therapy or temporary right ventricular endocardial pacing.

The electrocardiographic pattern of type I second degree AV block can also result from Wenckebach type conduction occurring within the His-Purkinje system, as illustrated in Figure 25. During 3:2 AV conduction in the presence of a fixed right bundle branch block pattern, a small increase in the P-R interval precedes a nonconducted P wave. The H-V interval increases from an initially abnormal value of 60 msec to 100 msec, indicating progressive conduction delay within the left bundle branch and the third P wave blocks within the His-Purkinje system. Patients exhibiting the findings illustrated in Figure 25 will also have intermittent periods of high degree (e.g., 2:1, 3:1) AV block within the His-Purkinje

Figure 24. Type I second degree AV block due to progressive conduction delay and block within the AV node.

Figure 25. Type I second degree AV block within the His-Purkinje system.

system, which accounts in part for their symptoms of fatigue, dizziness, and even syncope. Also, these patients almost invariably go on to develop complete AV block within the His-Purkinje system.

In the presence of a fixed bundle branch block pattern, the distinction, based solely on the ECG tracings, between type I second degree AV block occurring within the AV node and that of His-Purkinje origin may be quite difficult. In general, although not always, the increase in P-R interval from the first to the last of the conducted beats is significantly less in a His-Purkinje Wenckebach cycle than in an AV nodal Wenckebach cycle. However, when AV nodal Wenckebach type conduction is superimposed on a pre-existing first degree AV nodal block, the difference in P-R interval changes from the first to the last of the conducted beats may be of the magnitude seen with His-Purkinje Wenckebach cycles.

The least common site for the occurrence of Wenckebach type conduction is within the bundle of His itself. This phenomenon is characterized by the recording of two His deflections (H and H'), which signifies intra-His bundle conduction delay. As the P-R interval increases, the H-H' interval increases, and the nonconducted atrial impulse of the Wenckebach cycle is followed by only a single His deflection (H).

Type II Second Degree AV Block (Mobitz II)

Type II second degree AV block occurs less commonly than type I; it is almost always associated with a bundle branch block pattern and is a forerunner to complete AV block. The AV conduction ratio may be 3:2, 4:3, 5:4, and

so forth, and the P-R intervals preceding the nonconducted atrial beat are constant. His bundle recordings have consistently demonstrated that the site of block is within the His-Purkinje system. Figure 26 is a typical example of type II second degree AV block; a left bundle branch block pattern is present, and 3:2 AV conduction progresses to 2:1 AV block. The third P wave, which is unexpectedly blocked within the His-Purkinje system, is preceded by constant P-R intervals. A prolonged H-V interval of 76 msec in the presence of left bundle branch block indicates that a significant conduction delay also existed in the right bundle branch system.

In patients with type II second degree AV block, acceleration of the atrial rate by atropine, exercise, or atrial pacing generally leads to an increase in the degree of AV block within the His-Purkinje system. Lightheadedness, dizziness, fatigue, syncope, convulsions, and congestive heart failure are common symptoms and signs associated with type II AV block. The demonstration of type II AV block requires that a permanent ventricular pacemaker be inserted, because this form of block almost always progresses to complete AV block within a relatively short period of time.

During complete AV block, atrial impulses continue to block within the His-Purkinje system, and the ventricles come under the control of an idioventricular pacemaker discharging at a rate of 35 to 50 per minute (see Fig. 29). It is not unusual for patients with type II AV block which progresses to complete AV block to demonstrate 1:1 retrograde conduction during ventricular pacing at a rate faster than the sinus rate. This is called unidirectional block.

Figure 26. Type II second degree AV block in a patient with left bundle branch block and 3:2 AV conduction which progressed to 2:1 AV block. The third P wave is blocked within the His-Purkinje system.

Figure 27. 2:1 AV nodal block in a patient with normal QRS complexes.

2:1 AV Block

Like all other forms of AV block, 2:1 AV block may result from lesions in the AV node, bundle of His, or bundle branch–Purkinje system.

A fixed 2:1 AV block in the presence of normal QRS complexes is almost always due to AV nodal block, and the nonconducted P waves are not followed by bundle of His deflections (Fig. 27). The P-R interval of the conducted atrial impulses may be normal or prolonged. Uncommonly, 2:1 AV block with normal QRS complexes is due to block within the bundle of His itself. Each of the nonconducted atrial impulses is associated with a bundle of His deflection, and the P-R intervals of the conducted beats are normal.

In 2:1 AV block with a bundle branch block pattern, the localization of block by electrocardiographic recordings alone is difficult. In our experience, block within the His-Purkinje system is slightly more common than AV nodal block.

Third Degree AV Block

Third degree AV block (also referred to as complete AV block) may result from lesions located in the AV node, bundle of His, or bundle branch–Purkinje system.

In third degree AV nodal block (Fig. 28), atrial impulses are blocked within the AV node. The bundle of His usually emerges as the subsidiary or escape pacemaker, activating the ventricles at a rate of 40 to 60 per minute. Each QRS complex is preceded by a single His bundle deflection, and in general both the QRS complex and H-V intervals are the same as prior to the occurrence of AV block. Patients with complete AV nodal block and a junctional pacemaker (bundle of His) may remain asymptomatic for relatively longer periods of time, and therefore the mere presence of complete AV block is not an indication for pacemaker therapy. Junctional pacemakers generally increase their discharge rate in response to exercise or after administration of atropine.

Complete AV block within the bundle of His itself is characterized by nonconducted atrial impulses which are followed by a His bundle deflection (H) and QRS complexes which are preceded by His bundle deflections (H'). The QRS complexes may be normal or abnormal and the H'-V intervals normal (30 to 55 msec) or greater than normal. It is believed that the junctional pacemaker is located within the bundle of His but distal to the site of block. These patients may not demonstrate acceleration of their ventricular rates in response to exercise or atropine. This would not be surprising if the process which caused the intra-His bundle block also affected the autonomic innervation of the common bundle . In these cases the need for pacemaker therapy depends upon the patients' symptoms.

Complete AV block distal to the bundle of His is characterized by nonconducted atrial impulses which are followed by His bundle deflections and abnormal QRS complexes which are not preceded by His bundle deflections (Fig. 29). The subsidiary pacemaker is located somewhere within the bundle branch–Purkinje system, and its discharge rate is generally between 35 and 50 per minute. These patients are almost always symptomatic (fatigue, dyspnea, dizziness, syncope, congestive heart failure) and require permanent ventricular pacemaker therapy.

Functional or Physiologic AV Block

At sinus rates of 60 to 100 per minute, the spontaneous occurrence of various types of AV block usually represents an abnormal response of the AV conducting system. On the other hand, acceleration of the atrial rate in resting subjects, such as may occur with atrial flutter, with an ectopic atrial rhythm, or during electrical stimulation of the atrium, can result in various degrees of AV block which may be considered physiologic or functional in nature. Normally, the autonomic nervous system mediates a fine balance between atrial rate and AV nodal conduction. During exercise or other stressful situations, sympathetic stimulation simultaneously increases sinus

Figure 28. Third degree AV block. Atrial impulses are blocked within the AV node and dissociated from the ventricles. The latter come under control of a bundle of His pacemaker. H-V interval of 47 msec is within the normal range.

Figure 29. Third degree AV block within the His-Purkinje system. Nonconducted atrial impulses are followed by His bundle deflections. The wide QRS complexes come under control of a subjunctional pacemaker and are not preceded by bundle of His deflections.

rates and enhances AV nodal conduction so that there occurs little or no change in the P-R interval. During nonsympathetically mediated increases in atrial rate, the capacity of the AV node to transmit impulses to the ventricles is exceeded and a functional AV nodal block ensues.

Caracta, A. R., and Damato, A. N.: Significance of His bundle electrocardiography. In Fowler, N. O. (ed.): Cardiac Diagnosis and Treatment. New York, Harper & Row, 1976, pp. 979–1008.

Damato, A. N., Lau, S. H., and Bobb, G. A.: Cardiac arrhythmias simulated by concealed bundle of His extrasystoles in the dog. Circ. Res., 38:316, 1971.

Gallagher, J. J., Gilbert, M., Svensen, R. H., Sealy, W. C., Kassell, J., and Wallace, A. G.: Wolff-Parkinson-White syndrome. The problem, evaluation and surgical correction. Circulation, 51:767, 1975.

Gallagher, J. J., Svensen, R. H., Sealy, W. C., and Wallace, A. G.: The Wolff-Parkinson-White syndrome and the pre-excitation dysrhythmias. Medical and surgical management. Med. Clin. N. Am., 60:101, 1976.

Hoffman, B. F., and Cranefield, P. F.: Electrophysiology of the Heart. Mount Kisco, N. Y., Futura Publishing Company, 1976.

Narula, O. S.: His Bundle Electrocardiography and Clinical Electrophysiology. Philadelphia, F. A. Davis Company, 1975.

Rosen, K. M., Rahimtoola, S. H., and Gunnar, R.: Pseudo A-V block secondary to premature nonpropagated His bundle depolarizations. Documentation by His bundle recordings. Circulation, 42:367, 1970.

Wellens, H. J. J., Lie, K. I., and Janse, M. J.: The Conduction System of the Heart. Structure, Function and Clinical Implications. Philadelphia, Lea & Febiger, 1976.

364.3. ANTIARRHYTHMIC DRUGS

Several drugs, which may be administered singly or in combination, are available for the treatment of a variety of cardiac rhythm disturbances. Proper management of cardiac arrhythmias begins with a precise electrocardiographic diagnosis of the arrhythmia at hand. Equally important is knowledge of the clinical setting in which the rhythm disturbance is occurring. Prior to initiating therapy one should obtain the following information: Does the patient have heart disease, and, if so, to what extent? Are there initiating or contributing factors present which, if corrected, will either preclude the use of antiarrhythmic drugs or enhance their effectiveness (e.g., hypokalemia, hypoxia, acidosis, thyrotoxicosis, caffeine, amphetamines)? Does the patient have congestive heart failure or hypotension? Is this a recurrent arrhythmia, and, if so, what was the previous therapy and its effectiveness? Are there known intolerances to any antiarrhythmic drugs?

The effectiveness of a given drug regimen in treating arrhythmias will be enhanced if the physician has knowledge of the following aspects of a given drug: (1) sites(s) of action, (2) dosage, route, and rate of administration, (3) site of metabolism and route of excretion, (4) range of therapeutic plasma concentration, and (5) clinical and electrocardiographic manifestations of side effects or toxicity.

LIDOCAINE

This drug finds its greatest utility in the coronary care unit for the treatment of ventricular extrasystoles and ventricular tachycardia. It is ineffective in the treatment of atrial arrhythmias. Lidocaine is given initially as an intravenous bolus injection of 50 to 150 mg over a one- to two-minute period, followed by a constant infusion of 1 to 4 mg per minute. The pharmokinetics of lidocaine are such that following a single bolus injection there occurs within a few minutes a rapid decline in blood concentration to subtherapeutic levels. A constant infusion is used to maintain therapeutic blood levels between 0.5 and 5.0 μg per milliliter. As soon as it is established that the ventricular arrhythmia is under control, the infusion rate of lidocaine should be decreased to the minimal amount which will maintain control. Lidocaine is metabolized in the liver, and therefore patients who have liver dysfunction or decreased hepatic blood flow should receive lesser amounts of the drug and be more carefully observed for toxic effects.

Toxicity to lidocaine is not uncommon and is most frequently expressed as central nervous system effects. There include dizziness, paresthesias, confusion, agitation, muscle tremors, and seizures. Although toxic effects are most commonly seen when blood levels exceed 5.0 μg per milliliter, they may also be observed when blood levels are within the therapeutic range. This latter effect may be due to the accumulation of pharmacologically active metabolites of the drug.

PROCAINAMIDE

Procainamide is a very effective agent in the treatment of ventricular arrhythmias. When given intravenously, it is administered at a rate of 20 to 25 mg per minute until either the arrhythmia is abolished or a total of 1000 mg has been given. The width of the QRS complex should be monitored and the drug cautiously given after there is a 25 per cent widening over control values. If a 50 per cent widening of the QRS complex occurs without effect on the ventricular arrhythmia, one should stop the drug. After the acute intravenous therapy, a constant infusion of 1 to 5 mg per minute may be given. Most ventricular arrhythmias are controlled at serum concentrations between 4 and 8 mg per liter. Within this concentration range, toxic effects are minimal. Major toxicity begins to occur at serum concentrations above 8 mg per liter.

Procainamide can also be given orally on a long-term

basis for control of ventricular arrhythmias. In most clinical situations the drug is well absorbed from the gastrointestinal tract, with peak plasma concentrations occurring after one hour. In patients without significant cardiac, renal, or hepatic dysfunction, the serum half-life varies between 2 and 4 hours (mean, three hours). It has been demonstrated that dosing at an interval of every six hours produces wide fluctuations in plasma concentration, and therefore it is recommended that oral procainamide be given at intervals close to its half-life, i.e., every three to four hours. Some patients may need dosing at the shorter interval, whereas others demonstrate good control at a dosing schedule of every six or eight hours. N-acetylprocainamide (NAPA) is one of the metabolites of procainamide which has been reported to approximate the antiarrhythmic activity of the parent compound.

In urgent clinical situations, a priming dose of procainamide may be given in order to achieve adequate serum concentrations as quickly as possible. The loading dose is twice the three- to four-hour maintenance dose (i.e., load, 500 to 1000 mg). Forty to 70 per cent of the drug is excreted unchanged by the kidney, and therefore the dose may have to be modified in patients with renal disease. Side effects of procainamide include nausea, vomiting, fever, and skin rashes. The most troublesome side effect is the development of a lupus-like syndrome. Various reports indicate that between 20 and 75 per cent of patients taking procainamide develop positive ANA titers but only 5 to 30 per cent develop clinical symptoms. Symptoms usually remit with discontinuance of the drug. An ANA titer should be determined for each patient who is to receive prolonged procainamide therapy. If a positive titer develops, the drug should be stopped and a substitute drug given.

QUINIDINE

The electrophysiologic properties of quinidine are similar to those of procainamide. Quinidine appears to be more effective than procainamide against atrial arrhythmias but is equally effective against ventricular arrhythmias. Quinidine is primarily used as an oral agent; it may be administered intramuscularly and is rarely given parenterally. The primary indications for quinidine are (1) for the pharmacologic conversion of atrial flutter or fibrillation to sinus rhythm, (2) as prophylaxis in patients with paroxysmal atrial flutter, atrial fibrillation, or junctional re-entrant tachycardia, and (3) for suppression of ventricular arrhythmias.

Quinidine is rapidly and almost completely absorbed from the gastrointestinal tract. Absorption is better on an empty stomach. The drug is metabolized in the liver. Unchanged quinidine (25 to 50 per cent) and its metabolic products are excreted in the urine. The dosage of quinidine should be adjusted downward in patients who have liver dysfunction or renal disease. With short-acting preparations of quinidine, peak blood levels are achieved in one to three hours; long-acting preparations achieve peak levels in approximately four hours. Therapeutic blood levels range from 2 to 7 mg per liter. An average oral dose of quinidine is 400 mg every six to eight hours (range, 100 to 600 mg).

The electrocardiographic alterations resulting from quinidine are a prolongation of the QRS and Q-T intervals. These occur because quinidine increases conduction and refractoriness in the His-Purkinje system. Quinidine can be given to patients who have a pre-existing bundle branch block pattern.

Quinidine is vagolytic and as such can cause an increase in the sinus rate and enhance AV nodal conduction. It is this latter effect which requires that patients with atrial fibrillation or flutter be given digitalis prior to being given quinidine, lest the ventricular response increase to an undesirable level. In atrial flutter, the ventricular response may increase because quinidine both slows the atrial rate and enhances AV nodal conduction. Quinidine can cause hypotension by decreasing myocardial contractility and causing vasodilatation.

So-called quinidine syncope is a major but fortunately uncommon complication of therapy. Self-limiting episodes of ventricular tachycardia or ventricular fibrillation have been demonstrated to be a cause of quinidine syncope. Gastrointestinal toxicity includes anorexia, nausea, and vomiting. Diarrhea is the most common adverse effect. High blood levels may cause tinnitus, vertigo, and nausea (cinchonism). In a fair number of cases, quinidine causes thrombocytopenia.

PROPRANOLOL

Propranolol is a beta-adrenergic receptor blocking drug which has as its major electrophysiologic effects slowing of the sinus rate and AV nodal conduction time. As an antiarrhythmic agent the drug has its greatest usefulness in the following situations: (1) in cases of atrial fibrillation and atrial flutter in which the ventricular response cannot be controlled by digitalis alone or when digitalis is contraindicated, (2) as acute or prophylactic therapy in cases of AV junctional re-entrant tachycardias, and (3) for suppression of ventricular extrasystoles and ventricular tachycardia, especially those suspected of being due to excessive catecholamines or increased sympathetic tone. In most cases of ventricular arrhythmias, propranolol is not the first drug of choice.

Propranolol may be given orally or parenterally. It is almost completely absorbed form the gastrointestinal tract, with peak effect occurring in one to one and a half hours. Oral therapy is given every four to six hours. Since sympathetic tone varies considerably among individuals, the clinically effective dose varies from patient to patient (usual range, 20 to 80 mg four times per day). When given intravenously, the drug is administered at a rate of 1 mg per minute up to a maximum of 10 mg.* As with any intravenous therapy for cardiac arrhythmias, ECG and blood pressure monitoring should be performed.

Propranolol has a negative inotropic effect and may aggravate or precipitate heart failure in patients with borderline cardiac function. It may cause significant sinus bradycardia or hypotension or may intensify AV block. Beta-adrenergic blockade causes bronchial constriction, and therefore the drug is contraindicated in patients with bronchial asthma and chronic obstructive lung disease. Propranolol may mask the premonitory signs of hypoglycemia in patients with diabetes mellitus.

DIPHENYLHYDANTOIN†
(Phenytoin)

Diphenylhydantoin (DPH) is an anticonvulsant drug which has been shown to have cardiac antiarrhythmic

---

*See p. vi, Dosage Notice, immediately following Preface.
†Experimental drug for this purpose.

effects. Its effects on the electrophysiologic properties of the heart are similar to those of lidocaine and appear to be opposite to those of procainamide and quinidine. DPH has been shown to be effective against ventricular extrasystoles and tachycardia caused by digitalis and other agents. It is ineffective in converting atrial flutter or fibrillation to sinus rhythm. Effectiveness has been demonstrated in the treatment of atrial arrhythmias resulting from digitalis excess. DPH is not a first line drug; it is primarily used when other drugs have failed or when combination therapy is required. DPH may be given intravenously or orally. Intravenous administration should be at a rate of 20 mg per minute until (1) the arrhythmia is abolished, (2) 1000 mg has been given, or (3) serious side effects occur. Oral administration may be rapid or slow. To attain therapeutic blood levels rapidly by the oral route, 1000 mg is given within 24 hours, followed by 500 to 600 mg per day for two days. Thereafter, maintenance doses of 300 to 500 mg are given daily. If one starts by giving 300 to 500 mg per day, therapeutic blood levels will be attained in five to seven days. Therapeutic plasma levels are between 10 and 18 μg per milliliter. Toxic effects are generally seen at >20 μg per milliliter.

DPH is metabolized in the liver, and the dosage should be adjusted downward in patients who have liver dysfunction or decreased hepatic blood flow. The administration of usual doses of DPH in combination with isoniazid and aminosalicylic acid has resulted in toxic levels of DPH. Barbiturates increase microsomal enzyme activity, which accelerates the rate of DPH metabolism, causing diminished pharmacologic activity. Parenteral DPH may cause drowsiness, nystagmus, circumoral tingling, vertigo, nausea, and vomiting. Too rapid injection of DPH (>50 mg per minute) may cause cardiovascular collapse.

DISOPYRAMIDE

Disopyramide phosphate (Norpace) is an antiarrhythmic agent which has recently been approved for oral use. Its electrophysiologic actions appear to be similar to those of quinidine sulfate. Disopyramide is reported to be effective in the treatment of unifocal and multifocal ventricular extrasystoles and ventricular tachycardia. The usual adult dosage is 400 to 800 mg per day given in divided doses four times daily. Disopyramide is rapidly and almost completely absorbed from the gastrointestinal tract. Peak plasma levels are achieved within two hours of dosing. Therapeutic plasma levels are 2 to 4 μg per milliliter. Fifty per cent of the drug is excreted in the urine unchanged, and dosage should be lowered in patients with renal or hepatic impairment. The more common adverse effects are associated with the anticholinergic properties of the drug, which include dry mouth, urinary hesitancy or retention, constipation, and blurred vision. The drug should not be used in patients with glaucoma unless miotics are first given. Disopyramide may cause QRS widening and Q-T prolongation.

Benowitz, N. L.: Clinical applications of the pharmokinetics of lidocaine. Cardiovasc. Clin., 6:77, 1974.

Bigger, J. T., and Giardina, E. G. V.: Rational use of antiarrhythmic drugs alone and in combination. Cardiovasc. Clin., 6:103, 1974.

Koch-Weser, J.: Clinical application of the pharmokinetics of procaine amide. Cardiovasc. Clin., 6:63, 1974.

364.4. CARDIOVERSION OF ARRHYTHMIAS BY DC ELECTROSHOCK

DC shock applied externally to the chest wall is an effective method of converting several types of cardiac arrhythmias to sinus rhythm; these include atrial fibrillation, atrial flutter, paroxysmal atrial tachycardia, ventricular tachycardia, and ventricular fibrillation. AC cardioverters were originally used clinically but have been replaced by DC cardioverters. The advantages of DC cardioverters or defibrillators are as follows: (1) they are lighter in weight and more effective than AC defibrillators, (2) they can be made independent of line current and portable, and (3) the short duration of the electrical discharge (a few milliseconds) allows it to be delivered at a preset time within the QRS complex. This is called synchronized cardioversion. AC cardioverters produce sinusoidal pulses which deliver their energy over a period of 150 to 250 msec. Thus with AC cardioverters the ability to deliver a shock during the so-called vulnerable period of ventricles, and thereby to induce ventricular fibrillation, is greater than with DC cardioverters.

Cardioversion of supraventricular rhythms and ventricular tachycardia should always be performed in the synchronized mode. Input of an ECG signal into the defibrillator automatically programs it to discharge within the terminal portion of the QRS complex, thus avoiding the ventricular vulnerable period. It is extremely important to be sure that the synchronizer circuit is not activated when the defibrillator is used for the treatment of ventricular fibrillation. Since there are no QRS complexes generated during ventricular fibrillation, the activated synchronizer circuit will prevent the defibrillator from discharging.

Prior to cardioversion, patients should receive either thiopental or diazepam to create an amnesic state. Skin resistance must be decreased by the application of a suitable electrode paste or saline-soaked pads. Alcohol-soaked pads should never be used because passage of an electric current may cause them to burst into flames. Application of electrode paste should be limited to the diameter of the electrode paddles (3½ inches). One must avoid contact between the two areas of conductive material (bridging), as this will cause the electrical current to travel along the skin, causing burns and ineffectual cardioversion.

ATRIAL FLUTTER. Synchronized DC shock is considered by many to be the treatment of choice for atrial flutter. Sinus rhythm can be established in more than 90 per cent of patients. It is certainly the treatment of choice in those uncommon situations in which atrial flutter exists with 1:1 AV conduction. If a patient is receiving digitalis to slow the ventricular rate, it should be omitted for one or two days prior to electrical cardioversion. An oral dose of quinidine may be given one to three hours prior to cardioversion. Treatment of atrial flutter may begin with energy levels of 25 watt-sec (joules) and progressively increased until conversion occurs. The decision as to whether patients should receive long-term quinidine therapy to prevent future occurrences will depend upon the frequency of the episodes of atrial flutter and tolerance to the drug. In chronic or recurrent atrial flutter which is not prevented by quinidine, one may have to accept the persistence of the arrhythmia and maintain a suitable ventricular rate with the use of digitalis.

ATRIAL FIBRILLATION. Although most cases of atrial fibrillation can be converted to sinus rhythm, not all remain in sinus rhythm; nor should conversion be attempted in all cases of atrial fibrillation. Conversion by DC shock should be done immediately for those patients with the Wolff-Parkinson-White syndrome who have developed atrial fibrillation with rapid ventricular rates caused by conduction over the accessory pathway. Immediate conversion by DC shock should also be considered in the patient with atrial fibrillation with a rapid ventricular rate (>180 per minute) in whom significant hypotension, heart failure, or angina pectoris develops. Most other patients with atrial fibrillation can be treated with digitalis and/or propranolol for control of the ventricular rate, after which a decision for conversion to sinus rhythm can be made.

Conversion should not be attempted in the following: (1) Patients who have had established atrial fibrillation of several years' duration. (2) Patients in whom previous attempts to maintain sinus rhythm have been unsuccessful despite adequate prophylactic therapy with quinidine. (3) Patients with known sensitivity or idiosyncratic reactions to quinidine. (4) Patients with the bradycardia-tachycardia syndrome (sick sinus syndrome), in whom conversion of atrial fibrillation results in an inadequate sinus rate. (5) Patients with very large left atria. (6) Elderly patients (65 to 70 years of age).

Patients who are maintained in atrial fibrillation should be considered for anticoagulant therapy for the prevention of systemic embolization.

VENTRICULAR TACHYCARDIA. Drug therapy (e.g., lidocaine, procainamide) is the preferred method for treating ventricular tachycardia. Synchronized DC shock should be used for those patients who are resistant to conversion by drugs or in whom significant hypotension or shock is present. DC shock should be avoided in ventricular tachycardia due to digitalis toxicity. However, if DC shock must be used, one should begin with the lowest energy levels, i.e., 25 watt-sec. A lidocaine drip should be started and maintained during the postcardioversion period to prevent recurrences of ventricular tachycardia.

VENTRICULAR FIBRILLATION. Ventricular fibrillation should be immediately treated with 400 watt-sec energy levels. If anoxia and acidosis are present, it is more difficult to convert ventricular fibrillation and therefore these abnormalities must be corrected by adequate ventilation and $NaHCO_3$. If the initial one or two attempts at defibrillation are unsuccessful, basic life support measures should be applied while ventilatory and metabolic abnormalities are being corrected.

Ewy, G.: Cardiac arrest and resuscitation: Defibrillators and defibrillation. *In* Harvey, P. (ed.): Current Problems in Cardiology, Vol. II, no. 11. Chicago, Year Book Medical Publishers, 1978.

364.5. PACEMAKERS

The sick sinus syndrome and symptomatic AV block constitute the major reasons for insertion of cardiac pacemakers today. Much less frequently pacemakers are used in (1) control of drug-resistant ventricular tachycardia and (2) drug-resistant paroxysmal supraventricular tachycardia in which abrupt termination of the tachycardia is associated with a significant pause and symptoms prior to resumption of a sinus or escape rhythm.

Cardiac pacing may be performed by the transvenous method or by electrodes implanted directly onto the ventricular epicardium. Transvenous pacing may be temporary or permanent. In temporary transvenous pacing an electrode catheter is introduced into a peripheral vein and fluoroscopically positioned against the endocardium of the right ventricle. The proximal electrodes are connected to an external cardiac pacemaker which has an adjustable rate and milliamperage control. Temporary transvenous pacing is utilized (1) prior to the insertion of a permanent pacing system and (2) in situations in which the indication for pacing is judged to be reversible (drug-induced AV block or bradycardia) or possibly irreversible and progressive (AV and bundle branch blocks associated with myocardial infarction). Permanent transvenous pacing is performed under sterile surgical conditions. An electrode catheter is positioned in the right ventricle through a subclavian vein, and the proximal electrode terminals are attached to a pacemaker which is implanted subcutaneously.

Electrodes may be unipolar or bipolar. A unipolar lead-electrode system contains a single electrode in direct contact with the myocardium which is connected to the negative terminal of the pacemaker. The positive terminal functions as the indifferent electrode of the pacing system. In a bipolar lead electrode system, the electrodes are in close proximity to each other and are situated within or on the heart. Unipolar leads produce larger stimulus potentials on ECG tracings than do bipolar leads. In addition, unipolar leads are more sensitive to extraneous sig-

Figure 30. QRS-inhibited demand pacemaker functioning in both the pacing and sensing modes. Each paced QRS complex is preceded by a stimulus artifact. The stimulus interval is approximately 840 msec. The first two QRS complexes are paced beats. Following the second paced beat a single spontaneous QRS complex occurs approximately 720 msec after the last pacemaker discharge. The inherent beat is sensed by the pacemaker, which inhibits itself from firing. Absence of subsequent spontaneous activity results in the pacemaker functioning in a fixed mode. Sensing, inhibition, and subsequent pacing are repeated with the last two beats.

Figure 31. Sample tracing from a patient with a QRS-inhibited demand pacemaker. There is complete failure to capture, and only intermittent sensing. All QRS complexes are generated by the inherent heart rate, which varies between 1600 and 1720 msec. The stimulus interval of the pacemaker is 840 msec. The second spontaneous QRS complex, which occurs 40 msec before the expected discharge of the pacemaker, is sensed and inhibits the pacemaker. Thereafter, none of the QRS complexes are sensed and the pacemaker discharges at a fixed rate, but none of the stimuli capture the ventricles.

nals than are bipolar leads. In the event of a wire breakage, a bipolar lead system can be converted to a unipolar lead.

Cardiac pacing can be performed in the fixed or demand modes. In fixed rate cardiac pacing, the pacemaker is preset to discharge at a constant rate, irrespective of the inherent cardiac rate. The ability of fixed rate pacemakers to induce competitive rhythms which may cause tachycardia or fibrillation has discouraged their general use. Demand pacemakers may be QRS inhibited or QRS triggered. Both types of demand pacemakers are programmed to sense the inherent R-R interval (heart rate). In a QRS-inhibited demand pacemaker, the pacemaker will be inhibited from discharging a pacing stimulus if the inherent R-R interval is less than the preset firing rate of the pacemaker (stimulus to stimulus interval). It will also be inhibited if the interval from a paced or stimulated beat to a subsequent spontaneous beat is less than the preset firing interval (Fig. 30). If spontaneous ventricular activity is absent or consistently less than the preset firing rate, the demand pacemaker will essentially function as a fixed rate pacemaker (Fig. 31). QRS-triggered demand pacemakers are also programmed to sense the inherent R-R interval. However, when the R-R interval is less than the preset firing rate, these pacemakers discharge their stimulus within the spontaneously generated QRS complex. The pacemaker-generated stimulus is ineffectual because it occurs during the absolute refractory period of the ventricular myocardium. When the inherent R-R interval is greater than the preset firing rate of the pacemaker, the stimulus will be effective in eliciting a ventricular depolarization.

Temporary pacing as described above is usually not performed with the same catheter in place for more than five days, especially if phlebitis or local skin infection develops. If additional temporary pacing time is required, another vein with a new catheter will have to be used.

When failure to reliably pace occurs with the use of an external pacemaker, the physician should embark upon a systematic check of the pacing system: (1) Check to see that the proximal electrodes of the pacing catheter are secured within the positive and negative terminals of the external pacemaker. (2) Raise the milliampere level to ensure that it is above the minimum threshold for pacing. (3) Check for wire breaks on the externalized portion of the electrode catheter. (4) Check that the pacemaker batteries are not depleted. (5) Obtain appropriate x-rays of the chest to confirm location of the catheter.

A not infrequent complication of transvenous right ventricular pacing is dislodgment of the cardiac catheter from its endocardial pacing site. The design of newer

electrode catheters has helped to overcome this problem. Dislodgment results in failure to reliably capture or sense, or both. Perforation of the electrode catheter through the myocardium into the pericardial space is another cause for intermittent capture and sensing. Right ventricular apical pacing produces the electrocardiographic pattern of left bundle branch block with left axis deviation. A change from this pattern to one of right bundle branch block should suggest perforation of the electrode catheter and pacing of the left ventricle. Less commonly, failure to sense or capture is due to a wire break in the electrode catheter.

The development of newer battery energy sources has extended the functioning period of pacemaker power packs from two to five years before replacement is required. Nuclear-powered pacemakers are purported to last 20 years. After implantation of a permanent pacemaker, patients should be followed at monthly intervals for a few months, and thereafter the frequency of follow-up should be extended. The frequency of visits should be increased as the end of the expected life of the power source is approached. Transtelephonic monitoring has also been used for pacemaker surveillance.

Patients with cardiac pacemakers are subject to a wide variety of potential electrical dangers both in and outside the hospital. Patients with temporary transvenous electrode catheters are especially vulnerable to random current leakage, which, when bypassing the normally high skin resistance and delivered directly to the heart, may cause life-threatening ventricular arrhythmias. Malfunction of pacemakers may also occur from electromagnetic currents generated by electrocautery, diathermy, microwave ovens, television transmitting stations, or automobile ignitions. Skeletal muscle potentials have been reported to trigger the QRS sensing circuit of QRS-inhibited pacemakers and temporally suppress their function.

365. DISORDERS OF THE PERICARDIUM

Robert E. Whalen

365.1. INTRODUCTION

Claudius Galen first noted and named the pericardium in the second century A.D. He also recognized that the pericardium could be the site of inflammation in animals, that pericardial effusions had a deleterious

Etiology of Disorders of the Pericardium

I. Inflammatory
    A. Acute pericarditis
        1. Nonspecific "benign" or idiopathic
        2. Infections
            a. Viral
            b. Bacterial
            c. Tuberculous
            d. Fungal
            e. Others
        3. Myocardial infarction
            a. Acute myocardial infarction
            b. Postmyocardial infarction
        4. Postpericardiotomy or thoracotomy
        5. Post-traumatic
        6. Connective tissue disorders
        7. Allergic and hypersensitivity disorders
        8. Metabolic disorders
        9. Physical or chemical agents
    B. Chronic pericarditis (virtually all of the above)
II. Neoplastic disease
    A. Benign
    B. Malignant
        1. Primary
        2. Secondary
III. Congenital lesions of the pericardium
    A. Pericardial cysts and diverticula
    B. Partial or complete absence of the pericardium
IV. Disease of diverse or unknown etiology

effect on cardiac motion, and that the pericardium could be the site of tumor formation. Diseases of the pericardium typically present in one or more of three clinical forms: acute pericarditis, pericardial effusion, and pericardial constriction. Pericardial involvement may progress from inflammation to effusion and then constriction, or it may present as effusion or constriction without clinical evidence of preceding inflammation.

The pericardium may be the site of a variety of inflammatory, neoplastic, and congenital disorders. The incidence of such disorders, which are listed in the accompanying table, has changed markedly over the past several decades. This change stems from four major factors: the introduction of antibiotics, which has significantly decreased the incidence of bacterial involvement of the pericardium; the increasing clinical awareness of the involvement of the pericardium in various connective tissue diseases; the marked increase in the postpericardiotomy syndrome accompanying the advent of modern cardiac surgery; and the growing recognition of acute and delayed signs of pericardial involvement associated with myocardial infarction.

365.2. ACUTE PERICARDITIS

By far the most common initial manifestation of pericardial disease is acute pericarditis. This condition may be due to diverse causes. In many cases the same etiologic factors may persist over long periods of time and thus produce a recurrent, subacute, or chronic disorder.

ETIOLOGY. Nonspecific "Benign" or Idiopathic Pericarditis. This is perhaps the most common type of acute pericarditis in adults. The term benign should probably not be applied to this entity, because the symptomatology is certainly not benign and the disease can be accompanied by acute pericardial effusion and tamponade. The syndrome's designation is actually a reflection of our inability to determine an etiologic factor. For many years this syndrome has been attributed to either a viral agent or a hypersensitivity reaction, but there has been no effective proof of this. As detection and isolation techniques for viral diseases have been perfected and the skill of detecting other underlying diseases, such as connective tissue diseases and myocardial infarction, has improved, more and more cases of so-called idiopathic or nonspecific pericarditis have been removed from this category; but the cause of the rest remains unknown. Typically the syndrome occurs in late adolescence and early adulthood. It is often preceded by an upper respiratory infection days to several weeks before fever and precordial pain bring the patient to medical attention. The syndrome usually lasts one to several weeks, during which time the patient is mildly febrile and has varying degrees of precordial pain. Occasionally pericardial effusion may appear early, and sometimes it is the first sign of the syndrome. Although the acute symptoms may subside after a brief time, the patient may be left with easy fatigability for several months. This may reflect the fact that in virtually all cases of acute pericarditis there is some inflammatory response in the subepicardial myocardium, and there may be a greater degree of myocarditis than is recognized clinically. Exacerbations of the syndrome, particularly of precordial pain, are not rare and may occur sporadically for several months to years after the initial attack. The development of constrictive pericarditis is extremely rare. There are no classic differentiating laboratory studies, although the majority of patients have a mild leukocytosis. The electrocardiogram is almost always abnormal and shows the changes discussed under Laboratory Findings. Chest x-ray may show slight increase in cardiac size as compared to previous baseline x-rays; this may be due to either a small pericardial effusion or thickening of the inflamed pericardium. Pulmonary infiltrates are frequently noted, and pleural effusion may occur in one fourth of patients. In most cases bed rest and analgesics will produce relief of symptoms in one to two weeks. If these measures fail to produce relief of pain, various nonsteroidal anti-inflammatory agents, such as aspirin and indomethacin, have been effective. In patients with unusually severe and prolonged pain, adrenal corticosteroid hormone therapy may be indicated, but this should be undertaken only if bacterial infection can be excluded.

Infectious Pericarditis. Infections of proved etiology account for a significant number of cases of pericarditis. Various *viral agents* have long been suspected as causes for "idiopathic nonspecific" pericarditis. However, even with careful viral isolation studies, only a small percentage of cases have been demonstrated to be associated with viral infection of the pericardium or myocardium. The most common viral agent is coxsackievirus Type B; rarely, coxsackievirus Type A is the agent. Pericarditis has also been reported to be due to Type A echovirus, mumps, and infectious mononucleosis. The clinical course, physical findings, and method of treatment in proved cases of viral pericarditis are not significantly different from those discussed under Nonspecific "Benign" or Idiopathic Pericarditis. Although it has been suggested that diffuse myalgias, rubelliform rashes, and lymphadenopathy are more common in viral pericarditis than in idiopathic pericarditis, there have been insufficient viral studies in patients labeled as having idiopathic pericarditis to warrant this as being a diagnostic feature for separating the two entities, if indeed they are truly separate.

Bacterial infections of the pericardium may arise by direct extension of infection from foci in the thorax such as pneumonia or empyema. Less frequently bacterial pericarditis is caused by a septicemia which is initiated from a distant site of infection. The emergence of antibiotic-resistant strains of staphylococci, particularly in the hospital, has served to increase the frequency of this organism as a causative agent in relation to other previously classic bacterial causes for pericarditis. The unique susceptibility of the pneumococcus to penicillin has almost completely eliminated this as a cause for bacterial pericarditis, and cases are seldom seen unless treatment has been long delayed and the patient has empyema. A large number of other types of organisms have been implicated in the development of pericarditis, including the meningococcus, gonococcus, *Hemophilus influenzae,* and streptococcal organisms. Although gram-negative organisms are a relatively rare cause for acute pericarditis, their frequency has increased because of the development of antibiotic-resistant strains, particularly in patients having complications after cardiac surgery and in patients on immunosuppressive therapy for malignancies. *Pseudomonas, Proteus, E. coli* and *Klebsiella* have produced increasingly more difficult to treat pericardial infections in such patients. When typhoid fever was a scourge in earlier generations, involvement of the pericardium was recognized as a complication of this disease. Nontyphoidal *Salmonella* organisms are a very rare cause for pericarditis. Bacterial pericarditis rarely is the initial sign of infection and often appears only as a late complication of either untreated or poorly controlled bacterial infection. When it does appear, it may present with the classic signs of acute pericarditis and may eventuate in a pericardial effusion or constriction. However, it is important to recognize that the classic signs of acute pericarditis are present in probably less than half of patients with bacterial pericarditis, and therefore the diagnosis should not be discarded because of the absence of clinical signs of acute pericarditis. Laboratory signs are not significantly different from those seen in other forms of pericarditis except for the expected leukocytosis. Once the diagnosis is suspected, diagnostic studies must be initiated immediately, for time is of the essence if the infection is to be successfully treated. If suspicion is sufficient and diagnostic pericardial fluid cannot be obtained by pericardiocentesis, an exploratory thoracotomy should be performed promptly. If the diagnosis is not established either by pericardiocentesis or exploratory thoracotomy, a pericardiectomy, if feasible, or a pleuropericardial window procedure should be performed.

Although *tuberculous* involvement of the pericardium might justifiably be considered with the bacterial forms of pericarditis, it has earned a place of its own because of its prevalence in earlier decades and its propensity to produce constrictive pericarditis. Tuberculous pericarditis occurs predominantly in males, particularly in blacks, who have approximately ten times the incidence of the disease found in whites. Although tuberculous pericarditis may be the only evidence of the infection, it probably arises as a secondary manifestation of the disease rather than as a primary focus. Approximately half the patients with tuberculous pericarditis have evidence of previous or concurrent infection of the lung. In the acute phase it cannot be differentiated from other forms of infectious pericarditis. In the chronic phase it may have an insidious onset characterized more by systemic symptoms such as low grade fever and weakness. In the chronic form the progressive constrictive process may be its predominant manifestation. The disease must be considered in any patient presenting with acute pericarditis, pericardial effusion, or constriction. The diagnosis may sometimes be made by examination and culture of the pericardial fluid, although this is extremely difficult unless large volumes of pericardial fluid can be obtained. The diagnosis is more likely to be made by suitable pathologic examination and culture of pericardial tissue obtained at surgery.

TREATMENT. Evidence of old or active tuberculosis by chest x-ray or the presence of a positive tuberculin skin test in a patient who had a previous negative skin test not only heightens the likelihood of the diagnosis but should raise the question that antituberculous therapy should be started on clinical grounds alone. The effects of progressive tuberculous involvement of the pericardium are so devastating and the institution of antituberculous therapy is of such relatively low morbidity that on some occasions the clinician will feel forced to treat pericarditis of unknown etiology as though it might be tuberculous. When the diagnosis is likely on clinical grounds but cannot be proved by culture or pathologic studies, a more conservative approach with a combination of isoniazid and rifampin or ethambutol for 18 months, along with continued follow-up to be certain that there is no progression, may be indicated. If the index of suspicion is great and pericardiocentesis has not demonstrated an organism, a pericardiectomy, both to establish a diagnosis and to prevent future constriction, is frequently employed. When the diagnosis is established, triple therapy with isoniazid, streptomycin, and rifampin or ethambutol is indicated for 18 to 24 months. If the diagnosis has been made and antituberculous therapy has not eliminated signs of effusion or constriction in several months, a pericardiectomy should be performed.

Various *fungal disorders,* including histoplasmosis, coccidioidomycosis, actinomycosis, and nocardiosis, have been reported as etiologic agents in the development of pericarditis. Although these represent an extremely small number of cases, the possibility should be considered in patients who are uniquely susceptible to fungal infections, particularly those with lymphomas and leukemia and those who are undergoing immunosuppressant therapy for other systemic diseases. *Parasites* represent a very small but definite class of etiologic agents in the development of pericarditis. Infection with *Entamoeba histolytica* has been reported to produce pericarditis by hematogenous spread to the pericardium or by rupture of a hepatic cyst into the pericardial space. Although *Echinococcus* is a rare cause of pericarditis, over 100 cases of such involvement have been reported in the literature. Pericardial infection almost inevitably stems from initial invasion and cyst formation of the myocardium with rupture into the pericardial space.

Myocardial Infarction. Pericarditis associated with myocardial infarction may take two forms, and on occasion it may be difficult to be certain whether one is dealing with a late-appearing *acute pericarditis* or an early appearance of *postmyocardial infarction pericarditis.*

Acute inflammation of the pericardium frequently accompanies acute myocardial infarction, particularly if it is transmural. The clinical recognition of this, such as the development of consistent typical pericardial pain and a pericardial friction rub, is directly related to the frequency with which the patient is examined. With repetitive examination, signs may be recognized in at least two thirds of patients rather than the 20 per cent previously reported. The symptoms usually occur between the second and fifth days and rarely after the tenth day. The syndrome is thought to be due to an inflammatory response in the subepicardial region of the infarcted myocardium with some extension of inflammation to contiguous areas of the epicardium. It is almost inevitably a self-limited process and requires only analgesics or a nonsteroidal anti-inflammatory agent to control the symptoms. A pericardial effusion rarely presents a problem unless the patient has been anticoagulated. A second form of pericardial involvement occurs at any time from several weeks to several months after an acute myocardial infarction. This so-called *postmyocardial infarction pericarditis,* or *Dressler's syndrome,* is characterized by the onset of typical pericardial pain, particularly precipitated by changes in position or cough. It may be accompanied by fever and significant pericardial effusion. There may be a friction rub and systemic symptoms such as malaise and myalgias. Pericardial effusion may occur in such patients, particularly if they have received anticoagulants. The major differential diagnosis in such patients is the possibility of a recurrence of myocardial infarction, but the almost constant complaint of accentuation of symptoms by changes in body position, coughing, and inspiration, along with the presence of a pericardial rub without further evidence of infarction by ECG, serves to alert the clinician to the correct diagnosis.

TREATMENT. The syndrome is usually self-limited and can be treated with analgesics or nonsteroidal anti-inflammatory agents, but on occasion the syndrome may become so repetitive that it is necessary to rely on corticosteroid hormone therapy.

The Postpericardiotomy Syndrome. This has become a commonly recognized form of pericarditis. Although the incidence of the syndrome is reported to be approximately 10 per cent among patients undergoing cardiac surgery, it is undoubtedly higher than this, particularly if minor manifestations of the syndrome are taken into account. The exact cause of the syndrome is not understood. It has been suggested that a common denominator which ties together the pericarditis following myocardial infarction, cardiac surgery, and trauma to the pericardium is blood in the pericardium which produces an inflammatory response. However, it is clear that the presence of blood in the pericardium is not mandatory for the development of the syndrome, and there has been recent evidence to suggest that there may be a viral agent involved, perhaps arising from infection carried in the multiple transfusions often associated with cardiac surgery. The syndrome may occur as early as a week postoperatively, but frequently will not manifest itself until several weeks or months after surgery. Although the typical findings of acute pericarditis, such as fever, substernal chest pain, and a pericardial rub, usually are associated with the syndrome, it may appear with only one of these manifestations. Fever, typical ECG changes, and even an elevation of sedimentation rate may not accompany the

syndrome, and thus the absence of these abnormalities should not be used as evidence against the diagnosis of the postpericardiotomy syndrome. Actual entrance into the pericardium at surgery is not a necessity for the development of the syndrome, because it has been reported after thoracic surgery for pulmonary resection and repair of a hiatus hernia. It is frequently accompanied by a diffuse pleural reaction and associated small pleural effusions. Although the development of pericarditis several weeks postoperatively always raises the specter of a complicating postoperative bacterial pericarditis, the syndrome is almost invariably due to the postpericardiotomy syndrome rather than actual bacterial infection. However, it is important to keep in mind the possibility of a bacterial infection, particularly if the patient does not respond promptly to a brief course of anti-inflammatory agents.

Post-traumatic Pericarditis. Pericarditis may develop after both penetrating and nonpenetrating injury to the chest. The syndrome may appear early after a penetrating wound, and under these circumstances there is always concern that it may be due to bacterial infection of the pericardial space. The syndrome tends to occur weeks or even months after blunt trauma to the chest such as a steering wheel injury. Under these circumstances the concern about bacterial infection is less and one can move quickly with anti-inflammatory agents to suppress the symptoms.

Connective Tissue Disorders. These have become commonly recognized causes of pericarditis. In childhood the most common cause may be acute rheumatic fever. However, in the adult pericarditis is a relatively rare manifestation of acute rheumatic fever. In adults connective tissue disorders, such as systemic lupus erythematosus, rheumatoid arthritis, periarteritis, and, less likely, scleroderma, are much more frequent causes of pericarditis. Pericarditis may be the first sign of systemic lupus erythematosus and may precede other manifestations by months. It may be associated with a rapidly accumulating effusion which may present such a predominant and life-threatening clinical picture that other signs of the disease do not gain attention until the symptoms of pericarditis and effusion are controlled. Pericardial involvement has been noted in up to 40 per cent of documented cases of systemic lupus erythematosus. The diagnosis can be reasonably inferred when LE cells and anti-DNA antibodies are detectable in the blood. Steroid therapy is almost invariably necessary to control the symptoms of pericarditis. Clinical signs of typical acute pericarditis may be seen in approximately 3 per cent of patients with rheumatoid arthritis, even though autopsy series indicate that at least 10 per cent of patients with rheumatoid arthritis have an inflammatory response in the pericardium. Pericarditis is most commonly seen in patients with active rheumatoid disease, particularly those with rheumatoid nodules and markedly elevated titers of rheumatoid factor in serum. The pericarditis is seldom severe, but on rare occasions it can be accompanied by significant effusion. Examination of the pericardial fluid reveals a characteristic marked decrease in the concentration of glucose and elevated LDH enzyme levels as well as increased globulins and decreased complement values. Large round or oval multinucleated cells have been noted in the fluid and are thought by some to be pathognomonic of the disease. These "RA" cells contain cytoplasmic inclusion bodies thought to represent phagocytized rheumatoid factor complex. Other connective tissue disorders, such as periarteritis nodosa and scleroderma, as well as giant cell arteritis, have been reported to be associated with pericarditis less commonly. In particular, scleroderma more frequently involves the myocardium and is a rare cause of pericarditis.

Allergic and Hypersensitivity Disorders. Serum sickness, giant urticaria, and allergic responses to penicillin have been associated with pericarditis. In addition to penicillin, other drugs, including diphenylhydantoin, hydralazine, and procainamide, have been implicated in the development of pericarditis. With the renewed emphasis on prevention of cardiac arrhythmias following myocardial infarction and the consequent increased use of procainamide, a lupus-like syndrome involving the pericardium has been more frequently recognized after prolonged use of this drug.

Metabolic Disorders. Uremia and myxedema may provoke pericardial reactions. It has long been recognized that pericarditis, frequently with hemorrhagic pericardial effusions, may occur in the terminal phase of uremia; but before the advent of dialysis programs the incidence of this complication was relatively low, because the patient usually succumbed to renal failure before signs of pericarditis could develop. As many as 15 per cent of patients on dialysis programs may develop pericarditis. Indeed, one of the serious complications that must be watched for during long-term dialysis is the sudden development of a life-threatening pericardial effusion. The etiology of uremic pericarditis is not well understood. It has been seen to develop in patients well controlled with dialysis, but it has been noted that more frequent dialysis may lead to a remission in the pericarditis and pericardial effusion.

Cardiomegaly is not uncommon in hypothyroidism. In the majority of cases this cardiomegaly is due primarily to pericardial effusion. Effusions usually develop slowly and may become quite large with a minimum of symptoms. Hemodynamic embarrassment is rare. The condition responds promptly to thyroid replacement therapy.

Physical or Chemical Agents. The recent popularization of high dose radiation therapy for lymphomatous disease in the mediastinum has disclosed that the pericardium is more susceptible to radiation injury than had previously been thought. Acute pericarditis, pericardial effusion, and constriction have all been reported to follow high dose radiation to the mediastinum. This entity now is recognized as an uncommon but definite complication of radiation therapy, and congestive heart failure may result from either pericardial effusion or constriction, even as a late complication of therapy. Pericarditis is a rare complication of asbestosis and may be associated with a granulomatous thickening of the pericardium. It has also been suggested that irritation of the pericardium by urate crystals in patients with gout may on very rare occasions provoke pericarditis.

CLINICAL MANIFESTATIONS. The hallmark of acute pericarditis is the development of substernal chest pain, which is usually sharp and knife-like but may be a dull or oppressive sensation. The pain frequently is referred or radiates to other areas of the chest, particularly the left supraclavicular region. It may also be referred to the neck and shoulders, which may lead to an initial false impression that the symptom is primarily musculoskeletal in origin rather than due to acute pericarditis. Deep inspiration, rotation of the trunk, and coughing usually will precipitate the pain. Many patients find that it is accentuated and virtually intolerable when they lie on the back or the left side, but the pain can be partially alleviated by sitting up and leaning forward. Fever usually accompanies or initiates the pain and is often associated with other systemic symptoms, such as malaise, fatigue, and myalgias.

A characteristic physical finding in acute pericarditis is a pericardial friction rub. This leathery or scratchy sound may be heard over any portion of the anterior precordium, but it is most frequently heard low along the left sternal border. It may consist of one, two, or three components, presumably depending upon the extent of inflammatory involvement of the pericardium. When there is only a single component to the rub, it is confined to systole and may mimic a systolic cardiac murmur. Changes in the intensity and quality of the isolated systolic rub produced by variations in respiration and positions during auscultation will help differentiate a rub from a cardiac murmur. More commonly the pericardial rub has two or three components. When two components are heard, they occur during systole and diastole and are due to the rubbing of the inflamed epicardial surface against the parietal pericardial surface during systole and diastole. The presence of a third component to the rub, which is common, will eliminate any confusion as to whether the rub is due to an intracardiac murmur or pericardial inflammation. The third component of the rub is due to atrial contraction and occurs in the presystolic phase of the cardiac cycle. Frequently a rub may have a variable number of components, depending upon the position in which the patient is examined. Acute pericarditis is often accompanied by cardiac arrhythmias, which may be intermittent. The vast majority of arrhythmias are supraventricular arrhythmias, including frequent premature atrial contractions, paroxysmal atrial tachycardia, fibrillation, and flutter. This has been attributed to irritation and involvement of the sinus node, which lies close to the epicardial surface of the heart.

LABORATORY FINDINGS. Acute pericarditis is usually accompanied by a leukocytosis and an elevation in sedimentation rate, but these are by no means invariable. Chest x-ray may show a slight increase in cardiac size owing to either inflammatory thickening of the pericardium or a small pericardial effusion. In addition, there may be evidence of pleural involvement characterized by small pleural effusions. Pulmonary infiltrates also are common accompaniments. These changes reflect the fact that the inflammatory process involving the pericardium frequently will also involve the pleura. The electrocardiogram usually shows a typical pattern of S-T segment elevation without changes in the QRS morphology. The S-T segment elevation may last for weeks at a time, and frequently the elevation will show evolutionary changes with T wave inversion several days to weeks after the onset of the S-T segment changes. These electrocardiographic changes may be isolated to only several leads and are due to involvement of the subepicardial myocardium rather than involvement of the pericardium itself, because the pericardium is electrically silent. Serum levels of enzymes such as glutamic-oxaloacetic transaminase (SGOT) and lactic dehydrogenase (LDH) may be moderately elevated because there is inflammatory involvement of the subepicardial portion of the myocardium. Cardiac isoenzyme changes, including the presence of CPK-MB and LDH-1 greater than LDH-2 configurations, are less frequent but have been noted. The echocardiogram may show thickening of the pericardium and will often show a variable amount of pericardial effusion, as there is an almost inevitable increase in fluid in the pericardial space above the 25 to 35 ml normally present in the cavity.

DIFFERENTIAL DIAGNOSIS. When acute pericarditis presents in a young patient with sudden onset of sharp or grating substernal pain accentuated by changes in position and partially relieved by sitting up, plus a characteristic multicomponent rub and S-T segment elevation, the diagnosis is relatively simple. However, frequently the condition does not present in such a classic fashion; in such cases it is necessary to entertain other diagnoses, including acute myocardial infarction, pleurisy with or without pneumonia, pulmonary embolization, dissection of the aorta, pneumothorax, mediastinal emphysema, or an abdominal source for the complaint. Examination of serial electrocardiograms and serum cardiac isoenzyme levels will usually establish whether the primary process is due to myocardial infarction or pericarditis alone. The rub accompanying pleurisy which may raise the possibility of pericarditis is clearly related to and accentuated by the respiratory cycle and is usually heard diffusely over the chest or frequently in the lateral portions of the chest rather than in the precordial area. Pulmonary embolization may mimic pericarditis; but when further studies, such as serial chest x-rays, lung scans, and, if necessary, pulmonary arteriograms, are obtained, the differentiation becomes clear. Dissecting aortic aneurysm may simulate pericarditis and on occasion may actually be a cause for pericarditis owing to rupture of the base of the aorta, with a leak of blood into the pericardium which provokes a pericardial inflammatory reaction. However, the pain of dissection is usually more severe and unremitting than that of pericarditis and is usually noted in the infrascapular area, which is uncommon in pericarditis. Pneumothorax can be differentiated from pericarditis by physical examination which indicates absent breath sounds on the affected side if it is a large pneumothorax and by chest x-ray if it is not discernible by physical examination. Intra-abdominal events may produce pain which suggests acute pericarditis. Acute cholecystitis with referral of pain to the supraclavicular area must be considered. Pancreatitis can also produce a confusing picture suggestive of pericarditis. When there is inflammatory involvement of the diaphragm, there may be an associated small pleural effusion as well as nonspecific T wave changes. Splenic infarction may also provoke an inflammatory response in the diaphragm, and the pain may be referred to the left supraclavicular area, a favorite site for the referral of the pain of acute pericarditis.

365.3. PERICARDIAL EFFUSION

PATHOPHYSIOLOGY. Pericardial effusion, the accumulation of serous or serosanguineous fluid in excess of the normal 25 to 35 ml of lymphatic fluid in the pericardial space, may present in either acute or chronic form. It may be the first sign of acute pericarditis, and its severe hemodynamic consequences may actually obscure the classic signs of the underlying pericarditis. Although chronic pericardial effusion may be accompanied by a pericardial rub, the insidious development of this condition without other evidence of pericardial involvement may simulate progressive heart failure and, unless readily recognized, may lead to death, even though it is a readily treatable condition. An understanding of the pathophysiology of pericardial effusion makes the physical findings of this disorder more obvious and understandable. The circulatory effects of pericardial effusion are directly related to the rate at which the effusion develops. The sudden development of a pericardial effusion of several hundred milliliters of fluid may provoke profound hemodynamic changes, whereas the slower, more gradual development of pericardial effusion may be almost asymptomatic despite accumulations of several liters of fluid. The primary cause for the clinical and hemodynamic signs of pericardial effusion is the accumulation of fluid in the pericardium sufficient to prevent adequate filling of the cardiac chambers. Since venous inflow to the heart is markedly decreased, there is accumulation of blood in the venous system that is reflected in marked jugular venous distention and hepatic engorgement. If the process is chronic, there is usually peripheral edema as well. Jugular venous distention may be increased or at least unchanged by deep inspiration, a maneuver which usually decreases jugular venous pressure caused by increased venous return to the heart if no restriction to filling is present. In pericardial effusion deep inspiration may actually decrease venous filling of the ventricles and thus increase the volume of residual blood in the jugular veins, producing what has been called Kussmaul's sign. Since venous return to the heart is markedly diminished, cardiac output also falls, leading to a narrow pulse pressure and usually a reflex tachycardia.

CARDIAC TAMPONADE. The most severe complication of a pericardial effusion, no matter what its cause, is the development of cardiac tamponade. Cardiac tamponade is a classic example of the vicious cycle process in medicine. Accumulation of fluid in the relatively nondistensible pericardium initially limits cardiac filling and therefore cardiac output. As cardiac output declines, arterial pressure and coronary artery filling decrease. Coronary flow and thus myocardial function are further compromised by external pressure on the superficially lying coronary arteries. Eventually this decline in cardiac filling, decrease in cardiac output, fall in arterial and coronary artery filling pressure, and decreased coronary flow lead to severe myocardial ischemia, which initiates an even greater decline in myocardial function. Unless this cycle of events is contravened by elimination of the effusion, a fatal outcome is certain.

CLINICAL MANIFESTATIONS. A characteristic of a pericardial effusion is the presence of an abnormal paradoxical pulse. The paradoxical pulse is actually an exaggeration of a normal physiologic response. It is detected by determining the systolic blood pressure during inspiration and expiration. During normal inspiration the capacitance of the lung to accept blood volume is increased, and there is a decrease in venous return and a decreased filling pressure in the left heart. Thus left ventricular stroke volume falls, as does systolic blood pressure. The normal variation in systolic blood pressure between inspiration and expiration is in the range of 8 to 10 mm Hg. In the case of a pericardial effusion the systolic pressure may decline during inspiration to a point at which it is undetectable. In severe cases of pericardial effusion, this can be observed by simply palpating the peripheral pulse and noting a decrease in volume or complete absence of the pulse during inspiration. Although this finding is a prominent one in pericardial effusion, it is also a frequent accompaniment of chronic obstructive lung disease and cannot be used as a pathognomonic sign of pericardial effusion alone.

Dyspnea, tachycardia, distended jugular veins which do not decrease in size with inspiration, cyanosis, varying degrees of consciousness, and a rapid thready pulse with a frequently palpable decrease in the force of the peripheral pulse during inspiration warn of the presence of pericardial effusion. Examination of the lung fields may elicit Ewart's or Pins' sign, characterized by increased dullness, increased fremitus, and bronchial breath sounds at the base of the lung below the angle of the left scapula. These findings are believed to be due to compression of the lower lobe of the left lung by the distended pericardial sac. In large pericardial effusions percussion over the lower half of the sternum will reveal dullness caused by the underlying fluid in the pericardial sac, whereas under normal circumstances percussion over this region produces a resonant note. This sign may be obscured when there is obvious deformity of the anterior chest wall or emphysema, and it may be falsely present when there is marked obesity or right ventricular hypertrophy. Examination of the heart may reveal a quiet precordium with no palpable cardiac activity, but this is by no means the rule, and frequently significant pericardial effusions may be present with quite a distinct cardiac apex impulse. On auscultation the heart sounds may be normal or muffled, and there is frequently a pericardial rub even though the effusion may be a chronic one.

LABORATORY FINDINGS. The electrocardiogram may appear entirely normal, show generalized low voltage, reveal S-T segment elevation with or without T wave inversion, or demonstrate complete electrical alternans, which is characterized by a decrease in the size of the P, QRS, and T waves with alternate beats. Chest x-ray may show a normal-sized heart if the pericardial effusion is acute; but even in this situation, if previous chest x-rays are available, it will be apparent that there has been an increase in cardiac size.

In less acute situations the cardiac shadow may slowly enlarge and assume a pear shape. The normal contour of the left heart border may become straightened, and there may be a convex bulging of the right cardiophrenic junction. Signs of pulmonary congestion are variable. Cardiac fluoroscopy is suggestive but not definitive for the diagnosis if there is markedly decreased or no discernible cardiac pulsation and the epicardial fat line lies significantly inside the border of the presumed cardiac shadow. Further radiographic evidence of a pericardial effusion can be sought by placing a catheter in the right atrium and noting that the catheter tip cannot be passed to the lateral border of the right atrium, indicating that there is either a significant effusion or pericardial thickening between the lateral border of the right atrium and the lateral border of the cardiac shadow. This can be further confirmed by injection of contrast media, which will outline the chamber size in relation to the total cardiac shadow.

Similar conclusions can be drawn when carbon dioxide is injected into the right atrium while the patient is lying in the left lateral position and a lateral decubitus chest x-ray is obtained. Under these circumstances the radiolucent collection of carbon dioxide will be noted beneath the superiorly positioned lateral wall of the right atrium, and there will be a difference of greater than 10 mm between the superior dome of the carbon dioxide level and the border of the cardiac shadow. Since the development of echocardiography these invasive catheterization techniques are seldom warranted, because even small pericardial effusions can be detected with a high degree of accuracy with the echocardiogram. However, in rare cases in which the pericardial effusion is loculated, particularly in the space anterior to the heart, echocardiographic study may not be definitive and angiographic studies may be necessary.

TREATMENT: PERICARDIOCENTESIS. The ultimate proof of the diagnosis of pericardial effusion and also an often mandatory procedure to provide relief from cardiac tamponade is pericardiocentesis. This is accomplished by inserting a medium-sized needle high in the epigastrium in the angle formed between the left border of the xiphoid process and the lower left rib cage. After suitable local anesthesia, the exploring metal needle is connected by an insulated wire to the V lead electrode of the ECG. The needle is slowly advanced upward and slightly posterior in a line toward the medial third of the right clavicle. While the needle is being advanced, the electrocardiogram should be continuously monitored. Contact with the epicardium will be signaled by the development of marked S-T segment elevation on the electrocardiographic record. This procedure not only helps prevent puncture of the heart but also provides confidence that one has not perforated the heart if a frankly bloody pericardial effusion is encountered. In acute cases of tamponade such as can occur with aortic dissection or cardiac trauma, it may be impossible to ascertain whether one is draining the pericardial space or actually removing blood directly from a cardiac chamber. This quandary can usually be eliminated by making certain that there has been no evidence of a current of injury on the recorded V lead of the ECG. Once fluid is obtained by aspiration, it should be examined microscopically for the number and type of cells present and the presence of bacteria. The fluid should also undergo cytologic examination, be submitted for bacterial and tuberculous culture, and be analyzed for sugar and protein content, as well as LDH enzyme and rheumatoid factor if clinically indicated.

365.4. PERICARDIAL CONSTRICTION

PATHOPHYSIOLOGY. Constrictive pericarditis may be the last step in the process initiated by acute pericarditis and followed by a pericardial effusion. However, in many cases it develops insidiously without any previous evidence of pericardial disease, and its first manifestations are those suggestive of heart failure. The pericardium can become thickened, fibrosed, and eventually calcified in a remarkably short time. There are well documented cases of this whole process occurring in less than six months after the onset of bacterial or tuberculous disease involving the pericardium. The fundamental anatomic derangement which leads to the ultimate symptomatology of constrictive pericarditis is obstruction or constriction of either the cardiac chambers or the orifices of the great veins entering the heart. The constrictive process can be localized to isolated chambers of the heart and even small areas of the pericardium surrounding these chambers. Cases of localized constriction in the region of the outflow tract of the right ventricle have simulated subpulmonic stenosis. Isolated adhesions and constriction of the posterior portion of the epicardium have led to severe left ventricular dysfunction. The fundamental pathophysiologic process is one of inexorable decrease in cardiac filling, with consequent venous pooling in the periphery and decline in cardiac output. The process may be so slow that the onset of new symptoms is almost unrecognized by the patient and his physician. If the constriction is prolonged and generalized enough, there may be necrosis of myocardial tissue, and even eventual relief of the constriction will still not eliminate symptoms of heart failure because of residual myocardial damage.

CLINICAL MANIFESTATIONS. The classic clinical picture of constrictive pericarditis is the patient who appears emaciated with obvious venous distention in the neck, a potbellied appearance caused by ascites, and spindly, wasted, and often edematous extremities. The patient may be overtly dyspneic at rest or may complain only of dyspnea on exertion. Careful examination of the neck veins will demonstrate a prominent "Y" descent which corresponds with sudden brief right ventricular filling. Examination of the heart may reveal a quiet precordium with no palpable apical impulse, although this is by no means the rule. The heart sounds may be muffled, and frequently there is a prominent third heart sound occurring 0.09 to 0.12 second after the aortic closure sound. This so-called "pericardial knock" can easily be confused with the S_3 gallop associated with congestive heart failure. Atrial fibrillation is frequently encountered in the late stages of the disease. Hemodynamic deterioration of a patient with atrial fibrillation who has been given digitalis on the presumption that he has congestive heart failure should alert the clinician to the possibility of constrictive pericarditis. Administration of digitalis to the patient with rapid atrial fibrillation and heart failure should relieve signs of failure. However, the patient with constrictive pericarditis may be dependent for an effective cardiac output on a relatively rapid ventricular rate. When this ventricular rate is lowered by digitalis in a patient with atrial fibrillation, the patient is unable to increase ventricular filling and generate a greater stroke volume to maintain a normal cardiac output. Thus hemodynamic deterioration rather than improvement ensues.

LABORATORY FINDINGS. The electrocardiogram is almost invariably abnormal, with a decrease in QRS voltage, nonspecific S-T and T wave changes, and an irregular contour to the P waves. Chest x-ray will usually show a heart of smaller than expected or even normal size in view of the evidence of severe hemodynamic derangement. However, this is not invariable, and the diagnosis should not be discarded if the cardiac size is large, because much of this enlargement may be due to a markedly thickened pericardium. A characteristic of pericardial constriction is the presence of calcium in the pericardium, but this may not be seen on the standard chest x-ray because of technical factors. Thus if it is

suspected, overpenetrated x-rays of the heart in different views should be obtained. Careful fluoroscopy with image intensification will demonstrate calcification in over 75 per cent of cases of constrictive pericarditis. Echocardiography may play an important role in alerting the unsuspecting clinician that he is dealing with constrictive pericarditis rather than advanced heart failure. An echocardiogram which demonstrates a thickened pericardium, small ventricular chamber size, and increased atrial chamber size should raise the possibility of constrictive pericarditis. Cardiac catheterization provides a series of typical findings, but they are not absolutely diagnostic of constrictive pericarditis. The right atrial pressure may be seen to rise with inspiration, which is analogous to Kussmaul's sign seen in the jugular veins; the right atrial pressure tracing shows a typical "M or W" shape; and the right ventricular pressure demonstrates a so-called early diastolic dip and a late diastolic shoulder. The early diastolic dip conforms to the early rapid filling of the ventricle and is coincident with the sharp "Y" descent seen in the jugular venous pulse. There is a generalized equalization of all end-diastolic pressures in the chambers of the heart as well as in the pulmonary artery. Although these findings are typical, it should be noted that exactly the same findings can be observed in patients with cardiomyopathies, and thus their presence or absence should not be the sole determining factor as to whether a patient should undergo an exploratory thoracotomy or not. In occasional patients with subclinical constriction, these hemodynamic findings become evident only after they have received a rapid infusion of saline.

Angiography is frequently helpful in demonstrating that the cardiac chamber is markedly smaller than might be surmised from the total cardiac contour. Furthermore, an unusual downward tugging of the bifurcation of the opacified main pulmonary artery during systole has been noted and is presumably due to the flexible uninvolved pulmonary artery actually being tugged back toward the heart by the contracting ventricles that are encased in an immobile pericardial sac. Results of liver function studies are almost inevitably abnormal, and there may be hypoalbuminemia on the basis of both hepatic disease and a protein-losing enteropathy.

TREATMENT. The definitive treatment for constrictive pericarditis is a pericardiectomy. If delayed too long, the constrictive process may be so advanced that adequate stripping, particularly of the epicardial portion of the pericardium, cannot be accomplished, or there may have been such advanced degeneration of myocardial muscle that postoperative results are less than satisfactory. It should be noted that there are well documented cases of isolated epicardial constriction which is not apparent until the epicardium is actually dissected away from the myocardium itself. The prognosis for recovery from constrictive pericarditis is a function of the age of the patient, the severity of the fibrotic process, and the degree to which the patient's general medical condition has deteriorated before the pericardiectomy is performed. With the lowering of the operative mortality for pericardiectomy to the range of 5 per cent, particularly if done early, there is a general tendency now to operate at the first suggestion of constriction, particularly if the patient is known to have had a bacterial or tuberculous pericardial infection in the past.

365.5. NEOPLASTIC DISEASES

The pericardium may be the site of primary or metastatic tumors. Primary tumors are rare and may be generally classified into mesotheliomas, which encompass tumors that have previously been classified as fibromas and sarcomas, vascular tumors such as hemangiomas and lymphangiomas, pericardial cysts, lipomas, and tumors of heterotopic tissue such as bronchial cysts, teratomas, and dermoids. The pericardium is not a rare location for metastatic tumors. Metastatic tumors from the lung in men and the breast in women are the most common types encountered in the pericardium. Lymphomatous disease, particularly Hodgkin's disease, also may involve the pericardium. Occasionally involvement of the pericardium and its attendant restriction, either by tumor mass or effusion, may be the first sign of a malignancy. Pericardial effusion, which is often bloody, can be found with even small sized tumors and a small number of metastases.

365.6. CONGENITAL LESIONS OF THE PERICARDIUM

Congenital true pericardial cysts may be celomic, lymphangiomatous, bronchial, or teratomatous. These seldom produce significant clinical symptoms and usually come to light when a routine chest x-ray is obtained. The major problem they present is that of differentiation from a mediastinal tumor. They may gradually increase in size and necessitate an exploratory thoracotomy to rule out malignant disease. In addition to true congenital pericardial cysts, a diverticulum of the pericardium may occur. The diverticulum appears as a sharply outlined semicircular or oval area protruding from the cardiac silhouette, usually in the region of the right lower portion of the cardiac shadow. Such diverticula cannot be differentiated from a pericardial cyst without exploratory thoracotomy.

There may be a congenital complete or, less frequently, partial absence of the pericardium. When the defect is a partial one, it occurs on the left side of the pericardium in two thirds of the cases and is seen most frequently in males. Herniation of the heart, particularly the left atrial appendage through the defect, has been associated with recurrent syncope and, rarely, sudden death. The defect should be suspected when the left atrial appendage appears disproportionately prominent on chest x-ray. The diagnosis can be confirmed by inducing a pneumothorax which demonstrates a pneumopericardium in addition to the pneumothorax.

365.7. DISEASES OF DIVERSE UNKNOWN CAUSE

In addition to all the conditions discussed previously, the pericardium may be the site of involvement in a variety of other diseases. *Familial Mediterranean fever*, which involves various serous membranes, may also involve the pericardium. Although *sarcoidosis* more frequently involves the myocardium, granulomas can be found in the pericardium and on rare occasions may lead to signs of constrictive pericarditis. *Hydropericar-*

dium, which is an excessive accumulation of transudate in the pericardial cavity, may occur in conjunction with advanced cardiac or renal failure, as well as in association with inflammatory or malignant diseases which may obstruct lymphatic drainage from the pericardium. A *chylous pericardial effusion* may develop following traumatic rupture of the thoracic duct or in association with primary or metastatic malignant diseases which obstruct the thoracic duct. The pericardial fluid is milky white or brownish yellow, contains fat globules which can be visualized under the light microscope, and has markedly elevated triglyceride levels. *Cholesterol pericarditis*, which is characterized by an elevated level of cholesterol in the pericardial effusion and frequently by the appearance of a shiny or scintillating gold paint quality to the effusion, has been thought to be a separate clinical entity in the past. However, cholesterol pericarditis has been associated with a variety of disease states. Approximately one fourth of the cases reported have been associated with hypothyroidism. It is now thought that it is a manifestation of prolonged pericardial effusion with impairment of absorption of cholesterol from the chronically inflamed or scarred pericardium. There is subsequent gradual accumulation of large amounts of cholesterol crystals which give the effusion its unique appearance. Early treatment of hypothyroidism may produce a prompt elimination of the syndrome if the primary cause is hypothyroidism. However, if treatment is delayed in the case of hypothyroidism or if the condition is due to other causes, a pericardiectomy is the treatment of choice.

Bush, C. A., Stang, J. M., Wooley, C. F., and Kilman, J. W.: Occult constrictive pericardial disease: Diagnosis by rapid volume expansion and correction by pericardiectomy. Circulation, 56:924, 1977.

Cortes, F. M. (ed.): The Pericardium and Its Disorders. Springfield, Ill., Charles C Thomas, 1970.

Dressler, W.: The postmyocardial infarction syndrome. A report on forty-four cases. Arch. Intern. Med., 103:28, 1959.

Feigenbaum, H.: Echocardiography. *In* Pericardial Disease. Philadelphia, Lea & Febiger, 1976, p. 419.

Holt, J. P.: The normal pericardium. Am. J. Cardiol., 26:455, 1970.

Koontz, C. H., and Ray, C. G.: The role of coxsackie Group B virus infection in sporadic myopericarditis. Am. Heart J., 82:750, 1971.

Shabetai, R., Fowler, N. O., and Guntheroth, W. G.: The hemodynamics of cardiac tamponade and constrictive pericarditis. Am. J. Cardiol., 26:480, 1970.

Spodick, D. H.: Diagnostic electrocardiographic sequences in acute pericarditis. Circulation, 48:575, 1973.

366. DISEASES OF THE MYOCARDIUM

366.1. INTRODUCTION

Victor S. Behar

Myocardial failure may occur as the result of primary myocardial disease or secondary to hyperkinetic states or valvular or ischemic heart disease. The following chapters will deal with the primary myocardial diseases in which the basic pathology specifically involves the myocardium, thereby differentiating them from those caused by abnormalities of other cardiac structures. Much of the ambiguity surrounding the generalized term of cardiomyopathy stems from the inability of our predecessors to arrive at an etiologic diagnosis in patients with ill-defined heart disease. This frequently led them to the use of such terms as chronic myocarditis, myocardial degeneration, idiopathic myocardial hypertrophy, idiopathic cardiomyopathy, and noncoronary myocardial degeneration, to name a few. In many of the underdeveloped parts of the world, primary myocardial disease may account for 15 per cent or more of the patients with clinical heart disease. It has been estimated that in the United States, however, fewer than 1 per cent of cardiac deaths are due to primary myocardial disease. This may be a gross underestimate because of the difficulty in recognizing the disease as well as the tendency to attribute its etiology to a more common process such as coronary atherosclerosis.

The presentation and clinical course of patients with a cardiomyopathy are variable. The onset may frequently be silent and accompany an infectious disease with the development of a myocarditis manifest only by nonspecific electrocardiographic changes. These patients usually do not suffer any cardiac disability, and the persistence of the electrocardiographic abnormalities is variable. Although complete recovery is common with this type of presentation, patients may develop asymptomatic cardiomegaly, frequent bouts of congestive heart failure, systemic or pulmonary emboli, or rapid deterioration and sudden death.

The symptoms of a cardiomyopathy are not unlike those of other forms of heart disease. Weakness, fatigue, and dyspnea on exertion are the most frequent manifestations and are due to a low cardiac output. The signs and symptoms of right ventricular failure may occur soon after the development of left ventricular failure, and the combination appears to be more common than in other forms of heart disease. The low cardiac output may also produce peripheral cyanosis, falsely suggesting congenital heart disease. Although uncommon, chest pain may be suggestive of angina in character or due to an associated pericarditis. Right upper quadrant pain caused by congestive hepatomegaly is much more likely to occur and can be especially distressing during acute right ventricular decompensation. Palpitations are frequent and may be due to extrasystoles or arrhythmias, especially in acute myocarditis, alcoholic cardiomyopathy, or the familial cardiomyopathies.

The diagnosis of primary myocardial disease should be suspected in the young, normotensive individual with cardiomegaly or congestive heart failure in the absence of a prior history of congenital, valvular, or ischemic heart disease. The electrocardiogram characteristically demonstrates left ventricular hypertrophy, arrhythmias, or conduction defects. Because of the lack of etiologic information in the majority of these patients, it has proved useful to classify them by their pathophysiology into congestive, hypertrophic, and restrictive types.

In the congestive cardiomyopathies, there is systolic pump failure and dilatation of the left ventricle. These patients may remain asymptomatic for years, however, before developing congestive heart failure. On physical examination, there is frequently sinus tachycardia, pulsus alternans, and an enlarged apex beat with both atrial and ventricular gallop sounds. In addition, a murmur of mitral regurgitation is common, as is tricuspid regurgitation in the presence of right ventricular failure. The presence of Q waves on the electrocardiogram may falsely suggest myocardial infarction, making it

difficult to differentiate these patients from those with ischemic heart disease. In addition, conduction defects, including bundle branch block, bifascicular block, and sinoatrial node abnormalities, may be present. The chest x-ray demonstrates cardiomegaly and pulmonary congestion. The congestive type of cardiomyopathy may have the following causes: (1) infective, i.e., viral, bacterial; (2) metabolic, i.e., puerperal, endocrine, hemochromatosis, beriberi, amyloid; (3) heredofamilial neuromuscular diseases; (4) systemic diseases, i.e., collagen, sarcoid; (5) toxic, i.e., alcohol, heavy metals, drugs; (6) hypersensitivity reactions, i.e., serum sickness, postvaccinal; and (7) irradiation.

In hypertrophic cardiomyopathy, the pump function of the heart is usually maintained until late in the disease. The abnormal muscle reduces ventricular compliance and produces diastolic failure of the left ventricle with impaired diastolic filling. Outflow tract obstruction is common but not invariable. Although the majority of patients with this form of cardiomyopathy may be asymptomatic, others may complain of angina, dyspnea, syncope, or congestive heart failure. On physical examination, the classic findings include bisferious pulse, a bifid or trifid apical impulse, systolic ejection murmur, atrial gallop, and ventricular gallop in the presence of significant mitral regurgitation. This type of cardiomyopathy is most often familial and transmitted as an autosomal dominant trait. The clinical genetic marker is asymmetric septal hypertrophy (see Ch. 366.2).

Restrictive cardiomyopathies are rare and are most often due to an infiltrative process which frequently involves the endocardium. Pump function may be maintained and heart size normal, with symptoms being produced by restriction to ventricular filling. Although chest pain may be a presenting complaint, the majority of patients are asymptomatic and are referred because of an abnormal electrocardiogram or physical examination. Reduced ventricular compliance, secondary to the myopathic process, can simulate constrictive pericarditis because of the high venous pressure, rapid "y" descent, and loud early diastolic filling sound. In addition, at cardiac catheterization there may be an early diastolic dip in the right ventricular pressure recording, followed by a late diastolic plateau compatible with both restrictive and constrictive heart disease. When the restrictive process is disproportionately more severe on the left side of the heart, however, left ventricular end-diastolic, left atrial, and pulmonary artery pressures will be increased. Under these circumstances, the symptoms of pulmonary congestion may predominate. In constrictive pericarditis, there is equalization of diastolic pressures in all four chambers and normal pulmonary systolic pressure. This restrictive type of pathophysiology occurs in amyloidosis and less commonly in endomyocardial fibrosis of the African type and Löffler's fibroplastic eosinophilic endocarditis.

Goodwin, J. F.: Clarification of the cardiomyopathies. Mod. Concepts Cardiovasc. Dis., 41:41, 1972.

Mattingly, T. W.: Clinical features and diagnosis of primary myocardial disease. Mod. Concepts Cardiovasc. Dis., 30:677, 683, 1961.

Oakley, C. M.: Clinical recognition of the cardiomyopathies. Circ. Res., 35 (Suppl. II):II-152, 1974.

Perloff, J. K.: The cardiomyopathies — current perspectives. Circulation, 44:942, 1971.

Stapleton, J. F., Segal, J. P., and Harvey, W. P.: Clinical pathways of cardiomyopathy. Circ. Res., 35 (Suppl. II):II-168, 1974.

366.2. ASYMMETRIC SEPTAL HYPERTROPHY

Victor S. Behar

In recent years, asymmetric septal hypertrophy (ASH) has been identified as the unifying characteristic of the elusive disease which has been called idiopathic hypertrophic subaortic stenosis (IHSS), hypertrophic obstructive cardiomyopathy (HOCM), and muscular subaortic stenosis (MSS). Early accounts of this abnormality described marked hypertrophy of the left ventricular outflow tract with obstruction to ventricular ejection, leading ultimately to generalized ventricular hypertrophy. Our understanding of this disease progressed most rapidly with the advent of cardiac catheterization and echocardiography as diagnostic and research tools. These techniques have provided documentation of the unique clinical, physiologic, and pathologic characteristics of ASH. It was soon appreciated that patients with similar symptoms and physical findings may fall along a spectrum of hemodynamic abnormalities, ranging from severe resting gradients to gradients only with provocative maneuvers or to total absence of outflow tract obstruction. The confusion in this dynamic entity was greatly alleviated by the observation that the asymmetric septal hypertrophy, so readily seen at autopsy, can be visualized noninvasively during life through the use of echocardiography. The echocardiographic demonstration of a septal to posterior free wall ratio of 1.3 or greater provides a clinical marker for identifying patients with ASH independent of the existence of outflow tract obstruction (see accompanying figure). Although IHSS was originally felt to exist in both sporadic and familial forms, documentation of the latter was possible in only about 30 per cent of cases. The presence of asymmetric septal hypertrophy by echocardiogram throughout the entire spectrum of the disease provides a unique opportunity to study its pattern of inheritance. Such studies in first degree relatives of propositi illustrated that ASH is a genetic disease in almost all patients and is inherited as an autosomal dominant trait with a high degree of penetrance.

The most common clinical manifestations in symptomatic patients include dyspnea, angina, presyncope, syncope, paroxysmal nocturnal dyspnea, and palpitations. These symptoms bear a striking resemblance to those occurring in valvular aortic stenosis. However, in valvular aortic stenosis, syncope is associated with severe aortic valvular gradients, whereas patients with ASH and syncope frequently have little or no outflow tract gradients at rest. In addition, syncope in ASH is often postural in nature or produced after the cessation of exercise, whereas in valvular aortic stenosis syncope usually occurs during the actual performance of exercise.

On physical examination, a large "A" wave may be seen in the jugular venous pulse due to reduced distensibility of the right ventricle. The carotid arterial pulse is brisk and bifid in contour with a rapid initial rise followed by a mid-systolic dip and late systolic rise. This bisferious character of the pulse is most prominent in the presence of outflow tract obstruction. The heart is usually enlarged with a double apical impulse owing to presystolic expansion during atrial contraction. On auscultation, there is usually a loud atrial gallop. A parasternal thrill is frequently palpable and accompanies a holosystolic or systolic ejection murmur of variable intensity best heard at the left sternal border and apex. The second heart sound is usually normal but may be single or paradoxically split. A diastolic murmur is uncommon. A ventricular gallop may also be present at the apex. The variable intensity of the outflow tract murmur is due to its dependence upon the dimensions of the outflow tract and consequently the degree of obstruction during ventricular systole. Widening of the outflow tract with reduced obstruction occurs with an increase in end-diastolic volume, an increase in distending pressure during systole, or a decrease in the inotropic state of the myocardium. Increased obstruction occurs with opposite hemodynamic conditions. Because of these effects, the murmur classically increases in intensity during the Valsalva maneuver or upon assumption of the upright position; the murmur will decrease in intensity during leg raising and may completely disappear during squatting. Inhalation of amyl nitrite markedly increases the intensity of the murmur and outflow tract obstruction by its ability to decrease blood pressure and increase heart rate, as well as to increase the level of myocardial contractility. Other provocative maneuvers which increase outflow obstruction include postextrasystolic potentiation of the beat following a premature ventricular contraction, digitalis, nitroglycerin, isoproterenol, and exercise. Methoxamine or phenylephrine infusion and hypervolemia increase the dimensions of the outflow tract, thereby reducing or obliterating the gradient.

The electrocardiogram usually shows normal sinus

septum

1 cm

LV wall

Time motion echocardiogram of the left ventricle in idiopathic hypertrophic subaortic stenosis. The septal thickness is markedly increased, and the septal to posterior free wall ratio is abnormal at 3.5. In addition, the arrow identifies anterior motion of the anterior leaflet of the mitral valve during ventricular systole. The apposition of the septum and anterior mitral leaflet is responsible for the outflow tract obstruction.

rhythm and left ventricular hypertrophy. The occurrence of atrial fibrillation is an ominous sign because of the dependence of diastolic filling on atrial contraction. A short P-R interval, either with or without a delta wave and QRS prolongation characteristic of the Wolff-Parkinson-White syndrome, is not uncommon. Large Q waves may occur in more than half the patients, simulating a previous myocardial infarction. This has been attributed to abnormal septal depolarization.

The chest x-ray shows left ventricular enlargement, which is frequently manifest by a prominent "bump" along the anterolateral wall of the left ventricle as viewed in the frontal projection. Left atrial enlargement is less common. The aorta is usually not dilated, and the absence of aortic valvular calcification is helpful in excluding fixed valvular stenosis.

At cardiac catheterization, a resting gradient is frequently present within the left ventricular outflow tract or can be elicited with provocative maneuvers as described above. The gradient is labile and may vary on a beat-to-beat basis as well as during serial observations. Elevation of the left ventricular end-diastolic pressure is common. The angiocardiogram demonstrates marked thickening of the ventricular septum and left ventricular free wall. The papillary muscles are large and distort the shape of the ventricle, producing an hourglass configuration. Mitral regurgitation is common and is probably related to the altered geometry of the ventricle rather than deformity of the leaflets themselves. Systolic anterior motion of the anterior mitral leaflet is common and is thought to produce the outflow tract obstruction by its apposition to the hypertrophied septum. Systolic anterior motion of the anterior mitral leaflet may also be demonstrated by echocardiography (see figure) and correlates well with the presence of obstruction, on a beat-to-beat basis as well as during longitudinal studies and following surgery.

In patients with obstruction, the basic pathologic abnormality is felt to reside only in the asymmetric septum. The ventricular free wall is thickened but has a similar configuration to the chamber in patients with valvular aortic stenosis, suggesting that free wall hypertrophy is secondary to obstruction. Ultrastructural studies show bizarre cell-to-cell and intracellular abnormalities in the septum, with only rare cellular changes in the free wall. In nonobstructive patients, however, there are similar septal changes but a nonuniform distribution of free wall thickening associated with many disorganized and bizarre cells. This is interpreted as evidence that unlike obstructive ASH, in which the genetic defect is localized to the septum, the functional impairment in nonobstructive ASH is due to a diffuse expression of the genetic defect.

Although the echocardiographic finding of asymmetric septal hypertrophy and the histologic observations of myocardial fiber disarray are important morphologic features of this cardiomyopathy, recent studies have shown that they are not pathognomonic. ASH has been demonstrated in the normally developing heart and in the newborn. In addition, an abnormal septal to free wall ratio has been observed in approximately 20 per cent of patients with congenital heart disease primarily involving the right heart. Although a minor degree of ASH has been found in adult hearts with acquired right ventricular hypertrophy as well as in patients with coronary artery disease, the septal to free wall ratio on the echocardiogram generally does not exceed 1.3. The absence of ASH in first degree relatives of these patients indicates that this disproportionate septal hypertrophy does not represent genetically transmitted ASH. Focal zones of myocardial fiber disarray have also been observed in the normal heart and occur at the junction of the septum and free wall, as well as in the right ventricular infundibulum. Severe fiber disorganization has been found in congenital defects, characterized by hypertrophied ventricles, obliterated cavities, and outflow tract atresia, such as pulmonic atresia or the tetralogy of Fallot. These severe histologic abnormalities have not been found in acquired heart disease with right, left, or biventricular hypertrophy.

Relatively few patients with ASH are symptomatic. In the presence of symptoms the echocardiogram can be used to substantiate the diagnosis, and a trial of propranolol should then be attempted. Drugs such as nitroglycerin, digitalis, and diuretics should be avoided except for control of atrial fibrillation or the symptoms of congestive heart failure. As an important adjunct to therapy, patients should be taught to avoid the rapid assumption of the upright position, the Valsalva maneuver, and paroxysms of coughing. Approximately 10 to 15 per cent of symptomatic patients will not respond to medical therapy and will require surgery. Cardiac catheterization should be performed prior to surgery to document the severity of the resting or inducible gradient. The surgical procedure receiving greatest acclaim is that of left ventriculomyotomy and myectomy, which is performed through a vertical aortotomy while the patient is on cardiopulmonary bypass. Excellent symptomatic improvement has been reported in these patients with respect to dyspnea, angina, and syncope, but the amelioration of congestive heart failure has been somewhat disappointing. Postoperative hemodynamic studies in patients with obstruction at rest preoperatively have demonstrated complete abolition of the resting gradient in 90 per cent of patients, with the remainder having residual gradients of 25 mm Hg or less. Although mitral valve replacement has been advocated for the treatment of IHSS at some medical centers, the consensus suggests that valve replacement is not necessary even in the presence of significant mitral regurgitation, which has been found to regress clinically following left ventriculomyotomy and myectomy.

Braunwald, E., Lambrew, C. T., Rockoff, S. D., Ross, J., Jr., and Morrow, A. G.: Idiopathic hypertrophic subaortic stenosis. Circulation, 30 (Suppl. IV):IV-3, 1964.

Bulkley, B. H., Weisfeldt, M. L., and Hutchings, G. M.: Asymmetric septal hypertrophy and myocardial fiber disarray. Features of normal, developing, and malformed hearts. Circulation, 56:292, 1977.

Clark, C. E., Henry, W. L., and Epstein, S. E.: Familial prevalence and genetic transmission of idiopathic hypertrophic subaortic stenosis. N. Engl. J. Med., 289:709, 1973.

Henry, W. L., Clark, C. E., and Epstein, S. E.: Asymmetric septal hypertrophy. Circulation, 47:225, 1973.

Henry, W. L., Clark, C. E., Roberts, W. C., Morrow, A. G., and Epstein, S. E.: Differences in distribution of myocardial abnormalities in patients with obstructive and nonobstructive asymmetric septal hypertrophy (echo and gross anatomic findings). Circulation, 50:447, 1974.

Maron, B. J., Ferrans, V. J., Henry, W. L., Clark, C. E., Redwood, D. R., Roberts, W. C., Morrow, A. G., and Epstein, S. E.: Differences in distribution of myocardial abnormalities in patients with obstructive and nonobstructive asymmetric septal hypertrophy. Circulation, 50:436, 1974.

Morrow, A. G., Reitz, B. A., Epstein, S. E., Henry, W. L., Conkle, D. M., Itscoitz, S. B., and Redwood, D. R.: Operative treatment in hypertrophic subaortic stenosis. Circulation, 52:88, 1975.

366.3. FAMILIAL CARDIOMYOPATHY

Victor S. Behar

Although the term familial cardiomyopathy suggests a single disease entity, it more likely encompasses a variety of clinical and pathologic conditions. Included in this broad category are familial cardiomyopathy, asymmetric septal hypertrophy with or without obstruction, endocardial fibroelastosis, glycogen storage disease, Hunter's and Hurler's syndromes, and the heredofamilial neuromyopathic diseases.

FAMILIAL CARDIOMYOPATHY. Evans proposed the term familial cardiomyopathy in 1949 when he described three cases of heart disease in a single family. Clinically, the patients had palpitations, presyncope, congestive heart failure, or sudden death. Physical examination showed cardiomegaly and signs of left ventricular failure. The electrocardiogram showed extrasystoles, arrhythmias, and conduction abnormalities. At autopsy, there was generalized myocardial fibrosis and hypertrophy of the remaining myocardium. In addition, mural thrombi were present. The prognosis in young patients was worse than in adults, and death occurred from progressive congestive heart failure or was sudden. In recent years, the most frequent form of familial cardiomyopathy seen clinically is *asymmetric septal hypertrophy (ASH)*, either with or without left ventricular outflow tract obstruction. As described in Ch. 366.2, the unifying link in this disease is the demonstration of asymmetric septal hypertrophy either at autopsy or by echocardiography. Although it was originally felt that the disease could occur in either the sporadic or the familial form, echocardiographic studies in first degree relatives of patients with ASH demonstrate genetic transmission as an autosomal dominant trait. Most patients are asymptomatic, although angina, presyncope, syncope, and congestive heart failure may occur either with or without outflow tract obstruction.

ENDOCARDIAL FIBROELASTOSIS. Endocardial fibroelastosis is an obscure disease of unknown cause which may occur as an isolated lesion or in association with other cardiac anomalies. The occurrence of the isolated form in twins as well as siblings has suggested genetic transmission as an autosomal recessive trait. Endocardial fibroelastosis occurs in infancy and has no predilection for sex or race. The symptoms are usually dyspnea, orthopnea, wheezing, cyanosis, and failure to thrive. The course may be acute with rapid deterioration due to heart failure and death in several weeks, or chronic with remissions and exacerbations. Ninety per cent of patients are dead within one year because of heart failure, emboli, arrhythmias, or infection. The electrocardiogram shows left ventricular hypertrophy and, to a lesser extent, low voltage and conduction abnormalities. At autopsy, there is cardiomegaly with endocardial fibroelastosis involving all chambers, especially the left side of the heart. Grossly, the endocardium appears thickened, smooth, and porcelain white. The heart valves may be thickened and sclerotic in half the cases. The microscopic findings show increased amounts of endocardial ground substance with dense accumulation of elastic tissue and collagen at the junction with the subendocardium. Signs of inflammation and fibrous scarring of the myocardium are conspicuously absent. In addition, there is a periarterial adventitial hyperelastosis. The group of patients with associated cardiac anomalies may have aortic stenosis, mitral stenosis, coarctation of the aorta, ventricular septal defect, or the hypoplastic left heart syndrome. Although a genetic cause has been proposed, other suggested causes include maternal infection, fetal endocarditis, anoxia, or mechanical factors resulting from pressure or volume overload. Attention should be directed toward excluding associated cardiac anomalies and providing supportive therapy.

POMPE'S DISEASE. This severe form of glycogen storage disease, also known as Type II glycogenosis, is characterized by the generalized deposition of normal glycogen in the tissues and severe cardiomegaly. The defect is a deficiency of α-1,4-glucosidase and is transmitted as a single autosomal recessive gene. Clinically, the infant appears cretinoid with an enlarged tongue and has marked muscular hypotonicity and cardiomegaly. Hypoglycemia, ketosis, and hyperlipidemia do not occur, as in other types of glycogen storage disease. Tissue damage is thought to be due to progressive replacement by glycogen. The electrocardiogram shows left ventricular hypertrophy, and pathologically the interventricular septum is particularly involved and may produce outflow tract obstruction. Microscopic examination reveals glycogen-filled vacuoles, thought to be lysosomes.

HURLER'S SYNDROME AND HUNTER'S SYNDROME. Both these mucopolysaccharidoses may be associated with a cardiomyopathy. Hurler's syndrome is transmitted as an autosomal recessive trait and Hunter's syndrome by an X-linked gene. Hurler's syndrome is differentiated from Hunter's syndrome by its more severe clinical manifestations. They are characterized by the deposition of dermatan sulfate and heparan sulfate within cells and connective tissues. The cardiomegaly is generalized with involvement of the heart valves as well as the endocardium. In addition, there is intimal proliferation of the coronary arteries. Death is primarily due to congestive heart failure.

FABRY'S DISEASE. This is a sex-linked disorder characterized by deficient activity of α-galactosidase A. Males are primarily affected by this disorder, which results in the deposition of glycosphingolipids (chiefly globotriaosylceramide) in the walls of blood vessels, myocardium, and nerves. There is progressive cardiomegaly and death from left ventricular failure.

HEREDOFAMILIAL NEUROMYOPATHIC DISEASES. The nonmyotonic muscular dystrophies are frequently complicated by a cardiomyopathy. It is most common in the classic, rapidly progressive, sex-linked Duchenne's pseudohypertrophic form, which affects males in the first five years of life. The cardiomyopathy occurs in as many as 50 per cent of patients. The symptoms of heart failure are unusual in these patients because of their markedly diminished activity. On physical examination, it is common to hear atrial and ventricular gallop sounds as well as the murmur of mitral regurgitation. Cardiac chamber abnormalities are difficult to interpret by chest x-ray because of the severe thoracic abnormalities which are present. Cardiac involvement is most readily detected by the electrocardiogram. These changes include tall R waves in leads V_1 and V_3R, with an increased R/S ratio in V_1 together with deep Q waves in the standard limb leads and lateral precordial leads. Identical changes have been observed in female carriers of the dystrophy, who have also been demonstrated to have creatine phosphokinase abnormalities.

In addition, the electrocardiogram shows labile sinus tachycardia, premature atrial and ventricular extrasystoles, and atrial or ventricular tachycardia. Postmortem studies show selective scarring of the posterobasal left ventricle and the posteromedial papillary muscle. Noninflammatory degenerative changes have also been described in the arteries supplying the sinoatrial and atrioventricular nodes with sparing of the larger epicardial vessels.

Slowly progressive Duchenne's dystrophy (sex-linked recessive), limb-girdle dystrophy of Erb (autosomal recessive), and fascioscapulohumeral dystrophy of Dejerine and Landouzy (autosomal dominant) may also be associated with a cardiomyopathy, in decreasing order of frequency.

Myotonic muscular dystrophy is a heredofamilial multisystem disease which produces myotonia, muscle atrophy, myopathic facies, cataracts, frontal baldness, testicular atrophy, and a cardiomyopathy. The electrocardiogram is the most sensitive indicator of cardiac involvement and is abnormal in over half the patients. The electrocardiographic changes include sinus bradycardia, intraventricular and atrioventricular conduction disturbances, left axis deviation, low voltage, and supraventricular tachycardias. The conduction abnormalities may progress to complete heart block with Stokes-Adams attacks and sudden death. At autopsy, there is myocardial fibrosis and fatty infiltration.

Friedreich's ataxia is a neurologic heredofamilial disease characterized by ataxic gait, areflexia in the lower extremities, Babinski reflexes, sensory loss, scanning dysarthria, and skeletal deformities of the thorax. The cardiac symptoms include congestive heart failure and, less commonly, chest pain. The heart is clinically involved in 30 to 50 per cent of patients, although electrocardiographic changes may be present in as many as 90 per cent. These changes include sinus tachycardia, supraventricular tachycardias, and T wave inversion primarily involving leads I, II, AVF, and V_3 to V_6. In addition, left and right ventricular hypertrophy have been observed. Family members with the disease often show similar electrocardiographic changes. At autopsy, the heart demonstrates myocardial fiber hypertrophy, interstitial fibrosis, focal degeneration, and occasionally active necrosis. The coronary arteries may show atheromatous changes, and there is frequently medial degeneration and intimal hyperplasia in the small intramural vessels. Death is due to congestive heart failure or cor pulmonale secondary to the severe thoracic deformities.

Evans, W.: Familial cardiomegaly. Br. Heart J., 11:68, 1949.
Griggs, R. C.: Hypertrophy and cardiomyopathy in the neuromuscular diseases. Circ. Res., 35 (Suppl. II):II-145, 1974.
Perloff, J. K.: Cardiomyopathy associated with heredofamilial neuromyopathic diseases. Mod. Concepts Cardiovasc. Dis., 40:23, 1971.
Rosahn, P. D.: Endocardial fibroelastosis: Old and new concepts. Bull. N.Y. Acad. Med., 31:453, 1955.
Still, W. J. S.: Endocardial fibroelastosis. Am. Heart J., 61:579, 1961.

366.4. INFLAMMATORY OR INFECTIVE CARDIOMYOPATHY
(Myocarditis)

Victor S. Behar

The ubiquitous nature of myocarditis in a variety of infectious diseases makes it important to recognize.

Myocarditis may be associated with viral, bacterial, rickettsial, parasitic, fungal, or spirochetal disease, although with varying degrees of documentation. Myocarditis also may occur secondary to a systemic process such as a hypersensitivity reaction or connective tissue disease. The true incidence of myocarditis in the population is impossible to ascertain. Focal or diffuse myocarditis has been found to be relatively common in routine autopsy cases, ranging from 3.4 to 9.3 per cent. In addition, as many as one third of patients with common infectious diseases may have electrocardiographic abnormalities suggesting myocardial involvement. From these observations, it appears that myocarditis is most often silent and not accompanied by overt ventricular dysfunction. It has been postulated, however, that chronic cardiomyopathy may be a late manifestation of an acute myocarditis. It is well documented, for example, that such diseases as acute rheumatic carditis, Chagas' disease, and toxoplasmosis may progress to a stage of chronic fibrosis. Further credence is given to this postulate from observations that the incidence and severity of experimental myocarditis are increased by hypoxia, exercise, or concomitant exposure to bacterial toxins. In addition, treatment of experimental myocarditis with steroids may lead to diffuse myocardial abnormalities rather than focal lesions. One may speculate that factors such as these may select out patients with "silent" myocarditis to develop more extensive disease over time, leading ultimately to an "idiopathic" cardiomyopathy.

Myocarditis is frequently unrecognized either because of its subclinical nature or because of the severity of associated conditions. When symptomatic, the patient may complain of fever, palpitations, pleuropericardial pain, dyspnea, edema, or fatigue, or may die suddenly. The physical examination shows biventricular failure, including elevated venous pressure, cardiomegaly, soft first heart sound, ventricular gallop, mitral and tricuspid regurgitation, pulmonary rales, and congestive hepatomegaly. A pericardial friction rub is heard in the presence of an associated pericarditis. The electrocardiogram may show atrial and ventricular extrasystoles, arrhythmias, conduction disturbances, and ST-T wave abnormalities. Measurement of cardiac isoenzyme activities may be helpful in differentiating cardiac involvement from passive hepatic congestion.

Specific treatment is indicated for such conditions as rickettsial or *Mycoplasma pneumoniae* infections. The management of congestive heart failure includes digitalis, diuretics, and salt restriction. Short-acting digitalis preparations are recommended because of the propensity of these patients to develop digitalis toxicity. In addition, patients should be placed at bed rest and administered oxygen, if hypoxic, to reduce the deleterious effects of activity and hypoxia observed in experimental myocarditis. Lidocaine, quinidine, or procainamide may be necessary to control arrhythmias, but propranolol should be used with caution because of its negative inotropic effect. Although steroids may be of great benefit in acute rheumatic carditis, they should be used only as a last resort for infectious myocarditis because of the potential of more widespread myocardial disease as shown in the experimental model.

VIRAL MYOCARDITIS. Myocarditis without pericarditis is frequently caused by Group B coxsackieviruses. Group A coxsackieviruses are implicated much less often, as are echoviruses, measles, mumps, and poliomyelitis, as well as many others. Human infection with Group B coxsackievirus was first documented in neonatal infants and later in nursery epidemics, with the virus being recovered from the myocardium itself. Since then, coxsackievirus B heart disease has been identified in adults and is frequently associated with pericarditis. The only clinical manifestation may be electrocardiographic changes. Less commonly, cardiac enlargement and decreased exercise tolerance may occur. Idiopathic benign pericarditis, which is frequently associated with a myocarditis, is increasingly felt to represent coxsackievirus B disease.

Myocardial damage by a virus may result from its myocytolytic effect, through direct cellular invasion and multiplication, or by an autoimmune process. Microscopically, interstitial edema, round cell infiltration, loss of striations, and areas of necrosis are found. The newborn infant is particularly susceptible to viral myocarditis, which may be rapidly progressive, leading to congestive heart failure and death. In the adult, complete healing usually occurs, but chronic fibrosis may ensue. Although it has not been possible to isolate a virus in the chronic stage of the disease, studies in mice have shown continued inflammation and fibrosis well after disappearance of the virus from the myocardium. Through fluorescent antibody techniques, viral antigens have been identified in human cardiomyopathies, suggesting the possibility of a chronic, active process. Appropriate laboratory studies must be carried out during the acute or subacute stages in order to define the specific offending agent. These include viral isolation from pharynx and feces by tissue culture, and analysis of paired sera for type-specific IgM neutralizing or hemagglutination-inhibiting antibodies.

Poliomyelitis is frequently accompanied by myocarditis as manifest by conduction abnormalities and ST-T wave changes on the electrocardiogram. The significance of these changes is difficult to ascertain, however, as they may be due to concomitant brainstem disease, metabolic imbalance, or hypoxia. Cardiovascular collapse is a frequent cause of death in patients with bulbar poliomyelitis. The myocarditis is significantly more severe in these patients than in those dying of other polio-related causes. The myocardial lesions range from perivascular inflammation to diffuse myocardial involvement with edema, loss of striations, and fragmentation of myocardial cells. In addition, these patients appear to have more extensive involvement of the reticular substance in the medulla. A combination of vasoconstriction, mediated by the medullary lesion in bulbar poliomyelitis, and the extensive myocarditis may be responsible for the acute heart failure with pulmonary edema and cardiogenic shock.

Many other viruses in addition to coxsackievirus and poliomyelitis have been implicated in the production of myocarditis. These include measles, mumps, *Mycoplasma pneumoniae*, influenza, rabies, varicella, choriomeningitis, and infectious mononucleosis. Treatment of viral myocarditis is largely supportive and symptomatic. Since it appears that steroids may be responsible for more widespread inflammation during the early intracellular viral infection, they should be withheld initially and added later to inhibit the chronic inflammatory process. The efficacy of steroids in limiting chronic inflammation and subsequent fibrosis is still controversial.

BACTERIAL MYOCARDITIS.   Primary bacterial invasion of the myocardium is rare. It remains a grave complication, however, of bacterial endocarditis and may account for ventricular dysfunction because of myocardial microabscess formation. Later, during the reparative stage, ventricular dysfunction may result from chronic myocardial damage. The organisms most commonly involved are streptococci and staphylococci.

DIPHTHERITIC MYOCARDITIS.   Myocarditis is an ominous complication of *Corynebacterium diphtheriae* infection and accounts for the majority of deaths. The protein exotoxin responsible for many of the clinical manifestations of the disease is thought to interfere with the synthesis of polypeptide chains by inhibiting the transfer of amino acids from soluble RNA. In the myocardium, the oxidation of long-chain fatty acids is inhibited with resultant accumulation of triglycerides.

In a large compilation of patients with diphtheria, the over-all mortality rate has been reported as 11 per cent, whereas in those with an associated myocarditis the mortality rate may be as high as 60 per cent. The electrocardiogram is a sensitive histotoxic indicator of myocardial involvement and is abnormal in 20 to 40 per cent of patients by the second week of the disease. Clinically evident myocarditis, however, occurs in less than 10 per cent of cases. The prognosis for patients with P-R interval prolongation and T wave changes is excellent. Conduction disturbances which occur later in the illness have a poor prognosis, with reported mortality rates of 50 per cent for bundle branch block and 100 per cent for patients with complete heart block. Causes of death include congestive heart failure and arrhythmias. At autopsy, the hearts are dilated and flabby. Histologic examination reveals interstitial edema, fibrinoid degeneration and necrosis, and focal infiltrates of inflammatory cells. The treatment for diphtheria is prevention by immunization, antitoxin, and symptomatic therapy for the complications caused by myocarditis.

TOXOPLASMA MYOCARDITIS.   *Toxoplasma gondii* is a protozoan which infects humans as both a congenital and an acquired disease. The prevalence of *Toxoplasma* infection is highest in women of childbearing age and approaches 90 per cent in some areas of the world. The congenital form is thought to arise by transmission in utero and frequently results in abortion, premature birth, or neonatal death. Maternal infection in the first trimester of pregnancy is most likely to cause fetal infection with resultant central nervous system damage. Myocarditis is not prominent in congenital toxoplasmosis. The mode of transmission is unclear for the acquired form, and both domestic and wild animals have been implicated. In the adult, the disease is usually subclinical or mild and self-limiting. It is common for several members of the same family to be infected. Lethal disseminated toxoplasmosis may occur, however, and myocarditis or pericarditis is frequent in this situation. The disseminated form usually occurs in debilitated patients receiving cancer chemotherapy, irradiation, or steroids. The myocarditis is characterized pathologically by scattered areas of focal necrosis and inflammation. Intracellular organisms without surrounding inflammation are frequently observed in the myocardium, whereas other areas show severe inflammatory foci in the absence of the protozoan. The antemortem diagnosis is difficult and depends on the demonstration of the organism in tissue by animal inoculation or positive serologic tests. The latter include the Sabin-Feldman methylene blue dye test, hemagglutination, and fluorescent antibody tests. Although treatment is frequently unsatisfactory, the treatment of choice is combined pyrimethamine and sulfonamides, which act synergistically against the organism.

TRICHINOSIS. Although trichinosis is thought to be the most common helminthic infestation in man, the majority of patients are asymptomatic. Neurologic and myocardial involvement account for the fatalities. Symptoms of encephalitis begin during the stage of larval dissemination during the second week; more localizing neurologic signs begin during the encystment stage in the third week. Myocardial involvement, characterized by retrosternal chest pain, tachycardia, dyspnea, and congestive failure, usually begins after the third week. The electrocardiogram reveals nonspecific ST-T wave changes, conduction abnormalities, and extrasystoles. The majority of patients recover, but when death occurs it is usually between the fourth and eighth week. At autopsy, cardiomegaly, scattered areas of myocardial necrosis, and inflammatory infiltrates are found. Steroids appear to be beneficial for both the neurologic and cardiac complications.

TRYPANOSOMIASIS. Chagas' disease is produced by a protozoan, *Trypanosoma cruzi*, which is harbored by hematophagous insects more common in South and Central America. Although less than 1 per cent of infected individuals develop the acute form of Chagas' disease, approximately 30 per cent will develop chronic chagasic myocarditis 20 years after the initial infection. Acute Chagas' disease has a mortality rate of 1 per cent, largely resulting from myocarditis or meningoencephalitis, whereas approximately 20 per cent of those with the chronic myocarditis die within two years of diagnosis. Most cases of acute chagasic myocarditis are self-limited, and most patients recover with only transient cardiomegaly and minor electrocardiographic abnormalities. In patients with fatal cases, however, there is rapid deterioration due to congestive heart failure secondary to a panmyocarditis. Parasites are present in variable numbers within myocardial fibers, and there is extensive interstitial inflammation, necrosis, and hyaline degeneration. Toxic as well as immunoallergic mechanisms have been postulated. Chronic chagasic myocarditis manifests itself most commonly as a congestive cardiomyopathy and less often with restrictive signs and symptoms simulating constrictive pericarditis. The electrocardiogram classically shows right bundle branch block and S-T segment changes compatible with acute infarction. Right bundle branch block occurs in as many as 60 per cent of patients and is frequently associated with left anterior hemiblock, whereas left bundle branch block is rare. Premature ventricular contractions are common, as are ST-T wave changes and Q waves mimicking myocardial infarction. The diagnosis is made by demonstrating the organism in the patient's blood, culture, complement fixation test, or xenodiagnosis. Treatment is directed toward control of the arrhythmias and congestive heart failure.

GIANT CELL MYOCARDITIS. Idiopathic giant cell myocarditis is an uncommon disease of unknown cause that may present clinically as congestive heart failure, arrhythmias, or sudden death. All ages may be affected, and there is no predominance of either sex. Proposed causes include viral infection, autoimmune disease, and sarcoidosis. Histologically, there is interstitial edema with scattered areas of granulomatous lesions associated with fibrosis, multinucleated giant cells, plasma cells, lymphocytes, histiocytes, and fragments of degenerating myocardial fibers. In areas of myocardial necrosis, multinucleated giant cells are rare and polymorphonuclear cells are common. No other organs are involved. These observations by light microscopy and electron microscopy suggest that the process involves an unusual form of myocardial degeneration in which the multinucleated giant cells are myogenic in origin. The initiating cause of this degeneration is unknown, but of interest is the association with other diseases, including thymoma, myositis, thyroiditis, and systemic lupus erythematosus. There is no specific therapy, and the reports of results with steroids are conflicting.

Abelmann, W. H.: Myocarditis. N. Engl. J. Med., 275:832, 944, 1966.

Gleason, T. H., and Hamlin, W. B.: Disseminated toxoplasmosis in the compromised host. Arch. Intern. Med., 134:1059, 1974.

Gray, D. F., Morse, B. S., and Phillips, W. F.: Trichinosis with neurologic and cardiac involvement. Ann. Intern. Med., 57:230, 1962.

Hildes, J. A., Schaberg, A., and Alcock, A. J. W.: Cardiovascular collapse in acute poliomyelitis. Circulation, 12:986, 1955.

Hirschman, S. Z., and Hammer, G. S.: Coxsackie virus myopericarditis. Am. J. Cardiol., 34:224, 1974.

Ledbetter, M. K., Cannon, A. B., and Costa, A. F.: The electrocardiogram in diphtheritic myocarditis. Am. Heart J., 68:599, 1964.

Pyun, K. S., Kim, Y. H., Katzenstein, R. E., and Kikkawa, Y.: Giant cell myocarditis. Arch. Path., 90:181, 1970.

Rosenbaum, M. B.: Chagasic myocardiopathy. Prog. Cardiovasc. Dis., 7:199, 1964.

366.5. NUTRITIONAL CARDIOMYOPATHY

Victor S. Behar

Nutritional deficiencies have been known to produce as well as contribute to heart disease in virtually all parts of the world, although most commonly in the underdeveloped countries. In most instances, the precise cause remains unknown, and multiple factors no doubt exist.

Two identifiable forms of nutritional heart disease have been described in Africans. *Bantu hypokinetic heart disease* occurs in the adult Bantu with a poor nutritional background. The diet of those afflicted is primarily composed of carbohydrate and lacks protein and essential amino acids. No single food factor or vitamin has been identified. The patient has cardiomegaly and recurrent episodes of congestive heart failure. The circulation is described as "hypokinetic," and the cardiac output is usually between 1 and 2 liters per minute. In the early stages, the disease is reversible by the intake of a balanced diet. Without dietary therapy, the heart failure becomes intractable to conventional therapy and death is frequently sudden. At autopsy, there is cirrhosis of the liver with histologic features of hemochromatosis or cytosiderosis. The heart is dilated and hypertrophied, with mural thrombi seen on gross examination. Microscopically, there is interstitial edema and scattered areas of fibrosis, which at times may be extensive. Hemosiderin is not seen in the heart.

The second form of nutritional African heart disease is *kwashiorkor*, which is produced by a protein deficiency in infancy. The infant appears markedly cachectic with hepatomegaly and edema. With cardiovascular involvement, venous distention, decreased pulse pressure, cold extremities, and peripheral cyanosis occur. The heart is characteristically small both on chest x-ray and at autopsy. The histologic appearance is nonspecific. The electrocardiogram shows low voltage, and arrhythmias are uncommon. The Q-T interval is prolonged, and there are broad, deep ST-T wave changes. The severity of these findings is of prognostic value; they frequently revert to normal following adequate protein intake. Death is often sudden and unexplained.

Beriberi is responsible for the most common cause of nutritional heart disease in the world. The criteria for beriberi heart disease have been broadened since its first description in the Orient. The classic description was that of a hyperkinetic circulation with bounding and pistol shot pulses, predominant right heart failure with venous engorgement, flushing of the skin with peripheral vasodilation, and syncope or shock. In the Occidental form, there is usually biventricular failure, and the hyperkinetic aspects are masked or absent. The common denominator, however, is the low nutritional intake of vitamin B_1 (thiamin) and a high carbohydrate diet. The polished rice diet in the Orient accounts for this combination, whereas in the Western countries the disease occurs primarily in chronic alcoholics. It is an uncommon form of heart disease in alcoholics, however, but it may complicate the course and treatment of other organic types of heart disease. The electrocardiogram shows low voltage, nonspecific ST-T wave changes and prolongation of the Q-T interval. Conduction disturbances and arrhythmias are uncommon. Pathologically, the heart is markedly dilated, especially the right ventricle, and hypertrophied. Mural thrombi are not uncommon and may result in emboli. The histologic changes are nonspecific and include interstitial edema and hydropic degeneration, especially in the subendocardial myocardium.

The clinical diagnosis can be made in the presence of cardiomegaly, edema, increased venous pressure, peripheral neuritis or pellagra, and dietary deficiency of three months or greater, with improvement following thiamin therapy. The hemodynamic abnormalities of high cardiac output, low arteriovenous oxygen difference, and low peripheral vascular resistance return toward normal both acutely and chronically following the administration of thiamin. Digitalis and diuretics have also proved useful for the control of congestive heart failure.

Potassium deficiency produces characteristic abnormalities on the electrocardiogram. These include prolongation of the Q-T interval, depressed S-T segments, flattening of the T wave, and the appearance of large U waves. Prolonged hypokalemia in animals fed a diet deficient in potassium or made hypokalemic by the administration of desoxycorticosterone acetate has been shown to produce typical histologic changes in the kidneys as well as the heart. Similar histologic changes have been observed in humans with chronic steatorrhea following prolonged periods of hypokalemia. The myocarditis of potassium deficiency is characterized by an early focal infiltration of polymorphonuclear neutrophils surrounding normal myocardial fibers, and later by loss of muscle striations, necrosis, influx of inflammatory cells, and bands of fibrosis. Treatment is, of course, early potassium replacement in order to prevent the development of permanent changes and fibrosis.

ALCOHOLIC CARDIOMYOPATHY. This is a well known clinical entity characterized by congestive heart failure in the absence of a known cause for heart disease other than the presence of alcoholism. The dietary state of these patients is usually adequate, and there is no deficiency of thiamin or other essential nutrients. Chronic alcoholism may be defined as the daily intake of eight ounces of whiskey, one quart of wine, or two quarts of beer for five years or more. The clinical recognition of cardiomyopathy in patients with chronic alcoholism is usually not difficult and can be documented by hemodynamic abnormalities of ventricular function both invasively and noninvasively. With these techniques, it has been shown that patients with an alcoholic fatty liver in the absence of clinical evidence of cardiac involvement may also have significant depression of ventricular function. Studies in noncardiac chronic alcoholics reveal that the depressed resting level of ventricular function may be further depressed by the acute ingestion of ethanol in a moderate dose, but not following a low dose. However, normal subjects receiving a similar low dose, which produces nonintoxicating ethanol blood levels, showed significant transient depression of ventricular performance. These findings suggest that there is a myocardial adaptation to chronic alcohol use in which the threshold for myocardial depression is increased. Metabolic studies in animals and man during acute ingestion of ethanol in intoxicating amounts show a rise in the myocardial respiratory quotient followed by a return to control levels in 90 minutes. This is accompanied by a decrease in myocardial free fatty acid extraction and an increase in triglyceride uptake. Transient myocardial injury following ethanol administration has been demonstrated by an efflux of ions and transaminase in coronary sinus blood. It is therefore apparent that chronic ingestion of alcohol adversely affects the heart and that these changes are reversible prior to development of the overt cardiomyopathy of alcoholism.

The clinical manifestations are palpitations, secondary to extrasystoles and arrhythmias, followed by the symptoms of congestive heart failure and thromboembolic episodes. On physical examination, a resting tachycardia, cardiomegaly, atrial and ventricular gallop sounds, and the murmurs of mitral or tricuspid regurgitation are found. Other common signs of heart failure include venous distention, hepatomegaly, and edema. These signs of a hypokinetic circulation are readily differentiated from the hyperkinetic circulation of beriberi. The electrocardiogram shows distinctive T wave changes described as spinous (peaked), dimpled (shallow notch in Q-T segment), and cloven (cleft at summit of low T wave). The T waves may later become inverted, falsely suggesting coronary disease. In addition, there may be left ventricular hypertrophy, conduction disturbances, S-T segment depression, pathologic Q waves, and arrhythmias, including premature atrial and ventricular systoles as well as atrial fibrillation. The chest x-ray reveals cardiomegaly and pulmonary congestion.

At autopsy, there is marked cardiomegaly with both dilatation and hypertrophy. Mural thrombi are common. Histologic study shows hypertrophy of the myocardial fibers, increased glycogen and neutral lipid, interstitial edema, necrosis, and fibrosis. Electron microscopic studies of tissue obtained by endomyocardial biopsy following acute infusion of ethanol show severe alterations of myocardial cellular organelles. These changes include mitochondrial swelling with loss of its cristae and swelling of the sarcoplasmic reticulum.

In the natural course of alcoholic cardiomyopathy the three-year mortality rate exceeds 40 per cent after the development of symptoms. The prognosis is significantly better in those patients with a shorter duration of symptoms and those who are able to abstain from further alcohol ingestion. Prolonged bed rest has not substantially improved the long-term response to conventional therapy, which is largely supportive and symptomatic.

COBALT-BEER CARDIOMYOPATHY. In August, 1965, a bizarre cardiomyopathy became manifest in Quebec City, affecting heavy beer drinkers who were primarily males over the age of 25. The illness was fulminating with biventricular failure associated with polycythemia, low cardiac output, cyanosis, cardiomegaly, gallop rhythm, pericardial effusion, cardiogenic shock, and severe lactic acidosis. A similar disease occurred in Minneapolis and Omaha, as well as in several other cities throughout the world. The electrocardiogram in these patients showed sinus tachycardia, whereas arrhythmias were rare. A rightward shift of the P wave and QRS complex was observed, as were large Q waves simulating anterior myocardial infarction. The chest x-ray revealed cardiomegaly and signs of pericardial effusion. Serum glutamic oxaloacetic transaminase, lactic dehydrogenase, and creatine phosphokinase were markedly elevated. The mortality rate ranged from 40 to 45 per cent. At autopsy, electron microscopic studies of the heart showed dissolution of myofibrils, with loss of myofibrillar proteins and replacement by glycogen; abnormal and shrunken mitochondria, which contained large intramitochondrial vacuoles; and dilatation of the sarcoplasmic reticulum, with formation of large vesicles. The sarcolemma appeared to be intact. The thyroid gland demonstrated follicular hyperplasia and little or no colloid. These changes in the thyroid gland were an important clue in the final identification of cobalt as the toxic agent. Because of the extensive use of detergents in washing glassware, beer poured into glasses with residual detergent was unable to maintain its foam. Cobalt chloride was therefore added to the beer in order to stabilize the foam. The metabolic action of cobalt is to block the oxidation of pyruvate to acetyl-CoA and α-ketoglutarate to succinyl-CoA without affecting the synthesis of glycogen and triglyceride. The relative toxicity of cobalt on the heart is complicated by other factors such as duration of ethanol intake, dietary protein, thiamin deficiency, and pre-existing heart disease. Although the majority of survivors had a satisfactory recovery, residual electrocardiographic changes and chronic heart failure were not unusual. Since the removal of cobalt from beer, no additional cases have been reported.

Ahmed, S. S., Levinson, G. E., and Regan, T. J.: Depression of myocardial contractility with low doses of ethanol in normal man. Circulation, 48:378, 1973.

Akbarian, M., Yankopoulos, N. A., and Abelmann, W. H.: Hemodynamic studies in beriberi heart disease. Am. J. Med., 41:197, 1966.

Demakis, J. G., Proskey, A., Rahimtoola, S. H., Jamil, M., Sutton, G. C., Rosen, K. M., Gunnar, R. M., and Tobin, J. R.: The natural course of alcoholic cardiomyopathy. Ann. Intern. Med., 80:293, 1974.

Higginson, J., Gillanders, A. D., and Murray, J. F.: The heart in chronic malnutrition. Br. Heart J., 14:213, 1952.

McAllen, P. M.: Myocardial changes occurring in potassium deficiency. Br. Heart J., 17:5, 1955.

Morin, Y. C., Foley, A. R., Martineau, G., and Roussel, J.: Quebec beer-drinkers' cardiomyopathy: 48 cases. Can. Med. Assoc. J., 97:881, 1967.

Regan, T. J., Levinson, G. E., Oldewurtel, H. A., Frank, M. J., Weisse, A. B., and Moschos, C. B.: Ventricular function in noncardiacs with alcoholic fatty liver: Role of ethanol in the production of cardiomyopathy. J. Clin. Invest., 48:397, 1969.

Smythe, P. M., and Swanepoel, A.: The heart in kwashiorkor. Br. Med. J., 1:67, 1962.

366.6. CARDIAC AMYLOIDOSIS

Victor S. Behar

Cardiac amyloidosis is a disease of unknown cause characterized by the widespread tissue deposition of an amorphous hyaline-like substance. The disease is uncommon under age 40 and affects the sexes equally. The prevalence of amyloidosis in the general population is not known. Although patients with multiple myeloma may have an incidence of amyloidosis as high as 15 per cent, it occurs in less than 1 per cent of unselected cases at autopsy. The relationship of amyloidosis to the aging process is of particular interest, as it has been found in as many as 90 per cent of patients dying of senile dementia when specifically looked for in brain, heart, or pancreas.

There have been many attempts to classify amyloidosis; it appears most useful to divide them into the following groups: (1) primary amyloidosis (no coexisting disease), (2) myeloma associated amyloidosis, (3) secondary amyloidosis (coexisting, chronic inflammatory disease), (4) localized amyloidosis (single organ involvement), and (5) familial amyloidosis. Amyloidosis presents clinically most often with renal involvement, especially the nephrotic syndrome, congestive heart failure, carpal tunnel syndrome, sprue, peripheral neuropathy, or orthostatic hypotension. The most common symptoms are fatigue, weight loss, edema, dyspnea, and, to a lesser extent, hoarseness, paresthesias, or the carpal tunnel syndrome. Although the edema may be produced by either the nephrotic syndrome or congestive heart failure, the presence of dizziness, syncope, and orthostatic hypotension should suggest cardiac amyloidosis.

On physical examination, hepatomegaly, splenomegaly and macroglossia are usually found, the last being more common in patients with multiple myeloma. In addition, there may be lymphadenopathy, especially in the submandibular region, purpura, and skin lesions. The cardiac manifestations may simulate constrictive pericarditis because of impaired ventricular filling during diastole and include an elevated jugular venous pressure with a rapid "y" descent and an early diastolic filling sound. However, if the left heart is more severely involved, the signs of left heart failure may predominate.

The electrocardiogram shows low voltage, which may falsely suggest constrictive pericarditis, as well as Q wave abnormalities, which may be misinterpreted as old myocardial infarction. Supraventricular arrhythmias are frequently seen, as well as the entire spectrum of conduction abnormalities. Many investigators have made the observation that patients with cardiac amyloidosis are particularly susceptible to digitalis-induced arrhythmias, possibly because of the infiltration of amyloid in the perivascular region of the sinoatrial node.

Pathologically, the heart is increased in size and firm in consistency. Nodular lesions may be seen in the endocardium, valves, and pericardium. Histologic examination reveals diffuse interstitial infiltration of amyloid within the myocardium and in the blood vessels. Amyloid is identified by its distinctive green birefringence when stained with Congo red and examined under a polarizing microscope. In the electron microscope, the amyloid is seen to consist of rigid, nonbranching fibrils. In systemic primary amyloidosis these fibrils are identical to the variable portion of monoclonal Bence Jones protein. When Bence Jones proteins are subjected to pepsin digestion, amyloid fibrils are produced. This has led to the speculation that light chains produced by the plasma cells are precursors of the amyloid fibril, either being produced within the cell and secreted or being secreted to form the fibrils in the surrounding tissue. The association of Bence Jones protein and amyloidosis has been further substantiated by a report from the Mayo Clinic in which 50 per cent of their patients with primary amyloidosis were found to have a monoclonal protein in either the serum or urine. Similar monoclonal abnormalities were present in 89 per cent of patients with multiple myeloma–associated amyloidosis. The clinical diagnosis is proved by tissue biopsy from the rectum in over 80 per cent of patients, and in more than 90 per cent when tissue is obtained from the kidney, carpal tunnel, or liver. Two-year survival for patients with primary amyloidosis is 35 per cent, but only 10 per cent for those with amyloidosis associated with multiple myeloma. Congestive heart failure is the most common cause of death, and sudden death, presumably from arrhythmias, is also frequent.

Brigden, W.: Cardiac amyloidosis. Prog. Cardiovasc. Dis., 7:142, 1964.
Buerger, L., and Braunstein, H.: Senile cardiac amyloidosis. Am. J. Med., 28:357, 1960.
Cohen, A. S.: Amyloidosis. N. Engl. J. Med., 277:522, 1967.
James, T. N.: Pathology of the cardiac conduction system in amyloidosis. Ann. Intern. Med., 65:28, 1966.
Kyle, R. A., and Bayrd, E. D.: Amyloidosis: Review of 236 cases. Medicine, 54:271, 1975.

366.7. OTHER CARDIOMYOPATHIES

Victor S. Behar

ENDOMYOCARDIAL FIBROSIS. Endomyocardial fibrosis has been reported to be responsible for approximately 15 per cent of the cardiac deaths from heart failure in Uganda. The disease has also been reported in Celon and Sudan. No known cause has been defined, although increased consumption of African plantain, which is rich in serotonin, has been implicated, as well as persistence of the infantile form of fibroelastosis, hypersensitivity reactions, and inflammation caused by viral or parasitic disease. Both sexes and all age groups are affected. The manifestations are progressive biventricular failure with dyspnea, edema, ascites, and pain from hepatic congestion. Mitral regurgitation is common, and tricuspid regurgitation may occur in the presence of right ventricular failure. The signs of a restrictive cardiomyopathy are usually dominant both on physical examination and at cardiac catheterization, falsely suggesting constrictive pericarditis. The frequent occurrence of pulmonary hypertension, however, is strong evidence against constriction.

At autopsy, all chambers may show the endocardial and myocardial changes, but the ventricles are more severely involved. Microscopically, the endocardium demonstrates the presence of an acellular, hyalinized, fibrous tissue. These changes, together with granula-

tion tissue, extend into the inner one third of the myocardium. Mural thrombi are common despite the infrequent history of systemic emboli. There is no specific treatment for endomyocardial fibrosis other than the symptomatic management of congestive heart failure.

LÖFFLER'S FIBROPLASTIC ENDOCARDITIS. In 1936, Löffler reported a series of patients with progressive and refractory heart failure who had a febrile illness associated with a persistent eosinophilia and multiple systemic emboli. The mode of onset may be either acute, with abdominal, cerebral, or respiratory symptoms, or insidious, with a gradual decrease in exercise tolerance and a clinical picture simulating constrictive pericarditis. Mitral regurgitation is common, but murmurs of mitral stenosis and tricuspid regurgitation may also be heard. The electrocardiogram demonstrates low voltage with nonspecific S-T segment and T wave abnormalities. The chest x-ray shows pulmonary congestion and infiltrates as well as pleural effusions.

The acute phase of the disease is characterized by an eosinophilic arteritis involving the heart and other organs. In the late stages of the disease, the heart is enlarged and there is a leathery, grayish-white thickening of the endocardium which involves all chambers. The fibrosis extends into the myocardium as well as the papillary muscles and chordae tendineae, with resultant mitral and tricuspid valvular incompetence. The disease is inevitably fatal, and there is no specific form of therapy, although steroids have produced some improvement during the acute stage.

SARCOIDOSIS. Although clinical manifestations of cardiac involvement are unusual in sarcoidosis, postmortem studies have demonstrated parenchymal cardiac involvement in 20 per cent of cases. The patients with cardiac symptoms are frequently young or middle aged, with equal prevalence in males and females. There is almost always a known history of sarcoidosis. The clinical manifestations are most often palpitations, presyncope, or syncope; chest pain and congestive heart failure occur less often. Congestive heart failure is primarily due to cor pulmonale and not to direct myocardial involvement. The electrocardiogram demonstrates a high incidence of atrioventricular block, bundle branch block, ventricular ectopic beats, and ventricular tachycardia and fibrillation. Worsening of the arrhythmias has been noted during exercise testing. Death frequently occurs within six months of the onset of cardiac symptoms, and 75 per cent of patients are dead within two years. The cause of death is unexplained and sudden in approximately two thirds of patients. Arrhythmias and complete heart block, which occur in 30 per cent of patients, must, of course, be implicated. At autopsy, the typical lesion is a noncaseating granulomatous follicle composed of epithelioid cells and giant cells of the Langerhans type surrounded by a narrow zone of lymphocytes. Although many organs are involved, the lungs are frequently most severely affected, with progressive fibrosis leading to cor pulmonale. The myocardial lesions most often involve the left ventricle and the upper posterior part of the interventricular septum. The histologic lesions are variable but may be categorized as exudative, granulomatous, granulomatous plus fibrotic, and predominantly fibrotic. Although treatment is frequently disappointing, improvement in the recurrent arrhythmias has been observed with prednisone alone or in various combinations with procainamide, quinidine, and propranolol.

PERIPARTUM CARDIOMYOPATHY (PUERPERAL MYOCARDITIS). Peripartum cardiomyopathy is characterized by congestive heart failure in the last month of pregnancy or within five months of delivery in the absence of any pre-existing form of heart disease. The incidence is highest in multiparous blacks and is more common with increasing age, poor nutrition and prenatal care, toxemia, and multiple births. The onset of left ventricular failure occurs most often within the first three months post partum. The electrocardiogram may show left ventricular hypertrophy with inverted T waves, low voltage, and nonspecific ST-T wave abnormalities. The chest x-ray demonstrates cardiomegaly and pulmonary venous congestion.

Although the early prognosis is good, significant cardiac disability and death may ensue. The patients segregate into low risk and high risk groups, according to changes in heart size. In as many as 50 per cent of patients, heart size may return to normal within six months. In these patients, the persistence of gallop sounds, recurrence of heart failure, or recurrence of postpartum failure following subsequent pregnancies is rare. In the patients with persistent cardiomegaly, however, chronic heart failure and pulmonary or systemic emboli are common. Furthermore, in this poor risk group, subsequent pregnancies frequently result in worsening of symptoms and death. Long-term survival for these patients is approximately 15 per cent in five years.

Myocardial biopsy obtained within three months of the onset of heart failure shows myocardial hypertrophy and varying degrees of fibrosis. At autopsy, the heart is dilated and appears hypertrophied. Mural thrombi are common and frequently result in emboli. Histologically, there is myocardial hypertrophy, fibrosis, interstitial edema, and focal accumulation of lymphocytes.

No specific form of therapy is indicated other than the management of congestive heart failure. The risk of subsequent pregnancies is substantial, and the likelihood of carrying the pregnancy to term is reduced.

RADIATION MYOCARDITIS. In recent years, the goal of radiation therapy has increasingly been complete eradication of the malignancy. Cardiac injury is clinically apparent in approximately 5 per cent of patients receiving 4000 rads or more in the form of either orthovoltage or supervoltage. Patients receiving larger amounts of radiation, as in those undergoing retreatment therapy for Hodgkin's disease, have a much higher incidence of carditis. In the large series of patients treated at Stanford, 50 per cent of those receiving more than 6000 rads developed carditis, which in some cases was a severe pancarditis. Radiation heart disease is most commonly manifest in the form of pericardial disease, including acute pericarditis, chronic effusion, or chronic constrictive pericarditis. Less commonly, myocardial fibrosis may accompany pericarditis and has been observed to produce conduction disturbances, including bundle branch block and varying degrees of heart block, as well as ventricular dysfunction and mitral regurgitation. Of particular interest is the controversy that radiation injury produces premature coronary atherosclerosis. Indeed, there are many autopsy reports of patients dying in the second or third decade with extensive coronary artery disease and myocardial infarctions following radiation therapy. In addition to these clinical observations, there are experimental data that the changes induced in the dog aorta by radiation are very similar to those which occur during the normal aging process. Other studies in atherogenic animal models further substantiate the clinical observation in that more severe atheromatous lesions occur following exposure to high dose radiation. The microcirculation has also been shown to participate in the process of myocardial damage from radiation. Immediately following exposure, there is an acute and transient inflammatory exudate in all cardiac tissues. After a latent period, however, a focal cytoplasmic degeneration occurs in the endothelial cells of myocardial capillaries, followed by a proliferation of these cells in an apparent attempt to form new capillaries. Ischemia and diffuse myocardial fibrosis result from this gradual loss of the microcirculation.

With the advent of megavoltage therapy and innovative rotational techniques, more effective tumor doses can now be delivered and survival significantly prolonged. As a byproduct of this, however, the treatment of thoracic malignancy also results in more radiation to the heart, and because of the longer survival there is greater opportunity for the delayed effects of myocardial damage to occur. It is important to acknowledge the fact that although acute pericarditis may occur during the period of radiation treatment itself, it is more likely that the signs and symptoms of cardiac damage will occur after a variable latent period, frequently years. Thus the development of cardiac symptoms following a course of radiation therapy does not necessarily indicate recurrence of tumor in the myocardium but may be a manifestation of radiation disease of the heart.

DRUG-INDUCED MYOCARDITIS. Adriamycin, which closely resembles its parent compound daunorubicin, has been observed to produce cardiotoxicity during the treatment of far-advanced cancer. The cardiotoxicity is manifest as electrocardiographic changes or congestive heart failure. The electrocardiographic abnormalities occur in 10 per cent of patients and include sinus tachycardia, ST-T wave changes, and premature ventricular contractions. These are reversible upon discontinuance of the drug. An additional 10 per cent of patients develop intractable biventricular heart failure, with death within three weeks of the onset of symptoms. This appears to be dose related, with virtually all affected patients receiving more than 500 mg per square meter of Adriamycin. Impaired left ventricular function has been observed by noninvasive studies in patients receiving as little as 300 mg per square meter, and this technique should be useful in detecting subclinical cases of cardiotoxicity. These early changes are reversible, but the recovery time is directly related to the cumulative dose. The toxicity appears to be due to the aglycone metabolite of the drug.

Other drugs which may produce electrocardiographic changes or toxicity include the tricyclic antidepressants, phenothiazines, and emetine.

Cohn, K. E., Stewart, J. R., Fajardo, L. F., and Hancock, E. W.: Heart disease following radiation. Medicine, 46:281, 1967.

Davies, J. N. P.: Some considerations regarding obscure diseases affecting the mural endocardium. Am. Heart J., 59:600, 1960.

Demakis, J. G., Rahimtoola, S. H., Sutton, G. C., Meadows, W. R., Szanto, P. B., Tobin, J. R., and Gunnar, R. M.: Natural course of peripartum cardiomyopathy. Circulation, 44:1053, 1971.

Fajardo, L. F., and Stewart, J. R.: Pathogenesis of radiation-induced myocardial fibrosis. Lab. Invest., 29:244, 1973.

Lefrak, E. A., Pitha, J., Rosenheim, S., and Gottlieb, J. A.: A clinico-pathologic analysis of Adriamycin cardiotoxicity. Cancer, 32:302, 1973.

Matsui, Y., Iwai, K., Tachibana, T., Fruie, T., Shigematsu, N., Izumi, T., Homma, A. H., Mikami, R., Hongo, O., Hiraga, Y., and Yamamoto, M.: Clinicopathologic study on fatal myocardial sarcoidosis. Ann. N.Y. Acad. Sci., 278:455, 1976.

Rinehart, J. J., Lewis, R. P., and Balcerzak, S. P.: Adriamycin cardiotoxicity in man. Ann. Intern. Med., 81:475, 1974.

Stein, E., Stimmel, B., and Siltzbach, L. E.: Clinical course of cardiac saroidosis. Ann. N.Y. Acad. Sci., 278:470, 1976.

366.8.   TUMORS OF THE HEART

Robert E. Whalen

The heart itself can be the site of a host of primary as well as metastatic tumors. Almost every type of malignant tumor has been found in metastatic form in the heart, but by far the most frequent metastatic tumors include malignant melanomas, leukemia, and malignant lymphomas. Although metastatic tumors of the heart are more frequent than previously realized, they seldom play a significant role in the course of the patient. A large variety of primary tumors of the heart itself have been described, including myxomas, lipomas, fibromas, hemangiomas, lymphangiomas, mesotheliomas, and sarcomas.

The cardiac myxoma is the most frequent and also clinically the most significant primary tumor of the heart, for its discovery and treatment can be lifesaving, whereas its continued presence can be fatal. Myxomas can arise from the endocardial surface of any of the cardiac chambers, but 95 per cent of them arise in the atria, with at least 75 per cent of these arising in the left atrium. The classic location for a myxoma is the region of the fossa ovalis in the left atrium. Bilateral atrial myxomas have been reported. Myxomas have been reported from youth to old age, but most frequently they occur in the middle years. In most series there is a higher incidence among females. They usually present in one or more of three typical ways. The most frequent presentation, which is due to progressive enlargement of the tumor within the cardiac chamber, involves progressive decrease in exercise tolerance, increased dyspnea on exertion, and pulmonary or peripheral edema. Next, the first sign of a myxoma may be produced by occlusion of a major artery with fragments of the myxoma or thrombus previously lodged on the surface of the intracardiac myxoma. Cerebrovascular accidents and sudden ischemia to limbs from this mechanism often herald the presence of a myxoma. The last and least frequent manifestation of a myxoma is the development of systemic symptoms which may simulate acute rheumatic fever, bacterial endocarditis, systemic lupus erythematosus, or a fever of unknown etiology.

Myxomas are almost always accompanied by a regurgitant heart murmur, usually due to incompetence of either the tricuspid or the mitral valve produced by distortion of the valve leaflets. Less frequently the murmur of tricuspid or mitral stenosis may be the most prominent feature due to obstruction of either one of these orifices. The hallmark of the myxoma, frequently detected by auscultation, is a third heart sound which varies in time after the second heart sound. This "tumor plop" is due to the acceleration of the tumor mass through the atrioventricular valve and its impact against the ventricular wall. The presence of any of the aforementioned manifestations in the setting of a normal cardiothoracic ratio, particularly with atrial prominence by chest x-ray, should raise suspicion of a myxoma. The electrocardiogram may show atrial hypertrophy. The presence of a variable third heart sound by phonocardiography, the presence of either an elevated sedimentation rate or increased gamma globulin level, and the variable indentation of the barium-filled esophagus during systole under fluoroscopic observation should enhance suspicion.

The diagnosis of a myxoma is best confirmed by echocardiography, which provides a characteristic picture of the tumor mass as it moves from the atrium to the ventricle during diastole. Angiocardiography, formally the sine qua non for making the diagnosis, is seldom necessary. The life-threatening nature of a cardiac myxoma, the ease with which the diagnosis can be made by echocardiography, and the success of open heart surgery in eliminating the condition emphasize the importance of having a high index of suspicion when seeing a patient with symptoms suggestive of heart failure but with a normal heart size.

Fine, G.: Neoplasms of the pericardium and heart. In Gould, S. E. (ed.): Pathology of the Heart and Blood Vessels. Springfield, Ill., Charles C Thomas, 1968, p. 851.

Hardin, N. J., Wilson, J. M., Gray, G. F., and Gay, W. A.: Experience with primary tumors of the heart: Clinical and pathological study of seventeen cases. Johns Hopkins Med. J., 134:141, 1974.

Johnson, M. L., Sieker, H. O., Behar, V. S., and Whalen, R. E.: Echocardiographic diagnosis of a left atrial myxoma found attached to the free left atrial wall. J. Clin. Ultrasound, 1:75, 1973.

Peters, M. N., Hall, R. J., Cooley, D. A., Leachman, R. D., and Garcia, E.: The clinical syndrome of atrial myxoma. JAMA, 230:695, 1974.

Selzer, A., Sakai, F. J., and Popper, R. W.: Protean clinical manifestations of primary tumors of the heart. Am. J. Med., 52:9, 1972.

367.   DISEASES OF THE AORTA

Noble O. Fowler

367.1.   INTRODUCTION

The aorta begins just superior to the aortic valve and ends at the aortic bifurcation opposite the fourth lumbar vertebra. Diseases of the aorta cannot be entirely separated from diseases of the aortic branches. A pathologic process which involves both the aorta and its branches may provoke obstruction or occlusion of these branches and thereby call attention to the existence of aortic disease. For example, in the aortic root, obstruction of a coronary artery at its origin may be caused by aortic intimal disease, thus causing the pain of myocardial ischemia (angina pectoris). Takayasu's arteritis and syphilitic aortitis may represent examples of this mechanism. In a like manner, involvement of the aortic arch can lead to a constellation of symptoms known as the aortic arch syndrome. In this syndrome, obstruction of the orifice of the innominate or left common carotid artery can cause symptoms of cerebral ischemia or visual disturbance. Narrowing of the orifice of the innominate artery or left subclavian artery may cause ischemia of the upper extremities or syncope because of the "subclavian steal" syndrome. Thus patients with aortic atherosclerosis or Takayasu's arteritis may have attacks of syncope, transient pain or syncope with use of the arm with impaired blood supply, or transient monocular blindness. In the abdominal aorta, occlusion of the mesenteric arteries may lead to bowel ischemia with postprandial abdominal angina, or even to infarction of the bowel. Occlusion of a renal artery may lead to systemic hypertension through the Goldblatt mechanism, with increased renin production by the affected kidney causing activation of an alpha₂ globulin in plasma to angiotensin. Obstructive disease of the aorta may lead to absence or diminution of pulse in one or more areas; these include the carotid arteries, the subclavian or brachial arteries, and the femoral arteries. Extensive aortic intimal atherosclerosis may lead to cholesterol emboli or atheroembolism, which may cause transient cerebral ischemic attacks (TIA), renal insufficiency, pancreatitis, or cyanosis of one or more toes. Cholesterol emboli to the retinal arteries may be visualized by ophthalmoscopy.

There are other ways in which aortic disease may come to attention. When the aortic lumen is narrowed by disease, murmurs may be produced. Supravalvular aortic stenosis, aortic coarctation, and dissecting hematoma of the aorta each may produce a systolic murmur which is loudest downstream to the site of narrowing. On the other hand, when the aortic lumen is enlarged by aneurysm formation, the aneurysm may occasionally be appreciated on the chest wall or by physical examination of the abdomen; but more often it is detected because it produces pain, because it compresses other vital structures, or because it begins to leak, thereby causing bleeding and shock.

Many times aortic disease is discovered or evaluated more precisely by roentgenograms. Much of the length of the thoracic aorta can be studied by posteroanterior, oblique, and lateral roentgenograms of the chest without the use of contrast media. Although the sinuses of Valsalva are usually lost within the cardiac shadow, when the walls of an aneurysm are calcified, it may be possible to identify and evaluate the aneurysm precisely by plain radiograms, even though it is in the aortic sinuses. The employment of contrast medium increases the accuracy of evaluation of both the thoracic aorta and the abdominal aorta. Areas of narrowing of the lumen, irregularity of the lumen, and dilation of the aorta are thereby more accurately evaluated. Newer noninvasive methods of studying the aorta include echocardiography and dynamic radioisotope scanning (radioisotope aortogram). At present only the ascending thoracic aorta and the abdominal aorta can be studied accurately by echocardiography. In adults the remainder of the thoracic aorta lies too deep within the chest for good echocardiographic evaluation.

Moldveen-Geronimus, M., and Merriam, J. C., Jr.: Cholesterol embolization: From pathologic curiosity to clinical entity. Circulation, 35:946, 1967.

367.2. CONGENITAL DISEASES OF THE AORTA

Congenital diseases of the aorta are not rare in children. They are rather uncommon problems in adult life and will be considered briefly here.

SUPRAVALVULAR AORTIC STENOSIS. Eliot and Ed-

wards classify supravalvular aortic stenosis into three types: an hourglass form, a tubular form, and a fibrous diaphragm-like form. Supravalvular aortic stenosis may be associated with aortic intimal proliferation which may compromise the origin of the innominate artery or the left common carotid or subclavian artery. Thus blood pressure is often different in the two arms. The intimal process often involves the aortic valve as well, so that aortic insufficiency may occur. Coronary arterial stenosis also may occur. Supravalvular aortic stenosis is of two major etiologic backgrounds. One is the familial variety. In this variety mental deficiency and the characteristic facies are absent as a rule. The other variety is that associated with a characteristic facies, which consists of widely spaced teeth, dental malocclusion, full cheeks, elfin face, pug nose, and a wide mouth with pouting lips. Mental deficiency is usually present, and there is often a history of infantile hypercalcemia. In both varieties pulmonary arterial branch stenosis is a common associated disorder. Supravalvular aortic stenosis is diagnosed by left ventricular and aortic catheterization, which demonstrate the obstruction by showing a higher systolic pressure in the left ventricle and proximal ascending aorta than is found in the distal ascending aorta and aortic arch. The nature of the obstruction is shown more clearly by aortography. When the obstruction is sufficiently severe, it may be relieved by surgical operation.

COARCTATION OF THE AORTA AT THE AORTIC ISTHMUS. The most common variety of aortic coarctation consists of a narrowing of the isthmus of the aorta just distal to the left subclavian artery. This is a congenital disorder and is several times more common in males than in females. Occasionally the narrowing is proximal to the origin of the left subclavian artery. The ductus or ligamentum arteriosum may be inserted proximal or distal to the coarctation. The coarctation may be associated with patent ductus arteriosus. In some instances there is pulmonary hypertension and reversed flow of pulmonary arterial blood through the ductus arteriosus into the distal aorta beyond the coarctation, causing cyanosis of the lower extremities but not of the upper extremities. With aortic coarctation, the degree of aortic luminal narrowing varies greatly. At times the opening between the aortic arch and the ascending aorta is completely obliterated or only a few millimeters in diameter; in other instances the opening is 1 cm or more. The characteristic physical finding in this condition is hypertension in the upper extremities and low blood pressure and delayed pulse in the femoral arteries. The condition will rarely be overlooked if the blood pressure and pulse in the upper and lower extremities are compared in every patient with hypertension. Hypertension in these patients is usually not severe, and the blood pressure is usually of the order of 170/100 mm Hg. This is one variety of hypertension in which malignant hypertension is said not to occur.

The mechanism of hypertension in aortic coarctation is not clearly understood. The two principal theories are (1) that it is caused by mechanical blockage in the aorta and (2) that it is caused by impairment of renal blood flow. Studies of a limited number of patients have failed to show elevation of renal venous blood renin, thus failing to support the theory of restricted renal arterial blood flow as the cause of the hypertension.

Patients with aortic coarctation have collateral circulation between the aortic arch and the lower aorta. This is carried by three main routes: (1) the internal mammary arteries, which communicate through their anterior intercostal arteries with the posterior aortic intercostal arteries; (2) the internal mammary artery continuation, the superior epigastric artery, and anastomoses with the inferior epigastric branch of the external iliac artery; and (3) the anastomoses between subclavian artery branches and posterior aortic intercostal arteries around the scapula. In addition to the blood pressure differences between the upper and lower extremities, patients with aortic coarctation may have a murmur over the back caused either by the collateral circulation or by the obstruction in the aorta itself. The murmur caused by the narrowed aorta tends to be a systolic murmur when the opening is more than 3 mm in diameter; it may be continuous when the opening in the aorta is smaller than this. The collateral intercostal vessels may be seen or palpated over the posterior thorax. Approximately 50 per cent of patients with coarctation have a bicuspid aortic valve, and about 10 per cent have aortic insufficiency. Ventricular septal defect, subaortic stenosis, and congenital mitral stenosis are also found at times in patients with aortic coarctation. When the obstruction lies between the origins of the left common carotid and left subclavian arteries, the blood pressure is higher in the right than in the left arm. This is an uncommon occurrence. Ordinary radiologic examination of the chest tends to show bilateral notching of the inferior margins of the ribs between the third and tenth ribs. This notching is produced by dilation of the enlarged intercostal arteries which carry increased collateral flow. The aortic knob or arch is invisible on plain chest radiogram in approximately half the patients. A barium esophagram may show a so-called figure E or "reversed 3" sign. The upper esophageal compression is produced by prestenotic dilation of the aorta by the enlarged left subclavian artery and carotid arteries, and compression of the lower esophagus is produced by the poststenotic dilation of the aorta. The aortic coarctation can be best diagnosed and quantified by aortography.

Because of their associated difficulties and later complications, only a few patients with aortic coarctation have a normal life span, although many survive to adult life. Approximately 60 to 70 per cent of untreated patients die before 40 years of age. The common complications of this condition are congestive heart failure, bacterial endarteritis, aortic rupture or dissection, and bleeding intracranial berry aneurysms. The treatment ordinarily consists of surgical removal of the obstruction, except when there is severe pulmonary hypertension with reversal of blood flow through the patent ductus arteriosus.

PSEUDOCOARCTATION OF THE AORTA. This is probably a poor term. The aortic arch is elongated by hypertension or arteriosclerosis and is kinked downward in the region of the ligamentum arteriosum. This abnormality can resemble a mediastinal tumor or can be associated with a true aneurysm in this area. As a rule there is no true obstruction, and there is no blood pressure difference between the proximal aorta and the descending aorta. Subclinical true coarctation may exist in some instances.

COARCTATION OF THE ABDOMINAL AORTA. In addition to coarctation of the aorta at the usual site just distal to the left subclavian artery, coarctation may occur in the abdominal aorta. This lesion may be congenital, or it may be associated with Takayasu's syndrome (see Ch. 367.9). Coarctation of the abdominal aorta may involve the celiac axis, the mesenteric arteries, and the renal arteries. There may be associated hypertension because of the renal arterial involvement. Abdominal aortic coarctation is more common in women, whereas thoracic coarctation is more common in men.

Surgical Treatment. Ordinarily the diagnosis of coarctation of the aorta is in itself considered an indication for surgical correction. The preferable age for repair is between 8 and 12 years. However, when infants with coarctation have congestive heart failure which does not respond to medical management, surgical repair may be needed at that time. Surgical repair is generally not advisable in patients over the age of 50 years, because the operative risks are increased and the potential gain is less. In most patients repair can be done by resection of the coarctate area and end-to-end aortic anastomosis. In some, the coarctate area must be resected and a tubular prosthesis of Dacron inserted.

Results. In patients treated by experts in the field, the in-hospital mortality rate is low and should not exceed 2 per cent in uncomplicated cases. It is important, however, that the repair be done by an expert and not by an occasional cardiac surgeon. The early postoperative period may be complicated by abdominal pain and mesenteric arteritis. There is increasing evidence, from studies of James and Kaplan at the Cincinnati Children's Hospital, that hypertension is not completely relieved in many patients. These investigators found residual hypertension in 11 of 14 patients who were 9 to 22 years of age at the time of surgical repair. The failure to relieve hypertension is usually not due to an inadequate relief of the aortic narrowing. The mechanism of persistent postoperative hypertension is at present unknown.

ABSENCE OF THE AORTIC ARCH. The aortic arch may be absent or atretic. In this case the descending aorta is supplied with blood from the pulmonary artery through a patent ductus arteriosus. Thus there is unoxygenated blood entering the descending aorta, and there tends to be cyanosis and clubbing of the toes but usually not the hands — although the left hand may be involved. This is called differential cyanosis and clubbing. Whether or not the left hand is cyanotic depends upon the origin of the left subclavian artery. Associated defects are common. Among these are ventricular septal defect and aortic stenosis.

RIGHT-SIDED AORTIC ARCH. There are two basic types of right-sided aortic arch. In one, the aorta passes behind the esophagus and descends on the left. In this variety, associated congenital heart disease is less common (Knight and Edwards). When the arch remains on the right and descends to the right of the esophagus, additional congenital heart disease is usually present. The most common variety is tetralogy of Fallot; others include pulmonary atresia, tricuspid atresia, and truncus arteriosus. The right-sided aortic arch with a right-sided descending aorta is a common complication of tetralogy of Fallot and is found in approximately 25 per cent of patients with this disorder. It is also common in patients with truncus arteriosus. When right-sided aortic arch occurs as an isolated phenomenon, it may be mistaken for a mediastinal tumor. Right-sided aortic arch is a normal component of mirror-image dextrocardia. Isolated right-sided aortic arch is usually asymptomatic and can be recognized on plain roentgenogram or by demonstration of compression of the right side of the barium-filled esophagus. Knight and Edwards found that the right aortic arch was part of a double aortic arch pattern in 4 of 78 instances. Each arch gives rise to the common carotid artery on its side and then passes behind the esophagus to join the other arch, thus forming a vascular ring about the trachea and esophagus. Three of the four cases had an additional congenital cardiac anomaly. Dysphagia may be associated with double aortic arch or with right-sided aortic arch crossing behind the esophagus to descend on the left of the esophagus.

AORTIC ATRESIA. Aortic atresia may be associated with atresia of the aortic valve and, at times, with mitral atresia. This is part of the hypoplastic left heart syndrome and is not compatible with long survival. In this disorder the blood entering the left atrium through the pulmonary veins escapes into the right heart through the foramen ovale and then into the descending aorta through the patent ductus arteriosus from the right ventricle. The ascending aorta is extremely small, and carries blood in retrograde fashion from the patent ductus arteriosus to supply the coronary arteries. In patients with mitral atresia, blood enters the left ventricle and aorta from the right ventricle through a ventricular septal defect. In aortic atresia pulmonary venous pressure is high, tending to cause pulmonary edema. Death often occurs before the age of one week.

CONGENITAL AORTIC ANEURYSM. There may be a congenital aortic aneurysm of the sinus of Valsalva. These aneurysms involve either the right or noncoronary sinus in 90 per cent of instances. Those of the right aortic sinus usually project into the right ventricle, and those of the noncoronary sinus, into the right atrium. Aortic sinus aneurysms are difficult to see on plain roentgenogram of the chest unless they are calcified. They are recognizable, however, by echocardiography and by aortography. These aneurysms tend to rupture eventually, usually into the right atrium or ventricle where they produce a continuous shunt. The continuous shunt is associated with a continuous systolic and diastolic murmur, widening of the systemic arterial pulse pressure, and a tendency to heart failure. These conditions may be corrected surgically. The murmur of an aortic sinus aneurysm which has ruptured into the right heart resembles that of a patent ductus arteriosus except that, rather than being louder in the first and second left intercostal spaces like that of a patent ductus, it tends to be louder in the fourth and fifth left intercostal spaces near the sternum. As in other communications between the systemic circulation and the lesser circulation, the systemic arterial pulse pressure tends to be increased. It is said that these congenital aortic sinus aneurysms tend to rupture into the heart, whereas acquired syphilitic aneurysms in the same location tend to rupture into the pericardial sac. A similar condition is that of aortico–left ventricular tunnel in which there is a long tubular communication between the aortic sinus and the left ventricle. The unperforated aortic sinus aneurysm is usually asymptomatic but may cause cardiac conduction disturbances, myocardial ischemia due to coronary occlusion, or pulmonary stenosis or tricuspid insufficiency (Bulkley et al.).

Another congenital condition is that of aberrant right subclavian artery. It is said to occur in one of 200 individuals. In this condition the right subclavian artery is the last major branch of the aortic arch, rather than arising from the innominate artery as it does normally. It then passes behind the esophagus to reach the right arm. As a result the blood pressure may be lower in the right arm than the left; the pulse may be absent in the right upper extremity. These patients may have dysphagia produced by the pressure of the aberrant artery on the esophagus. The condition can be demonstrated by barium esophagram, which shows an oblique compression of the posterior esophagus. Aortography, of course, shows the condition more clearly. Rarely the aberrant right subclavian artery may be associated with coarctation of the aorta proximal to the left subclavian artery. In this condition arterial pulses tend to be feeble or absent in both upper and lower extremities.

Bulkley, B. H., Hutchins, G. M., and Ross, R. S.: Aortic sinus of Valsalva aneurysms simulating primary right-sided valvular disease. Circulation, 52:696, 1975.

Eliot, R. S., and Edwards, J. E.: Pathology of congenital heart disease. *In* Hurst, J. W., and Logue, R. B. (eds.): The Heart. Arteries and Veins. New York, McGraw-Hill Book Company, 1974, pp. 627–667.

James, F. W., and Kaplan, S.: Systolic hypertension during submaximal exercise after correction of coarctation of the aorta. Circulation, 49–50 (Suppl. II):27, 1974.

Knight, L., and Edwards, J. E.: Right aortic arch. Types and associated cardiac anomalies. Circulation 50:1047, 1974.

367.3. HEREDOFAMILIAL DISEASES OF THE AORTA

There are a number of heredofamilial disorders of connective tissue which may be associated with diseases of the aorta and its branches (McKusick). These conditions most commonly cause weakening of the aortic wall which may cause aneurysms, but at times there is occlusive aortic disease owing to thrombosis.

MARFAN'S SYNDROME. Marfan's syndrome, also known as arachnodactyly, is a heredofamilial disorder of connective tissue which may be associated with hydroxyprolinuria. Hydroxyprolinuria is neither a specific nor a constant finding, according to McKusick. The aortic lesion is characteristically that of cystic medial necrosis. The disease affects the blood vessels, the osseous skeleton, and the ligaments. Typically, arachnodactyly, increased height, ectopia lentis, and hypermobile joints are found. Abdominal hernia, pectus excavatum, and kyphoscoliosis are common. The principal cardiovascular manifestations are in the ascending aorta. The second most common cardiovascular abnormality involves the mitral valve. Occasionally, the tricuspid valve or the pulmonary artery is affected. Smaller arteries are usually not involved. The aortic lesion characteristically produces either sinus of Valsalva aneurysm or dilation of aneurysm in the ascending aorta above the sinuses. Its principal complications are dissecting aneurysm of the aorta, rupture of the aorta, and aortic insufficiency. Rarely, there is abdominal aortic aneurysm. The mitral valve involvement may cause mitral prolapse and mitral insufficiency.

EHLERS-DANLOS SYNDROME. This disorder is also known as cutis hyperelastica. Dissecting aortic aneurysm is a recognized complication. Also, there may be spontaneous rupture of the aorta or aortic rupture following slight trauma.

HOMOCYSTINURIA. Homocystinuria is a disorder which has some features in common with Marfan's syndrome. Ectopia lentis and disease of the aorta may occur in either condition. In homocystinuria more commonly there is occlusive disease of systemic arteries and veins. The coronary arteries may be occluded. Thrombosis of the terminal aorta may occur in this disorder. The elastica pattern of the aortic media is abnormal. It is uncertain whether aortic aneurysm is an essential part of this disease. In this disorder the enzyme cystathionine synthetase is lacking. Mental deficiency is common, whereas the patient with Marfan's syndrome usually has normal mental development.

OSTEOGENESIS IMPERFECTA. With osteogenesis imperfecta, deafness, fragilitas ossium, and blue sclerae are the common features. These patients often have a dilated aortic root and may suffer from aortic insufficiency. Mitral insufficiency is also a common cardiovascular manifestation.

MUCOPOLYSACCHARIDOSES. In these disorders, including Hurler's syndrome, Hunter's syndrome, and others, there may be gargoyle cells in the aorta. The principal involvement is of the aortic valve and coronary arteries. Aortic dilation and the aortic arch syndrome (see Ch. 367.9) have been described.

PSEUDOXANTHOMA ELASTICUM. Thrombosis of the terminal aorta has been described in this disorder, but its relationship to pseudoxanthoma elasticum is uncertain. Thrombotic occlusion involving coronary arteries and those of the extremities is a recognized complication. The iliac and femoral arteries may be smaller than normal, leading to impaired pulsations in the lower extremities and thus to confusion with coarctation of the aorta.

McKusick, V. A.: Heritable Disorders of Connective Tissue. 4th ed. St. Louis, C. V. Mosby Company, 1972.

367.4. EFFECTS OF AGING UPON THE AORTA

Arteriosclerosis affects the aorta more commonly in our civilization than in more primitive societies. The process tends to be progressively more severe as one proceeds down the descending aorta, in contrast to syphilitic aortitis, which is more pronounced in the ascending aorta just superior to the aortic valve. The process may lead to elongation or dilation of the aorta, producing an irregularity observed on chest radiogram. Commonly, in older patients one sees a calcific deposit in the aortic knob (arch). Roentgen evidence of aortic atherosclerosis includes calcification of the knob, increase in the width of the aorta, and unusual tortuosity or uncoiling. These changes are not seen in normal persons under the age of 30 years and in only 2.5 per cent of individuals under the age of 40 years (Felson). Extensive atherosclerosis involving the aortic intima may lead to ulcerative lesions with cholesterol deposits and to emboli. These emboli may consist of cholesterol or may arise from thrombi. There may be cholesterol emboli to the retinal arteries; emboli in the renal arteries may cause hypertension; peripheral emboli may cause impairment of femoral blood flow. Arteriosclerosis is believed to be the common cause of aortic aneurysm. Aortic aneurysms caused by arteriosclerosis are most common in the abdominal aorta just inferior to the renal arteries but may occur also in the thoracic aorta and in the abdominal aorta above the origin of the

renal arteries. Aortic arteriosclerosis causes loss of elasticity with decreased compliance during left ventricular ejection. Thus left ventricular work may rise with aging, contributing to a decrease of circulatory reserve with age.

Felson, B.: Chest Roentgenology. Philadelphia, W. B. Saunders Company, 1973.

367.5. INCREASED AORTIC DIMENSIONS

The enlarged aorta may increase in length or diameter or both. Increase in length usually reflects arteriosclerotic changes with aging. Increase in length may lead to an irregular margin, to apparent widening, or to kinking, tortuosity, or buckling. Increased diameter of the aorta may be generalized, as occurs in hypertensive disease, or localized. Localized increase of dimension may be called *ectasia* when of minor degree but more commonly is called *aneurysm*. Aneurysms of the aorta may be saccular or fusiform.

Aortic aneurysms are discussed in detail under the headings of the individual causative diseases. However, it is useful to summarize the relation of the location of an aneurysm to its etiology. Aortic aneurysms may be classified by etiology into congenital and acquired groups (DeBakey and Noon). By location, they are classified as follows: (1) ascending aorta, (2) aortic arch, (3) descending thoracic aorta, and (4) thoracoabdominal. Aortic sinus aneurysms are most commonly of congenital origin or due to Marfan's syndrome, syphilis, or infective endocarditis. Ascending aortic aneurysms are most commonly due to syphilis, Marfan's syndrome, aortic dissection, or cystic medial necrosis without the other features of Marfan's syndrome. Aortic arch aneurysms are most often due to syphilis, dissection, or Marfan's syndrome. An aneurysm of the descending thoracic aorta may be caused by syphilis, arteriosclerosis, or dissection. An aneurysm at the beginning of the descending aorta may be caused by trauma. Aneurysms of the abdominal aorta are most often caused by arteriosclerosis but may be the result of syphilis or the extension of aortic dissection from the thoracic aorta.

A number of other diseases may cause aortic aneurysms, which are usually smaller than those enumerated above and in varying sites. Among these is septicemia, which may cause mycotic aneurysms. Mycotic aneurysms may be caused by tuberculosis as well. Relapsing polychondritis may lead to aneurysm of either the thoracic or abdominal aorta. Localized aortic aneurysms often occur with Takayasu's aortitis and with giant cell aortitis.

ARTERIOSCLEROTIC AORTIC ANEURYSM. Arteriosclerotic aneurysms of the aorta, most common in the abdominal aorta, usually originate below the renal arteries. Arteriosclerotic aneurysms are most common in men over the age of 50 years. One study reported an autopsy incidence of 1.8 per cent of such aneurysms. Probably more than 95 per cent of abdominal aortic aneurysms are of arteriosclerotic origin. These aneurysms are most often discovered by roentgen examination of an asymptomatic patient. However, they may be discovered for the first time when the patient has pain — the pain may be in the back or the epigastrium, or may radiate to the flanks. Unfortunately, the first evidence of aneurysm may be that of rupture attended by the onset of severe and persistent pain and shock. Persistent abdominal pain of lesser severity may precede the more severe pain of aortic rupture.

ABDOMINAL AORTIC ANEURYSMS. Abdominal aortic aneurysms may be diagnosed by physical examination, but there are many possible errors. In obese or muscular patients or in those with small aneurysms, physical examination is unlikely to reveal the problem. On the other hand, abdominal aneurysm may be diagnosed in error. It is important to determine that there is actual increase in the width of the aorta and not merely a prominent aortic pulsation. Prominent pulsation of the abdominal aorta is common as a normal finding, especially in thin women with lax abdominal walls and lumbar lordosis. This often leads to the diagnosis of aneurysm by physical examination where none exists — "students' aneurysm." A prominent aortic pulsation may be due to an uncoiling of the aorta resulting from atherosclerosis or to aortic insufficiency or to a high output state producing an increased pulse pressure in the absence of aneurysm. Another pitfall in diagnosis is that a tumor overlying the aorta, such as pancreatic neoplasm, may appear to have an intrinsic pulsation and thus be mistaken for an aneurysm. Abdominal aneurysms may lead to ureteral obstruction with hydronephrosis. These aneurysms may also lead to consumption coagulopathy with diminished circulating platelets, reduced serum fibrinogen, and prolonged prothrombin time. A clue to the presence of aortic abdominal aneurysm may be that of cholesterol emboli to the smaller arteries of the feet and toes, leading to digital cyanosis and coldness.

Diagnosis. Roentgenograms of the abdomen may be helpful by showing calcification in the walls of the aneurysm. It is important to have lateral and oblique views in addition to anteroposterior views. Aortic wall calcification per se does not signify an aneurysm unless there is definite increase in the diameter of the aorta. The psoas shadow may be obliterated when rupture has occurred. Ultrasound scanning and radionuclide angiography may be useful in the diagnosis of abdominal aortic aneurysms. Aortography with radiopaque contrast medium is usually the diagnostic method of choice.

Prognosis. The prognosis of patients with abdominal arteriosclerotic aneurysms is generally considered poor, with only a small percentage of patients surviving for five years or more. The outlook is considered to be better when the lesion is less than 7.5 cm in diameter. However, it is difficult to know the true prognosis. Most patients who are operated upon and most patients who have been followed without operation were originally discovered because they had symptoms. The prognosis might conceivably be more favorable in patients who are symptomatic. Many unoperated patients had a poor prognosis because operation was considered inadvisable owing to an associated severe illness.

Surgical Treatment. Once the diagnosis of abdominal aortic aneurysm is made, one should in general recommend surgical replacement of the aneurysm even though the patient is asymptomatic. If the patient is having pain in relation to the aneurysm, replacement should be considered as an emergency. Surgical removal with insertion of a synthetic aortic graft of woven Dacron is the usual operative procedure. Aortic homo-grafts are no longer used because they tend to rupture at the line of anastomosis. However, late rupture at the suture line may be a problem even with synthetic grafts (Thompson et al.). There are two groups of patients in whom surgical resection might not be recommended. One is composed of those who are asymptomatic with aneurysms under 6 cm in diameter; the other group is patients who have some other life-threatening disease or who are extremely elderly and debilitated. Among the conditions which would be contraindications to resection are intractable heart failure, advanced renal failure, metastatic neoplasm, severe coronary artery disease with unstable angina pectoris or recent infarction, advanced cerebrovascular disease, and severe pulmonary insufficiency. In recent years the reported in-hospital mortality rate of abdominal aneurysm resection in several large series ranged from 5.3 to 9.5 per cent. It is greatly increased when there is severe cardiorenal disease or advanced age. The signs, symptoms, and treatment of thoracic aortic aneurysms are discussed in Ch. 367.7.

Bergan, J. J., and Yao, J. S. T.: Modern management of abdominal aortic aneurysms. Surg. Clin. N. Am., 54:175, 1974.

DeBakey, M. E., Beall, M. C., and Mattox, K. L.: Surgical treatment of diseases of the aorta and major arteries. *In* Hurst, J. W. (ed.): The Heart. 4th ed. New York, McGraw-Hill Book Company, 1978, Chap. 103.

DeBakey, M. E., and Noon, G. P.: Aneurysms of the thoracic aorta. Mod. Concepts Cardiovasc. Dis., 44:53, 1975.

Thompson, W. M., Johnsrude, I. S., Jackson, D. C., et al.: Late complications of abdominal aortic reconstructive surgery; roentgen evaluation. Ann. Surg., 185:326, 1977.

367.6. TRAUMATIC AORTIC DISEASE

The aorta may be damaged by nonpenetrating as well as penetrating trauma. The portion of the aorta most likely damaged by trauma is that lying just beyond the origin of the left subclavian artery. When the body is moving rapidly, followed by a sudden deceleration as in a fall or auto accident, differential rates of acceleration are greatest in this area because the aortic arch is relatively fixed by the root vessels. The second most common site of injury is the ascending aorta. The aorta may be lacerated or may rupture with either complete or almost complete transection. There may be a false aneurysm with extravasation of blood tamponaded by the mediastinal structure. Patients with nonpenetrating aortic trauma may have little or no external evidence of chest injury. In an acute setting, following decelerative-type injury, the patient may be in shock with a rapidly developing hemothorax — most commonly on the left side. Anuria and paraplegia, with absence of pulse in the femoral arteries and cold, pale lower extremities, are common. The initial findings thus simulate those of coarctation of the aorta. Arterial hypertension may be present as well. A routine chest radiogram may show widening of the mediastinum. A possible sequel is chronic traumatic aortic aneurysm, which may rupture during a period of days or years after the original injury. The characteristic location of an aortic traumatic aneurysm is distal to the origin of the subclavian artery (Fig. 1). The definitive diagnosis is made by aortography, and the treatment is that of surgical removal. Usually a graft replacement is employed in order to preserve aortic continuity.

Figure 1. Traumatic aortic aneurysm just distal to the subclavian artery. A, This posteroanterior roentgenogram demonstrates calcification in the aneurysm, which appears in the region of the aortic knob. B, Aortogram demonstrating opacification of the aneurysm, which lies just beyond the subclavian artery. (From Fowler, N. O.: Cardiac Diagnosis and Treatment, 2nd ed., 1977. With permission of Harper & Row, Publishers, Inc.)

367.7. SYPHILITIC AORTITIS AND SYPHILITIC HEART DISEASE

Syphilitic aortitis is the principal cardiovascular manifestation of syphilis. Syphilis does not ordinarily affect the cardiac valves, although the aortic valve commissures may be separated. Rarely, it may affect the myocardium. It may affect the coronary arteries more often, but usually only the proximal few centimeters of these vessels are involved. Thus the principal cardiovascular effect of syphilitic disease is aortitis with its complications of aortic insufficiency, angina pectoris, and aortic aneurysm. Syphilitic aortitis, as a rule, is a late lesion of acquired syphilis and is usually recognized 10 to 30 years after the initial primary chancre, but occasionally it occurs as early as a few years after the original infection. The disease characteristically produces aortic medial destruction with necrosis of smooth muscle and elastic tissue and periarterial inflammation with lymphocyte cuffing of the vasa vasorum. There is also intimal wrinkling with treebark formation and a tendency to narrow the lumen of the orifice of the coronary arteries, as well as to produce the dilation of the aortic root that leads to aortic insufficiency or aneurysm. At times, innominate artery aneurysm may occur, but more distal arterial aneurysms are unusual. The syphilitic process, in distinction to that of arteriosclerosis, is usually most intense in the aortic root and becomes less intense as one examines the more distal aorta. Congenital syphilis seldom produces aortitis. Because of the delay in clinical manifestations, patients with syphilitic aortitis are ordinarily more than 30 years of age when recognized clinically and are usually over 50 years of age when

syphilitic aneurysms are recognized. Uncomplicated syphilitic aortitis ordinarily produces no symptoms and may be recognized only at the autopsy table. It produces dilation of the aorta and perhaps calcification in the ascending aorta. The latter may be detected radiologically (Fig. 2).

SYPHILITIC AORTIC ANEURYSM. This lesion occurs most often in the ascending aorta. Aneurysms occur in 10 to 40 per cent of patients with syphilitic aortitis. Syphilitic aneurysms, once the most common cause of thoracic aneurysms, are much less commonly seen now than a few decades ago. Nearly half occur in the ascending aorta; 30 to 40 per cent of syphilitic aneurysms are found in the arch and 15 per cent in the descending thoracic aorta. Syphilitic aortic aneurysms may occur in the abdominal aorta but are distinctly uncommon in this location and especially so if there is no syphilitic aneurysm in the thoracic aorta. If the aneurysm involves the ascending aorta, aortic insufficiency is often present; rarely there is a visible pulsatile mass in the first and second right intercostal spaces with exaggerated pulsations of the right sternoclavicular joint or in the episternal notch. Chest pain, the most common symptom, may occur owing to rib, sternal, or vertebral erosion. The pain is usually substernal, in the dorsal spine, or at the side of the chest. It may extend to the neck, shoulders, lower back, or abdomen. Increasing intensity of pain is usually an ominous sign associated with impending rupture. A chest radiogram may demonstrate erosion of ribs and sternum by the aneurysm. Respiratory difficulty may indicate that the aneurysm is in the arch of the aorta; there may be a tracheal tug with hoarseness and a brassy cough because of recurrent laryngeal nerve paralysis. There may be Horner's

Figure 2. Calcification of the ascending aorta in syphilitic aortitis.

syndrome with ptosis, miosis, and decreased sweating on the left side of the face. There may be superior vena caval obstruction with distended nonpulsatile jugular veins, dyspnea, and collateral venous circulation over the thorax. Aneurysm in the aortic arch may produce compression of the left mainstem bronchus, with atelectasis of the left lung or of the left lower lobe. Hemoptysis may occur because of tracheal or bronchial ulceration. Hematemesis may indicate rupture into the esophagus. In the descending thoracic aorta, rarely the aneurysm may present as a pulsatile mass medial to, or inferior to, the angle of the left scapula. In these cases, vertebral erosion may occur. Cardiac enlargement does not occur because of aneurysm alone.

Radiologic studies are helpful in diagnosing thoracic aneurysm of any cause. When there is calcification in the ascending aorta, syphilitic aortitis is strongly suggested. A mass continuous with the aorta with calcification in its wall is very likely an aneurysm. When there is no calcification, then aortic aneurysm must be distinguished from other mediastinal masses, especially tumors of lymph nodes, dermoid cysts, thymic tumor, and substernal thyroid gland. Evaluation of pulsations of a mass by fluoroscopy is virtually worthless, because pulsatory movements transmitted into contiguous tumors are indistinguishable from those of intrinsic pulsations of the aorta. Conversely, aneurysms which are lined with thrombus may fail to show visible pulsations. Contrast or radionuclide aortography is the precise way of settling the diagnosis.

Course and Prognosis. Syphilitic aneurysms tend to rupture eventually. The rupture may take place into the right or left pleural space, into the trachea or esophagus, or into the pulmonary artery, where it produces a continuous murmur like that of patent ductus arteriosus. The aneurysm may rupture into the right heart, producing a continuous murmur like that described in Ch. 367.2. Laplace's law states that tension in walls of a cylinder is equal to the product of pressure times radius. Hence the tension in the wall of an aortic aneurysm is greater than that in the adjacent aorta. Because of its

tendency to expand according to Laplace's law and eventually to rupture, surgical resection of syphilitic aneurysms is recommended when feasible and when the patient does not suffer from some other disease which materially limits life expectancy.

Serologic studies of patients suspected of syphilitic aortitis may be misleading. The Kahn serologic test may be negative in as many as 23 per cent of patients with syphilitic aortitis. The VDRL test is said to be positive in 98 to 99 per cent of such patients but may be negative in patients over 65 years of age. The *Treponema pallidum* immobilization test may be positive when the VDRL test is negative and is especially useful when the patient is over 65 years of age or has had antisyphilitic therapy.

Antisyphilitic Treatment. For the patients who have cardiovascular syphilis, the Venereal Disease Control Advisory Committee has recommended that the patient receive benzathine penicillin, 2.4 million units intramuscularly weekly for three successive weeks, or aqueous procaine penicillin, 600,000 units intramuscularly daily for 15 days. There is no assurance that such therapy will allay the progression of syphilitic aortitis or aneurysm, as the weakened aortic wall continues to expand despite the absence of active infection.

Syphilis: Recommended Treatment Schedules, 1976. Center for Disease Control, Atlanta, Georgia. Ann. Intern. Med., 85:94, 1976.

367.8. DISSECTING ANEURYSM OF THE AORTA

Dissecting aneurysm of the aorta is also called dissecting hematoma of the aorta. The disease tends to occur in certain settings. It is most common in men of middle age with a background of hypertension, but is also found in the setting of Marfan's syndrome, cystic medial necrosis, or coarctation of the aorta and seems to be more common in pregnancy. Dissecting aneurysm may also occur in certain heritable disorders of connective tissue, including Ehlers-Danlos syndrome, and has been described as a complication of relapsing polychondritis. Its relationship to arteriosclerosis of the aorta is questionable. It probably bears no relationship to syphilitic aortitis, which may, in fact, offer some protection against the process because of the fibrosis of the aortic media which occurs in syphilis.

Ordinarily the dissection begins with an aortic intimal tear, followed by a dissecting channel in the media, followed in turn by a point of re-entry from the intima back into the aortic lumen or, occasionally, rupture through the adventitia. Thus a double-barreled aorta may be produced. Approximately 50 per cent of aortic dissections begin in the ascending aorta, 30 per cent in the aortic arch, and 20 per cent in the descending aorta. Dissecting aneurysm may be related to trauma, especially that produced by an angiographic catheter or aortic balloon catheter (Alpert et al.) striking an arteriosclerotic plaque in the aorta. A dissecting aneurysm may extend proximally to involve the aortic valve area, thus causing aortic valvular insufficiency; it may surround the coronary arteries, producing myocardial infarction; it may extend along the carotid sheath to cause hemiplegia. It may involve the blood supply to the spinal cord, leading to paraplegia and anesthesia below the level of involvement. It may involve the renal artery, thus aggravating pre-existing arterial hypertension. Hypertension may also be aggravated by a carotid artery involvement when it interferes with the carotid sinus baroreceptor response. Rupture into the pericardium may lead to cardiac tamponade and rapid demise.

HISTORY. Most dissecting aneurysms are associated with chest pain, which may radiate into the abdomen or into the back. The pain of aortic dissection must be distinguished from that of myocardial ischemia. The pain of ischemic heart disease seldom radiates to the back and infrequently extends below the diaphragm, so that those features should suggest the possibility of aortic dissection. In some patients, however, there is complicating myocardial infarction when a proximal aortic dissection involves the coronary arteries, and then the condition may masquerade as a case of myocardial infarction. When the patient with aortic dissection suffers from rupture into the pericardium, he may develop cardiac tamponade; on the other hand, when there is a gradual leak into the pericardial sac, the patient may appear to have unexplained pericarditis. Approximately 25 per cent of patients with aortic dissection are believed to develop aortic insufficiency. The sudden appearance of aortic insufficiency should raise the possibility of dissecting aneurysm even when pain is absent. Hemiplegia, paraplegia, or syncope may be the presenting features, as may the aortic arch syndrome (see Ch. 367.9). The prevalence of pain is believed to be about 70 per cent. Occasional patients appear with aortic insufficiency, a large heart, and heart failure without a history of an acute episode of aortic dissection.

PHYSICAL FINDINGS. The patient is often hypertensive and often complains of chest pain. The patient is most often a man between the ages of 40 and 60 years. When the process extends to involve the orifices of the femoral arteries or arteries to the head and neck, asymmetrical arterial pulses may be found. Although abnormal peripheral arterial pulses were found in 13 of 18 cases in one series of patients with aortic dissection, most series show that it is the minority of patients who have significant differences of pulse and blood pressure in the arms, legs, or carotid arteries. Possibly 25 per cent of patients develop aortic insufficiency. Either sternoclavicular joint may transmit an abnormal pulsation. Unilateral distention of the left external jugular vein results from pressure of the expanded aorta upon the left innominate vein. This sign suggests the possibility of aneurysm of the aorta. It is not specific for dissecting aneurysm, however, and may occur in a patient with an elongated and kinked arteriosclerotic or hypertensive aorta in the absence of aneurysm.

LABORATORY STUDIES. The electrocardiogram may be normal or may show left ventricular hypertrophy. It may show evidence of acute pericarditis. In approximately one case in six of one series, the electrocardiogram showed changes of myocardial infarction. The chest roentgenogram is very important in the study of patients, especially if there are serial studies. A change in the width of the aorta, especially involving the aortic arch, is very suggestive of dissection or of mediastinal bleeding. At times, the chest radiogram may show changes virtually specific for dissection by demonstrating a separation of more than a few millimeters between a calcified intimal plaque and the external border of the aorta. However, the majority of patients cannot be diagnosed from plain roentgenogram; aortography is usually required to make the diagnosis (Fig. 3). The

Figure 3. Aortogram: dissecting aneurysm. The arrow indicates line of separation between true and false channels. (Courtesy of Dr. Harold Spitz.)

aortographic features of dissecting hematoma are evidence of intimal tear, opacification of a false channel, and the indirect evidence of a false channel produced by narrowing of the original lumen. When the process involves the ascending aorta, echocardiography may be of value in showing thickening of the aortic wall.

The diagnosis requires a high index of suspicion. A patient thought to have myocardial infarction should be suspected of dissecting aortic aneurysm if the pain radiates to the back or into the abdomen, if the electrocardiogram shows no change or changes of pericarditis, and if the serum enzyme test results (especially the MB fraction of creatine phosphokinase) remain normal. Aortic dissection should also be considered when there is aortic insufficiency of recent onset or if there are impaired arterial pulses in the neck or extremities. Changes in aortic contour demonstrated by serial roentgenograms are highly suggestive. Once the suspicion of aortic dissection arises, the diagnosis may be proved in most cases by aortography. Uncommonly, when the dissection is entirely intramural, without either an entry or an exit channel, the aortogram does not show specific changes and the diagnosis can only be suspected from the unusual thickening of the aortic wall.

In one series described from Massachusetts General Hospital (Slater and DeSanctis), syncope with aortic dissection was usually caused by cardiac tamponade. There were differences between dissection involving the proximal ascending aorta and the distal dissection group when the descending thoracic aorta was involved. In 53 patients with proximal dissection, the patients tended to be younger and to have a significantly higher incidence of Marfan's syndrome or cystic medial necrosis. Anterior chest pain, pulse deficit, neurologic compromise, aortic insufficiency, and congestive heart failure were more common. With distal dissection, back pain was more common; hypertension and atherosclerosis were also more common. Chest radiograms almost always showed an abnormal aortic contour, although aortography was necessary to be certain of the diagnosis.

PROGNOSIS. The prognosis is poor in aortic dissecting aneurysm. If untreated, approximately 20 per cent of patients die within 24 hours and 27 per cent in 48 hours. A small percentage of patients with aortic dissection, probably less than 10 per cent, live for a year and may survive with chronic or even severe aortic insufficiency. With surgical resection of the diseased segment and aortic graft replacement, as many as 75 per cent may survive. The prognosis is better for either medical or surgical treatment when the dissection begins distal to the aortic arch. In this group, 50 per cent may survive the first three weeks even without modern therapy.

TREATMENT. Treatment may be either surgical or medical. Surgical management consists of resection of the involved segment and replacement with a prosthetic graft. Operative management is especially to be considered in the following circumstances: (1) when there is leaking from the dissection, which most commonly takes place into the left hemithorax or pericardium; (2) when the process is in the ascending aorta or arch; (3) when the cerebral circulation is compromised but not to a degree incompatible with recovery; (4) with severe heart failure caused by aortic regurgitation; (5) when there is evidence of continued dissection; (6) when pain and blood pressure cannot be controlled; and (7) when hypertension is absent.

Medical Management. Medical management involves control of hypertension and administration of drugs to lessen the systolic ejection force of the heart. Hypertension is controlled by such agents as trimethaphan (Arfonad) or, alternatively, intramuscular reserpine, 0.5 to 2 mg every six hours. One may also use oral or intravenous alpha methyldopa. The systolic blood pressure is reduced to 100 to 120 mm Hg. Along with these antihypertensive agents, oral propranolol is begun in a dosage of 10 to 40 mg four times daily so as to reduce the velocity of left ventricular ejection. In one series, 17 of 33 patients treated medically survived, and in another, 10 of 12. In the Peter Bent Brigham Hospital series, 26 of 31 patients with aortic dissection had contraindications to medical therapy; 17 of 22 did well after surgical correction. When dissection was limited to the descending aorta, none of 14 patients had contraindications to medical therapy, which was successful in each instance.

Medical management may be considered when the process is more than two weeks old. Resection of the dissected area, followed by grafting, may be carried out later when the condition of the patient is stabilized. Progressive enlargement of the aneurysm is an indication for surgical repair in patients who have received medical therapy. The majority can be brought through the acute phase of the illness alive. However, the long-term outlook in medically treated patients is questionable, and undoubtedly many of them will do better with surgical treatment once the condition has stabilized. Long-term antihypertensive therapy should be considered if indicated. This might include single drugs or combinations of methyldopa, propranolol, guanethidine, and diuretics as required.

Alpert, J., Bakhtan, E. K., Gielchinsky, I., et al.: Vascular complications of intra-aortic balloon pumping. Discussion. Arch. Surg., 111:1190, 1976.

Slater, E. E., and DeSanctis, R. W.: The clinical recognition of dissecting aortic aneurysm. Am. J. Med., 60:625, 1976.

367.9. MISCELLANEOUS FORMS OF AORTITIS AND THE AORTIC ARCH SYNDROME

The aorta may be affected by a number of inflammatory processes in addition to those previously described. In some instances the aortic involvement is caused by septicemia; in others, by inflammation of contiguous structures. In still others, the aortic disease is a part of the generalized disorder of connective tissue. The process may encroach upon the origin of the aortic arch vessels. Symptoms may arise owing to impairment of the blood supply to the areas supplied by these vessels, namely, the innominate artery, the left common carotid artery, and the left subclavian artery. This syndrome is called the aortic arch syndrome. Thus one may find cerebral ischemia, syncope, visual difficulties, claudication during exercise of the upper extremities, impairment of the pulse in the upper extremities, or intermittent claudication of the jaw muscles with chewing. The aortic arch syndrome may be produced by Takayasu's syndrome, by syphilis, by arteriosclerosis, or by dissecting aneurysm. The aorta may be involved by tuberculosis, usually as a result of inflammation of continuous tuberculous lymph nodes. Septicemia may lead to mycotic aneurysm of the aorta. This may be a complication of infectious endocarditis. Relapsing polychondritis may lead to aortic involvement, and aortic aneurysms occur fairly frequently in this condition. The aneurysms may involve both the thoracic and abdominal aorta. The aorta may be involved by idiopathic aortitis, a process which resembles syphilis anatomically but occurs in the absence of serologic or bacteriologic evidence of syphilis. This process may lead to calcification of the ascending aorta and even to calcification of the aortic and mitral valves. The aorta may be involved in rheumatic fever and in rheumatoid disease (Heggtveit et al.). Giant cell aortitis may occur. This syndrome is closely allied to temporal arteritis and polymyalgia rheumatica. It may lead to the aortic arch syndrome. In ankylosing spondylitis, 5 to 10 per cent of patients develop a proximal aortitis closely resembling syphilitic aortitis. Aortic regurgitation often occurs. The disease affects men nine times as often as women.

TAKAYASU'S SYNDROME. Takayasu's arteritis is a form of aortic involvement which appears to be much more common in females and in Japan, although increasing numbers of patients are being recognized in the United States. This syndrome has also been called "pulseless disease," but since there are other diseases which affect the arterial pulses similarly, this term should be either discarded or qualified. Nakao and associates reviewed 84 patients. They divided the patients into three types. One was the *aortic arch type* (they usually had stenosis or occlusion of branches of the aortic arch). Forty-seven patients, of whom 41 were women, were in this group. The second type was the *extensive type*, which involved the entire aorta and its branches. There were 27 cases in this group. The third type was the *descending thoracic and abdominal type*, of which there were ten patients, seven of them female. The first symptoms usually appeared between the ages of 11 and 48 years. In 66 of the 84 patients the first symptoms appeared between the ages of 11 and 29 years. Eleven patients had angina pectoris, presumably from coronary artery involvement. In the early stages of the disease dyspnea, cough, and edema may be present, only to disappear later. Twenty-seven patients had localized pain over the affected arteries, but only two had loss of arterial pulse. Fever was present in 17. Dizziness, syncope, headache, and impaired vision with claudication in the upper or lower extremities were commonly described. Thirty-four of 75 had slight anemia, and 46 of 76 had an increased erythrocyte sedimentation rate. C-reactive protein was present in 30 of 68. Aortographic studies were essential in confirming the diagnosis. In some, aortography showed localized aneurysms in each of the three types. In the aortic arch variety, extensive stenosis or occlusion of the proximal part of the aorta or aortic arch branches was found. This was present in all of 28 of the arch type and in most of the extensive type. Acquired coarctation of the aorta occurred occasionally. Six of 15 of the *extensive type* who were studied showed coarctation of the abdominal aorta, and eight of nine of the *descending thoracic and abdominal aortic type* showed abdominal aortic coarctation. Both the extensive and the descending aorta type frequently showed encroachment upon, and narrowing of, the lumen of the renal or mesenteric arteries (Fig. 4), and some showed femoral artery occlusion.

The patients commonly complained of arthralgia; carditis and high fever were not present. Five had erythema nodosum. Six of the patients in this report died; three died of left-sided heart failure, one had angina and pericarditis, and two died suddenly. Two died in less than a year from the onset of symptoms; two, in one to four years; and two, 20 to 29 years after the onset of symptoms.

Pathologic Lesions. Takayasu's disease is a segmental panaortitis, or panarteritis, characterized by cicatrization of all layers of involved arteries and dense bands of medial inflammatory cells. In advanced stages, the arteries become thick walled, rigid tubes, followed by luminal obliteration caused by superimposed thrombosis. There may be occlusive narrowing of the coronary ostia. The fibrous mural thickening exceeds that usually seen in other forms of aortic disease.

Treatment. Twenty-nine of the patients received adrenal corticosteroids; of these 29, 18 had remissions and 11 had no suppression of the inflammatory findings. Anticoagulants were used but were thought helpful in only one of 12 patients in whom they were used. Although a few of the patients had increased antistreptolysin "O" serologic titers or positive rheumatoid factor tests, none met the clinical criteria for either rheumatoid arthritis or acute rheumatic fever.

Heggtveit, H. S., Hennigar, G. R., and Morrione, T. G.: Panaortitis. Am. J. Path., 42:151, 1963.
Nakao, K., Ikeda, M., Kimata, S., et al.: Takayasu's arteritis. Clinical report of eighty-four cases and immunological studies of seven cases. Circulation, 35:1141, 1967.

367.10.   AORTIC OCCLUSION SYNDROMES

Occlusion of the terminal aorta at its bifurcation may be produced by traumatic severance, by arteriosclerotic thrombosis, or suddenly by embolism. The predisposing causes of emboli are most commonly atrial fibrillation, infective endocarditis, myocardial infarction, cardiomyopathy, prosthetic heart valves, ventricular or aortic aneurysm, and rheumatic mitral disease. Gradual occlusion of the terminal aorta is often well tolerated

Figure 4. Takayasu's aortitis in a 26-year-old black man. Thoracic (*A*) and abdominal (*B*) aortograms show dilation, irregularity, and wall thickening extending from proximal descending thoracic aorta to the abdominal aorta a few centimeters above the renal arteries. *A*, The cervical branches of the aortic arch are normal. *B*, There is a 30 per cent narrowing of the left main renal artery. The picture is consistent with Takayasu's arteritis. (Courtesy of Dr. Harold Spitz.)

without gangrene of the lower extremities, although the patient may have pain and claudication in the hips and thighs with exercise, and the male may suffer from impotence (Leriche's syndrome). Sudden occlusion of the aorta at its bifurcation is poorly tolerated, and immediate embolectomy is needed. Patients with this condition suffer from pain (but pain may be absent in as many as 50 per cent of instances), loss of the femoral pulses, coldness, pallor, and often ensuing gangrene of the lower extremities. Weakness or paralysis of the lower limbs, loss of deep tendon reflexes, and impairment or loss of sensation are usually present. Two instances seen within the last two years at the Cincinnati General Hospital were referred to neurologists because of sudden paraplegia. The diagnosis was originally overlooked because of failure to examine the femoral pulses. The superficial veins of the lower extremities are usually collapsed. The diagnosis is made clinically and confirmed by aortography. Without embolectomy, massive fatal gangrene of the lower extremities and pelvis is likely. With chronic aortic thrombotic occlusion at the bifurcation, a synthetic bypass graft is used to bridge the obstructed area, provided that the iliac and femoral arterial vascular beds are adequate. Endarterectomy may be employed alone when the process is quite localized, or combined with bypass grafting when the process is more extensive.

Fairbairn, J. R., II, Juergens, J. L., and Spittell, J. A., Jr.: Peripheral Vascular Diseases. 4th ed. Philadelphia, W. B. Saunders Company, 1972.

368. DISEASES OF THE PERIPHERAL VESSELS

Jay D. Coffman

368.1. PERIPHERAL VASCULAR DISEASES DUE TO ORGANIC ARTERIAL OBSTRUCTION

ARTERIOSCLEROSIS OBLITERANS

DEFINITION. Arteriosclerosis obliterans is caused by arteriosclerotic narrowing or obstruction of large and medium-sized arteries supplying the extremities; symptoms and signs are produced by ischemia.

ETIOLOGY. The etiology of arteriosclerosis is discussed in Ch. 474.

INCIDENCE. Arteriosclerosis obliterans is the leading cause of obstructive arterial disease of the extremities after age 30. The lower extremities are involved most commonly; the superficial femoral artery is affected by stenosis or obstruction in approximately 90 per cent of patients. The aortoiliac and popliteal areas are the next most common sites. The greatest incidence of superficial femoral and more distal arterial disease occurs in the seventh decade, but aortoiliac disease has its peak a decade earlier. The disease is more common in males than in females, especially before the menopause (about 9:1). Patients with diabetes mellitus develop arteriosclerosis obliterans more frequently and at an earli-

er age than nondiabetics. Diabetics have the same incidence of femoropopliteal disease but a greater frequency of vessel involvement between the knee and ankle than nondiabetics. In patients with isolated aortoiliac disease, high plasma cholesterol and total lipid concentrations are frequent findings, but diabetes mellitus is not.

PATHOLOGY. The stenotic or occlusive process is usually segmental, and surgical therapy depends on this characteristic; however, the intima also displays widespread arteriosclerotic changes proximal and distal to the segmental lesion. Although the occlusive or stenotic lesions causing symptoms are usually proximal to the knee, the incidence of concomitant lower leg arterial occlusions is high (45 per cent in some surveys) and rises steeply with increasing age. Of the vessels in the calf, the posterior tibial artery is most often affected. A specific lesion of arteriolar and capillary endothelial proliferation has been described in diabetes by some investigators but has not been found by others. In patients with diabetes the development of indolent ulcers in the presence of adequate pulses may be due to diabetic neuropathy and not to small vessel disease.

PATHOPHYSIOLOGY. Symptoms and signs are produced by inadequate oxygenation of the tissues distal to the arterial lesion, secondary to the decrease in blood flow or pressure at rest or during exercise. Large and medium-sized arteries must have a decrease in cross-sectional area of 70 to 90 per cent before a decrease in blood flow or pressure occurs at rest; during exercise a 60 per cent decrease may suffice. The critical stenosis diameter which decreases flow or pressure is dependent on the velocity of flow and therefore the peripheral resistance; the length of the stenotic segment has a lesser effect. Factors affecting peripheral resistance are discussed below. In patients who develop ischemic symptoms only during exercise, the calf blood flow may be normal at rest; however, during exercise the blood flow may stop or be abnormally slow. The decreased blood pressure in the arterial vasculature distal to the obstructing lesion allows the contracting muscle to obstruct arterial flow partially or completely during exercise. Also, if full vasodilatation (reactive hyperemia) is produced in an involved limb, the total blood flow is usually much less than in the normal limb.

Although all the vessels of a system contribute to its total resistance, the arterioles and precapillary sphincters are of greatest importance. Peripheral resistance is regulated reflexly by the sympathetic nervous system and locally by the formation of vasodilator metabolites. Activity of the sympathetic nervous system usually causes cutaneous vasoconstriction, thereby increasing peripheral resistance. This normal activity, i.e., reflex vasoconstriction when exposed to cold, can be harmful to an ischemic extremity. Removal of vasoconstrictor activity in an extremity results in vasodilatation. Blood vessels in skeletal muscle also are affected by sympathetic activity but only to a very limited extent during exercise when vasodilator metabolites are active.

Blood supply to the limb distal to an obstructing or stenotic arterial lesion is via collateral blood vessels. Most of these collaterals are present in the normal limb but unused until an obstruction occurs; many appear almost immediately after an acute arterial occlusion, but others form more gradually over a period of months. Little is known concerning the reactivity of the collateral vessels in man; in animals, exercise and systemic blood pressure elevation decrease collateral vessel resistance, whereas a decrease in systemic blood pressure increases collateral vascular resistance. Blood flow can be increased through collateral vessels in man by raising the systemic blood pressure.

CLINICAL MANIFESTATIONS. The most common symptom of arteriosclerosis obliterans is *intermittent claudication* (intermittent limping). The patient experiences cramping pain, tightness, numbness, or severe fatigue in the muscle group being exercised. The amount of exercise producing the pain is relatively constant in each patient, and the pain is relieved promptly by rest. In a few patients, pain may disappear on further walking, perhaps because of an unconscious slowing of gait. Intermittent claudication is most frequent in the calf muscles because femoral artery disease is so common. However, even in more proximal lesions (aortoiliac disease) the calf is the most common site of claudication because these muscles do the most work in walking. Low back, buttock, thigh, and foot claudication may also occur; the site of the symptoms localizes the obstructing lesion proximally.

Rest pain is the other important symptom of obstructive arterial disease. Rest pain is a grave sign indicating that the blood supply is not sufficient even for the small nutritional requirements of the skin. It may be localized to one or more toes but often has a stocking distribution. The latter distribution means that ischemic neuritis is not usually the cause of rest pain. Rest pain is worse at night and is relieved somewhat by dependency and by cooling.

Other symptoms of arteriosclerosis obliterans include coldness, numbness, paresthesias, and color changes in the involved extremity.

Examination of the patient with intermittent claudication reveals diminished or absent pulses distal to the site of obstruction. Although the dorsalis pedis pulse may be absent congenitally in more than 10 per cent of people, the posterior tibial pulse is absent in only 2 per cent, and both pulses in approximately 0.5 per cent. If pulses are palpable in the presence of an obstructive lesion, exercise will make the pulses disappear; this is often a valuable diagnostic test. The second important part of the examination is to listen with the stethoscope over the aorta and peripheral arteries. The presence of a systolic or continuous bruit usually indicates a proximal obstructive or stenotic lesion; a continuous bruit denotes a very low diastolic pressure distal to the obstruction and therefore an inadequate collateral blood flow.

Examination may also reveal signs of ischemia. Distal to an arterial obstruction, the limb is often cool when compared with the proximal part of the same extremity or the symmetrical part of the opposite extremity. Skin temperature may vary widely in health, and even profound coldness, if present in all extremities, particularly in a cool environment, may be physiologic. Severe coldness that persists in a warm environment is usually abnormal, and, if unilateral, definitely abnormal. A warm extremity with normal color but absent pulses means collateral blood flow is adequate. The involved extremity may also show color changes: pallor, owing to a markedly decreased blood flow; cyanosis, caused by a diminution in blood flow not sufficient to cause blanching of the skin; rubor, a persistent red or reddish-blue discoloration owing to injury from anoxemia of the cutaneous capillaries and venules. Trophic

changes may develop: the subcutaneous tissue becomes puffy and thickened; the skin becomes dry, atrophic, shiny, and tightly drawn with an absence of hair; and the toenails become hard, brittle, thickened, ridged, and deformed. Indolent ulceration and gangrene indicate severe local ischemia. Ischemic ulcers on the toes, and sometimes over the anterior and lateral lower calf, are usually quite painful and sensitive.

Isolated aortoiliac disease (Leriche's syndrome) produces a characteristic picture. Intermittent claudication of the low back, buttock, thighs, or calves may be present. Global atrophy of the limbs and pallor of the legs and feet are frequent findings. Other trophic changes are usually absent; if present, concomitant femoropopliteal disease is often found. Hypertension may be present in the upper extremities; impotence has been emphasized as a symptom but it is not frequent. All pulses are usually absent in the legs, but weak femorals may be felt if the collateral circulation is well developed or if the occlusive process is only partial. A systolic murmur is often heard over both femoral arteries and lower abdomen.

DIAGNOSIS. By careful palpation of pulses and auscultation for bruits, the diagnosis and site of obstruction or stenosis are easily determined in most patients. The presence of coldness, discoloration, and trophic changes indicates the degree of ischemia. A triad of tests can be used to evaluate the degree of ischemia and collateral circulation. With the patient supine, the involved limb is raised to a 45 degree angle. Normally the plantar surface remains pink; pallor indicates a deficient blood supply. If pallor occurs only after ankle exercise, the circulation is not as compromised. Then the patient sits up quickly, allowing the extremities to assume a dependent position, and flushing and filling of the veins of the feet are timed. Flushing should occur immediately; veins should fill in about 10 seconds. Flushing and venous filling times of greater than 20 and 30 seconds, respectively, denote a severely ischemic limb with inadequate collateral circulation. These tests should be performed in a warm room to rule out vasospasm; varicosities invalidate the venous filling time. The use of a Doppler velocitometer to measure systolic blood pressure in the dorsalis pedis and posterior tibial arteries with the pneumatic cuff on the thigh and then at the ankle is especially helpful in diagnosing obstructive disease (the pedal pressures should be equal to or higher than the brachial artery pressure) and its site. A pressure less than 30 mm Hg indicates very severe ischemia and often presages gangrene. In doubtful cases, the most sensitive test is the measurement of pedal arterial systolic blood pressure before and after exercise by use of a Doppler velocitometer. In patients with a pedal pressure similar to the brachial artery pressure, the pedal pressure below an obstructive lesion will fall to low levels for more than 30 seconds after exercise. Other tests include measurement of blood flow during exercise by the disappearance of a radioisotope (^{131}I, ^{133}Xe) from the involved muscle. During exercise the disappearance rate either falls to zero or is abnormally slow in claudicators compared with that in normal subjects. The postexercise disappearance rates are also usually abnormal in obstructive arterial disease. Postexercise or postischemic flow can also be measured with a plethysmograph, but there is some overlap of values between claudicators and normal persons.

The presence or absence of calcification by x-ray of

the extremities is usually meaningless. *Arteriography* is always performed if surgery is being considered to reveal the exact location and extent of the obstructive lesion and the collateral circulation.

Intermittent claudication may occur in *severe anemia* and in *McArdle's syndrome;* both are easily distinguished from arteriosclerosis obliterans by the presence of normal pulses. The pain of *arthritis* may radiate to the thighs or calves, but is present at rest and not usually worse with exercise. *Arterial embolism* pain does not develop as insidiously as arteriosclerotic ischemic symptoms. In occasional patients with *lumbar disc, spinal canal, or cauda equina disease,* pain may occur only with exercise; also vasospasm may be intense so that distal pulses cannot be felt. Usually neurologic signs are present or appear with exercise. Even large vessel pulsations may disappear in patients taking *vasoconstrictive drugs* (see Ergotism and Methysergide Toxicity in Ch. 368.2.); patients should be carefully questioned concerning the use of these drugs.

Ischemic ulcers resulting from arteriosclerosis obliterans must be differentiated from ulcers that occur in patients with hypertension (*Hines' ulcers*). In hypertensive ischemic ulcers, pulses in the leg and foot are normal, and signs of ischemia are absent elsewhere in the extremity. The hypertensive ulcer is most commonly located on the lateral aspect of the leg or ankle, but arteriosclerotic ulcers are usually on the toes. Hypertensive ulcers are more common in females and are extremely painful. They begin as a purplish plaque which develops into a hemorrhagic bleb; the bleb then ulcerates, leaving a lesion with purplish red margins.

PROGNOSIS. Often intermittent claudication is the first symptom of generalized arteriosclerotic vascular disease, and most patients die eventually from myocardial infarctions or cerebrovascular accidents. Seventy to 90 per cent of patients with femoral artery disease remain stable in their symptoms or improve over a nine-year follow-up period. If diabetes mellitus is present, the prognosis is grave, for progression of the disease almost always occurs. The prognosis after surgical revascularization appears good in large vessel (aortic or femoral artery) disease.

TREATMENT. If the patient has only intermittent claudication with a normal-appearing limb, he should be treated conservatively. He will be able to walk farther without pain if he slows his gait and loses excess weight. Tobacco should never be used in any form, for it causes cutaneous vasoconstriction via the sympathetic nervous system. The patient is advised to exercise frequently to the development of pain but to rest until the pain totally disappears. It is hoped that exercise will stimulate further growth of collateral blood vessels, but proof is lacking for this point. Recent studies indicate that treatment of hyperlipoproteinemias may prevent or improve arteriosclerotic lesions; they may be a contributing factor and should be sought and treated if present (see Ch. 532.7). Patients should protect their limbs from cold or trauma; careful attention to keep the skin scrupulously clean, dry, and soft is important. Even minor infections such as the dermatophytoses may produce problems. Toenail trimming should be done regularly and with care.

If the claudication is found to be progressively worse over a six-month to two-year observation period, if it interferes seriously with the patient's daily activity, or if even minor ischemic symptoms such as numbness or

paresthesias are present, *surgery* should be considered. Since the lesion is often localized and segmental, restoration of circulation beyond segmental stenotic or obstructive areas by graft bypass is the treatment of choice. Currently autogenous saphenous vein grafts are used most frequently because the incidence of thrombosis is less than with grafts made of synthetic materials. Often patch grafts are used on one portion of the vessel. Bypass grafts are favored over excision and graft replacement, because collateral circulation is not destroyed with the bypass method. Before a grafting procedure can be performed, arteriography must be done to determine that there are patent vessels below the obstruction ("good runoff"). However, connection of a graft to an "isolated" popliteal segment (no calf vessels patent) may produce good results with healing of trophic lesions. Vein grafts have been connected to distal arteries in the lower calf and foot with success in saving ischemic, even gangrenous, feet. In patients with aortoiliac disease who cannot undergo major surgery, subcutaneous axillofemoral or, if one femoral is patent, femorofemoral grafts have been a very successful innovation. In patients with more than one obstructing lesion in the vessels supplying an extremity, correction of the most proximal obstruction often produces relief of symptoms. Endarterectomy of an obstructed deep femoral artery in a limb with superficial femoral artery obstruction may supply enough collateral blood flow to allow a limb to survive. The success of a surgical attack on involved vessels is proportional to the size of the vessel involved; aortoiliac operations have a 90 per cent or better success rate; femoropopliteal, 70 to 80 per cent; and posterior tibial artery, 50 per cent.

If surgery cannot be performed because of poor runoff or other serious disease, and rest pain or gangrene is present, rest in bed is essential. The affected extremity should be kept 20 to 30 degrees below the horizontal, for the dependent position increases blood flow and pressure and occasionally is the only position the patient can tolerate. If edema is present, the extremity should be kept horizontal but never elevated. External local warmth, if used at all, is best applied by means of a thermoregulated cradle kept at a temperature below 38° C. Direct application of external heat should never be used, because ischemic tissue blisters and burns at much lower temperatures than normal tissue. Rest pain may require the use of sedatives and analgesics, even narcotics. Ulcers caused by ischemia are treated the same as rest pain; warm saline soaks should be used to keep the ulcer open, moist, and clean. Enzymatic debridement is not advised because of possible local allergic reactions. If infection is present, the appropriate systemic and local antimicrobial drug should be used as determined by culture and sensitivity tests.

Preganglionic lumbar sympathectomy may be performed to increased skin blood flow when rest pain or small areas of ulceration or gangrene are present. Before surgery, it must be demonstrated that the sympathetic nervous system is intact in the extremity, especially in diabetics in whom peripheral neuropathy sometimes produces an autosympathectomy. To assess sympathetic activity in an extremity, plethysmographic foot blood flow, toe pulse, or skin temperature may be measured before and after a procedure to remove sympathetic activity. Methods used to remove sympathetic activity are (1) a warm environment, (2) local anesthesia of sympathetic ganglia, (3) local anesthesia of appropriate mixed nerves, (4) spinal anesthesia, or (5) autonomic blocking agents. An increase in the parameter being measured after one of these procedures indicates that a sympathectomy may be beneficial. Sweating of the involved extremity is also an indication of sympathetic activity. Although superficial ulcers often heal after the operation, sympathectomy alone rarely improves intermittent claudication.

Arteriosclerotic *gangrene* often necessitates *amputation* of the limb. In the presence of gangrene with ascending infection (advancing lymphangitis, fever, and leukocytosis), antimicrobial chemotherapy is indicated. Prompt amputation must be considered, because the efficacy of the antimicrobial agents may be limited by the ischemia of the affected tissues and by local necrosis. The level of amputation is determined by palpable pulses and the presence of warm viable tissue of good color. The percentage of patients who become ambulatory after amputation is much higher with below-the-knee than above-the-knee operations.

Vasodilator drugs and agents are widely advertised but have little, if any, place in the treatment of arteriosclerosis obliterans. They are consistently ineffective in relieving intermittent claudication but may increase muscle or skin blood flow at rest in some patients. The efficacy of drugs with prolonged vasodilator action depends upon the degree to which structural disease has rendered the peripheral arteries rigid and incapable of dilatation; it has yet to be shown that they are active on the collateral vessels. Vasodilator drugs often lower systemic blood pressure so that flow to the ischemic limb may be decreased; even intra-arterial administration has been shown to decrease foot flow in some patients.

Long-term anticoagulation has also been recommended for treatment of arteriosclerosis obliterans, but conflicting results have been reported. Fibrinolytic therapy with intravenous streptokinase has been evaluated for chronic arterial occlusive disease, and a few patients, especially those with a recent onset of symptoms, have benefited.

Barndt, R., Jr., Blankenhorn, D. H., Crawford, D. W., and Brooks, S. H.: Regression and progression of early femoral atherosclerosis in treated hyperlipoproteinemic patients. Ann. Intern. Med., 86:139, 1977.

Coffman, J. D.: Peripheral collateral blood flow and vascular reactivity in the dog. J. Clin. Invest., 45:923, 1966.

Coffman, J. D., and Mannick, J. A.: An objective test to demonstrate the circulatory abnormality in intermittent claudication. Circulation, 33:177, 1966.

Coffman, J. D., and Mannick, J. A.: Failure of vasodilator drugs in arteriosclerosis obliterans. Ann. Intern. Med., 76:35, 1972.

Mannick, J. A., and Coffman, J. D.: Ischemic Limbs. New York, Grune & Stratton, 1973.

Schadt, D. C., Hines, E. A., Jr., Juergens, J. L., and Barker, N. W.: Chronic atherosclerotic occlusion of the femoral artery. JAMA, 175:937, 1961.

Verta, M. J., Jr., Gross, W. S., van Bellen, B., Yao, J. S. T., and Bergan, J. J.: Forefoot perfusion pressure and minor amputation for gangrene. Surgery, 80:729, 1976.

Young, D. F., Cholvin, N. R., Kirkeeide, R. L., and Roth, A. D.: Hemodynamics of arterial stenoses at elevated flow rates. Circ. Res., 41:99, 1977.

THROMBOANGIITIS OBLITERANS
(Buerger's Disease)

DEFINITION. Thromboangiitis obliterans is an obliterative vascular disease or syndrome, probably inflammatory in type, affecting chiefly the peripheral arteries and veins. Identified first as endarteritis obliterans (von Winiwarter, 1879), it was described more fully and given its present name by Buerger (1908).

INCIDENCE. All races are subject to thromboangiitis obliterans, but the greatest incidence is in the Ashkenazic Jews, of whom 20 in 100,000 develop the disease compared with 7 or 8 per 100,000 in the general population. The disease is also common in the Orient. The incidence of the disease in the United States has decreased markedly. Men are affected far more frequently than women, in a ratio of about 75 to 1. Thromboangiitis obliterans has been observed at all ages but occurs most frequently between 20 and 45.

ETIOLOGY. Although many agents, toxic and infectious, have been suggested, no etiology has received general acceptance. Cigarettes are used moderately or excessively by many, but not all, patients with thromboangiitis obliterans and have been thoroughly investigated as a causative agent, for smoking aggravates the disease. An increased skin sensitivity to tobacco has been reported by some investigators but not found by others. The higher carboxyhemoglobin levels observed in smokers have been proposed as an etiologic factor by increasing the affinity of hemoglobin for oxygen. A thrombotic etiology is supported by the reports of abnormal thromboplastin generation tests and higher levels of heparin precipitable fraction of fibrinogen in plasma in patients with thromboangiitis obliterans than in normal persons or patients with arteriosclerosis obliterans. A rise in adhesive platelet counts has also been described in the disease and apparently correlates with tobacco smoking.

Considerable skepticism has been expressed that this disease is an entity different from arteriosclerosis occurring in young people. Evidence has been presented that its clinical and pathologic pictures are specific; however, it may be a syndrome with more than one cause.

PATHOLOGY. The lesions are segmental in that diseased sections of arteries or veins are separated by normal areas. In the acute stage cellular proliferation of the intima is accompanied by the formation of red thrombi in small and medium-sized vessels, but the internal elastic lamina usually remains intact. Polymorphonuclear leukocytes, lymphocytes, and giant cells infiltrate all coats of the artery and extend into the thrombus. The formation of sterile microabscesses within the thrombi is a specific finding in this disease. Additional segments of artery or vein are involved acutely at intervals from days to years; hence, a single long artery may exhibit many stages, ranging from the acute picture to dense scar formation. Late stages cannot be distinguished pathologically from arteriosclerosis obliterans.

PATHOPHYSIOLOGY. The disease is characterized by alternating periods of activity and quiescence. Depending upon the time relation between the developing occlusion and compensation by collateral circulation, the onset and course vary from insidious to fulminant. Usually occlusion gradually outstrips the developing collateral circulation, and definite peripheral ischemia brings the patient under medical care within one to four years after the first mild symptoms appear. The disease often has an initially more active course of six to twelve years, and then advances much less rapidly; at this stage it is very difficult to differentiate from arteriosclerosis obliterans.

CLINICAL MANIFESTATIONS. The typical patient with thromboangiitis obliterans is a young male who smokes cigarettes, presents symptoms of peripheral vascular ischemia, and may have a history of thrombophlebitis. The lower extremities are affected most commonly, and the most frequent presenting complaint is persistent coldness of the limbs. The upper extremities are involved in more than 70 per cent of patients (sometimes without symptoms), the digital arteries being affected more frequently than the ulnar or radial. Raynaud's phenomenon, hyperhidrosis, and ulcers of the digits are common. In comparison with other vascular diseases, the pain is often excruciating. Migratory thrombophlebitis may precede or accompany arterial involvement and occurs in approximately 40 per cent of patients. Tender, red, elevated areas about 1 cm in diameter appear suddenly in the skin near the valves of small, superficial veins, and gradually disappear during two to three weeks, to be followed after irregular intervals by new lesions. Other symptoms and signs (intermittent claudication, rest pain, ulcers, gangrene) are the same as in arteriosclerosis obliterans except that femoral artery disease is less frequent and aortoiliac, rare. Thromboses of the mesenteric, coronary, cerebral, and renal arteries have been described but are uncommon.

DIAGNOSIS. The diagnosis may be suspected when a young male presents with peripheral vascular insufficiency and thrombophlebitis, but it can be definitely proved only by biopsy of an active lesion. The age group, sex, thrombophlebitis, frequent involvement of upper extremities, Raynaud's phenomenon, and normal blood cholesterol concentration and glucose tolerance test result help differentiate the disease from arteriosclerosis obliterans. Arteriography can be helpful in demonstrating normality of vessels between lesions, absence of atheroma, a characteristic tree root configuration of the collateral vessels around the point of abrupt occlusion, and asymptomatic involvement of the upper extremities. Since Raynaud's disease is rare in men, affects the upper extremities more severely, and usually does not obliterate arterial pulsation at the wrist or ankle, it should not be confused with Raynaud's phenomenon in thromboangiitis obliterans. Migratory thrombophlebitis without symptoms or signs of arterial involvement cannot be diagnosed as thromboangiitis obliterans unless histologic proof is obtained.

PROGNOSIS. The prognosis for life is good, but amputation of extremities is common, especially in the fulminant form. In the late stages, the prognosis and course are similar to arteriosclerosis obliterans.

TREATMENT. The treatment is the same as that outlined for arteriosclerosis obliterans, but it is imperative that tobacco never be used in any form. Nicotine produces transient vasoconstriction and probably favors extension of the disease. Bilateral preganglionic sympathectomy has been advocated for established, gradually advancing thromboangiitis obliterans, especially if vasospasm is prominent. This major operation is not indicated in mild cases responding well to medical treatment or in advanced cases with massive gangrene. Opinion is still divided concerning the usefulness of sympathectomy in this disease. In thromboangiitis obliterans resistance to infection is fairly high and collateral circulation usually good, so that minor amputations may be performed more safely than in arteriosclerotic gangrene.

Astrup, P., Hellung-Larsen, P., Kjeldsen, K., and Mellemgaard, K.: The effect of tobacco smoking on the dissociation curve of oxygen hemoglobin. Scand. J. Clin. Lab. Invest., 18:450, 1966.

Barker, N. W.: Diagnosis and treatment of thromboangiitis obliterans (Buerger's disease). Minn. Med., 39:303, 1956.

Craven, J. L., and Cotton, R. C.: Haematological differences between thromboangiitis obliterans and atherosclerosis. Br. J. Surg., 54:862, 1967.

Goodman, R. M., Elian, B., Mozes, M., and Deutsch, V.: Buerger's disease in Israel. Am. J. Med., 39:601, 1965.

McKusick, V. A., Harris, W. S., Ottesen, O. E., Goodman, R. M., Shelley, W. M., and Bloodwell, R. D.: Buerger's disease: A distinct clinical and pathologic entity. JAMA, 181:5, 1962.

Wessler, S., Ming, S. C., Gurewich, V., and Freiman, D. G.: A critical evaluation of thromboangiitis obliterans. N. Engl. J. Med., 262:1149, 1960.

Williams, G.: Recent views on Buerger's disease. J. Clin. Pathol., 22:573, 1969.

ARTERIAL EMBOLISM

DEFINITION. Fragments of centrally located thrombi or atheromatous material may embolize and occlude large or small peripheral blood vessels.

ETIOLOGY. Emboli usually originate from mural or valvular thrombi in the left side of the heart (atrium or ventricle), less commonly from an atheromatous ulcer in the aorta or a more peripheral artery, and from thrombi in aneurysms. Paradoxical emboli originate from venous thromboses, travel to the right side of the heart, and pass through a patent foramen ovale. Most emboli occur in association with myocardial infarction, atrial fibrillation associated with mitral valve disease, chronic congestive heart failure, cardiomyopathies, or endocarditis. With the advent of surgical replacement of heart valves, prostheses have become a common source of emboli. Emboli in the upper extremities often originate from a compressed subclavian artery in the thoracic outlet syndromes.

PATHOPHYSIOLOGY. Emboli lodge at bifurcations of arteries and at narrowed arteriosclerotic areas. The most common site is at the junction of the femoral artery with the profunda femoris; emboli at the origin of the iliac arteries from the aorta (*saddle emboli*) are also frequent. The embolus stops blood flow through the artery and is followed within a few hours by secondary progressive arterial thrombosis below and sometimes above the point of obstruction. Secondary vasospasm has been assumed to be an important factor causing ischemia of the affected extremity, but convincing experimental evidence has not been presented to support this theory. The amount of muscle and skin ischemia that occurs depends on the degree of collateral circulation development.

PATHOLOGY. Emboli from the heart or aneurysms show the same pathology as the parent thrombi. Emboli lodged in arteries usually organize by the ingrowth of connective tissue, and later recanalization may occur. However, fragmentation of the embolus before organization is not uncommon with fragments lodging in more distal vessels. Emboli that originate from friable, ulcerated atheromatous lesions produce either large vessel obstruction by amorphous debris or arteriolar and capillary blockage by a variable combination of cholesterol crystals and lipoid material. The cholesterol crystals incite an inflammatory response which leads to fibrosis and complete vessel obstruction.

CLINICAL MANIFESTATIONS. In approximately half of patients, there is the sudden onset of severe pain in the extremity distal to the site of embolization. The other cases have an insidious beginning over one to several hours; numbness and paresthesias may precede the pain. Pain is present in 80 per cent of patients and may become excruciating within one or two hours, particularly if the patient exercises the limb. Paresthesias occur in about 60 per cent of cases, and 20 per cent develop muscular weakness or actual paralysis. With an aortoiliac embolus, fainting, nausea, vomiting, and abdominal pain may precede a shocklike state.

Examination of the involved extremity reveals pallor and coldness, sharply demarcated distal to the site of embolization, viz., at the inguinal ligaments or sometimes as high as the umbilicus in saddle embolus, at the lower third of the thigh in femoral artery embolus, and at midcalf in popliteal artery embolus. Arterial pulses are absent below the embolus by palpation or oscillometry. In the arms, because of the easy palpability of the brachial artery, the site of embolus lodgment can be determined by the disappearance of the pulse. Occasionally there is tenderness directly over the embolus in an artery. The extremity may also show collapsed veins, decreased to absent reflexes and sensation, and weakness and paralysis. Later the initial pallor changes to a blotchy cyanosis. If collateral circulation is good, the extremity soon shows signs of improvement in color and temperature, but muscle tenderness and pitting edema may develop. If the collateral circulation is inadequate, massive gangrene follows with bleb formation, spotty vermilion discoloration of the skin, and mummification.

Large emboli from thrombi or amorphous atherosclerotic debris show the aforementioned picture. Smaller emboli may produce only local digital cyanosis with or without pain. Atheromatous microemboli (cholesterol crystals and lipoid material) may produce sudden leg pain, tender muscles, cool legs with pulses, petechiae, livedo reticularis, and plaquelike reddened elevations of the skin. Pedal pulses may disappear later in this syndrome. The spontaneous appearance of painful dusky discoloration of a toe or toes in the presence of pulses should suggest atheromatous microembolism.

DIAGNOSIS. The diagnosis of embolization is not difficult in the patient with the acute onset of a painful, ischemic extremity who demonstrates a source for embolus formation. Acute arterial thrombosis can be distinguished from an embolus only by the presence or absence of underlying etiologies; absent or decreased arterial pulsations in the opposite limb support a diagnosis of acute thrombosis. Patients with acute iliofemoral thrombophlebitis sometimes have no palpable pulses in the affected extremity and may show signs resembling those of arterial embolus. Detection of a feeble pulse by oscillometry, distended veins, and massive edema of the extremity helps rule out embolus. In patients with symptoms and signs of embolization or microembolization and normal pulses, angiography must be performed to look for ulcerative atherosclerotic lesions, aneurysms, or fibromuscular dysplasia in the proximal large vessels. Microembolization is often confused with polymyositis or polyarteritis nodosa; muscle biopsy may be necessary to demonstrate the cholesterol crystals.

PROGNOSIS. The prognosis in acute arterial embolization depends on several factors, including size of vessel affected, age of patient, collateral blood supply, and speed of treatment. The larger the artery involved, the worse the prognosis without surgical treatment. Gangrene is much more common after the age of 60 years, probably because of concomitant arteriosclerotic involvement of the blood vessels and collaterals. The development of collateral circulation is very important, for sufficient collaterals may save a limb without surgical

treatment. The presence of patent companion vessels, e.g., around the elbow, gives a favorable outlook. The earlier an embolus can be removed surgically, the better the prognosis for survival of the severely ischemic limb.

With any method of treatment, the mortality in most studies is usually greater than 20 per cent, owing to the underlying disease and recurrent embolization to vital areas. The incidence of embolus recurrence is very high. After either medical or surgical treatment, limb incapacity from muscle fibrosis with tendon shortening or intermittent claudication is common.

TREATMENT. Although embolectomy should restore the normal physiology and is strongly recommended in the surgical literature, conservative medical management often gives as good end results. The exception is emboli at the aortic bifurcation, when surgery is the optimal treatment. When the patient is first seen, treatment should be instituted to improve blood flow to the extremity, and a vascular surgeon should be immediately called in consultation. Anticoagulation with heparin should be started at once to prevent thrombus formation below and above the embolus, and further embolization (long-term anticoagulation is usually indicated to prevent recurrent emboli). Thrombolytic therapy with streptokinase may be valuable in acute embolization in about one third of patients; such therapy is given intravenously and must be followed by adequate anticoagulation (see Ch. 357.3). The limb should be positioned in 15 degree dependency and adequate analgesics given to relieve the pain. The affected limb should be kept comfortably warm, as in a thermoregulated (30 to 34° C) cradle, and the body and uninvolved extremities warmed in an effort to produce reflex vasodilatation in the involved limb. Every precaution should be taken to prevent burning during heat application; ischemic limbs burn at much lower temperatures than normal limbs. Lumbar sympathetic block by paravertebral injection of procaine or xylocaine has been recommended to relieve vasoconstrictor tone and vasospasm if present; if used, it should be performed before anticoagulation.

If conservative medical therapy is not effective in greatly improving the extremity in two to four hours and the underlying condition of the patient will allow surgery, embolectomy is indicated. Early diagnosis is essential, as the greatest success with embolectomy is within eight to ten hours of the incident. Embolectomy has been performed longer than 48 hours after the acute insult with some success, although less than with earlier operations. Muscle tenderness and edema often occur after embolectomy and may be mistakenly diagnosed as thrombophlebitis. In cases presenting with gangrene, amputation is usually necessary. In atheromatous embolization or emboli from aneurysmal thrombi, surgical attack on the proximal lesion may be successful in preventing further emboli; the use of anticoagulants in this situation has not been shown to be of value.

Amery, A., Deloof, W., Vermylen, J., and Verstraete, M.: Outcome of recent thromboembolic occlusions of limb arteries treated with streptokinase. Br. Med. J., 4:639, 1970.

Eliot, R. S., Kanjuh, V. I., and Edwards, J. E.: Atheromatous embolism. Circulation, 30:611, 1964.

Freund, U., Romanoff, H., and Floman, Y.: Mortality rate following lower limb arterial embolectomy: Causative factors. Surgery, 77:201, 1975.

Jacobs, A. L.: Arterial embolism in the limbs. Edinburgh, E. & S. Livingstone, Ltd., 1959.

Karmody, A. M., Powers, S. R., Monaco, V. J., and Leather, R. P.: "Blue toe" syndrome. Arch. Surg., 111:1263, 1976.

Silverblatt, C. W., Wasserman, F., and Wolcott, M. W.: Pulmonary artery embolism and paradoxical embolization. Arch. Intern. Med., 107:105, 1961.

Szekely, P.: Systemic embolism and anticoagulant prophylaxis in rheumatic heart disease. Br. Med. J., 1:1209, 1964.

Wessler, S., Sheps, S. G., Gilbert, M., and Sheps, M. C.: Studies in peripheral arterial occlusive disease. III. Acute arterial occlusion. Circulation, 17:512, 1958.

PERIPHERAL ARTERITIS AND GANGRENE IN SYSTEMIC INFECTIONS

Symptoms and signs of peripheral vascular disease, mild or severe, appear occasionally as complications in bacterial, viral, rickettsial, and fungal infections. Bacterial arteritis and abscess of the wall of an artery are uncommon complications of bacterial endocarditis and septicemias and may lead to hemorrhagic lesions or aneurysm formation. The rickettsial diseases, especially typhus and Rocky Mountain spotted fever, may cause endothelial proliferation of the arterioles, capillaries, and venules followed by degeneration and necrosis of the media; thrombosis of larger arteries may occur rarely. In infectious arteritis with direct vascular involvement, signs of subacute or acute arrest of peripheral blood flow occur with necrosis of skin and sometimes massive gangrene. However, peripheral ischemia may be transitory and, in large part, vasospastic. Gangrene of the extremities may follow acute infectious conditions, such as pneumonia and gastroenteritis, especially in children; the cause is unknown.

Tuberculosis of the peripheral arteries is rare, but occasionally metastatic infection or embolism produces panarteritis or endarteritis with fully developed tubercles in thrombosed vessels. Direct involvement by extension from adjacent tuberculous lesions, although common in centrally located vessels, is rare in the extremities.

Syphilis may diminish peripheral circulation by producing periarteritis, obliterative intimal hyperplasia, or panarteritis, but the media is much less affected than in the large arteries. True gummas have been found in the vessels of gangrenous limbs. Peripheral vascular complications of syphilis are more common in men than in women. Peripheral ischemia, vasospastic or organic, appears insidiously or suddenly, but gangrene is rare. Active antisyphilitic therapy usually arrests the acute progress of the disease and relieves vasospasm, but organic occlusion remains.

Collins, R. N., and Nadel, M. S.: Gangrene due to the hemolytic *Streptococcus* — a rare but treatable disease. N. Engl. J. Med., 272:578, 1965.

Derick, C. L., and Hass, G. M.: Diffuse arteritis of syphilitic origin. Am. J. Path., 11:291, 1935.

Koten, J. W.: Peripheral gangrene in infancy and childhood. Br. Med. J., 3:798, 1967.

Learmouth, G. E.: Gangrene of the lower extremities complicating scarlet fever. Can. Med. Assoc. J., 15:69, 1925.

Slaughter, W. H.: Symmetrical gangrene of malarial origin. JAMA, 86:1607, 1926.

SHIN SPLINTS AND ANTERIOR TIBIAL COMPARTMENT SYNDROMES

The anterior tibial compartment is a closed space in which the muscles and blood vessels are surrounded by nonexpanding fascia and bone. Swelling of the tissues in this compartment can cause mild to severe complications.

Shin splints is a frequently encountered syndrome of pain and discomfort in the lower anterior part of the leg after repetitive, unusual exertion. The syndrome is presumably a result of ischemia from an abnormally high tissue pressure compressing the blood vessels. It often occurs in athletes or dancers early in the season. The pain in the front of the legs occurs during or after exercise and is only slowly relieved by rest. Tenderness is most frequent at periosteal attachments of the muscles to the tibia or interosseous membrane. Mild swelling and a slight rise in local skin temperature may be present. When the pain is reproduced by repeated dorsiflexion of the foot against resistance, the anterior tibial muscles become very hard and bulge prominently; a pulsation may become visible over the front of the legs. Arterial pulses are normal. Treatment consists of rest of the muscles, supportive strapping, and a program of graduated exercise.

The *acute anterior tibial compartment syndrome* is a rare condition caused by the rapid onset of ischemic necrosis of muscles in the anterior tibial space. Swelling of the muscles compresses muscles, nerves, and blood vessels. The cause is usually unknown, but there is often a history of excessive exertion. The syndrome may occur after fractures of the tibia or fibula or restoration of blood flow to an acutely ischemic extremity. A dull, aching pain which becomes progressively severe is the major symptom; it is unrelieved by rest and sometimes by analgesics. Extreme tenderness is present over the entire anterior tibial compartment, and the fascia rapidly becomes tense and boardlike. The skin becomes glossy, erythematous, and edematous as muscle necrosis occurs; a slight fever and leukocytosis may be present. Loss of dorsiflexion of the great toe and foot then occurs, and sensation may be lost between the first and second toes (deep peroneal nerve compression). The dorsalis pedis pulse may be present or absent. Treatment must be immediate and involves surgical decompression of the anterior tibial compartment by fasciotomy. If treatment is delayed, complete necrosis of the muscles occurs with a resultant permanent footdrop.

A *chronic anterior tibial compartment syndrome* also has been described with pain similar to intermittent claudication in the front of the lower leg on severe exertion but not with ordinary walking. The discomfort disappears with rest. Tenderness is present over the entire compartment when the pain occurs; arterial pulses are normal. The syndrome is thought to be due to an abnormally small compartment. Treatment is usually unnecessary, but a fasciotomy will relieve the symptoms.

French, E. B., and Price, W. H.: Anterior tibial pain. Br. Med. J., 2:1290, 1962.

Reneman, R. S.: The anterior and the lateral compartmental syndrome of the leg due to intensive use of muscles. Clin. Orthop., 113:69, 1975.

Rorabeck, C. H., and MacNab, I.: The pathophysiology of the anterior tibial compartmental syndrome. Clin. Orthop., 113:52, 1975.

Slocum, D. B.: The shin syndrome. Am. J. Surg., 114:875, 1967.

368.2. PERIPHERAL VASCULAR DISEASE DUE TO ABNORMAL VASOCONSTRICTION OR VASODILATATION

RAYNAUD'S PHENOMENON AND DISEASE

DEFINITION. Raynaud's phenomenon is a syndrome characterized by paroxysmal, bilateral ischemia of the digits induced by cold or emotional stimuli and relieved by heat.

ETIOLOGY. Raynaud's phenomenon may be secondary to an underlying disease or anatomic abnormality, but the most common cause is *Raynaud's disease,* which is of unknown etiology. It is less common before puberty and after age 40 but may occur at any age. Women are affected more frequently than men (5:1). Raynaud concluded from his early studies (1862, 1874) that excessive sympathetic activity was responsible for the attacks, but Lewis found that the digital vessels were abnormally reactive to local cold. Since ischemic attacks can still be induced after sympathectomy, it may be concluded that there is a local fault in the blood vessels in Raynaud's disease which is aggravated by the normal degree of reflex sympathetic nervous activity. However, about a dozen cases of Raynaud's phenomenon associated with pulmonary hypertension have been reported, suggesting that a neurohumoral mechanism may be operative in causing both syndromes.

Raynaud's phenomenon may occur in occlusive arterial disease (thromboangiitis obliterans, arteriosclerosis obliterans, arterial emboli), collagen disease (especially scleroderma), after trauma (pneumatic hammer disease, injuries to pianists or typists), after gangrene from any cause, drug intoxication (ergot, methysergide), blood dyscrasias (cryopathies, cold hemagglutinins), and neurogenic lesions (thoracic outlet compression syndromes, carpal tunnel syndrome, poliomyelitis, syringomyelia, causalgia). In Raynaud's phenomenon from secondary causes, the syndrome is caused usually by irritation of the sympathetic nerves, pathologic alterations in the small blood vessels, or sludging and agglutination of red blood cells.

PATHOLOGIC PHYSIOLOGY. The paroxysmal ischemia of the digits is due to constriction of the digital and palmar or plantar arteries; initial pallor indicates that vasoconstriction involves the small cutaneous vessels. Later the digital capillaries and venules become dilated, and the slowed blood flow allows the hemoglobin to release more of its oxygen, producing cyanotic, cold digits. When the vasoconstriction is relieved, blood flow increases greatly (reactive hyperemia), imparting a red color to the previously ischemic digits. Total and capillary fingertip blood flow are smaller in patients with Raynaud's phenomenon and disease than in normal subjects. With a cooling stimulus, patients show a significant decrease in fingertip capillary flow not seen in normal subjects.

PATHOLOGY. In the early stages of the disease, the blood vessels are histologically normal. Later, in progressive cases, the intima is thickened and the muscular coats of the arteries are hypertrophied. Eventually thrombosis of small arteries may occur and focal gangrene of the digital tips may form, although elsewhere the arteries are still histologically normal or show only slight hypertrophy.

CLINICAL MANIFESTATIONS. In typical Raynaud's phenomenon, the fingers of both hands show well demarcated blanching on exposure to cold and then may turn cyanotic; sometimes only cyanosis occurs. During recovery, a bright red color (reactive hyperemia) replaces the cyanosis. During the ischemic phase, the digits are cold and numb. In the reactive hyperemia phase, throbbing pain, tingling, swelling, and a rise in skin temperature are found. The digits are affected to different levels in each patient (sometimes extending to the wrist), but the terminal phalanges are always most severely involved. Initially, attacks may be unilateral and involve only one or two digits, but they soon become bilateral and may be induced by emotional upsets as well as by cold exposure.

In Raynaud's disease, the onset is usually gradual with attacks only in the winter. Attacks may be rare, or they may occur several times a day; they may last a few minutes in mild cases to two hours or more in severe cases. They end spontaneously or can be terminated by immersing the hands in warm water. Between episodes, the digits are normal or, in severe cases, mildly cyanotic.

The hands alone are affected in half the cases, hands and feet in the remainder; nose, cheeks, ears, and chin are affected much more rarely. The course of the disease varies; after onset it may persist indefinitely in mild form, improve spontaneously, or become more severe. In the small number of cases that are progressive, the attacks become more frequent, persist during the summer, and last longer; finally, mild cyanosis may be present constantly.

Trophic changes appear in progressive cases, usually one to four years after onset. The fingers become thin and tapering and their skin smooth, shiny, less mobile, and eventually tightly stretched (sclerodactyly). The nails grow slowly and are ridged or curved. Recurrent infections, blisters, and small areas of local cutaneous gangrene appear on the fingertips, but gangrene of a whole digit is rare. The gangrenous areas are extremely painful and, on healing, leave tiny depressed scars.

DIAGNOSIS. Criteria which should be present in patients with Raynaud's phenomenon in order to diagnose Raynaud's disease include (1) absence of any disease or anatomic abnormality to which paroxysmal digital ischemia might be secondary; (2) well demarcated digital pallor or cyanosis occurring in intermittent attacks, induced by cold or emotion; (3) symmetrical or bilateral involvement of digits; and (4) gangrene, if present, usually limited to small areas of skin. Previously, presence of symptoms for two years with no evidence of an underlying cause had been considered a fifth diagnostic point; however, Raynaud's phenomenon may precede the diagnosis of scleroderma by many years. It is probably unsafe to diagnose the idiopathic disease in the presence of an elevated sedimentation rate or minor symptoms or signs suggestive of an underlying disease (arthralgias, telangiectasis). Raynaud's phenomenon is diagnosed by discovering an underlying disease or condition known to cause attacks.

Raynaud's disease and phenomenon are distinguished from acrocyanosis by the intermittency of attacks. The cyanotic, cold, and edematous limb affected by poliomyelitis or other diseases causing paralysis is also persistent in nature. The cause of sudden "bilateral gangrene of the digits" (Lewis), which appears rarely in children or young adults without previous attacks of discoloration and without cold exposure, is unknown. The fingers, toes, nose, and ears become permanently cyanotic, and within a few days gangrene develops in the distal phalanges of one or more fingers, often symmetrically and bilaterally. The gangrene is extensive and is due to sudden thrombotic occlusion of the final end branches of the digital arteries. The relationship of this syndrome to Raynaud's disease is uncertain, although typical cyclic color changes may appear during the healing stage.

PROGNOSIS. Mild cases of Raynaud's disease improve slowly or remain stationary for years, and the attacks, being few and avoidable, are merely an inconvenience. In a large series of cases, the disease caused no deaths and very little disability; amputations of terminal phalanges were necessary in only 0.4 per cent, and the phenomenon improved or disappeared in 46 per cent. The progressive form, with recurring infection and local gangrene, becomes increasingly painful and disabling, usually despite treatment, but only rarely results in the loss of more than the distal phalanges. The prognosis for secondary Raynaud's phenomenon depends on the underlying cause. Generalized scleroderma and rheumatoid arthritis, which are frequently associated with Raynaud's phenomenon, may produce extreme deformity and disability.

TREATMENT. Mild cases of Raynaud's disease with infrequent attacks limited to cold exposure, and without trophic changes or gangrene, may be relieved by reassurance, sedatives or tranquilizers, and protection from cold exposure. Smoking has been shown to produce cutaneous vasoconstriction, and the use of tobacco should therefore be avoided. Rauwolfia* products in continued small oral doses (reserpine, 0.25 to 0.5 mg daily) will often decrease the severity and frequency of attacks. Guanethidine* (10 to 40 mg daily) and alpha methyldopa* (1.5 to 2.0 grams daily) are also effective in treatment. If necessary, a vasodilator drug (tolazoline long-acting tablets, 80 mg every 12 hours) can be added to the therapeutic regimen. The addition of thyroid substances and androgens has been recommended but helps little, if any.

Vasoconstrictor tone caused by sympathetic nervous system activity is an important factor in bringing on and maintaining attacks of digital ischemia, whether or not the local arteries are abnormally reactive to cold. Removal of vasoconstrictor impulses by regional sympathectomy may be of benefit for the progressive type of Raynaud's disease with indolent ulcers or local gangrene. The success of the sympathectomy depends upon the extent to which the normal capacity for vasodilatation is preserved, as shown by the vasodilator response to body warming or sympathetic ganglion nerve block with lidocaine. In early Raynaud's disease of the lower extremities, lumbar sympathetic ganglionectomy gives complete relief of symptoms. For the upper extremity, preganglionic cervicodorsal sympathectomy is the operation of choice but usually is of temporary (six months to two years) benefit.

The treatment of Raynaud's phenomenon secondary to an underlying disease or anatomic abnormality is directed at the secondary cause. Sympathectomy is of little or no benefit in scleroderma or arthritis but may be helpful in Raynaud's phenomenon secondary to pneumatic hammer disease or causalgia (reflex sympathetic dystrophy).

Coffman, J. D., and Davies, E. T.: Vasospastic diseases: A review. Prog. Cardiovasc. Dis., 18:123, 1975.
Coffman, J. D., and Cohen, A. S.: Total and capillary fingertip blood flow in Raynaud's phenomenon. N. Engl. J. Med., 285:259, 1971.
Cosgriff, T. M., and Arnold, W. J.: Digital vasospasm and infarction associated with hepatitis B antigenemia. JAMA, 235:1362, 1976.
Farmer, R. G., Gifford, R. W., Jr., and Hines, E. A., Jr.: Raynaud's disease with sclerodactylia: A follow-up of seventy-one patients. Circulation, 22:13, 1961.
Gifford, R. W., Jr., and Hines, E. A., Jr.: Raynaud's disease among women and girls. Circulation, 16:1012, 1957.
Lewis, T., and Pickering, G. W.: Observations upon maladies in which the blood supply to digits ceases intermittently or permanently, and upon bilateral gangrene of digits; observations relevant to so-called "Raynaud's disase." Clin. Sci., 1:327, 1934.
McGrath, M. A., and Penney, R.: The mechanisms of Raynaud's phenomenon. Parts 1 and 2. Med. J. Aust., 2:328, 1974.
Tsur, N., Adar, R., Bechor, I., Bogokowsky, H., and Mozes, M.: Upper thoracic sympathectomy. Israel J. Med Sci., 9:53, 1973.

ACROCYANOSIS

Acrocyanosis (Croq, 1896; chronic acro-asphyxia, Cassirer, 1900) is a symmetrical cyanosis of the hands and, less commonly, the feet with few or no symptoms and no complications.

ETIOLOGY AND PATHOLOGY. It is primarily a vasospastic disturbance of the smaller arterioles of the skin of unknown cause, but is probably due to local cold sensitivity. When compared with normal digits, acrocyanotic digits have a heightened arteriolar tone at average room temperature. Secondary dilatation of the capillaries and the subpapillary venous plexus occurs, and the slower blood flow allows the hemoglobin to release a greater part of its oxygen content, accounting for the blue color. Acrocyanosis occurs without special age or sex incidence, and may be associated with various endocrine disorders or asthenias as well as with certain anxiety states. No specific pathology has been described.

CLINICAL MANIFESTATIONS. Patients usually present with an unevenly blue and red discoloration of the skin which may extend from the digits to the wrists and ankles but is most intense distally. The digits are also persistently cold and sweat profusely. Puffiness of the digits and mild hypesthesia may be present, but other trophic changes are rare. The cyanosis is intensified by cold or emotional upsets and is relieved by warmth.

DIAGNOSIS. Acrocyanosis can be distinguished from Raynaud's disease by the persistent nature of the discoloration. The presence of normal arterial pulses rules out obstructive arterial disease. Since the discoloration is limited to the hands and feet and disappears when the extremities are warmed, it should not be confused with various types of generalized cyanosis.

TREATMENT. Except for reassurance, treatment is usually unnecessary. Possible endocrine abnormalities should be investigated. To prevent reflex sympathetic vasoconstriction, general body protection from cold, as well as local measures, helps to decrease the intensity of the discoloration. For cosmetic reasons, vasodilator drugs (reserpine, 0.25 to 0.5 mg daily, or tolazoline long-acting tablets, 80 mg every 12 hours) may be used. Sympathectomy is helpful but seldom warranted.

Elliot, A. H., Evans, R. D., and Stone, C. S.: Acrocyanosis: A study of the circulatory fault. Am. Heart J., 11:431, 1936.
Larsson, Y.: The vasoconstrictor tone of the cutaneous arterioles in acroasphyxia, hypertension, and in the cold pressor test. Acta Med. Scand. (Supp. 206), 130:146, 1948.

*Experimental drug for this purpose.

Lewis, T., and Landis, E. M.: Observations upon the vascular mechanism in acrocyanosis. Heart, 15:229, 1930.

Lottenbach, K.: Vascular response to cold in acrocyanosis. Helv. Med. Acta, 33:437, 1966.

ERGOTISM AND METHYSERGIDE TOXICITY

DEFINITION. Intense vasoconstriction of small and large blood vessels, producing symptoms and signs of peripheral vascular ischemia, may result from the ingestion of ergot or methysergide.

ETIOLOGY. Ergotism results from the use of ergot-containing drugs or the ingestion of bread made from rye or wheat infected with the ergot fungus (*Claviceps purpurea*). It formerly occurred in epidemic form, but is now seen only sporadically (due to the fungus), or after the repeated administration of ergotamine (Gynergen, Cafergot) for migraine or pruritus or of ergot in abortion. Methysergide is a synthetic serotonin antagonist useful in the treatment of migraine headaches. Approximately 7 per cent of patients develop peripheral vascular symptoms or signs with methysergide ingestion, usually after large doses, although as little as 1 mg has caused symptoms in some patients.

PATHOPHYSIOLOGY AND PATHOLOGY. Both drugs induce large and small blood vessel vasoconstriction. Ergot induces vasoconstriction mainly by stimulation of the alpha adrenoceptors of vascular smooth muscle and can lead to thickening and fibrosis of the arterial wall resembling fibromuscular dysplasia. Secondary intimal hyperplasia and thrombosis may occur, resulting in gangrene. In methysergide toxicity, the arterial adventitia is markedly thickened by circular fibrous apposition. Its mode of action is unknown, but it does potentiate the effect of catecholamines on blood vessels.

CLINICAL MANIFESTATIONS. *Acute ergotism* produces diarrhea, colic, and vomiting, followed by headache, vertigo, paresthesias, convulsive seizures, and occasionally gangrene of the digits, nose and ears. It is rarely seen with the drug ingestion. In *chronic intoxications,* intermittent claudication, muscle pains, numbness, coldness and pallor of the digits, and even Raynaud's phenomenon may occur. Examination reveals only cool, pale digits or mottling of the skin with normal or decreased arterial pulsations; however, complete absence of medium- and large-vessel pulsations in the extremities may occur. Gangrene may develop in the severe cases. A similar picture of peripheral vascular ischemia may follow methysergide ingestion. Abdominal angina, angina pectoris, and cerebral ischemic symptoms have also been caused by these drugs. Methysergide has been implicated as an etiologic agent in periureteral or retroperitoneal fibrosis which can extrinsically obstruct arteries and veins.

DIAGNOSIS. The diagnosis is made from the history of drug ingestion associated with symptoms and signs of peripheral ischemia. Arteriography characteristically shows diffuse or segmental narrowing of large arteries and often very constricted distal vessels with collateral vessels present. Arteriosclerosis obliterans, Raynaud's disease, and acrocyanosis are differentiated from ergotism and methysergide toxicity by the history of drug ingestion and, if necessary, by arteriography.

PROGNOSIS. The prognosis is excellent if gangrene has not appeared before treatment and if drug administration is stopped.

TREATMENT. Treatment involves anticoagulation to prevent thromboses and the use of vasodilators, e.g., sodium nitroprusside, 50 μg per minute or more intravenously or intra-arterially,* to counteract the vasocontriction. Body warming is recommended to produce reflex vasodilatation in the involved extremities, but is often unsuccessful as is vasodilator drug therapy. With avoidance of the offending drug, the vasoconstriction usually subsides in one to three days. Sympathetic nerve block or sympathectomy may be necessary in pregangrenous or gangrenous cases.

Carliner, N. H., Denune, D. P., Finch, C. S., Jr., and Goldberg, L. I.: Sodium nitroprusside treatment of ergotamine-induced peripheral ischemia. JAMA, 227:308, 1974.

Graham, J. R.: Methysergide for prevention of headache. N. Eng. J. Med., 270:67, 1964.

Müller-Schweinitzer, E., and Stürmer, E.: Investigations on the mode of action of ergotamine in the isolated femoral vein of the dog. Br. J. Pharmacol., 51:441, 1974.

Rackley, C. E., Mengel, C. E., Pomerantz, M., and McIntosh, H. D.: Vascular complications with use of methysergide. Arch. Intern. Med., 117:265, 1966.

Regan, J. F., and Poletti, B. J.: Vascular adventitial fibrosis in a patient taking methysergide maleate. JAMA, 203:1069, 1968.

ERYTHROMELALGIA
(Erythermalgia)

DEFINITION. Erythromelalgia (Mitchell, 1878) is a rare syndrome of paroxysmal, bilateral vasodilatation of the feet and, less often, the hands, associated with burning pain, increased skin temperature, and redness of the skin.

ETIOLOGY AND PATHOLOGY. The cause is unknown. It has occurred as a hereditary affliction. Increased blood flow is usually present, but symptoms may occur in a limb in which the arteries are occluded by a blood pressure cuff. Therefore it is thought that there is a hypersensitivity of the skin to heat or tension. No uniform pathologic condition has been found, but data are scarce. The syndrome occurs without special age or sex incidence.

CLINICAL MANIFESTATIONS. The patient with erythromelalgia complains of attacks of bilateral burning pain, superficial or deep, involving circumscribed areas on the soles or palms, the entire foot or hand, or even the whole extremity. The attacks follow stimuli that normally induce only physiologic peripheral vasodilatation or engorgement such as local heat, a warm environment, exercise, standing, or simple dependency of the extremity. The onset is gradual, and symptoms may remain mild for years or may become so severe and continuous that total disability results. Examination during an attack (which may be produced by exposure to a 32 to 36° C environment) usually reveals that the affected skin is hot and red and often sweats profusely; arterial pulsations are normal. Trophic changes, gangrene, and ulceration do not occur, but swelling may be present.

The syndrome may be either idiopathic or secondary to polycythemia vera, hypertension, myeloproliferative diseases, or lupus erythematosus. The condition may precede the polycythemia by as long as 12 years. Secondary erythromelalgia occurs more commonly in an older age group, is more often unilateral, and produces pain of lesser intensity than idiopathic erythromelalgia.

---

*See p. vi, Dosage Notice, immediately following Preface.

DIAGNOSIS. Arteriosclerosis obliterans may produce localized and often unilateral burning pain and redness but, unlike erythromelalgia, is not associated with normal pulses or a rise in skin temperature. Neuritis, infectious ganglionitis, and poisoning by thallium, lead, or arsenic may produce painful peripheral hyperemia. Chronic inflammatory states produce in the skin a "susceptible state" with diminished capillary and arteriolar tone. Burning pain (erythralgia, Lewis) is then induced by mild grades of heat, cold, friction, and congestion that leave normal skin unaffected. A temporary reactive vasodilatation of the cutaneous vessels also normally occurs after prolonged exposure to cold in response to a histamine-like substance liberated by local tissue damage (Lewis). This is easily distinguished from erythromelalgia by the history.

TREATMENT. Attacks can be avoided or aborted by rest, elevation of the extremity, and cold application. Aspirin (0.6 gram orally) quickly relieves pain in some cases, and the remarkable response is of diagnostic value. Vasoconstrictor agents such as ephedrine (25 mg orally) may be useful; methysergide* (1 to 4 mg orally) has also produced relief. Even vasodilator agents (isoproterenol, nitroglycerin) have been reported to be helpful. Contrast baths, using heat below the threshold for pain, often afford considerable but temporary relief. Severe attacks require liberal doses of sedatives, and the therapy is generally unsatisfactory. Occasionally section or alcohol injection of peripheral nerve is required; sympathectomy has been successful in the treatment of three cases.

PROGNOSIS. The prognosis in idiopathic erythromelalgia is guarded, because the severe pain may become disabling. Prognosis of secondary cases depends on the underlying disease; treatment of the disease often relieves the symptoms.

Alarcon-Segovia, D., and Diaz-Jouanen, E.: Erythermalgia in systemic lupus erythematosus. Am. J. Med. Sci., 266:149, 1973.

Babb, R. R., Alarcon-Segovia, D., and Fairbairn, J. F., II: Erythermalgia. Review of 51 cases. Circulation, 29:136, 1964.

Catchpole, B. N.: Erythromelalgia. Lancet, 1:909, 1964.

Cross, E. G.: The familial occurrence of erythromelalgia and nephritis. Can. Med. Assoc. J., 87:1, 1962.

Lewis, T.: Clinical observations and experiments relating to burning pain in extremities and to so-called "erythromelalgia" in particular. Clin. Sci., 1:175, 1933.

368.3. PERIPHERAL VASCULAR DISEASES DUE TO EXPOSURE TO COLD

Exposure to cold induces vasoconstriction by a direct action on blood vessels and also by reflex sympathetic nervous system activity. Cold application to the forehead or to one extremity stimulates vasoconstriction in all extremities. The decreased blood flow and local anoxia may lead to tissue damage, depending on the degree and duration of exposure and the susceptibility of the patient.

Even brief exposure to nonfreezing cold is followed in sensitive persons by an exaggerated and prolonged type of reactive vasodilatation, low-grade edema, and tingling pain. Similar exposure in more susceptible pa-

tients produces pronounced edema of the angioneurotic or urticarial type on exposed areas; even mucous membranes may be involved on ingesting cold substances. A systemic reaction with increased pulse rate, decreased blood pressure, flushing of the face, and even syncope may accompany the edema. After swimming in cool water, this reaction has proved fatal in some instances. Familial cases of cold urticaria have been described; this is a milder condition not affecting mucous membranes. Histamine has been shown to be released and measurable in the blood and urine in the nonfamilial cases. The passive transfer of cold urticaria has been demonstrated with both IgE and IgM fractions of patients' serum. Diagnosis is made by exposure of a hand or arm to 12 to 14° C water; edema will develop during or after exposure. Antihistamines or cyproheptadine (Periactin, 4 mg three times a day) or repeated short episodes of cold exposure may be of use in the treatment of cold sensitivity, but protection of the patient from cold exposure is most important.

Bentley-Phillips, C. B., Black, A. K., and Greaves, M. W.: Induced tolerance in cold urticaria caused by cold-evoked histamine release. Lancet, 2:63, 1976.

Tindall, J. P.: Cold urticaria. Postgrad. Med., 50:133, 1971.

Wanderer, A. A., and Ellis, E. F.: Treatment of cold urticaria with cyproheptadine. J. Allergy Clin. Immunol., 48:366, 1971.

Wanderer, A. A., Maselli, R., Ellis, E. F., and Ishizaka, K.: Immunologic characterization of serum factors responsible for cold urticaria. J. Allergy Clin. Immunol., 48:13, 1971.

IMMERSION FOOT
(Trench Foot)

DEFINITION. Immersion foot is due to prolonged exposure of the extremities to water; syndromes characterized only by painful, swollen feet or hands to the more serious manifestations of muscle necrosis, ulceration, and gangrene may result.

ETIOLOGY. Although prolonged exposure (greater than 48 hours) to dampness or water is the important factor in the production of immersion foot, immobility and dependency of the lower extremities, constricting garments, chilling of the body, trauma, exhaustion, or dehydration, and, in some instances, semistarvation with deficient intake of protein and vitamins are often contributing causes. Two types, cold water and warm water immersion foot, exist and present different clinical pictures. The combination of wetness plus cold (not necessarily freezing) temperatures produces the most serious condition. Warm water injuries have been divided into warm water immersion foot and the more severe tropical immersion foot (paddy-field foot).

PATHOPHYSIOLOGY. The factors causing cold water immersion foot tend to decrease blood flow to the extremities. Vasoconstriction is caused by direct and reflex cold stimulation; actual cellular damage and the ensuing hyperemia are important in producing the clinical and pathologic picture. Persistent local anoxia leads to tissue necrosis and injures the capillary walls. Capillary filtration increases remarkably, and plasma and protein pass freely into the interstitial tissue, producing a tense edema. The resultant increased viscosity of the blood leads to stasis and occlusion of small vessels. The local anoxia may also produce wallerian degeneration of the nerves in the affected area.

---

*See p. vi, Dosage Notice, immediately following Preface.

Warm water immersion foot is thought to be caused by waterlogging and swelling of the stratum corneum together with abrasion from footwear. *Pseudomonas aeruginosa* can usually be cultured from the affected areas and may contribute by digesting human callus with its proteolytic enzymes. Tropical immersion foot may be caused by water entering the dermis through water-damaged stratum corneum.

PATHOLOGY. The early pathologic picture of the cold type has not been studied. In late stages, a nonspecific picture of vascular occlusion, desquamation of the skin, deep fibrosis, and superficial gangrene is seen. The nerves may be embedded in contracting fibrous tissue, and fibrosis of the media of arterioles and venules is present. Hyperhydration of the plantar stratum corneum is the only finding reported in warm water immersion foot. The pathologic features of tropical immersion foot are a lymphocytic infiltration, diapedesis of red blood cells, and swelling and proliferation of the endothelial lining of capillaries in the upper dermis.

INCIDENCE. Immersion foot is common in most wars. Non-Caucasians are thought to be more susceptible to the cold water type, perhaps on the basis of acclimatization.

CLINICAL MANIFESTATIONS. At the time of rescue from sea, or when first seen in trench warfare, cold water immersion foot often presents as pulseless, cold, red feet with a sock distribution of hypesthesia or anesthesia. The condition may develop insidiously with only numbness, paresthesias, and slight swelling as long as the tissues are supported by boots or shoes. As soon as the support is removed, edema, tingling, itching, and severe pain occur. The skin later becomes mottled yellow, blue or black. This is called the prehyperemic stage and lasts a few hours to a few days. A hyperemic stage follows, characterized by red, hot, dry feet, burning paresthesias, and intense pains, shooting or stabbing in nature. Pulses are now bounding. Edema increases with formation of blisters, which may weep serous fluid and then slowly heal. In severe cases, muscle weakness and wasting, ulcerations, and gangrenous patches develop. Gangrene is often superficial, and the necrotic skin sometimes sheds in large pieces, leaving healthy skin beneath. Even in the absence of gangrene, extensive exfoliation is common. This stage lasts one to ten weeks, depending on the grade of initial injury.

The recovery stage (posthyperemic) blends indistinguishably with the hyperemic stage; there is a return of vascular tone with restoration of normal skin color and temperature. Recovery may be complete in mild cases within two to five weeks, but severe cases often require three to twelve months. A few patients show late sequelae such as sensitivity to cold with Raynaud's phenomenon; general or marginal hyperhidrosis; paresthesias that are increased by warmth, dependency, or exertion; rigid toes caused by fibrosis of muscles; contracted joints in the feet and toes; or painful, indolent ulcers of the digits or their stumps.

Warm water immersion foot presents with painful and extremely tender feet, especially over pressure areas. Wrinkled, white, convoluted plantar surfaces and even maceration are seen on examination in the mild syndrome. In the more severe cases, called tropical immersion foot, pronounced erythema and edema of the ankles and dorsal aspects of the feet (boot area), fever, and femoral lymphadenopathy may occur. During healing, these patients develop diffuse ecchymoses, vesicles, and a maculopapular rash. Symptoms and signs subside within a week, usually leaving no residua.

PROPHYLAXIS. Drying of the feet overnight is the best method to prevent immersion foot. Avoidance of constricting clothing, prolonged dependency, or immobility; frequent rest periods; and several changes of clothes and boots will also help. If these conditions are impractical, application of silicone grease once a day may reduce the incidence of the affliction.

TREATMENT. In the prehyperemic stage of cold water immersion foot, bed rest and body warming are important. It is probably best to keep the extremities at heart level until pulses are present. Treatment of the hyperemic stage consists of complete bed rest, cooling of the hyperemic tissues to control pain and edema, keeping the body warm, elevation of the extremities above heart level, and correction of dietary deficiencies. If cleansing is necessary, light washing with dilute hexachlorophene solution may be used. Infected tissue and epidermophytosis should be treated with appropriate agents. For cooling, it may be sufficient to expose the extremities to room air, but sometimes electric fans with water sprays or ice bags are needed. With cooling, pain is usually relieved in a few hours, but in some instances it is necessary to discover an optimal temperature, because too low a temperature may again produce pain. Analgesics must be used. Tobacco smoking is prohibited. The patient is ready to walk when edema does not occur on dependency.

Sympathectomy has been helpful in the hyperemic stage but appears to improve late sequelae such as chronic painful ulcers, persistent vasospasm, and hyperhidrosis.

The treatment of warm water and tropical immersion foot involves bed rest with extremity elevation until edema and pain entirely disappear. Other measures are usually unnecessary; the symptoms and signs disappear in one to seven days.

Akers, W. A.: Paddy foot: A warm water immersion foot syndrome variant. Parts I and II. Milit. Med., 139:605, 1974.

Allen, A. M., and Taplin, D.: Tropical immersion foot. Lancet, 2:1185, 1973.

Lange, K., Weiner, D., and Boyd, L. J.: The functional pathology of experimental immersion foot. Am. Heart J., 35:238, 1948.

Montgomery, H.: Experimental immersion foot; review of physiopathology. Physiol. Rev., 34:127, 1954.

White, J. C.: Vascular and neurologic lesions in survivors of shipwreck. I. Immersion foot syndrome following exposure to cold. II. Painful swollen feet secondary to prolonged dehydration and malnutrition. N. Engl. J. Med., 228:211, 1943.

CHILBLAIN AND PERNIO

Chilblain and pernio (*erythrocyanosis*) occur commonly in patients, especially females, with a history of cool limbs in summer as well as winter. The etiologic and pathogenic factors are unknown, but the disease is seen only in cold, damp climates. However, it is much more frequent in England than in areas of the United States with comparable climates.

Acute chilblain occurs on the dorsum of the digits, hands, or feet as localized, warm, red, intensely pruritic swelling that may disappear spontaneously in a few days. Pernio is probably the same disease but involves the lower parts of the legs, especially in women who, because of their mode of dress, do not adequately protect their legs from cold weather. Rarely, indolent lesions, dull red or violaceous, proceed to painful bleb formation. The blebs contain blood-stained serous fluid and often lead to ulcer formation.

In some patients exposed repeatedly to cold, recurrent and chronic lesions, often appearing in crops, may develop. The lesions are erythematous and ulcerative and may leave residual scarring, fibrosis, and atrophy of the skin and subcutaneous tissues. The disease is more active during the cooler months and subsides in warm weather. Bilateral and symmetrical parts of the extremities are involved. This state is called chronic chilblain or pernio (erythrocyanosis frigida crurum).

Treatment is nonspecific. Corticosteroid creams may be used for itching and inflammation, antimicrobials for sepsis. Reserpine (0.25 mg orally daily)* has been reported to ameliorate the disease.

Eskell, J.: Reserpine in the treatment of chilblains. Practitioner, 189:792, 1962.

Lewis, T.: Observations on some normal and injurious effects of cold upon the skin and underlying tissues. II. Chilblains and allied conditions. Br. Med. J., 2:837, 1941.

McGovern, T., Wright, I. S., and Kruger, E.: Pernio: A vascular disease. Am. Heart J., 22:583, 1941.

Thomas, E. W. P.: Chapping and chilblains. Practitioner, 193:755, 1964.

FROSTBITE

DEFINITION. Frostbite is due to freezing of tissues which may result in damage to skin, muscle, blood vessels, and nerves.

ETIOLOGY. Superficial freezing of tissues evidently begins when the temperature of deeper tissues reaches about 10° C. During the Korean War, most cases of frostbite occurred at −6.5° C or below, after 7 to 18 hours' exposure. High winds, dampness, and general chilling of the body make frostbite more likely at above-freezing temperatures. Predisposing factors include any type of peripheral vascular insufficiency, improper clothing, exhaustion, and previous cold injury. Lack of acclimatization and geographic origin have also been implicated; the black race is more susceptible to frostbite. Most frostbite is of the slow freezing type, but a rapid frostbite (occurring in a few minutes) takes place at high altitudes with extremely low temperatures and has a predilection for the extremities rather than the face and ears.

PATHOPHYSIOLOGY. Whether actual tissue freezing or decreased blood flow from vasoconstriction is most important in producing cell injury is unknown. Damage is probably due to a combination of direct freezing with the formation of extracellular ice crystals, inducing dehydration of cells, and intense vasoconstriction. The vasoconstriction is due to direct cold exposure of the tissues but may also involve reflex vasoconstriction from chilling of other body areas. The reduced blood flow leads to capillary stasis and arteriolar and capillary thromboses. Capillary permeability is increased and results in edema formation.

PATHOLOGY. The pathologic findings vary with the stage of the disease and the depth of tissue affected. In early stages, low-grade vasculitis and inflammation are seen in all tissues. Later the skin is atrophied and may be keratinized, muscle is necrosed and shows waxy degeneration, arterioles and capillaries are thrombosed, and nerves demonstrate fibroblastic proliferation and neurolysis.

CLINICAL MANIFESTATIONS. The first indication of frostbite is often a sharp, pricking sensation that draws attention to a yellowish-white, numb area of hardened skin. However, cold itself produces numbness and anesthesia that may allow freezing of tissue without warning. When the freezing is superficial, thawing leads to local reddening and wheal and flare formation. When freezing involves deep tissues, subcutaneous edema occurs with thawing, followed by formation of vesicles and bullae. A hyperemic, reddish zone may be apparent between frozen and normal tissue. As the edema subsides in a day or two, necrosis and gangrene may become evident. However, it may take two to three months before final demarcation between viable and dead tissue can be ascertained. In the healing phase, a black eschar usually covers the area.

The traditional classification of frostbite has been from first to fourth degree, depending of the depth of tissue injury. Since the true extent of tissue damage cannot be judged on initial examination, a simpler classification of superficial and deep frostbite is more practical. The prognosis depends on the depth of freezing, as superficial cases usually have no sequelae, whereas deep freezing may end in amputation.

PROPHYLAXIS. Frostbite is preventable and occurs rarely among those who have been instructed how to protect themselves. Prophylactic measures include observance of each other for signs of frostbite; wearing adequate, loose fitting, dry clothing and mittens; exposure for only brief periods when exercise is not possible; and avoidance of smoking before and during exposure. Feet and socks should be kept dry.

TREATMENT. Superficial frostbite can be treated immediately by rewarming; affected areas on the face and ears can be warmed with the hands, hands can be placed in the axillae, or frostbitten parts can be warmed on the torso of a partner. Frostbitten areas should not be rubbed with snow or exercised.

Treatment of deep frostbite should be delayed until adequate facilities for rewarming are available. Therapy should always be very conservative, because the depth of tissue damage is difficult to ascertain, sometimes for months. It is best to rewarm the tissue as rapidly as possible in 40 to 44° C water. Massage, exposure to too high temperatures, and reactive hyperemia should be avoided because they tend to increase pain and edema. Analgesics usually are needed during rewarming. After rewarming, which usually requires about 20 minutes, the frostbitten area is exposed to room air (21 to 26° C). Although pressure dressings may be used, the open method with sterile surroundings is usually preferred. Vesicles, bullae, and eschars are left untouched. Antimicrobial drugs are indicated if infection is present. Tobacco smoking should be prohibited. Regional sympathectomy has been reported as beneficial, both clinically and experimentally, if performed at an optimal time of 24 to 48 hours after frostbite occurs. Sympathectomy may conserve tissue and lead to earlier demarcation, cessation of pain, and healing of tissue.

Eventual recovery is usually surprisingly good, the black eschar peeling off to leave normal tissue beneath.

*See p. vi, Dosage Notice, immediately following Preface.

Sensitivity to cold, paresthesias, and a predilection to repeated frostbite often persist. In severe frostbite, fibrosis of tissue may lead to disability, and gangrenous extremities may require amputation.

Golding, M. R., Martinez, A., DeJong, P., Mendosa, M., Fries, C. C., Sawyer, P. N., Hennigar, G. R., and Wesolowski, S. A.: The role of sympathectomy in frostbite, with review of 68 cases. Surgery, 57:774, 1965.

Lapp, N. L., and Juergens, J. L.: Frostbite. Mayo Clin. Proc., 40:932, 1965.

Meryman, H. T.: Tissue freezing and local cold injury. Physiol. Rev., 37:233, 1957.

Washburn, B.: Frostbite. What it is, how to prevent it, emergency treatment. N. Engl. J. Med., 266:974, 1962.

368.4. PERIPHERAL VASCULAR DISEASES DUE TO ABNORMAL COMMUNICATIONS BETWEEN ARTERIES AND VEINS

ARTERIOVENOUS FISTULA

DEFINITION. Arteriovenous fistulas are abnormal communications, single or multiple, between arteries and veins by which arterial blood enters the veins directly without transversing a capillary network.

ETIOLOGY. Arteriovenous fistulas created to facilitate renal dialysis are the most common fistulas. Acquired arteriovenous fistulas, usually single and saccular, may develop after a bullet or stab wound involving an artery and a contiguous vein, after vessel puncture (especially the vertebral artery), or after biopsy (especially the kidney). Fistulas of the iliac vessel may occur after surgery for intervertebral disc disease. Congenital fistulas are present from birth and are usually multiple; they result from defects in differentiation of the common embryologic anlage into artery and vein. There is no special sex incidence, and any part of the body may be involved. There is an association between large vessel congenital fistulas of the extremities and small cutaneous fistulas resembling angiomatoses.

PATHOPHYSIOLOGY. Arterial blood, following the path of least resistance, flows directly into the vein, bypassing the corresponding capillary bed. The arterial pressure is transmitted to the venous side of the fistula; the distal vein pressure is increased, but the proximal vein pressure may actually be negative during systole owing to the high velocity of blood flow. The elevated venous pressure leads to the development of varicose veins and venous stasis changes in the limb. Increased blood flow makes the tissues near the fistula abnormally warm, and diminished flow distal to the fistula may produce peripheral coldness and trophic changes. Large fistulas impose a burden on the heart; the cardiac output must be increased above normal by an amount proportional to the size of the fistula in order to maintain the general circulation. Total blood volume may be increased. The low peripheral resistance of the involved area tends to decrease diastolic and increase systolic and pulse pressures systemically. Large fistulas may lead to cardiac decompensation. Even the small fistulas created for renal dialysis induce a small increase in cardiac output and heart rate and occasionally have led to

heart failure. These fistulas have also led to ischemia or venous stasis and varicosities in the hand.

PATHOLOGY. In the region of the fistula, the intima and media of the involved veins become thickened, and newly developed elastic fibers appear. The arteries show a thinning of their walls with loss of elastic tissue and muscular fibers in the media.

CLINICAL MANIFESTATIONS. Patients complain of aching pain, edema, varicosities, or hypertrophied extremities. Occasionally, cardiac symptoms such as palpitation, substernal pain, and dyspnea on exertion are present. Examination reveals tortuous, dilated superficial veins in the extremity, and venous pulsation can be felt unless the fistula is small and deeply placed. In congenital fistulas, the skin temperature is usually elevated locally but decreased distal to the fistulas, although in acquired lesions, the temperature of the digits may be greater than in the opposite normal limb. A bruit and thrill are common over acquired fistulas; the bruit lasts throughout systole and diastole and has a coarse, machinery-like quality. The tissues near the fistula may be tender, edematous, and either red or slightly cyanotic. The circumference of the extremity is increased by edema or true hypertrophy, but bony structures are hypertrophied only if the fistula was present before epiphyseal closure. Stasis pigmentation and chronic indurative cellulitis with or without indolent ulceration may be present distal to the fistula. In contrast to the postphlebitic limb in which ulcers form around the medial malleolus, the ulceration of fistulas may affect the distal parts of the foot. Rarefaction of bone in the extremity may also occur. Temporary compression of the artery supplying a large fistula diminishes the heart rate (*Branham's sign*) and may be a helpful diagnostic sign.

DIAGNOSIS. If the diagnosis cannot be made from the clinical manifestations, other examinations may be helpful. The oxygen saturation of blood removed from proximal veins of an extremity with a fistula will be found to be greater than that of blood removed from corresponding veins in the opposite extremity. Arteriography will reveal the lesion, its location, and the number and size of communications. Edema of one or both extremities after surgery for intervertebral disc disease should suggest the possibility of a fistula. Thrombophlebitis and the postphlebitic extremity can be distinguished from fistulas by the oxygen studies and arteriography.

PROGNOSIS. The prognosis of acquired and single congenital fistulas is good after surgical repair. In acquired iliac vessel fistulas, congestive heart failure develops in two thirds of patients, and immediate repair is important. Without surgical repair, which is often not possible in multiple fistulas, the outlook is for a chronically swollen limb with varicosities, stasis pigmentation, and ulceration. Bacterial infection of acquired fistulas occurs but is rare.

TREATMENT. Single fistulas can be repaired surgically by re-establishing the continuity of the involved artery and vein walls by a variety of procedures (arteriorrhaphy, end-to-end suture, grafting). Ligation of the involved artery and vein leads to a high incidence of arterial and venous insufficiency of the extremity and should be avoided if possible. If the arterial supply depends upon a large anomalous artery, ligation of this vessel, followed by sclerosing injections of the dilated veins, may be effective. Multiple fistulas are much less amenable to surgery. Ulcers, edema, and pain may be relieved by wearing elastic bandages or stockings; pressure on the veins encourages blood flow to follow the arterial pathway. Amputation is required for large inoperable fistulas producing cardiac decompensation or gross deformity.

Binak, K., Regan, T. J., Christensen, R. C., and Hellems, H. K.: Arteriovenous fistula: Hemodynamic effects of occlusion and exercise. Am. Heart J., 60:495, 1960.

Johnson, G., Jr., and Blythe, W. B.: Hemodynamic effects of arteriovenous shunts used for hemodialysis. Ann. Surg., 17:715, 1970.

Lawton, R. L., Tidrick, R. T., and Brintnall, E. S.: A clinicopathologic study of multiple congenital arteriovenous fistulae of the lower extremities. Angiology, 8:161, 1957.

Nickerson, J. L., Elkin, D. C., and Warren J. V.: The effect of temporary occlusion of arteriovenous fistulas on heart rate, stroke volume, and cardiac output. J. Clin. Invest., 30:215, 1951.

Rossi, P., Carillo, F. J., Alfidi, R. J., and Ruzicka, F. F.: Iatrogenic arteriovenous fistulas. Radiology, 111:47, 1974.

Rusin, L. J., and Harrell, E. R.: Arteriovenous fistula: Cutaneous manifestations. Arch. Dermatol., 112:1135, 1976.

Wakim, K. G., and Janes, J. M.: Influence of arteriovenous fistula on the distal circulation in the involved extremity. Arch. Phys. Med. Rehabil., 39:431, 1958.

GLOMANGIOMA OR GLOMUS TUMOR

DEFINITION. Glomangioma or glomus tumor designates painful enlargement of a glomus body.

PATHOLOGY. The pathology consists of hypertrophy of the glomus body which contains an arteriovenous anastomosis with its associated smooth muscle coat, nonmyelinated nerve fibers, and connective tissue. Histologically, the lesion is encapsulated, occasionally diffuse but never invasive, and contains numerous epithelioid cells with no inflammatory cells.

CLINICAL MANIFESTATIONS. Glomus tumors are extremely tender but inconspicuous subcutaneous nodules which develop slowly during adult life. Pain may be present before the nodule becomes visible. They are found in various parts of the upper and lower extremities, but most frequently (30 per cent) beneath the fingernail. The diameter of the tumor is usually only a few millimeters. The nodule has a flat or slightly raised surface with reddish-blue to purplish discoloration. Excruciating burning or shooting pain, both local and referred up the extremity, occurs spontaneously or is produced by the slightest pressure. Hyperhidrosis, abnormal vasomotor activity, increased skin temperature, and tissue atrophy in the involved limb may be present. Heat, cold, and even contact with clothing may become intolerable so that protection is required continuously day and night. In glomus tumors beneath nails, a small excavation of the phalanx from erosion by the tumor can often be seen by roentgenography.

TREATMENT. Surgical excision leads to complete and immediate relief without recurrence.

Bailey, O. T.: The cutaneous glomus and its tumors — glomangiomas. Am. J. Path., 11:915, 1935.

Cooke, S. A. R.: Misleading features in the clinical diagnosis of the peripheral glomus tumor. Br. J. Surg., 58:602, 1971.

Horton, C., Maguire, C., Georgiade, N., and Pickrell, K.: Glomus tumors: An analysis of 25 cases. Arch. Surg., 71:712, 1955.

368.5. DISEASES OF THE PERIPHERAL VEINS

THROMBOPHLEBITIS

This subject is discussed in Ch. 357.2.

VARICOSE VEINS AND THE POSTPHLEBITIC SYNDROME

DEFINITION. Varicose veins are distended, tortuous veins with imcompetent valves. The postphlebitic syndrome denotes the chronically swollen extremity with trophic changes secondary to chronic venous stasis; despite the name, a previous history of thrombophlebitis is often not obtainable.

ETIOLOGY. Varicose veins are considered to be caused either by congenitally defective valves or by a condition that deforms valves or obstructs venous outflow over long periods of time. Varicosities resulting from congenital defects may develop early in life. Thrombophlebitis may lead to the formation of varicosities by deformation or destruction of venous valves and venous obstruction. Pregnancy, ascites, abdominal tumor, excessive weight or height, and prolonged weight bearing are all considered accelerating factors which cause increased venous pressures in the legs, distention of veins, and finally incompetency of valves. A generalized abnormality of the veins has been suggested as a predisposing factor. An increased forearm vein distensibility and a decreased amount of collagen and hexosamine in uninvolved veins have been demonstrated in patients with lower extremity varicosities; however, genetic evidence is not substantial. Since the majority of patients do not have obvious causes and varicose veins are an affliction of Western civilization, other factors in our society have been sought. The constipation associated with the Western countries' low-residue diet has been proposed as a frequent etiologic factor in varicosities. Emphasis is placed on the association of varicosities with hemorrhoids and diverticulosis, as a result of either increased intra-abdominal pressure during bowel movements or local pressure exerted by the bowel on intra-abdominal structures.

INCIDENCE. Varicose veins are very common, appearing in approximately 40 per cent of women; the incidence is less in men. The saphenous veins in the lower extremities are most frequently affected.

CLINICAL MANIFESTATIONS. The dilated, tortuous, sacculated varices are easily visible. Some patients with extensive superficial varicosities have no other symptoms or signs, but others have aching pain or easy fatigability of the calf muscles and edema after weight bearing. The edema usually disappears with bed rest overnight. Rarely the varicosities are so large that postural hypotension may result from pooling of blood in the lower extremities. When the communicating or deep veins are incompetent, symptoms and signs are more common. Chronic venous insufficiency is manifested by edema, which may later become fibrosed to produce a brawny induration. Extravasation of blood locally may cause a brownish pigmentation; an itchy, eczematoid rash may appear in the area. Finally the skin may ulcerate, producing an indolent, nonpainful lesion, usually above the medial malleolus near a palpable, incompetent communicating vein. This picture of chronic swelling and stasis dermatitis is called the postphlebitic syndrome. Arterial pulses are normal. When the deep venous system is blocked, pain similar to intermittent claudication may rarely occur.

DIAGNOSIS. The diagnosis can be made from the clinical picture. Retrograde flow of blood past incompetent valves can be demonstrated by the Trendelenburg test and its variations. The leg of the recumbent patient is elevated to empty the veins, and then a tourniquet is applied to occlude the superficial veins. The patient quickly assumes a standing position, the tourniquet is released, and the veins will become distended immediately if back flow is present. If two tourniquets are applied and left in place when the patient stands, filling of the saphenous veins between the tourniquets indicates an incompetent communicating vein. Application of the tourniquets to different levels on the limb can delineate exactly the sites of vein pathology. Venography may be used in doubtful cases or to be certain the deep venous system is patent. In a patient with varicosities and edema, other causes of edema, e.g., cardiovascular and renal disease, should be investigated.

PROGNOSIS. The prognosis for simple superficial varicose veins is good with treatment. Once the postphlebitic syndrome has developed, progressive disability usually can be expected despite treatment.

TREATMENT. Uncomplicated varicose veins respond well to support with elastic stockings or bandages to prevent progression. Panty girdles should never be worn. Frequent periods of elevation of the extremity above heart level, high ligation with stripping of the saphenous veins, and injection of sclerosing solutions may become necessary to prevent or treat the postphlebitic syndrome. However, since saphenous veins may be needed for arterial (coronary or peripheral) surgery, stripping should be performed only when absolutely unavoidable. Venous stasis ulcers are treated with sponge rubber pressure dressings or gelatin boots; local or systemic antimicrobials are indicated if infection is present. Sometimes the entire fibrosed area must be removed and a skin graft applied to heal an indolent ulcer.

Alexander, C. J.: The theoretical basis of varicose vein formation. Med. J. Aust., 1:258, 1972.

Burkitt, D. P.: Hemorrhoids, varicose veins and deep vein thrombosis: Epidemiologic features and suggested causative factors. Can. J. Surg., 18:483, 1975.

Fegan, W. G.: Conservative treatment of varicose veins. Prog. Surg., 11:37, 1973.

Hobbs, J. T.: The Treatment of Venous Disorders: A Comprehensive Review of Current Practice in the Management of Varicose Veins and the Post-thrombotic Syndrome. Philadelphia, J. B. Lippincott Company, 1977.

Mullarky, R. E.: The Anatomy of Varicose Veins. Springfield, Ill., Charles C Thomas, 1975.

Thurston, O. G., and Williams, H. T. G.: Chronic venous insufficiency of the lower extremity, Arch. Surg., 106:537, 1973.

Wood, J. E.: The Veins. Boston, Little, Brown & Company, 1965.

368.6. DISEASES OF THE PERIPHERAL LYMPHATIC VESSELS

Lymph is formed by the transudation of plasma through capillary walls into tissue spaces. The plasma that is not reabsorbed into the venular end of the capillaries is collected by a rich intercellular network of tiny lymphatic ves-

sels. These vessels possess semilunar valves and become larger as they convey lymph to the regional lymph nodes; then the lymph travels through trunk lymphatics to the thoracic duct and finally to the left internal jugular vein. In the extremities, there are superficial and deep lymphatic systems which probably are joined by communicating vessels. The flow of lymph depends on intrinsic, rhythmic contractions of the lymph vessels, muscular contraction, respiratory movements, and, to a certain extent, gravity. The lymphatic vessels are responsive to sympathetic nerve stimulation, but the functional significance of this is not known.

LYMPHEDEMA

DEFINITION. Lymphedema is a form of chronic unilateral or bilateral edema of the extremities caused by the accumulation of lymph secondary to abnormalities or blockage of the lymph vessels or pathologic conditions of the lymph nodes.

ETIOLOGY. Primary lymphedema may be a hereditary disease or may occur sporadically. Various classifications exist according to whether the lymphedema is present at birth (*congenital*), appears at or near puberty (*praecox*), occurs after age 35 (*tarda*), or is familial and congenital (*Milroy's disease*). The mode of inheritance is probably dominant but has not been thoroughly investigated. An increased incidence occurs in ovarian dysgenesis syndromes. Primary lymphedema affects females predominantly (about 8:1); the onset of the disease occurs before age 40 in more than 90 per cent of cases.

Secondary lymphedema is most commonly caused by inflammation and follows recurrent lymphangitis (see below). In tropical and subtropical regions, filariasis often leads to lymphedema. Neoplasms are the second most common cause either by invasion or compression of lymph vessels or nodes. Surgical removal of lymph nodes and the fibrosis that follows irradiation may also cause lymphedema. Secondary cases have no special sex incidence and are uncommon before age 40.

PATHOLOGY. Examination of primary lymphedematous limbs by lymphangiography has revealed aplasia, hypoplasia, or hyperplasia (varicosities) of the lymphatic vessels. The lymph nodes may also be aplastic or hypoplastic, producing an obstructive type of lymphedema. No specific pathologic picture has been correlated with the current classification system but the few cases of Milroy's disease examined have revealed aplasia (or absence) of the lymphatic vessels. There is some indication that lymphedema may be part of a generalized defect in lymphatic vessels. Patients with lymphedema have been reported to have chylous pleural effusions, chylous ascites, and even intestinal lymphangiectasis. A syndrome of yellow nails, recurrent pleural effusion, and lymphedema occurs and is believed to be secondary to lymphatic abnormalities in each area. Another familial syndrome of recurrent intrahepatic cholestasis and lymphedema exists, the cholestasis probably being caused by defective hepatic lymphatic vessels. In secondary lymphedema, innumerable small, irregular lymphatics are usually seen beside normal or tortuous, sometimes varicose, vessels.

CLINICAL MANIFESTATIONS. Primary lymphedema is usually gradual in onset and asymptomatic; the distal portion of the extremity or whole extremity, or even a portion of the trunk, may increase in size. The edema is soft and pitting at first and disappears with treatment but later becomes firm and nonpitting, and cannot be relieved completely by treatment. At this stage, the skin becomes thickened and resists wrinkling; hair follicles are prominent. The lower extremities are involved most often; about half the patients develop bilateral swelling. The edematous tissue is especially susceptible to episodes of lymphangitis and cellulitis, which add to the deformity.

Secondary lymphedema is seldom bilateral. Lymphedema of the inflammatory type follows recurrent episodes of lymphangitis. Each attack leaves more residual edema after the inflammation subsides. The skin finally becomes thick, coarse, folded, and hard so that the eventual deformity may be extreme (elephantiasis). Secondary lymphedema resuting from neoplasm and other noninflammatory causes produces painless swelling of an extremity. Painless swelling of an extremity in an elderly male must be considered secondary to carcinoma of the prostate until proved otherwise.

DIAGNOSIS. Painless chronic swelling of an extremity suggests the diagnosis of lymphedema. Differentiation from venous insufficiency may be made by the lack of prominent veins, stasis dermatitis, and ulceration; lymphangiography and venography may be necessary. Mixed lymphangiomatous and hemangiomatous malformations that cause enlarged limbs can be diagnosed by the obvious tumor mass. In lipodystrophy, lymphangiography is necessary to delineate the normal lymphatics displaced by the lipomatous masses.

PROGNOSIS. Primary lymphedema usually progresses inexorably to a chronically swollen limb or limbs despite treatment. However, the lymphedema associated with gonadal dysgenesis may disappear spontaneously in months to years. Secondary lymphedema caused by infection may be controlled with adequate treatment. The prognosis is that of the underlying disease in other causes.

TREATMENT. In primary lymphedema, the most important aim of therapy is to keep the involved extremities free of edema in order to prevent fibrosis and recurrent infection. Frequent elevation of the extremity (including sleeping with the extremity above the heart level), elastic support applying graded pressure from the foot or hand proximally, external pneumatic compression, low sodium diet, and diuretics are usually necessary. Recently, a group of drugs containing benzopyrones has been reported in uncontrolled studies to be useful in treating lymphedema; their main action may be to increase the lysis of accumulated proteins in the lymphedematous tissue. Local infection and obvious lesions, such as epidermophytosis, should be eradicated. Surgical attack in advanced cases with fibrosis and resistant edema (Kondoleon operation and its modifications) has produced some relief but is usually disappointing.

Dilley, J. J., Kierland, R. R., Randall, R. V., and Shick, R. M.: Primary lymphedema associated with yellow nails and pleural effusions, JAMA, 204:670, 1968.

Gough, M. H.: Primary lymphedema: Clinical and lymphangiographic studies. Br. J. Surg., 53:918, 1966.

Hall, J. G.: The flow of lymph. N. Engl. J. Med., 281:720, 1969.

Kinmonth, J. B.: The Lymphatics: Diseases, Lymphography and Surgery. Baltimore, Williams & Wilkins Company, 1972.

Piller, N. B., and Cloduis, L.: The use of a tissue tonometer as a diagnostic aid in extremity lymphedema; a determination of its conservative treatment with benzopyrones. Lymphology, 9:127, 1976.

Sigstad, H., Aagenaes, Ø., Bjorn-Hansen, R. W., and Rootwelt, K.: Primary lymphoedema combined with hereditary recurrent intrahepatic cholestasis. Acta Med. Scand., 188:213, 1970.

Smith, R. D., Spittell, J. A., Jr., and Schirger, A.: Secondary lymphedema of the leg: Its characteristics and diagnostic implications. JAMA, 185:80, 1963.

LYMPHANGITIS

DEFINITION. Lymphangitis is an acute or chronic inflammation, usually pyogenic, of the lymphatic vessels.

ETIOLOGY. In the majority of cases of lymphangitis the hemolytic *Streptococcus* is the infecting agent; second most common is the coagulase-positive *Staphylococcus*. The bacteria enter the skin via areas of local trauma, trichophytosis, or arterial ischemic or venous stasis ulcers, although a portal of entry cannot always be discovered. Infection then spreads by the lymphatic vessels to the local lymph nodes; an accompanying diffuse cellulitis of the extremity is often present. An immune response to previously present bacteria or their products has been postulated as a cause of lymphangitis when an organism cannot be isolated, but proof of this is lacking.

PATHOLOGY. Acute, subacute, or chronic inflammation is found in the subcutaneous tissues and regional lymph nodes.

CLINICAL MANIFESTATIONS. Attacks of lymphangitis may be ushered in by malaise, headache, nausea, vomiting, and shaking chills followed by fever. Systemic symptoms, however, may not be present. Red streaks appear in the affected extremity, originating at the portal of entry and following the pathway of lymphatic vessels. Regional lymph nodes are usually enlarged and tender. There may be a surrounding area of cellulitis with tenderness and red discoloration in the lower part of the extremity, which is usually swollen with a soft, pitting edema.

DIAGNOSIS. The clinical picture is usually typical and allows the diagnosis to be made easily. A leukocytosis is often present. The inciting organism should be sought by culturing the portal of entry if obvious or by needle puncture of the subcutaneous tissues. A difficult diagnosis to rule out is acute thrombophlebitis, especially when a diffuse cellulitis is present, for symptoms and signs are similar; it is often wise to administer therapy for both diseases simultaneously.

PROGNOSIS. For an initial attack in a limb without underlying disease, the prognosis with treatment is excellent. However, some patients have recurrent attacks, often mild, which can lead to the development of lymphedema. In recurrent cases, the limb may remain somewhat larger after each attack.

TREATMENT. Systemic antimicrobial drugs should be administered as indicated by culture (and sensitivity studies if necessary). If no organism is cultured, penicillin should be given because the *Streptococcus* is so commonly the etiologic agent. Drainage of any focus of origin is also extremely important. Adjunctive measures include rest, elevation of the extremity above heart level, and warm wet dressings. Possible fungal infections in the feet and causes of secondary lymphedema should be sought. When attacks subside, elastic support should be worn on the extremity for three months to prevent residual swelling. In recurrent cases, either with or without underlying lymphedema, prophylactic long-term antimicrobial therapy should be instituted. Lymphangitis is especially dangerous in the ischemic tissues of patients with obstructive arterial disease; only under these unfavorable conditions is prompt amputation sometimes required.

Babb, R. R., Spittell, J. A., Jr., Martin, W. J., and Schirger, A.: Prophylaxis of recurrent lymphangitis complicating lymphedema. JAMA, 195:871, 1966.

Edwards, E. A.: Recurrent febrile episodes and lymphedema. JAMA, 184:858, 1963.

PART XV
RENAL DISEASES

369. INTRODUCTION

369.1. STRUCTURE AND FUNCTION OF THE KIDNEYS

Barry M. Brenner

Maintenance of the volume, composition, and distribution of the body fluids is a function essential to the well-being, indeed the survival, of all animals. In man and other mammals, this homeostatic function is subserved largely by the kidneys. Although the kidneys operate primarily to maintain relative constancy of the *extracellular* environment, the continuous flux of water and solutes that takes place across all cell membranes during life also ensures that the kidneys regulate, albeit indirectly, the volume and tonicity of the *intracellular* compartment.

In adapting to this crucial task of maintaining a near-constant internal environment, the mammalian kidney has evolved a series of physiologic mechanisms which enable the organism to excrete the *surpluses* of water and nonmetabolized solute in the diet, as well as the nonvolatile nitrogenous end products of metabolism (e.g., urea, creatinine). Alternatively, when the organism is threatened with *deficits* of water or any of the major constituents of the body fluids, the kidney can lessen the excretion of these key substances, thereby minimizing the likelihood of profound dehydration or depletion of major solutes.

The purpose of this initial chapter is to review the basic structural and functional characteristics of the mammalian kidney, for only by understanding the elements of normal renal anatomy and physiology is it possible to adopt a rational and scientific approach to the broad clinical spectrum of renal disease discussed in the chapters that follow.

RENAL BLOOD FLOW

Under resting conditions in man, approximately 20 per cent of the cardiac output passes through the kidneys, paired organs comprising only about 0.5 per cent of the human body weight. The rate of blood flow, averaging some 400 ml per 100 grams of tissue per minute, is much greater than that observed in other vascular beds ordinarily considered well perfused, such as heart, liver, and brain. From this enormous blood flow, amounting to about 1 liter per minute, only a small quantity of urine is formed, about 1 ml in the same time period. The metabolic energy required for production of urine is great, amounting to some 10 per cent of basal oxygen consumption.

Blood enters each kidney through the *renal artery*, which divides to form the *interlobar* and then *arcuate* arteries. *Interlobular* arteries, derived from the latter, ex-

tend toward the cortex and give rise to *afferent arterioles*, each of which branches to form the *glomerular capillaries*. The latter fuse to form the *efferent arteriole*, usually of narrower diameter than the afferent arteriole. In the outer and mid-cortex, efferent arterioles divide soon after their origins into highly anastomotic *peritubular capillary plexuses*, which terminate in *venules* and, ultimately, veins that follow the course of the aforementioned arteries. In the juxtamedullary region of the inner cortex, however, the peritubular capillary plexuses differ from those elsewhere in the cortex, in that they give rise to long-looped vessels (*vasa recta*) which extend deep into the medulla. In man, the renal tubules associated with glomeruli located in outer and mid-cortex tend to have relatively short *loops of Henle*, so that all elements of the nephron derived from these glomeruli are confined to the cortex. By contrast, the tubules linked to juxtamedullary glomeruli have much longer loops, extending into the inner medulla in close apposition to the vasa recta.

Renal blood flow remains remarkably stable under normal physiologic conditions. This near-constancy of renal perfusion persists even when the perfusion pressure to the kidneys is varied over a wide range (e.g., 80 to 200 mm Hg). This property of the renal vasculature, termed *autoregulation*, derives from the ability of afferent and efferent arterioles (the major resistances to renal blood flow) to increase or decrease their vascular tone in response to directionally similar variations in perfusion pressure, thereby minimizing changes in total renal blood flow. Autoregulation is largely a property of the renal cortical circulation, a matter of some importance in view of the fact that 90 per cent or more of the total renal blood flow is distributed to cortical zones. The suggestion that variations in intrarenal blood flow distribution are an important mechanism in man for regulating renal excretion of sodium and water under physiologic conditions has not received general acceptance, although in all likelihood the often striking distortions of intrarenal blood flow distribution seen in certain diseases (e.g., outer cortical ischemia in cardiac or hepatic failure) may contribute to the fluid retention and edema seen in these disorders.

ELEMENTS OF GLOMERULAR AND TUBULAR FUNCTION

In man the formation of each milliliter of urine begins with the elaboration of about 125 ml of nearly protein-free plasma ultrafiltrate across the walls of glomerular capillaries. As the number of glomeruli is great, about one million in each kidney in man, the filtration rate of individual glomeruli is not large in absolute terms, only some 60 nl per minute. However, in terms of capillary wall permeability, this rate is enormous, exceeding that of other capillary networks by some two orders of magnitude, and amounting, in man, to about 175 liters per day. As mentioned above, renal blood flow rate averages about 1 liter per minute. Since erythrocyte packed cell volume is about 45 per cent, renal plasma flow rate equals roughly 550 ml per minute. The fraction of the total renal plasma flow that undergoes ultrafiltration is therefore ~125 ml per minute divided by ~550 ml per minute, or about 0.2 to 0.25. This quantity is referred to as the *filtration fraction*.

As the ultrafiltrate flows along the various segments of the renal tubules, it is modified by the removal of solutes and water by processes of *reabsorption*, as well as by addition of solutes which are *secreted* into the tubule lumen. *Proximal convoluted tubules* reabsorb about two thirds of the filtered water and sodium *isosmotically*, together with bicarbonate, glucose, and amino acids. Obviously this fluid cannot and does not remain in the cortical interstitium, but is taken up by the cortical peritubular capillaries, along with the lesser amounts of water and solute reabsorbed by other cortical nephron segments. Depending on the state of hydration of the organism, the final urine may be more or less concentrated than the plasma ultrafiltrate. In man, urine osmolality can range from less than 60 to more than 1200 mOsm per kilogram H_2O. Urinary dilution occurs in the *thick ascending limbs of Henle's loops,* segments which originate in the outer medulla, and whose epithelia are rich in aerobic transport enzyme systems. The concentrating process also resides in the medulla, and involves *loops of Henle* and *collecting ducts.* Normally, the inner medullary interstitium is very hypertonic to plasma. Hence, if the collecting ducts are water permeable (a function of the *antidiuretic hormone*), urine flowing in them toward the papillary tip will lose water and become concentrated. This reabsorbed water, together with solutes added through the concentrating mechanism, leaves the inner medulla by way of vasa recta.

The volume and composition of the final ureteral urine are thus the sum of several processes — filtration, reabsorption and secretion, dilution, and concentration. We will now analyze each of these processes in greater detail, based on an assessment of the operations of the various nephron segments.

GLOMERULAR FILTRATION

The initial event in the process of urine formation involves the separation of an essentially protein-free ultrafiltrate of plasma by the walls of the glomerular capillaries. As with capillaries elsewhere in the body, the rate of fluid filtration is determined by three factors: (1) the *balance of pressures* acting across the capillary wall — glomerular capillary *hydrostatic* and Bowman's space *oncotic* pressures tend to favor filtration, whereas glomerular capillary oncotic and Bowman's space hydrostatic pressures tend to retard filtration; (2) the *flow rate* of plasma entering the glomerulus; (3) the *permeability properties* and the *total surface area* of the filtering capillaries.

Decreases in glomerular filtration rate (GFR) will therefore occur if (1) glomerular hydrostatic pressure is reduced (i.e., as in hypotensive shock), (2) tubule and Bowman's space hydrostatic pressure are increased (ureteral obstruction), (3) plasma oncotic pressure rises to unusually high levels (hemoconcentration due to dehydration, multiple myeloma or other dysproteinemias), (4) decreased rates of renal (hence, glomerular)

blood and plasma flow (circulatory collapse, heart failure), and (5) reduced permeability and/or total filtering surface area (acute or chronic glomerulonephritis).

One of the most remarkable features of this filtration process is the extent to which the glomerular capillary wall discriminates among molecules of varying size. Molecules the size of inulin or smaller normally appear in glomerular ultrafiltrate in essentially the same concentrations as in plasma water, whereas the transport of substances of increasingly greater size diminishes progressively, normally approaching very low values as the size of serum albumin is approached. For this reason, all but the smallest plasma proteins are normally restricted from passage into Bowman's space. The *glomerular capillary basement membrane* and the *slit-like diaphragm* that connects adjacent epithelial cell foot processes on the urinary aspect of the glomerular capillary wall are believed to serve as the major barriers to protein filtration. With disruption of the integrity of these barriers, as seen in various forms of glomerular injury, plasma proteins gain access to the urine, with proteinuria often reaching massive proportions.

In addition to these mechanical barriers to protein filtration, it is now clear that *electrostatic* factors also normally operate to retard the filtration of plasma proteins, and especially albumin. The albumin molecule behaves as a polyanion in physiologic solutions, and is therefore retarded by the highly anionic glycoproteins that comprise the surface coats and substructure of the various component layers of the glomerular capillary wall. Of interest, these *fixed negative charges* on the capillary wall are known to be reduced in amount in many forms of glomerular injury, providing yet another explanation for the proteinuria seen in these conditions.

THE PROCESSING OF GLOMERULAR FILTRATE BY THE RENAL TUBULES

Large amounts of sodium salts are contained in the glomerular filtrate, as sodium is the chief osmotically active cation in the extracellular fluid. Most of the filtered fluid and sodium salts are reabsorbed by the renal tubule, leaving small and variable amounts, equivalent on a day-to-day basis to the quantities ingested, to reach the final urine.

Although many approaches have been employed to study the processing of glomerular ultrafiltrate as it flows along the tubule, our current understanding derives largely from direct measurements of transport across individual nephron segments. Since these segments are microscopic in size, microtechniques are required for their study, and of these, *micropuncture* and *microperfusion* have provided most of our current insights. Based on the results obtained with these techniques, we now recognize eight functionally distinct nephron segments, conveniently grouped as follows: proximal segments (convoluted, straight); limbs of Henle (descending and ascending thin limbs, thick ascending limb); distal convoluted tubule; and collecting segments (cortical collecting tubule, papillary collecting duct).

Sodium salts are reabsorbed throughout all segments, water from most. Just as the nephron segments are arranged in series anatomically, so too is the function of each segment dependent upon changes in the composition of tubule fluid brought about by transport processes that occurred in more proximal portions of the nephron.

PROXIMAL TUBULE. Convoluted and straight portions of this tubule segment reabsorb some two thirds of the glomerular filtrate, without changing the osmolality or sodium concentration of the unreabsorbed fraction. In other words, fluid reabsorption is *isosmotic*, and is coupled to the *active* transport of sodium. Most of the renal metabolic work and the high rate of oxygen consumption are linked to this active sodium transport.

In the early convoluted portion of the proximal tubule, bicarbonate is the principal anion accompanying the reabsorption of sodium. In consequence, the bicarbonate concentration in the tubule lumen falls, whereas that of chloride rises. These changes in luminal anion concentration are associated with concurrent changes in the polarity of the *transepithelial electrical potential difference*, which reverses from slightly negative (tubule lumen, relative to peritubular fluid) in the earliest proximal tubule segment to slightly positive in later segments. The reason for the reversal of voltage polarity is that the lumen negative voltage in the early segment is dependent upon the presence of glucose and/or amino acids in the lumen, and disappears when these solutes are completely reabsorbed. The positive voltage appears when the chloride concentration in the lumen rises to values in excess of that in peritubular fluid, thereby creating a *chloride diffusion potential*. Glucose, amino acids, and other organic solutes (e.g., lactate) are also extensively reabsorbed in the proximal convoluted tubule. The transport of sodium is critically dependent upon the co-transport of these organic substrates, probably in a manner analogous to that occurring in small intestine.

Sodium transport across proximal tubule cells involves a two-step process. Since the sodium concentration in the cell is lower, and the voltage more negative, than in either the tubule lumen or peritubular fluid, the movement of sodium from lumen to cell proceeds down an *electrochemical gradient*, and is therefore a *passive* process. Transport of sodium out of the tubule cell into the peritubular interstitial fluid of the renal cortex is believed to be an active, energy-dependent process, although the mechanism involved is not well understood.

The epithelium of the proximal tubule is highly permeable to water, sodium, and chloride, and the electrical conductance is also high. An *intercellular shunt pathway* is believed to provide the route for rapid permeation of these substances, and accounts for the relatively "leaky" nature of this epithelium. These shunts between adjacent cells have important consequences for the control of salt and water transport across the proximal tubule. For example, the existence of *lateral intercellular channels* provides the basis for an attractive theory to account for the reabsorption of water across the proximal tubule. According to this hypothesis, sodium salts enter tubule cells through the luminal brush border membrane, and then are transported from the cells into lateral intercellular channels. The salt concentration (and osmolality) within the channels thus exceeds that in adjacent tubule cells or in surrounding interstitium, thereby causing movement of water from tubule lumen and cell interior into the channels by osmosis. In consequence, the hydrostatic pressure within the channels rises, and, in turn, drives fluid from channels into the surrounding peritubular interstitium.

The rate of reabsorption of fluid from proximal convoluted tubules is sensitive to the effects of *physical factors*, i.e., the hydrostatic and colloid osmotic pressures acting across the walls of the peritubular capillaries. To appreciate the mechanisms involved, recall that within the kidney the processes of filtration and reabsorption involve separate capillary beds which are not only distinct, both functionally and anatomically, but are also connected in series. In the glomerular capillaries, fluid is filtered because the transcapillary hydrostatic pressure difference, ΔP, exceeds the opposing transcapillary oncotic pressure difference, $\Delta \Pi$. Since the plasma proteins in glomerular capillaries are concentrated by this ultrafiltration process, there is a marked rise in the *oncotic pressure* as plasma flows along the glomerular capillary network. This step-up in plasma oncotic pressure is transmitted largely unchanged to the peritubular capillaries via the efferent arterioles. These latter resistance vessels, however, cause a substantial drop in hydrostatic pressure, so that by the time plasma reaches the peritubular capillaries, $\Delta \Pi$ greatly exceeds ΔP. These Starling forces are now oriented in an *uptake* mode, in contrast to the filtration mode at the glomerulus, where ΔP exceeds $\Delta \Pi$. The extent to which $\Delta \Pi$ exceeds ΔP for the peritubular capillary network thereby provides a sensitive mechanism for modulating the over-all rate of reabsorption of fluid by the proximal tubules. Thus, when $\Delta \Pi$ falls or when ΔP increases, uptake of fluid by these capillaries is reduced. As a result, fluid is retained in the interstitial space, altering the hydrostatic pressure in the space, ultimately retarding the egress of fluid from the lateral intercellular channels. Without an adequate route of drainage, fluid in the channels leaks back into the tubule lumen, thus diminishing *net fluid reabsorption* by this tubule segment. The opposite is thought to occur in states which cause the value of $\Delta \Pi$ for the peritubular capillaries to increase (i.e., an increase in filtration fraction) or ΔP to decrease (enhanced efferent arteriolar tone). Under these circumstances, peritubular capillary uptake of reabsorbate is enhanced, leading ultimately to enhanced net fluid reabsorption by the proximal tubule.

LOOP OF HENLE. It is generally accepted that the formation of concentrated urine is the consequence of osmotic equilibrium of collecting duct fluid with a hypertonic medullary interstitium. The mechanism whereby the medullary osmolality is raised is not entirely clear; however, it is thought that the progressive increase in osmolality from the corticomedullary junction to the papillary tip is due to the operation of a *countercurrent multiplication system*.

Studies in animals in vivo show that fluid from *thin ascending limbs* is lower in osmolality than fluid obtained from *thin descending limbs* at comparable levels in the papilla. Furthermore, this hypotonicity of the fluid in ascending limbs is due not to net addition of water, but rather to net removal of solute, primarily sodium chloride. However, these studies did not define the nature of this salt reabsorptive process from the thin ascending limb. Indeed, because of inaccessibility, it is presently impossible to study entire lengths of thin descending and thin ascending limbs of Henle in vivo. Recently, however, in in vitro studies with the isolated tubule microperfusion technique, it has been possible to examine directly the salt, water, and urea transport characteristics of the rabbit thin descending limb of Henle, as well as the thin and thick portions of the ascending limb. The thin descending limb was found to be highly permeable to water but to be much less permeable to sodium and urea. Isotonic fluid enters thin segments of the descending limbs at the corticomedullary junction and equilibrates with the local hypertonic interstitium during its passage toward the papillary tip. This osmotic equilibration process, which has the effect of raising the sodium chloride concentration to very high levels by the hairpin turn of Henle's loop, occurs both by water abstraction and solute entry.

The principal site for active outward transport of sodium chloride has generally been taken to be the *thin ascending limb of Henle's loop*. The observation that the fluid within this segment is hypotonic to fluid in adjacent vasa recta and descending limbs at the same level is consistent with this view. Nevertheless, no direct evidence has yet been found to prove that this segment is capable of transporting sodium chloride actively. For this reason, it recently has been postulated that a concentration of NaCl lower in the thin ascending limb than in the surrounding interstitium could arise, provided that this segment is impermeable to water and that its permeability to sodium chloride is great enough to permit the passive outward diffusion of the salt at a rate sufficient to render hypotonic the fluid remaining behind. This possibility has recently received substantial experimental support.

When the tubule fluid enters the next segment of the nephron, the *medullary thick ascending limb of Henle's loop*, its relative and absolute amounts of sodium chloride and urea are lower and higher, respectively, than in the fluid entering the thin descending limb. The means for lowering salt concentration has already been discussed. The elevation in urea concentration appears to take place by two processes: (1) *abstraction of water* in excess of urea out of the thin descending limb of Henle, and (2) *net urea entry* (recycled from the collecting duct) into the thin descending and thin ascending limbs of Henle. With the microperfused isolated rabbit tubule preparation it has been shown that the voltage across the medullary thick ascending limb is oriented lumen positive (approximately +7 mV). This contrasts with the orientation of the voltage along other portions of Henle's loop which are typically lumen negative. This finding that the lumen of the thick ascending limb is electropositive, together with the finding that the sodium chloride concentration continues to decline as fluid travels along this medullary nephron segment, necessitates the conclusion that *chloride must be the actively transported moiety*. Since the permeability to sodium has been found to exceed that of chloride, the latter ion may be regarded as being transported by an *electrogenic pump*, whereas the bulk of the transported sodium moves by purely passive means, driven by the voltage. Besides generating hypotonic tubule fluid, the low water permeability of the thick ascending limb, coupled with extensive sodium and chloride efflux, gives rise to the high sodium chloride concentration of the outer medullary interstitium.

A Passive Equilibration Model of Countercurrent Multiplication. On the basis of the foregoing, a *pas-sive equilibration model* of countercurrent multiplication has been proposed to explain the production of concentrated urine. In this model it is envisaged that when the hypotonic fluid leaves the thick ascending limb of Henle's loop and courses through the distal tubule and cortical collecting tubule, it undergoes osmotic equilibration with the surrounding isotonic interstitium by virtue of water abstraction in the presence of antidiuretic hormone (ADH). The permeabilities of the thick ascending limb of Henle's loop and the distal convoluted tubule to urea are exceedingly low. Thus the urea concentration in the fluid entering the cortical collecting duct is extremely high and rises further as the collecting duct passes through the outer medulla. This progressive rise in urea concentration is the consequence of water removal, which, in turn, is secondary to the high salt concentration in the surrounding outer medullary interstitium. The high urea concentration in the collecting duct fluid persists until the fluid reaches the inner medulla where, because of a pronounced local increase in collecting duct permeability to urea, urea now diffuses down its concentration gradient into the papillary interstitium.

As already discussed, urea is recycled to a variable extent into thin descending and thin ascending limbs. In terms of the passive equilibration model, however, the main function of this high interstitial urea concentration is to exert an osmotic effect on thin descending limbs, favoring abstraction of water and raising the luminal concentration of sodium chloride. The thick ascending limb, in turn, is presented with a hypertonic fluid rich in sodium and chloride. Because the thin ascending limb is impermeable to water, slightly permeable to urea, and highly permeable to salt, the salt can diffuse down concentration gradients at rates faster than the inward diffusion of urea, leading to progressive dilution of the fluid as it flows toward the renal cortex. In combination, these processes appear to account for the progressive rise in the interstitial osmolality from the corticomedullary junction to the papillary tip.

In the intact animal, the fluid that leaves the thick ascending limb of Henle is low in sodium and chloride concentrations, and the concentrations of these ions are largely independent of the animal's state of hydration or diet. Were this fluid to be excreted without further modification, the urine would always be dilute. Usually, however, urine does not have these characteristics, but instead is altered further by the action of other ion transport processes located in more distal nephron segments.

DISTAL NEPHRON. The remainder of the nephron consists of several anatomically and physiologically discrete tubule segments which together account for a substantial fraction of the over-all reabsorption of sodium and chloride. Control of urinary dilution and concentration (i.e., water reabsorption) and the final modulation of net potassium and hydrogen excretion also occur in these distal segments. In addition, hormones such as ADH and *aldosterone* and a number of the clinically useful *diuretic drugs* exert major effects here.

In the *distal convoluted tubule*, water reabsorption is variable, depending on the state of hydration and, more specifically, on the presence or absence of ADH. In the absence of ADH, this and more distal nephron segments are essentially impermeable to water, so that the hypotonic fluid entering this segment is excreted as dilute urine. Indeed, continued salt reabsorption along the distal convoluted tubule results in further dilution of the urine in the absence of ADH. In the presence of ADH the permeability of the late portion of this segment to water increases, and as a result the osmolality of the late distal tubule fluid rises to a value close to that of plasma. Sodium chloride continues to be reabsorbed from the tubule lumen. Net sodium reabsorption proceeds uphill against moderately steep chemical and electrical gradients. In the absence of aldosterone the capacity of the epithelium of the distal tubule to lower the sodium concentration in tubule fluid is reduced.

The *cortical collecting tubule* possesses an extremely low permeability to water in the absence of ADH, whereas this permeability increases greatly in the presence of the hormone. The sensitivity of this segment to ADH appears to be more pronounced than that of the distal convoluted tubule. Urea permeability has been found to be low and remarkably *insensitive* to ADH. This unresponsiveness of urea permeability to ADH is considered essential to the efficient recycling of urea in the operation of the passive equilibration model of urine concentration discussed above. As with the distal

convoluted tubule, the cortical collecting tubule is capable of further net reabsorption of sodium.

The terminal segment of the distal nephron is the highly branched *papillary collecting duct*. Continued electrolyte transport in this segment results in the typically large differences of ion concentration that normally exist between urine and plasma. As in the cortical collecting tubule, sodium transport appears to be active because reabsorption proceeds against sizable electrochemical gradients. The rate of sodium transport in this segment depends on the diet, and on the load of sodium delivered from earlier segments, and is affected by the presence or absence of aldosterone. Water permeability increases markedly in the presence of ADH, an effect similar to that seen in the distal convoluted tubule and cortical collecting tubule. Importantly, the papillary collecting duct differs from these latter structures in that its permeability to urea increases dramatically in the presence of ADH. As noted above, the high water and urea permeabilities of the papillary collecting duct in the presence of ADH appear to be of fundamental importance to the formation of hypertonic urine.

A summary of the mechanisms believed to be involved in the production of concentrated urine is given in the accompanying figure.

Mechanism of urine concentration. There are three basic requirements for the loop of Henle to act as a multiplier: (1) countercurrent flow in ascending and descending limbs, (2) differences in water permeability of the two limbs, and (3) a source of energy. The lesser permeability of the ascending than descending limb to water is depicted by the darkened lines. The active reabsorption of chloride from the thick portion of the ascending limb (with sodium following passively) provides the source of energy. As a result of this NaCl reabsorption (process 1), the tubule fluid becomes dilute and the outer medullary interstitium hypertonic. As the fluid flows along the distal tubule and cortical and outer medullary portions of the collecting tubule, water is reabsorbed down its osmotic gradient (process 2, which takes place only when ADH is present in the circulation), causing the concentration of urea in the tubule lumen to rise. This rise in urea concentration is depicted schematically by the increase in lettering size. In the inner medulla, urea as well as water is reabsorbed from the papillary collecting duct (process 3). Although not shown, some of the reabsorbed urea re-enters the descending limb of Henle. This recycling causes urea to accumulate in high concentration in the medullary interstitium, thereby leading to the abstraction of water from the descending limb, as well as the progressive increase in luminal NaCl concentration (process 4). Finally, as the NaCl-rich fluid enters the water-impermeable thin ascending limb, NaCl diffuses into the surrounding medullary interstitium down its concentration gradient (process 5), resulting in a tubule fluid hypotonic to the surrounding interstitium. The extensive reabsorption of water along the collecting duct segment results in the elaboration of a highly concentrated final ureteral urine. (From Jamison, R. L., and Maffly, R. H.: N. Engl. J. Med., 295:1062, 1976. Reprinted by permission.)

FACTORS CONTROLLING RENAL SALT AND WATER EXCRETION

EFFECTIVE ARTERIAL BLOOD VOLUME. In man, it appears that the *effective arterial blood volume (EABV)* is a major physiologic factor which determines whether the kidneys retain or excrete sodium. Unfortunately, the term EABV is imprecise, both because it refers to that part of the total arterial blood volume (not yet exactly defined or measured) which is effective in stimulating volume receptors, and because the actual volume receptors have yet to be identified. Nevertheless, EABV becomes a useful operational concept. The determinants of EABV are (1) the extent of filling of the arterial circulation, governed largely by venous return and left ventricular cardiac performance, and (2) peripheral vascular resistance, which varies with compliance of the resistance vessels and the magnitude of the arterial runoff. In normal man, EABV correlates well with total extracellular fluid volume. Thus, when EABV is decreased by dehydration (i.e., salt and water loss due to profound vomiting or diarrhea) or by hemorrhage, venous return to the heart decreases, cardiac output falls, arterial filling is diminished, and EABV is further decreased. The response of the kidney is the same in the two instances — namely, renal retention of salt and water until extracellular fluid volume and EABV have been re-expanded to normal. In response to excessive salt intake, the opposite sequence ensues, in that venous return increases, leading to augmentation of cardiac output, arterial filling, and EABV. In consequence, the excretion of salt and water is increased until extracellular volume and EABV are reduced to normal.

The factor or factors that apprise the kidney of changes in EABV are not well understood, although a number of mechanisms are probably involved. The best defined are the Starling forces operating at the levels of the glomerular and peritubular capillaries, and the renin-angiotensin-aldosterone and antidiuretic hormone systems.

STARLING FORCES. In response to a fall in EABV, arterial blood pressure tends to fall, as does renal perfusion. There is evidence in animals and man to suggest that, in response to reduced renal perfusion pressure, renal (hence glomerular) plasma flow decreases more than does glomerular capillary hydrostatic pressure,* so that the resulting decline in GFR is proportionately less than the decline in renal plasma flow (RPF). The attendant rise in filtration fraction (GFR/RPF) serves to augment sodium and water reabsorption by the renal tubule, primarily because the higher filtration fraction leads to an elevation of peritubular capillary oncotic pressure, and hence a greater net force for peritubular capillary uptake of tubule reabsorbate. Thus in response to contraction of EABV, the glomerular and peritubular microcirculations act in concert to minimize renal fluid losses — by both lowering GFR and augmenting salt and water reabsorption by the tubules. Expansion of EABV leads to effects opposite to these. Thus an increase in renal perfusion leads not only to a rise in GFR but also to a proportionately greater rise in

renal plasma flow so that filtration fraction declines. The effect of the latter serves to suppress uptake of tubule reabsorbate into peritubular capillaries, thus causing natriuresis and diuresis and return of EABV toward normal.

RENIN-ANGIOTENSIN-ALDOSTERONE. Aldosterone is a steroid hormone capable of augmenting sodium reabsorption by the epithelial cells of the distal nephron. Variations in plasma aldosterone levels are therefore important in the regulation of renal sodium excretion. The major factor controlling aldosterone secretion is the plasma concentration of *angiotensin II,* a vasoactive octapeptide cleaved from an inactive precursor, *angiotensin I.* Formation of the latter from *angiotensinogen,* or *renin substrate,* is dependent upon the presence of *renin* — an enzyme synthesized and stored in the specialized granular cells of the renal *juxtaglomerular apparatus.* The latter is located at the site where each afferent arteriole comes in contact with the distal tubule of the same nephron. The juxtaglomerular apparatus is thus a major mechanism for controlling the rate of aldosterone secretion by the adrenal cortex. In response to a variety of stimuli initiated when EABV decreases, this apparatus secretes renin into the circulation via the adjacent afferent arterioles. One such stimulus, reduction in hydrostatic pressure in afferent arterioles, as occurs when EABV is contracted, augments renin release from the juxtaglomerular apparatus, imparting a *baroreceptor* function to this specialized cell complex. In addition, it has been suggested that a fall in the *rate of delivery* of sodium chloride to the *macula densa* region of the distal tubule, as occurs with EABV contraction, also leads to enhanced renin secretion by the juxtaglomerular apparatus. With expansion of EABV, on the other hand, the resulting increases both in afferent arteriolar blood pressure and in the rate of delivery of sodium chloride to the macula densa serve to suppress renin secretion and thereby adrenal aldosterone release.

ANTIDIURETIC HORMONE. In distal portions of the nephron, water reabsorption can be modulated independently of sodium, by virtue of the action of ADH to control the water permeability characteristics of these tubule segments. The factors governing the release of ADH from the neurohypophysis are therefore of great importance in determining the volume and osmotic character of the final urine, and thus, to a large extent, the state of hydration of the organism.

Neurohypophyseal ADH release is influenced both by osmotic and nonosmotic factors. In regard to the former, an ingested water load dilutes the osmotic concentration of all body fluids and leads to swelling of the bodies of specialized nerve cells located in the region of the hypothalamus — so-called *osmoreceptors* — which respond by inhibiting ADH release from the nerve endings in the posterior pituitary. In the absence of circulating ADH, the cells of the distal nephron become extremely impermeable to water, thereby facilitating excretion of the ingested water load. By contrast, a small increase in plasma tonicity, as occurs, for example, in response to excessive sweating in a hot climate, will lead to enhanced pituitary ADH release, which greatly increases the permeability of the distal nephron to water. As a result, the hypertonic medullary interstitium serves as an effective osmotic driving force for abstraction of water from terminal nephron segments, leading to the eventual excretion of a small volume of

---

*Maintenance of glomerular hydrostatic pressure is probably a consequence of the effects of catecholamines and angiotensin II to cause greater constriction of efferent than afferent arterioles.

highly concentrated urine. ADH release is also influenced to a major extent by nonosmotic factors. Of these, contraction of EABV is the most potent. Well defined volume receptors, located in the walls of the left atrium, carotid sinus, and aortic arch, respond to reduced perfusion of these critical areas by sending impulses, via the glossopharyngeal nerves, to the hypothalamus to augment ADH release. Expansion of EABV has the opposite effect — namely, to suppress ADH release.

OTHER FACTORS CONTROLLING RENAL SALT AND WATER EXCRETION. To account for the natriuresis that attends expansion of the extracellular fluid volume, many investigators have attempted to identify humoral inhibitors of tubule sodium reabsorption. No conclusive evidence has yet been provided for the existence of a *natriuretic hormone*, although several factors that appear to modify salt transport in various assay systems have been identified in plasma or urine of volume-expanded animals and man. It remains to be established whether a natriuretic hormone plays an important role in the regulation of sodium excretion in man, either in health or in disease. Likewise, whether *prostaglandins* or *catecholamines* play important physiologic roles in the renal regulation of salt and water homeostasis is unclear at present.

THE ROLE OF THE KIDNEY IN ACID-BASE HOMEOSTASIS

The pH of extracellular fluid in man is normally maintained within a narrow range, 7.36 to 7.44, despite day-to-day variations in the quantities of acid entering the body fluids from dietary and metabolic sources. These acids consume buffer, of which bicarbonate is the most important. Such buffering serves to minimize the changes in pH that would otherwise ensue. Nevertheless, the bicarbonate buffer system would be of little long-term benefit were it not for homeostatic mechanisms, for with unrelenting acquisition of nonvolatile acids from dietary and metabolic sources, the body buffers would eventually be exhausted and acidosis of lethal proportions would result. The kidneys normally ensure against this possibility by *regenerating* bicarbonate, thereby regulating the concentration of bicarbonate in the plasma.

One important contribution of the kidneys to maintenance of a normal plasma bicarbonate concentration is the virtually complete reabsorption (or *reclamation*, as it is often called) of the bicarbonate present in the glomerular ultrafiltrate. As discussed above, this is a process largely completed in the proximal tubule. The process of bicarbonate reclamation operates to reabsorb all the filtered bicarbonate below a critical serum concentration — *the bicarbonate threshold concentration* —which in man is normally about 26 mEq per liter, essentially identical to the concentration of bicarbonate in plasma. This mechanism prevents urinary wastage of bicarbonate. When plasma bicarbonate concentration rises above this threshold, renal reclamation is incomplete and the excess bicarbonate escapes into the final urine, enabling the plasma bicarbonate concentration to return to the threshold level. Even if all the filtered bicarbonate is reabsorbed, *metabolic acidosis* would still ensue if that fraction of the bicarbonate buffer system, consumed by entry of strong nonvolatile acids into the blood, were not regenerated.

Both the reclamation of filtered bicarbonate and the *regeneration* of new bicarbonate occur through the same mechanism in the tubule cell. In these cells, water is split to form H^+ and OH^-, the former secreted into the tubule lumen, probably in exchange for sodium. Under the catalytic influence of intracellular *carbonic anhydrase*, the OH^- ions combine with CO_2 to form bicarbonate, which moves across the peritubular cell membrane to join the pool of extracellular fluid bicarbonate. If the H^+ secreted into the tubule lumen combines with a filtered bicarbonate ion, H_2CO_3 is formed. Dehydration of the latter occurs in the proximal tubule lumen, again facilitated by carbonic anhydrase, which is also present in the brush border of this segment, and the CO_2 so formed diffuses from lumen to peritubular blood. *Thus a filtered bicarbonate ion is reclaimed.* Alternatively, secreted H^+ are also free to combine with *nonbicarbonate buffers* (e.g., phosphate or ammonia) in the tubule fluid, and be excreted in this form in the final urine. The bicarbonate ion, the other original product of the breakdown of H_2CO_3, formed within the tubule cell, enters the peritubular blood. *Thus a bicarbonate ion is regenerated.*

Hydrogen ions in the urine are primarily bound to buffers in an amount (the so-called *titratable acid*) equivalent to the amount of alkali required to titrate the urine to the pH of blood. It is usually not possible to excrete all the daily acid load as titratable acid alone. To serve as additional buffer the cells of the renal tubules are able to generate ammonia (NH_3) as a result of the hydrolysis of glutamine. NH_3 diffuses from these cells into the tubule lumen, where it combines with H^+ to form NH_4^+. As noted above, each mole of NH_4^+ excreted into the urine is associated with the regeneration of one mole of bicarbonate. *Ammoniagenesis*, a process which occurs within tubule cells, is believed to be responsive to the acid-base needs of the individual. Thus, when faced with an acute acid burden and an increased need for bicarbonate generation, the rate of renal ammonia synthesis increases sharply.

The quantity of hydrogen ions excreted as titratable acid and NH_4^+ is equal to the quantity of bicarbonate regenerated in tubule cells and added to the plasma. Under steady state conditions, the quantity of net acid excreted into the urine (the sum of titratable acid and NH_4^+ minus bicarbonate) must equal the quantity of acid gained by the extracellular fluid from all sources. *Metabolic acidosis* and *alkalosis* result when this delicate balance is perturbed — the former the result of insufficient net acid excretion, the latter due to excessive acid excretion.

A number of factors are known to modify the rate of secretion of H^+. Among the most important is the *carbon dioxide tension* (P_{CO_2}). The concentration of dissolved CO_2 in physiologic solutions varies directly with P_{CO_2}, and the concentration of H_2CO_3 is directly proportional to P_{CO_2}. Since all cell membranes are readily permeable to CO_2, changes in extracellular P_{CO_2} will be accompanied by equivalent changes in intracellular P_{CO_2}. Intracellular pH will therefore fall when extracellular P_{CO_2} rises (i.e., respiratory acidosis), resulting in an enhanced rate of H^+ secretion and excretion. The opposite responses are generally seen with reduced extracellular P_{CO_2}.

The rate of H$^+$ secretion is also critically dependent upon the state of *potassium balance*. This relationship again derives from the fact that H$^+$ secretion is dependent largely upon intracellular pH. Accordingly, when cells are relatively potassium deficient, intracellular pH falls and leads to enhanced H$^+$ secretion and a fall in urine pH. The opposite occurs in response to a net gain in intracellular potassium.

THE ROLE OF THE KIDNEY IN POTASSIUM HOMEOSTASIS

As with hydrogen ion, the concentration of potassium in extracellular fluid is normally maintained within relatively narrow limits, 4 to 5 mEq per liter. The importance of this close regulation is hardly surprising, in view of the profound effects of this cation on excitation and conduction in nerve and muscle. More than 95 per cent of total body stores of potassium resides in the intracellular fluid compartment, achieving an intracellular concentration of approximately 160 mEq per liter, and thus providing an effective osmotic force within the cell to balance that derived from sodium in the extracellular fluid.

The normal individual maintains external potassium balance by excreting an amount of potassium per day equivalent to the amount ingested, minus the relatively small quantities lost in stool and sweat. It is the kidney which primarily regulates body potassium homeostasis. Potassium is freely filtered at the glomerulus, although the amount excreted usually represents no more than about 20 per cent of the quantity filtered. Thus potassium must be extensively reabsorbed by the tubules. Nevertheless, under conditions of potassium loading, the excreted quantity may exceed substantially the quantity filtered, indicating that this cation can also be secreted by the tubules. Both transport mechanisms contribute to the over-all tubule processing of this ion under most physiologic circumstances. The great bulk of the filtered potassium is reabsorbed in the early portions of the nephron, about 70 per cent in the proximal tubule, and an additional 20 to 25 per cent in the loop of Henle. A potassium secretory process operates in the distal convoluted tubule and terminal nephron segments. The process is largely dependent on exchange of potassium for sodium, the reabsorbed sodium creating an electrical gradient across the tubule wall, lumen negative. Potassium ions are therefore free to diffuse from the cell interior into the distal tubule and collecting duct lumen, down this electrical gradient. Opposing this passive mechanism is an active process which serves to transport potassium from lumen to cell, so that the net flux of potassium at any point along the distal nephron is determined by the balance of these separate processes.

The rate of excretion of potassium is determined largely by four factors. One is the *circulating level of aldosterone*, which affects sodium reabsorption as well as potassium secretion. As noted above, as sodium is reabsorbed, a lumen-negative electrical potential is created across the tubule wall, which draws potassium (and H$^+$ as well) into the lumen. Hence, potassium secretion is dependent upon two operations: (1) delivery of adequate amounts of sodium salts to the distal nephron to permit an optimal rate of sodium reabsorption, and (2) the presence of sufficient levels of circulating aldosterone to stimulate sodium reabsorption, and thereby the electrical driving force for potassium secretion.

A second major influence on the potassium excretion rate is the *concentration of potassium within cells,* and in particular within tubule epithelial cells. Clearly, for any given rate of aldosterone secretion and distal delivery of sodium salts, a higher potassium concentration within cells of the distal nephron will augment potassium secretion, and vice versa. To a major extent intracellular concentration bears a close relation to total body potassium stores, so that an important influence of intracellular potassium concentration on the over-all rate of potassium excretion is highly desirable.

A third determinant of potassium excretion is the *absolute rate of flow of fluid* through distal tubules and collecting ducts. Finally, the *acid-base status* of the individual can also modify, to a large extent, the rate of potassium excretion. In general, *alkalosis* increases the renal secretion and excretion of potassium and *acidosis* depresses these responses. The effects of acid-base disturbances are mediated, at least in part, by changes in the intracellular concentration of potassium. In general, alkalotic states are associated with increases in cell potassium concentration, and thereby in potassium secretion. The opposite generally applies to acidotic states.

Barger, A. C., and Herd, J. A.: The renal circulation. N. Engl. J. Med., 284:482, 1971.

Brenner, B. M., Baylis, C., and Deen, W. M.: Transport of molecules across renal glomerular capillaries. Physiol. Rev., 56:502, 1976.

Brenner, B. M., Deen, W. M., and Robertson, C. R.: Glomerular filtration. *In* Brenner, B. M., and Rector, F. C., Jr. (eds.): The Kidney. Philadelphia, W. B. Saunders Company, 1976, p. 251.

Burg, M. B.: The renal handling of sodium chloride. *In* Brenner, B. M., and Rector, F. C., Jr. (eds.): The Kidney. Philadelphia, W. B. Saunders Company, 1976, p. 272.

Dirks, J. H., Seely, J. F., and Levy, M.: Control of extracellular fluid volumes and the pathophysiology of edema formation. *In* Brenner, B. M., and Rector, F. C., Jr. (eds.): The Kidney. Philadelphia, W. B. Saunders Company, 1976, p. 495.

Grantham, J. J.: Renal transport and excretion of potassium. *In* Brenner, B. M., and Rector, F. C., Jr. (eds.): The Kidney. Philadelphia, W. B. Saunders Company, 1976, p. 299.

Jamison, R. L., and Maffly, R. H.: The urinary concentrating mechanism. N. Engl. J. Med., 295:1059, 1976.

Malnic, G., and Giebisch, G.: Mechanism of renal hydrogen ion secretion. Kidney Int., 1:280, 1972.

369.2. MECHANISMS OF RENAL INJURY

Richard J. Glassock

The mechanisms of renal parenchymal injury are complex and diverse. They embrace abnormal immunologic processes, disturbances in coagulation, infection, biochemical and metabolic perturbations, vascular disorders, obstruction to urine flow, neoplasia, and trauma. Each of these mechanisms may interact with another to produce disease. Various segments of the nephron, the interstitium, or the vascular tree may be the principal target of these disturbances. The clinical expression of renal injury, e.g., acute renal failure, nephrotic syndrome, hypertension, will at least in part depend upon the primary locus of injury as well as the tempo of the pathogenetic process itself. Perhaps the best understood and most thoroughly investigated of the mechanisms of renal injury are those which involve aberrant immunologic processes, the so-called hypersensitivity diseases of the kidney.

IMMUNE-MEDIATED INJURY

It has been estimated that over 70 per cent of all the glomerulonephritides are the result of immunologic processes, largely based on the finding of deposits of immunoglobulin (Ig) and/or complement (C) during immunofluorescent studies of renal tissue. The importance of immunologic mechanisms in tubulointerstitial disease is also being increasingly appreciated. Several different mechanisms are recognized.

ANTI-TISSUE ANTIBODY–MEDIATED DISEASES. Anti-glomerular Basement Membrane Antibody Disease. In this circumstance, antibody, usually of the IgG class, is directed toward a native glomerular basement membrane (GBM) antigen. The antibody is usually host derived (autoantibody). The factors that terminate the natural tolerance to a native tissue antigen are presently unknown. Rarely, the antibody may be of exogenous origin. This mechanism has been well studied in experimental animals (nephrotoxic serum nephritis). Anti-GBM antibody–mediated nephritis is uncommon, accounting for less than 5 per cent of all glomerulonephritides. The antigen is believed to be a noncolla-

genous glycopeptide component of GBM, and the union of antibody and antigen occurs in situ. This antigen becomes readily available to the circulation and is uniformly distributed along the glomerular capillary wall. Thus the binding of circulating antibody is continuous and uninterrupted, giving rise to a "linear" pattern of deposited IgG upon immunofluorescent study of diseased renal tissue (see accompanying figure, A). "Linear" deposits of IgG may also occur in diseases in which anti-GBM antibody production and deposition have not yet been firmly established. For example, "linear" deposits of IgG, often accompanied by deposits of albumin in a similar distribution, frequently occur in diabetic glomerulopathy. Therefore "linear" deposits of IgG cannot be regarded as pathognomonic of anti-GBM antibody disease. Recovery of tissue-specific antibody activity in eluates from diseased renal tissue is a definitive test for the antibody nature of "linear" IgG deposits. As further proof, circulating anti-GBM antibodies may be detectable using indirect immunofluorescent or radioimmunoassay techniques.

The morphologic and clinical expression of anti-GBM antibody disease varies widely. At one extreme, the glomerular lesions are explosive, consisting of extensive extracapillary proliferation (crescents), rapidly progressive renal failure, and at times pulmonary hemorrhage (Goodpasture's syndrome). At the other end of the

Tissue sections reacted with fluorescein conjugated anti-human IgG. *A,* Glomerulus from a patient with anti-glomerular basement membrane antibody–mediated glomerulonephritis. Note the "linear" outline of the capillary walls. (Original magnification × 312.) *B,* Glomerulus from a patient with immune complex–mediated glomerulonephritis. Note the "granular" deposits of IgG along the capillary walls. (Original magnification × 312.) *C,* Tubulointerstitial area from a patient with anti-tubular basement membrane antibody–mediated nephritis. Note "linear" deposits. (Original magnification × 500.) *D,* Tubulointerstitial area of an immune complex–associated nephritis. Note irregular deposit in tubular basement membrane. (Original magnification × 500.)

spectrum, very mild renal disease, sometimes detectable only by renal biopsy and immunopathologic study, may be the only manifestation of anti-GBM antibody formation. The explanation for the variation in clinical and morphologic findings is obscure. Circulating levels of antibody do not correlate well with the severity or nature of the clinical or morphologic findings. The affinity and specificity of the antibody to basement membrane antigens or the mediators of inflammation, including complement (C), polymorphonuclear leukocytes, platelets, or coagulation processes, may contribute to the clinical expression of anti-GBM antibody disease.

The classic C sequence is frequently activated via the recognition by C1q of the in situ formed complex of anti-GBM antibody with the fixed tissue antigen. C activation leads to the generation of biologically active fragments with phlogistic, chemotactic, permeability-promoting, and vasoactive properties. These in turn may cause the release of vasoactive amines and peptides from cellular storage sites. Polymorphonuclear leukocytes and monocytes may be attracted to the sites of antibody deposition via C or Fc receptors and result in local basement membrane and cellular disruption. Sequential activation of the terminal C components may also lead to cytolysis of endothelial cells and exposure of the collagen matrix of GBM, thus resulting in localized platelet aggregation and fibrin formation. The binding of antibody to GBM may in itself evoke alterations of GBM structure and function independent of the effects of C activation and leukocytes.

Anti-tubular Basement Membrane Antibody Disease. The binding of antibody to the intrinsic antigens of tubular basement membranes (TBM) may also result in renal disease in a fashion similar to anti-GBM antibody disease. "Linear" TBM deposits may frequently be found in association with "linear" GBM deposits or in an isolated form, thus indicating that TBM contains antigens that are not necessarily shared by GBM (see figure, C). Circulating antibody to TBM may be found, and eluates of renal tissue have been shown to contain anti-TBM antibody activity. Studies in a variety of experimental animals have also indicated that there may be a substantial degree of individual specificity among TBM antigens (alloantigens), which may account for the production of anti-TBM antibody following allogeneic renal transplantation.

The binding of antibody to TBM may elicit both acute and chronic but progressive forms of tubulointer-stitial nephritis. Significant mononuclear (macrophage) infiltration is often observed in such lesions. Anti-TBM antibody–mediated disease in man is relatively uncommon. Examples include the acute hypersensitivity interstitial nephritis following methicillin administration and transplantation, as well as rare instances of idiopathic chronic tubulointerstitial nephritis.

Antibody to Other Native Constituents of Glomerular or Tubular Structures. Recently, the concept of anti-tissue antibody disease has been broadened considerably by an intensive exploration in experimental models of the possible role of antigens other than the classic noncollagen glycopeptide GBM or TBM antigens. It is possible, even likely, that a variety of potential antigens exist in normal glomerular and tubular structures (e.g., basement membrane, epithelial cells, mesangium) and that an autoantibody response to these antigens can lead to disease under appropriate circumstances. If these antigens are not uniformly distributed along the glomerular or tubular basement membranes, it follows that the pattern of Ig immunofluorescence may differ substantially from that of the classic "linear" deposits found when antibody is directed to the principal GBM or TBM glycopeptide. Perhaps the humorally mediated "hyperacute" rejection of renal allografts is an example of this mechanism of renal injury.

Antibody to Altered Tissue Antigens. Another form of immunologically mediated renal injury, presently better understood in experimental animal models than in man, is that which arises when an antigen, normally extrinsic to the kidney, is bound to basement membrane or other renal structures by biochemical or immunologic reactions. Once bound to tissue, this antigen then serves as an in situ focus for a host-derived immune response, one that may be directed to the bound antigen itself, rather than to the native renal structures. Theoretically at least, antigens that are not normally exposed to the circulation may also be uncovered by tissue injury and thus evoke a systemic antibody response. Examples of antigens that may bind to tissue include certain plant lectins, DNA, chemically reactive drugs and heterologous anti-GBM antibodies. Their participation in the process of injury may explain those human diseases in which Ig deposits are noted in glomerular or tubular basement membranes in the absence of circulating immune complexes or antibody to native basement membrane antigens.

CIRCULATING IMMUNE COMPLEX–MEDIATED DISEASES. Glomerular Disease. In this category, glo-

TABLE 1. Antigens Implicated in Human Circulating Immune Complex–Mediated Renal Disease

Antigens	Clinical Syndrome(s)
Exogenous	
Therapeutic agents	
Organic gold and mercury, penicillamine, foreign serum proteins	Serum sickness, nephrotic syndrome
Infectious disease	
Bacteria: nephritogenic streptococci, *Klebsiella*, pneumococci, staphylococci, *Salmonella*, *T. pallidum*, *Corynebacterium*, *P. acnes*	Acute nephritis, nephrotic syndrome
Viruses: hepatitis B, measles, Epstein-Barr, oncornavirus (retrovirus)	Vasculitis, acute nephritis, systemic lupus erythematosus (?) Nephrotic syndrome, acute nephritis
Parasitic: *P. malariae*, *Schistosoma mansoni*, *Toxoplasmia gondii*	Systemic lupus erythematosus
Endogenous	Acute nephritis with thyroiditis
Nuclear antigens (e.g., DNA)	Nephrotic syndrome with malignancy of colon, lung; melanoma
Thyroglobulin	Cryoimmunoglobulinemia, leukemia
Tumor-associated antigen (e.g., carcinoembryonic antigen)	Glomerulonephritis and autoerythrocyte sensitization
Immunoglobulins	Nephrotic syndrome in idiopathic membranous nephropathy and
Erythrocyte stroma	sickle cell disease
Renal tubule epithelial antigens	

merular and vascular structures of the kidney are damaged largely as a result of the deposition of circulating, soluble antigen-antibody complexes having no necessary immunochemical relationship to renal structures. Such immune aggregates may be formed by the reaction of antibody with any of a wide variety of antigens of exogenous or endogenous (autologous) origin (Table 1). This form of immunologic renal injury is much more common than that mediated by anti-tissue antibodies.

In order to generate soluble immune complexes, these antigens must be intrinsically immunogenic or acquire immunogenicity by an alteration in structure or binding to a carrier protein. Furthermore, the antigen must gain access to the circulation and remain for a period of time sufficient for reaction with antibody as it is formed and secreted. Immune complexes formed with multivalent antigens in antibody excess develop an extensive interconnecting lattice network and become essentially insoluble particulate material. Thus they readily undergo phagocytosis by the reticuloendothelial system and are not greatly available for deposition in the glomeruli or vessels of the kidney. Immune complexes formed at equivalence or in slight antigen excess tend to be of intermediate size, to remain in solution, and to localize in glomeruli and vessels. Immune complexes formed in large antigen excess tend to be quite small and very soluble, and to remain in the circulation for protracted periods of time with little avidity for tissue localization. IgG- and IgM-containing immune complexes formed at equivalence or in antibody excess fix C via recognition by C1q, the first component of the classic sequence of C activation.

The mechanism for glomerular or vascular deposition of circulating immune complexes is not completely understood. It may involve several important factors that are intrinsic to the immune complex itself, e.g., size, Ig class, and capability to fix C and induce the liberation of permeability factors such as histamine. Other factors are renal in origin, e.g., intraglomerular pressures and flow, Fc and C receptors, and possibly the ionic charge of the basement membrane. Circulating immune complexes may localize in various locations within the glomeruli, including the mesangium, between the endothelial cells and the GBM, within the basement membrane proper, and at the interface between visceral epithelial cells and the GBM. The precise explanation for differences in the site of deposition is not yet well understood. The size of immune complexes (a function of their antigen-antibody composition) and properties of the glomerular capillary wall itself appear to be important.

Immunofluorescent microscopy of renal tissue from patients with circulating immune complex-mediated disease reveals discontinuous, "granular" deposits (see figure, B) of Ig that are often accompanied by C components. The deposits also contain the relevant exogenous or endogenous antigen. This "granular" deposition of Ig and C is often taken as the hallmark of immune complex deposition. Once deposited within the glomeruli, immune complexes exist in dynamic equilibrium with circulating antigen and antibody. For example, if additional antigen is administered after an immune complex has been deposited, its solubility may be affected in such a way that the size of the deposited immune complex may decrease. Contrariwise, the size of immune complex deposits may increase further if additional antibody is administered.

Glomerular deposition of immune complexes will be relatively short lived and the disease will be potentially reversible if the source of the antigen is limited. This is best exemplified experimentally and clinically by acute serum sickness resulting from the parenteral administration of foreign (heterologous) serum protein antigens (tetanus antitoxin, snake antivenom). Initially, the administered serum proteins will equilibrate with the intra- and extravascular spaces and undergo slow metabolic degradation. Subsequently, as antibody formation and secretion begin, circulating immune complexes will be formed and the serum protein antigens will be removed from the circulation at an accelerated rate. As a balance is achieved between the amount of antigen and antibody, potentially phlogistic antigen-antibody complexes containing complement will be formed and deposited in various structures, including the glomeruli, blood vessels, joints, heart valves, lung, and spleen. Serum C levels will transiently decrease. Only a very small fraction of the resultant complexes will deposit within the glomerular structures and provoke an acute inflammatory reaction. The level of circulating immune complexes will decrease as all the administered antigen is removed from the circulation and not replenished by additional injections. As antibody excess develops, the immune complexes will be increasingly removed by the reticuloendothelial system. Ultimately, the inflammatory disturbance will subside as the deposited immune complexes are removed by phagocytosis and metabolism. Both the mesangial and epithelial cells of the glomerulus and infiltrating polymorphonuclear leukocytes and monocytes participate in the removal of immune complexes from glomerular deposits.

If antigen is administered repeatedly or if it is capable of replication (e.g., a bacterial, viral, protozoal, or autologous tissue antigen), the immune complexes will be formed in a state of antigen excess, and their circulation may be maintained at a persistent but variable level. Chronic disease may develop as a function of the size and nature of the antigen, the rate of its entrance into the circulation, the availability of antibody, and the propensity of a given complex to localize in a particular area of the glomerulus. Nearly every recognized form of altered glomerular morphology can occur as a result of such chronic, immune complex–mediated disease. When a load of circulating immune complexes is great and the capability of the reticuloendothelial system has been exhausted, lesions composed of extensive glomerular crescents and glomerular necrosis may develop explosively. When the immune complex load is small or intermittent and the size of immune complexes favors glomerular capillary wall localization, a slowly progressive chronic disease may ensue. Substantial amounts of immune complexes may be deposited in a variety of glomerular structures without evoking a clinically recognizable renal disease. Mediator systems similar to those described for anti-GBM antibody disease may be involved in tissue injury. Complement- and polymorphonuclear-independent mechanisms appear to be more important in glomerular than in extraglomerular vascular disease.

Tubulointerstitial Disease. Recent attention has focused on involvement of the peritubular capillary circulation and the tubule basement membrane in immune complex–mediated disease. Granular deposits of Ig and C components may be found along and within the TBM or peritubular capillaries in a variety of diseases (see figure, *D*). In most instances, similar granular deposits are found in the glomerular capillaries, but tubule-associated deposits alone can occur ocasionally. It is not well understood whether TBM and peritubular capillary deposits occur as a result of "spillover" from the glomerular circulation or because of the diffusion of antigens from the tubule cells toward the circulation with a resultant interaction with circulating antibody.

COMPLEMENT ACTIVATION–ASSOCIATED GLOMERULO-NEPHRITIS. In recent years a new group of glomerular disorders has been defined largely on the basis of association with prominent or isolated glomerular deposition of C3 or abnormalities of circulating levels of complement components, or both. Although the precise pathogenetic relationship of these phenomena to tissue injury has not been well established, it seems appropriate to consider them under the category of immunologically mediated glomerular diseases. The morphologic lesion typically associated with C activation is membranoproliferative glomerulonephritis (MPGN). This lesion is characterized by proliferation of mesangial cells and an increase in mesangial matrix with thickening of the peripheral capillary wall due to the interposition of mesangial cells. Under some circumstances, MPGN may be associated with glomerular C3 deposition without immunoglobulin deposition. Isolated C3 deposition may occur in the absence of deposits of early acting C components such as C1q, C4, and C2, thus suggesting involvement of the alternative pathway of C activation. In many cases isolated glomerular C3 deposition is accompanied by a distinct reduction of the plasma C3 level, with normal levels of C1q, C4, C2, circulating breakdown products of C3 and factors of the alternative pathway, increased C3 turnover, decreased C3 synthesis, and the presence of a circulating factor capable of cleaving native C3 in vitro (C3 nephritic factor or C3 NeF). Many but not all cases revealing this pattern of complement abnormalities demonstrate a unique ultrastructural lesion, consisting of transformation of the renal basement membranes (GBM, TBM, and Bowman's capsule) into an extremely electron-dense structure.

Since it has proved difficult to demonstrate experimentally that prolonged activation of C via the alternative pathway per se leads to glomerular damage, the demonstrable C abnormalities may be an epiphenomenon of a more basic but as yet obscure pathogenetic mechanism. Perhaps, as suggested by some, a pre-existing deficiency of C components may lead to defective mechanisms for processing potentially immunogenic environmental agents and thus predispose to the development of an immune complex–mediated renal disease. Such an explanation, however, could not account for the absence of immunoglobulin deposits in many of these lesions. Furthermore, several of the C components are determined by genes of the major histocompatibility complex (MHC) on chromosome 6. It is possible that the C abnormalities may be associated by linkage disequilibrium with certain genes in the immune response region of the MHC. This may predispose to aberrant immune responses to a variety of environmental or autologous tissue antigens.

CELL-MEDIATED IMMUNITY. The role of cell-mediated immunity (CMI) is well established in the rejection of human renal allografts, which serves as the prototype for cell-mediated renal injury. In allograft rejection, a subclass of T cells ("killer" T cells) specifically sensi-

tized to tissue alloantigens of the donor interacts to result in tissue damage. Insofar as other glomerular, vascular, and tubulointerstitial diseases are concerned, a primary role of cell-mediated immunity is far from established. Clearly, infiltration of the renal parenchyma by lymphocytes and monocytes cannot be taken as an index of involvement of cell-mediated immunity, as similar infiltrates may be observed in lesions unquestionably induced by humoral or nonimmune mechanisms. Nonetheless, certain tubulointerstitial diseases in man have prominent morphologic hallmarks of cell-mediated immunity, and occur in the absence of other signs of humoral immunity. The role of antibody-dependent cell-mediated tissue injury remains relatively unexplored in human renal disease.

It is possible that the structure and function of the kidney might be altered by cell-mediated processes without a direct cell-tissue interaction and without a requirement for invading cells. T cells are known to exert profound effects on the function of other cells and organs by virtue of their ability to secrete biologically active materials known as lymphokines. These substances exert potent cellular effects such as activation of proliferation, aggregation, inhibition of growth, and cytotoxicity. It is tempting to speculate that such secretory products may produce structural or functional glomerular alterations under some circumstances.

A possible candidate for the involvement of cell-mediated immunity in glomerular disease is a disorder known as lipoid nephrosis. This disorder is characterized by recurring episodes of self-limited heavy proteinuria. It is characterized morphologically by optically normal or minimally altered glomeruli, the absence of Ig and C deposits, effacement of the epithelial cell foot processes, and the absence of infiltration by mononuclear cells. Remission may occur during an intercurrent viral illness in which cell-mediated immunity is transiently depressed. Identical lesions may be found in Hodgkin's disease. A variety of studies have demonstrated in vitro abnormalities in cell-mediated immunity. Although these observations have led to some speculations, proof of a pivotal role of cell-mediated immunity in the pathogenesis of this disorder is lacking.

COAGULATION-INDUCED INJURY

A role of intravascular coagulation in renal disease is suggested by several lines of evidence: (1) the histochemical, ultrastructural, and immunofluorescent demonstration of proteins related to fibrinogen or fibrin (fibrin-related antigens, FRA) within the diseased glomeruli or vascular structures; (2) production of renal lesions by the induction of intravascular coagulation; (3) accelerated turnover of fibrinogen and/or platelets in some renal diseases; (4) accumulation of fibrin or fibrinogen degradation products (FDP) in the serum and/or increased excretion of such degradation products in the urine in renal disease and; (5) a beneficial effect of pharmacologic agents affecting coagulation on the morphology or clinical expression of certain renal diseases. An important unresolved question is whether the activity of the coagulation system is a major cause, a coincidental event, or merely the result of the renal damage.

Much of the evidence supporting a pathogenic role for coagulation in renal disease has been generated from studies of the Schwartzman-Sanarelli phenomenon in animals. This phenomenon is induced by giving two injections of bacterial endotoxin 18 hours apart. The first injection primes the animal, and the second injection is followed by massive disseminated intravascular coagulation (DIC) with extensive thrombosis in the vascular tree and the glomerular capillary bed that leads to renal cortical necrosis. Under some circumstances DIC may occur with a single injection of endotoxin (e.g., in pregnant and corticosteroid-treated animals). It is presumed that endotoxin disrupts the endothelial surfaces and leads to the activation of clotting factors and platelet aggregation. Endotoxin may also diminish glomerular fibrinolytic activity. The Shwartzman-Sanarelli reaction is polymorphonuclear leukocyte dependent but it does not require a fully active C system. Vasoactive amine– and angiotensin-induced vasoconstriction plays a role in the development of renal lesions, because adrenergic blockade and inhibition of angiotensin are protective. Low grade or intermittent intravascular coagulation may result in the development of morphologic glomerular lesions which encompass the entire spectrum seen in glomerulonephritis, with the possible exception of membranous glomerulopathy.

There are extensive interrelationships between coagulation and the immune system, including complement. The activation of factor XII (Hageman factor) also induces fibrinolysis, kinin generation, and activation of the first component of complement (C1). Plasmin generated in the process of fibrinolysis may also cleave C3 into C3b and C3a and thus initiate late-acting complement component activation via the alternative pathway. It is reasonably clear that antigen-antibody complexes which have fixed C1q or contain bacterial antigens can directly activate factor XII and thus initiate the intrinsic pathway of coagulation. Immune complexes may interact with basophils and platelets and lead to the aggregation and release of potentially inflammatory substances which facilitate the tissue localization of immune complexes. The fixation of antibodies on the glomerular basement membrane or the deposition of immune complexes in the glomerular capillary bed may disrupt the endothelial surface and expose the collagenous matrix of GBM to the circulation, leading to factor XII activation or platelet aggregation. Endothelial damage may be an extremely important factor involved in intraglomerular coagulation in glomerulonephritis.

The use of anticoagulants in experimental immunologic glomerular disease has led to conflicting results. Early studies employing mild forms of nephritis indicated a beneficial effect; however, more recent studies have indicated that anticoagulants (heparin or warfarin) have little effect in severe anti-GBM– and immune complex–mediated nephritis. Recently obtained evidence suggests that glomerular FRA deposition in glomerulonephritis with crescents may occur by thrombin-independent mechanisms, thus offering a potential explanation for the relative ineffectiveness of antithrombin agents in severe crescentic glomerulonephritis. Ancrod, a product of the pit viper venom which leads to fibrinogen lysis and thus bypasses a requirement for thrombin-induced coagulation, does seem to be effective in preventing crescent formation and leads to better preservation of renal function in experimental anti-GBM– and immune complex–mediated glomerulone-

phritis. Extracapillary proliferation (crescents) seems particularly dependent upon FRA deposition in Bowman's space. It is possible that the primary immunopathologic event itself is a sufficient insult to the glomeruli to evoke significant structural and functional alterations.

Despite these reservations, the features of a number of disorders do seem to indicate that intrarenal vascular coagulation may play a dominant role in their genesis. Examples include the hemolytic-uremic syndrome (childhood, adult, and postpartum forms), thrombotic thrombocytopenic purpura, and hyperacute or accelerated renal allograft rejection. Intrarenal vascular coagulation may also be involved in the renal injury observed in scleroderma, malignant hypertension, acute renal failure (acute tubular necrosis), and toxemia of pregnancy.

TOXIN-MEDIATED INJURY

Toxic nephropathy may be defined as a renal alteration produced by a chemical or biologic product or its metabolites. In the broadest sense, the term encompasses toxins of exogenous origin (e.g., lead, mercury, antibiotics), the toxic effect of abnormal concentrations of endogenous metabolites (e.g., oxalate, myoglobin, uric acid), and the damaging effects of physical agents (e.g., x-ray, heat). A classification of the major nephrotoxins is given in Table 2. The major mechanisms of toxin-induced injury include (1) direct cellular toxicity, including cell necrosis and interference with normal metabolic function; (2) intrarenal obstruction to urine flow owing to intraluminal crystallization or precipitation; (3) deposition of crystalline material in tubulointerstitial areas, leading to chronic inflammation; and (4) alteration of the renal macro- and microcirculation, including formation of glomerular ultrafiltrate. In addition, certain agents exert their toxic effect via hypersensitivity mechanisms, as discussed above. Certain properties of the kidneys render them particularly vulnerable to toxic injury — namely, a high blood flow–tissue mass ratio, an extensive endothelial surface area, a countercurrent mechanism for urine concentration leading to a high medullary solute concentration, trans-

TABLE 2. Classification of Major Nephrotoxins

Exogenous
  Metals
    Mercury, gold, silver, arsenic, lead, cadmium, uranium, lithium salts
  Solvents
    Carbon tetrachloride and other halogenated hydrocarbons, ethylene glycol
  Diagnostic agents
    Iodinated x-ray contrast media
  Therapeutic agents
    Antimicrobials (aminoglycosides, amphotericin B, sulfonamides)
    Analgesics (phenacetin, aspirin)
    Anesthetics (methoxyflurane)
    Hormones (vitamin D)
    Antineoplastics (methotrexate, cis-platinum, cyclophosphamide)
    X-irradiation
  Miscellaneous
    Elemental phosphorus, venoms, mushrooms, fluoride
Endogenous
  Uric acid
  Oxalate
  Pigments (myoglobin, hemoglobin)
  Bence Jones protein
  Hormones (e.g., parathyroid hormone)

cellular transport, alterations in pH and ionic strength in the distal nephron, ionic charge of GBM, and the ultrafiltering capacity of the glomerular capillary wall. These properties play an important role in determining the distribution of lesions seen after toxin exposure. Acute renal failure and chronic tubulointerstitial nephritis are common manifestations of toxin-mediated injury.

Several illustrative examples of toxic nephropathy may be cited. Excessive consumption of analgesic compounds leads to lesions initially confined to the renal papilla. Indeed, bland necrosis of the papilla is a major manifestation of this form of toxic nephropathy. The concentration of analgesics and metabolites in the lumina and interstitium of the papilla is increased by the countercurrent multiplication system. The relatively anaerobic environment of the deeper zones of the medulla and papilla contribute to their vulnerability in this form of toxic nephropathy.

Uric acid may crystallize in the distal nephron under conditions of high concentration and low pH. Such aggregates may lead to intranephronal obstruction and renal injury. High concentrations of urate or oxalate salts in the interstitial areas lead to crystallization and inflammatory changes. Some toxic agents, including nephrotoxic antimicrobials, halogenated hydrocarbons, and heavy metals, lead to a disturbance in formation of glomerular ultrafiltrate, in addition to exerting direct toxic effects on the tubule cells.

INFECTION-MEDIATED INJURY

Infections of the kidney and urinary tract lead to renal injury in a variety of ways. Direct invasion of renal tissue by viable organisms and the release of endotoxins or exotoxins result in direct tissue damage. The calling forth of cellular elements of inflammation leads to the localization of infection and to the formation of abscesses which may enlarge and compress adjacent renal tissue. Localized release of proteases, cathepsins, and other enzymes by the invading leukocytes may lead to the disruption of normal renal architecture, alterations of the renal microcirculation, and frank tissue necrosis when tissue oxygenation is already impaired. Vascular lesions induced by acute infections may ultimately lead to chronic ischemic changes. Urinary tract infection may interfere with normal urinary flow dynamics, thus predisposing to the stagnation of urine and stone formation. The integrity of the vesicoureteral valve may be altered by infection, thus leading to a free reflux of bladder urine and a high ureteric pressure during voiding, with pressure-induced changes in the calyceal architecture (see below). Certain infections, primarily tuberculosis, are noted for their tendency to produce cicatricial stenosis and obstruction in the upper urinary tract. Furthermore, some organisms (*Proteus* species) may degrade urinary urea into ammonia and CO_2, leading to a chronically elevated urinary pH and ammonia concentration. This alteration in urine composition predisposes to crystallization of magnesium–ammonium phosphate stones (struvite or infection stones), which may subsequently aggregate into casts of the calyceal system (staghorn calculi) and lead to significant degrees of obstruction and renal parenchymal damage. Infection of the urinary tract may lead to interference with certain specialized functions of

the kidney, most notably the ability to excrete maximally concentrated urine following water deprivation. Chronic bacterial infection of the urinary tract in the absence of associated disease (such as diabetes mellitus, analgesic abuse, or outflow obstruction) seldom leads to progressive parenchymal disease.

Remote infection of a viral, bacterial, protozoal, or helminthic nature (e.g., visceral abscesses, infective endocarditis, chronic hepatitis B, malaria, or toxoplasmosis) may result in renal damage indirectly by the formation of circulating immune complexes. These may deposit in the glomerular and vascular structures to evoke an array of morphologic changes and clinical syndromes.

HEREDITARY, BIOCHEMICAL, AND METABOLIC INJURY

Disordered biochemical and metabolic processes may lead to renal injury. These abnormalities may be the result of defective or excessive synthesis of a normal or abnormal structural component of renal tissue, the abnormal accumulation of metabolites in the kidney, or defects in the tubular transport or renal excretion of endogenous metabolites. Such alterations are frequently observed in the heredofamilial renal diseases. For example, diabetes mellitus is commonly complicated by progressive renal disease. These lesions are the consequence of the abnormal diabetic milieu, at least in part. The biochemical counterpart of the structural change seen in diabetic glomerular disease, i.e., increased thickness of the capillary basement membrane and increased production of mesangial matrix, is unknown. It has been suggested by some that it is due to accumulation of a collagen-related glycopeptide in basement membrane. Alport's syndrome (hereditary nephritis and deafness) may be another example of a biochemical lesion specifically affecting the structure and function of basement membranes. In this disease, renal basement membranes display a variety of ultrastructural lesions. Preliminary data indicate that the basement membrane of Alport's syndrome may be deficient in the noncollagen glycopeptide reacting with human autoantibodies to GBM.

Excessive accumulation of normal metabolites in the kidneys may at times result in damage. Fabry's disease, an X-linked lipid storage disease resulting from a generalized deficiency of ceramide trihexosidase (α-galactosidase A) leads to the deposition of a glycosphingolipid in the endothelial wall of vessels and in the epithelial cells of glomeruli. Deposition of amyloid in glomeruli may be another example of accumulation of an abnormal substance leading to disease. In cystinosis, the amino acid cysteine accumulates in cells of the reticuloendothelial system and the proximal tubule and in leukocytes. Such storage, or an independent but associated defect, leads to an anatomic lesion of the proximal tubule and disturbance of many functions of the proximal tubule such as glucose, phosphate, uric acid, and amino acid reabsorption.

Disordered transport of amino acids may lead to renal injury. For example, defective transport of cystine and basic amino acids in kidneys and intestines may lead to excessive excretion of poorly soluble cystine in the urine. Cystine crystalluria ensues and may ultimately be associated with urinary obstruction, infection, and renal parenchymal damage. In disorders of uric acid metabolism, salts of uric acid may accumulate in the interstitium of the kidney and provoke chronic interstitial nephritis or uric acid may crystallize within the tubule and cause obstruction.

Excessive excretion of the products of endocrine glands may result in renal damage from time to time. For example, nephrocalcinosis not uncommonly complicates primary hyperparathyroidism. Excessive elaboration of ACTH may lead to serious renal potassium wastage and kaliopenic nephropathy.

Although the mechanisms responsible for cystic diseases of the kidney are still largely unknown, they constitute an important group of hereditary disorders of the kidney and as such are likely to be the result of some biochemical defect. Polycystic kidney disease occurs in two forms. The adult form, transmitted as an autosomal dominant trait, is usually recognized in the fourth or fifth decades of life. The childhood form, transmitted as an autosomal recessive trait, is usually recognized in infancy. In adult polycystic kidney disease, the cysts are variable in size and involve the medullary collecting ducts and the cortical convoluted tubules. Cystic changes in the liver and pancreas and aneurysms of the cerebral circulation are associated abnormalities. In the childhood form, fusiform dilatation of the distal nephron occurs, leading to a relatively uniform array of cysts. Associated lesions include periportal hepatic fibrosis and biliary duct ectasia. Cysts chiefly involving the medulla are seen in the relatively benign medullary sponge kidney, in which cystic ectasia is present only at the tip of the papilla. By contrast, medullary cystic disease, occurring as either an autosomal dominant or recessive trait, pursues a relentlessly progressive course. In the latter disorder cysts are present throughout the medulla and at the cortical medullary junction, in association with progressive interstitial fibrosis and tubular atrophy of the outer cortex.

VASCULAR MECHANSIMS

Lesions of the renal circulation which lead to impairment of blood flow to renal tissue, if slowly developing and incomplete, may result in ischemic atrophy of the renal parenchyma and progressive interstitial and glomerular sclerosis. If they are rapid and complete, then tissue necrosis (i.e., infarction) develops. Such lesions may occur at any level of the renal circulation and may be bilateral or unilateral. They may be the result of an inflammatory disturbance (frequently immunologic or infectious in nature), the result of intrarenal vascular coagulation, secondary to embolization by clot or atheromatous debris, or due to poorly understood mechanisms often associated with chronically elevated arterial pressure and leading to endothelial proliferation, muscular hypertrophy, and luminal obliteration. Functional alterations in the renal microcirculation may underlie acute renal failure associated with toxin exposure or ischemic episodes. Weakening of the wall of vessels because of damage to elastic lamina may predispose to aneurysm formation. Impaired blood flow may also be due to alterations in the rheologic properties of blood (e.g., sickle cell disease, hyperviscosity) and not to intrinsic vascular disease. Sickle cell disease and trait may be associated with renal injury primarily because of

chronic or recurring disturbance of the renal circulation, principally in the medulla. The erythrocytes containing S hemoglobin may undergo sickle transformation during passage through the relatively hypoxic and hyperosmolar environment of the medulla. This intravascular sickling leads to a disturbance in the medullary circulation and to the impairment of the function of the deeper nephrons largely responsible for maximal urinary concentrating ability. At times the disturbance in the medullary circulation may be so severe as to lead to papillary necrosis.

OBSTRUCTIVE INJURY

Any process which impedes the normal flow of urine has the potential of inflicting renal injury. Intrarenal obstruction may occur consequent to crystallization or precipitation of urinary solutes (e.g., uric acid, Bence Jones proteins) or from extrinsic compression (e.g., edema, cysts). Extrarenal obstruction may be unilateral or bilateral and may develop at any site from the pelvocalyceal system to the tip of the urethra. Such obstruction may be consequent to a variety of conditions intrinsic (e.g., tumors, stones) or extrinsic (e.g., retroperitoneal fibrosis) to the urinary tract.

If obstruction to urine flow is abrupt, complete, and proximal to the ureterovesical junction, the formation of glomerular ultrafiltrate will practically cease, and pressures within the nephron usually will not rise above the difference between intraglomerular hydraulic pressure and the systemic oncotic pressure. As a result of increased intraluminal pressure, the tubules become increasingly permeable to urinary solutes. Permanent injury will not occur if such obstruction is relieved promptly and infection is absent. Longstanding obstruction leads to tubular atrophy and interstitial fibrosis with a permanent loss of renal function.

Slowly developing partial obstruction leads to progressive dilatation of the urinary tract and, depending upon the compliance of the system, less transmission of elevated pressure to the nephron. Nonetheless, chronic partial obstruction leads to defects in specific functions of the kidney, such as urinary concentrating ability and acidification. Progressive dilatation of the pelvocalyceal system and complicating infection ultimately lead to a loss of renal parenchyma. These changes begin in the deeper cortical nephrons and extend later to those in the outer cortex.

NEOPLASTIC INJURY

Under many circumstances the mechanism of neoplasm-induced renal injury is direct and obvious. Thus primary renal neoplasms (e.g., renal cell carcinoma) destroy parenchyma by direct invasion, interference with blood supply, or compression of adjacent normal tissue. Neoplasms originating at distant sites (metastatic carcinoma, lymphoma, leukemia) may also involve and damage renal tissue. Obstruction to urine flow may result from tumors originating at any site in the urinary tract.

Renal injury consequent to neoplastic disease may also be less obvious and indirect. Thus renal disease may result from the excessive elaboration by tumors of substances capable of inflicting tissue injury (e.g., para-thyroid hormone, Bence Jones protein, precursors of uric acid). Also, as previously noted, antibody responses to tumor-associated antigens may also lead to formation of potentially damaging circulating immune complexes.

Bricker, N. S., and Klahr, S.: Obstructive nephropathy. *In* Strauss, M. D., and Welt, L. G.: Diseases of the Kidney. 2nd ed. Boston, Little, Brown & Company, 1971, p. 997.

Heptinstall, R. H.: Interstitial nephritis. Am. J. Pathol., 83:214, 1976.

Kincaid-Smith, P.: Coagulation and renal diseases. Kidney Int., 2:183, 1972.

Maher, J. F.: Toxic nephropathy. *In* Brenner, B. M., and Rector, F. C. (eds.): The Kidney. Philadelphia, W. B. Saunders Company, 1976, p. 1355.

Morris, R. C., Jr., McInnes, R. R., Epstein, C. J., Sebastian, A., and Scriver, C. R.: Genetic and metabolic injury of the kidney. *In* Brenner, B. M., and Rector, F. C. (eds.): The Kidney. Philadelphia, W. B. Saunders Company, 1976, p. 1193.

Murray, T., and Goldberg, M.: Chronic interstitial nephritis: Etiologic factors. Ann. Intern. Med., 82:453, 1975.

Suki, W.: Renal involvement in leukemia and lymphoma. *In* Suki, W. N., and Eknoyan, G. (eds.): The Kidney in Systemic Disease. New York, John Wiley & Sons, 1976, p. 95.

Wilson, C. B., and Dixon, F. J.: The renal response to immunological injury. *In* Brenner, B. M., and Rector, F. C. (eds.): The Kidney. Philadelphia, W. B. Saunders Company, 1976, p. 838.

369.3.   THE MAJOR RENAL SYNDROMES

Roscoe R. Robinson

Diseases of the kidneys often present as one or more of a small group of clinical syndromes. The prompt recognition of these few syndromes therefore represents an important first step toward proper diagnosis and subsequent management. Their recognition, however, is the beginning and not the end of the diagnostic process; they should not be regarded as single or specific disease entities, and their presence should never be equated with any final determination of etiology. The same syndrome can be caused by several types of kidney disease, many of which may have multiple etiologies. Conversely, the same disease may well be seen in association with more than one of the major syndromes, either singly or in combination.

Eight major syndromes are primarily renal in origin: (1) an abnormal urinalysis alone in asymptomatic individuals, (2) the acute nephritic syndrome, (3) acute renal failure, (4) chronic renal failure, (5) nephrotic syndrome, (6) urinary tract infection, (7) urinary tract obstruction, and (8) defects of renal tubular structure or function. Other "syndromes," such as hypertension, urolithiasis, polyuria, and anemia, can also serve as the principal manifestations of underlying kidney disease, but they may have many causes that are not necessarily renal in origin. Hence the present chapter will deal only with those syndromes whose cause is almost always a primary or secondary disorder of kidney function. Greatest emphasis will be placed on a descriptive overview of the significance of various urinary abnormalities in asymptomatic patients who may otherwise seem healthy, because this "syndrome" or collection of findings is not described elsewhere. In all instances, additional detail can be obtained from subsequent chapters that deal with specific forms of kidney disease.

ABNORMAL URINALYSIS IN ASYMPTOMATIC AND APPARENTLY HEALTHY INDIVIDUALS

This "syndrome" is characterized by the presence of proteinuria, hematuria, pyuria, and casts, either alone or in combination, in patients who are asymptomatic and otherwise seem to be in the best of health. Such abnormalities are detected frequently on routine urinalysis, and they may occur in the absence of reduced renal function, hypertension, edema, urolithiasis, urinary tract infection or obstruction, or any other manifestation of kidney disease. When proteinuria, hematuria, and pyuria are coexistent, their presence is almost always indicative of underlying kidney disease; when one occurs alone, it may or may not be indicative of parenchymal renal disease.

PROTEINURIA.   The healthy kidneys can excrete up to 150 mg of total protein per 24 hours. The tetrabromphenol–citrate buffer qualitative test for urinary proteins ("dip-stick") may detect a total protein concentration as low as 10 to 15 mg per 100 ml. Hence a positive qualitative test can result if healthy urine is concentrated. In addition, there are a number of conditions, most of them transient, which may be accompanied by increased protein excretion in the absence of underlying kidney disease. These include vigorous exercise, fever, and various systemic or renal hemodynamic alterations such as congestive heart failure or transient renal ischemia of any cause. It can therefore be difficult to determine whether or not proteinuria is accompanied by underlying kidney disease, especially when proteinuria is small in magnitude (<1.0 gram per day) or an isolated finding in the absence of other signs of kidney disease.

Heavy proteinuria (>1.0 gram per day) is almost always indicative of kidney disease. Values greater than 3.0 to 3.5 grams per day are said to be in the "nephrotic" range and may precede the appearance of other manifestations of the nephrotic syndrome by weeks or months. The differential diagnosis of minimal degrees of proteinuria is far more difficult, particularly when proteinuria is present as an isolated finding. A uniform method of clinical classification is essential, and the serial collection test of Derow has proved to be useful. This test requires the timed and sequential collection of urine in the recumbent and quiet ambulatory postures during moderate antidiuresis. A measurement of specific gravity or osmolality and a qualitative test for protein are performed on each specimen. Three major patterns of proteinuria can be identified with the aid of repetitive testing over short periods of time: (1) "persistent" proteinuria during *both* the recumbent and upright postures; (2) "transient" postural proteinuria that is present inconstantly in the quiet upright ambulatory posture from day to day; and (3) "fixed" postural proteinuria that is demonstrable consistently during quiet upright ambulation whenever sought. These so-called "types" or "patterns" of proteinuria are nothing more than laboratory syndromes. They should not be viewed as a specific entity, as has sometimes been implied in the past. They may have many causes.

"Persistent" proteinuria, with or without other urinary abnormalities, is almost always indicative of some form of kidney disease. It may exist in 5 to 10 per cent of asymptomatic young adults whose qualitative proteinuria is first detected on casual routine urinalysis. Renal biopsy specimens may reveal the presence of a wide spectrum of morphologic alterations in as many as 80 per cent of such patients, ranging from glomerular to interstitial forms of kidney disease.

The clinical significance of postural forms of proteinuria is controversial. Traditionally, postural proteinuria has been regarded as a benign and transient condition of adolescence that is not associated with underlying kidney disease. This is almost certainly true in many instances, particularly in children. Other observations have suggested that it may well reflect the presence of early renal disease, at least in some patients. Once it has been established that proteinuria is "postural," it is wise to distinguish between that which occurs as an "isolated" finding, and that which is accompanied by other evidences of altered renal function. The minimal initial evaluation should include a search for antecedent evidences of renal or systemic disease, examination of the urine sediment, quantification of urine protein excretion, excretory urography, and a measurement of creatinine clearance. Renal biopsy is not performed routinely.

Postural proteinuria is usually discovered during a routine health examination, and the syndrome is especially common in adolescents or young adults; its incidence in older age groups has not been established. Its occurrence during subsiding acute nephritis or the nephrotic syndrome documents that it can and does occur in association with renal disease. Nevertheless, a detailed clinical examination is nonrevealing in most patients, i.e., this form of proteinuria usually occurs as an "isolated" clinical finding. Renal biopsy specimens from young adults with "fixed" postural proteinuria have shown unequivocal evidence of kidney disease in 8 per cent, subtle but definite structural alterations in 45 per cent, and normal renal histology in 47 per cent. Histologic observations in patients with "transient" postural proteinuria are so few that conclusions cannot be drawn.

The clinical significance of the aforementioned morphologic alterations is not clear. They may reflect an early manifestation of kidney disease, an expression of a healed form of antecedent disease, or an anatomic variant of normal. Resolution of this problem may well depend upon the results of long-term clinical follow-up studies. One ten-year follow-up study of young men with an initial diagnosis of fixed postural proteinuria has shown that 49 per cent still exhibited a qualitative pattern of proteinuria, but none of the patients had yet developed any evidence of renal functional impairment. The ten-year clinical outlook was therefore excellent in the group as a whole, but it must be remembered that the final outcome has not yet been established in those who still exhibited proteinuria. Continued follow-up will be required.

These results are not surprising in view of the initial heterogeneity of the renal lesions. The subtle or minimal histologic alterations may have reflected no more than nonpathologic structural defects; even among those that may have represented definite pathology, some may have already begun to heal and some may heal eventually, whereas others may progress with such indolence that clinical significance in terms of morbidity and mortality is not achieved within a lifetime.

Similar histologic observations are not available in patients whose postural proteinuria has been determined clearly to be transient. Most have felt that it is largely benign and that its prognosis is excellent. It may perhaps reflect nothing more than a transient exposure to environmental influences that are known to be accompanied by increased urine protein excretion, e.g., heat, cold, fever, or exercise. Even so, in view of the suggestion that the persistence or repetitive recurrence of *any* qualitative pattern of proteinuria may be of greater predictive prognostic value (in terms of underlying kidney disease) than the actual type of pattern itself, it is wise to regard even transient episodes of postural proteinuria with modest suspicion if they recur repetitively over a long period of time.

Treatment of postural proteinuria is not required, and restriction of physical activity is not beneficial. Follow-up evaluation at infrequent intervals is important following a thorough initial examination. Renal biopsy is not indicated unless there is a distinct change in clinical course (the appearance of urinary sediment abnormalities or renal functional impairment).

HEMATURIA. Although hematuria may occur during the course of nearly all forms of kidney disease, it is important to recognize that it may also serve as an indicator of hematologic, neoplastic, or other genitourinary tract disease. Hence its presence is a relatively nonspecific finding, and identification of its cause can be difficult.

It may appear as an isolated finding or in association with other, more specific signs and symptoms. Its coexistence with proteinuria and other abnormalities of the urine sediment enhances the likelihood of underlying kidney disease. It may appear intermittently or continuously, and it may be micro- or macroscopic. Hematuria per se is asymptomatic, although it may be accompanied by renal colic due to passage of ureteral clots.

Hematuria may originate at any point along the nephron or the genitourinary tract. Its origin cannot be established solely by examination of the urine. Instead, reliance must be placed on a detailed and thorough history and physical and laboratory examination. Even red blood cell casts themselves are a relatively nonspecific finding; certainly, their presence is indicative of an intrarenal source of hematuria, but their presence does not distinguish reliably between a glomerular origin and one at some other site along the nephron.

It is obvious that red blood cells must traverse an endothelial-epithelial barrier if they are to gain entrance into urine. The mechanism is not clear, except in those conditions in which anatomic integrity has been disrupted clearly (e.g., urolithiasis, neoplasia, trauma). The mechanism of entry is less clear in renal parenchymal disease, although in glomerular diseases it is assumed that red blood cells gain entrance to proximal tubule fluid via anatomic discontinuities of the glomerular capillary wall. Direct morphologic evidence of their apparent transglomerular passage has been presented recently.

Hematuria can occur during exposure to several environmental influences, including systemic infection, exercise, fever, and hypercatabolic states. The mechanism is unclear, but it is important to recognize that the diseased kidney may respond similarly if exposed to identical environmental stimuli. Hence in patients with kidney disease, increased microhematuria may not *necessarily* reflect progression or worsening of the disease process.

The specific conditions associated with hematuria are numerous. They include (1) those that are unrelated to kidney disease (e.g., hemoglobinopathies, coagulation disorders, exercise, systemic infection, heart failure); (2) those that are renal in origin; and (3) those that derive from lesions in the upper and lower genitourinary tract. The correct diagnosis is facilitated by the nature of other, more specific signs and symptoms.

On historical examination, a diagnosis of acute poststreptococcal glomerulonephritis can often be established easily. Conversely, an exact diagnosis may be more difficult if the history portrays little more than recurrent episodes of painless gross hematuria in the presence of normal renal function and no evidence of urolithiasis or urologic disease ("IgA" nephropathy, hereditary nephritis or Alport's syndrome, and benign familial recurrent hematuria should be considered as diagnostic possibilities). Special attention must therefore be directed toward taking a careful history, including an emphasis on age of onset, familial occurrence, exposure to nephrotoxins, antecedent infection, trauma, unusual physical activity, disorders of micturition, and signs and symptoms of systemic disease.

Laboratory evaluation should include a careful urinalysis. The presence of red cell casts implies a renal parenchymal origin of hematuria, and the need for urologic investigation may therefore be minimized. Conversely, urologic examination may be indicated when a definite diagnosis of renal parenchymal or systemic disease cannot be established. Other tests, including renal arteriography and renal biopsy, may be indicated if the results of antecedent examinations are nonrevealing.

LEUKOCYTURIA AND CYLINDRURIA. Leukocyturia is also a relatively nonspecific finding, although it admittedly serves to reflect the presence of some type of inflammatory disease of the kidneys or genitourinary tract. Its presence is perhaps most indicative of bacterial infection, but it can also be seen with some frequency in patients with other forms of inflammatory disease, e.g., glomerulonephritis, viremia, and chemical or irritative insults to the genitourinary tract. As with red cells, the urinary excretion of leukocytes can be increased by exposure to exercise or the injection of pyrogen.

On the average, leukocyturia can be said to exist when more than five cells are seen per high-power field in centrifuged urine. Pyuria may also be accompanied by the presence of clumps of leukocytes and leukocyte casts in the urine sediment. Leukocyte casts suggest the presence of parenchymal inflammation, whereas leukocytes in clumps are perhaps more suggestive of damage to the lower urinary tract.

The number and appearance of urinary leukocytes can be influenced by urine pH, osmolality, temperature, associated proteinuria and bacteriuria, and the interval between voiding and examination. Optimal preservation is achieved in an acid, hypertonic urine which has been refrigerated if examination cannot be carried out promptly.

Most urinary casts have been regarded traditionally as evidence of renal parenchymal injury. However, it must be remembered that no single type of cast is diagnostic of any specific disease entity. Red cell casts are perhaps most often indicative of glomerular injury, whereas white cell casts are suggestive of parenchymal inflammation. The exact significance of granular, epithelial, hyaline, and fatty casts is not always clear.

Recent evidence suggests that the matrix of most urinary casts is composed mainly of Tamm-Horsfall glyco-

protein derived from the renal tubular epithelium. That casts originate from within the renal parenchyma is clear. The usual urinary cast is probably formed most often within the distal nephron. So-called "broad" casts are almost certainly formed within the region of the collecting duct.

The presence of abnormal urinary casts is generally indicative of altered renal structure or function, or both, but it is not necessarily valid to assume that their number and type are indicative of the extent of injury. It must be remembered that both casts and cells must derive from nephrons that are still functional, at least in part. Hence a sediment replete with casts and cellular elements does not necessarily imply the presence of either irreversibility or end-stage disease. However, it must also be acknowledged that such a sediment *may* be consistent with extensive disease, although little of prognostic import can be inferred.

ACUTE NEPHRITIC SYNDROME

This syndrome represents the generalized clinical response to a number of acute inflammatory diseases of the nephron. It is characterized typically by the rather abrupt clinical appearance of varying degrees of peripheral edema with evidence of circulatory volume overload, hypertension, and hemodilution. Differing degrees of filtration rate reduction and azotemia may be noted, with or without oliguria or electrolyte disturbances. Urinalysis characteristically shows gross or microscopic hematuria, the sterile pyuria of a nonbacterial inflammatory process, proteinuria (usually less than 2 to 3 grams per day, but occasionally approaching values seen in the nephrotic syndrome), and cylindruria, including the presence of red blood cell casts. Such casts have long been considered a hallmark of the acute nephritic syndrome, but, as outlined earlier, their presence is not necessarily diagnostic. When oliguria occurs, the manifestations of the acute nephritic syndrome will blend with those of the syndrome of acute renal failure. Conversely, when the expression of an acute nephritic syndrome is limited mainly to an abnormal urinalysis and other manifestations are mild or subtle, it may be difficult to distinguish from the syndrome of abnormal urinalysis alone. Severe hypertension may be accompanied by headache, nausea, vomiting, and convulsions on occasion. Circulatory volume overload may be manifested by cardiac dilatation, pulmonary edema, and radiographic evidence of pulmonary congestion, orthopnea, rales, and venous distention. Cardiac output is usually normal or increased, and systolic flow murmurs are not uncommon. The patient may complain of nonspecific flank discomfort, and intravenous urography is unlikely to reveal anything more than decreased dye opacity in the outflow tract and a normal renal contour, albeit one that may be increased slightly in size. Fever, an elevated sedimentation rate, and alterations of serum complement activity, immunoglobulin concentrations, and other laboratory values may be seen, but such findings are perhaps more reflective of a specific etiology rather than a direct consequence of the syndrome itself.

Although the occurrence of an acute nephritic *syndrome* can almost always be equated with the presence of some type of acute *nephritis*, it must be recognized that the clinical expressions of acute nephritis may often extend beyond those of the acute nephritic syndrome, frequently including those of other major syndromes such as abnormal urinalysis alone, nephritic syndrome, or acute renal failure. Hence, at least in a semantic sense, one must be careful to distinguish between the characteristic manifestations of the acute nephritic syndrome (e.g., edema, circulatory volume overload, azotemia, proteinuria, and hematuria) and those of other syndromes that may also reflect the presence of an acute nephritis. Whatever syndrome is present, the specific manifestations of various individual types of acute proliferative nephritis may be seen in each of them, regardless of whether the clinical presentation is that of the acute nephritic syndrome, the nephrotic syndrome, an abnormal urinalysis alone, or a combination thereof (e.g., the transient hypocomplementemia of acute poststreptococcal glomerulonephritis).

The acute nephritic syndrome can be caused by almost any form of acute proliferative glomerulonephritis, whether it be generalized, focal and segmental, crescentic or noncrescentic, primary in origin or secondary to a systemic disease or process. The most common cause is probably the acute, generalized, and proliferative glomerulonephritis which follows a throat or skin infection with "nephritogenic" strains of Group A beta-hemolytic streptococci. The syndrome has also been described following other viral or bacterial infections, including infectious mononucleosis, measles, mumps, influenza, coxsackie- or echo-virus infections, ventriculoatrial infections, bacterial endocarditis, and pneumococcal pneumonia. It occurs with considerable frequency in membranoproliferative glomerulonephritis (Types I and II) and less often in patients with Henoch-Schönlein purpura and collagen vascular diseases such as systemic lupus erythematosus. Most important, it may serve as the initial manifestation of rapidly progressive glomerulonephritis of whatever type or cause (idiopathic, poststreptococcal, Goodpasture's syndrome with pulmonary hemorrhage, and, rarely, polyarteritis and Henoch-Schönlein purpura). It is the responsibility of the clinician to distinguish among these varied causes by searching for their characteristic features on history and physical or laboratory examination. Renal biopsy may be helpful.

ACUTE RENAL FAILURE

This is a very general term which can be used to describe any event in which renal function is suddenly impaired. An exact etiology is not implied. It may occur in the presence or absence of antecedent kidney disease, and it may be accompanied by anuria, oliguria (urine volume less than 400 ml per day), or the maintenance of a normal or even increased urine output ("nonoliguric" or "polyuric" acute renal failure). In any case, the relatively abrupt reduction of renal function is characterized by increasing azotemia over a short period of time (usually a few days) alongside the appearance of other biochemical and clinical manifestations of acute renal insufficiency.

Traditionally, the causes of acute renal failure have been divided into those that are prerenal, renal, or postrenal. These are discussed more fully in Ch. 372. However, it is only when acute renal failure is of renal origin that its cause can be ascribed to intrinsic renal damage. Such forms of renal injury include acute and rapidly progressive glomerulonephritis, acute interstitial nephritis, acute tubular necrosis, cortical necrosis, intrarenal obstruction such as that which may occur during hyperuricemic acute renal failure, and arterial or renal venous obstruction. The nature of the syndrome is such that it should always be considered to be reversible until proved otherwise. For this reason, attention must be directed toward the identification and correction of conditions that may sustain the impairment of renal function or otherwise retard its return to normality (e.g., hypotension, a deficit of extracellular fluid volume, congestive heart failure).

It can be difficult to distinguish between the syndromes of acute and chronic renal failure. A diagnosis of acute renal failure can be established most easily when rapid impairment of renal function occurs in a setting in which antecedent renal function was known to have been normal. Otherwise, one must depend upon such indirect indicators as an observed reduction of filtration rate over a short period of time or the maintenance of a relatively normal hematocrit in the presence of severe filtration rate reduction (a most unusual circumstance in chronic renal failure).

Measurements of renal size on echocardiography or a plain radiograph of the abdomen can be useful; most causes of acute renal failure are accompanied by renal shadows that are normal or slightly increased in size. The presence of small kidneys suggests a diagnosis of chronic renal failure; a finding of normal-sized kidneys is somewhat less useful, as they may coexist with either acute or chronic renal failure. Renal biopsy may again be useful in cautiously selected instances.

CHRONIC RENAL FAILURE

The pathophysiology and clinical manifestations of this clinical syndrome are discussed fully in Ch. 371. This syndrome is characterized by derangements of all aspects of renal function. Uremia is its end-stage hallmark. A diagnosis of chronic renal failure implies that it is the consequence of longstanding and progressive renal damage and that it is most likely irreversible.

The period over which chronic renal failure develops can range from a few months to many years. The term renal insufficiency is sometimes used to describe the presence of mild renal failure prior to the appearance of uremic symptoms. Evidence of longstanding renal failure can be provided by sequential measurements of a reduced or falling filtration rate over a period of at least several months, small renal shadows on echocardiography or plain radiographs of the abdomen, signs and symptoms of uremia (especially evidence of longstanding anemia or nocturia), and the presence of such complications as renal osteodystrophy. There are no reliable laboratory indicators of chronicity, although it is admittedly unusual to observe untreated chronic renal failure in the absence of severe anemia or hypocalcemia.

The syndrome of chronic renal failure can be caused by a myriad of parenchymal diseases of the kidneys. Once its presence has been established, its severity can be classified according to criteria developed by the Council on the Kidney in Cardiovascular Disease of the American Heart Association. Three categories of classification are used: one for signs and symptoms, one for the degree of functional impairment as reflected by estimates of filtration rate, and one for patient performance as an index of the degree of adaptation to the existence of a longstanding disease process.

NEPHROTIC SYNDROME

This syndrome is the consequence of sustained and heavy proteinuria (greater than 3.0 to 3.5 grams per day). It is characterized typically by peripheral edema, heavy proteinuria, hypoalbuminemia, and hyperlipidemia. It can occur in all age groups and in many clinical settings.

Perhaps most often, the patient first notices the gradual appearance of peripheral edema and/or weight gain. Urinalysis reveals the presence of heavy proteinuria, most of which is generally found to be albumin, and subsequent laboratory evaluation reveals the presence of hypoalbuminemia. More recently, it has been recognized that the syndrome may first present with moderate or heavy proteinuria alone and that edema and clear evidence of hypoalbuminemia may not appear until weeks or months later. In this circumstance, the full-blown syndrome has not yet developed and only a presumptive diagnosis can be made. More rarely, the detection of hyperlipidemia or an opalescent serum may provide the first clue to the presence of the syndrome. Hypertension and azotemia are not a part of the pure syndrome. However, it is not unusual for the nephrotic syndrome to coexist, at least to some degree, with other major renal syndromes such as acute and chronic renal failure or the acute nephritic syndrome, or even, if moderate to heavy proteinuria is its only manifestation, in the form of the syndrome of abnormal urinalysis alone in asymptomatic individuals.

In childhood, the great majority of patients exhibit minimal change or nil disease on any analysis of renal biopsy specimens. This "lesion" is generally responsive to corticosteroid therapy; hence it has become an increasing practice to institute such therapy prior to a consideration of renal biopsy. If the child is unresponsive to appropriate treatment with corticosteroids, renal biopsy has often revealed the presence of focal glomerular sclerosis in many such patients. In adults, at least in North America and Western Europe, the histopathologic lesions of minimal change disease, membranous glomerulonephropathy, proliferative and membranoproliferative glomerulonephritis, and a miscellaneous group of lesions (including focal glomerular sclerosis) have been found with roughly equal frequencies.

The clinical settings in which the nephrotic syndrome may occur are myriad. They include acute proliferative glomerulonephritis of varied etiology, rapidly progressive glomerulonephritis (Goodpasture's syndrome, poststreptococcal or idiopathic), chronic glomerulonephritis of differing types (membranous and membranoproliferative disease, focal glomerular sclerosis, "IgA nephropathy"), systemic diseases (Henoch-Schönlein purpura, systemic lupus erythematosus, mixed cryoglobulinemia, polyarteritis, neoplasia, diabetes mellitus, malignant hypertension, sickle cell disease, amyloidosis), constrictive pericarditis, renal vein thrombosis, congestive heart failure, exposure to specific "toxins" (drugs, heavy metals, and "allergens"), pregnancy, hemolytic-uremic syndrome, thrombotic thrombocytopenic purpura, renal transplant rejection, and others. Renal biopsy can be most useful in the evaluation of these patients.

URINARY TRACT INFECTION

This is perhaps the most common of all of the major renal syndromes. It is the consequence of the presence of significant numbers of pathogenic bacteria in the urinary tract, usually gram-negative organisms which derive from the gastrointestinal tract.

The clinical manifestations of this "syndrome" are varied. Actually, it is a group of syndromes rather than a single one. Its manifestations can range from those of an asymptomatic urinary tract infection to those of a destructive infectious process within the renal parenchyma which leads to chronic renal failure. Symptoms such as dysuria, urgency, frequency, fever, chill, and flank pain may all serve to indicate the presence of urinary tract infection. It is important to recognize that this syndrome can coexist with all the other seven clinical renal syndromes, either as a primary or secondary event.

Quantitative laboratory criteria for the diagnosis of "significant" urinary tract infection are now reasonably clear. Nevertheless, considerable difficulty still surrounds our attempts to distinguish between upper and lower tract infection, to relate the presence of infection to the sometimes obscure symptoms of the patient, to establish the relationship between antecedent urinary tract infection and the subsequent appearance of chronic interstitial nephritis, and to establish the long-term adequacy of a given program of treatment. Our ability to differentiate between upper and lower tract sites of infection has perhaps been improved by recent attempts to relate the site of infection to various humoral responses to bacterial infection (changes of serum antibody titers and the presence of an immunoglobulin coating or urinary bacteria may accompany renal parenchymal involvement). Lastly, more recent reexaminations have suggested that chronic interstitial nephritis may be an infrequent consequence of antecedent bacterial infection, at least in the absence of underlying structural abnormalities of the genitourinary tract or systemic diseases such as diabetes mellitus. At present, the major documented importances of urinary tract infection include its high incidence of discomfort and incapacitation with resultant loss of work, the need to exclude structural abnormalities of the genitourinary tract in its presence, its propensity to lead to urolithiasis or sepsis, and its ability to lead to further impairment of renal function (either directly or indirectly) when superimposed on already existent kidney disease.

URINARY TRACT OBSTRUCTION

This syndrome can be an important cause of chronic renal failure. Its initial clinical presentation may also encompass the syndromes of acute renal failure, urinary tract infection, or abnormal urinalysis alone. Its influences on renal function are variable, dependent upon its duration and whether it is bilateral or unilateral, partial or complete, and so forth. On the one hand, it may lead to progressive renal damage and end-stage kidney disease; on the other, its major manifestations may be limited solely to various radiographic and anatomic abnormalities without measurable impact on filtration rate.

Urinary tract obstruction can occur at any site along the outflow tract between the renal pelvis and the urethra. Bilateral acute ureteral obstruction can mimic the syndrome of acute renal failure, and its presence must always be sought in any patient with unexplained anuria. The intraluminal precipitation of crystals or protein within the nephrons of the renal parenchyma (e.g., the precipitation of uric acid crystals during acute hyperuricemia) is not always listed among the causes of acute obstruction, and its existence should be so acknowledged. Chronic obstructive uropathy has many causes ranging from urolithiasis to tumor, all of which are outlined fully in Ch. 382. It is important to recognize that the presence of chronic obstruction can be heralded by rather typical symptoms or by a complete lack thereof.

A diagnosis of lower tract obstruction is most often established first by the demonstration of urinary retention in the bladder or incomplete bladder emptying after micturition. Recently, a number of noninvasive techniques have been introduced to facilitate this diagnosis. Ultimately, urologic evaluation will most likely be necessary before the work-up can be completed. The symptoms of lower tract obstruction are often characterized by a slow urinary stream, dribbling after the completion of micturition, and hesitancy at its onset. A diagnosis of upper tract obstruction is most often established by the visualization of dilatation of the outflow tract proximal to a point of obstruction, cautiously utilizing intravenous high-dose urography as the first diagnostic step. Its causes and management are documented fully in Ch. 378 and 382.

DEFECTS OF RENAL TUBULAR FUNCTION

This category more properly encompasses a collection of separate conditions rather than a distinct clinical syndrome. It represents a constellation of disorders, many of which are familial or hereditary in origin, in which abnormalities of tubular structure or function dominate the clinical picture. Glomerular insufficiency, characterized by progressive filtration rate reduction, may occur in some but not all of them. Collectively, the clinical manifestations of these disorders are innumerable, largely reflecting the multiplicity of discrete functions of the renal tubule.

Anatomic defects include the cystic diseases of the kidneys such as medullary sponge kidney, isolated renal cysts, polycystic kidney disease, and microcystic disease of the renal medulla. Defects of renal tubular function include renal tubular acidosis (both proximal and distal), renal glucosuria, hypophosphatemia, aminoaciduria and hypouricemia, and nephrogenic diabetes insipidus. In sum, these defects reflect impaired renal tubular secretion, impaired reabsorption, or impaired renal tubular responsiveness to hormonal or other control systems.

Defects in proximal or distal hydrogen ion secretion can lead to impaired acid excretion and systemic acidosis; defects in the renal handling of potassium and urate may lead to altered plasma concentrations of those solutes. Defective glucose reabsorption may occur ˙ ne or in combination with other defects (altered acid ˙ tion and defective handling of phosphate, amino

acids, and uric acid). When the latter defects are seen collectively, they are often described as Fanconi's syndrome. Defective sodium reabsorption may be seen in microcystic disease of the renal medulla. Idiopathic hypercalciuria, at least in some patients, may well be due to defective reabsorption of calcium. Nephrogenic diabetes insipidus, leading to polyuria, is a general term which merely indicates that the renal tubule is unresponsive to vasopressin, either partly or completely. The condition may be familial or acquired.

Whatever the nature of the assumed functional disorder, it may sometimes be difficult to determine whether the defect is the consequence of an intrinsic alteration of renal tubular epithelial function, or the secondary manifestation of a normal response to an exaggerated control system. For example, idiopathic hypercalciuria could reflect either an intrinsic defect of renal tubular function or a normal response to secondary hyperparathyroidism consequent to the defective intestinal absorption of calcium. Similarly, renal tubular function may actually be intact, but increased excretion of a given solute may reflect nothing more than its increased concentration in plasma ("overflow" excretion). The evaluation of this family of disorders requires detailed insight into the physiologic nature and control of discrete tubular functions and their interrelationships. The clinical features and management of each such disorder are discussed fully in subsequent chapters.

AHA Council on the Kidney in Cardiovascular Disease: Criteria for the evaluation of the severity of established renal disease. Arch. Intern. Med., 128:304, 1971.

Derow, H. A.: The diagnostic value of serial measurements of albuminuria in ambulatory patients. N. Engl. J. Med., 227:827, 1942.

Glassock, R. J., and Bennett, C. M.: The glomerulopathies. In Brenner, B. M., and Rector, F. C. (eds.): The Kidney. Philadelphia, W. B. Saunders Company, 1976.

Howards, S. H., and Wright, F. S.: Obstructive injury. In Brenner, B. M., and Rector, F. C. (eds.): The Kidney. Philadelphia, W. B. Saunders Company, 1976.

Levinsky, N. G., and Alexander, E. A.: Acute renal failure. In Brenner, B. M., and Rector, F. C. (eds.): The Kidney. Philadelphia, W. B. Saunders Company, 1976.

Morris, R. C., McInnes, R. R., Epstein, C. J., Sebastian, A., and Schriver, C. R.: Genetic and metabolic injury of the kidney. In Brenner, B. M., and Rector, F. C. (eds.): The Kidney. Philadelphia, W. B. Saunders Company, 1976.

Robinson, R. R.: Proteinuria in asymptomatic patients. In Proceedings, 5th International Congress of Nephrology. Basel, S. Karger, 1974.

Thomas, V., Shelokov, A., and Forland, M.: Antibody-coated bacteria in the urine and the site of urinary tract infection. N. Engl. J. Med., 290:588, 1974.

369.4.   INVESTIGATION OF RENAL FUNCTION

D. N. S. Kerr

The common effects of disease on the renal parenchyma are increased excretion of protein and of the formed elements in urine, reduction in renal blood flow and glomerular filtration rate, impairment of tubular reabsorption and secretion, alteration in the secretion rates of erythropoietin and renin, and disordered metabolism of vitamin D. Renal prostaglandin secretion is altered in Bartter's syndrome; measurement of urinary and plasma prostaglandins is employed in its diagnosis but is otherwise a research tool. Plasma renin and angiotensin are studied almost exclusively in the investigation of hypertension. Measurement of plasma erythropoietin and 1,25-hydroxycholecalciferol is confined to a few research laboratories. Individual tubular functions, other than concentrating power, are tested in the investigation of renal tubular acidosis, other inherited and acquired tubular disorders, and renal calculous disease; the appropriate tests are discussed in the chapters dealing with these subjects.

PROTEINURIA. The urine of normal adults contains about 40 to 100 mg of protein per 24 hours during sedentary activity. The very low concentrations in normal urine are difficult to measure accurately, and the mean figure quoted varies widely. Conventionally the upper limit of normal is taken as 150 mg per 24 hours in the ambulant subject and 0.03 mg per minute during short periods of recumbency. The most sensitive screening test for urinary protein is the formation of a white cloud on heating filtered urine saturated with sodium sulfate and acidified with a few drops of 3 per cent acetic acid; this detects 5 to 10 mg per 100 ml as a faint trace. A definite positive with any clinical test therefore indicates a protein concentration higher than the normal subject should achieve at rest or during sedentary activity.

All such screening tests have a considerable observer error. The formation of a white cloud with 25 per cent salicylsulfonic acid is simpler than the heat test, and this compensates for its slightly lower sensitivity and for the false positives caused by radiographic contrast media in urine. The most popular test is the appearance of a green color on paper impregnated with bromophenol blue (Albustix, Labstix). It is more sensitive to albumin than to other urinary proteins and may fail to detect hemoglobin, myoglobin, and Bence Jones protein; it should therefore be used in conjunction with salicylsulfonic acid if anything other than glomerular proteinuria is suspected. It gives false positive results with high urinary pH (usually because of bacterial breakdown of urea) or heavy excretion of ascorbic acid (taken as the vitamin or as excipient in other medicines). However, if its limitations are recognized, it is a reliable test; patients taught to test their own urine (e.g., for recurrent nephrotic syndrome) seldom misinterpret it.

The four shades on the color scale of Albustix and Labstix correspond roughly to protein concentrations of 30, 100, 300, and 1000 mg per 100 ml, but the middle part of the range is unreliable. A more accurate quantitative test for proteinuria is needed but has proved elusive since it must measure a heterogeneous group of proteins in a very variable solvent. The reference Kjeldahl method is too tedious. A turbidimetric method, using salicylsulfonic acid and comparing the sample with an aqueous albumin standard, is very simple but it underestimates proteinuria, partly because it is insensitive to globulins. An automated biuret method is the most popular, but interfering substances must be removed and most urine samples concentrated for accurate results.

Normal urinary protein contains at least 30 components, the largest of which is a high molecular weight mucoprotein, called *Tamm-Horsfall protein*, which originates in the ascending limb of Henle's loop and the macula densa segment of the distal convoluted tubule. Precipitation of this protein in the distal tubule forms the matrix of renal casts. Other components include plasma proteins, with albumin the most prominent, and several proteins derived from the prostate and seminal vesicle. The normal glomerulus is a highly selective filter which virtually excludes from the urine plasma proteins above the weight of albumin. Smaller weight proteins such as β_2-microglobulin (11,800 daltons), retinol-binding protein (21,000), and light chains (22,500) are freely filtered at the glomerulus but largely reabsorbed in the tubule; they are present in trace amounts in normal urine and increased amounts when the tubules are damaged. The increased concentration in urine, relative to albumin, can be shown for all small plasma proteins by polyacrylamide gel electrophoresis of concentrated urine. Alternatively, albumin can be compared with a single small protein, usually β_2-microglobulin, by radioimmunoassay. This pattern is referred to as *tubular proteinuria*. The presence of larger molecular weight plasma proteins, such as IgG and α_2-macroglobulin, in urine indicates a "leaky" glomerulus. Albuminuria with an admixture of these larger proteins is called *glomerular proteinuria* and is the common finding in most renal diseases.

Isolated tubular proteinuria rarely exceeds 1 gram per 24 hours. It is an uncommon finding characteristic of congenital tubular disorders, Wilson's disease, Balkan nephropathy, and intoxication with cadmium, aminoglycosides, and other tubular poisons. It is found less constantly in hypokalemia, sarcoidosis, transplant rejection, and active pyelonephritis. Proteinuria in chronic pyelonephritis is usually glomerular. A combination of glomerular proteinuria and increased excretion of small plasma proteins, resulting from tubular damage, is found in late renal failure and in severe nephrotic syndrome.

Increased protein excretion occurs during heavy exertion. It is due partly to increased glomerular permeability and partly to impaired tubular reabsorption. It subsides rapidly and usually disappears within 24 hours but is a common cause of positive screening test results, particularly in children and young adults. Fever causes a tubular proteinuria which disappears as fever subsides, but febrile illnesses are also often accompanied by a more persistent glomerular proteinuria, attributed to immune-complex deposition. Emotional stress, operative trauma, exposure to extreme heat and cold, and cardiac failure can all cause proteinuria in previously normal subjects. It is often below 500 mg per 24 hours and rarely above 1 gram per 24 hours except in severe heart failure.

Proteinuria is detected in about 5 per cent of children and adolescents at school medical examinations; most of the "positives" prove to have benign exercise or postural proteinuria. Nearly all adolescents and about 50 per cent of young adults can produce proteinuria by adopting a lordotic position, e.g., bent backward over a chair. The proteinuria may be heavy but is of no pathologic significance. It is attributed to temporary obstruction of the renal venous outflow. About 5 per cent of adolescents and a few young adults develop proteinuria simply from standing erect. Postural or lordotic proteinuria is often benign (see Ch. 369.3).

Persistent proteinuria is always pathologic. Even if there is no other evidence of renal disorder, biopsy usually reveals glomerular or vascular disease, although often of a nonprogressive type. Glomerular proteinuria can be classified according to the "leakiness" of the glomerular filter. The normal glomerulus allows macromolecules to enter the urine in proportion to the logarithm

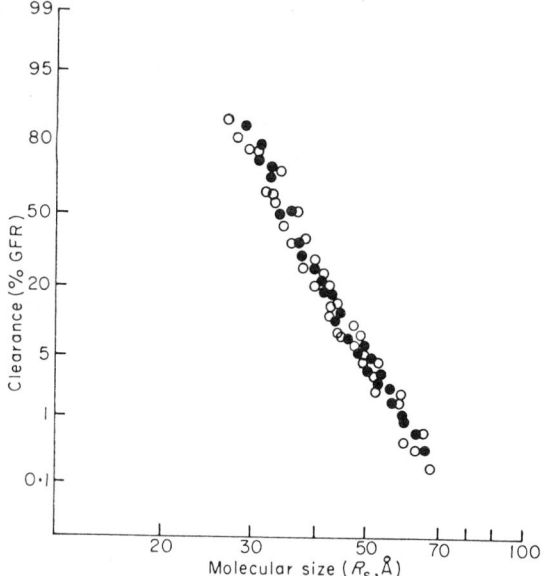

Figure 1. Relationship between the molecular size and the glomerular clearance of large polymers (○ = allyl-dextran; ● = polyvinylpyrrolidone) in normal rabbits. (From Hardwicke, J., et al.: Clin. Sci., 34:509, 1968.)

of their molecular size (Fig. 1). This relationship still holds approximately when the glomerulus becomes excessively leaky, but the slope of the graph varies. It is steep in nephrotic syndrome with minimal change so that only the smaller plasma proteins such as albumin enter the urine in detectable quantities (Fig. 2). In most

other glomerular diseases the graph is less steep and very large molecules such as α_2-macroglobulin can be detected in the urine. The slope of the graph can be estimated by measuring the clearance of two proteins, e.g., albumin and IgG. In practice the ratio of their clearances is simply calculated as a "selectivity index." The main value of this test is to confirm the diagnosis of childhood nephrotic syndrome with minimal change. Highly selected proteinuria makes a response to corticosteroids so likely that a renal biopsy may often be avoided.

URINE MICROSCOPY. Midstream urine should be collected with the same precautions as for culture. It should be examined with a well maintained microscope equipped with a variable illuminator and preferably a polarizer. A drop of fresh unspun urine should be examined first for bacteria and white cells. The urine should then be concentrated by centrifuging 10 ml at 3000 rpm for ten minutes and resuspending the sediment in the last 0.5 ml of urine, or by allowing the sample to stand in a test tube for half an hour and withdrawing the sediment with a Pasteur pipette. A drop of Sternheimer's stain can be added to aid identification of cells but is not essential. A well spread thick drop should be studied under low power for casts and crystals and the casts identified exactly by switching to medium power. A thin drop beneath a cover slip should be examined for red cells and white cells. These are readily confused with one another under low power, and even experienced observers have difficulty in distinguishing scanty red cells from oxalate crystals, talcum powder, and yeasts.

Red cells are normally excreted at a rate of about 150 to 300,000 per 24 hours, with an approximate upper limit of 1000 per minute in short collection periods. Only an occasional red cell should be seen during qualitative microscopy as described above. White cells are excreted at an average of about 70,000 per hour in both sexes, but this applies only to urine entirely free of vulval contamination, as shown by virtual absence of squamous epithelial cells. In contaminated urine leukocyturia cannot be interpreted unless it is very heavy. The upper limit of normal leukocyte excretion is 200,000 per hour, which yields one or two leukocytes per high power field in qualitative microscopy of a concentrated urine. Renal tubular cells appear in the urine in diseases such as tubular necrosis and after consumption of several drugs, notably aspirin. They can be distinguished from leukocytes when stained but are so similar in unstained preparations that they are usually counted as leukocytes.

Hyaline casts consist of precipitated Tamm-Horsfall protein only; they have a refractive index close to that of urine and are easily missed if the illumination is too high. Up to 10,000 per 24 hours are excreted by normal subjects, but at this rate only a very occasional one is seen in the thick drop. Numerous hyaline casts are seen in nearly all renal diseases which cause glomerular proteinuria. Most hyaline casts are of roughly constant diameter, corresponding to that of the convoluted tubule; but short, thick casts formed in the collecting duct and misshapen, long, and branching casts are seen in chronic renal disease. The description of thick casts as "renal failure casts" is an overinterpretation; they have no close correlation with renal function. Clear casts with angular ends and a tendency to fracture on bending are called waxy casts; they occur in renal disease,

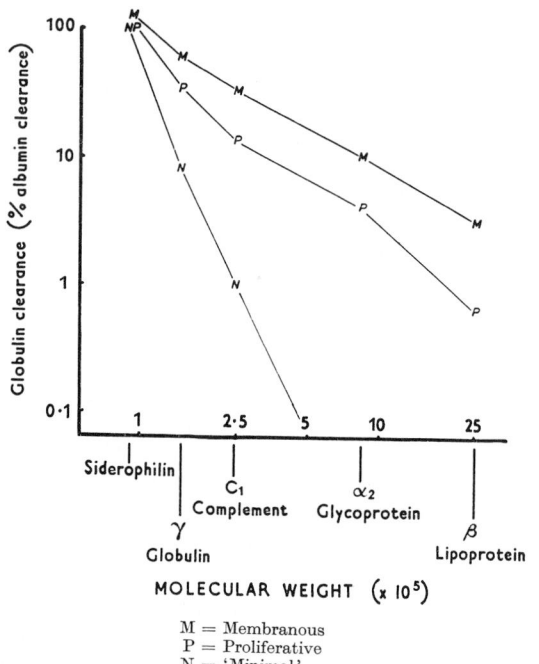

M = Membranous
P = Proliferative
N = 'Minimal'

Figure 2. Relationship between molecular weight and relative clearance of plasma proteins in three patients with nephrotic syndrome and different histology. In large series there is complete overlap between the results for membranous and proliferaglomerulonephritis but clear distinction from minimal e. (From Blainey, J. D., et al.: Quart. J. Med., 34:235, 1959.)

and their origin is uncertain. Numerous hyaline casts without any of the other varieties described below are seen in benign essential hypertension.

Granular casts are speckled due to the presence of albumin, immunoglobulin, and lipoprotein aggregates in a matrix of Tamm-Horsfall protein. Lightly speckled casts appear in normal urine after strenuous exercise or during fever; when present in the resting, afebrile subject, they nearly always indicate renal disease. Densely granular casts, which may appear almost black on microscopy, and which are readily confused with red cell casts if the granules are large, are always a sign of renal disease and are commonly found in active glomerulonephritis, lupus nephritis, malignant hypertension, amyloidosis, and diabetic nephropathy. Deeply pigmented granular casts are found in association with hemoglobinuria and in the brown urine that is often excreted in the early stages of acute renal failure. Bile-stained granular casts are excreted in large numbers by patients with obstructive jaundice, often without any other evidence of renal disease.

Red blood cell casts have greater diagnostic significance than any other variety. They usually indicate glomerular bleeding and are excreted in very large numbers in the acute phase of post-streptococcal nephritis or in rapidly progressive (crescent) nephritis. Smaller numbers are excreted in other forms of glomerulonephritis, notably in membranoproliferative, dense deposit, and the focal nephritis of Henoch-Schönlein syndrome, in polyarteritis, and in malignant hypertension. When packed with red cells they have a reddish tinge, but more often they contain a few red cells which give a greenish tinge under tungsten light. They can be distinguished from other cellular casts by the fact that the red cells are incorporated in the matrix; this can be confirmed by focusing up and down through the cast under medium or high power. *Leukocyte casts* are typical of acute pyelonephritis. They are not found in chronic interstitial nephritis with sterile urine, in which the deposit usually contains only a few leukocytes if the patient is normotensive. *Epithelial cell casts* are typical of acute tubular necrosis but are also common in glomerulonephritis and amyloidosis. *Fatty casts*, staining red with Sudan III and showing "Maltese crosses" in polarized light, accompany heavy proteinuria and are probably due to leakage of lipoproteins across the glomerular filter. Free fat globules and oval fat bodies — degenerate tubular cells in which "Maltese crosses" are best seen — are typical of nephrotic syndrome.

The recognition of casts is an important step in establishing the existence of renal disease. It is particularly helpful in distinguishing the proteinuria of renal disease from benign orthostatic proteinuria, and the investigation of hematuria, in which it indicates a probable renal source and the need to start investigation with pyelography and renal biopsy rather than cystoscopy. It is complementary to tests for proteinuria in seeking evidence of renal involvement in systemic disease. There would be fewer reports of "glomerular involvement with normal urinary deposit" if all authors had to certify that they had performed the microscopy in person and to detail the technique. Casts have some value as a sign of activity of disease, e.g., during the treatment of lupus nephritis. However, their prognostic value is limited. Excessive excretion of hyaline and lightly granular casts can continue for decades in inactive diseases such as treated essential hypertension,

gouty nephropathy, or nonprogressive glomerulonephritis. The disappearance of red cell and densely granular casts from the deposit as malignant hypertension is treated points to essential hypertension as the primary disorder; red cell casts strongly favor glomerulonephritis as the cause of acute renal failure; and red cell or epithelial cell casts in nephrotic syndrome make minimal change unlikely. Otherwise casts play only a minor role in differential diagnosis between renal disorders.

GLOMERULAR FILTRATION RATE. If a substance is filtered at the glomerulus in proportion to plasma water, and is not reabsorbed or secreted by the tubule, it can be used to estimate glomerular filtration rate (GFR) by the formula:

$$\text{GFR (clearance of marker substance)} = \frac{\text{excretion rate}}{\text{plasma level}}$$

The best established marker substance is *inulin*, a mixture of fructose polymers with an average molecular weight of 5200. It is a variable mixture of low solubility, it hydrolyzes to fructose during the boiling necessary to dissolve it, its measurement is difficult, and it requires about two hours of infusion before a stable plasma level is achieved. Accurate measurement of the excretion rate requires bladder catheterization or multiple voided samples over several hours, so it is clearly a research tool of limited value in the clinic. The need for urine collection can be eliminated if inulin is infused long enough to ensure that the plasma level is completely stable. The infusion rate is then assumed to equal excretion rate, the small extrarenal excretion of inulin being ignored.

Inulin has now been largely replaced by other substances which are nearly as good as markers of glomerular filtration and are easier to measure. ^{51}Cr-EDTA has been most fully studied; it has an extrarenal excretion of about 4 ml per minute in adults in health and disease. Other popular agents are [131/125]I-diacetrizoate, ^{125}I-iothalamate, and ^{99m}Tc-Sn-DPTA. All are given intravenously in a single shot, and the plasma level is followed by external counting over the heart; after an initial equilibration period, it falls exponentially and the slope of the line is a measure of GFR. Alternatively ^{125}I-iothalamate can be given subcutaneously to produce a roughly constant plasma level and urine collected between two plasma samples. Complete bladder emptying is checked by counting over the bladder. Both methods are acceptable to patients and have a reproducibility of ± 5 per cent. This is sufficient for clinical purposes since GFR is subject to a diurnal variation of ± 10 per cent, reaching its peak in the afternoon and its trough during the night, and is readily disturbed by exercise or emotional upset. However, since these methods are expensive and demand an extra visit to the medical physics department, they are not suitable for following the week-to-week fluctuations in renal disease.

For this purpose the most popular test has been the *endogenous creatinine clearance*. Plasma creatinine is virtually constant throughout the 24 hours, so a single plasma sample can be compared with a long urinary collection. The method can be used on outpatients provided that the instructions for collecting a 24-hour urine are stressed by the physician until the patient can recite them. However, creatinine clearance incorporates the errors of timing, bladder emptying, urinary washout, and measurement of plasma and urinary creatin-

Figure 3. Roughly linear decline in GFR with time in chronic renal disease. GFR was calculated from serum creatinine by the formula shown in the table.

ine, and it has proved poorly reproducible. In one careful study it varied by ± 27 per cent above a GFR of 30 ml per minute and ± 22 per cent below that figure. It overestimates GFR considerably and unpredictably in renal failure, in nephrotic syndrome, and after renal transplantation. Although force of habit maintains its popularity, it should eventually disappear from routine clinical practice. It will retain a role in those patients who are unsuitable for the radioactive methods (pregnant women, those with severe edema) or for indirect estimation of GFR from plasma creatinine (the obese, those with near normal renal function). When a single estimate of renal function is required, it should be performed on two or three consecutive 24-hour collections to cancel out bladder-emptying errors.

The *plasma creatinine* concentration is determined by the production rate, which is largely a reflection of muscle mass, and the excretion rate, which is roughly proportional to GFR. In a patient whose muscle mass is not changing rapidly, alterations in plasma creatinine are determined almost exclusively by changes in GFR; diet and fluid intake have very little effect. When plasma creatinine is greater than 1.0 mg per 100 ml (88 μmol per liter) its measurement presents few difficulties, and it is much more convenient than the creatinine clearance. It is therefore used by most nephrologists as their day-to-day guide to renal function. The relationship to GFR is hyperbolic; a large change in GFR produces a small change in plasma creatinine near the normal range, whereas a small change in GFR produces a large change in plasma creatinine in late renal failure. Since most patients with chronic renal disease lose GFR at a roughly constant rate (Fig. 3), a slow rise in plasma creatinine changes to a sharp upswing in the last few months of the illness, and this catches even experienced physicians off guard. It is one argument for converting plasma creatinine into an estimate of GFR and plotting the results, as in Figure 3.

The conversion requires an estimate of creatinine production which is made from body weight, age, and sex — three determinants of muscle mass. The accompanying table shows the formula of Cockcroft and Gault derived from 249 patients. A similar formula gave an estimate of GFR which agreed more closely with EDTA clearance than did measured creatinine clearance and had less than half the day-to-day variability. Calculation of GFR from plasma creatinine has two main uses: to follow the progress of chronic renal failure and to control drug therapy. For the former purpose many cli-

nicians do not bother to estimate GFR but merely plot the reciprocal of serum creatinine, which is proportional to GFR. However, the full calculation takes little more time and is preferable. Ideally it should be corrected for the extrarenal clearance of creatinine (probably into the gut), which is about 3 ml per minute on average. The correction is unimportant until terminal renal failure, when failure to apply it can cause an important overestimate of renal function. When drug therapy is required by the patient with renal impairment, an accurate, recent measurement of GFR is often unavailable, but plasma creatinine can be measured within an hour and used to calculate the required dose. The calculation is valid only if plasma creatinine is not changing rapidly, and this should be checked 12 to 24 hours after the start of drug therapy.

Plasma urea should no longer be used as the main guide to renal function. Under stable conditions of diet, lean body mass, and fluid intake it has a roughly hyperbolic relationship to GFR in the same manner as plasma creatinine, but the curve is distorted in late renal failure by a rise in urea clearance relative to GFR and by extrarenal removal of urea. Moreover stable conditions are not common in clinical practice, and plasma urea is readily affected by variations in protein intake and in net body catabolism or anabolism caused by trauma, infection, inactivity, refeeding, the anabolic phase after acute illness, and drug therapy, particularly with corticosteroids. Plasma urea falls during a water diuresis and fluctuates appreciably during the 24 hours under the influence of food and drink. However, plasma urea should still be measured as an index of the retention of those substances which are produced in response to protein ingestion. The ratio of plasma urea to plasma creatinine has some diagnostic significance. Plasma urea rises preferentially during water or sodium and water depletion, diuretic therapy, and heart failure, whereas plasma urea and creatinine rise together in established renal failure.

RENAL BLOOD FLOW. Renal blood flow can be measured as the clearance of a substance which is both filtered at the glomerulus and secreted by the tubule, so that it is cleared completely from the blood in one passage through the kidney. In health, para-aminohippurate (PAH) approaches this ideal, since 92 per cent of the circulating PAH is removed from blood traversing the kidney. It is easy to measure and it equilibrates rapidly so that prolonged infusion is not required. PAH clearance is therefore a useful test for studying renal blood flow in the normal, and it has been used to show that renal blood flow varies more widely than GFR with exercise and emotion but has

Formula for Calculating Creatinine Clearance from Serum Creatinine*

Males:

$$\text{Creatinine clearance (ml/min)} = \frac{(140 - \text{age in years}) \times \text{weight in kg}}{72 \times \text{serum creatinine in mg per 100 ml}}$$

$$= \frac{(140 - \text{age in years}) \times \text{weight in kg}}{0.82 \times \text{serum creatinine in } \mu\text{mole per liter}}$$

Females:
Same minus 15 per cent.

(A nomogram for converting serum creatinine to creatinine clearance is illustrated in the article by Kerr and Davison, 1975.)

*From Cockcroft, D. W., and Gault, M. H.: Nephron, 16:31, 1976.

about the same and parallel diurnal variation. However, in renal disease PAH extraction is often well below 92 per cent, so PAH clearance becomes an unreliable guide to renal blood flow unless a renal vein catheter is inserted to measure renal venous blood PAH, which is rarely justifiable. Similar criticisms apply to the use of $^{125/131}$I-hippuran clearance, which can be measured at the same time as GFR, if two different isotopes are selected and by the same techniques. These limitations are ignored in much current literature which reports the ratio "iothalamate clearance:hippuran clearance" as "filtration fraction." However, if the ratio is accepted as an empirical observation, it may still be useful in differential diagnosis; there is some evidence that a high "filtration fraction," so defined, is typical of renal transplant rejection and helpful in differentiating it from other causes of renal impairment in the post-transplant period.

CORRECTION FOR BODY SIZE. GFR and renal blood flow are both determined by body size, and surface area correlates with them better than other parameters such as height and weight in the adult. They are therefore corrected to a standard surface area of 1.73 square meters before comparison with the normal range. A nomogram for calculating surface area is published in Documenta Geigy. In infants under one year the GFR and renal blood flow are low in relationship to surface area, but this is probably a reflection of the high surface area of the infant rather than of a reduced renal reserve. On other criteria, e.g., using body surface area as standard, the GFR reaches adult proportions at about one month. Both GFR and renal blood flow rise in pregnancy, reaching a peak of about 150 per cent of nonpregnant normal at 36 weeks, and there is a corresponding fall in plasma creatinine starting early in pregnancy; plasma urea has a more pronounced fall because of anabolism. It is essential to compare results with the normal range for that stage of gestation (see Lindheimer and Katz). Glomerular filtration rate and renal plasma flow both decline with age. In men, mean GFR falls from about 125 ml per minute at age 40 to about 60 ml per minute at age 90 in a roughly linear manner but with a wide scatter. Normal ranges at different ages are illustrated by Wesson. The fall with age in women is not so well documented and probably slower.

URINARY CONCENTRATING POWER. The ability to concentrate the urine is impaired as the population of nephrons declines, and it is seldom worthwhile testing concentrating power at a GFR less than 30 ml per minute. It is reduced disproportionately in chronic pyelonephritis and particularly in analgesic nephropathy and has some value in differentiating them, and other diseases primarily affecting the medulla, from chronic glomerulonephritis. The concentration test has often been described as a sensitive index of early renal damage, but the reproducibility is so low, and the normal range so wide, that it cannot be more than a crude index. Its usefulness in detecting early disease is probably confined to patients obliged to take nephrotoxic analgesics, in whom a change in concentrating ability often precedes a fall in GFR or a change in the pyelogram.

To obtain maximal concentration reliably it is necessary to deprive the patient of fluid for more than 24 hours, which makes the test unpleasant, inapplicable to outpatients, and dangerous in renal failure. Three simpler tests are therefore used to give a rough idea of concentrating ability. (1) *Early morning urine.* If one or

more of several early morning samples, taken without special precautions, have an osmolality over 700 mOsm per kilogram, it is unlikely that there is an important defect in concentrating ability. (2) *The 16-hour test.* Fluid is withheld from 4 P.M. and a dry supper administered. The bladder is emptied at 10 P.M. and all samples collected until 8 A.M. Breakfast and morning drinks are not given until 8 A.M. One of the samples should have an osmolality of 700 mOsm per kilogram or over. (3) *Desmopressin test.* This has replaced the Pitressin test. Desmopressin is given intranasally in a dose of 40 μg at 5 P.M., and the last evening and first morning urines are tested. Omission of drinks in the evening increases the maximal osmolality only slightly and is probably unnecessary. Although 700 mOsm per kilogram is accepted conventionally as the criterion of normality in all these tests, the result should be corrected for age, since concentrating power declines with age even more rapidly than GFR. Healthy young adults consistently achieve over 800 mOsm per kilogram (mean over 1000) in the desmopressin test, whereas a result of 600 mOsm per kilogram is acceptable in those over 50.

Bröchner-Mortensen, J., and Rödbro, P.: Selection of routine method for determination of glomerular filtration rate in adult patients. Scand. J. Clin. Lab. Invest., 36:35, 1976.

Cockcroft, D. W., and Gault, M. H.: Prediction of creatinine clearance from serum creatinine. Nephron, 16:31, 1976.

Kerr, D. N. S., and Davison, J. M.: The assessment of renal function. Br. J. Hosp. Med., 14:360, 1975.

Lindheimer, M. D., and Katz, A. I.: Kidney Function and Disease in Pregnancy. Philadelphia, Lea & Febiger, 1977.

Monson, J. P., and Richards, P.: Desmopressin urine concentration test. Br. Med. J., 1:24, 1978.

Rutherford, W. E., Blondin, J., Miller, J. P., Greenwalt, A. S., and Vavra, J. D.: Chronic progressive renal disease: Rate of change of serum creatinine concentration. Kidney Int., 11:62, 1977.

Spencer, E. S., and Pedersen, I.: Hand Atlas of the Urinary Sediment. 2nd ed. Copenhagen, Munksgaard, 1976.

Wesson, L. G., Jr.: Physiology of the Human Kidney. New York, Grune & Stratton, 1969.

369.5. INVESTIGATION OF RENAL STRUCTURE AND REGIONAL FUNCTION

D. N. S. Kerr

PLAIN RADIOGRAPHY (Fig. 4). A straight roentgenogram of the kidneys, ureters, and bladder is referred to as a KUB. It is an essential preliminary to pyelography, revealing the presence of radiopaque calculi and nephrocalcinosis which may be confused on the subsequent pyelogram. It is often of value in estimating renal size; if the renal outlines are obscured by overlying bowel shadows, they can often be revealed by tomography. Renal size is roughly proportional to the cube of renal length, so it is conventionally measured as the length along the axis of the kidney. This gives a more reliable indication of renal volume than does any method of estimating renal area, since the latter is affected by the variable rotation of the kidney about its vertical axis. The left kidney is normally about 1 cm longer than the right. Kidneys with a partial or complete duplex collecting system are elongated. Charts showing the normal renal lengths at different ages are distributed by Kodak Ltd. and are available in most departments of radiology.

Figure 4. Plain radiograph of the renal tract showing nephrocalcinosis due to congenital oxalosis.

INTRAVENOUS (EXCRETION) UROGRAPHY (Fig. 5). The renal tract is displayed by the intravenous injection of a contrast medium. The main agents in current use are diatrizoate, metrizoate, and iothalamate. They are all iodine-containing compounds that are largely excreted by glomerular filtration and that produce an osmotic diuresis. They are injected slowly, over at least two minutes, to avoid the unpleasant flush that accompanies rapid injection. A film taken at the end of the injection, or after one minute, shows opacification of the renal parenchyma by contrast medium in the renal blood vessels and tubules, an appearance known as a nephrogram. If renal function is normal, the nephrogram fades rapidly and has almost gone at 30 minutes,

contrast enters the urine and outlines the calyces and pelves by two to five minutes, and the ureters and bladder are displayed over the following 30 minutes. It is usual to blow up air bladders under a compression belt in the second half of the procedure, to compress the ureters at the pelvic brim and distend the upper collecting systems to improve calyceal detail. Finally the patient is asked to void, and a postmicturition film of the bladder area is taken to estimate the residual bladder urine. Interference from bowel gas and feces can be reduced by administering a purgative the day before the procedure, and contrast is improved by withholding fluids for 6 to 12 hours to ensure a fairly concentrated urine. However, the latter is not essential with modern agents and is strongly contraindicated in diabetes, myelomatosis, and renal failure.

If renal function is impaired, the dose of contrast medium must be increased; it can be given as a drip infusion or a single slow injection as convenient. Late films should be taken over several hours, as the nephrogram and pyelogram develop more slowly than normal. Tomograms are essential to visualize the kidneys if GFR is reduced to a few milliliters per minute. Late films are required in two other situations: acute renal failure and suspected obstruction. In acute renal failure, resulting from acute tubular necrosis, a nephrogram may appear which persists for many hours or even days, although it is by no means a constant finding. The greatly distended pelvis of a hydronephrotic kidney may be invisible on the 30-minute film because the contrast medium excreted by a poorly functioning kidney is diluted in a large pool of urine. A dense pyelogram may be visible on films taken at 12 or 24 hours.

The major uses of intravenous urography are to demonstrate the calyceal clubbing and renal scarring of chronic pyelonephritis; the sloughed or cavitated papillae of analgesic nephropathy; the cavitated papillae and strictured ureters of tuberculosis; the distortion of renal outline and draining system caused by renal tumors, cysts, and polycystic disease; the filling defects produced by nonopaque calculi and epithelial tumors of pelves, ureters, and bladder; distention of ureters and pelves from obstruction or vesicoureteral reflux; trabeculation and enlargement of the bladder from obstruction; indentation of the bladder by an enlarged pros-

Figure 5. Intravenous pyelogram showing normal right kidney and small left kidney with renal scarring and outdrawing of the calyces due to chronic pyelonephritis. Outlined in pencil for clarity.

tate; and displacement of kidneys, ureters, or bladder by extrinsic tumors or retroperitoneal fibrosis. In addition, intravenous urography is used to investigate hypertension; for this purpose early and late films are taken to show the late appearance and disappearance of a dense pyelogram on the side of a unilateral renal artery stenosis. In renal failure the demonstration of smoothly contracted kidneys indicates chronic renal disease. The urogram gives a crude indication of the relative function of the two kidneys, but this can be better assessed by isotopic studies.

Modern contrast media are less toxic than their predecessors of ten years ago. Fatal reactions to injection occur in about 1 in 40,000 procedures. The procedure should be avoided in patients with known iodine sensitivity. Acute renal failure is a well recognized complication in patients with diabetes, myelomatosis, dehydration, and renal failure, and it may be a complication of vascular disease and hypoproteinemia. In these conditions the benefits of the investigation must be carefully weighed against its hazards and renal function should be monitored in the few days after urography. Male gonads should be protected by lead shielding, but the ovaries are inevitably irradiated. The procedure is avoided if possible in the second half of the menstrual cycle of women in the childbearing age, and during pregnancy.

One limitation of this very versatile investigation is its failure to show the site of complete urinary obstruction. For this purpose there are two alternatives: retrograde and antegrade pyelography.

RETROGRADE PYELOGRAPHY. Under cystoscopic control, thin catheters are passed up both ureters. They will often slip past the site of obstruction and can be left in situ after the procedure to provide temporary drainage pending surgery. The urine above the obstruction is aspirated for chemical, bacteriologic, and cytologic study and is replaced by contrast medium. The catheters are usually passed under general anesthesia, but the injection is best given with the patient awake so that overdistention, signaled by discomfort or pain, can be avoided.

Retrograde pyelography provides excellent calyceal detail, so it is sometimes used in the absence of obstruction to demonstrate, for instance, separation of a papilla or a small nonopaque stone, when the intravenous urogram is equivocal. However, its complications include renal colic, transient obstruction of the ureter by edema, perforation of the pelvis, intrarenal extravasation of the contrast, and introduction of infection into the upper urinary tract, plus the hazards of anesthesia and cystoscopy, so it should be used only on specific indications.

ANTEGRADE PYELOGRAPHY. A thin tube is passed over an exploring needle into the renal pelvis, via the renal substance. The technique is similar to that of renal biopsy under fluoroscopic control. Urine is aspirated for culture, cytology, and chemistry; contrast is injected to show the site of obstruction; and the tube is left in as a temporary nephrostomy until the obstruction is relieved.

There is sometimes difficulty in differentiating between a renal pelvis distended by previous obstruction and one which is obstructed now. A prone film should be taken, since an unobstructed "baggy" pelvis will sometimes empty in this position and display the full length of the ureter. An injection of furosemide may

demonstrate an obstruction at high urine flow which is absent at the slow urinary flow of urography after dehydration. After antegrade pyelography, obstruction can be assessed accurately by measuring pelvic pressure at varying flow rates.

RENAL ARTERIOGRAPHY (Fig. 6). The aorta is catheterized by the Seldinger technique; a guide wire is threaded up the femoral artery, through a needle, and a radiopaque catheter is passed percutaneously over the guide wire, which is then withdrawn. A translumbar needle can be passed directly into the aorta but is more hazardous and is employed only if the iliac vessels are blocked or excessively tortuous. Contrast medium, similar to that used for pyelography but in higher dose, is injected rapidly into the aorta to show the origins of the renal arteries and display accessory arteries. If necessary, the catheter is then turned into each renal artery for a direct injection to display the smaller renal arteries more clearly. This selective arteriography exposes the kidney to a higher concentration of contrast medium and carries a greater risk of producing acute tubular necrosis or of displacing atheromatous material and causing the more serious complication of atheroembolism. It should therefore be used only when inadequate detail is shown by the aortic injection.

The main function of renal arteriography is to display abnormalities of the main renal arteries and their branches: stenosis, aneurysm, arteriovenous aneurysm, obstruction by embolism, thrombosis, or traumatic rupture of the intima. It is also used to display the normal vasculature of a renal donor before transplantation and to distinguish rejection from vascular occlusion or ischemic death of the kidney in the recipient. It is sometimes required to display damage to the kidney by trauma or to show the site of brisk hemorrhage. It is the final court of appeal in deciding whether a renal mass is a tumor or a more benign lesion; a pathologic tumor circulation is usually pathognomonic. It is a pro-

Figure 6. Renal arteriogram showing pathologic circulation in a hypernephroma.

Figure 7. "B" mode ultrasonic scan through a mass replacing the upper pole of the kidney. Clear area free of echoes indicates that this is a fluid-filled cyst.

ture of a slice through the trunk, in which the kidneys and renal blood vessels are clearly distinguished from the surrounding perinephric fat. Contrast can be further improved by intravenous injection of one of the agents used for intravenous urography. CAT scanning has been used to display renal tumors and cysts, to show tumor growth along the renal veins, and to show hydronephrosis and renal trauma. With growing experience and improving technique it will probably replace some of the more invasive tests as the equipment becomes widely available.

ULTRASONOGRAPHY (Fig. 7). The B-mode ultrasonic scan shows a two-dimensional view of the kidney in any plane. The features are produced by reflection of ultrasound at tissue boundaries and back-scatter effects which depend on variations in tissue structure. It is most useful in demonstrating collections of fluid such as hydronephrosis, renal cysts, lymphoceles, and perinephric abscesses. Cysts are shown as clear spaces with no internal echoes. The usual routine for investigating a renal mass is as follows: plain radiography, intravenous urography and ultrasonography. Then, according to the results, cyst puncture and injection of contrast, to confirm a smooth cyst, or arteriography, to confirm a tumor, may be utilized. Ultrasonography is about as sensitive as intravenous urography in detecting polycystic disease; since it involves no known hazards, discomfort, or ionizing radiation, it is the preferable technique for screening asymptomatic relatives of known patients. It gives an excellent demonstration of the bladder and can be used to give rapid confirmation of bladder tumors suspected on pyelography.

cedure involving discomfort, hospital admission, about a 1 per cent risk of acute renal failure, and a risk of femoral hematoma and femoral arterial occlusion, in addition to the hazards of rapid injection of contrast medium. Major risk factors are advanced atheroma, diabetes, and renal impairment.

RENAL VENOGRAPHY. Renal vein thrombosis in infancy is a spontaneous event at about the time of birth or a complication of acute illness; clinical diagnosis and demonstration of a nonfunctioning kidney on intravenous urography are often sufficient. If confirmation is needed, a contrast medium can be injected into the vena cava to show loss of the negative shadow caused by the stream of nonopacified blood from the renal vein, on one side. In the adult renal vein thrombosis is usually a complication of nephrotic syndrome and is often incomplete or confined to the smaller branches. It is best sought by retrograde injection of contrast medium into the renal vein through a Seldinger catheter inserted via the femoral vein.

COMPUTER-ASSISTED AXIAL TOMOGRAPHY. The whole-body CAT scanner provides an impressive pic-

RENAL SCINTIGRAPHY (Fig. 8). A linear scanner will construct a picture of the kidneys after the injection of a suitable radiopharmaceutical. [197]Hg Chlormerodrin and ^{99m}Tc-iron–ascorbic acid are retained in the tubules of functioning nephrons. There they emit gamma rays at a nearly constant rate for many hours after the radionuclide has been cleared from the blood. The scanner moves back and forth over the renal areas, recording the counting rates and drawing a density pattern which reflects functioning tissue. Negative shadows indicate areas of nonfunctioning tissue such as cysts and tumors. This technique gives a good demonstration of renal position and size, even in patients with very poor renal function who produce indistinct urograms. It gives an approximate indication of the relative contri-

Figure 8. Normal renal scan.

bution of the two kidneys to renal function. It is useful in demonstrating renal masses. However, it requires a cooperative patient who can lie still for 20 minutes at a stretch, and the picture is blurred by the inevitable respiratory movement. It has been largely replaced by the gamma camera scan wherever the more expensive apparatus is available.

RENOGRAPHY. A renogram is a tracing of the radioactivity detected over a kidney after injection of a radiopharmaceutical, usually ¹²⁵I-hippuran. Since hippuran is filtered at the glomerulus and secreted by the tubule, it is rapidly taken up by functioning renal tissue. A single scintillation counter is placed over each kidney and shielded by a lead collimator from the rays emitted by other organs, particularly the liver. The renogram has three phases: (1) A rapidly rising curve as radio-hippuran reaches the kidney in the bloodstream. (2) A slowly rising curve as it is concentrated in the tubules and pelvis, reaching a peak at about three minutes if renal function and hydration are normal. (3) A falling curve as the radio-hippuran is cleared from the kidney and its drainage system. The field of view of the counter includes the blood perfusing tissues above and below the kidney; a better representation of renal function is obtained if this blood background is subtracted by computer. For this purpose a third counter is required over the heart or some other organ that does not concentrate hippuran.

The main uses of the renogram are to detect urinary obstruction and renal artery stenosis. If obstruction is present, there is a prolonged second phase, a late peak, and a slow fall. This pattern is particularly helpful in detecting unilateral obstruction, e.g., complicating pelvic neoplasms or gynecologic surgery. However, it can also occur with a dilated but unobstructed drainage system and, symmetrically, in acute tubular necrosis. Since renography causes much less radiation exposure than urography, it is used to follow the response to surgery for urinary obstruction. Renal artery stenosis causes a late peak and slow fall if renal function is well preserved, and a flattened curve if it is severely compromised. The renogram is complementary to the intravenous urogram in detecting this cause of hypertension.

GAMMA CAMERA SCANNING (Fig. 9). The gamma camera is a large sodium iodide disc, about 30 cm in diameter, which detects the gamma rays emitted by the kidney after injection of a radiopharmaceutical. A flash of light is emitted where a ray strikes the crystal, is picked up by a bank of photomultiplier tubes above it, and is reproduced as a bright dot on a cathode ray tube with the aid of a computer. Since gamma rays cannot be focused like light rays, a picture of the kidney is obtained by one of two techniques. For quick pictures of low resolution, a perforated lead disc is placed below the crystal, so that rays emitted by one area of kidney affect the crystal only at points immediately above it. For slower pictures (about five minutes of exposure time) of better resolution, a "camera lucida" image is obtained through a pinhole collimator. The latter technique is better for detecting structural lesions such as cysts, the former for functional studies. The gamma camera gives a good estimate of the relative contribution of the two kidneys to total renal function, with an error of about ± 5 per cent. Total radioactivity in each kidney is estimated at a time when all of it should be in renal blood and tubules, none having escaped in the urine, about two minutes after injection for hippuran. Normally each kidney should contribute 42.5 to 57.5 per cent of total function. If one kidney is causing hypertension, pain, hematuria, or urinary infection, a knowledge of its individual contribution to renal function is of great help in deciding between a reparative operation and nephrectomy. The other main application of the gamma camera is the study of renal transplant function. The initial scan helps differentiate vascular occlusion from tubular necrosis and rejection, in both of which renal perfusion is preserved, and serial scans distinguish the improving function of recovering tubular necrosis from the deteriorating function of untreated rejection.

The dose of iodine given in all radioisotopic studies, as well as the radiation dose, is well below that used in intravenous urography; sensitivity reactions are uncommon, with a mortality of about one per million procedures.

RENAL BIOPSY. Percutaneous renal biopsy is performed under local anesthesia except in small children

Figure 9. Gamma camera scan of two kidneys showing multiple negative shadows due to polycystic disease.

and confused adults. Light sedation is desirable, but the patient should be able to hold his breath reliably on request. The kidney is located by intravenous urography, with a marking grid on the back, fluoroscopy, or sonography. The presence of two functioning kidneys should be confirmed; biopsy of a single kidney is carried out only after careful consideration. The sample is usually taken from the lower pole. Two types of needle are in common use: (1) The Vim-Silverman and the disposable Tru-cut have a central cutting needle and an outer sheath which is slid over it. (2) The Menghini is a hollow needle with a cutting edge which is inserted and withdrawn rapidly with suction applied; results are similar with the two types. The patient rests for 24 to 48 hours, and pulse, blood pressure, symptoms, and color of urine are recorded. Visible hematuria occurs after 10 per cent of biopsies, and microscopic hematuria is invariable. Major complications are perinephric hematoma, prolonged or heavy hematuria, clot colic, ureteral obstruction, and formation of an arteriovenous aneurysm. Bleeding causes about one death and one nephrectomy in every 5000 procedures. It is a more difficult technique than liver biopsy and should be performed only by those who do it regularly and have access to a good renal pathology service.

The biopsy should be subdivided for all possible examinations, since this procedure should not be repeated unnecessarily. The cut should be made under a dissecting microscope to ensure that both parts contain glomeruli. One sample is preserved in glutaraldehyde for light and electron microscopy; the other is sectioned on the cryostat and stained with fluorescein-labeled antibodies to IgG, IgA, IgM, C3, fibrinogen, and other proteins as necessary, for fluorescence microscopy. If tissue is scanty and a second sample cannot be taken, the priority is (1) light microscopy, (2) fluorescence microscopy, (3) electron microscopy.

Renal biopsy has made many contributions to research but should be used for this purpose only under the strictest ethical control. Only the indications which influence the patient's management are listed here.

In *nephrotic syndrome* minimal change, which responds to corticosteroids, should be distinguished from the other major causes. Normal glomeruli on light microscopy and no staining for immunoglobulins, complement, or fibrinogen establish the diagnosis with near certainty. The demonstration of typical changes in the podocytes, and otherwise normal glomeruli, on electron micrographs really gilds the lily but is usually done because the diagnosis is so important. Membranous nephropathy should be identified because of its close association with neoplasm. Again, this can be done with some confidence on light and fluorescence microscopy, if typical spikes are shown on the basement membrane by silver-methenamine stain and there is strong granular fluorescence for IgG and C3 on the glomerular basement membrane. Electron microscopy may be needed to clinch the diagnosis in very early and late cases. Amyloidosis is often diagnosed on biopsy, and this may lead to the recognition of its primary cause. It can usually be shown by Congo red and methyl violet stains, or by polarized light, but demonstration of the typical fibrils on electron microscopy may be required.

In *acute renal failure* the distinction between tubular necrosis, acute glomerulonephritis, hemolytic-uremic

syndrome, and other disorders is largely made on light microscopic appearances. It is important to recognize some uncommon causes which respond to treatment but which do not recover with the usual conservative management of acute renal failure — notably lupus nephritis, polyarteritis, Wegener's granulomatosis, Goodpasture's syndrome, and other causes of crescent nephritis. Distinction between the last two is made on fluorescence microscopy: Goodpasture's syndrome is shown by linear fluorescence for IgG and C3 along the glomerular basement membrane; if there is fluorescence on the capillary wall in other causes of crescent nephritis, it is granular.

Following *renal transplantation* biopsy is of crucial importance in distinguishing acute rejection, chronic vascular rejection, recurrent glomerulonephritis, acute pyelonephritis, and tubular necrosis. The distinction rests heavily on light microscopy, but fluorescence microscopy is of some help in confirming recurrent nephritis.

In *systemic diseases* confirmation of renal involvement influences choice of treatment in systemic lupus and prognosis in systemic sclerosis, Henoch-Schönlein syndrome, and polyarteritis. If diagnosis is not in doubt, light microscopy provides most of the information, but demonstration of IgA deposition along capillary walls and in the mesangium is strong confirmation of Henoch-Schönlein nephritis.

In *genetic disease* demonstration of the typical findings of Fabry's disease or Alport's syndrome on light and electron microscopy aids genetic counseling.

In *glomerulonephritis* without nephrotic syndrome the provision of a firm histologic diagnosis seldom affects treatment at present. However, it is important in prognosis, in the recognition of the few forms with a high liability to recur after transplant, and in the conduct of controlled trials of therapy.

Britton, K.: Radionuclides in renal imaging. Br. J. Hosp. Med., 20:140, 1978.

Diaz-Buxo, J. A., and Donadio, J. V., Jr.: Complications of percutaneous renal biopsy: An analysis of 1000 consecutive biopsies. Clin. Nephrol., 6:223, 1975.

Maher, F. T.: Evaluation of renal and urinary tract abnormalities noted on scintiscans. Proc. Mayo Clin., 50:370, 1975.

Meadows, R.: Renal Histopathology. 2nd ed. Oxford, Oxford University Press, 1978.

Witten, D. M., Myers, G. H., Jr., and Utz, D. C.: Clinical Urography. 4th ed. Philadelphia, W. B. Saunders Company, 1977.

370. THE PATHOPHYSIOLOGY OF CHRONIC RENAL DISEASE

Neal S. Bricker

INTRODUCTION. Less than two decades ago, the pathophysiology of chronic renal disease would not have been assigned a chapter in a major textbook of medicine. Chronic renal disease had been recognized since the first third of the nineteenth century as a destructive process that converted the organized architecture of the normal kidney into a transfigured, scarred, and virtually unrecognizable vestige of its original form. It seemed a logical assumption that the deterioration in structure must be associated with a parallel deterioration in function. The abnormalities in function were assumed to be widespread and unpredictable. The organ thus, it was believed, was converted into an increasingly impotent aggregate of diseased nephrons, which became less and less capable of fulfilling its role as the prime defender of homeostasis.

The foregoing assumption not only lacked scientific validation, but, in a peculiar way, it served to discourage efforts to seek this validation. First, it seemed an inefficient and possibly futile exercise to try to establish a set of unified principles of pathophysiology that would apply with equal authority to the many different forms of chronic renal disease. Indeed, because of the diverse nature of the structural abnormalities, it was believed that the list of associated defects in function might differ greatly not only from one form of renal disease to another, but from one patient to another with the same disease. Second, there was a widely held feeling that even if one attempted to catalogue the functional abnormalities of the chronic renal diseases, the effort would prove self-defeating; for the requisite studies depended upon the ability to measure the key functions of the kidney reliably and sequentially in each of the different forms of chronic renal disease. The principal tools used by the renal physiologist to study the function of normal kidneys (clearance and micropuncture techniques) required inulin as a marker of glomerular filtration rate and para-aminohippurate as a marker of renal plasma flow; both markers were assumed to lose their validity in chronically diseased kidneys with disfigured nephrons. Thus the thesis that "so goes structure, so goes function" took on an "Alice in Wonderland" quality. It was true because it was true, and the scientific approach to validation was deemed to be an unscientific exercise.

Within the past 20 years, there has been a major change in concept. Inulin and para-aminohippurate (as well as other reference substances) have been shown to reflect function in the chronically diseased kidney and its constituent nephrons as accurately as in the normal kidney. Not only have clearance and micropuncture techniques been shown to be valid, but a growing armamentarium of other techniques, including the study of isolated perfused segments of single nephrons from chronically diseased kidneys, have been utilized in an accelerating search for new knowledge about the functional characteristics of the chronically diseased kidney. The picture that has evolved is not that of a cacophony of disorganized nephrons undergoing the transition from life to death. Rather, it is analogous to a large orchestral group in which the number of participating musicians is decreasing continuously, and some of the survivors are injured; but the smaller the group becomes, the greater is the effort made by each, and in the face of mounting adversity, the product continues to remain harmonious.

It thus *is* possible today to consider the pathophysiology of chronic progressive renal disease as a formal body of knowledge. Unifying principles have evolved that do apply with equal authority to the many different forms of chronic renal disease. Conceptually, the chronically diseased kidney is an organ which has responded to adversity in a remarkable fashion designed to protect the afflicted host. As nephrons are destroyed, the surviving units undergo a series of adaptations that, rather than exaggerating the abnormalities of body fluids, greatly minimize many of these abnormalities.

This chapter will deal with the impact of chronic renal disease on the biology of man. Consideration will be given to the effects of the pathologic abnormalities on the intrinsic functional properties of the surviving nephrons. However, more emphasis will be directed to the adaptations in the functions of these surviving nephrons. The latter will include a discussion of the nature of the adaptations and of their limitations. It also will address the evidence that these same adaptations that are responsible for prolonging life, often for years, may contribute to the symptoms and signs of the uremic syndrome. Finally, the possibility will be considered that the increasing level of knowledge about the pathophysiology of chronic renal disease may soon lead to major advances in our techniques of conservative management.

THE EFFECTS OF STRUCTURAL ABNORMALITIES ON INTRINSIC FUNCTIONAL INTEGRITY. There is considerable evidence that the surviving nephrons in the chronically diseased kidney remain functionally organized in the face of the pathologic alterations of the renal parenchyma. A summary of some of this evidence follows.

The Study of a Diseased Kidney and a Normal Kidney in the Same Host. An animal or a patient with unilateral renal disease and a contralateral nondiseased kidney provides several strategic advantages in the effort to understand effects of intrarenal lesions per se on the functional integrity of the nephrons in the involved organ. Because the reduction in nephrons is confined to one kidney, the total (bilateral) population of nephrons must always be at least 50 per cent of normal, and any distortions of the composition or volume of body fluids that might, in theory, alter renal function adversely in uremia would not occur. Moreover, any circulating factors that influence renal function, such as parathyroid hormone, antidiuretic hormone, natriuretic hormone, or aldosterone, should exist in the same concentration in the blood perfusing the nephrons of both diseased and normal kidneys. The arterial blood pressure and the serum protein concentration should also be identical bilaterally. Finally, at any moment the requirements for homeostasis of any constituent of the ECF are determined by conditions extant within the whole organism (i.e., the host); and theoretically each functioning nephron should share equally in discharging these requirements, whether it resides in the diseased or normal kidney. Thus as long as both organs are studied *simultaneously*, the normal kidney will provide a unique frame of reference with which the patterns of function of a diseased kidney can be compared.

The Bilateral Equality of "Glomerulotubular" (GT) Balance. A large body of data obtained from several species, including man, with unilateral or predominantly unilateral renal disease indicates that GT balance tends to remain equal bilaterally. Thus when glomerular function (expressed as glomerular filtration rate or GFR) is measured simultaneously with any one of a number of different tubular functions (expressed as a transport rate or clearance value), the ratio of GFR to the tubular function in the diseased kidney is closely comparable to the concurrent ratio in the contralateral control kidney. Thus if GRF in the diseased kidney is 85 per cent less than that of the control kidney, the values for a number of tubular functions in the diseased kidney will also be approximately 85 per cent less than those in the control organ.

The relevance of the preservation of bilateral equality of GT balance to the analysis of the functional integrity of the nephrons of the diseased kidney is well illustrated by studies of ammonia excretion. Ammonia is synthesized by the tubular epithelial cells of both proximal and distal segments of the nephron. The pathway is complex and depends upon a series of biochemical events that must proceed in orderly sequence, and upon the integrity and appropriate spatial orientation of at least several constituents of the epithelial cells. The process begins with the transport of substrate (principally glutamine) across the cell membranes lining both the luminal and the basolateral surfaces of the tubular cells. Glutamine then is converted to alpha-ketoglutarate through a series of steps involving intramitochondrial enzymes. In this process, NH_3 is liberated into the intracellular fluid. However, because NH_3 is such a very strong base (pK > 9), the great majority of NH_3 molecules are rapidly converted to NH_4^+. Moreover, some of the free NH_3 diffuses out of the cells into the peritubular capillary venous blood. Thus the rate of ammoniagenesis must be sufficiently great and precise to assure the diffusion of NH_3 in carefully regulated amounts across the *luminal* membrane of the cells into the tubular fluid. Within the tubules, the NH_3 molecules collide with hydrogen ions, also produced intracellularly and also transported across the luminal membrane. Ammonium ions thus are excreted in the final urine, thereby eliminating hydrogen ions from the body and replenishing bicarbonate ions in the extracellular fluid.

Thus ammoniagenesis occurs through much of the nephron; it involves a chain of interacting biochemical events and the juxtaposition of key subcellular organelles; and it must be responsive in the final analysis to the acid-base needs of the organism. If the pathologic abnormalities resident in the diseased kidney produce functional defects, precise measurements of GT balance for NH_3 should reflect these, and equal values for NH_3/GFR between diseased and contralateral control kidneys of animals or man would be unexpected and fortuitous. A prototypic experiment will be cited.

When a normal dog is made chronically acidotic to stimulate ammonia production maximally, NH_3/GFR values, as anticipated, are closely comparable bilaterally. If chronic renal disease is then induced in only one kidney and chronic metabolic acidosis is re-established, the effects on GT balance for ammonia are extremely interesting. In a representative dog, GFR in the diseased kidney fell markedly after the induction of disease (−65 per cent), whereas in the nondiseased kidney it rose modestly (+11 per cent). Ammonium excretion, on the other hand, fell somewhat less than GFR (−50 per cent) in the diseased kidney and rose more than GFR (+36 per cent) in the control. On initial inspection, these changes (−65, +11 to −50, +36) seem more suggestive of cacophony than harmony. However, the critical data are contained in the NH_3/GFR ratios, for they remained identical bilaterally. Therefore whatever stimulus induced a greater "hypertrophy" in ammoniagenesis than in GFR in the nephrons of the control kidney affected the residual nephrons of the diseased organ in an identical manner.

The Homogeneity of GT Balance. It is theoretically possible that the equality of clearance ratios between diseased and contralateral control kidneys could result from a fortuitous mix of nephrons with damaged tubules but relatively intact glomeruli (glomerular preponderance) and other nephrons in the same kidney

with tubular preponderance. The data on ammonia excretion make this explanation unlikely. So also does the fact that equality of GT balance has been found for a number of tubular transport systems located at different sites in the nephron in various types of chronic renal disease and in the several species studied.

A more direct approach to examining the homogeneity of GT balance in a whole kidney resides in a method called the "glucose titration." The concentration of glucose in the serum is increased (by intravenous infusion) in a stepwise fashion from normal to levels sufficiently high to exceed the reabsorptive capacity (or Tm). Because the glucose concentration in the glomerular filtrate of all nephrons must be identical, the *amount* of glucose filtered by any nephron will depend upon its GFR, and both the onset of glucosuria (the so-called "threshold") and the Tm will depend upon the balance between glomerular function and the function of the appended tubule. In a normal kidney, "small" glomeruli have "small" tubules, larger glomeruli, larger tubules, and the "titration curve" reveals a high level of homogeneity of GT balance (the latter is characterized by minimum "splay" in the curve).

In an animal with unilateral renal disease, any difference in GT balance for glucose among the constituent nephrons of the diseased kidney will result in a different "titration curve" from that obtained simultaneously from the contralateral organ. Thus, if there are nephrons with preferentially damaged tubules, glucosuria will occur earlier in the diseased than in the control kidney, whereas any nephrons with preferential impairment of glomerular filtration will require higher blood sugar levels to reach their Tm than will the nephrons in the healthy organ. Either form of glomerulotubular imbalance will distort the glucose titration curve. However, in both dogs and rats with unilateral chronic renal disease, the curves for the diseased kidneys have been identical to those for the contralateral control kidneys. Similar results have been obtained in bicarbonate titration studies and phosphate titration studies in animals with unilateral renal disease.

The question of homogeneity of GT balance in the chronically diseased kidney has also been approached by studying the individual nephrons of the diseased organ, using micropuncture techniques. Despite sampling limitations and the fact that data must be pooled from different animals in which the "setting" of GT balance for any solute may vary (see below), the majority of observations confirm the persistence of a high order of homogeneity of GT balance in the nephrons of diseased organs. Thus when one plots values for single nephron GFR (SNGFR) against fractional water (or sodium) reabsorption at any given point along the proximal tubule (expressed as a percentage of the total length), relative homogeneity of GT balance is evident. A similar plot comparing SNGFR with glucose reabsorption in the same nephrons demonstrates the same phenomenon.

In summary, homogeneity of GT balance in the diseased kidney, for many different tubular functions, remains relatively well preserved despite the inhomogeneity of structure of the renal parenchyma. The homogeneity cannot be explained by offsetting effects of nephrons with partially damaged glomeruli and normal tubules versus another group of nephrons with the reverse abnormality. Rather, the data require that if SNGFR changes in either direction, the change in a variety of tubular functions in the same nephron will be such that GT balance in that nephron will be similar to that of the composite group of nephrons. The data also would seem to require that if there is a primary alteration in a tubular function in given nephrons within a diseased kidney, there must be a series of feedback loops affecting SNGFR, and the unaltered tubular functions, that will maintain the setting of GT balance (for multiple tubular functions) in the afflicted nephron(s) in line with the rest of the nephrons.

Thus, if damaged nephrons contribute significantly to renal function, they neither set nor dominate the patterns of function of the involved kidneys. Rather, the damaged nephrons behave in concert with the remaining nephrons and retain normal mechanisms of integration of glomerular and tubular functions. This is the essence of the *intact nephron hypothesis*.

BEYOND HOMOGENEITY: THE MAGNIFICATION PHENOMENON. No matter how extraordinary a biologic phenomenon is the preservation of homogeneity of GT balance in a severely diseased kidney, the key to survival transcends this phenomenon; for survival depends not so much upon homogeneity of GT balance as upon the continual *resetting* of the level of GT balance as the disease advances.

The charge to the kidneys is to excrete from the body fluids the same amounts of many different substances as are acquired daily. In essence what comes in must go out regardless of how many nephrons there are. If such external balance is not maintained for any substance, that substance will be either retained or lost from the body.

The natural history of chronic renal disease is punctuated by a succession of disruptions of the equality between acquisition and excretion. Indeed, every time nephrons are destroyed (and GFR decreases permanently), everything that would have been excreted by the destroyed nephrons, at the time of their destruction, is retained. What happens following this retention accounts for the patient's ability to survive. With the retention of any solute that is actively regulated by the kidneys, the surviving nephrons must be reprogrammed to increase their rate of excretion of that solute. The change in excretion optimally should allow, first, for the elimination of whatever amount of the solute was retained when the nephron destruction occurred (even if the latter is so small as to be unmeasurable) and, second, for a permanent increase in the rate of solute excretion per nephron (assuming an unchanged rate of acquisition of the solute).

The adaptive increase in solute excretion rate per nephron occurs with differing degrees of efficiency for different solutes. Over-all, the adaptations are among the most elegant of all of nature's responses to biologic adversity.

For some solutes, of which urea and creatinine are the classic examples, there is no effective adaptation, and following each phase of nephron reduction the rise in serum concentration persists. It is because of this fact that each time GFR falls by 50 per cent, both urea and creatinine concentrations in the serum rise by approximately two-fold. For most other solutes, however, adaptation does occur. For certain of these, the increase in excretion rate per nephron which attends a permanent reduction in GFR is sufficiently precise to maintain normal serum concentrations, and thus to avert permanent solute retention, through most, but not all,

of the natural history of chronic renal disease. This pattern is exemplified by the adaptation in the excretion of phosphate, urate, and probably magnesium.

For a third group of solutes, the pattern of adaptation is characterized by the continuing ability to maintain external balance until virtually the agonal phases of chronic renal disease. Two of the most important solutes that can be regulated with this degree of precision are sodium and potassium.

The adaptations owe their existence to what we have called the "magnification phenomenon." The phenomenon is defined as follows: In response to a *fixed* perturbation of the extracellular fluid, occasioned by the addition to or loss from the ECF of one or more of the solutes that are excreted in a regulated manner, the excretory response per nephron will vary inversely with the number of nephrons. For example, a normal person, with two million nephrons and a GFR of 120 ml per minute, will form approximately 170,000 ml of glomerular filtrate per 24 hours; this filtrate will contain approximately 24,000 mEq of sodium. If the sodium intake in the diet is 120 mEq per day, each nephron must excrete an average of only *one out of every 200 sodium ions filtered*. On the other hand, in a patient with far advanced chronic renal disease, in whom the GFR is reduced to 2 ml per minute, slightly less than 3 liters of glomerular filtrate is formed per day and the total amount of sodium filtered is only about 400 mEq. To maintain external balance on the same daily sodium intake of 120 mEq, about 30 per cent of the filtered sodium must be excreted. Hence, in response to an identical perturbation of the ECF (i.e., the same salt intake), the end-organ response, expressed as fractional excretion of sodium (FE_{Na}) must be over 60 times as great in the patient with a GFR of 2 as in the normal person. Moreover, if sodium intake changes, for example, from 60 mEq on one day to 120 mEq on the following day, sodium excretion will change, in the normal person, from 0.25 to 0.50 per cent of the amount filtered. The achievement of balance requires the excretion of one additional sodium ion out of every *400* filtered. The same dietary change in the patient with a GFR of 2 ml per minute requires a change in FE_{Na} of 16 per cent (from 16 to 32 per cent); hence, not only is FE_{Na} 64 times as great on each of the two levels of salt intake; the *change* in FE_{Na} in the transition from one level of salt intake to the other also is 64 times as great.

But the magnification phenomenon must extend beyond the requirements for maintaining homeostasis and external balance for sodium. Consider what a representative nephron must do in the patient with a GFR of 2 ml per minute whose potassium intake falls from 80 to 40 mEq per day during the same two consecutive days that the sodium intake has risen from 60 to 120 mEq per day. At a serum potassium concentration of 4.5 mEq per liter, the total amount of potassium filtered in 24 hours is less than one fifth the amount ingested on the 80 mEq K diet. Thus on the higher K intake, potassium excretion must be approximately six times the amount filtered and, on the next day, at the same time that FE_{Na} rises from 8 to 16 per cent, K excretion must drop in half — to three times the filtered load.

BIOLOGIC CONTROL SYSTEMS. With each additional solute that is considered and with the knowledge that nephron destruction continues inexorably, the accomplishments of the surviving nephrons become ever more astonishing. The data seem virtually to mandate the existence of a series of solute specific biologic control systems. Each system would control one solute. It would perforce be capable of detecting very small (or very large) translocations from the steady-state occasioned by either the gain or loss of the solute from body fluids. It would possess the means of reversing the translocation by affecting either an increase or a decrease in the rate of renal excretion of the solute. It is implicit in the assumption that the biologic control systems are solute specific that each will exercise definitive control over only one substance; and despite any interdependencies in the transport of different ions (or nonpolar solutes), a biologic control system for sodium, responding to an increase in the intake of salt, must increase the excretion of *sodium* without altering, more than transiently, the regulated excretion of potassium, hydrogen, phosphate, or any other solute which demands independent control.

Although all the postulated biologic control systems have similar physiologic charges, the regulation of external balance, the different systems probably have a spectrum of modes of operation. For example, when the sodium contained in an average diet enters the extracellular fluid, it does so without producing any appreciable change in the sodium concentration of the serum. This relates to the fact that water is absorbed from the gut into the extracellular fluid, and additional water will move out of the cells if there is any persisting osmotic gradient. Hence the NaCl absorbed from the gut may be viewed as occurring isosmotically. The over-all effect is to expand ECF volume without changing the chemical concentration of the solute being detected. On the other hand, the amount of phosphorus absorbed into the blood on an average diet is equal to or greater than the total amount of inorganic phosphate circulating in the extracellular fluid. Thus the detector element for phosphorus must deal with a substantial rise in serum concentration (but no change in ECF volume). For potassium, and many other solutes, serum concentrations rise when the substance is ingested or produced metabolically; but the rate and degree of the respective increments vary widely, based upon the volume of distribution, rate of renal and nonrenal excretion, and metabolic rate. The gain or loss of water also will affect both the volume and the osmolality of the body fluids and the concentration of several ECF solutes.

If one works within the framework of the "detector, integrator, effector" model of a biologic control system, there may be multiple afferent stimuli arising simultaneously for a single substance, and the stimuli may not all convey identical information. For example, if there is sequestration of extracellular fluid in one extremity due to venous or lymphatic obstruction, fluid will accumulate in the affected extremity distal to the obstruction, and the input from the detector elements of the sodium control system within that extremity should favor an increase in sodium excretion. On the other hand, the sequestered fluid arises from the rest of the body, where detector elements would perceive a contraction of ECF volume and presumably would so "inform" an integrator element. The integrator element then would have to adjudicate and "instruct" the nephrons about any desired change in sodium excretion. It is not yet known whether control systems for solutes other than sodium possess "integrator elements"; but there probably is one for water, for there are many circumstances wherein osmolality and volume pose different requirements in regard to changes in water excretion.

The final component of a biologic control system is the effector element, which includes the nephron as the end-organ. There is firm evidence that a key "messenger" in the phosphorus control system is parathyroid hormone (PTH). There is also firm evidence that the messenger hormone which regulates nonosmotically obligated water excretion is the antidiuretic hormone vasopressin. Finally, there is growing evidence that a major messenger in the sodium control system may also be hormonal in nature — the natriuretic hormone. We believe therefore that there is a strong possibility that there also will be additional modulator hormones discovered within the foreseeable future and that, ultimately, each of the key solutes will be shown to have its own "effector" hormone.

THE "TRADE-OFF HYPOTHESIS." In advancing renal disease, if the average rate of enteric absorption of phosphorus remains relatively constant as the number of nephrons diminishes, the amount of phosphate requiring excretion per surviving nephron must increase progressively. The rise in phosphate excretion per nephron does occur, owing in large part to a continuing rise of circulating levels of PTH. In the case of the sodium control system, there also is evidence which suggests that the rate of production of natriuretic hormone may be increased in uremia, and it is possible that this hormonal change contributes to the magnification phenomenon for sodium. If other effector hormones are discovered, their rates of production and concentrations in the circulation also could increase as GFR falls.

The adaptations in solute excretion have been characterized properly as lifesaving in their impact and as a remarkable testament to nature's inherent ability to adapt to adversity. Yet there is another law of nature that appears also to apply to these adaptations. It is: "Nothing in nature is free." Is it possible that the cost of the adaptations in the patient with chronic renal disease is one, or many, of the adverse effects of the uremic syndrome? None of the traditional "uremic toxins," such as urea, organic acids, ammonia, or guanidinosuccinic acid, have been proved to be either a ubiquitous uremic toxin or even to produce a single major abnormality of the uremic state. On the other hand, patients with longstanding uremia develop severe skeletal manifestations of secondary hyperparathyroidism, and the high levels of PTH that produce these bone lesions appear to be involved in the adaptation in phosphate excretion. Thus at least one major abnormality might be explained as a trade-off. More recently, a growing list of uremic abnormalities, other than osteitis fibrosa, has been attributed to side effects or trade-offs of the high PTH levels. Among these are central nervous system abnormalities, including the abnormal electroencephalogram of uremia, prolongation of peripheral nerve conduction velocity, peripheral myopathy, ocular calcifications, sexual impotence, and even a part of the carbohydrate and lipid abnormalities of advanced uremia. A natriuretic hormone present in very high concentration in the blood of chronically uremic patients could inhibit sodium transport by many different cell types and thus, along with PTH, play a key role in the diverse and multiple system abnormalities of the uremic state.

IMPLICATIONS REGARDING THERAPY: "PROPORTIONAL REDUCTION" OF SOLUTE INTAKE. The so-called trade-off hypothesis arose almost entirely from studies designed to clarify the sequential events in the pathologic physiology of chronic renal failure. If it is true that the adaptations in nephron function exact a price from the patient, namely, a series of uremic abnormalities, then the study of pathophysiology could open wide the door to preventing these trade-off abnormalities, for all that would be required to prevent the trade-offs is to prevent the adaptations. The general approach centers on a concept termed "proportional reduction of solute intake." If the ratio between the intake of a solute and the number of nephrons available to accomplish the excretion of the solute were to be held constant throughout the course of chronic renal disease, by reducing the intake (or gastrointestinal absorption) in exact proportion to the fall in GFR, no adaptation would be required. If there were to be no adaptation, there would be no need for any increase in the blood level of any hormonal messenger component of a biologic control system involved in the adaptation. Finally, if the hormone is responsible for trade-off abnormalities, these should be prevented. One of the truly exciting prospects for the future is that certain trade-offs may actually increase the rate of nephron destruction, and studies now in progress will serve to determine the validity of this concept, and thus its importance, to patients afflicted with chronic progressive renal disease.

Bricker, N. S.: On the pathogenesis of the uremic state: An exposition of the "trade-off hypothesis." N. Engl. J. Med., 286:1093, 1972.

Bricker, N. S., Bourgoignie, J. J., and Weber, H.: The renal response to progressive nephron loss. *In* Brenner, B. M., and Rector, F. C., Jr. (eds.): The Kidney. 2nd ed. Philadelphia, W. B. Saunders Company, 1976, pp. 703–736.

Bricker, N. S., Klahr, S., Lubowitz, H., and Rieselbach, R. E.: Renal function in chronic renal disease. Medicine, 44:263, 1965.

Gottschalk, C. W.: Function of the chronically diseased kidney: the adaptive nephron. Circ. Res., 28:II–1, 1971.

Platt, R.: Sodium and potassium excretion in chronic renal failure. Clin. Sci., 9:367, 1950.

Smith, H. W.: The Kidney. Structure and Function in Health and Disease. New York, Oxford University Press, 1951.

371. CHRONIC RENAL FAILURE

D. N. S. Kerr

DEFINITION. Chronic renal impairment means any permanent depression of glomerular filtration rate (GFR). Impairment becomes "failure" when plasma biochemistry becomes substantially abnormal and symptoms appear — roughly at a GFR of 30 ml per minute. Chronic renal failure can be divided descriptively into early (GFR ca. 30 to 10 ml per minute), late (GFR 10 to 5 ml per minute), and terminal (<5 ml per minute) phases. Uremia becomes prominent in late chronic renal failure and life-threatening in the terminal phase.

ETIOLOGY. The major causes of chronic renal failure, and some of the minor ones, are listed in Table 1 in a manner intended to aid differential diagnosis. Diseases in the first group usually present with features of renal disease, although extrarenal manifestations such as tu-

TABLE 1. A Clinical Classification of the Causes of Chronic Renal Failure

1. Local causes:
Diseases in which the kidneys are predominantly involved and in which the presenting features are usually those of renal disease
    Proliferative glomerulonephritis
    Membranous glomerulonephropathy
    Chronic pyelonephritis
    Tuberculous pyelonephritis
    Renal calculi
    Congenital nephritis
    Polycystic disease
    Medullary cystic disease
    Renal hypoplasia
    Renal tubular acidosis
    Balkan nephropathy
    Upper urinary tract obstruction
        Hydronephrosis
        Retroperitoneal fibrosis
        Neoplasm

2. Lower urinary tract obstruction:
Presenting features often those of bladder dysfunction, but may present in renal failure
    Prostatic enlargement
        Adenoma
        Neoplasm
    Urethral stricture
    Urethral valves
    Bladder neck obstruction
    Neurogenic bladder

3. Systemic diseases and intoxications:
    a. In which renal failure is not infrequently a presenting feature
    Malignant essential hypertension
    Polyarteritis nodosa
    Disseminated lupus erythematosus
    Primary and secondary amyloidosis
    Analgesic overconsumption
    Potassium deficiency
    Hypercalcemia
    Cystinosis
    Oxalosis
    Consumption coagulopathies
        Hemolytic-uremic syndrome
        Thrombotic thrombocytopenic purpura
        Postpartum renal failure
    Lead or cadmium poisoning
    b. In which renal failure is usually a late feature or overshadowed by other manifestations
    Benign essential hypertension
    Atheroma
    Systemic emboli
        Subacute bacterial endocarditis
        Rheumatic heart disease
    Gout
    Diabetes
    Heart failure
    Cirrhosis

berculous epididymitis may provide a clue. Diseases in Group 2 will usually be identified by involvement of the bladder or of some other system, and those in Group 3b should be recognized readily from systemic manifestations, although renal failure may occasionally be a presenting feature. If a full history and physical examination fail to reveal a systemic cause for chronic renal failure, the most likely possibilities are in Groups 1 and 3a.

INCIDENCE AND PREVALENCE. In North America, Western Europe, and Australia about 100 to 150 persons per million per year contract chronic renal failure, of whom about 30 to 50 per million per year are deemed suitable for treatment by dialysis or/and renal transplantation. The causes of chronic renal failure in patients excluded from dialysis and transplantation are poorly documented: death certification statistics are hopelessly unreliable. A mass of data exists on the cause of renal failure in those accepted for treatment, who are predominantly children and adults up to the age of 60 or 65. The computer files of the renal failure registries have earned chronic renal failure the title of "best documented disease," but not all the data are reliable. Figures published up to about 1976 (including those in the last edition of this book) and all cumulative data exaggerate the contribution of glomerulonephritis; only a small minority of the earlier patients reported to the registries had histologic proof of the diagnosis.

Table 2 lists most of the important causes of chronic renal failure in children and adults, according to the Registry of the European Dialysis and Transplant Association. These figures, published in 1977 and based only on recent additions to the Registry's files, correspond closely to the author's experience except in the following respects: essential hypertension (included in renal vascular disease) is under-represented by a few per cent; the proportion of glomerulonephritis recognized as hereditary is too low in the Registry; and the importance of pyelonephritis is apparently exaggerated — it accounts for only 15 per cent of our patients on dialysis. However, the last difference is one of definition; in the Registry figures it clearly includes many patients with pyelonephritis secondary to other diseases such as renal calculi.

About 8 per cent of the Registry patients, and a slightly higher proportion of my own, have no better diagnosis than "chronic renal failure, cause unknown." They are predominantly adults who present in late chronic renal failure with severe, often malignant, hypertension and who have small fibrotic kidneys. Renal biopsy may be contraindicated and, if performed, may show only scarred "end-stage kidney" with severe hypertensive vascular change. The differential diagnosis between chronic glomerulonephritis, essential hypertension, and renal atheroma may be impossible, and it is better to admit ignorance than to distort the figures.

Gout does not figure individually in Table 2, although it is a fairly common disease which is often accompanied by renal impairment and which has been said to terminate in chronic renal failure in 18 to 30 per cent of cases. This is an overestimate based on selected hospital series before the widespread use of allopurin-

ol. The very few patients with gout who reach dialysis and transplant do so in middle or old age.

The European figures in Table 2 are very similar to those of other regions with reliable data except in one important respect. Analgesic nephropathy is apparently less common in North America, perhaps because of underdiagnosis in America, since the consumption of analgesics is similar to that in most of Western Europe, and much more common in Australia where it accounts for a quarter of all chronic renal failure.

INVESTIGATION OF CHRONIC RENAL FAILURE. Investigation has four objectives: recognition of the primary disease, assessment of the degree of renal failure, detection of any aggravating factors, and exploration of other medical and social problems which may have a bearing on the treatment of renal disease.

Recognition of the Primary Disease. It is the plea of every nephrologist that patients with chronic renal disease be referred early, when urography is particularly informative and renal biopsy can be performed without the hazards of uremia, hypertension, and small fibrotic kidneys. At this stage diagnosis of the primary disease is usually straightforward and worthwhile.

When the patient presents in late renal failure, exact diagnosis is more difficult and less rewarding. High dose urography, combined with tomography of the renal areas, will still provide invaluable information, but fine calyceal detail cannot be expected and renal biopsy is often uninformative, as indicated above. Nonetheless it is still important to establish or exclude a few diagnoses which call for specific treatment even in terminal renal failure or which influence decisions about renal transplantation. These diseases are listed in Table 3. Those conditions which recur in the graft (with the possible exception of oxalosis) are a smaller hazard to the transplant recipient than the risks of surgery, rejection, and immunosuppression, so they do not have a profound effect on therapeutic decisions. However, as transplant results improve, their existence will assume a growing importance.

Of the conditions that can be reversed at a late stage in chronic renal failure, the most important are analgesic nephropathy and urinary obstruction. Remarkable prolongation of life (10+ years on conservative treatment) can be achieved in many patients with analgesic nephropathy who can be persuaded to abandon their addiction and who have at least 8 or 10 ml per minute of GFR after correction of initial dehydration and urinary infection. The diagnosis is suggested by a history of headaches or arthritis, typically in a middle-aged woman, or may be prompted by the finding of calcified papillae, secondary calculi (radiolucent center and radiopaque rim) on the plain film, and scalloped kidneys, with cavitated papillae and "ring signs" caused by separated papillae. However, there may be no diagnostic features clinically or radiologically, and a careful analgesic history is an essential part of the workup of chronic renal failure. Denial of intake is common, and when suspicion is aroused it is essential to question the relatives and test the urine for metabolites of common analgesics.

Longstanding obstruction is rarely reversible at the stage of late renal failure. It is probably a disservice to the patient to attempt surgical correction of, for example, bilateral pelviureteral hydronephrosis or megaureter when these escape notice until the patient has renal failure. However, it is crucially important to de-

TABLE 2.   Causes of Chronic Renal Failure in Patients Starting Regular Dialysis in Europe in 1976*

	Adults	Children
Glomerulonephritis	38.4	37.9
Interstitial nephritis	20.0	16.9
Cystic kidney disease	8.3	9.0
Renal vascular disease	6.8	3.2
Analgesic nephropathy	2.7	—
Congenital hypoplasia	1.7	10.7
Other drugs	0.6	—
Hereditary nephropathy	0.4	7.8
Cortical necrosis	0.4	2.5
Other diseases	12.4	11.9
Uncertain	8.3	
	100%	100%

*From Jacobs, C., et al.: Proc. Eur. Dialysis Transplant Assoc., 14:2, 1977.

TABLE 3.   Diagnoses That Must Be Sought Even in Late Chronic Renal Failure

Potential for arrest or reversal of disease
  Analgesic nephropathy
  Recent obstruction
    Retroperitoneal fibrosis
    Malignant occlusion of ureters
    Calculous disease
    Lower urinary obstruction
  Systemic lupus erythematosus
  Goodpasture's syndrome
  Idiopathic crescentic glomerulonephritis
  Urinary infection
    Primary
    Secondary to obstruction, etc.
  Tuberculosis
  Gout
  Polyarteritis
  Wegener's granulomatosis

Likely to recur in renal graft
  Oxalosis
  Cystinosis
  ?Secondary amyloidosis
  Analgesic nephropathy
  Glomerulonephritis
    Dense deposit type
    ?Mesangiocapillary
    ?Membranous
    IgA-IgG (Berger's)
    Focal glomerulosclerosis

Possibly requiring surgical correction before transplant
  Lower urinary tract obstruction
  Vesicoureteral reflux
  Chronic or recurrent infection
    Chronic pyelonephritis
    Infected calculi
    Analgesic nephropathy
    Polycystic kidneys (some)

tect obstruction of recent origin (days, weeks, or months), of which the most important cause is retroperitoneal fibrosis. Withdrawal of drugs (if appropriate), ureterolysis, and steroid therapy can restore life-preserving renal function even when the patient presents in anuria. A similar benefit in renal function can be obtained in malignant obstruction of the ureters; but since the malignancy is usually inoperable, the diagnosis is sought more to prevent unnecessary prolongation of suffering than with cure in mind. The diagnosis is often missed through failure to perform a pelvic examination.

The rapidly progressive nephritides — those accompanying systemic lupus erythematosus, polyarteritis, Goodpasture's syndrome, and Wegener's granulomatosis, as well as the idiopathic variety — are partially reversible if treated as the patient approaches terminal renal failure, but results are disappointing once anuria has supervened; early diagnosis is essential and is discussed below.

The *history* in chronic renal failure should include a lifelong survey of renal complaints and of occupations and specific questions about drug consumption (analgesics, methysergide, vitamin D) and symptoms of urinary obstruction. The family history should explore renal disease, hypertension and its sequelae, gout, collagenoses, preeclampsia, and deafness.

The *physical signs* that should be sought include those of longstanding uremia (skin pigmentation and excoriation, brown arcs under the nail margins, tissue wast-

ing, neuropathy), hypertension (retinopathy, cardiac enlargement), atheroma (peripheral pulses, murmurs over large vessels), disturbed calcium metabolism (band keratopathy, pseudoclubbing, proximal muscle weakness), bladder obstruction (suprapubic dullness after micturition, poor stream during micturition), and collagenoses (rashes, joint deformity, arteritic skin lesions).

Investigations should include qualitative tests for glucosuria and hematuria and a quantitative test for proteinuria; urine microscopy and midstream culture; plasma or serum urea, creatinine, sodium, potassium, chloride, bicarbonate, urate, calcium, phosphate, alkaline phosphatase, total protein, and electrophoresis; and a straight roentgenogram of the urinary tract, with tomograms if necessary to define the renal outlines. Chest roentgenogram, electrocardiogram, serum magnesium, creatinine clearance, fasting plasma lipids, and test for HBsAg should be included in the initial screening, although not for the sake of differential diagnosis. High dose or infusion urography is often required to exclude obstruction; in the few patients in whom there is uncertainty about the presence of polycystic disease after clinical examination and pyelography, ultrasonography or renal scanning will usually provide a definite answer. The ultrasonogram is also helpful in the diagnosis of obstruction.

Glucosuria suggests diabetic nephropathy if heavy, but sufficient glucosuria to give a positive reaction with glucose oxidase sticks (Labstix, Testape) is a common accompaniment of heavy proteinuria from any cause. *Hematuria* is macroscopic intermittently in some patients with polycystic disease and may be heavy enough to cause smoky urine in crescentic glomerulonephritis, whatever its etiology. Microscopic hematuria heavy enough to cause a positive reaction for blood on Labstix is common in mesangiocapillary glomerulonephritis but rare in other nephritides at the stage of renal failure; it is also common in calculous disease and polycystic disease. Minor degrees of microscopic hematuria are found in all forms of glomerulonephritis leading to renal failure but are rare in chronic interstitial nephritis (unless there is an active urinary infection).

Proteinuria exceeding 3 grams per 24 hours is unusual in chronic interstitial nephritis, analgesic nephropathy, polycystic disease, urinary obstruction, calculous disease, and benign essential hypertension. It is usual or common in chronic proliferative glomerulonephritis, membranous glomerulonephritis, amyloidosis, diabetic nephropathy, polyarteritis, Wegener's granulomatosis, disseminated lupus erythematosus, and malignant hypertension. Glomerular proteinuria diminishes quantitatively as the GFR falls, but heavy proteinuria may still be encountered in terminal renal failure. Mild *hypoproteinemia* accompanies fluid overload in many forms of chronic renal disease; but severe hypoproteinemia (less than 5.0 grams per deciliter), particularly if accompanied by a nephrotic electrophoretic strip and hyperlipidemia, strongly suggests that heavy proteinuria has been present recently even if it is no longer demonstrable.

Red cell *casts in the urinary sediment* in chronic renal failure may suggest one of the more rapidly progressive forms of glomerulonephritis. They are plentiful in crescentic forms of glomerulonephritis whatever the etiology, and in the nephritides accompanying subacute bacterial endocarditis and similar infections. They can be found with a more diligent search in some patients with mesangiocapillary glomerulonephritis, polyarteritis, disseminated lupus erythematosus, and malignant hypertension. Numerous dense granular casts, and sometimes epithelial cell casts, are found in these conditions and in membranous glomerulonephropathy, diabetic nephropathy, and amyloidosis. Amyloid produces the most strikingly abnormal deposit of all, with an extraordinary density and variety of casts. Hyaline casts are found alone in patients with benign essential hypertension, even in renal failure.

Hyperchloremic acidosis accompanies urinary diversion into the bowel even when GFR is normal. If the lower urinary tract is intact, hyperchloremic acidosis in early renal failure should suggest chronic interstitial nephritis, analgesic nephropathy, or renal tubular acidosis of the genetic type. In late renal failure it can be found in many diseases.

Hypercalcemia may occur in secondary hyperparathyroidism, particularly in patients with a prolonged course through renal failure, but its presence should always raise the suspicion that hypercalcemia is the cause of the renal failure, not its effect.

Serum electrophoresis and a heat test for urinary Bence Jones protein will detect most cases of myelomatosis causing renal failure, but they will miss some and will also miss some patients with benign gammopathy causing primary amyloidosis or glomerulonephritis. A search for light chains by specific immunologic tests and for monoclonal peaks by immunoelectrophoresis is now an essential part of the screening of patients with chronic renal failure of obscure origin.

Very large kidneys in renal failure are typical of polycystic disease. Obstruction usually causes large or very large renal shadows. Renal failure with *kidneys of normal size* should alert the clinician to the possibility of acute renal failure or of a rapidly progressive lesion such as crescentic glomerulonephritis. Membranous glomerulonephritis, diabetic nephropathy, and amyloidosis have been regarded as causes of renal failure with normal-sized kidneys, but in practice there is usually considerable shrinkage in renal size by the stage of late renal failure. *Symmetrical small kidneys* with preservation of calyceal pattern suggest some form of glomerulonephritis, diabetic nephropathy, amyloid, or hypertensive nephrosclerosis. *Irregular scarring*, with clubbing and outdrawing of calyces, suggests chronic interstitial nephritis, with or without preceding calculous disease, or analgesic nephropathy. If the diagnostic features of papillary necrosis, listed above, are absent, these diseases cannot be differentiated radiologically.

Urinary infection is a common accompaniment of chronic pyelonephritis, calculous disease, analgesic nephropathy, and lower urinary tract obstruction. It is present in about 20 per cent of diabetics with chronic renal disease, and there is a modest increase in the incidence of urinary infection in polycystic disease. In all these conditions, urinary infection should be sought regularly and treated. Glomerulonephritis and most of the other diseases listed in Table 1 do not increase susceptibility to urinary infection.

Assessment of the Degree of Renal Failure. An initial measurement of GFR should be made by one of the techniques discussed in Ch. 369.4. Thereafter serial measurement of serum creatinine is the most useful and practical guide to change in renal function. For reasons discussed in Ch. 369.4, it is now common practice to calculate GFR from the serum creatinine, or to calculate the reciprocal of serum creatinine, and plot the results on a flow sheet or on ordinary graph paper.

Detection of Aggravating Factors. Glomerular filtration rate may be depressed by hypovolemia from sodium loss, resulting from a renal leak, vomiting, diarrhea, excessive sweating, or administration of diuretics. Sodium depletion should be considered in normotensive patients with chronic renal failure, particularly if they have postural hypotension. Temporary depression of GFR can also result from systemic infections, urinary infection, trauma, surgery, sudden reduction of long-standing hypertension, rapid rise in blood pressure, or administration of nephrotoxic drugs, including vitamin D analogues, calcium salts, and indigestion mixtures that can damage renal function by producing hypercalcemia. The production rate of urea and other metabolic end-products may be increased by excessive protein intake, tissue wasting from starvation, infection, trauma, surgery, resorption of hematoma, bleeding into the gut, and administration of corticosteroids or tetracyclines.

These aggravating factors should be sought and corrected when a patient is seen for the first time in chronic renal failure and on any subsequent occasion when he sustains a faster decline in renal function than would be expected from his primary disease.

It is possible that the decline in GFR caused by the primary disease may be accelerated by hyperphosphatemia which causes calcium phosphate deposition in the kidney. There are good reasons for controlling plasma phosphate at about 4.5 mg per 100 ml (1.4 mMol) in renal failure; higher concentrations should be regarded as correctable aggravating factors in renal failure.

Investigation of Other Medical and Social Problems. This is an essential part of the management of any chronic disease but is particularly important in guiding decisions about regular dialysis and renal transplantation. A social report should be obtained at the time of diagnosis and should be updated as the need for dialysis becomes imminent, so that rehousing and home adaptations can be planned well in advance. Family planning should be discussed and any sterilization procedures carried out before advanced renal failure adds to their hazards. They are best performed on the affected partner in young couples, since dialysis and transplantation still carry a five-year mortality of about 20 per cent in young adults, but vasectomy is a reasonable course for the healthy middle-aged husband of a woman in renal failure whose family is complete. Dental extractions should be carried out before uremia and heparinization add to their difficulty, and regular conservative dental care should be maintained thereafter. Indigestion should be thoroughly investigated and surgery for peptic ulcer considered before transplantation makes corticosteroid therapy necessary. Those centers which practice routine blood transfusion to improve the results of transplantation should plan the appropriate course. Tests for HBsAg should be carried out at regular intervals, particularly in those receiving transfusions, since the development of a carrier state for hepatitis B calls for a total recasting of the plan for dialysis and transplantation. A fistula should be inserted well before it is needed, so that it has time to enlarge.

A well organized, indexed case folder, with laboratory results on flow sheets or graphs and with a regularly updated problem list, is desirable in the management of any chronic disease, but is indispensable in managing chronic renal failure.

THE PATHOPHYSIOLOGY OF CHRONIC RENAL FAILURE. Chronically diseased kidneys often support life in reasonable comfort until 90 per cent of their glomerular filtration has been lost, and they maintain some sort of life until 97 to 99 per cent has gone. This implies that even in the late stages of disease the kidneys retain some ability to respond to the demands of the whole organism by varying the output of water and important solutes. The most popular explanation for this response of the diseased kidney to physiologic stimuli is the "intact nephron hypothesis" that most of the diseased nephrons seen in histologic preparations are nonfunctioning and that renal function depends on a remnant of surviving nephrons in which both glomerulus and tubule have escaped severe damage. In these nephrons, the glomerulus produces an increased volume of filtrate and the tubule hypertrophies to handle this extra filtrate. However, the additional solute load per nephron causes an osmotic diuresis similar to that produced by saline or mannitol infusion in the normal subject. Urine is produced at a nearly constant rate throughout the 24 hours, at an osmolality which is eventually fixed around 300 mOsm per kilogram (specific gravity about 1.010) — a state referred to as isosthenuria. This state becomes established when the GFR falls to about a quarter of normal. It causes nocturia, mild polyuria, and thirst.

The intact nephron hypothesis is clearly an oversimplification. Even the grotesquely deformed nephrons of the polycystic kidney continue to excrete insulin, and the same probably applies to other renal diseases. Those conditions in which medullary damage is a prominent feature — particularly chronic interstitial nephritis, analgesic nephropathy, and medullary cystic disease — are characterized by polyuria with hypotonic urine, suggesting that many functioning nephrons have lost their concentrating mechanism, and have other evidence of impaired distal tubular function.

A corollary of the intact nephron hypothesis is the "trade-off hypothesis" that homeostasis is only achieved in chronic renal failure by straining physiologic control mechanisms beyond their normal limits and exposing the organism to dangerous concentrations of hormones in the process. The one well documented example is the control of plasma phosphate. As GFR declines, the proportion of filtered phosphate excreted in the urine rises so that plasma phosphate remains normal. This is brought about by an increased secretion of parathyroid hormone (PTH), the plasma concentration of which rises above normal when GFR falls to about 30 ml per minute. High plasma PTH causes osteitis fibrosa and metastatic calcification, and according to some authors it contributes more widely to the uremic syndrome, particularly the neurologic features. The patient trades reasonable control of plasma phosphate for bone disease, vascular damage, and perhaps other ills. It has been postulated that there are similar trade-offs in the homeostasis of sodium and potassium, but the evidence so far is not convincing.

Water. Polyuria commonly accompanies isosthenuria. It reaches a peak while GFR declines through the range 25 to 5 ml per minute, and then gives way to oliguria in terminal renal failure except in a minority of patients with predominant medullary damage who remain polyuric even after they are established on regular dialysis. Thirst accompanies polyuria, and if the patient has free access to water, he will usually maintain his water balance with reasonable accuracy. The once popular practice of "pushing fluids" to reduce the plasma urea is unnecessary and potentially dangerous. Thirst is sometimes excessive because dryness of the mouth is common in renal failure; it may be due to overbreathing from acidosis or to an unexplained reduction in salivary flow. Large water loads are excreted more slowly than in the normal subject; hyponatremia follows their ingestion for several hours; convulsions are occasionally precipitated. Conversely, obligatory water loss through the kidney is increased, and patients are therefore sensitive to water deprivation, caused by drowsiness, vomiting, or surgery.

Sodium. Sodium excretion can only be varied over a restricted range in renal failure, and this narrows as GFR declines. The patient remains in reasonable health if his intake is adjusted to the ability of his kidneys to excrete, but he faces trouble if it is close to one of the extremes tolerated by normal persons. The hormonal mechanisms which maintain sodium homeostasis in health with remarkable little change in extracellular fluid (ECF) volume become inadequate as renal function declines. A patient placed on a sodium restricted diet, e.g., the traditional 22 mMol per day, is often unable to reduce his sodium output over the usual time scale. He goes into negative sodium balance and excretes a corresponding volume of water; his ECF volume, plasma volume, and GFR all fall. This has been attributed to the osmotic diuresis in his surviving nephrons which limits his response to normal hormonal controls. However, it has recently been shown that if sodium intake is reduced very gradually — over weeks or months rather than days — most patients with chronic renal failure can reduce renal sodium excretion below 10 mMol per day without substantial reduction in GFR. Clearly, sudden changes in sodium intake are undesirable; if the patient is normotensive on his chosen salt intake, it should not be changed without careful thought.

About 1 to 2 per cent of patients with early chronic renal failure have a urinary sodium leak which causes sodium depletion even on a normal salt intake. They are mainly sufferers from medullary cystic disease and analgesic nephropathy, but a few have obstructive uropathy, chronic interstitial nephritis, polycystic disease, and other renal diseases. They are typically normotensive or hypotensive at rest and have postural hypotension when sodium depleted; this sign often precedes the development of classic features of ECF depletion such as loss of tissue turgor and is an indication for a cautious trial of sodium repletion, which will usually cause a substantial fall in plasma urea.

Sodium retention is a far more common problem than sodium depletion in chronic renal failure. Typically there is an increase in ECF volume and intracellular sodium. If the patient is placed on a high sodium diet, he passes into positive sodium balance, further expanding his ECF and plasma volume and raising his GFR. A new equilibrium is achieved at the price of an overexpanded ECF which may be detectable as peripheral or pulmonary edema. Jugular venous pressure rises, the heart enlarges, a loud murmur of functional mitral incompetence appears, and there may be an early diastolic murmur which has been attributed to expansion of the aortic root, although one recent study suggests that it is often a sound of pericardial origin. The clinical picture is often interpreted as heart failure, and organic valve lesions are suspected erroneously. Less dramatic expansion of ECF is accommodated without overt edema; the overloaded subcutaneous tissue conceals the wasting of muscle and fat characteristic of chronic renal failure, giving the patient a false appearance of adequate nutrition, which is rapidly dispelled when his surplus fluid is removed at the start of regular dialysis.

A fortunate minority of patients remain normotensive when edematous, but the majority develop hypertension when their ECF is expanded. There is an initial rise in cardiac output, which may persist, followed by a rise in peripheral resistance. Sodium retention is the predominant cause of hypertension in chronic renal failure, although a substantial minority of patients have elevated plasma renin and angiotensin levels, particularly when their ECF volume is restored to normal by diuretic therapy or dialysis. About 5 to 10 per cent of patients in terminal renal failure have severe hypertension unresponsive to correction, or even contraction, of ECF volume and accompanied by extreme hyperreninemia. They respond well to bilateral nephrectomy at a considerable cost in operative morbidity and the handicaps associated with the anephric state.

Patients with the more common, sodium-responsive type of hypertension have increasing problems with blood pressure control as they progress into renal failure (Fig. 1). The normal subject excretes only 1 per cent of his filtered sodium in the urine. As GFR declines to a few milliliters per minute, this proportion must rise to 30 per cent if sodium balance is to be maintained — about the same sodium rejection as normal subjects achieve in maximal osmotic diuresis. Some patients fail to reach the goal unless helped by high dose loop diuretic therapy. Occasionally it is necessary to start regular dialysis earlier than would be required for control of uremia, in order to control sodium balance and blood pressure.

Sodium excretion is linked with that of calcium, magnesium, and phosphate, and all tend to move together in response to stimuli appropriate to one. The mechanisms are uncertain. High sodium intake and excretion probably exacerbate the negative calcium balance of chronic renal failure, constituting a further reason for moderate sodium restriction. However, the difficulties are considerable. Restriction of salt further reduces the palatability of a diet already restricted in phosphate, and possibly in potassium and protein, for an anorexic patient. It may be vitiated by the use of medicines such as magnesium trisilicate mixture NF and kaolin and morphine mixture NF, each of which adds 20 to 40 mMol per day to sodium intake in standard doses. Sodium bicarbonate may be needed for correction of acidosis. Although this sodium salt is well tolerated when given alone in renal failure, when it is added to a moderate sodium chloride intake it causes sodium retention. Dietary salt must therefore be curtailed again to compensate.

Potassium. As GFR declines, potassium excretion approaches, and may even surpass, filtered potassium. Nonetheless, for most of the course of chronic renal failure, plasma potassium remains normal or is only moderately elevated (Fig. 2). The ability to excrete a potassium load is diminished, and disastrous hyperkalemia can follow the injudicious administration of medications such as potassium citrate mixture or potassium-sparing diuretics. Intracellular potassium remains normal or low, but hyperkalemia causes the same cardiac abnormalities as in acute renal failure. Occasional patients complain of muscle weakness or paresthesias when plasma potassium reaches dangerous levels (over 7 mMol per liter), but the majority are unaware of the condition until cardiac arrest occurs. The only warning signs are those detected by electrocardiography — flattened P wave, widened QRS complex, and peaked T wave.

In late renal failure hyperkalemia becomes common (Fig. 2), and dangerous peaks of plasma potassium can be produced by trauma, surgery, anesthesia (particularly if depolarizing muscle relaxants are used), blood transfusion, or dietary intake. The use of instant coffee, fruit juice, meat and meat products, fried potatoes, soya flour, fruit, chocolate, peas, beans, and brown bread must be curtailed, and administration of ion exchange resins to increase fecal excretion of potassium may be necessary (though at some penalty in sodium or calcium retention).

Plasma potassium rises with acidosis and can be readily lowered by the administration of sodium bicarbonate. The cardiac effects of hyperkalemia are antagonized by raising plasma calcium with ain infusion of calcium gluconate.

About 2 per cent of patients in *early* chronic renal failure suffer from troublesome hyperkalemia. They are typically patients with a sodium leak, normotension, and hyperchloremic acidosis; some have hyporeninemia and hypoaldosteronism which respond poorly to physiologic stimuli. They often respond well to treatment with fludrocortisone.

Magnesium. Mild asymptomatic hypomagnesemia is seen occasionally in early renal failure (Fig. 3). It is due to increased fecal loss, which is accentuated by a high calcium diet, because calcium and magnesium compete for the same absorptive mechanism. Hypomagnesemia is accentuated by high dose diuretic therapy. It may prevent a satisfactory rise in plasma calcium when vitamin D analogues are administered.

Figure 1. Incidence of hypertension at various stages in chronic renal failure. Glomerular filtration rate is calculated from serum creatinine by formula (see text). (This figure and the next five are based on a survey of 202 patients with chronic renal failure at Newcastle upon Tyne, and are produced from Clinical Features of Chronic Renal Failure by Mishra and Kerr, *In* Proceedings of the XIII International Congress of Internal Medicine, Helsinki, 1976, by permission of the editor. Basel, Karger, 1976.)

Figure 2. Serum potassium at different stages in chronic renal failure.

Most patients in chronic renal failure have normal or moderately raised serum magnesium (Fig. 3), which seldom causes symptoms. Serum magnesium rises further in response to acidosis, tissue trauma, and the administration of vitamin D and its analogues, but very high levels causing drowsiness, coma, muscle weakness, and skin irritation (over 4 mMol) are nearly always due to the administration of magnesium salts as antacids, purgatives, or enemas (magnesium is well absorbed from the colon). The highest levels (over 8 mMol) and most dramatic symptoms are seen in patients on regular dialysis with "hard water syndrome" caused by failure of a water softener or deionizer.

Hydrogen Ion. Hydrogen ion excretion is impaired in two ways in chronic renal failure. There is a diminished capacity to excrete ammonia and a tendency to leak bicarbonate when the plasma bicarbonate level is restored to normal by infusion. When bicarbonate infusion is stopped, renal excretion of bicarbonate continues until plasma bicarbonate falls back to its previous level. This resetting of the plasma level at which a bicarbonate leak occurs is also encountered in primary hyperparathyroidism; in chronic renal failure it is partly but not wholly explained by the secondary hyperparathyroidism.

As renal failure progresses, urine becomes more acid, eventually reaching a pH of about 5 — close to the minimum achieved by normal subjects after acid loading. However, this does not imply normal urinary acid-ification, as the patient achieves this urine pH at a much lower plasma bicarbonate level than the normal subject. Urinary ammonia is lower than normal for the urinary pH, but titratable acidity is normal or only slightly reduced because the main buffers (monohydrogen phosphate and creatinine) are excreted in nearly normal amounts until very late in renal failure.

Respiratory compensation for the acidosis occurs in a predictable manner if there is no lung disease, the uremic subject behaving in the same manner as a normal subject ingesting ammonium chloride. Pa_{CO_2} falls by about 1.2 mm Hg (0.16 kPa) for every 1 mMol fall in plasma bicarbonate. This does not completely correct blood pH, which falls in a roughly linear relationship to the plasma bicarbonate, reaching the lower limit of normal (7.35) when the plasma bicarbonate is about 15 mMol. In terminal renal failure the plasma bicarbonate falls below 10 mMol and there is deep sighing (Kussmaul) respiration which produces a low Pa_{CO_2}, but blood pH is well below the normal range. Any interference with respiratory compensation by chest infection, pulmonary edema, heavy sedation, or coma leads to a rapid increase in the acidosis, and the plasma bicarbonate then ceases to be a reliable guide to the severity of the condition.

Rapid correction of extracellular acidosis by infusion of sodium bicarbonate or hemodialysis is followed by a respiratory alkalosis which persists for about 24 hours. Bicarbonate diffuses slowly into the CSF, which there-

Figure 3. Serum magnesium at different stages in chronic renal failure.

fore remains acid and continues to stimulate the respiratory centers on the anterior surface of the medulla, inappropriately lowering the Pa_{CO_2}.

In patients with predominant renal medullary damage resulting from analgesic nephropathy, calculous disease, and some cases of chronic interstitial nephritis and polycystic disease, ability to acidify the urine is lost in early chronic renal failure. Plasma bicarbonate is lower than would be expected for the GFR, and urinary pH is higher. This secondary renal tubular acidosis is of the distal tubular type due to inability of the distal tubule to maintain a high pH gradient between blood and tubular fluid. The fall in plasma bicarbonate is accompanied by a rise in plasma chloride which may exceed 110 mMol. When there is a reduced bicarbonate concentration in glomerular filtrate, some other anion must be reabsorbed with sodium. In early renal failure the readily available anion is chloride. Hyperchloremic acidosis therefore indicates impairment of hydrogen ion excretion greater than would be expected from loss of nephrons alone. A striking hyperchloremic acidosis is found after urinary diversion into the bowel, particularly the sigmoid colon, and is attributed to the action of bowel mucosa on retained urine, compounding the effect of the commonly associated chronic pyelonephritis. When acidosis develops in late renal failure, plasma chloride is usually normal or depressed, the anion concentration being made up by retained sulfate, phosphate, and other unidentified compounds.

Phosphate and Calcium. Phosphate excretion changes little as GFR falls, since there is a progressive fall in the proportion of filtered phosphate which is reabsorbed in the tubule. This is largely but not entirely the result of increased secretion of parathyroid hormone (PTH). Serum PTH rises above normal about the time GFR reaches 30 ml per minute and steadily climbs as the patient progresses into terminal renal failure. The immunologic methods of measuring PTH also detect its breakdown products, so the rise is exaggerated; but even after allowance for this, serum PTH reaches higher levels in renal failure than in primary hyperparathyroidism.

In spite of the compensatory mechanisms, plasma phosphate rises steeply in late renal failure (Fig. 4) unless dietary phosphate intake is severely curtailed. Milk, cheese, ice cream, meat and meat products, fish and shellfish, baking powder and cakes that incorporate it, bran, whole meal flour, and brown bread are all high in phosphate. It is difficult to construct a diet restricted in potassium and phosphate that still contains adequate first class protein and that patients will actually eat. Consequently moderate phosphate restriction is usually combined with the administration of aluminium hydroxide as gel or powder in doses of 0.5 to 2 grams three or four times a day with meals (the gels typically contain 4 to 5 per cent aluminium hydroxide weight for volume). Many patients find aluminium hydroxide difficult to swallow and nauseating, so it is often baked into cookies and similar preparations to be eaten as dietary supplements.

Despite its difficulty, phosphate restriction is one of the most important aspects of management in chronic renal failure. In experimental animals, and probably in man, if phosphate intake is reduced pari passu with the fall in GFR, hyperparathyroidism is prevented and the rate of decline of renal function is slowed. Hyperphosphatemia, in the presence of a normal or nearly normal plasma calcium, causes calcium phosphate deposition in soft tissues, including the kidney, where it contributes to the "vicious spiral" of declining renal function which seems to affect patients with a GFR below about 10 ml per minute, regardless of the cause.

In vitro, the parathyroid gland is not affected by the phosphate content of its perfusing fluid, provided that the ionized calcium concentration is kept constant. Consequently it is generally believed that hyperphosphatemia causes hyperparathyroidism by depressing serum ionized calcium, but there is a singular lack of experimental confirmation. Plasma phosphate correlates closely with serum PTH (as does plasma creatinine or any other measure of the severity of renal failure), but few authors have found any inverse correlation between serum total or ionized calcium and serum PTH. Patients can be observed to develop secondary hyperparathyroidism without ever having a low serum ionized calcium. Whatever the mechanism, there is no doubt that phosphate retention plays a crucial role in stimulating the parathyroids. They usually display chief cell hyperplasia, but mixed cell hyperplasia and adenoma formation are also common. The size and activity of the parathyroids correlate best with the duration of uremia.

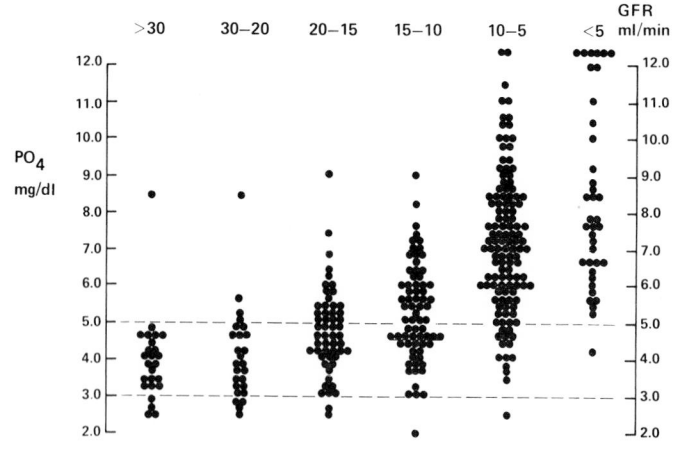

Figure 4. Serum phosphate at different stages in chronic renal failure.

Renal calcium excretion falls early in renal failure, before there is any drop in serum calcium, probably as a reflection of the fall in GFR. However, tubular calcium reabsorption also decreases, possibly as a result of high sodium concentration in tubular fluid, so that calcium excretion falls more slowly than the GFR. By the time that the GFR is about half normal, intestinal absorption of calcium is impaired, at least as judged by conventional tests. The defect is partly a delay in absorption, dietary calcium passing farther down the gut than normal to be absorbed in the ileum. Progressive impairment of calcium absorption occurs as renal failure advances, and in late renal failure there may be net intestinal excretion of calcium. At this stage, urinary calcium excretion has usually fallen to less than 100 mg per 24 hours, but over-all negative calcium balance is usual and is not corrected by regular dialysis, in spite of the virtual absence of urinary excretion, unless calcium is effectively infused into the patient by the use of a high calcium dialysate. Bone calcium content, estimated by bone densitometry or neutron activation, declines rapidly in late renal failure and during regular dialysis, at a rate of 1 to 10 per cent per annum.

Intestinal calcium absorption, calcium balance, and bone calcium content are all normalized by the administration of vitamin D or its analogues and metabolites dihydrotachysterol, 25-hydroxycholecalciferol (25-OHD), 1-α-hydroxycholecalciferol (1-α-OHD), and 1,25-dihydroxycholecalciferol (1,25-$(OH)_2$D). Serum 25-OHD, which reflects vitamin D intake and production in the skin, is normal in early renal failure, is low normal or depressed in late renal failure (probably reflecting anorexia and poor sunlight exposure), and is soon normalized during regular dialysis. Production of 1,25-$(OH)_2$D is depressed from early in renal failure; plasma levels are low or undetectable. It is uncertain whether this is entirely a result of the primary renal disease or whether it is at least partly due to hyperphosphatemia, which is a known inhibitor of 1,25-$(OH)_2$D production.

1-α-OHD is now freely available in Europe, and 1,25-$(OH)_2$D can be readily obtained on both sides of the Atlantic. They are both given in a dose of 0.25 to 2 μg per day by mouth, the higher dose being used for initial treatment and the lower for maintenance. They are interchangeable in action, since 1-α-OHD is readily metabolized by the liver to 1,25-$(OH)_2$D, except that the dose of 1-α-OHD must be increased if drugs that induce hepatic oxidizing enzymes are given simultane-

ously. They are preferred to the alternative drugs because they have a short biologic half-life, so that any hypercalcemia is reversed within a few days by withdrawal of the drug. In other respects, the actions of vitamin D, 25-OHD, and dihydrotachysterol appear to be almost identical to those of 1,25-$(OH)_2$D. A few authors prefer 25-OHD in the treatment of renal osteomalacia, but the evidence for its superiority is equivocal.

Serum calcium declines in renal failure (Fig. 5) and may reach dangerously low levels in late renal failure. Serum ionized calcium makes up an increased proportion of total serum calcium in the presence of acidosis, but even the ionized serum calcium is severely depressed in many patients with terminal renal failure. Tetany is surprisingly uncommon; it is occasionally precipitated by infusion of sodium bicarbonate into hypocalcemic patients and convulsions can then be precipitated, but the common muscle twitching and cramp of renal failure and uremic convulsions are unrelated to plasma calcium levels and are not helped by calcium administration. Cataract may develop rapidly if serum calcium is left untreated at very low levels (below 6 mg per deciliter; 1.5 mMol).

Figure 5 also shows that some patients maintain normal, or even elevated, serum total calcium levels in renal failure. When serum ionized calcium is measured routinely, hypercalcemia from secondary hyperparathyroidism is shown to be a more common problem. It is found mainly in patients with longstanding uremia and very large parathyroid glands. The administration of vitamin D analogues to such patients increases the hypercalcemia and precipitates metastatic calcification. Their plasma phosphate is difficult to control by diet, presumably because much of it is derived from dissolution of bone and muscle. They are best treated by subtotal parathyroidectomy or total parathyroidectomy and partial autotransplantation to the forearm.

Bone Disease. *Osteitis fibrosa* is characterized by increased osteoclastic and osteoblastic activity, more numerous Howship's lucanae, tunneling of trabeculae and cortical bone, and peritrabecular bone marrow fibrosis. It correlates closely with the size of the parathyroid glands and the circulating level of PTH. When well developed, it is revealed radiologically by subperiosteal erosions on the radial margins of the index and midfingers, and, when severe, by erosions on other bones, "pepper pot skull," "rugger-jersey spine" (density of the upper and lower margins of the vertebrae), and ero-

Figure 5. Serum calcium at different stages in chronic renal failure.

sions of the outer clavicles. In its severest forms it is accompanied by metastatic calcification in large and small vessels, in subcutaneous tissues, and around joints, with limb and skin ischemia, spontaneous rupture of tendons, and bone pain, deformity, and fracture. Metastatic calcification may be revealed first by band keratopathy — a crystalline white line just to the corneal side of the limbus, best seen by slit lamp but often visible with the +30 lens of the ophthalmoscope when the eye is viewed from the side. Accompanying conjunctivitis ("uremic red eye") is rare except in terminal renal failure or after overtreatment with vitamin D.

Osteitis fibrosa is almost universal in terminal renal failure; on bone biopsy it is found in about 90 per cent of patients starting regular dialysis, the exceptions being those with rapidly progressive disease and a short experience of uremia. However, only 30 per cent of patients have abnormal radiographs, and about 5 per cent have symptoms from their bone disease. It can be reversed by administration of vitamin D analogues and low phosphate diet in early renal failure, but is likely to recur in terminal renal failure when phosphate escapes from dietary control. It may be retarded for a year or two by regular dialysis but often recurs; few patients survive more than ten years on dialysis without requiring parathyroidectomy.

Osteomalacia affects about 30 per cent of patients starting regular dialysis, although only a small minority have severe symptomatic disease. It is recognized histologically by widened osteoid seams, which are distinguished from those of osteitis fibrosa by the absence of an ossification front. Radiologic features occur late and include pseudofractures (Looser's zones) — which should be sought on the femoral necks, pelvis, humeral necks, and scapulae but can occur almost anywhere — cortical striations, and complete fractures. Bone pain and proximal muscle weakness, with little wasting, well preserved reflexes and a waddling gait, are prominent features. Myopathy also occurs in secondary hyperparathyroidism but should always raise the suspicion of osteomalacia.

The cause of osteomalacia is obscure. It affects patients with renal hypoplasia, urinary obstruction, analgesic nephropathy, infected calculi, and other diseases with a tendency to acidosis but also with a prolonged course in uremia. Some authors have found low plasma 25-OHD levels in affected patients. Improvement has been reported with various vitamin D analogues, including 25-OHD and 1-α-OHD. Plasma alkaline phosphatase is consistently raised in renal osteodystrophy, reflecting the almost invariable presence of osteitis fibrosa, and its decline to normal is a good index of response to treatment.

Osteosclerosis: Thickening of bone trabeculae and sclerosis of certain sites such as the vertebral margins are common in renal failure and are difficult to reconcile with the negative calcium balance; they are presumably due to redistribution of bone.

Renal rickets: Growing children are particularly susceptible to renal osteodystrophy. If untreated, they develop clinical and radiologic features of rickets associated with gross deformity of long bones from continued weight-bearing. However, the histologic pattern in children is little different from that in adults, with osteitis fibrosa the predominant lesion, and the changes in the metaphysis are often those of osteitis fibrosa rather than true rickets. Treatment is similar to that of adults, but corrective surgery is more often required.

Sulfate. Sulfate is produced from the metabolism of sulfur-containing amino acids, approximately in proportion to protein intake. The plasma sulfate rises as GFR declines, roughly in parallel with plasma urea. Sulfate is not the direct cause of any known symptom of renal failure.

Trace Elements. Several trace elements are known to accumulate in renal failure, and it is likely that many others behave in the same way. The most dangerous yet recognized is aluminum. It is scarcely absorbed from the gut of the normal subject, but it probably accumulates with age, since, at least in animals, any which is absorbed is partially deposited in tissues. In renal failure it is more readily absorbed from the gut and less completely excreted by the kidney. Plasma aluminum shows a modest increase in late renal failure, and bone aluminum may be increased several-fold. Oral administration of aluminium hydroxide increases absorption, and this drug should only be given with meals to patients with an elevated serum phosphate. However, there is so far no evidence that it plays a major part in aluminum poisoning, and its benefits appear to outweigh its risks. Massive accumulation of aluminum, leading to dialysis encephalopathy and vitamin D resistant osteomalacia, occurs during dialysis against high-aluminum dialysate.

Fluoride similarly accumulates to a modest degree in late renal failure in fluoridated-water areas, and is readily absorbed from dialysate. No symptoms have been confidently attributed to fluoride accumulation in renal failure, but it is best avoided.

Urea and Ammonia. Urea diffuses into all body secretions. If the plasma concentration is very high, it occasionally crystallizes out of sweat, leaving "urea frost" on the skin. The breakdown of urea to ammonia in a dry and crusted mouth is one cause of the unpleasant, metallic taste and "uremic odor" of terminal renal failure.

In normal subjects about 20 per cent of the daily production of urea is secreted into the gut and broken down by bacteria to ammonia and carbon dioxide. The ammonia is reabsorbed and resynthesized into urea in the liver. A similar absolute amount of urea is catabolized in the gut in renal failure, and, contrary to earlier speculations, the ammonia is not resynthesized into protein to any significant degree. Blood ammonia is not elevated in renal failure unless there is simultaneous liver disease.

Urea production is curtailed by the administration of a low protein diet; but if this is a diet of the patient's own choosing, he develops negative nitrogen balance and other stigmata of protein malnutrition such as a fall in plasma albumin and transferrin. Nitrogen equilibrium can be maintained on a very low protein intake (18 grams per day) if first class protein (egg, milk, a little meat) is combined with protein-free cereals (Giovannetti diet) or if a similar protein-free base is supplemented with pure essential amino acids (plus histidine, which is virtually an essential amino acid in renal failure) or the ketoanalogues of essential amino acids (except lysine and threonine, which must be given intact). Any of these three approaches lowers plasma urea, sulfate, and usually phosphate, since the low protein diets are also phosphate deficient. They relieve nausea and vomiting in late renal failure and cause a modest rise (1 to 2 grams per liter) in hemoglobin. However, the change in diet from traditional food is so profound that long-term patient compliance is unusual, and most clinicians prefer to start dialysis a few months early rather than impose a strict diet in late renal failure.

Amino Acids and Protein. Protein depletion in renal failure can result from anorexia, dietary restriction, and proteinuria. The renal clearance of most amino acids increases when GFR falls below about 30 ml per minute, presumably because of impaired tubular reabsorption. There are substantial losses of amino acids and polypeptides during hemodialysis and peritoneal dialysis and of proteins during peritoneal dialysis. The plasma amino acid pattern is altered in late renal failure and remains abnormal during dialysis. Plasma levels of most of the essential amino acids are depressed, whereas those of most nonessential amino acids are elevated. There are abnormalities of amino acid concentration in intracellular fluid such as low threonine, valine, tyrosine, and carnosine. Most of these abnormalities of amino acid metabolism are ameliorated by administration of supplemental essential amino acids; but since these are expensive and rather unpalatable and no clinical benefit has been unequivocally shown from their use, they are usually prescribed only for patients with obvious malnutrition.

Uric Acid. A rise in plasma urate begins very early in chronic renal disease, but is so slight that the level becomes consistently abnormal only when the GFR falls to about 15 ml per minute. This stability of the plasma urate in the face of a normal production rate and a declining GFR is the result of increased distal tubular secretion of urate and increased uricolysis in the gut. In late renal failure there is a further increase in fractional urate clearance so that plasma urate rises less steeply than plasma urea or creatinine. Levels at least as high as those in gout are often encountered in late renal failure, but secondary gout is rare. It is a phenomenon associated with a few forms of renal disease (lead nephropathy and obstructive uropathy) in which plasma urate rises at an unusually early stage in renal failure.

Carbohydrates. Most patients with chronic renal failure display glucose intolerance, which is referred to as "uremic pseudodiabetes." Fasting plasma glucose may be normal or slightly elevated, but oral or intravenous glucose tolerance tests produce curves suggestive of mild diabetes. Fasting plasma insulin and insulin levels during glucose tolerance tests are higher than in normal subjects but appropriate to the raised plasma glucose concentrations. Severe hyperglycemia does not occur unless the patient is heavily overloaded with glucose, e.g., during peritoneal dialysis with high glucose solutions. Fructose and sorbitol tolerance are normal, suggesting that there is no defect in hepatic glycogenesis. The fall in plasma glucose in response to insulin injection is blunted, suggesting peripheral resistance to the action of insulin, particularly in skeletal muscle. However, if sufficient insulin is given, the patient in chronic renal failure displays hypoglycemia unresponsiveness; it is uncertain whether this reflects a defect in the breakdown of hepatic glycogen (stores of which are usually normal) or the prolonged half-life of insulin in uremia. The latter is largely due to loss of the normal renal degradation of insulin. It is responsible for the declining insulin requirements of diabetics who progress into renal failure.

Several known causes of glucose intolerance, including starvation, potassium depletion, and excessive secretion of growth hormone, can occur in renal failure, but they are seldom implicated in uremic pseudodiabetes. Hypercalcemia, secondary to hyperparathyroidism, causes tissue resistance to the action of insulin, but its contribution to glucose intolerance in uremia is uncertain. Earlier reports that hemodialysis and peritoneal dialysis corrected uremic pseudodiabetes have not been substantiated when the studies were repeated with specific methods for measuring dextrose, and it has been shown that there is considerable variation in glucose tolerance from week to week in uremia.

Plasma total and pancreatic glucagon are increased in fasting patients with chronic renal failure, and they rise abnormally high in response to glucose or alanine loads. This is largely due to loss of renal degradation of glucagon, a major breakdown pathway of this hormone. The glycemic response to injected glucagon is exaggerated in uremia but corrected by dialysis. These abnormalities of glucagon metabolism probably play a part in uremic pseudodiabetes.

Lipids. Atherogenic changes in the plasma lipids occur at all stages in the management of chronic renal failure. They probably act in concert with hypertension and hyperparathyroidism to produce the increased incidence of myocardial infarction, stroke, and peripheral vascular disease found in chronic renal failure. If proteinuria persists in chronic renal failure, it produces the lipid abnormalities of the nephrotic syndrome (raised plasma cholesterol, triglycerides, β and pre-β lipoproteins) in proportion to its severity. Even in the absence of proteinuria, chronic renal failure causes a type 4 hyperlipidemia (raised plasma triglycerides and pre-β lipoproteins) which persists during regular dialysis and is aggravated by the high calorie, high carbohydrate diet often given to such patients. It is probable that the use of acetate in dialysis fluid accentuates hypertriglyceridemia. After renal transplantation hypertriglyceridemia is corrected, unless the patient gains excessive weight, but is replaced by hypercholesterolemia and β lipoprotein increase (type 2a hyperlipidemia), probably as a result of corticosteroid therapy. At all stages of renal failure high density lipoprotein cholesterol is diminished.

The hyperlipidemia of all stages of renal failure responds to appropriate dietary measures (low carbohydrate for hypertriglyceridemia; low saturated fat, low cholesterol for hypercholesterolemia), but lipid-lowering agents such as clofibrate, nicotinic acid, and cholestyramine cause a high incidence of side effects and are best avoided unless there are facilities for monitoring drug levels.

Endocrine Function. In chronic renal failure plasma *renin* is normal or raised and responds to physiologic stimuli such as volume depletion and hyperkalemia, except in a few patients with hyperreninemia (see Sodium, above); plasma $1,25-(OH)_2D$ is low (see Bone Disease, above); and plasma *erythropoietin* is low for the level of hemoglobin, except in occasional patients with polycystic disease or hydronephrosis who develop polycythemia (see Anemia, below).

The kidney plays an important part in the degradation of many polypeptide and small protein hormones; loss of this catabolic pathway in chronic renal failure increases their half-life and prolongs their effect. Important examples include insulin, glucagon, and PTH (see Carbohydrates and Bone Disease, above). Plasma gastrin is elevated and probably contributes to the high incidence of peptic ulcer in chronic renal failure. Plasma vasoactive peptide hormone is raised, but secretin is normal.

The facial appearance in chronic renal failure is reminiscent of myxedema; plasma total thyroxine and triiodothyronine levels are reduced, whereas plasma thyroid-binding globulin is normal except in the presence of very heavy proteinuria, leading to overdiagnosis of hypothyroidism. However, plasma thyroid-stimulating hormone and free thyroxine and triiodothyronine levels are all normal; the true incidence of myxedema is probably no higher in chronic renal failure than in the normal population.

Sexual dysfunction is a major cause of misery in chronic renal failure. The onset of puberty is delayed by several years in children with renal insufficiency. In adult males, libido and potency decline in late renal failure, may be partially restored by regular dialysis, and improve considerably after transplantation. Reduced potency often persists throughout in middle-aged and elderly men. Plasma testosterone is consistently depressed, and plasma luteinizing hormone elevated, suggesting Leydig cell dysfunction. Poor spermatogenesis and elevated plasma follicle-stimulating hormone suggest similar dysfunction of the germ cells. The response of plasma gonadotropins to the LH-FSH-RH test is prolonged, but this may be due to slow clearance of the releasing hormone by the kidneys. Potency is seldom restored by testosterone administration.

In women, libido is depressed, ovulation suppressed, and amenorrhea common in late renal failure. However, contraception is advisable, since pregnancy can occur late in renal failure and is associated with decline in renal function, increased hypertension, slow fetal growth, and high fetal mortality. Pregnancy is usually uneventful for mother and fetus if the disease is static or slowly progressive, if blood pressure is normal at the start of pregnancy, and if serum creatinine is initially normal and shows the usual fall during the first trimester; it is increasingly hazardous if some of these conditions are not fulfilled.

Plasma prolactin is often raised in chronic renal failure and may play a role in the gynecomastia commonly seen in men in late renal failure and the first few months of dialysis. Suppression of prolactin secretion with bromocriptine has little effect on sexual function.

Uremic Toxins.   Many of the clinical features of chronic renal failure are explained by the perturbations of water, electrolyte, and hormone metabolism discussed in this chapter. The remainder compose the syndrome of *uremia,* which is attributed to retention of metabolic waste products. More than 300 compounds have been identified, at least as peaks on chromatograms, which accumulate in renal failure. Their concentrations rise roughly in parallel, so any of the features of renal failure are bound to correlate with the concentration of many different substances, and such correlations are no proof of cause and effect. Differential removal of some substances by diet or dialysis gives an idea of their role in causing uremia, and on this basis it is unlikely that many symptoms are due to accumulation of urea, creatinine, or uric acid. Other contenders for the role(s) of uremic toxin include guanidines, amines, phenols and phenolic acids, "middle molecules" (polypeptides with a molecular weight around 1100), myoinositol, polyamines, indoles, oxalic acid, cyclic AMP, and ribonuclease. None of these seems likely to explain more than one or two small facets of the syndrome.

CLINICAL FEATURES OF CHRONIC RENAL FAILURE AND THEIR MANAGEMENT.   The early stages of chronic renal disease are dominated by the manifestations of the primary illness, by proteinuria and its consequences, and by hypertension. Growth retardation in children, bone disease in patients with slowly declining GFR, and anemia are all features of early chronic renal failure, although they increase in incidence and severity in late renal failure. Most of the electrolyte derangements and hormonal changes discussed previously begin in early chronic renal failure (Figs. 2 to 5), but they seldom cause much morbidi-

ty or life-threatening complications until the GFR has fallen to 15 or 10 ml per minute. Most of the other clinical features described below occur predominantly in late renal failure.

In those countries where dialysis and transplant are freely available, many of these features can be avoided by plotting renal function and starting dialysis when the GFR has fallen to about 10 ml per minute, before the patient has suffered much morbidity or lost much time from work. In less fortunate countries, conservative treatment is continued until clinical features make dialysis essential. The clinician questions his patient at every visit and notes the onset of new features, not only for their own sake but also as warnings that the time for starting dialysis is fast approaching. The clinical features that have been discussed under Pathophysiology (bone disease, sexual dysfunction, electrolyte disturbance) will not be repeated here.

Hypertension.   Hypertension is present in half of all patients entering early chronic renal failure and 80 per cent of those starting dialysis (Fig. 1). Its causes are discussed under Sodium, above. The complications are similar to those of hypertension of any other cause, but a malignant phase and resistance to drug therapy are more common in renal failure than in essential hypertension. After the primary disease hypertension is the most important determinant of survival. Malignant hypertension causes a vicious spiral of declining renal function and worsening hypertension. The existence of a similar vicious spiral with lesser degrees of hypertension is widely assumed but poorly documented. Correction of hypertension seldom leads to an improvement in renal function and more often causes a fall in GFR. Nonetheless treatment of hypertension is mandatory to protect the patient from its extrarenal effects. The choice of drugs is similar to that in essential hypertension, except that note must be taken of the dependence of the drug on renal excretion.

Beta-blockers are common first choice drugs. Selective blockers such as atenolol, acebutolol, and metoprolol are theoretically preferable to nonselective blockers. Atenolol has the advantage of once-daily dosage, but it cumulates in renal failure and should be given in a small dose (not more than 50 mg per day) initially. Acebutolol has a major excretory pathway through the gut and can be given in normal dosage in renal failure (starting dose 200 mg twice daily). Propranolol (starting dose 20 to 40 mg three times a day) and oxprenolol (starting dose 40 mg three times a day) also have major extrarenal excretion. Presently, only propranolol and metoprolol are available in the United States.

The diuretics often given with beta-blockers in essential hypertension (e.g., bendrofluazide, cyclopenthiazide, chlorthalidone) are ineffective when GFR falls below about 20 ml per minute. Furosemide in increasing doses up to 1 gram per day retains its effectiveness in chronic renal failure, although the individual response is unpredictable. Hearing should be monitored in patients taking high dose furosemide.

The alpha-blocking drug prazosin or the vasodilator hydralazine is a reasonable third choice to add to a beta-blocker–diuretic combination. Prazosin should be started in a small dose (0.5 mg at night) and the patient warned to lie down if he experiences postural hypotension. This "first dose effect" usually wears off after the first few days. The dose can be increased to 2 to 6 mg three times a day. Hydralazine should be given in a dose up to 200 mg per day in two or three divided doses. Above that dosage there

Figure 6. Hemoglobin at different stages in chronic renal failure.

is an increasing incidence of allergic side effects (drug-induced lupus erythematosus).

Alternative drugs include methyldopa, which can be given in a starting dose of 125 mg three times a day and increased to a maximum of 500 mg four times a day. Increases beyond this dose seldom produce further benefit. Common side effects are drowsiness, thought blockage, and impotence. Postural hypotension is uncommon when methyldopa or beta-blockers are given alone but becomes increasingly common when diuretics or vasodilators are added. It is almost invariable with effective doses of the sympathetic blockers (guanethidine, bethanidine,* debrisoquine*), which is why they are now used as fourth-choice drugs when others have failed. Clonidine (initial dose 0.1 mg three times a day) is roughly interchangeable with methyldopa. It may cause less sexual disturbance, but has two additional side effects — dry mouth and severe rebound hypertension if the drug is stopped suddenly; it should be given only to patients who are reliable at taking their drugs and renewing their supply.

For patients who resist, or cannot tolerate, the usual drugs there are two last courts of appeal. Diazoxide is given in a rapid intravenous injection of 300 mg (which may be repeated up to four times daily) for hypertensive emergencies. Orally it is given in an initial dose of 50 mg three times a day, increasing to about 300 mg three times a day. The dose should be increased gradually and blood dextrose monitored frequently, as it causes hyperglycemia in some patients. Minoxidil* has similar actions without this liability to hyperglycemia, but it is not generally available. Both drugs cause excessive hair growth, which makes them unacceptable to women for long-term use.

Edema. Edema may be due to nephrotic syndrome or cardiac failure, but in chronic renal failure it is usually due to impaired renal excretion of sodium and water. Nephrotic syndrome is recognized by heavy proteinuria, severe hypoalbuminemia, and a nephrotic electrophoretic pattern. Heart failure and renal sodium retention are hard to distinguish, but the treatment is the same — dietary sodium restriction and diuretics. Cardiac glycosides are indicated in atrial fibrillation; digoxin cumulates in renal failure and should be given in about half the normal dose. Digitoxin can be given in normal dosage. Blood levels should be monitored. Their value is more dubious in normal sinus rhythm, and their hazards are increased if plasma potassium is oscillating over an abnormal range as a result of diuretic therapy and dialysis.

Pulmonary edema is a common complication of chronic renal failure, owing to disturbance of Starling forces in the lungs. The edema fluid has a high protein content. Clinical features are dyspnea, frothy sputum, basal crepitations, and "bat's wing" perihilar shadows on chest roentgenograms. Roentgenology is essential if the diagnosis is suspected, since severe edema can be present without physical signs. If treated early, the condition is readily reversible by high dose diuretics (250 to 500 mg furosemide intravenously in an infusion over one hour or in two slow injections) or by hemodialysis or peritoneal dialysis. The most dramatically effective treatment, if diuretics fail, is ultrafiltration through a dry dialyzer, which can remove 2 to 3 liters in one hour. Neglected or recurrent pulmonary edema causes thickening of lung septa and permanent reduction in diffusing capacity.

Anemia. Anemia is almost universal in late chronic renal failure (Fig. 6), so a patient with renal failure and a normal hemoglobin should be regarded as suffering from acute renal failure until proved otherwise. Patients with polycystic disease have higher hemoglobins than others with chronic renal failure at the same GFR, and a few develop polycythemia. Red cells are normochromic, red cell precursors in the marrow are normal or slightly increased, the reticulocyte count, when corrected for red cell count, is one to four times normal, and radioiron transit time through the marrow is normal or reduced. In each case the evidence of marrow activity is well below what would be expected for the degree of anemia. This marrow inactivity is partly, but not wholly, corrected by injection of erythropoietin, which is not available for clinical use. Anephric patients have lower hemoglobins than those who retain their diseased kidneys, but they can survive with a hemoglobin of around 6 grams per deciliter without transfusion. The bone marrow depression not accounted for by erythropoietin lack is presumed to be due to "uremic toxins," since it is often reversed by hemodialysis.

Iron deficiency can coexist with the anemia of renal failure, when it is revealed by the usual changes in absolute indices (low MCV, MCH, and MCHC) and responds to oral iron. Mild folate deficiency is suggested by raised leukocyte lobe counts and low red cell folate in chronic renal failure, but administration of folate has little effect.

When the plasma urea nitrogen concentration is above about 90 mg per deciliter (33 mMol), red cell life is shortened to about half normal and burr cells are seen on the blood film. Red cell life is restored to normal by adequate hemodialysis.

Anemia becomes a major cause of symptoms in renal

---

*Investigational drug in United States.

failure when the hemoglobin falls below about 7 grams per deciliter. Its effects are mitigated by a shift in the oxygen dissociation curve to the right due to an increased concentration of 2,3-diphosphoglycerate and other organic phosphates in the red cells. Its manifestations are pallor, raised jugular venous pressure, tachycardia, and wide pulse pressure accentuated by exercise and a systolic ejection murmur maximum over the pulmonary area, which is almost universal in late chronic renal failure. The murmur becomes louder when cardiac output is further increased by the insertion of an arteriovenous fistula, when it can readily suggest organic heart disease. Precipitation of severe angina is the symptom of anemia that most often calls for treatment.

The only effective drugs are androgens and anabolic steroids. Sustanon, a mixture of testosterone esters available in Great Britain, is given in a weekly intramuscular dose of 250 mg to men. (Testosterone cypionate [Depo-Testosterone], 100 or 200 mg per week, may be used in the United States.) A major, although rare, side effect of Sustanon is priapism, which usually starts during a nocturnal erection in the course of overnight dialysis. It causes a very uncomfortable three weeks, followed by permanent impotence. Sustanon will raise the hemoglobin by 10 to 20 grams per liter, which may be crucial to the patient with angina. Nandrolone decanoate, 50 to 100 mg intramuscularly every three weeks, has a similar effect in women; they should be warned to report masculinizing side effects such as hair growth and skin thickening as soon as they are noticed, for the voice change that follows is irreversible.

Transfusion can usually be avoided and was once banned with religious fervor. It is occasionally helpful to the patient with angina and is now thought to improve the chances of subsequent transplant. Small transfusions that do not overload the circulation (usually 200 to 500 ml of packed cells) do not affect renal function, but their effect is short lived since red cell life is shorter in uremics than in normals and marrow function is further depressed. Only blood meticulously screened for HbsAg, and preferably for HBcAb and cytomegalovirus, should be used.

Bleeding Tendency. A hemorrhagic tendency, manifested by epistaxis, menorrhagia, increased occult intestinal blood loss, and excessive bleeding or bruising after trauma, is common in late renal failure but seldom life threatening. Whole blood clotting time and prothrombin time are normal. Bleeding time is prolonged, although a sensitive test is necessary to demonstrate this. Total platelet count and life span are normal, but abnormalities of platelet function are thought to be responsible for the bleeding tendency. The proportion of sticky platelets is reduced, platelet aggregation with ADP and other agents impaired, the prothrombin consumption test abnormal, and platelet factor III availability decreased. These defects are largely corrected by hemodialysis and have been proposed as tests of adequate dialysis.

Plasma fibrinogen level is raised in chronic renal failure, particularly in patients with proliferative glomerular lesions. It is probably responsible for the raised ESR of chronic renal failure, which is out of proportion to the anemia. Plasma fibrinolytic activity is depressed but is corrected by hemodialysis. Fibrin degradation products can often be demonstrated in plasma, suggesting excessive intravascular deposition and removal of fibrin.

Bleeding in uremia is best controlled by local measures and adequate dialysis, with reduced heparinization, monitored by measurement of thrombin time or similar tests. Infusion of the fibrinolysis-inhibitor aminocaproic acid in an initial dose of 100 mg per kilogram of body weight over four hours is occasionally helpful when bleeding into the gut is not controlled by these measures.

Infection. Susceptibility to bacterial infection is believed to be characteristic of uremia, although this is hard to prove. Infection is certainly a cause of much morbidity in patients with chronic renal failure, and it remains one of the leading causes of death in patients treated by regular dialysis. The neutrophil count is normal in chronic renal failure and rises normally during infection, but the ability of the cells to ingest and kill bacteria is impaired. There is a steep fall in neutrophil count in the first half hour of dialysis with cellulose membranes and a rebound over the next four hours; leukocyte counts are mildly depressed in patients on regular dialysis, but there is wide overlap with the normal range. It is not known whether these changes affect resistance to infection.

The lymphocyte count is reduced in chronic renal failure. Total serum immunoglobulins are normal, unless altered by the primary disease or proteinuria, and the anamnestic response to antigens such as tetanus toxoid is normal, but the appearance of antibodies to new antigens is delayed and their titer low. The Mantoux and similar tests show impairment of delayed hypersensitivity, which is a mixed blessing; those with the most depressed reactions tolerate renal transplants well.

Colonization of the nose and other carrier sites with staphylococci is a common problem in patients with chronic renal failure which may reflect their exposure to the hospital environment rather than the uremic state. Chronic staphylococcal carriers are peculiarly susceptible to infection of shunts, fistulas, peritoneal catheters, and operation wounds, and local or systemic treatment of the carrier state is singularly ineffective. Superinfection with *Candida albicans* is very common in chronic renal failure and almost routine after renal transplantation. It affects the buccal mucosa, causing white plaques, which give way to painful ulcers and may spread to the esophagus, causing dysphagia. It is treated with amphotericin lozenges,* 10 mg sucked every hour, or/and with miconazole jelly* applied to the mouth every hour. Nystatin tablets or suspension, 500,000 units four hourly, should be given if there is a suspicion of intestinal candidiasis. Buccal "thrush" in chronic renal failure can be caused by bacteria, so it is essential to confirm the diagnosis by smear and culture.

Every effort should be made to identify the organism before starting antibacterial therapy. Blood culture is especially important, since septicemia is common in renal failure. If no portal of entry can be found, the arteriovenous fistula should be suspected. In staphylococcal carriers there is a good chance that the infectant is the organism carried in the nares. The loading dose of antibacterials is unchanged in renal failure. That statement is not strictly true of drugs which are rapidly excreted, such as penicillin G, but it is a good enough approximation for clinical purposes. The size or spacing of maintenance doses may be adjusted as described below under Drug Therapy. If the organism can be recognized with confidence, a narrow-spectrum antibacterial should be chosen where there is a choice on other grounds.

Gastrointestinal Symptoms. Dry mouth, metallic taste, and uremic odor can be helped a little by mouth toilet and chewing gum. Anorexia is a common early symptom, progressing to nausea, vomiting, and eventually continuous dry retching. Nausea and vomiting not explained by local disease are an indication for starting

---

*Not available in United States.

dialysis or, if this is unavailable, for temporary dialysis followed by a Giovannetti diet. Metoclopramide, 10 mg three times a day, or prochlorperazine, 10 mg three times a day, can be given orally or intramuscularly, or thiethylperazine, 10 mg by suppository, for temporary relief. All are likely to cumulate in renal failure and cause extrapyramidal side effects. A distressing tardive dyskinesia (uncontrolled facial grimacing) occurs early with metoclopramide in susceptible subjects. In the last resort stupor caused by large doses of chlorpromazine is preferable to the misery of continuous retching.

Diarrhea, resulting from uremic ulceration of the gut, is a very late manifestation of chronic renal failure. Most uremics complain of constipation; if they get diarrhea, it is because of their antibacterial or antihypertensive therapy. There is probably an increased incidence of hematemesis and melena in uremic patients even before they are subjected to heparinization for dialysis, owing to their susceptibility to peptic ulceration.

Nutrition and Growth. Wasting of fat and muscle, dry flaky skin, and straggly hair are common but not invariable features of late chronic renal failure. They are corrected by adequate dialysis and refeeding, although the average dialysis patient remains below average weight and retains a few biochemical stigmata of malnutrition even when encouraged to take a high protein diet.

Children even in early chronic renal failure have a slow growth rate. They are typically well below the third percentile for height and weight. Bone age is retarded, so potential for catch-up growth may be retained well after the usual age. Growth retardation is closely related to low calorie intake from anorexia, but attempts to correct it by feeding calorie supplements has merely reduced other food intake in proportion. Renal osteodystrophy aggravates stunting, and there is a modest improvement in growth when it is treated with vitamin D analogues. On regular dialysis growth rate improves, but there is seldom any catch-up growth. Much better results are obtained with a well matched transplant if it is implanted before puberty. Severe stunting is an indication for considering transplantation earlier than would be comtemplated on other grounds.

Pericarditis. Pericarditis was once the harbinger of death. It occurred in half the patients dying of renal failure, and they seldom survived its onset by more than two months. It is now a sign that hemodialysis has been delayed or ineffective and calls for urgent treatment. It is often precipitated by systemic viral or bacterial infection.

The onset is usually signaled by pain, which is often felt on the left side of the chest on inspiration for the first few hours but may be central from the start. Pain is frequently severe, mimicking myocardial infarction, but it may appear after the friction rub and disappear long after it. The friction rub is usually loud, generalized, and palpable, and it may persist when the pericardial cavity contains 0.5 liter of fluid and fatal tamponade is imminent. The important signs of tamponade are falling blood pressure and pulse pressure, paradoxical fall in blood pressure with inspiration, cold, poorly perfused extremities, and raised jugular venous pressure. Paradoxical movement of the neck veins is a late and inconstant sign. On chest roentgenograms the typical globular shape of the heart is seen in first attacks, but recurrent pericarditis produces a dense fibrous pericardium which alters little in shape as fluid accumulates. Electrocardiographic signs are inconstant and of no help in diagnosis. The diagnosis can be confirmed, the size of the effusion estimated, and the myocardial function judged by the echocardiogram. The fluid should be removed by paracentesis, repeatedly if necessary, and intensive dialysis maintained. The fluid is usually blood stained, with a hematocrit about half that of the circulating blood. Administration of indomethacin orally and instillation of corticosteroids locally have been advocated but without controlled trial. Recurrent effusion is treated by creating a pericardial window and fibrous constrictive pericarditis by complete pericardiectomy.

Other Cardiovascular Problems. Deposits of calcium phosphate are found in the heart in severe hyperparathyroidism, and calcium oxalate and urates are deposited during inadequate dialysis. Sudden cardiac arrest or arrhythmias may result from deposition in the conducting tissue.

Peripheral Neuropathy. Nerve conduction slows in chronic renal failure, falling to half normal in the legs in terminal renal failure; the arms are less affected. Diminished ankle jerks and reduced vibratory sense are found in about 20 per cent of patients starting dialysis, but spontaneous complaint is rare. Severe neuropathy leading to quadriplegia was a common complication in the early days of regular dialysis but is now rarely encountered. It began with numbness of the toes and tingling and burning in the feet and progressed with ascending anesthesia, areflexia, and finally paralysis. It was sometimes precipitated by infection, and it is likely that some cases were drug induced; nitrofurantoin was a common culprit in Britain. Neuropathy slowly improved with effective dialysis and was rapidly reversed by renal transplantation. An ischemic neuropathy, of mononeuritis multiplex type, can complicate falls in blood pressure during dialysis.

Patients with chronic renal failure who complain of tingling and numbness in fingers and toes are usually suffering from Raynaud's phenomenon, which is extremely common in renal failure and is exacerbated by the insertion of shunts and fistulas.

Myopathy. A proximal myopathy accompanies renal osteomalacia and, less commonly, osteitis fibrosa. It produces a waddling gait, difficulty in climbing stairs and mounting buses, and inability to work with the hands above the head. Wasting is slight and reflexes pathologically brisk.

Cramps. Muscle cramps in the calves, thighs, and flexors of the toes are common in early renal failure, particularly at night. They may also occur in the upper limbs and during the day, when they are precipitated by stretching, awkward posture, or repetitive movements such as knitting. Severe cramps are common during dialysis when fluid is rapidly removed, particularly if a low sodium dialysate is employed. Nocturnal cramps can be alleviated by a nightly dose of quinine sulfate, 300 mg orally.

Other Nervous and Muscular Symptoms. *Muscle twitching* affects single muscles or groups in late renal failure. It wakes the patient as he dozes off. When severe, it may prevent writing or holding a cup. *Flapping tremor* is due to a similar sudden involuntary relaxation of muscle groups. *Restlessness of the limbs* is another common complaint, probably of central origin. The whole limb must be moved to relieve an uncomfortable feeling which the patient has difficulty in describing and may refer to as pain. It may be accompanied by dysesthesias. In underdialyzed patients the syndrome may progress to generalized restlessness resembling hemiballismus. These features respond to dialysis, although they do not always disappear completely. As emergency treatment, diazepam, 10 mg intravenously, is effective and can be repeated every four hours.

Persistent *hiccup* is common in terminal renal failure, and it occasionally affects a patient at an earlier stage, exhausting him over the course of a few days. Heavy sedation with chlorpromazine will sometimes abort the attack.

Insomnia is common; although sometimes caused by pruritus or restless limbs, it may persist after these have been corrected. It is accompanied by lethargy during the day and may represent reversal of sleep rhythm. Nocturnal sedatives should be avoided as long as possible, and barbiturates and methaqualone should not be employed because, in addition to their other disadvantages, they induce hepatic enzymes and may aggravate bone disease. Nitrazepam in Britain or diazepam in the United States is the usual first choice drug. It does not cumulate in renal failure, but, like all drugs of this group, it is metabolized to compounds which do cumulate to very high levels. Although the metabolites of diazepam and its relatives are not as active as the parent compounds, they have some activity when in high concentration and have occasionally led to a state of pseudodementia.

Tiredness is almost universal in chronic renal failure, although the level at which it occurs is variable; some patients are active in business with a GFR of 10 ml per minute or even less. Its causes include sleep disturbance, anemia, hypertensive heart failure, myopathy, and drug side effects, but there is probably a specific effect of uremia which is noticeably relieved by the first one or two hemodialyses.

Mental fatigability begins in early chronic renal failure and is succeeded by loss of concentration, reduced performance at mental arithmetic and other demanding skills, impaired memory, and, in terminal renal failure, drowsiness, disorientation, stupor, and coma. Episodes of toxic psychosis are associated with infections and pericarditis in late renal failure. Electroencephalographic changes accompanying these mental disturbances are slowing of the dominant frequency, eventually to 2 or 3 waves per second, and sporadic spike potentials. The EEG and mental changes are rapidly corrected by adequate dialysis. However, if dialysis is performed too rapidly in a severely uremic patient, a disequilibrium syndrome of headache, vomiting, confusion, coma, and convulsions may be precipitated, probably as a result of cerebral edema following rapid change in plasma urea and sodium. It should be avoided by early or gentle dialysis; but if the risk is high, prophylactic anticonvulsants such as sodium phenytoin, 100 mg intramuscularly, should be given before dialysis.

Dialysis encephalopathy is a syndrome of speech disturbance, apraxia, myoclonic jerking, grimacing, convulsions, dementia, and a characteristic EEG abnormality which affects patients in some dialysis centers. It is almost certainly due to accumulation of aluminum from dialysis fluid and is discussed under Trace Elements, above.

Convulsions occur spontaneously in late and terminal renal failure. They are more common in patients with severe hypertension, and this is almost the exclusive cause in patients with early chronic renal failure. A few are precipitated by electrolyte disturbances such as water intoxication, hypocalcemia, and rapid correction of acidosis. They are usually of grand mal type, but some are jacksonian. They often recur in rapid succession and carry a formidable mortality from cardiac arrest during the anoxic phase or inhalation pneumonia. They should be treated much more seriously than ordinary epileptic fits, which rarely cause death. Emergency treatment is with intravenous diazepam, 10 mg intravenously, repeated as necessary to control the fits, or given by infusion. In the last resort it is better to anesthetize and ventilate the patient than to allow the fits to continue. Usually they can be controlled less drastically with intramuscular phenytoin, 100 mg every eight hours, and phenobarbital, 60 to 120 mg daily, once initial control has been gained with diazepam. Hypertension should be controlled simultaneously with diazoxide (as described under Hypertension, above).

Ocular Manifestations. The most important changes in the eye are those of hypertensive retinopathy. Visual acuity is impaired in the presence of papilledema, and some visual defect may persist, in which case the pale disc of optic atrophy will be seen when papilledema subsides. Large hemorrhages and exudates cause scotomas which seldom give rise to spontaneous complaint unless the lesion is at the macula. Control of hypertension is followed by disappearance of hemorrhages, soft exudates, and papilledema within a few weeks, but hard exudates may persist for many months.

Retinal detachment, usually of globular shape in the lower half of the eye, occurs in patients with severe hypertension, renal failure, and fluid overload. It sometimes resolves spontaneously but is more likely to do so if hypertension and fluid overload are corrected. Surgery may be required to close a retinal tear.

Pingueculae (lipid deposits under the conjunctiva) are common in renal failure, especially in patients with corneal and conjunctival calcification. Uremic red eye is discussed under Calcium, above.

Skin Manifestations. Pigmentation, particularly of sun-exposed areas, is common in chronic renal failure, particularly in dark-haired individuals. Pigmentation of the distal nail bed causes the brown nail arcs of renal failure. The pigment is partly melanin, partly lipochromes which accumulate in renal failure and darken on exposure to sunlight. Plasma melanophore-stimulating hormone is raised in renal failure, but its role in the pigmentation is uncertain. A reduced sebum secretion contributes to the dry skin of renal failure.

Pruritus is common in secondary hyperparathyroidism and responds to parathyroidectomy. Uremic itching when plasma $Ca \times PO_4$ product is normal is unexplained. Benefit has been claimed for treatment with ultraviolet light and for oral administration of cholestyramine, but further studies are needed to test these more rigorously; there is a large placebo response in itching.

Miscellaneous. *Wound healing* is delayed in uremia, and incisional hernia is common. Stitches should be retained for an extra week. *Pancreatitis* is common in renal failure. A modest rise in serum amylase can occur from renal failure alone. *Ascites* develops almost exclusively in patients who have had peritoneal dialysis at some time; the fluid has a high protein content. *Pleurisy* is usually secondary to pneumonia but has been described as a primary event in renal failure. *Hepatitis B* has a greatly increased liability to produce a chronic carrier state in renal failure; this is probably part of a generalized defect in mounting an immunologic attack on viruses. There appears to be an increased incidence of herpes zoster and recurrent facial herpes.

GENERAL MANAGEMENT OF CHRONIC RENAL FAILURE. This includes planned clinical and laboratory monitoring (discussed above under Investigation), the detec-

TABLE 4. Maintenance Dose of Antimicrobials in Renal Failure

Group 1. Mainly excreted or metabolized by nonrenal routes. Must be given in normal dosage for therapeutic effect.

    Fusidic acid
    Chloramphenicol

Group 2. Major pathway of nonrenal excretion or metabolism. Normal dosage schedule may be used for a day or two, but some reduction in dosage is desirable.

Methicillin	Erythromycin
Cloxacillin	Sulfadimidine
Flucloxacillin	Carbenicillin
Ampicillin	Doxycycline
Amoxycillin	Cephalexin

Group 3. Predominantly renal excretion. Some dosage reduction is desirable from the start. Space doses (of normal size) more widely than usual, but not more than 24 hours apart.

Penicillin G	Co-trimoxazole	Mecillinam
Cephaloridine	Nalidixic acid	Cephalexin
Cephalothin	Isoniazid	Cefuroxime
Lincomycin	Ethambutol	
Clindamycin	Rifampin	

Group 4. Mainly renal excretion and toxic effects during cumulation. Major adjustment of dosage required; daily monitoring of blood antibiotic concentration required.

Kanamycin	Vancomycin
Gentamicin	Para-aminosalicylate
Polymyxin B	Amphotericin
Colimycin	Amikacin
Streptomycin	Tobramycin

Group 5. Contraindicated in renal failure.

    Nitrofurantoin
    All tetracyclines except doxycycline
    Long-acting sulfonamides

tion and management of complications (discussed above), selection for dialysis and transplantation, and institution of these treatments at the correct time. A 40-gram high protein diet is usually instituted when uremic symptoms become troublesome if dialysis cannot be started forthwith. An aspect of growing importance is the management of drug therapy. Patients should be issued with a card which states that they are sufferers from chronic renal failure, and which lists the common drugs that should not be given in this state and to which the patient is allergic. The telephone number of the renal unit or local Drug Advisory Service should be provided so that practitioners can seek advice before prescribing drugs. Too often inquiries about the pharmacology of the drug are made after it has been given and has caused side effects. No drug should be given in renal failure without knowledge of its pharmacology and the effects of renal failure.

Drug Therapy in Renal Failure. Chronic renal failure can affect gut absorption of drugs (e.g., calcium salts), volume of distribution and regional blood flow (e.g., pancuronium, which has a protracted effect in renal failure), protein binding (e.g., phenytoin, diazoxide), or hepatic degradation. End-organ sensitivity may be altered, e.g., the bone marrow or the heart. Much the most common and most important effect of renal failure is loss of renal excretion of the drug or its active metabolites.

Sources of information on drug metabolism in renal failure are listed in the references below. If information is lacking, an intelligent guess can be made if the pharmacology in the normal is known. Water-soluble drugs are given by injection (e.g., penicillin G, gentamicin); they are usually excreted unchanged by the kidney and cumulate in renal failure. Lipid-soluble drugs are given by mouth and are metabolized in the liver; they do not cumulate in renal failure but their water-soluble metabolites do, so it is important to know whether these metabolites are active or toxic.

Table 4 lists some of the major antibacterials. They should be given with a normal loading dose but spaced maintenance doses as indicated in the table. Those with a narrow safety margin should be monitored by daily estimation of blood level and the dose schedule adjusted accordingly.

Drug Therapy in Renal Failure

Anderson, R. J., Gambertoglio, J. G., and Schrier, R. W.: Clinical Use of Drugs in Renal Failure. Springfield, Ill., Charles C Thomas, 1976.
Kerr, D. N. S. (ed.): Drug metabolism in chronic renal failure. Proc. Eur. Dialysis Transplant Assoc., 13:597, 1976.

Other Aspects of Chronic Renal Failure

Avram, M. M., Feinfeld, D. A., and Huatuco, A. H.: Search for the uremic toxin; decreased motor-nerve conduction velocity and elevated parathyroid hormone in uremia. N. Engl. J. Med., 298:1000, 1978.
Bergstrom, J. (ed.): Nitrogen and amino acid metabolism in uremia. Clin. Nephrol., 5:165, 1975.
Chesney, R. W., Moorthy, A. V., Eisman, J. A., Jax, D. K., Mazess, R. B., and DeLuca, H. F.: Increased growth after long-term oral 1α,25-vitamin D_3 in childhood renal osteodystrophy. N. Engl. J. Med., 298:238, 1978.
Danovitch, G. M., Bougiognie, J., and Bricker, N. S.: Reversibility of the "salt-losing" tendency of chronic renal failure. N. Engl. J. Med., 296:14, 1977.
Friedman, E. A., and Giordano, C. (eds.): Uremia. Kidney Int., Suppl. No. 8, June 1978.
Higgins, M. R., Grace, M., Ulan, R. A., Silverberg, D. S., Bettcher, K. B., and Dossetor, J. B.: Anemia in hemodialysis patients; changing concepts in management. Arch. Intern. Med., 137:172, 1977.
Holdsworth, S., Atkins, R. C., and de Kretser, D. M.: The pituitary-testicular axis in men with chronic renal failure. N. Engl. J. Med., 296:1245, 1977.
Pierides, A. M., Weightman, D., Goldfinch, M., Aljama, P., and Kerr, D. N. S.: Hyperlipidemia of regular hemodialysis and successful renal transplantation. Cardiovasc. Med., 3:185, 1978.

372. ACUTE RENAL FAILURE

Neal S. Bricker

DEFINITION. Acute renal failure is a clinical syndrome characterized by a sudden decrease in glomerular filtration rate, often to values of less than 1 to 2 per cent of normal. Acute renal failure is usually associated with oliguria (urine volumes of less than 400 ml per day), and is always associated with biochemical consequences of the reduction of glomerular filtration rate such as a rise in blood urea nitrogen (BUN), and serum creatinine concentrations. The occurrence of other abnormalities in body fluids such as metabolic acidosis, hyperkalemia, hyperphosphatemia, and hypocalcemia will depend upon the duration and severity of the renal failure, the nature and severity of any underlying injury or disease process, and the nature and intensity of treatment.

Acute renal failure so defined encompasses many different forms of disease with widely varying pathogeneses, natural histories, and prognostic implications. For example, a sudden decrease in glomerular filtration rate may occur in association with profound reduction in effective extracellular fluid volume or fall in blood pressure, and may be readily reversible by volume expansion or blood pressure elevation. More commonly acute renal failure is due to intrinsic disease of the renal parenchyma; but some forms are ultimately (albeit not immediately), reversible, and others are not. Finally, this syndrome may occur in consequence of urinary tract obstruction or occlusion of the renal arteries or veins.

Because of the diversity of etiologic and pathogenetic events which can culminate in acute renal failure; because recognition of the immediately reversible forms of the syndrome can lead to prompt restitution of normal renal function, whereas failure of recognition may lead to persistence of renal failure, increasingly severe manifestations of uremia, and, in some instances, permanent nephron destruction; because the syndrome is so frequently superimposed upon major injuries or serious systemic disease; and because a substantial percentage of patients will survive their disease if therapy is dedicated and skillful, this group of abnormalities stands among the most challenging problems in clinical medicine.

The discussion in this chapter will deal principally with one form of acute renal failure, *acute tubular necrosis*. Other types of the syndrome will be considered, but primarily as they relate to the differential diagnosis of acute tubular necrosis.

Acute tubular necrosis is defined as a special form of acute renal failure caused by an intrinsic abnormality of the renal parenchyma that is potentially reversible after an interval that typically ranges from several days to several weeks. Although the term acute tubular necrosis may not reflect accurately the basis of the lesion or even its pathologic concomitants, and although other names have been used or proposed (e.g., lower nephron nephrosis, tubulointerstitial nephritis, and vasomotor nephropathy), the designation acute tubular necrosis (or ATN) will be retained in this chapter because it remains the most commonly used expression, because none of the other terms have gained more widespread acceptance, and because none of the other terms reflect more accurately or comprehensively a unifying basis for the multiple forms of the syndrome. Acute tubular necrosis may follow exposure to a nephrotoxic drug or to a primary extrarenal injury or disease, especially when attended by hypotension and a sustained reduction in renal blood flow. Most characteristically there is a period of oliguria, followed by gradually increasing rates of urine flow, culminating in a period of polyuria. However, the oliguria is by no means a universal finding, and so-called "nonoliguric" or "high-output" acute renal failure or ATN is a well established entity. Recovery of renal function toward the pre-illness level characteristically (but not invariably) occurs in patients who survive the acute illness.

CAUSES OF ACUTE RENAL FAILURE. Acute Tubular Necrosis. NEPHROTOXIC DRUGS OR CHEMICALS. Acute tubular necrosis may follow exposure to a host of different chemical agents, some when administered in therapeutic doses. Sulfonamides and many of the commonly used antimicrobial drugs, including gentamicin, kanamycin, streptomycin and other aminoglycosides, colistin, cephaloridine, amphotericin, bacitracin, neomycin, vancomycin, and polymixin, have been incriminated as the causal agents in the induction of acute tubular necrosis. ATN has occurred after exposure to organic iodinated x-ray contrast media and after the use of the anesthetic methoxyflurane. It may also follow either accidental or intentional exposure to a variety of nephrotoxic agents. Included among these are organic solvents (especially carbon tetrachloride and tetrachloroethylene); ethylene and diethylene glycol; inorganic mercurials and other heavy metals, including bismuth, uranium, lead, and, rarely, organic mercurials; methyl alcohol; and massive doses of salicylates and paraldehyde. This subject is dealt with in greater detail in Ch. 379.

SYSTEMIC INJURY OR ILLNESS. Acute tubular necrosis may follow severe trauma such as crushing injuries or major operative procedures, especially when blood loss and/or hypotension occur. It may occur in association with rhabdomyolysis and myoglobinuria of any cause, including heat stroke and overdosage with heroin and probably intravenous methadone. It may also follow severe febrile illnesses, gram-negative or, less frequently, gram-positive sepsis, profound and sustained lactic acidosis, major losses of extracellular fluid volume, or major translocations of this volume, into gut, soft tissues, and skin (in burns). Acute tubular necrosis may develop in the course of complicated pregnancies, particulary when hemorrhage or hypotension occurs. It may follow an incompatible blood transfusion and, occasionally, intravascular hemolysis resulting from other mechanisms. In most of the foregoing entities, one or more of the following events frequently occur: (1) profound depletion of actual or effective extracellular fluid volume, (2) hypotension, or (3) hemoglobinuria or myoglobinuria.

ACUTE TUBULAR NECROSIS OCCURRING DE NOVO. Rarely, the disease occurs without known exposure to any nephrotoxic agent and in the absence of a detectable fall in blood pressure, obvious change in circulatory dynamics, loss or translocation of extracellular fluid volume, intravascular hemolysis, or myoglobinuria. Indeed, in very rare instances, it has been observed in the absence of any apparent predisposing illness or injury and in an apparently healthy individual.

Other Parenchymal Diseases. BILATERAL RENAL CORTICAL NECROSIS. Cortical necrosis may be diffuse or patchy. In the former instance, acute renal failure is severe, and may be characterized by total anuria. In patchy cortical necrosis, the severity of the renal failure will depend upon the extent of cortical destruction. Return of enough renal function to support life has been described in patients with bilateral cortical necrosis after prolonged periods of anuria or oliguria. The return of some renal function presumably relates to the survival and ultimate hypertrophy of juxtamedullary glomeruli and their attached nephrons. Survival with relatively good renal function is not infrequent in patients with patchy cortical necrosis.

GLOMERULITIS. Severe acute renal failure may be seen occasionally in poststreptococcal acute glomerulonephritis, particularly in the adult. Acute renal failure may also be seen in the acute glomerulitides associated with systemic lupus erythematosus, hypersensitivity angiitis, polyarteritis nodosa, rapidly progressive glomerulonephritis, Henoch-Schönlein purpura, Goodpasture's syndrome, thrombotic thrombocytopenic purpura, the hemolytic-uremic syndrome, and malignant nephrosclerosis. It may also be seen in accelerated scleroderma when the degree of actual glomerulitis is variable and the predominant site of involvement is in the small arterioles of the kidney.

PAPILLARY NECROSIS. Renal papillary necrosis appears classically in patients with diabetes mellitus, urinary tract obstruction (especially when accompanied by severe pyelonephritis), and sickle cell anemia, as well as in patients who have ingested excessive quantities of phenacetin and possibly other analgesic drugs. The severity of the renal failure, as well as the potential for ultimate recovery, will depend upon the number of renal papillae that escape destruction.

END-STAGE CHRONIC RENAL DISEASE. Acute renal failure may occur under two circumstances in patients with chronic progressive renal disease: (1) when the nephron population diminishes below a critical level and oliguria supervenes; and (2) when an acute complicating process (such as extracellular fluid volume depletion, acute glomerulitis, or urinary tract obstruction) results in a sudden but potentially reversible decrement in renal function from the previous steady-state level.

MISCELLANEOUS FORMS OF PARENCHYMAL INVOLVEMENT. Severe *hypercalcemia* may be associated with the rapid onset of acute renal failure. In most instances the rising BUN is accompanied by polyuria rather than oliguria; but occasionally, particularly with extremely high levels of serum calcium, urine volumes may fall to the oliguric range. *Hyperuricemia* can lead to acute renal failure when the plasma levels increase very rapidly and to concentrations in excess of 15 to 20 mg per 100 ml. The renal failure presumably is due to intrarenal obstruction caused by deposition of uric acid precipitates in collecting ducts and the renal papillae. Acute renal failure may occur during the course of *multiple myeloma.* In some instances this is the result of severe (but reversible) hypercalcemia; the disease may also follow a period of fluid deprivation of as little as several hours in duration. The fluids often are withheld for purposes of performing intravenous pyelography, in patients with Bence Jones proteinuria. The renal failure is presumed to be due to the inspissation of proteinaceous materials in the tubular lumina. There also appears to be an increased incidence of acute renal failure in patients with diabetic nephropathy subjected to fluid deprivation and intravenous pyelography. Whether the x-ray contrast media per se play a role in this form of the disease is not clear. Another cause which is being seen with increasing frequency is *homograft rejection* in transplanted kidneys. Treatment of the rejection often results in reversal of the acute renal failure. However, patients receiving transplanted kidneys, particularly from cadaveric sources, are also prone to the development of acute tubular necrosis.

Occlusion of the Renal Arteries or Veins. Acute interruption of the blood supply to the kidneys may occur after embolization, in situ thrombosis, or dissection of the aorta. For renal failure to occur, virtually the entire nephron population of both kidneys must be deprived of blood supply, and, with the exception of aortic surgery, when "sludge" may flow into both renal arteries during or after release of aortic clamping or extensive atheroembolization, arterial occlusion is an unusual cause of the renal failure. Bilateral renal vein thrombosis is also an unusual cause of the disease, especially in adults, for the involvement must be bilateral (if there are two kidneys), and the luminal occlusion must be complete or virtually complete.

Hemodynamic Alterations (Prerenal Azotemia). Prerenal azotemia is a reversible abnormality characterized by a functional reduction in glomerular filtration rate per nephron. The latter may be secondary to a decrease in mean arterial blood pressure and/or to intrarenal vascular adjustments initiated by marked depletion of effective extracellular fluid volume. This loss may be extracorporeal, or it may represent a sequestration of fluid in areas of the body such as the intestine (after major surgical procedures), or skin bullae (in burns). If prerenal azotemia is not recognized promptly and treated, it may lead to the development of acute tubular necrosis.

Hepatorenal Syndrome. Acute renal failure may occur in the course of severe hepatic failure, usually in association with incipient or overt hepatic encephalopathy. In some instances it is due to acute tubular necrosis; but it may also be due to the hepatorenal syndrome, an abnormality that is an entity in itself and clearly differentiable from acute tubular necrosis. The hepatorenal syndrome unfortunately appears to be almost always, if not always irreversible. The etiology and pathogenesis of the syndrome are unknown, and there are no characteristic pathologic changes in the kidneys. From a pathophysiologic point of view, the hepatorenal syndrome has functional characteristics (to be described under Pathologic Physiology) which correspond to those of prerenal azotemia and not those of acute tubular necrosis.

Urinary Tract Obstruction. For obstruction of the urinary tract to produce acute renal failure, the obstructing process must interfere with the flow of urine from the vast majority of nephrons. Thus if the obstructing lesion is at or above the ureterovesical junction, it must be bilateral if both kidneys are functioning.

PATHOGENESIS OF ACUTE TUBULAR NECROSIS. Several theories have been proposed for the pathogenesis of acute tubular necrosis. Each has its proponents, and there are at least some supporting experimental data in animals. But for each, contradictory evidence has also accrued; and for none is there universal acceptance.

The most prominently considered theories are the following: (1) *A profound reduction in glomerular filtration rate caused by renal vasoconstriction.* The decrease in glomerular filtration rate would be sufficiently severe to eliminate the great majority of nephrons from the urine-forming group, and would presumably affect the cortical nephrons preferentially. (2) *Obstruction of tubular lumina* secondary to inspissated debris. The debris may be composed of hemoglobin or myoglobin, of various plasma proteins, of Tamm-Horsfall mucoprotein, a substance found in normal urine, or of sloughed epithelial cells. (3) *"Back-leak" of tubular fluid into the renal interstitium* through areas of discontinuity in the tubular walls. The accumulation of tubular fluid in the interstitial spaces would result in obstruction of contiguous nephrons. Back-leak could occur with or without nephron obstruction and with or without a decrease in glomerular filtration rate per nephron. (4) *A profound reduction in glomerular filtration rate caused by structural alterations in the glomeruli,* leading to a reduction in glomerular permeability.

Essential to each of the four theories is renal vasoconstriction and/or tubular necrosis.

The first of the four theories is based upon vasoconstriction produced by activation of the renin-angiotensin system. All four theories would appear to require tubular necrosis or at least to have enhanced credibility by its presence. The tubular necrosis could occur as a primary and initiating event, or it could be secondary to angiotensin-mediated renal vasoconstriction.

The proponents of the *primacy* of angiotensin-induced renal vasoconstriction invoke the following sequence of events. Because of impaired sodium and water reabsorption in the proximal tubule, either the sodium concentration or the volume of the tubular fluid reaching the macula densa increases, and the sensors in the macula densa trigger an enhanced rate of release of renin from the juxtaglomerular granules (an alternative possibility is that the responsiveness of the macula densa per se becomes abnormal). The newly released renin, in turn, would lead to high local concentrations of angiotensin around the glomeruli and their arterioles. The angiotensin, finally, would produce vasoconstriction of the renal arterioles (primarily the afferent vessels). With the attendant decrease in renal blood flow, there would occur a sharp fall in glomerular filtration rate. To explain the first step in the sequence, the increase in "downstream" delivery of proximal fluid or sodium, damage to the tubular epithelial cells would be very helpful.

The proponents of tubular obstruction believe that the epithelial cells which are damaged secondary to tubular necrosis contribute to the luminal occlusion. In the "back-leak" hypothesis, damage to the epithelial cells and basement membranes would be required to account for the discontinuity of the tubular walls, and thus for the cycling of tubular fluid from nephron lumina into the interstitial spaces. Finally, a reduction in single nephron glomerular filtration rate secondary to impairment of glomerular permeability would become more credible were there to be associated tubular damage, for, as will be discussed under Pathologic Physiology, a decrease in glomerular filtration rate without a change in the integrity of tubular function should produce the physiologic changes of prerenal azotemia rather than those of acute tubular necrosis.

Although renin levels are elevated in most forms of experimentally induced acute renal failure in animals, neither the infusion of inhibitors of angiotensin nor immunization against renin has been found to protect against the development of acute renal failure. Thus theory number 1 does not provide a singular explanation for all forms of the disease. Unfortunately, tubular necrosis, which is important to all four theories of pathogenesis, is also found inconsistently in animal models, and, as will be noted below, in biopsy and necropsy studies in man, tubular necrosis is the exception rather than the rule. The problems of explanation continue, for neither tubular obstruction, "back-leak", nor pathologic changes in the glomeruli are universally observed. Hence, in at least some forms of experimental ATN, there is little evidence of widespread cast formation, of tubular dilation, or of increased intratubular pressure in individual surface nephrons. Each of these observations is difficult to reconcile with distal tubular obstruction. Moreover, although large molecules have been found to leak from tubular lumina into the interstitial spaces in some animal models of ATN, in other models neither inulin nor horseradish peroxidase back-leaks. Finally, direct measurement of glomerular filtration rate in individual surface nephrons of rats with the disease indicates that a primary, or at least a causal, reduction in filtration rate is not universal.

Unfortunately, the information about ATN in man is even less extensive than that in the experimental animal.

The ambiguity, in all probability, relates to the fact that many different techniques have been used to produce acute renal failure in the laboratory animal, and there may be differences in pathogenesis among these entities. Hence it is conceivable that angiotensin-induced renal vasoconstriction, tubular obstruction, back-leak of tubular fluid, and even, in some instances, pathologic changes in glomeruli may contribute either alone or in combination to the pathogenesis of acute renal failure in laboratory animals. But acute tubular necrosis in man also arises in a wide spectrum of circumstances and after a multiplicity of different insults, and it is equally conceivable that there is more than one pathogenetic pathway leading to the development of the human disease.

PATHOLOGY. On gross examination, kidneys with acute tubular necrosis may appear enlarged and swollen. On cut section they exhibit a pale cortex and a dark congested medulla. Microscopically the changes are largely confined to the tubules, and neither the glomeruli nor the vessels show consistent abnormalities. The changes in the tubular epithelia tend to be scattered and nonuniform, and in some cases no abnormalities can be seen on light microscopy. Usually, however, the proximal tubular epithelia tend to appear flattened, and mitotic figures may be seen. Frank necrosis may be observed in the proximal tubule, particularly after exposure to a nephrotoxic agent. In postischemic ATN, damage to epithelial cells, when it occurs, tends to be patchy, to occur in any portion of the nephron, but to be most concentrated in the area of the corticomedullary junction. The distal tubules may appear dilated, and the epithelia low and basophilic with dense staining nuclei and occasional mitotic figures. Casts of varying types often, but by no means invariably, appear within the distal segments of the nephrons. Tubular basement membranes may be disrupted in scattered areas in postischemic or non-nephrotoxic acute tubular necrosis, but this change is unusual when the disease is secondary to a nephrotoxic drug. Within several days of the onset of acute tubular necrosis, round cell infiltration and edema of the interstitial spaces occur in most cases. The edema can become pronounced in overhydrated patients.

Electron microscopic examination has revealed structural alterations in the mitochondria of tubular epithelial cells, loss of the microvilli in the proximal tubular epithelia, and loss of endoplasmic reticulum; there may also be disruption of continuity of the tubular basement membrane. However, the glomeruli have shown no consistent lesion that could provide a morphologic basis for a decrease in glomerular permeability.

PATHOLOGIC PHYSIOLOGY OF ACUTE TUBULAR NECROSIS. With normal renal function, less than 1 per cent of the water filtered at the glomeruli is ordinarily excreted in the urine, and only about 0.5 per cent of the filtered sodium is excreted on an average salt intake. In a typical patient with oliguric acute tubular necrosis, from 10 to 20 per cent of the filtered water and from 5 to 10 per cent of the filtered sodium are excreted. Considering the marked decrease in total kidney glomerular filtration rate, these increased *fractional* excretion rates are appropriate in direction; however, the changes are much less marked than in patients with chronic renal failure. For example, a patient with chronic uremia and a filtration rate of 1 ml per minute may excrete 50 per cent or more of the filtered water and sodium. The consequences of these excretory patterns are as follows: At a glomerular filtration rate of 1 ml per minute, the patient with acute tubular necrosis will typically excrete less than 300 ml of urine and less than 20 mEq of sodium per day, whereas the patient with chronic renal disease may excrete 1 liter or more of urine and as much as 100 mEq of sodium per day.

Two questions about the patterns of salt and water excretion in acute tubular necrosis thus emerge: (1) Are the increments in fractional salt and water excretion adaptive, and thus regulatory, in nature or are they fortuitous consequences of intrinsic damage to the tubular epithelial cells? (2) If the changes are adaptive, why are the responses not greater? Does it take more than a few days for the fully developed adaptations seen in chronic renal failure to develop; or do the functioning nephrons in acute tubular necrosis fail to respond to any extrarenal forces that help mediate the adaptations (e.g., parathyroid hormone for phosphate and possibly natriuretic hormone for sodium), either because the tubular epithelial cells are damaged or because single nephron glomerular filtration rate is too low? To date, answers to these questions are not available. However, the fact that patients with acute tubular necrosis do excrete a moderately high percentage of filtered water and filtered sodium (regardless of the mechanism) provides a clear explanation for "nonoliguric" tubular necrosis and for certain of the characteristics of the diuretic phase of the disease.

In most patients with the disease, the glomerular filtration rate (as estimated by endogenous creatinine clearance) drops to values of 1 ml per minute or less. Such patients are oliguric. However, in some patients the drop in the filtration rate is not as severe, and values may not fall below 3 to 5 ml per minute. Urea synthesis will still far exceed urea excretion, and the BUN will rise progressively. Creatinine and phosphate concentrations also will rise, and acidosis and hyperkalemia may develop. The patient thus may develop all the symptoms and signs of acute uremia. However, if 20 per cent of the filtered water is excreted at a glomerular filtration rate of 4 ml per minute, urine flow will be almost 1200 ml per day and sodium excretion may exceed 60 mEq per day. Hence there will exist a seeming paradox wherein the patient will present with stigmata of mounting uremia but with urine volumes that are not reduced, i.e., nonoliguric acute tubular necrosis.

A similar physiologic basis serves to explain the diuretic phase of oliguric ATN. If the glomerular filtration rate increases from 1 to 5 ml per minute (i.e., from 1440 to 7200 ml per 24 hours), the continued excretion of 20 per cent of the filtered water results in a rise in urine volume from 288 to 1440 ml per 24 hours. Despite the relatively high urine volume, however, the BUN (and creatinine concentrations) will rise until the glomerular filtration rate becomes high enough to allow for the filtration (and thus the excretion) of an amount of urea equal to that produced. The more catabolic the patient is, the higher must be the filtration rate (and the rate of urine flow) before the BUN will start to decline.

As the glomerular filtration rate increases progressively during the recovery phase of acute tubular necrosis, urine volumes may rise to very high levels. Three factors appear to have a profound influence on the magnitude of the diuresis. The first is the degree to which urea and other endogenous solutes accumulate in the blood during the oliguric phase. If urea is allowed to accumulate in body fluids rather than being removed by repeated dialysis, the retained solute will be excreted as the filtration rate rises toward normal. And because the urine remains isosmotic in acute tubular necrosis, every 300 mOsm of extra solute excreted will obligate the excretion of approximately a liter of water. If the BUN concentration is lowered by 20 mg per 100 ml in a 24-hour period via excretion in the urine, approximately 18 grams of urea (equal to 300 mOsm) will be excreted in a 70-kg man, and this will increase the 24-hour urine volume by about 1 liter.

The second factor that may influence the magnitude of the diuresis is the degree of expansion of extracellular fluid volume. If effective extracellular fluid volume is supranormal, natriuretic forces will be mobilized, and as the diuretic phase proceeds, the nephrons will respond to these forces and excrete an increasing fraction of filtered sodium and water. This phenomenon can lead to a vicious cycle wherein urine volume and solute excretion increase in consequence of fluid volume expansion, and the rate of fluid administration in turn is increased to keep up with the rising urine volumes.

The third factor which will influence importantly the magnitude of the diuresis is the rate of recovery of tubular reabsorptive capacity.

CLINICAL MANIFESTATIONS. When there is an inciting event, the onset of acute renal failure follows the insult by an interval varying from hours to as long as two days. The oliguric phase may last from a few hours to three or more weeks. However, as noted above, in some instances there is no oliguric phase, and in other patients the oliguria may persist for periods in excess of two months before renal function begins to improve. The diuretic phase lasts from a few days to a week or longer. The recovery phase is characterized by a progressive rise in glomerular filtration rate and restoration of renal responsiveness to the volume and homeostatic needs of the organism. With recovery, renal function is restored toward the pretubular necrosis level, but in most patients some permanent nephron loss probably occurs.

The presenting picture is usually that of an oliguric patient with a rising concentration of blood urea and creatinine. If the oliguria has been present for some period of time and if salt and water intake have continued unabated, or if an effort was made to restore normal renal function by overzealous fluid administration, salt and water retention, occasionally of massive proportions, may be present. Hyperkalemia may also be present when the patient is first seen. In untreated patients, the symptoms and signs of uremia may develop rapidly, and if there is an underlying injury or illness, the total constellation of clinical abnormalities will reflect the primary disease plus the superimposed manifestations of advancing uremia.

Uremia in acute tubular necrosis may affect many organ systems. *Gastrointestinal manifestations* include anorexia, nausea, and vomiting; if water must be restricted, thirst may become a disturbing symptom. *Central nervous system manifestations* include asterixis, subtle to overt changes in mentation (including organic psychosis), convulsions, and coma. *Cardiovascular changes* include an increase in cardiac output, presumably resulting from anemia and acidosis and, when present, hypervolemia, an increase in blood pressure in some patients, acute left ventricular failure in patients who are markedly hypervolemic, and pericarditis. Electrocardiographic changes are principally those of hyperkalemia and may include the successive development of tall peaked tent-shaped T waves, prolongation of the P-R interval, prolongation of the QRS interval, disappearance of P waves, and ultimately disintegration of the electrocardiographic pattern with a so-called sine wave appearance. For any given level of elevation of plasma potassium concentration, the cardiotoxic effects tend to be greater when either severe acidosis or hyponatremia is also present.

Therapy will exercise a profound influence on the clinical course of acute tubular necrosis. If dialysis is performed early and at frequent intervals, the patient may progress through the entire course of his illness with few symptoms or signs attributable to the renal failure and without the burden of severe dietary restrictions. If the patient is treated with optimal conservative therapy, but without dialysis, he will develop progressive manifestations of uremia, and moreover will be required to restrict markedly his fluid intake and protein intake. He also may require special treatment for preventing a dangerous rise in plasma potassium concentration. Owing to the high levels of blood urea and the difficulty in preventing volume overload in patients who are not dialyzed frequently enough, the diuretic phase will be more exaggerated. *In all instances the clinical course is influenced greatly by the nature and severity of any underlying illness or injury.* Patients with acute tubular necrosis need no longer die of uremia, but many, unfortunately, continue to die of the underlying abnormality that precipitated the renal failure.

During the recovery phase patients not infrequently exhibit reactive mental depression. They also may require a long period of recuperation, particularly if catabolism has been severe. Finally, at the end of the diuretic phase, body weight may be substantially less than the clinical estimate of dry weight. This reflects the fact that lean body mass often decreases far more than is suspected during the course of the illness, and the decrease is masked by unrecognized extracellular fluid volume expansion.

TREATMENT. The treatment of the renal failure in acute tubular necrosis is best accomplished by early and frequent dialysis. Either peritoneal or extracorporeal hemodialysis may be employed. If extracorporeal hemodialysis is preferred or is required because peritoneal dialysis is contraindicated, an arteriovenous shunt should be placed in an extremity at the beginning of the illness to facilitate dialysis on a daily or every-other-day basis. When frequent dialysis is employed, only modest salt and water restriction is needed, and a good caloric intake (at least 1500 calories in an adult), containing a moderate amount of protein, e.g., 40 to 60 grams per day, may be allowed in the diet. However, when dialysis is not used on a frequent basis, the amount of water, sodium, and potassium intake must be regulated with great care so as to minimize chemical and volumetric abnormalities of body fluids.

The standard principles of management in a patient who is not dialyzed repeatedly include fluid restriction sufficient to effect the loss of approximately half a pound of body weight per day. In general this amounts to the administration of 400 to 500 ml of fluid plus the amount lost in the urine and gastrointestinal tract. Excessive fluid administration carries the risk of inducing congestive heart failure and pulmonary edema. If the patient is able to take food by mouth, a diet providing approximately 2000 calories which is potassium and protein free and essentially sodium free is recommended; there are some observers, however, who favor the inclusion in the diet of a small amount of protein (ca. 20 grams per day), containing the minimal daily requirements of essential amino acids. If parenteral alimentation is necessary, it is the general practice to infuse dextrose (at least 100 grams per day) and vitamins; but both the caloric and nutritional requirements may be partially fulfilled by the infusion of essential amino acids or their keto analogues or by intravenous fat emulsions. When glucose is administered, it must usually be given as a hyperosmotic solution because of the requirement for fluid restriction. Precautions are required to prevent venous thrombosis and infection of the venous catheter.

Particular attention may be necessary to prevent the development of progressive hyperkalemia. The administration of a potassium-binding resin either by mouth or by enema two to four times daily will generally serve to prevent serious elevations of plasma potassium concentrations.* If marked hyperkalemia is present when the patient is first seen, intravenous glucose and insulin, sodium bicarbonate, or calcium chloride all will protect temporarily against the cardiotoxic effects of potassium. But potassium exchange resins and/or dialysis, both of which remove potassium from the body, should be initiated promptly to prevent the recurrence of hyperkalemia. Metabolic acidosis can generally be corrected and controlled by dialysis. If dialysis is not available, or the acidosis progresses despite dialysis, the administration of $NaHCO_3$ in carefully regulated amounts is indicated to keep the plasma bicarbonate concentration above 15 mEq per liter. Hyponatremia can best be prevented by restricting water intake (parenteral as well as oral) and can best be corrected by dialysis. *Hyponatremia should not be treated by the administration of hypertonic saline.* Anemia will develop routinely in the course of acute tubular necrosis, and ordinarily no effort should be made to maintain the hematocrit in excess of 20 volumes per 100 ml. If blood transfusion does become necessary because of a progressive fall in hematocrit or cardiovascular complications, packed red blood cells using fresh blood should be employed. In treating hemorrhage, fresh whole blood may be preferable. Hyperphosphatemia may occasionally become very pronounced, and may be attended by the development of hypocalcemia. The latter ordinarily does not produce manifestations of tetany; but if ionized calcium concentrations become reduced inordinately, as may occur if the patient becomes alkalotic from the infusion of bicarbonate in excessive amount or from vomiting, tetany and even seizures

---

*The resin generally used in the United States is a sodium cycle resin (Kayexalate), and in a standard dose of 15 to 60 grams per day over 30 mEq of Na may be released into the gastrointestinal tract. To obviate sodium retention, part or all of the resin may be given as a calcium cycle resin if the latter is available.

may develop. Hyperphosphatemia is best controlled by protein restriction and/or frequent dialysis, but the administration of phosphate-binding gels, e.g., aluminum hydroxide gel, 30 to 60 ml every six hours by mouth, may be of great value.

All drugs from antimicrobials to digitalis glycosides must be administered with full knowledge of their route of degradation and excretion, using serial measurements of blood concentrations whenever possible and indicated. Drugs which are not detoxified, metabolized, or excreted by the kidney may be given in full dosage. But these are the exception rather than the rule. Most drugs, including many antimicrobials, will have to be given in reduced amounts and at prolonged intervals. It is tragic indeed to have a patient recover from acute tubular necrosis only to have a permanent vestibular or auditory defect owing to streptomycin or kanamycin toxicity. Another aminoglycoside, gentamicin, may have serious nephrotoxic effects if the dosage and blood levels are not carefully controlled. Digoxin is the most widely recommended digitalis glycoside, although some authorities prefer digitoxin. If digoxin is employed, a digitalizing dose of 1.5 to 2.0 mg and a maintenance dose of 0.125 mg daily will provide a therapeutic effect without toxicity in most adult patients with acute tubular necrosis.

If the renal failure is treated satisfactorily, the outcome will depend in very large measure upon the treatment and the natural history of any underlying illness or injury. If the patient survives the extrarenal abnormalities, he may look forward to long-term survival even if the renal lesion proves to be irreversible, for in that instance he will become a candidate for either chronic hemodialysis or transplantation. Thus the intensity of treatment of a surgical wound, an area of necrotic tissue, or a burn should not be diminished because of the existence of acute tubular necrosis; quite the contrary: any delay in appropriate treatment may compromise the patient's chances of survival. Removal of necrotic tissue is, if anything, more urgent in the patient with acute renal failure than in the patient with normal renal function; and surgical procedures, even major ones, are not contraindicated if they are considered to have lifesaving importance. Finally, although prophylactic antimicrobial drugs are contraindicated, infection must be treated promptly with the correct drugs but with prorated dosages. In the same context, careful attention must be given to avoiding the introduction of secondary infection. Thus after the first few hours of observation, the use of a bladder catheter solely to monitor urine volumes is not justified, and intravenous catheters should be treated aseptically and rarely left in the same vein for more than three days. Skin care, with special attention to the prevention of pressure sores, is an essential component of rational and effective therapy.

DIFFERENTIAL DIAGNOSIS. The fact that the patient with acute tubular necrosis characteristically excretes a relatively large percentage of filtered salt and water may be very helpful in differentiating the disease from the oliguric states associated with volume depletion, hypotension with a readily reversible decrease in effective filtration pressure, acute glomerulitis, and the hepatorenal syndrome.

As indicated above, a normal person with an average salt and water intake will excrete less than 1 per cent of his filtered sodium and water. If extracellular fluid volume depletion occurs, the appropriate homeostatic response is to *decrease* salt and water excretion. With moderate degrees of volume depletion, this occurs without a fall in glomerular filtration rate. However, if the volume depletion is profound, and particularly if blood pressure falls, the glomerular filtration rate may fall markedly, in which case the patient will present not only with oliguria but with a rising level of BUN and creatinine. Thus he will fulfill the criteria for acute renal failure. But in contrast to the patient with acute tubular necrosis, the patient with volume depletion will typically excrete less than 5 per cent of his filtered water, and may excrete urine which is virtually free of sodium. A similar picture evolves early in the course of a severe glomerulitis and in the hepatorenal syndrome.

In most instances, acute tubular necrosis may be differentiated from prerenal azotemia, as well as from the other causes of acute renal failure, including acute glomerulitis and the hepatorenal syndrome, by relatively simple laboratory tests and knowledge of the underlying physiologic principles. The urine/plasma (U/P) creatinine ratio is (or should be) a readily available test for estimating the fraction of filtered water excreted. (It may be necessary to overcome the reluctance in some hospital laboratories to do emergency measurements of serum and urinary creatinine concentrations on a 24-hour basis. However, both analyses are simple to perform, and there is little justification for laboratory personnel being unwilling or unable to make the measurements). The accompanying table compares the U/P ratios with the fractional rate of water excretion. A U/P ratio of 10 indicates that approximately 10 per cent of the filtered water is excreted. A U/P ratio of 5 is equivalent to the excretion of 20 per cent of the filtered water, and a ratio of 2 signifies the excretion of 50 per cent of the filtered water. In acute tubular necrosis, creatinine U/P ratios typically range between 5 and 10, and rarely exceed 20. In prerenal azotemia, acute glomerulitides, and the hepatorenal syndrome, creatinine U/P ratios typically exceed 10, and often are well above 20. The urinary sodium concentration (U_{Na}) in acute tubular necrosis typically exceeds 20 mEq per liter, and in most patients ranges from 40 to 90 mEq per liter. In prerenal azotemia, acute glomerulitis, and the hepatorenal syndrome, U_{Na} is usually less than 20 mEq per liter, and often is less than 10 mEq per liter. Calculation of the fraction of filtered sodium excreted may also be very helpful. This value is equal to the U/P ratio for sodium divided by the U/P ratio for creatinine and expressed as a percentage. In acute tubular necrosis, 5 per cent or more of the filtered sodium typically is excreted; in

The Relationship Between Creatinine Urine/Plasma (U/P) Ratios and the Percentage of Filtered Water Excreted

Creatinine U/P ratio	Per Cent Filtered H_2O Excreted
100	1
50	2
20	5
10	10
5	20
2	50

prerenal azotemia, acute glomerulitis, and the hepatorenal syndrome, less than 5 per cent and often less than 2 per cent of the filtered sodium is excreted. In chronic end-stage renal disease, the values will depend upon the glomerular filtration rate and the salt intake; but at a glomerular filtration rate of 2 ml per minute and with an average salt and water intake (approximately 7 grams of salt and 1 liter of water per day), about 30 per cent of the filtered salt and water is excreted.

The creatinine U/P ratio, U_{Na}, and the U/P Na:U/P creatinine ratio are thus of help in the differential diagnosis of acute renal failure. But there are substantial gray zones where the patterns overlap, and these biochemical values must in all instances be viewed in light of historical and clinical findings. There are also sources of error in utilizing the biochemical values. One of these is that acute renal failure secondary to volume depletion may progress to acute tubular necrosis; and if the urine examined was produced prior to the advent of acute tubular necrosis, it will be low in sodium and have a high creatinine U/P ratio. Another source of error exists in a patient with true acute tubular necrosis in whom there is a profound stimulus to sodium retention. For example, in acute tubular necrosis associated with burns, the translocation of extracellular fluid into the affected areas results in a striking decrease in effective ECF volume. The patient thus may present with oliguria, a glomerular filtration rate below 1 ml per minute, a creatinine U/P ratio of less than 10, but virtually no sodium in the urine. A low U_{Na} has also been observed in acute tubular necrosis after major cardiac surgery and mercury poisoning.

Error in using the creatinine U/P ratio and U_{Na} may also occur in patients with glomerulitis, after the occurrence of compensation but before the filtration rate rises appreciably. After enough salt and water have been retained to expand extracellular fluid volume appreciably, natriuretic forces may be mobilized and fractional reabsorption of sodium (and water) in the urine-forming nephrons may be markedly depressed. Thus creatinine U/P ratios may fall below the 10 to 20 range and U_{Na} may be high. When acute renal failure is superimposed on advanced chronic renal disease, e.g., from volume depletion or either a recurrence or de novo occurrence of acute glomerulitis, the creatinine U/P ratio and the U_{Na} may both remain in the ATN, rather than the prerenal azotemic, range.

Other Aids in Differential Diagnosis. URINE VOLUME. Total anuria is very rare in acute tubular necrosis unless it is due to the ingestion of bichloride of mercury. Total anuria is seen in severe acute glomerulitis, bilateral cortical necrosis, and urinary tract obstruction. If there is a history of an abrupt change in urine volume from very low to high levels in a short period of time, or if there are alternating periods of oliguria and polyuria, obstruction is strongly suggested.

URINARY SEDIMENT. Red blood cell casts are unusual in acute tubular necrosis (but they occur) and are the rule in glomerulitides (but they may be absent). Qualitative measurements of protein in urine in the disease rarely exceed 1 to 2+ in acute tubular necrosis, whereas they often are 3 to 4+ in glomerulitides.

URINE OSMOLALITY. The osmolality of the urine is generally within 25 to 50 mOsm per kilogram of water of the serum or plasma value in patients with tubular necrosis. In patients with prerenal azotemia, glomerulitides, and the hepatorenal syndrome, the urine may occasionally be more hyperosmotic with respect to the plasma. *Consequently isosmotic urine is not of value in differential diagnosis, although hyperosmotic urine favors volume depletion, acute glomerulitis, and the hepatorenal syndrome, and virtually excludes acute tubular necrosis.*

RESPONSE TO MANNITOL, FUROSEMIDE, OR VOLUME EXPANSION. A limited increase in urine volume may occur in the disease after mannitol infusion, furosemide administration, or volume expansion. However, unless the increase is progressive and is attended by a substantial rise in glomerular filtration rate, repeated administration of either mannitol or furosemide or continuous infusion of a synthetic extracellular fluid solution is contraindicated in patients with acute renal failure of unknown variety. The differential diagnostic implications of a small increase in urine volume and sodium excretion after the administration of large doses of potent diuretics such as furosemide are not yet clear; but large increments in urine volume point away from the diagnosis of acute tubular necrosis.

PROGNOSIS. In uncomplicated cases of acute tubular necrosis, in which there is no serious underlying disease and treatment is optimal, survival rates in excess of 70 to 80 per cent are common. On the other hand, when there is a serious underlying disease or injury, the death rate exceeds 50 per cent, and in severely traumatized patients may exceed 70 per cent. Judging from the experience in the Vietnam war, as contrasted with the Korean war, the speedy evacuation of wounded and rapid treatment of blood loss and shock will substantially reduce the incidence of acute tubular necrosis; but unfortunately once it does develop, the mortality rate among wounded patients requiring hemodialysis remains at about 70 per cent.

PREVENTION. The likelihood of occurrence of acute tubular necrosis after a given insult is influenced by the composite physiologic adversities. Thus the better the supportive therapy, the lower should be the incidence of the disease. The war experience just cited supports this view.

The role of mannitol in preventing acute tubular necrosis is uncertain. Some observers have favored the view that administration of mannitol to an oliguric patient will confer a substantial degree of protection by eliminating the contribution of luminal obstruction to the disease. However, at the very least, obstruction is not a universal factor in its pathogenesis; moreover, it can be induced in the laboratory animal with myoglobinuria despite the presence of high rates of urine flow per nephron. Mannitol may also increase renal blood flow, and conceivably some protective effect could derive from this. But it seems most reasonable to confine the use of mannitol chiefly to patients in whom there is an increase in the creatinine U/P ratio and a decrease in urinary sodium concentration, but no evidence of hypervolemia. The mannitol should be administered only for a limited period of time and in an amount not to exceed 25 to 50 grams; if no substantial rise in glomerular filtration rate and/or urine flow occurs, its use should not be continued. The role of furosemide in preventing the development of acute tubular necrosis also has not been established, and repeated administration of high doses of this drug is contraindicated.

In patients with extracellular fluid volume depletion and oliguria, volume repletion should be effected as expeditiously as possible. When hypotension exists, this also should be corrected as rapidly as possible. The use of sodium bicarbonate intravenously in patients with intravascular hemolysis in an effort to prevent acute tubular necrosis is of dubious value.

The early recognition of urinary tract obstruction is of importance not only for the prompt reversal of acute renal failure, but also for the prevention of progressive nephron destruction. When obstruction is suspected in a patient with acute renal failure, either bladder catheterization or unilateral ureteral catheterization should be performed without delay.

Flamenbaum, W.: Pathophysiology of acute renal failure. Arch. Intern. Med., 131:911, 1973.

Franklyn, S. S., and Maxwell, M. H.: Acute renal failure. *In* Maxwell, M. H., and Kleeman, C. R. (eds.): Clinical Disorders of Fluid and Electrolyte Metabolism. New York, McGraw-Hill Book Company, 1972.

Levinsky, N. G.: Pathophysiology of acute renal failure. N. Engl. J. Med., 296:1453, 1977.

Merrill, J. P.: Acute renal failure. *In* Strauss, M. B., and Welt, L. G. (eds.): Diseases of the Kidney. Boston, Little, Brown and Company, 1971.

373. TREATMENT OF IRREVERSIBLE RENAL FAILURE BY TRANSPLANTATION AND DIALYSIS*

373.1. INTRODUCTION

Priscilla Kincaid-Smith

Renal transplantation and intermittent dialysis have become established as successful methods of treatment for irreversible renal failure over the last 10 to 15 years. There are few medical reasons for a definitive choice between dialysis and transplantation, and both offer reasonable success rates and good rehabilitation. From the patient's point of view a successful transplant offers a more independent life and avoids anemia, which is the major disadvantage of maintenance dialysis. Furthermore cadaveric transplantation is the only practical approach for a country wishing to accept and treat all medically suitable patients with irreversible renal failure and to avoid the allocation of very considerable financial and medical resources to treatment by dialysis.

An integrated program for patients with irreversible renal failure, utilizing both dialysis and transplantation, has evolved in the last few years. Such an approach is based on an initial choice made by patient and physician together. The medical commitment is to maintain the highest quality of life possible for each patient. Successful transplantation will usually remain the ultimate goal, but dialysis is carried out preferably in such a way that it can continue indefinitely if the need arises. Transplantation is carried out on optimally fit patients and is not regarded as a treatment for "failed" dialysis. Grafts are removed early if function is poor or deteriorating, and immunosuppression is not used to excess. Failed transplants are returned to dialysis to await another transplant should it be indicated. This integrated approach allows maximal use of available cadaver kidneys and in addition achieves an improved patient survival rate. This approach has resulted in a two-year patient survival of 80 per cent, four fifths of whom have a functioning cadaveric renal transplant (see accompanying figure).

Progress in clinical transplantation has proved disappointingly slow. Tissue typing assists the selection of living related donors but does not help in the majority of cadaveric donors. Organ preservation is now widely used and allows selective surgery and better preparation and selection of recipients. There has been a worldwide increase in patient survival, particularly in cadaveric transplantation (Table 1). Isolated units and some national programs, for example, that in Australia, report significantly better results than the worldwide experience.

THE PROBLEM OF IRREVERSIBLE RENAL FAILURE IN THE COMMUNITY

The provision of services to the community has been reviewed by Kerr. No country has yet reached an equilibrium in providing services for patients with irrevers-

Survival curves for patients who have been admitted to the dialysis and transplantation program at the Royal Melbourne Hospital (January 1970 to October 1974). The "integrated" curve dates from acceptance of 147 patients for hemodialysis and differs little from the patient survival following transplantation in 122 patients. Graft survival in these 122 patients is clearly lower, but when adequate dialysis facilities are available very few patients die because of transplant failure. The curve for patients treated in 1965 and 1966 represents both patient and graft survival because facilities did not permit early graft removal and return to dialysis. The numbers represent survivors at each time interval. (From Proceedings of the Sixth International Congress of Nephrology, Florence, 1975. Basel, S. Karger AG, 1976.)

*The assistance of Dr. T. H. Mathew in preparation of this chapter is gratefully acknowledged.

TABLE 1. Patient and Graft Survival, 1968 and 1971—
Primary Cadaveric Transplants (10th Report of Human Renal
Transplant Registry)

	One Year			
	% Living		% Functioning	
1968	58	(58)	46	(39)
1971	68	(88)	46	(69)

Royal Melbourne Hospital data are shown in parentheses.

ible renal failure in which the number of patients presenting for treatment equals those dying after treatment with dialysis or transplantation. It is notable that in Denmark and Australia, where cadaveric transplantation has been the major goal, twice the number of patients have been accepted for treatment and are alive as in countries where the major effort has gone toward dialysis.

The most significant factor in determining the need for facilities is the number of patients presenting for treatment. This number is age dependent, because renal failure is common above the age of 55. The other significant variable is "medical suitability." The criteria for medical acceptance have widened with experience, and there are now few absolute contraindications for either dialysis or transplantation. Estimates of the number of patients requiring treatment have varied from 25 to 75 per million per year, depending on the upper age limit. The figures of 35 per million of the population per year with an upper age limit of 55 and 50 per million per year for patients up to 65 years of age are probably accurate for most communities.

Utilizing published survival data for dialysis and transplantation and making reasonable assumptions in keeping with an integrated program, Kerr has calculated that approximate equilibrium could be achieved after 12 years (Table 2). These figures provide a valuable guide to physicians and administrators in planning the community requirements.

Transplantation costs approximately equal those of home dialysis in the first year but thereafter have been estimated to be a quarter of those of maintenance dialysis at home. Countries with transplantation as the major goal may therefore expect to save about US$500,000 per year per million of population (based

on Australian cost estimates applied to Table 2), compared with countries where the major goal is home dialysis.

A program based on cadaveric transplantation is dependent on an adequate supply of donor kidneys and a reasonable success rate. The Australian experience has proved encouraging in both these areas, with a donor procurement rate of 9 (18 kidneys) per million per year and a two-year graft survival of 62 per cent (see figure) with primary cadaveric transplants (compared to the Human Renal Transplant Registry report of 46 per cent). Factors contributing to the high donor procurement and graft success rate are discussed below.

PREVENTION OF IRREVERSIBLE RENAL FAILURE

A program which aims to treat irreversible renal failure in the community must include adequate provision for prevention. Irreversible renal failure can be prevented by the application of available methods of treatment to renal disease and improvement of present methods of treatment through research. All major renal units should include facilities for research and for adequate diagnosis and treatment of renal disease and renal failure at all stages. Even by applying present methods of prevention and treatment, the numbers requiring dialysis and transplantation may decrease substantially. Detection and treatment of asymptomatic bacteriuria and hypertension are very likely to reduce the numbers presenting with chronic renal failure. Glomerulonephritis is the most common cause of irreversible renal failure; although treatment of this condition has usually proved ineffective, promising results with newer forms of treatment, including immunosuppression and anticoagulants, have been reported. The encouraging results obtained using plasmapheresis in rapidly progressive forms of glomerulonephritis suggest that early diagnosis and referral of such cases might considerably reduce the numbers developing renal failure. Analgesic nephropathy, a totally preventable disease, is at present contributing 18 per cent of all patients presenting for dialysis and transplantation in Australia. This disease, which results from prolonged high doses of proprietary "over-the-counter" analgesic drugs, would disappear completely if abuse could be stopped by public education or if such preparations were available only on prescription.

TABLE 2. Approximate Equilibrium Population of Dialysis and Transplant Patients Expected from Current Survival Rates at Two Different Rates of Admission*

Treatment	Admission Rate 25 Million/Year		Admission Rate 50 Million/Year	
	Annual Cohort	Equilibrium Population	Annual Cohort	Equilibrium Population
Live donor graft	2.5	18	5	35
Home dialysis	18	32	22.5	40
Hospital dialysis	4.5	8	39	37
Cadaver graft	20	97	39	189
		155 million†		301 million†

*From Kerr, D. N. S.: Kidney Int., 3:197, 1973; with permission.
†The calculations are based on many simplifying assumptions and should be used only as a rough guide.

373.2. HEMODIALYSIS

Lee W. Henderson

The purification of blood by dialysis may be accomplished using either synthetic membranes (extracorporeal hemodialysis, commonly termed hemodialysis) or the biologic membrane lining the peritoneal cavity (peritoneal hemodialysis, commonly referred to as peritoneal dialysis). Both techniques rely on the process of diffusion down a concentration gradient and across the dialysis membrane that separates blood from dialysis fluid to effect desired adjustments in concentration and content of blood solutes. Although dialysis is most commonly applied in the treatment of renal parenchymal failure, it is also used to remove toxins or poisons or life-threatening excesses of total body water in the absence of renal failure when renal excretion of these substances is inadequate or compromised by prerenal factors.

The composition of the dialysis fluid determines the eventual composition of the plasma water. The degree to which equilibrium between plasma water and dialysis fluid is achieved is a function of the duration of treatment and the efficiency of the dialysis technique. The accompanying table lists the content and range of concentration of commonly used dialysis fluids. It should be noted that dialysis fluid is usually nothing more than a collection of the physiologically important electrolytes in concentrations comparable to those in normal plasma water. Hyperkalemia is a problem commonly requiring hemodialysis and, as such, potassium is usually left out completely or added in concentrations below those of normal plasma in order to steepen its concentration gradient across the membrane from "blood to bath" and hence expedite its removal. When treatment is more prolonged, of course, this important cation must be added to the bath in order to prevent hypokalemia. As most patients with acute or chronic renal failure have higher than normal total body sodium content, the dialysis fluid concentration of this cation is usually below physiologic, e.g., 132 to 138 mEq per liter. Bicarbonate ion tends to degrade to CO_2 and water with time and exposure of the dialysis fluid to the air; hence alkali equivalents that are nonvolatile are commonly used in dialysis fluid. At present acetate and, less commonly, lactate, both of which are swiftly metabolized on a mole for mole basis to bicarbonate, are used. The concentrations are higher than 25 mEq per liter because the bicarbonate present in plasma water is lost across the membrane into the dialysis fluid during treatment, and this quantity in addition to any deficit resulting from buffering metabolic hydrogen ion must be replaced. The value of 35 to 40 mEq per liter cited in the table has been arrived at rather empirically for the treatment of chronic renal failure and, at times, must be adjusted to accommodate special applications such as hemodialysis for drug overdose or acute renal failure in conjunction with abdominal surgery, nasogastric suction, and supernormal concentrations of plasma bicarbonate. Calcium and magnesium are present in concentrations comparable to their ionized fraction in plasma water. Chloride is used only as a balancing anion and will vary in parallel with the concentration of cations and reciprocally with the concentration of alkali equivalent in the bath. Glucose plays a major role in regulating the osmolality of peritoneal dialysis fluid and not infrequently is used in concentrations of 4250 mg per deciliter to enhance the removal of water. Extracorporeal hemodialysis relies more on hydrostatic than osmotic force to remove excess water, and hence glucose is not uncommonly absent from the bath. Solutes such as urea, creatinine, uric acid, poisons, or any solute not represented in the dialysis fluid will, of course, equilibrate across the membrane and be removed from the body via the dialysis fluid which is discarded. It should be noted that dialysis fluid used for extracorporeal hemodialysis usually contains both bacteria and pyrogen, unlike peritoneal dialysis fluid which is sterile, and its introduction into the blood may have serious clinical consequences. Hemodialysis, which works by diffusion, is unlike the human kidney that removes solutes by pressure filtration across the glomerular capillary wall. The human glomerulus, within relatively broad limits of solute molecular size, is not size discriminatory in its removal of solutes; i.e., creatinine at 113 daltons will be

Composition of Dialysis Fluid

Constituent	Common Concentration (Range), mEq per Liter
Sodium	133 (130–145)
Potassium	3 (0–5)
Calcium	3.5 (2.5–4.0)
Magnesium	1.5 (1.5)
Alkali equivalent (acetate, lactate)	37 (35–40)
Chloride	105 (98–106)
Glucose	(0–4250) mg/dl

removed at the same clearance rate as inulin, a test molecule of 5200 daltons. Hemodialysis, however, is always size discriminatory, with rapidly diffusing solutes such as urea (60 daltons) being more efficiently removed than larger ones.

PERITONEAL DIALYSIS

Peritoneal dialysis is simpler to conduct technically and requires only basic medical skills well within the grasp of the well informed internist-nurse team. Extracorporeal hemodialysis is technically demanding and should be restricted for use to the nephrologist-dialysis team. Specifically, peritoneal dialysis can be initiated by the internist. Access to the peritoneal space is accomplished either by using a disposable rigid catheter, or if repeated dialysis is anticipated, by use of a flexible silicone rubber catheter of slightly larger dimensions equipped with a Dacron velour cuff to permit the formation of bacteria-tight seals between the catheter and the abdominal wall. In either case, the catheter is placed through the anterior abdominal wall under local anesthesia. Satisfactory placement of a peritoneal catheter requires a modicum of experience. Common problems resulting from unsatisfactory placement are patient discomfort and difficulty in obtaining complete return of the administered dialysis fluid. A detailed description of the placement technique is commonly supplied with the catheters. With the catheter in place, sterile, pyrogen-free, warmed dialysis fluid is introduced in 1 to 2 liter aliquots, allowed to equilibrate (dwell), and subsequently drained and discarded. Two commonly used programs that give comparable clearance values for urea and creatinine are as follows:

(1) 2 liters dialysis fluid (gravity installation, usually over ten minutes)
   30-minute dwell time
   20-minute drain time
   or 2 liters per hour for 24 to 48 hours

(2) 1 liter of dialysis fluid (gravity installation, five minutes)
   20-minute dwell time
   10-minute drain time
   or 1 liter per hour for 24 to 48 hours

The latter program has the advantage of producing less restriction of diaphragmatic movement with a reduced risk of atelectasis and pneumonia, but it is considerably more demanding of personnel time.

Clearance rates for urea and creatinine with peritoneal dialysis are on the order of 20 to 35 ml per minute. Most artificial kidneys commonly achieve clearance figures for both solutes in excess of 100 ml per minute, a figure comparable in efficiency to the clearance of these solutes by a pair of intact human kidneys. Larger solutes (>500 daltons), not yet characterized biochemically, have been identified to be present in abnormally high concentrations in uremic plasma. The role of these "middle molecules" in the pathophysiology of uremia is as yet unclear. The peritoneal membrane, which has a smaller functional surface area than the artificial kidney, is on the order of 10 times more permeable for inulin (5200 daltons), a commonly used experimental middle molecule, than is cuprophan (the membrane common to most artificial kidneys). The clinical result of these differences in performance is still being evaluated. One difference, however, is the comparatively low incidence with peritoneal dialysis of problems arising from the too rapid restoration of abnormal serum solute concentrations to normal, seen at times with the extracorporeal technique. Fluid removal with peritoneal dialysis is also somewhat less rapidly achieved when compared with most artificial kidneys. However, because the treatment time with peritoneal dialysis is commonly 24 to 48 hours, rather than four to six hours as with the artificial kidney, the total amount of fluid removed per treatment may be higher with peritoneal dialysis. Negative fluid balance of 10 to 15 liters in 48 hours may at times be achieved with this technique, with few or no clinical signs or symptoms of hypovolemia. Maximal figures for an artificial kidney treatment of four to six hours are more nearly 5 to 7 liters, frequently with episodes of symptomatic hypotension.

At present fluid cycling machines are being marketed that warm, dispense, and discard dialysis fluid and keep records of dialysis fluid volume turnover. It is clear that they will have a major impact on this "labor-sensitive" procedure. At present, peritoneal dialysis is predominantly used for treating patients with acute rather than chronic renal failure. One reason for its limited use with chronic renal failure relates to the longer time per treatment required to accomplish reduction in urea and creatinine concentration to "satisfactory" levels. Judgments on what is "satisfactory" are changing, and this coupled with the new fluid cycling equipment may lead to increased popularity for chronic peritoneal dialysis. Prospective trials comparing the results of peritoneal and extracorporeal chronic dialysis have not yet been published, although several such studies are in progress.

EXTRACORPOREAL HEMODIALYSIS

Access to the vascular space is required for the dialysis of patients with acute renal failure and is usually accomplished by twin surgical cutdowns over an artery and vein at the wrist. Teflon-tipped cannulas of appropriate diameter are placed in each vessel, which is then tied distal to the point of placement. The silicone rubber tubing portion of the cannula is attached to the arterial and venous lines of the artificial kidney. At the conclusion of the procedure, the two silicone rubber tubes are connected and blood circulates directly from artery to vein, giving rise to the name "shunt" commonly applied to this form of vascular access. Blood flow rates through the artificial kidney of up to 350 ml per minute are commonly

Figure 1. Clearance of creatinine from whole blood is plotted against blood flow rate for an extracorporeal hemodialyzer. For blood flow rates of less than 200 ml per minute, clearance falls (i.e., flow limited). For flows above 200 ml per minute, increases in membrane area or permeability to creatinine are required to increase clearance (i.e., membrane limited).

achieved and, when not in use for dialysis, shunt flow rates are comparable or higher. Alternatively, access yielding satisfactory blood flow may be accomplished by using percutaneous vascular puncture with Seldinger equipment and specially designed catheters for this application in a manner analogous to catheter placement for radiographic diagnostic procedures. The femoral vessels are used, and two cannulas are placed. Extracorporeal hemodialysis may be conducted either artery to vein or with both cannulas in a single vessel at different levels so as to reduce admixture of the afferent and efferent bloodstreams. Somewhat less satisfactory is arterial puncture with any of the disposable sheathed needles that permit the placement of a flexible cannula in an artery (usually radial) with return of blood to one or more peripheral veins. The success of this latter technique depends upon the size of the cannula. Blood flow rates of 200 ml per minute may be obtained from a single well placed one and one-half inch 14-gauge needle in a patient with normal blood pressure. Attainable blood flow rates drop with increasing cannula length and/or smaller internal diameter. Central venous pressure lines are generally not satisfactory because they are too long. A blood flow rate of less than 200 ml per minute may impose an undesirably low upper limit on the clearance rate for small rapidly diffusing solutes such as potassium (cardiotoxicity) or urea (platelet malfunction) (Fig. 1).

For chronic renal failure the most desirable form of vascular access is provided by anastomosis of the radial artery and a forearm vein (usually side to side) in such a manner as to permit a significant component of the arterial blood to traverse the fistula into the vein. Hypertrophy of the veins in immediate continuity with the fistula provides large superficial thick-walled vessels with high blood flow rates at near arterial pressure for access, using a pair of short, wide (12 to 14 gauge) needles placed with standard percutaneous venipuncture technique. Equipment is now available that permits satisfactory perfusion of the dialyzer, using a single needle. The principle of operation may be understood by considering the analogous situation of air exchange through the trachea to the alveoli. Single needle operation through a forearm fistula may well become the common mode of vascular access. Recently, the development of synthetic vascular prosthetic material placed as a large bore arteriovenous connection that may be "venipunctured" has achieved considerable success as a second alternative for patients whose own vessels do not lend themselves to creation of a fistula. The surgical procedures for placing fistulas and shunts are truly lifesaving and should command the meticulous attention of a surgeon who is familiar with the rather considerable literature in this area. The surgeon should be prepared not only to carry out the initial procedure but also to join with the internist or nephrologist in follow-up of the subsequent course and possible complications. Inadequate flow, "steal" syndromes that compromise hand function or result in ischemic ulceration of the fingers, clotting, aneurysmal dilatations, and infection may all occur.

There are two components to an artificial kidney: the membrane package and the fluid cycler. Cuprophan, a particular form of cellulosic membrane, accounts for more than 90 per cent of artificial kidney membranes in use today. A vast majority of the remaining 10 per cent are cellulosic membranes made by other than the cuprammonium process. A variety of sterile disposable membrane formats (coil, hollow fiber, sheet) are available for hemodialysis. All formats share the features of presenting a substantial membrane surface area (usually 1 to 1.5 square meters, but ranging from 0.5 to 2.5 square meters), with minimal "blinding" by support structures and a very thin blood path (250 microns or less). Such a blood path reduces the total volume of blood in the extracorporeal circuit. In addition, a thin blood path results in a rapid flow of blood across the surface of the membrane and reduces stagnant fluid films or "unstirred" layers, that might otherwise develop and impede the transport of solutes into the bath by lengthening the diffusion path between the well mixed bulk phase of the two solutions. Figure 2 contrasts the solute clearance pattern of an artificial kidney with that of an intact normal human kidney. They are very different, with the artificial kidney removing small solutes better and larger solutes considerably less well than the human kidney.

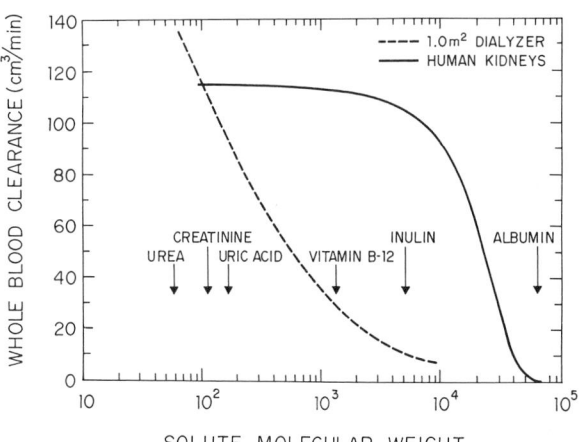

Figure 2. Whole blood clearance of solutes with increasing molecular weight is plotted for an artificial kidney and a pair of human kidneys. The artificial kidney clears small solutes (<100 daltons) more rapidly than the human kidney. Larger solutes, however, are progressively less well cleared.

The fluid cycler may either prepare dialysis fluid from good quality water and a concentrated solution of electrolytes "on line" at whatever flow rate is demanded (200 to 500 ml per minute) or deliver the appropriate flow rate from a large (100 to 150 liters) premade batch. "On-line" and, less conveniently, "batch" fluid cycling equipment may be centrally placed and scaled to deliver dialysis fluid to multiple dialysis stations, each with their separate membrane packages (central delivery system). All are designed to provide dialysis fluid to a membrane package with close monitoring for content and temperature. Many have blood leak detectors that indicate when red cells are present in the dialysis fluid leaving the membrane. Figure 3 is a diagram of an artificial kidney, showing the various components of such a system. It should be noted that extracorporeal hemodialysis is usually conducted with the patient anticoagulated with heparin. With peritoneal dialysis, in which small amounts of heparin may be added to the dialysis fluid, no systemic heparinization

Figure 3. The usual components of an artificial kidney are shown. Direction of flow for blood and dialysis fluid is indicated by the arrows. The quality control component monitors temperature and solute content (electrical conductivity). The water used in the preparation of dialysis fluid should be of high quality, e.g., treated by reverse osmosis.

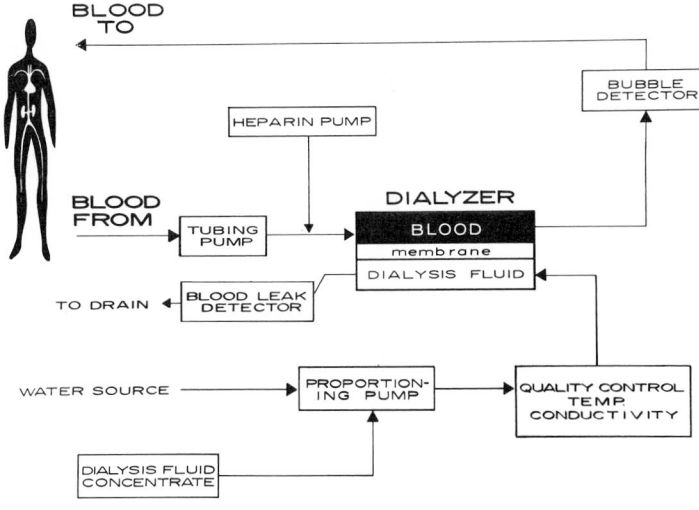

results owing to its large molecular size (slow diffusivity). When systemic heparinization is contraindicated and peritoneal dialysis should not be used, e.g., after recent abdominal surgery, regional heparinization may be used, with protamine sulfate introduced into the efferent blood line at a rate to precisely neutralize the heparin being added to the afferent line. Alternatively, lower than usual heparin doses may be used ("tight" systemic heparinization), relying on both dilution and metabolic degradation of the heparin returning in the efferent line to prevent significant systemic anticoagulation.

Patients with acute renal failure should be dialyzed promptly and aggressively so that severe and onerous restrictions of dietary protein and fluid intake are either not required or minimal. These patients frequently have wounds to heal and infections to overcome and as such need optimal nutrition. Biochemically, hemodialysis should be considered when the blood urea nitrogen concentration reaches 100 mg per 100 ml or the plasma creatinine level reaches 10 mg per 100 ml. The broad goal of treatment should be to hold the BUN and creatinine concentrations at or below these values while providing reasonable caloric and protein intake, i.e., 25 to 30 cal per kilogram per day and 1 gram per kilogram per day of protein. In addition, close monitoring of fluid balance and plasma potassium values with the use of modest fluid restriction and potassium-trapping resins should augment treatment by hemodialysis. Technical competence is at such a level that risks from hemodialysis treatment are very small. Therefore one should err on the side of more instead of less dialysis in the treatment of acute renal failure.

For patients with chronic renal failure, the decision must first be made as to whether or not maintenance dialysis is indicated. Arbitrary age limits and/or presence of disease entities that have been used in the past as criteria to withhold treatment are being liberalized daily, and it would behoove the well informed internist to identify the present criteria of acceptability for the hemodialysis units geographically convenient to his patients. There are now reports of small series in which successful maintenance dialysis has been conducted in the over 65 age group, in patients with disseminated lupus erythematosus and postcoronary artery bypass surgery. Although those with diabetic nephropathy do less well, they have nonetheless been chronically dialyzed with prolongation of life. Medical common sense will point away from sustaining life in patients with unrelenting disease that limits any reasonable human participation, e.g., metastatic cancer with bone pain, advanced cerebrovascular damage. At present, maintenance hemodialysis in the prepubertal child as an end in itself is not well considered because of the marginal results both physically and psychologically. As a holding measure for subsequent transplantation, it is highly appropriate.

When a maintenance hemodialysis program is indicated, the question of when to begin dialysis must be decided. Attitudes on this are changing in favor of beginning earlier in the course of chronic renal failure, i.e., before the occurrence of incapacitating malaise, nausea and vomiting, neuropathy, or pericarditis. In general, creatinine clearance of 5 ml per minute or less, coupled with malaise, may be sufficient to warrant starting treatment.

At present, federal reimbursement favors the more expensive in-center dialysis. However, it is clear that, for some, self-dialysis in the home is not only possible but preferable, both medically and logistically. It is hoped that time will change this administrative error and permit free selection of the best dialysis site by patient and physician without fiscal constraint (i.e., home, limited-care facility, or center).

ADEQUACY OF MAINTENANCE HEMODIALYSIS

At present there is no clear information which links uremic signs, symptoms, or pathophysiologic abnormalities with the presence of specific solutes in uremic plasma. It is clear that many abnormal solutes are present and that many normal solutes are there in abnormal concentrations. Application of methodology that separates these substances primarily by their molecular size, coupled with perceptive clinical and engineering analyses, has made it clear that traditional small molecular weight (<500 daltons) compounds such as urea, creatinine, and uric acid cannot account for the wide spectrum of uremic abnormalities clinically encountered, and that solutes of intermediate molecular weight (500 to 6000 daltons), so-called "middle molecules," may well contribute to the etiology of the uremic syndrome. Clear delineation of the abnormalities resulting from retention of solutes normally excreted in the urine has been confounded by the substantial endocrine and metabolic functions of the kidney that are lost in conjunction with diminished excretory function. At present, artificial kidney technology must address the problem of uremia empirically, with the guiding principle being to mimic the solute clearance pattern of the human kidney. By this standard, artificial kidneys in general use today perform well with respect to water and small solute removal, i.e., they fulfill the goals perceived by the original and early workers in the field. However, enthusiasm for the dramatic lifesaving results obtained with hemodialysis must be tempered with the realization that the well dialyzed patient with chronic renal failure is by no means normal even though he reports "feeling well." One need only identify the widely reported 5 to 10 per cent mortality per year, irrespective of patient age or sex, to know that present-day dialysis, no matter how prescribed, is incapable of restoring normality. A second and lower level of expectation for dialysis is to maintain the patient free of symptoms and signs of flagrant uremia (e.g., prevention of peripheral neuropathy, pericarditis, pleuritis). Average hemodialysis prescriptions empirically arrived at to achieve this for 70- to 80-kg patients on diets of reasonable protein, potassium, and caloric content are as follows: for extracorporeal hemodialysis, the application of 1 square meter of cuprophan membrane for five hours three times weekly at 200 to 300 ml per minute blood flow rates and 500 ml per minute dialysis fluid flow rate; for peritoneal dialysis, a weekly total of 30 to 40 2-liter exchanges. Application of larger membrane area packages for shorter treatment times and pharmacological manipulations of the permeability of the peritoneal membrane for more efficient dialysis are currently being explored. Tailoring of the dialysis prescription to the individual's needs is now carried out, based largely on body habitus, diet, pretreatment chemical values, and clinical response. The percentage of such patients who return to work successfully cannot be generally cited, as the range reported is so wide — 90 per cent for suburban middle class patients vs. near zero for populations drawn from urban ghettos.

It follows from what has been said that a well functioning kidney transplant results in a far higher quality of life than the very best maintenance hemodialysis. When the probability for such transplantation is present, i.e., availability of a well matched living related donor, this should be the primary therapy. When only donor kidneys of lower quality are available, the choice of direction is moot and requires a thorough exploration of the alternatives with the patient and his family. Figures for *kidney* mortality taken from the national transplantation registry should be compared with the results of the local transplantation and hemodialysis teams. Although these two modalities of treatment for chronic renal failure are used in a complementary manner, it should be noted that loss of a transplanted kidney does not automatically return a patient to maintenance hemodialysis. In the earlier days of transplantation, 20 to 30 per cent of patients would lose their lives from the complications of immunosuppression or infection when the transplant was lost. More recently greater conservatism in the prescription of azathioprine and steroids has been exercised. Awareness of the *patient* mortality figure for the surgical team considered will be important for the internist before advising the patient and his family about this difficult judgment.

MEDICAL COMPLICATIONS OF MAINTENANCE HEMODIALYSIS

HEMATOLOGIC.   There are numerous reasons for anemia to be part of the chronic uremic syndrome. Loss of synthetic capability by the kidney for erythropoietin, marrow depression, qualitative platelet defects with minor episodes of blood loss, and faulty gastrointestinal uptake of iron may all contribute. With the addition of extracorporeal hemodialysis, there is the added loss of blood left in the membrane package at the close of dialysis as well as iatrogenic losses, depending on the frequency with which blood chemistries are measured. Hematocrits in the 20 to 30 per cent range are common in the maintenance dialysis population. A small subset of patients may carry more normal values if the disease kidneys are in place, blood loss is kept minimal, and satisfactory iron stores are maintained. Synthetic erythropoietin is not yet available for therapy, but preliminary studies suggest that toxic marrow depression will block return to fully normal erythropoietic capability. Androgen-like synthetic steroids are currently undergoing trial, and time will be required to know which preparation is most effective and whether long-term negative side effects preclude their use. Transfusions of packed red cells are expensive and depress the marrow if used to bring hematocrit values to normal and, as such, should not be routinely employed for that purpose. Red cell transfusion should be saved for treating acute blood loss, e.g., from rupture of a dialysis membrane or to prepare for major surgery, e.g., transplantation. The concern about developing circulating preformed antibodies that would prejudice against successful transplantation as a result of exposure to foreign blood proteins has been tempered by new empirical information indicating that patients who are so exposed and then transplanted fare better in terms of sustaining kidney function. The mechanisms for this are not presently known. The risk of hepatitis must be weighed carefully in the decision to transfuse.

NEUROPSYCHIATRIC.   The presence of peripheral neuropathy has been used as an indication either that main-

tenance dialysis should be begun or that a given hemodialysis prescription was inadequate. Neither use is appropriate now, as irreversible neuropathy should be avoided. Measurement of motor nerve conduction velocity as performed at most hospitals is not done with sufficient skill to make it useful in judging subtle degrees of preclinical impairment and should not be relied on to guide the time of referral for hemodialysis.

Rapid reduction in the plasma concentration of small osmotically active solutes such as urea can result in a shift of water into the brain, causing brain edema and seizures. This disequilibrium syndrome is almost exclusively seen with extracorporeal dialysis in patients with acute renal failure and high (>180 mg per 100 ml) blood urea nitrogen values. Large membrane area, high efficiency dialysis equipment predisposes to this complication. Application of hemodialysis in patients early in the course of acute renal failure and reduced initial dialysis treatment times such that there is a less radical change in plasma solute concentrations will obviate this problem. Subdural hematoma without apparent antecedent trauma has been reported, presumably as a complication of the repeated systemic heparinization that this group of patients undergoes.

The heavy stress placed on patients maintained on hemodialysis and their families makes for a high incidence of depression, insomnia, and stress-related somatic complaints. How seriously this stress is felt by the patient may be judged by the suicide rate for this population, which is 100 to 400 times higher that among controls. "Dialysis dementia," a progressive and ultimately fatal encephalopathy of undetermined cause, may initially be misdiagnosed as a purely psychiatric disturbance. Facial grimacing, disturbed speech, and dementia may be present separately or together, and seizures may occur. Absence of focal signs may help distinguish this entity from subdural hematoma.

MUSCULOSKELETAL.   Muscle cramps of the lower extremities, analogous to the isolated "night cramps" in normal persons, occur during the course of extracorporeal hemodialysis, especially when large amounts of excess body water and electrolyte require a brisk rate of ultrafiltration to restore "dry weight" in the four- to five-hour treatment period. These cramps can be very painful and at times involve the upper extremities and abdominal musculature. Their mechanism is not well understood. Symptomatic relief may usually be obtained with hypertonic mannitol (12.5 grams) and/or sodium chloride solution given as an intravenous bolus.

Calcium malabsorption and faulty or absent conversion of vitamin D by the kidney to its active metabolites results in a pathophysiologic sequence involving profound chronic hyperparathyroidism with altered bone architecture (both osteitis fibrosa and osteomalacia) that at times may be crippling. The variability of this manifestation from one hemodialysis unit to another argues for local modulating features to this syndrome. At times, subtotal (or total with fragmented autotransplantation) removal of the parathyroid glands may be required when florid tertiary hyperparathyroidism occurs. Phosphate reduction, e.g., with orally administered phosphate binding gels, early in the course of renal failure should be an important ameliorating therapy, but it has yet to receive adequate clinical trials. Synthetic active vitamin D metabolites are undergoing clinical trial and will undoubtedly find an important place in management.

CARDIOVASCULAR.   Myocardial infarction and cerebrovascular accidents account for over half of the deaths in patients on maintenance hemodialysis. The high incidence of hypertension and accelerated atherogenesis contributes materially to this problem. Over half of the patients with end-stage renal failure on maintenance hemodialysis have hypertension, using >140 systolic and >90 diastolic mm Hg as the criteria for this abnormality. The common "lesion" appears to be an increase in peripheral vascular tone. All but a minority (5 to 10 per cent) of these patients can be controlled with sodium volume reduction and/or medications, but a saw-toothed pattern of blood pressure often results owing to the interdialytic sodium volume overload that these patients exhibit and the need for conservatism in drug management to prevent shock during hemodialysis when acute reductions in vascular volume may occur. Defective baroreceptor function with excessive lability of blood pressure in response to vascular volume changes may also be present as a subset of this group. The 5 to 10 per cent who fail to respond to conservative measures usually exhibit plasma renin values that are persistently above those obtained in normal volunteers. These patients at times show a further pressor response to sodium volume removal during hemodialysis. Bilateral nephrectomy has proved useful in ameliorating this form of hypertension.

Pericarditis is classically present at death if uremia is untreated. However, we now are finding pericarditis in isolated patients on "adequate" hemodialysis for reasons that cannot be identified. At times it is temporally related to stress, e.g., surgery, infection. The inflammation usually subsides with time, but may be complicated by pericardial tamponade or subsequent constrictive pericarditis. At times small epidemics of pericarditis spread through a hemodialysis unit, giving rise to the suspicion of an infectious rather than a toxic cause. Pericarditis is a life-threatening complication and should command close attention.

Congestive heart failure resulting from sodium volume overload is quite common in this population.

INFECTION. Blunted immunologic responsiveness and malfunctioning lymphocytes and polymorphs have all been demonstrated in patients with end-stage renal failure. Hemodialysis only partially restores these functions. Infection is the second most common cause of death in the maintenance hemodialysis population. Infections of the vascular access, whether it be shunt or prosthetic fistula, are particularly lethal. Slightly less so is infection of the peritoneal space. Early aggressive therapy is required, using either information from smears or "best guess" reasoning for the selection of antimicrobial agent. The altered kinetics of antimicrobial handling in this patient group and the unusual problems of infected prostheses that are required to remain in place for continued hemodialysis are persuasive arguments for seeking out experienced assistance in treating these problems. The maintenance hemodialysis population is particularly at risk for viral hepatitis (4.4 cases per 100 at risk). The disease is mild in its clinical manifestations, with a minority showing jaundice. However, the disease has proved to be infectious (3.4 cases per 100 at risk) and highly virulent to hospital staff, not infrequently resulting in death. Containment requires fastidious attention to sterile technique.

Barnes, B. A., et al.: The twelfth report of the Human Renal Transplant Registry. JAMA, 233:787, 1975.
Bricker, N. S.: On the pathogenesis of the uremic state: An exposition of the "trade-off hypothesis." N. Engl. J. Med., 286:1093, 1972.

373.3.   RENAL TRANSPLANTATION

Priscilla Kincaid-Smith

The value of renal transplantation in identical twins was established over 20 years ago; however, despite the surprising success of some of Hume's cadaver transplants in 1955, many years passed before transplantation became accepted as an effective means of treatment in chronic renal failure. Early deaths were mainly due to immunosuppressive methods, including total body irradiation; clinical success dates from the introduction of azathioprine in 1962. This drug remains the major immunosuppressive agent used in renal transplantation.

SELECTION AND PREPARATION OF PATIENTS

The selection of patients with irreversible renal failure who are suitable for renal transplantation poses few problems if adequate dialysis facilities exist and the invidious situation of competition for places is thus avoided.

Contraindications include old age, metastatic carcinoma, psychosis, active infection (e.g., tuberculosis), and severe cerebral, myocardial, or peripheral vascular disease. Patients with diabetes, inactive tuberculosis, coronary artery disease, multisystemic disease such as systemic lupus erythematosus, chronic obstructive lung disease, and peptic ulceration have all had successful transplants.

Age alone is not a contraindication to transplantation, because transplants have been performed in neonates and in those over the age of 80. Patient survival decreases in both low and high age groups. More important than chronologic age is the quality of life which can be achieved by the patient under consideration after a successful graft.

Transplantation in the very young poses problems relating to size vessels, lack of growth, and difficulties in social adjustment. Dialysis in this age group introduces further problems such as fluid and diet restriction and long hours of dialysis, and does not avoid the problems of growth and social adjustment. Children over age eight who weigh 20 kg or more pose fewer problems, and growth, sometimes with impressive spurts, has been reported.

In the congenital nephrotic syndrome transplantation appears to be "curative," whereas in hyperoxaluria the defect persists and has led to early graft loss.

There is no medical state for which dialysis is definitely indicated and transplantation not. Advanced vascular disease has been suggested as a contraindication to transplantation, but it is the most common cause of death on dialysis and makes blood vessel access difficult. Reported experience with hyperoxaluria patients on dialysis is poor, and survival in diabetes is worse than with transplantation.

Immunologic sensitization to transplantation antigens may make the selection of a suitable kidney difficult; but if an appropriate donor can be found, transplantation is not contraindicated.

The patient must be optimally fit at the time of transplantation in order to have every chance of surviving the stresses and complications of surgery, high steroids, and immunosuppression. Hypertension must be effectively controlled, the heart size returned toward normal, calcium and phosphate abnormalities rectified, anemia improved as far as possible, and infection eradicated. Preparatory surgery such as bilateral nephrectomy, ileal bladder construction, and peptic ulcer surgery may be necessary. Careful attention to patient preparation may be a major factor in the increased graft and patient survival rate achieved in some countries.

Bilateral nephrectomy carries a predictable morbidity and mortality and is only indicated when the patient's own kidneys may contribute to subsequent graft failure or death. Atrophic pyelonephritis and persistent active infection, as in some polycystic kidneys and in association with calculi, require bilateral nephrectomy. Patients with anti-GBM-antibody–mediated glomerulonephritis have been transplanted successfully with kidneys in situ. The case for leaving kidneys intact is compelling in an integrated program which may involve long periods on dialysis. This will significantly minimize anemia and fluid restriction and may permit clearance of "middle molecules" which may be of value.

DONOR PROCUREMENT

An adequate supply of cadaveric donors can be achieved only with cooperation and understanding between the public and physicians. To achieve HLA phenotype identical and ABO compatible cadaver donors for a pool size of 500 recipients and an average waiting time of six months, Kountz has estimated the necessity for 50 donors per month. This recruitment rate is not an unrealistic target even for large geographic areas, because Australia has consistently recruited one donor per month per 1.5 million of population in recent years.

Any patients under the age of 65 who have basically normal renal function and have no evidence of malignancy (excluding cerebral tumor) are potential donors. Systemic or urinary infection, severe hypertension, and renal disease are not acceptable in the donor. Urine flow should exceed 30 ml per hour up to one hour before death. Despite these liberal criteria, the vast majority of donors have in practice come from patients with head injuries or spontaneous intracerebral vascular catastrophes. Recent studies suggest that pretreatment of the donor with a large dose of cyclophosphamide may enhance graft survival. This aims to destroy passenger leukocytes in the graft which are thought to play an important part in rejection.

ORGAN PRESERVATION

Although kidneys can be successfully stored by simple flushing with a hyperosmolar solution followed by immersion in saline slush for 12 hours or more, pulsatile perfusion with oxygenated plasma at 10° C for 24 hours is associated with little deterioration in graft function. Both methods allow elective surgery at a time convenient to the patient and to the medical and surgical staff, as well as detailed cross-matching and tissue typing.

CADAVER VERSUS LIVE DONOR

There is a clear improvement in graft survival rate using living related donors with only one haplotype difference or no difference between donor and recipient. Experience with "HLA identical" siblings has been very good. If both haplotypes are nonidentical, results are no better than those of cadaveric transplantation, and most units no longer transplant in this situation.

The data in "HLA identical" siblings are so impressive that the results should be actively pointed out to families for their consideration.

The over-all trend is toward cadaveric transplantation.

HISTOCOMPATIBILITY TESTING

The human major histocompatibility complex (MHC) is located on the short arm of chromosome 6. This region codes for the major or most important transplantation antigens. There are at least four loci: HLA–A, B, C, and D. The gene products of the HLA–A, B, and C loci (the HLA–A, B, and C antigens) are expressed on the surface of nearly all cells and are detectable by serologic tests. The HLA-D antigens are expressed in significant amounts on a limited number of cell types, including B lymphocytes, monocytes, and endothelial cells. These antigens are responsible for the mixed lymphocyte reaction (MLR) by which they are detected. The relationship between the MLR-defined HLA-D antigens and a closely associated (? identical) serologically defined system of "B cell antigens" is currently under investigation.

Each individual inherits one chromosome 6 from each parent and thus has two HLA antigens expressed by each of the four HLA loci. The implications of this pattern of inheritance for transplantation are that in living related donor transplants the whole of one or both MHC complexes is shared by recipient and donor, whereas in cadaveric transplantation, matching is only for individual HLA antigens. The extreme polymorphism of the HLA system makes it very difficult to find an HLA-identical cadaveric donor for recipients. The chance of finding such a donor varies from 1:100 to more than 1:1,000,000. There is indirect evidence that the most important HLA antigens to match for are the D antigens, as these are the antigens first recognized as foreign by the host's immune system. The importance of the HLA–A, B, and C antigens is two-fold. First, they are the targets of the host's rejection reaction. Second, because of linkage disequilibrium, matching for HLA–A, B, and C antigens frequently results in accompanying HLA-D matching. Linkage disequilibrium, which means that the co-occurrence of antigens at one locus with those of another locus occurs more frequently than would occur by chance, is very strong within the HLA system. Until serologic detection of HLA-D antigens is freely available, the best that can be done is to attempt to match for the HLA–A, B, and C antigens.

Presensitization of the recipient against donor HLA–A, B, or C antigens must be avoided, as hyperacute rejection is an almost invariable consequence. This is detected as a positive "cross-match" between recipient serum and donor cells in the presence of complement. The sources of such presensitization are blood transfusion, pregnancies, and previous transplants. Blood transfusion has a paradoxical effect — it may enhance graft survival. The mechanism of this effect is not certain. It is suggested that blood transfusion provokes not only potentially deleterious presensitization against the

HLA–A, B, and C antigens, which is avoided by insisting that the cross-match be negative, but also the formation of antibodies against HLA-D, which by an unknown mechanism reduce the risk of allograft rejection. In making a decision to give potential cadaver transplant recipients blood transfusions which are not indicated on other grounds, it is important to remember that the development of presensitization will reduce their chances of transplantation.

PATHOLOGIC FEATURES OF REJECTION

Although intense cellular infiltration is a prominent feature in the unmodified rejection reaction seen in animals, this is not a prominent feature in patients in whom rejection is modified by treatment with steroids and azathioprine. The major lesions seen in renal allografts in man are in the vessels, and they involve all blood vessels from the main artery and vein to the glomerular capillaries and intertubular sinusoids.

Polymorphonuclear leukocytes may accumulate within the blood vessels of the allograft within minutes, and so-called "hyperacute" rejection, with very florid thrombotic vascular lesions, may develop within hours or days of grafting. Such patients may have preformed humoral antibody in their serum which conventional screening methods failed to detect. The vascular lesions of hyperacute rejection are similar to those occurring in acute and chronic rejection. The differences between the three are differences of degree and rate of progress, but the essential pathogenesis of lesions seen in vessels in serial percutaneous biopsies is similar. Platelet and fibrin thrombi may be demonstrated within vessels of all sizes in the acute stages, and the glomerular and vascular lesions seen months or years after transplantation represent the residual lesions that follow these thrombotic lesions. This process of "organization" may result in lesions which resemble atheroma and cause stenosis of the main renal artery. Intimal proliferation causes narrowing of interlobar, arcuate, and interlobular arteries and of arterioles. It has been shown that the cells which proliferate in the intima are smooth muscle cells and that their proliferation is stimulated by factors released from platelets. Glomerular capillaries show changes which closely mimic those of mesangiocapillary glomerulonephritis and make the distinction between late rejection and glomerulonephritis difficult.

Rejection poses the most danger during the first three months; subsequently severe acute rejection is rare, but episodes of rejection may occur as long as several years after transplantation. In a controlled trial, anticoagulation and antithrombotic drugs appear to affect the histologic lesions in vessels and glomeruli but have not shown any effect on graft function during the first three years.

NATURAL HISTORY OF PATIENTS WITH RENAL ALLOGRAFTS

Early Course

Although urine flow usually commences promptly with well-prepared live donor kidneys, a period of oliguria is common in cadaveric transplantation. Prompt urine flow will occur if warm ischemic times are kept to less than one hour and cold ischemic time is short. Early good renal function avoids dialysis and facilitates the early diagnosis of rejection, but initial oliguria does not alter the long-term outcome.

In the absence of complications, the patient may be ambulant on the second day and discharged from hospital between the fifth and tenth postoperative days. Daily outpatient attendance for review of renal function and detection of rejection and complications is essential during the first three to four weeks. Visits are gradually reduced in frequency to once a week at three months and once a month at a year and thereafter. Close and intense supervision in the first weeks and months is probably the major factor responsible for higher success rates in some programs.

Return to full activities is achieved in over 90 per cent of patients at about two months, and this coincides with the spontaneous restoration of a normal hemoglobin.

Rejection crises occurs in the majority of cadaver transplants and may even occur with identical sibling live donor kidneys. Although a number of techniques such as urinary FDP's, ^{131}I fibrinogen uptake, urinary enyzme levels, urine cell counts, hyperchloremia, induced lymphocyte transformation, urinary electrolyte patterns, and scanning techniques have all been suggested to give advance warning of rejection, alteration of renal function as judged by an elevation of the serum creatinine concentration remains the mainstay of diagnosis. A decrease in urine volume may precede the rise in creatinine. Fever, leukocytosis, local pain, and systemic symptoms are late features and correlate much better with a local complication such as a perirenal hematoma or a urinary leak.

The majority of rejection crises can be reversed by increased steroid dosage, and heparin may be of benefit.

It is important that immunosuppression and steroids should not be pushed to excess with consequent severe morbidity and mortality from infection and marrow depression. Azathioprine should be reduced in dosage when renal function is abnormal rather than increased. Consistent elevation of the serum creatinine above a level of 6 mg per 100 ml after the first four weeks results in high morbidity and mortality and is an indication for graft removal.

The best guide to graft prognosis is percutaneous renal biopsy, which is simple and safe owing to the fixed and superficial position of the kidney. The histologic appearance assists in the diagnosis of the cause of acute functional deterioration and may lead to the diagnosis of renal artery stenosis or obstruction if the histologic features of rejection are not sufficient to account for the deterioration in function.

Early Complications

PERSISTENT NONFUNCTION OF RENAL ALLOGRAFT. If the serum creatinine concentration is not falling a month after transplantation, severe rejection, major vessel thrombosis, or nonviability is likely and the graft should be removed, but obstruction to urine flow must always be excluded, and a biopsy is helpful before the graft is removed.

URINARY LEAKAGE. The incidence of urinary leaks leading to fistula formation or obstruction from a urine collection is only about 5 per cent if careful attention is paid to preserving ureteral blood supply and to surgical technique. Early surgical intervention in established urinary fistula reduces the morbidity from infection, although a fistula will usually close spontaneously in eight weeks.

LYMPHOCELE. Interruption of lymph channels during graft insertion may lead to lymph collections around the kidney or to fistula formation. Meticulous attention must be paid to ligation of all visible lymph channels at the time of initial operation. Marsupialization of the lymphocele into the peritoneal cavity may be necessary if leakage persists and collections recur.

URINARY INFECTION. Seventy-five per cent of all patients will have a urinary infection in the first three postoperative months, and in a few it will be recurrent. The patient who has reflux up the transplanted ureter often shows deterioration of function accompanying reflux and is at high risk from septicemia; but in the absence of reflux, infections are easily eradicated by conventional antimicrobial treatment.

VESICOURETERAL REFLUX. Reflux into the transplanted ureter, even in the absence of infection, reduces graft survival. The development of a mesangiocapillary lesion in glomeruli and associated progressive deterioration in renal function shows a high degree of correlation with the presence of vesicoureteral reflux. Segmental scars associated with dilated calyces may also develop in the presence of reflux. These may resemble the scars seen in children with vesicoureteral reflux.

HYPERTENSION. Hypertension may be difficult to control during severe acute rejection, and intravenous diazoxide administration may be necessary, in addition to oral medication with agents such as propranolol, prazosin, hydralazine, and alpha-methyldopa. The majority of successful cadaveric transplants are hypertensive, but control of the blood pressure is easily achieved. An increase in dose requirements or the development of severe hypertension is an indication for renal arteriography to exclude renal artery stenosis. Tight renal artery stenosis occurring just distal to the anastomosis is common, and correction may cure hypertension and improve renal function.

OTHER INFECTIONS. The patient receiving immunosuppressive agents is particularly liable to develop infections, most especially those fungal and viral infections for which man requires an intact T lymphocyte population to ensure an adequate resistance. Cytomegalovirus, herpes simplex and zoster, *Pneumocystis carinii*, *Listeria*, *Nocardia*, actinomycoses, and other unusual infections may be fatal. Most infections can be treated; early diagnosis, a high index of clinical suspicion, and sophisticated microbiologic facilities are essential for optimal results.

Bacteria are more likely to cause serious infection, and death from an overwhelming septicemia can occur within hours.

RESPIRATORY DISTRESS SYNDROME. A syndrome of progressive dyspnea, cyanosis with or without fine crepitations at the lung bases, an alveolar capillary block, and diffuse mottling and opacity on chest x-ray has been described. Progressive hypoxia with death in one to three weeks from presentation is the rule. The

suggestion that this "transplant lung" syndrome is immunologic in origin seems unlikely because pathogenic organisms such as *Pneumocystis carinii* and cytomegalic virus are almost always found, and an identical syndrome is seen in immunosuppressed patients without a renal transplant.

ASEPTIC NECROSIS OF BONE. This disabling complication usually affects the hip joint and may be bilateral. Its incidence correlates with prolonged or high doses of steroids.

OTHER STEROID COMPLICATIONS. Any of the well-recognized complications of steroid therapy such as peptic ulceration, diabetes, and cataract formation may develop after transplantation.

Late Course

The long-term prognosis for patients completing one year with normal or near normal renal function is excellent; however, there is a continuing slow rate of loss of grafted kidneys and mortality. Slow deterioration of renal function may be due to the chronic rejection, recurrence of glomerulonephritis, or other disease. In some patients the kidney is both histologically and functionally normal five or more years after a cadaver graft. Late mortality is predominantly due to degenerative vascular disease affecting coronary and cerebral vessels.

CHRONIC REJECTION. Progressive ischemia of the kidney caused by the vascular lesions affecting small and large vessels, along with glomerular capillary change identical to that seen in mesangiocapillary glomerulonephritis, characterizes chronic rejection. Deterioration of renal function is slow and occurs over several years.

RECURRENT GLOMERULONEPHRITIS. A true recurrence of an identifiable type of glomerulonephritis is unusual but has been described in focal glomerular sclerosis, membranous glomerulonephritis, antiglomerular basement membrane antibody-mediated glomerulonephritis, IgA-IgG glomerulonephritis, "dense deposit" disease, and hypocomplementemic mesangiocapillary glomerulonephritis, including lobular glomerulonephritis. Unless a histologic marker is present, it may be very difficult to separate changes caused by rejection from those of glomerulonephritis, particularly as the change is usually of the mesangiocapillary type. Some degree of mesangiocapillary change always accompanies rejection, and lesions identical with those of mesangiocapillary "recurrent" glomerulonephritis may occur in a patient who had chronic pyelonephritis or some other "nonglomerular" cause of end-stage renal failure. Transplantation is not contraindicated in any form of glomerulonephritis, because the incidence of significant "recurrence" is low in the first five years and deterioration in the function of the affected transplant is often slow. Sometimes the same morphologic lesion which recurs progresses much more slowly in the transplanted kidney than it did when it caused renal failure prior to transplantation.

MALIGNANCY IN THE TRANSPLANT RECIPIENT. There is little doubt that the incidence of malignancy is increased significantly in transplanted patients, presumably as a result of immunosuppression. There is a 5 to 6 per cent chance of a cancer developing within a few years of transplantation. Of reported cases 61 per cent have been epithelial in origin and 39 per cent mesenchymal. Skin, lip, and cervix have been the sites of the most common epithelial tumors, and reticulum cell sarcoma, often of the central nervous system, is the most common mesenchymal tumor. It appears that the risk of cancer is increased by 20 to 40 times. This complication may prove to be a major limiting factor in transplantation.

Treatment

Treatment regimens vary considerably from center to center. Azathioprine and steroids remain the major agents used for immunosuppression, although steroids may be avoided in "identical" sibling grafts, and cyclophosphamide is a reasonable alternative to azathioprine.

ANTILYMPHOCYTE SERA. Despite the experimental evidence of the effectiveness of antilymphocyte serum, its benefit to graft survival in man is less impressive. Controlled trials have shown a statistically significant improvement in survival, but the benefit is usually small. Recent evidence suggests that an antilymphocyte serum which is potent in preventing skin graft loss in primates confers greater benefit in terms of graft survival in man. If further trials confirm this benefit, antilymphocyte serum may become a standard method of treatment following transplantation.

FATE OF SECONDARY TRANSPLANTS. Although earlier results of multiple transplantation, particularly with repeated cadaveric donors, were disappointing, these appear to have improved. Isolated units achieve success rates as high as 75 per cent one-year graft survival, and the latest Australian Transplant Registry data show that there is only a 5 per cent difference between the survival of primary and secondary cadaveric renal transplants. The avoidance of disparate antigens which were present on the first kidney, careful cross-matching using donor spleen or lymph node cells which increase the sensitivity of the test, and an insistence on three or more shared antigens have increased second graft survival. In an integrated program in which home dialysis is available, the time needed to achieve these requirements in a second donor is not a problem. Splenectomy has now been shown in a large series to be ineffective in prolonging the function of a second transplant.

A. L. G. Therapy and Standardization Workshop, Behring Institute Mitteilungen No. 51, September 1972.

Gurland, H. J., Brunner, F. P., Chanther, C., Jacobs, C., Schärer, K., Selwood, N. H., Spies, G., and Wing, A. J.: Combined report on regular dialysis and transplantation in Europe, 1975. In Robinson, B. H. B., Vereerstraeten, P., and Hawkins, J. B. (eds.): Dialysis, Transplantation and Nephrology. Kent, Pitman Medical, 1976.

Kerr, D. N. S.: Provision of services to patients with chronic uremia. Kidney Int., 3:197, 1973.

Kincaid-Smith, P.: The pathogenesis of the vascular and glomerular lesions of renal allografts and their modification by antithrombotic and anticoagulant drugs. Alsian Ann. Med., 19:201, 1970.

Kountz, S. L.: Clinical transplantation — an overview. Transplant. Proc., 5:59, 1973.

Penn, I., and Starzl, T. E.: Immunosuppression and cancer. Transplant. Proc., 5:943, 1973.

Stewart, J. H., Topp, N. D., Martin, S., et al.: The costs of domiciliary maintenance dialysis. Med. J. Aust., 1:156, 1973.

Twelfth report of the Human Renal Transplant Registry. JAMA, 233:787, 1975.

374. GLOMERULAR DISEASE

374.1. INTRODUCTION

O. M. Wrong

Diseases which affect glomeruli display such important features in common that they can usefully be considered together and contrasted with diseases commencing in other parts of the kidney. Numerically, glomerular disease accounts for approximately half of the patients with severe renal disease seen in most communities and over two thirds of the patients accepted for renal displacement by units undertaking intermittent hemodialysis or renal transplantation.

Each glomerulus consists of a complex branching system of capillaries; thus, even though these capillaries are highly specialized, glomerular disease can be regarded as a form of capillary disease. In many forms of glomerular disease small blood vessels in other parts of the body are also diseased, but because the glomerular circulation is particularly vulnerable to pathologic insult the effects of renal damage may dominate the clinical picture. Many glomerular diseases, particularly the inflammations, are the result of antigen-antibody reactions; in others the glomeruli are infiltrated with abnormal deposits, e.g., diabetic renal disease, amyloid, Fabry's disease.

Most forms of glomerular disease are macroscopically diffuse, affecting equally the cortex of both kidneys, and one part of the cortex as severely as another. Consequently the small amount of material which can be removed by percutaneous renal biopsy usually yields a histologic picture which is representative of the kidneys as a whole, and this investigation has been valuable in both diagnosis and study of the natural history of glomerular disease. Histologically glomerular lesions may be *generalized* (i.e., involving all glomeruli), or *focal* (involving only some); within a glomerulus a lesion may be either *diffuse* (affecting the whole glomerulus) or *segmental* (affecting only a portion of the glomerulus). These topographic distinctions are of help in categorizing glomerular disease further.

PROTEINURIA. Increased loss of protein in the urine, in excess of the 30 to 130 mg per day excreted normally, is almost invariable in glomerular disease; it is a direct result of increased glomerular permeability to plasma proteins caused by the disease process. The amount of protein lost in the urine may be much greater than in other forms of renal disease; losses of more than 3 grams per day are rarely seen except in glomerular disease, and this finding therefore has great diagnostic value. The main urinary protein is always albumin, but variable amounts of other plasma proteins are also lost, depending on the type of disease. When urinary protein losses of more than 5 grams a day persist, hepatic synthesis may not be able to increase sufficiently to maintain the serum albumin concentration and hypoalbuminemic edema may result. The triad of proteinuria, hypoalbuminemia, and edema is known as *nephrotic syndrome,* and is discussed in detail in Ch. 374.2.

HYPERTENSION. Hypertension may complicate any form of renal disease, but is particularly common and severe in glomerular disease, although even here it is not invariable. It is now known that renal hypertension has at least two causes: (1) increased secretion of renin by the juxtaglomerular apparatus (JGA), and (2) increased extracellular fluid and blood volume caused by diminished renal ability to excrete salt and water, e.g., the "renoprival" hypertension that follows bilateral nephrectomy. Both factors play a part in the hypertension of glomerular disease, but their relative contributions differ from case to case. The JGA may be directly involved or rendered ischemic by the primary disease, and hypertension may be caused by the resultant hypersecretion of renin. When glomerular disease has resulted in renal failure, hypertension analogous to renoprival hypertension may develop simply from failure to excrete salt and water. The development of severe hypertension in glomerular disease is an ominous sign, as it leads to further damage from the effects of high blood pressure on the renal circulation. Prompt control of hypertension is therefore of vital importance in the care of such patients.

TUBULAR DEFECTS. Evidence of tubular dysfunction occurs early in the clinical course of many types of renal disease, e.g., analgesic nephropathy, polycystic disease, and obstructive uropathy. In such conditions renal acidosis, or renal wasting of sodium or water, may develop when there is still little reduction in glomerular filtration rate. In primary glomerular disease these defects are rarely seen until renal failure develops, with serum creatinine concentrations raised above 3 to 5 mg per 100 ml, and even then marked tubular abnormalities are rare. The acidosis is less severe than occurs in tubular syndromes with similar degrees of renal failure, and is not usually hyperchloremic in type. Urinary concentrating ability is impaired, but the defect is usually an obligatory isosthenuria rather than the hyposthenuria seen in some tubular syndromes. Experiments involving dietary sodium depletion have shown that patients with glomerular disease are often unable to reduce urinary losses of sodium as efficiently as normal subjects, but their obligatory losses are usually well below the amounts supplied by their diet, and it is exceptional for a sodium supplement to be required.

In clinical practice use of the aforementioned principles will usually distinguish glomerular disease from other forms of renal disease. However, it is frequently difficult to distinguish between different forms of glomerular disease, even with the assistance of all modern diagnostic laboratory aids. To some extent this is the result of artificial distinctions between so-called disease entities, which may represent merely groups of commonly associated clinical features, rather than the results of distinct etiologic processes. But the problem is also due to the very limited way in which glomeruli can respond to different pathologic insults, which means that the same histologic and clinical picture may result from several different pathologic processes.

374.2. NEPHROTIC SYNDROME

O. M. Wrong

DEFINITION. In the first half of this century the term *nephrosis*, introduced by Müller in 1905, was widely used in at least two quite different senses: (1) as a descriptive histopathologic term for renal disease without an inflammatory component, and (2) to describe the clinical picture caused by heavy urinary protein losses. Much confusion was caused by this double use, and as a result the word has been largely abandoned. By general agreement the term *nephrotic syndrome* has been adopted for the second of these meanings, and refers to the *clinical association of heavy proteinuria, hypoalbuminemia, and generalized edema*. It is further understood that the plasma albumin concentration is low as a result of urinary albumin loss, and the edema is the result of the altered Starling capillary forces caused by the consequent low plasma oncotic pressure. In general these criteria are not fulfilled unless at least 5 grams of protein a day is lost in the urine at some time in the course of the disease and the plasma albumin concentration is less than 3 grams per 100 ml.

The aforementioned definition does not include reference to renal excretory failure, to hypertension, or to hypercholesterolemia. At various times attempts have been made to include one or another of these features as obligatory items in the definition, particularly hypercholesterolemia. However, the advantages of simplicity are lost if the definition includes features not closely linked causally, such as hypertension and renal failure, or of which the mechanism is uncertain, such as hypercholesterolemia.

ETIOLOGY. The nephrotic syndrome has many causes. Table 1 shows those that have been fully substantiated. The list includes almost all recognized forms of glomerular disease, and *only* forms of glomerular disease, for urinary protein losses in other forms of renal disease are not gross enough to give rise to hypoalbuminemia. (It has sometimes been claimed that pyelonephritis can give rise to the nephrotic syndrome, but the

TABLE 1. Causes of Nephrotic Syndrome

Autoimmune forms of primary glomerular disease (see Table 2, Ch. 374.3)
Glomerular involvement in connective tissue diseases
  Systemic lupus erythematosus
  Polyarteritis
  Anaphylactoid purpura
  Goodpasture's syndrome
  Hemolytic-uremic syndrome
Familial nephritis
Congenital nephrotic syndrome
Glomerular involvement in other systemic diseases
  Quartan malaria
  Schistosomiasis
  Toxoplasmosis
  Secondary syphilis
  Accelerated hypertension
  Diabetic glomerulosclerosis
  Amyloidosis
Mechanical causes
  Renal vein thrombosis
  Constrictive pericarditis
  Obstruction of inferior vena cava
  Sickle cell anemia
Toxins
  Mercury, organic or inorganic
  Gold
  Allergy to pollen, insect bites, snake venom, plant toxins, vaccines
  Serum sickness
Drug hypersensitivity
  Trimethadione and paramethadione, perchlorate, probenecid, penicillamine, sulfonamides, etc.
Miscellaneous
  Toxemia of pregnancy
  Renal transplant

patients referred to have probably had glomerular disease complicated by pyelonephritis). The most important items in Table 1 are separately described in the text; in some of the others the glomerular morphology has not been fully established. There is some overlap between parts of the table; thus the nephrotic syndrome caused by various foreign proteins can be due to a proliferative glomerulonephritis or minimal change disease, and that seen in renal transplants may have either a proliferative or a membranous picture. Drug hypersensitivity may cause nephrotic syndrome as part of an allergic vasculitis (sulfonamides), an immune-complex glomerulonephritis (penicillamine), or minimal change disease (probenecid).

Many of the causes listed give rise to transient nephrotic syndrome which in itself is neither a diagnostic nor a therapeutic problem. Persistent nephrotic syndrome, on the other hand, is a major diagnostic and therapeutic problem to all who deal with renal disease. In Europe and North America about 75 per cent of cases are caused by three idiopathic types of glomerular disease — minimal change disease, membranous disease, and the various types of chronic proliferative glomerulonephritis. The frequency of these three types varies between centers, partly because of variations in classification of cases with mixed membranous and proliferative change, but in most centers miminal change disease causes the majority of cases in children and one fifth to one third of adult cases. The proliferative varieties of glomerulonephritis are slightly more common than membranous disease except in elderly men. The main causes of the disease in the remaining 25 per cent of nephrotics who do not have idiopathic glomerular disease are diabetic glomerulosclerosis, amyloidosis, various forms of focal glomerulonephritis (including lupus erythematosus and anaphylactoid purpura), and renal vein thrombosis.

CLINICAL MANIFESTATIONS. Generalized edema, often accompanied by ascites and pleural effusions, is the sine qua non of the nephrotic syndrome. The edema is primarily due to the reduced plasma oncotic pressure caused by hypoalbuminemia, but numerous other factors, such as salt intake and mineralocorticoid activity, contribute to its development, and because of these there is no predictable relationship between the amount of edema and the level of the plasma albumin. The sequence giving rise to edema is shown in Figure 1. In children gross edema of the face may develop early in the course of the disease, but in adults the legs are usually most affected. In severe cases the weight of the body may be increased by 50 per cent simply from accumulation of edema fluid. Pulmonary edema is unusual unless the glomerular disease causes severe renal excretory failure.

Hypertension is present in some patients, but its presence depends on the type of glomerular disease. The low plasma volume which results from a very low plasma albumin may occasionally cause severe vascular collapse with hypotension. Protein malnutrition caused by the high urinary losses may lead to muscle wasting (often obscured by the generalized edema) or growth retardation in children. Increased opacity of the nails (*leukonychia*) is often present, and occasionally it is possible to estimate how long the nephrotic syndrome has existed by the position of the discolored area.

Urine may be scanty while edema is accumulating, and contains more than 5 grams of protein a day. The

Figure 1. Sequence of main events giving rise to edema in the nephrotic syndrome. The cardinal clinical features of the nephrotic syndrome are shown in capitals.

feature of the urinary deposit and degree of renal impairment depend on the underlying glomerular pathology, but transient renal failure may occur from hypovolemia or tubular damage without implying a destructive glomerular disease. Children with nephrotic syndrome sometimes develop evidence of multiple renal tubular defects, with renal glycosuria, aminoaciduria, and a potassium-losing tendency.

Plasma albumin concentration is invariably reduced below 3.0 grams per 100 ml. The usual value is between 1.0 and 3.0 grams per 100 ml, but occasionally concentrations as low as 0.5 grams per 100 ml are seen; in such cases signs of hypovolemia (particularly postural hypotension) are common, and the edema is often resistant to treatment. The plasma proteins other than albumin may be normal, but electrophoresis often shows a decrease in alpha$_1$ and gamma globulins, and an increase in alpha$_2$ and beta globulins which is mainly due to increases in alpha-glycoprotein and beta lipoprotein. The concentrations of the relatively small molecular weight transferrin and ceruloplasmin are reduced, whereas fibrinogen concentrations are increased.

The other characteristic chemical change in the blood is hyperlipidemia. This involves not only cholesterol, the most easily measured plasma lipid, but all the major lipid components of plasma, including triglycerides and phospholipids. Plasma cholesterol may rise to

1500 mg per 100 ml, but the level of this and of the other lipids varies considerably, even in patients with the same type of nephrotic syndrome. Little prognostic or diagnostic value can be attached to the determination except that marked elevations appear to be less common in lupus erythematosus than in other forms of the nephrotic syndrome. The mechanism of the hyperlipidemia is obscure, but seems intimately linked to the low albumin concentration. Nephrotic hyperlipidemia carries an increased risk of premature generalized atheroma.

DIFFERENTIAL DIAGNOSIS. Two complex investigations, *renal biopsy* and *differential protein clearances*, have proved of great value in establishing the morphologic diagnosis in individual cases. Nephrotic syndrome is now one of the main indications for renal biopsy. The diseases that cause the syndrome are nearly always diffuse, so that needle biopsy yields a representative picture. The procedure is not usually technically difficult unless the kidneys are small, which is unusual. Frequently it is possible to base treatment and prognosis on the histologic findings. This matter is discussed under the various disease headings, and will not be further elaborated here.

The diagnostic value of differential protein clearances was largely established by Squire and his colleagues (for references, see under Minimal Change Glomerular Disease in Ch. 374.3). The principle is that the abnormal glomerulus in nephrotic syndrome permits the passage of increased amounts of protein, and that the selective pattern of this permeability varies in different diseases. Some glomerular diseases permit only the smaller proteins, e.g., albumin and transferrin, to escape in the urine (selective), whereas in others all the plasma proteins are found (nonselective). A crude idea of glomerular permeability can be obtained by electrophoresis of the urine; a highly selective proteinuria consists almost entirely of albumin with small peaks of alpha₁ and gamma globulin, whereas a nonselective proteinuria shows an electrophoretic pattern similar to that of normal plasma. However, electrophoresis is an unsatisfactory method for the study of glomerular selectivity, for the electrical charge and molecular weight of proteins are not closely related, and more satisfactory results can be obtained by measurement of individual proteins. A useful indication of selectivity, suggested by Cameron and Blandford, is the ratio of the clearance of IgG to that of transferrin; in highly selective proteinuria, values below 0.15 are obtained. The major cause of a highly selective proteinuria is minimal change glomerular disease, which carries a good prognosis and usually responds well to steroids. The forms of nephrotic syndrome likely to be confused with this disease, which have a much worse prognosis and do not satisfactorily respond to steroids, i.e., membranous and proliferative glomerular disease, show poor selectivity in their pattern of protein excretion. There appear to be only two exceptions to the general rule that a highly selective proteinuria indicates a good prognosis, and both are uncommon — congenital nephrotic syndrome, a rare disease, and occasional cases of renal amyloidosis.

TREATMENT. Glomerular Lesion. Treatment of the underlying glomerular disease of the common causes of nephrotic syndrome will be discussed under specific glomerular diseases. In general it is unsatisfactory, but exceptions will be mentioned as they arise.

Treatment of the Nephrotic Syndrome. Gross edema carries an appreciable morbidity and mortality, mainly from infection and the effects of immobility, and patients appear to be improved both physically and psychologically when treatment leads to its disappearance. But although the cause of the edema is the low serum albumin, there is no practicable way of increasing plasma albumin while urinary protein losses persist. *High protein diets* have been advocated for years; occasionally they cause a marginal increase in plasma albumin, but usually their only obvious effect is to increase urinary protein losses. Moreover, protein is the most costly item of the diet, and many patients are unable to take a high protein diet because of its expense. *Intravenous protein*, given as salt-poor human albumin, is occasionally of value in the treatment of hospital patients with circulatory collapse caused by hypovolemia, or to initiate diuresis in a patient with refractory edema, but it produces a transitory effect and is impractical for long-term treatment.

The most important factor in treatment is the proper use of *diuretics*. Except in cases of profound hypoalbuminemia, or when the syndrome is complicated by severe renal failure, edema can nearly always be controlled by diuretics alone. The diuretic regimen required varies from patient to patient; in general oral agents are best, and it is wise to start treatment with a relatively gentle drug, such as a thiazide, and only use the more powerful diuretics, e.g., furosemide, bumetanide, and ethacrynic acid, if initial treatment fails to produce diuresis. Potassium deficiency usually arises in patients given diuretics more than three times a week, and should be prevented by the simultaneous administration of potassium supplements or of potassium-sparing diuretics, such as spironolactone or amiloride; however, in renal failure potassium depletion is seldom a problem, and these measures should be avoided as they can precipitate hyperkalemia. Disappearance of edema can be hastened by combining diuretics with a low sodium intake (as low as 20 mEq per day), but this step is not usually necessary except in advanced renal failure.

Modern diuretics are now so efficient that there is no longer a place for local fluid removal by abdominal paracentesis or Southey's tubes, although occasionally benefit may be obtained by aspiration of pleural effusions if these do not disappear rapidly.

When assessing the progress of a patient with nephrotic syndrome, the most useful guides are the presence or absence of edema, body weight, 24-hour urinary proteins, and serum albumin concentrations; decisions regarding changes in treatment can be taken only with this information. Even when there is no effective treatment for the glomerular lesion per se, it is often found that proteinuria varies spontaneously over a wide range, and it may be possible to reduce or stop the use of diuretics as plasma albumin rises to a level at which edema no longer occurs. When diuretics are required, the mistake must not be made of pushing treatment to the point at which the patient suffers severe postural hypotension, and it may be good judgment to allow mild edema to persist, particularly when the serum albumin level is below 1.0 gram per 100 ml.

Nephrotic syndrome is usually a chronic state, and it is wise therefore to encourage patients to follow their normal activities as far as possible. Frequently the physician will be asked about possible risks of pregnancy.

The dangers depend largely on the nature of the underlying renal disease and the risk that because of this the pregnancy will be complicated by hypertension and placental insufficiency. Hypoalbuminemic edema does not per se contraindicate pregnancy (although edema frequently gets temporarily worse during pregnancy), and many women with nephrotic syndrome, particularly that resulting from minimal change glomerular disease, have completely normal pregnancies.

Cameron, J. S., and Blandford, G.: The simple assessment of selectivity in heavy proteinuria. Lancet, 2:242, 1966.

Denison, A. M., Lambie, A. T., Verth, A. H., and Cash, J. D.: Salt-poor human albumin in management of nephrotic syndrome. Br. Med. J., 1:481, 1974.

Edwards, K. D. G.: Antilipaemic drugs and nephrotic hyperlipidaemia. In Edwards, K. D. G. (ed.): Drugs Affecting Kidney Function and Metabolism. Basel, S. Karger, 1972, p. 370.

Robson, J. S.: The nephrotic syndrome. In Black, D. A. K. (ed.): Renal Disease, 3rd ed. Oxford, Blackwell Scientific Publications Ltd., 1972, p. 331.

374.3. GLOMERULONEPHRITIS

O. M. Wrong

DEFINITION. The term "glomerulonephritis" has usually been applied to forms of glomerular disease characterized by an inflammatory reaction, with leukocyte infiltration and cellular proliferation of the glomeruli. However, in recent years it has become clear that most forms of glomerular inflammation are caused by immune injury; this chapter has therefore been expanded to include some types of glomerular disease, e.g., minimal and membranous glomerulopathies, which strictly are not glomerular inflammations at all but also appear to be the results of immune glomerular injury.

ETIOLOGY.   Repeated attempts to isolate microorganisms from the lesions of glomerulonephritis have failed, and these diseases are not considered to be the direct result of bacterial invasion of the kidneys. It is more difficult to exclude the role of viruses, but at present there is no good evidence that any form of human glomerulonephritis is caused by the presence of viruses in the glomeruli.

The detailed pathogenesis of glomerulonephritis is still obscure, but there is considerable evidence that an antigen-antibody reaction plays a major part in initiating the glomerular lesions in most forms of glomerulonephritis. The evidence can be summarized as (1) demonstration by immunofluorescence and electron microscopy of complexes of antigen-antibody and complement either on or within the glomerular basement membrane in many forms of glomerulonephritis; (2) marked lowering of various fractions of serum complement in many cases; (3) experimental production of glomerular lesions resembling human glomerulonephritis by injections either of antikidney antibodies prepared from other species or of nonspecific antigen or antigen-antibody complexes.

Two main types of immune injury appear to be etiologically important in glomerulonephritis. In one of these, antibodies are directed against the glomerular basement membrane (anti-GBM nephritis) which becomes the seat of a reaction involving antigen (GBM), antibody, and complement, leading to polymorphonuclear infiltration, cellular proliferation, and fibrin deposition, with eventual crescent formation and oblitera-

Figure 2.   Linear glomerular deposition of IgG in a patient with Goodpasture's syndrome. (× 1050.) (Courtesy of Dr. D. J. Evans.)

tion of the glomerular space. Antibody (IgG) and complement can be shown by immunofluorescence to be deposited in a fine continuous line along the basement membrane of every capillary loop (Fig. 2). This type of immune injury appears to account for most cases of Goodpasture's syndrome and some cases of rapidly progressive proliferative glomerulonephritis and renal transplant nephritis.

The other and more common type of immune glomerular injury, immune complex disease (ICD), does not involve antibodies directed against renal tissues. The glomeruli are damaged by immune complexes which arise in the circulation from interaction of antibody with antigens of extrarenal origin. These complexes are deposited in the glomeruli in close relation to the basement membrane. Antigen-antibody complexes arising from relative antigen excess are particularly liable to cause glomerular injury, as they are relatively small and are not removed by the reticuloendothelial system as rapidly as larger complexes. Once deposited in the glomeruli, antigen-antibody complexes activate complement, leading to an acute inflammatory reaction, with polymorphonuclear

Figure 3.   Granular glomerular deposition of IgG in a patient with idiopathic membranous disease. (× 1050.) (Courtesy of Dr. D. J. Evans.)

TABLE 2.   Classification of Glomerulonephritis

1. Minimal change glomerular disease
2. Focal glomerulosclerosis
3. Idiopathic membranous glomerular disease
4. Proliferative glomerulonephritis
   a. Acute poststreptococcal glomerulonephritis
   b. Acute glomerulonephritis caused by other infections
   c. Glomerulonephritis in infective endocarditis
   d. Mesangiocapillary glomerulonephritis
   e. Focal glomerulonephritis with recurrent hematuria
   f. Other varieties of proliferative glomerulonephritis
5. Renal involvement in connective tissue diseases

infiltration and fibrin deposition. Immunofluorescent studies show irregular granular staining for gamma globulin and complement along the basement membrane (Fig. 3), a pattern distinct from the smoothly linear deposition seen in anti-GBM disease (Fig. 2). Under the electron microscope complexes appear as electron-dense masses arising from the basement membrane, usually on its epithelial surface. Examples of this type of glomerular disease are lupus nephritis (in which the antigen is DNA), poststreptococcal nephritis (streptococcal antigen), glomerulonephritis with glomerular deposition of Australia antigen, and the nephritis of both quartan malaria and infective endocarditis. However, in most cases of immune complex disease, it has not yet been possible to identify the responsible antigen.

It may eventually prove possible to devise a classification of glomerulonephritis entirely in immunologic terms, but this is not yet practicable. Renal immunology is still in its infancy, and there are many unanswered questions — for example, the role of deficiencies in the immune response of the host, the parts played by complement fixation and cell-mediated immunity, and the importance of damaged renal tissues as antigens promoting a further immunologic reaction. The classification used here (Table 2) is therefore based primarily on clinical and morphologic criteria.

Platelet aggregation in glomerular capillaries and fibrin deposition in the glomerulus and glomerular space occur in inflammatory forms of glomerular disease and potentiate immunologic damage. The presence of fibrin deposition can be suspected from the finding of fibrin degradation products in the urine; when intravascular coagulation is marked, and particularly when the renal disease is part of a generalized small vessel disease, fragmented and distorted red cells may appear in the peripheral blood and occasionally the full picture of a microangiopathic hemolytic anemia, with a lowered platelet count, increased platelet turnover, and reduced plasma fibrinogen concentration.

Logical therapeutic attempts to interrupt the immunologic processes responsible for glomerulonephritis, as well as their immediate consequences, have included cytotoxic drugs, such as the nitrogen mustards, cyclophosphamide, and azathioprine, to reduce antibody formation; plasma exchange to remove immune complexes and antibodies directed against the kidney; corticosteroids or other anti-inflammatory agents to reduce the effects of immune injury on the kidney; and anticoagulants to lessen platelet and fibrin deposition. Such rational forms of therapy have in general proved disappointing; the occasional successes are mentioned when appropriate.

Brain, M. C., Dacie, J. V., and Hourihane, D. O.: Microangiopathic haemolytic anaemia: The possible role of vascular lesions in pathogenesis. Br. J. Haematol., 8:358, 1962.

Germuth, F. G., and Rodriguez, E.: Immune Complex Deposit and Anti-basement Membrane Disease. Boston, Little, Brown & Company, 1973.
McCluskey, R. T.: Immunologic mechanisms in renal disease. *In* Heptinstall, R. H. (ed.): Pathology of the Kidney. 2nd ed. Boston, Little, Brown & Company, 1974, p. 273.
Peters, D. K.: The kidney in allergic disease. *In* Gell, P. G. H., Coombs, R. R. A., and Lachmann, P. J. (eds.): Clinical Aspects of Immunology. 3rd ed. New York, Oxford University Press, 1974, p. 1217.
Wilson, C. B.: Recent advances in the immunological aspects of renal disease. Fed. Proc., 36:2171, 1977.

MINIMAL CHANGE GLOMERULAR DISEASE
(Lipoid Nephrosis)

DEFINITION. This is a glomerular disease causing heavy proteinuria, characterized by absence of obvious histologic glomerular changes on light microscopy.

The term "lipoid nephrosis" was introduced by Munk in 1913, and refers to the presence of fat bodies in the urine and fatty change in the tubular cells. These changes are now known to be the result of a glomerular protein leak, but with the light microscope it is not usually possible to see glomerular abnormalities, and it was not until the advent of the electron microscope that glomerular changes were shown to be invariably present. Hamburger's suggestion that the term "minimal change" should be used to describe the glomerular lesions has been widely followed.

ETIOLOGY, INCIDENCE, AND PATHOLOGY. The frequent association with allergic conditions such as asthma and sensitivity to foreign proteins and the dramatic response induced by steroids have suggested to some that the condition is a form of IgE-mediated immune glomerular injury, but this has not been convincingly demonstrated.

The disease is most common in infancy and childhood, a fact largely responsible for the good prognosis of the nephrotic syndrome in childhood. The peak incidence is between three and four years, but no age is exempt. Males are affected more often than females, in a ratio of 3:2. In adults lymphoma elsewhere in the body, particularly Hodgkin's disease, has sometimes been reported in association with this type of renal disease, but the causal connection between the two conditions has not been explained.

Light microscopy usually shows no glomerular abnormalities, but there may be occasional small areas of glomerular proliferation or adhesions to Bowman's capsule. The tubules usually show protein casts and doubly refractile lipid vacuoles in the cells of the proximal tubule; edema of the interstitium is often present and may cause considerable renal enlargement. The electron microscope invariably shows changes in the glomeruli, consisting of swelling and fusion ("smudging") of the foot processes of the epithelial cells on the outer side of the basement membrane. The basement membrane itself usually has a normal appearance, but sometimes contains small vacuoles or shows irregular thickening.

Until recently the view was widely held that this form of renal disease represented an early form of glomerulonephritis which would eventually show destructive glomerular changes. This view is no longer tenable; serial renal biopsies have shown that the glomerular lesions do not usually progress; indeed, they disappear after a spontaneous or steroid-induced clinical remission. The few patients who do not remit appear to have a different condition to start with — either an early form of membranous glomerulopathy, which should be detected by electron microscopy, or focal glomerular sclerosis (described subsequently) which usually produces a nonselective proteinuria.

Despite the absence of gross changes in the basement membrane on light microscopy, it is likely that the protein leak is the result of change in the basement membrane itself. The change in the foot process is probably caused by the presence of protein within Bowman's space, for identical appearance can be produced in animals by intravenous injection of proteins which cross the glomerular filter. This histologic appearance is also a feature of other forms of glomerular disease with heavy proteinuria, and is in no way specific for minimal change glomerular disease, although here it is the only constant glomerular finding.

The permeability characteristics of the glomerulus in this disease have been well worked out (Squire, Blainey, Hardwicke, and Soothill). The urinary proteins consist almost entirely of the plasma proteins of lower molecular weight, particularly albumin (molecular weight 68,000) and transferrin (90,000), whereas plasma proteins of larger size, such as beta-lipoprotein (molecular weight up to 2,500,000) are almost completely absent. The same pattern of glomerular permeability can be demonstrated after intravenous injection of dextrans of different molecular sizes, when only the smaller molecules are found in the urine. The glomerular protein leak is thus highly selective, whereas in almost all other forms of glomerular disease the leak is nonselective, or poorly selective, in that plasma proteins of every molecular size are found in the urine.

CLINICAL MANIFESTATIONS. The most common first symptom is edema, which develops insidiously and often reaches mammoth proportions. Examination at this stage reveals all the characteristics of the nephrotic syndrome: heavy proteinuria (more than 5 grams per day), hypoalbuminemia, and usually hypercholesterolemia. The urine sediment contains hyaline, granular and fatty casts, and occasional red cells; red cell casts are not found. The plasma urea and creatinine concentrations are usually normal; however, azotemia is not uncommon in the early stages of the disease, and rarely transitory oliguric renal failure develops — perhaps the result of hypovolemia or obstruction of tubules by protein casts.

The disease has a remarkable tendency to remit. This may take place spontaneously, may follow systemic infections such as measles, or may result from treatment with steroids or cytotoxic drugs. Remissions are usually complete, with disappearance of all signs, but partial remissions with continuing mild proteinuria are also common. Relapses are unfortunately frequent, and may exactly replicate the initial attack. Repeated relapses may occur over a period of many years (over 20 years in one case personally known to the author) without deterioration in renal excretory function or the appearance of destructive changes in the glomeruli.

TREATMENT. The chief hazard lies in the complications of edema, particularly infection, which have been greatly reduced by modern diuretics and antimicrobial drugs. Before the advent of penicillin, pneumococcal peritonitis was a common cause of death, but this is now very rare. Treatment of edema is discussed in connection with the nephrotic syndrome. Two other hazards of the disease require mention. Hypogammaglobu-

linemia, owing partly to reduced synthesis and partly to urinary losses of gamma globulin, itself carries a risk of infection; hypercholesterolemia, as in other forms of nephrotic syndrome, may eventually lead to early atheroma and a predisposition to arterial thrombosis.

This is one of the very few forms of glomerular disease in which the underlying glomerular fault can be remedied by treatment. When given steroids or corticotropin (ACTH), most patients rapidly lose their proteinuria and all other signs, usually within two to six weeks of the start of treatment. Serial renal biopsies have shown that the glomerular foot processes simultaneously return to normal. It is not known how adrenal steroids exert this remarkable effect, and the dose required varies from case to case, usually being in the range of 20 to 60 mg of prednisolone, or equivalent, daily. Relapses often follow withdrawal of steroids, even when the dose has been reduced very gradually.

Treatment with steroids should not be lightly undertaken. It must be realized that this is the only form of nephrotic syndrome which shows a satisfactory response at all frequently, and that this treatment has definite dangers. The diagnosis should not rest on clinical manifestations alone, but should be based on the appearances of renal biopsy and on the finding of a highly selective proteinuria. In children, in whom high doses of steroids are less dangerous, and in whom most cases of nephrotic syndrome are caused by this process, it is justifiable to commence steroids without the evidence of renal biopsy or protein clearances, provided that treatment is gradually withdrawn if no effect is seen within six weeks. Conversely, in a few elderly patients, even those who have been shown by renal biopsy to have the disease, the risks of long-continued steroids, particularly peptic ulcer, may be greater than the risks of nephrotic syndrome, provided that edema can be satisfactorily controlled.

Once a decision is made to employ steroid treatment, it is wise to begin with a high dose, e.g., 60 to 80 mg of prednisolone per day in an adult, or 40 to 60 mg in a child. This should be maintained for three to six weeks and then reduced to a maintenance dose of one half to two thirds the original dose if a satisfactory response (disappearance or marked lessening of proteinuria) occurs; if not, the treatment should be gradually withdrawn. Maintenance treatment should be continued for three to six months; then periodic attempts can be made to reduce dosage further or stop altogether; if clinical relapse occurs, it will be necessary to increase the dose temporarily.

Troublesome side effects of steroids are common, but there is some evidence that they can be prevented or lessened by giving steroids on alternate days, without loss of therapeutic effect. It is unwise to regard complete abolition of proteinuria as the sole aim of treatment, for in some cases this requires an unacceptably high dose of steroids, whereas a much smaller dose will sufficiently lessen proteinuria to return the plasma albumin level to normal and so remove the risk of edema.

The most difficult patients to treat are those who become steroid dependent, relapsing as soon as the dosage is reduced or after intercurrent infections, yet developing severe side effects of steroid overdose. These patients are usually children, in whom retardation of growth is the most troublesome complication. In such cases ACTH may be preferable to steroids, because there is evidence that it has less effect in retarding growth. Alternatively, prolonged remission may be obtained by the use of cytotoxic drugs, of which cyclophosphamide and chlorambucil have been the most successful; because of the long-term risks of these drugs (particularly sterility and neoplasia), they should be reserved for patients whose disease cannot be controlled by steroids without unacceptable steroid toxicity, and whose nephrotic edema cannot be kept in reasonable bounds by diuretics.

Barratt, T. M., and Soothill, J. F.: Controlled trial of cyclophosphamide in steroid-sensitive relapsing nephrotic syndrome of childhood. Lancet, 2:479, 1970.

Black, D. A. K., Rose, G., and Brewer, D. B.: Controlled trial of prednisone in adult patients with the nephrotic syndrome. Br. Med. J., 3:421, 1970.

Connolly, M. E., Wrong, O. M., and Jones, N. F.: Reversible renal failure in idiopathic nephrotic syndrome with minimal glomerular changes. Lancet, 1:665, 1968.

Farquhar, M.: Ultrastructure of the nephron disclosed by electron microscopy. A review of normal and pathologic glomerular ultrastructure. In Metcoff, J. (ed.): Proceedings, 10th Annual Conference on the Nephrotic Syndrome. New York, National Kidney Disease Foundation, 1959, p. 2.

Hardwicke, J., and Soothill, J. F.: Proteinuria. In Black, D. A. K. (ed.): Renal Disease. 2nd ed. Oxford, Blackwell Scientific Publications, Ltd., 1967, p. 252.

Squire, J. R., Blainey, J. D., and Hardwicke, J.: The nephrotic syndrome. Br. Med. Bull., 13:43, 1957.

FOCAL GLOMERULOSCLEROSIS
(Segmental Hyalinosis)

DEFINITION AND PATHOLOGY. This form of glomerular disease is characterized by focal and segmental areas of glomerular sclerosis, usually commencing in the juxtamedullary glomeruli and gradually spreading to involve other parts of the kidney, with eventual renal failure. The condition has only recently been demarcated from other varieties of glomerulonephritis. The cause is obscure, but affected glomeruli have been shown to contain deposits of complement and gamma globulin. There is evidence that patients treated by renal transplantation may develop the disease in the transplanted kidney.

INCIDENCE AND CLINICAL COURSE. The incidence of the disease is unknown, for it is still frequently confused with minimal change glomerular disease, benign recurrent hematuria, and various other types of proliferative glomerulonephritis. It most commonly presents in children or adolescents, with nonselective proteinuria, often gross enough to cause nephrotic syndrome, or recurrent macroscopic hematuria. Renal biopsy may not sample the affected glomeruli, thus giving rise to a false diagnosis of minimal change glomerular disease. No treatment is known to definitely alter the course of the disease, but the progression to renal failure usually takes many years.

Churg, J., Habib, R., and White, R. H. R.: Pathology of the nephrotic syndrome in children. Lancet, 1:1299, 1970.

Newman, W. J., Tisher, C. C., McCoy, R. C., Gunnells, J. C., Kreuger, R. P., Clapp, J. R., and Robinson, R. R.: Focal glomerular sclerosis: Contrasting clinical patterns in children and adults. Medicine, 55:67, 1976.

IDIOPATHIC MEMBRANOUS GLOMERULAR DISEASE
(Epimembranous Nephritis)

DEFINITION. This is a glomerular disease of obscure cause, characterized by thickening of the capillary basement membrane, without cellular infiltration. The condition is often called "membranous glomerulonephritis," but this term is inappropriate inasmuch as there is no histologic evidence of glomerular inflammation.

ETIOLOGY, INCIDENCE, AND PATHOLOGY. The finding of granular deposits of IgG and complement on the thickened basement membrane has led to the suggestion that it is a form of immune-complex disease.

The disease affects all ages, but is most common in adults; males are affected more often than females, particularly in middle age and later life.

Histologically it can be recognized with the light microscope by a more or less uniform thickening of the capillary basement membrane of every glomerulus. This is often obvious in sections stained with hematoxylin and eosin, but is particularly apparent in thin sections (less than $2\ \mu$) stained with periodic acid–methenamine–silver. The thickening may be so marked that the capillary lumen is reduced in caliber or obliterated, but there is no increase in glomerular cellularity. Under the electron microscope the basement membrane is thickened, vacuolated, and irregular; arising from its epithelial side, under the fused foot processes of the epithelial cells, are electron-dense granules which can be shown by immunofluorescence (Fig. 3) to contain IgG and complement. These findings are very similar to those in some forms of proliferative glomerulonephritis, except for the absence of a cellular reaction, and the suggestion has been made that this is a similar type of immune-complex disease, but without involvement of cell-mediated immunity.

An association of membranous glomerular disease with malignancy arising outside the kidneys (especially bronchus and gut) has been reported, suggesting that in these cases the renal disease is caused by immune complexes of host antibody and tumor antigen.

The membranous form of glomerular disease is generally believed to be distinct from other forms, not merely a stage in the evolution of another process. This view is supported by serial renal biopsies, which have shown a worsening in the glomerular alterations with time but no real change in nature.

CLINICAL MANIFESTATIONS. Membranous glomerular disease usually presents with nephrotic syndrome, less often with asymptomatic proteinuria, renal hypertension, or chronic renal failure. All features of the nephrotic syndrome may be found, but the condition may be distinguished from minimal change glomerular disease by higher average age of patients, frequent presence of hypertension and renal failure, nonselective nature of the proteinuria, and rarity of clinical remission.

The disease runs a slowly progressive course; usually many years elapse before renal failure is a serious problem. Very occasionally a fulminant course is followed, oliguric renal failure developing within a few months of onset. No treatment is known to alter the course of the disease. Spontaneous clinical remissions do occur, and in about 25 per cent of patients they are complete and longlasting. When the disease is associated with carcinoma, remission may follow successful removal of the tumor.

Row, P. G., Cameron, J. S., Turner, D. R., Evans, D. J., White, R. H. R., Ogg, C. S., Chantler, C., and Brown, C. B.: Membranous nephropathy. Quart. J. Med., 44:207, 1975.

PROLIFERATIVE GLOMERULONEPHRITIS

DEFINITION. This term strictly covers all diseases in which cellular proliferation affects the glomeruli, but is most conveniently restricted to those in which renal involvement is not part of the vasculitis of a systemic disease such as lupus erythematosus.

ETIOLOGY. Until quite recently it was widely believed that most cases were poststreptococcal in origin. This view is now clearly recognized as incorrect; it is difficult to know the true proportion, but in adults less than 25 per cent appear to have disease of this cause.

The group is heterogeneous, but immune renal injury probably plays a part in all forms. Some cases of rapidly progressive disease show linear deposition of IgG and complement in the glomeruli, and are probably examples of anti-GBM nephritis. Immune-complex injury appears to be responsible for poststreptococcal nephritis, the nephritis caused by other acute infections and infective endocarditis, and that caused by chronic quartan malaria. In many other cases the immunofluorescent findings are those of immune-complex disease, but the nature of the antigen is unknown. Often patients come to medical attention late in the course of their disease, when evidence of the original immune glomerular injury can no longer be found.

Acute Poststreptococcal Glomerulonephritis

This is the best documented and most understood form of proliferative glomerulonephritis. Although its course is complex and variable, it does demonstrate almost all the possible features of glomerular disease, and therefore has served in the past as the usual starting point and reference in discussing glomerulonephritis. To some extent this emphasis has been unfortunate in that it has tended to delay recognition of the many forms of glomerulonephritis which are unrelated to the *Streptococcus* and are now becoming relatively more important because of the falling incidence of streptococcal infection. However, the disease is still common enough to deserve emphasis in its own right.

ETIOLOGY. In 1836 Richard Bright recognized that acute glomerulonephritis usually followed an infection, particularly scarlet fever. Since then scarlet fever has become much less common, and the incidence of postscarlatina nephritis has likewise fallen. It is now recognized that acute nephritis can follow streptococcal infection in any part of the body, although the pharynx is the usual site, and is unrelated to the production of erythrotoxin by the organism. Only certain strains of *Streptococcus* are "nephritogenic" (capable of initiating nephritis); all the offending organisms are Group A hemolytic streptococci, and the majority are of Type 12. Other less common nephritogenic strains are Types 1, 4, 25, 41, 49 (Red Lake strain), and 57; the last two have been incriminated in outbreaks of streptococcal pyoderma causing nephritis.

Symptoms of acute glomerulonephritis do not usually develop until 7 to 20 days after the streptococcal infection, by which time the patient appears to have recovered from the local infection. Transitory mild proteinuria and microscopic hematuria are common during the initial streptococcal infection, particularly in persons who subsequently develop clinical nephritis, but it is not clear whether these are the first manifestations of

nephritis or merely represent the urinary changes common in any severe infection.

Coincident with the development of nephritis there is a marked reduction in serum complement, apparently caused by its deposition in the kidney. Immunofluorescent studies during the acute stage of the disease show irregular staining for complement and gamma globulin, particularly IgG, within the glomeruli, and electron microscopy reveals electron-dense deposits, corresponding to this immunofluorescence, on the epithelial side of the glomerular basement membrane. These findings indicate that the disease is an immune-complex form of renal injury, but it is not known why only certain strains of streptococci can provide the necessary antigenic stimulus. Antigenic similarities between the glomerular basement membrane and *Streptococcus* have been demonstrated, but the weight of evidence is against this being a form of anti-GBM nephritis.

INCIDENCE. Acute poststreptococcal nephritis occurs in all parts of the world. Males are affected about twice as frequently as females. No age is exempt, but the disease is particularly common in children and adolescents, perhaps because of the increased risk of acquiring a streptococcal infection from exposure at school. In temperate climates it is most common in winter, when streptococcal infections are at their peak. The relationship of acute nephritis to certain streptococcal strains explains some epidemiologic features of the disease, such as its tendency to cause small epidemics in homes or schools, as well as the variations in incidence in persons known to have had streptococcal infections —from nil with a non-nephritogenic strain to as high as 40 per cent with a strain known to be nephritogenic. By contrast the incidence of rheumatic fever in those with streptococcal infections who have not previously had the disease is fairly constant at 2 to 3 per cent.

PATHOLOGY. The disease is rarely fatal, and most knowledge of its pathology comes from material obtained by biopsy. The occasional necropsy has shown symmetrical renal enlargement and pallor of the cortex. Histologically the glomeruli are nearly all similarly affected, with enlargement of the whole glomerulus and marked increase in the number of nucleated cells, consisting mainly of endothelial and mesangial cells and mononuclear leukocytes, although polymorphonuclears may also be found. Epithelial cell proliferation is usually not prominent. The glomerular lobules are swollen and relatively bloodless, with reduced capillary lumina and occasional necrotic and thrombosed capillary loops. The transitory renal failure of the acute phase of the disease is the result of these changes, rather than obliteration of Bowman's space by epithelial crescents.

During resolution the last feature to remain is hypercellularity, most marked in the vicinity of the glomerular stalk or mesangium, which may be detectable several months after apparently complete clinical recovery. This change, though typical of resolving poststreptococcal glomerulonephritis, does occur in some other forms of proliferative glomerulonephritis, and its presence cannot be regarded as conclusive evidence of an earlier poststreptococcal disease.

CLINICAL MANIFESTATIONS. Most patients have a fairly clear history of preceding streptococcal infection. Usually it is a pharyngitis which has been sufficiently severe to keep the patient away from school or work, but occasionally the infection lies elsewhere — for example, an otitis media, a leg ulcer, or a surgical wound. Sometimes the infection can only be demonstrated by a positive bacteriologic culture, or presumed from the finding of a raised antistreptolysin O titer.

The patient has usually recovered from the initial infection when manifestations of nephritis appear, some 7 to 20 days after onset of the original infection. The most common presenting symptom is *edema*, noted particularly in the face on first arising. *Hematuria* is also a common first symptom; usually the urine has a smoky brown color, but occasionally it is frankly blood stained. Less commonly the patient complains of *reduced urine output*, or of bilateral dull *loin pain*, which is probably caused by stretching of the renal capsules.

It is important to note that the edema present at the onset of the disease is invariably caused by fluid retention, which itself is the result of reduced renal excretion of salt and water. In an adult of average size the presence of generalized edema implies a weight gain of at least 5 kg. At this stage patients have not lost enough protein in the urine to develop hypoalbuminemic edema (nephrotic syndrome), although this complication may develop later; nor is there good evidence for the earlier views that the edema of acute nephritis is caused either by increased capillary permeability or by heart failure.

Vague *malaise, nausea,* and *headache* are common in acute nephritis, but fever is unusual, and patients do not usually feel really ill, although often distressed by the appearance of edema. In mild cases they may be quite asymptomatic; the disease may be picked up only by examining the urine of a person known to have had a recent streptococcal infection.

Physical examination usually shows generalized edema and mild hypertension of the order of 140 to 160 systolic, 90 to 110 diastolic. Very occasionally hypertension is severe, with retinal hemorrhages and exudates, papilledema, or hypertensive encephalopathy. In general, the degree of hypertension is in proportion to the amount of edema. Fluid retention, if marked, may lead to the signs of congestive cardiac failure, with cardiac enlargement and triple rhythm, venous engorgement, hepatic distention, and gross pulmonary and systemic edema.

Urinary output is usually reduced, although the reduction is often not noticed by the patient. Complete suppression of urine is rare, and indicates a very severe attack of nephritis; this complication may develop within a few days of the onset, or urinary output may gradually fall to nothing over several weeks. As might be expected, fluid retention is particularly severe in such cases, and unless rigid restriction of sodium and water has been instituted, edema and hypertension are particularly marked.

URINE. Urinary concentration is usually in the range of 350 to 600 mOsm per kilogram (corresponding to a specific gravity of 1.010 to 1.017) when correction is made for a protein content, but appears more concentrated because of the presence of red cells. Moderate quantities of protein are present, and occasionally mild renal glycosuria occurs. The urinary sediment contains large numbers of red cells and leukocytes, particularly the former, and a smaller number of renal tubular cells. Casts, particularly the granular variety, are also present; erythrocyte and hemoglobin casts indicate bleeding from the glomerulus and are particularly helpful in diagnosis.

LABORATORY TESTS. Mild renal failure, with plasma creatinine values of 1.5 to 4.0 mg per 100 ml, is very common in the initial stage of the disease. In the rare case of severe renal failure, the biochemical sequelae are similar to those of renal failure from other causes except that hyperkalemia seems particularly common, probably because these patients are usually previously fit and active young people who rapidly lose muscle mass during their illness.

A nephritogenic strain of *Streptococcus* can be cultured from the pharynx of many patients, except those treated with effective antimicrobial drugs, even when all clinical evidence of local infection has disappeared. Occasionally cultures taken from the throats of other members of the family will reveal the presence of a nephritogenic organism when this can no longer be cultured from the patient's own throat.

The serum antistreptolysin O titer is usually raised, indicating recent streptococcal infection, but the titer may fall rapidly to normal and so pass unnoticed, or it may not rise at all if the streptococcal infection is rapidly aborted by the use of antimicrobials. Unfortunately, as has been pointed out by Rammelkamp, not all nephritogenic strains of streptococci produce streptolysin O (nor do they invariably cause beta-hemolysis in culture), and so detection of the preceding streptococcal infection by this means may be difficult. The serum titer of type-specific antibody to streptococcal M antigen is more difficult to measure, but remains raised for considerably longer after a streptococcal infection (often for years), and has the added advantage of indicating whether an infection was caused by a strain known to be nephritogenic. A marked drop in serum complement is characteristic of acute poststreptococcal nephritis, but this finding is not diagnostic because it may occur in other forms of nephritis, e.g., systemic lupus erythematosus and the nephritis of bacterial endocarditis.

The erythrocyte sedimentation rate is moderately raised. The hemoglobin concentration is usually slightly reduced (to 11 to 12 grams per 100 ml) as a result of dilution.

COURSE AND PROGNOSIS. Diuresis usually starts 7 to 14 days after the onset of symptoms, and over the space of two days the patient loses edema and hypertension. Renal clearances and the plasma creatinine concentration return to normal, but microscopic hematuria and proteinuria persist longer, and may not disappear for weeks or months. During this period clinical relapses may occur, particularly at the time of other respiratory infections.

Occasionally urinary losses of protein during the first few weeks are sufficiently large to cause hypoalbuminemic edema, which at first reveals itself when renal excretory function improves and the expected diuresis does not materialize. Although the development of nephrotic syndrome is of grave import if it first appears after several months, its rapid appearance at this early stage of the disease does not necessarily carry a bad prognosis, and patients with this syndrome may recover completely within the next few weeks.

It is difficult to ascertain what proportion of patients recover completely, for hospital series are weighted by the more severe cases. Most estimates state that over 90 per cent of children and about 60 per cent of adults eventually make a full clinical recovery. These figures may be unduly pessimistic, because many of the published series have included patients, who, with the benefit of more recent advances of glomerular immunofluorescence and electron microscopy, might not now be classified as having poststreptococcal nephritis.

In the early years of this century, poststreptococcal nephritis in the acute stage caused death in about 5 per cent of patients. Death was usually due to pulmonary edema, the complications of hypertension, or intercurrent infections. Nowadays these complications can usually be prevented and most fatalities are the result of acute renal failure with anuria or severe oliguria. Patients can be kept alive by peritoneal dialysis or hemodialysis, and many so treated, particularly children, experience return of renal function after days or weeks. If renal recovery does not ensue or is inadequate to maintain life, and renal biopsy shows irrecoverable glomerular damage, they may be treated by intermittent hemodialysis or renal transplantation.

Unfavorable features which suggest that satisfactory recovery will not take place are (1) delayed or absent diuresis; (2) persistent renal failure; (3) persistent hypertension; (4) prolonged or increasing proteinuria, often leading to nephrotic syndrome; (5) a persistently lowered plasma complement; and (6) severe changes in the renal biopsy, particularly obliteration of Bowman's space by epithelial crescents and disappearance of glomerular capillaries.

Patients who recover from acute glomerulonephritis are not immune to second attacks, but these are uncommon because of the development of type-specific antibodies which protect against infection by the original strain of *Streptococcus* and exert an effect for many years. Some apparent second attacks of acute poststreptococcal glomerulonephritis are in reality exacerbations of a longstanding chronic glomerulonephritis.

DIFFERENTIAL DIAGNOSIS. The condition most easily confused with acute poststreptococcal nephritis is exacerbation of a subacute or chronic glomerulonephritis, with transitory hematuria and further reduction in renal function. Such exacerbations may be precipitated by many different infections, even those caused by viruses, but are particularly common after streptococcal infections; in the absence of previous evidence of renal disease, this situation closely resembles an initial attack of poststreptococcal nephritis. This diagnostic problem is now infrequent, probably because of the declining incidence of streptococcal infections.

The transient proteinuria and microscopic hematuria that accompany many severe systemic infections may also be mistaken for poststreptococcal nephritis, but these signs occur at the height of the infection and are not usually associated with other features of renal disease.

It may be difficult to distinguish acute poststreptococcal nephritis from other forms of acute glomerulonephritis, such as Henoch-Schönlein nephritis (which may also be precipitated by a streptococcal infection), systemic lupus erythematosus, the microscopic form of polyarteritis nodosa, recurrent focal nephritis with hematuria, and the nephritis of bacterial endocarditis. Here the physician will be guided by features suggesting systemic involvement and by evidence of recent streptococcal infection. Renal biopsy may also help by showing a glomerular lesion more focal than that of poststreptococcal nephritis.

Less often, acute poststreptococcal nephritis may be confused with primary malignant hypertension, with various forms of hemolytic anemia with hemoglobinuria, or with acute tubular necrosis, particularly when the latter is precipitated by a systemic infection.

TREATMENT. It has not been convincingly shown that any form of treatment alters the course of the glomerular lesion, but individual manifestations and complications frequently require treatment.

Infection. In the acute stage of nephritis, penicillin is usually given either by mouth or by injection to eradicate any remaining streptococcal infection. This treatment has much to commend it, but there is no evidence that it alters the subsequent evolution of the glomerular disease. Penicillin should also be used prophylactically to treat close contacts, particularly members of the family who may have contracted streptococcal infection from the patient, unless this possibility is excluded by bacteriologic tests. Oral penicillin V (phenoxymethyl penicillin, 250 mg twice a day) is often recommended after attacks of acute nephritis to reduce subsequent respiratory infections which might cause exacerbations of nephritis; it is best continued through the next winter season when streptococcal infections are more widespread. (The question of prophylaxis against streptococcal infections is further discussed in Ch. 129.)

Edema. Fluid retention during the oliguric phase of the disease should be prevented by careful attention to body weight. Salt and fluids should be restricted if edema is present or a weight gain of more than 2 to 3 kg occurs. In these circumstances oral fluids should be limited to no more than 500 ml per day, plus a volume equal to the urine output of the previous day, and dietary sodium should be reduced as far as possible, preferably to 20 mEq per day. If severe edema is already present, or develops despite these measures, a diuresis may occasionally be obtained by oral diuretics, particularly furosemide in doses of 40 to 1000 mg twice a day. Digitalis is ineffective, despite the presence of many classic features of congestive cardiac failure, because the circulatory troubles are due to excess of extracellular fluid, and not to a primary cardiac cause. In the rare case in which fluid overload threatens life and diuresis cannot be obtained by drugs, the excess fluid should be removed by dialysis.

Uremia. There is no convincing evidence that dietary protein influences the course of the glomerular lesion, but early in the disease it is wise to restrict protein intake moderately (40 to 70 grams per day) until it is clear that the patient is not likely to develop renal failure. Patients who do develop severe renal failure should be treated by more drastic protein restriction, with or without some form of dialysis, as described in Ch. 373.2.

Hypertension. If fluid retention is carefully controlled, there is usually no need to treat hypertension specifically. But the patient with severe fluid overload may require treatment for hypertensive encephalopathy with convulsions, or retinopathy with failing vision; in these emergencies parenteral hydralazine, reserpine, or diazoxide is the drug of choice.

Other Drugs. Steroids, anticoagulants, and cytotoxic drugs, either alone or in various combinations, have been used in the acute stage of the disease, particularly in patients with severe renal failure, but there is no good evidence that they alter the outcome.

Rest. In the acute stage of the disease bed rest is

advisable. The patient does not usually wish to be active, and the recumbent position facilitates diuresis. Once macroscopic hematuria, edema, and hypertension have disappeared and the plasma creatinine has returned to normal, the value of rest is uncertain. Many authorities recommend that bed rest continue as long as proteinuria is diminishing, but there is no evidence that this alters the course of the disease, and it may be impractical or economically disastrous for the patient whose proteinuria persists for months.

Continued Observation. Because of the difficulty in deciding when a patient has recovered from the disease, it is valuable to follow all patients until at least a year after the last clinical evidence of nephritis. Frequent determinations of blood pressure, urinary proteins and sediment, and plasma creatinine and creatinine clearances are the most useful indications of disease activity. The purpose of this follow-up is to observe any exacerbation of the disease, so that renal failure, nephrotic syndrome, or hypertension can be immediately recognized and treated. Acute urinary infections, which are not uncommon in such patients, can also be recognized and treated.

Bright, R.: In Osman, A. A. (ed.): Original Papers of Richard Bright on Renal Disease. London, Oxford University Press, 1937.

Dodge, W. F., Spargo, B. H., Travis, L. B., Srivastava, R. N., Carvajal, H. F., Debeukelaer, M. M., Longley, M. P., and Menchaca, J. A.: Poststreptococcal nephritis. A prospective study in children. N. Engl. J. Med., 286:273, 1972.

Heptinstall, R. H.: Pathology of acute glomerulonephritis. In Strauss, M. B., and Welt, L. G. (eds.): Diseases of the Kidney. 3rd ed. Boston, Little, Brown & Company, 1971, p. 405.

Levy, J. E., Salinas-Madrigal, L., Herdson, P. B., Pirani, C. L., and Metcoff, J.: Clinico-pathologic correlations in acute poststreptococcal glomerulonephritis. Medicine, 50:453, 1972.

Rammelkamp, C. H., and Earle, D. P.: Pathogenesis of chronic glomerulonephritis. In Ingelfinger, F. J., Relman, A. S., and Finland, M.: Controversy in Internal Medicine. Philadelphia, W. B. Saunders Company, 1966, p. 331.

Schwartz, W. B., and Kassirer, J. P.: Clinical aspects of acute poststreptococcal glomerulonephritis. In Strauss, M. B., and Welt, L. G. (eds.): Diseases of the Kidney. 3rd ed. Boston, Little, Brown & Company, 1971, p. 419.

Zabriskie, V., Utermohlen, V., Read, S. E., and Fischetti, V. A.: Streptococcus-related glomerulonephritis. Kidney Int., 3:100, 1973.

Acute Glomerulonephritis Caused by Other Infections

Frequently patients with acute glomerulonephritis show no evidence of a preceding streptococcal infection, even though in almost every other way their disease is typical of poststreptococcal nephritis. It is impossible to be sure that any patient has not had a streptococcal infection, and probably many of these patients have had an infection which cannot be detected in retrospect. However, it is now recognized that an acute glomerulonephritis may follow infections caused by microorganisms other than streptococci. It seems likely, from a consideration of the pathogenesis, that an acute immune complex type of nephritis in humans may, like the experimental model, be precipitated by exposure to a variety of foreign proteins, which need not be exclusively of infective origin.

When pneumococcal pneumonia was a common disease, before the advent of antimicrobial drugs, it was frequently reported to be a cause of acute glomerulonephritis. The disease was similar to the poststreptococcal variety, except that the latent interval was shorter and fluid retention and hypertension were less apparent. In most instances the possibility of a complicating strepto-

coccal infection was not adequately excluded, and there must be doubt as to the existence of such an entity.

Acute glomerulonephritis has also been reported after typhoid fever and diphtheria and after many virus infections such as mumps, measles, chickenpox, infective hepatitis, mononucleosis, and infections with echovirus and adenovirus. Although in many instances a complicating streptococcal infection has not been excluded, the number of these reports is so great that it is difficult to accept that they all represent cases of poststreptococcal nephritis. In several recent cases a renal biopsy has been obtained or the patient has come to necropsy, and glomerular changes very similar to those of poststreptococcal nephritis have been found.

The concept of an acute diffuse glomerulonephritis which results from nonstreptococcal infections has thus been established, but it should be emphasized that nephritis is much rarer after these infections than it is after infections with nephritogenic strains of group A streptococci.

The natural history of glomerulonephritis caused by other than streptococcal infections is not fully known. The disease appears to behave like poststreptococcal nephritis in that the majority of patients recover completely, but a few are left with a continuing process with progressive impairment of renal function, which may be complicated by nephrotic syndrome or severe hypertension.

Glomerulonephritis in Infective Endocarditis

The subacute glomerulonephritis that complicates endocarditis has often been regarded simply as a form of acute glomerulonephritis caused by streptococcal infection. This view is misleading for several reasons: (1) The viridans streptococci do not cause nephritis when they invade other parts of the body; (2) it has been increasingly realized, perhaps because of longer survival, that patients with other forms of infective endocarditis (e.g., pneumococcal, H. influenzae, and fungal) also develop glomerulonephritis. The usual alternative hypothesis, that the disease is caused by bacterial embolization to the glomeruli, would explain the focal type of glomerulonephritis which is sometimes seen, but not the more usual diffuse glomerulonephritis nor the fact that bacteria cannot be demonstrated in the glomeruli. Recent immunofluorescent and electron microscope studies have shown granular deposits of IgG and complement, and more rarely fibrin, in the glomeruli of patients with diffuse glomerulonephritis associated with endocarditis caused by a variety of organisms, findings strongly suggesting immune-complex disease.

Patients with infective endocarditis do not usually show evidence of glomerulonephritis until they have had infection for several weeks. The condition presents with hematuria and proteinuria, and less frequently with impairment of renal function, which is often first mistakenly attributed to severe cardiac failure and resulting reduced renal perfusion. Hypoalbuminemic edema and hypertension have not been features of most reports. Severe renal failure is seldom seen except in patients in the terminal stages of a prolonged endocarditis.

In most cases the diagnosis presents no serious difficulty because the symptoms and signs of the underlying endocarditis are prominent. Rarely this is not so, and the disease may be confused with diffuse forms of vasculitis, such as periarteritis or systemic lupus, because of fever and evidence of a systemic disease, necrotic and hemorrhagic skin lesions, or renal biopsy findings of a mixed focal and generalized glomerulonephritis. In such patients the true diagnosis may only be revealed by repeated blood culture, by the finding of splenomegaly, or by evidence of a cardiac lesion.

At present there is insufficient information on the natural history of the glomerulonephritis after successful treatment of the causative endocarditis, but it is unlikely that complete healing occurs in those with extensive glomerular disease.

Boulton-Jones, T. M., Sissons, J. G. P., Evans, D. J., and Peters, D. K.: Renal lesions of subacute infective endocarditis. Br. Med. J., 2:11, 1974.

Gutman, R. A., Striker, G. E., Gilliland, B. C., and Cutler, R. E.: The immune complex glomerulonephritis of bacterial endocarditis. Medicine, 51:1, 1972.

Mesangiocapillary Glomerulonephritis
(Membranoproliferative Glomerulonephritis)

DEFINITION. This disorder is a form of chronic glomerulonephritis, only recently demarcated, in which glomerular mesangial cells are increased and capillary walls are irregularly thickened. There is usually marked and persistent reduction in serum C3 complement.

ETIOLOGY AND PATHOLOGY. The reduction in complement is more persistent than in other forms of glomerulonephritis, and is not the result of deposition in the glomeruli, as it is unrelated to disease activity and persists after nephrectomy. There is evidence of an alternate pathway of C3 metabolism, caused by an abnormal factor of nonrenal origin (C3 "nephritic" factor, or C3 NeF) which in vitro breaks down C3 by a mechanism which does not involve the normal early components of complement activation. The fact that renal transplants can become affected by the disease suggests that a continuing systemic abnormality, perhaps involving the complement system, is responsible for the nephritis.

Immunofluorescence shows granular deposits of complement and properdin in glomerular capillaries; less often IgG and fibrin can be demonstrated. Histologic examination shows increased thickness of the basement membrane of peripheral glomerular capillaries, with some deposits on the endothelial sides of the basement membrane and narrowing of capillary lumina. Mesangial cells are increased in number, and their proliferation throughout the kidney may give the appearance of a lobular nephritis; there are occasional granulocytes.

CLINICAL MANIFESTATIONS. The disease has been reported in siblings, but most cases are sporadic. Older children and young adults are most often affected. Some patients have partial lipodystrophy, and patients with lipodystrophy and low serum C3 complement but no renal disease have also been reported. The glomerular disease may present with symptomless hematuria, proteinuria, or nephrotic syndrome, or rarely as an acute nephritis, although there is seldom a prior streptococcal infection. The course is slowly downhill, with episodes of hematuria and nephrotic syndrome, persistent hypocomplementemia, and gradual renal failure, apparently uninfluenced by any treatment. The average duration, from diagnosis to death or maintenance dialysis, is about ten years. In view of reports of involvement of renal homografts by the disease, maintenance

dialysis is preferable to transplantation as a form of renal replacement.

Lancet Annotation: Pathways in complement activation. Lancet, 1:473, 1973.

Peters, D. K., and Williams, D. G.: Complement and mesangiocapillary glomerulonephritis: The role of complement deficiency in glomerulonephritis. Adv. Nephrol., 4:67, 1974.

Focal Glomerulonephritis with Recurrent Hematuria
(Essential or Benign Hematuria)

The term *focal nephritis* has often been used in the European literature to designate a form of renal disease characterized by repeated attacks of profuse hematuria after systemic infection, leaving little residual renal damage. The renal lesion is a focal glomerular inflammation, but the disease clinically has little in common with other forms of focal glomerulonephritis, such as the renal lesions of polyarteritis or lupus erythematosus.

CLINICAL MANIFESTATIONS. The disease is most common in the second and third decades of life, and affects males much more frequently than females. Rarely other members of the family may be affected. The characteristic features are recurrent attacks of hematuria, which usually start about the age of puberty and continue at the rate of several a year for as many as 20 or 30 years. Attacks may occur without obvious precipitating cause, but most often follow a febrile illness or, less frequently, surgical operation or some strenuous unaccustomed exertion. Unlike poststreptococcal nephritis, hematuria may develop within a few hours of the evidence of systemic infection, and is seldom delayed more than two days; it is often heavier than that which occurs in poststreptococcal nephritis, and may be accompanied by renal pain. There is no constant relationship to group A streptococci or to any particular form of infection. Often the manifestations of the precipitating illness (usually an evanescent pyrexia and myalgia) are so slight that this cannot be diagnosed with certainty.

Even during the attack of hematuria it is unusual for hypertension, renal failure, or edema to develop, although the urinary deposit is characteristic of an acute glomerulonephritis. Renal biopsy discloses focal areas of glomerular proliferation, usually affecting only a segment of a glomerulus here and there. The glomerular lesions are similar to those of Henoch-Schönlein purpura, but are usually less diffuse, and, like them, they show immunofluorescence to IgA. Complement and IgG can also be shown, and the deposits tend to have a mesangial distribution.

PROGNOSIS. At first the urine clears completely after each attack, but in older patients mild proteinuria and microscopic hematuria may persist between attacks. The disorder is usually regarded as benign, because renal failure and hypertension do not commonly develop. However, occasionally these complications develop; more rarely still, the nephrotic syndrome is seen, and in such patients renal biopsy shows that the glomerular lesions, although still focal, have resulted in very severe glomerular destruction.

MANAGEMENT. The history is so distinctive that a diagnosis can usually be made with confidence from this alone. However, it is often valuable to demonstrate the characteristic histology by renal biopsy, either in order to reassure the patient that he has a form of renal disease that does not usually shorten life, or to put an end to repeated urologic investigations performed in an attempt to explain the hematuria.

Patients with the syndrome should be advised to avoid infections or any activities which they know are liable to precipitate an attack. Penicillin prophylaxis, to reduce bacterial respiratory infections, is often tried, but the results have been disappointing. The usual benign course of the condition does not justify routine use of steroids, nor is there any evidence that they influence the disease. Prolonged follow-up is advisable, because the course is not invariably benign and some of the long-term complications (e.g., hypertension and renal failure) require treatment.

Rapoport, A., Davidson, D. A., Deveber, G. A., Ranking, G. N., and McLean, C. R.: Idiopathic focal proliferative nephritis associated with persistent hematuria and normal renal function. Ann. Intern. Med., 73:921, 1970.

Roy, L. P., Fish, R. A., Vernier, R. L., and Michael, A. F.: Recurrent macroscopic hematuria, focal nephritis, and mesangial deposition of immunoglobulin and complement. J. Pediat., 82:767, 1973.

Other Varieties of Proliferative Glomerulonephritis

Many cases of proliferative glomerulonephritis do not fit clearly into one or other of the categories so far described. Although some are probably poststreptococcal in origin, this is no longer believed to be the cause in most cases.

EXTRACAPILLARY GLOMERULONEPHRITIS WITH EPITHELIAL CRESCENTS (Fig. 4). This type of glomerulonephritis is only rarely of poststreptococcal origin, and is often of anti-GBM type, showing linear glomerular immunofluorescence for IgG and complement. Epithelial proliferation leads to the formation of crescents which fluoresce for fibrin and obliterate Bowman's space. The course is often fulminating, justifying the title "rapidly progressive glomerulonephritis," but occasionally the disease appears to become stationary or only slowly progressive. Children are rarely affected, but the condition is a frequent type of glomerular disease at all other ages.

Clinical presentation is with hematuria, nephrotic syndrome, renal hypertension, or oliguric renal failure. No treatment is known to definitely alter the course of the disease; there is good rationale for the use of anticoagulants to reduce crescent formation, but there is no convincing evidence that they improve survival.

ENDOTHELIAL GLOMERULONEPHRITIS. When cells from within the glomerulus (endothelial and mesangial cells) proliferate, the histologic changes are those of a lobular nephritis, with fusion of glomerular capillary loops, but without marked adhesion formation between the visceral and parietal layers of Bowman's capsule. This pathologic picture is much more common than the extracapillary type of glomerulonephritis, but mixed types are also frequent. Some appear to be the result of a streptococcal infection, but in others this cause can be excluded with confidence.

The usual clinical presentations are with recurrent hematuria, nephrotic syndrome, or renal hypertension. Renal failure is not a prominent early feature, but it eventually develops after months or years as a result of progressive glomerulosclerosis. The disease frequently appears to remain unchanged for long periods, and renal function may even improve spontaneously, particularly in poststreptococcal cases. This is the histologic variety of glomerulonephritis to which the descriptive name *chronic glomerulonephritis* can most suitably be applied.

Although mixtures of types of glomerular disorders

Figure 4. Abundant crescent formation in a 13-year-old girl with rapidly progressive glomerular nephritis. No good history of streptococcal infection was obtained. (H & E; × 150.) (From Heptinstall, R. H.: Pathology of the Kidney. Boston, Little, Brown & Company, 1966.)

occur, in any one patient the renal condition usually runs true to type, the histology as shown by serial biopsies retaining its characteristics despite evolution of the disease.

In longstanding proliferative glomerulonephritis there may be little or no remaining cellular proliferation in the glomeruli, many of which are destroyed by fibrosis while the remainder show adhesions and segmental scarring. The atrophy of tubules rendered ischemic by glomerular destruction leads to gross renal shrinkage and distortion of renal architecture. Hypertensive damage, involving arterioles and arteries, is usually present and may lead to further ischemic atrophy. The final picture is difficult to distinguish from end-stage renal disease caused by other types of glomerular disease (e.g., membranous glomerular disease) and can even be confused with diseases which are not primarily glomerular, such as hypertensive nephropathy or chronic pyelonephritis.

Cameron, J. S.: The natural history of glomerulonephritis. *In* Black, D. A. K. (ed.): Renal Disease. 3rd ed. Oxford, Blackwell Scientific Publications, 1972, p. 295.

374.4. RENAL INVOLVEMENT IN CONNECTIVE TISSUE DISEASES

O. M. Wrong

Many generalized diseases of connective tissue may cause glomerular disease which may be difficult to distinguish, on either clinical or histologic grounds, from other forms of glomerulonephritis.

SYSTEMIC LUPUS ERYTHEMATOSUS. Some 50 to 75 per cent of patients with this condition develop renal disease at some time. It is an example of immune-complex glomerular injury, the complexes consisting of DNA (antigen), IgG, and complement. Glomerular involvement takes several forms: (1) segmental areas of glomerulitis, with hypercellularity and thickening of the basement membrane; (2) a membranous type of glomerulopathy without cellular proliferation; and (3) a diffuse proliferative glomerulonephritis with cellular proliferation, areas of glomerular necrosis, and crescent formation. These changes are not specific for lupus erythematosus, but their appearance in a patient with serologic and systemic evidence of that disease is sufficient to establish the cause of the glomerular lesion.

Renal involvement may be manifested clinically as a symptomless proteinuria which remains unchanged for months or years, with nephrotic syndrome, or with a severe progressive acute glomerulonephritis. Once renal failure has developed, the course is usually one of steady deterioration, leading to death in renal failure within a few months unless the patient is put on a renal replacement program. Steroids in high dosage (45 mg or more of prednisolone daily) have long been used in the treatment of active forms of lupus, and there is a strong impression that they are beneficial in lupus nephritis; patients with localized areas of glomerulitis do best, whereas there is little evidence of benefit in those with diffuse proliferative glomerulonephritis. Various cytotoxic drugs (especially the nitrogen mustards and azathioprine) have also been used, but there is no convincing evidence that they alter the course of the renal disease.

PERIARTERITIS NODOSA. Small arteries of the kidney may be affected, leading to macroscopic infarcts of the renal substance, or there may be the microscopic form first described by Davson, Ball, and Platt, in which glomerular arterioles and capillaries are involved, leading to a proliferative glomerulonephritis which closely resembles other types of this disease but usually shows a more segmental pattern.

Although the systemic manifestations of the disease may affect any organ of the body, skin involvement seems particularly common in those with renal disease, and is often manifested as small tender areas, 2 to 4 mm across, representing infarcts in the pulp of the fingers and toes. Subungual splinter hemorrhages, if numerous, may have the same significance. However, it is not uncommon for renal disease to be the sole clinical manifestation of a polyarteritis.

The renal presentation may be that of a repeated renal infarction with local pain and hematuria, of an acute oliguric nephritis, or of chronic glomerulonephritis with proteinuria and steady reduction in renal function. Renal hypertension is common.

Usually the course is progressive deterioration, particularly in those with the microscopic form of the disease. Large doses of steroids appear to halt the progress of the disease in a small proportion of cases, and steroid-induced remissions of several years have been recorded. Rarely the disease appears to become stationary spontaneously, or there may even be temporary periods of improved renal function.

WEGENER'S GRANULOMATOSIS. This entity is discussed in Ch. 68. The renal lesions may contain small granulomas in relation to blood vessels and glomeruli; otherwise the kidney disease cannot be distinguished from classic polyarteritis.

Although it may be months or years before the syndrome is complicated by renal involvement, the progression of the renal disease is usually rapid once it appears, leading to uremia within a few months. Steroids have been used in treatment, with little effect, but more recently encouraging results have been obtained with cytotoxic drugs, particularly cyclophosphamide, the renal disease either becoming stationary or showing actual improvement. No controlled trial of this treatment has been reported, but the course of the untreated renal disease is so uniformly bad that this treatment is worthy of trial.

ANAPHYLACTOID PURPURA (HENOCH-SCHÖNLEIN SYNDROME). In anaphylactoid purpura hematuria may be caused by bleeding from the mucosal surface of the ureters, bladder, or urethra. Occasionally, however, anaphylactoid purpura causes a true glomerulonephritis, which clinically resembles a poststreptococcal acute glomerulonephritis. This resemblance is enhanced if the disease follows a streptococcal infection, as is often the case. However, serum complement is not diminished, and renal biopsy shows focal rather than diffuse glomerulonephritis. The glomerular lesions are unusual in that they may show deposits of IgA on immunofluorescence, often accompanied by fibrin. It is generally believed, although the evidence is not convincing, that complete renal recovery is less common than after a poststreptococcal nephritis; but it must be remembered that recurrent attacks of anaphylactoid purupra are common, and the possibility of permanent renal damage may be greater for that reason. The course of the disease in patients whose glomerulonephritis does not resolve completely is very like that of other forms of glomerulonephritis, except that the nephrotic syndrome appears to be less common.

GOODPASTURE'S SYNDROME (LUNG PURPURA AND NEPHRITIS). Goodpasture's syndrome is a form of acute progressive glomerulonephritis accompanied by massive capillary hemorrhage into the lungs. The primary cause is unknown, but in most cases the glomerulonephritis appears to be caused by circulating anti-GBM antibodies (see Fig. 2) which also react with the basement membrane of the pulmonary alveoli. Histologically the renal lesion is difficult to distinguish from other forms of acute proliferative glomerulonephritis, except that it may initially show focal features. Within a few weeks the glomerular disease usually becomes generalized, with glomerular obliteration by epithelial crescents. The lungs show massive confluent alveolar hemorrhage, identical with that seen in the rare condition *idiopathic pulmonary hemosiderosis;* the pulmonary capillaries show patchy basement membrane changes, but it is usually difficult to see changes gross enough to account for the amount of blood in the alveoli.

No age is exempt, but the disease is most common in the second and third decades, and males are affected three or four times as often as females. A history of prior exposure to petroleum fumes has been found in some cases, and this has been suggested as an etiologic factor. The first symptom is usually recurrent hemoptysis, and only after days or weeks do manifestations of nephritis occur, most often hematuria. The pulmonary hemorrhage is often very severe, with symptoms and signs of acute blood loss; after repeated episodes an iron deficiency anemia may appear, owing to a sequestration of large amounts of iron in the lungs as hemosiderin. Occasionally the first manifestations are those of subacute glomerulonephritis, and only after several weeks does pulmonary hemorrhage indicate the presence of a generalized disease.

In most cases the renal lesion progresses rapidly to total glomerular destruction, often passing through a nephrotic phase, and leading to uremia within a few weeks or months of the onset of symptoms. Death may also result from pulmonary hemorrhage, either from asphyxia or acute blood loss. Treatment is usually without influence on the course of the disease; there have been reports of long remissions after treatment with steroids, and recently encouraging results have been reported from the use of cytotoxic drugs and plasma exchange. Hemorrhage into the lungs sometimes ceases after bilateral nephrectomy, and in patients in whom lung hemorrhage is life threatening this drastic form of treatment, combined with maintenance hemodialysis or renal transplantation, may have to be considered.

HEMOLYTIC-UREMIC SYNDROME. This affects infants and young children and, less frequently, young adults. It is characterized by thrombocytopenia, microangiopathic hemolytic anemia, and acute progressive renal failure. Histologically the renal lesion is a proliferative glomerulonephritis, less frequently a patchy cortical stenosis.

The hematologic manifestations appear to be secondary to vasculitis, which may be generalized or confined to the glomeruli. Minor degrees of the same blood changes are common in all forms of acute glomerulonephritis, or diffuse small vessel vasculitis, and for this reason many authorities do not accept the hemolytic-uremic syndrome as a separate disease entity, but regard it as a syndrome with many causes, including poststreptococcal nephritis and polyarteritis. However, because the condition has sometimes occurred in small local outbreaks and is much more common in some communities, e.g., Argentina and Chile, than in others, it has been suggested by some that there might be an infective basis.

The condition often starts with evidence of acute gastroenteritis with bloody diarrhea, but whether this is infective or due to vascular lesions in the bowel is uncertain. Fever, pulmonary symptoms, cutaneous purpura, and neurologic features (especially convulsions and coma) are common. It is difficult to ascertain in an individual case whether the diffuse organ involvement is caused by underlying vasculitis or by local hemorrhage resulting from the thrombocytopenia.

Renal involvement is shown by hematuria and the rapid development of oliguric renal failure, without clinical remissions. Milder cases occur, but when renal failure develops it seldom improves; the few recoveries that have been reported have often followed treatment with steroids or heparin.

Thrombotic thrombocytopenic purpura (TTP, Moschcowitz's syndrome) is a rare form of the syndrome characterized by widespread formation of platelet thrombi in small arteries and capillaries, including renal vessels; the consumption of coagulation factors which results causes a profound thrombocytopenia.

THE KIDNEY IN SYSTEMIC SCLEROSIS (SCLERODERMA). Although systemic sclerosis may affect the kidney, it is unusual among connective diseases in that it does not cause glomerulonephritis. Instead there is a slowly progressive obliteration of renal arteries of interlobular size or smaller, and of the renal arterioles, morphologically identical to the vascular involvement of other organs. Histologically the vascular changes closely resemble those of malignant hypertension and radiation nephritis. The usual clinical manifestations, if indeed there are any, include mild proteinuria, slowly progressive renal failure, and renal hypertension, which may be severe. Treatment of hypertension may be required, but otherwise there is no treatment for the renal lesion.

Benoit, F. L., Rulon, D. B., Theil, G. B., Doolan, P. D., and Watten, R. H.: Goodpasture's syndrome. A clinicopathologic entity. Am. J. Med., 37:424, 1964.
Clarkson, A., Lawrence, J., Meadows, R., and Seymour, A.: The haemolytic uraemic syndrome in adults. Quart. J. Med., 39:227, 1970.
Donadio, J. V.: Treatment of lupus nephritis. Nephron, 19:186, 1977.
Lieberman, E.: Hemolytic-uremic syndrome. J. Pediat., 80:1, 1972.
Lockwood, C. M., Rees, A. J., Pearson, T. A., Evans, D. J., Peters, D. K., and Wilson, C. B.: Immunosuppression and plasma exchange in the treatment of Goodpasture's syndrome. Lancet, I:711, 1976.
Meadow, S. R., Glasgow, E. F., White, R. H. R., Moncrieff, M. W., Cameron, J. S., and Ogg, C. S.: Schönlein-Henoch nephritis. Quart. J. Med., 41:241, 1972.
Pollak, V. E., Pirani, C. L., and Schwartz, F. D.: The natural history of the renal manifestations of systemic lupus erythematosus. J. Lab. Clin. Med., 63:537, 1963.
Wagner, L.: Immunosuppressive agents in lupus nephritis: A critical analysis. Medicine, 55:239, 1976.
Walker, W. G., Harvey, A. M., and Yardley, J. H.: Renal involvement in myeloma, amyloidosis, systemic lupus erythematosus, and other disorders of connective tissue. In Strauss, M. B., and Welt, L. G. (eds.): Diseases of the Kidney. 3rd. ed. Boston, Little Brown & Company, 1972, p. 825.

374.5.   HEREDITARY NEPHRITIS
(Alport's Syndrome)
O. M. Wrong

DEFINITION.   Hereditary nephritis is a form of hereditary renal disease, characterized histologically by glomerulonephritis and interstitial nephritis, frequently associated with nerve deafness.

GENETIC ASPECTS AND INCIDENCE.   The disease is inherited as an autosomal dominant. Males and females are approximately equally affected, but the disease usually takes a more serious form and is manifest at an earlier age in men. Patients with renal disease frequently have nerve deafness, and some members of the family may have deafness with normal renal function. Ophthalmologic defects, such as cataracts and lenticonus, occur less frequently.

Several hundred cases have been reported, but it is very difficult to make the diagnosis in sporadic cases or in families without deafness, and the true incidence is probably many times greater.

ETIOLOGY AND PATHOLOGY.   The nature of the underlying defect is unknown. Histologically the renal lesion may be a chronic proliferative glomerulonephritis, often with segmental glomerular lesions; in other patients the glomeruli appear normal, but there is an extensive interstitial nephritis which resembles pyelonephritis or analgesic nephropathy. Most writers have remarked on the fat-laden foam cells in the interstitium, but these are common in other forms of renal disease, and their presence cannot be regarded as diagnostic.

CLINICAL MANIFESTATIONS.   The first symptom is usually hematuria, often noticed in childhood, and frequently preceded by a systemic infection. Proteinuria is usually present, but is seldom severe enough to cause the nephrotic syndrome. Occasionally frank attacks of pyelonephritis occur, with positive urine cultures. The usual course is slow deterioration in renal function, often with hypertension, leading to renal failure in the third to fifth decade. Nerve deafness can develop at any age; initially it affects high tones predominantly, and may be unsuspected until revealed by audiometry.

DIAGNOSIS.   The diagnosis is often difficult because no single known feature of the disease is absolutely diagnostic. The most helpful features are nerve deafness in the patient or immediate relatives and familial renal disease. However, to be convincing, the family history should include more than one generation, for the presence of glomerulonephritis in several sibs might be the result of simultaneous infection with a nephritogenic *Streptococcus* during earlier childhood. Sporadic cases may be confused with other forms of chronic glomerulonephritis, with the syndrome of focal nephritis and recurrent hematuria described above, or with familial renal tubular defects which are occasionally associated with nerve deafness.

TREATMENT.   No treatment is known to alter the progress of the renal disease, but patients may require treatment for urinary infections, for renal hypertension, or for symptomatic renal failure.

Perkoff, G. T.: Hereditary chronic nephritis. *In* Strauss, W. B., and Welt, L. G. (eds.): Diseases of the Kidney, 3rd ed. Boston, Little, Brown & Company, 1971, p. 1275.

374.6.   RENAL CHANGES IN OTHER SYSTEMIC DISEASES
C. Craig Tisher

SARCOIDOSIS

Sarcoidosis, a granulomatous disease of unknown etiology and pathogenesis, is manifested by widespread involvement of virtually every organ system in the body, including the kidney. Renal involvement, frequently life threatening, is often treatable and therefore bears emphasis. The over-all incidence of renal involvement in sarcoid varies from 5 to 10 per cent in both children and adults.

The renal manifestations of sarcoid fall into three general categories: (1) direct granulomatous involvement of the parenchyma; (2) nephrocalcinosis and renal calculus formation, usually occurring in a setting of hypercalcemia or hypercalciuria or both; and (3) glomerulonephritis.

Granulomatous renal involvement is rarely accompanied by functional renal impairment in the absence of hypercalcemia or hypercalciuria or both. The histopathologic picture is that of an interstitial nephritis accompanying well localized granulomas. Immunofluorescence findings are generally restricted to the vasculature, where IgM and IgA immunoglobulins have been found in sites corresponding to hyaline deposits observed with light microscopy. When renal impairment is present, extensive granuloma formation accompanied by marked interstitial nephritis with attendant parenchymal destruction would appear to be the mechanism responsible. Findings on urinalysis include modest proteinuria, nonspecific cylindruria, and sterile pyuria, which are consistent with the presence of an interstitial nephritis. In most patients thus far reported with significant functional impairment, corticosteroid administration has resulted in some degree of initial improvement in both the creatinine clearance and the diminished urine concentrating ability when the latter has existed. The long-term outlook for such patients remains to be defined.

Renal disease secondary to disordered calcium metabolism is the most common form of involvement in sarcoid and occurs as a consequence of persistent hypercalcemia often accompanied by hypercalciuria. Nephrocalcinosis and nephrolithiasis complicate the abnormally elevated serum calcium concentration. In the absence of therapeutic intervention, renal involvement can intensify with the development of pyelonephritis, chronic pyelitis, hydronephrosis, and progressive renal failure. Histologically, there are no characteristic features which serve to distinguish the nephrocalcinosis associated with sarcoid from that of other conditions which also lead to nephrocalcinosis. Calcifications are distributed throughout the kidney, but often are present in greatest numbers in the medulla. Clinically, these patients present with signs and symptoms which are largely dependent upon the duration of the disorder, the extent of nephrocalcinosis and its sequelae, and the coexistence of either granulomatous involvement or glomerulonephritis. With minimal renal involvement, polyuria with or without azotemia may be the chief functional abnormality. Later, nephrocalcinosis may be severe and manifested by progressive renal failure with or without hypertension. Renal lithiasis may play the dominant role and lead to recurrent episodes of pyelonephritis, eventually ending in hydronephrosis and renal insufficiency. Aggressive treatment of the hypercalcemia is of paramount importance if serious and irreversible renal damage is to be avoided. Dietary restriction of calcium and vitamin D must be initiated. Excessive exposure to sunlight should be avoided. Corticosteroid administration is probably the treatment of choice, although chloroquine, sodium phytate, and inorganic phosphate may have therapeutic usefulness in some patients.

Glomerulonephritis is a relatively uncommon form of renal involvement in sarcoidosis. In 1951 Teilum first suggested a similarity between glomerular hyaline deposits in sarcoid and certain glomerular lesions in patients with systemic lupus erythematosus. Since that time a number of patients with glomerulonephritis associated with sarcoidosis have been recorded, most as isolated case reports. In 1972 McCoy and Tisher described six patients with glomerulonephritis associated with sarcoidosis, five of whom were nephrotic. Morphologic forms of glomerulonephritis that have been observed include endocapillary proliferative glomerulonephritis, crescentic proliferative glomerulonephritis, membranous glomerulonephritis, and end-stage chronic glomerulonephritis. Histologically, glomerulonephritis associated with sarcoidosis resembles the various primary forms of glomerulonephritis. Immunofluorescence studies have revealed the presence of immune complexes within the glomeruli. It is unclear whether the relationship between sarcoidosis and glomerulonephritis is causal or fortuitous. Although the etiology and pathogenesis of sarcoidosis are not yet established, this condition is thought to represent an altered immune response to one or more unidentified antigens. The spectrum of glomerular lesions observed in association with sarcoidosis closely mimics the spectrum encountered in lupus nephritis. The possible role of corticosteroids and immunosuppressive agents such as azathioprine and cyclophosphamide in the treatment of this form of renal involvement in sarcoidosis has not yet been established.

Longcope, W. T., and Freiman, D. G.: A study of sarcoidosis. Medicine, 31:1, 1952.

McCoy, R. C., and Tisher, C. C.: Glomerulonephritis associated with sarcoidosis. Am. J. Pathol., 68:339, 1972.

Teilum, G.: Glomerular lesions of the kidneys in sarcoidosis (Boeck's sarcoid). Acta Pathol. Microbiol. Scand., 28:294, 1951.

DIABETES MELLITUS

Nephropathy, neuropathy, and retinopathy are the three most devastating complications of the microangiopathy of diabetes mellitus. In approximately 50 per cent of patients with so-called juvenile onset diabetes mellitus, renal failure is the cause of death. In contrast, in patients in whom diabetes is first diagnosed after the age of 40, the major cause of death is obliterative arteriosclerosis of muscular arteries, especially occlusive disease involving the coronary arteries, whereas renal disease accounts for less than 10 per cent of all deaths. Although it is often stated that urinary tract infections occur with greater frequency in diabetic than nondiabetic patients, this is true only in the female population.

Papillary necrosis is frequently observed in the diabetic patient and is found in approximately 25 per cent of patients with diabetes and acute pyelonephritis.

In the juvenile diabetic, 10 to 15 years may elapse before functional renal impairment in the form of proteinuria first becomes manifest. Following the onset of proteinuria, however, the mean duration of life is approximately five years. Although the period preceding the onset of proteinuria may be quite variable in length, once evidence of functional renal deterioration occurs, little variation in the subsequent course is observed. The nephrotic syndrome occurs in approximately 10 per cent of diabetic patients. The sudden appearance of the nephrotic syndrome, however, especially in the young diabetic patient without previous evidence of functional renal impairment, should not be automatically ascribed to the patient's primary underlying disease, because such patients are not immune from other renal diseases which are also associated with the nephrotic syndrome and may be treatable.

Histologically, four rather distinctive lesions can be recognized in the glomeruli in addition to alterations in the thickness and configuration of the basement membranes of the peripheral capillary loops. These include the nodular and diffuse forms of intercapillary glomerulosclerosis, the capsular drop lesion, and the fibrin cap lesion. The nodular lesion, which was described by Kimmelstiel and Wilson in 1936, is pathognomonic of diabetes mellitus; the other lesions generally lack specificity. The lesion is an eosinophilic and periodic acid–Schiff (PAS) positive argyrophilic, homogeneous, largely acellular mass of variable size and is located in the mesangial or intercapillary regions of the glomerular tuft. As the nodules increase in size, there is a progressive encroachment on the patency of the adjacent capillaries which, when coupled with localized thickening of the basement membrane of the peripheral capillary loops, results in progressive occlusion of the capillary lumina and ischemia. Immunofluorescence microscopy has revealed the presence of immunoglobulins, various complement components, and fibrin within the glomeruli. However, localization of these plasma components is best explained to date on a nonimmunologic basis, probably occurring as a result of nonspecific trapping or secondary to basement membrane or mesangial dysfunction. Subintimal hyaline thickening of the arterioles is widespread in the diabetic kidney and often involves the efferent as well as the afferent arterioles. The presence of marked hyaline arteriolosclerosis even in the absence of glomerular lesions in a young patient with asymptomatic proteinuria should alert the clinician to the possible presence of diabetes mellitus. The best correlation between the severity of certain clinical parameters of this disease, such as proteinuria, hypertension, and reduction in glomerular filtration rate, and the histopathology is seen with the diffuse form of intercapillary glomerulosclerosis.

There is no specific treatment regimen currently available which is known to alter the natural history of the disease process. Treatment of progressive renal failure and control of secondary complications such as infection and hypertension are the same in this disease as in other forms of kidney disease associated with progressive renal failure. Repetitive dialysis and transplantation are being employed with increasing frequency in the diabetic patient with end-stage uremia.

Heptinstall, R. H.: Pathology of the Kidney. 2nd ed. Boston, Little, Brown & Company, 1974, p. 929.

Kimmelstiel, P., and Wilson, C.: Intercapillary lesions in glomeruli of kidney. Am. J. Pathol., 12:83, 1936.

Tisher, C. C., and McCoy, R. C.: Diabetes mellitus and the kidney. In Suki, W. N., and Eknoyan, G. (eds.): The Kidney in Systemic Disease. New York, John Wiley & Sons, 1976, p. 105.

SICKLE CELL DISEASE

Sickle cell disease occurring as a consequence of abnormal hemoglobin synthesis has several functional and anatomic abnormalities of the kidney. Functional alterations are found in both sickle cell disease and sickle cell trait, but anatomic abnormalities are more common in patients with sickle cell disease. The main renal abnormalities include defects in urine concentration and urine acidification, decrease in renal blood flow (RBF) and glomerular filtration rate (GFR) after the third decade of life, gross and microscopic hematuria, proteinuria, the nephrotic syndrome, papillary necrosis, and, on rare occasions, renal failure.

Histologically, dilatation and congestion of glomerular and peritubular capillaries are frequent findings. Cortical scars containing sclerotic glomeruli and atrophic tubules are often scattered through the parenchyma and represent the sequelae of localized cortical infarction. Abnormalities in the medulla include congestion and dilatation of the vasa recta and submucosal vessels and papillary necrosis. In most patients reported to date with the nephrotic syndrome, a typical membranoproliferative glomerulonephritis has been demonstrated.

The defect in urine concentration which is not associated with an inability to dilute the urine is a relatively early, albeit largely asymptomatic manifestation of both sickle cell disease and trait. In young patients multiple blood transfusions have been shown to reverse the defect transiently, suggesting that in the initial stages of the disease, before irreversible structural damage occurs, the defect is related in some way to the abnormal erythrocytes. The mechanism appears to be one of increased sickling secondary to the hypertonicity and the relative hypoxia of the medulla, which, in turn, leads to an increase in blood viscosity, a decrease in medullary blood flow, and subsequent functional disruption of the countercurrent system.

Painless, gross hematuria is a frequent complication of sickle cell hemoglobinopathy and is seen more commonly in those individuals with the trait. It has been estimated to occur in 20 to 30 per cent of patients with this hemoglobin abnormality and probably results from congestion, stasis, and dilatation of medullary and submucosal vasculature by sickled erythrocytes resulting in hypoxic damage, leading to loss of the integrity of the vessel walls. In some patients focal areas of papillary necrosis may also be important in the mechanism of hematuria. Unilateral bleeding is common, with left side involvement predominating. The abnormality is frequently recurrent, and is more common in the adult. In the renal medulla there are at least three factors present which have been shown in vitro to enhance sickling of abnormal erythrocytes. These include hypoxia, a hypertonic milieu, and a low pH. Treatment is generally directed toward minimizing the impact of these factors on sickling and includes alkalinization of the urine

and administration of diuretics such as furosemide or ethacrynic acid to establish a water diuresis and reduce the medullary tonicity. The use of intravenously administered distilled water in a dose of 500 ml given over a period of 15 minutes has also been shown to induce at least a transient cessation of hematuria. If such patients are adequately hydrated to assure a stable urine flow of approximately 100 ml per hour and have adequate renal function, distilled water can be administered intravenously with little or no danger of acute tubular necrosis resulting from the presence of free hemoglobin, which is occasionally released in small quantities during the procedure. Intravenously administered distilled water probably acts by causing the susceptible erythrocytes to swell, thereby decreasing the concentration of hemoglobin S below the critical concentration necessary for sickling, rather than having a direct effect on the renal medulla. The use of ϵ-aminocaproic acid has also been suggested in these patients, but must be undertaken with caution.

Papillary necrosis of widely varying severity is a frequent complication of sickle cell hemoglobinopathy, although it rarely leads to end-stage renal failure. The nephrotic syndrome, which occasionally complicates this disease, is most frequently observed in a histologic setting of membranoproliferative glomerulonephritis, although in a few instances renal vein thrombosis has been present. The pathogenesis of the glomerulonephritis remains unclear, but iron-bound protein complexes may play a role, possibly by initiating an immune-mediated glomerular injury. Corticosteroid therapy for treatment of the nephrotic syndrome in these patients has met with limited success. In the few patients who develop renal failure, repetitive dialysis therapy should be entertained despite the potential complications of hemolysis, thrombosis, and anemia.

Alfrey, A. C.: The renal response to vascular injury. In Brenner, B. M., and Rector, F. C., Jr. (eds.): The Kidney. Philadelphia, W. B. Saunders Company, 1976, p. 1145.

Friedman, E. A., Sreepadarrao, T. K., Sprung, C. L., Smith, A., Manis, T., Bellevue, R., Butt, K. M. H., Levere, R. D., and Holder, D. M.: Uremia in sickle cell anemia treated by maintenance hemodialysis. N. Engl. J. Med., 291:431, 1974.

Heptinstall, R. H.: Pathology of the Kidney. 2nd ed. Boston, Little, Brown & Company, 1974, p. 1151.

Knochel, J. P.: Hematuria in sickle cell trait. The effect of intravenous administration of distilled water, urinary alkalinization and diuresis. Arch. Intern. Med., 123:160, 1969.

Marynick, S. P., Ramsey, E. J., and Knochel, J. P.: The effect of bicarbonate and distilled water on sickle cell trait hematuria and in vitro studies on the interaction of osmolality and pH on erythrocyte sickling in sickle cell trait. J. Urol., 118:793, 1977.

MULTIPLE MYELOMA

Several structural and functional abnormalities of the kidney can be found in patients with multiple myeloma. Functional abnormalities include acute and chronic renal failure, defects in urine concentration and urine acidification, and several proximal tubular defects characteristic of the adult Fanconi syndrome. In addition to the presence of those lesions that are characteristic of the myeloma kidney to be described below, amyloid deposits and histologic evidence of acute and chronic pyelonephritis are often observed. Proteinuria occurs in over half of all patients with multiple myeloma, with Bence Jones proteins being the most common.

Myeloma cells are observed to infiltrate the kidney infrequently in this condition and even when present rarely cause any functional deterioration. These same cells can be identified in the urine sediment of some patients.

Histologically, the kidneys are usually enlarged in myeloma, but size can vary considerably. Glomeruli are generally normal in appearance, although mesangial thickening unrelated to amyloid deposition has been described. The eosinophilic laminated cast surrounded by an epithelial syncytium in distal convoluted tubules and collecting ducts is the most striking and characteristic alteration seen in the kidney in multiple myeloma. Several plasma components contribute to the casts, including kappa and lambda Bence Jones proteins, fibrinogen, albumin, and IgG immunoglobulin. Amyloid has also been demonstrated in the casts. Ultrastructural studies have revealed small rod-shaped crystals in proximal tubule epithelium which probably represent intracellular accumulation of Bence Jones protein. In many patients with multiple myeloma the presence of these inclusions has been correlated with those functional defects of the proximal tubule typical of the Fanconi syndrome. Immunofluorescence studies have confirmed the presence of kappa or lambda light chains in droplets within the tubular epithelium. Further evidence that excessive filtration, reabsorption, and catabolism of these light chains may be specifically associated with proximal and distal tubular dysfunction has been provided by studies in patients without multiple myeloma who produce excessive amounts of the light chain protein and exhibit similar defects in renal tubular function.

The progressive renal insufficiency observed in multiple myeloma is probably due to a combination of factors, including tubular obstruction with casts, tubular atrophy, interstitial nephritis, decreased RBF, hypercalcemia and nephrocalcinosis, and toxic injury to tubular epithelium secondary to abnormal protein accumulation, particularly kappa and lambda light chains. Superimposed amyloid deposition and pyelonephritis are also believed to contribute to the functional deterioration.

The hyposthenuria and polyuria are generally ascribed to hypercalcemia, which is often quite severe in multiple myeloma, and to destruction of collecting ducts, the site of action of vasopressin in the mammalian kidney. Reversal of the hypercalcemia through the administration of corticosteroids, osmotic agents such as mannitol, and the use of diuretics, including furosemide and ethacrynic acid, can reverse the urine concentrating defect in some patients.

Acute renal failure occasionally complicates the course of multiple myeloma and has been reported with apparent increased frequency after intravenous pyelography with certain contrast agents. However, other factors known to predispose individuals to acute tubular necrosis are often present, such as volume depletion, sepsis, and hypotension, thus casting considerable doubt on the specificity of the proposed etiology. Nevertheless, the use of intravenous contrast agents in these patients should be approached with caution, and adequate hydration should be maintained. The many agents employed to treat myeloma appear to have little effect on the progression of the renal lesions.

Limas, C., Wright, J. R., Matsuzaki, M., and Calkins, E.: Amyloidosis and multiple myeloma: A re-evaluation using a control population. Am. J. Med., 54:166, 1973.

Osserman, E. F.: Plasma-cell myeloma. II. Clinical aspects. N. Engl. J. Med., 261:952, 1006, 1959.

Walker, W. G., Harvey, A. M., and Yardley, J. H.: Renal involvement in myeloma, amyloidosis, systemic lupus erythematosus, and other disorders of connective tissue. In Strauss, W. B., and Welt, L. G. (eds.): Diseases of the Kidney. 2nd ed. Boston, Little, Brown & Company, 1971, p. 825.

AMYLOIDOSIS

Amyloidosis, a disease of unknown etiology and uncertain pathogenesis, is manifested by widespread organ involvement which includes the kidney. In the primary and secondary forms of amyloidosis, approximately 80 to 90 per cent of all patients will exhibit some type of renal abnormality, usually in the form of proteinuria. As many as 50 per cent of patients with renal amyloidosis will eventually develop the nephrotic syndrome, often after years of asymptomatic proteinuria. Renal amyloidosis is seen in approximately one quarter of those individuals with familial Mediterranean fever, one of the hereditary forms of amyloidosis. Renal failure is the leading cause of death in those afflicted patients. Amyloidosis is also seen in approximately 10 per cent of patients with multiple myeloma (see above), and is occasionally present in other types of malignant disease. Secondary amyloidosis with renal involvement occurring as a complication of several chronic illnesses, such as bronchiectasis, tuberculosis, osteomyelitis, syphilis, and rheumatoid arthritis, appears to be on the decline, undoubtedly reflecting better diagnosis and treatment of the underlying conditions. In addition to proteinuria and the nephrotic syndrome, other clinical features of renal amyloidosis that are occasionally seen include diabetes insipidus of the nephrogenic variety, renal tubular acidosis, and progressive renal failure. In the setting of the nephrotic syndrome, sudden worsening of edema and deterioration of renal function should lead one to suspect the presence of renal vein thrombosis, a complication of the disease which may respond to anticoagulant therapy.

The kidneys are usually enlarged in renal amyloidosis, and this finding in the clinical setting of chronic renal failure should alert the clinician to the possibility of this disease. Amyloid deposits in the glomeruli are found in the mesangium and along both the endothelial and epithelial aspects of the basement membranes of the peripheral capillary loops. Similar deposits are frequently observed along the basement membranes of tubules in the medulla, within the media and adventitia of arterioles and interlobular arteries, and infrequently within the medullary interstitium. The presence of glomerular amyloid is more common in the secondary forms of amyloid, with the exception of multiple myeloma in which the glomeruli are seldom involved. With the Congo red stain the amyloid deposits are orange-red and demonstrate a light green birefringence with polarized light. Other light microscopic stains for amyloid include methyl violet and thioflavine T. Electron microscopy of amyloid reveals the characteristic nonbranching fibrils, 80 to 100 Å in diameter, that are pathognomonic of the lesion. Immunofluorescence findings in this disease have been variable and of little diagnostic help.

Recent evidence suggests that amyloid fibrils are derived from at least two sources — immunoglobulin light chains and a nonimmunoglobulin protein, protein A, of undetermined etiology. The former is found more commonly in primary amyloidosis and the secondary form of amyloidosis associated with multiple myeloma. Amyloid fibrils derived from the proteolysis of protein A are found in other secondary forms of amyloid.

Attempts at treatment of renal amyloidosis have generally been unsuccessful, although in a single patient with primary amyloidosis and the nephrotic syndrome, combined therapy with penicillamine, melphalan, prednisone, and fluoxymesterone was associated with complete remission of the proteinuria and resolution of the amyloid previously present in the bone marrow. The use of corticosteroids alone is contraindicated for the treatment of the nephrotic syndrome in renal amyloidosis. Elimination of the precipitating cause in certain secondary forms of the disease may result in regression of the kidney infiltrates.

Cohen, H. J., Lessin, L. S., Hallal, J., and Burkholder, P.: Resolution of primary amyloidosis during chemotherapy. Studies in a patient with nephrotic syndrome. Ann. Intern. Med., 82:466, 1975.
Glenner, G. G., Ein, D., and Terry, W. D.: The immunoglobulin origin of amyloid. Am. J. Med., 52:141, 1972.
Heptinstall, R. H., and Joekes, A. M.: Renal amyloid: A report on 11 cases proven by renal biopsy. Ann. Rheum. Dis., 19:126, 1960.
Triger, D. R., and Joekes, A. M.: Renal amyloidosis — a fourteen-year followup. Quart. J. Med., 42:15, 1973.

DYSPROTEINEMIAS

Waldenström's Macroglobulinemia

Glomerular lesions consisting of IgM deposits within the capillary lumina and secondary amyloidosis represent the two most common renal lesions in Waldenström's macroglobulinemia. Clinically, kidney involvement is principally manifested by proteinuria, occasionally of the Bence Jones type, and hematuria. Acute renal failure is unusual. Interestingly, glomerular involvement with amyloid is seen more frequently in this disease than in multiple myeloma, and the presence of the nephrotic syndrome may be indicative of amyloidosis.

The glomerular lesions consist of eosinophilic thrombi within the capillary loops which are principally composed of IgM and, more rarely, kappa light chains. Interstitial infiltrates of plasma cells and lymphocytes in association with tubular atrophy are not uncommon. Current recommended therapy includes alkylating agents and plasmapheresis in selected patients.

Forget, B. G., Squires, J. W., and Sheldon, H.: Waldenström's macroglobulinemia with generalized amyloidosis. Arch. Intern. Med., 118:363, 1966.
Morel-Maroger, L., Basch, A., Danon, F., Verroust, P., and Richet, G.: Pathology of the kidney in Waldenström's macroglobulinemia: Study of sixteen cases. N. Engl. J. Med., 283:123, 1970.

Essential Cryoglobulinemia

Essential cryoglobulinemia, also referred to as mixed IgG-IgM cryoglobulinemia, is frequently associated with some form of renal involvement, usually a glomerulonephritis. It is estimated that 30 per cent of all patients with cryoglobulinemia fall into the essential category and manifest no underlying conditions such as autoimmune disease, infectious processes, or lymphoproliferative diseases. The renal involvement, which is seen in 20 per cent of the patients, may occur rather acutely and often follows exposure to cold or other stressful situations such as dehydration. In addition to overt glomerulonephritis, benign proteinuria or the nephrotic syndrome may be present. Clinical features of the illness other than renal involvement include fever, hepatosplenomegaly, purpuric and necrotizing skin lesions, and arthralgias. The IgG-IgM globulins possess rheumatoid activity, which may explain some of the aforementioned signs and symptoms of the disease.

Histologically, focal and generalized proliferative and membranous forms of glomerulonephritis have been observed. Eosinophilic intracapillary thrombi composed of IgG and IgM may also be present in the glomerular tufts. Immunofluorescence studies also reveal granular deposits of IgG, IgM, and C3 along glomerular capillary loops, providing support for an immune pathogenesis of the disease. Electron microscopy of the intracapillary deposits reveals a distinctive fibrillar pattern, which may represent a rather specific morphologic marker of glomerular disease associated with cryoglobulinemia.

Plasmapheresis has been employed to lower circulating IgG-IgM complexes with resultant reversal of the glomerular lesions. The efficacy of cytotoxic agents and corticosteroids has not been proved in clinical trials.

Brouet, J. C., Clauvel, J. P., Danon, F., Klein, M., and Seligmann, M.: Biologic and clinical significance of cryoglobulins. A report of 86 cases. Am. J. Med., 57:775, 1974.
Feiner, H., and Gallo, G.: Ultrastructure in glomerulonephritis associated with cryoglobulinemia. A report of six cases and review of the literature. Am. J. Pathol., 88:145, 1977.
Morel-Maroger, L., and Mery, J. P.: Renal lesions in mixed IgG-IgM essential cryoglobulinemia. In Villarreal, H. (ed.): Proceedings of the Fifth International Congress of Nephrology. Basel, S. Karger, 1972.

Benign Monoclonal Gammopathy

Patients with this entity exhibit a monoclonal elevation of serum immunoglobulin concentrations, including IgG, IgM, and IgA. These individuals are generally free of underlying diseases known to cause a rise in serum immunoglobulin levels such as malignancies, myeloma, infectious diseases, or macroglobulinemia. Renal involvement includes proteinuria, the nephrotic syndrome, and hematuria. Bence Jones protein has been found in the urine in a few patients. Severe renal failure is unusual in this population, but elevation of the BUN has been reported in many instances.

Histologically, PAS-negative eosinophilic deposits of immunoglobulins have been described in glomerular capillary loops which correspond to the particular Ig elevation in the patients' sera. Glomerular proliferation and amyloid deposition have also been reported. Crystalline structures, which undoubtedly represent immunoglobulins, have been observed with electron microscopy in glomerular mesangial and endothelial cells. A single case of membranous glomerulonephritis has been reported in this disease.

Morel-Maroger, L., and Verroust, P.: Glomerular lesions in dysproteinemias. Kidney Int., 5:249, 1974.
Waldenström, J.: The occurrence of benign, essential monoclonal (M type) non-macromolecular hyperglobulinemia and its differential diagnosis: IV. Studies in the gammapathies. Acta Med. Scand., 176:345, 1964.

375. VASCULAR DISORDERS OF THE KIDNEY

J. Caulie Gunnells, Jr.

375.1. RENAL INFARCTION FROM ARTERIAL THROMBI AND EMBOLI

Systemic hypertension or loss of functioning renal mass, or both, may occur as a result of vascular occlusions involving major or minor renal arteries or veins. Hypertension and renal failure occur more commonly following occlusive disease of the renal arterial than of the venous circulation. This chapter will be devoted primarily to the clinical consequences of acute renal arterial occlusive disease. The clinical features of renovascular hypertension are reviewed in detail in Ch. 361 and will therefore only be mentioned briefly as a concomitant of renal ischemia. In addition, since the end results of primary renal infarction from renal artery thrombi are essentially the same as those from renal emboli, these conditions will be considered together.

Not covered in this chapter are two forms of "functional" or "relative" renal ischemia leading to acute renal failure, usually without demonstrable intrinsic occlusive renal arterial lesions: acute tubular necrosis and acute renal cortical necrosis. These two widely different forms of acute renal failure incorporate unique alterations of the renal circulation and nephron function. They are discussed in detail in Ch. 372.

Renal infarction may be segmental or may involve the entire kidney. The degree or extent of ischemic injury reflects (1) the size and number of the renal artery or arteries involved, (2) the nature or type of vascular insult, (3) the extent of coexistent vascular or parenchymal renal disease, and (4) the presence and extent of capsular and collateral vessels. Fortunately, approximately 30 per cent of individuals have multiple main renal arteries, a well developed capsular circulation arising from vessels other than the main renal arteries, and a complex bifurcation of secondary and tertiary renal artery vessels. Therefore segmental rather than total renal infarction is a more common clinical event.

Renal arterial obstruction with infarction may occur as a result of thrombosis (superimposed on arteriosclerosis or fibrous dysplasia, aneurysm of the renal artery, aortic dissection, periarteritis nodosa, vasculitis, sickle cell disease, scleroderma, profound hypotension, and polycythemia) or embolism (mural thrombi or vegetations, cholesterol crystals or plaques, intravascular tumors [atrial myxoma], or foreign bodies). In addition, renal infarction is being recognized more frequently as a complication of severe trauma, with total interruption of the vascular supply to one or both kidneys. Therefore in the presence of extensive trauma, even in the absence of hematuria, it may be advisable to obtain early some diagnostic assessment of the integrity of the blood supply to the kidney.

CLINICAL PICTURE. The presence of total or segmental renal infarction is suspected with a history of flank pain or costovertebral angle tenderness, transient gross or microscopic hematuria, the recent onset of severe hypertension or the acceleration of prior hypertension, rapidly progressive renal failure without evidence of obstructive uropathy in the absence of other findings of coexistent parenchymal renal disease, signs and symptoms of severe peripheral vascular disease with an abdominal bruit, or evidence of abdominal aortic aneurysm.

Intravenous urography with nephrotomography may reveal absence of function in either one or both kidneys. Carefully performed midstream abdominal angiography with selective injection into each renal artery provides the necessary anatomic information concerning the extent and probable etiology of any demonstrable vascular occlusion. If indicated, catheterization of the renal veins for measurement of plasma renin activity may provide additional information relative to the presence or absence of renal ischemia and its contribution to any existent hypertension. This technique may have special value in segmental lesions of questionable clinical significance. The role of radioactive scintigrams, using the newer Anger camera techniques, deserves further investigation in the evaluation of these patients, because such procedures are not invasive and do not require the exposure of the patient to the potential toxicity of contrast media in the presence of a clinical setting in which rapidly deteriorating renal function may be important.

TREATMENT. In the presence of acute renal failure (oliguria or anuria), rapidly deteriorating renal function, or severe hypertension with the demonstration of renal infarction(s) secondary to thrombosis or embolus, endarterectomy or embolectomy should be considered and aggressively pursued with all attempts made to preserve or revascularize as much normal functioning renal tissue as possible. If there is coexistent vascular disease (i.e., aortic dissection), this should also be treated when possible. In the presence of emboli, the nature and source of the embolus should be determined, and in select cases concomitant anticoagulant therapy may be indicated.

The question arises as to the length of time that total renal artery occlusion may exist, with the hope of restoring some degree of renal function with subsequent operative intervention. Successful revascularizations (embolectomy, vascular bypass, and endarterectomy) of the kidney following oliguria and renal failure of up to 30 days' duration have been reported. The success of these surgical procedures depends upon the nature of the underlying lesion, coexistent vascular disease, and presence of collateral flow, together with the combined skill and experience of the surgeon and radiologist.

Besarab, A., Brown, R. S., Rubin, N. T., Salzman, E., Wirhlin, L., Steinman, T., Atlia, R. R., and Skillman, J. A.: Reversible renal failure following bilateral renal artery occlusive disease. JAMA, 235:2838, 1976.

Gulbrandson, R. N., Al-Bermani, J., and Gaspard, D. J.: Successful renal revascularization after prolonged nonfunction. JAMA, 238:2522, 1977.

Krumlovsky, F. A., Simon, N., Santhanam, S., del Greco, F., Roxe, D., and Pomaranc, M. M.: Acute renal failure. Association with administration of radiographic contrast material. JAMA, 239:125, 1978.

Perkins, R. P., Jacobsen, D. S., Feder, F. P., Lipchik, E. O., and Fine, P. H.: Return of renal function after late embolectomy. N. Engl. J. Med., 276:1194, 1972.

375.2. RENAL VEIN THROMBOSIS

The association of renal vein thrombosis and heavy proteinuria with clinical features of the nephrotic syndrome is well documented and dates to the observations of Rayer in 1837. Since then, many isolated cases and relatively large series of patients with renal vein thrombosis have been reported. However, only recently with the development and widespread use of newer and more sophisticated radiologic techniques has the relatively high frequency of renal vein thrombosis been appreciated ante mortem in patients with nephrotic syndrome. This observation, together with the correlation of histopathology from renal biopsy specimens, has led to changing concepts in the significance, pathogenesis, treatment, and prognosis of renal vein thrombosis.

Renal vein thrombosis may occur as a primary or secondary event, or as an acute or chronic process. In addition, it may be bilateral or unilateral and may involve the main or major renal vein, smaller renal venous radicles, or both. In the adult population the chronic and secondary variety is usually present and has been associated with heavy proteinuria. Most patients frequently exhibit all features of the nephrotic syndrome, regardless of the extent or location of anatomic involvement. The acute and primary variety almost always occurs in children, usually under the age of two years, and occurs in a clinical setting of an acute illness characterized by volume contraction, dehydration, gastroenteritis, and a fulminant, rapidly progressive, and often fatal clinical course with bilateral hemorrhagic renal infarction. The remainder of this discussion will be directed to the more common adult form of chronic renal venous thrombosis and its associated clinical features.

Renal vein thrombosis has recently been shown to be present in 33 to 50 per cent of patients with nephrotic syndrome secondary to membranous glomerulopathy and membranoproliferative glomerulonephritis. Renal vein thrombosis secondary to primary or coexistent renal disease is the most commonly encountered clinical variety of renal vein thrombosis in the adult population. In addition to its association with the two renal lesions mentioned, it is also very common in renal amyloidosis. There are also isolated reports of its association with the nephrotic syndrome of focal sclerosing glomerulopathy, systemic lupus erythematosus, and other infrequent forms of primary parenchymal renal disease. Renal vein thrombosis has been reported to occur with low frequency or to be absent in patients with minimal change or nil lesion nephrotic syndrome (lipoid nephrosis) and diabetic nephropathy. Renal vein thrombosis may also occur in association with thrombosis of the inferior vena cava and secondary involvement of the renal vein(s). It has also been observed to occur with intrinsic or extrinsic compression of the renal veins from neoplasm. In addition, renal vein thrombosis has been reported in association with congestive heart failure, pregnancy, constrictive pericarditis, trauma, and morbid obesity. As noted previously, renal vein thrombosis is rarely a primary event in the adult population.

CLINICAL SETTING. Clinical features of renal vein thrombosis are, for the most part, those of nephrotic syndrome — namely, massive edema and proteinuria.

On rare occasions, flank pain in association with gross or microhematuria may occur. Systemic hypertension is not uncommon. Rarely the patient may present with thromboembolism (pulmonary emboli) as the initial manifestation of renal vein thrombosis.

LABORATORY FEATURES. The urinalysis exhibits heavy qualitative proteinuria with quantitative protein excretion in the nephrotic range (see Ch. 374.2 for other biochemical features of the nephrotic syndrome). Attention has been directed toward two features of renal vein thrombosis; protein excretion is usually markedly increased, and there is a high incidence of initially decreased renal function, with a more rapid decline in glomerular filtration rate. A recent report has observed pyuria (without evidence of bacterial infection of the urinary tract), glycosuria, and hyperchloremic acidosis, and has presented evidence of a functional proximal tubular defect in patients with renal vein thrombosis.

Intravenous urography may demonstrate enlarged renal outlines with stretching of the calyces secondary to interstitial edema. The subsequent development of venous collaterals produces scalloping of the upper portion of the ureter. Conclusive anatomic diagnosis of renal vein thrombosis is best established by phlebography of the inferior vena cava and both renal veins. Diagnostic accuracy of phlebography may be improved by simultaneous injection of epinephrine into the renal artery to reduce vascular flow, thereby improving the quality of the films demonstrating renal venous filling.

HISTOPATHOLOGY. The major histologic features of renal vein thrombosis reflect the associated underlying renal disease as previously noted. However, several features have received emphasis: patients with renal vein thrombosis may show relatively more interstitial edema and fibrosis as compared to patients with identical varieties of primary renal disease but without associated renal vein thrombosis; a peculiar glomerular margination and stasis of leukocytes may be observed; and venous capillary thrombi are rare. However, fibrin deposition in some renal venous channels has recently been demonstrated by immunofluorescent techniques.

Glomerular evaluation by immunofluorescence and electron microscopic techniques has failed to yield specific or diagnostic changes in renal vein thrombosis, except as related to an underlying primary glomerular process, e.g., membranous glomerulopathy or membranoproliferative glomerulonephritis.

Histologic evaluation of the contralateral kidney in unilateral renal vein thrombosis has demonstrated similar or identical findings as in the ipsilateral kidney, thereby offering additional evidence as to the pathogenetic importance of the underlying primary renal disease, with renal vein thrombosis occurring as a probable secondary event.

PROGNOSIS. Patients with renal vein thrombosis and underlying primary parenchymal renal disease have a poorer prognosis than patients with similar forms of renal disease without renal vein thrombosis. They exhibit, as a group, a more rapid deterioration in renal function and greater degrees of proteinuria. In the absence of renal functional loss, the other most important factor in an unfavorable prognosis for these patients is the demonstration of existent or potential extrarenal thromboembolic episodes. Careful assessment for evidence of pulmonary embolization is of particular importance. It has been recommended that baseline noninvasive radioactive pulmonary scans be obtained in patients with renal vein thrombosis as an aid in establishing prognosis and making clinical decisions relative to therapy.

TREATMENT. To date the role of surgery in the treatment of chronic renal vein thrombosis has not been established. However, surgical therapy at an appropriate time may prove beneficial in the acute variety.

Anticoagulation remains the mainstay of therapy, primarily because of the ever-present threat of recurrent extrarenal thromboembolism. Unfortunately, treatment must be extended for long periods of time and is not without additional problems in patients with renal disease.

Adrenocortical steroids and cytotoxic drugs may be indicated for the underlying primary renal disease. However, in view of a possible thrombotic tendency in steroid-treated patients, their use in patients with renal vein thrombosis needs careful consideration.

Cade, R., Spooner, G., Juncos, L., et al.: Chronic renal vein thrombosis. Am. J. Med., 63:387, 1977.

Harrison, C. V., Milne, M. D., and Steiner, R. E.: Clinical aspects of renal vein thrombosis. Quart. J. Med., 25:285, 1956.

Llach, F., Koffler, A., Finch, E., et al.: On the incidence of renal vein thrombosis in the nephrotic syndrome. Arch. Intern. Med., 137:333, 1977.

Rosenmann, E., Pollak, V. E., and Pirani, C. L.: Renal vein thrombosis in the adult: A clinical and pathological study based on renal biopsies. Medicine, 42:269, 1968.

Trevor, P. A., Biava, C. G., Jacobs, R. P., et al.: Renal vein thrombosis in membranous glomerulopathy. Medicine, 57:69, 1978.

376. URINARY TRACT INFECTIONS AND PYELONEPHRITIS

Calvin M. Kunin

DEFINITION. The phrase urinary tract infection is a broad term used to describe both bacterial colonization of the urine and invasion of structures in any part of the urinary tract. Urine is ordinarily sterile. Colonization of the urine, that is, multiplication of large numbers of bacteria in the urine, is often difficult to distinguish from actual tissue invasion eliciting a host response, because of the frequent tendency of urinary tract infections to exhibit either few or no symptoms. This phenomenon is known as *asymptomatic bacteriuria.* At any given time, an individual may have bacteriuria alone, or bacteriuria with silent tissue invasion, or bacteriuria accompanied by signs of inflammation of the bladder (*cystitis*) or kidneys (*pyelonephritis*). Infections of the structures of the urinary tract are usually accompanied by colonization of the urine which bathes the kidney, ureter, bladder, and urethra. Thus bacteriuria is the most common denominator of urinary tract infections. Bacteriuria may be absent, however, when the infected focus is not contiguous with the urine as in early lesions of hematogenous pyelonephritis, when there is marked obstruction of the affected portion of the tract or when it is masked by antimicrobial therapy. Bacteriuria does not necessarily indicate that the patient has pyelonephritis or cystitis. Rather, it is an important and generally reliable laboratory finding that indicates an abnormal situation, reflecting either the presence of or potential for infection of the urinary tract. It is an excellent guide to early diagnosis and evaluation of therapy, because signs and symptoms of infection may be absent or disappear without bacteriologic cure.

The term *pyelonephritis* refers to immediate and residual effects of bacterial infection in the kidney. The clinical manifestations are generally conceived of as existing in two forms: *acute pyelonephritis,* an active pyogenic infection, usually accompanied by local and systemic symptoms of infection; and *chronic pyelonephritis,* wherein the principal manifestations are caused by the injury sustained in preceding active infections. Chronic bacterial pyelonephritis can be further subdivided into *active* and *inactive* forms. The *active* form usually occurs in patients with persistent infection *complicated* by a major abnormality of the voiding mechanism or with a persistent nidus of infection in renal or bladder calculi, in the prostate, or with continuous indwelling catheters. The *inactive* form consists of focal sterile scars of a past infection. Recurrent infection can result in multiple scars combined with active foci of infection.

There has been considerable controversy in the literature concerning the relation between episodes of urinary tract infection and the development of the shrunken scarred kidney of end-stage chronic bacterial pyelonephritis. It is now clear that, although in rare instances acute pyelonephritis *uncomplicated* by neurologic or obstructive lesions may leave residual focal scars, progression to a shrunken kidney is distinctly unusual, except in patients with diabetes, or unless "infection" stones develop and convert the patient to the complicated group. In contrast, paraplegics who require continuous indwelling urinary catheters frequently develop end-stage chronic active pyelonephritis.

Another confusing point is that many other noninfectious disease states can produce renal lesions that mimic those produced by active bacterial infection. The major characteristic of bacterial pyelonephritis observed on intravenous pyelography is blunting and distortion of the renal calyces and corresponding areas of focal cortical atrophy. Identical findings are observed in patients who, during childhood, suffered from severe grades of vesicoureteral reflux. This entity is termed *reflux nephropathy.* There is still considerable debate as to whether or not infection must accompany reflux to produce these lesions. Nevertheless, the combination of recurrent infection and reflux nephropathy can result in chronic active pyelonephritis. So-called "nonbacterial" pyelonephritis, in which there is no history of urinary tract infection but the patient has end-stage renal failure with scarred shrunken kidneys, may be the result of reflux nephropathy and not bacterial pyelonephritis. *Analgesic nephropathy* may result in papillary necrosis and may also mimic bacterial pyelonephritis on x-ray.

The normal urinary tract is free of bacteria except near the external urethral meatus. In both sexes, some organisms are normally present in the distal urethra. These are usually similar to the flora of the skin, and frequently consist of staphylococci and diphtheroids. Urine is a variable culture medium, depending upon pH, tonicity, and its constituents. High concentrations of urea, low pH, hyperosmolality, and products of dietary organic acids are generally unfavorable to bacteria. In addition, the dynamics of urine flow, or washout, and antibacterial properties of the lining membrane of the urinary tract appear to be important defense mechanisms.

The large bowel is considered to be the reservoir of most of the bacteria that invade the urinary tract because of the high frequency of coliforms found in urinary tract infection. Several possible pathways from the lumen of the intestine to the urinary passages and kidney can be postulated. The principal possibilities are the hematogenous, the lymphatic, and the "ascending" routes. The "ascending" pathway, involving migration of bacteria from the anus to the periurethral zone and through the urethra to the bladder, is the most favored at present. This route can be demonstrated experimentally, particularly in the presence of obstruction or of a foreign body. It also fits in well with the very much higher rate of urinary infections in the female, whose urethra is shorter than that of the male, and with the marked frequency of urinary infections associated with instrumentation of the urethra and bladder. Clear instances of the hematogenous origin of urinary infection have been demonstrated, particularly in the presence of staphylococcal or gram-negative bacteremia, but these are relatively less common.

PATHOLOGY. Knowledge of the pathologic process is meager because uncomplicated acute pyelonephritis does not lead to death. Nevertheless, on the basis of occasional chance opportunities and experiments in animals, it is possible to describe the probable form of the lesion with reasonable assurance. One or both kidneys may be affected. The lining of the renal pelvis and calyces is diffusely inflamed. Infection of the renal substance is usually confined to one or more wedge-shaped areas, the apices being in the medulla. In this zone of acute inflammation there are microabscesses, some of which may bulge under the capsule of the kidney, but rarely they rupture into the perinephric area, producing *perinephric abscess*. Collections of polymorphonuclear leukocytes can be seen in and around the lumina of the tubules throughout their length. The glomeruli are usually spared structurally, but may become functionless because the tubular part of the nephron is destroyed. The infectious process tends to remain confined within the originally involved segment of renal tissue and to subside gradually over a period of one to three weeks. As healing takes place, the area contracts, polymorphonuclear leukocytes are replaced by mononuclear cells, and scar tissue is deposited. Eventually a linear scar involving a streak of medulla and corresponding cortical tissue is all that remains. Remnants of glomeruli and tubules filled with a colloid-like material lie in this fibrous matrix.

A considerable amount of work has been done on the pathogenesis of pyelonephritis in laboratory animals. The kidney can be infected either by the intravenous route or by introducing bacteria into the urinary tract; the lesion is the same regardless of the route of inoculation. In order to infect the kidney by way of the bloodstream it is necessary to inject large numbers of bacteria, probably because only a minute proportion of the inoculum is trapped by the kidney. As a general rule, coliform bacteria, although the most common cause of human pyelonephritis, are incapable of infecting a normal kidney, although pathogenic strains of *Staphylococcus*, enterococcus, occasional strains of *Proteus,* and rare strains of coliform organisms will do so. In the presence of an obstructive lesion, however, the susceptibility of the kidney to infection by all these bacteria, including the coliforms, is greatly increased. Obstruction

has been produced by introducing artificial calculi into the bladder, by partial or complete ureteral ligation, or by mechanical injury of the kidney. Even small injuries of the medulla caused by needle puncture lead to obstruction of a few collecting tubules and localized susceptibility to infection. Experiments of this kind have demonstrated that bacterial multiplication begins in the medulla and then spreads into the corresponding area of cortex. It is thought, therefore, that infection spreads in retrograde manner from the obstructed collecting tubules in the medulla throughout the nephron. Characteristic wedge-shaped areas of acute pyelonephritis involving both medulla and cortex are also produced when small numbers of bacteria, e.g., 10 to 100 living organisms, are inoculated into the medulla. By contrast, as many as 100,000 coliform bacteria must be inoculated into the cortex in order to establish even local infection. A conspicuous feature of the areas of acute pyelonephritis produced in laboratory animals is lack of tendency for infection to invade neighboring, unobstructed areas of renal parenchyma. The process remains confined to the area of intrarenal hydronephrosis, eventually "burns out," and shrinks to a scar, leaving adjacent kidney unaffected. This seems compatible with acute pyelonephritis in man, wherein there is usually no measurable evidence of even temporary impairment of renal function other than a defect in concentrating ability. Evidence obtained in animals indicates that the medullary zone is the critical one from the standpoint of pathogenesis of acute bacterial infection. Factors that may be responsible include the following: (1) *Ammonia formation.* Evidence has been obtained that high local concentration of ammonia, as may be present when the body is dealing with an acid load, may be sufficient to inactivate complement, thus rendering ineffective a major defense mechanism against bacterial infection. (2) *Hypertonicity.* The unusual osmolarity in this area of the body may be sufficient to affect the activity of complement and phagocytes, as well as to permit survival of bacterial protoplasts. (3) *Differences in the blood supply.* The blood flow to the medulla is far less than that to the cortex and is a limiting factor in mobilizing leukocytes to the affected region.

CLINICAL MANIFESTATIONS. Symptoms of cystitis and urethritis include frequency of urination, burning pain on urination, and passage of cloudy, occasionally blood-tinged urine. The patient may complain of a foul odor to the urine, lassitude, and suprapubic discomfort. Fever and leukocytosis are rarely evident in urinary tract infection confined to the bladder and urethra; as a general rule, their presence should be looked upon as evidence of infection of the upper part of the tract. Nevertheless, absence of fever and leukocytosis does not by any means exclude the possibility of kidney involvement.

The clinical picture of acute pyelonephritis may be characteristic: sudden rise of body temperature to 38.9 to 40.6° C, shaking chills, aching pain in one or both costovertebral areas or flanks, and symptoms of bladder inflammation. Physical examination reveals tenderness in the region of one or both kidneys; at times a tender kidney may be detected by palpation. Laboratory tests show polymorphonuclear leukocytosis, and the urine is laden with leukocytes. Stain of the sediment reveals numerous bacteria, usually gram-negative bacilli, and culture confirms this. In a small proportion of cases blood culture is also positive. There are no signs of impaired renal function or of acute hypertension as is sometimes seen in acute glomerulonephritis.

In the absence of an obstructive lesion of the urinary tract, such as stone or tumor, this illness is self-limited, rarely lasting more than a week or ten days.

The clinical picture just described is easy to recognize and is seldom confused with anything else. Yet there must also be subclinical forms, because tests which differentiate "upper" (kidney) from "lower" (bladder) infection often indicate the presence of infection of the kidney in the absence of flank pain or fever. Procedures such as ureteral catheterization, bladder washout maneuvers, and search for antibody-coated bacteria are considered as research studies. Pyelonephritis at times presents with symptoms that do not point to the urinary tract. Dysuria may be lacking, and there may be no fever. There may only be backache, without demonstrable tenderness in the kidney region. Some patients have pain in either the upper or the lower abdomen, together with symptoms of disturbed gastrointestinal function. Others complain only of general fatigue.

Acute urinary tract infection, complicated by pyelonephritis, frequently arises in patients subjected to urethral instrumentation, especially the indwelling catheter. In such people the infection may take a fulminating course, with bacteremia and shock, and can in fact be the terminal event of prolonged illness. Gram-negative sepsis and bacteremic shock are described in Ch. 154.

Chronic active pyelonephritis is usually limited to patients with complicated infections (as described above). Patients often suffer from recurrent episodes of acute pyelonephritis or may have persistent smoldering infections which gradually result in end-stage renal failure. This process may persist for many years and be complicated by generalized debility, anemia of chronic infection, secondary amyloidosis, and, terminally, proteinuria and severe hypertension and its complications. Uncontrolled infection may lead to extension of infection into the surrounding renal fat pad and produce perinephric abscess. This may be exceedingly difficult to diagnose without use of radiologic and scanning procedures. It should be suspected when persistent flank pain, fever, and leukocytosis are unresponsive to otherwise adequate chemotherapy. Surgical drainage is usually required.

Course. The symptoms of inflammation of the urinary tract tend to disappear after several days even without bacteriologic cure. Recurrence of symptomatic infection is frequent in this group. Bacteriuria also tends to be highly recurrent. Persistence of fever and leukocytosis strongly suggest the presence of obstruction to flow of urine by stones or other mechanical means or a large renal or perinephric abscess. In the unobstructed female patient, recurrence is usually associated with reinfection with a new bacterial strain. Early recurrence, however, may be due to emergence of bacteria from a partially suppressed focus. Persistent infection with the same organisms should alert the physician to the presence of obstruction, calculus, or neurogenic lesions. Frequent follow-up examination of the patient's urine is essential to the management to be described below.

CONCEPT OF SIGNIFICANT BACTERIURIA. Bacteriuria literally means the presence of bacteria in the urine.

The concept of "significant bacteriuria" was introduced to distinguish between bacteria that are actually multiplying in the urine from contaminants in collection vessels, periurethral tissues, the urethra itself, and gross fecal or vaginal contamination. This separation can be accomplished by knowledge of the site and manner in which the urine is collected from the patient and enumeration of the number of organisms present in the sample. The criterion of 100,000 or more organisms per milliliter of urine for diagnosis of significant bacteriuria is an excellent *operational definition* when the clean voided method is used to collect specimens. It is based on the finding that contaminants will usually be present at numbers ranging from 1000 to 10,000 per milliliter. Organisms found in urinary tract infections grow well in urine; they usually achieve concentrations of greater than 100,000, and are often in the range of 1 to 10 million per milliliter. With proper instruction and cleansing, and prompt processing or refrigeration of specimens, it is usually not difficult to obtain reliable results by the clean voided method in both males and females. It is emphasized that, because the reliability of the method will differ with experience and care, it is often wise to avoid overdiagnosis by obtaining multiple specimens, particularly in the asymptomatic patient. Thus survey and screening procedures for bacteriuria generally require two or three consecutive positive specimens, indicating that the patient has "persistent significant bacteriuria." Bacterial counts lower than 100,000 per milliliter may occur in patients with true bacteriuria, but when the clean voided method is used, these counts can only be established as valid when shown to be persistent and when the same species of bacteria and preferably the same serotype can be repeatedly isolated. Bacterial counts are higher when urine is allowed to incubate for some time in the bladder. A first morning specimen is preferrred, but is not essential. Low or borderline counts may be due to dilution in a well-hydrated patient.

Aseptic methods of collection of urine such as from the renal pelvis or ureter, or by bladder puncture, *permit the diagnosis of significant bacteriuria regardless of the number of organisms found*, provided that the specimen is not contaminated prior to culture.

Screening for asymptomatic bacteriuria among females and treatment of this condition are based on the concept that urinary tract infections result in considerable morbidity, even though "uncomplicated" infection rarely results in end-stage renal disease. Screening of young girls is often the only means which permits early detection of correctable anatomic lesions such as severe grades of vesicoureteral reflux. Screening during early pregnancy and treatment of infection appear to prevent delivery of low birth weight infants. Urinary infections are too rare in boys and young men to warrant routine screening.

BACTERIOLOGIC FINDINGS. The species of bacteria most likely to be recovered in individuals with bacteriuria depends, for the most part, upon previous history of infection, receipt of antimicrobial therapy, hospitalization, and instrumentation of the urinary tract. In this respect, the bacterial flora found in individuals with asymptomatic bacteriuria is no different from that in cases of clinically obvious pyelonephritis. Enterobacteriaceae are by far the most common organisms identified. *E. coli* generally accounts for more than 80 per cent of all species recovered in so-called uncomplicated cases, whereas *Proteus, Klebsiella, Enterobacter, Pseudomonas aeruginosa*, enterococci, and *Staphylococcus aureus* are more likely to be found in patients who have had previous infection or instrumentation (the so-called complicated group). Occasionally, organisms such as *Serratia marcescens, Acinetobacter, Candida albicans,* and even *Cryptococcus neoformans* may be significant and produce disease in diabetics and in patients treated with corticosteroids and immunosuppressive agents. Diphtheroids, *Staphylococcus epidermidis,* and microaerophilic streptococci are highly suspect as contaminants. They usually will not be isolated on repeated culture. They should not, however, be dismissed if repeatedly recovered under optimal conditions of collection.

Despite the abundance of anaerobic flora in the gut, they are rare in urinary infections, owing to the poor growth of these organisms in urine.

Microscopic Methods. Rapid diagnostic methods are available either by preparation of a Gram stain of unsedimented urine and examination with an oil immersion lens, or by study of the centrifuged urinary sediment for bacteria, employing the high dry objective under reduced light with or without the addition of methylene blue. The Gram stain has been the most widely used of these methods and correlates about 80 to 90 per cent with quantitative culture. Examination of the unstained sediment as prepared for search for formed elements in the urine is very helpful. It is much less time consuming than preparation of a stained slide, and can be done in conjunction with the routine examination for formed elements. The criterion for a positive sediment is the presence of many (preferably more than 20) obvious bacteria. The presence of marked pyuria can mask bacteria in the sediment. Fresh urine is required, because crystals will also obscure the bacteria. If crystals do form, the urine should be warmed until they dissolve.

Ten or more leukocytes per high-powered field in the centrifuged specimen is usually accepted as representing pyuria. When inflammation of the bladder mucosa is intense, there may be some erythrocytes in the urine, and gross hematuria sometimes occurs. *Proteinuria* is not common in urinary infections.

EPIDEMIOLOGY AND NATURAL HISTORY. Extensive epidemiologic studies have provided information of the frequency of bacteriuria in various populations. Bacteriuria in the newborn period has been difficult to define because of problems inherent in collection, but information is being obtained with the widespread use of the bladder puncture method. Infection of the urinary tract in this age group may be part of a generalized, life-threatening gram-negative sepsis, and is more common in boys than girls. Symptomatic urinary infections, particularly among girls, are prominent in the preschool years, and are frequently associated with important obstructive or neurogenic lesions. Urologic investigation is extremely valuable in this age group. *It is mandatory in males of any age because of the high frequency of important structural abnormalities* found (valves, malformations, obstructive and neurogenic lesions). The prevalence of bacteriuria among schoolgirls is 1.2 per cent; it is only 0.03 per cent in boys of the same age. The incidence rate in girls is 0.4 per cent per year; it is linear with time throughout the school years and is unaffected by menarche. The cumulative frequency of

urinary infection in girls occurring at one time or another during the school years exceeds 5 per cent. Bacteriuria in girls is independent of socioeconomic status and race, and is not increased in diabetic girls. The prevalence of bacteriuria in females rises about 1 per cent per decade. Urinary infection is common after marriage. The "honeymoon cystitis" syndrome may be due to either infection or local irritation, and these should be clearly differentiated by culture. Bacteriuria in pregnancy varies from 2 to 6 per cent, depending upon age, parity, and socioeconomic groups. Early detection and treatment of bacteriuria in pregnancy will prevent the emergence of symptomatic infection. Elderly women may have frequencies of bacteriuria as high as 10 per cent; this rate may rise even higher in hospitalized patients, particularly diabetics. Bacteriuria in the male begins to appear in the "prostate" years, and is often initiated by instrumentation.

Role of Instrumentation. Persistent bacteriuria follows single catheterizations in relatively healthy individuals at a frequency of 1 to 2 per cent; the risk is much higher in the debilitated patient and in males with prostatic obstruction. With open indwelling catheter drainage bacterial colonization exceeds 90 per cent within three to four days. This may lead to life-threatening pyelonephritis and gram-negative sepsis. Fortunately, it is partially avoidable by (1) careful preselection of criteria for catheterization, and (2) use of aseptic closed drainage or antimicrobial bladder rinse during prolonged catheterization. The catheter should be removed as soon as it is no longer needed. (3) Intermittent self-catheterization may be of great benefit in patients with neurogenic bladders.

RENAL MEDULLARY NECROSIS
(Renal Papillary Necrosis, Necrotizing Papillitis)

Renal medullary necrosis is a severe complication of pyelonephritis — ischemic necrosis of the renal papilla and adjacent portions of the renal medulla. The lesion is most often, though not invariably, associated with severe acute and chronic pyelonephritis. It is especially common in patients with diabetes and pyelonephritis, about half the reported cases having involved such persons. Obstruction of the urinary tract is also a predisposing factor, aggravating infection in the kidney. Analgesic nephropathy is observed in individuals, particularly in Europe and Australia, who ingest large quantities of analgesic medicines for headache. Although phenacetin is a common ingredient, it has not proved to be the sole etiologic agent. The lesion is more common in women and may be complicated by urinary tract infection.

Although infection appears to be the most important factor in the pathogenesis of this lesion, there can be little doubt that the peculiarities of blood supply of the medulla must also be factors. This could help to explain the frequent occurrence of the lesion in patients with diabetes and generalized vascular disease, as well as the role of obstruction, which must impair the blood supply of this area.

The zone of necrosis may occur throughout the pyramid from the extreme tip as far proximally as the corticomedullary junction. Eventually this usually sloughs, so that chunks of necrotic tissue often migrate down through the urinary passages.

The clinical manifestations of renal medullary necrosis are intensification of symptoms of pre-existing pyelonephritis. There may be pain in the lumbar region, colicky pain along the ureteral radiation, and hematuria. Fever may be high. Manifestations of gram-negative bacteremia may supervene. This lesion should be considered always in elderly patients with diabetes who show rapid deterioration in clinical status with signs of active pyelonephritis and increasing renal decompensation.

The diagnosis can sometimes be made by finding pieces of renal medullary tissue in the urine sediment. Pyelography may also be of assistance: in addition to the scarring and asymmetry of chronic pyelonephritis, cavities and sinuses in the region of the papillae may be demonstrated.

Therapy should be directed toward control of infection and measures employed to improve the status of patients who have diabetes mellitus or who are habitual abusers of analgesic medicines.

MANAGEMENT. The therapeutic principles are similar for all urinary infections, including bacteriuria, cystitis, or pyelonephritis. *Recognition and relief of obstruction are essential.* Therapy is then directed to sterilization of the urine and careful follow-up to detect recurrence, using significant bacteriuria as a guide. Infections uncomplicated by obstruction or many previous episodes will generally respond to oral therapy with sulfonamides, tetracycline, ampicillin, nalidixic acid, cephalexin, co-trimoxazole (trimethoprim plus sulfamethoxazole), or nitrofurantoin. The last two drugs are particularly useful in recurrent infections because of relatively less frequency of emergence of resistant strains. The trimethoprim component of co-trimoxazole probably accounts for the remarkable efficacy of this combination in decreasing the colonization of the periurethral area by enteric gram-negative bacteria. Nitrofurantoin should not be used to treat systemic infection and is contraindicated in the presence of any degree of azotemia, because adequate concentrations cannot be achieved in the urine under these conditions. Oral preparations of carbenicillin are reserved for *Pseudomonas* infection. Drugs are selected on the basis of relative cost, side effects, and antimicrobial susceptibility, all of which may be highly variable. Antimicrobial susceptibility tests should be used to guide therapy of recurrent episodes. The initial attack is usually due to *E. coli*, which is sensitive to most of the commonly used agents. It may be treated "blindly" with a sulfonamide, ampicillin, or tetracycline with about equal probability of success; however, the widespread use of these agents for other infections has decreased their previous reliability. Bacteria should disappear within 24 to 48 hours even if pyuria and symptoms continue. It is important to recognize bacteriologic failure early and change to another drug. Generally, short courses of treatment, from 10 to 14 days, are quite adequate; short-term high-dose therapy, sometimes with parenteral agents such as ampicillin, a cephalosporin, or gentamicin, may be required in some instances of failure with lower doses or when the patient is too ill to receive an oral agent. Recurrence within a few weeks after treatment is usually due to persistence of the same focus, whereas later recurrence, particularly in females, is more often the result of reinfection. Highly recurrent infections may be managed by either very close follow-up and treatment of each episode or by prophylaxis with nitrofurantoin, co-trimoxazole, or nalidixic acid given as single bedtime doses. Urinary antiseptics such as methenamine mandelate or hippurate are less effective and *require an acid urine,* preferably at pH 5.5. This may be achieved by addition of a high protein diet, ammonium chloride, ascorbic acid, or methionine. Methionine is an effective acidifier, but it may have to be given in doses as high as 10 grams per day. The dose can be titrated downward by measuring urinary pH. They are best used *after* infection is eradicated by more effective drugs. They may occasionally be useful as "suppressive" agents in complicated infection, but their efficacy is very limited. Prophylaxis should not be given for more than three to six months if at all possible. Cessation of prophylaxis permits reassessment of the patient. Prophylaxis can then be reinstituted if infections frequently recur. The drug must be changed if bacteriuria persists or recurs during treatment. This usually means that an organism insusceptible to the agent is now colonizing the urine. *Prophylaxis is ineffective in patients with indwelling urinary catheters and will only lead to emergence of resistant bacteria.*

The patient should be instructed to drink fluids generously and void frequently. Double voiding in patients with vesicoureteral reflux is recommended. Voiding after intercourse is felt to decrease the chance of recurrent infection but bedtime use of prophylactic agents is probably more effective. *Frequent follow-up to detect silent recurrence* is the key to good management. Quantitative urine cultures ideally should be done once monthly for the first three months after each infection and then at three-month intervals for at least two years. Recurrence even after several years of freedom from infection is not uncommon in females.

Complex urinary infections, that is, those in the presence of obstructive uropathy, neurogenic bladders, or catheters, are exceedingly difficult to eradicate. The key to management is relief of obstruction or removal of foreign bodies. Intermittent catheterization has been shown to be of great benefit in patients with neurogenic bladders. Sepsis in these cases is usually precipitated by obstruction, which should be promptly relieved. Antimicrobial therapy is discussed in Ch. 154. *Bacteriuria in the aged* is frequent, usually uncomplicated, and highly recurrent. It should not be overzealously treated if simple measures fail, because toxicity and expense of therapy may outweigh the risk of disease.

Bailey, R. R.: The relationship of vesico-ureteric reflux to urinary tract infection and chronic pyelonephritis — reflux nephropathy. Clin. Nephrol., 1:132, 1973.

Bengtsson, U.: A comparative study of chronic non-obstructive pyelonephritis and renal papillary necrosis. Acta Med. Scand. (Suppl.), 388, 1962.

Kaye, D. (ed.): Urinary Tract Infection and Its Management. St. Louis, C. V. Mosby Company, 1972.

Kunin, C. M.: Detection, Prevention and Treatment of Urinary Tract Infections, 2nd ed. Philadelphia, Lea & Febiger, 1974.

Norden, C. W., and Kass, E. H.: Bacteriuria of pregnancy — a critical appraisal. Ann. Rev. Med., 19:431, 1968.

O'Grady, F., and Brumfitt, W.: Urinary Tract Infection. London, Oxford University Press, 1968.

Stamey, T. A., Condy, M., and Mihara, G.: Prophylactic efficacy of nitrofurantoin macrocrystals and trimethoprim-sulfamethoxazole in urinary infections: Biologic effects on the vaginal and rectal flora. N. Engl. J. Med., 296:780, 1977.

Thomas, V. L., Shelokov, A., and Forland, M.: Antibody-coated bacteria in the urine and the site of urinary tract infection. N. Engl. J. Med., 290:588, 1974.

377. RENAL DISEASE IN PREGNANCY

Thomas F. Ferris

Because pregnancy is occasionally associated with edema, hypertension, and proteinuria, pre-existent renal disease in a pregnant woman has traditionally been viewed with alarm. However, the majority of women with renal disease can, with proper medical care, have an uncomplicated pregnancy. In most women, pregnancy does not worsen renal disease or adversely affect the ultimate prognosis.

GLOMERULONEPHRITIS

The development of *acute glomerulonephritis* during pregnancy usually results in fetal death. Differentiation between acute glomerulonephritis and preeclampsia may be difficult if the disease occurs late in pregnancy, but the presence of microscopic hematuria with cellular and hyaline casts is most consistent with glomerulonephritis. The treatment of the disease is similar to that in the nonpregnant patient, with careful control of blood pressure and fluid balance. The danger of pregnancy in women with *chronic glomerulonephritis* is the increased incidence of preeclampsia. When proteinuria is the only manifestation of chronic glomerulonephritis, the incidence of preeclampsia is 35 per cent, with fetal survival around 80 per cent. If azotemia and hypertension precede the pregnancy, the incidence of preeclampsia rises to over 75 per cent, with fetal survival less than 40 per cent. The level of azotemia and hypertension best correlates with the risk of preeclampsia and fetal loss. Control of hypertension throughout pregnancy and careful observation of BUN, creatinine, and uric acid, particularly in the last trimester, are essential for a successful pregnancy. When preeclampsia develops early, termination of the pregnancy is indicated, because there is little chance for fetal survival in this group, and the renal disease may worsen.

NEPHROTIC SYNDROME

Although proteinuria may increase in nephrotics during pregnancy, probably because of the increase in glomerular filtration rate, there is no convincing evidence that the renal disease is worsened. The risk of pregnancy is similar to that in patients with chronic glomerulonephritis; with hypertension or azotemia the incidence of toxemia and fetal loss is increased. However, in nephrotics, birth weight correlates with serum albumin levels and severe hypoproteinemia often results in prematurity. Also infection, particularly of the urinary tract, may be more frequent, possibly because of the associated hypogammaglobulinemia. Thromboembolism during pregnancy and in the puerperium is more common in nephrotics, and conversely renal vein thrombosis may be a cause of the nephrotic syndrome developing in pregnancy. Venous stasis caused by the gravid uterus as well as the increase in clotting factors which occurs during pregnancy may predispose to development of both peripheral and renal vein thrombosis.

PYELONEPHRITIS

Acute pyelonephritis occurs in approximately 1 per cent of pregnant women, but in 30 per cent of women who have bacteriuria greater than 100,000 organisms per milliliter on their first prenatal visit. The incidence of bacteriuria is no greater in pregnancy, but the higher incidence of pyelonephritis is attributable to the dilatation of the urinary tract which occurs with pregnancy and which results in stasis and incomplete emptying. Two thirds of all cases of pyelonephritis during pregnancy can be prevented by treatment of asymptomatic bacteriuria. The relationship between asymptomatic bacteriuria, prematurity, fetal loss, and preeclampsia is unclear, because patients with chronic renal disease are more apt to have bacteriuria.

SYSTEMIC LUPUS ERYTHEMATOSUS

The course of systemic lupus erythematosus is varied during pregnancy. Most patients have either no change or an improvement in the symptoms of the disease. Aggravation of lupus seems to occur more frequently post partum. Whether this is a specific effect of the pregnancy or of demands made on the new mother is unclear. The course of lupus nephropathy during pregnancy is similar to that of chronic glomerulonephritis; patients with hypertension and azotemia preceding pregnancy have an increased incidence of preeclampsia, whereas patients with normal renal function usually have uncomplicated pregnancies.

POSTPARTUM RENAL FAILURE

The rapid development of renal failure has been reported to occur from one to ten weeks post partum with findings at autopsy of malignant nephrosclerosis. Evidence of intravascular coagulation is found in some patients with thrombocytopenia, fibrin degradation products in the serum, and findings on renal biopsy of intra-arteriolar and intraglomerular thromboses. The disease has been termed "postpartum hemolytic-uremic syndrome" by some; its cause may have a relationship to preeclampsia in which fibrin deposits are present in glomeruli and evidence of a consumptive coagulopathy is occasionally seen. There is some evidence that anticoagulant therapy may be of benefit in postpartum renal failure.

TOXEMIA OF PREGNANCY

Toxemia of pregnancy is a disease characterized by hypertension, edema, and proteinuria which occurs in late pregnancy and resolves following delivery. Historically, convulsions have been the hallmark of toxemia, and the disease has been divided into eclampsia (Greek, eclampsis: a sudden flash) and preeclampsia, based upon whether a convulsion has occurred. Although the presence of convulsions is usually indicative of severe disease, separating toxemia on this basis does not imply different causes, and may have no more validity than separating other hypertensive processes associated with convulsions, e.g., acute glomerulonephritis and malignant hypertension.

INCIDENCE. The disease occurs in 5 to 10 per cent of pregnancies, but the reported incidence depends upon criteria used to make the diagnosis and on the population studied. Hypertension alone has been reported to occur during the first pregnancy in 25 per cent of women in Great Britain. There is a bimodal frequency of the disease, with peak incidences in young primiparous women and in multiparous women over 35. Toxemia is more common with pre-existing renal disease, hypertension, and diabetes, with twin pregnancies, and in black women.

PATHOGENESIS. The cause of toxemia is unknown. Nonspecific changes have been described in the liver, brain, heart, and adrenals, but renal biopsies have demonstrated consistent findings. The glomeruli are swollen, and the glomerular lumen is occluded by cytoplasmic swelling of the endothelial cells. Electron microscopy may reveal focal basement menbrane thickening, and immunofluorescent studies have demonstrated fibrin deposits in glomeruli. These glomerular changes are distinctive for toxemia and are not seen in other hypertensive diseases.

The mechanism of the hypertension is unclear. Salt retention, caused in part by the reduction in glomerular filtration rate, might exacerbate the hypertension but alone would not cause it. The similarity of uterus and kidney in possessing the capacity to synthesize renin and prostaglandins is of interest, because there is clinical evidence to suggest uterine ischemia as a factor in the pathogenesis of toxemia. If renin is involved, the sequence of events resulting in hypertension has not been elucidated. Plasma renin is not elevated in toxemia, but since extracellular fluid expansion and increased sensitivity to angiotensin simultaneously occur, a "normal" renin value could be associated with renin-mediated hypertension. Any explanation of the pathogenesis of toxemia must account not only for hypertension but also for the renal pathology and central nervous system excitability which are disproportionate to the magnitude of the hypertension.

CLINICAL MANIFESTATIONS. The usual sequence of manifestations is edema and hypertension followed by proteinuria; occasionally proteinuria precedes hypertension. Because normal pregnancy is characterized by reduction in blood pressure, particularly in the second trimester, blood pressures higher than 130 systolic and 80 diastolic should be considered abnormal during pregnancy. Diastolic hypertension is more striking than systolic with toxemia, and systolic blood pressures greater than 180 to 200 mm Hg usually indicate that preceding hypertensive disease existed. Toxemia typically begins after the thirty-second week of pregnancy, but may occur as early as the twenty-fourth week, particuarly in women with pre-existing renal disease or hypertension. It can occur during the first trimester with a hydatidiform mole. The edema is similar to that seen in acute glomerulonephritis, with prominent distribution in the periorbital region, hands, and ankles. Headache, visual disturbances, and midepigastric pain are frequent symptoms. On funduscopic examination, segmental arteriolar narrowing and a wet glistening retina ("retinal sheen") are often seen. The presence of increased light reflex and tortuosity of the arterioles points to hypertensive disease having preceded the toxemia. Retinal hemorrhages and exudates are rare. The spinal reflexes may be hyperactive, and are important parameters to follow in assessing the degree of central

nervous system excitability. Proteinuria ranges from trace amounts to levels seen in the nephrotic syndrome, 5 to 10 grams per 24 hours. Microscopic examination of the urine may reveal a few red blood cells, but significant hematuria or pyuria is more consistent with the presence of a primary renal disease. Although reduction in glomerular filtration occurs with toxemia, azotemia is seldom prominent because of the increase in glomerular filtration accompanying pregnancy. The low blood urea nitrogen (9±2 mg per 100 ml) and creatinine (0.75±0.2 mg per 100 ml) in late pregnancy are indicative of this increase, and even with a 50 to 75 per cent fall in glomerular filtration, the blood urea nitrogen and creatinine can remain within the normal nonpregnancy range. A disproportionate reduction in urate clearance occurs in toxemia so that hyperuricemia usually precedes the development of azotemia.

TREATMENT. Prenatal care with particular attention to a rise in blood pressure during pregnancy is most important in preventing toxemia. Since pressures in excess of 125 systolic and 75 diastolic prior to the thirty-second week of pregnancy are associated with increase in fetal risk, blood pressures higher than this should be considered abnormal during pregnancy. Edema is common in pregnancy and as an isolated finding does not indicate toxemia. However, the development of edema with a rise in blood pressure usually marks the onset of the disease. With the onset of toxemia, bed rest, salt restriction, and sedation constitute the initial therapy, and when edema is present diuretics should be instituted. If hypertension does not abate, antihypertensive drugs should be instituted. For immediate control of the blood pressure intravenous hydralazine (Apresoline), 25 to 40 mg in 500 ml dextrose and water, or methyldopa (Aldomet), 500 mg, has been efficacious. For severe toxemia with diastolic pressure greater than 120 mm Hg, diazoxide, 300 mg rapidly given intravenously, is effective. Magnesium sulfate has been widely used in toxemia, because it has both a depressant effect upon the central nervous system and a mild antihypertensive action. Barbiturates are useful in controlling central nervous system hyperexcitability, and should be used if convulsions appear imminent. The definitive therapy is termination of the pregnancy, and, provided that the fetus is viable, this should be accomplished as soon as the patient's condition is stable. When fetal size makes viability of concern, control of the disease with antihypertensive drugs and diuretics may allow time for further fetal development. If proteinuria or azotemia persists despite therapy, delivery should be accomplished; there is little evidence that fetal growth occurs in the face of persistent toxemia. Eclampsia is sufficient reason for inducing delivery, because convulsions significantly increase maternal and fetal mortality.

PROGNOSIS. Maternal death with toxemia is now rare. Blood pressure usually returns to normal within two weeks after delivery, although the proteinuria may persist longer. However, women who develop toxemia have a higher incidence of hypertension in later life, and the role toxemia plays in its development has been a subject of concern and controversy. The unresolved question is whether toxemia causes subsequent hypertension or simply occurs more frequently in women with latent hypertension. In women having toxemia with a multiparous pregnancy, two findings favor an underlying hypertensive diathesis as a factor in the toxemia. First, the incidence of late hypertension is greater after multiparous than primiparous toxemia; indeed, in white women with eclampsia, a higher incidence of late hypertension can be demonstrated only after a multiparous toxemia. Second, the recurrence of toxemia with subsequent pregnancies is over 50 per cent after multiparous toxemia, but only 25 per cent in women developing toxemia with the first pregnancy.

Ferris, T. F.: Toxemia and hypertension. In Burrow, G. N., and Ferris, T. F. (eds.): Medical Complications During Pregnancy. Philadelphia, W. B. Saunders Company, 1975.

Sheehan, H. L., and Lynch, J. B.: Pathology of Toxaemia of Pregnancy. Baltimore, Williams & Wilkins Company, 1973.

378. INTERSTITIAL NEPHRITIS AND INTERSTITIAL NEPHROPATHY

Martin Goldberg

INTRODUCTION

As recently as a decade ago, bacterial infection of the kidneys was thought to be a major cause of chronic nonglomerular renal disease; hence the term chronic pyelonephritis. This entity was characterized by chronic inflammation and fibrosis involving primarily the renal interstitium and the structures passing through it, including the renal tubules and the renal vasculature. Because these changes resembled those seen in clinical and experimental conditions known to be due to bacterial infection, it was assumed by analogy that infection was the primary etiology of most conditions associated with these histopathologic alterations. When attempts were made to prove a consistent etiologic relationship between infection and chronic interstitial inflammation of the kidneys, they failed. Furthermore it has become apparent that many noninfectious conditions (see below) can produce identical histopathologic alterations even without evidence of concomitant infection. Several other observations have led to the conclusion that most cases of chronic interstitial renal disease in the adult (whether or not they are associated with inflammation) are *not* primarily caused by bacterial infections. Some of these facts are as follows: (1) only a minority of patients with interstitial disease have a clear previous history of acute renal infection; (2) there is little evidence to suggest that chronic bacteriuria per se (a risk factor for acute pyelonephritis) leads to chronic progressive renal disease with renal failure; and (3) some observations indicate that bacterial infection, when present, is usually preceded by another primary cause of chronic interstitial nephritis.

Hence, it is more useful to consider chronic interstitial nephropathy as a clinicopathologic syndrome in which the primary process involves the renal interstitium and related structures and with time is associated with a number of characteristic functional abnormalities. When associated with interstitial inflammation, this condition is best termed chronic interstitial nephritis, but frequently the pathologic process may involve only atrophy, sclerosis, or even neoplastic infiltration.

In these latter situations interstitial nephropathy (or tubulointerstitial disease) is a more appropriate term. The accompanying table provides an etiologic classification of the chronic interstitial nephropathies, including the common causes of chronic interstitial nephritis. Study of the table reveals that most of the causes of interstitial nephropathy are known conditions which are amenable to medical or surgical therapy. In fact it has been estimated that approximately 90 per cent of the cases of chronic interstitial nephritis are due to potentially remediable causes. This contrasts strikingly with chronic glomerulonephritis in the adult, in which commonly the precise etiology is unknown and specific therapy is lacking. The acute forms of interstitial nephritis are discussed in Ch. 369.2 and 376.

PATHOLOGY. Despite the varied causes, the pathology of the interstitial nephritis is generally nonspecific except in certain instances associated with obstruction or with infiltration by neoplastic cells or deposition of certain proteins (e.g., amyloid) or certain crystals (e.g., urate, oxalate, or calcium salts). Grossly, in the advanced stages, the kidneys are smaller than normal and usually irregular in outline, a manifestation of multiple scars. Dilatation of one or more calyces associated with overlying cortical scars is thought by some to be pathognomonic of bacterial infection, but this concept remains controversial.

Microscopically, there is typically a chronic inflammatory process of the interstitium involving mainly lymphocytes, plasma cells, and fibroblasts. These are associated with a heavy deposition of collagen and ground substance containing substantial quantities of mucopolysaccharide. The tubular cells are atrophic and flat, and the tubular configuration is distorted by surrounding fibrous tissue. These latter changes are often associated with dilated tubular lumens filled with eosinophilic casts. The tubular basement membranes are characteristically thickened. The glomeruli appear to be involved secondarily late in the disease process. Characteristically they are surrounded by a cuff of fibrous tissue, and the glomerular tuft undergoes fibrosis and hyalinization in the advanced stages. Involvement of the vasculature is variable, but in those patients with hypertension (approximately 50 per cent of patients with interstitial nephritis) arteriolar nephrosclerosis may be seen. Since most of the renal interstitium resides in the medulla, this structure and its papillae are heavily involved in a sclerosing and deforming process.

Etiologic Classification of Chronic Interstitial Nephropathies

1. Obstructive nephropathy
2. Toxic nephropathies (e.g., drugs [analgesics], heavy metals)
3. Metabolic nephropathies (e.g., intrarenal crystal nephropathy—urate, oxalate, hypercalcemia, hypokalemia)
4. Immunologic interstitial nephritis (e.g., systemic lupus erythematosus, transplant rejection, Sjögren's syndrome?)
5. Infiltrative disease of the interstitium (e.g., lymphoma, leukemia, myeloma, Waldenström's macroglobulinemia, amyloidosis)
6. Infectious interstitial nephritis (e.g., pyogenic [rarely a primary cause in the adult], tuberculosis, fungal)
7. Noninfectious granulomatous disease (e.g., sarcoidosis)
8. Physical and environmental factors (e.g., Balkan nephropathy, radiation nephritis)
9. Hereditary nephropathies (e.g., medullary cystic disease, congenital polycystic disease)
10. Vascular nephropathy (e.g., longstanding benign nephrosclerosis, chronic renal artery obstruction, sickle hemoglobinopathies)
11. Idiopathic

Occasionally frank papillary necrosis may occur, particularly in the nephropathy associated with overuse of analgesic drugs.

COMMON CLINICAL AND PATHOPHYSIOLOGIC MANIFESTATIONS. Despite the multiple causes of chronic interstitial renal disease, each of which may be associated with one or more specific clinical manifestations (e.g., hydronephrosis in obstructive uropathy, clinical gout in urate nephropathy, urinary stones in certain metabolic diseases), the clinical and laboratory features of the interstitial renal disease per se are remarkably similar. As already discussed, repeated episodes of acute infection are not common unless associated with another predisposing factor such as urinary tract obstruction. Furthermore, if a remediable or reversible factor can be removed or treated at any stage of the disease prior to the terminal phases, the condition has a remarkable propensity to stabilize, and progression may be arrested or retarded. Characteristically there are few symptoms and signs before the insidious onset of renal failure with its concomitant uremic syndrome. At this late stage anorexia, nausea, vomiting, fatigue, weight loss, and anemia appear, along with the other classic manifestations of end-stage renal disease (see Ch. 371). Prior to these late stages, the major manifestations of interstitial nephritis occur in certain laboratory tests (see below).

Hypertension is frequently present in advanced chronic interstitial nephritis, but it occurs less commonly than with chronic glomerulonephritis (approximately 50 per cent of cases in the former, compared to >80 per cent in the latter), and the severity of the hypertension appears to be less in primary interstitial disease than in glomerulonephritis. Occasionally chronic interstitial nephritis may be associated with episodes of acute hypotension due to sodium depletion and hypovolemia as a consequence of impaired renal conservation of sodium.

LABORATORY: URINALYSIS. The urine sediment usually contains no pathognomonic abnormalities. It may be entirely normal, but frequently it contains moderate numbers of red blood cells, white blood cells, and tubular epithelial cells. White blood cell casts may be present during active infection. Heavy proteinuria is not a characteristic feature. Dipstick examination usually reveals trace to 1+ proteinuria; 24-hour protein excretion is characteristically less than 2.5 grams and usually less than 1.5 grams. When present, the increased urinary protein contains a lesser fraction of albumin than in glomerulonephritis and a higher fraction of so-called tubular proteins such as lysozyme or beta-2 microglobulin, which are sometimes used as markers of tubular proteinuria.

RENAL FUNCTIONAL ABNORMALITIES AND THEIR PATHOPHYSIOLOGY. Although not diagnostic, certain changes in renal tubular function occur in chronic interstitial nephritis which are more characteristic and occur earlier than with chronic glomerulonephritis. Since a large portion of the involved interstitium is in the renal medulla, the structures in this region (the loop of Henle, vasa recta, interstitial cells, and collecting ducts) exhibit functional abnormalities relatively early in the course of the disease. Frequently evidence of dysfunction of the distal nephron is present with only moderate degrees of azotemia. The most important tubulointerstitial functional abnormalities in chronic interstitial nephritis are (1) impaired concentrating ability, (2) impaired renal conservation of sodium, (3) renal acidosis, often associated with hyperchloremia, and (4) impaired renal excretion of potassium and hyperkalemia even when oliguria or severe acidosis is absent.

Impaired Renal Concentrating Capacity. The normal concentrating mechanism requires not only the intactness of the specific structures involved, thin and thick limbs of the loop of Henle, cortical and medullary collecting tubules and ducts, and the vasa recta, but also a normal anatomic configuration of these structures in relation to each other and the medullary interstitium. Since the interstitial nephropathies primarily distort or displace the medullary architecture, the complex system responsible for generating the medullary concentration gradient is disorganized. This disorganization may occur with only minimal reduction in glomerular filtration rate (GFR). Hence, marked impairment in urine concentration (maximum urine osmolality [U_{max}] less than 500 to 600 mOsm per kilogram) after 12 to 16 hours of fluid deprivation is a common finding before severe azotemia occurs; when GFR reduction becomes moderate to severe (serum creatinine >6.0 to 7.0 mg per deciliter), the U_{max} is isotonic to plasma and may even be less than plasma despite the administration of vasopressin.

Impaired Renal Conservation of Sodium. Recent experimental observations indicate that the fine regulation of sodium excretion (under the influence of hormonal and other controlling factors) occurs in the terminal segments of the nephron, including the collecting system of tubules and ducts. Hence, it is not surprising that patients with chronic interstitial nephropathy exhibit "salt-wasting" relatively early in their disease. This usually means an inability to eliminate sodium from the urine or sharply reduce its excretion when dietary changes or pathophysiologic events require this homeostatic adaptation to prevent severe contraction of the extracellular fluid volume or hypovolemia. Hence, abrupt dietary sodium restriction is rarely indicated in these patients, since they characteristically cannot reduce sodium excretion below 50 to 75 mEq per day without experiencing the consequences of hypovolemia. Furthermore, such patients must be observed closely during bouts of intercurrent gastroenteritis in order to provide early replacement of fluid and electrolyte deficits which would tend to produce further deterioration of renal function.

Renal Acidosis. The distal nephron is important in the renal excretion of acid (hydrogen ions). In these segments hydrogen ions are secreted to react with the urinary buffers, ammonia, and monohydrogen phosphate. Also, the terminal nephron is a site for the addition of ammonia buffer into the tubular fluid. These processes are necessary to regenerate the bicarbonate buffer in body fluids which is consumed by the daily production of 60 to 80 mEq of hydrogen ions from the catabolism of proteins and the incomplete combustion of carbohydrates. Most evidence indicates that the major defect in acid excretion in patients with chronic interstitial nephritis is a reduction in ammonium excretion. This reduces the capacity of the kidney to eliminate "metabolic" hydrogen ions, leading to a decreased bicarbonate concentration in body fluids. As the acidosis develops, the renal tubules reabsorb a greater proportion of the filtered sodium as sodium chloride. Hence, hyperchloremic acidosis is typically observed; when azotemia is moderate (serum creatinine <4.0 mg per deciliter), the anion gap (the difference between the serum sodium concentration and the sum of the bicarbonate and chloride concentrations) may be normal, rising only in the advanced stages of the disease. This "tubular" acidosis of chronic interstitial nephritis is different, however, from classic renal tubular acidosis in that there is no major problem in secreting hydrogen ion against a gradient in the former condition. Hence, minimal urine pH is usually normal (<5.5).

Impaired Renal Excretion of Potassium. Hyperkalemia is not uncommonly found in patients with chronic interstitial nephritis. This not only is seen in the oliguric end-stages of the disorder (typical of all end-stage renal disease), but also may occur without oliguria. There are several mechanisms contributing to this abnormality which are secondary to impaired ability of the kidney to eliminate potassium. First, acute metabolic acidosis increases the rate of movement of potassium ions from cellular to extracellular fluid while concomitantly reducing the renal tubular secretion of potassium in the distal nephron. Since patients with interstitial nephropathy have a propensity for acidosis (see above), hyperkalemia is a frequent associated finding and may be rapidly corrected by the administration of alkali. Second, hyperkalemia may occur in these patients in the absence of both acidosis and oliguria. Two pathophysiologic mechanisms have been observed in some of these patients, the relative frequency and importance of which remain to be determined. In some patients, hyperkalemia has been associated with hyporeninemia and hypoaldosteronism (both unresponsive to sodium depletion). Hence mineralocorticoid deficiency due to either a primary abnormality in renal renin secretion or an abnormality in the adrenal response to changes in serum potassium appears to account for the hyperkalemia in this group. Interestingly, most subjects with interstitial nephritis in this category have had diabetes mellitus. In another group of patients, the hyperkalemia has been associated with an apparent intrinsic tubular defect in potassium secretion, unresponsive to endogenous and exogenous mineralocorticoid.

UROGRAPHY. The radiologic picture of the urinary tract is generally nonspecific. The specificity relates to some of the causes of the interstitial nephritis: e.g., hydronephrosis and hydroureter in obstructive uropathy, the occurrence of papillary necrosis in analgesic-associated nephropathy and sickle cell disease. Early in the course, the renal size and outlines may be normal, but bilaterally small kidneys are generally characteristic. The renal outlines are typically irregular due to cortical scar formation, and the calyces are frequently distorted and often dilated and blunted. Occasionally the urogram may be normal.

RENAL BIOPSY. As already stated, the histopathology of chronic interstitial nephritis is nonspecific with regard to etiology. Early in the course, the typical cortical biopsy specimen may show no abnormalities despite the presence of severe disease in the juxtamedullary and medullary areas. The most valuable use of renal biopsy is to exclude glomerulonephritis when this is a differential diagnostic problem (which is *not* commonly the case).

COURSE. The time course of chronic interstitial nephropathy is quite variable. If the primary cause can be treated *early* in the disease, progression is often retarded, and occasionally some improvement in renal function may occur. This is most dramatic in the relief of urinary tract obstruction. If the cause cannot be eliminated or the disease has progressed to an advanced stage, the subsequent rate of progression toward end-stage is often slower than occurs in chronic glomerulonephritis at comparable levels of renal dysfunction. Episodes of apparent acute deterioration of renal function can often be reversed by appropriate administration of fluids and electrolytes to treat hypovolemia, acidosis, or hyperkalemia.

TREATMENT. Specific therapy should be directed toward the primary causative factors (see below). In the presence of urinary infection, antimicrobial therapy is generally indicated as described in Ch. 376. An initial attempt should be made to eradicate the offending organisms. Often this is impossible, and a maintenance program designed to reduce the number of urinary pathogens may be in order. Management of hypertension and chronic renal failure (including dialysis and transplantation) is similar to that in other chronic renal diseases (see Ch. 361 and 371).

ETIOLOGIC TYPES OF CHRONIC INTERSTITIAL NEPHRITIS (see table)

Obstructive Nephropathy

Obstruction in the urinary tract distal to the renal papillae is the primary cause of more than half the interstitial nephritides. Obstruction may be due to a variety of congenital and acquired lesions that may occur from the ureteropelvic junction to the urethral meatus. Regardless of the cause, the mechanism of the structural renal damage and associated functional disorders is related to the increased pressure within the urinary tract transmitted to the nephrons within the kidney. When unilateral, the characteristic damage occurs to one kidney, but renal failure does not develop (except in cases of a solitary kidney); in bilateral obstruction renal failure is characteristic. Obstruction may be complete or partial, each of which produces different clinical syndromes. The primary event, obstruction to the flow of urine in the presence of continued urine formation by the kidney and ureteropelvic peristalsis proximal to the obstruction, is followed shortly by a rise in intraluminal hydrostatic pressure within the proximal ureters and pelvis. This is transmitted to the nephrons within the kidney, leading ultimately to a reduction in GFR. The magnitude of the fall in GFR depends on the completeness of obstruction and the magnitude of the pressure rise.

With acute obstruction, the dilatation of the ureters and the pelvocalyceal systems is only moderate; but with chronicity, atony and atrophy of the smooth muscle in the walls of the urinary structures occur, leading to the characteristic hydronephrosis and hydroureter. With chronic urinary obstruction both functional and morphologic deterioration occur within the intrarenal structures. GFR falls progressively and renal tubular abnormalities develop which are characteristic of those previously described for tubulointerstitial nephropathies in general: impaired concentrating ability, renal acidosis, hyperkalemia, and inability to conserve sodium. These functional changes are associated with tubular dilatation and atrophy predominantly in the medullary structures. The interstitium, edematous in the early stages, shows extensive fibrosis and varying degrees of infiltration by inflammatory cells. In the advanced stages, the medulla is completely scarred and atrophic, and this sclerosing and atrophic process progresses to involve the renal cortical structures.

Although all the aforementioned changes may result from obstruction alone, obstruction in the urinary tract is the single most important cause of chronic renal bacterial infection, such that the pathogenesis and rate of progression of the renal disease process are often due to a combination of pressure nephropathy and bacterial pyelonephritis. Frequently the infection is initiated by some form of diagnostic or therapeutic instrumentation of the urinary tract. The topic of obstructive nephropathy is discussed more extensively in Ch. 382.

Analgesic-Associated Nephropathy

(AAN)

In the past three decades increasing numbers of patients with chronic interstitial nephritis associated with the ingestion of large quantities of analgesic drugs have been reported from various parts of the world. Until the past decade, the importance of AAN as a cause of chronic renal disease in the United States was thought to be minor, but recent observations strongly suggest that this is not the case. In fact it is likely that AAN accounts for at least 6 per cent of all patients with chronic renal failure and at least 20 per cent of patients with interstitial nephropathies in the United States.

Absolute proof of the causal relationship between analgesics and renal disease is lacking, but circumstantial epidemiologic evidence as well as experimental studies in animals has convinced most observers that AAN is a specific entity with potentially important implications from the standpoint of public health and preventive medicine.

ETIOLOGY. In the earlier reports of AAN, phenacetin was implicated as the most important single nephrotoxic agent. Further clinical and experimental observations have strongly suggested, however, that nephrotoxicity and chronic renal disease are more likely to occur from ingestion of mixtures of aspirin and phenacetin (or related drugs such as acetaminophen) than from ingestion of either drug alone. The quantity of drugs required to produce renal damage is not known. Nevertheless the risk of developing renal disease appears to be higher following consumption of a cumulative dose of more than 1 kg of either aspirin or phenacetin (when taken in combination). This corresponds to ingestion of 6 or more tablets per day of most of the commonly available analgesic combinations for a period of three years or more. Actually, most patients with AAN have taken considerably more than this amount for longer periods of time when the disorder is first diagnosed by their physician.

PATHOGENESIS AND PATHOLOGY. Experiments in animals indicate that the major metabolic products of both aspirin and phenacetin are concentrated in the kidney. Further, acetaminophen (into which almost all phenacetin is converted within one hour of administration) accumulates in the renal medulla paralleling the normal medullary gradient for urea which is most concentrated at the papillary tip. Hypotheses have been proposed (but not yet proved) which suggest a synergistic toxic action of the metabolites of the two drugs. In this formulation, the phenacetin metabolites may produce oxidative damage to the medullary tissues, whereas salicylates simultaneously inhibit the major tissue defenses against oxidative damage (i.e., glucose-6-phosphate dehydrogenase).

The earliest morphologic changes occur in the inner medulla of the kidney and appear to be interstitial sclerosis (with minimal inflammation) and tubular degeneration and atrophy. With time focal areas of papillary and medullary necrosis develop, and occasionally the papillary tip may necrose entirely into the renal pelvis. Subsequently, the entire medulla undergoes a sclerosing and degenerative process, and at this stage there develops an infiltration with mononuclear inflammatory cells. The renal tubules undergo marked atrophy associated with thickening of their basement membranes. Finally the fibrotic and inflammatory process extends to the cortical interstitium. Secondarily marked degeneration and atrophy of the cortical structures develop, including ultimately periglomerular fibrosis, glomerular sclerosis, and arteriolar nephrosclerosis. At this late stage the kidney is grossly contracted and deformed with medullary and cortical scars.

Renal functional changes occur concomitantly with the pathologic alterations. Prior to the development of azotemia, the classic pathophysiologic changes of chronic interstitial nephritis may be manifest — especially fixed isosthenuria and a tendency toward a metabolic acidosis with a normal anion gap. The acidosis worsens with increasing renal insufficiency, and ultimately impaired renal sodium conservation may be an important feature.

CLINICAL MANIFESTATIONS. Analgesic-associated nephropathy characteristically occurs over the age of 30, and two thirds to three fourths of the patients have been women. Most patients attribute their ingestion of analgesics to headaches or backaches, and many feel that the drugs provide them with a significant "mood elevation." In fact, psychoneurotic problems are characteristic of this group of patients, particularly anxiety, depression, and hypochondriasis. Although a majority of the patients obtain these drugs directly as proprietary preparations, many receive them through prescriptions by physicians who are unaware that they are perpetuating the continued toxic exposure to the kidneys.

In most patients, the clinical manifestations are subtle or minimal until advanced renal failure develops. The patient with AAN may be seen by the physician for several reasons: for complaints concerning the original cause of the overuse of analgesics (e.g., headache, backache); acute urinary tract symptoms (e.g., colic, secondary infection, frequency, dysuria, hematuria); manifestations of chronic interstitial nephritis (e.g., nocturia, metabolic acidosis, salt wasting); manifestations of chronic renal failure (e.g., anemia, fatigue, uremia, hypertension); or manifestations of extrarenal effects of the continued analgesic overuse (e.g., gastrointestinal complaints, anemia).

The gastrointestinal disturbances (present in half the patients) include upper gastrointestinal bleeding secondary to gastritis or peptic ulcer, symptoms of peptic ulcer aggravated by the drugs, or nonspecific dyspepsia. A significant number of these patients have undergone gastrointestinal surgery.

Anemia is present in most patients with AAN and is not necessarily related to the degree of renal failure. It appears to be due to a combination of the toxic effects of phenacetin and similar drugs on the red blood cell to produce methemoglobinemia, the effects of chronic gastrointestinal blood loss, and the effects of uremia.

Hypertension, present in approximately half the patients, is typically mild and benign in character. It is usually discovered after the initial diagnosis of the renal disease.

A dramatic event which occurs at some time in a minority of patients with AAN is ureteral colic associated with passage of fragments of necrotic papillae. This is frequently associated with hematuria (gross or microscopic) and manifestations of acute pyelonephritis secondary to obstruction. Occasionally the patient may experience the passage of tissue which is a fragment of a necrosed renal papilla.

A troublesome and common characteristic of analgesic overusers is their reluctance to admit to the use of analgesics or to report the true amount of analgesic consumption. Such patient denial often occurs despite specific interrogation by the physician.

LABORATORY FINDINGS. Laboratory findings typically include evidence of azotemia and varying degrees of anemia. The latter may be normochromic, normocytic, or hypochromic microcytic with evidence of iron deficiency. Urinalysis is nonspecific and exhibits the characteristics of interstitial nephritis, as already discussed. Pyuria and hematuria are often unassociated with positive urine cultures. White blood cell casts in the sediment may be seen during a bout of acute pyelonephritis. Positive urine bacterial culture results are found in only approximately half of the patients at some point of their course. A substantial number of patients develop renal failure without any evidence of past infection despite multiple cultures of the urine.

DIAGNOSIS. The two most important elements in the diagnosis are the documentation of a history of ingestion of sufficient amounts of analgesics and the presence of a chronic interstitial nephritis unexplained by any other known pre-existing cause such as obstruction, stone disease, or gout.

As discussed, the history is frequently difficult to obtain because of denial characteristics of many of these patients. It is essential to speak with members of the family living in the same household or with the patient's pharmacist if the diagnosis of AAN is a possibility.

Evidence for papillary necrosis clinically or radiologically should significantly raise the suspicion of diagnosis of AAN. Other causes such as diabetes mellitus, obstructive uropathy, and sickle cell disease rarely are associated with passage of sloughed papillae.

Intravenous urography has been abnormal in as many as 90 per cent of these patients. Often it is nonspecific and shows calyceal distortion and clubbing associated with small kidneys. A common finding is the appearance of the radiopaque medium in tracts extending from the calyces; less often (20 to 40 per cent of patients) the classic radiologic findings of papillary necrosis (such as a "ring sign") may be seen.

PROGNOSIS AND TREATMENT. The natural history may be significantly influenced by the cessation of analgesic ingestion. Patients with renal disease who continue their drug consumption invariably develop progressive renal failure leading to end-stage disease over a period of five to ten years after initial diagnosis. It has been well documented, on the other hand, that ces-

sation of heavy analgesic use can result in prolonged periods of apparent stabilization of renal function in many patients with AAN (usually in those with a serum creatinine less than 5.0 mg per deciliter). In fact there have been some reports suggesting that, in a few patients, actual improvement in GFR with a fall in serum creatinine level may occur even with apparent end-stage disease. This knowledge emphasizes the importance of early diagnosis of AAN and insistence that the patient discontinue the chronic ingestion of analgesic combinations.

Chronic Gouty Nephropathy and Other Urate Nephropathies

This subject is also discussed in Ch. 379. Here, urate nephropathy will be briefly discussed as an example of an interstitial nephropathy with some commentary on pathogenesis.

Disturbances in renal function and abnormalities in renal morphology have been described in association with gout for centuries. Observations made in the past two decades indicate that abnormal urinalysis (mild proteinuria, hematuria, and pyuria) is present in the majority of patients with clinical gout. The incidence of renal failure (glomerular filtration rate <70 ml per minute) is present in a smaller but significant percentage of gouty patients, varying from 8 per cent in living patients with gout to 25 per cent in some autopsy series.

There is also ample clinical evidence to suggest that hyperuricemia associated with states of urate overproduction is associated with a significant incidence of chronic progressive renal disease (in addition to episodes of acute uric acid nephropathy, which is discussed in Ch. 380.4). These conditions include the myeloproliferative disorders, hypoxanthine-guanine-phosphoribosyl-transferase (HGPRT) deficiency, and, of course, gouty overproduction of urate.

Despite the impressive circumstantial evidence that gout or hyperuricemia and/or hyperuricosuria are damaging to the kidney, it is still widely debated whether gout per se is responsible for the renal damage or whether the commonly associated conditions such as hypertension, urate stone disease, urinary infection, or aging are the prime factors responsible for the nephropathy seen in gouty subjects.

PATHOLOGY AND PATHOGENESIS. In gouty patients with renal disease or in patients with urate overproduction states, the morphologic changes in the kidney are most commonly those of chronic interstitial nephritis, including interstitial round cell inflammation, fibrosis, tubular atrophy, glomerular sclerosis, and arteriolar nephrosclerosis. In addition, careful examination of the kidneys, especially prior to end-stage, reveals collections of crystals either in the medullary interstitium or in the lumens of the distal tubules and collecting system. The tubules are typically dilated proximal to the intraluminal deposits. These crystals consist of either sodium urate or uric acid, depending on the pH of the fluid in which they are deposited. In the medulla crystal deposits may be severe enough to form microtophi which are surrounded by inflammatory cells, including foreign body giant cells.

It is still debatable whether the interstitial crystals and microtophi originate from the blood supply and are therefore a direct consequence of the elevated plasma urate level plus local physiochemical factors, or whether they originate from the tubular deposits, passing into the surrounding interstitium through a rent in the damaged tubular wall. This is a critical issue to resolve because it may have a direct influence on prevention and treatment. For example, if blood-borne urate is the major causative factor, then therapy aimed at lowering plasma urate concentrations is most important. On the other hand, if the primary event in urate nephropathy (which secondarily leads to the interstitial changes) is intratubular deposition, then therapy should be directed primarily toward lowering the excreted load of urate.

Aside from the problems in urate metabolism contributing to renal damage in gout, there are other factors commonly also present which, in themselves, may contribute to the severity of the nephropathy. Uric acid or urate stones are prevalent in gouty patients, especially in overproducers and hence overexcreters of urate. In addition some data have suggested that the tendency toward stone formation is aggravated by the tendency of gouty subjects to have an inappropriately acid urine, possibly because of a defect in ammonium excretion. It is not clear whether this is a defect specific for gout or merely a nonspecific consequence of the interstitial nephritis. Stone disease is a condition known to predispose to obstruction in the urinary tract and to pyelonephritis. These factors undoubtedly contribute to irreversible structural damage and functional deterioration in many patients with gout. Hypertension, also common in gout, may also contribute to renal dysfunction, although by itself benign hypertension is an infrequent cause of chronic renal failure.

CLINICAL MANIFESTATIONS. Unless associated with the symptoms and signs of urinary stones, gouty or urate nephropathy is typically a slowly progressive chronic interstitial nephritis which is asymptomatic until the consequences of renal failure and/or hypertension are manifest. Urinalysis may reveal proteinuria which is rarely massive, although some observers have concluded that the quantity of protein excreted is occasionally greater than occurs in most interstitial nephropathies (sometimes reaching levels of 1 to 2 grams per day). Hematuria, pyuria, and bacteriuria are not infrequent findings. The remainder of the laboratory findings are typical of those already described for a chronic interstitial nephritis except for the abnormalities in urate metabolism. Aside from documenting hyperuricemia, it is wise to quantify the hyperexcretion of urate, since hyperexcretors are at increased risk for stone formation and probably also for the development of chronic intrarenal crystal deposition.

Intravenous urography and other imaging techniques generally reveal bilaterally small and often scarred kidneys when renal insufficiency is present, but these procedures are not diagnostic for urate nephropathy except to confirm the presence of obstruction or radiolucent stones.

DIAGNOSIS. Diagnosis of gouty or urate nephropathy is very difficult to make specifically. It is mainly based on circumstantial evidence, i.e., the presence of a chronic interstitial nephritis (unexplained by other known primary causes) in a patient with gout or a disorder associated with overproduction such as some of the blood dyscrasias. Renal biopsy is rarely helpful and generally not indicated because urate crystals are diffi-

cult to see with the standard pathologic preparations; furthermore, urate crystals may be observed in many other renal diseases not related to disorders of uric acid metabolism.

TREATMENT AND PREVENTION. This is a highly debatable area, depending upon the accuracy of one's concept of the pathogenesis. If hyperuricemia per se is the major contributing factor, then administration of allopurinol or probenecid to subjects with asymptomatic hyperuricemia from any cause would be indicated. There is, however, no evidence to date which clearly shows that asymptomatic hyperuricemia alone is associated with an increased incidence of renal disease.

For the present, a prudent approach to the problem would be to treat with allopurinol only those patients who demonstrate renal abnormalities attributable to disorders in urate metabolism such as uric acid–urate stone disease or hyperexcretion of urate (e.g., >0.8 gram per day) associated with renal functional deterioration. From a renal standpoint, probenecid administration has no established therapeutic role. In fact some patients may exhibit an increase in stone formation early in the course of therapy with this agent.

The other manifestations and complications of urate nephropathy are treated similarly to those of other interstitial nephritides.

Balkan Nephropathy

This peculiar disease has fascinated nephrologic and epidemiologic investigators since its description in 1942. It is a chronic progressive interstitial nephropathy of insidious onset and unknown cause, restricted to an area 120 by 30 miles in the rural area around the Danubian Gates tributaries. It occurs principally in farmers and their families living in the flat river bottom land of Yugoslavia, Rumania, and Bulgaria.

PATHOGENESIS AND PATHOLOGY. The disease has thus far defied exhaustive attempts at defining the etiology. Most of our scientific knowledge has been derived from epidemiologic observations. Although the data strongly suggest an environmental infectious or toxic factor, none has yet been specifically identified. Although it occurs in families, it is clearly an acquired disease. Families moving into the area may develop the disease, and relatives of involved individuals who leave the area early in life remain free of the disease. At least ten years of residence in the endemic area is required before the earliest manifestations develop, and it generally requires 20 years to develop clinical evidence of the full-blown renal disease. Therefore it is most frequent at ages 30 to 40 years. Females predominate in the younger age ranges (2:1), but in the older age of involvement the sex difference disappears. The characteristic renal lesion is progressive tubular atrophy with accompanying interstitial and subcapsular fibrosis and secondary glomerular hyalinization. Cellular infiltration is minimal. Ultimately the kidneys are grossly atrophic and fibrosed, weighing 40 to 60 grams. Some observers have described local deposition of immunoglobulins in the glomeruli. Recently, others have described virus-like particles in the cells of the nephron, and have suggested a pig coronavirus as a causal agent. The disease is said to be rare among Muslims, who avoid pigs, and in villages where no pigs are kept. The pathogenetic significance of these findings remains to be established.

CLINICAL MANIFESTATIONS, COURSE, AND PROGNOSIS. The earliest detectable abnormality is tubular proteinuria, manifested by an increase in beta-2-microglobulinuria (as a marker) and a urinary electrophoretic pattern containing spikes of alpha-1, alpha-2, beta, and gamma globulins. Total protein excretion rarely exceeds 1 gram per day. The urine sediment is generally unremarkable, containing granular casts and a few red and white blood cells per high power field. All these changes may occur prior to the development of any functional abnormalities and without symptoms.

The earliest functional disturbance is impaired renal concentrating capacity. Other evidence of tubular dysfunction may occur prior to renal failure and includes acidification defects (low ammonia excretion), general aminoaciduria, renal glucosuria, and an elevated urate clearance with hypouricemia. Ultimately the GFR begins to decrease, and an inexorable downhill course leading to uremia ensues. The duration of the entire course may vary from a few months to nearly ten years, with approximately half the patients dying in two years (unless dialysis is utilized). Overt dipstick-positive proteinuria is a late feature of the disease. Intravenous urography is nonspecific and reveals uniformly small kidneys. Hypertension is not a feature of the early phases of the disease, but may be severe in the terminal phase. There is no therapy known to alter the course of this disease.

One interesting associated finding is that about a third of the patients dying of the disease in Bulgaria and Yugoslavia have had papillomas and/or carcinomas of the renal pelvis, ureter, or bladder. These may be multiple or bilateral. It is possible, but not proved, that these neoplastic lesions have a common etiologic factor with the nephropathy.

Chronic (Nonobstructive) Pyelonephritis

Although significant portions of the renal disease chapters in previous editions of this textbook have been devoted to chronic pyelonephritis, the current status of this entity in the adult may be summarized by the following statement. Currently available evidence indicates that chronic progressive pyelonephritis due to bacterial infection of the kidney is a rare cause of chronic renal failure in the absence of obstruction or other primary causes of renal disease. It is true that acute pyelonephritis heals with some degree of scarring, and it is possible that in certain susceptible individuals the scar tissue may be excessive and could lead to significant deformity of the renal architecture. Multiple acute episodes followed by extensive scarring could theoretically lead to renal failure. Well-documented descriptions of this process in the adult are few in number. There is, however, some evidence suggesting that the growing kidney is more likely to develop deforming scars following acute infection than the mature kidney. Reports of postinfectious renal sclerosis and atrophy are more common in the pediatric literature, and it is likely that previous childhood infection is responsible for the occasional discovery of a unilateral contracted kidney sometimes seen on urography in the adult.

There have been numerous attempts to produce animal models of experimental chronic pyelonephritis, but none has been successful without also producing an obstructive lesion in the urinary tract or directly traumatizing the kidney. Some experimental work has suggested that certain bacterial antigens have persisted in the kidney after eradication of the primary infection. It has been proposed that this might initate a series of immunologic reactions in the kidney, leading to chronic renal disease. Unfortunately, these potentially interesting observations have not been confirmed. This mechanism could account for the causes of the small percentage of interstitial nephritides labeled as "idiopathic," but the solution to this problem requires further study.

Idiopathic Interstitial Nephritis

In approximately 10 per cent of patients with the clinicopathologic syndrome of interstitial nephritis, a cause cannot be discovered. There is nothing about the clinical manifestations, course, and prognosis in these patients that specifically differentiates them from other interstitial nephritides with known causes. It is likely that this percentage will decrease as our knowledge about exogenous (environmental) or endogenous (metabolic) nephrotoxins increases.

Apostolov, K., Spasic, P., and Bojanic, N.: Evidence of a viral aetiology in endemic (Balkan) nephropathy. Lancet, 2:1271, 1975.

Barlow, K. A., and Berlin, L. J.: Renal disease in primary gout. Quart. J. Med., 37:79, 1968.

Emmerson, B. T., and Row, P. G.: Editorial: An evaluation of the pathogenesis of the gouty kidney. Kidney Int., 8:65, 1975.

Freedman, L. R.: Urinary tract infection, pyelonephritis and other forms of chronic interstitial nephritis. In Strauss, M. B., and Welt, L. G. (eds.): Diseases of the Kidney. Boston, Little, Brown & Company, 1971.

Howards, S. H., and Wright, F. S.: Obstructive injury. In Brenner, B. M., and Rector, F. C., Jr. (eds.): The Kidney. Philadelphia, W. B. Saunders Company, 1976.

Kincaid-Smith, P. (ed.): Analgesic nephropathy. Kidney Int., 13:1, 1978.

Murray, T., and Goldberg, M.: Chronic interstitial nephritis: Etiological factors. Ann. Intern. Med., 82:453, 1975.

Suki, W. N., and Eknoyan, G.: Tubulo-interstitial diseases. In Brenner, B. M., and Rector, F. C., Jr. (eds.): The Kidney. Philadelphia, W. B. Saunders Company, 1976.

Wilson, D. R.: Renal function during and following obstruction. Ann. Rev. Med., 28:329, 1977.

Wolstenholme, G. E. W., and Knight, J. (eds.): The Balkan Nephropathy. Boston, Little, Brown & Company, 1967.

379.   TOXIC NEPHROPATHY

Bryan T. Emmerson

DEFINITION

Originally, the term toxic nephropathy was used to refer to acute renal damage from an exogenous poison. A cause and effect relationship between the toxin and the renal disease was usually obvious, the degree of renal damage was related to the dose of the toxin, and the damage was often reversible when the toxin ceased to act. The meaning was then extended to cover both acute and chronic processes. However, the establishment of an etiologic association between the toxic agent and the renal disease was often more difficult in the latter case, and required prolonged study of chronically exposed individuals. More recently, it has become clear that chemicals other than direct nephrotoxins may produce renal disease, so that the concept of a toxic nephropathy now includes any adverse alteration in renal function or structure caused by an exogenous chemical or abnormal body constituent. Thus renal damage caused by immunologically mediated reactions to foreign substances is classified with the toxic nephropathies. In such cases, the relationship between the causative agent and the renal disease is less clear and the development of the renal damage is less predictable because of the wide variations in the immune responsiveness of individuals. Moreover, remission is less likely to occur on removal of the initiating agent. The concept of toxic nephropathy also includes damage to the kidney by abnormal concentrations of normal body constituents, such as hypercalcemia, hyperuricemia, hypokalemia, and hypomagnesemia. These topics are dealt with elsewhere, and will not be considered further here. Renal damage from excessive analgesic consumption is such an important variety of toxic nephropathy that it, too, is dealt with in Ch. 378. The renal manifestations of drug-induced lupus erythematosus and the renal damage from drug-induced hemolysis, methemoglobinuria, or thrombotic thrombocytopenic purpura have also been excluded from detailed consideration in this chapter.

INCIDENCE

Incidence varies greatly in different parts of the world, depending in part on the number and variety of nephrotoxic agents in the environment. However, reported frequencies are rarely a reliable indication of true incidence. The diagnosis of a toxic nephropathy depends, first, upon awareness and, second, upon recognition of the causative agent; both may present major difficulties. Thus the early detection of renal damage by a putative nephrotoxin may be difficult because of the large functional reserve of the kidney and the lack of simple tests to demonstrate minor degrees of functional impairment. Once the nephrotoxic potential of a particular agent has become widely appreciated, further cases of nephrotoxicity relating to its use tend no longer to be reported. In different geographical areas, toxic nephropathy accounts for between 5 and 25 per cent of cases of acute renal insufficiency and failure. This incidence will change as new agents come into use, as their nephrotoxicity is recognized, and as their use subsequently declines, or as their intrinsic nephrotoxicity is modified, a pattern observed with the aminoglycoside antimicrobials.

SUSCEPTIBILITY OF THE KIDNEY TO TOXINS

Many factors contribute to the special susceptibility of the kidney to damage by chemicals, the major ones being its concentrating and excretory functions. The toxic effect of most substances depends upon the concentration achieved at the effector site, and high concentrations of toxic substances may occur during their excretion within tubular fluid and tubular epithelial cells. In the case of medullary damage, the countercurrent mechanism may also contribute. The volume of glomerular filtrate is large, and tubular epithelial cells have a high metabolic rate, transporting large amounts and a wide variety of substances (both endogenous and exogenous) during secretory and excretory processes. The flow rate and pH of the tubular fluid, as well as the presence of renal disease, may also affect the concentra-

tion of toxin to which tubular epithelial cells are exposed. These cells are particularly prone to damage during the period of neonatal development. The kidney is also liable to involvement in a broad spectrum of immunologically mediated disease, the fine structure of the glomerulus being important in determining the specific localization of immune complexes. When one considers the wide variety of substances absorbed from an increasingly complex environment and needing to be excreted (even large amounts of Worcestershire sauce are said to cause renal damage), it is perhaps surprising that the kidney is able to handle so many without developing lesions.

PATHOGENETIC MECHANISMS

In addition to the two mechanisms already mentioned, i.e., dose-related cytotoxicity and an immunologically mediated nephropathy, renal dysfunction caused by exogenous agents can result from prerenal or postrenal mechanisms. Thus disordered fluid and electrolyte balance or an anaphylactic reaction to a therapeutic agent may cause a reduction in renal blood flow and a corresponding fall in the glomerular filtration rate. Treatment with drugs which increase protein catabolism, such as the tetracyclines, can also contribute to nitrogen retention. Postrenal causes are relatively uncommon, the most important being tubular obstruction by sulfonamide or uric acid crystals, or ureteral obstruction from retroperitoneal fibrosis resulting from treatment with methysergide or practolol.

The usual and most important variety of toxic nephropathy is related to the cytotoxic effect of various exogenous protoplasmic poisons. The damage to the kidney is usually related to the degree of exposure and depends upon the concentration of the toxin to which the cell is exposed, both directly and during the concentration and transport processes involved in excretion. At the molecular level, the precise mechanism of cytotoxicity is complex and not well understood. When the concentration of toxin is low, only altered function of the involved cells may be apparent — in the proximal tubule by the Fanconi syndrome, and in the distal tubule by failure of concentrating capacity and acid excretion. If the concentration of toxin is high, on the other hand, necrosis of tubular cells may occur — in the proximal tubule leading to the syndrome of acute renal failure, and in the distal tubule leading to either nephrogenic diabetes insipidus or renal tubular acidosis. Disseminated intravascular coagulation may be superimposed on any of these acute processes as an additional pathogenetic mechanism. The concentration of some toxins may also be increased by the medullary countercurrent mechanism, which appears to be a factor in analgesic-induced papillary necrosis (see Ch. 378).

The recognition that immune mechanisms are involved in some varieties of renal damage from exogenous substances has been relatively recent. With some agents, information is insufficient to determine whether the renal damage is due to cytotoxic or to immune mechanisms, or whether both may be acting. Characteristic of an immune-mediated nephropathy is the fact that the extent of the renal damage is unrelated to the dose of the toxic agent and its development is less predictable. It is often associated with systemic manifestations of hypersensitivity and is likely to recur on a second exposure to the causative agent. Circulating antibodies to the causative agent may sometimes be demonstrable, and cell-mediated immune mechanisms may also play a pathogenetic role.

Hypersensitivity angiitis, sometimes with Henoch-Schönlein purpura, occurring as a reaction to an exogenous agent such as sulfonamide, may result in renal disease. Glomeruli may be involved when various processes leading to a glomerulonephritis are invoked as a response to an exogenous agent. Immune complexes, such as those occurring during gold therapy, may be deposited beneath, and induce a response on the part of, the epithelial cells of the glomerular capillary. It has been suggested that petroleum products may be involved in the genesis of Goodpasture's syndrome, in which circulating antibodies against glomerular basement membrane have been found. In drug-induced systemic lupus erythematosus, circulating immune complexes may cause damage to tubules as well as glomeruli. Damage to tubules may also be found in the presence of antibodies to tubular basement membrane. These have been said to develop following primary cytotoxic damage to tubular cells.

An immunologically mediated acute interstitial nephritis is also an important variety of toxic nephropathy. The best example is the reaction to methicillin, in which hematuria and deterioration of renal function occur. Kidney size is usually increased in acute cases. The characteristic histologic lesion consists of edema and infiltration of interstitial tissues, chiefly by lymphocytes and plasma cells, but also by eosinophils and occasional polymorphonuclear leukocytes, in the absence of interstitial fibrosis. Dilatation of tubules may be seen, occasionally with casts; there may also be degeneration and necrosis of tubular epithelial cells in the most severely affected areas with atrophy of tubules. Characteristically, the glomeruli and vessels are normal,

TABLE 1. Pathogenetic Mechanisms of Toxic Renal Damage

1. Concentration-dependent cytotoxicity, dose-related; superimposed acute renal failure and intravascular coagulation—e.g., metal-induced acute tubular necrosis or chronic nephropathy
2. Immune-mediated nephropathy
   a. With systemic hypersensitivity—e.g., methicillin-induced interstitial nephritis
   b. Without systemic manifestations—e.g., gold-induced glomerulonephritis or nephrotic syndrome
   c. Hypersensitivity angiitis—e.g., sulfonamide sensitivity
3. Prerenal: reduced renal blood flow or glomerular filtration rate—e.g., dehydration, anaphylactic reaction, hypotension
4. Postrenal: tubular or ureteric obstruction—e.g., crystal nephropathy, retroperitoneal fibrosis

whereas antibody to tubular basement membrane has been noted on immunofluorescence. Those agents, such as rifampin and phenindione, that can lead to prolonged anuria and impairment of renal function may cause histologic evidence of tubular atrophy and interstitial fibrosis as well as focal aggregations of lymphocytes and plasma cells.

The various pathogenetic mechanisms mentioned are not mutually exclusive, and various combinations may occur, as illustrated subsequently.

ASSOCIATED CLINICAL SYNDROMES

With such a wide variety of pathogenetic mechanisms, the clinical presentation may be extremely varied. The traditional toxic nephropathy following exposure to a poison is most likely to present with either tubular dysfunction or the syndrome of acute renal failure. If exposure has been prolonged, chronic renal failure may develop. The clinical manifestations of the immunologically mediated forms of renal disease include the nephritic syndrome, the nephrotic syndrome, and the

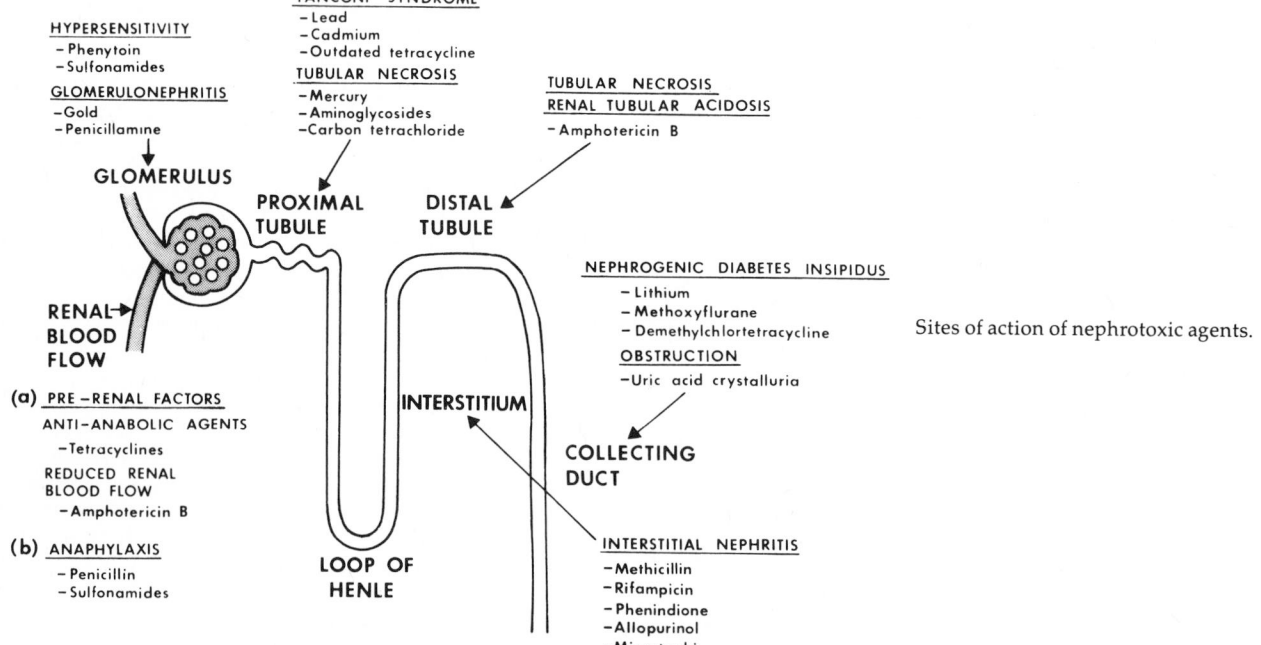

Sites of action of nephrotoxic agents.

acute or chronic renal failure of interstitial nephritis. Combinations of several of these syndromes may occur simultaneously or sequentially at different phases of exposure to a toxic agent. The recognition of any of the syndromes is greatly facilitated by information concerning renal function prior to contact with any potential nephrotoxin. The syndromes are included here to facilitate the subsequent consideration of particular nephrotoxic agents.

RENAL TUBULAR DYSFUNCTION. Although the clinical manifestations may vary widely, three syndromes are seen with toxic renal damage severe enough only to impair tubular function. (1) The Fanconi syndrome, a term used broadly to imply renal impairment in which tubular dysfunction is more severe than glomerular dysfunction. Its manifestations include glycosuria, aminoaciduria and phosphaturia, and sometimes hypokalemia. It is seen in several metal nephropathies, and in that caused by degraded tetracycline. (2) Impairment of urine concentrating capacity leading to nephrogenic diabetes insipidus with polyuria and polydipsia, as seen in nephrotoxicity caused by lithium, fluoride, and demethylchlortetracycline. (3) Impairment of acid excretion leading to renal tubular acidosis, as develops in the nephrotoxicity caused by amphotericin B.

ACUTE RENAL FAILURE. This may occur in varying degrees of severity, and may be detected only if one is alert to the possibility. In its milder form, slight proteinuria with an increased excretion of cells and casts in the urine may be found, with a fall in urine volume and the appearance of azotemia. An example of this may be seen in nephrotoxicity caused by the aminoglycoside antimicrobials. In its most acute form, such as that occurring after the ingestion of inorganic salts of mercury, the clinical pattern will be that of acute tubular necrosis with the early development of oliguria or anuria and a dramatic cessation of renal function (see Ch. 372). This is potentially reversible after removal of the causative agent. Although it might be supposed that the manifestations are due to direct tubular cytotoxicity, the same clinical syndrome may be seen when the tubular necrosis is mild as when it is severe, thereby suggesting that additional alternative pathogenetic mechanisms might be operating (Oken).

The syndrome of acute renal failure caused by acute interstitial nephritis usually presents with deterioration of renal function, often associated with oliguria, developing some days or weeks after exposure to the causative agent. Hematuria, either microscopic or macroscopic, and proteinuria are commonly seen, together with systemic manifestations such as fever, rash, arthralgia, eosinophilia, and sometimes disordered liver function. Mostly, the renal insufficiency is of moderate degree and is associated either with oliguria or with polyuria if the urine-concentrating mechanism is impaired. Remission usually occurs after withdrawal of the causative agent; however, if it is continued, the associated acute renal insufficiency may become chronic, leading to permanent renal impairment. Steroid therapy after withdrawal of the causative agent has appeared to hasten remission in some cases.

CHRONIC RENAL INSUFFICIENCY AND FAILURE. When caused by renal damage by toxic agents, the syndrome of chronic renal insufficiency will usually be indistinguishable clinically from that following renal damage of any other cause. The typical syndrome is described in Ch. 371. In some of these situations, there may be slowly progressive deterioration of renal function, even in the absence of continuing toxic concentrations of the initiating agent. In such cases, hypertension with consequent vascular sclerosis may be important in producing the progressive damage. Chronic lead nephropathy represents a typical example of this variety of toxic nephropathy.

THE GLOMERULONEPHRITIC SYNDROME. Glomerular involvement in an immune-mediated response to an exogenous toxin may present with the clinical features of a glomerulonephritis, with insidious proteinuria, hematuria, and nitrogen retention. When proteinuria becomes sufficient to induce hypoalbuminemia and edema, the nephrotic syndrome (see Ch. 374.2) may result. Typical examples occur with a wide variety of therapeutic agents, such as penicillamine, trimethadione, and gold, and with certain exogenous noxious agents such as snake venom, poison ivy, bee sting, or pollens.

Heptinstall, R. H.: Interstitial nephritis. A brief review. Am. J. Pathol., 83:213, 1976.

Maher, J. F.: Toxic nephropathy. In Brenner, B. M., and Rector, F. C., Jr. (eds.): The Kidney. Philadelphia, W. B. Saunders Company, 1976, p. 1355.

Méry, J-Ph., and Morel-Maroger, L.: Les néphrites interstitielles aiguës par hypersensibilité médicamenteuse. Ann. Med. Interne., 127:590, 1976.

Muehrcke, R. C., Volini, F. I., Morris, A. M., Moles, J. B., and Lawrence, A. G.: Acute toxic nephropathies: Clinical pathologic correlations. Ann. Clin. Lab. Sci., 6:477, 1976.

Oken, D. E.: Modern concepts of the role of nephrotoxic agents in the pathogenesis of acute renal failure. Prog. Biochem. Pharmacol., 7:219, 1972.

Singer, I., and Forrest, J. N.: Drug-induced states of nephrogenic diabetes insipidus. Kidney Int., 10:82, 1976.

SOME IMPORTANT NEPHROTOXINS

Antimicrobial and Chemotherapeutic Agents

Dose-related nephrotoxicity is generally greater if (1) even apparently minor renal insufficiency (such as occurs with increasing years, and which may not produce nitrogen retention) is present prior to therapy, (2) two potentially nephrotoxic agents are used together, or (3) exposure is prolonged. In the presence of preexisting renal disease, it may be possible to avoid nephrotoxicity by modifications of dosage which prevent the development of toxic serum concentrations.

AMINOGLYCOSIDES. These agents bind to renal tissue, and a large proportion of a given dose is rapidly excreted by the kidney. All are potential dose-related nephrotoxins which affect primarily the proximal tubule and present chiefly as acute renal insufficiency, sometimes with oliguria. Since nephrotoxicity is related to the serum concentration, the initial dosage regimen should be determined from a consideration of lean body weight and renal function and subsequently adjusted according to the measured serum concentrations of the aminoglycoside.

Streptomycin exhibits low nephrotoxicity, but renal function must be monitored in order to prevent accumulation of the drug and resulting ototoxicity. Neomycin, the most toxic aminoglycoside, is too toxic for parenteral use and is restricted to topical application or irrigation and to bowel sterilization by oral administration. Some neomycin is absorbed systemically from both these routes, however, and toxic serum concentrations may occur if renal excretory function is impaired.

TABLE 2. Some Common or Important Nephrotoxins

Antimicrobial and chemotherapeutic agents: Aminoglycosides (streptomycin, neomycin, kanamycin, gentamicin); cephalosporins (cephaloridine, cephalothin); colistimethate; penicillins (methicillin and ampicillin); sulfonamides; tetracycline, demethylchlortetracycline; rifampin, ethambutol; amphotericin B
Metallic salts: lead, cadmium, mercury, gold, uranium, copper, bismuth, thallium, arsenic and arsine, lithium
Therapeutic agents: phenindione, D-penicillamine, phenytoin, trimethadione, paramethadione, furosemide, streptozotocin, phenylbutazone, sulfinpyrazone, allopurinol, analgesics (salicylates and aspirin-phenacetin combinations)
Anesthetic agents: methoxyflurane, enflurane
Radiographic contrast media, especially those used in high concentration for angiography and cholecystography
Hydrocarbons and organic solvents: carbon tetrachloride, tetrachloroethylene, ethylene glycol
Osmotic agents: low molecular weight dextrans
Physical agents: radiation, heat stroke, electroshock
Miscellaneous: potassium bromate, carbon monoxide, snake and spider venom, mushroom poisoning

This list is not comprehensive and the omission of a substance does not imply the absence of nephrotoxicity.

Nephrotoxicity presents as acute renal failure, and eighth-nerve damage is also a major risk.

Kanamycin is the second most toxic aminoglycoside, and high serum concentrations can result in the typical picture of dose-related nephrotoxicity ranging from a mild decrease in renal function to acute tubular necrosis. It is particularly important to calculate dose carefully in relation to body size and renal function and to monitor renal function and serum concentrations of kanamycin during therapy.

Gentamicin is an aminoglycoside with great therapeutic value. Significant nephrotoxicity is relatively infrequent, occurring in less than 2 per cent of patients treated. Nonetheless, dosage should be calculated with care, and monitoring of serum gentamicin and creatinine and urea concentrations undertaken. The risk of renal damage may be increased by associated therapy with cephalosporins or diuretics. When acute tubular necrosis develops, hemodialysis may be needed, and, although the lesion is potentially reversible, recovery may be slow and incomplete.

Although the relative toxicity of the newer aminoglycoside antimicrobials, tobramycin and amikacin, has not been clearly established, it cannot yet be assumed that this is less than that of gentamicin. Accordingly, careful calculation of dose and monitoring of serum levels are important to minimize any risk of nephrotoxicity. Both are effectively removed by hemodialysis.

CEPHALOSPORINS. The original cephalosporin, cephaloridine, demonstrated dose-related nephrotoxicity. The newer cephalosporins, such as cephalothin, although certainly less nephrotoxic, may still on rare occasions induce renal damage in man. The nephrotoxic potential of cephalothin appears to be significantly less than that of even the newer aminoglycosides. There is relatively little information concerning the nephrotoxicity of the other new cephalosporins. Cephalosporins are rapidly excreted by tubular excretory mechanisms probably within the proximal convoluted tubule, and high concentrations are achieved within the tubular epithelial cells. Generally, nephrotoxicity seems to be dose related and to occur particularly if high dosage is used in patients with pre-existing renal disease. Although some reports have suggested that the lesion is an acute interstitial nephritis, immunofluorescence has

been negative and there has been no clear evidence of antibody production. Other factors promoting nephrotoxicity include concurrent diuretic therapy, dehydration or plasma volume depletion, and the simultaneous administration of aminoglycoside antibiotics.

There are many reports of nephrotoxicity during combined therapy with cephalosporins and gentamicin. It presents clinically as dose-related reversible acute renal failure. It is particularly likely in very ill patients with possible pre-existing renal disease exposed to high serum antibiotic concentrations for more than five days. Such concurrent administration follows the general rule of increased nephrotoxicity when two potential nephrotoxins are administered simultaneously.

SODIUM COLISTIMETHATE (POLYMYXIN E). All polymyxins must be regarded as potentially nephrotoxic; sodium colistimethate is the main one administered systemically to man. Even healthy volunteers demonstrated a fall in creatinine clearance during colistimethate therapy. Twenty per cent of patients treated with this drug showed features of a reversible dose-related nephrotoxicity within four days. This presented as hematuria, proteinuria, cylindruria, and oliguria; 2 per cent of patients ultimately developed acute tubular necrosis. Such nephrotoxicity occurred even with recommended doses; neurotoxicity resulting in respiratory insufficiency, paresthesias, and neuromuscular blockade was also seen. Nephrotoxicity was seen especially in overweight patients for whom it has been suggested that the risk might be lessened by a schedule relating the dosage to the square root of body weight. Colistimethate is removed by peritoneal dialysis but not by hemodialysis.

PENICILLIN DERIVATIVES. Penicillin preparations do not exhibit direct or dose-related nephrotoxicity. Renal damage may develop during an anaphylactic reaction to penicillin, particularly if hypotension occurs. There is also some evidence of a hypersensitivity type of angiitis developing after penicillin therapy which may affect the kidney, producing lesions in the glomerular tufts. However, the main renal lesion, associated in particular with the semisynthetic penicillins, is an acute interstitial nephritis of allergic origin. Although it is chiefly seen after methicillin therapy and occasionally after ampicillin therapy, it can probably be a rare complication of therapy with any of the penicillin derivatives. Methicillin nephropathy usually presents, some days after the beginning of treatment, with a rash and eosinophilia, with hematuria, which may be macroscopic, and with steadily progressive renal insufficiency. Sometimes eosinophils can be found in the patient's urine. Histologically, the glomeruli are normal and the tubules show only patchy changes, but there is interstitial edema with infiltration by lymphocytes, monocytes, plasma cells, and eosinophils. In some such cases, serum antibodies to the penicilloyl antigen have been detected, and immunofluorescence has been noted along both the tubular and the glomerular basement membrane. The postulated mechanism has been the development of an immune response to an antigen-protein complex resulting from the coupling of the penicilloyl hapten to a renal structural protein. Thus, although not conclusive, the evidence is suggestive of a cell-mediated type of immune response as the basis for methicillin-induced interstitial nephritis. Subsequent exposure to the same or a different penicillin has usually resulted in an exacerbation of the renal disease.

Apart from withdrawal of the causative agent and the standard management of the associated acute renal insufficiency, management of penicillin-induced acute interstitial nephritis has sometimes included therapy with prednisone and heparin. There are no good control studies to indicate whether such therapy is beneficial. However, histologic changes often persist for more than three months, so that in view of the postulated mechanism, therapy with prednisone would be justifiable in the more severe cases. Heparin should be considered if there is evidence of intravascular fibrin deposition.

SULFONAMIDES. Nephrotoxic reactions to the sulfonamides, relatively frequent during their early years of use, are now quite uncommon. There is probably no dose-related nephrotoxic effect. The main problem was related to crystallization of the sulfonamide within the renal tubules, leading to hematuria and an obstructive uropathy with oliguria and progressive renal failure. The tendency to crystallization of sulfonamides depended upon the sulfonamide concentration, the solubility of the particular compound, and the pH of the tubular fluid or urine. Thus crystallization is preventable by adequate hydration and maintenance of a dilute urine and by urinary alkalinization. The newer sulfonamides are appreciably more soluble, and the risk of sulfonamide crystalluria is low, although the necessity for a good urine flow rate during sulfonamide therapy cannot be overemphasized.

An allergic reaction to the sulfonamides is relatively common, unrelated to the dose used. Some of the manifestations resemble an acute interstitial nephritis; an immune complex glomerulonephritis has also been reported. In yet others, lesions have resembled a necrotizing angiitis. Such reactions were particularly associated with the use of the long-acting sulfonamides. The use of co-trimoxazole (trimethoprim-sulfamethoxazole) has not been associated with serious renal toxicity in patients with normal renal function.

TETRACYCLINE. The tetracyclines have a protein antianabolic effect which leads to elevation of the blood urea nitrogen concentration. This occurs even in normal subjects, but is a particular problem in patients with stable chronic renal failure in whom the excretion of the tetracycline is also delayed and its protein catabolic effect intensified. The tetracyclines also promote an increase in salt and water excretion which, in patients with chronic renal failure, leads to weight loss, acidosis, and a fall in the creatinine clearance. This can result in a marked deterioration of renal function and even death in subjects with pre-existing renal disease. Doxycycline has a half-life which is unchanged in chronic renal failure. Hence, although it has a slight antianabolic effect, it does not cause an exacerbation of renal failure in patients with renal disease and is the tetracycline of choice in this situation.

The consumption of outdated and deteriorated tetracyclines has caused a reversible Fanconi syndrome. This has been associated with glycosuria (sufficient at times to cause polyuria and weight loss), phosphaturia, and aminoaciduria, together with proteinuria which has varied from mild to considerable. There is often associated evidence of renal tubular acidosis, and the patients have usually shown hypokalemia, hypouricemia, and hypophosphatemia. Some have also had polyuria. These features have usually resolved within a month. The pathologic lesions have been primarily tubular, affecting both proximal and distal tubules, and are thought to be caused by the various degradation products of tetracycline, particularly epianhydrotetracycline. The change in the excipient used in tetracycline capsules has largely eliminated the risk of formation of such degradation products. Nonetheless, outdated tetracycline should be avoided.

Demethylchlortetracycline (demeclocycline) can cause impairment of renal concentrating power in normal subjects and can induce a reversible nephrogenic diabetes insipidus with polyuria and polydipsia. The effect is dose related and reversible. It is thought to act by inhibiting the generation of cyclic AMP and its action in promoting osmotic water flow through membranes. Its use has been associated with the development of nonoliguric renal failure in patients with cirrhosis.

ANTITUBERCULOUS AGENTS. Patients receiving therapy with rifampin may develop influenza-like symptoms of chills, malaise, vomiting, and fever, which are followed by oliguria, leading to acute renal failure. This often remits after rifampin is withdrawn. Most patients affected in this way have received a prior course of rifampin for between one and twelve months, and the syndrome has developed on starting a second course of the drug. Although the initial evidence suggested that the acute renal failure was related to an acute tubular necrosis produced by vasomotor mechanisms, the lesions have recently been regarded as fitting more an acute interstitial nephritis, and occasionally immunoglobulin deposits have been seen around the tubules. Some of these patients have also had positive Coombs' test results, and others a positive macrophage migration inhibition reaction. Anti-rifampin antibodies have been found in the serum of many affected patients, but have been absent in a few. However, these antibodies have also been demonstrated in serum from patients receiving regular daily therapy with rifampin in the absence of any complications. It is likely therefore that the renal lesions develop as a response to a critical level of antigen-antibody complex which occurs when rifampin therapy is intermittent. Clinical manifestations may vary from mild renal insufficiency to severe renal failure requiring dialysis.

The use of ethambutol has also been occasionally associated with an episode of acute renal failure which has remitted after withdrawal of the drug, only to leave persistent impairment of renal function in some cases. The pathologic changes suggested an interstitial nephritis, and, although this appears to be a rare development, observation of renal function during administration of ethambutol seems to be warranted. Ethambutol also causes hyperuricemia by lowering urate clearance, but this mechanism does not appear to be involved in the causation of the acute renal failure. Acute interstitial nephritis with allergic skin manifestations has, on rare occasions, been attributed to para-aminosalicylate.

AMPHOTERICIN B. This drug, used only in systemic fungal infections, causes nephrotoxicity in most patients. It is strongly protein bound, is not dialysable, and is slowly excreted from the body, largely by nonrenal routes. One of its earliest actions is to alter the permeability of cellular membranes. This effect on the luminal membrane of the renal tubular epithelium leads to a failure of hydrogen ion excretion and an increased urinary loss of potassium ions. Thus one of its earliest manifestations is the development of a distal type of renal tubular acidosis, with hypokalemia. A rise in the pH of the morning urine may be observed with the impairment of hydrogen ion excretion, and this will usually precede any fall in glomerular filtration rate. There is also a tendency to both uricosuria and phosphaturia, probably indicating proximal tubular damage, and there may be impairment of renal concentrating power similar to a nephrogenic diabetes insipidus. Of major importance, however, is the steady decrease in glomerular filtration rate, which is in proportion to the dose of amphotericin B administered and which has been attributed to renal vasoconstriction. This may progress to the syndrome of acute tubular necrosis. The associated renal insufficiency is potentially reversible at low dosage, and a slow recovery of function usually occurs. However, irreversible renal failure may develop with a sufficiently high dose. The histologic findings are primarily those of necrosis of both the proximal and distal tubules, together with a characteristic nephrocalcinosis in which calcium deposits are present within both tubules and the renal interstitium. Vacuolization of the smooth muscle cells in the media of arteries and arterioles has also been observed.

Because it is used chiefly in life-threatening situations, treatment may have to be continued despite developing nephrotoxicity. This may sometimes be mitigated by a reduction in the dose or in its frequency. In each case, the risk of nephrotoxicity must be weighed against the risk of the underlying disease. The varied sequelae of nephrotoxicity which have been described must be diagnosed early and corrected when possible. Correction may involve the early administration of potassium salts, alkali (usually in the form of sodium citrate), and fluids. Although a good urine volume should be maintained, there is no convincing evidence that the concurrent administration of mannitol reduces nephrotoxicity.

Appel, G. B., and Neu, H. C.: The nephrotoxicity of antimicrobial agents. N. Engl. J. Med., 296:663, 1977.

Bennett, W. M., Singer, I., Golper, T., Feig, P., and Coggins, C. J.: Guidelines for drug therapy in renal failure. Ann. Intern. Med., 86:754, 1977.

Burgess, J. L., and Birchall, R.: Nephrotoxicity of amphotericin B, with emphasis on changes in tubular function. Am. J. Med., 53:77, 1972.

Gary, N. E., Buzzeo, L., Salaki, J., and Eisinger, R. P.: Gentamicin-associated acute renal failure. Arch. Intern. Med., 136:1101, 1976.

Nessi, R., Bonoldi, G. L., Redaelli, B., and DiFilippo, G.: Acute renal failure after rifampicin: A case report and survey of the literature. Nephron, 16:148, 1976.

Oster, J. R., Epstein, M., and Ulano, H. B.: Deterioration of renal function with demeclocycline administration. Curr. Ther. Res., 20:794, 1976.

Whelton, A.: Antibacterial chemotherapy in renal insufficiency. A review. Antibiot. Chemother., 18:1, 1974.

Woodroffe, A. J., Thomson, N. M., Meadows, R., and Lawrence, J. R.: Nephropathy associated with methicillin administration. Aust. N.Z. J. Med., 4:256, 1974.

Metal Nephropathies

The pathogenesis of renal damage resulting from metals may be either by a direct, dose-dependent, and reversible toxicity or mediated by immune mechanisms. The spectrum of clinical manifestations will depend particularly on the acuteness and severity of exposure and its duration, and on the responses, particularly the immunologic responses, of the host. Any of the associated clinical syndromes may occur, although an acute interstitial nephritis is rare. Establishing an etiologic association between a metal and the renal lesion may be difficult enough in the acute nephropathies and may require extensive epidemiologic studies in the chronic nephropathies. The manifestations of the renal responses to the more important metals are shown below.

LEAD. Acute lead poisoning is probably the most common metal intoxication, especially in children. The frequency of its diagnosis depends upon an awareness of the possibility. Lead is chiefly absorbed through the gastrointestinal tract, although industrial absorption via the lungs is not uncommon and organic lead compounds may be absorbed through the skin. Lead paint is one of the most common sources, and lead can be absorbed either by children sucking fingers contaminated with lead paint and ingesting paint flakes or industrially during demolition of old buildings. Contaminated water, food, or utensils may cause sporadic lead poisoning. Contamination of "moonshine" produced in illicit lead-containing stills in the southern United States is a common source.

Acute lead poisoning is seen most frequently in the summer, possibly because of the enhancement of lead absorption by vitamin D. Acute lead intoxication may cause symptoms which at times are vague, but which may include intestinal colic, anemia, peripheral neuritis, or an encephalopathy with optic neuritis. The various indices of lead intoxication include an elevated lead content in whole blood and an increased excretion of lead in urine, together with features of consequent metabolic effects, notably the presence of coproporphyrinuria, an increased renal excretion of delta-aminolevulinic acid (ALA), and a reduction in the activity of erythrocyte ALA dehydratase. The kidney is frequently involved during acute lead intoxication, but symptoms may be few and specific search is often needed to demonstrate the acute nephropathy. Histologically, proximal tubular degeneration is seen, together with the presence of eosinophilic (acid-fast) intranuclear inclusion bodies. Swelling of the mitochondria is found with an impairment of their oxidative and phosphorylative functions. These intranuclear inclusions

TABLE 3.   Manifestations of Metal Nephrotoxicity

Metal	Acute Nephropathy		Chronic Nephropathy	Nephrotic Syndrome
	Tubular Necrosis	The Fanconi Syndrome		
Lead	+	+	+	0
Cadmium	+	+	+	0
Mercury	+	0	?	+
Gold	+	0	0	+
Uranium	+	+	+	0
Copper	+	+	+	0
Bismuth	+	+	+	0
Thallium	+	0	0	+

contain sulfhydryl groups and consist of a lead-protein complex. Such cells, still containing eosinophilic intranuclear inclusion bodies, may sometimes be detected in the urine during an acute lead nephropathy. Mild proteinuria is often found, with an increased excretion of casts. Glycosuria and aminoaciduria, manifestations of the Fanconi syndrome, are frequent. Nitrogen retention may be seen in more severe cases. The lesion, however, is usually reversible, and regeneration of the proximal tubular epithelial cells occurs.

With acute lead intoxication, prevention of further exposure alone will often cause a remission of many of the manifestations. Usually, however, parenteral treatment with calcium ethylenediamine-tetraacetate (EDTA) is desirable. This chelates the toxic lead, converting it into the relatively nontoxic lead-EDTA complex which is rapidly excreted by the kidney, thereby inducing a remission of the clinical and biochemical manifestations. However, the excretory capacity of the kidney for lead EDTA depends upon the glomerular filtration rate, so that the dose of calcium EDTA administered should be reduced in proportion to the creatinine clearance. In the presence of normal renal function, 1 gram of calcium EDTA given by infusion over six to eight hours each day for a period of five days can be given initially. Further similar courses may be administered as judged necessary by the various indices of intoxication mentioned above.

Long-continued low-grade exposure to lead may cause chronic lead nephropathy. Such exposure was seen particularly in Queensland, Australia, where acute lead poisoning was common in children until 1930, owing to the ingestion of powdered and flaking lead paint from weathered verandah railings. Careful epidemiologic follow-up subsequently established a greatly increased incidence of chronic renal disease in those children who had suffered from acute lead poisoning, and a positive correlation of the renal disease with increased lead stores in bone has incriminated lead etiologically. The prolonged ingestion of lead-contaminated water in Scotland has also been associated with raised blood lead concentrations, renal insufficiency, and hyperuricemia. A similar syndrome to that seen in Queensland has been detected among "moonshine" drinkers in the southern United States, where the "moonshine" has been prepared in stills with lead condensers. There are also occasional reports of chronic renal insufficiency following prolonged industrial exposure to lead, seen particularly, but not exclusively, in less developed countries. In Queensland, criteria for establishing a diagnosis of chronic lead nephropathy have been taken to include (1) the presence of uniform and equal contraction of both kidneys, (2) the presence of longstanding chronic renal disease with slow progression, (3) exclusion of an alternative cause for the renal disease, and (4) definite evidence of excessive past lead absorption. As continuing manifestations of lead intoxication were absent, evidence for the last-named aspect could be obtained either by demonstrating an increased content of lead in bone (usually skull bone) or by the presence of an increased excretion of lead in urine after a standardized dose (1 gram) of calcium EDTA. Those who developed their acute lead intoxication during childhood often had impairment of mental functions as well. Another associated feature in chronic lead nephropathy is the presence of disproportionate hyperuricemia and gouty arthritis; gout is

usually regarded as being rare in patients with chronic renal failure, whereas gout is seen in half the patients with chronic lead nephropathy. The disproportionate hyperuricemia in this condition is due to reduced renal excretion of urate. Pathologically, the kidneys show uniform granular contraction and fibrosis. The likely sequence of events includes severe renal damage with destruction of nephrons during the acute lead intoxication, followed by the disappearance of the damaged tissue during childhood and adolescence, the onset of hypertension in early adult life, and the gradual onset and progression of chronic renal failure with the development of the granular contracted kidneys.

The management of chronic lead nephropathy is essentially that of the conservative management of chronic renal failure. However, a much slower rate of progression may be expected than in glomerulonephritis, and the normalization of the plasma levels of urate, phosphate, and bicarbonate is desirable to minimize complications. Unless there are signs of acute lead intoxication, the administration of calcium disodium EDTA does not benefit the renal lesion. If it is to be given because signs of acute lead intoxication are present, the dose of calcium EDTA should be reduced in proportion to the reduced glomerular function.

CADMIUM. Cadmium can produce both an acute nephropathy with proximal tubular lesions and a chronic nephropathy. It has a high affinity for sulfhydryl groups, thereby damaging disulfide bonds and also leading to a disturbance of energy production at the cellular level which may lead to cellular necrosis. Cadmium is used in the metal plating industry and can be leached by acid from cadmium-plated containers or volatilized by heating, leading to acute respiratory symptoms. Because of the difficulty in the elimination of absorbed cadmium, measures to prevent absorption are of the greatest importance. Severe and acute exposure, which often occurs via the respiratory tract, may lead to renal tubular and cortical necrosis. Chronic cadmium poisoning occurs both in cadmium workers and in the nearby population following industrial contamination of large areas of the countryside. During this less severe exposure, a "tubular" proteinuria comprising low molecular weight proteins (between 15,000 and 40,000 daltons) is found. This urinary protein consists largely of β_2 microglobulins, immunoglobulin light chains, and lysozyme. Many persons from areas chronically polluted with cadmium are found to show this "tubular" type of proteinuria and also, in the early stages, aminoaciduria and glycosuria. Impaired concentrating ability and features of renal tubular acidosis may also occur. Some of these features may increase the tendency to form renal calculi, and persistent hypercalciuria may lead to a painful osteomalacia which, in Japan, is referred to as "itai-itai byo" or "ouch-ouch" disease. With continuing exposure, and often even without further exposure, progressive renal damage occurs. At this stage, the pathologic findings are similar to those in chronic lead nephropathy, but the presence of hypercalciuria and the absence of urate retention permit chronic cadmium nephropathy to be distinguished clinically from that caused by lead.

On diagnosis of cadmium intoxication, removal from exposure and reduction of cadmium intake are desirable when possible. The renal tubular acidosis and any other defects of tubular function may have to be compensated by specific supplements. There is concern for added nephrotoxicity from chelating agents in this condition, so that calcium EDTA should be used with great care, if it is to be used at all.

MERCURY. Mercury, probably the most nephrotoxic metal, causes cellular damage by combining with sulfhydryl groups of the mitochondrial membrane and by inhibiting sulfhydryl-containing enzyme systems. Mercurial compounds are used extensively in many industrial processes, and there have been areas of environmental contamination by mercurial waste. Mercurial fungicides applied to seed, intended for sowing but ingested, have caused outbreaks of acute intoxication. Ingestion is sometimes with suicidal intent. Mercurials were used in medicine as organic mercurial diuretics, as mercury-containing ointments and skin lotions, and as calomel; none is extensively used any longer. Absorption may occur from the skin or mucous surfaces or by inhalation, the last-named route being possible with metallic mercury.

Significant absorption of mercurial compounds may lead to systemic symptoms with circulatory collapse and oliguria. Acute ingestion of mercurial salts should be treated urgently by gastric lavage with a fluid containing milk and egg albumin, intended to combine with mercury, and charcoal may be added to adsorb any uncombined compound. Absorbed mercury is rapidly bound to renal tissue and is only slowly excreted. Oliguria develops early, at which time the urine is likely to show proteinuria with cellular casts and increased numbers of red and white cells. Occasionally glycosuria and aminoaciduria are seen, but the toxicity is such that these are only transient. Calcification of the necrotic proximal tubules occurs more commonly when this is due to mercury than to other metals. Regeneration of the tubules may occur, provided that the damage is not too great.

Because of its considerable toxicity, measures to prevent mercury intoxication are of great importance. Absorbed mercury is rapidly bound to protein, so that early treatment with dimercaprol (BAL) in full dosage should be commenced as soon as possible. This will have to be combined with early and frequent dialysis to remove the dimercaprol-mercury complexes which may not otherwise be eliminated if there is associated oliguria or anuria.

Mercurials have also been implicated in the nephrotic syndrome. This occurred particularly when organic mercurial diuretics were given to patients with preexisting renal disease. The proteinuria is glomerular in type, and symptoms of hypersensitivity may sometimes be detected. Light microscopy is frequently normal, but electron microscopy provides evidence of an immune-complex type of glomerulonephritis with epimembranous electron dense deposits, extension of the basement membrane between the deposits, and fusion of the epithelial foot processes. Removal from the mercury exposure will often produce a fall in the mercury excretion and a remission in the proteinuria.

Mercury has also been said to induce a chronic renal lesion, but the evidence is not strong that this can develop other than as a residual damage after an acute toxic nephropathy. Proteinuria has been recorded in workers with chronic exposure to mercury, and this has been observed to subside after removal from exposure. There are few pathologic or epidemiologic studies in such patients, and the lack of any relationship between exposure and response suggests that this might be a mild variety of immune complex glomerulonephritis such as has been considered above for the mercury-induced nephrotic syndrome. However, residents of Minimata Bay in Japan have suffered chronic organic mercurial exposure. Although this primarily caused neurologic disorders, affected persons showed low molecular weight tubular proteinuria. The demonstration of this type of proteinuria may therefore provide an early indication of renal damage from organic mercurials.

GOLD SALTS. Gold salts are used in the treatment of rheumatoid arthritis. Parenteral gold is initially bound to plasma proteins, but, with an increase in tissue binding, the amount of gold in the circulation steadily falls. Gold tends to accumulate particularly in the kidneys, where, in the first few days, it is seen chiefly in the proximal tubular epithelial cells. It is later present in the distal tubules and within interstitial macrophages, where it may persist for up to 30 years after its last administration.

Toxic reactions to gold result chiefly in dermatitis, bone marrow depression, or nephrotoxicity. The kidneys are involved in only a small proportion of such reactions, and renal damage usually manifests first either as microscopic hematuria or proteinuria. Mild proteinuria may remit despite continuation of therapy. Nephrotoxicity in the form of acute tubular necrosis with anuria may rarely be seen. The more common type of reaction, however, consists of the development of an immune complex glomerulonephritis, with proteinuria varying in degree from mild to sufficiently heavy to cause the nephrotic syndrome. Its development is not dose related. Intracytoplasmic gold inclusions are seen in proximal tubule cells, together with subepithelial deposits of electron dense material (presumably immune complexes) within the glomeruli with fusion of epithelial cell foot processes. However, gold is absent from the glomerular lesions. Subsequently, by a process of synthesis of basement membrane by the glomerular epithelial cells, the subepithelial deposits are displaced toward the endothelial side. Ultimately, these deposits may be eliminated and the basement membrane restored. Repair is usually incomplete, however, and the appearance is that of a chronic membranous glomerulonephritis, although this is of immune origin, rather than on a nephrotoxic basis as in chronic lead or chronic cadmium nephropathy.

URANIUM. Uranium is less nephrotoxic than either mercury or lead. Its chemical toxicity overshadows any associated radiation hazard. Accidental or industrial toxicity is rare in man because of the great care exercised with its use. After parenteral administration, it accumulates in the renal cortex and is excreted via the kidney. Acute or intense exposures may cause nephrotoxic tubular lesions, which may present either with acute renal failure or as specific abnormalities of tubular function. Workers exposed to uranium have shown aminoaciduria and glycosuria, but catalasuria is the most sensitive index of toxic tubular damage. Impairment of renal concentrating ability and acid excretion has been noted. There are few reports of chronic exposure in man, but prolonged high dosage in animals has led to granular contracted kidneys with cortical narrowing.

COPPER. Acute poisoning with copper salts occurs

during attempted suicide in some countries. Tubular degeneration and necrosis with acute renal failure are seen in the more severe cases, but it is difficult to tell whether this is a direct nephrotoxic lesion from copper or is secondary to the associated hemolysis, hemoglobinuria, and shock. Copper is nondialysable, and hemodialysis is of no value in its elimination; peritoneal dialysis may be of benefit.

Hepatolenticular degeneration (Wilson's disease), caused by a genetically determined reduction in ceruloplasmin, the copper-binding serum protein, is associated with deposition of copper in both the liver and the kidney. In the kidney, this results in areas of focal tubular necrosis corresponding with the sites of maximal copper deposition. The functional defects of the Fanconi syndrome are seen with tubular proteinuria, generalized aminoaciduria, phosphaturia, uricosuria, and distinctive hypercalciuria. Defective urinary acidification may also be present. Glomerular filtration rate steadily falls, although the fall rarely causes clinical symptoms. The chronic copper overload and the resultant functional tubular lesions are reversible by penicillamine therapy.

BISMUTH. Although bismuth is no longer used in the treatment of syphilis, soluble bismuth compounds may be taken either accidentally or with suicidal intent and have been administered in the treatment of warts. The kidney, which is the main excretory route for bismuth, retains bismuth tenaciously for long periods. Acute bismuth nephrotoxicity can lead to acute renal failure with tubular necrosis. Although potentially reversible, there is a high mortality. Less intense exposure may lead to the Fanconi syndrome with proteinuria, glycosuria, aminoaciduria, phosphaturia, uricosuria, and a salt-losing state. Refractile yellowish-brown inclusion bodies, usually intranuclear, may be found in the kidney for up to 30 years after exposure. Although dimercaprol (BAL) has been used in acute intoxications, experience with this use is limited and there is only limited evidence of a beneficial effect.

THALLIUM. Thallium is used chiefly as a rat poison or for denaturing alcohol. Although it is largely excreted by the kidneys and is concentrated in them, renal lesions are a relatively unimportant part of the syndrome of thallitoxicosis, which includes mental changes, peripheral neuropathy, loss of hair, and alimentary symptoms. Proteinuria is seen in such cases, and the urine also contains erythrocytes and granular casts. In more severe lesions, nitrogen retention with either oliguria or polyuria may develop. In such cases, toxic changes occur in the proximal convoluted tubules. One case of the nephrotic syndrome has been reported.

Potassium salts appear to promote renal elimination of thallium and have been used in association with diphenylthiocarbazone (dithizone) and diethyldithiocarbamate (dithiocarb) to increase its fecal and renal excretion. Although thallium is diffusible, the amount removed by hemodialysis is not large in comparison with that eliminated by other routes, and dialysis is probably best reserved for the management of any associated renal failure.

ARSENIC. The dramatic gastrointestinal manifestations of arsenical intoxication overshadow the associated toxic nephropathy. In its mildest form, the urine may contain protein, casts, erythrocytes, and leukocytes. Oliguria, nitrogen retention, and acute renal failure may develop, but it is difficult to differentiate the direct metal nephrotoxicity from that of any associated shock. In the presence of normal renal function, therapy with dimercaprol (BAL) is indicated. Arsenic is effectively removed by hemodialysis, and this should be used, either with or without dimercaprol, if the patient is oliguric or anuric. Arsine poisoning (AsH_3) is accompanied by impaired renal function, but this is due more to the associated hemolysis than to any direct nephrotoxic effect.

LITHIUM. Although renal toxicity from lithium has long been recognized, its importance has become apparent only since the more widespread appreciation of the value of lithium carbonate in serious affective disorders, such as the manic-depressive psychoses. Long-term therapy, even in doses yielding plasma lithium concentrations within the accepted safety range, can lead, in about 12 per cent of patients, to failure of renal concentrating capacity with polyuria and polydipsia. This is unresponsive to vasopressin and represents an acquired nephrogenic diabetes insipidus. The effect appears to be largely dose dependent and to be potentially reversible. Lithium is excreted from the body almost exclusively by the kidney. Patients who develop polyuria should not be allowed to become salt depleted, because this results in increased proximal tubular reabsorption of both salt and lithium, thereby leading to a tendency to a higher serum lithium concentration with associated features of systemic, particularly neurologic, toxicity. This nephrogenic diabetes insipidus has been associated with histologic evidence of damage to the epithelium of the distal convoluted tubules and the collecting ducts, but there is a stage when functional disturbances exist without evidence of histologic abnormality.

Adams, R. G., Harrison, J. F., and Scott, P.: The development of cadmium-induced proteinuria, impaired renal function, and osteomalacia in alkaline battery workers. Quart. J. Med., 38:425, 1969.

Emmerson, B. T.: Metals and the kidney. In Black, D. A. K. (ed.): Renal Disease. Oxford, Blackwell Scientific Publications, 1967, p. 561.

Emmerson, B. T.: Chronic lead nephropathy. Kidney Int., 4:1, 1973.

Kazantzis, G., Schiller, K. F. R., Asscher, A. W., and Drew, R. G.: Albuminuria and the nephrotic syndrome following exposure to mercury and its compounds. Quart. J. Med., 31:403, 1962.

Lindop, G. B., and Padfield, P. L.: The renal pathology in a case of lithium-induced diabetes insipidus. J. Clin. Pathol., 28:472, 1975.

Paulson, G., Vergara, G., Young, J., and Bird, M.: Thallium intoxication treated with dithizone and hemodialysis. Arch. Intern. Med., 129:100, 1972.

Törnroth, T., and Skrifvars, B.: Gold nephropathy prototype of membranous glomerulonephritis. Am. J. Pathol., 79:219, 1975.

Urizar, R., and Vernier, R. L.: Bismuth nephropathy. JAMA, 198:187, 1966.

Therapeutic Agents

Renal damage from therapeutic agents, although a rare occurrence, may develop unpredictably, usually as part of an abnormal immune response to a foreign substance. Features of an adverse drug reaction involving other organs, such as the skin or liver, may be found. Any of the associated clinical syndromes listed may occur, although those resulting from cytotoxic mechanisms occur least frequently. Many of the agents to be considered cause renal damage so rarely that monitoring of renal function is not indicated during their routine use.

PHENINDIONE. On rare occasions, patients treated with phenindione may develop an acute interstitial nephritis with acute renal failure. In such cases, dermatitis and hepatitis are often present, and the macrophage migration inhibition test may be positive. Some may present with the nephrotic syndrome. The severity of the renal failure varies greatly, but it may be prolonged and at times irreversible. When renal complications are recognized, the drug should be withdrawn and, if the renal lesion is severe, steroid therapy used.

D-PENICILLAMINE. D-Penicillamine, originally used in the treatment of hepatolenticular degeneration and in some metal intoxications, has recently been used more frequently for rheumatoid arthritis. Mild proteinuria occurs commonly, and this sometimes settles with lowering of the dose. However, the proteinuria may become heavy, and up to 30 per cent of patients develop the nephrotic syndrome. This, too, is potentially reversible on cessation of the drug, although remission may be delayed and incomplete in some patients. Renal complications force cessation of therapy in up to 20 per cent of patients.

The mechanism responsible appears to be an immunologic one, and examination of renal biopsies has shown electron-dense deposits, presumably of immune complexes, present on the epithelial surface of the glomerular basement membrane, together with fusion of the foot processes of the epithelial cells. IgG and complement have been identified in relation to these deposits. A rare complication of therapy has been the development of the syndrome of lung hemorrhage with nephritis. In such cases, the clinical picture has been of a rapidly progressive glomerulonephritis and the pathologic findings those of a focal proliferative glomerulonephritis, with prominent epithelial crescent formation. However, the linear immunofluorescence characteristic of Goodpasture's syndrome has not been present.

ANTICONVULSANTS. A hypersensitivity reaction to *phenytoin* (diphenylhydantoin) may involve the kidney, causing the syndrome of acute renal failure. Associated features have included skin lesions, varying from a rash to exfoliative dermatitis, and signs of hepatitis or myositis, which were sometimes accompanied by fever and lymphadenopathy. Some of the features have suggested an arteritis. The lesion is usually reversible on withdrawal of the drug, although sometimes steroid treatment has been needed.

Oxazolidinediones. Proteinuria, which may become heavy enough to induce the nephrotic syndrome, may occur in patients receiving trimethadione or paramethadione, sometimes after years of treatment. The proteinuria usually responds to withdrawal of the drug, but there is a wide variation in the rate of recovery, from a prompt fall to a gradual remission over six to twelve months. Some have remitted with continuing treatment at a lower dose. On light microscopy, the kidney has usually appeared normal, although occasional minor glomerular abnormalities have been found. Infiltration of the glomeruli with eosinophils has also been reported, suggesting an allergic reaction. In this case, immunofluorescence was negative for immunoglobulin and electron microscopy showed an irregular thickening and splitting of the glomerular basement membrane, which contained a variety of deposits different from those of membranous glomerulonephritis. Some patients with persistent disease have been treated successfully with steroids and immunosuppressive drugs, but in view of the recovery which occurs following simple withdrawal of the drug — albeit at a variable

rate — it is difficult to obtain clear evidence that such therapy changed the natural history of the disease. However, remission following withdrawal and steroid therapy has not been invariable, and renal failure and death have occurred.

DIURETICS. The thiazide diuretics, as well as furosemide and acetazolamide, have all on rare occasions been implicated in the etiology of allergic interstitial nephritis with acute renal failure. Sometimes there have been features of a hypersensitivity angiitis. However, the case for an etiologic association is not absolute, as many of the patients had also received other drugs; augmentation of nephrotoxicity may be involved.

PHENYLBUTAZONE. Renal lesions attributed to phenylbutazone have been seen after as little as 2 grams administered over a six-day period, and are due to a sensitivity mechanism. Although rare, they have presented either as acute renal failure (with or without oliguria), as acute interstitial nephritis, as membranous glomerulonephritis, or as an allergic angiitis, sometimes with manifestations of thrombotic thrombocytopenic purpura.

DRUGS ALTERING URATE CONCENTRATIONS. The potent uricosuric, *sulfinpyrazone*, has been reported to cause a typical acute interstitial nephritis which resolved on cessation of therapy. A second challenge with the drug caused a mild recurrence of the syndrome. Therapy with *allopurinol* has also been associated with the development of an acute interstitial nephritis, probably as a cell-mediated hypersensitivity response. In these cases there is often evidence of angiitis with skin lesions, fever, and eosinophilia, and the histologic findings are characteristic of acute interstitial nephritis. Glomerulonephritic lesions have been seen in some. Reactions to allopurinol have occurred in patients with previously normal renal function, but are more likely to occur in patients with pre-existing renal disease. The risk is probably less if a lower dose is used. Because of the severe associated nonrenal complications of fever, angiitis, and skin reaction, prednisone has usually been administered and has appeared to produce a more rapid improvement in renal function. However, therapy has often been needed for months, and earlier withdrawal has been followed by a relapse of fever and renal insufficiency. On occasion, despite steroid therapy, the renal insufficiency has been severe and prolonged and at times fatal.

STREPTOZOTOCIN. Streptozotocin, an anti-tumor agent used chiefly in malignant insulinomas because of its selective destruction of pancreatic β cells, is excreted in high concentration in the urine.

Mild proteinuria may be seen early, followed by a variety of tubular dysfunction. Glycosuria, phosphaturia, and uricosuria may occur as manifestations of the Fanconi syndrome, as well as renal tubular acidosis or nephrogenic diabetes insipidus. These may lead to azotemia and oliguric renal failure. In such cases, there is histologic evidence of proximal tubular necrosis, and cellular atypia with pleomorphism and hyperchromasia may be seen in the regenerating tubular epithelium. These lesions can develop in kidneys with previously normal function.

Bar-Khayim, Y., Teplitz, C., Garella, S., and Chazan, J. A.: Trimethadione-induced nephrotic syndrome. A report of a case with unique ultrastructural renal pathology. Am. J. Med., 54:272, 1973.

Flurane Anesthetics

Many anesthetic agents lead to a transient reduction in renal blood flow and glomerular filtration rate, but are not specifically nephrotoxic. The use of methoxyflurane and, to a lesser extent, enthrane as anesthetic agents has been associated with renal dysfunction in the immediate postoperative period. When this occurs, it presents as a vasopressin-resistant polyuric renal failure, which is usually transient and remits within 10 to 20 days. The loss of renal concentrating power with a persistently negative fluid balance leading to dehydration suggests damage to the distal nephrons. However, the initial polyuric phase may pass into a later oliguric phase with typical features of acute renal failure, which either may remit after weeks or months or may persist as chronic renal insufficiency for years. These developments are largely a reflection of the concentration and duration of administration of the anesthetic agent. The associated renal insufficiency varies greatly in severity, clinical presentation, and persistence.

Methoxyflurane is metabolized to fluoride and oxalate. Fluoride inhibits enzyme systems involved in sodium transport in the ascending limb of the loop of Henle and the early distal tubule. The threshold for nephrotoxicity is a plasma fluoride concentration of 40 or 50 μmole per liter, although lower concentrations have been associated with nephrotoxicity in patients with pre-existing renal disease. After methoxyflurane anesthesia, calcium oxalate crystals are frequently noted in the urine and, when toxicity occurs, intratubular and interstitial calcium oxalate crystals have been noted within the kidney. This oxalate deposition is thought to be relatively less important than the fluoride in the induction of renal damage. Histologic changes vary greatly, depending upon the stage and degree of toxicity. In the early stages, degeneration and necrosis of tubular epithelial cells and tubular dilatation are seen, whereas in those patients with persisting renal insufficiency increasing interstitial fibrosis is found.

Fluoride is rapidly excreted while the urine flow rate is good, so that a diuresis is important in prophylaxis. However, toxic levels may persist if oliguria occurs early. The finding of a high serum fluoride concentration in an oliguric patient therefore would support the early use of hemodialysis. Management otherwise is that appropriate for the stage of acute or chronic renal failure, with electrolyte and fluid supplements during the period of nephrogenic diabetes insipidus. The condition can be prevented by limiting the concentration and duration of methoxyflurane which is administered, particularly in subjects with even mild pre-existing renal disease, and by avoiding the simultaneous use of other potentially nephrotoxic drugs.

Gottlieb, L. S., and Trey, C.: The effects of fluorinated anesthetics on the liver and kidneys. Ann. Rev. Med., 25:411, 1974.

Radiographic Contrast Media

The major urographic and angiographic media in use are triiodinated benzoic acid derivatives — diatrizoate, iothalamate, and metrizoate. There is evidence that the methylglucamine salts have less endothelial toxicity than sodium salts and are preferable for coronary and cerebral angiography, whereas sodium salts are preferred for excretion urography. Occasional patients, particularly those with a history of allergy or asthma, may demonstrate idiosyncratic reactions to radiographic contrast media with widely varying manifestations, sometimes appearing as an anaphylactoid reaction and sometimes as acute renal failure. Their development is usually not dose dependent.

Although increasing amounts of contrast media are being used to provide better definition of the kidneys and urinary tract, the incidence of nephrotoxic reactions to these agents remains very low. The various contrast agents are excreted by glomerular filtration and are concentrated in the renal tubular fluid without active tubular secretion; the concentration in the urine may be up to 100 times that in the plasma. Toxicity is basically dependent upon the concentration of medium achieved at the cellular level. High dose excretion urography is only rarely associated with direct tubular toxicity, the risk of nephrotoxicity being related to (1) the state of hydration, (2) the presence of pre-existing renal disease and (3) the dose of contrast medium administered. Thus it is chiefly a risk in patients with diabetes or myeloma, in the presence of dehydration, stasis, or obstruction to urine flow, or when larger doses or repeated exposures occur to media with a high iodine content. Although dehydration seems to be the dominant factor in renal failure after urography in multiple myeloma, contrast media are better avoided in such patients if possible.

Nephrotoxicity is somewhat more of a hazard with selective renal angiography, although contrast agents are relatively nontoxic at ordinary concentrations. However, the renal vascular bed tends to react to high concentrations of contrast media by vasoconstriction (whereas in other vascular beds vasodilatation may occur), and this may lead to varying degrees of acute renal failure. A similar renal reaction may occur after cardiac angiography, especially in the presence of diabetic renal disease. The initial clinical manifestations of nephrotoxicity consist of microscopic hematuria with proteinuria and cylindruria, and this may pass into the typical syndrome of acute renal failure. In occasional cases, prolonged impairment of renal function has occurred. This nephrotoxicity has been attributed variously to altered renal hemodynamics and erythrocyte crenation and agglutination from the viscous hypertonic medium, tubular obstruction caused by dye-protein interactions, and direct toxicity to tubular epithelial cells. However, it may also develop when increased concentrations of contrast medium occur because of faulty placement of the intra-arterial catheter, reduced blood flow to a small kidney, injection of a branch artery, or wedging of a catheter tip in a narrowed renal artery, causing both delayed transit time of the dye and local renal ischemia. Many radiographic contrast agents are also uricosuric, and an acute uric acid nephropathy has been invoked. However, acute renal failure has occurred with these agents despite the maintenance of a vigorous diuresis and the prevention of a high urinary urate concentration, so that uric acid does not seem to have an etiologic role in any associated renal damage.

CHOLECYSTOGRAPHY. Contrast media, such as iopanoic acid and ipodate, which are used for oral cholecystography, or iodipamide and ioglycamate, which are used for intravenous cholangiography, have all on occasion been associated with the development of acute tubular necrosis, but the risk is much less with the newer agents. Dehydration is unnecessary in cholecystography and, because of the associated hazard, should be prevented, if necessary by prior water ingestion. The risk of nephrotoxicity is otherwise increased if multiple or repeated doses of contrast medium are given, if there has been a recent intravenous cholangiogram, if there is significant renal disease, or in the presence of hepatic disease with reduced hepatic excretion of contrast medium. The Dubin-Johnson syndrome is a contraindication to cholangiography.

Thus renal complications from radiographic contrast media may be minimized by using the lowest necessary dose of medium (especially if the normal route of elimination is impaired), together with the maintenance of a good urine flow rate. Should acute renal failure supervene, the management is that of this condition from whatever cause, and dialysis may be required.

Ansari, Z., and Baldwin, D. S.: Acute renal failure due to radio-contrast agents. Nephron, 17:28-40, 1976.

Ansell, G.: Adverse reactions to contrast agents. Scope of problem. Invest. Radiol., 5:374, 1970.

Grainger, R. G.: Renal toxicity of radiological contrast media. Br. Med. Bull., 28:191, 1972.

Mudge, G. H.: Some questions on nephrotoxicity of contrast agents. Invest. Radiol., 5:407, 1970.

Organic Solvents and Hydrocarbons

CARBON TETRACHLORIDE. Carbon tetrachloride is widely used as a solvent and dry cleaning fluid, occasionally in fire extinguishers, and rarely as a vermifuge. Absorption is usually by inhalation (this is aggravated by exposure in confined spaces) or following ingestion. Its toxicity is enhanced by alcohol, probably because of the increased activity of drug-metabolizing enzymes, leading to an increase in its conversion to ethylchlorformate. Being lipid-soluble, it is concentrated in tissue fat stores, the brain, and bone marrow. Either carbon tetrachloride itself or its metabolites have a direct toxic effect on the liver and kidney parenchyma, leading to centrilobular necrosis in the liver and degeneration of the proximal and, to a lesser extent, the distal tubular epithelium of the kidney.

The early clinical manifestations of intoxication involve the gastrointestinal and central nervous systems. Nausea, vomiting, and abdominal pain are common, and headache, confusion, convulsions, and coma may occur. A toxic hepatitis with jaundice is a later development. This is considered in further detail in Ch. 461.1. Renal complications may be delayed for up to a week and range from proteinuria, with microscopic hematuria and casts, to oliguria, passing into the full syndrome of acute renal failure. However, because of the associated hepatic disease, the rise in blood urea nitrogen is disproportionately low and the serum creatinine concentration should be used as the index of renal function. Bleeding tendencies may occur, caused by hypoprothrombinemia, disseminated intravascular coagulation, and hypofibrinogenemia. Carbon tetrachloride may be demonstrated in expired air or blood by infrared spectrophotometry. Trichloroethylene and tetrachloroethylene, although less toxic, may lead to similar renal complications.

Carbon tetrachloride is not dialysable. If exposure has been acute, removal to an area with adequate ven-tilation is essential. Management is like that of acute renal failure from other causes, including dialysis as indicated. The nephrotoxic lesion is potentially reversible following a single exposure, and the mortality in well managed cases is less than 20 per cent.

ETHYLENE GLYCOL. Ethylene glycol and its congeners are aliphatic alcohols used as freezing point depressants. They are potently nephrotoxic following ingestion, which usually occurs by error or in the search for an ethanol substitute. Initial symptoms are often encephalitic, with confusion, convulsions, and coma. A severe acidosis is often present at this stage. Features of myocarditis and myositis may become apparent and, prior to the development of oliguria, crystals of calcium oxalate may be seen in the urine, together with microscopic hematuria. When oliguria and anuria supervene, the clinical pattern is that of acute renal failure, which may remit or, if the damage has been severe enough, may pass into a chronic uremia. The pathologic findings result from the metabolism of ethylene glycol to oxalate and other toxic intermediates; the brilliant birefringent crystals of calcium oxalate are found in a wide variety of tissues. In the kidney, they are seen within the lumina of the proximal tubules, many of which also demonstrate tubular necrosis.

Ethylene glycol is dialysable so that early hemodialysis is indicated. As it is metabolized by alcohol dehydrogenase, its metabolism can be delayed by the simultaneous administration of ethanol (10 grams per hour). The most important aspect of management is the maintenance of a vigorous diuresis, using both mannitol and intravenous furosemide or ethacrynic acid. Acidosis should also be corrected. Institution of these measures soon after diagnosis or soon after the detection of hematuria with calcium oxalate crystalluria may prevent the development of acute renal failure, and this treatment may be needed for several days until all the ingested ethylene glycol has been metabolized. Should acute renal failure develop, therapy is essentially that of this condition with frequent hemodialysis. Ultimate prevention depends upon the widespread appreciation of its toxicity and the hazard of storage in improper containers.

HYDROCARBONS. Most toxins exert their primary effect upon renal tubules; however, it has recently been suggested that some hydrocarbon solvents may induce glomerular injury. Initially, Goodpasture's syndrome was linked with exposure to petroleum products, and more recently an increased incidence of exposure to inhaled hydrocarbon solvents has been reported in patients with proliferative glomerulonephritis and some other renal diseases with nonspecific types of glomerular disease. The proposed mechanism involves immune complex formation. Although the association remains of interest, causality has not yet been established.

Nielsen, V. K., and Larsen, J.: Acute renal failure due to carbon tetrachloride poisoning. Acta Med. Scand., 178:363, 1965.

Underwood, F., and Bennett, W. M.: Ethylene glycol intoxication. Prevention of renal failure by aggressive management. JAMA, 226:1453, 1973.

Osmotic Nephropathy and Low Molecular Weight Dextrans

Swelling and vacuolation of proximal tubular epithelial cells may be seen histologically in the severe glycosuria of diabetes, following the use of mannitol as a diuretic, or after the use of hypertonic sucrose to relieve cerebral edema. However, such lesions have no functional significance. On the other hand, the use of dextrans with a molecular weight of less than 60,000, with the aim of improving vascular flow, has not infrequently been associated with the development of oliguria and acute renal failure. Some of these patients have had acute allergic or anaphylactic reactions, and others have developed an acute hypersensitivity glomerulonephritis. Most of the persons who developed acute renal failure following the use of these low molecular weight dextrans, however, have had severe generalized vascular disease. It is therefore revelant that animal experiments have shown that anuria is likely to develop after their use when reduced perfusion of the kidney leading to reduced filtration pressure is present. These dextrans are readily filterable, and it has been noted that the concentration of the dextran which occurs in the tubules may promote plugging when there is slowing of flow. Thus in clinical practice, it is wise to limit the amount of dextran administration to 1 liter per day and to cease its administration if the urine flow rate is less than 1500 ml per 24 hours, or if the blood urea is more than 60 mg per 100 ml (10 mmol per liter). When renal complications are developing, the decline in urine flow rate is usually gradual and can be treated, and probably prevented, by a mannitol- or drug-induced diuresis. These are thought to act by preventing the development of high intratubular concentrations of dextran.

Feest, T. G.: Low molecular weight dextran: A continuing cause of acute renal failure. Br. Med. J., 2:1300, 1976.

Physical and Miscellaneous Agents

The development of radiation nephritis is now uncommon, being largely prevented by shielding the kidney during irradiation and control of the dose reaching the kidney during radiotherapy of malignancies near the kidney. Pathologically, the main lesion appears to affect the capillary endothelium of the glomeruli, possibly by interfering with its ability to produce the ground substance of the basement membrane. Subsequent death of these cells within two to three months is thought to cause local activation of the coagulation system and secondary vascular damage, leading to a response by mesangial cells and variable thickening and splitting of the glomerular basement membrane. Thus some glomeruli appear to be hyalinized, whereas some show fibrinoid necrosis and focal scarring. In addition, the epithelium and basement membranes of tubules are damaged, resulting in degeneration and collapse of tubules and diffuse interstitial changes which, in the acute phase, may consist of edema and, in the chronic stages, progressive fibrosis. Immunofluorescent studies are usually negative. Vascular lesions of the medium and small arterioles may also occur with intimal proliferation, degeneration of smooth muscle, fibrinoid necrosis, and thrombosis. The renal plasma flow falls steadily with doses of radiotherapy exceeding 400 rads, and there is also impairment of tubular function. At cumulative therapeutic doses of between 2000 and 2500 rads, a progressive decrease in glomerular filtration rate is found, and clinical manifestations are seen. These are usually not apparent until six to eight months or more

after the irradiation has occurred. The clinical pattern is variable, depending upon the severity of the lesion, and may range from a relatively acute renal dysfunction to the development of chronic renal damage. Hypertension, which may be either benign or, more frequently, severe, is a common development. In acute radiation nephritis, malignant hypertension is a major problem and there is a high mortality. The more chronic varieties show a moderate degree of proteinuria with impaired concentrating power and usually a steady decline in renal function unless malignant hypertension supervenes. Vigorous treatment of any associated hypertension is vital, but the management of the associated acute or chronic renal insufficiency does not differ from that of other causes. If only one kidney is involved and control of hypertension is difficult, nephrectomy may result in remission of the hypertension.

Potassium bromate is a common component of neutralizing solutions used for permanent waving. It can induce acute renal failure with persistent loss of hearing, an association also seen with aminoglycoside antimicrobials and occasionally reported with high dosage ethacrynic acid and furosemide. The renal lesion consists of an acute tubular necrosis with resulting severe interstitial fibrosis, usually followed by a slow recovery in renal function.

Absorption of sufficient ingested *paraquat* (a bipyridyl contact herbicide) can cause toxic damage to many tissues, including the kidneys, liver, and lungs. Emergency management should include its elimination (1) from the gut by lavage, the administration of adsorbents (Fuller's earth and bentonite), and purgation, and (2) from the bloodstream by hemodialysis, hemoperfusion through charcoal columns, and a forced diuresis.

Fairshter, R. D., Rosen, S. M., Smith, W. R., Glauser, F. L., McRae, D. M., and Wilson, A. F.: Paraquat poisoning: New aspects of therapy. Quart. J. Med., 45:551, 1976.
Keane, W. F., Crosson, J. T., Staley, N. A., Anderson, W. R., and Shapiro, F. L.: Radiation-induced renal disease. A clinicopathologic study. Am. J. Med., 60:127, 1976.

380.   OTHER SPECIFIC RENAL DISEASES

Robert W. Schrier

380.1.   NEPHROGENIC DIABETES INSIPIDUS

PATHOPHYSIOLOGY OF POLYURIC STATES ASSOCIATED WITH RENAL DISEASES. Polydipsia and polyuria may be due to several factors. Increased thirst and water intake may lead to polyuria. In this setting, the sequence of events leading to the polyuria includes (1) increased water intake, (2) a fall in plasma osmolality, (3) suppression of vasopressin release, (4) relative water impermeability of the collecting duct, and (5) increased solute-free water excretion. In the absence of increased water intake, polyuria may result from inadequate release of vasopressin (central or pituitary diabetes insipidus) or impaired concentration of urine by the kidney independent of the presence of adequate endogenous vasopressin (nephrogenic diabetes insipidus). The renal concentrating mechanism involves the following sequence of events:

1. Active chloride and passive sodium transport occurs in the water-impermeable portions of the nephron, including primarily the ascending limb of the loops of Henle. This process both dilutes the tubular fluid and establishes a hypertonic environment in the interstitium surrounding the medullary collecting duct.

2. Osmotic equilibration of fluid between the collecting ducts and hypertonic interstitium then occurs in the medulla and leads to a concentrated urine. This equilibration of water is dependent on the capacity of the medullary collecting duct to become water permeable in response to vasopressin.

Thus nephrogenic diabetes insipidus may be due to an impairment in the active transport mechanism in the water-impermeable ascending limb of Henle's loop or to failure of the medullary collecting duct to become water permeable in the presence of vasopressin. These effects may occur as a result of acquired renal diseases or a congenital defect.

PRESENTING COMPLAINTS. The presenting complaints of polydipsia and polyuria may be due to several different disorders in addition to nephrogenic diabetes insipidus. In many instances, the polydipsia is a secondary phenomenon which results as a consequence of a polyuric state which alters total body water and solute concentration. This stimulation of polydipsia occurs as a consequence of either a rise in plasma osmolality or a contraction of the extracellular fluid volume. As already discussed, patients with central or pituitary diabetes insipidus (vasopressin responsive) or nephrogenic diabetes insipidus (vasopressin resistant) may present with polydipsia and polyuria. Similarly, patients undergoing an osmotic diuresis, such as that which occurs in the hyperglycemic diabetic patient who is excreting large amounts of glucose, may present with polydipsia and polyuria.

In contrast, in other circumstances, the polydipsia may be the primary phenomenon which causes the polyuria. For example, some individuals have a primary polydipsia (compulsive water drinkers) or may have thirst stimulation secondary to serum electrolyte abnormalities such as hypokalemia and hypercalcemia. In both these settings, however, a renal resistance to the action of vasopressin (nephrogenic diabetes insipidus) may also be present.

Some characteristics of the polydipsia and polyuria may provide clues about the cause of the disorder. For example, the patient with primary polydipsia may relate a history of polydipsia and polyuria which is present primarily during the daytime. If so, polydipsia and polyuria may have a vague onset and vary in severity during the course of the disease. Individuals with this disorder are most often females who have a history of psychoneurotic or psychotic problems. In contrast, the individual with complete pituitary diabetes insipidus may complain of polydipsia and polyuria during the entire 24 hours each day. Such patients may relate a specific time and sudden onset of the polydipsia and polyuria which has persisted in a consistent pattern. Occasionally, however, large bladder capacities may develop in such patients which attenuate the nighttime complaints of polydipsia and polyuria. The patient with

nephrogenic diabetes insipidus may also exhibit polydipsia and polyuria throughout the entire 24-hour day. The onset of complaints, however, may be gradual. The magnitude of thirst and polyuria is less with acquired nephrogenic diabetes insipidus as compared to pituitary diabetes insipidus or primary polydipsia. In the latter two circumstances, the fluid intake and urine output frequently may exceed 4 to 5 liters per day. In contrast, most patients with acquired nephrogenic diabetes insipidus do not have polydipsia or polyuria greater than this degree. This is probably due to the degree of filtration rate reduction which frequently accompanies acquired nephrogenic diabetes insipidus. Congenital nephrogenic diabetes insipidus, which presents in young male children, may be associated with the excretion of large volumes of urine per day (10 to 12 liters).

ETIOLOGY. A number of renal diseases, drugs, and metabolic disorders have been associated with acquired nephrogenic diabetes insipidus. Perhaps the clearest mechanism for such a vasopressin-resistant state was evident in a reported patient in whom amyloid was shown to surround the medullary collecting ducts. In this instance, it was easy to conceive that vasopressin may not have exerted its normal response to increase the water permeability of medullary collecting ducts. However, in other causes of chronic renal failure, a similar relative unresponsiveness of the medullary collecting ducts to vasopressin may be present. Such a hyporesponsiveness of collecting ducts to vasopressin recently has been shown in vitro in nephrons from uremic animals. Most renal diseases that have been described in association with vasopressin-resistant hyposthenuria (acquired nephrogenic diabetes insipidus) primarily involve the renal medulla. Adult polycystic disease, medullary cystic disease, obstructive uropathy, sickle cell disease, Sjögren's syndrome, and chronic pyelonephritis are all such diseases. In addition to an impairment of the response of the collecting duct to vasopressin, these renal diseases may also have a diminished capacity of the ascending limb of Henle's loop to transport solute without water, and thus the creation of the hypertonic interstitium (osmotic driving force for passive reabsorption of water) is attenuated. Several drugs and metabolic disorders also may cause a nephrogenic diabetes insipidus. The main drugs known to interfere with the action of vasopressin include lithium, demeclocycline, and methoxyflurane. These pharmacologic agents probably interfere both with the effect of vasopressin to activate adenyl cyclase–mediated cyclic AMP (intracellular secondary messenger for vasopressin) and with the subsequent effect of cyclic AMP to initiate events leading to increased water permeability of the collecting duct epithelium. The effects of hypokalemia and hypercalcemia to cause nephrogenic diabetes insipidus have already been mentioned and will be discussed in more detail in Ch. 380.2 and 380.3.

LABORATORY FINDINGS. Polyuria may be associated with hypernatremia if urinary losses of solute-free water are not replaced. This is rarely the case if the subject is conscious, has accessible fluid to ingest, and has an intact thirst mechanism. These patients, however, are quite susceptible to water depletion if events supervene which impair the ingestion of adequate amounts of solute-free water, e.g., gastrointestinal disorders causing nausea and vomiting, or anesthesia.

A diminished plasma sodium concentration frequently accompanies the solute diuresis and polyuria associated with hyperglycemia in patients with diabetes mellitus. In the absence of adequate amounts of effective insulin, glucose remains in the extracellular fluid compartment (ECF), and the resultant ECF hyperosmolality causes osmotic water movement from the cell into the ECF compartment with the occurrence of hyponatremia. Nonketotic or ketotic hyperosmolar coma may occur in this setting. The presence of glucosuria is obviously pivotal to confirm this diagnosis. Although hyponatremia generally occurs in this setting, if the renal hypotonic losses caused by the osmotic diuresis predominate over the level of hyperglycemia, these patients may present with hypernatremia. This generally occurs in young individuals who have excellent renal function and thus large clearances of glucose. Other substances such as mannitol may cause hyponatremia by a similar movement of water from cells into the ECF volume and polyuria by inducing an osmotic diuresis. High protein gavage feedings also can lead to an osmotic diuresis and polyuria.

In addition to measuring plasma sodium, osmolality, and glucose in the polyuric patient, the presence of hypokalemia and hypercalcemia should be excluded as causes of this disorder. Renal function should be assessed by measurements of the serum creatinine and urea nitrogen concentrations. A careful assessment of the urine composition is critical in evaluating the patient with complaints of polydipsia and polyuria. Mannitol, glucose, and radiopaque dyes may cause an osmotic diuresis associated with a disproportionately high specific gravity as compared to urine osmolality. A urine osmolality below 100 mOsm per kilogram is characteristic of complete central diabetes insipidus or primary polydipsia, but less dilute urine (100 to 250 mOsm per kilogram) may occur with the polyuria associated with partial diabetes insipidus. With a pure water diuresis, as occurs with primary polydipsia or complete pituitary diabetes insipidus, the urinary sodium concentration is less than 10 mEq per liter, whereas it will be greater than 20 mEq per liter during an osmotic diuresis and in most patients with acquired nephrogenic diabetes insipidus. The definitive diagnosis of acquired nephrogenic diabetes insipidus requires demonstration that the renal concentrating defect is unresponsive to the administration of exogenous vasopressin.

THERAPY. The therapy for acquired nephrogenic diabetes insipidus should be aimed, if possible, at the primary disorder. Removal of the offending drug or the correction of hypokalemia or hypercalcemia should be undertaken. In the setting of chronic renal disease treatment is generally not feasible unless obstructive uropathy can be relieved. Infusion of mannitol or whole blood transfusions may reverse the renal concentrating defect in sickle cell anemia in the early stages, but in adults medullary infarctions cause an irreversible nephrogenic diabetes insipidus. Thiazide diuretics have been used effectively to produce volume depletion in the patient with congenital nephrogenic diabetes insipidus; this maneuver can enhance proximal fluid reabsorption and decrease required fluid intake. There are several factors involved in postobstructive diuresis, which is generally only marked following relief of bilateral obstruction. These factors include extracellular fluid volume expansion and an osmotic diuresis caused by retained sodium and urea, respectively. Postobstructive diuresis also may be due to defective renal tubular reabsorption of sodium and water as a result of tubular damage secondary to urinary tract obstruction. Such a diuresis can be perpetrated by the excessive administration of intravenous fluids. Hyponatremia, hypokalemia, and volume depletion must be avoided during fluid replacement therapy (as assessed by frequent evaluation of neck veins, skin turgor, mucous membranes, and postural changes of blood pressure and pulse).

The most important therapeutic factor is realization of the defect and prevention of the occurrence of negative fluid balances. For example, if maximal urinary osmolality is 200 mOsm per kilogram H_2O in a patient with chronic pyelonephritis who needs to excrete 600 mOsm of solute per day, the obligatory daily urinary losses are 3 liters exclusive of insensible losses. Thus one day of gastrointestinal upset and no fluid intake could be associated with a 3-kg weight loss and further impairment in renal function. Therefore the physician must educate the patient about such potential dangers associated with the diagnosis of acquired nephrogenic diabetes insipidus.

Berl, T., Anderson, R. J., McDonald, K. M., and Schrier, R.: Clinical disorders of water metabolism. Kidney Int., 10:38, 1976.

Carone, F. A., and Epstein, F. H.: Nephrogenic diabetes insipidus caused by amyloid disease. Am. J. Med., 29:539, 1960.

Hays, R. M., and Levine, S. D.: Pathophysiology of water metabolism. In Brenner, B. M., and Rector, F. C. (eds.): The Kidney, Vol. I. Philadelphia, W. B. Saunders Company, p. 553.

Kahn, M., Merrit, A. D., Wohl, M. J., and Orloff, J.: Renal concentrating defect in Sjögren's syndrome. Ann. Intern. Med., 56:883, 1962.

Schrier, R. W., and Berl, T.: Disorders of water metabolism. In Schrier, R. W. (ed.): Renal and Electrolyte Disorders. Boston, Little, Brown & Company, 1976, p. 1.

Singer, I., and Rotenberg, D.: Demeclocycline-induced nephrogenic diabetes insipidus. In vivo and in vitro studies. Ann. Intern. Med., 79:679, 1973.

Singer, I., Rotenberg, D., and Puschett, J. B.: Lithium-induced nephrogenic diabetes insipidus: In vivo and in vitro studies. J. Clin. Invest., 51:1081, 1972.

Tannen, R. L., Regal, E. M., Dunn, M. J., and Schrier, R. W.: Vasopressin-resistant hyposthenuria in advanced chronic renal disease. N. Engl. J. Med., 280:1135, 1969.

380.2. HYPOKALEMIC NEPHROPATHY

Potassium depletion of several weeks or months in duration may be associated with both functional and structural alterations of the kidney.

PRESENTING COMPLAINTS. Patients with chronic potassium depletion may present with polydipsia, polyuria, nocturia, and weakness. The muscle weakness may be severe, and quadriparesis and even quadriplegia can occur. Rhabdomyolysis and myoglobinuria may accompany severe potassium depletion, and the patient may present with acute renal failure. In this setting, the gastrointestinal (e.g., anorexia, nausea, vomiting) and central nervous system (e.g., depressed mentation, insomnia, inability to concentrate, irritability) symptoms of uremia may predominate. In other circumstances, the symptoms relating to the primary cause of the potassium losses may predominate. For example, abdominal pain, nausea and vomiting with chronic gastric outlet obstruction caused by peptic ulcer disease, chronic diarrhea with malabsorptive disorders, and renal calculi and bone disease with renal tubular acidosis may constitute the primary presenting complaints.

ETIOLOGY. Hypokalemic nephropathy can result from a wide variety of causes which lead to total body potassium depletion. A common setting is metabolic alkalosis. The saline-resistant causes of metabolic alkalosis and primary hypermineralocorticoidism include primary hyperaldosteronism, licorice ingestion, and Cushing's disease; saline-sensitive causes of metabolic alkalosis and secondary hyperaldosteronism include vomiting and diuretic abuse. However, the acid-base status is not a determinant, because hypokalemic metabolic acidosis with renal tubular acidosis or chronic diarrhea also may cause hypokalemic nephropathy.

LABORATORY FINDINGS. In addition to the low plasma concentration of potassium, a careful assessment of the acid-base status of the patient is helpful in the evaluation of the cause of potassium losses. Hypokalemic, hypochloremic metabolic alkalosis will be present with upper gastrointestinal losses of hydrochloric acid. In this setting, the urine may be alkaline or "paradoxically" acid if hydrogen ion secretion predominates in this potassium-depleted state. The urinalysis is generally normal but may reveal slight proteinuria and cylindruria. The serum creatinine and urea nitrogen concentrations are generally normal unless severe volume depletion or myoglobinuria-induced acute renal failure is present. Urine chloride concentration should be low (<10 mEq per liter), but even with volume depletion urine sodium concentration may not be low due to bicarbonaturia. In this setting of potassium and chloride depletion and bicarbonaturia, a urine pH of 7 to 8 should be present and the urine bicarbonate anions obligate the sodium cation. Thus urine sodium concentrations may be as high as 40 to 80 mEq per liter in the presence of volume depletion and a very low urine chloride concentration. Potassium depletion with chronic diarrhea and malabsorptive states or renal tubular acidosis presents with a normal "anion gap" metabolic acidosis, which may actually blunt the level of hypokalemia (owing to potassium shifts from the cell to ECF) despite severe potassium depletion. An evaluation of the urine potassium concentration is also very helpful in the setting of hypokalemia. If potassium losses have been present for several weeks and are of extrarenal origin, e.g., chronic diarrhea, the urine potassium concentration should be less than 20 mEq per liter. On the other hand, hypokalemia caused by renal potassium losses, e.g., metabolic alkalosis of vomiting, diuretic abuse, or primary hyperaldosteronism and renal tubular acidosis, is associated with urine potassium concentrations much higher than 20 mEq per liter. An exception may be the patient who has become potassium depleted secondary to diuretic abuse. Occasionally with severe potassium depletion in this setting, avid potassium reabsorption may occur distal to the site of diuretic action, or the diuretic agent may have been discontinued and on admission the urinary potassium concentration may be less than 20 mEq per liter even though the kidney was the source of the potassium losses.

If the patient has severe polydipsia and polyuria, the urinary osmolality will be less than 100 mOsm per kilogram or the specific gravity less than 1.005. Also, urinary sodium concentration falls during a water diuresis and may be very low in the absence of volume depletion.

The renal concentrating defect with hypokalemia is thought to involve a diminished renal medullary tonicity and perhaps a resistance of the collecting duct to the normal action of vasopressin. However, the renal concentrating defect which occurs with potassium depletion cannot totally account for the polyuria of 4 to 5 liters per day. For example, with hypokalemia, the urinary concentration after dehydration is never less than isotonicity, i.e., 300 mOsm per kilogram. Thus at this urine osmolality, a normal daily solute load of 600 mOsm would obligate only 2 liters or urine per day Because fluid intake is frequently greater than 2 liters, an effect of hypokalemia to stimulate thirst has been proposed and indeed has recently been shown to occur. Lastly, renal phosphate losses and hypophosphatemia have been described with hypokalemia; also, hypomagnesemia is not an uncommon accompaniment of hypokalemia.

HISTOLOGY. The functional abnormalities of hypokalemic nephropathy, i.e., renal concentrating defect, may occur without any obvious structural abnormalities. Nevertheless, in man the characteristic, but not pathognomonic, finding in hypokalemic nephropathy consists of multiple vacuoles in tubule epithelial cells. These vacuoles occur most frequently in the cells of the proximal tubule but also occur in the distal convoluted tubule. The vacuoles do not contain fat or glycogen, and they may relate to dilatation of normally apposed cell membranes or dilated cisternae of endoplasmic reticulum and basilar enfoldings of the cells. In most patients, however, vacuoles are not present and the tubular abnormalities are less specific and are limited to mild degenerative changes. The glomeruli and blood vessels of the kidney are generally normal. It has been suggested that prolonged potassium depletion may lead to irreversible lesions of interstitial fibrosis, scarring, and atrophy and also predispose to chronic pyelonephritis. However, the basis for suggesting these relationships is quite tenuous and uncertain.

THERAPY. The only indicated therapy in hypokalemic nephropathy is replenishment of the total potassium stores and treatment of the disorder causing the renal or extrarenal potassium losses. The functional abnormalities are generally then reversible within several weeks to months, whereas the structural abnormalities reverse within several months to a year.

Berl, T., Linas, S. L., Aisenbrey, G. A., and Anderson, R. J.: On the mechanism of polyuria on potassium depletion: The role of polydipsia. J. Clin. Invest., 60:620, 1977.

Gabow, P.: Disorders of potassium metabolism. In Schrier, R. W. (ed.): Renal and Electrolyte Disorders. Boston, Little, Brown & Company, 1976, p. 143.

Hollander, W., Jr., Winters, R. W., Bradley, J., Holliday, M., Williams, T. F., and Segar, W. E.: The renal lesions of electrolyte imbalance. I. The structural alterations in potassium-depleted rats. J. Exp. Med., 106:563, 1957.

Meuhrcke, R. C., and Rosen, S.: Hypokalemic nephropathy in rat and man. Lab. Invest., 13:1359, 1964.

Schwartz, W. B., and Relman, A. S.: Effects of electrolyte disorders on renal structure and function. N. Engl. J. Med., 276:383, 452, 1967.

Spargo, B. H.: Renal change with potassium depletion. In Becker, E. L. (ed.): Structural Basis of Renal Disease. New York, Hoeber Medical Division, Harper & Row, 1968.

Suki, W. N., and Eknoyan, G.: Tubulo-interstitial disease. In Brenner, B. M., and Rector, F. C. (eds.): The Kidney, Vol. II. Philadelphia, W. B. Saunders Company, p. 1113.

380.3. HYPERCALCEMIC NEPHROPATHY

PRESENTING COMPLAINTS. As with hypokalemic nephropathy, polydipsia and polyuria may provide the presenting complaints in patients with hypercalcemic nephropathy. The presence of other complaints depends on the duration and magnitude of hypercalcemia. Chronic hypercalcemia is associated with hypercalciuria, which may predispose to renal calculi. Severe hypercalcemia (15 to 20 mg per 100 ml) may present as a "hypercalcemic crisis" with rapidly progressive renal failure, oliguria, confusion, lethargy, and coma. Sudden elevation of blood pressure may accompany acutely severe hypercalcemia. Chronic hypercalcemia may be associated with renal impairment, azotemia, and symptoms of uremia. Hypercalcemic nephropathy may also lead to renal tubular acidosis, with renal tubular sodium and potassium wasting.

ETIOLOGY. Hypercalcemia of any cause may lead to hypercalcemic nephropathy. The most common cause is malignant disease; 10 to 20 per cent of patients will have primary hyperparathyroidism. In addition, hypercalcemia may be caused by various endocrine disorders, particularly hyperthyroidism (increased bone resorption) and adrenal insufficiency (increase in protein-bound calcium with volume depletion and increased intestinal calcium absorption with glucocorticoid deficiency). Approximately 20 per cent of patients with sarcoidosis have hypercalcemia, and its occurrence is not uncommon with multiple myeloma. Vitamin D intoxication and the milk-alkali syndrome are less frequent causes of hypercalcemic nephropathy. In the setting of malabsorption and postrenal transplantation, hypercalcemia may be related to excessive parathyroid activity. The terms autonomous and tertiary hyperparathyroidism have been used to describe this cause of hypercalcemia. These terms, however, are probably misnomers, as the parathyroid hormone levels are suppressible with calcium infusions. The hypercalcemia thus seems to be due to the continued output of hormone by the large number of cells in the hyperplastic glands. In acute renal failure associated with muscle necrosis, hypercalcemia may complicate the recovery phase of the disease.

LABORATORY FINDINGS. Symptomatic hypercalcemia relates to an increase in ionized calcium, the physiologic component of total serum calcium. If the clinical laboratory cannot measure ionized calcium, it can be estimated by noting the difference between total serum calcium minus protein-bound calcium. Each gram of albumin per 100 ml of plasma can be estimated to bind 1 mg of calcium. Hypercalcemia associated with the milk-alkali syndrome may be accompanied by metabolic alkalosis, whereas primary and secondary hyperparathyroidism may be associated with hyperchloremic metabolic acidosis. In most instances of primary hyperparathyroidism, however, hyperchloremia is present without evidence of acidosis. The serum phosphorus concentration also may be diminished in primary hyperparathyroidism; some investigators have suggested that a serum chloride to phosphorus concentration ratio in excess of 30 supports the diagnosis of primary hyperparathyroidism as the cause of the hypercalcemia. When the administration of thiazide diuretics is associated with hypercalcemia, the diuretics should be discontinued. Persistence of the hypercalcemia then suggests the diagnosis of primary hyperparathyroidism. As already indicated, there is an increase in serum creatinine and urea concentrations when hypercalcemia has caused acute or chronic renal impairment. A urine and serum electrophoresis also should be performed to exclude multiple myeloma or light chain disease as a cause of hypercalcemia and renal failure. Skeletal radiologic studies should be undertaken in search of evidence for primary hyperparathyroidism (subperiosteal resorption in phalanges or clavicles), bone metastasis, or multiple myeloma. On urinalysis, hypercalcemia of any cause may be associated with modest proteinuria, cylindruria, and white and red cells on examination of the sediment. If hypercalcemia occurs with immobilization, evidence of Paget's disease should be sought. With primary hyperparathyroidism an associated syndrome of multiple endocrine adenomatosis should be considered including Sipple's syndrome (hyperparathyroidism, medullary thyroid carcinoma, pheochromocytoma, and neuromas) and Wermer's syndrome (hyperparathyroidism and tumors of pituitary and pancreatic islet cells). A chest roentgenogram should provide evidence for sarcoid, tuberculosis, or bronchogenic (squamous) carcinoma, all of which may cause hypercalcemia without bone involvement. A plain roentgenogram of the abdomen with tomography may demonstrate renal calculi or nephrocalcinosis.

HISTOLOGY. The epithelium in both the collecting ducts and distal convoluted tubules demonstrates degenerative changes and often necrosis and calcification in hypercalcemic nephropathy. The earliest changes in the kidney of hypercalcemia occur in the mitochondria, which initially swell and then exhibit dark calcium granules. Calcium deposits are also demonstrable in the cytoplasm and basement membrane. Calcium casts occur in distal portions of the nephron with dilatation of proximal nephron segments, thus suggesting an element of luminal obstruction. Luminal obstruction may explain the tubular atrophy and interstitial fibrosis that occur with chronic hypercalcemia. In contrast to hypokalemic nephropathy, hypercalcemic nephropathy does not spare the glomeruli and blood vessels. In fact, calcification of vessels and glomeruli may lead to progressive scarring and loss of renal mass.

THERAPY. Hypercalcemic nephropathy is best treated by correcting the underlying disorder, such as treating the hyperthyroidism or adrenal insufficiency, removal of a parathyroid adenoma, cessation of thiazide diuretics, or ambulation of patient with Paget's disease with or without thyrocalcitonin therapy. Within one to two days, glucocorticoid hormone may be effective in lowering elevated serum calcium concentrations associated with sarcoidosis, vitamin D intoxication, multiple myeloma, and other malignancies. With the shorter duration of action of 1,25-dihydroxycholecalciferol, discontinuation of this drug may be adequate to treat an associated hypercalcemia. Hypercalcemia, caused by nonparathyroid humoral substances (prostaglandin-like) but without bone metastasis, may respond to inhibition of prostaglandin synthesis with indomethacin. The antitumor agent mithramycin may be used to lower severe hypercalcemia associated with malignancies if other treatments are ineffective. The dose of the drug used (25 μg per kg intravenously) is less than its antitumor dose, but hepatotoxicity and renal toxicity may occur nevertheless. Thus extreme caution is necessary, particularly in the patient who already has impaired renal or hepatic function.

In the presence of impaired renal function, salts of phosphorus should probably not be used to treat hypercalcemic nephropathy because of the danger of further nephrocalcinosis. If the renal impairment of hypercalcemic nephropathy is not too severe, furosemide administration with saline replacement of urinary losses may be used to lower the serum calcium concentration. However, with severely impaired renal function, hemodialysis with a calcium-free dialysis fluid is probably the treatment of choice if hypercalcemia is severe. The success of treatment depends on the severity and chronicity of hypercalcemia. With acute hypercalcemia, renal failure of recent onset may be totally reversible, but the functional changes with chronic renal failure and chronic hypercalcemia may not reverse for months after treatment or may be irreversible.

Duffy, J. L., Suzuki, Y., and Churg, J.: Acute calcium nephropathy. Early proximal tubular changes in the rat kidney. Arch. Pathol., 91:340, 1971.

Epstein, F. H.: Calcium and the kidney. Am. J. Med., 45:700, 1968.

Ferris, T., Kashgarian, M., Levitin, H., Brandt, I., and Epstein, F. H.: Renal tubular acidosis and renal potassium wasting acquired as a result of hypercalcemic nephropathy. N. Engl. J. Med., 265:924, 1961.

Goldsmith, R. S., and Ingbar, S. H.: Inorganic phosphate treatment of hypercalcemia of diverse etiologies. N. Engl. J. Med., 274:1, 1966.

Popovtzer, M. M.: Disorders of calcium, phosphorus, vitamin D, and parathyroid hormone activity. In Schrier, R. W. (ed.): Renal and Electrolyte Disorders. Boston, Little, Brown & Company, 1976, p. 167.

Singer, F. R., Neer, R. M., Murray, T. M., Keutmann, H. T., Deftos, L. J., and Potts, J. T.: Mithramycin treatment of intractable hypercalcemia due to parathyroid carcinoma. N. Engl. J. Med., 283:634, 1970.

Suki, W. N., and Eknoyan, G.: Tubulo-interstitial disease. In Brenner, B. M., and Rector, F. C. (eds.): The Kidney, Vol. II. Philadelphia, W. B. Saunders Company, p. 1113.

Suki, W. N., Yium, J. J., Von Minden, M., Saller-Herbert, C., Eknoyan, G., and Martinez-Maldonado, M.: Acute treatment of hypercalcemia with furosemide. N. Engl. J. Med., 283:836, 1970.

380.4. URIC ACID NEPHROPATHY

Acute uric acid nephropathy is a term used for the circumstances when acute elevations in serum uric acid occur and cause acute renal failure secondary to uric acid crystal blockade of collecting ducts, renal pelvis, or ureters. In contrast, gouty or urate nephropathy is a more chronic process in which the kidneys show evidence of arterial and arteriorolar disease, interstitial fibrosis and inflammation, loss of nephron units, and deposition of monosodium urate within the renal parenchyma. Uric acid nephrolithiasis is another cause of renal impairment. Neither of the last-named circumstances will be discussed here.

Acute uric acid nephropathy occurs during treatment of lymphoproliferative or myeloproliferative diseases with chemotherapy or radiation. In this setting, the treatment of lymphomas and leukemias reduces the number of white cells or mass of lymphoid or splenic tissue. Cellular destruction is associated with the release of nucleic acid, which is metabolized to uric acid. With this increase in the uric acid pool, the serum uric acid concentration may rise as high as 50 to 100 mg per 100 ml. The presenting symptoms of acute uric acid nephropathy relate to those of acute renal failure and uremia. Severe oliguria or anuria may occur with extreme elevations in the serum uric acid concentration.

LABORATORY FINDINGS. Acute renal failure secondary to any cause, particularly in association with hypercatabolism, may increase serum uric acid concentrations. However, it has been suggested that a urine uric acid to creatinine concentration ratio in excess of 1.0 indicates that hyperuricemia is the cause rather than

the consequence of the acute renal failure. With acute uric acid nephropathy, uric acid crystals may be seen in the urine sediment. Intravenous urography may show radiolucent masses of uric acid obstructing the ureters and renal pelvis. In the absence of such extrarenal masses, it is intraluminal obstruction by uric acid crystals within the medullary collecting ducts that is primarily responsible for acute renal failure. The precipitation of uric acid occurs mainly in the collecting ducts for several reasons. First, tubular acidification occurs in the distal nephron, and at a pH of 5 to 6 a large fraction of the uric acid ($pk_a = 5.5$) is the un-ionized and poorly soluble uric acid. Also, the collecting ducts are highly resistant structures where urine is concentrated, thus raising the uric acid concentration. In addition to uric acid crystals, modest proteinuria and red and white cells may be present in acute uric acid nephropathy. A spot urine uric acid to creatinine concentration ratio of greater than 1 suggests that the hyperuricemia caused the acute renal failure, whereas a value of less than 1 suggests that the hyperuricemia was a consequence of the acute renal failure.

THERAPY. The most important factor in acute uric acid nephropathy is prevention. In the setting of massive cell destruction, as occurs during treatment of lymphomas and leukemias, several means of preventing renal damage should be instituted. First of all, allopurinol therapy should be started. Allopurinol is a xanthine oxidase inhibitor which prevents the conversion of hypoxanthine and xanthine to uric acid. High doses of allopurinol (400 to 800 mg) may be required in this setting. In addition to allopurinol, other maneuvers constitute important preventive measures. Urinary alkalinization to a pH greater than 7 with sodium bicarbonate or the carbonic anhydrase inhibitor, acetazolamide, will convert the urine uric acid to the highly soluble urate anion. Perhaps even more important is the institution of a diuresis with mannitol or furosemide as urinary losses are replaced. The diuresis both decreases the uric acid concentration in the collecting ducts and increases the flow of tubule fluid through these structures.

If these prophylactic measures have not been instituted and acute uric acid nephropathy occurs, furosemide or mannitol may be effective early in instituting a diuresis. Cystoscopy with retrograde examination and irrigation has on occasion been effective in relieving ureteral or pelvic blockade and in instituting a diuresis. In the presence of anuria and severe renal failure, the only appropriate therapy is hemodialysis to lower the serum urate concentration as well as treating or preventing the uremic state.

Conger, J. D., and Falk, S. A.: Intrarenal dynamics in the pathogenesis and prevention of acute urate nephropathy. J. Clin. Invest., 59:786, 1977.

Conger, J. D., Falk, S. A., and Burke, T. J.: A micropuncture study of the early phase of acute urate nephropathy. J. Clin. Invest., 58:681, 1976.

DeConti, R. C., and Calabresi, P.: Use of allopurinol for prevention and control of hyperuricemia in patients with neoplastic disease. N. Engl. J. Med., 274:481, 1966.

Frei, E., III, Bentzel, C. J., Rieselbach, R., and Block, J. B.: Renal complications of neoplastic disease. J. Chron. Dis., 16:757, 1963.

Kelton, J., Kelley, W. N., and Holmes, E. W.: A rapid method for the diagnosis of acute uric acid nephropathy. Arch. Intern. Med., 138:612, 1978.

Kjellstrand, C. M., Campbell, D. C., II, Von Hartitzsch, B., and Buselmeier, T. J.: Hyperuricemic acute renal failure. Arch. Intern. Med., 133:349, 1974.

Muggia, F. M., Ball, T. J., and Ultmann, J. E.: Allopurinol in the treatment of neoplastic disease complicated by hyperuricemia. Arch. Intern. Med., 120:12, 1967.

Rieselbach, R. E., Bentzel, C. J., Cotlove, E., Frei, E., III, and Freireich, E. J.: Uric acid excretion and renal function in the acute hyperuricemia of leukemia: Pathogenesis and therapy of uric acid nephropathy. Am. J. Med., 37:872, 1964.

Steele, T. H., and Rieselbach, R. E.: The renal handling of urate and other organic anions. In Brenner, B. M., and Rector, F. C. (eds.): The Kidney, Vol. I. Philadelphia, W. B. Saunders Company, p. 442.

380.5. RENAL TUBULAR ACIDOSIS

Metabolic acidosis which is attributable to renal losses of alkali as sodium bicarbonate is termed renal tubular acidosis. When the renal tubular defect is not severe enough to cause metabolic acidosis, the condition is designated incomplete renal tubular acidosis.

CLASSIC OR DISTAL (TYPE I) RENAL TUBULAR ACIDOSIS (RTA)

In the patient with distal RTA, the urine pH remains high (>6.0) and bicarbonaturia persists despite severe degrees of metabolic acidosis. When the plasma concentration of bicarbonate is increased to normal by bicarbonate administration, neither the urinary pH nor urinary bicarbonate excretion increases greatly. Thus hydrogen ion secretion and bicarbonate reabsorption increase commensurately with elevations in filtered bicarbonate. Since 85 per cent of bicarbonate reabsorption occurs in the proximal tubule, this increased reabsorption of bicarbonate suggests an intact proximal tubular reabsorptive capacity. The dysfunction in renal acidification thus appears to reflect an inability of the distal nephron to generate and maintain a normally steep concentration gradient for hydrogen ion between blood and tubular fluid.

ETIOLOGY. Primary distal RTA generally becomes manifest during infancy or early childhood but may occur in early adulthood. In some cases, the disease is familial and occurs as an autosomal dominant condition with a variable degree of expression and greater penetrance in the female. There also appear to be nonfamilial, sporadic cases. A number of drugs may be associated with distal RTA, including amphotericin B, gentamicin, toluene (glue or paint sniffing), phenacetin, and lithium. Various autoimmune disorders also have been found to be accompanied by classic (distal) RTA. Among these disorders are Sjögren's syndrome, systemic lupus erythematosus, primary biliary cirrhosis, thyroiditis, and idiopathic hypergammaglobulinemia (cryoglobulinemia, hyperglobulinemic purpura, and familial hypergammaglobulinemia). Nephrocalcinosis of a variety of causes, including hyperparathyroidism, hyperthyroidism, vitamin D intoxication, medullary sponge kidney, Fabry's disease and idiopathic hypercalciuria, may be associated with distal RTA. Other diseases associated with distal RTA include sickle cell anemia, pyelonephritis, obstructive uropathy, renal transplantation, and hepatic cirrhosis.

PRESENTING COMPLAINTS. The initial clinical difficulty in primary classic RTA may be a disturbance in gait caused by abnormal skeletal growth and rickets. Growth retardation in children is common. Rickets and osteomalacia occur secondary to a high rate of phosphate excretion and hypophosphatemia. The metabolic acidosis contributes to the osteomalacia. Since hypercalciuria is a rather constant feature of distal RTA, patients may present with symptoms secondary to renal calculi, including renal colic and pyelonephritis. As a result of the impaired ability to secrete hydrogen ion, renal potassium wasting occurs and hypokalemia is not uncommon. The hypokalemia in RTA may be associated with muscle weakness and on occasion even quadriplegia, as well as a renal concentrating defect.

LABORATORY FINDINGS. A hyperchloremic, normal anion gap (Na $-[Cl + HCO_3] = 10–12$ mEq) metabolic acidosis suggests either renal tubular acidosis or gastrointestinal losses of alkali, e.g., diarrhea, pancreatic fistula. The history should differentiate between renal and gastrointestinal causes of normal anion gap metabolic acidosis. In distal RTA, hypokalemia with urinary potassium concentrations greater than 20 mEq per liter is a consistent laboratory finding. The urinary sodium concentration may be greater than 20 mEq per liter despite evidence of volume depletion, thus indicating some element of tubular sodium wasting. In distal RTA with volume depletion, hyperreninemia and hyperaldosteronism are generally present. Hypercalciuria (>300 mg per 24 hours) also is found consistently in distal RTA. To diagnose incomplete RTA an acid-loading test (0.1 gram of ammonium chloride per kilogram of body weight) is necessary. Within six to eight hours after this acid load, the normal subject should decrease urine pH below 5.4, and plasma bicarbonate concentrations should not fall.

TREATMENT. Therapy should be directed at a specific cause when possible. Otherwise, sufficient alkali to restore normal acid-base status should be administered. In contrast to patients with proximal (Type II) RTA, the amount of alkali necessary to treat distal RTA is modest (generally 1 to 3 mmoles per kilogram of body weight per day). With alkali administration, renal potassium losses may cease; otherwise, potassium supplements should be given. In children, more alkali may be needed to ensure growth; this increase in amount (5 to 14 mEq per kilogram of body weight) may be due to an increase in endogenous acid production accompanying the growth process or to larger renal bicarbonate losses. Normally in distal RTA, the fraction of filtered bicarbonate excreted is less than 3 per cent.

PROXIMAL (TYPE II) RTA

Another group of patients develops metabolic acidosis resulting from renal alkali losses secondary to an acidification defect in the proximal tubule. The fraction of filtered bicarbonate excreted in proximal RTA generally exceeds 15 per cent when plasma bicarbonate is maintained at a normal level. In proximal RTA, urinary pH is high and bicarbonaturia is present except when acidosis is severe. With severe acidosis bicarbonaturia disappears and urinary pH diminishes to a normal minimum (pH <5.4). With a lowered plasma bicarbonate level, the small filtered bicarbonate load can be reclaimed in the proximal tubule even in the presence of a diminution in the normal tubular capacity to reclaim bicarbonate. Thus the defect in hydrogen ion secretion and bicarbonate reabsorption in the proximal tubule is termed a "quantity-limited" variety of RTA. With a normal plasma concentration and filtered load of bicarbonate, a large quantity of bicarbonate escapes reabsorption and enters the distal nephron. Although in proximal RTA the distal nephron acidification process is normal, the large distal loads of bicarbonate exceed the limited capacity of the distal nephron to reclaim bicarbonate. Thus in proximal RTA, profound bicarbonaturia ensues during alkali administration to maintain plasma bicarbonate concentration at normal. Tubular dysfunctions accompanying proximal RTA may cause hyperaminoaciduria, glucosuria, increased phosphaturia, and uricosuria (Fanconi's syndrome).

ETIOLOGY. Various renal diseases may be accompanied by proximal RTA, including amyloidosis, multiple myeloma, renal transplantation, Sjögren's syndrome and medullary cystic disease. Drug-induced proximal RTA may be caused by acetazolamide, outdated tetracycline, streptozotocin, cadmium, and lead. Several genetic disorders, including cystinosis, Wilson's disease, hereditary fructose intolerance, Lowe's syndrome and tyrosinemia, are associated with proximal RTA. Secondary hyperparathyroidism with malabsorption and chronic renal failure also may suppress proximal tubular bicarbonate reabsorption and cause RTA. Primary-inherited or sporadic proximal RTA also occurs.

PRESENTING SYMPTOMS. Primary proximal RTA occurs chiefly in male infants and manifests primarily as metabolic acidosis and growth retardation. Renal potassium wasting and hypokalemia also occur; therefore muscle weakness, polyuria, and polydipsia may be initial complaints. The renal potassium wasting occurs secondary to the increased delivery of the bicarbonate anion to the distal tubule; thus correction of the acid-base status with bicarbonate does not correct the renal potassium wasting but actually makes it worse. In contrast to distal RTA, nephrocalcinosis and nephrolithiasis are not common accompaniments of proximal RTA. Renal losses of sodium, potassium, amino acids, phosphate, glucose, and uric acid may lead to chronic volume depletion with secondary hyperaldosteronism, malnutrition, failure to thrive, and osteomalacia.

LABORATORY FINDINGS. In contrast to distal RTA, the normal anion gap metabolic acidosis of proximal RTA may occur with an acid urine (pH <5.4) and no bicarbonaturia. This occurs when the acidosis is severe so that the lowered plasma and filtered bicarbonate allow adequate bicarbonate reabsorption in the proximal tubule, thus avoiding excessive delivery of bicarbonate to the normal distal acidification segment of the nephron. In proximal RTA, hypokalemia, hypocalcemia, hypophosphatemia, and hypouricemia may be associated with aminoaciduria and increased phosphate and uric acid clearance, as well as sodium and potassium wasting.

THERAPY. Treatment of the primary disorder associated with proximal RTA should be undertaken when feasible. If this is not possible, large quantities of alkali (5 to 10 mEq per kilogram of body weight per day) may be necessary to correct the acid-base disorder. Potassium supplements also will be necessary, and the amounts of potassium necessary may increase with bicarbonate therapy. With severe bone disease, vitamin D therapy may be indicated. Thiazide therapy may also be used to cause modest volume depletion, enhance proximal bicarbonate reabsorption, and diminish bicarbonaturia.

TYPES III AND IV RENAL TUBULAR ACIDOSIS

A hybrid of RTA with both distal and proximal acidification defects has been described and termed Type III RTA. Type IV RTA refers to some patients with chronic renal failure, metabolic acidosis, and RTA which occur despite relatively well preserved renal function (glomerular filtration rate greater than 25 ml per minute). In these patients, hyporeninemia and deficient secretion of aldosterone, but not cortisol, are invariably present. The renal conditions associated with this condition include diabetic nephropathy, pyelonephritis, interstitial nephritis, and nephrosclerosis. An occasional patient with glomerulonephritis has also been described. Adrenal disorders, e.g., Addison's disease, 21-hydroxylase deficiency, and 18-hydroxy-dehydrogenase deficiency, may cause Type IV RTA in the absence of renal impairment. The acidification defect in Type IV RTA appears to be due to a combination of effects, including decreased proximal bicarbonate reabsorption, a decrease in mineralocorticoid-mediated hydrogen ion secretion in the distal tubule, and the effect of hyperkalemia to decrease ammonium excretion.

Gill, J. R., Bell, N. H., and Bartter, F. C.: Impaired conservation of sodium and potassium in renal tubular acidosis and its correction by buffer anions. Clin. Sci., 33:577, 1967.

Kaehny, W. D.: Pathogenesis and management of metabolic acidosis and alkalosis. In Schrier, R. W. (ed.): Renal and Electrolyte Disorders. Boston, Little, Brown & Company, 1977, p. 79.

McSherry, E., Sebastian, A., and Morris, R. C., Jr.: Renal tubular acidosis (RTA) in infants: The several kinds, including bicarbonate-wasting, classic renal tubular acidosis. J. Clin. Invest., 51:4, 1972.

Morris, R. C., Sebastian, A., and McSherry, E.: Renal acidosis. Kidney Int., 1:322, 1972.

Sebastian, A., McSherry, E., and Morris, R. C., Jr.: On the mechanism of renal potassium wasting in renal tubular acidosis associated with the Fanconi syndrome (Type 2 RTA). J. Clin. Invest., 50:231, 1971.

Sebastian, A., McSherry, E., and Morris, R. C., Jr.: Metabolic acidosis with special reference to the renal acidoses. In Brenner, B. M., and Rector, F. C. (eds.): The Kidney, Vol. I. Philadelphia, W. B. Saunders Company, p. 615.

Sebastian, A., and Morris, R. C.: Renal tubular acidosis. Clin. Nephrol., 7:216, 1977.

380.6.   MISCELLANEOUS DISORDERS

In addition to protein and cellular elements, urine may contain lymph, lipid, or gas bubbles. *Chyluria* is the term used to describe lymph in the urine. With chyluria, the urine appears milky, either intermittently (postural) or constantly. The main constituent is triglycerides, but a colloidal suspension of albumin, lecithin, cholesterin, fibrinogen, and soaps is present, giving the urine the appearance of lactescent serum. The proteinuria may be in amount equal to the criteria for nephrotic syndrome (>3.5 grams per day). Chyluria may be secondary to lymphatic obstruction between the intestines and thoracic duct. Such obstruction may be due to tumors, fibrosis, trauma, and pregnancy. Filariasis (*Wuchereria bancrofti*) also may cause chyluria. In these settings, retrograde pyelography may demonstrate pyelolymphatic backflow. With chyluria, however, fat droplets are not present on microscopy. The differential diagnosis of chyluria includes pyuria and lipiduria.

Lipiduria is characterized by fat droplets that rise to the top on centrifugation. It may be associated with fractures, eclampsia, diabetes mellitus, and phosphorus arsenic, or carbon monoxide poisoning.

Pneumaturia is the passage of gas bubbles in the urine. It may result from a vesicovaginal or vesicoenteric fistula. Such fistulas may occur with pelvic infections, neoplasms, or surgery. A urinary tract infection with gas-forming bacteria such as *E. coli, A. aerogenes,* or yeast may cause pneumaturia. This cause of pneumaturia is most frequent in elderly female patients with diabetes mellitus. In pneumaturia, the urine may froth at the end of micturition, and the bladder may have a gas outline on roentgenographic study.

Caserta, S. J.: Description of chyluria: Report of a case. N. Engl. J. Med., 255:1239, 1956.

Tuller, M. A., Feuer, M. M., Schapira, H. E., and Ho, P-P.: Recumbent chyluria: Demonstration of unilateral renal-lymphatic communication. Am. J. Med., 33:951, 1962.

Yamauchi, S.: Chyluria: Clinical laboratory and statistical study of 45 personal cases observed in Hawaii. J. Urol., 54:318, 1945.

381. RENAL CALCULI

William C. Thomas, Jr.

Renal calculi are concretions consisting of crystals and a matrix of organic matter. Crystals usually constitute the predominant portion (>90 per cent) of the mass of most calculi, but those occurring as a consequence of urinary tract infections have a higher proportion of matrix material. Occasionally this latter type of calculus may be almost devoid of crystals. Renal calculi are to be distinguished from calcific deposits within the renal parenchyma. Such deposits occurring at sites of previous inflammation or degenerative change are designated by the term "nephrocalcinosis." Elsewhere in the text are specific presentations of a number of disorders often complicated by nephrolithiasis; this chapter is largely limited to a discussion of broadly applicable principles in the cause and management of renal calculi.

ETIOLOGY. General Factors. Our knowledge of the cause of various types of calculi is incomplete, but from available evidence it appears that a combination of factors rather than any single event is most often responsible for calculus formation. The likelihood and type of calculous disease is modified by geographic factors, sex, race, and probably diet. In the United States the incidence is greatest in the southeast, but there are other areas of the country where the incidence is also high. South Africa, parts of India, and Southeast Asia are regions where calculous disease also occurs with unusual frequency. In the southeastern United States "hard water" has been thought by some to be the important factor favoring calculus formation, but such a correlation fails to explain why calculi are infrequent in other hard water regions of the world. In India and Southeast Asia protein-poor, predominantly cereal diets have been considered to be of importance in the genesis of bladder calculi so common in children of these areas. Although these and other suggested explanations to account for the regional incidence of calculi have some attractiveness, none has sufficient investigative support to warrant complete acceptance.

Recurrent calculi composed of calcium oxalate and phosphate are relatively uncommon in women and rare in black people of either sex. The disproportionate occurrence of such calculi in white males is unexplained, but holds true even in the high incidence areas of the southeastern United States and South Africa. Women, however, are more susceptible than men to urinary tract infections. Thus women with magnesium-ammonium-phosphate or calcium-phosphate stones that develop as a complication of infection with urea-splitting organisms outnumber similarly affected men. Certain disorders predisposing to calculus formation, especially hyperparathyroidism, overcome the protective influence of sex or race, and this provides a diagnostic clue when searching for the cause of calculi in white women or black people.

There is an increased incidence of calcareous renal calculi in patients with small bowel disease or in those subjected to ileal resection. Patients who have undergone jejunoileal anastomosis in an effort to control morbid obesity are especially prone to develop calculi. It is now known that such patients usually have a significant hyperoxaluria as probably a most important factor favoring stone formation. Frequently these patients also have some degree of acidosis, presumably from loss of intestinal bicarbonate, and a consequent decrease in urinary citrate.

Although the hyperoxaluria of patients with disease of the small intestine may not be completely understood, considerable evidence now indicates that it is those patients with steatorrhea who are hyperoxaluric. Available data suggest that the binding of calcium by unabsorbed fatty acids within the intestinal lumen permits the increased absorption of ingested oxalate. Since oxalate is readily absorbed from the colon, it is not surprising that patients who have been subjected to a jejunoileal bypass procedure, and therefore are steatorrheic, are also markedly hyperoxaluric.

Structure and Composition of Calculi. Although all calculi must initially be small, it is the aggregation of crystals and matrix into a dense mass with subsequent growth to macroscopic size that accounts for their medical significance. The crystalline components of calculi are formed from the less soluble crystalloids predominant in the urine. It has not been determined whether the matrix component of calculi can be formed entirely from nonspecific proteinaceous material and cellular debris present in urine or consists of specific compounds, secreted by cells lining the urinary tract, that are important in promoting crystal growth and aggregation.

Examination of sectioned calculi usually reveals a distinct lamellar and sometimes radially striated organization. In most stones there is a small identifiable nidus around which the bulk of the calculus appears to have formed. In calcium oxalate stones, the most common variety, this nidus often consists of calcium phosphate, frequently in hydroxyapatite form. There is evidence that such a nidus may originate within the cells of the renal tubules or collecting ducts or beneath the papillary epithelium. As one means of stone formation, it has been suggested that extrusion of this type of nidus into the renal pelvis may promote apposition of crystals and matrix material from an appropriately saturated urine. There are other data, however, to indicate that the nidus of a stone need not be of specific composition. For example, calcium oxalate bladder stones in children of Southeast Asia regularly contain a core of acid urate crystals.

Crystalloids in Urine. Normal urine contains in solution a number of crystalloids, e.g., calcium, magnesium, phosphate, oxalate, and urate, at concentrations exceeding those achievable in water. The maintenance of this supersaturated state may be attributed to a number of factors. Urea, apparently by its interaction with water, increases the solubility of crystalloids, and the concentrations of sodium, potassium, chloride, and other soluble ions in urine also enhance the solution stability of the less soluble components. Organic acids, especially citrate, that form soluble chelates or complexes with calcium and magnesium are additional urinary constituents that promote the solubility of calcium or magnesium salts. One should be aware, however, that the potential of urinary organic acids to chelate metal ions is markedly decreased when urinary pH is low (<5.0).

In addition to the aforementioned factors that may account in part for the supersaturation of urine, specific inhibitors to the crystallization of calcium salts have been detected in urine and also in serum. A deficiency of these biologic "water conditioners" may be important in determining susceptibility to calculus formation. One of these constituents, inorganic pyrophosphate, has been studied in considerable detail. It is a product of intermediary metabolism and is present in serum at concentrations of 75 to 160 μg per 100 ml. Urinary excretion of pyrophosphate by subjects receiving diets free of dairy products ranges from 4 to 10 mg per day, and, within limits, the amount in urine varies directly with orthophosphate excretion. Although urinary pyrophosphate may be a protective constituent, the amount excreted is similar in calculous and normal subjects and is insufficient to account for the solution stability of calcium salts. Moreover, certain high-molecular-weight compounds in urine, possibly sulfated mucopolysaccharides, have the capacity to inhibit formation of calcium oxalate crystals, but as yet no information suggests the existence of a deficiency of such compounds in urine of calculous patients.

Indirect evidence indicates that urine of normal subjects contains still another inhibitor of crystal formation that is acidic, water soluble, and of low molecular weight. This compound is extremely potent in preventing crystallization of calcium salts, especially in the presence of small amounts of citrate. Whether this compound is a citrate derivative, such as phosphorylated citrate, has not been ascertained, but there is considerable evidence that patients with idiopathic calcareous calculi excrete less of this inhibitor than do normal subjects. Although conceptually quite relevant, the importance of a decreased excretion of this inhibitor of crystallization to the genesis of calcareous renal calculi remains uncertain. A number of investigators have observed that calcium-containing crystals form and aggregate more readily in urine from patients with calcareous calculi than in that from normal subjects. This difference is consistent with a deficiency of inhibitors of crystal formation in the urine of stone-formers.

The formation of renal calculi is dependent on the presence in urine of a supersaturation of crystalloids, but there must also be a component or nidus promoting the formation and aggregation of crystals. Whatever the initiating event, the growth of most calculi depends on the presence in urine of metastable concentrations of crystalloids. Such states of supersaturation may be achieved by various means; e.g., by increased excretion of specific crystalloids of limited solubility; decrease in urinary pH which converts urates to less soluble uric

acid; or infection with urea-splitting bacteria to release ammonia, which causes an increase in urinary pH and provides a setting for crystallization of complexes of magnesium-ammonium-phosphate or calcium phosphate. Furthermore, crystals of one type may promote formation of other types of crystals. For example, acid urate or calcium phosphate (brushite) crystals enhance crystallization of calcium oxalate. In addition to increased concentrations of crystalloids or alteration of urinary pH, reduced excretion of those urinary constituents that normally inhibit crystal formation would also induce a metastable state of crystalloids. This latter type of change is probably of more importance to the development of idiopathic calcareous calculi than is increased excretion of calcium or oxalate.

DIAGNOSIS. The medical history often provides important information. Infection as an etiologic or complicating factor is suggested by a history of fever preceding the initial episode of renal colic. Also, in postpartum women with calculi it is important to ascertain whether urinary tract infection occurred during pregnancy. Is there a family history of calculi? Genetic disorders such as renal tubular acidosis and cystinuria are expected in kindred, but idiopathic calcareous calculi may also occur in families. The occurrence of renal calculi in childhood may indicate the presence of a familial disorder, but infection or anatomic defects are more common causes in this age group. The contributory effect of intestinal disease to calculus formation was mentioned previously. A number of medications have been causally related to renal stone formation, and patients should be questioned about chronic use of medicines, particularly acetazolamide, absorbable alkali, silicates, allopurinol, or large amounts of ascorbic acid. The type of water used and unusual dietary habits are additional items of relevant information. A large intake of meat increases uric acid formation and excretion. Also, if the acid residue of ingested meat is not balanced by foods with an alkaline ash, such as vegetables, a high protein intake will increase urinary calcium excretion. Fruits or fruit juices, but especially tea, contain considerable amounts of soluble oxalate, and a large intake may increase calculus formation.

CLINICAL MANIFESTATIONS. Many patients with renal calculi are asymptomatic. Inflammation or infection resulting from calculi may lead to symptoms, but passage of a calculus into the ureter with resulting renal colic is the classic manifestation of calculous disease. Passage of small, sandlike concretions with relatively little pain is not uncommon, particularly with uric acid lithiasis and sometimes in patients with calcium oxalate stones. Gross hematuria, especially in the absence of accompanying renal colic and a demonstrable ureteral calculus, should be regarded with suspicion as possibly indicative of infection or a coexistent neoplasm. Microscopic hematuria, however, is quite regularly present in patients with calculi. The malingerer, feigning renal colic in order to obtain narcotics, may demonstrate considerable ingenuity in developing a convincing symptom complex.

LABORATORY FINDINGS. Careful examination of fresh urine provides immediate, valuable information. For example, an acid urine and urate crystals may be present in those with uric acid calculi, and octahedral crystals of calcium oxalate are frequent in patients with oxalate stones. A high urine pH (7.0 or higher) may signify infection or a renal tubular disorder. The presence of bacteria in fresh uncentrifuged urine usually indicates significant infection. As mentioned, microscopic hematuria is usual, and there may be few to many white blood cells. The pH of each freshly voided specimen of the patient's urine should be determined for 24 hours. Appropriately selected pH paper (pH range 4 to 9) is adequate for clinical purposes. If the pH is consistently high and infection is present (values between 8.5 and 9.0 always indicate infection), the pH determinations should be repeated after eradication of the infection. In normal persons receiving a diet of mixed composition, urine pH will usually be less than 6.0 at some time during the 24 hours. If this degree of acidity is not achieved, the presence of renal tubular acidosis is possible and should be confirmed by definitive tests. The occasional patient with uric acid stones may excrete unusually acid urine (pH 4.5 to 5.5), but most uric acid stone-formers do not excrete urine of such acidity.

A qualitative test for cystine should be performed at least once in every patient with radiopaque calculi, and freshly voided, concentrated urine is desired for this analysis. If positive, a quantitative analysis of the 24-hour excretion should be obtained. Although cystinuria is not a rare disorder, only a small proportion of cystinurics develop calculi.

A urine culture is indicated in the evaluation of patients with calculi. Of particular relevance to the problem of stone formation are infections with urea-splitting bacteria. It is pertinent to note that some strains of staphylococci are capable of splitting urea.

Although of limited clinical value, it is sometimes desirable to know the amount of calcium excreted per 24 hours by patients with radiopaque stones. This is conveniently done by having the patient abstain from dairy products (milk, cheese, and ice cream) for one or two days and then, while continuing the diet restriction, collect urine for one or two 24-hour periods. The calcium ingested with this regimen will usually be less than 300 mg per day, and the amount excreted by normal subjects will be less than 175 mg per 24 hours. With unrestricted diets urinary calcium values may be as much as 300 mg per 24 hours in normal subjects. Urinary calcium is increased in the majority of patients with calcareous calculi, but will be normal in patients whose primary problem is infection. Reliable oxalate analyses are not generally available, but, when possible, urinary oxalate should be measured in patients with calcium oxalate stones. The amount of phosphorus in urine reflects dietary phosphorus and is a useless measurement unless the amount ingested is accurately known.

In patients with calcareous calculi, serum analyses are required chiefly to establish the presence or absence of hypercalcemic states, particularly hyperparathyroidism or renal tubular acidosis. With the patient in a postabsorptive state, determinations of creatinine, carbon dioxide, chloride, uric acid, phosphorus, and calcium are sufficient. Abnormal values should be confirmed by repetition of the tests. The serum concentrations of bicarbonate and chloride may be normal in patients with mild renal tubular acidosis. Phosphorus concentrations in the sera of patients with idiopathic calcareous calculi are often slightly less than those of normal subjects, and uric acid values are frequently increased.

When the calculus is available, both its central and peripheral portions should be subjected to chemical or crystallographic (by x-ray diffraction) analysis. Much information as to cause and treatment may be gained from this.

RADIOLOGIC FINDINGS. A plain film of the abdomen or renal tomography in a patient properly prepared with laxatives is often informative, but contrast urography can also be helpful. Roentgenographic visualization of the urinary tract should be done promptly if an infected patient is suspected of having ureteral obstruction. Uric acid and the rare xanthine calculi are radiolucent and may be large or small. It is not uncommon for a patient with idiopathic calcareous calculi to have stones of mixed composition, e.g., uric acid and oxalate. A relatively small proportion as oxalate will induce radiopaqueness of a predominantly uric acid calculus. Also, it should be realized that patients with gout have an increased incidence of radiopaque oxalate stones.

Large or staghorn-shaped radiopaque calculi are usually the result of infection and are composed of magnesium-ammonium-phosphate or calcium phosphate, but cystine stones may achieve a similar size and configuration. In large calculi resulting from infection, detectable laminations are not uncommon. Calcium oxalate calculi are usually small (2 to 5 mm in diameter), dense, and frequently multiple. Such calculi in children may indicate the presence of oxalosis. When large (diameter greater than 10 mm), extremely dense (more dense than adjacent bone) stones are present in children or adults, hyperoxaluria should be suspected. The coexistence of nephrocalcinosis and renal calculi is not uncommon as a sequel of infection, but may also indicate the presence of medullary sponge kidneys, renal tubular acidosis, hyperparathyroidism, sarcoidosis, and rarely oxalosis.

Stones are often of mixed composition, particularly when infection has supervened; for example, at the center of a large calculus there may be either a radiolucent area composed of urates or a radiologically dense oxalate stone. The rare calculus consisting largely of matrix material may be barely visible radiologically.

Finally, roentgenographic visualization of the urinary tract may reveal anatomic abnormalities conducive to calculus formation. Obstruction, localized deformity, or medullary sponge kidneys are probably the most common such abnormalities.

TREATMENT. General. Avoidance of dehydration is important in calculous disease of all types, but especially in patients with cystinuria, those with a susceptibility to uric acid concretions, and those with urinary tract infections. To maintain continuously dilute urine usually requires a daily intake of approximately 4 quarts of liquids, which should be distributed throughout the 24 hours. Although dairy products are frequently omitted during test procedures, there are no data to suggest that continued avoidance is beneficial in reducing the incidence or growth of calcareous calculi in man. In contrast to the poor absorption of oxalate from vegetables, many foods and beverages (e.g., chocolate, tea, beer, fruits and fruit juices, cola drinks) contain significant amounts of oxalate in absorbable form. In patients with oxalate stones it is probably wise to limit the intake of these particular liquids to no more than 8 ounces daily until the specific role of diet in the pathogenesis of calculi is more fully delineated. The hyperoxaluria in patients with impaired function of the small intestine may be controlled by rigidly restricting oxalate or fat intake. Neither of these restrictions, which must be severe to be effective, is well accepted by patients. A practical approach to this problem has been to limit the intake of the aforementioned foods and beverages and to prescribe 2 to 4 grams of calcium daily, as calcium carbonate or calcium gluconate, in divided doses with meals. These calcium salts not only control the hyperoxaluria but also may correct the acidosis so often present in patients with malabsorption syndromes. To date, however, experience with this form of therapy is insufficient to know how effective it will be in preventing calculus formation.

Every effort should be made to eradicate infection promptly. For paraplegic patients, in whom the high incidence of calculi correlates with the presence of urinary tract infections, dramatic decreases in the occurrence of stones have been achieved by prompt and effective treatment of incipient infections. The size of ureteral calculi that can be passed spontaneously is surprising. Therefore it is often wise to delay instrumental intervention until it is certain that the calculus will not be extruded. In the absence of infection a high degree of or even complete ureteral obstruction may be well tolerated for a number of days without inducing permanent renal damage.

Specific. Details regarding the rationale for treatment of patients with cystinuria, renal tubular acidosis, and uric acid calculi are recorded in other parts of the text. Suffice it to say here that if treatment with absorbable alkali is to be instituted, the amount required varies, but for adults with normal glomerular filtration rates it is usually from 100 to 250 mEq of cation per day regardless of the salt used. For example, with sodium bicarbonate these amounts of cation are provided by 8.4 to 21.0 grams, respectively. Cystinurics to be treated in this manner require the larger amounts because of the need to maintain urinary pH in the range of 8.0. Dosage with alkali should be spaced equally throughout the 24 hours to ensure continuous control of urinary pH. Dietary habits will modify the amount of alkali required to achieve a particular urinary pH value. For example, a vegetarian may need very little alkali to maintain a urinary pH in the alkaline range, whereas the acid ash of a high-protein diet may impose a requirement for large amounts of alkali to compensate for the acid load.

Patients with single or very infrequent calcareous calculi that are passed without undue difficulty should be advised to drink copious amounts of liquid, but usually need not be considered candidates for continuous medicinal treatment.

Several largely empiric modes of therapy are currently in widespread use for patients with recurrent calcareous calculi. Each of these programs was devised in an effort to modify urine in a way that enhanced the solubility of the least soluble salts. Administration of divided doses of orthophosphates, usually as a neutral mixture of monobasic and dibasic salts, in amounts sufficient to provide 1500 to 2100 mg of phosphorus per 24 hours has been remarkably effective in preventing stone formation in uninfected patients with calcareous calculi of various causes. These phosphate salts are available in tablet or powder form, and effective treatment can be achieved by three equal doses at seven- to nine-hour intervals. Diarrhea is the major adverse symptom, but most males can tolerate the aforementioned doses. Amounts of phosphates providing less than 1500 mg of phosphorus are usually ineffective in preventing stone formation in males, but many females are adequately treated with 1200 mg of phosphorus per day. Potassium phosphates may be substituted for sodium salts in patients with hypertension. This form of therapy is contraindicated in patients whose renal function is impaired to the degree that there is inadequate excretion of a phosphate load. Phosphate administration induces an increased excretion of inorganic pyrophosphate, and possibly other phosphorylated inhibitors of crystal formation, and usually causes a modest reduction in urinary calcium. There is uncertainty, however, that these are the changes that account for the prevention of calculus formation by phosphates.

Hydrochlorothiazide administration, 50 mg twice daily, has proved effective in preventing stone formation in the majority of patients so treated. Thiazides reduce urinary calcium and augment magnesium excretion, but frequently cause symptomatic hypokalemia. Complete replacement of the potassium deficiency may lessen the effectiveness of this form of therapy. In calculous patients with hypertension or in those with a hyperactive intestinal tract, hydrochlorothiazide is often the therapy of choice. Magnesium oxide has been advocated for patients with oxalate stones on the basis that increased urinary magnesium promotes oxalate solubility, but published experiences with this form of therapy indicate it to be of limited effectiveness. In patients who form two types of stones, e.g., uric acid and calcium oxalate, it is often helpful to use allopurinol (200 to 300 mg daily) in addition to phosphates or hydrochlorothiazide. Such combined therapy is usually required to control calculus formation in those hyperuricemic patients who form calculi frequently, but allopurinol alone may be sufficient in the hyperuricemic patient who forms only an occasional calcareous calculus.

Patients with calculi caused by infection are the most difficult to manage. None of the regimens mentioned are effective in such patients. The infection should be treated, but it is difficult to prevent recurrence. In addition to control of infection, treatment directed to reducing the urinary phosphorus to several hundred milligrams per day has been used by a number of investigators. This program requires that the patient avoid dairy products and, to further decrease phosphate absorption, ingest 30 ml of aluminum carbonate gel or 45 ml of aluminum hydroxide gel after each meal and at bedtime. Caution must be exercised to guard against phosphate depletion with this regimen. It is usually impossible to eradicate a urinary tract infection as long as the patient harbors a magnesium-ammonium-phosphate stone. Meticulous surgical removal of such calculi followed by long-term appropriate antibiotic therapy is often the only effective means to cure the patient and prevent recurrence of calculi. Compounds that inhibit urease activity of bacteria should soon be available, and these compounds promise to be of real value in the treatment of patients with calculi resulting from infection with urea-splitting bacteria.

Boyce, W. H. (ed.): Symposium on renal lithiasis. Urol. Clin. North Am., 1:179, 1974.

Coe, F. L.: Treated and untreated recurrent calcium nephrolithiasis in patients with idiopathic hypercalciuria, hyperuricosuria, or no metabolic disorder. Ann. Intern. Med., 87:404, 1977.

Pak, C. Y. C. (guest ed.): Urolithiasis. Kidney Int., 13:341, 1978.

Thomas, W. C., Jr.: Renal Calculi. Springfield, Ill., Charles C Thomas, 1976.

Williams, H. E., and Prien, E. L., Jr.: Nephrolithiasis. *In* Avioli, L. V., and Krane, S. M. (eds.): Metabolic Bone Disease, Vol. 1. New York, Academic Press, 1977, p. 387.

382. OBSTRUCTIVE NEPHROPATHY*

Francis P. Muldowney

Back pressure arising from urinary tract obstruction may result in important structural and functional derangements of the kidney, and obstructive uropathy is one of the most frequent etiologic factors in patients presenting with unexplained uremia. Clinical progress may be deceptively slow or viciously accelerated, depending on whether obstruction is incomplete or complete, and especially on whether infection is also present. Since obstruction is clearly a remediable cause of kidney damage, accurate diagnosis and appropriate management assume considerable importance for restoration and preservation of renal function.

ETIOLOGY (see accompanying figure). The many causes of obstruction may be considered under three headings: those inside the lumen of the urinary conduit (intraluminal), those within the wall (intramural), and those causing pressure from outside. The accompanying table lists the major causes in each category. In unilateral (nonuremic) cases, the ureteropelvic junction is a common site of obstruction under all three etiologic headings. In bilateral (uremic) cases the most frequent causes are prostatic obstruction and urinary stone, comprising together some 55 per cent, with bladder tumor contributing a further 20 per cent. Retroperitoneal fibrosis is covered in detail in Ch. 71.2. A particular type of intraluminal obstruction is that seen in acute metabolic emergencies associated with intrarenal tubular blockage as in multiple myeloma with Bence Jones proteinuria, or

*The assistance of Mr. Daniel G. Kelly, F.R.C.S., in the preparation of this manuscript is gratefully acknowledged.

acute urate nephropathy during chemotherapy in malignant disease.

INCIDENCE AND PREVALENCE. Obstructive lesions of the urinary tract have been found in 3.8 per cent of a large series of routine autopsies. Corresponding figures from a population of uremic subjects at autopsy show a rise to fully 25 per cent, including those in whom obstructive uropathy was either a contributory or a major factor. A much higher relative incidence of obstructive versus other causes of renal disease is to be expected in particular at-risk age groups such as infants and children on the one hand (congenital strictures or ureteropelvic dysfunction) and elderly males (prostatic obstruction) on the other.

PATHOGENESIS AND PATHOLOGY. In slowly developing or partial obstruction gross dilatation of the renal pelvis and calyces may occur, especially when the impedance is situated high up — for example, at the ureteropelvic junction. In such cases, the distended sac may accommodate 2 to 3 liters of fluid, with a greatly thinned renal cortex, but clinical manifestations may be few. When infection has supervened, pyonephrosis with total destruction of renal parenchyma is the end result, usually with correspondingly severe clinical manifestations. When obstruction develops rapidly or is complete, distention of the renal pelvis and calyces is much less but intraluminal pressure above the level of obstruction may be very high. Correspondingly severe symptoms of loin pain, caused by distention of the renal capsule, or ureteral colic, caused by repeated ureteric peristaltic waves, are usually present. Occasionally, however, complete obstruction of one ureter may occur with very little evidence of back pressure or dilatation, resulting nevertheless in gradual total loss of renal function on that side if not relieved within four to six months. In general, the degree of renal damage is related to the duration of obstruction. In either situation, the occurrence of infection behind the obstruction, either blood-borne or introduced during diagnostic instrumentation, transforms the clinical picture into an acute pyrexial illness, accompanied by rapid destruction of renal tissue.

Infection is therefore an important determinant of the pathologic, functional, and prognostic picture. In lower

OBSTRUCTIVE NEPHROPATHY — CAUSES

Common sites of urinary tract obstruction.

Causes of Obstructive Uropathy

Intraluminal	Intramural	Extramural
Stone	Congenital:	Prostatic obstruction
Bladder tumor	Ureteropelvic dysfunction (10% bilateral)	Ureteropelvic juncture—vessels, bands, etc.
Papillary necrosis (diabetes)	Ureterovesical stricture (simple or ureterocele)	Aortic aneurysm
Clot	Bladder neck obstruction	Periureteral fibrosis
Ureteral tumor	Pinpoint meatus	Retroperitoneal tumor or nodes
Bence Jones proteinuria	Acquired:	Extraurinary growth (carcinoma of colon, diverticulitis)
Acute urate nephropathy	Urethral stricture	Pelvic tumor
	Ureteral stricture (tuberculosis, etc.)	Inadvertent ligature
	Neurogenic bladder dysfunction	

urinary tract lesions, infection tends to occur early in the disease but is often relatively slow in progression. In upper urinary tract lesions, infection may not occur until much later but runs a more rapidly destructive course. In either case, the most important factor predisposing to infection is instrumentation of the urinary tract, by bladder catheter, cystoscope, or ureteral catheter.

CLINICAL MANIFESTATIONS.　Obstructive nephropathy is one of the most important causes of that ubiquitous nephrologic problem, "unexplained uremia," and, as mentioned above, is present at least as a contributory factor in 25 per cent of such cases at autopsy. All patients presenting with renal failure, or in whom there is abrupt deterioration of renal function unexplained by their primary renal problem, should be carefully screened to exclude onset of obstruction.

Equally important is the mode of presentation in the form of recurrent urinary tract infection. Symptoms caused by complicating infection are commonly the presenting complaint with obstructive lesions at all levels. Persistent or recurrent urinary tract infection should always raise the suspicion of an obstructive lesion, even when specific localizing symptoms are absent.

In lower urinary tract lesions, the history of pattern of micturition provides an extremely useful guide to both diagnosis and treatment. Thus, for instance, a subject in whom rectal examination indicates apparently gross prostatic hypertrophy may nevertheless have minimal symptoms of urinary hesitancy or dribbling, and therefore does not merit further instrumentation or operation. On the other hand, a palpably normal prostate may give rise to severe obstructive symptoms by virtue of median lobe enlargement impinging inward on the prostatic urethra. In either case the history is of overriding importance.

Lower urinary tract obstruction — for example, in prostatic hypertrophy — is associated classically with hesitancy in commencing micturition, poor stream of urine, and inability to empty the bladder completely, with resulting stop-and-start urination and postmicturition dribbling. Sudden temporary urinary retention may result from vascular congestion of the prostate, e.g., after alcohol ingestion, with suprapubic pain caused by bladder distention. In chronic cases overflow incontinence from a distended bladder may produce deceptively large urinary volumes and thus cause suprapubic bladder enlargement to be overlooked. *Urine flow may be very large in such cases* owing to the associated defect in urinary concentrating ability producing hypotonicity.

Acute upper urinary tract obstruction of one or both ureters results in severe colicky pain referred to the groin, with associated symptoms of weakness and sweating. Chronic cases caused by gradually developing obstruction at the ureteropelvic junction present with dull pain in the renal angle but little or no severe colic. A minority of cases may obstruct one ureter without overt symptoms, with resulting silent loss of renal function on that side.

In some cases, development of high-renin hypertension or primary erythrocytosis may be the presenting features, leading to discovery of unsuspected unilateral hydronephrosis in, for example, pelviureteric obstruction.

DIAGNOSIS AND DIFFERENTIAL DIAGNOSIS.　Background etiologic factors such as family history of stone (cystinuria), arthritis (primary gout), lymphoma (secondary gout), drug therapy (periureteral fibrosis), diabetes (papillary necrosis), or neurologic disorders such as multiple sclerosis must be considered. Microscopic examination of the urinary sediment may reveal red cells, cystine or uric acid crystals, or rarely fragments of a necrosed renal papilla. Frequently, however, no specific abnormality is found in the urine. Physical examination may disclose loin tenderness or palpable renal swelling; careful suprapubic palpation and percussion will show a distended bladder. Rectal or vaginal examination may point to extraurinary growth.

Further investigation may then proceed along two lines — the assessment of glomerular filtration rate; and the definition of anatomic outlines of kidneys, ureters, and bladder. If serum urea or creatinine concentration is normal or only slightly raised, glomerular filtration rate (GFR) reduction even if present will not interfere with radiologic procedures such as intravenous pyelography, which may be pursued utilizing normal dosages of intravenous dye. If plasma urea or creatinine level is significantly raised, a more exact measurement of GFR may be made by measuring the disappearance rate of ^{51}Cr labeled EDTA from venous blood. This method circumvents the difficulty of conventional clearance measurements in the presence of temporary anuria or oliguria. Values less than 50 per cent of normal are clearly indicative of *bilateral* renal dysfunction. A "double-dose" of intravenous dye (i.e., 30 to 40 grams of iodine rather than the normal 15 to 30 grams) is needed if GFR is in the range of 70 to 25 ml per minute. Below this filtration level, doses of up to 42 grams may be given by bolus injection. In severely uremic cases, pyelography is best postponed until immediately after dialysis. The reduction in serum urea concentration with corresponding lessening of the osmotic diuresis per nephron allows better urinary concentration of the dye with correspondingly improved visualization. Utilizing this method, good visualization of the renal tract can be expected in 90 per cent of cases no matter how low the GFR. Retrograde pyelography is therefore almost never necessary. Certain extra precautions must, however, be taken to ensure useful results from intravenous pyelography. In addition to the conventional 5-, 10-, and 20-minute films, repeated late exposures over a period of 24 hours may show delayed nephrotomograms or dilated ureteral outlines. Nephrotomography is particularly useful in the definition of renal size and outline. Postmicturition films when feasible may show incomplete bladder emptying (residual urine) or prostatic encroachment.

While preliminary GFR assessment is taking place, a simple straight roentgenogram of the kidney-ureter-bladder area may give important information. A radiopaque stone may be seen along the line of the ureter, especially at the ureterovesical junction. Nonopaque stone (uric acid) is more difficult to exclude. In either case unilateral renal enlargement may be visible.

In order to obtain the maximal information, it is helpful to study the pyelogram films in a definite sequence, as follows:

Are two kidneys present?

Is there a difference in size?

Is there a delay in appearance of dye on one or other side?

Is there evidence of calyceal or pelvic dilatation?

Is there thinning, deformity, or shrinkage of the renal cortex?

Is there dilatation of the ureter and down to what level?

Is there displacement of the ureter medially (periureteral fibrosis) or laterally (aortic aneurysm or tumor)?

Does the bladder outline show a filling defect or deformity?

Does complete emptying of bladder dye occur after micturition?

Adequate answers to most of these questions can be supplied in 90 per cent of cases. Rarely, resort to cystoscopy may be necessary with or without retrograde ureteral catheterization and pyelography. Owing to the danger of introducing infection, these procedures are performed only when absolutely necessary for establishment of the diagnosis or with a view to operative treatment. If, for instance, prostatectomy has been decided upon, preliminary cystoscopy is essential in order to exclude associated asymptomatic pathology such as bladder tumor, diverticulum, or stone which may be present in 10 per cent of cases.

Percutaneous antegrade pyelography has been increasingly employed in recent years for obstructive problems in which retrograde catheterization is not possible. The technique has been developed mainly in radiology departments. A 20 or 22 gauge spinal needle or similar angiographic needle is inserted via the lumbar region into the renal pelvis under fluoroscopic or ultrasound guidance. Urine may thus be aspirated for microscopy and culture, and contrast medium introduced to delineate the pelvis, calyces, and ureter along its length. An additional advantage of the procedure is the possibility of leaving in situ a small balloon-tipped catheter as a nephrostomy drainage tube. Time is thus gained for further diagnostic or therapeutic procedures when necessary, as discussed below.

TREATMENT. The principles of treatment are to (1) relieve obstruction, (2) prevent infection, and (3) treat infection if present, with antimicrobial choice and dosage according to the degree of reduction of GFR (see Ch. 376). Surgical correction of obstruction is aimed at achieving comfort and preventing further damage to the threatened kidney. Before definitive relief of obstruction is attempted, it may be necessary in severely ill or uremic patients to employ dialysis with or without temporary external diversion of urine. Temporary diversion is useful when some doubt exists as to the ultimate viability of the kidney and when immediate radical relief of obstruction may appear hazardous. In some cases also the exact nature of the obstructing lesion may be in doubt for some time, e.g., whether prostatic enlargement is benign or malignant.

The decision to attempt surgical relief of obstruction must therefore be tempered initially by consideration of the aforementioned factors, and subsequently by other important aspects of the obstructive lesion itself such as its nature, location, and duration. Formerly, nephrectomy was commonly advised for unilateral cases, especially when infected, but such an approach obviously fails to provide for possible partial recovery of function on the affected side. Nephrectomy can now be advised only when extensive renal damage or pyonephrosis indicates an irrecoverable situation, especially when the remaining kidney might become involved in the destructive or infective process.

Urgent surgical relief is indicated for high-level lesions such as ureteral stone which is impacted, i.e., not moving spontaneously over a period of days. An initial attempt at dislodgment by cystoscopy and retrograde ureteral catheterization should be quickly followed, if unsuccessful, by direct open ureterolithotomy, because complicating infection must then be expected. Any other cause of recent *total* ureteral obstruction likewise demands surgical relief in order to restore function. "Recent" in this connection implies within the past four to six weeks or at most within four months, because total obstruction of longer duration is likely to have permanently destroyed the kidney.

Postponement of surgical intervention may be preferable in noninfected patients when obstruction is only *partial*, or when there is reasonable expectation of spontaneous relief. Time thus gained will help the eventual decision, based on the nature of the primary lesion. Even when infection is present, time may be gained in this way during which the response to antimicrobial therapy may be assessed. Such caution is particularly advisable in *lower* urinary tract disease, such as prostatic enlargement, in which eradication of infection may relieve many symptoms originally thought to be obstructive in origin. If significant residual bladder urine volumes (more than 100 ml) persist at this stage, however, surgery is indicated. The presence of infection in *high* urinary tract obstruction is a more urgent indication for surgical relief, because the complication of gram-negative septicemia represents a very serious hazard.

After relief of obstruction, whether by temporary external diversion or by definitive surgery, diuresis follows with rapid return to normal of blood urea and creatinine concentrations. The subsequent urinary flow may in some cases achieve massive proportions with considerable loss of solute, suggesting a diuresis of proximal tubular origin. Such a postobstructive diuresis is encountered especially in relatively chronic cases with evidence of increase in body sodium and water stores. Usually the diuresis with negative salt balance is self-limited and represents merely a restoration to normal of the previously expanded extracellular fluid volume and as such it does not require treatment. In a small minority, however, intravenous saline replacement may be necessary in this phase. Falling blood pressure or serum sodium concentration, or the occurrence of a secondary rise in serum urea or creatinine level, is an indication for fluid replenishment.

PROGNOSIS. Prognosis in obstructive nephropathy depends largely on whether treatment is instituted before irreversible damage has occurred. Without treatment, the subsequent natural history of the disorder is dependent on whether the obstructing lesion is complete or incomplete and unilateral or bilateral, and especially on whether infection is present. Complete blockage with infection can totally destroy the kidney(s) within days. Chronic partial blockage, as for example in congenital pelviureteral obstruction, may be consistent with many years without symptoms, but, if bilateral, is likely to present ultimately in the "unexplained uremia" category.

With treatment, much depends on the duration of obstruction prior to relief, and especially on whether infection has been present. Experimental data suggest that complete obstruction for one week results in a permanent 50 per cent reduction in GFR on the affected side. Obstruction of longer duration is associated with correspondingly more severe permanent damage. After three months gross GFR reduction is seen but with potential for partial recovery. Loss of maximal concentrating and acidifying ability may be a prominent residual tubular defect, but sodium excretion, although relatively high in the basal state, nevertheless responds normally to both volume expansion and mineralocorticoid administration, indicating preservation of tubular function. If the history suggests obstruction for longer than four to six months, recovery of function appears very unlikely. Operative interference is therefore not indicated unless complicating pyonephrosis, severe polycythemia, or developing high-renin hypertension supervenes.

Better, O. S., Arieff, A. I., Massry, S. G., Kleeman, C. R., and Maxwell, M. H.: Studies on renal function after relief of complete unilateral ureteral obstruction of three months' duration in man. Am. J. Med., 54:234, 1973.

Bricker, N. S., and Klahr, S.: Obstructive nephropathy. In Strauss, M. B., and Welt, L. G. (eds.): Diseases of the Kidney. 2nd ed. Edinburgh and London, Churchill/Livingstone, 1971.

Kerr, W. S.: Effects of complete ureteral obstruction in dogs on kidney function. Am. J. Physiol., 184:521, 1956.

Keuhnelian, J. G., Bartone, F., and Marshall, V. F.: Practical considerations from autopsies on azotemic patients. J. Urol., 91:467, 1964.

Legrain, M., Bitker, M., and Kuss, R.: Obstructive Nephropathy in Adults. Proc. 3rd Int. Cong. Nephrol. Washington, 2:336, 1966 (New York, Basel and Karger, 1967).

Muldowney, F. P., Duffy, G. T., Kelly, D. G., Duff, F. A., Harrington, C., and Freaney, R.: Sodium diuresis after relief of obstructive uropathy. N. Engl. J. Med., 274:1294, 1966.

Proca, E.: Errors and pitfalls in the management of acute urinary obstruction complicated by uraemia with special reference to stone. Br. J. Urol., 44:9, 1972.

Witten, D. M.: Case records of the Massachusetts General Hospital. N. Engl. J. Med., 295:1125, 1977.

383. CYSTIC DISEASES OF THE KIDNEY

Kenneth D. Gardner, Jr.

GENERAL CONSIDERATIONS

The renal cystic diseases are a group of heterogeneous disorders that share a single characteristic: cystic deformity of the kidney. They occur in infants, children, adults, and the elderly. They are a cause of significant morbidity and mortality, accounting for 5 to 10 per cent of end-stage renal disease among individuals who require renal transplantation or dialysis. Their management demands a practical understanding of human genetics, microbiology, and renal physiology, and a tolerant sensitivity to the intense pressures that some of these conditions bring to bear on individual patients, their families, and society through familial involvement and the costs of later-stage treatment.

Not all renal cystic diseases cause symptoms or signs. The simple or solitary cyst, for example, may remain silent during life, to be found incidentally during the course of routine postmortem examination. When renal cystic disease is the cause of morbidity, however, it usually presents with one or more of the symptoms and signs listed in Table 1. When renal disease occurs in an individual whose family history is positive for renal disease, early deaths, or premature deaths and abortions, or in an individual with multiple congenital anomalies, e.g., hypospadias or cryptorchidism, the likelihood that renal cysts are present in the patient is strengthened.

Cystic kidneys, like their noncystic counterparts, are susceptible to acquired renal disease. One must be especially alert to malignancy and tuberculosis, both of which may complicate several of these conditions.

The approach to definitive diagnosis of the renal cystic diseases depends heavily on radiographic and sonographic techniques. Cysts as small as 0.5 to 1.0 cm, depending on their location in the kidney, may be detected by modern sonographic techniques. Renal arteriography with tomography also has proved helpful in demonstrating renal cysts. Percutaneous cyst aspiration has a more restricted diagnostic application. Biopsy, open or percutaneous, also is often indicated, but when cysts are sparse or deep within the kidney, it may yield cyst-free tissue. Neither negative radiographic studies nor negative renal biopsy results rule out renal cystic disease with 100 per cent reliability.

In general, the renal cystic diseases have no specific treatment. Therapy is directed at control of symptoms and at complications, such as infection, when they occur.

CLASSIFICATION

Much disagreement has existed over the names and classification of individual renal cystic disorders. The discovery of a kidney with many cysts does not mean that the patient has *polycystic* kidney disease (PKD), or a congenital *multicystic* kidney (CMK). It means only that a kidney with multiple cysts has been found. In older literature, however, indiscriminate application

TABLE 1. Frequently Encountered Symptoms and Signs Among the Renal Cystic Diseases

Abdominal pain
Abdominal swelling
Palpable intra-abdominal mass(es)
Recurrent urinary tract infections
Hematuria (gross or microscopic)
Progressive renal failure
Anuria (rare)
Proteinuria <1 to 3 grams per day

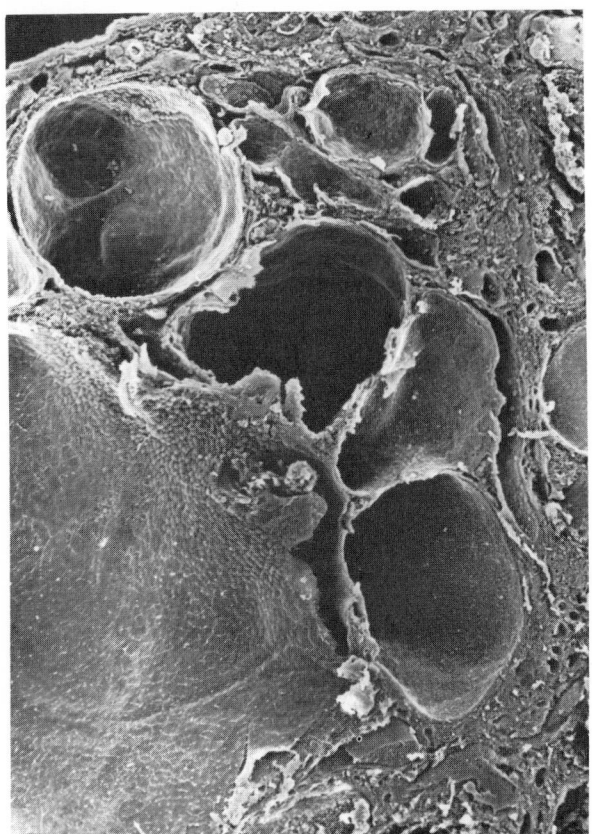

Scanning electron microscopic appearance of cysts in nordihydroguaiaretic acid–induced renal cystic disease in the rat. The massive distortion of normal renal architecture that is evident here is also found in cystic disorders of the human kidney. Experimental models provide ready access to in vivo and fresh postmortem kidneys for studies designed to answer such questions as what makes cysts form and why they enlarge. The degree of identity between models and human disease has not been established.

and interchange of these words has led to reports of PKD without familial involvement, unilateral PKD, PKD without progressive renal failure, and so on. Current usage and the necessity for clear communication dictate that the words *polycystic* and *multicystic* be reserved to describe those kidneys with multiple cysts that are encountered in the clinical entities of PKD and CMK, respectively. A many-cysted kidney under other circumstances should only be called many cysted.

The most workable current scheme of classification is that proposed by Bernstein (Table 2). It identifies seven major categories and includes heritable, congenital, and acquired conditions. Among them are six disorders that are relatively common and will be considered here in some detail: the simple cyst, multicystic dysplasia, infantile and adult polycystic kidney disease, medullary cystic disease, and medullary sponge kidney.

Bernstein, J.: A classification of renal cysts. *In* Gardner, K. D., Jr. (ed.): Cystic Diseases of the Kidney. New York, John Wiley & Sons, 1976, pp. 7–30.

SIMPLE CYST

With a frequency considered common but not well documented in numbers, the renal cortex may be the site of single or multiple simple cysts. These are thin-walled structures that usually bulge from the surface of the kidney and contain a sterile, clear ultrafiltrate of plasma. Evidently, they arise as a degenerative process, for they are most common in the elderly and very rare in the infant. Occasionally they reach prodigious size, with volumes of 3.5 and 23 (!) liters having been reported. Most frequently, simple cysts are asymptomatic and discovered incidentally during the course of pyelography or autopsy.

Simple renal cysts are of importance for at least two reasons. First, when multiple they may cause diagnostic confusion with the polycystic or multicystic kidney. Second, simple cysts may be the site of neoplasia.

Radiographically visible calcification in the wall of a simple renal cyst ("eggshell" calcification) is not reliable as evidence of a benign cystic lesion. Transcutaneous aspiration of a simple renal cyst, especially if its location is near the lower pole, is a relatively easy, safe procedure and can help distinguish between simple cyst and cystic neoplasm. It should be performed only when pyelography or sonography has established the presence of a definitely cystic renal mass. It is especially useful in the elderly or the severely ill patient, for whom the risks of arteriography or surgery may be increased.

Characteristically, fluid from the simple cyst contains nonmalignant cells on cytologic examination, is straw colored, and has low concentrations of lactic dehydrogenase (LDH), protein, and fat. Necrotic or cystic neoplasms, in contrast, contain fluid in which malignant cells and blood may be evident and whose concentrations of fat and protein are high. When cyst fluid is bloody, the odds are roughly one in three that carcinoma is present. LDH concentrations also are low in cystic malignancies but are high in the presence of inflammation.

After fluid removal, contrast medium may be injected into the cystic space. Simple cysts usually have a smooth wall and fill completely. Neoplastic cysts, in contrast, usually exhibit multiloculation, incomplete filling, and a shaggy or irregular lining.

TABLE 2. Classification of the Renal Cystic Diseases*

I. Renal dysplasia
   A. Multicystic dysplasia
   B. Focal and segmental cystic dysplasia
   C. Cystic dysplasia associated with lower urinary tract obstruction
   D. Familial cystic dysplasia
II. Polycystic disease
   A. Childhood polycystic disease
   B. Adult polycystic disease
III. Renal cysts in hereditary syndromes (e.g., in Meckel's syndrome, Zellweger's cerebrohepatorenal syndrome, Jeune's asphyxiating thoracic dystrophy, and cortical cysts in syndromes of multiple malformation
IV. Renal cortical cysts
V. Renal medullary cystic disorders
   A. Nephronophthisis–medullary cystic disease complex
   B. Medullary sponge kidney
VI. Miscellaneous parenchymal renal cysts
   A. Inflammation and necrosis
   B. Neoplasia
   C. Endometriosis
   D. Traumatic intrarenal hematoma
VII. Extraparenchymal renal cysts
   A. Pyelogenic cyst (pelvic diverticulum)
   B. Parapelvic cyst (lymphangiectasia)
   C. Perinephric cyst

*After Bernstein, J., *In* Gardner, K. D., Jr. (ed.): Cystic Diseases of the Kidney. New York, John Wiley & Sons, 1976, pp. 7–30.

Chynn, K. Y., and Evans, J. A.: Nephrotomography in the differentiation of renal cyst from neoplasm: A review of 500 cases. J. Urol.,
   83:21, 1960.
Devine, C. J., Jr., Buttarazzi, P. J., Devine, P. C., Fiveash, J. G., Jr.,
   and Poutasse, E. F.: Aspiration or exploration to confirm diagnoses
   of renal masses. JAMA, 204:758, 1968.
Jackman, R. J., and Stevens, G. M.: Benign hemorrhagic renal cysts.
   Radiology, 110:7, 1974.
Lalli, A. F.: Percutaneous aspiration of renal masses. Am. J. Roentgenol. Rad. Ther. Nucl. Med., 101:700, 1967.
Lang, E. K., Johnson, B., Chance, H. L., Enright, J. R., Fontenot, R.,
   Trichel, B. E., Wood, M., Brown, M., and St. Martin, E. C.: Assessment of avascular renal mass lesions: The use of nephrotomography, arteriography, cyst puncture, double contrast study and his-
   tochemical and histopathologic examination of the aspirate. South.
   Med. J., 65:1, 1972.
Spence, H. M., and Singleton, R.: Cysts and cystic disorders of the
   kidney: Types, diagnosis, treatment. Urol. Survey, 22:131, 1972.
Thornbury, J. R.: Needle aspiration of avascular renal lesions. Correlation of contrast medium injection with cytologic and arteriographic
   diagnosis. Radiology, 105:299, 1972.

CONGENITAL MULTICYSTIC KIDNEY
(CMK)

CMK or multicystic renal dysplasia may be encountered at any age. It is perhaps the most common cause
of an abdominal mass in infancy.

DEFINITION. *Renal dysplasia* is "a disturbance in
nephrogenesis that results in a conversion of all, a segment, or multiple microscopic foci of one or both kidneys to structures which do not recapitulate any stage
in normal nephrogenesis." Instead of kidneys, one
finds nests of normal renal tissue that are scattered
among cysts, variably differentiated mesenchyme,
weirdly branching tubules lined by atypical epithelium,
and foci of fatty, cartilaginous, and hematopoietic tissue.

ETIOLOGY. The majority of dysplastic (multicystic)
kidneys occur in association with obstruction. When
the entire kidney is involved, ipsilateral ureteral atresia
or stenosis is found in 90 per cent of cases. When a
segment of kidney is affected, drainage from the affected segment likewise is abnormal. This association
therefore implicates obstruction during development as
the causative mechanism of CMK.

CLINICAL MANIFESTATIONS. Bilateral diffuse involvement, because of the absence of functioning renal tissue, is incompatible with life. Unilateral or segmental
involvement is not, however, and such cases may go
undiscovered unless an abdominal mass is present or
infection, trauma, hemorrhage, or hypertension supervenes and leads to the diagnosis. Urinalyses and tests
of renal function are within normal limits in the affected adult. The roentgenographic picture is characteristic:
a nonfunctioning segment or mass of renal tissue to
which an arterial supply can be identified with difficulty if at all, and from which no continuity of ureteral
drainage can be demonstrated. Rim-like calcifications in
cyst walls strengthen the diagnosis.

INCIDENCE. Because of its frequently silent nature,
the true incidence of CMK is not known. Among reported cases, each sex and each kidney are affected
with equal frequency. A positive family history generally is absent, although scattered reports of involvement
in twins, siblings, and relatives have appeared.

DIAGNOSIS. In adulthood, the discovery of a CMK
usually is incidental to the workup of an abdominal
mass, intra-abdominal calcification, hypertension, recurrent urinary tract infection, or abdominal pain or

discomfort. Infants or children suffering from a variety
of teratologic syndromes may have renal dysplasia as
one abnormality. Usually involvement outside the kidney dominates the clinical picture in these cases, however, and the finding of renal dysplasia is of importance only to the geneticist and pathologist.

The segmental or unilateral forms of CMK occur only
rarely among several members of a given family. On
these grounds it is distinguished from PKD, which is
always bilateral and familial. Congenital unilateral hydronephrosis is a frequent cause of an abdominal mass
in children and is distinguished from CMK by the
usual persistence of residual renal function, a ureter
that is of normal caliber distal to the obstructed site
and a massively dilated pelvocalyceal system, and a
patent renal artery on the involved side. Among adults,
differentiation may be difficult between CMK and renal
agenesis. Renal function is absent in both. In renal
agenesis, retrograde pyelography shows only a small
stump of ureter or is unsuccessful because no ureteral
orifice can be found; no flank mass, renal artery, or
eggshell calcifications can be demonstrated. Ultimately
surgical exploration may be required to make the distinction.

PROGNOSIS AND TREATMENT. The prognosis of CMK
among adults is excellent. Malignant change has not
been reported. Should the involved kidney become infected or be traumatized, nephrectomy may be required.

Bernstein, J.: The morphogenesis of renal parenchymal maldevelopment
   (renal dysplasia). Pediat. Clin. North Am., 18:395, 1971.
Cussen, L. J.: Cystic kidneys in children with congenital urethral ob-
   struction. J. Urol., 106:939, 1971.
Greene, L. F., Feinzaig, W., and Dahlin, D. C.: Multicystic dysplasia of
   the kidney: With special reference to the contralateral kidney. J.
   Urol., 105:482, 1971.
Gur, A., Siegel, N. J., Davis, C. A., Kashgarian, M., and Hayslett, J.
   P.: Clinical aspects of bilateral renal dysplasia in children.
   Nephron, 15:50, 1975.
Kissane, J. M.: The morphology of renal cystic disease. In Gardner, K.
   D., Jr. (ed.): Cystic Diseases of the Kidney. New York, John Wiley
   & Sons, 1976, pp. 31–63.
Leonidas, J. C., Strauss, L., and Krasna, I. H.: Roentgen diagnosis of
   multicystic renal dysplasia in infancy by high dose urography. J.
   Urol., 108:963, 1972.
Newman, L., McAlister, W. H., and Kissane, J.: Segmental renal dys-
   plasia associated with ectopic ureteroceles in childhood. Urology,
   3:23, 1974.
Spence, H. M.: Congenital unilateral multicystic kidney: An entity to
   be distinguished from polycystic kidney disease and other cystic
   disorders. J. Urol., 74:693, 1955.

POLYCYSTIC KIDNEY DISEASE

In polycystic disease, the kidneys are characterized
by massive enlargement and a dramatic degree of cyst
formation. If ages at onset among patients with polycystic kidney disease are analyzed, two peaks are
found. In the minority of cases, diagnosis is made at
birth or during the first decade of life. In the majority
of cases, illness appears between the fourth and sixth
decades of life. These two kinds of polycystic kidney
disease are designated as *childhood* and *adult*. In addition to age at onset, they are distinguished by several
other characteristics.

Childhood Polycystic Disease

Childhood polycystic kidney disease (CPKD) can be
distinguished from the adult onset variety by at least
three groups of criteria: genetic, morphologic, and clin-

ical. The incidence of CPKD is not known. Among live births, estimates of its occurrence range between 1 in 6000 and 1 in 14,000. It has appeared in from 1 in 225 to 1 in 450 autopsies. The condition therefore is uncommon.

CPKD is considered to be inherited as a recessive trait, although the number of cases reported is relatively small.

Based on contact with kindreds in which a specific constellation of clinical signs seems to breed true, Blyth and Ockenden believe that four varieties of CPKD exist: *perinatal, neonatal, infantile,* and *juvenile.* Kidneys and liver are involved in both. The four variants are distinguished from one another by the extent to which either organ is affected and by differences in the evolution of clinical symptoms and signs.

In *perinatal* CPKD, massively enlarged and cystic kidneys are found at birth. Reduplication and proliferation of the lining of the intrahepatic bile ducts and minimal periportal fibrosis characterize the hepatic lesion. Renal failure causes death within weeks.

In the *neonatal* variant, patients present during the first month of life with less severe renal dysfunction. Although fewer nephrons are cystic, hepatic fibrosis and bile duct proliferation give the impression of more serious liver involvement. After months or several years, death from renal failure occurs.

The *infantile* variant is characterized by still more severe liver disease and less renal involvement. Instead of renal, hepatic signs may predominate. Patients with this variant present with nephromegaly, splenomegaly, and hepatomegaly. Death during late childhood or early adolescent years may occur either from portal hypertension or from chronic renal failure.

In the *juvenile* form, hepatosplenomegaly is the presenting characteristic. Patients are generally three to five years old. Only 10 per cent of nephrons are cystic, and azotemia does not occur. The characteristic signs and symptoms of juvenile polycystic kidney disease are those of liver failure with portal hypertension. Portacaval shunting has prolonged the lives of some individuals into their twenties.

Not everyone agrees with Blyth and Ockenden. For example, Lieberman and her associates think there is but one condition in which the less serious the renal lesion, the more apt the individuals are to live until hepatic fibrosis becomes clinically significant. At present there is insufficient evidence to settle this difference in opinion.

Typically the kidneys in CPKD when examined microscopically show greatly dilated collecting tubules that are interspersed between wedges of normal renal parenchyma. In kidneys from patients who have survived several years, the dilated tubules assume a more rounded, typically cystic appearance.

CPKD should be distinguished from adult-onset polycystic kidney disease and congenital multicystic kidney (CMK). The kidney in CPKD grossly has a smooth, rather than bosselated, surface. When the organ is cut, one sees fusiform, radially oriented rather than round cysts on the cut surface. Kidneys with the appearance typical of adult-onset polycystic kidney disease have been found infrequently in children and infants. Congenital multicystic kidney is almost never familial, may occur segmentally or unilaterally, and is a form of renal dysplasia. Thus it should be no problem to distinguish the two conditions clinically or pathologically.

In congenital hepatic fibrosis, hepatic fibrosis and renal cysts also occur. The renal cystic lesion is found in only half the cases. Renal cyst formation is mild. The hepatic lesion is one of periportal fibrosis and bile duct proliferation. Again, because of a relative lack of experience, there is continuing disagreement as to whether these cases can or cannot be distinguished from CPKD.

Adult Polycystic Kidney Disease

DEFINITION AND INCIDENCE. Adult polycystic kidney disease (APKD) is the most common form of renal cystic kidney disease in adults, aside from the simple renal cyst. It appears once in every 500 autopsies. It is responsible for renal failure in 5 to 7 per cent of patients coming to transplantation or dialysis. It is transmitted as a mendelian dominant trait. Typically, renal function is normal during the first few decades of life. Renal failure is attributed to progressive cyst formation and appears during the fifth decade of life, with terminal renal failure ensuing over the next ten years.

EPIDEMIOLOGY. Although the pathologic lesion characteristic of APKD has been recognized for a century, credit for recognizing the hereditary nature of the condition generally is extended to Cairns, a British urologist. He reported a single family with 84 members. Dalgaard has reported the largest number of families, 284, and his monograph remains the classic on APKD to date. Gene penetrance is 100 per cent by 80 years of age, meaning that if a genetically predisposed individual survives to that age, there is 100 per cent probability that polycystic kidneys will be present. In any affected family, renal failure tends to appear at about the same age. It appears that heritable factors influence not only the morphologic characteristics of APKD but also the temporal program of its evolution.

PATHOGENESIS AND PATHOLOGY. The pathogenesis of APKD is unknown. One early suggestion was that tubules in these kidneys were obstructed, either by "salts" of uric acid or by a failure of the two segments of nephrons to join properly during development of the kidney. Studies by Lambert and by Bricker and Patton demonstrated that most cystic nephrons in APKD were in communication with glomeruli and the final urinary space, making obstruction a far less attractive pathogenetic possibility. More recently, partial, not total, tubular obstruction and altered compliance of tubular basement membrane have been suggested. Whatever the pathogenetic mechanism, it has its effect over time in genetically preconditioned kidneys that originally appear grossly normal in structure and function.

The kidney from end-stage APKD is dramatically misshapen. It is variably enlarged, sometimes to the size of an American football. Its external surface is covered with countless numbers of cysts that are filled with yellow, white, brown, or black fluid. When examined microscopically, it appears that these cysts have compressed adjacent, otherwise normal renal tissue.

Analyses demonstrate that cystic contents have a composition that is characteristic of either proximal tubular or distal tubular fluid, suggesting that cyst walls continue to function in these kidneys.

CLINICAL MANIFESTATIONS. The classic clinical findings in APKD are a positive family history, bilateral flank masses, elevated blood pressure, and uremia. Flank pain is the earliest symptom. It begins months to years before detectable renal enlargement. Renal failure

then follows nephromegaly. This sequence of events —
discomfort, then deformity, then dysfunction — and
the impression one gets on microscopic evaluation that
cysts are compressing normal renal tissue have given
rise to the concept that cyst expansion is responsible
for renal failure in this entity.

Patients come to the attention of physicians because
of pain, bleeding, urinary tract infection, nephrolithiasis, or obstructive uropathy. Early an affected individual
may present with anuria caused by expansion of strategically located cysts to the point that urinary outflow
from otherwise functioning kidneys is obstructed.

Liver disease also occurs in APKD. However, it
differs dramatically from the hepatic lesion of CPKD.
Cyst formation, not hepatic fibrosis, can be demonstrated in up to 30 per cent of APKD cases. Rarely or never
is there evidence of hepatic dysfunction. Liver cysts are
demonstrated only because they are looked for by ultrasonography or radioisotopic scanning in known cases
of APKD. Cysts in other organs also can be found, although their frequency is far less. In approximately 10
per cent of cases, berry aneurysms in the cerebral circulation are present. A small percentage of cases of
APKD may first come to medical attention because of
cerebral vascular accidents.

DIAGNOSIS. Diagnosis of APKD rests on the presence of the clinical manifestations already discussed.
The family history is positive for renal disease in over
75 per cent of reported cases. Inattentiveness to history-
taking, inadequate autopsy data, and new mutations
are considered to account for failure to ascertain a positive family history in 100 per cent of cases. Depending
on the extent to which disease has progressed, any degree of abnormality may be found either on urinalysis
or in the level of azotemia. Massive proteinuria (>3
grams per 24 hours) is rare and should raise the possibility of complicating disease or an alternative diagnosis. In many cases, anemia is not marked, possibly because the APK retains significant erythropoietic
capability. Renal sodium wasting and nephrolithiasis
occur, but not with the severity or frequency seen in
medullary cystic disease or sponge kidney.

APKD must be differentiated from hydronephrosis,
pyelonephritis, renal neoplasm, and medullary sponge
kidney. Sonographic and radiographic techniques will
disclose bilateral massive cyst formation and enlarged
kidneys in APKD. Because polycystic kidneys may be
unusually susceptible to infection, retrograde pyelography is best avoided in making a diagnosis.

TREATMENT AND PROGNOSIS. Treatment is nonspecific and symptomatic. Complications should be treated
specifically. Renal transplantation and dialysis will prolong life once end-stage renal failure occurs. Genetic
counseling is of vital importance for affected individuals and their families. Because renal failure typically appears after the childbearing years, transmission of the
condition from generation to generation is assured. All
children of an affected individual are threatened by the
specter of renal failure later in life, even though only
one in every two on the average will actually be involved. Thus management of families with APKD requires participation not only of the physician but also
of the geneticist, social worker, surgeon, and often the
psychiatrist.

Blyth, H., and Ockenden, B. G.: Polycystic disease of kidneys present-
    ing in childhood. J. Med. Genet., 8:257, 1971.
Bricker, N. S., and Patton, J. F.: Cystic disease of the kidneys: A study

of dynamics and chemical composition of cyst fluid. Am. J. Med.,
    18:207, 1955.
Cairns, H. W. B.: Heredity in polycystic disease of the kidney. Quart.
    J. Med., 18:359, 1925.
Dalgaard, O. Z.: Bilateral polycystic disease of the kidneys: A followup
    study of 284 patients and their families. Acta Med. Scand., 158
    (Suppl 328), 1957.
Hartnett, M., and Bennett, W.: Extrarenal manifestations of cystic kid-
    ney disease. In Gardner, K. D., Jr. (ed.): Cystic Diseases of the
    Kidney. New York, John Wiley & Sons, 1976, pp. 201–219.
Lambert, P.: Polycystic disease of the kidney: A review. Arch. Pathol.,
    44:34, 1947.
Lieberman, E., Salinas-Madrigal, L., Gwinn, J. L., Brennan, L. P., Fine,
    R. N., and Landing, B. H.: Infantile polycystic disease of the kid-
    neys and liver: Clinical, pathological and radiological correlations
    and comparison with congenital hepatic fibrosis. Medicine, 50:277,
    1971.
Murray-Lyon, I. M., Ockenden, B. G., and Williams, R.: Congenital
    hepatic fibrosis — is it a single clinical entity? Gastroenterology,
    64:653, 1973.

NEPHRONOPHTHISIS–CYSTIC RENAL MEDULLA COMPLEX

DEFINITION.   A characteristic appearance of the kidney in this disorder gives the complex its name. There
is bilateral involvement. The kidneys are shrunken and
scarred, and contain a variable number of small intramedullary and corticomedullary cysts. Microscopically,
interstitial nephritis is present in varying degrees of severity among individual patients. Signs and symptoms
of the complex include a family history that is positive
for kidney disease, anemia, renal salt-wasting, failure
to thrive in children, and progressive renal failure.

INCIDENCE AND PREVALENCE.   Over the past 30 years,
more than 250 examples of the complex have been reported. Not all are typical. Renal cysts are not described
in some 15 per cent of cases. The family history is negative for renal disease in about 15 per cent. Renal salt-
wasting has been documented in fewer than 25 patients
although it has not universally been sought. The anemia which occurs does not appear to be disproportionate to the degree of renal failure.

EPIDEMIOLOGY.   Four variants of the complex can be
distinguished on genetic grounds: isolated cases, recessively inherited cases with or without retinal pathology, and dominantly transmitted disease. Sporadic cases
may reflect the occurrence of the complex in an only
child or a new mutation in the general population; or
medullary cysts might occur as an acquired rather than
a heritable trait in rare instances.

Approximately 50 per cent of reported patients describe instances in which a recessive mode of transmission appears most likely. There has been consanguineous mating in many families. Both sexes are equally
involved. Self-selection among involved families may
account for the fact that there is a tendency for a greater
than expected ratio of one affected to three unaffected
siblings. This variant is called *familial juvenile nephronophthisis.*

Retinal pathology, typically retinitis pigmentosa, and
recessive inheritance characterize an additional 17 per
cent of reported cases. This variant of the complex is
designated *renal-retinal dysplasia.*

In about 18 per cent of published cases, a dominant
pattern of inheritance is documented. Consanguinity
and retinal pathology have never been observed among
these individuals. This variant is designated *adult-onset
medullary cystic disease.*

Affected   individuals   with   dominantly   transmitted

disease are significantly older at the times of onset of renal failure and death. Among 34 published instances of recessively inherited disease, there was a mean age at onset of 10 years and a mean age at death of 14.4 years. In contrast, among 24 cases of dominantly inherited disease, the ages at onset and death were 28.4 and 31.7 years, respectively (p <0.001). Thus in the complex, as is the case in polycystic kidney disease, differing modes of inheritance are distinguished by differing ages at onset and death.

A defect in urinary concentrating ability has been reported in the parents or siblings of an affected individual on ten occasions. This evidence, tenuous as it is, raises the possibility that a heterozygous state of the complex exists.

PATHOGENESIS. Nothing is known of the pathogenesis of the complex. The disease has not recurred in transplanted kidneys, making it impossible to implicate a genetically determined, circulating, cystogenic nephrotoxin as its cause. Under light microscopy tubular atrophy, round cell infiltration, periglomerular fibrosis, and small noncortical cysts characterize the renal lesion. Involvement is always bilateral and symmetrical, even at the microscopic level. Microdissection reveals cyst formation along collecting tubules and loops of Henle but nowhere else along the nephron.

CLINICAL MANIFESTATIONS. Affected patients come to medical attention because of uremia or because the diagnosis has been made or is under consideration in a relative. Eighty per cent of patients present with nocturia, polyuria, polydipsia, and enuresis. Weakness, pallor, and disordered bone growth (in children) follow in descending order of frequency.

Hypertension is relatively infrequent, occurring in roughly one third of azotemic subjects. Its lower than usual incidence may be due to subclinical salt-wasting, but such a phenomenon has not been established among these patients as a group. In some patients, renal salt-wasting may reach tremendous proportions, exceeding 200 to 250 mEq of sodium per day. Renal function may transiently improve in these individuals when salt and water deficits are replaced.

The earliest clinical sign of involvement may be diminution of maximal urinary concentrating ability. It has been described in six instances in which other evidence of the complex ultimately evolved. More experience is necessary before the value of this test as a diagnostic tool can be established. Hair color has been touted as a helpful sign in diagnosing affected cases. In one series, affected individuals had red or blond hair. Because most other case reports do not indicate hair color, the validity of this sign also remains in doubt; in the author's experience, only four blonds and no redheads have been encountered.

Instances of the complex have been reported in patients with a horseshoe kidney, congenital hepatic fibrosis, and the Laurence-Moon-Biedl syndrome.

There are several negative features that distinguish the complex from other renal cystic disorders. Nephromegaly does not occur. Cyst formation is restricted to the kidneys; cysts (and aneurysms) are not found in other organs. Nephrocalcinosis and urolithiasis, with one exception, have not been reported. The urinalysis is remarkable for its lack of evident pathology, even in late uremia. Significant hematuria, proteinuria, cylindruria, and bacteriuria are decidedly unusual, so much so that when markedly abnormal urines are demonstrated repeatedly, alternative diagnoses should be considered.

DIAGNOSIS. Instances of the complex must be differentiated from all those conditions in which there is progressive and relentless azotemia and diminishing renal size. The family history that is positive for renal disease is helpful, especially if postmortem specimens of renal tissue from relatives disclose the typical cystic lesion. Renal arteriography with tomography has been helpful in making antemortem diagnoses, although small cysts can be missed. Similarly, renal biopsy, open or closed, is diagnostic when interstitial nephritis and cysts are found. Because cysts lie deep in the kidney substance, however, it is the more common experience to remove renal tissue without cysts. One is left, then, with the lesion of interstitial nephritis and all the diagnostic possibilities that it intimates.

TREATMENT AND PROGNOSIS. Genetic counseling, hemodialysis, and renal transplantation offer hope for prevention and for prolongation of life among affected individuals. As with adult polycystic kidney disease, individuals affected because of dominantly inherited disease often have procreated before becoming ill. No reliable means currently exists to differentiate affected from nonaffected children in these kindreds.

Renal salt-wasting should be treated with salt and water in amounts sufficient to maintain adequate blood volume and optimal renal function. Appropriate antibiotics should be used to treat recurrent urinary tract infection, but there is no evidence that they slow progression of the disease.

Fanconi, V. G., Hanhart, E., Albertini, A., et al.: Die familiäre juvenile Nephronophthise (die idiopathische parenchymatöse Schrumpfniere). Helv. Paediat. Acta, 6:1, 1951.

Gardner, K. D., Jr.: Juvenile nephronophthisis and renal medullary cystic disease. In Gardner, K. D., Jr. (ed.): Cystic Diseases of the Kidney. New York, John Wiley & Sons, 1976, pp. 173–185.

Mena, E., Bookstein, J. J., McDonald, F. D., et al.: Angiographic findings in renal medullary cystic disease. Radiology, 110:277, 1974.

Schimke, R. N.: Hereditary renal-retinal dysplasia. Ann. Intern. Med., 70:736, 1969.

Senior, B.: Familial renal-retinal dystrophy. Am. J. Dis. Child., 125:442, 1973.

Strauss, M. B.: Clinical and pathological aspects of cystic disease of renal medulla. Ann. Intern. Med., 57:373, 1962.

MEDULLARY SPONGE KIDNEY

Medullary sponge kidney (MSK) is a relatively common, roentgenographically diagnosed disorder of the intrapyramidal or intrapapillary segments of the renal collecting tubules, characterized by ectasia sometimes to the point of actual cyst formation.

Over 600 case reports of MSK have appeared in the literature. Estimates of its frequency in the general population range between 1 in 5000 and 1 in 20,000. It is found in approximately 1 in 200 individuals with urologic disease.

Infection, tubular obstruction, and heritable factors have been considered in the pathogenesis of MSK. Although evidence of chronic papillary infection is found in many patients, most authorities consider infection to be a secondary and not primary feature. The lesion is rare in infants and children, most cases having been reported in adults. Intraluminal deposits of uric acid are commonplace in children, but MSK is not. Therefore in utero obstruction of the distal nephron by "salts" is considered a remote possibility to account for the lesion. A role for heritable factors in the transmission of MSK is suggested by the facts that nine families are described in which MSK has affected two or more individuals (in one family, three consecutive generations were affected), and that instances of MSK are reported in association with other heritable diseases (e.g., the Ehlers-Danlos syndrome). Most authorities, however, consider MSK to be a congenital, not heritable, lesion.

Grossly the kidney in MSK is normal in size, but may be slightly enlarged (in 30 per cent of cases) when cystic changes are marked. The cut surface exhibits intrapyramidal cysts which contain calcareous deposits in approximately 50 per cent of cases. The cysts are, in fact, dilated collecting tubules. Any number from one to all renal pyramids in either or both kidneys may be affected. Microscopically, the most constant feature is a variably severe infiltration of the interstitium with inflammatory cells, usually most pronounced nearest the pelvis of the kidney.

Diagnosis of MSK is based on radiographic or clinical grounds. Many cases are identified incidentally, during the workup for hematuria, stones, recurrent urinary tract infection, or other conditions in which intravenous pyelography is indicated. During intravenous pyelography, contrast medium concentrates in the ectatic or cystic tubules. Calculi are located in the same regions. When one is careful to take films after the nephrographic phase and before pelvocalyceal filling is complete, contrast medium can be seen to fill the ectatic intrapyramidal tubules. As calyces empty, contrast medium persists in the ectatic intrapyramidal tubules. At present, there is not general acceptance that milder forms of MSK exist. For example, the *pyramidal blush*, which is seen frequently during routine pyelography, is considered by some to be an early stage of the MSK lesion; most radiourologists consider it an unrelated and perhaps even normal finding. The issue is unsettled at present.

When uncomplicated by stone formation or infection, MSK may go undetected. On the other hand, when complications intervene, debilitating disease and even renal failure may occur. Over two thirds of affected individuals with clinically overt disease have impairment in maximal urinary concentrating ability. Five instances of distal tubular renal acidosis have been reported, although in most patients with MSK the urinary acidifying ability is normal. Hypercalciuria occurs in 40 per cent of patients. Its mechanism has not been established. Renal salt-wasting in mild proportions also may be seen but does not reach the degree of severity noted in the nephronophthisis–cystic renal medulla complex.

In one large series, renal colic was the most frequent presenting complaint in complicated cases of MSK. Hematuria, either microscopic or macroscopic, and acute urinary tract infection together constituted the second most frequent set of presenting complaints. Renal failure and elevated blood pressure are unusual.

MSK has been reported in patients ranging in age from 3 weeks to 71 years of age. Involvement is equal between the two sexes. In one series, approximately 50 per cent of the patients had proteinuria and hyperuricemia.

Uncomplicated MSK follows a benign clinical course. Radiographic evidence of progression has been documented in fewer than 15 per cent of patients. Almost always it has consisted only of slight changes in the size or distribution of dilated collecting tubules. Among symptomatic patients, the disease runs a variable course. In one instance, there may be long periods free from symptoms; in a second, repeated hospitalizations for lithiasis or recurrent urinary tract infection may be required.

One patient in ten is regarded as having a poor prognosis. Partial or total nephrectomy, when the disease is unilateral, has been curable. However, the disease does progress asynchronously in the two kidneys in some instances. Therefore care must be exercised not to perform nephrectomy in an individual with asymmetric but bilateral involvement.

The list of differential diagnostic possibilities for MSK includes all those conditions in which nephrocalcinosis and nephrolithiasis occur: hyperparathyroidism, milk-alkali syndrome, multiple myeloma, sarcoidosis, tuberculosis, vitamin D intoxication, and so on. Among these possibilities, Ekström et al. consider hyperparathyroidism to be the most common. Renal papillary necrosis may mimic the appearance of MSK on excretory urography. In papillary necrosis, however, the clinical course usually is acute and occurs most frequently in patients with diabetes mellitus, sickle cell anemia, obstruction, analgesic abuse, and recurrent urinary tract infection. On pyelography, MSK can be confused with childhood polycystic kidney disease; differentiation can be made on clinical grounds. The experienced radiologist will have no difficulty distinguishing MSK from calyceal diverticula and calyceal cysts.

MSK has been reported to accompany a variety of other clinical diseases, including the Ehlers-Danlos syndrome, horseshoe kidney, ectopic kidney, and mongolism. MSK has accompanied congenital total hemihypertrophy in 17 instances; the lesion of MSK sometimes is on the same side as the hemihypertrophy and sometimes on the opposite.

The efficacy of stone-preventive measures in MSK has not been established; but on the grounds of "nothing ventured, nothing gained," it would appear worthwhile to institute them in patients with frequent episodes of urolithiasis.

Ekström, T., Engfeldt, B., Lagergren, C., et al.: Medullary Sponge Kidney. Stockholm, Almqvist and Wiksell, 1959.
Kuiper, J. J.: Medullary sponge kidney. *In* Gardner, K. D., Jr. (ed.): Cystic Diseases of the Kidney. New York, John Wiley & Sons, 1976, pp. 151–171.
Levine, A. S., and Michael, A. F.: Ehlers-Danlos syndrome with renal tubular acidosis and medullary sponge kidney. J. Pediat., 71:107, 1967.
Spence, H. M., and Singleton, R.: What is sponge kidney disease and where does it fit in the spectrum of cystic disorders? J. Urol., 107:176, 1972.

384. ANOMALIES OF THE URINARY TRACT

James F. Glenn

Anomalies of the genitourinary system are more common than congenital abnormalities of any other organ system, and it has been estimated that 10 per cent of the population will exhibit one or more significant congenital anomalies of the urinary tract. The various urinary tract congenital abnormalities to be enumerated below may or may not be of significance in themselves, but may induce complications of obstruction, stasis, infection, stone formation, and ultimate renal failure. In many cases, congenital abnormalities of the urinary tract are discovered only incidentally in the course of evaluation for other disease processes. In other instances, the congenital anomalies predispose to the complications which cause clinical symptoms and invite diagnostic evaluation.

KIDNEY

Total *bilateral renal agenesis* is a rare but recognized entity with characteristic oligohydramnios, Potter's facies, and pulmonary hypoplasia, death being due to the last-named problem. An identical syndrome is seen with bilateral multicystic kidneys or with complete lower tract obstruction and attendant renal dysplasia. *Solitary kidney* occurs when there is unilateral renal agenesis, perhaps once or twice in every one thousand live births, the result of failure of the renal bud, nephrogenic blastema, or vascular supply. *Hypoplastic kidney* may take several forms, including bilateral oligomeganephronic hypoplasia with mild azotemia as a rule, segmental hypoplasia, and the various forms of dysplasia associated with ureteral, bladder, or urethral obstruction. Renal vein thrombosis is usually a disease of neonates, but older children and adults can be affected. Various forms of renal cystic disease are seen in children and adults, including multicystic kidney (see Ureter, below); polycystic kidney, both the infantile and adult forms of which lead to renal failure; medullary cystic disease, a familial disorder leading to ultimate renal failure; medullary sponge kidney with attendant problems of stone formation; and cystic disorders with multiple anomalies.

True supernumerary kidney is exceedingly rare, whereas *"double kidney"* or duplication of the collecting system within a single renal substance is a common anomaly, often associated with partial or complete duplication of the ureter as well. Bilateral partial or complete duplications are often seen and usually have no significance, although with complete ureteral duplication there may be reflux — usually to the lower pole system — or obstruction — generally of the upper pole system — leading to complications of urinary infection.

Renal fusion anomalies are extremely interesting and include *horseshoe kidney*, in which the two renal masses are fused across the midline, usually at the lower pole but occasionally at the upper pole; *crossed fused ectopia*, in which the kidneys are connected lower pole to upper pole in S-shaped or sigmoid configuration; and *pelvic fusion*, which is referred to as "pancake kidney." Although most of these fusion anomalies cause no symptoms unless obstruction, infection, or stones supervene, horseshoe kidney may produce Rovsing's sign, abdominal pain on hyperextension which is thought to be due to compression of the renal isthmus against the great vessels in front of the spine.

Malrotation is the term applied to those kidneys which exhibit incomplete rotation as they ascend into the renal fossa, usually of no clinical significance. *Congenital ectopia*, usually unilateral, said to occur in 1 per cent of the population, reflects a pelvic position of some kidneys, and is probably due to abnormal blood supply which binds the developing kidney and prevents its ascent to the normal site.

Nephroptosis may be congenital, the kidney only loosely attached at its pedicle and within Garota's fascia, permitting marked downward excursion with the patient in the upright position. However, in most instances nephroptosis is observed following significant weight loss or multiple pregnancies with consequent loss of perinephric fat and other renal support. For the most part, the ptotic kidney will cause no symptoms, but on occasion there may be peaking of the ureter to cause transient urine outflow obstruction, or there may be transient compromise of renal blood flow through the attenuated vessels. Indeed, both severe abdominal pain and transient episodes of postural hypertension have been attributed to nephroptosis. At one time, it was the vogue to accomplish nephropexy in every instance of nephroptosis, but few such procedures are now performed, those only in instances in which there is reproducible pain with ptosis of the kidney or some other definitive reason for intervention. The very significant incidence of nephroptosis in patients suffering psychosomatic complaints necessitates very careful evaluation of this condition prior to surgical intervention, although the attendant complications of hypertension or hydronephrosis militate for surgical correction. Dietl's crisis may occur in association with nephroptosis or independently, the result of acute hyperhydration as seen with beer drinkers, the renal pelvis becoming overdistended and spastic, such acute hydronephrosis being reproducible by infusion pyelography in many instances.

Congenital hydronephrosis may be due to intrinsic ureteropelvic junction stricture, extrinsic compression by fibrous band or aberrant blood vessel, or intrinsic ureteromuscular deficit which inhibits normal peristaltic emptying of the renal pelvis. Evaluation is by intravenous and retrograde pyelography, and surgical correction — pyeloplasty — may be accomplished by a variety of satisfactory techniques.

BLOOD VESSELS

Minor variations in renal circulation may be seen in 25 per cent of the population, duality of arterial supply or venous drainage being the most common anomaly. The renal arteries may have aberrant origin or course, may produce ureteral or ureteropelvic junction obstruction, and may predispose to inadequate renal perfusion with renal hypoplasia. Renal artery aneurysm, usually located at the bifurcation of an artery, is a cause of hypertension and carries the risk of spontaneous rupture, particularly during pregnancy. Congenital arteriovenous fistulas are rare, but may predispose to hypertension. Anomalous vascularity of the kidneys is of most importance in relation to reconstructive renal surgery, nephrectomy for various causes, and renal transplantation.

URETER

The most important ureteral anomaly is complete duplication, as noted above (see Kidney), in which distal ectopia of the ureter from the upper pole may result in obstruction. Lateral vesical ectopia of the lower pole segment may predispose to reflux. Upper ureteral atresia or agenesis is most frequently associated with multicystic kidney, the primitive ipsilateral renal lobules becoming hydronephrotic with the "cluster of grapes" appearance, a congenital form of intrarenal hydrone- phrosis which is one of the most common causes of ab- dominal masses in neonates. Congenital malimplanta- tion of ureter or ureters into the urinary bladder is the primary cause of vesicoureteral reflux and the attendant complications of infection and potential compromise of renal function. Other ureteral malformations include ec- topia, ureterocele, megaloureter, congenital valves, bifid- ity, or diverticula.

BLADDER

Fortunately, congenital anomalies of the bladder are uncommon, but agenesis of the urinary bladder has been observed, along with hypoplasia, duplication, congenital diverticula and exstrophy (failure of closure), or cloacal exstrophy (involving the rectum as well). Neurogenic or neuropathic bladder may be associated with congenital neurologic disease such as meningo- myelocele or sacral agenesis. The more severe bladder anomalies may necessitate urinary diversion in infancy or childhood.

URETHRA

In the male, the most common urethral abnormality is hypospadias, the failure of distal development of the urethra with resultant proximal ventral urinary meatus and associated chordee or binding of the penis, neces- sitating one or more operative procedures for correc- tion. Epispadias, abnormal dorsal opening of the urethra, may be seen in both males and females, and may be associated with total incontinence or satisfacto- ry urinary control. Minor anomalies include urethral stenosis. Rare anomalies are urethral diverticula and megalourethra, the latter associated with developmental failure of the erectile bodies of the penis in the male.

Anderson, E. E., and Harrison, J. H.: Surgical importance of a solitary kidney. N. Engl. J. Med., 273:683, 1965.
Dees, J. E.: The clinical importance of congenital anomalies of the upper urinary tract. J. Urol., 46:659, 1941.
Glenn, J. F.: Fused pelvic kidney. J. Urol., 80:7, 1958.
Glenn, J. F.: Analysis of 51 patients with horseshoe kidney. New Engl. J. Med., 261:684, 1959.
Kelalis, P. P., et al.: Anomalies of the urinary tract. In Kelalis, P. P., and King, L. R. (eds.): Clinical Pediatric Urology. Philadelphia, W. B. Saunders Company, 1976, pp. 475–597.

385. TUMORS OF THE KIDNEY

James F. Glenn

Neoplasms or "new growths" of the genitourinary tract, both benign and malignant, account for up to one third of all tumors. Among the tumors of the urinary tract, renal tumors rank high as a cause of morbidity and mortality. Of greatest concern is the adult form of renal parenchymal malignancy, nephrocarcinoma.

CLASSIFICATION

Acknowledging that renal tumors may be of many types, authorities have devised almost unending clas-

sifications and subclassifications of morphologic and histologic characteristics, leading to proliferation of ter- minology without significant clinical impact. As an escape from the burdensome confusion imposed by elaborate classifications, it has been suggested that renal tumors of all sorts simply be subdivided into those which are benign and those which are malignant; unfortunately, this oversimplification fails for lack of recognition of the differing clinical import of the various neoplasms.

As a compromise between the simplistic and the complicated methods of classification, it has been pro- posed that a modified system be adopted which would subdivide renal tumors into six major categories: be- nign tumors, tumors of the renal pelvis, pyelorenal tumors, embryonic tumors, nephrocarcinoma, and other malignancies (see accompanying table). However, an even less complex and equally comprehensive ap- proach can be utilized: four distinct groups of tumors include *nephrocarcinoma, nephroblastoma, urothelial ma- lignancies,* and *other tumors.*

Glenn, J. F.: Renal parenchymal tumors. In Harrison, J. H., et al. (eds.): Campbell's Urology, Vol. II. Philadelphia, W. B. Saunders Com- pany, 1979.
Skinner, D. G.: Renal neoplasia. In Brenner, B. M., and Rector, F. C. (eds.): The Kidney. Philadelphia, W. B. Saunders Company, 1976, p. 1396.

NEPHROCARCINOMA

The adult form of renal malignancy is increasing in incidence; it is now said to afflict more than 7000 peo- ple annually in the United States, with the death rate from nephrocarcinoma rising from 1.8 per 100,000 in 1940 to approximately 2.8 per 100,000 in 1960. There is a marked difference in sex incidence; men afflicted with renal carcinoma outnumber women by two or three to one, supporting the concept that hormonal in- fluences may be involved in histogenesis of nephrocar- cinoma, even though the tumor has been reported in all age groups, including infants and prepubertal children. Although it is not known whether there is a familial tendency to nephrocarcinoma or a genetic predisposi- tion for it, certain species such as the leopard frog will exhibit virtually 100 per cent histologic evidence of spontaneous renal malignancies.

A Classification of Renal Tumors

1. Benign tumors
   Renal capsule
   Renal parenchyma
   Vascular tumors
   Cystic lesions, dysplasias, hydronephrosis
   Heteroplastic, mesenchymal tumors
2. Tumors of renal pelvis
   Benign papilloma
   Transitional and squamous cell carcinomas, adenocarcinomas
3. Pararenal tumors
   Benign
   Malignant
4. Embryonic tumors
   Nephroblastoma (Wilms' tumor)
   Embryonic, mesotheliomatous tumors
   Sarcomas
5. Nephrocarcinoma
   Renal cell carcinoma, adenocarcinoma, "hypernephroma"
   Papillary cystadenocarcinoma
6. Other malignancies
   Primary: mesenchymal, hemangiopericytoma, myeloma
   Secondary: metastatic lesions

PATHOLOGY. More than a century ago, pathologists tentatively concluded that solid tumors of the renal substance arose from tubular epithelium. Subsequent observers, including Grawitz (1883), confused the picture by introducing the concept that such tumors were of adrenal origin and represented rests within the kidney, "struma lipomatodes aberrata renis." Since it was thought that these cells derived from above the kidney, the term "hypernephroid carcinoma" or hypernephroma was widely employed. Subsequent terminology has included clear cell carcinoma, adenocarcinoma of the kidney, alveolar carcinoma, and Grawitz's tumor.

Nephrocarcinoma is usually unilateral in equal distribution, but may be bilateral or multifocal. It is firm and nodular with encapsulation, although there is often extension beyond the kidney itself. Normal renal cells vary widely in histologic characteristics, and, as might be anticipated, nephrocarcinomas exhibit a spectrum of cellular patterns. Most often, renal malignancies are glandular, acinar, or tubular in characteristics, and both papillary and cystic patterns are seen. Cells may vary from cuboidal to columnar to spindle shaped, and may be of the classically vacuolated "clear cell" variety or may display a granular pattern — the latter frequently associated with a more serious prognosis.

Grading on the standard Broders scale is often impossible, although the prognosis in a given patient may depend upon both grade and stage of disease. Most pathologists have adopted the practice of grading renal malignancies into well differentiated or poorly differentiated categories. The stage of nephrocarcinoma in which it is encountered and treated may have most significant impact upon prognosis, and a standardized staging system has been almost universally adopted:

Stage I: Tumor confined to kidney.
Stage II: Tumor confined to Gerota's space.
Stage III: Local spread.
  (A) Renal vein or vena caval involvement.
  (B) Local lymph node involvement.
  (C) Vascular and lymphatic involvement.
Stage IV: Advanced disease.
  (A) Adjacent organs involved.
  (B) Distant metastases.

CLINICAL MANIFESTATIONS. Nephrocarcinoma has often been called "the internist's tumor" because of its protean symptomatology and the frequent presentations suggesting systemic disease. The classic triad of signs and symptoms in renal tumor includes flank pain, palpable mass, and hematuria, although it is relatively uncommon for all these manifestations to occur simultaneously. Nearly two thirds of the patients with nephrocarcinoma will exhibit gross or microscopic hematuria, half will have some complaint of abdominal or flank pain, and about one third will exhibit a renal mass. Acute left varicocele, said to be pathognomonic of left renal tumor causing spermatic vein obstruction, is actually seen in only about 2 per cent of patients with renal malignancy. Metastatic disease, involving lung, liver, or bones, may be the presenting problem in as many as 10 per cent of patients with nephrocarcinoma.

Toxic systemic effects of nephrocarcinoma frequently include anemia, possibly resulting from erythropoietin deficiency or bone marrow depression. Fever of undetermined origin generally calls for a search for renal malignancy, as it is estimated that 15 to 20 per cent of patients with nephrocarcinoma exhibit fever, probably caused by endogenous production of pyrogens by the tumor. Hepatic dysfunction is observed as a toxic phenomenon in the presence of nephrocarcinoma, and both amyloidosis and peripheral neuropathies may be occasioned by immune mechanisms. Systemic endocrine effects in association with nephrocarcinoma are often recognized, including hypertension in as many as 10 per cent of patients with nephrocarcinoma, this possibly being due either to tumor production of renin or a renin-like substance or to mechanical vascular effects of the tumor such as arteriovenous fistula or compression of the renal pedicle. Erythrocytosis, seen in 2 to 4 per cent of patients with nephrocarcinoma, is due to a definite erythropoietin-like substance generated by the tumor; hypercalcemia, seen in 5 per cent or more of patients with nephrocarcinoma, is due to a tumor-produced parathormone-like substance. Additionally, renal tumors have been incriminated as producing both gonadotropins and glucagon, causing either masculinizing signs or protein-losing enteropathy.

DIAGNOSIS. All renal masses must be considered malignant until proved otherwise, but the diagnostic armamentarium offers great precision in differentiation. Infusion or high dose intravenous pyelography, particularly in combination with nephrotomography, will usually identify a renal mass, frequently with resolution of lesions as small as 1 or 2 cm in diameter. Poor renal function may sometimes demand retrograde pyelography for similar purposes. Ultrasonography offers a noninvasive and relatively accurate method of differentiating simple cysts form solid tumor, although such studies may be misleading in instances of cysts associated with tumor or hemorrhage within existing solid tumor. Computerized axial tomography (CAT scanning), now being employed with increasing frequency, increases diagnostic accuracy still further by noninvasive methods. However, the definitive diagnosis of nephrocarcinoma almost always demands angiography, both screening aortography and selective renal arteriography, demonstrating not only the characteristic neovascularity of the tumor but also the anatomic arrangement of the blood supply, important information in planning the surgical approach.

In the recent past, it has become popular to accomplish needle puncture of suspected benign renal cysts, aspirating cyst fluid for cytologic examination and injecting contrast for confirmation of the cystic configuration of the lesion. Needle puncture carries potential risk of hemorrhage, infection, or tumor spread, and it is most important to recognize that simple cysts often occur in association with nephrocarcinoma, the malignancy lying medial or adjacent to the cyst itself without invasion of tumor into the cyst cavity. Puncture of a suspected benign cyst should be undertaken only in consultation and collaboration with the urologic surgeon who will be responsible for the care of such a patient if surgery becomes necessary.

TREATMENT. Surgical extirpation offers the only known cure of nephrocarcinoma at present. The surgical approach for radical nephrectomy (removal of the kidney and perinephric fat with Gerota's fascia and regional lymphatics) may be dictated by size and location (upper pole or lower pole) of the tumor, as well as by the preference and experience of the urologist. The most commonly employed techniques are various forms of transabdominal exposure or the thoracolumbar approach, although variations on the standard lumbar approach may be applicable. The most critical factor is the amenability of the tumor to total removal. Direct extension (tumor thrombus) of nephrocarcinoma into the renal vein and the vena cava may necessitate cavotomy, but does not compromise potential curability if the tumor can be extracted intact. Tumor involvement of regional nodes or extension into adjacent organs seriously impairs prognosis.

Adjuvant therapy of nephrocarcinoma may take the form of radiation therapy, chemotherapy, or immunotherapy, although none of these modalities has been definitively demonstrated to enhance survival or cure. Radiotherapy may be accomplished preoperatively, as most nephrocarcinomas are radiosensitive. Postoperative radiation therapy in patients with residual disease may offer some prolongation of survival. Chemotherapy has been disappointing in general, although there are isolated reports of improvement with various drugs, frequently hormones; progestational agents, testosterone, and corticosteroids have been advocated and may afford subjective if not objective improvement in advanced metastatic disease, the most commonly employed drugs being Provera and Depo-Testosterone. Immunotherapy of nephrocarcinoma remains experimental, but the antigenicity and other propensities of renal carcinoma suggest that this may be a productive avenue of therapy in the future.

At this time, five-year apparent cure rates of 60 to 70 per cent may be anticipated, although delayed recurrence or manifestation of metastatic disease 20 years or more following extirpation of the primary lesion has been reported.

Ambrose, S. S., Lewis, E. L., O'Brien, D. P., III, Walton, K. N., and Ross, J. R.: Unsuspected renal tumors associated with renal cysts. J. Urol., 117:704, 1977.

Bloom, H. J. G., and Wallace, D. M.: Hormones and the kidney: Possible therapeutic role of testosterone in a patient with regression of metastases from a renal adenocarcinoma. Br. Med. J., 2:476, 1964.

Chisholm, G. B., and Roy, R. R.: The systemic effects of malignant renal tumors. Br. J. Urol., 43:687, 1971.

Gonzalez-Serva, L., Weinerth, H. L., and Glenn, J. F.: The minimal mortality of renal surgery. Urology, 9:253, 1977.

Holland, J. M.: Cancer of the kidney: Natural history and staging. Cancer, 32:1030, 1973.

Robson, C. J., Churchill, B. M., and Anderson, W.: The results of radical nephrectomy for renal cell carcinoma. J. Urol., 101:297, 1969.

NEPHROBLASTOMA

Embryonal carcinoma of the kidney or Wilms' tumor is now most commonly termed nephroblastoma. It is the most common solid tumor of a single site in infants and children, a malignancy exceeded in incidence only by the leukemias and by neuroblastoma, which may originate anywhere in neural tissue of the sympathetic chain. The peak incidence of nephroblastoma is at two to four years of age, although these tumors are recognized rarely in neonates and even more rarely in the aged.

Nephroblastoma most often presents as an abdominal mass, discovered incidentally by parents or an examining physician. Hematuria, gross or microscopic, is a late event, reflecting invasion of the urinary collecting system by the tumor, and is seen in only about 30 per cent of the patients. Abdominal pain, weight loss, anorexia, nausea and vomiting, and even intestinal obstruction may frequently accompany the tumor. Bilater-

al nephroblastoma may be encountered in 5 to 10 per cent of patients. Pulmonary metastases are most common, although metastatic involvement of local lymphatics, liver, and other soft tissues, as well as bone, may be encountered.

Diagnosis is generally made on a clinical basis with confirmation by intravenous pyelography. The most common abdominal masses in children are hydronephroses or multicystic dysplastic kidneys, but these entities generally do not exhibit appreciable pyelographic visualization, whereas nephroblastomas are almost universally opacified by pyelography. The collecting system of the involved kidney or kidneys is generally markedly distorted, and frequently massively displaced. Usually the differential diagnosis lies between nephroblastoma and neuroblastoma, this question being resolved in favor of the latter if any measurement of catecholamines or their derivatives discloses elevation. Obviously, other retroperitoneal masses such as neonatal adrenal hemorrhage, cysts, duplication of the renal collecting system, or retroperitoneal teratomatous lesion must be excluded. Ultrasonography and CAT scanning may be beneficial. Arteriography is usually not undertaken because of the increased risk of such vascular studies in infants and children, although inferior vena cavography may be extremely helpful in determining the extent of disease. Needle puncture is contraindicated in children.

The primary treatment of nephroblastoma is surgical removal. These tumors, often massive in size, almost always exhibit encapsulation and are relatively easily excised as compared with neuroblastoma, which is invasive in character. Nephroblastomas should be removed even in the presence of metastases, because adjuvant therapy will be more efficacious following removal of the primary bulk of tumor. The surgical approach is transabdominal, and it is desirable to visualize the contralateral kidney, the liver, and other organs to evaluate potential metastatic dissemination.

Nephroblastoma is radiosensitive, and radiation therapy may be employed preoperatively for shrinkage of a mass of tumor or postoperatively to the tumor bed if spillage has occurred. Selective chemotherapy is highly effective in nephroblastoma, the improvement in survival of children so afflicted being one of the success stories of modern chemotherapy. The drugs of choice are actinomycin D and vincristine. The prognosis in nephroblastoma continues to improve, with approximately 80 per cent two-year disease-free survival of all patients irrespective of stage or extent of disease at diagnosis. Clearly, children with extensive metastatic disease at diagnosis have a poor prognosis, but up to 60 per cent of these children may be alive without obvious disease after two years of treatment.

It is now clear that there are other primary renal malignancies of childhood in addition to nephroblastoma and the rarely encountered adult form of renal malignancy, nephrocarcinoma. A tumor quite similar in appearance to nephroblastoma is *congenital mesoblastic nephroma* or *fetal hamartoma*, usually presenting very early in infancy, rarely metastasizing, very rarely recurring following resection, and thus offering a much better prognosis than the usual nephroblastoma.

Casper, T. E., Osborne, R. W., Jr., Semerdjian, H. S., and Miller, H. C.: Urologic abdominal masses in infants and children. J. Urol., 116:629, 1976,

D'Angio, G. J., Evans, A. E., Breslow, N., Beckwith, B., Bishop, H.,

Feigl, P., Goodwin, W., Leap, L. L., Sinks, L. F., Sutow, W., Tefft, M., and Wolff, J.: The treatment of Wilms' tumor: Results of the National Wilms' Tumor Study. Cancer, 38:633, 1976.

Ehrlich, R. M., and Goodwin, W. E.: The surgical treatment of nephroblastomas (Wilms' tumor). Cancer, 32:1145, 1973.

Glenn, J. F., and Rhame, R. C.: Wilms' tumor: Epidemiological experience. J. Urol., 85:911, 1961.

Wigger, H. J.: Fetal hamartoma of kidney: A benign, symptomatic congenital tumor, not a form of Wilms' tumor. Am. J. Clin. Pathol., 51:323, 1969.

UROTHELIAL TUMORS

Nephrocarcinoma accounts for 85 per cent of renal malignancies, nephroblastoma for 5 or 6 per cent, and the various sarcomas for about 3 per cent; 7 or 8 per cent of the malignancies of the kidney arise in the urothelium. Occasional renal pelvic tumors may be benign papillomatous lesions, but most tumors primary to the renal pelvis are papillary transitional cell carcinomas, squamous lesions, or, rarely, adenocarcinomas.

Patients with urothelial tumors, benign or malignant, usually present with hematuria, gross or microscopic. Patients are most frequently free of any other signs or symptoms of disease unless the tumor has achieved sufficient size to cause obstruction or unless sloughing of tumor leads to passage of tissue with attendant renal colic. Occasionally there may be associated urinary infection. The diagnosis is generally established by intravenous pyelography; a filling defect in the collecting system may be identified by high dose techniques, nephrotomography, and simultaneous abdominal compression for satisfactory filling of the collecting system. Frequently, however, cystoscopic and retrograde pyelographic techniques may be necessary, utilizing not only retrograde contrast material but also air insufflation for definition of suspected intrapelvic abnormality.

In contrast to tumors of the renal substance, urinary cytology may be of great benefit in the diagnosis of urothelial tumors of the upper urinary tract. Freshly voided urine specimens obtained during the day and in the normally hydrated state are preferred to overnight urine collections. Precise and specific urine collections from the involved renal pelvis may be obtained by cystoscopic methods, introducing a ureteral catheter under fluoroscopic control. Similarly, brush biopsy of a suspected lesion may be obtained with a specially designed ureteral catheter.

Histologically, tumors of the renal pelvis tend to be of a low grade of malignancy, and spread of tumor beyond the confines of the kidney or ureter is uncommon. Local invasion and lymphatic involvement, however, are encountered more commonly than are distant metastases. Urothelial tumors tend to be multifocal, occurring not only in the renal pelvis but also in the urothelium of the ureter and urinary bladder as well as the urethra. There continues to be speculation as to whether such multifocal occurrence is due to spread by "seeding" or whether the multifocal character of these lesions represents multicentric cellular abnormality with malignant degeneration, possibly caused by urinary carcinogens.

The accepted treatment of choice is nephroureterectomy, removing the kidney and the entire ipsilateral ureter as well as a cuff of bladder. Subsequent followup cystoscopic examination at regular intervals is necessary because of the tendency for further urothelial tumors to develop. However, the low grade and low stage of malignancies of the renal pelvis and ureter have prompted many surgeons to undertake conservative surgery, on occasion removing simply the tumor or a segment of renal pelvis or ureter, an obviously desirable technique if dealing with a solitary kidney. Neither radiation therapy nor chemotherapy has any demonstrated value in the management of urothelial malignancies.

The prognosis with malignancies of the urothelium of the renal pelvis and ureter depends upon the extent of disease at the time of surgery. The patients with tumor confined to the urothelium and submucosa exhibit a 90 per cent five-year survival, although this diminishes markedly with muscular invasion, periureteral fat involvement, or extension beyond the ureter. With distant metastases, five-year survival is virtually nil.

Batata, M., and Grabstald, H.: Upper urinary tract urothelial tumors. Urol. Clin. North Am., 3:79, 1976.

Brown, H. E., and Roumani, G. K.: Conservative surgical management of transitional cell carcinoma of upper urinary tract. J. Urol., 112:184, 1974.

Grabstald, H., Whitmore, W. S., and Melamed, M.: Renal pelvic tumors. JAMA, 218:845, 1971.

OTHER TUMORS

Benign cysts are the most common and the most important of the other tumors of the kidney to be considered. Cysts constitute the principal differential diagnosis in assessing renal masses, and the various uroradiographic techniques available have been summarized above. Simple cysts may be single or multiple, are most common in elderly patients, and are probably most often due to retention of urine occasioned by tubular obstruction. They may cause obstruction to the calyces or renal pelvis, and often require surgical intervention for excision or marsupialization in treatment of symptomatic obstruction or discomfort. Other cysts include congenital polycystic disease and multicystic dysplasia. Hydronephrosis, resulting from ureteropelvic junction stricture or other form of outflow obstruction, constitutes a renal tumor or mass in the true sense, but does not represent neoplasia.

Benign tumors of the kidney include such relative rarities as fibroma of the renal capsule, lipoma, rhabdomyoma, leiomyoma, neurofibroma, and myxoma. Teratomas and dermoids have been described but are most often of pararenal origin.

Hamartoma or *angiomyolipoma* of the kidney is being discovered with increased frequency, undoubtedly because of improved diagnostic techniques. It may occur as an isolated lesion in the kidney or may be seen in association with tuberous sclerosis. Hypertension has been reported in association with renal hamartoma. The angiographic diagnosis may be difficult, as neovascularity is seen, suggesting malignancy, but the identification of the relatively lucent areas of fat in these tumors will often prove to be the diagnostic key. Removal of the tumor by wedge resection of the kidney, partial nephrectomy, or total nephrectomy is generally required.

Renal adenoma continues to cause some controversy. Histologically, renal adenoma and localized nephrocarcinoma may be indistinguishable, and it has been arbitrary practice among pathologists to classify those lesions of 2 or 3 cm in diameter as adenomas. On the other hand, authorities have concluded that renal adenomas can be distinguished from early nephrocarcinoma. If a conclusive diagnosis of adenoma could be achieved, surgery might be avoided, but in most instances it is necessary to proceed with nephrectomy because of the risk of malignancy.

Recently, benign functional tumors of the kidney have been reported, including a renin-secreting juxtaglomerular cell tumor and hemangiopericytoma. The latter lesion is generally thought to be benign, but in approximately 15 per cent of cases there have been local or distant metastases. These two lesions may or may not be associated with hypertension.

Finally, it must be remembered that the kidney is not uncommonly the site of metastatic disease. It is estimated that 20 per cent of patients with carcinoma of the lung will exhibit gross or microscopic evidence of renal metastases. If metastatic carcinoma in the kidney invades the collecting system, hematuria may result and may be the first manifestation of the underlying malignancy.

Other relatively rare lesions of the kidney include the various sarcomas, lymphoblastomas, nodular infiltration of multiple myeloma, and various malignant cystic dysplasias. Cerebroretinal angiomatosis of von Hippel–Lindau is often associated with renal lesions, frequently nephrocarcinoma.

MacCallum, D. K., Conn, J. W., and Baker, B. L.: Ultrastructure of a renin-secreting juxtaglomerular cell tumor of the kidney. Invest. Urol., 11:65, 1973.

Mullin, E. M., DeVere White, R., Peterson, L. J., and Paulson, D. F.: Bilateral renal carcinomas in von Hippel–Lindau disease. Urology, 8:475, 1976.

Murphy, G. P., and Mostafi, F. K.: Histologic assessment and clinical prognosis of renal adenoma. J. Urol., 103:31, 1970.

Ravich, L., Lerman, P. H., and Drabkin, J. W.: Metastatic disease to kidney from lung. Urology, 5:239, 1975.

Seabury, J. C., Jr., Ensor, R. D., and Wolfe, W. G.: Angiomyolipoma of the kidney: A benign tumor demonstrating neovascularization by arteriography: Report of two cases. J. Urol., 98:562, 1968.

Walsh, A.: Solitary cyst of the kidney and its relationship to renal tumor. Br. J. Urol., 23:377, 1951.

PART XVI
DISEASES OF THE DIGESTIVE SYSTEM

386. INTRODUCTION

Marvin H. Sleisenger

The chapters dealing with gastroenterology in this fifteenth edition of the Textbook consolidate the format used in the fourteenth edition published four years ago. We have found that a major division of topics according to organs within the system and a minor one along pathophysiologic lines have been well received. As in the preceding editions, appropriate attention, we believe, is also paid to normal function.

Both basic science and the technology of gastroenterology have advanced since publication of the fourteenth edition. We have tried to incorporate this new knowledge into the chapters which follow. In the former, there has been feverish activity in the study of gut hormones, particularly gastrin, but cholecystokinin (CCK), secretin, glucagon, and vasoactive intestinal peptides (VIP) have also received a large share of attention, and further work on gastrointestinal peptide (GIP), pancreatic polypeptide, and substance P has appeared. In terms of clinical gastroenterology, the highlight is the reliable measurement of serum gastrin and its application to the study of peptic ulcer. Of particular note is its usefulness in the diagnosis of gastrinomas associated with virulent peptic ulcer disease, the so-called Zollinger-Ellison syndrome. Although the control mechanisms for altering rates of secretion from these tumors are not completely understood, provocative tests with intravenous calcium and secretin (which paradoxically stimulates release of gastrin from these tumors) are extremely useful in the differential diagnosis of this disease.

An integrated scheme of the roles of CCK and secretin in the control of pancreatic secretion is emerging, but the measurement of these hormones in the blood is not yet reliable; further, rises in secretin postprandially in the blood are not detectable, yet there appears much evidence that supports its historic role in stimulating the flow of pancreatic juice.

Other nonbeta islet cell tumors of the pancreas oversecrete potent hormones and polypeptides; they may cause so-called "pancreatic cholera"; watery diarrhea, hypokalemia, and achlorhydria or hypochlorhydria (WDHA syndrome) are the outstanding clinical features. VIP is the principal substance released; other substances, including calcitonin, are also released. Severe diarrhea may also be caused by medullary carcinoma of the thyroid, usually associated with neural crest tumors. Calcitonin and prostaglandin are secreted in excess by the thyroid cancer and VIP by the associated neuroblastomas. The exact mechanism for these secretory types of diarrhea is unknown, but some attribute it to increased small bowel mucosal cell cyclic AMP, as in cholera. The same type of small bowel diarrhea, predominantly involving increase in cellular cyclic AMP, is

associated with infection by other organisms, particularly enterotoxigenic *E. coli*. It is likely that a number of viruses affecting the gastrointestinal tract behave similarly.

Recent work indicates that infection may cause chronic inflammatory bowel diseases such as Crohn's disease and ulcerative colitis. Some investigations indicate that viruses may be the etiologic agents; however, much remains to be done to confirm these preliminary data.

The theories which relate several gastrointestinal diseases to the diet are yet unproved but are provocative; these include the lack of fiber in the diet in the pathogenesis of diverticulosis of the colon and cancer of the colon. Although the associated conditions of either alcoholism or biliary tract disease remain prominent in the causation of acute and chronic pancreatitis, the exact mechanism still eludes explanation.

Despite dramatic advances in the therapy of peptic ulcer disease (see below), the pathogenesis of duodenal ulcer is still unknown; the etiology and pathophysiology for the genesis of such important disturbances as "dyspepsia" and irritable bowel syndrome are not understood. In part these disorders may reflect autoimmune central nervous sytem dysfunction, or they may be due to humoral agents (e.g., prostaglandin, serotonin). Nor have we yet an acceptable biologic explanation for the two principal diseases of the liver — chronic active (viral) hepatitis and alcoholic hepatitis and cirrhosis.

It is in the area of the technology of diagnostic procedures that the most discernible recent changes in gastroenterology have been noted. I am careful to avoid the word *advances*, because the contribution of these modalities to improved care, quality of life, and increased longevity remains to be proved. Nonetheless, they are with us and they require our attention and, even more important, our careful evaluation. They are the reasons for much of the rising cost of care of patients with gastrointestinal disorders and diseases. Among these procedures are flexible endoscopy, upper (esophagus, stomach, and duodenum) and lower (colon); they are referred to as upper gastrointestinal panendoscopy and colonoscopy, respectively. Since the student and physician in training will have the opportunity to see these procedures and since the policy of these chapters is to minimize descriptions of technique, they are mentioned in discussions of differential diagnosis for a number of diseases of the upper and lower intestines. The most dramatic use of upper endoscopy is for upper gastrointestinal bleeding, and the indications and possible benefits are described. Colonoscopy is increasingly used for diagnosis of cancer and excision of adenomatous polyps.

Other techniques include those used in differential diagnosis of jaundice, with particular reference to extrahepatic obstruction. These are endoscopic retrograde cholangiopancreatography and transhepatic cholangiography. The former is a combined endoscopic-radiologic method, and the latter is essentially radiologic. Both techniques demonstrate a dilated ductal system and points of obstruction; the former procedure also is useful in diagnosis of pancreatic disease that affects the main pancreatic duct and its tributaries. A diagnosis of lesions which cause such obstruction, particularly carcinoma of the pancreas, is also abetted by the new techniques of sonography and computerized axial tomography. Although small masses in the pancreas may be detected by either of these methods, rate of resectability of these cancers for cure is little changed. The role of arteriography in gastrointestinal diseases is becoming better defined; it is useful in the diagnosis of certain causes of massive gastrointestinal bleeding, particularly arterial bleeding from upper gastrointestinal lesions and colonic diverticula. It may also be used for therapy by either perfusion with vasconstrictive substances (decreasingly used) or embolization with autologous clot or other substance (increasingly used for gastric and duodenal arterial bleeding).

The major advance in therapy in gastroenterology since the last edition has been the use of H_2 blocking agents to suppress gastric acid secretion in the management of peptic ulcer disease. These agents — analogues of histamines — are very effective in reducing acid under all conditions: basically, following meals, and after various stimulants. Their use is now widespread and is based on the demonstrated efficacy in the healing of ulcer disease during their administration. However, problems remain. Insufficient time has elapsed to assess long-term toxicity; "rebound" ulcer following cessation of therapy is reported to be frequent; and the effect of pharmacologically active agents is always somewhat blunted by the problem of patient compliance. The emergence of the H_2 blockers has led to studies which have shown the efficacy of the more conventional aluminum-magnesium antacids for the treatment of ulcer disease. During the past five years a surgical procedure, the superselective or parietal cell vagotomy, has been further evaluated in the management of duodenal ulcer disease and has been found effective and essentially without undesirable side effects. Although the recurrence rate is higher than after more conventional forms of surgical management for duodenal ulcer,

the lack of side effects and safety of the procedure make it attractive.

The place of conjugated bile acids in the therapy of gallstone disease remains to be defined. The choice of therapy for gallstone disease in the operable patient is still operation by a skilled surgeon. The use of various agents in the treatment of chronic inflammatory bowel disease has been further evaluated, and the short-term usefulness of high dose steroids for acute exacerbations of both Crohn's disease and ulcerative colitis is confirmed. Long-term drug therapy for Crohn's disease is still unsatisfactory, but low dose steroids are marginally effective, and sulfasalazine reduces the recurrence rate of exacerbations of ulcerative colitis. Total colectomy for intractable ulcerative colitis, longstanding universal ulcerative colitis, or ulcerative colitis with complications appears more attractive with improving surgical technique and the emergence of new ileostomy procedures.

Dietotherapy in gastroenterology continues to rely mostly on the elimination diets, principally gluten for childhood and adult celiac disease and mild products for lactase deficiency. Dietotherapy for duodenal ulcer appears, on the whole, to be useless, except perhaps for the elimination of coffee and smoking; whether high fiber diets are the panacea for both the prevention and the management of patients with colonic diverticula remains to be demonstrated. The question of whether high fiber in the diet will reduce the incidence of colonic cancer likewise will not be answered for years. Management of chronic liver disease remains frustrating. Although use of steroids appears to increase longevity in chronic active hepatitis, the morbidity of this illness is still high. Nothing short of abstinence from alcohol and provision of an adequate diet can be used for liver injury caused by ethanol.

Finally, a word about hyperalimentation. We have not devoted a separate discussion to it in Part XVI, but it is discussed in detail in Ch. 476.3. Its usefulness in gastroenterology is demonstrated, but it is best used on a relatively short-term basis. It is invaluable in the preparation of depleted patients for surgery, or otherwise to tide patients over periods during which normal alimentation cannot be achieved. It is also being used for limited numbers of patients for sustaining life on a home treatment basis, but such therapy will require close scrutiny for proper evaluation of hazards, over-all cost, and other factors.

Section One   DIAGNOSTIC IMAGING PROCEDURES IN GASTROENTEROLOGY

Robert N. Berk

In the past decade several innovative techniques have been introduced in radiology for the detection of diseases of the gastrointestinal tract, liver, and spleen.

Acknowledgment: I wish to express my appreciation to Robert J. Stanley, M.D., and Stuart S. Sagel, M.D., Washington University School of Medicine, St. Louis, for providing the illustrations of computerized tomography.   R.N.B.

These remarkable new procedures have extended the diagnostic capability of radiologists far beyond that which was previously possible with conventional plain abdominal radiography and barium studies. At present, the technology involved in many of these modalities is advancing so rapidly that the full potential of the various procedures and their exact role in the diagnosis of intra-abdominal diseases have not yet been determined. These techniques include abdominal ultrasonography, computerized tomography, radionuclide scanning, visceral angiography, endoscopic retrograde cholangiopancreatography, and percutaneous transhepatic cholangiography.

387. ABDOMINAL ULTRASONOGRAPHY

Ultrasonography or echography employs sound waves in the range above human hearing which are generated by a piezoelectric crystal. The sound waves are reflected from tissue interfaces depending on differences in acoustical impedance. These echoes are recorded by the same crystal that generates the waves and are displayed as a cross-sectional image in longitudinal, transverse, or oblique planes (Fig. 1). The early instruments were capable of producing images only in black and white, whereas the new gray-scale scanners display the image in eight shades of gray, which permits more accurate characterization of the ultrasonic properties of tissues and better resolution of anatomic structures. Real-time scanning devices, similar to a fluoroscope except that ultrasound is used rather than x-rays, are now available. With these instruments motion, such as vascular pulsations, can be identified and studied.

Greater skill and effort are required to produce a sonography image with maximal diagnostic information than is necessary for conventional radiography. The operator must have exact knowledge of the diagnostic problem involved and must individualize each examination. However, sonography has the major advantage of being entirely noninvasive, and the ultrasound waves have no known harmful effects. Consequently, there are no risks involved in the examination. This offers the additional advantage that serial studies can safely be performed to follow the course of an illness and the results of treatment.

Figure 2. Ultrasound scan showing a bilobulated pancreatic pseudocyst (P). Longitudinal section made to the left of the midline and viewed with the patient's head on the observer's left. K, Kidney. Note the inflammatory debris in the dependent portion of the cyst (arrow).

Since ultrasound is transmitted poorly through air, gas in the intestinal lumen interferes with an adequate examination. This may be an insurmountable problem in patients with paralytic ileus. However, since sonography is not dependent on the presence of fat to identify the abdominal viscera as are procedures that use x-rays, diagnostic examinations can still be achieved in cachectic patients in whom there is a paucity of intra-abdominal fat.

Ultrasonography of the abdomen produces an image of a cross-section of the liver, gallbladder, pancreas, spleen, and kidneys. The examination is useful in the detection of intra-abdominal masses, which may be as small as 2 cm in diameter. Furthermore, it is usually

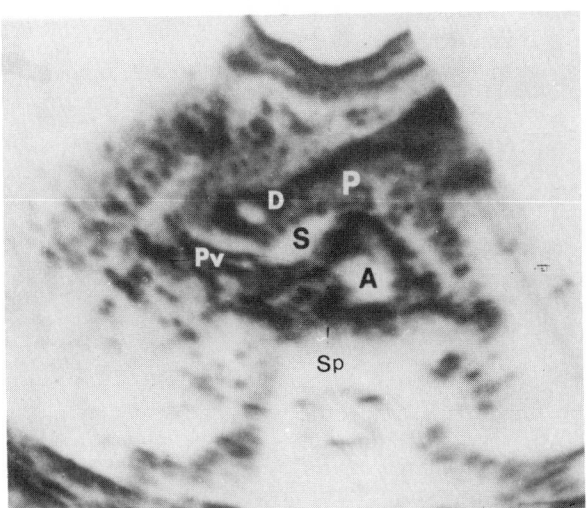

Figure 1. Normal ultrasound scan. Transverse section made at the level of the pancreas and viewed with the patient's right on the observer's left. A, Aorta; S, splenic vein; Pv, portal vein; D, common bile duct; P, pancreas; Sp, spine. A triangular portion of the right lobe of the liver is visible in front of the pancreas.

Figure 3. Ultrasound scan showing dilated bile ducts (D) in a patient with obstructive jaundice due to a gallstone. Longitudinal scan made to the right of the midline and viewed with the patient's head to the observer's left. The tubular structures are dilated bile ducts in the liver. The kidney (K) and diaphragm (arrows) are visible.

Figure 4.   Ultrasound scan showing a large aneurysm (A) of the abdominal aorta. Longitudinal scan made through the midline and viewed with the patient's head to the observer's left. The absence of internal echoes in the aneurysm and the good definition of the posterior border (arrow) indicate that it is fluid filled.

possible to distinguish between cysts and tumors. Fluid-filled structures such as cysts transmit ultrasound readily, so that there are few internal echoes and the posterior boundary of the mass is easily identified. Solid tumors transmit ultrasound poorly, internal echoes are evident, and the posterior margin of the lesion is not well defined. Consequently, ultrasonography is ideally suited for the identification of pancreatic pseudocysts, intra-abdominal abscess, and cysts of the liver and spleen (Fig. 2). Dilated bile ducts in the liver

in cases of obstructive jaundice, splenic and hepatic hematomas in patients with trauma, and aneurysms of the abdominal aorta can be visualized (Figs. 3 and 4). The gallbladder and gallstones can be recognized in patients in whom opacification of the gallbladder with cholangiography and cholecystography is impossible (Fig. 5). Solid masses such as carcinoma of the pancreas, hepatic metastases, and hepatomas can be detected. The diagnosis of pancreatitis can often be made by detecting diffuse enlargement of the pancreas. Finally, the presence of ascites can be readily established, even when only small amounts of fluid are present.

Asher, W. M., Parvin, S., Virgillo, R. W., and Haber, K.: Echographic evaluation of splenic injury after blunt trauma. Radiology, 118:411, 1976.

Doust, B. D., and Pearce, J. D.: Gray scale ultrasonic properties of the normal and inflamed pancreas. Radiology, 120:653, 1976.

Goldberg, B., Goodman, G., and Clearfield, H.: Evaluation of ascites by ultrasound. Radiology, 96:15, 1970.

Gonzales, E. K., Bradley, C. L., and Clements, J. L.: Pseudocyst formation in acute pancreatitis. Am. J. Roentgenol., 127:315, 1976.

Gosink, B. B., and Leopold, G. B.: Abdominal echography. Semin. Roentgenol., 10:299, 1975.

Leopold, G. R.: Pancreatic echography, a new dimension in the diagnosis of pseudocyst. Radiology, 104:365, 1972.

Leopold, G. R., and Asher, W. M.: Fundamentals of Abdominal and Pelvic Ultrasonography. Philadelphia, W. B. Saunders Company, 1975, pp. 217–229.

Leopold, G., Goldberger, L., and Bernstein, E.: Ultrasonic detection and evaluation of abdominal aortic aneurysms. Surgery, 72:939, 1972.

Leopold, G., and Sokoloff, J.: Ultrasonic scanning in the diagnosis of biliary disease. Surg. Clin. N. Am., 53:1043, 1973.

Maklad, N. F., Doust, B. D., and Baum, J. K.: Ultrasound diagnosis of postoperative intra-abdominal abscess. Radiology, 113:417, 1974.

Walls, W. J., Gonzales, G., Martin, N. L., and Templeton, A. W.: B scan ultrasound evaluation of the pancreas; advantages, and comparison with other techniques. Radiology, 114:127, 1975.

388.   COMPUTERIZED TOMOGRAPHY

Computerized tomography (CT) is a technique of radiography in which minor differences in x-ray absorption, not evident by conventional radiograph techniques, are made visible by computer processing of x-rays transmitted through the body. In 1969, Hounsfield originated the concept that the use of a computer would permit recovery of a large amount of information concerning soft tissues which had previously been lost because of superimposition of data and insensitivity of traditional methods of recording the radiographic image. He devised a method in which a cathode x-ray tube display of the processed information gives a gray scale image of a transverse section of the body (Fig. 6).

Anatomic definition is more precise with CT than with ultrasonography, but the equipment necessary for CT is extremely expensive, and the radiation dose is not inconsequential. Although intestinal gas does not interfere with CT scanning, absence of fat in malnourished patients impairs the quality of the CT image.

Like ultrasonography, CT is useful in the detection of hepatic metastases, cysts, and abscesses (Fig. 7). Tumors and cysts of the kidney and retroperitoneal lymphadenopathy and other masses can be identified. Pancreatitis produces diffuse enlargement of the pancreas, which is visible on the CT scan. Carcinoma of the pancreas has the same density as the normal pancreatic parenchyma, but the tumor can be recognized

Figure 5.   Ultrasound scan showing gallstones (f). Transverse section made at the level of the gallbladder and viewed with the patient's right on the observer's left. Sp, Spine. Note that the three faceted gallstones lie in the dependent portion of the gallbladder with the patient supine. The gallstones cast an acoustical shadow (A) because they transmit none of the ultrasound. The dotted line indicates intervals of 1 cm.

Figure 6. Normal computerized tomogram. Transverse section made at the level of the pancreas and viewed with the patient's right to the observer's left. A vertebra is visible posteriorly. The aorta and crura of the diaphragm are visible in front of the spine, and the kidneys (K) are evident laterally. The body and tail of the pancreas lie between the fluid-filled stomach (S) in front and the kidney posteriorly. The bile-filled gallbladder (thick arrow) lies in front of the liver. The second portion of the duodenum (thin arrow) is adjacent to the head of the pancreas.

Figure 7. Computerized tomogram in a patient with a hepatic abscess (arrow). Transverse section made at the level of the liver and viewed with the patient's right to the observer's left. The abscess is evident as a well-defined radiolucent mass in the liver (L). The spleen is also apparent (S).

Figure 8. Computerized tomogram in a patient with obstructive jaundice due to carcinoma of the pancreas. Transverse section made at the level of the pancreas and viewed with the patient's right to the observer's left. The spine and kidneys are evident posteriorly. The tubular structures are dilated (arrow), bile-filled bile ducts within the liver. There is a large mass (M) in the head of the pancreas.

Figure 9. Computerized tomogram in a diabetic patient with fatty infiltration of the liver. Transverse section made through the liver and viewed with the patient's right to the observer's left. The liver is abnormally radiolucent due to excessive fat so that the intrahepatic vascular tree is visible (arrow). The normal density of the liver is the same as that of the spleen (S).

by detecting focal enlargement of the pancreas and obliteration of adjacent fat planes (Fig. 8). At this time CT has only limited applicability in parenchymatous disease of the liver. However, nodularity in advanced cirrhosis and radiolucency in fatty infiltration of the liver can be identified (Fig. 9). CT plays a valuable role in differentiating jaundice caused by biliary obstruction from cholestasis caused by parenchymal disease. In the former, dilated bile ducts can be identified in the liver and in the porta hepatis (Fig. 8). Finally, the gallbladder can be seen on CT because of the difference in x-ray absorption between the hepatic parenchyma and bile (Fig. 6). Consequently, enlargement of the gallbladder and cholelithiasis can be identified.

In many cases, CT and ultrasonography are complementary diagnostic examinations. This is particularly true in diseases involving the liver, spleen, pancreas, and kidneys. However, the retroperitoneum is better evaluated with CT than with ultrasonography, whereas ultrasonography has advantages in the diagnosis of gallbladder disease and aneurysms of the abdominal aorta.

Alfidi, R. J., Haaga, J. R., Havilla, T. R., et al.: CT of the liver. Am. J. Roentgenol., 127:69, 1976.
Evens, R. G.: New frontiers for radiology, computed tomography. Am. J. Roentgenol., 126:1117, 1976.
Haaga, J. R., Alfidi, R. J., Zelch, M. G., et al.: Computer tomography of the pancreas. Radiology, 120:589, 1976.
Hounsfield, G. N.: Computerized transverse axial scanning (tomography). I. Description of system. Br. J. Radiol., 46:1016, 1973.
Stanley, R. J., Sagel, S. S., and Levitt, R. G.: CT of the body: early trends in application and accuracy of the method. Am. J. Roentgenol., 127:53, 1976.
Stephens, D. H., Hattery, R. R., and Sheedy, P. F.: CT of the abdomen; early experience with the EMI body scanner. Radiology, 119:331, 1976.
Stephens, D. H., Sheedy, P. F., Hattery, R. R. et al.: Computed tomography of the liver. Am. J. Roentgenol., 128:578, 1977.

389. RADIONUCLIDE IMAGING

Progressive improvements in radiopharmaceuticals and imaging devices in the past decade have resulted in increased accuracy of radionuclide imaging in the diagnosis of intra-abdominal disease. The degree of resolution of anatomic details of the nuclear medicine techniques is less than that of other radiographic procedures, but this disadvantage is offset by the lack of morbidity or mortality and the versatility of the radionuclide techniques.

Radiopharmaceuticals used for the evaluation of the liver include colloidal suspensions that undergo phagocytosis by the Kupffer cells (technetium-99m–labeled sulfur colloid) and substances that are excreted by the polygonal cells (iodine-131–labeled rose bengal). In addition, gallium-67 and indium-111-bleomycin are useful agents because of their tendency to concentrate in hepatic tumors and abscesses.

Liver scanning is useful to (1) evaluate the size, shape, and position of the liver; (2) diagnose hepatic masses such as tumors, abscesses, and hematomas; (3) estimate the extent of hepatocellular disease in such conditions as cirrhosis; and (4) determine the cause of jaundice (Figs. 10 to 12).

A major limitation in liver imaging with radionuclides is the difficulty inherent in detecting a small lesion of decreased uptake (cold spot) in a background of diffuse radioactivity in the normal tissue (Fig. 12). It is possible that in the future radiopharmaceuticals will be developed to label the abnormal tissue rather than the normal parenchyma, thereby increasing the resolution of the test. At present, lesions that are located at the periphery of the liver and those in the left lobe are more easily seen. The minimal resolution of the technique is approximately 1 cm in the left lobe and 2 cm in the right lobe. Even with the newer techniques, the over-all accuracy for detecting liver metastases is approximately 80 per cent. At present, combining radionuclide imaging with biomedical tests such as alkaline phosphatase, serum albumin, and serum glutamic oxaloacetic transaminase provides the best screening test for the detection of liver metastases.

Subphrenic abscesses are relatively easy to identify by combining liver and lung imaging in which the abscess produces a separation between the two visualized organs (Fig. 13). Gallium-67 scanning is a convenient supplement to the procedure and is particularly useful when a pleural effusion is a possible cause of the separation.

Iodine-131 rose bengal is useful to distinguish jaundice caused by hepatic parenchymal disease from that caused by obstruction of the biliary tract. In patients with high-grade obstructive disease of the biliary tract, there is increased concentration in the biliary tree and lack of excretion into the small bowel. The test is not

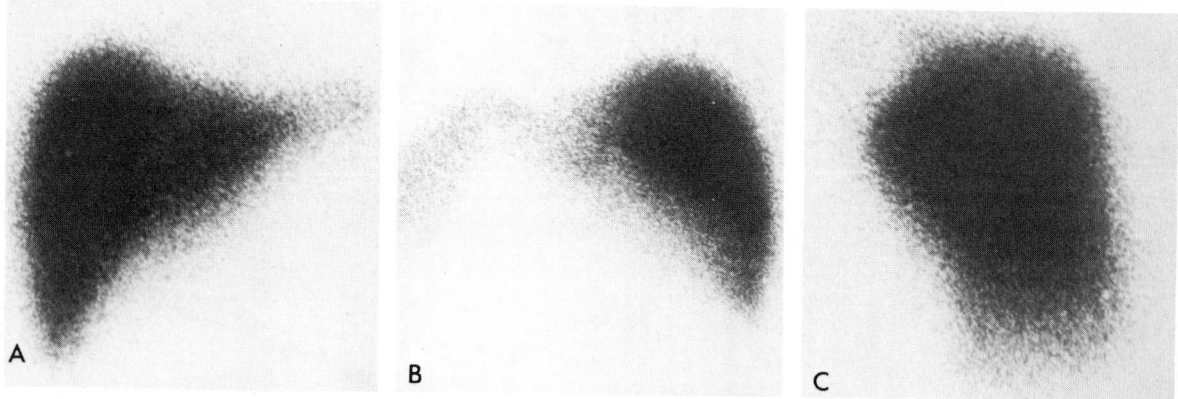

Figure 10.   Normal technetium-99m–labeled sulfur colloid radionuclide image. The normal liver is well seen. *A*, Anterior projection. *B*, Posterior projection. *C*, Right lateral projection.

Figure 11. Technetium-99m–labeled sulfur colloid radionuclide image showing a hepatoma in the right lobe of the liver. Note a mass in the right lobe of the liver and enlargement of the left lobe. *A*, Anterior projection. *B*, Posterior projection. *C*, Right lateral projection.

Figure 12. Technetium-99m–labeled sulfur colloid radionuclide image showing multiple metastases in the liver from carcinoma of the lung. Multiple "cold" areas are visible in the liver. Note also increased uptake in the bone marrow. *A*, Anterior projection. *B*, Posterior projection. *C*, Right lateral projection.

Figure 13. Combined liver-lung scan showing a subphrenic abscess. The examination was done with technetium-99m–labeled sulfur colloid and technetium-99m–labeled macroaggregated albumin. Note the separation between the right lung and the liver due to the abscess. *A*, Anterior projection. *B*, Posterior projection. *C*, Right lateral projection.

reliable in the presence of low grade obstruction. In these cases measurement of the urinary and fecal excretion of the radioisotope is a more accurate indication of biliary obstruction than the radionuclide image. Patients with parenchymal disease have generalized decreased concentration of the radiopharmaceutical in the liver.

Phagocytosis of technetium-99m–sulfur colloid by the spleen provides a valuable method for evaluating the spleen. This technique can be used to (1) determine the presence of splenomegaly, (2) detect accessory spleens, (3) diagnose a subcapsular hematoma, and (4) identify space-occupying lesions such as a cyst or tumor.

Pancreatic imaging can be done using ^{75}Se-selenomethionine. Methionine, an amino acid, localizes in the exocrine portion of the pancreas and reflects the metabolic activity of the gland. In carcinoma of the pancreas, there is decreased metabolism of methionine in the region of the tumor which produces a focal area of decreased uptake. However, wide variations in shape of the pancreas, irregular uptake of the isotope in the normal gland, and the superimposition of the liver which also concentrates the radiopharmaceutical limit the accuracy of the examination.

The affinity of technetium-99m–pertechnetate for gastric mucosa makes this radiopharmaceutical useful for the detection of Meckel's diverticula and ectopic gastric mucosa in the esophagus (Barrett's epithelium). Eighty-five per cent of symptomatic Meckel's diverticula contain functioning gastric mucosa, so the technique is useful in a high percentage of patients.

Braunstein, P., and Song, C. S.: Uses and limitations of radioisotopes in investigation of gastrointestinal diseases. Am. J. Dig. Dis., 20:53, 1975.

Freeman, L. M., and Rosenthall, L.: The role of radionuclide imaging in disease of the alimentary tract. Gastrointest. Radiol., 1:187, 1976.

Koenigsberg, J., and Freeman, L. M.: Multinuclide evaluation of hepatic mass lesions. Crit. Rev. Radiol. Nucl. Med., 113:152, 1975.

Lunia, S., Parthasarathy, K., Bakshi, S., and Bender, M. A.: Evaluation of 99mTc–sulfur colloid liver scintiscans and their usefulness in metastatic workup; review of 1424 studies. J. Nucl. Med., 16:62, 1975.

Lutsker, L., Koenigsberg, M., Meng, C., and Freeman, L. M.: The role of radionuclide imaging in spleen trauma. Radiology, 110:419, 1974.

Nagler, W., Bender, M. A., and Blau, M.: Radioisotope photoscanning of the liver. Gastroenterology, 44:36, 1963.

Rosenthall, L., Henry, J. N., Murphy, D. A., and Freeman, L. M.: Radiopertechnetate imaging of Meckel's diverticulum. Radiology, 105:371, 1972.

Winston, M. A., Guth, P., Endow, J. S., and Blahd, W. N.: Enhancement of pancreatic concentration of 75-Se-selenomethionine. J. Nucl. Med., 15:662, 1974.

390. VISCERAL ANGIOGRAPHY

Techniques for vascular catheterization, contrast materials, and radiographic equipment for visceral angiography have improved remarkably since the introduction of the Seldinger technique for the percutaneous insertion of a catheter into an artery or vein in 1953. The ability to perform subselective catheterization of intra-abdominal vessels and new methods to magnify the radiographic image have improved definition of vascular abnormalities. Procedures for interventional angiography have been devised in which selective occlusion of vessels can be accomplished through the arterial catheter for the control of gastrointestinal bleeding, preop-

Figure 14. Early arterial phase from a combined celiac and superior mesenteric artery angiogram in a patient with carcinoma of the pancreas. There is irregular encasement of the splenic (arrows) and left gastric arteries (triangle) indicative of invasion by carcinoma of the pancreas.

erative devascularization of tumors, and treatment of arteriovenous malformations. Progress in visceral angiography has led to pharmacoangiography, in which drugs are injected through the arterial catheter to enhance opacification, differentiate between normal and tumor vessels, control gastrointestinal bleeding, and treat hepatic metastases.

The introduction of ultrasonography and compu-

Figure 15. Late arterial phase from a subselective hepatic artery angiogram showing a highly vascular hepatoma of the right lobe of the liver. A large mass is apparent with abnormal vessels and pooling of contrast material. Contrast material also is visible in the pyelocalyceal structures of the right kidney.

Figure 16. Late arterial phase from a celiac artery angiogram showing a ruptured spleen. Irregular pooling of contrast material in the spleen is apparent in the upper pole with loss of the uniform sinusoidal opacification in the lacerated area.

Figure 17. Late arterial phase from a superior mesenteric artery angiogram showing pooling of contrast material in the lumen of the hepatic flexure due to hemorrhage from a colonic diverticulum (arrow). Opacification of the wall of the colon is evident, and there is faint visualization of the portal vein.

terized tomography has made it necessary to re-evaluate the role of visceral angiography in the diagnosis of tumors of the pancreas and liver. Arteriography is an invasive procedure associated with small but significant morbidity. Furthermore, the ability of angiography to detect pancreatic carcinoma in a curable stage and to differentiate it from pancreatitis has been disappointing (Fig. 14). Contrarily, angiography is obviously still a valuable tool for the diagnosis of vascular tumors of the liver such as angiomas, hemangioendotheliomas, benign hepatic adenomas, and most primary hepatomas (Fig. 15). The accuracy of angiography in the diagnosis of hepatic metastases depends on the vascularity of the metastases relative to the normal hepatic parenchyma. Metastases from hypernephromas and endocrine tumors tend to be hypervascular and are easily recognized compared to metastases from the pancreas, alimentary tract, and lung. Because of greater safety and relative simplicity, metastatic disease of the liver is best diagnosed by radionuclide scanning, ultrasonography, or computerized tomography. Angiography should be reserved for special situations in which the results of other procedures are not diagnostic.

Angiography is accurate in the diagnosis of splenic and hepatic rupture (Fig. 16). However, the introduction of peritoneal lavage for the detection of intraperitoneal bleeding has reduced the need for more complex diagnostic procedures. Nevertheless, the extent of liver injury can sometimes be evaluated more accurately by angiography than at surgery. In these cases, postoperative angiography is often indicated.

Emergency angiography is indicated for both localization and therapy in the management of patients with acute gastrointestinal bleeding (Fig. 17). Not only may bleeding sites be demonstrated by contrast medium extravasation, but also the hemorrhage may be stopped with infusions of vasoconstricting agents or by means of transcatheter vessel occlusion with blood clots and other materials. The intra-arterial infusion of vasopres-

sin is effective in controlling bleeding in 80 per cent of patients with gastric mucosal bleeding and in 60 per cent of those with bleeding duodenal ulcers. On the basis of present evidence it appears that intra-arterial infusion of vasopressin has no benefit over continuous low dose intravenous infusion of the drug in the control of bleeding from esophageal varices.

The majority of patients with massive rectal bleeding have hemorrhage from colonic diverticula, usually on the right side of the colon (Fig. 17). Following identification of the bleeding site by angiography, selective vasopressin infusion through the catheter acutely controls the hemorrhage in 90 to 95 per cent of patients.

Athanasoulis, C. A., Waltman, A. C., Novelline, R. A., Krudy, A. G., and Sniderman, K. W.: Angiography: Its contribution to the emergency management of gastrointestinal bleeding. Radiol. Clin. N. Am., 12:265, 1976.

Barr, J. W., Lakin, R. C., and Rosch, J.: Similarity of arterial and intravenous vasopressin on portal and systemic hemodynamics. Gastroenterology, 69:13, 1975.

Baum, S., Athanasoulis, C. A., and Waltman, A. C.: Gastrointestinal hemorrhage: Angiographic diagnosis and control. Adv. Surg., 7:149, 1973.

Baum, S., Rosch, J., Dotter, C.T., et al.: Selective mesenteric arterial infusions in the management of massive diverticular bleeding. N. Engl. J. Med., 288:1269, 1973.

Berk, R. N., and Wholey, M. H.: The application of splenic arteriography in the diagnosis of rupture of the spleen. Am. J. Roentgenol., 104:662, 1968.

Bookstein, J. J., Cholsta, E. M., Foley, D., et al.: Transcatheter hemostasis of gastrointestinal bleeding using modified autogenous clot. Radiology, 113:277, 1974.

Goldstein, H. M., Thaggard, A., Wallace, S., and Neiman, H. L.: Proscoline-augmented hepatic angiography. Radiology, 119:275, 1976.

Goldstein, H. M., Wallace, S., Anderson, J. H., Bree, R. L., and Gianturco, C.: Transcatheter occlusion of abdominal tumors. Radiology, 120:539, 1976.

Redman, H. C., Reuter, S. R., and Bookstein, J. J.: Angiography in abdominal trauma. Ann. Surg., 169:57, 1969.

Reuter, S. R., and Redman, H. C.: Gastrointestinal Angiography. Philadelphia, W. B. Saunders Company, 1972.

Wallace, S., Gainturco, C., Anderson, J. H., Goldstein, H. M., Davis, L. J., and Breem, R. L.: Therapeutic vascular occlusion utilizing steel coiled techniques. Am. J. Roentgenol., 127:381, 1976.

Figure 18. Normal endoscopic retrograde cholangiogram. The gallbladder, cystic duct, common hepatic duct, and common bile duct are visible. Note the endoscope with the tip positioned opposite the papilla of Vater. A catheter (arrow) has been inserted into the papilla of Vater under direct vision.

391.   ENDOSCOPIC RETROGRADE CHOLANGIO-PANCREATOGRAPHY

Endoscopic retrograde cholangiopancreatography (ERCP) is a new diagnostic modality which has been made possible by the development of the fiberoptic endoscope. With this instrument it is possible to insert a small catheter into either the common bile duct or the pancreatic duct through the papilla of Vater under direct vision. Radiographic contrast material can then be injected through the catheter under fluoroscopic control to opacify the biliary tree and/or the pancreatic duct (Fig. 18). Consequently, radiographic opacification of the biliary tree is possible when impaired liver function or common duct obstruction precludes successful opacification with oral cholecystography or intravenous cholangiography.

Complications associated with ERCP consist of pancreatitis and cholangitis and occur in less than 3 per cent of patients. The difficulty with the technique is that it requires an experienced endoscopist to cannulate the ducts successfully. Even in expert hands this may sometimes require several hours to accomplish. Most authors report a success rate of cannulating the relevant duct in 70 to 80 per cent of cases once the endoscopist has become experienced with the procedure.

Indications for ERCP include patients in whom biliary tract disease is suspected but not established by clinical laboratory or other radiographic techniques, patients in whom carcinoma of the pancreas is suspected, and those with chronic pancreatitis who are potential candidates for pancreatic surgery (Figs. 19 to 21). The procedure should not be performed in the presence of acute pancreatitis, positive hepatitis B antigen, recent myocardial infarction, or acute abdomen, or when the patient is uncooperative.

Carcinoma of the pancreas causes stenosis, occlusion, displacement, or serration of the pancreatic duct (Fig.

Figure 19. Endoscopic retrograde cholangiopancreatogram showing gallstones and a stricture (arrow) of the common bile duct. The patient had a previous cholecystectomy. Note the cystic duct remnant (arrow), mild dilatation of the common dile duct, and the normal pancreatic duct (curved arrow). The endoscope had been removed prior to the radiograph.

20). With chronic pancreatitis, the pancreatic duct may be irregularly dilated and intraductal calculi may be present. Extravasation of the contrast material may occur in patients with pancreatic pseudocysts or pancreatic ascites. Differentiation between pancreatitis and carcinoma of the pancreas is difficult, and the diagnosis of carcinoma is rarely made at a curable stage. The most important application of ERCP is to establish the

Figure 20. Endoscopic retrograde cholangiopancreatogram showing obstruction of the common bile duct due to bile duct carcinoma. Note the irregular obstruction of the common bile duct at the site of the tumor (broad arrow). The pancreatic duct is normal (thin arrow). The endoscope is visible with the tip positioned opposite the papilla of Vater.

Figure 21. Endoscopic retrograde cholangiopancreatogram showing narrowing of the common bile duct and irregular dilatation of the pancreatic duct due to chronic pancreatitis. Contrast material is present in a duodenal diverticulum (D) and in the fourth portion of the duodenum. Note saccular dilatation of the branches of the pancreatic duct and the smooth tapered appearance of the common bile duct (arrows).

Figure 22. Fine needle percutaneous transhepatic cholangiogram in a jaundiced patient showing marked dilatation of the biliary tree due to an obstructing gallstone in the common bile duct (arrowhead). The cystic duct (arrows) and intrahepatic ducts are dilated. The gallbladder is not filled.

presence, location, and cause of extrahepatic biliary tract obstruction. An obstructing gallstone may be visible in the common bile duct, or the duct may be occluded by carcinoma of the pancreas (Figs. 19 and 20). In either case, the procedure provides important information for the surgeon prior to operation.

Bilboa, M. K., Dotter, C. T., and Lee, T. G.: Complications of endoscopic retrograde cholangiopancreatography; a study of 10,000 cases. Gastroenterology, 70:314, 1976.

Blumgart, L. H., Cotton, P. B., Bruwood, R., et al.: Endoscopy and retrograde cholangiopancreatography. Gut, 13:1014, 1972.

Blumgart, L. H., Salmon, P. R., and Cotton, P. B.: Endoscopy and cholangiopancreatography in the diagnosis of patients with jaundice. Surg. Gynecol. Obstet., 138:565, 1974.

Cotton, P. B., and Blumgart, L. H.: Cannulation of the papilla of Vater via the fiberduodenoscope. Lancet, 1:53, 1972.

Kasugai, T., and Kuno, N.: Endoscopic pancreatocholangiography. I. The normal endoscopic pancreatocholangiogram. Gastroenterology, 63:116, 1972.

Loeb, P. M., Wheeler, H. O., and Berk, R. N.: Endoscopic retrograde cholangiopancreatography in the diagnosis of biliary tract disease. Surg. Clin. N. Am., 53:359, 1974.

Oi, I.: Fiberduodenoscopy and endoscopic pancreatography. Gastrointest. Endosc., 18:149, 1972.

Paul, R. E.: Endoscopic retrograde cholangiography. Semin. Roentgenol. 11:223, 1976.

Rohrman, C. A., Silvis, S., and Vennes, J.: Evaluation of the endoscopic pancreatogram. Radiology, 113:297, 1974.

Silvis, S., Rohrman, C. A., and Vennes, J.: Diagnostic accuracy of endoscopic retrograde cholangiopancreatography in hepatic, biliary and pancreatic malignancy. Ann. Intern. Med., 84:438, 1976.

392. PERCUTANEOUS TRANSHEPATIC CHOLANGIOGRAPHY

The introduction of the fine needle technique for percutaneous transhepatic cholangiography has made it possible to opacify the biliary tree safely in a high percentage of patients regardless of obstruction of the bile ducts. Consequently, the procedure is an important new tool for the evaluation of patients with jaundice in whom radiographic opacification of the biliary tree is not possible by oral cholecystography or intravenous cholangiography.

A flexible, 23-gauge needle with an outer diameter of 0.7 mm, 15 cm in length, is inserted into the liver percutaneously from the right midaxillary line. The tip of the needle is positioned in the hepatic parenchyma to the right of the twelfth thoracic vertebra under fluoroscopic guidance. Radiographic contrast material is injected slowly as the needle is withdrawn. Recognition of the site of contrast material deposition is readily made fluoroscopically. Contrast material in the hepatic parenchyma persists; contrast material in hepatic or portal venous radicles flows away rapidly; whereas contrast material in the bile ducts persists and moves slowly toward the porta hepatis. Insertion of the needle can safely be repeated several times if the bile ducts are not visualized on the initial trial. When the bile ducts are identified, contrast material is injected in sufficient quantities to fill the biliary tree and multiple radiographs are made.

Because the needle has an external diameter of only 0.7 mm, only a small hole is made in the liver capsule. In addition, the substance of the right lobe of the liver is used to tamponade any bile leakage from the bile ducts or bleeding from the portal or hepatic veins. Consequently, complications are rare and usually mild. Bacteremia with transient fever has been reported in 7 to 10 per cent and can be controlled with antimicrobial

Figure 24. Fine needle transhepatic percutaneous cholangio-gram in a jaundiced patient showing obstruction of the common bile duct due to carcinoma of the pancreas. Note the marked dilatation of the bile duct with the abrupt tapering at the point of obstruction (arrow).

Figure 23. Fine needle transhepatic percutaneous cholangio-gram in a jaundiced patient showing marked narrowing and displacement of the common bile duct (arrows) due to a large pseudocyst in the head of the pancreas. Marked dilatation of the intrahepatic bile ducts is evident. Contrast material is visible in the renal pelvis.

agents given systemically. Bile peritonitis or intraperi-toneal hemorrhage occurs in less than 2 per cent. Be-cause of the safety of the fine needle technique, imme-diate surgery following the procedure is unnecessary even when bile duct obstruction is present.

With the fine needle technique the success rate of opacifying the biliary tree is 100 per cent in patients with bile duct dilatation and between 60 and 80 per cent when the bile ducts are normal. The skill required

of the operator is modest compared to that necessary to perform retrograde endoscopic cholangiography. The time required to perform percutaneous cholangiography and the cost are considerably less.

Percutaneous cholangiography permits the differen-tiation of jaundice caused by obstruction of the bile duct from that caused by parenchymal disease and pro-vides valuable information for the surgeon concerning the cause, location, and extent of the biliary obstruction prior to surgery (Figs. 22 to 24).

Ferrucci, J. T., Wittenberg, J., Sarno, R. A., and Dreyfuss, J. R.: Fine needle transhepatic cholangiography: A new approach to obstruc-tive jaundice. Am. J. Roentgenol., 127:403, 1976.
Okuda, K., Tanikawa, K., Emura, T., et al.: Nonsurgical percutaneous transhepatic cholangiography; diagnostic significance in medical problems of the liver. Am. J. Dig. Dis., 19:21, 1974.
Redeker, A. G., Karvountzis, G. G., Richman, R. H., et al.: Percutane-ous transhepatic cholangiography: An improved technique. JAMA, 231:386, 1975.

Section Two DISORDERS OF MOTILITY

Marvin M. Schuster

393. NORMAL PHYSIOLOGY OF MOTOR ACTIVITY

Gastrointestinal motility is best understood not as a primary activity but as subserving the functions of the gastrointestinal tract and particularly its individual segments. Generally gastrointestinal function involves the absorption of fluid, nutrients, electrolytes, and trace metals. Motor action of the gastrointestinal tract assists these functions by presenting ingested material in a controlled manner to the various segments of the gastrointestinal tract for appropriate mixing, liquefaction, digestion, and absorption. Various areas of the gastrointestinal tract are separated into functional segments by sphincters. Each segment has a different type of motility to subserve its particular function. This variety of motor function in the different regions is reflected in a striking histologic, electrical, and motor diversity of smooth muscle in the different segments.

The esophagus serves solely as a conduit for transit of material from the oropharynx to the stomach. Its motor activity is peristaltic, resulting in immediate forward propulsion of material presented to it. The stomach, which serves to mix food and store it temporarily, has a complex motor activity which holds, grinds, and mixes material, thus subserving this function. The to and fro pendular movements and segmental contractions of the small intestine act to slow the forward progress of chyme and to facilitate its mixing with intestinal enzymes, while at the same time prolonging contact with the mucosal surface for improved absorption. The colon functions to dehydrate its contents and to store them until evacuation becomes socially convenient. The peristaltic activity which characterizes the esophagus and which automatically and efficiently propels material forward is rarely or never seen in the colon in its normal state, and indeed such activity would prove socially disastrous.

GASTROINTESTINAL SPHINCTERS. The sphincters which separate these segments also have specific properties which differ from each other, depending upon their individual function. Some features, however, are characteristic of all gastrointestinal sphincters. Sphincters have a resting pressure which is higher than the adjacent intestine on either side, and which therefore acts as a barrier to movement from either direction. Sphincters are characterized also by the fact that they relax in response to an appropriate stimulus, which is usually distention by intraluminal contents proximal to the sphincter. Some sphincters also assist in preserving a unidirectional flow from one segment to another by contracting in response to distention distal to the sphincter. This contraction provides a barrier which prevents reflux of material into the segment proximal to the sphincter.

In addition to generally shared characteristics, each smooth muscle sphincter has unique features which fulfill its specific function. The lower esophageal sphincter has the physiologic characteristics of a sphincter but eludes anatomic detection. The pylorus, with its concentrated bundle of circular muscle, has the anatomic configuration of a sphincter and some physiologic characteristics of a sphincter. The ileocecal sphincter has the appearance of a valve but behaves like a sphincter. The internal anal sphincter has both the anatomic and physiologic characteristics of a sphincter.

The upper esophageal (cricopharyngeal) sphincter helps separate the alimentary from the respiratory system because it normally is closed, except during swallowing. It prevents air from being aspirated into the esophagus during inspiration when intrathoracic pressure is negative and intraesophageal pressures are diminished. It also allows positive (peristaltic) pressures to develop within the esophagus during swallowing by occluding the upper esophagus to prevent exposure to ambient pressure. The lower esophageal sphincter prevents reflux of gastric acid contents from the stomach into the esophagus. The pylorus separates the stomach from the small intestine, allowing the stomach to mix food and propel only small amounts of the mixture in spurts into the intestine, while preventing reflux of alkaline bilious material from the duodenum into the stomach. The ileocecal sphincter serves as a barrier to prevent reflux into the ileum of colonic contents, which are putrefactive and heavily colonized by bacteria, and may also control ileal emptying. The anal sphincters prevent incontinence and assist with defecation.

ELECTRICAL CONTROL MECHANISMS FOR INTESTINAL MOTILITY. Smooth muscle electrical activity (myoelectric activity) controls contractile activity. A basic electric rhythm consisting of sinusoidal slow waves can be recorded from normal smooth muscle from the gastrointestinal tract. The slow wave is usually generated in the longitudinal muscle and spreads to the circular layer, although there is some dispute concerning this in the colon. Muscle contractions appear to be associated with rapid spike potentials that are superimposed on the slow wave. The maximal frequency of muscle contractions is determined by the frequency of slow waves for a particular area. A number of pacemaker sites exist throughout the alimentary tract, generating slow wave activity. Some known sites are the posterior stomach near the antrum, the duodenum, multiple areas along the small intestine, and a few areas within the colon, including one at the hepatic flexure. There is a decreasing gradient of slow wave frequency down the intestine which results in more rapid transit occurring in the proximal intestine than the distal.

NEURAL REGULATORY MECHANISMS. Intestinal motility is regulated by a number of factors, including intrinsic and extrinsic nerves derived from the sympathetic and parasympathetic outflow, osmoreceptors sensitive to the osmolarity of intraluminal contents, and gastrointestinal hormones. The cholinergic nervous system is dominant in the upper gastrointestinal tract and becomes less significant in the lower where the adrenergic system becomes more important.

HORMONAL CONTROL OF GASTROINTESTINAL MOTILITY. A number of gastrointestinal hormones are known to alter gastrointestinal motility. Gastrin stimulates nonsphincteric smooth muscle, increasing the force and frequency of contractions in the gastric antrum. It also causes contraction of the lower esophageal sphincter. Cholecystokinin (pancreozymin) stimulates the gallbladder to contract and also, at least in patients with the irritable bowel syndrome, the distal colon. A duodenal hormone, motilin, has a strong stimulating effect on the upper gastrointestinal tract. Among the known hormones which inhibit intestinal movements are secretin, glucagon, and gastric inhibitory polypeptide.

In malignant carcinoid, serotonin directly stimulates the smooth muscle of the small intestine but inhibits activity in the stomach and colon, which may in part account for the diarrhea associated with this syndrome.

394. RELATION OF SYMPTOMS TO DISORDERED MOTOR ACTIVITY

Many symptoms of gastrointestinal dysfunction are associated with motor disorders resulting from exaggeration, inhibition, or distortion of normal motor activity. Among these symptoms are pain, vomiting, dysphagia, regurgitation, bloating, diarrhea, constipation, and incontinence. "Functional" gastrointestinal disorders are the most common type encountered and, for the most part, are manifested by a motility disturbance without demonstrable organic basis or disease. Diffuse esophageal spasm and irritable bowel syndrome are examples. Symptoms often are triggered by stress and anxiety.

On the other hand, motor disturbances may be secondary to an underlying primary disorder. Reflux of acid from the stomach into the esophagus can produce esophagitis and, as a result, diffuse esophageal spasm. The abnormal innervation in achalasia of the esophagus and in aganglionic megacolon (Hirschsprung's disease) may be the direct cause of abnormal motility. Similarly, symptoms may result from motor abnormalities of the intestinal muscle itself (as in diffuse esophageal spasm, achalasia, and irritable bowel syndrome), or from motor abnormality of sphincters, as when reflux esophagitis occurs because of an incompetent lower esophageal sphincter or when incontinence occurs because of an incompetent anal sphincter.

Among the methods for studying intestinal motility, manometric techniques are the most sensitive but not always the most useful. These techniques measure pressures within the lumen of the intestine and the sphincter, and can measure pressure changes induced by contractions and relaxations of intestinal muscles or sphincters. Cineradiographic studies, using barium to outline the intestine, alone or in conjunction with manometric studies, have been useful in detecting disorders of gastrointestinal motility and in pointing toward causative mechanisms.

Recently electrical activity (myoelectric activity) has been recorded from intestinal smooth muscle, and this infant science is beginning to clarify some control mechanisms for gastrointestinal motility. In some instances correlations have been made between disordered myoelectric activity and intestinal disorders such as postgastrectomy syndromes and irritable bowel syndrome.

395. PATHOPHYSIOLOGY AND CARDINAL SYMPTOMS OF DISORDERED MOTILITY

Cardinal symptoms of disordered motility will be discussed as a unit rather than in sections specific to a particular intestinal segment, because they may represent a manifestation of motor disturbance in more than one area of the gastrointestinal tract or they may even derive from an extraintestinal disorder. For example, vomiting may occur because of psychologic factors or diseases involving the central nervous system, labyrinth, esophagus, stomach, duodenum, small or large intestine, or ingested toxins. Diarrhea can result from psychologic factors or from disease of the biliary system, pancreas, stomach, or small or large intestine.

395.1. PAIN

Three major types of abdominal pain are recognized: visceral, parietal, and referred. True *visceral pain* is usually due to disordered motor activity, as in the case of diffuse esophageal spasm, irritable bowel syndrome, intestinal obstruction, or biliary tract obstruction. The area in which visceral pain is experienced depends upon the intestinal segment involved. Esophageal pain is generally felt in the subxiphoid area. It is characterized as a squeezing tightness or as heartburn. When spasm is sufficiently pronounced and prolonged, there may be accompanying dysphagia.

Stomach pain is generally localized in the left hypochondrium and duodenal pain in the subxiphoid area or immediately to the right of it. An additional clue to duodenal involvement is tenderness on palpation over this area. Small bowel pain is poorly localized and is generally felt diffusely in the periumbilical region. Pain originating in the colon is experienced roughly at the area in which the involved colonic segment lies. This is true of the terminal ileum also, but whether this is because of its contiguity with colonic mesentery is unknown. Gallbladder pain is usually felt in the right upper quadrant, whereas pancreatic pain is felt more often in the lumbar region. Often visceral pain is crampy as opposed to parietal pain, which is more constant.

Parietal pain derives from inflammation of the parietal peritoneum. Any slight movement of the peritoneum may aggravate it. For this reason patients with peritonitis tend to lie perfectly still and are sensitive to any movement which jiggles the peritoneum. The test for rebound tenderness is an example of such a movement. In contrast, the person with true visceral pain frequently writhes, attempting to find a more comfortable position.

Pain may be *referred* from visceral organs or parietal surfaces by direct involvement of afferent nerve roots. Referral is along dermatome routes which share afferent neurons from distant sites. Referred pain may be felt in the skin or deeper tissues. Esophageal pain, when severe, may radiate to the neck or arms, or to the spine. Posterior radiation of duodenal ulcer pain usually represents penetration of the ulcer into the pancreas, rather than referral of pain along nerve routes. Gallbladder pain is referred classically to the intrascapular region. Pain from the distal colon may refer to the lumbar spine. The site of origin of pain can be inferred if compression over this site augments the pain both locally and at the referred site. The reverse is generally not true; compression over the referred point does not augment the pain at the original site. Hyperesthesia may be present over the involved dermatome.

IMPORTANT HISTORICAL FEATURES. In evaluating the diagnostic significance and therapeutic implications of pain, a number of historical features are important. (1) *Localization* (see above). (2) *Character* of the pain. Visceral pain resulting from disordered motor function is usually crampy except when ileus ensues, in which case the pain becomes constant. A gnawing distress that is different from pain is characteristic of peptic ulcer. (3) *Intensity* of pain. Pain from perforation of a viscus may be excruciating, as are gallbladder pain and the pain of pancreatitis. The more severe the pain, the more likely it is to be referred. (4) *Associated circumstances* (including precipitating and alleviating factors). Aggravation by anxiety and tension points to functional disorders such as irritable bowel syndrome and functional upper gastrointestinal disease. Relief by meals implies peptic ulcer, whereas aggravation by meals suggests an obstructive component or gastritis. Association with drugs such as aspirin, alcohol, phenylbutazone, or reserpine suggests gastric and duodenal inflammation or ulceration. Diffuse abdominal pain appearing 20 minutes to an hour after meals suggests the possibility of intestinal angina. Aggravation by positional factors such as bending or straining is noted in gastroesophageal reflux. History of previous ulcer operations may suggest dumping syndrome, afferent loop syndrome, or adhesions. (5) *Duration and frequency* of pain. Severe acute pain persisting for more than six hours often implies catastrophic events such as perforation, obstruction, or strangulation which require surgery. On the other hand, recurrent pain appearing one hour postprandially when the stomach is empty is a classic sign of peptic ulcer.

Biliary pain becomes progressively more intense with time but can be alleviated abruptly if a stone is passed, leaving a dull aching sensation in the right upper quadrant.

PHYSICAL EXAMINATION. The general physical appearance may indicate shock with perforated viscus, peritonitis, or strangulation. Auscultation may reveal evidence of ileus with absent bowel sounds in inflammatory conditions, or hyperperistalsis when obstruction is present. Bruits may suggest aneurysms or ischemic lesions. Palpation may reveal rigidity or extreme guarding and rebound tenderness when there is parietal involvement either directly or from perforation, strangulation, or obstruction. Distention of the capsule of the liver may produce diffuse right upper quadrant tenderness, which is aggravated when deep inspiration brings the liver and gallbladder against the examining finger. Gallbladder disease is more localized, and a distended viscus may be felt. Terminal ileal inflammation may reveal itself as a tender mass in the right lower quadrant, whereas in diverticular disease and irritable bowel syndrome a cord-like tender sigmoid may be felt in the left lower quadrant. Rectal and pelvic examination are mandatory and may help localize the tenderness as well as associated masses.

OTHER TESTS. In addition to the routine tests, special studies involving liver function and serum amylase are often indicated. Plain and upright films of the abdomen are often helpful in demonstrating areas of ileus or obstruction. Barium contrast x-rays are ordered as indicated for the specific area, and cine-esophagram may be helpful in detecting esophageal spasm. Cholecystography may demonstrate stones or nonvisualization of the gallbladder. Manometric studies of the esophagus and colon may reveal esophageal or colonic spasm. Endoscopic studies, including retrograde pancreatic cannulation, can detect inflammation as well as masses. Gallbladder motor activity can be evaluated by using intravenous cholecystokinin to contract the gallbladder.

395.2.   VOMITING

Vomiting, the forceful expulsion of stomach contents through the esophagus and mouth, occurs in three stages, each of which is characterized by a different type of gastrointestinal motor activity.

Nausea: Except with central nervous system lesions, nausea usually appears first as a premonitory symptom. The stomach becomes atonic, and duodenal tone increases. Duodenal contents may reflux into the stomach. These motor features are not essential for nausea, and they may be absent. A variety of stimuli, including psychic, central nervous system, labyrinthine, and visceral factors, may produce nausea.

Retching: During this stage gastric compression results from increased intra-abdominal pressure, spasmodic glottal closure, respiratory inspiration, forceful descent of the diaphragm, and contraction of extra-abdominal musculature, all of which increase intra-abdominal pressure at the same time that the distal stomach contracts and the proximal stomach relaxes.

Vomiting: During this stage the cardia becomes elevated, straightening out the esophagogastric junction, and the lower esophageal sphincter relaxes, permitting expulsion by the increased abdominal pressure of gastric contents into the relaxed esophagus. Aspiration of gastric contents is prevented by closure of the glottis.

CLINICAL TYPES OF VOMITING AND THEIR CHARACTERISTICS. Psychogenic vomiting typically occurs under tension and may have a regular pattern appearing early in the morning before school or prior to stressful tasks. Such vomiting, despite prolonged chronicity, produces no ill effects. Pernicious vomiting in anorexia nervosa usually occurs in young women with marked weight loss, amenorrhea antedating the weight loss, and secondary endocrine disturbances (see Ch. 475).

Irritative phenomena such as gastritis may be associated with nausea and vomiting which, like obstructive vomiting, tends to occur after meals. Emesis preceded by early satiety and a sense of fullness may indicate partial or complete obstruction. Frequently the vomitus consists of the undigested meal. Vomiting without antecedent nausea suggests central nervous system lesions and, in this instance, may be projectile in character. Fecal emesis implies a distal obstructing lesion in the ileum or large bowel. Gastric outlet obstruction caused by functional spasm or scarring from peptic ulceration may lead to postprandial vomiting, as may diabetic gastric atony or certain food allergies and drugs of many types, including digitalis. Early morning vomiting is seen in pregnancy, in metabolic states such as uremia, and in chronic alcoholism. Postprandial bilious vomiting preceded by borborygmus in a patient with a Billroth II operation is suggestive of the afferent loop syndrome. Vomiting of epidemic proportions may imply food toxins if a common food has been ingested within six hours of appearance of symptoms and the patients are afebrile. Infections also may affect large populations and are sometimes associated with headaches, myalgias, and fevers. Vomiting from motion sickness is usually preceded by a sense of extreme discomfort, nausea, lethargy, perspiration, and diminished desire to communicate. Vomiting can also be associated with Meniere's disease, migraine headaches, and endocrine disorders, including Addison's disease.

METABOLIC COMPLICATIONS OF VOMITING. The most common metabolic picture seen with prolonged vomiting is metabolic alkalosis associated with loss of potassium, chloride, and hydrogen ions in the vomitus. The hypokalemic syndrome consists of muscle weakness, constipation, polydipsia, nocturia, and decreased urinary concentration.

ESOPHAGOGASTRIC TRAUMA. Retching, especially with liquid material in the stomach, may induce forceful tears at the esophagogastric junction. Mucosal tears which bleed are known as the *Mallory-Weiss syndrome*, and esophageal perforations are recognized as *Boerhaave's syndrome*.

ASPIRATION PNEUMONITIS. Aspiration of gastric contents occurs more often in recumbent individuals who are elderly, are debilitated, or have neurologic impairment or diminished consciousness from trauma, drugs, or alcohol.

TREATMENT. Electrolyte imbalance should be corrected and the underlying cause treated whenever this is known. Symptomatic therapy includes medications, such as Dramamine, Bonamine, or Thorazine, which appear to act on several areas, including the chemoreceptor, whereas Tigan acts strictly on chemoreceptor zone. Compazine seems to be more effective than many of the other medications but carries with it the dangers of producing extrapyramidal side effects with doses higher than 40 mg a day, and therefore it should be used with caution.

395.3.   DISORDERS OF SWALLOWING

NORMAL SWALLOWING. Swallowing is voluntarily initiated under normal circumstances but can be triggered by stimulation of many areas in the mouth and pharynx. The act is customarily divided into oral, pharyngeal, and esophageal phases. Once initiated, whether voluntarily or reflexly, a series of autonomic reflexes ensues which propels the bolus through the esophagus and into the stomach (Fig. 1).

Figure 1. A composite of electromanometric recordings, showing simultaneous pressure changes throughout pharynx and esophagus during a single swallow. Read from left to right; interval between vertical lines = 1 second. P-E Sphincter = pharyngoesophageal sphincter. E-G Sphincter = esophagogastric sphincter or lower esophageal sphincter. (Adapted from Code, C. F.: An Atlas of Esophageal Motility in Health and Disease. Springfield, Ill., Charles C Thomas, 1958.)

During the initial phase of swallowing the tongue is elevated against the hard palate, propelling the bolus into the pharynx. Aspiration into respiratory passages is prevented by closure of the soft palate, glottis, and epiglottis. Pharyngeal muscle contraction is accompanied by synchronous relaxation of the cricopharyngeus (upper esophageal constrictor muscle), establishing a pressure gradient which propels the material into the upper esophagus. These two phases of swallowing, oral and pharyngeal, take place in less than a second. A peristaltic wave sweeps material down the esophagus, traversing the lower esophageal sphincter, which has relaxed, permitting material to enter the stomach. These reflexes are controlled by the fifth, seventh, ninth, tenth, and eleventh cranial nerves, which innervate the striated oropharynx and upper third of the esophagus as well as the smooth muscle comprising the lower two thirds of the esophagus. Motor innervation of the smooth muscle portion of the esophagus is cholinergic. Afferent visceral pain fibers course through sympathetic nerves.

Two normal types and one abnormal type of esophageal contraction are recognized. Primary peristalsis is initiated by deglutition as described above. Secondary peristalsis is similar to primary peristalsis but is initiated by local distention within the lumen of the esophagus, as for example under experimental conditions with balloon distention of the esophagus, or physiologically when bolus transit is delayed by obstructing lesions or spasm or when material is refluxed from the stomach into the esophagus. Tertiary esophageal contractions represent diffuse small purposeless contractions which are nonpropulsive. A fourth type of activity, diffuse esophageal spasm, will be described later.

The lower esophageal sphincter is under both neural and hormonal control, with the rapid responses being neurogenic. Motor stimulation is effected by both cholinergic and alpha-adrenergic innervation and motor inhibition by beta-adrenergic and nonadrenergic inhibitory fibers. *Gastrin* increases the contraction of lower esophageal sphincter by its action on postganglionic cholinergic nerves, and this effect is antagonized by secretin, cholecystokinin, and glucagon. Gastrin exerts its effect whether administered exogenously or induced endogenously by physiologic stimuli such as antral distention or alkalinization of gastric contents. Conversely, increase in intragastric acidity results in inhibition of gastrin release and diminution in lower esophageal sphincter contraction.

DYSPHAGIA. Dysphagia connotes difficulty in swallowing and is usually described as a sensation of food sticking in the esophagus. The point at which dysphagia is sensed may be at the level of obstruction, whether functional or mechanical, or may be referred to an area higher in the esophagus, never lower. Pain is not a characteristic of dysphagia. Pain occurring with swallowing is termed *odynophagia,* and is indicative of esophagitis from any cause. It is almost invariably experienced with monilial esophagitis.

True dysphagia, which always signifies organic disease, must be differentiated from *globus hystericus,* which is described as the feeling that there is a lump in the throat. There is no sensation or objective evidence of delay in transit of a swallowed bolus. Globus hystericus is considered to be a neurotic symptom without organic basis and is associated with anxiety and hysterical personality features.

Dysphagia may be due to a motor disorder or mechanical obstruction. The former is characterized by difficulty with both liquids and solids, whereas the latter begins characteristically with solids and, as the lumen is progressively compromised, there is increasing difficulty with soft and eventually liquid foods. Sudden onset of dysphagia may occur with obstructing lesions from a bolus of poorly chewed food.

PYROSIS (HEARTBURN). Pyrosis or heartburn consists of a substernal burning sensation which, when particularly severe, may be referred upward into the neck or posteriorly into the back. This symptom is usually due to esophagitis from reflux of gastric juice.

ERUCTATION (BELCHING). Belching refers to the retropulsion of air either from the esophagus or from the stomach through the esophagus. It is frequently a symptom of aerophagia (air swallowing) seen in intense, anxious individuals.

REGURGITATION. Regurgitation, like vomiting, involves the propulsion of material from the stomach into the mouth, but is distinguished from vomiting by the absence of nausea and by the small quantities of ejected material. Regurgitation from the stomach is often seen with gastroesophageal sphincter incompetence, especially if there is associated gastric outlet obstruction due to functional pylorospasm or constricting lesions. Regurgitation of acid peptic gastric contents is the usual mechanism for production of heartburn. Regurgitation of esophageal contents may occur from esophageal spasm, diverticula, or obstructive lesions of the esophagus such as strictures and tumors.

RUMINATION. The term rumination is derived from the habit that ruminant (cud-chewing) animals demonstrate of regurgitating food from the rumen (upper stomach) into the mouth, chewing it again and reswallowing it. This is an unusual symptom in humans. Generally one mouthful of material is regurgitated at a time into the mouth and then swallowed again. The symptoms generally occur shortly after meals, although a few patients can ruminate at will. The cause of the symptom is unknown, although it has been reported in neurotic individuals and also in starving populations. For many it is embarrassing socially and difficult to control. It is possible that sharp, perhaps involuntary, contractions of the extra-abdominal muscles and downward deflection of the diaphragm produce enough increased intra-abdominal pressure to bring small amounts of food into the mouth. One manometric study in a patient with voluntary ability to ruminate has shown that voluntary relaxation of the lower esophageal sphincter could occur for periods of up to three minutes. This, associated with contraction of voluntary muscle, could effect the retropulsion. Although reverse peristalsis has been described in ruminant animals, it has not been observed in humans. Some patients with this syndrome have severe psychoneurosis directly related to the perception of food, either because of problems with obesity or for other psychologic reasons.

395.4. DIARRHEA

For purposes of this discussion, diarrhea is defined as the excessively frequent passage of unformed stool. The symptom has many possible causes. Most acute diarrheas are of infectious origin or are stress related and, because they are self-limited, require no treatment.

ETIOLOGY. Diarrhea is generally divided into two types: *large volume* and *small volume* diarrhea. Large volume diarrhea implies hypersecretion, which is usually of small intestinal etiology. Secretory diarrhea can be assumed to be present if diarrhea persists in a fasting state. Increased secretion into the lumen generally is a response to infectious organisms such as cholera and pathogenic *E. coli,* vasoactive intestinal polypeptides, prostaglandins, peptide hormone–producing tumors such as medullary carcinoma of the thyroid, and islet cell tumors — all of which may result in increased intestinal propulsion owing to altered motility in addition to hypersecretion. Colonic hypersecretion can be induced by bile acids within the colon when significant ileal disease or resection interferes with ileal reabsorption of bile acids. This has been termed *"choleretic diarrhea."*

Large volume diarrhea also may result from an *osmotic* overload, as for example that produced by postgastrectomy syndrome, congenital chloridorrhea, and saline cathartics, or by undigested lactose caused by lactase deficiency. In contrast to secretory diarrhea, osmotic diarrhea should disappear when nothing is taken by mouth.

Small volume diarrhea (rapid colonic transit) is due to increased propulsive activity and is most commonly seen in irritable bowel syndrome. Antibiotic-associated diarrhea is caused by local mucosal inflammation. High levels of 5-hydroxytryptamine (serotonin) found in malignant carcinoid syndrome can produce hyperperistalsis of the small bowel and atony of the colon, resulting in diarrhea (Misiewicz et al., 1966). Partial intestinal obstruction may lead to compensatory hyperactive propulsive movements with intermittent diarrhea. Inflammatory disorders such as ulcerative colitis and Crohn's disease, radiation proctitis, and occasionally diverticulitis and ischemic proctitis may account for small volume diarrhea. Infectious diarrhea (e.g., shigellosis and salmonellosis) also may produce small volume frequent stools because of the local intolerance for distention. (Each of these disorders is discussed under its appropriate heading elsewhere in the text.) Urgency, often a more prominent symptom than pain, results from decreased compliance of the involved colon and often from exaggerated propulsive activity. When pain is experienced, it is generally in the lower abdomen, and mucus is often present. Adjacent pelvic inflammatory disease may produce colonic irritability as well. Tumors within the rectum also may induce hypermotility because of their "foreign body" distention effect. Hyperthyroidism generally results in increased frequency of stool without an appreciable change in its consistency. The cause of the diarrhea associated with systemic mast cell disease (urticaria pigmentosa) is not known.

DIFFERENTIAL DIAGNOSIS. Motor disturbance alone cannot explain large volume diarrhea. Abnormalities of absorption or secretion or both must be present. Historical features of importance are the patient's personality make-up, response to stress, and existing life stresses at the time of onset of symptoms. The diagnosis of irritable bowel syndrome or functional diarrhea is made on the basis not only of ruling out organic disease but also of positive personality, and stress-related features. Other factors of historical importance are exposure to laxatives, toxins, or allergens and history of similar disease within the community. Physical examination in irritable bowel syndrome may reveal a tender, cord-like sigmoid in the left lower quadrant. Tender masses may be felt in the right lower abdomen in Crohn's disease and the left lower quadrant with diverticular disease. There may be localized rebound tenderness. Fecal impaction with paradoxical diarrhea and overflow incontinence should be detected by digital examination.

Stools are examined for infectious agents, ova and parasites, and pus and food particles, and cultures are taken. Sigmoidoscopy may reveal inflammation of the rectum in inflammatory conditions or simply spasm of the rectum or rectosigmoid in the irritable bowel syndrome or diverticular disease. Barium enema may reveal ulcerations in cases of inflammatory bowel disease, may demonstrate abnormal motor patterns with exaggerated segmentation in irritable bowel syndrome, or may reveal diverticulosis with or without inflammation.

TREATMENT. Treatment demands electrolyte replacement and immediate withdrawal of the offending agent if this is known, as well as treatment of the underlying disorder. Symptomatic management of the motor disorder (rapid transit) should be withheld if possible for 24 hours if an infectious cause is likely, because there is evidence that such agents as Lomotil can prolong the course of shigellosis or salmonellosis (Merson, 1976). Glucose added to oral electrolyte solutions improves absorption, because glucose is actively absorbed and carries with it obligatory fluid and consequently electrolyte absorption. Because diarrhea is generally associated with decreased segmental (impeding) intestinal contractions, it is aggravated by gravitational factors when the patient is upright. Bed rest often provides symptomatic relief. Mild diarrheas may be treated with binding agents such as aluminum hydroxide gel, kaolin, pectin,

and bismuth. More serious diarrhea may require opiates, which act by increasing segmenting activity. Diphenoxylate (Lomotil), a synthetic derivative (given in 2.5- to 5-mg doses every four hours as long as diarrhea persists), can be helpful, as can deodorized tincture of opium, 5 to 10 drops given similarly. Camphorated tincture of opium (paregoric) can substitute for the aforementioned medication in 5-ml doses but may produce a sensation of esophageal burning. Codeine sulfate, 30 to 60 mg every four to six hours or more, is often extremely effective, but the physician must exert precautions to limit the dosage and the duration of treatment whenever possible. Even if chronic medication is required, intestinal tolerance does not develop as central nervous system tolerance does, and increasing dosage is not required to maintain efficacy. Hydrophilic colloids such as the psyllium seed derivatives and synthetic carboxymethylcellulose may be useful in decreasing the fluidity of the stool. These agents may be especially useful in patients with alternating constipation and diarrhea (as in irritable bowel syndrome), because hydrophilic colloids tend to soften hard stools and make watery stools more firm by binding water. The dosage is generally 1 tablespoon two or three times daily. Because additional bulk is produced, precautions should be taken if obstructive symptoms are present. Anticholinergic agents are rarely effective.

The timing of medications can best be adjusted to the individual patient's needs by having the patient keep a record of diarrheal episodes with correlations to other events such as stress and meals. When diarrhea occurs postprandially, medication should be given 30 minutes to an hour before meals so that maximal absorption will have occurred at the time of maximal needs. A general rule is that medication should be withdrawn as soon as the diarrhea appears to be under control.

395.5. CONSTIPATION

DEFINITION. For practical purposes constipation may be defined in relative terms as the infrequent and difficult passage of stool. Both frequency, which may be objective, and difficult passage, which is subjective, are relative concepts. The diagnosis of constipation is most readily established for a given individual on the basis of a significant change in frequency of stool along with increasing difficulty in passage. Consistency and size of stool are less diagnostic, because constipation can exist with difficult passage at infrequent intervals of hard small stools or voluminous soft stools. Few symptoms in medicine have been as injudiciously and incorrectly self-diagnosed by patients. One of the reasons for the frequent misdiagnosis and confusion is that the range of normality is extremely broad. In a healthy population stool frequency may vary between three times a day and two times a week without symptoms or apparent ill effects.

PATHOPHYSIOLOGY. Colonic motility studies by radiologic and manometric methods indicate two major motor disturbances leading to constipation: spasticity on the one hand and atonicity on the other. Spastic constipation, seen for example in irritable bowel syndrome, is often associated with hard, pellet-like stools. In atonic constipation, such as occurs with megacolon, stools may be voluminous and either hard or soft.

CAUSES OF CONSTIPATION. The most common form

of constipation, imaginary constipation, is based on public misconception, often enhanced by media advertisements extolling the virtues of "regularity," implying that a specified number of movements (usually one per day) represents the rigid limits of normal. This can lead to a secondary form of constipation resulting from abuse of laxative to achieve this imaginary goal. Laxative abuse results in excessive emptying of the colon, with a consequent delay in sufficient intraluminal distention to produce an urge. With this process of increasing desensitization, increasing laxative requirement ensues. Early coercive toilet training may engender retentive behavior on the part of the child, because toilet training generally occurs during a negativistic stage of human development. Sometimes extraneous events such as infections, imposed inactivity and bed rest, emotional factors, and travel produce temporary constipation, which can then be aggravated by psychologic reactions to symptoms or by unwise use of laxatives. The presence of painful anal conditions such as fissures may establish a vicious cycle, consisting of painful sphincter spasm, leading to constipation, which in turn leads to further fissuring and further pain. Medications such as ephedrine and anticholinergic drugs, bismuth, aluminum- and calcium-containing antacids, tricyclic antidepressants, ganglion blocking agents, and opiates may also induce this symptom. Constipation is one of the somatic manifestations of depression, which in turn is one of the more common disorders in society. Constipation may also result from neurotic fastidiousness with avoidance of public toilet facilities. In some instances constipation results from faulty habits which result from frequently suppressing the need to defecate because of time constraints. "Giant megacolon of the insane" has been attributed to indifference to sensation of a need to defecate, with resultant abnormal retention and colonic dilatation. Constipation also may result from mechanical obstruction of the intestine.

Controlled defecation mainly involves the use of voluntary musculature. This is achieved by glottal closure, rapid descent of the diaphragm, tightening of extra-abdominal musculature, and, initially, anal sphincter closure. This series of events increases intra-abdominal pressures, which ultimately inhibit the external anal sphincter and permit defecation. Neurologic or muscular disorders which produce diaphragmatic weakness or weakness of the abdominal musculature may interfere with defecation to a sufficient degree to induce constipation.

Neuromuscular and systemic disorders which affect the smooth muscle of the gastrointestinal tract may be determining factors in disorders such as myotonic dystrophy, scleroderma, and oculopharyngeal myopathy, Hirschsprung's disease results in a functional obstruction with dilatation proximal to the contracted aganglionic segment. Aganglionosis of the internal sphincter can produce constipation by interfering with the normal reflex relaxation of the internal anal sphincter which occurs as a prelude to defecation when the rectum becomes distended. Hyperparathyroidism can produce constipation, in part because of the effect of hypercalcemia on smooth muscle.

DIAGNOSIS. History. Primary local symptoms of constipation are those of the infrequent and often painful passage of hard stools. With excessive retention and abdominal distention, cramping pain may ensue. Complaints of headaches, lethargy, and anorexia may be elicited. Fever is sometimes reported after extremely long periods of retention, especially in children, who also may manifest irritability and hyperkinesis.

Physical Examination. Physical examination may reveal increased bowel sounds (except when ileus is present), tympany, and palpable masses in the descending and sigmoid colon. Digital examination reveals stool which, in the absence of aganglionic megacolon, extends to the anal sphincter itself. When aganglionic megacolon (Hirschsprung's disease) is present, the aganglionic segment is usually free of stool.

Endoscopy. Anoscopy and proctoscopy are necessary to rule out inflammatory anorectal conditions, tumors, and strictures. Excessive spasm noted on proctosigmoidoscopy suggests irritable bowel syndrome or diverticulosis. Melanosis coli (brownish mottling) can occur from laxative abuse, especially from laxatives containing emodin derivatives. Colonoscopy and barium enema may provide further help.

Motility Tests. Rectosphincteric manometric tests (see Megacolon in Ch. 399) are useful in differentiating idiopathic (acquired) megacolon from aganglionic megacolon (Hirschsprung's disease). Colonic motility studies may help differentiate atonic from spastic constipation by measuring compliance of the colon.

TREATMENT. Treatment is directed toward eradicating the underlying cause whenever this is known. Symptomatic therapy is used as an adjunct to specific therapy or as primary therapy when the cause is not apparent or is not amenable to specific therapy. Symptomatic therapy requires (1) the manual removal of impaction when present and cleansing enema; (2) re-establishment of the defecatory response to a convenient stimulus as rapidly as possible; and (3) substituting for the previous medication the mildest form of laxative in the lowest dose possible. Successful accomplishment of these goals requires re-education of the patient as well as his bowels. He must be given ample opportunity to reveal his attitudes and concepts and should be disabused of any misconceptions concerning "normal" bowel habits. He should be informed of the wide range of normality, should be instructed to develop an awareness of sensory urges and to respond to them whenever possible, and should be assisted in developing insight into neurotic attitudes that interfere with normal function.

Behavior Modification. One of the earliest socialization processes which humans undergo is that of learning bowel control. What is learned essentially is to suppress an automatic postprandial defecatory response. In many constipated persons this response is lost and must be re-established. A meticulous history indicating previous bowel habits can be quite helpful. An attempt is made to re-establish a stimulus-response pattern by instructing the patient to attempt to have a bowel movement shortly after breakfast or supper. If within ten minutes he is unsuccessful in having a voluntary movement, he is to take an enema to induce a movement. Remarkably rapid and successful results can be obtained in adults with short histories of constipation or in children with longer histories.

Activity. Exercise is advocated in order to promote colonic propulsion and to improve the tone of abdominal musculature which is required for defecation. Leg-raising exercises can help tone abdominal muscles and are especially helpful in postpartum constipation.

Diet. A diet is prescribed that is high in fiber, particularly bran. Sixteen grams of unprocessed miller's bran per day has been shown to be effective in increasing the frequency and size of stools. The flatulence and bloating that may result from this regimen generally last only two to three weeks but are intolerable enough to force discontinuation in about 15 per cent of patients. Water or fluid intake of more than 1500 ml per day is desirable. A careful history may indicate certain helpful foods such as prunes, figs, rhubarb, coffee, and milk which have a stimulant action for a particular patient.

Medication. Laxatives or cathartic medication should be avoided whenever possible and, when needed, used in the smallest doses possible as infrequently as possible. Periodic attempts are made to withdraw all laxatives gradually. Laxative medication may be considered under several categories:

BULK-FORMING AGENTS. Hydrophilic colloids derived from plants (psyllium seeds) or semi-synthetic polysaccharides and cellulose (carboxymethylcellulose) absorb water and swell, thus softening stools and providing bulk. This group of agents is particularly valuable in situations of alternating constipation and diarrhea, because absorbent qualities are useful under both circumstances. To achieve better mixing with stool as it is being formed, hydrophilic colloids should be prescribed with meals rather than at bedtime. Taken before meals they tend to suppress appetite, which may be desirable in obese individuals. Otherwise they should be prescribed after meals. Their absorbent and binding qualities may interfere with intestinal absorption of other medications given simultaneously.

WETTING AGENTS. Fifty to 200 mg of dioctyl sodium sulfosuccinate (Colace or Doxinate) softens stools by altering surface tension of liquids just as detergents do.

LUBRICANTS. Mineral oil, a poorly absorbed lubricant, prescribed in doses of 15 to 45 ml per day, is particularly helpful in the acute postoperative situation, but has disadvantages for long-term use because of interference with intestinal absorption of fat-soluble vitamins. The danger of aspiration should be considered in elderly patients who are bedridden or have swallowing disorders.

OSMOTIC AGENTS. Hypertonic phosphate or sulfate (magnesium sulfate or epsom salts) exerts an osmotic effect on both large and small intestine within six hours. Cholecystokinin release induced by these laxatives may further assist colonic emptying, as this hormone has a direct motor effect on colonic muscle and also produces contraction of the gallbladder. Bile salts thus released may stimulate colonic water secretion.

INTESTINAL STIMULANTS. Castor oil, anthracine derivatives (senna, cascara, rhubarb), phenolphthalein, and bisacodyl exert their action on the colon and are therefore slower to act. Prolonged administration of high doses of some of these agents can result in degeneration of the ganglion cells of Auerbach's plexus and consequent aggravation of constipation.

SUPPOSITORIES. Glycerin suppositories act by mechanically drawing water into the rectum. Vacuettes expand the rectum with carbon dioxide. Bisacodyl or senna suppositories stimulate smooth muscle locally or via ganglion cells. By virtue of their rapid effect, suppositories are useful for behavioral conditioning as well as for preparing for gastrointestinal and radiographic procedures.

ENEMAS. Enemas, too, have rapid onset of action and are useful on a short-term basis for reestablishment of gastroileocolic responses. For maximal results enemas should be administered with the patient lying on the left side and should be retained for five minutes or until a strong urge is felt.

Guiding Principle. A guiding principle of this form of therapy is that the goal of treatment is to end treatment by gradual withdrawal of all medications.

395.6. INCONTINENCE

MECHANISMS FOR MAINTAINING CONTINENCE. Fecal continence signifies the ability to retain bowel contents until evacuation becomes convenient. This requires intact neurosensory and motor innervation comprising an arc from a sensory receptive area with pathways to the central nervous system, a functioning efferent innervation, and a responsive neuromuscular target organ. Three basic mechanisms serve to provide for continence. These include the reservoir capacity of the colon, sensory stimulation, and sphincteric contraction.

A number of forces serve to keep the rectum empty in the resting state. First there is a reverse pressure gradient, with pressures within the rectum and sigmoid being of higher frequency and present for a longer time than in the sigmoid. In addition, the rectosigmoid flexures (two anterior and two posterior) serve to act as flap valves to retard the movement of stool when the subject is in the upright position. The spiral valves of Houston contribute further to sustain a column of stool, especially when this is solid. In addition, the rectum has the capacity of plastic adaptation, so that it adapts in a compliant fashion to gradual distention. This compliant capacity seems to be greatest in the distal 7 to 8 cm of rectum, and many of the sensory receptors reside here so that preservation of this segment is important for the maintenance of continence in operations which remove portions of the colon.

SPHINCTERIC CONTINENCE. The rectal outlet is guarded by two sphincters, the internal anal sphincter, which is composed of smooth muscle and innervated by the autonomic nervous system, and the external sphincter, which is composed of striated muscle with somatic innervation. The internal sphincter in its basal state is contracted, keeping the anal orifice closed and impeding progress of small amounts of material that enter the rectum in amounts insufficient to distend it. In addition, the contracted internal sphincter keeps the walls of the anorectal area collapsed, so that increase in intra-abdominal pressure further collapses the walls as pressures are transmitted against them. This prevents intrarectal material from reaching the highly sensitive anal receptory areas and thus prevents sensory stimulation. The external sphincter in its resting state is only minimally contracted but can respond reflexly to a number of events that call for increased resistance. The external sphincter reflexly develops increased tone under circumstances that threaten continence, e.g., when an upright position is assumed, or when intra-abdominal pressure is increased during coughing, laughing, or straining to lift a heavy object.

THE ROLE OF ANAL SENSORY RECEPTORS. The rectum proximal to the sphincter contains sensory receptors that are sensitive predominantly to stretch, whereas the anal canal itself contains a profuse network of various types of receptors that are capable of distinguishing the three physical states of matter — solids, liquids, and gases. Only when intraluminal material reaches the anal canal can this fine discrimination be made. The complex series of rectosphincteric reflexes provides the means for brief sensory stimulation without loss of continence. When material enters the rectum in amounts insufficient to distend it, the tonic contraction of the internal sphincter suffices to maintain continence and prevents material from reaching the afferent nerves in the anal canal, thus avoiding sensory stimulation. However, when quantities that are sufficient to distend it reach the rectum, the internal sphincter relaxes transiently, permitting brief contact of material with the sensitive receptors in the anal canal. Continence during this brief period is maintained by reflex transient contraction of the external sphincter. These sensory impulses reach cortical awareness, and appropriate action can be taken. Voluntary contraction of the external sphincter at this stage further preserves continence and often inhibits the rectal contraction above, providing for increased compliance. As the rectum adapts to a new and larger volume, the sensory stimulation diminishes and disappears until another stimulus recurs.

DISORDERS OF CONTINENCE (INCONTINENCE). Incontinence can result from interference at any level of this complex series of events. Disruption of the afferent arc by removal or diminution of the reservoir capacity resulting from operative resection, inflammatory disease, neurologic damage by local factors (such as spinal tumors and traumatic transections) or by systemic disease (such as diabetes mellitus, amyloidosis, and neuromuscular disorders), or local trauma to the sphincteric muscle itself (from fistula, abscess, or surgery) all can lead to incontinence.

Schuster, M. M.: Motor action of the rectum and anal sphincters in continence and defecation. In Code, C. F. (ed.): Handbook of Physiology, Section 6, Alimentary Canal, Vol. IV, Motility. Washington, D.C., American Physiological Society, 1968, pp. 2121–2146.

396. DISORDERS OF ESOPHAGEAL MOTILITY

STRIATED (PHARYNGOESOPHAGEAL) SEGMENT

Dysphagia caused by involvement of striated muscles of the pharnyx and esophagus can be due to neurologic diseases of the brain stem (bulbar palsy), bilateral corticobulbar tract (pseudobulbar palsy), or the striated muscle itself (polymyositis, myasthenia gravis, myotonic dystrophy, ocular myopathy, and sarcoidosis). These disorders result in high dysphagia, often associated with immediate regurgitation or aspiration of foods, especially fluids, into the respiratory passages. Mechanical compression from intrinsic or extrinsic lesions such as aneurysms, aberrant vessels (dysphagia lusoria), and enlarged thyroid may produce high dysphagia. Hypopharyngeal (Zenker's) diverticulum, which may be related to a hypertensive upper esophageal sphincter, is discussed in Ch. 401.

Fischer, R. A., Ellison, G. W., Thayer, W. R., Spiro, H. M., and Claser, G. H.: Esophageal motility in neuromuscular disorders. Ann. Intern. Med., 63:229, 1965.

Compression by Cervical Spine Spurs
(Forestier's Syndrome)

Hypertrophic spurs of cervical spine (C5 to C7) may produce dysphagia without symptoms related to the neck. Lateral cervical spine films demonstrate the osteophyte, and esophagram reveals posterior compression of the esophagus. The spur may impose an increased risk of laceration from endoscopy. Surgical resection of the spur is usually curative.

Beahrs, O. H., and Schmidt, H. W.: Dysphagia caused by hypertrophic changes in the cervical spine. Ann. Surg., 149:297, 1959.

Cricopharyngeal Achalasia

This is a motor disorder that involves the cricopharyngeal sphincter, producing difficulty in initiating swallowing. It is extremely rare. Motility studies of the esophagus demonstrate discoordination between pharyngeal contractions and sphincteric relaxation; cricopharyngeal relaxation occurs, but closure is premature. Esophagram may demonstrate a more than usual prominence of the cricopharyngeus muscle with hold-up of barium in the valleculae. There may be aspiration into the trachea. Cricopharyngeal myotomy may provide symptomatic improvement by decreasing intrasphincteric pressure. This syndrome may be associated with a hypopharyngeal (Zenker's) diverticulum (see Ch. 401).

Sideropenic Dysphagia
(Plummer-Vinson Syndrome, Paterson–Brown Kelly Syndrome)

This syndrome is characterized by high dysphagia seen usually in women of Scandinavian origin with hypochromic anemia. Dysphagia is thought to be due to an anterior esophageal web in some instances and to atrophy of the mucous membranes in the hypopharynx and pharynx in others. Dysphagia is referred to the upper esophagus and may be associated with occasional regurgitation. Associated symptoms are koilonychia, decreased serum iron, and achlorhydria. An anterior web indenting the esophagus can be seen on esophagram and occasionally at endoscopy. Differentiation from globus hystericus is made on the basis of presence of true dysphagia in the sideropenic disorder.

Dysphagia disappears rapidly after a single adequate dose of iron supplement or after dilatation by endoscopy. Careful follow-up is required because of an increased incidence of carcinoma of the pharynx or esophagus.

Jacobs, A., and Kilpatrick, G. S.: The Paterson-Kelly syndrome. Br. Med. J., 2:79, 1974.

SMOOTH MUSCLE (ESOPHAGOGASTRIC) SEGMENT

Esophagitis

DEFINITION AND PATHOGENESIS. Inflammation of the esophagus is a common gastrointestinal disorder and may be acute or chronic. Acute esophagitis is seen most commonly with reflux of acid peptic gastric juice secondary to an incompetent lower esophageal sphincter, or after prolonged nasogastric intubation. Reduced resting pressure of the lower esophageal sphincter is usually idiopathic but may be related to or aggravated by smoking, alcohol, or anticholinergic medications. Mechanical factors that increase intra-abdominal pressure, such as pregnancy, obesity, ascites, and occupations involving heavy lifting, may constitute aggravating features. Factors which inhibit gastrin release (increased acidity and anticholinergic drugs) or those which augment the release of secretin or cholecystokinin (fatty meals) may reduce lower esophageal sphincter pressures. Collagen vascular diseases associated with Raynaud's phenomena may also predispose to esophagitis because of incompetent lower esophageal sphincter. Chalasia in infants may result in reflux, which is difficult to recognize. Acute esophagitis is also encountered with lye ingestion, with infection by herpes or monilial organisms, and with central nervous system lesions or extensive body burns. Any of these causes, when persistent over a period of time, can result in chronic esophagitis.

CLINICAL MANIFESTATIONS. The most common complaint is that of heartburn, which is generally aggravated by truncal flexure, lying down, heavy meals, coffee, alcohol, or cigarette smoking. When pain is severe, a tight constricting sensation can be experienced radiating to the neck or down the arms. Bleeding may occur and may be vigorous but usually is occult, with the major presentation being that of hypochromic anemia. Patients may complain of acid eructation. Intermittent dysphagia is usually due to esophageal spasm, whereas progressive dysphagia implies development of an inflammatory stricture. Strictures develop in some patients without a prior history of heartburn, presumably because of insensitivity to inflammation. So-called *Barrett's esophagus* refers to heterotopic gastric mucosa lining the distal tubular esophagus. There is evidence that this may be a result as well as a cause of esophagitis and that with continued reflux the border of columnar mucosa travels proximally up the esophagus. Heterotopic gastric mucosa has been shown to be capable of secreting acid. Associated esophageal ulcerations are known as *"Barrett's ulcer."*

DIAGNOSIS. The diagnosis of esophagitis can be confirmed by esophagoscopy, with biopsy demonstrating inflammatory changes and neovascularization. Reflux etiology is best demonstrated by overnight recording of pH, with swallowed glass electrodes demonstrating increased periods of acid reflux. Bernstein's acid perfusion test is capable of demonstrating an acid-sensitive esophagus but is not direct evidence of reflux etiology. This test is performed by alternately dripping 0.1 normal HCl and normal saline into the esophagus without the patient's awareness of the material being infused. A positive response is represented by reproduction of pain with acid but not with saline. Esophageal motility studies performed during acid perfusion usually demonstrate diffuse esophageal spasm in patients who have a positive Bernstein test. Radiologic evidence of reflux is best obtained by the water siphon test. Under fluoroscopic vision after barium is swallowed into the stomach, water is swallowed. Barium can be seen to reflux from the stomach into the esophagus during deglutition in patients with incompetent sphincters. Acid sensitivity can also be demonstrated radiologically by comparing acid barium swallows with neutral barium swallows. When acid sensitivity is present, acid barium induces diffuse spasm, whereas neutral barium does not.

Underlying disorders such as collagen vascular disorders which impair lower esophageal sphincter competence should be ruled out. Differentiation from angina pectoris may be difficult, and both conditions may be present concurrently. Differentiation is based on the relationship of esophageal pain to position rather than exertion and is confirmed by reproduction of the pain during periods of acid reflux recorded with pH probes, or by acid perfusion test if the simultaneously obtained electrocardiogram is normal. The exercise stress test may be necessary to rule out cardiac factors. Nitroglycerin, being a smooth muscle relaxant, may alleviate esophageal spasm as well as coronary spasm and cannot therefore be used as a differentiating feature. Associated peptic ulcer may predispose toward reflux because of increased gastric acidity and sometimes because of gastric outlet obstruction. Gallbladder disease may also produce symptoms similar to those of esophagitis. When strictures are present, chemical burns should be ruled out. Carcinoma is distinguished on the basis of endoscopy with negative cytology and biopsy and radiologic appearance. Benign strictures are characterized by a smooth conical narrowing, as opposed to carcinomas, which have sharp, shelf-like margins. Barrett's esophagus is detected by biopsy, which must be carefully demonstrated to have been obtained from the tubular esophagus rather than in the stomach or hiatal hernia. The biopsy site can be localized by planting a silver neurosurgical clip at the time of biopsy and subsequently locating this by fluoroscopic observation of swallowed barium.

TREATMENT AND PREVENTION. The goal of both medical and surgical therapy is to prevent reflux. In addition, medical therapy is designed to neutralize as much as possible the gastric contents that reflux despite medical or surgical therapy. Nonabsorbable antacids are the backbone of medical therapy and are administered for two reasons: to neutralize refluxed material, and to increase the resting tone of the lower esophageal sphincter by stimulating exogenous gastrin release which results from alkalinization of gastric contents. Liquid antacids are preferable, especially in the early stages of treatment. Severe esophagitis is treated with hourly administration of 30 ml of antacid during waking hours. With continued improvement frequency of administration is decreased to four times a day, approximately an hour after meals and at bedtime and, in addition, whenever reflux symptoms appear. Anticholinergics are best avoided because they may dispose to reflux by decreasing gastric peristalsis, resulting in gastric retention. These drugs may also diminish lower esophageal sphincter contraction. Alginic acid (Gaviscon) may be helpful because it produces a foamy, slightly alkaline coating which floats on gastric contents. Urecholine, 25 mg four times a day, is prescribed if the more simple measures are unsuccessful. Urecholine exerts its effect by increasing lower esophageal sphincter contraction. Patients should be told of factors which predispose to reflux and instructed to avoid them. They are urged to eat small meals and to avoid lying down immediately after meals. Obese subjects should lose weight. Tight girdles or belts should be avoided. Patients should sleep with head and shoulders elevated at about a 20- to 30-degree angle. Fat intake should be reduced, and patients should abstain from alcohol and tobacco as much as possible. It is questionable whether topical anesthetics such as viscous xylocain or oxethazine (Oxaine-M) are more effective than antacid alone. Reports are conflicting as to whether cholestyramine taken in doses of 4 grams in one half glass of water after meals and at bedtime is useful in treating reflux of biliary material, especially after gastric surgery. The rationale for use of cholestyramine is its bile salt–binding qualities.

Surgery is reserved for the rare case of uncomplicated esophagitis that does not respond to medical management or for those strictures that do not respond to bougienage. Hiatal hernia is reduced when present, and an effective barrier to reflux is created surgically by augmenting sphincter pressures. This can be achieved by a number of mechanisms, including the wrapping of part of the stomach around the lower esophageal sphincter and anchoring the sphincter below the diaphragm within the abdomen. The results of medical management are usually excellent. Surgical treatment is also quite effective but is rarely required.

Skinner, D. B., and Hendrix, T. R.: Diagnostic tests. In Skinner, D. B., Belsey, R. H. R., Hendrix, T. R., and Zuidema, G. D.: Gastroesophageal Reflux and Hiatal Hernia. Boston, Little, Brown & Company, 1972.

Diaphragmatic Hernia
(Hiatal Hernia)

DEFINITION. A hiatal hernia refers to the protrusion of a portion of the stomach through the diaphragmatic hiatus into the chest. Herniation can occur through any number of weak spots at the diaphragm; most common are herniations through the foramen of Morgagni. Posterior herniations near the spine at the foramen of Bochdalek are rare variants. The classification which has the most practical clinical utility divides hernias into sliding hernias, in which the gastroesophageal junction is displaced upward into the chest, and paraesophageal (or rolling) hernias, in which the gastroesophageal junction remains in its normal position while portions of the stomach herniate into the chest by rolling up alongside the esophagus (Fig. 2).

PREVALENCE. Small, usually sliding hiatal hernias are commonly observed on gastrointestinal fluoroscopy, especially when maneuvers are performed to increase intra-abdominal pressures. Some radiologists maintain that under these conditions hiatal hernias can be demonstrated in the majority of the population. Most of these hernias are asymptomatic. More than three fourths of hernias are of the sliding type, the remaining being paraesophageal or mixed sliding-paraesophageal.

ETIOLOGY. Nontraumatic hernias may be congenital or acquired. The latter may not appear until adult life and may increase in size progressively with age. The congenital type results from a failure of the two diaphragmatic leaflets to fuse normally, whereas the acquired type results from herniation over a period of time through a weak area in the diaphragm. Herniation is much more common on the left side than on the right. Paraesophageal hernias are more frequent in women, especially the elderly. Sliding hernias may be associated with a "short" esophagus. In most instances this results from shortening caused by esophagitis and stricture rather than from congenital factors.

CLINICAL MANIFESTATIONS. Most hernias are asymptomatic. When symptoms are present, they are usually related to reflux esophagitis (see above). Hiatal hernia is not synonymous with gastroesophageal reflux, which is related more to sphincter incompetence than to any other factor. Reflux occurs without hiatal hernia, and conversely hiatal hernia can be present without reflux. When sphincter incompetence is present, a sliding hiatal hernia serves as an aggravating factor. Infants with large congenital hernias may succumb to respiratory embarrassment resulting from mechanical compression or pneumonia.

Symptoms related to the herniated pouch itself are generally mechanical, and are usually associated with the paraesophageal type or on rare occasions with large sliding hernias. Vague symptoms of intermittent abdominal or chest pain, dyspnea, and cardiovascular symptoms have been described, but proof that they are related to the hernia is often lacking. Incarceration may lead to sudden sharp substernal pain and symptoms of high gastrointestinal obstruction. This situation, although infrequent, constitutes a surgical emergency.

DIAGNOSIS. Presence of hiatal hernia is suspected on the basis of reflux symptoms or the mechanical symptoms mentioned above. Definitive diagnosis relies on radiologic demonstration of hernia. Because of the frequency of asymptomatic hernias, one should be as rigorous as possible in determining whether symptoms are in fact related to the hernia.

TREATMENT. Reflux symptoms are treated as noted under Esophagitis (see above). Medical management is effective for the great majority of symptoms associated with sliding hiatal hernias. Symptomatic paraesophageal hernias are less amenable to medical therapy and more often require a surgical approach. Emergency surgery is indicated for strangulation, perforation, or severe symptoms of esophageal obstruction or respiratory distress.

Diffuse Esophageal Spasm
(Corkscrew Esophagus, Curling)

DEFINITION. Diffuse esophageal spasm refers to strong nonpropulsive contractions over a large segment of the esophagus. It is a common disorder encountered most frequently in elderly patients.

ETIOLOGY AND PATHOGENESIS. This syndrome may be due to several causes, including gastroesophageal reflux and the aging process itself. The cause is frequently not known. Marked thickening of esophageal muscle may be present, and sometimes there may be a positive

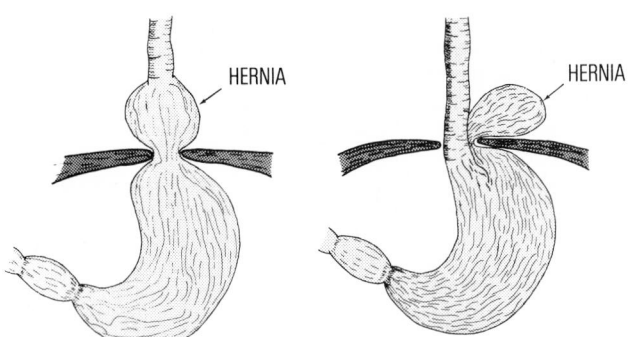

Figure 2. Sliding hiatal hernia (left) results when the esophagogastric junction and part of the stomach become displaced above the diaphragm. Paraesophageal ("rolling") hernia (right) results when the esophagogastric junction remains fixed in its normal intra-abdominal position, while a portion of the stomach is displaced into the chest.

Figure 3. Diffuse esophageal spasm.

strong spastic response to Mecholyl injection, suggesting that some instances may represent precursors of achalasia. Contractions can sometimes be triggered by swallowing.

CLINICAL MANIFESTATIONS. Symptoms are usually episodic and are frequently induced by swallowing or eating. They are often aggravated by tension and stress or by drinking cold liquids. Substernal chest pain and dysphagia are the most commonly encountered complaints. The pain, when severe, radiates through to the back and shoulder blades. Severe pain may be associated with pallor and perspiration, simulating coronary pain. Dysphagia may accompany chest pain or be dissociated from it. The dysphagia is typically episodic and not progressive. Weight loss may occur as a result of fear of eating.

DIAGNOSIS. Diagnosis is confirmed by x-ray examination and esophageal manometry (Fig. 3). Cinefluoroscopy may demonstrate a classic corkscrew appearance with pseudodiverticula produced by tertiary contractions and may reveal transient obstruction if a marshmallow is swallowed during the study. When gastroesophageal reflux is the precipitating factor, acid barium may induce spasm while neutral barium does not. Esophageal motility recordings may reveal diffuse spasm which is spontaneous or may show that swallowing or acid perfusion are precipitating factors. Some patients demonstrate positive responses to Mecholyl injection. These tests should be performed during a symptomatic stage because they may be negative during asymptomatic intervals.

TREATMENT AND PROGNOSIS. Since anxiety may induce or aggravate the symptoms, patients should be reassured that their disorder is benign. Precipitating factors such as cold liquids should be avoided, and a program of antacid and antireflux therapy instituted as a therapeutic trial, especially when acid sensitivity has been demonstrated (see Esophagitis). Sublingual nitroglycerin at the onset of an attack or prior to meals may give relief, as may longer acting smooth muscle relaxants such as Peritrate. Treatment with anticholinergic agents has generally proved disappointing. Patients with severe, unresponsive symptoms may derive benefit from forceful pneumostatic dilatation of the spastic segment, but this technique carries with it the risk of laceration. A long myotomy extending above the involved segment may be tried as a last resort if other measures fail. This operation requires a thoracotomy and produces good or excellent results in only two thirds of patients.

Bennett, J. R., and Hendrix, T. R.: Diffuse esophageal spasm: A disorder with more than one cause. Gastroenterology, 59:273, 1970.

Ellis, F. H., Olsen, A. M., Schlegel, M. F., and Code, C. F.: Surgical treatment of esophageal hypermotility disturbances. JAMA, 188:862, 1964.

Achalasia
(Cardiospasm, Aperistalsis, Megaesophagus)

DEFINITION. Achalasia is a chronic motor disorder that results from aperistalsis of the smooth muscle portion of the esophagus leading to functional obstruction proximal to the lower esophageal sphincter, which characteristically relaxes poorly. None of the current diagnostic labels is accurate and complete. The term achalasia connotes failure of relaxation of the lower esophageal sphincter and is inaccurate because the sphincter does relax, although incompletely. Cardiospasm emphasizes the hypertensive contraction of the sphincter, which at best is minimal, and the term ignores the basic underlying pathology in the body of the esophagus. Megaesophagus is anatomically descriptive but says nothing about the abnormal physiology; nor does it refer to impaired sphincter relaxation. The term aperistalsis ignores the sphincter disorder.

PREVALENCE AND EPIDEMIOLOGY. Achalasia, although uncommon, accounts for a large number of instances of esophageal obstruction. It can occur at any age but is most frequent between the ages of 20 and 50. There are no known familial, regional, or ethnic predisposing factors. The cause is unknown. The disorder is similar to Chagas' disease, which occurs in South America and results from degeneration of the ganglion cells in the myenteric plexus (see Ch. 194.3). The degeneration derives from infestation with trypanosomes and is associated with megacolon, megaloureter, megalobladder and cardiomegaly (see Megacolon in Ch. 399).

PATHOGENESIS. Degeneration of the nerve cells of Auerbach's plexus leads to aperistalsis and dilatation of the smooth muscle (lower two thirds of the esophagus) and incomplete relaxation of the lower esophageal sphincter. Resting pressures within the sphincter are normal or slightly elevated. This situation results in progressive dilatation of the esophagus with retention of fluids and food. As hydrostatic pressure increases to a point that exceeds the sphincteric resistance, small spurts of material are expelled into the stomach. A defect in cholinergic innervation can be demonstrated by the excessive spasm induced by Mecholyl (an acetylcholine analogue). This response is explained by Cannon's law of autonomic denervation, which states that end-organs deprived of their autonomic innervation respond in an exaggerated manner to neurohumoral stimulation. The lower esophageal sphincter is supersensitive to gastrin (but this effect appears to be mediated through postganglionic release of acetylcholine and therefore due to nerve degeneration) (Bennett, 1965).

A gradation of symptoms and signs suggests that various stages of achalasia exist and that some instances of diffuse esophageal spasm (see above) may represent an early phase of achalasia or a preachalasia syndrome. Two major types of achalasia are recognized: rigorous achalasia and a milder form which shows less dilatation and more segmental spasm both radiologically and manometrically, but in which lower esophageal sphincter relaxation is incomplete. The Mecholyl test is usually positive (Beckit et al., 1966; Sanderson et al., 1967). The more classic form of achalasia, which may represent a later stage, is characterized by marked sigmoid dilatation of the esophagus with little or no segmental spasm (Fig. 4).

CLINICAL MANIFESTATIONS. Dysphagia for both liquids and solids is the presenting complaint in 90 per cent of patients with classic achalasia. Progression may be so insidious that this symptom goes unnoticed until an advanced stage of obstruction has been reached. Close questioning of the patient or relatives may reveal that the patient has been an extremely slow eater for a long period. Patients often report increased difficulty eating when they are tense or in public places. They may drink fluid or swallow large gulps of air during meals in order to develop enough pressure to propel the material through the unrelaxing sphincter. Obstructive episodes may result from swallowing a bolus of poorly chewed food. Breath may be foul because of bacterial action on material retained within the esophagus, and there may be overnight staining of the pillow from overflow of esophageal contents. Aspiration pneumonia is a common complication. Substernal pain may occur especially after eating and is particularly common in patients with vigorous achalasia. Marked weight loss and nutritional deficiency may result.

DIAGNOSIS. Radiologic diagnosis is easily made on the basis of the markedly dilated tortuous esophagus which comes down to an elongated narrow sphincteric zone that has the appearance of a parrot's beak. There is no peristalsis in the body of the esophagus on cine-fluoroscopy or esophageal manometry. On occasion the dilated, fluid-filled esophagus can be seen behind the heart shadow on a chest film, and an air-fluid level may be noted. When tortuosity is sufficient to result in a plumber's trap effect, there is no gastric air bubble on the upright chest film. An epiphrenic diverticulum may be an associated finding.

Esophageal Motility Studies. Manometry reveals a normal cricopharyngeal sphincter but absence of peristalsis in the body of the esophagus, including the striated portion. When retained material is in the esophagus, there may be an increase in resting pressure within the body. Deglutition fails to induce peristalsis. Normal or increased pressures are noted within the lower esophageal sphincter, and swallowing produces incomplete or no relaxation. Intravenous Mecholyl induces marked esophageal spasm and severe pain. Because of the striking sensitivity to Mecholyl, small doses, beginning with 1 mg, should be used, with progressive increments as necessary. Diffuse spasm is noted with the vigorous form of achalasia.

Endoscopy demonstrates the markedly dilated esophagus with surprisingly little inflammation despite the chronic retention of secretions and ingested material.

Figure 4. Achalasia. Far advanced changes.

Unless the contour is extremely tortuous, the endoscope traverses the lower esophageal sphincter without difficulty, thus ruling out organic stricture or carcinoma. Cytology is negative.

Occasionally infiltrating carcinoma may produce a similar x-ray picture. Scleroderma affects only the smooth muscle portion of the esophagus, leaving normal contractions in the upper third as demonstrated by x-ray and manometry. Because scleroderma is associated with diminished pressures within the lower esophageal sphincter, reflux esophagitis may be noted.

TREATMENT AND PROGNOSIS. Forceful pneumostatic dilatation of the esophagus is the treatment of choice and should be performed early to avoid the development of marked dilatation that can ensue from chronic obstruction. To be successful, dilatation must be performed under fluoroscopic observation so that accurate placement of the dilator can be assured. Relief of dysphagia is obtained in 80 per cent of patients, only a few of whom will complain of reflux symptoms. Unfortunately in patients with vigorous achalasia, although forceful dilatation may relieve dysphagia, only one half of patients note relief of pain. The success of dilatation is attributable to its impairment of sphincter contraction, which permits esophageal emptying in the upright position even though aperistalsis persists.

When pneumostatic dilatation is unsuccessful or technically not feasible, sphincter pressure can be reduced surgically by a Heller myotomy. A surgical approach, however, is associated with a 15 per cent incidence of severe reflux esophagitis. Therefore antireflux measures should be taken postoperatively and may be wise as well for a short period after pneumostatic dilatation. Patients should be followed for recurrence of symptoms and may require additional pneumostatic dilatation after a number of years. The possibility of carcinoma should also be kept in mind to

Figure 5. A Schatzki ring is seen as a concentric web-like constriction in the distal esophagus.

explain recurrent obstructive symptoms, because the incidence of cancer is increased in patients with achalasia.

Hypertensive Lower Esophageal Sphincter

A rare entity characterized by marked increase in resting pressure and elongation of the lower esophageal sphincter high pressure zone has been described (Code et al., 1960). Esophageal peristalsis may be normal, or diffuse spasm may be present. Odynophagia or painful swallowing is the major complaint, and this is generally referred to the subxiphoid area when severe pain radiates through to the back. Combined cineradiographic studies demonstrate the hypertensive sphincter. Treatment is directed toward underlying emotional factors when detectable. Antispasmodics and sublingual nitroglycerin may be helpful. Pneumostatic dilatation or myotomy may be required if other measures fail and severity of symptoms warrants.

Lower Esophageal Ring

A thin web-like constriction at the lower end of the esophagus several centimeters above the diaphragm may be present in an asymptomatic form in up to 20 per cent of individuals fluoroscoped (Fig. 5). Symptoms appear when the diameter is smaller than 12 mm and are invariably present at less than 10 mm (Schatzki, 1963; Goyal et al., 1970). Symptoms are classically intermittent and related to eating solid foods. The complaints are those of intermittent dysphagia and lower substernal pain, which may be excruciating if a poorly chewed bolus becomes impacted at the lower esopha-

geal ring. A meat bolus may be disimpacted by mixing meat tenderizer (papaine), 1 to 2 teaspoons, in a glass of water to be sipped slowly every 10 to 15 minutes. This treatment is safe and will not harm the esophagus unless the impaction has been present for more than 24 hours, because there may then be some necrosis of the esophageal wall, and enzymatic digestion of the necrotic tissue may result in perforation.

Treatment involves careful instruction to the patient to eat slowly and to chew food well. He should be reassured of the benign nature of his disease. Brusk pneumostatic dilatation may be curative, or the ring may be cut surgically if medical management is unsuccessful and symptoms are severe.

Scleroderma
(Progressive Systemic Sclerosis)

Aperistalsis of the esophagus and diminished lower esophageal sphincter tone are noted in three fourths of patients with scleroderma. The aperistalsis is restricted to the smooth muscle (lower two thirds of the esophagus). Severe reflux esophagitis may result from incompetent sphincter combined with inability of the aperistaltic esophagus to clear the refluxed material. Perhaps because of the absence of spasm, reflux symptoms are infrequent and strictures may result. Because of reduced sphincter pressure the esophagus empties normally in the upright position. Radiographic and manometric studies demonstrate aperistalsis in the lower two thirds of the esophagus and impairment of lower esophageal sphincter. X-ray studies also can show reflux. Aperistalsis correlates more closely with the presence or absence of Raynaud's phenomenon than with other features of the disease (Stevens et al., 1964).

Diabetic and Alcoholic Neuropathy

Altered esophageal peristalsis can be demonstrated manometrically in diabetics and alcoholics with neuropathy, but motor abnormality does not correlate with clinical symptoms and most patients are asymptomatic.

Bayless, T. M. (ed.): Management of esophageal disease. Mod. Treatment, Vol. 7, No. 6, 1970.

397. DISORDERS OF GASTRODUODENAL MOTILITY

NORMAL MOTILITY

Gastric and duodenal motility will be considered together because of the interaction of these two organs to achieve their common goal of mixing food with digestive juices. The stomach when empty is collapsed and has feeble contractions. During states of hunger vigorous contractions begin at the pacemaker near the cardia and traverse the stomach at a frequency of three per minute. As food enters the stomach, the proximal stomach relaxes, a process called receptive relaxation. This accommodation to distention is so effective that no total change in intragastric pressure recurs. Vagal inhibitory neurons participate in the mediation of both receptive relaxation and an accommodation to distention. Postganglionic vagal stimulatory fibers initiate contractions by releasing acetylcholine, which depolarizes gastric smooth muscle. Postganglionic sympathetic nerves inhibit contraction by release of norepinephrine, which hyperpolarizes both the postganglionic cholinergic nerves and smooth muscle. The gastrointestinal hormones gastrin and cholecystokinin inhibit proximal contractions, decrease intragastric pressure, and retard gastric emptying both directly and by releasing neurotransmitters. Secretin, glucagon, and motilin also delay gastric emptying.

The primary motor action of the stomach is characterized by peristalsis, which serves to mix and churn food. As peristalsis reaches the distal antrum, this area contracts vigorously, as does the pylorus, thus favoring further mixing and preventing emptying of solid materials, but permitting fluid to pass into the duodenum. Solid material is propelled back into the stomach for further mixing and liquefaction. Partial depolarization of the smooth muscle cell is controlled by a slow wave potential (pacesetter potential) at a frequency of 3 cycles per minute. Spike potentials, or action potentials, produce complete depolarization and initiate contractions. In the distal stomach as in the proximal stomach, vagal nerves stimulate and sympathetic nerves inhibit contractions. Inhibitory vagal nerves have not been demonstrated in distal stomach. Gastrin stimulates peristalsis in the distal stomach while inhibiting the proximal stomach. Cholecystokinin and motilin also stimulate distal gastrointestinal contractions, whereas secretin, glucagon, vasoactive intestinal polypeptide, gastric inhibitory polypeptide, and bulbogastrone inhibit peristalsis. The pylorus contracts strongly, inhibiting gastric emptying and preventing duodenogastric reflux when acid, fatty meal, amino acids, or hypertonic solutions enter the duodenum. These effects may be mediated by cholecystokinin or secretin, both of which stimulate sphincter contraction, whereas exogenous gastrin inhibits their action. Until appropriately liquefied and mixed, food is retained in the stomach by the antral pump mechanism. Emptying of the stomach is delayed by osmoreceptors in the duodenum which prevent emptying of hypertonic material, and by receptors in the duodenum sensitive to fat and hydrogen ion. The gastrointestinal hormones, secretin and glucagon, released from the duodenum seem to be responsible in part for this action. Gastric distention augments gastric peristalsis by both vagal stimulation and gastrin release.

Kelly, K. A.: Gastric motility and health after gastric surgery. Viewpoints Dig. Dis., 8: March 1976.

PATHOPHYSIOLOGIC MOTILITY

Emotional factors may exert striking influences on gastric motility. Anxiety and hostility tend to augment activity, whereas fear, depression, and strong pain tend to reduce contractions and delay emptying. Hunger augments gastric peristalsis; nausea inhibits stomach contractions and stimulates duodenal spasm. Chronic gastritis and gastric ulcer may be associated with incompetence of pyloric muscle, resulting in a reflux of bile into the stomach.

Aerophagia

A small amount of air is swallowed with each deglutition. When excessive, air swallowing results in gastric distention, bloating, pain, increased belching, or rectal passage of flatus, termed *flatulence*. Aerophagia may result from anxiety or a compulsive habit and may reach striking proportions. It may also accompany hunger from decreased food intake or peptic ulcer and may represent an attempt to eliminate hunger contractions by distending the stomach. Frequent feedings or antiulcer management may alleviate symptoms which occur on this basis. Psychogenic aerophagia may respond to a supportive approach, combined with attempts to increase the patient's awareness of his symptoms. Chewing gum and carbonated beverages are interdicted. The patient is instructed to eat slowly. When frequent swallowing accompanies a dry throat, which itself may be a manifestation of anxiety, sucking on hard candy may be helpful. An object such as a pencil can be held between the teeth to keep the mouth open and prevent swallowing during heightened episodes of aerophagia. Patients should be warned against swallowing after taking deep sighs, which decrease intrathoracic pressure and may tend to suck air into the esophagus.

Acute Gastric Dilatation

ETIOLOGY. Gastric dilatation, previously a common postoperative feature associated with ileus, is less frequently encountered today because of postoperative decompression by nasogastric tube. Dilatation can be seen with profound compulsive aerophagia. Positive pressure respiratory assistance may produce dilatation with or without tracheostomy or endotracheal tubes. Acute dilatation may accompany diabetic acidosis as well as electrolyte imbalance, particularly hypokalemia. Chronic dilatation can be seen with obstructing lesions, diabetes (diabetic gastroparesis), collagen vascular disorders, or vagotomy. Chronic gastric dilatation may also be associated with neuromuscular disorders, anticholinergic therapy, hypothyroidism, or immobilization in body casts.

CLINICAL MANIFESTATIONS. The hypochondrium becomes distended and tympanitic, particularly on the left, and patients experience bloating or severe pain. Relief is obtained by belching or passing of flatus or nasogastric tube decompression. Mucosal bleeding may lead to "coffee ground" gastric contents.

TREATMENT. Effective decompression can be achieved by nasogastric aspiration while definitive treatment is directed toward the underlying cause. Electrolyte replacement, especially potassium, may be necessary.

Gastric Volvulus

Volvulus occurs with torsion of the stomach. Torsion may be along the longitudinal axis of the stomach (mesenteroaxial volvulus), in which case the greater curvature flips upward under the diaphragm, producing a 180 degree twist, while the esophagogastric junction and duodenum remain fixed. Organoaxial volvulus occurs when the upper part of the stomach twists in one direction and the distal portion in another.

ETIOLOGY. Etiology is unknown in most instances, but one fifth of patients have an associated diaphragmatic defect such as hiatal hernia or eventration of the diaphragm. Relaxation of the gastric ligaments is a prerequisite for volvulus to occur.

CLINICAL MANIFESTATIONS. Acute volvulus, which can result from or produce acute gastric distention, is associated with severe epigastric or left upper quadrant pain, often radiating to the back or thorax. Retching may occur, and the upper abdomen becomes distended. When there is compromise of blood supply, shock ensues. Chronic volvulus is more common than the acute type and is generally associated with milder symptoms of distention and bloating. Reflux symptoms may be present, as well as dysphagia caused by obstruction at the esophagogastric junction. Roentgenographic study reveals a double fluid level, one at the pyloric and the other at the cardiac end.

TREATMENT. Acute gastric volvulus is decompressed by nasogastric aspiration. Passage of the tube may be difficult, and there is a danger of esophageal perforation caused by obstruction. Chronic volvulus is treated with frequent small feedings and measures to decrease aerophagia. When symptoms are severe, surgical correction, including repair of diaphragmatic defects and gastropexy, may be necessary.

Pyloric Stenosis
(Gastric Outlet Obstruction)

ETIOLOGY AND PATHOGENESIS. Gastric outlet obstruction may occur transiently as a result of functional pyloric spasm or of mechanical obstruction from stenosis. Pyloric spasm also may occur because of adjacent duodenal gastric ulcer or gastritis. Carcinoma may also lead to outlet obstruction, but the most common cause is pyloric scarring and stenosis due to pyloric channel ulcer. Stenosis from hypertrophy of pyloric muscle occurs in two forms: congenital hypertrophic pyloric stenosis seen in infants, and adult hypertrophic pyloric stenosis seen in later life.

INCIDENCE. Congenital hypertrophic pyloric stenosis occurs in 2 per 1000 live births and is four times more common in males than in females. Familial incidence is noted, and the incidence in twins is 20 times that in single births. A spastic component to the hypertrophy exists; it disappears under anesthesia and frequently responds to anticholinergic drugs.

In adult hypertrophic pyloric stenosis the pyloric muscle is markedly thickened and elongated, but no inflammation or scarring is present. Symptoms often appear for the first time in middle or late life.

CLINICAL MANIFESTATIONS. Congenital hypertrophic pyloric stenosis is generally asymptomatic for the first five to ten days of life. From ten days to three weeks after birth, symptoms of regurgitation appear, followed eventually by projectile vomiting, weight loss, and dehydration without loss of appetite. Bile is not present in the vomitus. Prominent gastric peristalsis can be seen through the thin abdominal wall passing from left to right. The hypertrophied pylorus may be felt as a mass in the subxiphoid area. Adults generally present with epigastric distress, pain, and bloating, followed by nausea, vomiting, and weight loss.

DIAGNOSIS. The characteristic x-ray picture is that of an elongated, narrowed pylorus with a goose neck appearance. This is seen in both the congenital and adult forms. There may be an umbrella type of compression between the bile-filled duodenal bulb and the barium-

filled antrum. Gastroscopically, the hypertrophied muscle resembles the view of the cervix seen on pelvic examination and is therefore called the pyloric cervix sign.

TREATMENT. In patients with mild obstructive symptoms, medical management consists of parenteral rehydration as indicated, small feedings, and anticholinergic medication. When symptoms are more serious or if therapeutic response is not obtained within a week, pyloromyotomy (Ramstedt procedure) is performed. This consists of a longitudinal incision into the circular muscle. Muscle hypertrophy disappears after pyloromyotomy or in the milder cases after successful anticholinergic treatment. In adults pyloroplasty or resection of the hypertrophied muscle is generally required. Resection has the advantage of ruling out malignancy in adults when this is suspected.

Schuster, M. M., and Smith, V. M.: The pyloric cervix sign in adult hypertrophic stenosis. Gastrointest. Endosc., 16:210, 1970.

398. INTESTINAL OBSTRUCTION
(Ileus)

DEFINITION AND ETIOLOGY. Intestinal obstruction signifies impairment of cephalocaudad transit of intestinal contents. Obstruction is categorized under two broad etiologic headings: mechanical and adynamic (or paralytic). This classification carries therapeutic implications, because *mechanical obstruction* often requires correction by surgery, whereas adynamic ileus is approached medically. Extrinsic factors, including adhesions (often from previous operations or inflammation), and hernias are the most common cause of mechanical obstruction of small bowel, whereas intrinsic lesions such as cancer are the most common cause of large bowel obstruction. In infants and children congenital atresia or stenosis accounts for most intrinsic intestinal lesions, whereas in adults intrinsic narrowing is more often due to tumors or inflammatory strictures. Fecal impaction, meconium, and foreign bodies may also obstruct, as may gallstones, which usually lodge at the ileocecal sphincter. Intussusception and worms are uncommon causes.

Adynamic ileus occurs most commonly after operations or abdominal trauma, but may also result from chemical irritants (blood, bile, bacteria) electrolyte disturbances (such as hypokalemia), or vascular insufficiency (which may be either chronic or acute). The acute form is usually the result of arterial spasm, embolus, or thrombosis or of venous thrombosis. Other conditions, such as myocardial infarct, pneumonia, and spinal injuries, may result in ileus. Peritonitis produces generalized ileus, whereas more localized inflammation (biliary, pancreatic, or renal) may produce localized ileus.

PATHOGENESIS. The major effects of both mechanical and paralytic obstruction are intestinal distention and loss of fluid and electrolytes. If untreated by medical (intubation) or surgical decompression, distention tends to perpetuate itself by virtue of the intestinointestinal reflux described by Bayliss and Starling — a vicious cycle in which intestinal distention leads to further atony, which leads to further intestinal distention. In the early stage of mechanical obstruction hyperperistaltic waves may attempt to overcome the obstruction, but after a period atony ensues and the distinction between mechanical and paralytic ileus becomes difficult. When mechanical obstruction leads to perforation, an adynamic ileus is superimposed because of the ensuing peritonitis. Either form may lead to complications such as perforation, strangulation, volvulus, or gangrene. Distention is aggravated by swallowed air as well as by gas produced by bacteria which tend to multiply within the obstructed intestine. Increased intraluminal pressure may compromise mucosal blood flow, leading to necrosis and subsequent exudation of blood and plasma into the lumen while bacterial invasion and transport of toxins occur across the damaged mucosa.

Ileus results in serious interference with absorption of gas, both exogenous and endogenous, and of exogenous and endogenous intestinal fluids. Since the small bowel normally receives 8 or more liters of fluid per day, most of which is absorbed before reaching the colon, dehydration can occur even without vomiting as fluid leaves the vascular compartment and accumulates in the intestinal lumen. Especially if vomiting occurs, but even if it does not, this intraluminal accumulation of fluid leads to dehydration and loss from the extracellular fluid of sodium and chloride ions. A shift of potassium from intra- to extracellular compartment leads to hypokalemic alkalosis. Hypokalemia aggravates and perpetuates the ileus by inhibiting peristalsis, and the combination of hypovolemia and hypokalemia may lead to acute renal insufficiency even in the absence of arterial hypotension.

CLINICAL MANIFESTATIONS. The symptoms of mechanical obstruction depend to some extent on the degree of the obstruction and its duration. Characteristically the symptoms are those of crampy pain, either periumbilical or upper abdominal, and vomiting. Bowel sounds are hyperactive, high pitched, and tinkling, and coincide with painful cramps. Tympany may be present, but distention is not marked. Taut abdominal distention is more commonly encountered with colonic than with small bowel obstruction. The vomitus with distal obstructions may be fecal in character (fecal emesis). As the intestine dilates and becomes atonic, obstipation (absolute constipation without passage of gas or stool) ensues. Obstipation may be a later symptom occurring after the colon has emptied itself. With distal colonic obstruction, obstipation is an early complaint. As ileus and distention progress, the pain becomes less rhythmic and more continuous, there is increased tenderness, and rigidity of the abdomen and rebound tenderness may be noted. These signs plus increasing hypovolemia may suggest impending bowel necrosis, although an early definitive diagnosis of this is difficult. Tachycardia, fever, hypotension or shock, and leukocytosis are later signs suggesting necrosis.

Adynamic paralytic ileus is signaled by more distention than by obstipation, and the pain is less rhythmic than in mechanical ileus. There may be less guarding and tenderness. Vomiting is less pronounced, and bowel sounds are diminished or absent. Rectal examination can demonstrate extracolonic masses, intraluminal rectal obstructing lesions, and areas of tenderness within the pelvis.

DIAGNOSIS. Radiologic examination of the abdomen is vital to the diagnosis. Plain recumbent, upright, and lateral decubitus films are vital in determining whether the obstruction is located in small or large intestine. Air-fluid levels may be seen in the obstructed bowel in the upright and lateral decubitus positions. Small bowel obstruction results in a stepladder distribution of the loops of intestine. Jejunal obstruction is characterized by prominent valvulae conniventes, whereas ileal obstruction is not. Plain films may show distended haustra in colonic obstruction. Valvulae conniventes can often be distinguished from haustra because the valvulae traverse the entire lumen as a straight line, whereas haustra are asymmetric and do not extend across the entire lumen from one side to another. Barium contrast studies by mouth are to be avoided, but cautiously performed barium enema without preparation may be helpful in localizing the obstructed site if evidence indicates that it is in the colon.

Early laboratory findings include diminished urinary output and decrease in serum chloride and potassium, with rise in plasma bicarbonate, pH, and blood urea nitrogen. Hematocrit, urinary output, specific gravity, serum proteins, and BUN are all indicators of the state of hydration and hemoconcentration. Significant leukocytosis and grossly bloody stool warn of impending necrosis.

TREATMENT. The cornerstone of treatment is careful and repeated observation, with frequent reassessment of the clinical condition and laboratory features. The therapeutic plan is modified to deal with changing conditions. The primary goals of therapy are (1) fluid and electrolyte balance, (2) intestinal decompression, and (3) removal of the cause of obstruction. In some instances of adynamic ileus, a medical approach can achieve all three goals. In others, as well as when the obstruction is on a mechanical basis, initial decompression is achieved by medical intubation but definitive decompression and removal of the obstruction may require surgery. Often nasogastric aspiration is sufficient, because this removes air before it reaches the intestine.

Fluid replacement is aimed at replenishing depleted water, sodium, chloride, and potassium. This is first achieved by intravenous infusion of isotonic sodium chloride alternating with 5 per cent glucose if urine flow is adequate (over 50 ml per hour). Potassium replacement should not exceed 40 mEq per hour. Central venous pressure is monitored to assure adequate replacement as well as to avoid excessive overload, particularly in patients with compromised cardiovascular reserve. However, it is important to recognize that central venous pressure does not measure blood volume. Repeated observations are made of serum potassium and chloride as well as blood pressure, electrocardiogram, urinary output, and hematocrit. Caloric requirements approach 2000 calories per day. Alkalosis or acidosis should be corrected. Prostigmine, Urecholine, and parenteral pantothenic acid may be helpful in regaining tone after intubation but are dangerous in the face of mechanical obstruction. A barium enema may provide successful treatment for intussusception or volvulus by hydrostatic pressure. When fever, leukocytosis, or signs of peritonitis suggest perforation or strangulation, appropriate antimicrobials are administered to suppress growth of intestinal bacteria. Strangulation with impending gangrene demands surgery within six hours. Surgery is directed toward the underlying cause as well as removal of necrotic portions of the bowel.

When the underlying cause is ischemia of intestine, the obviously gangrenous portion is removed, leaving areas of questionable compromised blood supply. Twenty-four hours later a second operation is performed to determine whether these areas have regained normal appearance or whether more intestine must be resected to a line that obviously has good circulation.

PROGNOSIS. Prognosis depends on a number of factors. Necrosis, strangulation, and peritonitis seriously reduce chances for survival. These features in turn are influenced by the type of obstruction and its duration. Renal insufficiency or failure also imposes a poor prognosis, as do underlying vascular conditions, especially in the elderly. The outlook is worse for high than for low intestinal obstruction.

399. DISORDERS OF COLONIC MOTILITY

NORMAL MOTILITY

The colon functions to dehydrate its contents and store them until evacuation is socially convenient. Each of these three basic physiologic functions is subserved by a corresponding physiologic motor activity. Abnormality (pathophysiologic motility) of each activity is associated with corresponding clinical disorders. The primary motor activity of the colon, *segmentation,* consists of segmenting contractions which form simultaneously over long segments of colon and serve to impede the forward progress of intraluminal contents (Fig. 6). The segmenting contractions produce the haustral markings seen on barium enema. These contractions may remain present for minutes to hours. When they disappear they are replaced by others in the same area, with each new contraction approximately halfway between two old ones. As this process repeats itself over several hours, it results in a kneading of the colonic contents but does not result in forward propulsion. During the

process of dehydration the colon normally absorbs all except some 150 ml of the liter that has been presented daily to it by the ileum. Exaggerated segmentation results in excessive impedance, and constipation ensues. This type of motor hyperactivity is associated with clinical disorders such as irritable bowel syndrome and diverticulosis (Fig. 6). Diminished segmentation is seen in association with frequent diarrheal stools as in ulcerative colitis and is observed on the barium enema as a loss of the normal haustral contractions.

Compliance is the physiologic motor activity which provides for colonic storage function. A type of "plastic adaptation" occurs when the colon is gradually distended until a pressure is reached that initiates active colonic contractions. It is the active contraction that reaches sensory awareness and is felt as distention or urgency. Exaggerated compliance, seen in megacolon, results in colonic dilatation and prolonged retention of stool. Diminished compliance, seen in ulcerative colitis, decreases storage capacity, resulting in frequent passage of stools.

Evacuation results from a massive contractile movement at the proximal end of a bolus, producing forward propulsion. These massive propulsive movements are exaggerated in diarrheal disorders and diminished in constipation.

The aforementioned phenomena explain the apparent paradoxical motility of constipation and diarrhea. In diarrheal states motility is abnormally quiescent as segmental impeding activity is diminished. Increased mass propulsive movements are present, although these still are quite infrequent (a few per day) compared to the normal frequency of segmenting activity (a few per minute). Thus the over-all effect is one of general quiescence, with infrequent gross interruptions. In constipated states mass propulsive movements are diminished, although over-all colonic activity is usually increased because of the augmented segmenting, impeding activity which provides resistance to forward movement. An understanding of these basic physiologic principles is helpful in understanding not only disordered motility but also the response to drugs such as the opiates (codeine, paregoric) which, because they augment segmentation, are useful for the treatment of diarrhea.

As the stool is propelled into the normally empty rectum by mass movements, discomfort and urgency signal the need to defecate. This can be voluntarily inhibited by strongly contracting the external sphincter and relaxing diaphragmatic and abdominal musculature. Colonic compliance diminishes intraluminal pressure, and the sensation subsides until more material is propelled into the rectum.

To some extent the ileocecal sphincter regulates emptying from the ileum into the colon and acts to prevent reflux of colonic contents into the ileum. Distention proximal to the ileocecal sphincter results in relaxation of the sphincter, whereas distention of the colon distal to the sphincter results in augmented contraction. This situation favors unidirectional flow from ileum to colon.

Cholinergic (parasympathetic) nerve stimulation of the colon, as well as cholinergic agents and neostigmine, produces colonic contractions, whereas adrenergic stimulation causes inhibition. Anticholinergic agents may have a weak inhibiting activity, but their action is variable. Gastrin diminishes sphincter contraction. It is possible that the increased colonic activity

Figure 6. *A,* Segmented (haustral) contractions impede the progress of material through the intestine. *B,* Increased intraluminal pressures developed by segmental contractions can lead to diverticula which result from mucosal herniations. (After Painter, N. S., et al.: Gastroenterology, 49:169, 1965.)

which appears after eating is related to gastrin. Cholecystokinin stimulates and secretin inhibits both the basal motor activity of the sigmoid and cholecystokinin-induced motor activity. Neither cholecystokinin nor secretin influences motor activity of the rectum (Dinosa et al., 1973). Cholecystokinin is also a powerful stimulant in patients with irritable bowel syndrome. It is likely that what was formerly conceived to be a "gastrocolic reflex" (neural) is actually a gastroileocolic response to hormonal release.

Christensen, J.: The controls of gastrointestinal movements: Some old and new views. N. Engl. J. Med., 285:85, 1971.

IRRITABLE BOWEL SYNDROME

DEFINITION AND PREVALENCE. The irritable bowel syndrome is characterized by a triad of symptoms consisting of altered bowel habits, abdominal pain, and the absence of detectable organic disease. The altered bowel habits often refer to alternating constipation and diarrhea, although one of the two phases generally tends to predominate in a given patient.

The irritable bowel syndrome is the most common disorder encountered in gastrointestinal practice and may represent as much as 50 per cent of all gastrointestinal illness in countries like the United States. It is seen more often in women than men and usually occurs in younger persons, three fourths being between the ages of 20 and 50. Symptoms begin before age 20 in one fifth of patients. Many of the terms used to describe this disorder are inappropriate. Among them are *mucous colitis, adaptive colitis, nervous colon, spastic colon, unstable colon,* and *irritable colon.* Since it is not known whether the colon is exclusively involved in this disorder, it appears wise to refer to an irritable bowel rather than irritable colon. In any event, it is distinctly unwise to use the term "colitis," first, because no inflammation exists, and second, because this term is frightening to patients who associate "colitis" with inflammatory bowel disease. The very use of this term may have a deleterious effect on the course of the illness.

Painless diarrhea is sometimes considered separately from the irritable bowel syndrome, because it appears to be different in its precipitating factors, pathogenesis, and pathologic anatomy. For example, the hypertrophied circular muscle found in irritable bowel syndrome is not found with painless diarrhea, and painless diarrhea is more often directly associated with a precipitating stimulus such as emotional tension.

ETIOLOGY. Not only is the etiology of irritable bowel syndrome unclear, but it is probable that this syndrome includes a number of disorders for which specific causes may eventually be discovered. For example, prior to the recognition of lactose intolerance, many patients with lactase deficiency were diagnosed as having irritable bowel syndrome. In the future other patients with carbohydrate enzyme deficiency or maladaptation may be separated from this entity, but it presently appears that there will remain a group of patients with an abnormal neuromuscular irritability for whom the diagnosis is warranted.

Emotional and social stresses are usually present and are thought to be at least aggravating factors and perhaps even to play a causative role. Patients who live or have traveled in tropical areas may have symptoms which persist after attacks of dysentery, either amebic or bacterial.

The chances of irritable bowel syndrome continuing after acute dysentery are higher in patients who have psychologic disturbances.

PATHOGENESIS. Most physiologic investigations of irritable bowel syndrome have centered around motility studies, and the majority have been performed in the colon rather than the small bowel or other parts of the gastrointestinal tract. For this reason there is more information concerning the colonic motor disorder than other features. The colonic neuromuscular apparatus in patients with irritable bowel syndrome appears to be more sensitive than normal to a number of stimuli. Although basal pressures are not very different from normal, high spastic waves of contraction can be induced in patients with irritable bowel syndrome by a number of stimuli of diverse origins. Included are emotional stress, feeding, neostigmine, morphine, and balloon distention of the rectum. These exaggerated responses have been interpreted as implying an autonomic neuromuscular irritability. Recent studies of colonic myoelectric activity indicate an increased incidence of 3 cycles per second slow wave frequency in irritable bowel patients as opposed to the more characteristic 6 cycles per second in normal subjects. Colonoscopic, and occasionally morphologic, studies of the involved colonic musculature often demonstrate markedly hypertrophied circular muscle, especially in the rectosigmoid.

CLINICAL MANIFESTATIONS. Barium enema often shows exaggerated haustral contraction, and colonic motility recordings reveal episodic spastic waves of high amplitude. The haustral contractions retard the forward transit of stool and result in constipation. Constipated stools are often described as like marbles or pellets accompanied by passage of mucus. Patients with predominant diarrhea tend to have a colon more effaced and smooth in radiologic outline, although often contracted.

Although the clinical presentation varies greatly, a particular patient tends to have a pattern typical for him or her. Abdominal pain is the most common complaint, along with altered bowel habits, which may be constipation, diarrhea, or alternating constipation and diarrhea. Pain may be described as crampy, aching, stabbing, piercing, or excruciating, but the type and its location are characteristic for a given individual. Rarely is it periumbilical. Characteristically it does not interfere with sleep, even though it may persist for long periods during the day. Sometimes the pain is relieved by passing flatus, especially when gas is trapped in the hepatic or splenic flexures. When gas is present, stools may be expelled explosively, often triggered by a meal. Recent studies show increased sensitivity to gas and intolerance of it rather than increased quantities.

Associated symptoms often attributed to excessive vasomotor autonomic lability include excessive flushing, palpitation, weakness, lethargy, and headaches. Patients are often concerned about the possibility of malignancy, but weight loss is unusual unless severe depression is present. The course is completely benign.

PSYCHOLOGIC FACTORS. Psychiatric illness has been shown to precede gastrointestinal symptoms in the majority of cases, although this often goes unrecognized. Depression and hysteria are the most commonly associated psychiatric illnesses. Patients often rate between neurotic and normal on the Eysenck personality inventory test, implying a psychosomatic or psychophysiologic relationship.

Special personality traits have been attributed to patients with irritable bowel syndrome. They are described as being rigid, obsessive-compulsive people who retain tight controls over their impulses and are methodical, conscientious, precise, and punctual. It has been suggested that alternations in their symptoms represent shifts between psychologic holding back (maintaining control) and letting go in an aggressive, deprecatory way. Headaches usually accompany a controlled intellectual phase.

Controlled testing of responses to emotion in the laboratory shows that situations evoking hostility and anger result in augmentation of colonic motor activity, whereas circumstances leading to a feeling of hopelessness and giving up result in diminution of colonic motor activity. Based on our knowledge of the paradoxical motility of diarrhea (see above) and constipation, the implications of these findings are that patients with predominantly hostile and aggressive attitudes could be expected to suffer constipation, whereas the depressed patient who has given up is more likely to develop diarrhea.

PHYSICAL EXAMINATION. Physical findings are normal except for tenderness over the colon, usually the sigmoid, which can often be palpated as a thickened cord. Sigmoidoscopy shows no mucosal lesions but often demonstrates tenderness and spasticity. Excess mucus may be present, as well as some degree of hyperemia associated with spasm. *Melanosis coli* (brown pigmentation of mucosa) may indicate laxative abuse of the anthracine type, including cascara and senna. Barium enema may induce pain and segmental spasm in the sigmoid as well as exaggerated haustral contractions in patients with constipation, or may show effacement of the usual haustral markings in patients with diarrhea. Stool examination for ova and parasites is negative.

DIFFERENTIAL DIAGNOSIS. Differential considerations depend in part on the major manifestations of the syndrome and their location. Symptoms of diarrhea raise the possibility of thyrotoxicosis, malignant disease, carcinoid, Zollinger-Ellison syndrome, medullary carcinoma of the thyroid, parasitic infestation, and inflammatory bowel disease. Symptoms of constipation bring up consideration of hypothyroidism, hyperparathyroidism, and obstruction. The location of the pain dictates certain differential considerations. Hepatic flexure syndrome often mimics gallbladder disease. Mid-transverse colonic pain sometimes is confused with peptic ulcer or pancreatitis, and splenic flexure pain with heart disease or gastric disorder. Painful sigmoid spasm is sometimes difficult to differentiate from diverticular disease except on the basis of barium enema and colonoscopy.

TREATMENT. Because of its multifactorial nature, the irritable bowel syndrome is best treated by a holistic but individualistic approach. At the outset it must be recognized that prolonged treatment will be needed. The initial evaluation must be complete and thorough enough to convince both the patient and the examining physician of the accuracy of the diagnosis. An explanation to the patient that he has an illness related to bowel irritability is warranted, and cancer fears must be allayed. The patient should understand that he has a chronic disorder which is benign. The clinician must be sensitive to subtle symptoms of depression and responsive to the patient's need for support. Antidepressant medication is prescribed when depression is present. Milieu therapy is employed wherever feasible, assisting the patient to make his decision about appropriate changes in environmental factors. Spasmolytic drugs are prescribed, such as dicyclomine hydrochloride in 20-mg doses one hour before meals (to

reduce gastrocolic responses) and at bedtime. In elderly people subject to hypotensive episodes, 10-mg doses are appropriate. Pain may respond to a heating pad or, if severe, may require cautious use of Talwin or Demerol. Opiates should be avoided if possible because of potential addiction and because they augment colonic spasm. A diet high in bran and fiber is prescribed. Although it has not been established that high fiber diet is preventive or therapeutic, the evidence is suggestive enough to warrant its use. Studies have shown that increased dietary bran augments stool weight and increases the speed of transit, diminishes colonic pressures, alters lipid metabolism, and binds bile salts, metabolic ions, and vitamins. Hydrophilic colloids can be particularly helpful in patients who have alternating constipation and diarrhea, as these agents tend to soften the constipated stool and solidify the diarrheal stool. Gas-forming foods such as those in the legume and cabbage families are to be eliminated, as well as milk when there is suggestion of milk intolerance. (For further treatment of diarrhea and constipation see Ch. 395.4 and 395.5.) Cigarette smoking is discouraged.

Although the therapeutic implications have not yet been defined, it has been shown that 70 per cent of patients with spastic response to rectal distention can suppress this response with operant conditioning or biofeedback training, by observing the spasm which is present on manometric tracing. Finally, for extreme cases long myotomies have been performed in hopes of alleviating a functional distal obstruction caused by circular muscle hypertrophy.

PROGNOSIS. A life stress chart relating symptoms to daily events can be helpful in demonstrating correlations which would otherwise be missed. The disorder is a chronic, sometimes disabling one, and its symptoms will recur episodically. Above one third of patients will become symptom free, but the majority will continue to have intermittent symptoms. Patients with painless diarrhea show a much better prognosis than do those with pain. Those with a past history of dysentery also have a more favorable prognosis, whereas the presence of psychologic factors makes the prognosis worse. The influence of a major life change may be remarkable.

Chaudhary, N. A., and Truelove, S. C.: Irritable colon syndrome. Quart. J. Med., 31:307, 1962.

Hislop, I. G.: Psychological significance of irritable colon syndrome. Gut, 12:452, 1971.

Mendeloff, A. I., Monk, M., Siegel, C. I., and Lilienfeld, A.: Illness experience in life stresses in patients with irritable colon and ulcerative colitis. N. Engl. J. Med., 282:15, 1970.

Waller, S. L.: Irritable bowel syndrome: Clinical and pathophysiological features. Rendic. R. Gastroenterol., 3:80, 1971.

Young, S. F., Alpers, D. H., Norlan, C. C., and Woodruff, R. A.: Psychiatric illness and irritable bowel syndrome. Gastroenterology, 70:162, 1976.

MEGACOLON

DEFINITION. The term megacolon designates a colon that is increased in diameter over normal. Normal diameter varies, depending on age and size, but generally should be less than 6 cm for adults. The dilated colon is almost invariably associated with severe constipation. When extremely large stools are passed or when passage is an infrequent as every two to three weeks, colonic dilatation can be assumed. Two major types of megacolon are recognized: congenital or aganglionic megacolon and acquired megacolon.

Congenital Megacolon
(Aganglionic Megacolon, Hirschsprung's Disease)

Hirschsprung's disease is characterized by a large dilated colon proximal to a narrow segment in which the intramural ganglion cells of Auerbach's and Meissner's plexuses are congenitally absent, leading to abnormal motility in the narrowed segment, which therefore constitutes a functionally obstructing segment.

INCIDENCE. Aganglionosis occurs in approximately 1 in 5000 births. There is a 9:1 preponderance in males. A familial occurrence of 3.8 per cent has been noted. Down's syndrome is observed in over 2 per cent of cases, and other associated congenital anomalies have been reported.

PATHOGENESIS. The aganglionosis results from an arrest of the caudad migration of neural crest cells from the notochord during embryonic development. Therefore the aganglionic segment extends distally from a given point to and including the internal anal sphincter. Segments most commonly involved are the rectum and rectosigmoid, although aganglionosis can extend from the small bowel to the anus. Very short segments, involving only the internal anal sphincter, have been described. The aganglionic segment is persistently contracted, causing dilatation proximal to it. Megaloureter and megalobladder have also been reported.

CLINICAL MANIFESTATIONS. When symptoms appear within the first day or two of life, the presentation is that of intestinal obstruction with meconium ileus, marked abdominal distention, and obstipation. Later presentation is that of severe constipation, which in 80 per cent of patients with Hirschsprung's disease appears before the end of the first month of life. This later manifestation is characterized by abdominal distention, hard masses in the abdomen, poor nutritional state, growth retardation, and occasional episodes of enterocolitis with fever and diarrhea.

When aganglionosis affects only a very short segment of distal colon or is restricted to the internal anal sphincter, symptoms of constipation may not develop until late adolescence or early adulthood. Constipation then is progressive as opposed to the acute intestinal obstruction seen during infancy. The usual complaints are those of recurrent fecal impactions.

DIAGNOSIS. Neonatal obstruction must be differentiated from other causes of intestinal obstruction in infancy, including atresia, imperforate anus, and congenital bands. Symptoms which appear later usually require differentiation from various causes of acquired megacolon (see below).

Aganglionic megacolon is differentiated from acquired megacolon on the basis of history, physical examination, barium enema, rectosphincteric manometric studies, and biopsy. Patients with aganglionic megacolon rarely have fecal incontinence, whereas patients with acquired megacolon frequently do. Digital examination of the rectum reveals an empty rectal ampulla in half of patients with Hirschsprung's disease because of the functional distal obstruction. (In the absence of an aganglionic segment, stool is felt down to the anal verge.) Barium enema confirms the absence of stool in the rectal ampulla and demonstrates a narrowed distal segment in about 80 per cent of patients. Lateral films are the most effective means of radiologically demonstrating short involved segments. In acquired megaco-

lon dilatation extends to the sphincteric area. Pressure studies of the rectum and anal sphincter demonstrate an absence of normal relaxation of the internal sphincter in response to rectal distention (Fig. 7). Normal sphincter relaxation occurs in acquired megacolon. Full thickness biopsy of the rectal muscle obtained under general or spinal anesthesia demonstrates absence of ganglion cells in Meissner's submucosal plexus and Auerbach's myenteric plexus in Hirschsprung's disease but a normal complement of cells in acquired megacolon. The diagnosis of Hirschsprung's disease can be excluded on the basis of a punch or suction biopsy of the mucosa when Meissner's plexus cells are demonstrated. However, a failure to find ganglion cells may be attributable to technical factors, because detection of cells in the submucosal plexus is more difficult than in the myenteric plexus. Rectosphincteric manometric studies are sometimes the only means of demonstrating ultra short segment involvement, especially in those cases involving only the internal sphincter, because interpretation of muscle biopsy is difficult if muscle biopsies are taken from a point more distal than 1 or 2 cm above the sphincter. This is because the myenteric plexuses disappear at the sphincter, which is composed only of circular muscle and therefore has no intramural area at which ganglion cells normally aggregate. Biopsy is more accurate in acquired megacolon when ganglion cells can be demonstrated than in Hirschsprung's disease, in which they are absent, whereas barium enema

Transient Distention

HIRSCHSPRUNG'S DISEASE

Figure 7. *A*, Normal rectosphincteric reflexes. Transient rectal distention (arrows) produces reflex relaxation of the internal anal sphincter (upper tracing) and contraction of the external sphincter (lower tracing). (From Schuster, M. M., et al.: Bull. Johns Hopkins Hosp., 116:79, 1965.) *B*, Rectosphincteric reflexes in patient with Hirschsprung's disease. Internal sphincter relaxation is absent. (In this instance contraction occurs instead.) External sphincter reflex is normal. (With permission of the New England Journal of Medicine.)

is more useful in Hirschsprung's disease when a contracted segment can be demonstrated.

TREATMENT. Neonatal intestinal obstruction may require colostomy proximal to the aganglionic segment as a lifesaving measure. A more definitive surgical approach can be performed later when further growth has made the operation technically easier. In general the simplest approach is the best. This usually involves surgery even in short aganglionic segments. Short segment involvement is best treated by myectomy with resection of a thin strip of muscle which can provide diagnosis and treatment simultaneously. Longer segments may be treated by abdominal resection of the involved area proximal to the peritoneal reflection with myectomy below. Other operative approaches include resection of the entire aganglionic segment with coloanal anastomosis (Swenson procedure); a retrorectal end to side anastomosis of normal colon to rectum (Duhamel procedure), with resection of the aganglionic segment proximal to the peritoneal reflection; or resection of proximal aganglionic segment with mucosal denudation of the rectum, subsequently bringing normal colon into the lumen of the rectum, with serosa of normal colon approximated to mucosa of the rectum (Soave procedure). The incidence of complications of these procedures depends on the type of procedure, being least with a myectomy. Complications include impotence and incontinence. Most of the procedures lead to good results and are compatible with normal life.

Tobon, F., and Schuster, M. M.: Megacolon: Special diagnostic and therapeutic features. Johns Hopkins Med. J., 135:91, 1974.

Acquired Megacolon
(Idiopathic Megacolon, Psychogenic Megacolon, Secondary Megacolon)

ETIOLOGY AND INCIDENCE. The etiology of acquired megacolon is often indeterminate but may be secondary to any of the causes of constipation referred to in Ch. 395.5. Acquired megacolon may be assumed if there is evidence that megacolon did not exist on previous examination. Colonic dilatation is seen most often in children and in the elderly. It is quite possible that the acquired idiopathic megacolon of childhood and early adulthood derives from an organic cause which is presently unknown (1) because in this group of patients constipation begins before the age of one month in 30 per cent and before the first year of life in 60 per cent, (2) because there is a strong positive family history, and (3) because of inability to demonstrate psychogenic factors in many instances.

PATHOGENESIS. Pathogenesis in young patients appears different from that of the elderly, because constipation during the first month of life is often present in young patients with acquired megacolon but not in elderly patients. In young patients dilatation may involve only the distal colon, whereas the entire colon usually appears dilated in older patients.

CLINICAL MANIFESTATIONS. Encopresis (fecal incontinence) is present in almost half of the patients with idiopathic megacolon and may also be present in other acquired forms, but is absent in patients with Hirschsprung's disease. Personality disorders occur in about 60 per cent of patients with encopresis but are uncommon in patients who do not have encopresis. The history is often that of gradually progressive constipation, requiring larger and more frequent doses of laxatives.

Fecal impactions and overflow incontinence are common.

DIAGNOSIS. Primary causes are to be ruled out on the basis of symptoms and signs associated with these disorders. Primary underlying disorders include neurologic disease (parkinsonism, multiple sclerosis, spinal cord lesions, diabetic visceral neuropathy, Chagas' disease, and myotonic dystrophy), drugs (anticholinergic, antiparkinsonian, and phenothiazines), spasm caused by painful anal conditions (such as fissures, perirectal abscesses, and thrombosed hemorrhoids) mechanical obstruction, collagen vascular diseases (notably scleroderma), and metabolic disorders (such as hypothyroidism, hypokalemia, hypoparathyroidism, and lead poisoning). The major differential diagnosis in youth is that of aganglionic megacolon, and differentiation from this disorder has been discussed under Congenital Megacolon.

TREATMENT. Treatment, which is predominantly behavioral, involving bowel retraining, is generally more successful in younger than in older patients, even though colonic dilatation may be more dramatic in the young. After initial disimpaction, efforts are made to have the patient develop a stimulus-response pattern in relationship to meals by trying to have a voluntary movement five minutes after eating breakfast or supper. If a movement is not achieved within ten minutes, an enema is administered to initiate defecation. This process is repeated without variation every day or every other day until a bowel pattern is established. In the meantime laxatives are gradually withdrawn or replaced by more simple and milder medications. Hard stools are treated with wetting agents such as dioctyl sodium sulfosuccinate (Colace or Doxinate) in doses of 50 to 200 mg. Hydrophilic colloids such as carboxymethylcellulose may also be used, and a diet rich in fiber, bran, and prunes is prescribed. General exercises are encouraged, as well as leg-raising exercises to strengthen abdominal musculature. Of great importance are the assessment and management of psychologic factors. (For further details see Ch. 395.5.)

CHAGAS' DISEASE. Chagas' disease, caused by trypanosome infection, may lead to extensive destruction of ganglion cells and gross dilatation of the colon, esophagus, duodenum, urinary bladder, and heart (see Ch. 194.3). Destruction of 90 per cent of ganglion cells is required for clinical dilatation. The disorder appears predominantly in South America but has been described as far north as Texas. In sharp contrast to Hirschsprung's disease, in Chagas' disease it is the aganglionic viscera that are dilated.

DIABETIC DIARRHEA

An uncommon form of diarrhea is that seen in diabetics with visceral autonomic neuropathy and peripheral neuropathy. Suggestions of autonomic involvement include orthostatic hypotension, gastric atony, abnormal sweating, bladder or pupillary abnormalities, and impotence. Symptoms are attributed to degeneration of autonomic ganglia and dorsal nerve roots.

Diffuse watery diarrhea, frequently nocturnal, is usually episodic but may be continuous. Extreme urgency may awaken the patient from sleep, and there may be associated urinary or fecal incontinence. Mild steatorrhea may be present with normal pancreatic enzymes.

Positive findings on physical examination are those of orthostatic hypotension, pupillary abnormalities, and depressed peripheral deep tendon reflexes, particularly ankle jerk. X-ray examination may reveal gastric atony and rapid intestinal transit. Severity of symptoms need not correlate with severity of diabetes.

Treatment is difficult, frustrating, and frequently unrewarding. Vigorous diabetic control, although not uniformly successful, may be helpful in some instances. Antimicrobial treatment of intestinal bacterial overgrowth may be useful, especially when steatorrhea is present. Despite the annoying nature of the symptoms, the primary health hazard is not that of diarrhea but of the underlying diabetes.

PROCTALGIA FUGAX

A disorder of undetermined origin, proctalgia fugax consists of short-lived rectal pain, occurring episodically without demonstrable organic cause. Symptoms usually occur between puberty and age 60, in patients who are otherwise in excellent health; symptoms disappear by age 70. Some reports note a preponderance of males. Pain begins abruptly and may awaken the patient at night. It lasts from a few minutes to half an hour and is often excruciating. Described as sharp, cramp-like, gnawing, or grinding, it is located in the area of the rectum. Attacks may be precipitated by bowel movement, coitus, or mental fatigue. Mild attacks disappear spontaneously without residue, but severe attacks induce a weak, tired feeling. There are no associated intestinal disturbances such as altered bowel habit, tenesmus, or paresthesia. Patients have been noted on personality profiles to be anxious and perfectionistic, with a focus upon pain, while somatizing emotional conflicts to the gastrointestinal tract.

Rectal neuralgia is differentiated on the basis of longer duration of pain and its burning nature and radiation to the perineum, sacral region, and genitalia, as well as associated paresthesia and hyperesthesia. Coccygodynia is generally also of longer duration, and pain may be referred to the gluteal area. Rectal examination accentuates the pain, especially with movement of the coccyx. Rectal tabetic crises generally last for hours and are associated with positive serology.

TREATMENT AND PROGNOSIS. Firm upward pressure on the anus and hot sitz baths occasionally have been reported to provide some relief. Smooth muscle relaxants such as amyl nitrate and nitroglycerin and drugs such as quinine which affect striated muscle generally have proved ineffective. Psychotherapy may help the patient adjust to his illness and may relieve concern about cancer, but unfortunately it is not curative. Aside from being annoying and disruptive, the disorder does not affect the general state of health.

Pilling, L. F., Swenson, W. M., and Hill, J. R.: Psychologic factors of proctalgia fugax. Dis. Colon Rectum, 8:372, 1965.

INTESTINAL PSEUDO-OBSTRUCTION

DEFINITION. Intestinal pseudo-obstruction comprises a clinical and radiologic picture of acute or chronic intestinal obstruction for which no mechanical cause can be demonstrated.

ETIOLOGY. Known causes for acute pseudo-obstruction are renal failure, pancreatitis, pneumonia, congestive heart failure, spinal cord injury, and electrolyte imbalance. Chronic intestinal pseudo-obstruction may be idiopathic or associated with myxedema, scleroderma, hypo- or hyperthyroidism, celiac disease, peritonitis, amyloidosis, Chagas' disease, myotonic dystrophy, Hirschsprung's disease, or drug toxicity. When acute, the signs or symptoms disappear after treatment of the underlying disorder. Esophageal motility disturbances can be demonstrated by cineesophagram or manometric studies, which often reveal diminished esophageal peristalsis and incomplete lower esophageal sphincter relaxation. Duodenal myoelectric activity is normal in the basal state, but patients with chronic idiopathic intestinal obstruction do not demonstrate the normal increase of electric spike or motor activity in response to duodenal distention. This feature may account in part for disturbances in transit, because the intestine is capable of responding normally to exogenous neurohumoral stimulation (neostigmine and also secretin). The underlying disorder is unlikely to be due to primary impairment of smooth muscle but rather to a disorder of control mechanisms (Sullivan et al., 1977). The colon may be involved as well as the internal anal sphincter. In the idiopathic form the saccular pseudodiverticula, which can be seen with scleroderma of the small and large bowel, are not present. Some patients have abnormal sweating responses, suggesting the possibility of autonomic dysfunction. Histologic examination is often normal but may reveal mild inflammation and small round cell infiltration. Electron microscopic studies are nonspecific, and smooth muscle and ganglion cells are normal.

CLINICAL MANIFESTATIONS. Symptoms consist of intermittent abdominal pain, distention, and vomiting, which may be feculent. Diarrhea and steatorrhea may be present. With malabsorption weight loss occurs. Bowel sounds are diminished, and the abdomen is tympanitic to percussion. Plain films of the abdomen reveal distended loops of small intestine (and occasionally the colon) with air-fluid levels.

TREATMENT. Broad-spectrum antimicrobials may effect improvement in steatorrhea. In the secondary form treatment directed toward the underlying cause may be rewarding, but treatment of chronic idiopathic intestinal pseudo-obstruction is less successful. Intestinal decompression by long intestinal tube may be necessary during acute episodes of distention. Attempts at therapy with cholinergic medication and metoclopromide have been disappointing. Medical therapy has been ineffective in general. Surgical intervention is usually fruitless and should be avoided if possible.

Moss, A. A., Goldberg, H. I., and Brotman, M.: Idiopathic intestinal pseudo-obstruction. Am. J. Roentgenol., 115:312, 1972.

PSEUDO-OBSTRUCTION OF THE COLON
(Ileus of the Colon)

Colonic pseudo-obstruction, like intestinal pseudo-obstruction, is manifested by distention with clinical and radiologic findings suggesting mechanical obstruction, although no organic cause is detectable even by exploratory laparotomy. Etiologic considerations are similar to those of the more diffuse intestinal form. The symptoms are those of abdominal distention, crampy abdominal pain, constipation and diarrhea, and vomiting (which, in contrast to intestinal pseudo-obstruction, is not feculent). Symptoms are often intermittent. Cecostomy or ileostomy can prove lifesaving in instances of severe distention. In some instances minor small bowel dilatation is present. Approximately one fourth of patients die after repeated episodes, often from cardiovascular respiratory insufficiency. Cecal perforation is also a danger; this can be avoided by the diverting operation.

Pseudo-obstruction is to be distinguished from mechanical obstruction of the large bowel, which is more often due to malignant tumors, diverticulitis, or volvulus.

SMALL LEFT COLON SYNDROME

A rare cause of distal colonic obstruction is seen predominantly in newborn infants. Forty per cent of patients are offspring of insulin-dependent diabetic mothers. Barium enema reveals a uniformly small left colon from anus to splenic flexure, and ganglion cells are normal. Prognosis is generally good without surgical intervention.

Davis, W. S., and Campbell, J. B.: Neonatal small left colon syndrome. Am. J. Dis. Child., 129:1024, 1975.

400. GASTROINTESTINAL ALLERGY AND FOOD INTOLERANCE

DEFINITION.   There are two distinct types of allergy involving the gastrointestinal tract. Each is different from food intolerance, which can also affect the gastrointestinal tract.

Gastrointestinal allergy represents an antigen-antibody reaction in the gastrointestinal tract, usually as a result of ingested foods or drugs. Bacterial antigens may sometimes produce gastrointestinal allergy. Most cases appear to represent the immediate type of reaction, usually associated with antibodies that result in the release of a number of pharmacologic-reactive substances, including histamine. Reaction usually takes place within minutes after exposure to antigen (like hay fever and asthma). *Food allergy* may affect organ systems other than the digestive system, producing manifestations such as hives, eczema, asthma, rhinitis, and occasional central nervous manifestations. A family history of allergy is common in patients with food allergies and gastrointestinal allergies.

Quite different from these two conditions, and not related to immune hypersensitivity, is *food intolerance,* which may relate to the physical state of food, e.g., solid boluses producing obstructive symptoms in patients with esophageal strictures or cancer. Liquids may be regurgitated or aspirated in patients with neurologic impairment of the upper esophagus and cricopharyngeal muscle. Specific enzyme deficiencies occur in specific food intolerance (e.g., lactase deficiency produces intolerance of milk with distention, flatulence, and diarrhea). However, most food intolerance is poorly understood. Fatty food or spicy food intolerance is noted in many gastrointestinal disorders of diverse origins.

Specific causes for fatty food intolerance (such as pancreatic disease leading to insufficiency of lipase, or biliary tract obstruction resulting in poor emulsification of fats) are usually not present in these general conditions to account for the fatty food intolerance.

Some people and some families are more susceptible than others to bacterial fermentation of nonabsorbable carbohydrates such as raffinose contained in legumes. Bloating and gaseous distention may be quite distressful. Intestinal discomfort and distention following cabbage ingestion have been attributed to inhibition of intestinal motility by flavone compounds. Fatty foods may delay gastric emptying and produce some degree of gastric distention. Our present understanding of most of these complaints is meager.

CLINICAL MANIFESTATIONS.   Allergic phenomena may occur at any age after a period of sensitization and can affect any area of the alimentary tract from lips to anus. Initial symptoms, occurring within minutes of exposure to the allergens, consist of swelling, burning, and itching of the lips, mouth, and pharynx. Vomiting, abdominal pain and diarrhea may be severe. Endoscopic examination may show hives and marked spasm in the esophagus, stomach, and duodenum. Urticaria may also lead to dysphagia. The abdominal pain is often excruciating and crampy and may be related to edema. Mucus and blood may accompany severe diarrhea. More general manifestations include skin hives, asthmatic wheezing, arthralgia, and purpura.

DIAGNOSIS.   A personal and family history of allergy in conjunction with the aforementioned symptom complex should raise a suspicion of allergic response. Specific foods such as shellfish, eggs, and nuts are among the more common offenders. The diagnosis is more apparent if extraintestinal involvement is also present such as urticaria or asthmatic wheezing. The suspected offending agent may be confirmed as the culprit by skin testing, which, however, carries the danger of a generalized allergic response. Skin tests with food are less reliable than with inhaled antigens. Peripheral eosinophilia and eosinophilia in mucus discharge are suggestive.

Most helpful in defining the allergy is a food diary kept meticulously in conjunction with notation of symptoms. Also useful are elimination diets, which begin by eliminating all well known allergenic materials and gradually add one at a time. Confirmation is most valid if the material is reintroduced without the patient's knowledge, which may require instillation through a nasogastric tube. Folklore has a strong influence on the patient's concept of food tolerance, and many complaints are best handled by appropriate reeducation. Conditioning of the gastrointestinal tract and of preferences can be rapid and dramatic so that foods taken under adverse circumstances may subsequently be poorly tolerated, leading to motor disturbances such as gastric atony, delayed emptying, nausea, vomiting, or diarrhea.

TREATMENT AND PROGNOSIS.   If only one or two offending substances are responsible and the antigen is detected, elimination of this from the diet constitutes a cure provided that all sources of the antigen are known. More commonly, however, multiple allergies exist. Also, allergic responses may be superimposed upon other underlying disorders (such as milk intolerance in ulcerative colitis), in which case elimination of the offending substance may improve only one aspect, and sometimes this is a minor component of the illness. No satisfactory method of desensitization has been developed in food allergy. Parenteral epinephrine may be helpful for the acute attack, and spasmolytic agents may help alleviate hypermotility manifested by severe abdominal pain. Antihistamines, although not dramatically successful, may be beneficial, partly because of the sedation they produce. Interdermal injections of 0.5 to 1 ml of a 1:1000 solution of epinephrine may produce prompt relief of the acute severe abdominal attacks.

Ingelfinger, F. J., Lowell, F. C., and Franklin, W.: Gastrointestinal allergy. N. Engl. J. Med., 241:303, 1949.
Koch, J. P., and Donaldson, R. M., Jr.: A survey of food intolerances in hospitalized patients. N. Engl. J. Med., 271:657, 1964.

GASTROINTESTINAL ALLERGY IN CHILDREN

Childhood gastrointestinal allergy is most often attributable to cow's milk. The syndrome is characterized by diarrhea and colic developing a few days or weeks after the infant is placed on cow's milk. Vomiting, eczema, respiratory disease, and thrombocytopenia may be present. Frequently there is a strong family history of eczema, asthma, and rhinitis. Peripheral eosinophilia may be present, and there may be occult blood in the stools. Proctoscopy may reveal acute ulcerations indistinguishable from those of nonspecific ulcerative colitis. These disappear on withdrawal of the offending antigen (Freier and Kletter, 1970). In some children the allergy manifests itself by digestive symptoms alone. Withdrawal of milk results in prompt improvement and reinstitution of milk in recurrence of symptoms. Lactose intolerance must be considered and ruled out. Milk substitutes such as Nutramigen (hydrolyzed casein with corn oil and sucrose) are generally well tolerated. Soy bean substitutes may be helpful, but rarely infants are allergic to soy protein and may develop a picture identical to that of milk allergy. When this is suspected, soy must be eliminated.

401. DIVERTICULA OF THE INTESTINAL TRACT

DEFINITION. A diverticulum is a saccular outpouching of one or more layers of the walls of the intestine. Diverticula occur in all levels of the intestine from the hypopharynx to the sigmoid colon. With the exception of Meckel's diverticulum and possibly the solitary cecal diverticulum, all diverticula appear to be acquired herniations of mucosa and submucosa through defects in the muscle wall, and can often be shown to result from increased intraluminal pressure. High pressures are often related to excessive or disordered motility in the intestine immediately distal to the diverticula. The herniated diverticulum frequently appears at a weak point where arteries penetrate serosal and muscular layers. Diverticula are age related, appearing with increased frequency with age, possibly as a result of exposure to high intraluminal pressures throughout life. Diverticula are rarely encountered before the age of 30 and appear with increasing frequency and increasing numbers after the age of 50. Diverticula are most commonly encountered in the colon, especially in the sigmoid colon, which has higher intraluminal pressures than other areas.

ESOPHAGEAL DIVERTICULA

The customary division of esophageal diverticula according to the three major locations within the esophagus is a rational one, because the features characterizing each of these diverticula are distinctive. The three types are hypopharyngeal, mid-esophageal, and epiphrenic.

Hypopharyngeal (Zenker's) Diverticulum

This is the most common form of esophageal diverticulum. Although strictly speaking it is located in the hypopharynx rather than the esophagus, it is generally included among esophageal diverticula, because its pathogenesis is thought to be related to cricopharyngeal muscle pathology and its symptoms are often esophageal. Zenker's diverticulum is seen in 1 out of 800 upper gastrointestinal series. It affects males above the age of 60 and generally represents a pulsion herniation between fibers of the cricopharyngeal muscle. Motility studies reveal that the pulsion pressures derive from discoordination between pharyngeal contraction and cricopharyngeal sphincter relaxation. The sphincter appears to relax normally with swallowing but closes prematurely before pharyngeal contraction is completed.

Among the earliest symptoms are a sense of irritation or scratchiness in the throat. With time the sac increases in size until a bulge may be noted in the lateral neck. As the sac enlarges, dysphagia ensues, and spillage of diverticular contents into the pharynx and larynx may induce coughing or aspiration, leading to pneumonia, lung abscess, and bronchiectasis. Gurgling noises may be heard during swallowing, and regurgitation and choking occur. There may be a sense of fullness or a visible bulge in the neck with eating, and this can be decompressed by manual massage.

Ultimately compression may obstruct the esophagus enough to interfere with nutrition and result in weight loss. Diagnosis is made by barium study, preferably with cine-esophagram, with attention directed specifically at the hypopharyngeal and cricopharyngeal area. Endoscopy may be dangerous because of risk of perforation.

Definitive treatment involves correction of the motor abnormality by cricopharyngeal myotomy. When the diverticulum is large, this is performed in conjunction with resection of the diverticulum.

Mid-Esophageal Diverticulum

Although it is assumed by some that mid-esophageal diverticula result from traction caused by contiguous inflammation in the mediastinum, especially from inflamed lymph nodes, the few cases which have been studied manometrically show motor abnormalities distal to the diverticulum, and cine-esophagram often shows hold-up of a swallowed bolus (marshmallow). Some diverticula in this area may actually represent traction and have no demonstrable motor abnormality. Most patients are asymptomatic, but some with pronounced motor abnormality complain of intermittent dysphagia and occasional food impaction. The radiologic diagnosis may be confirmed endoscopically. Treatment is seldom needed, because the diverticula are usually small. Occasionally, therapy may be required for the distal motor disturbance (see Diffuse Esophageal Spasm in Ch. 396).

Epiphrenic Diverticulum

Epiphrenic diverticula occur a few centimeters proximal to the sphincter and can often be shown to relate to hypertensive lower esophageal sphincters with discoordinate relaxation (similar to the situation in Zenker's diverticulum). Hypertrophy of the lower esophageal sphincter muscle has been described. Epiphrenic diverticula also have been reported in association with achalasia. Most epiphrenic diverticula are asymptomatic, but occasionally large diverticula may produce overnight regurgitation of large amounts of fluid. Treatment is rarely required. In severe instances diverticulectomy and myotomy are performed. Those associated with achalasia are treated by myotomy for achalasia, because brusk pneumostatic dilatation may be hazardous under those circumstances.

Cross, F. S.: Esophageal diverticula: Related neuromuscular problems. Ann. Otol., 77:914, 1968.
Dorsey, J. M., and Randolph, D. A.: Long-term evaluation of pharyngoesophageal diverticulectomy. Ann. Surg., 173:680, 1971.
Goodman, H. I., and Parnes, I. H.: Epiphrenic diverticula of the esophagus. J. Thorac. Cardiovasc. Surg., 23:145, 1952.

GASTRIC DIVERTICULA

Diverticula of the stomach are rare, usually single, and most often asymptomatic. Three fourths appear high on the posterior wall of the stomach within several centimeters of the esophagogastric junction and the lesser curvature. Most of the others are located at the prepyloric area and result from obstructive disease, usually peptic or postoperative. A small percentage of diverticula are noted in the body of the stomach. The radiologic picture is usually distinctive enough to establish the diagnosis. Endoscopy with brush cytology can confirm the diagnosis or establish it in questionable cases and at the same time rule out malignancy. It is doubtful whether symptoms can be attributable to this lesion, although postural drainage and antacid therapy have been reported to be helpful for dyspeptic symptoms, postprandial fullness, pain, and vomiting for which no other cause can be determined. Bleeding from eroded mucosa is extremely rare, as is inflammation in the diverticulum. Reported success from surgical excision is difficult to evaluate.

DUODENAL DIVERTICULA

Small bowel diverticula are not uncommon and are usually encountered as an incidental finding on x-ray examination. The duodenum is the most common location, the medial surface of the second portion of the duodenum being the most frequent site. The duodenum is second in frequency only to the colon as a site of diverticulosis. These diverticula are unusual before age 30 and increase in frequency to 10 per cent above age 60. The majority are solitary, but about 20 per cent are multiple. When multiple, they are often associated with colonic diverticulosis. The duodenal bulb is rarely involved, pouches in this area being most frequently pseudodiverticula resulting from scarred retraction of portions of the duodenal bulb. They are an asymptomatic incidental finding on barium study in most instances, although some instances of postprandial distress, fullness, and pain in the epigastrium and right lower quadrant have been attributed to distention of

duodenal diverticula with intestinal contents. Relief may occur with vomiting or belching. A causal relationship to symptoms is difficult to establish. In rare instances hemorrhage and perforation with peritonitis have occurred and also obstructive jaundice caused by compression of perivaterian diverticula. Surgical resection is reversed exclusively for these demonstrated complications.

JEJUNAL AND ILEAL DIVERTICULA

Small bowel diverticula are uncommon, having an autopsy incidence of about 0.5 per cent. They increase in frequency with age and are more commonly found in the proximal than in the distal small bowel. They are usually multiple. Small bowel and colonic diverticulosis frequently coexist.

Four broad clinical manifestations exist: (1) By far the largest is the asymptomatic group. (2) Some patients have chronic dyspepsia with postprandial discomfort or pain, flatulence, or borborygmus. (3) Rarely, surgical complications such as obstruction, volvulus, perforation, intussusception, and hemorrhage may occur. (4) Multiple large diverticula may provide the setting for bacterial overgrowth caused by stagnation within the blind sacs and development of the "blind loop syndrome" (see Ch. 408).

Erect plain films of the abdomen may reveal air-fluid patterns, suggesting large mouth diverticula which can be confirmed by small bowel series. Treatment is rarely required. When macrocytic anemia and steatorrhea accompany blind loop syndrome, a broad-spectrum antimicrobial may be administered daily, and vitamin replacement, especially vitamin B_{12} and fat-soluble vitamins, is instituted.

Caplan, L. H., and Jacobson, H. G.: Small intestinal diverticulosis. Am. J. Roentgenol., 92:1048, 1964.

Meckel's Diverticulum

Meckel's diverticulum is the most common congenital anomaly of the alimentary canal and derives from incomplete obliteration of the yolk stalk (vitelline duct), resulting in a diverticulum at the antimesenteric margin of the ileum 30 to 90 cm from the ileocecal sphincter. This is a congenital diverticulum with all layers of the intestinal wall being present. Autopsies show an incidence of 1 to 2 per cent. It may contain ectopic glandular tissue — gastric, duodenal, pancreatic, or colonic. Twenty-five to 50 per cent of Meckel's diverticula are lined by gastric mucosa.

Most Meckel's diverticula are silent and are discovered only at autopsy. Symptoms usually occur in childhood and derive from the complications of diverticula. (1) *Bleeding*, the most common complication, usually develops from peptic ulceration in ectopic gastric mucosa, which is found in half of symptomatic patients (Rutherford and Akers, 1966). Bleeding is characteristically abrupt in onset, painless, and bright red or dark red when passed rectally. (2) Meckel's diverticulitis presents symptoms similar to those of acute appendicitis, usually in childhood. (3) Intestinal obstruction may result from an associated congenital band, volvulus around peridiverticular adhesions, or intussusception. (4) Perforation can result from foreign bodies, diverticulitis, or peptic ulceration.

DIAGNOSIS AND TREATMENT. Diagnosis is suspected

on the basis of the aforementioned symptoms or when symptoms of appendicitis appear before age two, because appendicitis is rare at this age, whereas one half of cases of Meckel's diverticulitis appear before age two. Resection is appropriate for symptoms or when Meckel's diverticulum is encountered at an operation, even if asymptomatic.

COLONIC DIVERTICULOSIS

PREVALENCE AND EPIDEMIOLOGY. Diverticula are encountered more often in the colon than in any other site. There is a definite increased incidence with aging. Colonic diverticula are rare before the age of 35 but increase progressively to reach a 50 per cent incidence above the age of 80. The increasing incidence with age suggests that muscle weakness may predispose to development of diverticulosis (Parks, 1969). Because of the high prevalence of colonic diverticula, and because the vast majority (80 per cent) remain asymptomatic, it is difficult to label simple diverticulosis as a disease. The term "diverticular disease" is a broad, general term which is appropriate to describe symptomatic diverticulosis (the symptoms usually being attributable to painful spasm) or the complications of diverticulosis such as diverticulitis resulting from minute or large perforations, hemorrhage, or obstruction.

PATHOGENESIS. Two broad categories of colonic diverticulosis are known. One type is thought to be related to chronic colonic spasm with increased intraluminal pressures and consequent hypertrophy of circular muscle in the vicinity of the diverticula. Manometric studies demonstrate excessively high spastic pressures in response to meals, cholinergic agents (such as neostigmine), and opiates (such as morphine). This is thought to be the physiologic basis for most of the diverticulosis which involves predominantly the sigmoid and descending colon. The spastic variety is thought to be the end result of the irritable bowel (spastic colon) syndrome. The second type, "simple massed diverticulosis," is characterized by multiple diverticula which are not associated with colonic spasm or muscle hypertrophy. Pathogenesis of this form is poorly understood.

The marked difference in prevalence in different countries has been attributed by some to dietary differences in fiber content of the diet, particularly bran. Diverticulosis is encountered 40 times more frequently in Western society than in the developing countries. This has been attributed to the higher crude fiber content of the native diet in developing countries than in Western countries, in which refined diets have eliminated much of the fiber. The protective effect of fibers is thought to be related to the increased intraluminal bulk and consequent increased diameter of the colon. Laplace's law relating to intraluminal pressures within cylinders states that for a given tension within the intestinal wall the pressures generated within the lumen are inversely proportional to the radius. The smaller the radius, the higher the pressures. This also may explain the predilection of the narrow sigmoid as the site of greatest involvement. The diverticula consist of mucosa and submucosa, which typically herniate through muscle wall at points of weakness where blood vessels penetrate from serosa to submucosa. The cause for the neuromuscular irritability which leads to spastic colon is not understood.

CLINICAL MANIFESTATIONS. No symptoms accompany diverticulosis in the majority of cases. Symptomatic diverticulosis is referred to as diverticular disease, and may result from painful colonic spasm associated with diverticula, from inflammation (diverticulitis), or from complications of inflammation such as perforation, obstruction, and hemorrhage. Diverticulitis and its complications are discussed in Ch. 414.2. The most common complaint in diverticular disease without inflammation is left lower quadrant pain, which may be mild or severe, steady or crampy, and which usually lasts from one day to a week. Eating and emotional tension frequently aggravate the symptoms, possibly by increasing spasm. Constipation may be present or alternating constipation and diarrhea. A tender sigmoid colon can be outlined by palpation as a sausage-shaped structure in the left lower quadrant. There is no rebound tenderness or abdominal rigidity, and the absence of inflammation is confirmed by the fact that there is neither fever nor leukocytosis. Bleeding from otherwise uncomplicated diverticulosis is usually brisk and may be massive but is almost invariably self-limited. Bleeding associated with diverticulitis is more often minimal or occult.

DIAGNOSIS. Asymptomatic diverticula are usually discovered incidentally on the basis of barium enema in search for other disorders. Painful diverticular disease is suspected on the basis of the manifestations just described, and confirmed by barium enema showing diverticulosis with colonic spasm that results in an asymmetrical sawtoothed pattern. In the elderly patient with this radiologic picture colonic cancer must be ruled out, because apple core lesions can be associated with diverticula proximal to them, presumably as a result of pressure build-up. Proctoscopy in diverticular disease is often painful and demonstrates rectosigmoid spasm. Diverticula rarely appear distal to the rectosigmoid, and their endoscopic detection therefore depends on the use of colonoscopy.

TREATMENT AND PROGNOSIS. The goal of treatment for the symptomatic patient with known diverticulosis is the prevention of symptoms and complications. Although the proposed therapeutic plan seems logical and some experiments suggest that it is effective, scientific proof based on hard data is not available. Treatment of asymptomatic diverticulosis is designed to increase stool bulk and to prevent constipation. To this end a high fiber diet containing 16 grams of bran per day is prescribed. Particulate matter such as grape seeds is probably best avoided. If unprocessed bran alone does not alleviate constipation, hydrophilic colloids or stool softeners are provided (see Ch. 395.5). The goals of the treatment of painful diverticular disease without inflammation are (1) to decrease intraluminal pressure by dietary means similar to that described above or by bulk laxatives; (2) to alleviate colonic spasm, which can often be achieved by local application of heat and by spasmolytic agents such as dicyclomine hydrochloride (Bentyl), 20 mg, or propantheline, 15 mg, one hour before meals and at bedtime; (3) to alleviate emotional stress by supportive therapy and use of sedatives and tranquilizers; and (4) to alleviate pain by using non-opiate analgesics (because opiates increase colonic spasm). In rare instances patients with severe muscle hypertrophy in the sigmoid colon may require surgical resection or long myotomy. Present evidence suggests that resection is the treatment of choice, because high intraluminal pressures recur after myotomy. Improvement is obtained in approximately two thirds of operated patients.

Although only 20 per cent of patients with known diverticulosis become symptomatic at some time during their lives, once symptoms appear there is frequent recurrence. Patients who have had one episode have at least a 25 or 30 per cent chance of recurrence, and those with two have a more than 50 per cent possibility of recurrence.

Connell, A. M.: Applied physiology of the colon: Factors relevant to diverticular disease. Clin. Gastroenterol., 4:23, 1975.

Fleischner, F. G.: Diverticular disease of the colon. New observations and revised concepts. Gastroenterology, 60:316, 1971.

Morson, B. C.: Pathology of diverticular disease of the colon. Clin. Gastroenterol., 4:37, 1975.

Painter, N. S., and Burkitt, D. P.: Diverticular disease of the colon, a 20th century problem. Clin. Gastroenterol., 4:3, 1975.

SOLITARY CECAL DIVERTICULUM

Solitary cecal diverticulum is probably congenital and usually consists of all three walls of the intestine. Most are asymptomatic and represent chance findings. Diverticulitis may present acutely, with symptoms suggesting appendicitis or Crohn's disease in children or young adults below 40. Conservative therapy consists of nasogastric aspiration and avoidance of oral intake. However, most symptomatic patients will undergo surgery because it is impossible to exclude appendicitis or carcinoma. Appendectomy should be performed at the same time if feasible.

Section Three   PEPTIC ULCER

402. PEPTIC ULCER: PATHOGENESIS AND PATHOPHYSIOLOGY

Morton I. Grossman

DEFINITION. Peptic ulcer is a sharply circumscribed loss of the tissue lining those parts of the digestive tract exposed to gastric juice containing acid and pepsin. These parts consist of the lower esophagus, the stomach, the upper intestine (usually only the first part of the duodenum), the small intestine adjacent to a surgically produced connection with the stomach, and those Meckel's diverticula that contain functioning gastric glands.

PATHOLOGY. Acute Lesions. Acute lesions must be clearly distinguished from chronic ulcers because they are different diseases. Acute lesions are almost always multiple and most are superficial, rarely extending through the muscularis mucosae. Lesions that do not extend through the muscularis mucosae are called erosions, whereas those that do penetrate this layer are called ulcers. Thus multiple acute lesions are mainly erosions, but chronic lesions are always ulcers.

Chronic Ulcers. When the unqualified term ulcer is used, chronic ulcer is meant. In contrast to acute lesions, chronic ulcers are usually single. About 4 per cent of patients with gastric ulcer and about 20 per cent of patients with duodenal ulcer have two ulcers at the same time (see accompanying figure). Gastric and duodenal ulcers occur in the same patient 20 times more frequently than would be expected by chance alone. The risk of a patient with gastric ulcer getting a duodenal ulcer within seven years is about 33 per cent, whereas the risk of a duodenal ulcer patient getting a gastric ulcer within this time is about 10 per cent.

The margins of chronic ulcers are thickened, rounded, and overhanging because of the excavation beneath them. Askanazy was the first to describe the four histologic zones of the ulcer floor: a surface layer of fibrin and pus, a narrow zone of fibrinoid necrosis, a zone of granulation tissue, and a cicatricial or fibrous zone. Chronic ulcers usually destroy the entire muscular coat.

During healing a single layer of epithelial cells covers the granulation tissue of the crater floor and then differentiates toward normal mucosa. There is no regeneration of muscle; a permanent scar in the muscular coat marks the site of a healed ulcer.

Gastritis. Chronic gastritis is present in the stomach of almost all patients with chronic gastric or duodenal ulcer. The proximal 80 per cent of the stomach has acid-secreting oxyntic glands; the distal 20 per cent has pyloric glands that produce gastrin but no acid. In patients with duodenal ulcer the gastritis is limited to the pyloric gland area and is mild. Gastric ulcers almost always are in mucosa involved by gastritis, and the extent of the gastritis influences the location of the ulcer. When gastritis is limited to the antrum, the ulcer tends to lie at the border of the antral mucosa with the oxyn-

Enlarged gastric rugal folds, along with increased gastric secretions, have produced a mottled appearance of the barium in the stomach. Two duodenal ulcers are present (open arrows). Thickened mucosal folds are present in the second portion of the duodenum and in the jejunum. The patient had the Zollinger-Ellison syndrome. (From Goldberg, H. I., *In* Sleisenger, M. H., and Fordtran, J. S. [eds.]: Gastrointestinal Disease. 2nd ed. Philadelphia, W. B. Saunders Company, 1978.)

tic mucosa at or near the lesser curve. When gastritis extends beyond the antrum to involve oxyntic mucosa, the ulcer tends to lie in this involved oxyntic mucosa near its border with normal oxyntic mucosa. Thus the greater the extent of gastritis, the higher in the stomach the ulcer tends to be and the lower acid secretion will be because of destruction of oxyntic mucosa by gastritis. The severity and extent of the gastritis do not change with healing of the ulcer. Histologically, chronic atrophic gastritis accompanying gastric ulcer is indistinguishable from the sporadic form common with advancing age but differs from the form associated with pernicious anemia; in the latter the antrum is spared, and antibodies to parietal cells and to intrinsic factor are often present.

Intestinal metaplasia is a common feature of the gastritis associated with gastric ulcer. The converse heterotopia, gastric mucosa in the duodenum, is equally common in patients with duodenal ulcer. In both instances the incidence is related to acid secretion: the higher the level of acid secretion, the greater the incidence of gastric heterotopia in the duodenum; the lower the level of acid secretion, the greater the incidence of intestinal heterotopia in the stomach.

PATHOGENESIS. Acid and pepsin are required for ulcer formation. Ulcers occur when there is an imbalance between acid-pepsin and mucosal resistance. Increased acid-pepsin secretion, decreased mucosal resistance, or the two acting together are ulcerogenic.

Epidemiology. Peptic ulcer is common, but there is much variation in frequency of occurrence from time to time and from place to place. In male Massachusetts physicians the lifetime prevalence of duodenal ulcer was 7.7 per cent and of gastric ulcer 0.9 per cent. The incidence rates peaked at 3.7 per thousand per year at age 55 to 64 for duodenal ulcer and at 1.4 per thousand per year at age 65 to 74 for gastric ulcer.

In a recent study in Denmark, the ratio of duodenal to gastric ulcers was 5.5 to 1 in men and 2.8 to 1 in women. In duodenal ulcer the ratio of men to women was 2.2 to 1, and in gastric ulcer 1.1 to 1.

The prevalence of peptic ulcer at autopsy is considerably higher than in clinical studies, probably because many ulcers never cause enough symptoms to lead to diagnosis. In an autopsy series from Leeds, England, the peak prevalence of ulcers plus scars was at ages 45 to 65, with rates of 27 per cent in men and 15 per cent in women.

In almost all parts of the world morbidity from duodenal ulcer is reported as more common than from gastric ulcer, but deaths from gastric ulcer equal or exceed those from duodenal ulcer. In a few populations, for unknown reasons, gastric ulcer has been reported to be more frequent than duodenal ulcer; examples are fishermen of a village in Norway and Indian miners high in the Peruvian Andes. Mortality rates for gastric ulcer (in deaths per 100,000 persons in the population) range from 30 in Japan to 3 in Israel, and for duodenal ulcer from 10 in Scotland to 0.5 in France. Mortality, prevalence, and incidence of new cases all show a higher rate in town than in country. However, high rates have also been reported from areas that are not industrialized such as South India, Assam, South Nigeria, and Uganda.

Duodenal ulcer was a rare disease before 1900. By 1914 it had become common in Europe and North America. The sharp rise in duodenal ulcer was accompanied by a modest increase in gastric ulcer. From 1914 to about 1955 they remained at a relatively constant level and then began to decrease. Whether the decrease is continuing is uncertain. Cohort analysis, following all persons born in the same year, shows that death rates steadily increased for cohorts born up to the year 1890, whereas death rates for cohorts born after 1890 steadily decreased.

Environmental Factors. Of the many environmental factors that have been suspected as possible contributing causes of peptic ulcer, the only one that has been adequately studied is *smoking*. Smokers have more ulcers, both gastric and duodenal, and higher morbidity and mortality rates from their ulcers than nonsmokers. The nature of the relation between smoking and ulcer is not understood. Smoking neither stimulates nor inhibits gastric acid secretion but does inhibit pancreatic bicarbonate secretion, and some have suggested that this is related to its ulcerogenic action.

Although a role of diet in ulcer causation is often hypothesized, there is as yet no direct evidence to incriminate either particular diets or elements of diets such as hot spices.

Duodenal ulcer is common among all social classes, but ulcer of the body of the stomach has a higher incidence in the poorer economic grades. Despite the persistent myth of the hard-driving executive's proneness to ulcer, occupational differences are in fact small.

Genetic Factors. Genetic factors contribute to both gastric and duodenal ulcer. Gastric and duodenal ulcers are inherited independently. Close relatives of gastric ulcer patients have three times the expected number of gastric ulcers, and close relatives of duodenal ulcer patients have three times the expected number of duodenal ulcers. Concordance for ulcer, i.e., presence of ulcer in the second twin if one twin has ulcer, is more common in monozygous than in dizygous twin pairs. There is strong evidence that the increased familial incidence of ulcer is due to genetic factors and not simply to a shared environment. Peptic ulcer is not a single disease but a number of disorders that are grouped together on the basis of the common clinical feature of an ulcer. Both gastric and duodenal ulcer are etiologically heterogeneous in regard to both genetic and nongenetic factors. No association of genes with ulcer of the body of the stomach has yet been identified. In duodenal ulcer abnormal frequencies have been demonstrated for genes affecting serum pepsinogen concentration, ABO blood groups, secretor status of blood group substances, and HLA antigens. Autosomal dominant transmission of elevated serum pepsinogen I concentration has been demonstrated in some families with a high incidence of duodenal ulcer. Each member of these families who had a duodenal ulcer also had elevated serum pepsinogen I concentration. Persons with blood group O are 1.4 times as liable to have duodenal or prepyloric ulcer as those with group A, B, or AB, and persons who are nonsecretors are 1.5 times as liable to these ulcers as those who are secretors. Group O nonsecretors are 2.5 times more liable than secretors of groups A, B, and AB. The excess of group O and nonsecretion is greater in patients with recurrent ulcers after operations than in unoperated patients. The basis for the association of duodenal ulcer with group O and nonsecretion is not yet known. The frequency of HLA antigen B5 was 2.9 times that of controls in white males with duodenal ulcer.

Psychosomatic Factors. Popular wisdom holds that ulcers are caused by "nerves." At least two notions are implied: (1) that persons who have certain psychic traits are prone to develop ulcers, and (2) that situations that produce psychic tension are likely to bring on ulcers. These hypotheses are awaiting definitive testing. Since it is well established that emotional factors can alter gastric function, it is plausible to hypothesize a role for these factors.

The most complete formulation of the interaction of psychic with other factors is that of Mirsky, whose postulates can be paraphrased as follows. The capacity to secrete acid and pepsin, of which serum pepsinogen level is an index, is genetically determined. Persons endowed with high capacity to secrete acid-pepsin also tend to have a psychic conflict between persistent infantile wishes to be loved and cared for and repudiation of these wishes by their adult sense of shame and pride. Persons who have this combined physiologic and psychic pattern (high acid-pepsin secretory capacity and conflict over dependency wishes) are predisposed to develop duodenal ulcer. Ulcer is most likely to develop when a social event or a series of such events causes an exacerbation of the basic psychic conflict. The mechanism by which the exacerbation of the conflict leads to ulcer is not known, but it probably is not through further increase in acid-pepsin secretion.

Ulcers Caused by Drugs. If all the drugs that cause ulcers when given in massive doses to animals were withdrawn from human use, the pharmacopeia would be noticeably thinner. The drugs strongly suspected of being ulcerogenic in man are salicylates, indomethacin, phenylbutazone, the various recently introduced aspirin substitutes such as ibuprofen, and glucocorticoids. Salicylates and indomethacin applied topically break the mucosal barrier to hydrogen ions. This cannot be the sole mechanism by which they produce ulcer in lower animals, however, because they are also ulcerogenic by the parenteral route and do not break the barrier when so given. All these drugs inhibit the synthesis of prostaglandins, and it is postulated that ulcers result from the loss of a protective action which prostaglandins exert on the mucosa.

The only drug with a highly incriminating dossier for ulcerogenesis in man is aspirin. It is implicated in peptic disease in two ways. First, there is strong but not conclusive evidence that major bleeding episodes, probably mainly from acute diffuse hemorrhagic lesions, may be provoked by ingestion of aspirin. Second, there is mounting evidence that chronic ingestion of aspirin can cause gastric ulcer. Aspirin-induced gastric ulcers occur in stomachs that do not have the atrophic gastritis so characteristic of nonaspirin ulcers.

Peptic Lesions Caused by Stress. The acute diffuse lesions brought on by stress are pathologically and clinically distinct from chronic peptic ulcer. Many different kinds of stress can cause the lesions. Some prominent examples are sepsis, advanced carcinomatosis, shock, severe trauma, surgery, extensive burns (so-called Curling's ulcer), and acute respiratory insufficiency. One category of stress lesions deserves separate mention, namely, those associated with brain injury (so-called Cushing's ulcer). Any acute brain injury, including surgical, traumatic, and cerebrovascular accidents, can cause the lesions. There is good evidence that hypersecretion of gastric acid and pepsin plays a role in stress lesions caused by brain injury, but hypersecretion has not been found in the other kinds of stress lesions. Although ischemia, breaking of the barrier to hydrogen ions, and mucus deficiency have been invoked in the pathogenesis of stress lesions, these are speculations without convincing supporting evidence. Hemorrhage is the main clinical manifestation of stress lesions; perforation occurs occasionally; pain is rare. Stress-related acute gastric lesions are a common life-threatening disease about which little is known.

Association with Other Diseases. The impression that two diseases appear together more frequently or less frequently than would be expected by chance must always be viewed skeptically, because it is easy to draw false conclusions about such associations from studies of nonrandom samples of broad populations. In a study of the entire population of Copenhagen County in Denmark, thereby avoiding the bias of unrepresentative samples, patients with gastric ulcer were found to have an excess of deaths from *chronic bronchitis* and *emphysema,* whereas patients with duodenal ulcer had an excess of deaths from *cirrhosis of the liver* and *cancer of the pancreas.* The mechanisms of these associations are not known. In hepatic cirrhosis hypersecretion of acid caused by a stimulant arising in intestinal mucosa and rendered more effective by bypassing the liver is postulated.

The incidence of gastric ulcer is apparently increased in patients with *rheumatoid arthritis,* and it seems likely that this is attributable to the ulcerogenic action of the drugs used for treatment.

Patients with *hyperparathyroidism* have a high incidence of duodenal ulcer. At least part of this association is due to the occurrence of both parathyroid tumor and gastrinoma in some patients with multiple endocrine adenoma. Since the diagnosis of gastrinoma may not always be obvious, the question of whether patients with hyperparathyroidism without gastrinoma also have an increased incidence of duodenal ulcer must be regarded as unanswered.

PATHOPHYSIOLOGY. Mucosal Resistance. Since most gastric ulcers and many duodenal ulcers occur in patients who do not have increased gastric secretion, a decrease in resistance of the mucosa to acid-peptic injury is presumably involved. Unfortunately, the factors that determine mucosal resistance have not yet been clearly identified. Some suggested contributory factors include mucosal blood flow, regeneration of epithelium, secretion of mucus, and integrity of the barrier to back-diffusion of hydrogen ions.

Gastric mucosa, like all tissue, requires adequate blood supply to remain intact. Although impaired blood supply is a theoretical possibility as a contributor to ulcerogenesis, there are no clues suggesting that it is so implicated. This same statement can be made for most factors that have been suggested as being involved in ulcerogenesis.

The epithelium of the entire gastrointestinal tract is rapidly replaced. It is estimated that the surface cells of the human stomach are replaced every four to six days. Good methods for measuring mucosal regeneration rate in man are available, but these have not yet been applied to the study of patients with peptic ulcer. Patients with atrophic gastritis have an increased rate of cell shedding from the gastric surface as measured by the rate of appearance of DNA in gastric washings; this also applies to the atrophic gastritis associated with gastric ulcer.

The notion that mucus somehow protects the mucosa against damage by acid-pepsin is very old and still widely held, but there is no known biologic or physicochemical basis for such an action. Some sulfated mucosubstances inhibit peptic activity, but these do not occur in human gastric juice or gastric mucosa. The interstices of a gel of mucus are too large to offer significant resistance to diffusion of hydrogen ions or pepsin. The methods presently available have not shown any defect in secretion of mucus in patients with ulcer.

Back-Diffusion. Acid secreted into the gastric lumen diffuses back into the mucosa very slowly provided that the mucosa is normal; the leakback rate is only a few per cent of the maximal rate of acid secretion. This is spoken of as a "barrier" to back-diffusion. A variety of chemical agents, some arising in the body, others ingested, can break this barrier and allow markedly increased rates of back-diffusion of acid. Bile acids are endogenous barrier breakers. Exogenous barrier breakers likely to enter the human stomach include alcohol, salicylates, and oxethazaine. To break the barrier the chemical must enter the mucosa. If the agent is ionizable, it must be in its un-ionized lipid-soluble form to enter the mucosa; for example, aspirin must be in acid solution. Manifestations of a broken barrier include decrease in the electrical potential difference across the gastric mucosa and increased bidirectional permeability to sodium with increased accumulation of sodium in the gastric lumen. As acid diffuses through the broken barrier, it causes additional damage manifested by leakage of interstitial fluid and plasma into the gastric lumen and bleeding.

The locus of the barrier to back-diffusion of hydrogen ions is not known. Because Hollander used the term "mucous barrier" and Davenport used the term "mucosal barrier to hydrogen ions," it is commonly assumed that these two are the same barriers. There is no evidence that mucus has anything to do with the barrier to hydrogen ions.

Gastric Acid Secretion. CAPACITY TO SECRETE ACID. The capacity to secrete acid is determined mainly by the number of parietal cells in the gastric mucosa, and this is mainly genetically determined. The capacity to secrete acid can be estimated by measuring the response to a high dose (such that a higher dose would not give a greater response) of a stimulant such as gastrin, pentagastrin, histamine, or betazole, which all give about the same highest attainable response.

Secretory capacity is less in women than in men, a difference partially accounted for by difference in body size. Secretory capacity declines with age, presumably because of increasing incidence of gastritis that destroys acid-secreting cells.

REGULATION OF GASTRIC SECRETION IN MAN. Three substances activate the parietal cell to secrete acid: the endocrine substance *gastrin*, which reaches the parietal cell by way of the blood; the neurocrine substance *acetylcholine*, which is released at the parietal cell by postganglionic endings of the vagus nerve; and the paracrine substance histamine, which diffuses across intercellular spaces from its cell of origin in the lamina propria to the parietal cell.

Gastrins. Scattered among the mucous cells of the pyloric glands are specialized cells, the G-cells, that produce gastrin and store it in granules.

Gastrin occurs in several molecular sizes. Gastrins with chain lengths of 14, 17, and 34 amino acid residues, designated G14, G17, and G34, have been isolated and chemically identified by Gregory. Each of these occurs in sulfated and nonsulfated forms. Pentagastrin, β-Ala-Trp-Met-Asp-Phe-NH$_2$, a synthetic peptide that contains the last four amino acids of gastrin, is widely used as a stimulant for gastric acid secretion in diagnostic testing.

In antral mucosa the predominant form of gastrin is G17, whereas in blood plasma after eating the most abundant form is G34. The greater abundance of G34 in plasma can be accounted for at least in part by its slower removal; the half-time of G34 is six times longer than that of G17. A six times higher blood level of G34 than of G17 is needed to give equal rates of acid secretion.

The richest source of gastrin is antral mucosa. The concentration of gastrin in the mucosa of the duodenal bulb is 10 to 20 per cent that in antral mucosa, and much lower concentrations are found in more distal intestine.

Small amounts of gastrin are released by the cephalic phase of feeding. The main stimulant for gastrin release is the topical action of protein digestion products on the antral mucosa, presumably by a direct action on the luminal microvilli of the G-cells. All modes of gastrin release are enhanced by atropine, indicating that there is a cholinergic inhibitory mechanism. It is not known whether the cephalic vagal release of gastrin is cholinergic and atropine resistant or noncholinergic.

The concentration of gastrin in antral mucosa is normal in patients with duodenal ulcer and decreased in patients with gastric ulcer. In patients with duodenal ulcer serum gastrin concentration is normal in the fasting state and greater than normal after feeding. In patients with gastric ulcer both fasting and postprandial concentrations of serum gastrin are increased. The increased gastrin responses to meals in duodenal and gastric ulcer subjects are due mainly to a component other than G17, probably G34 but not yet positively identified.

All kinds of vagotomy (truncal, selective, proximal gastric) cause an increase in serum gastrin, both fasting and after feeding. Antrectomy causes a modest decrease in fasting serum gastrin level.

Acetylcholine. The postganglionic cholinergic nerves to the parietal cell are activated by vagal impulses and by so-called short reflexes that are completed within the wall of the stomach. Vagal activation occurs as a result of stimuli acting in the head (cephalic phase) and in the stomach (gastric phase). Cephalic stimuli include chewing, tasting, and swallowing food (as in sham feeding), the sight, smell, or thought of food (conditioned relex), hypoglycemia induced by insulin, and interference with glucose utilization by nonmetabolizable analogues such as 2-deoxyglucose. Gastric distention initiates both long vagovagal reflexes and short intramural relexes; the long reflexes are more effective.

The vagus nerve influences gastric secretion in at least three ways: (1) direct cholinergic stimulation of parietal cells, (2) release of gastrin, and (3) sensitizing the parietal cell to stimulation by gastrin and other stimulants. After vagotomy the highest attainable response to gastrin is reduced and the dose of gastrin needed to get that reduced response is increased. Antrectomy, removal of the major source of gastrin, reduces the response to vagal stimulation and to other stimulants such as gastrin and histamine. Antrectomy and vagotomy augment each other's effects. For example, the highest attainable response to histamine is about 40 per cent of the preoperative level with vagotomy alone, about 50 per cent with antrectomy alone, and about 20 per cent with the two together.

Histamine. The mast-like cells of the lamina propria of the gastric mucosa store histamine and release it near the parietal cells. Isolated parietal cells respond weakly to histamine, acetylcholine, or gastrin given singly, whereas the responses are greatly enhanced when histamine is given with either of the other two stimulants. It is postulated that in the intact mucosa histamine is always present in amounts too small to stimulate alone but great enough to amplify the responses to other stimuli. Another postulate is that acetylcholine and gastrin release histamine. Either of these postulates could explain why histamine H_2-receptor antagonists such as cimetidine inhibit not only histamine but other forms of stimulation as well.

Other Factors. Partially digested protein bathing the intestinal mucosa stimulates gastric acid secretion. Release of gastrin is not great enough to account for this effect, so other unidentified hormones from intestinal mucosa are postulated. A part of the effect is probably due to absorbed amino acids, because intravenous infusion of amino acids stimulates acid secretion.

Caffeine and theophylline stimulate gastric acid secretion, an action that may be secondary to inhibition of breakdown of cyclic AMP.

Inhibition. Release of gastrin is inhibited by acid bathing the antral mucosa. When antral pH is 1.5 or lower, all forms of gastrin release are almost totally suppressed.

Acid, fat, and hypertonic fluids bathing the intestinal mucosa inhibit gastric acid secretion. The neural and hormonal mechanisms involved in these effects have not been identified. Secretin and cholecystokinin are weak inhibitors of acid secretion, so they are unlikely to contribute significantly to physiologic regulation of acid secretion.

GASTRIC ACID SECRETION IN PATIENTS WITH ULCER. Normal adults have on average about one billion parietal cells and can secrete about 22 mmol of acid per hour. The corresponding values for duodenal ulcer are 1.9 billion and 42 mmol and for gastric ulcer 0.8 billion and 18 mmol. The variations around the means are very large, so there is much overlap between these groups. However, on average, patients with chronic duodenal ulcer secrete more acid than normal subjects both at rest and in response to stimuli. At all times, day and night, in the fasted and fed states, the acidity of the gastric contents and of the first 5 to 10 cm of duodenum is greater than normal.

POSTULATED ABNORMALITIES IN ULCER PATIENTS. The increased average rate of secretion in patients with duodenal ulcer could be due to one or more of these factors: (1) increased capacity to secrete, (2) increased responsiveness of acid-secreting cells, (3) increased drive to acid secretion, and (4) decreased inhibition of secretion. These factors are not entirely independent. For example, gastrin not only drives secretion but also stimulates growth of mucosa. Acetylcholine drives secretion and sensitizes to other stimuli; whether it also stimulates growth of mucosa is not known. Of these factors, increased capacity to secrete is the one most clearly involved in the hypersecretion seen in duodenal ulcer. Increased capacity to secrete

acid is present long before the duodenal ulcer appears and stays relatively constant during exacerbations and remissions. There is some evidence that increased sensitivity to stimulation by gastrin is also present. There is also some evidence for increased drive in the form of greater than normal increments in serum gastrin after feeding, but the relative importance of this factor is not yet clear. Defective inhibitory mechanisms may contribute to hypersecretion. For example, acidification of a test meal causes less suppression of gastrin release and of acid secretion in duodenal ulcer patients than in controls.

Basal acid secretion rate divided by maximal rate can be used as an index of basal "drive." In both duodenal ulcer patients and controls, this fraction increases as basal rate increases, indicating that some unidentified factor other than maximal capacity is a major determinant of high basal rates.

A popular notion holds that the hypersecretion of duodenal ulcer is caused by excessive vagal activity. The only evidence in support of this idea is that the hypersecretion is eliminated by vagotomy. However, since vagotomy decreases the response to all forms of stimulation, the decrease in secretion that follows vagotomy cannot be accepted as proof that vagal overactivity caused the hypersecretion. There is no satisfactory method for measuring vagal "tone."

Impaired release of secretin or impaired capacity of the pancreas to secrete bicarbonate could contribute to the increased duodenal acidity seen in patients with duodenal ulcer. However, there is no convincing evidence for impaired secretin release, and capacity to secrete bicarbonate is actually increased, proportionately to the increased capacity to secrete acid.

In gastric ulcer associated with duodenal ulcer, the secretory pattern tends to be like that of duodenal ulcer. The higher in the stomach the gastric ulcer is located, the lower the secretory capacity; ulcers near the pylorus give secretory patterns like duodenal ulcer, whereas those near the cardia show marked hyposecretion. The decrease in acid secretion in gastric ulcer can be accounted for mainly by the associated gastritis that causes loss of parietal cells, but increased back-diffusion may also contribute.

Pepsins. Seven pepsinogens belonging to two immunochemical groups occur in human gastroduodenal mucosa. Group I pepsinogens are limited to mucous neck cells and zymogen cells of the oxyntic gland area, and Group II pepsinogens are present in these cells and also in the mucous cells of pyloric glands and Brunner's glands. Group I and II pepsinogens are present in blood plasma, but only Group I is found in normal urine.

There is a strong correlation between capacity to secrete acid and capacity to secrete pepsin and also between capacity to secrete acid and pepsin and concentration of pepsinogen in blood. Determination by radioimmunoassay of the concentration of Group I pepsinogens in blood serum is a convenient and accurate method of assessing the secretory capacity for acid and pepsin.

The major stimulants for acid secretion, gastrin and acetylcholine, are also the major regulators of pepsin secretion. The ratio of pepsin to acid is higher in cholinergically stimulated gastric juice (e.g., insulin hypoglycemia) than in that evoked by gastrin. The increase in gastric secretion in patients with duodenal ulcer and the decrease in patients with gastric ulcer involve both acid and pepsin.

Duodenogastric Reflux. Du Plessis (1965) offered the suggestion that reflux of bile from the duodenum into the stomach may be an important factor in the pathogenesis of gastric ulcer. Patients with gastric ulcer do reflux duodenal contents into the stomach more often and in larger amounts than controls, both in the fasting and fed states, but the overlap between controls and gastric ulcer patients is great. Over the short term this reflux leads to breaking of the gastric barrier to back-diffusion of hydrogen ion, and over the long term it is presumed to lead to gastric atrophy, factors that may make the mucosa less resistant to ulceration. Further studies are needed to assess fully the role of this factor.

Gastric Emptying. There is a tendency for rapid emptying of a mixed meal in patients with duodenal ulcer, but the overlap with normal subjects is great. Some patients with duodenal ulcer or with gastric ulcer have markedly impaired gastric emptying. This impairment of emptying cannot always be accounted for by anatomic narrowing of the gastric outlet, and its pathogenesis is not well understood.

403. PEPTIC ULCER: CLINICAL AND ENDOCRINE ASPECTS

John H. Walsh

CLINICAL MANIFESTATIONS

SYMPTOMS. In many patients the diagnosis of peptic ulcer disease may be suspected by history alone. Epigastric pain is the cardinal symptom. The location and character of the pain, its temporal pattern, and factors that aggravate or relieve it produce a characteristic clinical picture.

Location. Typical ulcer pain is epigastric, near the midline. The pain may be so sharply localized that the patient will indicate its site by pointing with one finger. The pain of both duodenal and gastric ulcer is localized in the epigastrium, so it is not possible to localize the ulcer by the location of pain. The pain of uncomplicated ulcers does not radiate to the back, nor does it radiate substernally unless accompanied by gastroesophageal reflux.

Character. The pain may be described as burning, gnawing, cramping, boring, or aching, or as a sensation of pressure, heaviness, or hunger. It may be mild or severe. It may fluctuate in intensity but usually achieves maximal intensity for periods lasting minutes rather than hours. The pain is not aggravated by body movement. The difficulty many patients have in describing the nature of the pain is probably due to its visceral origin.

Temporal Relationships and Pain Relief. The time course of the pain helps differentiate it from pain of other diseases. Usually, ulcer pain appears in clusters of days to weeks, interspersed with pain-free intervals of weeks to months. Thus chronicity and periodicity are typical of ulcer symptoms. During periods between attacks, many patients are completely free of ulcer pain, but a minority have almost daily episodes of low grade epigastric discomfort. The pattern of recurrent attacks may continue for many years without significant change; the pain may become more frequent or severe, or in some patients it may diminish and finally disappear after a few years.

The daily pain pattern roughly parallels the normal time course of gastric acidity. Pain is usually absent in the morning, when gastric secretion is low, and immediately after meals, when acid is buffered by food. It tends to become most severe several hours after meals and at bedtime, when acid secretion rates are relatively high and gastric contents are unbuffered. Likewise, measures which reduce intragastric acidity (antacids, food, nasogastric suction) typically relieve the pain. Recent studies have shown that pain is relieved as effectively by placebo as by antacid, casting some doubt on the theory that acid and pepsin are the main determinants of peptic ulcer pain. In some patients with gastric ulcer food may produce transient worsening of the pain followed by relief.

Associated Symptoms. Nausea and/or excessive salivation may accompany peptic ulcer pain. Anorexia may occur in patients with gastric ulcer. Spontaneous vomiting is an occasional symptom, more commonly associated with gastric than with duodenal ulcer. These symptoms are relatively rare.

These features of pain just described are typical of uncomplicated peptic ulcer disease. Some patients may never experience pain and are found to have an ulcer only after they present with a complication of their disease. Development of a complication also may lead to a change in the character of the pain. As determined by endoscopic observations, resolution of pain commonly precedes actual healing of ulcers. Atypical symptoms are more common in children and in elderly patients with peptic ulcer disease.

PHYSICAL EXAMINATION. Epigastric tenderness, although frequently present, is seldom marked, and is nonspecific. In fact, the general physical examination is of little help in establishing the diagnosis of uncomplicated peptic ulcer disease.

DIFFERENTIAL DIAGNOSIS. Any disease producing epigastric pain must be differentiated from peptic ulcer disease. Disease of only a few abdominal organs (stomach, liver, gallbladder, and pancreas) produces pain in this area. Pain arising from the small intestine, large intestine, and bladder is felt lower in the abdomen. Pain arising in the gastroesophageal region and esophagus is usually felt in the subxiphoid area and retrosternally.

Pain from intrathoracic structures may also be referred to the epigastrium, e.g., in pleuritis, myocardial infarction, or pericarditis. These diseases are usually not confused with peptic ulcer disease. The pain they produce tends to be acute rather than chronic, constant rather than episodic, not related to meals or relieved by antacids, and usually associated with other manifestations not characteristic of ulcer disease.

Pain arising from the esophagus (usually from peptic esophagitis or peptic ulcer disease of the esophagus) may exhibit some features typical of peptic ulcer pain such as temporal relation to meals and relief by antacids. Lower esophageal pain, although occasionally epigastric, is usually felt as retrosternal "heartburn." Esophagitis is usually accompanied by symptoms of regurgitation of gastric contents which are accentuated by straining or by assuming a horizontal position. However, many patients have both esophagitis and ulcer. It is important to distinguish the symptoms due to each of these conditions.

Epigastric pain produced by intra-abdominal diseases not involving the stomach or duodenum can usually be distinguished easily from peptic ulcer disease. Acute cholecystitis may produce epigastric pain or pain in the right upper quadrant with rapid onset and duration of hours to days, and is frequently accompanied by tenderness over the gallbladder and fever. There is often a history of previous attacks of biliary colic. Acute pancreatitis frequently produces epigastric pain, but the pain usually radiates to the back, and is aggravated by changes in position. Moreover, in either acute cholecystitis or pancreatitis, signs of acute abdominal inflammation (fever, direct and rebound tenderness, abdominal distention, or ileus) are typical and are not found in uncomplicated ulcer disease.

Malignant Ulcer. In the United States most gastric ulcers are benign, but the possibility of malignant gastric ulcer must be considered in every patient with gastric ulceration. Appropriate studies are discussed in Ch. 404. Duodenal ulcers are almost never malignant.

Duodenitis. Inflammation of the duodenal mucosa is frequently found in conjunction with active duodenal ulcer. It may also be found in patients with typical ulcer symptoms but without demonstrable ulcers. Such patients may have gastric hypersecretion, radiologic evidence of coarse duodenal folds, and histologic evidence of mononuclear infiltration and microscopic ulceration. Patients with duodenitis later may develop frank duodenal ulcer disease; this therefore may be a stage in the natural history of ulcer disease in some patients. Symptomatic duodenitis may also arise from eosinophilic or granulomatous infiltration of the duodenum.

Gastritis. In addition to gastritis associated with ulcer disease (see above), several forms of chronic gastritis may affect the stomach. Chronic superficial gastritis, atrophic gastritis, and gastric atrophy increase in frequency with age and sometimes are associated with epigastric symptoms but seldom produce a well defined pattern resembling peptic ulcer. Diseases infiltrating the wall of the stomach (carcinoma, lymphoma, granulomatous gastritis caused by Crohn's disease, eosinophilic granuloma, sarcoidosis, tuberculosis, or syphilis) may produce ulcer-like symptoms. Such symptoms are found in about a third of patients with adult hypertrophic pyloric stenosis and are relatively common in patients with Menetrier's disease (hypertrophic gastropathy associated with protein loss into the gastrointestinal tract). Most of these are rare. Their diagnosis depends on exclusion of peptic ulcer disease and demonstration of characteristic pathology by radiographic, endoscopic, and/or histologic examination.

Functional Dyspepsia. Functional dyspepsia may cause symptoms resembling those found in peptic ulcer disease but with no demonstrable pathologic lesion and with a prognosis free of complications of ulcer disease. It is more common in women. The disorder is characterized by chronic and recurrent symptoms of epigastric distress. Pain-free intervals tend to be of short duration. Antacids frequently produce either partial or complete relief of epigastric pain, but food is likely to aggravate the distress. Often the pain is poorly localized, and the patients complain of "gas." Nausea, vomiting, and pain may occur in the morning before breakfast. Nocturnal pain is less frequent than in ulcer disease.

The distinction between functional dyspepsia and peptic ulcer disease may be impossible by history alone. It is a diagnosis of exclusion, made only after careful radiographic and endoscopic examinations have excluded peptic ulcer disease.

ENDOCRINE HYPERFUNCTION AND ULCER DISEASE

Zollinger-Ellison Syndrome

One syndrome in which it has been established without doubt that ulcer disease is caused by hormonal excess is the Zollinger-Ellison syndrome. This is characterized by peptic ulcer or occasionally by diarrhea without ulcer, gastric acid hypersecretion, and a gastrin-secreting tumor, usually originating in the pancreas, which causes hypergastrinemia. The role of gastrin in this syndrome was proved by chemical isolation of gastrin from such tumors and by bioassay of gastrin in serum and tumor extracts from patients. Gastrin radioimmunoassay has provided additional information about the pathogenesis and has permitted identification of many additional cases.

The Zollinger-Ellison syndrome occurs in all age groups but is diagnosed most often between the third and fifth decades. The proportion of patients with ulcer disease who have the syndrome is unknown, but it is probably less than 1 per cent.

The predominant symptom is abdominal pain, which may be similar to that of ordinary ulcer disease or may be more severe. Intervals without pain tend to be shorter. Pain is present in more than 80 per cent of patients and usually has been present for a year or more before the diagnosis is established. Other prominent symptoms include diarrhea, vomiting, melena, hematemesis, and weight loss. Recurrent ulceration after ulcer operation is unfortunately too often the first evidence of the disease. Some patients do not exhibit florid symptoms or may not have marked hypergastrinemia on a single determination and may be difficult to distinguish from those with ordinary ulcers.

In approximately three fourths of patients with the Zollinger-Ellison syndrome, there is an ulcer in the duodenal bulb or immediate postbulbar area. Ulcers in the distal duodenum or proximal jejunum are very suggestive but are found in less than one fourth of patients. Other radiologic features helpful in the diagnosis are hypertrophic gastric folds, increased quantities of gastric juice, dilatation of the duodenum and jejunum, mucosal edema, and irregularity in the small intestine. Occasionally there is a gastric ulcer.

The diarrhea associated with the Zollinger-Ellison syndrome is due to massive hypersecretion and can be relieved by nasogastric aspiration or by total gastrectomy. The large amount of acid delivered into the upper intestine causes mucosal damage and increased intestinal motility. In addition, gastrin exerts an effect on the intestinal mucosa, decreasing absorption of salt and water, and also affects intestinal motility. The diarrhea is frequently accompanied by steatorrhea. Responsible factors include inactivation of pancreatic lipase and precipitation of conjugated bile salts at low intraluminal pH as well as direct damage of the mucosa by acid.

The gastrin-secreting tumors, or gastrinomas, responsible for the Zollinger-Ellison syndrome are usually small and may be difficult to find at operation or even at postmortem examination. They are most commonly located in the pancreas where they originate in the islets, but they may also arise in the duodenum. Metastasis and occurrence of multiple primary tumors are common, so that the chances of locating a single benign operable tumor are probably less than one in ten.

ASSOCIATION WITH OTHER ENDOCRINE TUMORS. Individuals with the Zollinger-Ellison syndrome frequently have other endocrine abnormalities. The most common associated syndrome is *hyperparathyroidism*, which is found in about 20 per cent of patients with the disease. Hyperparathyroidism may greatly affect the gastric secretory pattern. Hypercalcemia has been shown to release tumor gastrin and to increase acid secretion. Conversely, correction of hypercalcemia by parathyroidectomy may result in transient or prolonged decreases in serum gastrin and acid secretion and periods of clinical remission. Other endocrine tumors found in the Zollinger-Ellison syndrome may be in the pituitary, adrenal, ovary, or thyroid. The abnormality may be carcinoma, single or multiple adenomas, or diffuse hyperplasia. The islet cell tumors may produce other substances such as insulin, glucagon, and ACTH.

A familial form of the Zollinger-Ellison syndrome associated with other endocrine tumors was first described by Wermer. Several families have been described subsequently. There is autosomal dominant transmission with high but variable expressivity. The same pattern of glandular involvement and pathology is found as in the sporadic cases of multiple endocrine neoplasia.

DIAGNOSIS. The diagnosis of the Zollinger-Ellison syndrome may be suggested by ulcer symptoms refractory to ordinary medical treatment, by radiologic findings, by recurrence of ulcer after an ulcer operation, or by the finding of an increased serum gastrin concentration. Gastric secretion is usually found to be excessive. Suspicion should be aroused when basal secretion is greater than 10 mEq HCl per hour in an unoperated patient or greater than 5 mEq per hour in a patient with previous gastric surgery for ulcer. Confirmation of the diagnosis in most patients can be made by measurement of fasting serum gastrin concentration, with levels greater than 500 pg per milliliter in the presence of acid hypersecretion. When fasting serum gastrin values are equivocal (100 to 500 pg per milliliter), further evidence for the presence of gastrinoma may be obtained by demonstration of exaggerated increases in serum gastrin in response to intravenous secretin, which normally inhibits gastrin release, and intravenous calcium, which normally is a very weak stimulant of gastrin release. Conversely, patients with gastrinoma typically have minimal serum responses following ingestion of a protein meal, whereas patients with hypergastrinemia caused by hyperactivity of antral gastrin cells have large increases in serum gastrin following a meal. Some patients with ordinary duodenal ulcer appear to have an exaggerated postprandial release of gastrin. It is not clear whether there is a separate group of patients with hypergastrinemia due to antral gastrin-cell hyperplasia with autonomous release of gastrin not susceptible to acid inhibition.

Hypergastrinemia is often associated with low rates of gastric acid secretion in patients with intact antral mucosa. Very high serum gastrin levels are common in

patients with atrophic gastritis, including many of those with pernicious anemia. Serum gastrin values may be increased after surgical vagotomy without antral resection. Hypergastrinemia also is found in approximately 20 per cent of patients with severe renal failure, but seldom associated with peptic ulcer or gastric hypersecretion. Pathologic hypergastrinemia, associated with acid hypersecretion, may occur in the syndrome of isolated retained antrum after attempted antrectomy and gastrojejunostomy. Moderate increases in serum gastrin may occur with gastric outlet obstruction.

TREATMENT. The usual treatment of the Zollinger-Ellison syndrome is total gastrectomy. Medical therapy with the histamine H_2-receptor antagonist cimetidine has been highly effective in the short-term management of these patients. The duration of cimetidine effect may be prolonged by addition of anticholinergic drugs if necessary, and higher than normal therapeutic doses of cimetidine may be required for optimal management. The role of medical versus surgical therapy of Zollinger-Ellison syndrome requires evaluation. Preliminary studies suggest that medical management may be the preferred treatment in many patients. If operation is indicated, total gastrectomy should be performed. Less extensive resections often lead to recurrent ulceration, frequently in the immediate postoperative period, which may be complicated by bleeding, perforation, and death. In less than 10 per cent of the patients, it is possible to resect a single tumor and cure the disease.

404. PEPTIC ULCER: DIAGNOSIS

Jon I. Isenberg

RADIOGRAPHY. Radiography remains the most commonly used technique for the diagnosis of peptic ulcer disease. Ulcers may rarely be visualized on standard abdominal radiograms if air is trapped in the crater. Barium sulfate suspension is usually used as the radiopaque contrast material for routine gastrointestinal radiography. In patients with suspected perforated ulcers, an absorbable water-soluble contrast agent is used instead of barium sulfate. Air contrast films help to clearly define the mucosal pattern of the upper gastrointestinal tract. Delayed films, taken about one hour after ingestion of barium, may demonstrate a collection of barium within an ulcer which was not seen on the initial fluoroscopic examination.

For certainty of diagnosis, the ulcer niche should be seen on more than one x-ray film. When an ulcer is viewed in profile, the niche appears as a collection of contrast material which extends beyond the confines of the gut wall. When the ulcer niche is seen en face, it appears as a puddle of barium, often surrounded by a halo and/or radiating folds to the ulcer. The halo is due to surrounding mucosal and submucosal edema.

Ulcers of the esophagus usually occur within the lower half (Fig. 1). Ulcer and diverticulum of the esophagus may have similar radiographic appearances. Esophagoscopy (see below) can distinguish one from the other. The presence of an esophageal ulcer, particularly with an accompanying esophageal stricture, should suggest the possibility that the lower esophagus

Figure 1. B. H., a 44-year-old housewife with intermittent dysphagia for four years and burning midepigastric pain, recurring after meals and during the night, for eight months. Esophagoscopy revealed chronic esophagitis with stricture; biopsies did not demonstrate neoplasia. The roentgenogram demonstrates an ulcer crater in the esophagus. Antacid therapy facilitated healing, and the dysphagia subsided.

is lined with columnar epithelium, Barrett's syndrome. Almost all ulcers in the lower columnar, Barrett's, esophagus are visualized on radiography. Long linear ulcers in the squamous mucosa associated with peptic esophagitis often are not seen on x-ray.

The great majority of gastric ulcers (approximately 85 per cent) occur in pyloric gland mucosa at or near the junction with oxyntic gland mucosa. Approximately 85 per cent of gastric ulcers occur on the lesser curvature of the stomach. About 90 per cent of endoscopically visualized gastric ulcers are seen on upper gastrointestinal series.

Gastric ulcers vary in diameter from less than 1 cm to greater than 10 cm. Nearly 80 per cent of gastric ulcers are less than 2 cm in widest diameter. When seen in profile, a narrow density may surround the neck of the ulcer; this is due to an undermined margin of gastric mucosa which produces a narrow ring around part or all of the ulcer (Hampton's line). A thicker radiolucent density often surrounds a benign ulcer, the ulcer "collar," caused by edema and inflammation of the adjacent mucosa (Fig. 2). Although these radiographic changes tend to be more common with benign ulcers, they may rarely be seen in ulcerating gastric cancers.

Gastric ulcers may not be visualized because (1) the ulcer may be shallow and barium may not collect within it, (2) there may be mucus or blood within the ulcer crater, (3) the edematous margins around the ulcer may occlude the mouth of the ulcer, (4) the positions used may not throw it into profile, or (5) the patient may be too large or may be unable to permit adequate radiographic examination.

Approximately 4 per cent of all gastric ulcers seen on gastrointestinal radiograms are malignant. Radiographic

features which tend to distinguish benign gastric ulcer from gastric cancer include the following: (1) most benign ulcers extend beyond the confines of the gastric wall, whereas gastric cancers tend to occur within the confines of the gastric wall; (2) benign ulcers tend to be round or ovoid, whereas cancers often are irregular in shape; (3) benign ulcers usually have a smooth base, whereas the base of a cancer may be nodular; (4) the gastric folds radiate to the lip of a benign ulcer, whereas there may be not radiating folds around a cancer, or the folds may be blunted and stop some distance from an ulcerating cancer; and (5) the stomach around a benign ulcer is usually pliable and has normal motility, whereas the wall around a cancer is often rigid. Also, some ulcerating carcinomas may "heal" radiographically. Since some ulcerating cancers may resemble benign gastric ulcers, other studies, such as endoscopy, biopsy, and cytology (see below), assist in distinguishing benign gastric ulcer from gastric cancer.

Benign gastric ulcers within the body of the stomach may produce infolding of the gastric wall opposite the ulcer. With healing of the ulcer, this cleft or incisura in the gastric contour may persist, producing an "hourglass stomach."

Figure 2. A benign ulcer of the lesser curvature is surrounded by an ulcer collar — the broad lucent band resulting from edema at the ulcer orifice. Gastric mucosal folds radiate from this mass of edema. (From Goldberg, H. I., *In* Sleisenger, M. H., and Fordtran, J. S. [eds.]: Gastrointestinal Disease. 2nd ed. Philadelphia, W. B. Saunders Company, 1978.)

Figure 3. Edematous folds radiate from a pinpoint ulcer of the posterior duodenal wall (arrows). Compression of the duodenal bulb by the radiologist produced the best roentgenographic demonstration of this ulcer. (From Goldberg, H. I., *In* Sleisenger, M. H., and Fordtran, J. S. [eds.]: Gastrointestinal Disease. 2nd ed. Philadelphia, W. B. Saunders Company, 1978.)

More than 90 per cent of duodenal ulcers are located within the duodenal bulb (Fig. 3). Rarely, ulcers may be located in the postbulbar area as well as the more distal duodenum and proximal jejunum. Approximately 85 per cent of endoscopically visualized duodenal ulcers (see below) are seen on upper gastrointestinal series (Fig. 4).

In the absence of a definite ulcer niche, radiographic findings which suggest duodenal ulcer disease include (1) spasm of the duodenal bulb; (2) eccentricity of the pyloric channel; (3) a persistent fold (i.e., incisura) extending across the duodenal bulb; (4) loss of the superior or inferior fornix of the duodenal bulb; (5) persistent spasm and/or fibrosis of the duodenal bulb, producing a "cloverleaf" or other kind of deformity; and (6) distortion of the duodenal mucosa, suggesting edema, heterotopic gastric mucosa, or large duodenal folds. It is often difficult, if not impossible, to determine radiographically if there is an active ulcer in a scarred and deformed duodenal bulb. Giant duodenal ulcers (i.e., greater than 2 cm in diameter) may not be radiographically apparent, because they tend to simulate the normal superior or inferior fornix of the duodenal bulb (Fig. 5).

False-positive radiographic findings of duodenal ulcer may be due to ectopic pancreatic tissue with a minor pancreatic duct in the duodenal bulb, regional enteritis involving the duodenum, varicosities of the pancreaticoduodenal vein, carcinoma of the pancreas extending into the duodenum, and pancreatitis or cholecystitis producing inflammation of the adjacent duodenal mucosa.

ENDOSCOPY. In the diagnosis of peptic ulcer disease, endoscopy is valuable in differentiating esophageal ulcer from diverticulum, defining the bleeding site in upper gastrointestinal hemorrhage (see Ch. 407), differentiating benign from malignant gastric ulcers, differentiating recurrent ulcer from surgical deformity, and determining the presence or absence of organic disease in patients with ulcer symptoms but normal upper gastrointestinal x-rays (so-called x-ray negative dyspepsia). In a scarred deformed duodenal bulb, duodenoscopy

may demonstrate an ulcer not seen on radiographic study. In patients with clinical findings and radiographic evidence of duodenal ulcer, confirmation of the presence of an ulcer with endoscopy does not assist in diagnosis or treatment. Duodenoscopy may reveal hyperemia, friability, or erosions of the duodenal bulb (findings suggestive of duodenitis) without an ulcer.

Figure 4. A small ulcer (arrow) has produced deformity of the duodenal bulb. Flattening of the superior surface of the bulb has resulted from edema and spasm. The superior and inferior recesses of the base of the bulb appear as diverticular outpouchings, so-called pseudodiverticula. (From Goldberg, H. I., *In* Sleisenger, M. H., and Fordtran, J. S. [eds.]: Gastrointestinal Disease. 2nd ed. Philadelphia, W. B. Saunders Company, 1978.)

Figure 5. The arrows outline an oval-shaped, irregular barium collection at the site of the duodenal bulb. Serial roentgenograms demonstrated the same unchanging configuration. A giant duodenal ulcer occupied the entire bulb in the surgical abdomen. (From Goldberg, H. I., *In* Sleisenger, M. H., and Fordtran, J. S. [eds.]: Gastrointestinal Disease. 2nd ed. Philadelphia, W. B. Saunders Company, 1978.)

The pathophysiologic significance of duodenitis is not fully understood. Some studies suggest that it is a precursor of duodenal ulcers, whereas others do not. The natural history of duodenitis needs to be studied.

With current endoscopic techniques almost all ulcers of the esophagus and stomach can be seen, and approximately 85 per cent of radiographically demonstrated duodenal ulcers are seen. Conversely, about 10 to 15 per cent of duodenal ulcer craters seen endoscopically are not demonstrated radiographically. Mucosal lesions such as esophagitis, gastritis, and duodenitis are usually not seen on radiographic study but can be diagnosed endoscopically, particularly with corroboration by directed endoscopic biopsy.

Viewed through the endoscope, a benign gastric ulcer is usually round or ovoid and has a clear whitish base and a hyperemic border; the gastric folds radiate to the edge of the ulcer crater. Gastric cancers are often irregular in shape, have a necrotic hemorrhagic and nodular base, are surrounded by nodularity, and have clubbed folds radiating toward the cancer but stopping short of the ulcerated area. Multiple deep biopsies of the rim or direct brush cytology often establishes a histologic or cytologic diagnosis of cancer.

An unresolved question is whether all patients with gastric ulcer should have endoscopy and biopsy of the ulcer. At present it seem appropriate to perform endoscopy, biopsy, and gastric cytology on all patients with gastric ulcers in whom there is any clinical or radiographic suspicion that the ulcer may be malignant. Those with radiographically benign-appearing gastric ulcers should be treated medically for six to twelve weeks. If the ulcer fails to heal, endoscopy, biopsy, and gastric cytology should be performed.

SECRETORY TESTS. For generations gastric secretory tests have been performed in patients with acid-peptic diseases. The following are some generalizations regarding both basal and pentagastrin- or betazole-stimulated gastric acid secretion: (1) patients with gastric ulcers of the body of the stomach tend to secrete subnormal amounts of acid; (2) patients with duodenal ulcer or prepyloric ulcer secrete more acid than normal; (3) patients with gastrin-secreting tumors of the pancreas (i.e., gastrinoma, Zollinger-Ellison syndrome) tend to secrete more acid than duodenal ulcer patients. These generalizations refer to the "average patient" in each group. It must be emphasized that there is considerable overlap between groups. Also, some patients with gastric retention, systemic mastocytosis (see Ch. 574.4), and large small intestinal resection may secrete large amounts of gastric acid and pepsin.

Although there is a wealth of information on gastric secretion in both healthy subjects and patients with peptic ulcer disease, measurement of acid secretion in an individual patient very rarely assists the physician in either diagnosis or management. The reason for this is that measurement of gastric acid secretion is neither sensitive nor specific in the diagnosis of upper gastrointestinal diseases. Therefore, under what circumstances may secretory tests be helpful? In those patients in whom there is a high index of suspicion of gastrinoma (Zollinger-Ellison syndrome), the finding of markedly elevated basal and stimulated secretion would support this diagnosis. In patients with fasting hypergastrinemia, measurement of basal and stimulated acid secretion will distinguish those with appropriate hypergastrinemia secondary to absent or low rates of acid secretion (e.g., postvagotomy, gastric atrophy, pernicious anemia) from those with increased gastric secretion and inappropriate hypergastrinemia (e.g., gastrinoma, gastric retention, antral G-cell hyperfunction). Some have suggested measurement of basal and stimulated gastric acid secretion in patients with recurrent ulcer because a small percentage will have gastrinoma or retained gastric antrum. However, serum gastrin determination in recurrent ulcer patients is more sensitive and specific (see Ch. 403). Measurement of gastric acid secretion is also insensitive and nonspecific in distinguishing benign gastric ulcer from gastric cancer. About 80 per cent of patients with gastric cancer secrete acid, and a small percentage of benign gastric ulcer patients do not secrete acid. Therefore more direct methods (e.g., endoscopy, biopsy, and cytology) are more helpful in distinguishing one from the other.

Two additional situations in which secretory studies are often performed but have not been shown to be useful include (1) x-ray-negative dyspepsia, in which acid secretion is similar to normal, and (2) following vagotomy, to determine which patients have an increase in acid secretion in response to insulin-induced hypoglycemia (i.e., Hollander test), therefore suggesting persistent vagal innervation to the stomach. One to two years after vagotomy about 70 per cent of postvagotomy patients respond to insulin, but only one in seven will develop recurrent ulcer. Also, a small percentage of those who do not respond to insulin-induced hypoglycemia will develop ulcer recurrence. Because the insulin test has so little predictive value as to who will develop an ulcer recurrence, it is not routinely indicated following vagotomy.

405. PEPTIC ULCER: MEDICAL THERAPY

Jon I. Isenberg

The four goals of therapy of peptic ulcer are to relieve symptoms, to increase the rate of ulcer healing, to prevent complications, and to prevent recurrences. A host of drugs have been used to treat ulcer patients. Unfortunately, there are only a few recent double-blind studies that have studied drug efficacy on pain and healing in this common disease. Since the medical treatment of esophageal, gastric, and duodenal ulcer is similar, the following applies to all forms of peptic ulcer disease except when stated otherwise.

ANTACIDS. In the United States, approximately $110 million is spent on antacids each year. Recently, a one-month double-blind study in outpatients with endoscopically proved duodenal ulcer demonstrated that seven daily 30-ml doses of a magnesium-aluminum hydroxide liquid antacid, equivalent to 144 mEq of antacid, produced ulcer healing in almost 80 per cent of patients. Ulcer healing in the placebo-treated group was about 45 per cent, significantly less than the antacid-treated patients. In a single study antacids were no better than placebo in hospitalized gastric ulcer patients. This may be secondary to the effect of hospitalization, which may have obviated any additional effect of antacids. Liquid antacids have not been compared with placebo in outpatients with gastric ulcer.

Interestingly, in a number of studies, antacid and placebo have produced similar degrees of pain relief. Whether antacids protect the patient from ulcer complications or recurrences has not been adequately tested.

The rationale for the use of antacids in treating ulcer is as follows: (1) ulcer disease very rarely occurs in the absence of gastric acid and pepsin; (2) peptic activity decreases markedly at pH greater than 3.5; (3) the incidence of experimental ulcers in animals can be decreased by antacids; and (4) ulcer disease usually resolves with surgical therapy, which decreases gastric acid and pepsin secretion.

Most commercially available antacids consist of mixtures of magnesium, aluminum, or calcium compounds. Factors that influence the in vivo efficacy of an antacid include the neutralizing capacity of the antacid, the rate of reaction with acid, the rate of gastric acid secretion, and the rate of gastric emptying.

Sodium Bicarbonate. Sodium bicarbonate is a potent, rapidly acting antacid. It is completely absorbed and so presents the body with a load of sodium and alkali. With normal renal function the body can tolerate the excess alkaline and sodium load. In patients with decreased renal function or salt retention, the alkaline and sodium load may lead to alkalosis and an increase in total body sodium and water. Because sodium bicarbonate is water soluble, it leaves the stomach rapidly, thus producing only transient intragastric alkalization. Because of the risk of alkalosis and its relative inefficacy, sodium bicarbonate is no longer used in the treatment of ulcer disease.

Calcium Carbonate. Calcium carbonate is a potent, rapidly acting antacid. In the duodenum most of the calcium is converted into poorly absorbed calcium carbonate, calcium phosphate, and calcium soaps, less than 10 per cent being absorbed from the gut. Calcium-containing antacids may cause hypercalcemia. Also, oral calcium antacids produce an increase in acid secretion after their buffering effect has been fully utilized. This has been called "acid rebound." The calcium-induced increase in acid secretion is probably mediated in part by an increase in serum gastrin and in part by a direct effect of calcium on the parietal cells. It occurs only after calcium-containing antacids, not with noncalcium antacids. Repeated oral doses of calcium may produce an increase in serum calcium, phosphate, creatinine, and bicarbonate. Long-term ingestion of calcium carbonate plus sodium bicarbonate may result in the milk-alkali syndrome (see Ch. 555). Since there are many available noncalcium antacids which do not have the untoward effects of calcium but are effective antacids, most experts believe that calcium-containing antacids should not be used in the treatment of acid-peptic diseases.

Magnesium Hydroxide. Magnesium hydroxide is a potent antacid that reacts rapidly with hydrochloric acid. Magnesium trisilicate reacts with hydrochloric acid more slowly than magnesium hydroxide. Approximately 5 to 10 per cent of the ingested magnesium is absorbed from the gut and excreted by the kidneys. In patients with decreased renal function, serum magnesium level can increase and rarely may produce hypotension and respiratory arrest. Within the gut, magnesium compounds act as cathartics, so they can seldom be used as the sole antacid.

Aluminum Hydroxide. Aluminum hydroxide reacts with hydrochloric acid to form aluminum chloride. The neutralizing capacity of aluminum hydroxide preparations varies widely; some are effective, whereas others are ineffective antacids. In the gut aluminum hydroxide and aluminum chloride bind phosphate, producing nonabsorbable aluminum phosphate. Chronic ingestion of aluminum hydroxide can decrease serum and total body phosphate. It is therefore of therapeutic benefit in patients with chronic renal insufficiency and hyperphosphatemia. The adsorptive properties of aluminum hydroxide may decrease absorption of other agents (e.g., tetracycline, bile salts).

Fordtran found that in vitro buffering capacity correlated well with in vivo postprandial antacid activity. Patients with high levels of gastric acid secretion, "hypersecretors," tend to require larger amounts of antacid than low secretors to achieve a similar degree of neutralization. Because antacids rapidly leave the empty stomach, the effect of antacids in the fasting patient is transient, lasting about 10 to 20 minutes. However, when adequate amounts of antacids are administered one hour after a meal, they are disbursed in the meal and regenerate the buffering capacity of the meal itself. Therefore their effect lasts up to three hours.

In patients with duodenal ulcer, antacids should be given in doses of approximately 120 to 140 mEq (e.g., 30 ml of Mylanta II, 60 ml of Maalox, Riopan, Aludrox) one and three hours after each meal and before bed for one month, and then discontinued. In gastric ulcer patients, who generally secrete less acid than duodenal ulcer patients, doses should be about one half of those listed above, but administered on the same time schedule. Patients with gastroesophageal reflux and esopha-

Figure 6. Structure of histamine; a histamine H₂-receptor antagonist, cimetidine; and a histamine H₁-receptor antagonist, chlorpheniramine. Note that cimetidine and histamine both have an imidazole ring, whereas cimetidine has modification of the side chain. Also note that chlorpheniramine has modification of the ring structure with no significant changes of the side chain.

geal ulcer can be treated similarly to gastric ulcer patients. In those ulcer patients requiring sodium restriction (e.g., congestive heart failure, cirrhosis with ascites, hypertension), low sodium-containing antacids should be prescribed (e.g., Riopan).

HISTAMINE H₂-RECEPTOR ANTAGONISTS. James W. Black and associates described this new class of drugs in 1972. The standard "anti-allergic" antihistamines (e.g., diphenhydramine) do not inhibit gastric acid secretion, but instead inhibit the effect of histamine at other sites such as bronchial and ileal smooth muscle. These "anti-allergic" antihistamines are referred to as histamine H₁-receptor antagonists. The H₂-receptor antagonists (Fig. 6) are potent inhibitors of gastric acid secretion and have little or no effect on histamine H₁-receptor sites.

Cimetidine is the H₂-receptor antagonist currently available for treatment of patients with duodenal ulcer and massive gastric acid hypersecretion (e.g., Zollinger-Ellison syndrome, systemic mastocytosis). Cimetidine inhibits all forms of gastric acid secretion. Three hundred mg of oral cimetidine almost totally abolishes basal gastric secretion for approximately four hours, and inhibits meal-stimulated gastric acid secretion by about 75 per cent for three hours. Cimetidine is significantly more effective than anticholinergics (e.g., propantheline bromide), which inhibit meal-stimulated secretion by only 30 per cent (see below).

Cimetidine is well absorbed from the small intestine and excreted largely unchanged by the kidneys. Therefore in patients with renal failure the dose must be decreased by approximately one half. Cimetidine is re-

moved during either hemodialysis or peritoneal dialysis. In normal and ulcer subjects the circulating half-life of cimetidine is approximately two hours. Importantly, cimetidine does not alter gastric emptying or pancreatic bicarbonate or water secretion.

In a number of clinical trials cimetidine has been shown to heal approximately 70 to 80 per cent of duodenal ulcers over a one-month treatment period, similar to an intensive course of antacids (see above), and significantly better than placebo.

Over-all, duodenal ulcer pain has been better relieved by cimetidine than by placebo. Recent studies suggest that cimetidine is superior to placebo in expediting gastric ulcer healing. Current evidence suggests that cimetidine is effective in decreasing symptoms in patients with gastroesophageal reflux; however, results of clinical trials are not yet available in patients with esophageal ulcer.

In Great Britain both 1.2 grams of cimetidine daily and a single 400-mg nocturnal dose of cimetidine have been shown to be superior to placebo in preventing duodenal ulcer recurrences.

Thus far, cimetidine has no recognized severe toxicity in man. However, the following untoward effects have been reported: (1) Gynecomastia has been reported in a few patients receiving chronic cimetidine therapy. The mechanism for gynecomastia is not fully understood, but in part may be related to cimetidine increasing serum prolactin. (2) There has been a slight but significant increase in SGOT, SGPT, and creatinine with chronic cimetidine treatment. The increase is usually not above the upper limits of normal. (3) Serum gastrin increases more after a meal plus cimetidine than after a meal plus placebo. The postprandial increase in serum gastrin produced by cimetidine is undoubtedly due to decreased gastric acid secretion, resulting in prolonged neutralization of the gastric antrum. Therefore the acid-induced inhibition of gastrin release is delayed in the presence of cimetidine. Whether prolonged postprandial hypergastrinemia has a detrimental effect in man is not known. Gastrin, however, has a trophic effect on the parietal cell mass; hence, it is conceivable that prolonged cimetidine-induced hypergastrinemia may increase the number of parietal cells and ultimately increase gastric secretion. (4) Metiamide, a precursor of cimetidine, contained thiourea and produced agranulocytosis in approximately 1 per cent of the patients. Cimetidine contains cyanoguanidine in place of the thiourea radical. In two patients receiving chronic cimetidine a transient decrease in the number of circulating granulocytes developed. Whether this is directly related to cimetidine treatment, to other drugs the patients were receiving, or to other explanations is not known. The frequency of granulocytopenia requires study in large numbers of patients receiving cimetidine. (5) In experimental animals chronic cimetidine administration is associated with testicular Leydig cell tumors, and is also associated with a decrease in prostatic size. Whether there is a human counterpart of these phenomena is not known. (6) Finally, studies are in progress to determine whether the effects of cimetidine diminish with long-term treatment.

Cimetidine and large doses of antacid result in equivalent gastric neutralization and similar rates of duodenal and gastric ulcer healing. Since antacids are free of significant untoward side effects, it seems reasonable at present to prescribe them as the initial form of therapy. In patients unable to comply with antacid treatment, 300 mg of cimetidine with each meal and before bed is indicated for up to eight weeks of treatment. Cimetidine is not yet approved in the United States for patients with gastric ulcer or as chronic treatment in duodenal ulcer patients. Patients with a duodenal ulcer recurrence should be treated with either antacid or cimetidine as outlined above. Cimetidine treatment has been demonstrated to be of marked beneficial effect in patients with gastrinoma (see Ch. 403).

ANTICHOLINERGIC DRUGS. Anticholinergics block the action of acetylcholine on postganglionic nerve sites. They have been used in the treatment of ulcer to decrease acid and pepsin secretion. They also decrease salivary, bronchial, sweat, and pancreatic secretion, increase heart rate, produce mydriasis, decrease gastric and intestinal motility, and decrease urinary bladder tone and strength of contraction. There is not convincing evidence that any anticholinergic has a selective action on a specific target.

Since anticholinergics are less potent inhibitors of gastric secretion than either large doses of antacids or cimetidine, their use alone is not recommended in ulcer patients. They should not be used in patients in whom the anticholinergic effect may be harmful, as in patients with narrow-angle glaucoma, prostatism, gastroesophageal reflux, gastric retention, or chronic bronchitis. Importantly, anticholinergics plus cimetidine have an additive inhibitory effect on gastric secretion. Therefore in the future they may be shown to be more effective in combination than either one alone in ulcer healing.

DIET. Although bland diets have been used in the treatment of ulcer disease for the past 70 years, there is no evidence that a bland diet is more effective than a regular diet in ulcer healing, prevention of complications, or recurrence. During flare-ups of ulcer distress patients often restrict their diets to bland food, although there is no evidence that this reduces symptoms or shortens the attack.

In patients with ulcer disease, hourly milk and cream produced a lower intragastric pH (i.e., more acid) than three regular meals. In addition, excessive milk and cream with antacid may be a factor in the pathogenesis of the milk-alkali syndrome, coronary artery disease, and atherosclerosis.

There is no evidence that spices in moderate amounts are ulcerogenic or alter the course of ulcer healing or frequency of recurrence. Also, the texture of the diet, soft versus rough, seems unimportant in ulcer pathogenesis or therapy. Since caffeine is a stimulant of acid secretion, caffeine-containing beverages (including cola drinks) should probably be excluded from the diet in ulcer patients. Interestingly, decaffeinated coffee and caffeine-containing coffee produce equivalent increases in gastric acid secretion. Concentrated spirits (e.g., whiskey, gin) are capable of damaging the gastric mucosa, and may be involved in the pathogenesis of acute gastric erosions. Excessive alcohol intake should be curtailed in ulcer patients. Whether moderate intake (e.g., 1 to 2 ounces per day) has a harmful, beneficial, or no effect on ulcer healing is not known.

Bedtime snacks which will stimulate acid secretion while the patient is sleeping should be avoided. Food should not be used as an antacid, because the neutralization produced by food is always followed by increased secretion.

HOSPITAL CARE. In a single study, admission of gastric ulcer patients to hospital increased the rate of ulcer healing when compared to outpatient management. The cost of prolonged hospital care is almost prohibitive. It is recommended therefore that patients with suspected or demonstrated gastric ulcer be admitted for a brief period to expedite careful evaluation of the ulcer by radiography, endoscopy with biopsy, and, if available, gastric cytology. Medical therapy can be initiated during that time and continued on an outpatient basis.

Serial radiograms or endoscopies of a gastric ulcer should be obtained at four- to six-week intervals for up to 12 weeks. The ulcer should completely heal within this period. For those patients in whom the ulcer does not heal, surgery is usually indicated. Surgery is also recommended for the patient with second or third gastric ulcer recurrences (see Ch. 406). The recurrence rate of gastric ulcer following antrectomy is less than 2 per cent.

OTHER TREATMENTS. Colloidal Bismuth. Recent studies in Great Britain indicate that tripotassium dicitratobismuthate is superior to placebo in expediting gastric or duodenal ulcer healing in man. It does not alter gastric secretion. The mechanism of action of tripotassium dicitratobismuthate is not known, but it is postulated to form a "protective layer" over the ulcer base. It has no severe recognized toxicity in either animals or man. Colloidal bismuth is not yet approved for use in the United States.

Prostaglandins. Prostaglandins of the E and A class are potent inhibitors of gastric secretion. The natural prostaglandins are rapidly inactivated within the stomach. However, a number of synthetic prostaglandin analogues (e.g., 16,16-dimethyl prostaglandin E_2, 15(S)-15-methyl prostaglandin E_2) are effective orally. Their antiulcer action in animals is primarily due to their inherent cytoprotective effects, and less to their antisecretory effects. Untoward effects with high doses of prostaglandin in man include diarrhea, abdominal cramps, and uterotonia. Preliminary studies in human beings suggest that some prostaglandins may be effective in treatment of gastric or duodenal ulcer, but further clinical and toxicity studies are required. The prostaglandins are not approved for use in ulcer patients in the United States.

Carbenoxolone Sodium. Carbenoxolone sodium has been shown to increase healing rates in ambulatory gastric ulcer patients. A delayed release form designed to release the drug in the duodenal bulb has been shown to increase the healing rates in duodenal ulcer patients. The mechanism of action is not known. It does not alter gastric secretion. Postulated mechanisms include an increase in the production, viscosity, and glycoprotein content of mucus, and prolongation of the life span of gastric mucosal cells. Carbenoxolone sodium is structurally similar to aldosterone and often causes salt and water retention. Because of its untoward effects and the lack of evidence that it is superior to other forms of ulcer therapy, it has not been approved for use in the United States.

Sedation. Sedation has not been shown to be of definite value in the treatment of patients with peptic ulcer, and therefore is not routinely recommended. In patients with severe anxiety the addition of tranquilizers seems reasonable. Recently, the tricyclic antidepressant trimipramine has been reported to be more effective than placebo in expediting duodenal ulcer healing. It does not have potent antisecretory effects, and its mechanism of action is not known. Trimipramine has not been approved for use in ulcer patients in the United States, and further clinical trials are needed.

Interdiction of Smoking. The incidence of gastric and duodenal ulcer is greater in cigarette smokers than in nonsmokers. Discontinuation of smoking has been shown to increase ulcer healing rates in some studies, whereas in others no differences were noted between those who stopped smoking and those who continued. Since there are no beneficial effects of smoking, and since discontinuation may expedite ulcer healing and possibly prevent recurrences, ulcer patients should be encouraged to stop smoking.

Gastric Irradiation. Irradiation of the oxyntic gland portion of the stomach produces a decrease in acid secretion usually lasting less than one year. In some patients prolonged hypochlorhydria is produced. At present, gastric irradiation is employed only in those rare elderly patients who are unresponsive to medical therapy and in whom surgery carries a substantial risk of mortality.

406. PEPTIC ULCER: COMPLICATIONS AND SURGICAL TREATMENT

James H. Meyer

COMPLICATIONS

HEMORRHAGE. Hemorrhage afflicts about 15 to 20 per cent of ulcer patients, being two to three times more common than perforation or obstruction. Duodenal ulcers bleed slightly more often than gastric ulcers; duodenal ulcers along the posterior duodenal wall or postbulbar ulcers bleed more frequently than anterior duodenal ulcers. Hemorrhage is usually from a major artery eroded by the ulcer and less commonly from smaller vessels in granulation tissue of the ulcer.

About 25 per cent of patients with bleeding ulcers have never recognized ulcer symptoms previously. In almost all patients hemorrhage is manifested by melena; but three patients in four (fewer with duodenal ulcer) experience hematemesis as well. Diaphoresis, pallor, palpitations, lightheadedness, mental confusion, and syncope are symptoms of associated hypotension which arises either as a direct result of blood volume loss or from a vasovagal reaction to sudden loss of blood.

Other than ulcer, the only common causes of upper gastrointestinal bleeding are acute gastric *mucosal lesions* (diffuse or localized, spontaneous or drug induced) and *esophageal varices.* Less common causes include *bleeding esophagitis, Mallory-Weiss tears, benign* (leiomyoma) or *malignant* (gastric carcinoma, lymphoma) *tumors, eosinophilic gastritis, milk allergy* (in children), and a variety of *rare vascular lesions* (hereditary hemorrhagic telangiectasia, phlebectasia of the jejunum, pseudoxanthoma elasticum, periarteritis, Ehlers-Danlos syndrome). Spontaneous upper gastrointestinal hemorrhage may accompany severe coagulation defects associated with underlying disease or anticoagulant therapy. As a diagnostic tool, the physical examination is helpful primarily in providing clues to bleeding lesions other than peptic ulcer, especially esophageal varices (e.g., hepatosplenomegaly, ascites, jaundice) and vascular abnormalities.

Upper gastrointestinal hemorrhage carries a significant mortality (about 10 per cent in ulcer disease). Therefore any patient experiencing melena, with or without hematemesis or associated symptoms or hypotension, should be admitted to hospital immediately for observation and treatment. The over-all approach to the patient with upper gastrointestinal bleeding is discussed in Ch. 407.

Treatment. The program includes resuscitation as needed, reduction of gastric acidity, and continuous evaluation of the patient with the expectation that surgical intervention may be required. It is desirable that both physician and surgeon follow the patient's progress from the outset.

Many physicians prefer to treat the patient with continuous nasogastric aspiration as long as bleeding continues. When properly employed (proper tube placement, periodic venting), this procedure empties 90 to 95 per cent of secreted acid from the stomach and is therefore an adequate treatment. The appearance of blood in the gastric aspirate may also serve as an index of recurrent or continued bleeding. Alternatively, the patient may be treated with frequent antacids either from the outset or after the nasogastric tube is removed when bleeding has stopped. Most physicians prefer not to use anticholinergic drugs during hemorrhage, because these obscure signs of recurrent bleeding (they produce sustained tachycardia and diminish hyperactive bowel sounds which often indicate fresh blood in the gut).

If more than 3000 ml of blood is required for resuscitation, mortality increases significantly and is especially high if this quantity of blood is required in the first 48 hours. Emergency surgery is indicated in a patient who requires transfusion at a rate in excess of 3 units per day for the first 24 to 48 hours to maintain a stable circulation, once antecedent losses have been replenished. When bleeding has stopped under medical management but major hemorrhage subsequently reappears in spite of continued treatment, surgery should be undertaken, because it is likely that further medical treatment will not be successful and it is known that continued medical treatment in this situation carries a high mortality. Under these policies 15 to 30 per cent of bleeding ulcer patients will require emergency surgery.

Until recently, the traditional form of emergency surgery had been subtotal gastrectomy, usually with ligation or removal of the bleeding ulcer. Since the early 1960's, surgeons have favored the use of vagotomy plus pyloroplasty with ligation of bleeding vessels, citing lower mortality because of the speed and ease with which this operation can be performed. Retrospective analyses of mortality rates of these two operations in the bleeding patient are to date inadequate to substantiate the superiority of vagotomy plus pyloroplasty. Both operations effectively stop acute bleeding in 92 to 95 per cent of patients who are bleeding from a single, discrete ulcer, but are much less effective in stopping bleeding in patients with multiple stress ulcers.

Prognosis. Death from bleeding ulcer is more frequent in patients over 50 years of age. Bleeding gastric ulcers are more apt to be lethal than bleeding duodenal ulcers for two reasons: (1) patients with gastric ulcers are older than patients with duodenal ulcers, and (2) regardless of age, gastric ulcers tend to bleed more profusely than duodenal ulcers. Most forms of associated cardiovascular disease other than benign hypertension (ischemic or valvular heart disease, cor pulmonale) adversely affect the prognosis, as does any severe associated disease. It is not known whether earlier surgery in these higher risk patients would reduce mortality, because those patients are also the ones with higher operative mortality.

Thirty to 50 per cent of patients surviving the first hemorrhage without operative intervention will bleed again; the severity of the subsequent hemorrhage bears no relationship to the severity of the first episode. Continued morbidity (recurrent hemorrhage, intractable ulcer pain, subsequent perforation) is the rule in up to 70 per cent of ulcer patients who have bleeding. It is not clear whether surgery (emergent or elective) in the bleeding duodenal ulcer patient will significantly reduce recurrent bleeding. For the most part this is due to bleeding from recurrence of ulcer after surgery.

IMPAIRED GASTRIC EMPTYING ("OUTLET OBSTRUCTION"). This complication is seen in 5 to 10 per cent of ulcer patients. In the majority of cases (80 per cent), it appears as a complication of duodenal ulcer disease, usually of long duration. Gastric ulcers, most frequently prepyloric, are the second most common cause. Although pyloric channel ulcers may cause gastric outlet obstruction, ulcers at this site are infrequent.

In ulcer disease, impaired gastric emptying may develop as the result of narrowing of the lumen by fibrosis and/or inflammatory tumor around the ulcer. However, in many cases gastric motor dysfunction, associated with inflammation around the ulcer or with gradual dilatation of the stomach and stretching of gastric muscle beyond optimal force/length characteristics, plays a dominant role. Impaired gastric emptying is thus potentially reversible to the extent that gastric motor dysfunction can be corrected or that luminal narrowing by inflammation can be reduced with healing.

In the initial phases, mechanical outlet obstruction is usually not complete. However, ingested materials and gastric secretions gradually accumulate to produce gastric dilatation. With gastric dilatation, the patient begins to experience symptoms of constant epigastric fullness and discomfort, anorexia, morbid aversion to food, and nausea. Vomiting (spontaneous or induced) may relieve these symptoms. The whole process tends to develop insidiously over days or weeks. The eventual development of protracted vomiting, usually of copious amounts of undigested food, brings the patient to the physician.

In the typical case the diagnosis is easily made by the history. However, about one fourth of patients with impaired gastric emptying never vomit before seeking medical attention, presumably because they have reduced their oral intake to an amount that can be emptied. In this minority the diagnosis is usually discovered during an upper gastrointestinal series which reveals a large, dilated stomach filled with solid and liquid material in spite of the customary overnight fast prior to the examination. In most patients physical examination confirms recent weight loss and evidence of dehydration. Abdominal distention and tenderness are rarely noted, and bowel sounds are normal. A gastric succussion splash may be elicited in about half the patients. Diagnosis suspected on the basis of historical and physical findings can be quickly confirmed by placement of a large-bore orogastric (Ewald) tube; aspiration of 300 ml or more of gastric contents three or more hours after the last meal indicates gastric outlet obstruction.

Patients with gastric outlet obstruction must be admitted to hospital for treatment. The goals are fourfold: (1) correction of fluid and electrolyte deficits, (2) gastric decompression, (3) intensive ulcer treatment, and (4) surgery if obstruction persists.

In the face of protracted vomiting and no effective oral intake, fluid and electrolyte depletion may be profound. Extracellular fluid and plasma volume deficits may be reflected by orthostatic hypotension, prerenal azotemia, elevated hematocrit, and abnormally low central venous pressure. Some degree of metabolic alkalosis and hypokalemia is common. The latter may accentuate gastric motor dysfunction. These deficits must be rapidly corrected; they contribute to continued morbidity and may be responsible for increased surgical mortality.

There are two sources of electrolyte loss in gastric outlet obstruction: (1) hydrochloric acid and lesser amounts of sodium and potassium chloride are lost with the gastric juice which is vomited or removed by tube; and (2) considerable amounts of sodium and potassium are lost in the urine. For every H^+ ion lost in the gastric juice, one Cl^- ion is similarly lost and one HCO_3^- ion enters the circulation. During the early phases of obstruction, bicarbonate entering the bloodstream is cleared from the urine as $NaHCO_3$, and chloride losses are minimized by renal tubular reabsorption. At this stage the urine is characteristically alkaline and contains appreciable sodium, but is low in chloride. In effect, the kidney converts an HCl loss from the stomach to a net NaCl loss from the body (Na^+ lost in urine, Cl^- lost in gastric juice), and in this way metabolic alkalosis is minimized. However, as the body's deficit in NaCl mounts, secondary hyperaldosteronism intervenes. As a result, much more filtered Na^+ is reabsorbed by the renal tubules. Some is absorbed in exchange for K^+, and more is absorbed in exchange for H^+ secreted by the tubules. For every H^+ secreted by the renal tubules, one HCO_3^- enters the bloodstream. At this stage the urine is characteristically low in both sodium and chloride, but may contain significant amounts of potassium and may be paradoxically acidic. In effect, the kidney is no longer compensating for gastric losses; H^+ and Cl^- losses from the stomach are now aggravated by H^+ and Cl^- losses from the kidney. Sustained metabolic alkalosis, hypochloremia, and hypokalemia result.

Reversal of this sequence of events is accomplished by infusion of 0.15N NaCl intravenously. Potassium replacement as KCl may be started once an adequate urinary output has been established. Enough saline has to be given (1) to replenish continued gastric losses and (2) to replace antecedent sodium and chloride deficits. The adequacy of this replacement can be judged (1) by disappearance of orthostatic hypotension and return of venous pressure to normal, (2) by reappearance of an alkaline urine with a rising sodium concentration, and (3) by rising chloride concentration in the urine. As these changes take place, prerenal azotemia, metabolic alkalosis, and hypokalemia should disappear.

In the meantime gastric decompression is instituted to eliminate gastric dilatation and restore motor tone.

This is accomplished by continuous nasogastric aspiration once the stomach has been lavaged free of solid debris through a large-bore tube. Usually a period of 72 hours is adequate to restore gastric tone. Continuous gastric aspiration, by removing secreted gastric acid, is also an effective treatment for active ulcer disease. This treatment thus serves to reduce inflammatory edema around the ulcer and thus may help relieve the cause of the obstruction. With good management, fluid and electrolyte disturbances will have been corrected by 72 hours as well.

The end of the first 72 hours thus represents a point of reappraisal. If the nature of the obstructing lesion is in doubt at this time, an upper gastrointestinal series may be obtained to establish the diagnosis. This examination will also provide some indication as to how well the preceding treatment has restored gastric emptying. Some physicians assess gastric emptying by the saline load test. If more than 400 ml remains in the stomach 30 minutes after instilling 750 ml of isotonic saline, emptying is impaired. If the stomach does not empty, further medical treatment is unlikely to be effective, and surgery should be considered. If emptying is adequate, the patient may be begun on oral liquids and antacids. However, for the next several days continuous assessment of gastric emptying must be performed. If the patient has more than 300 ml gastric residual at bedtime (four hours after the last intake) or more than 200 ml after an overnight fast, or if the saline load test is abnormal, gastric emptying is still impaired and surgical treatment is indicated.

About 25 per cent of obstructed patients will require surgery by these criteria. Of those who escape surgery in a given episode, 15 per cent will have a recurrent episode of obstruction, frequently requiring surgery.

PERFORATION. Any peptic ulcer may erode through the muscular and serosal walls of the viscus in which it is located. If such erosion establishes a communication between the lumen of the viscus and the surrounding body cavity, allowing spillage of luminal contents into this cavity, perforation has occurred. If, on the other hand, the transmural erosion is sealed by surrounding visceral structures or peritoneum before spillage of luminal contents supervenes, the ulcer is said to have penetrated.

Free perforation occurs in about 5 to 10 per cent of ulcer patients. About 90 per cent of these perforations arise from a duodenal ulcer, usually in the anterior duodenal wall. Nine per cent arise from gastric ulcers and the remainder from perforated malignant gastric ulcers or perforated marginal ulcers after subtotal gastric resection. Free perforation is almost always heralded by sudden onset of intense, usually generalized and constant abdominal pain. Usually these dramatic symptoms follow years of intermittent ulcer-like pain, but in about 25 per cent of patients ulcer pain preceding the perforation will have been noted for less than three months, and 7 per cent of patients with perforation have never recognized ulcer symptoms previously. Perforation may occur at any age (peak incidence is the fifth and sixth decades), and age-specific rates of perforation increase throughout life, even though ulcer disease generally remits in older life. Elderly patients who perforate may not experience intense symptoms, so the diagnosis may not be appreciated. Ten per cent of patients who perforate hemorrhage at the same time.

Physical examination usually confirms the diagnosis suspected on historical grounds. Generalized direct and rebound tenderness, board-like rigidity of the abdominal musculature, and diminished or absent bowel sounds resulting from reflex ileus are signs of generalized peritonitis which accompanies perforation. Swallowed air escaping through the perforation into the abdominal cavity may result in loss of normal hepatic dullness on percussion; this can be visualized radiographically under the diaphragm on upright or lateral abdominal films in 75 to 80 per cent of patients who have perforated. In the absence of a typical history, signs of generalized peritonitis from perforated ulcer could be ascribed to any abdominal catastrophe (e.g., rupture of a volvulus, diverticulum, gallbladder, or appendix; fulminant pancreatitis). Moreover, escaping luminal contents are occasionally confined to the upper abdomen or lesser sac or are spilled down the right gutter into the right lower quadrant; in these situations signs of peritonitis may be localized rather than generalized, so the condition may be misdiagnosed. In practice, however, the diagnosis of perforated ulcer is made correctly about 90 per cent of the time.

Peritonitis associated with perforation produces dehydration owing to fluid loss into the peritoneal cavity. Leukocytosis and fever also reflect peritonitis, but the latter is not a common sequel to perforation treated quickly. Serum amylase is often elevated as the result of perforation.

Three forms of treatment are available: (1) medical treatment, which consists of carefully monitored continuous nasogastric aspiration to allow the perforation to seal, (2) simple surgical closure of the perforation, and (3) surgical closure of the perforation combined with an operation for the ulcer disease. Medical treatment, *when properly managed,* is as safe and effective as surgical closure. However, surgical closure permits direct inspection of the abdominal cavity, minimizing errors in diagnosis. Consequently, surgical closure is the preferred treatment. Patients who perforate after long-standing ulcer symptoms continue to experience significant morbidity from ulcer disease after simple closure of the perforation. For this reason, most surgeons undertake definitive ulcer surgery at the time of closure of a perforation in patients with a longstanding ulcer history, provided that the circumstances permit a more extensive procedure.

PENETRATION. Ulcers which penetrate are usually refractory to medical treatment. Posterior duodenal ulcers are most likely to do this. The complication is heralded by a change in pain pattern. Classically visceral ulcer pain takes on somatic characteristics felt in the back, chest, or lateral abdomen. Often pain becomes constant and is no longer relieved by food or antacids. Some ulcers which penetrate into the head of the pancreas may cause localized pancreatitis and elevation of serum amylase. Definitive treatment for penetrating ulcer is surgical.

SURGICAL TREATMENT

INDICATIONS FOR ELECTIVE SURGERY FOR PEPTIC ULCER. Although medical therapy promotes the healing of an acute ulcer, we do not know whether sustained medical treatment can significantly alter the long-term course of ulcer disease. For the relapse-prone patient who experiences significant cumulative morbid-

Outcome of Elective Operation for Duodenal Ulcer in Patients Followed Three to Eight Years*

Operation	Ulcer Recurrence (%)	Postprandial Symptoms (%)†	Weight Loss	Diarrhea (%)
Subtotal gastrectomy	2–5	36–40	++	7
Truncal vagotomy and antrectomy	0–3	34–39	++	20–23
Truncal vagotomy and drainage	7–15‡	21–40	+	25–26
Proximal gastric vagotomy	1–22§	0–14	+	0–14

*Results compiled from three randomized studies: Br. Med. J., 2:781, 1968; Ann. Surg., 172:547, 1970; Surg. Gynecol. Obstet., 137:387, 1973; and a recent review of proximal gastric vagotomy: Ann. Surg., 184:659, 1976.

†Highest percentage of patients with any of several varieties of postprandial distress.

‡Some studies indicate even higher recurrence after ten years of follow-up.

§Data from less than five years of follow-up in eight studies indicate recurrence in fewer than 8 per cent of patients; the high estimate of 22 per cent comes from one study.

ity attended with economic loss and periods of absence from his life's pursuits, surgical treatment is an alternative, but unfortunately the operations available are all associated with continued postoperative morbidity in a significant number of patients (see accompanying table). Moreover, although surgery cures the ulcer in a high proportion of patients (see below), no guarantee can be made in the individual case. For these reasons, the decision to operate electively for intractable ulcer disease must be carefully considered by patient, physician, and surgeon. The problem is to decide whether morbidity under medical management is likely to be greater than that which arises after surgery. Only a few guidelines can be offered to aid this decision.

Duodenal Ulcer. A period of observation under medical supervision is required to judge the virulence of duodenal ulcer disease in any individual patient. A significant number (probably about 25 per cent) of patients will experience only a single symptomatic episode of duodenal ulceration which responds adequately to medical treatment; clearly these patients do not require surgery. Symptomatic recurrences more often than biannually indicate that the patient suffers from a severe form of the disease and that surgical treatment should be considered, but other factors must be taken into account as well. Among these factors is the disability produced by each recurrence. The personality of the patient must also be considered, for there is some evidence that a poorly motivated patient (as evidenced by poor work records antedating the ulcer disease or poor social adjustment) is more likely to experience postoperative morbidity. Only a minority of duodenal ulcer patients present with less equivocal indications for surgery: duodenal ulcer secondary to gastrinomas (see above), penetrating duodenal ulcers (see above), and giant duodenal ulcers. These are frequently refractory to medical treatment and are prone to complications, so surgical treatment is appropriate. Also, the development of one or more complications alters the prognosis; surgery may be required to treat these complications as they arise, or may be subsequently elected because the patient has demonstrated by the development of these complications that he has severe ulcer disease.

Gastric Ulcer. A similar line of reasoning applies to the patient with gastric ulcer. Recurrence is common (up to 40 per cent in two years), and morbidity from frequent recurrence is high. However, the problem of gastric ulcer differs from duodenal ulcer in two respects: (1) In gastric ulcer healing poorly under medical treatment, the possibility arises that the lesion is an ulcerated cancer. However, present-day techniques of endoscopy plus endoscopically directed biopsy and/or exfoliative cytologic examinations are 90 to 95 per cent

accurate in distinguishing a malignant from a benign gastric ulcer, so in current practice doubt about malignancy is rarely an issue. Rather, it is the expected continued morbidity from an unhealed benign gastric ulcer that prompts surgery. (2) The patient with gastric ulcer tends to be older and may suffer from diseases associated with aging which alter operative risks and thus may influence the decision concerning surgery.

TYPES OF SURGICAL TREATMENT. Duodenal Ulcer. Three types of operation are commonly employed for duodenal ulcer: (1) *subtotal gastrectomy*, in which 75 to 80 per cent of distal stomach is removed and gastrointestinal continuity is restored by an anastomosis between the gastric remnant and the jejunum; (2) *truncal vagotomy and "drainage,"* a procedure in which the vagus nerve trunks are cut and the outlet of the stomach is widened by either a pyloroplasty or a gastroenterostomy; and (3) *truncal vagotomy and antrectomy*, which consists of cutting the vagus nerves, removing the distal 50 per cent of the stomach, and reestablishing gastrointestinal continuity by gastroduodenostomy or gastrojejunostomy. "Drainage" is performed to prevent gastric stasis, which tends to occur after truncal vagotomy.

All three traditional operations are associated with some degree of postoperative morbidity (see table). Truncal vagotomy plus pyloroplasty requires no gastric resection, less operating time, and no intestinal transection, thus reducing the possibility of postoperative leakage from an intestinal suture line; consequently, this operation has been preferred in situations in which surgical risks are great. Nevertheless, chronic postoperative symptoms are as severe after vagotomy plus drainage as after vagotomy plus antrectomy, which has much lower rate of ulcer recurrence; as a result, truncal vagotomy plus antrectomy is being chosen for elective operations for duodenal ulcer in otherwise healthy patients. In elective surgery, operative mortality for each of these three operations is less than 2 per cent.

A new operation, *proximal gastric vagotomy*, has been utilized extensively in Europe and increasingly in the United States. In this procedure vagal nerve fibers to the proximal stomach are individually transected, leaving innervation to the antrum intact, and no drainage procedure is employed. This operation reduces the rapid gastric emptying which results from the other procedures and the frequency and severity of chronic postoperative symptoms (see table). Even though this operation requires special training of the surgeon and may turn out to have as high a recurrence rate as truncal vagotomy plus pyloroplasty, the apparent marked reduction in postoperative morbidity would warrant its increasing use.

Gastric Ulcer. For gastric ulcer, the traditional surgical treatment is distal gastrectomy with gastroduodenostomy. In most instances this resection removes the ulcer; with high gastric ulcers it may be combined with a wedge resection of the ulcer or biopsies of the ulcer margins to ascertain the benignancy of the ulcer. Some have proposed that vagotomy and drainage be used for gastric ulcer. However, gastric ulcer recurrences are more frequent after this procedure than after distal resection.

CHRONIC POSTOPERATIVE MORBIDITY. Prandial and Postprandial Symptoms. *Early satiety* (intense feeling of fullness before finishing a meal, experienced by 36 to 60 per cent of patients) and *bilious vomiting* (in 13 per cent) shortly after eating are complaints encountered after all three operations. The "dumping" syndrome, a symptom complex which includes any or all of the following: nausea, vomiting, abdominal cramps, borborygmi, flatulence, diarrhea, diaphoresis, palpitations, tachycardia, lightheadedness, and flushing, may be experienced while eating or immediately afterward, especially after meals high in sugar content. The syndrome is believed to arise from the rapid entry of hyperosmolar liquids into the gut. It is experienced in mild form by about 20 per cent of operated patients, but is troublesome in only about 7 per cent. Somewhat later postprandially (two to four hours), some patients (about 10 per cent) may experience *hypoglycemia* and symptoms thereof. Such patients exhibit abnormally rapid rises in both serum glucose and insulin concentrations, thought to be related to rapid entry of glucose into the gut. All three operations accelerate the passage of liquid material into the gut.

These symptoms are usually more prominent in the first month after surgery and diminish as time passes. They may be ameliorated by use of frequent small feedings taken without liquids and the avoidance of sugar in the diet (sugar is the most osmotically active dietary component).

Nutritional Problems. Some weight loss is common, particularly after resective procedures. Frequently weight loss is associated with reduced caloric intake as the result of early satiety or the desire to minimize postprandial symptoms. However, about a quarter of the patients have mild steatorrhea, which may also contribute to malnutrition. Anemias occur in 20 to 50 per cent of patients, particularly after resection. Anemias usually appear more than five years after surgery; usually they reflect deficiency in iron, occasionally in folate or vitamin B_{12}. Osteomalacia may appear many years after subtotal gastrectomy.

Recurrent Ulceration. When the ulcer recurs in a duodenum left in continuity with the stomach, as after vagotomy and drainage, symptoms are typical of duodenal ulcer. However, when a recurrent ulcer arises at a gastrojejunal anastomosis ("marginal ulceration"), symptoms may be atypical. Pain frequently occurs in the left upper quadrant but may appear anywhere in the abdomen; marginal ulcers are refractory to medical treatment, frequently bleed, and occasionally perforate. Appropriate treatment is surgical. In patients who have had a subtotal gastrectomy, the treatment consists of a vagotomy. In patients who have had a prior vagotomy without resection, the treatment is antrectomy, often with attempts to cut more vagal fibers.

Postvagotomy Diarrhea. Although postcibal diarrhea may be associated with the dumping syndrome after any of the procedures, a different form of diarrhea is seen in about one in four patients who have had a vagotomy (see table). This diarrhea tends to be episodic, lasting a day or two, and during such episodes may continue during periods of fasting. In only a few patients is it disabling. For these few patients treatment with opiates or anticholinergics has been tried but has not been uniformly successful. Recent controlled trials indicate that cholestyramine may be helpful in reducing the diarrhea. The cause of postvagotomy diarrhea is unknown.

Rare Mechanical Problems. These include stomal obstruction, partial afferent loop obstruction, intermittent jejunal intussusception, gastro- or jejunocolic fistulas, and gastric bezoars. They arise almost exclusively in resected patients with gastrojejunal anastomoses.

Section Four
GASTROINTESTINAL BLEEDING

407. GASTROINTESTINAL BLEEDING

David H. Law

TYPES OF BLEEDING. Bleeding may be manifested by *hematemesis* (vomiting of blood, either bright red or brown and precipitated, resembling coffee grounds), by *melena* (the passage of tarry black, sticky stool), or by *hematochezia* (the passage of fresh red blood per rectum). Bleeding, however, may be only occult, with normal-appearing stools which on chemical determination are shown to contain blood.

DEGREE AND EFFECTS OF BLEEDING. The pathophysiologic effects which result from gastrointestinal blood loss give rise to many of the symptoms and signs which have been shown to be of clinical importance in determining the presence and the severity of bleeding. In large part, however, this response to blood loss is unrelated to the site or cause of the bleeding, depending more upon the *rate* and *extent*.

After acute massive bleeding, typified by loss of greater than 1500 ml or 25 per cent of the circulating blood volume within a period of minutes to hours, cardiac output and systolic blood pressure decrease, followed by decrease in diastolic blood pressure and increased pulse. Blood pressure responses occur first in the form of orthostatic hypotension. Pulse rate seems to be a less accurate parameter, even at a time when orthostatic hypotension is clearly evident, but it usually does rise. Compensatory vascular responses include constriction of the arterial bed with skin pallor, decreased splanchnic blood flow, and decreased renal blood flow with relative maintenance of cerebral and cardiopulmonary vascular systems. Vascular complications may include acute tubular necrosis, mesenteric vascular insufficiency with bowel infarction, and centrilobular necrosis of the liver. With continued acute blood loss, cerebral blood flow is embarrassed and there may be confusion, progressing to obtundation. Early electrocardiographic changes of T wave flattening or inversion and possibly S-T segment depression document insufficiency of coronary blood flow. Most of the early changes respond to correction of the diminished plasma volume, using blood transfusions or other plasma expanders such as electrolyte solutions or dextrans. If, however, blood loss continues unabated, the secondary effects of *shock* — increasing anoxia, cellular dysfunction, and acidosis — may lead to death. The mortality from massive gastrointestinal bleeding varies from 5 to 50 per cent, depending upon the cause of the hemorrhage and the age and condition of the patient.

More gradual compensatory physiologic mechanisms, including antidiuretic hormone and aldosterone release, act to re-establish intravascular volume, with a resultant drop in hematocrit and hemoglobin concentration. This plasma restoration begins rapidly, and up to one half the total compensation may occur within 8 to 12 hours. However, depending upon the patient's state of hydration, age, ability to resorb fluid lost into the gut, and rate of both oral and parenteral fluid repletion, this process may continue for 48 to 72 hours. For these reasons hematocrit and hemoglobin concentration values may be misleading during acute bleeding episodes. By recognizing these responses, the reduction in blood volume can be estimated and a logical sequence of diagnostic studies outlined to define the source of bleeding.

The degree of blood loss is the single most important parameter to be defined when a patient presents with gastrointestinal bleeding. This will establish the relative emergency of the problem and set the diagnostic and therapeutic pace to follow. Although the clinical history is often nondiagnostic, it will provide useful information in about one third of the cases and should be thoroughly evaluated.

Examination of the patient provides the best means of assessing severity of acute blood loss based on the responses previously outlined. As a general rule, blood pressure less than 100 mm Hg or a pulse rate exceeding 100 per minute in an otherwise normotensive patient indicates a 20 per cent volume depletion. Associated pallor and/or postural hypotension lends support to this estimate. A pulse rate increase of 20 per minute or orthostatic blood pressure decreases of greater than 10 mm Hg further suggest acute blood loss in excess of 1000 ml.

LOCALIZATION AND SITE. In the acute situation, several points of history may be useful in finding the site of bleeding. (1) Hematemesis indicates bleeding from above the duodenal-jejunal junction, whereas passage of red blood per rectum is most frequently associated with a bleeding site below the ligament of Treitz and usually from the colon. (2) The onset of hematemesis after forceful vomiting suggests the Mallory-Weiss syndrome or even esophageal rupture. (3) Typical abdominal pain may suggest peptic ulcer or reflux esophagitis. (4) Stress ulcers may occur hours to days after trauma, severe burns, or surgical procedures. (5) Associated diseases may suggest the source of gastrointestinal hemorrhage; i.e., alcoholism is associated with bleeding from gastritis and varices; arthritis is associated with salicylate and other drug ingestion which may cause gastritis; diverticulosis may bleed massively; emphysema carries an increased risk for development of peptic ulcer; and cirrhosis and peptic ulcer suggest sources of blood loss. (6) Past surgical procedures may suggest a bleeding site such as marginal ulcer or aortointestinal fistula. (7) Medications and toxins (analgesics such as salicylates and indomethacin, adrenocortical steroids and phenylbutazone, antihypertensives, and alcohol) may be associated with bleeding. Qualitative characteristics of bleeding, such as the presence of clots or bright red, mahogany, or coffee-ground material, have little quantitative significance but may help localize bleeding to a given area of the gastrointestinal tract.

The *physical examination*, in addition to demonstrating the nonspecific signs of blood loss, may reveal lesions which suggest a specific cause of the bleeding. One should inspect the orpharynx and skin for vascular lesions, dermatoses, or tumorous lesions. Relevant vascular lesions include the telangiectasia of Osler-Weber-Rendu disease, blue rubber bleb nevi, Henoch-Schönlein purpura, and spiders or caput medusae of cirrhosis. Skin changes characteristic of Ehlers-Danlos syndrome, pseudoxanthoma elasticum, scurvy, and the phenotype of Turner's syndrome all may be clues. The dermatoses, pyoderma gangrenosum or erythema nodosum, suggest underlying inflammatory bowel disease, and skin changes of scleroderma, amyloidosis, carcinoid syndrome or the Peutz-Jeghers syndrome suggest a specific cause for bleeding. Acanthosis nigricans may be found with occult malignancy of the gastrointestinal tract. Finally, tumorous lesions of Gardner's syndrome, neurofibromatosis, or Kaposi's sarcoma necessitate a search for neoplasia in the bowel. Hepatosplenomegaly, adenopathy (especially Virchow's node), the presence of a rectal or abdominal mass, and overt congenital anomalies may also suggest a site of bleeding.

LABORATORY STUDIES. Immediate *laboratory* evaluation should include a white blood cell count, hematocrit, hemoglobin, blood urea nitrogen, and evaluation for bleeding diathesis. An abrupt leukocytosis up to 20,000 per cubic millimeter and an outpouring of platelets may be seen with acute hemorrhage. A nasogastric tube should be inserted to estimate the amount and character of blood in the stomach, and guaiac tests performed on gastric contents. A hemoglobin level of less than 11 grams per 100 ml and a blood urea nitrogen (BUN) greater than 40 mg per 100 ml, in an otherwise normal patient, indicate a blood loss greater than 1000 ml. Blood in the upper intestine is reflected in an increased level of BUN with essentially no effect on serum creatinine. With cessation of bleeding, the BUN returns to normal within two to three days.

MANAGEMENT. It is important to stress that management of·the patient with massive bleeding frequently does not permit the luxury of a thorough diagnostic search. Immediate steps must be taken to minimize morbidity and mortality. The most important single aim in the management of *emergent* bleeding is the maintenance of an adequate blood volume. This requires adequate access to the venous system. With massive bleeding or shock, central venous or pulmonary artery pressure monitoring and measurement of hourly urinary output in an intensive care unit may be the most accurate and efficient guides in determining the need for increasing or decreasing subsequent plasma expansion. This is especially true for the high risk patient (e.g., age over 50; associated renal, pulmonary, or cardiac disease; presence of acidosis). Simultaneously with typing and cross-matching of blood for transfusion, some form of *plasma expander* should be infused — normal saline, Ringer's lactate, or even 5 per cent dextrose solution may be used initially, but dextran or plasma may be more effective while awaiting the arrival of whole blood and/or blood products. After establishment of intravenous access, a large-bore tube should be passed into the stomach. Blood in the gastric aspirate confirms a bleeding site proximal to the ligament of Treitz; however, failure to find blood does not exclude this possibility. If blood is present, one should continuously lavage the stomach with ice water or saline, using an Ewald tube, until the returns are free of clots and clear. In addition to controlling hemorrhage, this may minimize vomiting and monitor the activity of bleeding. The patient with suspected esophageal variceal hemorrhage constitutes a special problem and will be discussed separately.

The use of vasoconstrictor drugs should be considered when bleeding is massive, but great care must be taken in the presence of hypertensive or arteriosclerotic cardiovascular disease. Intravenous infusion over 20 minutes of 20 units of vasopressin, diluted in 100 ml of 5 per cent dextrose in distilled water, may be effective for diffuse lesions of gastritis, or duodenitis. Continuous or hourly infusions of antacids adequate to maintain the intragastric pH at 4.5 may lead to cessation of bleeding. If bleeding is massive and endoscopy fails to reveal the lesion or one is unable to clear the stomach of blood, angiography may identify the site and permit direct selective arterial infusion of vasoactive agents (0.2 unit per minute of Pitressin, or equivalent amounts of epinephrine) to control the hemorrhage. Experimental approaches using various types of embolization (e.g., autologous clot or Gelfoam) show promise for controlling arterial hemorrhage, and studies are currently underway to evaluate the effectiveness of H_2 histamine blockers (cimetidine) in the acute treatment of various lesions in which peptic activity plays a role.

SPECIFIC DIAGNOSTIC TECHNIQUES. The clinical decision as to the diagnostic use of endoscopy or x-ray should be based on skills of the immediately available personnel. If peptic ulcer seems the most likely probability after considering all factors, a barium contrast study of the esophagus, stomach, and upper intestine would most likely yield a diagnosis, while minimizing diagnostic risks. Evidence suggesting the Mallory-Weiss syndrome, gastritis, or portal hypertension is an indication for *panendoscopy* as the *initial* diagnostic procedure if an experienced endoscopist is available. The availability of a wide selection of flexible fiberoptic instruments for direct visualization of the esophageal, gastric, and duodenal mucosa has greatly enhanced the detection of lesions responsible for gastrointestinal bleeding. It is the most reliable procedure for diagnosing mucosal disorders of the esophagus, stomach, and duodenum. Although skilled endoscopy in the emer-

gent setting can be performed with minimal patient risk and provide accurate diagnostic information, it should be emphasized that optimal visualization requires proper timing of the procedure, a clean stomach, and a relaxed, cooperative patient. These conditions are best accomplished when the patient's clinical situation is stable. It is also important to note that there are as yet no adequate studies to demonstrate that early endoscopy significantly changes mortality rates from gastrointestinal bleeding.

Emergency radiologic evaluation requires close cooperation between the primary care physician and a well-informed radiologist with a preplanned course of action and special arrangements to avoid delays or untoward risks while the patient is away from his room. Cinefluoroscopy, air contrast study of the stomach, and hypotonic duodenography have increased the sensitivity of this procedure, but, are much more difficult in the patient with emergent bleeding.

As noted above, if routine studies are negative and the rate of blood loss is greater than 0.5 ml per minute, celiac and mesenteric angiography may be useful by showing puddling of contrast agent at the site of hemorrhage within the bowel and permitting the infusion of vasoactive drugs. This approach, however, requires a skilled, trained angiographer.

When all the aforementioned studies are nondiagnostic and very active bleeding persists, small intestinal intubation with sequential aspirations of the intestinal content may localize the bleeding site. Barium contrast study may then be performed through the tube to document a lesion at the site of bleeding. This test is most useful for locating obscure bleeding sites between the ligament of Treitz and the ileocecal valve, such as small bowel tumors, ulcers, Meckel's diverticula, or vascular anomalies.

The terminal ileum is often seen during reflux from a barium enema and may show terminal ileitis, an infrequent cause of massive gastrointestinal bleeding. Colonic diverticula are increasingly frequent with age and therefore cannot necessarily be implicated as the cause of bleeding when they are visualized by barium contrast study. They are, however, a common cause of massive lower gastrointestinal bleeding. In this situation, as well as with vascular anomalies of the colon, selective inferior mesenteric arteriography may reveal the precise site of hemorrhage.

On occasion emergency surgical intervention must be considered for the patient with shock caused by uncontrollable massive hemorrhage. In addition, certain patients with gastrointestinal bleeding have an increased mortality, suggesting the need for early surgery, such as those who rebleed while hospitalized with good medical management and those older than 60.

In the setting of *nonemergent bleeding*, a more deliberate plan, involving detailed history, physical examination, and selected special studies, including endoscopy and complete radiologic survey of the gastrointestinal tract, may be undertaken. Since bleeding may not be evident, laboratory data may be necessary to establish bleeding and to define its source. Inspection and chemical tests (i.e., guaiac) of fresh stool are important in assessing the presence and extent of nonemergent gastrointestinal bleeding. Vomitus and gastric and small bowel aspirates, in addition to stools, should be tested for the presence of occult blood in patients suspected of bleeding. When the aforementioned radiologic and endoscopic studies are nondiagnostic and persistent active bleeding is suspected, small intestinal intubation or passage of a weighted umbilical tape that will reach the small bowel may demonstrate the bleeding site.

Portal hypertension with gastrointestinal bleeding constitutes a special problem and is the most critical hazard to patients with portal hypertension. Approximately one third of cirrhotic patients die from this complication. When the patient with massive gastrointestinal bleeding also has portal hypertension, initial management should follow the guidelines noted above and be carried out in an intensive care area if available. Management is complicated by the frequent association of multisystem disease with renal, central nervous sytem, clotting mechanism or cardiac, and fluid and electrolyte abnormalities. Panendoscopy should be performed to establish that varices are, indeed, the site of blood loss, because at least one fourth of the patients with esophageal varices who present with gastrointestinal hemorrhage may be bleeding from another source. Treatment directed at the bleeding varices includes vasopressin and mechanical tamponade. Intravenous Pitressin, 20 units diluted in 100 ml of isotonic saline or dextrose, should be delivered over a 20- to 30-minute period and repeated at one- to two-hour intervals as indicated. If this fails to control hemorrhage, esophageal tamponade, using a Sengstaken-Blakemore or Linton tube, is indicated. Regardless of which tube is used, ultimate survival with minimal morbidity depends on close supervision and strict attention to detail of the method. Complications of balloon tamponade include asphyxiation from tracheal obstruction by the balloon, aspiration, esophageal erosions, and rupture. Rarely should the tube remain inflated over 48 hours. The immediate aim of therapy is to control hemorrhage, and this is possible in the majority of cases. Failure to control bleeding by tamponade may indicate that varices are not the source of bleeding.

Ultimate therapy to prevent rebleeding is directed at elective surgical decompression of the portal system, because operative mortality approaches 70 per cent when emergent surgery is required to control variceal bleeding. The most important criteria for selecting a successful surgical candidate relate to the patient's age and hepatic function. A serum albumin above 3.0 grams per 100 ml, bilirubin less than 3.0 mg per 100 ml, sulfobromophthalein retention less than 20 per cent, prothrombin time less than four seconds elevated, absence of ascites, and a liver biopsy showing only minimal fatty metamorphosis and absence of alcoholic hepatitis in the presence of cirrhosis are the most important criteria to consider when selecting the ideal surgical candidate. Mortality and morbidity of shunt surgery seem related directly to abnormalities of these parameters reflecting hepatic reserve. Thus after emergent gastrointestinal hemorrhage has been controlled, an intensive nutritional and rehabilitation program is essential to improve liver function in preparation for surgery. This may require up to three months to achieve maximal benefit.

Bleeding diathesis, although infrequently a cause of massive gastrointestinal hemorrhage, may complicate bleeding esophageal varices or be present in patients with blood dyscrasias, vascular abnormalities, or multiple systemic diseases which present with gastrointestinal bleeding. When the history, physical examination, or clinical course suggests such a possibility, the sequence of diagnostic studies should include expert hematologic consultation and the appropriate laboratory tests to detect these disorders and dictate appropriate therapy.

Baum, S., and Nusbaum, M.: The control of gastrointestinal haemorrhage by selective mesenteric arterial infusion of vasopressin. Radiology, 98:497, 1971.

Brick, I. B., and Jeghers, H. J.: Gastrointestinal hemorrhage. N. Engl. J. Med., 253:458, 511, 555, 1955.

Conn, H. O., Ramsby, G. R., Storer, R. H., et al.: Intra-arterial vasopressins in the treatment of upper intestinal hemorrhage: A prospective, controlled clinical trial. Gastroenterology, 68:211, 1975.

Isenberg, J. I., Walsh, J. H., and Grossman, M. I.: Zollinger-Ellison syndrome. Gastroenterology, 65:140, 1973.

Pitcher, J. L.: Safety and effectiveness of the modified Sengstaken-Blakemore tube: A prospective study. Gastroenterology, 61:291, 1971.

Schille, K. F. R.: Truelove, S. C., and Williams, D. J.: Hematemesis and melena with special reference to factors influencing the outcome. Br. Med. J., 2:7, 1970.

Sleisenger, M. H., and Fordtran, J. S. (eds.): Gastrointestinal Disease. 2nd ed. Philadelphia, W. B. Saunders Company, 1978, Chapters 11, 36–39, 46–56.

Section Five
MALABSORPTION

408. MALABSORPTION

Marvin H. Sleisenger

The malabsorption syndrome is a constellation of symptoms and signs that are the result of abnormal fecal excretion of fat (steatorrhea) and of varying degrees of malabsorption of fat-soluble vitamins as well as carbohydrate, protein, minerals, other vitamins, and water.

MECHANISM OF NORMAL ABSORPTION

In view of the wide range of absorption defects that can be involved, each instance of the malabsorption syndrome must be analyzed against the background of the processes of *normal* absorption. Accordingly, a brief review of the processes of normal absorption is presented at this time.

During absorption, the end products of digestion must leave the intestinal lumen, traverse the mucosal cells, enter the terminal branches of the vascular and lymphatic vessels, and thus gain entrance into the general circulation. Before penetrating the cell membrane, they must pass through an "unstirred water layer" which may influence absorption. Two mechanisms, acting separately or together, are important in this process: *active transport* and *passive transport*. Both of these are presumed to take place in relationship to a hypothetical cell membrane. Strictly defined, *absorption* means greater lumen to plasma unidirectional flux; *secretion* is the reverse.

Passive transport is the passage of a molecule across a membrane barrier according to chemical concentration and electrical gradients. (Examples are the absorption of fatty acids, water, and bile salts in the jejunum. It requires no energy and is not saturable. A kind of passive transport is "solvent drag," by which ions are simply carried across by water moving into the cell. *Active transport* requires metabolic work with expenditure of energy that results in a net movement of substances against a chemical or electrical difference. An important characteristic of active transport is that the transport mechanism is "saturable," since the rate levels off as luminal electrochemical activity of the ion increases.

FAT ABSORPTION. Intraluminal Phase. Sixty to 100 grams of fat is eaten daily by adults, principally as triglycerides containing long-chain fatty acids. This triglyceride must be digested (i.e., hydrolyzed) and solubilized intraluminally before absorption. Absorption, in turn, consists of uptake and transport, both processes requiring normally functioning mucosal cells.

The stomach plays a role in fat digestion. It reduces the size of particles and, by slowly emptying its acid chyme into the duodenum, ensures not only a normal rate of absorption but also an adequate stimulation for the flow of bile and pancreatic juice.

The initial intraluminal event in the jejunum is hydrolysis of triglyceride into two fatty acids and a residual β monoglyceride by *pancreatic lipase;* this enzyme, contained in high concentration in secreted pancreatic juice, is activated at the alkaline pH of the upper jejunum. Its action is facilitated by pancreatic *colipase.*

At a critical concentration, conjugated bile acids, contained in bile provided by contraction of the gallbladder, form small spheres with detergent properties. These molecules are *amphiphils* with a portion polar and water soluble and a portion nonpolar and fat soluble. The polar (aliphatic) region makes the polymolecular aggregate water soluble. At its hydrophobic center are monoglycerides and fatty acids and the fat-soluble vitamins, A, D, and K. This complex is known as a mixed micelle. Di-and triglycerides remain in an oil phase until hydrolyzed to monoglycerides and fatty acids.

Micelle formation may be impaired in several ways: *inadequate hydrolysis* of triglyceride to monoglyceride and fatty acids (as in pancreatic insufficiency); *dilution* of pancreatic lipase (after subtotal gastrectomy); or *deficiency of conjugated bile acids* (as in bacterial overgrowth, cholestatic liver disease, or biliary tract obstruction, or after resection of distal ileum).

Cellular Phase. The monoglycerides, fatty acids, and hydrophobic vitamins of micelles cross the membrane, a lipophilic structure, and the conjugated bile acids remain in the lumen to form more micelles, eventually to be actively absorbed in the ileum and returned to the liver for re-excretion into bile. Normally more than 95 per cent of the total bile acid pool, 4.0 grams, is reabsorbed during each enterohepatic cycle, and each day the pool is circulated four times. Thus only about 400 mg of bile acid is lost in the feces, the amount synthesized in the liver daily.

Although exact figures are not available, a considerable amount of fat may be absorbed in the absence of bile, indicating that the process is not entirely dependent upon micelles. The question of ileal absorption of fat has not been resolved. The rate of absorption of both free fatty acids and glycerides is determined mainly by both chain length and degree of saturation of the fatty acids involved.

The major site for fat absorption is the upper jejunum. For normal function, at least 90 cm of this segment must be free of bacterial overgrowth and must contain normal villi and patent lymphatics. These are the conditions for the uptake and transport of lipid which are phases of fat absorption. Triglycerides (neutral fat) after emulsification with fatty acids and bile salts *may* be absorbed unhydrolyzed, but apparently only in small quantity. Indeed, 80 to 90 per cent of neutral fat is either partly or completely hydrolyzed.

Conjugated bile acids also help to activate intracellular enzymes, which are required for resynthesis of fatty acids and monoglyceride into triglyceride, a necessary step in chylomicron formation. A fatty acid binding protein (FABP) carries fatty acids to the smooth endoplasmic reticulum where activation to fatty acid CoA, joining of fatty acids with monoglyceride, and esterification to triglyceride take place. In the mucosal cells, molecules of triglyceride coalesce into large particles which are then coated with small amounts of protein, cholesterol and phospholipid, thus becoming β-lipoproteins, called chylomicrons. These exit via the base of the cells, enter the lacteals whence they pass into the mesenteric lymphatic system, the thoracic duct, and, finally, the vena cava. Long-chain fatty acids (i.e., 10 or more C atoms) undergo this process. In the mucosal cells some fatty acids are incorporated into phospholipids.

Medium-chain triglycerides with fatty acids of length C6 to C10, are better absorbed than long-chain triglycerides because they are more completely hydrolyzed by pancreatic lipase, being split at the β position as well, with release of three medium-chain fatty acids. Also, medium-chain triglyceride forms micelles more readily. Thus this lipid is more readily prepared for absorption than the long-chain triglycerides. Unsplit medium-chain triglyceride also appears to be taken up by cells (30 per cent of an oral dose) and is hydrolyzed by mucosal lipase, releasing fatty acids. Further, medium-chain fatty acids pass directly into the portal venous system without re-esterification. This independence of mucosal re-esterification and of the lymphatics is thought to be advantageous in patients with intestinal mucosal disease. Obviously, medium-chain triglyceride may be extremely useful in the therapy of patients with malabsorption syndrome, and its indications and usefulness will be discussed under Treatment (see Table 5).

Absorption of *cholesterol* appears to depend upon its separation from protein and release from fatty acid esters through hydrolysis by pancreatic esterase. The intestine also synthesizes cholesterol as well as very low density lipoproteins. Dietary vitamin A, largely in ester form, undergoes hydrolysis in the intestinal lumen to the free alcohol. The absorption of cholesterol, free vitamin A, and vitamins D, E, and K requires bile salts.

PROTEIN AND AMINO ACID ABSORPTION. Gastric pepsin may partially hydrolyze dietary protein; however, this action is almost entirely due to pancreatic proteolytic endopeptidases such as *trypsin, chymotrypsin,* and *elastase. Trypsinogen,* as well as precursors of the other endopeptidases, is activated by a mucosal enzyme, *enterokinase,* released by presence of food in the duodenum. *Trypsin* is liberated and, in turn, continues to activate trypsinogen as well as the other pancreatic endopeptidases. These substances attack the interior of the protein molecules, yielding oligopeptides which are further split by exopeptidases such as *carboxypeptidase.* Neutral and basic amino acids are released, as well as small peptides, di- to hexa-, in large quantities. These peptides enter the brush border where they are hydrolyzed by amino peptidases sequentially, releasing the constituent amino acids; some di- and tripeptides, however, enter the cells and are split into their constituent amino acids by cytosol peptidases. Indeed, amino acid absorption is greater after administration of some dipeptides than with equimolar mixtures of amino acids.

Amino acids liberated intraluminally or within the brush border are transported across the cell membrane actively, i.e., by a process which consumes energy. It is Na^+ dependent to a varying degree. Thus neutral amino acids are more dependent and basic amino acids less so. Both types, however, are absorbed rapidly. Other active carriers operate for movement of glycine (which also is transported as a neutral amino acid), hydroxyproline, and proline; and for the dicarboxylic amino acids, aspartic and glutamic. Di- and tripeptides also enter the cells by an active transport mechanism. Resynthesis of protein from absorbed amino acids takes place to a limited extent in the mucosa; the liver, however, is the predominant site for such synthesis.

Most amino acids pass quickly into the blood, however, and enter the general "metabolic pool." The liver is the principal organ for their metabolism.

CARBOHYDRATE ABSORPTION. Dietary carbohydrate consists of starch and two disaccharides, sucrose and lactose. Amylose and amylopectin are the principal starches — long chains of connected (C1-C4) glucose molecules which are split in the duodenum by pancreatic amylase at these 1 to 4 α glucose-glucose linkages. Amylose is cleaved to yield maltose and maltotriose; amylopectin, however, yields molecules, α-limit dextrins, containing some branch points (C6-C1) present sequentially in amylopectin which are not split by the enzyme.

Maltose, maltotriose, α-limit dextrins, and other dietary disaccharides, sucrose and lactose, are split further by specific brush border *disaccharidases* into their component hexoses: glucose-glucose, glucose-fructose, and glucose-galactose, respectively.

The rate of absorption of hexoses in descending order is galactose, glucose, fructose. Glucose and galactose are actively transported, as is fructose, whose absorption was thought to be "facilitated" by a poorly understood carrier. Xylose shares the same transport system with glucose and galactose but not so avidly.

Transport of glucose and galactose depends upon a process requiring both energy and Na^+. Possibly glucose and Na^+ bind to a carrier protein in the microvilli, and thus glucose moves into the cell. Na^+ then moves out of the cell via the so-called "Na^+ pump" mechanism. This driving force enables glucose and galactose to be absorbed against a concentration gradient. Na^+ also increases cellular permeability for glucose, although glucose may be transported at low concentrations of Na^+.

VITAMIN B$_{12}$ ABSORPTION. Vitamin B$_{12}$ absorption is dependent upon the presence of intrinsic factor, a glycoprotein (50,000 to 60,000 m.w.) contained in gastric juice. Vitamin B$_{12}$ is bound to intrinsic factor, and the complex in turn is bound to a specific ileal receptor. In some unknown manner, after several hours, vitamin B$_{12}$ becomes "unbound" and passes into the blood. Whether uptake is energy dependent is not settled. Calcium ion is required for uptake of the vitamin B$_{12}$– intrinsic factor complex as well as a substance in pancreatic juice which somehow facilitates its absorption. Alterations in bacterial flora, such as are observed in the bacterial overgrowth syndrome (see below), lead to decreased absorption of vitamin B$_{12}$ that, in most instances, can be reversed by the administration of broad-spectrum antimicrobial drugs. In some manner these bacteria bind the vitamin B$_{12}$.

FOLIC ACID ABSORPTION. Dietary folic acid is in the form of polyglutamate conjugates of pteroylglutamic acid. About 1000 μg, as contained in yeast, liver, and green vegetables, is ingested daily in the Western world. Pteroylpolyglutamates are sequentially cleaved at the cell surface, yielding glutamates, which are reduced and methylated within the mucosa, yielding active forms, particularly 5-methyl tetrahydrofolate, which is a necessary coenzyme for synthesis of purines, pyrimidines, and DNA. The mode of transport of pteroylmonoglutamate into the cell is thought to be active.

WATER AND ELECTROLYTE ABSORPTION. Water and electrolyte absorption takes place in the small intestine. *Water* moves across the membrane passively, i.e., secondary to osmotic gradients. However, under certain circumstances it can move against a gradient without requiring energy. The rate of water absorption in the small gut is five to ten times that in the stomach. To some extent, also, water follows the active transport of glucose and electrolytes, moving with them to maintain isotonicity of intraluminal contents. The small intestine usually absorbs over 7 liters of water per day.

Sodium transport is in part an active process and is linked to an exchange with H^+ in both jejunum and ileum. A similar exchange mechanism for C1' and HCO_3' exists only in the ileum. The sites of these exchanges in the cell are not known, but the exchanges are certainly mediated by carriers. It is also believed from in vitro studies that a Na^+ pump mechanism may be operative. In man, Na^+ transport is enhanced by absorption of glucose in the jejunum, either via this mechanism or by being "dragged" into the cell by the water in which glucose is carried. Some Na^+ also moves passively, i.e., down a gradient across the mucosa. Potassium movement seems to be passive, diffusing from the lumen proximally and into the lumen distally.

The amount of water and sodium absorbed represents the difference between influx from lumen to blood and efflux in the reverse direction. This net flux is diminished by hypertonicity of the intraluminal solution and is increased by hypotonicity. Changes in concentration of sodium in the lumen depend on relative rates of exchange of both sodium and water between blood and lumen.

During diarrhea, sodium concentration increases with increasing stool volume, and beyond 3 liters approaches values close to that of plasma. Conversely, potassium concentration progressively decreases.

CALCIUM AND IRON ABSORPTION. Calcium is absorbed actively in the duodenum. The transport is facilitated by *parathyroid hormone* and, principally, by *vitamin D,* and is inhibited by deprivation of this vitamin. The active form of vitamin D involved in the process is a kidney metabolite, *1,25-dihydroxycholecalciferol* (1,25 dehydroxy D_3). In vivo calcium absorption depends also upon pH and concentration of phosphates and fatty acids. Vitamin D absorption is necessary for calcium absorption, because 1,25-dihydroxy D_3 stimulates synthesis of a calcium-binding protein which is a key substance in the active transport of the cation.

Iron, 0.5 to 1.0 mg daily, is absorbed *actively,* in an amount sufficient for normal hematopoiesis and five to eight times this amount in people who are iron deficient. Absorption is a two-step process, principally in the duodenum, of uptake and transfer; the former is dependent upon oxidative metabolism. The latter, probably the rate-limit step, involves movement of Fe through the serosa to the circulation where it is bound to a globulin, *transferrin,* which transports it to tissues, particularly the liver. Iron absorption is diminished in chronic infection and by prior administration of large amounts of iron, and apparently is increased in pregnancy as well as iron deficiency. Animal hemoglobin is an important source of iron in the human, and is absorbed most rapidly, followed by Fe^{++}, then Fe^{+++}. After ingestion, hemoglobin is split in the upper gut; heme is readily absorbed, from which iron is split within the cell by heme oxygenase. It passes thence into the circulation where it is bound by iron-binding protein. Some iron is released from heme intraluminally and is taken up directly by the cells.

In human subjects, absorption of inorganic iron depends upon its release from dietary compounds to which it is originally bound. Absorption of both Fe^{+++} and Fe^{++} is enhanced by chelation with ascorbic acid, carbohydrates, and amino acids at the pH of normal gastric juice. These complexes remain soluble at the alkaline pH of the duodenum where iron is absorbed. Diminished iron absorption is associated with achlorhydria, because an acid pH is needed to solubilize ferric iron for chelation with ascorbic acid and other substances, in which form it is absorbed. Ferrous iron may also, however, be chelated at an alkaline pH. Over-all, iron absorption is regulated by the state of repletion, content of iron in absorbing cells, and factors affecting erythropoiesis. The influence of gastric and pancreatic juice proteins which bind iron is still uncertain.

CAUSES OF THE MALABSORPTION SYNDROME

The principal diseases and disorders that may give rise to the malabsorption syndrome are listed in Table 1. These conditions are discussed in detail in a subsequent portion of this chapter and are presented only in brief outline at this point. They can be divided conveniently into seven categories, based upon pathologic and pathophysiologic considerations.

TABLE 1. Classification of Malabsorption Syndrome

I. Category 1: Defective Intraluminal Hydrolysis or Solubilization
   A. Primary pancreatic insufficiency
   B. Secondary pancreatic insufficiency
   C. Deficiency of conjugated bile acids
   D. Bacterial overgrowth (bile acid deconjugation)
      1. Blind loops
      2. Multiple strictures and jejunal diverticula
      3. Fistulas
      4. Postgastrectomy
      5. Scleroderma and pseudo-obstruction
II. Category 2: Mucosal Cell Abnormality and Inadequate Surface
   A. Primary mucosal cell disorders
      1. Disaccharidase deficiency and monosaccharide malabsorption
      2. Abetalipoproteinemia
      3. Vitamin B_{12} malabsorption
      4. Cystinuria and Hartnup disease
   B. Small bowel disease
      1. Celiac disease
      2. Whipple's disease
      3. Nongranulomatous ileojejunitis
      4. Allergic and eosinophilic gastroenteritis
      5. Amyloidosis
      6. Small bowel ischemia
      7. Crohn's disease (granulomatous enteritis)
   C. Inadequate surface
III. Category 3: Lymphatic Obstruction
   A. Lymphoma
   B. Tuberculosis and tuberculous lymphadenitis
   C. Lymphangiectasia
IV. Category 4: Infection
   A. Tropical sprue
   B. Acute infectious enteritis
   C. Parasitoses
V. Category 5: Multiple Defects
   A. Subtotal gastrectomy
   B. Distal ileal resection, disease, or bypass
   C. Radiation enteritis
VI. Category 6: Unexplained
   A. Hypogammaglobulinemia
   B. Carcinoid syndrome
   C. Hypothyroidism
   D. Diabetes mellitus
   E. Mastocytosis
   F. Hyperthyroidism and hypoadrenocorticism
VII. Category 7: Drug-Induced Malabsorption
   A. Cholestyramine
   B. Colchicine
   C. Irritant laxatives
   D. Neomycin
   E. p-Aminosalicylic acid
   F. Phenindione

CLINICAL MANIFESTATIONS

The signs and symptoms of the malabsorption syndrome include weight loss, anorexia, abdominal distention, borborygmi, muscle wasting, and passage of abnormal stools that are characteristically light yellow to gray, greasy, and soft. In many instances frequent movements are noted, but occasionally there is only one very bulky stool per day. In addition, edema, ascites, skeletal disorders, peripheral and circumoral paresthesias, tetany, and, rarely, convulsions may be observed.

The clinical features that result from deficiencies of fat-soluble vitamins include hyperkeratosis follicularis (vitamin A); bleeding, particularly ecchymoses and hematuria (vitamin K); and bone pain or fractures (vitamin D) (Table 2). Deficiencies of the vitamin B complex are manifested by glossitis, cheilosis, muscle tenderness, peripheral neuritis, and dermatitis (Table 2). The symptoms of the malabsorption syndrome may be intermittent or low grade, so that medical attention is not

TABLE 2. Correlation of Laboratory Data with Absorptive Defects and
Signs and Symptoms of the Malabsorption Syndrome

Clinical Features	Laboratory Evidence	Pathophysiology
Muscle wasting; small stature; edema	↓ Serum albumin	*Impaired protein metabolism* ↓ Absorption ↓ Intake ↑ Enteric loss ?Impaired synthesis
Skeletal deformity; pain fractures	X-ray: demineralization; collapsed vertebrae	
Weight loss; pale, bulky stools	↑ Fecal fat ↓ Serum cholesterol, carotene	*Impaired absorption and excess loss of:* Fat
Paresthesias; tetany; + Chvostek; Trousseau; bone pain; fractures	↓ Serum Ca^{++}; ↓ or normal PO$_4$′′′; ↑ alkaline phosphatase; x-ray: Looser's lines, Milkman's fractures; ↑ osteoid seams; ↓ serum Mg^{++}	Fat-soluble vitamins and calcium Vitamin D, calcium, magnesium
Bleeding: ecchymoses, hematuria	↑ Prothrombin time with response to vitamin K	Vitamin K
Hyperkeratosis follicularis	↓ Serum carotene, vitamin A tolerance	Vitamin A
(ANEMIAS) Paresthesias; neuropathy	Macrocytic anemia; megaloblastosis; ↓ serum B$_{12}$ and ↓ absorption B$_{12}$	Vitamin B$_{12}$
(GLOSSITIS)	Macrocytic anemia; megaloblastosis; ↓ serum folic acid	Folic acid
Koilonychia	Microcystosis, hypochromia; ↓ serum iron and ↓ saturation iron binding protein; ↓ iron in marrow	Iron
Dehydration; nocturia	↓ Plasma volume	Water
Muscle cramps, weakness	↓ Serum Na$^+$	Sodium
Muscle flaccidity, weakness; ↓ tendon reflexes, arrhythmias	↓ Serum K$^+$; EKG abnormalities	Potassium
Cheilosis; neuritis; dermatitis, glossitis; muscle weakness	↑ Urinary I3AA, Indican; ↓ serum B$_{12}$, folic acid	Vitamin B complex; folic acid vitamin B$_{12}$
Abdominal distention, flatulence; diarrhea	Low to flat oral glucose tolerance curve; ↓ absorption d-xylose; ↓ oral lactose tolerance; ↓ or absent rise of blood glucose after oral sucrose; ↓ or absent rise of blood reducing substances after oral galactose; fluid levels on x-ray; stools: acid pH, + Clinitest	Impaired hydrolysis of disaccharides, particularly lactose and sucrose, or ↓ absorption of monosaccharides and amino acids

sought for a very long time — more than 35 years in some instances of adult celiac disease. Unfortunately, many of these patients whose malabsorption is mild escape diagnosis and suffer subtle changes for years. They do not exhibit obvious manifestations of malabsorption; they are chronically fatigued, lack drive, and may have symptoms of chronic depression. Further, they may lose weight only during the early months of illness and then will stabilize at a lower level.

In those with more severe malabsorption, the secondary manifestations may often overshadow the intestinal complaints. For example, patients with *adult celiac disease* may seek aid for bleeding or for skeletal pain or fractures. In many patients, weakness, fatigue, dyspnea, or dizziness, all caused by anemia, may be the presenting symptoms. Borborygmi and abdominal distention, which increase during the day and are often not relieved by defecation, are among the most common complaints. An extreme degree of such distress is frequently noted in patients with *scleroderma* of the small intestine.

Cramping lower abdominal pain is noted in a large number of diseases of malabsorption, usually preceding loose bowel movements, and thus does not distinguish between the various entities. Persistent or severe cramping, pain, periumbilical or right lower quadrant, not relieved by movements is frequently seen in patients with *Crohn's disease* and, with stricturing and obstruction, may become chronic and associated with distention and emesis. Diffuse periumbilical pain is often suffered by patients with *nongranulomatous ileojejunitis, lymphoma, eosinophilic gastroenteritis, radiation enteritis, amyloidosis,* and, occasionally, *adult celiac disease.* Patients with *chronic pancreatitis* usually suffer recurrent

deep epigastric pain that radiates to the midback; in patients with *lymphoma* of the small intestine and mesentery, the pain may be cramping (obstruction) or steady and intense (local invasion or spread).

Patients with malabsorption owing to *ischemia* of the small gut often also have periumbilical or midabdominal cramping pains 20 to 30 minutes after meals and often other evidence of widespread arteriosclerosis, or have chronic atrial fibrillation. Those with *hypogammaglobulinemia* may have other historic evidences of immunoglobulin deficiency (repeated infections, or even symptoms suggesting malignancy). *Eosinophilic gastroenteritis* may be highlighted by a specific "food allergy" or by a history of skin, nasopharyngeal, bronchial, or other allergy. Virulent peptic ulcer disease (*Zollinger-Ellison syndrome*) will usually highlight the history of malabsorption caused by gastric hypersecretion. Diarrhea associated with carbohydrate will be noted from childhood in those with *disaccharidase deficiency* or *monosaccharide malabsorption.* Surgical scars and associated histories will highlight cases of *massive resection, gastrectomy* and *ileal resection, bypass procedures,* and *blind loops.* Those with *enteroenteric* or *enterocolic fistulas* as well have a long history of inflammatory disease, usually Crohn's disease, or malignancy. Hepatobiliary tract disorders will have features of chronic obstruction of the common bile duct or of chronic intrahepatic disease.

Physical examination early in the course may be unimpressive, with perhaps only some smoothness of the edges of the tongue or minimal abdominal distention. Later it will reveal one or more evidences of malnutrition and multiple vitamin deficiencies: pallor, diffuse brownish pigmentation of the skin but not of the

mucous membranes, hyperkeratosis, petechiae or ecchymoses, muscle wasting, edema, abdominal distention, skeletal deformity (particularly kyphosis), positive
Chvostek and/or Trousseau signs, glossitis, cheilosis,
impaired vibration sense, deep muscle pain, and clubbing of the fingers. In addition, signs of various underlying diseases may be noted: an abdominal mass
(*lymphoma, regional enteritis*); fixation or severe limitation of joint movement and thickened skin (*sclero-
ma*); facial flush and hepatomegaly (*carcinoid syndrome*);
puffed facies, bradycardia, and hair loss (*hypothyroidism*); proptosis, thyromegaly, tachycardia, and tremor
(*hyperthyroidism*); arthritis or skin rashes (*hypogammaglobulinemia*); nasopharyngeal congestion, skin rash, and
wheezing (*eosinophilic gastroenteritis*); butterfly rash and
splenomegaly (*systemic lupus erythematosus*); neurologic impairments (*abetalipoproteinemia*); diminished or
absent peripheral arterial pulsations, skin lesions (particularly diabetic dermopathy), cataracts, and absent or
diminished deep tendon reflexes or other evidences of
diabetic neuropathy or retinopathy (*diabetes mellitus*);
lymphadenopathy, arthritis, and signs of pulmonary
disease (*Whipple's disease*); enlarged tongue and hepatosplenomegaly (*amyloidosis*); urticaria pigmentosa, flushing, and pruritus (*mastocytosis*).

The malabsorption syndrome may be fatal, owing to
the nature of the underlying disease (*lymphoma, pancreatic carcinoma, progressive scleroderma,* or *granulomatous
enteritis*) or to the complications of malabsorption,
which include superimposed infection, hypokalemia, or
progressive inanition.

PATHOPHYSIOLOGIC BASIS FOR CLINICAL MANIFESTATIONS

In Table 2 may be seen the correlation between various absorptive defects and vitamin deficiencies, the
clinical signs and symptoms, and the abnormalities of
the routine laboratory tests in the malabsorption syndrome. Rarely does a patient manifest all the findings
listed in Table 2, but many patients will exhibit many
of them.

**IMPAIRED PROTEIN METABOLISM: WEIGHT LOSS,
EDEMA.** Protein metabolism, reflected by decreased
muscle mass and lowered serum protein levels, is impaired for several reasons. Synthesis may be below normal owing to defective protein absorption, diminished
intake, or associated liver disease. Catabolism or
breakdown is accelerated because of inadequate intake
and absorption of carbohydrate. Decreased serum albumin may result also from abnormal loss of protein into
the lumen of the gut, so-called *protein-losing enteropathy*. Such loss is usually associated with diseases that
cause malabsorption by lymphatic obstruction or in
which there is an inflammatory mucosal lesion, although it has also been reported in *adult celiac disease*
(see below). *Hypogammaglobulinemia*, both congenital
and acquired, has also been associated with steatorrhea, but the defective fat absorption cannot be related
directly to low plasma globulins.

The emaciation and weakness may be extreme (Fig.
1). The finding of hypotension and diffuse pigmentation makes the picture closely resemble severe *adrenal
cortical insufficiency*. Hypokalemia as well as partial atrophy may underlie muscle weakness.

CLINICAL EFFECTS OF STEATORRHEA. Excess loss of

Figure 1. Extreme wasting in a patient with adult celiac disease (nontropical sprue).

fat in the stool deprives the body of substantial
numbers of calories and contributes greatly to weight
loss and malnutrition. Perhaps the irritative effect of
unabsorbed long-chain (C18) fatty acids which are hydroxylated contributes to the diarrhea with its severe
losses of water, electrolytes, and other nutrients. In addition, binding of calcium by fatty acids contributes to
hypocalcemia. It also leads to hyperabsorption of oxalate, ordinarily precipitated as calcium oxalate, resulting in calcium oxalate kidney stones, particularly in patients with massive small bowel resections. Flatulence,
fluid in loops of small intestine, and abdominal distention may be related to both diminished fat absorption
and excessive carbohydrate fermentation. Failure to absorb fat-soluble vitamins A, D, and K also results in a
variety of serious symptoms as recorded in Table 2.

**VITAMIN D DEFICIENCY: HYPOCALCEMIA AND SKELETAL
DISEASE IN MALABSORPTION SYNDROME; HYPOMAGNESE-
MIA.** Low serum calcium results from failure of normal
absorption owing both to vitamin D deficiency and to
chelation of calcium by unabsorbed fatty acids. Symptoms caused by depression of unbound or "ultrafilterable" calcium of the blood range from paresthesias of
extremities and circumoral area to carpopedal and
laryngeal spasms and muscle cramps. When levels are
extremely low, the patient may even convulse. Clinically, hypocalcemia may be demonstrated by *Chvostek*
or *Trousseau signs*. Obviously, the defect in calcium absorption involves more than deficiency of vitamin D,
particularly its metabolite, 1,25-dihydroxy D_3, active in
calcium absorption, because the return of serum calcium
to normal in patients with adult celiac disease who are on
a gluten-free diet is more rapid than may be attributed to
the action of this vitamin.

Low levels of serum calcium stimulate parathyroid
activity. Increased secretion of parathormone raises the
level of blood calcium both by direct effect upon bone
and by a renal mechanism. These processes lead to demineralization — *osteomalacia*. Osteomalacia principally
affects the spine, rib cage, and long bones, with or
without fractures (Milkman's fractures), and may cause
extreme pain, particularly of the spine, pelvis, and legs.

In patients with poor protein nutrition, in part
caused by malabsorption or protein-losing enteropathy
(see below), particularly postmenopausal women and
elderly men, the demineralization process is aggravated
by *osteoporosis* or failure to deposit bone matrix.

Hypomagnesemia may also be noted in the malabsorption syndrome, causing symptoms that are identical
with those of hypocalcemia. Differentiation is accomplished by the finding of lowered serum magnesium

and by disappearance of symptoms only after administration of magnesium chloride or sulfate. Hypomagnesemia may also dramatically reduce the responsiveness of the parathyroids to hypocalcemia. Indeed, correction of magnesium deficiency may be essential to restoration of normal calcium by action of the parathyroid glands.

VITAMIN K DEFICIENCY: BLEEDING DIATHESIS IN MALABSORPTION SYNDROME. As noted, *bleeding*, particularly subcutaneous, nasal, urinary, vaginal, and occasionally, gastrointestinal, is not uncommon in the malabsorption syndrome and may be the principal symptom. Defects in coagulation result from deficiency of plasma prothrombin owing to impaired absorption of fat-soluble vitamin K.

VITAMIN A DEFICIENCY. In the malabsorption syndrome *hyperkeratosis follicularis* may be noted, but *nyctalopia* is very rare.

VITAMIN E DEFICIENCY. Although plasma vitamin E levels are often depressed in malabsorption, no specific signs or symptoms may be attributed to it.

MANIFESTATIONS OF ABNORMAL CARBOHYDRATE ABSORPTION. The abnormal carbohydrate absorption results in diminished glycogen stores in liver and muscle. Also, intraluminal fermentation of sugars contributes greatly to abdominal distention and flatulence. Failure to hydrolyze disaccharides, particularly lactose *(disaccharidase deficiency)*, results in watery diarrhea as well as these local abdominal complaints (see below). Bacterial conversion of unabsorbed carbohydrate yields volatile fatty acids which may cause diarrhea by inhibiting water and sodium absorption by the colon.

ANEMIA. Deficiency of vitamin B_{12} or folic acid may cause a macrocytic anemia with a megaloblastic bone marrow, whereas iron deficiency will cause a microcytic hypochromic anemia. With deficiency of vitamin B_{12}, folic acid, and iron, anemia with mixed features will be present. The former type is seen in *tropical sprue*, after *resection* of, or *disease* in, a large segment of the *terminal ileum*; rarely, in pancreatic insufficiency; in *"primary" malabsorption of vitamin B_{12}* (defective ileal receptor); and in conditions in which there is bacterial overgrowth in the upper small intestine — *"blind loops,"* jejunal diverticulosis, enteroenteric or *enterocolic fistulas*, and *multiple small bowel strictures*. In contrast to pernicious anemia, in these conditions simultaneous feeding of intrinsic factor does not improve vitamin B_{12} absorption. In those cases caused by bacterial overgrowth as well as in tropical sprue, normal absorption of vitamin B_{12} may be restored by oral administration of a broad-spectrum antimicrobial drug — tetracycline, oxytetracycline, or ampicillin (1.0 gram daily) for 10 to 14 days (Table 3). Indeed, a brisk reticulocytosis may be noted in three to four days. Impaired absorption of vitamin B_{12} and megaloblastosis may also be noted occasionally in patients with *adult celiac disease.*

FOLIC ACID DEFICIENCY. Folic acid deficiency may also underlie *megaloblastosis* and *anemia*. As there is often an associated deficiency of vitamin B_{12}, diagnosis may be established only by the finding of low serum folic acid levels (less than 5.0 ng), or of a reticulocytic response to administration of minimal daily effective dosage (0.05 to 0.5 mg parenterally). Usually, however, folic acid deficiency is corrected by adequate diet or oral supplementation.

GLOSSITIS AND PERIPHERAL NEUROPATHY. *Glossitis* and *peripheral neuropathy* can in part be attributed to deficiency of vitamin B_{12}. Since combined system disease may be induced or exacerbated by administration of folic acid, *vitamin B_{12} stores in tissues must be replenished before administration of folic acid alone for megaloblastic anemia.*

IMPAIRED IRON ABSORPTION. Iron absorption may be subnormal except when the malabsorption syndrome is due to uncomplicated pancreatic insufficiency. Most often the iron deficiency is caused by poor absorption owing either to mucosal disease or to inability to release inorganic iron from organic compounds. However, occult blood loss may contribute to the anemia. Iron deficiency anemia is very common in *adult celiac disease* and may be noted also in the later stages of *tropical sprue*. When associated with deficiencies of folic acid and vitamin B_{12}, iron deficiency may not become apparent until these substances are repleted. Incorporation of iron into young marrow red blood cells requires both folic acid and vitamin B_{12}.

DIMINISHED ABSORPTION OF WATER AND ELECTROLYTES. Common in the malabsorption syndrome are *dehydration, weakness,* and *hypotension*. Large amounts of water and electrolytes are lost if diarrhea is severe or if stools are very loose or bulky. Absorption of water in adult celiac disease is slower than normal; the small intestine, in fact, secretes water and sodium. Thus diuresis after a water load is delayed. Thus patients with steatorrhea often have nocturia. *Hyponatremia* not caused by renal loss responds readily to administration of sodium, and symptoms of "low salt" — weakness, leth-

TABLE 3. ^{60}Co-Vitamin B_{12} Absorption (Schilling)

	Megaloblastic Anemia Associated with:					
Result after:	Pernicious Anemia and Total Gastrectomy	Adult Celiac Disease*	Blind Loop Syndrome	Primary Malabsorption of Vitamin B_{12}	Tropical Sprue	Pancreatic Insufficiency*
	... Absorption ...					
Vitamin B_{12}	Low	Low-normal or low	Low	Low	No change	Normal-low†
Vitamin B_{12} + intrinsic factor	Normal	No change	No change	No change	No change	No change
Vitamin B_{12} after antimicrobial therapy	Low	No change	Normal	No change	Normal or low	No change
Vitamin B_{12} after gluten-free diet	No change	Normal	No change	No change	No change	No change
Vitamin B_{12} + bicarbonate	No change	No change	No change	No change	No change	Normal‡
Vitamin B_{12} + pancreatic extract	No change	No change	No change	No change	No change	Normal‡

*Rare in adult celiac disease: very rare in pancreatic insufficiency.
†Rare to be low.
‡Very rare.

argy, nausea, cramps — rapidly disappear. *Hypokalemia*, if severe, causes muscle flaccidity and cardiac arrhythmias.

VITAMIN B COMPLEX DEFICIENCY: DERMATITIS, NEURITIS, AND CHEILOSIS. Although *glossitis, neuritis* (peripheral neuropathy), and *dermatitis* in the malabsorption syndrome have been attributed to deficiency of B vitamins, proof of impaired absorption of these substances (vitamins B_1, B_2, and B_6) is not at hand. Perhaps deficiency results from metabolic action of abnormal bacterial flora that ordinarily do not inhabit the small bowel. However, conclusive demonstration of this mechanism also is lacking, particularly in *adult celiac disease*. Moreover, administration of vitamin B complex ($B_{1, 2, 6, 12}$) does not always cure the glossitis, which may be partially due to iron deficiency.

DIAGNOSIS

Although the spectrum of clinical symptoms and signs of malabsorption syndrome is broad, those with mild chronic illness display one or more important clinical or laboratory abnormalities. A high index of suspicion of the diagnosis is essential for those with minimal complaints and seemingly normal-appearing stools. Unfortunately, there is no short cut to diagnosis of the syndrome and, equally important, of its underlying cause.

The clues to diagnosis of the malabsorption syndrome are the history, symptoms, signs, and laboratory abnormalities listed in Tables 2, 3, and 4 that relate to malabsorption of fat and other substances, particularly fat-soluble vitamins, proteins, iron, and vitamin B_{12}. The average patient will complain of rather bulky, light-colored stools, often with increased frequency (but not necessarily so), abdominal distention, and variable weight loss, and will also show laboratory evidence of impaired absorption. However, special diagnostic attention must be tendered those with subtler histories and findings and especially those who complain principally of bleeding tendency or of some skeletal disability, chiefly pain. Other features commonly seen in many diseases of this syndrome include *hypotension, abdominal distention, diffuse brownish pigmentation,* and *clubbing* of the fingers and toes.

It is not usually difficult to establish solely by clinical examination that the malabsorption syndrome is present. Much more precise information as to *which* absorption defects are present is necessary, however, if the physician is to treat the illness successfully. In large measure, this essential information can be obtained only by the proper use of a number of laboratory procedures.

Laboratory Diagnosis

The pathophysiologic basis for the abnormal findings of the laboratory tests has been described and is presented in Table 2. The particular values of the individual tests in arriving at a diagnosis are considered in Table 4. The essential diagnostic tests, excluding routine blood studies (complete blood count, determination of Ca^{++}, K^+, and prothrombin time), include measurement of 72-hour stool fat and serum carotene, d-xylose absorption, tests of pancreatic function, tests for bacterial overgrowth, roentgenographic study of

small bowel, vitamin B_{12} absorption, and biopsy of the small intestine.

MEASUREMENT OF STOOL FAT: SERUM CAROTENE. Because the most important feature in diagnosis of the malabsorption syndrome is steatorrhea, accurate measurement of fecal fat is extremely important. The only reliable method is the chemical analysis of a 72-hour stool collection, the patient ingesting 80 to 100 grams of fat per day. Normal excretion in these circumstances is 6.0 grams or less per 24 hours (Table 4).

This test is essential for diagnosis, because only in the so-called primary mucosal cell abnormalities (except for abetalipoproteinemia) is fat absorption normal (Table 1). Steatorrhea, however, does not indicate into which category of malabsorptive disorders the patient falls. If fecal fat is elevated, a roentgenographic study of the small intestine as well as a d-xylose test must be performed. Increasingly, small bowel biopsy is being done routinely if pancreatic disease is unlikely. Finally, determinations which reflect bacterial overgrowth (intestinal stasis) are required either when the roentgenographic studies display a *blind loop, jejunal diverticula, strictures, enteroenteric* or *enterocolic fistula,* or the marked intestinal stasis of *scleroderma,* or when the biopsy is normal.

Depressed levels of serum carotene will usually be found in patients with steatorrhea. This test is useful in "screening" those in whom the malabsorption syndrome is suspected.

d-XYLOSE ABSORPTION (Table 4). During recent years, absorption of d-xylose, a pentose, has been measured in the study of malabsorption. Twenty-five grams is given orally; if the patient does not vomit, has no delay in gastric emptying, is well hydrated, and has normal kidney function, 4.5 grams or more will be excreted in a five-hour collection of urine. It is absorbed actively like glucose, but its metabolism is not as rapid as that of glucose, and its renal excretion does not depend upon a threshold. As a measure of carbohydrate absorption, it is more reliable than an oral glucose tolerance test. In patients over 60, renal excretion diminishes; in such individuals, as well as in patients with delayed gastric emptying, liver disease with ascites, or renal disease, blood levels are measured and should reach 20 mg per 100 ml in two hours.

Although the fate of about half of the 50 per cent of the 25.0 gram oral load which is absorbed normally is unknown, it is clear that excretion in five hours is significantly diminished (less than 3.0 grams) with intestinal *disease* affecting particularly the *jejunum,* after *massive resection,* and in marked *bacterial overgrowth,* presumably owing to bacterial action. The procedure thus serves to separate these patients from those with pancreatic insufficiency and from normal subjects. d-Xylose absorption has occasionally been found to be abnormal in *pancreatic carcinoma* with metastatic involvement of the small intestine.

Normal d-xylose absorption is strong evidence against the diagnosis of *adult celiac disease.* An abnormal result, however, casts strong doubt upon the diagnosis of *pancreatic insufficiency.* The test is also valuable in gauging the effect of therapy when pretreatment values have been low.

TESTS FOR UNABSORBED CARBOHYDRATE. In disaccharidase deficiency following massive small intestinal resection or in bacterial overgrowth syndrome (see below), unabsorbed carbohydrate is broken down by

TABLE 4. Laboratory Tests Commonly Employed to Study Malabsorption

	Normal Values	Malabsorption Syndrome*
Serum:		
Albumin	4.0 to 5.2 grams/100 ml	Diminished
Carotene	0.06 to 0.4 mg/100 ml	Diminished, particularly in small bowel disease
Calcium	9.0 to 10.5 mg/100 ml	Diminished, particularly in small bowel disease
Cholesterol	150 to 250 mg/100 ml	Diminished
Potassium	3.5 to 4.7 mEq/L	Diminished
Magnesium	1.7 to 2.0 mEq/L	Diminished
Vitamin B_{12}	100 to 700 $\mu\mu g$/ml	Diminished, particularly in tropical sprue and bacterial overgrowth
Folic acid	5 to 21 ng/ml	Diminished, particularly in small bowel disease
Plasma:		
Prothrombin time	Control value	Elevated
Tolerance tests:		
d-Xylose (25 grams orally)	Urinary excretion of 4.5 grams or greater per 5 hours	Diminished in diseases of the mucosa, particularly celiac disease, and in intestinal stasis (normal in pancreatic insufficiency)
Glucose (100 grams orally)	35 mg over fasting plasma level	"Flat curve" in celiac disease and diseases of intestinal wall and in monosaccharide malabsorption
Lactose (50 to 100 grams orally) (2.0 grams/kg in children)	Rise in blood glucose of 20 mg/100 ml	Low to flat curve in primary lactose deficiency, celiac disease, and diseases of the intestinal wall
Sucrose (100 grams orally)	Rise in blood glucose of 20 mg/100 ml	Low to flat in celiac disease and disease of intestinal wall
Vitamin B_{12} (μc ^{60}CO B_{12})	> 7% urine excretion/24 hours	Decreased with intestinal stasis, ileal dysfunction, or resection
Stool fat:		
Chemical determination (80–100 grams fat daily)	< 6 grams/24 hours	Increased
Miscellaneous:		
5-Hydroxyindolacetic acid (urinary excretion)	1.7 to 8.0 mg/24 hours	9 to 20 mg in adult celiac disease; 30 to 600 mg in metastatic carcinoid syndrome
Indole-3-acetic acid (urinary excretion)	Less than 18 mg/24 hours	
Indican (urinary excretion)	Less than 100 mg/24 hours	Elevated in bacterial overgrowth and ileal dysfunction
Bile acid breath test	Minute amounts of $^{14}CO_2$/4 to 8 hours	

*Usual findings. Some values for serum tests may be normal in some patients, e.g., carotene, calcium, and vitamin B_{12} in pancreatic insufficiency and calcium in tropical sprue.

bacterial enzymes with formation of H_2 and volatile fatty acids. Measured breath H_2 is increased after ingestion of poorly absorbed sugars, e.g., unlabeled lactose in lactase deficiency, in which disorder breath $^{14}CO_2$ is also increased if ^{14}C-lactose is given.

PANCREATIC FUNCTION. Evaluation of pancreatic function by measurement of volume and bicarbonate concentration of duodenal aspirates after appropriate stimulation or concentration of enzymes after a test meal is in order if the d-xylose test is normal and roentgenographic study of the small intestine is normal or equivocally so. It is clearly indicated if biopsy is normal and there is no other apparent disease or disorder. Subnormal response strongly indicates pancreatic insufficiency or pancreatic ductal obstruction, although normal values do not exclude these possibilities.

TESTS FOR BACTERIAL OVERGROWTH. The increasing clinical importance of bacterial overgrowth as a cause for malabsorption syndrome has stimulated development of tests which directly and indirectly indicate the presence of this condition. It may be present in a large number of diseases in which there is either small bowel stasis or contamination by lower gut organisms. These tests include the *bile salt breath test*, measurement of *urinary tryptophan metabolites*, and direct *culture* of jejunal aspirates.

Bile Acid Breath Test. The so-called "bile acid breath test" is enormously helpful in diagnosis of malabsorption caused by diseases or disorders in which bile acid deconjugation is abnormal. These include diseases of bacterial overgrowth and ileal dysfunction (diseases or absent long segment or terminal ileum). In either situation, bacteria (small intestinal in the former situation and colonic in the latter) will deconjugate a significant amount of orally administered ^{14}C glycine-cholate before it is absorbed; the released ^{14}C glycine will be further metabolized by bacterial enzymes to $^{14}CO_2$ which quickly diffuses into the circulation and is breathed out. Normally, only a minute quantity of $^{14}CO_2$ is detectable in four to six hours; however, when bacteria are present in the small gut or conjugated bile acid reabsorption by the terminal ileum is subnormal, $^{14}CO_2$ excretion in breath is elevated tenfold or more after ingestion of ^{14}C glycine-cholate.

Tryptophan Metabolites. The measurement of two urinary metabolites of L-tryptophan, indican and 5-hydroxyindolacetic acid (5-HIAA), has been valuable in diagnosis of diseases of bacterial overgrowth and of ileal dysfunction (diseases, bypassed or absent terminal ileum) and of adult celiac disease. Elevated urinary levels of indoxylsulfate (indican) are found in virtually all diseases in which intestinal stasis is present or the terminal ileum is diseased or absent (greater than 100 mg per 24 hours). Return toward normal values may follow administration of broad-spectrum antimicrobials over a one- to two-week period.

The normal range of 5-hydroxyindolacetic acid is up to about 8.0 mg per 24 hours. In *adult celiac disease*, however, the urinary level is elevated — 9.0 to 15.0 mg — reflecting perhaps an increased amount of circulating 5-hydroxytryptamine or serotonin. Treatment with a gluten-free diet restores normal excretion of this substance. Except for the metastatic *carcinoid* syndrome, in which levels are greatly elevated (300 to 500 mg per 24 hours), or *Whipple's disease,* in which an elevated level (15 mg per 24 hours) has been reported in several instances, excretion of this substance is usually normal in the various disorders which may cause the malabsorption syndrome.

The significance of these findings is not clear, but they indicate abnormal metabolism of tryptophan. Most likely this is related in some way to stasis and bacterial overgrowth, but also, as shown by appropriate loading tests with tryptophan, to a deficiency in vitamin B_6, which is necessary for its normal metabolism. The role of indolacetic acid in the pathophysiology of the malabsorption is not known, but there is evidence that it may have a suppressant effect upon the bone marrow.

Culture of Jejunal Aspirates. Techniques for culture of jejunal aspirates for fastidious anaerobic bacteria (clostridia, fusiforms, bacteroides) are increasingly available for diagnosis of intestinal stasis (bacterial overgrowth). Usually, the upper small intestine appears bacteria free in about one third of normal subjects; in the remainder, gram-positive or facultative anaerobes are present (lactobacilli and enterococci) in concentrations of 10^1 to 10^3 organisms per gram of content. Coliforms may be transiently present but rarely exceed 10^3. Normally, the terminal ileum has concentrations of organisms approaching 10^5 to 10^8 per gram, and these include gram-negative coliforms and bacteroides. In the colon enormous concentrations of anaerobes — bacteroides, lactobacilli, and clostridia — are usually present. When these organisms, particularly bacteroides and lactobacilli (but also clostridia and coliforms), luxuriate in the small intestine, the so-called bacterial overgrowth syndrome results (see Bacterial Overgrowth).

Cultures of aspirates may now be obtained via sterile polyethylene tubes. Precise microbiologic technique for anaerobic organisms must, however, be practiced or the exercise will be futile.

ROENTGENOGRAPHIC STUDIES. Diagnosis of the malabsorption syndrome may be facilitated by recognition of changes in the roentgenograms of the small bowel which point to bacterial overgrowth and include *strictures* or *fistulas, blind loops* usually from previous surgery (Fig. 2), or marked *stasis,* as in scleroderma. Dilatation of the proximal jejunum with "flocculation" and "scattering" of barium, slight coarsening of valvulae conniventes, and rather oddly shaped collections called "moulage," point strongly to *adult celiac disease* (Fig. 3). The factors underlying these changes are not completely understood but include some disturbance of motility or the effect of overproduction of mucus, caused perhaps in both instances by the collection in the gut of irritating substances such as fatty acids. Such changes, but particularly disordered transit and markedly thickened folds, may be noted in *Whipple's disease. Amyloidosis, radiation enteritis, hypoproteinemia, Zollinger-Ellison syndrome,* and *eosinophilic enteritis* may also be responsible. Small mucosal nodules may be noted in so-called *lymphoid nodular hyperplasia* associated with hypogammaglobulinemia and giardiasis. Differential diagnosis of various malabsorption states by roentgenographic examination of the small bowel, however, is often most difficult unless a characteristic finding for an underlying disease (e.g., tumor, stricture, or blind loop) is

Figure 2. Small bowel series showing postoperative terminal ileum (arrow on left) and ileotransverse colostomy stoma (between arrows on right). Note the blind loop.

evident. Some roentgenographic changes associated with *chronic pancreatitis* or *cancer of the pancreas* include diffuse calcification or displacement of the stomach by a pseudocyst in the former condition and widening of the duodenal loop or distortion or destruction of mucosal folds in the latter (see Ch. 410.3 and 411).

VITAMIN B_{12} ABSORPTION. Vitamin B_{12} absorption is tested after intramuscular administration of 1000 μg by oral administration of radioactive vitamin B_{12} and measurement of the excretion in the urine over a 24-hour period. Greater than 7 per cent of the administered dose should be excreted. The absolute values depend upon dose of labeled B_{12}.

Abnormal results are found after *resection* of the *terminal ileum,* extensive and severe *terminal ileal disease,* and *bacterial overgrowth.* It is also abnormal in *pernicious anemia,* after *total gastrectomy,* in some patients with *pancreatic insufficiency,* or in a very rare person with abnormal or *defective ileal* mucosal cell *receptors* for B_{12}. Ampicillin, 1.0 gram daily for two weeks, will usually restore vitamin B_{12} absorption in bacterial overgrowth to normal. On the other hand, administration of the test substance with intrinsic factor will yield a normal result in patients with pernicious anemia and after total gastrectomy, but not after extensive resection of the terminal ileum or in pancreatic insufficiency. In the latter condition bicarbonate or pancreatic extract may be required (see Table 3).

JEJUNAL HISTOLOGY. Histologic study of jejunal mucosa obtained by suction biopsy technique has further aided differential diagnosis of the malabsorption syndrome. The procedure is easily performed with one of several available tubes (Rubin tube or Crosby capsule). Prothrombin time must be normal. Characteristic findings have been associated with *celiac disease* in both children and adults and in *tropical sprue, Whipple's disease, amyloidosis,* and *eosinophilic gastroenteritis.* In some instances alterations may be noted in diffuse nongranulomatous *ileojejunitis,* in *lymphoma,* after *gastrectomy,* in *hypogammaglobulinemia* with steatorrhea, in patients with intestinal *lymphangiectasia* associated with protein-losing en-

Figure 3. Small bowel roentgenographic series in patient (M.S.) with adult celiac disease. *A*, Before treatment. *B*, Six weeks after elimination of gluten from the diet. Note that the severely disordered pattern has improved.

Figure 4. Jejunal mucosa of patient (F. G.) with adult celiac disease. *A*, Before treatment (60 ×). *B*, Twenty-eight months after elimination of gluten from the diet. Note the regeneration of the villi and the return toward normal of the columnar epithelium (60 ×).

teropathy who have dilated lacteals, and in individuals with *radiation enteritis, mastocytosis,* or severe *drug reactions.* Fat-laden epithelial cells are found in *abetalipoproteinemia.* Certain parasites, namely, *Giardia lamblia* and *Coccidioides immitis,* have also been found on biopsy.

A section of normal jejunal mucosa from a specimen obtained by suction biopsy is shown in Figures 4 and 5. The villi are long, delicate, and frondlike; the lining columnar epithelium is regular with basal orientation of nuclei. The crypts are normal, and cellular infiltration of the lamina propria is minimal. Proper interpretation of jejunal histology, it must be emphasized, depends upon correct (perpendicular) sectioning of the specimen, which, in turn, requires correct mounting before fixing.

The jejunal histology in *adult celiac disease and tropical sprue* is strikingly abnormal. In evaluation of small bowel biopsies from such patients, particular attention must be directed to configuration of the villi, morphology of the epithelial cells with their brush border, and the degree of the chronic inflammatory cell infiltration. The severity of changes may be graded from mild to moderate to severe. In the *severe* group (total villous atrophy) the changes consist of complete flattening of the mucosal surface without detectable villi or, at best, only very short and broad villi. Generally, there is a dense infiltration of chronic inflammatory cells and disorganization of the epithelial cells with a sparse brush border (Figs. 4 and 5). In the *mild* group (partial villous atrophy), the villi are formed but still are shorter and broader than normal. In some areas the villi approach normal in all respects. The epithelial cells

Figure 5. Comparison of dissecting microscopy and light microscopy of jejunal biopsy specimens. *A,* Finger-like villi vs. *B,* normal villous pattern. *C,* Leaflike villi vs. *D,* normal villous pattern. *E,* Convolutions vs. *F,* partial villous atrophy. *G,* "Mosaics" vs. *H,* total villous atrophy. *E* through *H* are specimens from patients with adult celiac disease.

with brush border generally may be nearly normal and the cellular infiltration is mild. In the *moderate* subdivision (subtotal villous atrophy), changes ranging between those of the mild and severe groups are noted (Fig. 5).

The degree of infiltration of the lamina propria and of alteration of the epithelial cells is proportional to the extent of villous atrophy. The brush border frequently appears intact in the crypts, although it is disorganized and sparse near the midportion and tip of the villus. Although the severity of the lesion varies considerably among patients, the variation within a limited region of the proximal jejunum in a single patient is minimal; however, definite differences between the samples from more distant locations in the same patient have been noted. Total villous atrophy, although characteristic of celiac disease, is not specific. Occasionally, it may be noted in *tropical sprue,* and, in patchy fashion, in *bacterial overgrowth syndrome, infectious gastroenteritis, kwashiorkor, giardiasis, lymphoma,* or *Whipple's disease;* it has also been reported in *diffuse nongranulomatous ileojejunitis* (often "ulcerative"), as well as in patients with *congenital hypogammaglobulinemia* in whom plasma cells are absent in the lamina propria. Some of the last-named will respond to a gluten-free diet and thus have adult celiac disease as well; the same coincidence may be noted in patients with *diabetes mellitus* after *gastrectomy,* and in *Sjögren's syndrome, mastocytosis, jejunal diverticulosis,* and even *cystic fibrosis.* The classic findings are also present in so-called *collagenous sprue,* in which there is also a broad band of collagen between surface cells and lamina propria.

Changes of this nature have also been noted (but not responsive to gluten elimination) in patients with *eosinophilic gastroenteritis,* in some *parasitoses,* and in *intestinal ischemia, dermatitis herpetiformis, soy bean sensitivity, radiation enteritis, tuberculosis, viral enteritis,* and conditions caused by *colchicine* and *neomycin.* Mild inflammatory cell infiltration of the lamina propria has been noted in biopsies from patients with bacterial overgrowth. Specific diagnosis may also be made in *strongyloidiasis, capillariasis,* and *coccidiosis.*

In *Whipple's disease* the diagnosis may be made by the demonstration of macrophages laden with periodic acid–Schiff staining material in lymph nodes or in the lamina propria of the intestinal wall. In addition, total villous atrophy may be noted (Fig. 6). Electron microscopic studies during the active phase of the disease have revealed membranous structures, which may represent an infectious agent outside the macrophages. Deposits of amyloid have been found in the submucosa of the jejunum in patients with *amyloidosis,* particularly within the walls of arterioles.

In the past few years examination of fresh biopsy specimens under the dissecting microscope has yielded information about a number of diseases of the small intestine associated with malabsorption. The normal patterns of *finger-like villi* and *leaf-like villi* are seen in Figure 5. The former are jejunal, and the latter are also normally present in the duodenum and upper jejunum. Epithelial convolutions usually indicate disease and, on histologic examination, correspond to *partial villous atrophy.* A most extreme change is noted with total villous atrophy, with *"mosaics"* or *"brain patterns"* as the picture under the dissecting

microscope. Examples of this classification are presented in Figure 5.

DIFFERENTIAL FEATURES AND TREATMENT OF INDIVIDUAL FORMS OF THE MALABSORPTION SYNDROME

Because the presenting clinical picture includes a wide range of symptoms — bulky stools, flatulence, distention, anorexia, weight loss, weakness, glossitis, paresthesias, bleeding, bone pain — a careful history is of extreme importance in differential diagnosis. Particular attention must be paid to bowel habits in childhood, family history, previous illnesses and surgical operations, and dietary habits (including consumption of alcohol). A history of symptoms commonly associated with diseases that might underlie the malabsorption must be sought. Valuable clues may also be derived from a careful physical examination. In this way diagnosis of *tropical sprue, adult celiac disease, Whipple's disease, hypothyroidism, hyperthyroidism, hypoparathyroidism, scleroderma, lymphoma,* and other disorders which may underlie malabsorption is facilitated.

The malabsorption syndrome must be differentiated from a wide variety of conditions characterized by a bleeding diathesis, by skeletal pain with or without fracture, by evidence of vitamin B deficiency and extreme malnutrition, or by chronic diarrhea. Diagnosis of the malabsorption syndrome as a cause for these symptoms and signs must first, however, be based upon demonstration of abnormal fat absorption.

As the patient with the malabsorption syndrome may have extreme weight loss, weakness, hypotension, and diffuse pigmentation, differentiation from *Addison's disease* must be made. Abnormalities of serum calcium, carotene, or plasma prothrombin and impaired absorption of fat and xylose indicate the presence of the malabsorption syndrome (Table 4). Addison's disease may be excluded by the responsiveness of the adrenal gland to an intravenous infusion of corticotropin. However, it must be stressed that patients very severely, acutely, and chronically ill with malabsorption syndrome, particularly *celiac disease,* may have evidence of hypoadrenocorticism.

The principal distinctive features of the individual forms of the malabsorption syndrome are discussed according to the seven categories of Table 1.

As there are numerous conditions that can produce the malabsorption syndrome, its treatment must be individualized. In contrast to the often gratifying response to dietotherapy shown by patients with *adult celiac disease,* or to antimicrobials by patients with *Whipple's disease, diseases with bacterial overgrowth,* and *tropical sprue,* successful management of malabsorption resulting from various other diseases or alterations of the gastrointestinal tract is often difficult. Dosage schedules for agents used in the treatment of malabsorption syndrome are listed in Table 5.

Category 1: Defective Intraluminal Hydrolysis or Solubilization

PRIMARY PANCREATIC INSUFFICIENCY. Pancreatic insufficiency results from *chronic relapsing pancreatitis, carcinoma of the pancreas,* or *cystic fibrosis,* or occurs *after extensive resection* of the gland. In the first three instances, it is due to extensive parenchymal destruction and/or obstruction of the major ductal system. In chronic pan-

Figure 6. Jejunal biopsy from a patient with Whipple's disease. Periodic acid–Schiff stain. Note macrophages laden with stained material in the lamina propria.

**TABLE 5.   Representative Dosages for Agents Used in Management of
Patients with the Malabsorption Syndrome**

1. CALCIUM
   Oral: Calcium gluconate (91 mg Ca^{++}/gram), 1 to 5 grams three times daily
   Intravenous: Calcium gluconate injection. U.S.P. 10 per cent solution (9.1 mg Ca^{++}/ml), 10 to 30 ml administered slowly intravenously depending upon response
2. MAGNESIUM
   Oral: Magnesium sulfate (8 mEq/gram), 1.0 to 6.0 grams daily in divided dosage
   Intramuscular: (20% sol.) 10 ml two or three times daily
   Intravenous: Magnesium sulfate, 0.5 per cent solution, up to 1000 ml at a rate not faster than 1.0 mEq/minute
3. IRON
   Oral: Ferrous gluconate, 0.6 gram three times daily
   Intramuscular: (Imferon). Must be calculated according to severity of anemia. Detailed instructions accompany preparation.
4. FAT-SOLUBLE VITAMINS
   a. VITAMIN A
      Oleovitamin A capsules, U.S.P. (25,000 units per capsule), 100,000 to 200,000 units daily in severe deficiencies; maintenance, 25,000 to 50,000 units daily.
   b. VITAMIN D
      Synthetic oleovitamin D, U.S.P. (10,000 U.S.P. units vitamin D/gram), 30,000 units daily; increase dosage as necessary to raise serum calcium to normal. Dosage varies considerably depending on response as determined by level of serum calcium and urinary calcium.
   c. COMBINATION A AND D VITAMINS
      Concentrated oleovitamins A and D, U.S.P. (50,000 to 65,000 U.S.P. A units and 10,000 to 13,000 U.S.P. D units/gram) may be used rather than separate preparations.
   d. VITAMIN K
      Oral: Menadione, U.S.P., 4 to 12 mg daily. Vitamin K$_1$ tablets (Mephyton), 5 to 10 mg daily.
      Intravenous: (Bleeding episodes—acute situations.) Vitamin K$_1$ (Mephyton), 50 mg ampule. Administer 50 mg slowly over 10-minute period. Repeat in 8 to 12 hours if prothrombin time has not returned to normal.
5. FOLIC ACID, U.S.P. (5 mg tablets)
   Dose: Initial, 10 to 20 mg daily
   Maintenance, 5 to 10 mg daily
6. VITAMIN B$_{12}$ INJECTION, U.S.P. (15 μg/ml)
   Dose: Initial, 30 to 60 μg daily for two to three weeks
   Maintenance, 100 μg monthly
   If combined system disease is present, a more intensive program is indicated.
7. VITAMIN B COMPLEX
   Any multivitamin preparation that contains daily requirements (thiamine 1.6 mg, riboflavin 1.8 mg, and niacin 20 mg). Use two or three tablets daily. Intramuscular preparations are available for severe deficiencies.
8. PANCREATIC SUPPLEMENTS, ORAL
   Recently these agents have been shown to be more effective when given at 6 to 12 regular intervals during the day rather than at meal times.
   a. *Pancreatin,* U.S.P. (0.3 gram tablet), 6 to 18 grams daily.

   b. *Viokase* (0.3 gram tablet), 4 to 12 grams daily in divided doses at meals or hourly per day.
   c. *Cotazym* (0.3 gram capsule), 4.0 to 12.0 grams daily, divided doses at meals or hourly per day.
9. BROAD-SPECTRUM ANTIMICROBIALS
   Oral: Chloramphenicol, tetracycline, or oxytetracycline (0.25 gram), 1.0 gram per day in divided doses for 10 to 14 days; ampicillin (0.25 gram), 2.0 to 4.0 grams per day in divided doses; kanamycin (0.5 gram), 2.0 to 4.0 grams per day in divided doses; sulfisoxazole (0.5 gram), 1.0 to 2.0 grams daily in divided doses; lincomycin (0.25 gram), 1.0 to 2.0 grams daily. Repeated courses often necessary or administration for three to four days each week indefinitely.
10. HUMAN ALBUMIN, SALT POOR (0.25 gram/ml)
    Intravenous administration of 50 to 100 grams each day for three to seven days to elevate a severely depressed serum albumin level
11. GLOBULIN, IMMUNE SERUM (0.165 gram/ml)
    Intramuscular injection of 0.05 ml/kg each three to four weeks in patients with hypogammaglobulinemia and recurrent infection.
12. CORTICOTROPIN AND ADRENOCORTICOSTEROIDS
    a. Corticotropin, 30 to 40 units intravenously each day, 10 to 21 days or longer for severely ill patients.
    b. Prednisolone or prednisone, 30 to 60 mg orally each day as needed; 5.0 to 15.0 mg maintenance dose.
13. ANTIDIARRHEAL AGENTS
    Oral: Diphenoxylate hydrochloride (2.5 mg), 5.0 mg twice or three times daily. Deodorized tincture opium, 10 drops twice to three times per day. Propantheline (15.0 mg), 30 mg twice or three times daily.
14. CHOLESTYRAMINE, ORAL RESIN
    4.0 gram dose, three to six times daily, before feedings.
15. CALORIC SUPPLEMENTATION
    Oral: (a) Medium-chain triglyceride (MCT). "Home or Hospital Mix" (MCT: 45 per cent calories; caseinate, 15 per cent; dextrose, 40 per cent). Ingredients homogenized with H_2O to one liter (MCT: 75 mg; caseinate, 60 grams; dextrose 160 grams). Keep at 20°C for one year. Defrost day's formula each morning; give three ounces at meals; gradually increase between-meal feedings to six ounces. Portagen (MCT: 45.0 grams fat/quart; 30 cal/oz; 10 per cent carbohydrate). Formula mix. Prepare according to instructions. Give 16 oz every day.
    (b) Vivonex, 80 grams = 300 cal: 90.8% CHO; 0.7% fat; 8.5% amino acids, plus minerals and electrolytes. Dissolve in 100 ml water. Feed up to 480 grams q.d.
    Intravenous: * Prepare solution of approx. 0.9 cal/ml: 20% dextrose and 5% fibrin hydrolysate (w/v). Give 1500–3000 ml q.d. Increase amounts cautiously. Solution contains electrolytes, including PO_4'''
16. DRUGS FOR PARASITES
    Oral: Thiabendazole (25 mg/kg/day). Strongyloidiasis, two to three days: *Capillaria philippensis,* 30 days. *A. duodenale, N. americanus,* 25 mg/kg/day twice daily for two days.
    Oral: Metronidazole (0.25 gram), 0.25 gram three times daily for 7 days for *Giardia lamblia.*
    Oral: Bephenium (5 gram packet). *A. duodenale,* one packet twice for one day; *N. americanus,* one packet twice daily for three days.

---

*See Table 6 for intravenous hyperalimentation formula.

---

creatitis with malabsorption (see Ch. 410.3), the patient is frequently diabetic, the gland is often calcified, and frequently, but not always, there is a history of recurrent attacks of inflammation. Occasionally the dominant symptoms of *carcinoma of the pancreas* are those of malabsorption rather than pain, anorexia, or jaundice. *Cystic fibrosis* is most often clinically apparent in early childhood; however, the digagnosis is often made in young adults.

Whatever the cause of pancreatic insufficiency, failure of lipolysis results in moderate to severe steatorrhea, depending to some degree on the amount of gland remaining. Patients with this disease may show evidence of deficiency of either vitamin B$_{12}$ or fat-soluble vitamins. In contrast to adult celiac disease, d-xylose absorption is normal in pancreatic insufficiency except in the unusual instance of carcinoma of the pancreas that has invaded the

small intestine. As noted earlier, the diagnosis of pancreatic insufficiency is facilitated by analysis of duodenal fluid after stimulation of the pancreas.

SECONDARY PANCREATIC INSUFFICIENCY. Since pancreatic lipase is inactivated at an acid pH, conditions characterized by excessive gastric acid secretion, such as non-β islet cell tumor of the pancreas (Zollinger-Ellison syndrome) or massive small bowel resection, are associated with significant steatorrhea. A low pH in the upper small gut also precipitates bile salts and causes mild histologic abnormalities. Recent studies show that dilution of pancreatic hydrolytic enzymes because of rapid gastric emptying is responsible for an apparent pancreatic insufficiency after subtotal gastrectomy and pyloroplasty with vagotomy.

DEFICIENCY OF CONJUGATED BILE ACIDS. Insufficient

concentration of conjugated bile acids in the upper intestine, caused by severe liver disease or prolonged extrahepatic biliary tract obstruction, diminished bile acid pool, or significant reduction of conjugated bile acids resulting from bacterial overgrowth (see below), diminishes hydrolysis of neutral lipid and results in steatorrhea. The pathophysiologic mechanism is subnormal concentration of conjugated bile acids necessary for micelle formation.

Distal *ileectomy,* severely *diseased terminal ileum,* or *ileal bypass* (surgical or via cholecystocolonic fistula), by disrupting the enterohepatic circulation of conjugated bile acids, also causes steatorrhea, the degree proportional to the length of the resected, diseased, or bypassed segment (about 8 to 15 grams per 24 hours for distal 100 cm). Bile acid pool is diminished, the critical level of conjugated bile acids is not achieved in the jejunum, and micellar solubilization of lipid diminishes. Further, since bile acid absorption is subnormal, these substances make contact with colonic mucosa, inhibiting water and salt absorption, particularly in the ascending colon. Diarrhea — three to six loose to soft movements per day — results. When less than 100 cm of terminal ileum is involved, both the steatorrhea and diarrhea are mild. Patients with distal ileectomy generally lose from 15 to 30 grams of fat in stools per day. This large degree of steatorrhea may be due in small part to loss of absorptive function of the ileum, although it is likely that the diminished bile acid pool is mainly responsible.

Decreased conjugated bile acid pool is also notable in primary or *secondary biliary cirrhosis;* that the steatorrhea in these cases is due to liver disease is supported by disappearance of malabsorption with improvement of liver function. It is surprising, however, that the steatorrhea of complete biliary tract obstruction is moderate, indicating other mechanisms for absorption in addition to proximal uptake of micellar lipid. Malabsorption of fat in *postnecrotic* (macronodular) or *portal* (micronodular) *cirrhosis* is usually mild unless *chronic pancreatitis* (usually caused by alcohol) is also present.

BACTERIAL OVERGROWTH (INCREASED BILE ACID DECONJUGATION). For many years, steatorrhea and vitamin B_{12} deficiency anemia have been clinically and experimentally associated with alterations in the anatomy of the small intestine, particularly surgically created *"blind" loops; enteroenteric, enterocolic,* or *gastrojejunocolic fistulas; afferent loop stasis* after subtotal gastrectomy and gastrojejunostomy; or *chronic obstruction* caused by adhesions or strictures, *jejunal diverticula,* or diseases with *motor abnormalities* such as scleroderma and pseudo-obstruction.

The common denominator in all conditions is bacterial overgrowth, which results from stasis in a segment of small bowel caused by anatomic factors, motor abnormalities, or contamination of small bowel by large bowel content. Concentration of anaerobic organisms greater than 10^7 per milliliter, particularly *bacteroides, clostridia,* and *lactobacilli,* is responsible for impairment of intraluminal solubilization of hydrolyzed lipid. Bacteria play a role in the malabsorption of *tropical sprue,* and after *subtotal gastrectomy* and Billroth II gastrojejunostomy. Overgrowth rarely is responsible for malabsorption in the diarrhea of *diabetic neuropathy.* These patients may also have severe diarrhea as well as steatorrhea, possibly owing to impairment of Na^+ and water absorption by hydroxy fatty acids which result from bacterial action on unabsorbed fatty acids; also, volatile fatty acids, products of fermentation of sugars and amino acids, may cause diarrhea by inhibiting water and salt absorption by the colon.

The mechanism of the malabsorption of vitamin B_{12} and fat caused by bacterial overgrowth is clear. Vitamin B_{12} is utilized by multiplying anaerobic organisms. Fat absorption is impaired by deconjugation of bile acids by bacterial enzymes. The decline in concentration of conjugated bile acids below a critical level impairs micelle formation, reducing uptake of lipid by the mucosa. Concentration of free bile acids is increased intraluminally; their absorption from the proximal small gut by passive diffusion is rapid, and their serum levels are elevated; these compounds may also inhibit cellular resynthesis of triglycerides. Observations on patients with bacterial overgrowth indicate that less than 20 per cent of intraluminal fat is in a micellar phase 45 minutes after ingestion of a lipid meal (normal: more than 50 per cent). Since hydrolysis of fat is not impaired, steatorrhea is principally the result of impaired micelle formation.

Although the jejunal villi are not entirely normal in jejunal biopsy specimens of patients with bacterial overgrowth, demonstrating some infiltration of the lamina propria with lymphocytes, plasma cells, and occasionally polymorphonuclear cells, along with mild blunting, the appearance is strikingly different from the picture in adult celiac disease.

"Blind" Loops. A loop of intestine is "blind" either when it is disconnected from the main stream (rare) or when intestinal contents may gain access to it but not readily egress from it. An example would be a partly defunctionalized terminal ileal loop that has been partially excluded by either side-to-side or end-to-side ileotransverse colostomy (Fig. 2). Stasis and overgrowth of bacteria take place with subsequent invasion of the upper small intestine.

Multiple Strictures and Jejunal Diverticula. Strictures result from diffuse *granulomatous ileojejunitis, tuberculosis,* or *x-radiation* therapy. Frequently these patients have crampy abdominal pain, bloating, and other symptoms of progressive luminal narrowing, as well as other evidences of their underlying diseases. Most multiple jejunal diverticula are probably acquired. Stasis of intestinal content in these pockets of bowel leads to bacterial overgrowth. It is thought that such patients usually are achlorhydric.

Fistulas. Fistulas may complicate gastric or intestinal neoplasm or granulomatous enteritis, involving stomach, small gut, and colon (gastrocolic), small gut and colon (enterocolic), or loops of small gut (enteroenteric). Malabsorption may also, of course, result from exclusion of significant lengths of absorbing surface from the main stream by large fistulas (gastroileostomy).

The diagnosis is greatly aided by a history of previous chronic enteric disease or of surgical procedure. Roentgenographic examination will often establish the diagnosis by the demonstration of one of these diseases or alterations. Frequently, however, the cause may not be demonstrated.

The megaloblastic anemia commonly associated with the "blind loop" syndrome will, unlike pernicious anemia, respond to the administration of broad-spectrum antimicrobial drugs. After 10 to 14 days of such therapy (ampicillin, 1.0 gram daily in divided dose), absorption of vitamin B_{12} is usually, but not always, restored to normal (Table 5). In contrast to those with pernicious anemia and many with *jejunal diverticula,* these patients usually secrete hydrochloric acid.

Postgastrectomy. Afferent loop stasis after gastrectomy and gastrojejunostomy (Billroth II) is a cause for steatorrhea and malabsorption and may be due in part to bacterial contamination of the afferent loop (see Category 5).

Scleroderma and Pseudo-Obstruction. Although a disturbance of esophageal motor function is the most common gastrointestinal manifestation of scleroderma, severe involvement of the small bowel may cause malabsorption. Atrophy of the smooth muscle of the gut, submucosal fibrosis, and damage to the myenteric plexuses severely impair or abolish peristalsis. The resulting intermittent ileus may simulate closely the picture of complete intestinal obstruction. Severe involvement of the small intestine is usually associated with esophageal involvement, thickening of the skin, or other evidence of disseminated sclerosis, e.g., soft tissue calcification, telangiectasia, pulmonary diffusion defect, so that diagnosis is not difficult. Jejunal biopsy reveals normal villi, but there may be an increased number of inflammatory cells in the lamina propria.

Bacterial overgrowth is the principal factor in the steatorrhea and malabsorption of most patients with scleroderma involving the small intestine. As with the esophagus (see Ch. 396), small bowel smooth muscle is atrophic and is replaced with fibrous tissue. Motility is severely impaired; stasis and bacterial overgrowth result. Culture of small bowel content of such patients may yield a heavy growth of anaerobic organisms.

Pseudo-obstruction of the small and large intestine is a rare condition, reflecting an abnormality of gut smooth muscle function, and characterized by periodic episodes of prolonged ileus. It is chronic in some patients and may be associated with malabsorption resulting from bacterial overgrowth.

Treatment of Defective Intraluminal Hydrolysis

PRIMARY PANCREATIC INSUFFICIENCY. Replacement of digestive enzymes and insulin is important in the treatment of patients with *primary pancreatic insufficiency.* Among the available sources of enzymes are a commercial pancreatic extract, pancreatin, U.S.P.; a preparation containing whole raw pancreas, Viokase; and one containing hog pancreas extract, Cotazym. Doses of these preparations are listed in Table 5; occasionally, it may be necessary to increase the recommended amounts. Replacement therapy may be more effective when it is given in divided doses at regular intervals six times daily or even hourly during the day than when it is limited to mealtimes. Some patients with primary pancreatic insufficiency do not absorb vitamin B_{12} normally, a defect that may not be corrected by giving bicarbonate alone; pancreatic extracts, however, will increase absorption to normal.

SECONDARY PANCREATIC INSUFFICIENCY. Hypersecretion of acid caused by *non-β islet cell tumor* (Zollinger-Ellison syndrome) is best treated by total gastrectomy (see Ch. 406); after *massive small bowel resection,* hypersecretion may appear and be relieved by vagotomy and pyloroplasty. Both conditions, however, may be successfully treated with adequate doses of an H_2 blocker, cimetidine, and adding an anticholinergic drug may further help in the Zollinger-Ellison syndrome. Fortunately, hypersecretion is transient in most patients after massive small bowel resection. Relative pancreatic insufficiency after surgery for peptic ulcer disease (subtotal gastrectomy, pyloro-

plasty and vagotomy) also should be treated with pancreatic extract (Table 5).

DEFICIENCY OF CONJUGATED BILE ACIDS. Cases in which insufficient bile reaches the intestine pose a difficult problem in treatment. If possible, *cholecystocolonic fistulas* or chronic *obstruction* of the *biliary tree* should be corrected surgically. The keystone of medical management is a balanced diet without restriction of fat. For patients with chronic *cholestatic liver disease* it is important to provide calcium and fat-soluble vitamins A, K, and D in adequate amounts (Table 5). The demineralization of bone in patients with prolonged biliary obstruction results from osteoporosis and osteomalacia. Adequate supplements of vitamin D and calcium not only may prevent further osteomalacia but also may increase calcium deposition. More recently, a synthetic compound, 1α-OH-D_3, has been effectively used in patients with vitamin D deficiency and demineralization. Because inactivity contributes to the skeletal demineralization, maximal ambulation must be encouraged.

BACTERIAL OVERGROWTH (BILE ACID DECONJUGATION). Absorption of vitamin B_{12} and of fat is impaired with *intestinal strictures, fistulas, blind loops,* and multiple *jejunal diverticula.* The surgical correction of the strictures, fistulas, or blind loops may effect a permanent cure and is therefore the therapy of choice.

In some patients with malabsorption syndrome associated with either *subtotal* (Billroth II) or *total gastrectomy* or *scleroderma,* long-term antimicrobial therapy should be undertaken. Ampicillin, 1.0 gram per day, should be given for 10 to 14 days, and intermittently every other day for three days each week thereafter (Table 5). Chloramphenicol, also in a daily dosage of 1.0 gram, may be used in situations in which the risks of drug toxicity seem clearly to be outweighed by the potential dangers of the disease. Many of these patients, similar to those with bacterial overgrowth from other disorders, require continuous treatment. Rotation of antimicrobial drugs may be advisable in an effort to avoid the emergence of drug-resistant microbial populations. Aspiration of jejunal contents for cultures and periodic drug susceptibility determinations are necessary for therapeutic guidance. If organisms are not susceptible to the more usually employed drugs, courses of kanamycin (2.0 to 4.0 grams daily orally) may be given. All these drugs should be used in a rotational scheme. Occasionally, some patients with recurrent *Crohn's disease* and strictures or fistulas, in whom the surgical approach is not feasible, will have to be managed in a similar fashion.

In addition to the assessment of clinical response, efficiency of antimicrobial therapy may be judged by the return of the bile salt breath test and urinary indican to normal or nearly normal levels.

USE OF MEDIUM-CHAIN TRIGLYCERIDES (Table 5). Feeding preparations of medium-chain triglycerides, composed of fatty acids with six to ten carbons, appears to be valuable in a number of diseases that cause malabsorption, including those associated with defective intraluminal hydrolysis or solubilization of fat (see above).

Medium-chain triglycerides are most effective in those with pancreatic insufficiency who are also being given supplements of pancreatic enzymes (see above) and in patients with deficiency of conjugated bile salts (particularly biliary tract obstruction or bile fistulas).

Indication for medium-chain triglycerides is also strong in situations in which no specific therapy for malabsorption is available, such as after massive *small bowel resection* (short gut syndrome), *lymphatic obstruction*, and *biliary atresia*. Medium-chain triglycerides are a useful adjunct in malabsorption for which specific therapy is available (*celiac disease, bacterial overgrowth, Whipple's disease, parasitism,* and *tropical sprue* — all of which will be discussed in detail later in this chapter).

Category 2: Mucosal Cell Abnormality and Inadequate Surface

Primary Mucosal Cell Disorders

DISACCHARIDASE DEFICIENCY AND MONOSACCHARIDE MALABSORPTION. Inability to split disaccharides because of disaccharidase deficiency (lactase or sucrase and isomaltase) may be primary or secondary. The primary type of *lactase deficiency* is either familial (very rare, fatal) or congenital with an autosomal dominant inheritance. Symptoms may appear during infancy, childhood, or adulthood. Primary lactase deficiency (as well as other primary disaccharidase deficiencies) is not associated with any discernible alteration of the villi or their brush borders which contain these enzymes. Bacterial fermentation of unsplit lactose produces lactic and other organic acids which increase osmotic load with water entering the lumen. Diarrhea, cramping abdominal pain, borborygmi, and flatulence result from ingestion of milk and milk products. Weight loss and steatorrhea are usually mild and appetite is good, although infants and children may not thrive well. This pathophysiologic concept applies equally to *sucrase deficiency* when sucrose is ingested.

Lactase deficit is by far the most common, particularly in blacks, and is more common in Orientals than in whites. Dietary deficiency of lactose is not the cause. Adults diagnosed as having irritable colon syndrome (see Ch. 399) may be deficient in jejunal lactase. The reason for the clinical appearance of the disorder in adulthood is not clear; it is also occasionally unmasked after subtotal gastrectomy. Since no disease of the mucosal cells is evident, the deficiency is thought to be primary, but its clinical development is somehow acquired.

Diagnosis of lactase deficiency may be made by the measurement of blood glucose after the oral administration of lactose (Table 4). A rise of less than 20 mg per 100 ml is abnormal, and if the patient's blood glucose rises normally after he ingests a mixture of glucose-galactose of equal amount, lactase deficiency is extremely likely. Diagnosis may be confirmed only by the finding of low lactase activity in a jejunal biopsy specimen. Occasionally, these patients have lactosuria after administration of 50 grams of lactose during the lactose tolerance test.

Treatment of primary lactase deficiency is elimination of milk and milk products from the diet. It often dramatically relieves all symptoms. It may also be beneficial to patients with the secondary variety of deficiency.

Depression of lactase activity is also secondary to certain diseases affecting the brush borders of jejunal mucosal cells, such as *celiac disease;* but it is also found after *massive* small bowel *resection* and in *nonbacterial jejunitis, infectious diarrhea of childhood, Giardia lamblia infection, Whipple's disease, cystic fibrosis,* and *Crohn's disease.*

Deficiency of *sucrase* is rare; it is associated with deficiency of isomaltase. Recent studies indicate that it is a homozygotic deficiency affecting perhaps as many as 2 in 1000 individuals in the population. Symptoms include watery diarrhea and borborygmi, usually from infancy,

and are caused by ingestion of sucrose and sucrose-containing foods. Secondary sucrase deficiency may often accompany secondary lactase deficiency.

Diagnosis of sucrase deficiency may be made by failure of blood glucose to rise at least 20 mg per 100 ml after ingestion of 100 grams of sucrose. Treatment may be either elimination or marked reduction of sucrose, dextrins, and starches from the diet.

Congenital *glucose-galactose malabsorption* is present from birth and is exacerbated by all sugars broken down to these hexoses. Diagnosis is made by failure of these children to absorb either of these substances. Treatment consists of feeding fructose or fructose precursor–containing foods.

ABETALIPOPROTEINEMIA (ACANTHOCYTOSIS). Abetalipoproteinemia is a disease characterized by a morphologic defect of erythrocytes, "spiny red cells," low to absent serum beta-lipoproteins, very low serum cholesterol, and, in some instances, mild steatorrhea, ataxia, nystagmus, motor incoordination, and retinitis pigmentosa. The cause of the disease is unknown, but it is related to an inability of the mucosal cells to invest lipid with a protein envelope necessary for entry to the lacteals. The severity varies — in milder cases, no steatorrhea or neurologic defects occur. Substitution of medium-chain triglycerides for ordinary triglycerides has led to weight gain in some patients, because the component fatty acids enter the portal, not the lacteal, system.

VITAMIN B$_{12}$ MALABSORPTION. Very rarely, primary malabsorption of the vitamin B$_{12}$–intrinsic factor complex is noted, perhaps owing to absence of a specific but unidentified "receptor" in the ileal mucosa. These patients have been shown to have adequate intrinsic factor, normal ileal histology and calcium concentration, and alkaline pH. Treatment is monthly injections of vitamin B$_{12}$ intramuscularly (Table 5).

CYSTINURIA AND HARTNUP DISEASE. Rarely, patients may have genetic disorders of intestinal transport of amino acids. In *cystinuria* dibasic amino acids are involved — cystine, arginine, lysine, and ornithine; in *Hartnup disease,* neutral amino acids — e.g., phenylalanine and leucine. Tryptophan deficiency leads to nicotinamide deficiencies with rash, dementia, and ataxia. These patients are cured with adequate oral nicotinamide or adequate oral protein, because they absorb small peptides normally.

Intraluminal Small Bowel Disease

These diseases include *adult celiac disease, Whipple's disease, nongranulomatous ileojejunitis, eosinophilic gastroenteritis, amyloidosis, small bowel ischemia,* and *Crohn's disease.*

ADULT CELIAC DISEASE. An important cause of chronic malabsorption in temperate climates is adult celiac disease (gluten enteropathy, celiac sprue, nontropical sprue). In some undemonstrated way, dietary gluten is related to this disease. Perhaps the intestinal mucosa of these patients is damaged by acidic peptides contained in the gliadin fraction of this substance, either because of a deficiency or absence of specific peptidases or, more likely, by an immunologic reaction to them unrelated to enzyme activity. The process affects the mucosa principally with villous atrophy, columnar to cuboidal change of absorbing cells, and infiltration of the lamina propria with plasma cells and lymphocytes. Jejunum is more affected than ileum. The extent of this lesion may be roughly correlated with clinical severity.

Patients in this group have an abnormal incidence either of a history of childhood celiac disease or of evidence of the disease in relatives. The high incidence of HLA-B8 and -DW3 in these patients suggest a genetic predisposition. Further, individuals with congenital IgA deficiency are predisposed to this disease.

Commonly, the symptoms of celiac disease disappear in later childhood and in adolescence, despite continued malabsorption. Although the clinical remission is sometimes permanent, the classic features of adult celiac disease may appear during the third to sixth decades. The patients then may present with a spectrum of disability, ranging from mild discomfort and diarrhea with perhaps some anemia to severe illness with an extreme degree of malabsorption, foul-smelling diarrheal stools, skeletal disorders, bleeding phenomena, and symptoms of hypocalcemia. There are no pathognomonic physical signs in this disease. There may be all degrees of malnutrition, as evidenced by muscle wasting and edema (Fig. 1). Hypotension and abdominal bloating are very common. Occasionally, there are clubbing of the fingers and pigmentation similar to that of Addison's disease. Signs and symptoms of celiac disease and their pathophysiologic bases are noted in Table 2.

Roentgenography of the small bowel gives findings that are characteristic but not specific. Frequently the only change is an altered pattern with some dilatation of proximal loops of small bowel and minimal coarsening of the jejunal folds. More severe impairment is manifested by marked dilatation of small bowel segments and clumping of the barium meal, with a waxy cast appearance of bowel segments (the "moulage" sign) (Fig. 3). As mentioned previously, the routine laboratory studies used in establishing the presence of the malabsorption syndrome are not specific.

Better techniques in diagnosis of adult celiac disease are measurement of d-xylose absorption and study of jejunal histology. Indeed, the diagnosis is untenable unless total or nearly total villous atrophy is found. Vitamin B_{12} absorption is usually normal, but may be depressed if disease is extensive, involving the ileum. Other interesting findings, aside from those in Table 2, include frequent elevation of serum IgA and depression of IgM, along with reduced numbers of IgA-containing plasma cells in the biopsy.

A *trial of dietotherapy* may be important diagnostically in these patients. That the vast majority of adult celiac disease patients will respond favorably to an adequate gluten-free diet has been well established, and no other condition will respond so dramatically or so completely. Although clinical remission well within two months of institution of this therapy is the rule, some patients may require six to twelve months or even longer.

Treatment of Celiac Disease. The basis for the use of the gluten-free diet in adult celiac disease lay in observations of its beneficial effects (in children initially) in celiac syndrome. Laboratory as well as clinical data strongly indicated that these patients cannot tolerate cereals with high gluten content. Thus when wheat, rye, oats, and barley are eliminated from the diet, diarrhea and steatorrhea cease, appetite improves, and rapid weight gain ensues. (Conversely, the introduction of gluten or gliadin into a histologically normal segment of small bowel causes mucosal inflammation with villous atrophy within 12 hours, associated with diarrhea and steatorrhea.)

The gluten-free diet excludes all cereal grains except rice and corn. To follow this diet, all labels must be carefully scrutinized to eliminate completely products that contain wheat, rye, barley, and oats as "fillers" (e.g., ice cream, salad dressings, canned foods, condiments, candy). As substitutes for the usual grains, rice, corn, and soy flours may be used. A wheat starch flour (Cellu Products Company) is available. Beer and ale must be avoided, because they contain cereal residues; however, whiskies can be used, because the offending agent is not contained in the distillate. All other foods, except milk and milk products if they cause symptoms owing to lactase deficiency, are permitted, including fats. In general, the diet should be well balanced and high in protein. The complete diet is available in standard nutrition texts.

A substantial majority of the patients with adult celiac disease have responded to this diet, showing symptomatic improvement within a few days or a week, although a rare patient may require as long as 12 months. Weight gain has been so striking that patients have voluntarily restricted their caloric intake. The fact that a complete clinical remission with return to normal of pertinent blood components can be obtained in the majority of cases is significant, because previous treatment programs were usually only incompletely effective (Fig. 7). Follow-up biopsies demonstrate return to normal of mucosal histology in 50 per cent of patients who maintain that they adhere strictly to their diet, and marked improvement in most others. Complete restoration of villi and of the columnar epithelium in one patient is shown in Figure 4. Repeated biopsies in a minority of patients, however, reveal little or no improvement. It is difficult to ascertain whether they are ingesting some gluten; the physician should, however, also suspect other diseases which are associated with non-gluten-sensitive villous atrophy (*hypogammaglobulinemia,* particularly with *Giardia lamblia; lymphoma; dermatitis herpetiformis; collagenous sprue; Whipple's disease;* and *diffuse nongranulomatous ileojejunitis*). In these conditions villous atrophy is patchy. Absorption of d-xylose returns to normal, as does urinary excretion of 5-hydroxyindolacetic acid, within a few weeks of elimination of gluten. Steatorrhea diminishes remarkably in all instances, but fat absorption returns completely to normal only in those patients who carefully eliminate all gluten. It must be noted, however, that a rare patient will not respond (see below).

Corticosteroids have been shown to produce significant improvement in adult celiac disease without entirely correcting the steatorrhea or biochemical abnormalities. These agents should be used for long-term therapy only in cases refractory to the gluten-free diet, for impaired protein metabolism and osteoporosis are troublesome features in this chronic condition.

Occasionally, a patient with adult celiac disease is critically ill, with severe diarrhea, wasting and anorexia, and serious protein and electrolyte depletion. There may also be bleeding, tetany, and edema. This situation demands a rigorous therapeutic regimen, employing intravenous vitamin K and calcium as well as infusions of salt-poor albumin (Table 5). It is in this clinical situation that corticosteroids may be lifesaving by greatly stimulating the appetite and perhaps by increasing absorption. Initially, corticotropin, 30 units, should be given intravenously over an eight-hour period daily. After 10 to 14 days, either prednisolone or prednisone, 60 mg a day, may be substituted. Simultaneously, a gluten-free diet should be offered, and, as the patient's condition improves, drug therapy should be discontinued by gradual reduction in dosage over three to four weeks. These patients should remain on such dietotherapy permanently. Supplements (vitamin D and K, calcium, iron, folic acid, B-soluble vitamins, and vitamin B_{12}) are gradually withdrawn as clinical and chemical improvement proceeds; the program is set by results of reported essential laboratory determinations and personal observations.

Special Considerations and Complications of Adult Celiac Disease. Lymphoma and Carcinoma. The incidence of primary small bowel lymphoma and carcinoma in patients with adult celiac disease is high, about 13 per cent in a large collected series, with lymphoma contributing 10 per cent. Abdominal pain, weight loss, bleeding, obstruction, and perforation are the cardinal clinical features of this fatal complication. It is believed that lymphoma is more common in those not treated with a gluten-free diet. Relapse in those who have responded, associated with suggestive symptoms, should alert one to the possibility.

Small Bowel Ulceration. Nonmalignant ulcers of the jejunum and ileum may complicate celiac disease, and are manifested by exacerbation of severe diarrhea, abdominal pain, fever, and severe hypoproteinemia secondary to protein-losing enteropathy (see below). Perforation, bleeding, and/or obstruction are late manifestations.

Neurologic Complications. A syndrome similar to subacute combined degeneration of the spinal cord is noted early in celiac disease, despite remission with a gluten-free diet and no vitamin B_{12} deficiency (see Ch. 285 to 292).

Celiac Disease and the Skin. *Dermatitis herpetiformis* may be associated with patchy villous atrophy of the duodenum and upper jejunum; this abnormality does not extend beyond the proximal foot or so of the small gut, perhaps explaining why malabsorption in these patients is mild or even absent. Response to a gluten-free diet is poor, and instillation of gluten into the gut causes no inflammatory response as it does in gluten enteropathy. Partial and total villous atrophy have also been noted in *psoriasis*.

A rare patient with adult celiac disease who does not respond entirely to the diet may also have relative *pancreatic insufficiency*, i.e., the release of secretion and CCK is diminished. These patients require oral pancreatic extract (Table 5).

Collagenous Sprue. This disease resembles adult celiac disease in that it has the identical histologic picture, but it is not responsive to gluten elimination. Later, collagen is extensively deposited in the lamina propria beneath the epithelium.

Hyposplenism. Recent studies indicate that an occasional patient will have splenic atrophy with hyposplenism and diminished immunologic response to antigens.

WHIPPLE'S DISEASE. In Whipple's disease, or lipophagic intestinal granulomatosis (intestinal "lipodystrophy"), there is a heavy infiltration of the intestinal wall and lymphatics by macrophages filled with glycoprotein. It is a generalized disease with steatorrhea as its principal feature, and it occurs predominantly in males in the fourth to seventh decades.

It may be difficult to differentiate this entity from other serious to fatal causes of malabsorption, particularly *lymphoma* and *tuberculosis*. Several manifestations such as polyserositis and postprandial pain are seen in all three diseases. However, nondeforming arthritis is most characteristic of Whipple's disease and is frequently the initial complaint. When gastrointestinal symptoms occur,

Figure 7. Appearance of patient (M. S.) with adult celiac disease. *A,* Before treatment. Note wasting and edema. *B,* Six weeks after elimination of gluten from the diet.

the disease usually progresses rapidly with marked diarrhea, weight loss, weakness, and symptoms of anemia and deficiencies of fat- and water-soluble vitamins. Physical findings that suggest this disorder include lymphadenopathy, found in 40 per cent of the patients, and the various manifestations of polyserositis. Fever may be noted in about one third of the patients. Indefinite plastic or doughy abdominal masses have been described in approximately one quarter of the patients. The most consistent findings in the routine laboratory studies are anemia and an increased sedimentation rate; eosinophilia is occasionally present. Classically, steatorrhea is severe, with d-xylose absorption depressed and thickened folds. The roentgenographic findings in the small bowel are nonspecific, usually showing a "sprue-like pattern."

The diagnosis of Whipple's disease can be verified either by peripheral lymph node biopsy or, when this is normal, by biopsy of a mesenteric lymph node at laparotomy. Diagnosis may be established by identification of macrophages containing periodic acid–Schiff positive material in jejunal biopsy specimens obtained perorally (Fig. 6). Patchy villous atrophy may also be noted; thus identification of the engorged macrophages is crucial. Electron microscopic studies have revealed bacilliform bodies in and near these macrophages that may be infectious agents. Recent studies suggest that a pleomorphic organism is involved. Infiltration of the lamina propria also causes enlargement of villi and thickening of the submucosa.

Treatment of Whipple's Disease. Antimicrobial drugs by mouth are effective in treating Whipple's disease. Indeed, present information indicates that continuous treatment with penicillin G, 0.25 gram four times daily, or broad-spectrum antimicrobials, tetracycline or ampicillin, always brings about remission. The dose of tetracycline or ampicillin is 1.0 gram daily. The duration of therapy with antimicrobials is determined by the clinical response. Present data indicate that such treatment should be maintained indefinitely; otherwise, symptoms may return. Histologic as well as clinical improvement is noted after a period of weeks to months, with loss of diarrhea, reappearance of appetite, and tremendous gain of weight. The PAS-positive material slowly disappears from the mucosa, and the bacilliform bodies are no longer visible on electron microscopy. When remission has been sustained for nine months to one year, antimicrobial agents may be given intermittently, i.e., every other day or for three consecutive days each week (Table 5).

The symptoms of Whipple's disease may respond to corticosteroid therapy, as do those of other diseases characterized by arthritis and polyserositis, but the over-all result of such treatment is not satisfactory. Present evidence strongly indicates that only 40 per cent of patients achieve remission of the disease for two to six months while receiving corticotropin or corticosteroids, and, in the majority, the disease relapses on cessation of such therapy. Many patients, particularly those whose illness is in a terminal phase, do not respond at all. The desperately ill patient should be given both corticotropin intravenously, 40 units daily, *and* parenteral antimicrobial agents until the improvement of the patient permits withdrawal of the former agent.

NONGRANULOMATOUS ILEOJEJUNITIS. Steatorrhea and malabsorption may result not only from the complications of Crohn's disease *(strictures, fistulas,* or *massive resections)* (see Ch. 413.2), but also from nongranulomatous involvement of a large segment of the small intestine, particularly the jejunum. The small intestine is diffusely inflamed; mesenteric nodes are slightly enlarged, and serosal lymphatics are dilated. Although the mucosa is heavily infiltrated with inflammatory cells and has patchy ulcerations, the wall is not thickened as in Crohn's disease, nor are there strictures or fistulas.

The onset of this latter illness is abrupt, and signs and symptoms of malabsorption may predominate in a matter of one to two weeks. A daily remittent fever (39 to 40.5° C), abdominal cramping pain, usually periumbilical, and frequent watery stools are common complaints. Splenomegaly, occurring in 20 per cent of these patients with fever, may suggest an initial diagnosis of abdominal lymphoma. Usually, diffuse inflammatory changes are noted in roentgenograms of the small bowel. Stenotic segments and fistulas are not usually seen. The small bowel pattern may be indistinguishable from that of a wide variety of conditions associated with the malabsorption syndrome. Laboratory findings of help in the differential diagnosis are elevation of the leukocyte count and rapid fall in serum albumin to the range of 1.5 to 2.5 grams per 100 ml. Diagnosis is usually made either by the response to treatment or by surgical exploration (see Ch. 413.2).

Treatment of Nongranulomatous Ileojejunitis. In diffuse nongranulomatous ileojejunitis, corticosteroids may have a dramatic effect upon the clinical symptoms, including those that are due to malabsorption. Steatorrhea will diminish or cease; serum calcium, carotene, and plasma prothrombin concentration will return to normal. Serum albumin, often severely depressed to levels of 1.5 to 2.5 grams per 100 ml by "weeping" of serum protein into a large segment of inflamed gut, so-called protein-losing enteropathy (see below), likewise rises as the inflammation subsides. These improvements, as indicated by laboratory tests, accompany the disappearance of fever as well as the increase in appetite, weight, and strength. Although such a therapeutic result is most salutary, it may not, unfortunately, be permanent. Recurrence is frequent, with progress of the disease in localized areas.

The consensus is that such patients, often acutely ill with fever and diarrhea, respond best to intravenous corticotropin, 40 units daily, given over an eight-hour period for 10 to 14 days. The oral corticosteroid preparations are used after corticotropin in the more serious cases and may be the principal therapeutic agents throughout the course of the less severe cases. The initial dose range in either instance is 40 to 60 mg of prednisone or prednisolone daily. The dose is gradually tapered over a week or longer to a maintenance level of 10 to 30 mg daily. The day-to-day clinical response best regulates the dose of drug at this stage of treatment. Broad-spectrum antimicrobials are not useful except in the presence of septic complications. Unfortunately, some of these patients have a relentless, refractory course and die of bowel perforation or intercurrent sepsis in two to three months, and the long-range outlook for permanent remission of this disease in those who initially respond is likewise not good.

ALLERGIC AND EOSINOPHILIC GASTROENTERITIS. Some patients are seen with malabsorption, varying degrees of gastrointestinal bleeding, and protein-losing enteropathy; their small gut mucosa is infiltrated by eosinophils and is edematous but shows no vasculitis. The involvement in many instances is principally mucosal. In some patients, in whom the stomach is also involved, the deeper layers of the gut, including serosa, are infiltrated. In a minority of instances in adults, the disease appears to be a response to an allergen such as milk protein, meat, or even fruit. Even in the absence of an offending agent, these patients have histories of hay fever, eczema, and asthma, particularly in childhood, or other food idiosyncrasies.

The symptoms — cramping pain, diarrhea, weight loss, nausea, fever, and a degree of malabsorption — are related to the location and extent of the disease in the small bowel. Fat loss in stool is about 15 to 20 grams per day. If the stomach is also involved, epigastric pain, vomiting, and bleeding are common. Frequently, the patients have allergies, particularly hay fever and asthma, and many have urticaria as well as diarrhea after eating certain foods (milk, egg, cereal, meat). Marked eosinophilia is a constant finding and is greater than 20 per cent. The disease tends to be chronic with recurrent symptoms. Roentgenographic examination often reveals a nonspecific "malabsorption pattern" with coarsened folds of jejunum. Occasionally, narrowed segments may be seen. Hypoproteinemia caused by protein-losing enteropathy may be severe and may be associated with marked edema and ascites. Iron deficiency anemia resulting from occult gastrointestinal bleeding is common in children. Disease of the stomach, particularly antral, may cause hematemesis.

Another form of this disease is so-called *eosinophilic granuloma*, in which the process consists of localized nodular or pedunculated infiltrative eosinophilic lesions (involving the submucosa and muscle layer) without allergy or peripheral eosinophilia. *Eosinophilic gastroenteritis* may also involve the serosa of the bowel as well as peritoneum, with ascites the predominant manifestation.

Treatment of Eosinophilic Gastroenteritis. Effective therapy consists of withdrawal of offending foods, particularly milk for children and fish or a particular meat in some adults. In more ill patients, prednisone, 20 to 40 mg daily orally with gradual tapering to a low maintenance dose, will bring remission of major symptoms and decrease of eosinophilia. With remission, edema and infiltrate of the jejunal mucosa also disappear in patients with no involvement of deeper layers. In patients with brisk bleeding from the stomach, surgery may have to be performed. Laparotomy, for severe pain or bleeding resulting from transmural small bowel disease, reveals thickened loops of jejunum, involved antrum, and enlarged mesenteric nodes. Biopsy differentiates this disease from granulomatous enteritis and tuberculosis. In the majority of patients the clinical picture, typical history, eosinophilia, obvious allergies, and response to treatment are sufficient to exclude *acute diffuse nongranulomatous ileojejunitis, Crohn's disease, lymphoma,* and *celiac disease.* Transoral jejunal biopsy will also be helpful.

AMYLOIDOSIS. Either the primary or the secondary form of the disorder may affect the gastrointestinal tract and cause malabsorption. Diffuse crampy pain and ileus are the most frequent abdominal symptoms. In the primary form of the disease, cardiac failure, macroglossia, and renal disease may be noted, but the Congo red test is negative. Roentgenographically, amyloidosis is characterized by dilated loops of bowel, occasionally with thickening of the jejunoileum and slow passage of the barium meal through the intestines. The diagnosis is made by tissue study. Gingival or rectal biopsies are frequently positive in *primary amyloidosis*, particularly when the disease is associated with myelomatosis; liver biopsy, although hazardous, may also establish the diagnosis. Biopsy of the liver or bowel at laparotomy may be necessary in some instances. Diagnosis may also be made from specimens of jejunal mucosa obtained by transoral suction biopsy.

In *secondary amyloidosis,* the presence of a chronic inflammatory illness and hepatosplenomegaly suggests the diagnosis. Congo red tests may show greater than 90 per cent retention of the injected material by the tissues.

Treatment is supportive, because the disease is too extensive for resection. If it is secondary to chronic infection or granulomatous disease, successful management of the underlying disorder may be helpful, although it is unlikely.

SMALL BOWEL ISCHEMIA. Chronic ischemia of the small bowel, caused by atherosclerosis of the celiac, superior, and inferior mesenteric arteries, may occasionally cause malabsorption, presumably because of impairment of mucosal cell function. No histologic damage, however, has been demonstrated in such instances (see Ch. 416).

The blood supply to the small intestine is occasionally severely compromised in patients with so-called collagen vascular disease, particularly *periarteritis nodosa* and *systemic lupus erythematosus.* Although malabsorption syndrome has been reported in these diseases, the documentation is unclear; *Degos' disease,* characterized by necrotic skin lesions and vasculitis of the small gut, may also cause malabsorption, although the far more serious and common clinical manifestation is infarction of the gut. A necrotizing type of arteriolitis leading to ulceration and perforation of the small gut is a serious form of vascular complication of the collagen vascular diseases.

CROHN'S DISEASE. This important disease of the small bowel may cause malabsorption in a number of ways: by extensive damage to the mucosa; by multiple strictures (bacterial overgrowth); by fistulas between small bowel and colon (bacterial overgrowth); or by necessitating ileectomy (defective solubilization and loss of absorptive surface) or massive resection (inadequate surface and defective solubilization). Bacterial overgrowth and defective solubilization are discussed in Category 1 above; inadequate surface, a portion of Category 2, is discussed below. The clinical picture of diffuse Crohn's disease of the small intestine is discussed in Ch. 413.2. It is sufficient here to emphasize that an important part of this picture is the signs and symptoms of malabsorption, the range and severity of which are proportional to the extent (length of bowel involved), to severity (i.e., complications) of the disease, and to the type and extent of surgery which may have been performed.

Inadequate Surface

Most absorption takes place in the duodenum and first 90 cm of the jejunum. Clinical studies of patients who have had extensive resection of the small intestine indicate that survival is now reasonably certain with 90 to 120 cm of remaining normal small bowel, and is possible with shorter segments provided that caloric intake is adequate. This length of jejunum is sufficient for normal carbohydrate absorption and, in most instances, for maintenance of positive nitrogen balance. The postoperative course is influenced by the site of resection — jejunum or ileum. Thus vitamin B_{12} absorption will be subnormal if a large length of ileum has been removed; conversely, sacrifice of a corresponding amount of jejunum will more seriously impair absorption of fat, calcium, and folic acid.

During the past decade, *jejunoileal bypass* has been performed on morbidly obese patients to achieve weight loss. The common procedure is the so-called "14 and 4," in

TABLE 6. Protein Hydrolysate Solutions: Contents Per Unit and Variations*

Ingredient (mEq Unless Otherwise Indicated)	Hydrolysate Solution 900	Hydrolysate Solution 900 with Added Sodium	Hydrolysate Solution 900 with Insulin	Hydrolysate Solution 900 with Insulin and Added Sodium	Hydrolysate Solution 900 Low Potassium	Hydrolysate Solution 900 Low Potassium with Added Sodium
Protein equivalent (grams)	23.4	23.4	23.4	23.4	23.4	23.4
Nitrogen, utilizable (grams)	2.7	2.7	2.7	2.7	2.7	2.7
Dextrose (grams)	230.0	230.0	230.0	230.0	230.0	230.0
Total calories (no.)	887	887	887	887	887	887
Potassium	36	36	36	36	12	12
Sodium	31	61	31	61	31	61
Magnesium	6	6	6	6	6	6
Calcium	4.5	4.5	4.5	4.5	4.5	4.5
Calcium (mg)	90	90	90	90	90	90
Phosphate	25	25	25	25	15	15
Chloride	18.8	33.8	18.8	33.8	18.8	33.8
Acetate	14	37	14	37	8	23
Insulin (units)	None	None	15	15	None	None
Vitamins	B-group vitamins and ascorbic acid are added to each unit daily; vitamins A, D,† and E‡ are added in addition to the B-group vitamins and ascorbic acid to each unit 1 day a week.					

*From Giovanoni, R., *In* Fischer, J. E. (ed.): Total Parenteral Nutrition. Boston, Little, Brown & Company, 1976.
†As ergocalciferol.
‡As *dl*-alpha tocopheryl acetate.

which 14 inches of proximal jejunum is anastomosed to 4 inches of terminal ileum. The proximal end of excluded bowel is closed, and the distal end is anastomosed to colon. The effect of this procedure is a marked malabsorption identical to that which follows massive resection of small bowel (see below). Although enormous losses of pounds ensue in most patients — usually 25 to 45 per cent of preoperative weight in one to two years — some undesirable sequelae, not related to intestinal deficiency, are observed. These include hepatic dysfunction, arthritis, motor disturbances (colonic pseudo-obstruction) of the gut, and oxalate stores in the kidneys. Care must always be taken to replete inevitable losses of water, electrolytes, calcium, magnesium, and vitamins caused by the inevitable diarrhea which follows the operation (Table 5).

The three common causes for extensive resection of large segments of the small intestine are (1) *recurrent regional enteritis*, (2) *mesenteric vascular disease*, particularly thrombosis of the superior mesenteric artery, and (3) *malignant processes* involving the blood supply of the small bowel.

TREATMENT. Inadvertent surgical *jejunocolostomies* or *gastroileostomies*, which sidetrack large segments of small intestine, must be corrected surgically as soon as possible.

The patient who has had an *extensive resection of the small intestine*, nearly always right colon, ileum, and part of distal jejunum, requires continuous and meticulous medical care. For weeks or even for one or two months, nutrition may adequately be maintained by intravenous hyperalimentation which employs fluids containing adequate calories, protein, minerals, and vitamins. Usually, 3 liters daily may satisfy nutritional requirements for an adult (Table 6). Certain complications may attend such therapy, and the physician must be aware of them. They are due to necessity for catheterizing the subclavian vein (sepsis, thrombosis, hemo- or pneumothorax). Hyperosmolar, hyperglycemic dehydration, or hypophosphatemia may also ensue. The patient's fluid and electrolyte balance must, of course, be meticulously monitored on a daily basis.

Oral feedings should be initiated as soon as possible, preferably containing substances which require minimal hydrolysis and are easily absorbed. Such refined preparations as Vivonex have been useful, because they contain simple sugars and amino acids; however, as with all hypertonic preparations, diarrhea may be aggravated.

For periods of up to 12 months postoperatively, the remaining segment of intestine will show progressive improvement in absorptive capacity, associated with elongation and dilatation. It is important to remember that, since the amount of fat absorbed is proportional to the amount presented to the absorbing surface, the maximal intake of fat that does not cause symptoms is desirable. Regardless of which segment or its part — ileum or jejunum — remains, the diet should be high in protein, and frequent feeding (six times daily) should be recommended and may consist in part of protein and amino acids (Table 5). Vitamins A, D, and K and the B-complex vitamins as well as calcium, iron, and magnesium may be given orally, except in those instances in which adequate replacement is possible only by the parenteral route (Table 5). In general, a high protein intake will adequately maintain the serum albumin; however, occasionally, infusions of salt-poor albumin must be given.

Supplementation of the diet by medium-chain triglycerides (see above; Table 5) has been of distinct benefit to patients with massive small bowel resection, diminishing diarrhea and helping to stabilize weight by improving fat absorption; however, it must be noted that weight gain attributable principally to medium-chain triglycerides in these patients is slight. Drugs that decrease intestinal motility, such as diphenoxylate hydrochloride (5.0 mg twice or three times daily), anticholinergics (propantheline, 15 to 30 mg twice to three times daily), and/or small doses of tincture of opium (10 drops twice to three times daily) may help reduce diarrhea (Table 5).

Category 3: Lymphatic Obstruction

LYMPHOMA. The malabsorption syndrome secondary to lymphoma of the small bowel and mesentery may be clinically and roentgenographically identical to the classic picture of adult celiac disease. Several features, however, suggest the correct diagnosis. The symptoms of this disease are likely to be of much shorter duration and to include crampy abdominal pain and fever. Lymphadenopathy and hepatosplenomegaly do not appear until late in the course. Although intramural small bowel masses may be present in some cases, the roentgenographic study of the intestine generally does not reveal them. Unexpectedly, the usual therapeutic measures, such as diet, fat-soluble vitamins, and vitamin B_{12}, may lead to a temporary clinical and laboratory remission. The incidence of malabsorption syndrome caused by small bowel lymphoma is difficult to ascertain. It appears that as many as 10 per cent of patients with adult celiac disease may develop lymphoma. Although lymphatic obstruction is important in the pathophysiology of steatorrhea in lymphoma, widespread disease of the intestine will also contribute significantly to the malabsorption.

The diagnosis is usually established by laparotomy necessitated by some complication of the underlying disease, such as bleeding, perforation, or obstruction. In some patients, the diagnosis may be made from jejunal tissue obtained by peroral biopsy. The average duration of this illness after onset of symptoms is 13 months, despite resection and roentgen therapy.

Primary intestinal lymphoma, with malabsorption, may be a chronic condition in certain parts of the world, particularly in the Middle East in young Arabs and Sephardic Jews, and in Mexico. The clinical picture strongly resembles adult celiac disease in terms of chronicity and jejeunal villous atrophy; however, most of these patients do not respond to elimination of gluten, and peroral biopsies will show evidence of lymphoma in the majority. In contrast to primary lymphoma of the small bowel with malabsorption in North America and Europe, which carries a prognosis of death one to two years after onset of symptoms (despite surgery, radiation, and chemotherapy), the young Middle Easterners may live with their disease for as long as ten years. Lymphoma also complicates *α-chain disease* in which heavy chains of IgA are produced excessively.

Treatment. Treatment of lymphoma of the small bowel and mesentery includes local resections as well as radiotherapy, and possibly therapy with chlorambucil and steroids or cyclophosphamide when the disease is disseminated. Despite this program, the course is frequently progressive, the average duration of life after onset of symptoms being one to two years. In these patients, continuous supportive therapy (high caloric diet, iron, vitamins, calcium, as needed) is frequently helpful and may result in successful maintenance of the patient's activity over a period of months. Indeed, these patients have also improved when given low-fat diets with vitamin and mineral supplementation.

INTESTINAL TUBERCULOSIS AND TUBERCULOUS LYMPHADENITIS. Tuberculosis may result in a malabsorption syndrome through involvement of the mesenteric lymph nodes, although in some cases there may be associated disease of the intestinal wall. It is extremely rare in the United States, and it occurs almost always in persons with a history of severe pulmonary or lymph node tuberculosis.

Fever, palpable abdominal masses, a positive tuberculin skin test, evidence of old or recent disease on chest roentgenography, and calcification of mesenteric and pelvic lymph nodes on flat film all suggest the diagnosis, which may be confirmed by culture of sputum or gastric juice. Rarely, stool culture may be useful, but only if the

other secretions are demonstrably free of tubercle bacilli. Roentgenographic studies, both barium enema and small bowel series, are particularly helpful when there is also deformity of the ileocecal segment resulting from hyperplastic lesions. Rarely, there may be diffuse small bowel abnormalities, such as coarsening of the folds, stricture formation, and edema, which suggest ileojejunitis. At times, exploratory laparotomy with node or bowel biopsy is necessary for diagnosis (see Ch. 168.6 and 168.12).

Treatment. Tuberculous involvement of the mesenteric lymph nodes should be treated by chemotherapy, as set forth in Ch. 168.12. A high caloric diet should be employed with calcium and vitamins as indicated. When there is an associated hyperplastic ileocecal tuberculosis with partial obstruction, appropriate local resection may be necessary.

LYMPHANGIECTASIA. In addition to the diseases just discussed, several other conditions may rarely cause the malabsorption syndrome by lymphatic blockade. These include *primary lymphangiectasia*, a genetically determined disease characterized by mild to moderate diarrhea, mild steatorrhea, and protein-losing enteropathy (see below), certain *protozoan diseases* (see Category 4), *the reticuloendothelioses, metastatic tumor* to the mesenteric nodes, and *neoplastic invasion of the main lymphatic channels* in the retroperitoneal tissues.

Category 4: Infection

TROPICAL SPRUE. Tropical sprue can be differentiated from adult celiac disease. The disease occurs primarily in persons residing in certain areas of the Far East, India, and the Caribbean. Both nutritional deficiencies and bacterial contamination of the small gut appear to play causative roles. This disease responds to administration of broad-spectrum antimicrobial drugs, suggesting, but not proving, that infection is responsible. Histologic changes suggestive of tropical sprue may be noted in individuals newly arrived in the tropics; such changes may often be associated with an acute enteritis and a variable degree of malabsorption. Although the remarkable clinical improvement that follows folic acid therapy strongly suggests a vitamin deficiency, tropical sprue is not seen in some areas of the world where the population has a marginal or even inadequate diet; conversely, it has been noted in people with adequately "balanced" diets.

Clinically, three phases of the disease have been described. In the initial phase the patient complains only of fatigue, asthenia, and bulky stools. After weeks to months, the second phase of malnutrition is noted. Weight loss is prominent. Glossitis, stomatitis, cheilosis, and hyperkeratosis are observed in varying degrees. Moderate prothrombin depletion is present but is rarely associated with bleeding. Manifestations of impaired calcium absorption are not usually clinically apparent in patients with tropical sprue, in contrast to those with adult celiac disease. Iron deficiency anemia follows depletion of iron stores. Hypoalbuminemia with edema may be a late manifestation of this disease. Some laboratory criteria of impaired absorption are present (Table 4). The third stage is characterized by anemia and megaloblastosis and the symptoms of full-blown severe malabsorption described earlier in this chapter, although diarrhea may not be prominent. However, the clinical spectrum is wide — steatorrhea mya be minimal, glossitis absent, and megaloblastosis inconstant. This inconsistent picture may indicate various causes.

Laboratory investigation reveals mainly steatorrhea and megaloblastic anemia. Small bowel roentgenographic findings and histologic changes of the jejunum are the same as those in adult celiac disease except that *total villous atrophy* is not as commonly encountered in tropical sprue. In many tropical areas, however, asymptomatic individuals often have histologic abnormalities suggestive of tropical sprue, making tissue diagnosis very difficult. Other routine laboratory studies, including d-xylose absorption, are also comparable in the two diseases. The gluten-free diet is ineffective.

Treatment for Tropical Sprue. The therapy for this disease is very effective. The similarity of tropical sprue to pernicious anemia, particularly in its hematologic aspects, prompted the use of liver extract, folic acid, and vitamin B_{12}, and remissions have also been noted with antimicrobial drugs, a low-fat, high-protein diet, and migration to a temperate climate. Administration of a broad-spectrum antimicrobial (tetracycline, 1.0 gram daily by mouth) along with 10 mg of folic acid daily is the best treatment and frequently brings remission, with disappearance of diarrhea and glossitis and gain in appetite and weight. However, response may be slow in some patients, and normal absorption and jejunal histology may not be noted for six months or longer. Parenteral vitamin B_{12} should be given for two months (Table 5). For those not responding completely within six months of treatment with antimicrobials and folic acid, therapy should be continued for as long as absorption continues to improve.

When remission has been achieved, 5.0 mg of folic acid daily is the maintenance therapy. In the presence of achlorhydria, addition of vitamin B_{12} to the regimen should be considered unless absorption of ^{60}Co B_{12} is normal (Table 5). If absorption of vitamin B_{12} remains subnormal after remission, monthly injections should be given.

ACUTE INFECTIOUS ENTERITIS. Bacterial and viral infections may cause transient but severe malabsorption. Patients with this condition have steatorrhea and may have diminished xylose absorption. The serum calcium as well as the plasma prothrombin concentration may be depressed. Serum proteins may fall rapidly, largely owing to abnormal rate of loss into the inflamed gut. With recovery, absorption returns to normal. Agents responsible, often in epidemics, include shigellae, enteropathic *E. coli*, *V. cholerae*, *V. parahaemolyticus*, some salmonellae, *C. perfringens*, staphylococci, *Yersinia*, and enteroviruses. (Details of diagnosis and treatment of these disorders are discussed in the appropriate chapters of Part IX.)

Treatment. These patients may recover without specific antimicrobial therapy, provided that fluids and electrolytes have been rapidly and adequately replaced. Such infections are apt to attack patients who travel to tropical countries or are debilitated, or who have had abdominal surgery, particularly those also given broad-spectrum antimicrobials. Patients severely ill with salmonellosis (septicemia) may require treatment with broad-spectrum antimicrobials (see Ch. 153). The keystone of therapy for all infectious enteritis is rapid and complete replacement of fluid and electrolytes. Acidosis, hypokalemia, and hyponatremia are often severe (see Ch. 154).

PROTOZOAN AND HELMINTHIC DISEASES. Protozoan or helminthic diseases are a common cause of malabsorption in many tropical areas and are particularly associated with malnutrition. Because tropical sprue is also endemic in many of these countries, it is often difficult to assign a cause for malabsorption, especially in view of the histologic changes (blunting of villi, cellular infiltration of the lamina propria) which are present in many asymptomatic individuals who are malnourished with or without parasites. Some of these patients with mild to moderate steatorrhea (10 to 15 grams per 24 hours), however, have malabsorption syndrome caused by *hookworm, strongyloidiasis, Capillaria philippensis, coccidiosis, giardiasis,* and *tapeworm infestations.* Parasites must be isolated and identified, and response to therapy, clinically, biochemically, and histologically, must be forthcoming before definite etiologic attribution of the malabsorption and malnutrition to parasitic infection can be made. (For details of diagnosis and treatment of parasitoses, see the relevant chapters of Part X.)

Patients with *Giardia lamblia* infection of the small bowel may suffer from malabsorption, particularly individuals with *subtotal gastrectomy; hypogammaglobulinemia* often associated with so-called "nodular lymphoid hyperplasia"; *tropical sprue;* or *severe malnutrition,* particularly in children. Thus the role played by the parasite is not completely clear despite demonstration of its invasion of the mucosa and report of some improvement in absorption after treatment with quinacrine (0.1 gram three times daily for one week). Recent evidence indicates that villous atrophy which is associated with the giardiasis of hypogammaglobulinemia is reversed with effective therapy for the parasite (see below, Category 6). In all doubtful cases it is wise to treat the patient (Table 5).

Category 5: Multiple Defects

SUBTOTAL GASTRECTOMY. Steatorrhea and malabsorption after subtotal gastrectomy and gastrojejunostomy (Billroth II) or total gastrectomy are attributable to (1) loss of reservoir function with rapid emptying and dispersion of food through the small intestine, thereby diluting the normal output of pancreatic enzymes; or (2) stasis with bacterial contamination of the afferent loop of a Billroth II gastrojejunostomy. Deficiency of vitamin B_{12} will inevitably follow total gastrectomy, the lag period being determined by the liver store of the vitamin.

Treatment. Administration of ox bile extract is not helpful, probably because of its high content of unconjugated acids. As yet no preparation of pure conjugated bile acids is available for treatment. Pancreatic extracts may be tried in selected cases, although when given alone they have not produced consistent improvement. However, when pancreatic extract is combined with broad-spectrum antimicrobials (ampicillin or tetracycline, 1.0 gram per day in divided dosage, or lincomycin, 1.0 to 2.0 grams per day), in the treatment of patients after Billroth II operations, fat absorption may improve. These results indicate that in some patients bacterial contamination—probably originating in the afferent loop—plays an important etiologic role in the malabsorption syndrome that follows this procedure. Conversion of Billroth II to Billroth I has been reported to reduce steatorrhea in some patients.

Patients who have undergone Billroth II procedures should receive a high-calorie diet rich in protein, with frequent feedings containing as much fat as can be tolerated, in order to maintain good nutrition. After a total gastrectomy, 30 to 100 μg of vitamin B_{12} intramuscularly must be given monthly. Calcium, iron, and the fat-soluble vitamins may be added to this regimen as needed or when diarrhea or steatorrhea is so severe that deficient absorption of these substances may be anticipated (Table 5).

DISTAL ILEAL RESECTION, DISEASE, OR BYPASS. As noted, resection, often required for *Crohn's disease* or *vascular insufficiency, ileal bypass* for *obesity,* or extensive ileal disease causes deficiencies of vitamin B$_{12}$ and bile salts. Malabsorption is also in part due to loss of the reserve capacity of the ileum for absorbing fat, a function which would be carried on if proximal fat absorption were impaired by deficiency of bile salts.

Vitamin B$_{12}$ should be replaced parenterally, as in pernicious anemia. If the megaloblastic anemia that appears does not respond entirely to vitamin B$_{12}$, folic acid should be added to the regimen (Table 5).

Treatment with cholestyramine, a bile salt–binding resin, is indicated and will often ameliorate the diarrhea caused by the effect of unabsorbed bile acids upon the colon. However, it may increase steatorrhea by further diminishing the bile acid pool. No replacement therapy for the bile acid deficiency is currently available clinically. Steatorrhea will be reduced, however, by feeding medium-chain triglycerides in place of dietary lipid (Table 5). Studies of the effect of potent pancreatic extracts and/or antimicrobials (broad-spectrum) are not available.

RADIATION ENTERITIS. A few patients who receive high dosage x-ray therapy to the abdomen will develop a malabsorption syndrome on the basis of radiation injury to the bowel. It is difficult to assess how much of the defect in absorption is attributable to the arterial damage, mucosal inflammation, or atrophy. Since the reaction to injury is slow, symptoms do not appear for weeks to months after exposure. In the usual patient, villous damage, mucosal and submucosal edema, and cellular infiltration are the main features and repair follows. However, larger doses cause ulceration of the mucosa and endarteritis of submucosal vessels with transmural necrosis, followed by scarring with strictures and permanent loss of function. Thus malabsorption is principally due to disease of the small bowel wall; however, in some instances stasis caused by obstruction (*bacterial overgrowth*) contributes, and in others *lymphatic obstruction* (and perhaps ileal dysfunction) may contribute. Fibrosis and stricture are occasional sequelae of severe reaction, causing obstruction, usually chronic. Jejunal biopsy may reveal patchy villous atrophy.

Category 6: Unexplained

HYPOGAMMAGLOBULINEMIA. The role of intraluminal immunoglobulins, particularly IgA, in maintaining the structure and function of the intestinal tract is not known, because their antibacterial activity as antibodies is minimal. Patients with hypogammaglobulinemia may, however, have steatorrhea and diminished d-xylose absorption, but the precise incidence is not known. Although the number of cases so documented is small, it is steadily growing. Evidence at hand indicates that most (if not all) of these patients have a deficiency of both plasma IgA and IgG and of intestinal IgA. Some patients have only plasma IgA ("selective") deficiency. IgM may be increased in serum and intestine in patients with selective IgA deficiency. The intestinal histology in diffuse hypogammaglobulinemia reveals normal histology or patchy villous atrophy, but *plasma cells are absent* and lymphocytes are reduced in all cases. Occasionally, it shows so-called "nodular lymphoid hyperplasia," and rarely it causes a granulomatous lesion. A high percentage of these patients

with malabsorption will have *Giardia lamblia* infestation of their intestinal fluid, and in some the organism invades the mucosa. This infection is often associated with either villous atrophy or nodular lymphoid hyperplasia and appears to be present in a high percentage of these patients with steatorrhea. Although anaerobic bacteria may be present in the upper small bowel, their role in the pathogenesis of the steatorrhea is not proved. Other abnormalities include splenomegaly and gastric atrophy.

Treatment. Of those with villous atrophy, a rare patient will have a good to excellent response to the gluten-free diet. Antimicrobial drugs and injections of gamma globulin appear to be ineffective. The key to successful management appears to be eradication of giardiasis with atabrine or metronidazole (Table 5). Symptoms remit, absorption improves (including d-xylose), and villi regenerate. As noted above, patients with *celiac disease* have normal or elevated serum IgA, depressed IgM (one third), and normal IgG levels and have reduced IgA plasma cells and increased IgG and IgM plasma cells in the lamina propria.

METASTATIC MALIGNANT CARCINOID SYNDROME. The presenting symptoms of this disease may be those of malabsorption. Steatorrhea may be caused by an increased production of 5-hydroxytryptamine (serotonin), which markedly increases gastrointestinal motility and thus impairs absorption. Other explanations for diarrhea and steatorrhea in this disease include lymphatic obstruction of the mesentery of the small bowel by tumor and ileal dysfunction. Treatment is that used for carcinoid syndrome in general. Methysergide (8.0 to 12.0 mg per day, orally) and cyproheptadine (80 mg per day in divided doses) have been reported to decrease diarrhea in this disease. Small doses of tincture of opium, however, seem most effective for the diarrhea. Parachlorphenylalanine, which inhibits hydroxylation of tryptophan to 5-HTP, has been effective in controlling diarrhea; however, side effects may preclude its general use. (See Ch. 551.)

HYPOPARATHYROIDISM AND PSEUDOHYPOPARATHYROIDISM. Steatorrhea and deficient parathyroid function are associated. The mechanism by which parathormone is involved in fat absorption or transport is unknown. Symptoms of malabsorption may be the earliest manifestation of deficient parathyroid function. With vitamin D$_2$ therapy, diarrhea decreases, steatorrhea disappears, serum carotene and albumin levels rise, vitamin B$_{12}$ absorption increases, and the roentgenographic appearance of the small bowel becomes normal. Diagnosis of hypoparathyroidism as a basis for malabsorption may be established by measuring parathormone levels or by changes in urinary phosphate excretion after intravenous infusions of parathormone or calcium (see Ch. 552.3). Mild malabsorption (fecal fat about 10 grams per 24 hours) has been reported in pseudohypoparathyroidism. Parathormone in some way facilitates the effect of vitamin D upon calcium absorption by the intestinal tract. In pseudohypoparathyroidism the end organs, including the gut, are not responsive to parathormone. The effect of hypocalcemia per se upon intestinal absorption is not known.

Treatment. Administration of vitamin D and calcium will correct hypocalcemia and improve fat absorption as well as other manifestations of disease.

DIABETES MELLITUS. Patients with longstanding diabetes mellitus may have severe diarrhea (see Ch. 399). Some with diarrhea will also have steatorrhea and malabsorption, and these patients are usually not well controlled by dietotherapy or insulin, or both, and a high percentage also have some evidence of neuropathy. In these patients, the intestinal difficulty may be due to involvement of the autonomic innervation of the small bowel, because they also have orthostatic hypotension, inability to perspire, and impotence. Changes in the microbial flora or mesenteric vascular insufficiency may also contribute to the malabsorptive state. An occasional response to broad-spectrum antimicrobials supports the former hypothesis; however, careful bacteriologic studies of intestinal contents in a group of patients with diabetic neuropathy and diarrhea reveal that bacterial overgrowth is a rare cause for the steatorrhea of diabetic neuropathy. Although exocrine function is usually normal in diabetes, some patients have *pancreatic insufficiency*, for which replacement therapy should also be given (Table 5) (see Ch. 410.3). An increased incidence of *adult celiac disease* has also been reported in diabetics.

MASTOCYTOSIS. Patients with overproduction of mast cells suffer not only from urticaria pigmentosa, but also from gastrointestinal symptoms. Perhaps the latter result from overproduction of histamine and perhaps of serotonin as well. Malabsorption is rare in these individuals. The lamina propria of the jejunal mucosa may or may not be infiltrated with mast cells; villi may be absent or stunted. Whether fat absorption is also impaired because of gastric hypersecretion or increased intestinal transit has not been determined.

HYPERTHYROIDISM AND HYPOADRENOCORTICISM. Some patients with hyperthyroidism have steatorrhea. The pathogenesis is not understood. Steatorrhea is due in part to excessive intake of fat in the diet (more than 120 grams per day). Successful therapy returns fat absorption to normal. Likewise, steatorrhea has been found in patients with Addison's disease in whom replacement therapy has corrected it.

TABLE 7. Classification and Therapy of Diseases Associated with Enteric Loss of Plasma Protein

Disease	Therapy
A. Mucosal ulceration:	
Gastric carcinoma	
Gastric lymphoma	
Multiple gastric ulcers	Surgical resection
Colon cancer	
Granulomatous enteritis	
Diffuse nongranulomatous ileojejunitis	Corticosteroids
B. Mucosal disease without ulceration:	
Rugal hypertrophy	Resection, if local
(Menetrier's, etc.)	Gluten elimination
Celiac disease	Antimicrobials; folic acid
Tropical sprue	Antimicrobials
Whipple's disease	Elimination diet; steroids
Allergic gastroenteropathy	Antimicrobial drugs
Bacterial or parasitic enteritis	
Gastrocolic fistula	Resection
C. Lymphatic abnormalities:	
Capillaria philippensis	Thiabendazole
Primary lymphangiectasias	Low-fat diet or medium-chain triglycerides
Lymphenteric fistula	Resection
Lymphoma	Chemotherapy
Constrictive pericarditis	Pericardiectomy
Tricuspid valvular disease	Rx of heart failure

Category 7: Drug-Induced Malabsorption

Some commonly used drugs may cause malabsorption. *Cholestyramine*, in doses of 12.0 or more grams per day, by binding bile salts renders them inactive in the process of fat solubilization and causes mild steatorrhea (7.0 to 15.0 grams of fat per day). *Colchicine* ingestion leads to mild malabsorption of fat (about 9.0 grams of fat per day), protein, and d-xylose by affecting epithelial cell replication and function. Certain *irritant laxatives*, presumably by markedly increasing transit, likewise may cause mild steatorrhea. *Neomycin*, frequently administered to patients with severe hepatic disease, causes steatorrhea, increased fecal loss of nitrogen, and impaired d-xylose absorption. The degree of malabsorption is dose related and may be noted with as little as 4.0 grams per day. It causes some blunting of villi and of their absorptive cells, reduces hydrolysis of fat, and precipitates bile salts. *Bacitracin, tetracycline, polymyxin,* and *kanamycin* may also cause malabsorption. Large doses (twice normal) of *p-aminosalicylic acid* lead to mild steatorrhea and decrease in absorption of d-xylose. *Phenindione*, an anticoagulant, may also cause steatorrhea. Anticonvulsants such as *diphenylhydantoin* in some way cause folic acid deficiency, as do *oral contraceptive* agents.

MALABSORPTION SYNDROME AND ENTERIC LOSS OF PROTEIN
(Protein-Losing Enteropathy)

Hypoalbuminemia without liver disease, inadequate protein intake, or albuminuria may be due to excessive loss of serum protein into the intestine. This loss has been noted in patients with mucosal ulceration of the stomach, small bowel, or colon; with mucosal disease without ulceration; or in lymphatic obstruction (Table 7). Intestinal lymphatic dilatation without obvious cause (lymphangiectasia, Fig. 8) is associated with abnormal enteric protein loss in some patients whose illness was previously termed "hypercatabolic hypoproteinemia." Many of these patients, regardless of the cause for plasma protein leakage, have some degree of malabsorption.

Edema or ascites, or both, secondary to hypoalbuminemia may overshadow enteric symptoms and, indeed, underlie presenting symptoms in patients with so-called *protein-losing enteropathy*. Most of these patients have specific diseases of the intestine. Thus the syndrome has been reported with gastric diseases such as *giant hypertrophic rugae* (Ménétrier's disease), *giant gastric ulcer, gastric cancer,* and *eosinophilic granuloma of the stomach.* A variety of inflammatory diseases of the small and large intestines are also associated with this syndrome: *Crohn's disease of the small intestine and colon; nongranulomatous ileojejunitis; acute infectious enteritis; ulcerative colitis; celiac disease, tropical sprue, lymphoma* of the small intestine, and *Whipple's disease;* and *lymphangiectasia* secondary to known causes such as *lymphoma* or *tuberculosis* or *Crohn's disease.*

Allergy to milk protein and, in rare cases, to cereals or even meat may underlie *protein-losing enteropathy* by affecting the small intestine. Biopsy is normal or shows mild infiltration of the lamina propria with eosinophils; the disorder usually begins in childhood; it is characterized by hypoproteinemia and edema; an iron deficiency anemia is common, as is diarrhea; eosinophilia

Figure 8. Jejunal biopsy demonstrating dilated lacteals of lymphangiectasia associated with protein-losing enteropathy.

is a prominent feature. This condition may well be a milder form of *eosinophilic gastroenteritis* in which both protein-losing enteropathy and malabsorption may be more serious (see above). Infestation with a roundworm, *Capillaria philippensis,* has been described in the Philippines; it causes diarrhea, protein-losing enteropathy, and malabsorption, and proves fatal in two to four months unless vigorously treated (Table 7) (see Ch. 213.2).

CLINICAL PICTURE. As noted, the clinical picture may be dominated by signs and symptoms of hypoproteinemia. In most instances, the patient complains of some abdominal symptoms related to the underlying disease.

DIAGNOSIS. The diagnosis of protein-losing enteropathy should be suspected in any patient with low serum albumin who has normal liver function and does not have an abnormal amount of protein in the urine. The abnormal loss may be confirmed by abnormal fecal excretion of ^{51}Cr after intravenous injection of ^{51}Cr albumin or by a rapid decay curve after intravenous ^{51}Cr chloride or ^{131}I-albumin.

TREATMENT (Table 7). Since therapy may be very successful, accurate diagnosis is extremely important. Resection of localized granuloma or ulcers of the stomach and bowel, or of localized giant gastric rugae, may lead to complete cessation of enteric protein loss. Patients with adult celiac disease and those with allergic gastroenteropathy who are sensitive to milk protein or other substances will respond to elimination of gluten or milk or other offending agents from the diet. Patients with intestinal lymphangiectasia of congenital origin respond to reduction of dietary fat to very low levels — 5 grams or less — or to administration of medium-chain triglycerides in place of dietary fat. These regimens will usually reverse the abnormal protein loss in this disease, and may lessen it in any disease that obstructs lymphatics. Protein loss resulting from *acute nongranulomatous ileojejunitis,* as well as *Crohn's disease* and *ulcerative colitis,* may disappear during therapy with corticosteroids, or, in the case of *viral enteritides,* with spontaneous recovery from the infection. *Acute bacterial enteritis* caused by *Shigella* or *Salmonella, Whipple's disease, enteric tuberculosis,* and instances of excessive protein loss associated with bacterial overgrowth in the small intestine ("blind loop

syndrome") all may respond to appropriate antimicrobial therapy. *Capillaria philippensis* is said to respond to thiabendazole, 25 mg per kilogram per day for 30 days (see Ch. 213.2). A similar effect has likewise been reported in enteric lymphoma after x-radiation and treatment with chlorambucil (Table 7).

Protein-losing enteropathy may be associated with *chronic constrictive pericarditis,* presumably caused by mediastinal lymphatic obstruction. Pericardiolysis or parietal pericardiectomy will alleviate or even completely reverse this enteric loss. Also, effective treatment of severe *right heart failure,* particularly that associated with tricuspid insufficiency, may alleviate protein-losing enteropathy.

PROGNOSIS OF MALABSORPTION SYNDROME

The outlook for the patient with malabsorption syndrome depends upon both the nature of the underlying disease and the institution of appropriate therapy. (Proper treatment, of course, implies correct diagnosis.)

Specific threapy for patients with adult celiac disease (gluten-free diet) and effective antimicrobial agents for tropical sprue are available. Intelligent replacement therapy for those with deficient digestion (*gastrectomy, hepatobiliary disease, pancreatic insufficiency, massive resection* of the small intestine, or *ileectomy*) often alleviates the major symptoms (Table 5).

Whipple's disease now appears entirely manageable, and perhaps even reversible, with the use of broad-spectrum antimicrobial agents and adrenal steroids. The malabsorption of diffuse *nongranulomatous ileojejunitis,* involving large segments of the small intestine, may be completely abolished by administration of adrenal steroids or corticotropin. Likewise, isoniazid, streptomycin, and ethambutol or rifampin may be effective in *tuberculosis enteritis.* Elimination of an offender in the diet and use of corticosteroids are an effective combination against *eosinophilic gastroenteritis.*

The correction of conditions in which intestinal anaerobic microbes play an important role may be accomplished by appropriate surgery, such as resection of fistulas or strictures, or by administration of broad-spectrum antimicrobial drugs. In either case, a normal or nearly normal state of health may be achieved.

The prognosis for patients with malabsorption associated with endocrine disorders is good. The patient with intestinal *scleroderma* or with *diabetes mellitus* who has neuropathy and bacterial overgrowth may be helped by the intermittent administration of antimicrobial drugs. Vitamin D and calcium will restore absorption toward normal in cases of *hypoparathyroidism.* Appropriate management of *hyperthyroidism* will reverse abnormal fat absorption, as will replacement therapy for *Addison's disease.* Specific treatment for *Giardia lamblia* will likely cure the malabsorption of the patient with *hypogammaglobulinemia.*

Because of the nature of the underlying disease, the outlook is not hopeful for a number of patients with malabsorption syndrome. These are the patients with advancing *biliary cirrhosis;* complicated *relapsing pancreatitis;* extensive *Crohn's disease* associated with recurrent fistulas, strictures, and mutilative surgery; progressive *scleroderma* of the intestine; *lymphoma* of the small bowel and mesenteric lymph nodes; and progressive *occlusive disease* of the *superior mesenteric artery*. Prognosis for those who have undergone *massive resection* of the small intestine — at once or in stages — is now vastly improved, however, because of intravenous hyperalimentation programs, improved feeding regimens of foods containing protein hydrolysates, and more potent antimicrobial drugs to treat infection. Therapy for *protein-losing enteropathy* is remarkably good if the correct diagnosis is made (Table 7).

On the whole, the prognosis for the malabsorption syndrome is optimistic, provided that the specific abnormality is identified and appropriate corrective measures are instituted.

Losowsky, M. S., Walker, B. E., and Kelleher, J.: Malabsorption in Clinical Practice. Edinburgh and London, Churchill, Livingstone, 1974.

Perera, D. E., Weinstein, W. M., and Rubin, C. E.: Small intestinal biopsy. Hum. Path., 6:157, 1975.

Sleisenger, M. H., and Brandborg, L. L.: Malabsorption. Philadelphia, W. B. Saunders Company, 1977.

Sleisenger, M. H., and Fordtran, J. S. (eds.): Gastrointestinal Disease. 2nd ed. Philadelphia, W. B. Saunders Company, 1978, Chapters 4–5, 12–16, 60–75, 92, 108.

Section Six DISEASES OF THE PANCREAS

Frank P. Brooks

409. INTRODUCTION

The principal diseases of the exocrine pancreas are inflammatory (pancreatitis), neoplastic (carcinoma) or degenerative, secondary to an abnormal secretion (cystic fibrosis), in origin. The etiology of pancreatitis and carcinoma of the pancreas is unknown; yet if chronic alcoholism could be reduced, there would probably be a substantial fall in the number of patients with pancreatitis. Cystic fibrosis is a heritable disease seen in homozygotes. Advances in supportive therapy have changed the age distribution from almost exclusively a disease of infancy and childhood to one that includes an increasing number of adults.

410. PANCREATITIS

410.1. INTRODUCTION

Histologic evidence of inflammation of pancreatic exocrine tissue in the form of focal collections of inflammatory cells is a rather common finding at autopsy and is without clinical significance. Acute diffuse inflammation associated with necrosis, hemorrhage, and/or edema is usually accompanied by the clinical syndrome of acute pancreatitis but may be found unexpectedly at autopsy in patients with other diseases such as acute hepatic failure. Chronic inflammation of the exocrine pancreas is characterized by fibrosis, atrophy of the acinar tissue, and cystic dilatation of the ducts. Loss of exocrine function leads to maldigestion with resulting malabsorption, particularly of fat, with steatorrhea.

The clinical course of pancreatitis falls into five general categories; acute pancreatitis occurring as an isolated episode, recurrent attacks of acute pancreatitis with apparent complete recovery between episodes (acute recurrent pancreatitis), acute pancreatitis followed by the development of chronic pancreatitis, chronic pancreatitis without recognized episodes of acute pancreatitis, and chronic pancreatitis with superimposed episodes of acute pancreatitis (chronic relapsing pancreatitis). Figure 1 is a diagrammatic representation of these syndromes. The great reserve capacity of the pancreas makes it impossible to determine clinically that the pancreas is histologically normal between attacks, and the lack of specific sensitive indicators of acute pancreatitis probably results in overlooking mild episodes of acute pancreatitis. Nevertheless, the Marseilles Classification points out important characteristics of the natural history of pancreatitis which should be considered in evaluating the results of treatment.

410.2. ACUTE PANCREATITIS

DEFINITION. Acute pancreatitis is characterized by acute onset of epigastric pain in the absence of physical signs of peritonitis together with evidence of systemic disease such as fever, malaise, hypotension, nausea,

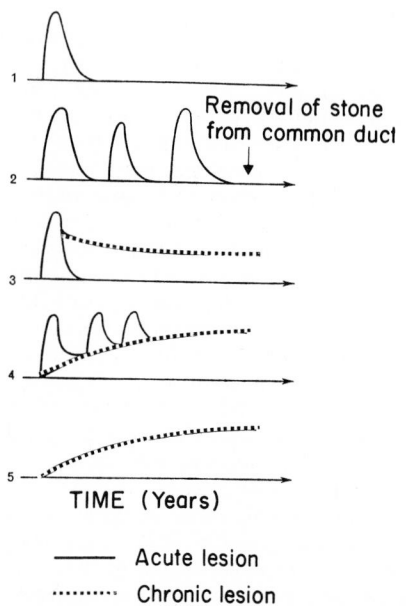

Figure 1. Diagrammatic representation of the clinical course of pancreatitis in relation to the inflammatory lesion in the pancreas. (Modified from Benhamou, J. P. and Sarles, H.: Foie Pancreas Voies Biliaires. Paris, Flammarion Médecine, 1972, p. 121.)

TABLE 1.   Etiologic Factors in Acute Pancreatitis

1. Mechanical factors
   a. Gallstones and diseases of the biliary tract
   b. Tumors of the pancreas and ampulla of Vater: duodenal diverticula
   c. Duodenal obstruction: postgastrectomy, Crohn's disease
   d. Endoscopic retrograde cholangiopancreatography
2. Tissue injury
   a. Infections and infestations: viruses, bacteria, parasites
   b. Toxins: ethyl alcohol, methyl alcohol, scorpion venom
   c. Medications: glucocorticoids, oral contraceptives, thiazide
      diuretics, azathioprine, acetaminophen
3. Circulatory factors: atheromatous embolism, periarteritis nodosa,
   lupus erythematosus, atherosclerosis, shock
4. Endocrine factors: hyperparathyroidism, pregnancy
5. Metabolic factors: hyperlipidemia, hereditary pancreatitis
6. Immunologic factors: hypersensitivity, post–kidney transplantation
7. Trauma: postoperative, abdominal trauma
8. Idiopathic

and vomiting. The pathology is a spectrum from edema to hemorrhagic necrosis with dissolution of most of the gland. The gross findings at laparotomy, when characteristic, are the most reliable criteria for the diagnosis, but mild forms of the disease can be overlooked easily. There is no specific laboratory diagnosis.

ETIOLOGY. In most patients with acute pancreatitis, the etiology is unknown. However, in the majority, factors known to be associated with acute pancreatitis will be present (Table 1). In about 25 per cent of patients, no recognizable factors can be identified. Physicians with experience in inner city or veterans hospitals find that the great majority of patients with acute pancreatitis abuse alcohol, but this is not the case in some other populations. Multiple acute attacks are the rule in "alcoholic pancreatitis," and it is impossible to exclude continuing chronic pancreatitis between attacks.

Disease of the biliary tract is present in about half the patients with acute pancreatitis, although there is evidence that this may be decreasing in contemporary practice. Of these, about 90 per cent have stones in the gallbladder or common bile duct. The remainder have stenoses of the ampulla of Vater or noncalculous cholecystitis. The mechanism by which gallstones precipitate acute pancreatitis is uncertain, but gallstones were recovered in the stools within ten days of the onset of the attack of acute pancreatitis in about 90 per cent of patients with gallstones and acute pancreatitis. This suggests that partial obstruction in the biliary and pancreatic duct may have occurred, although the common channel theory does not appear applicable to many patients. It is not uncommon to find gallstones and alcohol abuse both present in older patients, but alcoholic pancreatitis usually occurs at a younger age.

About 3 per cent of patients with carcinoma of the pancreas or ampulla will have an attack of acute pancreatitis. Periampullary duodenal diverticula are sometimes responsible for acute pancreatitis. Obstruction of the duodenum either following gastric resection or in patients with Crohn's disease of the duodenum may cause acute pancreatitis. Endoscopic retrograde cholangiopancreatography, if carried out with sufficient pressure, will cause pancreatitis.

Viral infections, including group B coxsackievirus, can be expected to be significant etiologic factors in about 5 to 10 per cent of patients with acute pancreatitis, as documented by rises in agglutination titers. About 10 per cent of patients dying with acute hepatic failure have acute pancreatitis. In mumps about 15 per cent of patients probably have mild pancreatitis. Bacterial pancreatitis is unusual. Parasitic infestations such as *Ascaris* and *Echinococcus* may be important causes of acute pancreatitis in some parts of the world.

In large urban centers in the United States and in South Africa, the majority of acute attacks of pancreatitis appear to be alcohol related. No satisfactory animal model for acute pancreatitis has been produced with alcohol alone. Alcohol given acutely inhibits pancreatic secretion but may have an excitatory effect in chronic alcohol abusers. By contrast, methyl alcohol poisoning is associated with acute pancreatitis in a high percentage of patients. Scorpion bites may cause pancreatitis. The venom is a stimulant to pancreatic secretion in animals.

The importance of medications in causing acute pancreatitis is difficult to evaluate, so much of the evidence is based upon temporal relationships in small numbers of patients. However, in the interest of protecting patients from a second exposure, information should be sought in the history regarding the use of glucocorticoids, oral contraceptives, thiazide diuretics, furosemide, azathioprine, and acetaminophen. The acute pancreatitis that occurs in about 5 to 6 per cent of patients receiving a kidney transplantation may be related to corticosteroids or azathioprine.

Circulatory factors in acute pancreatitis may be very important, especially in elderly patients when shock is superimposed upon severe atherosclerosis. Atheromatous embolism is an unusual cause of acute pancreatitis. Pancreatitis occurs rarely in patients with periarteritis nodosa and lupus erythematosus.

Endocrine factors are significant in a small number of patients with acute pancreatitis. About 6 per cent of patients with pancreatitis can be shown to have hyperparathyroidism. It usually takes the form of recurrent acute pancreatitis and may be the first presenting evidence of the hyperparathyroidism. The relationship of acute pancreatitis to diabetes mellitus is uncertain, but it is important to recognize that patients may have both diabetic ketoacidosis or nonketotic hyperosmolar coma and acute pancreatitis. Acute pancreatitis is an unusual complication of pregnancy, usually in the last trimester.

Hyperlipidemia may be both a consequence of alcoholic pancreatitis and a factor in the etiology of acute pancreatitis in nonalcoholic patients with hyperlipidemia of Types I, IV, and V. Most convincing are reports in which patients have had no further episodes of pancreatitis when placed on low fat diets. Hereditary pancreatitis occurs in families, most often at an early age. An associated aminoaciduria may or may not be present. Acute pancreatitis as a manifestation of hypersensitivity is very rare, but, as noted, immunosuppression in patients with renal transplants or fulminant hepatitis may play a role. Antibodies to pancreatic tissue may be found in the blood during acute pancreatitis, but they are probably secondary to the disease.

Traumatic pancreatitis is secondary to abdominal surgery or to abdominal trauma, most often from an automobile steering wheel. This accounts for about 5 per cent of patients with acute pancreatitis, and may be increasing. Operations on the biliary tree and stomach are the most common surgical procedures, but only about 1 per cent of patients develop clinical acute pancreatitis postoperatively.

INCIDENCE AND EPIDEMIOLOGY. Considering the uncertainties of the clinical diagnosis of acute pancreatitis,

Figure 2. The exocrine-endocrine partition of enzyme secretion under physiologic conditions (left) and when the isthmus of the acinus is blocked by secretions (right). (From Wanke, M.: Experimental acute pancreatitis. Curr. Topics Pathol., 52:72, 1970.)

perhaps the best evidence of the incidence of pancreatitis is the death rate. This is 1.3 per 1000 of population, which is about equivalent to the death rate from acute appendicitis. In Rochester, Minnesota, over the decades from 1940 to 1960, 151 patients with a clinical diagnosis of pancreatitis were identified. Acute pancreatitis exceeded chronic pancreatitis in the ratio of 3:1. Biliary tract disease was an etiologic factor in 37 per cent and alcohol abuse in 19 per cent. By contrast, in Göteborg, Sweden, by the early 1970's alcohol had replaced biliary tract disease as the major etiologic factor in patients dying with acute pancreatitis. There was no difference between binge drinkers and steady consumers of alcohol. In Sweden also the incidence of alcohol abuse was 70 per cent in a group of patients with acute pancreatitis compared to 22 per cent in a control population. At the Manchester Royal Infirmary, acute pancreatitis accounted for about half the admissions for pancreatitis. Of these, half were admitted with their first attack of pancreatitis with an average age of 56 years, whereas of those with more than one attack the average age was 48 years.

PATHOPHYSIOLOGY. The dominant theory of the mechanism of acute pancreatitis is that active proteolytic enzymes gain access to the pancreatic tissue, leading to autodigestion of the pancreas. The normal directions of transport of pancreatic enzymes and the hypothesis of events in acute pancreatitis are shown in Figure 2. There is a normal endocrine-exocrine secretion of enzymes by the pancreatic acinar cells documented by levels of amylase, lipase, and trypsin in plasma as well as pancreatic juice. Under normal circumstances, proteolytic enzymes, including phospholipase A in pancreatic juice, are present as inactive precursors. In addition, protein inhibitors of the proteolytic enzymes are present. On entrance into the duodenum, the brush border enzyme enterokinase converts trypsinogen to trypsin. Trypsin in turn catalyzes the further conversion of trypsinogen to trypsin as well as the activation of proelastase and phospholipase A. In experimental models these two enzymes seem to duplicate the necrosis of blood vessels and the destruction of cell membranes seen in acute pancreatitis. Activation of trypsin has been noted in pancreatic juice collected from the

pancreatic ducts associated with attacks of pancreatitis. The mechanism by which activation of enzymes occurs is unknown. Reflux of bile, pancreatic proteolytic enzymes, and bacteria at sufficiently high pressures into the pancreatic duct will cause pancreatitis experimentally, as will enterokinase injected into the duct. Increases in permeability of the ductal mucosa will initiate experimental pancreatitis. Figure 2 suggests that obstruction in the ducts has a similar effect.

Increased permeability of the blood vessels leads to losses of plasma to the intercellular fluid space of up to 2 liters per day. The blood volume can be reduced by a third, and this can result in clinical signs of shock. Collections of blood, digested tissue, and pancreatic secretion may burrow along tissue spaces into the gastrohepatic ligament and retroperitoneally into the lesser peritoneal sac and flank. Peritoneal effusions occur, and there may be varying degrees of paralytic ileus. In the most severe forms secondary infection may lead to the production of pancreatic abscesses and septicemia. In milder forms the disease does not progress beyond the stage of pancreatic edema, and resolution may occur within two weeks.

CLINICAL MANIFESTATIONS. In acute pancreatitis, the clinical syndrome may vary from mild abdominal pain to circulatory collapse. Pain is present in 90 per cent of patients. Typically, the onset is acute, sometimes within a few hours of a large meal or at the end of a drinking bout. It is most commonly felt in the epigastrium (60 per cent) but may occur in other parts of the abdomen. In about half the patients, there is radiation of the pain to the back. In a third of the patients, the pain is diffuse and may not be possible to localize. It is usually constant rather than intermittent. The pain can be among the most severe encountered in medical practice, or it may be relatively mild, depending upon severity of the disease. Lying in one position, particularly supine, seems to make the patient more uncomfortable, so that frequent shifts in position are common. Flexing the trunk may give some relief. Patients usually require opiates rather than salicylates or codeine for relief. There may be a moderate elevation in temperature. In from 10 to 70 per cent of patients hypotension or shock is present, depending upon the severity of the disease. Tachycardia is usual. Tenderness is common, but localized muscle spasm is unusual. In about half the patients the abdomen will be distended, with diminished to absent bowel sounds. Signs of pleural effusion, especially on the left side, may be detected in about 10 per cent of patients. An abdominal mass is found in about 20 per cent of patients, and this can be expected to disappear slowly about half the time. Pancreatic pseudocysts are detected by ultrasound examination in 10 to 20 per cent of patients, and pancreatic abscesses occur in about 5 per cent of patients. Other complications include acute renal failure in 5 per cent, respiratory failure in 5 to 10 per cent (including a peculiar form of acute pulmonary edema resulting from increased capillary permeability), jaundice caused by compression of the common bile duct or associated liver disease in 10 per cent, hematemesis caused by a variety of lesions in 3 per cent, mental confusion to mania in 8 per cent, and diabetic coma in 1 per cent.

Uncommon events are tetany caused by hypocalcemia, cutaneous lesions resembling erythema nodosum but caused by fat necrosis, and polyarthritis. The course of the disease is variable. The over-all mortality

TABLE 2. Serum Amylase, Urinary Amylase and C.A./C.C. Ratio Data of 177 Patients with Acute Pancreatitis*

	Number	Serum Amylase (mg %)	Urinary Amylase (mg %)	C.A./C.C. (%)
Acute pancreatitis	177			
Mean		852	2491	14.5†
S.D.		200	683	6.5
Calculated range		452–1252	1128–3854	1.5–27.5
Observed range		216–4150	620–12,000	0.8–71.8
Proposed upper limit normal range		200	1200	4.0

*From Dreiling, D. A., et al.: Am. J. Gastroenterol., *61*:290, 1974.
†Statistically significant at 1 per cent level.

is around 10 per cent. Patients who die succumb during the first week in shock, or later from complications. In mild forms the pain may subside in two to three days with rapid improvement in the patient's general condition. As a general rule, acute pancreatitis associated with biliary tract disease is more severe and carries a higher mortality. Alcoholic pancreatitis presents with recurrent acute episodes of a less severe nature.

LABORATORY STUDIES. The most important test currently available is determination of blood amylase. Most laboratories report results in terms of reducing sugars (Somogyi units) or dye units. An elevation of serum amylase to over 1000 units per 100 ml usually means acute pancreatitis and more likely the form associated with biliary tract disease. Unfortunately, most acute alcoholic pancreatitis is associated with values in the range of 250 to 500 units per 100 ml, which is the same range for many other acute abdominal diseases such as perforated peptic ulcer, perforated gallbladder, or ruptured tubal pregnancy. There is no correlation with the severity of the disease; indeed, fatal acute pancreatitis can occur in the face of normal values. Two major sources of difficulty are the rapid clearing of amylase from the blood and the fact that the usual technique determines a variety of isoamylases of which the major one in normal serum is derived from the salivary glands. Pending development of reliable rapid clinical methods for measuring pancreatic isoamylase, additional help can be obtained by measuring amylase in the urine. Probably at present, the most sensitive and specific test is the amylase-creatinine clearance ratio. Table 2 shows a comparison of serum and urine amylases and the ratio of amylase to creatinine clearance. The calculation for the latter is shown at the bottom of this page.

In acute pancreatitis, for unknown reasons the renal tubular reabsorption of amylase is significantly reduced. Elevations of the clearance ratio, although not completely specific, offer the best means of distinguishing hyperamylasemias unrelated to acute pancreatitis. Some patients have an elevated macroamylase detectable by electrophoretic techniques in the serum and by high serum amylase but normal urine amylase. Elevations of the serum lipase are confirmative. An amylase of 300 units in a sample of peritoneal or pleural fluid is usually diagnostic, if above the serum level. The blood leukocyte count is moderately elevated, between 10,000 and 30,000 per cubic millimeter. Hypocalcemia occurs

in 10 to 30 per cent of patients, but the level of calcium should be considered in relation to the serum albumin level. Presumably the calcium enters bone and is precipitated as calcium soaps, but the mechanism is controversial. Serum calcium values below 7 mg per 100 ml indicate a poor prognosis. Hypomagnesemia and hypokalemia may occur, and metabolic acidosis is seen in severely ill patients. Elevations of blood alkaline phosphatase occur particularly in gallstone pancreatitis (in which a transient rise to over ten times normal values can be seen), and modest elevations in the serum transaminases are frequent. Hyperglycemia occurs in about half the patients with acute pancreatitis, with glycosuria in about 25 per cent. Hyperglycemia persists in only 1 to 5 per cent. Hyperlipidemia is present in about 10 per cent of patients with acute pancreatitis, and tends to disappear as the disease subsides. Electrocardiographic changes may occasionally be worrisome in differentiating acute myocardial infarction. A positive test for methemalbumin in the serum is not specific for acute hemorrhagic pancreatitis. X-ray examinations may be helpful in the diagnosis of other intra-abdominal diseases such as a perforated viscus, but the sentinel loop and colon cutoff signs are relatively uncommon. Ultrasound is useful in the diagnosis of pancreatic pseudocyst and other pancreatic masses. Pancreatic stimulation with secretin, provocative serum amylase, and endoscopic retrograde cholangiopancreatography should not be done in acute pancreatitis.

DIAGNOSIS. The cornerstone in the diagnosis of acute pancreatitis is the combination of abdominal pain and elevated amylase. If gallstone disease, alcoholism, or other known etiologic factors are present, the diagnosis should be considered with particular care. Elevated amylase levels in peritoneal fluid or a pleural effusion may be helpful. Occasionally laparotomy will be necessary because of the uncertainty of ruling out intra-abdominal disease for which surgery would be lifesaving. The major errors in diagnosis come from failing to consider that acute pancreatitis may accompany other diseases such as gallstones, excessive reliance on the serum amylase, and failure to consider the diagnosis in patients presenting with alcoholic intoxication, shock, or diabetic coma. The differential diagnosis includes perforated viscus, mesenteric vascular disease, volvulus, ruptured spleen, acute appendicitis, acute calculous cholecystitis, small bowel obstruction, dissecting an-

$$\frac{A.C.\%}{C.C.} = \frac{\text{Amylase conc in urine}}{\text{Amylase conc in serum}} \times \frac{\text{Creatinine conc in serum}}{\text{Creatinine conc in urine}} \times 100$$

eurysm, nephrolithiasis, and acute porphyria. An important factor is the rapid changes in the course of acute pancreatitis which requires a vigilant watch on the patient.

TREATMENT. There are few measures of proved value in the treatment of acute pancreatitis. Medical treatment is generally preferred because the disease is either mild and spontaneously subsides or severe with a significant mortality after operation. Nevertheless, if one could identify those patients who will progress to the severe form of the disease with major complications, one might be tempted to engage in at least a controlled trial of laparotomy with drainage and/or peritoneal lavage. A few bold surgeons have performed pancreatectomy but without a controlled trial. Nasogastric suction in moderately severe acute pancreatitis, antibiotics, aprotinin (Trasylol), and glucagon have failed to influence the course of the disease in controlled trials. Nevertheless, most experienced clinicians follow the principle of "resting" the inflamed organ by stopping oral intake; providing intravenous fluids, especially colloids such as albumin, as necessary to maintain an effective blood volume; relieving pain, preferably with meperidine but often with morphine if necessary; and maintaining nasogastric suction. Anticholinergics are not of proved value. If gallstones are present, cholecystectomy should be done when the patient's condition permits. Common duct stone will require surgical removal. If alcohol is a factor, abstinence should be encouraged. Persistent pseudocysts in symptomatic patients should be drained, usually internally into the stomach. Respiratory failure may require positive pressure breathing.

PROGNOSIS. Acute pancreatitis related to gallstones carries a significant mortality but an excellent prognosis of freedom from subsequent attacks if the gallstones can be treated surgically. Alcoholic pancreatitis carries a lower mortality but a discouragingly high incidence of recurrence of acute attacks or progression to chronic pancreatitis. Factors indicating severe disease with a higher mortality are age over 55 years, blood sugar >200 mg per 100 ml, white blood cell count >16,000, lactic dehydrogenase >350, and SGOT >250 units on admission. During the first 48 hours of treatment, a fall in hematocrit of greater than 10 per cent, a serum calcium <8 mg per 100 ml, an anion base deficit >4 mEq per liter, an increase in BUN >5 mg per 100 ml, an arterial P_{O_2} <60 mm Hg, and an estimated fluid sequestration >6 liters indicate severe disease.

PREVENTION. The challenging fact for physicians remains that if the problem of chronic alcoholism could be solved, the prevalence of acute pancreatitis would be cut by at least 50 per cent.

Forell, M. M.: Pankreas. Handbuch der inneren Medizin. Dritter Band, Verdauungsorgane, Teil 6. Berlin, Springer-Verlag, 1976.
Long, W. B., and Brooks, F. P.: Acute pancreatitis. In Brooks, F. P. (ed.): Gastrointestinal Pathophysiology. 2nd ed. New York, Oxford University Press, 1978.
Warshaw, A. L.: Acute pancreatitis. Viewpoints Dig. Dis., Vol. 9, No. 5, November 1977.

410.3.   CHRONIC PANCREATITIS

DEFINITION. Chronic pancreatitis is characterized by the progressive replacement of pancreatic acinar tissue with fibrous tissue, with relative preservation of the islets of Langerhans. This results in a decrease in pan-

creatic exocrine secretion until the luminal phase of digestion becomes inadequate and dietary triglyceride cannot be split to monoglyceride and free fatty acids. The normal absorption of fat can no longer occur and steatorrhea results. The course of the disease may be punctuated by episodes of acute pancreatitis and pain, or the pain may be relatively constant. The end stage of chronic pancreatitis is pancreatic insufficiency when little acinar tissue remains and the number of islets is also reduced.

ETIOLOGY. As in the acute disease, it is rare that a specific cause for chronic pancreatitis can be found. Patients with the syndrome of protein malnutrition known as kwashiorkor develop an atrophy of the pancreas with pancreatic insufficiency but do not experience abdominal pain in acute crises. With treatment pancreatic function returns to normal. Most of the etiologic factors in acute pancreatitis can lead to chronic pancreatitis, but alcohol abuse stands out as an even more prominent factor, especially now that the diagnosis of biliary tract disease as a cause of acute pancreatitis is pursued vigorously and treated. (Gallstone disease is associated more often with recurrent attacks of acute pancreatitis.) Carcinoma of the pancreas may present as pancreatic insufficiency; hyperlipidemia, hyperparathyroidism, and hereditary pancreatitis may present as chronic relapsing pancreatitis. Inadvertent ligation of the pancreatic duct during surgery for ulcer disease is an unusual cause of pancreatic insufficiency.

PATHOPHYSIOLOGY. The acinar tissue is replaced by fibrous tissue, with relative sparing of the islets of Langerhans. Cystic dilatation of the ducts occurs. Calcification of the pancreas occurs at times with stones within the lumens of the ducts. Ligation of the pancreatic duct in animals reduces the absorption of dietary fat by about 50 per cent. This is due to lack of lipase activity in the duodenum and failure of micelle formation, which in turn results in inability to solubilize fat in the aqueous milieu of the small intestine. Unfortunately, the amount of lipase secreted in response to amino

Figure 3. The relationship of lipase outputs to 24-hour fecal fat excretion. Values above horizontal dashed line indicate steatorrhea. The shaded area represents lipase outputs less than 15 per cent of normal. EAA 1D = intraduodenal amino acid infusion. (From DiMagno, E. P., and Go, V. L. W., In Gambill E. E.[ed.]: Pancreatitis. St. Louis, C. V. Mosby Company, 1973, p. 27.)

Figure 4. Posture assumed by patient with pain of chronic pancreatitis. (From Gambill, E. E. [ed.]: Pancreatitis. St. Louis, C. V. Mosby Company, 1973, p. 97.)

acids in the small intestine or exogenous cholecystokinin (CCK) must be reduced to 10 per cent of normal before steatorrhea appears (Fig. 3). Protein digestion is also impaired, and the amount of protein nitrogen in the stool increases. Malabsorption of fat-soluble vitamins results in easy bruising and bleeding from mild trauma. Precipitation of calcium as soaps in the intestine contributes to calcium malabsorption. In some patients (about a third), malabsorption of vitamin B_{12} occurs. Glucose intolerance with insulin-dependent diabetes is a late manifestation of chronic pancreatitis. Chronic administration of alcohol over years to rats and dogs has produced lesions of the pancreas characterized by protein precipitations in the ducts and dilatation of ducts. The protein known as lactoferrin has been found

in association with the precipitates. Chronic alcohol consumption also alters the pancreatic secretory response to the hormones secretin and CCK. Protein concentrations and outputs increase with long-term alcohol consumption in animals.

CLINICAL MANIFESTATIONS. Patients fall into three groups: (1) those who sustain repeated attacks of abdominal pain similar to but usually milder than (2) those who have the acute form with gradual development of pancreatic insufficiency, and (3) those who have a steady progression of pancreatic insufficiency with or without chronic pain. The pain in chronic pancreatitis is usually less severe than in the acute disease. The patient usually continues to eat and notes that the pain is worse after eating. Radiation to the back is more common, and flexing the trunk to obtain relief is characteristic (Fig. 4). Addiction to codeine, meperidine, or morphine is common. With time there is a tendency for the pain to abate, but when present it is usually present for days at a time. Nausea and vomiting are not uncommonly associated. A history of years of alcohol abuse is frequently obtained. As the disease advances, the patient may complain of bulky, foulsmelling stools with oil droplets in the toilet water. The stool is light colored and pasty, but the patient may or may not complain of diarrhea. Physical examination shows evidence of weight loss, but the patient may fall within the limits of normal body weight. During an attack of pain there is usually slight fever and upper abdominal tenderness but not localized muscle spasm. A mass may be felt in the abdomen, representing either an acute inflammatory pancreatic swelling or a pseudocyst. About half of such masses disappear spontaneously. Jaundice may be noted. Hematemesis may occur from varices in the esophagus due to portal hypertension or other sources of upper gastrointestinal bleeding such as gastric erosions. In patients with alcohol-induced calcific pancreatitis in South Africa, the dominant presentation is either pain or symptoms of insufficient pancreatic exocrine or endocrine function. A summary of the presenting symptoms and signs is shown in Figure 5. Calcific pancreatitis is more often related to alcohol than is noncalcific pancreatitis. A comparison of the clinical manifestations in the two groups of patients is shown in Figure 6. Pseudocyst formation, gastrointestinal bleeding, and jaundice occur as in acute pan-

Figure 5. Dominant clinical presentation in 172 patients with alcohol-induced calcific pancreatitis. (From Marks, I. N., and Bank, S., *In* Bockus, H. L. [ed.]: Gastroenterology, Vol. III. 3rd ed. Philadelphia, W. B. Saunders Company, 1976, p. 1054.)

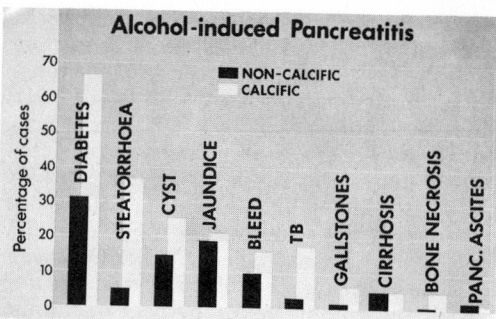

Figure 6. Complications and associated features in calcific and noncalcific alcohol-induced pancreatitis. (From Marks, I. N., and Banks, S., *In* Bockus, H. L. [ed.]: Gastroenterology, Vol. III. 3rd ed. Philadelphia, W. B. Saunders Company, 1976, p. 1060.)

creatitis. The incidence of pulmonary tuberculosis in chronic pancreatitis in the United States is probably substantially less than in these data from South Africa. Bone infarcts are often asymptomatic but spectacular radiographic evidence of calcium deposits during pancreatitis. Pancreatic ascites occurs most often in patients with pseudocysts. The fluid contains high concentrations of pancreatic enzymes.

LABORATORY STUDIES. During acute exacerbations, patients with chronic relapsing pancreatitis may show elevations of serum amylase and lipase as do patients with acute pancreatitis until the progression of damage and chronic disease reduces the pancreatic acinar tissue to a level at which the source of enzyme is no longer sufficient for endocrine secretion. Eventually, serum pancreatic isoenzyme determinations may make a low level of enzyme diagnostic of pancreatic insufficiency, but with present techniques the serum enzymes are of little value in well developed chronic pancreatitis. Determination of pancreatic secretion of bicarbonate after stimulation by secretin is an important method of detecting a reduced pancreatic parenchymal mass in patients who do not have calcification of the pancreas. Gastric content must be separated from duodenal content. The standard dose of secretin is 1 clinical unit per kilogram of body weight. This is submaximal for most patients. In the absence of perfusion with a marker, the volume of duodenal content recovered is quite variable and cannot be corrected for secretion escaping down the intestine. The coefficient of variation is smallest for bicarbonate concentration. Values less than 70 mEq per liter indicate impaired secretory capacity. Unfortunately, this is a relatively insensitive measure and the maximal bicarbonate output is a more sensitive indicator of secretory mass. An output of bicarbonate less than 10 mEq per 20 minutes is indicative of decreased secretory mass. A volume less than 80 ml per 20 minutes indicates obstruction or decreased secretion. Enzyme determinations after secretin stimulation have not proved to be of clinical importance. Cholecystokinin-pancreozymin (CCK-PZ) is not currently available for general use in the United States. Several potentially improved techniques are under study, including direct cannulation of the pancreatic duct by endoscopic retrograde cholangiopancreatography, use of a maximal stimulating dose of secretin, infusions of secretin rather than bolus injections, use of markers to verify the extent of

fluid lost into the small intestine, and determination of enzyme outputs after stimulation with pure forms of CCK-PZ. Determination of the trypsin concentration in duodenal content after a liquid test meal (the Lundh meal) correlates well with the secretin test in established chronic pancreatitis, but its sensitivity in mild forms is still uncertain. Neither procedure can be considered to be reliable in differentiating chronic pancreatitis from carcinoma of the pancreas.

Pancreatic calcification can be seen on survey films of the abdomen in from 25 to 35 per cent of patients with chronic relapsing pancreatitis. Conventional barium meals will show encroachment and displacement of the stomach and duodenum in a minority of patients. Cholangiography may show long tapering structures of the distal common bile duct in its course through the pancreas and duodenum. Endoscopic retrograde cholangiopancreatography is an important procedure in the diagnosis of chronic pancreatitis and of pseudocysts of the pancreas. The characteristic finding in chronic pancreatitis is the "chain of lakes" appearance of the pancreatic duct resulting from alternating strictures and dilatation. However, in about 30 per cent of patients with chronic pancreatitis, the pancreatogram has been normal. Once contrast medium has demonstrated a pseudocyst, the injection should be stopped without filling the cyst, because acute attacks of pancreatitis have followed further contrast injection.

Ultrasound and computerized tomography have made the diagnosis of pseudocyst much easier for both the patient and physician. Different types of pancreatic cysts are shown in Figure 7. The ability of these modalities to detect enlargement of the pancreas and its significance in chronic pancreatitis await further data. Arteriography is considered in Ch. 411.

DIAGNOSIS. Patients with chronic pancreatitis usually present with abdominal pain or with symptoms of

Figure 7. Schematic representation of cysts of the pancreas. *A,* Intrapancreatic retention cysts in calcific pancreatitis. *B,* Intra- and extrapancreatic retention cysts in calcific pancreatitis. *C,* Intrapancreatic pseudocysts with and without communication with the duct of Wirsung after acute pancreatitis. *D,* Extrapancreatic pseudocyst with and without communication with the duct of Wirsung after acute pancreatitis. *E,* Cystadenocarcinoma. *F, Echinococcus* cyst of pancreas. (From Hess, W., *In* Forell, M. M. [ed.]: Handbuch der Inneren Medizin, dritter Band, sechster Teil, funfte Auflage, Pankreas. Berlin, Springer-Verlag, 1976, p. 979.)

malabsorption (see Ch. 408). Those with pain may be labeled as malingerers, drug addicts, or neurotics. The presence of calcification in the pancreas or a subnormal secretory response to exogenous secretin points to the pancreas as a source of the pain. Ultrasound may show enlargement of the pancreas or a pseudocyst. Endoscopic retrograde cholangiopancreatography may be diagnostic. Differentiation from carcinoma of the pancreas on occasion can be made only by cytology or biopsy. Conventional barium meals may show displacement and encroachment on the stomach or duodenum by the inflamed pancreas. Glucose intolerance is present in two thirds of the patients but is not specific. Posterior penetrating duodenal ulcer may produce a localized pancreatitis with pain. Duodenoscopy should show the ulcer.

Patients with malabsorption must be differentiated from those with adult celiac disease and Crohn's disease. In pancreatic insufficiency, the patient rarely loses as much weight as in true malabsorption, although the degree of steatorrhea may be 20 to 30 grams per day. The d-xylose absorption test will be normal, and a small bowel biopsy will exclude celiac disease. Impaired endogenous release of CCK after a Billroth II gastric resection or in celiac disease may complicate the diagnosis unless exogenous stimulation is used.

Occasionally hyperparathyroidism may present as chronic pancreatitis. Traumatic pancreatitis with fistula formation may progress to chronic pancreatitis. Pancreatic pseudocysts shown by ultrasound help in the identification of chronic relapsing pancreatitis.

TREATMENT. The treatment of pancreatic insufficiency is relatively simple and effective, i.e., the use of 20 grams of pancreatic extract with each meal. If this fails to control the foul, bulky stools, it is likely that gastric acid secretion is inactivating the enzymes in the pancreatic extract. Sodium bicarbonate, 2.5 grams, may be added 30 minutes after meals or the histamine-2 antagonist cimetidine may be given as 300 mg one half hour before meals to inhibit acid secretion. Insulin should be used with caution to avoid hypoglycemia, particularly in alcohol abusers.

The major unsolved problem in treatment of chronic pancreatitis is relief of pain. Anticholinergics such as propantheline, 15 mg before meals, may be tried, but there are no controlled studies to document their effectiveness. Antacids may be given in 1-ounce quantities after meals to inhibit secretin release, but again this is without proved value. Nonaddictive analgesics such as acetaminophen or acetylsalicylic acid may give relief initially, but all too often they lead to the use of codeine, meperidine, and morphine. Surgical procedures for the relief of pancreatic pain are also far from satisfactory. Pancreatography should demonstrate the site of strictures and obstruction in the ducts, and a procedure can be chosen to relieve the obstruction, e.g., distal pancreatectomy and anastomosis of the duct to the jejunum, the Puestow procedure of filleting of the pancreas and anastomosis along the length of the duct to the jejunum. In the absence of localized obstruction, there is an increasing tendency to remove large amounts of the pancreas such as a 95 per cent pancreatectomy, leaving only a rim of tissue in the head. None of these surgical procedures have been evaluated in a randomized controlled fashion.

PROGNOSIS. In some patients the pain disappears spontaneously as the fibrosis and atrophy of the pancreas progress. In others it appears to be responsive to a program of pancreatic rest. Abstinence from alcohol, although rarely achieved, is thought by most to be effective, although there are a few dissenting observations. The malabsorptive features of pancreatic insufficiency can be controlled with substitution therapy. Results of surgical procedures for pain are controversial but appear to be better with more radical operations. Drainage of pancreatic pseudocysts into the stomach provides satisfactory relief in the majority of patients.

Cotton, P. B.: Cannulation of the papilla of Vater by endoscopy and retrograde cholangiopancreatography. Gut, 13:1014, 1972.

Donowitz, M., Kerstein, M. D., and Spiro, H. M.: Pancreatic ascites. Medicine, 53:183, 1974.

Fontana, G., Bolondi, L., Conti, M., Plicchi, G., Gullo, L., Caletti, G. C., and Labo, G.: An evaluation of echography in the diagnosis of pancreatic disease. Gut, 17:228, 1976.

Gambill, E. E.: Pancreatitis. S. Louis, C. V. Mosby Company, 1973.

Haaga, J. R., Alfidi, R. J., Zelch, M. G., Meany, T. F., Boller, M., Gonzalez, L., and Jelden, G. L.: Computed tomography of the pancreas. Radiology, 120:589, 1976.

Regan, P. T., Malagelada, J. R., DiMagno, E. P., Glanzman, S. L., and Go, V. L. W.: Comparative effects of antacids, cimetidine and enteric coating on the therapeutic response to oral enzymes in severe pancreatic insufficiency. N. Engl. J. Med., 297:854, 1977.

Snape, W. J., Jr., Long, W. B., Trotman, B. W., Marin, G. A., and Czaja, A. J.: Marked alkaline phosphatase elevations with partial common bile duct obstruction due to calcific pancreatitis. Gastroenterology, 70:70, 1976.

411. CARCINOMA OF THE PANCREAS

DEFINITION. Most carcinomas of the pancreas are adenocarcinomas arising in the epithelium of the ducts. At least three clinical syndromes are seen in patients with this tumor: chronic pain, jaundice, or malabsorption, depending in part upon the location of the tumor. Jaundice is a prominent feature of carcinoma of the head of the pancreas. Severe pain and the malabsorption syndrome are more characteristic of carcinoma of the body and tail. Carcinoma of the head of the pancreas accounts for two thirds of the patients. The ratio of carcinoma of the head, body, and tail is 8:2:1.

INCIDENCE AND EPIDEMIOLOGY. Carcinoma of the pancreas as a cause of death in men now ranks fourth among cancers in the United States. The ratio of men to women is about 2:1. The peak age incidence is 55 years. This appears to be the result of a true increase in incidence. It surpasses carcinoma of the stomach in some areas. In general, the increase in carcinoma of the pancreas has been accompanied by a decrease in carcinoma of the stomach. No localized geographical areas of increased incidence have been identified.

Risk Factors. Cigarette smoking, more than 10 to 20 per day, and diabetes mellitus appear to be associated with an increased risk of developing the disease, although the increase is relatively modest, two to three times. The relationship to chronic pancreatitis is less convincing. Localized areas of pancreatitis in a pancreas containing an adenocarcinoma are not uncommon, but clinical acute pancreatitis is unusual, and in the case of chronic pancreatitis there is always the question of a carcinoma having been present from the beginning. Carcinoma of the pancreas can be produced in experimental animals by known carcinogens, but its relationship to environmentally induced cancer is uncertain. Cellular changes in ductal epithelium can be found in the pancreas of patients with frank carcinoma and may represent precancerous lesions.

PATHOPHYSIOLOGY. Carcinoma of the pancreas invades and obstructs ducts, invades nerve sheaths, and enters blood vessels and lymphatics as well as spreading to adjacent organs by contiguous extension. Obstruction of the pancreatic ducts causes pain and maldigestion and malabsorption of fat. Obstruction of the common bile duct produces jaundice. Involvement of regional lymph nodes may also cause jaundice by obstruction at the porta hepatis. Distant metastases are common. Invasion of the portal and splenic veins may cause portal hypertension. Carcinomas of the pancreas are among those tumors associated with the production of peptide hormones such as ACTH, parathormone, ADH, and MSH. Diabetes mellitus is present in about 30 per cent of patients.

CLINICAL MANIFESTATIONS. Carcinoma of the head of the pancreas leads to jaundice in about 85 per cent of patients. It is of the obstructive type with bile in the urine and pruritus. It is usually unremitting. Pruritus is common. The liver is often enlarged, and in about 25 per cent of patients the gallbladder is palpable (Courvoisier's sign). In some patients, a hemolytic component of the jaundice may be present, particularly in patients with serum bilirubins above 30 mg per 100 ml. Dark urine is the first sign usually noted by the patient; friends and relatives may note yellow sclera or skin. Weight loss of more than 5 pounds is almost universally present.

The issue of "painless jaundice" as a sign of carcinoma of the head of the pancreas has been resolved in favor of some discomfort or distress in the abdomen being present in the majority of patients, although they may not volunteer the complaint of pain. However, the characteristic feature of boring abdominal pain, radiating to the back, relieved by flexing the trunk or by analgesics, and growing worse at night, is more often seen in the absence of jaundice of a significant degree and more frequently in patients with carcinoma of the body of the pancreas. These are the patients who may be diagnosed as having functional disease, low back pain, or narcotic addiction until late in the course of the disease. The syndrome of portal hypertension with esophageal varices, splenomegaly, and ascites may be seen in patients in whom the tumor invades the portal and splenic veins. At times the patients present with distant metastases as the first evidence of the disease, such as involvement of the lung or liver. Carcinoma of the pancreas ranks high on the list of possible primaries when a histologic diagnosis of metastatic adenocarcinoma, primary source unknown, is obtained.

Occasionally patients present with the malabsorption syndrome, including weight loss, steatorrhea, and signs of deficiencies of fat-soluble vitamins. The development of jaundice in a patient with adult type diabetes mellitus may be a clue. Upper gastrointestinal bleeding is a rare presenting manifestation of pancreatic carcinoma. Symptoms of depression appear to occur more frequently in patients with pancreatic carcinoma than would be expected by chance alone. Subcutaneous fat necrosis, splenomegaly, and thrombophlebitis are unusual findings on physical examination.

DIAGNOSIS. In the patients with obstructive jaundice, carcinoma of the pancreas should be considered as a possible cause, especially in the absence of symptoms of biliary colic or previous biliary tract surgery. Abdominal pain, especially when radiating to the back and not relieved by food, alkalis, or a bowel movement, which persists beyond two to three weeks in patients who are middle aged or older should be considered as a possible manifestation of pancreatic carcinoma. Malabsorption syndromes should be studied quickly to differentiate those patients with primary maldigestion from those with intestinal mucosal disease (see Ch. 408). The major difficulty comes in the differentiation from chronic pancreatitis.

LABORATORY STUDIES. The serum bilirubin must reach levels of 2 to 3 mg per 100 ml before clinical jaundice is apparent, particularly when lighting conditions are poor and in black patients. The division between direct and indirect reacting serum bilirubin in obstructive jaundice is about 50 per cent. Bile (bilirubin or bile salts) will be present in the urine. The serum transaminases will be less than two to three times normal. The serum alkaline phosphatase, leucine amino peptidase, and 5'-nucleotidase will be elevated more than two times normal in most patients. The prothrombin time may be prolonged but should return to normal with treatment with vitamin K. Examination by ultrasound or computerized axial tomography will detect gallstones and enlargement of the pancreas in most patients. Data on precise accuracy are still being accumulated. A barium meal will detect displacement of the stomach or invasion of the duodenum. In the presence of a duodenal mass, endoscopic retrograde pancreatography would be the first choice if available. Otherwise, percutaneous transhepatic cholangiography with the Chiba (skinny) needle is the preferred procedure. The finding of an obstructive lesion at the lower end of the common bile duct is an indication for laparotomy. Histologic diagnosis of carcinoma may be made by biopsy of the lesion of pancreas or by biopsy of lymph nodes or secondaries in the liver. Needle biopsy of the pancreas is being performed more frequently now, with an acceptably low incidence of complications such as pancreatic fistula.

In patients with persistent abdominal pain, the first step is the demonstration of disease in the pancreas. Ultrasound and computerized tomography are the least invasive measures. Barium meal may show displacement of contiguous organs. Determination of duodenal secretion volume and bicarbonate concentration and output after the intravenous administration of 1 clinical unit per kilogram of secretin (preferably relatively pure) will detect significant reductions in pancreatic mass if the bicarbonate concentration is less than 70 mEq per liter or the output less than 10 mEq per 20 minutes. Trypsin concentrations in the duodenum after a test meal (Lundh meal) are an alternative measurement. Evidence of pancreatic disease should lead to an attempt to determine the specific diagnosis. Two techniques may provide a tissue diagnosis: direct needle biopsy guided by ultrasound findings, and cytology of material obtained directly from the pancreatic duct during secretin stimulation by endoscopic retrograde cholangiopancreatography. Indirect evidence of high diagnostic reliability can be obtained by endoscopic retrograde cholangiopancreatography or arteriography. Localized obstruction of ducts and encasement of arteries or obstruction of the splenic vein are the most reliable signs of pancreatic carcinoma. Justification for such procedures, as opposed to proceeding directly to laparotomy, is the notorious unreliability of the surgeon's palpating hand in evaluating the difference in texture of the pancreas and the continued reluctance of many surgeons to perform biopsy of the pancreas.

For the other less common clinical syndromes associated with carcinoma of the pancreas, the physician must have a high index of suspicion and direct efforts at establishing the diagnosis as indicated above. Serum amylase determinations are of little value. A diabetic type of glucose tolerance curve will be found in two thirds of patients late in the disease.

DIFFERENTIAL DIAGNOSIS. Gallstone disease is by far the most common and important consideration in the differential diagnosis. Cholecystography often fails because of nonvisualization, but ultrasound and computerized tomography may show stones or an enlarged gallbladder. The differentiation of extrinsic from intrinsic mucosal gastrointestinal lesions is a perennial problem for the radiologist, but fortunately endoscopy with biopsy is often helpful. Chronic pancreatitis and carcinoma of the pancreas can be indistinguishable by sonography, arteriography, endoscopic retrograde cholangiopancreatography, and palpation at laparotomy. Biopsy and cytology remain the only completely valid means of differentiation, and even this holds true only when the diagnosis of carcinoma is made. The diagnosis of an intestinal cause of malabsorption syndrome should not be made without confirmation by small bowel biopsy or without histologic evidence of disease in surgical biopsy. Cystadenomas and pancreatic cystadenocarcinomas are uncommon causes of pancreatic mass lesions. Arteriography may be very suggestive in the latter, as they are usually very vascular. Portal hypertension should not be attributed to primary liver disease without confirmation by biopsy if possible. Pancreatic function tests do not reliably differentiate carcinoma from chronic pancreatitis. Carcinoembryonic antigen is found in the serum of both patients with carcinoma of the pancreas and those with chronic pancreatitis. It may have some value in the follow-up of patients after surgery.

The combination of a mass on ultrasonography, the secretory response to CCK, and endoscopic retrograde cholangiopancreatography give the highest percentage of correct diagnoses in carcinoma of the pancreas. Since this is the order of invasiveness, they should be done in that order. This procedure will identify correctly about 90 per cent of patients with pancreatic carcinoma and also 90 per cent of the patients without carcinoma. Surgical exploration and/or biopsy will be required for final diagnosis.

PROGNOSIS. The five-year survival of patients with carcinoma of the pancreas has been so poor that some physicians have abandoned hope of curative surgical procedures. This does not seem justified until the newer diagnostic aids have been adequately tested for their ability to detect operable lesions.

TREATMENT. The merits of the Whipple procedure (duodenopancreatectomy) versus total pancreatectomy are still debated. Bypass procedures may improve symptoms but contribute little to prolonging survival. Chemotherapy and radiotherapy have some claims for benefit, but adequately controlled trials are only now being done. Adenocarcinoma of the papilla of Vater carries a definitely better prognosis after resection than does carcinoma of the pancreas, but the preoperative

differential diagnosis may be difficult. Until better results can be obtained, it seems appropriate to inform the patients and their families of the alternatives and to consider their opinions carefully in arriving at a decision.

Barkin, J., Vining, D., Miale, A., Jr., Gottlieb, S., Ridlhammer, D. C., and Kalser, M. H.: Computerized tomography, diagnostic ultrasound, and radionuclide scanning; comparison of efficacy in diagnosis of pancreatic carcinoma. JAMA, 238:2040, 1977.

Bookstein, J. J., Reuter, S. R., and Martel, W.: Angiographic evaluation of pancreatic carcinoma. Radiology, 93:757, 1969.

DiMagno, E. P., Malagelada, J. R., Taylor, W. F., and Go, V. L. W.: A prospective comparison of current diagnostic tests for pancreatic cancer. N. Engl. J. Med., 297:737, 1977.

Morgan, R. G. H., and Wormsley, K. G.: Cancer of the pancreas. Gut, 18:580, 1977.

Silvis, S. E., Rohrmann, C. H., and Vennes, J. A.: Diagnostic accuracy of endoscopic retrograde cholangiopancreatography in hepatic, biliary, and pancreatic malignancy. Ann. Intern. Med., 84:438, 1976.

Smith, E. H., Bartrum, R. J., Jr., Chang, Y. C., D'Orsi, D., Lokich, J., Albruzzese, A., and Dantono, J.: Percutaneous aspiration biopsy of the pancreas under ultrasonic guidance. N. Engl. J. Med., 292:825, 1975.

412. CYSTIC FIBROSIS OF THE PANCREAS

(Mucoviscidosis)

DEFINITION. This is a generalized disease of exocrine secretions inherited in an autosomal recessive pattern and expressed clinically only in homozygotes. It is one of the most commonly inherited abnormal genes. The abnormality in secretion includes electrolytes, proteins, and glycoproteins and results in a viscid secretion which produces obstruction in ductal systems. The primary target organs are the lungs, pancreas, and gastrointestinal tract (including the liver).

INCIDENCE. The disease occurs in about 1 in 2000 live births. Heterozygotes are represented in 2 to 5 per cent of the population. There has been a steady increase in the number of patients surviving to adult life. Projections reach up to 50,000 adults with cystic fibrosis in the United States by 1985.

ETIOLOGY. The basic defect in cystic fibrosis is unknown. Much effort has been expended in searching for humoral factors related to the disease, including substances which might impair the function of cilia, but the results are controversial. Attempts to identify heterozygotes by a variety of determinations have also not been successful.

PATHOPHYSIOLOGY. The initial presentation in childhood is often that of meconium ileus: small intestinal obstruction caused by a mass of viscid secretions and meconium. The sugar side chains of the glycoproteins of intestinal secretions are abnormal, with increase in fucose and decrease in sialic acid. Complexes of calcium and glycoproteins have been found. Impaired bronchial drainage as a result of viscid secretions leads to bronchiectasis and repeated respiratory infections and eventually to respiratory failure resulting from necrosis and fibrosis of the pulmonary alveoli. In the pancreas, viscid secretions produce chronic pancreatitis. The islets of Langerhans remain intact. A deficiency of pancreatic exocrine secretion leads to malabsorption of fat and steatorrhea. Impaired glucose tolerance, when present, is probably due to fibrosis disrupting the ducts. A similar process in the bile passages causes a secondary biliary cirrhosis with portal hypertension and esophageal varices. Recent studies showed a substantial increase in bile acid excretion in the stools of patients with cystic fibrosis who had steatorrhea. Bile has been shown to be lithogenic, and patients with cystic fibrosis have an increased incidence of gallstones. Although not of much clinical significance, the changes in salivary secretions give suggestions as to the pathophysiology of other exocrine glands. The concentrations of sodium and chloride are significantly greater in patients with cystic fibrosis. Similar changes in sweat are the basis of a diagnostic test.

CLINICAL MANIFESTATIONS. Chronic pulmonary disease with cough, wheezing, and repeated respiratory infections is the most common clinical syndrome. The sputum may resemble that of patients with bronchiectasis. The chest is hyperresonant, there is impaired movement of the diaphragm, and clubbing of the fingers may develop. Chronic paranasal sinus infection, with postnasal drip and formation of polyps, is common. Pancreatic insufficiency results in the passage of large, bulky, foul-smelling stools and abdominal cramps. Secondary biliary cirrhosis with portal hypertension leads to presentation with hepatomegaly and bleeding from esophageal varices in about 2 per cent of patients with cystic fibrosis. Adults are now being found with a syndrome resembling meconium ileus. Partial bowel obstruction occurred in 7 per cent of patients with cystic fibrosis seen at the Mayo Clinic. Only 2 to 3 per cent of men with cystic fibrosis who reach adulthood are fertile because of defective development of the wolffian duct.

DIAGNOSIS. The majority of adults have a history of the disorder in childhood with repeated respiratory infections. Pancreatic insufficiency and secondary biliary cirrhosis may not be recognized until early adult life. The family history may be helpful. Sweat electrolytes and duodenal drainage after stimulation of the pancreas with secretin are the most helpful laboratory tests. The demarcation of normal from abnormal sodium concentrations in sweat is not as clear in adults as in childhood (>60 mEq per liter), giving rise to periodic claims of high incidence of cystic fibrosis in patients with pulmonary emphysema. In comparison to those with other forms of chronic pancreatitis, those with cystic fibrosis respond to stimulation with secretin and CCK with a nearly normal enzyme output but impaired volume and bicarbonate output. Chest roentgenograms usually show evidence of chronic pulmonary infection. A mass in the right lower quadrant and findings of mechanical intestinal obstruction should suggest the adult equivalent of meconium ileus in young adults with cystic fibrosis.

TREATMENT. Meticulous attention to pulmonary toilet and administration of broad-spectrum antimicrobials have slowed the ravages of pulmonary infections. Pancreatic extracts given with meals usually control the symptoms of steatorrhea. Medium-chain triglycerides may be helpful in keeping up caloric intake in some patients. Surgical relief of intestinal obstruction in meconium ileus may be required, and portosystemic shunts may be indicated to control bleeding from esophageal varices.

PROGNOSIS. As stated, the prognosis for patients with cystic fibrosis has improved remarkably in recent years, largely because of improved treatment of respiratory infections.

Hadorn, B., Zoppi, G., Shmerling, D. H., Prader, A., McIntire, I., and Anderson, C. M.: Quantitative assessment of exocrine pancreatic function in infants and children. J. Pediat., 73:39, 1968.

Matseshe, J. W., Go, V. L. W., and DiMagno, E. P.: Meconium ileus equivalent complicating cystic fibrosis in postneonatal children and young adults. Report of 12 cases. Gastroenterology, 72:732, 1977.

Rosenlund, M. L., and Lustig, H. S.: Young adults with cystic fibrosis. Ann. Intern. Med., 78:959, 1973.

Stern, R. C., Stevens, D. P., Boat, T. F., Doershuk, C. F., Izant, R. J., and Matthews, L. W.: Symptomatic hepatic disease in cystic fibrosis: Incidence, course, and outcome of portal systemic shunting. Gastroenterology, 70:645, 1976.

Stern, R. C., Boat, T. F., Doershuk, C. F., Tucker, A. S., Miller, R. B., and Matthews, L. S.: Cystic fibrosis diagnosed after age 13. Ann. Intern. Med., 87:188, 1977.

Warwick, W. J., and Pogue, R. E.: Cystic fibrosis. An expanding challenge for internal medicine. JAMA, 238:2159, 1977.

Watkins, J. B., Tercyak, A. M., Szczepanik, P., and Klein, P. D.: Bile salt kinetics in cystic fibrosis: Influence of pancreatic enzyme replacement. Gastroenterology, 73:1023, 1977.

Section Seven INFLAMMATORY DISEASES OF THE INTESTINE

413. CHRONIC INFLAMMATORY DISEASES OF THE INTESTINE

Henry D. Janowitz

413.1. INTRODUCTION

Chronic inflammatory bowel disease includes a group of disorders characterized by acute and chronic inflammatory changes in all portions of the small and large intestines. The best and oldest known is *ulcerative colitis*, an inflammatory disease confined to the colonic mucosa and submucosa. Equally well characterized now is *regional enteritis*, an inflammatory disease involving the entire wall of a portion of the small gut. This process may involve ileum and colon (*ileocolitis*), or any portion of the colon alone with a similar granulomatous pathologic process. These separate groups (*regional enteritis, ileocolitis,* and *granulomatous colitis*) are now designated as *Crohn's disease* (after the author who, with his colleagues Ginzberg and Oppenheimer, described regional enteritis precisely) to avoid confusion and without commitment to any etiologic theory.

413.2. REGIONAL ENTERITIS
(Crohn's Disease of Small Bowel)

DEFINITION. Regional enteritis is a chronic inflammatory disorder of the intestinal tract of unknown origin which may appear at any site but characteristically involves the terminal ileum (hence its original name, "terminal ileitis"). Clinically, regional enteritis is a diarrheal disease often associated with fever, abdominal pain, weight loss, abdominal masses, and anal or perianal lesions. The disease is also characterized by the frequent formation of enteric fistulas or sinus tracts. Characteristically regional enteritis produces linear ulcers and deep fissures in the gut; inflammation (characterized by aggregations of inflammatory cells and sarcoid-like granulomas) may extend through the full thickness of the bowel wall.

ETIOLOGY.   Forty-six years after its original description (in 1932), regional enteritis remains a disease of unknown origin, although considerable search has been made for causes. No recognized infectious agent has been isolated, although the resemblance of its histopathology to that of noncaseating tuberculosis was noted early. Tremendous interest and effort are being expended in the search for a transmissible agent. Several viral candidates have been proposed, but none has been accepted. The psychosomatic approach to this disorder has evoked little interest and little supportive research and documentation. Much recent heavy emphasis has been on investigations of the immunologic reactivity of patients with Crohn's disease. No characteristic or significant alterations in serum immunoglobulins have been described. Impaired cutaneous responses to tuberculin, stressed in the earlier literature, are not supported by recent studies. We have noted an absolute lymphopenia in some patients. With a widely accepted test of delayed hypersensitivity, 70 per cent of patients are not sensitized to dinitrochlorobenzene. Further evidence of depressed lymphocyte immunologic competence has been obtained by several groups who have shown that the circulating lymphocytes have a diminished response in vitro to phytohemagglutinin, suggesting impairment of thymic derived lymphocytes associated with diminished numbers of T lymphocytes. This depressed responsiveness was present in an equal number (40 per cent) of patients with ulcerative colitis as well. Controversy exists regarding immunologic cross-reactivity between sarcoidosis and Crohn's disease. The active international standard Siltzbach-Chase Kveim antigen does not give a positive skin reaction in patients with Crohn's disease. The significance of the important observation that tissues from Crohn's disease introduced into several animal species, especially the footpad of the mouse, induce granulomas is confused by current controversy regarding the specificity of this response both with control material and with tissue from ulcerative colitis colons. However the hypothesis that Crohn's disease may be due to a transmissible agent, one with a long latent period, in a susceptible population, one with an immunologic defect, seems most attractive at present.

INCIDENCE, PREVALENCE, AND EPIDEMIOLOGY.   Epidemiologic studies tend to lump all forms of Crohn's disease into one, regardless of the location of the disease, and have the added difficulty of separating Crohn's disease of the colon from ulcerative colitis. It has its highest incidence in the United States, is thought to be infrequent in Central Europe, and is recorded frequently in Britain and the Scandinavian countries. It appears to be seen only infrequently in Africa, Asia, and South America.

Variable *incidence rates* (rate of occurrence of the dis-

ease per 100,000 persons at risk per year) have been reported. In the Baltimore study of patients over 20 years of age which utilized hospital cases only, the incidence in males was 2.5 and in females 1.2, for an average of 1.8. In the Oxford study of Evans and Acheson (1967), the incidence for both men and women was approximately 1.0.

Evidence regarding *prevalence* (all the patients affected with this disease at any one moment per 100,000 persons at risk) is difficult to obtain. Based on 36 reports, Mendeloff has estimated the range of prevalence as between 20 and 40 per 100,000 population. Fragmentary evidence suggests that the incidence of Crohn's disease may be rising in the western world.

There is no significant difference in regard to sex. In contrast to ulcerative colitis, Crohn's disease under age six appears to be rare but is rising. The first incidence mode can be seen to occur between 15 and 20, with a second mode at age 55 to 60. In the United States, blacks and Indians are at low risk. Evidence has been accumulating that the incidence of inflammatory bowel disease in Jewish patients is strikingly higher than in the non-Jewish populations. In Baltimore, in Crohn's disease, the rate was six times higher for Jewish males and three times higher for Jewish females than the rates for non-Jews. Although these higher rates in Jews might be due to social, dietary, or genetic factors, current epidemiologic studies offer no explanation. There is a slight preponderance of urban over rural setting for Crohn's disease. Nevertheless, exhaustive study of socioeconomic status, for the United States, has demonstrated no significant difference for patient and control populations. Perhaps farmers are less vulnerable because of some occupational factor.

GENETICS.   Since the search for an exogenous (environmental) etiology in Crohn's disease has been fruitless so far, recent attention has been devoted to the problem of genetic susceptibility. No simple mendelian genetic mechanism has been forthcoming. A considerable number of family aggregations have been reported, the most frequent combination being two affected siblings, with parent (more often mother) and child combination a close second. This evidence may argue more for common environmental factors than for genetic influence. The literature contains no reference to a husband and wife both being affected, and studies on twins (concordance has been recorded in seven pairs of monozygotic twins) do not contribute to the solution of this problem. Family incidence of Crohn's disease is low; 1 in 15 to 1 in 50 patients have an affected first-degree relative. Although this incidence in first-degree relatives is higher than in the general population, lack of control data limits this interpretation. The association of Crohn's disease with other disorders of an inherited nature is pertinent. In one series eczema and hay fever were particularly common, possibly pointing to a genetically controlled immunologic mechanism. A stronger association exists with *ankylosing spondylitis* and its associated HLA antigen B27, which has hereditary features and which may appear before the clinical manifestations of the bowel disease. The association of Crohn's disease and ulcerative colitis within families is well recorded, but the uncertainties of this relationship do not advance our understanding. An interesting and curious feature in families with these diseases is that the index patient with Crohn's disease often has relatives with ulcerative colitis, whereas many series with families of ulcerative colitis patients have no relatives with Crohn's disease. One conclusion is that the genetic influence on etiology is likely to be polygenic, alleles at several different loci providing a genotype which determines susceptibility or resistance to environmental factors, although a virus-like maternal factor is a possibility.

PATHOLOGY. All areas of the gastrointestinal tract may be involved in regional enteritis, including rare lesions of the oral cavity and esophagus. Lesions of the stomach and duodenum occur more frequently, and the terminal ileum is the most common site of the disease. Although isolated regional jejunitis does occur, combined lesions of ileum and jejunum are more frequent. The lesion in the colon is discussed in Ch. 413.4. The *perirectal fistula* should be considered an integral part of Crohn's disease of the small bowel because of its frequency. All layers of the small intestine are involved, as are the regional lymph nodes. The bowel wall is remarkably thickened and rigid. Skip areas of disease are frequently seen with intervening normal bowel. Loops of affected small intestine may be adherent; frequently fistulas exist between these adherent loops. In addition, sinus tracts may extend into a thickened and inflamed mesentery, producing an inflammatory mass. Fistulas from the ileum to cecum and/or sigmoid are very common, but others may reach to the skin (often in old operative scars, occasionally to the navel), bladder, ureter, vagina, flank, and even the right hip joint. Frequently perianal inflammation arising in the crypts of Morgagni leads to anal and perirectal fistulas. An inflammatory mass may encase the ureter, producing ureteral obstruction and hydronephrosis. Superficial discrete ulcers which extend to form confluent linear ulcerations are characteristic of the macroscopic appearance of the intestinal mucosa, as are deep fissures which may extend through all coats and serve as the basis of fistulas. Recent studies have emphasized the presence of aphthous ulceration of the mucosa as the earliest pathologic lesion. Microscopically, aggregations of inflammatory cells involving all layers predominate, with the sarcoid granuloma most characteristic when present. Such granulomas are noncaseating collections of epithelioid cells (large mononuclear phagocytes) and multinucleated giant cells whose nuclei are arranged around the periphery or collected at the poles of the cell (Langerhans type) (Fig. 1). When a large number of sections are searched, granulomas have been found in the bowel wall in up to 75 to 85 per cent of patients.

Figure 1. Regional enteritis. Submucosa of ileum, showing noncaseating granulomas with multinucleated giant cells. Hematoxylin and eosin stain, × 150.

The regional lymph nodes, often containing granulomas, are enlarged owing to nonspecific reactive changes. In one series, 38 per cent of lymph nodes contained granulomas, and in 63 per cent granulomas were present in the bowel wall. Further, 20 per cent of nodes may have this lesion without granulomas present in the bowel. Not all areas of the bowel and all regional nodes are equally affected in the same specimen.

A few available ultrastructural studies have not contributed to pathologic understanding or differential diagnosis but have confirmed the curious finding of neuronal hyperplasia in the mesenteric plexus.

PATHOGENESIS. An acute inflammatory reaction in the ileum has been well documented (albeit with little histologic confirmation), but most studies have demonstrated its disappearance without any of the sequelae of Crohn's disease, so that the transition from acute to chronic forms of regional enteritis is not recorded. Bacteriologic and serologic evidence has associated some cases of acute ileitis with infection with the bacteria *Yersinia enterocolitica*, formerly known as *Pasteurella X*. (We need, however, to distinguish this situation from lymphoid hyperplasia of the ileum, frequently seen in the small bowel x-rays of youngsters studied for abdominal pain.)

Since all portions of the gastrointestinal tract from mouth to anus may participate in the pathologic process, an important question is the extent of dissemination. It is extremely rare to obtain characteristic pathologic changes in jejunal biopsies of patients with regional ileitis, and we have never had a positive rectal biopsy in patients with ileitis except when a local rectal or anal lesion was also present. Resected specimens show few lesions 6 cm beyond the edge. Although some scattered microscopic lesions have been noted in grossly normal colon adjacent to classic regional ileitis, in general the disease is localized and segmental rather than universal; however, some investigators have recently stressed the presence of more widespread nonspecific histologic and physiologic alterations. Any scheme of pathogenesis must take into account other histologic features of this disease: hyperplastic reactive lymph nodes, the development of granulomas in regional nodes or in ectopic lymph follicles, inflammatory reactions in lymphatics and perilymphatics, ectasia of lymph channels, and the development of submucosal lymphedema secondary to obstructed lymphatics. Although the pathologic process may spread from ileum to adjacent large bowel by extension along sinus tracts with fistula formation, retrograde extension over any long segment does not occur in the absence of surgical intervention. Repeated surgical experience has demonstrated that in portions of the involved ileum excluded from the intestinal stream, completely diverting "bypass" operations lead quite regularly to subsidence of the inflammatory reaction and to recurrence of the pathologic process most frequently in the new "terminal ileum." One might postulate from this line of evidence that the exciting agent of the tissue reaction in Crohn's disease may be present in the intestinal stream, moving down and becoming more concentrated as it reaches the ileocecal area. Delay behind the ileocecal sphincter and above the anal sphincter favors its absorption and entry into submucosal lymphatics and lymphoid tissue with the characteristic tissue response in these loci.

CLINICAL MANIFESTATIONS. The classic presentation

of regional enteritis is that of a young person, in his or her late teens or early twenties, who has not been feeling well for an ill-defined time but whose indisposition has suddenly worsened. Whereas the past history may have included an occasional episode of cramps and diarrhea frequently ascribed to dietary indiscretions or "nerves," the patient now complains of more constant abdominal pain and more persistent diarrhea. The pain is most frequently cramping and periodic, and is often worse after eating; it is confined principally to the right lower quadrant; occasionally it radiates into the right upper thigh. At times it is more persistent, dull, and annoying. The stools become more frequent, small, and loose to watery, often waking the patient at night as well, but are free of gross blood. Appetite clearly declines, and parents become alerted and alarmed by the obvious weight loss, which may be considerable. Often there is a low-grade fever—usually, however, not recorded at home. There may be a history of a recent appendectomy (performed for right lower quadrant pain and tenderness) or a slowly healing perirectal abscess.

Histories of some "allergic" phenomena, including pollen sensitivities and possibly intolerance to milk, seem to be present more frequently than by chance, but no obvious association with other so-called "immune" diseases exists. There may be a history of recurrent crops of aphthous ulcers of the mouth which not only may plague the patient but may also herald an acute exacerbation. Less frequently, persistent fever, malaise, and anorexia may overshadow the abdominal complaints, and the patient may be labeled as having "fever of unknown origin" or rheumatic fever (especially in the younger child). Failure of sexual and somatic development may be the sole clinical feature.

Less frequent is the patient who presents with fecal fistula in the unhealed scar of an appendectomy, or persistent mucopurulent drainage from the wound. Equally striking are the extraintestinal clinical manifestations of regional enteritis. These include joint symptoms, ranging from fleeting *arthralgias* to obvious *arthritis* and tender, swollen, hot joints, particularly knees and ankles. Backaches may also precede intestinal symptoms, later found to be due to *ankylosing spondylitis*. Skin manifestations include *erythema multiforme*, and especially the painful *erythema nodosum* of shins and feet and the rarer *pyoderma gangrenosum*. An intense *conjunctivitis* (often phlyctenular in nature) and *uveitis* and *iritis* with eye pain and visual disturbances may also accompany an underlying chronic intestinal inflammatory disorder. Except for ocular involvements, these extraintestinal manifestations parallel the intensity of the bowel symptoms. Less frequent concomitants include biliary colic caused by *cholelithiasis*, and renal colic associated with either showers of uric acid crystals in the urine or the presence of mixed, especially oxalate, *kidney stones*. Malabsorption may also be obvious clinically.

Although the presentation thus far appears to stress the youth of patients, the symptoms may begin at any age; indeed, there seems to be a bimodal distribution, with a second peak in the forties and fifties. A frequent and distressing clinical manifestation is delayed reappearance of general and intestinal symptoms after surgical intervention. Such clinical behavior heralds the discovery of recurrent enteritis, readily confirmed radiographically.

PHYSICAL EXAMINATION. Physical examination often reveals a well-developed young adult, with some evidence of recent weight loss, moderate pallor, and lassitude. Clubbing of the phalanges is usually not present unless there is extensive involvement of jejunum and ileum, or of ileum and colon. A large number of patients have either a palpable loop of thickened inflamed ileum or a clear-cut mass in the right lower quadrant. Pedal edema may be present. The cutaneous, joint, and eye manifestations cited above may be present. Examination of the rectal area may disclose nothing abnormal or may reveal a perianal or perirectal abscess; evidence of the prior surgical attempts to treat perirectal abscesses and fistulas; or, in patients with colonic involvement, the curious florid indolent ulcers of the anus which often make rectal examination difficult. Proctoscopy demonstrates a normal mucosa except in those with Crohn's disease of the rectum and anus. In children, evidence of retarded growth and delayed secondary sexual characteristics may be striking.

LABORATORY STUDIES. Laboratory findings may include evidence of a mild to moderate anemia; the white cell count is usually normal except in the presence of suppuration. Lymphopenia may be present. Albuminuria is rare and may indicate renal amyloidosis. The stools may reveal the existence of occult blood. The erythrocyte sedimentation rate, a crude but useful index of disease activity, is elevated, at times paralleled by marked thrombocytosis. The serum albumin may be lowered, and often the gamma globulin fraction is elevated. Occasionally elevated blood uric acid levels in both females and males are present. Minor abnormalities in liver function tests may indicate the presence of fatty liver; more marked elevation in serum alkaline phosphatase or SGOT or SGPT determinations indicates the associated pericholangitis seen more frequently in ulcerative colitis and ileocolitis. Serum vitamin B_{12} levels and the Schilling test of vitamin B_{12} absorption may be abnormal, and variable amounts of unabsorbed fat can be detected by measuring fecal fat in a 72-hour collection (see Ch. 408); however, anorexia often precludes adequate fat intake, making this determination meaningless. The d-xylose test, a measure of carbohydrate absorption, is usually within normal limits except when the jejunum is involved.

MECHANISMS OF DISEASE MANIFESTATIONS. The weight loss in regional enteritis is due in large part to failure of caloric intake, with a smaller contribution from failure of absorption. The reduced caloric intake derives mainly from loss of appetite but also from the generally restrictive diets that physicians recommend or patients adopt. The diarrhea of regional enteritis may arise from a multitude of causes: (1) failure of diseased ileum to resorb bile salts can result in excessive passage of bile salts into the colon where these products inhibit colonic fluid and electrolyte resorption; (2) loss of small bowel absorbing surface, as the result of disease or surgical resection, may produce general malabsorption with increased fecal output; (3) partial intestinal obstruction (caused by intestinal stenosis or mechanical obstruction from inflammatory masses or adherent loops of bowel) may produce diarrhea either as a result of excessive net secretion of fluid and electrolytes by dilated proximal bowel or as a result of intestinal stasis and bacterial overgrowth (see Ch. 408); and (4) lactase deficiency may be accentuated by the impaired nutritional status of these patients, because all brush border enzymes are decreased in the patients who are most ill (see below).

ABSORPTIVE DEFECTS. Fat malabsorption is correlated with the length of inflamed or resected ileum, the incidence of steatorrhea increasing in those with more than 90 to 100 cm involved or resected. The mechanism is ascribed to the loss of bile salts (failure to be reabsorbed) in this portion of the gut, with resultant reduction of the bile salt pool and thus hepatic secretion of the bile salts needed for proper micelle formation and pancreatic lipase activity. This reduction in the bile salt pool and resultant secretion of "lithogenic" bile also accounts for the increased incidence of gallstones. Bacterial overgrowth in those with stenosis, stricture, fistulas, or surgically created blind loops may also contribute to steatorrhea by deconjugating bile salts needed for fat absorption. Carbohydrate absorption is usually quite normal (at least as measured by the d-xylose test) except in patients with jejunitis, or in those with stricture formation and consequent overgrowth of luminal bacteria which may metabolize this sugar. Lactose maldigestion secondary to intestinal lactase deficiency is seen in some patients, many of whom have themselves eliminated milk and milk products from their diets; the diarrhea of lactase deficiency in such patients arises from (1) the osmotic effects of unabsorbed lactose and (2) a lowered colonic pH (from bacterial breakdown products of lactose) which inhibits colonic water and electrolyte resorption. Vitamin B_{12} malabsorption is related to the loss of normal ileal absorptive mechanism. When the length of involved or resected ileum exceeds 90 cm, the Schilling test is abnormal in all; thus malabsorption of vitamin B_{12} is correlated with fat malabsorption. The increased incidence of gallstones is ascribed to the alteration in bile salt pool and the secretion of "lithogenic" bile secondary to failure to reabsorb bile salts in the ileum (see Ch. 408).

RENAL CALCULI. Urinary uric acid crystals are more common in these patients. Several defects are believed responsible for this finding: (1) some patients have hyperuricemia, thought to result from increased catabolic rates; (2) the urine is more frequently acid, perhaps reflecting excessive loss of bicarbonate in the diarrheal stools; and (3) loss of excessive stool water results in the formation of a more concentrated urine. Some patients have in addition increased levels of blood uric acid, presumed to be associated with breakdown of tissue. Other types of renal calculi likewise appear to be correlated with fluid loss through the gut. The recognition of increased oxalate excretion in the urine and presence of oxalate stones has revealed a new metabolic complication. Hyperoxaluria now appears to result from increased intestinal absorption of dietary oxalate secondary to diminished absorption of calcium in the presence of steatorrhea.

CLINICAL COMPLICATIONS. Despite their frequency, certain manifestations of the disease are considered as complications. These include *local suppurative complications,* arising from extension of sinus tracts into the adjacent mesentery and giving rise to right lower quadrant abscess formation. These sinus tracts may also extend into the right psoas region, giving rise to a psoas syndrome of low backache, pain in the right upper thigh, and flexion deformity with limp. Healing takes place by a marked fibrotic reaction with narrowing of the intestinal lumen and *stricture formation,* ac-

counting for the paradoxical increase in crampy abdominal pain with subsidence of systemic symptoms. The syndrome of incomplete intestinal obstruction rarely leads to complete obstruction unless there is a complicating local abscess or an impacted foreign body, usually of dietary origin (e.g., corn kernels, berries, peach pits). *Free perforation* of the ileum is reported with increasing frequency in recent years; usually, however, perforation of the bowel is confined by surrounding tissues and leads to sinus formation. *Massive hemorrhage* occurs in less than 5 per cent of patients with Crohn's disease of the small intestine, occasioned at times by stercorous ulceration proximal to a stenotic area. *Fistulization* may be considered an integral part of the basic disease; however, fistulas to the urinary bladder deserve some additional comment. Passage of frank feces through the urethra is quickly recognized by the patient. The passage of air or gas through the urethra, however, may require detailed specific inquiry by the physician. (This is also true of the passage of gas from the vagina.) Despite the frequently expressed fear of ascending urinary tract infections in the presence of an ileovesical fistula, patients tolerate this condition surprisingly well.

Renal Complications. *Uric acid* and *oxalate stones* have already been stressed. Right *hydronephrosis* and *hydroureter* from obstruction caused by a retroperitoneal inflammatory mass usually create few symptoms, and the urine is rarely infected. *Renal amyloidosis* is more common in Crohn's disease than in ulcerative colitis. The writer has seen five instances in a series of 17 patients dying of ileitis in which the renal amyloid contributed to death.

Although *carcinoma* of the ileum or jejunum is rare, the 46 reported instances of adenocarcinoma in longstanding Crohn's disease of the ileum, especially in excluded intestine, suggest that this is more than a matter of chance. Cancer in a "bypassed" loop is even more treacherous to diagnose, because these segments are almost always stenotic.

Neurologic Complications. Neurologic complications in the form of "startle reactions," tetany, and grand mal seizures, have been observed, usually on the basis of electrolyte and fluid disturbances, mainly hypocalcemia and hypomagnesemia. The clinical setting is one of a patient with profuse diarrhea, receiving steroids and intravenous fluids free of magnesium. We have seen a few patients with concurrent multiple sclerosis, one of whom had a diffuse vasculitis. Three of our younger patients suffered thrombosis of the middle cerebral artery without evidence of atherosclerosis, which may be related to thrombocytosis.

DIAGNOSIS. The history of malaise, anorexia with weight loss, and abdominal pain, especially in the right lower quadrant associated with increasing nonbloody diarrhea, together with the finding of thickened loops of intestine or a mass in the right lower quadrant, makes the diagnosis of Crohn's disease of the small bowel highly probable. The finding of an anal lesion or perirectal abscess or fistula or a cutaneous fistula increases the certainty of this diagnosis. Short of resection of bowel for histologic confirmation, characteristic x-ray findings in the small bowel (Fig. 2) confirm the diagnosis. Although the pathology of early regional enteritis may be insufficient to make the disease evident on barium contrast meal, patients with Crohn's disease should not be treated without x-ray confirmation. If the

Figure 2. Involvement of terminal ileum in regional enteritis. Note narrowing of lumen with hoselike configuration of ileal contours.

terminal ileum fails to visualize on barium enema examination because of failure of the barium to reflux from colon into ileum, an upper gastrointestinal series with small bowel follow-through is indicated. Failure to visualize adequately the terminal ileum with barium by mouth is the most frequent reason for the failure to find radiographic confirmation of a strong clinical impression. The characteristic x-ray finding is segmental involvement of the bowel, most frequently the terminal ileum; at times, several segments of the ileum may be separated by "skip areas" of normal intervening bowel. Thickened, edematous mucosa with a "cobblestone" appearance reflects the submucosal cellular aggregates. Aphthous ulceration may be demonstrated on occasion. Narrowing of the lumen, the so-called "string sign," represents a functionally contracted irritable segment, or, in a later stage of the disease, fibrotic stenosis. Progressive thickening of the bowel wall stiffens the loops, which may be widely separated because of the thickened swollen mesentery, agglutinated by serosal inflammatory changes, or draped over a right lower quadrant inflammatory mass. The presence of sinus tracts and fistulas to adjacent loops of small or large bowel, especially the cecum or sigmoid colon, are classic findings. With the development of stenosis, dilatation of proximal loops of gut appears, together with pseudodiverticula. In the less common ileojejunitis, similar changes are found throughout contiguous loops of jejunum and ileum.

Rectal biopsy is rarely of use diagnostically except when amyloidosis is suspected or an obvious anal lesion is present. Biopsy of the perirectal fistula may reveal the characteristic granuloma.

DIFFERENTIAL DIAGNOSIS. The differential diagnosis includes *acute appendicitis, appendiceal abscess, cecal diverticulitis* with localized perforation, *ovarian carcinoma, carcinoma* of the *cecum* invading the ileum, *lymphosarcoma, Hodgkin's disease, lymphoid hyperplasia, ileocecal tuberculosis, ileal carcinoid,* and the *"backwash" ileitis* of ulcerative colitis. In diagnosis of regional jejunitis, *nod-*

ular lymphoid hyperplasia with dysgammaglobulinemia, the *erosive jejunitis* of *Zollinger-Ellison syndrome,* nonspecific *erosive jejunitis,* and *metastatic melanocarcinoma* must be considered. The differential diagnosis for *regional ileojejunitis* includes *nodular lymphoid hyperplasia* with dysgammaglobulinemia, *lymphosarcoma,* the *diffuse nonerosive ileojejunitis* reported on occasion in patients with *sprue, diffuse nongranulomatous ileojejunitis,* and prior *severe ischemia* of *small intestines.*

Of this list only a few diseases present real problems. *Acute appendicitis* may be extremely difficult to separate from an acute episode of regional ileitis in the absence of an antecedent history of bowel problems. Exploration is the method of choice if any doubt exists; current experience justifies removal of the normal appendix to prevent confusion in the future if the cause of the patient's syndrome is Crohn's disease of the ileum; fecal fistulas arise mainly from unsatisfactory surgical technique in manipulating the ileum, not from the appendiceal stump. Extremely rarely, Crohn's disease may be confined to the appendix. Patients with known Crohn's disease of the ileum only rarely develop acute appendicitis.

Appendiceal abscess frequently cannot be distinguished from regional enteritis with right lower quadrant mass, and the roentgenographic findings in the ileum may mimic ileitis. Occasionally the disappearance of the abscess and clearing of ileal x-ray changes under the influence of antimicrobial drugs may resolve this clinical dilemma.

Lymphosarcoma usually occupies longer segments than the ileum, often extending across the ileocecal valve; although the appearances are similar in some respects, roentgenograms usually show no luminal narrowing as noted in regional ileitis. Further, and most important, the clinical picture is quite different.

Ileocecal tuberculosis is a rare disease in the United States and therefore rarely considered in the differential diagnosis in patients without pulmonary tuberculosis. However, this diagnosis is important to consider in patients with pulmonary tuberculosis and ileocecal disease, or in areas of the globe where tuberculosis—especially milk-borne tuberculosis—is very common. At times the differential diagnosis cannot be made except at laparotomy. A negative tuberculin test in a patient with ileal disease is more likely found with Crohn's disease than with tuberculous enteritis. Moreover, tuberculous enteritis most often involves ileum and cecum; thus patients with disease confined to the ileum most often have Crohn's disease, but since ileocecal disease is found both in granulomatous colitis and in tuberculous enteritis, the distribution of the lesions is rarely helpful in distinguishing these two diseases.

Carcinoid of the ileum usually presents no problem, except when it is invasive, and the x-ray appearance may resemble regional enteritis. The innocuous *lymphoid hyperplasia* of the ileum seen in young patients is easily distinguished from the acute inflammatory changes seen in regional enteritis. This is true also of the roentgenographic changes of *nodular lymphoid hyperplasia* with dysgammaglobulinemia.

Some special problems arise in patients with known regional enteritis. The problem of right lower quadrant suppuration and appendicitis has been discussed. The coexistence of ileitis and cancer of the right ovary and/or cecum has tripped the unwary. One must be alert for the development of *adenocarcinoma* of the *ileum* in the stenotic phase of ileitis, or in patients who have had "bypass" operations in the past.

"Backwash ileitis" is a poor but widely used term to describe the changes in a short segment of terminal ileitis associated with universal ulcerative colitis, and diagnosed by barium enema. It should be distinguished from regional enteritis and does not represent clinically significant disease. It probably represents a direct extension of the associated ulcerative colitis through a patulous ileocecal valve, and is confined to the mucosal surface. It is easily separated from classic regional ileitis, but its distinction from ileocolitis of the Crohn variety may be difficult at times.

Eosinophilic gastroenteritis is also important in the differential diagnosis, especially of ileojejunitis. This illness, usually associated with a significant blood and tissue eosinophilia representing a response in some to a dietary allergy, may present with diarrhea, malabsorption, and protein-losing enteropathy. The stomach, duodenum, and entire small bowel may be involved alone or in various combinations. Although it is superficially similar to Crohn's disease, the intestinal films do not present with the characteristic infiltrated thickened loops of the latter disease; further, strictures and fistula are not present.

TREATMENT. There is no known specific therapy for this disorder. Accordingly, treatment is essentially supportive. It is empirical; its efficiency is still undetermined; and it involves review of the patient's activity, dietary intake, life style, and personal habits. It also requires consideration of a number of drugs currently employed in the management of ileitis and imposes important decisions regarding the necessity of surgical intervention. It also requires an awareness of the mortality rate, ranging from 5 to 18 per cent.

Medical Management. All approaches to the medical management of the patient with regional enteritis begin with an awareness of the high rate of recurrence (up to 90 per cent in some series) after operation. Accordingly, the current therapeutic stance of most experienced clinicians in this field is one of surgical conservatism unless the patient cannot be managed medically in the presence of a continuously unfavorable course or some of the more dramatic complications.

Although it has yet to be shown that prolonged rest favorably affects this illness, management of the patient must begin with an evaluation of the patient's energy balance. Caloric intake usually being suboptimal, some restriction of energy expenditure is clearly in order. This is an individual matter, but all patients must establish and accept some limitations of activity. Although the physician must avoid being arbitrary, he will have to be firm in some situations.

Efforts to improve the patient's nutritional status are necessary and difficult. The victim of this illness must be encouraged to take a well-balanced, high caloric, high protein diet. Care must be taken to discourage food faddism and avoid arbitrarily conceived medical dietary advice. The patient's ability to tolerate milk and milk-containing products should be the criterion for lactose intake rather than a lactose tolerance test. Most patients have already established their tolerance by the time they see the physician. In the presence of profuse diarrhea or stenotic lesions, some reduction of the noncaloric residue of the diet is prudent. In the patient with stenotic areas of the bowel, the use of such nonresidue diets as Vivamex or Flexical is rational.

However, long-term use is rendered difficult by patient refusal, osmotic diarrheal effects, and cost. For patients with marked reduction in absorptive mucosal surface, medium-chain triglycerides are a reasonable supplement; however, they are often of limited use because of patient reluctance to ingest the oil (free from any lactose fillers) owing to the induction of diarrhea. Vitamin supplementation is rational in view of the restricted food intake of many patients (see Table 5 in Ch. 408). In markedly depleted patients, especially those with diffuse small bowel disease, or in children with retarded growth, total parenteral nutrition can be helpful, especially in preparation for operation in those with localized Crohn's disease.

The anemia of enteritis is rarely due only to vitamin B_{12} deficiency and iron deficiency from bleeding but rather to the effects of the chronic illness on bone marrow synthesis. When there is significant loss of the ileum vitamin B_{12} replacement is required. Oral iron preparations seem to be tolerated poorly by these sick individuals, and a parenteral form such as Imferon is useful.

The symptomatic treatment of abdominal pain, cramps, and diarrhea is an integral part of management. Judicious and temporary use of analgesics, anticholinergics, and opiates is very frequently required. The overuse of deodorized tincture of opium, codeine, or the diphenoxylate and atropine combination (Lomotil) may lead to dependence and addiction.

Antimicrobial Therapy. Antimicrobial drugs modify the symptoms and course of ileitis very little. Local suppurative complications involving gram-negative organisms of the bowel require the appropriate drug; ampicillin, in doses up to 4 grams daily by mouth or 4 to 6 grams intravenously, provides an acceptable regimen. When stenosis, stricture, or surgical bypass with blind loops or small bowel to colon anastomoses leads to intestinal overgrowth with colonic organisms, tetracycline (0.25 gram every four to six hours) may be helpful in treating the attendant vitamin B_{12} deficiency and/or steatorrhea (see Ch. 408). At present some experienced clinicians use ampicillin and/or tetracycline for long-term maintenence therapy with some enthusiasm despite the absence of convincing evidence of usefulness from controlled trials.

For a long time the relatively poorly absorbed sulfonamide derivatives, succinylsulfathiazole and phthalylsulfathiazole in doses of 1.0 to 3.0 grams every six hours were commonly prescribed. More recently, salicylazosulfapyridine (Azulfidine) in doses of 1.0 to 2.0 grams every six hours is the drug more widely used. This sulfonamide whose metabolites are concentrated in the intestinal tissues is a relatively poor antimicrobial agent. The mechanism of its limited usefulness in ulcerative colitis is not known. Its value in Crohn's disease has been demonstrated in a short (four-month) course in moderately sick patients. Its value in maintenance therapy to prevent relapse or protection after operation has not been demonstrated. Adverse reactions to this drug, which include nausea, headache and vomiting, skin rashes, high fever, leukopenia and agranulocytosis, hemolysis, and occasional jaundice, may occur in up to 15 to 20 per cent of patients. Recent studies relate the majority of toxic reactions to the serum levels of sulfapyridine achieved in those taking 4 or more grams daily. Since sulfapyridine is acetylated after absorption and conjugated as a glucuronide in the liver before being excreted in the urine, the majority of patients with adverse effects phenotypically acetylate slowly. It has recently been suggested that its active moiety is its 5-aminosalicylic acid component.

Anti-inflammatory Agents: Corticotropin (ACTH) and Adrenal Corticosteroids. Because these anti-inflammatory agents affect the course of ulcerative colitis favorably, and because ileitis and ulcerative colitis have certain non-intestinal manifestations (arthritis, uveitis, erythema nodosum), adrenocorticosteroids, especially prednisone, are now also widely used in these diseases. They improve the patient's sense of well-being and often stimulate his capricious and depressed appetite. It is doubtful, however, that they have been shown to influence the long-term course of the illness for the better, and they do not affect the histopathology of the disease. Indeed, their hazards impose serious limitations for their long-term use. Yet prednisone is widely used in an attempt to induce remissions in this disorder. The National Cooperative Crohn's Disease Study did indicate that four months of prednisone was superior to placebo but not to azulfidine in the moderately sick patient. Most clinicians, especially pediatricians, aim at an every-other-day dosage schedule. Occasionally, in some desperately ill patients, especially those with diffuse ileojejunitis or recurrent enteritis after multiple resections, the use of corticotropin intravenously (25 units every eight hours continuously) may be more helpful than the conventional doses of prednisone, 40 to 60 mg daily or on alternate-day schedules. However, enthusiasm for corticosteroids must be tempered by the realization that in at least one good recent study a higher than expected mortality for Crohn's disease was related in part to prolonged corticosteroid therapy; however, the series included many patients who were extremely ill.

Immunosuppressive Therapy. Azathioprine (Imuran) was introduced for the therapy of Crohn's disease with fistulas in 1969. Although the National Cooperative Crohn's Disease study found four months of azathioprine to be of no value and the incidence of pancreatitis disturbing, a considerable number of other controlled trials have supported a place for this drug even if only for its steroid sparing and occasional dramatic effect, especially on fistula closure. In daily doses of 1.0 to 1.5 mg per kilogram, this writer has observed no catastrophes when the white blood count remained above 3500. Immunosuppression requires at least 8 to 12 weeks' therapy, and the long-term undesirable effects of this therapy are unknown. Although only patients with renal transplants have thus far been reported to develop lymphomas while being treated with azathioprine, the possible risks of therapy must be balanced against possible untoward effects.

Surgical Therapy. The early expectation that surgical excision would lead to a permanent cure in regional ileitis was soon followed by an era of disillusion based upon increasing evidence of recurrence. Recognition of the limited value of steroid and other current therapy, however, has refocused attention on the effects of surgical therapy. Whether judged by clinical recurrence or reoperation rates, Crohn's disease involving the ileum or ileum and colon has an inexorable tendency to return. When studied by actuarial methods, the cumulative recurrence rate (the ratio of the number of patients experiencing a recurrence during the follow-up year to the number of patients who are at risk for that year) is depressingly high whatever the type of operation used. In our own series, and in some others, this rate was 50 per cent by five years, and more than 75 per cent by ten; our data for 15 years were 91 per

cent for clinical recurrence and 85 per cent for reoperation. The recurrences are usually on the ileal side of the ileocolonic anastomosis; although in some the recurrences are solely radiographic, in others clinical severity parallels the original disease. Since as many as half of the surgically treated patients are faring well at the end of five years, this form of treatment should not be deprecated, especially in the young person when growth and education are critical.

If surgery is elected, the operation of choice is resection of the diseased ileum with an ileoascending colostomy to preserve the right colon for water absorption. These patients may have some period of watery diarrhea after resection with removal of the ileocecal valve. This often responds to bile salt binding therapy with cholestyramine (Questran, 1 to 4 grams daily in divided doses). The mortality and morbidity of this procedure is no higher than that from the older bypass operation (side tracking of the involved ileum with exclusion), and eliminates the risk of the late development of neoplasm in the excluded loop. When a suppurative complication in the right lower quadrant makes resection hazardous, especially an abscess or inflammatory mass encroaching on the right ureter, a bypass operation is to be preferred. Few factors are known to influence recurrence rate after surgery. The rate is higher in patients whose symptoms first appeared below the age of 40, and is higher the more extensive the involvement of the small bowel.

The indications for surgery are the obvious ones of intestinal obstruction, massive hemorrhage, and fistulization to the bladder. An internal fistula between adjacent loops of bowel or an intra-abdominal mass per se does not necessarily indicate surgery. A cutaneous fistula, often after exploratory laparotomy and appendectomy, may on occasion close under medical treatment but usually requires surgery. The more difficult clinical problem is the patient who fails to improve or deteriorates under our current supportive management. This patient can be remarkably helped, albeit often temporarily, by resection. On occasion, severe or nonhealing perirectal fistulas are an indication for resection of proximal ileal disease.

PROGNOSIS. Regional enteritis is a disease of quite variable course. It has the interesting characteristic of not spreading in a retrograde fashion in the absence of surgery. Extension to sigmoid or cecum by fistulization, however, is common. Over-all, mortality ranges from 5 to 18 per cent; however, it is from 4 to 12 per cent when related to the ileitis itself. In view of current unsatisfactory medical therapy, it is not surprising that the majority of patients ultimately come to operation, many of whom have multiple procedures. Thus in one surgical center, of 332 patients with Crohn's disease (large as well as small bowel), 295 sooner or later were submitted to surgical treatment, with an operative mortality of 5.8 per cent.

Crohn, B. B., Ginzberg, L., and Oppenheimer, G. D.: Regional ileitis: A pathologic and clinical entity. JAMA, 99:1323, 1932.

Gerson, C. D., Cohen, N., and Janowitz, H. D.: Small intestinal absorptive function in regional enteritis. Gastroenterology, 64:907, 1973.

Janowitz, H. D., and Sachar, D. B.: New observations in Crohn's disease. Ann. Rev. Med., 27:269, 1976.

Monk, M., Mendeloff, A., Siegel, C., and Lilienfeld, A.: An epidemiological study of ulcerative colitis and regional enteritis among adults in Baltimore. I. Hospital incidence and prevalence, 1960 to 1963. Gastroenterology, 53:198, 1967. II. Social and demographic factors. Gastroenterology, 56:847, 1969.

Strickland, R. G., and Sachar, D. B.: The immunology of inflammatory bowel disease. In Glass, G. B. J. (ed.): Progress in Gastroenterology, Vol. III. New York, Grune & Stratton, 1977, pp. 821–838.

413.3.   ULCERATIVE COLITIS

Ulcerative colitis is an inflammatory disease of unknown cause which involves the mucosa of the colon. Confined in some patients to the rectum, involving the left colon in many, it may also involve the entire colon. Its onset may be acute and fulminant, and its course often continues chronically in an intermittent or continuous form. Diarrhea is a common symptom and bleeding is an almost constant concomitant symptom, because friability in the mucosa is an integral feature of the illness. Although ulcerative colitis is capable of the most startling resolution and reversal, the more typical course is one of unpredictable recurrences. Thus like the more recently defined Crohn's disease, ulcerative colitis constitutes an enigmatic clinical entity.

INCIDENCE, PREVALENCE, AND EPIDEMIOLOGY. Estimating the incidence and prevalence of ulcerative colitis is difficult. Most estimates are based on studies of hospitalized patients. Some patients — particularly those with disease confined to the rectosigmoid colon (ulcerative proctitis) — have such mild symptoms that they are not commonly hospitalized and hence are not accounted for in such surveys. Also, physicians are reluctant to examine and investigate thoroughly patients with mild chronic diarrhea or children with diarrheal disorders; thus some of these patients may have undiagnosed ulcerative colitis. Finally, granulomatous colitis (Crohn's colitis) cannot always be distinguished on clinical grounds from ulcerative colitis.

Incidence rates (rate of occurrence of the disease per 100,000 persons at risk per year): In a study of the Oxford area, the incidence was 7.3 for females and 5.2 for males, for an average of 6.5. In a Baltimore study of hospitalized patients over 20 years of age, the corresponding figures were 5.2 and 3.9, for an average of 4.6. To these figures should be added the incidence of ulcerative proctitis, which may range from 3 to 6.

Prevalence (all the patients affected with this disease per 100,000 persons at risk): In the United Kingdom, the data suggest that for each patient admitted to a hospital for the first time with ulcerative colitis, there were 12 patients at large in the population with the same disease. The range of prevalence for this disease has been estimated for proctitis as 40 to 80, and for ulcerative colitis as 35 to 70.

Although inflammatory bowel disease as a whole is being increasingly recognized, there is no evidence to support impressions of increasing incidence of ulcerative colitis. In the United States, between 200,000 and 400,000 persons have been estimated to suffer from the disease, with between 25,000 and 30,000 new cases each year. In almost all series there is a preponderance of females over males. The first peak of incidence occurs between the ages of 20 and 25, as in Crohn's disease. Again, almost all series show a second rise in incidence in the decade from age 50 to 60. Kirsner and coworkers have suggested that this second peak may be related to mesenteric vascular disease. In the Baltimore study the urban black population was one third as likely to have ulcerative colitis as the white population. Among veterans of World War II in England and the United States, the incidence of ulcerative colitis among Jewish patients was two to four times greater than might be expected. In the Baltimore study the frequency of ulcerative colitis among Jews was 3.5 times the rate for non-Jews. Although impressions exist that the ulcerative colitis population has a higher socioeconomic and educational status than the general population, careful analysis does not confirm this.

GENETICS. As with Crohn's disease, there is no simple mendelian genetic mechanism operative. Aggregation of families includes both ulcerative colitis and Crohn's disease; the incidence of familial disease is higher for Crohn's disease alone than for ulcerative colitis alone. In a recent study from Chicago, only 4 per cent of the control population had a family history of such bowel disease, whereas 11 per cent of those with chronic inflammatory disease had a family history of the same. Jews dominated this group and with onset at significantly lower age (under age 20). Ulcerative colitis has been recorded in eight pairs of monozygotic twins with concordance in five. The association of *ankylosing spondylitis* with ulcerative colitis is similar to that of Crohn's disease. It may be that these two diseases have different environmental causes but occur in the same families because the genotypes determining susceptibility have genes in common.

ETIOLOGY. In the more than 100 years since Samuel Wilks separated nonspecific ulcerative colitis from epidemic forms of dysentery, many etiologic agents and concepts have been advanced. None has been convincingly demonstrated. No virus, bacterium, or protozoon has been shown to be specifically related to the disease. Occasionally after an epidemic of bacillary dysentery, a few individuals will be left with chronic ulcerative colitis, but this occurs in only a small minority. The disease occurring simultaneously in husband and wife is extremely rare, indicating that an environmental agent alone is not responsible; however, the presence of lymphocytotoxins in some spouses and household contacts again raises the possibility of such an agent. The relatively isolated dramatic response of the disease to withdrawal of milk from the diet has always raised the question of specific allergic factors.

Since all experienced clinicians have been impressed with exacerbation of ulcerative colitis in the setting of tensions, conflicts, and anxiety of their patients, much emphasis has been placed on the role of psychosomatic factors in initiating and perpetuating this disorder. George Engle, the most persuasive recent investigator of this aspect, has stressed the obsessive-compulsive immaturity of these patients and the dependency on parent or parent surrogate figures, and emphasized the "hopeless and helpless" reaction they experience at the loss of these figures by death, rejection, or removal. In similar approaches it is assumed that disturbances in secretory, vascular, and motor responses are mediated through the autonomic nervous system. Why only the colon should respond is obscure. More recently, these concepts have been both challenged and ignored by workers in the field. In the Baltimore study, in which the control population (patients with the irritable colon syndrome) and those with ulcerative colitis were meticulously interrogated for psychosomatic factors in their history, the results did not demonstrate that patients with inflammatory bowel disease had unusual health histories or significantly more of those factors which could be interpreted as evidence of life stresses and failure to adapt to them; indeed, there were more such factors in the patients with the irritable colon syndrome. Attention should also be paid to the failure of experienced clinicians to document the transition of the irritable colon syndrome into ulcerative colitis. However, the relatively crude investigative techniques used in these studies do not meet the criticism of more sophisticated psychiatrists. The inconclusive reports of the results of psychologic therapy cannot be interpreted in terms of etiology. Although the psychosomatic concept remains unproved, this does not gainsay the need to understand the emotional setting in which ulcerative colitis appears and exacerbates.

Immunologic mechanisms now occupy the forefront of investigations into the etiology, encouraged both by the concomitant presence of manifestations of hypersensitivity states such as *erythema nodosum, arthritis,* and *uveitis* and by the response to steroid therapy. More than 15 per cent of patients have high titers of circulating antibodies against colonic epithelial mucopolysaccharide antigens, and against certain cross-reacting bacterial lipopolysaccharide antigens, especially those of *E. coli* 014. These antibodies can bind to intestinal epithelial cells in vitro. But it has never been possible to demonstrate that these antibodies possess cytotoxic activity, or even that these antibodies are bound to colonic tissue in vivo. Anticolon antibodies also have been found in clinically healthy relatives of colitis patients, and classic ulcerative colitis has been reported in a patient with agammaglobulinemia. There is presently no evidence that anticolon or cross-reacting antibacterial antibodies in ulcerative colitis play any pathogenetic role in the disease. Individual patients with ulcerative colitis may have elevated serum levels of immunoglobulins and of secretory IgA in particular, in the presence of longstanding disease; but as a group, ulcerative colitis patients have no statistically different serum immunoglobulin levels or patterns from the general population, nor is there any consistent correlation between immunoglobulin patterns and disease severity. There is, however, some evidence to suggest that circulating immunoglobulins might be sequestered in diseased bowel, because a fall in concentration can be demonstrated across inferior mesenteric artery and vein during active disease. Moreover, serum IgM has been shown to rise acutely after bowel resection, but this is now interpreted as an acute phase reactant. Formation of antigen-antibody complexes in ulcerative colitis consumes the C1q component of complement. Pathologic processes might bind or catabolize immunoglobulins in diseased tissue in ulcerative colitis and initiate the formation of circulating immune complexes. Although no role has been identified for immunoglobulins in pathogenesis, circulating immune complexes could underlie such extracolonic manifestations as arthritis or erythema nodosum.

Lymphocytes from patients with ulcerative (and granulomatous) colitis are cytotoxic to intestinal epithelial cells in vivo and in vitro. There is also a cytopathic IgM antibody in the serum of patients with ulcerative colitis that confers this property upon normal lymphocytes. Neither lymphocyte cytotoxicity nor circulating cytopathic antibody reflects a basic underlying immune disorder in ulcerative colitis, because both disappear very rapidly when the inflamed colon is removed.

A considerable number of patients with inflammatory bowel disease manifest a variety of defects in their cellular immune systems, including depressed in vitro lymphocyte responses to phytohemagglutinin and depressed peripheral blood T lymphocyte counts. About half of our patients demonstrated cutaneous anergy to dinitrochlorobenzene, which was not present in spouses or first-degree relatives, and which persisted in Crohn's disease subjects but disappeared in ulcerative colitis patients after resection of diseased tissue.

Transmission studies of ulcerative colitis, using human colon injected into a variety of animals, remain in a confused state at present; they require systematic confirmation.

PATHOLOGY AND PATHOGENESIS. In contrast to the characteristic histopathologic features of Crohn's disease, the pathologic changes in ulcerative colitis are even more nonspecific. Throughout its course ulcerative colitis generally remains a disorder of the mucosa and submucosa of the colon. Under unusual circumstances the histopathologic process may extend through the muscular layer to reach the mucosa and may penetrate through the serosa.

The increasing use of rectal biopsy has made it possible to document the early pathologic features. The earliest lesion appears to involve the base of the crypts of Lieberkühn in the form of infiltration with polymorphonuclear leukocytes at the tip of the crypts with degenerative changes in the overlying epithelial cells. This is followed by the development of crypt abscesses with extension of the polymorphonuclear infiltrate into the crypts and necrosis of the crypt epithelium. A more heterogeneous cellular inflammatory reaction supervenes, involving lymphocytes, plasma cells, mast cells, and eosinophils, with vascular dilatation and engorgement. These so-called microabscesses of the crypts may next coalesce and separate the overlying mucosa from the lamina propria and its blood supply, producing ulceration of the mucosal surface and even its denudation. The extension of crypt abscess and ulceration results in the formation of residual islands of mucosa with undetermined edges. These fragments of epithelial tissue constitute the pathologic basis of *pseudopolyps.* Concurrent healing leads to some collagen deposition, but fibrosis is not prominent. Hypertrophy of the muscularis mucosae may also develop. Ineffective healing and regeneration lead to the presence of thin atrophic epithelium. These features are far from specific; similar changes have been described in a variety of infectious colitides, including *shigellosis* and *gonococcal infection,* and even in *amebic colitis.* However, the chronic recurrent nature of the changes, especially the crypt abscesses, and the development of either the atrophic mucosa or the multiple pseudopolypoid reactions are quite characteristic. Shortening of the bowel with narrowing of the lumen, loss of haustrations, and stricture formation in chronic cases appear to result infrequently from fixed fibrotic changes but more often from spasm and hypertrophy of the muscularis mucosae, which may account for their reversibility on occasion. Such reversals stand in marked contrast to the course of luminal narrowing in Crohn's disease.

In more severe forms the inflammatory necrotizing process may extend through all coats of the colon, leading to the clinical situation known as *toxic megacolon.* Here all elements are involved in the inflammatory reaction, and a vasculitis (swelling of the vascular endothelium, inflammatory changes in vessel walls, necrosis of blood vessels, and local thrombosis) is prominent. The inflammatory changes in the neural elements (especially ganglion cells) and musculature of the colon may account for the characteristic dilatation in toxic megacolon. The extension of the pathologic process to the serosa, with deep ulceration through the muscular walls, together with loss of tone, sets the stage for free or walled-off perforations, more frequently diagnosed than found at laparotomy.

Grossly, the anatomic extent of the process differs widely. Perhaps as many as half the patients have the disease limited to the rectum alone, *ulcerative proctitis,* whose microscopic pathology in no way is different. Of the remainder, perhaps less than half involve the rectum and the left side of the colon from sigmoid to most of the descending colon. About one third of all patients have universal colitis. In about one fifth of the patients with involvement of the entire colon there is some superficial disease in the terminal ileum for a distance of 8 to 12 inches. The pathologic nature of "segmental colitis" involving portions of the right colon with significant ileal disease is that of Crohn's disease or regional (granulomatous) enterocolitis.

CLINICAL MANIFESTATIONS.   The wide diversity of clinical presentations is part of the highly variable course of this disease. Its onset may be most insidious or of catastrophic abruptness. In some patients (perhaps half) the initial symptoms of malaise, mild lower abdominal discomfort with slight increase in frequency, and softening of the stool with small amounts of blood are vaguely recalled. In another quarter of patients, the onset is more intense and more easily dated, often related by the patient to an upper respiratory infection, a "stomach virus," or a specific emotional trauma. More intense lower abdominal cramping pain, an increased number of loose to watery stools containing blood and often waking the patient at night, and mild systemic symptoms of easy fatigability and low-grade fever are characteristic of this moderately severe group. Perhaps in 15 per cent of patients there is an onset with profuse bloody diarrhea, high fever up to 39.5 to 40° C, and severe abdominal diffuse pain. Such a sudden onset with fever and frequent bowel movements has been shown to portend a grave outcome.

Paralleling the diversity of the mode of presentation is the variability of the clinical course. A very small group will have but one attack and go into prolonged remission for years. The majority will have a chronic intermittent course with asymptomatic remissions between recurring attacks. The remainder (perhaps 5 to 15 per cent) will have a chronic, continuous, progressively relentless course. The outlook for survival after any episode is directly related to its severity. In an attack of mild disease the patient has few stools and lacks tachycardia, fever, and loss of appetite, whereas the patient with severe disease has severe bleeding, fever, anemia, and lowered serum albumin. Patients with mild disease rarely die, but as many as 35 per cent of those with severe attacks may die.

Those with mild colitis may also have vague lower abdominal distress, minor variations in the number and consistency of stools, and small amounts of rectal bleeding. This group of patients have few or no constitutional symptoms, except for perhaps a slight falling off of appetite. The patients usually continue their full activities, and if bleeding is not stressed, their symptoms may be interpreted as part of the irritable colon syndrome. Although in some the pathologic process is confined to the rectum or rectosigmoid, the mucosa of the entire colon may be involved as demonstrated by colonoscopy. The group with the more limited distal disease, "ulcerative proctitis" or "idiopathic proctitis," may have all the attendant clinical features, both local and extraintestinal, as the more diffuse variants. Usually, however, the effects of illness are not striking, and reassuringly it tends to remain localized. Further, the immediate and long-term mortality in this variant is negligible and the risk of cancer is much reduced.

Immediate in intensity, morbidity, and mortality between the "proctitis" variety and the severe form which may be fulminant and catastrophic is the group whose

disease is moderate, about one quarter of patients. Diffuse lower abdominal pain, increasing number of stools both by day and — more troublesome — by night, tenesmus, more marked rectal bleeding than in the mild form, some anorexia, and low-grade fever (37 to 37.5° C) are associated with disinclination to carry on usual activities.

The most dramatic and frightening presentation of ulcerative colitis is the severe disease which fulminates. Without any antecedent history, or in the first attack, or in the chronic course of mild and moderately severe ulcerative colitis, the illness begins explosively with high fever, profuse bleeding, marked diarrhea with profuse watery stools, associated with diffuse abdominal crampy pain, and prostration. With the extension of the pathologic process throughout all the coats of the colon, marked dilatation of the colon, "toxic dilatation" or "toxic megacolon," supervenes (Fig. 3). Death in an acute attack of ulcerative colitis is most frequent in this group.

In ulcerative colitis, as in Crohn's disease, certain extraintestinal manifestations may accompany the disease and parallel the "colitis" activity; areas affected include skin (erythema nodosum and pyoderma gangrenosum), eye (iritis and conjunctivitis), joints (migratory and polyarthritic), and mouth (stomatitis and aphthous ulcers). History-taking in the ulcerative colitis patient does not reveal any strikingly associated diseases except ankylosing spondylitis. In contrast to Crohn's disease, these extraintestinal manifestations rarely precede the intestinal symptoms.

PHYSICAL EXAMINATION.   In the mild forms, examination usually reveals no significant findings. In the more severe forms the physical examination reveals the ill, dehydrated, acutely or chronically sick and feverish patient. There may be diffuse abdominal tenderness, but except in patients with "toxic megacolon" or perforation, there is no evidence of peritonitis, localized or general. Direct visceral tenderness on pressure over the inflamed colon may be difficult to distinguish from peritoneal irritation. The spleen is rarely palpable. The skin, eye, and joint

Figure 3. Dilatation of the transverse colon in fulminating ulcerative colitis.

manifestations can at times all be present. Clubbing of the fingers and toes is rare in the absence of small bowel involvement.

LABORATORY STUDIES.   Routine studies reveal a degree of blood loss which may be profound. Marked leukocytosis is usually present, as high, indeed, as 35,000 to 40,000. Remarkable increases in platelets may also be recorded in these same patients, and may play a role in thromboembolic phenomena and parallel the rapid erythrocyte sedimentation rate. A hemolytic anemia may occur, usually in those receiving salicylazosulfapyridine (Azulfidine), but a Coombs-positive autoimmune hemolytic anemia may be present unrelated to sulfonamides. A prolonged prothrombin time may result from associated liver damage, or from the effects of antimicrobial drugs on intestinal bacterial synthesis of vitamin K. A reduction in platelets and fibrinogen levels may document disseminated intravascular coagulation. Fluid, electrolyte, and serum losses lead to marked reduction in levels of serum potassium and albumin. Blood zinc levels may decline in those receiving ACTH or total parenteral nutrition. The flat film of the abdomen usually reveals some gas in the colon, and allows visualization of the thickened edematous colonic wall.

MECHANISMS OF DISEASE MANIFESTATIONS.   Rectal bleeding arises from friability of the colonic mucosa and deeper ulceration. The cause of this friability (manifested by the elicitation of bleeding when the surface is gently stroked at sigmoidoscopy with a cotton swab, a pathognomonic feature of the disease) is undetermined, although some evidence suggests increased local concentration of fibrinolysins. The anemia is secondary to blood loss, usually grossly visible; on occasion, however, occult bleeding may continue from the friable mucosa. Chronic colonic bleeding may give rise to *iron deficiency anemia*. Azulfidine-related and rare idiopathic hemolytic anemias also contribute to the anemia. Hypoalbuminemia ensues as the result of colonic loss of serum albumin from altered, more permeable mucosa, although diminished protein intake (caused by loss of appetite) and, rarely, liver disease contribute to a limited extent. The diarrhea, which may be profound, results from the inability of the damaged colonic mucosa to reabsorb water and sodium and from the increased secretion of potassium.

DISTURBANCES IN COLONIC MOTILITY.   The colon is primarily a storage or reservoir organ, and the motility waves ordinarily recorded from it (designated types I, II, and III) are of low amplitude and are believed to have a segmenting, restraining, or mixing function. The "mass movement" activity of the colon which results in evacuation and defecation is associated with the normal, rarely occurring, large amplitude type IV wave, which may reach 80 to 100 cm of water pressure. Colonic pain and frequency of rectal evacuation in ulcerative colitis have been associated with a marked increase in type IV activity; there is also some increase in type I and lack of type III (increase in tone superimposed on type I or II). The net effect is a reduction in segmenting but an increase in propulsive motility.

DIAGNOSIS.   Ulcerative colitis is a syndrome — a constellation of clinical features — an abnormal, inflamed colonic mucosa (demonstrated by sigmoidoscopy and barium enema) and a characteristic histologic substrate (demonstrated by rectal biopsy). Since the disease by definition is mucosal in location, the sigmoidoscopic examination is the single most important diagnostic tool, and will establish the diagnosis in 95 to 98 per cent of cases, because the rectosigmoid is almost universally involved. On occasion the lesion is patchy, and the rectum

may not be clearly involved (often as a result of local steroid therapy); in these few instances colonoscopy, which is dangerous in the acutely inflamed colon of the sick patient, may be useful. On sigmoidoscopy the earliest changes are edema and hyperemia of the mucosa, which give the granular appearance. This is followed by the development of such fragility that gentle wiping with cotton, or the pressure of the instrument alone, leads to bleeding. This finding is the most characteristic. The colon bleeds spontaneously as well. Discrete ulcerations are not seen frequently on sigmoidoscopy, but the mucopurulent, slightly foul exudate is characteristic. Pseudopolyps are also hallmarks (Fig. 4). In most the diagnosis can be easily made by sigmoidoscopy; in some cases, however, the findings are extremely subtle, with friability the only positive finding. Here rectal biopsy may be helpful, with cellular infiltration, crypt abscesses, and atrophic epithelium (denudation of glands, evidence of previous mucosal ulceration). When the sigmoidoscopic examination is positive, there is little point in rectal biopsy except for serial study of the course of the patient; however, when the sigmoidoscopic lesion is equivocal, biopsy may be helpful in the differential diagnosis from Crohn's disease, and in diagnosis of concomitant amebiasis and amyloidosis.

RADIOLOGIC FINDINGS.   Examination of the colon by barium enema is needed to determine the extent of disease for permanent recording, and to detect such complications as stricture, polyps, or cancer. Care must be used in the selection of patients for this examination. In the desperately ill patient, it is not only necessary but dangerous. The preparation of the colon for examination is also a serious concern. Cathartics and laxatives should not be used; rather, reliance is placed on several days of low-residue diet and gentle saline or tapwater enemas.

In the *acute stage* the roentgenographic findings are secondary to edema, ulceration, and alterations in motility. Spasm with narrowing and incomplete filling is associated with secretions within the lumen. Ulcerations are tiny and produce serrations along the contour of the filled bowel or small spicules in the film after evacuation. The bowel wall is fuzzy, and as ulceration proceeds "collar button"–like projections appear. In the *moderate* or *moderately severe stage*, the roentgenographic features are due to

Figure 4.   Diffuse ulcerative colitis with pseudopolyposis.

Figure 5. Evacuation film of colon of same patient as in Figure 4.

continued ulceration, beginning fibrosis, and epithelial regeneration, and pseudopolyps are the prominent features (Fig. 5). The results are shortening of the bowel, rigidity, and narrowing of the bowel lumen. The haustral markings, which are often missing in the normal left colon, disappear throughout. Some of the alterations in the shape of the colon are secondary to smooth muscle hypertrophy rather than collagen deposition. In this stage a patulous ileocecal valve allows visualization of the terminal ileum, which may (in 5 to 15 per cent of cases) have minimal involvement of the mucosa without narrowing of the lumen. In some patients early in the disease the barium enema may be entirely within normal limits. In others with "proctitis" the retrorectal space, which is increased owing to spasm and fibrosis of the rectal segment of the colon, may be the only evidence that this area has been involved in an inflammatory reaction.

DIFFERENTIAL DIAGNOSIS. Clinical presentation, the sigmoidoscopic findings, and the roentgenographic appearance usually establish the diagnosis with a high degree of accuracy. Yet certain other syndromes present real problems. Some acute *infectious colitides*, particularly shigellosis, may mimic the picture of acute fulminant colitis but usually are not chronic. The patient with the *irritable bowel syndrome* may have lower abdominal distress, intermittent cramps, and diarrhea. However, fever, the systemic symptoms, night stools, and bloody evacuations are absent, and a normal sigmoidoscopy establishes the difference authoritatively. *Amebic colitis* may be distinguished with some difficulty from acute ulcerative colitis, although the conventional teaching is that the ulcerations of amebic infection are larger and separated by islands of intact mucosa. If direct aspirates of the lesions fail to disclose the motile trophozoites, rectal biopsy may help by demonstrating them in the tissue. The patient with classic *ischemic colitis* is usually over 50 years of age, and has evidence of atherosclerotic vascular disease. However, *infarction of the colon* may be seen in young women taking oral contraceptive pills. The clinical picture of abrupt onset of lower abdominal pain, crampy in nature, fever, and rectal bleeding may mimic the acute onset of fulminant colitis, but the course with progression to gangrene or resolution with stricture formation helps to distinguish it. The typical x-ray features of intramural hemorrhage and edema with "thumbprinting" also help. But the occasional involvement of the rectosigmoid by ischemic colitis adds to the complexity of the differential diagnosis, because the proctoscopic features resemble nonspecific "proctitis." *Radiation colitis,* usually seen after radium treatment for carcinoma of the cervix, and occasionally seen in men after radiation and abdominal lymph node dissection for cancer of the testicle, presents with disturbances of bowel movements and bleeding at a variable time after the original exposure. Distinction from the other nonspecific forms of colitis may be difficult, but the history is all-important. The acute enterocolitis which may occur after a large number of broad-spectrum antimicrobial agents is discussed in Ch. 414.4. *Gonococcal infection* of the rectum should also be considered in the male homosexual population. *Lymphogranuloma venereum* may simulate all the specific and nonspecific forms of proctitis. Positive Frei and complement fixation tests, together with presence or history of inguinal buboes, help establish this diagnosis. *Cancer of the colon* and *diverticulitis of the sigmoid colon* may on occasion have a few clinical features in common with ulcerative colitis, but sigmoidoscopy and barium enema examination usually resolve the question. The interesting and important differential diagnosis of *ulcerative colitis* and *Crohn's disease of the colon* is discussed in Ch. 413.4.

TREATMENT. Medical Therapy. It must be recognized that ulcerative colitis is a disease with an extremely variable course and with no known specific therapy. The aim of therapy is therefore supportive: in the acute episode to reduce the still significant mortality (up to 35 per cent in severe cases), and in the chronic forms to induce and maintain remissions and reduce the number, severity, and duration of exacerbations. Therapy thus includes the establishment of a good relationship between patient and physician in view of the disturbing nature of this illness to recur, correction of nutritional deficits, the restoration of fluid and electrolyte equilibrium, replacement of blood loss, and symptomatic relief of pain and diarrhea.

General Symptomatic Therapy. In all but the mildest forms, a period of restricted energy expenditure with appropriate rest periods is useful, especially if accomplished in a stable supporting environment. The diet should be adequate in total calories, contain enough protein to replace the losses caused by colonic leak and offset the effects of fever, and be palatable enough to appeal to the capricious appetite of these sick patients. Granted that no convincing evidence exists regarding the widely prescribed unpalatable low residue diet, it seems rational during episodes of marked rectal frequency to limit the amount of calorically insignificant cellulose residue of the diet proffered to the already irritated, inflamed colon. There is much anecdotal and a little scientific evidence that some patients dramatically improve on a diet from which cow's milk is excluded. This can be related only in part to intestinal lactase deficiency, but the patient's prior experience should guide the decision to withdraw milk and its products. The place of total parenteral nutrition in ulcerative colitis is uncertain for the acutely ill patient, but may be useful in preparing the chronically depleted one for operation. Massive blood loss requires adequate blood replacement. The anemia of chronically ill patients is in part due to iron deficiency of chronic bleeding, to hemolysis, and to bone marrow failure to incorporate iron. The intolerance of a considerable number of patients to oral iron preparations is genuine, and the use of parenteral iron in the form of dextrose iron complex (Imferon) is justified. Although some apprehension is justified regarding the use of anticholinergics and opiates for the control of pain and diarrhea, because they may play a role in precipitating toxic dilatation of the colon, the judicious use of these agents is valuable on the basis of clinical experience. Tincture of belladonna (15 drops), codeine (15 to 30 mg), deodorized tincture of opium (6 to 10 drops), paregoric (4 to 8 ml), or Lomotil (2.5 to 5 mg) before meals and at bedtime gives the patient considerable comfort.

Antimicrobial Therapy. Salicylazosulfapyridine (Azulfidine) is discussed in Ch. 413.2. This sulfonamide was introduced, however, for the treatment of ulcerative colitis, and in the opinion of most experienced clinicians it has a place in the management of milder forms of ulcerative colitis. The sulfonamide may be the sole drug used in treating patients who have mild disease and who are ambulatory. For those ill enough to be put to bed or hospitalized, however, it is inadequate. When used for those with mild disease, 2 to 8 grams in divided doses is prescribed; in view of the high percentage of patients developing nausea and anorexia or headache, it is wise to begin with smaller doses, or to add an antihistaminic to the regimen. Some clinicians are more comfortable with the use of other, non- or poorly absorbed sulfonamides in this group of patients.

In the sicker patients there is a place for maintenance therapy with the sulfonamide as well as for those who have gone into remission on corticosteroid therapy. In mild or moderately severe disease in remission, Azulfidine in doses of 2 grams per day is more effective in preventing relapses than are corticosteroids. Azulfidine has no place in the fulminatingly ill patient. Other antimicrobials also have no place in the management of ulcerative colitis except in the presence of toxic megacolon and suppurative complications.

Corticotropin (ACTH) and Adrenocorticosteroids. Corticotropin and corticosteroids were introduced into the therapy of ulcerative colitis on the assumption that their anti-inflammatory actions would be useful, especially because certain associated lesions of ulcerative colitis (*arthritis, uveitis,* and *erythema nodosum*) often responded to these compounds, and in the hope of reducing the colonic mucosal inflammatory reaction. Also, these agents stimulate appetite and elevate the patient's mood. Early studies revealed that a short course of cortisone induced an increased incidence of remission of this disease, but the effect was short lived and the long-term benefits have not been demonstrated. Yet the introduction of corticotropin and steroid therapy with newer analogues of cortisone (prednisone or prednisolone) represents an advance in the management of the severe and the moderately severe attack.

In the mild forms, especially in those patients whose disease is confined to the rectosigmoid and distal colon, rectal instillations of steroids are of distinct use in inducing remissions, and their continued intermittent use may maintain remissions. Plastic disposable enema units containing 100 mg of hydrocortisone hemisuccinate or 20 to 40 mg of prednisolone phosphate are commercially available. This form of treatment may be used nightly as a retention enema until remission occurs, and maintained by instillation two to three times weekly. There is good evidence that these instillations may reach large sections of the colon (up to the hepatic flexure). The main effects are local, but some steroids are absorbed and the degree of adrenocortical suppression is minimal. In universal ulcerative colitis and

in those sick enough to be hospitalized, rectal steroid therapy does not appear to be sufficient as the sole form of treatment.

In the moderately ill patient systemic oral steroids are the current drugs of choice. Forty to 60 mg of prednisone or its equivalent is a reasonable initial dose which should induce marked improvement and/or remission within two weeks, at which point it should be slowly tapered. In some patients the remission may be only partial and steroid therapy must be continued. Supplementation with Azulfidine at this point may be wise in the weaning period as well as for maintenance. Stepwise reduction in oral steroids should be continued while clinical well-being is maintained at a reasonably low dose. In view of the serious hazards of long-term corticosteroid therapy, which includes *profound suppression of endogenous adrenal activity, muscle weakness* and *wasting, osteoporosis* and *vertebral collapse, hypertension, diabetes, cosmetic deformities* with their attendant *psychologic disturbances, psychosis,* and *growth retardation* in children, doses above 15 to 20 mg should not be prescribed for longer than six to eight weeks. Although alternate-day therapy minimizes the incidence of undesirable side effects, the suppressive effect on symptoms is also lessened.

In the acutely ill patient with the fulminant presentation, intravenous therapy with corticotropin or corticosteroids is the best current method of management. There is a clinical impression that corticotropin is superior to corticosteroids in this group; this judgment has, however, little supportive objective evidence. In these gravely ill patients corticotropin should be given by continuous intravenous drip, 25 to 40 units per eight-hour period. If there is any question of adrenal responsiveness, intravenous hydrocortisone in doses of 100 mg given over each eight-hour period may be substituted. Fluid overload, sodium retention, and hypokalemia must be meticulously prevented. If a remission is to be achieved, it usually will be obvious within seven to ten days; it is hazardous to continue such therapy beyond 14 days. Failure of discernible response should lead to prompt colectomy at this point. If the expected clinical improvement occurs, the intravenous dose should be gradually reduced and supplemented by orally administered steroids. Dosage in turn is then gradually tapered until the patient can either be weaned or maintained on not more than 15 to 20 mg of prednisolone per day. The regimen may be supplemented in some by Azulfidine at this time.

Other complications of steroid therapy further limit the enthusiastic use of these compounds: *retinopathy, chemosis of lids, adrenocortical insufficiency* from too rapid withdrawal of the drug, or *inadequate adrenocortical reserve* which may persist for months after their use. These agents may mask signs and symptoms of *sepsis* and *colonic perforation.* There is much discussion as to whether high-dose corticotropin or prednisone therapy in the acutely ill patient increases the likelihood of perforation. Certainly in such circumstances the usual clinical signs and symptoms may be concealed. Demonstration of the preservation of liver dullness and measurement of abdominal girth should be part of the daily routine examination of this group of acutely ill patients. The activation of peptic ulcer and the precipitation of massive upper gastrointestinal hemorrhage are further reasons for close observation. Large doses of antacids, avoiding those containing magnesium which may aggravate the diarrhea, are widely and perhaps rationally used; their effectiveness in preventing ulceration and bleeding, however, is unproved. Cumulative experience supports the view that the mortality has been reduced considerably since the introduction of steroids, especially in the moderate to severe group in their acute attacks. It remains to be proved that the long-term outcome has been significantly altered. The earlier use of colectomy appears to be of major importance.

Immunosuppressive Therapy. Immunosuppressive therapy with 6-mercaptopurine (Purinethol) or its metabolite Azathioprine (Imuran) has been used for a number of years for some patients not responsive to steroids or sulfonamides, or in an effort to reduce the dose of steroids needed to induce remission. There are few well controlled trials with azathioprine in ulcerative colitis, but those available suggest that this drug may exert some beneficial effects and allow for the reduction of steroid dosage. However, its toxic effects on the bone marrow, its long-term unknown effects, and its teratogenic and possibly even carcinogenic potential must limit its use, especially as colectomy offers a safe and permanent cure.

Disodium cromoglicate (Aarane), which inhibits mast cell degranulation and suppresses immediate hypersensitivity reactions, has been tried with some success in chronic ulcerative proctitis, given by mouth and locally by enemas; however, this compound is not yet available in the United States in appropriate dosage forms.

Psychotherapy. All who deal with patients with ulcerative colitis recognize the importance of the supportive role that the physician must play in this labile illness; indeed, most doctors act out their psychotherapeutic role intuitively. It is difficult to find convincing evidence that more fomal psychotherapy by psychiatrists or lay analysts alters the long-term course of the illness. Despite this gap in knowledge, there is an obvious place for recommending psychotherapy for those patients and their families in whom personality problems and distorted interpersonal relationships exist. It is more difficult to decide whether all patients should have some exploration of possible psychic conflicts. If this is undertaken, the psychiatrist should be one who has experience with this illness and sensitivity to the often fragile psychic structures of these patients. There is little place for psychotherapy for the patient who is acutely ill. In general, psychotherapy should be reserved for the more quiescent interval phases of the disease.

COMPLICATIONS. Local Complications. These include the development of *anal fissures, rectal prolapse,* and *hemorrhoids* and are to be related to the intensity of the diarrhea. *Perianal abscess* and *fistulas* are rare in ulcerative colitis in contrast to Crohn's disease. *Rectovaginal fistulas,* however, may appear and do not heal with local surgical measures. The pseudopolyps carry with them no prognostic significance. They may disappear completely and have no relation to the development of cancer. *Massive hemorrhage* occurs in about 5 per cent of patients. Rapid replacement of blood and restoration of circulating blood volume are the initial factors in treatment. Hypoprothrombinemia should be corrected by ingestion or injection of vitamin K. Although most patients will respond to medical management, an occasional patient may require colectomy, because the bleeding is from diffuse areas of the mucosa. At times inferior mesenteric arteriography may reveal a more discrete site of bleeding. The colectomy must be total to control bleeding; failure to remove the rectal stump usually requires further emergency surgery. *Strictures of the colon* occur in a little less than 10 per cent of patients, and are rarely of such magnitude as to compromise the intestinal lumen. They usually develop in the rectum or transverse colon, are of variable lengths, and may appear at any

time in the course of the disease. They are not important symptomatically, because they only rarely cause abdominal cramping pain and obstipation. They require attention, because their differentiation from cancer is often difficult. *In fact, it is wise to consider every stricture in ulcerative colitis as carcinomatous until proved otherwise.* Exploratory laparotomy was the only method until recently, but colonoscopy and biopsy have been helpful when the strictured area can be thoroughly visualized and multiple biopsies taken.

Cancer of the Colon. The incidence of cancer of the colon is strikingly higher in patients with ulcerative colitis than in the control population, and contributes significantly to the colitis-related death rate. Current evidence relates this incidence to the duration of the colitis, rather than its activity, and to the extent of the colon involved. The risk of cancer rises regularly in all patients with the duration of the disease. After 10 years the cumulative risk of cancer in all patients is about 5 per cent, and at 20 years it is 25 per cent. In children it has been estimated that 3 per cent of those who develop the disease in childhood will have cancer of the colon after 10 years and 20 per cent per decade thereafter. The risk rises strikingly after the first decade of disease in children and after the second decade in adults.

The extent of colonic involvement with colitis plays an important role in determining the risk of subsequent cancer development. In proctitis it does not differ significantly from that in the control population. The incidence in left-sided colitis is lower than in universal colitis, but, in our experience, significantly increased over the control population. In universal ulcerative colitis the incidence may approach 13 per cent at 15 years, 25 per cent at 20 years, and 40 per cent at 25 years. Since childhood colitis is usually universal in type, this factor influences the high rate of malignancy. Most cancers of the colon are in the rectum; however, in ulcerative colitis they tend to be more uniformly distributed. Such cancers may, however, involve any segment of the colon, the transverse colon being the second most common location. The survival rate after surgery for cancer complicating ulcerative colitis is lower than for cancer unrelated to ulcerative colitis. One reason is that cancer in ulcerative colitis is frequently multicentered (10 to 15 per cent). Clearly the population at greatest risk are those with universal colitis of more than 10 years' duration. Although prophylactic colectomy has been advocated for this group, no consensus exists at present on this point; however, yearly colonoscopy and barium enema examinations are widely proposed. The search for "precancerous" changes on biopsy may be more rewarding, although the significance of "dysplasia" on rectal or colonoscopic biopsy remains controversial. At present the value of serum carcinoembryonic antigen (CEA) levels in the diagnosis of malignancy in this disease has not been established, because levels are elevated in 30 per cent of patients with inflammatory bowel disease.

Toxic Megacolon. At any time in the course of ulcerative colitis the patient may become gravely ill with the signs of systemic toxicity and marked dilatation of the colon. Although much ingenuity has been expended in establishing the criteria for defining this distention, usually the colon is more than 6 cm in width on the flat plate of the abdomen. This drastic episode coincides with extension of the previous mucosal inflammation through all coats of the colon, with evidence of involvement of neural and vascular components. Factors which decrease muscular tone or increase intraluminal pressure may be important in precipitating an episode of colonic dilatation: barium enema examination, injudicious use of opiates and anticholinergic drugs, or hypokalemia. In some patients no obvious triggering mechanism, except worsening of the pathologic process, can be found. Clinically, this is the most dramatic episode in all the variegated course of ulcerative colitis.

The patient is gravely ill, with high fever and rapid pulse, and dry. He complains of abdominal pain which may be continuous, and the abdomen is markedly distended. The previous diarrhea may cease abruptly. The abdomen is diffusely tender and ominously silent. Marked leukocytosis, hypokalemia, and a precipitous fall in serum albumin are usually present. The flat film reveals dilatation of all the colon or a segment, usually the transverse colon, and the edematous ragged colonic mucosa can be seen with the air contrast. If the colon has freely perforated, air may be seen under the diaphragm. Diffuse peritonitis and localized perforation are frequently overdiagnosed because of direct visceral tenderness elicited by pressure on the inflamed serosa of the dilated colon.

The diagnosis is made on the basis of the history of ulcerative colitis, acute worsening of the clinical picture, systemic toxicity, and dilatation of the colon on clinical and radiologic evidence. A few patients, however, will present initially with this condition. Barium enema examination should be avoided, and gentle proctoscopy in bed will make the diagnosis if the antecedent history of ulcerative colitis is not present.

Therapy of acute toxic dilatation of the colon should be intensive and meticulous. Correction of fluid and electrolyte deficits, especially of potassium, is needed. Anemia, hypoalbuminemia, and decreased circulatory blood volume require correction. Steroids are the therapy of choice, and if the patient has been on previous corticosteroids, corticotropin or hydrocortisone in large doses is used as outlined above (25 to 40 units of corticotropin or 100 mg of hydrocortisone, given over the course of each eight-hour period by intravenous drip). No decisive evidence at present allows us to choose one over the other. Since there is probably localized suppuration which has extended to the serosa, intravenous antimicrobial therapy is in order: ampicillin in doses of 8 to 12 grams daily intravenously is usually ordered. Daily flat film and physical examination two or three times a day are required. In view of the usual accompanying small bowel ileus, long-tube intubation should be promptly instituted along with cessation of feedings, anticholinergics, and opiates. The response to this vigorous form of therapy must be evaluated daily in terms of the patient's systemic improvement and regaining of colonic tone in terms of the distention of the colon clinically on flat film. The first 48 to 72 hours will usually indicate whether the hoped-for improvement is indeed beginning to take place. Failure to respond by the fourth or fifth day should lead to prompt subtotal colectomy (avoiding the trauma of the abdominoperineal resection in those desperately ill patients) and ileostomy. On occasion preliminary cecostomy or transverse colostomy has helped by decompressing the colon. The surgical difficulties in handling the thin, distended, often perforated colon should not be underestimated, even if performed by experienced surgeons, and the postoperative periods are often stormy, including localized or generalized peritonitis, walled-off abscesses, and the ominous iliofemoral thrombophlebitis. The mortality of toxic megacolon has been markedly reduced in recent years, in part because of steroid therapy and better systemic management, but probably in major part because of earlier surgical intervention. Of those who recover on current medical programs, the majority usually come to surgery during the next year because of persistent activity of the disease. An interesting clinical variant is the occasional patient who has a "subacute," perhaps a "chronic," megacolon, in contrast to the terribly sick "toxic" patient, whose clinical course is more indolent, although similar.

Perforation of the Colon. Perforation of the colon is most likely to occur in the course of toxic dilatation, and is rare simply in the course of an acute attack. As noted, it is presumably the result of extension of the inflammatory ulcerative process through all layers of the bowel. Since the vast majority of these sick people are already receiving large doses of steroids, recognition is difficult, although sudden clinical worsening with increasing abdominal distention and tenderness of the colon may arouse suspicion. Obliteration of liver dullness must be sought for at all times, and the presence of free air under the diaphragm on x-ray examination makes the diagnosis. Surgical intervention is urgently required and colectomy indicated. Rarely, an episode of perforation may not be recognized and the patient survives; the perforation is documented later by an abdominal film showing free air in the peritoneal cavity.

Extracolonic Complications. As with Crohn's disease, a number of extracolonic complications or manifestations are part of the clinical syndrome. The *arthritis* may be severe, migratory, and accompanied by synovial swelling affecting knees, elbows, and ankles; however, the serologic factors of rheumatoid arthritis are missing, and there is no residual deformity. *Ankylosing spondylitis* and *sacroiliitis* occur with higher frequency than might be expected. *Iritis* and *uveitis* are correlated with the degree of clinical colitis. Of the skin manifestations, *erythema nodosum* and *pyoderma gangrenosum* are the most common. The incidence of kidney stones is highest in those with ileostomies. The hepatic complications include *fatty infiltration, pericholangitis* and *chronic active hepatitis*, and, rarely, *sclerosing cholangitis* and its associated *carcinoma of the bile ducts*. It is not known at present whether colectomy improves liver function or structure. Massive peripheral or pelvic thrombophlebitis, especially *iliofemoral venous thrombosis*, is a grave complication, and may be related to marked thrombocytosis.

SURGICAL THERAPY. Colectomy is curative in ulcerative colitis, at the cost of life with an ileostomy. The marked reduction in mortality from colectomy and the recent improvement in the quality of life with an ileostomy now makes colectomy an acceptable form of treatment for the patient with ulcerative colitis. Whether done in one or two stages, most experts agree that preservation of the rectum is not possible in this disease, although ileoproctostomy (with or without active disease in the rectum) still has a few advocates. However, subsequent ileal dysfunction, intestinal obstruction, ileostomy prolapse or retraction, delayed healing of the perianal wound, and fear of psychogenic or neurogenic impotence present realistic limitations to the overenthusiastic use of surgery. The clearest indications for immediate surgery are those complications for which no other therapy is available: massive uncontrollable hemorrhage, perforation of the colon, cancer of the colon, a stricture which cannot be distinguished from cancer, and medically unresponsive toxic dilatation. Close behind this group are the patients in a severe acute attack, which carries with it the highest mortality risk. This is the group which has until recently been usually treated with two to three weeks of intravenous steroids at high dosage plus massive antimicrobial therapy. Although continued disease activity, protein and electrolyte depletion, serious anemia, and localized suppuration make surgical intervention at this stage somewhat risky, it is the best choice. Some proponents of early surgery have advocated intervention after four to five days if the patient has not clinically shown remission in this period of time. Although this point of view has yet to be unequivocally established, the trend of modern therapy is toward earlier intervention in the acutely ill patient. Moreover, there is probably little disagreement at present that the patient with intractable pyoderma gangrenosum and probably also persistent or serious uveitis should undergo colectomy. No solid evidence exists, however, that colectomy improves serious liver disease.

A decision for surgery in the patient with persistent symptomatic disease, sufficiently severe to prevent normal function, is indicated, especially for those who require unacceptably high levels of steroids (greater than 20 mg of prednisone daily) for suppression of symptoms. In others the decision for colectomy is more difficult, especially with childhood disease. These patients suffer a lower survival rate with or without malignancy, and growth and sexual maturation are retarded. Colectomy should be recommended for such children who are chronically ill, despite the reluctance and anxiety of both family and physician, but only after a period of medical trial, possible not longer than two years, at a time of early pubertal development with retarded bone age.

The most difficult problem is the risk of cancer in the patient who has had the disease for ten years or more, either quiescent or with minimal medical therapy. Those with only rectal involvement have little risk and can be followed with barium enema, proctosigmoidoscopy, and colonoscopy. It is those with universal and left-sided colitis who raise the question of prophylactic colectomy. As indicated, no firm trend is visible at present. It should be pointed out that the development of the "continent" ileostomy of Kock of Sweden with its internal pouch and avoidance of an external mechanical appliance may simplify the decision in borderline patients.

Edwards, F. C., and Truelove, S. C.: The course and prognosis of ulcerative colitis. I. Short term prognosis. Gut, 4:299, 1964. II. Long term prognosis. Gut, 4:309, 1964.

Engle, G. L.: Studies of ulcerative colitis. III. The nature of the psychological processes. Am. J. Med., 19:231, 1955.

Greenstein, A. J., Janowitz, H. D., and Sachar, D. B.: The extraintestinal complications of Crohn's disease and ulcerative colitis: Study of 700 patients. Medicine, 55:401, 1976.

Marshak, R. H., Korelitz, B. I., Klein, S. H., Wolf, B. S., and Janowitz, H. D.: Toxic dilatation of the colon in the course of ulcerative colitis. Gastroenterology, 38:165, 1960.

Sparberg, M., Genonessy, J., and Kirsner, J. B.: Ulcerative proctitis and mild ulcerative colitis: A study of 220 patients. Medicine, 45:391, 1966.

413.4. CROHN'S DISEASE OF THE COLON

(Granulomatous Colitis)

DEFINITION. Crohn's disease of the colon is a chronic inflammatory disease of the colon of unknown origin, characteristically of young adults, most frequently involving the proximal colon and its adjacent terminal ileum. Although any and all portions of the colon alone may be involved, it classically spares the rectum.

Crohn's disease of the colon alone comprises at present the smallest segment of this disease. A diarrheal disease of insidious onset and progressive course, it usually has little tendency to rectal bleeding, great tendency to fistulize both internally and externally, and, frequently, significant anal and perianal lesions. The characteristic pathology includes confluent linear ulceration, intramucosal fissuring, aggregates of mononuclear inflammatory cells, and epithelioid granulomas within the bowel wall or regional lymph nodes (hence the term granulomatous colitis). Because of similarities of clinical course, pathology, tendency to recur after resection, and coexistence with regional enteritis (Crohn's disease of the ileum), Crohn's disease of the colon is considered the same disease. The term "ileocolitis" is reserved for simultaneous involvement of the ileum and colon. The distinction from ulcerative colitis may be difficult on occasion, but this does not obliterate their differences and the therapeutic consequences of such differentiation.

SEPARATION OF ULCERATIVE COLITIS AND CROHN'S DISEASE OF THE COLON. The year after the original description of regional enteritis, Colp described a patient with involvement of both ileum and cecum and demonstrated that the ileocecal valve is no barrier to the development of this process in the colon. Despite sporadic papers, it was not until 1960 that it became apparent that Crohn's disease could occur frequently in the colon as well as in the small bowel and could be differentiated from ulcerative colitis. The clinical and pathologic characteristics of Crohn's disease of the small bowel and ulcerative colitis are presented in Ch. 413.2 and 413.3, respectively.

The features which distinguish ulcerative colitis and Crohn's disease of the colon should be emphasized: In Crohn's disease the small bowel is also involved in up to 80 per cent of cases; the lesion is segmental, sparing the rectum in perhaps more than half the patients; and fistulas are extremely frequent — all in marked contrast to ulcerative colitis. Clinically, in Crohn's disease rectal bleeding is a much less frequent occurrence, severe perianal and perirectal disease is often florid, free perforation and toxic dilatation are rarer, and development of cancer is rarer. In contrast to the mucosal pathology of ulcerative colitis, all coats are involved in Crohn's disease, with marked thickening and a high percentage of granulomas in the bowel wall and regional lymph nodes. Finally, in therapeutic contrast to ulcerative colitis, excision in Crohn's disease of the colon is often followed by recurrences in the small bowel. Our inability to differentiate these two entities even when adequate histologic material is present (in perhaps 15 per cent of cases) does not argue for their identity. The colon has a limited repertoire of tissue responses to injury, and other disorders are still to be separated from this group of inflammatory diseases, ischemic colitis being the most recently segregated entity.

INCIDENCE AND DISTRIBUTION OF LESIONS. The available data regarding the incidence and prevalence of Crohn's disease have been cited in Ch. 413.2. Despite the increasing recognition of this entity, the impression that the incidence of Crohn's disease of the colon rivals that of ulcerative colitis appears erroneous. Of over 600 patients with inflammatory colonic disease sick enough to require ileostomy and colectomy in the writer's series, less than 10 per cent had Crohn's disease of the colon.

The colon may be involved in Crohn's disease in one of several ways. The least significant is by way of fistula formation from a contiguous loop of small bowel which is the site of regional enteritis. This is relatively trivial, because the disease does not appear to spread, and the colonic area heals when the small bowel is resected and the fistula closed. Second, the colon may become involved only after an anastomotic operation for regional ileitis, and almost always directly adjacent to the anastomosis. More important, the colon alone may exhibit the disease. Finally, the colon and small bowel are simultaneously the seat of the pathologic process, with continuity of disease in the colon, and occasionally normal segment intervenes. When the colon is involved, less than 20 per cent of patients have the lesion confined to that organ; 80 per cent have disease in the ileum. Over-all, about two thirds of Crohn's disease involves the small bowel alone. The anal involvement in Crohn's disease of the colon is noteworthy. It may be in the form of edematous anal tags, chronic fissuring, anorectal fistulas, and indolent undermining ulceration. About 75 per cent of patients with Crohn's disease of the colon and 25 per cent of those with Crohn's disease of the small bowel have an anal lesion at some time in the course of this illness.

PATHOLOGY. The pathology of Crohn's disease of the colon and rectum is fundamentally that of Crohn's disease of the small intestine. Because of the interest and difficulty at times of distinguishing colonic involvement from ulcerative colitis, some additional points should be mentioned. In contrast to ulcerative colitis, Crohn's disease is a discontinuous process, sparing the rectum generally in more than half the instances and involving the terminal ileum in a very high percentage of cases. Intense vascularity is characteristic of ulcerative colitis, not of Crohn's disease. Muscular shortening of the colon in ulcerative colitis contrasts with the fibrosis and stricturing of Crohn's disease. Pseudopolyp formation is characteristic of ulcerative colitis. External and internal fistulas are the hallmark of Crohn's disease, including such unusual sites as the stomach; the only fistula characteristic of ulcerative colitis is rectovaginal fistula.

The microscopic characteristics of both diseases have also been described under their respective categories. Ulcerative colitis is primarily a mucosal disease; Crohn's disease involves all layers. The aphthous ulcers of the mucosa in Crohn's disease have been mentioned in Ch. 413.2. In Crohn's disease, in contrast to ulcerative colitis, fissuring is prominent, as well as aggregates of mononuclear inflammation and sarcoid granulomas in the bowel wall and regional lymph nodes. In biopsies of the rectum in Crohn's disease of the colon we have found about 10 per cent to have these granulomas when no gross lesion was visible on sigmoidoscopic or barium enema examination. Ultrastructural studies have disclosed no characteristic findings of these granulomas. Although crypt abscesses are not specific for ulcerative colitis, they are a prominent pattern in its histopathology, in contrast to Crohn's disease of the colon. The latter may also exist in a colon with sigmoid diverticular disease, and the clinical and radiographic features are as difficult to assign to each component as are the pathologic findings.

Cancer as an important feature of the natural history of ulcerative colitis has already been emphasized; even in the small bowel in Crohn's disease, the incidence of adenocarcinoma is more frequent, especially in the bypassed ileum. Although cancers have been observed in colons which are the seat of Crohn's disease, the data at present do not allow any firm statistical statement regarding the risk of cancer development; our own studies suggest an increased risk — not, however, of the dimensions of ulcerative colitis.

CLINICAL MANIFESTATIONS. Crohn's disease of the colon, like Crohn's disease of the small bowel, begins in young adult life. About a third of the writer's patients had their first manifestations between 16 and 20 years of age. In comparison with ulcerative colitis, an acute fulminant presentation is rare, toxic dilatation is rarer, and free perforation, rarest. Onset is usually slow and insidious, with diarrhea as the principal symptom in the majority of patients. The stools are small, frequent, and soft but not necessarily watery; some patients may be constipated, especially if they have anal lesions. Over three quarters of the patients lose weight. Crampy abdominal pain of a diffuse nature is prominent. Gross bleeding is noted only in less than half the patients; indeed, important rectal bleeding is most unusual except in the presence of rectal involvement. The history of a perirectal abscess or fistula often precedes the obvious clinical onset by years. *Aphthous stomatitis, arthralgias* and *arthritis, uveitis, pyoderma gangrenosum* and *erythema nodosum*, and backache caused by *ankylosing spondylitis* and *sacroiliitis* are secondary manifestations, as in the other variants of inflammatory bowel diseases.

PHYSICAL EXAMINATION. In contrast to those with regional ileitis, patients with Crohn's disease of the colon rarely have a palpable right lower quadrant mass, even when the ileum is involved. Clubbing of the fingers and curvature of the nails may be present. Edematous perianal skin tags and perirectal fistulas may be noted.

DIAGNOSIS. Confirmation of the clinical suspicion of Crohn's disease of the colon depends upon sigmoidoscopic or colonoscopic and barium enema examination, and, on occasion, upon the small bowel series. In half the cases, the sigmoidoscopic examination is negative; in the others it may reveal an edematous mucosa, mucoid secretions, or a cobblestoned surface. At times discrete linear ulcers may be seen. In contrast to ulcerative colitis, however, bleeding from a friable mucosa is not present. Diagnosis may be suggested by biopsy findings.

The roentgenologic features are the same as in regional enteritis of the small bowel, i.e., segmental involvement with normal skip areas, longitudinal ulcerations, fissures, eccentric involvement, pseudodiverticula, strictures, internal fistulas, and sinus tracts (Fig. 6). In early cases nodular defects or irregularity of the contour of a short segment of colon may be the only findings, and may be obscured on the filled films. At times the evacuation films or examination of the colon from above may be the only way of documenting these changes. Strictures, as in ulcerative colitis, are difficult to distinguish from cancer; when the entire colon is diffusely involved in a symmetrical fashion, and when the ileum is normal, it may be impossible to distinguish Crohn's disease of the colon from ulcerative colitis by x-ray examination.

DIFFERENTIAL DIAGNOSIS. The important conditions which must be differentiated from Crohn's disease of the colon include *ulcerative colitis, cancer* of the *colon, tuberculosis* of the *ileocecal area, amebiasis*, and, rarely,

Figure 6. Crohn's colitis. Note involvement of terminal ileum as well as right side of colon.

radiation enteritis and *colitis.* When a left-sided colonic segment is the site of disease, *ischemic colitis* and *sigmoid diverticulitis* are the disorders which must be distinguished. The intramural abscess of diverticulitis and the longitudinal submucosal ulceration of Crohn's disease are similar on barium enema, but the very long tracts are more characteristic of Crohn's disease.

THERAPY. Current approaches to therapy of Crohn's disease of the colon reflect the perspective of experience with Crohn's disease of the small bowel. The unpredictable course of the disease, the significant reduction in longevity, and the high rate of recurrence of surgically treated ileitis have engendered a cautious view of therapies available at present for Crohn's disease of the colon. All the modalities of medical treatment for ileitis are used in Crohn's colitis: general supportive measures, nutritional supplements, sulfonamides (especially Azulfidine), antimicrobials, steroids (corticotropin and adrenocorticosteroids), and immunosuppressives (azathioprine [Imuran]). Even more than in regional ileitis, the therapeutic value of all these methods remains to be demonstrated in repeated sound controlled clinical trials, although the National Cooperative Crohn's Disease Study has shown that treatment for four months with prednisone and azulfidine was superior to azathioprine and placebo in an outpatient population followed for the next 18 months. When multiple enteric and cutaneous fistulas lead to marked malnutrition and malabsorption, hyperalimentation with a central venous catheter may be effective.

Surgical intervention is clearly indicated for those complications for which no medical therapy exists: perforation, cancer, obstruction resulting from stricture,

massive hemorrhage, and fistulization into stomach, duodenum, and bladder. The more difficult decisions concern those patients who are not able to carry out their usual daily activities and those who require more than 20 mg of prednisolone daily to suppress their symptoms over a period of months. Almost 75 per cent of patients ultimately come to surgery. Since considerable controversy exists at present regarding the fate of patients with total extirpation of the colon for Crohn's disease, the decision is by no means easy in sick patients. Diversionary ileostomy in the hope of resting an inflamed colon and possibly even subsequently utilizing this organ has become discredited. When the disease is segmental and especially since the left colon and rectosigmoid are free in at least half the patients, resection and anastomosis with sigmoid or rectum is the operation of choice. The rate of recurrence in these localized extirpations clearly resembles the rate of recurrence of Crohn's disease of the ileum alone (approaching 50 per cent in five years). In the writer's experience, of 67 patients with Crohn's colitis, 31, or 46 per cent, had significant recurrences in the ileum after ileostomy and colectomy, 8 required multiple operations, and 6 had severe nutritional deficits. This experience is not paralleled by all observers. In some series recurrences have been observed in none or only 3 per cent. A review of the experience at St. Mark's Hospital in London indicated four recurrences in 56 patients (7 per cent), but others have reported as many as 16 recurrences in 37 patients treated similarly. These differences may relate in part to the extent to which the ileum is involved; in our group almost all had the ileal involvement. Accordingly, some delay in deciding on colectomy seems warranted. Even the most vigorous proponents of ileostomy and total colectomy grant that the patients with Crohn's disease of the colon have a higher rate of stomal dysfunction and ileitis than patients with ulcerative colitis, and all observers agree that ileostomy plus total excision is less likely to lead to recurrence and reoperation than are anastomotic procedures.

Greenstein, A. J., Sachar, D. B., Pasternack, B. S., and Janowitz, H. D.: Reoperation and recurrence in Crohn's colitis and ileocolitis: Crude and cumulative rates. N. Engl. J. Med., 293:685, 1975.

Korelitz, B. I., Present, D. H., Alpert, L. I., Marshak, R. H., and Janowitz, H. D.: Recurrent regional ileitis after ileostomy and colectomy for granulomatous colitis. N. Engl. J. Med., 287:110, 1972.

Lindner, A. E., Marshak, R. H., Wolf, B. S., and Janowitz, H. D.: Granulomatous colitis, a clinical study. N. Engl. J. Med., 269:379, 1963.

Ritchie, J. K., and Lockhart-Mummery, H. E.: Nonrestorative surgery in the treatment of Crohn's disease of the large bowel. Gut, 14:263, 1973.

414. OTHER INFLAMMATORY DISEASES OF THE INTESTINE

Marvin H. Sleisenger

414.1. ACUTE APPENDICITIS (INCLUDING THE ACUTE ABDOMEN)

DEFINITION. Appendicitis is acute inflammation of the vermiform appendix. It is rare before the age of two and reaches a peak incidence in the second and third decades. The vast majority of patients are between the ages of 5 and 30. Although incidence of the disease declines after the age of 40, the annual incidence is about 1.5 per thousand for males and 1.9 per thousand for females between the ages of 17 and 64. The disease is important because it is common and curable; it therefore constitutes the most important entity in the differential diagnosis of the acute abdomen.

PATHOLOGY. Usually, the appendix is swollen, hyperemic, warm, and covered with exudate. However, in the early stages it may appear only slightly discolored and, in the late stages, gangrenous with perforation. Microscopically, the picture ranges from some acute inflammatory cells in the lumen and mucosa to acute inflammatory changes transmurally with superficial mucosal ulcerations; in advanced stages, one or more perforations may be noted, particularly in patients over the age of 60.

ETIOLOGY AND PATHOGENESIS. The initiating event in acute appendicitis appears to be obstruction, followed by increased intraluminal pressure, reduced venous drainage, thrombosis, hemorrhage, edema, and bacterial invasion of the wall. As the process proceeds, the appendiceal artery (an end artery) becomes occluded as a result of the inflammation, and venous stasis and perforation result.

Calculi are thought to be the most common cause of the initial obstruction. Indeed, about one third of inflamed appendices contain a radiologically demonstrable calculus, as compared with 2.7 per cent of normal ones. In turn, about a third of these are visible on plain films of the abdomen preoperatively, whereas they may be seen in only 1 per cent of a control population. The incidence of gangrene and perforation is significantly higher also in appendices which contain calculi. The nidus for these calculi is inspissated fecal material which is covered by a calcium phosphate–rich mucus; inorganic salts precipitate, hardening the calculus and increasing the likelihood for obstruction. Fecaliths are more common in populations eating a low fiber diet. It must be stressed, however, that two thirds to three quarters of patients with proved acute appendicitis do not have calculi. In these patients, obviously, an alternative pathogenetic mechanism must be responsible. Obstruction by parasites, lymphoid hyperplasia associated with viral infections, and twisting of the appendix by adhesions have all been incriminated. An additional theory is malfunction of a valve system at the entrance of the appendix. Thus it is likely that the etiology of acute appendicitis is multiple.

CLINICAL PICTURE AND DIAGNOSIS. The history of appendicitis is of short duration in the vast majority of cases — between 12 and 48 hours from onset to hospitalization. Over 95 per cent complain of *pain* at onset, classically referred to the epigastric or periumbilical areas and later localizing in the right lower quadrant. This sequence, however, is not found in all patients and is notably absent in *retrocecal appendicitis.* Further, a significant number will not localize clearly to the right lower quadrant, the pain being either diffuse or in the lower abdomen. In *pelvic appendicitis* the pain may be in the left lower quadrant. When retrocecal, the pain may be referred to the thigh or right testicle. Dysuria is present frequently in both types of appendicitis.

Pain referred to the mid-epigastrium is due to stretching of the organ during early inflammation; ini-

tially it is vague and mild, but it gradually increases over about four hours and may be colicky. It tends to subside, and when the process has reached the serosa and the peritoneum, it localizes over the site of disease. In some patients distress appears to be alleviated at the time of perforation; after perforation, localization of pain will depend on whether or not the process is quickly walled off locally. Thus if the spreading infection is not contained, generalized abdominal discomfort of variable severity will result. *Anorexia* and *nausea* (with or without vomiting) are the second and third most frequent symptoms. In almost all instances, pain precedes the appearance of these other complaints. About 10 per cent of patients will have constipation; diarrhea is relatively infrequent. Temperature usually ranges between 38 and 38.6° C; higher levels usually indicate perforation.

PHYSICAL EXAMINATION. The findings on physical examination differ widely and depend not only upon the stage of the inflammation but also upon the age of the patient. Tenderness to palpation is the most common and most reliable sign; indeed, without it, diagnosis is unlikely. It is usually confined to McBurney's point (one finger) in the right lower quadrant, corresponding to the usual location of the organ. However, although rectal tenderness is present in about one third of patients, it may be so severe as to indicate pelvic peritonitis and thus probable *pelvic appendicitis.* On initial examination in a minority of patients, a mass may be felt in the right lower quadrant or in the pelvis or transrectally. Three quarters of patients will have unquestionable localized tenderness with localized rebound. Generalized rebound tenderness indicates diffuse peritonitis. Bowel sounds may be present or absent; absence associated with distention and generalized rebound tenderness is consistent with perforation and diffuse peritonitis.

On occasion, tenderness may be elicited in the case of retrocecal appendicitis by stretching the psoas by hip extension. Very rarely, because of the odd location of the appendix, tenderness may be in the right upper quadrant or even the left lower quadrant.

Laboratory studies consistently show a leukocytosis with an increase in polymorphonuclear cells — over 10,000 per cubic millimeter and greater than 75 per cent, respectively. Urinalysis is usually normal; however, about 15 per cent of patients have either a slight amount of protein or mild pyuria or hematuria. Presence of a calcified fecalith in the right lower quadrant on flat film of the abdomen is helpful, but its absence has no meaning in the diagnosis. Other findings on flat film include possible obliteration of the right psoas shadow, right lower quadrant sentinel loop ileus, and a right lower quadrant soft tissue mass with or without gas bubbles; with perforation and generalized peritonitis, fluid in the peritoneal cavity and obliteration of the peritoneal lines may be noted.

DIFFERENTIAL DIAGNOSIS OF APPENDICITIS AND OF THE ACUTE ABDOMEN. Appendicitis is first on the list of conditions causing acute abdominal pain which require surgery or immediate consultation with a surgeon. Here a few principles regarding the acute surgical abdomen in the setting of the differential diagnosis of acute appendicitis will be reviewed.

Pain Characteristics. Conditions associated with pain of sudden onset include *perforated viscus* or *acute ischemia;* occasionally, the onset of pain in *acute small* *bowel obstruction, choledocholithiasis,* and *ureteral obstruction* may also be abrupt. The more gradual onset of pain usually indicates an inflammatory lesion, including appendicitis. However, the pain of diffuse *inflammatory bowel disease* is not localized as it is in appendicitis, except as a consequence of perforation or fistulization in Crohn's disease.

The type and radiation of the pain also help in differential diagnosis. For example, evidence of irritation of the diaphragm may be found on the right in *acute cholecystitis* and on the left in *acute pancreatitis;* sudden severe pain referred to the tips of the shoulders, associated with diffuse intra-abdominal pain and, later, distention, is more typical of perforated viscus, particularly *peptic ulcer. Ureteral obstruction* causes pain which is frequently referred to the genitalia or groin. Steady continuous pain is more characteristic of inflammation, as in appendicitis; on the other hand, intermittent or crampy pain is more characteristic of *obstruction of a hollow viscus* such as the gallbladder or small bowel.

It is important again to stress that pain precedes nausea and vomiting in *appendicitis;* on the other hand, vomiting may be an early symptom of *acute cholecystitis or acute pancreatitis.* Bile-stained vomitus associated with acute cramping upper abdominal pain suggests *small bowel obstruction;* blood in the vomitus points toward a mucosal lesion proximal to the third portion of the duodenum. Relief of pain by vomiting suggests *gastric outlet obstruction.* Vomiting, of course, may accompany any intra-abdominal conditions, particularly if the patient has ileus or generalized peritonitis.

Physical Findings. Physical examination of the patient with an acute abdomen is of great importance, and the range of findings expected in acute appendicitis has been discussed. Localized tenderness and temperature elevation associated with continuing pain over a period of hours reflect either *localized peritonitis,* with or without perforation, or *vascular necrosis* of an ischemic organ. In such instances, the temperature is approximately 38.5 to 39.5° C. Higher temperatures are more often associated with urinary tract infections or bacterial pneumonias. A continuing rising pulse rate likewise indicates the possibility of gangrene or perforation of a viscus.

Careful examination of the abdomen is of extreme importance in differential diagnosis. *Diffuse peritonitis* is reflected by resistance of movement and change in position because of accentuation of pain; on the other hand, colic caused by *obstruction* of bile ducts, ureter, or small bowel early in its course is associated with restless movement. Later, in biliary tract and small bowel obstruction, infection and compromise of the blood supply may ensue and will cause the appearance of signs of localized tissue necrosis and peritonitis. The abdomen should be carefully examined for scars of previous surgery which may now underlie an *intestinal obstruction* caused by adhesions; hernias must be sought. A succussion splash indicates marked *gastric outlet obstruction.*

In examining the patient with an acute abdomen, the physician should palpate in that quadrant which is farthest removed from the site of distress. The important findings which indicate a surgical condition include persistent localized tenderness with unequivocal rebound, indicating localized peritonitis, and guarding. Guarding must be interpreted circumspectly, because it

may be voluntary or involuntary. If it is the latter, underlying peritoneal irritation is likely. Generalized involuntary guarding is a classic finding for a perforated intra-abdominal viscus. The presence of an abdominal mass not previously noted, particularly when associated with other findings of inflammation, gangrene, or perforation, is very strong evidence for a surgical condition. Likewise, free air in the abdominal cavity, as evidenced by distention, absence of bowel sounds, and absence of liver dullness in the setting of acute abdominal pain, reflects a perforated viscus. Bowel sounds may be more active and high pitched in early obstruction or continuously active in diffuse acute inflammation (nonsurgical) of the small bowel. With increasing distention of small bowel loops, the sounds become less frequent and more high pitched. Bruits are an important finding, because they may reflect the presence of *arterial aneurysms,* the dissections of which may be the cause for the abdominal pain.

Rectal examination is crucial in differential diagnosis. Unequivocal tenderness indicates pelvic inflammation, and a mass usually reflects the presence of an abscess. As noted above, this examination often reveals positive findings in acute appendicitis. A glove specimen of stool must always be examined for occult blood. In females with acute abdominal pain, pelvic examination is essential to complement a careful gynecologic history.

Laboratory Aids in Diagnosis. The laboratory examination, consisting of urinalysis, complete blood count, serum electrolytes, BUN and creatinine, and x-ray examination of the abdomen and chest, is essential in differential diagnosis of the acute abdomen.

A *polymorphonuclear leukocytosis* strongly substantiates an acute intra-abdominal process with inflammation or necrosis; a low hematocrit reflects a disorder which is also capable of bleeding — *mucosal ulcerations, intestinal carcinoma, ischemia,* or *dissecting aneurysms.* An elevated hematocrit and BUN suggest dehydration, usually caused by vomiting and deficient fluid intake.

Urinalysis is vital in differential diagnosis, because the presence of pyuria, particularly white cell casts and bacteria on the smear of urinary sediment, is strong evidence for urinary tract infection and interdicts surgical exploration. Microscopic hematuria (numerous red cells) suggests stone or tumor of the genitourinary tract; red cell casts, on the other hand, suggest glomerulitis. A few scattered white and red cells may be seen in the sediment of about 20 per cent of patients with acute appendicitis.

Important blood chemistries are *serum amylase,* elevation of which usually reflects acute pancreatitis; however, it may not be elevated in chronic relapsing pancreatitis, and it is elevated in other conditions such as *perforated peptic ulcer, strangulated obstruction* of the small bowel with perforation, and both *acute cholecystitis* and *acute common duct obstruction.*

Roentgenographic Studies in the Acute Abdomen. Roentgenologic examinations of importance include chest films, flat film of the abdomen, intravenous cholangiogram, and intravenous pyelogram. The flat and upright films of the abdomen may be specific for diagnosing free air in the peritoneal cavity, reflecting a perforation of a hollow viscus; in supporting the diagnosis of acute small bowel obstruction; in indicating the likelihood of calculus disease of either gallbladder or urogenital tract; of outlining a large obstructed stomach; and of revealing a variety of soft tissue masses which may reflect cysts or abscesses. Collections of extraintestinal gas often point to abscesses; occasionally, the biliary tree may be outlined by air, thus revealing a fistula to bowel. Diffuse calcification of the region of the pancreas indicates chronic pancreatitis. As noted, calculi in the right lower quadrant may help in the diagnosis of acute appendicitis. Flat film of the abdomen also may yield findings characteristic of acute pancreatitis, including "sentinel" loops and a "cut-off" of the colon. A routine chest x-ray is essential in order to reveal free intraperitoneal air under the diaphragm, to demonstrate pneumonia, or to show an elevated diaphragm on the left with or without pleural effusion and partial atelectasis as noted in acute pancreatitis, or on the right, reflecting subphrenic abscess.

The more special radiographic tests which may be of help in the differential diagnosis include an intravenous cholangiogram to evaluate the possibility of biliary tract obstruction and inflammation; cholangiographic demonstration of the gallbladder renders the diagnosis of acute cholecystitis highly unlikely. Intravenous pyelogram may establish the patency of the urinary tract or, conversely, establish ureteral obstruction or hydronephrosis unilaterally. Examination of the upper gastrointestinal tract with non-barium-containing radiopaque substances (Gastrografin) may help in the diagnosis of perforated ulcer.

Important in the differential diagnosis of acute appendicitis are those nonsurgical conditions which cause acute abdominal pain. These conditions may be excluded by appropriate attention to history, physical examination, and the laboratory studies enumerated in the preceding paragraphs. Chief among these are *pyelonephritis, pneumonia, pulmonary infarction, acute myocardial infarction,* and *pericarditis,* all of which may present with acute upper abdominal pain. Acute distention of the liver and its capsule resulting from *acute right heart failure* may simulate *acute cholecystitis; acute hepatitis,* viral or toxic (including alcohol), may closely simulate acute biliary tract disease. In these instances, however, an enlarged tender liver will be felt. Further, serum SGOT determinations will be markedly elevated (it is well to remember, however, that acute obstruction of the common duct with cholangitis may transiently raise SGOT to levels of a thousand units or more for 24 to 48 hours).

Systemic diseases, such as *sickle cell disease, acute intermittent porphyria, tabes dorsalis, heavy metal poisoning,* and *diabetic neuropathy,* all may present pictures simulating an acute surgical abdomen. Appropriate tests for sickling, for excretion of porphobilinogen (Watson-Schwartz test), for urinary lead, and for other evidences of syphilis or diabetes greatly aid in ruling out these conditions.

Acute pancreatitis, still considered a nonsurgical condition unless caused by common bile duct obstruction, usually presents with pain of many hours' to days' duration, associated with a history suggestive of biliary tract disease or indicative of acute and chronic alcoholism, and in its early stages abdominal tenderness is usually localized to the epigastrium. Markedly elevated plasma amylase (within 48 hours of onset) or elevated urinary amylase-creatinine clearance (>3 per cent) will help establish the diagnosis.

Special Considerations of Age in Differential Diag- nosis of Acute Appendicitis. Great care must be extended to establish the diagnosis of this condition in the very young and very old. Children with diffuse abdominal pain which is preceded by anorexia, nausea, and vomiting and often associated with diarrhea are more likely to have *acute infectious gastroenteritis. Acute mesenteric adenitis,* presumably caused by viral illnesses and often associated with diffuse abdominal pain, is frequently confused with acute appendicitis in children. The difficulty is in those patients in whom there is some right lower quadrant tenderness and slight elevation of the white count. In such instances a diagnosis must be established at operation, because it is far safer to undertake a negative exploration than to neglect removal of an acutely inflamed appendix. The clarity of all signs and intensity of symptoms are diminished in the elderly. Thus pain and tenderness may be minimal and temperature only slightly elevated despite perforation or even abscess. These patients tend to perforate early.

In young females diagnosis is confused by problems in the reproductive system, such as *ruptured graafian follicles, twisted ovarian cysts, ectopic pregnancies, dysmenorrhea, ruptured endometrioma,* and *acute pelvic inflammatory disease. Ruptured ectopic pregnancy* is usually of dramatic suddenness and is often associated with shock and massive blood loss; these findings in a pregnant woman make the diagnosis virtually certain. The *ruptured graafian follicle* is noted in midcycle; fever and leukocytosis are uncommon. Tenderness on moving of cervix on vaginal examination points toward a *twisted ovarian cyst,* the pain of which is out of proportion to the general well-being of the patient. *Gonococcal salpingitis* may be difficult to establish, because endocervical smears may be negative for the organism. Usually, however, the pain is more diffuse and tenderness not so well localized as in appendicitis. However, in questionable instances, exploration must be performed.

The differential diagnosis of appendicitis in the elderly may also be difficult. The classic picture is seldom noted, the history may be inadequate or misleading because of infirmity or the effects of medication, and the appendix perforates early. Findings on physical examination are usually not as dramatic, and, despite complications, fever may only be slightly elevated. Accuracy in diagnosis of patients over 60 years of age is below 70 per cent, and the incidence of perforation without a localized or generalized peritonitis at surgery is nearly 70 per cent — more than twice as high as all other age groups combined.

In elderly patients the principal problems in differential diagnosis are *cholecystitis, diverticulitis, mesenteric thrombosis, intestinal obstruction, incarcerated hernia,* and *perforated ulcer.* In these individuals it is well simply to recognize that one is dealing with a surgical abdomen, because, as stated, it is difficult to be clinically accurate in establishing acute appendicitis.

Right-sided acute diverticulitis may simulate acute appendicitis in every respect. In a few instances, *left-sided diverticulitis* may localize tenderness to the right lower quadrant, because the sigmoid is often more redundant in the elderly, and an excessively mobile loop may come to rest on the right side of the abdomen. In such instances, the patient also may have symptoms suggestive of diverticulitis, such as an episode of diarrhea associated with cramping or steady lower abdominal pain, slight temperature elevation, and, later, evidence of moderate to complete large bowel obstruction. When differential diagnosis is difficult, a cautious barium enema may help greatly in excluding acute diverticulitis as the cause of the problem.

Conversely, elderly patients must not be subjected to the risk of exploration falsely. Accordingly, all efforts should be extended to make certain that *acute myocardial* or *pulmonary infarction, pneumonia,* or other systemic disease or toxin is not responsible for acute abdominal pain simulating appendicitis.

TREATMENT. Unless strongly contraindicated, the only therapy for acute appendicitis is surgical removal of the appendix. Since mortality correlates with perforation and, except in elderly patients, perforation correlates with duration of symptoms, early diagnosis and appendectomy are essential for the lowest acceptable morbidity and mortality for the disease. When surgery is performed early in the disease in an otherwise healthy individual, mortality is only slightly above that for general anesthesia. In view of these facts and since the diagnosis is often difficult to make early in the course of disease, some normal appendices will inevitably have to be removed. To avoid the catastrophe of unoperated-upon acute appendicitis, normal appendices may have to be removed in 20 to 25 per cent of patients.

In patients in whom complications have already occurred prior to surgery, necessary measures to correct dehydration and combat infection must be instituted. If perforation is very likely or suspected, continuous nasogastric suction should be instituted. Those patients with temperatures higher than 39° C and with findings indicative of localized abscess or generalized peritonitis should be given broad-spectrum antimicrobials, usually high-dose penicillin and gentamicin or high-dose ampicillin.

The surgical approach, i.e., whether the usual transabdominal or other, to institute drainage of an established abscess is a decision for the surgeon to make. In those patients with obvious acute appendicitis for whom no surgeon is available, the patients may be treated with head-up position of the bed, intravenous fluids, broad-spectrum antimicrobial drugs, and nasogastric suction. The chance for recovery in otherwise healthy individuals with this program is surprisingly good.

MORBIDITY AND MORTALITY OF SURGERY. Over-all, about 15 per cent of patients with acute appendicitis develop complications postoperatively; this figure is 35.6 per cent in those with perforation and localized peritonitis at the time of surgery and is 70 per cent in those with perforation and generalized peritonitis. The complications include *wound infection, intra-abdominal abscess,* mechanical *small bowel obstruction, fecal fistula,* and, much more rarely, *intraperitoneal hemorrhage. Pylephlebitis* is extremely rare (one in a thousand). In the elderly, of course, mortality is increased by the usual cardiovascular, pulmonary, renal, and cerebral complications.

The over-all mortality of acute appendicitis is now less than 1 per 100,000 population. It ranges from 0.18 to 1.6 per cent and is due principally to the interrelated factors of age and perforation. Indeed, mortality over the age of 60 ranges from 6.4 to 14 per cent. The cause of death in this group may be attributed equally to septic and nonseptic complications.

SPECIAL CONSIDERATIONS. Incidental Appendectomy. In view of the decreasing risk of appendicitis with advancing age and the extremely low risk of developing

acute appendicitis, it is difficult to advocate elective appendectomy during laparotomy (for example, at age 37 years the risk is 0.0431 for males and 0.369 for females). Nevertheless, if the procedure should be performed, the patient, as in any other operation, should be fully informed of what was done.

Prophylactic Appendectomy. At present all data indicate that there is no place for prophylactic appendectomy. The one possible exception may be a move of indefinite duration to an area where neither adequate medical care nor surgical care is available on the part of an individual known to have a fecalith in the region of the appendix.

Cope, Z.: The Early Diagnosis of the Acute Abdomen. 14th ed. London, Oxford University Press, 1972, pp. 48, 62.

Law, D., Law, R., and Eiseman, B.: The continuing challenge of acute and perforated appendicitis. Am. J. Surg., 131:533, 1976.

Lewis, F. R., Holcraft, J. W., Boey, J., and Dunphy, J. E.: Appendicitis. A critical review of diagnoses and treatment in 1000 cases. Arch. Surg., 110:677, 1975.

Schrock, T. R.: Acute appendicitis. In Sleisenger, M. H., and Fordtran, J. S. (eds.): Gastrointestinal Disease. 2nd ed. Philadelphia, W. B. Saunders Company, 1978, p. 1825.

Thorbjarnarson, B., and Loehr, W. J.: Acute appendicitis in patients over the age of sixty. Surg. Gynecol. Obstet., 125:1277, 1967.

Way, L. W.: Abdominal pain and the acute abdomen. In Sleisenger, M. H., and Fordtran, J. S. (eds.): Gastrointestinal Disease. 2nd ed. Philadelphia, W. B. Saunders Company, 1978, p. 394.

414.2. DIVERTICULITIS

DEFINITION. Diverticulitis of the colon is a complication of diverticulosis defined as a micro- or macroperforation of a diverticulum. The etiology and pathogenesis of this complication are not clear; however, it is thought that increased segmental pressure causes a weakened area in the wall to perforate. There is no evidence for vascular occlusion or obstruction by stool as the cause.

CLINICAL PICTURE. The predominant clinical symptoms of diverticulitis are *pain* and *fever.* The pain is usually prominent and is frequently constant. Most commonly, it is localized in the left lower quadrant, because the sigmoid and descending colons are the sites of the largest number of diverticula. Occasionally, the patient will have a brief period of diarrhea or a few loose stools, and only rarely is rectal bleeding noted with diverticulitis. When the perforation and sepsis are of sufficient magnitude, the patient may also have chills with fever as high as 39 to 39.5° C. Usually, however, the fever is low grade, between 38 and 39° C.

Although the pain may be somewhat intermittent and even colicky at onset, it usually becomes steady and is of the same quality as noted in acute appendicitis. Indeed, acute diverticulitis has often been referred to as "left-sided appendicitis." The patient may present for examination after only a few hours or, when the situation is not so severe, after a few days of lingering but nagging left lower quadrant pain and low-grade fever.

Physical examination is extremely important in establishing the diagnosis. Since the process usually quickly involves the serosal surface and peritoneal cover, tenderness will be marked, and, as in acute appendicitis when the process has reached the peritoneal surface, will be both direct and rebound, though localized. Frequently, a tender mass may be discerned. When present for more than a few days, this mass may be astonishingly firm, even hard, and the distinction grossly from carcinoma is almost impossible. Rectal examination also will be painful, because inflamed bowel is often within reach of the finger;

also, a mass may be palpable if a sizable abscess has formed.

In some instances the patient will present with complications of diverticulitis: *dysuria, pyuria,* and *pneumaturia,* all related to involvement of the urinary bladder. In extreme instances, the inflammatory process has perforated into the bladder; symptoms may be due to large collections of pus, not only adjacent to the colon but also in the pelvis or under the diaphragm. Often the presenting symptom in these instances is simply septic fever; however, some patients will initially complain only of *pneumaturia* or *dysuria.* Rarely, the diverticulum perforates freely. In this instance the signs of free perforation are evident; that is, distention of the abdomen, generalized rebound tenderness, and absent bowel sounds.

DIAGNOSIS. Diagnosis of diverticulitis should be suspected particularly in patients with known diverticula who present with fever, leukocytosis, and signs of pericolic and peritoneal inflammation in the left lower quadrant. The diagnosis is even more likely if a mass is palpable. Fever between 38.5 and 39° C is also compatible with the diagnosis; when the process is more extensive and with formation of a *pericolic abscess* and its complications, the temperature is usually over 39° C, and the white count is proportionately higher. Urinalysis will reflect varying degrees of involvement of the urinary tract by this septic process; that is, with mild ureteral irritation a few red and white cells may be seen in the urinary sediment, but with direct involvement of the ureter or invasion of the ureter or the bladder by a pericolic abscess, the urine may be frankly septic and contain large numbers of red cells. Witnessing a patient pass gas on urination is also a sign, in the presence of other findings, that diverticulitis is the probable underlying diagnosis.

Some patients suffer much left flank pain owing to *hydronephrosis* resulting from obstruction of the ureter by a *pericolic abscess.* An intravenous pyelogram shows no function or an obstructed kidney on the left.

The use of x-rays is of crucial importance in the diagnosis, especially flat film of the abdomen. Evidence of pericolic perforation and abscess formation may be suspected from collections of air and fluid in the left lower quadrant; free air may be seen under the diaphragm in instances of free perforation, and with complete sigmoid obstruction the dilatation of the proximal colon down to the point of the obstruction affords important information.

Sigmoidoscopy should be carefully performed. Air insufflation should not be used, and the importance of the examination is to exclude other conditions (see below). Usually, diverticulitis per se produces no abnormalities on sigmoidoscopy except an undue amount of spasm at the rectosigmoid junction.

Clinicians debate the advisability of using a barium enema in the diagnosis of diverticulitis, particularly in its acute phase. The concern is that the increased intraluminal pressure may produce further complications. The history, physical examination, and laboratory information are sufficient to make the clinical diagnosis in the vast majority of instances, and barium enema should await some subsidence of the acute phase of the illness. The single exception to this dictum is in those instances in which the clinical picture does not permit distinguishing between *acute ischemic colitis* of the left colon and sigmoid diverticulitis.

The roentgenographic features characteristic of diverticulitis are the presence of barium outside a diverticulum, the delineation of a pericolic mass, or the demonstration of a fistula originating in the colon. In some instances the distinction between diverticulitis and carcinoma may be difficult. The presence of irregularity, thickening, or even a sawtooth appearance of the bowel is not sufficient to make the diagnosis of diverticulitis, because these are typical for diverticula without perforation.

After diagnosis of diverticulitis has been established, intravenous pyelography should be done to ascertain whether or not obstructive involvement of the urinary tract is present, particularly on the left side. In some instances, as noted above, urinary symptoms may be the predominant feature, and radiographic examination of the urinary tract may have to be performed early.

DIFFERENTIAL DIAGNOSIS. **Diverticulosis.** For many years symptoms of *diverticulosis* have been attributed incorrectly to diverticulitis. *Diverticulosis* may periodically be associated with marked local tenderness, a palpable sigmoid loop, and some degree of large bowel obstruction, and thus the picture suggests diverticulitis. However, such patients do not have fever, the localized tenderness gradually recedes, the white count is not elevated, and there is no evidence of involvement of contiguous organs. Barium enema will reveal an irregular luminal contour with a narrowed sigmoid, possibly even a so-called "sawtooth" appearance of the mucosa. Barium must be noted outside the diverticulum, a fistula seen, or evidences of a pericolic or intramural mass detected before the diagnosis of diverticulitis is definitely made.

Carcinoma of the colon must be distinguished from diverticulitis because of similarity of age during which both diverticulitis and cancer of the colon appear. The differential diagnosis is especially difficult, because diverticulitis also often causes luminal narrowing with partial or complete bowel obstruction, may be associated with mild rectal bleeding, and may appear rather insidiously. Chronic obstruction, more persistent rectal bleeding, and weight loss are more characteristic of *cancer,* whereas localized tenderness with rebound, leukocytosis, and fever support the diagnosis of diverticulitis. In some cases, however, it may be impossible to distinguish the two conditions, especially when the barium enema has features common to both; that is, a mass, luminal irregularities, and partial obstruction. The matter can only be settled at exploratory laparotomy. In those instances in which the signs and symptoms of obstruction rather rapidly recede, repeat barium enema will reveal marked improvement only in the patient with diverticulitis. In the event that a suspicious defect remains, exploration will have to be done.

Crohn's disease of the colon may be difficult to exclude in the face of marked luminal narrowing or multiloculated channels parallel to the bowel wall on x-ray. Clinically, although both may exhibit pain, partial obstruction and lower abdominal mass, some rectal bleeding, fever, and leukocytosis, the history preceding the inflammatory event is usually markedly different. The patient with Crohn's colitis usually will have had previous episodes of lower abdominal pain, fever, and diarrhea, and it is unusual for such patients to present for the first time with advanced localized colonic disease.

Sigmoidoscopy may be crucial in making the differential diagnosis if the rectum is involved with granulomatous disease. Also, evidence elsewhere in the bowel of granulomatous disease, such as cobblestoning, long intramucosal sinus tracts, and skip areas, will help in the differential diagnosis (see Ch. 413.4).

Ischemic colitis of the left colon in elderly patients may present with signs and symptoms of bowel necrosis and localized peritonitis which are difficult to distinguish from diverticulitis. In these instances, gross rectal bleeding is prominent, and a barium enema is of crucial importance, because so-called "thumb printing" will be found in ischemic colitis, especially in the area of the splenic flexure and descending colon (see Ch. 416).

TREATMENT OF DIVERTICULITIS. The patient is given nothing by mouth, and continuous nasogastric suction is instituted if signs of obstruction are present or if the patient is nauseated. Appropriate intravenous fluid is administered. Broad-spectrum antimicrobials should be given to cover gram-positive cocci and gram-negative bacilli; e.g., high-dose penicillin and gentamicin or ampicillin. Clindamycin should be added if sepsis is severe or if anaerobic *Bacteroides* (*B. fragilis*) has been isolated from a drainage site or is suspected when therapy with other antimicrobials is ineffective. Some favor chloramphenicol in the latter situation.

As noted above, an intravenous pyelogram should be performed early if the clinical picture suggests urinary tract infection or left ureteral obstruction. Surgical consultation must be obtained early in all cases in which a mass is palpable or when there is suspicion of peritonitis or involvement of a contiguous organ.

Most patients respond well to this type of therapy with abatement of the fever, tenderness, and evidence of partial obstruction. Long-term therapy becomes identical with that for diverticulosis (see Ch. 401).

INDICATIONS FOR SURGERY. Surgical intervention is necessary for the complications of diverticulitis such as an *enlarging mass* despite therapy, *generalized peritonitis, persisting intestinal obstruction,* or the development of a *fistula.* Elective surgery is indicated for recurrent attacks of diverticulitis and for the inability to exclude a carcinoma as the cause for persisting deformity after recovery from the acute phase.

Botsford, T. W., and Zollinger, R. M.: Diverticulitis of the colon. Surg., Gynecol. Obstet., 128:1209, 1969.

Dean, A. C., and Newell, J. P.: Colonoscopy in the differential diagnosis of carcinoma from diverticulitis of the sigmoid colon. Br. J. Surg., 60:633, 1973.

Loeb, P. M.: Diverticular disease of the colon. *In* Sleisenger, M. H., and Fordtran, J. S. (eds.): Gastrointestinal Disease. 2nd ed. Philadelphia, W. B. Saunders Company, 1978, p. 1745.

Small, W. P., and Smith, A. N.: Fistula and conditions associated with diverticular disease of the colon. Clin. Gastroenterol., 4:171, 1975.

414.3.   RADIATION ENTEROCOLITIS

Damage to the small intestine and colon may result from radiation therapy for abdominal and pelvic malignancy.

INCIDENCE. Incidence of severe radiation injury varies between 2.5 and 25 per cent of patients treated with radiotherapy for pelvic and intra-abdominal malignancy. Minor degrees of damage are common, as evidenced by impaired ileal absorption of conjugated bile acids in many women who are irradiated for pelvic cancer. It is noted most commonly after the total dosage exceeds 5000 rads. Transient histologic inflammatory change may, however, be found in the rectal mucosa of nearly 75 per cent of individuals receiving such therapeutic irradiation.

PATHOGENESIS AND PATHOLOGY. Radiation damage results from interference with cell replication. Such damage may follow dosage of less than 5000 rads in patients being treated concomitantly with 5-fluorouracil, Adriamycin, bleomycin, or actinomycin D. Damage to the

mesothelial cells of the small submucosal arterioles results in varying degrees of occlusion and mucosal transmural necrosis. Accordingly, hyperemia and ulceration of the mucosa are frequent. With extreme damage, diffuse edema is followed by extensive fibrosis with multiple strictures and irreversible damage.

The pathologic changes range from diminution of crypt cell mitosis, shortening of the villi of the small intestine to varying degrees of hyperemia, edema, and inflammatory cell infiltration of the mucosa. Mucosal thickness decreases. Progress of damage is marked by crypt abscesses, sloughing of epithelial cells, and, later, mucosal ulcerations, diffuse or localized, are found. Two to 12 months after radiotherapy, the damage to the blood vessels becomes prominent. In these instances, repair of acute damage does not ensue. The mucosa and submucosa become progressively ischemic and fibrotic. *Abscesses* and *fistulas* may form with sinus tracts between loops of intestine and between intestine and neighboring organs.

CLINICAL PICTURE. Symptoms may appear early, that is, during the first or second week of therapy, or late, that is, six months or more after completion of therapy. Early, diarrhea and mild rectal bleeding may appear, resembling ulcerative colitis. Sigmoidoscopy reveals an edematous mucosa which may be friable; in more extreme instances, the acute changes also reveal a patchy or diffusely necrotic mucosa.

Later, symptoms of radiation include gross rectal bleeding, decrease in stool caliber, and progressive difficulty in defecation with marked constipation, all indicating severe rectal involvement. Small intestinal symptoms result from either fibrosis and obstruction or fistulization and abscess formation. If the damage is especially diffuse, malabsorption may be noted, as described in Ch. 408.

DIAGNOSIS. Diagnosis of radiation enteritis is suspected with any of the aforementioned symptoms in patients who have received significant radiation. Sigmoidoscopy shows a picture which ranges from variable degrees of edema to a markedly inflamed and necrotic mucosa. Multiple telangiectases are common, as is rectal stricture. Since most cases are fairly clear cut, biopsy is usually not indicated.

Barium studies of the intestine are not specific and range from changes of diffuse edema and spasm to diffuse fibrosis with strictures, fistulas, and ulceration in more severe cases. Thus the picture may resemble localized malignancy in the colon or diffuse granulomatous disease in the small intestine. Long strictured areas may also be noted, however, in the colon.

Differential diagnostic usefulness of small vessel angiography to the intestine in radiation enteritis remains to be confirmed.

TREATMENT. Improving methods for monitoring radiotherapy will probably reduce the incidence of this complication; however, the increasing incidence of malignancy and of the efficacy of radiotherapy will probably increase the total number of such patients.

Symptoms caused by early reaction consist of mild diarrhea and perhaps some minimal bleeding which can be managed with the judicious use of tranquilizers, anticholinergic drugs, local analgesics, and warm sitz baths. Recent studies indicate that an elemental diet free of gluten, milk protein, and lactose may benefit patients with early radiation reaction. If rectal bleeding is prominent, treatment with steroid retention enemas should be initiated as in ulcerative colitis (see Ch. 413.3). If the bleeding is more significant, transfusions may be required and even, possibly, surgery. Rectal strictures may be dilated, provided that it is early in their course and they are not extensive. Lubricants and stool softeners are often helpful; however, the progress to symptomatic occlusion of the lumen may necessitate proximal colostomy. Fistulas should be resected and abscesses drained. Resection of bowel and anastomoses are hazardous in view of the impaired blood supply.

In patients with malabsorption, treatment is as outlined in Ch. 408.

PROGNOSIS.   Prognosis depends on the extent and degree of damage, the age of the patient, the course of the underlying malignancy, and whether or not the patient has systemic vascular disease. Unfortunately, extensive disease of the colon usually means significant disease in the small intestine. The prognosis is guarded in those with ulceration, fibrosis, or fistulas in whom repeated resections or other major surgical procedures must be carried out. In such cases, age and cardiovascular status are also crucial determining factors.

DeCosse, J. J., Rhodes, R. S., Wentz, W. B., Reagan, J. W., Dwarken, H. J., and Holden, W. D.: The natural history and management of radiation-induced injury of the gastrointestinal tract. Ann. Surg., 170:369, 1969.

Earnest, D. H., and Trier, J. S.: Radiation enteritis and colitis. *In* Sleisenger, M. H., and Fordtran, J. S. (eds.): Gastrointestinal Disease. 2nd ed. Philadelphia, W. B. Saunders Company, 1978, p. 1736.

Newman, A., Katsaris, J., Blendis, L. M., Charlesworth, M., and Walter, L. H.: Small intestinal injury in women who have had pelvic radiotherapy. Lancet, 2:1471, 1973.

Weisbrot, I. M., Liber, A. F., and Gordon, B. S.: The effects of therapeutic radiation on colonic mucosa. Cancer, 36:931, 1975.

414.4.   PSEUDOMEMBRANOUS ENTEROCOLITIS

Pseudomembranous enterocolitis is an inflammatory disease of the small and large bowel; occasionally it involves either the small bowel or the large bowel exclusively.

ETIOLOGY AND PATHOGENESIS.   This disease is often seen in patients with underlying serious illness and in the postoperative period with intestinal obstruction. In some instances it is associated with recovery of *Staphylococcus aureus* from intestinal contents, but the exact relationship of the organism to the disease is not clearly defined. Shock or ischemia of the intestine may also play a role in the pathogenesis of this entity. Often it is due to the toxins of a clostridial organism, *C. difficile*, which attends or follows the use of broad-spectrum antibiotics, particularly clindamycin and lincomycin.

PATHOLOGY.   The involved bowel is covered with yellowish-green membranous plaques which may become confluent. The changes in the mucosa range from mild edema to marked friability and ulceration. The "membrane" is made up of fibrin, mucus, and a variety of mononuclear and polymorphonuclear cells; staphylococci may also be seen in clusters in the increasingly rare case of staphylococcal disease. Mucosal ulcerations may be scattered, and the submucosal tissue is edematous and congested. In its advanced stage, the intestine is completely covered with the membrane, and the underlying bowel exhibits extensive necrosis and ulceration.

CLINICAL PICTURE.   The onset ranges from gradual to abrupt, with fever from 38 to 40° C, associated with watery diarrhea containing mucus, pus, and, on occasion, blood. The amount of fluid lost may be extreme, and dehydration and metabolic acidosis may be prominent.

DIAGNOSIS.   The disease should be suspected when the symptoms described appear in particular settings described above. The stool may reveal clusters of gram-positive cocci, suggesting *S. aureus*. In most patients who have received clindamycin, lincomycin, or, rarely, other antimicrobial agents, culture of stool or exudate will yield *C. difficile*. Sigmoidoscopy reveals yellowish-white plaques covering an erythematous mucosa which, in severe cases of diarrhea, is also friable and may be ulcerated. Flat film of the abdomen yields nondiagnostic findings; occasionally barium will outline plaques.

TREATMENT.   Attention must be first paid to dehydration and electrolyte imbalance which includes hyponatremia and hypokalemia. As in enterotoxic diarrhea, enormous amounts of fluid may be required — 10 to 15 liters in 24 to 36 hours. Potassium must be replaced before bicarbonate may be given for acidosis.

Shock must be combated with intravenous fluids, pressor agents, and 100 mg of prednisolone per 24 hours intravenously. Steroids are not indicated after correction of shock. If large clusters of staphylococci are seen on fecal smear, then appropriate antimicrobial agents such as methicillin or cephalothin should be given; if the patient is sensitive to penicillin, erythromycin, 2 to 4 grams intravenously per day, should be administered. In those whose disease begins while on antimicrobial drugs, these agents must be withdrawn and vancomycin, 0.5 gram intravenously slowly twice daily, must be given while results of culture are awaited. If *C. difficile* is isolated, such treatment should be given for ten days. After the initial 48 hours of therapy, attention must be paid to replacement of protein which has been lost into the intestine by administration of salt-free albumin (50 to 100 grams per 24 hours). In some patients ileostomy or colonic exclusion may be required.

PROGNOSIS.   Except for rapidly diagnosed and properly treated patients with *C. difficile* or *S. aureus*, the mortality is extremely high in pseudomembranous enterocolitis, 15 to 20 per cent. The reason is that this disease is often superimposed upon an already serious clinical situation. If fluid and electrolyte balance is quickly restored and blood pressure returns to normal with increasing urinary output and cessation of diarrhea, the prognosis is good. Such signs are usually noted within 72 hours. Complete recovery with disappearance of the membrane may require weeks.

Alpers, D. H.: The pseudomembranous enterocolitides. *In* Sleisenger, M. H., and Fordtran, J. S. (eds.): Gastrointestinal Disease. 2nd ed. Philadelphia, W. B. Saunders Company, 1978, p. 1715.

Editorial. Antibiotic-associated colitis. A progress report. Br. Med. J., 1:669, 1978.

Saylor, J. L., Anderson, C. B., and Tedesco, F. J.: Pseudomembranous colitis treated with completely diverting ileostomy. Arch. Surg., 111:596, 1976.

Tedesco, F. J.: Clindamycin-associated colitis: A review of the clinical spectrum of 47 cases. Am. J. Dig. Dis., 21:26, 1976.

414.5.   PRIMARY NONSPECIFIC ULCERATION OF THE SMALL INTESTINE

This inflammatory disease of unknown etiology is rare, although in a majority of instances it is attributable to ingestion of enteric-coated potassium chloride. Such ulceration may also be associated with *vascular disease, central nervous system disease, infection, trauma,* and *malnutrition.*

The clinical picture consists of symptoms of small bowel

obstruction and, more rarely, perforation or bleeding. Earlier, the patient reveals periumbilical colicky pain and perhaps nausea and vomiting.

If the patient has small bowel obstruction, the findings associated with this condition would be noted. Distention, diffuse tympany, absence of liver dullness, and generalized tenderness with rebound may be found on examination if the ulcer has perforated.

Laboratory investigation is normal unless the patient has been bleeding or has had protracted vomiting; plain films of the abdomen are of great value if small bowel obstruction is present. Barium contrast studies in the uncomplicated cases are most often unrevealing, although in rare instances ulceration and narrowing in the jejunum may be noted.

Treatment for the disease is surgical with resection of the involved segment. Postassium supplements (if prescribed) in such patients should always be given in liquid form.

NONGRANULOMATOUS DIFFUSE ILEOJEJUNITIS AND EOSINOPHILIC GASTROENTERITIS

Diffuse nongranulomatous ileojejunitis and *eosinophilic gastroenteritis* are described in Ch. 408. *Tuberculous enteritis* and *enterocolitis* are discussed in Ch. 168.6.

Brandborg, L. L.: Other infectious, inflammatory and miscellaneous diseases. *In* Sleisenger, M. H., and Fordtran, J. S. (eds.): Gastrointestinal Disease. 2nd ed. Philadelphia, W. B. Saunders Company, 1978, p. 1076.

Greenberger, N., and Gryboski, J. D.: Allergic disorders of the intestine and eosinophilic gastroenteritis. *In* Sleisenger, M. H., and Fordtran, J. S. (eds.): Gastrointestinal Disease. 2nd ed. Philadelphia, W. B. Saunders Company, 1978, p. 1228.

Jeffries, G. H., Steinberg, H., and Sleisenger, M. H.: Cronic ulcerative (nongranulomatous) ileojejunitis. Am. J. Med., 44:47, 1968.

Klein, N. C., Hargrove, M. D., Sleisenger, M. H., and Jeffries, G. H.: Eosinophilic gastroenteritis. Medicine, 49:299, 1970.

Leinbach, G. E., and Rubin, C. E.: Eosinophilic gastroenteritis: A simple reaction to food allergens. Gastroenterology, 59:874, 1970.

Section Eight VASCULAR DISEASES OF THE INTESTINE

Robert K. Ockner

415. ANATOMY, PHYSIOLOGY, AND PATHOPHYSIOLOGY OF THE MESENTERIC CIRCULATION

The abdominal viscera receive their blood supply from three relatively large arteries which originate on the ventral aspect of the aorta. The most cephalad of these, the celiac axis, arises at the level of the twelfth thoracic or first lumbar vertebra, i.e., approximately at the insertion of the median arcuate ligament of the diaphragm (Fig. 1). Its subdivisions supply the liver and biliary structures (hepatic artery), spleen (splenic artery), and the stomach (left gastric and gastroepiploic, short gastrics, and branches of the gastroduodenal, including the right gastroepiploic). The pancreaticoduodenal arcades provide important anastomotic connections between the hepatic branch of the celiac artery and the superior mesenteric artery in the region of the second portion of the duodenum; branches of these arcades also supply the pancreas and duodenum.

The second major visceral artery, the superior mesenteric, arises from the aorta just caudal to the celiac (Fig. 2). In addition to its pancreaticoduodenal anastomoses with the celiac arterial system, branches of the superior

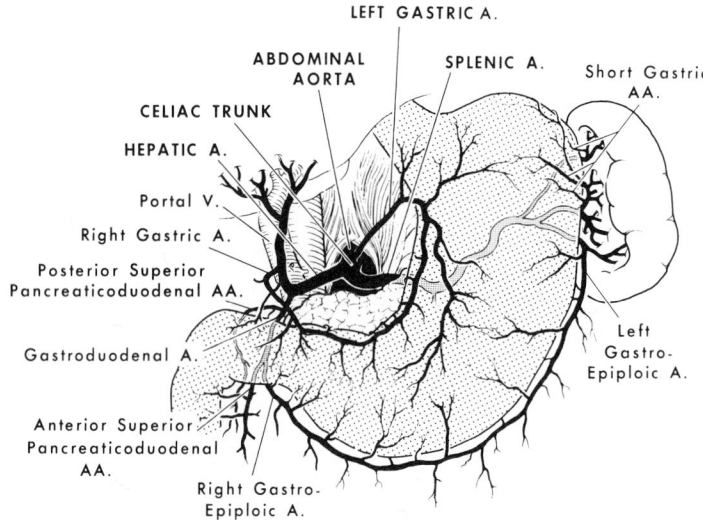

Figure 1. Arterial supply to the stomach and duodenum, showing major branches of the celiac axis and the superior portion of the pancreaticoduodenal arcades. (From Ockner, R. K., *In* Sleisenger, M. H., and Fordtran, J. S. [eds.]: Gastrointestinal Disease. 2nd ed. Philadelphia, W. B. Saunders Company, 1978.)

LEFT GASTRIC A.
ABDOMINAL AORTA
SPLENIC A.
Short Gastric AA.
CELIAC TRUNK
HEPATIC A.
Portal V.
Right Gastric A.
Posterior Superior Pancreaticoduodenal AA.
Gastroduodenal A.
Left Gastro-Epiploic A.
Anterior Superior Pancreaticoduodenal AA.
Right Gastro-Epiploic A.

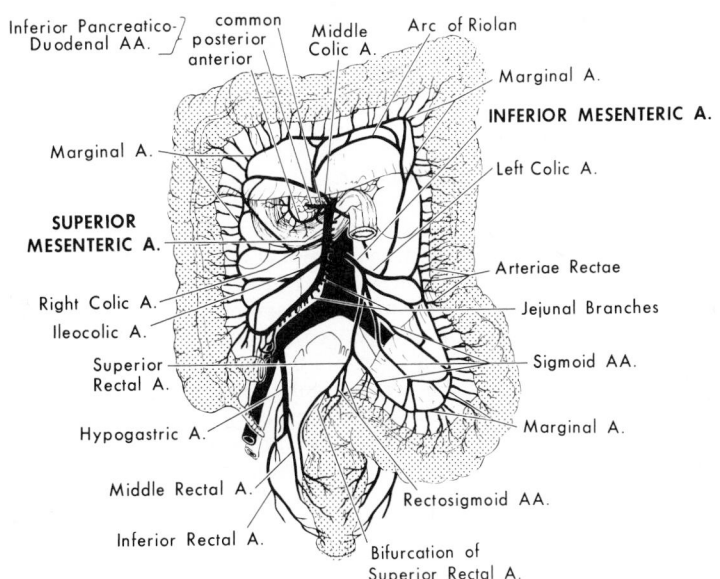

Figure 2. Arterial supply to the small and large intestines, showing the inferior portion of the pancreaticoduodenal arcades and the anastomoses between superior and inferior mesenteric arteries (arc of Riolan or "meandering mesenteric," and the marginal artery). (From Ockner, R. K., *In* Sleisenger, M. H., and Fordtran, J. S. [eds.]: Gastrointestinal Disease. 2nd ed. Philadelphia, W. B. Saunders Company, 1978.)

mesenteric artery supply those portions of the small and large intestines between the distal duodenum and the distal transverse colon.

The third visceral branch of the aorta is the inferior mesenteric artery. This vessel, the smallest of the three, arises at the level of the third lumbar vertebra and supplies the distal transverse and descending colon, sigmoid, and proximal rectum. Its branches connect with those of the superior mesenteric artery via the arc of Riolan ("meandering mesenteric artery") and the marginal artery (Fig. 2), and with the inferior and middle rectal branches of the hypogastric (internal iliac) arteries.

These abundant interconnections among the three major visceral arterial systems (i.e., the celiac axis and the superior and inferior mesenteric arteries) permit the formation of collateral channels in the event that occlusive vascular disease develops. As a result, it is not uncommon for slowly developing complete or nearly complete occlusions of a single vessel to be associated with little in the way of clinical sequelae.

The intestinal microcirculation is of major importance in controlling vascular perfusion, and the arteriole is the principal local determinant of resistance. Arteriolar resistance is increased by vasoconstrictors such as α-adrenergic stimulators, vasopressin, angiotensin II, and digitalis glycosides. Vasodilators include cholinergic stimuli, β-adrenergic agonists, locally produced metabolites, prostaglandins, and exogenous hormones, including pentagastrin, cholecystokinin, and glucagon. Mesenteric blood flow increases during feeding, but the role of endogenous gastrointestinal hormones in this response has not been established. With prolonged arteriolar vasoconstriction, there may occur a secondary increase in mesenteric blood flow, the so-called "autoregulatory escape"; the mechanism is not fully understood. The precapillary sphincter controls entry of blood into the villous capillaries and therefore is an important determinant of mucosal oxygenation. However, it does not significantly affect over-all mesenteric vascular resistance or flow.

Available evidence suggests that vasopressin, norepinephrine, and digitalis glycosides cause constriction of both the arterioles and the precapillary sphincters, resulting in both diminished intestinal blood flow and oxygen consumption. In contrast, recent animal studies suggest that epinephrine, which also diminishes total flow, does not appear to affect oxygen consumption or the precapillary sphincter. This "protective effect" of epinephrine on mucosal oxygen delivery was blocked by propranolol, suggesting that the precapillary sphincter is particularly responsive to β-adrenergic stimuli. Oxygenation of the villus may also be affected by a countercurrent exchange between the central villous arteriole and the surrounding venules. Under conditions in which blood flow is diminished, the countercurrent exchange is especially efficient, and delivery of oxygen to the mucosa may be even further compromised. This may account in part for the particular sensitivity of the mucosa to ischemic injury in low-flow states.

Several other factors may determine the adequacy of intestinal oxygenation and the possible development of ischemia in a given clinical situation. These include the abruptness of a vascular occlusion (more gradually occlusive processes may permit development of collaterals), the size and configuration of a vessel (emboli most commonly enter the large, obliquely situated superior mesenteric artery), and the site of a localized occlusive process (vasculitis involving arteriae rectae or intramural arteries may cause ischemia of a limited segment of intestine).

416. CHRONIC INTESTINAL ISCHEMIC SYNDROMES

ABDOMINAL ANGINA. This is an uncommon syndrome of postprandial epigastric or midabdominal pain caused by relative bowel ischemia. It usually occurs 15 to 30 minutes after eating, i.e., at a time when intestinal blood flow and oxygen demand normally increase, and persists for one to two hours. The syndrome is almost invariably associated with extensive atherosclerosis affecting two or more of the major visceral arterial trunks. Clinically, in addition to the history of pain, patients exhibit marked weight loss. Although the over-all picture may suggest a diagnosis of advanced malignancy, careful questioning will usually elicit a fear of pain, which the patient has learned to associate with eating, resulting in diminished food intake. History and physical examination often provide evidence of atherosclerotic disease affecting other vessels, but the presence or absence of an abdominal bruit is of little help. Establishment of the diagnosis, which must be strongly suggested by the history, requires exclusion of other potentially confusing intra-abdominal pathology and the demonstration, by arteriography, of significant (i.e., more than 50 per cent) narrowing of at least two of the three major visceral arteries. If the occlusive lesions are close to their takeoff from the aorta, then surgical correction is possible in most patients. Revascularization results in significant relief of symptoms, but the long-term effects of surgery on the natural history of the disease and on survival have not been established conclusively.

Because a significant number of patients with bowel infarction give an antecedent history of abdominal angina, correct diagnosis and treatment of this disorder are essential. It must be emphasized, however, that in the absence of a convincing history, a positive arteriogram alone does not establish the diagnosis, because advanced but asymptomatic occlusive vascular disease is not uncommon.

CELIAC COMPRESSION SYNDROME. This more recently described syndrome, the validity of which is the subject of considerable skepticism, is characterized by vague, intermittent epigastric pain, occasionally associated with other nonspecific gastrointestinal symptomatology. There is no clear relation to meals, but it may represent visceral ischemia caused in this instance by isolated narrowing of the celiac axis. Most cases have been ascribed to celiac axis compression by the adjacent median arcuate ligament of the diaphragm, but excess neurofibrous tissue of the celiac ganglion and intimal stenosis have also been incriminated. The patients are for the most part relatively young women who are otherwise healthy, without evidence of atherosclerotic disease or other significant abdominal pathology. An epigastric bruit, failing to radiate inferiorly, has been a common finding. Celiac arteriography will successfully demonstrate the narrowing, and in many cases reconstructive or bypass surgery has been effective in relief of symptoms. Despite these favorable reports, however, the diagnosis should be made only with caution, because similar degrees of celiac axis narrowing have been found incidentally (autopsy or angiography) in a substantial number of asymptomatic subjects, because follow-up studies of operated patients have been disappointing, and because of persisting uncertainty as to why this lesion should be associated with pain in the presence of an adequate collateral circulation. (It has been suggested that the pain is not ischemic, but rather arises in the celiac ganglion itself.) For these reasons, surgery for this syndrome should be reserved for those patients with prolonged, disabling symptoms in whom other pathology has been excluded. The need for additional follow-up data cannot be overemphasized.

417. ACUTE INTESTINAL ISCHEMIC SYNDROMES

ACUTE BOWEL INFARCTION: MESENTERIC ARTERIAL OCCLUSION. Occlusion of the superior mesenteric artery may be asymptomatic if it evolves slowly enough to permit the formation of adequate collaterals, as noted above. More sudden occlusions, however, are associated with ischemic infarction of some or all of the supplied bowel. Most commonly, advanced atherosclerotic disease is responsible, but the syndrome may also occur in dissecting aneurysm, systemic vasculitis of all varieties, use of oral contraceptives, hypercoagulable states, and, rarely, without apparent explanation. Among causes of bowel infarction, the true incidence of arterial thrombosis is not certain, but it may be less common than previously thought in view of the increasingly recognized importance of nonocclusive infarction (see below).

The clinical presentation of massive intestinal infarction (occlusive or nonocclusive) is often misleading. In its advanced stages, the associated abdominal pain, signs of intestinal obstruction, fever, leukocytosis, volume depletion, peritonitis with bloody abdominal fluid, hematemesis, and rectal bleeding are "classic" and render the diagnosis obvious. Earlier in the course, however, abdominal findings may be minimal, gastrointestinal bleeding may be absent, and the far less specific features of leukocytosis, pain, and confusional state may dominate the clinical picture. Bowel sounds not only may be present, but may be hyperactive. The history is usually not helpful, but evidence of pre-existing "abdominal angina" (see above) or other conditions predisposing to thrombosis may aid in the evaluation of the problem.

The early diagnosis of bowel infarction therefore depends upon a high index of suspicion and exclusion of other conditions likely to present as an acute abdomen. The demonstration of mesenteric vascular occlusion by abdominal angiography does not necessarily mean that the patient has an acute bowel infarction, because in many patients advanced occlusive disease is asymptomatic. On the other hand, the demonstration of *patent* vessels may serve to exclude *surgically correctable* vascular disease as a cause of bowel infarction, although this finding does not exclude nonocclusive infarction (see below).

Initial therapeutic efforts should be supportive, i.e., correction of fluid and electrolyte imbalance (including administration of blood, plasma, or albumin as needed), cardiopulmonary support, and broad-spectrum antimicrobial drugs. Unoperated, massive bowel infarction carries essentially a 100 per cent mortality rate. Unfortunately, since many patients with this diagnosis are poor surgical risks because of age, advanced vascular disease affecting other vital organs, or poor general condition resulting from delay in diagnosis, surgery itself may contribute to a fatal outcome. As a rule, however, operation should be undertaken as soon as the patient is in optimal condition, because time is of the essence. At surgery, infarcted bowel should be resected and, if large vessel thrombi are present and the patient's condition permits, corrective vascular surgery (bypass or endarterectomy) may be attempted. Because it is often difficult to define accurately the limits of viable bowel, many surgeons have recommended a "second look" operation after 24 hours, in order to resect any additional nonviable intestine. It should be recognized, however, that even under the best of circumstances, massive bowel infarction carries a mortality rate of at least 60 to 70 per cent, except in those cases caused by emboli (see below), in which a somewhat more favorable prognosis may be expected.

In some patients, especially those with mesenteric vasculitis (e.g., as may occur in lupus erythematosus, polyarteritis, dermatomyositis, rheumatoid vasculitis, and Henoch-Schönlein purpura), infarction may be segmental, it may not conform to the distribution of major arteries, and vascular occlusion may not be demonstrable angiographically. Since these patients occasionally require surgery for intestinal gangrene and perforation, they must be monitored accordingly; however, these complications are less common than with major vessel occlusions, and the acute episode may subside spontaneously. Subsequent barium contrast studies may show segmental submucosal edema and hemorrhage. In these patients surgery is not necessary unless development of a stricture causes intestinal obstruction.

MESENTERIC ARTERY EMBOLISM. As noted, arterial emboli to the splanchnic viscera most commonly lodge in the superior mesenteric artery. They usually arise from endocardial mural thrombi or vegetations, atrial myxomas, valvular prostheses, or atherosclerotic plaques in the proximal aorta, either spontaneously or during angiography. The condition is associated with diseases (e.g., mitral stenosis) which occur in a somewhat younger population than that at risk for occlusive or nonocclusive infarction, and because of this and the fact that its dramatic clinical presentation often leads to earlier diagnosis, embolic disease carries a somewhat more favorable prognosis. Classically, a patient with mitral stenosis will experience the sudden onset of severe periumbilical pain, followed by vomiting and diarrhea. Evidence of embolism to cerebral or peripheral arteries may be present. Initially bleeding may be absent and bowel sounds present, but ultimately the picture progresses, if untreated, to one identical with that of advanced occlusive infarction. Angiography may demonstrate mesenteric artery occlusion in the absence of a collateral circulation. Treatment consists of urgent exploration, with embolectomy and resection of infarcted bowel, followed by a "second look" procedure. It is important to note that there are well-documented cases in which early embolectomy has obviated the need for bowel resection, although a transient malabsorption syndrome may result.

NONOCCLUSIVE INTESTINAL INFARCTION. This syndrome presents clinically in a manner quite similar to that of occlusive infarction, but only more recently has its frequency been appreciated. Characteristically but not invariably, it occurs in a setting in which systemic anoxia, hypotension, congestive cardiac failure, or severe dehydration impairs the delivery of adequately oxygenated blood to the bowel, even though the splanchnic vessels themselves are patent. Many of these patients are receiving digitalis glycosides, but an etiologic role for these agents is not established. The mucosa, being most sensitive to oxygen deprivation, undergoes hemorrhagic necrosis first, but necrosis of the entire bowel wall usually supervenes. At surgery or autopsy, ischemic lesions may not conform to the distribution of major arterial supply routes. Experience is accumulating with the potential usefulness of mesenteric angiography in the diagnosis and management of this highly lethal condition. Angiography, as noted, will serve to exclude surgically approachable large vessel occlusions; it also may demonstrate narrowed major branches and arcades and impaired filling of intramural vessels. Administration of vasodilator substances has been suggested as a means of restoring intestinal vascular perfusion. However, treatment is otherwise the same as that of thrombotic infarction, i.e., supportive therapy and, as soon as feasible, surgical resection of infarcted bowel.

ISCHEMIC COLITIS. The large bowel is subject to most of the same problems associated with impaired blood supply which affect the small intestine, and many of the same pathophysiologic, diagnostic, and therapeutic principles apply. Thus occlusive or nonocclusive infarction may be widespread or segmental, and may be caused by injury or removal of the inferior mesenteric artery during aortic surgery, or associated with hypercoagulable states, atherosclerosis, vasculitis, amyloid, and oral contraceptive use. Perforation and peritonitis may require surgical intervention, with resection of infarcted bowel. Reconstructive surgery of the inferior mesenteric artery is not generally feasible. However, patients may present with a self-limited episode characterized by left-sided abdominal pain, fever, leukocytosis, and passage of bloody stools. The potential confusion resulting from this superficial resemblance to acute ulcerative colitis may be compounded by sigmoidoscopic findings which also suggest ulcerative colitis. Sigmoidoscopy, however, may disclose a normal mucosa, or one which shows discrete ulcers or blue-black hemorrhagic submucosal blebs or nodules. All or part of the colon may be involved, but the process usually affects the region of the splenic flexure or recto-sigmoid. Angiography has not proved generally useful in the management of patients with ischemic colitis. For those patients in whom surgery is not indicated, barium contrast studies performed after subsidence of the acute phase disclose mucosal edema and hemorrhage, as reflected by a sawtooth irregularity or by so-called "thumbprinting." Eventually, the healing process is often associated with scar and stricture formation, and surgery may be required at a later date because of partial obstruction.

The true incidence of ischemic colitis is difficult to estimate, but its presence should be suspected in any patient over 50 who first presents with what clinically resembles acute ulcerative colitis, as well as in younger individuals who are at increased risk.

MESENTERIC VENOUS THROMBOSIS. This condition is less frequent than either mesenteric artery occlusion or nonocclusive intestinal infarction. It can occur in association with hypercoagulable states, polycythemia, portal venous stasis, tumor infiltration, sepsis, trauma, or oral contraceptive use, after renal transplantation, and occasionally without evident cause. It may present abruptly, as an acute bowel infarction, but in some patients it may develop over a period of up to two weeks in association with vague abdominal symptoms. Physical findings are nonspecific, but 80 per cent of patients are found to have serosanguineous ascites. Gastrointestinal bleeding is common later in the course. Preoperative angiography may suggest the diagnosis by showing a prolonged arterial phase and failure to opacify the venous system. At surgery infarcted bowel is resected and anticoagulation is instituted to minimize the chances of recurrence during the first postoperative weeks. The prognosis is more favorable than that of arterial occlusion and nonocclusive infarction.

418. MISCELLANEOUS DISORDERS

INTRAMURAL INTESTINAL HEMORRHAGE. Bleeding into the wall of the intestine may occur as the result of spontaneous or iatrogenic hypocoagulable states (e.g., anticoagulant therapy), localized hemorrhagic infarction (e.g., vasculitis), or as the result of blunt abdominal trauma. Patients usually present with abdominal pain and exhibit variable findings suggestive of intestinal obstruction and bleeding. A significant obstructive picture is especially common in those patients who sustain upper abdominal trauma, resulting in the formation of a large intramural hematoma in that portion of the duodenum which is fixed retroperitoneally. Barium studies show the "stacked coins" or "thumbprint" appearance typical of submucosal bleeding.

In most patients, intramural hemorrhage can be managed conservatively, including appropriate treatment of the underlying causative factors and nasogastric suction when indicated. In those patients with high-grade or unremitting intestinal obstruction, or in whom signs of peritonitis develop (suggesting perforation), surgery is necessary.

ABDOMINAL AORTIC ANEURYSM. Pathologic dilatation of the abdominal aorta is usually due to advanced atherosclerosis, and most commonly affects that segment distal to the origin of the renal arteries. Mild degrees of dilatation (i.e., 4 to 5 cm or less) are rarely symptomatic or associated with significant morbidity or mortality. Aneurysms larger than 6 to 7 cm, however, and those of any size which are increasing in caliber or causing symptoms (usually because of erosion of adjacent vertebrae) constitute serious threats to life. Such aneurysms may lead to a rapid exsanguination, by rupturing into the bowel, the free peritoneal cavity, or the retroperitoneal space. Since the operative mortality under these urgent conditions is unacceptably high, such high-risk aneurysms should be resected electively (see Ch. 367).

PARAPROSTHETIC-ENTERIC FISTULA. This syndrome is an important complication of the presence of a prosthesis in the abdominal aorta or other retroperitoneal artery. It is characterized by massive abrupt or intermittent gastrointestinal bleeding, and may present between 21 days and 14 years after surgery. It usually results from deterioration of the vascular suture line because of infection or local ischemia, and erosion into adjacent bowel. Untreated, the syndrome is fatal in 40 to 75 per cent of cases. Because its preoperative diagnosis is extremely difficult, patients with gastrointestinal bleeding who have abdominal arterial prostheses should be regarded as having a paraprosthetic-enteric fistula until proved otherwise, and as candidates for urgent surgery.

SUPERIOR MESENTERIC ARTERY SYNDROME. An uncommon syndrome of postprandial upper intestinal obstruction has been attributed to compression of the third portion of the duodenum between the superior mesenteric artery anteriorly and the fixed retroperitoneal structures posteriorly. Such patients generally have lost weight or are of the "asthenic habitus"; in children, it is associated with rapid growth in the absence of corresponding weight gain, or with fixed hyperextension of the spine by a cast. Barium contrast studies show duodenal distention, and the differential diagnosis includes generalized disorders of intestinal motility such as scleroderma. Relief of symptoms may be afforded by assumption of the knee-chest or prone position, or the use of small feedings or chemically defined liquid diets with the patient lying prone or on the left side after eating. In refractory cases, duodenal bypass or mobilization reportedly has been effective.

VASCULAR MALFORMATIONS. Hemangiomas of the small intestine are very uncommon vascular tumors found throughout the bowel, particularly the jejunum. They assume clinical importance as one cause of gastrointestinal bleeding of undetermined source. These lesions are most reliably diagnosed by abdominal angiography. Telangiectasias may also be causes of gastrointestinal bleeding, and may be associated with mucocutaneous telangiectasias (Osler-Weber-Rendu disease) or Turner's syndrome.

VASCULAR ECTASIAS OF THE COLON. Vascular abnormalities of the cecum and ascending colon not associated with vascular lesions in skin or other viscera have been increasingly recognized as important causes of lower gastrointestinal bleeding, especially in patients over 60 years of age. They consist of ectatic areas of the mucosal microvasculature, especially the capillaries and venules, associated with dilatation of submucosal veins. Recent evidence suggests that the primary abnormality is chronic obstruction of the submucosal veins as they penetrate the muscularis, and that these lesions are neither congenital malformations nor neoplasms (angiomas). It has also been suggested that they may develop as the consequence of chronic mucosal ischemia. By means of special techniques, such lesions have been demonstrated in a significant number of resected right colon specimens from older patients who have no history of gastrointestinal bleeding. The basis for the apparent association of bleeding from colonic vascular ectasias with aortic stenosis is not known. The lesion may be diagnosed by angiography, which may demonstrate a late-emptying dilated tortuous intramural vein, a vascular tuft filled by a prominent artery, or an early filling vein. However, many smaller lesions will not be demonstrable angiographically. Colonoscopy has been reported to reveal their presence, but the over-all accuracy of this approach is not known. The clinical importance of this lesion is potentially great, because it may be quite common in the older population generally, and may account for a large number of those patients with unexplained lower gastrointestinal bleeding, including some in whom bleeding has been attributed to right colon diverticula. Right hemicolectomy is indicated in those patients who have bled without other obvious cause and in whom ectasias are demonstrated.

Boley, S. J. (ed.): Vascular Disorders of the Intestine. New York, Appleton-Century-Crofts, 1971.
Boley, S. J., Sammartano, R., Adams, A., Dibiase, A., Kleinhaus, S., and Sprayregen, S.: On the nature and etiology of vascular ectasias of the colon. Degenerative lesions of aging. Gastroenterology, 72:650, 1977.
Bond, J. H., Levitt, D. G., and Levitt, M. D.: Quantitation of counter-

current exchange during passive absorption from the dog small intestine. J. Clin Invest., 59:308, 1977.

Bowen, J. C., Pawlik, W., Fang, W-F., and Jacobson, E. D.: Pharmacologic effects of gastrointestinal hormones on intestinal oxygen consumption and blood flow. Surgery, 78:515, 1975.

Lanciault, G., and Jacobson, E. D.: The gastrointestinal circulation. Gastroenterology, 71:851, 1976.

Lundgren, O.: The circulation of the small bowel mucosa. Gut, 15:1005, 1975.

Novelline, R. A., Waltman, A. C., Athanasoulis, C. A., and Baum, S.: Recent advances in abdominal angiography. Adv. Intern. Med., 21:417, 1976.

Ockner, R. K.: Vascular diseases of the bowel. *In* Sleisenger, M. H., and Fordtran, J. S. (eds.): Gastrointestinal Disease. 2nd ed. Philadelphia, W. B. Saunders Company, 1978, p. 1889.

Pawlik, W., Shepherd, A. P., Mailman, D., and Jacobson, E. D.: Effects of ouabain on intestinal oxygen consumption. Gastroenterology, 67:100, 1974.

Williams, L. F., Jr.: Vascular insufficiency of the intestine. Gastroenterology, 61:757, 1971.

Section Nine DISEASES OF THE PERITONEUM, MESENTERY, AND OMENTUM

Robert K. Ockner

419. DISEASES OF THE PERITONEUM

ANATOMY AND PHYSIOLOGY. The peritoneum is a continuous mesothelial membrane which lines the abdominal cavity and covers its contained viscera. This structure forms a closed sac, except at the entry of the fimbriated ostia of the fallopian tubes, and consists of two anatomically distinct but contiguous portions. The *visceral* peritoneum encloses those organs which are entirely intraperitoneal, including the mesenteries by which they are suspended, whereas the *parietal* peritoneum lines the walls of the abdominal cavity (including the undersurface of the diaphragm and the pelvis) and the retroperitoneal organs (including the duodenum, ascending and descending colon, pancreas, kidneys, and adrenals). The two portions of the peritoneal membrane also differ in blood supply and innervation. The visceral peritoneum is supplied by the splanchnic arterial system, and its venous drainage enters the portal vein. In contrast, the parietal peritoneum receives branches of arteries which nourish the abdominal wall and diaphragm, and its venous drainage is by way of systemic veins. The visceral peritoneum does not contain pain receptors, and afferent stimuli are transmitted via the visceral autonomics. The parietal peritoneum, on the other hand, is supplied by spinal nerves which also innervate the abdominal wall. As a result, irritation of the parietal peritoneum produces well-localized somatic pain (which may be referred to other sites in the same dermatome); in contrast, irritation of the visceral peritoneum produces a much less well-defined discomfort which is often poorly localized. The diaphragmatic portion of the peritoneum is supplied by the phrenic nerve (spinal roots C3 to C5) centrally and, in its more peripheral portions, by the intercostal nerves. As a result, pain caused by diaphragmatic irritation may be referred either to the shoulder or to the thoracic or abdominal wall.

The peritoneal surface is a semipermeable membrane, and allows for the passive diffusion of water and solutes between the abdominal cavity and the subperitoneal vascular (blood and lymphatic) channels. In general, water and solutes of molecular weight less than 2000 are absorbed from the peritoneal cavity via the blood vascular system; larger molecules and particulate substances enter the lymphatics. Movement of particles from the peritoneal cavity into the subdiaphragmatic lymphatics is facilitated by specialized areas of contact between the parietal peritoneum and the underlying lymphatics. In these areas, discontinuities exist between the peritoneal mesothelial cells and the lymphatic endothelial cells; basement membranes are scanty or absent. As a result, particles of substantial size (e.g., red blood cells) move freely from the abdominal cavity into the subdiaphragmatic lymphatics, a process which may be facilitated by respiratory motion of the diaphragm itself.

Water and electrolytes equilibrate rapidly (i.e., within two hours) between the blood vascular compartment and the free peritoneal cavity. *Net* fluid movement from the abdominal cavity into the plasma occurs at a maximal rate of approximately 30 to 35 ml per hour. This figure applies not only to the normal man but also to patients with portal hypertension and ascites; this rate cannot be exceeded despite vigorous diuresis; rather, such diuresis only serves to remove fluid from other body compartments, and may cause hypovolemia.

DIAGNOSIS. Because of the wide diversity of diseases of the peritoneum, few generalizations can be made regarding history and physical examination. Abdominal pain and ascites may be present, as may other less specific complaints of fever, nausea, and vomiting, depending on the nature and localization of the process. Diagnosis of known or suspected peritoneal disease is therefore greatly dependent upon special techniques, including routine radiology, ultrasonography, computerized tomography, abdominal paracentesis, peritoneal biopsy, peritoneoscopy, and exploratory laparotomy.

Radiographically, ascites may be manifest by haziness and separation of bowel loops on plain abdominal films. Otherwise, peritoneal disease reflects itself only indirectly. For example, an inflammatory process resulting in scar formation may cause angulation, separation, or narrowing of intestinal loops or evidence of mucosal edema (owing to obstruction of lymphatic or venous channels) on barium contrast studies. If ascites is present, abdominal paracentesis is essential in order to establish its cause (see below). Ultrasonography and computerized tomography may be useful in demonstrating relatively small amounts of peritoneal fluid, and especially in distinguishing free fluid from cystic masses. Computerized tomography also has been successful in demonstration of peritoneal implants and in examination of the retroperitoneum. Peritoneal biopsy, particularly with the Cope needle, is a relatively simple and safe bedside technique which may yield a positive diagnosis of neoplastic or infectious causes in 50 to 60 per cent of cases. Peritoneoscopy, performed under the proper circumstances by a physician experienced in this technique, can be accomplished with little morbidity or mortality. A successful examination may obviate the need for exploratory surgery and may permit biopsy under direct vision of involved portions of the peritoneum or liver. If a diagnosis cannot be made in a patient with obvious peritoneal disease by means of the aforementioned procedures, exploratory laparotomy may be necessary.

ASCITES

The accumulation of fluid within the peritoneal cavity may result from several different pathophysiologic mechanisms. These include (1) increases in the permeability of the peritoneal capillaries (e.g., in neoplastic and inflammatory diseases of the peritoneum) and (2) diminished plasma colloid osmotic pressure (e.g., severe hypoalbuminemia of any cause). An elevation in portal venous pressure alone (i.e., in the absence of hypoalbuminemia) is ordinarily not adequate cause for ascites formation, as evidenced by its relative infrequency in portal vein thrombosis not associated with hypoalbuminemia or liver disease. A third important mechanism for ascites formation is elevation of the hydrostatic pressure within the hepatic sinusoids. This may result from any of the conditions associated with *postsinusoidal portal hypertension*, including *cirrhosis, hepatic vein or inferior vena cava obstruction*, and advanced *congestive heart failure* or *constrictive pericarditis*. In these conditions, elevated sinusoidal pressure increases the movement of protein-rich plasma filtrate from the sinusoid into the space of Disse and the hepatic lymphatics. Although much of the fluid ultimately enters the thoracic duct, hepatic lymph may be lost directly from the surface of the liver into the free peritoneal cavity. This mechanism undoubtedly accounts for the not infrequent finding that patients with postsinusoidal portal hypertension of any cause, including cirrhosis and congestive failure, may have ascites with an unexpectedly high protein concentration, despite the fact that its formation may be considered to represent "transudation" rather than "exudation" in the usual sense.

Ascites formation in the cirrhotic, and in other situations in which plasma volume or renal vascular perfusion is abnormal, may be aggravated by renal retention of sodium and water. It seems unlikely, however, that these latter factors alone are sufficient for the formation of ascites, because neither primary hyperaldosteronism nor increased antidiuretic hormone secretion is associated with ascites formation in the absence of other contributing factors.

EVALUATION OF ASCITES FLUID. Although laboratory analysis of fluid removed from the abdominal cavity may not provide a specific etiologic diagnosis, no patient with ascites can be considered to have been properly evaluated without this examination. Fluids with protein concentrations exceeding 2.5 grams are usually regarded as "exudates," whereas those with lower concentrations are designated "transudates." Although this classification is useful, exceptions in both directions occur not infrequently. Thus cases of neoplasm or infection of the peritoneum in association with "transudative" fluids and of cirrhosis and congestive heart failure in association with "exudative" protein levels are numerous and well documented. For this reason, ascites fluid protein concentrations must be interpreted only in the context of all other clinical and laboratory findings. Other chemical determinations may be helpful, including amylase (markedly elevated in pancreatic ascites), glucose (often less than 60 mg per 100 ml in neoplastic ascites), and triglyceride (in excess of plasma concentrations in chylous ascites). Bloody ascites strongly suggests neoplasm, especially benign and malignant tumors. Elevated leukocyte counts (in excess of 250 per cubic millimeter) suggest peritoneal irritation, e.g., neoplasm or infection. The differential leukocyte count is of help in that a very high percentage of lymphocytes strongly suggests tuberculous peritonitis. Cytology is an essential part of the examination and may be expected to yield accurate results in more than half the cases. Ascites fluid should be cultured for routine pathogens, acid-fast bacilli, and fungi.

DIFFERENTIAL DIAGNOSIS OF ASCITES. Although a wide variety of disease processes may be associated with the presence of ascites, more than 90 per cent of patients with this complication are found to have cirrhosis, neoplasm, congestive heart failure, or tuberculosis. For purposes of classification, causes of ascites may be divided into diseases not involving the peritoneum on the one hand (Table 1) and diseases of the peritoneum on the other (Table 2). Of those cases not associated with peritoneal disease, *cirrhosis* is by far the most

TABLE 1.   Causes of Ascites Not Associated with Peritoneal Disease*

I. Portal hypertension
  A. Cirrhosis
  B. Hepatic congestion
    1. Congestive heart failure
    2. Constrictive pericarditis
    3. Inferior vena cava obstruction
    4. Hepatic vein obstruction (Budd-Chiari syndrome)
  C. Portal vein occlusion
II. Hypoalbuminemia
  A. Nephrotic syndrome
  B. Protein-losing enteropathy
  C. Malnutrition
III. Miscellaneous
  A. Myxedema
  B. Ovarian disease
    1. Meigs' syndrome
    2. Struma ovarii
    3. Ovarian overstimulation syndrome
  C. Pancreatic ascites
  D. Bile ascites
  E. Chylous ascites
  F. Urine ascites and dialysis-associated ascites

*From Bender, M. D., and Ockner, R. K., *In* Sleisenger, M. H., and Fordtran, J. S. (eds.): Gastrointestinal Disease. 2nd ed. Philadelphia, W. B. Saunders Company, 1978.

TABLE 2. Diseases of the Peritoneum*

I. Infections
   A. Acute peritonitis
   B. Tuberculous peritonitis
   C. Fungal diseases
     1. Candidiasis
     2. Histoplasmosis
     3. Coccidioidomycosis
     4. Cryptococcosis
   D. Parasitic diseases
     1. Schistosomiasis
     2. Enterobiasis
     3. Ascariasis
     4. Strongyloidiasis
     5. Amebiasis
II. Neoplasms
   A. Secondary malignancy
   B. Primary mesothelioma
   C. Pseudomyxoma peritonei
III. Miscellaneous
   A. Vasculitis
   B. Granulomatous peritonitis
     1. Sarcoidosis
     2. Crohn's disease
     3. Starch peritonitis
   C. Familial paroxysmal peritonitis
   D. Eosinophilic gastroenteritis
   E. Whipple's disease
   F. Gynecologic disease
     1. Endometriosis
     2. Deciduosis
     3. Gliomatosis
     4. Leiomyomatosis
     5. Dermoid cyst
     6. Melanosis
   G. Splenosis
   H. Sclerosing peritonitis
   I. Peritoneal lymphangiectasia
   J. Peritoneal loose bodies and cysts
   K. Peritoneal encapsulation

*Modified from Bender, M. D., and Ockner, R. K., *In* Sleisenger, M. H., and Fordtran, J. S. (eds.): Gastrointestinal Disease. 2nd ed. Philadelphia, W. B. Saunders Company, 1978.

common; it is considered in Ch. 465.2. *Portal hypertension* caused by diseases of the heart and great veins accounts for a substantial number of patients with ascites of obscure origin. Included in this group are patients with *congestive heart failure, constrictive pericarditis,* and *inferior vena cava* and *hepatic vein obstruction (Budd-Chiari syndrome).* Clinically, patients with these conditions may not be readily distinguishable from those with hepatic cirrhosis; a high index of suspicion is necessary, and special procedures may be required in order to establish or exclude the diagnosis. Hypoalbuminemia of any cause, including nephrotic syndrome and protein-losing enteropathy, may be associated with a classically "transudative" ascites.

Various endocrine conditions may be associated with ascites. These include *myxedema,* in which the fluid is typically protein rich, and *diseases* of the *ovary,* among them *Meigs' syndrome,* in which transudative ascites is associated with ovarian fibroma or cystadenoma, struma ovarii, and "ovarian overstimulation" syndrome.

Ascites associated with pancreatic disease usually occurs in the presence of chronic *pancreatitis* and *pseudocyst.* The most common etiologic factors are alcohol and trauma. The ascites fluid amylase concentration is elevated, often to very high levels. Drainage of the pseudocyst and repair of duct injury often have been effective in managing this complication, particularly in traumatic cases. In the chronic alcoholic with pancreatic ascites, a trial of conservative management is indicated

before surgery is undertaken. Leakage of bile may be associated with the development of *bile ascites,* a condition for which surgical repair of the biliary tract is usually necessary. This situation is not necessarily associated with the fulminant clinical picture of fever, leukocytosis, and peritonitis, i.e., *bile peritonitis,* which appears to result from superimposed infection.

Chylous ascites is due to the presence of lymph lipoproteins and chylomicrons in the peritoneal cavity. These lipid-rich particles impart a turbidity to the fluid which facilitates its diagnosis. However, not all turbid abdominal fluids are "chylous." Establishment of the diagnosis requires direct evidence that the turbidity is indeed due to neutral lipid, a determination best made by analysis of the fluid for triglyceride concentration; alternatively, solvent extraction (ether or chloroform) which results in clearing of the fluid may be taken as presumptive evidence for the diagnosis. Other turbid abdominal fluids may be due to cellular debris, and are designated *"pseudochylous"* ascites, a condition occasionally associated with abdominal neoplasm or infection. The differential diagnosis of truly chylous ascites depends upon its chronicity and the age of the patient. *Chronic chylous ascites* in adults is caused in over 80 per cent of cases by abdominal neoplasm, usually *lymphoma,* with associated obstruction and disruption of the abdominal lymphatics resulting from extensive lymph node involvement. *Acute chylous ascites* ("chylous peritonitis") is associated with abrupt onset of abdominal pain. In some cases, this syndrome is due to *trauma, intestinal obstruction,* or *rupture* of a *chylous cyst,* but a specific etiologic diagnosis may not be possible even at laparotomy. In children, congenital malformations of the lymphatics, including intestinal *lymphangiectasia,* account for a higher proportion of the cases of chylous ascites.

Urine ascites may result from trauma to the urinary tract, high grade obstruction caused by posterior urethral valves in the neonate, or renal transplantation. Ascites also may occur in a few patients maintained on *chronic hemodialysis.* The cause of this is not defined, but it appears to reflect a number of factors, including prior peritoneal dialysis or infection, fluid overload, hypertension, poor nutrition, or hypoalbuminemia. Management is not totally satisfactory, and aggressive dialysis, nephrectomy for hypertensive patients, and renal transplantation offer the best possibilities for relief.

INFECTIONS OF THE PERITONEUM

Acute Peritonitis

Although this syndrome may result from a chemical irritation or "burn" of the peritoneal surface (as in severe acute pancreatitis), most cases are due to *bacterial infection.* Most commonly, enteric organisms enter the peritoneal cavity through a necrotic defect in the wall of the intestine or other abdominal viscus resulting from *obstruction, infarction, neoplasm, foreign body,* or primary inflammatory disease such as *fulminant ulcerative colitis. Perforated peptic ulcer* and *ruptured appendix* are particularly frequent causes. If unchecked, bacterial contamination of the peritoneum results in a "spreading peritonitis," leading ultimately to marked exudation of protein-rich fluid into the abdominal cavity, paralytic ileus, and reflex spasm of the overlying abdominal musculature. The systemic consequences of this cata-strophic event are predictable. Loss of fluid from the vascular compartment into both the free peritoneal cav-ity and the bowel lumen results in volume depletion and hemoconcentration; these factors, together with the possible systemic effects of the bacterial infection itself, may lead to shock and oliguria. The latter may progress to acute tubular necrosis.

Despite its often dramatic presentation, recognition of acute peritonitis may be difficult in those patients in whom the clinical manifestations are masked or sup-pressed. This applies particularly to the elderly and to those receiving corticosteroids, as, for example, in the treatment of acute ulcerative colitis. In these patients, a particularly high index of suspicion is necessary, and the only *early* manifestation may be a rise in pulse rate or unexplained hypotension. Diagnosis in such situa-tions may depend upon the radiographic demonstration of free air in the peritoneal cavity and upon aspiration of abdominal contents to confirm the presence of poly-morphonuclear leukocytes and bacteria. Fortunately, the peritoneum is often able to confine inflammatory processes of this type. As a result, acute peritonitis may be restricted to one portion of the abdomen and may not spread or become generalized.

Management of peritonitis includes restoration of fluid and electrolyte imbalance; the administration of fresh frozen plasma or albumin is often required. An-timicrobial therapy and nasogastric suction should be instituted. Analgesics are often necessary, but their premature use may hinder proper evaluation of the pa-tient. The decision to operate must be individualized. In those patients who are seen early after a recognized perforation of a viscus and who are good operative can-didates, surgery usually should be undertaken as soon as feasible. However, in a few patients (particularly those who are very poor operative risks), it may be de-sirable to attempt to control the process nonoperatively and to encourage its localization by means of antimi-crobial drugs and other conservative measures. Local-ized abscesses so formed may be drained later, when circumstances are more favorable.

Subphrenic Abscess

Particularly challenging problems in diagnosis and treatment are posed by the collection of pus in one of the more or less well-defined tissue spaces inferior to the diaphragm and adjacent to the liver, stomach, spleen, and lesser sac. Most often, subphrenic abscess develops secondary to other septic and inflammatory processes in the abdomen, especially *ruptured appendix* or *diverticulum, infected gallbladder, perforated ulcer* with bacterial contamination, *pancreatitis, penetrating abdomi-nal wound,* or extension of an *intrahepatic abscess* beyond the liver capsule. It may also complicate surgi-cal treatment of one of these conditions.

Clinically, the picture usually suggests a septic proc-ess, with malaise, fever, and pain, and leukocytosis. The subphrenic location is often not obvious, but may be suggested by a history of one of the aforementioned antecedent events, by direct clinical evidence such as the location of pain, elevation or impaired motion of the diaphragm, or by x-ray evidence of a pleural effu-sion associated with a subdiaphragmatic air-fluid level. Diagnosis may be facilitated by means of ^{67}gallium scanning, ultrasonography, and computerized tomogra-phy.

Antimicrobial therapy usually suppresses the process and helps to contain it, but may also obscure its recog-nition. Definitive therapy consists of surgical drainage.

Spontaneous ("Primary") Peritonitis

Bacterial peritonitis may also occur in the absence of an acute intra-abdominal precipitating factor. In this circumstance, the offending organism may not be en-teric, and the syndrome is more likely to occur in pa-tients who have pre-existing ascites, impaired immun-ologic defenses, or a cause for bacteremia such as localized infection elsewhere in the body or indwelling catheters. A well-recognized example of this circum-stance is the child with nephrotic syndrome and ascites who develops primary peritonitis, but urinary tract in-fection may now be a more common predisposing fac-tor in children. The mortality rate associated with this entity has diminished considerably during recent dec-ades because of the availability of antimicrobial drugs.

More common is spontaneous bacterial peritonitis in patients with advanced, decompensated *cirrhosis* and *ascites*. This syndrome may occur in up to 10 per cent of such patients, and although enteric organisms (par-ticularly *E. coli*) are most often cultured, pneumococci and streptococci are frequent offenders. The cause of the syndrome is not known; perforated viscus, pneu-monia, biliary tract infection, and other local sites of bacterial infection cannot be implicated. Possibly, the cirrhotic liver with spontaneous portal-systemic shunt-ing is less effective in clearing bacteria from the portal blood, but this would not explain the occurrence of nonenteric organisms. The syndrome may be recog-nized by the sudden onset of abdominal pain, fever, and leukocytosis, occurring in the setting of decompen-sated cirrhosis and ascites. Blood cultures are positive in 75 per cent of cases; abdominal fluid usually yields a positive culture and contains an elevated number of polymorphonuclear leukocytes. Although appropriate antimicrobial therapy may afford a satisfactory bacterio-logic response in the majority of patients, the over-all mortality rate remains very high. A few patients have been described in whom ascites fluid cultures were positive in the absence of other clinical features of the syndrome; such patients probably should be treated with antimicrobial agents.

Other Infections

Tuberculous peritonitis is discussed in detail in Ch. 168.11. It should be emphasized that this disorder may present in a variety of ways, ranging from an acute ab-domen to an insidiously developing, otherwise unex-plained ascites resembling (or associated with) cirrho-sis. Accordingly its presence should be suspected in all patients with ascites, with or without an apparently ad-equate cause. Fewer than half of the patients have ac-tive disease elsewhere in the body, and tuberculosis skin testing and appropriate cultures of ascites fluid for tubercle bacilli should be regarded as routine in the evaluation of ascites. The diagnosis is strongly suggest-ed by a high percentage of lymphocytes in the abdomi-nal fluid, and may be confirmed by means of a positive culture, peritoneal biopsy, laparoscopy, or, if necessary, exploratory laparotomy. The very satisfactory response of this condition to appropriate chemotherapy adds to the importance of early diagnosis.

Fungal and parasitic diseases may be associated with

peritoneal involvement and, occasionally, with ascites. These disorders, including *histoplasmosis, candidiasis, coccidioidomycosis, cryptococcosis, ascariasis, amebiasis,* and *schistosomiasis,* are quite uncommon, but deserve consideration in otherwise unexplained cases of peritoneal disease with or without ascites.

TUMORS OF THE PERITONEUM

Secondary malignancy is the most common form of neoplastic involvement of the peritoneum. More than 75 per cent of such tumors are *adenocarcinomas,* but peritoneal involvement by *sarcomas, lymphomas, leukemias, carcinoids,* and *multiple myeloma* has been described. Ascites formation in these patients appears to result from the combination of increased capillary permeability and obstruction of channels which drain the peritoneal cavity by way of the subdiaphragmatic lymphatics. The clinical picture is usually that associated with advancing malignancy, including weakness and weight loss, and variable complaints referable to the abdomen such as pain, distention, nausea, or vomiting. Radiographic findings may include angulation, fixation, or displacement of intestinal loops, or submucosal edema reflecting lymphatic obstruction. On abdominal paracentesis, the fluid obtained usually has a high protein content (more than 2.5 grams per 100 ml); cellular composition is variable, and occasionally the fluid is grossly bloody. The diagnosis is reliably made in most patients by means of cytology or peritoneal biopsy, but peritoneoscopy or surgical exploration occasionally may be necessary.

Treatment of this condition involves the intraperitoneal administration of antitumor agents, including alkylators, antimetabolites, or radioactive isotopes. Unfortunately, the prognosis of patients in this advanced stage of malignancy is poor. Intra-abdominal quinacrine has occasionally been successful in producing a fibrous serositis, thereby obliterating the free peritoneal space and reducing further fluid exudation, but the usefulness of this approach is limited by the frequent occurrence of fever, nausea, vomiting, and abdominal pain.

Primary Mesothelioma

This rare primary tumor of the peritoneum is most common in males over age 50, and is associated with the gradual onset of abdominal pain and distention, nausea, vomiting, weight loss, and development of ascites. Cytology or peritoneal biopsy reveals a variable histopathology in which epithelial and mesenchymal elements are combined, and for this reason differentiation from other malignancies may be difficult. It has been suggested on epidemiologic grounds that exposure to asbestos fibers may play an etiologic role in the development of this tumor. This conclusion is based on the association, in most patients, with environmental exposure to asbestos fibers and evidence of pulmonary asbestosis, including "asbestos bodies" in the lungs. Because of evidence that these so-called "asbestos bodies" are nonspecific and may occur in up to 50 per cent of the general population, the importance of asbestos in the etiology of this tumor is uncertain (see Ch. 348.6). A significant number of patients with peritoneal mesothelioma have a similar process affecting the pleura. The prognosis of the disease is exceedingly poor, averaging one to two years' survival after diagno-

sis. Chemotherapy and radiation therapy have generally been unsuccessful, but more intensive treatment programs are being evaluated.

Pseudomyxoma Peritonei

Classification of this rare disorder as a tumor is a matter of some uncertainty, because in many cases it appears to arise as a complication of certain relatively benign processes, including mucocele of the appendix. On the other hand, its neoplastic nature is suggested by a high incidence of cellular atypia in carefully examined pathologic specimens, as well as by evidence for low-grade malignancy in a high percentage of those patients in whom the syndrome develops subsequent to *mucinous cystadenomas* of the *ovaries.* The syndrome is characterized by abdominal distention resulting from the accumulation of a mucinous, gelatinous, translucent material. Most cases seem to originate as an outgrowth of pre-existing mucinous cystadenomas and cystadenocarcinomas of the ovary and mucocele of the appendix, but other tumors of the genitourinary tract or gastrointestinal tract may be associated with the process.

The condition usually presents as an increase in abdominal girth, with little in the way of other clinical signs of disease. At surgery, the abdominal cavity is found to contain gelatinous material existing in a variety of states, including cystic masses, lying freely without apparent attachment, or anchored to the peritoneal surface.

If the tumor is indeed malignant, it appears to be of low grade and rarely metastasizes. As a result, the course of the disease is prolonged and is characterized by recurrent episodes of intestinal obstruction and fistula formation. The most promising therapeutic approach at present appears to be one which combines surgical removal of the ovary, appendix, and as much mucin as possible, with intraperitoneal instillation of an alkylating agent.

Miscellaneous Diseases of the Peritoneum

The peritoneal membrane may be affected by a wide variety of systemic diseases, including *systemic lupus erythematosus* (see Ch. 52) and other "collagen vascular" diseases, *Whipple's disease* (see Ch. 408), and *sarcoidosis* (see Ch. 65). Eosinophilic ascites may complicate eosinophilic gastroenteritis or other causes of peripheral eosinophilia. Several other unusual conditions affecting the peritoneum have been described (Table 2), including lesions associated with gynecologic disorders, splenosis, sclerosing peritonitis, mesothelial hyperplasia and metaplasia, peritoneal lymphangiectasis, and peritoneal loose bodies, cysts, and encapsulation.

Bender, M. D., and Ockner, R. K.: Diseases of the peritoneum, mesentery, and diaphragm. *In* Sleisenger, M. H., and Fordtran, J. S. (eds.): Gastrointestinal Disease. 2nd ed. Philadelphia, W. B. Saunders Company, 1978, p. 1947.

420. DISEASES OF THE MESENTERY AND OMENTUM

MESENTERIC INFLAMMATORY DISEASE. This syndrome includes a spectrum of conditions ranging from acute inflammation to a chronic fibrosing process associated with intestinal obstruction, ascites, and steator-rhea. Included are such conditions as "*mesenteric panniculitis*" and "*retractile mesenteritis*." The cause of this syndrome is not known, but it is believed to represent the sequel to some inciting event such as trauma, infection, or ischemia in the mesentery. Fat necrosis occurs, evoking an inflammatory reaction with subsequent scarring and granuloma formation.

The condition is most commonly seen in males in late adulthood. The acute syndrome ("mesenteric panniculitis"), which constitutes the presentation of 60 per cent of cases, is characterized by recurrent abdominal pain, weight loss, nausea, vomiting, and fever. In most patients, a tender abdominal mass is palpable; leukocytosis may or may not be present. The remaining 40 per cent of cases are identified by the discovery of a mass on examination or at surgery. Radiographic examination is nonspecific, showing the effects of an abdominal mass and variable scarring, which include displacement and separation of intestinal loops, with angulation, stenosis, and extrinsic compression. In some patients the condition evolves into a more chronic process ("retractile mesenteritis"), characterized by continuing pain, fever, weight loss, and various signs of intestinal obstruction, ascites, and steatorrhea.

At surgery, the small bowel mesentery is found to be the principal site of involvement; it is thickened and fibrotic, particularly at the root. Microscopically in *mesenteric panniculitis*, there is infiltration of adipose tissue by foamy macrophages and lymphocytes, with fat necrosis, fibrosis, and calcification. In *retractile mesenteritis*, the thickening and fibrosis are more pronounced, and there is less evidence of acute necrosis and inflammation. Infrequently, the mesocolon or parietal peritoneum may be involved, or the process may occur in association with retroperitoneal fibrosis.

Although long-term experience with this syndrome is limited, most patients seem to have a prolonged survival; most become asymptomatic after a period of months to years, whereas a minority exhibit the more chronic symptoms noted above. The role of corticosteroids is uncertain; although they may be effective in the management of those patients in whom acute symptoms predominate, there is no evidence that they affect the long-term prognosis or progression of the disease. In 15 per cent of patients, malignant lymphomas develop; the basis for this apparent association is not known.

MESENTERIC CYSTS AND TUMORS. Mesenteric cysts usually develop as the result of anomalies in the mesenteric lymphatic system, but may also consist of enteric or urogenital epithelium or celomic mesothelium. They may spontaneously wax and wane in size, and usually do not present symptomatically in patients less than 10 years of age. Symptoms are related to the size and position of the cyst, which on physical examination is nontender, round, and mobile. Spontaneous rupture, hemorrhage, or infection may occur, but these complications are unusual. Treatment consists of surgical excision.

Mesenteric tumors are rare and usually arise from the cellular elements normally present in the mesentery. They include *fibromas, myxomas, lipomas,* and other less common neoplasms of mesenchymal or neural origin. Most are well differentiated, low-grade *fibrosarcomas* which produce symptoms such as pain, weight loss, abdominal mass, and compression of adjacent organs. They may be treated successfully by surgical excision. Others are more highly malignant and may metastasize distally. *Mesenteric lymphoid tumors* also occur, and certain of these have been associated with unexplained abnormalities in iron metabolism with hypochromic microcytic anemia.

Tumors of the omentum, unlike those of the mesentery, are chiefly muscular in origin (*leiomyomas, leiomyosarcomas*). About 40 per cent of these are malignant and cause symptoms by virtue of local invasion and development of an abdominal mass; distant metastasis is unusual.

Bender, M. D., and Ockner, R. K.: Diseases of the peritoneum, mesentery, and diaphragm. *In* Sleisenger, M. H., and Fordtran, J. S. (eds.): Gastrointestinal Disease. 2nd ed. Philadelphia, W. B. Saunders Company, 1978, p. 1947.

Section Ten NEOPLASTIC DISEASES OF THE ALIMENTARY TRACT

421. INTRODUCTION

Lloyd L. Brandborg

Gastrointestinal cancer comprises 20 per cent of all cancers and accounts for 30 per cent of cancer deaths. In a single year in the United States there are about 133,000 new cancers and 97,000 deaths from cancers of the digestive organs. Cure rates of digestive organ cancer have remained constant for several decades. "Early" diagnosis and more effective treatment have not been achieved.

Striking geographic differences occur in the incidence of various gastrointestinal malignancies. There has been a marked decrease over the past several decades in carcinoma of the stomach in the United States. Carcinoma of the pancreas is increasing. Carcinoma of the colon has remained constant. Gastric carcinoma declines in migrants from countries with a high incidence to those with a low incidence, suggesting that environmental factors play a significant role in its causation. Carcinoma of the colon is virtually unknown in rural Africa, but the incidence in black people in the United States equals that in the white population. None of the factors identified in epidemiologic studies have been shown to cause any of the cancers of the gastrointestinal tract. Tantalizing clues are provided which require further intensive investigation.

Hereditary and genetic factors have been examined. There is an increase in gastric carcinoma in patients having blood group A, in pernicious anemia, and in patients having Lewis group specific substances, either Le[a] or Le[b] or both in saliva. Some families have been described with inordinately high incidences of carcinoma of the stomach or colon. Except for these patients and those with inherited multiple polyposis of the colon, gastrointestinal cancer does not have a familial distribution.

The symptoms of gastrointestinal cancer are not specific. Such phenomena as pain, bleeding, intestinal obstruction, weight loss, fever, or anemia should lead to a search for gastrointestinal malignancy. Most symptomatic gastrointestinal malignancies may be detected by roentgenographic, endoscopic, and cytologic techniques.

Specific chemical and serologic tests for gastrointestinal malignancy are not available. As the techniques become more sensitive, many of these tests become less specific. An example is the occurrence of carcinoembryonic antigen (CEA, see below) in many patients with nonmalignant disease.

Currently, surgery offers the main hopes for cure of gastrointestinal cancer. It may also provide palliation. Preoperative irradiation therapy in gastrointestinal carcinomas may increase resectability and improve prognosis. Some advances have been made in combination drug therapy of gastrointestinal malignancy. Increased response rates and increase in survival have been observed (see below). Combined therapy with 5-fluorouracil and irradiation has improved response rates and survival in gastric carcinoma.

Silverberg, E.: Cancer statistics, 1977. Ca, 27:26, 1977.

422. NEOPLASMS OF THE ESOPHAGUS

Lloyd L. Brandborg

CARCINOMA OF THE ESOPHAGUS

ETIOLOGY. Although the etiology of carcinoma of the esophagus is not known, a number of clinical conditions are associated with an increased incidence of the condition. Patients with *lye damage* of the esophagus have a 1000 times higher risk of developing carcinoma of the esophagus than the general population. Patients with *achalasia* have a reported incidence from 2 to up to 19 per cent. It is presumed that these lesions result from "irritation" caused by retention of esophageal contents. Whether successful brusk dilatation or myotomy, by virtue of eliminating stagnation, decreases the occurrence of carcinoma is not known. *Sideropenic dysphagia* is characterized by esophageal webs in the region of the cricopharyngeus, buccal mucosal atrophy, and a high incidence of carcinoma. This condition occurs most often in Scandinavia, particularly in northern Sweden, predominantly in elderly women. A strikingly high incidence of esophageal carcinoma occurs in some families with *tylosis*, an inherited disorder characterized by marked thickening of the skin of the hands and feet.

A statistical correlation exists between esophageal carcinoma and the use of cigarettes and alcohol. Atypical esophageal epithelium has been observed in the esophagus of smokers examined at autopsy. In view of the widespread use of cigarettes and alcohol, it is surprising that esophageal carcinoma is not more common.

Adenocarcinoma of the esophagus has been described in association with a columnar-lined esophagus (Barrett's esophagus). Adenomatous polyps, a lesion considered to be precancerous, have also been observed in some of these patients.

INCIDENCE AND PREVALENCE. The incidence of carcinoma of the esophagus is 5.8 per 100,000 in whites and 20.5 per 100,000 in nonwhites in the United States. Each year this amounts to 6800 new cases of esophageal cancer and 6400 deaths. Carcinoma of the esophagus is responsible for approximately 2 per cent of cancer deaths in the United States.

EPIDEMIOLOGY. The differences in geographic distribution of carcinoma of the esophagus are so striking throughout the world that it has been concluded that some environmental factors must have a role in etiology. The incidence in the United States in whites is 5.8 cases per 100,000 population per year, whereas in southern Rhodesia it is 157, in Transkei in South Africa it is 357, and in Kazakhstan in Asia it rises to 547 cases per 100,000 population. Statistical associations include long-term ingestion of very hot beverages, climate, vegetation, agriculture, trace metals in soils, and background irradiation. Genetic differences and chemicals in the diet may possibly contribute.

PATHOLOGY. Approximately one half of esophageal carcinomas occur at the level of the arch of the aorta, one third just above the esophagogastric junction, and the remainder in the hypopharynx and proximal esophagus.

If carcinomas arising in the cardia and fundus of the stomach are excluded, virtually all malignancies of the esophagus are squamous cell carcinomas. The gross appearance of carcinoma of the esophagus varies from hard, fibrotic infiltrative lesions to friable, exophytic papillary lesions. They are frequently ulcerated.

Eosphageal carcinoma spreads by local invasion and lymphatic metastases. Microscopic lymphatic spread is common. These tumors frequently involve adjacent structures. The distal lesions invade the stomach and the left gastric and celiac lymph nodes. Extension into the diaphragm, vertebral bodies, pericardium, and heart is not rare. Lesions of the middle and upper third extend into the trachea and bronchi and may involve the lungs and occasionally the recurrent laryngeal nerves.

Hematogenous metastases are less common than lymphatic extension and usually affect the liver, lungs, bones, and kidneys.

CLINICAL MANIFESTATIONS. Carcinoma of the esophagus is unusual under the age of 40. The peak incidence occurs in the decade between the ages of 60 and 70. In most countries, males are afflicted approximately twice as often as females.

The most common symptom is progressive dysphagia. There is first difficulty in swallowing solid food, followed by inability to swallow semisolid foods and, finally, liquids. Occasionally, sudden esophageal obstruction occurs with a bolus of food that could have been easily swallowed a few days previously. Pain with swallowing, odynophagia, is due to extension of the tumor beyond the wall of the esophagus. It is located substernally, tends to be constant, is not always associated with swallowing, and is dull or burning. Occasionally, it may be felt in the back.

Other symptoms are due to chronic obstruction, extension of the tumor into adjacent organs, and hemorrhage. Brisk hemorrhage is uncommon (5 per cent of patients); however, occult bleeding is common.

Chronic obstruction leads to aspiration of secretions and undigested food, with severe coughing episodes and penumonia; eating may become virtually intolerable. Food intake is reduced with ensuing weight loss. Regurgitation during the night, bad breath, bad taste, and thirst are frequent. Fever is common, usually because of pulmonary infection.

Symptoms of metastatic spread depend upon the organs involved. Involvement of the phrenic nerve or diaphragm may lead to unremitting hiccups. Extension into the trachea and bronchi produces coughing, infection, and tracheal or bronchoesophageal fistulas. Perforation into the mediastinum causes mediastinitis and empyema. Extension into the pericardium and heart causes pericardial effusions. A rare but dramatic symptom is exsanguinating hemorrhage caused by erosion into the aorta. Involvement of the recurrent laryngeal nerve will cause hoarseness. With distant metastases, patients may have jaundice, abdominal discomfort, ascites, cyanosis, dyspnea, and bone pain.

DIAGNOSIS. *Every* patient with dysphagia should be investigated for carcinoma of the esophagus. The first procedure is a careful roentgenologic examination under fluoroscopic control (Fig. 1). Careful attention should be paid to the fundus of the stomach and cardia. Cineradiography is useful in detecting disordered motility. The most usual radiographic finding is a circumferential, irregular narrowing of the esophagus which is often ulcerated. There is slight or no dilatation proximal to the tumor. The mucosal folds are destroyed. In some smoothly tapering lesions, the differential diagnosis between benign stricture and carcinoma may be extraordinarily difficult.

Fiberoptic endoscopy permits direct visualization, biopsy, and directed cytology of esophageal cancers. Correct pretreatment diagnoses may be expected in virtually 100 per cent of visualized lesions utilizing both biopsy and cytology. Multiple biopsies and cytologic preparation should be obtained. If these procedures do not yield a diagnosis and malignancy is still suspected, lavage cytology performed by skilled technicians and interpreted by interested physicians will provide a correct diagnosis of malignancy, when present, in 95 per cent or more of subjects.

DIFFERENTIAL DIAGNOSIS. Only a few diseases may be confused with carcinoma of the esophagus. Most important is peptic *esophagitis* with *stricture* (see Ch. 396). Although most patients have a history of pyrosis, some have only a short history of dysphagia with little discomfort. The roentgenographic appearance may mimic malignant neoplasm. Eosphagoscopy with biopsy and cytology and lavage cytology will establish the benign nature of the stricture in virtually every patient.

The history of intermittent dysphagia in *achalasia* is much more characteristic than in carcinoma of the esophagus, which has a gradual increase in severity. Total obstruction is uncommon. The esophagus is dilated, often massively, and patients with achalasia may have symptoms of aspiration. The diagnosis may be made on a chest x-ray by finding a wide, mediastinal

Figure 1. Extensive, sessile, ulcerated carcinoma of the esophagus.

mass with a fluid level. The usual radiographic appearance is that of megaesophagus with a sharply tapering "beak" at the gastroesophageal junction. Test dilatation with a Hurst dilator has only a transient holdup at the cardioesophageal junction, whereas in malignancy the dilator usually cannot be passed. Manometric studies reveal absent peristaltic waves, a high pressure in the sphincter zone, and failure of the sphincter to relax in response to a swallow. The Mecholyl test is positive; however, a rare patient with carcinoma of the fundus or cardia which closely resembles achalasia radiographically may also have a positive Mecholyl test. Further, achalasia and carcinoma may coexist. (See Ch. 396.)

In *lye stricture*, the history of ingestion of caustic is usually clear; however, elderly patients may have ingested lye in childhood and not remember it. Because of the malignant potential of lye strictures, these patients should be followed periodically with roentgenologic examination, endoscopy, and exfoliative cytology.

TREATMENT AND PROGNOSIS. Patients with cervical and high thoracic esophageal carcinoma should receive high voltage irradiation therapy. Five-year survival of 15 to 20 per cent may be obtained. Patients with carcinoma of the middle third and distal third of the esophagus have a miserable prognosis when treated with irradiation therapy or surgery alone. Five-year cure ranges between 0 and 5 per cent. Operative mortality for esophagectomy is between 15 and 20 per cent. Adenocarcinoma of the distal esophagus and proximal stomach should be treated surgically.

Preoperative irradiation, 4500 to 5000 rads, through planned fields intended to encompass the tumor with 5-cm margins will improve resectability. This approach has resulted in two-year survival of 23 per cent and five-year survival of 14 per cent.

Chemotherapy of esophageal carcinoma is disappointing. Bleomycin, given at a dosage of 10 to 15 units per square meter intravenously or intramuscularly, one to two times weekly, has produced a response rate of 17 per cent. Unfortunately, responses are short lived, and increased survival has not been shown. The major toxicity is pulmonary, and fatal pulmonary fibrosis may result. Skin eruptions, mucositis, anorexia, nausea, and fever are common.

Supervoltage irradiation is preferable to major bypass or resectional surgery for palliation in incurable patients. Two thirds of such patients will have significant relief of dysphagia for two months or longer. Median survival is seven months, with 7 per cent of patients living two years or more. Those patients failing irradiation should have an endoscopically placed prosthetic tube. Obstruction may be relieved for some weeks or even months. Although nutrition may be improved, these tubes may migrate through the tumor, erode into the mediastinum, or become occluded with tumor. Gastrostomy alone should not be done in patients with total obstruction caused by carcinoma of the esophagus. This only prolongs these patients' misery. They are unable even to swallow their own secretions, and have repeated pulmonary infections. If esophageal patency cannot be maintained by irradiation therapy with or without prosthetic tubes, these patients should be allowed to die with some dignity.

Marks, R. D., Jr., Scruggs, H. J., and Keene, M. W.: Preoperative radiation therapy for carcinoma of the esophagus. Cancer, 38:84, 1976.

Pearson, J. G.: The present status and future potential of radiotherapy in the management of esophageal cancer. Cancern, 39:882, 1977.

Prolla, J. C., Reilly, R. W., Kirsner, J. B., and Cockerham, L.: Direct-vision endoscopic cytology and biopsy in the diagnosis of esophageal and gastric tumors: Current experience. Acta Cytol., 21:399, 1977.

Radigan, L. R., Glover, J. L., Shipley, F. E., and Shoemaker, R. G.: Barrett esophagus. Arch. Surg., 112:486, 1977.

Wara, W. M., Mauch, P. M., Thomas, A. N., and Phillips, T. L.: Palliation for carcinoma of the esophagus. Radiology, 121:717, 1976.

OTHER NEOPLASMS OF THE ESOPHAGUS

Carcinosarcomas

Carcinosarcomas are rare tumors of the esophagus. They tend to be polypoid and contain both carcinomatous and sarcomatous tissue. Exfoliative cytology may reveal both malignant sarcomatous and epithelial cells. Biopsy with histologic examination is probably more accurate. These tumors tend to be radiosensitive and

should be treated with irradiation therapy if they are not resectable.

Malignant Lymphoma

Malignant lymphoma confined to the esophagus is extremely rare. The usual symptoms are either dysphagia or odynophagia. The roentgenographic appearance resembles monilial esophagitis. If the diagnosis can be established by exfoliative cytology or biopsy, irradiation therapy is the treatment of choice.

Leiomyomas

Leiomyomas are the most common benign neoplasms of the esophagus. Most often they cause no symptoms and are an incidental finding either at autopsy or surgery. They are usually less than 2 cm in diameter. They are intramural, extramucosal tumors and produce a smooth indentation in the esophagus on roentgenographic examination. Rarely, they may be "polyps" with a stalk. Even when they attain huge size, they may not produce symptoms. Rarely, patients have dysphagia and may even bleed. With large lesions, the diagnosis may be suspected by seeing a spherical mediastinal mass on chest x-ray. There is no evidence that leiomyomas undergo sarcomatous degeneration. The treatment of symptomatic esophageal leiomyomas is enucleation of the tumor. Resection is rarely necessary.

423. MALIGNANT NEOPLASMS OF THE STOMACH

Lloyd L. Brandborg

Ninety-five per cent of gastric neoplasms are malignant and 5 per cent benign. The most common benign neoplasm is the *leiomyoma*, which is usually an incidental finding at surgery or autopsy. The next most common is the *hyperplastic polyp*. Other benign neoplasms of the stomach are exceedingly rare.

With the decreasing incidence of *adenocarcinoma* of the stomach in the United States and a constant incidence of gastric *lymphoma*, the proportion of malignant lymphomas has increased and possibly accounts for as many as 10 per cent of gastric malignancies. The other major malignant neoplasm of the stomach is the *leiomyosarcoma*, which accounts for about 1 per cent of gastric malignancies.

CARCINOMA OF THE STOMACH

ETIOLOGY. In spite of numerous experimental studies and epidemiologic investigations, a causative agent or agents responsible for carcinoma of the stomach remain elusive.

Genetic factors have been associated with an increased incidence of carcinoma of the stomach. Several families have been described with an unusually high occurrence. Studies of gastric carcinoma in twins have shown a higher frequency in monozygotic than in dizygotic twins. There is a 10 per cent increase in blood group A in gastric cancer patients when compared with suitable controls. Patients with pernicious anemia have been estimated to have a 10 per cent chance of developing gastric cancer. In these patients blood group A is also increased. Lewis group specific substances, either Le[a] or Le[b] or both, have been found in saliva in all patients with gastric carcinoma who have been examined. In the normal population 7 per cent of subjects are Lewis negative. These genetic factors are not etiologic, because the vast majority of subjects having them do not develop gastric carcinoma. They may be predisposing factors in response to other etiologic agents.

Gastric polyps are rare lesions. The introduction of fiberoptic polypectomy has led to a reclassification of gastric polyps. About three fourths of them are hyperplastic lesions, composed of normal mucosal components, and these appear to have no neoplastic potential. Adenomatous polyps account for fewer than 10 per cent of polypoid tumors in the stomach. Invasive carcinoma or carcinoma in situ derived from polypoid lesions occurs only in adenomas and villous adenomas. Villous adenomas of the stomach are exceedingly rare. They seem to have a malignant potential similar to those occurring in the colon. Microinvasion of carcinoma in situ has been observed in adenomas not associated with invasive carcinoma elsewhere in the stomach. Metastases have not been seen. Regenerating epithelium in the vicinity of acute inflammation and granulation tissue may be difficult to differentiate from carcinoma in situ. Misinterpretation of these regenerating cells may lead to a diagnosis of carcinoma in situ when it is not warranted.

Chronic atrophic gastritis may be divided into two categories based on the distribution of pathology and autoimmune serologic tests. Type A gastritis has a positive test for parietal cell antibody, elevated serum gastrin levels, diffuse fundal gland atrophy, and severe impairment of gastric acid secretion. Type B gastritis is negative for parietal cell antibody, the serum gastrin level is low, and the antrum is involved in the pathologic process. Gastric acid secretion is variably impaired. Type B gastritis is four times more prevalent than Type A. Gastric carcinoma may develop in both, but Type B seems to be a more important precursor. Pernicious anemia occurs almost exclusively in Type A gastritis. Other unknown factors are essential for the development of gastric carcinoma, as most patients with either type of gastritis do not develop it.

Patients with adult pernicious anemia have an increased incidence of gastric carcinoma. They are achlorhydric and achylic, and have intestinalization of their gastric mucosa and a high incidence of benign adenomas. Despite all these abnormalities, most of them do not develop carcinoma of the stomach.

Peptic ulcer of the stomach has been thought to be a precursor of carcinoma of the stomach. The finding of malignant cells in the margins of the ulcers has been offered as evidence. It is more likely, however, that ulcer in this circumstance develops as a result of peptic digestion of a small carcinoma. Further, virtually all such lesions have been described in patients secreting hydrochloric acid. Possibly neoplastic tissue is more susceptible to digestion than the surrounding mucosa. Although a benign gastric ulcer may degenerate into a malignant one, such an event must be extremely rare.

Previous surgery for benign peptic ulcer appears to be associated with an increase in carcinoma of the stomach. Several large reviews have shown that surgery for benign duodenal ulcer disease increases the risk of carcinoma in these patients. Carcinoma in association with duodenal ulcer is otherwise rare. The etiology and pathogenesis of gastric cancer in this situation are unknown. Possibly reflux of intestinal and pancreatic secretions into the gastric remnant may contribute. The interval between surgery for benign ulcer disease and the appearance of carcinoma of the stomach varies from 6 to up to 37 or more years. Any patient who develops gastric symptoms after several years of good health after surgery for benign peptic ulcer deserves a thorough investigation for malignancy.

EPIDEMIOLOGY. Striking geographic differences characterize the incidence and death rates from carcinoma of the stomach. The highest rates occur in Japan and Chile and the lowest in Egypt, Malaysia, and Nicaragua. Despite the marked differences, no environmental or dietary factor has been identified as being causative. Factors which have been found to be related to a high incidence include low socioeconomic status, urban dwelling, smoked fish in the diet, presence of carcinogens such as benzpyrene in barbecued meat or heated fats, background irradiation, trace metals in soil, types of soil, climate, and occupation.

INCIDENCE AND PREVALENCE. A striking and unexplained decrease in mortality from carcinoma of the stomach has occurred over the past five decades, from 33 per 100,000 population in 1930 to 7 to 8 per 100,000 population in the 1970's. During the same interval, five-year cure rates have improved from 7 per cent to 9 per cent of all patients treated. These apparent small gains may be attributed to blood transfusion, better understanding of fluid and electrolyte therapy, better anesthesia, and the introduction of antimicrobial drugs.

Carcinoma of the stomach is twice as common in men as in women. This ratio tends to be maintained in all countries for which cancer statistics exist. In the United States the incidence in both men and women is approximately twice as high in blacks and Orientals as it is in whites. Carcinoma of the stomach has been observed in all age groups, but is most common in patients between the ages of 50 and 69.

PATHOLOGY. Carcinomas may be found at any site within the stomach. They may be divided into four gross classifications: polypoid, ulcerated noninfiltrating, ulcerated infiltrating, and the diffuse infiltrating varieties. (This classification corresponds to the Borrman classification.) The rare superficial spreading carcinoma is not included in the preceding classification. Most gastric carcinomas are adenocarcinomas of widely varying histology. The histology ranges from well-differentiated adenocarcinoma to mucoid carcinoma to undifferentiated carcinomas which may be difficult to differentiate from sarcomas. Two types of growth pattern are easily recognizable. One type includes expanding carcinomas which grow en masse and by expansion, forming discrete tumor nodules. The other type is infiltrative carcinoma, in which tumor cells invade individually. The expanding carcinomas have a better prognosis than the infiltrating varieties.

Carcinoma of the stomach spreads by direct invasion and lymphatic channels. The pancreas, liver, and transverse colon are often invaded by tumor. Tumors in the proximal stomach often invade the esophagus for variable distances. The distensibility of the esophagus may be restricted. If the neural plexuses are invaded, these cancers may mimic achalasia. Extension across the pylorus from distal lesions is uncommon.

Probably lymph node metastases appear early. The local perigastric, preaortic, porta hepatis, and mediastinal nodes are frequently involved. Malignant deposits are frequently found in nodes in the hilum of the spleen and in the spleen itself. Occasionally metastases to the left supraclavicular space occur (Virchow's node), probably through the thoracic duct. Peritoneal implants are frequent, occurring in one third of patients coming to autopsy. In women the ovaries may have metastases, the so-called Krukenberg tumors.

Hematogenous metastases most often involve the liver, lungs, and bone. Pulmonary metastases may appear as a pneumonitis or as discrete masses, or may resemble miliary tuberculosis.

CLINICAL MANIFESTATIONS. The mass survey studies in Japan have clearly shown that "early" gastric carcinoma confined to the mucosa does not produce symptoms. Most carcinomas of the stomach seen in the United States are already advanced. Symptoms are the result of ulceration, obstruction, necrosis, and disorders of gastric motility caused by tumor invasion.

Weight loss is the most common symptom and occurs in up to 96 per cent of patients. Approximately 70 per cent of patients have pain of variable intensity. Some patients have a mild and vague discomfort. Approximately 25 per cent of patients describe the pain as being similar to that of peptic ulcer. The pain may or may not be relieved by food or antacids. In a few patients it is of long duration. If the cancer has invaded the pancreas, pain may be referred to the back. The pain may be described as pressure sensations, fullness, aching, bloating, indigestion, dyspepsia, or gas pains. Some patients have pain immediately after eating. In others there is no apparent relationship to the ingestion of food.

Approximately 50 per cent of patients have vomiting. This usually implies pyloric obstruction, but occurs with carcinomas at any location within the stomach. Anorexia occurs in about 25 per cent of patients. The degree of weight loss often cannot be related to a reduction of food intake. Early satiety occurs in about 10 per cent of patients and is a fairly constant symptom in linitis plastica but may also occur with relatively small tumors.

Other gastrointestinal symptoms are changes in bowel habits such as constipation or diarrhea. Dysphagia is common with carcinoma of the fundus and cardia. A few patients may have odynophagia, and some have pyrosis. Gross hematemesis and melena are unusual, each occurring in 10 per cent of patients. Occult bleeding, on the other hand, is extremely common.

Other symptoms resulting from gastric carcinoma are unusual fatigability and symptoms of anemia such as dyspnea, dizziness and fainting, pallor, angina pectoris, and burning of the tongue. Some patients may have eructations, bad breath, and hiccups, and a few discover an abdominal mass. Peritoneal implants may cause ascites. Metastases in the liver or to the porta hepatis may produce jaundice. Bone pain may be the result of either pathologic fractures or invasion of the periosteum. Carcinomas may perforate and mimic perforated peptic ulcer.

PHYSICAL EXAMINATION. Only 45 to 50 per cent of patients with advanced gastric carcinoma have a palpable mass. Hepatomegaly is common but does not always indicate metastatic disease. Twenty per cent of patients will be emaciated or cachectic. Abdominal tenderness is noted in only 20 per cent of patients. Five per cent of patients have palpable peripheral lymph nodes caused by the metastases. Metastatic disease may also be manifest by hard nodular livers and palpable nodules on rectal examination. Rarely, a tumor nodule may be palpated or even seen in the umbilicus. Ascites is present in a few patients owing to hepatic or peritoneal metastases. Jaundice may be seen with metastases to the porta hepatis or liver.

DIFFERENTIAL DIAGNOSIS. A number of other diseases may produce symptoms similar or identical to gastric carcinoma. The most important is benign *peptic ulcer. Cholelithiasis, pancreatitis, pancreatic neoplasm,* or *coronary artery disease* and other neoplasms of the stomach should be considered. Appropriate investigation will establish the correct diagnosis in most patients.

LABORATORY STUDIES. The anemias of gastric carcinomas are of several varieties. Approximately two thirds of patients will have a hypochromic microcytic anemia. Macrocytic anemia caused by vitamin B_{12} or folate deficiency is not rare. A normochromic normocytic anemia may appear without bone marrow metastases. Occult blood is present in the stool in only about 45 per cent of patients on a single determination; when the stool is repeatedly tested, the percentage is much higher.

Gastric analysis is mandatory in every patient with a gastric ulcer. Ideally, the tube should be placed under fluoroscopic control with the tip in the middle of the antrum. If a fluoroscope is not readily available, the tube should be passed 55 to 60 cm from the nares. The secretagogue should be pentagastrin, 1 to 6 μg per kilogram intramuscularly. An ulcerating lesion in an achlorhydric patient is virtually pathognomonic of a malignant neoplasm. Presence of acid in no way excludes a diagnosis of cancer.

ROENTGENOLOGIC DIAGNOSIS. Roentgenologic examination will detect 95 per cent of gastric lesions. The radiologist must procure good mucosal detail to avoid overlooking small lesions. One of the more difficult differential diagnoses is between malignant and benign ulcers. In some ulcers, this distinction may be impossible. Some features which favor malignant ulcer are effacement of folds and abnormal mucosal folds, a niche in a notch (an ulcer within an ulcer), an ulcer with a flat wavy base, and a triangular-shaped wide-based ulcer. Linitis plastica is characterized by loss of distensibility of the stomach and absent or marked reduction of motility. Other malignant lesions are characterized by rigidity, mucosal distortion, irregular and enlarged mucosal folds, and fixed filling defects. An ulcer within a mass is characteristic of carcinoma of the stomach (Fig. 2). Some ulcers have features of both benignancy and malignancy.

GASTROSCOPY. Fiberoptic endoscopy with directed biopsy and cytology will yield a diagnosis of malignancy in the vast majority of cases. It may be impossible in some lesions to obtain a tissue or cytologic diagnosis. These include recurrent or infiltrative cancers, location in the cardia or antrum, and linitis plastica. Often the nature of these lesions is apparent from the gross appearance. In some lesions it may be technically impossible to obtain tissue because of the location. A minimum of ten biopsies should be taken from each lesion if technically possible. With the end-viewing instru-

Figure 2. Carcinoma of the stomach. The tumor has involved the entire antrum and produced a characteristic filling defect and mucosal destruction. An ulcer within the mass is indicated by the arrow.

ments, it may be impossible to biopsy the proximal edge of an ulcerating lesion. It is not possible to sample the entire stomach when early carcinoma may not be grossly recognizable. Still or motion picture photography through the fiberoptic endoscope provides a permanent record of the gross appearance of the lesion (Fig. 3).

EXFOLIATIVE CYTOLOGY. If the directed biopsies and cytologies do not provide a tissue diagnosis and malignancy is still suspected, lavage cytology is indicated if available.

Lavage cytology is superior to abrasive instruments. The highest accuracy has resulted from the utilization of chymotrypsin as a mucolytic enzyme. Lavage cytology provides a total mucosal "biopsy." In laboratories regularly performing gastric exfoliative cytology, accuracy ranges from 90 to 95 per cent in patients with proved malignancy, and cancer is falsely diagnosed in less than 1 per cent of patients with benign disease. The diagnosis rendered by the responsible physician should include only three possible categories: (1) malignant cells present with an interpretation of cell type, (2) no malignant cells present, and (3) unsatisfactory test which must be repeated after appropriate cleansing of the stomach.

Figure 3. Four gastric lesions photographed with the gastrocamera (reproduced from 5 mm color transparencies). A, Adenocarcinoma (arrow) seen on the posterior aspect of the stomach near the incisura angularis. B, Benign gastric ulcer (arrow) from a tangential view, showing the incisura angularis with the antral region to the left and fundus to the right. The edematous rolled margins of the ulcer surround the typical necrotic center; there is no evidence of neoplasia. C, This adenomatous polyp (arrow) in the gastric antrum had bled persistently, causing the patient to become severely anemic. The 5 to 6 mm lesion was seen in only one of several carefully performed upper gastrointestinal series. Its size, shape, and smooth contours are consistent with the subsequently proved diagnosis of adenoma. D, Leiomyoma (arrow) on the posterior wall of the body of the stomach lying above the incisura angularis. Note the obviously submucosal character of this lesion and its typical umbilication by an apical ulcer.

USE OF ALL TECHNIQUES. All available techniques should be used in gastric cancer suspects. Overconfidence in one method to the exclusion of others is to be avoided. The application of roentgenologic, gastroscopic, and cytologic methods affords the greatest benefit to the patient under consideration. If all these techniques indicate a benign lesion, the patient with gastric ulcer warrants a trial of medical therapy. However, it is mandatory that these patients be repeatedly examined to ensure ulcer healing.

TREATMENT. The only curative therapy for gastric carcinoma is surgical excision. The type and extent of the procedure must be left to the discretion of the surgeon. Polypoid carcinoma may be treated with a limited gastrectomy if no evidence of metastasis is present. Antral lesions may be treated by a subtotal gastrectomy, including the regional lymph nodes in the vicinity of the tumor. Patients with cancer of the cardia and fundus should have a proximal gastrectomy. Super-radical gastrectomy, in which all areas of *predicted* metastases are removed, was advocated in the past, but these procedures double surgical mortality and actually decrease cure rates. Total gastrectomy is almost never indicated for treatment of gastric carcinoma. Palliative resection is indicated for patients with incurable disease. Even though survival may not be improved, these patients may derive considerable benefit from relief of obstruction and hemorrhage and from improved nutrition.

Combination drug chemotherapy has been shown to increase response rates in gastric carcinoma and to prolong survival. Regimens which have been effective are combinations of 5-fluorouracil (5-FU) plus mitomycin C; 5-FU plus BCNU; and 5-FU, mitomycin C, and cytosine arabinoside. Adriamycin as a single agent has produced objective responses in about one third of patients. Combination therapy with methyl-CCNU, 175 mg per square meter, given on day 1, plus 5-FU, 300 mg per square meter per day, given by rapid intravenous injections on days 1 through 5, has increased response rates and survival. The program is repeated every seven weeks. It is necessary to determine leukocyte and platelet counts twice weekly following therapy. These drugs should be administered by physicians skilled in their use because of danger of serious toxicity.

Patients with inoperable gastric adenocarcinoma may respond to high voltage irradiation therapy. Six thousand rads, given at 150 to 200 rads daily, has resulted in an 11 per cent three-year survival and 7 per cent five-year survival. This is nine to ten months longer than for untreated patients. 5-Fluorouracil, at a daily dose of 15 mg per kilogram for three days at the initiation of irradiation therapy, plus a total dose of 3500 to 4000 rads, administered at a rate of 900 to 1200 rads per week, increases mean survival to 13 months, compared with six months in placebo-treated patients. Twelve per cent survived more than five years. Irradiation is also useful in controlling hemorrhage.

PROGNOSIS. Advanced carcinoma of the stomach has a dismal prognosis. Sixty-five per cent of patients subjected to surgery are found to be incurable. Fewer than 10 per cent of all patients with the disease can be cured. Factors which favor a more favorable prognosis are a long history as opposed to a brief history. The gross appearance of the tumor is related to prognosis. The polypoid tumors and the ulcerating but noninfil-

trating tumors have the best prognosis, and the ulcerated, infiltrating, and diffuse infiltrating varieties have extremely low cure rates. Superficial spreading carcinoma, which is usually diagnosed cytologically, and carcinoma of the stomach confined to the mucosa have cure rates in the order of 90 to 95 per cent.

OTHER NEOPLASMS OF THE STOMACH

Lymphoma

Malignant lymphoma may be confined to the stomach. With the decreasing incidence of carcinoma, it assumes an increasingly important proportion of gastric cancers. *Reticulum cell sarcoma* and *lymphosarcoma* are the most common types. *Hodgkin's disease, giant follicular lymphoma,* and *plasmacytoma* may also involve the stomach primarily. The symptoms of malignant lymphoma are similar to carcinoma except that some patients have a history similar to that of peptic ulcer, sometimes for as long as several years. Men and women are equally affected. The peak incidence is between the ages of 40 and 60. Anemia, overt bleeding, and marked weight loss are somewhat less frequent than with carcinoma of the stomach.

There are no distinctive roentgenographic or gastroscopic appearances to permit differentiation from carcinoma. Exfoliative cytology is diagnostic in up to 90 per cent of patients. It is possible to differentiate reticulum cell sarcoma, lymphosarcoma, and Hodgkin's disease by cytologic criteria. Few data are available for fiberoptic endoscopic biopsy and directed cytology. The few reports available suggest that the diagnosis may be made in 80 to 90 per cent of patients by directed biopsy. The yield with brushing cytology has been disappointing, approximately 20 per cent detection.

Treatment consists of resection of the tumor followed by irradiation therapy. The surgeon should attempt to excise as much tumor tissue as possible even if it cannot be resected in toto. Some patients who have been deemed inoperable and treated with radiation alone have had long survival. Cure rates, as judged by five-year survival, are 50 per cent in patients treated with surgery followed by irradiation therapy.

Leiomyosarcoma

The history of patients with leiomyosarcoma is similar to that of patients with carcinoma of the stomach; however, bleeding is more common, particularly massive hemorrhage, because these tumors are frequently ulcerated. Metastatic spread tends to be confined to the abdomen. Treatment is wide surgical excision. Five-year survival after surgery is 40 per cent and is dependent upon the degree of anaplasia of the tumor rather than its size.

Dekker, W., and Tygat, G. N.: Diagnostic accuracy of fiberendoscopy in the detection of upper intestinal malignancy. A follow-up analysis. Gastroenterology, 73:710, 1977.

Domellöf, L., and Janunger, K G.: The risk for gastric carcinoma after partial gastrectomy. Am. J. Surg., 134:581, 1977.

Gunderson, L. L.: Radiation therapy: Results and future possibilities. Clin. Gastroenterol., 5:743, 1976.

Lim, F. E., Hartman, A. S., Tan, E. G. C., Cady, B, and Meissner, W. A.: Factors in the prognosis of gastric lymphoma. Cancer, 39:1715, 1977.

Ming, S-C.: Gastric carcinoma. A pathobiological classification. Cancer, 39:2475, 1977.

Moertel, C. G.: Chemotherapy of gastrointestinal cancer. Clin. Gastroenterol., 5:777, 1976.

Moertel, C. G, Mittelman, J. A., Bakemeier, R. F., Engstrom, P., and Hanley, J.: Sequential and combination chemotherapy of advanced gastric cancer. Cancer, 38:678, 1976.

Seifert, E., and Elster, K.: Gastric polypectomy. Am. J. Gastroenterol., 63:451, 1975.

Strickland, R. G., and Mackay, I. R.: A reappraisal of the nature and significance of chronic atrophic gastritis. Am. J. Dig. Dis., 18:426, 1973.

Tomasulo, J.: Gastric polyps. Histologic types and their relationship to gastric carcinoma. Cancer, 27:1346, 1971.

Winawer, S. J., Posner, G., Lightdale, C. J., Sherlock, P, Melamed, M., and Fortner, J. G.: Endoscopic diagnosis of advanced gastric cancer. Factors influencing yield. Gastroenterology, 69:1183, 1975.

424.   BENIGN NEOPLASMS OF THE STOMACH

Lloyd L. Brandborg

ADENOMA

Adenomas of the stomach are generally seen in patients over the age of 50. Ninety-five per cent of patients with adenomas have achlorhydria, and they occur in 2 per cent of patients with achlorhydria. The incidence in pernicious anemia varies widely from series to series and may be as high as 20 per cent in these patients.

Probably most adenomas of the stomach are asymptomatic. The most common symptom is a nondescript upper abdominal pain. It is not related to food, is described as a dull ache and occasionally gnawing sensation, and is not relieved by antacids or food. Rarely, nausea and vomiting may be present. Overt hemorrhage is unusual, but the tumor may bleed occultly.

The physical examination is usually normal. In a few patients the signs of iron deficiency anemia are present. A palpable abdominal mass caused by adenoma is virtually never found.

The roentgenographic appearance of gastric adenoma is that of a spherical filling defect often on a stalk of variable length. Fiberoptic endoscopy is more sensitive than radiology in detecting small polypoid lesions. It also assists in differentiating the nature of these lesions and permits biopsy and cytologic examination. Endoscopy frequently detects several gastric polyps when one is identified on roentgenologic examination.

If it is highly likely that a patient's symptoms are due to gastric adenoma, therapy is local excision, including the stalk. Because of the low potential of malignancy, polyps less than 2 cm in diameter may be followed annually with cytologic examination and endoscopy. Polyps larger than 2 cm in diameter, particularly if they are sessile, have a higher probability of being malignant. If surgical contraindications are not present, these lesions should be locally excised.

LEIOMYOMA

Although leiomyomas are the most common benign tumors found in the stomach at autopsy, they are rarely responsible for clinical symptoms. Intramural, extramucosal tumors, they occur with equal frequency in men and women and are seen most often in subjects between the ages of 40 and 60. Most are between 1 and 2 cm in diameter, but they can attain huge size. Evidence of previous ulceration of the mucosa overlying the tumor is found in as many as 60 per cent of cases.

The most important symptom of gastric leiomyoma is bleeding. Usually it is occult and leads to iron deficiency anemia, but on occasion it may be massive. Some patients may also complain of epigastric burning or gnawing pain and anorexia.

The roentgenographic features are those of an intramucosal, usually spherical, intramural mass projecting into the lumen of the stomach. An ulceration may be detected within the mass. Gastroscopically, the tumor is covered by a normal but somewhat stretched mucosa with flattened rugae. The central ulcer is visible if present.

Symptomatic leiomyomas should be treated by local excision or limited gastrectomy. Prognosis is excellent.

MISCELLANEOUS BENIGN TUMORS

Other benign tumors occurring in the stomach are rare. They include lipomas, tumors of neural origin, angiomas, hemangiopericytoma or glomus tumors, granular cell myoblastoma, and carcinoid tumors. These lesions are extramucosal intramural tumors. They can usually be observed unless symptomatic. Local excision is usually curative.

Cox, A. J., Jr.: Pathology. *In* Harkins, H. N., and Nyhus, L. M. (eds.): Surgery of the Stomach and Duodenum. 2nd ed. Boston, Little, Brown & Company. 1966.

425.   NEOPLASMS OF THE SMALL INTESTINE

Thomas F. O'Brien, Jr.

Primary neoplasms of the small intestine which are of clinical importance arise from the epithelial, muscular, vascular, and lymphatic components of the small intestine. Thus *adenomas, adenocarcinomas, leiomyomas, leiomyosarcomas, hemangiomas,* and *lymphomas* represent the most frequently observed tumors of the small intestine.

MALIGNANT NEOPLASMS

TYPES. *Adenocarcinomas, lymphomas,* and *leiomyosarcomas* are the three most common primary malignancies of the small intestine. Adenocarcinoma occurs with the greatest frequency and leiomyosarcoma with the least.

ETIOLOGY. Very little is known or hypothesized about the etiology of small intestinal malignancy. Dietary factors do not appear to play an important role in the development of adenocarcinoma, and no major differences in incidence have been observed among population groups. Chronic small bowel disease, however, may represent a predisposing factor, because *celiac sprue* and chronic *regional enteritis* appear to be associated with a disproportionate number of primary small bowel malignancies. Chronic parasitism has been suggested as a predisposing factor toward the development of primary small bowel lymphoma which is seen frequently in the Mediterranean basin and South America.

The plasma cells which compose this tumor secrete large quantities of the α-chain component of IgA.

INCIDENCE. Primary small intestinal malignancies are rare. Excluding carcinoids, they represent only 1 to 2 per cent of all malignant gastrointestinal neoplasms.

PATHOLOGY. More than 90 per cent of the *adenocarcinomas* of the small intestine are located in the duodenum, and most lie within 20 cm of the ligament of Treitz. The lesions are usually annular in configuration and reveal a moderate degree of differentiation under the microscope. More than half the patients will show extension to or beyond regional lymph nodes at the time of initial diagnosis.

All varieties of lymphoma may arise primarily in the small intestine, although *reticulum cell sarcoma* is by far the most common. *Lymphomas* tend to involve the more distal portions of the jejunum and ileum and rarely arise in the duodenum.

Leiomyosarcomas of the small intestine may arise in any portion of the small intestine; however, the jejunum and ileum are the usual sites. They tend to be bulky tumors, exceeding 5 cm in diameter. Central necrosis is a common feature. Metastatic spread occurs primarily by the blood-borne route or by direct extension, rather than lymphatically.

CLINICAL MANIFESTATIONS. Malignant primary tumors of the small intestine are usually discovered in persons over 50 years of age. Lymphomas of the small intestine, however, tend to occur at a somewhat earlier age than adenocarcinomas or leiomyosarcomas. Men are afflicted with a frequency more than double that of women. Abdominal pain, malaise, anorexia, weight loss, and bleeding are common presenting symptoms. Although prodromal symptoms are usually present, sudden obstruction of the small intestine may be the first manifestation of a small bowel malignancy. A small bowel tumor, when palpable on physical examination, is almost invariably malignant. Free perforation is an important clinical manifestation of the sarcoma.

DIAGNOSIS. Most primary small intestinal malignancies are identified by radiographic examination of the small bowel. Certain roentgenologic features characterize the various histologic types. Annular lesions of short length are typically found with an *adenocarcinoma* (Fig. 1). Longer, ulcerating lesions producing so-called aneurysmal dilatation of the lumen favor lymphoma. Diffuse small bowel involvement suggesting a malabsorption syndrome is a less common manifestation of lymphoma. *Leiomyosarcomas* are bulky tumors which displace adjacent bowel loops.

Visceral angiography has become a valuable tool in identification of malignant small bowel tumors. The source of blood supply is an important clue in the differential diagnosis of benign and malignant lesions. Benign tumors are invariably fed by a branch of the gastroduodenal or superior mesenteric artery. Blood supply from a renal or lumbar artery (parasitic blood supply) is characteristic of a malignant lesion.

TREATMENT. Surgery is required for the majority of patients with primary small bowel malignancies. Although in two thirds of the patients the disease will have spread at the time of surgical intervention, the procedure is usually indicated for relief of obstruction, control of hemorrhage, and alleviation of pain.

Radiation therapy, alkalating agents, and nitrogen mustard, together with corticosteroids, often prove effective for some patients with lymphoma. 5-

Figure 1. Adenocarcinoma of the duodenum, close-up view. The characteristic features of a small bowel adenocarcinoma are demonstrated here. Note the "shelving" edges at the proximal portion of the tumor. The central lumen shows destruction of the normal mucosal pattern with ulceration (arrow). (From O'Brien, T. F., Jr., *In* Sleisenger, M. H., and Fordtran, J. S. [eds.]: Gastrointestinal Disease. 2nd ed. Philadelphia, W. B. Saunders Company, 1978.)

Fluorouracil and its derivatives have not proved to be beneficial in most instances.

PROGNOSIS. Prognosis in primary bowel malignancy is dependent to some extent upon location, histology, and duration of disease. Under favorable circumstances five-year survivals of 20 per cent have been reported with adenocarcinoma, 60 per cent with lymphoma, and up to 50 per cent with leiomyosarcomas.

BENIGN NEOPLASMS

The small intestine may give rise to a variety of benign small bowel tumors. Among these are *adenomas*, *leiomyomas*, *lipomas*, *fibromas*, and *hemangiomas*. Of these, the *leiomyoma* is the most important of the group to the clinician. They may arise at any level of the small intestine but favor the jejunum. Central necrosis with ulceration, resulting in severe hemorrhage, is a characteristic feature of the leiomyoma.

Hemangiomas are much less frequently found than adenomas or leiomyomas. They, too, are clinically important because of their propensity to bleed.

CLINICAL MANIFESTATIONS. Benign small bowel tumors occur with equal frequency in men and women and are usually symptomatic in persons above 50 years of age. Colicky abdominal pain caused by luminal obstruction or intussusception is the predominant symptom. Massive gastrointestinal hemorrhage is suggestive of a leiomyoma. Benign small bowel tumors are rarely palpable.

DIAGNOSIS. Barium contrast studies of the small intestine and visceral angiography represent the principal diagnostic methods. A small bowel series occasionally demonstrates localized intussusception, an important clue that the lesion is benign.

TREATMENT AND PROGNOSIS. Surgical excision is the treatment of choice for virtually all symptomatic primary benign small bowel tumors. Prognosis is excellent with resection.

426. NEOPLASMS OF THE LARGE INTESTINE

Thomas F. O'Brien, Jr.

CARCINOMA OF THE LARGE INTESTINE

INCIDENCE AND PREVALENCE. Colorectal cancer is the second most common malignancy of the adult population in the United States (excluding skin cancer). It is exceeded only by lung cancer among males and breast cancer among females. Malignancies of the colon and rectum are responsible for approximately 15 per cent of all adult cancer deaths, resulting in an annual fatality rate of 16 to 18 patients per 100,000 population. A similar incidence has been noted in Great Britain, France, Germany, New Zealand, and a number of other countries which share an urbanized Western culture. In sharp contrast is a considerably reduced incidence in Japan, rural Africa, India, and a number of Latin American countries.

ETIOLOGY. The etiology of malignant tumors of the colon and rectum remains unknown. At least three factors must be considered in the development of large intestinal neoplasms, namely environmental factors, heredity, and pre-existing disease.

Environmental Factors. The contrasting prevalence of the disease among different cultures has led to increasing speculation that environmental factors, such as exposure to ingested carcinogens, play a primary role in pathogenesis. Considerable differences in dietary patterns exist between populations with high and low rates of large intestinal cancer. For example, those in cultures with a low incidence of large bowel cancer consume diets containing a large amount of plant fiber. Conversely, diets in areas where colon cancer is more prevalent tend to contain large amounts of highly refined carbohydrates and are generally low in fiber content. Perhaps related to these dissimilarities in diet are the significant differences in colonic bacterial flora which exist between the two groups. High fiber content diets produce bulky stools containing principally aerobic organisms (enterococci, streptococci), whereas the compact, small volume stools of low residue diets contain principally anaerobic organisms (bacteroides). Furthermore, it has been shown that some anaerobic organisms have the capacity metabolically to transform certain innocuous substances, such as bile acids, into potentially carcinogenic compounds. The latter phenomenon, together with the relatively prolonged colonic transit time of the small-volume stool, could lead to extended contact time between carcinogen and large bowel epithelium. Although unproved, this hypothesis is both popular and plausible.

In further support of the environmental theory is the observation that individuals from a "low-cancer" culture, such as native Japanese, develop large intestinal malignancies with an incidence similar to Americans when they establish residence in the United States and adopt Western dietary patterns.

Hereditary Factors. Genetic factors appear to play a primary role in several varieties of inherited colorectal neoplasms to be discussed.

FAMILIAL POLYPOSIS. Familial polyposis is inherited as an autosomal dominant trait. Multiple polypoid adenomas of the colon become apparent in patients be-tween the ages of 10 and 15 years. In untreated cases, colorectal cancer will develop in 75 to 80 per cent of the patients. Unfortunately, some 40 per cent of index cases already have a malignancy at the time of original diagnosis. The identification of such an index case should prompt a thorough survey of all immediate family members with the usual diagnostic methods (see below). Subtotal colectomy with ileoproctectomy should be recommended to all asymptomatic patients in whom multiple polyps are present. The remaining rectal tissue, although subject to the development of polypoid adenomas and adenocarcinomas, can be inspected regularly with a proctoscope and suspicious lesions removed locally. The preservation of rectal function is desirable and more easily acceptable to asymptomatic patients.

GARDNER'S SYNDROME. Gardner's syndrome consists of multiple polyps of the small and large intestines associated with osteomas and soft tissue lesions. This disorder is also transmitted as an autosomal dominant trait. A variety of soft tissue lesions are seen, including sebaceous cysts, lipomas, fibromas, leiomyomas, and occasionally fibrosarcomas. These soft tissue tumors may occur in the skin, in subcutaneous tissues, or in a variety of mesenteric or retroperitoneal locations. Colorectal carcinoma occurs in these patients with a high frequency, similar to that observed in familial polyposis; however, the malignancies tend to develop at a later age in life. Prophylactic subtotal colectomy with ileorectal anastomosis is the treatment of choice.

FAMILY COLONIC CANCER WITHOUT POLYPS (THE CANCER FAMILY SYNDROME). Several kindreds have been described in which there is an unusual frequency of colonic cancer. The neoplasms tend to occur at an early age, and polyposis is *not* a feature. Pedigree studies suggest that the mode of inheritance is via an autosomal dominant trait.

PEUTZ-JEGHERS SYNDROME. Mucocutaneous pigmentation, primarily involving the buccal mucosa, perioral and periorbital skin, and distal extremities, characterizes this variety of gastrointestinal polyposis. The syndrome is transmitted by a single mendelian dominant trait responsible for both the melanin deposits and the polyps. Histologically, the latter are hamartomas rather than adenomas. In the great majority of cases the polyps are distributed primarily in the jejunum and ileum, although gastric polyps occur in approximately 25 per cent of cases, and colorectal polyps are seen in 30 to 50 per cent. The risk of associated gastrointestinal malignancy is small, of the order of 3 per cent of cases. In a recent review, it was reported that 15 of 125 female patients with Peutz-Jeghers syndrome had developed ovarian tumors. The wide distribution of the gastrointestinal polyps and the low incidence of associated malignancy make prophylactic bowel resection unrealistic.

TURCOT SYNDROME. This extremely rare condition features the association of malignant tumors of the central nervous system and familial polyposis. To date, only a single kindred has been described. No rational therapeutic management program has developed because of the insufficient case material.

CRONKHITE-CANADA SYNDROME. Diffuse gastrointestinal polyposis, alopecia, pigmentation, and onychotrophia characterize this syndrome. Diarrhea, hypoproteinemia, edema, and cachexia are important additional clinical manifestations. Patients with this syndrome have usually been in their fifth and sixth decades of

Figure 2. Adenomatous polyp, sigmoid colon (arrow).

life, and there is no predominant sex distribution. Although colorectal malignancy has not been associated with the polyposis, rapidly progressive cachexia and a fatal outcome are characteristic.

Predisposing Diseases. CANCER RISK AND POLYPOID ADENOMAS. Whether small (less than 1 cm), histologically benign polypoid adenomas (Fig. 2) represent the earliest stage of an eventual colorectal cancer has not been established with certainty. On the one hand, they appear to be commonly present in adults. In a large autopsy series in which meticulous inspection of the large bowel was carried out, adenomas were demonstrated in approximately three fourths of all those examined. On the other hand, their common association with adenocarcinoma of the colon, both hereditary and nonhereditary varieties, makes them suspect, especially by authorities such as Morson. In support of the hypothesis of their premalignant nature is the report by Gilbertsen that interval proctosigmoidoscopy and polypectomy reduced the expected incidence of colorectal cancer in a large series of patients so treated.

From the clinical standpoint, the question of the premalignant nature of polypoid adenomas is moot. Improved techniques for air contrast barium studies of the colon and fiberoptic colonoscopy have permitted ready identification of adenomas down to 0.5 cm or smaller in size. Malignant changes are rarely identified in polyps less than 1 cm in diameter, yet are found with increasing frequency (up to 3.5 per cent) in polyps larger than 2 cm. Most authorities therefore recommend colonoscopic polypectomy for polyps measuring greater than 1 cm. As this practice gains wider acceptance, one should expect a reduction in the incidence of colorectal carcinoma if the polyp-carcinoma sequence hypothesis is valid.

ULCERATIVE COLITIS. The development of colorectal carcinoma at a greatly increased rate in patients with chronic ulcerative colitis appears well established. Approximately 5 per cent of patients with prolonged disease develop this serious complication. At least three parameters appear important when considering the risk of malignancy in these patients: the duration of the disease, the age at initial onset of the disease, and the extent of colonic involvement with the disease. The majority of patients in whom ulcerative colitis is complicated by malignancy have usually had universal involvement of the colon by the inflammatory process, and their disease has been present in excess of 15 years on the average.

So-called childhood ulcerative colitis, with onset at less than 14 years of age, appears to have an unusual incidence of colonic carcinoma. An analysis of almost 400 cases from the Mayo Clinic places the cancer risk at 20 per cent for each 10 years of duration beyond the initial decade. This carcinogenic risk of longstanding ulcerative colitis makes duration of disease the most important single consideration in the decision for colectomy. To date there is insufficient evidence to establish a relationship between granulomatous-segmental colitis (Crohn's disease) and colorectal carcinoma.

PATHOGENESIS. Normal and Abnormal Cellular Kinetics. Radiothymidine-labeling studies of cellular proliferation in the colon have shown important differences between normal epithelium and areas of neoplasia. Mitosis of colonic epithelial cells is normally limited to a regeneration zone in the lower two thirds of the crypts of Lieberkühn. Newly formed epithelial cells then migrate to the mucosal surface over a period of approximately 72 hours, and are finally shed into the lumen in about 96 hours. No appreciable cellular division takes place once the cell has begun its journey out of the crypt. However, when surface epithelial cells of laboratory animals are exposed to chemical carcinogens, they begin to show considerable mitotic activity. Eventually polypoid adenomas develop which are histologically similar to those observed in humans. Parallel isotopic studies in humans with hyperplastic colonic neoplasms and ulcerative colitis have confirmed that increased cellular proliferation occurs within the superficial epithelium of these lesions. Such studies support the theory that environmental carcinogens play an important role in colorectal neoplasms.

PATHOLOGY. The majority of rectal and colonic malignancies are adenocarcinomas. In a series of more than 50,000 cases of large intestinal malignancy, 86 per cent were adenocarcinoma in type. *Carcinoids, squamous cell carcinoma, leiomyosarcoma, adenoacanthoma,* and *lymphoma,* as a group, accounted for only 2 per cent of the total. The remainder were undifferentiated or poorly differentiated carcinomas. Multiple primary tumors within the colon are noted in approximately 5 per cent of patients at the time of initial diagnosis.

The distribution of large intestinal malignancies is similar in most large series. Approximately 15 per cent arise in the cecum and ascending colon, 10 per cent are distributed along the transverse colon, 5 per cent occur in the descending colon, 25 per cent occur in the sigmoid, and 45 per cent arise in the rectum. Metastatic spread may occur by direct invasion of surrounding tissues, by way of the regional lymphatics, or by multiple peritoneal implants. The liver is the principal site of major organ metastasis, with the lungs, brain, bones, and other viscera less frequently involved.

Microscopically, adenocarcinomas of the large intestine show a poorly formed acinar architecture, containing small amounts of mucus. A small number, perhaps 5 per cent, show considerable mucus production and have been assigned the term *mucoid adenocarcinoma.* Paradoxically, the well-differentiated mucoid carcinoma has a rather poor prognosis.

CLINICAL MANIFESTATIONS. Carcinoma of the colon and rectum is primarily a disease of later life. Although sporadic cases may be observed in any age group, the disease occurs with increasing frequency above the age of 55 years and reaches its peak incidence beyond 65 years of age. Males and females develop tumors above the rectum with approximately equal frequency, whereas males predominate in rectal cancer.

The presenting clinical manifestations of colorectal cancer are primarily determined by the location of the tumor. Approximately 75 per cent of all large intestinal malignancies occur within, or distal to, the sigmoid colon. Characteristically, tumors in these locations grow circumferentially, producing some degree of bowel obstruction. For this reason a significant change in bowel pattern is reported by the majority of the patients. Common symptoms include increasing constipation or alternating constipation and diarrhea, usually accompanied by colicky lower abdominal pain.

Most tumors in this location have ulcerating surfaces, and because of their proximity to the rectum, visible blood is usually observed by the patient. When the tumors arise within or near the rectum, more severe obstipation, tenesmus, and visible blood are nearly always reported and pencil-shaped stools are frequently observed.

In contrast, carcinomas arising in the cecum and ascending colon usually do not produce obstructive symptoms. Growths in this area often assume a polypoid configuration and may reach considerable size prior to discovery. Blood loss is typically occult, and is rarely observed by the patient. Frequently it is the symptoms of profound anemia which bring the patient to the physician. Quite often the tumor has metastasized to the liver at the time of initial examination, and jaundice, right upper quadrant pain, or a mass lesion may be noted.

Tumors arising in the middle third of the colon present with variable symptomatology. Vague discomfort, nonspecific dyspepsia, or colicky pain with gross or occult blood loss may be reported by the patient. Weight loss is variable, but when it exceeds 10 per cent or more of the patient's usual weight it usually indicates a poor prognosis.

DIAGNOSIS. The diagnosis of a large intestinal malignancy is usually suggested by the patient's history. In addition, it must be strongly considered in all patients beyond the age of 45 years with unexplained anemia. A primary lesion in the large intestine must also be ruled out in those patients who present with evidence of metastatic liver disease such as jaundice and hepatic enlargement.

On physical examination, palpation of the abdomen may reveal a mass lesion, but this is highly variable and depends in large part upon the size of the tumor, degree of obesity, and location of the tumor in relationship to pelvic bony structures. Digital and proctoscopic examination of the rectosigmoid usually reveals two out of three lesions arising below the pelvic peritoneal reflection. The physician should be alert to those cutaneous manifestations suggestive of a familial syndrome associated with colorectal cancer. Superficial forceps biopsy of the lesion can usually be obtained safely by an experienced physician and will lead to rapid histologic confirmation of the diagnosis. Reluctance toward biopsy on the grounds of tumor dissemination is not justified. Comparative five-year survival studies of patients with and without circulating malignant cells after

surgical manipulation have demonstrated that their presence is without prognostic significance.

Lesions beyond the reach of the proctoscope are best revealed by barium contrast radiographic examination. Typical lesions in the sigmoid colon produce a sharply demarcated narrowing of the lumen usually not exceeding 8 to 10 cm in length. The "napkin ring" or "apple core" appearance with shelving edges is a most characteristic radiographic feature (Fig. 3). Tumors arising in the cecum often assume polypoid rather than annular configuration and may be obscured by excessive barium filling of the cecum. In suspicious cases, when an annular lesion is not demonstrated, an air contrast barium enema can be diagnostic. The introduction of heavy density barium suspensions for air contrast examinations has considerably improved the resolution of smaller polypoid lesions, even those measuring 0.5 cm and less. A carcinoma lying within an area of massed diverticula can easily be overlooked, and repeat studies with special emphasis to the area of interest should be performed in suspicious cases.

Fiberoptic Colonoscopy and Sigmoidoscopy. In the past decade, significant advances have been made in the development of versatile fiberoptic instruments which permit both detailed inspection and operative manipulation of the large intestine. The longer instruments, measuring from 105 to 185 cm in length, permit visualization of the entire colon to the ileocecal valve. This can be accomplished more than 80 per cent of the time by a skilled colonoscopist. The safety of the procedure appears well established, provided that the examination is performed by an experienced endoscopist. Complications of bleeding and perforation occur in well under 1

Figure 3. Carcinoma of the colon. This annular lesion in the ascending colon has produced a typical appearance of mucosal destruction and overhanging margins.

Figure 4. Polypoid adenoma on a stalk as seen through a fiberoptic endoscope. This lesion can be readily removed by snare electrocautery.

per cent of those examined, and the over-all mortality to date has been negligible, including patients who have biopsy or excisional procedures. Colonoscopy with snare cautery polypectomy is currently the method of choice for the removal of clinically significant polypoid adenomas (Fig. 4).

Fiberoptic colonoscopy is not a substitute for standard radiographic examinations, as the cost, availability of expertise, and complications would be prohibitive. Nevertheless, several studies have led to the development of clear-cut indications for diagnostic colonoscopy. These include (1) x-ray abnormalities which cannot be resolved by a repeat study; (2) chronic gastrointestinal blood loss in which radiographic examinations are unrevealing; (3) interval re-evaluation of an anastomotic site following segmental resection for malignancy; and (4) selected patients with chronic inflammatory bowel disease (CIBD).

In the last-named instance, colonoscopy with or without biopsy may be useful in distinguishing chronic ulcerative colitis from Crohn's disease of the colon in equivocal cases. In addition, for some patients with CIBD it may be necessary to establish the limits of involvement. Studies to date indicate that approximately two thirds of patients with CIBD will have more widespread disease than is indicated on radiographic examination.

Colonoscopy is not recommended for active lower gastrointestinal bleeding or for acute inflammatory lesions such as diverticulitis. Colonoscopy has not been helpful in the differential diagnosis of chronic abdominal pain. Shorter fiberoptic instruments (length 65 cm) have been developed and designated as "flexible sigmoidoscopes." These instruments can be passed beyond the usual reach of the rigid sigmoidoscope, even by less experienced individuals. It would appear that the combination of flexible sigmoidoscopy and a well-done air contrast barium enema will considerably reduce the necessity for total fiberoptic examination of the colon.

Screening for Colorectal Cancer. The common occurrence of colorectal cancer, together with the potential for cure of early-detected lesions, has led to a search for effective and acceptable methods of mass screening. Radiographic and endoscopic procedures do not appear to be patient acceptable or cost effective. Occult blood testing, on the other hand, has been shown to be both acceptable and reliable in two large studies. Commercially prepared, guaiac-impregnated paper slides (Hemoccult) are prepared by the patient from stool specimens taken on three successive days. During the test period, the patient consumes a meat-free, high roughage diet, beginning at least one day prior to the preparation of the first slide. Ascorbic acid (vitamin C) must not be taken, because it leads to a false-negative result. Approximately 1 to 2 per cent of screened patients will have one or more positive slides. Of this group, approximately 12 to 14 per cent will have previously undetected colorectal cancer. Forty to 50 per cent of those with positive tests will have polypoid adenomas measuring more than 0.5 cm. Such screening is highly recommended for all individuals over 40 years of age.

Exfoliative cytology, although advocated by Papanicolaou more than 20 years ago, has not gained wide acceptance in the diagnosis of colorectal cancer. Several series, however, have demonstrated a high degree of diagnostic accuracy for the method. A correct cytologic diagnosis is established in 80 to 95 per cent of patients with malignancy. The percentages of false-positive and false-negative reports are small in these series. Underutilization of the technique is probably accounted for by the belief that satisfactory specimens are difficult and unpleasant to obtain. In practice, however, quite satisfactory cytologic material may be obtained by a simple saline lavage of the colon preceded by several days of an elemental diet and a strong cathartic the night before the collection of the specimen.

Carcinoembryonic Antigen (CEA). A tumor-associated antigen, referred to as CEA, can be demonstrated in the serum of over 95 per cent of patients with disseminated colonic carcinoma and approximately 20 per cent of patients with localized disease. The CEA appears to be a glycoprotein with a molecular weight of approximately 200,000. In general, serum levels appear to be elevated in proportion to the mass of tumor tissue present. Serum levels of CEA below 2.5 ng per milliliter are clearly normal, whereas values which exceed 5.0 ng per milliliter are stongly suggestive of underlying disease (see below). Levels between 2.5 and 5.0 ng must be considered indeterminate, especially if underlying inflammatory disease is present.

The early promise of specific serologic diagnosis of large intestinal malignancy by means of the CEA has not been sustained.

Positive tests can be obtained in a significant percentage of other gastrointestinal diseases, both malignant (hepatoma and gastric, pancreatic, and small bowel carcinomas) and nonmalignant (alcoholic cirrhosis, pancreatitis, and ulcerative colitis). Positive CEA tests have also been reported in lung cancer, breast cancer, prostatic cancer, neuroblastoma, and osteogenic sarcoma. These findings cast much doubt on the utility of the CEA as a screening test for colorectal cancer. The test may be useful in postoperative cases, because elevated levels tend to fall with successful resection. A return to elevated values is indicative of recurrent or disseminated disease.

DIFFERENTIAL DIAGNOSIS. Malignancies of the large intestine must be differentiated from other diseases which present with an abdominal mass. rectal bleeding, colicky abdominal pain, or a change in bowel habit. A number of diseases may produce these symptoms either singly or in combination. Included in the differential diagnosis are *diverticulosis coli*, with or without diverticulitis; inflammatory bowel diseases, including *ulcerative colitis* and *proctitis* and *ileocolitis* of the Crohn variety; and *benign tumors* (most frequently polypoid adenomas).

On rare occasions *pelvic endometriosis* may mimic a primary large bowel cancer. In this instance, usually the age, sex, and relationship of the rectal bleeding to menstrual flow are important differential diagnostic features in the history.

The finding of hemorrhoidal varices should not be accepted as sufficient explanation for rectal bleeding in any patient, especially in those over 45 years. Proctoscopy should be performed routinely in all patients with rectal bleeding, and radiographic studies should be obtained in most instances.

TREATMENT AND PROGNOSIS. Surgical Resection. Most patients with colorectal carcinoma require surgical resection of the primary tumor. The operation may be either curative or palliative in intent. A palliative resection is justified when lower bowel obstruction is imminent, even though known metastases are present. In a series of over 1800 cases from the University of Minnesota, the over-all five-year survival of patients with colorectal carcinoma was approximately 30 per cent. Patients with rectal carcinoma generally showed a poorer prognosis than those with tumors of other segments of the colon. Patients without lymph node involvement, whose surgery took place between 1958 and 1963, showed a five-year survival of 43.5 per cent for carcinoma of the rectum and 62.5 per cent for other colonic cancers. The operative mortality for rectal carcinoma was more than twice that for higher lesions.

Rectal Fulguration and Radiotherapy. The higher operative mortality and poorer prognosis for rectal cancer have led to several innovations in therapy. Rectal fulguration and/or local radiation therapy have been successfully employed by some as an alternative mode of therapy for selected patients.

Chemotherapy. There has been disappointingly little progress in the development of effective chemotherapeutic agents for colorectal carcinoma. 5-Fluorouracil (5-FU) remains the most widely used agent. Objective tumor regression occurs in approximately 20 per cent of the treated patients. The rather slow cellular doubling time of colorectal cancers has been offered as an explanation for the general unresponsiveness to chemotherapeutic agents.

Some are cautiously optimistic that immunotherapy may play a role in future treatment. The identification of tumor-specific antigens within human neoplastic colon cells justifies the hope that specific antibodies can be developed and directed against the neoplastic tissues.

VILLOUS ADENOMAS

The villous adenoma is a special form of colonic neoplasm with interesting gross anatomic, histologic, physiologic, and clinical features. Villous adenomas occur with much less frequency than polypoid adenomas (ratio 1:9), and are usually seen in patients in the seventh decade of life. Grossly, the tumors are broad based, usually measuring more than 4 cm in transverse diameter, and consist of numerous frond-like projections. The majority are in the rectum and rectosigmoid portion of the colon. Those which can be reached by digital examination are very soft to palpation and appear velvety on proctoscopy. The epithelial cells of these tumors are abundant in mucin, and patients with villous adenomas often note considerable mucoid content in their stools. In rare instances a villous adenoma will secrete considerable volumes of fluid, rich in potassium, leading to severe hypokalemia.

In the microscopic evaluation of these tumors a clear distinction between atypical focal hyperplasia and carcinoma in situ can be very difficult for the pathologist. Such foci of cellular atypia can be found in up to 50 per cent of all villous adenomas upon careful serial sectioning. It is very unlikely, however, that 50 per cent of the lesions advance to infiltrating adenocarcinoma. The unpredictable course, together with frequently distressing clinical symptoms, dictates complete surgical excision whenever possible.

Devroede, G. J., Taylor, W. F., Sauer, W. G., Jackman, R. J., and Stickler, G. B.: Cancer risk and life expectancy of children with ulcerative colitis. N. Engl. J. Med., 285:17, 1971.

Gilbertsen, V. A.: Proctosigmoidoscopy and polypectomy in reducing the incidence of rectal cancer. Cancer, 34:936, 1974.

Griffiths, J. D., McKinna, J. A., Rowbotham, H. D., Tsolakidis, P., and Salisbury, A. J.: Carcinoma of the colon and rectum: Circulating malignant cells and five year survival. Cancer, 31:226, 1973.

Margulis, A. R., and Burhenne, H. J.: Alimentary Tract Radiology. St. Louis, C. V. Mosby Company, 1973.

Morrissey, J. F.: Gastrointestinal endoscopy. Gastroenterology, 62:1241, 1972.

Morson, B. C.: Genesis of colorectal cancer. Clin. Gastroenterol., 5:505, 1976.

Sleisenger, M. H., and Fordtran, J. S. (eds.): Gastrointestinal Disease. 2nd ed. Philadelphia, W. B. Saunders Company, 1978.

Winawer, S. J., and Sherlock, P.: Detecting early colon cancer. Hosp. Prac., March, 1977, p 49.

Section Eleven   OTHER DISEASES OF THE COLON, RECTUM, AND ANUS

David L. Earnest

427.   INTRODUCTION

Certain diseases of the colon are not conveniently classified with other vascular, motor, malignant, or inflammatory conditions. In general, these miscellaneous colonic diseases are uncommon, often of uncertain etiology, and frequently perplexing to diagnose and treat. Although x-ray studies are helpful in their evaluation, mucosal biopsy specimens obtained by sigmoidoscopy or colonoscopy, procedures which are discussed in detail in Ch. 425, can significantly contribute to early correct diagnosis. A pedunculated or sessile mucosal mass may be biopsied with either punch or cutting forceps. Biopsy of an ulcerating lesion should be taken at its margin and should include some normal tissue. A suction biopsy tube can be used when there is diffuse mucosal disease. This instrument is especially useful if the abnormality is located above the peritoneal reflection, because the use of conventional biopsy forceps for small mucosal lesions 12 to 14 cm or more above the pectinate line always carries the potential hazard of bowel perforation. Tissue specimens should be mounted on a piece of monofilament mesh with the mucosal side up and then placed in a fixative solution. Proper orientation of the tissue on the mesh may facilitate diagnostic interpretation by making it easier to section the specimen perpendicular to the mucosa.

Edling, N. P. G., Ekloff, O., Kistner, S., and Lagarlof, F.: Correlation of findings at barium enema examination, rectoscopy and biopsy of the rectum. Acta Radiol., 4:536, 1966.

Gear, E. V., and Dobbins, W. O., III: Rectal biopsy. A review of its diagnostic usefulness. Gastroenterology, 55:522, 1968.

428.   COLITIS CYSTICA SUPERFICIALIS AND PROFUNDA

There are two types of benign, cystic, mucus-filled lesions of the colonic mucosa: *colitis cystica superficialis* and *colitis cystica profunda*. The superficialis type occurs predominantly in patients with pellagra and may develop at a time when typical skin lesions are absent. It has also been described in a few cases of adult celiac disease. Diarrhea is frequently the presenting symptom. The condition is characterized by very small mucus-filled cysts which lie superficial to the muscularis mucosae of the colon. Grossly, the cysts appear on the mucosal surface as thousands of minute gray blebs from which mucus can be expressed. Treatment with niacin or tryptophan for the underlying pellagra is curative.

In colitis cystica profunda the cysts are located below the muscularis mucosae and occasionally appear to "invade" the muscularis propria. They are filled with ba-sophilic mucoid material and are lined by colonic epithelium, showing varying degrees of pressure atrophy. Pathologically, colitis cystica profunda must be differentiated from mucus-producing adenocarcinoma. Misdiagnosis has resulted in extensive cancer surgery for this benign condition.

The pathogenesis of cyst formation is uncertain. Congenitally ectopic mucosa may be responsible. However, communications between the cyst and the bowel lumen have been demonstrated, suggesting a weakness in the muscularis mucosae which allows herniation of mucosal epithelium into the submucosa. Another possibility is downgrowth of colonic epithelium during the healing process into areas of inflammatory ulceration. The frequently obtained history of preceding severe diarrhea or dysentery supports an inflammatory origin.

Cramping lower abdominal pain, rectal tenesmus, and mild diarrhea associated with blood and mucus in the stool are the most consistent symptoms. If palpated on rectal examination, the cystic lesion usually has a rubbery firm consistency and is not adherent to surrounding tissue. It may be sessile or polypoid and have either normal or ulcerated overlying mucosa. The lesions are most often located on the anterior rectal wall within 12 cm of the anal verge. Sigmoidoscopy may demonstrate that the mucosa overlying the mass appears normal or congested, edematous or ulcerated, or even contains an umbilication on the intraluminal protrusion. A nodular irregularity in the bowel wall may be the only radiologic abnormality on barium enema and may stimulate a large differential diagnosis. Biopsy of one of the cystic nodules should settle the diagnostic dilemma. Treatment consists of local surgical excision. There are no reports of recurrence in uninvolved intestine.

Epstein, S. E., Ascare, W. A., Ablow, R. C., Seaman, W. B., and Lattis, R.: Colitis cystica profunda. Am. J. Clin. Pathol., 5:186, 1966.

Farman, J., Dallemand, S., Robinson, T., and Keokane, M. F.: Colitis cystica profunda, an unusual solitary tumor. Dis. Colon Rectum, 17:565, 1974.

Tedesco, F. J., Summer, H. W., and Kassens, W. D.: Colitis cystica profunda. Am. J. Gastroenterol., 65:339, 1976.

429.   PNEUMATOSIS CYSTOIDES INTESTINALIS

Pneumatosis cystoides intestinalis is characterized by multiple gas-filled cysts in the submucosa or subserosa of both the small intestine and the colon. The mesentery and omentum may also be involved. The majority of cases with involvement of the small intestine are in patients between ages 25 and 50 years who have either chronic obstructive pulmonary disease or peptic ulcer with some degree of pyloric obstruction. Pneumatosis cystoides intestinalis has also been reported in patients who have mesenteric vascular occlusion, necrotizing enterocolitis, chronic mucosal inflammatory diseases, lymphosarcoma of the intestine, perforated diverticula, collagen disorders (especially scleroderma), Whipple's disease, abdominal trauma, and intestinal parasites; in those who have ingested caustic agents; and in those who have had recent surgical bowel anastomosis. Fewer than 2 per cent of patients with pneumatosis cystoides intestinalis have no evidence of other gastrointestinal abnormality.

The exact cause of the gas-filled cysts is unknown. It is postulated that air, forced into tissue spaces around an ulcer or from rupture of a pulmonary bleb, dissects along facial planes into the retroperitoneal space and out along blood vessels in the mesentery to the intestinal subserosa. Patients with pneumatosis in the wall of the rectum and sigmoid colon usually have undergone previous sigmoidoscopy. Presumably air entered the rectosigmoid wall through a small mucosal tear. The origin of pneumatosis in association with the varied other conditions listed above is less clear. Analysis of gas in the cysts usually demonstrates a composition similar to atmospheric air: 70 to 90 per cent nitrogen, 3 to 20 per cent oxygen, 0 to 15 per cent carbon dioxide, and traces of methane.

The gas-filled cysts may vary in size from a few millimeters to several centimeters and grossly look like multiple lymphangiomas or even multiple sessile polyps. Microscopically, the gas cysts are lined by a layer of endothelial cells which have a tendency to coalesce to form giant cells. A progressive fibrotic reaction may develop and ultimately obliterate the cyst. Because the cysts do not communicate with the bowel lumen, cyst rupture does not result in peritonitis except in ischemic bowel disease when pneumatosis of the intestinal wall is produced by invading bacteria.

Pneumatosis cystoides intestinalis usually produces no specific symptoms. It is often an incidental finding during radiologic examination of the abdomen or intestine. Nevertheless, lower abdominal cramping pain, recurrent diarrhea, rectal bleeding, tenesmus, and partial bowel obstruction have all been described in patients with colonic pneumatosis. In addition, pneumatosis should be considered in the patient who presents with vague abdominal discomfort and free air under the diaphragm on x-ray examination, and who has no other evidence for a perforated viscus.

The most useful way of establishing the diagnosis is by barium x-ray examination of the small bowel and colon. Pneumatosis involving the rectosigmoid area can be recognized during sigmoidoscopy as pale bluish soft masses which protrude into the lumen and often collapse when biopsied.

When pneumatosis involves the small bowel, often no specific treatment is necessary except for the underlying or primary disease. The value of correct diagnosis is mainly in preventing unnecessary surgery. However, if there is severe tenesmus, bleeding, pain, or partial intestinal obstruction associated with the pneumatosis cystoides intestinalis, hospitalization and treatment are indicated. Medical treatment should be attempted first. It is based on the premise that persistence of the gas cysts in the bowel wall implies that gas in the cyst is replenished at a rate equal to or exceeding the rate of gas resorption by the surrounding tissues. Diffusion of the gas across the wall of the cysts depends in part on the partial pressure of gases in the intestinal lumen,

cystic spaces, and capillary blood. Since the predominant gas in the cysts is nitrogen, prolonged breathing of oxygen reduces the partial pressure of other gases in blood and thereby promotes diffusion of gas from the cystic spaces. An arterial oxygen tension of 200 to 350 mm Hg should be achieved for optimal results. The patient should be closely monitored for evidence of developing oxygen toxicity. Complete resolution of the cysts usually occurs by the end of a week. They may recur but usually respond to repeat oxygen therapy. If evidence of oxygen toxicity develops or the cysts do not resolve, surgery may be necessary. Unfortunately, pneumatosis may recur and become more extensive after resection. If surgery is performed, the rectum should be spared, because pneumatosis in the rectum usually regresses after resection of more proximally involved colon.

Andrade, S., and Andrade, V. H.: Intestinal pneumatosis. Presentation of five cases. Am. J. Proctol., 19:39, 1968.

Down, R. H. L., and Castleden, W. M.: Oxygen therapy for pneumatosis coli. Br. Med. J., 1:493, 1975.

Forgacs, P., Wright, P. H., and Wyatt, A. P.: Treatment of intestinal gas cysts by oxygen breathing. Lancet, 1:579, 1973.

Nelson, S. W.: Extraluminal gas collections due to diseases of the gastrointestinal tract. Am. J. Roentgenol., 115:225, 1972.

430. ENDOMETRIOSIS

Endometriosis refers to the presence of extrauterine endometrial tissue and the clinical sequelae produced by its normal function in an abnormal site. It is a disease of the reproductive period, with peak incidence between the ages of 30 and 40 years. It is uncommon in the 20's and, rarely, may produce symptoms after menopause. Intestinal involvement with endometriosis is usually greatest in those parts of the bowel that are pelvic in location, especially the rectosigmoid colon.

It is uncertain exactly how the heterotopic endometrium reaches the subserosa of the bowel wall. Theories which have been advanced to explain this include a congenitally ectopic location, reflux of endometrial cells through the fallopian tubes, and lymphatic or hematologic dissemination of endometrial cells capable of heterotopic growth and maturation. This last explanation would help explain the rare cases of endometriosis involving the lungs, pleura, eyes, arms, and legs. Despite the reason for its abnormal location, under hormonal influence there is maturation, slough of the surface endometrial epithelium, and bleeding as occurs in the uterine cavity. Debris generated from this process may produce pressure necrosis of adjacent tissue, resulting in progressive dissection of the endometriosis through both subserosa and muscularis of the bowel wall. The mucosa is seldom penetrated, a fact which explains why periodic intraluminal intestinal bleeding infrequently occurs from endometriosis. Rectal bleeding should prompt evaluation for another disease. A large bulky intramural lesion can develop which contains areas of fibrosis and marked smooth muscle hyperplasia. This firm mass, known as an endometrioma, can produce luminal obstruction, especially in the sigmoid colon.

Symptoms of endometriosis include dysmenorrhea, menometrorrhagia, intermenstrual pelvic pain, sterility, dyspareunia, and low backache. Involvement of the rectosigmoid colon is usually signaled by cyclic cramping pains in the rectum and occasionally mild tenesmus.

Endometriosis of the more proximal colon is usually asymptomatic. Implants on the small intestine are often discovered incidentally during abdominal surgery. Bowel obstruction may develop from endometriosis at any level of the intestinal tract owing to fibrous adhesions, stenosis from fibrosis, or volvulus.

Clinical diagnosis of intestinal endometriosis primarily requires a high index of suspicion. The first diagnostic maneuver should be a thorough pelvic examination with combined rectovaginal palpation. Tender nodules with irregular induration in the cul-de-sac are suggestive of rectosigmoid endometriosis. Repeated pelvic examination later in the menstrual cycle should demonstrate some variation in character of the lesion. When a mass is palpable in the free portion of the sigmoid colon and none in the cul-de-sac, the diagnosis of endometriosis is much less certain. Radiologic, sigmoidoscopic, and mucosal biopsy findings may not significantly contribute to the diagnosis. Persisting uncertainty about a constricting rectosigmoid lesion, especially in an older woman, should prompt needle biopsy or surgical exploration to exclude adenocarcinoma.

The therapy of symptomatic intestinal endometriosis lies between watchful waiting, hormonal therapy, surgical excision, and castration. Treatment must be individualized and flexible during the course of the disease. Mildly symptomatic patients are best managed by analgesics, antispasmodics, and sedatives. Less than half of patients with rectosigmoid involvement will ever have severe symptoms. Significant difficulty from appendiceal, cecal, or small bowel endometriosis is even less frequent. If further treatment is necessary, progestin therapy occasionally produces regression and even disappearance of symptomatic colonic endometriosis. Recently, an antigonadotropic agent, Danzol, has been used to decrease pituitary-ovarian stimulation, and thereby cyclic changes in the endometriosis tissue. Such attempts at hormonal treatment should be undertaken with gynecologic consultation. The results of hormonal therapy may be inconstant, and if symptoms are not promptly alleviated, obstructing lesions should be excised.

Boles, R. S., and Hodes, P. J.: Endometriosis of the small and large intestine. Gastroenterology, 34:367, 1958.

Gray, L. A.: The management of endometriosis involving the bowel. Clin. Obstet. Gynecol., 9:309, 1966.

Ranney, B.: The prevention, inhibition, palliation and treatment of endometriosis. Am. J. Obstet. Gynecol., 123:778, 1975.

Spjut, H. T., and Perkins, D. E.: Endometriosis of the sigmoid colon and rectum. Am. J. Roentgenol., 82:1070, 1959.

431. MALAKOPLAKIA

Malakoplakia is a rare granulomatous disease of unknown cause which usually affects the urinary tract but which has also been reported in the colon, retroperitoneum, and stomach. It is characterized pathologically by the presence of histiocytes containing peculiar intracytoplasmic dark, round laminated inclusions called Michaelis-Gutmann bodies. These inclusions are PAS positive, stain for both calcium and iron, and appear to be a cellular reaction to breakdown products of bacteria. An intracellular abnormality of the macrophage phagolysosomes is thought to result in defective digestion of phagocytosed bacteria, especially *E. coli*. In addition, an abnormality in circulating monocytes, but not neutrophils, has recently been described which can be corrected by administration of cholinergic agonists.

Colonic malakoplakia is most often noted as an incidental finding in elderly debilitated patients and is usually histologically associated with coexisting malignancy such as adenocarcinoma of the colon. An abnormal delayed immune response has also been found in these patients. Fever, diarrhea, hematochezia, and even death have occurred in patients with only intestinal malakoplakia. Reported x-ray findings are not diagnostic. When visualized at sigmoidoscopy, areas of malakoplakia may vary from soft grayish-tan nodular lesions with serpiginous borders to confluent superficial ulcerations. Correct diagnosis is made by histologic examination. Because of its known high association with cancer, the discovery of malakoplakia in an intestinal biopsy should prompt further evaluation for colonic carcinoma.

Treatment of intestinal malakoplakia is difficult and often unsuccessful. In the urinary bladder the disease has been successfully treated with streptomycin, para-aminosalicylic acid, and isoniazid. Excision or fulguration may be tried for localized disease. A provocative recent case study reports successful treatment of an otherwise unresponsive case by use of the cholinergic drug bethanechol chloride.

Abdou, N. I., Chaiyakiati, N., Sagawa, A., Ragland, C., et al.: Malakoplakia: Evidence for monocyte lysosomal abnormality correctable by cholinergic agonist in vitro and in vivo. N. Eng. J. Med., 297:1413, 1977.

Dockerty, M. B.: Primary malakoplakia of the colon. Mayo Clin. Proc., 47:114, 1972.

Gonzales-Angulo, A., Corral, E., Garcia-Torres, R., and Quijano, M.: Malakoplakia of the colon. Gastroenterology, 48:383, 1965.

Lewin, J., Harell, G. A., Lee, A. S., and Crowley, L. G.: Malacoplakia. An electron microscopic study: Demonstration of bacilliform organisms in malacoplakic macrophages. Gastroenterology, 66:28, 1974.

Lou, T. Y., and Teplitz, C.: Malakoplakia: Pathogenesis and ultrastructural morphogenesis — a problem of altered macrophage (phagolysosomal) response. Hum. Pathol., 5:191, 1974.

432. MELANOSIS COLI, CATHARTIC COLON, AND SOAP COLITIS

The use of "irritant" purgatives has been associated with at least three colonic abnormalities: *melanosis coli, cathartic colon,* and *soap colitis.*

MELANOSIS COLI

Melanosis coli is an abnormal black or brown discoloration of the colonic mucosa which has been compared in appearance to tiger or crocodile skin or cross-section of nutmeg. The discoloration is due to brownish-black pigment in large mononuclear cells or macrophages in the lamina propria of the mucosa. The pigment may be distributed throughout the entire colon but is mainly found in the cecum and rectum. The coloration is usually most intense just inside the anal sphincter and less dark higher in the sigmoid, and is usually discovered quite unexpectedly during sigmoidoscopy. Melanosis pigment has also been found in the appendix, in mesenteric lymph nodes, in the terminal ileum, and in the liver. The pigment granules have histo-chemical staining characteristics of both melanin and lipofuscin. Its exact origin, however, is uncertain.

Melanosis coli is considered to be an entirely benign condition associated with fecal stasis and the regular use of anthracene cathartics such as cascara sagrada, senna, aloe, and frangula. The pigment has been noted as soon as four months after the onset of taking cascara preparations and may disappear after the laxative is discontinued.

By itself, melanosis coli produces no specific symptoms and has no known unfavorable long-term prognostic significance. However, a few patients with carcinoma of the colon have also had melanosis coli. It is uncertain how many of them actually took laxatives. Without an accompanying history of anthracene laxative abuse or fecal stasis, the presence of malanosis coli probably warrants radiologic evaluation for an occult colonic neoplasm.

CATHARTIC COLON

Cathartic colon occurs predominantly in women who have taken irritant laxatives (cascara sagrada, senna, aloe, podophyllin, castor oil, phenolphthalein, calomel) for a period of at least 15 years. It is a radiologic diagnosis characterized by loss of haustral markings, with lengthy inconstant areas of constriction having long tapering margins. At fluoroscopy, the distensibility of the narrowed segments can be demonstrated, excluding a stricture. The terminal ileum and ascending colon are most commonly involved, although the abnormality may extend to the lower descending colon. The radiologic differential diagnosis includes chronic ulcerative colitis, granulomatous colitis, and amebic colitis. An adequate medical history and examination of the stools for amebae will help exclude these differential possibilities. There should be no history of recent fever, recurrent diarrhea, or the passage of mucus or blood in stool. Sigmoidoscopic findings should be normal.

Very little is known about the pathophysiology resulting from chronic laxative abuse which produces cathartic colon. Gross examination of the bowel wall shows excessive submucosal fat and muscular atrophy. Silver impregnation stains of the myenteric plexus demonstrate abnormalities similar to those produced in experimental animals by large doses of senna. Senna causes contraction of colonic musculature, apparently by contact stimulation of the submucosal and subsequently intermuscular plexus. Therefore prolonged cathartic use may induce abnormalities in neural pathways regulating colonic motor activity. Indeed, advanced cases of cathartic colon have shown loss of colonic myenteric neurons and replacement of associated ganglia by Schwann cells.

The pathologic significance and sequelae of cathartic colon remain poorly defined. Treatment begins by enforced discontinuation of all irritant cathartics. In some patients, normal colonic motor function will return, but usually only after many months. The main problem is management of ensuing constipation. This should be treated by use of a bulk-forming hydrophilic mucilloid, emollient laxatives, and, if necessary, an occasional enema. In particularly resistant cases, subtotal colectomy has produced mixed results.

SOAP COLITIS

The use of cleansing "soapsuds" enemas may produce a spectrum of symptoms from slight discomfort to severe prostration. The colonic mucosal reaction also varies from mild irritation to frank necrosis. Severe reactions have usually occurred in cases in which a concentrated soap solution was administered. Symptoms, which begin within a few hours after the enema, may include severe abdominal cramps, abdominal distention, mucorrhea and serosanguineous diarrhea. Hypovolemia and acute hemoconcentration can result from rapid exudation of fluid into the colon. Hypokalemia may develop when exudation of colonic mucus is massive. On abdominal examination, the transverse and descending colon are usually tender to palpation. Sigmoidoscopy demonstrates severe spasm, edema, hyperemia, and occasionally in severe cases hemorrhagic mucosal necrosis. Barium enema may also demonstrate marked spasm along with abnormal massive propulsive movements and diffuse submucosal edema of the colon.

Despite the severe symptoms, most patients recover from this serious illness with treatment consisting of close observation, careful replacement of fluid and electrolytes, and possibly administration of broad-spectrum antimicrobial drugs.

SYSTEMIC EFFECTS OF CATHARTIC ABUSE

Some patients who chronically abuse cathartics may develop initially baffling symptoms and metabolic abnormalities, including chronic thirst and hyperaldosteronism resulting from volume depletion. Hypokalemia may develop from intestinal potassium loss with the watery stool and renal potassium loss caused by excess aldosterone effect. In turn, potassium deficiency can lead to alkalosis and a renal tubular concentrating defect which enhances the tendency to dehydration and thirst. Profound muscular weakness may accompany the hypokalemia. These symptoms respond to withdrawal of the laxative and potassium replacement.

A main difficulty in treatment of such patients is often initial consideration of the diagnosis, because many of them deny both excessive laxative use and the presence of diarrhea. An underlying personality disorder is often found, and successful management requires both the science and the art of medicine.

Fleischer, N., Brown, H., Graham, D. Y., and Delena, S.: Chronic laxative-induced hyperaldosteronism and hypokalemia simulating Bartter's syndrome. Ann. Intern. Med., 70:791, 1969.

Ghadially, F. N., and Parry, E. W.: An electron-microscope and histochemical study of melanosis coli. J. Path. Bact., 92:313, 1966.

Pike, B. F., Phillips, P. J., and Lauson, E. H.: Soap colitis. N. Engl. J. Med., 285:217, 1971.

Sladen, G. E.: Effects of chronic purgative abuse. Proc. Royal Soc. Med., 65:288, 1972.

Smith, B.: Effect of irritant purgatives on the myenteric plexus in man and the mouse. Gut, 9:139, 1968.

Steer, H. D., and Colin-Jones, D. G.: Melanosis coli: Studies of toxic effects of irritant purgatives. J. Pathol., 115:119, 1975.

Wittoesch, J. H., Hackman, R. J., and McDonald, J. R.: Melanosis coli: General review and a study of 887 cases. Dis. colon Rectum, 1:172, 1958.

Ziter, F. M.: Cathartic colon. N.Y. State J. Med., 67:546, 1967.

433. FECAL IMPACTION AND STERCORAL ULCER

Incomplete evacuation of feces for an extended time may lead to formation of a large firm mass of stool in the distal colon and rectum known as a fecal impaction. The large irregular mass of feces cannot be expelled from the dilated rectosigmoid through the disproportionately small anal canal. Fecal impactions most often occur in children who have undiagnosed megacolon or psychiatric problems, in elderly, debilitated, or sedentary persons, and in patients with painful anal diseases such as hemorrhoids, fissures, and cryptitis.

A sensation of rectal fullness, lower abdominal discomfort, headache, mild anorexia with weight loss, and a general sense of ill-being are the most commonly reported symptoms. Liquid stool above the fecal mass can expand the already distended colon and pass around the impaction, thus preventing complete obstruction. Unfortunately, this watery stool is occasionally interpreted as diarrhea, and the patient is improperly treated with constipating agents. The true diagnosis could be easily made by rectal examination. On physical examination, the impaction may be felt as a large firm mass in the left lower abdomen. Bimanual abdominorectal examination should be done to best palpate the fecal bolus. The impaction may not be located in the rectal ampulla but instead lodged in the sigmoid colon beyond complete reach of the examining finger, and may feel like a smooth but irregular mass in the intestinal wall. Firm pressure against the mass produces a persisting indentation that will not occur with a polyp or a carcinoma.

Treatment of large fecal impactions with enemas alone is usually not sufficient. Initially, small pieces of a large impaction in the rectum should be removed digitally. Thereafter, warm water or saline enemas may be given as well as mineral oil orally. More proximal sigmoid impactions can be broken up by advancing a large bore rubber tube through a sigmoidoscope into the fecal mass and gently flushing small amounts of water through the tube. An enema containing 15 to 20 per cent water-soluble x-ray constrast material may be useful because the hypertonic iodinated material can penetrate the fecal mass and, with osmotic equilibration, produce fragmentation of the firm stool. Enemas containing 0.5 ounce of 1 per cent dioctyl sodium sulfosuccinate in 4 ounces of water may also be helpful. Warm oil enemas are unnecessary and may produce burns of the heat-insensitive colonic mucosa. Enemas containing a dilute (5 to 10 per cent) solution of hydrogen peroxide have been used, but this technique risks rupture of an already distended colon by the liberated gas. Dilatation of the anus under anesthesia to allow removal of the impaction is occasionally necessary.

Fecal impactions have on occasion been associated with development of hernia, recurrent volvulus, megacolon, rectal prolapse, dystocia, and intestinal obstruction. More common significant complications include urinary tract obstruction, spontaneous perforation of the colon, and stercoral ulcer. Progressive enlargement of the rectosigmoid by the impaction can compress the ureters near the ureterovesical junction or elevate the bladder, producing marked angulation of the urethra. The resulting obstruction may present as symptomatic urinary tract infection.

Spontaneous perforation of the colon in patients with fecal impaction usually occurs during attempts by the patient to pass the fecal mass. Unfortunately, vague lower abdominal pain often precedes physical findings of a perforated viscus by only a few hours. More commonly, colonic perforation associated with fecal impaction is iatrogenic and occurs during sigmoidoscopy or attempted disimpaction. The development of fever, abdominal pain or distention, or shock after a disimpaction procedure should immediately alert one to this possibility. Treatment requires surgical closure of the perforation, drainage, and antimicrobial agents. Unless the disorder is diagnosed and treated early, mortality is high.

Since fecal impaction most frequently complicates other illnesses and may itself create new and serious problems in clinical management, preventive measures are important. These consist of the use of stool-wetting and bulk-forming drugs, mild laxatives, and a recording of stool frequency, with periodic rectal examination if constipation or small volume watery stool develops.

Stercoral ulcers in the rectum and colon likely result from pressure necrosis produced by a large fecal mass. The ulceration has a dark yellow-gray to greenish-purple irregular outline. Microscopically, there is little acute inflammatory reaction around the necrotic center. The ulcer usually heals rapidly after removal of the fecal mass. Chronic stercoral ulcers occasionally can be asymptomatic. Complications are bleeding and perforation. Perforation, occurring either spontaneously or during disimpaction, can result in a localized abscess or suppurative peritonitis.

Andrews, N. L.: Impactions of the rectum and colon. Am. Surgeon, 21:1147, 1962.

Culp, W. C.: Relief of severe fecal impactions with water soluble contrast enemas. Radiology, 115:9, 1975.

Grinvalsky, H. T., and Bowerman, C. I.: Stercoraceous ulcers of the colon. Relatively neglected medical and surgical problem. JAMA, 171:1941, 1959.

Huttunen, R., Heikkinin, E., and Larmi, T. K. I.: Stercoraceous and idiopathic perforations of the colon. Surg. Gynecol. Obstet., 140:756, 1975.

Lal, S., and Brown, G. N.: Some unusual complications of fecal impaction. Am. J. Proctol., 18:226, 1967.

Suckling, P. V.: The ball-valve rectum due to impacted feces. Lancet, 2:1147, 1962.

434. NONSPECIFIC OR SOLITARY ULCER OF THE COLON

Discrete, usually single, ulcerations of unknown cause may develop in any segment of the colon or rectum. The ulceration may vary from 5 mm to 4 or 5 cm with slightly raised edges that sharply demarcate it from surrounding normal mucosa. The cecum, ascending colon, and rectosigmoid colon are the most frequent locations. Symptoms and clinical course of the ulceration vary, depending on the segment of colon involved. Nonspecific ulceration in the cecum or ascending colon frequently presents with right lower abdominal pain. Fever and leukocytosis may be present, and a tender mass may develop. Gross bleeding is uncommon. The usual initial differential diagnosis includes *appendicitis, pelvic inflammatory disease, ovarian disease,* and *tuberculous* or *idiopathic regional enteritis.* Perforation of the cecum with peritonitis is a frequent complication.

The sigmoid colon is the second most common site of nonspecific ulceration. The diagnosis is seldom made prior to surgery. Chronic lower abdominal pain, constipation, recurrent rectal bleeding, and a high incidence of perforation characterize the ulcer in this location. Misdiagnosis of *diverticulitis* is common. An inflammatory mass may develop, and surgery may eventually be required to exclude *carcinoma.*

In contrast to the acute symptoms of nonspecific ulceration elsewhere in the colon, solitary ulcer of the rectum is a more chronic condition which tends to be resistant to therapy. Dull pain in the rectum or left iliac fossa, which is increased during defecation, and the passage of small amounts of bloody mucus with stool are typical symptoms. Massive bleeding is unusual. The shallow rectal ulceration frequently occurs 7 to 10 cm above the anal margin and is usually demarcated from normal mucosa by a narrow area of hyperemia. The lesion may be round, have an irregular outline, or even be linear. A symptomatic preulcer, hyperemic, or "granular" phase can antedate the actual crater.

Correct diagnosis of nonspecific ulcer of the colon requires a high index of suspicion. The yield of positive x-ray findings, even if a definite ulcer is present, decreases from right to left colon. Since cancer is usually the most serious differential diagnostic possibility, surgery is often employed to solve the dilemma. Benignity can be established by biopsy and cytologic study of tissue obtained at sigmoidoscopy or fiberoptic colonoscopy, and surgery avoided. However, if healing of ulcers in the cecum or sigmoid colon is not progressive, the ulcer should be excised to prevent complications.

In contrast, nonspecific ulcers of the rectum may remain static for years. Their extreme chronicity is matched by resistance to local or systemic treatment. However, perforation and serious bleeding from rectal ulcers are uncommon, and thus nonsurgical attempts to relieve mild symptoms are indicated, using stool softeners, local anesthetic suppositories, and periodic reexamination. Spontaneous healing of a chronic rectal ulcer may occur even after many years. For severe symptoms, surgical excision is curative.

Butsch, J. L., Dockerty, M. B., McGill, D. B., and Judd, E. S.: Solitary nonspecific ulcer of the colon. Arch. Surg., 98:171, 1969.
Madigan, M. R., and Marson, B. C.: Solitary ulcer of the rectum. Gut, 10:871, 1969.
Sleisenger, M. H., and Fordtran, J. S. (eds.): Gastrointestinal Disease. 2nd ed. Philadelphia, W. B. Saunders Company, 1978.

435. NONSPECIFIC ULCERATIVE PROCTITIS

Patients may present with rectal bleeding, tenesmus, and occasionally a mucosanguineous anal discharge and are found to have inflammation of the rectal mucosa with a clearly demarcated upper border above which the mucosa is normal. Histologic changes in tissue from rectal biopsy are usually compatible with ulcerative colitis, but barium enema and colonoscopy demonstrate no abnormality of the colon above the rectum. This disease, ulcerative proctitis, appears to be a localized milder form of generalized ulcerative colitis, but with a better prognosis (see Ch. 413.3). The age of onset parallels that for typical ulcerative colitis but with increased incidence in the late 20's. Typically the patient presents with rectal bleeding which is seldom severe. A change in bowel pattern is also common, both diarrhea and constipation being frequent complaints. Patients who complain of diarrhea often describe a normal stool volume but frequent passage of a mucoid or mucosanguineous discharge. Systemic symptoms such as fever, malaise, and weight loss are usually absent. Diagnosis is confirmed by sigmoidoscopy and rectal biopsy demonstrating typical changes of ulcerative colitis, but limited only to the rectum. Barium x-rays should confirm absence of abnormality in the remainder of the colon and small intestine. Differential diagnosis includes radiation proctitis, bacillary dysentery, amebiasis, lymphogranuloma venereum, gonorrheal proctitis, chemical or mechanical irritation, and proctitis resulting from gold therapy for rheumatoid arthritis. A detailed medical history, appropriate cultures, microscopic examination of the mucoid discharge, mucosal biopsy, and the Frei test should help exclude these differential possibilities.

Treatment of mild cases is usually limited to sedatives and stool softeners. Rectal bleeding and tenesmus may respond to poorly absorbable sulfur preparations given orally and rectal administration of adrenocorticosteroids in either enema or suppository form. Systemic corticosteroid administration is not indicated.

In general the disease runs a relapsing course, three or four symptomatic episodes a year being usual. In contrast to diffuse ulcerative colitis, the complications of arthritis, uveitis, and pyoderma gangrenosum are not seen. Development of carcinoma of the rectum, even in longstanding cases, is rare. Occasionally rectal stricture may occur. Fewer than 15 per cent of patients with this disease will progress to diffuse ulcerative colitis.

Farmer, R. G., and Brown, C. H.: Ulcerative proctitis: Course and prognosis. Gastroenterology, 51:219, 1966.
Folley, J. H.: Ulcerative proctitis. N. Engl. J. Med., 282:1362, 1970.
Sparberg, M., Gennessey, J., and Kirsner, J. B.: Ulcerative proctitis and mild ulcerative colitis: Astudy of 220 patients. Medicine, 45:391, 1966.

436. DISEASES OF THE ANUS

GENERAL CONSIDERATIONS

Functionally, the most important parts of the anus are the neural innervation and muscular elements composing the internal and external anal sphincters which maintain rectal continence. Anal sphincter dysfunction without perianal disease, a history of prior anal surgery, or evidence of more generalized neurologic disease should prompt evaluation for rectal carcinoma. Although various reconstructive techniques appear to improve some patients with anal incontinence, surgery should be considered only after the cause of sphincter dysfunction has been thoroughly investigated. In general, anal and perianal diseases produce disproportionately great symptoms when compared with the extent of tissue involved. In this chapter, a number of anal diseases are discussed briefly to acquaint the reader with diagnostic possibilities.

HEMORRHOIDS

Hemorrhoids or piles are varicosities of the hemorrhoidal venous plexuses. External hemorrhoids occur below the anorectal line and are covered by pain-sensitive anal skin. Thrombosis or rupture of the vein leads to a small, very tender, tense, bluish lump which can be seen in the anal canal. For mild symptoms, conservative treatment is usually effective and consists of hot sitz baths, stool softeners, a recumbent position if possible, and avoidance of straining or strenuous work. Anti-inflammatory drugs such as phenylbutazone appear to shorten the symptomatic course. Extremely painful thrombosed hemorrhoids may be incised and the clot removed if seen within the first 24 hours. Relief of the severe pain is often dramatic. Small anal skin tags may be left after resolution of the acute process. If the pile ruptures, the clot should be removed or the area excised.

Internal hemorrhoids are varicosities of the superior and middle hemorrhoidal veins above the anorectal line and are covered by relatively pain-insensitive mucosa. These hemorrhoids tend to prolapse during defecation and usually become symptomatic by bleeding. A mucoid anal discharge is common with chronic prolapse and can irritate the anal skin. Bleeding from hemorrhoids is often noted by the patient as streaks of blood on the outside of stool or on toilet tissue. It is usually intermittent. Prolonged or excessive bleeding can result in iron deficiency and anemia. Use of an astringent suppository and the conservative treatment outlined above are often adequate treatment. Nonsurgical management for recurrently symptomatic internal hemorrhoids is now common and includes cryosurgery, rubber band ligation, and injection of sclerosing agents. Surgical therapy may be indicated for recurrent bleeding, protrusion, thrombosis, ulceration, infection, or coexistent severe pruritus ani. Surgery should be avoided in patients with only moderately symptomatic hemorrhoids who have portal hypertension, incurable cancer, intractable heart disease, or persistent hemorrhoidal symptoms for less than six months post partum. Rectal bleeding should not be attributed to hemorrhoids without complete anorectal examination.

ANORECTAL ABSCESS AND FISTULA IN ANO

Patients with a rapidly developing painful anal mass may have an abscess in the perianal and perirectal tissue. After diagnosis, proper treatment requires surgical drainage. *Perianal abscess* occurs superficially, adjacent to the anal opening and below the anorectal ring. Severe throbbing pain is the major symptom. An *ischiorectal fossa abscess* involves deeper tissue of the buttocks and presents with perirectal discomfort and fever. Digital examination of the lower part of the rectum will demonstrate a tender mass bulging into the lumen. A *submucous abscess* extends upward in the submucous space above the anal valves. It may cause fever and dull

rectal pain with no visible perianal abnormality except occasionally a purulent rectal discharge. A *pelvirectal abscess* arises from a primary infection elsewhere in the pelvis and usually presents with systemic toxic symptoms. An *anorectal abscess* may develop as a complication of acute hemorrhoids, an anal fissure, or injections into the anorectal area. A *tuberculous anorectal abscess* often presents as a gradually enlarging perianal or ischiorectal mass with less pain than that caused by a similar acute infection.

After an acute infection in the anorectal area, a chronic suppurative process may develop and form a *fistula in ano*. This fistula is a tract of chronic granulation tissue which connects two epithelial surfaces, either cutaneous or mucosal, and may have several external openings. The main symptom is persistent or intermittent drainage which soils the patient's clothing and leads to soreness and pruritus in the perianal area. Treatment requires complete surgical excision of the fistulous tract.

ANAL FISSURE

An anal fissure is a painful, usually elliptical ulceration of unknown cause which is commonly located posteriorly in the midline of the anal orifice and may extend into the anal canal as far as the pectinate line. Early, the fissure appears as a simple slit in the anal skin, but secondary changes soon develop, the most striking of which is a swelling at the lower end of the fissure known as a sentinel pile. If untreated, the ulceration can "erode" down to the internal sphincter muscle. Chronic spasm of the sphincter and postinflammatory fibrosis can produce a fibrotic, tightly contracted anal opening. Pain, especially with defecation, is the main symptom. Bleeding is usually only modest, but can be severe.

Most fissures heal spontaneously. Dilatation of the spastic sphincter, hot sitz baths, local analgesics, and stool softeners give good results in most cases. When the ulceration is deep enough to expose the sphincter muscle fibers, surgical therapy is usually required. Acceptable surgical treatment includes partial or complete sphincterotomy.

PRURITUS ANI

Pruritus ani refers to perianal itching which is frequently intense. In early cases, the primary rugae of the anus may be edematous and red. The skin is often moist and macerated. Multiple excoriations are evidence of frequent scratching. Later the perianal skin may become thickened or lichenified and have increased pigmentation. Superficial ulcers may be present, and with extreme chronicity leukoplakia may develop.

In evaluating the cause of pruritus ani, dermatologic abnormalities such as *seborrheic dermatitis, atopic eczema, psoriasis, lichen planus, neurodermatitis,* and *contact dermatitis* must be excluded. Involvement of the perianal skin with fungal or yeast infection, or parasitic infestation such as scabies or pinworm, may produce intense pruritus. Pruritus ani may also complicate many of the so-called surgical diseases of the anus such as *prolapsed hemorrhoids, prolapse of the rectum, benign* or *malignant tumors of the rectum,* or *chronic anal fissure* or *fistula.* An increase in perianal moisture from chronic diarrhea or vaginal discharge may also play a causative role. Finally, many patients with idiopathic pruritus ani have been shown to have an abnormally alkaline anal discharge. This may produce a chemical dermatitis and alter perianal skin resistance to normal bacterial flora.

Treatment of pruritus ani should begin with an exclusion of correctable underlying causes. A large number of idiopathic cases are cured by strict anal hygiene. Anesthetic ointments, abrasive toilet tissue and clothing, constipation or diarrhea, and gas-producing foods should be avoided. The use of bland soap, dusting powders (zinc, starch, or boric acid), and hydrocortisone or betamethasone cream is often helpful. In cases of idiopathic pruritus ani, oral administration of capsules of *Lactobacillus acidophilus* or malt soup extract (Maltsupex) has been shown to normalize the alkaline anal discharge and lead to improvement in symptoms.

ANAL MALIGNANCY

The most common malignant tumor of the anus is *squamous cell carcinoma.* Treatment of this widely metastasizing lesion requires radical surgical excision. *Intraepithelial squamous cell* carcinoma or Bowen's disease may present as an irregular reddish plaque. Wide local excision is usually adequate therapy. *Basal cell carcinoma* of the anus produces a superficial ulcerating lesion. *Paget's disease* may involve the perianal dermal apocrine sweat glands and present as an anal mass. Since both of these tumors do not metastasize widely, excisional biopsy is usually adequate.

Malignant melanomas of the anus are highly lethal, but fortunately rare. Initially, a small melanoma may be interpreted as a hemorrhoid by both patient and physician. Later the tumor becomes more polypoid and tends to ulcerate. Wide excision biopsy of a suspect lesion should be done immediately when the diagnosis is considered. Radical surgery for an advanced melanoma does not seem to improve survival.

PROCTALGIA

There are several conditions in which the main symptom is anorectal pain and for which there is no obvious cause, even after full proctologic examination.

Coccygodynia refers to pain in the coccyx area. This is thought to be due to tonic spasm of the levator ani, coccygeal, and pyriform muscles and to result from trauma to the coccyx. Diagnosis is made by eliciting pain during palpation of these muscles and movement of the coccyx. Treatment consists of improved sitting posture, warm sitz baths, massage of the spastic muscles, and systemic analgesics or tranquilizers which have a muscle relaxant property such as diazepam.

Proctalgia fugax is a rectal pain syndrome which frequently awakens the patient at night and most commonly occurs in young men. Most patients describe the discomfort as a severe cramping rectal pain unassociated with straining efforts. The pain usually lasts 30 to 45 minutes. Spasms of a segment of the levator ani muscle may be the source of the pain, but the true cause is unknown. Various recommended treatments have included hot sitz baths or warm water enemas, passing flatus or stool, sublingual nitroglycerin, and firm pressure upward against the anus. In many patients the symptoms respond to no treatment but resolve spontaneously after a period of months or years.

The *puborectalis syndrome* is characterized by chronic constipation, rectal tenesmus, and pain during and after defecation. This is thought to result from hypertrophy and spasm of the puborectalis muscle sling. Diagnosis is made on rectal examination by finding a constricting tender muscular ring at the upper end of the anus. Conservative treatment includes anal dilatation prior to defecation and the use of stool softeners. If this treatment is unsuccessful, surgical resection of a small segment of the puborectalis sling is usually curative without producing anal incontinence.

Tumors of the *cauda equina* of the spinal cord may also produce anal pain. Examination of the anus will demonstrate a weak sphincter and a small perianal area of diminished cutaneous sensation. Transient *sigmoidorectal intussusception* may also produce rectal pain which is difficult to diagnose.

Section Twelve DISEASES OF THE GALLBLADDER AND BILE DUCTS

Lawrence W. Way

437. INTRODUCTION

Biliary disease in adults includes congenital, metabolic, neoplastic, infectious, and parasitic conditions which cause considerable morbidity and pose challenging diagnostic problems to the clinician. Symptomatic cholelithiasis and its complications alone are responsible for over 500,000 operations in the United States annually, entailing great financial and emotional cost for

the affected patients. Fortunately, improvements have recently been made in techniques of diagnosis and therapy.

PHYSIOLOGY. Bile, an alkaline isotonic fluid (pH 7.8), is a mixture of the secretion of hepatocytes and the duct epithelial cells and has the composition given in Table 1. The volume of bile ranges from 500 to 1500 ml per day, depending on the amount and kind of food ingested. The greatest fraction of the bile volume is

TABLE 1. Average Composition of Human
Gallbladder Bile (Gram/100 ml)

		% Total Solids
Lipids { Bile acids	12.00	
Lecithin	3.00	91
Cholesterol	0.50	
Bilirubin	0.15	
Protein	0.10	
Potassium	0.05	9
Calcium and magnesium	0.06	
Chloride	0.08	
Bicarbonate and phosphate	0.04	

produced by the hepatocytes and correlates directly with output of bile salts.

Bile salts are synthesized by hepatocytes from cholesterol by a process whose rate-limiting step involves the action of the enzyme 7 α-hydroxylase. The two *primary bile salts*, cholate and chenodeoxycholate, are conjugated before secretion with either glycine or taurine to improve solubility. After entering the gut, bile salts aid in fat absorption, and then are mostly reabsorbed in the ileum. Those that reach the colon are partially converted by bacteria to the secondary bile salts, deoxycholate and lithocholate. About 30 per cent of the newly formed secondary bile salts are absorbed from the colon, conjugated in the liver, and excreted in bile. Lithocholate is also sulfated during hepatic transfer and thereafter is poorly absorbed, but deoxycholate continues to recycle within the enterohepatic circulation. The actual composition of bile is 40 per cent cholate, 40 per cent chenodeoxycholate, 18 per cent deoxycholate, and 2 per cent lithocholate, each conjugated with glycine or taurine in a ratio of 3:1. Other than bile salts, the major solids in bile are cholesterol and phospholipid (mainly lecithin). There is a close correlation between the output of bile salt and lecithin and, to a lesser extent, between bile salt and cholesterol. Whether the cholesterol and lecithin originate from hepatocyte microsomes or the canalicular membrane is not settled.

Intestinal reabsorption of bile salts, which is about 95 per cent complete for a single passage, occurs by passive diffusion throughout the gut and (more importantly) by active transport within the terminal 100 cm of ileum. The reabsorbed bile salts are largely bound to albumin in portal blood, and are then almost completely cleared in a single passage through the liver. The bile salt pool, normally 1.5 to 3.0 grams, passes through the liver and gut more than twice during each meal, producing six to eight cycles daily (i.e., each day about 20 grams of bile salt enters the duodenum). During an average day involving three meals, the bile salt pool is in continuous motion until at night the stomach and bowel are empty and the gallbladder fills. Conservation of bile salts in this *enterohepatic circulation* is so efficient that only 20 per cent of the daily secretion of bile salts must be replaced by newly synthesized molecules.

If the efficiency of the enterohepatic conservation is impaired by conditions such as a biliary fistula, Crohn's disease, or ileal resection, hepatic synthesis of bile salts increases, but the maximal synthetic rate (5 grams per day) may be insufficient to restore intraluminal concentrations to normal if external losses exceed this amount.

In the gut biliary lecithin is broken down to lysolecithin and fatty acid, and cholesterol is excreted unab-

sorbed; thus none of the biliary solids other than bile salt has an enterohepatic circulation.

The second component of bile, the ductular secretion, is generated by an active transport process which is stimulated by secretin, cholecystokinin, and gastrin, with vagal tone acting as a sensitizing influence. Ductular secretion results from active transport of Na^+ and HCO^- and seems to be useful in maintaining the alkalinity of bile.

Under basal conditions, tonic contraction of the sphincter of Oddi diverts hepatic bile from the common duct into the gallbladder where it is concentrated by active absorption of Na^+, Cl^-, and HCO_3^- and passive return of H_2O. The absorptive mechanism is capable of concentrating gallbladder bile at a rate of 10 per cent of its volume per hour. The concentration of bile salt may exceed 200 millimoles per liter, and since the gallbladder holds 40 ml, 8 millimoles (equivalent to 3 grams of cholic acid) or the entire bile salt pool can be sequestered here during prolonged fasting.

Cholecystokinin, released from the intestinal mucosa by fat, amino acids, and H^+, stimulates gallbladder contraction and simultaneous relaxation of the choledochal sphincter, emptying gallbladder contents into the duodenum. Basal pressures in the biliary ducts and gallbladder are 10 to 15 cm H_2O. After eating, gallbladder pressure rises to 25 to 30 cm H_2O, slightly exceeding ductal pressure.

Bile salt molecules are amphophils, possessing water-soluble and fat-soluble poles. In an aqueous medium, they are distributed randomly, until a critical concentration (about 2 millimolar) is reached, at which point spontaneous aggregation forms multimolecular structures called micelles. In micelles, the bile salt molecules line up with their hydrophilic portions facing the solvent (water) and their hydrophobic portions facing each other. The hydrocarbon center of the micelle can incorporate biliary lecithin and cholesterol, and the entire aggregate remains water soluble. The addition of lecithin, a water-insoluble compound, enhances the ability of bile salt micelles to incorporate other lipids. The ultimate cholesterol-carrying capacity of bile depends on the relative amounts of bile salt and lecithin (Fig. 1).

GALLSTONES

In Western cultures about 75 per cent of gallstones are composed principally of cholesterol (*cholesterol gallstones*) and 25 per cent of calcium bilirubinate (*pigment gallstones*). Cholesterol stones are usually yellow or brown, and round or faceted. They may be single or multiple, and most range in size from 1 mm to 3 to 4 cm (although one of the largest on record measured over 17 cm in its longest diameter). Pigment stones are usually black, under 1 cm, and irregular in shape, and tend to crumble and flake when handled. Over-all, about 15 per cent of gallstones are radiopaque, and of radiopaque stones about two thirds are pigment stones and one third are cholesterol stones. The symptoms caused by gallstones are the same regardless of the chemical composition of the stone, and to a large extent regardless of the size of the stones.

CHOLESTEROL GALLSTONES. Cholesterol makes up from 50 to 100 per cent of the weight of cholesterol gallstones, the remainder consisting of bile salt, bilirubinate, calcium, and other unidentified solids. Cholesterol

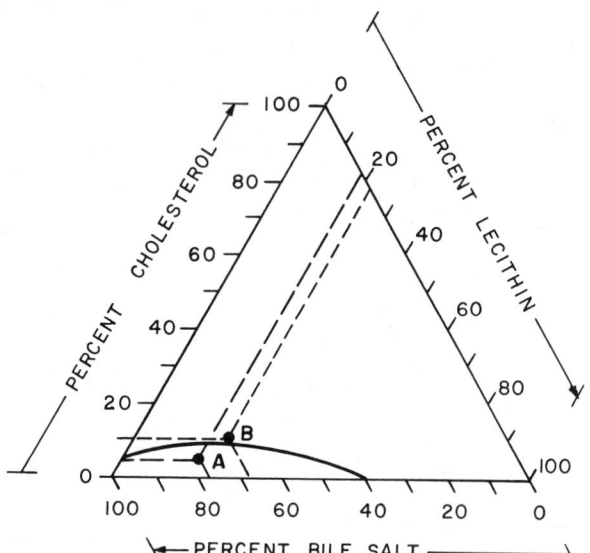

Figure 1. Phase diagram for plotting different mixtures of bile salt, lecithin, and cholesterol. The curved line represents the boundary of the micellar zone for aqueous solutions containing 4 to 10 per cent solids. Any mixture, such as A, falling within this area contains all its cholesterol in solution. Any mixture, such as B, falling outside this area has excess cholesterol as a precipitate or supersaturated solution. The points A and B actually depict the average composition of gallbladder bile obtained by Admirand and Small from normal persons and patients with cholesterol gallstones, respectively.

gallstones affect three times as many women as men, the difference beginning at puberty and declining after menopause. The incidence is higher with multiparity and with use of birth control pills, all of which suggests an etiologic role for female sex hormones. The incidence in blacks, whites, and American Indians increases in that order, so that at the upper extreme about 75 per cent of American Indian women over age 25 and 90 per cent of those over age 60 are affected. The incidence of gallstones in blacks in Africa is much lower than in blacks in Western cultures. Cholesterol, which is insoluble in water, is normally carried in bile within bile salt micelles. A prerequisite to cholesterol gallstone formation is an excess of cholesterol in relation to micella carrying capacity, a circumstance that could result from decreased bile salt or increased cholesterol concentrations.

Figure 1 is a phase diagram on which any aqueous mixture of bile salt, lecithin, and cholesterol can be represented by a point indicating the molar percentage each contributes to total solids. In vitro tests show that the cholesterol of mixtures which fall in the lower left area of the triangle exists in stable micellar solution. Outside this area cholesterol forms a supersaturated solution or precipitates. The particular micellar zone depicted in Figure 1 pertains to solutions ranging from 4 to 10 per cent solids, which is comparable to bile.

Plotted on this diagram, bile of patients with gallstones tends to have relatively more cholesterol than that of normal persons, and simultaneous sampling from the gallbladder and hepatic ducts of patients with gallstones shows that bile is supersaturated with cholesterol as it emerges from the liver, implicating the hepatocytes rather than the gallbladder as the cause of the abnormality. Gallstone patients have a total bile salt pool of 1.0 to 1.5 grams, about half normal, and their hepatocytes have decreased amounts of the enzyme 7 α-hydroxylase. These observations suggest that diminished bile salt secretion is a factor in the genesis of lithogenic bile in many patients. Another factor, particularly associated with obesity, is increased cholesterol secretion. Biliary cholesterol is not derived from plasma or dietary cholesterol, but is newly synthesized within the hepatocytes.

The relationship between cholesterol and bile salt output is such that when bile salt secretion drops, the cholesterol : bile salt ratio climbs and the bile assumes greater lithogenicity. During fasting bile salts are sequestered in the gallbladder, hepatic secretion drops, the rate of cholesterol secretion persists, and the bile becomes more lithogenic. Supersaturation produced in this way is common in humans regardless of the presence of gallstones.

The aforementioned observations account for the production of lithogenic bile but do not explain why all persons with abnormal bile do not form stones, why stone formation occurs mainly in the gallbladder, and why cholecystectomy is curative. The gallbladder must be important in the genesis of gallstones, possibly by supplying a nidus for crystallization (a small particle of bile pigment or mucoprotein can be found in the center of most stones), a mucoprotein lattice for further cholesterol deposition and stone growth, and an area of stasis to facilitate precipitation. Apparently the more supersaturated the bile, the more likely it is that gallstones will develop, but other initiating factors must have quantitative importance.

PIGMENT GALLSTONES. Pigment stones are composed of calcium bilirubinate, inorganic solids, and unidentified organic solids. Pigment stones are more common than cholesterol stones in the elderly. The incidence is the same in men and women, and in blacks and whites, but American Indians are rarely affected.

There is no relationship of pigment stones to obesity, and the saturation of bile for cholesterol and size of the bile salt pool are normal in patients with pigment stones. In Western cultures, the concentration of unconjugated bilirubin is increased in the bile of people with pigment stones. Although cirrhosis and hemolytic diseases predispose to the development of pigment stones, these conditions are absent in most patients.

In the Orient, invasion of the ducts by parasites (*Clonorchis sinensis, Ascaris*) may be an initiating factor in some patients. The bile in parasitic disease becomes secondarily contaminated with *E. coli,* which produces β-glucuronidase that deconjugates bilirubin. The deconjugated bilirubin, being much less soluble, precipitates with calcium.

DISSOLUTION OF GALLSTONES BY CHENODEOXYCHOLIC ACID

Chenodeoxycholate (CDC), 20 mg per kilogram per day orally, will dissolve most radiolucent cholesterol gallbladder stones within one to two years. CDC causes the bile to become unsaturated by lowering cholesterol output and by expanding the bile salt pool and increasing bile salt secretion. Ursodeoxycholate has a similar effect, but cholate does not. CDC is ineffective for pigment stones and radiopaque stones, and also when the

Figure 2. In the absence of obstruction there are no symptoms or active infection from bacterial contamination of bile. Obstruction, indicated by the arrow, produces either jaundice alone or cholangitis, depending on the original bacteriologic status of the duct.

gallbladder does not opacify on oral cholecystography. If treatment is stopped, gallstones return in some patients. Fear of toxic effects of the bile salt on the fetal liver has led to exclusion of women capable of bearing children from this therapy. A nationwide clinical trial to determine the efficacy and safety of CDC treatment is in progress. Because of the aforementioned exclusions, only 15 per cent of patients with gallstone disease now being treated by cholecystectomy are potential candidates for dissolution therapy. Screening for gallstones followed by prophylactic therapy might be feasible, but the costs of such a program would be enormous, and whether the results in improved health would justify such a program is debatable.

PATHOPHYSIOLOGY OF GALLSTONE DISEASE

Obstruction caused by a stone is the primary cause of all manifestations of gallstone disease. Obstruction of the cystic duct by gallbladder stones distends the gallbladder, producing biliary colic. If the obstruction persists, acute cholecystitis may ensue. The intermediary steps from obstruction to acute inflammation are discussed later. Whether complications such as empyema, perforation, and hydrops of the gallbladder develop depends on whether secondary infection occurs. Cholecystectomy cures cholecystitis, but cholecystostomy, which only relieves the obstruction, will eliminate all the clinical manifestations of the disease.

Obstruction of the common duct may produce pain, jaundice, pruritus, infection, and biliary cirrhosis, and, as with gallbladder disease, surgical procedures that decompress the duct upstream from the stone eliminate these manifestations. The situation in the ductal system differs from that in the gallbladder, however, because when ductal pressure exceeds about 25 cm per H_2O, bile is refluxed from the smallest ductules into hepatic venous blood. Pressures in this range and even higher commonly accompany mechanical obstruction and are probably aggravated by infection. Regurgitation of ductal bacteria into the systemic circulation may explain why cholangitis is often accompanied by chills, positive blood cultures, and high fever. Fortunately, obstruction by calculus is rarely complete, because the combination of high-grade obstruction and infection (as in suppura-

tive cholangitis) may produce profound sepsis (Fig. 2). It is also fortunate that neoplasms, which uniformly give almost complete obstruction, occur most often in patients with sterile bile.

With unrelieved ductal obstruction, biliary cirrhosis gradually develops. About three months is the shortest time in which cirrhosis occurs; as might be expected, the earliest cases follow neoplastic (high-grade) obstruction. On the average, biliary cirrhosis from choledocholithiasis or biliary stricture takes five to seven years to develop.

438. CLINICAL EVALUATION OF JAUNDICE

So many tests are now available to study jaundice (Table 2) that they must be ordered selectively to avoid unnecessary morbidity, delay in reaching the correct diagnosis, and costly overtesting. In general, tests should not be ordered unless the results would possibly affect the patient's management; knowing more about the patient's disease is not an a priori necessity. After

TABLE 2. Tests for Evaluation of Jaundice

Clinical findings: signs and symptoms
Liver function tests (see Ch. 453)
Intravenous cholangiogram
Oral cholecystogram
Ultrasound scan
Liver biopsy
Upper gastrointestinal x-rays
Gastroduodenal endoscopy
Hepatic scan (^{99m}Tc)
Transhepatic cholangiogram
Endoscopic retrograde cholangiogram (ERC)
Peritoneoscopy
Angiography
Diagnostic laparotomy
Gallium scan
Minilaparotomy
CT scan
Radionuclide excretion scans
Transjugular cholangiogram

an initial evaluation, including clinical examination and a standard set of laboratory tests, each additional special test should usually be chosen based on the results of the last test.

The most important objective is to differentiate between surgical (obstructive) and medical causes of the jaundice. Although helpful in selected cases, details regarding the exact cause and configuration of obstructing lesions are not regularly of value to the surgeon preoperatively and usually can be quickly determined at laparotomy.

The approach to the patient will differ depending on whether the disease is acute and changing or has been present for more than a week or two and is stable. Unexplained jaundice of four weeks or more will prove to be caused by obstruction in about 75 per cent of cases. The initial clinical findings supplemented by measurement of serum SGOT, alkaline phosphatase, bilirubin, prothrombin time, and albumin will give a fairly certain diagnosis in over half of all jaundiced patients. Examples include viral hepatitis in a young person, most cases of acute or chronic alcoholic liver disease, and jaundice caused by hemolysis. Special tests will not be needed in these situations.

In an acute evolving illness it is often best to observe the course of the disease for a day or two. Ultrasound examination may be obtained at this early stage and may demonstrate gallstones or dilatation of the ducts. Uncontrolled cholangitis is the only condition associated with jaundice that requires urgent treatment. If the patient appears to have cholangitis, antimicrobials should be given; if a response is not observed, emergency surgery may be required. This sequence, however, is relatively uncommon.

If acute jaundice resolves, as it often does in patients with choledocholithiasis, an oral cholecystogram or, if the patient has had a previous cholecystectomy, an intravenous cholangiogram, can be obtained. If gallstones are demonstrated, no further preoperative workup is generally needed.

When the course of the disease is apparent, an estimate should be made of whether the patient is more likely to have medical or surgical jaundice. If the patient is thought to have hepatic parenchymal disease but some of the features are atypical, a liver biopsy should be considered.

Additional information concerning the presence of an obstructing lesion may be obtained from ultrasound or CT scans, and from transhepatic (THC) or retrograde endoscopic (ERCP) cholangiograms. Only rarely will all four of these tests be indicated in any patient. To demonstrate duct dilatation, ultrasound is equally as accurate as CT scans and much less expensive. For direct cholangiography, THC is most often the best technique because it is simple and easy to learn, it is inexpensive, and it more adequately delineates the proximal (hepatic) side of the lesion, the area of greatest interest to the surgeon. ERCP may be preferable, however, when THC is contraindicated because of abnormal coagulation, when THC is unsuccessful, or when there is a specific need also to obtain a pancreatogram.

Other than to prove the presence of an obstructing lesion, preoperative delineation of ductal anatomy by direct cholangiography is useful to the surgeon in the following conditions: (1) biliary stricture, (2) proximal biliary tumors (e.g., Klatskin tumor), and (3) other proximal obstructions (e.g., sclerosing cholangitis). Details of ductal anatomy are not generally useful preoperatively in patients with (1) gallbladder stones, (2) common duct stones, (3) periampullary neoplasms, and (4) other distal obstructions.

Arteriograms, peritoneoscopy, ^{99m}Tc-liver scans, CT scans, and gallium scans may be indicated for specific purposes but should not be performed routinely. For example, a combination of ultrasound and ^{99m}Tc-liver scans is the best approach to detect focal liver lesions (e.g., tumors, abscesses). A CT scan may be useful if the results of these first two are equivocal. Arteriograms may be of value to differentiate a hepatic tumor from a cystic lesion and to gauge the extent of a tumor (although the reliability of the latter is poor). Peritoneoscopy may be the most accurate way to stage an abdominal tumor preoperatively, although staging is not often useful if laparotomy would be indicated regardless of the extent of the disease. CT scans, in general, have proved to be of disappointing reliability and much less cost effective than ultrasound scans. So far, the ability of CT scans to demonstrate small pancreatic tumors is virtually nil.

Transjugular cholangiography, minilaparotomy, and radionuclide excretion scans are at present of questionable usefulness under any circumstances.

Finally, visual inspection of the upper abdomen by the surgeon nearly always gives more information about the spread of tumors than do liver scans, CT scans, or arteriograms, and high quality cholangiograms can usually be obtained during laparotomy with little difficulty.

439. ROENTGENOLOGIC EXAMINATION

Because biliary disease usually results from obstructive lesions, radiologic techniques, if successful in outlining the system, are often diagnostic. Direct and indirect methods are available, and the diagnostic strategy often revolves around the choice and timing of these procedures.

Plain roentgenograms can demonstrate the 10 to 15 per cent of gallstones which contain sufficient calcium to be radiopaque, but the relationship of the stones to the gallbladder or bile ducts is not always obvious. Emphysematous cholecystitis, air in the bile ducts, and calcium in the wall of the gallbladder also have diagnostic appearances on plain films.

For *oral cholecystography,* the patient swallows tablets of iopanoic or tyropanoic acid, which are then absorbed from the gut, excreted in bile, and concentrated in the gallbladder. If the gallbladder is opacified, stones in its lumen are shown as radiolucent defects (Fig. 3). The gallbladder may not be opacified if the drug is not taken, if absorption by the gut or excretion by the liver is faulty, if the cystic duct is blocked, or if the diseased gallbladder mucosa cannot concentrate the bile. Oral cholecystography is the simplest and least expensive way of verifying gallstone disease in patients without acute symptoms. If hepatic and intestinal function are normal, nonopacification is 95 per cent reliable in indicating gallbladder disease.

Intravenous cholangiography (IVC) relies on hepatic excretion in a concentration sufficient for ductal opacifi-

Figure 3. Oral cholecystogram, showing gallstones. In this case the stones are considerably less distinct on the supine than on the upright film (inset), where they float as a layer.

cation of intravenously injected sodium or methylglucamine iodipamide. The procedure is used principally to identify common duct stones in patients who previously had a cholecystectomy and to verify acute cholecystitis (an opacified duct and nonopacified gallbladder are diagnostic). The disadvantage of intravenous cholangiography is that even with perfect liver function the concentration of contrast medium in bile is barely above the threshold level; tomography must be used routinely, and, even so, false-negative results are common in choledocholithiasis. When the bilirubin exceeds 3.0 mg per 100 ml, the study is rarely successful and, because of its high cost and the occasional allergic reaction, should usually be deferred.

Transhepatic cholangiography (THC) involves direct percutaneous puncture of an intrahepatic duct by a needle inserted through the eighth or ninth right intercostal space into the center of the liver. An abnormal clotting mechanism, ascites, and severe cholangitis are contraindications. If a duct is entered, water-soluble contrast medium is injected through the needle, and roentgenograms are obtained. Transhepatic cholangiography has proved particularly valuable in diagnosing biliary stricture and neoplastic obstruction of the bile ducts. A technically successful study can be obtained in nearly all patients with dilated ducts and in most patients with normal-sized ducts.

Endoscopic retrograde cholangiography (ERCP) involves cannulation of the ampulla of Vater via the duodeno-

scope (Fig. 4). With experience, the duct can be entered successfully in about 80 per cent of attempts. Concomitant pancreatography is often possible.

Both THC and ERCP are usually contraindicated in active cholangitis because as ductal pressure increases during injection of the contrast material, severe uncontrollable sepsis may be produced. Patients undergoing either of these procedures should usually be premedicated with antimicrobial agents regardless of whether there is a history of cholangitis.

Ultrasound of the biliary tree may demonstrate gallstones or dilatation of the intrahepatic ductal system. The finding of gallstones is highly reliable (false positives are uncommon), but in about 15 per cent of cases stones will be missed by this technique. Inability to identify the gallbladder is usually due to thick scarring and contraction of the wall about a lumen full of stones. Ductal dilatation usually indicates distal obstruction by neoplasm, stricture, or stone. The correlation between dilatation and obstruction is inexact because (1) the ducts may be dilated from previous disease although currently unobstructed, (2) cirrhosis or cholangitis may stiffen the ducts enough to prevent dilatation, and (3) lesions characterized by intermittent obstruction (e.g., common duct stones, stricture) may have undilated ducts if the patient is examined after the duct has spontaneously decompressed.

440. ASYMPTOMATIC GALLSTONES

In the absence of a population survey to determine the prevalence of gallstones, the exact percentage of asymptomatic cases, estimated now at 30 to 50 per cent of all patients with gallstones, can only be guessed at

Figure 4. Retrograde cholangiopancreatogram, showing a large gallstone in a dilated common duct and a normal pancreatic duct. (Courtesy of Dr. Jack Vennes.)

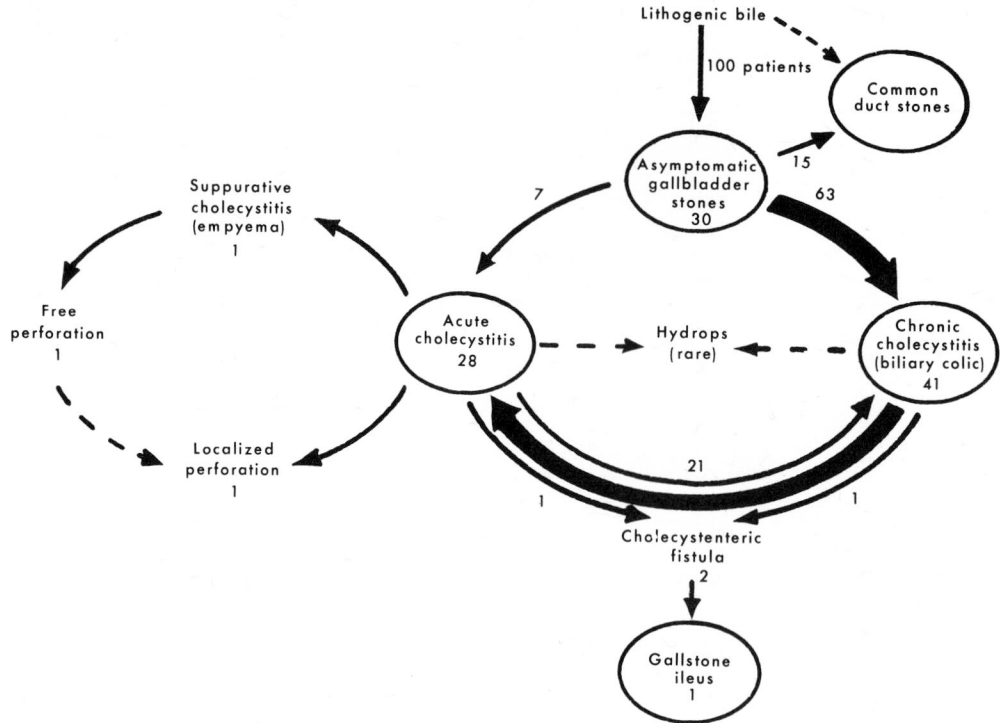

Figure 5. Natural history of cholecystolithiasis. The major clinical syndromes are contained in the ovals, and the numbers represent the approximate percentage of patients with gallstone disease who present in that way.

(Fig. 5). Of the total estimated pool of gallstone patients in the United States, about 1.5 per cent are treated each year by cholecystectomy. Since the mortality of gallstone disease with the present plan of management, i.e., essentially treating only those who present with symptoms, is reasonably low, with a few exceptions asymptomatic patients may be followed expectantly and surgery advised only if symptoms develop. Asymptomatic patients for whom prophylactic cholecystectomy is generally recommended are (1) diabetics, because their mortality from acute cholecystitis is 10 to 15 per cent; (2) patients with nonfunctioning gallbladders or large (more than 2 cm diameter) stones, because their incidence of complications is considerably higher; and (3) patients with calcified gallbladders, because this change is so often associated with carcinoma of the gallbladder. Altogether these groups constitute less than half the patients with asymptomatic gallstones. At least three quarters of the asymptomatic patients who later become symptomatic will first experience episodes of biliary colic, and at that point cholecystectomy can be performed electively.

441. CHRONIC CHOLECYSTITIS AND BILIARY COLIC

The term chronic cholecystitis is often used to denote the clinical condition of symptomatic (nonacute) cholecystolithiasis. A better term, however, is biliary colic, as there is only a loose relationship between the pathologic findings in the gallbladder wall and the clinical manifestations of gallstone disease. Chronic chole-

cystitis without gallstones is even more uncommon than acute cholecystitis without gallstones.

A wide spectrum of patients is included. In some patients the gallbladder appears grossly normal, the mucosa is slightly thinned, and the wall contains minor amounts of patchy scarring and cellular infiltration. Oral cholecystograms nearly always opacify the gallbladder and demonstrate its stones. Many patients have colic, but in others the symptoms are often vague, such as flatulence or food intolerance, and they sometimes persist after cholecystectomy.

In other patients the gallbladder is more severely affected, often the result of previous attacks of acute cholecystitis. The signs of resolved inflammatory disease consist of thickening of the wall by scar, adhesions to adjacent viscera, and patchy replacement of the mucosa by granulation tissue or collagen. In advanced cases the gallbladder may be so shrunken as to be almost unrecognizable. Nonopacification is frequent on oral cholecystograms, biliary colic is the principal symptom, and relief is more predictable after cholecystectomy. There is a great deal of overlap between these two extremes of the clinicopathologic spectrum.

Cholesterolosis, present in about 5 per cent of cases, gives the mucosal surface a streaked appearance, a condition which has been called "strawberry gallbladder." The changes are due to cholesterol located within clusters of large foamy macrophages in the submucosa. Cholesterolosis is occasionally seen without gallstones, in which case it may be asymptomatic or associated with biliary colic.

CLINICAL MANIFESTATIONS. The most specific symptom of chronic cholecystitis is biliary colic, a severe, cramplike pain located in the epigastrium or right upper quadrant. It is caused by gallbladder contraction during transient obstruction of the cystic duct by a gallstone. Onset of pain takes only a few minutes; it quickly reaches a plateau in intensity and after an hour or more subsides gradually. The pain of biliary colic usually does not wax and wane like intestinal colic. Even after the acute episode has resolved, a vague residual ache or soreness may remain. The absence of tenderness, muscular guarding, a palpable mass, fever, and leukocytosis distinguishes biliary colic from acute cholecystitis. Many patients have simultaneous referred pain located in the back at the level of the scapula. Vomiting may accompany the attack. The timing of attacks of biliary colic most often is unpredictable, but in some cases attacks may be related to ingestion of an especially large or fatty meal. Attacks may occur as seldom as once every few years or as often as daily.

Considerably less reliable from the diagnostic standpoint are dyspepsia, fatty food intolerance, flatulence, heartburn, and belching. Although these symptoms may be the result of chronic cholecystitis, they often occur in persons with normal gallbladders.

Hydrops, in which the lumen of the gallbladder contains mucus and gallstones, may develop from cystic duct obstruction in either chronic or acute cholecystitis. Hydrops produces constant discomfort in the right upper quadrant and a palpable mass without the clinical findings of acute cholecystitis.

DIAGNOSIS. Oral cholecystograms will demonstrate the gallstones in about two thirds of patients, but in others the gallbladder does not opacify. In the latter case, a second dose of the cholecystographic agent should be given and the x-rays repeated; if nonopacification persists and liver function and intestinal absorption are normal, gallbladder disease can be inferred. An alternative approach with a nonopacified gallbladder is to obtain an ultrasound scan to demonstrate the gallstones. It should be remembered, however, that false-negative results are fairly common with ultrasound. Because of the expense and risks of allergic reactions, an intravenous cholecystogram is not usually warranted to study the average patient with a nonopacified gallbladder, but may be ordered selectively in puzzling cases. In about half the cases in which they are present, gallbladder stones are missed by an intravenous cholangiogram that opacifies the gallbladder.

About 2 to 3 per cent of adequately opacified oral cholecystograms are false negative, either because the stones are too small to be seen or because they are of the same radiographic density as the contrast medium. The diagnosis can often be made in these patients by examining an aliquot of bile obtained from an orally placed duodenal tube for the presence of cholesterol crystals or bilirubinate precipitate. In the presence of what seems to be biliary colic, a positive duodenal drainage test permits cholecystectomy to be performed with confidence that the patient will obtain symptomatic relief. On gross examination cholesterolosis is the principal finding in the gallbladder of some of these patients.

DIFFERENTIAL DIAGNOSIS. The other common causes of chronic abdominal symptoms, such as *peptic ulcer* and *pancreatitis*, may have manifestations similar to those of chronic cholecystitis. Radicular pain from *spinal lesions* may mimic biliary colic, and vertebral films, or, in some instances, myelograms of the T6-T8 segment may be indicated. Angina pectoris may cause pain thought to be abdominal, just as biliary colic may be felt in the precordial region. Postprandial pain or discomfort may result from the *irritable colon syndrome* or from *adenocarcinoma* of the *right colon*.

TREATMENT. Dietary changes, anticholinergics, and antacids have no effect on the course of the disease, but they sometimes provide symptomatic relief for a while. Cholecystectomy is the treatment of choice. Cholecystolithotomy was tried at one time in patients whose gallbladders were normal in function and appearance, but gallstones recurred in most within a few years of surgery. At operation the common bile duct is inspected, operative cholangiograms are obtained, and the common duct is explored if there is evidence of choledocholithiasis.

COMPLICATIONS. *Choledocholithiasis* is the most common complication, affecting about 15 per cent of patients with cholecystolithiasis. The incidence of common duct stones increases with advancing age.

About two thirds of patients with *acute cholecystitis* have previously had symptomatic chronic cholecystitis. The complication of acute cholecystitis is more common in the elderly and in patients with large gallstones.

Mirizzi's syndrome results from gradual extrusion of a large gallstone from the gallbladder into the common duct. The cystic duct enlarges to accommodate the advancing stone, which eventually comes to reside in a common cavity comprising the residual gallbladder lumen, cystic duct, and common duct. Obstructive jaundice may develop.

Calcification of the *gallbladder*, an uncommon condition, is of special significance because of its frequent association with carcinoma of the gallbladder. Whether it can be considered truly premalignant is not clear. The diagnosis is usually obvious when the abdominal x-ray shows an eggshell rim of calcium in the gallbladder wall.

Adenocarcinoma of the gallbladder is found mainly in elderly patients with cholelithiasis, most of whom have had biliary symptoms for many years.

PROGNOSIS. Cholecystectomy relieves biliary colic and is about 80 per cent successful in eradicating other kinds of preoperative complaints (e.g., dyspepsia or flatulence). Loss of the gallbladder does not impair gastrointestinal function.

The mortality of elective cholecystectomy is under 0.5 per cent, and most of the postoperative deaths follow cardiac and respiratory complications in elderly patients with pre-existing disease of these organs. The *postcholecystectomy syndrome* is discussed in Ch. 451.

442. ACUTE CHOLECYSTITIS

Acute cholecystitis usually presents with acute right subcostal pain and tenderness. Obstruction of the cystic duct by a gallstone is usually the cause, and cholelithiasis is present in 95 per cent of patients.

A variety of caustic agents produce cholecystitis when injected into gallbladders of animals, but the relation of this kind of experiment to the human disease is obscure. Filling the gallbladder of a dog with concentrated bile and obstructing the cystic duct, however, also produces acute inflammation, presumably an effect of the bile salts. In control experiments, if the gallbladder is empty or distended with physiologic saline solution instead of bile, cystic duct obstruction is tolerated without inflammation.

As in other biliary diseases, bacterial infection is secondary to the obstruction rather than a primary factor. Bacteria are present as contaminants in the gallbladders of about 25 per cent of patients with chronic cholecystitis. Early in acute cholecystitis the gallbladder bile is positive in 50 per cent of cases, but within a week after onset the figure reaches 90 per cent. Although infection is secondary, it is ultimately responsible for the most serious sequelae of acute cholecystitis — empyema and perforation.

Acalculous cholecystitis, accounting for 5 per cent of cases, is more common in men and in patients with unrelated sepsis. Some cases have been associated with prolonged fasting after major trauma, e.g., war injuries or surgical operations remote from the biliary system. At operation the bile is viscous and full of sludge. Perforation is more frequent, and the outcome is generally worse than in acute gallstone cholecystitis.

Primary gallbladder infection by *Salmonella typhosa* was responsible for some cases of acalculous cholecystitis in the past when typhoid fever was more prevalent. *Polyarteritis nodosa* has occasionally been implicated.

PATHOLOGY. Subserosal edema, mucosal ulcerations, and submucosal hemorrhages are the earliest pathologic findings. The inflammatory process usually evolves slowly in contrast to that in appendicitis or diverticulitis (other conditions involving an obstructed diverticulum), probably because the bacterial population within the gallbladder is relatively sparse at the moment of ductal obstruction. Cellular infiltration of the wall becomes prominent only after three to four days, reaching its greatest intensity at the end of the first week. During the second week, patchy mural gangrene and small intramural abscesses appear, the edema becomes organized, and the first signs of collagen deposition appear. Resolution of the acute changes takes another week or more.

The term *empyema* denotes a pus-filled gallbladder which clinically is characterized by a septic form of acute cholecystitis. On gross examination the condition tends to be overdiagnosed, because gallbladder mucus containing precipitated calcium closely resembles pus. *Gangrene* and *perforation* are most common in the fundus where the blood supply is meager, or in the infundibulum where stones impact. With perforation, gallbladder contents may spill into the free abdominal cavity (bile peritonitis) or may be confined by adhesions (pericholecystic abscess). Sometimes an adherent viscus is penetrated, making a *cholecystenteric fistula* through which the gallstones and pus may be discharged. If a large gallstone reaches the intestine and blocks its lumen, the presenting complaints are those of small bowel obstruction, i.e., *gallstone ileus.*

Chronic obstruction of the cystic duct causes *hydrops* (mucocele), a condition in which the gallbladder is distended with uninfected mucus (white bile). Hydrops may result either from resolved acute cholecystitis or from cystic duct obstruction without inflammation.

CLINICAL MANIFESTATIONS AND DIAGNOSIS. The attack begins with abdominal pain that mounts gradually in severity. The pain is usually located in the right subcostal region from the start, but it sometimes begins in the epigastrium or left upper quadrant and then shifts to the region of the gallbladder as inflammation progresses. Two thirds or more of patients have had previous attacks of biliary colic. Early in the attack the patient may expect the symptoms to subside spontaneously as had happened before with similar pains, and medical aid is often not sought until 48 hours or more. Referred pain may be experienced in the back at the scapular level.

Anorexia, nausea, and vomiting are present in the average case, but the vomiting is rarely severe enough to be confused with bowel obstruction and is generally less than in acute pancreatitis. In the absence of complications, chills are rare; their presence should suggest suppurative cholecystitis or associated cholangitis. Fever is also moderate, reaching an average of 38° C in the absence of complications.

The right subcostal region is tender to palpation, and involuntary muscle spasm generally exists which limits the examination. If the patient takes a deep breath while the subhepatic area is being palpated, tenderness is suddenly worse and inspiratory arrest is produced (*Murphy's sign*).

In somewhat more than a third of the patients, a distended, tender gallbladder can be felt as a distinct mass, which often is located farther to the right than the normal gallbladder. The presence of the palpable gallbladder is an important finding which generally clinches the diagnosis in an otherwise typical case. The gallbladder cannot be felt in the rest of the patients because of obesity, rigidity of the abdominal wall, or a deep subhepatic location, or because it is small and shrunken from previous inflammation. Other related conditions characterized by a tender mass in the same area are *pericholecystic abscess,* acute cholecystitis complicating *carcinoma* of the *gallbladder, torsion* of the *gallbladder,* or the rare case of gallbladder distention in *obstructive cholangitis* (e.g., suppurative cholangitis and Oriental cholangiohepatitis).

About 20 per cent of patients with acute cholecystitis are slightly jaundiced. This is sometimes due only to edema of the nearby common duct; however, two thirds of jaundiced patients will have a mechanical cause such as *common duct stones* or, less often, a *biliary tumor.*

After hospitalization, improvement is usually noticeable within the first 12 to 24 hours, and the signs and symptoms gradually subside over three to seven days. Oral feedings can usually be resumed after a few days. Persistent severe pain after hospitalization, a rise in temperature or leukocyte count, development of shaking chills, and the appearance of more severe local or generalized abdominal tenderness all indicate progression of the disease and suggest the need for emergency operation.

Empyema (suppurative cholecystitis) can produce systemic toxicity and may herald perforation. After empyema develops, if the infection is subsequently controlled with antimicrobial drugs, the large tender gallbladder may remain palpable for several weeks, and return of well-being is similarly prolonged. The leukocyte count is 10,000 to 15,000 per microliter or even higher with complications. Mild rises in bilirubin, alkaline phosphatase, and transaminases are frequent.

Roentgenograms of the abdomen may show calcified gallstones or an enlarged gallbladder. An ultrasound examination is probably the simplest and most reliable method of detecting gallbladder stones in these patients. Oral cholecystograms will not opacify during an acute attack and are diagnostically unreliable because of unpredictable absorption and excretion of the contrast agent. Except in patients who become asymptomatic rapidly, oral cholecystograms should not be scheduled until four to six weeks after the attack; the rate of nonopacification remains high even then.

Intravenous cholangiograms (IVC) may give useful information if liver function is good, and may be ordered if more information would be useful for clinical management. This situation usually occurs in a patient for whom an early operation would be appropriate, but in whom an enlarged gallbladder cannot be felt on physical examination. If on IVC the gallbladder fills, the diagnosis of acute cholecystitis is essentially excluded; if the ductal system is demonstrated but the gallbladder does not opacify, the diagnosis is confirmed. More difficult to interpret is the situation in which neither gallbladder nor ducts are shown. If the bilirubin level is normal and the upper abdominal pain and tenderness are typical, most patients will turn out to have acute cholecystitis as suspected.

DIFFERENTIAL DIAGNOSIS. *Acute pancreatitis, acute appendicitis,* and *perforated peptic ulcer* are the conditions which most often cause major problems in differential diagnosis. In acute cholecystitis the serum amylase may rise to 1000 per 100 ml or more. Furthermore, acute cholecystitis and acute pancreatitis may coexist. Intravenous cholangiography may be helpful because the gallbladder usually opacifies in acute pancreatitis.

In women, gonococcal perihepatitis *(Fitz-Hugh–Curtis syndrome)* may be mistaken for acute cholecystitis, but adnexal tenderness is usually present on pelvic examination, a cervical smear usually reveals gonococci, and the patients are younger, often have higher fever, and are in less distress than would be expected in cholecystitis. Shoulder pain and a friction rub over the liver, common in the Fitz-Hugh–Curtis syndrome, are not found in uncomplicated acute cholecystitis.

Acute hepatitis, either *viral* or *alcoholic,* sometimes produces marked right upper quadrant pain and tenderness. A history of recent binge drinking, high SGOT levels, and liver biopsy aid differentiation. *Pneumonitis, pyelonephritis,* and *cardiac disease* have all on occasion produced acute pain suggestive of cholecystitis.

TREATMENT. Most patients with acute cholecystitis will improve with either expectant treatment or cholecystectomy performed during the acute attack. In general, the decision regarding the kind of treatment should include the following considerations (Fig. 6): (1) whether the diagnosis is secure, (2) whether biliary complications have occurred or appear imminent, and (3) the over-all condition of the patient (operative risk).

Upon admission to the hospital, nasogastric suction should be started and fluid requirements given intravenously. Vomiting and fasting before hospitalization often cause dehydration, which must be corrected. In many elderly patients, the acute biliary condition has aggravated pre-existing cardiac, pulmonary, or renal disease, and these systems must be evaluated and treated appropriately. Diabetes mellitus must be sought, because it heralds a more ominous prognosis if surgery is delayed.

If the patient is first seen shortly after symptoms began, and if local signs and symptoms are mild, antimicrobial therapy need not be given. Antimicrobials are of principal value to treat suppurative complications. Ampicillin, cephalosporin, or tetracycline is adequate, except in patients with empyema or perforation in whom cephalosporin plus gentamicin or kanamycin would be preferable.

A preponderance of opinion considers cholecystectomy to be the optimal therapy for acute cholecystitis. This does not imply an emergency operation. The workup should proceed deliberately to confirm the diagnosis and to prepare the patient by procedures such as correcting fluid deficits. Cholecystectomy should then be scheduled for the next routine operating day.

Many clinicians, however, still prefer to follow an expectant regimen for the average case, reserving surgery during the acute attack for patients with complications and for those who become worse or fail to improve while being observed. For patients who respond to nonoperative management, interval cholecystectomy is generally recommended four to eight weeks later. Although nonoperative therapy is still common practice, about 25 per cent of patients managed in this way require urgent operation for worsening disease, the patient ultimately loses about 40 more days off work or away from his usual activity, several thousand dollars more in medical expenses results from the second hospitalization, and the over-all success of this approach is no different from a policy of early operation for suitable patients. The following remarks indicate how patients are managed on a policy of early operation.

In about 30 per cent of cases, the patient is a good surgical risk, the diagnosis is obvious within 12 to 24 hours, and cholecystectomy can be scheduled promptly. Another 30 per cent are good surgical candidates, but the

Figure 6. Scheme for managing patients with right upper quadrant pain and tenderness who are thought to have acute cholecystitis. This scheme is based on a policy of early operation for appropriate patients.

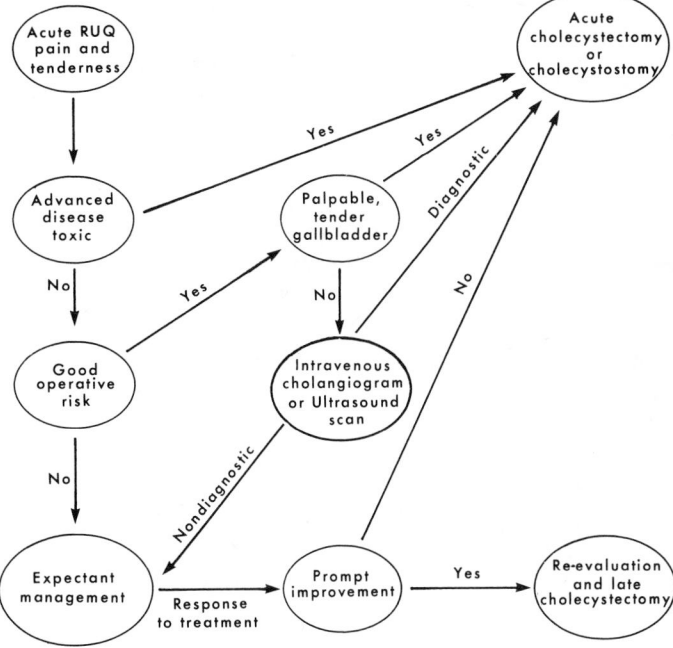

gallbladder cannot be felt. In this situation the diagnosis should be regarded as tentative, because 10 to 15 per cent of patients whose only finding is tenderness will have some other condition. An ultrasound scan or IVC should be performed preoperatively to verify the clinical impression.

Another third of patients will have serious coexistent cardiac, respiratory, or other disease whose treatment takes precedence. The cholecystitis should be treated expectantly while correcting the other problems. Progression of local abdominal findings requires continued reevaluation, balancing the risks of operation with the risks of continued delay.

About 10 per cent of patients require emergency surgery for complications present on admission or which appear later during observation and medical management. When emergency operation becomes necessary, *cholecystostomy* may be preferable to cholecystectomy in the seriously ill patient. In this procedure, the fundus is incised, stones and pus are removed from the lumen, and a catheter secured in the lumen is brought out through the abdominal wall and placed to gravity drainage. As in draining any abscess, this procedure allows the acute infection to resolve. Patients who recover should usually have a cholecystectomy six to eight weeks later. Those who continue to be poor surgical risks may be followed expectantly if postoperative cholecystography shows that the gallbladder and common duct contain no residual stones. If stones are present, surgery will be needed to avoid further acute attacks. In seriously ill patients, the cholecystostomy tube can be left in place indefinitely.

Postoperatively it may be possible to extract residual gallbladder or common duct stones with flexible forceps or snares passed through the cholecystostomy fistula. The procedure is difficult to perform, and success is unpredictable.

After the cholecystostomy tube is removed from a patient whose biliary system contains no calculi, within the first year about 50 per cent of patients develop new stones and additional symptoms. Recurrent disease is less common after one year.

COMPLICATIONS. In *emphysematous cholecystitis,* a variant of acute cholecystitis, gas of bacterial origin can be seen in the gallbladder lumen and adjacent tissues. Clinically, emphysematous cholecystitis causes the same signs and symptoms as acute cholecystitis. Men are affected twice as frequently as women, about 30 per cent of patients have diabetes mellitus, and the gallbladder is acalculous in about half the cases. Gas does not develop until 24 to 48 hours after the attack begins, at which time a radiolucent halo outlines the lumen and an air-fluid level may be seen on upright films. Subserosal and then pericholecystic emphysema appear with time. Differential diagnosis of the x-ray findings includes *cholecystenteric fistula, appendiceal* or *subhepatic abscess,* and, rarely, *lipomatosis* of the *gallbladder.* In about half the cases the gas-forming organisms are clostridia, and the rest are *E. coli,* streptococci, and others. Treatment is the same as for acute cholecystitis in general, but the somewhat more aggressive nature of emphysematous cholecystitis and the association with diabetes mellitus mean that prompt surgery is usually required.

Empyema and *perforation* are usually manifested by greater sepsis and more marked abdominal signs. Perforation may take any of three forms: (1) free perforation into the abdominal cavity, (2) localized (contained) perforation

with pericholecystic abscess, and (3) perforation into another viscus with fistula formation.

Free perforation, which has a 25 per cent mortality, is fortunately the least common type. It usually occurs early in the attack, often within the first three days, suggesting that when gangrene develops this quickly it cannot be walled off by adjacent viscera. Clinically, free perforation causes toxicity with high temperatures (greater than 39° C), leukocytosis over 15,000 per μl, and diffuse abdominal tenderness and rigidity. In more than half the cases, the correct diagnosis is unsuspected until laparotomy or autopsy, because a clear-cut history of preliminary right upper quadrant pain is often lacking. Treatment consists of intravenous antimicrobial therapy and emergency laparotomy with cholecystectomy.

Localized perforation most often appears in the second week of the attack at the peak of the inflammatory reaction. The diagnosis should be suspected with increasing local signs, especially when a mass suddenly appears. In most cases cholecystectomy can be performed; but in a severely ill patient, cholecystostomy and drainage of the abscess may be wiser.

Fistula formation usually involves the nearby second portion of the duodenum or, less commonly, the colon, jejunum, stomach, or common bile duct. Rare fistulas have entered the renal pelvis or bronchus, or through the abdominal wall (empyema necessitatis). After intestinal fistulization the contents of the gallbladder are discharged into the gut, often aborting the acute attack. Clinically, the fistula itself may not be suspected because it produces no unique findings; many are discovered incidentally during a later cholecystectomy. In the absence of biliary obstruction a cholecystenteric fistula is not necessarily of pathophysiologic significance. Cholecystocolonic fistulas may cause malabsorption from diversion of bile, or from heavy bacterial contamination of the upper gut. If a particularly large gallstone enters through the fistula, it may obstruct the intestine, a condition called *gallstone ileus* (see Ch. 443).

PROGNOSIS. The mortality of 5 to 10 per cent is almost confined to patients over 60 years of age with serious associated disease. Suppurative complications are more common in the elderly, who can tolerate them least. In most instances, localized perforation can be managed satisfactorily at operation. Free perforation is considerably more ominous (25 per cent mortality), but is rare.

In patients who are treated expectantly, recurrent biliary symptoms are so common that an elective cholecystectomy should be planned in most cases. Another acute attack is not unusual during the month or two of waiting.

443. GALLSTONE ILEUS

Gallstone ileus is intestinal obstruction caused by a gallstone lodged in the intestinal lumen. The stone, passing through a cholecystenteric fistula, most often enters the gut in the duodenum, less commonly the jejunum, ileum, colon, or stomach. Although it is often assumed that the initial event responsible for fistula formation is an attack of acute cholecystitis, only 30 per cent of patients with gallstone ileus give a history of recent right upper quadrant pain, and usually the clinical picture is that of bowel obstruction only.

After entering the gut, the gallstone moves downstream until it becomes too large for the intestinal lumen to accommodate. Obstruction is usually caused by gallstones over 2.5 cm in diameter, and because the lumen becomes progressively smaller aborally, the ileum is the final point of obturation in most cases. Typically, the patient's symptoms are intermittent at first as the stone transiently obstructs and then dislodges, passing further along. This has been termed "tumbling obstruction," the brief periods of respite sometimes leading patient and physician to expect a spontaneous resolution of the symptoms. Eventually, however, vomiting, pain, and distention persist.

If the stone lodges in the duodenum, the diagnosis may be especially difficult in the absence of distention, hyperactive peristalsis, or x-ray findings of small bowel obstruction. Another uncommon variant is gallstone ileus of the large bowel. In these cases, the stone may have entered via a cholecystocolonic fistula or, less often, after traversing the entire small bowel. Obstruction of the colon, rare because its lumen is so wide, most often occurs when diverticulitis has narrowed the sigmoid.

Women are more often affected than men, and the average age is about 70 years. As a cause of intestinal obstruction, gallstone ileus is relatively uncommon but should always be high on the list in elderly patients, especially when incarceration in an external hernia is absent and there has been no previous laparotomy which might have produced adhesions.

On physical examination the findings are those of small bowel obstruction. Sometimes the large stone can be felt as a mass on abdominal, vaginal, or rectal examination, but it is rarely correctly identified.

Roentgenograms usually show air in the biliary tree if the films are carefully examined, and in some cases the radiopaque gallstone can be seen in its unusual location. Otherwise, the films are typical of bowel obstruction. Sometimes a gastrointestinal series is performed for the diagnosis of partial obstruction, revealing the cholecystoduodenal fistula.

Treatment consists of removing the obstructing gallstone through a small enterotomy and examining the proximal gut carefully to ensure that a second stone is not left which could produce an immediate recurrence. It is generally wise to leave the biliary disease undisturbed initially, because elderly patients tolerate long procedures poorly, and nothing much is gained by repairing the fistula primarily.

Postoperatively, if the patient has symptoms of biliary disease, an elective cholecystectomy may be scheduled several months later. Many patients become asymptomatic and the fistula closes spontaneously; for them, expectant management is best. About 50 per cent will require cholecystectomy.

The mortality rate, 15 to 20 per cent, remains high because of delay in diagnosis and the fragile state of cardiopulmonary function in elderly patients.

444. CHOLEDOCHOLITHIASIS AND CHOLANGITIS

In Western countries choledocholithiasis is usually the result of passage into the common duct of gallstones formed in the gallbladder. Once in the common duct, the stones may pass into the duodenum, but the frequency of this event is not known and is rarely observed with certainty. The less common primary duct stone is usually associated with bile stasis caused by secondary dilatation of the duct from longstanding obstruction by stones, stricture, or ampullary stenosis. About 15 per cent of patients with gallbladder stones have concomitant choledocholithiasis. The incidence is higher in elderly patients and in patients who seek medical care late. In rare instances choledocholithiasis is found in the absence of gallbladder stones; in such a case it is assumed that all the gallbladder stones escaped into the duct.

CLINICAL MANIFESTATIONS. The natural history of choledocholithiasis is only vaguely known. Available data suggest that 30 to 40 per cent of patients are asymptomatic at the time of diagnosis, implying a relatively benign course in many cases. Obstruction by stones of the biliary or pancreatic ducts may produce any of the following syndromes: biliary colic, jaundice (without pain), cholangitis, pancreatitis, or a combination of these (Fig. 7). Secondary hepatic effects of persistent obstruction include biliary cirrhosis or hepatic abscesses.

Intermittent cholangitis, consisting of biliary colic, jaundice, and fever and chills (*Charcot's triad*), is the most common presenting symptom complex; in the absence of previous biliary surgery it is almost diagnostic in the Western Hemisphere of choledocholithiasis. Intermittency of symptoms is quite characteristic, a manifestation of intermittent partial obstruction. Whenever pain, chills with fever, and jaundice fluctuate together over a span of a few days or a week, cholangitis from biliary obstruction is almost certainly the cause. In a typical attack chills may precede the other symptoms, and dark urine from bilirubinuria may follow after a day or so. The pain, located in

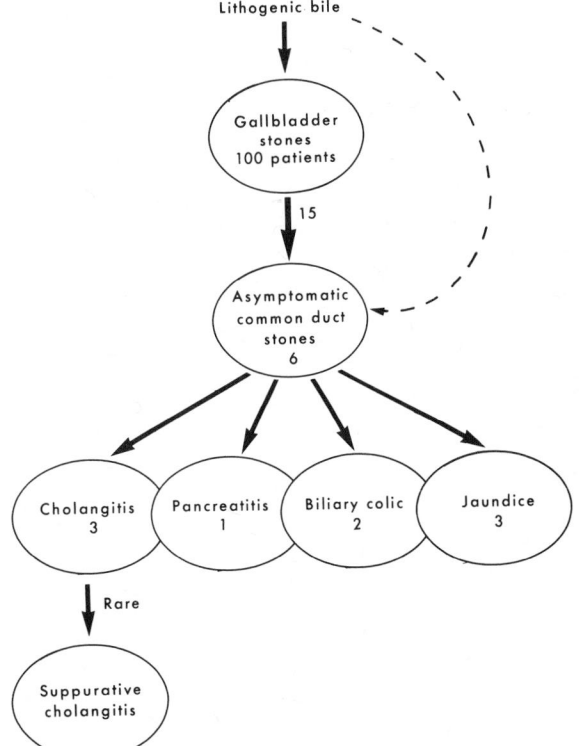

Figure 7. Natural history of choledocholithiasis, indicating that this complication affects about 15 per cent of patients with gallstone disease and that in most cases the common duct stones originate in the gallbladder. Most patients acquire one of the syndromes in the ovals at the bottom, but many probably remain asymptomatic.

the epigastrium or right upper quadrant, is indistinguishable from biliary colic caused by gallbladder stones and is steady, dull, and cramplike in quality. Pain may be referred to the upper back or even the precordium, occasionally suggesting coronary artery or esophageal disease.

The severity of the systemic reaction, i.e., fever and chills, varies widely from the usual mild transient illness to overwhelming sepsis with shock (see Suppurative Cholangitis, below). In the average case, the temperature rises to 38.5 to 40° C, preceded by chills and positive blood cultures. Localized tenderness in the subcostal region may be associated with extreme guarding and rigidity, but more often the local findings are minimal and are distinctly less severe than in acute cholecystitis. In most cases of common duct obstruction by stones, chronic inflammation and scarring of the gallbladder prevent it from becoming distended, as often occurs with periampullary malignancies. This serves as the basis for *Courvoisier's law:* a distended, nontender gallbladder in a jaundiced patient signifies neoplastic obstruction of the bile duct.

LABORATORY STUDIES. In cholangitis the leukocyte count averages 15,000 μl but may go much higher in severe cases. Bilirubin values are usually in the range of 2 to 4 mg per 100 ml, and are uncommonly higher than 10 mg per 100 ml. Elevated serum alkaline phosphatase, leucine aminopeptidase, and 5'-nucleotidase levels indicate extrahepatic obstruction. The SGOT generally remains below 200 units, but values of 500 are not rare, and a few cases have been reported in which it has transiently exceeded 1000 units. In these instances the prompt drop within 48 hours and associated tenfold increase in LDH allows differentiation from serum hepatitis.

DIFFERENTIAL DIAGNOSIS. The same conditions considered for the patient with chronic cholecystitis must be excluded for biliary colic caused by ductal calculi. In patients who have had a cholecystectomy, differentiation between choledocholithiasis and biliary stricture as the cause of cholangitis usually depends on radiologic demonstration of the ducts. When the presenting syndrome is painless cholestatic jaundice, other causes, especially *periampullary* and *biliary neoplasms,* must be considered. With neoplastic obstruction the bilirubin averages about 18 mg per 100 ml and rarely fluctuates. Although jaundice from stones may be as intense, the bilirubin is characteristically less than 10 mg per 100 ml and it rises and falls episodically. The diagnosis of *intrahepatic cholestasis* from causes such as drugs, viral hepatitis, or pregnancy should in most cases be reached by exclusion only after opacification of normal bile ducts by direct or intravenous cholangiography. Gallstone disease is common in cirrhosis, so choledocholithiasis and alcoholic liver disease may coexist.

Common duct stones may cause *acute pancreatitis* indistinguishable clinically from that resulting from alcohol or other causes and unaccompanied by specific signs of biliary disease. Pancreatitis caused by biliary calculi, despite numerous attacks, rarely progresses to pancreatic calcification, chronic pain, and pancreatic insufficiency, as so often occurs in the alcoholic variety. As a rule, gallstone disease should be searched for radiologically in every patient with acute pancreatitis, because further attacks can be avoided if the gallstones are removed.

TREATMENT. The potential seriousness of cholangitis warrants hospitalization for diagnosis and treatment in most cases. After blood cultures are drawn, antimicrobial drugs effective against enteric organisms are given by the parenteral route. At present cephalosporin or ampicillin

for mild attacks or either of these drugs plus gentamicin or kanamycin in severe infection has a good chance of controlling the infection. There is no rationale for choosing antimicrobial drugs based on their excretion in bile, because the block responsible for cholangitis also affects hepatic secretion. Failure to obtain a rapid response may mean that the organisms were not susceptible to the initial drugs, justifying the addition of another drug or a shift from the initial regimen based upon the results of cultures and drug susceptibility tests. The margin between mild and severe illness is small; antimicrobial therapy should be expected to control the acute attack within 48 to 72 hours, and if there is no improvement or worsening after this period, emergency surgery must be considered seriously.

More than 90 per cent of cases respond satisfactorily to treatment and allow an orderly attempt at diagnosis. If oral cholecystography or an ultrasound scan has already demonstrated gallbladder stones, laparotomy is indicated, and additional studies aimed at demonstrating the ductal pathology are usually not necessary. In patients with jaundice, acute pancreatitis, or upper abdominal pain who have had a cholecystectomy in the past, an ultrasound scan should be performed; an intravenous cholangiogram can be obtained if the bilirubin is below 3 or 4 mg per 100 ml, or direct opacification can be attempted by percutaneous transhepatic or, preferably, retrograde endoscopic cholangiography. Both kinds of direct cholangiography are potentially hazardous in active cholangitis and should be postponed until infection is well controlled, proceeding then only under the protection of antimicrobial therapy.

Surgical exploration and choledochotomy should be scheduled after the diagnosis of choledocholithiasis has been made. If the gallbladder is present, cholecystectomy is done, and the common duct is opened and emptied of stones. A T tube is usually left in the duct to decompress biliary pressure in the postoperative period and to provide a route for additional cholangiograms a week or so later.

In patients with advanced disease, the common duct may be so packed with hundreds of stones that it is dilated to 3 cm or more in diameter. Rarely, the intrahepatic ducts become markedly dilated and contain innumerable stones, making complete extraction technically impossible. In either of these situations recurrent or persistent choledocholithiasis is almost certain unless a choledochoduodenostomy, sphincteroplasty, or Roux-en-Y choledochojejunostomy is performed to create a wide conduit between the duct and intestine through which residual stones can pass.

Selected patients with choledocholithiasis who previously have had a cholecystectomy may sometimes be satisfactorily treated by *transendoscopic sphincterotomy.* Using the side viewing duodenoscope, a wire is passed into the bile duct and the sphincter divided by electrocautery. Common duct stones 1 cm or smaller will usually pass into the duodenum. This technique is usually unsuccessful with large stones or when the common duct is greatly dilated. Bleeding and pancreatitis are the principal complications, and the mortality of the procedure is about 1 per cent.

RETAINED COMMON DUCT STONES. The methods for detecting duct stones at operation are about 95 per cent reliable, which means, unfortunately, that a few are overlooked only to be discovered on postoperative T tube cholangiograms. There are two approaches to eliminate residual stones without another laparotomy. Neither method should be tried until four to six weeks postoperatively. One technique depends on the ability of bile salt solutions and mono-octanoin (glyceryl-one-mono-octanoate) to dissolve cholesterol gallstones. The technique with bile salts is to infuse sodium cholate (150 mM) into the T tube at 30 ml per hour until the stone is gone. Oral cholestyramine must be given to prevent diarrhea from the large amount of bile salt delivered to the intestine. Mono-octanoin, which is about equally as successful as cholate but avoids the potential of diarrhea, is infused at 5 to 10 ml per hour. Care must be exercised to avoid producing pressures in the duct greater than 30 cm H_2O during infusion of either solvent. The retained stones disappear in about two thirds of patients within a two-week treatment period. There is no known solvent effective against pigment stones.

Instrumental extraction, an alternative technique, is somewhat simpler, faster, and about equally successful. Under image intensification fluoroscopy the T tube is pulled out, a Dormia ureteral basket is passed into the duct, and the stone is grasped and withdrawn. The best approach usually is to try instrumental extraction first and dissolution if that fails. If neither mechanical extraction nor chemical dissolution is successful, transendoscopic sphincterotomy may allow the stone to pass into the duodenum. If that technique is contraindicated or unsuccessful, reoperation is usually necessary.

PROGNOSIS. With accurate diagnosis and treatment, choledocholithiasis is cured by cholecystectomy and choledocholithotomy. Recurrent ductal stone formation is rare except as noted when the duct has become markedly dilated.

SUPPURATIVE CHOLANGITIS

The severest form of cholangitis, variously termed *suppurative* or *obstructive cholangitis,* involves the same causative factors as the "nonsuppurative" form but differs in that obstruction is complete, ductal contents become purulent, and clinically the manifestations of sepsis overshadow those of cholestasis. Hypotension and mental changes, such as lethargy or confusion, appear in addition to right upper quadrant pain, chills, fever, and jaundice. Because infection in the face of the high-grade obstruction progresses so rapidly, the serum bilirubin does not reach very high levels before the patient becomes moribund from sepsis. Costly delays in diagnosis are frequent, a consequence of failure to recognize the significance of mild icterus and abdominal pain in a patient with sepsis. All but a few cases are complications of choledocholithiasis, the others occurring with biliary stricture or neoplastic obstruction.

Laboratory tests reveal evidence of cholestasis with bilirubin values between 2 and 5 mg per 100 ml and elevated serum levels of alkaline phosphatase, 5'-nucleotidase, leucine aminopeptidase, and SGOT. The leukocyte count varies from normal to 40,000 per microliter.

Tenderness is present to palpation in the right upper quadrant, but rigidity is rare. In some cases secondary cholecystitis develops, and an enlarged tender gallbladder may be found on abdominal examination.

An ultrasound scan may show dilated bile ducts. Transhepatic or retrograde cholangiography would be extremely hazardous, and intravenous cholangiograms are unsuccessful. Therefore diagnosis rests on recognizing the evidence of biliary obstruction and its relationship to the sepsis, and on verifying the initial impression by an ultrasound scan.

After initial resuscitation, consisting of intravenous infusions, antimicrobial drugs, and measures to restore cardiac, pulmonary, or renal function, decompression of the duct by emergency laparotomy or transendoscopic sphincterotomy offers the only hope of saving the patient. Hypoglycemia has been found in some patients whose depressed cerebral function seemed to improve with infusion of hypertonic glucose solutions.

At surgery when choledochotomy is performed, pus often squirts from the duct owing to the high pressure. If the patient's condition permits, thorough exploration can be performed to correct the obstruction by removing stones, repairing a stricture, or bypassing a tumor. Insertion of a T tube proximal to the obstruction is sufficient in patients who are unable to tolerate a longer operation, but sometime later it will be necessary to perform a second, more definitive procedure before the T tube can be removed.

The mortality is about 50 per cent, resulting from septic shock, renal failure, acute hepatic insufficiency, or a combination of these complications.

445. BILIARY STRICTURE

Biliary stricture, except in rare instances, results from surgical injury to the duct and usually follows cholecystectomy rather than procedures on the duct itself such as deliberate choledochotomy for common duct exploration. In some cases the surgeon may recognize the injury and attempt its repair. Often, however, it is not identified at the primary operation, and the first sign of trouble postoperatively might be excessive escape of bile along drains or the appearance of jaundice or cholangitis. A few noniatrogenic examples of biliary stricture stem from external trauma or scarring produced by choledocholithiasis.

Injury to the duct that is identified immediately or within a few days can sometimes be repaired without serious consequences. The patient who has signs of partial biliary obstruction and intermittent cholangitis weeks or months after cholecystectomy is the one who presents challenges for diagnosis and treatment. The symptoms closely resemble those of choledocholithiasis, the obvious clue being a history of previous cholecystectomy or attempt at repair of a stricture.

Leukocytosis and laboratory evidence of cholestasis parallel the clinical manifestations. The jaundice or cholangitis is generally mild and transient, and infection generally responds promptly to antimicrobial therapy.

Intravenous cholangiograms may be obtained if the bilirubin drops below 3 mg per 100 ml. Otherwise, transhepatic or retrograde cholangiograms will be necessary.

With persistent obstruction over several years, secondary biliary cirrhosis develops, and portal hypertension may give rise to bleeding esophageal varices, or hepatic failure may ensue gradually. In other cases, uncontrolled sepsis results in multiple intrahepatic abscesses and death.

Differential diagnosis must include all the various causes of obstructive jaundice and cholangitis, but in most cases the major consideration is *choledocholithiasis.* A useful differential feature is that the initial symptoms of stricture nearly always begin within two years of the cholecystectomy, whereas a symptom-free interval longer than this is common with residual or recurrent common duct stones.

In all but a few cases an attempt should be made to repair the stricture surgically by creating a new unobstructed conduit between normal duct on the hepatic side of the lesion and the proximal intestine. Direct end-to-end anastomosis of the duct after excising the lesion is rarely as satisfactory a method of reconstruction as choledochoduodenostomy or choledochojejunostomy to a Roux-en-Y jejunal segment. Loss of the duodenal end of the duct and choledochal sphincter with the last two operations is of no physiologic significance. By diverting alkaline bile from the duodenum, choledochojejunostomy predisposes slightly to peptic ulcer disease, but the problem is not of sufficient magnitude to weigh heavily in the choice of procedure unless the patient already has a peptic ulcer.

The over-all success rate of these operations is about 75 per cent, but it is important to note that even when there has been one or more previous failures, the odds still favor a good result after another try. For this reason, it is rarely wise to keep a patient with a known stricture indefinitely on a regimen of intermittent antimicrobial drugs for symptoms. The obstruction invariably produces cirrhosis or uncontrollable infection, and the opportunity to obtain a real cure is lost.

The mortality of 10 per cent is from the complications mentioned above.

446. UNCOMMON CAUSES OF BILE DUCT OBSTRUCTION

The following inventory briefly covers several uncommon causes of common duct obstruction manifested clinically by jaundice, colic, cholangitis, or a combination of these. *Pancreatic* and *duodenal tumors* are covered in Ch. 411 and 425, respectively. Other causes rarely encountered are compression by *neoplastic* or *inflammatory paraductal lymph nodes* and *duodenal Crohn's disease*.

Choledochal cysts occasionally produce their initial clinical manifestations in adults, presenting with jaundice, cholangitis, and, in some, a right upper quadrant mass consisting of the cyst full of stones. Diagnosis may require transhepatic cholangiography or may not be obvious until operation. The most definitive surgical procedure is excision of the abnormal duct, followed by Roux-en-Y jejunal anastomosis to the stump of the hepatic duct. The simpler cystenteric anastomosis may be preferable in some situations.

Caroli's disease consists of saccular intrahepatic bile duct dilatation which in most cases becomes symptomatic in patients between the ages of 20 and 50 owing to intrahepatic stone formation and cholangitis. Two forms are recognized: one a disease of the ducts only, and the more common type which is associated with hepatic fibrosis and medullary sponge kidney. The latter patients often have complications of portal hypertension before cholangitis or obstructive jaundice appears. Antimicrobial therapy may control attacks of cholangitis, and surgical procedures to facilitate ductal emptying or to extract stones may help in some cases, but the intrahepatic anomaly cannot

be definitively corrected. Rarely the left lobe alone is involved, and lobectomy is curative.

Hemobilia presents with the triad of biliary colic, obstructive jaundice, and occult or gross intestinal bleeding. Most cases are caused by hepatic injury from external trauma with secondary bleeding into the ductal system, usually beginning several weeks after the trauma. Hemobilia is occasionally caused by *biliary* or *hepatic neoplasms*, ductal rupture of an *hepatic artery aneurysm, hepatic abscess*, or *biliary calculus*. A few cases have followed percutaneous needle biopsy of the liver. Inflammatory hemobilia has been reported mostly from the Orient, where it accompanies *biliary parasitism (Ascaris lumbricoides)* or *cholangiohepatitis*. The diagnosis can be verified preoperatively by selective hepatic arteriography. Treatment may require hepatic artery ligation for hemobilia secondary to trauma, but for the other types direct surgical management of the lesion is usually necessary.

Pancreatitis can produce transient jaundice by obstruction of the distal common duct where it is encased by pancreatic tissue. Prolonged obstruction can result from pressure by a pseudocyst or entrapment in severe pancreatic scarring from chronic pancreatitis. Diagnosis may be difficult in alcoholic patients in whom elevated bilirubin values are usually attributed to hepatic parenchymal disease. Jaundice resulting from pressure by a pseudocyst is best treated by internal drainage of the cyst, leaving the bile duct alone. Jaundice resulting from chronic pancreatitis requires choledochoduodenostomy or Roux-en-Y anastomosis of jejunum to the gallbladder or bile duct.

Most *duodenal diverticula* arise within 1 to 2 cm of the hepatobiliary ampulla, and in some patients the common duct empties directly into a diverticulum. Duodenal diverticula may obstruct the common duct by anatomic distortion of its duodenal entry, by diverticulitis, or by an enterolith (of bile acids) in the sac. Even in jaundiced patients most duodenal diverticula are only incidental findings, but when definite proof implicates them in ductal obstruction, either choledochoduodenostomy or Roux-en-Y choledochojejunostomy is simpler treatment than attempting to excise the diverticulum or surgically to enlarge its entry into the duodenum.

Echinococcosis, by rupture of an hepatic cyst into the ducts, can give rise to biliary colic, jaundice, and cholangitis. Treatment involves surgical removal of the obstructing hydatid debris and daughter cysts from the ducts and excision of the parent cyst from the liver after attempting to sterilize its contents with silver nitrate (0.5 per cent), sodium hypochlorite (0.05 per cent), or hypertonic saline (30 per cent) solution. The practice of injecting formalin into the hepatic cysts is no longer used, because in patients with a biliary communication serious damage to the bile ducts and even death have occurred.

Ascariasis may produce colic, jaundice, and cholangitis by a worm which invades the bile ducts through the choledochal sphincter from the duodenum. The worm eventually dies, but in some cases not until after depositing ova. Air is sometimes seen in the ducts, presumably entering through the sphincter with the ascarid. Treatment entails antimicrobial drugs and then piperazine after the acute symptoms are controlled. If progressive cholangitis occurs despite antimicrobial therapy, common duct exploration and extraction of the parasite may be necessary. After the nonsurgical regimen, follow-up intravenous cholangiograms should be obtained to verify that no worms remain in the duct; if residual defects are present, they should be surgically removed.

Throughout coastal regions of the Orient, from Japan to Malaysia, many persons of low socioeconomic status are affected by *Oriental cholangiohepatitis*, a form of chronic recurrent cholangitis caused by calcium bilirubinate stones formed primarily within the bile ducts. Among the various etiologic possibilities are the effects of parasites in the ducts (especially *Clonorchis sinensis* and *Ascaris lumbricoides*), diet (low in fat and animal protein), and excessive bilirubin excretion. In some regions, ova or fragments of adult parasites have been demonstrated within the center of the stones, but the disease has also been reported in populations without heavy parasitic infestation. Within the ducts, *Clornorchis* is especially capable of inciting ductal inflammation and scarring. Whatever the initial event, there is good evidence that β-glucuronidase, produced in the bile by secondarily invading *E. coli*, hydrolyzes bilirubin diglucuronide which then precipitates as sludge and stones of calcium bilirubinate.

Acute cholangitis is the usual presenting syndrome. Subcostal abdominal tenderness is present, and the gallbladder, which contains stones in only 20 to 30 per cent, is usually palpable, or even visible on abdominal inspection. Strictures sometimes develop in the hepatic ducts, leading to further stasis and intrahepatic stone formation. In advanced cases, one (usually the left) or both lobar ducts may become honeycombed with cysts or abscesses, producing atrophy of the hepatic parenchyma. Laboratory abnormalities consist of leukocytosis, elevated serum bilirubin (2 to 10 mg per 100 ml), and elevated serum alkaline phosphatase. During symptomatic episodes neither plain films nor oral or intravenous cholangiograms will demonstrate the pathology.

Most acute cases can be controlled with antimicrobials, but severe toxicity, fever (39 to 40°C), or septic shock mandates emergency laparotomy in as many as 30 per cent. If nonsurgical management is initially successful, transhepatic cholangiograms can be used later to outline the ducts.

The common duct stones should be removed through a generous choledochotomy. If it is impossible to empty the intrahepatic ducts, transhepatic lithotomy or even lobectomy may be required if there is unilateral lobar atrophy or abscess formation. Recurrence of choledocholithiasis is almost certain unless the junction between duct and intestine is surgically enlarged by sphincteroplasty, choledochoduodenostomy, or Roux-en-Y choledochojejunostomy.

Sclerosing cholangitis, a rare condition of unknown etiology, consists of benign nonbacterial chronic inflammatory narrowing of the bile ducts. The entire ductal system may be involved, or, less commonly, the process may be confined to the extrahepatic or intrahepatic portion. Males predominate in a ratio of 3:1, and the peak incidence occurs in the third and fourth decades. About one third of the cases are associated with *retroperitoneal fibrosis, Riedel's thyroiditis, regional enteritis*, or especially *ulcerative colitis*. When both are present, the severity of sclerosing cholangitis and ulcerative colitis is not correlated, and colectomy has an uncertain effect on the biliary disease.

The initial complaint may be jaundice or pruritus, although both eventually appear in most cases. There may be mild upper abdominal pain and sometimes fever, but a clinical picture resembling bacterial cholangitis is uncommon in the absence of previous surgical exploration of the ducts. Hepatomegaly is the only abdominal finding until late when secondary cirrhosis produces ascites or splenomegaly.

Jaundice may be constant or fluctuating, and bilirubin values are usually in the range of 2 to 10 mg per 100 ml. The alkaline phosphatase is quite high and remains elevated despite variations in clinical manifestations. Antimitochondrial antibodies are absent. Other liver function tests are normal until late in the illness when hepatic failure develops.

Transhepatic cholangiography or retrograde endoscopic cholangiography is required to establish the diagnosis preoperatively. The x-rays show diffuse irregular ductal narrowing with only a tiny residual lumen in the most severely involved areas. When considering the differential diagnosis, a short stenosis (1 to 2 cm) of the duct more likely represents a neoplasm or traumatic stricture than sclerosing cholangitis. Other causes of persistent cholestatic jaundice must be considered, especially *primary biliary cirrhosis, drug cholestasis*, and *neoplastic ductal obstruction*.

The effectiveness of surgical dilatation of the duct in improving the course of the disease is not conclusively proved, but the striking relief and even permanent remissions that occasionally result support this approach. At operation the lumen is identified, often a tedious process, and then dilated with progressively larger probes. An operative cholangiogram should be obtained to show the extent and severity of involvement, and as large a T tube as possible should be placed in the duct and left there for several months. Since differentiation from scirrhous biliary malignancy may be difficult even at operation, a biopsy of the duct should be obtained in all cases, and even then the pathologist may have trouble distinguishing sclerosing cholangitis from neoplasm.

Many experts favor postoperative administration of systemic corticosteroids for 6 to 12 months. After surgery which introduces a few bacteria and a foreign body, short courses of antimicrobial therapy can be given to hasten their resolution. Cholestyramine may be useful for pruritus at any stage of the disease.

Significant palliation follows surgery in many cases, but is not often permanent. Some patients seem to recover completely; most have episodic remissions and exacerbations over five to ten years, during which time secondary biliary cirrhosis develops. Death may follow uncontrollable biliary sepsis with hepatic abscesses, liver failure, or bleeding from esophageal varices.

447. CARCINOMA OF THE GALLBLADDER

About 6000 people in the United States die each year from carcinoma of the gallbladder, a number equal to the mortality from benign disease of the biliary tract. Gallbladder cancer accounts for 1 per cent of all cancer deaths and 3 per cent of gastrointestinal malignancies. Women outnumber men by 3 to 1, and the average age is 70. Because 85 per cent of cases occur in patients with gallstones, cholelithiasis is thought to be etiologically important; gallbladder cancer develops in fewer than 1 per cent of patients with cholelithiasis.

All but a few gallbladder carcinomas are adenocarcinoma, the remainder being squamous cell carcinoma. The earliest spread is usually by metastasis to the hilar lymph nodes and hepatic parenchyma and by direct extension to the liver and hilar structures. Distant metastases appear relatively late.

The patients present clinically in one of the following ways: (1) unremitting deep jaundice from common duct and hepatic involvement; (2) acute cholecystitis, usually with a palpable mass; (3) chronic cholecystitis with intermittent right upper quadrant pain; and (4) advanced disseminated carcinoma. The diagnosis is not often considered preoperatively, but in some instances clinical clues are present. In about two thirds of patients a mass can be felt, and in one third there is local tenderness. Gallbladder symptoms in patients 70 years or older are associated with carcinoma in about 10 per cent. In all but a few cases, the oral cholecystogram does not opacify, and even when it does, the tumor can rarely be demonstrated. Because the tumor becomes surgically incurable before it has grown very large, there is a strong correlation between presence of a palpable mass and incurability. More than half the patients have had chronic biliary symptoms for several years, and presumably earlier cholecystectomy in these would have avoided the development of carcinoma.

Surgery is indicated in most patients if for no more than diagnosis. Pathologic studies indicate that all apparent tumor would be removed in 25 per cent of cases by cholecystectomy, resection of a rim of adjacent liver, and dissection of the common duct lymph node chain. It is important that cases suitable for this procedure, especially relatively small tumors found incidentally during cholecystectomy for gallstone disease, not be overlooked. In some cases palliative procedures will relieve jaundice. Most cures have resulted from excision of the gallbladder with a tumor so small that it was unsuspected by the surgeon. Most patients live for only a few months after the diagnosis.

448.   BENIGN TUMORS AND PSEUDOTUMORS OF THE GALLBLADDER

This is a heterogeneous group of uncommon lesions with uncertain clinical significance. The roentgenographic appearance may be distinctive, especially for adenomyomatous hyperplasia, but often is not. A pathologic classification is presented in Table 3.

Adenomatous hyperplasia, consisting of mucosal thickening, may be focal or diffuse. Gallstones are present in some cases. The diagnosis cannot be made by x-ray.

Adenomyomatous hyperplasia, the most common lesion, has sometimes been called *adenomyomatosis, diverticulosis, cholecystitis glandularis proliferans*, or *cholecystitis cystica*. Focal, segmental, and diffuse forms exist, but the first of these is by far the most common. Most pathologists agree that the lesion is not neoplastic; the absence of cases in children argues against a congenital origin. Located invariably in the fundus, the focal form consists of a thick button of smooth muscle invaded by cystic mucosal glands and punctuated by a central umbilication. Some cases are associated with episodic pain that can be cured by cholecystectomy, but most often adenomyomatosis produces no symptoms.

Cholesterol polyps are a focal form of cholesterolosis consisting of submucosal histiocytes stuffed with cholesterol and located at a villous tip. Interestingly, diffuse cholesterolosis rarely gives rise to cholesterol polyps. The polyp is attached to the mucosa by a fragile stalk which can

TABLE 3.   Benign Tumors and Pseudotumors of Gallbladder — Classification

Benign pseudotumors:
1. Mucosal hyperplasia
    a. Adenomatous
    b. Adenomyomatous (adenomyoma)
2. Polyps
    a. Inflammatory
    b. Cholesterol
3. Mucosal heterotopia
4. Miscellaneous
    a. Fibroxanthogranulomatous inflammation
    b. Parasitic
    c. Other

Benign tumors:
1. Epithelial
    a. Adenoma, papillary
    b. Adenoma, nonpapillary
2. Supporting tissue
    a. Hemangioma
    b. Lipoma
    c. Leiomyoma
    d. Granular cell tumor

easily be broken. This has engendered speculation concerning a possible role for cholesterol polyps in the genesis of some cholesterol gallstones. Cholecystectomy is indicated if the patient has abdominal pain and no other apparent cause.

Papillary and *nonpapillary adenomas* are the only true benign neoplasms of the gallbladder seen with any frequency. Although the other lesions mentioned above clearly have no neoplastic potential, several cases of carcinoma have been reported in association with adenomas. It is doubtful, however, that many malignancies could arise in this way, because adenomas are rare compared with carcinoma of the gallbladder.

449.   MALIGNANT BILE DUCT TUMORS

The main cause of early morbidity from tumors of the bile duct is biliary obstruction with gradual hepatocellular damage or secondary hepatobiliary infection. Except for a rare squamous cell tumor, bile duct malignancies consist of adenocarcinoma with either a scirrhous or a papillary pattern. Grossly, three types of pathologic presentations occur: focal stricture, diffuse thickening, and nodular mass. The first two varieties can easily be mistaken for a benign process, such as post-traumatic stricture or sclerosing cholangitis. To further complicate differentiation, some tumors are so marked by desmoplasia that tumor cells may be hard to find in the extensive collagen stroma. In many cases, spread is confined to local lymph node metastases or hepatic invasion for months or years before there is more widespread abdominal or systemic involvement. The common hepatic duct or common bile duct is the site of origin in about two thirds of the cases. The eponym *Klatskin tumor* is often used in the United States to refer to adenocarcinoma at the bifurcation of the common hepatic duct. By contrast with carcinoma of the gallbladder, cholelithiasis is found in only one third of patients, and men slightly outnumber women. The average age at diagnosis is 70 years. A number of cases have been reported in younger patients with ulcerative colitis, and since some of these had previously undergone colectomy, it is thought that elimination of the ulcerated colon is not protective. Exposure to the chemical carcinogens benzidine, 3,3-dichlorobenzidine, and M-toluene-diamine has been etiologically implicated in some cases. Japanese- and Mexican-Americans are more often affected than whites in the United States. In the Orient, infestation with *Clonorchis sinensis* probably contributes to the higher incidence of *intrahepatic cholangiocarcinoma.*

CLINICAL MANIFESTATIONS. The typical patient presents with unremitting deep jaundice, mild deep-seated upper abdominal pain, and weight loss. Pruritus is reported by many, usually after the jaundice, but preceding it in some cases. Diarrhea, presumably from steatorrhea, is reported by some. Pain, which affects over half the patients, is not of an intensity or character to be confused with biliary colic. In the absence of previous surgery, fever and chills are rarely present. Hepatomegaly without splenomegaly is found on abdominal examination. Tumors of the common duct sparing the cystic duct generally produce in addition to jaundice a distended nontender palpable gallbladder (Courvoisier's law). Otherwise, the abdomen is unremarkable, because palpation of the tumor itself is almost never possible. Most patients have occult blood in the stool.

The serum bilirubin exceeds 10 mg per 100 ml in most cases, with a mean value of around 18 mg per 100 ml. The alkaline phosphatase is raised and SGOT may be slightly elevated, although rarely higher than 200. Serum proteins are most often normal. The prothrombin time may be depressed but responds to parenteral vitamin K. Serum cholesterol averages about 400 mg per 100 ml.

Ultrasound or CT scans show dilatation of the intrahepatic bile ducts. Transhepatic cholangiography demonstrates the site of the block and marked ductal dilatation. Only benign stricture of the duct is likely to create a similar radiographic picture, but if the patient has had no previous biliary surgery, benign stricture can be excluded.

Diagnostic confusion most often involves *primary biliary cirrhosis* and *jaundice* produced by *various drugs.* In neither of these does the bilirubin generally reach such high levels as with biliary tumors. Xanthelasma, found often with primary biliary cirrhosis, is only rarely seen with neoplastic obstruction. Antimitochondrial antibodies can be demonstrated in the serum of patients with primary biliary cirrhosis and are usually absent in those with neoplastic obstruction.

Choledocholithiasis and *biliary stricture* are less likely to present with steady deep jaundice and weight loss. The clinical finding in these conditions is fluctuating, milder jaundice, usually associated with fever. Transhepatic cholangiograms may exclude calculous obstruction or stricture.

TREATMENT. Unfortunately, complete excision of the tumor is not usually possible, because unexpendable anatomic structures are involved early despite the slow growth of most biliary tumors. Nevertheless, a few cures can be expected when radical surgery is judiciously employed; and with new techniques for re-establishing bile flow, palliation is of increasing importance.

With proximal lesions, the findings at surgery consist of a collapsed gallbladder and a small common duct. Not infrequently patients with tumors of the hepatic duct are subjected to at least one "negative" laparotomy before the problem is recognized. This could be largely obviated if operative cholangiograms that include the intrahepatic system were considered essential in abdominal exploration for jaundice.

Distal lesions require radical pancreaticoduodenectomy (Whipple procedure) for complete removal. Because the operation has a 15 per cent mortality, it should rarely be performed if tumor would be left behind. Tumors of the supraduodenal duct are sometimes amenable to complete resection. Those of the left hepatic duct require a left hepatectomy, but secondary involvement of the right hepatic duct means this is rarely possible.

For most cases the goal is palliation. Distal tumors can be bypassed by cholecystojejunostomy or other types of biliary-enteric anastomosis. For tumors at the junction of the hepatic ducts (Klatskin tumors) a polyethylene tube is placed in the duct to maintain bile flow by spanning the tumor; the hepatic end is brought out directly through the liver substance, and the duodenal end is brought out through a choledochotomy (the U-tube technique). In this way the tube can be replaced later without reoperation when debris begins to plug the lumen, as usually happens after six months or so. Holes in the intraductal portion of the tube allow bile to reach the gut from the liver.

PROGNOSIS. Cure is achieved in no more than 5 to 10 per cent, and survival is usually less than one year. If biliary drainage can be maintained, patients may survive for five to six years, even continuing their regular employment. Death eventually results from hepatic replacement with tumor or intrahepatic sepsis from recurrent ductal obstruction.

450. BENIGN TUMORS OF THE BILE DUCTS

The rare benign tumors of the bile ducts present with obstructive jaundice. *Papilloma*, the predominant morphologic type, is often multifocal and therefore difficult to cure. The next most common, *adenoma*, is more often localized. If the patient is an acceptable candidate, radical excision of the extrahepatic ducts is preferable to local currettement or limited resection.

451. POSTCHOLECYSTECTOMY SYNDROME

After cholecystectomy, a small percentage of patients continue to have significant abdominal symptoms. It was originally thought that in some cases this postoperative disability might result from the absence of the gallbladder; hence the name postcholecystectomy syndrome. To avoid cholecystectomy, cholecystolithotomy was tried for chronic cholecystitis by several groups of surgeons, but an unacceptably high incidence of recurrent gallstones and persistent symptoms stimulated a return to cholecystectomy.

In most patients, the explanation for continued postoperative symptoms is that the gallstone disease was not the cause of their preoperative complaints. Patients with biliary colic, a symptom rather specific for chronic cholecystitis, are more often relieved than those with the vague symptoms of fatty food intolerance, dyspepsia, or flatulence. Success of cholecystectomy also correlates with the extent of pathologic change in the gallbladder wall; patients with persistent symptoms more often had minimal scarring and a functioning gallbladder.

In others, postcholecystectomy complaints can be attributed to overlooked organic disease, especially *choledocholithiasis, pancreatitis, peptic ulcer,* or *irritable colon syndrome.* These possibilities must be investigated by appropriate studies.

Last is a group of clinical entities whose clinical significance, incidence, or even existence in some instances remains in dispute. *Stenosis of the sphincter of Oddi* (ampullary stenosis), *biliary dyskinesia, neuroma of the cystic duct stump,* and other cystic duct remnant lesions are the main examples.

Renewed interest in *ampullary stenosis* has followed the development of methods to perform sphincterotomy transendoscopically. Other than definite signs of common duct obstruction, no reliable diagnostic criteria have yet been presented for this condition. The visual appearance of the sphincter alone is insufficient. A provocative test has been used which involves injecting morphine (10 mg) and Prostigmin (1 mg) intramuscularly and using pain and a rise in serum amylase levels as positive indications of ampullary stenosis. The results of this test, however, do not correlate with sphincter of Oddi pressures, and the test is sometimes positive in normal subjects. Whether sphincter pressures measured transendoscopically will be any more reliable for diagnosing ampullary stenosis has yet to be determined. Clinicians should remain skeptical about the presence of this condition when the principal finding is abdominal pain. The diagnosis is more secure in patients with pancreatitis, cholangitis, recurrent choledocholithiasis, and a dilated bile duct, whose sphincter appears tight on x-ray and will only accept a small probe. Treatment consists of division of the sphincter at operation or transendoscopically.

Convincing evidence has been submitted to document the importance of each of the aforementioned conditions in specific cases, but as a group they are all uncommon. It should be appreciated in the management of patients with chronic abdominal pain that, in the absence of objective findings, exploratory laparotomy has a low rate of success for diagnosis and that surgical correction of minor variations in the gut anatomy usually fails to cure.

General

Schein, C. J.: Acute Cholecystitis. New York, Harper & Row, 1972.
Sleisenger, M. H., and Fordtran, J. S. (eds.): Gastrointestinal Disease. 2nd ed. Philadelphia, W. B. Saunders Company, 1978.

Specific

Adson, M. A.: Carcinoma of the gallbladder. Surg. Clin. North Am., 53:1203, 1973.
Blumgart, L. H., Carachi, R., Imrie, C. W., Benjamin, I. S., and Duncan, J. G.: Diagnosis and management of post-cholecystectomy symptoms: The place of endoscopy and retrograde choledochopancreatography. Br. J. Surg., 64:809, 1977.
Bodvall, B.: The postcholecystectomy syndromes. Clin. Gastroenterol., 2:103, 1973.

Bulow, S., Kronborg, O., and Lund-Kristensen, J.: Reappraisal of surgery for suppurative cholecystitis. Arch. Surg., 112:282, 1977.
Classen, M., and Ossenberg, F. W.: Progress report. Non-surgical removal of common bile duct stones. Gut, 18:760, 1977.
Foulk, W. T.: Congenital malformations of the intrahepatic biliary tree in the adult. Gastroenterology, 58:253, 1970.
Forker, E. L.: Mechanisms of hepatic bile formation. Ann. Rev. Physiol., 39:323, 1977.
French, E. B., and Robb, W. A. T.: Biliary and renal colic. Br. Med. J., 3:135, 1963.
Gregg, J. A., Taddeo, A. E., Milano, A. F., McCartney, A. J., Santoro, B. T., Frager, S. H., and Capobianco, A. G.: Duodenoscopy and endoscopic pancreatography in patients with positive morphine prostigmine tests. Am. J. Surg., 134:318, 1977.
Grundy, S. M., Metzger, A. L., and Adler, R. D.: Mechanisms of lithogenic bile formation in American Indian women with cholesterol gallstones. J. Clin. Invest., 51:3026, 1972.
Gunn, A., and Keddie, N.: Some clinical observations on patients with gallstones. Lancet, 2:7771, 1972.
Hofmann, A. F.: The enterohepatic circulation of bile acids in man. Adv. Intern. Med., 21:501, 1976.
Keighley, M. R. B., Drysdale, R. B., Quoraishi, A. H., Burdon, D. W., and Alexander-Williams, J.: Antibiotic treatment of biliary sepsis. Surg. Clin. North Am., 55:1379, 1975.
Kingston, R. W., and Windsor, C. W. O.: Flatulent dyspepsia in patients with gallstones undergoing cholecystectomy. Br. J. Surg., 62:231, 1975.
Koch, H., Rosch, W., Schaffner, O., and Demling, L.: Endoscopic papillotomy. Gastroenterology, 73:1393, 1977.
Longmire, W. P., Jr., McArthur, M. D., Bastounis, E. A., and Hiatt, J.: Carcinoma of the extrahepatic biliary tract. Ann. Surg., 178:333, 1973.
McArthur, P., Cuschieri, A., Sells, R. A., and Shields, R.: Controlled clinical trial comparing early with interval cholecystectomy for acute cholecystitis. Br. J. Surg., 62:850, 1975.
Metzger, A. L., Adler, R., Heymsfield, S., and Grundy, S. M.: Diurnal variation in biliary lipid composition: Possible role in cholesterol gallstone formation. N. Engl. J. Med., 288:333, 1973.
Mujahed, Z., Evans, J. A., and Whalen, J. P.: The nonopacified gallbladder on oral cholecystography. Radiology, 112:1, 1974.
Pereiras, R., Jr., Chiprut, R. O., Greenwald, R. A., and Schiff, E. R.: Percutaneous transhepatic cholangiography with the "skinny" needle. A rapid, simple, and accurate method in the diagnosis of cholestasis. Ann. Intern. Med., 86:562, 1977.
Prian, G. W., Norton, L. W., Eule, J., Jr., and Eiseman, B.: Clinical indications and accuracy of gray scale ultrasonography in the patient with suspected biliary tract disease. Am. J. Surg., 134:705, 1977.
Saharia, P. C., Zuidema, G. D., and Cameron, J. L.: Primary common duct stones. Ann. Surg., 185:598, 1977.
Schoenfield, L. J.: Stone dissolution and the national cooperative gallstone study. Dig. Dis., 22:1115, 1977.
Schwartz, S. I.: Primary sclerosing cholangitis. Surg. Clin. North Am., 53:1161, 1973.
Small, D. M., and Rapo, S.: Source of abnormal bile in patients with cholesterol gallstones. N. Engl. J. Med., 283:53, 1970.
Soloway, R. D., Trotman, B. W., and Ostrow, J. D.: Pigment gallstones. Gastroenterology, 72:167, 1977.
Terblanche, J., and Louw, J. H.: U tube drainage in the palliative therapy of carcinoma of the main hepatic duct junction. Surg. Clin. North Am., 53:1245, 1975.
Thistle, J. L., and Hofmann, A. F.: Efficacy and specificity of chenodeoxycholic acid therapy for dissolving gallstones. N. Engl. J. Med., 289:655, 1973.
van der Linden, W., and Sunzel, H.: Early versus delayed operation for acute cholecystitis. Am. J. Surg., 120:7, 1970.
Way, L. W.: Retained common duct stones. Surg. Clin. North Am., 53:1139, 1973.
Way, L. W., Admirand, W. H., and Dunphy, J. E.: Management of choledocholithiasis. Ann. Surg., 176:347, 1972.
Way, L. W., and Dunphy, J. E.: Biliary stricture. Am. J. Surg., 124:287, 1972.
Wenckert, A., and Robertson, B.: The natural course of gallstone disease. Gastroenterology, 50:376, 1966.

Section Thirteen DISEASES OF THE LIVER

Graham H. Jeffries

452. MECHANISMS OF HEPATIC DISEASE

An understanding of the pathophysiology of liver disease provides the basis for a rational clinical approach to the patient. The chapters that follow will review selective aspects of the biochemical and regulatory functions of the liver, the pathophysiology of clinical manifestations of liver disease, and the differential diagnosis and treatment of diseases of the liver.

JAUNDICE

Jaundice or *icterus* refers to a yellow discoloration of the skin or sclerae by bilirubin. Jaundice is usually apparent when the serum concentration of bilirubin exceeds 2 to 3 mg per 100 ml. Mucous membranes, colored by capillary blood, usually appear icteric only when serum bilirubin levels are considerably elevated. In patients with longstanding jaundice of the obstructive type, the skin may assume a greenish hue that is due in part to melanin pigmentation.

Bilirubin Metabolism

PRODUCTION. Bilirubin is a yellow tetrapyrrol pigment derived from heme-containing proteins. The hemoglobin of red blood cells is the major source of bilirubin (80 to 90 per cent). Normally, senescent red cells that have survived in the circulation for approximately 120 days are taken up by macrophages in the reticuloendothelial system (R-E system), and their hemoglobin is degraded to bilirubin. Biliverdin is an intermediate in the reactions that separate iron and protein (globin) from the molecule and open the tetrapyrrol ring at the α-methene bridge. The iron released from hemoglobin is stored in the R-E cells or is reutilized for heme synthesis.

When there is hemorrhage into tissues, the extravasated red cells are engulfed by macrophages which accumulate at the site of hemorrhage; the color changes of a subcutaneous hematoma reflect the conversion of hemoglobin to bilirubin.

Hemolytic disease states are usually accompanied by hyperplasia of the R-E system and an increased R-E cell production of bilirubin. When hemolysis is intravascular and hemoglobin is released into the blood, the pigment may be cleared by hepatic parenchymal cells or alternatively excreted by the renal glomeruli and reabsorbed by renal tubule cells; these parenchymal cells also have the capacity to degrade hemoglobin to bilirubin.

Small amounts of bilirubin are derived from the breakdown of hemoproteins other than hemoglobin — e.g., myoglobin and cytochromes. In studies on the incorporation of N^{15}-labeled glycine into the fecal pigment *stercobilin* (urobilin) that is derived from bilirubin, a small fraction (10 to 20 per cent) of labeled bile pigment was excreted within a few days of isotope administration. This "early-labeled" bile pigment is derived from the degradation of cytochromes, particularly in the liver, and from hemoglobin which escapes incorporation into peripheral red blood cells.

TRANSPORT AND DISTRIBUTION. Unconjugated bilirubin is a lipid-soluble molecule with minimal solubility in aqueous solution at the pH of plasma. The transport of bilirubin from the R-E cells and its subsequent distribution is determined by binding with plasma albumin; each albumin molecule has the capacity to bind two molecules of bilirubin. Unconjugated bilirubin, which is strongly albumin bound and thus nondialyzable, is not filtered by renal glomeruli and is not excreted in the urine. Conjugated bilirubin (see below) is water soluble and dialyzable from albumin solutions; in patients with obstructive jaundice and conjugated hyperbilirubinemia, the pigment is filtered and excreted in the urine. In patients with jaundice, bilirubin equilibrates between the intravascular and extravascular albumin pool. In the extravascular space, the pigment will distribute between tissue and plasma protein binding sites. Lipid-soluble, unconjugated bilirubin binds preferentially to albumin, and does not diffuse into cells other than the liver unless albumin binding sites are saturated (see Kernicterus in Ch. 454). The cerebrospinal and intraocular fluids do not become icteric in jaundiced patients.

HEPATIC UPTAKE AND EXCRETION. The transfer of bilirubin from plasma to bile can be divided into four steps: (1) passage from sinusoidal blood across the liver cell membrane, (2) concentration in the liver cell, (3) conjugation to diglucuronide, and (4) secretion into the bile canaliculus. The passage of bilirubin from albumin-bilirubin complexes in plasma across the plasma membrane into the liver cell is facilitated by low molecular weight binding proteins, designated Y and Z, in the liver cell cytoplasm. These intracellular binding proteins also bind other organic anions. In the liver cell, bilirubin is conjugated to form bilirubin diglucuronide. Conjugation with glucuronic acid is catalyzed by a microsomal enzyme, *glucuronyl transferase*, in the presence of uridine diphospho-glucuronic acid, and converts nonpolar, lipid-soluble, unconjugated bilirubin to a polar, water-soluble compound, which is excreted in bile.

The secretion of conjugated bilirubin from the liver cell across the membrane lining the bile canaliculi is an active process which is probably carrier mediated. *Conjugation of the pigment is a prerequisite for its secretion into the bile.* Normal bile contains only trace amounts of unconjugated bilirubin, and in the absence of bilirubin glucuronyl transferase (see Crigler-Najjar syndrome in Ch. 454), the bile is colorless, and bile pigment is excreted by unidentified metabolic pathways.

Although conjugated bilirubin and bile salts are

transported into the bile canaliculus by independent mechanisms, the rate of bilirubin secretion in bile is modulated by bile salt secretion. In patients with draining T tubes in the common bile duct following cholecystectomy, the output of conjugated bilirubin was related linearly to bile salt output; one third of bilirubin excretion was bile salt independent, and two thirds was bile salt associated.

INTESTINAL DEGRADATION. Bacterial enzymes in the distal small intestine and colon convert conjugated bilirubin to colorless urobilinogens, which are excreted predominantly in the feces but are partly reabsorbed in the ileum and colon. Reabsorbed urobilinogen is either cleared by the liver and re-excreted in bile or excreted in the urine.

Pathophysiology of Jaundice

Hyperbilirubinemia with jaundice may be due to one or several mechanisms that include excessive pigment production, reduced hepatic uptake or conjugation of bilirubin, or decreased excretion of the conjugated pigment.

EXCESSIVE BILIRUBIN PRODUCTION. *Hemolysis,* an excessive rate of red blood cell destruction, is the most common mechanism of excessive bilirubin production. In the normal subject, the low serum bilirubin concentration predominantly in the unconjugated fraction reflects the efficient hepatic clearance of the pigment. Hepatic bilirubin excretion may increase to maximal levels when pigment production is increased by hemolysis, but the serum concentration of bilirubin (predominantly unconjugated) rarely exceeds 3 to 5 mg per 100 ml unless hepatic excretion is impaired by reduced blood flow, impaired hepatocellular function, or ductal obstruction.

In some patients with unconjugated hyperbilirubinemia, bile pigment may be excreted in excess of the amount derived from peripheral red cell destruction. This is typical of thalassemia and pernicious anemia, but is sometimes unassociated with hemolytic disease. *Ineffective erythropoiesis* may account for excessive bilirubin production and jaundice in these patients. Although the "early-labeled" pigment excreted in bile is partly derived from the metabolism of heme enzymes (cytochromes) in the liver, there is currently no evidence that jaundice may result from increased hepatic metabolism of cytochromes.

REDUCED HEPATIC UPTAKE OF BILIRUBIN. A defect in the transfer of plasma bilirubin to the liver cell may explain the unconjugated hyperbilirubinemia in *Gilbert's syndrome* (see Ch. 454), after recovery from acute *viral hepatitis,* in congestive heart failure and after portacaval shunt surgery. Certain drugs may also competitively interfere with bilirubin uptake (iodopanoic acid, novobiocin).

REDUCED HEPATIC CONJUGATION OF BILIRUBIN. Bilirubin conjugation with glucuronic acid is essential for normal bilirubin excretion. A deficiency or inhibition of glucuronyl transferase activity causes unconjugated hyperbilirubinemia. *Neonatal jaundice* is commonly due to immaturity of the hepatic excretory system, particularly in premature infants. In the *Crigler-Najjar syndrome* (see Ch. 454), glucuronyl transferase activity is congenitally absent, the serum concentration of unconjugated bilirubin reaches high levels, and brain damage caused by deposition of pigment in the basal ganglia

(kernicterus) is usual. Rare patients have survived to adulthood.

Inhibition of glucuronyl transferase activity by a steroid excreted in maternal milk is an unusual cause for neonatal jaundice.

REDUCED EXCRETION OF CONJUGATED BILIRUBIN. The excretion of conjugated bilirubin into the bile canaliculus is an active transport process which may be impaired by a variety of processes. In the *Dubin-Johnson* and *Rotor syndromes* there is a congenital defect in hepatic excretion of conjugated bilirubin and other organic anions including sulfobromophthalein (BSP); the normal excretion of conjugated bile salts in these patients suggests a separate transport pathway. Impaired excretion may result from hepatocellular injury as in *virus hepatitis,* or may be due to *drugs* that interfere with cell metabolism or increase the permeability of the biliary tree (methyl testosterone, estrogens), compete for excretion in bile, or damage bile ductules (chlorpromazine). Inflammatory, granulomatous, or neoplastic *infiltration* of the liver and extrahepatic *bile duct obstruction* by gallstone, stricture, or carcinoma commonly interfere with bile excretion. The mechanism by which water-soluble, conjugated bilirubin enters the plasma in patients with impaired hepatic excretion is uncertain. The pigment either may be transferred across the liver cell directly into sinusoidal blood or may diffuse from bile ductules or canaliculi when the permeability of the biliary system is modified by disease.

Classification of Jaundice

Patients with jaundice may be subdivided clinically into two groups in which serum bilirubin is either predominantly unconjugated or conjugated. *Unconjugated hyperbilirubinemia* is due to excessive production, reduced uptake, or reduced conjugation of pigment, whereas *conjugated hyperbilirubinemia* may result from hepatocellular or biliary tract disease. The terms *hemolytic jaundice, hepatocellular jaundice,* and *obstructive jaundice* of intra- and extrahepatic types *(intra- and extrahepatic cholestasis)* are often used to describe these types of jaundice. *Cholestasis* refers to reduced bile flow and reduced excretion of bile constituents; pathologically, there is usually evidence of bile stasis with bile plugs in the canaliculi. Several of the mechanisms discussed previously may be responsible for jaundice in a particular patient. As an example, in acute viral hepatitis mild hemolysis may increase bilirubin production; parenchymal cell damage may impair uptake, conjugation, and excretion of pigment; and intrahepatic cholestasis resulting from disruption of bile canaliculi or inflammation may reduce bile excretion.

Fecal and Urinary Excretion of Bile Pigments

Unconjugated bilirubin, tightly bound to albumin and relatively nonpolar, cannot be dialyzed from plasma and does not pass the glomerular filter; jaundice with unconjugated hyperbilirubinemia is thus *acholuric.* Bilirubin diglucuronide, less avidly bound to plasma albumin, is partly dialyzable from plasma, and is excreted in the urine by glomerular filtration. In the presence of complete biliary obstruction, the urinary excretion of conjugated bilirubin will be equal to bilirubin production, and serum levels will stabilize at 15 to 25 mg per 100 ml; when bilirubin excretion is limited by both hepatobiliary and renal disease, higher serum bilirubin levels will result.

The quantity of bile pigment excreted as urobilinogens in feces and urine is a reflection of the amount of bilirubin in the bile, the bacterial conversion of bilirubin to urobilinogens, and the capacity of the liver to excrete urobilinogen absorbed from the intestine. *Fecal urobilinogen* is increased by excessive bilirubin production, and is reduced when hepatobiliary disease impairs bilirubin excretion or when bacterial conversion of bilirubin to urobilinogens is inhibited by antimicrobial therapy. *Urinary urobilinogen* is increased when greater amounts of urobilinogen are absorbed from the intestine or when parenchymal liver disease impairs the hepatic excretion of this pigment. Reduced urinary levels suggest cholestasis or impaired renal function.

PHYSICAL CHANGES OF THE DISEASED LIVER

Liver enlargement is usually an indication of disease. A normal liver displaced by a depressed diaphragm or a Riedel lobe must be considered in the differential diagnosis. An increase in liver size may reflect changes in liver cells (infiltration with fat or glycogen, or an increase in the smooth endoplasmic reticulum), cholestasis (intrahepatic or extrahepatic), venous congestion, inflammation (hepatitis) or abscess formation, cellular infiltration (macrophages in Gaucher's disease, granuloma in sarcoidosis, hematopoietic cells in extramedullary hematopoiesis, tumor cells in primary or secondary neoplasms), or fibrosis with regeneration (cirrhosis in the alcoholic). A *small liver* is characteristic of massive or multilobular necrosis with parenchymal collapse, and macronodular cirrhosis. The *consistency* of the liver may indicate the nature of the underlying disease. Infiltration and fibrosis cause induration; palpable *nodules* may be neoplasm, cysts, abscesses, or regeneration nodules. *Tenderness* may be due to acute enlargement or inflammation, and may be elicited by direct palpation or by percussion over the right lower ribs. Expansile *pulsation* of the congested liver results from tricuspid regurgitation. Vascular *bruits* over the liver may be due to arteriovenous fistulas, vascular tumors, or pressure on the aorta by an enlarged liver. *Friction rubs* are usually associated with neoplastic infiltration of the liver capsule and peritoneum, but may be due to peritonitis.

PORTAL HYPERTENSION

The normal flow of blood through the liver approximates 1.5 liters per minute (25 per cent of the cardiac output); portal venous inflow from the splanchnic circulation contributes approximately 1 liter per minute, and the hepatic artery 0.5 liter per minute. Portal venous and hepatic arterial blood combine in the periphery of the hepatic sinusoids and flow centrally to the central vein and hepatic venous system. Hepatic blood flow is normally phasic with a pressure gradient between portal vein and inferior vena cava of 0 to 5 mm Hg.
Portal hypertension, an increased pressure gradient across the liver (>10 to 12 mm Hg), may be due to an increased splanchnic blood flow, or to an increased resistance to blood flow through the liver.

An increase in splanchnic blood flow may be due to *arteriovenous fistulas*, either congenital or secondary to ruptured splenic or hepatic artery aneurysms. Massive *splenomegaly* in patients with *hematologic disorders* (polycythemia vera, agnogenic myeloid metaplasia, lymphoma, or leukemia) is sometimes associated with portal hypertension; both an increase in splenic blood flow and infiltration of hepatic sinusoids by hematopoietic cells or tumor cells contribute to the elevation of portal pressure. In patients with *tropical splenomegaly*, portal hypertension is also secondary to an increased splenic blood flow. Although an increase in splenic blood flow through arteriovenous shunts may contribute to portal hypertension in some patients with cirrhosis, the increase in vascular resistance across the liver is the major factor causing portal hypertension in these patients.

An increase in vascular resistance in the portal system is the most common cause for portal hypertension. The obstruction to blood flow may be localized to one or several sites: (1) prehepatic lesions of the splenic and/or portal veins; (2) intrahepatic, presinusoidal lesions which obstruct blood flow through the terminal branches of the portal vein; (3) parasinusoidal and postsinusoidal lesions which obstruct blood flow through sinusoids and hepatic vein tributaries; or (4) posthepatic lesions of the major hepatic veins. *Splenic and portal venous obstruction* is usually due to thrombosis complicating neoplasm (particularly pancreatic carcinoma), local inflammatory disease (including pancreatitis and abscess), conditions predisposing to thrombosis (e.g. polycythemia vera), abdominal surgery, and cirrhosis. In patients with cirrhosis, portal vein thrombosis may be a complication of portal hypertension or hepatoma. *Intrahepatic, presinusoidal portal obstruction* results from fibrosis within the portal triads. This is a common lesion in schistosomiasis. In patients with congenital hepatic fibrosis and in chronic arsenic or vinyl chloride toxicity, fibrosis may be confined to portal triads with preservation of the normal lobular architecture. Presinusoidal obstruction may also be due to biliary cirrhosis, Wilson's disease, and hepatic infiltration with neoplasm or granulomas. *Parasinusoidal and postsinusoidal obstruction* is usually seen in patients with acute alcoholic hepatitis or cirrhosis. Inflammation and fatty infiltration of the hepatic parenchyma may also impair sinusoidal blood flow. In veno-occlusive disease, inflammation and thrombosis of hepatic vein tributaries cause a postsinusoidal obstruction. *Posthepatic obstruction* of hepatic veins *(the Budd-Chiari syndrome)* is caused by thrombosis, by neoplastic obstruction (particularly hepatoma), or by congenital webs.

Manifestations

The manifestations of portal hypertension are *splenomegaly,* the development of a *collateral circulation,* and *ascites.*

SPLENOMEGALY. Splenic enlargement is commonly due to venous congestion, but may also result from lymphoid hyperplasia and cellular infiltration. The spleen is not always palpable in patients with portal hypertension, and, conversely, an enlarged spleen does not necessarily imply that a patient with liver disease has portal hypertension. Splenomegaly in cirrhotic patients is usually associated with an increased splenic artery blood flow.

PORTAL-SYSTEMIC COLLATERAL VESSELS. Collateral veins draining from the portal to the systemic venous system develop in response to an *increased pressure gradient* at sites of anastomosis between portal and systemic veins — in the esophagus and lower rectum, in the falciform ligament, in the retroperitoneal space, and in adhesions between the visceral and parietal peritoneum.

Esophageal collateral vessels between the left gastric and azygos veins develop as tortuous, dilated, thin-walled submucosal veins that may extend from the fundus of the stomach to the midesophagus (*esophageal* and *gastric varices*). Collateral vessels between the inferior mesenteric and internal iliac veins may form *hemorrhoids*. Collaterals from the left branch of the portal vein through patent umbilical or paraumbilical veins in the falciform ligament to the anterior abdominal wall may form a *caput medusae* — dilated, tortuous veins radiating from the umbilicus with centrifugal blood flow to epigastric, lateral thoracic, and saphenous vessels. A *venous hum* may be audible at the umbilicus (Cruveilhier-Baumgarten syndrome). These subcutaneous collaterals are most prominent when the patient is erect, and their origin from the portal system may be proved by showing that the glucose content of variceal blood exceeds that of peripheral venous blood during glucose absorption.

Acute upper gastrointestinal *bleeding from esophageal varices* is the major complication of portal hypertension.

ASCITES. Ascites is an accumulation of lymph in the peritoneal cavity. Hepatic and intestinal lymph normally drains through the thoracic duct into the left subclavian vein. Ascitic fluid accumulates when hepatic and intestinal lymph is formed in amounts that exceed the capacity of the thoracic duct to drain lymph from the abdomen. Two factors, *portal hypertension* and a *lowered plasma colloidal osmotic pressure*, contribute to the increased transudation of fluid from hepatic sinusoids and splanchnic capillaries in patients with liver disease. A third factor, *increased plasma aldosterone* concentration, augments sodium and water retention by promoting distal renal tubular reabsorption of sodium.

Portal hypertension caused by hepatic venous outflow tract obstruction (hepatic vein occlusion or cirrhosis), with *increased hepatic sinusoidal pressure*, is a major factor that determines the *selective* accumulation of fluid in the peritoneal cavity of patients with liver disease. Large volumes of hepatic lymph drain from congested sinusoids through dilated hilar lymphatic vessels to the thoracic duct, or may leak from lymphatic vessels in the capsule and hilum of the liver into the peritoneal cavity. In some patients, the ascitic fluid may be chylous due to the leakage of intestinal lymph containing chylomicrons.

Portal hypertension without sinusoidal hypertension rarely causes ascites unless acute bleeding from esophageal varices precipitates hypoalbuminemia and stimulates aldosterone secretion. (See Hepatic Schistosomiasis in Ch. 460.)

Hypoalbuminemia with a lowered plasma colloidal osmotic pressure increases fluid transudation from hepatic sinusoids and splanchnic capillaries, and thus augments lymph flow from these congested vascular beds. Hypoalbuminemic patients without portal hypertension, however, develop ascites only as a manifestation of fluid accumulation in dependent parts, as in the nephrotic syndrome.

In cirrhotic patients with ascites there are increased urinary excretion and plasma concentration of *aldosterone,* owing in part to an *increased adrenal secretion* of aldosterone and in part to *reduced hepatic metabolism* of the hormone. Although it has been shown that inferior vena caval obstruction proximal to the hepatic veins in the dog stimulates aldosterone secretion, the exact mechanism of *secondary hyperaldosteronism* in patients with cirrhosis and portal hypertension has not been defined. A relative pooling of blood in the splanchnic bed with reduced renal blood flow may be the primary stimulus for the release of *renin* from the juxtaglomerular cells in the kidney and the subsequent secretion of salt-retaining hormone; it has been shown, however, that the elevated plasma levels of renin in patients with cirrhosis and ascites are depressed by beta-adrenergic blocking drugs, whereas aldosterone levels remain unchanged. Stimuli which normally cause aldosterone release (bleeding, infection, and diuretic therapy) will augment the secondary hyperaldosteronism of liver disease.

Ascites in patients with cirrhosis is sometimes precipitated by *bacterial peritonitis (E. coli, Strep. pneumoniae, M. tuberculosis)* or *tumor* invasion of the peritoneal cavity. These complications must be considered in the differential diagnosis (see below).

The clinical manifestations of ascites are increasing *abdominal distention* with *weight gain* and an associated *decrease in urine output*. Distention of the abdominal wall may cause pain over the lower ribs at the insertion of the abdominal muscles, and may promote the formation of umbilical and inguinal hernias. On physical examination there may be *shifting dullness, a fluid wave,* and *elevation of the diaphragms.* Ascitic fluid may leak through the diaphragm to create a *pleural effusion;* this is more often seen on the right than on the left. The urinary excretion of sodium is considerably decreased and may be less than 1 mEq in 24 hours, whereas urinary potassium excretion is increased.

NEUROPSYCHIATRIC ABNORMALITIES ASSOCIATED WITH LIVER DISEASE

The neuropsychiatric manifestations of acute alcohol intoxication, prolonged excessive use of alcohol, alcohol withdrawal, vitamin deficiency in alcoholics, and head injury are often encountered in patients with cirrhosis. These are considered in Ch. 250. *Wilson's disease* (see Ch. 537) is important in the differential diagnosis of chronic active hepatitis or cirrhosis in young patients.

Hepatic Coma and Precoma
(Hepatic Encephalopathy, Portal-Systemic Encephalopathy)

Patients with acute or chronic liver disease may develop a *metabolic encephalopathy* characterized by a variable disturbance of consciousness, psychiatric changes, a flapping tremor with hyperreflexia and increased muscle tone, hyperventilation with respiratory alkalosis, and a typical fetor.

PATHOGENESIS. Hepatic coma is associated with impaired hepatic detoxification of endogenous and exogenous substances and variable shunting of portal venous blood through collateral vessels into the peripheral circulation. There may be an accumulation of toxic substances which impair cerebral function or a lack of substances which are necessary for cerebral function. Of the several factors that may contribute to this metabolic encephalopathy, changes in *ammonium metabolism* have been studied most extensively. An increase in blood ammonium concentration parallels the severity of neuropsychiatric changes in cirrhotic patients with *chronic* encephalopathy after portacaval anastomosis. This increase in blood ammonium concentration resulting from enteric absorption of ammonia formed by bacterial deamination of amino acids or urea hydrolysis may be the major biochemical change that precipitates dysfunction of the central nervous system. In patients with *acute* hepatic coma, however, disturbances of ammonium metabolism may be of lesser importance, and blood ammonium levels may be normal.

Other agents which may impair central nervous system function in cirrhotic patients include *short chain fatty acids* (from the diet or from bacterial metabolism of carbohydrate) and bacterial metabolites of protein and amino acids, particularly *biogenic amines* (octopamine) which may function as false neurotransmitters.

The central nervous system of the patient with liver disease may be more susceptible to a variety of metabolic insults. Thus *hypoxia, electrolyte* and *acid-base imbalance, infection,* and *depressant drugs* may each contribute to metabolic encephalopathy in these patients. Although there may be changes in the serum concentration of electrolytes, elevation of blood ammonium concentration, and/or altered blood pH in patients with hepatic coma, these changes do not necessarily parallel electrolyte and pH changes and ammonium concentrations in the central nervous system. These changes *within the brain* are of primary importance in precipitating encephalopathy; alkalosis, which favors the diffusion of ammonia across the blood-brain barrier, increases ammonia toxicity. In patients with hepatic encephalopathy, there is a decrease in cerebral metabolism and oxygen utilization. There is evidence in animal experiments that ammonia inhibits oxidative phosphorylation and the maleate-aspartate hydrogen shuttle in the brain, and depresses the concentration of phosphocreatine, adenosine triphosphate, glutamate, and aspartate.

CLINICAL FEATURES. The neuropsychiatric changes in hepatic encephalopathy are nonspecific. One of the more characteristic features of the metabolic encephalopathy associated with liver disease is its *rapid fluctuation. Disturbances of consciousness* may range from mild lethargy to deep coma. *Personality changes,* with depression or euphoria, irritability, anxiety, and paranoid features, together with a loss of concern for person or property, are evident. Intellectual function is variably impaired with *memory loss, inability to concentrate,* and a loss of the capacity for abstract thought. Speech may be slow and slurred, with a loss of modulation, and writing deteriorates; there may be dysphasia, perseveration, and apraxia. The common neurologic changes are asterixis, a "flapping" tremor of the outstretched hands, an increase in muscle tone, hyper-reflexia with clonus — often with flexor plantar responses — and ataxia. Hyperventilation causes respiratory alkalosis. The electroencephalogram shows the nonspecific changes of metabolic encephalopathy; high amplitude delta waves (2 to 3 per second) replace normal alpha waves.

Fetor hepaticus is a characteristic sweet, musty odor of the breath attributed to the excretion of mercaptans,

particularly dimethylsulfide. Mercaptans produced by bacterial degradation of methionine escape hepatic detoxification and are excreted in excessive amounts in cirrhotic patients.

The *clinical course* of hepatic encephalopathy varies with its pathogenesis. In patients with *fulminant hepatitis* there is a rapid progression; mania and convulsions may precede the development of decerebrate rigidity and terminal deep coma. In patients with cirrhosis, encephalopathy may be acute or chronic and of varying severity. Chronic encephalopathy usually improves with therapy (see below), but may progress to permanent neuropsychiatric syndromes (paraplegia, dementia) over a period of years.

CLINICAL MANIFESTATIONS RESULTING FROM IMPAIRED HEPATIC DETOXIFICATION

The liver cell is the major site of detoxification of many drugs and exogenous substances and of endogenous substances, including hormones. In general, by processes of oxidation, reduction, hydrolysis, or conjugation, mediated by enzymes in the smooth endoplasmic reticulum, relatively lipid-soluble substances are converted to water-soluble compounds that may be excreted in bile or urine. Several agents (e.g., phenobarbital) stimulate the hepatic metabolism of drugs; prolonged phenobarbital administration is associated with hyperplasia of the smooth endoplasmic reticulum and an increase in activity of the hepatic microsomal drug metabolizing enzyme systems. Changes in drug metabolism induced by agents which activate microsomal metabolism, as well as genetically determined differences in drug metabolism (e.g., slow and fast acetylation), are of major clinical importance.

CHANGES IN DRUG METABOLISM IN LIVER DISEASE. Liver disease may modify drug metabolism through several mechanisms. *Changes in the plasma binding* of drugs (e.g., by lowered serum albumin levels) will modify the concentration of free drug in plasma and will thus affect drug distribution, action, and clearance. *Decrease in hepatic blood flow* (e.g., following a portacaval shunt) will depress the clearance of those agents that are rapidly extracted by the liver, but will not modify the clearance of poorly extracted agents. *Parenchymal cell damage* (e.g., in viral hepatitis) or *decrease in parenchymal cell mass* (e.g., in cirrhosis) is usually associated with a decreased capacity to metabolize drugs. *Cholestasis,* either intrahepatic or extrahepatic, will reduce the hepatic clearance of drugs that are normally secreted in bile; the hepatic metabolism of drugs, however, may remain unaffected by cholestasis.

Conventional tests of liver function correlate poorly with changes in drug clearance and metabolism in patients with liver disease. Agents that are metabolized or excreted by the liver should be administered cautiously to patients with liver disease, and drug therapy should be guided by the clinical response and by measurements of blood levels of the agent.

ENDOCRINE CHANGES. The liver has a dual role in the metabolism of hormones. Several plasma proteins, alpha globulins, which bind hormones in the plasma, e.g., *thyroxine-binding protein, transcortin,* are synthesized by the liver; hormone activity may be influenced by protein binding in the plasma. Thyroxine and adrenal and gonadal steroid hormones are conjugated in the liver and partly excreted in bile. Conjugation forms polar, water-soluble molecules that have an enterohepatic circulation and are finally excreted in the urine.

Endocrine abnormalities in patients with liver disease may be due to malnutrition or chronic illness, to specific lesions of the endocrine glands (iron infiltration in hemochromatosis), or to altered hepatic metabolism, conjugation, and excretion of hormones by the diseased liver. Disturbances of gonadal function are particularly common in alcoholic patients with or without cirrhosis. In males, there may be *hypogonadism*, with small testes, reduced libido and impotence, *gynecomastia*, and delayed development or regression of secondary sex characteristics. Depressed plasma levels of unbound 17β-hydroxy-androgens (particularly testosterone) with normal plasma levels of unbound estradiol have been documented in these patients with gynecomastia. The changes in hormone levels in the male alcoholic with cirrhosis suggest both primary testicular failure and a depression of hypothalamic-pituitary regulatory function. In females there may be delayed menarche, oligomenorrhea, or amenorrhea with subnormal breast development. Normal cyclic hormonal activity is disturbed, and cessation of ovulation leads to sterility.

Cutaneous *striae, acne,* and *hirsutism* with truncal obesity and moon facies may suggest *Cushing's syndrome*. Although plasma cortisol levels may be slightly elevated in these patients, the urinary excretion of hydroxy- and ketosteroids is either normal or subnormal.

The appearance of some alcoholic patients with cirrhosis may suggest *hyperthyroidism*. There may be a tremor, peripheral vasodilatation with sweating, tachycardia, and a slight stare. The plasma level of thyroxine is usually normal in these patients.

NUTRITIONAL AND METABOLIC ABNORMALITIES IN LIVER DISEASE

Weight loss may be due to malabsorption, reduced caloric intake in patients with anorexia, or increased tissue catabolism in acutely ill febrile patients. The chronic alcoholic, deriving a major fraction of his calories from alcohol, consumes a diet that may be deficient in protein, folic acid, ascorbic acid, B vitamins, and minerals. Although body weight may be maintained by alcohol and carbohydrate, *muscle wasting* with progressive weakness is usual. *Hypokalemia*, magnesium deficiency, or alcoholic *myopathy* may accentuate muscle weakness in some patients.

CARBOHYDRATE METABOLISM. The liver has a central role in regulating blood sugar levels. During carbohydrate absorption, the monosaccharides glucose, fructose, and galactose are taken up from portal venous blood by liver cells, phosphorylated in the presence of specific hexokinases, and converted to glycogen or metabolized through pyruvate and Krebs cycle intermediates. During periods of fasting, or with secretion of epinephrine and glucagon, glycogenolysis or gluconeogenesis maintains or increases blood sugar levels.

Symptomatic *hypoglycemia* may occur in liver disease when hepatic glycogenolysis and gluconeogenesis are impaired. When liver glycogen stores are depleted by fasting, the ingestion of alcohol, which inhibits gluconeogenesis, may precipitate hypoglycemia (*alcoholic hypoglycemia*). Lowered blood sugar levels also result from massive hepatic necrosis (fulminant hepatitis) or a deficiency of enzymes necessary for glycogenolysis (glycogen storage diseases).

Diabetes mellitus in patients with cirrhosis is often due to associated pancreatic disease (chronic alcoholic pancreatitis, or hemochromatosis), or may be coincidental. Portal-systemic shunting is associated with a higher frequency of diabetes mellitus; plasma glucagon levels are significantly elevated in these patients. Cirrhotic patients often have an abnormal glucose tolerance curve owing to a reduced rate of glucose uptake and release from the diseased liver. Normal fasting blood sugar levels, with prolonged hyperglycemia and late hypoglycemia after a glucose load, are characteristic.

TRIGLYCERIDE METABOLISM. Postprandially, dietary triglyceride enters the circulation as a lipid emulsion (chyle) from the thoracic duct (fatty acids of chain length greater than C10), or passes directly as fatty acid into the portal venous blood (fatty acids of chain length less than C10). During periods of fasting, free fatty acid (FFA) is mobilized from peripheral fat depots and circulates as an albumin-FFA complex. Plasma FFA or triglyceride entering the liver cell is stored as triglyceride droplets, incorporated into plasma lipoproteins and thus transported to peripheral depots or catabolized to ketone bodies for peripheral utilization.

Triglyceride accumulates in the liver whenever there is excessive peripheral mobilization of fat (e.g., in uncontrolled diabetes mellitus) or when liver cell injury prevents the normal metabolism of triglyceride (e.g., in carbon tetrachloride or yellow phosphorus poisoning). A fatty liver is commonly found in obese subjects, in patients with protein-calorie malnutrition (kwashiorkor), in diabetics, and in alcoholics. The disturbances in triglyceride metabolism caused by acute and chronic alcohol ingestion are discussed in Ch. 465.2.

CHOLESTEROL AND BILE ACIDS. Cholesterol synthesized in the liver is incorporated into plasma lipoproteins, excreted directly into bile, or converted to primary bile acids.

Plasma lipoproteins, containing varying amounts of cholesterol (both free and esterified), phospholipid, triglyceride, and specific proteins are synthesized by the liver and intestinal epithelium. Cholestasis causes an increase in plasma cholesterol concentration; this is associated with an increase in high density lipoprotein with a high content of cholesterol and phospholipid. This does not cause a lipemic serum. Liver failure with impaired hepatic synthesis depresses serum concentrations of lipoprotein and cholesterol.

Cholesterol is excreted in bile as a micellar solution with conjugated bile salt and phospholipid. Changes in the concentration of these compounds may lead to the formation of gallstones (see Ch. 440 to 444).

The primary bile acids (cholic and chenodeoxycholic acids) are synthesized from cholesterol and are secreted in bile as their glycine and taurine conjugates (bile salts). These conjugated bile salts undergo an enterohepatic circulation with active reabsorption from the distal small intestine and efficient clearance from portal venous blood during a single passage through the liver. Between 20 and 30 grams of conjugated bile salts are thus excreted in bile and reabsorbed daily; the daily fecal loss of bile acids (approximately 1 gram) is balanced by resynthesis from cholesterol.

The conjugated bile salts have important functions that depend on their detergent properties. In the bile they permit the formation of soluble micelles containing cholesterol; in the intestinal lumen they activate pancreatic lipase and form mixed micelles with monoglyceride and long-chain fatty acids, thus facilitating the absorption of fat and fat-soluble vitamins.

The concentration of bile salts in the peripheral blood is very low in normal fasting subjects, and increases slightly after a meal. When the hepatic clearance of bile salts is depressed by cholestasis, parenchymal cell injury, or portal-systemic shunting, peripheral blood levels are increased.

Liver disease may be complicated by *malabsorption* when biliary secretion of conjugated bile salts is insufficient to promote the formation of lipid micelles in the jejunum. The duration of malabsorption in patients with acute liver disease may be too short to cause deficiency states other than *hypoprothrombinemia* owing to malabsorption of vitamin K. In patients with chronic cholestasis (primary and secondary biliary cirrhosis, Ch. 465.2) steatorrhea may cause diarrhea and weight loss, and malabsorption of fat-soluble vitamins A, D, and K may lead to night blindness, bone demineralization, and hypoprothrombinemia.

PROTEIN METABOLISM. The liver cell contains enzyme systems that permit the synthesis of nonessential amino acids, synthesis of cellular and plasma proteins from amino acids, catabolism of plasma protein and amino acids, and conversion of ammonia to urea.

Amino acids derived from digested dietary proteins are absorbed in the upper small intestine, enter the portal venous blood, and are almost completely cleared by the liver to be catabolized or utilized in protein synthesis. During periods of fasting, amino acids are converted to pyruvate and phosphorylated hexose intermediates, which support gluconeogenesis and provide a source of glucose for brain metabolism.

Perfusion studies have shown that the liver is responsible for the synthesis of plasma proteins, with the exception of the immunoglobulins and factor VIII. The factors which control protein synthesis are not well understood. Experimental studies suggest that the colloidal osmotic pressure of plasma has a regulatory function; albumin synthesis is depressed in laboratory animals or isolated liver preparations when the colloidal osmotic pressure of plasma is increased with dextran or gamma globulin. Adequate nutrition is essential for normal plasma protein synthesis; liver perfusion studies have shown that amino acids exert a specific role in activating albumin synthesis, whereas ethanol has a depressant effect.

The sites of plasma protein degradation and the factors which regulate this are unknown. Studies with labeled albumin indicate that catabolism is in proportion to the total albumin pool. Catabolism by the liver, kidney, and gastrointestinal tract is well documented, but explains only a fraction of the total albumin catabolized daily.

Plasma proteins maintain the colloidal osmotic pressure of plasma, play a vital role in the transport of many substances (including iron, vitamin B_{12}, hormones, hemoglobin, bilirubin, and nonesterified fatty acids), and maintain normal blood clotting mechanisms. The clinical manifestations of depressed plasma protein synthesis include *hypoproteinemia* with *edema* and prolonged *prothrombin time* with increased risk of *bleeding*. Excessive urinary excretion and elevated plasma levels of amino acids are manifestations of severe hepatocellular failure, particularly fulminant hepatitis.

Acute or chronic liver disease may reduce the capacity of the liver to synthesize urea from ammonia; elevated peripheral blood ammonia levels correlate with impaired urea synthesis, particularly when the ammonia load is increased by gastrointestinal bleeding or a high protein intake.

HEMATOLOGIC ABNORMALITIES

Anemia in patients with liver disease may be due to *blood loss* or *excessive destruction* and/or *reduced formation* of red cells. Changes in red cell morphology may reflect specific deficiency (iron or folic acid) or may result from changes in the lipid composition of the red cell membrane. Red blood cells from patients with cholestasis have an increased surface area related to the reversible accumulation of cholesterol from the plasma; these cells have a lowered osmotic fragility, and appear as target-cells on stained smears. Severe hemolysis in the alcoholic with liver disease may be associated with the appearance of poikilocytes (burr-cells) on peripheral smears.

Bleeding from the nose, upper gastrointestinal tract (esophageal varices, erosive gastritis, or peptic ulcer), or rectum (hemorrhoids) may precipitate acute anemia or chronic iron deficiency anemia. In the absence of blood loss, iron deficiency is uncommon in patients with liver disease; an increase in total body iron with hemosiderosis is more usual, particularly in alcoholic patients with pancreatic disease. The pathogenesis of this secondary hemosiderosis is not known.

Uncompensated hemolysis is the most common cause of chronic anemia in patients with liver disease. Chronic, low-grade hemolysis in patients with splenomegaly is due to sequestration of red blood cells in the cortex of the congested spleen. Red cell production may fail to compensate for this increased destruction, particularly during periods of hepatic decompensation, so that the patient may exhibit a normochromic and sometimes macrocytic anemia with a normal reticulocyte count, reduced serum levels of haptoglobin, an increased serum level of unconjugated bilirubin, and a bone marrow showing cellular hyperplasia. Severe hemolytic anemia may be associated with hyperlipemia in alcoholic hepatitis (*Zieve's syndrome*) (see Ch. 465.2), but a causal relationship between the hyperlipemia and hemolysis has not been established. Acute viral hepatitis may precipitate hemolysis in patients with *glucose-6-phosphate dehydrogenase (G-6-PD) deficiency*; particularly high serum concentrations of bilirubin usually result.

A *deficiency of folic acid* may lead to a severe macrocytic anemia with *megaloblastic* bone marrow in alcoholic patients with liver disease. An inadequate vitamin intake, together with alcohol inhibition of folic acid utilization, contributes to the anemia. Treatment with a normal diet containing folic acid or with folic acid supplements corrects this deficiency. Rarely, a normochromic normocytic anemia may be due to *pyridoxine deficiency*.

Although *thrombocytopenia* (platelet counts less than 200,000 per cubic millimeter) and *granulocytopenia* (WBC counts <4000 per cubic millimeter) may be associated with anemia in patients with liver disease and congestive splenomegaly, these abnormalities are rarely complicated by serious bleeding or infection. Severe thrombocytopenia and fatal aplastic anemia have been reported as complications of acute viral hepatitis.

Clotting abnormalities in patients with acute or chronic liver disease result from reduced synthesis of blood-clotting factors or their increased consumption. Many of the factors active in blood clotting — factors V, VII, IX, X, prothrombin, and fibrinogen — are synthesized by the liver. A lowered plasma concentration of these proteins, measured by blood-clotting tests (see Ch. 519), may be due to *malabsorption of vitamin K* which is required for the synthesis of prothrombin and factors VII, IX, and X, or may reflect *impaired hepatic protein synthesis*. Vitamin K malabsorption results from obstructive jaundice. Hepatic parenchymal disease, either acute or chronic, depresses the synthesis of clotting factors. The capacity of liver cells to produce fibrinogen appears to exceed that of other clotting factors, so that fibrinogen levels are often maintained when other clotting factors are deficient; fibrin polymerization, however, is often abnormal in patients with severe liver disease. *Intravascular coagulation* with consumption of clotting factors, thrombocytopenia, and the appearance of fibrin split products in the plasma is a complication of fulminant hepatitis, decompensated cirrhosis, and metastatic cancer.

IMMUNE PHENOMENA IN LIVER DISEASE

Hypergammaglobulinemia is a common manifestation of *chronic active hepatitis, idiopathic cirrhosis,* and *primary biliary cirrhosis*. The gamma globulin increase is *polyclonal*, involving all classes of immunoglobulin (IgA, IgM, and IgG), although in primary biliary cirrhosis IgM may be increased selectively. Hypergammaglobulinemia is often associated with positive serologic tests for syphilis, heterophil antibody, antinuclear antibody, antimitochondrial antibody, and LE cell phenomena. Furthermore the titers of antibody against bacterial and viral antigens may be increased. The increase in circulating immunoglobulin in patients with liver disease usually reflects disease activity, particularly in chronic active hepatitis. The liver is usually infiltrated with lymphocytes and plasma cells in areas of parenchymal cell necrosis.

The role of *immunologic mechanisms* in the *pathogenesis* of chronic liver disease has not been fully established. Immune phenomena may be secondary to the release of antigens from damaged liver cells, or, alternatively, local immunologic processes (both humoral and cell mediated) may play an active role in destroying liver cells. The association between chronic liver disease, chronic thyroiditis, and Sjögren's syndrome suggests that autoimmune phenomena may indeed be important in pathogenesis (see Ch. 465). Depression of *serum complement* levels in patients with chronic liver disease cannot be correlated with immune phenomena, but appears to be related to impaired hepatic protein synthesis.

CARDIOVASCULAR CHANGES

Hepatocellular failure is often associated with an *increase* in *cardiac output* manifested by tachycardia, a precordial ejection systolic murmur, and peripheral vasodilatation. The cause for these circulatory changes is not known.

Some patients with cirrhosis exhibit central *cyanosis* with arterial oxygen unsaturation. In patients with portal hypertension, this may be due to portopulmonary venous shunts that bypass the pulmonary capillaries, or may

result from increased blood flow through dilated pulmonary vessels and arteriovenous communications.

The plasma volume is usually normal or increased in cirrhotic patients prior to diuretic therapy. When patients with ascites are treated with diuretic agents, brisk diuresis is often accompanied by a fall in plasma volume which is particularly marked when fluid loss exceeds the volume of fluid mobilized from the ascitic pool. Hypovolemic shock may be a terminal complication of cirrhosis, precipitated by massive bleeding, by infection (especially gram-negative septicemia), or by paracentesis. Metabolic acidosis with hyperkalemia and hyponatremia is a terminal event.

CHANGES IN RENAL FUNCTION

There are many causes for impairment of renal function in patients with liver disease. Many agents may cause acute cellular injury in both liver and kidneys; these include *hepatotoxins* (carbon tetrachloride, *Amanita phalloides*), *infectious agents* (leptospirosis, infectious hepatitis virus; see below), and *hypoxia* (shock). *Metabolic disease* may damage both organs; in Wilson's disease the deposition of copper in the tissues is associated with cirrhosis and impaired tubular reabsorptive function with glycosuria, aminoaciduria, and hypouricemia.

In patients with cirrhosis and ascites several factors modify renal function. There may be a physiologic response to secondary hyperaldosteronism with sodium retention and potassium excretion, reversed by aldosterone-blocking drugs (see below). Abnormal excretion of a water load usually accompanies cirrhosis with ascites.

HEPATORENAL SYNDROME. This term refers to the functional renal failure which is a common terminal event in patients with cirrhosis and ascites, and a less common complication of obstructive jaundice after surgery. Progressive azotemia with hyperkalemia and hyponatremia, a reduced creatinine clearance, and progressive oliguria with a concentrated urine free of protein and formed elements and low in sodium are usually observed. Spontaneous recovery is rare. At postmortem examination, no significant pathologic changes are present in the kidneys.

The functional renal failure in patients with cirrhosis and ascites has been attributed to a decrease in renal blood flow resulting from hypovolemia after vigorous diuresis, abdominal paracentesis, or massive bleeding. Alternatively, increased renal rein pressure caused by increased intra-abdominal pressure was suggested as a mechanism. Although hypovolemia will contribute to renal failure, these mechanisms do not explain this syndrome. Studies of renal blood flow by isotope scanning and by renal arteriography have demonstrated an intrarenal shunting of blood with reduced cortical perfusion in cirrhotic patients with ascites and reduced creatinine clearance. Vasoconstriction of cortical vessels reduces glomerular perfusion, although total renal blood flow may remain normal. The agents which cause cortical vasoconstriction have not been identified, but it is known that sympathetic blocking agents do not restore cortical flow.

When a cirrhotic patient with ascites develops the hepatorenal syndrome, increasing jaundice results from decreased bilirubin excretion in the urine, and azotemia with increased blood ammonia levels usually precipitates hepatic coma.

CUTANEOUS MANIFESTATIONS OF LIVER DISEASE

PRURITUS. Patients with obstructive jaundice (both intrahepatic and extrahepatic cholestasis) may suffer from generalized itching. This is unrelated to the intensity of jaundice; patients with primary biliary cirrhosis may develop severe pruritus prior to the onset of jaundice, whereas deeply jaundiced patients with hepatocellular failure may remain asymptomatic. The hypothesis that pruritus results from retained bile salts is consistent with the therapeutic effect of cholestyramine; itching is controlled when the binding of bile salts in the intestine lowers plasma levels. A recent study, however, showed that there was no correlation between pruritus and the concentration of bile salts in the plasma or skin of patients with cholestasis. Thus the pathogenesis of pruritus remains undefined.

PIGMENTATION. An increase in *melanin pigmentation* of the skin is typical of chronic obstructive jaundice (biliary cirrhosis) and in hemochromatosis. The pathogenesis is not known.

SPIDER ANGIOMAS (VASCULAR SPIDERS). These cutaneous lesions, found in areas drained by the superior vena cava, have a central pulsating arteriole from which small vessels radiate over an area 1 to 10 mm in diameter. Multiple lesions may appear and disappear during the course of both acute and chronic liver disease, but are most numerous when liver disease is chronic and progressive. Small arterial spiders are also seen in normal subjects, and often appear during pregnancy. Their pathogenesis is not known.

PALMAR ERYTHEMA. Cutaneous erythema, maximal over the thenar and hypothenar eminences and the pulp of the fingers and less often seen on the soles of the feet, is due to local vasodilatation with increased blood flow. The cardiac output is usually increased in patients with prominent palmar erythema.

Other changes in the hands include *Dupuytren's contractures* in patients with cirrhosis associated with alcohol ingestion, *clubbing* of the nails in patients with biliary cirrhosis, and white, opaque nails with loss of lunulae in hypoalbuminemic patients.

XANTHOMAS. Prolonged obstructive jaundice with elevation of serum lipoprotein may be associated with deposits of lipid, predominantly cholesterol, in macrophages in the dermis or subcutaneous tissue. Flat lesions (*xanthelasma*) are common on the eyelids, on the neck, and in the palm creases, as yellow, slightly raised, soft deposits. Tuberous lesions, more common over areas exposed to pressure, are firm, nodular, and slightly yellow. These lesions may appear when serum cholesterol levels exceed 450 mg per 100 ml for several months, and may disappear when serum cholesterol levels falls below that value.

NONSPECIFIC SYMPTOMS IN PATIENTS WITH LIVER DISEASE

Many symptoms in patients with liver disease are also common manifestations of nonhepatic disorders. It is often impossible to determine whether these symptoms are primarily due to liver disease or whether they result from extrahepatic effects of the primary noxious agent. The prodromal symptoms of acute viral hepatitis — malaise, weakness, unusual fatigability, anorexia, fever, myalgia, and headache — are good examples. Although these symptoms are nonspecific, they are often helpful in differential diagnosis.

FEVER. Fever is common in patients with acute liver disease and is usually due to tissue necrosis, infection, or drug hypersensitivity. In patients with acute metabolic encephalopathy, fever may be due to dysfunction of central thermoregulatory mechanisms. This usually occurs in fulminant hepatitis and in the alcoholic with a severe withdrawal reaction (delirium tremens).

ABDOMINAL PAIN. Abdominal pain may be localized to the right upper quadrant and may result from inflammation or stretching of the pain-sensitive capsule of the liver. Epigastric or midabdominal pain may be due to associated peptic ulcer disease, acute gastritis, or pancreatitis. Stretching of the abdominal wall by tense ascites may cause pain over the lower costal margin.

453. DIAGNOSTIC PROCEDURES

TESTS OF LIVER FUNCTION

Many biochemical tests have been used to estimate liver function. In interpreting tests of liver function one must remember that no test is diagnostic of specific liver lesion, that many tests may be normal in the presence of liver disease, and that factors other than liver disease may cause abnormal tests.

SERUM BILIRUBIN. Spectrophotometric measurement of the amount of diazo-pigment formed by the van den Bergh reaction after one minute in the absence of alcohol gives an estimate of the *direct-reacting* serum bilirubin concentration; this is approximately equal to the serum concentration of *conjugated bilirubin*, which is diazotized in the absence of alcohol. When alcohol is added in the van den Bergh reaction, unconjugated bilirubin is able to react with the diazo reagent, and the total concentration of bilirubin (direct plus indirect reacting) in the serum is estimated. Normal serum contains less than 0.2 mg of direct-reacting pigment and less than 0.8 mg of indirect-reacting pigment per 100 ml. Measurements of serum bilirubin (direct-reacting and total) are helpful in separating diseases associated with unconjugated bilirubinemia from those causing predominantly conjugated hyperbilirubinemia, but are of no value in differentiating jaundice resulting from hepatocellular disease from extrahepatic cholestasis. Serial determinations of serum bilirubin concentration provide a more accurate measure of the impairment of bilirubin excretion during the course of liver disease than can be gained by a clinical assessment of the degree of jaundice.

Tests for *bilirubin in the urine* are helpful in differentiating jaundice caused by unconjugated hyperbilirubinemia; only conjugated bilirubin is excreted in the urine. Bilirubin may be excreted in the urine when the elevation of serum bilirubin is insufficient to cause jaundice.

URINARY AND FECAL UROBILINOGEN. Urinary excretion of urobilinogen increases when the amount of urobilinogen absorbed from the intestine is increased by excessive pigment production or when hepatic excretion of urobilinogen is impaired by liver disease. Normally, urobilinogen can be detected in urine diluted to 1 in 16. *An increase in urinary urobilinogen excretion in the absence of increased fecal excretion of pigment is a very sensitive indicator of liver disease.* A quantitative measurement of the 24-hour fecal excretion of urobilinogen is of diagnostic value in hemolytic states and in patients with biliary tract disease. An increased fecal excretion of urobilinogen confirms that there is excessive bilirubin production, and a total absence of urobilinogen in the stool indicates complete biliary tract obstruction owing to atresia or neoplasm.

SERUM BILE ACIDS. The concentration of primary (cholic and chenodeoxycholic) and secondary (deoxycholic and lithocholic) bile acids in peripheral blood serum can now be measured by sensitive and specific radioimmunoassay and chromatographic methods. During periods of fasting, when the bile acid pool is retained in the gallbladder, the low bile acid levels in peripheral blood reflect the minimal levels in portal blood and efficient hepatic extraction (70 per cent for chenodeoxycholic acid, and 90 per cent for cholic acid). Following a meal, when gallbladder emptying causes the enterohepatic cycling of bile salts, peripheral blood levels of bile acid increase above fasting levels. When the hepatic extraction of bile acids is impaired by cholestasis, parenchymal cell injury, or portal-systemic shunting in patients with liver disease, there is an increase in the fasting and postprandial levels of bile acids in the peripheral blood, and delayed clearance of an intravenously injected bile acid load. The changes in peripheral blood levels of bile acids provide a very sensitive but nonspecific test for liver disease; many patients with normal conventional tests of liver function exhibit elevated bile acid levels.

SULFOBROMOPHTHALEIN SODIUM (BROMSULPHALEIN, BSP) CLEARANCE. The measurement of the hepatic clearance of this organic, anionic dye is a very sensitive test of liver function. Injected BSP, bound by plasma proteins (albumin and alpha globulin), is cleared by the liver and excreted in bile. BSP excretion by the liver depends on the selective uptake and concentration of dye by Y and Z binding proteins in the liver cell and the rate-limiting active transport of both unconjugated and glutathione-conjugated BSP into the bile canaliculi. BSP clearance varies with bile salt excretion, and can be increased experimentally by intravenous infusion of bile salt which augments excretion by increasing canalicular bile flow.

In the standard liver function test, the amount of BSP retained in the plasma is measured 30 or 45 minutes after an intravenous injection of the dye (5 mg per kilogram of body weight). The normal subject excretes more than 90 and 96 per cent of the injected BSP in 30 and 45 minutes, respectively. A reduced plasma clearance of BSP (increased retention of dye in the plasma) may result from changes in hepatic blood flow as in congestive heart failure or portal vein thrombosis, from reduced ability of liver cells to concentrate or excrete the dye as in hepatocellular injury and metabolic abnormalities, or from obstruction to bile flow in intrahepatic and extrahepatic cholestasis. Thus abnormal BSP excretion does not indicate a specific hepatic lesion.

The dye should be injected with care, because leakage outside the vein causes severe pain and tissue necrosis.

Although the standard BSP test is a sensitive measure of liver function, the maximal capacity of the liver to excrete the dye is not measured. The maximal capacity of the liver to concentrate and to excrete BSP may be estimated by measuring plasma clearance when infusions of the dye are given. Either of these maxima may be reduced when all other tests of liver function remain normal. In some patients with liver disease, the maximal excretion rate of the dye may be reduced when hepatic storage is normal or increased.

ALBUMIN. Normal levels of plasma albumin are maintained by an equilibrium between hepatic synthesis and degradation or loss. When synthesis is reduced in liver disease, the serum albumin concentration and the total body albumin pool decrease until a new equilibrium is established between synthesis and degradation. In view of the slow rate of albumin degradation (the half-time of plasma albumin degradation varies between 12 and 18 days), the serum concentration of albumin does not immediately reflect rapid changes in liver function, but decreases slowly when synthesis is impaired. In patients with cirrhosis, a depressed level of serum albumin reflects reduced synthesis and/or distribution of the albumin pool in an expanded extravascular space (ascitic fluid).

GLOBULINS. Changes in the concentration of the serum globulins can be assessed by salt fractionation or by electrophoresis of serum. *Alpha and beta globulin* concentrations increase in patients with infection or obstructive jaundice and decrease when hepatocellular failure impairs their synthesis. The serum concentration of the *immunoglobulins* increases when antibody production is stimulated by exogenous or tissue antigen. Although immunoglobulin synthesis is not a function of the hepatic parenchymal cell, measurements of serum gamma globulin concentrations are helpful in diagnosis. Extreme hypergammaglobulinemia suggests a diagnosis of chronic active hepatitis or active cirrhosis. Positive tests for antinuclear and smooth muscle antibody and LE cell reaction are frequent in patients with chronic active hepatitis, whereas antimitochondrial antibody tests are usually positive in patients with primary biliary cirrhosis (see Ch. 465.1 and Primary Biliary Cirrhosis in Ch. 465.2).

The serum *flocculation tests* are nonspecific tests in which the plasma proteins are precipitated or flocculated by a variety of agents. Positive tests depend on relative changes in the concentration of several plasma proteins and are not specific for liver disease.

BLOOD-CLOTTING TESTS. Tests of blood coagulation provide a sensitive measure of hepatic synthetic function. The relatively short half-life (two to four days) of several of the blood-clotting factors leads to a rapid change in the one-stage prothrombin time when synthesis is depressed by acute parenchymal liver disease. In acute hepatitis, the prothrombin time is a valuable guide to the severity of parenchymal damage; marked prolongation of the prothrombin time (greater than 20 seconds) is an early reflection of massive necrosis. Whenever clotting tests are used to measure liver function, possible deficiency of vitamin K resulting from malabsorption should be first excluded by parenteral therapy.

CHOLESTEROL. Changes in serum cholesterol concentrations reflect changes in serum lipoprotein. In cholestasis, when cholesterol and bile acid excretion are impaired but cholesterol synthesis is normal, serum cholesterol concentrations increase with the appearance of an abnormal lipoprotein (lipoprotein X). When hepatic lipoprotein synthesis is impaired by hepatocellular disease, serum cholesterol concentrations fall. A parallel decrease in the fraction of serum cholesterol in the esterified form (normally two thirds) results from decreased hepatic synthesis and plasma activity of the esterifying enzyme, lecithin–cholesterol acyltransferase.

SERUM ENZYMES. A large number of enzymes normally concentrated in the liver (and other tissues) are also present at low activity in the plasma. The level of enzyme activity in the plasma is determined by the rate of release from cells and the rate of clearance from plasma, in addition to the presence of activators or inhibitors in the plasma. Three patterns of abnormal plasma enzyme activity which depend on differences in enzyme synthesis and release are seen in patients with liver disease.

1. *Increased enzyme activity due to release from damaged liver cells.* Enzymes present in high concentration in the liver cell are released with damage to parenchymal cells. These enzymes include the *transaminases* and *dehydrogenases* which are measured routinely in clinical laboratories. The wide tissue distribution of these enzymes limits their specificity in localizing the site of cell damage unless other diagnostic criteria are used concomitantly or unless the elevation of serum enzyme is of such degree that liver cell damage could be the only source. In *acute hepatitis,* serum transaminase levels are usually elevated to levels in excess of 500 IU, but the degree of enzyme elevation correlates poorly with the extent of liver cell necrosis seen on liver biopsy. In patients with fulminant hepatitis, progressive clinical deterioration is often accompanied by a fall in serum enzyme activity (see Ch. 456). In *chronic active hepatitis,* the level of serum transaminase reflects the activity of the disease process and is a useful guide to therapy with corticosteroids (see Ch. 465.1).

2. *Increased enzyme activity due to de novo synthesis by liver cells and/or bile ducts with release into plasma.* The serum levels of alkaline phosphatase, 5'-nucleotidase, and leucine aminopeptidase are increased in patients with cholestasis — either intrahepatic or extrahepatic. Experimental studies have shown that the increase in serum alkaline phosphatase activity after bile duct ligation is due to the release of enzyme that is newly synthesized in the liver. The level of serum alkaline phosphatase is of no value in the differential diagnosis of obstructive jaundice. When the origin of the serum alkaline phosphatase is uncertain (serum enzyme activity may be derived from bone, intestine, or liver), the hepatic origin of the enzyme can be confirmed by measurement of serum 5'-nucleotidase or leucine aminopeptidase activity; these enzymes are more specific for liver disease. Alternatively, the isoenzyme of hepatic origin can be separated from bone and intestinal isoenzymes by polyacrylamide gel electrophoresis or heat inactivation; hepatic alkaline phosphatase is more heat stable than bone alkaline phosphatase. In the *absence of jaundice,* an elevated alkaline phosphatase suggests early cholestasis or hepatic infiltration by tumor or granuloma; patients with lymphoma, however, may have elevated levels of hepatic alkaline phosphatase without liver infiltration, and, conversely, early metastatic disease of the liver may not be associated with an increase

in enzyme activity. A normal alkaline phosphatase in a jaundiced patient with conjugated hyperbilirubinemia is usually indicative of parenchymal cell disease.

3. *Decreased serum enzyme activity due to impaired hepatic synthesis.* The serum level of some enzymes may decrease in patients with impaired synthesis. These enzymes include *ceruloplasmin,* a copper-containing oxidase, and lecithin–cholesterol acyltransferase, an enzyme which normally esterifies plasma cholesterol. These enzymes are not routinely measured as tests of liver function.

PATTERNS OF ALTERED LIVER FUNCTION IN PATIENTS WITH LIVER DISEASE. Multiple and serial tests of liver function often provide patterns of disturbed function that are of greater diagnostic value than individual tests. In *cholestasis,* an increase in conjugated bilirubin is associated with elevation of the serum alkaline phosphatase and 5'-nucleotidase and an increase in serum cholesterol when the cholestasis is prolonged. Serum transaminase levels are only mildly increased (<200 units), and hepatic synthetic function remains normal with normal serum albumin and clotting factor levels (when vitamin K has been administered parenterally). When *cholestasis is accompanied by parenchymal cell necrosis,* hyperbilirubinemia and elevated serum alkaline phosphatase levels will be associated with greater elevations of serum transaminases. *Parenchymal cell injury or necrosis* is reflected by the release of enzymes into the serum (SGOT >500 IU), variable depression of hepatic synthetic function with depression of clotting factor levels and hypoalbuminemia, and impaired hepatic excretory function with bilirubinemia and normal or slightly increased levels of alkaline phosphatase. A *reduced liver cell mass* without active inflammation or parenchymal cell necrosis may depress hepatic metabolic, synthetic, or excretory function without causing changes in serum enzymes. The *immunologic activity* associated with chronic active liver disease is usually associated with hypergammaglobulinemia and positive serologic tests.

NEEDLE BIOPSY OF THE LIVER

Percutaneous needle biopsy of the liver by an intercostal approach under local anesthesia is a simple, safe bedside procedure that provides a tissue diagnosis of liver disease without subjecting the patient to the greater risk of general anesthesia and laparotomy with open surgical biopsy.

INDICATIONS. Needle biopsy of the liver is of proved value in the following situations:

1. In the differential diagnosis of jaundice, hepatic enlargement, and splenomegaly.

2. In the differential diagnosis of unexplained fever. A liver biopsy may suggest or establish the diagnosis of *miliary tuberculosis,* sarcoidosis, brucellosis, or neoplasm.

3. To assess the degree of hepatic fibrosis in chronic hepatitis and cirrhosis, to evaluate the course of hepatitis and acute liver disease, and to estimate hepatic stores of iron in hemochromatosis.

CONTRAINDICATIONS. The risk of complications (bleeding, bile peritonitis) after liver biopsy is increased in the following circumstances:

1. In patients who are uncooperative or who cannot control movements of the diaphragm, e.g., with severe recurrent cough.

2. In patients with bleeding disorders, with clotting defects (prothrombin time elevations greater than two to three seconds over control), or with vascular tumors in the liver. The risk of bleeding following the procedure may be reduced by platelet transfusion or infusions of fresh frozen plasma to restore a normal prothrombin time.

3. In patients with severe cardiopulmonary disease that would be a contraindication to surgery should a biopsy complication ensue.

4. In patients with prolonged jaundice, probably extrahepatic in origin.

COMPLICATIONS. Needle biopsy of the liver is usually painless, but is occasionally followed by right pleuritic chest pain referred to the shoulder; a transient pleural friction rub may be audible at the site of biopsy. Serious complications include *hemorrhage* from the biopsy site and leakage of bile from dilated intrahepatic bile ducts or gallbladder, with *bile peritonitis;* this is usually a complication of extrahepatic obstruction. The incidence of these major complications should be less than 0.1 per cent.

PROCEDURES USED TO DIAGNOSE BILIARY TRACT DISEASE

The *radiographic procedures* used to visualize the biliary tree depend on the hepatic excretion of radiopaque dye (*oral cholecystography* and *intravenous cholangiography*) or on the direct injection of contrast agents into the bile ducts either at operation (*operative cholangiography*) or after cannulation of the ampulla via the duodenoscope (*retrograde duodenoscopic cholangiography*) or by needle (at *peritoneoscopy,* or by *percutaneous transhepatic* and *transvenous* transhepatic approaches). These procedures are described in Ch. 387 to 392. Examination of duodenal bile (*biliary drainage*) and the *secretin test* are of value in the differential diagnosis of obstructive jaundice. They are discussed in detail in Ch. 411.

The hepatic excretion of the most commonly used oral cholecystographic agent, *iopanoic acid,* involves a sequence that is similar to the excretion of bilirubin. In the plasma, iopanoic acid is albumin bound. Excretion depends on diffusion across the liver cell membrane, concentration in the liver cell by binding to Y and Z proteins, conjugation with glucuronide to form a water-soluble complex, and active transport of the glucuronyl conjugate into the bile canaliculi. Impaired excretion of iopanoic acid should thus be expected in patients with malabsorption, parenchymal liver disease, or cholestasis.

DIAGNOSTIC PROCEDURES IN PORTAL HYPERTENSION

Esophageal varices may be demonstrated roentgenographically by a *barium swallow,* although *esophagoscopy* is a more accurate method for their identification.

Portal venous pressure can be measured indirectly by inserting a needle into the splenic pulp or by wedging a catheter in a branch of the hepatic vein. Comparative studies have shown that portal vein pressures measured directly through a catheter in the umbilical vein correspond to pressures recorded from wedged hepatic vein catheters in patients with cirrhosis. Measurement of wedged hepatic vein catheter pressure has the advantage of providing baseline inferior vena cava pressures. Portal

pressure measurements are of value in establishing the presence of portal hypertension when this is in doubt in patients with splenomegaly or ascites. An elevated pressure is consistent with the diagnosis of chronic liver disease rather than presinusoidal portal vein obstruction. Repeated pressure measurements provide evidence of changes in portal pressure which may be of prognostic value; with recovery from acute alcoholic hepatitis, a fall in portal pressure suggests a better prognosis than a stable or rising pressure which reflects progressive fibrosis. The degree of pressure elevation does not appear to indicate the risk of hemorrhage from esophageal varices or the prognosis after portacaval shunt surgery.

The portal circulation can be visualized roentgenographically by *selective celiac arteriography* or by injection of contrast material into the spleen (*transsplenic venography*) or directly through the catheterized umbilical vein. The portal vein and collateral circulation should be demonstrated before portacaval shunt surgery is performed.

LIVER SCANNING

When compounds that are concentrated in the liver (either by parenchymal or Kupffer cells) are labeled with gamma-emitting isotopes and injected intravenously, their uptake by the liver can be assessed by surface scanning. ^{131}I-labeled rose bengal, ^{198}Au colloidal gold, and ^{99}technetium have been used. Space-occupying lesions (cysts, abscesses, or tumors) appear as filling defects. In patients with cirrhosis, hepatic uptake is decreased and irregular and splenic uptake may be increased. A liver scan is of value in providing evidence of a space-occupying lesion when this was not evident clinically. A liver biopsy should be performed to confirm the pathologic diagnosis; the biopsy needle may be directed to the site of infiltration demonstrated by the scan. Serial liver scans may be of value in documenting the response of a patient with metastatic neoplasm to therapy.

454. METABOLIC DISORDERS

Inborn errors of metabolism may cause chronic liver disease. In some of these conditions specific enzyme defects have been demonstrated (glycogen storage diseases [see Ch. 531.4], galactosemia [see Ch. 531.3]), whereas in others the underlying metabolic abnormality has not yet been defined (idiopathic hemochromatosis [see Ch. 489], Wilson's disease [see Ch. 537], Gaucher's disease [see Ch. 533.2]).

DISORDERS OF BILIRUBIN METABOLISM. Knowledge of several metabolic disorders has contributed greatly to an understanding of bilirubin metabolism and excretion.

Unconjugated Hyperbilirubinemia. Acholuric jaundice with unconjugated hyperbilirubinemia in the absence of other signs of anemia or liver disease may be due to one of the following conditions:

1. *Compensated hemolysis* in which increased red cell production masks excessive red cell destruction. This abnormality may be suggested by lowered serum haptoglobin concentrations and increased fecal urobilinogen and reticulocyte counts, but can be confirmed only by direct measurement of red cell survival using tagged erythrocytes. An increase in bilirubin production alone is insuf-

ficient to account for the unconjugated hyperbilirubinemia in patients with compensated hemolysis. Studies of bilirubin clearance using labeled bilirubin indicate that these patients also have a delayed clearance of pigment; the excessive bilirubin load unmasks this excretory defect (see Gilbert's syndrome, below).

2. *Excessive bilirubin production without hemolysis* ("shunt hyperbilirubinemia"). This is a rare condition in which abnormal catabolism of hemoglobin in red cell precursors in the bone marrow results in excessive pigment production (early-labeled bilirubin) and increased fecal urobilinogen excretion; peripheral red cell survival is normal.

3. *Idiopathic unconjugated hyperbilirubinemia (Gilbert's syndrome).* Mild unconjugated hyperbilirubinemia (usually less than 3 mg per 100 ml) without hemolysis or excessive bilirubin production is commonly recognized in healthy young subjects. Jaundice may be intermittent with exacerbations during intercurrent illness and particularly during periods of fasting. The absence of physical abnormalities, normal liver function tests, and normal liver histology exclude a diagnosis of viral hepatitis. Family studies suggest an autosomal dominant inheritance.

A defect in the hepatic uptake of unconjugated bilirubin from plasma has been documented by a depressed plasma clearance of labeled unconjugated bilirubin in patients with Gilbert's syndrome. In some patients, excessive bilirubin production from compensated hemolysis accentuates the excretory defect. Although the transport defect in Gilbert's syndrome is usually confined to unconjugated bilirubin, a partial deficiency of UDP glucuronyl transferase activity in some patients and variable defects in the uptake and excretion of BSP and indocyanine green in other patients suggest that the syndrome is heterogeneous.

It has been observed that fasting increases serum levels of unconjugated bilirubin in patients with Gilbert's syndrome; in normal subjects there is also a slight increase within the normal range. Although this phenomenon has not been explained, the response to fasting and refeeding may be of diagnostic value in some patients. Phenobarbital lowers serum bilirubin levels in Gilbert's syndrome; increases in microsomal enzyme activity and in the concentration of binding proteins in the liver cell may increase bilirubin clearance.

4. *Parenchymal liver disease* may be associated with unconjugated hyperbilirubinemia. This has been recognized in patients during recovery from viral hepatitis. Other abnormal tests of liver function (positive flocculation tests, mildly abnormal BSP) and histologic changes on liver biopsy suggest hepatitis in these patients. Unconjugated hyperbilirubinemia in patients with congestive heart failure, or after portacaval shunt surgery for portal hypertension, reflects reduced hepatic blood flow and bilirubin clearance.

5. *Impaired bilirubin conjugation.* A defect in bilirubin conjugation is usually manifest during the neonatal period, and may be due to immaturity of the liver, inhibition of glucuronyl transferase, or deficiency of this enzyme.

a. *The immature liver* of the premature infant exhibits a reduced level of glucuronyl transferase activity. It has not been established, however, that this is the primary cause for physiologic jaundice; there may be other defects in the excretory mechanism.

b. *Prolonged neonatal jaundice in breast-fed infants* may be due to inhibition of glucuronyl transferase activity by an abnormal steroid (pregnane-3α-20β-diol) excreted in the mother's milk. Jaundice is maximal during the second to third week, and subsides rapidly if breast feeding is discontinued, or over a four- to eight-week period with continued breast feeding.

Transient neonatal hyperbilirubinemia, described in successive infants of several mothers, has been related to the presence of an inhibitor of glucuronyl transferase in the maternal plasma during pregnancy. Several of these infants developed kernicterus.

c. *The Crigler-Najjar syndrome* (congenital, nonhemolytic, unconjugated hyperbilirubinemia with glucuronyl transferase deficiency). This syndrome, characterized by severe jaundice, usually from birth, is transmitted in some patients as an autosomal recessive defect (Type I), and in others as an autosomal dominant (Type II). Type I patients with the autosomal recessive defect are deeply jaundiced (mean bilirubin levels 25 to 31 mg per 100 ml) and develop kernicterus. Their bile is colorless, and phenobarbital administration does not lower the serum level of unconjugated bilirubin. The autosomal dominant defect in Type II patients may cause less severe hyperbilirubinemia so that some patients survive to adulthood without kernicterus. When phenobarbital is given to these patients, the serum bilirubin concentration falls dramatically; this effect may be due to induction of glucuronyl transferase activity.

The homozygous *Gunn rat*, deficient in glucuronyl transferase, provides a laboratory model of the Crigler-Najjar syndrome.

Kernicterus (Bilirubin Encephalopathy). This neurologic complication of severe unconjugated hyperbilirubinemia usually develops in the jaundiced infant during the first week of life with the appearance of spasticity, leading to head retraction, opisthotonos, muscle twitching, or convulsions. The infant may die during the neonatal period, whereas survivors exhibit mental retardation and spastic paraplegia with athetosis.

Normally, the binding of unconjugated bilirubin by albumin restricts pigment diffusion into tissue cells. However, when the concentration of unconjugated bilirubin exceeds the albumin-binding capacity (approximately 20 mg of bilirubin per 100 ml of plasma in the normal infant), unconjugated bilirubin is free to diffuse into tissues; the lipid solubility of the pigment enhances its diffusion across cell membranes and the blood-brain barrier. Depression of the plasma albumin level, the administration of drugs which bind albumin and thus displace bilirubin (sulfonamides and salicylate), and metabolic acidosis all predispose to kernicterus. The biochemical mechanism for bilirubin encephalopathy has not been well defined.

Preventive therapy depends on the early recognition and treatment of conditions that may cause severe hemolysis in the newborn (ABO and Rh incompatibility or red cell enzyme defects). Infection and metabolic acidosis should be treated vigorously, and drugs which bind bilirubin should be avoided. Phototherapy (exposure to light of wavelength 440 mμ) may reduce the level of serum bilirubin by converting the tetrapyrrole pigment to colorless products with alternate pathways of excretion. Exchange transfusion is indicated when the serum bilirubin rises to dangerous levels; in sick premature infants with depressed albumin binding, serum bilirubin levels in excess of 10 mg per 100 ml plasma may be unsafe.

The Dubin-Johnson Syndrome. This is a familial (autosomal recessive) metabolic disorder caused by impaired hepatic excretion of certain organic anions into the bile. Jaundice is associated with an increased serum level of conjugated bilirubin and bilirubinuria. The Dubin-Johnson syndrome is more commonly diagnosed in females than in males, and often presents with jaundice during pregnancy when the hepatic excretory defect is accentuated by hormones. Jaundice is usually intermittent, and exacerbations are often associated with mild right upper quadrant abdominal pain. There is no hepatic enlargement. The excretion of oral cholecystographic agents is impaired so that the normal biliary system often cannot be visualized. Although BSP is concentrated and conjugated normally in the liver cell, biliary excretion of the dye is impaired, and large amounts of conjugated BSP passing back into the plasma may elevate the two-hour plasma BSP level above the 45-minute value. Patients with the Dubin-Johnson syndrome do not suffer from pruritus, and there is no evidence for abnormal biliary secretion of the conjugated bile salts. In contrast to the retention of conjugated bilirubin and BSP, serum alkaline phosphatase levels are usually normal. There is a characteristic abnormality of coproporphyrin excretion in the Dubin-Johnson syndrome; coproporphyrin I rather than coproporphyrin III is the predominant urinary coproporphyrin.

The diagnosis of the Dubin-Johnson syndrome is established by needle biopsy of the liver. Macroscopically the fresh liver tissue is black, and microscopically there are deposits of melanin-like pigment in the parenchymal cells, particularly in the centrilobular areas. The Kupffer cells do not contain pigment, the bile canaliculi are normal, and the liver is free of fibrosis or inflammatory infiltrate. Recent studies on mutant Corriedale sheep with a similar defect in organic anion transport and liver pigmentation suggest that the pigment may be an oxidation product of metanephrine glucuronide, an epinephrine metabolite normally excreted in bile but poorly excreted by these animals and by patients with the Dubin-Johnson syndrome. The hepatic pigment accumulates with increasing age in both conditions.

The more important considerations in managing patients with this disorder of bilirubin metabolism are the reassurance that the abnormality is benign and leads to no disability or reduction in life expectancy and the avoidance of unnecessary biliary tract surgery.

The Rotor Syndrome. This rare autosomal recessive syndrome of mild conjugated hyperbilirubinemia without hepatic pigmentation was formerly considered to be a variant of the Dubin-Johnson syndrome. Differences in the excretion of BSP and coproporphyrin suggest that these are separate syndromes. Patients with the Rotor syndrome exhibit normal gallbladder filling on oral cholecystography, have delayed excretion of BSP without a late plasma rise in conjugated pigment, and have the same abnormalities of urinary coproporphyrin excretion as other patients with hepatobiliary disease.

455. ACUTE VIRAL HEPATITIS

Acute viral hepatitis is a common acute inflammatory disease of the liver caused by at least two strains of hepatotropic virus. *Type A hepatitis* (formerly called infec-

tious or short-incubation hepatitis) is due to hepatitis A virus (or viruses), and *Type B hepatitis* (formerly called serum, post-transfusion, or long-incubation hepatitis) is due to hepatitis B viruses.

ETIOLOGY. Early attempts to isolate the viruses of human hepatitis, to propagate them in tissue culture, or to transmit them to laboratory animals were unsuccessful, and knowledge of these agents was thus limited. Information relating to the viral etiology of human hepatitis was based on indirect evidence derived from studies of epidemic hepatitis and from human transmission experiments. Hepatitis A and B were both shown to be caused by filterable agents that were relatively resistant to heat and chemical disinfectants. Epidemiologic and clinical studies suggested differences in the biologic properties of the two viral agents. "Infectious hepatitis" was believed to be transmitted by the fecal-oral route in the majority of patients in both endemic and epidemic outbreaks. Experimental studies suggested a short incubation period of two to six weeks, with the appearance of the infective agent in both blood and feces during the prodromal and early icteric phases of illness. Infection conferred immunity against further attacks of "infectious hepatitis," but did not protect against "serum hepatitis" infection. "Serum hepatitis" was considered to be transmitted only by parenteral inoculation of infected blood or blood products with a long incubation period of six weeks to six months. The infective agent was thought to be confined to the circulation and not excreted in feces. The transmission of disease by transfusion of blood from healthy donors indicated a prolonged carrier state.

Identification of Hepatitis A Virus. Virus-like particles, 27 nm in size, have been identified by immune electron microscopy in the stool of volunteers infected with hepatitis A; these particles appeared several days before tests of liver function became abnormal, and disappeared with the onset of jaundice. Similar virus particles recovered from the livers of marmosets infected with human type A hepatitis were shown to be neutralized by antibody to hepatitis A (anti-HA). Specific immune adherence and complement fixation tests for anti-HA have now been developed, using hepatitis A antigen (HAAg) from the liver of infected marmosets. Hepatitis A infection is associated with a rise in anti-HA titer within one to four weeks of the onset of clinical illness, and persisting high titers for years thereafter.

Identification of Hepatitis B Virus. Hepatitis B virus antigen was first identified in the serum of an Australian aboriginal, and was initially called Australia antigen. Hepatitis B virus (HBV) has been identified by electron microscopy in the serum of patients with HBV infection. The virus particle (Dane particle) is 42 nm in diameter with a central core and surface capsid. The virus core contains DNA and DNA polymerase activity and has distinct antigenic characteristics as hepatitis B_{core} antigen (HB_cAg). Capsid antigen, designated as hepatitis $B_{surface}$ antigen (HB_sAg), has distinct immunologic subtypes D and Y. HB_cAg and HB_sAg promote the formation of their corresponding antibodies, anti-HB_c and anti-HB_s. An additional antigen-antibody system, e-antigen and anti-e, has recently been identified with the hepatitis B virus.

HB_cAg and HB_sAg have been identified by immunofluorescent and immunoelectronmicroscopic methods in the nuclei and cytoplasm, respectively, of liver cells from patients who were chronic HB_sAg carriers. HB_sAg has been identified in peripheral blood serum as 20 nm spheres or filaments without the central virus core; this antigen is readily identified by immunodiffusion, complement fixation, and radioimmunoassay techniques.

EPIDEMIOLOGY. Hepatitis A. Transmission of the hepatitis A virus is usually by the fecal-oral route, although infusion of infected blood obtained from viremic donors may cause sporadic infection. There is no clinical, epidemiologic, or serologic evidence of a chronic hepatitis A carrier state in man; thus infection depends on exposure to virus from an acutely infected subject. The occurrence of both sporadic and epidemic hepatitis depends on the distribution of infected material and the susceptibility of the exposed population. Thus poor sanitation, overcrowding, and exposure of a nonimmune population will contribute to an epidemic situation with a high frequency of infection in the young. Adults without previous exposure to hepatitis A infection are particularly at risk when traveling in or moving to an area of high endemic infection with poor sanitation. Explosive epidemics have been described after fecal contamination of drinking water and milk, and several epidemics have been attributed to the ingestion of raw or steamed shellfish which concentrate the virus in contaminated sea water. The common epidemics in institutions that house small children — orphanages, schools, and homes for the mentally retarded — reflect the exposure of a nonimmune population to many cases of anicteric or preicteric infection. Clinical and serologic evidence has now documented that hepatitis A virus can be transmitted not only from man to primates but also from infected primates to animal handlers.

Hepatitis B. PARENTERAL TRANSMISSION. Transmission of hepatitis B virus by the parenteral route is well documented. This is a hazard among recipients of transfused blood (particularly blood from paid donors), pooled plasma, fibrinogen, factor VIII concentrate, and vaccines contaminated with human serum (e.g., yellow fever vaccine during World War II). Inoculation with minute amounts of infected blood may transmit hepatitis B virus infection; inadequately sterilized syringes, hypodermic needles, dental and surgical instruments, tattoo needles, and razors have all been implicated in the transmission of infection. A high frequency of parenteral drug abuse is a major cause for infection in the young adult population; in one study, 39 per cent of heroin addicts entering a treatment program had positive tests for HB_sAg.

The development of immunologic methods for the detection of HB_sAg and anti-HB_s has led to major advances in the understanding of hepatitis B infection and provides a means for reducing infection, particularly among recipients of transfused blood. Tests for HB_sAg identify many carriers of the hepatitis B virus; between 1 and 2 per cent of paid donors were found to be HB_sAg positive, whereas volunteer blood donors have a hepatitis carrier rate of between 1 and 2 per 1000. A majority of patients transfused with HB_sAg positive blood either develop HBV infection (either anicteric or icteric) or exhibit a rise in the titer of anti-HB_s in their serum. The frequency of post-transfusion hepatitis B infection is significantly decreased when transfused blood is derived from volunteer rather than paid donors and when HB_sAg positive blood is discarded.

VERTICAL TRANSMISSION (MOTHER TO INFANT). Studies on the infants of mothers who suffered from hepatitis B infection during the last trimester of pregnancy or during the immediate postpartum period have shown a high frequency of neonatal infection. Studies on the perinatal transmission of hepatitis B infection in a large population of HB_sAg positive maternal carriers suggest that the risk of vertical transmission of infection is greatest when the mother has a high titer of HB_sAg, is e-antigen positive, and has transmitted hepatitis to previous children. Maternal carriers who were e-antigen negative with anti-e did not transmit hepatitis B. In view of the high incidence of the hepatitis B carrier state in some African and Asian populations, vertical transmission may be of considerable epidemiologic importance.

NONPARENTERAL TRANSMISSION. In epidemiologic studies, Krugman and coworkers showed that hepatitis B infection could be transmitted by nonparenteral (fecal-oral) as well as by parenteral routes. Although the high concentration of HBV in blood favors parenteral transmission, it has also been shown that HB_sAg is present in oropharyngeal secretions, in seminal fluid, in urine, and in stool of patients with hepatitis B infection. This excretion of hepatitis B antigen provides opportunities for the nonparenteral transmission of infection, but the factors that determine such transmission by individual HB_sAg positive carriers are still poorly defined. Among relatives of HB_sAg positive prospective blood donors, serologic evidence of hepatitis B infection (positive tests for HB_sAg or anti-HB_s) was ten times more frequent than in relatives of HB_sAg negative blood donors. This familial clustering of hepatitis B infection may be determined by genetic factors, by vertical transmission, or by nonparenteral transmission. The high frequency of serologic evidence of hepatitis B infection among homosexual males (30 to 50 per cent) provides strong evidence for venereal transmission, but the frequency of infection among the spouses of HB_sAg carriers was no higher than among other family members.

NOSOCOMIAL TRANSMISSION. Hospital personnel, particularly operating room staff, dialysis unit staff, and laboratory technicians who handle blood, have an increased risk of accidental parenteral exposure to hepatitis B virus. Serologic evidence of previous hepatitis infection was found in 16.8 per cent of health care personnel and in only 8.7 per cent of a control group matched for age, sex, and socioeconomic status. There is evidence of a similar increased risk of hepatitis B infection among dentists. What is the risk of hepatitis B transmission from HB_sAg positive hospital personnel or dentists to their patients? Several outbreaks of hepatitis B have been traced to oral surgeons who were HB_sAg carriers, but documentation of transmission of hepatitis B from health care personnel to patients has been documented in only a single instance; an inhalation therapist with a severe exudative dermatitis on both hands transmitted hepatitis B to two patients. The increased risk of hepatitis transmission during dental surgery may be decreased by the routine use of operating gloves. Further information about the factors that determine the risk of hepatitis transmission from healthy HB_sAg carriers is necessary before this risk can be eliminated.

TRANSMISSION BY INSECT VECTORS. HB_sAg has been detected in mosquitoes and bedbugs collected from West Africa, where there is a high incidence of endemic hepatitis B infection. In one study, six of nine insects were antigen positive. Antigen persisted for several weeks in naturally or experimentally infected bedbugs. Although not yet documented, arthropod transmission of hepatitis B virus is possible in tropical areas.

PATHOLOGY. The hepatic lesion in uncomplicated viral hepatitis (both hepatitis A and B, whether anicteric or icteric) is characterized by parenchymal cell degeneration and necrosis, proliferation of Kupffer's cells, inflammatory cell infiltration, and cell regeneration. Parenchymal cells throughout the lobule, and particularly in centrilobular areas, undergo rapid necrosis so that the cell cords are disrupted. Degenerating liver cells either show *ballooning* of their cytoplasm or hyalinize to form *acidophilic bodies* that may exhibit pyknotic nuclei. Cell necrosis is closely followed by cell regeneration; this may be recognized by the appearance of cells in mitosis and by large cells with multiple hyperchromatic nuclei. An increased number of macrophages containing a yellow, acid-fast pigment (lipofuscin) accumulate at sites of cell necrosis. Numerous lymphocytes, plasma cells, and polymorphonuclear cells, both neutrophil and eosinophil, also accumulate focally at sites of cell necrosis in the lobules and in the portal areas.

Although necrosis disrupts the normal cell cords, the reticulum framework surrounding the hepatic sinusoids is preserved, and cell regeneration restores normal lobules. During the recovery phase an increased number of fibroblasts with collagen may appear in the portal areas, together with proliferating bile ductules; these changes, together with the inflammatory cell infiltrate, disappear with full recovery.

Dilated bile canaliculi containing bile plugs, particularly in centrilobular areas, and bile staining of parenchymal cells reflect impaired bile secretion in jaundiced patients. This may be due to a disruption of bile canaliculi by parenchymal cell necrosis, or it may result from a change in the composition of bile due to cell injury.

Rarely, viral hepatitis may cause more extensive zones of parenchymal cell necrosis bridging adjacent portal triads and/or central veins with collapse of the normal reticulum framework. This lesion has been termed *bridging necrosis* when it involves a single lobule, or *multilobular necrosis* when adjacent lobules are affected. *Massive hepatic necrosis,* usually associated with fulminant hepatitis, is associated with widespread necrosis. The term *acute yellow atrophy* refers to the shrunken, bile-stained liver in which zones of collapsed reticulum and sinusoids lie between islands of surviving cells.

Although complete recovery can be anticipated in patients with typical focal necrosis, more extensive necrosis may lead to liver failure and death, or to chronic disease with fibrosis. Massive necrosis in patients with fulminant hepatitis is usually fatal. In patients who survive, liver cell regeneration may restore normal liver structure and function or may result in a macronodular cirrhosis. Bridging or multilobular necrosis has a variable clinical course. Of 52 patients who exhibited this lesion on liver biopsy, 4 died with fulminant hepatitis, 6 died after a subacute illness of several weeks, and the remainder survived the acute illness; of the survivors, 7 exhibited the clinical and histologic features of chronic active hepatitis, 5 had residual abnormalities of liver function with cirrhosis documented by biopsy in 2, and 28 recovered with normal liver function but with biopsy evidence of inactive cirrhosis in 9 of 19 subjected to repeat liver biopsy.

There is evidence that *chronic active hepatitis* (see Ch. 465.1) may complicate hepatitis B infection. This condition usually has an insidious onset, but may also follow icteric hepatitis with bridging or multilobular necrosis.

Extrahepatic Lesions in Viral Hepatitis. Extrahepatic lesions are relatively common in patients with hepatitis B infection. The presence of large amounts of viral antigen (Dane particles and HB_sAg) in the blood for extended periods provides a unique opportunity for the formation of *immune complexes* that may be deposited in the skin, in serous membranes, in blood vessels, and in the renal glomeruli. Immune complexes containing HB_sAg and anti-HB_s have been identified in *mixed cryoglobulinemia, polyarteritis nodosa,* and *membranous glomerulonephritis.* Virus-like particles have been demonstrated by electron microscopy in degenerating synovial cells and in the endothelium of blood vessels in synovial biopsies from two patients with acute arthritis complicating hepatitis B infection; direct cell injury by virus may also be responsible for some of the extrahepatic lesions.

CLINICAL MANIFESTATIONS. Acute viral hepatitis (Type A or B) is commonly a mild disease without jaundice, particularly in those with relative immunity from previous infection, or in infants and children. Infection may be followed by a mild illness without clinical evidence of hepatitis; a rise in viral antibody titer or transiently positive test for HB_sAg may be the only evidence of infection. In many subjects exposed to either of the viral agents, there is evidence of hepatitis without jaundice — *anicteric hepatitis.* Icteric hepatitis is usually a short, uncomplicated illness, but sometimes has a prolonged course (*chronic persisting hepatitis*). Acute exacerbations may follow partial recovery, or *recurrent hepatitis* may follow complete recovery. When a clinical picture of cholestasis is the dominant abnormality, the term *cholestatic hepatitis* is used. In jaundiced patients with hepatitis A infection, the risk of *fulminant hepatitis* with massive necrosis is less than 1 per cent. The risk of bridging, multilobular, or massive hepatic necrosis in patients with hepatitis B infection is increased in elderly patients, in diabetics, and in patients with severe illness, particularly neoplasms, which have required surgery and transfusion.

The clinical features of each of these variants of viral hepatitis will be discussed below. *Fulminant hepatitis* and *chronic active liver disease* are discussed in Ch. 456 and 465.1, respectively.

Anicteric Hepatitis. The symptoms of anicteric hepatitis are similar to those of many other viral infections; the onset of disease may resemble the prodromal (preicteric) period of icteric hepatitis. The diagnosis is suspected only in epidemic situations, in patients exposed to known infection, or in those who develop tender enlargement of the liver. A diagnosis is confirmed by liver function tests and liver biopsy. There is often slight hyperbilirubinemia with an increase in urinary urobilinogen and bilirubin and BSP retention. The serum enzyme changes are most helpful in diagnosis; serum transaminase and dehydrogenase levels are elevated, and serum alkaline phosphatase and 5'-nucleotidase may be slightly increased. On liver biopsy, the hepatic lesion is indistinguishable from that of icteric hepatitis except for the absence of bile stasis.

Icteric Hepatitis. THE PREICTERIC PHASE. The preicteric phase of nonspecific constitutional and gastrointestinal symptoms varies in duration from a few days to several weeks. It is usually abrupt in onset in patients with hepatitis A and often of insidious onset with hepatitis B; these symptoms may mimic those of other viral infections of the respiratory or gastrointestinal tract. *Fever* is usually most pronounced at the onset, and may be accompanied by a shaking chill; it is unusual, however, for shaking chills to be recurrent, although fever may persist until the early icteric phase. *Anorexia, weakness, headache,* and *myalgia* are common symptoms; there may be a striking loss of taste for cigarettes. Right upper quadrant pain with local tenderness and muscle spasm may simulate an acute abdominal emergency. Joint pains or acute migratory arthritis and urticarial or erythematous maculopapular rashes are sometimes seen, particularly in patients with hepatitis B infection. During this preicteric phase, the liver may become enlarged and tender, and the urine may become discolored with bilirubin.

THE ICTERIC PHASE. Gastrointestinal symptoms — anorexia, nausea, and vomiting with right upper abdominal discomfort — usually increase during the early period of increasing jaundice, the liver becomes more enlarged and tender, and the spleen may be palpable. Fever usually subsides a few days after the onset of jaundice. Within a few days of hospitalization and bed rest, nausea subsides, and the appetite improves in most patients. Typically, the patient is maximally jaundiced within two weeks, and thereafter clinical jaundice and serum bilirubin levels gradually return to normal within six weeks. Hepatic enlargement may subside with symptomatic improvement, but often persists during the icteric period. The maximal changes in urinary and fecal bilirubin excretion coincide with maximal serum bilirubin levels.

In patients with *cholestatic hepatitis* jaundice is usually more severe and prolonged and accompanied by *pruritus*. Liver enlargement usually persists during the period of jaundice, whereas hepatic tenderness is usually observed early in the acute illness. *Diarrhea* may be due to the cathartic action of nonabsorbed fatty acids.

Some patients with otherwise typical acute viral hepatitis may remain icteric with hepatic enlargement and abnormalities of liver function for a period of several months. A liver biopsy is indicated in such patients to confirm a diagnosis of *chronic persisting hepatitis;* the histologic features of typical viral hepatitis in spite of the prolonged clinical course indicate an excellent prognosis for full recovery.

Occasionally there may be acute exacerbations with anorexia, nausea, recurrent liver enlargement, and tenderness and jaundice after partial recovery from the initial icteric illness. Such exacerbations are sometimes precipitated by vigorous physical activity, and usually resolve promptly without long-term complications.

THE CONVALESCENT PHASE. The convalescent phase, leading to complete recovery and resumption of normal activity, may last for several weeks or months. During this period variable tiredness and malaise with mild hepatic tenderness may persist. These symptoms may be quite troublesome to the patient. They are often precipitated by unaccustomed activity and may be accompanied by mild elevation of serum transaminase levels and minimal BSP retention.

LABORATORY FEATURES. The hemoglobin and hematocrit are usually normal early in the illness, but mild hemolysis and repeated venipuncture for laboratory tests may cause anemia later in the course of the acute disease. A normal or reduced white cell count, with atypical mononuclear cells (virocytes) on smear, is usual during the preicteric and early icteric periods. The erythrocyte sedimentation rate is slightly increased. Aplastic anemia is an unusual complication of acute viral hepatitis. Thrombocytopenic purpura is occasionally seen, as in other viral illnesses. Evidence of acute hemolysis, usually with deep jaundice, may be secondary to a red cell defect, particularly G-6-PD deficiency.

The urine contains an increased amount of both urobilinogen and bilirubin in the early icteric period; bilirubinemia increases with increasing jaundice, whereas urinary urobilinogen excretion decreases to minimal levels when jaundice is maximal. Minimal proteinuria with microscopic hematuria, pyuria, and granular casts during the early icteric period may reflect the renal abnormalities that have been demonstrated on renal biopsy.

During the icteric period both direct- and indirect-reacting bilirubin are almost equally elevated in the serum, but during the convalescent period indirect bilirubinemia may persist (see Gilbert's syndrome in Ch. 454). Serum transaminase (glutamic-oxaloacetic or glutamic-pyruvic) levels, maximally elevated in the late prodromal or early icteric periods, may exceed 500 to 1000 IU. These increased enzyme levels may be sustained during the icteric period but usually fall toward normal during the icteric period. Serum elevations of alkaline phosphatase, 5'-nucleotidase, and leucine aminopeptidase are usually minimal and return to normal during the late icteric period. In patients with *cholestatic hepatitis* the increases in serum alkaline phosphatase, 5'-nucleotidase, and conjugated bilirubin are usually more prominent than the rise in serum transaminase levels. Serum cholesterol levels will increase in these patients. The typical changes in plasma proteins include a slight decrease in albumin and a late increase in gamma globulin, and the flocculation tests may be abnormal late in the prodromal period and return to normal during convalescence. The increase in gamma globulin levels in patients with acute hepatitis or in patients with *chronic persisting hepatitis* is considerably less than that seen in patients with *chronic active hepatitis* (see below). BSP retention decreases to normal levels during the convalescent period.

In hepatitis B infection, tests for HBV antigens (HB$_c$Ag, e-antigen, and HB$_s$Ag) are usually positive during the preicteric and early icteric phases of illness. HB$_c$Ag usually disappears from the blood earlier than HB$_s$Ag. The majority of patients become HB$_s$Ag negative with the appearance of anti-HB$_s$ during the early recovery phase. A minority of patients remain HB$_s$Ag positive and anti-HB$_s$ negative; these patients may become healthy carriers without liver disease, or may develop chronic hepatitis — either chronic persisting or chronic active hepatitis. The development of the chronic carrier state, with or without liver disease, is more common when infection is acquired early in life, or when the immunologic reaction to infection is modified by disease (e.g., in patients with chronic renal failure or following renal transplant). Serologic tests for hepatitis A infection (anti-HA) have not been developed as routine tests in clinical laboratories.

DIAGNOSIS. During the prodromal period, symptoms may suggest some other viral infection — *influenza* or *gastroenteritis*. Abdominal pain may mimic *acute cholecystitis, pneumonia,* or *acute appendicitis*. In the icteric patient, other causes for jaundice must be considered; *drug-induced or toxic hepatitis* is usually indicated by a history of drug exposure, but cannot be clearly differentiated by the preicteric symptoms from viral hepatitis. Choledocholithiasis with obstruction is suggested by a history of calculous disease, biliary colic, predominant cholestasis with pruritus, high alkaline phosphatase levels with only slight increases in transaminase, and signs of bacterial infection — shaking chills and polymorphonuclear leukocytosis. *Infectious mononucleosis* with hepatic involvement is distinguished by lymphadenopathy, pharyngitis, and a positive *heterophil* test. *Leptospirosis* is usually accompanied by headache and photophobia, signs of meningeal irritation with abnormal cerebrospinal fluid, persisting fever, leukocytosis, and proteinuria or renal insufficiency.

It is important to exclude an exacerbation of chronic liver disease with jaundice; *acute alcoholic hepatitis* or *chronic active hepatitis* may present with jaundice (see below).

A percutaneous liver biopsy is of diagnostic value whenever the clinical picture is atypical. Lesions of extrahepatic obstruction, chronic active hepatitis, acute alcoholic hepatitis, or active cirrhosis can be distinguished from the changes of acute viral hepatitis.

Hepatitis types A and B cannot be differentiated by clinical, biochemical, or histopathologic findings. Infection by hepatitis B virus is established by specific serologic tests (see above); positive tests for HB_cAg or HB_sAg indicate acute or chronic infection, whereas the presence of anti-HB_s suggests previous infection. When a patient with acute hepatitis has negative tests for HB_sAg and anti-HB_s, it is sometimes assumed that the illness is due to hepatitis A, but other viruses may also be responsible; unequivocal diagnosis of hepatitis A requires specific serologic evidence.

MANAGEMENT OF ACUTE VIRAL HEPATITIS. Hospitalization of patients with acute viral hepatitis is indicated during the early icteric phase when symptoms are severe (e.g., severe vomiting) or when there is clinical evidence at the time of diagnosis of serious illness, particularly manifestations of fulminant hepatitis. High risk patients — pregnant, diabetic, elderly, or those with complicating disease — should also be observed in hospital. Patients treated at home should be advised with respect to diet, alcohol intake, physical activity, and measures to reduce their infectivity. The routine precautions to reduce cross-infection in hospital are those applicable to enteric diseases, plus careful disposal of needles and syringes. During the early symptomatic period frequent careful clinical observation and assessment of liver function are necessary for early recognition and treatment of fulminant hepatitis. Liver function tests should be performed as often as is necessary to assess the patient's progress; a daily estimation of the prothrombin time after parenteral vitamin K_1 (10 mg intramuscularly) is valuable in detecting a sudden deterioration in liver function. A daily measurement of caloric intake is also helpful in assessing the patient's progress.

A liver biopsy should be performed if the diagnosis is not firmly established on the basis of clinical, biochemical, and serologic findings, or if an atypical course suggests progression to chronic disease.

Rest. The value of rest in acute viral hepatitis is suggested by the remission and exacerbation of symptoms that follow bed rest and physical activity, respectively. Nevertheless, the only controlled study on the effect of rest and activity in infectious hepatitis indicated that enforced rest was of no value in therapy and that activity did not cause complications, lengthen the course of the disease, or lead to chronic residual abnormalities. This controlled study was carried out on military personnel who were young and fit and who, irrespective of therapy, suffered no mortality or long-term sequelae that could be attributed to the viral hepatitis. In a civilian population of varied age, with other disease states complicating viral hepatitis infection, there are significant morbidity and mortality from bridging, multilobular, or massive necrosis. *Complete bed rest during the acute phase of viral hepatitis may protect some of these patients from these complications.* Until there is further information relating to a civilian population, it is recommended that all icteric patients rest in bed during the early symptomatic period when it may be difficult to assess the severity of illness; limited physical activity

should be permitted during the period of jaundice when the patient is otherwise asymptomatic.

Diet. During the preicteric and early icteric periods, a poor appetite and nausea or vomiting may limit food intake. The patient should be served and encouraged to eat those foods that appeal to him. For some patients, it is possible to increase the caloric content of the breakfast when they have difficulty in eating other meals. If a total intake of 2000 calories daily is not maintained, intravenous glucose supplements should be given.

Corticosteroids. Randomized clinical trials of corticosteroid therapy in patients with severe or fulminant hepatitis have shown that these agents are of no benefit in increasing patient survival. Thus steroid therapy is no longer recommended in acute hepatitis. (The use of corticosteroid therapy in chronic active hepatitis is discussed in Ch. 465.1.)

Sedatives. The plasma clearance of sedative agents may be depressed when the activity of microsomal drug metabolizing enzymes is reduced by acute liver injury; thus the plasma clearance and metabolism of diazepam and meperidine are markedly depressed in patients with acute hepatitis. Oxazepam may be the ideal sedative in these patients; its distribution, plasma binding, plasma clearance, and excretion remain normal in acute hepatitis.

Surgery. All surgical procedures should be deferred to the postconvalescent period if possible. There is evidence that abdominal surgery under general anesthesia increases the risk of bridging or multilobular necrosis.

MANAGEMENT OF THE HEPATITIS B CARRIER. The routine screening of blood donors and patients with liver disease for HB_sAg has raised special problems in the management and education of subjects who may be otherwise perfectly healthy. When a person is found to be HB_sAg positive, it should be confirmed that a chronic carrier state exists by repeated tests. If tests of liver function are abnormal, a liver biopsy is advised to define the nature of the associated liver disease. If there are no clinical manifestations of liver disease and liver function tests are normal, liver disease is very unlikely. The healthy HB_sAg carrier should be excluded from donating blood and should be advised to maintain careful personal hygiene.

PROPHYLAXIS. Immune globulins (ISG), prepared by cold ethanol fractionation of large pools of human plasma, contain varying amounts of antibody against hepatitis A and B viruses. A high titer of anti-HA is assured by the prevalence of anicteric hepatitis in the young. The titers of anti-HB_s in ISG usually exceed 1:64; specific immunoglobulin with a high titer of anti-HB_s (hepatitis B immune globulin [HBIG]) is prepared from sera of donors with anti-HB_s, and has been used in several clinical trials.

Hepatitis A. It is well established that ISG administered before or within two weeks of hepatitis A exposure will reduce the frequency of acute illness. Eighty to 90 per cent of those who develop hepatitis have an anicteric or asymptomatic infection which confers active immunity.

Pre-exposure prophylaxis is recommended for travelers who plan to reside in tropical or developing countries; for periods less than three months, a single dose of ISG, 0.02 ml per kilogram intramuscularly, is recommended, whereas for periods in excess of three months a larger dose of 0.05 ml per kilogram should be repeated every four to six months. Those exposed to nonhuman primates, particularly chimpanzees, should receive a prophylactic dose of ISG, 0.05 ml per kilogram every four months.

Postexposure prophylaxis with ISG is recommended within two weeks for those who have close personal contact with a hepatitis A patient; this should include household contacts and contacts within closed institutions such as prisons and facilities for the mentally retarded. Prophylaxis is not recommended for school and hospital contacts unless there is evidence of an outbreak of disease.

Hepatitis B. Immune globulin containing anti-HB$_s$ (either ISG or HBIG) has been shown to be of significant value in pre-exposure prophylaxis of patients and staff in hemodialysis units and in children admitted to institutions for the mentally retarded, as well as in postexposure prophylaxis of spouse contacts of hepatitis B patients, of infants born to HB$_s$Ag positive mothers, and of medical personnel accidentally inoculated with contaminated needles.

Pre-exposure prophylaxis is recommended only under conditions in which there is repeated exposure to HBV and appropriate environmental measures to limit infection cannot be implemented; prophylaxis with ISG, 0.05 to 0.07 ml per kilogram at four-month intervals, should be combined with routine serologic monitoring for HB$_s$Ag and anti-HB$_s$ so that those who acquire anti-HB$_s$ by infection can be removed from the program of prophylaxis.

Postexposure prophylaxis is recommended for those who are accidentally exposed to contaminated needles; HBIG in a dose of 0.05 to 0.07 ml per kilogram within seven days of inoculation and again after four weeks is suggested. ISG should be given in the same dose if HBIG is not available. Infants born of mothers who are HB$_s$Ag positive should be protected with ISG (0.5 ml per kilogram) or HBIG (0.13 ml per kilogram) within one week of birth.

456. FULMINANT HEPATITIS

Fulminant hepatitis (acute hepatitis with coma) resulting from extensive hepatic necrosis may be due to *toxic liver injury* (e.g., carbon tetrachloride toxicity or acetaminophen overdosage), *hypersensitivity reactions* to therapeutic agents (e.g., halothane sensitivity), or *viral hepatitis*. In the case of toxic liver injury, the lesion is predictable and dose related; in the case of hypersensitivity reactions, the development of liver disease is unpredictable unless there has been a previous sensitivity reaction to the drug. Fulminant hepatitis may be caused by viruses A or B; predisposing factors have not been well documented, but the risk of infection during late pregnancy in malnourished patients is high.

PATHOLOGY. When a diagnosis of fulminant hepatitis is suspected by the clinical course, a percutaneous liver biopsy is often precluded by the risk of bleeding caused by clotting abnormalities; the pathologic features are usually defined at postmortem examination. The liver is usually smaller than normal with a soft consistency and red-brown discoloration — thus the term *acute yellow atrophy*. Microscopically, there is confluent necrosis with disappearance of parenchymal cells, leaving a residual framework of collapsed reticulin, hepatic sinusoids, Kupffer cells, and inflammatory cells. Parenchymal cells surrounding portal tracts may be spared, or may exhibit evidence of degeneration or regeneration. The surviving Kupffer cells are usually hypertrophied and contain a yellow pigment — lipofuchsin. In portal areas, proliferation of bile ducts is commonly observed, and infiltration with inflammatory cells is usual. *Massive hepatic necrosis* usually leads to early death. *Bridging, multilobular, or severe zonal necrosis* may also cause hepatic coma. These lesions may extend, with death of the patient, or regeneration of parenchymal cells may permit survival. In surviving patients, parenchymal collapse with fibrosis or the development of chronic active hepatitis may lead to cirrhosis, or rapid parenchymal cell regeneration may restore normal hepatic architecture.

Pathologically, it is not possible to differentiate the hepatic lesions caused by toxic injury, drug hypersensitivity, or viral hepatitis.

CLINICAL MANIFESTATIONS. In patients with fulminant hepatitis, the preicteric period is usually brief with severe symptoms, particularly abdominal pain, vomiting, and high fever. The clinical features which suggest a fulminant course are as follows: (1) High fever, severe abdominal pain, and vomiting which persist for several days after the initiation of bed rest. (2) A sudden decrease in the size of the liver. (3) Neuropsychiatric changes of early hepatic encephalopathy, including drowsiness, irritability, insomnia, and confusion. (4) Severe prolongation of the prothrombin time (more than 20 seconds with control of 12 seconds) with or without bleeding (uncorrected by parenteral vitamin K). (Serum bilirubin and transaminase levels do not reflect the severity of illness; patients may die in hepatic coma during the early icteric period, or may become deeply jaundiced, while serum transaminase levels often fall during the period of clinical deterioration.) (5) The appearance of ascites during the acute illness.

The complications of acute liver failure include *hypoglycemia; bleeding* caused by deficient clotting factors; *disseminated intravascular coagulation*, which may accentuate liver cell necrosis; *acute hepatic encephalopathy* (described in Ch. 452) with terminal depression of medullary centers; *pneumonia* secondary to aspiration; *septicemia* with portals of entry at the sites of intravenous catheter lines, the gut, or urinary system; and terminal *renal failure* (hepatorenal syndrome).

MANAGEMENT. The patient with fulminant hepatitis requires intensive nursing care with monitoring and support of vital functions. In the comatose patient, a cuffed nasotracheal or tracheostomy tube should be inserted to prevent aspiration and to ensure adequate ventilation, with respirator support if necessary. Continuous intravenous infusion of glucose solution is required to prevent hypoglycemia in a patient who has no hepatic glycogen stores and has depressed glyconeogenesis. Fluid and electrolyte balance should be achieved by accurate measurement of intake and output. In the absence of hepatic plasma protein synthesis, plasma albumin levels can be maintained by intravenous infusion of solutions of salt-poor albumin. Deficiency of clotting factors can be partially corrected by infusion of fresh-frozen plasma. Although there is evidence for disseminated intravascular coagulation in patients with fulminant hepatitis, treatment with heparin has not been of benefit in limited clinical trials. The agitated, hyperactive patient should be restrained to prevent injury and should be sedated with small doses of diazepam (5 mg by intravenous injection); heavy sedation will deepen coma. General measures to treat hepatic coma are indicated (see Hepatic Coma in Ch. 465.2).

High dose corticosteroid therapy does not increase survival of patients with fulminant hepatitis and is no longer recommended.

A variety of measures designed to support the patient in acute liver failure have been described. These include *exchange transfusion, plasmapheresis, charcoal hemoperfusion, polyacrylonitrile-membrane hemodialysis, cross-perfusion* with a human volunteer or primate, or *extracorporeal perfusion* through a mammalian liver. Although published reports suggest that these measures may restore consciousness in some patients and thus prolong life, it has not been established by randomized controlled trials that any of these procedures are of benefit in reducing mortality. In the one prospective controlled study, exchange transfusion was of no benefit in decreasing mortality. Studies in experimental canine hepatitis showed that infusion of immune serum improved the survival of infected animals. Treatment of patients with fulminant viral hepatitis, type B, with plasma containing hepatitis B antibody has been evaluated, however, in a randomized, double-blind controlled study and found to be of no benefit.

Recovery from fulminant hepatitis depends on liver cell regeneration; currently there are no measures known to potentiate liver regeneration in these patients. The better prognosis for recovery in children probably relates to a greater regenerative capacity; any measures which prolong survival and increase the chance of liver cell regeneration should be used in treatment.

457. HEPATITIS DUE TO OTHER VIRUSES

The viruses of yellow fever, rubella, cytomegalic inclusion disease, and herpes simplex may cause hepatitis. Yellow fever is discussed in Ch. 102.2. Infection with *rubella, cytomegalic inclusion virus,* and *herpes simplex* may cause *neonatal hepatitis* with jaundice and hepatosplenomegaly. Rubella and cytomegalic inclusion viruses are transmitted transplacentally, whereas herpes virus infects the infant during delivery. Hepatitis resulting from these viral agents may be part of a generalized disease.

Many viral illnesses may be accompanied by minor, nonspecific changes in liver function (positive flocculation tests and slight transaminase elevation). There may be hyperplasia of Kupffer's cells and infiltration with mononuclear cells in portal areas — nonspecific reactive hepatitis.

VIRAL HEPATITIS, NON-A, NON-B

Immunologic evidence now indicates that the majority of patients who develop acute hepatitis following blood transfusions are infected with an unidentified agent; their sera remain Hb_sAg negative and exhibit no serologic response indicative of hepatitis A, hepatitis B, cytomegalovirus, or Epstein-Barr virus infection. This infection appears to have an incubation period of approximately six weeks and causes a milder illness than that due to hepatitis B virus.

INFECTIOUS MONONUCLEOSIS

Infectious mononucleosis is a systemic disease which is commonly associated with liver disease (see Ch. 89). Jaundice is unusual, although hepatic enlargement with mild

tenderness is often seen. The disturbances of liver function are those associated with hepatic infiltration: an elevation of the serum alkaline phosphatase, 5'-nucleotidase and leucine aminopeptidase, and BSP retention. Serum transaminase levels may be slightly elevated. Histologically, there is mononuclear infiltration predominantly in the portal areas with minimal evidence of cell necrosis.

No case of chronic liver disease has been proved to result from an attack of infectious mononucleosis.

This disease must be considered in the differential diagnosis of acute viral hepatitis. An atypical mononuclear cell reaction is common to these diseases, but tests for heterophil antibody, Epstein-Barr virus, and cytomegaloviruses differentiate them.

458. LIVER DISEASE ASSOCIATED WITH BACTERIAL INFECTIONS

In bacterial infection, liver disease may result from the effect of bacterial toxins on cell metabolism, changes in liver blood flow caused by endotoxin, shock or fever, localization and multiplication of bacteria in the liver, or the effect of antimicrobial agents.

Severe infections, particularly intraperitoneal, may cause obstructive jaundice with conjugated bilirubinemia, increased alkaline phosphatase, and minimal elevation of serum transaminase. In the absence of demonstrable lesions of the extrahepatic biliary system and normal operative cholangiograms, the jaundice in these patients is due to intrahepatic cholestasis resulting from unknown toxic factors.

Gram-negative septicemia with shock may cause acute hypoxic necrosis of the liver with jaundice as a terminal manifestation. The liver may be enlarged and tender. In *typhoid fever* there is focal necrosis of liver cells with acute and chronic inflammatory cell infiltration. An elevation of serum transaminases reflects parenchymal cell injury. In *leptospirosis,* jaundice is usually disproportionally greater than other evidence of liver involvement; the associated renal disease may impair urinary excretion of conjugated bilirubin.

Although the mucocutaneous lesions are most prominent features of *secondary syphilis,* liver disease is well documented. Hepatic enlargement with mild jaundice and elevated levels of alkaline phosphatase and transaminase in the serum are associated with polymorphonuclear infiltration of the portal tracts. Hepatic *tuberculosis* is discussed in Ch. 168.7.

459. ACUTE LIVER ABSCESS

Amebic abscesses are discussed in Ch. 196.

Pyogenic organisms which cause liver abscess may reach the liver by the biliary system (cholangitis), the portal venous system (portal pyemia in patients with appendicitis or umbilical sepsis), or arterial blood (staphylococcal septicemia or bacteremia from distant foci); by direct spread from contiguous structures (empyema of gallbladder or subphrenic abscess); or by penetrating wounds. Infection complicating biliary tract disease — *suppurative (ascending) cholangitis* — is now the most common cause for liver abscesses; the early diagnosis and treatment of acute appendicitis and umbilical sepsis in the newborn have decreased the frequency of abscess caused by pylephlebitis. The responsible organism for liver abscess reflects the source of infection; cholangitis is usually due to enteric organisms, particularly *E. coli*, anaerobic streptococci, and *Bacteroides* species. Abscesses formerly regarded as being sterile probably harbored anaerobic organisms which were not isolated because of inadequate anaerobic transport and culture techniques. Abscesses are more often multiple than solitary and involve the right lobe more frequently than the left. A decreasing frequency in the young and increasing frequency in the elderly reflect the decreasing morbidity after appendicitis and the greater relative frequency of abscesses caused by biliary tract disease.

The *clinical manifestations* of liver abscess are the result of sepsis and the presence of a space-occupying lesion(s) in the liver. *Paroxysmal fever* with *chills* and a *polymorphonuclear leukocytosis* are usual; a liver abscess should be considered in the differential diagnosis of persistent unexplained fever (FUO). Blood cultures are positive in approximately 50 per cent of patients. Gastrointestinal symptoms and abdominal signs are often nonspecific and include anorexia, nausea, epigastric or right upper quadrant pain, and liver enlargement with tenderness. Jaundice may not be an early clinical finding unless there is associated biliary tract obstruction.

Abnormalities of liver function reflect associated biliary tract disease and focal inflammatory disease in relation to the lesion. In the absence of biliary tract obstruction, serum alkaline phosphatase levels are usually only mildly elevated, and transaminase levels are often normal. A decrease in synthesis and an increased catabolism of albumin cause hypoproteinemia in the majority of patients. An enlarging liver abscess may elevate the diaphragm or may be associated with a pleural effusion.

DIAGNOSIS. The diagnosis of liver abscess is made too frequently at postmortem examination in patients who did not have the benefit of treatment. When symptoms and signs suggest the possibility of a liver abscess, the presence of a space-occupying lesion must be confirmed by *liver scanning* or by *ultrasound*. Selective *celiac arteriography* is of value in differentiating avascular (cysts and abscesses) and vascular (primary or metastatic neoplasms) space-occupying lesions in the liver. Amebic liver abscesses should be diagnosed by appropriate serologic tests (see Ch. 196); the clinical manifestations of pyogenic and amebic liver abscesses are similar.

TREATMENT. *Surgical drainage* of pyogenic liver abscess is usually recommended as the treatment of choice. Preoperative *antimicrobial therapy* to cover gram-negative and anaerobic organisms should be continued postoperatively until bacteriologic studies have identified the causal organism and specific drug therapy can be provided. There have been no clinical trials to determine whether antimicrobial therapy alone without surgical drainage is as effective as the surgical approach in treating liver abscesses; multiple small abscesses may be less accessible to the surgeon.

COMPLICATIONS. The major complications of liver abscess are septicemia and rupture of the abscess into the pleural space or peritoneum to produce an *empyema*, *subphrenic abscess*, or *generalized peritonitis*.

460. PROTOZOAN OR HELMINTHIC DISEASE OF THE LIVER

Parasites that commonly invade the liver include amebae (*E. histolytica* and malarial parasites), *schistosomes* (*S. mansoni*), flukes (*Clonorchis sinensis, Fasciola hepatica*), and tapeworms (*Echinococcus granulosus*). These diseases are discussed in Part X.

HEPATIC SCHISTOSOMIASIS. Hepatic involvement in patients with *Schistosoma mansoni* results from portal seeding with ova that lodge in the portal areas and stimulate an inflammatory reaction with fibrosis. In acute schistosomiasis, the response to ova liberated two to eight weeks after infection is often associated with fever, diarrhea, hepatic and splenic enlargement, and intense eosinophilia. Transient abnormalities of liver function include increases in serum alkaline phosphatase and transaminase. In the later stage of hepatic parasitism, portal fibrosis interferes with hepatic blood flow and causes a presinusoidal portal hypertension, splenomegaly, and a collateral portal-systemic circulation. Bleeding from esophageal varices is a major complication. Liver function is usually good, so that patients may tolerate recurrent bleeding very well and do not usually develop ascites unless bleeding or malnutrition lowers serum albumin concentrations. Surgical decompression of the portal system by portacaval or splenorenal shunting is effective in preventing recurrent bleeding from esophageal varices, but it has not been established by prospectively controlled clinical trials that shunt surgery prolongs the life of these patients.

The diagnosis of hepatic schisotomiasis is established by demonstrating ova on liver biopsy; examination of "squash" preparations in glycerol is more helpful than routine histologic examination. The presence of ova in the stools or rectal biopsy of a patient with portal hypertension and splenomegaly suggests this diagnosis (see Ch. 210).

461. TOXIC AND DRUG-INDUCED LIVER DISEASE

461.1. TOXIC HEPATITIS

A *hepatotoxin* is defined as an agent that causes liver injury in both man and animals in a predictable manner. Liver injury is dose related and is usually manifest after a relatively short latent period. Hepatotoxins may cause liver cell necrosis or biochemical changes with necrosis; these changes may be manifest by impaired formation of bile, disturbances of lipid metabolism with fat accumulation, or altered enzyme activity. Some hepatotoxins may exert their effect indirectly by interfering with hepatic blood flow (*Senecio* alkaloids in veno-occlusive disease).

With elimination of a number of industrial hazards, exposure to hepatotoxins other than alcohol (ethanol) is now usually accidental or suicidal. Hepatotoxic agents are not often used pharmacologically unless the therapeutic dose is considerably less than the toxic dose, or unless therapy, despite toxic side effects, may still benefit the patient. Immunosuppressive agents and certain agents used in the chemotherapy of cancer may be hepatotoxic.

Poisoning by several hepatotoxic agents is discussed in Part IV.

CARBON TETRACHLORIDE LIVER INJURY

The hepatotoxicity of carbon tetrachloride is believed to be due to the formation of toxic metabolites which bind to microsomal proteins. The increase in carbon tetrachloride toxicity after alcohol ingestion in man and laboratory animals has been related to an increase in the activity of drug metabolizing enzymes with increased formation of toxic metabolites; phenobarbital also increases carbon tetrachloride toxicity in laboratory animals.

The clinical features of carbon tetrachloride liver injury are similar to those of acute viral hepatitis, but with a shorter symptomatic preicteric period and with more rapid recovery, unless massive necrosis causes early death or renal tubular necrosis leads to irreversible or fatal renal failure.

The symptoms that follow inhalation or ingestion of the agent are predominantly gastrointestinal, with *anorexia, nausea* and *vomiting,* and right upper quadrant *pain* with *tender hepatomegaly* preceding the onset of jaundice. In many patients there may be hepatic enlargement with acute elevation of serum transaminase levels without jaundice. Acute renal failure is often a more prominent manifestation of poisoning.

Pathologically, there is centrilobular necrosis without inflammation during the period of maximal liver injury, followed rapidly by regeneration of parenchymal cells and hyperplasia of Kupffer's cells. Complete restoration of structure and function follows recovery from a single exposure. There is some evidence, however, that repeated exposure may sometimes lead to cirrhosis of the liver.

The management of acute liver failure caused by carbon tetrachloride is discussed in Ch. 456.

LIVER INJURY DUE TO ALCOHOL

Experimental studies in man and animals have shown that alcohol (ethanol) is a direct hepatotoxin. All the lesions of alcoholic liver disease in man have been produced by feeding alcohol to baboons for periods up to four years; these lesions included fatty infiltration, alcoholic hepatitis, fibrosis, and cirrhosis. A nutritious diet did not protect these animals from developing liver disease.

The clinical and pathologic manifestations of alcoholic liver disease are discussed in detail in Ch. 465.2.

SEX HORMONES AND THE LIVER

Methyl testosterone and C-17 alkyl substituted steroids (norethandrolone) may cause *intrahepatic cholestasis* with conjugated hyperbilirubinemia, reduced clearance of BSP (with normal hepatic uptake and conjugation), and increased serum alkaline phosphatase and 5'-nucleotidase activity. This effect is dose related in man, causes no permanent liver damage or acute

parenchymal cell necrosis, and is reversible. This type of cholestasis may be due to a change in the permeability of the biliary tree to bile salts.

Peliosis hepatis has been described as a complication of long-term therapy with androgenic-anabolic steroids; this lesion consists of blood-filled spaces of varying size in the hepatic parenchyma. Liver enlargement usually precedes changes in liver function; patients with extensive lesions may exhibit severe impairment of liver function with jaundice, hypoalbuminemia, and prolonged prothrombin time. Liver failure or bleeding from a ruptured cyst may contribute to the patient's death. The pathogenesis of the peliosis hepatis lesion has not been well defined, but it has been suggested that focal areas of parenchymal necrosis are replaced by blood. Patients on long-term therapy with androgenic-anabolic steroids should be screened for changes in liver function; if peliosis hepatis is diagnosed early by liver biopsy, withdrawal of the steroid may prevent progressive disease. Hepatomas may also complicate high dose anabolic steroid therapy.

During the third trimester of normal pregnancy there may be increases in serum cholesterol, alkaline phosphatase, and 5'-nucleotidase with reduced clearance of BSP. Occasionally, impaired hepatic excretory function may cause jaundice that recurs in subsequent pregnancies — *recurrent jaundice of pregnancy.* Recent studies have shown that natural estrogens reduce hepatic BSP clearance. It is probable that the physiologic changes in liver function during the third trimester of pregnancy are due to hormone effects on the liver. These observations are of particular interest in view of the recent reports that hormones given to suppress ovulation may occasionally cause hepatic dysfunction.

The association of liver cell adenomas with oral contraceptive use is discussed in Ch. 467.

ACETAMINOPHEN LIVER INJURY

Self-poisoning with excessive doses of acetaminophen is now recognized as a relatively common cause for centrilobular liver necrosis with severe hepatitis in Great Britain. Therapeutic doses of acetaminophen cause no liver injury, because potentially toxic metabolites are rapidly conjugated with glutathione to nontoxic compounds. Excessive doses of acetaminophen (particularly with blood levels in excess of 300 μg per milliliter four hours after drug administration) exhaust the available glutathione, and toxic metabolites which bind covalently to microsomal protein accumulate and cause liver cell necrosis. In animal experiments, the glutathione precursors, cysteine and cysteamine, protect against liver injury caused by acetaminophen. In clinical trials, cysteamine hydrochloride administered intravenously within ten hours of acetaminophen ingestion was effective in reducing the severity of liver injury; this therapy was associated with severe gastrointestinal side effects (anorexia, nausea, and vomiting). N-acetylcysteine, available as a 10 or 20 per cent sterile solution, is effective orally and better tolerated than cysteamine. This agent is currently under clinical trial.

ISONIAZID HEPATITIS

Prospective studies in tuberculin-positive patients receiving isoniazid revealed that between 10 and 20 per cent developed transient elevations of serum transaminase activity (usually less than 100 IU). Clinically overt liver disease occurs in approximately 1 per cent of patients, and is indistinguishable clinically, biochemically, and pathologically from acute viral hepatitis. The onset of symptoms is usually during the first 12 weeks of treatment but may be delayed for up to a year. Jaundice is preceded by gastrointestinal symptoms (anorexia, nausea, vomiting, or abdominal discomfort) in more than half the patients, and by symptoms suggestive of a viral illness (fever, myalgias, or arthralgias) in 35 per cent. With cessation of drug therapy there is usually prompt resolution of the liver disease, but in approximately 10 per cent of patients the liver disease is fulminant and fatal.

Factors that influence the hepatotoxicity of isoniazid include the patient's age and acetylator phenotype. Isoniazid hepatitis is rare in patients under 20 years of age and increases in incidence with increasing age. Patients who have survived liver injury are more often rapid acetylators of the drug who may thus produce a higher concentration of toxic metabolites. In animals, the hepatotoxicity of isoniazid and acetylisoniazid is increased by phenobarbital; this is accompanied by increased formation of metabolites that covalently bind to liver macromolecules.

It is recommended, in patients over the age of 35, that the prophylactic use of isoniazid be restricted to those with a high risk of developing active tuberculosis. The drug should be immediately discontinued when symptoms suggest the possibility of liver disease, or when biochemical monitoring (SGOT test at intervals of two to four weeks) shows evidence of liver injury. Early cessation of therapy may reduce the severity of liver disease and decrease mortality from this complication.

461.2. LIVER DISEASE DUE TO HYPERSENSITIVITY DRUG REACTIONS

Liver injury after drug therapy is more often due to a *hypersensitivity reaction* than to a hepatotoxic effect. In contrast to hepatotoxic reactions, the hypersensitivity reaction is quite unpredictable unless a previous reaction has been recorded, is not dose related, follows a variable latent period after drug exposure, cannot be reproduced in experimental animals, and may be associated with other manifestations of hypersensitivity (skin rash, fever, eosinophilia).

Drug hypersensitivity reactions involving the liver may be minor local manifestations of a generalized reaction, e.g., minor changes in liver function in patients with exfoliative dermatitis, or may be the predominant manifestation of the reaction. The common hepatic lesions are *intrahepatic cholestasis* and *parenchymal cell necrosis*. The former is illustrated by reactions to *chlorpromazine,* and the latter by reactions to halothane or *alpha-methyldopa.*

CHLORPROMAZINE JAUNDICE

Approximately 1 per cent of patients treated with this phenothiazine develop a hypersensitivity reaction with intrahepatic cholestasis and jaundice. A greater number of patients develop changes in excretory function without jaundice. Early symptoms, beginning acutely usually within one to four weeks of initial drug exposure, or within a few days of repeated challenge, include *nausea, vomiting,* and *epigastric pain* often associated with *fever, lymphadenopathy, skin eruptions,* and *arthralgias.* The liver becomes enlarged and variably tender. Jaundice is obstructive in type with severe pruritus, dark urine, and pale stools, and tests of liver function reflect predominant *cholestasis* with conjugated hyperbilirubinemia and increased serum alkaline phosphatase, 5'-nucleotidase, and cholesterol levels. The serum transaminase levels may be elevated in the range of 100 to 200 IU. The white blood count may be normal or slightly elevated, with peripheral eosinophilia.

On liver biopsy, intrahepatic cholestasis, with bile plugs in dilated bile canaliculi and bile staining of parenchymal cells, and variable periportal infiltration with mononuclear and eosinophil cells are the predominant findings. There may be minimal centrilobular necrosis of liver cells.

Jaundice usually subsides within a few days or weeks of onset, with complete recovery, but occasionally chronic intrahepatic cholestasis may develop in spite of cessation of drug therapy. The clinical features in these patients may be similar to those in primary biliary cirrhosis, but periportal fibrosis is less severe, and eventual recovery without cirrhosis is usual.

TREATMENT. There is no specific therapy. The offending agent should be discontinued and avoided thereafter. Cholestyramine, 2 to 4 grams orally before meals, may relieve pruritus with lowering of serum bile acid levels. Vitamin K should be given parenterally if malabsorption causes an increase in prothrombin time. Corticosteroids are of little benefit either in relieving jaundice or in reducing pruritus.

HEPATITIS AFTER ANESTHESIA WITH FLUORINATED AGENTS

Acute liver disease, clinically and pathologically similar to viral hepatitis, is an uncommon complication of anesthesia with the fluorinated agents *halothane* and *methoxyflurane.* The mechanism of liver injury appears to be a *hypersensitivity reaction.* Liver disease is more common with repeated exposure to the anesthetic agent, and recurrent episodes have shorter latent periods between exposure and onset of symptoms; recurrent hepatitis has been well documented in several anesthetists after occupational exposure to halothane. Immunologic phenomena in patients with hepatitis after halothane exposure include peripheral eosinophilia, a transiently positive test for antimitochondrial antibodies in serum, and stimulation of cultured peripheral lymphocytes by halothane.

Several etiologic factors should be excluded before postoperative liver necrosis is attributed to an anesthetic agent; these include *hypoxia, hypotension, postoperative sepsis, biliary tract disease, viral hepatitis* (either coincidental or after transfusion), and *reactions to other drugs.* It is difficult to establish a diagnosis of hepatitis caused by anesthetic exposure with any degree of certainty unless there is a history of acute liver disease after previous exposure to the agent.

The treatment of patients with hepatitis caused by anesthetic agents is similar to that of acute viral hepatitis (see Ch. 455 and 456). When a patient has recovered from halothane or methoxyflurane hepatitis, further exposure to these anesthetic agents should be avoided.

METHYLDOPA HEPATITIS

Hepatitis is a rare complication of methyldopa therapy; it is unpredictable, unrelated to drug dosage, and not reproducible in experimental animals. Like isoniazid hepatitis, methyldopa hepatitis is clinically, biochemically, and pathologically similar to acute viral hepatitis but with a higher mortality. Liver disease usually occurs within four weeks of initial drug therapy, and jaundice is preceded for one to two weeks by prodromal symptoms of fever, malaise, fatigue, anorexia, nausea, vomiting, and weight loss. When a patient is rechallenged with methyldopa following recovery from hepatitis, the recurrent liver disease is usually of earlier onset and more severe. The abnormalities of liver function are those of parenchymal cell injury; cholestasis is rarely the predominant abnormality. Tests for antinuclear antibodies and LE cells are sometimes positive, suggesting an immunologic reaction. The hepatic lesion may be focal necrosis with inflammation, or may be more extensive with bridging, multilobular, or massive necrosis. In some patients, the clinical and pathologic changes are suggestive of chronic active hepatitis. Early withdrawal of methyldopa therapy before the onset of jaundice permits rapid recovery; continued drug therapy or rechallenge with methyldopa may lead to massive necrosis. Although patients have been treated with corticosteroids, there is no evidence that this therapy is of benefit. Patients with liver failure should receive the general supportive therapy discussed under fulminant hepatitis. Careful clinical and biochemical monitoring during the first eight weeks of methyldopa therapy should be effective in preventing severe liver disease.

462. FATTY LIVER

Fat accumulation in the liver (fatty liver) may be a physiologic response to an increase in lipid mobilization from peripheral fat, e.g., during early starvation, or may result from several disturbances of lipid transport and metabolism in a variety of disease states. Excessive lipid in parenchymal cells may arise from one or more of three sources: (1) the diet, (2) peripheral fat depots, and (3) hepatic synthesis. Lipid from any of these sources may accumulate when the supply is increased, or when a decrease in hepatic oxidation of fatty acids or reduced lipoprotein synthesis and release diminishes the clearance of lipid from the liver.

In *starvation*, free fatty acids are mobilized from adipose tissue, and are in part esterified in the liver to triglyceride. This physiologic response is probably the mechanism for the fatty infiltration of the liver observed in many patients after acute and chronic illnesses. In *protein malnutrition (kwashiorkor),* extreme fatty liver may be related to fat mobilization from depots (free fatty acid concentrations in serum are elevated), and in part to impaired lipoprotein synthesis. In *obese patients,* an excessive accumulation of fat in the liver may be a reflection of the general increase in the triglyceride stores. *Diabetic ketoacidosis,* with excessive mobilization of depot fat, is usually accompanied by liver enlargement caused by fat. In

each of these conditions the major clinical manifestation of fatty liver is hepatic enlargement; tenderness usually accompanies acute enlargement. *BSP retention* may be the only abnormality of liver function.

In several conditions fatty liver may be associated with severe derangement of liver function. This is particularly the case when fat accumulation is due to toxic injury causing decreased fatty acid oxidation or impaired lipoprotein synthesis. In *carbon tetrachloride* or *phosphorus* poisoning, fat accumulation is one manifestation of toxic liver injury. Large intravenous doses of *tetracycline* (usually more than 1 gram daily), particularly in pregnant women, have caused liver failure and death; a fine fatty vacuolization of the liver cells is the major pathologic change in the liver. In two syndromes, fatty liver is accompanied by severe encephalopathy with high mortality; the clinical picture is that of fulminant hepatitis. *Fatty liver of pregnancy* usually presents with vomiting, abdominal pain, and jaundice during the last month of pregnancy; bleeding, premature labor, renal failure, and coma with convulsions rapidly lead to death. The serum bilirubin and alkaline phosphatase elevations suggest severe cholestasis; disturbances of the clotting mechanism reflect impaired synthesis of clotting factors. *Reye's syndrome* is a fulminant childhood illness in which a panlobular fatty liver is associated with acute encephalopathy. The presenting symptoms are usually those of a severe encephalopathy with an agitated delirium and vomiting. Liver enlargement is usual, but jaundice is rare. The encephalopathy may proceed rapidly to coma with decerebrate posturing and cerebral edema with midbrain herniation and death. Severe hypoglycemia may precipitate convulsions. Epidemiologic studies during an outbreak in 1973–1974 showed that 88 per cent of patients, with a mean age of 11 years, suffered from an upper respiratory illness during the preceding two weeks; this coincided with an epidemic of influenza B. Sporadic cases among younger children followed a variety of viral illnesses, including varicella. The morphologic and biochemical changes in the liver of patients subjected to liver biopsy correlate with the laboratory features of the illness and probably parallel the changes that occur in other organs. Liver glycogen stores are depleted, cell membranes are disrupted and permit leakage of enzymes with serum transaminase elevation, and mitochondrial damage is accompanied by lowered levels of the urea cycle enzymes, ornithine transcarbamylase, and carbamyl phosphate synthetase. An increased protein and amino acid catabolism with reduced urea synthesis causes an increase in blood ammonia. Both the neurologic and liver lesions are reversible if cerebral edema can be controlled. Treatment of mild disease (Grade I and II encephalopathy) requires only intravenous glucose and maintenance of fluid and electrolyte balance. Patients with severe encephalopathy require intensive care with endotracheal intubation, exchange transfusion, and monitoring of intracranial pressure. *Small bowel bypass surgery* (particularly jejunocolic shunts) for the treatment of extreme obesity is often complicated by fatty infiltration of the liver with progressive impairment of liver function or the development of cirrhosis. These changes may be secondary to protein malnutrition caused by malabsorption and bacterial overgrowth in the intestine. Serial liver biopsies should be performed in these patients to monitor histologic changes.

The most common form of toxic liver injury leading to fatty infiltration of the liver is that due to *alcohol (ethanol) ingestion* (see Ch. 465.2).

Treatment of the underlying cause of fatty liver, e.g., correction or protein malnutrition, or withdrawal from alcohol, is usually effective in lowering the fat content of the liver. In patients with acute severe liver injury associated with encephalopathy, measures used in the management of patients with fulminant hepatitis have been applied with variable success (see Ch. 456).

463. THE LIVER IN ACUTE HEART FAILURE AND SHOCK

Hypoxia secondary to reduced liver blood flow may cause centrilobular parenchymal cell necrosis. This often complicates *acute congestive heart failure* or *hypotension* of any cause. The liver may be enlarged and tender if the central venous pressure is raised. The predominant clinical manifestations are those of the underlying cardiovascular disease, which determines both therapy and prognosis. The biochemical features of liver disease in patients with heart failure may be those of liver cell necrosis with enzyme release from damaged liver cells, or intrahepatic cholestasis when excretory function is impaired by decreased perfusion. A decrease in the synthesis of plasma proteins often causes hypoprothrombinemia and increases the sensitivity to anticoagulant drugs. In shock, the serum transaminase levels are sometimes markedly elevated but return quickly to normal levels with restoration of normal blood flow and parenchymal cell regeneration. Deep jaundice may be a terminal event in patients with prolonged shock.

464. HEPATIC VEIN OCCLUSION

(Budd-Chiari Syndrome)

Occlusion of the hepatic veins is a rare condition usually caused by *tumor infiltration* (hepatoma, metastatic tumor) or *thrombosis* of the vessels. This may be a local lesion, or may extend from the inferior vena cava. *Polycythemia vera* is one of the more common causes of thrombosis of these veins. The major clinical manifestations of this condition are *hepatic enlargement*, with *pain* and *tenderness*, and *ascites*. In the acute form, hepatic vein occlusion is characterized pathologically by centrilobular congestion and necrosis of the adjacent parenchyma. A needle biopsy of the liver should establish the diagnosis when hepatic congestion resulting from an increase in central venous pressure has been excluded. The obstruction may be subacute or chronic when ascites and portal hypertension are the major clinical problems. *Hepatic venography* by direct injection of contrast material into a hepatic catheter is the most valuable technique for establishing the diagnosis.

Patients with chronic hepatic vein occlusion usually respond to a diuretic program (see Ascites in Ch. 465.2). Polycythemia vera should also be treated vigorously (see Ch. 492.1).

465. CHRONIC LIVER DISEASE

465.1. CHRONIC ACTIVE HEPATITIS

Chronic active hepatitis is characterized pathologically by a normal lobular architecture in which fibrous septa extend from enlarged portal tracts into the parenchyma, disrupting the liver cell plates adjacent to the portal zones and separating off rosettes of parenchymal cells. Piecemeal necrosis of liver cells adjacent to the expanding portal zones, infiltration of the portal areas with eosinophils, lymphocytes and plasma cells, and focal necrosis and inflammation within liver lobules are present in varying degrees and reflect the "activity" of the lesion. Progressive destruction of the normal lobular architecture with proliferation of fibroblasts in expanding portal areas and nodular regeneration of parenchymal cells may ultimately lead to cirrhosis in untreated patients.

PATHOGENESIS. Chronic active hepatitis is a disease process of diverse etiology. In the majority of patients, a specific etiologic factor has not been identified, but in others, chronic hepatitis B infection or drug reactions are of etiologic importance. The relative frequency of chronic hepatitis B infection as a cause for chronic active hepatitis in a given population will vary with the incidence of infection in that population. In some patients with hepatitis B infection, chronic active hepatitis may follow acute viral hepatitis, but in the majority there is no history of acute infection with jaundice. *Immunologic mechanisms*, either humoral or cellular, may play an important role in the pathogenesis of chronic active hepatitis irrespective of the primary etiology. In patients who are HB_sAg negative, there may be an autoimmune reaction to a specific lipoprotein antigen localized on the plasma membrane of liver cells; these patients have circulating antibodies to liver-specific lipoprotein, immunoglobulin G is bound to the membrane of liver cells, and their peripheral lymphocytes bearing Fc-receptors are cytotoxic to liver cells. In patients with chronic active hepatitis who are HB_sAg positive, the localization of HB_sAg to the surface membrane of liver cells may be responsible for liver cell injury either by antibody or by immunologically stimulated cells bearing Fc-receptors. Although there have been no immunologic studies to confirm this, it is possible that chronic active hepatitis associated with drug therapy (oxyphenisatin or methyldopa) may be related to the localization of drug or metabolite on the liver cell membrane where it acts as an antigen.

Immunologic phenomena are a prominent feature of patients with idiopathic (or autoimmune) chronic active hepatitis. Hypergammaglobulinemia parallels disease activity, and the patient's serum may contain a variety of autoantibodies which lack organ specificity; these include antinuclear, anti-DNA (native), antimitochondrial, and anti–smooth muscle antibodies. These antibodies are uncommon in patients with HB_sAg positive chronic active hepatitis. The increased frequency of other diseases considered to have an immunopathologic basis, both in patients with idiopathic chronic active hepatitis and in their close relatives, provides further support for an autoimmune pathogenesis; Sjögren's syndrome, thyroid disease, and fibrosing alveolitis with pulmonary diffusion defects are commonly associated diseases. Studies on serum complement levels in patients with chronic active hepatitis have revealed that depressed complement levels are related to impaired hepatic protein synthesis and do not reflect immunologic activity.

The association of HB$_s$Ag negative chronic active hepatitis with the HLA-B8 antigen suggests that genetic factors play a role in the development of this disease.

CLINICAL MANIFESTATIONS. Chronic active hepatitis is a disease with a wide clinical spectrum and insidious onset; it may be clinically silent for long periods, as in patients who present as asymptomatic blood donors and are found to be HB$_s$Ag positive with elevated SGOT levels; patients with more active disease may present with symptoms suggestive of acute hepatitis with malaise, arthralgias, anorexia, and low-grade fever. Amenorrhea commonly results from disturbances of endocrine function. On physical examination, the patient may exhibit signs of both acute and chronic liver disease; these include jaundice, spider angiomas, liver enlargement with variable tenderness, and splenomegaly. The presence of ascites or manifestations of portal hypertension suggests that cirrhosis is already established. The important laboratory features of chronic active hepatitis are changes in *serum transaminase* levels and *hypergammaglobulinemia*, because it has been shown that these tests reflect the activity of the disease — the extent of liver cell necrosis and the degree of associated round cell infiltration in the liver. Patients who present with clinical manifestations of acute hepatitis and subsequently exhibit elevated levels of serum transaminase and gamma globulin for periods in excess of ten weeks are likely to be suffering from chronic active hepatitis or bridging zonal necrosis. The prognosis of patients with extreme hyperglobulinemia (gamma globulin levels greater than twice normal) and with five- to ten-fold elevations of serum transaminase (SGOT) persisting without improvement over a ten-week period is extremely poor without therapy; more than a third of these patients die within a period of six months. When disease activity is minimal, patients may remain well for long periods. Increases in the level of serum bilirubin and alkaline phosphatase caused by intrahepatic cholestasis and depression of plasma albumin and clotting factor levels caused by impaired hepatic plasma protein synthesis are variable features of advanced disease.

DIAGNOSIS. The diagnosis of chronic active hepatitis should be confirmed by percutaneous *liver biopsy* whenever there is clinical or laboratory evidence of this disease. It is important to differentiate chronic active hepatitis from other liver diseases, particularly *chronic persisting hepatitis* which has a favorable prognosis for full recovery without therapy. The degree of irreversible liver damage — cirrhosis — can be determined only by morphologic studies. In all patients with chronic active hepatitis, potential etiologic factors should be fully evaluated, i.e., exposure to drugs and the presence of circulating HB$_s$Ag or anti-HB$_s$. Wilson's disease must be excluded by slit lamp examination of the eyes for Kayser-Fleischer rings, and by measurements of serum ceruloplasmin levels and urinary copper excretion; acute liver disease in these patients may mimic chronic active hepatitis.

Patients with chronic active hepatitis and cholestasis may be difficult to differentiate from those with active primary biliary cirrhosis. Although tests for antimitochondrial antibody may be positive in some patients with chronic active hepatitis, the titer is usually low in contrast to the high titers seen in patients with primary biliary cirrhosis. The patients with primary biliary cirrhosis do not respond to treatment with corticosteroids; but if this diagnosis is uncertain, a trial of therapy is indicated.

TREATMENT. It has been established by controlled clinical studies that corticosteroids increase the survival of *symptomatic patients with severe chronic active hepatitis*. In the Mayo Clinic study, patients with biochemical and histologic evidence of severe disease (SGOT levels five- to ten-fold elevated, and gamma globulin more than two-fold increased for periods of ten weeks) were treated with prednisone (20 mg daily), a combination of prednisone (10 mg daily) with azathioprine (50 mg daily), azathioprine (100 mg) alone, or placebo; treatment with prednisone or prednisone with azathioprine was significantly more effective than azathioprine alone or placebo in inducing clinical remission and prolonging survival. The frequency of drug-related side effects is less in patients on a combined regimen of prednisone (10 mg daily) with azathioprine (50 mg daily) than in patients receiving higher maintenance doses of prednisone (20 mg daily). Thus the combined drug regimen is recommended, particularly in patients with relative contraindications to steroid therapy (e.g., with diabetes mellitus) or in those who develop complications during steroid therapy. Although treatment with a single dose of prednisone on alternate mornings is effective in inducing a clinical and biochemical remission in patients with chronic active hepatitis, there is biopsy evidence that this regimen may not be effective in preventing disease activity and progression.

The duration of corticosteroid therapy should be determined by the clinical, biochemical, and histologic response. The goal of therapy is to induce remission of active hepatitis; the patient should be asymptomatic, with normal or minimally elevated SGOT (less than twice normal) and normal gamma globulin levels, and with resolution of inflammation and liver cell necrosis on liver biopsy; this end result can be anticipated in approximately two thirds of patients treated for one to three years. When complete remission is established, corticosteroids can be slowly withdrawn and discontinued; subsequent relapses usually occur within six months and require further therapy.

Although treatment with prednisone or prednisone and azathioprine is clearly indicated in symptomatic patients with severe chronic active hepatitis, the decision whether to treat a patient with low-grade activity, e.g., a patient with mild symptoms and minimal elevation of SGOT and gamma globulin, may be difficult. Guidelines derived from controlled clinical trials are not available, and the potential benefit from corticosteroid therapy may be exceeded by the risks of long-term therapy.

PROGNOSIS. With adequate therapy, remission of active disease with restoration of normal liver morphology or with residual inactive cirrhosis is achieved in approximately two thirds of patients. Approximately 20 per cent of patients with severe chronic active hepatitis, particularly those who are HB$_s$Ag positive, fail to respond to steroid therapy and die with liver failure caused by progressive cirrhosis within a period of one to three years. The long-term prognosis of patients with chronic active hepatitis of low-grade activity has not been defined.

465.2. CIRRHOSIS OF THE LIVER

DEFINITION AND CLASSIFICATION. The cirrhotic liver is one in which the normal lobular architecture is destroyed by bands of fibrous tissue which separate nodules of regenerated liver cells (regeneration nodules). Clinically, patients with cirrhosis usually present with symptoms that relate to the primary etiology (e.g., chronic active hepatitis or manifestations of excessive alcohol intake) or with complications of cirrhosis (e.g., ascites, bleeding from esophageal varices, or hepatic coma). At the time of diagnosis, major etiologic factors causing chronic liver disease may be evident (e.g., documented hepatitis progressing to *chronic active hepatitis, excessive alcohol intake,* or *chronic biliary tract obstruction),* but in many patients the etiology is never defined. Macroscopic and/or microscopic examination of liver tissue is necessary to establish the diagnosis of cirrhosis, but the pathologic changes in the liver may be the end-stage of several alternative processes which are not always evident at the time of autopsy examination.

In this chapter an *etiologic* classification is used; alternative terminology for cirrhosis will be referred to in the text.

1. Posthepatitic and idiopathic cirrhosis.
2. Alcoholic cirrhosis.
3. Metabolic cirrhosis (hemochromatosis and Wilson's disease).
4. Biliary cirrhosis (primary and secondary).
5. Schistosomal fibrosis.
6. Cardiac cirrhosis.

Hemochromatosis is discussed in Ch. 489, Wilson's disease in Ch. 537, and schistosomal fibrosis in Ch. 210.

POSTHEPATITIC AND IDIOPATHIC CIRRHOSIS (POSTNECROTIC CIRRHOSIS)

PATHOGENESIS. It has been shown by serial liver biopsy studies that acute viral hepatitis (usually type B, either icteric or anicteric), toxic hepatitis complicated by bridging or multilobular necrosis, or chronic active hepatitis may lead to a macronodular cirrhosis. In many nonalcoholic patients there is no history to suggest previous viral or toxic hepatitis; i.e., the cirrhosis is idiopathic (cryptogenic). Undiagnosed chronic active hepatitis may be responsible for the cirrhosis in the majority of these patients. Idiopathic cirrhosis is sometimes associated with chronic ulcerative colitis; it has been suggested but not proved that chronic pericholangitis resulting from portal bacteremia may cause cirrhosis in these patients.

PATHOLOGY. The liver in posthepatitic or idiopathic cirrhosis is typically shrunken, with irregular large regeneration nodules and broad zones of fibrous tissue. Pathologically, this is referred to as *macronodular (postnecrotic) cirrhosis.* During the phase of *progressive (active) cirrhosis* after bridging or multilobular necrosis or chronic active hepatitis, there may be microscopic evidence of cell degeneration and regeneration, and mononuclear infiltration (both lymphocytes and plasma cells) is prominent in the zones of fibrosis. Intrahepatic cholestasis with bile plugs in dilated bile canaliculi varies with the degree of jaundice, and bile duct proliferation is usual.

CLINICAL MANIFESTATIONS. The progressive cirrhosis that follows chronic active hepatitis is often associated with malaise, weakness, anorexia, and jaundice. The patient often has a low-grade fever, and multiple spider angiomas may be seen. The liver is sometimes enlarged and tender, but is more typically shrunken and associated with increased percussion resonance over the right lower costal margin; the spleen may be slightly or massively enlarged. Ascites or peripheral edema may complicate portal hypertension or hypoalbuminemia, and increased bruising may be due to hypoprothrombinemia. Manifestations of disturbed endocrine function — acne, striae, gynecomastia, and amenorrhea — are particularly common in juvenile patients with active cirrhosis. Hypergammaglobulinemia parallels the degree of lymphocytic and plasma cell infiltration in the liver, and may be accompanied by serologic abnormalities. Chronic intrahepatic cholestasis with jaundice, hypercholesterolemia, and high alkaline phosphatase levels sometimes mimics primary biliary cirrhosis. It is not unusual for the biochemical evidence of hepatocellular failure to exceed the clinical evidence of this condition.

The only clinical manifestations of compensated idiopathic cirrhosis may be the cutaneous stigmata of chronic liver disease and splenic enlargement. In these patients, ascites, hepatic coma, and bleeding from esophageal varices may be late complications.

TREATMENT. Patients with chronic active hepatitis should be treated with corticosteroids to induce clinical remission. When cirrhosis is already established in these patients (confirmed by liver biopsy), corticosteroids will not reverse the existing cirrhosis, but by suppressing continued destructive activity they may prevent progression of the liver disease (see Ch. 465.1). Corticosteroid therapy is not indicated in patients with inactive posthepatitic cirrhosis.

The management of the complications of cirrhosis is discussed later in this chapter under treatment of portal hypertension, ascites, and hepatic coma.

CIRRHOSIS IN THE ALCOHOLIC

PATHOGENESIS AND EPIDEMIOLOGY. The incidence of cirrhosis in the United States parallels the consumption of alcohol. Little is known, however, of the factors that determine individual susceptibility to cirrhosis; these would explain why many persons with a chronic heavy intake of alcohol do not develop liver disease; both genetic and dietary factors may be of importance. Some insight into the problem of liver disease in the alcoholic has been gained from experimental studies on the effect of alcohol (ethanol) on liver metabolism.

The Effects of Alcohol (Ethanol) on the Liver. Both in man and in laboratory animals, alcohol ingestion is associated with two prominent morphologic changes: the accumulation of fat (triglyceride) in parenchymal cells and degeneration of cell organelles (visible as *alcoholic hyaline*–eosinophilic cytoplasmic inclusions). These changes may result from a direct *hepatotoxic effect of alcohol* rather than a deficiency of dietary factors;

they are seen when alcohol is substituted for carbohydrate in an adequate diet.

The pathogenesis of cirrhosis in the alcoholic was not clarified by earlier studies in laboratory animals; in the rat, prolonged administration of alcohol caused fatty infiltration and parenchymal cell degeneration, but these lesions did not progress to cirrhosis. Recent studies in baboons fed alcohol for periods of nine months to four years have reproduced all the pathologic lesions of human alcoholic liver disease.

PATHOLOGY. The liver in *acute alcoholic hepatitis* is enlarged and firm, and on microscopic examination the parenchymal cells are distended with droplets of fat, and may contain eosinophilic cytoplasmic inclusions (alcoholic hyaline). Central veins show early fibrosis, and centrilobular areas may be replaced by zones of *hyaline sclerosis,* a lesion which undergoes subsequent fibrosis and may contribute to the development of portal hypertension. There is variable inflammatory cell infiltration in portal areas and throughout the parenchyma, and bile stasis occurs in jaundiced patients.

Cirrhosis in the alcoholic is usually of the *micronodular type,* with small uniform regeneration nodules separated by fibrous bands containing mononuclear cells and proliferating bile ductules. The pathologic changes of acute alcoholic hepatitis — inflammation, cell degeneration, and infiltration with fat — are often seen in the cirrhotic liver. Occasionally the cirrhosis is of the *macronodular type,* with coarse, irregular regeneration nodules and broad intervening bands of fibrous tissue.

CLINICAL MANIFESTATIONS. A patient with *acute alcoholic hepatitis* may seek medical help because of *abdominal pain* caused by acute hepatic enlargement, gastritis, or pancreatitis; *vomiting,* with or without *hematemesis,* caused by gastritis, ulcer, or sometimes esophageal varices; *jaundice; abdominal swelling* with ascites; or because of symptoms caused by head injury, alcohol withdrawal, or thiamin deficiency.

On admission to hospital, the patient is usually *febrile* and *dehydrated* and has an alcoholic fetor. An *enlarged, firm, tender liver* and abdominal distention with *ascites* and *jaundice,* with prominent spider angiomas and palmar erythema, are typically present. The early hospital course is often complicated by *delirium tremens.* Intense jaundice with *pruritus* in febrile patients may simulate extrahepatic biliary tract obstruction.

Liver function tests reveal conjugated hyperbilirubinemia, elevated serum transaminase levels (50 to 300 units), variable increases in alkaline phosphatase activity, and normal or depressed levels of albumin and clotting factors. The serum cholesterol concentration may be increased, normal, or depressed. *Hypokalemia* often results from increased urinary excretion of potassium. *Hyperuricemia* resulting from depressed urinary excretion of uric acid parallels lactic acidosis. Anemia may be due to bleeding or *hemolysis; acute severe hemolysis* is sometimes associated with *hyperlipemia* (Zieve's syndrome).

Cirrhosis in the alcoholic may present insidiously with anorexia, fatigue, and weakness, and a gradual onset of jaundice and ascites, or may present acutely with one or several major complications: acute upper gastrointestinal *bleeding,* sudden onset of *ascites,* liver failure with *jaundice* or *coma,* or symptoms of hepatic *carcinoma.* When the cirrhotic patient shows manifestations of acute alcoholic hepatitis, the term *florid cirrhosis* is often used. In the absence of these complications the

only stigmata of cirrhosis may be a firm, enlarged, nontender liver with or without splenomegaly, and the cutaneous manifestations of chronic liver disease.

In *compensated cirrhosis* the only abnormalities of liver function may be mild BSP retention and an increased urinary excretion of urobilinogen. With progressive decompensation, serum protein concentrations fall, and hyperbilirubinemia and BSP retention increase. Serum enzyme levels are usually only slightly elevated.

DIFFERENTIAL DIAGNOSIS. In the differential diagnosis of acute alcoholic hepatitis other causes for acute jaundice must be considered, i.e., *viral hepatitis, extrahepatic obstruction,* and *drug reactions.* Infection should be considered in the febrile patient, although fever may be due to cell necrosis. In the compensated cirrhotic, an enlarged, firm liver may be suggestive of infiltrative disease. A needle biopsy of the liver usually resolves these differential diagnostic problems.

When cirrhosis is complicated by bleeding, ascites, or coma, other causes for these complications must be excluded. In cirrhotic patients, acute upper gastrointestinal *bleeding* may come from esophageal varices; but acute gastric erosions, peptic ulcer, and neoplasm must also be considered. Esophagoscopy, gastroscopy, and roentgenologic evaluation of the esophagus, stomach, and duodenum are necessary to establish the site of bleeding (see Ch. 407). Although *ascites* is usually due to portal hypertension with hypoalbuminemia, *constrictive pericarditis, bacterial peritonitis* (especially *tuberculous*), and *intra-abdominal neoplasm* must also be considered. Measurement of the venous pressure and a diagnostic paracentesis with analysis for protein, enzymes, bacteria, and cells are of value in differential diagnosis. In tuberculous peritonitis the protein concentration of ascitic fluid may exceed 2.5 grams per 100 ml and the ascitic fluid white cell count usually exceeds 250 per cubic millimeter, with lymphocytes predominant. Malignant effusions are often hemorrhagic, with a protein content greater than 2.5 grams per 100 ml and elevated lactic dehydrogenase activity; malignant cells may be found on cytologic examination.

TREATMENT. Long-term abstinence from alcohol is the single major factor that may modify the course of liver disease in the alcoholic. With abstinence, liver function may return to normal after an episode of acute alcoholic hepatitis, and minimal hepatic fibrosis may persist without progression. When cirrhosis is well established and portal hypertension with esophageal varices complicates the liver disease, abstinence from alcohol may not prolong the patient's survival.

Patients with *acute alcoholic hepatitis* should be treated with bed rest, alcohol withdrawal, and a diet containing adequate proteins, vitamins, minerals, and calories. Intravenous infusions of 5 per cent glucose, with potassium, magnesium, and vitamin supplements, may be needed by the febrile, dehydrated patient. Oral supplements of ferrous sulfate (0.3 gram three times a day) or folic acid (5 mg daily) should be given to correct anemia caused by iron or folic acid deficiency. Salt intake should be restricted to 1 gram per 24 hours in patients with ascites, and fluid intake and output should be monitored with daily weights. On this regimen clinical and biochemical improvement is usual within two to three weeks, and is accompanied by a spontaneous diuresis and disappearance of ascites unless portal hypertension is already established by fibrosis.

In a series of controlled clinical trials, corticosteroid

therapy was not shown to be of benefit in patients with acute alcoholic hepatitis. In five studies the over-all mortality in steroid-treated patients was 37 per cent, as compared to a mortality of 42 per cent in those receiving placebo.

TREATMENT OF THE COMPLICATIONS OF CIRRHOSIS

PORTAL HYPERTENSION WITH UPPER GASTROINTESTINAL BLEEDING. In the early management of bleeding, treatment is directed toward restoring blood volume and controlling the bleeding at the same time that diagnostic efforts are made to determine the site of bleeding. The alcoholic patient may bleed from *acute gastric erosions, peptic ulcer,* or *esophageal varices;* appropriate therapy depends on the site of bleeding. The several measures that may be used to control bleeding in cirrhotic patients include gastric lavage with ice water, local gastric hypothermia using an esophagogastric balloon, intravenous infusions of Pitressin, esophageal tamponade with an inflated balloon, or direct surgical procedures. *Lavage* with ice water is unlikely to control esophageal bleeding, but may be effective when bleeding is from gastric erosions. Infusions of Pitressin (20 units intravenously in 10 minutes) constrict the splanchnic arterioles, reduce splanchnic blood flow, and lower portal venous pressure. Bleeding from varices may thus be temporarily controlled. Similar results may be achieved without systemic side effects by continuous infusion of vasoconstrictor drugs into the superior mesenteric artery, selectively catheterized. *Esophageal tamponade* (with a Sengstaken esophageal tube) may be the only nonoperative procedure that will control massive bleeding from esophageal varices. The disadvantage of this procedure is the many complications that result from tamponade: asphyxia resulting from upward displacement of the balloon, aspiration, and esophageal erosion by pressure necrosis. These complications, however, will be minimized by using an additional smooth bore tube attached to the Sengstaken tube for aspiration of secretions proximal to the balloon and by tracheal intubation with a cuffed endotracheal tube.

Several surgical procedures have been recommended to control bleeding from esophageal varices. These include direct ligation of varices, transection of the esophagus with division of varices, esophagogastric resection, splenectomy, and splenorenal or portacaval anastomosis. Each procedure carries a high risk in the poor-risk patient with hepatic decompensation. The surgical procedure of choice is a *portacaval anastomosis,* which controls bleeding by lowering portal pressure; with the subsequent disappearance of esophageal varices, recurrent bleeding is unusual.

A portacaval anastomosis is recommended for the good-risk patient with documented bleeding from esophageal varices, unless bleeding has been precipitated by acute alcoholic hepatitis. In the latter instance, portal pressure may return to normal, and varices may disappear upon recovery from acute hepatic decompensation and resolution of hepatic inflammation and fatty infiltration. When esophageal bleeding complicates hepatocellular failure, surgery is contraindicated even when medical therapy is ineffective in controlling hemorrhage. There is no evidence that a prophylactic portacaval shunt is of value in prolonging the life of a patient with portal hypertension and esophageal varices that have not bled. Although prophylactic shunt surgery reduces the risk of subsequent variceal hemorrhage, the complications of surgery — hepatic encephalopathy and hepatic failure — result in considerable morbidity.

Of the several portal-systemic shunt procedures that have been described, the distal splenorenal shunt, which selectively decompresses the esophageal varices without draining mesenteric blood from the liver, may be the procedure of choice. Although this operation is probably more likely to be associated with shunt thrombosis caused by a low flow rate, the risk of progressive liver failure following operation may be considerably decreased.

ASCITES. When ascites complicates acute alcoholic hepatitis, therapy aimed at improving liver function usually leads to a spontaneous diuresis as the portal pressure falls toward normal and serum albumin levels rise. Sodium intake should be restricted to 1 gram daily, and diuretics should be used with caution.

When ascites is of longer duration and is associated with sustained portal hypertension and hypoalbuminemia, diuretic agents together with a restricted intake of sodium may be necessary to control sodium and water retention. Water intake may need to be restricted to a volume that equals insensible losses plus urine output in patients who fail to excrete a fluid load. The sole use of diuretic agents that act principally on the proximal tubule (mercurials and chlorothiazides) is contraindicated. These agents do not counteract the effect of aldosterone on the distal tubule; not only are they ineffective diuretics in cirrhotic patients with secondary hyperaldosteronism, but they also augment potassium loss and may precipitate *hypokalemic alkalosis* with hepatic coma in spite of oral potassium supplements.

To promote an *effective* and *safe* diuresis, an *aldosterone blocking agent* should be given in combination with one of the aforementioned diuretic agents. Spironolactone (50 to 200 mg daily) with hydrochlorothiazide (50 to 100 mg daily) is recommended. Oral potassium supplements (KCl in cherry syrup, 1 gram three times a day) may be necessary during the initial two to four days of combined drug therapy to prevent hypokalemia. Whereas edema fluid can be mobilized rapidly during diuresis, the maximal rate at which ascitic fluid can be removed by diuresis in the cirrhotic is approximately 900 ml per 24 hours. In patients free of peripheral edema, the rate of diuresis should not produce a daily weight loss in excess of 0.5 kg; if diuresis is more rapid, there will be a fall in plasma volume.

The complications of diuretic therapy include the following: (1) *Hyperkalemia* often results from the use of aldosterone-blocking drugs in patients with impaired renal function. (2) *Hyponatremia* may be associated with an abnormal distribution of sodium between the intracellular and extracellular fluid pools in patients with an increased total body sodium, with disproportionate water retention, or with sodium depletion after prolonged diuresis. (3) *Azotemia* may be due to contraction of the extracellular fluid pool or a decrease in glomerular blood flow owing to intrarenal shunting of blood. (4) *Hepatic encephalopathy* may follow rapid diuresis or disturbances of pH and electrolyte balance. These complications will be reduced if serum electrolyte concentrations and urinary electrolyte excretion are measured frequently during therapy. Diuretics should be discontinued when neuropsychiatric symptoms complicate rapid diuresis or electrolyte imbalance, and no attempt should be made to mobilize all ascitic fluid by prolonged therapy that increases the risk of complication without benefit to the patient. When long-term diuretic therapy is necessary to control ascites, diuretics should be given intermittently rather than continuously.

When ascites is associated with severe hypoalbuminemia, intravenous infusions of salt-poor albumin (50 to 100 grams daily) may potentiate a diuresis, but pulmonary edema caused by an expanded plasma volume must be avoided.

Paracentesis with removal of less than 1000 ml of ascitic fluid should be performed for diagnostic purposes, but is now rarely indicated for therapy of ascites except when impaired renal function prevents safe or effective diuretic therapy. Ascitic fluid should then be removed slowly through a small plastic catheter, and salt-poor human albumin (50 to 200 grams) should be infused intravenously over a period of 12 to 24 hours to prevent hypovolemia and shock that may result from a shift of fluid from the intravascular compartment into the peritoneal cavity.

HEPATIC COMA. When a cirrhotic patient develops hepatic encephalopathy it is important to identify the precipitating cause. It may be due to gastrointestinal bleeding; fluid and electrolyte imbalances and pH disturbances, particularly during diuretic therapy; the administration of depressant drugs, both analgesic and sedative; intercurrent infection with fever; or increased dietary intake of protein. In the treatment of hepatic coma, gastrointestinal bleeding and infection must be controlled, depressant drugs withheld, and disturbances of fluid, electrolyte, and acid-base balance corrected. In all patients, measures that lower blood ammonium concentration by reducing enteric bacterial breakdown of amino acids and urea should be instituted. These measures include dietary *protein restriction* (complete in the comatose patient, or partial — 20 to 40 grams — in patients with mild encephalopathy), *cathartics* (magnesium citrate, 240 ml twice daily), *enemas* to clear the intestine of its nitrogenous content, and *neomycin* (4 to 6 grams daily by mouth or by nasogastric tube) to reduce the bacterial flora.

Patients with chronic hepatic encephalopathy, who usually have extensive portal-systemic shunts, may be helped by long-term restriction of protein intake to 40 grams and the administration of neomycin, 2 to 3 grams daily. Lactulose, a disaccharide that is not absorbed but is metabolized by intestinal bacteria to organic acids, is effective in lowering the blood ammonia levels of patients with chronic encephalopathy; the unabsorbed sugar produces an osmotic diarrhea, and ammonia is retained in the fecal content at the acid pH.

A surgical approach to the management of the patient with chronic hepatic encephalopathy is excision or exclusion of the colon; the complications of surgery in chronically ill patients usually balance the potential benefit of removing a bacteria-laden gut.

BILIARY CIRRHOSIS

Primary biliary cirrhosis (chronic nonsuppurative destructive cholangitis) is a disease of unknown etiology. *Chronic intrahepatic cholestasis* is associated with progressive periportal fibrosis and chronic inflammation. Cirrhosis with nodular regeneration is a late pathologic finding. Although hypersensitivity reactions to drugs sometimes cause prolonged intrahepatic cholestasis, there is no evidence that acute intrahepatic cholestasis leads to primary biliary cirrhosis. It has been suggested that the primary lesion may be an injury to small bile ducts; these are often absent in liver biopsy specimens taken early in the course of the disease, but regenerate in the cirrhotic liver. Patients with primary biliary cirrhosis may exhibit hypergammaglobulinemia with circulating antibodies reactive against mitochondria (antimitochondrial antibody), but the significance of immunologic phenomena has not been established.

In *secondary biliary cirrhosis,* bile duct obstruction with or without infection causes periportal inflammation with progressive fibrosis, parenchymal cell destruction, and nodular regeneration.

CLINICAL FEATURES. Primary biliary cirrhosis is most often diagnosed in women aged 40 to 60. The earliest symptom may be generalized *pruritus.* Jaundice with dark urine and pale stools and cutaneous xanthomas appear later with increasing intrahepatic cholestasis. At the time of onset of symptoms, the liver is usually firm and enlarged, and the spleen is palpable. Liver function tests at this time reflect cholestasis with good hepatocellular function; alkaline phosphatase, 5'-nucleotidase, and cholesterol levels may be markedly elevated, whereas serum albumin levels remain normal. During the period of maximal cholestasis the manifestations of malabsorption may become evident: *weight loss, diarrhea* with pale bulky stools, *bleeding* resulting from hypoprothrombinemia, and collapse of vertebrae and *pathologic fractures* with bone demineralization caused by malabsorption of vitamin D and calcium. *Xanthomas* usually appear when the serum cholesterol level exceeds 450 mg per 100 ml. Acute upper gastrointestinal bleeding is more often from a duodenal ulcer than from esophageal varices; a reduced flow of alkaline bile with normal gastric acid secretion may contribute to peptic ulcer. It has been suggested that excessive copper deposition in the liver resulting from impaired biliary excretion may be responsible for progressive liver failure in these patients. The increase in copper stores is occasionally associated with the development of Kayser-Fleischer rings.

The terminal stage of biliary cirrhosis is one of hepatocellular failure with rising serum bilirubin levels, a decrease in serum albumin and cholesterol with disappearance of xanthomas, and the onset of ascites.

DIFFERENTIAL DIAGNOSIS. The diagnosis of primary biliary cirrhosis must always be confirmed by liver biopsy and cholangiography (percutaneous, retrograde, or operative). Stenosing cholangitis, extrahepatic bile duct obstruction resulting from stone or stricture, and carcinoma involving the major extrahepatic or intrahepatic bile ducts should be excluded. The presence of antimitochondrial antibody is of diagnostic importance — patients with acute extrahepatic biliary obstruction do not exhibit this antibody.

TREATMENT. Supplements of fat-soluble vitamins should be given to prevent or correct deficiency caused by malabsorption. Vitamin K_1, 5 to 10 mg, vitamin A 10,000 units, and 25-hydroxy–vitamin D, 100 to 200 μg, should be administered daily by mouth. *Pruritus* may be relieved by methyltestosterone or norethandrolone, 10 mg twice or three times daily, but these agents increase the jaundice. The bile acid sequestrant resin, *cholestyramine*, 8 to 12 grams daily in divided doses, is effective in relieving pruritus, lowering serum cholesterol levels, and reducing xanthomas when cholestasis is incomplete. Patients with duodenal ulcer or with complications of cirrhosis should be treated appropriately as outlined elsewhere.

Preliminary controlled studies suggest that treatment with d-penicillamine may be of long-term benefit in decreasing the progression of liver disease.

PROGNOSIS. Asymptomatic patients who are diagnosed by screening biochemical tests have an excellent prognosis and may never develop icteric disease. Symptomatic patients have an average life expectancy of five years after the onset of jaundice. With supportive therapy the patient will be more comfortable and will suffer fewer complications during this period.

CARDIAC CIRRHOSIS

Chronic congestive heart failure with valvular heart disease and tricuspid incompetence or constrictive pericarditis may cause progressive fibrosis extending peripherally from centrilobular to portal areas. Regeneration nodules are not prominent. Fat may accumulate in hypoxic cells.

The liver is usually firm, with tenderness and an increase in size during more severe episodes of heart failure. Hepatic pulsation may be detected with tricuspid insufficiency. The changes in liver function are those of acute hepatic congestion, but hypoalbuminemia may be more severe when there is excessive enteric leakage of plasma protein. (See Ch. 408.) Although chronic congestive heart failure may raise the portal venous pressure, a portal-systemic collateral circulation, e.g., esophageal varices, does not develop in the absence of an increased pressure gradient between these systems.

466. CONGENITAL HEPATIC FIBROSIS

Congenital hepatic fibrosis is a variant of polycystic disease. Broad bands of fibrous tissue containing bile ducts surround the liver lobules and obstruct portal blood flow. Splenomegaly, portal hypertension, and bleeding from esophageal varices are the usual presenting manifestations in childhood or adolescence. With normal liver function these children usually tolerate recurrent bleeding and portacaval shunt surgery better than patients with cirrhosis. In adults, *polycystic disease of the liver* may cause massive liver enlargement without interfering with liver function. The complications include hemorrhage into a cyst with abdominal pain and bleeding from esophageal varices.

467. INFILTRATIVE DISEASE OF THE LIVER

HEPATIC GRANULOMAS

Hepatic granulomas are most commonly due to *sarcoidosis* and *tuberculosis*, but also occur in beryllium

poisoning, brucellosis, fungal and parasitic infections, and Hodgkin's disease.

In sarcoidosis there are noncaseating granulomas, with mononuclear, epithelioid, and giant cells, and variable fibrosis. In patients with pulmonary tuberculosis or miliary tuberculosis, hepatic granulomas are particularly common. Small lesions may exhibit no caseation, and no organisms may be demonstrated; but larger lesions may have a central area of caseation.

Granulomatous disease of the liver may be associated with enlargement of the liver and BSP retention with elevation of alkaline phosphatase and 5'-nucleotidase without jaundice. A needle biopsy of the liver should be performed to establish the diagnosis of granulomatous disease. This is particularly helpful in the diagnosis of miliary tuberculosis in an ill, febrile patient without typical radiologic changes in the chest.

BENIGN TUMORS OF THE LIVER

Hemangiomas are the most common benign tumors of the liver. Capillary hemangiomas may be associated with *hereditary telangiectasias*. Cavernous hemangiomas are usually small (1 to 2 cm) and solitary. Rarely, large lesions may rupture and cause intraperitoneal bleeding.

Adenomas of the liver, particularly large symptomatic tumors that have presented with abdominal pain, intraperitoneal bleeding, or as a palpable abdominal mass, have increased in frequency during recent years. These have been associated with the long-term use of oral contraceptive agents. Regression following cessation of hormone therapy and recurrence following resection in patients who continued therapy provide strong support for this association. The adenomas described in patients who were not receiving oral contraceptive agents were usually smaller, and were rarely symptomatic.

SECONDARY CARCINOMA OF THE LIVER

Primary carcinomas of the lung, gastrointestinal tract, and breast are the most common neoplasms that metastasize to the liver. Abdominal swelling or pain and jaundice are the presenting symptoms, but the liver is usually massively enlarged with multiple nodules before jaundice develops. The earlier biochemical manifestations of hepatic metastases are BSP retention and elevations of serum alkaline phosphatase and 5'-nucleotidase. Needle biopsy of the liver is helpful in providing a tissue diagnosis of secondary carcinoma, and may save the patient from the discomfort of an exploratory laparotomy. External radioisotopic scanning of the liver after the intravenous injection of a gamma-emitting radioisotope that is concentrated in the liver may be helpful in localizing large metastases that appear as "cold" areas in the surface scan. The presence of hepatic metastases from carcinomas of the colon and pancreas is usually associated with positive tests for carcinoembryonic antigen (CEA) in the serum; false-positive tests have been reported in patients with decompensated alcoholic liver disease.

SARCOMAS OF THE LIVER

Hepatic infiltration with lymphoma, lymphosarcoma, or Hodgkin's disease is usually a manifestation of disseminated disease. Firm liver enlargement and bio-chemical evidence of intrahepatic cholestasis suggest, but are not necessarily diagnostic of, hepatic infiltration. Jaundice is more often the result of hepatic infiltration than invasion of the extrahepatic bile ducts by tumor; jaundice caused by intrahepatic cholestasis may develop, however, in the absence of liver infiltration. Splenomegaly is commonly associated with hepatic involvement in Hodgkin's disease. Percutaneous liver biopsy is less effective than biopsy through a peritoneoscopy in establishing the presence of liver involvement.

Angiosarcoma of the liver has been documented as a late complication of occupational exposure to vinyl chloride. Portal hypertension caused by hepatic fibrosis may precede the development of this neoplasm.

PRIMARY CARCINOMAS OF THE LIVER
(Hepatoma)

Hepatic carcinoma usually complicates cirrhosis of the liver; it has a higher incidence in postnecrotic cirrhosis and hemochromatosis than in Laennec's cirrhosis. This lesion should be suspected whenever a cirrhotic patient exhibits unexplained clinical deterioration with enlarging liver, right upper quadrant pain, or sudden onset of ascites. A vascular bruit may be heard over these tumors. Hypoglycemia is sometimes a prominent clinical manifestation. Changes in liver function include a rising alkaline phosphatase and elevated lactic dehydrogenase. A laboratory manifestation of hepatoma is the appearance of a fetal plasma protein, alpha-fetoprotein, in the plasma; sensitive radioimmunoassay techniques have recently detected this protein in the plasma of patients recovering from hepatitis. Hepatomas localized to one lobe of the liver have been excised successfully on several occasions, but usually cirrhosis and invasion of hepatic veins or local spread prevent surgical therapy.

Hepatoma can be produced with a high degree of regularity in several species of laboratory animals by injection of minute doses of the microtoxin known as *aflatoxin*. This substance is produced by *Aspergillus* growing on peanut (groundnut) meal that has been stored in appropriately hot, humid conditions. The incidence of hepatoma in man has long been known to show a marked geographic variation, and there is a correlation between the localities where hepatoma is the most frequently occurring carcinoma and the particular complex of circumstances that favors the production of aflatoxin. Obviously, it cannot be stated as yet that hepatoma in man is caused by aflatoxin, but this possibility that hepatoma is thus environmentally induced is being actively pursued in epidemiologic. clinical, and laboratory studies. The association of positive HB_sAg tests in patients with hepatoma in tropical and developing countries has also suggested that chronic viral hepatitis B infection may play an etiologic role in the development of this neoplasm.

General

Davidson, C. S.: Liver Pathophysiology. Its Relevance to Disease. Boston, Little, Brown & Company, 1970.

Scheuer, P. J.: Liver Biopsy Interpretation. London, Balliere, Tindall and Cassell, Ltd.,

Schiff, L.: Diseases of the Liver. 4th ed. Philadelphia, J. B. Lippincott Company, 1975.

Sherlock, S.: Diseases of the Liver. 5th ed. Oxford, Blackwell Scientific Publications, 1975.

Manifestations of Liver Disease

Berk, P., Bloomer, J. R., Howe, R. B., and Berlin, N. I.: Constitutional hepatic dysfunction (Gilbert's syndrome). A new definition based on kinetic studies with unconjugated radiobilirubin. Am. J. Med., 49:296, 1970.

Bissell, D. M.: Formation and elimination of bilirubin. Gastroenterology, 69:519, 1975.

Kaplan, M. M.: Alkaline phosphatase, N. Engl. J. Med., 286:200, 1972.

LaRusso, N. F., Hofmann, E. F., and Korman, M. G.: Validity and sensitivity of an intravenous bile acid tolerance test in patients with liver disease. N. Engl. J. Med., 292:1209, 1975.

Reynolds, T. B., Ito, S., and Iwatsuki, S.: Measurement of portal pressure and its clinical application. Am. J. Med., 49:649, 1970.

Rothschild, M. A., Oratz, M., and Schreiber, S. S.: Albumin metabolism. Gastroenterology, 64:324, 1973.

Scheuer, P. J.: Liver biopsy in the diagnosis of cirrhosis. Gut, 11:275, 1970.

Shand, D. G.: Drug disposition in liver disease. N. Engl. J. Med., 296:1527, 1977.

Acute Liver Disease

Chalmers, T. C., Eckhardt, R. D., Reynolds, W. E., Cigarroa, J. G., Jr., Deane, N., Reifenstein, R. W., Smith, C. W., and Davidson, C. S.: The treatment of acute infectious hepatitis. Controlled studies of the effect of diet, rest, and physical reconditioning on the acute course of the disease and on the incidence of relapses and residual abnormalities. J. Clin. Invest., 34:1136, 1955.

Chalmers, T. C., and Alter, H. J.: Management of the asymptomatic carrier of the hepatitis-associated (Australia) antigen. N. Engl. J. Med., 285:613, 1971.

Duffy, J., Lidsky, M. D., Sharp, J. T., Davis, J. S., Person, D. A., Hollinger, F. B., and Min, K-W: Polyarthritis, polyarteritis and hepatitis B. Medicine, 55:19, 1976.

Gregory, P. B., Knauer, C. M., Kempson, R. L., and Miller, R.: Steroid therapy in severe viral hepatitis. A double-blind, randomized trial of methyl-prednisolone versus placebo. N. Engl. J. Med., 294:681, 1976.

Klatskin, G., and Kimberg, D. V.: Recurrent hepatitis attributable to halothane sensitization in an anesthetist. N. Engl. J. Med., 280:515, 1969.

Krugman, S., Friedman, H., and Lattimer, C.: Viral hepatitis, type A. Identification by specific complement fixation and immune adherence tests. N. Engl. J. Med., 292:1141, 1975.

Mitchell, J. R., Zimmerman, H. J., Ishak, K. G., Thorgeirsson, U. P., Timbrell, J. A., Snodgrass, W. R., and Nelson, S. D.: Isoniazid liver injury: Clinical spectrum, pathology and probable pathogenesis. Ann. Intern. Med., 84:181, 1976.

Public Health Service Advisory Committee on Immunization Practices: Immune globulins for protection against viral hepatitis. Center for Disease Control, Morbidity and Mortality Weekly Report, 26:425, 1977.

Redeker, A. G., and Hamahiro, H. S.: Controlled trial of exchange-transfusion therapy in fulminant hepatitis. Lancet, 1:3, 1973.

Rimland, D., Parkin, W. E., Miller, G. B., and Schrack, W. D.: Hepatitis B outbreak traced to an oral surgeon. N. Engl. J. Med., 296:953, 1977.

Sabbaj, J., Sutter, V. L., and Finegold, S. M.: Anaerobic pyogenic liver abscess. Ann. Intern. Med., 77:629, 1972.

Schweitzer, I. L., Dunn, A. E. G., Peters, R. L., and Spears, R. L.: Viral hepatitis B in neonates and infants. Am. J. Med., 55:762, 1973.

Sherlock, S.: Halothane hepatitis. Gut, 12:324, 1971.

Sherlock, S.: The course of long incubation (virus B) hepatitis. Br. Med. Bull., 28:109, 1972.

Snodgrass, P. J., and DeLong, G. R.: Urea-cycle enzyme deficiencies and an increased nitrogen load producing hyperammonemia in Reye's syndrome. N. Engl. J. Med., 294:855, 1976.

Vittal, S. B. V., Thomas, W., Jr., and Clowdus, B. F.: Acute viral hepatitis. Course and incidence of progression to chronic hepatitis. Am. J. Med., 55:757, 1973.

Chronic Liver Disease

Blitzer, B. L., Mutchnick, M. G., Joshi, P. H., Phillips, M. M., Fessel, J. M., and Conn, H. O.: Adrenocorticosteroid therapy in alcoholic hepatitis. A prospective, double-blind, randomized study. Dig. Dis., 22:477, 1977.

Boyer, J. L., and Katskin, G.: Patterns of necrosis in acute viral hepatitis. Prognostic value of bridging (subacute hepatic necrosis). N. Engl. J. Med., 283:1063, 1970.

Conn, H. O.: A rational approach to the hepatorenal syndrome. Gastroenterology, 65:321, 1973.

Conn, H. O., Lindenmuth, W. W., May, C. J., and Ramsby, G. R.: Prophylactic portacaval anastomosis. Medicine, 51:27, 1972.

Gabuzda, G. J.: Cirrhosis, ascites and edema. Clinical course related to management. Gastroenterology, 58:546, 1970.

Golding, P. L., Smith, M., and Williams, R.: Multisystem involvement in chronic liver disease. Studies on the incidence and pathogenesis. Am. J. Med., 55:772, 1973.

Klatskin, G.: Hepatic tumors: Possible relationship to use of oral contraceptives. Gastroenterology, 73:386, 1977.

Lieber, C. S.: Hepatic and metabolic effects of alcohol. Gastroenterology, 65:821, 1973.

Maddrey, W. C., and Boitnott, J. K.: Drug-induced chronic liver disease. Gastroenterology, 72:1348, 1977.

Ray, M. B., Desmet, V. J., Bradburne, A. F., Desmyter, J., Fevery, J., and DeGroote, J.: Differential distribution of hepatitis B surface antigen and hepatitis B core antigen in the liver of hepatitis B patients. Gastroenterology, 71:462, 1976.

Rubin, E., and Lieber, C. S.: Fatty liver, alcoholic hepatitis and cirrhosis produced by alcohol in primates. N. Engl. J. Med., 290:128, 1974.

Schenker, S., Breen, K. J., and Hoyumpa, A. M.: Hepatic encephalopathy; current status. Gastroenterology, 66:121, 1974.

Sherlock, S., and Scheuer, P. J.: The presentation and diagnosis of 100 patients with primary biliary cirrhosis. N. Engl. J. Med., 289:674, 1973.

Soterakis, J., Resnick, R. H., and Iber, F. L.: Effects of alcohol abstinence on survival in cirrhotic portal hypertension. Lancet, 2:65, 1973.

Summerskill, W. H. J., Korman, M. G., Ammon, H. V., and Baggenstoss, A. H.: Prednisone for chronic active liver disease: Dose titration, standard dose, and combination with azathioprine compared. Gut, 16:876, 1975.

PART XVII

DISEASES OF NUTRITION

468. NUTRIENT REQUIREMENTS

Nevin S. Scrimshaw

GENERAL CONSIDERATIONS

The nutrient intakes recommended by most national and international organizations are defined as the amounts sufficient for the physiologic needs of virtually all healthy persons in a population. Conceptually, they are intended to cover the mean plus two standard deviations, although the data for actually calculating a standard deviation are rarely available. It is important for the physician to recognize that existing recommended dietary allowances for nutrients do not cover the additional needs that arise from microbial disease, trauma, advanced malignancies, disorders of the gastrointestinal tract, or metabolic diseases and abnormalities. Moreover, the intake recommended for any one nutrient presupposes that the requirements for energy and for all other nutrients are fully met.

Persons receiving less than the recommended allowance are not necessarily malnourished; it depends on their individual requirements, on the margin of safety inherent in the recommendation, and on whether other deficiencies are more limiting. On the other hand, persons consuming the recommended allowance are not necessarily adequately nourished. The presence of disease may interfere with absorption, increase utilization, or accelerate loss of an essential nutrient. This should be taken into account in prescribing diets for persons with acute or chronic disease. Moreover, imbalance among nutrients can render inadequate an intake which would otherwise be ample.

The 1974 Recommended Dietary Allowances of the Food and Nutrition Board (FNB) of the National Academy of Sciences are given in Table 1. They differ from those of the United Kingdom and FAO/WHO in their higher recommendations for calcium and ascorbic acid and slightly lower recommendations for calories.

The following nutrients have been established as necessary dietary constituents for man under physiologic or pathologic conditions.

NECESSARY NUTRIENTS

CALORIES. The body requires a source of energy to maintain the normal processes of life and to meet the demands of activity and growth. Calorie requirements depend mainly on body size, basal metabolic rate, activity, age, sex, and environmental temperature. Clinical diseases associated with calorie deficiency are marasmus in children and cachexia in adults. A 70-kg male requires approximately 70 calories per hour under basal conditions and up to 600 calories per hour for very heavy muscular work, so that activity levels largely determine gain or loss of weight on a given diet. Carbohydrate and protein furnish about 4 calories per gram, alcohol about 7, and fat about 9. The report of the Joint FAO/WHO Expert Committee on Energy and Protein Requirements (1973) provides more detailed information.

PROTEIN. Proteins in the diet vary in their usefulness, depending on the availability of their essential amino acids, mainly those eight that cannot be synthesized within the body in the proportions needed for making new tissue. When protein is severely deficient relative to calories, kwashiorkor develops.

Protein requirements have two components: sufficient amounts and proportions of the essential amino acids, and adequate additional nitrogen from any utilizable source. The latter comes from both the dietarily dispensable amino acids and those essential amino acids present in excess of requirements. If the diet does not supply adequate calories, dietary protein will be utilized to meet energy needs at the expense of fulfilling requirements for protein. Protein requirements are increased by microbial disease, trauma, and most other pathologic states.

Protein requirements are expressed in terms of reference protein, which, in theory, is 100 per cent absorbed and utilized. Only egg and milk approach this ideal, and then only under the conditions of severe negative nitrogen balance used for conventional measurement of net protein utilization (NPU). Recommended dietary allowances for protein must be expressed in terms of the quality of the protein of the actual diet. At intakes adequate for maintenance, net utilization of egg and milk protein drops to about 60 per cent. Thus utilization of protein is generally no greater than about 40 per cent in the animal protein–containing diets of industrialized countries, and less with diets of poorer quality. After animal protein, those best utilized are from legumes, oilseeds, rice, oats, and Opaque-2 corn. Most other cereal proteins are of relatively poor quality.

CARBOHYDRATES AND FATS. Carbohydrates supply dietary energy and are necessary constituents of a balanced and palatable diet. There is no fixed requirement for carbohydrates, however, since they can be completely replaced as energy sources in the diet by protein and fats. Fats supply more than twice the energy of carbohydrate and protein per gram, and thus contribute a concentrated source of calories as well as palatability in the diet. The actual requirement for fat, however, is limited to a minute quantity of linoleic, linolenic, or arachidonic acid — all polyunsaturated fatty acids. Deficiency of these in young children leads to defective growth and scaly skin.

Fat-Soluble Vitamins

VITAMIN A. Vitamin A (retinol) is essential for integrity of mucosal surfaces and is required in the form of its aldehyde for vision, particularly in dim light. Avitaminosis A results in skin and eye lesions and reduced

TABLE 1. Food and Nutrition Board, National Academy of Sciences–National Research Council Recommended Daily Dietary Allowances,* Revised 1974 Designed for the Maintenance of Good Nutrition of Practically All Healthy People in the U.S.A.

	Age (Years) From Up to	Weight (kg)	Weight (lbs)	Height (cm)	Height (in)	Energy (kcal)†	Protein (grams)	Fat-Soluble Vitamins — Vitamin A Activity (RE)‡§	Vitamin A Activity (IU)	Vitamin D (IU)	Vitamin E Activity¶ (IU)	Water-Soluble Vitamins — Ascorbic Acid (mg)	Folacin (µg)	Niacin†† (mg)	Riboflavin (mg)	Thiamin (mg)	Vitamin B6 (mg)	Vitamin B12 (µg)	Minerals — Calcium (mg)	Phosphorus (mg)	Iodine (µg)	Iron (mg)	Magnesium (mg)	Zinc (mg)
Infants	0.0–0.5	6	14	60	24	kg × 117	kg × 2.2	420§	1400	400	4	35	50	5	0.4	0.3	0.3	0.3	360	240	35	10	60	3
	0.5–1.0	9	20	71	28	kg × 108	kg × 2.0	400	2000	400	5	35	50	8	0.6	0.5	0.4	0.3	540	400	45	15	70	5
Children	1–3	13	28	86	34	1300	23	400	2000	400	7	40	100	9	0.8	0.7	0.6	1.0	800	800	60	15	150	10
	4–6	20	44	110	44	1800	30	500	2500	400	9	40	200	12	1.1	0.9	0.9	1.5	800	800	80	10	200	10
	7–10	30	66	135	54	2400	36	700	3300	400	10	40	300	16	1.2	1.2	1.2	2.0	800	800	110	10	250	10
Males	11–14	44	97	158	63	2800	44	1000	5000	400	12	45	400	18	1.5	1.4	1.6	3.0	1200	1200	130	18	350	15
	15–18	61	134	172	69	3000	54	1000	5000	400	15	45	400	20	1.8	1.5	2.0	3.0	1200	1200	150	18	400	15
	19–22	67	147	172	69	3000	54	1000	5000	400	15	45	400	20	1.8	1.5	2.0	3.0	800	800	140	10	350	15
	23–50	70	154	172	69	2700	56	1000	5000		15	45	400	18	1.6	1.4	2.0	3.0	800	800	130	10	350	15
	51+	70	154	172	69	2400	56	1000	5000		15	45	400	16	1.5	1.2	2.0	3.0	800	800	110	10	350	15
Females	11–14	44	97	155	62	2400	44	800	4000	400	12	45	400	16	1.3	1.2	1.6	3.0	1200	1200	115	18	300	15
	15–18	54	119	162	65	2100	48	800	4000	400	12	45	400	14	1.4	1.1	2.0	3.0	1200	1200	115	18	300	15
	19–22	58	128	162	65	2100	46	800	4000	400	12	45	400	14	1.4	1.1	2.0	3.0	800	800	100	18	300	15
	23–50	58	128	162	65	2000	46	800	4000		12	45	400	13	1.2	1.0	2.0	3.0	800	800	100	18	300	15
	51+	58	128	162	65	1800	46	800	4000		12	45	400	12	1.1	1.0	2.0	3.0	800	800	80	10	300	15
Pregnant						+300	+30	1000	5000	400	15	60	800	+2	+0.3	+0.3	2.5	4.0	1200	1200	125	18‡‡	450	20
Lactating						+500	+20	1200	6000	400	15	80	600	+4	+0.5	+0.3	2.5	4.0	1200	1200	150	18	450	25

*Reprinted from Recommended Dietary Allowances. 8th revised edition. Washington, D.C., National Academy of Sciences, 1973. The allowances are intended to provide for individual variations among most normal persons as they live in the United States under usual environmental stresses. Diets should be based on a variety of common foods in order to provide other nutrients for which human requirements have been less well defined. See text for more detailed discussion of allowances and of nutrients not tabulated.

†Kilojoules (KJ) = 4.2 × kcal.

‡Retinol equivalents.

§Assumed to be all as retinol in milk during the first six months of life. All subsequent intakes are assumed to be one half as retinol and one half as β-carotene when calculated from international units. As retinol equivalents, three fourths are as retinol and one fourth as β-carotene.

¶Total vitamin E activity, estimated to be 80 per cent as α-tocopherol and 20 per cent other tocopherols. See text for variation in allowances.

**The folacin allowances refer to dietary sources as determined by *Lactobacillus casei* assay. Pure forms of folacin may be effective in doses less than one fourth of the RDA.

††Although allowances are expressed as niacin, it is recognized that on the average 1 mg of niacin is derived from each 60 mg of dietary tryptophan.

‡‡This increased requirement cannot be met by ordinary diets; therefore the use of supplemental iron is recommended.

resistance to infection (see Ch. 473.1), and hypervitaminosis A is equally serious (see Ch. 473.6).

Vitamin A is found preformed in animal tissue, and the beta-carotene of green and yellow vegetables is converted in the body to vitamin A with an efficiency of about 50 per cent. There are several other forms of carotene that have some activity but are still less efficiently utilized. One international unit (IU) is equivalent to 0.3 μg of retinol, or 6 μg of beta-carotene.

VITAMIN D. Vitamin D is essential at all ages for maintenance of calcium homeostasis and skeletal integrity. It can be acquired by ingestion of vitamin D_2 (ergocalciferol) or D_3 (cholecalciferol) and by exposure to certain ultraviolet wavelengths of light that convert 7-dehydro-cholesterol in the skin to vitamin D_3.

One IU of vitamin D is 0.025 μg of pure vitamin D_3. Excessive amounts of vitamin D (of the order of 1000 to 3000 IU per kilogram per day are potentially dangerous and may lead to hypercalcemia and attendant complications.

Most foods of animal origin have some vitamin D activity, and 1 quart of vitamin D–fortified milk supplies the daily requirement.

VITAMIN E. The earliest evidence of vitamin E deficiency differs with the species, but eventually the hematopoietic, muscular, vascular, and central nervous systems are affected. The normal resistance of red blood cells to rupture by oxidizing agents is also markedly reduced in vitamin E deficiency. One IU of vitamin E is 1 mg of synthetic *dl*-alpha-tocopherol acetate. Recommendations are based on the formula IU = 1.25 × body weight in kg.$^{0.75}$

Abundant vitamin E is supplied by salad oils, shortening, margarine, fruits and vegetables, and whole-grain products. However, high intakes of polyunsaturated fatty acids may increase requirements sufficiently to induce a deficiency of this vitamin.

VITAMIN K. The K family of vitamins occurs throughout nature and is required in microgram amounts by man and certain animals to maintain prothrombin and other clotting factors. The average diet apparently contains adequate amounts of vitamin K, and additional amounts are supplied by the gastrointestinal flora. Thus few malnourished human beings have presented findings indicating inadequate dietary vitamin K. Because of the lack of reliable information, a daily allowance for this vitamin has not been established. A group of older adults experimentally depleted of vitamin K were found to require slightly more than 0.03 mg per kilogram of body weight intravenously to obtain normal blood clotting.

(For the clinically important states in which deficiency of vitamin K develops, see Ch. 521.l.)

Water-Soluble Vitamins

ASCORBIC ACID (VITAMIN C). Ascorbic acid has many biochemical functions in the body and is essential for normal wound healing and resistance to infection. Man, higher apes, and the guinea pig lack the metabolic pathway to synthesize adequate amounts of ascorbic acid, and in these species a lack of sufficient dietary ascorbic acid leads to scurvy. Benefits have been claimed, but not substantiated, for high doses of ascorbic acid. The minimal daily intake of ascorbic acid to prevent scurvy in the adult is about 10 mg, but this does not allow tissue saturation. Ascorbic acid is fur-

nished by fruits, particularly citrus fruits, as well as by most fresh vegetables. (For more information on ascorbic acid deficiency, see Ch. 473.5.)

BIOTIN. Biotin is essential for the activity of many enzyme systems in bacteria, animals, and, presumably, man. Biotin deficiency does not occur naturally in man because the vitamin is so widely distributed in all common foods. Experimental biotin deficiency in man, induced by feeding the metabolic antagonist avidin found in egg white, results in the development of serious clinical and pathologic changes. These include scaly dermatitis, pallor, extreme lassitude, anorexia, muscle pains, insomnia, precordial pain, and slight anemia.

CHOLINE. Choline serves as a source of labile methyl groups in the body, and in addition is a constituent of several compounds necessary for nerve function and lipid metabolism. Choline is generally considered to be an essential nutrient in the diet, although human choline deficiency has not been demonstrated. The average mixed diet consumed by persons in industrialized countries has been estimated to contain 500 to 900 mg per day of choline, mostly from egg yolk, vegetables, and milk. Beef liver contains about 0.6 per cent choline.

FOLACIN. Folacin coenzymes function in the transfer of single carbon units in a number of intracellular metabolic processes, particularly in the synthesis of purine and pyrimidine ribotides and deoxyribotides and in amino acid interconversions. A folacin deficiency may arise from inadequate dietary intake, impaired absorption, excessive demands by tissues of the body, and metabolic derangements. Megaloblastic anemias resulting from folacin deficiency have been recognized with increasing frequency (see Ch. 479), and respond promptly to folacin administration. Folacin also reverses the anemia of vitamin B_{12} deficiency, but does not arrest the associated nerve degeneration. The intake of food folacins depends on the highly variable amount destroyed by cooking. Folic acid (phenylmonoglutamic acid) and folacin (tetrahydropteroyl glutamic acid) occur in a wide variety of foods of animal and vegetable origin, particularly in glandular meats, yeasts, and green leafy vegetables.

NIACIN. The term "niacin" is generic for both nicotinic acid and nicotinamide. Nicotinamide functions in the body as a component of two important coenzymes that are primarily concerned with glycolysis, tissue respiration, and fat synthesis. Tryptophan is a precursor of niacin in man, and the efficiency of conversion is such that an average of 60 mg of dietary tryptophan is equivalent to 1 mg of niacin. Good dietary sources of niacin are liver, other meats, fish, whole-grain cereals and enriched breads, dried peas, nuts, and peanut butter.

PANTOTHENIC ACID. Pantothenic acid is of biologic importance because of its incorporation into CoA, on which acylation and acetylation and other interactions depend. Pantothenic acid deficiency induced in human volunteers by feeding the metabolic antagonist omega-methylpantothenic acid, together with a deficient diet, resulted in serious clinical signs and symptoms within a few months. An important feature of the syndrome produced by pantothenic acid deficiency was reduced antibody formation. Neuropathy associated with low serum pantothenic acid has been observed in alcoholic patients habitually consuming extremely poor diets. A daily intake of 5 to 10 mg is probably adequate for children and adults. Ordinary cooking does not cause excessive losses of pantothenic acid, and the vitamin is so widely distributed in plant and animal tissues that deficiency does not occur spontaneously in human populations.

Food sources include organ meats, egg yolk, peanuts, plants of the cabbage family, and whole grains. Other meats, vegetables, milk, and fruits also contain moderate amounts of pantothenic acid.

RIBOFLAVIN. Riboflavin functions as a coenzyme or active prosthetic group of flavoproteins concerned with the oxidative processes. The requirement for riboflavin is related to body size, metabolic rate, and rate of growth. Deficiency of riboflavin produces lesions in mucous membranes, most easily seen in the tongue, lips, and cornea (see Ch. 473.2).

Riboflavin is soluble in water. It is widely distributed in all leafy vegetables, in the flesh of animals and fish, and in milk, but may be destroyed when food is exposed to sunlight or cooked.

THIAMIN. Thiamin functions in carbohydrate metabolism as a coenzyme in the decarboxylation of alpha-keto acids and in the utilization of pentose in the hexose monophosphate shunt. Thiamin deficiency leads to beriberi, still seen among populations subsisting primarily on rice; but in the industrialized countries, signs of thiamin deficiency are limited almost entirely to chronic alcoholics (see Ch. 473.4).

Thiamin is widely distributed in foods and readily available. It is soluble in water, sensitive to oxidation, and destroyed rapidly by heat in neutral or alkaline solutions. Roasting and stewing of meat may reduce the thiamin content by 30 to 50 per cent, and vegetables may lose 25 to 40 per cent in cooking.

It has been generally assumed that thiamin need is related to caloric intake, particularly to those calories derived from carbohydrate. Although dietary fat does "spare" thiamin to some extent, the reduction in requirement appears to be small. Because it is possible that older persons use thiamin less efficiently, it is deemed advisable to recommend that a thiamin intake or 1 mg per day be maintained by older adults, even when they are consuming less than 2000 calories daily.

VITAMIN B_6. Vitamin B_6 in the form pyridoxal phosphate or pyridoxamine phosphate has been shown to function in carbohydrate, fat, and protein metabolism. Vitamin B_6 is a collective term for a group of naturally occurring pyridines that are metabolically and functionally interrelated, namely, pyridoxine, pyridoxal, and pyridoxamine. Phosphorylated pyridoxal and, to a lesser extent, pyridoxamine are coenzymes for many of the enzymes of amino acid metabolism. Pyridoxine deficiency has occurred in children fed a proprietary formula in which the B_6 content was largely destroyed as a result of changes in the sterilization process. Symptoms were restlessness and irritability, and some developed convulsions. Pyridoxine deficiency may be responsible for anemia in adults.

Good dietary sources are liver, other meats, whole-grain cereals, soybeans, peanuts, corn, and many vegetables.

VITAMIN B_{12}. Vitamin B_{12} is essential for the normal functioning of all cells, but particularly those of the bone marrow, nervous system, and gastrointestinal tract, because it facilitates reduction reactions and participates in the transfer of methyl groups. Its chief importance seems to be in nucleic and folic acid metabolism. Deficiency of vitamin B_{12} results in the development of megaloblastic anemia and signs of degeneration of the long tracts of the spinal cord. Sore tongue, paresthesias, and amenorrhea may also be present (see Ch. 292 and 479).

Cyanocobalamin is the principal one of several compounds with vitamin B_{12} activity. As little as 1.0 μg daily will cure most cases of megaloblastic anemia resulting from deficiency of this vitamin, but will not replenish liver stores. In a dose of 0.5 μg more than 70 per cent is absorbed, but as the dosage of vitamin B_{12} increases, absorption gradually decreases to 30 per cent in a dose of 5 μg. Vitamin B_{12} occurs predominantly in foods of animal origin, with very little present in vegetables. Nevertheless, except in vegetarians, deficiency states are likely to arise only as a result of superimposed infections, malabsorption, or lack of intrinsic factor (pernicious anemia).

Mineral Elements

CALCIUM. Calcium is a major mineral constituent of the body and makes up about 1.5 to 2.0 per cent of the body weight of the mature human, more than 99 per cent of it in bones and teeth. Active processes of bone formation and resorption constantly exchange calcium with body fluids. The small proportion of calcium distributed in body fluids and tissues contributes importantly to other functions, such as blood coagulation, neuromuscular irritability, muscle contractility, and myocardial function. Calcium is incompletely absorbed, and phytate, oxalate, and fatty acids of the diet form nonionized or poorly soluble calcium complexes, further interfering with intestinal absorption. Calcium requirements are increased during periods of growth, and in pregnancy and lactation, but intestinal absorption is more efficient as need increases.

Good sources of calcium include milk and most other dairy products, shellfish, egg yolk, canned sardines and salmon (with bones), soy beans, and many green vegetables. Adequate vitamin D is required for efficient absorption of calcium.

COPPER. Copper-containing proteins in the body include ceruloplasmin, erythrocuprein, hepatocuprein, cerebrocuprein, cytochrome-C oxidase, tyrosinase, and monoamine oxidase. Copper depletion of a degree severe enough to cause hypocupremia has been observed in a few patients with iron deficiency anemia and edema, kwashiorkor, sprue, and the nephrotic syndrome. Anemia, neutropenia, and bone changes caused by copper depletion have been reported in Peruvian children.

A copper intake of 2 mg per day appears to maintain balance in adults, and an intake of 0.08 mg per kilogram per day is recommended.

Copper is widely distributed in foodstuffs, and a diet of even mediocre quality contains more than the recommended amount. The richest sources are liver, kidney, shellfish, nuts, raisins, and dried legumes. Milk is poor in both copper and iron.

FLUORIDE. Fluoride is incorporated into the structure of teeth and bone, and is necessary for maximal resistance to dental caries. In areas where natural water supplies do not contain this amount, the addition of fluoride to bring the concentration to 1 part per million has proved to be a safe, economical, and efficient way to reduce the incidence of dental decay. In communities where fluoridation has been introduced, the incidence of tooth decay in children has been decreased up to 50 per cent or more. The range of safety in fluoride intake is wide enough for safe accommodation to normal fluctuations in the fluoride content of foods among populations with fluoridated water supplies, without risk of inducing the first indication of an excess — slight mottling of the enamel. Some natural water supplies contain sufficient fluoride to induce mottling of the enamel, but no other associated adverse effects have been found (see Ch. 564).

IODINE. Iodine is an integral part of the thyroid hormones thyroxine and triiodothyronine, which have important metabolic roles. Dietary iodine deficiency leads to thyroid enlargement (goiter) as a result of increase in size and number of the epithelial cells in the gland (see Ch. 546.6).

Balance studies in adults indicate a daily requirement of 50 to 75 μg of iodine, approximately 1 μg per kilogram. Sources of iodine are food and water, but in large sections of the world the amount of iodine in the water supply and locally produced foods is too low to meet human needs without hypertrophy and hyperplasia of the thyroid gland. Although today's wide diversification in the origin of foodstuffs has reduced the problem in many countries, iodization of salt is a desirable and effective measure of ensuring an adequate iodine intake for all segments of the population.

IRON. Iron is an essential constituent of hemoglobin and a variety of enzymes. An absolute deficiency owing to a low dietary intake, or a relative deficiency owing to high body losses of iron, results in the development of microcytic anemia and other clinical signs (see Ch. 481.1). Iron deficiency with or without anemia also appears to reduce the work capacity of adults and to impair performance of children on some tests of learning and behavior.

Iron is widely distributed in both animal and vegetable foods, but intake estimates based on food iron values in food composition tables are of limited value. Foods lose iron during preparation, gain iron from cooking vessels or from other contamination, or have much of the iron in poorly utilized bound forms.

MAGNESIUM. Magnesium appears to activate the enzymes that catalyze the transfer of phosphate from ATP to a phosphate receptor, or from a phosphorylated compound to ADP. It appears to be associated with thermoregulation, neuromuscular contraction, and protein synthesis. Magnesium deficiency disease in man is similar to hypocalcemic tetany, and is reversed by administration of magnesium sulfate. Low serum magnesium levels have been observed in a variety of clinical conditions, including alcoholism, diabetes, malabsorption syndromes, kwashiorkor, neuromuscular conditions associated with parathyroid disease in surgical patients on restricted dietary regimens or parenteral feeding, and in patients receiving diuretic therapy.

Magnesium is widely distributed in ordinary foods. For example, cocoa, nuts and soy flour, barley, lima beans, corn, whole wheat flour, and oatmeal all contain over 100 mg per 100-gram edible portion.

CHROMIUM, COBALT, MANGANESE, MOLYBDENUM, SELENIUM, AND ZINC. Direct evidence for the essentiality of these trace or microelements in human nutrition is generally difficult to obtain, although deficiency signs can be induced experimentally in animals. Clear evidence that an element is required by mammals has pro-

vided a reliable index of a human requirement. Identification of elements in normal human enzyme systems has also afforded substantial evidence of a nutritional requirement.

There is evidence that *chromium* is a required nutrient. Continuing investigations of the relationship of this element to carbohydrate metabolism suggest its possible role in human nutrition.

Cobalt is an integral part of vitamin B_{12}. It is found in most common foods, and is readily absorbed from the gastrointestinal tract. Cobalt deficiency in man is unknown.

Manganese is an essential element, needed for normal bone structure, and is a part of enzyme systems that occur in man. A human deficiency has not been demonstrated, nor a recommended dietary allowance established.

Molybdenum and selenium have been shown to be essential in laboratory animals, and may also function nutritionally in man. There are insufficient data to establish a recommended dietary allowance. The close parallel of the functions of selenium and vitamin E in laboratory animals suggests a need for an evaluation of selenium in man.

Zinc has been recognized as an essential element in the nutrition of animals and humans, and there is some evidence for the occurrence of zinc deficiency in man under some circumstances. Patients exhibiting anemia, hepatosplenomegaly, short stature, hypogonadism, and geophagia have responded to zinc therapy when tissue levels of zinc and zinc intakes were low.

A mixed diet may be expected to supply adequate amounts of these microelements, and the risk of a deficiency in the United States is slight. Green leafy foods, fruit, whole grains, organ meats, and lean meats usually serve as generous sources of these elements.

At high levels of intake, all the elements are known to cause injury and to interfere with the utilization of other elements. Supplements should be used with caution and only with clear evidence of deficiency.

Beaton, G. H., and McHenry, E. W. (eds.): Nutrition: A Comprehensive Treatise, Vol. II: Vitamins, Nutrient Requirements, and Food Selection. New York, Academic Press, Inc., 1964.

Canadian Bulletin on Nutrition, Vol. 6, No. 1, Dietary Standard for Canada. Ottawa, Department of Public Printing and Stationery, March, 1964.

Department of Health and Social Security: Recommended Intakes of Nutrients for the United Kingdom (Report of the Panel on Recommended Allowances of Nutrients). Department of Health and Social Security Reports on Public Health and Medical Subjects No. 120. London, Her Majesty's Stationery Office, 1969.

Food and Agriculture Organization of the United Nations: Calorie Requirements: Report of the Second Committee on Calorie Requirements. FAO Nutritional Studies, No. 15. Rome, Italy, FAO, 1957. (Third printing, 1965.)

Food and Agriculture Organization of the United Nations/World Health Organization: Report of an FAO/WHO Expert Group, Rome, Italy, 23 to 30 May, 1961. Published jointly by FAO and WHO, FAO Nutrition Meetings Report Series No. 30 and World Health Organization Technical Report Series No. 230. Rome, FAO, 1962.

Food and Agriculture Organization of the United Nations/World Health Organization: Requirements of Vitamin A, Thiamin, Riboflavin and Niacin; Report of a Joint FAO/WHO Expert Group, Rome, Italy, 6–17 September, 1965. FAO Nutrition Meetings Report Series No. 41, World Health Organization Technical Report Series No. 362. Rome, FAO, 1967.

Food and Nutrition Board, National Research Council: Recommended Dietary Allowances, eighth revised edition, 1974. Publication 2216. National Academy of Sciences, 1974. Washington, D.C., Printing and Publishing Office, National Academy of Sciences.

World Health Organization: Energy and Protein Requirements. Report of a Joint FAO/WHO ad hoc Expert Committee. WHO Technical Report Series No. 522 and FAO Nutrition Meetings Report Series No. 52. Geneva, World Health Organization, 1973.

469. ASSESSMENT OF NUTRITIONAL STATUS

Nevin S. Scrimshaw

The physician should always look for the clinical signs suggestive of nutritional disease in his patients. Inspection of those body areas in which signs of deficiency are most likely to be detected — the hair, eyes, lips, mouth, and skin of the face, neck, and arms — can be part of any examination, no matter how cursory, because neither formal examination facilities nor disrobing is essential. Suspicions aroused by clinical examination can then be verified by medical and dietary history and appropriate biochemical tests.

A manual of procedures developed primarily to guide surveys of the assessment of nutritional status in populations was prepared by a committee of experts convened in 1962 by the World Health Organization (WHO, 1963). The publication *Nutritional Assessment in Health Programs* provides more detailed guidelines.

CLINICAL EXAMINATION: INSPECTION AND MEASUREMENT. The over-all nutritional appearance of each patient should be appraised before examination of specific areas. This will indicate whether a person has excessive pallor, generalized skin lesions, or other indications of unsatisfactory health, possibly related to diet. Although simple inspection also reveals obvious overweight and underweight in individuals, weight for height is a more reliable means of discrimination. Similarly, a gross subjective estimate of subcutaneous fat can be obtained by pinching a double fold of skin over the outer surface of the upper arm (midtriceps region), but skin calipers provide a more precise estimate.

Hair. Protein malnutrition causes the hair to change color and become fine, dry, and brittle. Characteristically, the hair of persons with severe protein deficiency can be pulled out of the scalp without discomfort; whole tufts of hair come out readily by the roots. Since the hair is brittle, the tips also break off easily. In whites, Indians, and Orientals who normally have brown or black hair, the change to a lighter color is readily detected, but without knowledge of prior hair color it might be thought to be genetic. The hair of blacks tends to become reddish in cases of protein deficiency before becoming lighter. In persons with naturally light and fine hair, the change is more difficult to detect.

Eyes. Both vitamin A and riboflavin deficiencies are known to affect the eyes. The xerophthalmia caused by avitaminosis A begins with a dryness of the bulbar conjunctiva, loss of the light reflex, lack of luster, and decreased lacrimation. It may proceed to keratomalacia, which is a softening of the cornea, and lead to ulceration, perforation, rupture, and destruction of the cornea. The final result is a scarred, opaque cornea and a sightless eye.

Bitot spots are often associated with vitamin A deficiency, although they cannot be regarded as specific to it. They appear as frothy, irregular, white or light yellow spots from 1 to several millimeters in diameter, most often on the conjunctiva lateral to the cornea. A small Bitot spot may consist of only a few tiny bubbles visible in the triangles, especially the outer ones. Both photophobia and the inability to see in dim light may be due to vitamin A deficiency.

The circumcorneal injection seen in riboflavin deficiency consists of penetration of the corneal limbus by the subconjunctival arterioles that normally terminate within 0.5 mm of the limbus. However, proliferation and congestion of the blood vessels in the sclerae and their extension into the clear corneal tissue is by no means pathognomonic of riboflavin deficiency. Excessive exposure to sunlight, smoke, dust, and other irritants is a recognized factor. Ariboflavinosis may also produce a moist, red lesion of the external angles of both eyes.

Skin. The areas of the skin most affected by nutritional deficiency usually are those most exposed to the environment. The skin of the face, neck, arms, and legs, and over pressure points such as the elbows, knees, and ankles is most likely to show positive findings in nutritional deficiencies.

Dyssebacea refers to a series of disturbances of the sebaceous glands characterized by increased oiliness, dermatitis, fissuring, and exfoliation. For positive identification, the lesion must be red and moist. In riboflavin deficiency, it occurs at the external angles of the eye, the nasolabial fold, and behind the ears, and may appear in other skin folds of the body. The nasolabial lesions should not be confused with acne in adolescents or with the irritation from nasal discharge in small children.

Xerosis, or generalized dryness of the skin, is thought to be characteristic of vitamin A deficiency, but is difficult to evaluate in the individual because the appearance of the skin is influenced so much by bathing habits and exposure to dust and sunlight. The follicular hyperkeratosis widely ascribed to vitamin A deficiency consists of a "goose flesh" appearance which is not altered by temperature or brisk rubbing, and is most prominent on the skin of the outer forearm and thigh. Fully developed lesions consist of symmetrically distributed, rough, horny papules formed by keratotic plugs projecting from hypertrophied hair follicles; they make the skin look and feel like coarse sandpaper. Several well conducted therapeutic trials have failed to demonstrate any relationship between this hyperkeratosis and vitamin A deficiency, even when dietary fat is sufficient, and its specific etiology is not yet understood.

It is important to differentiate follicular hyperkeratosis from the perifolliculitis of ascorbic acid deficiency. The latter consists of perifollicular congestion, swelling, and, eventually, hypertrophy of the follicles. Only in this late stage is the skin rough to the touch. Other skin changes observed in severe ascorbic acid deficiency include petechiae, purpura, and hematomas. Because of increased capillary fragility, they are readily caused by a blood pressure cuff, shoes, or accidental bruising. Obviously, other factors increasing capillary fragility or interfering with blood clotting could cause these phenomena.

The cutaneous lesions of pellagra vary because of differences in the degree of deficiency, natural skin color, and conditioning factors, but they are sufficiently characteristic to be diagnostic in many instances. The most common chronic form is thickening, inelastic, fissured, and deeply pigmented areas of skin where exposed to sunlight or covering pressure points. Eventually, the skin in affected areas becomes dry, scaly, and atrophic. Erythema upon exposure to sunlight is an acute manifestation, with subsequent vascularization, crusting, and desquamation out of proportion to the precipitating exposure. In intertriginous areas a common, acute, but highly nonspecific reaction is redness, maceration, abrasion, and superimposed infection. Heat friction and poor personal hygiene contribute importantly to these signs. The symmetrical distribution of pellagrous lesions over skin exposed to sunlight and over pressure points is the most characteristic feature. Casal's necklace is a virtually diagnostic distribution of pellagrous dermatitis which sharply follows the neckline when a low-necked dress or an open shirt collar is habitually worn outdoors by persons on a niacin-tryptophan–deficient diet.

In severe protein deficiency, the skin of the legs, arms, and thighs shows marked pitting edema (which is a sine qua non of the diagnosis), and a dermatosis characterized by hyperkeratosis, hyperpigmentation, and desquamation. Although often similar in appearance to the lesions of pellagra, they are not limited to the exposed areas, and often extend to the thighs and lower trunk.

Neck. Endemic goiter resulting from a deficiency of iodine available to the thyroid gland usually can be detected by inspection and palpation (see Ch. 546.6).

Mouth. The mouth is one of the areas most sensitive to nutritional deficiencies, but the changes are nonspecific, confusing, and difficult to evaluate. Pallor of the lips and mucous membranes, like pallor of the skin and fingernails, may be a consequence of anemia, but its clinical appraisal is so subjective as to be of little value unless the anemia is severe. The stomatitis which may be a consequence of riboflavin deficiency has already been mentioned. Angular scars may be the result of past episodes of acute ariboflavinosis, but may also be wholly non-nutritional in origin. Poorly fitting dentures are a common cause.

The gums may reflect any of a variety of nutritional deficiencies, but the changes are difficult to differentiate from those resulting from local irritants and poor hygiene. This is especially true because neglect of both diet and oral hygiene are likely in the same individual. Marginal gingivitis and periodontal disease are reported to be common in persons whose diets are deficient in ascorbic acid, but attempts to prove such a relationship by ascorbic acid therapy have been failures. On the other hand, engorged, dark red, and bleeding gums are characteristic of scurvy.

Marginal and generalized gingivitis may also be found associated with deficiencies of vitamin A, niacin, and riboflavin. The problem is that many factors may play a causal role simultaneously so that the experimental correction of a single factor, even if contributory, does not necessarily effect a cure. General improvement of both diet and oral hygiene is usually required.

Marked hypertrophy of the filiform and fungiform papillae of the tongue is more frequently seen in populations in which vitamin B deficiencies, particularly of thiamin and riboflavin, are present. Papillary atrophy is also sometimes related to niacin or iron deficiency. Both nutritional megaloblastic anemia and the microcytic anemia of iron deficiency result in a smooth tongue. A markedly furrowed, so-called scrotal tongue is a possible manifestation of vitamin A deficiency.

Impression of the teeth on the borders of the tongue may be due to the edema resulting from protein deficiency as well as to defective dentures and a variety of other causes. When protein deficiency is the cause, edema is likely to be present in the extremities as well.

Nutritional deficiencies may also cause changes in the color of the tongue, although they are usually difficult to evaluate. Reddening, either generalized or limited mainly to the distal third, may be associated with sprue. It affects first the tip and lateral margins, but may progress to include not only the entire tongue but all of the oral mucous membranes as well. A beefy red glossitis resembling raw beefsteak most frequently represents a deficiency of niacin, but other B vitamin deficiencies may be involved. Riboflavin deficiency is probably most often responsible for the purplish discoloration known as magenta tongue. Patchy areas of paler discoloration give rise to the name "geographic" tongue, which has no nutritional significance.

Teeth. The frequency and severity of dental caries are increased by a diet relatively high in soluble carbohydrates and decreased by adequate fluoride and phosphate intake. Any severe dietary deficiency in infancy and early childhood will delay tooth eruption and contribute to malposition of teeth. Malposition resulting from retarded mandibular development is a common sequela of early protein deficiency.

In children of many underdeveloped countries, a so-called hypoplastic line across the upper primary incisors has been described, in which a yellow or brown pigment becomes deposited. This is followed by the development of caries on the labial surface of the teeth. Subsequently, the teeth may break off along this line. A nutritional or febrile insult in the neonatal period is a probable cause.

Fluorosis, occurring in regions where the fluoride content of the water supplies is above about 2 to 6 parts per million of fluoride in drinking water, is characterized by mottled enamel and chalky white patches distributed over the surface of the teeth. In some cases, the entire tooth surface may be dull white and lusterless. Although cosmetically undesirable, the lesion is harmless, and such teeth are usually resistant to caries.

Edema. Edema of the lower extremities is characteristic of protein deficiency, and may also be seen in acute beriberi. In severe cases it becomes generalized.

EVALUATION OF SIGNS. The signs suggesting nutritional deficiency are easier to evaluate and more specific in children than in adults. In adults, lesions from other causes, such as aging and repeated trauma, and confusing signs such as pinguecula, pterygium, and geographic tongue, are more likely to be present. The clinical signs that suggest more or less strongly the possibility of a nutritional deficiency are summarized in Table 2.

It must be emphasized again that the aforementioned signs are largely nonspecific. Moreover, they are more reliable in the assessment of nutritional status of population groups than of single individuals. Excellent color illustrations will be found in several of the references listed at the end of this chapter.

It should be clear from the foregoing that clinical examination alone will rarely be sufficient to establish a definite diagnosis. Many of the signs are so nonspecific that they cannot be relied upon in a given individual even when appropriate for population surveys. A medical history and confirmatory dietary and biochemical data are required when clinical examination raises the question of nutritional deficiency in the individual.

TABLE 2. Suggested Guide for Interpretation of Clinical Signs*

Dietary Obesity Excessive weight Excessive skin folds Excessive abdominal girth	Sensory loss and motor weakness Calf-muscle tenderness Cardiovascular dysfunction Edema
Undernutrition Lethargy, mental and physical Low weight in relation to height Diminished skin folds Exaggerated skeletal prominences Loss of elasticity of skin	*Niacin Deficiency* Pellagrous dermatosis Scarlet and raw tongue Tongue fissuring Atrophic lingual papillae Malar and supraorbital pigmentation
Protein-Calorie Deficiency Disease Edema Muscle wasting Low body weight Pyschomotor change Dyspigmentation of the hair Thin, sparse hair Moon face Flaky paint dermatosis Areas of hyperpigmentation	*Vitamin C Deficiency* Spongy and bleeding gums Folliculosis Petechiae Ecchymoses Intramuscular or subperiosteal hematoma Epiphyseal enlargement (painful)

Vitamin A Deficiency
Xerosis of skin
Follicular hyperkeratosis
Xerosis conjunctivae
Keratomalacia
Bitot's spots
	Vitamin D Deficiency
	1. *Active rickets* (in children)
	  Epiphyseal enlargement (over 6 months of age), painless
	  Beading of ribs
	  Craniotabes (under 1 year of age)
	  Muscular hypotonia
	2. *Healed rickets* (in children or adults)
	  Frontal and parietal bossing
	  Knock-knees or bow legs
	  Deformities of thorax
	3. *Osteomalacia* (in adults)
	  Local or generalized skeletal deformities

Riboflavin Deficiency Angular stomatitis Cheilosis Magenta tongue Central atrophy of lingual papillae Nasolabial dyssebacea Angular palpebritis Scrotal and vulval dermatosis Corneal vascularization	*Iron Deficiency* Pallor of mucous membranes Koilonychia Atrophic lingual papillae
Thiamin Deficiency Loss of ankle jerks	*Iodine Deficiency* Enlargement of the thyroid *Excess of Fluorine (Fluorosis)* Mottled dental enamel

*Adapted from World Health Organization Technical Report Series No. 258, Expert Committee on Medical Assessment of Nutritional Status. Geneva, WHO, 1963, pp. 59–61.

PHYSICAL METHODS COMPLEMENTARY TO CLINICAL EXAMINATION. Although routine roentgenographic studies are rarely possible, or indeed required, it is valuable to carry out roentgenographic examinations if physical signs and other circumstances suggest that rickets, osteomalacia, infantile scurvy, beriberi, fluorosis, or protein-calorie malnutrition is present.

The test of dark adaptation is sometimes used as a measure of vitamin A deficiency. It is, however, difficult to perform, and is influenced by factors other than vitamin A. The same appears to be true of electroretinography.

BIOCHEMICAL TESTS. A single biochemical determination, if accurate, may decisively confirm or deny the nutritional origin of an uncertain complex of clinical signs. Here again, biochemical measures vary in their reliability and specificity. Serum levels of vitamin A and ascorbic acid are quite useful, although very low levels may be present for some time before lesions appear.

For the B vitamins, blood serum levels are relatively insensitive, and measurement of thiamin, riboflavin, and niacin excretion in 24-hour urine samples is recommended.

Total serum protein and serum albumin are decreased markedly in protein deficiency, but only when the deficiency has progressed to the point at which it is beginning to be clinically evident. The ratio of urea to creatinine has been recommended as a measure of the loss of lean body mass in protein-calorie malnutrition. Anemia is also a laboratory-based diagnosis. A tentative guide to the interpretation of selected biochemical data is given in Table 3. It should be noted that most biochemical measures show only the current state of the patient, so that chronic nutritional lesions are possible even in those with normal serum levels of various nutrients.

Beaton, G. H., and McHenry, E. W. (eds.): Nutrition: A Comprehensive Treatise. Vol. III. New York, Academic Press, 1966.

Christakis, G. (ed.): Nutritional assessment in health programs. Am. J. Public Health. 63: Suppl. 1–82, 1973.

Davidson, S., Passmore, R., and Brock, J. F.: Human Nutrition and Dietetics. 5th ed. Edinburgh, Churchill Livingstone, 1972.

Jelliffe, D. B.: The Assessment of the Nutritional Status of the Community. World Health Organization Monograph Series No. 53. Geneva, World Health Organization, 1966.

Jolliffe, N.: Clinical Nutrition. 2nd ed. New York, Hoeber Medical Book, Harper & Brothers, 1962.

Sauberlich, H. E., Dowdy, R. P., and Skala, J. H.: Laboratory tests for assessment of nutritional status. Crit. Rev. Lab. Clin. Sci., 4:215, 1973.

World Health Organization Technical Report Series No. 258: Expert Committee on Medical Assessment of Nutritional Status. Geneva, World Health Organization, 1963.

TABLE 3.   Tentative Guide to the Interpretation of Selected Biochemical Data Useful in the Appraisal of
Nutritional Status of Adults*

	Deficient (High Risk)	Low (Medium Risk)	Acceptable (Low Risk)
Serum protein: grams/100 ml	<6.0	6.0–6.4	>6.5
Serum albumin (electrophoretic method): grams/100 ml	<2.8	2.8–3.4	>3.5
Nonessential/essential amino acid ratio (NE/E)†	<3.0	3.0–2.0	>2.0
Urea/creatinine ratio‡	<6.0	6.0–12.0	>12.0
Hemoglobin: grams/100 ml sea level			
Men	<12.0	12.0–13.9	>14.0
Women§	<10.0	10.0–11.9	>12.0
Hematocrit % (sea level)			
Men	<37	37–43	>44
Women§	<31	31–37	>38
Serum ascorbic acid: mg/100 ml	<0.20	0.20–0.29	>0.30
Plasma retinol: μg/100 ml	<10	10–19	>20
Thiamin, urinary excretion μg/gram creatinine	<27	27–65	>66–129
Riboflavin, urinary excretion μg/gram creatinine	<27	27–79	>80
N-methylnicotinamide, urinary excretion mg/gram creatinine	<0.5	0.5–1.59	>1.6–4.29
Pyridoxine, urinary excretion μg/gram creatinine	<20	–	>20
Serum folacin ng (mμg)/ml¶	<3.0	3.0–5.9	>6.0
Red cell folacin¶	<140	140–159	>160
Serum vitamin B$_{12}$ pg ($\mu\mu$g)/ml	<150	150–200	>200
Serum vitamin E (α-tocopherol) level, mg/100 ml (levels will vary according to method of analysis)	<0.50	0.50–0.70	>0.70

*Adapted from Sauberlich, H. E., Dowdy, R. P., and Skala, J. H.: Crit. Rev. Lab. Clin. Sci., 4:215, 1973.
†Value depends upon the analytical method employed and the procedure used to calculate the ratio.
‡These values are considered exceedingly tentative in view of the effect of age and the wide range of values reported in the literature.
§Nonpregnant, nonlactating.
¶Guidelines should be regarded as tentative and must be considered in terms of the microbiologic assay procedure employed. Values are based on the use of *Lactobacillus casei* as the test organism.

470.   NUTRITION AND INFECTION

Nevin S. Scrimshaw

Malnutrition in man is inseparable from the occurrence and effects of microbial disease. Infection precipitates nutritional disease in the malnourished, and malnutrition worsens the consequences of infection. The interaction between the two is synergistic. Both are major health problems wherever poverty and ignorance result in poor dietary habits as well as inferior environmental sanitation and personal hygiene. The World Health Organization monograph *Interactions of Nutrition and Infection* provides extensive documentation for the statements and conclusions of this chapter.

EFFECT OF INFECTION ON NUTRITIONAL STATUS

GENERAL. One of the earliest and most constant consequences of infection is loss of appetite and a decrease in the amount of food tolerated. Another is the almost universal tendency to change the diet to one that is more liquid and higher in carbohydrates at the expense of foods that are good sources of protein and other essential nutrients. This is a particularly common practice in the feeding of young children in less developed areas. Often milk as well as solid food is removed from the diet in favor of starchy gruels and cooking water from cereal grains or plant leaves when a child has diarrheal disease or other acute infections. In addition, therapeutic agents such as purgatives may reduce intestinal absorption, or antimicrobial drugs may interfere with intestinal synthesis of some nutrients. The direct influence of fever in increasing both basal metabolism and the loss of nutrients in sweat must also be taken into account. Sweat losses may amount to as much as 4 grams of nitrogen per day, together with significant quantities of electrolytes and iron.

PROTEIN. Acute infections cause a stress response qualitatively the same as that observed in states of pain, anxiety, fear, and other psychologic stress. The stress reaction, mediated by cortisone and insulin, mobilizes amino acids from skeletal muscle and other tissues from which they can be spared for gluconeogenesis in the liver. This is necessary because in man the contribution of liver glycogen to maintain blood glucose is relatively limited. The stress reaction undoubtedly arose to enable individuals to fight, flee from sudden danger, or recover from wounds and infections, regardless of the timing of meals. However, it necessarily depletes the body of protein because the amino acids thus mobilized are deaminated to provide the carbons of glucose, and the nitrogen is excreted in the urine, largely as urea.

Nitrogen losses during severe infectious diseases have long been recognized and can be equivalent to the nitrogen of 2 or 3 kg of muscle during the acute phase of the illness. It is now clear that even such mild infections as vaccination against smallpox and immunization with the 17-D strain of yellow fever vaccine, as well as tonsillitis, otitis media, bronchitis, and localized abscesses, will also provoke this stress reaction.

The duration of the metabolic effect of stress depends upon the nature and extent of the precipitating cause. If the stress is of short duration, it may be balanced by an increase in nitrogen retention during the succeeding 24 hours. The catabolic period associated with an infectious disease episode, however, is likely to last for several days, and the anabolic period of increased nitrogen retention is at least two to three times longer even when the protein intake is sufficient for recovery. After the acute stress is over, dietary amino acids are normally returned to the depleted tissues; hence protein intakes above maintenance levels are required at this time for repletion to occur.

In individuals already depleted by low levels of protein intake, the urinary loss of nitrogen measured during stress is less than that observed in those who are well nourished. Nevertheless, increases in urinary loss of nitrogen during minor infections have been found even in experimental subjects receiving a nitrogen-free diet.

In infections associated with diarrhea, reduced absorption of nitrogen and other nutrients adds to the nutritional consequences. However, even in severe diarrheal disease the drop in nitrogen absorption may be only 10 to 15 per cent, and seldom exceeds 50 per cent. *Thus it is worthwhile to continue feeding persons with diarrhea even though stool volume may be increased.*

With so many factors adversely affecting protein nutritional status during infectious disease, it is not surprising that in underdeveloped countries the protein deficiency disease kwashiorkor is commonly precipitated by diarrheal disease, measles, or other infections in children who are already in a precarious nutritional state. Similarly, infections, especially of a chronic nature, are responsible for much of the protein deficiency seen in adults.

VITAMINS. Blood levels of vitamin A are reduced in acute infections. Diarrheal and other infectious diseases, particularly measles, are frequently responsible for precipitating xerophthalmia and keratomalacia in children receiving diets deficient in vitamin A. It is probable that most clinical cases of avitaminosis A follow an acute infection. The absorption of vitamin A has been found to be reduced by severe *Giardia lamblia* infections. It is probable that other intestinal infections have this effect when sufficiently severe.

As was observed among prisoners of war of the Japanese during World War II, clinical beriberi is frequently precipitated in thiamin-deficient individuals by an infectious episode. The synthesis of thiamin and other B vitamins by intestinal bacterial flora may also be affected by both intestinal infections and chemotherapy.

Spontaneous respiratory infections have been found to induce megaloblastic anemia in monkeys maintained on a diet low in folic acid. Also, the dietary intake of folic acid is not low enough to account for the megaloblastic anemia seen in many patients with complicating infections.

Well confirmed is the appetite of the fish tapeworm, *Diphyllobothrium latum*, for vitamin B_{12}. These tapeworms are a significant cause of anemia in people infected from eating raw fresh-water fish, a common custom in Scandinavia and among persons of Scandinavian descent in the United States.

The role of infections in lowering serum ascorbic acid and increasing urinary excretion of this vitamin has been demonstrated by many experimental studies in guinea pigs. In poorly nourished children, otitis media, pneumonia, pyelonephritis, and other infections have long been recognized as precipitators of scurvy. Malaria, typhoid fever, influenza, measles, tuberculosis, and vaccination against smallpox are among other specific infections reported responsible for the appearance of scurvy in vulnerable children.

MINERALS. Early in an infectious episode there is a sharp decrease in blood levels of iron and zinc. It is

well recognized that hookworm infection, if sufficiently severe, causes enough loss of blood to produce microcytic-hypochromic anemia even when dietary intakes of iron appear adequate. This may also occur with urinary or intestinal blood loss caused by schistosomiasis. Increased losses of calcium and phosphorus have been reported for tuberculosis in both guinea pigs and man. Losses of sodium, chloride, potassium, and phosphorus, which are sometimes severe enough to cause death, occur in diarrhea of infectious origin.

EFFECT OF MALNUTRITION ON INFECTION

There are large numbers of laboratory, clinical, and field observations which demonstrate that the severity and outcome of infection are frequently worsened by malnutrition. The prevalence of diarrheal disease, both upper and lower respiratory infections, and some other types of microbial disease is also influenced by malnutrition. Moreover, much of the high infant and preschool mortality in developing countries attributed to microbial disease would not occur in well nourished children. The relative influence of the various potential mechanisms whereby nutritional deficiencies influence resistance to infectious disease under field conditions is not really known. The following must be considered.

THE IMMUNE RESPONSE. Humoral Antibodies. Nutritional interference with humoral antibodies specific for infectious agents has, until recently, received the most attention because severe deficiencies of protein, vitamin A, ascorbic acid, riboflavin, thiamin, pantothenic acid, biotin, and niacin-tryptophan in laboratory animals have long been known to interfere with antibody formation. A number of studies confirm that serious protein deficiency in man can interfere with formation of antibodies, as, for example, in children with untreated kwashiorkor. In human volunteers, antibody formation has been suppressed by inducing metabolic deficiencies of pantothenic acid or pyridoxine by feeding the corresponding antimetabolites, desoxypyridoxine and omega-methylpyridoxine. The same effect has been observed in cases of severe pellagra and moderately severe deficiency of several of the B vitamins. It is clear from field studies of preschool children, however, that resistance to infection can be reduced by degrees of malnutrition that do not seem to affect antibody formation, although sufficient to impair growth and development.

Cell-Mediated Immunity. The immune system can be divided into two fundamental cellular components — the bone marrow–derived B cells responsible for antibody formation, and the thymus-derived T cells that are essential components in the defense against infectious agents. T cells function as killer, effector, or helper cells. Cell-mediated immunity (CMI) induction and expression depend on T cells. It has recently been recognized that CMI can be affected in man by relatively mild degrees of protein-calorie malnutrition, by iron depletion, and probably by other nutrient deficiencies. One manifestation of this is delayed cutaneous hypersensitivity to skin test antigens such as streptokinase-streptodornase, mumps, *Candida*, trichophyton, and tuberculin. Ability to develop contact allergy to 2,4-dinitrochlorobenzene is another reliable indicator of the integrity of the T cell immune system. Delayed lymphocyte transformation response in vitro to phytohemagglutinins and other mitogenic stimuli is another manifestation.

PHAGOCYTIC ACTIVITY. The *macrophages and microphages of the reticuloendothelial system* are important protectors of the body against microbial diseases, particularly those caused by bacteria. Although of B cell origin, they may be potentiated by T cell activities. Nutritional deficiency can reduce both the number and the phagocytic capacity of these cells. Children with kwashiorkor have little or no leukocyte response to superimposed infections. Macrophage activity is decreased in the presence of vitamin A, ascorbic acid, thiamin, and riboflavin deficiency in laboratory animals. A decrease of *granulocytes* in the intestinal wall with reduced myeloperoxidase activity necessary to kill ingested bacteria has been described in rats with protein or iron deficiency. Both animal studies and clinical observations of folic acid deficiency have shown production of phagocytes in mammalian bone marrow to be depressed to the extent of nullifying the effect of protective antibodies.

TISSUE INTEGRITY. The integrity of the skin, mucous membranes, and other epithelial tissues helps to prevent entry of the infectious agent. Various pathologic changes occur in tissues, depending on the type and severity of the nutritional deficiency. Mucous secretions may be reduced or absent, mucosal surfaces may become easily permeable, changes may take place in intercellular substance, or there may be epithelial metaplasia, edema in underlying tissues, and accumulation of cellular debris to form a favorable culture medium for the infectious agent. Deficiencies in vitamin A, ascorbic acid, thiamin, riboflavin, niacin, and protein are especially likely to cause tissue changes that lower resistance.

WOUND HEALING AND COLLAGEN FORMATION. How long an infection will be disabling depends on how rapidly it can be localized and contained. Nutritional deficiencies affect not only tissue integrity but also wound healing, fibroblastic response to trauma, walling off of abscesses, and collagen formation. In protein-deficient rats, the walls of induced sterile subcutaneous abscesses were much thinner than those of spontaneous or induced abscesses in well nourished animals. The fibroblastic response in the deficient rats was markedly reduced, and as a result fatal septicemia frequently developed.

Ascorbic acid intake must be adequate for synthesis of the amino acids from which collagen is formed, particularly hydroxyproline and hydroxylysine, which are almost unique to collagen.

NONSPECIFIC RESISTANCE FACTORS. There is little evidence of the importance of various nonspecific mechanisms of resistance to infection such as those requiring properdin, interferon, or lysozymes, although all would appear vulnerable to nutritional deficiencies.

DESTRUCTION OF BACTERIAL TOXINS. Most of the destruction of bacterial toxins or resistance to them in the animal host occurs as the result of the toxins combining with specific antibodies. There is some evidence from experiments in animals that other mechanisms may exist as well. For example, rats suffering from deficiencies of B vitamins or vitamin A are more susceptible than controls to diphtheria toxin, even though antitoxin titers and rate of disappearance of injected toxin are similar in the two groups.

INTESTINAL FLORA. Changes in the intestinal flora induced by diet can influence susceptibility to some intestinal pathogens. In kwashiorkor, there is a tendency for the bacteria of the lower intestinal tract to appear at a higher level. In milder degrees of protein malnutrition it seems likely that intestinal organisms that are not normally pathogenic to the well nourished host may cause diarrhea. Changes in gastrointestinal motility secondary to malnutrition may also play a role in the severity of protozoal and helminthic infections.

ENDOCRINE BALANCE. Prolonged adrenocorticotropic hormone (ACTH) or cortisone therapy increases the spread of many infections, presumably by inhibiting local inflammatory reactions at the site of bacterial proliferation. These observations may have a bearing on the question of how malnutrition influences resistance to infection, since protein deficiency, caloric deprivation, and a number of other nutritional deficiencies influence endocrine balance.

Chung, A., and Viscorová, B.: The effect of early oral feeding versus early oral starvation on the course of infantile diarrhea. J. Pediat., 33:14, 1948.

Gallin, J. I., Kaye, D., and O'Leary, W. M.: Serum lipids in infection. N. Engl. J. Med., 281:1081, 1969.

Law, D. K., Dudrick, S. J., and Abdou, N. I.: Immunocompetence of patients with protein-calorie malnutrition. Ann. Intern. Med., 79:545, 1973.

Scrimshaw, N. S.: Protein deficiency and infective disease. *In* Munro, H. N., and Allison, J. B. (eds.): Mammalian Protein Metabolism, Vol. II. New York, Academic Press, 1964, Chap. 23, p. 569.

Scrimshaw, N. S., Taylor, C. E., and Gordon, J. E.: Interactions of Nutrition and Infection, World Health Organization Monograph Series No. 57. Geneva, World Health Organization, 1968.

Smythe, P. M., Brereton-Stiles, G. G., Grace, H. J., Mafoyane, A., Schonland, M., Coovadia, H. M., Loening, W. E. K., Parent, M. A., and Vos, G. H.: Thymolymphatic deficiency and depression of cell-mediated immunity in protein-calorie malnutrition. Lancet, 2:939, 1971.

Taylor, P. E., Tejada, C., and Sánchez, M.: The effect of malnutrition on the inflammatory response as exhibited by the granuloma pouch of the rat. J. Exp. Med., 126:539, 1967.

471. KWASHIORKOR, MARASMUS, AND INTERMEDIATE FORMS OF PROTEIN-CALORIE MALNUTRITION

Nevin S. Scrimshaw

DEFINITION. The clinical spectrum of protein-calorie deficiency ranges from forms characterized only by growth retardation to the extremes of kwashiorkor and marasmus. Kwashiorkor results from a deficiency of protein relative to calories, is found in children whose caloric intake is adequate and even excessive, or may be superimposed on varying degrees of protein-calorie deficiency. When protein and calories are limited to about the same degree, the clinical condition that develops is marasmus.

PATHOGENESIS. The various forms of protein-calorie malnutrition are of major public health significance in most underdeveloped countries. They result from diets that are quantitatively and qualitatively inadequate in individuals with superimposed stress, usually episodes of infectious disease. A deficient diet results in turn from varying combinations of low food production, inadequate preservation and distribution of foods, restricted purchasing power, poor food habits, and deficient knowledge of the relation between diet and health. The excessive incidence of infectious disease is a consequence of poor environmental conditions, inadequate knowledge of epidemiologic factors, poor personal hygiene, and insufficient health services.

The clinical result depends on the severity and duration of the nutritional deficiencies of protein and calories, on the relative importance of the deficiency of protein to that of calories, on the nature and severity of other associated nutritional deficiencies, on the age of the person affected, and on the presence of other complications. The mild and moderate forms in children, frequently unrecognized or misinterpreted, are primarily characterized by inadequate growth and development. In adults they reduce work performance and resistance to infection.

Mild to Moderate Protein-Calorie Malnutrition in Children. Retarded growth is greatest in the first two years of life, when dietary inadequacy and frequency of infections are most pronounced. Insufficient or improper supplementation of breast feeding is usually a factor. After weaning, the usual diet is cereal grains, starchy roots, overdiluted milk, or even cornstarch. Often such a regimen not only fails to provide the needed calories but also is deficient in many essential nutrients, particularly proteins of high biologic value.

Not until the third to fifth year of life is the usual child in underdeveloped countries permitted an adult type of diet. The period of greatest dietary inadequacy coincides in general with increased exposure to an unsanitary environment and a greater frequency of diarrheal and parasitic diseases, measles, whooping cough, and other diseases of childhood. By the time children enter school this critical period of high morbidity from infection is largely past because of an acquired immunity and better nutrition.

The assumption that reduced growth of children in underdeveloped countries is due more to environmental than to genetic factors is supported by observations of children of different races living under similar adverse conditions. Conversely, well nourished children of the same genetic origins usually follow the growth pattern of well fed North American or European children in a healthy environment.

The shorter limb-to-trunk ratio often observed in poorly nourished populations is caused mainly by primary or secondary malnutrition during the period when growth, particularly of the long bones, is normally rapid in the young child. There is also x-ray evidence that such children have retarded ossification of centers in their wrists and hands. Children with early growth retardation experience a parallel impairment of psychomotor development that persists at least through the school years, although the latter stems partly from social deprivation.

Mild to Moderate Protein-Calorie Malnutrition in Adults. The consequences of the mild to moderate chronic protein-calorie malnutrition common among adult populations has been little studied. Adaptation to insufficient calories includes low weight for height and reduced caloric expenditure. Accordingly, it is probable that it seriously reduces work capacity and thereby contributes to the low social and economic development in these areas. The effects of such malnutrition on resistance to stress, particularly that resulting from infectious disease, also needs further attention. Pregnant

and lactating women are a particularly vulnerable segment of adult populations of underdeveloped countries. Many women do not gain a normal amount of weight during pregnancy, and average weights of their children at birth are generally at least 200 to 300 grams lighter than those of well nourished mothers. Associated with this lower birth weight is higher neonatal and perinatal mortality as well as higher morbidity and poorer growth in infancy. The consequences of repeated pregnancy and lactation on poorly nourished mothers have received too little attention. It is noteworthy that such women look older than their chronologic age.

MARASMUS

The extremely low calorie diets responsible for the syndrome of marasmus are obviously also deficient in proteins and many other essential nutrients. Because calories are so inadequate, the child utilizes amino acids from the skeletal muscles and other less essential tissues for gluconeogenesis in addition to energy from fat deposits. Growth stops, but the amino acids and other nutrients liberated from the child's tissues permit a continuing synthesis of serum albumin, enzymes, and other essential metabolites, and no serious metabolic disturbances are observed.

The child with marasmus is emaciated owing to a loss of subcutaneous fat, extreme muscle wasting, and atrophy of most organs. Although the liver and other essential organs are much reduced in size, histologic changes are minimal. Despite the apt description of being reduced to "skin and bones," the child remains clinically alert, and maintains an appetite.

KWASHIORKOR

CLINICAL CHARACTERISTICS. Clinically, the syndrome of kwashiorkor presents a pitting edema varying from a mild form localized in feet and ankles to severe, generalized edema, with eyelids swollen shut. Movement of the extremities may be limited, and fluid accumulates in the peritoneal cavity. Patients are usually extremely apathetic, with a weak, monotonous cry if disturbed. Anorexia is frequently severe; diarrhea is an almost constant finding. The characteristic alterations of the skin resemble the dermatosis of pellagra, with which they have been mistakenly identified. The lesions are pigmented, dry, hyperkeratotic, and sometimes excoriated. They may vary in size from small patches to large, confluent areas. They are most numerous where subject to irritation, especially in the perineal region. They frequently occur on the extremities and face, and may extend to the trunk.

Normally curly hair becomes dry, fine, brittle, and straight. It is easily pulled out or may even fall out. It may become reddish, yellowish, or even white. These pigmentation changes are often observed in stripes, indicating successive periods of normal and abnormal hair growth. The extremities are frequently cold and cyanotic. The abdomen may be distended owing to flaccid abdominal muscles and ascites. Hepatomegaly is sometimes found.

BIOCHEMICAL ALTERATIONS. Protein. Low total serum protein is a diagnostic characteristic. It is due

Figure 1. Edema and skin lesions in child with kwashiorkor. (Courtesy of Institute of Nutrition of Central America and Panama.)

almost entirely to a low level of albumin, and is sometimes partially obscured by a relatively high level of gamma globulin resulting from a concurrent infectious process. There is a tendency for the beta globulin fraction to be both relatively and absolutely decreased; a relative increase in the alpha$_2$ globulin has also been found. Studies with ^{127}I-labeled albumin indicate that the lowering of this fraction is due to a decrease in rate of synthesis and not to abnormal catabolism.

Total α-amino nitrogen in plasma is abnormally low because most amino acids are present in decreased amount. The greatest reductions are in tryptophan, cystine, valine, tyrosine, and methionine. Low levels of urea in both blood and urine indicate decreased protein metabolism. The synthesis of antibodies is also inhibited. A very marked increase in the proportion of urinary nitrogen excreted as purine derivatives has been taken as evidence of cellular breakdown in kwashiorkor. Other abnormal substances in the urine indicating impairment of important metabolic pathways are β-aminoisobutyric acid and ethanolamine.

Although the liver protein concentration in kwashiorkor is greatly reduced by fat, it is not decreased in absolute amount in relation to body size. However, a lowered ratio of nitrogen to deoxyribonucleic acid has been reported, suggesting a true loss of protoplasmic nitrogen. In any case, the level of nitrogen in the liver of children with kwashiorkor is markedly decreased over that for normal children of the same age. There is also a marked loss of muscle nitrogen in kwashiorkor, the degree depending largely upon the severity of preexisting marasmus.

Lipids and Carbohydrates. All the lipid fractions that have been determined in the blood of children with kwashiorkor, including neutral fat, fatty acids, phospholipids, and cholesterol, have been found to be low, and levels of these substances rise rapidly in the course of treatment. An increase in fat content of the

liver, found by gross and microscopic examination, is another diagnostic criterion. In true marasmus, on the other hand, the amount of liver fat is decreased. Blood glucose levels are generally low. Although glucose tolerance is sometimes reduced, and a diabetic type of glucose tolerance curve is observed, this is not an invariable feature of the disease.

Enzymes. In acute kwashiorkor, lipase, trypsin, and amylase activities in the duodenal secretion are lowered almost to zero, and marked reductions in serum pseudocholinesterase, amylase, carbonic anhydrase, and alkaline phosphatase are recognized characteristics. The activity of these enzymes returns rapidly to normal with the administration of an adequate diet. Alkaline phosphatase levels, however, show a slight further drop before rising with therapy.

The activity of a number of enzymes has also been measured in liver obtained by needle biopsy from children with kwashiorkor. The outstanding finding is a decrease in xanthine oxidase activity per unit of protein, although cholinesterase and D-amino acid oxidase activity are also definitely lowered. Alkaline phosphatase activity in the liver is generally increased. These findings suggest that, although the activity of many key enzymes is maintained even in the presence of extreme protein deficiency, some are sufficiently affected to initiate the train of events culminating in death.

Vitamins. Levels of vitamin A and carotene in the serum of children with kwashiorkor are extremely low. It was assumed that this was due to low intake of vitamin A, until studies demonstrated that children with acute kwashiorkor upon admission to the hospital did not have an increase in serum vitamin A after a 75-mg oral dose of vitamin A palmitate. After three to five days of intensive protein therapy, however, a similar dose gave the same sharp increase in serum vitamin A that is found in normal children. It was also found that, in most cases, serum vitamin A levels rose with protein therapy, even when the diet contained no carotene or vitamin A. Analysis of liver biopsy material demonstrated that this phenomenon occurred whenever there were adequate stores of vitamin A in the liver, and that in those few cases in which there was gross depletion of vitamin A, administration of protein alone produced no serum response. From this and similar studies, it appears probable that the *transport* of vitamin A and possibly of vitamin E, which also occurs in abnormally low amounts in blood plasma of children with kwashiorkor, is inadequate because of the lack of a protein carrier.

Blood levels of thiamin and riboflavin are within normal limits. Even though the pigmented skin lesions superficially resemble those of pellagra, there is no evidence of niacin deficiency. The urinary excretion of N-methylnicotinamide, in cases in Central America at least, is within normal limits. Levels of serum ascorbic acid are relatively low, but are not in the range commonly associated with clinical deficiency. No significant alterations of levels of vitamin B_{12} in the blood have been found.

Electrolytes and Other Minerals. Potassium depletion is a major biochemical characteristic of kwashiorkor, and is a direct consequence of the protein deficiency. Other electrolyte changes are secondary to diarrhea (a symptom almost always present in kwashiorkor) or vomiting. Interpretation and correction of electrolyte changes in kwashiorkor are complicated by the abnormal distribution of water and the severe degree of potassium depletion. Magnesium deficiency may occur and lead to tetany.

ENDOCRINE FUNCTION. On the basis of observed normal adrenal cortex function in marasmus and decreased glucocorticoid production in kwashiorkor, the hypothesis has been proposed that the severe restriction of calories in children in whom marasmus develops results in increased production of ACTH by the anterior pituitary gland, which in turn stimulates the adrenal cortex to produce more corticosteroids. These hormones assure catabolism of muscle and other labile proteins sufficient to furnish amino acids to the liver for gluconeogenesis and likewise provide the liver with amino acids for synthesis of essential proteins. This mechanism does not operate when the child receives a diet with enough calories to meet minimal energy needs even though it is extremely deficient in proteins. Under these circumstances, children do not mobilize amino acids from muscle and instead present the serious metabolic disturbances of protein deficiency without much further muscle wasting. The result is kwashiorkor.

OTHER PHYSIOLOGIC CHANGES. In the marasmic type of kwashiorkor seen in Central America, a relatively small heart, which rapidly increases in size with treatment, is found upon radiologic examination. Electrocardiographic findings have consisted of low voltage and minor abnormalities, including alterations in the T wave and changes in rhythm. To judge by the volume of feces excreted by children with kwashiorkor, these children suffer from a malabsorption syndrome which is not completely corrected even after some weeks of treatment. Good digestion and absorption of proteins still take place during the acute state, but fat is poorly handled at first. Although fat absorption improves very rapidly as the child recovers, some degree of steatorrhea persists even into late recovery. Despite the

marked histologic alterations in the liver, the common tests for liver function have been found to give results within normal limits, with the possible exception of sulfobromophthalein retention, which is frequently high.

Electroencephalographic studies have shown diminished voltage and excessively slow rhythmic activity. Some authors have also reported abnormal focal activity and other alterations. These abnormalities tend to disappear as recovery progresses.

PATHOLOGY. The main pathologic alterations in kwashiorkor include fatty changes in the liver, of the large droplet type, beginning in periportal areas of the lobule and extending progressively to the central vein. The pancreas and endocrine glands become atrophic, along with marked atrophy of the intestinal mucosa, to give changes like those in primary malabsorption. The skin shows atrophy of the epidermis, with varying degrees of hyperkeratosis and parakeratosis.

COEXISTING DEFICIENCIES. The clinical manifestations of protein-calorie malnutrition are further complicated by the presence of other nutritional deficiencies. Vitamin A deficiency with severe ocular lesions is frequent in both marasmus and kwashiorkor. Concurrent deficiencies of components of B vitamins, particularly riboflavin, are also common. The mild normocytic, normochromic anemia attributable to protein deficiency is often complicated and becomes much more severe because of simultaneous deficiencies of iron, vitamin E, folic acid, and other hematopoietic factors of the B vitamins. A recent report suggests that vitamin E deficiency is sometimes responsible. Dehydration and serious electrolyte imbalance are usual because of the coexisting diarrhea.

TREATMENT. The correction of dehydration and associated electrolyte imbalance and the treatment of infections are the immediate demands in management of protein-calorie malnutrition. The basic requirement, however, is a diet providing all essential nutrients. Three to 4 grams of protein of high biologic value and 100 to 140 calories per kilogram of body weight are useful in children with kwashiorkor, and up to 200 calories per kilogram in those with marasmus.

PREVENTION. The prevention of protein-calorie malnutrition depends upon teaching mothers the importance of feeding their young children properly. Efforts should be made to increase the availability of low-cost protein foods suitable for feeding to infants and young children, ensuring that the mother can obtain them through either commercial channels or welfare programs. There must also be effective public health measures for reducing the burden of infectious disease in vulnerable populations.

Béhar, M., Viteri, F., and Scrimshaw, N. S.: Treatment of severe protein deficiency in children (kwashiorkor). Am. J. Clin. Nutr., 5:506, 1957.

National Academy of Sciences–National Research Council: Pre-School Child Malnutrition: Primary Deterrent to Human Progress. An International Conference on Prevention of Malnutrition in the Pre-School Child, Washington, D.C., December 7–11, 1964. NAS–NRC Publication No. 1282, 1966.

Scrimshaw, N. S., and Béhar, M.: Protein malnutrition in young children. Science, 133:2039, 1961.

Scrimshaw, N. S., and Béhar, M.: Malnutrition in underdeveloped countries. N. Engl. J. Med., 272:137, 193, 1965.

Viteri, F., Béhar, M., Arroyave, G., and Scrimshaw, N. S.: Clinical aspects of protein malnutrition. *In* Munro, H. N., and Allison, J. B. (eds.): Mammalian Protein Metabolism. Vol. II. New York, Academic Press, 1964, Chap. 22, p. 523.

Waterlow, J. C., and Alleyne, G. A. O.: Protein malnutrition in children: Advances in knowledge in the last ten years. Adv. Protein Chem., 25:117, 1971.

Waterlow, J. C., Cravioto, J., and Stephen, J. M. L.: Protein malnutrition in man. Adv. Protein Chem., 15:131, 1960.

472. UNDERNUTRITION, STARVATION, AND HUNGER EDEMA

Nevin S. Scrimshaw

When a person's caloric intake is far below his daily energy expenditure, he must either bring the two into balance by reduced activity or draw upon his own tissues for energy. Initially, tissue fat is a major energy source, but protein is also required as a source of amino acids for gluconeogenesis. Cahill has shown that after several weeks of fasting, dependence on endogenous amino acids decreases, because even the central nervous system can then utilize fatty acids.

Once adipose tissue has been exhausted, lassitude, loss of ambition, hypotension, collapse, and death follow if the caloric intake deficit continues. The late stages of this syndrome are also observed in anorexia nervosa, terminal carcinoma, and other wasting diseases.

Keys provides the most comprehensive review of the world literature on starvation, and adds important experimental observations of his own. Others have described severe malnutrition in the prisons and concentration camps of World War II and famines in many parts of the world.

Dependent edema often accompanies severe, prolonged undernutrition (starvation). The edema is soft and pitting, and usually disappears when the person is recumbent for some time, as during sleep. The causes of the edema are not entirely clear. Hypoproteinemia (specifically hypoalbuminemia, thus lowering the colloid osmotic pressure) is frequent but by no means invariable. Loss of fat and muscle, leaving a "loose sack" of skin with fluid filling the empty spaces, has been thought of as a contributing phenomenon. Diminished renal blood flow and glomerular filtration resulting from diminished cardiac output would presumably lead to sodium retention and edema.

Treatment of starvation demands caution. *In all forms of severe undernutrition, refeeding must be instituted slowly.* Overeating was a cause of shock and death of concentration camp victims at the end of World War II. The same is true for nutritional treatment of patients severely undernourished because of non-nutritional disease, e.g., esophageal carcinoma. Sudden flooding of the intestine with rich food through a feeding jejunostomy or gastrostomy may produce shock and death.

Benedict, F. G.: A Study of Prolonged Fasting. Carnegie Institute of Washington, Publication No. 203, 1915.

Keys, A.: The Biology of Human Starvation. Minneapolis, University of Minnesota Press, 1950.

Mollison, P. L.: Observations on cases of starvation at Belsen. Br. Med. J., 1:4, 1946.

Owen, O. E., Morgan, A. P., Kemp, H. G., Sullivan, J. M., Herrera, M. G., and Cahill, G. F., Jr.: Brain metabolism during fasting. J. Clin. Invest., 46:1589, 1967.

Young, V. R., and Scrimshaw, N. S.: The physiology of starvation. Sci. Am., 225:14, 1971.

473. DEFICIENCIES OF INDIVIDUAL NUTRIENTS: VITAMIN DISEASES

Nevin S. Scrimshaw

473.1. HYPOVITAMINOSIS A (INCLUDING XEROPHTHALMIA AND KERATOMALACIA)

ETIOLOGY AND DISTRIBUTION. The term vitamin A is used to include all compounds having vitamin A activity, but requirements are now expressed by the Food and Agriculture Organization and World Health Organization in terms of crystalline vitamin A_1 alcohol (retinol). The international unit, still used in many countries, is equivalent to 0.3 μg of retinol (or 0.344 μg of retinyl acetate) or to 0.6 μg of the provitamin beta-carotene. The recommended intake for adult males is 1000 μg of retinol per day, and for adult females, 800 μg, increasing to 1000 μg during pregnancy. During lactation 1200 μg of retinol per day is recommended. For children the recommendations are estimated from expected body weight for age, ranging from 420 μg per day at three to five months of age to the adult levels. Requirements are not influenced by physical activity or climate, but any pathologic condition that interferes with fat absorption is likely to impede vitamin A absorption, and infections can increase vitamin A needs.

Signs and symptoms of hypovitaminosis A are particularly common in Indonesia and most other countries of Southeast Asia and the Indian subcontinent, but are seen at least occasionally in nearly all economically underdeveloped countries. They are most often precipitated by infectious disease in infants and young children who already suffer from chronic malnutrition. Sporadic cases occur among particularly underprivileged infants in most of the industrialized areas of the world.

CLINICAL MANIFESTATIONS; PATHOLOGY AND PATHOLOGIC PHYSIOLOGY. The best known and generally the earliest physiologic effect of hypovitaminosis A is the loss of night vision (nyctalopia). The retinal rods responsible for vision in dim light contain a light-sensitive pigment, rhodopsin, an aldehyde of vitamin A that breaks down to retinene when light strikes a rod. In vitamin A deficiency rhodopsin regeneration fails.

Xerophthalmia is a dryness of the only transparent epithelial structures of the body that are exposed to air and light. The conjunctiva is affected earlier and more constantly than the cornea. Typical is a fatty dryness, most pronounced at the thickened wrinkles of the corners; the eye loses its porcelain aspect and looks muddy-greasy, like oil paint.

Bitot spots are often present, ranging in severity from a few tiny air bubbles visible on the exposed conjunctiva between the corneal rim and limbus, to a frothy white coating that overflows onto the cornea. The meibomian glands sometimes enlarge to look like a string of beads along the margin of the eyelids. The cornea is more resistant, but becomes hazy, rough, and dry and insensitive to touch. Punctate superficial infiltrations or small erosions may be seen on the surface. As the disease progresses to *keratomalacia*, one of these erosions may enlarge rapidly, with protrusion and eventually prolapse of the iris and loss of the lens. Sometimes there is a rather sudden spongy swelling and melting down of the cornea, a colliquative necrosis, with subsequent shrinkage of the eyeball (Fig. 2).

The skin becomes dry as the sebaceous glands become covered with keratin, so that secretions are diminished. *Phrynoderma*, an elevated papular lesion caused by plugging of the mouth of the hair follicles with a dense keratotic mass together with hyperplasia of the epithelium lining the plugged follicles, has been mistakenly listed as a sign of vitamin A deficiency. This condition is not necessarily associated with low serum levels of vitamin A, and does not respond to prolonged vitamin A therapy. Moreover, it is different from the follicular lesion of vitamin A deficiency in laboratory animals, in which the upper third of the hair follicles contains loose keratin and becomes dilated.

The small intestine is the main site of the conversion of active forms of carotene to vitamin A and its absorption. Therefore, when the intestine is affected by diseases such as sprue, fibrocystic disease of the pancreas, lymphomas, or lipodystrophy (Whipple's disease), hypovitaminosis A is likely to result. The liver contains 90 per cent of vitamin A stores, but these may be markedly reduced in some hepatic diseases.

Lowered dietary intake of preformed vitamin A or of an active carotene precursor is the most obvious and common factor in hypovitaminosis A, but any condition interfering with the intestinal absorption and conversion of carotene to vitamin A and its transport to the liver will contribute to deficiency of this vitamin. Surgical removal of sections of the small bowel and excessive consumption of mineral oil are in this category. So are massive intestinal infections with *Giardia lamblia* and probably also ascaris and hookworm. Severe protein deficiency (kwashiorkor) decreases the availability of transport protein. Dried skim milk fed to protein-deficient children in Indonesia increased the frequency of xerophthalmia, presumably by removing the limitation of protein and calories on growth and thereby increasing the need for vitamin A which the milk did not contain.

TREATMENT.   Treatment consists of administration of therapeutic amounts of vitamin A, correction of the pattern of dietary intake, and, in cases of secondary deficiency, therapy of the underlying disease. In young children without serious eye involvement, the daily oral administration of 3000 μg of retinol is recommended. When there is reason to suspect that dietary fat, including the fat-soluble vitamin A, is not properly absorbed, the new water-miscible vitamin A preparations are indicated rather than fish liver oil. If no response is observed, or signs of keratomalacia are present, daily doses of 15,000 to 25,000 μg of retinol should be given intramuscularly for the first week in an attempt to prevent permanent impairment of vision. Improvement

Figure 2.   *A*, Keratomalacia in four year old boy. *Left eye:* Perforation of cornea, through which lens has escaped, with drop of vitreous substance visible on lower lid. *Right eye:* Necrosis of cornea with small ulcer. *B*, Bitot spot on transparent conjunctiva, nine year old child. *C*, Xerosis conjunctivae, showing Bitot spot and dryness of mucosal folds, four year old boy. *D*, Xerophthalmia with subtotal leukoma, after measles with perforating xerosis of cornea, in three year old child. (Courtesy of Dr. H. A. P. C. Oomen.)

may be seen within a week, but maximal healing may take many weeks. If the lens is intact, residual corneal scarring can sometimes be treated by transplant.

When hypovitaminosis A is associated with protein deficiency, dietary protein alone will bring a prompt increase in serum vitamin A levels if the stores in the liver are adequate. Conversely, if protein deficiency is present, hypovitaminosis A will not respond to treatment with the vitamin alone owing to the lack of transport protein.

PREVENTION.   Primary prevention depends upon assuring a diet with adequate vitamin A activity to meet all body needs and to maintain good stores of vitamin A in the liver. Foods of animal origin such as dairy products containing butter fat, egg yolk, liver, and fish liver oils are excellent sources. Sufficient quantities of the provitamin beta-carotene and other active carotenoids are also found in many vegetables and fruits. For populations in tropical and less developed countries, most of the vitamin A activity in the diet can come from fruits such as the mango and papaya. African palm oil, used in cooking in many parts of the world, is rich in vitamin A activity.

When processing has reduced the vitamin A activity of a food or when substitute foods of lower vitamin A content are introduced, fortification may be indicated. For example, margarine is routinely fortified with 10,000 IU of vitamin A per pound because it replaces butter, a good source of this vitamin. Similarly, skim milk for human consumption should be fortified with water-miscible vitamin A, because all vitamin A activity has been removed with the cream. Synthetic breakfast drinks replacing natural fruit juices can be made good sources of vitamin A.

Prevention of deficiency secondary to other disease requires measures to control the primary cause. Most important will be environmental sanitation and other public health measures to reduce the prevalence of infections.

Federation of American Societies for Experimental Biology: Nutritional Disease, Proceedings of a Conference on Beriberi, Endemic Goiter and Hypovitaminosis A, held at Princeton, New Jersey, June 1–5, 1958. Fed. Proc. 17:Part II, Supplement No. 2, 1958, pp. 103–143.

McLaren, D. S.: Malnutrition and the Eye. New York, Academic Press, 1963.

Scrimshaw, N. S., Taylor, C. E., and Gordon, J. E.: Interactions of Nutrition and Infection. World Health Organization, Monograph Series No. 57. Geneva, World Health Organization, 1968.

RICKETS AND OSTEOMALACIA

See Ch. 558.

ENDEMIC GOITER

See Ch. 546.6.

473.2.   ARIBOFLAVINOSIS

ETIOLOGY AND DISTRIBUTION.   The intake of riboflavin must be low for many months before symptoms become evident. Among persons whose diets contain limited riboflavin, the disease often appears during periods of physiologic stress such as pregnancy and lactation, and during the rapid growth of childhood. Ariboflavinosis is so commonly associated with diets deficient in niacin and protein that for years it was considered part of the pellagra syndrome.

Characteristic deficiency signs appear in persons on deficient diets for three to eight months, depending upon the exact level of riboflavin and individual variation.

Low urinary riboflavin excretion levels and mild clinical signs of ariboflavinosis are common among the low-income populations of developing countries. Moderate to severe ariboflavinosis is usually seen only in association with other deficiency diseases such as pellagra and kwashiorkor. In the industrialized countries it is likely to be one of the deficiencies seen in alcoholics and persons with longstanding infections, malignancies, and other chronic debilitating diseases.

CLINICAL SIGNS.   Early symptoms of ariboflavinosis are soreness and burning of the lips, mouth, and tongue, and photophobia, lacrimation, burning, and itching of the eyes. The lesions of the lips may progress so that fissures extend from the angles of the mouth for a centimeter or more, and the lips themselves may appear dry and chapped. Shallow ulcerations and crusting sometimes develop. Neither the cheilosis nor the angular stomatitis is pathognomonic of riboflavin deficiency, because similar lesions may result from deficiency of niacin, iron, or pyridoxine.

The seborrheic type of dermatitis has a scaly, greasy appearance and is associated with erythema. Hard sebaceous plugs or fine filiform comedones may be seen over the bridge of the nose and on the malar prominences and chin. Dermatitis of the scrotum and vulva may also appear. In some instances, the redness, scaling, and desquamation of the skin of the scrotum extend to adjacent areas of the thigh which become raw and weeping.

The tongue in ariboflavinosis is characteristically purplish red or magenta and often has deep fissures. The papillae may be swollen, flattened, or mushroom shaped, giving a pebbled appearance. In chronic deficiency the papillae may become atrophic. The glossitis of riboflavin deficiency cannot be clearly differentiated from that caused by lack of niacin, folic acid, or vitamin B_{12}.

Eye signs responding to administration of riboflavin include diffuse inflammation of the conjunctivae, and red, swollen eyelids with a sticky exudate. Photophobia may be intense. Injection and proliferation of the capillaries of the limbic plexus may develop.

BIOCHEMICAL FUNCTION.   Riboflavin functions as a coenzyme of the active prosthetic group of flavoproteins concerned with oxidative processes. Among these are cytochrome-c reductase, D- and L-amino oxidases, succinic dehydrogenase, diaphorase, and xanthine and aldehyde oxidases.

The concentrations of free riboflavin, flavin mononucleotide, and flavin dinucleotide in plasma can be readily measured, but are not reliable indicators of deficiency, nor are white or red blood cell levels of riboflavin any more specific. Either 24-hour urinary excretion of riboflavin or the excretion four hours after subcutaneous administration of 1.0 mg will be found reduced in those whose diets have been deficient in riboflavin for an extended period. Less than 50 mg in 24 hours or 20 μg in the four hours after the test dose indicates that prior intake has been inadequate.

PREVENTION AND TREATMENT. Prevention requires a diet that includes foods that are rich sources of riboflavin such as milk, liver, other meats, eggs, and many green and yellow vegetables. For treatment, an adequate diet should be prescribed, and 5 mg of riboflavin given orally twice a day. Symptoms disappear in a few days, and the lesions clear up in a few weeks. In general, it is better to give a multivitamin preparation in treating ariboflavinosis because of the frequency of simultaneous deficiency of other B vitamins. When signs suggestive of such deficiencies are present, therapeutic doses of the appropriate vitamins should also be given.

Goldsmith, G. A.: The B vitamins: Thiamine, riboflavin, niacin. *In* Beaton, G. H., and McHenry, E. W. (eds.): Nutrition: A Comprehensive Treatise. Vol. II. New York. Academic Press, 1964, Chap. 2, p. 145.

473.3. PELLAGRA

ETIOLOGY AND DISTRIBUTION. Although pellagra is caused by a primary dietary deficiency of niacin, the adequacy of dietary niacin is influenced by the quantity and quality of dietary protein, and particularly by the availability of tryptophan, which is a metabolic precursor of niacin. The term "niacin" is generic for both nicotinic acid and nicotinamide. One niacin equivalent is defined as 1 mg of niacin or 60 mg of tryptophan. The minimum required to prevent pellagra is 4.4 mg of niacin or niacin equivalent per 1000 kcal per day, and a recommended allowance of 6.6 niacin equivalents per 1000 calories per day allows for individual variation.

Pellagra is traditionally associated with maize (corn) diets because this cereal grain has a low tryptophan as well as niacin content. It does not occur, however, where maize diets are supplemented with sufficient legume protein, as they are in Central America. It is still seen in the Yucatan peninsula of Mexico where the raising of henequen, maguey, hemp, or sisal takes most of the land, and in corn-eating populations of several Middle Eastern and African countries, notably in Egypt and Lesotho. In the 1930's it was still common in the southern United States among low-income groups whose diets consisted mainly of pork fat and hominy grits made from degerminated corn, but the disease has now disappeared from the United States except in alcoholics. Until recently it was still seen among corn-eating populations of rural Yugoslavia, Rumania, and Greece.

The pellagra common in Indian populations subsisting on a diet of jowar (millet, *Sorghum vulgare*) is reported to be influenced by the relative excess of leucine as well as the low tryptophan and niacin of this cereal. Diets containing protein of animal origin or vegetable proteins of good quality contain enough tryptophan to prevent pellagra even when niacin intakes are low.

Experimental niacin-tryptophan deficiency in human subjects duplicates most but not all of the features of pellagra as it occurs in populations, because in the latter there are nearly always other complicating diseases and deficiencies. Pellagra in the industrialized countries at present is generally a result of the vitamin- and protein-deficient diets of chronic alcoholics.

Deficiency of folic acid probably accounts for the frequency of megaloblastic anemia in pellagra. The cheilosis, angular stomatitis, proctitis, scrotal dermatitis, and vaginitis may be more related to concomitant deficiency of riboflavin (vitamin B_2) or vitamin B_6 than to that of niacin. The neurologic and mental symptoms, especially the cord degeneration sometimes found, could possibly be caused by poor vitamin B_{12} absorption. Reversible achlorhydria often occurs. The peripheral neuropathy and occasional mental changes, suggesting Korsakoff's psychosis, are possibly due to concomitant deficiency of thiamin or pyridoxine. Because fatty liver may be present, deficiency of protein and especially of choline and methionine must also be considered.

Pellagra is encountered in patients with cirrhosis of the liver, chronic diarrheal disease, diabetes mellitus, and neoplasia. Prolonged infectious diseases, such as tuberculosis, or thyrotoxicosis may lead to deficiency owing to an increase in niacin requirement. Pellagrous dermatitis has also been reported in patients with malignant carcinoid, a rare tumor which may convert as

Figure 3. Modern pellagra. Egypt and the Balkans. (Courtesy of Dr. William J. Darby.)

much as 60 per cent of the body's tryptophan to serotonin instead of the usual 1 per cent. Decreased food intake and diarrhea presumably contribute to the development of pellagra in this condition.

CLINICAL MANIFESTATIONS. The early signs of pellagra are nonspecific and include lassitude, anorexia, weakness, digestive disturbances, and often anxiety, irritability, and depression. As the deficiency progresses, soreness of the tongue gives way to severe inflammation of mucous membranes manifested by glossitis, stomatitis, esophagitis, diarrhea, urethritis, proctitis, and vaginitis. The mouth may be so painful that it is difficult to take even liquids, and the mucous membranes become bright red. The tongue is scarlet and swollen, with atrophy of the papillae. Not surprisingly, severe weight loss ensues.

The chronic dermatitis of pellagra may be difficult to distinguish from extensive exposure to dust and sunlight. It varies with the acuteness and severity of the deficiency state. At the earlier, acute stages it resembles sunburn. In chronic pellagra, which has developed more slowly, skin changes include thickening, scaling, hyperkeratinization, and pigmentation. Either type will usually be found on areas of skin exposed to sunlight — the backs of the hands and forearms, the anterior surfaces of the feet and lower legs, and the face and neck. Lesions following the sharp neckline of a dress or an open shirt are known as Casal's necklace. Other areas which may be involved are the axillae, groin, perineum, genitalia, elbows, knees, and skin under the breasts.

The early nonspecific psychic and emotional changes of early pellagra may, with increasing severity, progress to disorientation, delirium, and hallucination. The dementia may be hyperactive and manic or apathetic, lethargic, and stuporous. Other sensory and neurologic abnormalities and acute encephalopathy have been described in some cases. Anemia from associated deficiencies is common.

BIOCHEMISTRY AND PATHOLOGY. Nicotinamide functions in the body as the component of two important coenzymes, DPN (diphosphopyridine nucleotide) and TPN (triphosphopyridine nucleotide), which are functional groups in intracellular oxidation-reduction enzyme systems necessary for tissue respiration, glycolysis, and fat synthesis. In endemic pellagra the combined excretion of the niacin metabolites, N^1-methylnicotinamide and pyridone, seldom exceeds 2 grams daily.

The skin lesions are hyperkeratotic, often with vesicles containing erythrocytes, fibrin, and melanin pigment. Microscopic examination reveals atrophy of the sebaceous glands and hair follicles and degeneration of the peripheral nerves of the skin. Pathologic changes have also been reported in the brain, spinal cord, and peripheral nerves. Mucous membranes show inflammation and atrophy.

TREATMENT AND PREVENTION. The treatment of pellagra is a diet adequate in niacin and tryptophan and the administration of therapeutic doses of the vitamin. The best food sources of niacin are yeast, liver, lean meat, poultry, peanuts, and legumes. Potatoes, other vegetables, and whole wheat cereal and bread are fair sources. Most of these are also good sources of tryptophan as well. Although milk and eggs contain little niacin, they are also protective against pellagra because of their high tryptophan content. Enrichment of cereal flours with niacin and other B vitamins is a simple and inexpensive way of ensuring an ample intake of these nutrients.

In severe deficiency, niacinamide may be given in divided doses of 50 to 100 mg to a total of 300 to 500 mg for the first few days and then decreased to 150 mg daily. When circumstances make oral administration difficult, niacinamide can also be given intramuscularly in a dose of 100 mg three times daily. In advanced pellagra, bed rest is essential, and calorie intakes up to 3500 per day may be required. Acute symptoms improve within a few days, but several weeks of therapy may be required for complete recovery. Because concurrent deficiencies of other B vitamins are generally present, a multivitamin tablet containing 5.0 mg each of thiamin, riboflavin, and pyridoxine should be given daily in the treatment of pellagra. Associated anemia may require either folic acid or iron therapy.

Goldsmith, G. A.: The B vitamins: Thiamine, riboflavin, niacin. *In* Beaton, G. H., and McHenry, E. W. (eds.): Nutrition: A Comprehensive Treatise. Vol. II. New York, Academic Press, 1964, Chap. 2, p. 161.

Goldsmith, G. A., Sarett, H. P., Register, U. D., and Gibbens, J.: Studies of niacin requirements in man. I. Experimental pellagra in subjects on corn diets low in niacin and tryptophan. J. Clin. Invest., 31:533, 1952.

Spies, T. D.: Niacinamide malnutrition and pellagra. *In* Jolliffe, N. (ed.): Clinical Nutrition. 2nd ed. New York, Hoeber Medical Book, Harper & Brothers, 1962, Chap. 18, p. 622.

Spies, T. D., Aring, C. D., Gelperin, J., and Bean, W. B.: The mental symptoms of pellagra. Their relief with nicotinic acid. Am. J. Med. Sci., 196:461, 1938.

473.4.   BERIBERI

ETIOLOGY AND DISTRIBUTION. Beriberi occurs mainly in countries where polished rice provides a diet low in thiamin and high in carbohydrate. Among prisoners subsisting largely on polished rice in Japanese prison camps during World War II, beriberi developed when the thiamin supply was less than 0.3 mg per 1000 nonfat calories, with the acute episode usually precipitated by dysentery or other infectious disease. Deficiency signs may be anticipated when dietary intakes are less than 0.2 mg per 1000 calories, and intakes of 0.5 mg or more per 1000 calories are recommended. Because it is possible that older persons utilize thiamin less efficiently, they should maintain an intake of 1.0 mg per day, even when they are consuming less than 2000 kcal daily. The allowance of 0.5 mg per 1000 calories also applies to pregnant and lactating women and to children.

Beriberi is still seen occasionally in the rice-eating populations of Southeast Asia and the Indian subcontinent, and infantile beriberi has actually increased in some villages where newly introduced gasoline mills more completely separate the germ from the endosperm than does traditional hand-pounding. It has been described in some populations of Brazil and Africa among persons consuming cassava as the primary source of calories. It may also occur in association with pathologic states that interfere with the ingestion or absorption of food, and it is the most important of the B vitamin deficiencies common to alcoholism. Wernicke's syndrome is often associated with beriberi. Korsakoff's psychosis found among alcoholics is closely related to it (see Ch. 287).

CLINICAL CHARACTERISTICS. The great majority of

cases of beriberi are of the mild, subacute form, in which paresthesias and altered reflexes are the most characteristic findings. The muscle groups involved seem related to the length of the nerve controlling them, the amount of work they do, and possibly their blood supply. Laborers complain of disturbances of the lower legs, women more often of sensations in the fingers; other distributions can be related to the occupational use of muscle groups. Fullness or tightening of the muscles and fatigue pains resembling those of muscle ischemia are prominent, and, especially at night, muscle cramps occur.

In well developed cases, tachycardia is present, and the heart is enlarged. The edema may be generalized and massive or minimal without clear relation to the severity of the other symptoms. The most common characteristics of acute beriberi in prisoners of the Japanese in World War II were persistent tachycardia, symmetrical foot and wrist drop associated with muscle tenderness, mild disturbances of sensation over the outer aspects of the legs and thighs, and in patches over the abdomen, chest, and forearms. Most of these signs and symptoms have been reproduced experimentally in 30 to 120 days in adult subjects on thiamin intakes from 0.075 to 0.2 mg per 1000 calories.

The acute fulminating form of beriberi has been called shoshin; it is dominated by circulatory insufficiency. The milder forms may develop into this often fatal type, but more often it is of sudden onset. When nerve lesions develop early, the heart is saved from extreme insufficiency because the patient is forced to rest. In terminal cases, severe dyspnea and violent palpitations of the heart allow the patient no rest, and precordial pain may be intense. The patient tosses and turns about violently and complains of heaviness, constriction, oppression, and sometimes actual pain over the epigastrium. The moans and shrieks of the patient are distorted by the coincident hoarseness and sometimes aphonia. Pupils are dilated, and respirations are frequent and superficial. The liver and heart are enlarged and the heart action tumultuous. Cyanosis is obvious, and the pulse is weak but regular.

The chronic, dry, atrophic type — with wrist drop and foot drop — is generally found only in older adults. They no longer show the biochemical changes characteristic of acute beriberi, nor do they respond satisfactorily to therapy.

The beriberi seen in *infants*, particularly from one to four months of age, is associated with poor thiamin content of, and possibly abnormal metabolites in, the breast milk of mothers subsisting on a rice diet. It begins with vomiting, restlessness, pallor, anorexia, and insomnia, and evolves variously. In acute infantile beriberi, the infant develops cyanosis, dyspnea, and running pulse with cardiac crises which are often fatal. If the process is more chronic, the symptoms are vomiting, inanition, anorexia, aphonia, opisthotonos, edema, oliguria, constipation, and meteorism. A subacute form that may evolve into either the acute or chronic type is also described. The infant develops puffiness, vomiting, oliguria, abdominal pain, dysphagia, aphonia, and even convulsions. These forms are not really distinct, and the signs and symptoms may be present in almost any combination. Case fatality is very high unless treatment is given.

BIOCHEMISTRY AND PATHOLOGY. Pyruvic acid tends to accumulate in the tissues in severe thiamin deficiency. Because thiamin pyrophosphate is a coenzyme in the reaction, reduced transketolase activity can be detected in the red blood cells of persons consuming diets low in thiamin. Urinary excretion of thiamin of 0 to 14 μg in 24 hours has been reported in beriberi, and early signs have been observed with excretions of less than 40 μg in 24 hours.

The pathology of thiamin-deficient states ranges from maximal disturbance of function with minimal histologic abnormalities in acute, severe deficiency to minimal biochemical changes and well defined peripheral nerve lesions in chronic deficiency. In fatal cases, hypertrophy of the heart is a constant finding.

Degeneration is found not only in peripheral but also in cerebrospinal nerves, in terminal branches of the vagus and phrenic nerves, and sometimes in the spinal cord and fibers of the posterior root. In Wernicke's encephalopathy, histologic changes are found chiefly in the mamillary bodies, the related walls of the third ventricle, and the aqueduct and tegmentum of the medulla.

TREATMENT AND PREVENTION. The treatment of beriberi consists of a balanced diet plus the administration of 5.0 to 10.0 mg of thiamin three times daily. In severe beriberi the thiamin should be given parenterally for the first few days, but oral administration is satisfactory for the treatment of most cases. Delay in the treatment of Wernicke's syndrome may result in cardiac death or in permanent cerebral damage with signs of Korsakoff's syndrome. Because other B vitamin deficiencies are often present in beriberi, a multivitamin preparation is also advisable.

The biochemical lesions are rapidly reversed, but structural defects require long recovery periods. Signs of heart failure disappear within a few days; within a few weeks the heart returns to normal size, and electrocardiographic abnormalities disappear. In longstanding cases of advanced neuropathy, complete restoration to normal may be impossible, although improvement may continue for many months.

Prevention requires an increase in the intake of thiamin for persons consuming rice diets. Parboiling causes the thiamin to pass into the grain so that it is not removed in the milling process. In practice, efforts to encourage parboiling or the use of home-pounded and undermilled rice have not been successful. Enrichment of rice at the mill with thiamin, riboflavin, and niacin has not been adopted by those countries needing it most. A generally improved diet, containing foods which are good sources of thiamin, and extensive distribution of synthetic thiamin are the measures that have been most effective in Asia.

Federation of American Societies for Experimental Biology: Nutritional Disease, Proceedings of a Conference on Beriberi, Endemic Goiter and Hypovitaminosis A, held at Princeton, New Jersey, June 1–5, 1958. Fed. Proc., 17: Part II, Supplement No. 2, September, 1958, pp. 3–56.

Goldsmith, G. A.: The B Vitamins: Thiamine, riboflavin, niacin, *In* Beaton, G. H., and McHenry, E. W. (eds.): A Comprehensive Treatise, Vol. II. New York, Academic Press, 1964, Chap. 2, p. 109.

Spillane, J. D.: Nutritional Disorders of the Nervous System. Baltimore, Williams & Wilkins Company, 1947.

Weiss, S., and Wilkins, R. W.: The nature of the cardiovascular disturbances in nutritional deficiency states (beriberi). Ann. Intern. Med., 11:104, 1937.

473.5. SCURVY

ETIOLOGY AND DISTRIBUTION. Most mammals are able to synthesize ascorbic acid from glucose by way of glucuronic acid. Man, other primates, and guinea pig lack the enzyme required for conversion of gluconate to ascorbate. If dietary intake of ascorbic acid ceases for several months, clinical scurvy develops. Scurvy has most commonly occurred in the spring in temperate climates or at the end of the dry season in tropical ones, because of the relative lack of fresh fruit and vegetables during the preceding months and because several months are required for the disease to become manifest. Although now rare, the disease is still seen in exceptional circumstances, and the treatment is specific and effective. The minimal daily requirement for ascorbic acid is controversial. A group of British volunteers remained in good health and had normal wound healing on a daily intake of 10 mg for almost a year, although plasma and leukocyte ascorbic acid contents were very low. In a notable human experiment by Crandon, under controlled conditions with complete deficiency of the vitamin, the plasma level of ascorbic acid fell to zero by the forty-first day, but abnormal hair and hair follicles appeared only after four months. Perifollicular hemorrhages were not evident until after five months on the experimental diet. Subjective symptoms of a less specific nature — fatigability and anorexia — preceded the appearance of objective signs.

BIOCHEMISTRY AND PATHOLOGY. The effect of ascorbic acid on enzymes depends on its properties as either a strong reducing agent or the source of peroxide from its oxidation with air. It is a reactant in such well defined enzyme systems as hydroxylation to form norepinephrine, 5-hydroxylation of tryptophan, tyrosine oxidase, and a number of others. In the oxidation of p-hydroxyphenylpyruvic acid, it protects the enzyme involved from inhibition by its substrate, a necessary function when large amounts of tyrosine are being metabolized. It is also a specific reductant of the ferric ion in its transfer from plasma transferrin to liver ferritin.

It is needed also for the conversion of proline to hydroxyproline and the synthesis of chondroitin sulfate in the ground substance of collagen; hydroxyproline is an amino acid found only in collagen. Ascorbic acid is a necessary component of the mucopolysaccharides of ground substance. In the vitamin's absence, defective ground substance is formed, and can be seen by electron microscopy to have lost its characteristic periodicity. At any rate, scar tissue does not form. Ascorbic acid is involved in the preservation of folinic acid, the reduced form of folic acid. Perhaps this contributes to the occasional macrocytic anemia seen in scurvy by diminishing the amount of folinic acid available. There is no good evidence that ascorbic acid is itself required for erythropoiesis.

The pathologic changes in scurvy are predominantly in the mesenchymal tissues of the body, especially in collagen, growing bones, teeth, and blood vessels. In growing bones the histopathology of scurvy is distinctive: a suppression of the orderly growth process and of the normal calcification of the cartilage matrix. In addition, hemorrhages may be found in the interior of the bone at the cartilage-shaft junction, together with fractures of the minute columns of cartilage matrix and, at times, dislocation, separation, or impaction of the epiphyses.

Subperiosteal hemorrhages are relatively uncommon in the adult but frequent in infantile scurvy. Loosening of the periosteal attachment leads to capillary bleeding, which may dissect the periosteum free over a large area. Most frequently these subperiosteal hemorrhages are found at the lower end of the femur, the upper end of the humerus, both ends of the tibia, and the costochondral junctions of the middle ribs.

Capillaries in the skin become fragile, and petechiae, ecchymoses, and hematomas result. Hemorrhages into the gums lead to swelling, tissue friability, and even gangrene.

The teeth become loose because of resorption of alveolar bone. In children the teeth also show abnormalities of development, with poorly formed matrix and porous dentine.

The laboratory detection of this deficiency or confirmation of the clinical diagnosis of scurvy requires measurement of the plasma or leukocyte concentration of ascorbic acid, or the urinary excretion of the vitamin with or without a "loading" test. With low levels of dietary ascorbic acid intake, plasma ascorbic acid levels fall sharply, but even levels below 0.2 mg may be associated with a wide range of tissue saturations, from 0 to approximately 50 per cent. At this level of nutriture, the white blood cell–platelet ascorbic acid level is most useful. It will average 20 to 30 mg per 100 ml in a well nourished subject, and on an ascorbic acid–free diet will decrease to 0 to 2 mg per 100 ml in three to five months. Clinical scurvy usually appears shortly thereafter.

CLINICAL MANIFESTATIONS. Malaise, weakness, and lassitude are early and constant symptoms. Shortness of breath and aching in the bones and joints follow. The most distinctive physical sign and one of the earliest is perifollicular hemorrhage, usually in hyperkeratotic hair follicles, appearing particularly on the posterior thighs, anterior forearms, and abdomen. The hairs become fragmented, coiled, and buried in the follicles.

Petechiae are characteristic features of fully developed scurvy, and are usually most prominent in the same hair-bearing areas and in dependent parts of the body. Scorbutic petechiae are usually larger and more purplish than those in other forms of purpura, for example, in thrombocytopenia. Similarly, a tourniquet produces petechiae that are typically large and dark in color, appearing mostly on the hair-bearing areas of the forearm rather than on the flexor surface usually examined.

As scurvy becomes more advanced, ecchymoses appear, first at areas of irritation, pressure, or trauma. The "saddle area" and posterior thighs are the most frequent locations. Larger hemorrhages occur later in subcutaneous tissue, muscles, or joints, but are uncommon in the viscera, heart, or brain. Gums become swollen, inflamed, and "spongy," bleed easily, and are usually infected. Gum changes are less pronounced in edentulous subjects.

Figure 4. Ecchymoses, petechiae, and perifollicular hemorrhages on legs of patient with scurvy.

In untreated disease of long duration, postural hypotension and syncope are common. They may be part of the preterminal state in which vomiting and frank hypotension occur, resembling an Addisonian crisis.

Anemia, normocytic or macrocytic, with resultant pallor, is frequent. Two major causes of anemia must be considered. First, and most important, is the blood loss into the skin and deeper tissues or, uncommonly, into the gastrointestinal tract. Second is the possibility that dietary intake of folic acid may also be deficient. Many foods are important sources of both folic acid and ascorbic acid, and the two deficiencies may potentiate one another.

Most cases of scurvy seen in infancy (*Barlow's disease*) develop 6 to 12 months after the institution of artificial feeding. A few examples have been reported in infants considerably younger, but in these instances the mothers habitually subsisted on a diet inadequate in ascorbic acid. The concentration of ascorbic acid in human milk, invariably higher than that in maternal plasma, closely reflects the mother's intake.

Loss of appetite, listlessness, and irritability are early and insidious signs of infantile scurvy. The bony lesions and subperiosteal hemorrhages lead to tenderness, swelling, and evidence of pain on movement. Bleeding into the costochondral junctions of the ribs is noted externally as swellings — the "scorbutic rosary." Purpura and gum changes are similar to those in the adult except that pre-existing gum infection is less common.

SIGNIFICANCE OF ASCORBIC ACID IN CLINICAL MEDI-CINE. Although scurvy is now a rare disease, in several important clinical situations the state of ascorbic acid nutrition is a significant consideration. Resistance to infection is reduced in ascorbic acid deficiency, and microbial diseases have long been recognized to precipitate scurvy in individuals on borderline intakes of this vitamin.

Healing of wounds is defective in scurvy because of poor collagen formation. Experimentally deficient subjects fail to form new collagen in experimental wounds until the vitamin is administered. Delayed healing of wounds, postoperative breakdown of incisions, and delayed union of fractures may sometimes be at least partly the result of unrecognized but severe ascorbic acid deficiency. It is also known that extensive trauma and infectious diseases lower the plasma concentration of the vitamin. Ascorbic acid appears to be transported to wounds soon after injury, its concentration rising there as the plasma concentration falls, perhaps because the vitamin is needed for new ground substance and collagen formation.

Patients with thermal burns may develop ascorbic acid deficiency, especially when the burns are extensive and deep. Large doses of the vitamin may be necessary to maintain even low-normal plasma concentrations. Such deficiency leads to delayed healing of burns and impaired skin graft "takes."

Attention to nutrient intake, including that of ascorbic acid, is an essential part of the medical care of many illnesses. For example, the diet prescribed for peptic ulcer may be almost free of ascorbic acid, a situation which favors bleeding rather than healing.

TREATMENT AND PREVENTION. Small amounts of ascorbic acid will promptly reverse the florid clinical manifestations of scurvy. Even in severe scurvy, 100 mg per day for several days, accompanied by a normal diet, usually produces rapid cure. Because retention is high in the deficient state, this is also sufficient to restore the normal 4- to 5-gram body content of the vitamin in a few weeks.

Prevention requires a diet containing adequate ascorbic acid. The vitamin is present in most fresh fruits and vegetables, and in liver. Citrus fruits are particularly good sources. Synthetic ascorbic acid is chemically identical, and is very cheap.

Attention must be paid to the prevention of infantile scurvy, for the disease continues to occur sporadically in the United States in spite of our knowledge of prevention. At least 2 ounces of orange juice or its ascorbic acid equivalent should be given to all infants after the first month.

When extensive wounds, fractures, or chronic infections are treated, supplementary ascorbic acid should be given if any reasonable doubt exists regarding previous nutrition with this vitamin. Patients with deep and extensive burns may require large amounts of ascorbic acid (200 to 500 mg daily) to maintain measurable blood concentrations.

Crandon, J. H., Lund, C C., and Dill, D. B.: Experimental human scurvy. N. Engl. J. Med., 223:253, 1940.

Levenson, S. M., Green, R. W., Taylor, F. H. L., Robinson, P., Page, R. C., Johnson, R. E., and Lund, C. C.: Ascorbic acid, riboflavin, thiamin, and nicotinic acid in relation to severe injury, hemorrhage and infection in the human. Ann. Surg., 124:840, 1946.

Sebrell, W. H., Jr., and Harris, R. S. (eds.): The Vitamins: Chemistry, Physiology, Pathology, Methods. New York, Academic Press, 1967. (See Chapter 2, Ascorbic Acid, p. 305.)

Woodruff, C. W.: Ascorbic Acid, *In* Beaton, G. H., and McHenry, E. W. (eds.): Nutrition, a Comprehensive Treatise, Vol. 2, New York, Academic Press, 1964, p. 265.

473.6.   HYPERVITAMINOSIS A AND D

Vitamin A is not normally excreted except during disease states. Therefore, massive doses may lead to increased storage in the liver and hepatomegaly. Toxicity from hypervitaminosis A brought on by eating polar bear liver has been reported since 1596 by Arctic explorers. A 500-gram polar bear liver may contain over nine million IU of vitamin A, more than twenty times the total normal liver reserves in man. Toxic symptoms are drowsiness, irritability, severe headache, and vomiting within a few hours after ingestion. Acute hypervitaminosis A was reported in an infant given a single dose of 300,000 IU. Drowsiness, hydrocephalus with protrusion of the fontanel, and vomiting ensued 12 hours after administration. Hepatosplenomegaly, hypoplastic anemia, leukopenia, precocious skeletal development, clubbing of the fingers, and coarse, sparse hair have been reported from long-continued high doses in children. Most symptoms, but not the hepatomegaly and abnormal bone growth, clear with discontinuation of the vitamin.

Overdosage of any form of vitamin D is dangerous. The syndrome of hypervitaminosis D is characterized by hypercalcemia and by generalized calcinosis (deposition of calcium phosphate in a matrix of mucoproteins) affecting joints, synovial membranes, kidneys, myocardium, pulmonary alveoli, parathyroid glands, pancreas, skin, lymph glands, arteries, conjunctivae and cornea of the eyes, and the acid-secreting portion of the stomach. In advanced stages, demineralization of the bones will occur.

The exact borderline between tolerable and noxious doses is not known. Certainly the continuous ingestion of 150,000 IU per day may result in symptoms. It is possible that some infants may show hypercalcemia on relatively small doses of 2500 to 4000 IU per day. Retardation of linear growth in children has been reported with 1800 IU per day. Complete recovery usually occurs when vitamin D is temporarily withdrawn. Treatment should include lowering of the calcium intake and a generous fluid intake.

Dam, H., and Sondergaard, E.: Fat-soluble vitamins. *In* Beaton, G. H., and McHenry, E. W. (eds.): Nutrition, A Comprehensive Treatise. Vol. II. New York, Academic Press, 1964, pp. 34–35.

Sebrell, W. H., Jr., and Harris, R. S. (eds.): The Vitamins: Chemistry, Physiology, Pathology, Methods. Vol. I. 2nd ed. New York and London, Academic Press, 1967.

Stimson, W. H.: Vitamin A intoxication in adults. Report of a case with summary of the literature. N. Engl. J. Med., 265:369, 1961.

474. OBESITY

Edwin L. Bierman

Obesity is the most common disorder of metabolism in man and is also one of the oldest documented metabolic disturbances in recorded history. A limestone statuette dating from the Stone Age has been unearthed which appears to be the most ancient example of obesity, antedating the development of agriculture by about 10,000 years. Similar historical evidence for obesity is found in Egyptian mummies and Greek sculpture. This abnormality has persisted throughout the centuries, which have been characterized by markedly different environmental stresses and dietary habits. However, the problem of obesity has dramatically increased since the evolutionary advantage of the ability to efficiently store energy as fat has been dissipated in modern affluent societies. Thus caloric excess and sedentary habits have led to an increased prevalence of obesity and its life-shortening consequences, including cardiovascular disease, diabetes, and hypertension.

DEFINITION AND MEASUREMENT. Obesity can be defined as excess adipose tissue. However, it is still not clear whether obesity represents a "disease" or a common clinical manifestation of a group of disorders like anemia or hypertension. The definition of obesity is necessarily arbitrary, since body weight (or more accurately, quantity of body fat) is continuously distributed in populations with no clear dividing line between individuals who are obese and those who are thin. A definition of obesity could be made more easily if there were a distinct point at which a clear influence of obesity on morbidity and mortality begins. This is not the case, however, since there is a continually progressive excess mortality for increasing degrees of overweight. Moreover, the metabolic, physiologic, and pathophysiologic consequences appear to increase continuously with the degree of deviation above average weight.

Although it is the simplest index of obesity, body weight is not always the best reflection of the relative proportion of adipose tissue in the body or of total adipose mass. The latter needs to be determined or estimated if exact knowledge of the degree of excess adiposity is desirable. Weight adjusted to body size gives a better indication than body weight alone. For clinical purposes, per cent ideal body weight (relative weight) based on the readily available Metropolitan Life Insurance Company tables usually gives a close approximation of the degree of adiposity (Table 1). For common use, obesity can be defined as that body weight over 20 per cent above mean ideal body weight.

TABLE 1.   Desirable Weights for Men and Women According to Height and Frame, Ages 25 and Over*

Height (in Shoes)	Weight in Pounds (in Indoor Clothing)		
	Small Frame	Medium Frame	Large Frame
Men			
5 ft 2 in	112–120	118–129	126–141
5 ft 3 in	115–123	121–133	129–144
5 ft 4 in	118–126	124–136	132–148
5 ft 5 in	121–129	127–139	135–152
5 ft 6 in	124–133	130–143	138–156
5 ft 7 in	128–137	134–147	142–161
5 ft 8 in	132–141	138–152	147–166
5 ft 9 in	136–145	142–156	151–170
5 ft 10 in	140–150	146–160	155–174
5 ft 11 in	144–154	150–165	159–179
6 ft 0 in	148–158	154–170	164–184
6 ft 1 in	152–162	158–175	168–189
6 ft 2 in	156–167	162–180	173–194
6 ft 3 in	160–171	167–185	177–199
6 ft 4 in	164–175	172–190	182–204
Women			
4 ft 10 in	92–98	96–107	104–119
4 ft 11 in	94–101	98–110	106–122
5 ft 0 in	96–104	101–113	109–124
5 ft 1 in	99–107	104–116	112–128
5 ft 2 in	102–110	107–119	115–131
5 ft 3 in	105–113	110–122	118–134
5 ft 4 in	108–116	113–126	121–138
5 ft 5 in	111–119	116–130	125–142
5 ft 6 in	114–123	120–135	129–146
5 ft 7 in	118–127	124–139	133–150
5 ft 8 in	122–131	128–143	137–154
5 ft 9 in	126–135	132–147	141–158
5 ft 10 in	130–140	136–151	145–163
5 ft 11 in	134–144	140–155	149–168
6 ft 0 in	138–148	144–159	153–174

*Prepared by the Metropolitan Life Insurance Company. Derived primarily from data of the Build and Blood Pressure Study, 1959.
†1 inch heels for men and 2 inch heels for women.

A variety of methods for assessment of total body fat, such as body density, x-ray, distribution of fat-soluble gases, total body water, and total body potassium-40, have been used for research purposes. In addition, a variety of anthropometric measurements (limb and trunk diameters and circumferences, skin-fold thicknesses) have been used to derive regression equations that correlate closely with per cent body fat.

However, elaborate techniques are usually not necessary to quantify body fat for clinical purposes. The weight/height^2 index (body mass index) is the most useful anthropometric measurement and the simplest to obtain; it de-emphasizes the effect of stature on body weight and also correlates closely with adiposity. Subscapular and triceps skin-fold thickness measurements using inexpensive skin-fold calipers also provide an accurate and simple guide. On the basis of population studies, it has been suggested that triceps skin-fold thickness greater than 23 mm in men and 30 mm in women should be defined as obesity.

PREVALENCE AND EPIDEMIOLOGY. A large proportion of Western populations is obese. In the United States, using a definition of obesity based on triceps skin-fold thickness, approximately 20 per cent of middle-aged males and 40 per cent of middle-aged females are obese. In cross-sectional population surveys, the prevalence of obesity increases with age, reaching a peak by age 50 in males and somewhat later in females. The lower prevalence of obesity in older age groups may reflect the higher mortality at earlier ages associated with obesity-related diseases; hence fewer obese individuals are found among the elderly.

Cultural influences and socioeconomic status have a strong influence on the prevalence of obesity. As Stunkard has pointed out, every social factor studied has been correlated with obesity, and thus there are many determinants. Socioeconomic status, based on occupation, education, and income, showed a particularly strong inverse correlation with obesity among women, i.e., the lower the socioeconomic status, the higher the prevalence of obesity.

PATHOGENESIS. Clinical Types. Although it has been clear for some time that there are two clinical types of obesity, there has been little metabolic or physiologic evidence until recently to support such a concept. In one type (lifelong obesity), patients give a characteristic history. Although generally of normal birth weight, they tend to have been heavier as children, to have a large spurt in weight gain during puberty, and (in females) to give a history of gaining weight with each successive pregnancy. These individuals usually have tried all available methods and fads promoted for caloric restriction and weight reduction to no permanent avail. After successful weight loss regardless of the program, they usually return gradually to approximately their prereduction level of overweight as though it were preset. These individuals also tend to be grossly obese (more than 150 per cent of ideal body weight) adults.

The other clinical type (adult-onset obesity) is much more common and represents "middle-age spread." These individuals give a history of being thin or of average weight until age 20 to 40, when weight gain associated with a more sedentary existence begins. This type of weight gain in adult life is extremely common and is seen in most affluent populations.

A possible explanation for weight gain during adult life that does not appear to be tenable is a decrease in basal energy utilization with aging. Basal oxygen consumption decreases only slightly during adult life. Body composition is changing, however, even at constant body weight. There is a larger proportion of body fat and a smaller proportion of lean body mass with age, so that basal oxygen consumption in terms of lean body mass (predominantly muscle and bone) may actually be constant with age. Therefore adult-onset obesity simply may reflect an imbalance between caloric intake and utilization because such individuals do not reduce their caloric intake with age appropriately for their change in body composition. Ahrens has calculated that the daily caloric requirement for weight maintenance of adults decreases 43 calories per decade per square meter of surface area for males and 27 calories per decade per square meter for females.

These two broad clinical types of obesity were recognized early by Albrink, who proposed that adult-onset obesity is mainly central in location (the "middle-age spread"), whereas lifelong obesity might be peripheral as well as central. For peripheral localization of adiposity, skin-fold thickness of the forearm or the triceps is measured and compared with skin-fold thickness over the tip of the scapula. Weight gain during adult life is significantly correlated with costal, scapular, and, to a lesser extent, triceps skin-fold thickness but not with ulnar skin-fold thickness. Thus forearm fat is minimally influenced by adult-onset obesity, whereas adipose tissue of the trunk is most influenced by weight gain during adult life.

Pathophysiology. A possible pathophysiologic basis for these clinical observations was first proposed by Bjurulf, who suggested that some forms of obesity might be due to increased numbers of cells. Proof of this hypothesis was provided by the elegant experiments of Hirsch and his coworkers, who measured the cellularity of adipose tissue sampled by needle aspiration biopsy. They demonstrated that grossly obese humans (lifelong) characteristically have an increase in adipose cell number as well as adipose cell size. After weight reduction, adipose cell size shrinks, but hypercellularity remains fixed.

Adult-onset obesity (after age 20) appears to be characterized predominantly by adipose cell hypertrophy, with no increase in cell number. Adipose cell number appears to be fixed very early in life. In studies with rats, animals subjected to overnutrition before weaning maintained larger numbers of adipose cells throughout life than did litter mates subjected to undernutrition prior to weaning. Weight changes during adult life did not influence the cell number of these animals. Studies in man also have shown that adipose cell number is determined early in life. In the nonobese, two periods of adipose cell proliferation have been identified: in the first two years and again just prior to puberty. In obese children, adipose cell number increases throughout childhood.

This has profound implications with regard to the effect of feeding patterns during infancy and early childhood on the subsequent development of lifelong obesity. It has been shown that excessive weight gain within the first six months of life is correlated with overweight at the age of six to eight years, and thus it appears that the rapidity of weight gain in infancy is a better guide to the risk of obesity in later years than is the weight of the parents. Although less than a third of obese adults were overweight children, most overweight children become obese adults. Those adults who were obese in childhood had a larger number of fat cells than in those whose obesity was of late onset. The familial aggregation of obesity, then, could be in part explained by a familial aggregation of eating patterns, particularly in early life. There also appears to be some genetic influence, since body weights of identical twins are correlated more closely than are those of fraternal twins.

Experimental Obesity. Support for the concept of two types of obesity has been derived from studies of experimental obesity in man by Sims and coworkers. They force-fed volunteers to produce 20 to 30 per cent increments in weight associated with central distribution of excess fat, which was predominantly due to an increase in adipose cell size without a change in adipose cell number. Prompt, spontaneous reversal of excess fat and cell size was achieved at the end of the experimental forced feeding. Thus there appears to be no change in adipose cell number during adulthood despite changes in body weight.

Studies of experimental obesity in animals also lend some support to these concepts. Genetically transmitted obesity in rodents is characterized by adipose cell hyperplasia as well as hypertrophy, whereas experimentally induced obesity, such as that obtained by destruction of the ventromedial nucleus of the hypothalamus, is associated with hypertrophy alone. The only experimental manipulation that produces a significant change in adipose cell number in adults is a change in very early infantile nutrition. A summary of these two broad general categories of obesity is given in Table 2. All obesity is hypertrophic because the adipose cells are enlarged, but only certain individuals have adipose hyperplasia. Massive obesity is usually of the juvenile onset, lifelong hyperplastic type.

ETIOLOGY. Possible factors in the pathogenesis of adipose cell hypertrophy are listed in Table 3. No primary biochemical lesion of adipose tissue has ever been firmly documented as a cause of generalized obesity in man. Also, little is known of the etiologic basis for adipose cell hyperplasia. Genetic factors play a role, but their mechanism remains unknown. Estrogen-androgen balance also appears to influence the site and amount of adipose tissue deposition, since women and prepubertal children have a higher proportion of subcutaneous fat than men.

Only in rare instances of hypothalamic obesity in man, in which damage to the ventromedial hypothalamic nucleus occurs as a result of tumor or trauma, can an etiology be defined and, with surgical removal of the tumor, obesity cured. This hypothalamic center appears to regulate the deposition of adipose tissue triglyceride. Formerly its role as an appetite or satiety center was emphasized, and when it was destroyed its role was related to obesity in man because inappropriate hyperphagia sometimes occurred. Recent studies, however, have shown that experimentally induced hypothalamic lesions alter insulin levels and lipogenesis independent of changes in food intake. Anomalous insulin secretion after hypothalamic injury in man has also been observed. Possibly it can be linked to the development of obesity in such individuals. In any event, the relevance of experimental animal models whose obesity has been produced by injuring the hypothalamus to the common types of human obesity is open to question.

Cerebral and emotional influences on eating patterns as well as cultural influences and socioeconomic status surely play a role in obesity, but, aside from overt psychiatric disturbances, the general role of altered behavioral patterns in the etiology of obesity has been difficult to define, and a specific type of personality associated with obesity has not been distinguished. No less important, habit and environment also appear to influence appetite regulation. In simplest terms, a non-obese individual eats when hungry, stimulated by internal cues presumably related to physiologic appetite regulation, whereas an obese person eats because it is time to eat and the food is appetizing (external cues).

TABLE 2. Types of Obesity

	Hyperplastic	Hypertrophic
History	Lifelong	Adult-onset
Fat distribution	Peripheral and central	Central ("middle-age spread")
Adipose cellularity	Increase in cell number and cell size	Increase in cell size only
Insulin resistance	Related to cell size	Related to cell size
Metabolic consequences	Related to cell size	Related to cell size
Long-term response to treatment	Poor	Fair

TABLE 3. Possible Factors in the Pathogenesis of Obesity (Adipocyte Hypertrophy)

Excessive lipid deposition
  Increased food intake
  Hypothalamic lesions
  Adipose cell hyperplasia
  Hyperlipogenesis
Diminished lipid mobilization
  Decrease in lipolytic hormones
  Defective adipose-cell lipolysis
  Abnormality of autonomic innervation
Diminished lipid utilization
  Aging
  Defective lipid oxidation
  Defective thermogenesis
  Inactivity

As shown by ingenious "black box" feeding experiments in which subjects fed themselves through an automatic liquid formula–dispensing device without being able to monitor the amount of intake, if food is not readily available or is not appetizing, an obese individual will actually consume far fewer calories than will his thin control counterpart.

Metabolic Abnormalities. Regardless of the cause or type of obesity, the metabolic consequences are predictable. They appear to relate directly to fat cell size, and virtually all metabolic disturbances that have been observed are inducible with weight gain and reversible with weight reduction. Thus, although numerous hormonal imbalances have been described in obesity, they are likely to be consequences of rather than causes of the obese state (Table 4).

The metabolic alteration with the most profound influence is the acquired resistance to the action of insulin on glucose utilization by fat and muscle cells. Insulin resistance associated with adiposity has been demonstrated both in vivo and in isolated fat cell systems. Muscle metabolism also presumably plays an important role in the insulin resistance of obesity. One of the consequences of this resistance to the action of insulin appears to be a feedback compensatory hyperinsulinism. The beta cells of the pancreatic islets are stimulated by an unknown mechanism to produce more insulin, and beta-cell hypertrophy eventually results. The signal is as yet unknown but may be neuronal or hormonal, or may involve small changes in glucose, fatty acids, or specific amino acids. In any case, the result is an increase in circulating insulin levels (both basal and in response to a variety of stimuli), which is directly related to the degree of adiposity and is reversible with weight reduction. It is not simply a matter of body weight or lean body mass that is associated with hyperinsulinemia, since very muscular individuals who are heavy do not appear to have hyperinsulinism. It has recently been shown that circulating levels of insulin regulate their own receptors on cell surfaces. Thus obesity has been associated with fewer numbers of insulin receptors on muscle, liver, and adipose cell surfaces, thereby further contributing to insulin resistance and impaired glucose utilization by cells.

The emergence of adult-onset diabetes mellitus in the population is profoundly influenced by the degree and duration of obesity. One concept is that prolonged hyperinsulinism might lead to beta-cell "exhaustion" in those individuals who are genetically susceptible. As is well known, when the pressure is off after successful

TABLE 4. Metabolic and Endocrine Consequences of Obesity

Decreased sensitivity to insulin (muscle, adipose tissue)
Hyperinsulinemia
Decreased glucose tolerance, hyperglycemia
Hyperaminoacidemia
Hypertriglyceridemia
Hypercholesterolemia
Decreased growth hormone responses
"Resistance" to ketosis
Increased 17-hydroxycorticoid excretion

weight reduction, glucose intolerance is reversed. Thus glucose intolerance in the obese adult may represent "high-output failure," in which the beta cell has failed to compensate fully for the degree of peripheral insulin resistance associated with adiposity. Abnormal growth hormone regulation has been associated with obesity (lack of a normal rise with starvation, hypoglycemia, or arginine stimulation), but the significance of this finding and its relation to the glucose intolerance of obesity is not understood. These changes in insulin and growth hormone regulation in obesity can be found even in early childhood.

Fatty acid mobilization from adipose tissue appears to be less affected by insulin resistance and is considered to be normal in simple obesity. There is little evidence that decreased lipolysis, or resistance to normal fat-mobilizing stimuli (hormonal, neuronal), plays an etiologic role in obesity (Table 3).

Lipoprotein lipase (the enzyme in adipose tissue responsible for assimilation of fatty acids contained in circulating triglyceride-rich lipoproteins) appears to be sensitive to the availability of insulin, and its activity is increased in hypertrophic adipose cells. Whether this leads to further increased deposition of dietary and endogenous fat in adipose tissue in obesity is presently unknown.

Another metabolic consequence of obesity is hypertriglyceridemia, which may result in part from the associated hyperinsulinism. Triglyceride levels in populations are correlated with relative body weight, with skin-fold thickness, and particularly with weight gain in adult life. In a variety of studies circulating insulin levels are consistently correlated with triglyceride levels, and insulin is one of the factors involved in endogenous triglyceride-rich lipoprotein secretion by the liver. In obese individuals, both hyperinsulinism and hypertriglyceridemia are reversible with weight reduction. Both hyperinsulinism and increased endogenous triglyceride production rates have been produced with overfeeding in an experimental animal model for obesity, the desert sand rat. The role of obesity in determining serum lipid levels is suggested by the finding that age-related curves of relative body weight, plasma triglycerides, and plasma cholesterol in comparable population groups are superimposable.

Serum cholesterol levels are less closely linked with obesity, but a significant relationship exists. This could be explained in part by the observation that the cholesterol production rate appears to be related to the degree of adiposity. This relationship may be linked to the increased propensity of obese individuals to develop gallstones.

The influence of obesity on glucose and lipid levels also may be related to the increased tendency of the obese to develop all the complications of atherosclero-sis. Thus obesity, altered carbohydrate and fat metabolism, and atherosclerosis appear to be linked.

CLINICAL MANIFESTATIONS. The pathophysiologic consequences of obesity lead to a variety of clinical manifestations and aggravate or predispose to a number of common diseases (Table 5). The net result is a progressively rising over-all mortality rate with increasing degrees of obesity. Furthermore, for many of the diseases listed in Table 5, obese individuals have higher death rates than their thin counterparts affected by the same disorder.

Every major organ system appears to be involved. In the *cardiovascular system*, obesity is associated with four major risk factors for atherosclerosis, i.e., hypertension, diabetes, hypercholesterolemia, and hypertriglyceridemia. Therefore it is not surprising that obese individuals have more atherosclerotic manifestations, particularly angina pectoris, and are more prone to sudden death. The effect of obesity in predisposing to atherosclerosis may be mediated by these factors rather than by more direct mechanisms related perhaps to nonspecific myocardial lesions or hemodynamic factors (increased oxygen consumption, blood volume, cardiac output, stroke volume, and cardiac work).

There is a close correlation between blood pressure levels and obesity in most populations. (In the markedly obese individual with large subcutaneous fat deposits in the arm, blood pressure measurements should be made with a large leg cuff which more accurately reflects arterial levels.) A large portion of the increased death rate of obese individuals may be a direct or indirect consequence of hypertension (e.g., cerebrovascular accidents). Several factors have been implicated in the association between obesity and hypertension, including hemodynamic alterations resulting from increased blood volume and the need for increased perfusion of excess adipose tissue and lean body mass, and increased salt intake accompanying increased food consumption. Increased stroke volume and left ventricular hypertrophy often result. Obese individuals appear to respond to antihypertensive management as do their nonobese hypertensive counterparts with an improvement in morbidity and mortality from cerebrovascular complications.

In the *respiratory system*, alveolar hypoventilation associated with massive obesity eventually leads to carbon dioxide retention (Pco_2 values consistently above

TABLE 5. Diseases Associated with Obesity

Cardiovascular disease
  Atherosclerotic
  Hypertensive
  Cor pulmonale
Hypertension
Pulmonary disease
Diabetes mellitus, adult-onset
Fatty liver
Cholelithiasis and cholecystitis
Arthritis
  Osteoarthritis
  Gout
Varicose veins and thromboembolism
Intertriginous dermatitis
Hernias, ventral and diaphragmatic
Endometrial carcinoma
Toxemia of pregnancy
Amenorrhea and oligomenorrhea

48 mm Hg), daytime somnolence, chronic fatigue, dyspnea, and personality changes (the obesity-hypoventilation syndrome or pickwickian syndrome, named after a character in Dickens' *Pickwick Papers*, Fat Joe, who fell asleep at the most inopportune moments). The syndrome is initiated by the increased work of respiration necessary to move the ponderous thoracic wall and abdomen and is associated with decreased compliance of the thorax. Hypoxia, secondary polycythemia, pulmonary hypertension, and eventually cor pulmonale with cardiopulmonary failure ensue. Many of these abnormalities can be partly reversed by weight loss. Although the full-blown syndrome is seen in only grossly obese adults, milder pulmonary functional abnormalities can be detected with lesser degrees of obesity, including reduction in vital capacity and expiratory reserve volume, and ventilation-perfusion disturbances resulting in mild decreases in arterial oxygenation. All these abnormalities contribute to the increased surgical risk in obesity associated with use of general anesthetics.

Obesity is the single important factor associated with the emergence of *diabetes mellitus* in both Westernized and non-Westernized populations throughout the world. In the United States more than 80 per cent of adult-onset diabetics are more than 20 per cent overweight. The duration rather than the degree of obesity in individuals is more closely correlated with glucose intolerance. As indicated, certain genetically prone individuals may not be able to sustain the chronic oversecretion of insulin necessary to overcome the insulin resistance of obesity, and although absolute circulating insulin levels after carbohydrate intake may be higher than in thin individuals, they may not be high enough to compensate for the extra demand resulting from adiposity. Again, weight reduction may be dramatically successful in reducing the hyperglycemia of the adult diabetic and is the treatment of choice; however, the influence of weight gain and loss on the associated microangiopathy of diabetes is unknown.

Gastrointestinal symptoms are frequent in the obese and are usually nonspecific (bloating, dyspepsia). Diaphragmatic hernias may become symptomatic. Fatty liver is common, with associated abnormalities of liver function being detectable in as many as 85 per cent of obese patients. The incidence of cholesterol-rich gallstones is strikingly related to the degree of obesity, particularly among women. Women below the age of 50 with cholelithiasis average 25 pounds heavier than women without gallstones. The mechanism presumably relates to the supersaturation of bile with cholesterol resulting from the overproduction and increased excretion of cholesterol in obesity. Weight reduction will reduce the saturation of bile with cholesterol after a new stable lower weight is achieved. However, during the period of active weight loss, bile remains supersaturated, apparently because of increased mobilization of cholesterol from large adipose tissue stores. Thus continuous weight loss–weight gain cycles characteristic of many obese patients during their lifetime may be a potent predisposing condition for gallstone formation.

The incidence of several types of *arthritis* is increased among the obese. In populations, uric acid levels are directly related to the degree of overweight, and the prevalence of gouty arthritis is increased in obesity. Gouty arthritis may also be precipitated during treatment of obesity with carbohydrate-deficient ("ketogen-

ic") fad diets (see Treatment) presumably related to the hyperuricemia resulting from the competition between ketone acids and uric acid for renal excretion. Osteoarthritis is also more common and severe, particularly in the spine and other joints that bear the brunt of excess weight bearing.

In addition to the arterial lesions of atherosclerosis, *varicose veins* are common, as is venous stasis and edema. This contributes to the increased postoperative morbidity caused by thrombophlebitis and pulmonary embolism in obesity.

Flabby and redundant *skin* associated with excessive subcutaneous fat produces moist folds, resulting in a propensity to fungal and yeast skin lesions (intertriginous dermatitis, particularly in the axillae, in the perineal region, and under the breasts).

Women who are obese tend to have irregular *menses* and increased morbidity associated with *pregnancy* and again after childbearing ceases. The incidence of toxemia of pregnancy and hypertension is increased. Obstetric risk is higher due to longer duration of labor, larger babies, more cesarean sections, and higher anesthetic risk. Later in life, there are more uterine fibroids and an increased risk of development of endometrial cancer directly related to the degree of obesity. The large adipose mass is associated with both increased estrogen storage and increased conversion of adrenal androgens to estrone, which may result in increased chronic hormonal stimulation of the uterus.

Surgical risk is in general greater in obesity. Mortality figures for a variety of surgical procedures may be two- to three-fold higher for the obese than for the non-obese. Contributing factors include increased anesthetic risk, technical difficulties and longer duration of procedures, and increased atelectasis, wound infection, and thrombophlebitis postoperatively.

DIFFERENTIAL DIAGNOSIS. Less than 1 per cent of obesity can be ascribed to an identifiable cause or aggravating factor (Table 6). There is no rationale for the use of the popular diagnostic terms "exogenous" and

---

TABLE 6.   Differential Diagnosis of Obesity*

Endocrine syndromes
  Hypothyroidism
  Hyperadrenocorticism
  Hypogonadism
  Insulinoma
  Polycystic ovaries (Stein-Leventhal)
  Pseudohypoparathyroidism
Hypothalamic syndromes
  Tumors
    Craniopharyngioma
    Others
  Trauma
  Inflammatory disease
  Increased intracranial pressure
  Pseudotumor cerebri
  Empty sella syndrome
  Adiposogenital dystrophy
  Prader-Willi syndrome
  Laurence-Moon-Biedl syndrome
Multiple lipomatosis
Partial lipodystrophy
Drugs
  Cyproheptadine
  Phenothiazine

*An identifiable cause such as any of those listed above is present in less than 1 per cent of cases.

"endogenous" obesity, which have no pathophysiologic meaning.

Endocrine lesions as specific primary causes of adiposity are relatively uncommon. It is clear, however, that hormones influence fat deposition. This may involve a general effect on adipocyte metabolism throughout the body (e.g., insulin, thyroid hormone) or characteristic regional effects (e.g., glucocorticoids, estrogen). Hyperinsulinism can lead to adiposity, as exemplified by patients with insulinoma. However, individuals with this tumor are rarely markedly obese.

Although much attention has been given to hypothyroidism and milder degrees of "hypometabolism" as a cause of obesity, and vast quantities of thyroid extract have been administered for treatment, there is little evidence for deficiency of thyroid hormone secretion or action as a primary cause in most cases. Most of the weight gain associated with the development of myxedema is due to the accumulation of fluid rather than to adipose mass. Furthermore, the administration of thyroid hormone to obese patients may result in a loss of lean body mass exceeding the loss of fat and in increased appetite. Circulating thyroid hormone levels, thyroidal radioiodine uptake, and Achilles reflex time are usually normal.

The fat deposition associated with hyperadrenocorticism (Cushing's syndrome) is characteristic. Helpful diagnostic clinical features, in addition to fat distribution, that distinguish the much more common obese individual with mild hypertension and glucose intolerance from obesity secondary to adrenal hypersecretion include thick rather than thin skin, pale rather than purplish striae, absence of plethora and polycythemia, preservation of muscle strength, and absence of osteoporosis. Laboratory tests are also helpful. Higher than normal urinary excretion rates of hydroxycorticoids and an increase in cortisol turnover may be present, but these changes correlate with the increase in lean body mass associated with obesity. Blood cortisol levels tend to be normal in obesity and are suppressible, and the diurnal rhythm in adrenal steroid secretion appears to be maintained.

Gonadal deficiency certainly is not a common cause of obesity. Although in animals it has been shown that castration is often followed by obesity, this association has been much less prominent in man. Nevertheless, it has been observed to occur, particularly when the castration is performed after puberty. Moreover, some eunuchoid males are found to be somewhat obese and tend to lose some of the obesity after the administration of testosterone. Women with the Stein-Leventhal syndrome tend to be obese. Presumably the obesity results from the secretion by the ovary of steroids with actions similar to those of some of the adrenal steroids.

Hypothalamic syndromes are rare causes of obesity in man. Bray has recently collected a series of these patients and found that they were of the hypertrophic type but characterized by unusually high insulin levels. In the case of gross lesions found in the vicinity of the hypothalamus, e.g., craniopharyngioma or lesions caused by trauma, obesity associated with hypogonadotropic hypogonadism, and in some instances with diabetes insipidus, is part of the syndrome. It is not clear to what extent impairment of the secretion of hypothalamic pituitary releasing factors might contribute to the obesity.

Obesity rarely may be present in early childhood as part of a variety of congenital syndromes such as adiposogenital dystrophy (Fröhlich's syndrome), Prader-Willi syndrome, Laurence-Moon-Biedl syndrome, and pseudohypoparathyroidism. The cause of the obesity in these syndromes remains unknown, although structural or functional hypothalamic defects have been postulated.

Unusual distributions of adiposity can occur. Partial lipodystrophy is a rare variation of congenital lipodystrophy (lipoatrophy), in which subcutaneous fat is totally absent from a portion of the body and hypertrophied in the remainder. In multiple lipomatosis, a familial disorder characterized by localized, discrete, subcutaneous fat deposits throughout the body, stored triglyceride in lipoma cells (indistinguishable from the more usual adipose tissue cells) appears to be unavailable for mobilization even during starvation.

TREATMENT. In general, obesity can be treated by reduction of caloric intake or increase of caloric expenditure, or both. In special circumstances, particularly as applied to lifelong obesity, surgical techniques to decrease gastrointestinal adsorption of food and to decrease fat storage capacity by resection of large amounts of tissues have been used. Weight loss can be achieved by caloric restriction, regardless of the nature of the diet. The amount of weight loss depends largely on the degree of negative energy balance that is attained. Unfortunately, oxygen consumption declines in parallel with weight loss, making it more difficult to maintain a steady degree of weight loss over the long term.

Diet. Although there have been many suggestions that the macronutrient composition of the calorically restricted diet is important for successful weight reduction, there is no firm evidence that a calorie is anything more or less than a calorie, regardless of the food source from which it is derived, despite the popularity of many calorically unbalanced "fad" diets. The rate of weight loss on low calorie diets high in protein is the same as the rate on diets high in fat or high in carbohydrate. Previous observations that indicated less rapid weight loss with high-carbohydrate, low-calorie diets have been attributed to short-term treatment in which changes in salt and water balance obscure changes in weight. It is apparent that an obese individual has a marked propensity to retain sodium during weight reduction and that this tendency is transiently exaggerated by carbohydrate in the diet. Meal frequency may play a role in the degree of success; frequent feedings may be more likely to prompt weight loss than less frequent consumption of larger loads which may lead to abnormal eating patterns, such as the night-eating syndrome. Although obesity may be more common in individuals who eat less frequently, there is no evidence of an effect of feeding frequency on the rate of weight loss in obese subjects studied in a metabolic ward. Total starvation has been promoted as a rapid route to achieve or start weight loss. However, the additional metabolic and other consequences of prolonged total starvation, such as unexplained anemia, body potassium depletion, hyperuricemia, gout, ketosis, lactic acidosis, liver function abnormalities, arrhythmias, hypotension, and, rarely, sudden death, have limited the utility of this form of treatment. Furthermore, it has been shown that the additional weight loss achieved by total starvation or carbohydrate-deprived diets over that achieved by a 600 to 800 mixed calorie diet is achieved by a selective loss in lean body mass rather than by additional loss of fat mass. The protein-modified fast may minimize this loss, but does not influence the other side effects of starvation. Thus a minimal quantity of protein and carbohydrate in weight reduction diets appears necessary, although the body has an unusual capacity to conserve nitrogen. In principle, it is clear that the aim of a weight reduction diet should be to keep normal body composition as well as to attain normal weight. There is no evidence to support the superiority of any form of low-calorie diet over that of any other. Thus a practical dietary recommendation for long-term management of obesity would be 15 to 20 cal per kilogram of ideal body weight, containing 20 per cent protein, 45 per cent carbohydrate, and 35 per cent fat calories. Substitution of one or more meals each day by fixed composition liquid formulas appears to have contributed to successful initiation of weight loss in many individuals. However, unbalanced formulations, such as the high protein, "protein-sparing" formula, appear to be associated with the same untoward consequences as seen with total starvation and other carbohydrate-deprived regimens. When psychologic problems appear prominent, emotional support may be necessary. The success of weight reduction groups for many individuals indicates that support of the "group therapy" type may be a useful adjunct.

Exercise. The most common method for promoting caloric expenditure in obese individuals is increased exercise. Obese patients, particularly adolescent females, are consistently less active than are thin individuals. In practice, obese individuals on weight reduction diets tend spontaneously to decrease their activity further, perhaps to compensate for decreased caloric intake in an attempt to preserve their fat mass. Exercising animals appear to gain less weight than do free-eating sedentary controls as a result of both an increase in caloric expenditure and a decrease in food intake. Exercise results in a significant decrease in the percentage of body fat, with a proportional increase in lean body mass. Thus exercise does appear to influence both body composition and food intake and should be part of reducing regimens. Exercise alone, however, does not appear to be an effective means of weight reduction, since the caloric equivalent of most activities is easily nullified by small amounts of food intake.

Drugs. Appetite suppressants (usually amphetamine derivatives) are of limited utility, because their effect is transient and rarely leads to more than a 10 per cent weight reduction. Inasmuch as the treatment of obesity is lifelong, such drugs have no demonstrable role in the long-term management of obesity. However, since neural regulation of adipose mass appears likely, future development of drugs altering such mechanisms holds promise. Thyroid extract has been widely used to increase oxygen consumption of obese patients regardless of whether they suffer from hypothyroidism or "hypometabolism." Studies of body composition have shown that the accelerated weight loss from superimposition of thyroid extract on a low-calorie diet is due to a differential loss of lean body mass rather than to loss of fat tissue. Numerous other medications have been promoted for ability to achieve weight loss in obese individuals. Evaluation of these becomes a problem, because the routine of frequent physician visits, weight measurement, emotional support, medication, and diet itself promotes weight loss, and it is difficult to ascribe success to a particular medication. Furthermore, weight loss may result predominantly from loss of fluid, as with the widely dispensed diuretics, rather than from loss of adipose mass.

Surgery. An ileal bypass operation is being used as a radical form of treatment of severe and refractory obesity in an attempt to lessen morbidity and early mortality. This procedure was devised to eliminate the function of a sufficient length of jejunum and ileum to cause weight loss without producing clinical steatorrhea. The distal ileum is essentially completely bypassed. Unfortunately, bypass surgery has, in several instances, caused massive fatty changes in the liver, cholestasis, fibrosis, interstitial inflammation, and fatal hepatic necrosis. Other complications include high operative mortality, severe crippling diarrhea, electrolyte imbalance, arthritis, and oxalate renal stones. At present, caution in use of this experimental procedure is warranted. There is some rationale for adipectomy in the management of lifelong obesity, since the disorder is characterized by adipose cell hyperplasia. Experimental studies in animals, however, lead to little optimism, because excision of large adipose deposits has been followed by compensatory hypertrophy of remaining fat cell mass.

Behavior Modification. Since there are differences in the feeding behavior of obese and thin individuals, the newer methods of behavioral control have been applied to overeating. Short-term success in small groups of patients has been reported, and this approach appears to have promise, particularly as an adjunct to other forms of therapy.

PROGNOSIS. Over-all mortality rates are higher in untreated obesity. Insurance company figures suggest that for 45-year-old men averaging about 30 per cent overweight, death rates are 40 per cent higher than those for all insured men. For any degree of obesity, the mortality risk is higher for males than females and is greater for obesity occurring at a younger rather than an older age. These higher mortality rates can be reversed with weight reduction.

Unfortunately, successful weight reduction over the long term is difficult to achieve. The prognosis for treatment of obesity appears to vary with the clinical type. Lifelong obesity is frustrating to treat and leads to grief on the part of both physician and patient. In view of the poor results after long-term follow-up of a variety of dietary weight reduction schemes (which may be very successful in the short term), this form of obesity may be virtually irreversible. It is a common experience in obesity clinics that less than 5 per cent of the grossly (presumably lifelong) obese patients ever attain normal weight, and few can maintain a short-term weight loss in excess of 40 pounds. The long-term prognosis after ileal bypass surgery is as yet unknown.

On the other hand, the more common adult-onset obesity should be amenable to treatment, so that most of the metabolic and pathophysiologic consequences of enlarged adipose cell mass and its associated excess mortality can be reversed.

PREVENTION. As with hypertension, most obesity is "essential," because definable, preventable, and treatable causes rarely can be identified. However, focus on the most refractory form of obesity, hyperplastic or juvenile-onset, should produce additional insights leading to more effective prevention. It is premature to suggest to physicians who struggle ineffectively with grossly obese patients that the breakthrough is here at last; if only the excessive replication of fat cells during some critical period in infancy could be prevented, adult obesity might be averted. However, on the basis of present evidence, it appears that obesity must be prevented in childhood if there is to be an impact on obesity in the adult.

Thus it can no longer be assumed that most obesity is simply the result of overeating and that every fat person is an overfed normal one. Most slightly overweight adults are fundamentally normal, but have eaten a little too much and exercised much too little. The grossly overweight patient who has had the problem from early childhood suffers from a disorder that is not well understood and is unsuccessfully treated.

Alexander, J. K., and Peterson, K. L.: Cardiovascular effects of weight reduction. Circulation, 45:310, 1972.

Bierman, E. L., Bagdade, J. D., and Porte, D., Jr.: Obesity and diabetes: The odd couple. Am. J. Clin. Nutr., 21:1434, 1968.

Bierman, E. L., Porte, D., Jr., and Bagdade, J. D.: Hypertriglyceridemia and glucose intolerance in man. Horm. Metab. Res., Suppl. 2:209, 1970.

Bray, G. (ed.): Obesity in Perspective. Fogerty International Center Conference on Obesity. Washington, D.C., U.S. Government Printing Office, 1975.

Bray, G. A., and Gallagher, T. F., Jr.: Manifestations of hypothalamic obesity in man. A comprehensive investigation of 8 patients and a review of the literature. Medicine, 54:301, 1975.

Bray, G. A., et al.: Obesity: A serious symptom. Ann. Intern. Med., 77:795, 1972.

Czech, M. P., Richardson, D. K., and Smith, C. J.: Biochemical basis of fat cell insulin resistance in obese rodents and man. Metabolism, 26:1057, 1977.

Hirsch, J., and Batchelor, B.: Adipose tissue cellularity in human obesity. Clin. Endocrinol. Metab., 5:299, 1976.

Howard, A. (ed.): Recent Advances in Obesity Research. London, Newman Publishing Ltd., 1975.

Keys, A., Aravanis, C., Blackburn, H., Van Buchem, F., Buzina, R., Djordjevic, B. S., Fidanza, F., Karvonen, M. J., Menotti, A., Puddu, V., and Taylor, H.: Coronary heart disease: Overweight and obesity as risk factors. Ann. Intern. Med., 77:15, 1972.

Knittle, J. L., Ginsberg-Fellner, F., and Brown, R. E.: Adipose tissue development in man. Am. J. Clin. Nutr., 30:762, 1977.

Mann, G. V.: Influence of obesity on health. N. Engl. J. Med., 291:178, 226, 1974.

Sims, E. A. H., Danforth, E., Jr., Horton, E. S., Bray, G. A., Glennon, J. A., and Salans, L. B.: Endocrine and metabolic effects of experimental obesity in man. Recent Prog. Horm. Res., 29:457, 1973.

Sturat, R. B., and Davis, B.: Slim Chance in a Fat World: Behavioral Control of Obesity. Champaign, Ill., Research Press, 1972.

475. ANOREXIA NERVOSA

Gerald F. M. Russell

DEFINITION. Anorexia nervosa is a prolonged illness principally affecting young girls after puberty. It is characterized by severe weight loss which is self-induced, amenorrhea, and a specific psychopathology.

HISTORICAL NOTE. Sir William Gull described anorexia nervosa in 1868 and 1874 and concluded that "the want of appetite is due to a morbid mental state." This he attributed to the wiles of young women whom he considered "specially obnoxious to mental perversity." He advised that "the patients should be fed at regular intervals, and surrounded by persons who would have more control over them, relations and friends being generally the worst attendants." For a long time, confusion resulted from the concept of "Simmonds' cachexia," which embodied the mistaken view that panhypopituitarism usually caused loss of weight and wasting. Thus much needless effort was spent on the differential diagnosis of these two disorders which do not resemble each other.

ETIOLOGY. The cause of anorexia nervosa is unknown. Little is known about genetic aspects: morbidity is higher among sisters of patients (6.6 per cent), and concordance for the illness has been described in identical twins, but these observations are also explicable by the similarity of the home environment. Anorexia nervosa used to be considered a rare illness. However, a five-fold increase in incidence was reported in Malmö, Sweden, by Theander when he compared the 1950's with the 1930's. Similar observations in Britain have led to the hypothesis that culturally determined attitudes might lead to the illness. In recent years the upper social class bias for anorexia nervosa has tended to disappear. The incidence of new cases ranges from 0.6 to 1.6 per 100,000 of the whole population, but the prevalence among the schoolgirls around puberty may be as high as one in a hundred. The usual age of onset is 14 to 17 years, but it can be earlier (10 to 13 years) or later (up to 40 years). The illness is at least ten times more frequent in girls than in boys.

PSYCHOPATHOLOGY AND PATHOGENESIS. Anorexia nervosa is usually thought to be a disorder of psychogenic origin. The illness can also be viewed as a disorder of the feeding and endocrine functions normally controlled by the hypothalamus. It is recommended to consider simultaneously the mental and bodily disturbances in anorexia nervosa so as to comprehend their interaction as far as is possible.

The evidence for a psychogenic origin of anorexia nervosa is strong. Patients emphasize that they cannot eat because they feel guilty after eating, or are fearful that they will be unable to stop and hence will become unbearably fat. Psychodynamic explanations stress the role of disturbed family relationships, and of the powerful emotional conflicts of puberty and adolescence which often distress the patients. The proposal that a disturbance of body image underlies the illness (Bruch) has received experimental support from the finding that patients tend to overestimate the width of their own body (Slade and Russell). Food intake is primarily determined by the patient's impression of the size of her own body. Because this impression is a distorted one, she imagines herself to be already too fat, and starves herself so as to acquire what she considers to be more desirable proportions. The ensuing weight loss paradoxically increases her faulty perception of her body shape; hence the patient's abnormal attitudes to food and body size lead to the self-perpetuation of the illness.

It was originally postulated that anorexia nervosa was associated with a hypothalamic disorder on the grounds that destruction of the "feeding centers" in animals causes refusal of food. The impaired thermoregulation in anorexia nervosa is an example of a hypothalamic disturbance, but it is corrected when the patient's weight is restored to normal and is therefore secondary to the malnutrition. The strongest evidence for a primary hypothalamic disorder is the failure in the function of the hypothalamic–anterior pituitary–gonadal axis. Gonadotropins (FSH and LH) are not released from the anterior pituitary, the ovarian production of estrogens ceases, and ovulation fails to occur. Researches have shown that there is a reversible hypothalamic disturbance interfering with the secretion of gonadotropin-releasing hormone from the hypothalamus and hence a diminished release of FSH and LH. The patient with anorexia nervosa reverts to a 24-hour secretory pattern of gonadotropins resembling that of normal prepubertal and pubertal girls in whom the plasma levels of FSH and LH are higher during sleeping than waking hours (Boyar and Katz). It has also been shown that in the malnourished patient the hypothalamus fails to respond to a course of clomiphene or to a three-day course of ethinyl estradiol, either of which is followed in normal women by a peak rise of LH in the plasma. As the patient regains weight, the recovery of endocrine function follows a definite sequence. First, there is a gradual increase in the levels of gonadotropins; the anterior pituitary also responds to administered LH-releasing hormones by releasing FSH and LH. Next, a return of the negative feedback effect of estrogens can be shown: directly with a course of ethinyl estradiol which causes lowering of plasma LH levels, or indirectly with clomiphene (blocking the negative feedback action), which causes a rise in basal plasma LH levels. The positive feedback effect of estrogens is last to return and can be demonstrated directly with a three-day course of ethinyl estradiol, or indirectly with a seven-day course of clomiphene, either of which is followed by a peak rise in plasma LH. This final stage of recovery may be delayed, even after the patient's weight has returned to normal (Wakeling et al.) but is necessary for the resumption of cyclical menstruation and ovulation. The persistence of abnormal endocrine function in anorexia nervosa is probably also dependent in part on the patient's abnormal mental state. For example, the immature 24-hour secretory pattern with increased plasma LH levels during sleeping hours has been found in patients who are only slightly underweight but still display anorexic attitudes leading to overeating and self-induced vomiting. It also appears that a complete response to administered estrogens (with a positive feedback effect) is less likely to occur if there has not been an improvement in the psychologic disorder. These findings, together with the early onset of amenorrhea which may precede weight loss, indicate that the endocrine disorder is not wholly due to malnutrition.

A simplified diagram (Fig. 1) serves to emphasize the complexity of the interactions between the psychologic disorder, the endocrine disturbances, and the malnutrition in anorexia nervosa. The thickness of the lines reflects the strength of the evidence in support of each interaction. The best established pathways are those of the mental disorder causing a reduced food intake and weight loss (a), which in turn cause the endocrine disturbance and amenorrhea (b). It is also probable that weight loss and malnutrition worsen the mental disorder (c). The adverse effects of the patient's abnormal mental state on her endocrine and menstrual function support pathway (d). The original postulate that a disorder in the hypothalamic control of food intake might underlie the food refusal of anorexia nervosa is represented by the dotted line (e). It must be conceded that there is no direct evidence in support of this mechanism or for the postulated link (f), representing the neural effects of a hypothalamic disorder in molding mental function so as to give rise to faulty attitudes to eating and body size. Nevertheless it is clear that self-perpetuating disturbances play an important part in anorexia nervosa.

CLINICAL MANIFESTATIONS. The illness usually begins in a girl aged 14 to 17 years. Her previous personality may have been normal. In some patients, however, there may be a preceding history of food fads or difficulty in making friendships; other signs of maladjustment are excessive tidiness or fears of meeting strangers or of taking school examinations. Loss of weight may be the first feature noticed by the parents, who draw the patient's attention to it. She is likely to explain the weight loss as the result of dieting for the purpose of improving her figure. Menstruation will have ceased by the time there has been a significant loss of weight, or this may happen as the first feature of the illness. There is often a change in the girl's temperament, consisting of impatience, irritability, and depression. She may become preoccupied with schoolwork or indulge in solitary exercises, thus withdrawing from her customary social life. The loss of weight can be very rapid, with a fall from 55 kg (121) pounds) to 35 kg (77 pounds) within two to three months. This is achieved mainly by avoiding carbohydrate-containing foods, but self-induced vomiting, the abuse of purgatives, and excessive exercising, in various combinations, may accelerate the loss of weight. The patient's life becomes unhappy and constricted. If she had a boyfriend, she loses interest in him and avoids any sexual contact. Relations with members of the family become strained. Parents may react to their daughter's food refusal by alternately pleading with her and trying to force her to eat. Food refusal leads to malnutrition which may persist for months or even years. The patient subsists on a diet of vegetables, fruit, and cheese, and avoids bread, potatoes, cakes, and sugar. On some days she may take only black coffee. In severe cases the patient presents a pitiable sight of emaciation, apathy, weakness, and severe depression. There is a risk of death from suicide or complications of malnutrition—infections, potassium depletion, or hypothermia.

In spite of progressive malnutrition, the patient may reject her parents' entreaties to see a doctor, and she

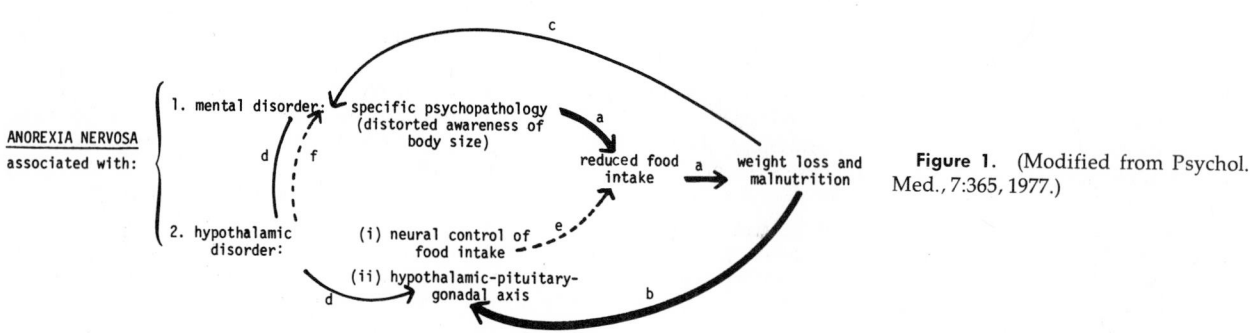

Figure 1. (Modified from Psychol. Med., 7:365, 1977.)

minimizes the extent of her dieting. When she does agree to seek help, she is likely to deny that she is unwell or admit only to insomnia, constipation, sensitivity to cold, or some depression of mood.

The clinical picture may change in some patients whose illness is of long standing. They may complain of distressing preoccupations with food which lead to orgiastic bouts of overeating, followed by self-induced vomiting. Their weight tends to rise and may be only slightly below the optimal level. Menstruation may also return. Occasionally the illness manifests itself from the onset in this way, especially in older women (in their twenties) who may have married and even had children.

Mental Examination. Examination of the patient's mental state may reveal a variety of disturbances. There may be depression and agitation; compulsive features may be prominent, such as elaborate feeding rituals and the counting of calories eaten daily; hysterical mechanisms may account for her assertion that she is eating well, whereas at the same time she hides food surreptitiously or vomits in secret. In addition, however, more specific psychologic abnormalities will be present. Their central theme is the patient's fear of becoming fat as a result of "losing control over eating." To play safe she resolves to remain thin and sets herself a sharply defined weight threshold above which she is unwilling to rise, defending her chosen weight as "right" for her. She may betray an abnormal sensitivity about the shape and size of her body, saying that fat would go to her stomach (hips, thighs, or some other part of the body). She may overestimate her weight and maintain, with all sincerity, that she eats large amounts of food. In an extreme case she may deny that she is thin, or even state that she is fat in spite of obvious emaciation. The patient's distorted awareness of her size can be tested by getting her to estimate the width of her body at various levels. Her estimate is liable to exceed her actual measurements by as much as 50 per cent. Patients may offer a variety of other reasons for their reluctance to return to a normal weight, or they may conceal their abnormal attitudes which nonetheless become explicit by their behavior when they are under observation in hospital.

Physical Examination. Physical examination will reveal the signs of severe malnutrition in a young girl who has developed secondary sex characteristics. The malnutrition is of a calorie-deficiency type. The disappearance of subcutaneous fat leads to gaunt, hollow facial features; bony prominences stand out sharply, the limbs are reduced to sticks, the belly is flat, the breasts shrunken, and the buttocks wasted. The hands and feet remain cold and blue, even when the room temperature is warm. The central body temperature may be reduced by 1° C. The blood pressure is low (e.g., 90/60), and the heart rate is slow (50 to 60). The skin is dry, and there is an excessive growth of dry, downy hair over the nape of the neck, cheeks, forearms, and legs (lanugo hair), changes attributed to a follicular keratosis. In older patients purpuric patches resembling senile purpura may appear over the dorsum of the hands, the forearms, and the legs after minor knocks.

In patients who vomit, dehydration ensues, together with a marked fall in the level of serum potassium (e.g., to 1.4 mEq per liter), a reduction in serum sodium, and hypochloremic alkalosis. These complications may lead to muscular weakness, tetany, and electrocar-diographic abnormalities; epileptic seizures may occur; chronic potassium depletion may lead to urinary infections and renal failure. Serum cholesterol levels may be raised. Carotenemia may follow a high intake of carrots or spinach, and causes a yellow pigmentation of the palms and soles. Vitamin deficiencies occur only rarely.

Endocrine Changes. Patients who are wasted show a fall in the plasma levels of LH, FSH, and estrogens. A course of clomiphene fails to raise the low plasma LH levels. Specific measures of thyroid function fall within the normal range. Plasma levels of growth hormone and cortisol are normal or elevated, and can be raised further by the administration of insulin. Most of the physical abnormalities disappear when the malnutrition is corrected. An exception to this recovery is the disorder of gonadotropin activity, as described above.

Side Effects of Refeeding. Peripheral edema may occur, especially when the diet has a high content of salt, water, and carbohydrates which cause water retention. A moderate normochromic normocytic anemia may result from hemodilution, or a more severe anemia may result from hemolysis or temporary hypoplasia of the bone marrow; occasionally, moderate iron deficiency anemia may occur. Acute dilatation of the stomach is a rare complication of too rapid refeeding.

Anorexia Nervosa in the Male. The illness in the male is rare, but resembles closely that in the female. The onset occurs around the time of puberty. The young boy rapidly loses weight as a result of avoiding carbohydrate-containing foods. Like the female, he expresses a fear of becoming fat, and resorts to a similar abnormal behavior of food refusal, possibly with vomiting, purgation, or exercising to excess. Because of the later age of physical maturation in the male, there is a greater risk of malnutrition causing retardation of growth and delayed puberty. The malnutrition is more likely to be of a type combining a deficiency of calories and proteins. The endocrine disorder in the male is analogous to that in the female. Urinary gonadotropins and blood LH levels are low; the urinary output of testosterone is reduced. Questioning will elicit loss of recently acquired sexual interest and potency. As in the female, these hormonal abormalities can be slowly reversed by treatment resulting in weight gain.

TREATMENT. There is no specific treatment; nevertheless the general management of patients is crucial and rewarding. The approach is essentially empirical; the treatments used are those which have been found to be effective in practice. The immediate aim is to treat the patient's malnutrition, which can become severe and dangerous. Even during the early stages of treatment it is desirable to try altering abnormal attitudes, for the course of the illness is much affected by the psychologic state. Thus treatment is best administered in a psychiatric unit, but it is essential that there should be good nursing facilities. The long-term aim of treatment is to reduce the duration of the illness and prevent relapses.

Short-Term Treatment. SECURING THE PATIENT'S COOPERATION. The first need is to obtain as much cooperation from the patient as possible, notwithstanding her denial of illness. By the time there has been severe loss of weight, admission to hospital is the only certain way of restoring her nutrition to normal. The doctor's skills must therefore be focused on persuading the patient to come into hospital. Compulsory admission is best avoided whenever possible, because the patient's continued cooperation is essential throughout the course of the illness, which may last for a few years.

NURSING TREATMENT.   The refeeding of the patient is best achieved by skilled nurses. After having assessed the severity of the feeding disorder, the nurse should try to establish a good relationship with her patient, one based on trust but not dependent on giving way to the patient's abnormal wishes to avoid food and weight gain. This is best achieved by the nurse asking the patient to look upon her as a person whom she can trust to decide on the amount of food to be eaten each day, and who will not allow her to become fat. The patient is told frankly that because of her illness she will be tempted to be deceitful about eating, vomiting, or taking purgatives. The nurse thus explains that close supervision will be necessary at first to reduce the strength of these temptations. Complete bed rest is seldom necessary for more than a few days, but it may facilitate a close watch being kept. The patient must be observed throughout every meal, and the nurse will cajole her into finishing all the food put on her plate. The avoidance of self-induced vomiting can be difficult. It requires round-the-clock nursing supervision, limiting the fluid intake to 1.5 liters daily, preventing access to the toilet for at least two hours after meals, and removal of vomit-bowls. The use of purgatives should also be stopped. As soon as the patient gains weight, she is complimented on her improved looks and is encouraged to use cosmetics and buy new clothes suitable for a person of normal weight. The nurse will decide on a judicious balance between restrictions and privileges, in collaboration with the medical staff. The balance is gradually altered in favor of added privileges which will be viewed by the patient as rewards for continuing progress.

DIET.   No special diets are needed. The patient is given her own choice of food so long as she does not exclude carbohydrate-containing foods. To begin with, the food intake should be 1500 calories daily; within seven to ten days she should be persuaded to accept full meals totaling 3000 to 5000 calories daily. Concentrated foods may be used to achieve this high intake (e.g., Complan, Metrecal, or Carnation breakfast food) by adding them to milk. Potassium supplements do not remedy the hypokalemia unless vomiting is controlled, and then they become unnecessary.

ADDITIONAL MEASURES.   The nursing care described should be viewed as a form of *psychologic treatment* embodying the principles of psychotherapy and behavior therapy. Formal psychotherapy has only a limited place during the early stages of treatment.

Large doses of chlorpromazine are sometimes advocated to reduce the patient's resistance to eating, but they can be dangerous in undernourished patients, and are seldom necessary. In very agitated patients the nursing task can be facilitated by administering moderate, divided doses of chlorpromazine up to a total of 300 mg daily. There is no place for tube feeding. It is doubtful whether a modified leukotomy is ever justified. Weight gain can be achieved by conservative treatment, and the risk of suicide is increased after leukotomy.

ASSESSMENT OF PROGRESS.   The patient is weighed daily before breakfast, and this provides the best check on her progress. A weight gain of up to 28 pounds (12.7 kg) in eight weeks should be possible. Figure 2 shows an 18-year-old patient before treatment and nine weeks later when she had gained 18.3 kg. The patient should be seen to maintain a healthy weight for about two weeks before being discharged from hospital.

Long-Term Treatment.   There is less known about the efficacy of long-term treatments. After discharge from hospital, it is necessary to provide outpatient supervision. Psychotherapy should be directed to whatever emotional problems have been identified in the patient and her family. Even when a normal weight is

Figure 2. Photographs of the same patient on admission (*A*) and at the completion of treatment, nine weeks later (*B*). (From the Bethlem and Maudsley Gazette, Spring/Summer, 1977.)

maintained, amenorrhea may persist for months or years. When the patient is eager to resume normal menstruation, one or two courses of clomiphene (50 to 100 mg daily for seven days) may be effective, but only when body weight has been restored to a normal level. In the event of a serious relapse, readmission to hospital will be necessary.

PROGNOSIS. The short-term prognosis is usually excellent. Treatment should lead to a return to a normal weight; at the same time, the majority of patients show a marked improvement in their mental state. Deaths from malnutrition should not occur.

The long-term prognosis is more problematical. Relapses requiring readmissions occur in about half the patients. The illness often lasts two to three years or even longer. In a follow-up of severely ill patients who had been treated at least four years previously, 40 per cent had recovered, 27 per cent had menstrual irregularity or a moderately low body weight, 29 per cent had serious weight loss with amenorrhea, and 5 per cent had died. Poor prognostic signs are a later age of onset (early twenties as opposed to early teens), or an illness which has lasted more than five years. Even in these patients, however, good results can still be obtained from energetic treatment. In many patients the prognosis is good — their health returns to normal and they may marry and can bear children.

Boyar, R. M., and Katz, J.: *In* Vigersky reference (see below), p. 177.
Bruch, H.: Eating Disorders: Obesity, Anorexia Nervosa and the Person Within. New York, Basic Books, 1972.
Gull, W. W.: Anorexia nervosa (apepsia hysterica, anorexia hysterica). Trans. Clin. Soc. London, 7:22, 1874.
Mecklenburg, R. S., Loriaux, D. L., Thompson, R. H., Anderson, A. E., and Lipsett, M. B.: Hypothalamic dysfunction in patients with anorexia nervosa. Medicine, 53:147, 1974.
Russell, G. F. M.: Anorexia nervosa: Its identity as an illness and its treatment. *In* Price, J. H. (ed.): Modern Trends in Psychological Medicine. 2d ed. London, Butterworth & Co. (Publishers) Ltd., 1970.
Russell, G. F. M.: The management of anorexia nervosa. *In* Robertson, R. F. (ed.): Symposium — Anorexia Nervosa and Obesity. Edinburgh, The Royal College of Physicians, 1973.
Slade, P. D., and Russell, G. F. M.: Awareness of body dimensions in anorexia nervosa: Cross-sectional and longitudinal studies. Psychol. Med., 3:188, 1973.
Theander, S.: Anorexia nervosa. A psychiatric investigation of 94 female patients. Acta Psychiatr. Scand., Supplement 211, 1970.
Vigersky, R. A. (ed.): Anorexia Nervosa: A Monograph of the National Institute of Child Health and Human Development. New York, Raven Press, 1977.
Wakeling, A., DeSouza, V., and Beardwood, C. J.: *In* Vigersky reference (see above), p. 199.

476. NUTRITIONAL MAINTENANCE AND DIET THERAPY IN ACUTE AND CHRONIC DISEASE

Philip Felig

476.1. INTRODUCTION

Diseases resulting from deficiencies of specific nutrients in the diet are well recognized and have been covered in detail in Ch. 473. Except in underdeveloped areas of the world, problems of nutritional homeostasis in hospitalized patients are generally a secondary consequence rather than a cause of disease processes. The normal intake of nutrients may be interfered with in a variety of inflammatory, septic, or malignant disorders as a result of anorexia or vomiting, in association with primary disturbances of the gastrointestinal tract, and in the postoperative state. Nutritional maintenance also poses a problem in patients placed on therapeutic diets designed to limit the intake of calories, carbohydrate, protein, sodium, or potassium. Generally attention is focused on correcting the primary disorder, and little concern is attached to over-all nutritional requirements, since most patients are expected to tolerate limited periods of subnutrition without difficulty. Considerations of nutritional factors are often limited to providing vitamin supplements, with little attention to caloric and nitrogen balance. It is noteworthy, however, that sepsis secondary to debilitation, in the form of terminal bronchopneumonia, is a major cause of death in hospitalized patients. The sequence of events in such patients is often as follows: primary disease (e.g., uremia, malignancy, ulcerative colitis) → poor nutrition and protein catabolism → depletion of body protein reserves (i.e., muscle) → weakness of respiratory muscles → atelectasis → pneumonia → death. In less severe circumstances, failure of adequate nutrition may prolong convalescence, predispose to infection, and interfere with wound healing.

An important goal in the medical management of disease is thus the maintenance of normal body composition in the face of reduced intake, increased metabolic requirements, or disordered metabolic machinery. From a practical standpoint nutritional considerations become an integral aspect of the therapeutic decision process in patients during short-term or long-term parenteral feeding, particularly when an anabolic response is necessary, and in patients on restrictive diets. To understand the principles underlying such nutritional interventions, it is first necessary to consider body composition in healthy subjects prior to the onset of illness, the metabolic response to nutritional deprivation in normal man, and the accelerated catabolism observed in disease states.

476.2. FUEL HOMEOSTASIS IN HEALTH AND DISEASE

BODY COMPOSITION. Normal man may be considered not only in terms of his constituent organ systems, but also with respect to his underlying fuel reserves. The energy resources available in a 70-kg man are shown in Table 1. Body fat, comprising 15 to 25 per cent of body weight, constitutes the primary fuel depot,

TABLE 1. Body Composition and Fuel Reserves in a Normal 70-kg Man

Fuel	Tissue	kg	% Body Weight	Energy Value (kcal)
Fat	Adipose tissue	11–17	15–25	100,000–150,000
Protein	Primarily muscle	8–12	12–17	32,000–48,000
Carbohydrate	Liver glycogen	0.070	<1	280
	Muscle glycogen	0.200	<1	800
	Blood glucose	0.020	<1	80

each gram providing 9 kcal. Smaller amounts of calories are available in the form of protein (4 kcal per gram), whereas carbohydrate stores (4 kcal per gram) are calorically insignificant. The enormity of fat stores relative to other nutrients is readily apparent. Furthermore, an increase in body weight, such as occurs in obesity, involves little change in the quantity of protein of carbohydrate but is associated primarily with an increase in fat. Thus a 25 per cent gain in weight is accompanied by a doubling in body fat. In contrast, weight loss, as observed in chronic debilitated states, involves a substantial reduction in body protein as well as fat. The ability to withstand a debilitating illness is accordingly reduced in the already wasted patient.

SHORT-TERM STARVATION. In individuals of normal weight or in those who are obese, even under circumstances of heavy exercise or the increased demands engendered by severe injury (Table 2), the magnitude of body fat stores is such that they might be expected to meet the total energy needs during periods of total starvation extending at least two months. However, it is not the depletion of fat which is the limiting factor in survival during food restriction. Death caused by starvation is a consequence of protein loss and generally occurs when one third to one half of total protein stores has been depleted. The continuous, obligate utilization of protein in the face of more plentiful fat reserves is a consequence of three factors: (1) protein constitutes the sole source of noncarbohydrate precursors which can be converted to glucose, inasmuch as net glucose synthesis from fatty acids does not occur in mammalian tissue; (2) certain tissues are obligate consumers of glucose; and (3) carbohydrate reserves (particularly liver glycogen) are extremely limited (Table 1) and are dissipated in less than 24 hours of starvation.

During short-term starvation the brain is the major site of glucose utilization. Glucose is consumed by the brain at a rate of 100 to 150 grams per day and undergoes terminal oxidation to CO_2 and water. Smaller amounts of glucose (50 to 75 grams) are converted to lactic acid by the formed elements of the blood, the renal medulla, and muscle tissue. The bulk of the energy requirements of muscle, heart, and visceral tissues are not dependent on glucose utilization (in either the fed state or starvation), but are met by the oxidation of free fatty acids mobilized from adipose tissue, and ketone acids formed in the liver in association with fat oxidation.

Since, as noted above, liver glycogen stores are limited to less than 100 grams, hepatic glycogenolysis can sustain brain glucose requirements for less than 24 hours. Synthesis of glucose from noncarbohydrate precursors (gluconeogenesis) consequently begins in the

immediate postabsorptive state (10- to 12-hour fast). Amino acids, particularly large amounts of alanine, are released from muscle tissue and are taken up by the liver where they are converted to glucose. The rate of protein breakdown is approximately 60 to 75 grams per day, resulting in the appearance fo 10 to 12 grams of nitrogen in the urine (6.25 grams N per gram of protein). Since muscle tissue is about 75 to 80 per cent water, this rate of protein catabolism results in a loss of approximately one half pound (200 to 300 grams) of lean body mass per day. A more rapid rate of weight loss reflects either a loss of body fluids (diuresis) or a catabolic state (see below).

The primary hormonal modulators of the gluconeogenic and ketogenic response to short-term starvation are insulin and glucagon. Fasting evokes a prompt decrease in serum insulin and a rise in circulating levels of glucagon. These hormonal changes, particularly the fall in insulin, provide the signal which stimulates lipolysis in adipose tissue and augmented gluconeogenesis by the liver. Insulin does not disappear entirely from the circulation; the small amounts remaining probably serve to prevent the massive ketogenesis and gluconeogenesis observed in diabetic ketoacidosis.

The catabolic processes precipitated by starvation may be dramatically altered by providing minimal amounts of carbohydrate. Administration of 100 grams of carbohydrate (400 calories) in the absence of other foodstuffs results in a marked diminution in urinary nitrogen losses to as little as 2 to 3 grams per day. This protein-sparing effect of calorically insignificant amounts of carbohydrate is of prime consideration in determining the composition of fluids administered to patients in whom food intake must be withheld for short periods (see below). Two points deserve emphasis regarding carbohydrate intake in otherwise fasted individuals: (1) increasing the carbohydrate content above 100 grams does not increase the protein-sparing effect; (2) positive nitrogen balance (anabolism) cannot be achieved unless an exogenous source of protein is provided as well.

LONG-TERM STARVATION. As fasting continues beyond several days, a series of adaptations occurs designed to limit the rate and magnitude of protein breakdown. Total glucose utilization decreases as the brain consumes ketone bodies as an alternative oxidative fuel. Since less glucose is required, gluconeogenic processes are curtailed, and the outflow of alanine and other amino acids from muscle is greatly reduced. Urinary nitrogen excretion falls to as little as 3 grams per day, reflecting the catabolism of no more than 20 grams of protein and depletion of less than 100 grams of lean body mass. The expendable nature of fat as compared to protein is indicated by the fact that 95 per cent of caloric needs are met by combustion of free fatty acids and ketone bodies. The patient in this circumstance is on an "endogenous high-fat diet" in which protein breakdown continues, but at a greatly reduced rate. The precise signal (?hormonal) triggering this decrease in protein catabolism has not been identified.

CATABOLIC STATES: INFLAMMATION, SEPSIS, TRAUMA. The orderly adaptive processes directed at minimizing protein losses in prolonged or short-term starvation are predicated upon the absence of significant underlying disease. In association with acute or chronic inflammation, sepsis, or trauma (burns, injuries, or surgery), the response to nutritional deprivation is

TABLE 2.   Caloric Expenditure in Normal and Disease States

Normal Activity	Calories/kg Body Weight/Day	Disease States
Bed rest	25	Bed rest
Light exercise (light housework, office work)	30–35	Fever of 39.4 C
Moderate exercise (industrial work, heavy housework)	35–40	Peritonitis, sepsis
Heavy exercise (construction work, farm work)	40–45	Extensive burns

characterized by an accelerated rate of protein catabolism. The magnitude of the catabolic response is related in part to increases in energy expenditure. Oxygen consumption is increased by fever at a rate of 15 per cent per degree Celsius. Thus a fever of 39.4° C results in a 25 to 30 per cent elevation in energy requirements (Table 2). In addition to the effects of fever, the nature of the underlying disease or injury will influence caloric expenditure. The trauma associated with elective surgery causes no increase in basal oxygen consumption. In contrast, compound fractures or severe infections (e.g., peritonitis) are associated with an increase of 50 per cent, whereas extensive body burns are followed by elevations of 100 per cent above normal (Table 2). These increased demands for energy are met by an accelerated rate of protein dissolution. Urinary nitrogen losses in the poorly fed patient with an extensive inflammatory process may amount to 25 grams per day (more than twice the rate observed in uncomplicated starvation), reflecting the breakdown of over 150 grams of protein and resulting in a loss of more than 1 pound per day of lean body mass. The origin of the protein loss is primarily muscle, inasmuch as the integrity of visceral tissues (e.g., liver) is maintained. Although the fate of the amino acids mobilized from muscle has not been precisely defined, recent studies by Kinney suggest that this rapid loss of protein is coupled with an accelerated rate of gluconeogenesis. This increased production of glucose may serve to meet the needs of reparative tissues such as fibroblasts and phagocytes.

The over-all metabolic picture thus contrasts markedly with that which occurs in prolonged starvation in normal subjects. Oxygen consumption, protein dissolution, and gluconeogenesis are all accelerated. Even more striking is the dissimilarity in the response to glucose administration. In contrast to the protein-sparing effects of minimal amounts of carbohydrate in starvation, administration of 100 to 400 grams of glucose fails to influence substantially the course of protein breakdown. Positive nitrogen balance or even a substantial reduction in net nitrogen losses is achieved only by providing an exogenous source of amino acids as well as sufficient calories (in the form of carbohydrate and/or fat) to meet the increased energy demands of catabolic states.

ACCELERATED STARVATION: ALCOHOLIC KETOACIDOSIS, ALCOHOL-INDUCED HYPOGLYCEMIA, AND ALCOHOL-INDUCED HYPOMAGNESEMIA. The response to nutritional deprivation in normal man not only is directed at minimizing protein losses but also involves a limitation of ketone acid (beta-hydroxybutyrate and acetoacetate) production so as to avoid metabolic acidosis. In addition, continuous production of glucose assures the maintenance of blood glucose concentrations above the hypoglycemic range. During periods of total starvation extending for several days to weeks in healthy subjects, ketone acid accumulation in blood does not exceed 8 mM per liter, serum bicarbonate remains above 14 mEq per liter, and blood glucose concentration remains above 50 mg per 100 ml. In contrast, in alcoholic patients, particularly after binge drinking and protracted vomiting, starvation-induced metabolic acidosis (caused by excessive ketone acid accumulation) and/or hypoglycemia may be observed. Clinically, patients with alcoholic ketoacidosis present in a comatose state or are alert but appear acutely ill and have rapid, deep respirations. Arterial pH is reduced to less than 7.2,

and an increased anion gap is observed. In about 25 per cent of cases the blood glucose level is less than 50 mg per 100 ml. The nature of the metabolic acidosis is often not recognized or is mistakenly attributed to lactate, since the semiquantitative nitroprusside reaction for ketones (Acetest, Ketostix, Ames Co.) is often only faintly positive. The failure to detect the extent of ketonemia is due to the high ratio of betahydroxybutyrate (which is not detected in the nitroprusside test) to acetoacetate. The mechanism whereby alcohol accelerates the ketotic response to starvation involves augmented lipolysis and probably altered intramitochondrial oxidative pathways. In most instances a prompt clinical response follows the administration of parenteral fluids containing glucose.

Alcohol-induced hypoglycemia is observed in circumstances in which liver glycogen stores have been depleted by a period of one or more days of food abstinence or vomiting. Alcohol interferes with glucose homeostasis by inhibiting hepatic gluconeogenesis from lactate, pyruvate, and amino acids. This effect is mediated by changes in cytoplasmic redox (i.e., an increase in hepatic NADH) that accompany the metabolic degradation of alcohol. The hypoglycemic action of alcohol therefore does not become apparent until glycogen stores have been exhausted, and maintenance of the glucose supply to the brain is solely dependent on gluconeogenic processes. Consequently, this disorder is most likely to be encountered in the chronic alcoholic who has been eating poorly or has had protracted vomiting. In addition to the usual signs and symptoms of hypoglycemia, alcohol hypoglycemia is frequently accompanied by hypothermia. In contrast to insulin-induced hypoglycemia, glucagon is ineffective in raising the blood sugar level since glycogen reserves have already been depleted. As in the case of ketoacidosis, patients promptly respond to infusion of glucose.

Alcohol also accelerates electrolyte deficiencies induced by poor food intake, particularly with respect to magnesium. Under normal circumstances it is extremely difficult to induce magnesium deficiency by dietary deprivation, as the renal conservation of magnesium is very efficient. Ethanol, however, interferes with renal tubular reabsorption of magnesium, leading to relatively rapid depletion of body magnesium stores and the development of hypomagnesemia. Vomiting, diarrhea, and secondary hyperaldosteronism accompanying hepatic cirrhosis may also contribute to hypomagnesemia in the chronic alcoholic. Clinical manifestations include irritability, tetany (identical to that observed with hypocalcemia), and convulsions. Magnesium deficiency also interferes with parathormone secretion as well as tissue responsiveness to this hormone, and thus frequently results in hypocalcemia. Abstinence from alcohol, dietary intake of magnesium-containing foods, and (in symptomatic patients) the slow intravenous administration of magnesium (16 to 32 mEq per day) results in normalization of serum magnesium concentration.

476.3. PARENTERAL NUTRITION

The problem of assuring nutritional maintenance or minimizing losses in body composition in association with acute or chronic disease is particularly challenging in patients in whom feeding via the gastrointestinal route is precluded. Until recently the primary focus in parenteral nutrition has been mainly on water and electrolyte replacement with little emphasis on meeting total caloric and protein requirements. The development of new techniques involving the infusion of markedly hypertonic solutions containing glucose and amino acids (parenteral hyperalimentation) or isotonic fat emulsions has revolutionized the field of parenteral nutrition. Weight gain and positive nitrogen balance are now attainable goals in patients fed intravenously. However, total parenteral nutrition is not without morbidity (as noted below, a variety of infectious and metabolic complications have been described), and consequently is not indicated for all patients in whom oral or tube feeding cannot be maintained. The factors determining the composition, tonicity, and volume of fluid to be administered will depend in large part on whether feeding via the intravenous route must be sustained for a relatively brief period of up to a week or whether one is dealing with a prolonged period of parenteral alimentation. In the former instance the goal is primarily to minimize losses in body composition, whereas in the long-term situation the objective is positive caloric and protein balance to facilitate repair and healing of inflamed or traumatized tissue and to hasten convalescence.

SHORT-TERM INTRAVENOUS NUTRITION. In the patient requiring intravenous feeding for a period of several days, treatment is directed at providing sufficient carbohydrate to meet cerebral glucose requirements without depleting liver glycogen stores. In this manner, the need for gluconeogenesis and its attendant dissolution of body protein is minimized. Simultaneously, the glucose infusion prevents the fall in serum insulin levels which would otherwise occur in a nonfed individual, thereby inhibiting the development of starvation ketosis. These protein-sparing and antiketogenic effects are achieved with as little as 100 grams of carbohydrate, which may be infused over 24 hours as 2 liters of a 5 per cent dextrose solution. The net effect of the conventional glucose infusion is not one of stimulation of glucose uptake by muscle or fat tissue, but inhibition of hepatic glycogenolysis and replacement of the liver (by the infusion) as the source of glucose for brain oxidative requirements. Such an infusion doubles circulating insulin levels (as compared to the five- to ten-fold increase observed after a carbohydrate meal) and elevates blood glucose by 15 to 30 mg per 100 ml. Increasing the amount of glucose infused above 100 grams per day will not further reduce the small degree of protein catabolism which persists in nonfed patients, unless one achieves caloric balance by administering markedly hypertonic solutions (see below).

An alternative form of carbohydrate available in commercial parenteral fluids is fructose. There is no evidence, however, that fructose has any advantage over glucose. Furthermore, rapid administration of large amounts of fructose (0.5 gram per kilogram per hour) can result in the development of lactic acidosis.

In addition to meeting nutritional needs, the major goal in short-term intravenous therapy is the maintenance of fluid and electrolyte balance. Basal fluid requirements may be estimated at 2000 ml per day, which consists of (1) 800 ml to provide for insensible losses via the lungs and skin and sensible losses as sweat, and (2) 1200 ml to maintain a reasonable urine output. The electrolyte requirements are in the form of sodium and potassium. Although the urine will become free of sodium after five to eight days of total sodium restriction, negative sodium balance (and the possibility of plasma volume contraction) will prevail during this interval if exogenous sodium is not provided. The usual intake of sodium in the diet is 4 to 6 grams (174 to 261 mEq), which is ingested as 10 to 12 grams of NaCl. Sodium depletion can be readily prevented in normal man by infusing 500 ml of isotonic (0.9 per cent) sodium chloride containing 77 mEq of NaCl. Potassium supplementation is also necessary, because there is an obligatory daily loss of about 40 mEq per day.

The total carbohydrate, fluid, and electrolyte requirements during short-term intravenous therapy may thus be met with the following daily infusion regimen: 1500 ml of 5 per cent dextrose in water containing 40 mEq KCl; and 500 ml of 5 per cent dextrose in isotonic (0.9) per cent) saline.

It should be noted that this regimen is designed to meet basal fluid and electrolyte requirements in patients without cardiac or renal failure and does not take into account pre-existing deficits or abnormal losses. For the modifications necessary to meet problems of hydration and electrolyte imbalance, see Ch. 530.

LONG-TERM INTRAVENOUS NUTRITION (TOTAL PARENTERAL NUTRITION, PARENTERAL HYPERALIMENTATION). In circumstances requiring long-term intravenous nutrition, particularly in debilitated patients, the optimal goal is positive nitrogen balance and weight gain. The infusion program outlined above for short-term therapy is obviously nutritionally inadequate in that it provides only 400 calories and no amino acids. Although protein hydrolysates have been available for over 30 years, a major problem has been the provision of parenteral means of an adequate amount of calories (2500 or more calories per day) to promote anabolism. Fat emulsions providing 9 calories per gram are potentially the most efficient energy source; however, there is some controversy whether fat is as effective as carbohydrate in promoting nitrogen balance (see below). Ethyl alcohol (7 calories per gram) is also a relatively efficient source of calories, but the toxic effects associated with infusion of alcohol limit its usefulness. The achievement of caloric balance by infusion of carbohydrate (4 calories per gram) necessitates the infusion of massive amounts of isotonic or moderately hypertonic fluid (6 liters of a 10 per cent solution), or, alternatively, the infusion of hypertonic solutions (20 to 25 per cent or four to five times the tonicity of plasma). The former regimen results in problems of fluid overload, whereas the latter approach leads to thrombosis of peripheral veins. These difficulties in providing adequate calories were solved by Dudrick and his colleagues with their introduction of parenteral hyperalimentation, a technique involving placement of a catheter in the superior vena cava followed by infusion of a hypertonic glucose–amino acid mixture.

Indications. The following disorders are likely to benefit from this form of therapy: (1) Gastrointestinal disorders, particularly chronic inflammatory bowel disease (regional enteritis, ulcerative colitis) complicated by fistula formation; the "short bowel syndrome" after extensive intestinal resection; and congenital lesions of the gastrointestinal tract amenable to surgical repair. (2) Extensive body burns and traumatic injuries in which caloric requirements are markedly increased. In such cases parenteral nutrition may be used as a supplement to oral feeding. (3) Acute renal failure. Over-all mortality and duration of azotemia have been demonstrated to decrease in patients with acute renal failure treated with a mixture of glucose and 1.8 per cent essential amino acids.

It should be emphasized that neither the presence of an acute focal, septic condition nor the requirement to "put the alimentary tract at rest" is a sufficient indication for this form of treatment.

Composition of Solutions. A variety of hypertonic glucose and amino acid mixtures are currently available in commercial form. The solution to be administered is generally prepared by mixing 500 to 600 ml of the commercial protein hydrolysate or synthetic amino acid mixture with 400 to 500 ml of 50 per cent dextrose. The resulting solution should provide 900 to 1200 calories per liter. The recommended concentrations of nutrients and electrolytes in the infusate are shown in Table 3. Inasmuch as commercial preparations vary markedly in their content of sodium, potassium, and phosphate, supplemental electrolytes may have to be added to the infusate to achieve desired concentrations. Particular attention should be focused on administration of adequate phosphate, inasmuch as the phosphate requirement in parenterally alimented patients may exceed the 40 mEq per day recommended in patients fed via the oral route. The concentrations of nutrients shown in Table 3 do not apply to patients in renal failure or with congestive heart failure. In the former circumstance, a sodium-free solution containing only essential amino acids (1.8 per cent) is employed. In cardiac failure the sodium content of the infusate is reduced to 20 mEq per liter or less.

Solution Administration and Patient Management. Because of the hypertonicity of the infusate, rapid dilution of the infusion mixture by high blood flow is necessary to prevent phlebitis or thrombosis. Consequently total parenteral nutrition necessitates administration of nutrient solutions through a catheter in the superior vena cava. The latter may be cannulated via an infraclavicular percutaneous subclavian vein puncture. Alternatively, a surgical cutdown may be performed with exposure of a peripheral vein through which the catheter is threaded to the superior vena cava. Strict asepsis must be used in inserting and maintaining catheters. The dressing over the puncture site should be changed every two to three days and an antibiotic ointment reapplied.

The solution is initially administered at a rate of 2 liters per day, and thereafter is gradually increased to 3 liters per day. In dealing with a markedly catabolic

state, 4 to 5 liters may be administered. The solution should be infused at a constant rate over the entire 24-hour period.

Complications. Total parenteral nutrition is not without risk to the patient. The reported complications relate to either infection or metabolic disorders.

SEPSIS. This is the most frequently observed complication; it may occur in 25 per cent or more of patients. Fungemia caused by *Candida albicans* accounts for half the cases, with the remainder attributable to *Staphylococcus aureus* and *Klebsiella aerobacter*. In most instances the organism can be cultured from the catheter tip, implicating the catheter as the source of sepsis. Factors which may predispose to sepsis are prior antimicrobial use, the nutrient content of the infusate (which may serve as growth medium), and possible adverse effects of hypertonicity on phagocytic function. The incidence of septicemia may be reduced by placing an on-line membrane filter of 0.22 μ pore size in the infusion apparatus, frequent changing of the catheter, and meticulous care of the skin puncture site.

HYPERGLYCEMIA. In patients with normal pancreatic islet cell function, the dextrose-rich infusate invokes a hyperinsulinemic response wich permits disposal of the administered glucose load without the development of hyperglycemia in excess of 200 mg per 100 ml. In patients with a predisposition to diabetes, the islet cell response is inadequate and hyperglycemia and glycosuria develop. In some instances this may take the form of *hyperglycemic nonketotic hyperosmolar coma* in which the blood glucose reaches levels of 1000 mg per 100 ml and is accompanied by dehydration, azotemia, obtundation, and occasionally seizures. Such patients should be treated with rapid-acting insulin intravenously and large volumes of water containing 2.5 per cent glucose. The development of a severe hyperosmolar state can generally be prevented by frequent monitoring of the urine and blood glucose levels and by administering insulin in doses of 10 to 20 units to patients with persistent hyperglycemia (above 200 mg per 100 ml) and glycosuria.

POSTINFUSION HYPOGLYCEMIA. If the intravenous infusion is suddenly dislodged or discontinued, a rapid fall in blood glucose occurs which may reach hypoglycemic levels. Presumably this is due to persistence of hyperinsulinemia and suppression of counter-regulatory hormones (glucagon, epinephrine, growth hormone, cortisol). This complication may be avoided by maintaining a constant infusion rate and by switching to a solution containing 5 per cent glucose several hours before terminating the infusion.

HYPOPHOSPHATEMIA. A decline in serum phosphate concentration to levels less than 1 mg per 100 ml is almost uniformly observed after hyperalimentation with phosphate-free solutions for periods of seven to ten days. Accompanying the hypophosphatemia is a decline in red cell levels of 2,3-diphosphoglycerate and an increase in red cell oxygen affinity as indicated by a left-shift in the oxygen dissociation curve. The clinical picture consists of circumoral paresthesias, obtundation, hyperventilation, and, in severe cases, seizures and coma. The hypophosphatemia is not due to urinary losses but is probably a consequence of shifts in body phosphate. Insulin-mediated glucose uptake in muscle and liver brought about by the hypertonic glucose infusion is accompanied by phosphate deposition in these tissues. This redistribution apparently occurs at the ex-

TABLE 3. Nutrient Concentration in Hypertonic
Solutions Used in Total Parenteral Nutrition*

Glucose	200–250 grams
Protein hydrolysate or synthetic amino acids	30–50 grams
Calories	920–1200 kcal
Sodium	40–50 mEq
Potassium	30–40 mEq
Calcium	5–10 mEq
Magnesium	4–8 mEq
Phosphate	15–20 mEq
Multivitamin concentrate†	2 ml

*Expressed per liter of infusate.
†Vitamin K and folic acid which are not present in the multivitamin concentrate are administered by intramuscular injection.

pense of plasma and red cell phosphate reserves. The syndrome may be prevented by adding phosphate supplements to the nutrient solution; in debilitated patients the requirement may be as high as 20 to 25 mEq per liter.

HYPERCHLOREMIC ACIDOSIS. In patients receiving synthetic amino acid mixtures rather than protein hydrolysates, the concentration of cationic amino acids (histidine, arginine, lysine) is substantially greater than that of metabolizable anions as reflected in a large cation gap. These cationic amino acids contribute hydrogen ions (thereby lowering blood pH) and chloride to body fluids upon conversion to urea or incorporation into peptide chains. The resulting effect is hyperchloremic metabolic acidosis. This syndrome may be prevented by adding a portion of the sodium supplements to the infusate in the form of bicarbonate rather than chloride when using synthetic amino acid mixtures.

HYPERAMMONEMIA. Abnormally elevated concentrations of blood ammonia have been reported in premature infants and in adults with liver disease receiving infusions containing casein or fibrin hydrolysates. It is probably due to an inability to metabolize preformed ammonia which may account for as much as 8 to 10 per cent of the total nitrogen content in protein hydrolysate solutions. This complication can be prevented or minimized by utilizing synthetic amino acid mixtures in patients with liver disease and in premature infants.

ESSENTIAL FATTY ACID DEFICIENCY. In occasional patients receiving long-term fat-free parenteral nutrition, a syndrome has been observed characterized by scaly skin lesions, hair loss, and poor wound healing. The biochemical findings consist of a decrease in plasma concentrations of linoleic and arachidonic acids and an increase in 5,8,-11-eicosatrienoic acid. Administration of soy bean oil emulsion has been shown to reverse the chemical findings and correct the biochemical abnormalities.

Fat Emulsions for Intravenous Nutrition. As noted above, the low caloric density of carbohydrate necessitates use of hypertonic solutions for long-term total parenteral nutrition and consequently dictates the need for a central venous catheter with its attendant risks of infection. Fat emulsions have the inherent advantage of permitting administration of 1000 calories per liter of infusate as an isotonic solution which may be infused via a peripheral vein. The initial clinical experience with fat emulsion prepared from cottonseed oil was, however, disappointing because of toxic reactions, including fever, anemia, thrombocytopenia, hepatosplenomegaly, and jaundice. The introduction of a soy bean oil emulsion has provided a safe means of administering, via a peripheral vein, a calorie-rich solution which is isotonic. The experience with the soy bean oil emulsion in Europe has indicated its efficacy (when combined with amino acids) in promoting positive nitrogen balance. In the United States, where such solutions have only recently become available for use, the experience has been less uniform. Although positive nitrogen balance has been achieved in many patients receiving combined fat emulsion and amino acids, in at least some septic patients the fat emulsion has been less effective than hypertonic glucose in promoting protein anabolism. Nevertheless, fat emulsions are useful as an adjunct to regimens containing hypertonic glucose for the treatment or prevention of essential fatty acid deficiency.

Isotonic Amino Acids. Blackburn and colleagues have demonstrated that peripheral infusions of isotonic amino acids in a dose of 100 grams per day are an effective means of reversing the nitrogen wasting observed in starvation or in postoperative patients following elective surgery. Since such patients must be fed intravenously for only short periods and inasmuch as glucose-containing solutions will reduce (but not eliminate) protein catabolism, the actual amount of protein sparing achieved by isotonic amino acids is relatively small. The precise indications for and advantages of intravenous infusions of isotonic amino acids remain to be established.

476.4. DIET THERAPY

Diets are employed in the care of the sick for the following purposes: (1) to regulate (either decrease or increase) the total caloric intake; (2) to restrict (or less frequently augment) the content of specific nutrients, such as protein, fat, sodium, or potassium; (3) to provide foods which are bland in flavor, as in patients with peptic ulcer disease; (4) to reduce fiber content, as in disorders characterized by chronic diarrhea; (5) to eliminate specific foods, as in allergic conditions; and (6) to modify the consistency of foods, as in "soft" or "liquid" diets. Here we will consider specific conditions (diabetes, obesity) and diets in which the treatment program is restrictive in total calories and/or specific nutrients (protein, carbohydrate, sodium, potassium). The dietary treatment of hyperlipidemias is described in Ch. 474.

In prescribing a diet it is important to recognize not only the therapeutic goals but also the likelihood of patient acceptance. The patient's likes and dislikes as well as cultural, sociologic, and economic factors must all be considered. For example, the high protein, low carbohydrate diet advocated by some in the treatment of obesity has been referred to as a "rich man's diet," since the cost of a diet made up primarily of foods high in protein content (meat, fish) may be prohibitively expensive. On the other hand, diet treatment based on an extremely restrictive protein content (20 grams) may fail because the basic unpalatability and limited food selection result in noncompliance.

A second factor to be considered in the make-up of a diet is the influence of restriction of one nutrient on the availability of other dietary components. A diet which is extremely low in sodium (250 mg) requires restriction in protein intake inasmuch as unlimited ingestion of milk or meat will increase the sodium content of the diet. The use of such a diet for the patient with chronic congestive heart failure may contribute to mobilization of edema fluid, but at the expense of a depletion in lean body mass. Similarly, a diet low in protein (20 to 40 grams) as used in cirrhotic patients with portal-systemic shunting and in renal disease will generally be calorically inadequate. Caloric balance can only be achieved by means of a very high intake of carbohydrate in the form of concentrated sweets, which may cause difficulty if there is an associated diabetic tendency. Deficiencies in vitamins are also likely to occur on severely restrictive diets but are more readily corrected by giving a single multivitamin tablet daily.

A third principle requiring emphasis is the requirement for precision in nomenclature and the need for close communication between the physician and dietician. The term "diabetic diet" has no meaning as such. However, a prescription for a 1900-calorie, 200-gram carbohydrate, 80-gram protein, and 90-gram fat diet is readily interpretable. Similarly, a "low salt diet" does not specify the precise level of sodium restriction as indicated by a "500-mg sodium diet." Few physicians have adequate knowledge of nutrition to construct a palatable and effective diet. On the other hand, the dietician, even when given a precise diet order, may not be aware of the therapeutic priorities for a particular patient. Communication between the physician and dietician will permit the minor modifications which may transform an unpalatable regimen into an acceptable program. For example, in the case of the patient in chronic renal failure on a restricted protein, sodium, and potassium intake, it is important for the dietician to know which nutrient may be most safely liberalized so as to improve patient acceptance without imposing serious difficulties in over-all management.

THE NORMAL DIET. In prescribing a therapeutic diet it is useful to begin by considering the normal diet. In an individual with a stable body weight and no marked shifts in body fluid, caloric intake equals caloric expenditure. As indicated in Table 2, the caloric requirements in a 70-kg man engaged in moderate activity are approximately 2500 to 2800 calories per day. In the "average" diet consumed in the United States, 15 per cent of these calories are derived from protein, 45 to 50 per cent are in the form of carbohydrate, and the remaining 35 to 40 per cent are derived from fat.

The normal diet can also be defined in terms of the relative contributions of six basic food groups (Table 4). Each of these basic food groups has a specific content of calories, protein, fat, and carbohydrate. In addition, for each of these groups an "exchange list" may be prepared, in which all of the specific food items of approximately equal carbohydrate, protein, and fat value are grouped. In this manner it becomes relatively simple to determine which foods are to be eliminated or reduced when intake of a specific nutrient is restricted. For example, it is clear

that a diet low in protein entails a restriction in milk and meat. It is also obvious that a reduction in total calories can be achieved by substituting nonfat milk for whole milk and by restricting fat intake, while increasing vegetables (group A) as desired. It should be noted that certain vegetables such as potatoes, beans, peas, and corn are placed in the "bread group" because of their relatively high content of carbohydrate. The use of exchange lists, which is the fundamental tactic employed by the dietician in constructing a specific diet, is also extremely helpful to the patient in that it allows variety in food choices while maintaining specific nutritional guidelines.

DIABETES MELLITUS. The fundamental role of diet in the management of diabetes is well recognized. Nevertheless, the specific principles involved in diet therapy have been poorly understood. The generally held notion is that carbohydrate is bad for people with diabetes and that a "diabetic diet" is a carbohydrate-restricted diet. In fact, the major emphasis in diet treatment in the diabetic should be directed at the following points in decreasing order of priority:

1. Regulation of total caloric intake so as to achieve an ideal body weight. For the maturity-onset diabetic in whom the incidence of obesity is 60 per cent or more, this generally entails a reduction in caloric intake. The importance of weight reduction in these patients is based upon the fact that obesity results in resistance to endogenous insulin; this is reversed by a return to ideal weight. With restoration to normal weight, the demand for endogenous insulin is reduced and an improvement in glucose tolerance will ensue. In contrast to the obese, maturity-onset diabetic, a hypercaloric intake is indicated in the thin, wasted insulin-dependent diabetic, particularly in childhood. Such patients require an increase in calories to restore body fat and protein and to permit normal growth.

TABLE 4. Nutritive Values for Food Groups*

Food Group	Serving	Weight (grams)	Calories	Carbo-hydrate (grams)	Fat (grams)	Protein (grams)	Sodium (mg)	Potassium (mg)
1. Milk								
Whole milk	1 cup	240	170	12	10	8	120	335
Nonfat milk	1 cup	240	80	12	–	8	120	335
Low-sodium milk	1 cup	240	170	12	10	8	7	600
2. Meat								
Lean meat or fish	3 oz	90	219	–	15	21	75	300
Egg	1	50	73	–	5	7	60	65
3. Vegetables								
Group A†	½ cup	100	2–8	–	–	0.5–2.0	9	100–250
Group B‡	½ cup	100	35	7	–	2	9	100–200
4. Fruits	½ cup	100	40	10	–	0–1.0	2	75–250
5. Bread§								
Regular	1 slice	30	68	15	–	2	120	30
Low-sodium	1 slice	30	68	15	–	2	5	30
Low protein and low electrolyte	1 slice	30	68	17	–	0.1	9	3
Potatoes	1 small	100	68	15	–	2	4	407
Spaghetti	½ cup	100	68	15	–	2	1	61
6. Fat								
Butter, unsalted	1 tsp	5	45	–	5	–	–	–
Butter, salted	1 tsp	5	45	–	5	–	50	–

*Based on the Manual of Diets, Departments of Dietetics, Hospital of St. Raphael, Veterans Administration Hospital, and Yale–New Haven Hospital, New Haven, Connecticut, 1972.

†Includes all vegetables not listed in Group B or classified in "bread" group.

‡Beets, carrots, onions, green peas, turnips, squash.

§Includes high carbohydrate vegetables (potatoes, beans, and corn), cereals, and noodle products.

2. The total carbohydrate content of the diet should not be disproportionately restricted, but the intake of concentrated sweets (candies, table sugar, pastries) should be limited. There is no compelling evidence that isocaloric reduction in the carbohydrate content to 30 per cent results in improvement of the diabetic state. Such an approach may be deleterious in the long run, because the calories not taken as carbohydrate are generally made up in the form of a high fat intake which may have an adverse effect in accelerating atherosclerosis. Once the appropriate caloric intake has been determined, approximately 45 per cent of the calories should be provided in the form of carbohydrate. An exception is the diabetic with a carbohydrate-inducible (Type III or Type IV) form of hyperlipidemia, in whom a low carbohydrate, high fat intake is indicated (see Ch. 532.5). To avoid marked swings in the blood glucose concentration, particularly in insulin-dependent diabetics, simple sugars in the form of concentrated sweets should be avoided. Instead the carbohydrate in the diet should be primarily in the form of complex carbohydrates or starches (such as potatoes, beans, bread, and noodle products), because the glucose derived from these foods is released more slowly into the bloodstream.

3. Day-to-day regularity of food intake with respect to total consumption of calories and carbohydrates and with regard to the timing of meals is of importance in insulin-dependent diabetics so as to prevent insulin-induced hypoglycemia. An increase in the number and frequency of feedings in the form of a midmorning, afternoon, and bedtime snack is also helpful in this regard. The regularity and frequency of feedings are predicated on the fact that, in contrast to the normal subject in whom insulin secretion is dictated by food ingestion, the insulin-dependent diabetic must match his food intake to the continuing action of injected insulin. The consistency in the pattern of food ingestion does not apply on those days in which there is a marked increase in caloric expenditure as a consequence of moderate to severe exercise. In normal subjects exercise causes an inhibition in beta cell secretion, resulting in a fall in endogenous insulin levels which permits an increase in hepatic glucose output. In the diabetic subject receiving insulin injections such homeostatic changes in circulating insulin levels will not occur in response to exercise. Here, extra food should be taken so as to meet the needs of contracting muscles and to prevent hypoglycemia.

Dietary management in diabetes must be related to the two primary types of the disease. In the obese, adult-onset diabetic the primary goal is a hypocaloric intake and weight reduction. In the insulin-dependent diabetic the major dietary objective is regularity of food ingestion so as to prevent hypoglycemia. Despite the simplicity of these principles, less than 50 per cent of the diabetic population adheres to the recommended dietary regimen. Poor understanding on the part of the patient as well as the physician with respect to dietary goals and tactics is frequently responsible for failure. Often the basic prescription is clearly an error and unsuitable for the specific patient. For example, to many physicians a "diabetic diet" almost by definition means an 1800-calorie intake. Such a diet in a vigorous, nonobese 160-pound insulin-dependent diabetic is obviously too restrictive and is likely to have adverse consequences: (1) the patient will not follow the diet and will supplement his intake, generally with concentrated sweets, resulting in marked swings in the blood glucose; or (2) he may stick to the diet but will develop hypoglycemic episodes and/or lose weight. An 1800-calorie diet is equally inappropriate in the 180-pound, 5 foot 2 inch, 50-year-old, sedentary, noninsulin-dependent diabetic woman, in whom the major objective should be weight reduction by means of a more limited caloric intake.

Diet treatment is also useful in the prevention of diabetes. The most important nutritional factor contributing to the development of diabetes is obesity, irrespective of the ratio of individual foodstuffs in the diet. The notion that an increased intake of concentrated carbohydrate is in itself a major causative factor in diabetes has not been substantiated. Thus in patients with a predisposition to diabetes (e.g., strong family history; mothers with a history of large babies), the emphasis should be on *total caloric regulation* so as to prevent obesity rather than on disproportionate restriction in carbohydrate intake.

OBESITY. The situation in which diets are most commonly used in the general population is in obesity (see Ch. 474). A wide variety of "fad" diets have been heralded in the lay press (water diet, grapefruit diet, the low carbohydrate "diet revolution," etc.). Unfortunately none of these provides more rapid weight loss or a greater likelihood for long-term success than is achieved by more conventional caloric restriction. To be particularly condemned is the practice of restricting carbohydrate intake to virtually zero while permitting unlimited ingestion of fat. Such a diet will cause ketosis and hyperuricemia and will result in weight loss only so long as total calories as well as carbohydrate are restricted. On the other hand, if fat intake is increased to high levels, weight loss will not occur, and the tendency toward hyperlipidemia may be exaggerated. Another potentially dangerous regimen is the so-called "protein-sparing modified fast." With this diet the total oral intake consists of approximately 100 grams of protein, which is often recommended as a liquid formula containing low quality, collagen protein. Some deaths have been reported in obese patients on this regimen; hypokalemia causing arrhythmias has been the proposed explanation of these deaths. There is no convincing evidence that patients are more likely to maintain weight loss after the "protein-sparing modified fast" as compared to conventional hypocaloric regimens. Furthermore, partial isocaloric replacement of protein by carbohydrate does not impair nitrogen balance or lipolysis, yet reduces the urinary losses of potassium, sodium, and calcium. Hypocaloric diets consisting solely of protein should thus be used with extreme caution and with careful monitoring and replacement of electrolyte losses.

Generally, the most appropriate dietary approach to obesity is to restrict total caloric intake to 1000 to 1400 calories per day, while maintaining the protein contribution at 20 per cent or more. In this manner the amount of bulk in the diet is increased, thereby prolonging the amount of time spent on eating and providing the patient with more oral gratification.

A major cause for the failure of diet treatment in obesity is the patient's loss of motivation because of his expectation of totally unrealistic results (e.g., continued weight reduction at a rate of 4 pounds or more per week). It is therefore imperative that the following points be stressed to the patient: (1) Weight loss is most rapid in the first one to two weeks as a consequence of an initial (hypocaloric-induced) diuresis. (2) Subsequent weight loss will be dictated by the caloric value of the tissue lost (adipose tissue) and the extent of negative caloric balance. (3) Adipose tissue has a caloric value of 3500 calories per pound. (4) It is unlikely that on a long-term basis intake can be adequately restricted and/or activity substantially increased to achieve a negative caloric balance of greater than 500 calories per day. (5) The expected rate of weight loss should therefore be no greater than approximately 1 pound per week.

PROTEIN-RESTRICTED DIETS. Protein, as noted above, contributes approximately 15 per cent of the total calories consumed in the American diet. The daily intake of protein by healthy adults in the United States varies between 70 and 125 grams, averaging about 100 grams. Diets in which protein content is restricted to 60 grams or less are frequently used in the treatment of chronic renal failure (see Ch. 371) and to a lesser extent in the management of patients with cirrhosis of the liver complicated by portal hypertension. In these conditions the concomitant requirement to limit the intake of sodium and (in patients with renal disease) restrict the ingestion of potassium complicates the over-all nutritional approach.

Since it has long been recognized that dietary protein contributes to the endogenous pool of urea, diets low in protein have been advocated in the treatment of acute or chronic renal disease for over 50 years. The nutritional management of renal disease gained impetus, however, after the classic observations by Giordano and Giovannetti in the early 1960's that patients with chronic renal failure achieved symptomatic relief, a decrease in blood urea nitrogen, and positive nitrogen balance when essential amino acid requirements were met by providing no more than 20 grams of dietary protein. This limited intake of nitrogen could be either in the form of natural foods containing proteins of high biologic value or a synthetic mixture of essential amino acids. The principle is that with adequate calories and minimal requirements for essential amino acids, retained nitrogen, principally in the form of urea, can be used for the synthesis of nonessential amino acids which are then incorporated into tissue proteins. In this manner the accumulation of urea is reduced, and, to the extent that breakdown products of nitrogen metabolism contribute to the symptoms of uremia (nausea, vomiting, anorexia), clinical improvement is obtained. The extrarenal metabolism of urea and its incorporation into protein have subsequently been confirmed by a variety of techniques. In fact, recent data indicate that urea utilization can be further stimulated and dietary nitrogen requirements can be further reduced by feeding patients the alpha-keto analogues of the essential amino acids.

Despite its rational basis and initially enthusiastic reception, the over-all usefulness and frequency of implementation of the Giordano-Giovannetti diet are currently rather limited. It was early recognized that dietary manipulation provided symptomatic relief but in no way improved underlying renal function. Second, the increasing use of dialysis and renal transplantation programs lessened the need for purely symptomatic maneuvers. Third, implementation of the diet has proved to be extremely difficult with respect to food preparation and patient acceptance.

In addition to restricting total protein intake, the success of the Giordano-Giovannetti diet depends on two additional constraints: (1) the protein ingested must be of high biologic value; and (2) the caloric intake must be maintained at 2000 to 3000 calories per day. The biologic value or quality of food proteins is an index of the efficiency with which these foodstuffs can be used for anabolic processes and is dependent on the amounts and ratios of the constituent essential amino acids. Proteins such as eggs, meat, fish, and milk are of high biologic value since they can

meet the essential amino acid requirements when supplied in minimal quantities. In contrast, bread, cereals, fruits, and vegetables contain significant amounts of protein (Table 4), but are lacking in one or more essential amino acids and consequently are of low biologic value. Formulation of a 20-gram protein diet thus involves the administration of one egg (or 1 ounce of meat, cheese, or fish) plus three fourths of a cup of milk (to provide 14 grams of high quality protein) plus one serving each of a fruit and vegetable. To provide the patient with an adequate amount of calories without increasing protein content, it is necessary to add to the diet low-protein bread, biscuits, and noodle products which are specially prepared from wheat starch (rather than wheat flour). A major problem is the lack of palatability and difficulty in preparation of such a diet. The result is poor compliance and often an angry, frustrated patient with a limited caloric intake and progressive wasting of lean body mass.

To meet the twin goals of symptomatic improvement plus maintenance of body protein reserves in chronic renal disease, a more moderate degree of protein restriction than that in the 20-gram protein diet is generally recommended. In *symptomatic* patients (i.e., patients with nausea, anorexia, or vomiting) in whom glomerular filtration rate (GFR) is between 5 and 10 ml per minute, dietary management consists of a 40-gram protein intake, composed primarily of high quality protein. In patients with a GFR below 5 ml per minute who fail to achieve relief with a 40-gram intake, the 20-gram protein diet is used while awaiting initiation of dialysis treatment or transplantation. The 20-gram protein diet should be used on a long-term basis only in circumstances in which dialysis is unavailable or impracticable. Institution of chronic dialysis treatment should not be delayed solely because a symptomtic response has been obtained while the patient is on a 20-gram protein intake. In patients on dialysis treatment, the recommendations regarding dietary protein content vary from 40 to 80 grams per day. The general trend at present is toward more liberalized protein intake so as to ensure adequate caloric ingestion and avoidance of wastage of lean body tissue.

In addition to reducing protein ingestion, a restriction in sodium (see below) and potassium content of the diet is generally necessary in patients with renal failure. The average intake of potassium in the normal diet is 3000 mg per day. In renal failure potassium ingestion is generally reduced to levels of 1000 to 2000 mg. Because potassium is so widely distributed in foods (Table 4), restriction in potassium becomes an important factor limiting the palatability and choice of foods. Since fruits and vegetables are quite variable with respect to their potassium content, diet planning is facilitated by grouping these foods on the basis of their potassium content (Table 5). It should be noted that the number of permissible foods can be increased by extracting their potassium content during preparation. For example, the potassium content of potatoes is 407 mg per serving when prepared in the usual manner, but is greatly reduced by cutting the potatoes into small pieces and boiling in a large volume of water. The caloric value of the protein-potassium restricted diet may be increased with such carbohydrate-rich foods as hard candies, honey, jams, jellies, and granulated sugar. However, chocolate candies should be avoided because of their potassium content.

SODIUM RESTRICTION. The intake of sodium in the normal diet ranges between 4 and 6 grams (174 to 261 mEq) per day, ingested primarily in the form of sodium chlo-

TABLE 5. Potassium Content of Fruits and Vegetables

Fruits	Vegetables
Group I (less than 100 mg; average 75 mg)	Group I (100–150 mg)
Applesauce, cranberries, pears (canned), pineapple (canned), blueberries (canned)	Lettuce, cucumber, onions, cabbage, carrots (canned), corn (canned)
Group II (100–150 mg)	Group II (150–200 mg)
Apples (raw or juice), grapefruit, cherries, tangerine, watermelon, pineapple juice, grape juice, peaches (canned)	Carrots (raw or cooked), celery, beets, turnips, asparagus (canned), mushrooms (canned)
Group III (150–200 mg)	Group III (200–250 mg)
Oranges (raw or juice), grapes, grapefruit juice, fruit cocktail	Tomatoes (fresh, canned, or juice), asparagus (fresh or frozen), broccoli, cauliflower, lima beans, spinach
Group IV (greater than 200 mg)†	Group IV (over 250 mg)†
Apricots (canned), bananas, cantaloupe, dates, honeydew melon, prunes (raw or juice), raisins	Potatoes, artichokes, Brussels sprouts

*Potassium content is given per serving (½ cup or small size for raw fruits such as apples, oranges, and pears) and is based on the Manual of Diets, Department of Dietetics, Hospital of St. Raphael, Veterans Administration Hospital, and Yale–New Haven Hospital, New Haven, Connecticut, 1972.
†Fruits and vegetables in Group IV are generally omitted in potassium-restricted diets.

ride. The sources of sodium in the diet include naturally occurring sodium in foods (Table 4) and sodium added to foods. Among the foods rich in natural sodium are the milk, egg, and meat groups, particularly organ meats and shellfish. Bread is another important source of sodium (160 mg per slice) because of the addition of sodium chloride in its preparation. Sodium is also added in the canning and freezing of vegetables, as a preservative in the form of sodium benzoate, and as a seasoning in the form of monosodium glutamate. An additional important source of sodium is table salt used at the time of cooking or eating. Each teaspoonful of table salt provides 2000 mg of sodium.

A restricted sodium intake is employed in the management of edematous states such as congestive heart failure, cirrhosis, and renal disease (nephrotic syndrome and oliguric renal failure), and in the treatment of hypertension. Since it is the sodium ion rather than chloride which must be limited in these conditions, and inasmuch as sodium may be present in the diet in a variety of forms (e.g., bicarbonate, glutamate, benzoate, propionate, or chloride), it is inappropriate to characterize diets in terms of *salt* intake. Instead the diet prescription should designate the precise number of *milligrams of sodium* to be provided each day. In general one of four categories of sodium restriction is employed: 2000 to 4000 mg, 1000 mg, 500 mg, and 250 mg.

The 2000 to 4000 mg (87 to 174 mEq) sodium diet represents a mild degree of sodium restriction which is attained by (1) elimination of table salt and sodium-rich seasonings added at meal times and (2) avoidance of salted foods such as pretzels, potato chips, processed meats (e.g., bacon, sausages), and salty fish (anchovies, sardines). Small amounts of salt may be used in cooking with this diet. This level of sodium restriction is useful as a maintenance diet in subjects in whom a diuresis has already been achieved.

A reduction in sodium intake to 1000 mg (43 mEq) requires, in addition to the measures outlined above, the elimination of salt in cooking and the avoidance of canned or frozen fruits and vegetables, unless specially processed as low-sodium dietetic foods. The ingestion of foods con-

taining significant amounts of sodium such as regular bread and milk must be limited, generally to three slices and 1 pint per day, respectively. This level of sodium intake is often used when therapy is initiated in edematous patients.

In patients with severe refractory edema, it may be necessary to reduce the level of sodium intake to 500 mg (22 mEq) or less to effect a diuresis. This degree of restriction in sodium (500 mg) requires avoidance of all the foods omitted in the 1000 mg diet, substitution of low sodium bread for regular bread, and strict limitation in the intake of allowable foods (particularly meat, fish, eggs, and milk) to carefully measured amounts. A further reduction in sodium intake to 250 mg (11 mEq) is achieved by substituting low-sodium milk for regular milk. Because of the restriction in choices and amounts of food involved in such diets, it is difficult to maintain an adequate caloric or protein intake or to provide sufficient palatability to assure patient compliance. Consequently, severe sodium restriction (250 or 500 mg diets), particularly on a long-term basis, should be employed only for patients who are clearly refractory to more moderate degrees of sodium restriction.

Bar, R. S., Gorden, P., Roth, J., Kahn, C. R., and De Meyts, P.: Fluctuations in the affinity and concentration of insulin receptors on circulating monocytes in obese patients. Effects of starvation, refeeding, and dieting. J. Clin. Invest., 58:1123, 1976.

Blackburn, G. L., and Bistrian, B. R.: Nutritional care of the injured and/or septic patient. Surg. Clin. North Am., 56:1195, 1976.

Fulop, M., and Hoberman, H. D.: Alcoholic ketosis. Diabetes, 24:785, 1975.

Hansen, L. M., Hardie, W. R., and Hidalgo, J.: Fat emulsion for intravenous administration: Clinical experience with Intralipid 10%. Ann. Surg., 184:80, 1976.

Hyne, B. E. B., Fowell, E., and Lee, H. A.: The effect of caloric intake on nitrogen balance in chronic renal failure. Clin. Sci., 43:679, 1972.

Kinney, J. M., and Felig, P.: The metabolic response to injury and infection. *In* DeGroot, L. (ed.): The Metabolic Basis of Endocrine Disease. New York, Grune & Stratton, in press.

Long, J. M., Wilmore, D. W., Mason, A. D., and Pruitt, B. A., Jr.: Effect of carbohydrate and fat intake of nitrogen excretion during total intravenous feeding. Ann. Surg., 185:417, 1977.

Saudek, C. D., and Felig, P.: The metabolic events of starvation. Am. J. Med., 60:117, 1976.

West, K. M.: Diet therapy of diabetes: An analysis of failure. Ann. Intern. Med., 79:425, 1973.

PART XVIII
HEMATOLOGIC AND HEMATOPOIETIC DISEASES

477. INTRODUCTION

Ralph L. Nachman

This edition includes several new and exciting advances in clinical hematology. Much of the new knowledge is directly applicable to the diagnosis and treatment of patients with hematologic disease and originated from the discipline of molecular biology — particularly appropriate, since modern molecular biology began only three decades ago with the observations of Pauling and associates on sickle cell hemoglobin. The increase in complexity and sophistication has given rise to new subspecialties within general hematology. We now have "superspecialists," such as red cell enzymologists, hemoglobinopathy experts, chemotherapits, and coagulationists. Despite this fragmentation, it is important to note that hematologic symptoms, signs, and laboratory abnormalities frequently accompany common clinical disorders in internal medicine. A careful and detailed history and physical examination are still essential prerequisites for adequate evaluation of a clinical hematologic problem. Although some clinical hematologic disorders require complicated laboratory procedures before a final diagnosis can be established, it is clear that these studies must be performed as part of an evaluation of all aspects of the patient's illness, and not as an investigation of a single organ system.

Clinical hematology is a unique model for a cell biology–oriented approach to the pathophysiology of human disease. Thus diseases of the blood and blood-forming organs can be divided into disorders affecting primarily erythrocytes, leukocytes (including lymphocytes, monocytes, and tissue macrophages), and platelets.

In the fetus the liver is the primary site of hematopoiesis; between the fourth and eighth month of gestation the spleen participates in this function. Toward the seventh month of gestation the bone marrow becomes the principal organ of hematopoiesis. Normally the bone marrow is the only active site of hematopoiesis three weeks after birth. Under conditions of hematologic stress the spleen and liver may revert to their fetal function and become sites of extramedullary hematopoiesis, as in agnogenic myeloid metaplasia. At birth the bone marrow is uniformly active. During growth less of the marrow medullary cavity is required to meet physiologic demands, and the long bones contain increasing amounts of fat. The flat bones of the pelvis, rib cage, and vertebrae, where hematopoiesis remains most active, also contain a certain amount of fat. The area occupied by this marrow fat is actually a reservoir into which active marrow may expand should need arise for an increase in hematopoiesis.

Erythrocytes, leukocytes, and megakaryocytes develop from a common precursor stem cell. These multipotential stem cells, which have been termed colony forming units (CFU), give rise to precursor cells committed to erythroid, myeloid, or megakaryocytic differentiation. The circulating humoral agents, erythropoietin, granulopoietin, and thrombopoietin, regulate the rate of production of erythrocytes, leukocytes, and platelets from committed stem cell precursors. At present, granulopoietin and thrombopoietin are less clearly defined than is erythropoietin.

Under normal conditions the quantity of circulating red cells, white cells, and platelets is maintained within relatively narrow limits by adjustments in the rate of their production. Control of erythropoiesis is mediated mainly through alterations in tissue oxygen tension. The sensor mechanisms that directly control granulocyte production and platelet production have not as yet been elucidated.

A decrease in levels of circulating blood cells occurs in association with many clinical disorders. Thus anemia should be considered as a clinical sign and not as an isolated diagnostic entity. A decrease in red cell mass can result from hemorrhage, decreased marrow production, a defect in maturation (as seen in vitamin B_{12} deficiency), or an increase in the rate of red cell destruction. Symptoms such as headache, weakness, fatigue and dyspnea on exertion, angina, and claudication will vary with the severity of the anemia and, more importantly, the duration of time involved in development of the anemia. Thus it is not uncommon to encounter patients suffering from pernicious anemia with hematocrits of 10 to 15 per cent who are completely asymptomatic at rest. This represents a state of compensation for a significant loss of erythrocyte mass developed over a long period of time.

Neutropenia means a reduction in circulating neutrophils. Agranulocytosis is a term often used to designate a severe degree of neutropenia. Granulocytopenia refers to a reduced number of all granulocytes — including neutrophils, eosinophils, and basophils. Decrease in the circulating leukocyte mass can result from inadequate proliferation in the marrow, diminished mobilization from marrow stores, shifts of cells from the circulating to the marginal leukocyte pool, or excessive loss by utilization of leukocytes in the tissues. The risk of infection is slight when the neutrophil count exceeds 1000 per cubic millimeter, but below 500 cells per cubic millimeter it is greatly increased.

The term thrombocytopenia refers to a reduction in the number of circulating platelets. This can result from decrease in marrow megakaryocytes, decrease in the survival of circulating platelets, sequestration of platelets in an enlarged spleen, or dilution of circulating platelets by excessive transfusion with platelet-poor stored blood.

Overproduction of blood cells may lead to significant clinical abnormalities. In polycythemia there is a marked increase in viscosity of the blood; in leukemia there is organ infiltration and altered leukocyte function; in thrombocythemia, thrombosis and/or hemorrhage can occur. These states of cellular overproduction may be due to primary bone marrow disorders such as polycythemia vera, or they may result from a secondary effect on bone marrow function, as in the reactive thrombocytosis observed in malignancies and following acute hemorrhage. In recent years it has become apparent that qualitative cellular abnormalities may be the underlying cause of clinical disease. For example, in chronic granulomatous disease of childhood, neutrophils are present in normal numbers and can ingest bacteria in a normal fashion. However, the neutrophils are unable to kill many species of bacteria following phagocytosis. This is related to the inability of the cells of these patients to produce superoxide radicals in the phagocytic vacuole; thus bacteria remain viable in the leukocytes. Elucidation of this and similar leukocyte disorders has greatly increased our knowledge of intracellular bactericidal mechanisms. The neutrophil generates H_2O_2, which, in the presence of halide and the lysosomal enzyme myeloperoxidase, kills phagocytized bacteria. Diseases involving other qualitative defects in neutrophil function, such as chemotaxis and phagocytosis itself, have also been reported.

In the laboratory, accurate blood counts and careful morphologic characterization of cells in the peripheral blood and bone marrow remain the foundation of hematologic diagnosis. Every physician should be able to evaluate a peripheral blood smear. All too frequently the blood smear is employed solely to obtain a differential count. Additional information, such as red cell morphology, size and estimate of platelet number, and evaluation of the lymphocyte population, can provide crucial information regarding the patient's diagnosis and clinical course. For example, distortions of erythrocyte morphology are commonly seen in disseminated intravascular coagulation.

Bone marrow aspiration and biopsy have now become common procedures and are mandatory in many hematologic disorders. Since hematologic tissue can be obtained with relative ease, many hematologic diagnostic laboratory tests have been developed in recent years. Nevertheless, these tests should be selected thoughtfully, with appropriate consideration to expense. The effort required to identify a specific clinical entity in the setting of a broad differential diagnosis of blood diseases should bear some reasonable relationship to economic realities. Thus whether total body computerized transaxial tomography should be used for routine staging of a lymphoma is questionable.

The treatment of hematologic disorders ranges from highly specific remedies to broad palliative measures. Administration of iron to patients with unequivocal iron deficiency anemia, and of vitamin B_{12} to patients with classic pernicious anemia, will correct the hematologic abnormality completely. The underlying problem, however, must be clarified and dealt with. For example, iron deficiency in an adult may reflect gastrointestinal bleeding, and the source of blood loss should be found. Adult pernicious anemia is due to a deficiency of intrinsic factor, and this deficiency is permanent. However, the clinical disorder is cured by parenteral replacement of the deficient vitamin, since it cannot be absorbed in the absence of intrinsic factor.

Chemotherapy of the leukemias and lymphomas has made major strides in recent years. Combination chemotherapy and newer concepts of induction, consolidation, and maintenance have led to significant prolongation of survival and even "cures" in acute lymphocytic leukemia of childhood. Radiation therapy and combination chemotherapy have also prolonged survival significantly in Hodgkin's disease.

Modern blood banking techniques have greatly facilitated the application of transfusion therapy. The use of blood components for transfusion has largely replaced whole blood. Currently whole blood is used primarily for replacement of blood loss following trauma or extensive hemorrhage. Blood products including packed erythrocytes, platelet concentrates, and leukocyte concentrates are being used in increasing quantities. In addition, the use of cryoprecipitate in hemophilic patients and of gamma globulin for prophylaxis and replacement therapy in certain immune deficiencies has helped revolutionize the therapy of many hematologic disorders.

Section One   THE ANEMIAS

478.   INTRODUCTION

M. C. Brain

The function of the red blood cell is the transport of oxygen from the capillaries in the lungs to the systemic capillaries of the tissues and the facilitation of carbon dioxide transport from the tissues to the lungs. In physiologic terms, anemia can be regarded as a reduction in oxygen transporting capacity of the blood. The normal response to increased demand by the tissues for oxygen is met by an increase in cardiac output; thus the symptoms of anemia first become apparent on exercise. Since oxygen is transported by the red blood cell in combination with hemoglobin, the principal protein constituent of the cell, anemia can be most simply and practically defined as a lowering of the hemoglobin concentration of the blood below the normal range for a population of comparable age and sex. However, the definition of anemia solely in terms of whole blood hemoglobin concentration makes several assumptions. First, the whole blood hemoglobin concentration does not take into account the influence of changes in plasma volume, nor does it provide information on the concentration of hemoglobin within the red blood cells, although the latter can be determined from knowledge of the cell count and the packed red cell volume or hematocrit. Second, and physiologically of greater importance, the definition of anemia in terms of hemoglobin concentration might be thought to imply that the hemoglobin concentration is the sole determinant of oxygen delivery by the red blood cells. Recent work on the regulation of the affinity of hemoglobin for oxygen has shown this not to be true. A number of factors are known to influence hemoglobin-oxygen affinity and hence both the amount and rate at which oxygen is released from red blood cells at the lowered partial pressure of oxygen in the systemic capillaries. These factors include blood pH, temperature, the concentration of hemoglobin within the red blood cell (the mean corpuscular hemoglobin concentration [MCHC]), the red blood cell concentration of organic phosphates (principally 2,3-diphosphoglycerate [DPG] and, to a lesser extent, adenosine triphosphate [ATP], which are products of red cell metabolism, and the presence of genetically determined substitutions in key positions in the polypeptide chains of the hemoglobin molecule. All these factors may either increase or reduce hemoglobin-oxygen affinity and thereby enhance or diminish the amount and rate of oxygen release. Thus the physiologic consequences of anemia must reflect the hemoglobin concentration of the blood and the hemoglobin-oxygen affinity of red blood cells in the circulation. Whereas the hemoglobin concentration of the blood can be readily and rapidly determined, the measurement of hemoglobin-oxygen affinity is less simple. However, changes in hemoglobin-oxygen affinity caused by variations in pH and the MCHC can be readily calculated, as can the effects of DPG and ATP if the concentrations of these compounds in the red blood cell are known. Although changes in hemoglobin-oxygen affinity are rare and are therefore of less clinical importance than changes in hemoglobin concentration, it is important to be aware that they exist, because they may modify the physiologic effects of anemia.

An understanding of the pathologic and physiologic factors which give rise to anemia and its consequences requires an appreciation of the following: (1) the structure and function of the normal red blood cell, (2) the formation of red blood cells in the bone marrow and the factors which regulate erythropoiesis, (3) the disorders which influence the quantity and/or the normal constitution of red blood cells produced by the bone marrow, (4) the factors which influence the distribution and/or survival of red blood cells within the circulation, and (5) the disorders which result in loss of erythrocytes from the circulation.

The mammalian red blood cell is remarkable in that it carries out its function after loss of the nucleus which determined and controlled the synthesis of its constituents. The nucleus is normally extruded from the cell as it enters the circulation by passing into the venous sinuses of the bone marrow. For the first few days after entering the circulation the red blood cell retains cytoplasmic organelles, including mitochondria and ribosomes, and ribonucleic acids, and can be identified with supravital dyes which stain these constituents. The filamentous or reticulin-like pattern of the stained structures gave rise to the term *reticulocyte* for these cells. Once the mitochondria and ribosomes are lost, the cell's capability to synthesize proteins ceases. Thereafter the mature red blood cell has only a limited capacity to reconstitute membrane lipid and other non-lipid cytoplasmic constituents. As a consequence it has a finite life span of approximately 120 days. The main-

tenance of normal numbers of red blood cells in the circulation is thus dependent on their continuous production from precursor cells in the bone marrow. In an adult approximately 1×10^6 red cells are released from the bone marrow every second. In anemia the number of circulating red blood cells depends upon the capacity of the bone marrow to increase the number produced to compensate for the loss from the circulation — a response which requires time for the precursor cells to proliferate and which will be ultimately restricted by the limitations imposed by the bony skeleton upon expansion of the bone marrow within it.

The mature red blood cell is a highly deformable cell which in the resting state assumes the shape of a biconcave disc with an average diameter of 8.4 μ. The biconcave shape is primarily determined by the inherent physical strains within the membrane in relation to the ratio of membrane surface area to volume of the cell. The remarkable deformability of the red blood cell which results in its behaving more like a "fluid drop" than as a solid particle accounts for the low viscosity of blood at high flow rates despite the high proportion of red blood cells present in blood. Furthermore, the deformability enables the cell to pass repeatedly through the capillaries of the microcirculation, some of which have a diameter of 3 μ or less. Reduction in deformability resulting from a change in shape, from loss of membrane surface area relative to volume, or from a change in solubility or stability of hemoglobin with the formation of intracellular inclusions predisposes the red blood cell to selective sequestration in the microcirculation, especially in the spleen, and can lead to shortened survival in the circulation.

Hemoglobin comprises approximately 95 per cent of the dry weight of the red blood cell and on average 34 per cent of the wet weight, the remainder being made up of water, anions, cations (principally potassium), glucose, phosphorylated glycolytic intermediates (principally 2,3-diphosphoglycerate which is present in the same molar concentration as hemoglobin), glutathione, adenosine and pyridine nucleotides, and the enzymes responsible for the metabolism of glucose to lactic acid. Glucose is metabolized by two linked metabolic pathways. The principal functions of the Embden-Meyerhof pathway include the formation of ATP, which is utilized in maintenance of the normal cation content of the red blood cells through ATP-dependent transport mechanisms, in maintenance of membrane lipid composition, and in cell shape; the maintenance of optimal concentrations of DPG; and the reduction of methemoglobin. The hexose monophosphate shunt, the subsidiary pathway of glucose metabolism, is responsible for maintaining glutathione in a reduced state and thereby in protecting the cellular constituents (notably hemoglobin) from oxidative denaturation.

The hemoglobin within the red blood cell is formed of spheroidal molecules of a molecular weight of 64,458. Ninety-seven per cent of the molecule consists of the polypeptide chains of globin, and 3 per cent of the heme groups. Each molecule is formed from four subunits, comprising two pairs of identical polypeptide chains, to each of which is attached a heme group partially buried in the outer aspect of the molecule. In the red blood cells of adults, 97 per cent of the hemoglobin is made up of two α and two β chains and is designated *hemoglobin A. Hemoglobin A₂*, consisting of two α and two δ chains, forms 2 per cent, and *hemoglobin F*, formed from two α and two λ chains, provides the remaining 1 per cent. Hemoglobin F is the principal hemoglobin in the red blood cells of the fetus, and is gradually replaced by hemoglobin A with the onset of β chain synthesis in the last trimester of pregnancy. Hemoglobin F levels fall from birth and reach adult levels by the end of the first year of life. For the red blood cell to contain a normal concentration of hemoglobin requires balanced synthesis of both the α and β chains and of the heme groups by the erythroblasts in the bone marrow. Disorders of hemoglobin constitution and/or concentration within the red blood cell can arise through abnormalities of synthesis either of the globin (polypeptide chain) or of heme groups. Disorders of the constitution of the globin chains are not usually associated with major reductions in the amount of hemoglobin synthesized. Although many genetic variations in the primary amino acid structure of hemoglobin molecule have been recognized, they only become clinically important when such substitutions are at critical sites in the molecule, thereby influencing the function, solubility, or stability of the molecule. Normal hemoglobin A has recently been shown to be accompanied by small proportions of glycosylated derivatives which confer more rapid electrophoretic mobility. One of these minor derivatives, hemoglobin A_1C, resulting from the attachment of a hexose to the normal β chain, has been shown to be elevated in patients with poorly controlled diabetes mellitus. Deficient hemoglobin synthesis within the erythroblast can result from failure or imbalance of the synthesis of the polypeptide chains (the thalassemia syndrome), or through disturbances of heme synthesis, commonly caused by lack of iron, and more rarely caused by disorders in the porphyrin synthetic pathway.

The red blood cell formed in the bone marrow is the final stage in a sequence of cell divisions arising from a common multipotential hematopoietic stem cell. This common hematopoietic stem cell gives rise to a number of committed stem cells from which develop the erythroid, granulocyte, and megakaryocyte cell lines. The committed stem cells form a self-regenerating stem cell pool, as well as giving rise to differentiated erythroblasts which undergo three mitotic divisions during the course of maturation to the late normoblast and finally through extrusion of the nucleus to the reticulocyte. The time taken between an erythropoietic stimulus and the outpouring of reticulocytes from the bone marrow is approximately five days. It has long been recognized that anemia or hypoxia stimulates increased erythropoiesis. The response is mediated through the action of a specific erythropoiesis-stimulating hormone, *erythropoietin*. Erythropoietin is a relatively heat-stable glycoprotein with a molecular weight of between 40,000 and 70,000. It has been shown experimentally that erythropoietin stimulates the erythroid stem cell to undergo mitosis and accelerates the rate of cell division of the developing erythroblasts. Raised levels of erythropoietin have been demonstrated in the serum and urine of anemic patients. The primary stimulus to its release into the circulation has been shown to be hypoxia. There is much evidence to suggest that the kidneys are the principal site of erythropoietin formation or release. Destruction or removal of the kidneys is associated with diminished erythropoiesis; yet other organs and tissues must be responsible for erythropoietin formation, because erythropoiesis

continues in anephric patients and erythropoietin has been detected in their serum. Although hypoxia is the principal stimulus to erythropoietin release, clinical evidence indicates a greater erythropoietic response to hemolytic anemia than to comparable anemia resulting from blood loss. Thus the products of red blood cell destruction may provide an additional stimulus to erythropoietin release.

The continuous formation of red blood cells from precursor cells in the bone marrow is dependent upon both normal bone marrow function and the stimulus of erythropoietin. The recent development of methods which have enabled erythropoiesis to be maintained in culture in vitro has led to the recognition of two precursor cells which vary in their response to erythropoietin and in the size of the erythroid colonies produced. These techniques have demonstrated a regulatory role of T lymphocytes and of androgens and thyroid hormones. Disorders of red blood cell formation can arise from diminution of the number of pluripotent hematopoietic stem cells, as in aplastic or hypoplastic anemias, or from disturbances in maturation of the committed erythropoietic stem cell, as in isolated red cell asplasias. In acute and chronic leukemias the disorder of stem cell differentiation will adversely affect erythropoiesis. Similarly, infiltration of the bone marrow by malignant cells arising from other organs or the progressive sclerosis of the bone marrow in myelosclerosis will reduce erythropoiesis. In the latter circumstance, hematopoiesis, including erythropoiesis, may be undertaken at *extramedullary sites* in the body such as the liver and spleen. Erythropoiesis is quantitatively reduced in acute and chronic infections, by chronic inflammatory disorders such as rheumatoid arthritis, and by renal failure. It is influenced by the nutritional status of the individual, being particularly affected by deficiencies of vitamin B_{12}, folic acid, iron, and protein. Vitamin B_{12} and folic acid are essential cofactors in the synthesis of DNA. Deficiency of either one results in impairment of cell division with formation of megaloblasts, macroerythroblasts with defective nuclear maturation, and production of large red blood cells (*macrocytes*). Conversely, deficiency of heme, through lack of iron or as a consequence of defects in the heme synthetic pathway, by impairment of hemoglobin synthesis results in the production of *hypochromic microcytic* (small) red blood cells. Defective hemoglobinization of the red blood cell is also a feature of the defective hemoglobin synthesis resulting from imbalanced globin synthesis of the thalassemia syndromes. Disorders of red blood cell maturation within the bone marrow, whether caused by disorders of cell division as in the megaloblastic anemias or by defective hemoglobin synthesis, are associated with *ineffective erythropoiesis*, a considerable proportion of the abnormal erythroblasts undergoing phagocytic destruction within the bone marrow and therefore failing to gain entry to the circulation. The extent of ineffective erythropoiesis can be assessed by measurement of the rate of clearance of radioactive iron from the plasma and of the proportion of the radioactive iron entering the circulation in labeled hemoglobin. In ineffective erythropoiesis there is rapid clearance of radioactive iron from the plasma, but only 20 to 40 per cent of the iron enters the blood compared with the 70 to 90 per cent in normal subjects. Ineffective erythropoiesis can also be assessed by the early excretion of ^{14}C-carbon monoxide and ^{14}C-stercobilin derived from the catabolism of newly synthesized heme after the administration of ^{14}C-glycine. This latter method has shown that even in normal subjects a small proportion of the newly synthesized heme is catabolized to bilirubin, which may reflect the rapid turnover of nonhemoglobin heme proteins in the liver. In ineffective erythropoiesis the proportion of newly synthesized heme which is catabolized and the products excreted are greatly increased.

Red blood cells entering the circulation are normally uniformly distributed within the circulation, and the hematocrit of the venous blood corresponds closely to the whole-body hematocrit derived from simultaneous measurements of the red blood cell and plasma volumes. The distribution of red blood cells within the circulation is influenced by the spleen. Reticulocytes, until they mature, are preferentially sequestered within the spleen. In conditions which cause massive enlargement of spleen, such as the congestive splenomegaly of portal hypertension, the proportion of red blood cells sequestered may be greatly increased. The sequestration of red blood cells in the spleen together with the associated increase in plasma volume can result in a lowering of the red blood cell count and hematocrit in the venous blood to produce an apparent anemia, although the red blood cell mass may be normal or only slightly below normal.

Red blood cells normally survive in the circulation for 120 days. The degree of anemia caused by shortened red blood cell survival is governed by the rate of the hemolysis and the ability of the bone marrow to compensate. Hemolytic anemia can usually be recognized by the association of an anemia, in the absence of evidence of blood loss, with an increase in the catabolism of hemoglobin, as reflected by unconjugated hyperbilirubinemia, increased excretion of urobilinogen in the urine, lowered levels of haptoglobin in the serum, and a persistent increase in the absolute reticulocyte count, the consequence of the compensatory erythropoiesis by the bone marrow. Minor degrees of hemolysis accompany many disorders associated with ineffective erythropoiesis. Shortened red blood cell survival may be due to abnormalities inherent to the cell, such as congenital or familial disorders of the membrane, metabolism, or hemoglobin, or may be brought about by the action of extrinsic or environmental factors in the circulation. The latter include the effects of plasma factors (antibodies), the action of drugs or toxins, or changes in the vascular environment through which the red blood cells circulate. The extrinsic factors influencing red blood cell survival in general tend to be acquired rather than congenital or familial in etiology. But this distinction is not always valid, because congenital disorders of metabolism or of hemoglobin may

predispose the cell to deleterious action of extrinsic agents such as oxidative drugs.

Loss of red blood cells from the circulation through frank or occult hemorrhage is a common cause of acute or chronic anemia, the degree of anemia reflecting the magnitude and duration of the blood loss and the reduction in body iron stores through loss of hemoglobin from the body. Thus chronic blood loss rapidly produces iron deficiency, with consequent impairment of erythropoiesis by the bone marrow.

The normal range of red blood cell values in adults is shown in Table 1.

The values of the red blood cell count, hemoglobin concentration, and packed cell volume in children between the ages of three months and puberty are approximately 10 to 20 per cent lower than the adult values, the difference being more marked in younger children. The differences between the sexes become apparent only at puberty. The lower values in children probably reflect the diminished affinity of hemoglobin for oxygen in children. Thus the lower red blood cell count and hemoglobin concentration meet the normal physiologic needs for oxygen transport.

CLASSIFICATION

Anemias can be classified according to the etiology of the disorder giving rise to anemia (Table 2) or in relation to the morphologic appearance and quantitative abnormality of red blood cell size (mean corpuscular volume [MCV]), hemoglobin content (MCH), and hemoglobin concentration (MCHC). Any attempt at classification is at best somewhat arbitrary, because in many disorders the degree of anemia and the morphologic appearance of the red blood cell are consequences of the effects of both the primary cause and the erythropoietic response by the bone marrow. Furthermore, it is difficult to combine a logical pathophysiologic classification with the expected frequency with which the various etiologies may be encountered, the latter being influenced by the age, racial background, socioeconomic factors, and geographic location of the population encountered.

A classification of anemia on the basis of red blood cell morphology, as seen in the peripheral blood smear and supported by the quantitative measurements of cell size (MCV) and hemoglobin content and concentration (MCH and MCHC), can provide a valuable indication as to the possible etiologic mechanisms (Table 3). The introduction of automatic equipment for the rapid and accurate enumeration of red blood cells and determination of the MCV, MCH, and MCHC has greatly enhanced the diagnostic value of these measurements.

TABLE 1.   Red Cell Values in Adults: Normal Range

	Men	Women
Red blood cells	5.11 ± 0.38	$4.51 \pm 0.36 \times 10^{12}$/l
Hemoglobin	15.5 ± 1.1	13.7 ± 1.0 g/dl
Packed cell volume	46.0 ± 3.1	40.9 ± 3.0 l/l
Mean corpuscular volume	90.0 ± 4.8	90.4 ± 4.8 fl
Mean corpuscular hemoglobin	30.2 ± 1.8	30.2 ± 1.9 pg
Mean corpuscular hemoglobin concentration	33.9 ± 1.2	33.6 ± 1.1 g/dl
Reticulocytes absolute	0.2 to 2.0	0.2 to 2.0×10^9/l

TABLE 2.   Anemias: Etiologic Classification

I. Principally caused by impaired production
  A. Disturbances of the proliferation and differentiation of stem cells
    1. Aplastic anemia: idiopathic; due to physical or chemical injury (radiation, benzol, lead, or cytotoxic and other drugs such as chloramphenicol, phenylbutazone, etc.)
    2. Pure red blood cell aplasia
    3. Anemia of chronic renal failure
    4. Endocrine deficiency (pituitary, thyroid, adrenal, or testicular hormones)
  B. Disturbances of proliferation and maturation of differentiated erythroblasts
    1. Defective DNA synthesis (vitamin B_{12}, folic acid, and metabolic defects in purine and pyrimidine metabolism)
    2. Defective hemoglobin synthesis
      a. Deficient globin synthesis (thalassemia)
      b. Deficient heme synthesis (iron deficiency)
      c. Sideroblastic anemia
    3. Protein malnutrition
    4. Anemia of chronic infections or inflammatory or neoplastic disease
    5. Myelophthisic anemias due to bone marrow infiltration or replacement (leukemias, myelofibrosis, Hodgkin's disease, multiple myeloma, metastatic carcinoma, etc.)
II. Principally caused by shortened red blood cell survival (increased rate of destruction)
  A. Intrinsic or red blood cell abnormalities
    1. Membrane disorders
      a. Inherited disorders of cell shape; spherocytosis, elliptocytosis, stomatocytosis
      b. Inherited disorders of membrane lipid synthesis
      c. Paroxysmal nocturnal hemoglobinuria
    2. Disorders of red blood cell metabolism
    3. Congenital or inherited enzyme deficiencies
    4. Disorders of hemoglobin (globin) structure, solubility, and stability (sickle cell anemia, hemoglobin C disease, unstable hemoglobins, etc.)
  B. Extrinsic or extraerythrocytic abnormalities
    1. Plasma factors
      a. Antibody mediated destruction
      b. Disturbance of cholesterol or plasma lipids (abetalipoproteinemia, liver disease)
    2. Physical factors (cardiac, microangiopathic, burns)
    3. Chemical or toxic agents (copper, lead, oxidative drugs: dapsone, phenacetin)
    4. Bacterial or other organisms: (Cl, welchii, malaria)
    5. Reticuloendothelial sequestration (splenomegaly)
III. Anemia of blood loss (acute or chronic)

The classification shown in Table 3 fails to include much additional information which can be obtained from examination of stained blood smears. Quantitative data with the emphasis on mean values cannot reflect variations in cell shape, size, or hemoglobin content or cell staining such as the polychromasia indicative of reticulocytosis. Only examination of the stained smear can lead to the recognition of intracellular inclusions such as *Howell-Jolly bodies* (nuclear remnants indicative of splenectomy or splenic dysfunction), *Pappenheimer bodies* (granules of hemosiderin), *punctate basophilia* (a feature of disorders of hemoglobin synthesis often seen in lead poisoning and in thalassemia), and malarial parasites. Disturbances of cell size *(anisocytosis)*, shape *(poikilocytosis)*, and staining can lead to the recognition of congenital or acquired causes of spherocytosis, of elliptocytosis, or of stomatocytosis. Poikilocytosis is a frequent accompaniment of disordered erythropoiesis, and is associated with disorders of hemoglobin synthesis as in iron deficiency or thalassemia. The abnormal shape of the *sickle cell* was recognized long before the molecular pathology of the sickle cell anemia was understood. Likewise, *target cells* in the absence of macrocytosis may suggest the presence of hemoglobin C; when mi-

crocytosis is present, thalassemia; and when macrocytosis is present, liver disease. The presence of *red blood cell fragments* in the presence of hemolysis suggests a cardiac or microangiopathic mechanical hemolysis. Variation in hemoglobinization of erythrocytes can suggest partial response to iron therapy, be compatible with recent blood transfusion, or be a feature of the sideroblastic anemias. The recognition of megaloblastic anemia when associated with iron deficiency may not be accompanied by macrocytosis; however, the presence of multilobed polymorphonuclear leukocytes may provide the clue to an underlying vitamin B_{12} or folate deficiency. The knowledge of the differential white cell count and platelet count can lead to the recognition of hypoplastic anemias, myelophthisic anemias, and leukemic disorders. Further information may be derived from examination of the reticulocyte preparation in the detection of *Heinz bodies* (precipitated denatured hemoglobin) and *hemoglobin H bodies* (β_4 inclusions). It may be helpful to examine a diluted wet preparation of blood in determining the nature of shape changes which can arise from the drying of conventional stained smears. Finally, the presence of intense rouleaux formation may indicate the presence of a paraprotein, whereas frank agglutination can point to the presence of cold-agglutinating antibodies.

Although knowledge of the red blood cell count, hemoglobin concentration, and MCV, MCH, and MCHC provides valuable information as to whether an anemia is macrocytic, normocytic, or microcytic, examination of the blood film can often give a more specific indication of the etiology of the disorder. This in turn can lead to further diagnostic investigations of erythropoiesis, such as a bone marrow biopsy, or of disorders of red blood cell membrane, metabolism, or hemoglobin, including the detection of antibodies on the membrane surface, or to evidence of frank or occult blood loss by appropriate inquiry or investigation.

PRINCIPLES OF THERAPY

As in all conditions, the principles of the treatment of anemia are primarily dependent on recognition of the cause of an anemia and, when possible, the correction of the cause with appropriate treatment. Consideration of the classification of the etiology of anemia provides a useful framework on which to base the principles of treatment. When a cause for aplastic or hypoplastic anemia can be identified, exposure to the agent or

TABLE 3.   Anemias: Morphologic Classification

1. Macrocytic (MCV 93 cu mm)
  a. Megaloblastic erythropoiesis (deficiency of vitamin B_{12} or folic acid)
  b. Liver disease and obstructive jaundice
  c. Reticulocytosis
2. Normocytic
  a. Acute blood loss before reticulocytosis
  b. Hemolytic anemia when not associated with spherocytosis
  c. Anemia of chronic disease
3. Microcytic and hypochromic
  a. Iron deficiency
  b. Thalassemia
  c. Sideroblastic anemia

agents should cease and an incriminated drug should never again be given to the patient. Heavy metals may be excreted in response to appropriate chelating agents. A patient with severe aplastic anemia who is under age 30 and who has a histocompatible donor, preferably of the same sex, should be considered a suitable subject for bone marrow transplantation. Transfusion of blood should be avoided prior to transplantation, and, if required, should be provided from an unrelated donor. In older patients or in patients for whom no compatible donors are available, the principal measures are supportive with red cell, platelet, and, if required, white cell transfusions. Erythropoiesis may be improved by androgenic steroids. Renal failure and endocrine deficiencies should be treated appropriately.

The cause of megaloblastic anemia should be sought and appropriate replacement therapy with either vitamin B_{12} or folic acid given. Neither of these vitamins should be prescribed without clear-cut indications. Among these indications is the folate deficiency associated with increased requirement for this vitamin in pregnancy and in the erythropoietic response to hemolytic anemia. Iron therapy should be given when anemia is recognized as being due to iron deficiency resulting either from inadequate intake or increased demand, as in pregnancy, or from blood loss. Patients with sideroblastic anemia may respond to treatment with pyridoxine. Iron therapy should be avoided in patients with anemia of other causes such as thalassemia or sideroblastic anemia, in both of which the hypochromic anemia may be mistaken for iron deficiency; nor should iron be given to patients with chronic hemolytic anemia. In all these disorders iron therapy can lead to tissue damage through iron overload. In the secondary anemias caused by infective or inflammatory disorders or metastatic neoplastic disease, the anemia only responds to the treatment of the underlying disease. The same is true for the myelophthisic anemias caused by marrow infiltrations. In hemolytic anemias treatment with corticosteroids may be indicated, depending upon the nature of the hemolysis, and splenectomy may be indicated when there is evidence that the spleen is playing a major role in red blood cell destruction. Anemia caused by acute blood loss and the anemias which fail to or cannot be expected to respond to specific hematinics may require blood transfusions. It must be recognized that blood transfusions are not without the risk of serious and sometimes fatal reactions, and that multiple transfusions increase the risk of both serum hepatitis and iron overload. Except for replacement of acute blood loss, the risk of circulatory overload and of transfusion reactions can be reduced by transfusing red blood cell concentrates from which the plasma has been removed. There is little cause to give blood transfusions if the hemoglobin is greater than 10 grams per 100 ml or to endeavor to maintain the hemoglobin above that level. Blood transfusions should be given after a full cross-match, including an indirect Coombs test, has established that the blood to be transfused is compatible. However, in patients with life-threatening autoimmune hemolytic anemia, the most compatible blood should be given despite the presence of a positive indirect Coombs test, because the survival of the transfused cells is likely to be no shorter than that of the patient's own red blood cells, and death from anemia can be prevented until more specific treatment with corticosteroids and/or splenectomy becomes effective.

Finch, C. A., and Lenfant, C.: Oxygen transport in man. N. Engl. J. Med., 286:407, 1972.

Gordon, A. S.: Regulation of Hematopoiesis. Vol. 1, Red Cell Production. New York, Appleton-Century-Crofts, 1970.

Harris, J. W., and Kellermyer, R. W.: The Red Cell Production, Metabolism, Destruction: Normal and Abnormal. 2nd ed. Cambridge, Mass., Harvard University Press, 1970.

Williams, W. J., Beutler, E., Erslev, A. J., and Rundles, R. W. (eds.): Hematology. 2nd ed. New York, McGraw-Hill Book Company, 1977.

Wintrobe, M. M., Lee, G. R., Boggs, D. R., Bithell, T. C., Athens, J. W., and Foerster, J.: Clinical Hematology. Philadelphia, Lea & Febiger, 1974.

479. MEGALOBLASTIC ANEMIAS

Victor Herbert

DEFINITION. The megaloblastic (Greek: megas=large + blaste=germ) anemias or macro-ovalocytic anemias are characterized by a common morphology of giantism of every proliferating cell and an underlying common biochemical defect of slowed DNA synthesis. Classically, the diagnosis of megaloblastic anemia is made when the first-visit evaluation of a new patient reveals anemia, often with pancytopenia, and the peripheral blood smear reveals the progeny of a megaloblastic bone marrow, namely, macro-ovalocytic red cells, granulocytes whose nuclei are hypersegmented ("hypersegmented polys"), and giant platelets. Although megaloblastic anemia is a single *morphologic* entity, the underlying slowed DNA synthesis may result from any of a wide variety of causes. Thus the *diagnosis* of megaloblastic anemia is usually very easy, but the *differential diagnosis* of underlying cause and therefore *proper therapy* rest on determination of the precise etiologic classification into which the patient fits.

Pernicious anemia is *not* a synonym for megaloblastic anemia. It is that etiologic subcategory of megaloblastic anemia which is due to inadequate intrinsic factor secretion of uncertain etiology (Table 1).

ETIOLOGIC CLASSIFICATION AND PATHOGENESIS. In about 95 per cent of cases, megaloblastic anemia proves to be a nutritional anemia (or, more broadly, a nutritional pancytopenia) caused by deficiency of vitamin B_{12}, folic acid, or, in some cases, both. Classification therefore usually falls in one of the six etiologic categories common to all nutritional deficiencies: inadequate ingestion, absorption, or utilization, and/or increased requirement, excretion, or destruction. Table 1 presents an etiologic classification of the causes of slowed DNA synthesis and therefore of the megaloblastic anemias, and Figures 1 and 2 present the flow charts of vitamin B_{12} and folate metabolism which provide the nutritional, physiologic, and biochemical underpinnings on which much of the etiologic classification rests.

As indicated in Figure 1, food vitamin B_{12} is liberated from its bonds by gastric acid and gastric and intestinal enzymes. The freed B_{12} (of which there is less when there is no gastric acid) attaches to salivary and gastric B_{12} binders (called "R binders" or cobalophilins because of their strong affinity for B_{12}) and to the intrinsic factor (IF), a glycoprotein of molecular weight about 50,000 secreted by gastric parietal cells, and the B_{12}-IF complex dimerizes and passes with B_{12}–binder complexes into the ileum, where it is plastered onto specific brush border receptors for the IF-B_{12} complex in the presence of ionic calcium and a pH of more than 7, at

TABLE 1. Etiologic Classification of Megaloblastic Anemias: a Tabular Lexicon

I. *Vitamin B_{12} Deficiency* (normal B_{12} body stores last 3 to 6 years after cessation of B_{12} absorption, but 20 to 30 years after cessation of only B_{12} ingestion, because of continuation of reabsorption of the 3 to 6 μg of B_{12} excreted daily in bile):

A. Inadequate ingestion
  1. Poor diet (lacking microorganisms and animal foods, which are the sole B_{12} sources)
    a. Strict vegetarianism (eating no meat, fowl, seafood, eggs, milk, or any products thereof)
    b. Chronic alcoholism (no B_{12} or folate in hard liquor) (folate deficiency occurs first, and is more common, partly because body stores of B_{12} last much longer than those of folate)
    c. Poverty, religious tenets (Hinduism, Seventh-Day Adventism, certain Catholic orders), dietary faddism
B. Inadequate absorption
  1. Gastric disorder, producing inadequate or absent secretion by gastric parietal cells of intrinsic factor
    a. Addisonian pernicious anemia (PA) (PA is that form of B_{12} deficiency disease due to inadequate intrinsic factor secretion of uncertain etiology)
      (1) Hereditary absence of normal intrinsic factor secretion; absent secretion at birth (circulating antibody to intrinsic factor never present) (supports theory that antibody only occurs when antigenic stimulus is produced by intrinsic factor which enters bloodstream from damaged parietal cells and is recognized as foreign by the immunologic surveillance system); rare
      (2) Congenital production of defective intrinsic factor molecule (one published case)
      (3) Autoimmunity-associated gastric atrophy. These patients almost always have nondiagnostic-for-PA circulating parietal cell antibody, which is index only of past or present gastric damage and *not* of amount of intrinsic factor secretion (circulating diagnostic-for-PA antibody to intrinsic factor is always present under age 21; there is a gradual decrease in measurable antibody, so that by age 65 only two thirds of cases present with measurable circulating antibody to intrinsic factor)
        (a) Juvenile pernicious anemia (usually presents between ages 3 and 14)
        (b) Hereditarily determined degenerative gastric atrophy (gradually progressing with increasing age) (almost half of all adult PA cases fall in this category)
        (c) Acquired gastric atrophy as the end result of superficial inflammatory gastritis; superficial gastritis with atrophy (almost half of all adult PA cases fall in this category, which includes acquired gastric damage related to iron deficiency, alcohol, etc.)
        (d) Endocrine disorders (hypothyroidism, polyendocrinopathy, etc.) associated with gastric damage
    b. Gastrectomy
      (1) Total
      (2) Subtotal (approximately 20% develop PA within ten years after surgery, associated with atrophy of remaining parietal cells)
        (a) Proximal
        (b) Distal
    c. Lesions which destroy the gastric mucosa (ingested corrosives, linitis plastica, etc.)
    d. Intrinsic factor inhibitor in gastric secretion
      (1) Antibody to intrinsic factor (in saliva or gastric juice)
        (a) "Blocking" antibody (attaches to intrinsic factor so as to block ability of intrinsic factor to take up B_{12})
        (b) "Binding" antibody (attaches to intrinsic factor at site distal to site of B_{12} attachment)
  2. Small intestinal disorder (affecting ileum, which is the main site of B_{12} absorption)
    a. Gluten-induced enteropathy (childhood and adult celiac disease); idiopathic steatorrhea; nontropical sprue
    b. Tropical sprue (B_{12} is often the first nutrient to be subnormally absorbed and the last to return to normal absorption)
    c. Regional enteritis
    d. Strictures or anastomoses of the small bowel, other "stagnant bowel" syndromes

  e. Intestinal resection
  f. Malignancies and granulomatous lesions involving the small intestine
  g. Other conditions characterized by chronically disturbed intestinal function
  h. Drugs damaging B_{12} absorption
    (1) Para-aminosalicylic acid (PAS) (therapy of tuberculosis)
    (2) Colchicine (therapy of gout)
    (3) Neomycin (antimicrobial)
    (4) Ethanol (societal)
    (5) Metformin (and other biguanide oral antidiabetic agents)
    (6) Oral contraceptive agents?
  i. Specific malabsorption for vitamin B_{12}
    (1) Due to long-term ingestion of calcium-chelating agents (ionic calcium required for B_{12} absorption)
    (2) Due to inadequately alkaline pH in ileum (Zollinger-Ellison syndrome, pancreatic disease, etc.) (pH > 6 required for B_{12} absorption)
    (3) Unknown causes (absence of intestinal receptors for B_{12}-intrinsic factor complex? absence of "releasing factor"?)
      (a) Congenital (Imerslund-Gräsbeck syndrome) (receptors probably functioning)
      (b) Acquired (forme fruste of sprue?) (receptors absent or nonfunctioning)
  3. Competition for vitamin B_{12} by intestinal parasites or bacteria
    a. Fish tapeworm (*Diphyllobothrium latum*) (decreasing in Finland because of pollution of fresh water killing the host fish)
    b. Bacteria: The blind loop syndrome (B_{12} adsorbing bacteria)
  4. Pancreatic disease (normal pancreatic exocrine secretion of trypsin and bicarbonate required for normal B_{12} absorption)
C. Inadequate utilization
  1. Vitamin B_{12} antagonists
    a. Substituted B_{12} amides and anilides (experimental agents)
    b. Cobaloximes (experimental agents)
  2. Congenital or acquired enzyme deficiency or deletion
    a. Methylmalonyl-CoA mutase
    b. Methyltetrahydrofolate-homocysteine methyltransferase
    c. B_{12a} reductase
    d. B_{12r} reductase
    e. Deoxyadenosyltransferase
    f. Other enzyme reduction or deletion
  3. Abnormal B_{12}-binding protein in serum, irreversibly binding B_{12} and making it unavailable to tissues
    a. Increased TC I and/or TC III glycoprotein (myeloproliferative disorders) ("granulocyte-related" B_{12} binders)
    b. Increased TC II protein (liver disease) ("liver-related" B_{12} binders)
    c. Other abnormal B_{12} binding (a glycoprotein in some hepatoma cases, etc.)
  4. Inadequate serum B_{12}-binding protein (congenital or acquired)
    a. TC II protein (lack produces megaloblastic anemia) (it delivers B_{12} to blood cells, as transferrin delivers iron)
    b. TC I glycoprotein (lack not known to produce megaloblastic anemia) (it is mainly a storage protein for B_{12}, somewhat akin to ceruloplasmin for copper)
    c. TC III (large amounts produced in vitro by granulocytes)
  5. Protein malnutrition?
  6. Malignancy?
  7. Liver disease?
  8. Renal disease?
  9. Thiocyanate intoxication?
D. Increased requirement (normal adult daily requirement from exogenous sources is 0.1 μg)
  1. Hyperthyroidism
  2. Increased hematopoiesis?
  3. Infancy (increased requirement for growth)
  4. Parasitization
    a. By fetus
    b. By malignant tissue?
E. Increased excretion
  1. Inadequate B_{12}-binding protein in serum (inadequate TC II particularly?)
  2. Liver disease (inadequate storage capacity for B_{12})
  3. Renal disease?

F. Increased destruction
  1. By pharmacologic doses of ascorbic acid

II. Folic acid deficiency (normal folate body stores will last only 3 to 6 months after cessation of folate ingestion or absorption):
  A. Inadequate ingestion
    1. Poor diet (lacking unprocessed fresh, uncooked, or slightly cooked food) (or fruit juices) (folates are heat labile)
      a. Nutritional megaloblastic anemia
        (1) Tropical
        (2) Nontropical
        (3) Scurvy (diets poor in vitamin C are also poor in folate)
      b. Chronic alcoholism with or without cirrhosis
  B. Inadequate absorption (affecting upper third of small intestine, which is the main site of folate absorption) (since most food folates are in polyglutamate forms, biliary and intestinal gamma glutamyl conjugases are necessary to split off excess glutamates to make folates absorbable)
    1. Malabsorption syndromes
      a. Gluten-induced enteropathy (childhood and adult celiac disease) (idiopathic steatorrhea, nontropical sprue) (coincident B_{12} malabsorption rare)
      b. Any other chronic functional or structural disorder involving the upper small intestine
        (1) Tropical sprue (coincident B_{12} malabsorption almost invariably present)
        (2) Associated with herpetic and other skin disorders
      c. Drugs
        (1) Diphenylhydantoin (Dilantin) (anticonvulsant)
        (2) Primidone (anticonvulsant)
        (3) Barbiturates
        (4) Oral contraceptive agents (?)
        (5) Cycloserine (tuberculosis)
        (6) Ethanol (societal)
        (7) Metformin (diabetes therapy)
        (8) Dietary amino acid excess of glycine and/or methionine
        (9) Nitrofurantoin? (antimicrobial)
        (10) Glutethimide? (sedative)
        (11) Cholestyramine
        (12) Salicylazosulfapyridine (Azulfidine)
    2. Specific malabsorption for folate
      a. Congenital nonconjugase defects (four cases published)
      b. Acquired nonconjugase defects
      c. Inadequate biliary or intestinal conjugase
      d. Conjugase inhibitors (such as are contained in some beans)
    3. Blind loop syndrome (folate-greedy bacteria) (more commonly, bacteria make folate and actually raise serum folate level of host)
  C. Inadequate utilization (metabolic block)
    1. Folic acid antagonists (dihydrofolate reductase inhibitors)
      a. 4-amino-4-deoxyfolates (Chemotherapy, immunosuppression, psoriasis)
        (i.e., methotrexate)
      b. 2,4-Diaminopyrimidine
        Pyrimethamine (Malaria, toxoplasmosis)
        Trimethoprim (Antibacterial)
      c. Triamterene (Diuretic)
      d. Diamidine compounds (*Pneumocystis carinii*, protozoacidal)
        (i.e., pentamidine isethionate)
    2. Diphenylhydantoin and possibly other anticonvulsants (possibly block cell uptake or use of folate)
    3. Enzyme deficiency
      a. Congenital
        (1) Formiminotransferase
        (2) Dihydrofolate reductase
        (3) Methyltetrahydrofolate transmethylase
        (4) Other enzymes (some secondarily affect folate)
      b. Acquired
        (1) Liver disease
          (a) Formiminotransferase
          (b) Other enzymes
    4. Vitamin B_{12} deficiency (reduces folate uptake and retention by cells)
    5. Alcohol (both specific and nonspecific damage to folate metabolism)
    6. Ascorbic acid deficiency (increased hematopoiesis associated with bleeding reduces folate stores) (may also decrease ability of body to retain folates in their metabolically active reduced state)
    7. Dietary amino acid excess (glycine, methionine)
  D. Increased requirement (normal adult daily requirement from exogenous sources is 50 μg)

    1. Parasitization
      a. By fetus (especially in multiple and twin pregnancies)
      b. By malignant tissue (especially lymphoproliferative disorders)
      c. By breast-fed infant
    2. Infancy (increased requirement for growth)
    3. Increased hematopoiesis (hemolytic anemias; chronic blood loss [including scurvy])
    4. Increased metabolic activity (hyperthyroidism, chronic temperature elevations)
    5. Lesch-Nyhan syndrome
    6. Drugs (L-Dopa?)
  E. Increased excretion
    1. Vitamin B_{12} deficiency? (? of obligatory excretion of folate in urine and bile) (possible inability to reabsorb methylfolate excreted in bile, because B_{12} required for it)
    2. Liver disease?
    3. Kidney dialysis
    4. Chronic exfoliative dermatitis
  F. Increased destruction
    1. Oxidant in diet?

III. Interference with purine ring synthesis and interconversion of purine bases:
  A. Purine antagonists
    1. 6-Mercaptopurine (6-MP)   Chemotherapy, immunosuppression
    2. Thioguanine   Chemotherapy, immunosuppression
    3. Azathioprine   Immunosuppression
  B. Enzymatic defects in ability to make purine nucleotide from preformed bases
    1. Lesch-Nyhan syndrome (there is an associated increased requirement for folate, which is needed at two steps in the increased de novo biosynthesis of purine)

IV. Interference with pyrimidine synthesis:
  A. Pyrimidine antagonists
    1. 5-Fluorouracil (5-FU)   Chemotherapy
      (blocks thymidylate synthetase)
    2. 6-Azauridine   Chemotherapy, psoriasis
  B. Enzymatic defects in ability to make pyrimidine
    1. Hereditary oroticaciduria (not responsive to therapy with vitamin B_{12} or folic acid, but responsive to yeast extract or its active ingredients, uridine or the pyrimidine nucleotides, cytidylic and uridylic acids)

V. Inhibition of ribonucleotide reductase (cytidylic to deoxycytidylic acid):
  A. Cytosine arabinoside (inhibits DNA polymerase also)   Chemotherapy, antiviral
  B. Hydroxyurea   Chemotherapy, psoriasis
  C. Iron deficiency: iron is required for ribonucleotide reductase, but it is not yet established that lack of iron can produce megaloblastosis; some workers have reported hypersegmented polys in iron deficiency which disappear with iron therapy, but coincident folate deficiency has not yet been excluded fully
  D. Procarbazine (depolymerizes DNA)

VI. Inhibition of protein synthesis:
  A. L-Asparaginase   Chemotherapy

VII. Mechanism unknown:
  A. Benzene   Solvent
  B. Azulfidine   Ulcerative colitis
  C. Arsenic   Poison
  D. Pyridoxine-responsive megaloblastic anemia (only about 10% of patients with pyridoxine-responsive sideroblastic anemia have megaloblastic morphology)
  E. Thiamin-responsive megaloblastic anemia (one case reported)
  F. Megaloblastoid anemias (differentiated from megaloblastic anemias by bizarre morphology, including marked polyploidy, few to no orthochromatic megaloblasts, tendency to hyposegmentation, and sometimes karyorrhexis in nucleated red cells)
    1. Di Guglielmo's syndrome (erythremic myelosis) (a myeloproliferative disorder usually presenting as refractory anemia and eventuating in death from "erythroleukemia" or myelogenous leukemia); preleukemia
    2. Occasional cases of polycythemia vera and other myeloproliferative disorders
    3. Occasional cases of aplastic anemia (which cases may subsequently develop myeloproliferative disorders)
    4. Occasional cases of miliary tuberculosis (in such cases, the megaloblastoid marrow is often accompanied by monocytosis and leukopenia or leukocytosis)

Figure 1. Flow chart of vitamin B_{12} metabolism.

which pH pancreatic proteases partially degrade R protein and enable B_{12} to become exclusively bound to IF. The vitamin is absorbed and transported in the bloodstream, attached to the B_{12}-delivery protein, transcobalamin II (TC II, B_{12}-binding beta globulin), to be rapidly delivered to the liver, hematopoietic system, and other proliferative cells. Some B_{12} attaches in an apparently permanent fashion to granulocyte-related serum B_{12}-binding glycoproteins (TC I, a β_{12}-binding alpha globulin, and TC III, a B_{12}-binding globulin which moves with approximately the speed of transferrin on electrophoresis at pH 8.6). Normally, when a sample of blood is drawn, plasma B_{12}-binding protein is found to be approximately one third saturated with B_{12}, almost none of which is on TC II. Of the unsaturated B_{12}-binding protein, approximately 90 per cent is TC II. TC II delivers B_{12} to cells in an ionic calcium- and pH-dependent manner similar to the delivery of B_{12} to the brush border of the ileal cell by IF. The liver is the main storage organ for B_{12} in man, normally containing about 1 μg B_{12} per gram of liver, and there is a large enterohepatic circulation of the vitamin. It is this which explains why vitamin B_{12} deficiency occurs so slowly in vegetarians (whose enterohepatic circulation of B_{12} is usually intact) and relatively rapidly when B_{12} absorption (and therefore reabsorption) is shut off.

As indicated in Figure 2, food folates are predominantly in polyglutamate form. Prior to absorption, the excess glutamates must be split off by conjugases (gamma-glutamyl carboxypeptidases) present in bile and intestine; this process is variably inhibited by inappropriate pH (optimal pH for conjugase action is 4.6) and by conjugase inhibitors in beans, yeast, and some other foods. Once deconjugated, folate is absorbed primarily across the upper third of the small bowel, mainly as reduced monoglutamate, but partly as pteroylglu-

tamic acid (PGA). The absorption of 5-methyl tetrahydrofolate (5-methyl THF) does not appear to be B_{12} dependent. Dilantin and certain other drugs inhibit folate absorption at step 2 in Figure 2. After absorption, folate is transported, mainly as 5-methyl THF, probably by a carrier protein, to cellular sites of utilization. Vitamin B_{12} appears necessary to get 5-methyl THF across cell walls (or to retain it in the cell once absorbed), step 5 in Figure 2, and this vitamin B_{12}–dependent cell uptake (or cell retention) of folate helps explain why patients with uncomplicated vitamin B_{12} deficiency have a "pile-up" of folate in serum, resulting in a high serum folate and a low red cell folate. The "folate trap" in vitamin B_{12} deficiency consists in this folate "pile-up" due largely to inability to convert body folate stores (which are mainly methyl THF) to metabolically usable tetrahydrofolate (THF) because this conversion (step 6 in Fig. 2) is vitamin B_{12} dependent. Normal total body folate stores are in the range of 5 to 10 mg, about half of which is in the liver. There is an enterohepatic circulation of about 100 μg folate daily.

The defective DNA synthesis is due to inadequate thymidylate synthesis (step 11 in Fig. 2). Folate deficiency directly reduces the amount of 5,10-methylene THF available for thymidylate synthesis, and vitamin B_{12} deficiency reduces production of 5,10-methylene THF by blocking utilization of 5-methyl THF (at step 6 in Fig. 2) and possibly by directly reducing synthesis of thymidylate synthetase.

INCIDENCE AND PREVALENCE. Dietary vitamin B_{12} deficiency megaloblastic anemia is common among vege-

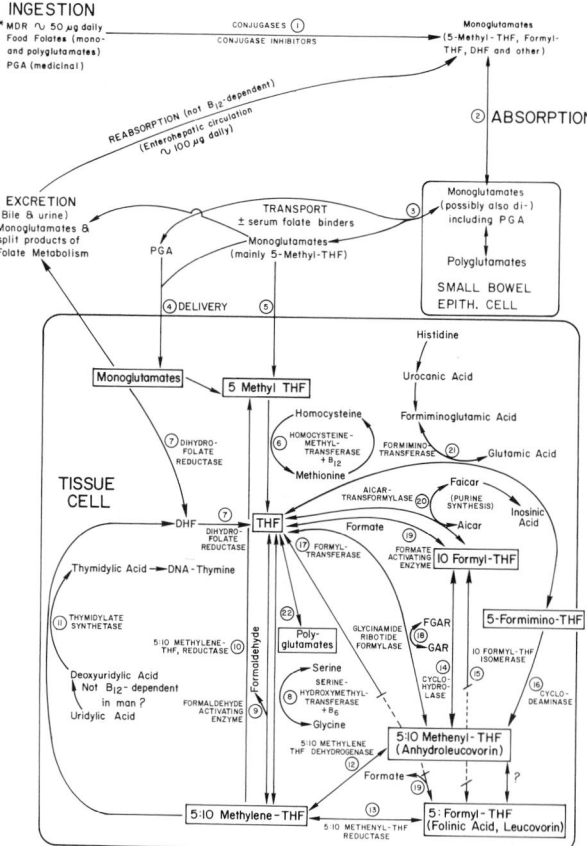

Figure 2. Flow chart of folate metabolism.

tarians because animal protein is the sole source of the vitamin. Conversely, it rarely occurs among meat eaters because the vitamin is almost indestructible by cooking or other processing. On the other hand, dietary folate deficiency megaloblastic anemia occurs in about one third of all the pregnant women in the world ("megaloblastic anemia of pregnancy") despite the fact that folate is found in nearly all natural foods, because folate is heat labile and is rapidly destroyed by extensive cooking, especially of finely divided foods such as beans and rice. Any pregnant women whose daily diet contains neither a fresh uncooked fruit nor a fresh lightly cooked vegetable, and all of whose food is heated at 100° C for periods in excess of 15 minutes, can be assumed to have folate deficiency until proved otherwise. Dietary folate deficiency is also present in over 90 per cent of hard-liquor alcoholics, a majority of wine and beer alcoholics, and about half of narcotic addicts, because these groups waste little money on solid food.

Pernicious anemia (megaloblastic anemia caused by inadequate secretion of gastric intrinsic factor) is age related, with an approximate incidence of 1 per million persons at ages 6 months to 1 year, 1 per 10,000 at ages 1 to 10, 1 per 5000 at ages 30 to 40, and a progressive increase in frequency thereafter so that the incidence is approximately 1 per 200 persons at ages 60 to 70. When statistics are corrected for age, there appears to be a predilection for young black females, and also a predilection for following by some years the incidence of gastric atrophy with its consequent histamine-refractory achlorhydria, which is present in about 15 per cent of people between ages 40 and 60, 25 per cent between ages 60 and 70, and 30 per cent over the age of 70. Age of onset of pernicious anemia is earlier when there are immune disorders present other than just circulating antibody to intrinsic factor.

Megaloblastosis caused by subnormal intestinal absorption of vitamin B_{12} (often with associated folate deficiency) is almost always present in active tropical sprue, which is endemic in the Caribbean and Southeast Asia, and has been most studied in Puerto Ricans, Haitians, Vietnamese, Pakistanis, and Indians, but is also found in other nationals from these two geographic regions. For unknown reasons, a person born in an endemic sprue region who gets sprue may have remissions and exacerbations of the disease throughout life; recurrences are seen in such persons even after they have been in a temperate zone and apparently symptom free for up to 20 years. For this reason, when a person born in Puerto Rico develops megaloblastic anemia in the continental United States, he should be considered to have tropical sprue until proved otherwise. Subnormal absorption of vitamin B_{12} is also present in the majority of patients with regional enteritis, and is also present in a majority with chronic pancreatic disease.

HEMATOLOGIC AND OTHER PATHOLOGY. The pathology of megaloblastic anemia is generated by slowed DNA synthesis per unit time, and this is observed in all proliferating cells. Normally, cells capable of reproducing themselves are in the resting state (i.e., 1 unit of DNA) most of the time. When they reproduce, they do so by rapidly doubling their DNA, dividing, and returning to the resting state. Thus at any instant 100 such normal cells may contain 101 units of DNA (99 cells with 1 unit each plus 1 cell which is about to divide and has rapidly doubled its DNA to do so). Unlike

such normal cells, at any given instant few megaloblastic cells are resting, because nearly all are engaged in a slowed attempt to complete doubling their DNA, with frequent arrest in the S (synthesis) phase and lesser arrest in other phases. Thus the amount of DNA observed per cell may be almost 2 units, so that instead of the hypothetical 101 units of DNA per 100 normoblastic cells, there may be close to 200 units of DNA per 100 megaloblastic cells. This largely explains the apparent anomaly that megaloblastic cells are seen under the microscope to have larger than normal nuclei with *increased DNA content* and yet they have biochemically *defective DNA synthesis*. Megaloblasts have an even larger cytoplasm than nucleus, as compared with normal cells, because, although their synthesis of DNA is impaired, their ability to synthesize RNA is usually relatively unimpeded. This disparity or nuclear-cytoplasmic dissociation or asynchrony, as it is variously termed, is reflected in the finely particulate nuclear chromatin ("young nucleus," or nucleus with retarded maturation) of the erythroid megaloblasts at all stages of their development, even when hemoglobin is clearly visible in the cytoplasm ("old cytoplasm"), easily differentiating them from normoblasts with their coarsely clumped "old" nuclear chromatin.

Another striking feature of megaloblastic hematopoiesis is the megaloblastic myelopoiesis, manifested most dramatically by the presence of many giant metamyelocytes, whose increased DNA is eventually packaged in an increased number of mature neutrophil lobes.

The evolutionary biochemical and hematologic sequence in development of folate deficiency is indicated in Figure 3; the sequence in development of vitamin B_{12} deficiency is similar, but is measured in years rather than months.

When there is concomitant iron deficiency, as is often the case in pregnancy, various malabsorption syndromes, and alcoholism, and in about a third of cases of pernicious anemia, the erythroid megaloblastosis and macrocytic "overcolored" erythrocytes may be masked by the countervailing tendency of iron deficiency to produce microblasts and hypochromic microcytic erythrocytes. The result may be "intermediate megaloblasts" (cells halfway between megaloblasts and normoblasts) in the bone marrow, and in the peripheral blood both red cell forms may be present ("dimorphic

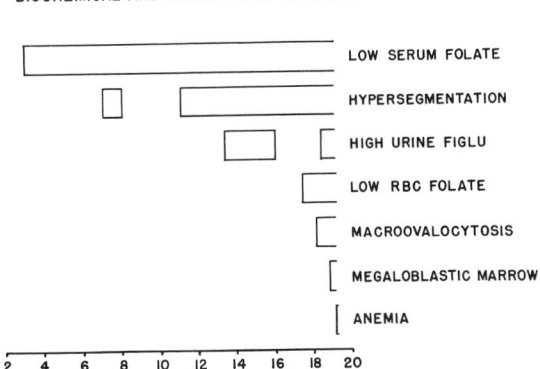

DIETARY FOLIC ACID DEPRIVATION IN MAN:
BIOCHEMICAL AND HEMATOLOGIC SEQUENCE OF EVENTS

LOW SERUM FOLATE
HYPERSEGMENTATION
HIGH URINE FIGLU
LOW RBC FOLATE
MACROOVALOCYTOSIS
MEGALOBLASTIC MARROW
ANEMIA

WEEKS

Figure 3. Biochemical and hematologic sequence of events in folate deficiency.

anemia"), or one may dominate. The myeloid megaloblastosis in the bone marrow and the hypersegmented polymorphonuclear leukocytes ("hypersegmented polys") in the peripheral blood are not masked by iron deficiency, and they provide the morphologic key to the existence of vitamin B₁₂ or folate deficiency even in the presence of severe iron deficiency.

Hypersegmentation can be a crucial clue to covert folate deficiency despite normal serum and red cell folate levels in patients with "uncomplicated" iron deficiency. Such patients have abnormal lymphocyte "dU suppression" tests, and after three to six weeks of treatment with iron alone their normoblastic erythroid bone marrow converts to megaloblastic.

"Hypersegmented polys" are sought by either the simple "rule of fives" (i.e., if more than five of 100 neutrophils have five or more lobes, hypersegmentation is present) or the more elaborate "lobe average" (i.e., count the number of lobes in 100 "polys" and divide by 100; the normal lobe average is 3.00 ± 0.25; hypersegmentation is present if the lobe average is greater than 3.5; normally 20 to 40 per cent of "polys" have two lobes, 40 to 50 per cent have three lobes, and 15 to 25 per cent have four lobes; a substantial increase in percentage with four or more lobes means megaloblastosis, congenital hypersegmentation, or chronic renal disease). As Figure 3 indicates, in incipient megaloblastic anemia, hypersegmentation is present prior to the appearance of an obviously megaloblastic bone marrow or anemia. When the peripheral blood smears of all new patients are screened on a routine basis for hypersegmentation, one third of those found to have it are subsequently proved to have early vitamin B₁₂ or folate deficiency, with low serum vitamin level but no anemia and no clinical suspicion of the diagnosis. The "twenty per cent rule" (i.e., if less than 20 per cent of 100 neutrophils have two or less lobes, hypersegmentation is present) is particularly useful when there are few or no "polys" with more than five lobes.

The megaloblastic anemias are due to ineffective erythropoiesis, and as such they have both a hemolytic component and an iron overload pathologic picture. The increased intramedullary "fetal" death rate of the erythroid cells is dramatically illustrated by the frequent finding of up to 25 per cent reticulocytes among the bone marrow erythrons but 1 per cent or less in the peripheral blood, the high serum lactate dehydrogenase, and the modestly elevated serum bilirubin. Ineffective utilization of iron results in increased saturation of the iron-binding capacity and increased iron stores; this is so prominent that when a patient presents with megaloblastic anemia and normal rather than elevated serum and bone marrow iron, often with an elevated total iron binding capacity, one should suspect iron deficiency, and should repeat the measurements of serum and bone marrow iron a month after vitamin therapy to determine whether overt iron deficiency has now been unmasked.

Megaloblastosis with underlying defective DNA synthesis is present in all proliferating cells; this is almost as striking in epithelial cells, particularly those of the alimentary tract and vagina, as in hematopoietic cells. This defective DNA synthesis results in a variable degree of secondary atrophy in epithelial cells of the tongue, stomach, and small intestine. It is this atrophy which produces secondary failure of gastric intrinsic factor secretion in one third of patients with tropical sprue, secondary failure of intestinal absorption of vitamin B₁₂ in about half of patients with primary failure of intrinsic factor secretion, and the variety of other vicious cycles whereby vitamin B₁₂ deficiency results in secondary decreased absorption of folate (and B₁₂) and folate deficiency results in secondary decreased absorption of vitamin B₁₂ (and folate). These secondary malabsorption phenomena disappear after a variable period of vitamin therapy.

In addition to the defective DNA synthesis common to all megaloblastic anemias, a primary defect of unknown cause in ability to synthesize myelin is present only in vitamin B₁₂ deficiency. This results in the insidious development of demyelinating vitamin B₁₂ deficiency neuropathy, often beginning in peripheral nerves and progressing to involve the posterior and lateral columns of the spinal cord (variously called subacute combined degeneration, combined system disease, posterolateral sclerosis, and funicular degeneration) and the cerebrum ("megaloblastic madness"). (See Ch. 292.)

CLINICAL MANIFESTATIONS. Infrequently, the patient with megaloblastic anemia presents with bleeding caused by the thrombocytopenia, or infection caused by the leukopenia, but usually the presentation is with one or more of the symptoms of a gradually developing and slowly progressive anemia: easy fatigability, weakness, tiredness, shortness of breath, occasional faintness (particularly on suddenly arising from a recumbent or sitting position), headache, palpitations, and syncope. Before such symptoms are brushed off as "neurotic" (which they frequently prove to be), laboratory testing for anemia should be carried out, consisting at the least of determination of hematocrit (and/or hemoglobin) and examination of peripheral blood smear morphology.

If the patient has vitamin B₁₂ deficiency and a good diet supplying adequate folate to substantially mask the hematologic picture, he may have no anemia and only slight morphologic evidence of megaloblastosis, and may present as a neurologic or neuropsychiatric problem, with paresthesias (especially numbness and tingling in the hands and feet) and diminished vibration and/or position sense (with loss of perception of 256 vps preceding by many months loss of perception of 128 vps, and loss of position sense in the index toes preceding by many months loss of position sense in the great toes). Examination with a "256" tuning fork may reveal compete loss of vibration sense from toes to iliac crest bilaterally before any loss of perception of vibration of a "128" tuning fork.

The classic neurologic disorder associated with vitamin B₁₂ deficiency is combined system disease (subacute combined degeneration). Usually slow and insidious in onset, it is characterized by degeneration of the dorsal and lateral columns of the spinal cord, with paresthesias of the hands and feet, ataxia of the legs with variable spasticity and weakness, and eventual paraplegia. The classic symptoms are symmetrical paresthesias (numbness, tingling, burning) in feet and/or hands, followed by unsteadiness of gait associated with loss of position sense, manifested by inability to detect passive movements of the great toes. Prior to the appearance of deficits in the great toes, there may be inability to detect passive movements of the index toes. Knee and ankle jerks may be diminished or lost, or the knee jerks increased; extensor plantar responses, indicating damage to the spinal cord, commonly occur. Mental changes are variable, may include paranoid ideation and depression, and may be sufficiently severe to mimic paranoid schizophrenia or senility. (British workers have referred to this phenomenon as "megaloblastic madness"). Ataxis paraplegia similar to that resulting from vitamin B_{12} deficiency results from any kind of damage to the dorsal or lateral columns of the spinal cord, as may occur with multiple sclerosis or chronic meningeal syphilis.

Subjective neurologic dysfunction, such as irritability, forgetfulness, and sleeplessness, occurs not only with vitamin B_{12} deficiency but even more frequently with folate deficiency. Such subjective stigmata are of limited differential diagnostic value in separating the two vitamin deficiency states; when caused by folate deficiency, these stigamata disappear dramatically within 24 hours of the start of folate therapy.

Occasionally, a chronic alcoholic with megaloblastic anemia caused by folate deficiency is erroneously diagnosed as having vitamin B deficiency because he has neurologic damage, including impaired position and vibration sense. However, associated thiamin deficiency in the alcoholic produces peripheral neuropathy mimicking that caused by vitamin B_{12} deficiency. Confusion may also arise in patients with folate deficiency and diabetes mellitus, because diabetic neuropathy may also mimic the neuropathy resulting from vitamin B_{12} deficiency.

The skin may have a lemon-yellow cast owing to the combination of pallor from anemia and low-grade icterus from the hemolytic component of the disorder. The "classic" pernicious anemia patient still appears as described by Addison in 1855:

The countenance gets pale, the whites of the eyes become pearly, *the general frame flabby rather than wasted*; the pulse perhaps large but remarkably soft and compressible, and occasionally with a slight jerk, especially under the slightest excitement. There is an increasing indisposition to exertion with an uncomfortable feeling of faintness or breathlessness on attempting it; the heart is readily made to palpitate; the whole surface presents a blanched, smooth and waxy appearance: the lips, gums and tongue seem bloodless; *the flabbiness of the solids increases*; the appetite fails, extreme languor and faintness supervene, breathlessness and palpitation being produced by the most trifling exertion or emotion; some slight edema is probably perceived about the ankles. The debility becomes extreme; the patient can no longer arise from his bed; *the mind occasionally wanders*; he falls into a prostrate and half torpid state, and at length expires. *Nevertheless, to the very last, and after a sickness of perhaps several months' duration, the bulkiness of the general frame and the obesity often present a most striking contrast to the failure and exhaustion observable in every other respect.*

The parts of Addison's classic description which do not fit folic acid deficiency states as generally as those caused by vitamin B_{12} deficiency have been italicized. In folate deficiency, emaciation is more common than flabbiness, and diarrhea is more common than the constipation often seen in vitamin B_{12} deficiency.

About one third of patients with megaloblastic anemia have splenomegaly, but this may be observable only on abdominal radiography, because the spleen exceeds two to three times normal size in less than 10 per cent of cases. Moderate hepatomegaly may also be present.

A smooth or sore tongue is frequent, owing to megaloblastosis of the cells of the papillary surface. Almost

TABLE 2. Separating Vitamin B_{12} Deficiency from Folate Deficiency: Laboratory Differential Diagnosis

Before therapy only:

1. Serum vitamin B_{12} (microbiologic: *Euglena gracilis, Escherichia coli, Lactobacillus leichmannii,* etc.) (radioassay); normal: 200–900 pg/ml
2. Serum folate (*Lactobacillus casei*) (radioassay); normal: 7–16 ng/ml
3. Erythrocyte folate; normal: >150 ng/ml
4. Methylmalonate in urine; ↑ usually means B_{12} deficiency
5. Formiminoglutamate (FIGLU) (FGA) and urocanate in urine after oral histidine load; ↑ in B_{12} deficiency, folate deficiency, liver disease
6. "dU suppression" test (i.e., in vitro therapeutic trial) on bone marrow cells

Before or after therapy:

7. Gastric analysis: acid, pepsin, quality, quantity, intrinsic factor (IF) content
8. Tests of radio-B_{12} absorption (radioactivity in stool, plasma, liver, whole body, or urine) after physiologic dose (0.5–2 µg) of radio-B_{12} orally*
   a. Urine (Schilling test)
      Stage 1: Radio-B_{12} orally + 1000 µg "cold" B_{12} IM, followed by 24-hour urine collection, another 1000 µg "cold" B_{12} IM, another 24-hour urine collection (normal result: >5% in 48-hour urine) (2 µg dose)
      Stage 2: Repeat Stage 1, but this time mix IF with radio-B_{12} before administering to patient (normal result: >5% in 48-hour urine) (2 µg dose)†
      Stage 3: See text
9. Circulating antibody to human IF; normally absent
10. "dU suppression" test on lymphocytes (may remain abnormal up to two months after the start of therapy)
11. Lymphocyte folate (may be low as long as lymphocyte "dU suppression" test remains abnormal)

---

*If there has been loss of gastric acid and enzymes, the patient may be unable to free vitamin B_{12} from food, but may still have intrinsic factor secretion. In this circumstance, Doscherholmen and his colleagues have shown that absorption of radioactive vitamin B_{12} from food (i.e., radioactive eggs) is subnormal, but absorption of free vitamin B_{12} is normal.

†A subnormal result in a Stage 2 test may be due to disorder primarily in the small bowel (or pancreas) or may be secondary to vitamin B_{12} deficiency resulting from primary gastric disorder. The test should be repeated a month or more after vitamin therapy. If Stage 2 has reverted to normal, the small bowel disease was secondary rather than primary.

10 per cent of patients have hyperpigmentation, often most marked in the palmar creases, but occasionally in bizarre patterns such as occur with Addison's disease, sometimes with vitiligo. Occasionally low-grade fever is present.

LABORATORY FINDINGS AND DIFFERENTIAL DIAGNOSIS. *Primary* laboratory findings include macro-ovalocytic anemia, leukopenia (with "hypersegmented polys"), thrombocytopenia (with giant platelets), and megaloblastic bone marrow. Reticulocyte count below 1 per cent is common with vitamin B_{12} deficiency, and that of 1.5 to 8 per cent is common with folate deficiency. *Secondary* findings include reduced haptoglobin, hyperbilirubinemia, increased fecal stercobilin, elevated serum lactate dehydrogenase, formiminoglutamic aciduria (found not only in primary folate deficiency but also in primary vitamin B_{12} deficiency and primary liver disease), high serum iron and high saturation of transferrin, loss of gastric acid and abnormal liver function, and intestinal absorption tests. Megaloblasts are usually present in the buffy coat of centrifuged peripheral blood.

An elevated MCV does not mean megaloblastosis unless the red cells are oval as well as large. About a quarter of patients with an elevated MCV have large red cells caused by hypothyroidism, hypoplastic anemia, hemolytic anemia, sideroblastic anemia, neoplasia, liver disease, or other conditions producing large but not oval red cells.

A serum B_{12} level below 100 pg per milliliter is essentially diagnostic for primary vitamin B_{12} deficiency and *both* a serum folate of less than 3 ng per milliliter and a red cell folate below 150 ng per milliliter are diagnostic for primary folate deficiency. (Low serum folate alone may occur long before tissue folate depletion, and low red cell folate occurs also in primary vitamin B_{12} deficiency, because B_{12} is necessary to keep methylfolate in red cells). One caveat: when the serum levels of both vitamins are low, the primary deficiency may be of just one, with resultant intestinal megaloblastosis producing malabsorption and therefore secondary deficiency of the other. For example, in megaloblastic anemia of pregnancy, both vitamin levels may be low, but treatment with only folic acid results in gradual rise to normal of the serum B_{12} level. Normal red cell folate may be present despite folate deficiency because of lag in replacing normal with low folate red cells as pregnancy develops, because of the presence of high folate cells (reticulocytosis or transfused cells), or because of iron deficiency.

Methylmalonic aciduria occurs only in vitamin B_{12} deficiency and not in folate deficiency.

Absence of intrinsic factor in the gastric juice on in vitro assay is essentially diagnostic for pernicious anemia. One caveat: primary intestinal malabsorption of B_{12} or folate deficiency may produce secondary loss of intrinsic factor secretion; this will return to normal after vitamin therapy. Gastric juice pH greater than 5 and viscidity plus a volume of less than 25 ml in the 45 minutes after histamine stimulation all suggest pernicious anemia.

In vivo tests for detection of vitamin B_{12} malabsorption involve feeding 0.5 to 2 μg of the vitamin, labeled with ^{56}Co (half-life, 77 days), ^{57}Co (half-life, 270 days), ^{58}Co (half-life, 71 days), or ^{60}Co (half-life, 5.26 years), and measuring the amount absorbed by the amount of radioactivity in either stool, urine, blood, liver, or whole body. The test is divided into three stages: (1) Feed radio-B_{12} alone. Subnormal absorption means gastric or ileal dysfunction. It need not be done if in vitro radioassay for intrinsic factor is carried out. (2) Feed radio-B_{12} plus intrinsic factor concentrate. Subnormal absorption means ileal dysfunction, but does not rule out concomitant gastric dysfunction. (3) Only done if second stage is subnormal: Feed antimicrobial (or anthelmintic) for appropriate period, then feed radio-B_{12}. A normal result means that the patient had blind loop syndrome (or fish tapeworm). When pancreatic dysfunction is suspected, the third stage consists in feeding the radio-B_{12} with added bicarbonate or pancreatin, or both. When drug-induced B_{12} malabsorption is suspected, the third-stage test is carried out after withdrawal of the offending agent.

Every patient in whom tests reveal gastric or intestinal malabsorption of B_{12} that is not of a clear single cause should have the tests repeated after therapy with B_{12} (or after therapy with folic acid, if deficiency of folic acid is present). Vitamin B_{12} deficiency is a vicious-cycle disease (as is folic acid deficiency); severe deficiency of either B_{12} or folic acid may produce a variable degree of gastric and/or intestinal damage, and therefore may itself produce a variable degree of secondary reduction of gastric secretion of intrinsic factor and/or ileal ability to absorb B_{12} (and/or intestinal ability to ab-

sorb folate). This secondary malabsorption of B_{12} or folate is corrected by therapy.

Repetition of tests after therapy will establish which damage was secondary (i.e., a result of deficiency of B_{12} or folic acid) and which was primary (i.e., a lesion not produced by deficiency of B_{12} or folate). The B_{12} deficiency of a patient with regional enteritis may produce secondary gastric damage which may reduce intrinsic factor secretion; this secondary gastric damage may be corrected by B_{12} therapy. Conversely, the B_{12} deficiency of a patient with pernicious anemia may produce secondary ileal damage and resultant malabsorption of a test dose of B_{12} fed with intrinsic factor; this secondary ileal damage may be corrected by B_{12} therapy. Additionally, the B_{12} deficiency of either patient may make the malabsorption worse owing to his primary lesion.

Circulating antibody to intrinsic factor is present in two thirds of patients with pernicious anemia and, when found, is essentially diagnostic. Less than 10 per cent saturation of serum vitamin B_{12} binding capacity is also essentially diagnostic.

The dU suppression test on bone marrow cells aspirated from the patient is diagnostic for folate deficiency if a deficit in deoxyuridine suppression of radioactive iododeoxyuridine incorporation into DNA is found, and is corrected in vitro by pteroylglutamic acid (PGA) or methylfolate; it is diagnostic for vitamin B_{12} deficiency if corrected by B_{12} but not by methylfolate. This "therapeutic trial in the test tube" is the laboratory equivalent of the classic clinical trial discussed below. Because circulating mature lymphocytes are impervious to vitamin B_{12} and folic acid, the dU suppression test on lymphocytes can reveal a past deficiency of vitamin B_{12} or folic acid up to two months after the start of vitamin therapy. The test can also reveal occult folate deficiency in patients with dominant iron deficiency, as can measurement of lymphocyte folate level.

THERAPY. *Therapeutic trial* is diagnostic for vitamin B_{12} or folate deficiency. Such trial is carried out by giving the patient a diet devoid of foods high in vitamin B_{12} and folate, i.e., devoid of all fresh uncooked fruits and vegetables, fruit juices, nuts or other uncooked natural foods, and liver. After ten days on such a diet, and while continuing the diet, the patient is then treated with 1 μg of vitamin B_{12} parenterally daily if vitamin B_{12} deficiency is suspected, and with 50 to 100 μg of folic acid parenterally daily if folic acid deficiency is suspected. Unless hematopoiesis is suppressed by infection, uremia, chloramphenicol, alcohol, or some other chronic systemic disease or drug, approximately three days after the start of therapy reticulocytosis will appear and will reach a peak at approximately seven days (range: five to twelve days) after the start of the daily vitamin therapy. The lower the initial red count, the higher the reticulocyte peak. The hemoglobin will gradually rise, and by approximately seven days after the start of therapy the white cell and platelet counts will rise to normal. The platelet count will usually, and the white count will in 10 per cent of cases, exceed normal before falling back into the normal range. It is important that the therapeutic trial vitamin dose not be larger than the aforementioned, to avoid "nonspecific" response (Fig. 4).

Immediate therapy is advisable in patients with megaloblastosis accompanied by anemia so severe as to be associated with dyspnea, congestive failure, and occasionally angina. Such symptoms, when found, usually

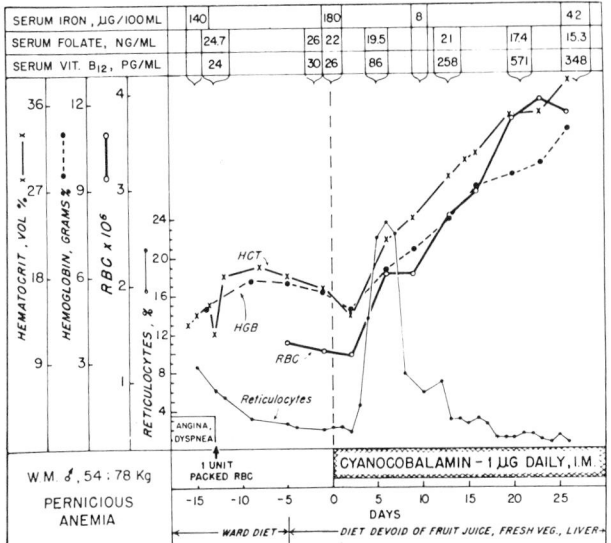

SERUM IRON , μG/100ML	140		180		8			42	
SERUM FOLATE, NG/ML	24.7		26	22	19.5		21	17.4	15.3
SERUM VIT. B₁₂, PG/ML	24		30	26	86		258	571	348

Figure 4. Therapeutic trial with 1 μg of vitamin B₁₂ daily. Note the "spontaneous" reticulocytosis present on admission (more frequent in folate deficiency), the termination of angina and dyspnea by a single unit of packed red blood cells (RBC), the initial high serum iron and folate, and their fall on vitamin B₁₂ therapy.

occur in association with a hematocrit below 15 per cent. Rapid and dramatic relief of these symptoms may be obtained by administration of packed cells into one arm, accompanied by withdrawal of a slightly lesser quantity of whole blood from the contralateral arm. Venous pressure should be monitored, and only that amount of whole blood removed which is necessary to prevent elevation of the venous pressure. Packed cells may be given at the rate of 1 unit per five minutes by interposing a three-way stopcock and a 50-ml syringe between the bottle or bag of packed cells and the vein, drawing the packed cells from source into the syringe and then injecting into the vein. Using the three-way stopcock, venous pressure can be monitored and whole blood drawn off as required. In this procedure, packed cells with a hematocrit of approximately 80 are going into one arm while whole blood with a hematocrit of less than 15 is coming out the same or the other arm; there is therefore no dangerous sudden rise in circulating blood volume to induce the irreversible congestive failure so dreaded when chronically anemic patients are given packed cells or whole blood in the conventional manner.

Immediate therapy with vitamin B₁₂ and/or folate is advisable in patients with severe megaloblastic anemia and bleeding associated with platelet levels below 50,000 per cubic millimeter of blood or associated with infection accompanied by leukopenia with a white cell count below 2000 per cubic millimeter of blood. Immediate therapy with vitamin B₁₂ and/or folate is also advisable in patients with severe infection, coma, severe disorientation, marked neurologic damage, severe liver disease, uremia, or other markedly debilitating illness complicating the deficiency of vitamin B₁₂ and/or folate. When one of these reasons makes necessary immediate vitamin therapy before establishing the etiologic diagnosis, such therapy should be given intramuscularly with a minimum of 30 μg (1 ml) of vitamin B₁₂ (cyanocobalamin) and 1 mg (1 ml) of folic (pteroylglutamic) acid, followed by 1 tablet (1 mg) of folic acid by mouth

daily for a week and a minimum of 30 μg of vitamin B₁₂ by intramuscular injection daily for a week. The fall in serum potassium in the first week after commencing therapy is rarely of clinical significance and does not require therapy. There is a slow increase in whole body potassium with treatment which parallels the increase in red cell mass.

After a week of therapy to carry the patient from the critical state to a state of well-being, all vitamin therapy should be stopped if necessary to make an etiologic diagnosis. However, with a combination of foresight and laboratory facilities, blood will have been obtained from the patient immediately on admission and prior to treatment, and diagnosis of vitamin B₁₂ and/or folate deficiency will have been made from determination of the serum and erythrocyte levels of these vitamins, supplemented by the various tests which may be performed even when the patient is in a treated state. Initial therapy for inadequate absorption of vitamin B₁₂ is 30 μg (or more) of cyanocobalamin daily for a week, or every other day for a total of five doses, to help replenish the body stores, followed by a minimum of 30 μg monthly. This quantity is not adequate to sustain complete normality and allows morphologic damage of moderate degree to persist; therefore a monthly injection of 100 μg of cyanocobalamin is preferable, because it will sustain in complete remission all patients with uncomplicated vitamin B₁₂ deficiency.

Monthly maintenance therapy must be carried out for life in the patient whose inadequate absorption of B₁₂ is due to lack of intrinsic factor secretion or to a noncorrectable structural or functional lesion of the ileum. Although there is no evidence that greater or more frequent therapy has any value, it has become general practice to give patients with neurologic damage 250 μg or more of vitamin B₁₂ once or twice weekly for several months followed by similar doses once or twice monthly for another year. Neurologic damage resulting from vitamin B₁₂ deficiency, when of behavioral nature such as paranoia, may improve very rapidly (even within 24 hours) after the start of therapy. Objectively ascertainable neurologic damage, such as loss of position and/or vibration sense, improves more slowly, and there may be return of ability to perceive 128 vps before return of ability to perceive 256 vps, as well as return of ability to perceive passive motion of the great toes before return of ability to perceive passive motion of index toes. *Any neurologic damage which has not been corrected at the end of approximately one to one and a half years may be considered to be irreversible.* Neurologic damage caused by vitamin B₁₂ deficiency begins as inability to make myelin, followed by gradual deterioration of the axon, followed by deterioration of the nerve head. This process occurs very slowly and is reversible until the nerve head deteriorates.

Oral therapy with large doses of vitamin B₁₂ (500 to 1000 μg daily) should only be used when the patient with B₁₂ malabsorption refuses parenteral therapy. Although there is usually sufficient diffusion-absorption from such doses to maintain patients in remission, this is not always reliable.

Oral therapy with vitamin B₁₂–intrinsic factor complexes should not be used, because such preparations are valueless to patients with structural or functional disorders of the small bowel and produce unreliable absorption of B₁₂ in patients with pernicious anemia, many of whom become refractory owing to development in the gut wall of local antibody to intrinsic factor.

"Shotgun" antianemia preparations may actually harm the patient, because they may obscure the real nature of the anemia. For example, response to folic acid in a patient with megaloblastic anemia secondary to gastric carcinoma may obscure and delay the correct diagnosis.

The only recommended use of low (5 μg) daily dose oral B_{12} maintenance therapy is in the management of vegetarians who refuse to eat any animal matter.

Satisfactory clinical and hematologic remission may be obtained in any patient with uncomplicated vitamin B_{12} deficiency disease by daily parenteral administration of only 1 μg of vitamin B_{12} for ten days. Larger doses simply allow more rapid repletion of body stores. Initial therapy with doses of cyanocobalamin greater than 1 μg daily is desirable only when the vitamin B_{12} deficiency is complicated by other debilitating illness. Parenteral amounts of vitamin B_{12} greater than 30 μg daily have no proved therapeutic advantage, although it is possible that larger daily doses may result in slightly more rapid repletion of body stores. However, the percentage of the injected dose of vitamin B_{12} excreted in the urine rises logarithmically as the quantity of cyanocobalamin injected rises above 30 μg daily.

The most frequent complications of vitamin B_{12} deficiency, especially that caused by pernicious anemia, are infections, especially of the genitourinary tract, and variable degrees of congestive failure. These should be managed appropriately. Since the incidence of carcinoma of the stomach in patients with pernicious anemia is approximately three-fold higher than chance, this entity should be looked for at yearly intervals.

In patients with chronic pancreatic disease, the intrinsic factor mechanism may not be operative and may be enhanced by feeding sodium bicarbonate, pancreatin, or trypsin. Pancreatic proteolytic enzymes free B_{12} from R proteins so that the B_{12} can bind to IF. Bicarbonate raises intestinal pH so that IF can better compete with R proteins for B_{12}.

Initial therapy with larger doses of pteroylglutamic acid than 0.1 mg daily is desirable when the folate deficiency state is complicated by conditions which may suppress hematopoiesis (infection, uremia, tumor; active inflammatory lesions such as rheumatoid arthritis, ulcerative colitis, or hepatitis; chloramphenicol or alcohol administration), or conditions which increase folate requirements (pregnancy; hypermetabolic states; states of increased hematopoiesis such as occur with hemolytic anemia or protracted blood loss). Therapy should then be 0.5 to 1 mg of pteroylglutamic acid daily.

There is no evidence that doses greater than 1 mg daily have greater efficacy than does 1 mg. Additionally, loss of folate in the urine becomes roughly logarithmic as quantities of administered pteroylglutamic acid exceed 1 mg. It is possible that the use of larger daily doses, especially if given in several spaced doses each day, may more rapidly replete the body folate stores, but the value of such rapid replenishment is uncertain.

When folate deficiency is due to malabsorption rather than inadequate ingestion, parenteral therapy is preferable initially, and maintenance therapy is preferably with 500 to 1000 μg (0.5 to 1.0 mg) of PGA daily rather than 100 μg (at least until further studies support the current impression that PGA is well absorbed even when the patient is only poorly capable of absorbing other nutrients [such as food folates]).

The best maintenance therapy for dietary folate deficiency is correction of the diet rather than permanent supplementation. Such correction often simply requires less prolonged cooking of the same foods the patient has always eaten, because prolonged cooking destroys folates. In other instances, such correction involves switching from canned to fresh fruits and vegetables, because the canning process may destroy 50 to 95 per cent of food folate.

Summary of Response to Therapy. Objective and subjective improvement occurs within a few days and a sense of well-being often within a day of the start of therapy with the lacking vitamin. Within 48 hours, the bone marrow returns sharply toward normoblastic. Reticulocytosis begins within two to five days after therapy is started and usually reaches its peak on about the fifth to twelfth day. The shape and height of the reticulocyte curve depend on the dose of vitamin B_{12} or folic acid, the route of its administration, and the severity of the anemia. At approximately the time the reticulocytes reach their peak, the leukocytes and platelets will have risen to normal levels. Serum iron is usually elevated in untreated patients and falls abruptly within one to two days after starting therapy. This fall is to iron deficiency levels, but does not represent iron deficiency unless it persists past three weeks after the start of vitamin therapy. This sequence of events should be followed by obtaining a blood count just prior to the start of therapy and a reticulocyte count at least once every two days from then until the reticulocyte peak has passed, plus a hemoglobin or hematocrit determination at weekly intervals for the first month and then every two weeks for the next month or two. If hematologic recovery does not follow the outlined response pattern, then either the diagnosis is wrong or complications suppressing hematopoiesis are present. Since almost half of patients with megaloblastic anemia have iron deficiency, which may be undiagnosable in some cases prior to vitamin therapy, patients with megaloblastic anemia should be re-evaluated for iron deficiency a month after the start of vitamin therapy. Conversely, because covert folate deficiency frequently occurs in iron-deficient patients, such patients should be re-evaluated for folate deficiency two months after the start of iron therapy.

Allen, R. H., Seetharam, B., Podell, E., and Alpers, D. H.: Effect of proteolytic enzymes on the binding of cobalamin to R protein and intrinsic factor. In vitro evidence that a failure to partially degrade R protein is responsible for cobalamin malabsorption in pancreatic insufficiency. J. Clin. Invest., 71:47, 1978.

Babior, B. N. (ed.): Cobalamin: Biochemistry and Pathophysiology. New York, John Wiley & Sons, 1975.

Beck, W. S.: Erythrocyte disorders — anemias related to disturbance of DNA synthesis (megaloblastic anemias). In Williams, W. J., Beutler, E., Erslev, A., and Rundles, R. W. (eds.): Hematology. 2nd ed. New York, McGraw-Hill Book Company, 1977, p. 300.

Carmel, R., and Johnson, C. S.: Racial patterns in pernicious anemia: Unusual age of onset and intrinsic factor prevalence in black women. N. Engl. J. Med., 298:647, 1978.

Colman, N.: Folate deficiency in humans. In Draper, H. H. (ed.): Advances in Nutritional Research, Vol. 1. New York and London, Plenum Press, 1977, p. 77.

Das, K. C., and Herbert, V.: The lymphocyte as a marker of past nutritional status: Persistence of abnormal lymphocyte deoxyuridine (dU) suppression test and chromosomes in patients with past deficiency of folate and vitamin B_{12}. Br. J. Haematol., 38:219, 1978.

Das, K. C., Herbert, V., Colman, N., and Longo, D. L.: Unmasking covert folate deficiency in iron-deficient subjects with neutrophil hypersegmentation: dU suppression tests on lymphocytes and bone marrow. Br. J. Haematol., 39:357, 1978.

Food and Nutrition Board, National Research Council: Folic Acid: Biochemistry and Physiology in Relation to the Human Nutrition Requirement. Washington, D.C., National Academy of Sciences, 1977.

Herbert, V.: Detection of malabsorption of vitamin B$_{12}$ due to gastric or intestinal dysfunction. Semin. Nucl. Med., 2:220, 1972.

Herbert, V.: Drugs effective in megaloblastic anemias. In Goodman, L. S., and Gilman, A. (eds.): The Pharmacological Basis of Therapeutics. 5th ed. New York, The Macmillan Company, 1975, p. 1324.

Herbert, V., Colman, N., and Jacob, E.: Nutritional overview; megaloblastic anemias. In Gordon, A. S., Silber, R., and LoBue, J. (eds.): The Year in Hematology — 1977. New York and London, Plenum Press, 1977, p. 549.

Herbert, V., Colman, N., and Jacob, E.: Folic acid and vitamin B$_{12}$. In Goodhart, R. S., and Shils, M. E. (eds.): Modern Nutrition in Health and Disease. 6th ed. Philadelphia, Lea & Febiger, 1978.

Herbert, V., and Tisman, G.: Effects of deficiency of folic acid and vitamin B$_{12}$ on central nervous system function and development. In Gaull, G. (ed.): Biology of Brain Dysfunction, Vol. 1. New York and London, Plenum Press, 1973, p. 373.

Hoffbrand, A. V. (ed.): Symposium on Megaloblastic Anaemia. Clin. Haematol., 5:471, 1976.

Jerzy Glass, G. B.: Gastric Intrinsic Factor and Other Vitamin B$_{12}$ Binders. Biochemistry, Physiology and Relation to Vitamin B$_{12}$ Metabolism. Stuttgart and New York, Thieme Verlag and Intercontinental Medical Book Corp., 1974.

Kass, L.: Pernicious Anemia. Philadelphia, W. B. Saunders Company, 1976.

Rosenberg, L. E.: Disorders of propionate, methylmalonate, and cobalamin metabolism. In Stanbury, J. B., Wyngaarden, J. B., and Fredrickson, D. S. (eds.): The Metabolic Basis of Inherited Disease. 4th ed. New York, McGraw-Hill Book Company, 1978, p. 411.

Rowe, P. B.: Inherited disorders of folate metabolism. In Stanbury, J. B., Wyngaarden, J. B., and Fredrickson, D. S. (eds.): The Metabolic Basis of Inherited Disease. 4th ed. New York, McGraw-Hill Book Company, 1978, p. 430.

Sauer, H., and Wilmanns, W.: Cobalamin dependent methionine synthesis and methyl-folate-trap in human vitamin B$_{12}$ deficiency. Br. J. Haematol., 36:189, 1977.

Stebbins, R., Scott, J., and Herbert, V.: Drug-induced megaloblastic anemias. Semin. Hematol., 10:235, 1973.

Youngdahl-Turner, P., Rosenberg, L. E., and Allen, R. H.: Binding and uptake of transcobalamin II by human fibroblasts. J. Clin. Invest., 61:133, 1978.

Zittoun, J., Marquet, J., and Zittoun, R.: Effect of folate and cobalamin compounds on the deoxyuridine suppression test in vitamin B$_{12}$ and folate deficiency. Blood, 51:119, 1978.

480. NORMOCHROMIC NORMOCYTIC ANEMIAS

480.1. ACUTE HEMORRHAGIC ANEMIA

Elmer B. Brown

DEFINITION. Acute hemorrhagic anemia caused by loss of a large volume of blood may result from trauma, ulcerative lesions, abnormal blood vessels, or coagulation defects; it may occur from a severed blood vessel, from the gastrointestinal, respiratory, or genitourinary tracts, into a large muscle mass, or into various body cavities such as cysts or the pleural, peritoneal, and retroperitoneal spaces. The hemorrhage is grossly evident except when blood is lost into the gastrointestinal tract, body cavities, or tissues. Clinical manifestations vary with the size, rate, and site of the hemorrhage, with the lesion responsible for the bleeding, and with the state of consciousness of the patient.

CLINICAL MANIFESTATIONS. The manifestations of acute severe hemorrhage are remarkably consistent regardless of the underlying cause, because they depend on the volume of blood lost. As outlined in the accompanying table, the loss of as much as 500 ml of blood in five minutes usually produces only trivial effects on the circulation without changes in blood pressure or pulse rate. Withdrawal of a liter of blood often produces no fall in blood pressure in the recumbent subject, although if he sits up or attempts to walk, tachycardia occurs, the blood pressure often falls, and consciousness may be lost. When apprehension is added to the loss of even small amounts of blood, syncope caused by a vasovagal reaction may occur. Loss of 1500 to 2000 ml of blood leads to a fall in right atrial pressure, diminished cardiac output, hypotension, and a rapid, thready pulse. Additional symptoms are prostration, restlessness, thirst, tachypnea and air hunger, pallor with cold clammy skin, sweating, pounding headache, and frequent syncope. Rapid blood loss of greater than 40 per cent of the patient's blood volume leads to shock, the risk of renal tubular necrosis, myocardial infarction, and a high risk of death unless immediate replacement therapy is initiated. However, a previously healthy person may survive the gradual loss of as much as 50 per cent of his blood volume over a period of 24 hours. Hemorrhage into pleural, peritoneal, or retroperitoneal spaces usually causes pain, fever, and signs of serosal inflammation; bleeding into muscles may also produce marked limitation of motion.

DIAGNOSIS. Initial assessment of the degree of hemorrhage may be difficult. When associated with multiple trauma, the amount of swelling surrounding the area of a wound correlates roughly with the amount of blood lost. Wounds of the thigh involving large muscles may be associated with a blood loss of 2500 ml or more. With gross disruption of tissues, as in gunshot or automobile injuries, the size of the wound correlates fairly well with the degree of blood loss — for an area of tissue damage the size of the patient's hand, loss of approximately 10 per cent of the patient's blood volume should be assumed. Upper gastrointestinal bleeding can be roughly quantitated by the fact that frank hematemesis indicates a large hemorrhage (usually more than 25 per cent of the blood volume), whereas melena alone indicates a much smaller blood loss. Generalizations of this type are important, because the initial hematocrit does not adequately reflect the size of the hemorrhage. Blood vessels of the skin and muscles constrict in an attempt to compensate for the decreased

Clinical Manifestations of Acute Blood Loss

Volume of Blood Lost		Clinical Manifestations
% of Blood Volume	ml*	
10	500	Usually none; rarely vasovagal syncope
20	1000	Few changes supine; upright or with exercise, tachycardia and mild hypotension are often present
30–40	1500–2000	Marked postural hypotension and tachycardia; central venous pressure, cardiac output, and arterial blood pressure are reduced; pulse is thready; skin is cold and clammy; thirst, air hunger, headache, and syncope are frequent
50	2500	Severe shock, often leading to death

blood volume and to provide blood flow and adequate oxygen supply for vital organs. Replacement of plasma from endogenous sources is slow. The initial changes in blood counts after hemorrhage reflect the mobilization of platelets and leukocytes from marginated storage pools. Thrombocytosis to levels approaching 1 million per cubic millimeter may occur within an hour; a polymorphonuclear leukocytosis with white cell counts as high as 20,000 to 30,000 occurs within two to three hours. Metamyelocytes, myelocytes, and nucleated red blood cells often appear in the peripheral blood after severe hemorrhage. Replacement of plasma volume by fluid from the extravascular space is a relatively slow process, with the limiting factor being the rate at which albumin and other proteins are mobilized. After loss of 10 per cent of the blood volume, about half of the lost red cells and plasma are replaced by plasma alone after 24 hours. Loss of about 20 per cent of the blood volume requires 24 to 60 hours for restoration of the normal blood volume as reflected by a decreasing hematocrit for two or three days. Loss of red blood cell mass causes decreased tissue oxygenation only partially compensated for by adjustments in cardiovascular dynamics. Tissue hypoxia by a still unknown mechanism triggers erythropoietin production with measurable increases in plasma levels of this hormone within six hours. Increased levels of 2,3-diphosphoglycerate in circulating erythrocytes contribute to a shift of the hemoglobin oxygen dissociation curve for more efficient tissue oxygenation. Erythropoietin-stimulated erythropoiesis causes a fall of the plasma iron during the two to five days required for marrow stem cells to proliferate and mature into circulating reticulocytes to expand the red cell mass. Some reticulocytes are released prematurely from the marrow in response to hemorrhage, and their numbers increase to peak levels of 10 to 15 per cent after seven to ten days. Since reticulocytes are larger than mature erythrocytes, the mean corpuscular volume (MCV) rises (approximately 1 fl for each per cent of increase in reticulocyte count) and polychromatophilic macrocytes are seen in Wright-stained blood films. Depending on the size of the hemorrhage and the adequacy of iron stores, the red cell volume and hematocrit are restored to normal in about five or six weeks. Elevated platelet counts and leukocytosis have usually returned to the normal range within three to five days. Bleeding into the gastrointestinal tract produces an elevation of the blood urea nitrogen which may be accentuated if renal function is impaired. Resorption of blood from body cavities or tissues results in increased production of unconjugated bilirubin and may be associated with mild jaundice; iron released from hemoglobin bled into tissues is reutilized for new erythropoiesis.

TREATMENT. Treatment should be directed at stopping the hemorrhage, combating shock, and restoring blood volume. The patient should be kept warm and quiet; sedation and analgesics may be required. It is essential to begin an infusion through a needle or catheter of adequate bore to permit rapid fluid replacement, and this will sometimes require a surgical cutdown to find collapsed veins. The choice of solutions for initial replacement therapy depends on how critical the patient's condition is and what solutions are available. Most quickly available for rapid expansion of plasma volume are noncolloid electrolyte solutions (e.g., iso-

tonic saline and Ringer's lactate) or dextran solutions, either a 10 per cent solution of low molecular weight dextran in isotonic saline (dextran 40, with an average molecular weight of 40,000) or a 6 per cent solution of high molecular weight dextran (dextran 70, with an average molecular weight of 70,000). Dextran 40 has the advantage of increasing the plasma volume by one to two times the amount infused, but is more rapidly cleared in the urine. Its effect is rapidly dissipated during the succeeding 12 hours, and in a few patients it may precipitate acute renal failure. Dextran 70 is cleared more slowly and sustains the plasma volume expansion for 24 to 48 hours. Both may produce circulatory overload, which can usually be avoided by administering the first 500 ml rapidly and the remainder more slowly with frequent monitoring of central venous pressure. When volumes of dextran solution in excess of 1000 ml are used, interference with platelet adhesiveness and coagulation mechanisms may accentuate bleeding. Plasma protein solutions and 5 per cent albumin in saline have the advantage of predictable volume expansion with physiologic materials, but carry the disadvantages of relatively high cost, slower time for reconstitution, and with plasma solutions, the risk of hepatitis. Noncolloid electrolyte solutions such as isotonic saline or Ringer's lactate may be given quickly in acute emergencies for support of blood volume, but since they are rapidly distributed throughout the intravascular and extravascular compartments they must be supplemented with blood or colloid solutions. Use of fresh whole blood, packed erythrocytes, or saline-resuspended, concentrated red blood cells requires typing and cross-matching that cause too great a delay for routine use in the initial treatment of life-threatening hemorrhage. Use of un-cross-matched universal donor blood cannot be condoned except in extreme emergencies. Rarely is red cell depletion so severe that blood transfusions cannot wait for careful cross-matching. Blood transfusions supplement initial volume expansion with dextran or other colloidal solutions and are the mainstay of the definitive treatment of acute hemorrhage. When bleeding is due to absence of platelets or coagulation factors, transfusion of fresh whole blood or concentrates of blood components is essential and may be lifesaving. With prolonged bleeding requiring replacement of more than 5000 ml of stored blood within 48 hours, thrombocytopenia caused by transfusion of nonviable platelets may cause bleeding. Anticipation of this complication as well as the risks of severe uncontrolled bleeding may favor early surgical attempts to identify and correct the cause of bleeding from gastrointestinal or other obscure sites. After the emergency is over, provision of a high protein diet and iron by mouth are indicated to replace the stores depleted by blood loss; no other supplements are needed.

Adamson, J., and Hillman, R. S.: Blood volume and plasma protein replacement following acute blood loss in normal man. JAMA, 205:609, 1968.

Collins, J. A., and Ballinger, W. F.: The treatment of shock. In Ballinger, W. F., Rutherford, R. B., and Zuidema, G. D. (eds.): The Management of Trauma. Philadelphia, W. B. Saunders Company, 1973, Chapter 3.

Harris, J. W., and Kellermeyer, R. W.: The Red Cell. Production, Metabolism, Destruction: Normal and Abnormal, Revised ed. Cambridge, Harvard University Press, 1970, Chapter 4.

Mollison, P. L.: Blood Transfusion in Clinical Medicine. 5th ed. Oxford, Blackwell Scientific Publications, 1972.

480.2. ANEMIA ASSOCIATED WITH INFECTION AND CHRONIC SYSTEMIC DISEASES

(Simple Chronic Anemia, Anemia of Chronic Disorders)

Elmer B. Brown

DEFINITION. The anemia of infection and many chronic disorders is usually mild and nonprogressive in severity. It develops over a period of one to two months, is usually normochromic normocytic, and is characterized by decreased plasma iron, decreased transferrin iron-binding capacity, decreased bone marrow sideroblasts, increased reticuloendothelial iron deposits, mild hemolysis, and relative bone marrow failure. The occurrence of anemia in association with chronic disease of multiple etiologies makes the selection of an appropriate descriptive name difficult. The term "anemia of chronic disorders" may be the least restrictive for anemia underlying cancer, lymphomas, connective tissue disorders, hepatic, renal and endocrine disorders, fractures and tissue injury, and chronic viral and suppurative infections. Other types of anemia, such as those related to blood loss, iron or vitamin deficiency, or hemolysis, may accentuate and complicate the underlying anemia of a chronic disorder. By its widespread association with many chronic diseases this anemia is the most common form seen in hospital populations, and it is frequent in the population at large.

ETIOLOGY AND PATHOGENESIS. The mechanism can generally be framed in terms of three basic abnormalities: (1) moderate shortening of erythrocyte life span; (2) failure of the bone marrow to increase erythropoiesis sufficiently to compensate for the mild hemolytic anemia; and (3) an unexplained impairment of iron release from reticuloendothelial cells throughout the body. Examination of the interaction of these three basic abnormalities is essential before special features of anemias associated with specific diseases can be defined.

Decreased erythrocyte life span is of moderate degree and requires measurements with special erythrocyte labeling techniques; half-time survival of ^{51}Cr-tagged cells is reduced from a normal range of 30 ± 3 days to about 20 to 25 days. In absolute terms, erythrocyte survival is about 80 days instead of the normal 120 days. Cross-transfusion experiments have shown normal survival of red cells from anemic patients transfused into normal recipients, whereas cells from normal subjects transfused into the patient show decreased survival indicative of an extracorpuscular factor responsible for the decreased erythrocyte life span. Whether this unidentified factor acts in the plasma or adversely influences other portions of the erythrocyte's environment has never been defined.

Ordinarily, this mild degree of hemolysis would be compensated for by greater erythropoietic activity of the bone marrow which can increase red cell production six to eight times the normal rate. However, erythropoiesis in patients with chronic disorders rarely increases more than two-fold; as a result, production of red cells falls behind destruction until a new balance is reached at mildly anemic levels. Normally the body responds to tissue hypoxia of anemia by increasing the output of erythropoietin which stimulates the differentiation of marrow stem cells into erythroblasts and speeds their maturation to circulating erythrocytes. One might suppose, under conditions of chronic disease, that either the stimulation of erythropoietin production is defective or the marrow is incapable of responding to this hormone. Experimental evidence indicates that erythropoietin levels are low and that the marrow is quite capable of responding to erythropoietin when injected in pure form or when stimulated by external hypoxia or cobalt administration. Thus the block to an appropriate erythropoietic response seems to be an insensitive "thermostat," failing to stimulate erythropoietin release in response to slowly developing anemia. The precise mechanism of this defect is unknown.

The third basic abnormality common to the anemias of chronic disorders is the impairment of iron release from reticuloendothelial cells. Normally, senescent erythrocytes are removed from the circulation by reticuloendothelial cells which digest hemoglobin, free its iron from the heme ring, and release it to plasma transferrin for transport to the marrow and reutilization in erythropoiesis. Within hours after infection or injury a block occurs to the normal release of iron by the reticuloendothelial cells, as evidenced by a precipitous fall in plasma iron concentrations. Further experimental evidence for this block was obtained by injecting ^{59}Fe-labeled, heat-damaged red cells that are rapidly cleared by reticuloendothelial cells and measuring the release and reutilization of ^{59}Fe into newly formed erythrocytes. Normal subjects reutilize 55 to 70 per cent of the ^{59}Fe for hemoglobin synthesis, whereas patients with anemia of chronic disorders utilize less than 40 per cent. As a result of this block to normal iron flow, there is a buildup of ferritin and hemosiderin in reticuloendothelial cells in the bone marrow and throughout the body. The paucity of iron available for erythropoietic cells in turn leads to decreased numbers of marrow sideroblasts and other evidence of iron-deficient erythropoiesis. The three basic abnormalities are balanced so that the resultant anemia is mild and self-limiting. However, if blood loss, red cell fragmentation, or immune hemolysis increases the rate of red cell loss, if folate or vitamin B_{12} deficiency further decreases erythropoietic response, or if iron deficiency accentuates the block to iron flow, the anemia may be much more severe.

Various diseases have additional specific etiologic factors that might profitably be examined separately from the basic abnormalities that characterize the anemia of chronic disorders.

Renal failure is usually accompanied by anemia which may be quite severe. Anemia correlates roughly with the elevation of blood urea nitrogen, although a more nearly linear relationship exists between elevated BUN and decreased red cell life span. The factor or factors in uremic plasma that damage erythrocytes and cause anemia have not been identified, although many substances have been suggested. In some patients mechanical trauma and increased fragmentation of red cells lead to severe hemolytic anemia when renal failure is associated with accelerated hypertension or various types of hemolytic-uremic syndrome. Other patients with renal failure have hemorrhagic tendencies caused by decreased numbers and function of platelets.

Deficiency of folate and iron aggravates the *anemia of*

patients undergoing dialysis; folate is dialyzable and is lost into the dialysis bath, whereas iron is lost with blood in the dialysis coil. Since approximately 90 per cent of erythropoietin originates in the kidney, either directly or through a renal activating system, progressive renal disease leads to decreased erythropoietin production. In addition, the presence of uremia may blunt the bone marrow's response to the reduced amounts of erythropoietin released by damaged kidneys; dialysis may salvage some of the effectiveness of the available erythropoietin and cause amelioration of the anemia.

Rheumatoid arthritis in the active phase is frequently accompanied by the anemia of chronic disorders. A unique feature is the microscopic bleeding into the inflamed joints that leads to massive accumulation of iron in the hyperplastic synovial tissue. Sequestration of several hundred milligrams of iron in hypertrophied synovium may contribute to an iron deficiency state superimposed on the anemia of inflammation. Bleeding induced by the gastrointestinal irritation of aspirin, corticosteroids, and other anti-inflammatory therapeutic agents may further accentuate the iron deficiency.

Cancer in its later stages is almost always accompanied by the anemia of chronic disorders. Frequently there is no correlation between the degree of anemia and the extent of the tumor. Bone marrow invasion by cancer is often associated with the release of immature leukocytes and nucleated erythrocytes, but the extent of marrow metastases correlates poorly with the degree of anemia. Substances released from necrotic cancer cells and the red cell fragmentation from fibrin strands in vessels narrowed by tumor invasion have been postulated to explain the hemolytic anemia in cancer. Bleeding from tumors of the alimentary or genitourinary tracts or from vascular lesions of the skin causes hemorrhagic or iron deficiency anemia, and the inanition leading to calorie, protein, and vitamin deficiency accentuates the underlying simple chronic anemia.

Liver disease is associated with various complications in addition to the underlying anemia of chronic disorders. The increased plasma volume of cirrhosis may give an exaggerated impression of anemia when the concentration of erythrocytes is measured by hematocrit and hemoglobin determinations. Bleeding related to peptic ulcers, varices, and deficient coagulation factors may produce rapid blood loss anemia or slowly developing iron deficiency. Alcohol depresses erythropoiesis acutely and leads to folate deficiency anemia because of inadequate intake and defective absorption of the vitamin. Erythrocyte abnormalities — thin macrocytic target cells or burr cells — may contribute to the decreased red cell survival. Hypersplenism frequently associated with portal hypertension of liver disease also accentuates the hemolytic anemia of chronic disorders.

Endocrine disorders, including thyroid, pituitary, and adrenal insufficiency, are associated with a normochromic normocytic anemia most severe in hypothyroidism. Presumably these endocrine deficiencies lead to decreased erythropoietin production. In the case of *hypothyroidism* the diminished need of the tissues for oxygen leads to an adaptive partial atrophy of the erythron. Frequently, coexistent iron, folate, and especially vitamin B_{12} deficiencies are present with the anemia of hypothyroidism.

CLINICAL MANIFESTATIONS. The symptoms are primarily those of the underlying disease. As the anemia is mild and develops slowly, the patient can adjust to it with minimal accentuation of fatigue, dyspnea, and palpitations. When bleeding or hemolysis complicates the underlying anemia of chronic disorders in patients with leukemia, lymphoma, or chronic renal failure, symptoms of anemia may be disabling and lead to coronary insufficiency and congestive failure. Pallor, tachycardia, cardiac dilatation, and low-grade sustained fever are nonspecific signs common to many types of chronic anemia.

DIAGNOSIS. The anemia of chronic disorders is usually normocytic normochromic (MCV 87 to 103 fl and MCHC 32 to 36 grams per deciliter), but may be normocytic hypochromic or even microcytic hypochromic. When microcytosis or hypochromia is present, it is usually milder than that seen in well-developed iron deficiency anemia. The hematocrit usually remains constant in a range between 25 and 39 per cent at full development of anemia after six to eight weeks. Erythrocyte morphology is unremarkable except for burr cells of uremia and some types of cancer and the thin, flat macrocyte of chronic liver disease. Reticulocytosis or polychromasia indicative of increased erythropoiesis is rare. Leukocytes and platelets are normal unless they reflect changes related to the underlying disease. Bone marrow morphology on Wright-stained specimens shows no specific abnormality; changes related to the underlying disease may include increased numbers of plasma cells in cirrhosis or rheumatoid arthritis and leukemic or tumor cell infiltration. Prussian blue stains for iron in bone marrow disclose decreased numbers of erythroid precursors with iron granules (sideroblasts), whereas reticuloendothelial cells show increased hemosiderin deposits. Plasma iron and total iron-binding capacity are both reduced; the per cent saturation of transferrin is normal or low. Serum ferritin levels are normal or increased. Differentiation from the plasma iron changes of iron deficiency anemia may be difficult; the major difference is a tendency toward increased transferrin concentration and absence of stainable marrow iron in iron deficiency. When iron deficiency and the anemia of chronic disorders occur together, the rise in transferrin usually seen in iron deficiency is blunted; absent marrow hemosiderin and low serum ferritin concentrations are the key diagnostic observations. Despite the underlying hemolysis, the serum bilirubin is usually normal unless there is associated liver dysfunction. Hemolysis is usually detectable only by special red cell survival measurements.

TREATMENT. The only effective therapy is that directed toward correction of the underlying disease. Since the anemia typically is mild and nonprogressive, no attempt at correction may be necessary. When symptoms of underlying heart disease are triggered by anemia, transfusions with packed erythrocytes to a hematocrit of 30 to 35 per cent may be temporarily beneficial. Attempts to stimulate erythropoiesis by administration of cobalt have been abandoned because undesirable side effects outweigh the modest improvement of the anemia. Androgenic steroids may be effective in some patients with cancer or chronic renal disease. Purified erythropoietin is not yet available in sufficient amounts for adequate clinical trials. Corticosteroids frequently ameliorate the anemia of rheumatoid arthritis and other connective tissue diseases; they may also be beneficial in treatment of complicating immune hemolysis. No means has been found to bypass the block to iron flow in the anemia of chronic disorders. Since colloidal iron preparations given parenterally must be processed by the reticuloendothelial cells before iron is made available to transferrin, the colloidal iron is blocked as effectively as that from senescent erythrocytes. When bleeding causes superimposed iron deficiency, giving iron by mouth or parenterally will restore hemoglobin levels to those of the underlying chronic disorder, but not back to normal. Similarly, folate deficiency of alcoholic cirrhosis will respond to folate therapy by partial correction of anemia.

Cartwright, G. E.: The anemia of chronic disorders. Semin. Hematol., 3:351, 1966.

Harris, J. W., and Kellermeyer, R. W.: The Red Cell. Production, Metabolism, Destruction: Normal and Abnormal. Cambridge, Mass., Harvard University Press, 1970.

Kimber, C., Deller, D. J., Ibbotson, R. N., and Lander, H.: The mechanism of anaemia in chronic liver disease. Quart. J. Med., 34:33, 1965.

Strandberg, O.: Anemia in rheumatoid arthritis. Acta Med. Scand. [Suppl.], 454:1, 1966.

Williams, W. J., Beutler, E., Erslev, A. J., and Rundles, R. W. (eds.): Hematology. 2nd ed. New York, McGraw-Hill Book Company, 1977.

480.3. APLASTIC ANEMIA

M. C. Brain

DEFINITION. Aplastic or hypoplastic anemia is a term applied to a group of disorders characterized by a reduction in all the cellular elements of the blood (pancytopenia), and associated with hypocellularity of the bone marrow. The degree of pancytopenia reflects the severity of the disorder and determines the prognosis. Less severe pancytopenia is present in hypoplastic anemia than in aplasia of the bone marrow. Bone marrow aspiration or biopsy may on rare occasions yield a hypercellular or normocellular specimen. Such a finding usually is due to the chance sampling of a residual focus of marrow showing normal or increased cellularity. The presence of such foci of normal or increased cellularity is additional indication of the fundamental defect in hematopoietic stem cell proliferation and differentiation; for although capable of giving rise to differentiated cell lines in the small foci, the stem cells seem incapable of repopulating the hypoplastic areas of the bone marrow. The widespread nature of the hypocellularity can be confirmed by isotopic scanning techniques and by the finding at necropsy of a diffusely hypocellular fatty marrow throughout the normal hematopoietic skeleton. Evidence for the ability of these hypocellular areas to maintain normal hematopoiesis has come from the demonstration that the whole bone marrow can be repopulated with active hematopoiesis after successful bone marrow transplantation.

The term aplastic anemia is descriptive. It is reasonable therefore, in the light of present knowledge, to recognize a form of failure of hematopoiesis which may be associated with a hypercellular marrow — ineffective hematopoiesis. However, it must be noted that certain bone marrow toxins which are known to produce aplastic anemia, such as benzol, may also give rise to pancytopenia with a hypercellular marrow exhibiting ineffective hematopoiesis. It is also reasonable to draw a distinction between the pancytopenia associated with aplastic anemia, through a presumed abnormality of the pluripotent stem cell, and the isolated reductions in red cells, granulocytes, or platelets, through failure of proliferation and differentiation of the committed stem cells which give rise to the principal cell lines. The disorders of formation of isolated cell lines probably reflect the action of toxic agents or of immune mechanisms on the differentiation of committed rather than the pluripotent stem cells. Support for such a distinction has come from the knowledge gained of the factors stimulating and regulating the growth of differentiated cells from human bone marrow in vitro. Thus granulopoiesis is dependent upon the production by monocytes of a colony-stimulating factor. Recently it has been shown that erythropoiesis in vitro is dependent not only on the stimulation of erythropoietin but also on the presence of T lymphocytes. The latter observation is consistent with the recognized association of pure red cell aplasia with immunologic disorders and thymic tumors, and suggests that lymphocytes may facilitate normal erythropoiesis as well as potentially impeding erythropoiesis through aberrant immunologic mechanisms.

Aplastic anemia may develop without an apparent or recognized cause; may follow exposure to ionizing radiation or a variety of chemical agents, including drugs, either known to be potentially toxic to hematopoiesis or recognized to have this effect only occasionally; or may be of familial or constitutional etiology, becoming manifest in childhood or early adult life. The clinical course is influenced by the severity of the pancytopenia, especially by the degree of leukopenia or thrombocytopenia. If severe infective or hemorrhagic complications do not take place, or can be prevented, the patient may survive for a number of months or occasionally years. Rarely, complete or partial remissions may take place.

In selected patients successful bone marrow transplantation may result in a complete recovery, such that the disorder can be regarded as cured.

ETIOLOGY. A general classification of the etiology of aplastic anemia is given in Table 1. The exact cause of aplastic anemia is often obscure. In the majority of patients no etiologic agent can be incriminated with certainty, and these are described as idiopathic. A small proportion of the idiopathic group occur in childhood or in early adult life; when associated with other congenital abnormalities and a history of aplastic anemia in other members of the family, their separate designation as to the constitutional type of aplastic anemia (*Fanconi's anemia*) is warranted. The majority of idiopathic cases are presumed to be acquired, and although no etiologic agent may be incriminated, this designation does not preclude

TABLE 1. Etiologic Classification of Aplastic Anemia

Idiopathic
    Familial or constitutional (Fanconi's anemia)
    Acquired
Secondary
    Physical or chemical agents
        Ionizing radiation
        Drugs (cytotoxic; normally noncytotoxic)
        Nonpharmacological chemicals
    Infections
        Viral hepatitis
        Bacterial: miliary tuberculosis
    Metabolic
        Pancreatitis
        Pregnancy
    Immunologic
        Antibody mediated
        Graft versus host reaction
    Neoplastic
        Myelophthisic
        Paroxysmal nocturnal hemoglobinuria

exposure to some unrecalled or unrecognized environmental agent. In patients with secondary aplastic anemia in whom a history can be obtained of exposure to chemical or physical agents known to adversely affect the hematopoietic stem cell, or when the onset was preceded by an event known to be associated with aplastic anemia, the exact causal relationship between the implicated agent or agents to the fundamental disturbance of hematopoiesis often remains obscure.

It seems likely that the disorder of the pluripotent hematopoietic stem cell which results in failure of replication and/or differentiation may be due to somatic mutation with alteration of the controlling mechanisms governing cell replication and differentiation. Support for such a concept has come from the recognition of increased frequency of breaks in the chromosomes of patients with Fanconi's anemia, and from the increased incidence of such patients developing leukemia. Additional support for such a hypothesis has come from the well recognized association between paroxysmal nocturnal hemoglobinuria (PNH) and aplastic anemia. PNH may precede the development of aplastic anemia; or patients with hypoplastic anemia may produce a small proportion of red blood cells with increased susceptibility to complement lysis, or may in the course of recovery from a hypoplastic anemia produce a large proportion of such abnormal red blood cells, and in consequence develop the classic features of PNH. It seems likely that the alteration in the regulatory mechanism governing stem cell replication in aplastic anemia is somewhat analogous to the modification in the regulatory mechanisms in cells implicit in the loss of control of replication in malignant diseases. Such a hypothesis would be consistent with the view that the cellular changes giving rise to aplastic anemia, as in malignant diseases, are the outcome of possibly one or more somatic mutations, and may reflect both genetic predisposition and the impact of environmental factors.

An alternative hypothesis is that in some patients aplastic anemia may be due to an immunologic mechanism. Support for this has come from the demonstration that lymphocytes from the bone marrow and peripheral blood of patients with aplastic anemia inhibit erythropoiesis and granulopoiesis of bone marrow cells in culture in vitro both from the patients and from normal subjects. Further support has been provided by recognition that immunosuppressive therapy for bone marrow transplantation has led to recovery of bone function when a graft has been rejected. In the absence of a suitably matched donor, treatment with immunosuppressive drugs has been followed by remission.

The agents which are known or are thought to cause aplastic anemia can be divided into two broad categories. The first category includes those that predictably produce bone marrow damage if the magnitude or duration of exposure is sufficient to cause cytotoxicity. These include exposure to ionizing radiation from x-rays, radioactive elements, or nuclear explosions; chemical agents such as benzol; and the wide variety of drugs used in the treatment of malignant disease (antimetabolites such as 6-mercaptopurine, 5-fluorouracil, cytosine arabinoside, and methotrexate; alkylating agents such as cyclophosphamide, melphalan, busulfan, chlorambucil, and nitrogen mustard; natural products such as the vinca alkaloids, actinomycin D, bleomycin, Adriamycin, and daunorubicin; and synthetic compounds such as BCNU and CCNU). All these agents act by interfering with DNA synthesis, structure, or replication. The second category contains agents which have been recognized as being associated with aplastic anemia in only a small proportion of the population exposed to them. The incidence of aplastic anemia in the second category is so low that a considerable period of time has usually elapsed before the adverse reaction has been sufficiently widely recognized and reported for it to be appreciated as being a statistically significant risk. Drugs are the most common agents in this second category. Chloramphenicol, phenylbutazone and its related compounds, and gold are widely recognized as potential causes of aplastic anemia. Inquiry as to exposure to drugs must include both drugs prescribed by physicians and drugs that can be purchased without prescription, including analgesics, hypnotics, and antihistamines. Inquiries should be made and evidence sought for the possibility of self-administration or abuse of mood-changing drugs, or the inhalation of organic solvents for the same purpose. When no history of drug ingestion can be established, the incrimination of possible etiologic agents may be exceedingly difficult, because many chemical compounds in common daily use contain benzene derivatives or allied compounds which must be regarded with suspicion. Many such chemicals are used as solvents in common household cleaning agents, in dyes and paints, in insecticides and fertilizers, and in industrial processes, and have been identified in animal feed supplements in which the manufacturing processes or biologic degradation may have resulted in toxic products being derived from relatively nontoxic precursors. Despite the frequent difficulty in establishing a definite etiologic agent, it is important that a full and detailed inquiry be made of the patient and relatives as to the possible exposure at work or in the home to potentially toxic chemicals, through a detailed history of daily activities and hobbies. Occasionally aplastic anemia may follow infections, and is a rare but recognized complication of viral hepatitis. As yet, this intriguing association remains unexplained.

Since its introduction in 1948, *chloramphenicol* became recognized as the drug most commonly associated with aplastic anemia. The drug achieved rapid and widespread popularity with physicians by virtue of its range of antimicrobial activity and the ease with which it could be administered. In 1952, a number of reports were published associating chloramphenicol with aplastic anemia, an association which was directly responsible for the establishment of a registry of drugs giving rise to aplastic anemia and other adverse hematologic reactions. A report published in 1965 and 1967 by the Registry on Adverse Reactions showed that of 771 cases of pancytopenia, 338 (44 per cent) followed the use of chloramphenicol, and that in 154 (20 per cent) chloramphenicol was the only drug taken in the preceding six months. Although the risk of developing pancytopenia and aplastic anemia after chloramphenicol is approximately 1 in 20,000 to 30,000, this is about 13 times greater than the risk of idiopathic aplastic anemia in the population as a whole. Awareness of the risk has resulted in a considerable and commendable reduction in the prescribing of chloramphenicol, partly through the increasing availability of other broad-spectrum antimicrobials of comparable activity and ease of administration. It is now generally accepted that chloramphenicol should be prescribed only in specific and serious infections in which it can be shown to be the *only* agent suitable on the basis of antimicrobial sensitivity testing. However, awareness of the hazards of this serious complication of chloramphenicol differs in different countries, and there are still countries where it is widely prescribed or may even be obtained without prescription. The higher incidence of aplastic anemia in certain countries may reflect relative lack of control over the availability of this drug, or lack of awareness of its hazards. Thus with increasing air travel the risks of exposure to chloramphenicol may persist despite the adverse publicity and the application of more stringent indications for its use.

There are two independent types of bone marrow toxicity produced by chloramphenicol. It is well established that this drug induces a dose-related reversible bone marrow lesion characterized by maturation arrest and vacuolization in early erythroid cells, reticulocytopenia, and ferrokinetic changes indicative of suppressed erythropoiesis. This reversible effect results from inhibition of mitochondrial protein synthesis and consequent mitochondrial injury. These changes appear to be quite distinct from the much rarer and devastating complication of aplastic anemia, which may not be dose dependent or even directly temporally related to exposure to the drug. There is some evidence that the bone marrow aplasia may occur on the basis of a genetically determined predisposition to toxicity involving the DNA synthetic pathway. Thus exposure to chloramphenicol may be the second of two mutagenic steps giving rise to this disorder, analogous to the recognition of two mutagenic events in the transformation of malignant cells. Although knowledge as to the mechanism of the reversible pharmacologic toxicity of chloramphenicol on the bone marrow may ultimately throw light on the mechanism of marrow aplasia, it must be emphasized that currently these two mechanisms appear to be distinct, that the onset of aplasia cannot be predicted, and that it is not readily reversible. Thus the only way to avoid the calamitous consequences of aplastic anemia is not to expose a patient to chloramphenicol.

Although the association of aplastic anemia with drugs other than chloramphenicol is now well recognized, the low incidence and the fact that, as mentioned already, it is common for patients with aplastic anemia to give a history of exposure to a number of potentially toxic agents make it difficult to calculate the possible risk with any accuracy. However, phenylbutazone and its derivatives were the second most frequently recorded drugs in the AMA Registry, having been administered alone or concomitantly with an apparently innocuous agent to 27 patients and having been associated with other potentially toxic agents in a total of 52 patients (6.7 per cent). Other drugs include the hydantoin analogues used in treatment of epilepsy, sulfonamides, sulfonylureas, gold compounds, organic arsenicals, potassium perchlorate, and quinacrine. At least 50 other drugs have been implicated, and many of them are chemically related to drugs established as being associated with aplastic anemia. Among those obtainable without prescription are a wide variety of antihistamine preparations. In addition, salicylamine, widely available as a sedative without prescription, has been reported as being associated with aplastic anemia in three patients.

Benzol and a wide variety of *aromatic hydrocarbons* derived from the refining of petroleum and coal products are included in many cleaning solvents and form the basis of many compounds used in the petrochemical and plastic industries. Aplastic anemia has been reported following exposure to aromatic hydrocarbons by siphoning gasoline from gas tanks. The widespread use of these compounds in dyes, solvents, insecticides, cements, glues, and fingernail polish, and as diluents to paints, varnishes, and lacquers as thinners and paint removers, makes the risk of exposure of the general population very considerable. Furthermore, in many instances the relative purity of organic solvents is unknown and significant amounts of benzene may be present. Aplastic anemia is recognized to follow ingestion of benzene or trinitrotoluene or exposure to Stoddard solvent, widely used in the automobile industry as a cleaning agent.

Aplastic anemia is a recognized complication of "glue-sniffing," and many of the glues and cements may contain benzene or bezene derivatives.

Insecticides such as gamma benzene hexachloride (lindane), chlordane, and chlorophenothane (DDT) have been associated with aplastic anemia and have been reported in the AMA Registry. Many of these organic insecticides are used suspended in petroleum solvents which may contain benzene.

Aplastic anemia has been associated with *hepatitis* in more than 50 patients. The onset of aplastic anemia usually occurs two to six months after an episode of viral hepatitis has resolved. The nature of the etiologic relationship between hepatitis and aplastic anemia is unclear. The viral etiology of the hepatitis has seldom been established. Furthermore, it is well recognized that many agents capable of producing aplastic anemia are also hepatotoxic; thus the hepatitis and the aplastic anemia may have a common etiology. Even when the viral nature of the hepatitis is established, the possibility remains that hepatic dysfunction may itself increase the risk of aplastic anemia through impaired or abnormal handling of potentially marrow-toxic agents.

The etiology of *pure red cell aplasia* can, like that of aplastic anemia, be divided into constitutional and acquired forms. More than 100 cases of chronic erythroid hypoplasia and aplasia have been described in childhood. The onset may be at birth but is more commonly recognized within the first two years of life. The occasional occurrence of the disorder in a sibling has suggested that a genetic or inherited abnormality may be present. A metabolic defect in the handling of tryptophan has been described in some of the affected children. The children go into remission either spontaneously or in response to adrenal steroid administration. Acquired red cell aplasia may occur as an acute transient episode, particularly in children with congenital hemolytic anemia. This disorder, most frequently reported in hereditary spherocytosis, is thought to be due to suppression of erythropoiesis in association with viral illnesses and may reflect a direct action of viruses on erythropoiesis or may be a consequence of an immunologic response to a viral infection. The recognition of this disorder in association with chronic hemolytic anemia probably reflects the dramatic onset of anemia caused by the cessation of erythropoiesis in association with an increased rate of hemolysis, and may indicate an increased susceptibility of an active erythropoietic bone marrow to a variety of toxic agents. Pure red cell aplasia in the adult is associated with thymic tumors in about 30 to 50 per cent of patients. The presence of a thymoma and the response of these patients to thymectomy or adrenal steroid or immunosuppressive treatment have suggested that the selective disturbance of erythropoiesis is due to an immunologic mechanism. Support for this has come from demonstration in some patients of antibodies which react against erythroid precursor cells, or from the direct cytotoxic action of the patient's lymphocytes on erythroid precursor cells in culture in vitro. More recent evidence of the importance of T lymphocytes for erythroid colony formation in vitro suggests that these cells may have an important stimulatory function in normal erythroid development, as well as potentially having adverse effects on erythroid maturation. Although anti-erythropoietin antibodies have also been demonstrated, the presence of high levels of erythropoietin in the serum of these patients makes it unlikely that this is a primary mode of action.

INCIDENCE. Idiopathic aplastic anemia is rare and occurs predominantly in children and young adults of either sex. The incidence of secondary aplastic anemia is directly related to the size of the population exposed to the causal factor. Increasing use of atomic energy and of radioactive isotopes and x-rays in both industry and medicine has increased the risks of exposure to ionizing radiation. However, the widespread recognition of this hazard makes it unlikely that aplastic anemia caused by ionizing radiation will increase except through war, nuclear accidents, or negligence. Nevertheless numerous cases of aplastic anemia resulted from the two atomic bombs exploded over Japan in 1945, and the risk of aplastic anemia from accidents occurring through the proliferating use of atomic energy and the dangers of atomic warfare is ever present. The incidence of secondary aplastic anemia caused by drugs and other toxic chemicals is difficult to estimate with accuracy. Careful monitoring of adverse reactions to drugs should detect this complication of new drugs earlier than was the case with chloramphenicol. The increasing use of cytotoxic drugs in malignant disease and to produce suppression of the immune system in a wide variety of disorders, along with the use of methotrexate in treatment of psoriasis, has greatly increased the risk of the development of hypoplastic or aplastic anemia as a complication of treatment. In patients exposed to phenylbutazone, the incidence rises with age. The relative preponderance of women reflects the use of this and related agents in the treatment of rheumatoid arthritis. The incidence of pure red cell aplasia depends on whether the disorder is constitutional or acquired. Acquired pure red cell aplasia in the adult is mainly seen in middle age. There is a significant preponderance of females over males when pure red cell aplasia is associated with thymoma, whereas males exceed females when a thymoma cannot be demonstrated.

PATHOLOGY AND PATHOGENESIS. The peripheral blood count reveals a reduction in all cellular elements, with the lowering of the red cell count, packed red cell volume, and hemoglobin concentration and a reduction in the total circulating white cells, particularly those of the granulocyte series, although absolute monocytopenia is usually present. The platelet count is invariably reduced and may be very low. The anemia is usually normochromic but may be slightly or definitely macrocytic with red blood cells showing some slight changes in size and shape. The reticulocytes vary from 0 to 5 per cent, but the absolute count is usually subnormal. The reticulocytes may be large and immature, possibly reflecting a response of the remaining erythroid cells to an increased erythropoietic stimulation with a shorter bone marrow transit time. The presence of nucleated red blood cells in the peripheral blood is unusual and implies some other disorder of hematopoiesis. Granulocytopenia is an invariable feature and is of importance in relation to the

immediate prognosis, because a granulocyte count of less than 500 per cubic millimeter puts a patient at great risk from infectious complications. The monocyte count is usually reduced, and lymphocytopenia is a common finding. It is unusual to find immature cells of the granulocytic or lymphocytic cell lines in the peripheral blood; such a finding is likely to suggest that the disorder of hematopoiesis is due to subacute leukemia rather than hypoplastic or aplastic anemia.

The peripheral blood findings reflect the disordered hematopoiesis in the *bone marrow*. Specimens of marrow are usually aspirated without difficulty or pain and consist of fat spaces with few cellular elements. Occasionally bone marrow aspiration reveals a normocellular or hypercellular specimen, which probably reflects the chance aspiration of a sample with residual normal activity. To confirm the diagnosis, aspiration should be carried out at other sites. Further information regarding the over-all cellularity of the bone marrow can be obtained from the histology of needle or trephine biopsies. The relative proportions of different cellular elements in the bone marrow seen on aspiration or on biopsy can vary from patient to patient. Both the degree of cellularity and the relative involvement of the different cell lines may reflect the nature and severity of the action of the toxic agent inducing the disordered hematopoiesis. Although increases in precursor cells may be present, suggesting a "maturation arrest," or may be accompanied by changes in the chromatin pattern of the erythroid precursors with some megaloblast-like features, an absolute increase in blast cells is uncommon. The presence of an increase in granulocyte precursors and a reduction in cytoplasmic granules within maturing cells may make the distinction between aplastic anemia and subacute myelocytic leukemia difficult. However, the absence of an increase in the proportion of blast cells in the peripheral blood or bone marrow and the presence of a hypoplastic or aplastic marrow at other sites usually enable a distinction to be made between aplastic anemia and subacute leukemia. When the patient has received multiple blood transfusions, hemosiderosis of the marrow may be present and in due course will involve other organs, notably the liver, spleen, and heart. Enlargement of the liver and spleen may be due to hemosiderosis, because extramedullary hematopoiesis is uncommon. Other pathologic changes are related to the infectious and hemorrhagic complications which are frequently encountered during the course of the illness and are the usual causes of death.

The mechanism by which exposure to irradiation or chemical agents induces aplastic anemia is incompletely understood. Ionizing radiations and radiomimetic drugs are thought to inhibit mitosis, probably by causing disturbances of DNA structure, synthesis, or replication. The antimetabolites used in treatment of malignant disease either interfere with the formation of purines or nuclei acids or, in the case of vinca alkaloids, inhibit chromatin separation through interaction with spindle proteins. Although exposure to radiation or cytotoxic drugs characteristically produces a transient depression of hematopoiesis, the persistent disorder of hematopoiesis characterizing aplastic anemia implies a more fundamental defect in stem cell proliferation and differentiation. A similar distinction must be drawn between the transient, reversible, and dose-related disturbance of hematopoiesis due to chloramphenicol, and the more fundamental and probably dose-unrelated disturbance of hematopoiesis seen in aplastic anemia caused by chloramphenicol. Whereas as the former can be considered as being due to direct or metabolic effect on cell maturation, aplastic anemia would appear to implicate some more fundamental derangement of the genetic information necessary for stem cell proliferation and differentiation.

Exposure to irradiation may be followed by persistent disorders of the chromosomal structure of lymphocytes which may be detected months or years after the irradiation exposure. In aplastic anemia of any cause, the level of fetal hemoglobin in the erythrocytes produced by the bone marrow may be increased, suggesting some persistent derangement of the control of globin chain synthesis. Although initial results suggested that a high hemoglobin F might be a good prognostic sign, this interpretation has been questioned. In Fanconi's anemia, in which some as yet unknown inherited influence can result in the appearance of aplastic anemia in childhood or early adult life, chromatin breaks and other disturbances of the karyotype have been described. Furthermore, abnormalities of the red cell enzymes have also been recognized. The common association of Fanconi's anemia with developmental abnormalities affecting the structural position of the kidneys and radiologic evidence of abnormalities of the bony skeleton suggests the presence of some fundamental derangement of genetic factors influencing development, although the causal relationship between these abnormalities and the subsequent development of aplastic anemia is as yet unexplained.

Still further support for the view that a fundamental disturbance of stem cell structure and function is the basis for aplastic anemia comes from the association between aplastic anemia and *paroxysmal nocturnal hemoglobinuria*. Hypoplastic or aplastic anemia may develop as a complication of PNH, or a small proportion of the red blood cells in aplastic anemia may show the increased susceptibility to complement lysis characteristic of PNH. The PNH red blood cells may be found at the onset or during recovery from aplastic anemia and may be associated with frank hemolytic anemia. Since the membrane disorder characterizing PNH can be shown to be present in red blood cells, granulocytes, and platelets, it is probable that the membrane disorder in all the blood cell lines is due to proliferation of a modified stem cell. In pure red cell aplasia there is an isolated failure of differentiation of the erythroid cell line which may reflect different susceptibilities of the various hematopoietic cell lines to agents capable of inducing aplastic anemia. A variety of drugs may induce transient erythroid hypoplasia and, in the case of chloramphenicol, may be associated with morphologic changes in erythroid precursors, whereas pure red cell aplasia is ill understood and appears to represent a more fundamental disorder of erythroid differentiation. Pure red cell aplasia, as its name indicates, is a failure of differentiation of committed erythroid precursor cells. It seems probable that the mechanisms disturbing differentiation of a committed cell line, as in this disorder and in agranulocytosis, differ from the primary stem cell defect in aplastic anemia. The association of pure red cell aplasia with thymoma suggests that there is an immunologic mechanism involved. There has been recent evidence that in aplastic anemia the lymphocytes from the bone marrow and peripheral blood of some patients can suppress both erythropoiesis and granulopoiesis of normal bone marrow in vitro, and that removal of the lymphocytes from an aplastic marrow results in improved cell colony formation by aplastic bone marrow in culture. These initial observations may necessitate a funda-

mental reconsideration of the relative importance of defective stem cell function and immunologic mechanisms, including the role of suppressor lymphocytes in the pathogenesis of aplastic and hypoplastic anemias.

CLINICAL MANIFESTATIONS. The symptoms are related to the rapidity of onset and the extent to which the different hematopoietic cell lines are affected. Acute aplasia induced by ionizing radiation or by cytotoxic drugs can develop rapidly, and in such circumstances the symptoms are predominantly due to the infective or hemorrhagic complications of severe granulocytopenia or thrombocytopenia. Anemia, unless it is due to some underlying disease, develops more insidiously, although gastrointestinal hemorrhage or an increase in menstrual blood loss or uterine bleeding can aggravate it. When the granulocyte and platelet counts are at levels which provide some protection against infection and spontaneous hemorrhage, the presenting symptoms are usually those of anemia: pallor, fatigue, dyspnea, and tachycardia on exertion. Severe granulocytopenia may be accompanied by infections of the skin and oral and rectal mucosa, with development of painful ulceration at these sites which may cause difficulties in swallowing and defecation, or by urinary tract infections. Thrombocytopenia is usually associated with bleeding into the skin from mucous membranes and spontaneous bleeding from gums, nose, vagina, or rectum, or with occult intestinal blood loss. Occasionally patients appear to tolerate severe thrombocytopenia without serious bleeding except at sites subjected to minor trauma. Intracerebral or subarachnoid hemorrhage may take place and is one of the causes of death. However, it is often remarkable how long patients survive with an increased hemorrhagic tendency caused by thrombocytopenia before this serious complication occurs.

The principal findings on physical examination relate to the changes that result from anemia, the infective or hemorrhagic complications. At the onset physical examination may be unremarkable apart from petechiae of the skin at the sites exposed to undue pressure and on the lower limbs. Larger bruises may be present at the sites subjected to trauma, including venipuncture. Examination of the optic fundi often reveals flame-shaped hemorrhages and occasional Roth spots. The extent of the retinal changes is frequently related to the degree of anemia as well as to the severity of the thrombocytopenia. It is unusual for the spleen to be enlarged at any stage of the disease; indeed, the finding of splenic enlargement usually suggests the presence of some other disorder causing pancytopenia. Severe anemia is accompanied by tachycardia, cardiac enlargement, a systolic heart murmur, and signs of congestive cardiac failure. In the later stages of the disease, particularly when multiple transfusions have been given, increased pigmentation of the skin and enlargement of the liver and spleen may indicate the development of hemosiderosis. Infective complications can be accompanied by chronic ulceration of the oral and rectal mucosa, and can give rise to fever. Hectic fever and rigors are usually due to widespread infections, which in the absence of a granulocyte response may be accompanied by few localizing symptoms or signs. Neurologic signs may be present when hemorrhagic or infective complications involve the brain, spinal cord, or peripheral nerves.

DIAGNOSIS. Pancytopenia is a cardinal feature of aplastic anemia, and although the blood count may vary, it is unwise to make the diagnosis unless there is severe depression of all cellular elements at some stage in the disease.

The degree of anemia may vary, depending upon when the patient is seen and the relationship of the blood count to previous transfusions. The morphology of the red cells in peripheral blood smears is usually normal, but slight or moderate macrocytosis and anisocytosis may be present. There is usually a reticulocytopenia, although because of the degree of anemia the percentage of reticulocytes may be normal, and an absolute reticulocyte should be calculated. The presence of an increased reticulocyte count should lead one to suspect development of PNH. It is unusual for nucleated red cells to be present in the peripheral blood; when found, some other disorder of hematopoiesis should be considered. The total white cell count is usually low, and an absolute granulocytopenia is a feature. The severity of the granulocytopenia is of considerable immediate prognostic significance, because of danger of infective complications. The neutrophil granulocytes may be deficient in granules. Metamyelocytes, myelocytes, and blast cells are rarely found; if present they suggest the presence of leukemia rather than aplastic anemia. The absolute monocyte and lymphocyte counts are often depressed in severe cases. Thrombocytopenia is frequently present and may be severe. Large and bizarre-shaped platelets may be present in the blood smear. Severe thrombocytopenia is associated with prolonged bleeding time and a positive test for capillary fragility, but neither of these tests is of diagnostic value, and they do not warrant the discomfort they may produce for the patient. Coagulation tests are usually normal. Bone marrow aspiration and biopsy should be carried out and may be performed safely if attention is paid to aseptic techniques and to the prevention of subsequent hemorrhage by application of firm pressure to the site of aspirational biopsy for 15 or 20 minutes. Aspiration is achieved with little pain. The specimen often contains adequate numbers of fragments, although diluted with blood. A needle or trephine biopsy is helpful in the assessment of over-all cellularity. Smears from the bone marrow aspirate usually reveal marked hypocellularity of the marrow fragments with a predominance of recticulum cells, mast cells, lymphocytes, and plasma cells. Cells of the myeloid series are often grossly reduced in numbers, and those that are present are usually at the promyelocyte and myelocyte stages of maturation. Megakaryocytes may be absent or very infrequent. Erythroid precursors may be more numerous than those of the myeloid series, and, although usually normoblastic, may show abnormal nuclear maturation with megaloblastic features. Iron can usually be demonstrated in the reticulum cells and may be greatly increased if the patient has received blood transfusion.

The serum iron level is usually elevated, and the total iron binding capacity of the serum is reduced. Ferrokinetic studies usually reveal a diminished rate of plasma iron clearance and turnover and marked diminution of iron utilization. External scanning of distribution of iron or technetium into organs and the skeleton has shown that most of these isotopes are taken up by the liver rather than by the bone marrow. The levels of erythropoietin in plasma and excreted in the urine are high and often exceed values found in patients with comparable degrees of anemia. The levels of fetal hemoglobin (hemoglobin F) may be increased. Except for the association with paroxysmal nocturnal hemoglobinuria, evidence for shortened red blood cell survival caused by hemolysis is usually absent and of little value in the presence of frank or occult hemorrhage.

The diseases most likely to be confused with aplastic or hypoplastic anemia are those which lead to pancytopenia by other mechanisms. They include subacute leukemia or preleukemia and other forms of myelophthisic anemia.

The greatest diagnostic difficulty may be encountered in distinguishing between a hypoplastic anemia and subacute or subleukemic myelocytic leukemia. The presence of increased numbers of blast cells and of myelocytic precursors in the bone marrow can usually enable the distinction to be made, as can the finding of blast cells and other immature cells in the peripheral blood. The distinction usually becomes apparent during the course of the illness when a more obviously leukemic blood picture may develop. The distinction between a preleukemic state and a true aplastic anemia is sometimes rendered difficult by the development of an acute myelocytic leukemia in a patient who has had aplastic anemia for many months or years. The finding of enlargement of the spleen or lymph nodes, generalized bone tenderness, or radiologic evidence of bone destruction should lead one to doubt the diagnosis. It is unusual for the levels of immunoglobulins to be raised, and the finding of a monoclonal protein in the serum should arouse suspicion. Infiltration of the bone marrow by metastatic malignancy, metastasis or plasma cells, Hodgkin's disease, lymphosarcoma, or myelofibrosis, all of which can cause a myelophthisic anemia, can usually be recognized by the cellular infiltration seen in bone marrow aspirations or on bone marrow biopsy.

TREATMENT. The treatment of aplastic anemia has changed radically in the past few years because of the success of bone marrow transplantation. In a child or adult under age 40 with severe aplastic anemia (as defined by having two of the following features: corrected reticulocyte count of less than 1 per cent; granulocytes less than 500×10^6 per liter; platelet count less than 20×10^9 per liter) for whom there is an HLA-compatible donor, bone marrow transplantation must now be regarded as the treatment of choice. The success of this procedure is governed (1) by avoiding or preventing graft rejection, and (2) by minimizing or preventing graft-versus-host disease (GVHD). Graft rejection has been found to be minimal in those patients showing a negative reaction in mixed leukocyte cultures, indicating an absence of prior sensitization of the recipient to the donor's white cells, and in those receiving more than 3×10^8 marrow cells per kilogram. Graft-versus-host disease has been absent or minimal in patients receiving bone marrow from a sibling donor of the same sex and in patients who had not become refractory to random donor platelet transfusions.

These observations are of importance in the selection of patients to undergo bone marrow transplantation, as the greatest success can be predicted for those who have an HLA-compatible sibling donor of the same sex and who have not received blood transfusions in the past. If blood transfusions have to be given, blood from random donors and not family members should be used, and should if at all possible be avoided until HLA-typing of family members has established whether bone marrow transplantation is feasible. The risk of immunization will be reduced if frozen red cells are available to be used to correct anemia; if not, packed cells are preferable to whole blood. Platelet and granulocyte transfusions may be required to overcome life-threatening thrombocytopenic bleeding and/or for proved systemic infections.

If a patient with severe aplastic anemia has an HLA-compatible donor and has not required blood transfusion, an endeavor should be made to have such a patient referred to a center with experience in performing bone marrow transplantation. It must be recognized that successful bone marrow transplantation necessitates immunosuppressive therapy and that for several weeks until engraftment takes place the patient is at risk from hemorrhage and infection caused by thrombocytopenia and granulocytopenia. However, these risks can be minimized by platelet and granulocyte transfusions, the latter being best provided by the donor. The direct medical costs and the need to have the donor readily available during the acute phase are self-evident and must be borne in mind when discussing this procedure with the patient and family members. Nevertheless, bone marrow transplantation in those patients for whom a compatible donor is available has radically altered the immediate prognosis.

In the exceedingly rare circumstance of aplastic anemia being present in one of identical twins, bone marrow transplantation should not be accompanied by either rejection or GVHD unless it is due to an immune mechanism and can be regarded as capable of curing the disorder.

HLA-compatible donors can only be expected to be found among siblings in 25 per cent of families, and bone marrow transplantation is less successful in patients over 40. Thus at best in only 15 per cent of all patients with aplastic anemia is bone marrow transplantation likely to be feasible.

In the majority of patients with aplastic anemia more conventional principles of treatment still apply. It is important to recognize and, whenever possible, to prevent further exposure to any implicated causative agent, and then to endeavor to prevent hemorrhagic infective complications and anemia by appropriate blood component transfusion therapy in the hope that the patient may go into remission.

Whenever possible, all drug therapy should be discontinued unless specifically indicated, as in the treatment of malignant diseases, including leukemia. Only in the case of heavy metals, such as gold, are measures directed toward increasing excretion of the toxic agent from the body likely to be helpful. The patient should be advised against coming into contact with organic solvents in any form and should take only those drugs specifically prescribed.

The general supportive measures required are determined by the severity of the pancytopenia. An ambulatory patient will often tolerate an anemia of 8 grams per deciliter, and therefore blood transfusion is indicated only when anemia is more severe than this or when hemorrhage or intercurrent infections result in fall in the hemoglobin concentration below this level. Blood should be given as packed cells which have been stored for less than seven days, and care should be taken in the cross-matching procedure, because it is not uncommon for the patient to develop group-specific antibodies and anti-leukocyte antibodies after receiving multiple transfusions. The risk of development of anti-leukocyte antibodies is minimized if reconstituted frozen red cells are available. Transfusion of platelet concentrates is indicated to control hemorrhagic complications when the platelet count falls to 10 to 20 $\times$ 10^9 per liter. If possible, platelets transfused should be blood group compatible; platelets can be shown to have improved survival if drawn from an HLA-compatible donor. The use of platelet transfusions is best reserved for control of serious thrombocytopenic bleeding, as the development of antibodies so often limits their effectiveness when given on a regular or prophylactic basis. When severe granulocytopenia is accompanied by blood-borne bacterial infections, transfusion of granulocytes obtained by using a white cell separator or by filtration techniques may enable an infection which is not responding to appropriate antimicrobial therapy to be brought under control. Granulocytes so prepared have a very short survival and therefore can only be used to combat serious infective complications.

Apart from these measures, meticulous care should be given to the acutely ill pancytopenic patient with regard to prevention of infection by scrupulous attention to aseptic techniques in setting up intravenous infusions, by regular four-hourly oral hygiene, and by protection of the skin, particularly at pressure points. At no time should intramuscular injections be given, because the hematoma at the site of injection impedes the absorption of a drug and greatly increases the risks of the introduction of infection at the injection site. The principal benefit of isolation procedures may be to constantly remind those looking after the patient of the risks of inappropriate procedures. Microbial cultures should be obtained from all infected lesions, and blood cultures should be performed whenever the patient's condition suggests a systemic infection. Antimicrobial therapy should be given after cultures have been taken and should be modified in the light of the sensitivity of the organisms cultured. It is not uncommon for patients with granulocytopenia to have serious infections with bacteria or fungi which in other circumstances would not be regarded as pathogens. Prophylactic administration of antimicrobial drugs is of doubtful benefit and may predispose to infection with resistant organisms.

There is little evidence that adrenal corticosteroids influence the degree of pancytopenia or the prognosis. Transient remissions have been documented, but these may reflect the natural history of the disease. Steroids may lessen the bleeding caused by thrombocytopenia and may occasionally reduce the fever in patients unresponsive to antimicrobial therapy. In view of uncertainty as to the beneficial effects of adrenal steroids, it may be warranted to give prednisone or prednisolone in a dose of 20 mg per day for a trial period of one or two months. The possible benefits of adrenal steroid administration must be weighed against the known side effects and the greater risk of bacterial infections. Likewise, there is no evidence that splenectomy is beneficial; it should be considered only after multiple blood transfusions associated with enlargement of the spleen and evidence that the survival of the transfused cells is significantly reduced. The immediate risks of hemorrhage and splenectomy have been reduced with increasing availability of platelet transfusions, but any benefit must be balanced against the risk of increased susceptibility to bacterial infections that have followed splenectomy, particularly when associated with persistent hematopoietic disorders.

A variety of drugs have been used to enhance the hematopoietic activity of the bone marrow. There is no evidence that administration of vitamin B$_{12}$ is of benefit; indeed, the fact that this has to be given as an intramuscular injection is a contraindication. Occasionally patients may become deficient in folic acid, but this is unlikely to take place if the patient is able to tolerate an adequate diet. Treatment with iron is contraindicated, because it will further add to the iron overload induced by multiple blood transfusions.

There is evidence in children that the combined use of

androgens and steroids in patients with constitutional aplastic anemia (Fanconi's anemia) or acquired aplastic anemia may be accompanied by partial or complete remission of the anemia, although the response of the granulocytes or platelets tends to be less satisfactory. Both in children and in adults several studies have suggested that androgen therapy does not influence the immediate or long-term prognosis. Nevertheless, in occasional patients with aplastic anemia convincing evidence has been presented of an androgen-dependent response of anemia and, to a lesser extent, of granulocytopenia and thrombocytopenia. It therefore seems reasonable to try androgen therapy for a period of three to six months in the hope that a partial remission may be induced or that transfusion requirements may be reduced. The oral synthetic testosterone oxymetholone (2 to 4 mg per kilogram per day) is the drug of choice, because it has fewer side effects than intramuscular injections of testosterone enanthate (3 to 10 mg per kilogram once a week). Liver function tests should be performed regularly on all patients receiving androgen therapy because cholestatic hepatitis may develop. In the absence of a remission in two or three months the drug should be discontinued, because the side effects of hepatotoxicity, fluid retention, hirsutism, clitoral enlargement, and pelvic discomfort in women do not justify their continued use.

Evidence that some patients who have received immunosuppression in preparation for bone marrow transplantation, and in whom graft rejection has taken place, but who have nevertheless gone into remission, has suggested that immunosuppressive therapy may be of benefit in patients with severe aplastic anemia refractory to all other modes of treatment. In one such patient the administration of cyclophosphamide (30 mg per kilogram per day intravenously for four days) was followed by a remission. These observations suggest that in patients refractory to more conventional treatment a trial with intravenous or oral cyclophosphamide (100 mg daily or on alternate days, depending on the severity of the pancytopenia) may be worth trying.

In patients with pure red cell aplasia and radiologic evidence of a thymoma, surgical excision of the thymic tumor has been associated with remission of approximately half the cases. These patients may benefit from the use of adrenal steroids, although the dose required to maintain a remission may be too high to be tolerated by the patient without producing serious side effects. The evidence that pure red cell aplasia may have an autoimmune basis has led to the use of immunosuppressive drugs, such as cyclophosphamide, and a few patients seem to have successfully responded to such treatment. It is thus worthwhile giving a course of treatment with this drug at a dosage which does not induce severe depression of the granulocyte or platelet counts. There is evidence that splenectomy is of benefit to patients with pure red cell aplasia.

PROGNOSIS.   The immediate prognosis is related to the severity of the pancytopenia and the degree of bone marrow aplasia. In patients with severe aplastic anemia as defined earlier, median survival is approximately four months. The initial survival may be improved with the increased availability of platelet and granulocyte transfusions and through the use of antimicrobial drugs in overcoming bacterial infections. Patients with less severe pancytopenia may survive for a number of years despite persistent anemia, granulocytopenia, and thrombocytopenia. Spontaneous or drug-induced remissions may take place and are most likely to be seen in patients with mild pancytopenia and moderate hypercellularity of the bone

marrow. Further studies of the role of lymphocytes in suppressing hematopoiesis with the bone marrow in culture in vitro may lead to improved selection of patients likely to respond to immunosuppressive therapy. Death usually results from infective or hemorrhagic complications. Hemosiderosis of the heart and liver may be a late sequel in patients requiring repeated blood transfusions.

Acensa, J., Pahura, R., Kagan, W., Hanesen, J., Moore, M., and Good, R.: Aplastic anemia: Evidence for an immune mechanism. Lancet, 1:669, 1976.

Azen, E. A., and Shahidi, N. T.: Androgen dependency in acquired aplastic anemia. Am. J. Med., 63:320, 1977.

Baran, D. T., Griner, P. F., and Klemperer, M. R.: Recovery from aplastic anemia after treatment with cyclophosphamide. N. Engl. J. Med., 295:1522, 1976.

Gill, P. J., Amare, M., and Larsen, W. E.: Pure red cell aplasia: Three cases responding to immunosuppression. Am. J. Med. Sci., 273:213, 1977.

Hoffman, R., Zanjani, E. D., Lutton, J. D., Zalusky, R., and Wasserman, L. R.: Suppression of erythroid-colony formation by lymphocytes from patients with aplastic anemia. N.Engl. J. Med., 296:10, 1977.

Lewis, S. M.: Aplastic anaemia. In Hardisty, R. M., and Weatherall, D. J. (eds.): Blood and its disorders. Oxford, Blackwell Scientific Publications, 1974, p. 1113.

Li, F. P., Alter, B. P., and Nathan, D. G.: The mortality of acquired aplastic anemia in children. Blood, 40:153, 1972.

Lynch, R. E., Williams, D. M., Reading, J. C., and Cartwright, G. E.: The prognosis in aplastic anemia. Blood, 45:517, 1975.

Storb, R., Prentice, R. L., and Thomas, E. D.: Marrow transplantation for treatment of aplastic anemia. An analysis of factors associated with graft rejection. N. Engl. J. Med., 296:61, 1977.

Storb, R., Prentice, R. L., and Thomas, E. D.: Treatment of aplastic anemia by bone marrow transplantation from HLA sibling donors. Prognostic factors associated with graft-versus-host disease and survival. J. Clin. Invest., 59:625, 1977.

Thomas, E. D., Buckner, C. D., and Storb, R.: Current status of bone marrow transplantation for aplastic anemia and acute leukemia. Blood, 49:671, 1977.

Tso, S. C., Chan, T. K., and Todd, D.: Aplastic anaemia: A study of prognosis and the effect of androgen therapy. Quart. J. Med., 46:513, 1977.

480.4.   SIDEROBLASTIC ANEMIA

M. C. Brain

The sideroblastic anemias are a heterogeneous group of disorders in which a normocytic or slightly macrocytic anemia is accompanied by ineffective erythropoiesis and defective hemoglobin synthesis, manifested by hypochromasia of a proportion of red cells in the peripheral blood, with the finding of *ringed sideroblasts* in the bone marrow. Ringed sideroblasts are nucleated red blood cell precursors, often showing defective hemoglobinization, which can be shown on iron staining to have a perinuclear ring distribution of iron-staining granules. The perinuclear distribution of the iron distinguishes this disorder from the increase in iron-staining granules which may be seen in megaloblastic anemias and in thalassemia. Electron microscopy has shown that nonferritin iron is located between the cristae of the perinuclear mitochondria. A distinction must be made between the normal accumulation of ferritin clumps in the cytoplasm of the developing erythroblast, which is associated with the finding of a few, rarely more than three, iron staining granules in the cytoplasm, and the iron-loaded mitochondria in sideroblastic anemia, in which 40 to 70 per cent of the normoblasts in the bone marrow are ringed sideroblasts. The presence of ringed sideroblasts may be suspected when basophilic granules are observed in hypochromic

TABLE 2. Sideroblastic Anemias: Classification

1. Primary
   a. Acquired sideroblastic anemia in adults (synonyms: chronic refractory anemia with sideroblastic bone marrow, refractory normoblastic anemia, sideroachrestic anemia, refractory sideroblastic anemia)
   b. Hereditary (sex-linked) sideroblastic anemia
2. Pyridoxine-responsive sideroblastic anemia
3. Secondary
   a. Sideroblastic anemia associated with rheumatoid arthritis, polyarthritis, carcinoma, myelofibrosis, leukemia, multiple myeloma, hereditary and acquired hemolytic anemias, malabsorption syndromes, or chronic alcoholism
   b. Drug-induced: isoniazid, cycloserine, and other antituberculous drugs
   c. Lead poisoning

erythroblasts in Romanovsky-stained preparations. Studies of heme and globin synthesis have demonstrated that the defective hemoglobin synthesis is due to failure of incorporation of iron into protoporphyrin to form heme. Increased levels of erythrocyte protoporphyrin may be found, and the defective hemoglobin synthesis observed in vitro can be corrected by the provision of heme. The sideroblastic anemias may be classified as in Table 2.

Primary acquired sideroblastic anemia is considered to be due to an acquired disorder of the heme synthetic pathway. It has been thought by some workers to be a variant of erythroleukemia, as a proportion of patients may subsequently develop either erythroleukemia or a subacute myeloid leukemia. Support for the hypothesis that it is a variant of preleukemia has come from the recognition of abnormalities in the activity of red cell enzyme unrelated to the heme synthetic pathway, suggesting that more than one abnormality in cellular function is present. Sideroblastic anemia may be one manifestation of a broader group of acquired dyserythropoietic anemias. This type of sideroblastic anemia occurs most frequently in men and women late in life, and has no distinguishing clinical features. Hereditary sex-linked sideroblastic anemia is a rare familial disorder transmitted as a sex-linked recessive abnormality. The precise metabolic defect is still incompletely understood and may be due to a defect in one of the enzymatic steps in the protoporphyrin synthetic pathway, leading to a deficiency in protoporphyrin or in heme synthetase, the enzyme responsible for the insertion of iron into protoporphyrin. Anemia occurs in early childhood and presents problems analogous to the chronic anemia caused by defective globin chain synthesis which characterizes thalassemic syndromes. However, it requires blood transfusions less commonly but, as in thalassemia, the chronic anemia and enhanced dietary iron absorption can lead to development of hemosiderosis of the liver and myocardium.

Pyridoxal phosphate functions as a coenzyme in the synthesis of delta-aminolevulinic acid, the product of the first synthetic step in porphyrin synthesis. Pyridoxal-responsive sideroblastic anemias may thus arise as an unexplained primary disorder; in alcoholism, in which the formation of pyridoxal phosphate from pyridoxine may be impaired; or as a consequence of isoniazid therapy, a drug which is a metabolic antagonist of pyridoxine. Sideroblastic anemia may also be due to pyridoxine deficiency as a complication of severe malabsorption syndromes. In patients in whom there is pyridoxal phosphate deficiency caused by ethanol ingestion, malabsorption, or drug antagonism, the anemia responds to the administration of physiologic concentrations of pyridoxal phosphate. Patients with acquired pyridoxine-responsive anemia not apparently caused by isoniazid ingestion or ethanol occasionally respond to pharmacologic doses of pyridoxine. The biochemical explanation for this is as yet unclear. Still other patients have been described who appear to respond to crude liver extract and may have a fundamental disorder of tryptophan metabolism. The sideroblastic anemia that results from lead poisoning is due to inhibition of delta-levulinic acid dehydrase and ferrochetalase (heme synthetase), important steps in heme synthesis.

The degree of anemia may vary but is usually in the range of 7 to 8 grams of hemoglobin, with a lowered mean cell hemoglobin concentration. The red cells may show a varying degree of hypochromasia, and not uncommonly there may be a dimorphic blood picture with a varying proportion of normochromic normocytic cells with hypochromic microcytic red cells. Macrocytosis and a moderate degree of poikilocytosis may be present. The red cells may contain Pappenheimer bodies, demonstrable as iron-containing siderocytes on iron staining. Basophilic stippling is a feature of lead poisoning. The absolute reticulocyte count is usually reduced. The leukocyte and platelet counts are usually normal. The plasma iron and transferrin saturation are either normal or high. As mentioned earlier, the diagnosis is made on examination of the bone marrow which shows erythroid hyperplasia, defective hemoglobinization, and increased iron both in the marrow fragments and in the developing erythroblasts. The erythroblasts may show megaloblastic features and the associated defective maturation of white cell precursors. These changes are usually indicative of an accompanying folate deficiency, which can be confirmed by finding a low serum folate level. Myelopoiesis is usually normal, although an increase in blast cells and early precursor cells of the myeloid series may point to an associated subacute myeloid leukemia.

It is not uncommon for acquired sideroblastic anemia in the adult to be confused with iron deficiency anemia, although the high serum iron and the presence of iron in the bone marrow preclude this diagnosis.

Treatment should be directed toward correcting a folate deficiency when it is present and vitamin B_{12} deficiency has been excluded. A trial of pyridoxine of 50 mg a day for two to four weeks is indicated. A variable response may take place to either folate and/or pyridoxine treatment. Patients have been reported who only respond to pyridoxal phosphate given parenterally. Blood transfusions may be required when the hemoglobin level falls to below 8 grams per 100 ml and when symptoms or complications caused by anemia are present. The blood transfusion requiements may increase and will tend to exacerbate iron overload. Iron treatment by any route is absolutely contraindicated. When sideroblastic anemia is due to a drug, removal of the agent or treatment with pyridoxine can result in complete recovery. Except in those patients in whom the anemia is associated with a subacute leukemia, the prognosis in terms of survival is good, although chronic anemia usually persists.

Cartwright, G. E., and Deiss, A.: Sideroblasts, siderocytes and sideroblastic anemia. N. Engl. J. Med., 292:185, 1975.

Catovsky, D., Shaw, M. T., Hoffbrand, A. V., and Dacie, J. V.: Sideroblastic anaemia and its association with leukaemia and myelomatosis: A report of five cases. Br. J. Haematol., 20:385, 1971.

Khaleeli, J. P., Keane, W. M., and Lee, G. R.: Sideroblastic anemia in multiple myeloma: A preleukemic change. Blood, 41:17, 1973.

Valentine, W. N., Konrad, P. N., and Paglia, D. E.: Dyserythropoiesis, refractory anemia, and "preleukemia": Metabolic features of the erythrocytes. Blood, 41:857, 1973.

White, J. M.: Haem and pyridoxine metabolism: The sideroblastic and related refractory anaemias. In Hardisty, R. M., and Weatherall, D. J. (eds.): Blood and Its Disorders. Oxford, Blackwell Scientific Publications, 1974, p. 798.

480.5. MYELOPHTHISIC ANEMIA

M. C. Brain

The term myelophthisic anemia is applied to those anemias accompanied by the presence of nucleated red cell precursors and immature white cells in the peripheral blood (leukoerythroblastic anemia) resulting from a disturbance in the microarchitecture of the bone marrow brought about by infiltration of the bone marrow by abnormal cells or progressive fibrosis of the bone marrow, as in myelosclerosis. The disorder occurs when the bone marrow is extensively invaded or replaced with leukemic cells, the plasma cells of multiple myeloma, metastatic carcinoma or sarcoma, Hodgkin's disease and other malignant lymphomas, infectious or noninfectious granulomas, or lipid storage cells. Carcinomas of the breast, lung, prostate, stomach, kidney, and thyroid and neuroblastomas are most frequently associated with metastatic infiltration of the bone marrow. Extramedullary hematopoiesis can often be demonstrated at necropsy and can give rise to massive enlargement of the spleen and liver in a patient with a chronic myelophthisic anemia such as myelosclerosis.

The anemia may be moderate to severe; the white blood cell count may be elevated or depressed; and the platelet count may be normal or increased, but is more commonly reduced. A degree of anemia is often unrelated to the extent of bone marrow infiltration, suggesting that there is a more fundamental disturbance of hematopoiesis than can be accounted for by the extent of bone marrow infiltration. Survival of red cells may be reduced.

The clinical manifestations are usually those of the underlying disease, although not infrequently a myelophthisic anemia may be the presenting feature in a patient with widespread metastasis from a small primary tumor which may itself have given rise to few symptoms or signs. Bone pain may be severe, and may be either generalized or localized to the site of pathologic fractures. Symptoms may arise from the severity of the anemia, and bleeding may be associated with the thrombocytopenia. In patients with widespread metastatic adenocarcinoma, activation of coagulation within the blood can contribute to the thrombocytopenia and may rarely be associated with a microangiopathic hemolytic anemia. Enlargement of lymph nodes and the liver may be a manifestation of the underlying malignant disease; enlargement of spleen usually reflects the duration of the anemia and the extent of extramedullary hematopoiesis.

Myelophthisic anemia should be suspected whenever nucleated red blood cell precursors are found in the peripheral blood in association with a normocytic anemia and in the absence of other obvious disorders of hematopoiesis. In patients with known malignant diseases, the apearance of nucleated red cells in the blood is highly suggestive of bone marrow infiltration. In patients with moderate anemia the red blood cells show few morphologic changes. The presence of teardrop cells is suggestive of myelofibrosis, and when anemia is marked there may be greater degrees of poikilocytosis, polychromasia, and basophilic stippling. The blood picture may be complicated by a concomitant hypochromic anemia resulting from iron deficiency, by gastrointestinal blood loss, or by macrocytosis caused by folate deficiency in myelofibrosis. The reticulocyte count may be normal or increased. The total leukocyte count is often elevated, and usually exhibits a left shift with the presence of myelocytes and metamyelocytes. The platelet count will vary with the extent of the disease; large and bizarre platelets and occasionally megakaryocytic nuclei may be seen. The diagnosis of myelophthisic anemia is made by the finding of abnormal cells in the bone marrow. Aspiration of this may be difficult or, indeed, unsuccessful, or at best may yield a specimen containing few or no fragments diluted with blood. Owing to the focal nature of the infiltration, a normal actively hematopoietic bone marrow may be obtained. Nevertheless, all the slides should be surveyed extensively for presence of malignant cells; not infrequently these are found in small groups. A needle or trephined biopsy of the bone marrow is very helpful in the assessment of hematopoiesis, the recognition of bone marrow infiltration, and the demonstration of an increase in reticulin and fibrosis by silver stains characteristic of myelofibrosis. Bone marrow aspiration and biopsy may have to be carried out at more than one site before the diagnosis can be made with certainty. The diagnosis of the cause of myelophthisic anemia depends upon the identification of the underlying disease. The differential diagnosis of myelophthisic anemia includes other disorders which can cause a leukoerythroblastic anemia. The blood picture in idiopathic myelosclerosis or agnogenic metaplasia is very similar. However, this disorder usually runs a slowly progressive course with marked or massive splenomegaly. Occasionally the onset is more acute with severe pancytopenia and a more rapid course, leading to the designation of such patients as having *acute* or malignant myelosclerosis. Both the acute and chronic forms of myelosclerosis are characterized by a marked fibrosis with dense reticulum fibers in bone marrow biopsies.

Treatment and prognosis depend upon the cause of the myelophthisic anemia. Improvement in the anemia and disappearance of the leukoerythroblastic anemia has been reported following the regression of metastatic malignant disease with treatment. In most patients myelophthisic anemia is a feature of the terminal phase of metastatic malignancy when blood transfusion and palliative therapy may be all that is warranted.

Eriksson, S., Killander, J., and Wadman, B.: Leuco-erythroblastic anaemia in prostatic cancer — report of two cases with complete haematological remission. Scand. J. Haematol., 9:648, 1972.

Laszlon, J.: Anemias associated with marrow infiltration. In Williams, W. J., Beutler, E., Erslev, A. J., and Rundles, R. W. (eds.): Hematology. 2nd ed. New York, McGraw-Hill Book Company, 1977.

Wintrobe, M. M., Lee, G. R., Boggs, D. R., Bithell, T. C., Athens, J. W., and Foerster, J.: Secondary forms of myelofibrosis. In Clinical Hematology. 7th ed. Philadelphia, Lea & Febiger, 1974, p. 1786.

481. HYPOCHROMIC ANEMIAS

Elmer B. Brown

481.1. IRON DEFICIENCY ANEMIA

DEFINITION. Iron deficiency anemia occurs when the supply of iron is inadequate to support optimal erythropoiesis. In its fully developed form it is characterized by hypochromia and microcytosis of the circulating erythrocytes, low plasma iron, low transferrin saturation, and marked depletion of bone marrow and other body iron stores.

PREVALENCE. Throughout the world iron deficiency is almost certainly the most common cause of anemia. In parts of Africa and Asia, where marginal dietary intake and excessive iron loss owing to intestinal parasites occur together, more than 50 per cent of the population may suffer from iron deficiency anemia. Variable figures of the incidence of iron deficiency have been reported from surveys in temperate countries. Reasons for variation include the criteria used for detecting borderline iron deficiency as well as the nature of the population sampled in terms of age, sex, economic status, and local environmental factors. Fewer than 3 per cent of men are affected in most population surveys; 10 to 30 per cent of all women may show signs of iron deficiency; and 10 to 60 per cent of pregnant women and infants in the first year of life have iron deficiency anemia. Much more information is needed to define precisely the prevalence of iron deficiency in representative geographic and socioeconomic cross sections of the United States.

IRON METABOLISM. Iron is essential to human life because of its central role in the heme molecule that permits oxygen and electron transport. Every cell in the body contains some iron.

Distribution. The body's iron can be divided into two main compartments: (1) an essential, functional component composed of hemoglobin, myoglobin, enzyme and cofactor iron, and plasma transport iron, and (2) a nonessential storage component made up predominantly of ferritin and hemosiderin, not required for health but providing a reserve of iron readily mobilizable into the essential functional compartment in time of need.

In the normal adult man there is about 50 mg of iron per kilogram of body weight, approximately 80 per cent of which is in the functional compartment and 20 per cent in a storage form. Women, with a reduction in red cell mass and hemoglobin concentration as well as smaller iron stores, have a body iron concentration of about 40 mg per kilogram. Total body iron ranges between extremes of 2 and 6 grams in small women and large men. These differences are reflected in the amount and percentage distribution of iron in the body (Table 1). Approximately 85 per cent of the functional iron in the body is present in the red blood cells as hemoglobin, which contains 0.34 per cent iron by weight. Divalent iron in each of the four disc-shaped heme groups carefully positioned in the pocket of coiled globin chains binds oxygen reversibly for transport to all tissues. Oxidation of the iron to the ferric

state (as in methemoglobin) causes hemoglobin to lose its capacity to carry oxygen. Myoglobin, one fourth the size of hemoglobin and with one iron atom per molecule, accounts for about 15 per cent of the functional iron. It is present in concentrations of 0.9 to 2.2 mg per gram dry weight of human muscle; cardiac muscle contains consistently less myoglobin than skeletal muscle. Myoglobin functions as a reservoir of oxygen for muscle metabolism. A small but extremely important component of body iron is that bound to transferrin. Approximately half of the transferrin iron is in extravascular tissue fluids while a more easily measured fraction is circulating in the plasma in transit from sites of hemoglobin destruction, iron absorption, or storage depots to the bone marrow and other areas of utilization. Lactoferrin, an iron-binding protein of milk, mucosal tissues, and leukocytes, is similar to transferrin structurally but appears to function in the body's defense against bacterial infection by binding iron essential to bacterial growth. Iron present as an integral part of various enzymes or as a cofactor constitutes a small but important part of the functional iron compartment. Iron enzymes may be classified as heme-proteins (cytochromes a, a_3, b, b_5, c, c_1, P-450, cytochrome c oxidase, catalase, peroxidases, tryptophan pyrrolase, lipoxidase, and homogentisic oxidase) and iron-flavoproteins cytochrome c reductase, NADH dehydrogenase, xanthine oxidase, succinate dehydrogenase, and acyl CoA dehydrogenase). Iron as an essential cofactor is required by aconitase, ribonucleotide reductase, and succinic dehydrogenase. Most of these enzymes function as reversible donors or acceptors of electrons and are critical to the metabolism of every cell in the body.

Nonessential storage compounds that account for the remaining body iron are ferritin and hemosiderin. Ferritin, composed of a large, water-soluble, crystalline protein surrounding micelles of iron (up to 20 per cent by weight), is a ubiquitous compound found in many tissues of the body but predominantly in liver parenchymal cells and reticuloendothelial cells of the liver, spleen, and bone marrow. Hemosiderin is a water-insoluble protein with higher concentrations of iron (up to 35 per cent by weight) that is readily identified by Prussian blue staining of tissues. Since the iron in

TABLE 1. Distribution of Iron in the Body

Compartment	Iron Content (grams)		Fraction of Total Body Fe (%)	
	Men	Women	Men	Women
Functional				
Hemoglobin	3.050	1.700	71.8	73.5
Myoglobin	0.430	0.300	10.1	13.0
Enzymes	(?) 0.010	0.010	0.2	0.4
Transferrin	0.008	0.006	0.2	0.2
Subtotal	3.498	2.016	82.3	87.1
Storage				
Ferritin-hemosiderin	0.750	0.300	17.7	12.9
Total	4.248	2.316	100.0	100.0

Values are based on data from various sources. Assumptions include a body weight for men of 80 kg, blood volume of 70 ml per kilogram, and Hgb of 16 grams per deciliter; for women the values used were a weight of 55 kg, blood volumes of 65 ml per kilogram, and Hgb of 14 grams per deciliter.

these compounds is readily mobilizable for use by the essential functional iron compounds, there is wide variation in their amounts and percentage of total body iron.

Absorption. Iron absorption assumes great importance in human iron metabolism, because iron balance is regulated by controlled absorption rather than by excretion. Despite intensive investigation, many facets of the mechanism and control of iron absorption remain unexplained or controversial. Current information suggests that iron entering the stomach in various organic compounds of food is digested to soluble ferric salts that may be either reduced to ferrous ions or chelated in either the ferrous or ferric valence state to maintain stability and promote absorption. The presence of hydrochloric acid in the stomach is not essential for iron absorption, although an acid milieu prevents the formation of insoluble complexes of ionized iron. Other unidentified iron-stabilizing substances in gastric secretions — possibly mucoproteins — promote iron absorption. Entry of iron at the brush border of mucosal cells appears to be mainly by passive diffusion; exit from the cells to the plasma transferrin probably requires metabolic energy for active transport. Most of the iron destined to enter the bloodstream traverses the mucosal cell rapidly in the form of small molecules. Attempts to identify specific mucosal iron carrier substances have been unsuccessful. Likewise, efforts to identify subcellular fractions in the sequence of iron transfer across the mucosal cell have added little to our understanding of the precise process of iron absorption. Older theories implicating mucosal ferritin as a carrier of iron and the key to regulation of iron absorption through a "mucosal block" mechanism have been abandoned. The small quantities of ferritin in intestinal mucosal cells appear to function as a storage compound to accept a proportion of iron in excess of the rapid transport capacity. The ferritin is then lost when the cells are desquamated at the end of their three- to five-day life span. Luminal factors modifying the form in which iron is presented to the mucosal cell play an important role in the amount of iron that can be absorbed. Sugar, sorbitol, cysteine and other amino acids, ascorbic and succinic acids, mucoproteins, and various other components of the dietary constituents or intestinal secretions tend to stabilize iron in a soluble form and to promote iron absorption. Phytates, phosphates, carbonate, oxalate, pancreatic bicarbonate, and gastroferrin bind iron as relatively insoluble complexes and decrease iron absorption. The means by which the body's need for increased or decreased iron absorption is transmitted to the mucosal cell have not been completely defined. Multiple signals, including mucosal cell iron concentration, local hypoxia, tissue iron stores, rate of erythropoiesis, plasma transferrin saturation, plasma iron turnover, and humoral factors, have been suggested, but without compelling evidence for any precise mechanism.

Measurement of iron absorption has progressed from the tedious and cumbersome dietary iron balance studies to the use of radioactive iron with determination of unabsorbed iron in the feces, absorbed radioactivity in the circulating red blood cells, or total body radioiron using sensitive whole body counters. Studies of iron absorption can be divided conveniently into two groups: (1) those using simple iron salts such as ferrous sulfate or ferric chloride which give information applicable to the behavior of iron given therapeutically; and (2) those measuring the absorption of iron from foods.

Ferrous salts are better absorbed than ferric compounds, and various agents such as ascorbic and succinic acids and sorbitol enhance iron absorption. Other substances such as phytates, phosphates, and various antacid preparations bind iron and diminish its absorption. Maximal absorption occurs in the duodenum and upper jejunum where the villous surface is maximal and in which the luminal contents are acid or neutral; there is progressively less absorption distally from a more alkaline environment, although the potentiality for some iron absorption exists throughout the length of the gut from the stomach to the rectum. Iron absorption from mucosal cells is via intestinal capillaries with little lymphatic participation, and is virtually complete within several hours after ingestion. Uptake of iron is undirectional without any back-flux except for iron lost into the gut lumen by desquamation of mucosal cells. There is no enterohepatic circulation. Small doses of iron are absorbed from the duodenum by an active process; with large doses of iron, passive diffusion occurs. Increasing the ingestion of simple iron salts results in increasing absorption of iron until toxicity becomes the limiting factor. Conditions associated with increased iron absorption include iron deficiency, hemolytic and sideroblastic anemias, hypoxia, cobalt and erythropoietin administration, hemochromatosis, cirrhosis and portacaval shunts, some types of pancreatic insufficiency, and the later stages of pregnancy. Decreased iron absorption is present in patients with iron overload, erythroid hypoplasia, generalized malabsorption states, malignant, infectious, and inflammatory diseases, and achlorhydria.

Less information is available about the absorption of food iron. Attempts have been made to classify the "availability" of iron in various foods by its release after incubation in digestion mixtures or by its ability to increase hemoglobin formation in anemic animals or human subjects. These efforts have been relatively unsuccessful. Radioactive iron biosynthetically incorporated into various foods or added as a simple salt to dietary food mixtures has allowed comparison of dietary iron absorption with that of simple iron salts. From these studies it was learned that heme iron is absorbed differently from various nonheme iron compounds in the diet. Heme is taken up by the mucosal cell where the porphyrin ring is split open to make iron available to the body. Heme iron absorption is not influenced by dietary composition (ascorbic acid, phytates, or phosphates) as is the case with nonheme iron compounds. Furthermore, the nonheme iron compounds of food behave as a single pool in their absorption characteristics and can be labeled with a single radioiron salt. ^{55}Fe labeling of heme (intrinsic tag) and $^{59}FeCl_3$ for labeling of nonheme vegetable components (extrinsic tag) have allowed the precise measurement of the absorption of complex dietary iron mixtures. Results of this type of study indicate that iron in meat (primarily heme) is better absorbed (12 to 20 per cent) than iron from vegetable sources (primarily nonheme) (Fig. 1). Iron from vegetable sources is absorbed to a variable extent — about 1 to 7 per cent of usual doses in a meal — with substances such as phytates accounting for the diminished absorption. Rice and spinach are at the lower end of the absorption scale, whereas wheat and soybean iron are better absorbed. When mixtures of foods ap-

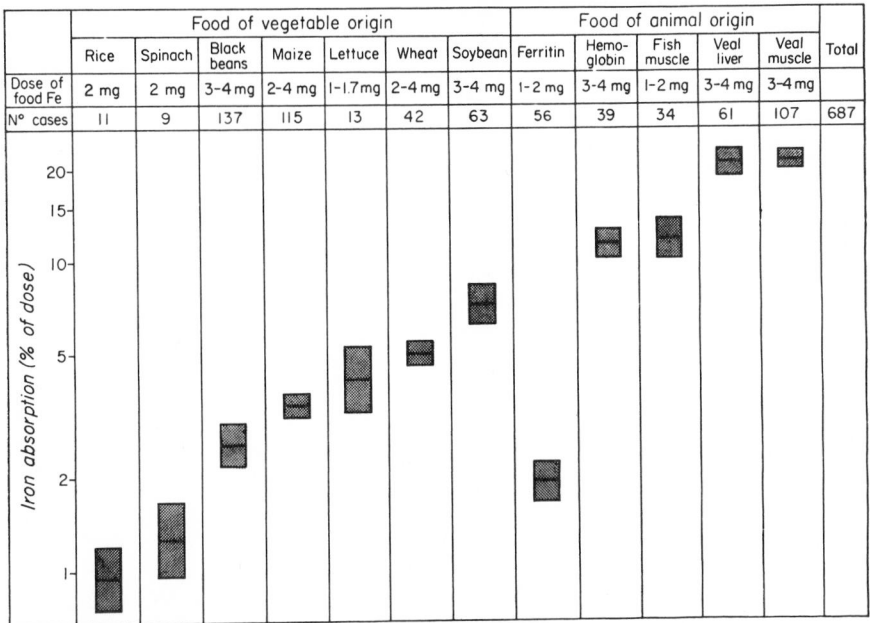

	Food of vegetable origin							Food of animal origin					Total
	Rice	Spinach	Black beans	Maize	Lettuce	Wheat	Soybean	Ferritin	Hemo-globin	Fish muscle	Veal liver	Veal muscle	
Dose of food Fe	2 mg	2 mg	3-4 mg	2-4 mg	1-1.7mg	2-4 mg	3-4 mg	1-2 mg	3-4 mg	1-2 mg	3-4 mg	3-4 mg	
N° cases	11	9	137	115	13	42	63	56	39	34	61	107	687

Figure 1. Iron absorption from food biosynthetically labeled with radioactive iron. (From Layrisse, M., *In* Kief, H. [ed.]: Iron Metabolism and Its Disorders. Amsterdam, Excerpta Medica, 1975, p. 26.)

proximating these of usual diets are given, the percentage of iron absorption from the total mixture is similar to that of the least well-absorbed vegetable source, except for the heme component whose absorption is uninfluenced by other dietary components. Of importance in the consideration of food iron supplementation to prevent iron deficiency is the finding that diets containing foods with little heme (meat) and with a predominance of poorly absorbed vegetable iron sources, such as rice, impart their poor iron absorbability to the supplementary iron salt irrespective of the compound used.

Transport. Iron is transported in plasma bound to a specific carrier protein, transferrin. This β-globulin of about 80,000 molecular weight is synthesized in the liver and has an eight- to ten-day half-time in plasma; the 7 to 15 grams present in the body is almost equally distributed in the extravascular and intravascular spaces, with plasma concentrations varying from 215 to 350 mg per deciliter. At least 19 genetic variants have been described, but all that have been studied appear to be identical in their iron-binding properties. Transferrin can bind two atoms of ferric iron per molecule in the presence of carbonate or bicarbonate. Binding of iron to transferrin receptor sites is a random process in vitro, and there is no exchange of iron from one molecule to another. The two iron-binding sites on the transferrin molecule differ in their uptake and release of iron in vitro. Whether these differences are important in the delivery of iron to various tissues in vivo remains controversial. Measurement of functional iron-binding capacity rather than direct determination of transferrin is employed clinically. Iron is present in equal amounts in plasma and serum; normal values range from 60 to 160 μg per deciliter, with a mean of 120 for men and 110 for women. Plasma transferrin is normally about one third saturated and the total plasma iron-binding capacity is 280 to 400 μg per deciliter. Plasma iron shows a diurnal variation, with morning values about 30 per cent higher than those in the eve-

ning. Menses, exercise, or normal meals have no appreciable effect on plasma iron concentrations. Highest concentrations are seen during reproductive years in both sexes, with a modest decline in old age. Variations in plasma iron and iron-binding capacity are seen in a variety of disorders, as illustrated in Figure 2.

Small amounts of ferritin of low iron concentration circulate in plasma and can be measured by sensitive immunoradiometric assays. The origin and function of plasma ferritin are obscure; its contribution to plasma iron transport is uncertain. Normal values range from 12 to 250 μg per liter, with a mean of 123 for men and 56 for women. The concentration of plasma ferritin is less than 10 μg per liter in iron deficiency, whereas in iron overload high values are proportional to increased tissue iron storage.

Ferrokinetics. Since the pioneering studies of the

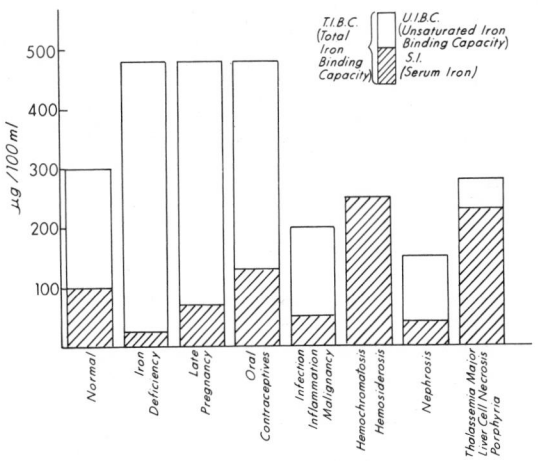

Figure 2. Representative serum iron and iron-binding capacity values in a variety of conditions.

kinetics of iron transfer were published by Huff and coworkers in 1950, there have been many refinements in technique that have added much to the precision of measurement and the complexity of mathematical analysis, but little to the clinical interpretation of ferrokinetic data. Measurement of plasma radioiron clearance and erythrocyte utilization are simple, useful tests available to any clinician with access to radioisotope facilities. If more sophisticated interpretation of deranged iron metabolism in a variety of diseases is desired, computer evaluation of prolonged plasma iron disappearance curves and external monitoring over liver, spleen, and sacrum are needed. By this type of analysis a number of compartments with various rates of iron interchange can be identified with analyses too complex for routine use. However, useful basic information is obtained by measuring the rate of disappearance of radioactive iron bound to plasma transferrin after intravenous injection and its subsequent incorporation into circulating erythrocytes 7 to 14 days later (Figs. 3 and 4). Plasma radioiron disappearance, measured at 10- to 15-minute intervals and plotted semilogarithmically, is linear with a half-time of disappearance normally between 60 and 120 minutes. More rapid disappearance rates (shorter half-time values) are found in iron deficiency and conditions with increased erythropoiesis such as polycythemia vera and hemolytic anemias. Slow rates of radioiron disappearance indicate erythroid hypoplasia from various causes. By extrapolating the plasma iron disappearance line back to zero time, one may obtain a close estimate of plasma volume by dividing the total count rate of the injected radioiron by the count rate at time zero. Calculation of the plasma iron turnover rate (PITR) requires only the additional measurement of plasma iron concentration. The formula for this calculation is shown at the bottom of this page. The PITR reflects changes in two variables, the size of the plasma iron pool and the rate of disappearance of ^{59}Fe from plasma. Normal values of PITR range from 25 to 40 mg per day. Increased PITR is observed in patients whose plasma radioiron disappearance is rapid and whose plasma iron values are normal or increased, e.g., hemolytic states and ineffective erythropoiesis with values four to ten times normal. Decreased PITR is seen in some patients with hypoplastic anemias, infection, or uremia or after irradiation when slow plasma radioiron disappearance rates are combined with normal or low plasma iron values. In iron deficiency anemia, in which there is rapid radioiron disappearance and low plasma iron values, the PITR is usually normal.

Measurement of the utilization of radioiron incorporated into hemoglobin of red cells during the one to two weeks after a plasma radioiron clearance study provides valuable information about the effective production of erythrocytes compared to total erythropoiesis reflected by the PITR. Iron utilization is calculated from the radioactivity in 1 ml of packed red cells multiplied by the red cell volume (calculated from the previously determined plasma volume and the hematocrit) divided by the count rate of injected radioiron, and is expressed

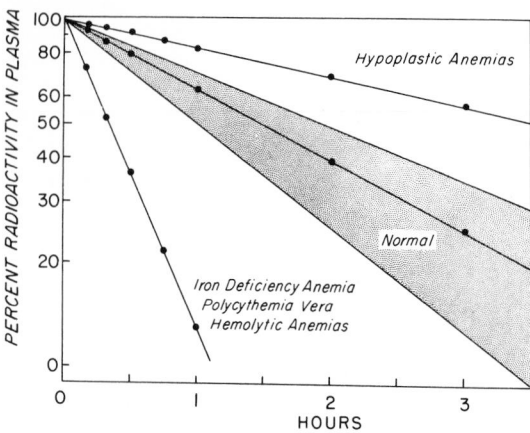

Figure 3. Plasma radioiron disappearance curves for normal subjects and for patients with increased and decreased erythropoiesis.

in percentage terms. Normally 70 to 90 per cent of the injected radioiron can be accounted for in circulating cells two weeks after injection. Decreased radioiron utilization reflects decreased erythropoiesis with extreme reductions in aplastic anemia. Radioiron utilization to levels slightly above the normal range occurs sooner in iron deficiency or polycythemia. Complex intermediate curves reflecting rapid red cell production and destruction may be seen in various hemolytic anemias.

Storage. Iron in excess of the needs for hemoglobin, myoglobin, and essential intracellular enzymes is stored as ferritin and hemosiderin. Major sites of storage iron are hepatic parenchymal cells, reticuloendothelial cells of the bone marrow, liver, and spleen, and a poorly defined store in skeletal muscle. The immediate source of most reticuloendothelial iron stores is hemoglobin iron conserved from the breakdown of red cells at the end of their life span. Hepatic parenchymal iron comes from plasma transferrin. Accurate measurement of diffusely distributed iron stores is difficult. Qualitative estimates are usually based on histochemical appraisal of bone marrow or liver hemosiderin deposits. More quantitative estimates can be obtained from measurement of iron excreted into the urine after injections of deferoxamine or other chelating agents; chelate iron mobilization correlates closely with the amount of iron mobilized by phlebotomy before iron deficiency anemia supervenes. Minute amounts of ferritin circulating in plasma are related to the amount of iron stores, and plasma ferritin measurement provides another means of determining body iron stores. One μg per liter of plasma ferritin is equivalent to approximately 8 mg of storage iron. Estimates of storage iron in normal adults have decreased in recent years to an average in men of 750 mg (range 200 to 1400 mg) and an average in women of 300 mg (range 60 to 500 mg). Approximately 65 per cent of storage iron is normally in the form of ferritin; the remainder is hemosiderin. In disorders of iron overload the proportion of hemosiderin increases progressively. Both storage forms are readily mobilized

$$\text{PITR (mg/day)} = \frac{0.693}{^{59}\text{Fe T/2 (hrs)}} \times \text{mg Fe/ml plasma} \times \text{plasma vol (ml)} \times 24 \text{ hrs}$$

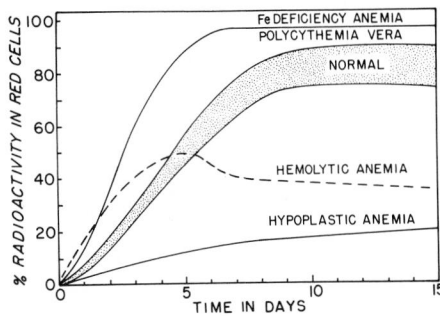

Figure 4. Patterns of radioiron utilization in peripheral erythrocytes for normal subjects and for patients with various disorders with increased or decreased erythropoiesis.

in response to need such as bleeding. Regulatory mechanisms controlling the buildup and mobilization of iron stores are poorly understood. Mobilization is frequently interfered with by infection, inflammation, and malignancy.

Excretion. The body has a limited capacity to excrete iron except by means of hemorrhage. Normally, excretion balances absorption, because most of the iron released from hemoglobin of senescent red blood cells is conserved and reutilized. Total daily excretion amounts to slightly less than 1 mg for men and postmenopausal women. Of this amount approximately 0.1 mg is excreted in the urine, and about 0.6 mg in the feces from mucosal cell desquamation, bile, and small amounts of blood loss; the remainder is lost from skin as desquamated cells and in sweat. Approximately 0.5 mg of iron is present per milliliter of blood. With normal menstrual blood losses of 25 to 60 ml monthly, this normal bleeding accounts for an additional 12 to 30 mg of iron lost monthly, or 0.4 to 1.0 mg per day, in women during their reproductive years. Iron loss occurs in pregnancy and delivery in amounts totaling more than 500 mg. Obligatory daily iron losses are about 50 per cent less than normal in patients with iron deficiency anemia.

Requirements. Since iron absorption must balance excretion for the body's iron stores to stay in balance, one may construct a table of iron requirements for different physiologic states (Table 2). In addition to the exceptional stresses on iron balance imposed by menstrual losses and pregnancy, one must also add the needs related to growth. These needs of iron to build hemoglobin, myoglobin, and other intracellular iron compounds are greatest at growth spurts of infancy and adolescence. An increment of 0.5 mg per day is an acceptable estimate in the absence of precise measurements.

These requirements of iron to meet special circumstances can be translated into terms of nutritional iron intake to prevent a negative balance from occurring. Assuming that absorption of iron from food mixtures normally averages about 10 per cent, the figures for dietary iron intake can be derived (Table 2). Iron concentrations of foods in most Western diets are related to calories, with about 6 mg of iron per 1000 calories. Although iron absorption may increase to about 20 per cent with the onset of iron deficiency, it is obvious that pregnant women can hardly eat enough food to provide for their markedly increased iron needs and that they, with many menstruating women and adolescent girls, are likely to fall behind in meeting dietary iron needs.

PATHOGENESIS. Iron deficiency develops because of one or a combination of the following factors: inadequate dietary iron intake, malabsorption, blood loss, or repeated pregnancies. Since excretion of iron is limited, assigning the cause of iron deficiency in adults to inadequate intake or malabsorption implies chronicity measured in years. More important are iron losses which occur most often from the gastrointestinal tract of men and from abnormal menstrual bleeding in women. A convenient way to consider these causes of iron deficiency is to divide them into two categories — low intake and high output.

Low Intake. Restrictions of dietary iron because of economic, religious, or cultural considerations lead to iron deficiency in many parts of the world. Economic and religious factors weigh heaviest in underdeveloped nations, whereas in the United States one might cite the inadequate meals of weight-conscious young women and mothers caught up in the harried pace of rearing children. In old age, absent or ill-fitting dentures combined with apathy, inactivity, and financial restrictions reduce the intake of foods with high iron nutritive value. Continual refinement and cleanliness of our food supplies combined with the use of noniron cooking vessels may have the undesired effect of reducing our iron intake. Assimilation of iron is often reduced owing to interaction of phytates from cereals, phosphates, and other substances in the foods we eat. Malabsorption of iron rarely if ever occurs as an isolated absorptive defect, but is present in sprue syndromes and is associated with iron deficiency. (Surprisingly, the steatorrhea of pancreatic insufficiency allows normal or even increased iron absorption.) Abnormal gastrointestinal motility secondary to gastrectomy or to a variety of causes for diarrhea is usually associated with decreased iron absorption. Patients with achlorhydria have inefficient absorption of food iron, and cannot increase iron uptake effectively when they become iron deficient.

High Output. Identification of the site of blood loss responsible for high output iron deficiency may be quite difficult. One reason for this difficulty is that increased menstrual blood loss, the single most common cause of iron deficiency in temperate countries, is often not recognized, and is difficult to quantitate. The best estimates of the frequency and extent of menorrhagia in randomly selected women indicate that the normal menstrual flow (25 to 60 ml) is exceeded in about 20 per cent of women, with occasional blood losses as high as 500 ml per month.

TABLE 2. Estimated Dietary Iron Requirements

	Absorbed Iron Requirement, mg/Day	Daily Food Iron Requirement,* mg/Day
Normal men and nonmenstruating women	0.5–1.0	5–10
Menstruating women	0.7–2.0	7–20
Pregnant women	2.0–4.8	20–48†
Adolescents	1.0–2.0	10–20
Children	0.4–1.0	4–10
Infants	0.5–1.5	1.5 mg per kg‡

*Assuming 10 per cent absorption.
†This amount of iron cannot be derived from diet and should be met by iron supplementation in the latter half of pregnancy.
‡To a maximum of 15 mg.

Unfortunately, predictions of menstrual loss by the patient's account of the number and saturation of tampons and sanitary napkins and the number of days of flow are only partially successful. Contraceptive pills of the combined estrogen-progesterone type reduce menstrual blood loss by 50 to 60 per cent, whereas intrauterine devices tend to increase menstrual blood loss. Iron loss associated with pregnancy is easier to estimate and totals about 500 mg. Unless iron supplementation is provided, repeated pregnancies are almost invariably accompanied by iron deficiency.

Blood loss from the alimentary tract is frequently occult and intermittent, and may elude careful search with a battery of sophisticated techniques. In a recent study no demonstrable source of blood loss could be found in 16 per cent of patients with gastrointestinal bleeding. In those whose bleeding could be explained, the cause was hemorrhoidal bleeding in 10 per cent, salicylate ingestion in 8 per cent, peptic ulceration and hiatus hernia in 7 per cent each, diverticulosis in 4 per cent, neoplasm in 2 per cent, and a sprinkling of additional cases of esophageal varices, hemorrhagic gastritis, regional enteritis, ulcerative colitis, hemorrhagic telangiectasia, and intestinal polyps. Hookworm and other intestinal parasites are important causes of blood loss and iron deficiency in many countries. Blood donation — which must be specifically inquired about — doubles the amount of iron that must be absorbed when only three pints are removed per year. Blood removed for diagnostic studies from patients undergoing prolonged or repeated hospitalization is a cause for iron deficiency that can easily be overlooked. Rare causes of excess iron loss include the hemosiderinuria from chronic intravascular hemolysis of paroxysmal nocturnal hemoglobinuria and cardiac prostheses, and the iron that is trapped in the lungs of patients with pulmonary hemosiderosis. One cannot overemphasize the dictum that iron deficiency anemia in the adult man and the postmenopausal woman is due to blood loss until proved otherwise.

The sequence of changes in slowly developing iron deficiency is fairly predictable. Initially iron stores in reticuloendothelial and parenchymal cells are mobilized to provide for functional iron needs. When demands for functional iron cannot be met from the stores, a signal of some sort is transmitted to the intestine to increase iron absorption. Transferrin concentration increases while the plasma iron concentration falls as demands of the bone marrow exceed the supply of iron released from senescent erythrocytes and intestinal absorption. Anemia appears when the supply of iron restricts erythropoiesis. Distorted cells reflecting skipped divisions and hypochromic cells reflecting insufficient iron for heme synthesis gradually replace the normal cells of the circulating blood. Later, increased cell division or more severe maturation defects lead to microcytosis and dyserythropoiesis of the fully developed iron deficiency anemia. The extent of the depletion of cell enzyme iron is variable in different tissues sampled in man, and little is known of the rate of these changes.

CLINICAL MANIFESTATIONS. Iron deficiency anemia is accompanied by a wide diversity of symptoms. Some patients have no awareness of ill health despite marked anemia which may be recognized by chance examinations. Symptoms usually appear insidiously, and their onset is difficult to date. The gradual development of iron deficiency often allows remarkable adaptation, and may permit strenuous work with few symptoms. At the other extreme, marked tiredness, easy fatigability, dyspnea on exertion, palpitations, headache, irritability, paresthesias, lightheadedness, and other vague symptoms may trouble patients with borderline or mild anemia.

Examination usually discloses pallor, although on casual observation this finding may not be noticed. A peculiar greenish appearance of the skin of young girls, vividly described by careful observers before 1900 and termed chlorosis, has mysteriously disappeared. Vitiligo is a rare skin change in blacks. Angular stomatitis — most marked in edentulous patients — frequent papillary atrophy, and varying degrees of glossitis comprise the oral lesions associated with iron deficiency. Dysphagia resulting from postcricoid esophageal webs or strictures, associated with hypochromic anemia and achlorhydria, and most frequently seen in middle-aged women — the Paterson-Kelly or Plummer-Vinson syndrome — is rare in the United States, but is fairly common in the British Isles and Scandinavia. Whether this syndrome is due to iron deficiency or some associated disorder is not known. Multiple gastrointestinal complaints, such as anorexia, pyrosis, flatulence, nausea, eructation, and constipation, are common in association with iron deficiency. Occasionally bizarre cravings for cornstarch, ice, clay, and other substances may appear. These forms of pica are especially common in iron-deficient black women, but probably have a worldwide distribution. Gastritis, which is reversible after iron therapy, and permanent gastric atrophy have been described in numerous gastroscopic investigations of iron-deficiency patients. Whether these gastric lesions are cause or effect of iron deficiency is debatable. Spoon nail (koilonychia) is the most advanced abnormality of the nails and is becoming very rare. Often, milder nail changes such as thinning, brittleness, lusterless appearance, longitudinal ridging, and flattening accompany prolonged iron deficiency, and are associated with depletion of cysteine in the nails. The frequent suggestion that these epithelial changes are related to the severity or chronicity of iron deficiency anemia may be questioned because of their virtual absence in patients with severe, lifelong iron deficiency owing to hookworm infestation. An attractive but unproved hypothesis is that the epithelial changes may reflect a chronically depressed intake of iron (and possibly other substances) rather than chronically increased loss of iron from bleeding.

Severe anemia often leads to cardiac dilatation, the occurrence of hemic murmurs, and, in older patients, the development of congestive heart failure. Enlargement of the spleen to slightly below the costal margin is observed in about 10 per cent of patients, and recedes after treatment. Claims of aggravation of menorrhagia by iron deficiency anemia and improvement after treatment are difficult to substantiate. Numbness and tingling without objective neurologic abnormalities are reported by about 25 per cent of patients. Extremely rare are the papilledema and increased pressure of cerebrospinal fluid that may be confused with intracranial tumors. Infants often show marked irritability and present difficulties in feeding.

LABORATORY FINDINGS. A number of laboratory procedures facilitate the identification of iron deficiency anemia. A well-stained blood film shows small erythrocytes (microcytosis) poorly filled with hemoglobin (hypochromia) with marked variation in size (anisocytosis) and shape (poikilocytosis). Mean corpuscular volume is less than 80 fl, and mean corpuscular hemoglobin concentration is less than 30 grams per deciliter. Since the introduction of the Model S Coulter electronic counter into many hematology laboratories, the mean corpuscular hemoglobin concentration in iron deficiency anemia has been observed to be in the low normal range. The explanation for this seems to be that the volume of the erythrocytes, calculated from their number and degree of interference with the electrical field across the aperture through which they pass, is different from that measured by packing in a high speed centrifuge. Erroneous estimates of packed cell volume occur because of increased plasma trapping between distorted iron-deficient cells. Thus to identify iron deficiency, the key measurement to note in the printout of the Model S Coulter Counter is the mean cell volume. Plasma iron concentration is usually less than 80 μg per deciliter, associated with a total plasma iron-binding capacity of more than 400 μg per deciliter. Transferrin saturation (the product of plasma iron divided by total iron-binding capacity multiplied by 100) is 15 per cent or less. Plasma ferritin concentration is less than 10 μg per liter. Examination of bone marrow particles shows normoblastic erythroid hyperplasia; sideroblasts and hemosiderin in macrophages are absent when the marrow particles are stained for iron. Defective heme synthesis is associated with elevated erythrocyte protoporphyrin concentration and decreased plasma bilirubin. Reticulocytes are present in normal numbers except for elevations secondary to recent hemorrhage. Erythrocyte osmotic fragility is decreased, reflecting the diminished hemoglobin concentration. The life span of erythrocytes is usually normal, although shortened survival has been reported. Thrombocytosis in the range of one million platelets per cubic millimeter, or, less often, thrombocytopenia, both of which return to normal after iron therapy, may be observed. Abnormalities of the leukocytes are rare and are usually confined to slight leukopenia and occasional hypersegmented neutrophils. Unfortunately there is no practical laboratory test to measure depletion of tissue enzyme iron.

TREATMENT. The two objects of treatment of iron deficiency anemia are (1) to replace the blood and tissue iron deficits, and (2) to recognize and, if possible, correct the underlying cause. Despite the vast array of therapeutic preparations containing iron, simple ferrous salts (ferrous sulfate, ferrous gluconate, and ferrous fumarate) given by mouth remain the mainstay of treatment for iron deficiency anemia. Large doses of ascorbic or succinic acid will increase iron absorption but only to a small extent that hardly warrants the extra expense. The addition of other substances found in "shotgun" mixtures such as copper, cobalt, molybdenum, intrinsic factor, and various B vitamins is of no benefit. The use of these shotgun hematinics must be condemned, because they may obscure the correct diagnosis as indicated by a response to iron alone; further, they encourage sloppiness in diagnosis, and they are unnecessarily expensive. Enteric-coated and delayed-release iron preparations are poorly designed to exploit the fact of maximal absorption in the upper gastrointestinal tract. All too often their delay in iron release serves to dump the metal in the lower intestine, in which absorption is greatly diminished. When iron medication is prescribed in tablet form, the physician should warn the patient to keep the tablets out of reach of small children to reduce the danger of severe iron intoxication. Suitable warnings on the label and the use of child-proof containers will further reduce this risk.

A total daily dose of iron in the range of 180 to 240 mg provides for maximal rates of hemoglobin regeneration in adults. Three or four tablets of ferrous sulfate (60 mg of

elemental iron) or ferrous fumarate (66 mg of iron) provide the requisite daily dose. Ferrous gluconate, with only 36 mg of elemental iron per tablet, requires a dosage of six tablets per day. These iron preparations are given in equal doses with or after meals and with a snack at bedtime. The advantage of increased absorption of iron salts taken on an empty stomach is often overweighed by the undesirable side effects of gastrointestinal irritation.

Approximately one patient in ten will experience unpleasant side effects such as nausea, epigastric pain, abdominal cramps, diarrhea, or vomiting of sufficient severity to require discontinuation of treatment. No effective iron preparation is free from causing gastric or intestinal irritation. Gastric symptomatology is dose dependent, and may be minimized by a gradual buildup of the iron dose during the first three days of treatment. A few patients are completely unable or unwilling to take iron by mouth; patience and understanding on the part of the physician can keep this group small. Treatment with iron should be continued for four to six months and even longer in the face of recurrent bleeding. Restoration of iron stores to provide a buffer against recurrent iron deficiency is a slow process.

Infants and toddlers are best treated with liquid iron preparations. Infants should receive a total of 60 to 90 mg of iron daily in water or fruit juices. Ferrous sulfate is available in concentrated drops containing 15 mg of iron per 0.6 ml, as a syrup with 30 mg of iron per 5 ml, or as an elixir with 44 mg of iron per 5 ml. Transient staining of the teeth by liquid iron preparations can be prevented by using a dropper or a straw. Most children weighing 35 to 75 pounds can satisfactorily take iron tablets in half the adult dosage; larger children usually receive adult doses of iron.

Response to adequate doses of iron given to a patient with iron deficiency anemia is quite predictable (Fig. 5). An initial sense of well-being is often observed within 48 hours. This improvement appears to be more than a psychologic effect from taking medications, as infants often lose their irritability and begin to eat better. Because this response occurs before any change in blood values is measurable, it has been attributed, without any real evidence, to replenishment of some vital cellular iron compound. The height of the reticulocyte peak and the rate of hemoglobin regeneration are proportional to the severity of the anemia; maximal daily rates of hemoglobin regeneration are 0.3 gram per deciliter.

Failure to respond to iron given by mouth should call forth the following considerations: (1) the patient failed to take the iron as prescribed; (2) the patient did not have iron deficiency anemia, and re-evaluation of the diagnosis is necessary; (3) blood loss exceeded new blood formation; (4) intercurrent infection, inflammation, or malignancy interfered with the response to iron; (5) the patient was unable to absorb the iron; and (6) an ineffective iron preparation was administered.

Parenteral administration of iron should be reserved for the following indications: (1) patients with malabsorption syndromes; (2) the relatively small group of patients who are unable or unwilling to take iron by mouth, including some people with ulcerative colitis, regional enteritis, and colostomies; (3) selected patients who prove unreliable in taking their prescribed iron; and (4) some patients with chronic uncorrectable bleeding with iron loss in excess of that which can be replaced by the oral route. Two satisfactory preparations are available for parenteral use. Both iron dextran (Imferon) and iron sorbitex (Jectofer) contain

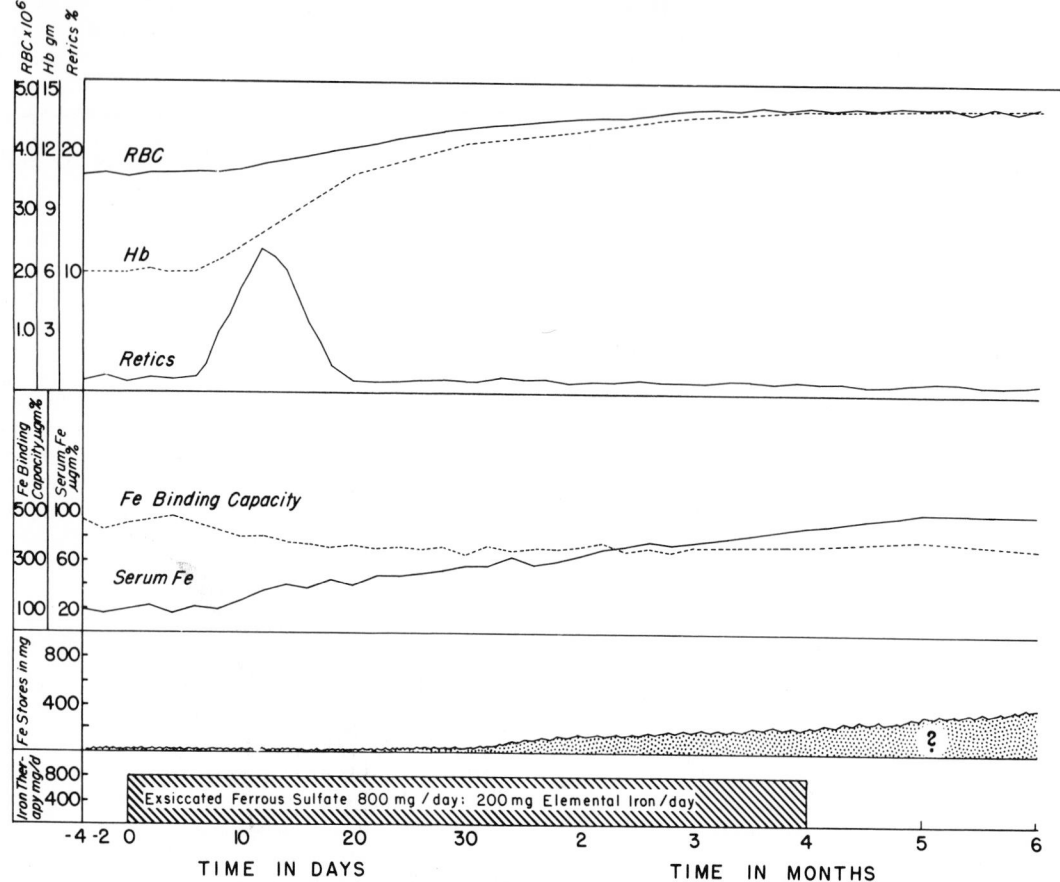

Figure 5. Schematized response to iron therapy. Reticulocytes begin to rise about the fifth to seventh day after iron therapy is started, reach a peak between the tenth and fourteenth days, and then fall to normal levels. Hemoglobin level begins to increase on about the seventh to tenth day. From four to eight weeks are required before normal values are attained. No accurate data are available to describe the reappearance of storage iron; its reaccumulation may be slower than shown; hence the question mark.

50 mg of iron per milliliter. Iron sorbitex should be administered only by intramuscular injection, but iron dextran can be given by either the intramuscular or the intravenous route. The technique of deep intramuscular injections is important. The skin at the injection site (preferably the buttock) should first be displaced laterally before the needle is inserted into the muscle, so that reflux of the dark brown iron solution along the injection path, causing skin staining, can be prevented. After a test dose of 0.5 ml, 2 to 5 ml doses are given daily into alternate extremities until a calculated total dose is administered. Intravenous injection of iron dextran is reserved for patients in whom insufficient muscle mass or the discomfort of massive and prolonged intramuscular therapy precludes the intramuscular route. Usually iron dextran is injected undiluted in a dose of 2 to 5 ml per day, although the total dose may be diluted in 250 to 1000 ml of isotonic saline and infused during a two-hour period without untoward reactions. Dosage is calculated by the following formula: Normal Hgb (grams per deciliter) − patient's Hgb × 0.255 = iron dose in grams. This formula provides sufficient iron to replace the circulating hemoglobin deficit plus a 50 per cent excess for creation of tissue stores. Side effects such as local pain, lymphadenitis, headache, dizziness, fever, urticaria, arthralgias, myalgias, and hypotension occur in about 5 per cent of patients; rare fatal anaphylactic reactions have been reported. Urine that turns black on stand-

ing and urinary irritation may occur after injections of iron sorbitex, because one third of the dose is excreted into the urine, a fact that should be considered in total dose calculations.

Preventive iron therapy for groups prone to develop iron deficiency (infants, pregnant women, and blood donors) requires special consideration. Fortification of foods with iron salts seems a reasonable and fairly effective way to improve the iron intake of infants. Iron enrichment of bread remains a hotly debated subject both in terms of its efficacy in preventing iron deficiency of groups at special risk and in terms of risks of eventual iron overload in other groups. Pregnant women should be given iron during the last half of pregnancy, after the early period of "morning sickness" that might erroneously be attributed to the iron tablets and influence the patient's subsequent willingness to take this medication. One tablet of ferrous sulfate (60 mg of iron daily) is sufficient to provide for the extra iron needs of pregnancy. For repeated blood donors the dose of iron will depend on the rate of donation — one to three tablets daily may be required.

PROGNOSIS. Prognosis in iron deficiency can only be applied to the underlying disorder causing the anemia. A vastly different prognosis is expected in a patient with a bleeding carcinoma of the alimentary tract and another with hemorrhoids. Patients rarely die of iron deficiency anemia itself, but they often die of the underlying cause.

Recurrence of iron deficiency anemia after treatment is common; one third of women and one fourth of men have a recurrence in extended follow-up studies. These recurrence rates emphasize the importance of identifying and correcting the cause of iron deficiency.

Bothwell, T. H., and Finch, C. A.: Iron Metabolism. Boston, Little, Brown & Company, 1962.
Committee on Iron Deficiency: Iron deficiency in the United States. J.A.M.A., 203:407, 1968.
Fairbanks, V. F., Fahey, J. L., and Beutler, E.: Clinical Disorders of Iron Metabolism. New York, Grune & Stratton, 1971.
Gross, F. (ed.): Iron Metabolism — An International Symposium. Berlin, Springer-Verlag OHG, 1964.
Halberg, L., Harwerth, H.-G., and Vanotti, A. (eds.): Iron Deficiency. Pathogenesis, Clinical Aspects, Therapy. New York, Academic Press, 1970.
Harris, J. W., and Kellermeyer, R. W.: The Red Cell. Production, Metabolism, Destruction: Normal and Abnormal. Cambridge, Mass., Harvard University Press, 1970.
Moore, C. V.: Iron nutrition and requirements. Scand. J. Haematol. (Series Haematologica), 6:1, 1965.
Williams, W. J., Beutler, E., Erslev, A. J., and Rundles, R. W. (eds.): Hematology, 1977. New York, McGraw-Hill Book Company, 1977.
Wintrobe, M. M.: Clinical Hematology. 7th ed. Philadelphia, Lea & Febiger, 1974.

481.2. HYPOCHROMIC ANEMIAS NOT CAUSED BY IRON DEFICIENCY

Hypochromic anemia occurs predominantly when hemoglobin synthesis is interfered with out of proportion to defects in erythrocyte proliferation. Biosynthetic abnormalities have been identified at one or more stages of protoporphyrin synthesis, iron incorporation into the heme ring — the prime defect in iron deficiency anemia — or globin synthesis. Compared to iron deficiency anemia, these disorders of hemoglobin synthesis are rare. As a group they can be differentiated from iron deficiency anemia by increased body iron stores with increased hemosiderin in marrow particles, the presence of sideroblasts and siderocytes, and increased plasma iron and transferrin sautration. Special distinguishing features are included with the following list of these disorders. (1) By far the most common of the hypochromic anemias not caused by iron deficiency are thalassemia and its variants resulting from interaction with abnormal hemoglobins. The basic defect is in the synthesis of globin chains. Thalassemia and its variants can be distinguished from iron deficiency by hemoglobin electrophoresis and detection of elevated levels of hemoglobins A_2 and F. (2) Homozygous Hgb-C disease and Hgb-S-D are hypochromic anemias readily identified by appropriate hemoglobin electrophoresis. (3) Sideroblastic anemias can be subdivided into congenital, acquired, and pyridoxine-responsive categories. They share the common features of disordered heme synthesis with prominent ringed sideroblasts observable on iron staining of bone marrow particles. Electron microscopy discloses the siderotic granules to be diffuse iron aggregates in the intercristal spaces of mitochondria surrounding the nucleus of an erythrocyte precursor. Abnormalities in tryptophan metabolism and partial improvement of the anemia after pyridoxine or crude liver extract administration, as well as a high rate of leukemic transformation, have been reported in this group of disorders. (4) Chronic lead intoxication produces a hypochromic anemia resulting from defective hemoglobin synthesis. Stippling of erythrocytes and abnormal urinary excretion of coproporphyrin and aminolevulinic acid distinguish this disorder from iron deficiency, although in young children whose lead poisoning is due to pica of lead-based paint the two disorders may coexist. (5) Inadequate delivery of iron from plentiful stores to the marrow for hemoglobin synthesis has been observed in rare instances, such as in a child with congenital absence of transferrin, in pulmonary hemosiderosis, and in older people with an unexplained block in the release of iron from reticuloendothelial sites of hemoglobin catabolism.

Williams, W. J., Beutler, E., Erslev, A. J., and Rundles, R. W. (eds.): Hematology. 2nd ed. New York, McGraw-Hill Book Company, 1977.
Wintrobe, M. M.: Clinical Hematology. 7th ed. Philadelphia, Lea & Febiger, 1974.

Section Two HEMOLYTIC DISORDERS

482. INTRODUCTION

Wendell F. Rosse

By "hemolytic anemia" is meant the clinical state in which the life span of the red cell in the circulation is curtailed and the cell is destroyed before its usual 90 to 120 days of survival. The shortening of the red cell life span may be due to a variety of causes, and hemolytic anemia should be considered a symptom and not a diagnosis. As such, a reason for its presence must be sought.

The causes of hemolysis are many and can be classified in a number of ways. A simple categorization (see accompanying table) divides them into those which are congenital and those which are acquired. Those which are congenital in general result in an intrinsic (intracorpuscular) defect in the red cell which, either of itself or in conjunction with some environmental modification, leads to the premature destruction of the cell. These defects are of the membrane, of the contained hemoglobin, or of the enzyme systems responsible for internal homeostasis of the cell.

The acquired causes of hemolysis are usually not due to an intrinsic abnormality (the exceptions are the acquired dysplastic membrane alterations) but rather are due to some alteration of the initially normal red cell by extrinsic (extracorpuscular) factors. Such factors include antibodies, toxins, altered metabolites, and altered hemodynamics leading to fragmentation. These acquired factors are usually ultimately derived from some "exogenous" cause, which may or may not be known. In some cases, the "exogenous" cause may be another definable disease. For instance, immune hemolytic ane-

Classification of Hemolytic Disorders

I. Hemolytic anemia due to congenital abnormalities
  A. Membrane defects
    1. Spherocytosis
    2. Elliptocytosis
    3. Stomatocytosis
  B. Enzyme deficiencies
    1. Defect in Embden-Meyerhof pathway of glycolysis
      a. Hexokinase
      b. Glucose phosphate isomerase
      c. Phosphofructokinase
      d. Fructosediphosphate aldolase
      e. Triosephosphate isomerase
      f. Diphosphoglyceromutase
      g. Phosphoglycerate kinase
      h. Pyruvate kinase
    2. Deficiency in enzyme activity related to the hexose monophosphate shunt pathway
      a. Glucose-6-phosphate dehydrogenase
      b. Phosphogluconate-dehydrogenase
      c. Glutathione reductase
      d. γ-Glutamyl-cysteine synthetase
      e. Glutathione peroxidase
  C. Hemoglobinopathies—qualitative defect in alpha or beta chains of globin
    1. Aggregating hemoglobins (S, C, D, I)
    2. Unstable hemoglobins (Zürich, Köln, etc., with Heinz body formation)
  D. Thalassemias—quantitative deficiency in synthesis of alpha or beta chains (may be combined with qualitative defect)
  E. Other types
    1. Low ATP concentration
    2. High ATP concentration
    3. ATPase deficiency
    4. Erythropoietic porphyria
    5. Increased red cell lecithin
II. Hemolytic anemia due to acquired abnormalities
  A. Immunologic alteration of the membrane
    1. Warm-reacting antibodies
      a. Alloimmune
        (1) Transfusion reactions
        (2) Hemolytic disease of newborn
      b. Autoimmune
    2. Cold-reacting antibodies
      a. Cold agglutinin syndrome
      b. Paroxysmal cold hemoglobinuria
    3. Drug-induced antibodies
  B. Traumatic alteration of the membrane
    1. Microangiopathic—intravascular clotting hemolysis
    2. Cardiac valvular hemolysis
    3. March hemoglobinuria
  C. Dysplastic alteration of the membrane
    1. PNH
    2. Other myelodysplasias
  D. Chemical alteration of the membrane
    1. Drugs
    2. Poison and toxins
      a. Venoms
      b. Vegetable toxins
    3. Metabolic products and abnormalities
      a. Liver failure
      b. Hypophosphatemia
    4. Infectious agents and products
      a. Parasitism of the red cell
      b. Clostridial infections
      c. Other infections
  E. Hemolysis due to abnormal sequestration of normal red cells by the reticuloendothelial system
    1. Hypersplenism
    2. Histiocytic medullary reticulosis

mia is often seen in patients with systemic lupus erythematosus or chronic lymphocytic leukemia. In other cases, the cause may be iatrogenic, as in drug-induced hemolysis and fragmentation hemolysis caused by heart valve prosthesis.

Thus when considering the causes of acquired hemolytic anemia, due care must be taken to consider other disease syndromes which may be causally related to the hemolytic process.

Whatever the cause of hemolysis, the erythropoietic elements of the bone marrow may be able to increase the rate of red cell production to compensate for the diminution in the life span so that the hematocrit is not decreased; such a state is called *compensated hemolytic anemia*. On the other hand, the maximal erythropoietic activity of the normal bone marrow (about 6 to 10 times the normal erythropoietic activity) may be insufficient to compensate for the degree of red cell destruction, or the erythropoietic potential of the bone marrow may be curtailed by a wide variety of causes, e.g., lack of elements necessary for erythropoiesis, replacement of the bone marrow by nonerythropoietic elements. The hemolytic anemia is then *uncompensated*. Both the amount of red cell destruction and the degree of the resulting anemia are highly variable.

CLINICAL SYNDROMES. In general, the clinical syndromes which result from hemolysis will vary somewhat according to the cause of the process. There are, however, certain elements common to all anemias and some specific to hemolytic anemias. As in anemia of any cause, the patient may exhibit a variable degree of fatigue, weakness, pallor, and, if the anemia is severe, cardiovascular compromise, including orthostatic hypotension, tachycardia, and faintness. Many patients with hemolytic anemia have mild jaundice. Since the spleen is the prime organ of destruction of red cells, it is not infrequently increased in size. Other signs and symptoms specific to specific causes of hemolytic anemia will be discussed subsequently.

LABORATORY SIGNS. The laboratory indications of hemolysis reflect primarily the results of hemolysis and secondarily the results of the compensating increased erythropoiesis. In actual fact, the latter set of signs is the more useful in the initial appreciation of the presence of hemolysis. Reticulocytosis and erythroid hyperplasia of the bone marrow are both valuable clues, particularly when blood loss and recovery of the marrow from injury are not the cause of the increased red cell production.

The reticulocyte count should be interpreted in the light of the degree of anemia and of knowledge concerning life span of this young red cell. Erythropoiesis is controlled so that the degree of marrow hyperplasia is as commensurate as possible with the need for additional red cells. Thus for very low hematocrit and hence very great need, maximal erythroid hyperplasia results. For lesser need, lesser hyperplasia is called for. Thus the reticulocyte count should be higher for the more severely anemic than for the less severely anemic patient.

Normally, the reticulocyte exists for four days, from the time the nucleus is ejected until the disappearance of the last remnant of intracellular material which will identify the red cell as a reticulocyte. Two of these days are spent in the marrow, one in the spleen, and one in the circulation. Since the normal red cell survives about 100 days, the normal reticulocyte count represents the daily input of new cells into the circulation. However, when the marrow is working overtime to compensate for anemia, the reticulocyte is not allowed to spend two full days in the marrow. It enters the circulation shortly after the ejection of the nucleus and, in severe cases, even before the nucleus is ejected. This results in an increase of the time a reticulocyte spends in the circulation, with the result that the reticulocyte count may be disproportionately high for the number of cells delivered to the circulation.

As noted above, hemolytic anemia may be accompanied by an inability of the marrow to respond with maximal erythropoietic activity. In this case, the reticulocyte count may be much lower than one would expect for the degree of anemia, and relative marrow hypoplasia, as well as hemolysis, may contribute to the anemia.

Examination of the peripheral blood may reveal red cells which are distinctive for particular causes of hemolysis. These include the distinctive *sickle cells* of sickle cell anemia; *schistocytes*, which are cell fragments in such shapes as helmets or triangles, and which possess sharp points at the site of fragmentation; *spherocytes*, which are small cells lacking in central pallor; *acanthocytes*, which are small crenated cells with irregular projections on the surface; *target cells*, red cells somewhat larger than normal with a spot of hemoglobin in the center of the area of pallor; and *Heinz body–*containing cells, which show, with special stains, membrane-associated globules of denatured hemoglobin. The reasons for each of these morphologic abnormalities will be apparent in the discussion of the specific syndromes. It is important to remember that many patients with hemolytic anemia will not have red cells with a characteristic morphology.

Specific signs of hemolysis largely result from the extracellular presence of hemoglobin or its catabolic products. Although overt hemoglobinemia does not occur often, evidence that some hemoglobinemia occurs is almost always present; this is manifest by a diminution of the *serum haptoglobin*, the protein which binds hemoglobin in the serum and delivers it to the liver. This diminution is the result of the catabolism of the hemoglobin-haptoglobin complex. When the level of hemoglobin in the plasma exceeds the capacity of haptoglobin to bind to it, hemoglobinuria may result. Hemoglobin is absorbed in the proximal tubule of the kidney and is there catabolized to hemosiderin, which may also appear in the urine. If all the filtered hemoglobin is reabsorbed, hemosiderinuria without hemoglobinuria will result. Such instances of overt hemoglobinuria are usually present in the so-called "intravascular" forms of hemolysis. Hemoglobinuria is then frequently accompanied by increase in the serum *lactic acid dehydrogenase* (LDH), with a predominance of the fast-moving isoenzyme band.

The heme of hemoglobin is catabolized to bilirubin and carbon monoxide. In the presence of a normally functioning liver, small increases in unconjugated bilirubin may occur during excessive hemolysis. The total body hemoglobin, the capacity of the liver to conjugate bilirubin, and the rate of hemolysis all determine the degree of elevation. With a normally functioning liver, the level seldom rises above 3.5 to 4 mg per cent, even in severe hemolysis. When liver function is deranged, even by such minor anomalies as Gilbert's syndrome, the level of bilirubin may rise strikingly. The urinary and fecal catabolites of bilirubin (e.g., urobilinogen, stercobilin) are of little value in assessing the presence of hemolysis. Detailed studies of bilirubin metabolism may be used to demonstrate the excessive production of these hemoglobin catabolites, but these studies are not practical for clinical use.

During the catabolism of a molecule of heme, one molecule of carbon monoxide is evolved; this is the only source of this compound in the body. Techniques have been evolved which measure the endogenous production of carbon monoxide and relate that to the rate of destruction of heme. These tests are relatively simple and have the advantages of requiring no radioisotopes and being performed in a single day. They have the disadvantage that ineffective erythropoiesis (destruction of cells prior to their circulation) also results in the release of carbon monoxide, and carbon monoxide from this source cannot be distinguished from that due to hemolysis.

The most definitive means of demonstrating hemolytic anemia is measurement of the red cell life span. This is most often done by labeling the red cells with chromium-51 and reinjecting them. The rate of disappearance of the isotope from the blood is assessed over a period of 5 to 15 days. Normally, half of the chromium will have disappeared from the blood in 24 to 30 days. If hemolysis is present, this is shortened. At the same time one may assess the sequestration of the labeled cells in the spleen by counting the radioactivity over that organ and comparing it to that of other parts of the body. This may identify the spleen as a site of destruction.

Other isotopic methods (e.g., diisopropylfluorophosphate [^{32}DFP], glycine-2-^{14}C) have been used to study the red cell life span; they are less practical than the ^{51}Cr technique.

DIAGNOSIS OF THE CAUSE OF HEMOLYTIC ANEMIA. Once the presence of hemolysis has been established, there remains the need to determine its cause. There are many reasons for premature destruction of the red cells (see table), so that care and perspicacity must be used to try to decide why the patient has hemolytic anemia.

The following series of questions may be useful in unraveling the cause of hemolysis in a given patient:

1. Is the hemolysis recent in onset, or did it occur at an early age? Is there a family history of such hemolytic episodes? If there is evidence that the patient had hemolysis for a long period of time, particularly if during childhood, and if there is a family history of anemia, the cause is more likely to be an intrinsic defect of the red cell. If the hemolysis is acquired and has a definable time of onset, it is more likely to be an extrinsic defect.

2. Does the patient belong to an ethnic group which has a high incidence of hemolytic anemia? The incidence of glucose-6-phosphate dehydrogenase deficiency and hemoglobinopathies among blacks and thalassemia among Greeks and Italians is sufficiently high to merit consideration of these causes in these patients, particularly if there is any corroborating evidence.

3. Does the patient have any other condition commonly associated with hemolytic anemia? Patients with chronic lymphocytic leukemia or systemic lupus erythematosus frequently have immune hemolytic anemia. Patients with heart valve replacement frequently have fragmentation hemolysis. Patients taking certain drugs may have hemolysis because of the drug. Many further examples could be cited. Thorough knowledge of these associations is useful in diagnosing the cause of hemolytic anemia.

4. Does the patient have a spleen sufficiently large to account for the hemolysis? Is the enlargement due to the hemolytic process or some other cause?

5. Are there distinctive red cells present in the pe-

ripheral blood? Some of these are described above. Ability to look at the blood film knowledgeably is important in the diagnosis of hemolytic anemia.

6. Is there evidence of a major component of intravascular hemolysis, such as hemoglobinuria? The syndromes which result in hemoglobinuria are relatively few and include paroxysmal nocturnal hemoglobinuria, paroxysmal cold hemoglobinuria, rarely other forms of immune hemolysis, transfusion reactions, and fragmentation hemolysis.

When all else fails and no clues are perceived, then it is unfortunately necessary to proceed directly to the laboratory tests without much guidance.

Although the answers to the questions posed above may give clues to the diagnosis of hemolytic anemia, it is usually necessary to verify or clarify a suspicion with laboratory tests. In general, the tests selected should be guided by the hypotheses which result from analysis of the answers to the questions. For instance, if spherocytes are present on the blood film, one may wish to perform the osmotic fragility test to verify their presence, as well as the direct antiglobulin (Coombs) test and autohemolysis tests to distinguish immune hemolytic anemia and hereditary spherocytosis.

When no clues are given by the aforementioned considerations, then a series of screening tests must be performed. The number and identity of these may vary from physician to physician; the list offered here is the one used by the author:

1. The direct antiglobulin (Coombs) test.
2. Hemoglobin electrophoresis at pH 8.6 and pH 6.8.
3. Glucose-6-phosphate dehydrogenase and pyruvate kinase screening tests.
4. Ham (acidified serum lysis) test for paroxysmal nocturnal hemoglobinuria.

If the answer is not given by the results of these tests, then the cause of the hemolytic anemia is probably rare and unusual, and its detection will be outside the purview of the general internist and perhaps even the expert hematologist.

THERAPY OF HEMOLYTIC ANEMIA. The correct therapy of hemolytic anemia depends upon its cause. For this reason, the search for the cause is of the greatest importance. Other than the ensuing anemia, no effects from the hemolysis itself result, except in hemolytic disease of the newborn, in which the accumulation of unconjugated bilirubin, caused both by the effects of hemolysis and by the inability of the liver to conjugate well, results in the accumulation of unconjugated bilirubin in the plasma. This may cross the blood-brain barrier, injuring certain structures of the nervous system (particularly the basal ganglia) and causing permanent damage, a syndrome called *kernicterus*. In the adult, the liver is able to conjugate bilirubin sufficiently well that the total quantity of unconjugated bilirubin seldom rises above 5 mg per cent unless there is an abnormality of liver function. Further, the adult brain is not subject to damage by unconjugaged bilirubin.

Transfusion. Transfusion may be necessary if the anemia becomes sufficiently severe as to interfere with physiologic processes. Since surgery and pregnancy provide additional strain upon the circulatory system, patients with chronic hemolytic anemia undergoing these may require transfusion. As in other forms of anemia, one should be guided by physiologic needs rather than absolute values of hematocrit or hemoglobin.

When the hemolysis is due to "autoimmune" disease, compatibility testing prior to transfusion may be difficult because the patient's serum frequently contains an antibody which will react with cells of many potential donors. The danger of transfusion in these cases lies not in the incompatibility with the autoantibody but in the possibility of simultaneous presence of an alloantibody which may be present in sufficiently high concentration to result in a severe hemolytic reaction. These problems should be investigated thoroughly, and every attempt should be made to give the safest transfusion possible. However, it must be borne in mind that often no completely compatible blood may be found and yet transfusion may be lifesaving.

Splenectomy. The spleen is thought to be one of the normal sites of destruction of red cells. Neither the exact signal given for the destruction of the effete red cell nor the mechanism by which it is destroyed is known. Some have proposed that reduction in surface sialic acid content may be responsible; others have suggested that autoantibodies may arise to coat the aging cells.

The spleen is also the site of entrapment of cells which are not deformable. This is brought about by the peculiar filtering mechanism of the lining of the splenic sinuses. The fenestrations in this lining are only 3 to 5 μ across; red cells must deform in order to penetrate these fenestrations. If they cannot, they are trapped behind in the cords of Billroth.

Those cells which contain inclusions that are themselves not deformable may be trapped behind these fenestrations. Thus Howell-Jolly bodies (chromosomal remnants present in the red cell after the nucleus has been ejected) are picked out by spleen through this sieving mechanism. Anyone lacking splenic function will have these small inclusions. Heinz bodies, which are masses of denatured hemoglobin, may form in certain types of hemolytic anemia; these are usually picked out by the spleen but may persist if made in excessive numbers. Certain intracellular remnants, such as iron-containing Pappenheimer bodies, mitochondria, and remnants of the ribosomes responsible for hemoglobin formation, are not picked out by the spleen.

The normal spleen entraps a small proportion of the normal red cells going through its interstices. When the spleen becomes enlarged, the proportion of red cells sequestered there may be markedly increased. As a result of their entrapment, they may undergo metabolic changes which lead to their destruction; these metabolic changes may be due to hypoxia, decreased glucose, or other undefined abnormalities as the result of the static circulation. Thus hemolysis may result from what is called anatomic hypersplenism. The causes of the enlarged spleen which results in this syndrome are many, including portal hypertension, lymphoma, mild proliferative disorders, and infectious disease.

Cells which are less deformable than normal are likewise not able to penetrate the fenestrations of the wall of the sinus. The reticulocyte membrane is less deformable than the normal membrane and is trapped in the spleen for approximately one day of its total life span. Since the reticulocyte normally circulates for a single day in the peripheral blood, removal of the spleen will thus double its circulating life span and double the reticulocyte count without an increase in the delivery of cells to the periphery (see above).

The red cells in many forms of hemolytic anemia are less deformable than normal. Often, this is the result of shape change such as the spherocytosis seen with hereditary spherocytosis and autoimmune hemolytic anemia. Occasionally a change in shape is accompanied by changes in the internal viscosity of the cells, as in sickle cell disease. In other instances, there may be abnormalities in deformability of the membrane caused by conditions such as hypophosphatemia.

A function of the spleen apparently involves initiation of immune reactions. As the result of its filtering action, bacteria are filtered from the blood. These bacteria are then processed, and initial antibody formation occurs. It has been shown in some animals that splenectomy abrogates ability to mount a primary response to intravascular organisms. These same animals are, however, able to mount a response to antigens from bacteria injected subcutaneously and thus primarily processed by regional lymph nodes. Thus it is felt that patients who have undergone splenectomy are at some risk of attack by blood-borne organisms. This is particularly true in the young, presumably because of the importance of the spleen in mounting primary immune responses. Since the spleen appears to be functionally incompetent at a very early age in patients with sickle cell disease, this is thought to play a role in the great proportion of deaths attributable to pneumococcus and *Hemophilus influenzae*. The threat of overwhelming sepsis apparently diminishes rapidly after five to ten years of age, and, although occasionally adults are subject to the same problem, particularly those who have compromised immunologic systems from other diseases, the incidence is clearly less than in splenectomized children.

For these reasons, there has been a controversy over the danger of splenectomy in hemolytic anemia in childhood. Most authorities now agree that it is best to postpone splenectomy until at least five years of age if possible. When splenectomy must be performed before that time, and perhaps even afterward, parenteral vaccination with antigens of the pneumococcus should be given.

The spleen is also a site of brief entrapment for platelets and provides a reservoir which apparently is readily accessible for these important elements. Following splenectomy, particularly when anemia persists, there may be a striking increase in the total platelet count. This may be temporary as the body readjusts by its usual homeostatic mechanisms, or it may persist. Although it has long been felt that this may be harmful in that it could lead to thromboses, more recent observations suggest that in fact it is relatively harmless, in contrast to the thrombocytosis in the myeloproliferative disorder essential thrombocythemia. The difference lies in the degree of thrombocytosis (rarely over 1 to 1.5 million in secondary thrombocytosis, frequently higher in thrombocythemia) as well as in abnormalities of the platelets in patients with essential thrombocythemia.

Splenectomy itself is a relatively benign operation unless the spleen is of massive size. Great care should be taken to prevent abscess formation, atelectasis, and other complications. The effects of splenectomy can be beneficial, but its use should be judicious.

483. HEMOLYSIS DUE TO INTRACORPUSCULAR ABNORMALITIES

Harry S. Jacob

483.1. INTRODUCTION

Unlike acquired hemolytic anemias, in which environmental stresses cause shortened red cell survival, erythrocytes from patients with congenital hemolytic anemias are usually intrinsically defective. The ultimate proof of intrinsic abnormality requires cross-transfusion studies in which the suspect cells are labeled with an appropriate radioactive material, such as ^{51}Cr–sodium chromate, and then infused into a normal recipient; an excessively rapid disappearance of circulating radioactivity (red cells) is noted. Although such a test defines this class of disorders, the risk of transfusion-induced hepatitis has reduced its utility. Instead, careful history-taking frequently provides ample support for suspicion that congenital hemolytic anemia involving an intrinsic red cell abnormality is present. Thus a history of similar disorders in several members of the patient's family is often elicitable. In addition, these disorders are usually present from birth, so that childhood episodes of jaundice and anemia are frequently noted in a careful system review. Finally, since such patients suffer lifelong overproduction of bilirubin, signs and symptoms of cholelithiasis often occur at a uniquely early age.

Having suspected a congenital hemolytic disorder, one should consider whether abnormalities of the erythrocyte membrane or its cytoplasm are at fault. The erythrocyte membrane must serve both as a semipermeable barrier to cations (with sodium, potassium, and calcium being the most important in considerations of normal red cell viability) and as a flexible envelope which must provide the cell sufficient deforming capacity to allow for its journeys through small capillaries — many with smaller diameters than those of the erythrocytes themselves. In addition, a unique filtering apparatus exists in the spleen in which the vascular wall separating cords from sinusoids is fenestrated; cordal erythrocytes must pass through this "filter," the apertures of which are smaller by half than the diameter of the intact erythrocyte, to escape splenic sequestration and destruction. This suggests that deformability is an important determinant of red cell survival, and much interest has recently centered on elucidation of intrinsic (and acquired) abnormalities in membrane flexibility as they may relate to hemolytic processes.

The cytoplasm of erythrocytes is constituted of hemoglobin and of enzymes required for cellular production of energy (mainly in the form of adenosine triphosphate [ATP]) and of reducing capacity (mainly stored as NADPH). Genetic deficiencies of single such enzymes frequently lead to shortened red cell survival and congenital hemolytic anemia, whereas mutations in the molecular structure of hemoglobin can also produce diminished survival, particularly when the mutant hemoglobin manifests abnormal solubility. Thus hemoglobins which tend to gel (hemoglobin S or sickle hemoglobin), to precipitate (as in certain unstable hemoglobinopathies), or to crystallize (hemoglobin C) cause premature red cell destruction, probably by diminishing cellular deformability. Although the nature of the intrinsic defects in congenital hemolytic anemia may differ widely, cellular destruction in these disorders generally occurs in reticuloendothelial organs, such as the spleen and liver, rather than intravascularly.

483.2. MEMBRANE ABNORMALITIES

HEREDITARY SPHEROCYTOSIS
(HS)

DEFINITION. This condition is inherited as an autosomal dominant disorder and is found throughout the world; however, its incidence seems highest in northern Europeans, in whom rates of 1 in 5000 have been reported. The disorder is characterized by the presence in peripheral blood smears of numerous abnormally shaped red cells which are generally spheroidal, lacking the usual central pallor of normal biconcave discocytes. Blood smears obtained after splenectomy, which produces virtually complete remission of hemolysis, may contain large numbers of spiculated (acanthocytic) cells as well.

CLINICAL MANIFESTATIONS. Three different modes of presentation are commonly encountered. Generally children are only minimally anemic most of the time, because increased marrow production of erythrocytes matches the increased destruction rates, so that the hemolytic process is well compensated. However, without warning, or frequently during intercurrent infections, bone marrow function diminishes and the young patient becomes rapidly and severely anemic to levels which on occasion produce congestive heart failure; these so-called "aplastic crises" are observed usually during the first six years of life. Often, however, the compensatory increase in bone marrow function is well enough maintained so that patients go undiscovered until adulthood. With time, splenic enlargement, which is detectable in the great majority of patients, tends to worsen progressively with attendant increase in hemolytic rate and less efficient compensation. Although episodic worsening of unconjugated hyperbilirubinemia (secondary to increased hemoglobin catabolism) occurs at all ages, adults frequently present with sudden onset of more severe jaundice — now caused by conjugated hyperbilirubinemia. The explanation is that bilirubinate gallstones, a manifestation of many chronic hemolytic processes, are commonly encountered in young adult HS patients, and since such stones are usually small, they tend to enter and occlude the common bile duct. Finally, some patients escape detection until old age, when bone marrow function normally becomes sluggish; previous compensation of hemolysis now wanes, and anemia becomes obvious and frequently dangerous. This normal senescent process is exacerbated in many elderly patients by concomitant folic acid deficiency because of the increased folate requirements attendant on chronic increased marrow turnover; this combination may produce severe anemia with congestive heart failure.

In addition to these more common manifestations, chronic ulceration of ankle skin occurs in 10 to 15 per cent of adult patients. Rarer but potentially interesting syndromes which coexist with HS have also been described. Since the erythrocyte membrane is abnormal in this disorder (see below), the occurrence of abnormality in nonhematologic tissues invites speculation that defects in membrane composition might be more generalized. The coincident syndromes include (1) spinal cord dysfunction, producing a multiple sclerosis–like illness; (2) unconjugated hyperbilirubinemia which continues despite correction of hemolysis by splenectomy, suggesting the diagnosis of Gilbert's syndrome; and (3) an unusual coincidence of familial myocardiopathy with HS in several recently examined families.

DIAGNOSIS. Spherocytosis, which is usually evident in peripheral blood smears, strongly suggests the diagnosis, particularly in patients with childhood hemolytic anemia and history of similar abnormalities in other family members. The red cells are somewhat dehydrated and thereby have elevated MCHC levels. In fact, an observed MCHC above 36 is itself strong evidence of HS, although it should be noted that patients may acquire spherocytosis with similarly elevated MCHC during episodes of particularly severe immune hemolytic anemia.* The most useful confirmatory test for HS is assay of osmotic fragility. This test, which measures the amount of hemolysis suffered by red cells placed in a gradient series of hypotonic solutions, is rendered even more specific for HS if suspect whole blood is incubated for 24 hours at 37° C before the fragility assay; hereditary spherocytes markedly increase in osmotic fragility when so stressed, compared with the minimal increase manifested by normal cells. By increasing incubation time to 48 hours, one notes excessive spontaneous hemolysis of hereditary spherocytes in their own plasma — the so-called "autohemolysis test." Characteristically, this excessive autohemolysis is markedly lessened by addition of large amounts of glucose to the incubated cells.

When the diagnosis of HS is established, close relatives should be investigated for unsuspected disease. These same tests are frequently useful in uncovering mildly affected new patients. However, it should be noted that gene penetrance is low in this disease, and both parents of established HS patients are completely normal in 5 to 20 per cent of families. Nonetheless, other close relatives may be affected when the parents seemingly are not.

PATHOGENESIS. Spherocytes are less deformable than normal biconcave discocytes. This single characteristic is probably the most critical to the hemolytic process and makes the spleen the specific organ of entrapment and destruction. The spleen — in fact, a filter — contains a unique microvasculature in which 1 to 3 μ diameter holes perforate the membrane which separates splenic cords from splenic sinusoids. Hereditary spherocytes are unable to undergo the marked deformation required for 7 μ erythrocytes to traverse these constraining apertures, and thus they become sequestered and ultimately destroyed by splenic cord ma-

---

*Spherocytosis on blood smears can also be seen (along with fragmented erythrocytes) in microangiopathic hemolytic anemias, in severely burned patients, and in those with overwhelming clostridial bacteremia. In the last-named case this is due to the detergent action on red cell membranes of phospholipases released by clostridial organisms.

crophages. This intrinsic red cell abnormality is exacerbated by the acidotic environment of the splenic red pulp — an environment which suppresses erythrocyte glycolytic metabolism and thus reduces ATP production. Since ATP is somehow required for maintenance of normal membrane flexibility, its deficiency worsens the already existing stiffness of spherocytes and renders them even less likely to escape from the splenic cords. The underlying cause of the decreased flexibility of hereditary spherocytes is not completely understood, but evidence is accumulating that some structural protein of the erythrocyte membrane may be defective in HS. Most attention in this regard has been given to two filamentous proteins, *spectrin* (a myosin-like protein) and a topographically related one, *actin*. Although rigorous evidence of mutation in one or another of these two muscle-like moieties has not yet been provided, a spherocytic hemolytic anemia has recently been described in inbred mice in which erythrocytes lack spectrin.

In addition to its stiffness, the hereditary spherocyte membrane is hyperpermeable to sodium ions, which serves to promote intracellular sodium accumulation, particularly when metabolic energy production (ATP) flags. Water is accumulated concomitantly with sodium, resulting in cellular swelling, which, in turn, further jeopardizes the escape of stressed spherocytes through the apertures of the splenic microvasculature.

TREATMENT. Although the point is somewhat controversial, many hematologists advise that splenectomy be performed in virtually all patients, with surgery delayed until the age of six if possible. Conversely, some physicians choose to postpone splenectomy in mild cases because compensation seems excellent. However, the later increased likelihood of cholelithiasis and the progressive splenomegaly with increasing hemolysis, which occurs later in life at a time when bone marrow compensation is diminishing, suggest that such conservative decisions should be infrequently made. In the pediatric age group an excellent growth spurt and feeling of well-being are commonly noted following splenectomy. Nevertheless, children seem to be particularly at risk to develop pyogenic infections (particularly with pneumococci and *H. influenzae*) following splenectomy for any cause. Thus the use of prophylactic antimicrobial agents (generally penicillin, 250 mg twice daily) in all nonhypersensitive, splenectomized patients is strongly urged; this prophylaxis should be continued for at least two years following the surgery and perhaps for longer periods in small children. The need for lifelong prophylaxis following splenectomy is uncertain. Use of polyvalent pneumococcal polysaccharide vaccine could also be considered.

An interesting complication of splenectomy, albeit rare, provides insight into spleen physiology. On occasion a small spleen remnant is inadvertently left in the abdomen at the time of splenectomy. By a process evidently akin to work hypertrophy, this remnant may grow after several years into a full-sized spleen, and hemolysis, which has been in complete remission, may recur. Regeneration is documented by splenic scan, and re-splenectomy becomes necessary.

Transfusions are rarely required, except in the aplastic crises seen in some children. Until splenectomy can be accomplished, folic acid therapy (1 mg three times a day) is suggested in order to prevent deficiency of this vitamin, which is excessively utilized in HS (and other

chronic hemolytic syndromes) to sustain increased bone marrow proliferative activity. Finally, no patient should be diagnosed and treated for HS without also making a careful search for the disorder in close family members. It is particularly tragic when severe anemia of HS occurs in elderly, poor-operative-risk patients who might have been discovered earlier by such epidemiologic concern.

HEREDITARY ELLIPTOCYTOSIS

Hereditary elliptocytosis is closely allied to hereditary spherocytosis in most respects. However, red cells tend to be oval or elliptical rather than spheroidal, and only about 10 per cent of affected patients manifest significant shortening of red cell survival. It is only in this small proportion that osmotic fragility abnormalities, similar to those of HS, can be detected. Diagnosis is made by blood smear examination, and the defect appears to be inherited as an autosomal dominant trait. The close association with HS is particularly noted in some families in which some members have blood smears typical of hereditary spherocytosis, whereas other members appear to have elliptocytosis. Furthermore, recent evidence suggests that the hereditary elliptocyte membrane also may possess abnormal spectrin or actin structural proteins — an implication made previously for hereditary spherocytes. In those patients who manifest hemolysis, the spleen is the specific site of sequestration and destruction, and splenectomy induces long-term remission. However, it is stressed that splenectomy is rarely required in this very mild syndrome.

HEREDITARY STOMATOCYTOSIS AND OTHER RARE MEMBRANE ABNORMALITIES

Stomatocytosis is characterized by red cells with a linear, slit-like area of central pallor as seen on stained films and of bowl-shaped erythrocytes when perceived in wet preparations. Several different membrane abnormalities probably underlie stomatocytic shape, and most of these produce very mild or no hemolysis. Moderate increases in red blood cell membrane permeability to cations (particularly sodium and potassium) have been discerned in many affected persons. A recent interesting study demonstrated that stomatocytes from some families are corrected in shape, cation permeability, and ^{51}Cr erythrocyte survival when their membrane constituents are cross-linked by various bifunctional reagents. Such corrections suggest that an abnormality in protein-protein interactions in the red cell membrane may underlie the disorder, at least in some patients. There is other evidence that abnormal membrane structure is involved; (1) rare erythrocytes which completely lack membrane Rh antigens (Rh null cells) appear stomatocytic, and (2) typical stomatocytes can be experimentally generated by intercalating various amphiphilic reagents into normal red cell membranes.

Other rare intrinsic abnormalities which presumably affect erythrocyte membranes produce red cells with aberrant water content. Thus swollen, water-logged red cells ("hydrocytosis") and, conversely, dehydrated, shrunken red cells ("desiccocytosis") have been reported in rare patients with severe congenital hemolytic anemias. In both situations, it is inferred that abnormalities in membrane cation and, secondarily, water permeability reflect inborn errors in structural elements of the erythrocyte membrane. Finally, three families with "hereditary pyropoikilocytosis" have been described. Red cells from affected patients are bizarrely shaped, generally appearing shrunken and dehydrated. The disorder derives its name from the fact that the abnormal red cells hemolyze when heated to temperatures 2 to 3° C below that required to hemolyze normal cells (50° C). Since, when purified, the structural membrane protein, spectrin, melts at exactly 50° C, it has been suggested that this protein is mutant (and thus denatured at lower than normal temperatures) in hereditary pyropoikilocytes; rigorous evidence of this, however, is still unavailable. The hemolytic anemia associated with this intriguing abnormality may be severe and only moderately improved by splenectomy.

483.3. ENZYME DEFICIENCIES

The accompanying figure demonstrates the pathways of glycolysis in the mature human erythrocyte, with lines drawn under the names of enzymes thus far demonstrated to be deficient in various families with congenital hemolytic states. Although in many cases the

exact mechanism by which enzyme deficiency produces hemolysis is only partially understood, that a relationship between enzyme deficiency and shortened red cell survival occurs is well documented in most instances. Normally, red cells metabolize about 90 per cent of incorporated glucose anaerobically through the Embden-Meyerhof pathway — the major products of which are adenosine triphosphate (ATP) and 2,3-diphosphoglycerate (2,3-DPG). ATP acts to preserve membrane flexibility and thus is critical in providing necessary deformability for erythrocytes to flow through the microvasculature. It is not surprising that deficiencies of Embden-Meyerhof pathway enzymes frequently engender premature sequestration and destruction of erythrocytes in reticuloendothelial organs, such as the spleen and liver. The other product of glycolysis, 2,3-DPG, influences the binding of oxygen to hemoglobin, so that abnormalities in the Embden-Meyerhof pathway may alter oxygen delivery to tissues quite apart from inducing shortened red cell survival. About 10 per cent of glucose is metabolized by erythrocytes through the hexose monophosphate shunt, the sole producer of the reducing substance NADPH. Thus deficiencies of enzymes in this pathway produce red cells with a propensity to be damaged by various oxidative stresses — particularly those imposed by certain pharmacologic agents.

DEFECTS IN EMBDEN-MEYERHOF PATHWAY GLYCOLYTIC ENZYMES

Several enzymes involved in the anaerobic pathway of glycolysis in red cells have been identified since 1962, and deficiencies in several have been found to produce congenital hemolytic anemia in various families. Pyruvate kinase (PK) deficiency is the most frequently encountered example of this relatively uncommon group of disorders and was the first to be described. The pattern of inheritance is autosomal recessive in most of the glycolytic enzyme–deficient hemolytic anemias, and the deficiency may be manifest in nonhematologic tissues producing coincident abnormalities such as neurologic dysfunction.

In PK deficiency, heterozygote parents are hematologically normal but can be detected by erythrocyte enzyme assay. Hemolyzing homozygotes usually have unimpressive blood smears, although crenated spheres are sometimes seen. As with most of the other glycolytic enzyme deficiencies, moderate to marked hemolytic anemia occurs and is readily apparent in most patients during childhood. A strong family history, the occurrence of premature gallstones, and splenomegaly all mimic the manifestations of hereditary spherocytosis (HS); however, splenomegaly is generally not as marked as in HS. Several mutant PK enzymes which produce hemolytic anemia have now been described; since many have altered substrate affinities, enzyme assay conditions, particularly substrate concentrations, must be varied to document the deficiency in some patients. The osmotic fragility test is not particularly helpful, although autohemolysis (hemolysis after 48 hours of sterile incubation) is generally abnormally increased; but unlike the situation in hereditary spherocytosis, such hemolysis is not thwarted by glucose supplementation. This simple screening test (and the lack of spherocytes on blood smears) helps differentiate PK de-

Pathways of glycolysis in mature human red cell (modified from Valentine).

Abbreviations: ATP = adenosine triphosphate; ADP = adenosine diphosphate; NADP = nicotinamide-adenine dinucleotide phosphate (TPN); NADPH = reduced nicotinamide-adenine dinucleotide phosphate (TPNH); G-6-P = glucose-6-phosphate; 6-PG = 6-phospho-3-ketogluconate; Pentose-5-P = pentose-5-phosphate; GSH = reduced glutathione; GSSG = oxidized glutathione; F-6-P = fructose-6-phosphate; F-1,6-P = fructose-1,6-phosphate; DHAP = dihydroxyacetonephosphate; G-3-P = glyceraldehyde-3-phosphate; P_i = inorganic phosphorus; 1,3-DPG = 1,3-diphosphoglycerate; 2,3-DPG = 2,3-diphosphoglycerate; 3-PG = 3-phosphoglycerate; 2-PG = 2-phosphoglycerate; PEP = phosphoenol pyruvate.

ficiency from HS, the other common congenital hemolytic anemia of childhood. The definitive test for PK deficiency is assay of enzyme activity in red cell hemolysates. This assay should be done in evaluating all childhood hemolytic anemias, especially when blood smears are relatively normal and when family (particularly sibling) histories are positive for other cases of possible hemolytic anemia. A useful associated observation which suggests PK deficiency is the finding of increased levels of erythrocyte 2,3-DPG. The PK enzymatic step is beyond the 2,3-DPG synthetic one and, thus, with PK deficiency 2,3-DPG tends to accumulate. Since this important glycolytic intermediate may increase oxygen delivery from hemoglobin to tissues, anemic PK-deficient patients may be less handicapped than expected from consideration of hemoglobin levels alone. Relatively simple assay methods for the PK enzyme and for 2,3-DPG are now available in many clinical laboratories.

Hemolysis in PK deficiency is generally attributed to impaired glycolysis with concomitant deficient ATP generation. Actual documentation of ATP deficiency and the exact mechanism by which such deficiency might lead to shortened red cell survival are still not available, however. It does seem likely that the small population of crenated spherocytes which are generally seen in PK-deficient blood smears are destined for rapid destruction in reticuloendothelial tissues, and similar-appearing cells are experimentally produced by raising red cell intracellular calcium levels in vitro; this suggests that PK deficiency may promote excessive calcium loading in red cells. Since ATP is constantly required to pump intracellular calcium outward — a process which generally maintains intracellular calcium levels at $1/100$ those of the extracellular plasma — its sluggish production in PK deficiency may produce the stiffened, dehydrated echinocytes (spiculated cells) characteristic of this disorder. Since reticulocytes, but not mature red cells, still contain viable mitochrondria, which are efficient organelles for producing ATP by oxidative phosphorylation, they are presumably somewhat protected from lysis in this disorder. However, entrapment of PK-deficient cells — even reticulocytes — in the acidotic and anaerobic splenic environment probably diminishes their ATP production. This may explain why reticulocyte levels may strikingly increase in PK deficiency following splenectomy, despite the partial amelioration of the hemolytic rate produced by the operative procedure. That is, in the absence of the spleen, mitochrondial ATP production in reticulocytes permits their relative metabolic advantage to be expressed as increased survival time. However, it must be emphasized that splenectomy is much less effective than in hereditary spherocytosis, and should be recommended, after infancy, only for severely affected patients, generally those requiring transfusions. All patients harboring PK-deficient red cells should be given folic acid supplementation (1 mg three times a day), and family members should be screened for heterozygosity and genetically counseled.

Numerous other red cell glycolytic enzyme deficiencies which lead to sporadic congenital hemolytic anemia in families have also been described, but are rare occurrences. A recent compendium of these deficiencies and their coexisting nonhematologic consequences (i.e., neurologic dysfunction) has been published (Jaffe). Any patient with a congenital hemolytic process should

have assays performed of all the glycolytic enzymes — assays which are currently available in only a few research laboratories throughout the world; however, these laboratories have been generous in performing the needed measurements on shipped blood specimens. After PK deficiency the next most commonly encountered of the red cell glycolytic abnormalities is hexokinase deficiency, a particularly instructive pathophysiologic error. Hexokinase is the first enzyme in red cell glycolysis, so that its deficiency decreases several glycolytic intermediates. Indeed, 2,3-DPG levels are low (in contrast to high levels with PK deficiency), and thus oxygen delivery to tissues is probably particularly inefficient. Interesting support for this surmise has been provided by the finding that patients with hexokinase deficiency have poorer exercise tolerance than those with PK deficiency despite similar levels of anemia.

DEFICIENCY IN ENZYME ACTIVITY RELATED TO THE HEXOSE MONOPHOSPHATE (HMP) SHUNT PATHWAY

Glucose-6-Phosphate Dehydrogenase (G-6-PD) Deficiency

The enzyme G-6-PD initiates the HMP shunt pathway, which normally consumes about 10 per cent of the glucose metabolized by the red cell. By this pathway NADPH, the major reducing compound synthesized by the red cell, is generated. Thus cells deficient in G-6-PD (or, more rarely, any of the other enzymes of the HMP shunt pathway) are hypersusceptible to damage by various oxidative stresses. When undefended oxidation occurs, a sequence of damage to erythrocyte constituents can be discerned. First, ferrohemoglobin is oxidized to ferrihemoglobin (methemoglobin); next, the thiol compound, glutathione, which is present in large amounts in intact red cells, is oxidized; finally, with the loss of this important thiol buffer, sulfhydryl groups of the globin chains of hemoglobin become oxidized, which, in turn, eventuates in denaturation of these chains into precipitates termed "Heinz bodies." Such precipitates assume coccoid shapes and frequently attach to the inner surface of the red cell membrane; there, presumably by limiting deformability, they cause premature cell destruction. It is important to recognize that any red cell can be oxidatively damaged if stress is great enough. For example, certain oxidant drugs such as phenylhydrazine are extremely potent and cause hemolytic anemia in normal individuals; in fact, this agent was previously used therapeutically to decrease red cell mass in patients with polycythemia vera. In contrast, patients harboring red cells with a deficiency in one or another HMP shunt enzyme hemolyze when exposed to normally innocuous doses of oxidant compounds.

Investigations into the mechanism of hemolysis associated with HMP shunt pathway abnormalities constitute one of the more exciting chapters in clinical research. During the Korean War approximately 15 per cent of black American soldiers given the prophylactic antimalarial drug primaquine developed explosive hemolytic anemia. Intensive study of this extraordinary circumstance eventually showed that 10 to 15 per cent of black American males harbor red cells deficient in G-6-PD. Deficiency is inherited as a sex-linked trait, and the gene coding for G-6-PD has been proved to be located on the X chromosome. Thus the defect is fully expressed in male hemizygotes and female homozygotes, but is generally only minimally manifest in female heterozygotes. In such heterozygotes, two populations of red cells have been demonstrated by histochemical methods — normal and G-6-PD–deficient cells in varying proportions. This "mosaicism" constituted the first proof that one of the two X chromosomes (with its constituent genes) is randomly inactivated in somatic cells of females.

Several different qualitative mutations in the G-6-PD enzyme which lead to quantitative deficiency (probably through accelerated in vivo enzyme inactivation) have been discovered in nearly all ethnic groups. Highest incidences of deficiency occur in malaria endemic areas, suggesting that, as with sickle cell anemia, red cell G-6-PD deficiency has somehow protected against fatal varieties of malaria, and thus has been positively selected by this parasitization. Recent evidence suggests that protection might accrue from the fact that the malaria parasite itself imposes an oxidative stress on the red cells it invades. G-6-PD–deficient red cells, being unable to withstand this oxidative stress, prematurely hemolyze, foreshortening the required intraerythrocytic period for parasite maturation and propagation.

There are two common red cell G-6-PD isozymes. Type A, which moves rapidly under starch gel electrophoresis conditions usually used to characterize the enzyme, is found in about 30 per cent of American blacks, including most of those who are enzyme deficient; Type B moves electrophoretically more slowly and is found in about 70 per cent of black and in nearly all whites.

MANIFESTATIONS IN BLACKS. The most common type of G-6-PD deficiency is found in blacks; about 10 per cent of American blacks, 8 to 20 per cent in West Africa, but only 2 per cent of South African Bantus harbor deficient red cells. Enzyme activity is reduced to about 15 per cent of normal in hemizygous males, whereas in heterozygous females levels range from normal to those nearly as deficient as in hemizygotes; in the latter females, random inactivation of the X chromosomes carrying normal G-6-PD genes has by chance evidently been excessive. Red cell survival is virtually normal in G-6-PD–deficient blacks unless the patients are subjected to oxidative stress, usually imposed by derivatives of several commonly utilized drugs; in addition, certain infections (pyogenic and infectious hepatitis) as well as diabetic ketoacidosis can also trigger hemolytic episodes in these patients. More than 40 drugs have been found to produce hemolysis in G-6-PD–deficient persons. These include the antimalarial drugs primaquine and quinine (the latter, it should be noted, is also used in popular beverages), antipyretics and analgesics such as phenacetin (commonly) and aspirin (only in large doses), the nitrofurans (such as Furadantin), sulfones, many sulfonamides, para-aminosalicylic acid, probenecid, quinidine, and water-soluble analogues of vitamin K, to name but a few. In addition, mothballs, which contain naphthalene, are not infrequently ingested by children who may develop explosive hemolysis if G-6-PD deficient. In fact, severe acute hemolytic episodes have been reported in black infants simply exposed to diapers stored in mothballs.

Hemolytic episodes induced by oxidant drugs in G-6-PD–deficient patients may be exacerbated or, in fact,

triggered de novo by unrelated medical conditions. Thus bacterial infections can lead to hemolysis, perhaps because the oxidant compound hydrogen peroxide, which is generated by phagocytizing white cells, impinges on neighboring G-6-PD–deficient red cells. In addition, an acquired inefficiency in red cell HMP shunt metabolism occurs in some patients who become uremic; thus excessive hemolysis may occur in G-6-PD–deficient blacks for obscure reasons.

Regardless of the triggering event, the kinetics of hemolysis are similar in G-6-PD–deficient blacks given oxidant drugs. Following a lag period of approximately two to three days, explosive destruction of red cells occurs. Elevated methemoglobin levels and the occurrence of Heinz bodies are frequently, but not always, perceptible indicators of oxidative damage, often having disappeared by the time hemolysis is obvious. Frequently, circulating red cells appear on blood smears with apparent pieces missing from their perimeters; presumably these missing portions originally contained Heinz bodies which were pitted in the constraining filtration apertures of the spleen; thus such morphology suggests that oxidative hemolysis is occurring; indeed, similarly scalloped cells may be regularly seen in patients with normal red cell HMP shunt metabolism who are given large doses of the oxidant drugs Azulfidine (in ulcerative colitis) or dapsone (in dermatitis herpetiformis). Hemoglobinemia and hemoglobinuria are usually of moderate degree during the explosive episode, but typically hemolysis is limited in duration, since only relatively old cells are vulnerable. That is, the more nearly normal G-6-PD activity found in younger red cells, which become more abundant in the circulation in response to hemolysis, protects them from excessive oxidative damage. Consequently, the red cell count may return to normal even though administration of the offending drug is continued, and diagnosis of the deficiency by assay of red cell enzyme activity may be difficult during this equilibrium phase when reticulocytosis is marked. Confirmation of the clinical diagnosis often must await the return to normal of the red cell age distribution.

MANIFESTATIONS IN OTHER POPULATIONS. G-6-PD deficiency in populations other than blacks is usually more severe, with red cell enzyme activity in most cases in the range of 0 to 5 per cent of normal. In addition, reduced G-6-PD activity is frequently observed in leukocytes and platelets, as well as red cells, in these patients. At least 100 different forms of G-6-PD have been demonstrated among white and Oriental populations by precise biochemical characterization of the enzymes. Greeks, Sardinians, Chinese, and Thais are populations with particularly frequent (1 to 10 per cent) incidences of G-6-PD deficiency. Deficient patients may manifest moderate chronic hemolytic anemia in the absence of drugs which can become dangerously severe with extrinsic oxidative challenge. In addition, hemolysis may worsen during episodes of acidosis, uremia, and infection. Generally, the spleen is not enlarged and osmotic fragility studies are normal. As might be expected, splenectomy is not useful in this disorder. Favism is a special type of G-6-PD–deficient hemolysis, and is observed almost solely in Mediterranean patients with the deficiency. This acute hemolytic disorder occurs after ingestion of Italian broad (fava) beans or, on occasion, after inhalation of pollen from the plant *Vicia faba* by patients with Mediterranean variety G-6-

PD–deficient red cells. The hemolytic episode may be severe enough to cause death and occurs even in female heterozygotes. It has been speculated that two genes are necessary for favism to occur — one coding for G-6-PD deficiency, and the other for a unique type of metabolic degradation of a fava bean constituent which renders it especially oxidant. During the acute episode Heinz bodies are frequently seen in blood smears, as is methemoglobinemia.

G-6-PD–deficient white infants, particularly when premature, seem particularly prone to develop neonatal jaundice caused by excessive hemolysis. In addition, marked potentiation of hemolysis with dangerous hyperbilirubinemia may occur if the deficient newborn is inadvertently given water-soluble synthetic vitamin K preparations (even if these drugs are administered to the mother before delivery). In fact, in Hong Kong it has been reported that G-6-PD deficiency is the most common cause of severe neonatal jaundice leading to kernicterus. The propensity to develop marked neonatal jaundice in G-6-PD deficiency may reflect the fact that other red cell enzymes utilized in the defense against oxidative stresses, such as glutathione peroxidase, are also evidently somewhat diminished even in normal infant red cells.

PREVENTION OF G-6-PD DEFICIENCY HEMOLYSIS. It is estimated that at least 100 million persons in the world have red cell G-6-PD deficiency, so that efforts to screen populations at high risk, using one of many simple screening tests for this deficiency, should be encouraged. Screening performed when the patient is well can serve to forewarn both patient and physician of hypersusceptibility to oxidant drugs. This seems particularly relevant, since many deficient patients reside in areas where prophylactic antimalarials are commonly employed, and some of these (e.g., chloroquine) are less liable to cause hemolysis than others (e.g., primaquine).

Other Deficiencies Related to the HMP Shunt Pathway

Deficiency of 6-phosphogluconate dehydrogenase has been described, although its relationship to hemolysis is not yet clear. Glutathione reductase deficiency has also been described in several patients, although it now seems clear that this deficiency is rarely or never inherited, but instead is commonly caused by dietary riboflavin lack. This vitamin is a constituent of the coenzyme FAD, required for glutathione reductase activity, and its therapeutic administration ameliorates the red cell defect in virtually all patients. Absent red cell glutathione with an associated chronic hemolytic state has been reported to be due to genetic deficiency in either of the two enzymes involved in the synthesis of this important thiol compound — i.e., with γ-glutamylcysteine synthetase or glutathione synthetase deficiencies. With deficiency of the latter enzyme chronic neurologic disease may occur, but the causal relationship between the degenerative neurologic abnormality and the enzyme deficiency has not yet been established. Although a relatively mild hemolytic state has been reported to be due to glutathione peroxidase deficiency, the fact that most normal newborns harbor red cells with diminished levels of this enzyme makes it uncertain whether true genetic deficiency occurs.

ACQUIRED HYPERSUSCEPTIBILITY OF NORMAL RED CELLS TO OXIDATIVE STRESS. Patients with certain diseases of the gastrointestinal tract, particularly those leading to intestinal stasis, often harbor red cells that are hypersusceptible to oxidative stress. Overgrowth of bacteria in the small intestine may in some way be etiologic, as such patients frequently lose their oxidant hypersusceptibility when treated with nonabsorbable antimicrobials. It seems likely that the not uncommon hemolytic episodes noted when ulcerative colitis patients are treated with sulfonamides, such as Azulfidine, may reflect this bacterial-induced reduction in red cell oxidant defense mechanisms; the nature of the putative bacterial toxins remains to be elucidated. An analogous, and frequently overlooked, hemolytic anemia occurs in patients with dermatitis herpetiformis who are given sulfones, such as dapsone. Since patients with this dermatologic condition frequently suffer from coexistent small intestine disease, hemolysis probably reflects oxidant hypersensitivity — a suggestion supported by the finding of scalloped (Heinz body–pitted?) red cells under these circumstances. Finally, a small proportion (10 to 25 per cent) of uremic patients acquire a defect in red cell HMP shunt activity. As with bacterial toxins, the nature of the uremic toxin is currently unknown. Affected patients are prone to hemolyze during hemodialysis, particularly if exposed to various oxidants, such as chloramine, commonly used to purify urban water supplies. In addition, the use of sulfonamides in the treatment of genitourinary infections in patients with chronic renal failure should be considered a potential exacerbator of the anemia suffered by such patients.

483.4. OTHER INTRACORPUSCULAR ABNORMALITIES

The hemoglobinopathies and thalassemias, many of which are associated with hemolytic anemia, are considered in Ch. 485. Individual patients have been described with congenital hemolytic anemias caused by various other intrinsic red cell abnormalities. Thus a family manifesting increased membrane lecithin is an example of an intrinsic defect in red cell lipid homeostasis. An intriguing recent report of a family with chronic hemolytic anemia in which red cells contain *excessive* adenosine deaminase attests to the importance of ATP in red cell integrity. In affected patients the excessive deamination of adenosine evidently lowers the availability of this purine for synthesis of ATP, which, in turn, is relatively deficient; red cell survival concomitantly diminishes. A congenital hemolytic anemia associated with pyrimidine nucleotidase deficiency is easily suspected in that basophilic stippling of red cells is striking in peripheral blood smears. In this condition pyrimidines accumulate intracellularly because of the deficiency of pyrimidine nucleotide catabolic enzyme. The accumulated material or the ribosomes containing it evidently precipitates into basophilic-staining particles.

Finally, a large proportion of patients with erythropoietic porphyria have hemolytic anemia which may be partially relieved by splenectomy. It is presumed that the excessive porphyrins of this disease act as free radical generators which produce oxidative damage to red cells not unlike that noted with oxidant drug ingestion in G-6-PD–deficient patients.

General References

Dacie, J. V.: The Haemolytic Anaemias: Congenital and Acquired, Part 1. 2nd ed. New York, Grune & Stratton, 1960.

Harris, J. W., and Kellermeyer, R. W.: The Red Cell. Production, Metabolism, Destruction: Normal and Abnormal. Revised ed. Cambridge, Mass., Harvard University Press, 1970, pp. 447-593.

Specific Hemolytic States

Beutler, E.: Abnormalities of the hexose monophosphate shunt. Semin. Hematol., 8:311, 1971.

Jacob, H. S.: Pathologic states of the erythrocyte membrane. In Weissmann, G., and Clarborn, R. (eds.): Cell Membrane Biochemistry, Cell Biology, and Pathology. New York, H. P. Publishing Company, 1975, pp. 249-256.

Mentzer, W. C., Lubin, B. H., and Emmons, S.: Correction of the permeability defect in hereditary stomatocytosis by dimethyl adipimidate. N. Engl. J. Med., 294:1200, 1976.

Oski, F. A., Marshall, B. E., Cohen, P. J., Sugerman, H. J., and Miller, L. D.: Exercise with anemia: The role of the left-shifted or right-shifted oxygen-hemoglobin equilibrium curve. Ann. Intern. Med., 74:44, 1971.

Valentine, W. N.: Hereditary enzymatic deficiencies of erythrocytes. Introduction. Deficiencies associated with Embden-Meyerhof pathway and other metabolic pathways. Semin. Hematol., 8:307, 348, 1971.

484.   HEMOLYSIS DUE TO ACQUIRED ABNORMALITIES

Wendell F. Rosse

484.1.   INTRODUCTION

Hemolysis not resulting from congenital intrinsic defects of the red cell itself may be caused by a variety of acquired abnormalities. Except in the cases of acquired membrane defects caused by dysplasia, the red cell is formed normally and the cause of the premature destruction is acquired or encountered during circulation. In most cases, these acquired lesions alter the membrane immunologically, physically, or chemically. The general manifestations of the hemolytic anemia resulting from acquired causes do not differ from those for hemolysis resulting from intracorpuscular lesions, which are discussed in Ch. 483.

484.2.   IMMUNOLOGIC ALTERATION OF THE MEMBRANE

Alteration of the red cell membrane by immunologic reactions is one of the more common mechanisms by which the life span of the red cell may be shortened. These immune processes are usually initiated by IgG or IgM immunoglobulins; the diagnosis often depends upon demonstration of an antibody on the cells or in the serum of the patient.

Antibodies may sometimes be demonstrated by their ability to agglutinate the cells. This is effected by the fixation of one antigen binding site of the antibody molecule on one cell and the other on a different cell. When several cells are thus bound together, an agglutinate forms. IgM molecules are able to do this readily, because they are large enough to bridge the distance imposed by forces responsible for mutual repulsion of the red cells (the "zeta potential"). Many IgG antibod-

ies cannot agglutinate red cells suspended in saline because the molecule is too small to bridge this distance. Their presence on the red cell surface is often detected by the addition of antibodies directed against antigens present on the antibody molecules (*antiglobulin reaction; Coombs' reaction*). These heterologous antibodies are able to react with IgG antibodies on two red cells, thus linking the cells and forming the agglutinate. This reaction has immeasurably increased our ability to define immunologic reactions involving red cells. The "direct" antiglobulin test detects antibody or components of complement (see below) on the patient's red cells; the "indirect" antiglobulin test detects antibody in the patient's serum.

The mechanisms by which immune reactions effect hemolysis depend upon the nature of the antibody, its interaction with antigen, and its ability to fix complement. When most IgG antibodies interact with red cell antigens, an area changes in the heavy chain portion of the molecule which permits it to interact with receptor sites on phagocytic cells, neutrophils, and macrophages (monocytes). The red cell may thus be held in place, and the whole cell or a portion of the membrane may be ingested; the remaining membrane may reseal across the defect, and the resulting cell fragment is capable of escaping from the phagocyte. Since it has lost more membrane than contents, the remainder of the red cell must assume the shape of a spherocyte.

The spleen plays an important role in hemolysis by this mechanism. A portion of the blood delivered to the spleen enters the pulp, where the cells coated with IgG antibody are in prolonged contact with macrophages. Further, to regain the circulation, the cells must pass through 2 to 4 μ fenestrations in the lining of the sinus. Because they are less deformable, spherocytes cannot pass and are trapped in the macrophage-rich cords of Billroth. However, even when the spleen is removed, if sufficent antibody is present, the cells may be destroyed in other parts of the phagocytic system.

Antibodies may fix complement, which may also play a role in the destruction of the cell. The complement sequence is initiated when two IgG antibody molecules or one IgM antibody molecule react with two antigen sites in close proximity to one another. This fixes a molecule of the first component of complement (C1), which acts upon the fourth component (C4) which may be then firmly affixed to the red cell surface. The second component, also activated by C1, is affixed to the fourth component, and this combination is able to activate a third component (C3) which is also fixed to the membrane. The fixed, active C3b molecule may interact with membrane receptors on phagocytic cells different from those interacting with IgG. This immune adherence may lead to phagocytosis, but usually complement is a weak stimulus for the reaction. However, the presence of even relatively small amounts of C3b on the membrane markedly enhances IgG antibody–mediated destruction. Immune adherence is reversed or prevented when the C3b molecule is digested by a serum enzyme, leaving a small, inactive fragment (C3d) attached to the membrane. It is this fragment which is usually detected by anti-C3 antiserum in an antiglobulin (Coombs) reaction like that used to detect IgG antibodies.

The active C3b molecule on the red cell membrane is able to propagate the complement sequence; if the sequence is successfully completed, disruption of the membrane occurs and intravascular hemolysis follows. This completion of the complement sequence is singularly inefficient on normal human red cells, and therefore marked intravascular hemolysis is uncommon in immune hemolytic anemia.

The hematologic manifestations and the mechanism of destruction depend in large part upon the properties of the antibody initiating the immune reaction. Although many classifications could be constructed according to the various properties of the antibodies, it has been found most convenient to classify the syndromes by whether the antibody is able to react with the cell at body temperature (*warm-reacting antibodies*) or only at reduced temperatures (*cold-reacting antibodies*).

Antibodies may also be classified as isoimmune and autoimmune. The former arise in response to antigens not present on the red cells of the patient. Autoimmune antibodies react with antigens of the patient's own red cells. This distinction is usually relatively simple to make in the untransfused patient, because the direct antiglobulin test will be negative if the antibodies are isoimmune and positive if the antibodies are autoimmune. In complex clinical situations in which transfusion has taken place, this distinction may be more difficult.

HEMOLYSIS DUE TO WARM-REACTING ANTIBODIES

Warm-reacting antibodies are those capable of reacting with red cell antigens at 37° C. They may or may not fix complement, depending upon the spacing of the antigen sites with which they interact and the immunoglobulin subclass of the antibody. In some instances, the antibody is not readily detectable on the red cell membrane by the antiglobulin test, but fixed complement components indicate that the immune reaction has taken place.

Hemolysis Due to Isoimmune (Alloimmune) Antibodies

Transfusion Reactions

See Ch. 488.

Hemolytic Disease of the Newborn

Hemolytic disease of the newborn is due to the transplacental infusion of isoimmune antibodies from the mother to the infant when the infant's red cells have an antigen against which they may react. The antibody is, in most instances, formed in the mother in response to the prior transplacental transfer of "incompatible" red cells from that infant or previous infants, with the resultant production of isoimmune antibodies; occasionally, prior transfusion may be the cause of maternal sensitization. Hemolytic anemia in the infant results from the interaction of the maternal antibody which has crossed the placenta and the infant's red cells.

CLINICAL MANIFESTATIONS. The clinical manifestations are dependent in part upon the degree of sensitization of the mother, the immunoglobulin class of the antibody, and the antigen with which the antibody is reacting. In its most severe manifestations, the infant is born with anasarca, marked anemia, and hepatosplenomegaly; such infants rarely survive. In other instances, marked hemolytic anemia with jaundice may result. The anemia may persist for days to weeks. If appropriate treatment is instituted quickly, the resultant outcome is usually good; in some instances of marked sensitization, the infant is delivered prematurely in order to institute treatment. Where there is lesser sensitization, the extent of hemolytic anemia may be minimal.

DIAGNOSIS. Hemolytic disease of the newborn is usually diagnosed by finding a positive direct antiglobulin test with the cells of the infant. The antibody may be eluted and its specificity determined. Occurrence of the illness may be anticipated by demonstration of an isoantibody in the mother's serum before birth where a rising titer may be assumed to indicate increasing sensitization and therefore increased chance of severe hemolysis. In some instances, prenatal hemolytic anemia is diagnosed by examination of the amniotic fluid for bilirubin-like catabolic products.

PREVENTION AND TREATMENT. The chief complications of hemolytic disease of the newborn are anemia and excessive bilirubinemia, which may lead to kernicterus. The standard treatment is exchange transfusion. More recently, exposure of the infant to ultraviolet light has been shown to lower the bilirubin level and reduce the number of exchange transfusions needed.

Since most of the transplacental infusion of fetal cells into the mother occurs at birth, it has been found possible to prevent sensitization of the Rh_0 (D) negative mother to the Rh_0 (D) antigen by injection of a large quantitiy of the anti-Rh_0 (anti-D) antibody shortly after parturition. Any cells that have leaked from the fetus to the mother are destroyed by the injected antibody, and sensitization of the mother does not occur. This preventive treatment does not work if the mother has been previously sensitized by other pregnancies or by transfusion.

Hemolysis Due to Autoimmune Antibodies

When the antibody is directed against an antigen on the red cells of the host (autoimmune hemolytic anemia), the warm-reacting antibodies are usually IgG; although IgM and IgA antibodies have been described, their pathogenetic role is unclear. In approximately two thirds of cases, the IgG antibodies fix complement; when complement is not fixed, the antibody usually has specificity for the Rh locus or one of its antigens.

The hemolytic anemia which results may vary greatly in intensity. Usually the amount of hemolysis is related to the amount of antibody detectable on the red cell surface, but this is not always the case. In approximately one instance in fifty, immunoglobulin may not be detected on the red cell surface (*Coombs-negative immune hemolytic anemia*). In general, an antibody fixing complement probably causes a greater degree of hemolysis than one which does not.

In approximately one third of cases there may be no other manifestation of disease, except perhaps for immune thrombocytopenia. In the remaining half to two thirds of the instances, an underlying disease may be defined at the time of the initial diagnosis or during the clinical course. The most common diseases associated with immune hemolytic anemia of the warm antibody type are *chronic lymphocytic leukemia, lymphoma,* and *systemic lupus erythematosus*. It may be seen with other diseases of the immune system such as the *Wiskott-Aldrich syndrome, agammaglobulinemia,* and *malignant thymoma,* as well as a variety of syndromes such as *rheumatoid arthritis, systemic sclerosis,* or *ulcerative colitis.*

CLINICAL MANIFESTATIONS. The degree of hemolysis varies from patient to patient. In its classic presentation, immune hemolytic anemia is rapid in onset. The anemia can be so severe as to be fatal if not competently treated. The spleen is frequently enlarged and may vary in size according to the degree of hemolysis. The liver is less commonly enlarged. Jaundice and pallor are usually present. The peripheral blood frequently shows spherocytosis and marked reticulocytosis; however, considerable hemolysis can take place in the absence of overt spherocytes. The white blood count may be elevated slightly. Hemoglobinemia may be chemically detectable, but hemoglobinuria is rare. There are few other manifestations associated with the anemia itself, although, if it is secondary to some underlying disease, symptoms of that disease may be manifest.

DIAGNOSIS. The diagnosis usually depends upon the demonstration of immunoglobulins or components of complement on the red cells of the patient. This is best done with specific antisera containing only antibodies against IgG or the inactive fragment of the third component of complement (C3d). Tests with these reagents may reveal the presence of either or both on the surface (Table 1). When complement alone is found, further efforts must be made to demonstrate the antibody. Cooling the cells to 4° C may reveal an IgG antibody on the surface (*cold-detectable antibody*) capable of reacting with the cell at 37° C but detectable only at reduced temperature. An antibody of low affinity may be detected in the serum, using papainized normal cells to increase the interaction of the antigen and antibody. The antibody may rarely be IgM or IgA, and specific anti-IgM or anti-IgA antisera may be needed to reveal its presence. The antibody may be cold reactive or drug related, and appropriate steps will be needed to reveal its presence, as described later in this chapter.

TREATMENT. The initial treatment of autoimmune hemolytic anemia caused by IgG warm-reacting antibodies is prednisone. In general, 1 mg per kilogram per day in divided doses is sufficient for initial therapy. If response to this dose of the drug is seen in elevation of the hematocrit, the amount of prednisone being administered can be rapidly tapered to approximately 0.3 mg per kilogram per day. Thereafter the dose may be tapered more slowly, at about the rate of 5 mg per day each month. Often, in immune hemolytic anemia of childhood, remission occurs and prednisone may be omitted entirely; however, in adults, this is unusual, and great caution must be used in discontinuing prednisone completely. Many patients will maintain total remission on 2.5 to 10 mg per day; alternate-day dosage appears to be as good as daily dosage and is attended by less severe side effects.

The mode of action of prednisone is not clear but appears to be multiple. Evidence has been adduced that it causes the removal of antibody from the red cell membrane when given in high doses. This effect appears to account for many of the instances of rapid remission obtained with the drug. In addition, it appears to suppress the production of antibody in two to three weeks in those patients achieving remission which can be maintained on small doses. Finally, it is thought that prednisone can interfere with sequestration of cells by the reticuloendothelial system. The basic mechanism of any of these actions is not known.

If prednisone is unsuccessful in initial therapy or if the dose of prednisone required to maintain remission is too high, other measures must be sought. In general, these consist of *immunosuppression* by other drugs (azathioprine, 100 to 150 mg per day; cyclophosphamide, 50 to 100 per day) or splenectomy. *Splenectomy* is generally preferred in younger patients, whereas in older patients immunosuppression may be wiser. If one of these treatments fails to bring about an adequate remission, the other method may be required. Seldom is the process resistant to a combination of prednisone, immunosuppression, and splenectomy.

Transfusion may be necessary during the acute hemolytic phase of the disease. This is often attended by difficulty because of problems in obtaining complete compatibility by testing; however, if it is clinically indicated, a transfusion that is not completely compatible is preferable to having the patient succumb to the anemia. The best chance of a proper cross-match is obtained if the antibody is isolated, either from eluates or from the serum, to determine whether specificity exists and, if it does, in selecting units of blood which are compatible. If the specificity cannot be identified, the blood bank is often obliged to test the patient's serum against all units of blood available of the appropriate type to determine which are optimal. When this procedure is carefully performed, few transfusion reactions will occur; however, one must be cautious about the simultaneous presence of isoantibody in addition to the autoimmune antibody.

TABLE 1. Types and Significance of Direct Antiglobulin (Coombs) Tests Using Specific Antiglobulin Antisera

Type	I	II	III
Anti IgG	+	+	−
Anti C3d	−	+	+
Occurs in:			
Idiopathic warm antibody	Yes	Yes	Uncommon
Chronic lymphocytic leukemia	Yes	Yes	Uncommon
Systemic lupus erythematosus	No	Yes	Yes
Cold agglutinin disease	No	No	Yes
Paroxysmal cold hemoglobinuria	No	No	Yes
Hemolytic disease of newborn			
Anti-Rh	Yes	No	No
Anti A or B	Yes	Yes	No
Drug-induced			
α-Methyldopa	Yes	Rare	No
Penicillin and cephalosporins	Yes	Rare	No
Others	No	No	Yes

HEMOLYSIS DUE TO COLD-REACTING ANTIBODIES

Cold-reacting antibodies are those unable to react with antigen at 37° C. This means that the mode of destruction cannot be mediated by antibody (see above); since these antibodies are able to fix complement, complement is responsible for the hemolysis.

Cold Agglutinin Syndrome

The cold agglutinin syndrome is due to antibodies, usually IgM, which are able to act at reduced temperature and cause agglutination of the red cells. The presence of the antibody is readily demonstrable in the serum of the patient; the serum may on occasion be diluted several thousand fold and still be able to agglutinate red cells.

The antigens with which these antibodies interact are of three general sorts, called "I", "i," and "Pr." The *"I" antigens* are those which are most strongly expressed on adult cells; the *"i" antigens* are most strongly expressed on cells of newborn infants and of rare adults; the *"Pr" antigens* are equally well expressed on both cells and are destroyed by neuraminidase (Table 2). The antigens are polysaccharide in nature, and some of them appear to be related to the polysaccharides of the ABH and Lewis groups.

The maximal temperature at which the antibody interacts with the red cell is variable. Since the interaction in vivo of antigen and antibody depends upon lowering the temperature of the blood below 37° C in the peripheral areas (arms, legs, and appendages), those antibodies which are able to interact at higher temperatures will, in general, have a greater opportunity to cause hemolysis than those which react only at lower temperatures.

CLINICAL MANIFESTATIONS. The clinical manifestations of the cold agglutinin syndrome are due to two phenomena: (1) intravascular agglutination, which occurs when blood is cooled in peripheral parts of the body, and (2) hemolytic anemia, which occurs consequent upon the fixation of complement. Upon exposure to cold, patients with cold agglutinin syndrome may note that the hands, ears, nose, or feet may turn purple and become painful; this process is rapidly reversed upon rewarming and is distinguished from Raynaud's phenomenon in that there is no blanching phase and little evidence of hyperemia. If the symptoms of agglutination are sufficiently severe, pain may result upon breathing cold air or eating cold food, or from so small a stimulus as holding a glass of ice water.

The hemolytic anemia which accompanies cold agglutinin syndrome is rarely severe. Usually the patient has moderate hemolytic anemia which is exacerbated during the winter. The spleen may or may not be enlarged. Spherocytosis is usually absent. If the patient is exposed to severe chilling, he may have a sudden bout of hemolysis with consequent hemoglobinemia and hemoglobinuria. When the antibody has a high thermal am-

plitude, the anemia may be severe even when the patient is carefully protected from the cold.

Cold agglutinin syndrome is seen in two major clinical settings: (1) *chronic cold agglutinin disease* of the elderly and (2) *postinfectious cold agglutinin syndrome.* Chronic cold agglutinin disease of the elderly is characterized by a gradual onset of symptoms and a chronic course. The antibody seen is usually monoclonal and is nearly always of the κ light chain type. Some patients with this syndrome have been found to have lymphoma when the antibody is anti-i.

Postinfectious cold agglutinin syndrome usually follows infection with *Mycoplasma pneumoniae* (in which case the antibody is anti-I) or *infectious mononucleosis* (in which case the antibody is often anti-i). Antibodies in these instances are not monoclonal, as in the chronic idiopathic type, but may be restricted in their molecular variation. The antibodies in infectious mononucleosis are highly variable; some may even be IgG. Although most patients with either *Mycoplasma* infection or mononucleosis may have a rise in the titer of the cold agglutinins in their serum, reaching a peak two to three weeks after onset of the illness, clinically manifest hemolytic anemia is uncommon, usually appearing only when the amount of antibody is very great. The course of the illness is self-limited, and all manifestations usually disappear within two to three months.

DIAGNOSIS. The presence of cold agglutinins is often suspected by casual observation of an anticoagulated sample of blood at room temperature. The sample may appear to be coagulated or show marked clumping, which disappears when warmed to 37° C. This is more rigorously tested by diluting the serum and testing it against normal adult and newborn cells; in some instances dilutions as high as 1 in 100,000 may cause agglutination.

The patient's cells invariably have on them relatively large amounts of C3d, giving a Type III direct Coombs test (see Table 1). The hemolytic ability of the antibody may also be tested by appropriate in vitro reactions.

TREATMENT. The treatment of chronic cold agglutinin disease is usually simplified if the patient is able to avoid cold exposure during the winter months. This may require near-incarceration in heated rooms and wearing heavy, warm clothes. Sometimes it may require traveling to warmer climates. If this is insufficient or not possible, treatment with chlorambucil (2 mg per day) has been suggested. In general, little or no benefit results from treatment with prednisone or splenectomy.

Paroxysmal Cold Hemoglobinuria

Paroxysmal cold hemoglobinuria was the first hemolytic disease to be specifically defined. It formerly was encountered in patients with syphilis; it now more commonly occurs as an autoimmune or postviral disease. The antibody is IgG in type and reacts with the P blood group antigen which is possessed by nearly all red cells. For reasons not clearly understood, the antibody is able to effect marked lysis by complement. This is detectable clinically by episodes of hemoglobinemia and hemoglobinuria after exposure to cold and is detected in vitro by the *Donath-Landsteiner test*, by which the syndrome is frequently diagnosed. In some instances, the syndrome may be so severe as to threaten life; this usually occurs after viral infection in children. Paroxysmal cold hemoglobinuria is treated by

TABLE 2.   Classification of Cold Agglutinin Antibodies

	Anti-I	Anti-i	Anti-Pr
Relative reaction with adult and fetal red cells	Adult>fetal	Adult<fetal	Adult=fetal
Effect of enzyme treatment of red cells on reaction	Increases	Increases	Abolishes
Primary chronic cold agglutinin syndrome	Yes*	No	Yes*
Secondary to:			
Malignancy			
Lymphoma	No	Yes*	?
Adenocarcinoma	Yes*	No	?
Infection			
M. pneumoniae	Yes†	No	?
Cytomegalovirus	Yes†	No	?
Infectious mononucleosis	Yes†	Yes†	?

*Monoclonal.
†Oligo- or polyclonal.

protection from exposure to cold, by prednisone, and by cyclophosphamide, just as any other IgG antibody syndrome.

HEMOLYSIS DUE TO DRUG-INDUCED ANTIBODIES

Immune hemolysis initiated by drugs is not uncommon. There are basically two types: (1) "autoimmune" hemolytic anemia, in which the drug induces an antibody which reacts with antigens normally present in the red cell, and (2) "immune" hemolytic anemia, in which the antibody formed is directed against the drug and the red cell is lysed as a consequence of the interaction between antibody and drug. In this latter group, the drug may be firmly fixed to the red cell membrane (*haptene-like reaction*) or only loosely attached to the membrane ("*innocent bystander*" *reaction*).

"Autoimmune" drug-induced hemolysis is almost exclusively due to a single drug, α-methyldopa (Aldomet), although L-dopa and mefanemic acid have been implicated as well. After taking the drug for at least two to three months, about 5 to 10 per cent of all patients will have a positive direct antiglobulin (Coombs) test (DCT) caused by the presence of IgG antibody directed against components of the Rh complex locus; complement is almost never fixed (Type I DCT). Antibody may be detected in the serum without addition of the drug to the test. In most patients, little if any hemolysis will result, but in a small proportion of patients taking the drug, significant hemolysis occurs. The syndrome produced is that of warm-reacting IgG antibody with spherocytosis, splenomegaly, and response to prednisone therapy, if its use becomes necessary. When the drug is stopped, the antibody usually disappears within two to three months, and the direct antiglobulin test reverts to negative. The reason a drug should stimulate production of an antibody capable of reacting with autologous red cell antigens is not clear.

Many drugs serving as haptenes apparently stimulate the production of antibodies. These antibodies may be capable of destroying red cells as a result of their reaction with the drug. In some cases, the drug may be firmly attached to the red cell, as in the case of penicillin; in those instances, the IgG antibody will also be detectable on the red cell surface in the direct antiglobulin test. Since relatively small amounts of antibody are attached, complement is usually not fixed (Type I DCT). In other instances, the drug is not firmly attached to the red cell. However, the interaction of drug and antibody results in the activation of complement at the red cell surface. If sufficient complement is fixed, hemolysis results, as outlined above. Since the initial steps of the immune reaction are not firmly associated with the red cell, antibody will not be detected on the direct antiglobulin test. In these reactions, the red cell has been called an "innocent bystander"; some doubt has been raised as to its complete innocence in this reaction.

Numerous drugs have been implicated in an "innocent bystander" reaction: *Fuadin* (an antischistosomal agent), *sulfonamides, quinidine, chlorpropamide,* and *thorazine,* to name a few. When the "innocent bystander" reaction is responsible for hemolysis, only complement will be present on the patient's cells (antibody having been washed away during the prepara-

tion of the cells for the test) (Type III DCT), and the indirect antiglobulin test will be positive only when the responsible drug is present in the reaction mixture.

484.3. HEMOLYSIS DUE TO TRAUMATIC ALTERATION OF THE MEMBRANE

The membrane of the normal red cell is readily deformable but with limits to its elasticity. When sufficient shear stress is placed upon the cell, it undergoes progressive deformation and, eventually, membrane rupture. The amount of shear stress required has been estimated at about 3000 dynes per square centimeter. Such stresses do not occur in the normal circulation, because the vessels of the circulatory system are designed to allow the smooth passage of the blood, and the turbulence of the blood passing through the normal heart does not generate forces of this magnitude. However, such shear stress forces may be generated when abnormalities occur in the circulatory system, and fragmentation of the red cells may result. The characteristic red cell fragments resulting from this phenomenon are called *schistocytes*; these usually have sharp points and have been called *"helmet" cells, "triangle" cells,* and other similar names.

Fragmentation within the circulation occurs in two general clinical situations: (1) when intravascular fibrinous coagulation or abnormalities of the vessel walls in small arterioles cause irregularities upon which red cells may be fragmented, much as cells may be fragmented by being pushed through a fine wire screen, and (2) when alterations in the heart and major vessels occur such that turbulence and other factors yield shear stress forces sufficient to fragment the red cells.

HEMOLYSIS DUE TO ABNORMALITIES OF THE MICROCIRCULATION
(Microangiopathic Hemolytic Anemia)

The first clear-cut description of fragmentation hemolytic anemia in patients in whom abnormalities of the arterioles could be demonstrated was in 1963 by Brain, Dacie, and Hourihane. They named the syndrome "microangiopathic hemolytic anemia." The mechanism of this hemolysis was soon elucidated, using an artificial circulatory system. If blood was pumped through a bed of fibers of sufficiently small diameter so that the red cells could be looped over the fibers like clothes hung on a clothesline (without clothespins) and if sufficient force were applied as pressure, the cells were severed by the strand much as a wire cheese knife cuts cheese. Since the opposite sides of the membrane were brought into the apposition, they were sometimes able to reseal and the fragment was able to float away.

Fragmentation in vivo results when threads of sufficiently small size (usually fibrin) occur in the arteriolar side of the circulation where the blood pressure provides sufficient force to fragment the cells. Table 3 lists some of the clinical states in which this occurs. There is a greater or lesser degree of intravascular coagulation. When the primary defect appears to be arteriolar damage, the amount of intravascular coagulation demonstrable by a diminution in procoagulants may be small or even absent. On the other hand, when intravascular

TABLE 3.   Causes of "Microangiopathic" Fragmentation Hemolysis

Vascular abnormality predominant:
1. Thrombotic thrombocytopenic purpura (hemolytic-uremic syndrome)
2. Renal lesions
   a. Malignant hypertension
   b. Glomerulonephritis
   c. Transplant rejection
   d. Preeclampsia
3. Vasculitis
   a. Polyarteritis nodosa
   b. Rocky Mountain spotted fever
   c. Wegener's granulomatosis
4. Vascular anomalies
   a. Giant cavernous hemangioma (Kasabach-Merritt syndrome)
   b. Arteriovenous fistula
Intravascular coagulation predominant:
1. Septicemia with shock
2. Abruptio placentae

coagulation is the major event and occurs on both the arteriolar and venous sides, marked diminution in procoagulants may be present with only minor amounts of fragmentation hemolysis.

CLINICAL MANIFESTATIONS.   The degree of hemolysis may vary, depending upon the underlying process. Fragmentation hemolysis occurs in malignant hypertension, usually only when renal failure and papilledema are present; pathologically the kidneys usually show fibrinoid necrosis. The fragmentation hemolysis in carcinoma is usually seen only in adenocarcinoma and then only when metastatic; the degree of hemolysis may be considerable. The hemolysis in vasculitic lesions (e.g., Rocky Mountain spotted fever, periarteritis nodosa, Wegener's granulomatosis) is generally relatively minor, and the major manifestations are those of the underlying disease.

DIAGNOSIS.   The diagnosis of fragmentation hemolysis is made by the demonstration of schistocytic forms in the peripheral blood. Evidences of intravascular hemolysis (increased plasma hemoglobin and lactic acid dehydrogenase, urine hemosiderin, and, perhaps, urine hemoglobin) are usually present. Ancillary evidence may include evidence of disseminated intravascular coagulation (see Ch. 521.5).

TREATMENT.   Treatment of fragmentation hemolysis depends in large part on the management of the underlying lesion. Reduction in blood pressure in malignant hypertension will reduce the rate of fragmentation hemolysis. Resolution of the septic shock or the Rocky Mountain spotted fever will also end the hemolytic episode. Irradiation or removal of vascular abnormalities (giant hemangioma, traumatic arteriovenous fistula) will usually end the hemolytic process. In those instances in which intravascular coagulation plays a major role, treatment with heparin may be of value. Heparin does not appear to be of value in widely metastatic carcinoma.

HEMOLYSIS DUE TO ABNORMALITY OF THE HEART AND GREAT VESSELS
(Traumatic Cardiac Hemolytic Anemia)

Abnormalities of the heart and great vessels may lead to such degrees of turbulence that fragmentation may occur. The resultant hemolytic anemia is in general mild. Fragmentation hemolysis has been described in aortic stenosis, ruptured sinus of Valsalva, congenital stenosis of the aorta, traumatic arteriovenous fistula,

marked aortic regurgitation, and marked tachycardia. In general, only lesions of the left side of the heart and general circulation lead to traumatic fragmentation hemolysis, because only on that side are the shear stress forces of sufficient strength.

When prosthetic devices are inserted into the heart or great vessels, fragmentation hemolysis is frequent. In one large series, 60 to 80 per cent of all patients with prosthetic aortic or mitral valves demonstrated clinically significant hemolysis. Patients with both aortic and mitral prostheses are more likely to have hemolysis than are those with only one.

A frequent cause of severe hemolysis is regurgitation around the outside of the valve owing to poor seating; this is particularly common in prosthetic aortic valves. The material of which the valve is composed is of some importance; cloth-covered valves tend to give more hemolysis than others, and those with steel balls show less hemolysis than those with Silastic balls. When variance of the Silastic ball occurs, increased hemolysis may result. In general, increased hemolysis occurs in situations of increased turbulence, as when large quantities of blood are forced through small apertures by high pressure.

Fragmentation hemolysis may also occur after surgery for correction of the ostium primum defect with a patch. In certain instances, the defect in the mitral valve is insufficiently closed, and blood regurgitates forcefully against the patch. When this occurs, epithelialization of the patch may be prevented, and since the surface is relatively rougher than the endothelium, the forceful jet of blood may create forces sufficient to fragment the cells.

CLINICAL MANIFESTATIONS.   The degree of hemolysis is variable from patient to patient, depending upon the underlying abnormality. In a given patient the amount of hemolysis tends to vary with the cardiac output. Hence patients tend to have more hemolysis during the day when active than at night. If the patient becomes markedly anemic, in compensation the cardiac output is raised and the degree of hemolysis may increase. This may be manifest to the patient as increasing hemoglobinuria.

As in all chronic intravascular hemolysis, considerable iron is lost into the urine as hemosiderin and hemoglobin. Hence the patients may become iron deficient, thus suppressing erythropoiesis. This will lead to more severe anemia, which will lead to an increase in cardiac output and thus more severe hemolysis.

TREATMENT.   All patients with evidences of fragmentation hemolysis ought to be given iron supplementation (ferrous sulfate, 300 mg three times a day). When the degree of hemolysis is severe, parenteral iron therapy with iron-dextran may be needed. Transfusion may be required. However, if chronic transfusion is necessary, some consideration should be given to replacement of the valve if, as is usually the case, some defect in the valve placement is present. When hemolysis is due to a patch on an ostium primum defect, it may be necessary to replace the patch and further to replace the mitral valve so that regurgitation against the patch does not occur.

In those instances of traumatic fragmentation hemolysis in which no prosthesis has been inserted, the hemolysis is usually not severe enough to require treatment.

MARCH HEMOGLOBINURIA

March hemoglobinuria was first described in 1881 in an infantryman in the Prussian army who, after long marches, noted passage of dark urine. Since that time, many instances of hemoglobinuria occurring after running or after repeated trauma to some part of the body have been described. *Marathon runners* commonly demonstrate this syndrome, especially those with a stomping gait or those who run barefoot or in poorly cushioned shoes. *Karate experts* who practice their art by repeatedly striking their hand against hard surfaces, *pelota players*, *bongo drummers*, and *patients who strike their heads* repeatedly against the wall have all been found to have hemolysis as a result of their particular activity.

The red cells do not appear to be abnormal. The hemolysis apparently occurs because the red cells are forceably smashed within the microcirculation when the body part is struck against a hard surface or object. The cells may be popped like a balloon, and schistocytes are rarely or never seen. The syndrome can be stopped by altering the activity so that forceable striking of a body part does not occur; e.g., marathon runners may be advised to use cushioned shoes or to alter their gait.

CLINICAL MANIFESTATIONS. The patient commonly notes dark urine immediately after the activity; it generally clears by the second or third voiding. Anemia seldom occurs, and no other serious side effects, save for the fright of seeing dark urine, have been noted.

484.4. HEMOLYSIS DUE TO ACQUIRED DYSPLASTIC ALTERATION OF THE MEMBRANE

In most acquired hemolytic syndromes, the red cell is made normally and the defect which leads to its destruction is acquired. However, in certain acquired diseases of the bone marrow, the red cells which are produced by the marrow have an abnormal membrane and as a result do not survive normally in the circulation. Frequently, other manifestations of the dysplastic process, particularly ineffective erythropoiesis, are more obvious and the hemolysis is not readily recognized. Thus the red cells in megaloblastic anemia of whatever cause do not survive normally, but the other effects of megaloblastosis are so great that the anemia is not usually classed as "hemolytic." Similarly, the red cells of such syndromes of dysplastic erythropoiesis as myelofibrosis, sideroblastic anemia, and some forms of leukemia and preleukemia also do not survive normally. These syndromes are discussed in detail elsewhere.

PAROXYSMAL NOCTURNAL HEMOGLOBINURIA

Paroxysmal nocturnal hemoglobinuria (PNH) is an acquired complex disorder of dysplastic blood cell production which is usually classed among the hemolytic anemias, since that is one of its chief manifestations. It results from the abnormal proliferation of a clone of defective stem cells whose product cells are characterized by an abnormality in the interaction of the membrane with the components of hemolytic plasma complement. This abnormal interaction results in either destruction or dysfunction of these cells.

The disease is characterized by red cells which are hemolyzed more readily by complement, no matter how it is activated, than are normal cells. This results in a syndrome of variable severity, depending upon the proportion of affected cells and the degree of their abnormality. In addition to normal or normal-like cells (PNH I cells), there may be two kinds of abnormal cells: (1) PNH II cells, which require about one fourth as much of serum complement for an equal degree of lysis as normal cells, and (2) PNH III cells, which require one fifteenth as much. Both kinds of abnormal cells fix much greater amounts of the third component of complement for a given degree of complement activation than normal cells. In addition, PNH III cells are more readily lysed by the terminal complex of complement.

These three kinds of cells occur in various combinations and proportions in patients with PNH. Most patients have PNH I and PNH III cells. The proportion of abnormal cells may range from less than 2 per cent to greater than 90 per cent. Since the abnormal cells are readily lysed in the circulation, the degree of lysis is in large part a reflection of their number. When there are many such cells, the classic manifestations of PNH are present: hemoglobinuria, which is worse during the night and which may occur in paroxysms lasting several days, and marked hemosiderinuria; marked anemia may also be present. When fewer abnormal cells are present, the paroxysms of hemoglobinuria may occur only rarely, frequently only following infections. When very small proportions of abnormal cells are encountered, chronic hemolytic anemia alone, not characterized by hemoglobinuria, may be seen. In nearly all patients there is loss of iron through hemosiderinuria, and patients frequently become iron deficient.

Patients with PNH are also subject to thrombotic episodes in unusual sites. Hepatic vein thrombosis, frequently insidious in nature; cerebral vein thrombosis; splenic vein thrombosis; and portal vein thrombosis may be encountered. This is thought to be due to the abnormal interaction of the platelet membrane with plasma complement. The resulting excessive fixation of C3 to the platelet membrane results in activation of the PNH platelet.

Patients with PNH are also subject to infections; in part this may be due to granulocytopenia, but it may also be due to a functional disability of the abnormal granulocytes.

Patients with PNH may have episodes of abdominal pain, particularly during hemolytic crises. These may be related to small thromboses or perhaps to spasm of smooth muscle. The latter manifestation is demonstrated in the esophagus and results in a marked retrosternal discomfort in patients with severe hemolysis. Episodes of severe low back pain of unknown cause may also be seen in these patients.

LABORATORY MANIFESTATIONS. The degree of anemia is highly variable, as is the degree of reticulocytosis, which is often less than expected for the degree of anemia. Many patients are thrombocytopenic and/or granulocytopenic during part of their illness. In some cases these abnormalities are clearly due to residua from aplastic anemia; in others the bone marrow shows hyperplasia of the appropriate precursors, suggesting that the circulatory cells are being destroyed.

The abnormalities of the red cells, and thus the diagnosis, are demonstrated by activating complement by any of a number of ways in the presence of the red cells. Normal red cells will not be hemolyzed, whereas the abnormal red cells of patients with PNH will. Complement may be activated by the alternative pathway through the acidification of the serum (*Ham's test*), by any of a number of techniques using antibodies, or by reduction in the ionic strength through the substitution of sucrose for salt (*sucrose lysis test*). Of these, Ham's test is the most widely used and is the most specific; the only false positives are in the rare and easily discriminated form of congenital dyserythropoietic anemia called hereditary erythroblastic multinuclearity with a positive acidified lysis test (HEMPAS). When the population of abnormal red cells is extremely small, Ham's test as usually performed may not detect it; the sensitivity of this test may be increased by addition of magnesium. The sucrose lysis test is more sensitive but less specific; false-positive reactions are not infrequently encountered. The tests using antibody, particularly the complement lysis sensitivity test, are the most accurate and sensitive; they delineate not only the proportion of abnormal cells but also their degree of abnormality.

Because of the marked intravascular hemolysis, hemosiderinuria is nearly always present, and hemoglobinuria may likewise be seen. The plasma lactic acid dehydrogenase may be elevated.

INCIDENCE. The syndrome is unusual but not rare. The diagnosis must be sought in anyone with chronic hemolytic anemia, pancytopenia, hemosiderinuria, unusual venous thromboses, and unusual painful episodes. The peak incidence is in young adulthood, although children five years old and adults over 75 have had the disorder.

COURSE. The course is generally long lasting and often eventful. Episodes of hemolysis frequently follow infections and can be life threatening in severely affected patients. Thrombotic episodes, particularly of the hepatic veins, are the most dreaded consequence of the disease. These are especially frequent following surgery or pregnancy. Chronic renal failure is uncommon but does occur.

TREATMENT. The treatment of PNH is symptomatic, since the replacement of the abnormal clone of stem cells by bone marrow transplantation is not practical in most cases.

Most patients with PNH become iron deficient; when replenished with iron, they may have an episode of increased hemolysis. This is due to the sudden delivery to the peripheral blood of a number of young cells which are susceptible to hemolysis. This can be prevented by prior transfusion or by treatment with prednisone (see below).

Many patients with PNH appear to have an increase in the hematocrit in response to androgens, usually given as fluoxymesterone or oxymetholone in doses of 10 to 50 mg per day. This treatment is particularly useful for those patients with an element of erythroid hypoplasia. One must be careful of the hepatic complications of such therapy.

Prednisone is able to diminish the occurrence of hemolysis in patients with PNH by an unknown mechanism. Unfortunately, the doses required are greater than can be sustained on a long-term basis. Hence, patients with severe hemolysis may benefit from alternate-day dosage of prednisone (15 to 40 mg every other day). On the day the prednisone is not taken, more hemolysis will occur. It is to be emphasized that daily dosages of prednisone in this amount must be avoided except for short intervals during hemolytic crises.

Transfusion of whole blood may be accompanied by hemolysis of the patient's cells. This may be due to the presence of small amounts of activated complement in the transferred plasma. This reaction can largely be prevented by infusing washed cells or cells which have been frozen and reconstituted.

Patients with PNH who are having acute or chronic thrombosis must be anticoagulated. The use of heparin has been said to be accompanied by hemolytic reactions. However, if heparin is used in a sufficiently high dose, this apparently does not occur. Coumadin derivatives may be used without difficulty. Patients with such problems should be treated with prednisone as outlined above.

PROGNOSIS. PNH is a chronic disease with a highly variable outcome. It has been estimated that half the patients will be dead within ten years of diagnosis; on the other hand, many patients have survived for very long periods of time. Among these, a proportion may lose their abnormal PNH clone; this is particularly true for those in whom this syndrome arose as a result of aplastic anemia. In any event, recognition of this syndrome and appropriate care of the symptoms are of paramount importance in survival.

484.5. HEMOLYSIS DUE TO CHEMICAL ALTERATION OF THE MEMBRANE

During the normal circulation of red cells, the red cell membrane is not appreciably altered in such a way as to effect hemolysis until 120 days are reached. However, certain alterations in the environment have been defined which can alter the red cell membrane and shorten the life span of the red cells.

DRUGS

Drugs and other chemicals may diminish the life span of the red cell in several ways: (1) they may interact directly with the membrane of the normal cell, resulting in abnormalities which lead to hemolysis; (2) they may stimulate the formation of antibodies which then lead to the destruction of the red cell; or (3) they may effect certain reactions which are not usually toxic for the normal red cell but are injurious to red cells deficient in detoxifying mechanisms, usually related to deficiencies of the hexose monophosphate shunt. Since these deficiencies are usually on a congenital basis (e.g., glucose-6-phosphate dehydrogenase deficiency), this form of hemolysis is considered in Ch. 483.

Drugs which cause hemolysis directly are few in number, because this effect is readily detected and the drugs are not used. *Amphotericin* may do so by its ability to interact with lipids of the membrane. Certain lipid solvents may interact with the membrane and bring about its dissolution. This form of hemolysis is probably rare.

TOXINS AND POISONS

Toxic substances ("poisons") may bring about hemolysis by alteration of the membrane. These substances may be of animal origin, as in the case of hemolysis after snake bites or spider bites (see Ch. 33.9 and 36). In the former, phospholipases are thought to release the lipids of the membrane and destroy its integrity. Hemolysis, if present at all, is only a minor part of the complex clinical syndrome.

Some vegetable poisons such as *castor beans* and certain *mushrooms* may cause hemolysis. The mechanism of this has not been delineated. Certain minerals may also cause hemolysis, the best known of which is *copper*. This is thought to be the cause of the hemolysis which occasionally occurs in Wilson's disease. Its role has been very clearly demonstrated in patients undergoing dialysis in which the medium became so alkaline that copper salts were dissolved from the machine. The precise mechanism of its action is not clear; it may have to do with the fact that the copper ion is able to bind to the membrane sulfhydryl groups. Patients with *arsenical* intoxication sometimes have hemolytic anemia. Again, interference with the membrane structure is probably the cause, although the details have not been ascertained.

METABOLIC PRODUCTS AND ABNORMALITIES

The milieu in which the red cells circulate may be altered by failure of one of the excretory organs. When this occurs, some of the accumulated abnormal metabolites may alter the red cell membrane and result in hemolysis. With *liver failure*, commonly secondary to cirrhosis or alcoholic hepatitis, the red cells may become markedly overloaded with cholesterol. This at first leads to a spreading of the membrane, resulting in target cells which have a normal life span. However, if the process is further exaggerated and if the ratio of cholesterol to phospholipids is altered, the membrane may become markedly abnormal, and a *spur cell*, a contracted, irregular cell fancifully resembling a spur for horses, may result. When this occurs, marked intravascular hemolysis may result.

Some patients with renal failure also exhibit hemolysis. The precise nature of the accumulated metabolite which is responsible for this phenomenon has not been demonstrated. In some instances, the defect may be demonstrated by an abnormal autohemolysis (sterile incubation) test.

In patients in whom the serum phosphate falls to less than 1.0 mg per cent, the intracellular phosphate of the red cell may fall sufficiently to deplete the cell of ATP. This results in "stiffening" of the membrane, with the result that the cell is readily lysed. Such diminution of phosphate levels occurs in malnutrition, especially in alcoholism, and in the overuse of phosphate-binding antacids.

INFECTIOUS AGENTS

Hemolysis is a frequent accompaniment of infections. This may be due to the fact that the infectious agent invades the red cell and directly effects its lysis. This most commonly occurs in malaria, particularly by *Plasmodium falciparum*. The sudden release of merozoites may result in sufficient hemolysis to cause hemoglobinuria *(blackwater fever)*. The bacterial organism *Bartonella* may also invade the red cells and cause hemolysis.

Infections with clostridial organisms causing gas gangrene may result in marked hemolysis; instances of hemolysis of all circulating red cells have been recorded. This is thought to be due to alteration of the membrane phospholipids by enzymes elaborated by the organisms, but this has not been proved. The red cells show marked spherocytosis, and readily apparent evidences of intravascular hemolysis are present. The occurrence of this complication usually indicates a very poor prognosis, although instances of recovery have been reported when the infection is adequately treated.

In other instances of infection of various sorts (e.g., *Salmonella, Neisseria, E. coli, D. pneumoniae*), hemolysis of a less dramatic degree may occur in the absence of evidence of immunologic reaction on the red cell membrane. This has been thought, as in the case of the clostridial infection, to be due to alteration of the membrane by the organism or some product elaborated by it; this theory remains to be proved.

484.6.   HEMOLYSIS DUE TO OVERACTIVITY OF THE RETICULOENDOTHELIAL SYSTEM

Red cells are presumably destroyed normally in the reticuloendothelial system, although the causes and the details of this destruction are not known. In certain instances, overactivity of the reticuloendothelial system, resulting from either anatomic alteration or malignancy of its cells as in histiocytic medullary reticulosis, has been thought to cause premature destruction of normal cells.

HYPERSPLENISM

See Ch. 513.

Immune Hemolytic Anemia

Garratty, G., and Petz, L. D.: Drug-induced immune hemolytic anemia. Am. J. Med., 58:398, 1975.
Jensen, K. G., and Killmann, S. A. (eds.): Aspects of the autoimmune hemolytic anemias. Series Hematol., 7:303, 1974.
Pirofsky, B. M.: Autoimmunization and the Autoimmune Hemolytic Anemias. Baltimore, Williams & Wilkins Company, 1960.
Pruzanski, W., and Shumak, K. H.: Biologic activity of cold-reacting autoantibodies (Parts 1 and 2). N. Engl. J. Med., 297:538, 583, 1977.
Rosse, W. F.: Correlation of in vivo and in vitro measurements of hemolysis in hemolytic anemia due to immune reactions. Prog. Hematol., 8:51, 1973.
Swisher, S. N. (ed.): Immune hemolytic anemias. Semin. Hematol., 13:247, 1974.
Worlledge, S. M.: Immune drug-induced haemolytic anaemias. Semin. Hematol., 6:181, 1969.

Paroxysmal Nocturnal Hemoglobinuria

Jensen, K. G., and Killman, S. A. (eds.): Paroxysmal nocturnal hemoglobinuria. Series Hematol., 5:1, 1972.
Rosse, W. F.: Paroxysmal nocturnal hemoglobinuria in aplastic anemia. Clin. Haematol., in press.
Rosse, W. F., Logue, G. L., Adams, J., and Crookston, J. H.: Mechanisms of immune lysis of the red cells in hereditary erythroblastic multinuclearity with a positive acidified serum lysis test (HEMPAS) and paroxysmal nocturnal hemoglobinuria (PNH). J. Clin. Invest., 53:31, 1974.
Sirchia, G., and Lewis, S. M.: Paroxysmal nocturnal hemoglobinuria. Clin. Haematol., 4:199, 1975.

Fragmentation Hemolysis

Brain, M. J.: Microangiopathic hemolytic anemia. Ann. Rev. Med., 21:133, 1970.
Bull, B. S., Rubenberg, M. L., Dacie, J. V., and Brain, M. C.: Microangiopathic haemolytic anaemia: Mechanisms of red-cell fragmentation. Br. J. Haematol., 14:643, 1968.
Crexells, C., Aerichide, N., Bonny, Y., Lepage, C., and Campeau, L.: Factors influencing hemolysis in valve prostheses. Am. Heart J., 84:161, 1972.
Davidson, R. J. L.: March or exertional hemoglobinuria. Semin. Hematol., 6:150, 1969.
Marsh, G. W., and Lewis, S. M.: Cardiac hemolytic anemia. Semin. Hematol., 6:133, 1969.

485. HEMOGLOBIN, THE HEMOGLOBINOPATHIES, AND THE THALASSEMIAS

C. Lockard Conley

485.1. INTRODUCTION

The primary role of the red cells is transport of oxygen, a function made possible by the hemoglobin within the erythrocytes. The amount of oxygen delivered by fully oxygenated blood is dependent not only on the hemoglobin content and rate of flow but also on the affinity of the hemoglobin for oxygen at existing oxygen tensions. The effectiveness of hemoglobin in oxygen transport is the result of its variable oxygen affinity, a unique property dependent upon the tetrameric structure of the hemoglobin molecule.

The major hemoglobin component of the normal adult (Hb A) contains four polypeptide chains, two alpha chains each with 141 amino acid residues, and two beta chains each with 146 residues; it is designated $\alpha_2\beta_2$. A heme group containing an iron atom is affixed to each chain. A minor component comprising 2 to 3 per cent of the hemoglobin is designated Hb A_2, consisting of alpha and delta chains ($\alpha_2\delta_2$). The predominant hemoglobin of the fetus and newborn (Hb F) contains pairs of alpha and gamma chains ($\alpha_2\gamma_2$). Current evidence indicates that the gamma, delta, and beta globin genes are tightly linked on chromosome 11, and the nonlinked alpha globin genes are on chromosome 16. There are two pairs of gamma chain genes, differing in the codon that determines the amino acid residue in position 136; therefore normal persons have two types of gamma chains, one with glycine and the other with alanine as the 136th residue. The alpha globin gene also is duplicated, at least in some populations, so that normal persons have four alpha chain genes. There are multiple differences in amino acid sequences of beta, delta, and gamma chains, but the physiologic properties of the hemoglobins are similar. The fashion in which the globin chains and their heme groups are bonded together provides the iron atoms with precisely the environment necessary for reversible combination with oxygen. As oxygen is bound successively to each of the four iron atoms, stereochemical changes occur in the hemoglobin molecule that cause an increased affinity of the remaining iron atoms for oxygen. The sigmoid oxygen dissociation curve is the graphic representation of these relationships. Because of these allosteric effects, hemoglobin is fully oxygenated in the lungs even if the alveolar oxygen tension is appreciably less than normal; as oxygen is unloaded in the tissues, progressive reduction in the oxygen affinity of the hemoglobin provides for maximal delivery of oxygen with little change in oxygen tension.

485.2. OXYGEN AFFINITY OF THE RED CELLS

Pure hemoglobin has too high an affinity for oxygen to release appreciable amounts at normal tissue oxygen tensions. Within the red cell the oxygen affinity of the hemoglobin is modified by several mechanisms. Hydrogen ions stabilize the deoxy-state of hemoglobin, lessening affinity (Bohr effect). Carbon dioxide binds to hemoglobin and decreases its affinity for oxygen. Both these reactions facilitate release of oxygen in the capillaries. Certain phosphate compounds within the red cells significantly reduce the oxygen affinity of hemoglobin. Of these, 2,3-diphosphoglycerate (DPG) occurs in highest concentration (almost 1 mol per mol of hemoglobin), and is most important in regulation of oxygen dissociation. The deoxy-conformation of hemoglobin permits binding of DPG to the beta chains, stabilizing this conformation and lessening oxygen affinity. Fetal hemoglobin binds less DPG than Hb A; therefore the oxygen affinity of red cells containing Hb F is higher than that of normal adult red cells, even though the oxygen dissociation curves of purified Hb A and Hb F are similar. The position of the oxygen dissociation curve is expressed as the P_{50}, the oxygen tension required to half-saturate the hemoglobin with oxygen. The P_{50} of the blood of the fetus and newborn is reduced, and the oxygen dissociation curve is shifted to the left of the adult curve.

Each red cell produces its own DPG, an intermediate in glycolytic metabolism. DPG increases when there is a persistent rise in intracellular pH or in the proportion of deoxyhemoglobin, conditions influenced by the environment of the erythrocyte. Anemia or anoxia causes the concentration of DPG within normal erythrocytes to rise. When normal red cells are transfused to anemic patients, the DPG level of the transfused red cells increases, demonstrating that the effect is initiated by extracellular mechanisms. In addition, alterations of DPG concentration may result from intrinsic disorders of the metabolism of the red cell; for example, in erythrocyte pyruvate kinase deficiency, DPG is usually elevated. The presence of DPG is largely responsible for reducing the oxygen affinity of the hemoglobin within normal red cells to a value appropriate for release of oxygen at tissue oxygen tensions. When the concentration of DPG rises, oxygen affinity is lessened, so that more oxygen is released in the tissues without a change in the tissue oxygen tension. This phenomenon is significant in adaptation to anoxia and anemia. In persons acclimatized to low oxygen tensions, as at high altitude, values for DPG are high, assuring that relatively large amounts of oxygen are released at tissue tensions even though the arterial blood is not fully saturated. The remarkable ability of patients with chronic severe anemia to tolerate extremely low concentrations of hemoglobin in the blood is largely attributable to the high values of DPG in the erythrocytes, permitting release of greatly increased amounts of oxygen per red cell at normal tissue oxygen tensions. These adaptive changes are promptly and effectively regulated, the oxygen affinity of red cells changing within hours after the onset of anemia or anoxia. Pathologic states that cause increased oxygen affinity of the blood impair oxygen delivery. The increase of oxygen affinity of hemoglobin produced by carbon monoxide poisoning and methemoglobinemia may be more important than the reduced oxygen carrying capacity in producing clinical effects.

485.3. ABNORMALITIES OF HEMOGLOBIN

Abnormalities of hemoglobin may involve the heme group with its iron atom, the globin moiety, or both. Oxidation of the iron to form methemoglobin or displacement of oxygen by carbon monoxide causes serious but reversible impairment of hemoglobin function. Certain toxic agents and drugs (e.g., nitrates, sulfonamides, phenylhydrazine) may produce methemoglobin or sulfhemoglobin and may denature and precipitate hemoglobin, an irreversible reaction. Modifications of globin may occur in other acquired disorders. In diabetics a minor hemoglobin fraction, Hb A_{1c}, tends to be increased, reflecting the average degree of hyperglycemia over a period of weeks. Hb A_{1c} is normal hemoglobin modified by postsynthetic glycosylation, an irreversible in vivo reaction in which hexose structures are bound to the beta chains. Quantification of hemoglobin Hb A_{1c} has been proposed as a measure of the adequacy of the control of diabetes. In some patients with lead poisoning the hemoglobin may contain a small component with abnormal electrophoretic mobility. An increased concentration of Hb F may occur in several acquired conditions, including pregnancy, aplastic anemia, leukemia, myeloproliferative disorders, and hemolytic anemias. In these conditions the augmented levels of Hb F are limited to a minority of the red cell population (F cells). Hb A_2 may be increased in megaloblastic anemia and decreased in iron deficiency. Hb H (β_4) sometimes appears in the red cells of patients with certain myeloproliferative diseases, notably erythroleukemia.

The *heritable hemoglobinopathies* are genetically determined disorders of hemoglobin synthesis, of which there are two principal types. In one group there are structural abnormalities of the globin polypeptides. In the other, the *thalassemias*, there is impaired synthesis of globin chains usually not associated with a structural abnormality. More than 300 structural variants of hemoglobin have been discovered. The most common abnormality is a single amino acid substitution in one type of polypeptide chain, a change that can be explained in almost all instances by replacement of one nucleotide in an RNA codon. Thus the abnormality of sickle hemoglobin can be attributed to a change in a single purine base in the codon which specifies the sixth amino acid of the beta chain, with the result that glutamic acid is replaced by valine. Rarely two amino acid substitutions occur within a single polypeptide chain, as in Hb C Harlem. In certain abnormal hemoglobins, including Hb Freiburg and Hb Gun Hill, amino acid residues are missing from a globin chain, an abnormality that can be accounted for by loss of one or more codons ("deletion" of part of a gene) during nonhomologous crossing-over of genes. The hemoglobins Lepore have as their nonalpha chains polypeptides consisting of the amino-terminal portion of the delta chain and the carboxy-terminal portion of the beta chain, an abnormal structure that can be explained by loss of DNA from portions of closely linked genes with formation of a "fusion" gene. Hb Kenya contains the amino-terminal sequence of the gamma chain and the carboxy-terminal segment of the beta chain. Hb Constant Spring contains elongated alpha chains, an abnormality that can be explained by a mutation affecting a terminator codon. Hb Wayne also has elongated alpha chains, but resulting from a "frame shift" mutation attributable to deletion of a single nucleotide base of a codon. Hb McKees Rocks has a shortened beta chain, probably the result of a mutation producing a "nonsense" codon.

Thalassemia is a generic term for a heterogeneous group of inherited disorders of hemoglobin synthesis manifested by retarded production of specific types of globin chains. The synthetic defect in most forms of thalassemia is associated with deficiency of messenger RNA. In some instances the primary abnormality has been identified as deletion of globin genes (e.g., the alpha globin gene is deleted in some types of alpha thalassemia), but in other types of thalassemia the genes are present and the abnormality must be at the transcriptional or later stages. The abnormal peptide chains of the Lepore hemoglobins are synthesized at a slow rate. Similarly, abnormal peptides formed as a consequence of mutations in chain terminating codons (e.g., Hb Constant Spring) are produced slowly. In both cases a thalassemic disorder is the result. In beta thalassemia increased production of gamma chains partially compensates for the deficit of beta chains; therefore the erythrocytes contain a larger than normal fraction of Hb F, which is heterogeneously distributed among the red cells. *Hereditary persistence of fetal hemoglobin* is an anomaly in which Hb F is present in the red cells throughout life without anemia. Several forms have been described. In one type occurring in about 1 in 1000 American blacks, beta and delta chains are not produced at all because of deletion of closely linked genes. Compensation for the deficit is achieved by synthesis of gamma chains. The heterozygous carrier has about 25 per cent Hb F in each red cell. The homozygote has exclusively Hb F but no anemia or other clinical manifestations. Why Hb F is produced in fully compensating amounts in hereditary persistence of fetal hemoglobin but not in delta-beta thalassemia, also caused by deletion of globin genes, is unknown.

The hemoglobinopathies are inherited as autosomal codominant traits; heterozygous carriers have both the normal and the abnormal hemoglobin in each red cell. The normal component almost always constitutes the larger fraction. The genes that determine the structure of one class of globin chains are alleles; thus a person heterozygous for Hb S and Hb C, both of which contain abnormalities of the beta chain, has no Hb A and transmits one or the other but never both of the abnormal hemoglobins to each child. Thalassemia is inherited as if closely linked to the structural gene for the same chain. The alpha and beta chain genes segregate independently; accordingly a person heterozygous for both Hb G Philadelphia (an alpha chain variant) and Hb S (a beta chain variant) may transmit either, both, or neither of the abnormal hemoglobins to a child.

Hemoglobinopathies occur as a result of genetic mutations. Very high gene frequencies for harmful mutants are maintained in some areas of the world, presumably by strong selection pressures. Heterozygosity for Hb S appears to protect infants against the lethal effects of falciparum malaria, accounting for the maintenance of a high frequency of this deleterious abnormality in Africa. What selective advantage is conferred by Hb C in West Africa, by Hb E in Southeast Asia, and by thalassemia in several parts of the world is unknown. New mutations account for a surprising number of the unstable hemoglobins; in these cases the abnormal hemoglobin may not be detected in other members of the family.

485.4. CLINICAL SYNDROMES ASSOCIATED WITH HEMOGLOBINOPATHIES

Substitutions of amino acids in the globin chains do not necessarily cause untoward effects, and most of the known abnormal hemoglobins are not associated with disease, at least in heterozygous carriers. Two types of clinically important abnormalities have been identified: (1) Replacements on the surface of the molecule may cause abnormal *intermolecular* reactions, phenomena which explain the pathologic effects of Hb S and Hb C. Individual molecules function satisfactorily, and the peculiar interactions between molecules tend to occur only with the high intraerythrocytic concentrations of the abnormal hemoglobin found in homozygotes. Therefore the disease appears to be recessively inherited. When a red cell contains two major hemoglobin components (e.g., Hb S and Hb C), interactions may occur that importantly influence the pathologic effects. (2) Replacements in critical areas of the molecule may lead to *intramolecular* abnormalities with resultant alteration in oxygen binding or in molecular stability. These effects are manifested in heterozygotes, and in some the homozygous state presumably would be lethal.

Amino acid substitutions are likely to impair molecular function or stability when they occur in the area in which the heme group is attached, when they distort the conformation of the molecule, or when they occur at points of interaction between the polypeptide chains. The net result may be formation of methemoglobin, alteration of oxygen affinity, denaturation of the hemoglobin, or a combination of these effects.

Many of the known hemoglobin variants were discovered because of abnormal electrophoretic mobility under usual conditions of measurement. The electrophoretic method continues to be useful, but many amino acid substitutions do not alter net charge on the molecule and may be electrophoretically neutral. A number of abnormal hemoglobins have the same electrophoretic pattern, and some clinically important variants appear normal when studied by electrophoresis. The method therefore has important limitations in the detection as well as in the recognition of mutant hemoglobins. Other types of investigation, including detailed analysis of the functional properties of the hemoglobin, may be required for identification.

SICKLING DISORDERS

The single amino acid substitution in the beta chain in Hb S, located on the surface of the molecule, has no significant effect on oxygen affinity or molecular stability. It causes a unique *intermolecular* reaction in which molecules of deoxygenated Hb S align in spirally arranged polymers, forming insoluble fiber-like structures which distort the erythrocyte, increase its rigidity, and thereby cause the sickling deformation. The attractive forces between molecules operate only at short distances, so that the sickling phenomenon is markedly influenced by the concentration of deoxygenated Hb S in the red cell. Conditions influencing the intracellular concentration of deoxyhemoglobin, in particular oxygen tension and pH, are critical determinants of the degree of sickling. Sickling may be enhanced by the low oxy-gen affinity of the red cells of patients with sickle cell anemia; the low affinity is attributable in part to elevated values of 2,3-DPG and in part to the high concentration of hemoglobin in irreversibly sickled cells. Sickling is not instantaneous when hemoglobin is deoxygenated, so that duration of exposure of red cells to low oxygen tension is also a conditioning factor. Whether intravascular sickling occurs depends on local conditions of blood flow, oxygen tension, pH, and the oxygen affinity of the hemoglobin; on the concentration of Hb S in the red cell; and on the presence in the erythrocyte of another hemoglobin which may interact with Hb S to lessen or enhance sickling. Except for irreversibly sickled cells, the production of which seems to be correlated with severity of disease, erythrocytes quickly resume their normal shape when the hemoglobin is reoxygenated.

Manifestations of disease attributable to Hb S are caused by intravascular sickling of partially deoxygenated erythrocytes. The rigid sickle cells tend to be tangled, trapped, and fragmented in small vascular channels; in addition, the cell membrane is damaged by the recurring sickling distortion. Both factors shorten red cell survival with predominant destruction of erythrocytes within the RE system. The unyielding elongate and crescentic cells increase the viscosity of the blood, retard flow, occlude small blood vessels, and produce infarcts and other lesions as a result of local anoxia.

Sickle Cell Anemia

DEFINITION. Sickle cell anemia, the clinical expression of homozygosity for Hb S, is a serious disease characterized by unrelenting hemolytic anemia, recurrent episodes of pain and fever, and pathologic involvement of many organs. Affected persons, predominantly blacks, have obtained the mutant gene from both parents. About 8 per cent of American blacks are heterozygous carriers, so that approximately 1 in 600 blacks is expected to be homozygous at the time of conception; the actual prevalence of sickle cell anemia is lower because of its high mortality. First described by J. B. Herrick in 1910, the disease is of unique historic significance. Study of the sickling phenomenon led Hahn and Gillespie in 1927 to discover that the distortion of the red cells is related to the state of oxygenation of the hemoglobin. Pauling and his associates in 1949 demonstrated the existence of an abnormal hemoglobin and developed the concept of "molecular" disease. Subsequently the investigation of Ingram showed that the abnormality in Hb S is limited to a single amino acid substitution within a polypeptide chain of globin. These discoveries initiated an unprecedented era of scientific advancement, with rapid evolution of knowledge pertaining to molecular biology, genetics, and pathophysiology.

CLINICAL MANIFESTATIONS. Manifestations of the disease appear after the newborn period, when Hb F is replaced by Hb S. Persistent hemolytic anemia, although usually severe, is remarkably well tolerated and is not often the cause of the presenting symptoms. Many patients lead reasonably normal lives, at least for long intervals, and may be capable of a surprising amount of physical exertion. Much of the havoc of the disease is related to the periodic occurrence of disabling "crises," acute self-limited episodes of pain and fever, usually incapacitating but often not associated with increase in the degree of anemia. Precipitating factors may not be apparent; but attacks tend to occur at night, on exposure to cold, or during infections, times at which erythrostasis may be enhanced. Pain frequently is experienced in the bones and large joints of the extremities and in the back. Agonizing pain of great severity may be localized to a single area, involve multiple sites, or have a migratory character. Episodes tend to subside within a few days, but some patients have more persistent grumbling discomfort. Dramatic episodes of severe abdominal pain and fever simulate acute appendicitis and other urgent intra-abdominal disorders.

Most patients have a characteristic asthenic habitus with disproportionately long extremities and "spider" fingers, probably as a result of delayed closure of epiphyses. Growth tends to be retarded and sexual maturation delayed; fertility is reduced. Pregnancies often are concluded successfully, although fetal loss and maternal morbidity and mortality are increased. Susceptibility to infection is enhanced. Pneumococcal infections, including meningitis, occur with increased frequency in children, probably because of decreased serum opsinizing activity related to an abnormality of the properdin pathway. A unique predisposition to salmonellal osteomyelitis is a remarkable feature of the disease, but staphylococcal osteomyelitis also occurs. Chronic ulcers of the legs, overlying the malleoli, tend to occur at puberty or later. Multisystemic involvement is caused principally by ischemia resulting from anemia, erythrostasis, and vascular occlusions. Segmentation of blood flow can be seen in conjunctival vessels. Peripheral vascular occlusions in the retina may cause infarctions, neovascularization, vitreous hemorrhage, and retinal detachment. Many symptoms are referable to infarction of bones and bone marrow. In infancy the earliest manifestation may be the "hand-foot" syndrome, a painful swelling of the hands or feet, associated with appearance on roentgenograms of rectangular deformities of metacarpals, metatarsals, and phalanges. Later avascular necrosis of the femoral or humeral heads may cause permanent disability. Bone involvement is readily seen in dental films, which show radiolucency, abnormal trabeculation, and infarcts. Similar changes, with widening of marrow cavities and elevation of the periosteum, may be seen in other bones. Osteoporosis of the spine may be associated with a "fish" deformity of the vertebrae.

Repeated episodes of pneumonia tend to occur, sometimes in conjunction with painful crises. Infarction of the lung is responsible for many pneumonia-like illnesses. Pulmonary vessels are occluded by masses of sickled erythrocytes or by emboli arising in veins or in infarcted marrow. Rarely, repeated emboli lead to cor pulmonale. The heart is enlarged, and the dilated chambers and accelerated circulation give rise to impressive murmurs. These are most often systolic; they simulate the murmurs of valvular heart disease. Electrocardiographic abnormalities are not unusual. Congestive heart failure, uncommon in childhood, becomes more frequent as age advances. Vascular lesions in the nervous system may produce focal or multifocal neurologic manifestations, sometimes with convulsions. Hemolytic jaundice is persistent, and the chronic overproduction of bilirubin predisposes to formation of gallstones, cholecystitis, and obstruction of the biliary tract. The liver is usually enlarged. Erythrostasis in hepatic sinusoids may cause necrosis of liver cells, leading to episodes of marked jaundice with high levels of conjugated bilirubin and aberrations of liver function tests, suggesting both hepatocellular damage and intrahepatic biliary obstruction. Damage to the liver may cause chronic hepatic dysfunction, and the end result may be a peculiar form of cirrhosis. In addition to these disorders hepatitis may be acquired through blood transfusions. The spleen is enlarged in infancy, but infarctions lead to its shrinkage to a fibrous remnant, and splenomegaly is rare in adults. Even when enlarged the spleen does not function normally, probably a factor in the increased susceptibility to infection. Hyposthenuria is the most common evidence of renal dysfunction. Pyelonephritis is increased in frequency and is a serious problem for some patients, contributing to the development of renal failure. Infarcts of the kidney or papillary necrosis may cause hematuria, and recurrent infarction may lead to progressive renal insufficiency. The nephrotic syndrome occurs more often than would be expected by chance and is sometimes associated with renal vein thrombosis. Priapism may lead to permanent deformity and impotence.

Anemia is normocytic, with hemoglobin concentrations ranging between 5 and 10 grams per 100 ml. The reticulocyte count persistently exceeds 10 per cent, and polychromatophilia, stippling, and target cells are usual; siderocytes and Howell-Jolly bodies may be seen. The sickled erythrocytes observed in the stained blood smear are irreversibly sickled cells and may not be numerous, but in blood deoxygenated with sodium metabisulfite virtually all the red cells are sickled. Hemolytic jaundice is associated with a slight increase in the plasma hemoglobin because of intravascular destruction of some cells. Thrombocytosis and leukocytosis tend to persist and increase during crises, when leukocyte counts of more than 20,000 per cubic millimeter are common. The bone marrow is hyperplastic with a predominance of erythroid precursors. At times necrotic marrow can be aspirated from areas of acute bone pain. Profound anemia may be the result of "aplastic crises," transient episodes of retarded erythropoiesis associated with reticulocytopenia; these occur most often in association with infections. Folate deficiency, attributable in part to the high folate requirement of chronic hemolytic anemia, may lead to a superimposed megaloblastic anemia.

DIAGNOSIS. In typical cases the diagnosis is readily established by the demonstration of hemolytic anemia, positive sickling preparation with sodium metabisulfite, and the abnormal mobility of the hemoglobin on electrophoresis. Anemia may be overlooked in blacks, and the dramatic nonhematologic manifestations can be misleading. Recurrent joint pain and striking cardiac abnormalities often suggest rheumatic fever. Differentiation between the painful abdominal crises and other intra-abdominal disorders may be extremely difficult. Differential diagnosis of marked jaundice in patients with sickle cell anemia may require meticulous evaluation, including liver biopsy in appropriate cases. Limitations of the electrophoretic method should be recognized. Sickle cell anemia is clearly distinguished from sickle cell trait by this procedure in untreated patients, but after transfusions the patterns may be similar. The electrophoretic pattern of hemoglobin in untreated sickle cell anemia may be indistinguishable from that of other disorders, including sickle cell–thalassemia, sickle cell–hemoglobin D disease, sickle cell–hereditary persistence of fetal hemoglobin, and homozygous sickle cell anemia with heterozygosity for hemoglobin Memphis or alpha thalassemia, disorders which tend to be less severe. A patient with sickle cell anemia who is the heterozygous carrier of Hb G Philadelphia, an innocuous alpha chain variant, has an electrophoretic pattern of hemoglobin resembling that of sickle cell–hemoglobin C disease. Accordingly, proof of diagnosis may require family studies and additional analysis of the hemoglobin. Special investigations are warranted when the clinical disorder is atypical, e.g., when splenomegaly persists into adult life, when anemia is mild or absent, or when the disease is unusually benign.

PROGNOSIS. The disease in the past has had a high mortality rate in early childhood, few patients reaching adult life. Recent decades have seen progressively increasing longevity, and increasing numbers of patients survive beyond the age of 50. This improvement in outlook is not attributable to advances in specific therapy, but is largely the result of better nutrition and more adequate prevention and treatment of infections. Infection remains the most common cause of death. Aplastic crises are a serious threat to life if not treated promptly. Death may result from renal or hepatic insufficiency, cardiac failure, or vascular occlusions in the nervous system. Widespread intravascular sickling is found in some patients dying suddenly or during a painful crisis. The clinical spectrum of the disease is broad, and mild cases of sickle cell anemia are increasingly recognized. Some older patients have chronic anemia but have not had the characteristic symptoms associated with the disease.

TREATMENT. Specific therapy is not available. The painful episodes are self-limited; accordingly they appear to respond to a variety of therapeutic measures, but convincing evidence of efficacy is lacking. None of the drugs or agents reported to shorten a crisis has stood the test of a properly conducted controlled trial. The lesions underlying the painful crisis are related to ischemia and infarction, and there is no proof that unsickling the red cells will relieve pain after the crisis has occurred. A promising approach to treatment of sickle cell disease is the long-term use of an agent that modifies the hemoglobin molecule in such a way as to lessen the tendency to sickling. An effective and nontoxic agent has not as yet been found. Severe pain justifies the use of narcotics, with care to avoid respiratory depression. Narcotic addiction attributable to appropriate therapy is rare, because the painful episodes are too short to induce dependence. Hydration should be maintained by use of intravenous fluids as needed during the crisis. Careful attention should be given to oxygenation of the blood in patients with pulmonary lesions, with administration of oxygen in appropriate concentrations when the arterial oxygen tension is reduced. Patients with sickle cell anemia should continuously receive supplemental folic acid (1.0 mg per day). Infections, common in patients with sickle cell anemia, are often coincident with or mistaken for a sickle cell crisis. They should be diligently sought and promptly treated. Since pneumococcal infection represents a special hazard in this disease, administration of polyvalent pneumococcal polysaccharide vaccine appears promising. Transfusions may be lifesaving in aplastic crises and in the shock of abdominal crises, but their use in other situations should be considered carefully. Administration of usual volumes of blood raises the hematocrit value without markedly diluting the sickle cells, increasing the viscosity of deoxygenated blood and potentially enhancing the production of vascular occlusions. Partial exchange transfusions are effective in preventing crises when about 50 per cent of the red cells are replaced by normal erythrocytes. This procedure is particularly useful in preparing patients for surgical operations, and may be used in other critical situations. Leg ulcers tend to heal with conservative measures, particularly when anemia is corrected by transfusions and during bed rest; however, they often recur even after grafting procedures. When anesthesia is administered, good ventilation and high oxygen tensions in the inspired gas mixture should be maintained. Surgical procedures can be safely performed in patients in good general condition. Renal transplants have been successful in a few cases. Nevertheless, major elective procedures such as removal of asymptomatic gallstones appear to be unjustified. Most patients with sickle cell anemia have severe psychosocial problems, and dealing with these is an essential part of effective management. Excessive invalidism is to be avoided. With proper support, many patients can be educated and employed.

Sickle Cell Trait

Persons heterozygous for hemoglobin S are said to have sickle cell trait, with rare exceptions innocuous and not associated with anemia. In some areas of Africa more than 30 per cent of blacks carry the mutant gene. The prevalence is much lower in the populations of the Mediterranean area, the Middle East, and India. About 8 per cent of American blacks are affected. Each erythrocyte contains both Hb S and Hb A, and all the red cells sickle when deoxygenated; but the concentration of Hb S in the red cells is sufficiently low that intravascular sickling does not occur at physiologic oxygen tensions. Clinical manifestations may appear when unusual circumstances foster intravascular sickling. Hemolytic anemia simulating sickle cell anemia has been encountered in heterozygous carriers of Hb S with severe anoxemia caused by congenital heart disease. Infarction of the spleen may occur during travel in unpressurized aircraft. In a few instances sudden death has been attributed to sicklemia, but documentation of the role of the sickle cells is not adequate. Hyposthenuria is relatively common. Unilateral renal hematuria may appear without demonstrable cause and may persist for weeks; it usually ceases without relation to therapeutic efforts, none of which is clearly effective. Recurrent gross bleeding may originate in either kidney, and nephrectomy is contraindicated. Hematuria attributable to sickle cell trait is rare, and other causes should always be sought. Infection of the urinary tract in pregnancy is reported to be increased in frequency in women with sickle cell trait. Accurate recognition of the sickle cell trait requires demonstration of the sickling phenomenon in addition to the electrophoretic abnormality of the hemoglobin. Carriers are discovered only as a result of routine testing or surveys, and should be assured of the trivial nature of the abnormality as well as its genetic implications.

Other Heterozygous Sickling Disorders

Persons heterozygous for hemoglobin S and for another abnormality of either the alpha or beta chain may have no evidence of disease. Thus persons heterozygous for Hb S and Hb J (an innocuous beta chain variant) have no Hb A in their red cell hemolysates, yet appear perfectly well. In certain other heterozygous states intravascular sickling of red cells is enhanced by the additional genetic abnormality.

Sickle cell–thalassemia resembles sickle cell anemia but is generally less severe, with atypical features including relatively mild anemia and persistent splenomegaly. It occurs predominantly in persons of black or Mediterranean ancestry. The beta thalassemia gene lessens production of Hb A, which occurs in low proportion. Electrophoresis of hemoglobin shows that the predominant hemoglobin is Hb S, with smaller fractions of Hb A and Hb F; sometimes, as in sickle cell–beta⁰ thalassemia, Hb A cannot be detected and family studies are required to differentiate the disorder from sickle cell anemia.

Sickle cell–hemoglobin C disease occurs in American blacks at birth with about one fourth the frequency of sickle cell anemia. Anemia tends to be mild, and some patients are asymptomatic. Splenomegaly is usual and may persist to old age; but atrophy of the spleen attributable to infarction occurs in some cases. The disease has special importance because of its predominantly nonhematologic manifestations. Symptoms may be referable to the eye, where peripheral vascular occlusions in the retina cause retinal avascularity and neovascular proliferations; these tend to bleed, producing vitreous hemorrhages with subsequent fibrosis and retinal detachment. Pain and dysfunction of the hip or shoulder are caused by avascular necrosis of capital epiphyses, especially the femoral head. Acute abdominal pain after anesthesia or during flight in unpressurized aircraft is the result of infarction of the spleen. Gross unilateral renal hematuria is not uncommon. Pregnancy may be complicated by severe anemia, infarcts of bone, and pulmonary emboli; but in many instances pregnancy is uncomplicated. Diagnosis is suggested by examination of the blood smear in which almost all the red cells are target forms. Electrophoresis of hemoglobin shows two major components, Hb S and Hb C; Hb A is absent.

Sickle cell–hemoglobin O Arab disease is much less common but more severe than sickle cell–hemoglobin C disease, with which it is easily confused because Hb C and Hb O Arab have the same electrophoretic mobility on usual conditions of measurement. The blood smear resembles that of sickle cell anemia. Hb C and Hb O Arab can be differentiated by electrophoresis on agar gel at low pH.

Sickle cell–hemoglobin D Punjab disease has many of the features of sickle cell anemia and may be incapacitating because of vascular occlusive lesions, although anemia tends to be less severe. The rarity of the disease, its predominant occurrence in white persons, and the nonhematologic presenting manifestations obscure the diagnosis. Standard electrophoretic methods yield a pattern indistinguishable from that of sickle cell anemia, but Hb D separates from Hb S on agar gel at low pH.

DISORDERS ASSOCIATED WITH HEMOGLOBINS C, D PUNJAB, AND E

Homozygous hemoglobin C disease is an uncommon disorder occurring in blacks. Affected persons have few

symptoms, but the spleen is enlarged. Chronic hemolytic anemia is rarely severe and is often discovered incidentally. Hb C ($\alpha_2\beta_2$ $^{6\ glu\to lys}$) is relatively insoluble, causing increased rigidity of the red cells with fragmentation and accelerated destruction. The blood film contains populations of target cells and microspherocytes, the latter representing older fragmented cells. *Hemoglobin C–thalassemia* causes a similar disorder. Heterozygosity for Hb C, *hemoglobin C trait,* occurs with high frequency in some areas of West Africa and in 2 to 3 per cent of American blacks. Some target cells are seen in the blood smear without anemia or other evidence of disease.

Homozygous hemoglobin D Punjab disease is a rare disorder causing mild or moderately severe anemia with numerous target cells in the blood smear. Hb D Punjab ($\alpha_2\beta_2$ $^{121\ glu\to gln}$) occurs in India but also in many other parts of the world, and several instances of the disease have been encountered in white families. Hemoglobin D–thalassemia resembles the homozygous disorder but can be differentiated by family studies. Persons heterozygous for Hb D alone have no hematologic abnormalities.

Homozygous hemoglobin E disease is manifested by mild microcytic and normochromic anemia, usually without splenomegaly. Large numbers of target cells are seen in the blood smear. The disease has been encountered with considerable frequency in Orientals. Persons heterozygous for Hb E ($\alpha_2\beta_2$ $^{26\ glu\to lys}$) and beta thalassemia have a more severe anemia, and the spleen is usually enlarged. The high frequency of the genes for Hb E and various types of thalassemia in Southeast Asia has led to the appearance of some complex genetic disorders, e.g., hemoglobin E–alpha thalassemia disease, in which affected persons appear to have the characteristics of hemoglobin H disease in addition to hemoglobin E. Heterogeneity of the hemoglobin E diseases is related in part to the diversity of genetic factors.

485.5. HEMOLYTIC ANEMIAS CAUSED BY UNSTABLE HEMOGLOBINS

Congenital hemolytic disorders attributable to unstable hemoglobin molecules have been discovered in widely scattered cases (Table 1). Affected persons are the heterozygous carriers of the abnormal hemoglobin, and homozygotes are unknown. The structural abnormality of the hemoglobin predisposes to intraerythrocytic denaturation and precipitation. The severity of the hemolytic process is related to the degree of instability of the hemoglobin molecules. Some patients present with chronic anemia of varying severity, jaundice, and splenomegaly. Others are so mildly affected that there is no anemia and the red cells may appear normal. Persons with Hb Zürich have a compensated mild hemolytic disorder without anemia except after administration of sulfonamides or during infections, when fulminant hemolytic anemia may occur. Drug-induced hemolytic episodes have been described in carriers of several other unstable hemoglobins, including Hb Torino, Hb Köln, Hb Shepherd's Bush, and Hb Hasharon. Hb Köln causes chronic hemolytic anemia, with recurring bouts of more severe anemia, jaundice, and

TABLE 1. Unstable Hemoglobins That May Produce Hemolytic Disorders

Abnormal Hb	Structural Change		Abnormal Hb	Structural Change	
*Hirosaki	alpha 43	phe → leu	Sydney	beta 67	val → ala
*Torino	alpha 43	phe → val	*Mizuho	beta 68	leu → pro
*Hasharon	alpha 47	asp → his	*Seattle	beta 70	ala → asp
Russ	alpha 51	gly → arg	*Christchurch	beta 71	phe → ser
Rovigo	alpha 53	ala → asp	Bushwick	beta 74	gly → val
Ann Arbor	alpha 80	leu → arg	Shepherd's Bush	beta 74	gly → asp
Etobicoke	alpha 84	ser → arg	St. Antoine	beta 74, 75	gly, leu deleted
Setif	alpha 94	asp → tyr	*Atlanta	beta 75	leu → pro
*Bibba	alpha 136	leu → pro	Bryn Mawr	beta 85	phe → ser
Leiden	beta 6 or 7	glu deleted	Tours	beta 87	thr deleted
Saki	beta 14	leu → pro	*Borås	beta 88	leu → arg
Sögn	beta 14	leu → arg	*Santa Ana	beta 88	leu → pro
Belfast	beta 15	trp → arg	*Sabine	beta 91	leu → pro
Lyon	beta 17, 18	lys, val deleted	Gun Hill	beta deletion of 5 residues	
Freiburg	beta 23	val deleted		between 91 and 95	
Moscva	beta 24	gly → asp	*Istanbul	beta 92	his → gln
Riverdale-Bronx	beta 24	gly → arg	*Newcastle	beta 92	his → pro
*Savannah	beta 24	gly → val	Djelfa	beta 98	val → ala
Volga	beta 27	ala → asp	*Köln	beta 98	val → met
Genova	beta 28	leu → pro	*Nottingham	beta 98	val → gly
St. Louis	beta 28	leu → gln	Rush	beta 101	glu → gln
Tacoma	beta 30	arg → ser	Camperdown	beta 104	arg → ser
*Abraham Lincoln	beta 32	leu → pro	*Casper	beta 106	leu → pro
*Castilla	beta 32	leu → arg	Tübingen	beta 106	leu → gln
Philly	beta 35	tyr → phe	Peterborough	beta 111	val → phe
Mequon	beta 41	phe → tyr	*Madrid	beta 115	ala → pro
*Hammersmith	beta 42	phe → ser	Khartoum	beta 124	pro → arg
Louisville	beta 42	phe → leu	J Guantanamo	beta 128	ala → asp
Niteroi	beta 42-45	phe, glu, ser deleted	*Wien	beta 130	tyr → asp
			Leslie	beta 131	gln deleted
Okaloosa	beta 48	leu → arg	North Shore	beta 134	val → glu
*Tochigi	beta 56-59	gly, asn, pro lys deleted	Altdorf	beta 135	ala → pro
			Hope	beta 136	gly → asp
Duarte	beta 62	ala → pro	*Coventry	beta 141	leu deleted
Bičetre	beta 63	his → pro	*Olmstead	beta 141	leu → arg
*Zürich	beta 63	his → arg	Cranston	beta chain elongated	
J Calabria	beta 64	gly → arg	Tak	beta chain elongated	
Toulouse	beta 66	lys → glu	*Poole	gamma 130	trp → gly
*Bristol	beta 67	val → asp	*H	alpha₂ beta₂ → beta₄	

Unstable hemoglobins known to have caused moderately severe or severe anemia are designated by asterisks. Some (e.g., Hb Zurich, Hb Hasharon) have been associated with anemia only during febrile illness or administration of sulfonamides. Others are not known to have produced anemia, but it is quite possible that anemia might occur during administration of oxidant drugs.

dark urine; splenectomy has sometimes appeared to have a beneficial effect. Other unstable hemoglobins are not associated with distinguishing clinical features. Mild methemoglobinemia accompanies the hemolytic process in some instances, and the variant hemoglobin may have abnormal oxygen affinity. Increased oxygen affinity in Hb Zürich appears to have no clinical importance; reduced oxygen affinity in Hb Seattle is thought to increase anemia by lessening the stimulus for compensatory erythropoiesis. Diagnosis of unstable hemoglobin disorders is suggested by demonstration of precipitates of denatured hemoglobin (Heinz bodies) in the red cells, using supravital stains such as crystal violet. In patients with Hb Zürich these may appear during hemolytic episodes as large globular inclusions. Heinz bodies are seen in many of the red cells of patients with Hb Köln after splenectomy. They can be demonstrated in other cases by incubating red cells with brilliant cresyl blue, a redox dye. The abnormal hemoglobin tends to precipitate when hemolysates are heated at 50 to 60° C, or incubated at 37° C in 17 per cent isopropanol, a valuable test. The mean corpuscular hemoglobin concentration of the red cells may be somewhat low and the proportion of Hb A₂ increased as a result of preferential loss of the abnormal hemoglobin from the red cells. The electrophoretic mobility of he-

moglobin is abnormal in only about half the variants. The urine may be darkened by a dipyrrole pigment thought to originate from heme groups dislodged from unstable hemoglobin molecules. Treatment is usually not required. Severe anemia has improved in some patients after splenectomy.

485.6. DISORDERS CAUSED BY HEMOGLOBINS WITH ABNORMAL OXYGEN AFFINITY

Cyanosis is caused by methemoglobinemia in the heterozygous carriers of the hemoglobins M. A firm bond between the iron atom and the substituted amino acid in the globin chain maintains the iron permanently in the ferric state. The concentration of methemoglobin is not sufficiently high to cause major symptoms. In some instances there is an associated mild hemolytic disorder. Cyanosis resulting from methemoglobin formation occurs in carriers of certain unstable hemoglobins, notably Hb Freiburg and Hb St. Louis. Carriers of Hb Kansas and Hb Beth Israel also display cyanosis, in these cases caused by an increased concentration of deoxyhemoglobin in the blood in capillaries and venules; low affinity for oxygen facilitates unloading of oxygen in the tissues, a phenomenon without apparent harmful effects (Table 2).

Erythrocytosis (polycythemia) is the clinical expression of numerous abnormal hemoglobins with increased oxygen affinity (Table 3). These rare variants cause one form of familial polycythemia without leukocytosis, thrombocytosis, or splenomegaly. Hematocrit values of some heterozygotes have exceeded 65 per cent, and homozygotes are unknown. Impaired release of oxygen activates the erythropoietin mechanism, producing the compensatory erythrocytosis. These hemoglobins should be sought by direct measurement of oxygen affinity in cases of unexplained erythrocytosis; electrophoretic mobility of the variant hemoglobin is not always abnormal.

485.7. THE THALASSEMIA SYNDROMES

Two major categories of thalassemia are recognized: *alpha thalassemia*, caused by retarded production of alpha chains of globin, and *beta thalassemia*, caused by retarded production of beta chains. Since Hb F contains alpha chains, the fetus is affected by alpha thalassemia. Beta thalassemia becomes apparent after the newborn period, when Hb F is replaced by Hb A. Impaired hemoglobin synthesis causes anemia and microcytosis. In addition, unbalanced production of globin chains leads secondarily to accumulation of uncombined alpha chains in beta thalassemia and to formation of the abnormal molecules γ_4 (Hb Bart's) and β_4 (Hb H) in alpha thalassemia; these tend to precipitate within red cells, hastening their destruction. Much of the cell damage involves the erythrocyte precursors in the marrow. There is pronounced heterogeneity of the clinical disorders, largely resulting from a multiplicity of genetic mechanisms.

HOMOZYGOUS BETA THALASSEMIA

DEFINITION. Homozygous beta thalassemia is the inherited disorder described by Cooley and Lee in 1925 and subsequently known as Cooley's anemia, Mediterranean anemia, target cell anemia, or thalassemia major. Occurring most often in persons of Mediterranean ancestry, the disease is characterized by profound anemia, marked hepatosplenomegaly, and premature death, often in childhood.

CLINICAL MANIFESTATIONS. Anemia appears after the newborn period and thereafter is severe, with marked pallor and mild to moderate hemolytic jaundice. Growth and development are impaired. The spleen and liver become tremendously enlarged. Deformation of the bones, particularly those of the head, contributes to the characteristic "Mongoloid" facies, and distorts the mouth and disturbs the alignment of the teeth. Roentgenograms show a "hair-on-end" appearance of the skull, enlargement of other marrow cavities with thinning of cortical bone, and abnormalities of trabeculation related to the marked hyperplasia of marrow. Cardiac enlargement and failure are explained by the anemia and by the deposition of large amounts of iron in the myocardium. Hemosiderosis is largely the result of the many transfusions required to maintain life, but an additional factor is enhanced absorption of iron from the gastrointestinal tract. The hypochromic microcytic red cells are flattened and distorted, usually with numerous target and stippled forms and variable numbers of nucleated erythrocytes, polychromatic cells, and reticulocytes. Inclusion bodies consisting of denatured alpha globin can be demonstrated in normoblasts and reticulocytes when stained with methyl violet. Leukocytosis may be marked and persistent. Much of the hemolytic activity appears to be intramedullary with resulting ineffective erythropoiesis. Serum iron is elevated with increased saturation of iron-binding protein. The proportion of Hb F is usually between 20 and 60 per cent, but values as high as 90 per cent may occur. Hemoglobin A_2 is increased when expressed as a fraction of Hb A.

TREATMENT AND PROGNOSIS. With frequent transfusions and appropriate prevention and treatment of infections, life may be improved and prolonged. Massive deposition of iron is often the cause of cardiac failure and death. Folic acid, 1.0 mg per day, should be given to provide for the enhanced requirement. In selected cases splenectomy is beneficial when the spleen is actively sequestering red cells, but there is a danger that susceptibility to infection may be enhanced. Chelating agents such as deferoxamine mesylate have been used in an effort to reduce iron stores. Substantial amounts of iron can be removed by continuous parenteral administration of deferoxamine with concomitant oral administration of ascorbic acid. Whether long-term use of this or other methods is safe and effective has not been determined.

HETEROZYGOUS BETA THALASSEMIA

Heterozygous beta thalassemia (thalassemia minor) is manifested by mild anemia, usually with microcytosis,

TABLE 2.   Abnormal Hemoglobins That Produce Cyanosis

Abnormal Hb	Structural Change		Mechanisms
M Boston	alpha 58	his → tyr	Abnormal bond stabilizes iron in ferric state, producing methemoglobin
M Iwate	alpha 87	his → tyr	
M Saskatoon	beta 63	his → tyr	
M Milwaukee	beta 67	val → glu	
M Hyde Park	beta 92	his → tyr	
Freiburg	beta 23	val deleted	Unstable hemoglobin predisposes to methemoglobin formation
St. Louis	beta 28	leu → gln	
Kansas	beta 102	asn → thr	Reduced oxygen affinity causes increased deoxyhemoglobin
Beth Israel	beta 102	asn → ser	

TABLE 3. Some Abnormal Hemoglobins That May Cause Erythrocytosis (Polycythemia)

Abnormal Hb	Structural Change		Estimated P_{50} Whole Blood (mm Hg)*
Chesapeake	alpha 92	arg → leu	20
J Capetown	alpha 92	arg → gln	20
Suresnes	alpha 141	arg → his	17
Olympia	beta 20	val → met	21
Helsinki	beta 82	lys → met	23
Creteil	beta 89	ser → asn	13
Vanderbilt	beta 89	ser → arg	15
Malmö	beta 97	his → gln	11
Wood	beta 97	his → leu	14
Kempsey	beta 99	asp → asn	11
Radcliffe	beta 99	asp → ala	12
Yakima	beta 99	asp → his	12
Ypsilanti	beta 99	asp → tyr	—
Brigham	beta 100	pro → leu	19
Alberta	beta 101	glu → gly	16
Heathrow	beta 103	phe → leu	11
San Diego	beta 109	val → met	16
Little Rock	beta 143	his → gln	12
Syracuse	beta 143	his → pro	11
Osler	beta 145	tyr → asp	10
Bethesda	beta 145	tyr → his	13
McKees Rocks	beta 145	tyr → term	10
Ranier	beta 145	tyr → cys	11
Hiroshima	beta 146	his → asp	13

*The P_{50} of normal blood is approximately 26.6 mm Hg.

hypochromia, stippling, and target cells. Most frequent in Mediterranean populations, it is widely distributed throughout the world, occurring not rarely in blacks and less often in white persons from northern Europe. Symptoms are unusual, but some persons have anemia of moderate severity associated with jaundice and splenomegaly. Red cell abnormalities, which are variable and sometimes hardly detectable, are associated with resistance to osmotic lysis. Genetic heterogeneity is suggested not only by the clinical variability but also by differences in proportions of hemoglobins in hemolysates. Typically Hb A_2 is increased to about 5 per cent, sometimes with a slight increase in Hb F. Thalassemia minor is discovered during routine examination of blood smears or by detection of a low MCV using an electronic cell counter. It is often mistaken for iron deficiency anemia. In thalassemia minor the microcytic red cells are uniformly of small size as measured by a size-distribution analyzer; in contrast there is a more heterogeneous distribution of red cell sizes in iron deficiency. Lead poisoning may be suggested by the numerous stippled cells, or other iron-refractory microcytic anemias may be considered. Diagnosis is supported by demonstration of the same blood abnormality in other members of the family. An elevated level of Hb A_2 is confirmatory.

Heterozygous beta thalassemia occurs in about 1 per cent of American blacks, who are so mildly affected that the red cell abnormality is rarely noted. Even homozygous beta thalassemia is relatively mild in blacks. Thalassemia comes to attention most often in patients who are heterozygous for an additional hemoglobinopathy, as in sickle cell–thalassemia or Hb C thalassemia.

ALPHA THALASSEMIA

Two principal types of alpha thalassemia disease are recognized, and in addition there are two types of asymptomatic carriers. The four groups are thought to correspond to the number of functional alpha globin genes.

Hydrops fetalis with Hemoglobin Bart's is the most severe form, in which alpha chains are not produced at all, presumably because of deletion of both pairs of alpha chain genes. In the fetus Hb F cannot be synthesized, and the unpaired gamma chains combine to form Hb Bart's, which is unstable and has such a high oxygen affinity that it is nonfunctional. Death occurs in utero or at birth, the infant presenting the features of hydrops fetalis. The disease has been encountered almost exclusively in Southeast Asia.

Hemoglobin H disease is a less serious form of alpha thalassemia, apparently occurring when only one of the four alpha globin genes is functional. Insufficient alpha chains are produced to pair with the normal output of gamma and beta chains; as a result Hb Bart's as well as Hb F is produced in early life; later, Hb H and Hb A are synthesized. Hb H, like Hb Bart's, is unstable and has a high oxygen affinity. Hemoglobin H disease is characterized by splenomegaly and chronic hemolytic anemia, which may become worse during administration of sulfonamides. Hb H has unique electrophoretic properties and is precipitated to form Heinz bodies on incubation of blood with brilliant cresyl blue. Hemoglobin H disease has been encountered among populations of the Mediterranean, the Middle East, and Asia. Sporadic cases have appeared in northern Europe, but blacks are rarely affected. Many patients are carriers of Hb Constant Spring. Patients with Hb H disease typically have one parent with alpha thalassemia$_1$, the other with alpha thalassemia$_2$.

Asymptomatic carriers of *alpha thalassemia$_1$* (alpha$^+$ thalassemia) are thought to have two functional alpha globin genes. They have mild microcytosis and abnormalities of the red cells similar to those of heterozygous beta thalassemia, but Hb A_2 and Hb F are normal.

Silent carriers of *alpha thalassemia$_2$* (alpha^0 thalassemia) probably have three functional alpha globin genes. Their red cells appear normal.

Bunn, H. F., Forget, B. G., and Ranney, H. M.: Human Hemoglobins. Philadelphia, W. B. Saunders Company, 1977.

Diggs, L. W.: Sickle cell crises. Am. J. Clin. Pathol., 44:1, 1965.

Herrick, J. B.: Peculiar elongated and sickle-shaped red corpuscles in a case of severe anemia. Arch. Intern. Med., 6:517, 1910.

Lehmann, H., and Huntsman, R. G.: Man's Haemoglobins. 2nd ed. Oxford, North-Holland Publishing Company, Ltd., 1974.

Lessin, L. S., and Jensen, W. N. (eds.): Sickle cell symposium. Arch. Intern. Med., 133:529, 1974.

Pauling, L.: Abnormality of hemoglobin molecules in hereditary hemolytic anemias. Harvey Lecture, 1953–1954, p. 216.

Weatherall, D. J., and Clegg, J. B.: The Thalassemia Syndromes. 2nd ed. Oxford, Blackwell Scientific Publications, 1972.

486. METHEMOGLOBINEMIA AND SULFHEMOGLOBINEMIA

Ernst R. Jaffé

METHEMOGLOBINEMIA

DEFINITION. Methemoglobinemia occurs when the concentration of methemoglobin within circulating erythrocytes is increased above the normal level of about 1 per cent. Since the abnormal pigment is intracellular, methemoglobinemia is perhaps a misnomer, but methemoglobincythemia and methemoglobinia are too clumsy, and convention dictates the use of the former term. Methemoglobin (ferrihemoglobin, hemiglobin, ferric protoporphyrin IX-globin) is defined as an oxidation product of hemoglobin in which the sixth coordination position of ferric heme is bound to a water molecule (acid form) or to a hydroxyl group (alkaline form), each with its characteristic optical spectrum. Because of the additional positive charge, the sixth coordination position of iron is no longer available to bind molecular oxygen reversibly.

ETIOLOGY AND PATHOGENESIS. The intracellular environment of hemoglobin is such that some oxidation of heme iron might be expected. Although the intrinsic structure of hemoglobin shields the iron against oxidation, metabolic processes are also normally active to protect hemoglobin against oxidation or irreversible denaturation and to reduce any methemoglobin which is formed to hemoglobin. An increase in the concentration of methemoglobin above the normal level can result from (1) the presence of a hemoglobin with an abnormal structure that makes it more susceptible to oxidation and/or unsuitable for reduction, (2) deficiency in the ability to reduce methemoglobin, and (3) exposure to drugs or chemicals which increase the rate of oxidation beyond the protective and reductive capacities of the cell. Whereas the first two mechanisms are associated with inherited disorders, the latter occurs in toxic or acquired methemoglobinemia.

Hereditary Methemoglobinemia Due to an Abnormal Hemoglobin (Hemoglobin M) (see Ch. 485). Substitution of tyrosine for histidine occurs at or across from the heme-binding site in the α chains of hemoglobin M Iwate and M Boston and in the β chains of hemoglobin M Hyde Park and M Saskatoon. Glutamic acid replaces valine in the β chain of hemoglobin M Milwaukee-1 one helical turn away from, but still facing, the heme iron. These alterations in the primary structure of hemoglobin increase the tendency of the heme iron to be oxidized and/or stabilize the methemoglobin form so that the normal mechanism for the reduction of methemoglobin is ineffective. Thus the methemoglobinemia

does not respond significantly to conventional therapy (see below). As with other abnormal hemoglobins, hemoglobin M is transmitted as a codominant characteristic. Only heterozygotes for hemoglobin M have been identified, presumably because the homozygous state would be incompatible with life. Because only one pair of chains (either α or β) of a hemoglobin M is affected, and in the oxidized state, the concentration of methemoglobin does not exceed 25 to 30 per cent. Since α chains are already present in large amounts at birth, M hemoglobins with α chain substitutions are usually apparent immediately, whereas β chain abnormalities are often not manifest until later.

Hereditary Methemoglobinemia Due to a Deficiency in the Ability to Reduce Methemoglobin. The reduction of methemoglobin in human erythrocytes depends, primarily, on the activity of a reduced nicotinamide adenine dinucleotide (NADH or DPNH)–dependent methemoglobin reductase system. This system utilizes NADH generated by glyceraldehyde-3-phosphate dehydrogenase in the Embden-Meyerhof pathway of glycolysis to reduce cytochrome b_5 which, in turn, reduces methemoglobin to hemoglobin. Three other pathways capable of reducing methemoglobin are present in human erythrocytes, but are much less important: nonenzymatic reduction by ascorbic acid or reduced glutathione (GSH) and a reduced nicotinamide adenine dinucleotide phosphate (NADPH or TPNH)–methemoglobin reductase system, which requires an artificial electron carrier, such as methylene blue, to become effective in reducing methemoglobin. Significant methemoglobinemia is not observed in scurvy, glucose-6-phosphate dehydrogenase deficiency, marked GSH deficiency, or NADPH–methemoglobin reductase deficiency. Although other defects in the metabolic pathways of erythrocytes theoretically might lead to methemoglobinemia, they have not been identified.

The limited ability of erythrocytes from patients with hereditary methemoglobinemia not due to an abnormal hemoglobin to reduce methemoglobin in vitro has been demonstrated in numerous investigations. In most cases, this handicap has been traced to decreased activity of the NADH–methemoglobin reductase system. Methemoglobinemia as high as 40 to 50 per cent results from the accumulation of spontaneously formed methemoglobin in the absence of the normal mechanism for reduction. Data from family and biochemical studies are consistent with an autosomal codominant mode of inheritance. Marked deficiency in activity is seen in erythrocytes of affected homozygous patients, whereas approximately half normal activity is usually evident in cells from acyanotic, asymptomatic heterozygous subjects. At least 12 different electrophoretic variants of NADH–methemoglobin reductase have been demonstrated; several are associated with only slight decreases in activity. Altered kinetic properties and differences in stability have also been reported for some variants. Thus, as is true for hemoglobin, glucose-6-phosphate dehydrogenase and other enzymes, multiple aberrations in the NADH–methemoglobin reductase system apparently exist, some with and some without functional consequences.

Toxic (Acquired) Methemoglobinemia. Methemoglobinemia occurs when oxidative stress overwhelms the protective capacities of erythrocytes and exceeds the ability of the cells to reduce methemoglobin. The heme iron may be oxidized directly by ferricyanide, ferric tartrate, bivalent copper, chromate, chlorate, certain quinones, alloxans, and some dyes with a high oxidation-reduction potential. Nitrite, a powerful reducing agent and one of the most common methemoglobin-forming compounds, produces methemoglobinemia by a reaction that is not completely understood, but that may involve the generation of intermediate complexes between hemoglobin and nitrite redox products. Nitrates, upon conversion to nitrites, especially in the gastrointestinal tract of infants, can lead to toxic methemoglobinemia. Erythrocytes of newborns also are less able than adults' cells to protect hemoglobin against oxidation and to reduce methemoglobin, owing to decreased activities of NADH–methemoglobin reductase and other enzymes. More complex reactions are postulated to explain the methemoglobin-forming properties of aromatic amino and nitro compounds (acetanilid, phenacetin, nitrosobenzene, phenazopyridine, primaquine, sulfonamides, prilocaine, benzocaine) and of aniline dyes in laundry marks and wax crayons. These compounds may be converted to metabolites which either act as direct oxidants or participate in a coupled oxidation with oxyhemoglobin. In the latter reaction, generation of superoxide anion, hydrogen peroxide, peroxyhemoglobin, or free radicals is thought to be involved in the formation of methemoglobin. In addition to producing methemoglobinemia, some of these agents also can induce alterations which lead to hemolysis, especially in erythrocytes deficient in glucose-6-phosphate dehydrogenase activity.

INCIDENCE AND PREVALENCE. Although hereditary methemoglobinemia is rare, over 450 probable cases have been recorded. It is impossible to determine accurately how many are the result of a deficiency in NADH–methemoglobin reductase activity and how many are due to hemoglobin M. Patients in whom complete biochemical studies have not been performed, but whose chronic methemoglobinemia responds to therapy, presumably have had an abnormality in erythrocyte metabolism. Most of these patients probably have a deficiency in NADH–methemoglobin reductase activity; about 250 examples can be cited. The abnormality has a worldwide distribution and is particularly prevalent in inbred populations.

The M hemoglobins also have a worldwide distribution with about 200 examples. Although many patients are of Northern European origin, a number have been reported form Japan, and the patient with hemoglobin M Hyde Park was a 77-year-old black man.

There have probably been thousands of instances of acquired methemoglobinemia, but most have been transient and either clinically insignificant or coincidental complications of another disease. The chronic methemoglobinemia ("enterogenous cyanosis") which is believed to result from the absorption of nitrites produced in a gastrointestinal (or urinary) tract persistently infected with nitrite-producing bacteria is extremely rare. More than 700 cases of toxic methemoglobinemia have been reported in infants fed formulas prepared with well-water containing high concentrations of nitrate; the mortality has been as high as 10 per cent. The anticipated increase in susceptibility to toxic methemoglobinemia of individuals heterozygous for NADH–methemoglobin reductase deficiency is seen in such subjects while receiving primaquine, chloroquine, or diaminodiphenylsulfone as malarial chemoprophylaxis.

CLINICAL MANIFESTATIONS. The characteristic clinical picture of hereditary methemoglobinemia is presented by a patient with diffuse, persistent slate-gray cyanosis, often present from birth and not associated with clubbing of the fingers or evidence of cardiopulmonary disease. Concentrations of methemoglobin of 10 to 25 per cent are tolerated without apparent ill effect, but levels of 30 to 40 per cent may be associated with mild exertional dyspnea and headaches. These patients are really more blue than sick.

Toxic methemoglobinemia, especially if it develops rapidly, will produce symptoms of anoxia. Levels of 20 to 30 per cent methemoglobin are accompanied by dyspnea, tachycardia, headache, fatigue, fainting, nausea, anorexia, and vomiting. Some of these symptoms may reflect direct toxic effects of the causative agent. Lethargy and stupor may appear with methemoglobin concentrations above 55 or 60 per cent. The lethal concentration probably is greater than 70 per cent.

The decreased oxygen-carrying capacity resulting from untreated hereditary methemoglobinemia is sometimes associated with a mild compensatory erythrocytosis. This is often not as great as expected and is not observed with M hemoglobins. Segregation of methemoglobin in a population of older erythrocytes in NADH–methemoglobin reductase deficiency and counteracting intramolecular interactions have been invoked to explain the absence of erythrocytosis. The heme groups of the normal hemoglobin chains in the M hemoglobins retain their capacity to bind oxygen, and normal oxygen affinities are observed with hemoglobin M Saskatoon and Hyde Park. The oxygen affinity, however, is decreased in hemoglobin M Boston, Iwate, and Milwaukee-1. This looser binding of oxygen may facilitate delivery to the tissues and may make an erythrocytosis unnecessary. In toxic methemoglobinemia, the methemoglobin not only decreases the available oxygen-carrying pigment but also increases the affinity of the unaltered hemoglobin for oxygen, thereby further impairing the delivery of oxygen and enhancing symptoms.

Systemic effects usually do not occur in hereditary methemoglobinemia. The association of severe mental retardation has been noted in 21 children from 12 different families with NADH–methemoglobin reductase deficiency, perhaps caused by a generalized disorder not limited to the erythrocytes. Toxic methemoglobinemia may be associated with hemolysis, central nervous system depression, hepatic damage, or renal dysfunction, depending upon the causative agent or associated disease.

DIAGNOSIS. Methemoglobinemia should be considered, even if only briefly, in the differential diagnosis of cyanosis. About 5 grams of deoxyhemoglobin per 100 ml of blood are required to produce visible cyanosis, but a comparable discoloration is produced by 1.5 to 2 grams per 100 ml of methemoglobin and by about 0.5 gram per 100 ml of sulfhemoglobin (see below). The greater visible effect of these abnormal pigments is due to the alterations in the absorption spectra. Blood which contains more than about 10 per cent methemoglobin (or sulfhemoglobin) appears unusually dark red or even brown, and does not change color upon vigorous shaking with air. Addition and mixing of a few drops of 10 per cent NaCN or KCN results in the rapid formation of bright red cyanmethemoglobin, but has no effect on the color of sulfhemoglobin.

Determination of the absorption spectrum is required

to define the nature of the abnormal pigment. Acid methemoglobin has a characteristic spectrum with peaks at 502 and 632 mμ that disappear upon the addition of cyanide. Sulfhemoglobin has a peak at 620 mμ that is not altered by cyanide. The absorption spectra of methemoglobin M variants differ from those of normal methemoglobin with displacement of the peaks at 502 and 632 mμ toward lower wavelengths. Sulfhemoglobin, however, may be difficult to differentiate from methemoglobin M. The rate of formation of a complex with cyanide, the resulting absorption spectrum, and the electrophoretic migration of the methemoglobin form of hemoglobin M variants often differ from those of normal methemoglobin and help to establish the diagnosis.

NADH–methemoglobin reductase deficiency can be detected by a simple spot test, but confirmation of the diagnosis requires assay of this enzyme system in a hemolysate.

A careful history should provide clues to possible toxic methemoglobinemia. Parent-to-child transmission of congenital cyanosis should suggest the possibility of a hemoglobin M, whereas unexplained cyanosis in siblings but not in parents or offspring is more consistent with NADH–methemoglobin reductase deficiency.

TREATMENT. With toxic methemoglobinemia, concentrations of 20 to 30 per cent will disappear spontaneously in 24 to 72 hours after exposure to the offending agent terminates. More vigorous therapy is indicated if unconsciousness, stupor, or methemoglobinemia greater than 40 per cent supervenes. Oxygen administration and hemodialysis or exchange transfusion to remove the toxic agent may be helpful. Methylene blue, 1 to 2 mg per kilogram given intravenously during five minutes, will often correct the methemoglobinemia within 30 to 60 minutes. Repeated doses may be needed. Toxicity from methylene blue is uncommon, but doses over 15 mg per kilogram may cause hemolysis in infants. Individuals with glucose-6-phosphate dehydrogenase deficiency may respond suboptimally, and may develop hemolysis. Since neither methemoglobin M nor sulfhemoglobin will respond to methylene blue administration, failure to observe a significant change in color should alert the physician to the possibility of these abnormal pigments. Ascorbic acid has no place in the management of toxic methemoglobinemia because the rate at which it reduces methemoglobin is so much slower than that of the normal intrinsic mechanism.

Hereditary methemoglobinemia resulting from NADH–methemoglobin reductase deficiency usually does not require treatment except for cosmetic reasons. Intravenous methylene blue will reduce the methemoglobinemia rapidly, and daily oral administration of 100 to 300 mg will maintain the concentration below 10 per cent. Somewhat less effective is oral administration of ascorbic acid, 500 mg daily, to maintain the concentration of methemoglobin between 5 and 13 per cent. Despite good control of methemoglobinemia, therapy does not influence the mental retardation suffered by some patients.

Since the causal abnormality in the M hemoglobins resides in the structure of the hemoglobin, no effective form of therapy has been discovered.

PROGNOSIS AND PREVENTION. Methemoglobinemia, as an isolated alteration, does not have an adverse effect on the life expectancy of the patient or on the life span of the erythrocyte. The prognosis in toxic methe-

moglobinemia, once the acute episode is over, depends upon the precipitating circumstances. Toxic methemoglobinemia can be avoided by careful supervision of potential methemoglobin-producing drugs and chemicals, including thorough laundering of diapers to remove excess aniline dyes.

SULFHEMOGLOBINEMIA

Sulfhemoglobin, an incompletely characterized pigment not normally present, arises from the interaction of hemoglobin with soluble sulfides, especially hydrogen sulfide, in the presence of an oxidizing agent, usually hydrogen peroxide. Sulfhemoglobinemia is caused by the same aromatic amino drugs (acetanilid, phenacetin) that are associated with toxic methemoglobinemia. Why some patients develop methemoglobinemia and others have sulfhemoglobinemia is unknown. The concentration of GSH in the erythrocytes of some of the latter patients is elevated, perhaps because of activation of the erythrocytes' glutathione synthetase. Sulfhemoglobinemia may occur in patients with "enterogenous cyanosis," and has been attributed to the absorption of H_2S from the diseased gastrointestinal tract. The effect of sulfhemoglobin on the life span of human erythrocytes is uncertain, but many patients with sulfhemoglobinemia also have hemolysis. Since sulfhemoglobin cannot bind oxygen, the clinical effects are similar to those of methemoglobin. Sulfhemoglobin cannot be converted to hemoglobin, and there is no effective treatment. The pigment disappears when the erythrocytes containing sulfhemoglobin leave the circulation.

Cumming, R. L. C., and Pollock, A.: Drug-induced sulphaemoglobinaemia and Heinz body anaemia in pregnancy with involvement of the foetus. Scott. Med. J., 12:320, 1967.

Jaffé, E. R., and Hsieh, H.-S.: DPNH-methemoglobin reductase deficiency and hereditary methemoglobinemia. Semin. Hematol., 8:417, 1971.

Kiese, M.: Methemoglobinemia: A Comprehensive Treatise. Cleveland, CRC Press, 1974.

Schwartz, J. M., and Jaffé, E. R.: Hereditary methemoglobinemia with deficiency of NADH dehydrogenase. In Stanbury, J. B., Wyngaarden, J. B., and Fredrickson, D. S. (eds.): The Metabolic Basis of Inherited Disease. 4th ed. New York, McGraw-Hill Book Company, 1978, p. 1452.

487. HEMOGLOBINURIA

Hugh Chaplin, Jr.

DEFINITION AND MECHANISM. Hemoglobinuria (the presence of free hemoglobin in the urine) is a sign of a variety of pathologic states and not a disease entity in itself. Hemoglobin generally finds its way into the urine by filtration from the plasma; uncommonly, it may be released from red cells which lyse within the kidney or urinary outflow tract. Normal human plasma contains an alpha$_2$ globulin, haptoglobin, present in amounts sufficient to bind 75 to 175 mg of hemoglobin per 100 ml of plasma. The tightly bound hemoglobin-haptoglobin complex, which has a molecular weight above 280,000, is not filtered by the normal glomerulus but is metabolized independent of the kidney at a linear rate of approximately 10 mg per 100 ml of plasma per hour. The total plasma hemoglobin binding capacity of the average normal adult, e.g., 3 liter plasma volume, is $125 \times 30 = 3750$ mg of hemoglobin, the amount contained in 11 ml of red blood cells. When hemoglobin entering the total plasma pool exceeds this relatively modest amount, the pigment exists free in the plasma, and is either metabolized or filtered into the urine and excreted. During metabolism of free plasma hemoglobin, some of the heme moiety is split from the parent molecule and binds to albumin, forming methemalbumin, which is readily distinguishable chemically and spectroscopically from free hemoglobin and hemoglobin-haptoglobin complex, and which is relatively slowly metabolized over 24 to 48 hours. Normal plasma also contains a beta globulin, hemopexin (50 to 100 mg per 100 ml), which selectively binds free heme in equimolar amounts.

It has been puzzling that free hemoglobin (molecular weight 66,000) should pass so readily into the glomerular filtrate when albumin (molecular weight 60,000) is filtered so poorly. It is known that under physiologic conditions oxyhemoglobin in dilute solution partially and reversibly dissociates into two alpha beta dimers each with a molecular weight of about 32,000. Studies by Bunn et al. suggest that it is this phenomenon occurring in the glomerulus that is responsible for the increased filtration of hemoglobin into the urine. The kidney has a limited capacity for tubular reabsorption of filtered hemoglobin; free hemoglobin will be excreted in the urine when the plasma free hemoglobin concentration exceeds 15 to 25 mg per 100 ml.

OCCURRENCE. Hemoglobinuria Following Intravascular Hemolysis. Lysis of red cells within the circulation may occur under a variety of circumstances. The plasma will appear pink or red (free and haptoglobin-bound hemoglobin) or brown (methemalbumin). Alloimmune hemolysis occurs in relation to transfusion when the patient's plasma contains antibodies to donor red cell antigens. Hemolytic transfusion reactions usually involve incompatibility within the ABO system, but may occur within the other blood group systems, especially when complement-binding antibodies are involved, e.g., anti-Jk^a. Repeated transfusion of group A, B, or AB recipients with group O "universal donor" blood may result in alloimmune hemolysis of the recipient's red cells owing to the cumulative effect of donor alloantibodies. Autoimmune hemolysis, particularly when complement components are part of the erythrocyte-autoantibody complex, may result in massive hemoglobinemia (as in "cold" autoimmune hemolytic anemia and in the rare condition of paroxysmal cold hemoglobinuria). It should be emphasized here that hemoglobinemia is not an inevitable accompaniment of severe allo- and autohemolysis; when red cell destruction occurs primarily extravascularly, i.e., by phagocytosis within the reticuloendothelial system (especially in the spleen), plasma hemoglobin levels will be low, and haptoglobin levels may be only minimally depressed. Severe hemoglobinemia has also occurred in relation to certain drug-antibody-erythrocyte complexes, as in patients sensitized to Fuadin and quinidine. A number of intrinsic red cell defects may result in massive intravascular hemolysis under appropriate conditions. The most striking example is the poorly understood cell membrane defect in patients with paroxysmal nocturnal hemoglobinuria (PNH); also important are the enzyme-deficient cells, e.g., cells deficient in G-6-PD, which may lyse massively when exposed to sufficient concentrations of oxidant drugs or to

components of the fava bean. Rarely, mechanical damage to red cells, as in severe microangiopathic hemolytic states or after extensive body surface burns, may cause gross hemoglobinemia; physical damage also accounts for the hemoglobinemia that accompanies many extracorporeal perfusion procedures. A number of snake and spider venoms contain enzymes that provoke rapid red cell lysis (lecithinase in the venom of the brown recluse spider, reported mainly in the south central United States). Massive destruction of red cells may result from direct erythrocyte parasitism in falciparum malaria. Hypotonic red cell lysis follows the intravenous infusion of distilled water, and may occur inadvertently when water is used to irrigate the bladder during exposure of the vascular prostatic bed in the course of transurethral resection procedures. A rare but interesting condition, "march (or exertional) hemoglobinuria," has been described, wherein hemoglobinuria follows prolonged exercise (usually, running) in susceptible individuals. Because of the variety of conditions under which this poorly understood phenomenon has been reported, it is likely that multiple factors may be responsible for its occurrence. The condition is clearly distinguishable from myoglobinuria.

Hemoglobinuria Originating in the Urinary Tract. Hemoglobinuria may accompany infarction of the kidney. Presumably, red cells lyse in the infarcted tissue, and the liberated hemoglobin "leaks" into the urinary outflow tract directly; cytoscopy reveals the unilateral origin of the pigmenturia. Rarely, when hematuria occurs coincident with a very dilute urine (specific gravity less than 1.006), hypotonic lysis of the cells occurs within the collecting system. In neither of the aforementioned conditions is hemoglobinemia found, and plasma haptoglobin levels are normal.

CLINICAL MANIFESTATIONS AND IMPLICATIONS. Hemoglobinemia and hemoglobinuria, when induced by the experimental infusion of hemoglobin, when occurring from nonimmune causes, and when unaccompanied by shock or dehydration, are generally asymptomatic and benign phenomena. Stroma-free hemoglobin administered intravenously has no demonstrable effect on renal function. Red cell stroma is known to have coagulant properties; signs of mild disseminated intravascular coagulation and mild transient impairment of inulin and creatinine clearances have been observed in monkeys receiving large amounts of hemoglobin-free autologous stroma intravenously. Nonetheless, massive hemoglobinuria occurring in patients with PNH and in human subjects mistakenly given distilled water intravenously has not been associated with renal impairment.

By contrast, hemoglobinuria can be associated with severe renal damage following a major antigen-antibody reaction, e.g., incompatible transfusion. Pathogenesis of the renal failure is not altogether clear. In some instances, renal vascular insufficiency may result from disseminated intravascular coagulation secondary to liberation of thromboplastic substance by lysed red cell membranes and activation of coagulation by complement involved in the erythrocyte-alloantibody reaction. Furthermore, since hemoglobin and its breakdown products are relatively insoluble when in high concentration and at acid pH, precipitation of hemoglobin products in renal tubules will be favored by conditions that result in reduced urine volume and acid urine pH, e.g., shock, dehydration. The extent to which tubular obstruction by hemoglobin casts contributes to oliguric renal failure is controversial; there is considerable experimental evidence for passive backflow or leakage of tubular fluid proximal to points of tubular obstruction. That hemoglobinuria per se is not necessarily the cause of renal shutdown after transfusion reaction has been demonstrated by Schmidt et al., who observed renal failure after the infusion of hemoglobin-free incompatible red cell stroma.

DIAGNOSIS. Investigation of suspected hemoglobinuria should include studies of the plasma as well as of the urine. Plasma obtained at the time of active intravascular hemolysis will be pink or red; free hemoglobin and haptoglobin-bound hemoglobin (in acute hemolysis) will be demonstrable by electrophoretic, spectrophotometric, and gel filtration methods. If a blood sample is not obtained until 18 to 48 hours after intravascular hemolysis has ceased, the plasma will have a brown discoloration, and the only heme-containing pigment present will be methemalbumin, demonstrable spectroscopically by Schumm's test (appearance of a sharply defined band at 558 mμ after treatment with one tenth volume of concentrated ammonium sulfide).

During acute hemoglobinuria, the freshly voided urine will be pink, red, or deep port wine in color, depending on the hemoglobin concentration. Over a period of hours (whether in the bladder or during storage after voiding) the color turns brownish red or almost black owing to the formation of reduced hemoglobin, methemoglobin, acid hematin, and other breakdown products. Differential diagnosis should include hematuria, myoglobinuria, porphyrinuria, bilirubinuria, melanuria, betaninuria (beet pigment sometimes excreted in urine), alcaptonuria (darkens only after storage and at alkaline pH), and red discoloration by the pigmented excretory products of drugs (e.g., phenazopyridine, rifampin). Hematuria can be quickly ruled out by centrifugation of the specimen. Several techniques employing benzidine reagents (which react with the iron-containing heme portion of the molecule) will help rule out porphyrinuria, bilirubinuria, melanuria, alcaptonuria, and drug-related pigmenturia, each of which can be separately identified by appropriate laboratory tests. Benzidine reagents will not, however, make the important distinction between hemoglobinuria and myoglobinuria, because they react with the heme groups of both molecules. The excretion of myoglobin in the urine should be suspected on clinical grounds when pigmenturia follows extreme excessive exercise (especially in the untrained individual who complains of severe postexercise muscle pain and weakness) and infarction of, or trauma to, a large muscle mass (crush syndrome). Although there are minor spectroscopic differences between hemoglobin and myoglobin, differentiation of these pigments is made easier by two physicochemical properties of myoglobin. Myoglobin does not bind to haptoglobin, and, because of its small molecular size (molecular weight 17,500), is rapidly excreted in the urine. Therefore during acute myoglobinuria, the plasma will be only slightly discolored or normal in appearance, and plasma haptoglobin levels will be normal. Second, hemoglobin is essentially insoluble at 80 per cent saturation with ammonium sulfate, whereas myoglobin remains in solution under these conditions. Thus the addition of 2.8 grams of ammonium sulfate to 5 ml of benzidine-positive red-brown urine will result in precipitation of the abnormal pigment if hemoglobinuria is present. Rarely, both pigments may occur together in the urine and may be identified by a variety of immunologic, electrophoretic, or gel filtration techniques.

Chronic hemoglobinuria, even at levels too low to discolor the urine, is always accompanied by *hemosiderin granules* in the urinary sediment. The hemosiderin is formed within tubular cells after reabsorption of hemoglobin, and is either released from the cells or appears within cells sloughed into the outflow tract. The brown granules are readily identified by the Prussian blue reaction with potassium ferrocyanide. Hemosiderinuria is a common accompaniment of many chronic hemolytic states, and is occasionally seen in patients with hemochromatosis. When hemolysis is sufficiently prolonged and severe (as in PNH), the cumulative loss of hemoglobin and hemosiderin in the urine may lead to frank iron deficiency.

TREATMENT. Therapy must be directed to the primary cause of the red cell lysis that is ultimately responsible for the hemoglobinuria. Assurance of adequate urine volume (by maintenance of adequate systolic blood pressure and good hydration) is essential. Special measures of importance in treating acute hemoglobinuria of alloimmune origin or under any circumstances, e.g., shock, in which acute renal shutdown is threatened are described in detail in Ch. 488.

Allison, A. C., and Rees, W.: The binding of hemoglobin by plasma proteins (haptoglobins). Br. Med. J., 2:1137, 1957.
Birndorf, N. I., Lopas, H., and Robboy, S. J.: Disseminated intravascular coagulation and renal failure. Production in the monkey with autologous red cell stroma. Lab. Invest., 25:314, 1971.
Blondheim, S. H., Margoliash, E., and Shafrir, E.: A simple test for myohaemoglobinuria (myoglobinuria). JAMA, 167:453, 1957.
Bunn, H. F., Esham, W. T., and Bull, R. W.: The renal handling of hemoglobin. I. Glomerular filtration. J. Exp. Med., 129:909, 1969.
Ham, T. H.: Hemoglobinuria. Am. J. Med., 18:990, 1955.
Rabiner, S. F., Helbert, J. R., Lopas, H., and Friedman, L. H.: Evaluation of a stroma-free hemoglobin solution for use as a plasma expander. J. Exp. Med., 126:1127, 1967.
Schmidt, P. J., and Holland, P. V.: Pathogenesis of the acute renal failure associated with incompatible transfusions. Lancet, 2:1169, 1967.

Section Three
TRANSFUSION REACTIONS

488. TRANSFUSION REACTIONS

Hugh Chaplin, Jr.

GENERAL CONSIDERATIONS

The true frequency of untoward reactions to transfusions of whole human blood is unknown. Incidences varying from 10 per cent to less than 0.2 per cent have been reported; the wide variation reflects principally the care with which the observer followed the recipients and the strictness of the criteria employed for defining reactions. A conservative estimate would be that 2 per cent of all transfusions are accompanied by some sort of unfavorable response. Thus with approximately 8 million units of whole blood administered annually in the United States, at least 160,000 recognizable reactions can be expected.

Caution must be exercised against erroneous diagnoses of transfusion reactions. Most of the symptoms of transfusion reactions are nonspecific (see accompanying table). Patients who receive transfusions are often seriously ill with disorders which themselves may be responsible for the acute onset of chills, fever, shock, or jaundice. The temporal association of the transfusion with the onset of symptoms certainly constitutes presumptive evidence of cause and effect, but important errors in patient care may result if wisdom and restraint are not exercised to assure a comprehensive consideration of possible causes other than transfusion.

Several complications of transfusions do not strictly qualify as transfusion "reactions," and thus are not included in the table. Among these are the development of *transfusion hemosiderosis* in the chronically anemic patient who receives a great many transfusions (usually more than 50) over a period of months or years, and the possible prejudicial effect of *sensitization to blood donor histocompatibility antigens* with respect to subsequent homograft survival. Another complication is the *transmission of diseases* such as syphilis, malaria, and hepatitis. The value of immune serum globulin (ISG) as prophylaxis against transmission of serum hepatitis (type B viral hepatitis, HBV) has been controversial. In mid-1976, a joint statement by the Committee on Viral Hepatitis (National Academy of Sciences) and the Public Health Advisory Committee on Immunization Practices noted that antibody titers against HB surface antigen were regularly detectable in commercial samples of ISG manufactured after 1972 (in contrast to prior samples) and that administration of such ISG (5 ml intramuscularly) had reduced the clinical severity and complications of HBV infection when the virus inoculum was small and the exposure either percutaneous or oral. Hepatitis B immune globulin (HBIG) has recently been licensed and shown to provide significantly greater protection against HBV infection than the lower titer ISG. It is expensive, and its use should probably be reserved for circumstances in which exposure has been relatively great.

An additional recognized complication of transfusion is the *"postperfusion syndrome,"* an infectious mononucleosis–like illness occurring in 5 to 10 per cent of patients approximately one month after open-heart surgery. Possible causes include transmission of infectious mononucleosis or cytomegalovirus organisms via the transfusions, or transient graft versus host reactions secondary to donor leukocytes (principally lymphocytes).

There are several *complications of massive transfusion* (usually more than 3000 ml to an adult recipient within 12 hours). Citrate toxicity may occur, particularly during rapid intra-arterial transfusion or in patients with hepatic insufficiency or shunt bypass of the portal venous circulation. At citrate concentrations higher than

Categories of Transfusion Reactions

Cause of Reaction	Common Symptoms	Frequency	Shock	Prognosis
Contaminated blood	Chills, fever, headache, backache, delirium, bloody vomitus, and diarrhea	Rare	Yes ("red shock")	Serious
Bacterial pyrogens	Chills, fever, headache, malaise	Rare	No*	Good
Circulatory overload	Dyspnea, cough, hemoptysis, tachycardia	Rare	Rare*	Good
Air embolism	Sudden onset of cough, cyanosis, syncope, convulsions	Rare	Yes	Serious
Allergy	Itching, urticaria, fever, angioneurotic edema, bronchospasm	Common	No*	Good
Red cell incompatibility: intravascular hemolysis, extravascular hemolysis	Chills, fever, headache, backache, hemoglobinemia, hemoglobinuria, oliguria, jaundice	Moderate	Yes	Serious
Sensitivity to:				
Donor leukocytes	Chills, fever, headache, malaise, confusion	Common	Rare*	Good
Donor platelets	Chills, fever, headache, malaise, confusion	Rare	Rare*	Good
Donor plasma (IgA)	Anaphylaxis, collapse, chest pain	Rare	Yes	Serious
Unexplained (febrile)	Chills, fever, headache, malaise	Common	No*	Good

*Although shock is absent or rare as a general feature of these types of reactions, in the seriously ill or injured patient shock may be precipitated by the added stress of the transfusion reaction.

100 mg per 100 ml, skeletal muscle tremors may occur, along with prolongation of the QT segment of the electrocardiogram. Cardiac arrest may result if the citrate concentrations rise even higher. The manifestations of citrate intoxication can be prevented or eliminated by the simultaneous administration of calcium gluconate into another vein. Two other complications of massive transfusion are related to changes that take place in blood during storage in the blood bank. A hemorrhagic diathesis may develop, caused principally by the absence of viable donor platelets in blood stored more than 24 to 48 hours, even under ideal blood bank conditions. Depletion of the patients' own platelets by preceding massive blood loss is thus not compensated by the transfusion of viable donor platelets, and thrombocytopenia develops. Other causes for hemorrhagic tendency are deficiencies of labile plasma coagulation factors in stored donor blood. Abnormal bleeding may occur on this basis in an adult who receives more than 8 to 10 successive units of stored blood in less than 24 hours; the complication can be largely prevented if every fourth unit of blood given within a 12- to 18-hour period is a "fresh" unit, i.e., drawn within three to four hours of administration. A unit of fresh-frozen plasma may be substituted at the same intervals if the patient's platelet count is adequate. A less frequent complication of massive transfusion of stored blood is the occurrence of clinically significant hyperkalemia in the recipient. During storage donor red blood cells continuously lose potassium ion; thus the concentration of potassium in the suspending donor plasma will average 15 to 20 mEq per liter after two weeks of storage and 25 to 30 mEq per liter after three weeks. The danger of hyperkalemia is increased in the presence of impaired renal function. When renal insufficiency is known to exist, transfusion should employ blood stored less than five to seven days, and packed red cells should be used, whenever possible.

MECHANISMS OF REACTIONS

CONTAMINATED BLOOD. The transfusion of banked blood contaminated by endotoxin-producing bacteria (usually gram-negative rods that grow well at refrigerator temperature) may give rise to extremely serious reactions in the recipient, with a fatal outcome likely in more than 50 per cent of the patients. Death usually results from profound and persistent vascular collapse. In addition to the symptoms listed in the table, a characteristic feature is the occurrence of "red shock"; i.e., unlike the more common hypovolemic shock in which peripheral vasoconstriction results in cold, gray, clammy skin, endotoxin shock may be accompanied by marked peripheral vasodilatation so that the skin is dry, warm, and pink. Thus it is essential that blood pressure be measured frequently in patients suspected of having reactions to contaminated blood, because dangerous hypotension may coexist with an outward appearance that belies the severity of the circulatory collapse.

Fortunately, with current blood banking procedures, contamination of stored blood rarely occurs. It is also fortunate that the diagnosis of significant bacterial contamination can be established within ten minutes. A small sample of residual donor blood from the container or tubing used for administration is centrifuged

lightly (500 rpm for two to three minutes); a drop of the supernatant plasma is smeared, fixed by heating, and Gram stained. Unless most oil immersion fields contain several clearly definable organisms, contamination can be disregarded as the primary cause of the reaction. If the blood is cultured to confirm the diagnosis, incubation should be carried out at 30° C as well as at 37° C, because some contaminants will not grow at temperatures as high as 37° C.

Because of the extreme gravity of reactions owing to contaminated blood, rapid institution of comprehensive supportive therapy is essential. Intravenous therapy should include sufficient vasopressor drug to maintain the systolic pressure above 100 mm of mercury, corticosteroids (200 mg of hydrocortisone), broad-spectrum antimicrobials in high dosage, and additional whole blood if the estimated blood loss has not been corrected. Special measures to mitigate renal complications are discussed later.

PYROGENIC REACTIONS. The term "pyrogenic reactions" should be reserved for reactions related to the presence of demonstrable bacterial pyrogens (endotoxins) in the infused blood or in the transfusion equipment. Now that commercially manufactured pyrogen-tested disposable transfusion equipment is widely employed, the frequency of pyrogenic transfusion reactions has diminished strikingly. When parenteral therapy equipment does contain pyrogens, febrile reactions are "epidemic" among patients receiving intravenous infusions, and the aid of a specialized laboratory qualified to demonstrate the presence of bacterial pyrogens should be sought. Treatment is symptomatic.

CIRCULATORY OVERLOAD. The onset of acute left-sided heart failure during transfusion may reflect actual hypervolemia caused by administration of excessive amounts of blood to a patient whose volume deficit has been seriously overestimated. Even in the absence of hypervolemia, pulmonary edema may be precipitated by the too rapid administration of blood to a patient who is profoundly anemic (hemoglobin concentration less than 4 to 5 grams per 100 ml) or in cardiac failure. A further cause for the symptoms of circulatory overload may be the presence of mechanical circulatory obstruction, e.g., mitral or aortic valve disease. Whatever the cause, treatment consists of slowing the rate of transfusion (cessation if necessary), changing to packed red blood cells, and digitalization. Rarely, a small phlebotomy is required. When there is reason to be concerned about possible circulatory overload in an elderly or severely anemic patient, or in one suffering from either cardiac or renal insufficiency, venous pressure should be monitored at frequent intervals during transfusion.

AIR EMBOLISM. Air embolism is rarely encountered as a life-threatening cause of transfusion reaction except when blood is being administered under air pressure after massive exsanguination. The accident occurs when all the blood in the container into which air has been pumped has been delivered and air is allowed to flow into the patient. This complication has been largely eliminated with the increasing use of plastic blood containers to which external pressure can be safely applied without the possibility of air infusion (provided that air has not inadvertently got into the bag, e.g., during prior component preparation). When air embolism has occurred, the administration tubing should be immediately clamped and the patient turned on his left side in the head-down, feet-up position so that air in the right ventricle floats away from the pulmonary outflow tract.

ALLERGY. Allergic reactions are relatively common and are generally mild (hives, bronchial wheezing, and congestion of mucous membranes). Treatment is symptomatic (antishistaminics). The drugs should be administered directly to the patient; under no circumstances should they be added to the container of blood. Marked angioneurotic edema or anaphylaxis may require prompt parenteral administration of epinephrine, vasopressor drugs, and corticosteroids.

RED BLOOD CELL INCOMPATIBILITY. Incompatibility within the ABO system, with the resultant destruction of donor cells by alloantibodies in the recipient's circulation, is the most common cause of life-threatening reactions in contemporary transfusion practice. These preventable transfusion accidents almost always occur because of technical or logistic errors — the use of faulty techniques of blood typing and improper identification of blood samples, donor bottles, and patients. When the recipient's blood contains potent allohemolysins, acute intravascular hemolysis of the donor cells occurs. When the plasma hemoglobin concentration exceeds the hemoglobin binding capacity of the recipient's plasma (normally 75 to 175 mg of hemoglobin per 100 ml of plasma), *hemoglobinuria* occurs. Whereas many patients tolerate severe hemoglobinuria, e.g., paroxysmal nocturnal hemoglobinuria, without serious impairment of renal function, intravascular hemolytic reactions are potentially dangerous, especially when accompanied by shock, because of the possible development of oliguria, anuria, and uremia. For possible mechanisms of the renal failure, see Ch. 487.

When donor red blood cell destruction occurs predominantly extravascularly, as for example in the presence of RH antibodies demonstrable only by the indirect antiglobulin (Coombs) reaction, hemoglobinemia is generally much less severe, and jaundice is a more prominent feature, reflecting reticuloendothelial cell destruction of antibody-coated donor erythrocytes sequestered from the circulation predominantly in the spleen and/or liver.

Although the occurrence of an acute hemolytic transfusion reaction can generally be suspected on the basis of the symptoms and signs shown in the table, a special problem is presented by *anesthetized patients*, in whom the only sign of serious hemolytic reaction may be oozing of blood at the operative site. The bleeding tendency, which is often accompanied by severe transient thrombocytopenia, is generally thought to be the consequence of disseminated intravascular coagulation in response to thromboplastic substances liberated from the hemolyzing cells and activation of coagulation by activated complement components involved in the alloantibody-erythrocyte reaction. Transient activation of the fibrinolytic system may also contribute to the bleeding.

To determine quickly whether acute intravascular hemolysis has occurred, a blood sample is drawn from the patient into a clean, dry syringe or a syringe rinsed with physiologic saline. The blood is mixed with an anticoagulant by repeated gentle inversion (with care to avoid foaming, which causes in vitro hemolysis) and immediately centrifuged. If the plasma is obtained within two to eight hours of massive intravascular lysis, it will appear frankly pink or red. Plasma examined 12 to 48 hours after intravascular lysis is more apt to be brown, reflecting the presence of methemalbumin, which can be demonstrated spectroscopically by Schumm's test (appearance of a sharply defined band at 558 mμ after treatment with one tenth volume of concentrated ammonium sulfide). When donor red blood cell destruction has been largely extravascular, the plasma will show increased indirect-reacting (unconjugated) bilirubin; peak levels generally occur four to six hours after the transfusion.

To ascertain the basis for incompatibility, blood freshly drawn from the recipient should be sent immediately to the blood bank along with the donor blood container so that a thorough serologic review can be carried out. Along with the conventional retesting of the recipient's serum for the presence of antibodies against donor erythrocytes, such a review should include search for antibodies in the donor plasma that might cause destruction of the patient's cells, or cells of the other donors in the case of multiple transfusions.

In addition to general supportive measures therapy of acute hemolytic transfusion reactions should be especially directed to minimizing possible renal complications (see below).

Delayed hemolysis of donor cells may occur early (24 to 48 hours) or late (one to four weeks) after transfusion. Early delayed reactions may be severe (with intravascular hemolysis) and represent secondary immune responses to donor antigens to which the recipient had been previously sensitized but to which antibody levels were below detection in the pretransfusion crossmatch. Late delayed reactions represent primary alloimmunization and are usually mild. Red blood cell destruction generally occurs by an extravascular mechanism, and is manifested principally by jaundice and progressive anemia. The latter signs may be severe if the patient has been massively transfused and develops alloantibody to a high prevalence donor antigen. The indirect and direct antiglobulin tests will be positive initially, simulating an autoimmune hemolytic process. The anemia, if severe, may be treated safely by further transfusion, provided that serologic investigation has clarified the cause of the erythrocyte destruction so that repetition may be avoided.

DANGEROUS UNIVERSAL DONOR. A special instance of hemolytic transfusion reaction is the destruction of the group A, B, or AB patient's cells by high-titer alloantibodies in the plasma of a group O donor blood. In modern practice, every effort is made to screen group O donor bloods so as to detect those with dangerously high titers of alloantibodies. Except under emergency conditions, group O blood should be given to A, B, or AB recipients only if screening tests have defined the blood as "low titer." When a "dangerous universal donor" reaction does occur, its severity is usually tempered by the dilution effect of the recipient's plasma volume, the neutralizing effect of soluble group-specific A or B substance (or both) in the recipient plasma, and the large recipient red cell mass. Nonetheless, hypotension, hemoglobinemia, hemoglobinuria, and renal shutdown may result. Clinical management is similar to that described above for hemolytic reactions resulting from destruction of donor cells.

When an A, B, or AB recipient must be transfused with multiple units (4 or more) of low-titer group O whole blood, a cumulative effect of donor alloantibodies may result in relatively slow extravascular destruction of the patient's red blood cells. Jaundice and progressive anemia are the chief signs. If the patient requires further transfusion, it is advisable to continue with low-titer O blood and to resume type-specific blood only after two weeks have elapsed from the time of multiple Group O transfusions.

A special category of "dangerous donors" consists of those whose plasma contains alloantibodies (which may be of any blood group specificity) as a result of multiple prior transfusions or incompatible pregnancies, the latter usually associated with evidence of hemolytic disease of the newborn. In most blood banks, donor alloantibodies against red cells will be detected by routine screening of all donor sera against commercially available cells containing all the clinically important erythrocyte antigens. Even when such screening has not been performed, the donor alloantibodies will be detected if a sensitive technique is employed for the minor cross-match.

SENSITIVITY TO DONOR LEUKOCYTES, PLATELETS, OR PLASMA. Transfusion reactions in this category are observed in patients who have had multiple previous exposures to the homologous antigens either by repeated transfusions or by pregnancies. The aid of an experienced serologic laboratory should be sought to demonstrate the presence in the patient's plasma of antibodies to donor leukocytes, platelets, and plasma proteins. The majority of such reactions are caused by recipient sensitization to donor *leukocytes;* symptoms appear within 30 to 90 minutes from the start of transfusion and subside over the succeeding four to eight hours. Treatment is symptomatic. The reactions can be prevented by several effective procedures for removing leukocytes from the blood prior to transfusion. In addition, there have been increasingly frequent reports that *donor* plasma containing antileukocyte antibodies active against recipient white cells may cause an anaphylaxis-like reaction with hypotension, tachycardia, prolonged fever (up to 48 hours), tachypnea, cyanosis, and x-ray findings of "allergic pneumonia." Eosinophilia is sometimes observed. Treatment is symptomatic. Although antibodies to donor *platelets* are commonly demonstrable in multitransfused recipients, symptomatic reactions to the platelets in a single unit of transfused blood rarely or never occur. Reactions may be observed when a sensitized recipient receives multiple platelet concentrates in a single infusion. Shulman has described a rare form of delayed post-transfusion thrombocytopenia representing a complex immune response to incompatible donor platelets. The patients are generally multiparous women; profound thrombocytopenia develops five to seven days after transfusion and may persist for up to six weeks thereafter. Steroid therapy has been ineffective, but there are several reports of prompt termination of thrombocytopenia after exchange transfusions. An additional complication of platelet transfusion has been observed in severely leukopenic sensitized recipients; immediately after transfusion of multiple HLA-incompatible platelet concentrates, leukopenia becomes more profound and may not recover to pretransfusion values for 48 to 72 hours. Finally, dangerous acute post-transfusion thrombocytopenia may result when the plasma from multitransfused donors contains antibodies to recipient platelets. Rare but extremely serious anaphylactic reactions have been observed in recipients whose sera contain antibodies to donor *IgA globulin.* The patient's own serum generally lacks IgA globulin, and anti-IgA antibodies are invariably demonstrable by hemagglutination methods and occasionally also by immunoprecipitation. Marked anxiety, collapse, and unconsciousness may occur immediately upon receipt of as little as 2 to 5 ml of donor plasma; measures to combat anaphylaxis must be undertaken immediately. Because the reactions may be provoked by such small amounts of IgA globulin, prevention requires either transfusion of blood from donors known to lack IgA or extensive washing of donor red cells to accomplish virtual elimination of residual donor plasma.

UNEXPLAINED FEBRILE REACTIONS. These continue to make up a large proportion of the febrile reactions observed on a busy hospital service. Incompatibility between recipient's plasma and donor's red cells, white cells, platelets, and plasma cannot be demonstrated, nor can pyrogens be detected. There have been several well documented reports of symptomatic reactions associated with rapid destruction of donor red cells in the absence of any evidence of incompatibility by an elaborate battery of in vitro serologic tests. Therefore transfusion reactions that remain unexplained should not be comfortably dismissed as "idiopathic" but should stimulate persistent diagnostic investigation. Until the cause is found, the patient remains prey to recurring reactions with all subsequent transfusions.

MANAGEMENT OF RENAL COMPLICATIONS

A patient who has experienced severe hemorrhage with actual or impending hypovolemic shock, or who is suffering from bacteremia, may be precipitated into more severe circulatory collapse by any of the transfusion reactions described above. Under these circumstances the hazard of oliguric renal failure is ever present. The hazard is greatly increased when the reaction is of the acute alloimmune hemolytic variety, in which renal vascular damage and precipitation of hemoglobin in the renal tubules may occur.

The following recommendations for treatment of threatened or actual renal failure complicating transfusion reactions are based in general on a program developed by Barry and Crosby at the Walter Reed Medical Center. Urine flow, as a reliable indicator of renal function, is an important guide to management, and such measures as may be necessary should be taken to assure accurate measurement of urine volume at hourly intervals. The objective of treatment is to maintain a urine flow of at least 100 ml per hour until the effects of the reaction have subsided. Systolic blood pressure should be maintained at a sufficient level (above 100 mm of mercury) to assure adequate renal perfusion. Excessive elevation of blood pressure is to be avoided because of accompanying renal vasoconstriction.

As soon as the reaction has occurred, 20 grams of mannitol as a 20 per cent aqueous solution should be infused intravenously during a five-minute interval. This dose should initiate diuresis in the patient capable of responding to mannitol. In the event of an acute hemolytic reaction, the infusion of 45 mEq of sodium bicarbonate subsequent to the test dose of mannitol may be indicated. Because some of the urine obtained at the end of the first hour may have been in the bladder before the reaction, an additional one-hour collection should be obtained to enable reliable evaluation of the patient's response to mannitol. If the urine flow is greater than 40 ml per hour, intravenous fluid containing approximately 50 mEq of sodium per liter as chloride or bicarbonate, e.g., 300 ml normal saline plus 700 ml 5 per cent dextrose in water, should be administered in sufficient volume to match the desired urine flow (100 to 150 ml per hour) until the possibility of renal injury is past and the patient is able to take oral fluids in sufficient volume to maintain satisfactory urine flow. The original dose of mannitol may be repeated whenever urine flow drops below 100 ml per hour for any two-hour period, but not more than 150 grams of mannitol should be administered in any 24-hour period.

Alternatively, diuresis may be attempted by the injection of 80 to 120 mg of furosemide (in an adult), which theoretically could have the additional beneficial effect of causing a redistribution of renal blood flow resulting in increased flow in the renal cortex. Furosemide may be repeated every six to eight hours. Coincident parenteral administration of sufficient fluid and electrolyte to ensure against hypovolemia and electrolyte depletion is essential, as described above for mannitol.

The use of full dose heparin to ameliorate postulated intravascular coagulation within renal cortical vessels must be considered controversial at this time. It could only be effective if administered very early in the course of a hemolytic reaction (i.e., immediately upon the onset of symptoms) and it carries the manifest hazard of promoting bleeding in a patient who may already be in danger of hemorrhagic complications.

If the patient does not respond to the aforementioned measures and renal shutdown has become established, Barry and Crosby recommend the following:

1. Restriction of fluid intake to 500 ml plus visible output per 24 hours.

2. Provision of 100 grams of carbohydrate per day at a constant rate to avoid periods of hypoglycemia and to decrease catabolism.

3. Control of hyperkalemia by the administration of 15 to 30 grams of sodium polystyrene sulfonate resin every six hours by mouth or by rectum.

4. Transfer of the patient within the first few days of oliguria to a renal center. Prior to transport, any ECG abnormality associated with hyperkalemia should be corrected by the infusion of 25 per cent glucose in distilled water containing 25 units of regular insulin and 200 ml of 10 per cent calcium gluconate per liter. An infusion rate of 3 ml per minute or more may be re-

quired during the first 30 minutes to return the electrocardiogram to normal. Thereafter, during transportation, rates of 0.25 to 1 ml per minute will usually protect the patient from cardiac arrest.

SUBSEQUENT TRANSFUSION OF THE REACTION-PRONE PATIENT

There is always an increased hazard in transfusing a recipient who has had a previous transfusion reaction. Therefore the indications for subsequent transfusions in these patients should be subjected to especially critical scrutiny, and transfusion should be avoided whenever possible. On the other hand, the added hazard should not engender indecision and delay, to the detriment of the patient. Informed of the possible causes for transfusion reactions, supported by the results of thorough investigation of previous reactions in the patient, and possessing a variety of sensitive cross-matching procedures as well as methods for separating donor blood to provide only the components actually needed by the patient, the physician can proceed with confidence to meet such a patient's transfusion needs. The transfusion should be administered slowly, and the patient should be watched especially carefully to detect the earliest signs of recurrent reaction so that the procedure can be discontinued if serious symptoms develop.

Barry, K. G., and Crosby, W. H.: The prevention and treatment of renal failure following transfusion reactions. Transfusion, 3:34, 1963.

Bjerrum, O. J., and Jersild, C.: Class-specific anti-IgA associated with severe anaphylactic transfusion reactions in a patient with pernicious anemia. Vox Sang., 21:411, 1971.

Chaplin, H., Jr., and Cassell, M.: The occasional fallibility of in vitro compatibility tests. Transfusion, 2:375, 1962.

Committee on Viral Hepatitis (National Academy of Sciences) and Public Health Service Advisory Committee on Immunization Practices: Perspectives on the control of viral hepatitis, type B. Morbidity and Mortality Weekly Report (supplement), Center for Disease Control, 25:3, 1976.

Dorner, I., Moore, J. A., Collins, J. A., et al.: Efficacy of leukocyte-poor red blood cell suspensions prepared by sedimentation in hydroxyethyl starch. Transfusion, 15:439, 1975.

Greenwalt, T. J., Chaplin, H., Polesky, H. F., et al.: General Principles of Blood Transfusion. 3rd ed. Chicago, American Medical Association, 1977.

Shulman, N. R., Marder, V. S., Hiller, M. C., et al.: Platelet and leukocyte isoantigens and their antibodies: Serologic, physiologic and clinical studies. Prog. Hematol., 4:222, 1964.

Ward, H. N.: Pulmonary infiltrates associated with leukoagglutinin transfusion reactions. Ann. Intern. Med., 73:689, 1970.

Section Four
HEMOCHROMATOSIS

489. HEMOCHROMATOSIS
(Iron Storage Disease)

Thomas H. Bothwell

DEFINITIONS. An increase in the quantity of storage iron in the body is called *hemosiderosis* or *siderosis,* and it may be relative or absolute. A relative siderosis occurs in any anemia not due to blood loss and simply represents an internal distribution of the body's iron, with less in the red cell mass and more in stores. Siderosis may also be localized to certain organs; in idiopathic pulmonary hemosiderosis it is the lung and in paroxysmal nocturnal hemoglobinuria, the kidneys. Such conditions are examples of *focal siderosis.* When the total body iron content is increased, the extra iron is laid down in storage compounds and the condition is called absolute siderosis or *iron overload.* The term *hemochromatosis* implies the presence of massive generalized iron deposits in parenchymal tissues, together with evidence of fibrotic changes and functional impairment in the most severely affected organs.

PATHOGENESIS. The amounts of iron normally absorbed and excreted daily are small, being about 1.0 mg in men and 1.5 mg in menstruating women. Any variations in absorption that do occur are directed toward maintaining a normal body iron content. There are three basic ways in which excessive amounts of iron can accumulate in the body.

First, there are conditions in which mucosal behavior is abnormal and amounts of iron are absorbed that are inappropriate to body needs. This occurs in idiopathic hemochromatosis, in which a daily absorptive rate of no more than 3 to 5 mg extending over half a lifetime is enough to account for the eventual development of massive iron overload with its attendant pathologic sequelae. The tendency to absorb iron excessively in the condition is inherited, but the exact mode varies in different families. The most common is an intermediate one, with homozygotes developing severe iron overload and heterozygotes developing minor derangements in iron metabolism. Inappropriate absorption of iron has also been noted in certain anemias, being a feature of thalassemia major and of other refractory anemias. The common denominator in such "iron-loading" anemias appears to be increased but ineffective erythropoietic activity. Excess iron absorption has also been noted sometimes in liver disease, especially that associated with alcohol abuse, and in porphyria cutanea tarda, but why this should be so is not known.

A second cause of iron overload is too much iron in the diet. When large amounts of absorbable iron reach the lumen of the upper small intestine, the mucosal mechanism for excluding unwanted iron is overwhelmed, and excessive quantities are absorbed. This occurs most commonly in South African blacks who brew fermented drinks in iron containers. The iron in these drinks is well absorbed, and as a result iron overload of varying degrees is found in the majority of adult men, with a small proportion exhibiting fully developed hemochromatosis. Other potential sources of excessive iron in the diet are medicinal tonics and red wine.

Finally, there are situations in which iron is introduced into the body by another route. Multiple transfusions are used in the management of hypoplastic and other forms of refractory anemia. Each unit of blood contains approximately 200 mg of iron, and massive quantities of the metal can be introduced by this means. Since the body's capacity to excrete iron is very limited, subjects on regular transfusion therapy accumulate large amounts.

The eventual outcome in an individual patient can be modified by several factors. Caloric intake and hence iron intake tend to be greater in males, whereas menstruation and pregnancies increase iron losses in females. As a result, clinical manifestations of idiopathic hemochromatosis are four times more common in males than in females and occur at a younger age. Approximately a third of patients presenting clinically with the disease give a history of excessive intake of alcohol. There are several reasons for this association. As mentioned previously, some alcoholic beverages, such as red wines, contain appreciable amounts of iron. Alcohol also stimulates iron absorption. Finally, the hepatotoxicity of alcohol and iron are almost certainly additive. A similar interplay between genetic and environmental factors is seen in the hemochromatosis that occurs as a complication in thalassemia major. Such subjects have an inherent tendency to absorb increased amount of iron. In addition, they receive multiple blood transfusions and in the past have often been subjected to misguided therapy with oral iron.

PATHOLOGY. Approximately one quarter of the 3 to 4 grams of iron normally present in the body is stored in the liver and reticuloendothelial system as a soluble complex, ferritin, and as a closely related but insoluble golden-brown compound, hemosiderin. In hemochromatosis the total body iron content is usually increased to between 20 and 40 grams, most of the extra iron being deposited as hemosiderin. Concentrations are greatest in the parenchymal cells of the liver and pancreas, but significant deposits are also present in other endocrine organs and in the heart. Varying degrees of fibrosis occur in affected organs, and cirrhosis of the liver is almost invariably present. Deposits in the reticuloendothelial system are relatively scanty in the genetic disorder idiopathic hemochromatosis, but are often heavy after multiple transfusions and are also prominent in the dietary iron overload that occurs in South African blacks. The degree to which the iron from transfused blood is redistributed from reticuloendothelial cells depends on the activity of the erythroid marrow and the plasma iron level. Redistribution, with offloading onto parenchymal cells, is particularly liable to occur when there is a hyperplastic erythroid marrow and when the transferrin of plasma is saturated with iron. Why reticuloendothelial deposits are such a feature of the dietary iron overload occurring in South African blacks is unknown. A similar distribution has, however, been noted in animals given large amounts of oral iron. The cellular localization of the iron is important, because parenchymal deposits are noxious to tissues, whereas iron in reticuloendothelial cells seems to be harmless.

CLINICAL MANIFESTATIONS. Idiopathic hemochromatosis is usually regarded as a model of the effects of the slow accumulation of large amounts of iron in parenchymal tissues. Symptoms commonly develop between the ages of 40 and 60 years, and presenting clinical features relate to one or more of a number of organs. The most prominent are skin pigmentation, diabetes mellitus, hepatomegaly with symptoms of hepatic dysfunction, cardiac failure, and evidence of hypogonadism.

Over 90 per cent of patients show bronzing of the skin owing to excess quantities of melanin. In half of them hemosiderin is also present, which gives the skin a slaty-gray appearance. Pigmentation is most prominent on the exposed parts. Although firm hepatomegaly is almost invariably present, liver function in the absence of associated alcoholism is often surprisingly good. Hepatic failure with coma can, however, be precipitated by intercurrent infections and other acute insults. The spleen is enlarged in about 50 per cent of patients, but complications as a result of portal hypertension are not common. Hepatoma may occur as a complication in older patients.

Diabetes is present in the majority of subjects and may be mild or severe; insulin, occasionally in large doses, is usually needed for its control. Complications, such as nephropathy, neuropathy, and peripheral vascular disease, occur in about 20 per cent of patients. It has been customary to ascribe the diabetes to inadequate islet cell function, as a result of iron deposits in the pancreas. This is, however, not the only factor, since insulin levels are often normal. In addition, the prevalence of diabetes is high in the relatives of affected individuals, and this is not related to the presence of iron overload.

Arrhythmias and refractory cardiac failure occur in a number of affected persons and are particularly troublesome in younger patients. Sexual impotence, testicular atrophy, and sparsity of body hair are present in more than 50 per cent of patients and are usually due to a deficient production of trophic sex hormones by the anterior pituitary. An arthropathy involving both large and small joints occurs in about a third of patients. Chondrocalcinosis is present in a number of them and can be associated with attacks of acute synovitis. A polyarthritis may also occur, but its relationship to the iron deposits present in the joints is not clear.

The symptom complex that is such a characteristic feature of idiopathic hemochromatosis is sometimes found in other forms of iron overload. For example, cirrhosis and diabetes have been reported both in South African blacks and in subjects who have had many transfusions; cardiac failure is also common in the hemochromatosis that occurs in thalassemia major. Other complications of excessive iron deposits have been recognized in South African blacks. Ascorbic acid deficiency and osteoporosis are both common in affected individuals, and there is some evidence that the iron overload is a causal factor in their occurrence.

DIAGNOSIS. The diagnosis is not difficult when the classic tetrad of skin pigmentation, liver disease, diabetes, and heart failure is present. In fact, the combination of any two of these should alert the physician. Laboratory tests are required to confirm the diagnosis. The best screening test is the measurement of the plasma iron concentration and the plasma iron-binding capacity. In the absence of intercurrent infection or complicating hepatoma, the plasma iron is usually greater than 200 μg per deciliter, and the transferrin is virtually completely saturated. It must be emphasized that this test does not define the degree of iron overload, since the plasma is often saturated with iron both in affected relatives prior to the accumulation of significant stores and in patients with hypoplastic anemias and anemias resulting from ineffective erythropoiesis. Insight into the amount of parenchymal iron present can be gained in several ways. The first and most recent is the estimation of the concentration of ferritin circulating in the serum. The serum ferritin mirrors the size of the body iron stores; in normal subjects values vary between 50 and 200 μg per liter, whereas in untreated idiopathic hemochromatosis the concentrations are usually several thousand μg per liter. A second way of diagnosing the degree of overload is to inject chelating agents such as desferrioxamine (Desferal) and measure the quantity of iron passed in the urine, since it has been established that this is positively correlated with the size of the iron stores. With an intramuscular dose of desferrioxamine of 10 mg per kilogram, a normal person excretes less than 2 mg of iron over the next 24 hours, whereas subjects with idiopathic hemochromatosis usually excrete more than 10 mg. The test is particularly useful in distinguishing between idiopathic hemochromatosis and alcoholic cirrhosis with only moderate iron overload. Liver biopsy provides the final proof, with evidence of heavy parenchymal iron deposits together with a fibrous reaction. The amount of connective tissue varies from a fine portal tract fibrosis to frank macronodular cirrhosis. Further important information can be obtained by chemical estimation of the concentration of iron present in a needle biopsy specimen.

It is important to emphasize that the physician's role extends beyond the diagnosis and treatment of affected patients. With up to half of siblings showing a predisposition to develop varying degrees of iron overload, it is essential that they be located and treated prior to the accumulation of massive quantities of iron. Ideally several screening tests should be done, including the serum iron and total iron-binding capacity, the serum ferritin, and the measurement of urinary iron excretion after the administration of desferrioxamine.

TREATMENT AND PROGNOSIS. Apart from the management of complications such as diabetes and heart failure along conventional lines, the specific treatment is to remove the iron as rapidly as possible. This objective is normally achieved by repeated phlebotomies. The 200 to 250 mg of iron removed in each pint of blood creates a deficit that leads to the mobilization of a similar quantity of iron from the body's stores. Weekly phlebotomies are tolerated well by most patients, and hemoglobin levels greater than 11.0 grams per deciliter are often maintained with venesection programs that are even more vigorous. As the stores diminish, there is a steady decrease in the concentrations of serum ferritin. Once the stores are exhausted, venesections are continued at less frequent intervals to prevent reaccumulation of the iron. Successful removal of all the iron deposits, which is heralded by a drop in the plasma iron concentration, may occur only after weekly venesections have been carried out for two years or more. Provided that the patient is eating a well balanced diet, no specific supplementation is required. When venesections are not feasible (e.g., in thalassemia), intramuscular desferrioxamine can be given on a daily basis in a dose of 0.5 to 1.0 gram. Although such therapy diminishes to some extent the rate at which iron accumulates and retards the development of hepatic fibrosis, its effects, if any, on the long-term prognosis are not known. Currently other more aggressive forms of chelation therapy are being tested.

COURSE AND PROGNOSIS. Without therapy, idiopathic hemochromatosis is a fatal disease. Death usually results from cardiac failure in younger patients and from liver disease or its complications in older ones. Some subjects succumb to an acute abdominal crisis followed by shock. Although the cause has not been definitely established, it may result from gram-negative bacteremia. In one recent study, life table data showed that the percentage survival 5 and 10 years after diagnosis in untreated patients was only 18 and 6, respectively; in patients treated by venesection the compara-

ble figures were 66 and 32 per cent, respectively. Such therapy is associated with gain in weight, increased sense of well-being, regression of skin pigmentation, and improvement in hepatic and cardiac function; insulin requirements are also often reduced. The arthropathy is, however, not affected, and hepatoma can still occur as a late complication.

Bergsma, D., Cerami, A., Peterson, C. M., and Graziano, J. H. (eds.): Iron Metabolism and Thalassemia. New York, Alan R. Liss, Inc., 1976.

Bomford, A., and Williams, R.: Long term results of venesection therapy in idiopathic haemochromatosis. Quart. J. Med. N S, 45:611, 1976.

Bothwell, T. H., and Finch, C. A.: Iron Metabolism. Boston, Little, Brown & Company, 1962.

Charlton, R. W., Bothwell, T. H., and Seftel, H. C.: Dietary iron overload. Clin. Haematol., 2:383, 1973.

Fairbanks, V. F., Fahey, J. L., and Beutler, E.: Clinical Disorders of Iron Metabolism. 2nd ed. New York, Grune & Stratton, 1971.

Grace, N. D., and Powell, L. W.: Iron storage disorders of the liver. Gastroenterology, 67:1257, 1974.

Halliday, J. W., Russo, A. M., Cowlishaw, J. L., and Powell, L. W.: Serum-ferritin in diagnosis of haemochromatosis. Lancet, 2:621, 1977.

Iron. Subcommittee on Iron, Committee on Medical and Biologic Effects of Environmental Pollutants, Assembly of Life Sciences, National Academy of Sciences, Washington, D.C., 1977, p. 196.

Section Five   POLYCYTHEMIA

Allan J. Erslev

490.   INTRODUCTION

Polycythemia is the commonly used designation for conditions in which the red blood cell count and its associated parameters, hemoglobin concentration and hematocrit, are increased above normal. Since such conditions can be caused by a decrease in plasma volume as well as by an increase in red cell mass, polycythemias are subdivided into *relative* polycythemias characterized by a normal red cell mass and *absolute* polycythemias characterized by an increased red cell mass (Fig. 1). Relative polycythemias are most commonly found associated with dehydration and cannot be considered as true hematologic disorders, whereas absolute polycythemias are caused by a sustained overactivity of the erythroid component of the bone marrow. This overactivity may be part of a neoplastic dysfunction of the bone marrow as in polycythemia vera, or it may be a compensatory response to tissue hypoxia as in secondary polycythemia. This compensatory response may in turn be appropriate and adjust for general tissue hypoxia or inappropriate and reflect excessive production of erythropoietin.

491.   RELATIVE POLYCYTHEMIA

A decrease in plasma volume with unchanged red cell mass is the hallmark of dehydration polycythemia, and is seen in a wide variety of conditions associated with excessive fluid loss or deficient fluid intake. In

such conditions, the hematocrit is a most useful gauge of the extent of dehydration. A high hematocrit in an acutely ill patient should rarely suggest the need for extensive hematologic workup but rather for immediate fluid replacement.

The diagnostic and therapeutic problems are considerably greater when patients who are not ill and do not suffer from an obvious fluid imbalance are found to have a hematocrit in the polycythemic range (more than 53 per cent at sea level) but a normal red cell mass. In 1952, Lawrence and Berlin first clearly separated these polycythemias from absolute polycythemia and, because of the more than normal anxiety and worry experienced by their patients, suggested that the plasma volume deficiency was caused by "stress." Similar polycythemias had been described many years before by Gaisböck, and he had related the polycythemia to the frequent coexistent hypertension. Other problems characteristic of stress and middle age such as overweight, hypercholesterolemia, and arteriosclerosis were added, and the designation *"stress polycythemia"* was almost accepted as a pathophysiologic entity. However, serious reservations have been raised as to the validity of this concept. First of all, it is important to be circumspect when evaluating the normality of the measured red cell mass. It can be measured accurately in milliliters either directly with labeled red cells or indirectly by measuring plasma volume and body hematocrit (body hematocrit = venous hematocrit × 0.93), but it is difficult to express in meaningful terms. It is most often expressed per kilogram of body weight, but because of great variations among normals in body composition, height, and surface area the normal values have a wide range (males: 27 to 34 ml per kilogram; females: 18 to

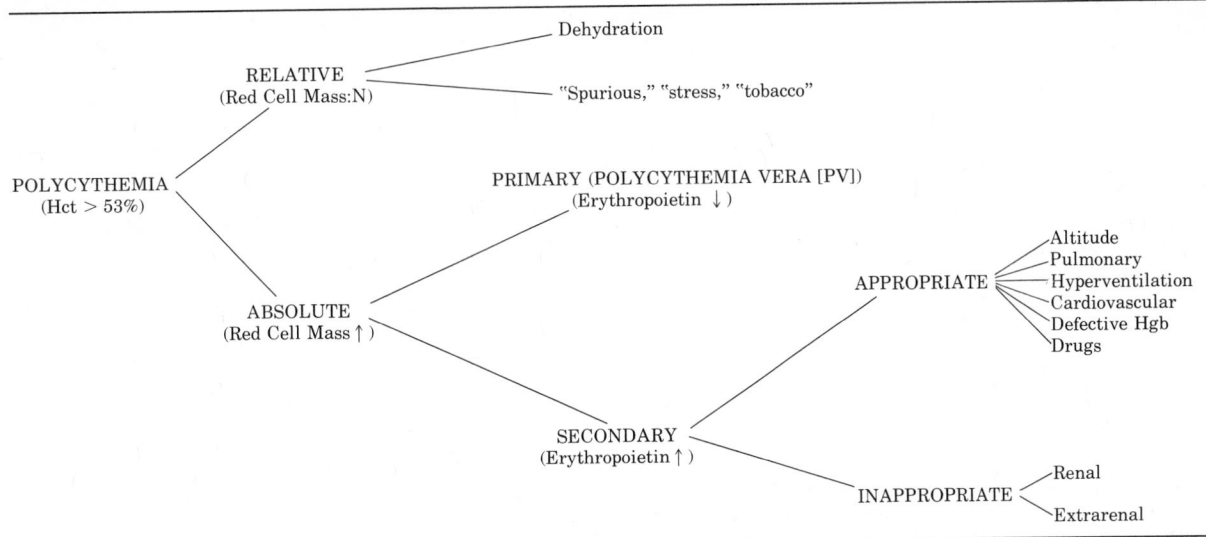

Figure 1. Classification of the polycythemias.

28 ml per kilogram). This problem has led Wasserman and his coworkers to propose that in many cases relative polycythemia with a "normal" red cell mass and no evidence of fluid imbalance is really "spurious" and merely represents a fortuitous combination of a low normal plasma volume and a high normal red cell mass.

Still, this fortuitous combination does appear more commonly in the obese, hypertensive, and "stressed" middle-aged man than in other individuals. Hypertension per se has been shown by Chrysant and coworkers to cause a contraction of plasma volume, but probably of more importance is the recent proposal that an increase in hematocrit can be caused by excessive smoking. Carbon monoxide in inhaled smoke will change a proportion of hemoglobin to carbon monoxide hemoglobin and shift the oxygen dissociation curve of the remaining hemoglobin to the left, leading to impaired oxygen transport and tissue hypoxia. This in turn will cause a mild secondary polycythemia, but the absolute increase in the red cell mass is often too slight to be appreciated when expressed per kilogram of obese body weight. Furthermore, carbon monoxide or perhaps nicotine will have a mild diuretic effect, reducing the plasma volume to low normal levels and aggravate the hematocrit increase caused by carbon monoxide hemoglobin. Smith and Landow have recently shown that the discontinuation of smoking can cure "stress" polycythemia, and it seems more and more likely that this nebulous cause will have to be replaced by smoking.

The symptoms are negligible and, if present, can usually be related to other effects of an immoderate middle age life style. However, a high hematocrit and the associated hyperviscosity of blood can cause concern to both physician and patient. Although attempts made to relate risk of heart attack or strokes to hematocrit have been inconclusive, it may still be advisable to reduce all potential problems in this coronary-prone age group. If the patient is an incorrigible heavy smoker, judicious phlebotomies maintaining the hematocrit at around 50 per cent may at least reduce anxiety and benefit the blood donor program.

Brown, S. M., Gilbert, H. S., Krauss, S., and Wasserman, L. R.: Relative polycythemia: A non-existent disease. Am. J. Med., 50:200, 1971.

Chrysant, S. G., Frolich, E. D., Adamopoulos, P. N., et al.: Pathophysiologic significance of "stress" or relative polycythemia in essential hypertension. Am. J. Cardiol., 37:1069, 1976.

Lawrence, J. H., and Berlin, N. J.: Relative polycythemia — the polycythemia of stress. Yale J. Biol. Med., 24:498, 1952.

Smith, J. R., and Landow, S. A.: Smokers' polycythemia. N. Engl. J. Med., 298:6, 1978.

492. ABSOLUTE POLYCYTHEMIA

PATHOLOGIC PHYSIOLOGY. The clinical manifestations of absolute polycythemia are in general related to the expanded blood volume and to the increased blood viscosity. Bone marrow hyperactivity, although responsible for the expanded red cell mass, is often more difficult to appreciate. A doubling of the red cell mass, for example, will cause a symptomatic increase in the volume and viscosity of blood, but the responsible doubling in the rate of red cell production is reflected by relatively insignificant increases in bone marrow volume, erythroid-myeloid ratio, reticulocyte counts, or serum iron turnover. The consequent doubling in red cell destruction will likewise not be symptomatic and rarely will increase bilirubin or LDH concentration in plasma beyond their wide normal range.

The increased volume of circulating blood leads to vascular expansion and venous engorgement and in turn to the characteristic ruddy cyanosis of skin and mucous membranes, to headaches, tinnitus, and a feeling of fullness in the head and neck, and to frequent nasal and gastric bleedings. The increased viscosity has more subtle effects on the cardiovascular system, and although total blood viscosity may be extremely high, patients rarely experience the same cerebral hyperviscosity symptoms as observed in macroglobulinemia. Nevertheless, the increase in blood viscosity can cause an increase in peripheral resistance and in turn a decrease in blood flow and cardiac output and an impaired oxygen transport to the tissues. Fortunately, polycythemia is associated with an increase in both viscosity and blood volume, and dilated vessels will reduce viscous drag and improve oxygen transport. Blood volume and blood viscosity are usually carefully balanced in favor of oxygen transport. Occasionally, however, as in chronic mountain sickness, the hematocrit and viscosity exceed the adjusting effect of vascular dilation, and in such instances the oxygen transport becomes seriously curtailed, resulting in a vicious circle of tissue hypoxia, further increase in red cell production, further increase in viscosity, and further aggravation of tissue hypoxia. Thrombosis may occur in such conditions, but otherwise thromboses are unusual in mere red cell polycythemias despite the increase in viscosity.

492.1.   PRIMARY POLYCYTHEMIA
(Polycythemia Vera)

Polycythemia vera (PV) is characterized by a sustained but inappropriate overproduction of erythrocytes leading to an absolute increase in the circulating red cell mass. It is associated with varying degrees of overproduction of granulocytes and thrombocytes; thus a true "polycythemia" with corresponding bone marrow and splenic hyperplasia is the hallmark of its fully developed form. The bone marrow and circulating cells appear morphologically normal but display chromosomal and functional characteristics suggesting that PV ultimately is caused by proliferation of abnormal hematopoietic clones.

PV is often designated as *Vasquez-Osler disease*, from the two clinicians who independently described it in the years 1892 and 1903. Since then it has been the popular subject of numerous clinical descriptions and pathophysiologic hypotheses, primarily because it is a fairly common disease with very dramatic manifestations.

At the time PV was first recognized as a clinical entity, the polycythemia observed at altitude was believed to be caused by a stimulating effect of hypoxia on the bone marrow. Consequently, the first hypothesis attempting to explain the pathogenesis of PV involved such bone marrow hypoxia. Eventually, this was found to be invalid both for PV and for altitude polycythemia, and subsequent studies have shown clearly that the two conditions are pathogenetically different. Specifically, the physiologic erythropoietic hormone, *erythropoietin*, which is elevated in altitude polycythemia, is low or absent in PV, suggesting an autonomous overproduction of red cells rather than a response to generalized or localized hypoxia.

The autonomous overproduction of erythrocytes as well as of granulocytes and thrombocytes has recently been related to an acquired stem cell dysfunction. Under physiologic conditions, each of the differentiated blood cell lines is derived from a pool of undifferentiated but committed stem cells, which in turn are derived from a single pool of multi- or pluripotential stem cells, CFU-S (Fig. 2) (Lajtha, 1975). These latter stem cells are normally inactive and merely serve as a potential backup for more specialized and committed stem cells. Using the X-linked glucose-6-phosphate dehydrogenase

HEMATOPOIESIS

Figure 2.   Outline of the cellular kinetics of the bone marrow. The stem cell pool consists of multi- or pluripotential stem cells (colony-forming units — spleen, or CFU-S), which under normal conditions are resting but, if required, are capable of differentiating into committed, unipotential stem cells belonging to each of the three major cellular lines. Unipotential stem cells destined to become erythroid (burst-forming units — erythroid, or BFU-E) respond to erythropoietin, by proliferation and further differentiation until they reach a state of development (colony-forming units — Erythroid, or CFU-E) at which erythropoietin will initiate blast transformation to proerythroblasts. Unipotential stem cells destined to become megakaryocytic (colony-forming units — Megakaryocytes, or CFU-M) will also proliferate, mature, and eventually undergo blast transformation in response to a "poietin." However, the nature of this "poietin" has not been resolved yet. The stem cells destined to become granulocytes (colony-forming units — Culture, or CFU-C) will proliferate, mature, and eventually undergo blast transformation in response to a colony-stimulating factor or CSF acting as a "granulopoietin." After blast transformation the differentiated proerythroblasts and myeloblasts will multiply and mature until they are not capable of further division (reticulocytes, myelocytes). They will remain in the bone marrow for a few more days before being released into the circulation. The megakaryoblasts will not proliferate but undergo endomitoses until platelets peel off the abundant cytoplasm. In the peripheral blood all red cells circulate, while granulocytes are divided into marginated and circulating cells and platelets into stored and circulatory cells.

as a marker, Adamson, Prchal, and their coworkers have shown that PV probably is a clonal disease originating from a single multipotential stem cell. They observed that the fibroblasts of two polycythemic women, heterozygous for the A and B isoenzymes, were, as expected, composed of a mosaic of A and B cells. However, the red cells, granulocytes, and platelets contained only one isoenzyme, Type A, as if they all were derived from a single Type A stem cell. They furthermore observed that bone marrow from these women cultured in the absence of erythropoietin would spontaneously grow out erythroid colonies, in sharp contradistinction to normal bone marrow which only produces erythroid colonies if erythropoietin is present. These autonomous colonies were all made up by Type A cells. When erythropoietin was added, the number of Type A colonies increased, but now type B colonies also appeared. They concluded that the bone marrow of patients with PV is composed of PV clones, which, although autonomous, can be further stimulated by erythropoietin, and of normal erythropoietin-dependent clones. The presence of excess leukocyte alkaline phosphatase in granulocytes and of functional impairment of thrombocytes suggests that the clone responsible for excess cellular production is not only autonomous but also abnormal. Consequently, the hematopoietic overproduction observed in PV is today best explained on the basis of the emergence of abnormal, autonomous clones of multipotential stem cells.

The agent or event responsible for the formation of these abnormal clones is as unknown in PV as in other clonal hematologic disorders. It is primarily a disease of middle or old age, with a slight preference for males of Jewish ancestry. However, a family history of PV or other hematologic disorder is rarely obtained. It is equally rare to obtain a history of a significant exposure to toxic chemicals or to x-ray radiation. A viral etiology, although frequently suspected, has not been substantiated. In mice, several viruses (Friend's and Rauscher's) can cause polycythemia, but their relationship to PV in humans is extremely tenuous.

CLINICAL MANIFESTATIONS. PV may remain asymptomatic for a prolonged period of time. Mild headaches and "high color" are often disregarded until a routine blood count discloses an elevated hematocrit. When symptomatic, the symptoms can usually be referred to the hypervolemia and hyperviscosity of the increased red cell mass and to platelet dysfunction.

Headaches, dizziness, tinnitus, vertigo, and blurred or abnormal vision appear to be caused by hypervolemia. Venous thrombosis with distant embolization is usually related to the combined effect of hyperviscosity and platelet dysfunction; nosebleedings, spontaneous bruising, and bleeding peptic ulcers are usually related to the combined effect of hypervolemia and platelet dysfunction. Pruritus can be an intolerable symptom and is often aggravated after hot baths or showers. It is believed to be caused by histamine release from excessive granulocyte turnover.

Plethora or ruddy cyanosis of the face, hands, and mucous membranes and engorgements of the conjunctival and retinal veins are usually present with hematocrits above 55 per cent. Ecchymoses may also be noticed, but the most consistent abnormal finding on physical examination is a palpable spleen. Splenomegaly is present in about three fourths of patients when first seen and may be even more frequent if spleen size is assessed by isotope scanning. The spleen is firm and nontender and contains large amounts of extramedullary tissue. Although the spleen may contribute all types of mature cells to circulating blood, its size and extramedullary function are more closely related to excessive granulo- and thrombopoiesis than to erythropoiesis. The liver may also participate in extramedullary blood formation, but overt hepatomegaly is usually a late phenomenon associated with the final myeloproliferative phase. Bone tenderness and bone pain, especially in the ribs and in the lower part of the sternum, can be quite pronounced and usually reflect bone marrow hyperplasia.

LABORATORY FINDINGS. The laboratory findings are dominated by the consequences of bone marrow hyperactivity. The red cell count is always increased and often to a greater degree than the hemoglobin concentration and hematocrit percentage. Consequently, the MCV is usually low, reflecting a low serum iron and iron stores depleted by phlebotomies and blood loss. The hematocrit percentage, although less elevated than the red cell count, is probably the best parameter to follow through remissions and relapses. It reflects directly the viscosity of circulating blood, and it provides a visible although not always accurate gauge of total red cell mass and total plasma volume. A hematocrit at sea level of greater than 53 per cent defines polycythemia. When between 53 and 60 per cent this polycythemia can be either relative or absolute, but when in excess of 60 per cent it almost always signifies an absolute polycythemia with expanded red cell mass. Nevertheless, a direct measurement of the red cell mass should be obtained for diagnostic and prognostic purposes in almost all patients with polycythemia. The plasma volume in PV seems to have no direct relation to the red cell mass, since it has been reported to be less than normal, normal, and greater than normal. The life span of circulating red cells is usually normal in the early years of the disease, despite the presence of splenomegaly, but eventually bone marrow erythropoiesis becomes more ineffective, with the appearance of nucleated red cells, anisocytes, poikilocytes, and short-lived red cells in the circulating blood. Erythropoietin titers in plasma and the 24-hour urine excretion of erythropoietin are, as expected, close to zero. However, as mentioned under differential diagnosis, these potentially valuable tests are difficult to carry out and evaluate.

The concomitant increase in granulocytes in peripheral blood is moderate at first but may take on leukemoid proportions. Early myeloid forms can be seen, and when associated with nucleated red cells and red cell shape changes they indicate transformation from effective bone marrow hyperplasia to ineffective myeloid metaplasia. The increase in granulocyte turnover is reflected by high muramidase content in serum and urine and by high transcobalamin I and III levels (usually recognized by high serum vitamin B_{12} concentration). Circulating granulocytes regularly show increased concentrations of leukocyte alkaline phosphatase. This is of unknown functional significance but is an important differential diagnostic feature, since it can distinguish PV with excessive granulocytosis from chronic granulocytic leukemia in which the granulocytes have a low concentration of alkaline phosphatase.

The circulating platelets are increased in about 50 per cent of early cases and occasionally can be counted in the millions. Such increases in number have been used

TABLE 1. Absolute Polycythemia

	Polycythemia Vera	Secondary
RBC, Hgb, Hct	Increased	Increased
Red cell mass	Increased	Increased
MCV	Decreased	Normal
Serum iron	Decreased	Normal
Erythropoietin	Decreased	Increased
White blood count	Increased	Normal
Platelet count	Increased	Normal
Spleen size	Increased	Normal
Transcobalamin I and III	Increased	Normal
B_{12}	Increased	Normal
Muramidase	Increased	Normal
Leukocyte alkaline phosphatase	Increased	Normal
Platelet function	Decreased	Normal
Bone marrow cellularity	Increased	Normal
Bone marrow megakaryocytes	Increased	Normal

to explain the tendency to develop venous thrombosis, but the concomitant hemorrhagic tendency has been more difficult to explain. However, the platelets produced are neither morphologically nor functionally quite normal (Berger et al., 1973). Megathrombocytes and large megakaryocyte fragments may be seen on the blood smear, and a number of functional impairments have been noted such as a decrease in platelet factor III, decreased adhesion to glass beads, and decreased aggregation after exposure in vitro to ADP or thrombin. Furthermore, the firmness and stability of clotted PV blood is less than normal, presumably because each volume of blood contains a relatively small volume of plasma and its associated coagulation proteins.

The bone marrow is hyperplastic, with a decrease in fat cells and a decrease in macrophage iron. Since myelopoiesis and erythropoiesis are often increased together, the M:E ratio is fairly normal. However, megakaryocytes may be present in sheets and can provide an important diagnostic clue. A bone marrow biopsy can be of value in disclosing the extent of myelofibrosis. Cytogenetic changes have been found in almost 50 per cent of untreated patients, but no consistent abnormality has been noted (Wurster-Hill et al.).

Since patient are most often in an age group associated with the onset of many illnesses, it is important to separate random laboratory abnormalities from those specific for PV. A moderate increase in uric acid, lactic dehydrogenase, and indirect bilirubin can be related to increased granulocytes and erythrocyte turnover, but most other abnormalities unearthed by our extensive laboratory screens are probably unrelated. However, a low glucose and a high potassium must always be looked at with suspicion, since excess glucose consumption and excessive cellular release of potassium may occur in PV blood samples waiting for laboratory processing.

DIFFERENTIAL DIAGNOSIS (see Tables 1 and 2). The diagnosis of PV rests on finding an increased red cell mass unassociated with excessive erythropoietin production and a concomitant increase in granulocyte and thrombocyte production.

A hematocrit of higher than 53 per cent at sea level without obvious fluid imbalance should lead to a red cell mass determination. If elevated, erythropoietin titers should ideally be measured in order to rule out secondary polycythemia. Unfortunately, the routine bioassay for erythropoietin in plasma is quite crude

with a lower limit of sensitivity of 50 mU per milliliter and will not separate normal levels (5 to 20 mU per milliliter) from PV levels (<5 mU per milliliter) or from levels in secondary steady state polycythemia (20 to 50 mU per milliliter). Bioassay of plasma concentrates, however, can be used to demonstrate these differences. An assay of a urine concentrate can be used to measure 24-hour erythropoietin excretion, a measure which also can be used to separate PV (<2 U excretion a day) from secondary polycythemia (>5 U excretion a day). The current development of a highly sensitive radioimmunoassay promises to make a test available which should be able to separate secondary from primary polycythemia.

In the meantime, however, we must rule out secondary appropriate and inappropriate polycythemia by other tests. The measurement of arterial oxygen tension and saturation may help rule out pulmonary or cardiac polycythemia, the determination of P_{50} may help rule out genetic hemoglobin abnormalities, and the examination of an IVP may help rule out renal cysts or tumors. In regard to arterial gas studies, it must be realized that patients with PV often have oxygen saturations slightly below normal, and borderline changes in both saturation and tension are of little differential diagnostic importance.

The concomitant increase in granulocyte and thrombocyte turnover in PV are most easily appreciated from peripheral blood counts. However, splenomegaly, muramidase, and B_{12} measurements may give additional hints as to the presence of generalized myeloid overactivity. Although splenomegaly caused by extramedullary hematopoiesis is present in 75 per cent of patients with PV, it is important to rule out the presence of a splenic cyst by means of an isotope scan and to rule out old malaria, splenic vein thrombosis, or other causes of splenomegaly. An elevated leukocyte alkaline phosphatase measurement may help in separating PV from chronic myeloid leukemia as well as from secondary polycythemia.

An unusual condition, *primary erythrocytosis*, is characterized by an autonomous increase in red cell production almost identical with that observed in PV but without any associated granulocyte or thrombocyte changes. It is often familial and may be a genetic variant of the general myeloproliferative syndrome.

COURSE. PV is often an easily managed disease which may stay asymptomatic for 10 to 15 years with little more therapy than occasional phlebotomies. How-

TABLE 2. Diagnostic Criteria for Polycythemia Vera Utilized by the Polycythemia Vera Study Group

Category A
  A1. Increased red cell mass (measured with ^{51}Cr-labeled red cells):
      Male > 36 ml per kg
      Female > 32 ml per kg
  A2. Normal arterial oxygen saturation > 92 per cent
  A3. Splenomegaly
Category B
  B1. Thrombocytosis: platelets > 400,000 per mm
  B2. Leukocytosis: white count > 12,000 per mm (in absence of fever or infection)
  B3. Elevated leukocyte alkaline phosphatase score >100 in absence of fever or infection
  B4. Elevated serum vitamin B_{12} or unbound B_{12}-binding capacity: B_{12} >900 pg per ml; $UB_{12}BC$ >2200 pg per ml

Diagnosis of PV is acceptable if A1, A2, and A3 are present or if A1, A2, and two parameters of category B are present.

ever, catastrophic complications may occur at any time, and all patients need regular checkups in order to keep blood counts at as normal levels as possible. Thrombosis and hemorrhage occur in about one half of poorly managed patients, ranging from minor peripheral thromboses and dermal ecchymoses to life-threatening cerebral, coronary, and abdominal vascular occlusions and intestinal hemorrhages. Peptic ulcer bleedings are particularly common and may be initiated by vascular mucosal ischemia, leading to peptic ulcerations. Elective surgery can be extremely hazardous because of the associated immobilization and postoperative elevation of platelet count, and in general should not be contemplated until the blood counts have been brought under control.

After years of uneventful management, many cases of PV will "burn out" and be replaced by a picture resembling myelofibrosis and myeloid metaplasia. The bone marrow becomes densely infiltrated with fibrotic tissue, the liver and spleen increase in size, and examination of peripheral blood reveals anemia with many early and abnormal red cells, granulocytosis with early myeloid elements, and thrombocytosis with many large and peculiarly sized platelets. In about 10 per cent of all cases this phase progresses into acute leukemia. This is most often of the myelomonocytic variety but may have the characteristics of lymphoblastic leukemia. This transformation was initially believed to be related to treatment with radioactive phosphorus, but recent studies have shown that patients treated with alkylating agents such as chlorambucil and busulfan also develop acute leukemia. Even untreated patients may succumb from this complication, suggesting that it is an integral part of the natural history of the disease and merely accentuated by the use of radiomimetic agents.

TREATMENT. The initial treatment for a newly diagnosed patient with PV is phlebotomy. Reduction of the hematocrit to below 53 per cent will usually be associated with a reduction in red cell mass to a level at which hypervolemia and hyperviscosity no longer pose a threat. This decompression should be carried out cautiously with no more than a single 500 ml bloodletting every two to three days. Subsequent phlebotomies are aimed at maintaining the hematocrit below 50 per cent. In the beginning, phlebotomies may have to be carried out frequently, but when iron deficiency becomes more pronounced, the low MCV will tend to keep the hematocrit low despite brisk red cell production, and eventually the iron deficiency will help retard red cell production as well.

Symptoms of iron deficiency, such as weakness and tiredness, may occur especially if solicited by excessive questioning by the physician. Since these symptoms are nonspecific, they should be tested with a careful monitored trial on iron before they are used as a reason for abandoning a simple phlebotomy regimen.

The presence of a substantial increase in platelet count (i.e., in excess of 1 million per cubic millimeter) should generate some concern and ought to be treated. Furthermore, excessive splenic enlargement, bony tenderness, pruritus, hyperuricemia, and poor veins also indicate the need for additional treatment. These treatments consist either of radioactive phosphorus or of various alkylating agents.

Radioactive phosphorus (^{32}P), preferably given intravenously in doses of 3 to 5 mC, has a solid reputation of causing a balanced and smooth reduction in bone marrow activity, with no immediate side effects. However, ^{32}P has been suspected of causing acute leukemia in a considerable number of cases. Alkylating agents are usually given by mouth, busulfan in doses of 4 to 6 mg a day and chlorambucil in doses of 6 to 8 mg per day. They also cause a predictable decrease in hematopoietic activity, but their immediate side effects are believed to be more capricious and difficult to manage than those associated with ^{32}P treatment. Busulfan, for example, can occasionally cause an almost irreversible thrombocytopenia and severe pulmonary fibrosis. On the other hand, the alkylating agents are thought not to be as leukemogenic as ^{32}P. These assumptions have been challenged recently, and it now appears that both regimens can induce and maintain smooth remissions and that both are equally leukemogenic.

Because of the long expected survival, chemotherapy and radiotherapy should be used sparingly, especially in view of the numerous reports on the emergence of second malignancies in patients with prolonged exposure to radiomimetic agents.

Therapy of the thrombotic and embolic complications involves use of anticoagulants, anti-platelet aggregating agents, and myelosuppressive drugs. The treatment of the final "burned out" myelofibrotic phase can be extremely difficult. The spleen may become large and mechanically symptomatic, the granulocytes may approach leukemic values, and the hematocrit may gradually decrease to levels demanding transfusions. Androgen therapy may ameliorate the anemia, but chemotherapy is often ineffective in the treatment of extramedullary myelopoiesis. Splenectomy is hazardous because of the postoperative thrombocytosis, and a trial of splenic radiation is preferable if spleen size becomes a major problem. The treatment of the acute leukemia which occurs in 10 per cent of patients is most difficult, and agents used in the management of acute myelomonocytic leukemia are often ineffective. A trial of vincristine and prednisone is probably indicated if everything else fails, but the prognosis is grim.

Throughout the many years of management, attention must be paid to good general medical and emotional support. Many diseases of middle and old age can complicate the course and must be recognized and treated. However, with good management and prevention of hypervolemia, hyperviscosity, and thrombocytosis, an asymptomatic life span of 15 to 20 or more years can and should be anticipated.

Adamson, J. W., et al.: Polycythemia vera: Stem-cell and probable clonal origin of the disease. N. Engl. J. Med., 295:913, 1976.

Erslev, A. J.: The clinical usefulness of erythropoietin measurements. *In* Fisher, J. W. (ed.): Kidney Hormones. 2nd ed. London, Academic Press, 1977, p. 571.

Erslev, A. J., and Weiss, L.: Structure and function of the bone marrow. *In* Williams, W. J., Beutler, E., Erslev, A. J., and Rundles, R. W. (eds.): Hematology. New York, McGraw-Hill Book Company, 1977, p. 57.

Glass, J. L., and Wasserman, L. R.: Primary polycythemia. *In* Williams, W. J., Beutler, E., Erslev, A. J., and Rundles, R. W. (eds.): Hematology. New York, McGraw-Hill Book Company, 1977, p. 624.

Lajtha, L. G.: Haemopoietic stem cells. Br. J. Haematol., 29:529, 1975.

Landow, S. A.: Acute leukemia in polycythemia vera. Semin. Hematol., 13:33, 1976.

Prchal, J. F., Adamson, J. W., Murphy, S., Steinman, L., and Fialkow, P. J.: Polycythemia vera: The in vitro response of normal and abnormal stem cell lines to erythropoietin. J. Clin. Invest., 61:1044, 1978.

Wasserman, L. R.: The treatment of polycythemia vera. Semin. Hematol., 13:57, 1976.

Wurster-Hill, D., et al.: Cytogenetic studies in polycythemia vera. Semin. Hematol., 13:13, 1976.

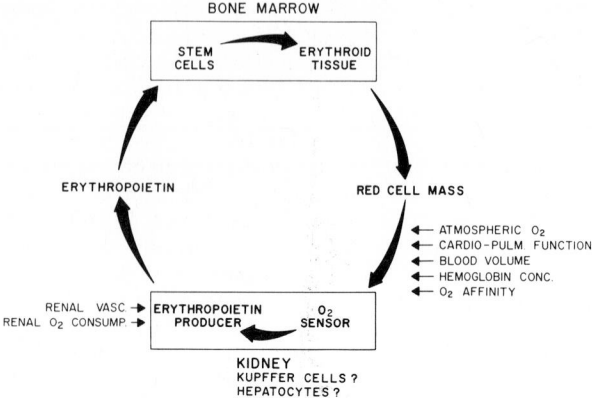

Figure 3. Outline of feedback system regulating the size of the circulating red cell mass. Signals are transmitted from the bone marrow to the kidney via oxygen carried by red cells and from the kidney to the bone marrow via erythropoietin. The oxygen sensor in the kidney transmits signals to erythropoietin-producing cells, and it appears that similar oxygen sensors and erythropoietin producers are present in the hepatocytes or the Kupffer cells of the liver.

492.2. SECONDARY POLYCYTHEMIA

The existence of a relationship between hypoxia and polycythemia was first noted by Dennis Jourdanet, a French physician, who in the 1860's practiced in the highlands of Mexico. He noticed that his surgical patients had thick, slowly running blood, and he related this to the thin air and the low oxygen content of arterial blood. At the turn of the century, Friedrich Miescher elaborated on this observation and concluded that the bone marrow must be stimulated directly by low arterial oxygen pressure. However, the demonstration of a renal erythropoietic hormone in the 1950's established that the effect of hypoxia on the bone marrow is indirect and mediated by this hormone, aptly named *erythropoietin*. Subsequent studies have led to the hypothesis that the size of the red cell mass is maintained within normal limits by a feedback control system operating between the kidney and the bone marrow (Fig. 3). When this feedback system is perturbed by impaired oxygen delivery to a renal oxygen sensor, erythropoietin-producing cells initiate the development of a compensatory and appropriate secondary polycythemia. Occasionally, those cells are activated locally, resulting in the development of an inappropriate secondary polycythemia.

APPROPRIATE SECONDARY POLYCYTHEMIA

HIGH ALTITUDE. About 25 million people live and toil at altitudes in excess of 3000 m, and experience has shown that man can readily adapt to altitudes of up to 4300 m or an atmospheric pressure of two thirds normal. Permanent settlements above this altitude are few in number, with the highest known, Aucanquilcha in Chile, at 5400 m, and with an atmospheric pressure of one half normal probably representing the upper limit of sustained physiologic adaptation. Above this level, transient visits are possible, but so far no climber has scaled Mt. Everest at 8848 m and one third normal at-mospheric pressure without the use of supplemental oxygen.

At sea level, oxygen is transported quite easily from atmospheric air to the tissues along a steep pressure gradient from 160 mm mercury in air to 40 mm at the venous end of the tissue capillaries. At an altitude of 5400 m with an oxygen pressure of 80 mm, the gradient is obviously more shallow, especially since the all-important oxygen pressure in the capillaries has to be maintained at about 40 mm in order to prevent destructive tissue anoxia. To overcome the effect of a shallow oxygen gradient the acclimatized individual depends primarily on hyperventilation and polycythemia. Hyperventilation will reduce dead space and enlarge the alveolar diffusing area and thereby more effectively bring atmospheric oxygen in contact with alveolar capillaries. Polycythemia will increase the oxygen carrying capacity of circulating blood and thereby permit extraction of needed oxygen in the tissues with relatively little deoxygenation of blood and little decrease in oxygen pressure. An increase in cardiac output with a greater perfusion of the tissues will of course also permit needed oxygen extraction with a relatively small decrease in the oxygen content and oxygen pressure of capillary blood. However, the added work load on a vital and vulnerable organ makes this an unacceptable device for chronic acclimatization. A shift of the oxygen dissociation curve to the right could likewise provide more oxygen for the tissues with only a minimal reduction in the capillary oxygen tension. However, a shift to the right would also impair oxygen loading in the lungs at low atmospheric pressure, and direct measurement of the oxygen dissociation curve of high altitude dwellers has not disclosed a significant shift from normal. Actually, animals indigenous to high altitudes, such as llamas and vicuñas, have oxygen dissociation curves shifted to the left, suggesting that at least for these superbly acclimatized animals oxygen loading in the lungs takes precedence over oxygen unloading in the tissues. In these animals tissue oxygen transport is facilitated by increased capillary density and by increased concentrations of myoglobin, but whether acclimatized human beings also use these facilitating devices has not been resolved. Anyhow, the over-all compensatory effect of hyperventilation and polycythemia in fully acclimatized individuals living at atmospheric air pressure of from two thirds to one half normal is such that they do not experience more tissue hypoxia than that needed to mobilize and maintain these adaptive measures.

Clinical Features. Barrel chest and ruddy cyanosis are the two most characteristic features of high altitude dwellers. Vascular engorgement resulting from blood volume expansion can be observed in conjunctivae, mucous membranes, and skin and may contribute to headaches and nosebleedings and to the remarkable capacity of Sherpas to walk barefooted and sleep on ice and snow. Splenomegaly is unusual and, if present, should suggest a complicating unrelated disease.

The hematocrit is above 53 per cent, and the red cells are usually normochromic and normocytic with a normal life span. The red cell mass is increased above normal, but the plasma volume usually remains unchanged. The white blood cells and platelets are numerically and functionally normal (Table 1).

In some cases altitude acclimatization cannot be

maintained but merges into hypervolemic decompensation — so-called "chronic mountain sickness," or Monge's disease. This disorder is characterized by increasing cyanosis and plethora, mental deterioration, and right-sided heart failure with hepatosplenomegaly, edema, and ascites. The hematocrit is increased out of proportion to the altitude, and the resulting hyperviscosity is in part responsible for the cerebral and cardiovascular decompensation. The reason for the excessive rate of red cell production appears to lie in a suppressed respiratory center, causing hypoventilation despite increasing hypoxia and hypercapnia. Therapeutic phlebotomy and oxygen may provide relief, but a temporary stay at sea level is usually needed for cure.

PULMONARY DISEASE. Chronic obstructive pulmonary disease with hypoxemia and hypercapnia ("blue bloaters") is associated with secondary polycythemia but rarely as severe as that observed in a corresponding hypoxemia caused by altitude. In some cases a concomitant increase in plasma volume may conceal the increase in red cell mass, but in most cases the absolute increase in red cell mass is suboptimal. This could be due to chronic respiratory acidosis reducing tissue hypoxia by shifting the oxygen dissociation curve to the right, or it could be due to a reduced bone marrow responsiveness to erythropoietin as observed in patients with chronic inflammatory or infectious disease. Despite the compensatory nature of the polycythemia, a high hematocrit may cause sluggish blood flow and a tendency to thrombosis. Phlebotomy is usually indicated when the hematocrit is in excess of 60 per cent.

ALVEOLAR HYPOVENTILATION. Central or peripheral impairment of ventilatory function also causes arterial hypoxemia, cyanosis, and secondary polycythemia. Its two most colorful variants are Monge's chronic mountain disease and the "pickwickian syndrome." In the latter the ventilatory burden of obesity is aggravated by unresponsiveness of the respiratory center to hypoxemia and hypercapnia, resulting in the proverbial somnolent cyanosis of Mrs. Wardle's boy Joe.

CARDIOVASCULAR DISEASE. Right to left shunt in congenital heart disease is characteristically associated with cyanosis, clubbing, and secondary polycythemia ("blue babies"). In acquired heart disease with congestive failure the red cell mass is often increased moderately, but the hematocrit is rarely increased above normal because of the simultaneous expansion in plasma volume.

DEFECTIVE HEMOGLOBIN. Chronic carbon monoxide poisoning may be associated with secondary polycythemia resulting from both inactive carbon monoxide hemoglobin and increased oxygen affinity of the remaining normal hemoglobin. Although such poisoning has been observed occasionally in workers exposed to excessive carbon monoxide fumes, it has been recognized recently that it also involves chain smokers. In these individuals carbon monoxide may cause a mild increase in the red cell mass and for unknown reasons a mild decrease in plasma volume, resulting in an over-all increase in the hematocrit. Although these individuals have been thought to have relative polycythemia as a result of "stress," it seems much more likely that they have a true secondary polycythemia caused by defective oxygen transport.

Acquired methemoglobinemia may also cause a mild secondary polycythemia, but hereditary changes in the hemoglobin molecule are a more frequent cause. In some cases, amino acid substitutions occur in the heme pockets, causing cyanotic methemoglobinemia which, if not associated with hemolysis, will result in a secondary polycythemia. In others the amino acid substitution occurs in the contact area between the alpha and beta chains, interfering with the conformational changes which normally facilitate oxygen release from the hemoglobin molecule. The resulting high oxygen affinity leads to noncyanotic tissue hypoxia and secondary polycythemia. Both alpha chain substitutions (Hb Chesapeake, Hb Capetown) and beta chain substitutions (Hb Yakima, Hb Rainier) have been found among the more than 25 variants described. In some, the charge difference between the normal and its substituted amino acid makes it easy to identify the hemoglobin as abnormal. In others, however, the charge is electrophoretically silent, and more sophisticated methods must be used to recognize the responsible hemoglobinopathy. However, such studies should be carried out in polycythemic patients with a family history of polycythemia and with increased oxygen affinity of their hemoglobin. (See Ch. 485.)

DRUG-INDUCED. Cobalt, testosterone, and of course erythropoietin are the only chemicals or drugs with a predictable capacity to stimulate red cell production and cause secondary polycythemia. Cobalt was once used extensively as a hematinic agent in patients with refractory anemia, but although the effect on hemoglobin concentration was often gratifying, the side effects were troublesome. Of more importance, however, was the slow realization that the erythropoietic effect probably was caused by an inhibition of the cellular oxidative metabolism. Since an increase in red cell production which merely compensates for a drug-induced cellular hypoxia does not appear to justify the use of such a drug, cobalt is seldom used now.

Testosterone and its many natural and synthetic derivatives will stimulate red cell production in many patients with aregenerative anemias and will in some cases cause a pronounced secondary polycythemia. They are used in many dialysis centers to augment red cell production of patients with chronic renal disease and can often decrease or eliminate transfusion requirements. The action of androgenic steroids on the erythroid tissue appears to be dual. They will stimulate the production of both renal and extrarenal erythropoietin, and they will sensitize erythroid precursor cells to the effect of erythropoietin. In some patients androgens will also stimulate granulocyte and platelet production, and they have been used with varying success in the treatment of aplastic anemia.

Erythropoietin, the true erythropoietic hormone, will as expected cause polycythemia in laboratory animals if administered over a prolonged period. The successful purification, identification, and mass production of this hormone will undoubtedly lead to the inclusion of a very effective and desirable erythropoietic agent in our therapeutic armamentarium.

INAPPROPRIATE SECONDARY POLYCYTHEMIA

In the absence of bone marrow dysfunction and general tissue hypoxia, the presence of an absolute polycythemia should suggest inappropriate erythropoietin production, either renal or extrarenal. Unfortunately, the diagnosis must be made by exclusion, since an accurate assessment of the site and magnitude of erythropoietin production is still not possible.

RENAL DISORDERS. Partial obstruction of a renal artery should in theory cause renal ischemia and excessive renal erythropoietin production. Only in a few cases, however, has renal artery stenosis been observed to cause secondary polycythemia. More frequently secondary polycythemia has been found in association with intrarenal vascular obstruction, e.g., in kidney transplants undergoing chronic rejection.

In patients with hypernephroma, secondary polycythemia is a well recognized although quite rare complication. This finding has led to the concept of inappropriate erythropoietin production by hypernephroma cells. However, a number of completely different tumors, both malignant (Wilms') and benign (fibroma), have also been associated with excessive red cell production, rendering a neoplastic origin of erythropoietin less likely. The fact that solitary renal cysts, polycystic disease, and hydronephrosis also may be found in association with polycythemia suggests that the erythropoietin is derived from normal renal tissue rendered hypoxic from the pressure of space-occupying lesions. A definite answer to this pathogenetic question cannot be provided as yet because of our inability to assay tissue extracts for erythropoietin. However, from a clinical point of view, every patient with suspected secondary polycythemia should have a thorough renal workup to rule out the presence of a benign or malignant erythropoietin producing or inducing lesion.

EXTRARENAL DISORDERS. In the adult about 10 per cent of erythropoietin is produced by extrarenal tissue. During fetal life, however, these tissues appear to make most of the circulating erythropoietin, and it is at birth that the production switches to the kidney. The extrarenal site of production is believed to be the liver, either the hepatocytes or the Kupffer cells. In this regard, it is of great interest that regenerating hepatic cells, as observed experimentally after partial hepatectomy and clinically after hepatitis, appear to release extrarenal erythropoietin. Furthermore, 10 per cent of patients with hepatoma have been shown to have increased rates of red cell production, occasionally leading to pronounced secondary polycythemia. This could suggest a reversal to fetal metabolism in regenerating and neoplastic hepatocytes. Further studies of these illnesses may provide information about extrarenal production of erythropoietin which could be of future importance for patients with chronic renal disease in which renal production of erythropoietin is failing.

Cerebellar cystic adenomas and large uterine myomas have also been associated with secondary polycythemia. In some of these, mechanical interference with the respiratory center or with the renal supply of blood may play a causative role, but in others erythropoietin has been isolated from the tumors themselves. Secondary polycythemia has also been found in patients with pheochromocytomas, aldosterone-producing tumors, and Cushing's disease; but until we have a reliable radioimmunoassay for erythropoietin, the pathogenesis of these polycythemias must remain in question.

Finch, C. A., and Lenfant, C.: Oxygen transport in man. N. Engl. J. Med., 286:407, 1972.

Frisancho, A. R.: Functional adaptation to high altitude hypoxia. Science, 187:313, 1975.

Jourdanet, D.: De l'anémie des altitudes et de l'anémie en général dans ses rapports avec la pression de l'atmosphère. Paris, Bailliere, 1863.

Penaloga, D., and Sime, F.: Chronic cor pulmonade due to loss of altitude acclimatization (chronic mountain sickness). Am. J. Med., 50:728, 1971.

Shahidi, N. T.: Androgens and erythropoiesis. N. Engl. J. Med., 289:72, 1973.

Smith, J. R., and Landow, S. A.: Smokers' polycythemia. N. Engl. J. Med., 298:6, 1978.

Stephens, A. D.: Polycythemia and high affinity haemoglobins. Br. J. Haematol., 36:153, 1977.

Thorling, E. B.: Paraneoplastic erythrocytosis and inappropriate erythropoietin production. Scand. J. Haematol., Supp. 17, 1972.

Thorling, E. B., and Erslev, A. J.: The effect of some erythropoietic agents on the "tissue" tension of oxygen. Br. J. Haematol., 23:483, 1972.

Zwillich, C. W., Sutton, F. O., Pierson, D. J., Creagh, E. M., and Weil, J. V.: Decreased hypoxic ventilatory drive in the obesity-hyperventilation syndrome. Am. J. Med., 59:343, 1975.

Section Six DISEASES OF THE WHITE BLOOD CELLS

493. NEUTROPHIL FUNCTION

S. J. Klebanoff

The primary function of the neutrophilic polymorphonuclear leukocyte is the phagocytosis and destruction of microorganisms, and this functional specialization is reflected in its unique morphologic and biochemical characteristics. The neutrophil develops in the bone marrow, beginning with the pluripotential stem cell and continuing through the committed stem cell and a series of morphologically recognizable precursors to the fully segmented mature cell. The bone marrow myeloid cells consist of an actively dividing marrow precursor pool made up, in order of develop-

ment, of myeloblasts, promyelocytes, and myelocytes and a marrow granulocyte reserve consisting of nondividing, maturing metamyelocytes, band cells, and fully segmented mature cells (Fig. 1). Transit time through the bone marrow is about nine days, and mature neutrophils exit into the circulation at a rate of approximately 1.5×10^9 cells per kilogram of body weight per day. Administration of endotoxin, etiocholanolone, or glucocorticosteroids increases the blood neutrophil count owing in part to the discharge of cells from the marrow granulocyte reserve.

The total blood granulocyte pool consists of actively circulating cells which are sampled during venipuncture, in equilibrium with a marginated group of cells which are sequestered or marginated along the walls of small blood vessels. Exercise and agents such as epinephrine or glucocorticosteroids can reduce margina-

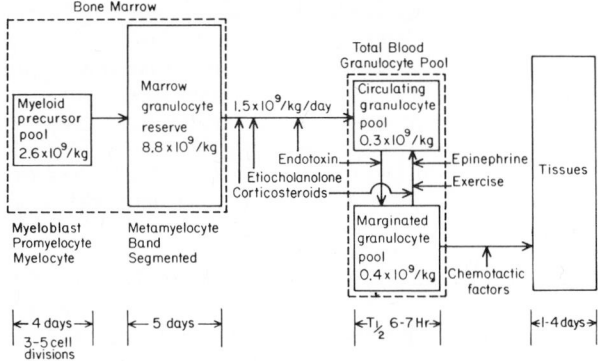

Figure 1. Schematic representation of neutrophil kinetics. (Adapted from Klebanoff and Clark, 1978.)

tion and thus increase the peripheral blood count. The life span of the peripheral neutrophil is relatively short; its mean half-life in the circulation is six to seven hours, and its extravascular life span is a few days. Some of the cells which leave the circulation are removed by the fixed macrophages of the liver and spleen. The remainder pass into the tissues or migrate to areas of direct contact with the environment (oral cavity, bronchotracheal tree, cervical canal).

The neutrophil response to microbial invasion can be divided into several stages: mobilization, adherence, chemotaxis, phagocytosis, intracellular killing, digestion, and extracellular release (Fig. 2). Neutrophils are discharged from the bone marrow in large numbers, producing a leukocytosis, and margination and adherence of the mobilized cells to the vessel wall are accentuated in areas of inflammation. The neutrophil extends pseudopods between the endothelial cells of small venules, opening up a passageway through which it passes. The channel immediately closes behind it, and the neutrophil migrates by ameboid movement along an increasing concentration gradient of a specific chemotactic agent or agents, directly to the site of microbial invasion. This process requires major alterations in cell shape; the "deformability" of granulocytes increases with maturation.

A large number of factors are chemotactic for neutrophils. Those of possible physiologic significance include the following: (1) Low molecular weight (approximately 1000) factors formed by most bacteria which act directly on neutrophils. (2) Complement (C)-derived factors (C3a, C5a, C567) formed either by activation of

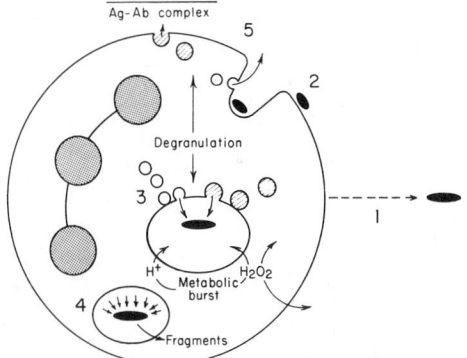

Figure 2. Schematic representation of the neutrophil response: (1) chemotaxis; (2) phagocytosis; (3) microbicidal activity; (4) digestion; (5) extracellular enzyme release.

complement or by proteolytic cleavage of individual complement components (C3, C5) by enzymes released by bacteria, leukocytes, or damaged tissues. Complement is activated by certain microbial cell wall components (e.g., endotoxin) in the absence of antibody and by complexes formed when microbial antigens react with specific antibody, with activation occurring either by the classic pathway involving the first three functional complement components, C1, 4, and 2, or by the alternative (properdin) pathway which bypasses these early components. C5a, a 15,000 molecular weight fragment of C5, is the predominant chemotactic factor in activated serum. Proteolytic cleavage can release both C5a and a low molecular weight (approximately 6000) fragment of C3, C3a. (3) Leukocyte-derived chemotactic factors, which include agents from neutrophils, from macrophages, and from lymphocytes exposed to specific antigens or nonspecific mitogens (lymphocyte-derived chemotactic factor, LDCF). (4) Factors formed as a consequence of Hageman factor activation, which include kallikrein, plasminogen activator, and low molecular weight fibrinogen or fibrin cleavage products. (5) Other factors such as N-formylmethionyl peptides, an oxidation product of arachidonic acid (12-L-hydroxy-5,8,10,14-eicosatetranoic acid, HETE), collagen degradation products, cyclic nucleotides, and prostaglandins.

The chemotactic stimulus brings the neutrophil into direct contact with the microorganism, and phagocytosis rapidly follows. A number of virulent organisms resist phagocytosis by virtue of the nature of their capsular material. These organisms are ingested when they can be trapped against a surface by the leukocyte (surface phagocytosis) or when the antiphagocytic nature of the capsular material is neutralized. Substances which react with particles to render them more susceptible to phagocytosis are termed opsonins. They may be heat stable or heat labile. IgG antibodies to surface antigens function as heat-stable opsonins. They attach to the bacterium through the antibody combining site on the $F(ab')_2$ portion and to receptors on the phagocyte through the Fc portion of the antibody molecule. The heat-labile opsonins are derived largely from complement. They are polyspecific and are not dependent on previous exposure to the organism. C3 when activated (C3b) attaches both to the bacterial cell wall and to neutrophil surface receptors. In general, antibody and complement combine to prepare the particle for ingestion, antibody serving both to identify the invading organism and to initiate adjacent complement activation. The sequential and circumferential interaction between cell receptors and opsonins distributed over the entire bacterial surface, together with the gelation and contraction of submembranous actomyosin microfilaments, results in the movement of the pseudopods around the particle until engulfment is complete. The membranous stalk which connects the vacuole to the cell surface fuses and ruptures, and the particle is set free in the interior of the cell, isolated from the extracellular environment in a vacuole lined by the invaginated cell membrane.

Phagocytosis initiates a sequence of morphologic and biochemical events which result in the death of most ingested organisms. The most important morphologic feature of the mature neutrophil is the abundance of membrane-bound cytoplasmic granules. At least two granule populations exist. Dense, relatively large granules which stain reddish purple with azure dyes (azurophil or primary granules) develop in the promyelocyte. These granules, which contain myeloperoxidase, elastase, cationic proteins, and a number of acid hydrolases, are primary lysosomes. During the myelocyte stage smaller, less dense granules are formed which contain lactoferrin, collagenase, lysozyme, and, in some species, alkaline phosphatase. These specific or secondary granules are free of acid hydrolases and thus are not lysosomes in the strict sense of the term. No further granule formation occurs beyond the myelocyte stage. Approximately three fourths of the granules of the mature neutrophil are of the specific (secondary) variety, and the remainder are azurophil (primary) granules. The granules adjacent to the phagocytic vacuole fuse with the vacuole, the common membrane ruptures, and the granule contents are discharged into the vacuolar space. Both granule types participate in the degranulation process.

The metabolic machinery of the neutrophil is geared primarily to the production of energy (ATP) for chemotaxis and phagocytosis and to the production of oxygen radicals and H_2O_2 for microbicidal activity (Fig. 3). Energy production is dependent on glycolysis; it occurs in the absence of oxygen. Phagocytosis, however, is associated with a burst of oxygen consumption and much or all of the extra oxygen consumed is converted to H_2O_2 via a superoxide anion intermediate. This respiratory burst is associated with the emission of light (chemiluminescence). Glucose oxidation via the hexose monophosphate (HMP) shunt, reduction of nitroblue tetrazolium (NBT) to insoluble blue formazan, conversion of iodide to organic form (iodination), degradation of thyroid hormones, and binding of estrogens are all markedly increased by phagocytosis. Glycogen, which is present in large amounts in the neutrophil as particulate deposits, is broken down at an accelerated rate, and lactic acid production and phospholipid turnover also are increased.

Studies of the enzymic mechanisms responsible for the metabolic burst have focused on the oxidase responsible for the increased oxygen consumption and H_2O_2 production and on the link between this oxidase and the activation of the HMP shunt. The first two enzymes of the HMP shunt, glucose-6-phosphate dehydrogenase (G-6-PD) and 6-phosphogluconate dehydrogenase, reduce NADP to NADPH, and the continued activity of the shunt is dependent upon the reoxidation

of NADPH. There are two prevalent views: (1) Oxygen is converted to H_2O_2 by NADH oxidase, an enzyme which utilizes the NADH formed in the glycolytic pathway, and the H_2O_2 so formed activates the HMP shunt by a sequence of reactions, the oxidation of GSH by glutathione peroxidase and the reduction of GSSG by glutathione reductase, which result in the reoxidation of NADPH. (2) An NADPH oxidase is activated which meets the total requirements of the metabolic burst–increased oxygen consumption, H_2O_2 formation, and NADPH oxidation. The oxygen radicals and H_2O_2 formed by these or other mechanisms are released into the phagocytic vacuole where they exert a microbicidal effect (see below), whereas cytoplasmic components are protected from excess H_2O_2 by the glutathione system and by catalase and from the superoxide anion by superoxide dismutase.

A variety of antimicrobial agents are released into the phagocytic vacuole. Some require oxygen, whereas others are effective under anaerobic conditions. Among the oxygen-dependent systems is one which consists of myeloperoxidase, H_2O_2, and a halide. Myeloperoxidase is discharged into the vacuole during the degranulation process, H_2O_2 is generated either by leukocytic metabolism or by certain ingested microorganisms (e.g., streptococci, pneumococci), and the halide requirement can be met by chloride ions, which are present in excess, and the small amounts of iodide absorbed as such or released by the deiodination of the thyroid hormones. When iodide is the halide employed, iodination of the microorganism occurs. The products of oxygen metabolism (H_2O_2, superoxide anion, hydroxyl radicals, singlet oxygen) also have antimicrobial activity in the absence of myeloperoxidase. The oxygen-independent antimicrobial systems include the acid pH of the vacuolar contents, lactoferrin, lysozyme, and the granular cationic proteins.

Ingested organisms vary in their sensitivity to the intravacuolar microbicidal systems. Some organisms (e.g., pneumococci) are susceptible to acid, whereas others (e.g., lactobacilli) are acidophilic; some are readily lysed by lysozyme, whereas most organisms resist the action of this enzyme; some organisms (e.g., streptococci, pneumococci) secrete H_2O_2 or acid into the vacuolar space, and this contributes to their own destruction, whereas others contain catalase or superoxide dismutase and thus resist H_2O_2- or superoxide-dependent systems. The level and variety of the antimicrobial systems endow the neutrophil with an overkill capacity which allows it to function adequately despite a decrease in the activity of one of the systems. The death of the ingested organisms is followed by their digestion to low molecular weight fragments by acid hydrolases.

Although the neutrophil primarily serves a protective function, tissue damage may result from the release of toxic agents into the extracellular fluid because of cell disintegration, leakage during phagocytosis, or secretion when leukocytes are in contact with antigen-antibody complexes on a nonphagocytizable surface. Neutrophil-mediated injury is seen in the Arthus and Shwartzman reactions and in experimental immune complex disease. In man, it may contribute to the tissue damage in acute glomerulonephritis, polyarteritis nodosa, rheumatoid or gouty arthritis, and transplantation rejection.

Figure 3. Neutrophil metabolism: (1) glucose-6-phosphate dehydrogenase and 6-phosphogluconate dehydrogenase; (2) NADPH oxidase; (3) glutathione reductase; (4) glutathione peroxidase; (5) NADH oxidase.

Cline, M. J.: The White Cell. Cambridge, Mass., Harvard University Press, 1975.

Gallin, J. I., and Wolff, S. M.: Leucocyte chemotaxis: Physiological considerations and abnormalities. Clin. Haematol., 4:567, 1975.

Klebanoff, S. J.: Antimicrobial mechanisms in neutrophilic polymorphonuclear leukocytes. Semin. Hematol., 12:117, 1975.

Klebanoff, S. J., and Clark, R. A.: The Neutrophil: Function and Clinical Disorders. Amsterdam, Elsevier/North-Holland Biomedical Press B.V., 1978.

Murphy, P.: The Neutrophil. New York, Plenum Medical Book Company, 1976.

Stossel, T. P.: Phagocytosis. N. Engl. J. Med., 290:717, 774, 833, 1974.

494. NEUTROPHIL DYSFUNCTION SYNDROMES

S. J. Klebanoff

Metchnikoff over 70 years ago proposed that the destruction of microorganisms by "microphages" is essential to the host defense, and the increased incidence of infection in severe neutropenia or agranulocytosis fully supports this thesis. What has become apparent within the past decade is that neutrophils may be present in adequate numbers in the bloodstream, yet still be unable to perform their function adequately. Defects in neutrophil adherence, chemotaxis, phagocytosis, microbicidal activity, and mixed defects have been described (see accompanying table).

DEFECTS OF ADHERENCE

The emigration of neutrophils from the bloodstream is initiated by adherence to the vessel wall. In vitro methods for the study of leukocyte adherence, involving the sticking of the cell to a glass or nylon surface, have been described. Decreased adherence has been reported in diabetes, myelogenous leukemia, and after administration of alcohol, prednisone, or aspirin. A transient increase in leukocyte adherence is associated with the granulocytopenia observed following the initiation of hemodialysis.

Functional Classification of Neutrophil Dysfunction Syndromes

Defect of adherence
Defect of chemotaxis
  Cellular defect
  Defect in chemotactic factor generation
  Serum inhibitor
    Directed against the cell
    Directed against the chemotactic factor
Defect of phagocytosis
  Cellular defect
  Humoral (opsonic) defect
Defect of degranulation
Defect of microbicidal activity
  Defect in oxidative metabolism
    Chronic granulomatous disease (CGD)
      X-linked
      Autosomal
    Familial lipochrome histiocytosis
    Severe leukocytic G-6-PD deficiency
  Myeloperoxidase deficiency
    Hereditary
    Acquired
Mixed defects
  Chédiak-Higashi syndrome

DEFECTS OF CHEMOTAXIS

Decreased chemotaxis may result from a cellular defect in which the leukocytes do not respond appropriately to a normal chemotactic stimulus, from a serum defect in which activation of the patient's serum fails to generate normal amounts of chemotactic factors, or from the presence of an inhibitor of chemotaxis in serum directed either against the cells or the chemotactic factor. A combined cellular and serum defect may exist. Chemotaxis is evaluated in vivo by the *skin window* technique, in which coverslips, applied to areas of abraded skin, are replaced at intervals and the cells which have adhered to their undersurface are stained and counted. The cells which enter the lesion during the first six hours are predominantly neutrophils, after which mononuclear cells predominate. In vitro methods include measurement of migration toward a chemoattractant on a plastic surface under agarose gel or use of the *Boyden chamber.* The latter consists of two compartments separated by a membrane filter. The leukocytes present in one compartment migrate through pores in the filter under the influence of a chemotactic agent and are counted.

A cellular defect in chemotaxis has been described in healthy neonates and in some patients with the Chédiak-Higashi syndrome (see below), diabetes, rheumatoid arthritis, severe thermal injury, juvenile periodontal disease (periodontosis), severe infection with toxic granulation of neutrophils, graft-vs-host disease following bone marrow transplantation, neutrophil actin dysfunction, congenital ichthyosis, hypophosphatemia, severe hypogammaglobulinemia, Down's syndrome, the lazy leukocyte syndrome, or hyperimmunoglobulin E. The *lazy leukocyte syndrome* is characterized by low grade fever, neutropenia, recurrent gingivitis, stomatitis and otitis media, a cellular defect in chemotaxis and random mobility, and impaired release of granulocytes from the bone marrow. A number of patients with *hyperimmunoglobulin E*, recurrent, generally staphylococcal infections, and allergic disorders such as eczema, asthma, or urticaria have a cellular chemotactic defect. *Job's syndrome*, for example, is characterized by recurrent "cold" staphylococcal abscesses, eczematous dermatitis, high IgE levels, a cellular defect in chemotaxis, and, in some instances, hyperkeratotic nails, hyperextensible joints, and periodontal disease.

A serum defect in the generation of complement-derived chemotactic factors is seen in complement component deficiencies, immunoglobulin deficiencies, neonates, systemic lupus erythematosus, and diabetes. Patients with hereditary Hageman factor or prekallikrein deficiency have abnormalities in the formation of the Hageman factor–dependent chemotactic agents, kallikrein and plasminogen activator. Cell-directed inhibitors of chemotaxis are found in the serum of some patients with thermal injury, neoplasms, Wiskott-Aldrich syndrome, IgA myeloma, and in other isolated cases. Chemotactic factor–directed inhibitors are normally present in serum. Increased levels are found in some patients with anergy (Hodgkin's disease, lepromatous leprosy, sarcoidosis) and alcoholic liver disease. Reduced levels are found in α_1-antitrypsin deficiency.

DEFECTS OF PHAGOCYTOSIS

Decreased phagocytosis may be due to a cellular defect or to a deficiency or dysfunction of either immunoglobulin or complement resulting in decreased opsonic activity. A cellular defect in phagocytosis has been described in some patients with diabetes mellitus, systemic lupus erythematosus, rheumatoid arthritis, autoimmune neutropenia, hypophosphatemia, leukemia, juvenile periodontal disease (periodontosis), and neutrophil actin dysfunction. The sera of patients with hypo- or agammaglobulinemia have decreased levels of heat-stable opsonins, and patients with complement deficiencies have decreased levels of heat-labile opsonins, resulting in an increased susceptibility to infection by encapsulated bacteria.

C3 deficiency with decreased opsonic activity is seen in systemic lupus erythematosus and progressive glomerulonephritis. Neonates, particularly with low birth weight, have decreased serum opsonic activity related either to C3 deficiency or to lack of transplacental transfer of IgM. Hereditary defects involving C3 include homozygous C3 deficiency and hypercatabolism of C3. The latter has been subdivided into Type I associated with a deficiency in C3b inactivator (C3b INA) and Type II caused by enhanced C3 cleaving activity in the patient's serum and associated with lipodystrophy and glomerulonephritis. The patient's serum is deficient in a number of complement-mediated functions, namely, bactericidal activity and opsonic activity, and in the generation of chemotactic factors, resulting in an increased susceptibility to infection with pyogenic bacteria. The administration of normal serum or, in some instances, purified C3 produces a temporary increase in C3 levels with restoration of the complement-mediated functions. *C5 dysfunction* is found in infants with a syndrome consisting of generalized seborrheic dermatitis, intractable severe diarrhea, recurrent local and systemic infections, usually with gram-negative organisms, and marked wasting and dystrophy (*Leiner's syndrome*). Total hemolytic complement activity is normal, as is the level of the individual complement components. However, dysfunction of C5 is indicated by inability of the serum to opsonize particles dependent on C5 for optimal opsonization and reversal of this defect with purified C5. The generation of chemotactic factors in serum is defective in some patients.

The serum in *sickle cell disease* is deficient in heat-labile opsonins for pneumococci. It has normal levels of immunoglobulin, total complement, and the opsonic components of complement (C3, C5), and a defect in alternative pathway activation of complement to form opsonins has been proposed. Decreased splenic clearance resulting from functional splenectomy also contributes to the decreased resistance to the pneumococcus in sickle cell disease. *Tuftsin*, a tetrapeptide fragment of IgG (L-threonyl-L-lysyl-L-prolyl-L-arginine) which stimulates phagocytosis, is decreased following splenectomy and in hereditary tuftsin deficiency.

DEFECTS OF DEGRANULATION

A degranulation defect with impaired release of granule constituents has been reported in the Chédiak-Higashi syndrome (see below) and in some patients

with leukemia. The enlarged "toxic" granules associated with severe infection also may be functionally abnormal. Selective deficiency of granule populations was detected in leukemia and in other isolated cases.

DEFECT OF MICROBICIDAL ACTIVITY

A defect of microbicidal activity is indicated by impaired microbial killing which cannot be accounted for by a decrease in phagocytosis. It can be caused by decreased oxidative metabolism (chronic granulomatous disease), by myeloperoxidase deficiency, or by granule dysfunction (e.g., Chédiak-Higashi syndrome). In some conditions in which a microbicidal defect has been described (e.g., leukemia, malnutrition, thermal injury, iron deficiency), the pathogenesis is less well characterized.

CHRONIC GRANULOMATOUS DISEASE

DEFINITION. Chronic granulomatous disease (CGD) is characterized by repeated and severe infection affecting lymph nodes, skin, lung, liver, bone, and many other tissues. *Staphylococcus aureus*, certain gram-negative bacteria, and fungi are the predominant pathogens. Tissue examination reveals multiple abscesses and granulomas and characteristic lipid-filled macrophages. The neutrophils (and monocytes) of these patients fail to kill certain ingested bacteria or fungi normally, and this is correlated with impaired leukocyte metabolic activity.

INCIDENCE. CGD is a rare disease generally found in infants and children, but also seen in young adults. The most common form exhibits *X-linked* transmission. The affected children are males, and the mother and approximately 50 per cent of female siblings are carriers. There is also a variant (or variants) of CGD with *autosomal* inheritance.

PATHOLOGY. Miliary abscesses, varying from a few millimeters to several centimeters in diameter with occasional large abscesses, are seen on gross examination. Although any tissue may be involved, liver, spleen, lung, and lymph nodes are particularly susceptible. Patchy areas of hemorrhage and necrosis are common. Microscopic examination reveals evidence of an acute and a chronic inflammatory response. An influx of polymorphonuclear leukocytes with abscess formation is seen, particularly in early lesions. Granulomas are a prominent feature, with areas of central necrosis surrounded by numerous plasma cells, lymphocytes, macrophages, and a few multinuclear giant cells. Tissue macrophages may be large, with a foamy or vacuolated cytoplasm containing a characteristic yellow-brown lipid material. The organisms most commonly found in the lesions are staphylococci, enteric bacilli (*Klebsiella-Aerobacter* organisms, *Escherichia coli*, *Serratia marcescens*, *Pseudomonas*, *Proteus*, and *Salmonella*) and certain fungi (*Candida*, *Aspergillus*). The possibility of CGD should be considered in all children with nocardiosis. Conspicuous by their rarity or absence from the lesions are β-hemolytic streptococci, pneumococci, *Hemophilus influenzae*, and *Mycobacterium tuberculosis*.

PATHOGENESIS. CGD is characterized by impaired host defense against certain microorganisms. Immunoglobulin levels are normal or elevated, and delayed hypersensitivity is unimpaired. Leukocytosis, with a high proportion of neutrophils, is characteristic of CGD as it is of infection in the general population. The peripheral neutrophils are morphologically indistinguishable from normal cells, although toxic granulation may be seen with longstanding infection. Chemotaxis and phagocytosis are unimpaired; however, the neutrophils do not kill normally those microorganisms generally found in the lesions. Other organisms (e.g., streptococci, lactobacilli, pneumococci) are readily killed by the patient's cells. This microbicidal defect is associated with a marked decrease in the phagocytosis-induced metabolic burst. The role of H_2O_2 deficiency in the microbicidal defect is emphasized by the improvement in microbicidal activity in vitro on the introduction of H_2O_2 into the cell. Indeed, those organisms which are killed well by CGD leukocytes generate H_2O_2, and thus replace the defective leukocytic H_2O_2-generating system with H_2O_2 of microbial origin. Different intraleukocytic molecular lesions have been described to account for the microbicidal defect. They include leukocyte NADH oxidase deficiency, NADPH oxidase deficiency, and, in some female patients, glutathione peroxidase deficiency. Neutrophil dysfunction is also associated with a severe leukocytic deficiency of glucose-6-phosphate dehydrogenase, which is discussed later in this chapter. A newly described antigen, K_x, related to the common Kell antigens, is absent from the leukocytes of male patients with X-linked CGD. This antigen is absent from erythrocytes in the Kell phenotype designated McLeod, and when it is absent from both erythrocytes and leukocytes the McLeod phenotype coexists with CGD.

A decrease in intraleukocytic microbicidal activity results in the prolonged intracellular survival of ingested organisms. These sequestered organisms are protected from certain antimicrobials and from extracellular microbicidal systems, and multiplication and dissemination occur. The organisms spread via the lymphatics and the bloodstream to the second line of defense, the fixed cells of the mononuclear phagocyte system. Lymphadenopathy and hepatosplenomegaly result. It is not known whether a defect exists in the fixed macrophage; however, its precursor, the blood monocyte, has decreased microbicidal activity. The fixed macrophages are unable to control the spread of infection, and miliary abscesses and septicemia result.

DIAGNOSIS. Any patient with severe staphylococcal, gram-negative, or fungal infections since childhood who has normal or elevated immunoglobulin and WBC levels and normal delayed hypersensitivity should be suspected of having CGD. The diagnosis can be made with confidence by neutrophil function tests. A defect in leukocyte microbicidal activity associated with normal phagocytosis is suggestive of CGD. The microorganism employed in the test is important, because the defect is selective, affecting staphylococci, gram-negative pathogens, and certain fungi. The diagnosis is confirmed by one of a number of tests which detect the defect in the phagocytosis-induced metabolic burst, specifically oxygen consumption, glucose 1-^{14}C oxidation, superoxide anion production, H_2O_2 formation, chemiluminescence, NBT reduction, iodination, thyroid hormone degradation, or estrogen binding. The diagnosis of the carrier state in female siblings of patients with X-linked CGD should be attempted for purposes of genetic counseling. The female carrier of the abnormal X chromosome has two populations of granulocytes, one with normal metabolic and microbicidal activity and a second with the same defect as affected children (Lyon hypothesis). When the leukocytes of carriers are treated as a single population, intermediate activity in the neutrophil function tests is observed. Two populations of cells are seen in procedures (slide NBT test, radioautographic iodination test) which detect activity in individual cells.

CLINICAL MANIFESTATIONS. CGD is characterized by repeated, severe, and widespread infections. Chronic suppurative lymphadenitis is the most common feature, with cervical lymphadenitis often its first manifestation. Enlargement of the inguinal, axillary, mesenteric, and mediastinal nodes also occurs regularly. The initial and most striking feature in some patients is a refractory eczematoid dermatitis, particularly around the eyes, nose, mouth, and other body orifices. Stomatitis, conjunctivitis, and persistent rhinitis occur with regularity. Wounds often are infected. Pneumonitis is seen in most patients, although it may be a late manifestation. The lesion progresses from a patchy bronchopneumonia with hilar node enlargement to massive consolidation, involving the entire lobe or lung. Lung abscesses are common, and pleural effusion and empyema may occur. A distinctive roentgenologic finding in some patients is discrete, usually round, homogeneous areas of consolidation ("encapsulating" pneumonia). The pulmonary lesions run a protracted course, leading in some instances to progressively increasing pulmonary insufficiency and death. Hepatosplenomegaly is a consistent feature of the disease. Liver scans may reveal focal lesions, either abscesses or sterile granulomas. Chronic subphrenic abscesses occur frequently. Osteomyelitis, often at multiple sites, is common. The metacarpal and metatarsal bones are particularly susceptible; however, the large bones may also be involved. A feature of the osteomyelitis of CGD is absence of sclerosis and complete healing with long-term antimicrobial therapy. Gastrointestinal manifestations include persistent, often bloody diarrhea, nausea, anorexia, and abdominal pain. Perianal and perineal abscesses with fistula formation occur frequently. Pigmented lipid histiocytes and granulomas with giant cells are seen in rectal biopsies. Pericarditis may occur, and anemia, either hypochromic microcytic or normochromic normocytic, is found in almost all patients.

Female carriers of X-linked CGD are generally healthy. Unequal X inactivation may result in a preponderance of defective cells and in an increased incidence of infection. This, however, is rare in proved carriers. A chronic lupus-like illness, sometimes limited to the skin lesions of discoid lupus but on other occasions characterized by a more systemic disease, with arthralgia, cutaneous manifestations of lupus erythematosus, photosensitivity, fever, Raynaud's phenomenon, and recurrent stomatitis, has been noted in several CGD carriers. Tests for antinuclear antibodies are negative.

THERAPY. The treatment of CGD remains the vigorous treatment of infection, namely, antimicrobial administration and surgical drainage or excision. Both should be instituted promptly and antimicrobial administration maintained until healing is complete. Surgical excision of circumscribed suppurative lesions, e.g., lymph nodes, is preferable to incisional drainage, because the latter heals slowly with seeding at other sites. There are two considerations in the choice of antimicrobial agent: (1) sensitivity of the microorganism and (2) ability of the antimicrobial to reach and destroy the intracellular organisms. Viable microorganisms sequestered within intact leukocytes are protected from the lethal effects of many antimicrobials. The preferred antimicrobial based on sensitivity should be used despite poor penetrance, to combat extracellular organisms. Rifampin, which readily penetrates into leukocytes, is effective against sensitive intracellular staphylococci in vitro and in animal models, but has not yet been proved effective in man. If used, it should be in conjunction with other antimicrobials to minimize the development of resistance. Continuous antimicrobial therapy with nafcillin or sulfisoxazole during periods of remission has been advocated. Granulocyte transfusion may be beneficial for life-threatening infections, and on one occasion marrow transplantation has been employed successfully.

Whole blood transfusions may be required when the anemia is severe. The coexistence of CGD and the very rare Kell phenotypes, Kell null (K_o) or McLeod, has been observed in a number of patients. Such patients are sensitized by transfusions with blood containing Kell antigens, making subsequent transfusions difficult. The Kell phenotype of patients with CGD should be determined, and those with either K_o or McLeod phenotypes should not be transfused unless a compatible blood is available or the clinical situation warrants the risk of sensitization. Most patients with CGD have normal Kell antigens.

PROGNOSIS. In some patients, the disease is apparent within the first year of life and progresses relentlessly, with remissions measured in weeks or months to death within the first decade. In others, there is a relatively late onset and long periods of remission measured in years.

Variants of Chronic Granulomatous Disease

Variants of CGD have been described which can be separated from "classic" CGD by clinical and/or laboratory findings but which have in common a leukocytic microbicidal defect caused by decreased oxidative metabolism.

FAMILIAL LIPOCHROME HISTIOCYTOSIS. Three female siblings have been described with splenomegaly, pulmonary infiltration, hypergammaglobulinemia, arthritis, and an increased susceptibility to infection. The most striking histologic feature was the presence of numerous large, pigmented, lipid-filled histiocytes. The patients had a neutrophil microbicidal and metabolic defect similar to that of CGD. This condition differed from "classic" CGD, not only in sex affected but also in the late onset of symptoms, absence of a chronic granulomatous response, and occurrence of arthritis.

SEVERE LEUKOCYTIC GLUCOSE-6-PHOSPHATE DEHYDROGENASE DEFICIENCY. Patients with glucose-6-phosphate dehydrogenase (G-6-PD) levels which are 20 per cent of normal or greater do not have an increased incidence of infection and have leukocytes with normal metabolic and microbicidal activity. This includes all patients with the common African Gd A$^-$ variant of G-6-PD deficiency who have normal leukocyte G-6-PD activity and most patients with the Mediterranean Gd B$^-$ variant who have a partial deficiency of leukocyte G-6-

PD. Patients with leukocyte G-6-PD levels of 5 per cent of normal or below, however, have neutrophil dysfunction and increased susceptibility to infection. The leukocyte abnormality differs from the more common variants of CGD in that the decrease in hexose monophosphate shunt activity is not reversed by methylene blue. Further, the metabolic and microbicidal defect is not as severe, which correlates well with the milder clinical course. The patients with neutrophil dysfunction also have chronic nonspherocytic hemolytic anemia.

MYELOPEROXIDASE DEFICIENCY

Neutrophils in a normal human blood smear contain an abundance of peroxidase-positive granules. Myeloperoxidase (MPO) deficiency is indicated by a decrease in this peroxidase reaction. It may be hereditary or acquired.

HEREDITARY MPO DEFICIENCY. In this condition there is complete absence of MPO from neutrophils and monocytes, whereas the eosinophil peroxidase is present in normal amounts. The leukocytes are otherwise morphologically indistinguishable from normal cells. Genetic studies suggest autosomal recessive inheritance. Some patients have increased infections with *Candida* or bacterial pathogens, whereas others are in good health. MPO-deficient leukocytes have decreased fungicidal and bactericidal activity despite normal phagocytosis, although the defect is not as severe as in CGD. Iodination and chemiluminescence also are decreased; however, in contrast to CGD, there is no decrease in phagocytosis-induced NBT reduction, oxygen consumption, superoxide production, glucose C1 oxidation, or formate oxidation; indeed, the metabolic burst appears to be increased.

ACQUIRED MPO DEFICIENCY. Acquired MPO deficiency may involve all or a portion of the neutrophils; myeloperoxidase may be undetectable or decreased in amount, and the deficiency may be permanent or temporary. It has been observed in some patients with severe untreated bacterial infection, in acute encephalitis lethargica (von Economo), in a few patients with refractory megaloblastic anemia, and in some patients with acute myelogenous leukemia, chronic myelogenous leukemia with blast-cell transformation, or myelomonocytic leukemia. When tested, the microbicidal defect in the isolated leukocytes was comparable with that found in hereditary MPO deficiency.

THE CHÉDIAK-HIGASHI SYNDROME

The Chédiak-Higashi syndrome is a rare autosomal recessive disease characterized by the presence of giant lysosome-like granules in all granule-containing cells. Animal homologues of the human disease have been detected in Aleutian mink, Hereford cattle, beige mice, Persian cats, and a killer whale. Less than 100 cases have been described in man, with a roughly equal proportion of males and females. Its main clinical features are (1) partial oculocutaneous albinism with photophobia, rotatory nystagmus, and hair with a characteristic silken sheen when exposed to light; (2) repeated febrile episodes resulting chiefly from staphylococcal infection of the skin, lungs, and upper respiratory tract; and (3) a lymphoma-like "accelerated phase," characterized by widespread tissue infiltration by lymphoid and histiocytic elements, lymphadenopathy, hepatosplenomegaly, neutropenia, hypogammaglobulinemia, hemolytic anemia, bleeding tendency caused by thrombocytopenia and coagulation factor deficiencies, and peripheral neuropathy.

The diagnosis of the Chédiak-Higashi syndrome is made by demonstration of giant granules in circulating leukocytes. In the bone marrow, abnormally large, pleomorphic, azurophil (primary) granules are seen in promyelocytes which undergo a series of fusions to form giant granules containing myeloperoxidase and acid phosphatase. The specific (secondary) granules develop normally. The bone marrow neutrophil reserve is low, and neutropenia is common, particularly in the accelerated phase when lymphocytic infiltration of the bone marrow is apparent. The presence of giant granules in mature neutrophils is associated with some impairment in function. Chemotaxis, as measured by migration into a skin window in vivo or by the response to a preformed chemotactic agent in vitro, is decreased. Phagocytosis and the related metabolic burst are unimpaired; indeed, an increase in the initial rate of phagocytosis has been reported. However, degranulation with the release of the contents of the giant granules into the phagocytic vacuole is delayed or absent, resulting in delay in the killing of some bacterial species. A microtubule polymerization defect related to abnormal cyclic nucleotide levels has been described. These abnormalities in neutrophil function combine to increase the susceptibility of the patients to pyogenic infections. The partial albinism is a consequence of the abnormal distribution of melanin in giant melanosomes, and the neurologic manifestations are associated with a lymphohistiocyte infiltration in the region of the degenerated peripheral nerves. Giant lysosomes are seen in both peripheral and central nervous system elements.

TREATMENT. The infections generally respond to conventional antimicrobial therapy, and the anemia and hemorrhagic tendency to multiple blood or platelet transfusions. In one patient, defective neutrophil function was returned to normal by the administration of ascorbic acid. The low serum folic acid levels and megaloblastic bone marrow changes can be corrected by folic acid therapy. Treatment of the accelerated phase with combined vincristine and prednisone administration has been advocated. Death usually occurs within the first two decades owing to infection but less commonly to hemorrhage or to the extensive lymphocytic infiltration of the accelerated phase.

Baehner, R. L.: Microbe ingestion and killing by neutrophils: Normal mechanisms and abnormalities. Clin. Haematol., 4:609, 1975.

Blume, R. S., and Wolff, S. M.: The Chédiak-Higashi syndrome: Studies in four patients and a review of the literature. Medicine, 51:247, 1972.

Good, R. A., Quie, P. G., Windhorst, D. B., Page, A. R., Rodey, G. E., White, J., Wolfson, J. J., and Holmes, B. H.: Fatal (chronic) granulomatous disease of childhood: A hereditary defect of leukocyte function. Semin. Hematol., 5:215, 1968.

Karnovsky, M. L.: Chronic granulomatous disease—pieces of a cellular and molecular puzzle. Fed. Proc., 32:1527, 1973.

Klebanoff, S. J., and Clark, R. A.: The Neutrophil: Function and Clinical Disorders. Amsterdam, Elsevier/North-Holland Biomedical Press B.V., 1978.

Quie, P. G.: Pathology of bactericidal power of neutrophils. Semin. Hematol., 12:143, 1975.

Snyderman, R., and Pike, M. C.: Disorders of leukocyte chemotaxis. Pediat. Clin. North. Am. 24:377, 1977.

495. THE LEUKOPENIC STATE

Dane R. Boggs

Leukopenia is defined as a reduction in the total number of leukocytes in the blood, usually to less than 4.0×10^9 per liter. It is a laboratory observation of little diagnostic significance unless absolute numbers of specific types of cells are calculated from an accompanying differential cell count. Each of the leukocytes, neutrophils, lymphocytes, monocytes, eosinophils, and basophils constitutes a separate and distinct system (systems, in the case of lymphocytes) with respect to function and to control of production and distribution. Since neutrophils are the most common blood leukocytes, leukopenia usually reflects neutropenia. Neutropenia may be an isolated finding or may be accompanied by lymphopenia and/or decreased numbers of other leukocytes, particularly in patients with induced or idiopathic aplastic anemia. Lymphopenia may occur as an isolated finding but usually does not result in leukopenia. Reduced numbers of monocytes, eosinophils, or basophils may be observed in certain conditions, but such reduction usually is not detected in "routine" laboratory examination, for when the usual 100-cell differential count is employed, failure to observe one of any of these cells is within the normal distributional error of the count.

NEUTROPENIA

The lower limit for neutrophil concentration in the blood of whites is approximately 2.0×10^9 per liter. In blacks it is somewhat lower, approximately 1.5×10^9 per liter. Normal values for other leukocytes as well as for red cells and platelets apparently are similar in the two groups.

KINETICS OF NEUTROPHILS. The production of neutrophils is limited to the bone marrow of normal postnatal man. They are released to the blood for a brief sojourn from which they enter tissues and body cavities or areas of inflammation.

The marrow compartment can be divided into a proliferative (mitotic) compartment and a postmitotic compartment. As with any cellular system in which cells are regularly lost, a stem cell is a necessary component of cell renewal. Normal hematopoietic stem cells must have two essential characteristics: ability to divide and reproduce themselves (self-replication), and ability to differentiate into mature blood cells. The ultimate hematopoietic stem cell is totipotent for all blood cells, including lymphocytes, but data from animal studies suggest that the systems ordinarily are maintained from stem cells which are descendants of the totipotent cell but of more restricted pluripotency. The cell which produces colonies of neutrophils in vitro in semisolid media (CFU-C) is the prime candidate for the immediate stem cell for neutrophils. This is probably a true stem cell, although evidence for self replication is indirect. The CFU-C requires colony-stimulating factor (see below) to initiate and sustain growth of the colony and is pluripotent for at least monocytes and neutrophils. The myeloblast is the earliest morphologically recognized neutrophil precursor, but whether there is direct conversion of CFU-C to myeloblasts or whether there are intermediate cellular steps between the CFU-C and the myeloblast is unknown.

The morphologically recognized mitotic compartment is divided, somewhat arbitrarily, into myeloblasts, promyelocytes, and myelocytes. The promyelocyte stage is defined by the synthesis of primary granules, peroxidase-positive lysosomes. The myelocyte stage is recognized by the synthesis of secondary granules and by the nucleolus becoming inapparent under light microscopy. The generation time of cells in the mitotic compartment is approximately 24 hours, and there are somewhere in the order of five multiplicative divisions in this compartment. Thus for each myeloblast produced from the stem cell compartment, approximately 32 maturing cells emerge five days later.

When the metamyelocyte stage is reached, cell division ceases and maturation proceeds through the band stage, culminating in the segmented neutrophil (seg). Bands and segs are released readily to the blood, although segs are released preferentially. Release of more than an occasional cell less mature than bands is unusual unless there is intrinsic disease of the bone marrow. Therefore the compartment of bands and segs constitutes the marrow neutrophil reserve which is called upon to supply an increased demand for blood neutrophils prior to an increase in neutrophil production. The transit time through the postmitotic compartment normally is six to ten days, so that the time from the myeloblast stage to emergence into the blood of a segmented neutrophil is about two weeks. However, under conditions of extreme demand for neutrophils this transit time can be reduced to four to five days.

The blood is a rapid-transit, one-way street for neutrophils. The average time spent in the blood is but ten hours, and loss from the blood is in a random fashion; that is, a neutrophil which has just entered the blood from the marrow is as likely to leave it as one which has been in circulation for some time. The major site for egress from the blood is unknown. Approximately half the neutrophils in the blood are not circulating freely but are stuck to or rolling along the walls of capillaries or postcapillary venules (marginated neutrophils). Thus the blood compartment is divided into two pools, the circulating and the marginal pool, but exchange between the two can be almost instantaneous.

Systems regulating the rate of production and the distribution of neutrophils are incompletely understood. The prime candidate for a major regulator of production is *colony-stimulating factor*. This glycoprotein is necessary for the growth of neutrophil colonies in vitro in semisolid media and for their growth in liquid culture. A major source of colony-stimulating factor is monocytes and their progeny, the macrophages, and stimulated lymphocytes. However, firm proof that it plays a physiologic in vivo role is lacking. A role for an inhibitor in controlling production has been suggested in certain studies. Excessive numbers of mature neutrophils can be shown to be inhibitory in certain circumstances. If neutropenia is induced in man or in other experimental animals, the rate of release of mature cells from the marrow storage pool to the blood is rapidly accelerated. This is mediated by an increase in the concentration of *neutrophil-releasing factor* in plasma. Releasing factor probably has no direct effect upon the rate of production. Thus it seems likely that regula-

tion of this system is probably much more complex than erythroid regulation by erythropoietin.

ETIOLOGY. Neutropenia can accompany many diseases, can be produced by a variety of drugs, or can occur as a congenital or an idiopathic acquired syndrome. It can result from one or a combination of four mechanisms: decrease in the size of the production pool; ineffective production with cell death in the marrow; shift or "pseudo" neutropenia, in which the circulating pool is depleted but the marginal pool is within normal limits, giving a total blood pool within the lower limits of normal; or an increased rate of loss of blood neutrophils, to the point that the marrow cannot compensate by an increase in production. Simple examination of the blood and bone marrow often allows one to infer the kinetic cause of neutropenia. If anemia is not present, the myeloid-to-erythroid ratio in a marrow aspirate gives information whether production is increased or decreased. Frequently bands and segs are virtually absent in marrow aspirates from patients with neutropenia despite an abundance of metamyelocytes and earlier precursors. This is often referred to as *"maturation arrest,"* a very misleading term, since this picture simply reflects the release of a band to the blood as soon as it is formed owing to increased demand for cell release. In this circumstance the ratio of bands to segs in the blood is increased. If the marrow and the band-seg ratio in the blood are normal, "pseudo" neutropenia should be suspected. An intravenous infusion of 0.1 mg of epinephrine results in an acute demargination of most neutrophils. If such an infusion results in an increase in circulating cells of 2×10^9 per liter or more, a diagnosis of "pseudo" neutropenia is strengthened. However, caution must be exercised in considering "pseudo" neutropenia as a diagnosis. There is a positive correlation between the ratio of marginal to circulating pools and the severity of neutropenia. The relative increase in size of the marginal pool as the size of the circulating pool decreases may represent a physiologic mechanism.

Neutropenia Induced by Drugs or Physical Agents. This is probably the most common cause of neutropenia. It is predictably produced by certain drugs (or physical agents such as x-irradiation), most notably those used in cancer chemotherapy, and occurs unpredictably and idiosyncratically in occasional patients exposed to any of more than 100 different drugs. The dose-related marrow toxins interfere with cell production in general, so in many instances decreased production of neutrophils is accompanied by decreased production of other blood cells.

Idiosyncratic neutropenic reactions to drugs may be the result of decreased production or increased destruction. Chlorpromazine and related compounds are the classic offenders as regards decreased production, and amidopyrine can be considered the index drug producing increased destruction of blood neutrophils. Two different forms of production defects may be induced in occasional (perhaps 1 in 1200) patients exposed to chlorpromazine. In one form blood neutrophils suddenly disappear, and examination of the marrow reveals an absence of recognizable precursors. When the drug is stopped, neutrophil production is resumed within a day or two, suggesting that the stem cell system was not affected. Re-exposure to the drug results in almost immediate loss of cell production, but in most instances closely related phenothiazines do not produce the syndrome. In other patients a mild degree of neutropenia develops, and examination of bone marrow in such patients indicates that production is decreased but not abolished. If the drug is continued at the same dosage, neutropenia persists but usually does not worsen. If the dosage is increased, neutropenia may become more severe, and when the drug is stopped many weeks may pass before blood neutrophils gradually return to normal. In many instances closely related phenothiazines also produce neutropenia. If the use of chlorpromazine or related compounds is clearly indicated, the latter form of neutropenia is not a contraindication for their use, although blood counts should be monitored frequently after neutropenia is detected. There is evidence to suggest that patients who develop neutropenia in response to chlorpromazine have an innate abnormality in DNA synthesis in neutrophil precursors.

Amidopyrine (and other drugs such as sulfonamides) may act as a hapten and lead to formation of antineutrophil antibodies. Moeschlin demonstrated that when such patients had recovered, a single dose of amidopyrine eliminated blood neutrophils in a few hours and that the plasma of such neutropenic patients produced neutropenia when infused into normal subjects. In animal experiments, injection of antineutrophil antibody destroys not only blood neutrophils but also marrow cells, although most of the mitotic pool is spared. Thus marrow examination in patients with this or other forms of antibody-induced neutropenia may reveal an increased production pool, but increased metamyelocytes may not be present as might be expected in response to increased destruction of mature cells.

Sudden and transient increase in the ratio of marginated to circulating neutrophils resulting in "pseudo" neutropenia develops during the early phase of hemodialysis as well as in other instances in which blood is exposed to cellulose or various plastics. This appears to be the result of activation of complement, which in turn results in pulmonary margination of neutrophils, and the neutropenia persists for less than an hour.

Neutropenia Associated with Various Diseases. A wide spectrum of diseases result in neutropenia, but only a few will be discussed as examples of various mechanisms: the acute leukemias, infections, rheumatoid arthritis, vitamin B_{12} deficiency, and congestive splenomegaly with cirrhosis of the liver.

In the acute leukemias neutropenia is almost always present at diagnosis, as are anemia and thrombocytopenia, and this represents decreased normal cell production. It seems likely that production from the stem cell compartment is reduced due to faulty recognition of the leukemic compartment as if it were an expanded normal stem cell compartment. In acute myeloblastic or promyelocytic leukemia there is increased production of those precursors by the leukemic stem cell clone, but only a few are able to mature into segmented neutrophils, and even these segs are functionally abnormal.

A variety of infections induce neutropenia by several different mechanisms. While neutrophilia is anticipated with pneumococcal pneumonia, otherwise normal patients with extensive disease may develop neutropenia. This represents utilization of so many neutrophils in the pneumonic exudate that the marrow reserve is exhausted and has long been recognized as a grave prognostic sign. Neutropenia secondary to loss of cells in infected areas obviously is much more common in patients with underlying disease of the marrow than in otherwise normal patients. Mild neutropenia is a common finding in typhoid fever but is not indicative of a poor prognosis. Mild neutropenia is common with malaria and with a variety of viral infections such as measles, influenza, and infectious mononucleosis. The kinetic mechanism has not been studied in most circumstances, but in malaria it is a "pseudo" neutropenia due to an increase in the marginal–circulating pool ratio.

In occasional patients with rheumatoid arthritis, splenomegaly and severe neutropenia develop (Felty's syndrome). Although it is generally assumed that this is due to the development of an antineutrophil antibody, firm proof for this thesis is lacking. The kinetic pattern leading to neutropenia is highly variable. Rate of loss of blood neutrophils is accelerated in some patients and normal in others, and the marrow mitotic pool size varies from less than normal to 10 times normal. Splenectomy may or may not be beneficial but can be tried, especially if the patient has experienced a severe infection.

Congestive splenomegaly, as occurs secondary to cirrhosis of the liver, may produce neutropenia as well as anemia and thrombocytopenia. This appears to be secondary to neutrophil destruction in the abnormal spleen. Blood neutrophil turnover rate is markedly accelerated, and the marrow mitotic pool is increased in size. Splenectomy eliminates neutropenia but is almost never indicated for this purpose. Under ordinary circumstances the spleen is not an important site of neutrophil destruction, so why it should become so when congested is unclear. It should be kept in mind that the congested spleen produces anemia and thrombocytopenia primarily by sequestering the cells without much increase in their rate of destruction.

Deficiency of vitamin B_{12} or folic acid often is associated with neutropenia. This is due to ineffective neutrophil production in which the marrow production pool is increased in size but intramedullary cell death is occurring. The mature cells produced are abnormally large and hypersegmented, and in B_{12} (not in folic acid) deficiency they have defective bactericidal capacity.

Congenital Neutropenia. These syndromes have been described under many terms, but at present at least ten separate types of congenital neutropenia can be distinguished. Probably the most common is a transient neonatal neutropenia due to placental passage of maternal antibody directed against fetal neutrophils. This occurs when the mother has been exposed to neutrophils of the antigenic type of the fetus (different from her own) during a previous pregnancy or by transfusion. There are at least three forms of dominantly inherited neutropenia, but all three are usually benign and rarely lead to life-threatening infection. The most common is due to a modest decrease in production accompanied by a decrease in stem cells in marrow. Neutrophil counts rarely are below 0.5×10^9 per liter and may reach normal limits when patients become adults. A second form, described to date only in Arabs, is similar except that marrow stem cells are increased. The third is characterized by severe neutropenia with almost complete absence of marrow neutrophil precursors and virtually no detectable neutrophil stem cells. However, monocyte production is increased, and presumably monocytosis in excess of 2×10^9 per liter protects these patients against infection. The most severe form of congenital neutropenia is that originally described by Kostman (1956). Recessive inheritance has appeared to be likely in some patients, and neutrophils are virtually absent from the blood. Marrow stem cells are increased, as are myeloblasts and promyelocytes, but more mature cells are reduced markedly. Some but not all patients can transiently produce mature cells in response to severe infection, so there may be two forms of this disease. Whether the defect is one of true maturation arrest at the promyelocyte stage or of intramedullary destruction of maturing neutrophils is unknown. All patients yet described have died of infection before reaching adulthood. Neutropenia with excessive numbers of segmented neutrophils in the marrow has been described, and this apparent defect in release of cells has been termed *myelocathexis. Cyclic neutropenia* has been present at birth as a familial or sporadic occurrence. Neutrophils decline to 0 in the blood at regular intervals, usually every three weeks, and then return to normal levels within a few days. Monocytes, platelets, and reticulocytes cycle also, although not in phase with the neutrophils, and the cycling of blood cells reflects cyclical changes in production. Severe infections may accompany the neutrophil nadir, but most patients survive these if vigorously treated until the neutrophils reappear. Recessively inherited cyclic neutropenia is found in the gray collie dog, in which the disease represents a stem cell defect. The affected dog can be cured by a marrow transplant from a normal littermate, whereas marrow transplant from affected to normal littermate transmits the disease. Very rarely congenital neutropenia may be a "pseudo" neutropenia. Congenital neutropenia in association with pancreatic insufficiency has been reported, as has severe neutropenia associated with severe immunologic deficiency.

Other Forms of Neutropenia. Unassociated with any apparent underlying disease or toxic exposure, neutropenia can occur as an isolated blood abnormality or as a part of such syndromes as aplastic anemia. Instances of isolated neutropenia may be due to decreased production or to increased destruction with increased production, or may be cyclic. The term "chronic benign neutropenia" has been applied to a number of patients with idiopathic acquired neutropenias. If this is to be considered a syndrome, then it probably exists in two forms. In certain patients it is due to decreased production and mimics the most common form of dominantly inherited neutropenia almost exactly. In some of these it may be inherited but not detected before adulthood. In other patients, the production pool is expanded and stem cells are increased, suggesting that neutropenia is due to increased destruction of cells. Antineutrophil autoantibodies have been detected in some patients with neutropenia resulting from increased destruction.

CLINICAL MANIFESTATIONS. Bacterial infections and oral ulceration are the only manifestations which can be attributed to neutropenia in most instances. However, when neutropenia is of very sudden onset and due to rapid destruction of cells, as with amidopyrine sensitivity, severe but transient chills, fever, and malaise may be present in the absence of infection. The most commonly infected sites are the lungs, the oropharyngeal cavity, and the perianal area. In general, the infecting organisms are those which commonly produce acute bacterial infections, but there are certain special features of infection in neutropenic patients. It is important to recognize that infection is often more virulent

once it begins in patients with neutropenia in comparison to normal individuals. The absence of infection-localizing properties of the neutrophil may result in septicemia within a few hours of the onset of a seemingly minor infection. Furthermore, lanthanic septicemia, septicemia in which there is no demonstrable portal of entry, is not uncommon. Poor localization can change the characteristic appearance of infections so that staphylococcal skin infections may mimic erysipelas rather than appearing as furuncles. Pneumonic infiltrates may not appear as dense as usual owing to reduced neutrophil exudation. Pyelonephritis may not be recognized, because the usual clue of increased urinary neutrophils may be absent. Mouth ulcers are somewhat mysterious as to their cause. In most instances culture of these lesions does not suggest an infectious cause, and they are much more common with some syndromes such as cyclic neutropenia than with others such as Felty's syndrome.

The frequency and severity of infection varies remarkably among the various types of neutropenia and correlates poorly at best with the severity of neutropenia. However, within any type of neutropenia, life-threatening infections usually are found in patients with less than 0.5×10^9 per liter. Ancillary abnormalities undoubtedly contribute to the liability to infections associated with neutropenia. For example, when blood neutrophils are virtually absent secondary to vigorous cancer chemotherapy, the majority of patients will become infected unless neutrophils recover within two weeks. On the other hand, it is not unusual for a patient with Felty's syndrome or with severe congenital neutropenia to remain uninfected for months and sometimes for years with virtually no blood neutrophils. There are a number of possible explanations for the different frequency of infection in these conditions. The patient whose marrow is poisoned by cancer chemotherapy also has a damaged lymphoid and monocyte system, and the integrity of his serosal surfaces may be interrupted.

TREATMENT. Unless a treatable underlying disease is present or unless there is a causative drug or toxin which can be withdrawn, little can be done to alter neutropenia. Obviously a prompt and correct diagnosis followed by proper antimicrobial treatment of an infection is mandatory. Lithium produces an increase in neutrophil production in patients with a normal bone marrow, but preliminary trials of its use in various forms of neutropenia are not promising. Therapy with adrenal glucocorticosteroids may lead to an improvement in neutropenia, but this is the result of reducing the rate of egress from the blood. As a consequence the patient is potentially more susceptible to infection than he was initially. Therefore steroids are contraindicated unless an antineutrophil antibody is present, in which case at least transient improvement has resulted from such therapy. Splenectomy has been tried in virtually all types of neutropenia (except drug-induced neutropenia), but it has proved beneficial only in some patients with Felty's syndrome.

Allogeneic *marrow transplantation* is an accepted form of therapy for patients with severe aplastic anemia, assuming that a sibling matched with the patient for all major histocompatibility loci is available as a donor. Mortality from the allogeneic transplant procedure is of the order of 50 per cent, so this is acceptable therapy only if death from the disease being treated is anticipated. Therefore of the idiopathic acquired and congenital forms of neutropenia, allogeneic transplantation would be clearly indicated only in patients with congenital neutropenia plus severe immune deficiency. It would be of interest to determine if Kostman's type of congenital neutropenia could be cured by marrow transplantation, but as noted previously the nature of the defect is unclear. If a patient with severe acquired neutropenia, apparently caused by decreased production, were fortunate enough to have a normal identical twin, then infusion of the twin's marrow would represent a reasonable therapeutic trial. Autologous marrow transplantation is under study as a potential means of reducing the duration of neutropenia (pancytopenia) induced by vigorous chemotherapy of certain cancers. Dimethyl sulfoxide is added to marrow prior to freezing in liquid nitrogen, and the stem cells remain viable when the marrow is unfrozen. Thus large volumes of marrow are aspirated from the patient, frozen, and then reinfused following chemotherapy.

Neutrophil transfusion is of benefit as ancillary therapy of the infected, neutropenic patient. Controlled clinical trials have demonstrated superior survival of infection in neutropenic patients, primarily patients with acute leukemia, who were given such transfusions. Neutrophil transfusions given on a daily basis during the period of severe pancytopenia following allogeneic marrow transplantation also have been shown to provide prophylactic protection against infection in a controlled trial. However, despite the modest benefit provided by this procedure, it is attended by multiple problems and as yet is far from a "routine" part of the expected activity of most blood banks. The short blood half-time of normal neutrophils and their relatively small numbers in the blood of normal donors presently preclude "replacing" neutrophils in a neutropenic patient as is done with red cell and is possible with platelet transfusion. In many instances there is no detectable increase in circulating neutrophils following infusion of 10^{10} allogeneic neutrophils, the minimal number considered of possible benefit to an adult. Collection requires processing of approximately the equivalent of the total blood volume of the donor by use of either continuous or discontinuous centrifugation technique or by passing blood through fibrous filters to which neutrophils adhere and from which they subsequently can be eluted. The procedure is safe for most donors, as is evident from the lack of untoward reactions in donor populations at many centers. However, there are three causes of continuing concern regarding donor safety. Steroids often are given to the donor to raise blood neutrophil levels and increase efficiency of collection, and even a single large dose of steroid is potentially hazardous. Hydroxyethyl starch is used as a red cell sedimenting agent to facilitate neutrophil separation in centrifugal collection techniques, and the long-term effects, if any, of retention of this starch by the donor are unknown. During the early phase of filtration collection, complement is activated, which in turn leads to sudden margination of large numbers of neutrophils in the pulmonary circulation, a similar phenomenon to that already discussed for hemodialysis. This poses a potential hazard owing to elevation in pulmonary artery pressure, particularly if the donor has pre-existing pulmonary disease. For these reasons many centers limit donors to concerned family members or friends of the patient.

The donor must be connected to the collecting apparatus for two to four hours, and most consider at least five consecutive days of transfusion as minimal acceptable therapy. Consequently the procedure is very expensive in time and money for personnel, as well as in equipment cost. Recipients should be tested for the presence of preformed antibodies against the potential donor's leukocytes, since their presence probably not only negates the usefulness of the transfusion but also increases the likelihood of transfusion reaction, consisting of fever, chills, malaise, and sometimes dyspnea. The major histocompatibility loci (HLA) match of donor and recipient may be important, as there is evidence to suggest that the post-transfusion increment in neutrophil concentration is higher when donor and recipient are matched at two or more of the four HLA sites than when they are completely mismatched. This constitutes another reason for preferring family members as donors.

Sterile environments markedly reduce the probability of infection in neutropenic patients. In many instances all detectable bacteria and fungi can be eliminated by vigorous skin and mucous membrane antisepsis and by administration of nonabsorbable antimicrobials, with the patient either in complete barrier isolation ("life island") or in a room with a laminar flow filtration system. The psychologic stress of such isolation is considerable, and most find that a constantly visible attendant is needed. Expense of maintaining patients in such environments is considerable.

If drugs with a long pharmacokinetic half-life are suspected of being the cause of neutropenia, efforts should be made to accelerate their removal from the body. If the drug is in circulation, plasmapheresis should be considered; if gold is suspected of being the offending agent, British anti-lewisite (BAL) should be given. Plasmapheresis may prove of benefit in any form of antibody-induced neutropenia in which the antigen is no longer present.

Approach to and Management of Patients with Neutropenia. Once neutropenia is detected, an intensive search for its cause must be initiated by history and by physical and laboratory examination. When it is secondary to an underlying disease, the disease usually will be detected easily. However, in rare instances, diseases such as those of the collagen vascular system, infectious mononucleosis, or rheumatoid arthritis may result in neutropenia in the absence of other overt signs of disease. Thus tests for anti-DNA, anti-Epstein-Barr virus, and rheumatoid factor should be done. Most patients with Felty's syndrome have longstanding rheumatoid arthritis, but occasionally it precedes development of arthritic symptoms and signs.

A detailed history of drug ingestion and chemical exposure should be taken. If medically feasible, *all* drugs should be discontinued. Reduction in the use of household cleansers, solvents, and paints, as well as cosmetics, is advised, and when possible, a change to an agent of different chemical composition is advised. There is no proof that most drugs, cleansers, or cosmetics will produce neutropenia. However, it is possible that any compound could be toxic to a rare individual. For instance, if chloramphenicol produced aplastic anemia in 1 of 200,000 persons so treated instead of 1 in 20,000 to 60,000, it would never have been recognized as causative.

A careful differential count of the blood and a marrow aspirate should be done by the physician. If blood abnormalities other than neutropenia are present, a needle biopsy of marrow should be done in addition to the aspirate to determine cellularity and to search for fibrosis or tumor in bone marrow. Neutropenia as an isolated blood finding is almost never indicative of primary diseases of marrow, so the biopsy, which is more expensive and more painful than an aspirate, need not be done in that circumstance. If the myeloid-to-erythroid ratio is reduced or if the biopsy appears hypocellular, one can be reasonably certain that decreased production is the cause of neutropenia. If the M-E ratio is normal or increased, then increased destruction should be considered the possible cause of neutropenia and antineutrophil antibodies should be searched for. In the differential count of the neutrophil series, bands and segs often are reduced well below their normal percentage of the total series, reflecting early release to the blood and depletion of the storage compartment. If bands and segs constitute more than 25 per cent of the neutrophil compartment, then the integrity of marrow release mechanisms should be tested. Endotoxin or adrenal glucocorticosteroid infusion or etiocholanolone injection will lead to accelerated release of bands and segs, detectable by their increased concentration in blood. If the marrow appears normal and the band-seg ratio in the blood is normal, "pseudo" neutropenia should be suspected and an epinephrine test done as previously outlined.

Neutropenia per se is not an indication for hospitalization unless it is necessary for diagnostic studies. If a patient is going to become infected, microorganisms in the general environment are preferable to those found in hospitals. However, the patient should be instructed to call with any fever or any evidence of infection and should immediately see the physician if any signs and symptoms of infection develop. Emphasis should be placed on scrupulous hygiene, particularly of oral and anal areas. Prophylactic antimicrobial agents should not be used.

If there is evidence of infection, culture of blood and urine and any visible lesion should be obtained, and a combination of antimicrobial drugs with a broad spectrum of activity should immediately be started, using the intravenous route of administration. If a causative organism is isolated, therapy should be altered to the agent with the narrowest spectrum to which the organism is sensitive. Superinfections are common in neutropenic patients, and it is desirable to change their bacterial flora as little as possible. If the patient is no better after three days of therapy and the cause of infection has not been found but the patient does not appear critically ill, it probably is advisable to stop therapy and reculture. However, if the patient is no better in two to three days and does appear critically ill, a program of neutrophil transfusion should be begun. Addition of amphotericin B should also be considered, especially in patients with acute leukemia, since *Candida* infections are common and most are not diagnosed during life. In patients with any chronic form of neutropenia, neutrophil transfusion should be limited to intractable life-threatening infections, since development of alloantibodies may limit their subsequent usefulness. If the patient has an HLA identical sibling as an available donor, a more liberal attitude toward transfusion might be taken.

DECREASE IN OTHER TYPES OF LEUKOCYTES

LYMPHOPENIA. Acute, transient decrease in blood lymphocytes to less than 1.5×10^9 per liter is very common, occurring with almost any form of stress, be it an acute bacterial infection or a traumatic injury. This type of lymphopenia may be mediated by increased secretion of adrenal glucocorticosteroids. Lymphocytes recirculate from blood to lymphoid tissue to blood, and steroids change the recirculatory pattern, redistributing lymphocytes but having no apparent effect on rates of production or destruction of normal lymphocytes, at least when given in moderate doses for relatively brief periods. When normal subjects are given steroids, blood lymphocytes are reduced within two hours, but even if the drug is continued, they return to normal within two days.

Chronic lymphocytopenia is less common. It is observed in patients with diseases characterized by defective cellular immunity such as Hodgkin's disease or congenital immune deficiency syndromes, and it presumably reflects a reduction in the total number of thymic-derived (T) lymphocytes in the body. Vigorous cancer chemotherapy and particularly radiotherapy may lead to lymphopenia. Blood lymphocytes may remain reduced for a year or more after completion of a course of x-irradiation.

MONOCYTOPENIA. Monocytopenia is occasionally observed as the only abnormality in the blood of a subject, but nothing is known of its cause or its consequences. Similarly, patients have been observed in whom a scan of several smears failed to reveal either any *eosinophils* or *basophils*, but whose blood was otherwise unremarkable. Acute eosinopenia is a well known accompaniment of a wide variety of acute stresses. All three of these blood cells are affected by the same dose-related toxins which affect the neutrophil system.

Bishop, D. R., Rothstein, G., Ashenbrucker, H. E., et al.: Leukokinetic studies. XIV. Blood neutrophil kinetics in chronic steady-state neutropenia. J. Clin. Invest., 50:1678, 1971.

Boggs, D. R.: The kinetics of neutrophilic leukocytes in health and disease. Semin. Hematol., 4:359, 1967.

Joyce, R. A., Boggs, D. R., and Chervenick, P. A.: Neutrophil kinetics in hereditary and congenital neutropenias. N. Engl. J. Med., 295:1385, 1976.

Joyce, R. A., Boggs, D. R., Hasiba, U., and Srodes, C. H.: Marginal neutrophil pool size in normal subjects and neutropenic patients as measured by epinephrine infusion. J. Lab. Clin. Med., 88:614, 1976.

Moeschlin, S.: Immunological granulocytopenia and agranulocytosis (clinical aspects). Sang, 26:32, 1955.

Morley, A. A., Carew, J. P., and Baikie, A. G.: Familial cyclical neutropenia. Br. J. Haematol., 13:719, 1967.

Pisciotta, A. V.: Immune and toxic mechanisms in drug-induced agranulocytosis. Semin. Hematol., 10:279, 1973.

Wintrobe, M. M., Lee, R. E., Boggs, D. R., Bithel, T., Athens, J. W., and Foerster, J.: Clinical Hematology. 7th ed. Philadelphia, Lea & Febiger, 1974.

496. LEUKEMOID REACTIONS

Richard T. Silver

A leukemoid reaction is defined as a clinical syndrome in which changes are found in the peripheral blood suggesting leukemia. Usually, the white blood cell count is elevated, but a picture resembling leukemia may develop even when the white blood cell count is normal or reduced.

The most important distinction between a leukemoid reaction and leukemia is that the former is not an unregulated proliferation of leukocytes but an expression of a bone marrow response to some underlying cause. Thus the peripheral blood and bone marrow abnormalities return to normal when the cause has disappeared. Leukemoid reactions involve any of the white blood cells and can occur in a variety of diseases caused by bacterial and viral infections, allergy, inflammatory disease, poisoning, drugs, and malignancy, and during or after diverse acute conditions such as physical and emotional stimuli, hemolytic anemia, hemorrhage, and burns. It is unclear why certain leukemoid reactions are seen in some patients and some diseases and not in others. Leukocyte stimulatory and maturation factors and leukocyte kinetics are not well defined. Different types of leukemoid reactions occur with the same frequency as those cells which appear in the peripheral blood. Thus neutrophilic leukemoid reactions are most frequent; lymphocyte and then eosinophilic leukemoid reactions are next most common; and monocytic leukemoid reactions are relatively infrequent.

Neutrophilic leukemoid reactions are associated with neutrophilic granulocytic hyperplasia in the marrow. Such increases in neutrophilic leukocytes are seen, for example, in certain types of acute bacterial infections, acute hemolytic anemias, and metastatic disease of the bone marrow. Often, there is shift toward immaturity in both the marrow and the peripheral blood, for increased numbers of metamyelocytes and myelocytes are observed. Vacuoles and heavy, coarse granules may be seen in the cytoplasm of the granulocytes. Differentiation of a neutrophilic leukemoid reaction from chronic granulocytic leukemia is difficult if based only upon microscopic examination of the peripheral blood and bone marrow. Abnormalities suggestive but not diagnostic of chronic granulocytic leukemia include an increased platelet count (and correspondingly increased megakaryocytes in the marrow), increased numbers of circulating basophils and eosinophils, slight marrow fibrosis, and complete obliteration of marrow fat spaces. Anemia is less helpful in differentiating a benign from a malignant elevation of the white blood cell count, because it may be related either to the leukemia or to the disease causing the leukemoid reaction. Much more useful is the leukocyte alkaline phosphatase (LAP) score of the mature neutrophils in the peripheral blood. It is difficult to attribute an elevated white blood cell count to a leukemoid reaction unless there is a significant increase in the LAP score, whereas in the typical case of chronic myeloid leukemia, the LAP score is low. Of course, in a leukemoid reaction the Philadelphia chromosome is absent, whereas in CML it is present. Striking elevations of serum B_{12} and its binding proteins which are found in chronic granulocytic leukemia are rarely seen in neutrophilic leukemoid reactions, and this test can be helpful in differential diagnosis.

Leukemoid reactions should be readily distinguishable from acute granulocytic leukemia, even though a the latter disease the LAP score may also be increased. In a leukemoid reaction, the marrow shows relatively good preservation of erythropoiesis and granulocytes in all stages of maturation. There is no diffuse replacement of normal cellular elements by abnormal, immature cells as occurs in acute leukemia. *Auer rods,* usually considered strong morphologic evidence for acute granulocytic leukemia, have been reported in leukemoid reactions associated with disseminated tuberculosis.

Eosinophilic leukemoid reactions are often seen in parasitic, allergic, neoplastic, dermatologic, and collagen vascular diseases and in drug reactions. They are accompanied by eosinophilic proliferation in the marrow with a shift toward immaturity, and eosinophilic myelocytes and metamyelocytes may be observed. Eosinophilic (granulocytic) leukemia is indeed a rare clinical entity. Thus when a patient is observed with a high white blood cell count and a predominance of eosinophils, the condition is far more likely to represent a benign proliferation. It is noteworthy that eosinophils do not have alkaline phosphatase activity. Hence, in contrast to neutrophilic cells, eosinophilic leukemoid reactions and chronic eosinophilic leukemia cannot be distinguished by using the LAP determination. (See Ch. 72.)

Leukemoid reactions involving lymphocytes are seen, for example, in whooping cough, chickenpox, and infectious mononucleosis. In these conditions, the peripheral blood contains an increased number of lymphocytes, many of which are atypical and are known as "virocytes." There is considerable morphologic heterogeneity in contrast to the singular lymphocyte type seen in acute lymphocytic leukemia. The cytoplasm is vacuolated, and the cell border is serrated and wavy. Nuclear configuration and staining characteristics range from dark, clumped chromatin to lighter and more open or vesicular patterns. Most often, the bone marrow does not show a marked increase in lymphocytes or suppression of erythropoiesis or thrombopoiesis. Therefore marrow examination may be quite useful in excluding acute lymphocytic leukemia. Helpful distinction in diseases such as infectious mononucleosis, for example, may be made by utilizing serologic tests such as the heterophil reaction.

Striking increase in number of peripheral blood monocytes occurs infrequently, and rarely should cause difficulty in distinction from myelomonocytic or monocytic leukemia. Monocytosis has been seen in disseminated tuberculosis, in syphilis, in brucellosis, in other granulomatous diseases, in infectious diseases such as subacute bacterial endocarditis, in malignancy, in some collagen vascular diseases, and during marrow recovery after the vigorous use of chemotherapeutic drugs.

No therapy is required for a leukemoid reaction per se, although obviously the underlying condition should be appropriately treated. In those few but difficult instances in which it is initially impossible to distinguish a leukemoid reaction from leukemia, specific treatment must be deferred until the situation has clarified. The premature use of potent drugs in a patient without a primary hematologic malignancy is far more hazardous than deferring the onset of chemotherapy in a patient who subsequently proves to have leukemia.

497. THE ACUTE LEUKEMIAS

James F. Holland

DEFINITION. The acute leukemias are a group of neoplasms which are manifest in the bone marrow. They are characterized by cells analogous to, and often individually indistinguishable by light microscopy from, normal immature hematopoietic cells. In the untreated state, acute leukemic cells enter the blood, where they usually become the predominant leukocyte, and invade other organs. The untreated disease leads to death after a brief and stormy illness, rarely lasting more than a year. Therapy has markedly altered prognosis, however, and the name "acute" as distinguished from "chronic" leukemia is no longer wholly descriptive.

Acute myelocytic leukemia arises from the marrow hematopoietic stem cell or its progeny; the term subsumes several subtypes of leukemia: *myeloblastic leukemia, promyelocytic leukemia, myelomonocytic leukemia, acute myelocytic leukemia* that is none of the foregoing, and *erythroleukemia.* Special forms of acute myelocytic leukemia often occur as the terminal events of chronic myelocytic leukemia, polycythemia vera, and myelofibrosis. Acute "pure" *monocytic leukemia* (Schilling) is characterized by monoblastic proliferation which can be distinguished cytochemically. Acute leukemias apparently derived from eosinophilic, megakaryoblastic, plasmablastic, and mast cells, although uncommon, display unique characteristics as well as some features in common with the other acute leukemias of marrow origin.

Acute lymphocytic leukemia arises in lymphoid tissue and is ordinarily first manifest by its presence in marrow. In some instances thymic infiltration precedes overt marrow disease, but it is not known whether the initial leukemogenic event in man is usually extramedullary. Many instances of lymphosarcoma of various cell types culminate in an acute leukemic phase which bears some resemblance to acute lymphocytic leukemia.

Acute leukemias and related lymphoreticular neoplasms occur throughout the vertebrate animals; examples are even known in some invertebrates. In the mouse, the species most extensively studied, a single transplanted leukemic cell can give rise to the full-blown disease. Removal of lymphoid target organs, such as thymus and spleen, causes a much higher frequency of acute myelocytic leukemia after leukemogenic viral infection than ordinarily would be the case. This indicates that host factors may in large part determine the type of leukemia which evolves.

ETIOLOGY. The etiology of human leukemia has not been established. It is known that leukemias and related sarcomas of pike, chicken, mouse, cat, cow, monkey, and gibbon are caused by RNA virus infection. Viruses have also been associated with leukemia in viper, rat, guinea pig, hamster, pig, deer, horse, dog, and baboon. In inbred laboratory mice transmission may occur through the germ line. Some selectively inbred strains such as AKR eventually develop leukemia in nearly every mouse. Mice may harbor and transmit the incorporated leukemic virus without manifestations of leukemia, allowing it to become apparent in progeny as if sui generis. In pike, chicken, hamster, cat, cow, and gibbon, horizontal leukemia or sarcoma *viral transmission* has been conclusively proved. The risk of neoplasm in healthy cats after known viral infection has been shown to be several hundred-fold higher than in the general cat population.

When analyses are made of all cases of human acute leukemia, clusters in space and time cannot be conclusively shown. Rare anecdotal instances of contact transmission are provocative. Leukemic families have been reported in which several offspring have been affected.

In one such family, fibroblasts from surviving members showed increased susceptibility to transformation in vitro by SV 40 virus, a suggestive analogy to ease of induction of the neoplastic state in vivo.

Radiation leukemogenesis in man is well known. Radiologists sustained nearly ten-fold the death rate from leukemia of other physicians before the widespread use of protective measures. Survivors of atomic bombings, patients who formerly were x-irradiated for spondylitis, and those who received therapeutic doses of ^{131}I for thyroid cancer all showed increased incidence of acute myelocytic leukemia. Patients with multiple myeloma, Hodgkin's disease, or other cancers, who were previously treated with alkylating agents, with or without x-irradiation, have increased frequency of acute myelocytic or acute histiocytic leukemia.

Chronic benzene exposure is leukemogenic in mice and can cause human acute myelocytic leukemia. Anecdotal data on other aromatic solvents suggest their possible human leukemogenicity, but less widespread use. Acute myelocytic leukemia has been reported after marrow aplasia induced by chloramphenicol and by phenylbutazone.

A few *constitutional diseases* lead to disproportionate frequency of acute leukemia. In trisomy 21 *(Down's syndrome)* both acute lymphocytic and acute myelocytic leukemia are increased. *Bloom's syndrome* characterized by chromosomal fragility and rearrangements, the pancytopenia of *Fanconi's syndrome,* and *idiopathic aplastic anemia* are sometimes followed by acute myelocytic leukemia. *Paroxysmal nocturnal hemoglobinuria* probably represents a clonal stem cell disorder, first manifest by production of abnormal erythrocytes, culminating occasionally in acute myelocytic leukemia.

None of these data on family clusters, radiologic initiation, chemical induction, or constitutional predisposition are inconsistent with the possibility of underlying viral leukemogenesis in man. Available molecular biologic data from human experiments are essentially congruent with observations made in the known viral leukemias of mice. The discovery of an RNA-instructed DNA polymerase (reverse transcriptase) in the avian sarcoma and murine leukemia viruses was a monumental step. This enzymatic activity provides an explanation for the mechanism of transcribing oncogenic information from the RNA of an infecting virus into DNA polymers. Such heteropolymers can be incorporated into the host cell DNA, thereby introducing a heritable template for transcription in daughter cells. This provides information to maintain the neoplastic state and, under proper circumstances, to make new virus. The enzyme has been found in high concentration in every RNA oncogenic virus studied.

An RNA-instructed DNA polymerase has also been found in virtually every instance of fresh human acute leukemic cells, and commonly in preleukemic states and in leukemic patients in remission. A DNA transcript prepared from the RNA of a murine leukemia virus underwent partial hybridization with RNA from human leukemic cells. This suggests that the human RNA had itself been transcribed from a DNA codon similar to the nucleic acid sequences of mouse leukemia.

An antibody to the purified reverse transcriptase of a known primate sarcoma virus cross-reacted with and inactivated the human enzyme, suggesting their near identity. In extracts of human acute leukemic cells, a virus-like particulate is found on centrifugation in a sucrose gradient, corresponding to the known density of murine leukemogenic viruses. On rupture of this particulate, reverse transcriptase activity is released. In the presence of labeled deoxynucleotide triphosphates, and using the RNA of the particulate as template, a DNA transcript is synthesized similar to the DNA transcribed from known primate sarcoma virus. In other experiments, the labeled transcribed DNA specifically hybridized with segments of DNA in human leukemic cells, but not in normal cells. This implies that nucleic acid sequences in the particular RNA template had been transcribed from sequences uniquely found in the DNA of the leukemic cell. Nucleotide sequences complementary to those found in baboon endogenous virus, gibbon leukemia virus, and mouse leukemia virus have all been found in human leukemic DNA.

In two pairs of identical twins, each with one normal and one leukemic member, the patients' DNA's contained segments that hybridized with DNA transcribed from the 70s RNA recovered from particulates in the leukemic leukocytes. The normal twins had no such particle-related sequences in the DNA of their leukocytes. These data support the concept that the leukemia-associated DNA sequences were inserted after twinning, and not through the germ line.

These data, taken together, provide strong molecular biologic support consistent with but not sufficient to establish the viral etiology of human leukemia. Infectivity of the isolated particulate remains to be demonstrated. Since there is no proof of utility of laboratory animals or in vitro systems for this purpose, reservations must still be held until this investigative impasse is surmounted. The appearance of leukemia in normal male donor cells transplanted into two female leukemic recipients could be due to viral induction, but may also be explained in other ways.

PATHOGENESIS. The recognizable leukemogenic event may precede clinical disease by many years. The time of appearance of the first leukemic cell and the interim behavior of the population of leukemic cells can only be inferred from data in man obtained during evident leukemia, or from animal models. Under the conditions of marrow crowding inherent in the fully developed leukemic state, the thymidine labeling index is substantially lower for leukemic blasts than for normal myeloblasts. This indicates that a large proportion of cells are not entering the DNA synthetic phase during the availability of labeled thymidine. It is clear evidence that many leukemic blasts are dividing slowly if at all. The largest leukemic myeloblasts or lymphoblasts are the cells which have the highest frequency of labeling. These large blasts mature, partially, to smaller blasts.

In some experimental murine leukemias, the doubling time progressively lengthens as the population density of cells becomes greater, thus deviating from exponential growth. This could be a result of lengthening of the cell cycle, cell death, and an increasing number of cells that do not divide. Some nondividing cells are sterile, whereas others may again be recruited into the mitotic cycle. Early in the pathogenesis of the human acute leukemic process, cells might divide more rapidly than normal cells, but this is usually not true when the disease has become advanced enough to measure.

Acute leukemic cells generally lack the appropriate metabolic programming for the physiologic aging that dictates leukocyte death or loss from the body across membrane surfaces. Such cells therefore accumulate, and, relatively deprived of or insensitive to whatever mechanisms control normal hematopoietic cell population size, they become an ever-increasing tumor that "spills over" into the blood. Normal immature hematopoietic cells are ordinarily excluded from the blood, perhaps because their nondeformability precludes traversing the interstices of the marrow sinusoids. Leukemia, in its literal sense, occurs late in the disease. The reason why immature acute leukemic cells eventually appear in the blood is not known; it probably depends on complex interactions with or invasion of the sinusoidal wall.

Myeloblasts demonstrate positive staining reactions for peroxidase and Sudan black which are negative in *lymphoblasts* and *monoblasts*. Myeloblasts do not stain, or at most have diffuse cytoplasmic periodic acid–Schiff (PAS) staining, whereas lymphoblasts often show large, coarse granules with this stain. Fluoride inhibits esterase activity of monoblasts for naphthol AS-D acetate, but not that of myeloblasts. Electron microscopic studies often show dissociation in nuclear and cytoplasmic age and other ultrastructural characteristics which distinguish leukemic blasts from other types of hematopoietic cells.

On direct preparations made from bone marrow, about half the patients with acute leukemia have a normal *karyotype*. This establishes that grossly visible chromosomal abnormalities are not essential in the pathogenesis. The half of patients with acute lymphocytic leukemia and half of those with acute myelocytic leukemia who have abnormal karyotypes (hyperdiploid for acute lymphocytic leukemia, hypo-, pseudo-, and hyperdiploid for acute myelocytic leukemia) are of great significance in studying pathogenesis. In acute myelocytic leukemia karyotypic abnormalities are nonrandom, with trisomy 8 or translocation of chromosomal pieces between numbers 8 and 21 the most common. In both major forms of acute leukemia, the aneuploid modal chromosome pattern disappears when a complete remission of the disease is achieved and is replaced by a normal karyotype. On relapse of the disease, the original leukemic karyotype reappears, almost without exception. This indicates that the acute leukemias are clones of abnormal cells, rather than abnormally functioning normal cells. This distinction has great importance when devising a therapeutic strategy.

The fact that cells are fundamentally abnormal does not preclude their demonstrating many normal characteristics, including maturation, albeit impaired. Leukemic cells form much smaller colonies of granulocytes and macrophages in semi-solid culture media than do normal marrow cells, and then only in the presence of a glycoprotein colony-stimulating factor. Since the colony-stimulating factor(s) also enhance normal colony growth and are found in abundant quantity in the urine of some patients with acute myelocytic leukemia, a possible role of this bioregulatory substance in the evolution and pathogenesis of the leukemic state has been postulated.

The maturing granulocytes in acute myelocytic leukemia may have abnormal size and distribution of specific granules, sometimes appearing as a regional haze of eosinophilic dust. *Auer bodies* are highly refractile cytoplasmic rods derived from coalescence of azurophilic granules. They are seen in some of the myeloblasts or promyelocytes of about one third of patients with acute myelocytic leukemia. Rarely, these nearly pathognomonic markers are also seen in mature polymorphonuclear neutrophilic granulocytes of acute myelocytic leukemia, demonstrating that maturation has occurred in some cells. The granulocytes of acute myelocytic leukemia show diminished migration across capillary membranes; this test also returns to normal during remission when granulocytes derive from the euploid stem cells.

In *acute lymphocytic leukemia*, it is commonplace to see different stages of lymphoid maturation in the marrow, up to and including lymphocytes morphologically indistinguishable from normal. The degree of immaturity of the predominant acute lymphocytic leukemic cell in the marrow is of prognostic importance. Patients do not reach remission as frequently, or survive as long, if their lymphoblasts contain large amounts of cytoplasm or two nucleoli (or one very prominent one). These simple quantifiable characteristics are more reproducible than more complex cytomorphologic analyses. Lymphoblasts show high terminal nucleotidyl transferase activity, an enzyme lacking in myeloblasts.

Leukemic lymphoblasts from 22 to 28 per cent of patients display T cell antigens on their surface. Rosettes with sheep erythrocytes or reactions with antisera raised against T cells occur in 10 to 90 per cent of the cells from such patients. Only 3 to 4 per cent of acute leukemias display immunoglobulin synthesis and receptors for activated C'3 complement, indicating their B cell origin. The cells from approximately 70 per cent of patients show neither T nor B cell antigens. Although other cytologic features are not discriminating, staining for acid phosphatase is significantly more intense in T cells than in the common acute lymphocytic leukemia. B cell leukemia may resemble lymphosarcoma cell leukemia.

The proliferation of acute leukemic cells in the marrow impairs normal hematopoiesis, even at population densities of leukemic cells when mechanical crowding alone cannot be responsible. One explanation relates this to inhibition of normal hematopoiesis by a hypothetical biochemical product of the leukemic cells. Alternatively, the affected cell in acute myelocytic leukemia may in fact be the early progenitor cell whose progeny are the stem cells for myeloblasts, erythroblasts, megakaryoblasts, monoblasts, and probably marrow fibroblasts. Leukemic proliferation of one cell might be associated with concomitant abnormalities of the other progeny, including hypoplasia. This interpretation would help explain the abnormalities in erythrocyte maturation commonly seen in acute myelocytic leukemia, which in the extreme are called *erythroleukemia*. In its end stages the natural evolution of erythroleukemia is for a clonal selection to myeloblastic proliferation. Megakaryocytes in acute myelocytic leukemia are also often bizarre in appearance and maturation, and their derived platelets may be abnormal.

Leukemic cells invade tissues; infiltration with enlargement of spleen, liver, and lymph nodes is common in all types of acute leukemia. Central nervous system leukemia, characterized by infiltration of the pia and arachnoid, occurs in about half the patients with acute lymphocytic leukemia and less frequently in acute myelocytic leukemia, in which it is found nearly exclusively among patients with myelomonocytic morphology.

Central nervous system leukemia ordinarily becomes clinically manifest only in patients whose early death from hematologic manifestations of disease has been prevented by therapy. Leukostasis, infiltration of vascular walls, invasion into surrounding tissues, and hemorrhage occur particularly at high myeloblast counts, and may account for rapid death when the vessel is in the brain substance. Infiltrates of skin, testes, serosal membranes, and bone may be prominent, particularly in leukemia escaped from chemotherapeutic control. Enlargement of liver and kidney may also occur without infiltration by leukemic cells.

Acute myelocytic leukemic cells, particularly in promyelocytic leukemia, may secrete a vitamin B$_{12}$–binding protein in large quantity, accounting for high serum levels of B$_{12}$. Acute myelocytic leukemic cells, particularly those with monocytoid characteristics, may secrete *muramidase*. This low molecular weight lysosomal enzyme, also known as lysozyme, may appear in the urine, leading to tubular damage and renal insufficiency. Elevated serum levels of the enzyme have been reported prognostically favorable for chemotherapeutic response. In promyelocytic leukemia, and occasionally in other types of acute myelocytic leukemia, secretion of plasminogen-activating substances accounts for the frequent (but not invariable) syndrome of disseminated intravascular coagulation, fibrinolysis, and major hemorrhage.

EPIDEMIOLOGY. The annual incidence per million of acute myelocytic leukemia is quite constant from birth throughout the first ten years at about ten cases. A slight peak in late adolescence occurs, and the incidence remains at a nearly constant 15 per million until age 55, after which the incidence progressively rises to 50 at age 75. This suggests some ubiquitous agent and cumulative injury.

The incidence of acute lymphocytic leukemia is sharply different. There is a peak incidence from two to four years reaching 50 per million annually, falling to 20 or less by age eight until puberty, when the rate declines to about 10. The incidence remains below 10 until age 65, when it again climbs to about 15 per million at age 75. These data are not inconsistent with an infectious disease with greatest susceptibility in childhood.

Numerous clusters of leukemia have been reported, although it has not been persuasively demonstrated that they occur more frequently than by chance. In three separate series, however, coincidences in time (within 60 to 75 days) and space (within 1 kilometer or 1 mile) have been seen in a total of 15 pairs of children less than six years old, sufficiently frequently to make their occurrence by chance improbable (P <0.01). Of the 30 children involved, 27 were under four years. These occurrences, taken in conjunction with the virologic data aforementioned, are compatible with a contagious infectious origin of acute lymphocytic leukemia of young childhood. Prospective search for continuous clustering in large cities has not been successful.

Clinically, approximately 80 to 90 per cent of children with acute leukemia have acute lymphocytic leukemia, and 80 to 90 per cent of adults with acute leukemia have the acute myelocytic varieties.

CLINICAL MANIFESTATIONS. The symptoms and signs of acute leukemia relate to decrease or disordered function of normal hematopoietic cells, and to tumefaction by leukemic cells.

Anemia. Asthenia, pallor, headache, tinnitus, dyspnea, angina, edema, and congestive heart failure may all indicate anemia. The anemia may result in part from diminished erythropoiesis; excessive hemolysis and blood loss are also often contributory. Evidence of specific antibody mediated hemolysis (positive Coombs test) is uncommon. Erythrocytes may show considerable variation in size and shape. Normoblasts and erythroblasts are common in the peripheral blood in erythroleukemia, but occasional nucleated red cells can also be seen in other types of acute leukemia.

Hemorrhage. Oozing gums, epistaxis, petechiae, ecchymosis, menorrhagia, melena, and excessive bleeding after tooth extraction are common initial manifestations of coagulation disorder in acute leukemia. Retinal hemorrhages, subarachnoid bleeding, and gross hematuria are rare initial manifestations, but may occur later. In nearly all instances the abnormal hemostasis can be correlated with decrease in circulating thrombocytes. Hemorrhagic manifestations are uncommon when circulating levels are above 50,000 per microliter; below this level, hemorrhage is inversely related to platelet count. Most thrombocytopenic bleeding occurs when platelets are 20,000 per microliter or less. Increased intravascular pressure (venous occlusion or dependency) augments the appearance of petechiae. Sepsis markedly accentuates thrombocytopenic bleeding, not only locally as in hemorrhagic pneumonia, but also systemically.

In promyelocytic leukemia, thromboplastic substances released from the cells can initiate disseminated intravascular coagulation which leads to activation of normal fibrinolytic systems and the appearance of fibrin split products in the blood. Massive ecchymosis and exsanguinating hemorrhage can occur if not promptly treated.

Infection. Acute leukemia is sometimes first recognized by the occurrence of a respiratory infection from which the patient never fully recovers. Bacterial infections are frequent before therapeutic control is attained: dental infections, sinusitis, bronchitis, pneumonia, perirectal abscess, urinary tract infections, paronychiae, and skin infections. Infections appear to be attributable to absolute granulocytopenia and, to some extent in acute myelocytic leukemia, to impaired function of the granulocytes present. Fever without recognizable infection is also common in acute leukemia, but this is always a diagnosis by exclusion. Every new fever in an acute leukemic patient could be the beginning of a bacterial infection with potential life-threatening consequences. Early, diligent, and repeated search is required before accepting an interpretation of "leukemic fever."

Infiltration. Lymphadenopathy, particularly of the cervical nodes in children, may be the first sign of the disease. It is often generalized. Splenomegaly is present in most patients with acute lymphocytic leukemia, and in about half of those with acute myelocytic leukemia. Hepatomegaly is usually present. T cell acute lymphocytic leukemia is characterized by anterosuperior mediastinal (thymic) enlargement, extensive lymphadenopathy of large size, hyperleukocytosis, more frequent meningeal involvement, and predominance in males. Bulging interdental papillae are highly characteristic of acute monocytic or myelomonocytic leukemia. Tumefaction in bone may lead to bone or joint pain and tenderness. These are common in children, and the disease may present as a limp or protective restriction of motion. Confusion of acute leukemia with acute rheumatic

fever was once common. Subepiphyseal decalcification in children and small areas of osteolysis may be recognized on x-ray films.

A diagnosis can be long delayed by failure to obtain a blood count. Pancytopenia without recognizably abnormal leukocytes is found in a small proportion of patients, the so-called aleukemic leukemia. Granulocytopenia with a normal number of circulating lymphocytes may occur in any kind of acute leukemia. Ordinarily, however, the peripheral blood contains immature myelocytic or lymphocytic cells, and the leukocyte count is elevated owing to the abnormal cells, sometimes in excess of 100,000 per microliter.

A suspicion or presumption of acute leukemia necessitates an examination of the bone marrow, because a diagnosis ordinarily cannot be established with certainty on peripheral blood findings alone. If cells are not obtained in adequate quantity (a circumstance that occurs from entrapment in reticulin fibers or cellular "packing"), a needle biopsy is also required. Other causes of hematologic disorders which mimic acute leukemia must be excluded. Among these are toxic cytopenias, isolated or multiple, and conditions such as infections, neoplasms, or marrow infiltrations that may lead to leukocytosis and to immature cells in the peripheral blood. The most commonly confused disorders are infectious mononucleosis, hematogenous tuberculosis, and drug-induced myelotoxicity. Drug-induced marrow aplasia may be succeeded by a marrow filled with myeloblasts. This normal cohort of repopulating cells matures in a few days, thus establishing the differential diagnosis.

Preleukemia is a term which has been applied to patients with symptoms and findings suggesting acute myelocytic leukemia but whose diagnosis cannot be established on the basis of the evidence then available. Refractory anemia of uncertain etiology is a common precursor. The marrow may be hypo-, normo-, or hypercellular. The change of marrow differential to a younger cell type, ordinarily with peripheral leukocytosis, may come suddenly after years of desultory mild illness. Adequate studies have not been performed to establish if karyotypic or other characteristics of neoplasia are always present from the beginning, although clonal abnormalities have been found before frank leukemia in some patients.

THERAPY. The treatment of acute leukemia is aimed at eradication or at least marked destruction of the tumor, and at supporting the patient through manifestations of the disease per se, its complicating disorders, and the effects of therapy. The strategy of antileukemic treatment is conveniently divided into remission induction, sustaining or maintaining the remission, reinforcement of the remission, treatment of central nervous system disease, and, on an investigational basis, immunotherapy. Conversion of leukemic to nonleukemic normal cells has not been achieved in vivo.

The possibility of cure of acute lymphocytic leukemia has become realistic. Although not yet at this level of accomplishment, chemotherapy of acute myelocytic leukemia is better than a few years ago, and several five-year survivors without evident disease are known. Before undertaking the induction treatment of patients with acute leukemia, the conscientious physician should establish that he has the most current information, drugs, and professional resources available. Since the therapy has been progressively improving, much important information is embodied in current research undertakings. Several drugs of great usefulness have not yet been released from investigational status. Many supportive services are not available except in large centers participating in leukemia research. For these reasons, care of an acute leukemia patient should be carried out by a physician in cooperation with the closest leukemia center. Strategy can be planned and induction accomplished there, and the patient can be managed by his own physician during remission. This participation in ongoing research is also critical to continued progress toward universally curative therapy.

Single drug treatments of acute leukemia have largely given way to combinations of therapeutic procedures tailored to different body burdens of leukemic cells. Induction treatments are effective in abruptly lowering the leukemic population but are less effective in prolonging remissions. Drugs of value in maintaining remissions are somewhat less active in inducing them. Experimentally, immunotherapy is known to be ineffectual when leukemic populations are sizable.

Classification of Response. After therapeutic reduction of leukemic infiltration of the marrow, restitution of normal elements occurs. Clinical improvement and survival correlate well with disappearance or decrease of detectable leukemic infiltration and return of normal hematopoiesis. For convenience, codification systems have been devised for marrow (M), peripheral hematologic data (H), physical status (P), and symptomatic status (S).

In the best remission, the marrow is classified as M_0, indicating no recognizable abnormality in any constituent. When the blast cells are less than 5 per cent by Wright's stain, it is difficult if not impossible to be certain a blast cell is leukemic and not a normal myeloblast. M_1 allows up to 5 per cent blasts and M_2 up to 25 per cent blasts; M_3 and M_4 are more abnormal. In similar fashion, the hematologic values in the peripheral blood can be classified as H_0, indicating no abnormalities whatever in erythrocytes, leukocytes, or platelets; H_1, for minor variations within the range of normal; and H_2, H_3, and H_4, for more pronounced departures from normal. Similar rating scales exist for physical abnormalities (P) and symptomatic manifestations (S). These allow classification of individuals for clinical purposes into those with complete remission (M_1, H_1, P_1, S_1, or better), partial remission (all values 2 or better), improvement, no change, and progression.

Acute Lymphocytic Leukemia. Induction of remission is sucessfully accomplished in 85 per cent or more of children with vincristine and prednisone. The use of daunorubicin, methotrexate, 6-mercaptopurine, or asparaginase during this induction period has not consistently increased the induction frequency. The sequence of events includes a rapid fall in leukemic cells in the peripheral blood, often beginning within 48 hours. Leukopenia usually ensues, which is not ordinarily a cause for alteration in dose during vincristine and prednisone administration. In 7 or 14 days the population of leukemic cells in the bone marrow is noticeably decreased and the marrow cellularity is less. By 28 days half of children have less than 5 per cent leukemic cells remaining in their marrow, and a brisk erythroid hyperplasia is often present. Repopulation of the marrow with normal hematopoietic cells follows. The appearance of increasing platelet counts and granulocyte counts in the blood precedes return of marrow

entirely to normal and is a favorable prognostic sign of an oncoming remission.

Administration of E. coli asparaginase immediately after the vincristine and prednisone administration significantly lengthens the subsequent remission duration without serious addition to the toxicity which simultaneous daily administration entails.

The prognosis for T cell and B cell leukemias is more grave than for the non-T non-B cell common disease in most series. Although T cell leukemia is initially responsive to the same chemotherapy, remissions are short.

MAINTENANCE. Combined use of 6-mercaptopurine and methotrexate delays the emergence of resistant clones of cells. The probability of a single cell being or becoming refractory to both drugs simultaneously is much less than for a single drug, thereby accounting for some of the benefits which accrue to combination chemotherapy. Although immunosuppression exists during this drug regimen, attempts to change the dose and schedule of the combination, allowing for periods of immunologic recovery during the intermittency, have not proved superior to the uninterrupted administration of both drugs.

REINFORCEMENT. During remission maintenance, reinforcement with one or two doses of vincristine plus prednisone for one or two weeks has been applied every four to 12 weeks. Reinforcement has been proved of value when contrasted to maintenance chemotherapy alone. Cyclophosphamide and daunorubicin have not been beneficial for reinforcement.

CENTRAL NERVOUS SYSTEM TREATMENT. Central nervous system leukemia is rare early in the disease. CNS leukemia became clinically frequent only after systemic manifestations of the disease yielded to control, precluding early death. Without specific treatment to the central nervous system, nearly half of affected children develop infiltration of the meninges and brain substance, often as the first manifestation of relapse, giving rise to headaches, irritability, vomiting, personality change, meningismus, papilledema, cranial nerve palsies, and, in young children, separation of the cranial sutures. The failure of systemic treatment to control the central nervous system manifestations probably results from sanctuary of the leukemic cells beyond the blood-brain barrier where drug concentrations are substantially lower. Because of the high frequency of CNS manifestations, regional treatment for central nervous system leukemia with intrathecal methotrexate has been applied effectively before the clinical syndrome emerges. This therapy decreases the central nervous system manifestations and improves the duration of the hematologic remission as well. Intravenous infusions of high dose methotrexate have also elevated cerebrospinal fluid drug concentrations to therapeutic levels.

The early administration of cranial radiation (2400 rads in 12 treatment days) to include the entire brain, retinas, and upper cervical cord has slightly further reduced the appearance of CNS leukemia in patients treated with systemic chemotherapy at standard doses plus intrathecal methotrexate. Late effects on the developing brain include calcification and atrophy or underdevelopment; controlled studies in progress suggest that cranial radiotherapy may be dispensable.

TREATMENT DURATION. The optimal duration of treatment for patients with acute lymphocytic leukemia is not well established. Some patients have sustained

CANCER AND LEUKEMIA GROUP B
SURVIVAL OF ACUTE LYMPHOCYTIC LEUKEMIA
IN CHILDREN UNDER 20 1956-1977

———————	5601	39/ 39	MED= 6 MOS
— — — — —	5702	299/301	MED= 6 MOS
··············	6005	148/151	MED=13 MOS
··············	6307	50/ 52	MED=25 MOS
—·—·—·—	6313	177/183	MED=18 MOS
—··—··—	6601	229/265	MED=28 MOS
—·—··—·	6801	349/475	MED=32 MOS
··············	7111	329/642	MED=50 MOS
— — — —	7411	153/481	MED NOT REACHED
	7611	12/205	MED NOT REACHED

Figure 1. Successive improvement of survival in studies of Cancer and Leukemia Group B in chemotherapeutic programs begun between 1956 and 1977. The numerator represents the number who have died and the denominator the number entered on study. Each protocol contained several alternative therapeutic choices allocated at random. Note the truncated logarithmic ordinate.

long-term remissions on particular regimens. Relapses in patients on these same regimens have almost always occurred within three years. Some investigators thus terminate chemotherapy after three years of treatment, whereas others are engaged in study programs which allocate patients at random to continue or terminate treatment after five years. Premature termination might, of course, lead to relapse, whereas adverse effects of unnecessary continuation would be cumulative toxicity and immunosuppression, leading to opportunistic infections or possibly to reinduction of leukemia through a repetition of the leukemogenic stimulus. Long-term freedom from disease has been produced in approximately 50 per cent in recent protocols of several research groups.

Immunotherapy, using allogeneic leukemic myeloblasts and the BCG strain of tubercle bacilli, has been successful in reports by Mathe and colleagues. Seven of 20 patients repetitively treated with these immunologic stimuli after a short chemotherapeutic course have remained in remission for ten or more years. Unfortunately, this experience has not been duplicated elsewhere. This appears related in part to failure to reproduce the exact experimental design and in part to the progressive success of chemotherapy, which has pre-empted investigators' attention. Intensive immunotherapy with leukemia cells and other immunostimulatory materials after intensive prolonged chemotherapeutic induction has been equally successful as and less toxic than chemotherapeutic maintenance.

In children who fail to remain disease free, relapse of the leukemia can be detected in the marrow weeks or months before it is apparent in the peripheral blood. Reinduction into remission with vincristine and prednisone is ordinarily successful, but sustaining the remission with the drugs from which the child has just relapsed, or with new drugs, becomes progressively more difficult, and after a shorter remission florid leukemia reappears. Death usually comes during the florid uncontrolled leukemic state, although some children die of intercurrent fungal, viral, protozoal (*Pneumocystis*), and bacterial infections while in remission.

Acute Myelocytic Leukemia in Adults. The chemotherapy of acute myelocytic leukemia is more difficult than that of acute lymphocytic leukemia. Drugs known to affect the leukemic myeloblast also affect the normal myeloblast. Selective toxicity is heavily dependent on differences in kinetics of the leukemic and normal populations. Indeed, at the outset in florid leukemia, the population of normal myeloblasts is diminished or absent; normal hematopoietic stem cells, through unknown mechanisms, are apparently in prolonged G_1 or in G_0 cell cycle status. The leukemic population is primarily in cell cycle, however. Because of this kinetic difference, maximal therapeutic advantage appears to derive from treatment programs of relatively short duration, five to ten days, which seriously injure the cycling leukemic population before substantial numbers of normal stem cells enter the cycle. In the hiatus before a second course of treatment is administered, two to four weeks after the initiation of the first course, recovery of antibody synthesis and cellular immunologic functions is recognizable. It is presumed that the normal hematopoietic stem cell pool is similarly replenished, thus explaining the avoidance of irreversible marrow aplasia. Failure of remission induction or eventual relapse is ascribable to cells in the leukemic population which are, or become, relatively insusceptible to the drugs which can be given within the tolerance of nonlethal toxicity. Second remission induction can be accomplished with different drug regimens in a minority of patients.

Age is a significant determinant of successful induction frequency in acute myelocytic leukemia; patients over 60 fare worse in virtually every study. This is not inherently a difference in the susceptibility of leukemic cells, but is rather due to a lesser recovery of normal stem cell functions and decreased resiliency in withstanding the nearly invariable complications of the induction phase.

Cytosine arabinoside, a highly specific inhibitor of the "S" or DNA synthetic phase of the cell cycle, can cause 20 to 35 per cent complete remissions of acute myelocytic leukemia. Given in combinations with other active antileukemic drugs, the remission rates reach 50 to 80 per cent. Cytosine arabinoside must be given frequently daily or by continuous infusion, to ensure that drug is present at some time during the S phase of each leukemic cell in cycle. Effective combinations of cytosine arabinoside with thioguanine, cyclophosphamide, and, most successfully, the anthracycline antimicrobial drugs daunorubicin or Adriamycin have been reported. Some investigators also add vincristine and prednisone. Induction can be achieved in the majority of patients under 60 years of age with a single course of seven days of cytosine arabinoside and three days of daunorubicin (other regimens often require two or three repeated courses). For patients over 60 the "7 and 3" regimen is more effective and less toxic than two courses

Figure 2. Successive improvement of survival in patients of any age with acute myelocytic leukemia in studies of Cancer and Luekemia Group B begun between 1967 and 1975. The numerator represents the number who have died and the denominator the number entered on study. The progressive improvement is similar to studies in acute lymphocytic leukemia in the early years.

of shorter duration, and about one third reach remission.

The continuous drug administration regimens so useful in maintaining remission in acute lymphocytic leukemia of childhood are without equivalent impact in acute myelocytic leukemia of adults. Remissions can be sustained by intermittent courses resembling the induction treatment, or by rotating cycles of active agents in combinations. Median remission duration is 10 to 18 months on different programs, with second remissions, if they occur, of short duration. Twenty per cent survive at 30 months, a change from 2 per cent a decade ago. Central nervous system leukemia is substantially less common than in acute lymphocytic leukemia, in part because of earlier demise from systemic disease and in part because myelomonocytic leukemia is only a segment of acute myelocytic leukemia. Intrathecal methotrexate or intrathecal cytosine arabinoside given in combination with cranial irradiation is temporarily effective in controlling manifestations.

The majority of patients with acute myelocytic leukemia show blastogenesis when their lymphocytes are incubated in vitro with their autologous leukemic cells. This is a manifestation of immune cellular recognition. Competence of the efferent immunologic arm is demonstrable by delayed skin hypersensitivity to leukemic cell membranes. Complete immunologic responses are detectable in animal leukemias, and are subject to augmentation with immunotherapy. Many studies of immunization of patients with acute myelocytic leukemia in remission, using repeated BCG and allogeneic leukemic cell inoculations, have appreciably prolonged survival without significant prolongation of the first remission duration. This effect may thus relate to ease of reinduction and altered risk of fatal infections.

Allogeneic myeloblasts desialated by incubation with *Vibrio cholerae* neuraminidase immediately prior to intradermal injection in multiple sites to patients with acute myelocytic leukemia in remission evoke a powerful immunologic response. Repeated courses of chemoimmunotherapy as maintenance therapy have led to

significant prolongation of remission duration and survival compared to concurrent controls.

Less Common Acute Leukemias. Acute lymphocytic leukemia in adults can be effectively treated with nearly as good induction results as in children, using the programs for this disease outlined previously. Vincristine and prednisone induction, asparaginase intensification, 6-mercaptopurine and methotrexate maintenance with vincristine and prednisone reinforcement, and intrathecal methotrexate therapy with cranial irradiation have produced 70 per cent remission rates lasting four years in 30 per cent. Investigators whose programs for acute myelocytic leukemia of adults include vincristine and prednisone have treated adults with acute lymphocytic leukemia similarly, and have reported equally good induction results.

Acute myelocytic leukemia in children is even more responsive than the adult disease to the identical treatments.

The subvarieties of acute myelocytic leukemia have rates of response which are not importantly different from unclassified acute myelocytic leukemia, except for promyelocytic leukemia, which is particularly sensitive to daunorubicin. No in vitro or in vivo tests are sufficiently developed to predict reliably which drugs will be best for which tumor.

Supportive Measures. Massive leukemic cellular destruction releases a sudden load of purines to be oxidized to urate. This can lead to hyperuricemia and to urate nephropathy with uremia. If this possibility appears likely because of leukocytosis or organ infiltration with leukemic cells, short-term prophylaxis with a xanthine oxidase inhibitor such as allopurinol is appropriate.

Anemia is common and erythrocyte replacement is necessary to keep levels of hemoglobin above the threshold of physiologic dysfunction, at least above 7 grams per 100 ml. Thrombocytopenic bleeding should be prevented. The value of prophylactic platelet administration to preclude hemorrhage has been clearly demonstrated. Optimal platelet survival occurs when the genetic mismatch between donor and recipient is minimal. A sibling, particularly one who is HLA identical, is the best repetitive donor. Random donors are also of value, however, and enough platelets should be administered to protect against hemorrhage during the critical hypoplastic phase before remission ensues if the platelet count is less than 30,000 per microliter. Platelets which have been separated by flotation centrifugation survive longer and are required less frequently than those which are precipitated and resuspended.

Prevention of infection is of great significance. Barrier isolation with sterile filtered air circulating in a laminar flow pattern essentially eliminates exposure to exogenous airborne infection, and the likelihood of serious and fatal infections should thereby be decreased. Although most investigators have combined this isolation with oral nonabsorbable or systemic antimicrobial administration, equivalent effects have also been reported in patients isolated without prophylactic antimicrobial administration.

The nature of many serious infections depends upon the prevalence of particular organisms selected by the prior use of antimicrobial drugs in the hospital environment. In hospitals where extensive use has been made of antimicrobial drugs, *Pseudomonas* and *Enterobacter* infections outnumber infections caused by staphylococci and *E. coli,* the ordinary organisms in hospitals where extensive antimicrobial drug use has not been practiced. Opportunistic infections from fungi, *Pneumocystis carinii,* or cytomegalovirus may occur in granulocytopenic or immunodepressed patients who are protected against bacterial infection by early use of antibacterial drugs.

In the presence of granulocytopenia, new symptoms, signs, or unexplained fever require vigorous and immediate action. If infection is suspected, appropriate cultures and other diagnostic tests should be made and treatment started before results are returned. Evolving insusceptibilities in hospital organisms dictate the antimicrobials to be used which provide broad and effective coverage for gram-positive organisms and the likely spectrum of gram-negatives. Cephalothin or clindamycin has largely superseded ampicillin or methicillin, and is widely used for broad-spectrum coverage. Gentamicin and carbenicillin may be added if the suspicion of *Pseudomonas* is particularly strong. The antimicrobial regimen can be discontinued or changed early, if the initial clinical impression proves incorrect.

When visceral infection occurs in the presence of granulocytopenia, mortality is high despite treatment with antimicrobials, unless marrow recovery occurs nearly simultaneously, with the consequent return of granulocytes. Transfusion of allogeneic normal donor granulocytes, collected by differential centrifugation or by filtration leukophoresis on nylon filters with subsequent elution, has proved a component of major effectiveness in the treatment of sepsis during granulocytopenia. Recovery of transfused granulocytes is best when donated by histocompatible sibling donors, but even granulocytes from random donors in adequate quantity, more than 10^{10} daily for several days, can cause significant improvement in survival from serious infections.

Baxt, J., et al.: Leukemic-specific DNA sequences in leukocytes of the leukemic member of identical twins. Proc. Natl. Acad. Sci. U.S.A., 70:2629, 1973.

Clarkson, B. D.: Acute myelocytic leukemia in adults. Cancer, 30:1572, 1972.

Cronkite, E. P.: Kinetics of leukemic cell proliferation. *In* Dameshek, W., and Dutcher, R. (eds.): Perspectives in Leukemia. New York, Grune & Stratton, 1968, pp. 158–186.

Currie, G.: Prognostic significance of serum lysozyme in adult acute myelogenous leukaemia. Lancet, 1:835, 1976.

Ellison, R. R.: Acute myelocytic leukemia. *In* Holland, J. F., and Frei, E., III (eds.): Cancer Medicine, 2nd ed. Philadelphia, Lea & Febiger, 1979.

Henderson, E., and Jones, B.: Acute lymphoblastic leukemia. *In* Holland, J. F., and Frei, E., III (eds.): Cancer Medicine. 2nd ed. Philadelphia, Lea & Febiger, 1979.

Holland, J. F., and Bekesi, J. G.: Comparison of chemotherapy with chemotherapy plus VCN-treated cells in acute myelocytic leukemia. *In* Terry, W. D., and Windhorst, J. D. (eds.): Immunotherapy of Cancer: Present Status of Trials in Man. New York, Raven Press, 1978.

Holland, J. F., and Glidewell, O.: Chemotherapy of acute lymphocytic leukemia of childhood. Cancer, 26:1480, 1972.

Holland, J. F., and Glidewell, O.: Survival expectancy in acute lymphocytic leukemia. N. Engl. J. Med., 287:769, 1972.

Lee, S. L., Kopel, S., and Glidewell, O.: Cytomorphological determinants of prognosis in acute lymphoblastic leukemia of children. Semin. Oncol., 3:209, 1978.

Todaro, G. J., and Gallo, R. C.: Immunological relationship of DNA polymerase from human acute leukaemia cells and primate and mouse leukaemia virus reverse transcriptase. Nature, 244:206, 1973.

Yates, J. W., and Holland, J. F.: A controlled study of isolation and endogenous microbial suppression in acute myelocytic leukemia patients. Cancer, 32:1490, 1973.

Yates, J. W., Wallace, H. J., Jr., Ellison, R. R., and Holland, J. F.: Cytosine arabinoside and daunorubicin therapy in acute myelocytic leukemia. Cancer Chemother. Rep., 57:485, 1973.

498. THE CHRONIC LEUKEMIAS

Charles M. Huguley, Jr.

498.1. CHRONIC GRANULOCYTIC LEUKEMIA

(Chronic Myelocytic Leukemia [CML], Chronic Myeloid Leukemia, Chronic Myelogenous Leukemia)

DEFINITION. Chronic granulocytic leukemic (CGL) is characterized by abnormal proliferation of immature granulocytes — neutrophils, eosinophils, and basophils — in the blood, the bone marrow, the spleen, the liver, and sometimes other tissues.

ETIOLOGY. The etiology of chronic granulocytic leukemia remains obscure. Epidemiologic studies have been essentially negative with the exception of two well-established factors: exposure to ionizing radiation and chronic exposure to benzene. There is no evidence for a viral etiology. A specific genetic predisposition appears improbable.

The relationship to ionizing radiation was first suggested by the increased incidence of chronic granulocytic leukemia among radiologists who practiced in the era before careful shielding. Later an increased frequency of the disease was found in patients with ankylosing spondylitis treated by radiation to the entire spine and in the Japanese population exposed to a single massive dose of radiation from atomic bomb explosions. There is also a demonstrated increase in CGL among workers with chronic occupational exposure to benzene, mostly among those who had previously experienced acute hematologic damage from the chemical. A relationship to other myelotoxic chemicals and drugs such as chloramphenicol and phenylbutazone is not established. There is no association with other cancer.

INCIDENCE AND PREVALENCE. Chronic granulocytic leukemia accounts for about 20 per cent of all leukemia in the United States, about 15 cases per million population per year. The disease is rare below age 20, slowly rises in incidence to about age 60, and then remains high. It is equally common in males and females.

PATHOLOGY. The essential feature is accumulation of granulocytic precursors in the blood, marrow, and spleen. The marrow is usually completely cellular, and 80 to 90 per cent of the cells are granulocytes. The distribution of granulocytes shows only a slight shift toward immaturity. In the early stages megakaryocytes are nearly always strikingly increased. Needle biopsy of the marrow will reveal some degree of fibrosis with positive stain for reticulin in about 25 per cent of cases. This fibrosis tends to become progressively more severe, and many patients end with a marrow picture similar to that of myelofibrosis. In a moderate percentage of patients there are cells closely resembling Gaucher cells. The spleen is usually very much enlarged. Its normal architecture is replaced by extramedullary myelopoiesis, including not only granulocytes but also erythroblasts and megakaryocytes. Infarcts are common. The liver is often enlarged, although not massively. There are infiltrations with myeloid cells but usually not much damage to the liver cells. Other tissues are usually not involved early.

Although the numbers of granulocytes in the marrow, blood, and spleen are greatly increased, the mitotic index is usually lower than normal, because the mean generation time of immature cells is longer. An exchange of cells between the marrow, the blood, and the spleen has been demonstrated.

About 80 to 90 per cent of patients with chronic granulocytic leukemia exhibit an abnormal chromosome called the Philadelphia chromosome (Ph[1]). This abnormality results from the deletion of a long arm from chromosome number 22. It is generally found to be translocated rather than lost, usually to number 9. When present the Ph[1] chromosome is usually found in all metaphases observed in the marrow, including erythroid precursors and megakaryocytes as well as granulocytes. It is not found in lymphocytes, skin, or connective tissue, indicating that the Ph[1] chromosome is an acquired abnormality of a common stem cell for granulocytes, red cells, and megakaryocytes. There is controversy whether a normal clone of these cells persists in a suppressed state. It has been possible by vigorous therapy to repopulate the marrow with cells lacking the Ph[1] chromosome in a moderate percentage of patients, usually partially, occasionally completely. Although this normal population has usually persisted for only a short time, the achievement does give some hope of a potential for the eventual eradication of the abnormal cell. For the moment, the significance is not known.

Eventually 60 to 80 per cent of patients will develop a transformation into a pattern indistinguishable from acute granulocytic leukemia. This change is called the *"blast crisis."* The pathologic manifestations are those of acute granulocytic leukemia. In perhaps a quarter of cases, however, the presence of the enzyme terminal deoxynucleotidyl transferase suggests a lymphoid origin of the blast cell. Occasionally a blast transformation will occur in extramedullary sites, particularly in lymph nodes, producing a histologic pattern resembling sarcoma. The demonstration that such cellular infiltrations contain the Ph[1] chromosome proves that the cells are immature granulocytes rather than other cells. Such tumors have been called *chloromas* or *granulocytic sarcomas.*

CLINICAL MANIFESTATIONS. Sometimes the disease may be diagnosed at an early stage by an incidental blood count. More commonly the patient experiences insidious onset of fatigue, sometimes accompanied by anorexia and weight loss. There may be fullness or heaviness in the left upper quadrant, or the discovery of a mass in that region may bring the patient to the doctor. More rarely, the physician is consulted because of the manifestations of anemia, pain in the splenic region secondary to a splenic infarct, hemorrhagic or thrombotic manifestations, or an attack of gout.

The spleen is palpable in nearly all patients at the time of diagnosis and is often quite large, frequently extending beyond the umbilicus. If there has been a recent splenic infarct, the organ may be tender and a rub may be heard. The liver is also palpable. Less commonly it is possible to elicit sternal tenderness. Lymphadenopathy is rare. In short, the typical patient has relatively minor symptoms, and the usual physical finding is splenomegaly.

The essential laboratory abnormality is leukocytosis. The patient who presents with symptoms will characteristically have more than 75,000 WBC per cubic milli-

meter, and the count may exceed 500,000. The differential white cell count shows a spectrum of immature granulocytes similar to that seen in normal bone marrow. Myeloblasts rarely exceed 5 per cent of the count. Eosinophils and basophils are increased in percentage, which means a striking absolute increase. Monocytes may also be increased.

Anemia of varying degree may be present, but seldom unless the white cell count exceeds 50,000 per cubic millimeter. About half of all patients at the time of diagnosis will have thrombocytosis which may be associated with bleeding as well as thrombotic manifestations. Some patients present initially with thrombocytopenia, and as the disease progresses thrombocytopenia becomes increasingly frequent.

The bone marrow is as described under Pathology.

Alkaline phosphatase activity in the mature neutrophils is strikingly decreased. Uric acid is elevated. The serum vitamin B_{12} level is high, as is the B_{12} binding protein transcobalamin I. The level of serum lactate dehydrogenase is considerably elevated in CGL.

DIAGNOSIS. Leukocytosis with the characteristic shift to immaturity of the granulocytes and the increase in eosinophils and basophils suggests the diagnosis of chronic granulocytic leukemia. The presence of splenomegaly in most cases will serve to distinguish CGL from leukemoid reactions, although not from other myeloproliferative syndromes. The determination of the leukocyte alkaline phosphatase activity in mature neutrophils is an important test, since it is nearly always very low in untreated CGL and usually very high in leukemoid reactions and other myeloproliferative disorders.

A bone marrow aspiration and needle biopsy are mandatory. The presence of the Ph[1] chromosome is important confirmatory evidence of the diagnosis. Those patients who have Ph[1]-negative CGL can expect an atypical course with a poor prognosis. Myelofibrosis with myeloid metaplasia can closely mimic CGL, and a special stain of the biopsy section for reticulin fibers may be necessary for the distinction. A further confusion is the occasional presence of some fibrosis at the time of diagnosis in an otherwise typical CGL.

In the unusual case identified by a routine blood count, the diagnosis may at first be difficult. Sometimes patients are seen who have a persistent leukocytosis of 15 to 20,000 WBC per cubic millimeter with a mild shift toward immature forms. At this point the neutrophil alkaline phosphatase may not be much reduced. Many months may elapse before the more characteristic findings of the disease appear.

TREATMENT. Chronic granulocytic leukemia is remarkably easy to control until complications develop. Benzene was first used a century ago. Later, arsenic in the form of Fowler's solution was found to be effective. With the advent of radiotherapy, it was shown that the disease was readily responsive to radiotherapy directed to the spleen or to the whole body. Later radiophosphorus ^{32}P also proved effective. More recently it has been demonstrated that extracorporeal irradiation of the blood will control the disease.

With the advent of chemotherapy it was readily shown that most of the agents which produce leukopenia and are effective against any tumor are also effective against CGL. Busulfan has been found to be the drug which combines effectiveness with ease of use and is the standby of treatment. Dibromomannitol, phenylalanine mustard, and hydroxyurea are also effective.

Standard treatment consists of oral administration of busulfan (Myleran). It is available in 2-mg tablets, and the dose is 6 mg daily. The blood count must be monitored at weekly intervals and the dose adjusted as indicated. The fall in the white count is usually steady after about two weeks. A safe rule is to halve the dose of busulfan as soon as the white count has halved. If the white count falls more gradually and smoothly, the original dose may be maintained until the count is in the neighborhood of 15,000 per cubic millimeter. In any event therapy should cease when the count reaches this level, because there is a tendency for the decline to continue for a week or two after the busulfan is discontinued. Once the white cell count plateaus, it is advisable to resume busulfan in a reduced dose (2 to 4 mg daily) in order to bring the count down somewhat below 10,000 per cubic millimeter. The dose will then have to be titrated, ordinarily between 2 mg every other day and 4 mg daily in order to maintain a normal white blood cell count until the spleen is no longer palpable and the platelet count is normal. Control of the leukocyte count is achievable in over 90 per cent of patients. In perhaps 60 to 70 per cent it is possible to eradicate splenomegaly and have the platelet count, the hemoglobin, and the white cell differential return to normal, thus eradicating diagnostic features of the disease. At this point the leukocyte alkaline phosphatase may return to normal but the Ph[1] chromosome will persist.

Once control has been established, it is possible to maintain it by continuous treatment with busulfan at a low dose. Most hematologists, however, will stop treatment and observe. The remission may last for many months. Treatment can be restarted at some arbitrary level of white cell count, say 50,000 per cubic millimeter, before any untoward manifestations appear. Such inductions of remission can be repeated many times, although there is a tendency to require more drug and more time to attain less complete control and a shorter duration. Eventually it will be easier to maintain control by continuous treatment than to go through reinduction at short intervals. Maintenance requires careful monitoring not only of leukocytes but also of platelets at intervals of two weeks because of occasional sudden development of toxicity from which recovery is often slow.

Other manifestations of busulfan toxicity usually occur with prolonged treatment and include the development of amenorrhea in females or aspermia in males and a dark pigmentation of the skin. These patients may develop a rare syndrome resembling Addison's disease but not accompanied by evidence of adrenal insufficiency. In addition, the so-called "busulfan lung," a fibrosing process, is a serious complication only partially relieved by steroid therapy.

COMPLICATIONS. Anemia, when present, is attributable to crowding of the marrow and responds to control of the leukemia. Thrombocytosis may be accompanied by thrombotic complications. Bleeding may be associated with either thrombocytosis or thrombocytopenia which may be due to disease or to treatment. The mature neutrophils of CGL have been shown to be effective in control of infection when transfused into granulocytopenic recipients. Infection is not a usual complication of CGL.

The untreated patient, or one in florid relapse with high leukocyte count and large spleen, has an elevated uric acid and greatly elevated uric acid excretion. This will be exaggerated by the destruction of leukocytes after treatment, which occasionally causes precipitation of uric acid in the renal tubules and anuria. Therefore it is advisable to administer allopurinol, 100 mg three times a day, during the initial weeks of treatment.

About 25 per cent of patients with CGL will have some degree of fibrosis of the marrow at the time of diagnosis. This tends to progress and occasionally develops into a picture indistinguishable from myelofibrosis. At this point the hypocellularity of the marrow makes continued chemotherapy difficult, and the prognosis is poor. Another unusual outcome is development of a refractory state to chemotherapy. It becomes no longer possible to control the white cell count without producing unacceptable thrombocytopenia. Hydroxyurea or 6-mercaptopurine may be somewhat more effective than busulfan at this stage.

PROGNOSIS. The patient in remission ordinarily leads a normal life for an indefinite period. Once a change takes place in the character of the disease, prognosis is very poor. As might be expected in a chronic disease affecting older people, patients with CGL often die of unrelated illnesses. Some 60 to 80 per cent of patients with CGL will develop a "blast crisis." The change most often occurs suddenly, presenting the usual manifestations of acute leukemia. Sometimes it is insidious and is preceded by anemia or pancytopenia or unexplained fever for some weeks. The clinical picture is most commonly indistinguishable from acute granulocytic leukemia except that treatment is even less frequently successful. In perhaps a quarter, the new "blasts" will contain terminal deoxynucleotidyl transferase or show morphologic evidences to suggest acute lymphocytic leukemia. It is currently thought advisable to treat such patients with vincristine and prednisone in the manner of childhood acute lymphocytic leukemia. Recent reports of survival of patients with chronic granulocytic leukemia do not indicate an improved survival over the series of untreated patients reported by Minot in the 1920's. The median survival is between 2½ and 3½ years, and the range is between one and ten years. It is somewhat paradoxical that the most easily controlled of all malignant conditions treated with chemotherapy has been so refractory to efforts at improving survival. Nevertheless, the quality of life is strikingly improved by treatment and is approximately normal until the appearance of the blast crisis. No means of preventing this complication is yet known. There is no clear evidence that any treatment accelerates or delays its onset. This failure has cast a pall of pessimism over all attempts at controlling chronic granulocytic leukemia. However, a recent clinical study has succeeded in eliminating the Ph[1] chromosome and repopulating the marrow with normal cells. The demonstration that there is indeed a clone of normal cells in the marrow suggests the possibility that the abnormal clone can indeed be destroyed and that some cases of chronic granulocytic leukemia may be curable.

The immediate outlook for patients with chronic granulocytic leukemia is excellent. The major manifestations of the disease can be controlled in nearly all patients, and in the majority the blood counts and splenomegaly can be reverted to normal. However, within one to ten years, usually two to four years, complications will develop as described which lead to death within a few months.

Dowling, M., Jr., Haghbin, M., Gee, T. J., Wakonig-Vaar Tara, T., and Clarkson, B.: Attempt to induce true remissions in chronic myelocytic leukemia (CML). Am. Soc. Clin. Oncol., April 1973 (Abst. No. 50).

Ezdinli, E. Z., Sokal, J. E., Crosswhite, L., and Sandberg, A. A.: Philadelphia-chromosome-positive and -negative chronic myelocytic leukemia. Ann. Intern. Med., 7:175, 1970.

Galton, D. A. G.: Chemotherapy of chronic myelocytic leukemia. Semin. Hematol., 6:323, 1969.

Gralnick, H. R., Harbor, J., and Vogel, C.: Myelofibrosis in chronic granulocytic leukemia. Blood, 37:152, 1971.

Haut, A., Abbott, W. S., Wintrobe, M. M., and Cartwright, G. E.: Busulfan in the treatment of chronic myelocytic leukemia. The effect of long-term intermittent therapy. Blood, 37:152, 1971.

Huguley, C. M.: Chronic granulocytic leukemia: Prognostic factors and criteria of response. In Staquet, M. J. (ed.): Cancer Therapy: Prognostic Factors and Criteria of Response. New York, Raven Press, 1975, p. 107.

Stryckmans, P. A.: Current concepts in CML. Semin. Hematol., 11:116, 1974.

Tjio, J. H., Carbone, P. P., Whang, J., and Frei, E., III: The Philadelphia chromosome and chronic myelogenous leukemia. J. Natl. Cancer Inst., 36:567, 1966.

498.2.   CHRONIC LYMPHOCYTIC LEUKEMIA

(Chronic Lymphatic Leukemia)

DEFINITION. Chronic lymphocytic leukemia (CLL) is characterized by accumulation in the lymphoid organs, bone marrow, and blood of long-lived cells with uniform appearance similar to that of the small lymphocyte. There is mild to severe immunologic deficiency characterized by hypogammaglobulinemia.

At present the whole subject of the lymphoproliferative diseases, including chronic lymphocytic leukemia, is in process of re-evaluation, stimulated by the increasing sophisticaiton of our knowledge of the immune system and the role of the lymphocyte and the relation of lymphocyte function and morphology. This knowledge is being applied to the classification and identification of the lymphoproliferative disorders. CLL is characterized by "well-differentiated lymphocytes," and in nearly all cases tested the cells have had the characteristics of B cells (see Ch. 38). Several other leukemic lymphoproliferative diseases have been distinguished from CLL. These include "hairy-cell" leukemia or leukemic reticuloendotheliosis and Sézary's syndrome, a T cell disorder. More difficult to distinguish at times is the "lymphosarcoma-cell leukemia" which might more properly be called poorly differentiated lymphocytic leukemia, the leukemic manifestation of poorly differentiated lymphocytic lymphoma.

ETIOLOGY. Epidemiologic studies have given very little insight into the etiology of chronic lymphocytic leukemia. It is clear that exposure to ionizing radiation is not a factor. It is also clear that genetic factors play some role, as evidenced by the occasional appearance of multiple cases of CLL within a family. CLL is comparatively rare in Japanese, even among Japanese living in the United States. There has been no evidence of a relationship to any chemical carcinogen or to oncogenic viruses.

INCIDENCE AND PREVALENCE. Chronic lymphocytic leukemia accounts for about 30 per cent of all leukemia in the United States and has an incidence of about 20 cases per million population per year. The disease is unusual below age 45, but thereafter it rises rapidly to age 65 and then remains high. The disease is nearly twice as frequent in males as females.

PATHOLOGY. Chronic lymphocytic leukemia must be considered as a leukemic form of well-differentiated lymphocytic lymphoma. It is not possible to distinguish between the lymph node pathology in the two variants or in Waldenström's macroglobulinemia. The normal architecture is replaced by a sea of small lymphocytes. Lymph nodes are characteristically enlarged. The spleen is usually enlarged but seldom to a conspicuous degree. Infarction is uncommon. Its architecture is similarly replaced by monotonous infiltration of small lymphocytes. The liver may be enlarged and demonstrates a lymphocytic infiltration which is often minimal and may be either diffuse or nodular. The bone marrow is involved. In early cases this may be patchy, and a bone marrow aspirate may be hypocellular without a particularly large number of lymphocytes, whereas a biopsy will show nodules of lymphocytes interspersed in normal marrow. Later the marrow becomes almost completely replaced with lymphocytes to the detriment of granulocytes, erythrocytes, and megakaryocytes, yielding a so-called "packed marrow" syndrome. Other organs may be involved, in particular the gastrointestinal tract and the skin.

CLINICAL MANIFESTATIONS. In at least a quarter of patients with CLL, symptoms are absent and the diagnosis is suggested by a blood count obtained as part of a routine examination or for the diagnosis of some other illness. In other patients there is insidious onset of noncharacteristic symptoms, and in some the first sign of the disease is a complicating infection. There may be a vague feeling of malaise with easy fatigability. Sometimes there is loss of appetite and weight or a low-grade unexplained fever associated with night sweats. In an appreciable percentage of patients, with or without other symptoms, the physician will be consulted because enlarged lymph nodes or spleen have been observed by the patient. More rarely, bleeding manifestations bring the patient to the physician. Although generalized leukemia cutis may occur, it is rare. Nevertheless, skin manifestations are common. They may take the form of nonspecific leukemids represented by scattered papular or vesicular lesions, often intensely pruritic. These must be distinguished from hyperreactivity to insect bites or a generalized herpes simplex infection. Herpes zoster occurs frequently and may become generalized. Smallpox vaccination may produce a very severe local lesion, and it may go on to generalized vaccinia. The expanding lesions in the marrow encroach upon the bone, leading to demineralization and sometimes to collapse of vertebrae. (The use of steroids in treatment will aggravate demineralization.)

The blood picture is characterized by an absolute lymphocytosis composed mostly of uniform, small, mature-appearing lymphocytes. There will be some large lymphocytes, perhaps with a cleaved nucleus or nucleoli. Smudge cells are common. Early in the disease the absolute number of granulocytes is normal. There is often no thrombocytopenia or anemia at the time of diagnosis. The total white count is usually more than 20,000 but not usually more than 100,000. An occasional patient will have a normal or low white cell count consisting of the same type of abnormal lymphocytes. Most authorities would include such patients within the group of CLL. Examination of the marrow reveals an infiltration with small lymphocytes similar to those in the blood. The marrow may be difficult to aspirate, and a needle biopsy will demonstrate the infiltration of lymphocytes. In more advanced disease, the marrow will be packed with lymphocytes at the expense of the normal myeloid cells. At this point there will be neutropenia, thrombocytopenia, and anemia.

In CLL the rate of production of lymphocytes is little, if any, above normal. The abnormal cells are especially long lived so that they accumulate. They are of the B cell type, characterized by a monoclonal immunoglobulin coating. These abnormal B cells do not respond appropriately to antigen stimulation, and antibody formation is diminished.

Hypogammaglobulinemia is characteristic of the disease, and it increases in severity as the disease progresses. This leads to an increased susceptibility to infection which is the major cause of morbidity in patients with CLL. In advanced disease all patients will have hypogammaglobulinemia with a reduction in normal immunoglobulins. T cells are normal or reduced in absolute numbers, and the percentage reacting to antigen or phytohemagglutinin stimulation is low. Impairment of cell-mediated immune functions may result. There may also be "immunologic excess" with a polyclonal hyperglobulinemia or a monoclonal hyperglobulinemia, usually IgM. Hyperimmune phenomena may occur such as a positive Coombs test, often with hemolytic anemia, or a hyperreactivity to insect bites.

Although the serum uric acid concentration is usually normal, it may be elevated in rapidly progressive cases or after treatment.

DIAGNOSIS.   The diagnosis of CLL depends upon examination of the blood and marrow, as described under Pathology. Lymph node biopsy will show a diffuse, well-differentiated lymphocytic lymphoma. Lymphadenopathy and splenomegaly are usually present. Either may be massive but usually is not. Studies at the time of diagnosis should include careful history with an attempt to identify the earliest manifestations of the disease. There should be special examination of the skin, lymph nodes, liver, and spleen. The patient must have a complete blood count, including reticulocytes and platelet count, and a bone marrow examination. A needle biopsy of the marrow as well as the aspirate is desirable.

Other studies should include chest film, bilirubin, direct Coombs test, and studies of liver and kidney function. Determination of total protein and serum electrophoresis is important. An abnormal electrophoretic pattern should be studied by immunoelectrophoresis to identify a monoclonal peak.

TREATMENT.   Many forms of treatment have been effective, but in the past all have been of somewhat limited value. Since we have no clear evidence that treatment has led to an improved survival, many hematologists believe that only the symptomatic patient should be treated.

Many patients (up to half) have the diagnosis of CLL made incidental to examinations carried out for other reasons. These patients may exhibit no morbidity from the disease and may show no progression for many years. Patients with "active" disease, by contrast, may be defined as those who have one or more of the following: unexplained weight loss, unexplained fever of more than two weeks' duration, rapidly enlarging or painful lymph nodes or spleen, anemia, thrombocyto-

penia, or such complications as hemolytic anemia, recurrent infections, or skin involvement. Active disease is an indication for treatment.

CLL is an accumulative disease of slowly proliferating but long-lived lymphocytes. The key to treatment with present modalities is the gradual reduction of the tumor cell burden while inducing minimal toxicity to normal marrow cells. If doses are spaced so as to permit recovery of the rapidly recuperating normal cells between doses, there will be a stepwise reduction in lymphocytes which cannot replenish themselves rapidly. The appropriate agents should be those to which lymphocytes are especially sensitive and which have just as great an effect on resting cells as upon proliferating cells. Such agents are ionizing radiation, alkylating agents, and the corticosteroids. These, alone or in combination, have been shown to be especially effective for CLL. An effective technique used investigatively is the direct removal of lymphocytes through leukapheresis. This noncytotoxic procedure leads to mobilization of lymphocytes from the spleen and lymph nodes so that the blood lymphocytosis tends to remain high until the involved tissues shrink. A similar effect follows the irradiation of blood extracorporeally as it is pumped through a grid and also after the administration of prednisone.

Radiation has been given as splenic irradiation, extracorporeal irradiation, and total body irradiation, and also as radiophosphorus. Recently total body radiation has been revived with excellent results reported.

Chlorambucil has been the most extensively used alkylating agent and has achieved a higher response rate with less toxicity than others. The standard treatment has been chlorambucil (Leukeran, 2-mg tablets) orally in a daily dose of 12 mg. My recommendation, which differs from that of the manufacturer, is to administer the drug in a large single dose of 0.8 mg per kilogram once every two weeks, at bedtime with an antiemetic. Over a period of six months the response rate is as good as with daily administration and the hematologic toxicity is considerably less. Several studies have demonstrated the greater effectiveness of a combination of chlorambucil and prednisone over either alone. My recommendation is to give chlorambucil every two weeks as described together with prednisone, 80 mg daily for five days. This may avoid some of the adverse effects of long-term daily steroid therapy in infection-prone patients.

Treatment should be maintained in an individually titrated dose for at least six months and certainly until maximal effect appears to have been achieved. This may require as long as a year. During this time careful monitoring of blood counts for hematopoietic toxicity will necessitate counts weekly until stability is achieved and then at least every four weeks. Treatment can then be stopped until the evidences of active disease return. A majority of patients will require constant treatment. It has not been shown that continuation of regularly spaced titrated therapy to the patient in complete remission is more effective than treatment administered as needed.

COMPLICATIONS.   Most complications have already been mentioned. About 20 per cent of patients will develop an autoimmune hemolytic anemia. Not infrequently hemolysis may be precipitated by treatment. It will usually respond well to prednisone. If the disease is then controlled with chlorambucil, the hemolytic anemia may not recur. Nonhemolytic anemia and sometimes the thrombocytopenia and neutropenia of advanced disease may be helped by the administration of an androgen. Fluoxymesterone in a dose of 10 mg three times daily has often been quite effective.

Infections require specific and vigorous treatment. The regular administration of gamma globulin has not been shown to be effective in preventing infections.

PROGNOSIS. Extensive tumor registry data indicate that patients diagnosed since 1955 have fared better than those diagnosed previously in the same hospitals. Although these data correspond to the introduction of chlorambucil, it may be that longer survival should be attributed to wider availability of blood banks, introduction of better antimicrobial drugs, the use of prednisone for treatment of hemolytic anemia and thrombocytopenia, and earlier diagnosis. Series reported from centers particularly interested in the care of patients with chronic lymphocytic leukemia seem to show a much better median survival (on the order of five to six years) than do series of patients derived from tumor registry data which indicate a median survival of less than four years. The difference may be artifactual in that referral centers tend to attract patients whose disease was discovered in the indolent phase because of routine yearly examinations, whereas district hospitals may handle a higher proportion of patients who have only sought help when symptoms had interfered with ability to work.

It has become obvious that staging of the patient at the time of diagnosis is very important from a prognostic standpoint and especially if therapeutic trials are to be compared. Rai has devised a simple plan which has been very useful. Successive stages are characterized by an additional finding of increasingly severe prognostic import. Stage 0 has lymphocytosis only; Stage I adds lymphadenopathy; Stage II, splenomegaly and/or hepatomegaly; Stage III, anemia; and Stage IV, thrombocytopenia. Several series have been analyzed according to this system. Patients in Stage 0 have enjoyed an extraordinarily long survival with a median of ten years. Stages I and II have a similar and intermediate prognosis with a median of four to eight years, whereas Stages III and IV can expect only one to three years. The median survival of a particular series is related to the proportion of patients in early stages.

Whole body irradiation or some combination of chlorambucil and prednisone will produce a satisfactory response in 70 to 85 per cent of previously untreated patients. A "complete remission" — i.e., eradication of lymphadenopathy, splenomegaly, and hepatomegaly; restoration to normal of the total and differential white blood cell counts, the red blood cell count, and platelet count; and the reduction of marrow lymphocytosis to less than 30 per cent — will be obtained in 10 to 40 per cent. Patients reported to have improved to the status of "complete remission" have enjoyed long remissions and a median survival considerably lengthened over that expected. In some of those tested, the immunoglobulins have been restored to normal. These reports should give us hope that a more aggressive attack upon the disease may lead to better survival than we have obtained in the past.

Cutler, S. J., Axtell, L., and Heise, H.: Ten thousand cases of leukemia: 1940–62. J. Natl. Cancer Inst., 39:993, 1967.
Han, T., Ezdinli, E. Z., Shimaoka, K., and Desai, D. V.: Chlorambucil

vs. combined chlorambucil-corticosteroid therapy in chronic lymphocytic leukemia. Cancer, 31:502, 1973.
Huguley, C. M., Jr.: Treatment of chronic lymphocytic leukemia. In Cancer Treat. Rev., 4:261, 1977.
Johnson, R. E. Total body irradiation of chronic lymphocytic leukemia. Cancer, 37:2691, 1976.
Pangalis, G. A., Nathwani, B. N., and Rappaport, H.: Malignant lymphoma, well differentiated lymphocytic. Its relationship with chronic lymphocytic leukemia and macroglobulinemia of Waldenström. Cancer, 39:999, 1977.
Rai, K. R., Sawitsky, A., Cronkite, E. P., Chanana, A. D., Levy, R. N., and Pasternack, B. S.: Clinical staging of chronic lymphocytic leukemia. Blood, 46:219, 1975.
Silver, R. T.: The treatment of chronic lymphocytic leukemia. Semin. Hematol., 6:344, 1969.
Zimmerman, T. S., Godwin, H. A., and Perry, S.: Studies of leukocyte kinetics in chronic lymphocytic leukemia. Blood, 31:277, 1968.

499. MYELOPROLIFERATIVE DISORDERS

Richard T. Silver

499.1. INTRODUCTION

The bone marrow, an organ diffusely spread throughout the bones of the body, consists of several different cell types that are strikingly different with regard to their physiologic roles. Depending upon the stimulus, a normal marrow response is unique and selective, occurring, for example, with an elevated white blood cell count after a pyogenic infection or with an elevated platelet count after hemorrhage. These reactions are self-limited, for the marrow reverts to its normal status once the provocative stimulus subsides. The myeloproliferative disorders refer to certain diseases in which the marrow and sometimes hematopoietic stem cells in extramedullary sites proliferate more or less en masse. This proliferation is self-perpetuating, thus resembling a neoplastic disease, and results in common clinical, hematologic, biochemical, and morphologic characteristics. The concept of the myeloproliferative syndrome as a spectrum of disease with transitions from one form to another has achieved a certain popularity. There is a wide difference of opinion, however, as to which disease should be included in the "myeloproliferative disorders," and a few hematologists find the term neither precise nor productive. Most would include in this group of diseases chronic granulocytic leukemia, polycythemia vera, myelofibrosis with myeloid metaplasia, and essential (idiopathic) thrombocythemia. At the onset of these illnesses, despite predominant proliferation of one cell type, there is evidence that the marrow *is* reacting en masse. Thus, for example, patients with chronic granulocytic leukemia initially may have an increased platelet count or even an increased red cell count in addition to an elevated white blood cell count. When first diagnosed, patients with polycythemia usually have, in addition to an increased red cell mass, elevations of white blood cell and platelet counts. Most patients with chronic myeloproliferative disorders have increased reticulin fibers in the bone marrow, presumably reflecting mesenchymal cell proliferation which reaches its greatest expression in the disease myelofibrosis with myeloid metaplasia (agnogenic myeloid metaplasia). All these illnesses involve the spleen as well as marrow. In some cases at diagnosis the bone marrow biopsy in the four conditions may be indistinguishable. Alterations are also seen in the levels of serum uric acid, vitamin B_{12} and its binding proteins, and leukocyte alkaline phosphatase activity. The terminal episode in many of these patients is often a disease resembling acute granulocytic leukemia.

The caveat regarding the myeloproliferative concept clearly relates to causation. The *Philadelphia chromosome*, the hallmark of about 90 per cent of the cases of chronic granulocytic leukemia, has not been found in the other diseases of the myeloproliferative group. Moreover, there is no current reason to indicate a common cause for these diseases. Although myelofibrosis may be seen in end-stage patients with polycythemia vera and chronic granulocytic leukemia, it is unlikely that this is the same disease as the idiopathic form. The similarities seen in these disorders may be explained on the basis of the limited manner in which the marrow can express itself in different disease states. Finally, transitions of chronic granulocytic leukemia and agnogenic myeloid metaplasia to polycythemia vera or idiopathic thrombocythemia are difficult to document.

In summary, whereas the term "myeloproliferative disorder" in a restricted sense is useful to refer to certain chronic proliferative diseases of the marrow which share certain characteristics, it should not embrace all the malignant hematologic disorders known to man.

Dameshek, W.: Some speculations on the myeloproliferative syndrome. Blood, 6:372, 1951.
Glasser, R. M., and Walker, R. L.: Transitions among the myeloproliferative disorders. Ann Intern. Med., 71:284, 1969.
Myeloproliferative Disorders of Animals and Man. Proceedings of the Eighth Annual Hanford Biology Symposium at Richland, Washington, May 20–23, 1968, edited by W. J. Clarke, E. B. Howard, and P. L. Hackett, U.S. Atomic Energy Commission, published June 1970.

499.2. AGNOGENIC MYELOID METAPLASIA

DEFINITION AND PATHOGENESIS. The degree of confusion and controversy regarding the etiology, pathogenesis, and treatment of agnogenic myeloid metaplasia (*myelofibrosis with myeloid metaplasia* or *myelofibrosis with extramedullary hematopoiesis*) has been proportional to its polysyllabic length. No wonder this entity has been described in the hematologic literature under at least 35 additional names, ranging from *leukoerythroblastic anemia* to *pseudoleukemic-pseudoerythremic myelosis*. In order to understand this disease it is helpful to review the meaning of some terms constituting the name of this disorder. *Agnogenic* is derived from the Greek *agnostos* meaning unknown. *Myeloid*, as a general hematologic term, refers either to myeloid (or granulocytic) cells or to the marrow as a whole. In this disease it should be interpreted as referring to the marrow. *Metaplasia* is characterized by the proliferation of cells which are not usually histologically or functionally important in an organ or tissue. Therefore the term agnogenic myeloid metaplasia can be redefined as the causally unknown proliferation of cells which normally arise from the bone marrow in organs and tissues which are not usually involved in blood cell formation. What is *extramedullary hematopoiesis*? In the early devel-

opmental stages of the human embryo, hematopoiesis is a function of embryonic connective tissue or mesenchyme. Erythrocytes are first formed in the blood islands of the yolk sac, followed by active hematopoiesis in the liver, spleen, and lymph nodes. Intramedullary blood formation within the bone marrow cavity has its onset at about the fifth month of gestation, and by the eighth month the marrow is the principal site of hematopoiesis as extramedullary (outside the marrow) hematopoiesis gradually subsides. At birth, significant extramedullary blood cell formation no longer exists. Nevertheless, the mesenchymal cells originally responsible for hematopoiesis persist throughout life. Normally inactive, they nevertheless retain their embryonic potential, and under a variety of stimuli they are capable of resuming active hematopoiesis. When the mesenchymal cells of the spleen and liver resume blood formation, once again there is extramedullary hematopoiesis (or myeloid metaplasia), for now there is production of marrow cells by organs not usually concerned with hematopoiesis. Such formation of blood outside the marrow cavity may occur secondary to a variety of clinical conditions, including, for example, severe hemolytic anemias, Hodgkin's disease, metastatic neoplasms to the marrow, irradiation, and infections such as tuberculosis, or may occur after poisoning of the bone marrow by fluorine, phosphorus, benzol, or strontium. In some patients with chronic granulocytic leukemia or polycythemia vera, myeloid metaplasia or extramedullary hematopoiesis occurs in association with fibrosis of the marrow during the course of the illness and/or as a consequence of therapy. In a certain number of patients the cause of the myeloid metaplasia is unknown; thus the term *agnogenic* myeloid metaplasia. This occurrence is most commonly (but not always) associated with fibrosis of the marrow; thus the term *myelofibrosis*.

CLINICAL MANIFESTATIONS. Agnogenic myeloid metaplasia (AMM) occurs primarily in the older age groups. Nearly two thirds of the cases occur between the ages of 50 and 70 years, about equally in men and women. Symptoms may be of several years' duration, are usually insidious in onset, and are referable to anemia or to abdominal discomfort owing to splenic enlargement. Deafness caused by otosclerosis has been reported in 10 per cent of cases. Less often, migratory bone pain and symptoms of gouty arthritis may occur. The spleen is almost always enlarged when the patient is first seen, and without this physical finding the diagnosis on clinical grounds must be held suspect. The liver is palpable in approximately two thirds of the cases, and this finding may be associated with mild liver function test abnormalities. Hepatomegaly without splenomegaly does not occur in AMM. When an enlarged liver without splenomegaly is found in a patient with proved extramedullary hematopoiesis, a diagnosis of *secondary* myeloid metaplasia is almost certain. Extramedullary hematopoiesis is frequent in lymph nodes, but rarely accounts for significant nodal enlargement.

LABORATORY FINDINGS. Severe degrees of anemia are uncommon when the patient is first seen. Usually the hemoglobin ranges between 9 and 13 grams per 100 ml. The white blood cell count is elevated in about half the patients, normal in one third, and low in the remainder. The leukocyte alkaline phosphatase score is variable, but usually it is normal or increased. The Philadelphia chromosome, the hallmark for the typical case of chronic granulocytic leukemia, is absent. Karyotypic abnormalities have occasionally been reported in AMM, although the majority of studies have been negative. A peripheral blood smear shows striking changes; typically there is a shift toward granulocyte immaturity, even with the appearance of a few myeloblasts and progranulocytes. The presence of these immature cells does not imply a shortened survival time. Marked changes in the red cells include variations in size and shape and teardrop forms. Polychromatophilia and nucleated red cells are characteristic. Acquired Pelger-Hüet cells are often observed. The reticulocyte count is usually elevated and reflects either dyspoiesis or hemolysis. The platelets may appear large and bizarre and may be increased, normal, or low in number. Megakaryocyte fragments may be seen. In summary, a peripheral smear showing teardrop poikilocytosis, leukoerythroblastic forms, and giant platelets or megakaryocyte fragments is highly suggestive of AMM. Normal or slightly elevated serum levels of vitamin B_{12} and its binding proteins have been reported in AMM, but a clear separation between the extremely high values in chronic granulocytic leukemia (CGL) and AMM is usually apparent. Radioactive iron studies reflect ineffective erythropoiesis and decreased red cell formation in medullary and extramedullary sites. Radioactive chromium-51 studies demonstrate shortened red cell survival in the majority of cases. Most likely this is due to hypersplenism, because the Coombs test is rarely positive and tests for red cell enzyme deficiencies are inconclusive. Coagulation abnormalities are frequent and are attributed to qualitative and quantitative platelet dysfunction, deficiencies of clotting factors manufactured in the liver, and fibrinolysis.

The frequency of radiographic evidence of *osteosclerosis* in patients with AMM has ranged from 30 to 70 per cent and may be severe enough to be recognized on a routine chest x-ray in about one third of the cases. The distribution of osteosclerosis is primarily in the axial skeleton where changes are most apparent in the vertebrae, ribs, clavicles, pelvis, scapulae, and metaphyseal ends of the femur and humerus. Bones distal to the elbow and knee are rarely involved. Osteosclerosis of the skull may occur. The most frequent radiographic finding is a "ground-glass appearance" of the bones with loss of definition of individual trabeculae.

In almost every case (even when the marrow is very cellular) the bone marrow aspiration yields a "dry tap," but this finding must not be used as sole evidence for diagnosis. A closed needle biopsy can be readily obtained from the posterior iliac crest. If not, then an open surgical biopsy should be performed. In more than 90 per cent of the cases, the marrow shows fibrosis, and in some, osteosclerosis which is marked by the formation of broad irregular bone lamellae. Islands and clumps of megakaryocytes may remain. In a small but significant percentage of cases, the marrow at the time of diagnosis may be hypercellular, although the architecture in these instances is disorganized. When panhyperplasia occurs, the marrow findings may not be distinguishable from the histologic changes seen in polycythemia vera. Granulocytic hyperplasia is never found to the degree that occurs in chronic granulocytic leukemia. Striking increase in the amount of reticulin fibers is demonstrated by silver impregnation stain and may be found even before the classic increase in collagenous tissue is observed. Although the sine qua non for the diagnosis rests on the demonstration of myeloid metaplasia in the liver or spleen, the risks involved in biopsying these organs are rarely justified.

COURSE. As the disease progresses, the spleen gradually enlarges, and so may the liver. Anemia becomes more severe in degree and may be complicated by iron deficiency owing to blood loss or, more rarely, to folic acid deficiency. Bacterial infections occur more frequently and can be a major contributing factor leading to death. Of particular importance is the association of tuberculosis with myelofibrosis, and this infectious disease should be excluded. Nearly all patients have elevated levels of serum uric acid, and attacks of gouty arthritis may develop. Within the past decade, the association of portal hypertension and ascites has been reported in a significant percentage of patients with AMM. Thrombosis of the hepatic vein and the development of the Budd-Chiari syndrome have been recognized. It has been suggested that portal hypertension is a manifestation of both high portal blood flow and a relative obstruction of portal flow at the hepatic sinusoidal level.

TREATMENT AND PROGNOSIS. No treatment affects the basic fibrosis of the marrow, and no form of therapy has been shown to prolong life. Survival time in AMM is difficult to state with assurance because of the problem of accurately determining the onset of the illness. Suggested estimated median survival times are approximately ten years from onset of disease and five years from diagnosis, although there is considerable heterogeneity with both shorter- and longer-lived survivors. Insofar as AMM can thus be a disease of long duration, presently no specific treatment should be undertaken unless the patient becomes symptomatic. All patients should receive at least 200 to 400 mg of *allopurinol* daily in order to avoid the complications of elevated serum uric acid levels. If a patient becomes symptomatic from anemia, *androgens* may be employed, although the high doses used to stimulate erythropoiesis lead to excess fluid accumulation and to masculinizing effects in women. Doses of testosterone enanthate, 600 mg weekly intramuscularly, or oxymetholone, 50 to 100 mg daily by mouth, can be used. Treatment must be continued for 6 to 12 weeks to evaluate its efficacy. It seems most effective in women whose spleen had been removed prior to the onset of therapy or in whom it had not been massively enlarged. Treatment becomes less impressive in patients with more advanced disease. The hemolytic anemia which is most often due to hypersplenism rarely responds to *corticosteroids*. In those patients who initially present with markedly elevated platelet counts, *busulfan* in a dose of 4 mg per day, followed by lower doses as the platelet count falls, may be instituted. In most cases, busulfan cannot be used for definitive reduction in spleen size, because prohibitive degrees of suppression of erythropoiesis and thrombopoiesis result. *Radiation therapy* to the spleen rarely produces meaningful reduction in spleen size, and the dose required often causes severe leukopenia, anemia, and thrombocytopenia. Treatment of bleeding complications depends upon cause. In patients with platelet deficiencies, the use of adrenocortical steroids and fresh platelet transfusions has produced good temporary relief. Although *splenectomy* is not automatically interdicted in patients with AMM, it should be reserved for those individuals with severe hemolytic anemia, thrombocytopenia and clinical bleeding, portal hypertension, or mechanical symptoms secondary to splenomegaly. It has been suggested that women are better candidates for splenectomy than men. Nevertheless, the postoperative morbidity of splenectomy is significant. Striking thrombocythemia after splenectomy, with thrombosis and hemorrhage, may develop. Often there is further gradual enlargement of the liver, and recurrent hemolysis and thrombocytopenia may occur owing to sequestration by the liver.

In summary, one cannot be categorical about the therapy of AMM, and each treatment modality has its significant attendant risks. On the other hand, future studies may show that earlier treatment, including splenectomy, of the relatively asymptomatic patient may alter the heretofore slow but nevertheless inexorable course of the illness.

Gardner, F., and Nathan, D.: Androgens and erythropoiesis. Further evaluation of testosterone treatment of myelofibrosis. N. Engl. J. Med., 274:420, 1966.

Silver, R. T., Jenkins, D., and Engle, R. L.: Use of testosterone and busulfan in the treatment of myelofibrosis with myeloid metaplasia. Blood, 23:341, 1964.

Silverstein, M. N.: Agnogenic Myeloid Metaplasia. Acton, Mass., Publishing Science Group, Inc., 1975.

Ward, H. P., and Block, M. H.: The natural history of agnogenic myeloid metaplasia (AMM) and a critical evaluation of its relationship with the myeloproliferative syndrome. Medicine, 50:357, 1971.

Section Seven
LYMPHORETICULAR NEOPLASMS

500. INTRODUCTION

Paul P. Carbone

Neoplasms of the reticuloendothelial system are characterized as myeloproliferative or lymphoreticular. The myeloproliferative disorders include erythroid, myeloid, and megakaryocytic neoplasms that start in the bone marrow and only secondarily invade other tissues of the reticuloendothelial system (lymph nodes, spleen). Lymphoreticular neoplasms arise in lymphocytic cells, reticulum cells, or primitive precursor cells. The lymphocytic cells, primarily involved in immune reactions, are either T cells (thymus derived) or B cells (bone marrow derived). Malignant diseases of lymphoid cells, referred to as lymphoproliferative disorders, may be associated with immune disturbances or monoclonal gammopathies. Reticulum cells, referred to as histiocytic or macrophage cells, form the background population of all lymphoreticular tissues. The lymphoreticular cells are located primarily in lymph nodes, thymus, spleen, and liver, but components of the lymphoreticular system are also found in the submucosal areas of the respiratory and gastrointestinal tracts as well as in the marrow. Although these cells morphologically appear to be distinct from lymphocytic cells, on the basis of immunologic markers they are likely to be B cells.

Lymphoreticular tumors may become clinically apparent as single or multiple tumors in the lymph nodes, spleen, or gastrointestinal tract and may or may not involve the bone marrow. Since lymphocytes and macrophages also normally occur in the peripheral blood, lymphoreticular tumor cells may circulate. The term malignant lymphoma commonly refers to patients who present predominantly with solid tumors and must be further classified as to cell type, i.e., histiocytic, lymphocytic, or Hodgkin's. Since the tumor cells may exhibit different degrees of differentiation, i.e., well differentiated or poorly differentiated, that affect prognosis and response to therapy, subclassification for differentiation also is important. Occasional patients have such primitive cells that the terms stem cell and Burkitt's tumor are applied to indicate less differentiated populations In the lymph node or tissue section, two populations of malignant cells may occur simultaneously with neoplastic lymphocytic and histiocytic components, and the term mixed lymphomas is used. As mentioned above, there may not be distinctly different cells immunologically. When the marrow and peripheral blood manifestations are prominent, as contrasted to tumor or nodal enlargement, the term leukemia or leukemic phase is applied. Thus in patients with lymphoreticular neoplasms, one sees a complete spectrum from localized tumors only to multiple tumors, leukemia, and mixtures. The presentation at the time of diagnosis reflects only a point in time, and the natural progression — untreated or after ineffective therapy — is toward dissemination.

Two other points deserve mention in understanding these disease processes. First, the cell type and disease progression may change with time to a less differentiated state. Patients with relatively well differentiated tumors may have subsequent biopsies that indicate less differentiation and even a stem cell–like picture. This is important to appreciate, because therapy may need to be changed drastically in form or intensity. A second point relates to the identification of the pattern of lymph node involvement. The term giant follicle lymphoma, originally proposed by Brill and Symmers, referred to a *benign* form of involvement. Subsequent investigators recognized the fact that some of these patients did indeed die of cancer and that nodular involvement (follicular) occurred in patients with Hodgkin's disease, lymphocytic lymphoma, and, rarely, histiocytic lymphoma. Data from several centers indicate that the involvement pattern of follicular or diffuse can be applied to most histologic subtypes except Burkitt's tumor. In general, the prognoses of nodular forms are better than those of corresponding histologic varieties with diffuse patterns.

The current approach to classification of lymphoreticular neoplasms, as well as the previously applied terms, is shown in the accompanying table. The use of this classification and the appreciation of chronologic

Classification of Lymphoreticular Neoplasms*

Proposed Name	Old Name
Lymphoma, lymphocytic type, well differentiated	Lymphosarcoma
Lymphoma, lymphocytic type, poorly differentiated	
Lymphoma, histiocytic type	Reticulum cell sarcoma
Lymphoma, mixed lymphocytic-histiocytic type	Mixed lymphoma
Lymphoma, undifferentiated pleomorphic type	Stem cell lymphoma
Lymphoma, undifferentiated Burkitt type	Stem cell lymphoma

*From Berard, 1972. All varieties except Burkitt's may be classified as nodular or diffuse.

changes in cell type should clear up many of the previous difficulties with confusing names that encompassed grossly different prognostic categories.

The diagnosis of lymphoreticular neoplasms must always be based on an adequate tissue biopsy. Occasionally, multiple biopsies may be needed before the decision as to pathologic classification can be definitively made. Imprint preparations as well as cytochemical studies will help clarify the specific cell type and degree of differentiation. More recently, specific markers of the cell surface such as immunoglobulin receptors, complement receptors, immunoglobulin fluorescence, or rosette cell formation have classified cell variants that heretofore were difficult or impossible to categorize. Current histologic variants may in fact be lymphocytic cells but with cytologic variations. Electron microscopy studies may also be helpful in identifying the nature of the cell involved in the malignant process.

Besides insisting on adequate tissue for diagnosis, the physician responsible for the patient's care must work in concert with the clinical pathologist, nuclear medicine specialist, radiologist, and surgeon to establish the extent of disease. This process is known as staging. The complete extent of staging procedures has not been determined. One must do a careful history and physical examination, asking for symptoms, examining all nodal areas, determining liver and spleen involvement, and searching for abdominal or testicular masses. Careful examination of the oropharynx is a necessity, because much lymphoid tissue is located in those regions. In addition to routine laboratory studies, radioisotope scans (particularly bone and ^{67}Ga studies), bone marrow biopsy, x-rays of chest and abdomen, intravenous pyelograms and lymphograms are all helpful in evaluating the extent of disease. Further emphasis on evaluating liver involvement has shown that liver function tests and even closed hepatic biopsies can be misleading. To achieve a greater degree of accuracy, laparoscopy with several direct biopsies of the liver and laparotomy have been used. Diagnostic laparotomy has been adopted by many centers because of the opportunity to do biopsies of other suspicious abdominal areas and to perform a splenectomy. In patients with Hodgkin's disease the spleen if involved seems to predict liver spread. The more extended procedures also aid in the shaping of radiotherapy fields to fit the specific pattern of involvement. The use of laparoscopy and laparotomy has demonstrated that often mesenteric or periportal lymph nodes may be involved but would not be included in the usual radiotherapy port. Since patients with lymphoreticular disorders tend to be older than patients with Hodgkin's disease and generalized dis-

ease is more common, these additional staging procedures must be justified on the basis of risk and morbidity in relation to possible therapeutic benefit. In general, the use of more extended surgical procedures to stage patients must be justified on the basis that the findings will have significant influence on approaches to therapy.

DIFFERENTIAL DIAGNOSIS.   The major considerations in the differential diagnosis of lymph node enlargement include infections, reactive lymphadenopathy, and other neoplastic illnesses. Principal among the infectious causes are diseases such as infectious mononucleosis, tuberculosis, syphilis, toxoplasmosis, cytomegalovirus infection, and many pediatric viral illnesses. Reactive hyperplasias of the lymph nodes may accompany acute or chronic infections of the extremities or throat, particularly after vaccinations. Lymphadenopathy has also been associated with diphenylhydantoin administration. Nonlymphoreticular neoplasms characteristically spread to local lymph nodes only. A careful search of the oropharynx and mucosal surfaces may reveal a primary cancer that should be biopsied rather than the neck nodes. Breast cancer may present as lymph node enlargement in the axilla with a small primary tumor in the breast that may escape initial evaluation. Occasionally, diffuse adenopathy with histologic features of a lymphoma can be seen in association with immunoglobulin abnormalities characteristic of Waldenström's macroglobulinemia. Differentiation between a primary macroglobulinemia and a lymphoma with paraproteinemia may be difficult. Immunoglobulin M paraproteinemia with lymphoma occurs in the diffuse varieties more often than in the nodular forms. Examination of the marrow may reveal the characteristic lymphoid plasma cell along with the hyperviscosity, purpura, and bleeding tendency in patients with macroglobulinemia.

501.   NON-HODGKIN'S LYMPHOMAS

Thomas E. Davis

The non-Hodgkin's lymphomas are a heterogeneous group of malignant neoplasms which arise from lymphoid components of the immune system. These disorders are histopathologically distinct from Hodgkin's disease and include the following subtypes: lymphocytic, histiocytic, mixed histiocytic and lymphocytic, pleomorphic (or stem cell type), and Burkitt's tumor (Burkitt's tumor is described in Ch. 502).

ETIOLOGY.   The cause of the non-Hodgkin's lymphomas is unknown. Although viruses have been shown to be associated with lymphoid tumors in several animal species, efforts to isolate infectious etiologic agents in humans have been unsuccessful. An increased frequency of lymphocytic lymphomas and Hodgkin's disease has been reported in survivors of the atomic bomb explosions in Japan. Patients with genetic or acquired disorders associated with immune deficiency are known to be predisposed to lymphoid malignancy. The genetic disorders include ataxia telangiectasia, the Wiskott-Aldrich syndrome, congenital sex-linked agammaglobulinemia, and the Chédiak-Higashi syndrome. The acquired disorders associated with an increased frequency of lymphoid malignancy include acquired hypogammaglobulinemia, Sjögren's disease, and certain of the autoimmune syndromes. In addition, patients with renal allografts and others receiving long-term immunosuppressive therapy have an increased incidence of malignant lymphoid neoplasms.

EPIDEMIOLOGY. In the United States, the non-Hodgkin's lymphomas are approximately twice as common as Hodgkin's disease. There were an estimated 14,500 new cases in 1977, representing 2 per cent of all new cancer diagnoses. The non-Hodgkin's lymphomas can occur in individuals of any age, although they are rare in children younger than two years and become increasingly frequent with advancing age. Worldwide there are striking variations in the incidence of certain types of non-Hodgkin's lymphoma. There is a high incidence of Burkitt's tumor among children in central Africa. Several investigators have observed an increased frequency of intestinal lymphoma associated with immunoglobulin abnormalities among individuals in the Middle East.

PATHOLOGY. The diagnosis and classification of a lymphoma must be based on careful evaluation of biopsy material. However, in certain instances it may be difficult to distinguish benign from malignant disorders. Misinterpretations with respect to histopathologic subclassification are also common. Frequently the distinction between leukemia and lymphoma cannot be made on the basis of biopsy alone. For these reasons, it is important in each case to integrate the biopsy findings with clinical information obtained from the patient's history, physical examination, peripheral blood, bone marrow, and other laboratory studies.

The non-Hodgkin's lymphomas have traditionally been classified according to their morphology under the light microscope. Most of the terminologies used to describe and classify these disorders were proposed long before the remarkable developments in immunology of recent years. It is now recognized that the immune system can be subdivided into several distinct populations of cells with varied physiologic functions. These cell populations can be distinguished on the basis of electron microscopy, cytochemistry, cell surface receptors, and functional characteristics. As newer techniques in immunology have been applied to the study of the non-Hodgkin's lymphomas, several new classification systems have been suggested. However, the ultimate value of these remains to be demonstrated. The ideal classification system should have three characteristics: (1) it should provide information that is clinically relevant in terms of predicting response or prognosis; (2) it should establish criteria sufficiently distinctive to yield reproducible results when applied by expert pathologists; and (3) it should be consistent with modern concepts of immunobiology. In the United States, the most widely utilized classification is the one originally proposed by Rappaport in 1966. This has been found by many investigators to be both clinically relevant and reproducible, although it does not incorporate some of the newer concepts regarding lymphocyte differentiation. This classification, with minor modifications, is presented in the table in Ch. 500. Characteristic histopathologic sections are shown in the accompanying figure.

The Rappaport classification is based upon two morphologic features: the cytologic characteristics of the cell populations and the histologic pattern of lymph node involvement. In general, patients with nodular involvement have a better prognosis then patients with a diffuse histologic pattern.

Lymphocytic, Well Differentiated Type. This variety of non-Hodgkin's lymphoma is characterized by a relatively homogeneous infiltrate of small, normal-appearing lymphocytes. The histologic pattern is identical to that of chronic lymphocytic leukemia. Well differentiated lymphocytic lymphoma may present either with focal lymph node enlargement or with generalized lymphadenopathy and splenomegaly. The bone marrow is usually involved. A monoclonal gammopathy may occur without appreciable numbers of plasmacytoid lymphocytes in the histologic sections. The disease most commonly occurs after the fifth decade and tends to be slowly progressive. Chronic lymphocytic leukemia, Waldenström's macroglobulinemia, and well differentiated lymphocytic lymphoma appear to represent different manifestations of a fundamentally similar disorder, namely, the proliferation of well differentiated B lymphocytes. Nevertheless, these entities differ sufficiently from each other in terms of laboratory features, natural history, prognosis, and other clinical aspects to justify their continued separation as distinct clinicopathologic entities. In young persons, these diseases are uncommon and a proliferation of normal-appearing lymphocytes is more frequently associated with a reactive process or occasionally with Hodgkin's disease of the lymphocyte predominant type.

Lymphocytic, Poorly Differentiated Type. In adults, these tumors arise primarily in the lymph nodes and are composed of cells which exhibit considerable variation in size, configuration, and degree of differentiation. The histology may be either nodular or diffuse. Patients with a nodular pattern of involvement have few symptoms at the time of presentation, and their prognosis is considerably better than that of patients with a diffuse histologic pattern. Although the bone marrow is frequently involved, only 5 to 10 per cent of adults with poorly differentiated lymphocytic lymphoma develop frank leukemia. Children most commonly present with abdominal, retroperitoneal, or mediastinal disease. A nodular histologic pattern is exceedingly rare. Progression to acute leukemia is very common in children, and involvement of the central nervous system occurs frequently.

Histiocytic Type. Although the malignant cells in histiocytic lymphoma resemble histiocytes morphologically, they are presently considered to be derived from lymphoid elements. These malignant cells tend to be large and irregular with relatively abundant cytoplasm which is frequently acidophilic. In certain instances, the cells may be multinucleate and difficult to distinguish from Reed-Sternberg cells. There may be increased reticulin associated with individual cells, but this feature is not a diagnostic criterion. The histologic pattern may be either nodular or diffuse. Histiocytic lymphoma occurs predominantly in adults, with increased frequency in the older age groups. Patients may present with either localized or widespread lymphadenopathy. However, extranodal presentations are more common with this disease than with the lymphocytic lymphomas. On the other hand, the bone marrow is involved in less than 10 per cent of the patients at the time of presentation, and progression to frank leukemia is rare.

Mixed Histiocytic-Lymphocytic Type. This variety

of non-Hodgkin's lymphoma is characterized by a mixed population of malignant cells, with the larger cells resembling histiocytes and the smaller ones appearing more like poorly differentiated lymphocytes. The histologic pattern is usually nodular at the time of presentation. In most cases, there is evolution with time and treatment, to a pattern of diffuse histiocytic lymphoma. This disease occurs predominantly in older adults who typically seek medical attention because of generalized lymphadenopathy.

Undifferentiated or Pleomorphic Type. These tumors are composed of undifferentiated cells which vary widely in size and may include bizarre giant forms. Subsequent differentiation to lymphocytic or histiocytic types may occur. These should not be confused with Burkitt's tumor, in which the malignant cells also lack evidence of cytologic differentiation but have a uniform and characteristic appearance in tissue sections and imprints.

Two disorders which share certain clinical and pathologic features with the non-Hodgkin's lymphomas deserve brief mention, although their position in the classification of lymphoid neoplasia remains to be clarified. *Angioimmunoblastic lymphadenopathy* is a systemic disease characterized by lymphadenopathy, hepatosplenomegaly, and constitutional symptoms. Anemia, lymphocytopenia, and polyclonal hypergammaglobulinemia are frequently present. The histologic picture is benign, consisting of immunoblasts, plasma cells, and proliferation of small vessels. Although the disease is responsive to therapy with prednisone or cytotoxic agents, the median survival is only three years. In about one third of the patients, transformation to a malignant lymphoblastic lymphoma may be observed on repeated biopsies or at autopsy. *Malignant lymphoma with a high content of epithelioid histiocytes* ("Lennert's lymphoma") resembles the diffuse, mixed cell lymphoma of the Rappaport classification. However, this entity can be distinguished morphologically by the presence of epithelioid cell clusters scattered throughout the stroma. Constitutional symptoms and bone marrow involvement are common. Patients respond poorly to chemotherapy, and the median survival is short.

CLINICAL MANIFESTATIONS. The most common clinical manifestation of non-Hodgkin's lymphoma is painless enlargement of one or more peripheral lymph nodes. The average patient has been aware of the enlarged lymph nodes for several months before consulting a physician. Systemic symptoms of fever, night sweats, or weight loss are usually not prominent. Anterior mediastinal adenopathy occurs infrequently as contrasted with Hodgkin's disease, in which 50 to 70 per cent of patients manifest mediastinal involvement. Lymphoid structures throughout the body may be involved, including the tissue within Waldeyer's ring and preauricular, epitrochlear, or mesenteric lymph nodes. Palpable *splenomegaly* occurs in about 20 per cent of the patients and is more frequently observed in the lymphocytic varieties.

Approximately one third of the patients with non-Hodgkin's lymphoma initially present with extranodal disease. This is most common in patients with diffuse histiocytic lymphoma and occurs infrequently in patients with nodular lymphocytic lymphoma. The *gastrointestinal tract* may be the primary site of disease or may be involved as part of a more generalized process. The stomach and small intestine are most often involved, although the pancreas is frequently found to be infiltrated at autopsy. Primary histiocytic lymphoma of the stomach may be confused with carcinoma. Symptoms and signs of gastrointestinal involvement include malabsorption, obstruction, perforation, and bleeding.

Hepatic enlargement and jaundice are uncommon presenting manifestations, but percutaneous biopsy will demonstrate liver involvement in about 20 per cent of patients. Further diagnostic procedures to evaluate the liver, including peritoneoscopy and laparotomy, increase the yield of positives to about 50 per cent. Jaundice, when it occurs, is usually caused by tumor infiltration of the liver, but in certain cases it may be due to extrahepatic biliary obstruction.

Although *impaired renal function* may occur secondary to direct parenchymal infiltration, it is more often due to obstruction of the urinary outflow. Other causes of renal dysfunction in patients with non-Hodgkin's lymphoma include compression of the renal vascular supply, hypercalcemia, hyperuricemia, amyloidosis, and radiation nephritis. Cardiac involvement is frequently noted at autopsy, but clinical manifestations are unusual. Primary lymphomas of the lung are rare, whereas secondary spread to the lungs is more common. Primary lymphomas also have been reported to occur in the bone, thyroid, testes, female genital organs, and salivary glands. Diffuse histiocytic lymphoma is the most commonly observed histologic pattern in patients with these extranodal presentations. Primary lymphomas of bone usually appear as lytic lesions and most frequently involve the femur, tibia, humerus, scapula, or pelvis.

A, Normal lymph node (×11). Nodal architecture clearly shows nodules, germinal centers, and sinuses, particularly under capsule.

B, Diffuse lymphoma (×7). The normal nodal architecture is completely obliterated by a diffuse infiltrate of lymphoid malignant cells. The capsule, although intact here, can be disrupted with tumor cells extending outside the lymph node.

C, Nodular lymphoma (×7). The nodal structure is replaced by large nodules of malignant cells. The subcapsular area reveals fibrosis characteristic of an inguinal lymph node.

D, Well differentiated lymphocytic lymphoma (×600). The malignant cells are small and uniform, with minimal cytoplasm, compact nuclear chromatin, and absence of mitoses.

E, Poorly differentiated lymphocytic lymphoma (×600). The cell size varies, particularly nuclear size with occasional mitoses. The nuclei are often irregular in shape. The nuclear chromatin is finely dispersed.

F, Mixed lymphocytic-histiocytic lymphoma (×600). Two morphologic populations of cells are clearly seen, small irregular lymphoid cells and large histiocytic cells with prominent nuclei.

G, Histiocytic lymphoma (×600). The cells are large and irregular, with clearly evident cytoplasm and large nucleoli.

H, Undifferentiated, non-Burkitt (×600). The pleomorphic cells are large and lack clear histologic differentiation with primitive nuclear pattern. A large multinucleate cell is also seen.

(Illustrations were kindly supplied by Dr. Costan Berard, Head, Hematopathology Section, Laboratory of Pathology, National Cancer Institute.)

The most common *neurologic manifestation* of lymphoma is spinal cord compression resulting from extradural tumor. Meningeal involvement is unusual in adults, generally a late manifestation of the disease. In children, central nervous system involvement is much more common, occurring in about 25 per cent of patients. Parenchymal brain involvement is rare, but has been noted to occur in patients with renal allografts.

The non-Hodgkin's lymphomas may occur as primary *skin* tumors. More frequently the skin is involved as part of a more generalized disease process. *Sézary's syndrome*, a T cell variant of the non-Hodgkin's lymphomas, is characterized by chronic erythroderma with diffuse infiltration of the dermis and characteristic abnormal lymphocytes in the peripheral blood.

Bone marrow is invaded in about one third of the patients with non-Hodgkin's lymphoma, but the incidence of this varies considerably among the different histologic types. The bone marrow biopsy may be positive at the time of presentation in more than half the patients with diffuse well differentiated lymphocytic lymphoma or nodular poorly differentiated lymphocytic disease.

Most patients with lymphoma have normal peripheral blood counts early in their clinical course. However, nearly 50 per cent will develop *anemia* as their disease progresses. The causes of anemia include marrow replacement, hypersplenism, autoimmune hemolytic anemia, hemorrhage, and marrow hypoplasia resulting from chemotherapy or irradiation. The peripheral white blood counts are usually normal, but lymphocytosis may occur, particularly in association with well differentiated lymphocytic lymphoma. A small number of characteristic notched or cleft cells may be seen in the peripheral blood of patients with nodular, poorly differentiated lymphocytic lymphoma. The conversion to a frank *leukemic phase* is uncommon in adults, but may occur with any of the histologic varieties of lymphoma. In children, leukemic conversion is observed in about 25 per cent of the patients.

STAGING. After establishing the diagnosis of non-Hodgkin's lymphoma, the next responsibility of the physician is to obtain an adequate assessment of the extent of disease. Careful staging prior to the initiation of therapy is important for several reasons: (1) to provide an estimate of prognosis, (2) to aid in the selection of an appropriate treatment program, and (3) to establish a precise point of reference which will later permit accurate assessment of the response to therapy. A standardized system of diagnostic procedures and descriptive terminology is also important in facilitating the comparison of therapeutic results among patients treated in different medical centers with a variety of treatment programs.

The continuing evolution in the staging of Hodgkin's disease over a period of 40 years culminated in the adoption of the Ann Arbor staging classification in 1971. This classification system, shown in Table 1, has also been widely applied to the staging of the non-Hodgkin's lymphomas. The Ann Arbor system has proved to be of exceptional value in the management of patients with Hodgkin's disease. However, the prognosis of patients with non-Hodgkin's lymphoma is influenced to such an important degree by the histologic classification that the Ann Arbor staging system is of limited clinical value. As an example, certain patients who present with what appears to be a localized form

TABLE 1. Ann Arbor Staging Classification

Stage I:	Involvement of a single lymph node region (I) or a single extralymphatic site (IE)
Stage II:	Involvement of two or more lymph node regions on the same side of the diaphragm (II) or a solitary extralymphatic site and one or more of lymph node areas on the same side of the diaphragm (IIE)
Stage III:	Involvement of lymph node regions on both sides of the diaphragm (III), accompanied by spleen involvement (IIIS), or by solitary involvement of an extralymphatic organ or site (IIIE) or both (IIISE)
Stage IV:	Diffuse involvement of extralymphatic sites with or without lymph node enlargement

Clinical stage and pathologic stage defined for each patient; extranodal sites are designated by specific denominators; presence or absence of symptoms is designated B or A, respectively

of diffuse histiocytic lymphoma may develop rapidly fatal disease progression in spite of intensive treatment. Conversely, many patients with nodular lymphocytic lymphoma that is widespread at the time of initial presentation may experience a very indolent clinical course for several years with only a minimum of therapy. Despite these limitations, the Ann Arbor classification does provide a standardized system of terminology which has facilitated the comparison of therapeutic results among patients treated in different medical centers.

The staging procedures currently recommended for patients with non-Hodgkin's lymphoma are shown in Table 2. These must include a careful clinical history and a thorough physical examination, with a description of all superficial lymph nodes and of the lymphoid structures within Waldeyer's ring. It is also important to obtain chest x-rays, complete blood counts, and serum chemistry determinations. In recent years, the use of more invasive staging procedures has become increasingly common. These procedures include lymphangiography, bone marrow biopsy, percutaneous liver biopsy, peritoneoscopy, and exploratory laparotomy. Widespread use of these techniques has demonstrated that the likelihood of detecting occult lesions increases in proportion to the diagnostic effort employed. Several studies have indicated that the incidence of Stage I or II disease may be about 20 to 30 per cent in patients with a diffuse histologic pattern and as low as 10 per cent in patients with nodular lymphoma.

The *retroperitoneal lymphangiogram* is a major tool in the evaluation of patients with non-Hodgkin's lymphoma. In this procedure, a radiopaque dye is injected into the small lymphatics of the foot under pressure. The dye is taken up by the abdominal lymph nodes and can then be seen in roentgenograms of the abdomen for several months afterward, permitting assessment of treatment response. False-negative studies occur in only

TABLE 2. Staging Procedures

1. History and physical examination
2. Chest x-rays and tomograms as indicated
3. Complete blood counts
4. Liver function tests, serum electrophoresis, BUN, and creatinine
5. Bone marrow biopsy
6. Lower extremity lymphogram
7. Intravenous pyelogram
8. Bone and liver scans
9. Laparoscopy
10. Laparotomy when indicated

15 per cent of the patients with non-Hodgkin's lymphoma, and false-positive findings are even less common. The lymphangiogram is positive at the time of presentation in 75 to 90 per cent of patients with a nodular histologic pattern. At staging laparotomy, most of these patients will have additional sites of subdiaphragmatic involvement. A normal lymphangiogram does not exclude subdiaphragmatic disease. Involvement of the spleen and mesenteric lymph nodes occurs in about half the patients with nodular lymphoma who have a normal lymphangiogram. The lymphangiogram is initially positive in approximately 50 per cent of the patients with a diffuse histologic pattern. At laparotomy, most of these patients will also have additional foci of disease in the spleen, mesenteric lymph nodes, or liver. However, patients with diffuse histology and negative lymphangiogram rarely have subdiaphragmatic involvement.

In recent years, *exploratory laparotomy and splenectomy* have been widely employed in the staging evaluation of patients with Hodgkin's disease. These studies have demonstrated that Hodgkin's disease usually presents with an orderly pattern of involvement. Data obtained from meticulous surgical staging can serve as an important guide to therapy, particularly in the selection of appropriate radiotherapy fields. In patients with non-Hodgkin's lymphoma, the indications for exploratory laparotomy are far less certain and the routine use of this staging technique cannot be recommended. A sequential approach to staging would appear to be the most reasonable strategy in these patients. In the majority of patients with nodular lymphoma, biopsy of the bone marrow along with percutaneous liver biopsy or peritoneoscopy will yield evidence of disseminated disease. In patients with either nodular or diffuse lymphoma, a positive lymphangiogram is so frequently associated with involvement outside the usual nodal irradiation fields that a decision to employ systemic therapy may be based upon the positive lymphangiogram alone. Exploratory laparotomy would appear to be of value in the selection of therapy only for patients with Stage I or II disease in whom the bone marrow biopsy, lymphangiogram, and closed liver biopsy are negative. The potential clinical benefits of laparotomy must also be weighed against the expected complications of this procedure, which may be increased in elderly patients or in patients with associated medical illnesses. If the treatment program will not be influenced by laparotomy regardless of the findings, then surgical exploration is not justified.

TREATMENT. The most effective modalities for the treatment of non-Hodgkin's lymphoma are irradiation and chemotherapy. Historically, surgery was employed not only to establish the diagnosis but also to remove localized tumor masses. However, surgery alone rarely resulted in long-term control of the disease.

Radiotherapy. The non-Hodgkin's lymphomas are generally considered to be among the most radiosensitive human neoplasms. It is frequently possible to achieve permanent control of individual tumors with doses of irradiation in the range of 3500 to 5000 rads. However, the curative potential of radiotherapy is severely limited by the fact that the vast majority of patients present with widely disseminated disease. Most authorities would agree that radiotherapy alone is the treatment of choice only for carefully staged patients with localized disease. Approximately 60 per cent of

patients with Stage I disease and 30 per cent with Stage II disease will be relapse-free at five years following radiotherapy. The use of total nodal radiotherapy does not appear to have improved these figures.

Extralymphatic structures are involved in about one third of the relapses which occur following radiotherapy. It is also common for relapses to occur in lymph nodes located outside the fields normally used for total nodal radiotherapy. These patterns of relapse have suggested that it may not be possible to improve cure rates through the refinement of conventional radiotherapy methods. An alternative approach utilizing *total body irradiation* has been proposed by several investigators. With this technique, about 15 rads is administered to the entire body twice a week until a total of approximately 150 rads is delivered or until severe hematopoietic depression occurs. This total dose of 150 rads is far below the doses of 3500 to 5000 rads delivered within conventional radiotherapy fields. However, the total body technique has the advantage of reaching sites of occult disease which must be excluded from conventional fields. Total body irradiation has most frequently been employed in patients with advanced lymphocytic lymphoma whose potential for cure with either chemotherapy or conventional radiotherapy is very low. Nevertheless, about 80 per cent of previously untreated patients have achieved a complete remission. This technique is now being compared with chemotherapy or conventional radiotherapy in prospective clinical trials.

Palliative radiotherapy continues to play an important role in the management of bulky masses and in the control of specific symptoms. In patients with advanced disease, lymphomatous masses may encroach on vital structures, resulting in serious morbidity. Obstruction of the ureters, bowel, or upper airway, as well as extradural compression of the spinal cord, represents a medical emergency. In these clinical situations, radiotherapy may be very effective in relieving symptoms and preventing irreversible damage. Radiotherapy to the brain combined with intrathecal chemotherapy is useful in controlling meningeal involvement.

Chemotherapy. The non-Hodgkin's lymphomas are highly responsive to a wide variety of chemotherapeutic agents. The response rates and major toxicities of the most effective drugs are shown in Table 3. In the past, most patients with advanced disease were treated with single agents. A high percentage of these patients exhibited an objective response to chemotherapy, but complete responses were uncommon. Patients who achieved only a partial response to treatment with a single drug generally relapsed within six months, in spite of maintenance therapy. Patients with nodular lymphomas exhibited a higher rate of complete response, as well as a longer duration of remission and survival, when compared to patients with diffuse lymphomas.

Combination chemotherapy was introduced into the treatment of patients with non-Hodgkin's lymphomas in the late 1960's. The goal of combination drug treatment was to improve the complete response rate without increasing the degree of bone marrow suppression. Several of the more effective drug combinations that have been developed over the past ten years are shown in Table 4. Each of these combinations contains three or more of the most active single agents. The use of combination chemotherapy has increased the rate of complete remission to between 40 and 80 per cent, de-

TABLE 3. Response Rates and Major Toxicities of the Single Agents*

Drug	Response Rate (%) Lymphocytic	Response Rate (%) Histiocytic	Major Toxicities
Nitrogen mustard	50–70	40–50	Bone marrow suppression; nausea and vomiting
Cyclophosphamide	50–70	50–70	Bone marrow suppression; nausea and vomiting; cystitis; alopecia
Chlorambucil	40–60	20–30	Bone marrow suppression
Prednisone	60–80	20–30	Fluid retention; diabetes; psychosis; increased susceptibility to infection
Vincristine	40–65	40–80	Peripheral neuropathy; paralytic ileus; alopecia
Vinblastine	15–25	20–35	Bone marrow suppression; nausea and vomiting; peripheral neuropathy; alopecia
Procarbazine	40–50	20–35	Bone marrow suppression; nausea and vomiting
Adriamycin	35–50	50–65	Bone marrow suppression; nausea and vomiting; cardiomyopathy; alopecia
Bleomycin	30–40	30–40	Fever and chills; stomatitis; dermatitis; pulmonary fibrosis; alopecia
BCNU, CCNU, Me-CCNU	20–30	25–35	Bone marrow suppression; nausea and vomiting
Imidazole-carboxamide	20–25	10	Bone marrow suppression; nausea and vomiting
Methotrexate	15–25	15–25	Bone marrow suppression; stomatitis and enteritis; dermatitis
Cytosine arabinoside	20–25	15–20	Bone marrow suppression

*Modified from Bonadonna, G., et al.: Eur. J. Cancer, *12*:661, 1976.

pending on the histologic subtype. In general, patients who achieve a complete response experience a longer median survival than nonresponding patients or those who achieve only a partial response. The long-term results of several chemotherapy trials have suggested that some patients with diffuse histiocytic, nodular histiocytic, and nodular mixed cell lymphomas may be cured with drug combinations. In one series, for example, 10 of 11 complete responders with diffuse histiocytic lymphoma were alive and free of disease from 26 to 105 months following the completion of treatment. The im-

pact of combination chemotherapy on the survival of patients with lymphocytic lymphomas is not as clear. Although 80 per cent of these patients may achieve complete remission with drug combination, relapses continue to occur as late as five years after completion of treatment. Several more years of observation will be required to determine whether a small fraction of patients with lymphocytic lymphoma might have been cured as a result of combination chemotherapy.

Combined Radiotherapy and Chemotherapy. The most common sites of relapse following chemotherapy

TABLE 4. Representative Drug Combinations

Reference	Drug Regimen		Response (%)	Complete Response (%)
Bagley (1972)	Cyclophosphamide Vincristine Prednisone	400 mg/M² PO days 1–5 1.4 mg/M² IV day 1 100 mg/M² PO days 1–5 } Repeat q 3 wks	91	57
McKelvey (1976)	Adriamycin Vincristine Prednisone	80 mg/M² IV day 1 1.4 mg/M² IV day 1 100 mg PO days 1–5 } Repeat q 3 wks	88	61
Stein (1974)	Cyclophosphamide Vincristine Procarbazine Prednisone	600 mg/M² IV days 1 and 8 1.4 mg/M² IV days 1 and 8 100 mg/M² PO days 1–10 40 mg/M² PO days 1–14 } Repeat q 4 wks	82	68
McKelvey (1976)	Cyclophosphamide Adriamycin Vincristine Prednisone	750 mg/M² IV day 1 50 mg/M² IV day 1 1.4 mg/M² IV day 1 100 mg PO days 1–5 } Repeat q 3 wks	92	71
Berd (1975)	Cyclophosphamide Vincristine Methotrexate Cytosine arabinoside	1500 mg/M² IV day 1 1.4 mg/M² IV days 1,8,15 120 mg/M² PO + Leucovorin weekly × 8 (day 22–71) 300 mg/M² IV weekly × 8 (day 22–71) } Repeat q 12 wks	100	60
Rodriguez (1977)	Cyclophosphamide* Adriamycin* Vincristine Prednisone Bleomycin†	750 mg/M² IV day 1 50 mg/M² IV day 1 1.2 mg/M² IV days 1 and 5 100 mg PO days 1–5 15 units IV days 1–5 } Repeat q 3 wks	92	66

*Starting dose to be reduced by 20 per cent for patients with prior extensive radiotherapy or hypocellular bone marrow (<20 per cent).
†Dose to be reduced to 4 units per square meter on days 1 and 5 for patients older than 60 years.

are the documented sites of initial involvement. Conversely, the most likely sites of relapse following radiotherapy are unirradiated nodal and extranodal sites remote from the area of initial involvement. Therefore it would appear reasonable to manage patients with Stage I, II, or III disease by treating the sites of documented involvement with irradiation and the sites of clinically occult disease with chemotherapy. Several controlled clinical trials designed to test this hypothesis are now in progress. At present, none of these has provided evidence that the combination of radiotherapy and chemotherapy is superior to either modality alone. However, judgment regarding the ultimate value of combined therapy should be reserved until more information becomes available.

Recommended Therapy. The proper management of any patient with non-Hodgkin's lymphoma generally requires close collaboration between attending physician, medical oncologist, experienced pathologist, radiation therapist, and, frequently, skilled surgeon. The final therapeutic decision must take into account the histologic type of lymphoma, the pattern of lymph node involvement, the state of disease, and the general medical condition of the patient.

Although the therapy of patients with non-Hodgkin's lymphoma is presently undergoing rapid evolution, certain basic recommendations appear to be valid. Patients with Stage I or II diffuse, well differentiated lymphocytic lymphoma may be treated with involved-field radiotherapy alone, although most will ultimately relapse after a long disease-free interval. Patients with this histologic subtype who present with Stage III or IV disease should probably be treated with chlorambucil alone, since their clinical course is usually quite indolent.

Patients with Stage I or II disease of the other histologic varieties should be treated with radiotherapy alone, unless they are candidates for controlled clinical trials of combined-modality therapy. When the primary site of involvement is in the peripheral lymph nodes or in extranodal sites outside the abdomen, radiotherapy is generally given to the involved fields and to adjacent normal lymph nodes. For patients with localized disease in the abdomen, consideration should be given to techniques which can deliver irradiation to the whole abdomen. The use of total nodal radiotherapy or total body irradiation has not been shown to enhance the cure rates in patients with Stage I or II disease.

Patients with Stage III or IV diffuse histiocytic, nodular histiocytic, or nodular mixed lymphomas should be treated aggressively with a drug combination of the types listed in Table 4. These patients are potentially curable if they achieve complete remission with their initial chemotherapeutic program.

There is considerable variation of opinion regarding the optimal therapy for patients with Stage III or IV nodular lymphocytic lymphoma. Certain highly selected patients whose disease was asymptomatic at the time of initial presentation have been followed without any treatment for periods up to several years. Although complete response rates have been reported to be higher with combination chemotherapy, the use of sequential single agent therapy appears to yield equivalent median survival figures. Long-term remissions have also been reported with total body irradiation, although, again, median survival does not seem to have been improved with this technique.

Patients with Stage III or IV diffuse, poorly differentiated lymphocytic lymphoma should probably be treated with combination chemotherapy. The average clinical course of these is not as indolent as that of patients with nodular lymphocytic disease. On the other hand, it has not yet been demonstrated that a significant percentage will be cured as a result of combination chemotherapy.

SELECTED CLINICAL PROBLEMS. The rapid turnover of tumor cells in patients with non-Hodgkin's lymphoma may result in the production of increased quantities of uric acid. Treatment with either chemotherapy or irradiation may further increase the size of the uric acid pool owing to metabolism of nucleic acids released during rapid tumor cell destruction. *Acute uric acid nephropathy* was once a relatively common complication of initial therapy. For this reason, it is currently recommended that allopurinol, a metabolic inhibitor of xanthine oxidase, be administered routinely at the start of therapy, along with enough fluids to ensure an adequate urine output. Patients with non-Hodgkin's lymphoma are also at *increased risk of infection* because of immune disturbances resulting from therapy or induced by the disease itself. Infectious complications must be adequately diagnosed prior to the initiation of antimicrobial therapy, since they are frequently caused by unusual organisms. These include herpes zoster, cytomegalovirus, *Cryptococcus, Candida, Listeria, Nocardia, Pneumocystis,* and *Toxoplasma.* Most of the modern chemotherapy and radiotherapy regimens are safe enough for administration to outpatients and are not designed to produce severe bone marrow depression. However, platelet and white cell transfusions should be available for the occasional patient who develops severe pancytopenia during the course of treatment.

PROGNOSIS. The outlook for many patients with non-Hodgkin's lymphoma has improved in recent years. This improvement has not resulted from the introduction of new treatment methods. It has occurred gradually as our understanding of lymphoid neoplasia has increased, and as the available treatment methods have been refined and applied with greater precision. It is now possible to identify a group of patients with localized disease who can be cured with radiotherapy alone. It is also possible to define a group of patients with advanced disease who can be cured with chemotherapy alone. The challenge for the future is to integrate the best available radiotherapy techniques and chemotherapy regimens to improve the management of patients who presently cannot be cured with either modality. This will require effective collaboration between medical oncologists and radiotherapists in the implementation of well-designed, prospective clinical trials.

Bagley, C. M., Jr., DeVita, V. T., Jr., Berard, C. W., and Canellos, G. P.: Advanced lymphosarcoma: Intensive cyclical combination chemotherapy with cyclophosphamide, vincristine, and prednisone. Ann. Intern. Med., 76:227, 1972.

Banks, P. M., and Berard, C. W.: Lymphoreticular disorders; malignant proliferative response; lymphoma: Histopathology of the malignant lymphomas. In Williams, W. J., Beutler, E., Erslev, A. J., and Rundles, R. W. (eds.): Hematology. New York, McGraw-Hill Book Company, 1977, p. 1026.

Berd, D., Cornog, J., DeConti, R. C., Levitt, M., and Bertino, J. R.: Long-term remission in diffuse histiocytic lymphoma treated with combination sequential chemotherapy. Cancer, 35:1050, 1975.

Bonadonna, G., Lattuada, A., and Banfi, A.: Recent trends in the treatment of non-Hodgkin's lymphoma. Eur. J. Cancer, 12:661, 1976.

Carbone, P. P., and DeVita, V. T.: Malignant lymphoma. In Holland, J. F., and Frei, E., III (eds.): Cancer Medicine. Philadelphia, Lea & Febiger, 1973, p. 1302.

Jones, S. E., and Godden, J. (eds.): Proceedings of the conference of non-Hodgkin's lymphomas. Cancer Treat. Rep., 61:935, 1977.

McKelvey, E. M., Gottlieb, J. A., Wilson, H. E., Haut, A., Talley, R. W., Stephens, R., Lane, M., Gamble, J. F., Jones, S. E., Grozea, P. N., Gutterman, J., Coltman, C., Jr., and Moon, T. E.: Hydroxyldaunomycin (Adriamycin) combination chemotherapy in malignant lymphoma. Cancer, 38:1484, 1976.

Rodriguez, V., Cabanillas, F., Burgess, M. A., McKelvey, E. M., Valdivieso, M., Bodey, G. P., and Freireich, E. J.: Combination chemotherapy ("CHOP-Bleo") in advanced (non-Hodgkin) malignant lymphoma. Blood, 49:325, 1977.

Stein, R. S., Moran, E. M., Desser, R. K., Miller, J. B., Golomb, H. M., and Ultmann, J. E.: Combination chemotherapy of lymphomas other than Hodgkin's disease. Ann. Intern. Med., 81:601, 1974.

502. BURKITT'S LYMPHOMA

Paul P. Carbone

Burkitt's lymphoma has attracted a great deal of interest because of its unique geographical distribution, response to treatment, and epidemiologic features highly suggestive of an infectious origin. The clinical and pathologic features were originally described by Dennis Burkitt, a British surgeon, in East Africa in 1958. Burkitt's lymphoma also occurs in the United States, South America, and New Guinea. In Africa, Burkitt's lymphoma accounts for over 80 per cent of all childhood lymphomas; the incidence in the United States is not known, but more than 200 cases have been reported. The features of the disease and response to treatment are quite similar in Africa and in the United States.

ETIOLOGY AND PATHOGENESIS. Burkitt's observations suggested that there were climatic restrictions for expression of this disease in Africa. These were weather and terrain conditions conducive to malaria, i.e., adequate rainfall and lack of freezing temperatures. Epidemiologic studies have confirmed these initial observations as well as time-space clustering of cases, further suggesting a viral etiology. Serologic and virologic studies of Burkitt's lymphoma in Africa have indicated that the Epstein-Barr virus (EBV) was associated with 90 per cent of the cases. In the United States only 44 per cent are associated with elevated EBV titers. More recently, EBV has been proposed as the cause of infectious mononucleosis and possibly as a passenger virus in Burkitt's lymphoma. Malaria has also been associated with Burkitt's lymphoma, because those places that have eliminated malaria do not have a high incidence of this tumor. Malaria has been implicated as a possible co-carcinogen, i.e., priming the reticuloendothelial system, or as an immunosuppressive agent. Reverse transcriptase (RNA-dependent DNA polymerase) and Rauscher virus material have been found in some tumors. Despite all these associations, the cause of Burkitt's lymphoma and the causes of its peculiar distribution have not been uncovered.

PATHOLOGY. Burkitt's lymphoma, histologically, contains undifferentiated lymphoid cells of uniform size. Burkitt's lymphoma has the membrane markers characteristic of a B cell with IgM heavy chains on the surface. The nuclei are round and vesicular with prominent nucleoli. The cytoplasm is basophilic with small vacuoles shown to contain fat by special stains. Large histiocytes ingesting tumor debris are scattered throughout the section. The cells can be differentiated from other lymphomas by their characteristic large size and lack of differentiation.

CLINICAL FEATURES. The tumor affects primarily children. The average age in Africa is 9 years, as compared to 12 years in the United States. Males are slightly more prone to develop the disease than are females. The clinical history of illness is short. In Africa, the most common presenting features relate to facial tumors (60 per cent). Abdominal masses occur in 30 per cent, usually as a result of ovarian, mesenteric, or retroperitoneal tumors. Peripheral adenopathy, splenomegaly, and/or hepatomegaly are rarely the main presenting features. Neurologic manifestations, such as paraplegia, cranial nerve paresis, and/or meningeal involvement, occur less frequently (10 per cent). In American patients abdominal manifestations predominate (75 per cent), and less than 25 per cent present with primary localized involvement elsewhere. Hematologic manifestations, such as marrow involvement and/or frank leukemia, are rare in contrast to other childhood lymphomas.

Because these tumors grow rapidly and because they involve the kidneys or obstruct the ureters, hyperuricemia and azotemia are common. The serum LDH may be extremely elevated and is of prognostic value; generally, high abnormal values that do not fall are associated with the poorest results. Metabolically, the tumor produces large amounts of lactic acid, and lactic acidosis may be an added complication. After chemotherapy, tumor lysis may be so rapid that hyperkalemia may be fatal unless treated prophylactically by maintaining high fluid volumes and frequent serum K^+ determinations.

DIAGNOSIS. The diagnosis can be established only by biopsy, because many of the clinical features, even in endemic areas, can be mimicked by other lymphomas, acute granulocytic leukemia (chloromas), and pediatric solid tumors such as Wilms' tumor, retinoblastomas, embryonal rhabdomyosarcomas, and neuroblastoma. Cytologic material should be prepared by touching a freshly cut surface of the tumor to the glass slides and then staining with standard hematologic techniques.

In the absence of the classic jaw tumor, Burkitt's lymphoma may not be suspected. The surgeon may first encounter the disease in the abdomen at laparotomy because of an expanding mass or intestinal obstruction. Attempts should be made to debulk the tumor as much as possible, because this may improve the over-all prognosis. Additional staging procedures include intravenous pyelogram, bone survey, bone marrow biopsy, lumbar puncture, lymphograms, and ^{67}gallium scans. It must be emphasized, however, that the tumor grows so fast that undue delay may be deleterious to the patient's eventual prognosis. Clinical staging schemes have generally acknowledged the good prognosis of facial tumors and limited abdominal disease. Conversely, central nervous system and bone marrow involvement convey a poor prognosis.

MANAGEMENT AND PROGNOSIS. Even in the localized cases, chemotherapy plays a major role in management. Cyclophosphamide has been the major therapeutic agent. Despite rapid response and apparent clinical remissions with this or with combination programs, many of these patients will relapse. More recently, Ziegler and coworkers have employed high dose chemotherapy with autologous marrow transplantation.

When complete remission has been achieved, maintenance treatment has not been shown to be of value. X-ray therapy has not been useful in this disease except for treatment of obstructive symptoms. Ninety per cent of all patients achieve complete disappearance of tumor. About 30 per cent of these patients never relapse. The disease in one third of the remaining patients recurs early or produces central nervous system manifestations. These patients have a poor prognosis and will die usually in six months. The remainder have late recurrence (after six months) after a complete response. Characteristically, they respond to the same initial treatment. As mentioned above, care must be taken to prevent or manage the metabolic complications, particularly hyperuricemia, lactic acidosis, and hyperkalemia.

The long-term survival with Burkitt's lymphoma both in the United States and in Africa is extremely good, about 50 to 60 per cent. Best results are obtained in those patients with localized disease. Extensive abdominal disease or liver, central nervous system, or bone marrow involvement carries the poorest prognosis. Despite the strong evidence for tumor-associated antigens and spontaneous regressions in some patients, immunotherapy with BCG and/or allogenic tumor cells has not been shown to be better than chemotherapy alone.

Burkitt, D., and O'Conor, G. T.: Malignant lymphoma in African children: Clinical syndrome. Cancer, 14:256, 1966.
Cohen, M. H., et al.: Burkitt's tumor in the United States. Cancer, 23:1259, 1969.
Ziegler, J. L., et al.: Burkitt's lymphoma — a model for intensive chemotherapy. Semin. Oncol., 4:317, 1977.
Ziegler, J. L., and Magrath, I. T.: Burkitt's lymphoma. Pathobiology Annual 129. New York, Appleton-Century-Crofts, 1974.

503. HODGKIN'S DISEASE

Saul A. Rosenberg

DEFINITION AND HISTORY. Hodgkin's disease can be defined as a malignant disease, usually arising in the lymph nodes, with a histopathologic appearance which includes characteristic giant cells in an appropriate cellular background. The affliction has challenged clinicians and investigators because of its unknown etiology, its clinical and histopathologic features suggesting a granulomatous infection as well as neoplasia, the extreme variability of its microscopic and clinical picture, its peculiar associated immunologic abnormalities, and its frequent responsiveness to modern therapeutic approaches, which can result in cure of the disease.

In the absence of a known etiology or satisfactory animal model, it can be challenged that the characteristic giant cell of Hodgkin's disease, the so-called Reed-Sternberg cell, identifies a single disease entity. Nonetheless, considerable information and literature have supported the clinical value of considering Hodgkin's disease as a disease which can be variable yet reasonably predictable in its expression.

Thomas Hodgkin's name has been immortalized for his description, in 1832, of seven patients with a fatal illness in a report entitled On Some Morbid Appearances of the Absorbent Glands and Spleen. On later histopathologic review, Fox confirmed only two of Hodgkin's cases, but on clinical grounds suggested that a third patient of the original seven belonged to the entity now bearing Hodgkin's name.

Although numerous names have been given to this disease, such as *lymphogranuloma, lymphogranulomatosis, lymphadenoma*, and *malignant granuloma*, the name of Hodgkin's disease, initially suggested by Sir Samuel Wilks, has now received international recognition. Many pathologists have contributed to the characterization of this disease, but Dorothy Reed and Carl Sternberg are given credit for the clearest description of the virtually pathognomonic giant cell which bears their names.

ETIOLOGY AND PATHOGENESIS. The cause of Hodgkin's disease is unknown. Athough various etiologic agents, including bacteria, protozoa, and viruses, have been proposed, none have withstood the tests of time and confirmation. The problem of secondary invaders in the infection-susceptible patient with late-stage Hodgkin's disease has plagued the efforts of investigators for almost a century. The very nature of Hodgkin's disease, whether infectious in the usual sense or neoplastic, has long been a controversy and remains unsettled. The finding of aneuploidy and marker chromosomes in cells from Hodgkin's disease tissue is preliminary evidence that Hodgkin's disease is a true neoplasm. Whether this holds for all clinical and histologic types of the disease remains to be determined.

It is not yet established which, if any, of the mononuclear cells in tumor tissue are malignant or premalignant. There is preliminary evidence suggesting that the Reed-Sternberg cell is derived from a B lymphocyte and conflicting evidence that the giant cell is phagocytic and derived from monocyte-histiocyte precursors. There is good evidence that the Reed-Sternberg cell is surrounded by T lymphocytes, and early tumor involvement is found in the T lymphocyte zones of lymph nodes and the spleen.

Any view of the cause of Hodgkin's disease must take into account the wide variety of histopathologic and clinical pictures, the usual rarity of neoplastic-appearing giant cells, the signs of an inflammatory reaction, the frequent infection-like symptoms, its anatomic predilections, its characteristic immunologic deficiencies, and its peculiar epidemiologic characteristics.

EPIDEMIOLOGY. In the United States the annual incidence of Hodgkin's disease is 35 per million for white males and 26 per million for white females, with an annual death rate of 23 per million and 13 per million, respectively. Nonwhites have a somewhat lower reported incidence than whites in all age groups, although the rates approach each other in the age range between 35 and 59 years. Hodgkin's disease has an unusual bimodal age-specific incidence curve, with one mode at ages 15 to 34 and another after the age of 50. The disease is distributed throughout the world, but the incidence peaks differ somewhat for various regions, e.g., absence of the first age mode in Japan.

Approximately 60 to 65 per cent of reported patients are male; 85 per cent of children with disease at age ten or younger are male, but between ages 15 and 35 the sex incidence is about the same.

Occurrence of the disease in two or more members of the same family has been documented in numerous reports and studies. Although the data are inadequate, it is likely that close relatives of patients with Hodgkin's disease experience a slightly increased risk of developing the disease. Observations suggesting a higher incidence of Hodgkin's disease among close unrelated contacts of those with the disease have been made.

PATHOLOGY. The minimal requirement for the pathologic diagnosis of Hodgkin's disease is the presence of characteristic giant cells of the Reed-Sternberg type in

TABLE 1. Histopathologic Classification
of Hodgkin's Disease

Relative Frequency (%)	Jackson and Parker	Rye, 1965	Relative Frequency (%)
5–10	Paragranuloma→	Lymphocyte predominance	10–15
80–90	Granuloma<	→Nodular sclerosis	40–70
		→Mixed cellularity	20–40
5–10	Sarcoma——→	Lymphocyte depletion	5–15

an appropriate histologic setting. The morphologic findings, however, can be very diverse.

The most reliable characteristics of the Reed-Sternberg cell are the large inclusion-like nucleoli and the double or multiple nuclei of large size. Mononuclear forms are also found in typical lesions of Hodgkin's disease, but cannot be considered as reliably diagnostic. The Reed-Sternberg cells may vary considerably in appearance, depending on the type of histologic response and category. The distinctive multinucleated giant cells associated with the nodular sclerosis variety are presumed to be variants of the Reed-Sternberg cell, with abundant pale eosinophilic cytoplasm, well-defined cellular borders in lacuna-like spaces (in formalin-fixed tissue) with small to medium-sized nucleoli, and an unusual hyperlobation.

Cells indistinguishable from, or closely resembling, Reed-Sternberg cells may be found in conditions other than Hodgkin's disease. The appropriate cellular and architectural environment for these cells is required to permit the diagnosis of Hodgkin's disease.

The Rye histopathologic classification, proposed in 1965, has largely replaced the older Jackson and Parker classification. The relative frequency of the subgroups of these classifications is shown in Table 1. The major advantage of the Rye classification lies in recognition of the important subgroup of nodular sclerosis described by Lukes and his colleagues.

CLINICAL MANIFESTATIONS. The presenting and subsequent clinical manifestations of patients with Hodgkin's disease can be extremely varied and considerably influenced by therapy.

A typical onset is in the observation, usually by the patient, of a painless, enlarging mass, most commonly in the neck (Fig. 1), but occasionally in the axilla or inguinal-femoral region. Upon examination this is found to be a discrete, rubbery, painless lymphadenopathy, frequently with surrounding enlarged lymph nodes. In other instances, a chest roentgenogram, taken for a routine purpose, demonstrates mediastinal node enlargement; examination may then disclose lower cervical lymphadenopathy, which had not been noticed by the patient. Although these typical presentations may occur at any age with any histopathologic type, these patients are usually between 15 and 35 years of age and have the histologic variety of nodular sclerosis.

As the typical asymptomatic patient is evaluated more thoroughly with available diagnostic methods, the anatomic extent of disease is usually more widespread than was apparent on physical examination. In particular, mediastinal enlargement is found on routine or detailed radiologic examination, para-aortic node involvement is noted on lower extremity lymphography, or

splenic involvement is found at exploratory laparotomy in significant numbers of such patients (Figs. 2 to 4).

Occasionally the lymphadenopathy makes itself known to the patient or his physician by producing local symptoms of pain, lymphatic or venous obstruction of an extremity, vena caval obstruction, or airway narrowing. The duration of lymphadenopathy prior to diagnosis is extremely variable. Some patients report that a particular mass had been present for several years, even waxing and waning in size. Typically several weeks to several months elapse between the time of the patient's first observation and the diagnostic biopsy.

Another group of patients with Hodgkin's disease have unexplained and persistent fever and/or night sweats as initial symptoms. Fatigue and weight loss may be associated complaints as these symptoms become more severe and prolonged. These patients tend to be in the older age group, are more often male than female, and, when evaluated, are found to have more widespread disease than the typical patient presenting without symptoms. Occasionally, in older patients, usually past the age of 40, the systemic symptoms are severe, often with associated anemia, but the lymphadenopathy is minimal. Extensive diagnostic efforts may be required to uncover the cause of the symptoms, including lymphography, bone marrow and liver biopsies, or even exploratory laparotomy. In rare cases, the diagnosis is not made before a postmortem examination. These older patients, with predominant systemic symptoms at the onset, usually show the histologic varieties of mixed cellularity or lymphocyte depletion.

Figure 1. Typical asymptomatic left supraclavicular lymphadenopathy in a young man with Hodgkin's disease.

Figure 2. Typical intrathoracic lymphadenopathy in a patient with Hodgkin's disease prior to therapy.

Occasional patients with Hodgkin's disease have intermittent evening fever lasting several days, alternating with afebrile periods lasting days or weeks. Usually, the fever gradually becomes more severe and more continuous. This *cyclic fever* has been labeled as the *Pel-Ebstein* or *Murchison* type and is rarely a presenting manifestation of the disease.

Pruritus, usually generalized and severe, is another characteristic systemic symptom of Hodgkin's disease. It may appear as a mild localized symptom, but, if caused by Hodgkin's disease, it usually progresses and becomes generalized. The pruritus may be the only systemic symptom in the otherwise typical presentation of a young person. Generalized severe pruritus may occur in patients with lymphoma other than Hodgkin's disease and in other medical and dermatologic conditions, but its presence should always suggest Hodgkin's disease. Its cause is unknown.

Rarely, patients complain of *pain* in the region of Hodgkin's disease sites within a few minutes *after drinking alcoholic beverages*. Although this is very suggestive of Hodgkin's disease, it is not diagnostic. Its mechanism is not known.

A wide variety of other symptoms may initially call the attention of the patient and his physician to the disease. These same problems occur more commonly as the course of the disease progresses.

The *clinical course* of the disease can be extremely variable. In addition, almost all patients receive treatment that may profoundly affect the course, sometimes resulting in apparent cure, and in many instances resulting in complications that become difficult to separate from the disease itself.

In the typical young patient with Hodgkin's disease, the disease progresses at a variable rate, over a period of months or years, to involve lymph nodes adjacent to those initially involved. In time, if not adequately controlled, typical extensions beyond the lymph nodes

occur. There may be intrathoracic problems with compression of the airway or great veins, involvement of the pleura and/or pericardium with resultant effusions, increasing pulmonary parenchymal involvement, or local osseous involvement of sternum, clavicle, ribs, or vertebrae (Fig. 5).

It is not uncommon for patients with early disease, apparently localized to the neck, to develop disease in the lymph nodes in the upper para-aortic region and/or spleen. Later, even the young patient with an initially favorable prognosis may develop widespread problems, as if there has been a loss of defense mechanisms. At this stage the *bone marrow* may become focally and then diffusely involved (Figs. 6 and 7), with eventual marrow failure. Multiple *osseous lesions* may occur, usually of an osteoblastic or mixed osteoblastic and osteolytic radiologic appearance. These often produce pain, but rarely fractures. The *liver* may become progressively affected, diffuse infiltration of the portal spaces causing serious and even fatal hepatic dysfunction and laboratory features of intrahepatic biliary obstruction. Liver involvement in Hodgkin's disease is closely, or even uniformly, associated with disease in the spleen. Peripheral *neuropathies* as a direct result of tumor growth and epidural cord compression are seen increasingly as the disease progresses.

In time, virtually all patients with Hodgkin's disease develop severe systemic symptoms as their disease progresses beyond control. High continuous fever, drenching night sweats, malaise, fatigue, anorexia, and weight loss are all characteristic of the terminal picture of Hodgkin's disease. Generalized pruritus is seen in a

Figure 3. Abnormal lymphogram due to Hodgkin's disease before (left) and after (right) MOPP chemotherapy.

Figure 4. Hodgkin's disease involving the spleen, evident only on cut section of the spleen removed at diagnostic laparotomy.

proportion of patients during their course but is not uniform in its appearance. Selected aspects of some of the clinical problems of patients with Hodgkin's disease require emphasis.

Hematologic Abnormalities. It is especially difficult to separate the effects of therapy for Hodgkin's disease from the effects of the disease itself on hematologic parameters. Anemia of a moderate degree may be found in patients who present with widespread disease, often associated with systemic symptoms. This is usually with normal indices, normal or low reticulocyte count, and a negative Coombs test. When analyzed in detail, there may be shortened red blood cell survival with inadequate marrow response, as is also seen in patients with advanced cancer or chronic infection. Excluding effects of therapy, which can greatly aggravate the situation, some patients develop profound anemia occasionally at the onset, but more commonly during the

course of the disease. This may be due to extensive bone marrow invasion, hypersplenism, or, rarely, a Coombs-positive hemolytic picture. Often, combinations of these are responsible for the most severe anemias.

Bone marrow involvement by Hodgkin's disease can only rarely be demonstrated by the usual marrow aspirate technique and examination of marrow smears. The process is focal, often associated with fibrosis, and can be discovered more readily by a marrow biopsy performed with a large-bore needle or open surgical technique (Figs. 6 and 7).

The erythrocyte sedimentation is commonly elevated in patients with active disease, and sometimes it may be the only evidence that the disease has been inadequately treated or that clinical recurrence is imminent. Numerous other laboratory abnormalities have been thought to be correlated with disease activity. These include elevations of serum alpha-2-globulin, fibrinogen, haptoglobin, copper, zinc, and ceruloplasmin; depression of serum iron and iron-binding capacity; elevation of leukocyte alkaline phosphatase; and increase in urinary hydroxproline and muramidase.

In the untreated patient, or if therapy has been minimal, moderate to marked neutrophilic leukocytosis and thrombocytosis are characteristic of active, symptomatic Hodgkin's disease. Occasionally, the granulocytosis may be so marked as to suggest chronic granulocytic leukemia. More careful study, however, usually demonstrates that this is a "leukemoid" reaction. Eosinophilia of a mild degree is not uncommon, but occasionally it is moderate or marked, tending to occur in patients with severe and longstanding pruritus. Absolute lymphopenia, even in untreated patients, is seen in a small percentage of cases and, when present, is a poor prognostic sign. Absolute lymphocytosis rarely if ever is seen in Hodgkin's disease and should always suggest an error in diagnosis. Reed-Sternberg cells have been described in the peripheral blood in studies employing special techniques, but they are seldom seen with usual hematologic techniques.

Acute myelomonocytic leukemia has been described as a rare late occurrence in patients with Hodgkin's disease. Although its exact incidence and cause are not established, it is being described more frequently as more patients are surviving a longer period of time. It may be that the leukemia is caused, in part, by the aggressive treatment programs utilizing irradiation and combination chemotherapy, which also have been re-

5 19 75

Figure 5. Advanced intrathoracic Hodgkin's disease with lung involvement prior to therapy.

Figure 6. Focal bone marrow involvement by Hodgkin's disease evident only by biopsy. (Low power magnification.)

sponsible for the improved cure rates. However, the incidence of acute leukemia is approaching 5 per cent for patients at risk for seven or more years following combined modality treatment. The acute myelomonocytic leukemia frequently presents with a picture of pancytopenia and bone marrow hypoplasia many months or several years after the patient had recovered from the acute effects of the Hodgkin's disease treatment program. The condition may be difficult to diagnose and is especially difficult to treat.

Immunologic Abnormalities. The observation that patients with Hodgkin's disease frequently fail to develop a delayed type of skin reaction to tuberculin, even in the presence of active tuberculosis, has stimulated considerable study and speculation. Patients with Hodgkin's disease, even when apparently well, have a

higher frequency of cutaneous anergy than is observed in a control population.

Numerous studies have confirmed that patients with Hodgkin's disease have a defect in delayed hypersensitivity. In general, the more widespread and advanced the clinical extent of the Hodgkin's disease, the more complete is the loss of this immunologic reaction. The therapy used for Hodgkin's disease contributes to the immunologic deficiencies observed. However, despite the immunosuppressive effects of therapy, partial recovery of parameters of delayed hypersensitivity has been observed as disease activity has been controlled.

It remains to be determined whether the defect in cellular immunity is uniformly observed in Hodgkin's disease, and thus may be of etiologic importance, or is a result of the disease and its therapy. Techniques of

Figure 7. Extensive bone marrow involvement by Hodgkin's disease evident only by biopsy. (Medium power magnification.)

measuring cellular immunity are not yet sufficiently precise to be certain. It appears that the more sensitive the test, the more frequently it is abnormal, even in limited disease and prior to therapy.

The relatively well patient with Hodgkin's disease cannot be shown to be more susceptible to infections of any kind, even though he may be anergic to the usual skin tests. As the disease progresses with greater use of radiotherapy, chemotherapy, corticosteroids, and antimicrobials, bacterial, viral, and mycotic infections become more frequent. However, this is not substantially different from other hematologic and immunologic diseases in the late stages.

SELECTED CLINICAL PROBLEMS. *Epidural tumors* occur in Hodgkin's disease and other lymphomas. These may be seen in patients with otherwise favorable prognosis and must be recognized and managed as a medical emergency. Any patient who complains of back or neck pain, numbness, tingling or weakness of an extremity, or bladder or bowel dysfunction should be carefully examined for a transverse *spinal cord* or *cauda equina lesion*. This will require the cooperative efforts of neurologic, neurosurgical, radiologic, and radiotherapeutic consultants.

The problem of the *pulmonary infiltrate* in Hodgkin's disease is especially challenging. Involvement of the lungs is common, but its appearance is variable and must be distinguished from radiation effects, partial lung collapse, drug reactions, and especially the wide variety of pulmonary infections which occur in these patients. In some situations the therapeutic significance of these lesions is so great that a diagnostic thoracotomy is justified.

Virtually all patients with uncontrolled Hodgkin's disease who succumb to their disease will have episodes of serious infections. These occur most frequently during the later stages of the disease and are associated with the more intensive use of therapy, especially of myelosuppressive drugs, irradiation, and corticosteroids.

At the turn of the century, tuberculosis was so prevalent in patients with Hodgkin's disease that a causal relationship was proposed. Since tuberculosis has come under relative control in the United States and elsewhere, this infection is only rarely observed to coexist with Hodgkin's disease and is only rarely a cause of death in these patients. Although bacterial infections are commonly identified and respond to the modern use of antimicrobials, other infections complicate the later clinical course.

Fungal infections, especially of the lungs and meninges, with almost any organism but especially *Cryptococcus*, are encountered in most series of patients with hematologic neoplasms, especially when corticosteroids are employed. *Pneumocystis carinii* and toxoplasmosis are being recognized with increasing frequency and must be sought, because effective therapy is now available. Viral infections, especially herpes zoster and cytomegalovirus infection, have frequently been described.

DIAGNOSTIC EVALUATION. The progress being made in the treatment of Hodgkin's disease has paralleled the improvement in techniques for identifying the extent of the disease in the untreated patient. In view of the current choices of therapy, it is essential that all patients with Hodgkin's disease be evaluated completely by physicians experienced with the disease before therapeutic decisions are made.

A careful history and physical examination are essential to uncover characteristic systemic symptoms and to describe all the lymph node areas of the body. Not all palpable lymph nodes are pathologic in the sense that they contain Hodgkin's disease. However, if there are suspicious lymph nodes which, if involved, would change the therapeutic approach, biopsy should be done for confirmation. The lymphoid tissues in the oropharynx and nasopharynx should be evaluated by a skillful examiner. The size of the liver and spleen must be determined as carefully as possible. The bones should be examined for areas of tenderness.

Radiologic examinations should include routine chest films and, if abnormal, whole lung tomography. This allows better definition of mediastinal, hilar, and paravertebral adenopathy and pulmonary involvement. Lower extremity lymphography is important in all patients, unless pulmonary function is seriously limited. Lymphography is valuable in preparation for exploratory laparotomy, for planning of radiotherapy fields, and especially for follow-up evaluations of the important retroperitoneal lymph nodes. Bone scans complemented by selective skeletal x-rays are desirable to detect osseous lesions. Routine blood cell counts and determination of sedimentation rate, serum alkaline phosphatase, and urinalysis and evaluation of renal function are the minimal laboratory studies required for evaluation. Bone marrow biopsy, using a needle or an open technique, should be performed in all patients with advanced lymph node involvement and those who have significant peripheral blood count depressions, elevated serum alkaline phosphatase, osseous or bone scan abnormalities, or systemic symptoms.

Exploratory laparotomy and splenectomy are widely employed to identify and confirm the presence of Hodgkin's disease in the abdomen. Studies have demonstrated that approximately half the patients with clinical enlargement of the spleen do not have histologic involvement of that organ; conversely, in approximately one patient in four, spleens of normal size have demonstrable foci of Hodgkin's disease. The identification of involvement of the liver by Hodgkin's disease is especially difficult. It is unusual for marked and obvious liver involvement to occur early in the course of the disease. Abnormalities of liver function tests, including borderline elevations of the serum alkaline phosphatase and other enzymes, modest hepatomegaly, and nonspecific hepatic scan abnormalities, may all be misleading. These abnormalities may occur nonspecifically, especially in patients with systemic symptoms, and histologic verification of hepatic involvement should be sought. Conversely, liver involvement can be demonstrated, although rarely, at laparotomy, with no laboratory abnormalities thought to be characteristic of that condition.

The role of diagnostic laparotomy and splenectomy is undergoing re-evaluation because of the occasional severe post splenectomy bacterial infections which are seen and because of the more frequent use of chemotherapy programs in the initial management of Hodgkin's disease. The purpose of the laparotomy is *diagnostic*, and primarily for identifying Hodgkin's disease in the spleen. There are secondary benefits of reducing required irradiation fields when treating the spleen, for attempting to preserve ovarian function by means of an oophoropexy when pelvic irradiation is to be utilized in young women, and for improving the peripheral blood counts in the occasional patients with mild or serious hypersplenism. However, if the primary management program will not be modified significantly by the diagnostic information obtained at laparotomy, the procedure should not be routinely performed.

The advances in diagnostic ability and the results of detailed study of patients early in their course provide strong evidence that Hodgkin's disease presents in relatively orderly patterns of involvement, suggesting a unifocal origin. Before the distribution of disease has been altered by treatment, the lymph node involvement is not a random affair, but nodal disease occurs in contiguous regions (or those directly connected by lymphatic channels, such as the low neck and upper paraaortic lymph nodes) in 90 per cent or more of the cases when a second node group is involved.

Staging in Hodgkin's Disease. There have been several attempts to classify the extent of the disease, in previously untreated patients, to provide useful prognostic and therapeutic indicators. All the proposals acknowledge the poor prognostic significance of widespread disease and of systemic symptoms. The importance of an accepted staging classification in any disease is to facilitate the selection of appropriate treatment programs, to give an estimate of prognosis, and to permit a valid comparison among medical centers for evaluation of their therapeutic results and investigative programs. The classification of disease by stage in current use is the one agreed upon at the Ann Arbor Conference and is shown in Table 1 of Ch. 501. The *E-lesion* or extranodal site of Hodgkin's disease is an important contribution of the Ann Arbor classification. Involvement by Hodgkin's disease of tissues such as the lung, bone, pleura, and pericardium when limited in extent, so that it can be encompassed safely by full doses of irradiation, is still relatively favorable and must be distinguished from widespread extranodal Stage IV disease, which has a poorer prognosis and different therapeutic implications.

TREATMENT. The treatment and results of therapy for patients with Hodgkin's disease have changed radically since about 1940. These have resulted from the diagnostic advances described previously, the considerable improvement in the availability and techniques of supervoltage radiotherapy, and the dramatic effectiveness of combination chemotherapy programs. The entire philosophy of the management of these patients has changed from accepting their inevitable fatal outcome to realizing that every patient has a reasonable potential for cure.

Radiotherapy. The basic concepts of modern radiotherapy for Hodgkin's disease were enunciated years ago by the Swiss radiotherapist René Gilbert and were effectively put into practice during the kilovoltage era by Vera Peters, and later, utilizing megavoltage apparatus, by Henry S. Kaplan and others.

The major considerations which determine the success of radiation therapy are the radiation dose per field, the extent of the fields employed, and the beam energy. It is inappropriate to employ kilovoltage x-rays in a curative attempt for a patient with Hodgkin's disease. Doses of 3500 to 4500 rads are required to relatively large fields to effect permanent eradication of any given site. Because of the limitations of present diagnostic methods in determining the true extent of the disease, lymphoid regions adjacent to known disease or contiguous via lymphatic channels are usually treated to full dose to achieve the best results. Modern equipment and methods permit the treatment of most of the commonly involved lymphoid tissues in two or three large single fields, the "mantle" or supradiaphragmatic field and the "inverted-Y" below the diaphragm. Extended field, so-called total lymphoid or total nodal radiotherapy should not be attempted by radiologists who do not devote their entire time to radiation therapy.

Data are available which support this philosophy and type of therapy for all carefully studied patients with Stages IA, IIA and IIIA disease, in which 60 to 90 per cent of the patients can be cured with irradiation alone. There is more controversy over the indications for therapy for patients with Stages IB and IIB disease and those with limited extranodal disease (the E-lesion of Ann Arbor). However, irradiation should always be utilized in those disease settings as the primary treatment program. The utilization and timing of chemotherapy programs along with or following the irradiation remains controversial, and additional studies will be required before firm recommendations can be made.

Chemotherapy. Chemotherapy has developed significantly since the initial experience with nitrogen mustard during World War II. Successful palliation now can be obtained in the majority of patients. Not infrequently, treatment with one agent will eliminate all evidence of Hodgkin's disease, but inevitably the disease recurs. No documented instance of apparent cure by single drug chemotherapy is on record. It is therefore not justifiable to utilize chemotherapy as initial treatment for patients with localized disease who have a chance for cure by intensive radiotherapy or to use palliative chemotherapy programs for patients with more advanced disease who may be cured by combination chemotherapy.

The major chemotherapeutic agents used in the treatment of Hodgkin's disease are the alkylating agents, the vinca alkaloids, procarbazine, the nitrosoureas, Adriamycin, and bleomycin. In addition the corticosteroids are often included in combination chemotherapy programs. The drugs will be discussed individually, and only several of the more established combination chemotherapy regimens will be described.

The principal alkylating agents are mechlorethamine (nitrogen mustard, HN-2), chlorambucil (Leukeran), cyclophosphamide (Cytoxan), alkeran (Melphalan), and thiotriethylenephosphoramide (thio-tepa). *Nitrogen mustard* has the advantage of rapid action, but it must be given intravenously and causes brief but occasionally severe nausea and vomiting. The average duration of benefit is two to three months after a single dose when used as a single agent. The advantage of *chlorambucil* and *alkeran* is that they may be given orally, and their effect may be titrated more readily against both tumor and bone marrow response.

Cyclophosphamide is a good drug for Hodgkin's disease. Its gastrointestinal toxicity is mild, and it may be used intravenously or orally. An advantage is its lesser toxicity for blood platelet formation. However, it causes alopecia in many patients in whom administration of the drug is carried to the point of marrow toxicity, and hemorrhagic cystitis occurs in 10 to 20 per cent of patients with long-term administration.

Vinblastine provides significant objective improvement for the majority of patients with Hodgkin's disease. Although oral preparations have been tested, the clinically available form of the drug must be given intravenously. It is well tolerated, granulocytopenia being its major toxic effect. There is little or no depression of the platelet count when usual doses are used. The drug is usually given at weekly intervals when used as a single agent. Although pronounced leukopenia may develop, rapid recovery is the rule. In some patients, injections may be spaced at two to four-week intervals after the initial response is obtained. With maintenance therapy, the disease may be kept in remission for many months, occasionally for several years. *Vincristine* probably has a similar range of effectiveness to the closely related vinblastine. At the doses usually employed it has only minimal myelosuppressive effects, and thus its usefulness in combination chemotherapy regimens which employ several marrow toxic drugs. The dose-limiting toxicity of vincristine is its neurotoxicity. This is usually a sensory and motor peripheral neuropathy of the extremities, but many other neurologic toxic manifestations may occur. Alopecia may also be seen. *Procarbazine*, which is probably an alkylating agent, has definite activity against Hodgkin's disease. A high proportion of patients experience objective benefit for at least a short time. Its bone marrow toxicity is similar to that of nitrogen mustard, affecting all the formed elements. When used as the third sequential drug for Hodgkin's disease, as a single agent, the responses have been relatively short in duration, averaging two or three months, and marrow suppression may be prolonged.

Several *nitrosoureas* are available and have activity as single agents in treating Hodgkin's disease. BCNU are the initials for Lomustine, which must be given intravenously, and can palliate approximately 40 per cent of patients who relapse after the alkylating agents and vinca alkaloids. CCNU, a related drug, is available as Carmustine and can be given by mouth. Both drugs produce brief severe nausea and vomiting, but their most serious toxicity is delayed bone marrow suppression. The nadir of peripheral blood count depressions may not be seen before four to six weeks, and a second course of treatment is not ordinarily given before that time.

Adriamycin is a potent anti-tumor antibiotic which has definite activity in patients with Hodgkin's disease. It is used primarily in drug combinations after initial treatment programs have failed. In addition to bone marrow toxicity, nausea and vomiting, alopecia and potential aggravation of irradiation effects, Adriamycin has serious cardiac toxicity which must be monitored closely.

Bleomycin is a useful antimicrobial with good single agent activity in treating Hodgkin's disease. It has minimal myelosuppression, its major toxicity being an acute febrile reaction, sometimes with hypotension and rarely with anaphylaxis. Chronically the drug produces serious pulmonary fibrosis and skin changes.

There is no doubt that objective regression of Hodgkin's disease is observed in some patients treated with *corticosteroids*. However, the general experience is that the responses are brief in duration and overshadowed by the serious toxic effects of steroids, which are particularly distressing in leukopenic patients. The corticosteroids have been employed in combination drug programs, because they are not myelosuppressive.

Combination Chemotherapy. In recent years there has been great interest in the use of combinations of chemotherapeutic agents. It is possible to achieve greater cell destruction when drugs that do not have overlapping toxicity can be combined at relatively full dosage. The most successful and widely tested combination has been developed at the National Cancer Institute and consists of six two-week cycles of therapy with nitrogen mustard, vincristine, procarbazine, and prednisone —the so-called MOPP program. Since two-week rest periods intervene between successive cycles, the entire course requires six months. Although this is a prolonged and occasionally difficult therapeutic program, complete suppression of evidence of Hodgkin's disease can be obtained in 70 to 80 per cent of previously untreated patients. The value of this approach has been the high percentage of complete regression of disease and of long disease-free intervals without maintenance therapy.

Between 40 and 60 per cent of patients who have obtained a documented complete remission have not had a recurrence of their disease for five years following the cessation of chemotherapy. It has been very rare for patients to suffer a relapse after five years, and these individuals can be considered cured by the chemotherapy.

Other combination chemotherapy programs have had equal success in inducing high complete remission rates. Prednisone is probably not necessary in the MOPP program. But no properly randomized study has established the superiority of other regimens to MOPP in the duration of disease control, and therefore it should be utilized whenever possible.

Combination chemotherapy programs for patients who fail to respond to the MOPP regimen or who relapse after MOPP remissions are being developed. The most widely used is the ABVD program of Bonadonna, which utilizes Adriamycin, bleomycin, vinblastine, and DTIC, an imidazole carboxamide. These salvage drug programs can induce complete remissions in approximately half the patients treated, but their curative potential is not yet established.

Combination Radiotherapy and Chemotherapy. Attempts to combine irradiation and chemotherapy in the treatment of Hodgkin's disease were initiated soon after the discovery of nitrogen mustard and continue. It is logical to assume that combination chemotherapy, effective in curing a significant proportion of patients with evident disease, should be even more effective for occult disease which might be present after radiation therapy. Similarly, the chemotherapy programs for patients with advanced Stage IV disease should be more effective if irradiation were used to reduce or eliminate the major tumor masses. Both approaches have been successfully employed in inducing very high complete remission rates for almost all stages of the disease. The combination chemotherapy can effectively replace the wide radiation fields usually used for patients with Stages IA and IIA disease, provided that the evident tumor is treated appropriately. Significant improvement in survival rates as a result of combined modality treatment programs have not yet been clearly demonstrated. In part, this is due to the long period of up to ten years or more required to establish the survival benefit. In addition the success, even in terms of cure which can be achieved for patients who relapse after irradiation programs, has diminished the apparent advantage of improved initial complete remission rates following combined modality treatment. It may be more acceptable to treat patients more conservatively at the onset of the disease, reserving the more difficult chemotherapy and combined modality programs for those patients who relapse after established low morbidity irradiation programs.

The complications and morbidity of the current treatment of Hodgkin's disease are considerable. These are partially listed in Table 2. These problems can be minimized by experienced teams of physicians who work together to achieve the excellent cure rate now possible, avoiding overtreatment.

Recommended Therapy. The recommended therapy for a patient with Hodgkin's disease must be individualized. Considerations of age, extent of disease, prior therapy, and availability of modern skills in radiotherapy and chemotherapy are important in making therapeutic decisions. However, the improving results of aggressive therapy after accurate clinical evaluation and staging in the untreated patient must be acknowledged. Although the value of some therapeutic regimens remains to be established, in terms of survival the recommended therapeutic approaches for the previously untreated patient with various stages of Hodgkin's disease are listed in Table 3. Estimated results are expressed as the percentage of patients likely to achieve a disease-free interval of five years. Careful evaluation and observation of a high proportion of patients, perhaps 90 or 95 per cent, who have survived free from relapse for five years show them to be clinically cured of their disease. Trials are being conducted to further improve these results or to reduce the morbidity of therapy. These newer approaches are also listed in Table 3.

PROGNOSIS. Hodgkin's disease can no longer be accepted as a uniformly fatal disease. The advances in histopathologic classification and diagnostic evaluation and the selection of appropriate aggressive therapy are resulting in a continuous improvement in over-all survival.

Survival figures and prognostic factors which were accepted 20 or even 10 years ago are not acceptable today. This is dramatically demonstrated by comparing over-all survival figures for all patients seen, not only from individual institutions but from public health reports.The five-year survival rate has increased from ap-

TABLE 2. Major Long-Term Complications of the Treatment of Hodgkin's Disease

1. Radiation pneumonitis
2. Radiation carditis
3. Radiation-induced hypothyroidism
4. Radiation bone growth abnormalities in children
5. Chemotherapy-induced male sterility
6. Bone marrow hypoplasia
7. Acute myelomonocytic leukemia, especially after combined modality therapy

proximately 25 to 50 per cent over the past 20 years. In many institutions the five-year survival rate exceeds 75 per cent, and in a few centers has reached 85 per cent, for all patients seen with the disease.

Even prognostic variables are being obscured by modern aggressive therapy. Such important factors as histology, stage of the disease, and presence of systemic symptoms, for example, are becoming less significant as the therapy has become more successful.

Within the context of the foregoing considerations, certain prognostic indicators can be re-emphasized. In general, the more widespread the disease, the poorer the prognosis. Patients with systemic symptoms as defined by the Ann Arbor Conference have a poorer prognosis than those without symptoms, independent of the extent of disease. Patients with the histologic varieties of mixed cellularity and lymphocyte depletion have a much shorter survival, on the average, than those with lymphocyte predominance and nodular sclerosis. All series show that female patients survive longer than males. Patients over the age of 40 have a poorer prognosis than children and younger adults. An important observation is that limited involvement of nonlymphoid structures does not indicate a poor prognosis.

The prognostic variables described above are not completely independent of each other. For example, systemic symptoms are correlated with the extent of disease, and the histologic type is correlated with the sex of the patient. Nonetheless, these prognostic variables are of practical value in considering the management of each patient and in evaluating the relative success of various therapeutic approaches.

Table 3 presents a reasonable estimate of prognosis, recommended therapy, and current appropriate investigative approaches for the various stages of Hodgkin's

TABLE 3. The Treatment of Hodgkin's Disease (February, 1978)

Ann Arbor Pathologic Stage	Recommended Therapy	Estimated Five-Year Disease-Free Survival (%)	Experimental Therapy
IA, I_EA, IIA, II_EA	Subtotal nodal radiotherapy	90	Limited radiotherapy ± combination chemotherapy; combination chemotherapy alone
IB, I_EB, IIB, II_EB	Total lymphoid radiotherapy	75	Total lymphoid radiotherapy + combination chemotherapy
IIIA, III_EA, III_SA	Total lymphoid radiotherapy	60	Combination chemotherapy ± total lymphoid radiotherapy
IIIB, III_EB, III_SB	Combination chemotherapy	40	Total lymphoid radiotherapy + combination chemotherapy
IVA, IVB	Combination chemotherapy	20–40	Total lymphoid radiotherapy + combination chemotherapy

disease, as of February, 1978. That such estimates and recommendations must be dated is testimony to the fact that the understanding and management of patients with Hodgkin's disease are dynamic and gratifying endeavors.

Bonadonna, G., Zucali, R., Delana, M., and Valagussa, P.: Combined chemotherapy (MOPP or ABVD) — radiotherapy approach in advanced Hodgkin's disease. Cancer Treat. Rep., 61:769, 1977.

DeVita, V. T., Jr., Lewis, B. J., Rozencweig, M., and Muggia, F. M.: The chemotherapy of Hodgkin's disease, past experience and future directions. Cancer, 42:979, 1978.

DeVita, V. T., Serpick, A. A., and Carbone, P. P.: Combination chemotherapy in the treatment of advanced Hodgkin's disease. Ann. Intern. Med., 73:881, 1970.

Jacobs, C., Portlock, C. S., and Rosenberg, S. A.: Prednisone in MOPP chemotherapy for Hodgkin's disease. Br. Med. J., 2:1469, 1976.

Kaplan, H. S.: Hodgkin's Disease. Cambridge, Mass., Harvard University Press, 1972.

Prosnitz, L. R., Farber, L. R., Fisher, J. J., Bertino, J. R., and Fisher, D. B.: Long term remissions with combined modality therapy for advanced Hodgkin's disease. Cancer, 37:2826, 1976.

Rosenberg, S. A., Kaplan, H. S., Glatstein, E. J., and Portlock, C. S.: Combined modality therapy of Hodgkin's disease: A report on the Stanford trials. Cancer, 42:991, 1978.

Rosenberg, S. A., and Kaplan, H. S.: Hodgkin's disease and other malignant lymphomas, Calif. Med., 113:23, 1970.

Symposium: Obstacles to the Control of Hodgkin's Disease, Rye, N.Y. Cancer Res., 26, 1966.

Symposium: Staging in Hodgkin's Disease, Ann Arbor, Mich. Cancer Res., 31, 1971.

Section Eight EOSINOPHILIC GRANULOMA AND RELATED SYNDROMES

Philip H. Lieberman

504. INTRODUCTION

Eosinophilic granuloma is a benign disorder characterized by infiltrates of mononuclear cells which probably belong to the mononuclear-phagocyte system and eosinophils. The term "eosinophilic granuloma" has been used in the past for several unrelated disorders such as diffuse or polypoid eosinophilic enteritis or cystitis. The original descriptions of eosinophilic granuloma were those of bone lesions, and many statistical facts about the disease relate to the large number of osseous cases in the literature.

The study of eosinophilic granuloma has been complicated by a complex terminology having its origin in the empiricism of yesteryear. "Histiocytosis X" or, more recently, "histiocytosis" is an old concept which refers to a spectrum of diseases encompassing both the benign disorder, eosinophilic granuloma, and malignant lymphomatous diseases. The concept of "histiocytosis X" has been challenged on clinical, historical, and histologic grounds. The classic triad of the Hand-Schüller-Christian syndrome — namely, exophthalmos, diabetes insipidus, and bone destruction — may be found in eosinophilic granuloma as well as in other disorders such as carcinoma and malignant lymphoma. Hand-Schüller-Christian disease has been redefined over the years and, as used today, is probably synonymous with the more exact description "multifocal eosinophilic granuloma." The use of the terms "histiocytosis Type I" to indicate a fatal disorder with nonspecific histology and "histiocytosis Type II" as a synonym for multifocal eosinophilic granuloma is of little help.

505. EOSINOPHILIC GRANULOMA

The prototype lesion, eosinophilic granuloma of bone, consists of aggregates of mature eosinophils and mononuclear cells as described above. Varying degrees of necrosis are encountered, as well as multinucleated giant cells, common in many bone lesions. In areas of suppuration, foamy histiocytes are not uncommon. There may be some fibrosis, especially when the lesion is healing. Serial biopsies do *not* show a progression of the typical eosinophilic and mononuclear cell mixtures to a lipid phase followed by healing fibrosis, as was originally thought. More commonly, the lesion heals by direct fibrosis. Because of the benign clinical course there have been relatively few studies of soft tissue lesions. Most of the latter studies have been of accessible sites such as skin, vulva, and gingiva. Much has been written about skin lesions in this disorder, with attempts to classify benign versus malignant forms on the basis of skin or mucous membrane histology. We have not found such biopsies to be helpful in this respect. In our experience, isolated eosinophilic granuloma of lymph nodes or salivary glands has had the same benign course as the osseous cases despite unsubstantiated statements to the contrary in the literature. There has been recent increasing interest in primary pulmonary lesions. Because of the benign course of eosinophilic granuloma of bone, relatively few pulmonary biopsies have been recorded in such cases. Resolution of small lung infiltrates has been attributed to transient bouts of pneumonitis healing spontaneously or healed by antimicrobial therapy. It may be possible that the use of chemotherapy in typical cases of multifocal eosinophilic granuloma has kept eosinophilic granuloma of the lung from being much of a problem. Nevertheless, primary eosinophilic granuloma of the lung is recognized as an entity in its own right and is capable of causing severe disability or death secondary to progressive fibrosis and interference with pulmonary function.

Eosinophilic granuloma of bone has a higher incidence in males and occurs most frequently in children and young adults but is occasionally seen as late as the sixth and seventh decades of life. Eosinophilic granuloma of soft tissue may be seen somewhat more frequently in adults, and the male to female predominance is not quite as significant in these cases. Of particular importance is whether the lesions are *unifocal* or *multifocal*. In the latter instance one must expect a chronic disease state with generalized manifestations. If a unifocal bone lesion is found and is verified by bone scan or the somewhat less useful skeletal x-ray survey, and if no secondary lesions develop within 12 months, one can be reasonably certain that the process is limited and that no further defects will develop. Unifocal bone lesions are found in long or flat bones, frequently in the calvarium or femur in children and not infrequently in ribs in adults. Multifocal lesions may involve any site, but are less frequent in the hands and feet. Bone pain and swelling are common presenting complaints, and pathologic fractures may occur. Many of the patients have otitis externa, recurrent bouts of otitis media, and mastoiditis. Ulcerative gingival lesions and loosening of posterior and later anterior teeth secondary to erosions of jaw bones, accompanied by severe pain, focal infection, and malnutrition, are not uncommon. The concept of "triggering factors" such as the smoking of tobacco or other substances or the ingestion of possible allergens becomes most plausible when one is dealing with oral lesions.

Laboratory studies have been rather disappointing. Blood counts are generally within normal range, except for a slight shift to the left in differential counts when the patient develops secondary infections. Eosinophilia is not uncommon. Serum lipid levels (including IgE levels) and tests of cellular immunity (dinitrochlorobenzene and tuberculin skin tests) have occasionally been abnormal but usually are within normal limits. Almost invariably studies of stools for ova and parasites have not been helpful. Occasional cases of infection by uncommon mycobacteria have been reported, but these are most unusual. Viral studies are lacking in most of these cases. Careful history often reveals an allergic background. The periodicity of disease with attacks of hepatosplenomegaly, adenopathy, and disability is impressive. The patient may have transient or permanent diabetes insipidus at the onset of disease, or it may develop at a later date. Diabetes insipidus may be due to granulomatous involvement of the hypothalmus and adjacent areas. Despite the chronicity of the disease with periodic bouts of frequent severe illness, these patients almost all recover; some will have residual orthopedic, dental, or pulmonary defects. Persistent diabetes insipidus may also be a problem.

The pathogenesis of eosinophilic granuloma is unknown. In almost all cases of eosinophilic granuloma, it has been possible to identify the rod- or tennis racket–shaped cytoplasmic granules first identified ultrastructurally in Langerhans cells of the epidermis. These Langerhans (Birbeck) granules are believed to arise by inversion of the plasmalemma and may represent structural membrane changes secondary to antigenic

Electron micrograph showing a mononuclear cell characteristically found in eosinophilic granuloma. Arrows indicate two of the numerous Langerhans-type granules found in these cells. (× 10,800.) Inset: Langerhans granules. (× 128,000.)

challenge. The ubiquitousness of Langerhans cells in squamous epithelia of many parts of the body, dermis, and lymph nodes and reports of their presence in numerous benign conditions (e.g., pityriasis rosea, Ehlers-Danlos syndrome, subacute sclerosing panencephalitis, dermatopathic lymphadenitis, vitiligo) as well as in benign and malignant tumors of various types (Vernon et al.) probably reflect a reactive rather than neoplastic role for these cells. It is possible that the finding of Langerhans cells in some instances may reflect the presence of normal structures in skin and lymph nodes. The presence of Langerhans cells, eosinophilic reactions, high frequency of allergic background in patients, and the recent studies of eosinophilia and its suppression by many of the therapeutic agents used in this disorder all suggest that the disease is reactive rather than neoplastic and may have an immunologic basis.

506. LETTERER-SIWE SYNDROME

The Letterer-Siwe syndrome, as formally defined by Abt and Denenholz, consists of (1) marked splenomegaly with moderate to considerable enlargement of the liver; (2) hemorrhagic diathesis; (3) lymphadenopathy; (4) localized tumefactions over bones (may be diagnosed radiologically); (5) secondary anemia with normal or somewhat diminished leukocyte count, normal differential count, and unremarkable platelet count; (6) splenic aspirates, containing increased numbers of non-lipid-containing macrophages; (7) no familial or hereditary disposition; (8) occurrence exclusively in infants; (9) acute onset unrelated to infection; downhill course, with duration from a few weeks to several years; (10) unknown etiology; and (11) generalized hyperplasia of non-lipid-storing macrophages in various organs. These criteria have been variously altered by authors throughout the years, but they are nonspecific and have included both benign and malignant disorders, causing much confusion. After eliminating various infectious diseases, nonspecific case reports, "familial Letterer-Siwe disease," or hemophagocytic reticulosis, which may be due to maternal hematopoietic grafts (Blennow et al.), graft versus host disease, and combined immunodeficiency syndromes, one is left with a group of malignant neoplasms principally characterized by the presence of histiocytic elements. On purely morphologic grounds, these disorders probably represent unusual forms of malignant lymphoma. It is probable that the Letterer-Siwe syndrome or disease and eosinophilic granuloma are independent entities. If it is true that eosinophilic granuloma may represent an immunologic response to an unknown etiologic agent, one would expect that the picture of eosinophilic granuloma might occur not only in rare lymphomatous disorders but also in other disorders, as, indeed, has been the case.

507. FURTHER NOTES ON TERMINOLOGY

It should be pointed out that, in addition to the inadvisability of using expressions such as "histiocytosis X"

and the "histiocytoses," the terms "reticuloendotheliosis" and "reticulosis" likewise do not belong in the lexicon of the modern clinical. The term "reticuloendotheliosis" was intended to describe proliferation of reticuloendothelial cells giving rise to circulating monocytes, thus being analogous to the terms "myelosis" and "lymphadenosis" used to describe disorders of the bone marrow and lymph nodes, respectively (Symmers). The term "reticulosis" was introduced by Letterer as a synonym for reticuloendotheliosis. The use of these terms has caused confusion. "Reticulosis" has unfortunately become synonymous with malignant lymphoma in some parts of the world, and "reticuloendotheliosis" (and later "histiocytosis") has been used to describe not only the disorders under discussion in these chapters but also various lipid storage diseases and infectious granulomas.

508. TREATMENT*

Three factors must be considered before therapy: (1) histology of lesions; (2) distribution of lesions (unifocal or multifocal; lung, oral, or elsewhere); and (3) definition and elimination of possible aggravating agents (e.g., smoking of tobacco and other substances).

The following suggestions for therapy are not meant to be used in cookbook fashion. The care of these patients is complex and should be carried out under the guidance of experienced therapists.

MANAGEMENT OF UNIFOCAL (SOLITARY) EOSINOPHILIC GRANULOMA OF BONE

1. Bone scan to determine extent of disease.
2. Open biopsy for exact diagnosis.
3. Curettage (with or without bone chip packing).
4. Supervoltage radiation therapy to local "hazardous" sites such as cervical vertebrae or weight-bearing bones (300 to 600 r TD fractionated). Such noncancericidal dosages arrest progression of lesions and stimulate repair. High dosage radiotherapy can lead to tissue damage with resultant poor healing.
5. Supportive therapy, e.g., bed rest as indicated, a brace or cast to protect collapsed vertebra. (See below for diabetes insipidus.)
6. Surgery: (a) to relieve cord compression; (b) partial mastoidectomy if indicated; (c) skin grafts if necessary.
7. Observation for development of other lesions, which usually occur within the first 12 months after diagnosis. Patients with lesions in the mandible, mastoid, facial or orbital bones, and ilium are more likely to develop further disease. Monthly or more frequent history and physical examination. Focal x-rays of sites of known involvement six months after biopsy if indicated. If necessary, repeat x-rays of known lesions or suspicious new lesions every six months for one to two years.

MANAGEMENT OF MULTIFOCAL EOSINOPHILIC GRANULOMA

1. Bone scan to determine extent of disease and to help select most acceptable biopsy site.

---

*The author is indebted to Dr. Charles Ray Jones for help in the preparation of this material.

2. Open biopsy for exact diagnosis.

3. Chemotherapy is essential in management to prevent prolonged disease and to lessen morbidity and permanent deformity. This non-neoplastic disorder can best be treated with drugs used in cancer chemotherapy. Bone marrow depression is *not* necessary to achieve desired effect. Methotrexate, prednisone, and vinblastine used judiciously by experienced physicians can lead to resolution of the disease process.

Preferred therapy for acute phase: Methotrexate — children under 5 years: 1.25 mg by mouth every day for three months; children over 5 years and adults: 2.5 mg by mouth, every day for three months. *Note:* Never exceed 2.5 mg per day. If signs of hematologic or mucosal toxicity develop, stop therapy. Resume with dosage every other day when abnormalities clear. Prednisone — 30 mg per square meter by mouth every other day in three divided doses, for three months. *Note:* Never exceed 60 mg per day. If hypertension, diabetes mellitus, or mental problems develop, stop medication. When abnormalities clear, resume with half dosage every other day.

Alternative therapy for acute phase: Vinblastine, 0.1 mg per kilogram intravenously every week for five weeks. Prednisone 30 mg per square meter by mouth every other day in three divided doses, for five weeks.

Maintenance therapy: Methotrexate, same dosage as for acute phase every other day for three months. Prednisone, 15 mg per square meter by mouth every other day in two divided doses for three months. *Note:* If lesions regress and no new lesions develop, continue maintenance therapy for three consecutive days of the week and then withhold medication for four days, for a total course of therapy of one year.

4. Supervoltage radiation therapy to local "hazardous" sites, 300 to 600 r TD fractionated. There should be a prompt response, especially if radiation is administered after chemotherapy is initiated.

5. Antimicrobial agents — used to treat otitis externa, mastoiditis, and sinusitis.

6. Surgery — for cord compression, to relieve mastoid problems, and to excise calvarial lesions eroding through skin.

7. Supportive therapy: (a) maintain good nutrition; (b) whole blood transfusion when indicated; (c) bed rest, casts, braces, as indicated; (d) physical therapy as indicated; (e) *reassurance* that the process is not neoplastic and that the patient will be able to regain normal life.

8. Diabetes insipidus: Pitressin tannate in oil and/or Diapid insufflation in conventional dosages (see Ch. 544.2).

MANAGEMENT OF ORAL EOSINOPHILIC GRANULOMA

1. Dexamethasone elixir (used as a mouth rinse), three times a day until lesions begin to resolve.

2. Treatment for multifocal eosinophilic granuloma.

MANAGEMENT OF PULMONARY EOSINOPHILIC GRANULOMA

1. Treat as multifocal eosinophilic granuloma.

2. Beclomethasone dipropionate, inhalations (100 μg) given two times a day. Indications of response: decreased sedimentation rate, decreased alpha-1-antitrypsin, x-ray evidence of clearing (tomography), improved pulmonary function studies.

MANAGEMENT OF VULVAR EOSINOPHILIC GRANULOMA

1. Topical steroid cream.

2. If no response or multiple lesions, use therapy for multifocal eosinophilic granuloma.

MANAGEMENT OF THE LETTERER-SIWE SYNDROME (WHEN PRESENTING AS HISTIOCYTIC LYMPHOMA)

See Ch. 501.

Abt, A. F., and Denenholz, E. J.: Letterer-Siwe's disease. Splenohepatomegaly associated with widespread hyperplasia of non-lipoid-storing macrophages; discussion of the so-called reticuloendothelioses. Am. J. Dis. Child., 51:499, 1936.

Beeson, P. B., and Bass, D. A.: The Eosinophil. Philadelphia, W. B. Saunders Company, 1977.

Blennow, G., Berg, B., Brandt, L., Messeter, L., Low, B., and Soderstrom, N.: Haemophagocytic reticulosis. A state of chimerism? Arch. Dis. Child., 49:960, 1974.

Lichtenstein, L.: Histiocytosis X. Integration of eosinophilic granuloma of bone, "Letterer-Siwe disease," and "Schüller-Christian disease" as related manifestations of a single nosologic entity. Arch. Pathol., 56:84, 1953.

Lieberman, P. H., Jones, C. R., Dargeon, H. W. K., and Begg, C. F.: A reappraisal of eosinophilic granuloma of bone, Hand-Schüller-Christian syndrome and Letterer-Siwe syndrome. Medicine, 48:375, 1969.

Symmers, W. S. C.: The lymphoreticular system. In Wright, G. P., and Symmers, W. S. C. (eds.): Systemic Pathology, Vol. I. London, Longmans, Green & Company, 1966, Chap. 5.

Vernon, M. L., Fountain, L., Krebs, H. M., Horta-Barbosa, L., Fuccillo, D. A., and Sever, J. L.: Birbeck granules (Langerhans' cell granules) in human lymph nodes. Am. J. Clin. Pathol., 60:771, 1973.

Wolff, K.: The Langerhans cell. Curr. Probl. Derm., 4:79, 1972.

Section Nine PLASMA CELL DYSCRASIAS

Elliott F. Osserman

509. INTRODUCTION

DEFINITION AND TERMINOLOGY. The term "plasma cell dyscrasia" is employed to encompass the wide range of pathologic conditions and biochemical abnormalities considered to represent unbalanced proliferative disorders of the cells that normally synthesize and secrete gamma (immuno-) globulins. The extent of the proliferative abnormality in the various plasma cell dyscrasias ranges from apparently autonomous, malignant proliferation (neoplasia) in typical multiple myeloma to apparently benign and stable dyscrasias manifested principally by their associated gamma globulin abnormalities. The plasma cell dyscrasias are characterized by (1) the proliferation of plasma cells in the absence of an identifiable antigenic stimulus; (2) elaboration of electrophoretically and structurally homogeneous, monoclonal, "M-type" (myeloma, macroglobulinemia) gamma globulins and/or excessive quantities of comparably homogeneous polypeptide subunits of these proteins, i.e., Bence Jones proteins, H-chains; and (3) commonly, an associated deficiency in the synthesis of normal immunoglobulins.

The major clinical patterns associated with plasma cell dyscrasia are listed in Table 1. Certain of these categories, such as myeloma, macroglobulinemia, amyloidosis, and heavy chain diseases, have sufficiently well defined clinical patterns to permit precise diagnostic classification. With increasing use of electrophoresis, however, many cases of M-type gamma globulin abnormalities are being found that apparently do not represent typical plasma cell myeloma or primary Waldenström's macroglobulinemia at the time of initial study. The fact that some of these patients ultimately develop clinically typical myeloma or macroglobulinemia is well documented, but there are many cases (of the order of 20 to 30 per cent of patients with M-type gamma globulin abnormalities) that almost certainly do not belong in the diagnostic categories of myeloma or primary macroglobulinemia. Various designations have been given to these cases, including premyeloma, essential hyperglobulinemia, essential benign hyperglobulinemia, essential macroglobulinemia, idiopathic or essential cryoglobulinemia, the dysgammaglobulinemic syndromes, idiopathic or essential monoclonal gammopathy, paraimmunoglobulinopathy, and others. The probable inaccuracies of all these terms are evident.

It is recommended that the inclusive term "plasma cell dyscrasia" be used, modified by the clinical pattern, e.g., myeloma, Waldenström's macroglobulinemia, or amyloidosis, when this is overt and evident. When no recognizable clinical pattern is associated with the finding of an M-type protein, the condition is classified as a plasma cell dyscrasia of unknown significance ("PCDUS") because the ultimate course is not presently predictable. However, many, if not all, of the diagnostic categories listed in Table 1 overlap. Thus either amyloidosis can be the predominant feature of a

TABLE 1.   Plasma Cell Dyscrasias

Clinically overt forms, with distinctive clinical and pathologic features:
  Plasma cell myeloma (multiple myeloma, myelomatosis, "solitary" and multiple plasmacytomas, plasma cell leukemia)
  Waldenström's (primary) macroglobulinemia
  γ Heavy chain (Franklin's) disease
  α Heavy chain (Seligmann's) disease (abdominal "lymphoma")
  μ Heavy chain disease
  Amyloidosis (Pattern I and Mixed Pattern I and II amyloidosis)
  Lichen myxedematosus (papular mucinosis, lichen amyloidosus)

Clinically occult (asymptomatic or presymptomatic) forms
  Plasma cell dyscrasia of unknown significance (PCDUS)
    Associated with chronic inflammatory and infectious processes, e.g., osteomyelitis, tuberculosis, chronic biliary tract disease, pyelonephritis, rheumatoid arthritis, chronic pyoderma, etc.
    Associated with nonreticular neoplasms, particularly cancers of the bowel, biliary tract and breast
    Associated with neurologic manifestations, particularly polyneuropathy, subacute sclerosing panencephalitis (SSPE), amyotrophic lateral sclerosis (ALS), and myopathies
    Associated with lipodystrophies, particularly Gaucher's disease, familial hypercholesteremia, and xanthomatosis
  Transient plasma cell dyscrasias
    Associated with drug hypersensitivity, sulfonamides
    Associated with (presumed) viral infections
    Associated with cardiac surgery: valve prosthesis

plasma cell dyscrasia, in which case the diagnosis of "primary amyloidosis" is commonly, although inappropriately, applied, or the amyloid infiltrates can occur in association with otherwise typical myeloma. Also, a given case can progress from an asymptomatic status, i.e., plasma cell dyscrasia of unknown significance, to symptomatic myeloma, macroglobulinemia, amyloidosis, and so forth. Accordingly, the categories listed in Table 1 are tentative and somewhat indefinite diagnostic groupings in many instances.

In a significant percentage of cases the finding of an M-type protein abnormality is associated with another chronic disease such as recurrent cholecystitis and cholelithiasis, a chronic infection (particularly tuberculosis), or a nonreticular neoplasm (particularly rectosigmoid and biliary carcinoma). *These associations may not be coincidental,* but may represent plasma cell dyscrasias related to and possibly induced by these diverse chronic reticuloendothelial stimuli. For this reason, it is considered useful to document the associations by designations such as "plasma cell dyscrasia associated with chronic biliary tract disease" or "plasma cell dyscrasia associated with adenocarcinoma of the rectosigmoid."

PATHOGENESIS OF PLASMA CELL DYSCRASIAS. Although the etiologic factors responsible for production of plasma cell dyscrasias in man are still unknown, it is possible that some clues may have been provided by studies of experimental plasma cell tumors in mice. These studies have established the importance of genetic factors with the demonstration of the particular susceptibility of the inbred C_3H mouse strain and the F^1 hybrids of CBA × DBA/2 mice to develop plasma cell tumors spontaneously. In an effort to document genetic factors, chromosome studies have been carried out in several of these murine tumors as well as in human myeloma and macroglobulinemia, but thus far no consistent karyotypic abnormalities have been documented.

The *interdependence of genetic and carcinogenic mechanisms* is apparent in the interesting group of experimental *plasma cell tumors* that have been induced in BALB/c strain mice. A variety of plasma cell neoplasms can be induced in this strain by the intraperitoneal implantation of plastics, mineral oil–adjuvant mixtures, and mineral oil alone. The importance of genetic mechanisms is evident from the particular susceptibility of the BALB/c strain to develop plasma cell tumors in response to these forms of chronic peritoneal (reticuloendothelial) irritation. Significantly, strain C_3H mice, which develop spontaneous plasma cell tumors, are *not susceptible* to the induction of these tumors by intraperitoneal adjuvants and the like. With many other experimental tumors the intimate interaction of genetic factors, oncogenic viruses, and chemical and physical carcinogens has been established.

CYTOLOGY. The synthesis of specific proteins is the principal and probably the sole function of plasma cells. The abundant cytoplasmic RNA is responsible for the characteristic basophilia and pyroninophilia of plasma cells, and the highly developed Golgi apparatus is responsible for the typical paranuclear "halo" or clear zone. Electron microscopy of plasma cells has shown that the cytoplasmic RNA is organized in the form of granules (ribosomes) attached to a highly developed network of endoplasmic reticulum. All these structural features have now been related to the complex functions of protein synthesis and secretion. The nucleus of the plasma cell with its characteristically clumped chromatin (DNA) contains the genetic information that determines the structure of the protein to be synthesized. The synthesis of ribosomal RNA is carried out on DNA localized in the nucleolus. Messenger RNA's, which determine the structure of the specific proteins to be synthesized on these ribosomes, are derived from the nonnucleolar DNA's.

The different classes of immunoglobulins are synthesized and secreted by different cells. A single cell may under certain conditions synthesize two types of immunoglobulins (e.g., IgG and IgM) either simultaneously or sequentially, but most studies have indicated the synthesis of only one type of immunoglobulin by a single cell. Immunohistochemical studies, using fluorescein-labeled antisera specific for each of the immunoglobulin groups, have generally shown IgG globulin synthesis in typical, mature, Marshalko-type plasma cells. IgA globulin has been localized in cells with relatively more abundant and vacuolated cytoplasm but still having the major features of plasma cells; IgM synthesis has been related to a population of somewhat smaller cells with proportionately less cytoplasm. These cells have been variously classified as lymphocytoid-plasma cells, plasmacytoid-lymphocytes, atypical plasma cells, and atypical lymphocytes.

Typical, ovoid plasma cells with eccentric nuclei, clumped chromatin, prominent nucleoli, paranuclear halo, and basophilic cytoplasm are widely distributed in lymph nodes, spleen, marrow, intestinal wall, and other tissues and organs. They constitute less than 5 per cent of the normal bone marrow population but increase significantly in association with infection, sensitivity reactions (particularly serum sickness), collagen diseases, cirrhosis, parasitism, and certain neoplasms. In these conditions, the increase in plasma cells includes both "typical" and "atypical" forms (including multinucleated cells and cells with prominent nucleoli), and there are *no reliable morphologic criteria to distinguish these reactive plasmacytic populations from the cells that are found in the plasma cell dyscrasias.*

NORMAL IMMUNOGLOBULINS AND THE PARAPROTEINS OF THE PLASMA CELL DYSCRASIAS. Figure 1 is a schematic summary of the present working hypothesis relating the synthesis of individual gamma globulin molecules (1, 2, 3, 4 . . . n) to specific plasmacytic clones. The normally broad, polydispersed serum gamma globulin peak represents the balanced synthesis of small quantities of a very large and presently indeterminate

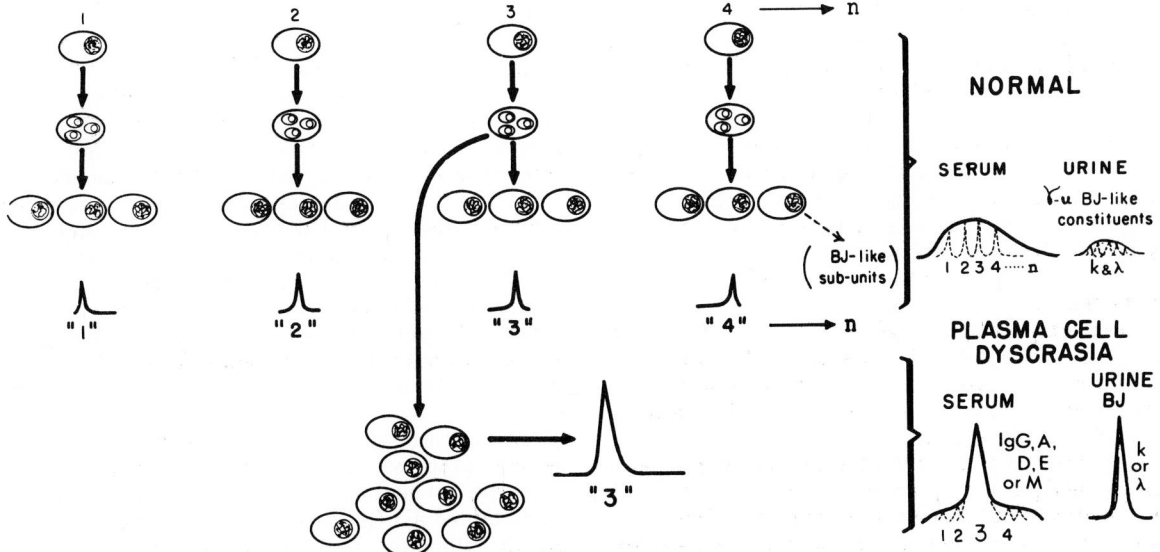

Figure 1. Schematic representation of the clonal hypothesis of immunoglobulin synthesis and the derangements in protein synthesis associated with plasma cell dyscrasias.

number (n) of individual and specific gamma globulin molecules by specific plasma cell populations. Normally, most of the proteins synthesized by these cells are complete immunoglobulin molecules, and there is only a small quantity of incomplete polypeptide subunits elaborated. These incomplete proteins, designated "gamma-u," are low molecular weight constituents (M.W. 20,000 to 25,000) and closely resemble Bence Jones proteins. Because of their small molecular size, gamma-u polypeptides are rapidly excreted by the kidney. Normally, 20 to 40 mg of gamma-u is excreted per 24 hours.

A plasma cell dyscrasia is considered to represent the excessive proliferation of a single clone of plasma cells, resulting in the synthesis of large quantities of a single protein related to one of the major classes of immunoglobulins and/or the synthesis of excessive quantities of a constituent polypeptide subunit of one of these proteins, usually of the Bence Jones type.

The proteins elaborated in the plasma cell dyscrasias have been shown to be very closely related and structurally similar to the normal immunoglobulins. As large quantities of these single proteins are synthesized in the plasma cell dyscrasias, they are more suitable for structural studies than the heterogeneous and polydispersed normal immunoglobulins. Significantly, much of our present knowledge regarding the structure and properties of normal immunoglobulins has been obtained from studies of the M-type paraproteins.

The biochemical and physiologic properties of the presently recognized immunoglobulins, IgG, IgA, IgD, IgE, and IgM globulins, are presented in Ch. 38. In typical multiple myeloma, approximately 70 per cent of the serum "spikes" are IgG, 28 per cent are IgA, and 2 per cent are IgD. There have been only four cases of IgE myeloma reported to date. Bence Jones proteins, which represent free light chains, are elaborated in large quantities and excreted in the urine in approximately 50 per cent of cases of myeloma. Bence Jones proteins have molecular weights in the range of 20,000 to 25,000 but are commonly excreted as disulfide-bonded or hydrogen-bonded dimers. In any given case of plasma cell dyscrasia with Bence Jones proteinuria, the Bence Jones protein is *either* Type κ *or* Type λ, in contrast to excretion of small quantities of *both* Type κ and Type λ constituents in normal urine. In those cases of plasma cell dyscrasia in which there is synthesis of both an M-type serum paraprotein and a Bence Jones–type protein, the Bence Jones protein is apparently identical to the constituent light chains of the corresponding serum paraprotein. This evidence is interpreted as indicating that a portion of the abnormal cells has retained the capacity to elaborate complete molecules with light and heavy chains, whereas others are capable of synthesizing only one of the constituent polypeptide subunits, i.e., light chains.

In recent years much evidence has been obtained that the proteins elaborated in the plasma cell dyscrasias are "true" antibodies elaborated in great quantitative excess as a consequence of the proliferative abnormality. Thus many human and mouse myeloma proteins and macroglobulins have been found to interact with a variety of synthetic haptens, polysaccharides, lipids, and bacterial antigens. The present consensus is that some of these reactions are probably cross-reactions between these proteins and ligands which are structurally related but not identical to the true antigens. We have re-

cently described a flavin-binding monoclonal IgG in a patient with myeloma who also exhibited xanthoderma and xanthotrichia. The IgG isolated from the serum was bright yellow and was approximately 70 per cent saturated with riboflavin. This observation has raised the potentially important possibility that other M-type immunoglobulins may also have bound-but-colorless haptens already attached. Investigations are presently underway to identify the true antigens to which the myeloma proteins are directed, and this will unquestionably shed light on the pathogenic mechanisms responsible for plasma cell dyscrasias in man.

ELECTROPHORETIC PATTERNS OF SERUM AND URINARY PROTEINS IN THE PLASMA CELL DYSCRASIAS. As a result of the more general use of electrophoresis, increasing numbers of cases of plasma cell dyscrasia are being documented by the electrophoretic demonstration of M-type serum or urinary protein abnormalities, or both. These M-type abnormalities (see Figs. 3 and 4) are best appreciated by comparison with the patterns of normal serum and urine and the serum in certain disease states affecting the reticuloendothelial system generally (Fig. 2). The electrophoretic analyses illustrated were performed by the Spinco cellulose acetate method, which is now routinely employed in most clinical laboratories. For diagnostic purposes, the *contours of electrophoretic patterns are more significant* than the precise quantitation of individual peaks. A careful appraisal of the contours of each peak, particularly distinguishing a *diffuse gamma elevation* from an M-type spike, in conjunction with a rough quantitative comparison of the patient's serum albumin, alpha-1, alpha-2, beta, and gamma globulins with a normal serum pattern will yield most of the clinically important information offered by this method.

In Figure 2, the normal serum pattern shows the characteristically broad contour of the major slow gamma peak, sometimes referred to as gamma-2, and a small secondary peak in the fast gamma region (between gamma and beta), which at times is designated gamma-1. The gamma-1 peak is detectable by cellulose acetate electrophoresis in most but not all normal sera. It is not resolved as a distinct peak by filter paper electrophoresis. The gamma-1 peak has been related to the faster migrating IgA and IgM globulins.

The electrophoretic pattern of the normal urinary proteins in Figure 2 shows albumin to be the major constituent, with lesser quantities of alpha, beta, and gamma globulins. Because of the extremely low concentration of protein in normal urine, the sample must be concentrated 50- to 100-fold by dialysis against 25 per cent dextran or polyvinylpyrrolidone (PVP) prior to electrophoresis. As in the case of serum proteins, the clinically important abnormal urinary proteins are detected as changes in the contours of the pattern and the relative concentrations of albumin and proteins of alpha, beta, and gamma mobility. Serial quantitation of 24-hour urinary protein excretion is useful for evaluating therapy but is not of particular importance diagnostically.

As illustrated in the lower patterns in Figure 2, the general suppression of plasmacytic function associated with the congenital and acquired forms of hypogammaglobulinemia is reflected in a *broad decrease* in gamma globulin, and conversely, the generalized hyperactivity of the reticuloendothelial system associated with certain chronic infections, cirrhosis, collagen dis-

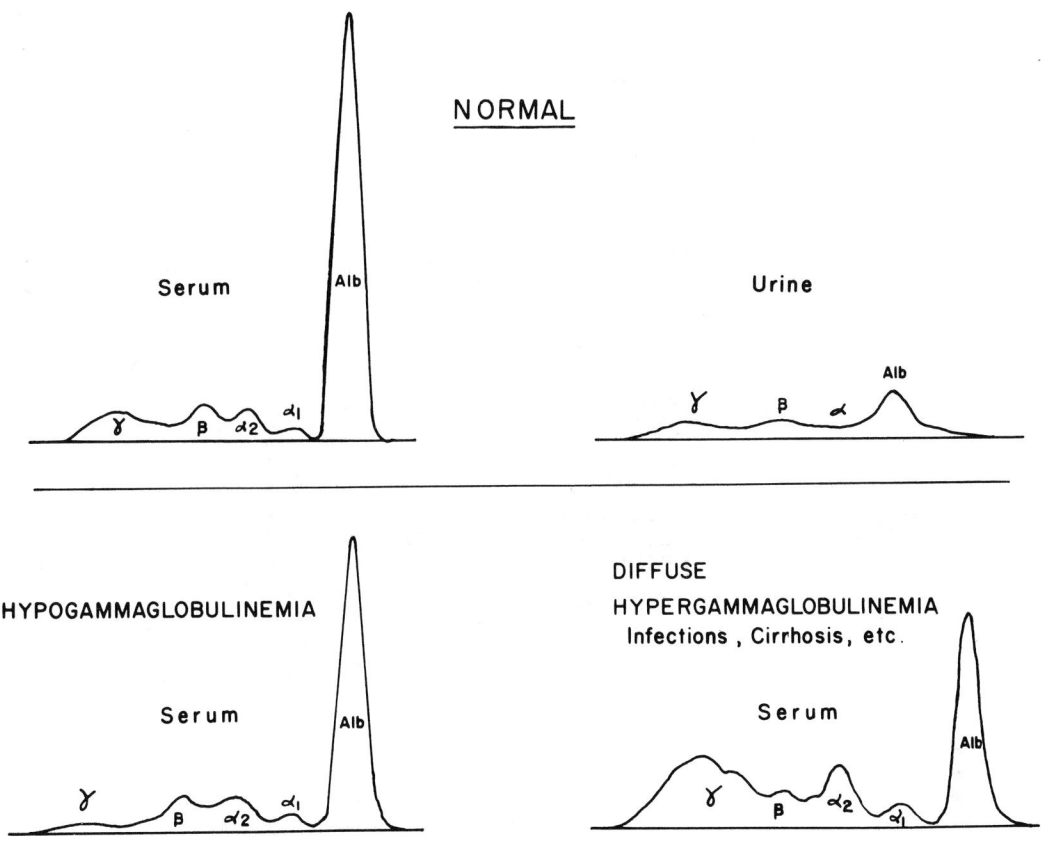

Figure 2. Representative electrophoretic patterns (Spinco, cellulose acetate system). *Top,* Normal serum and normal urinary proteins (concentrated 50×). *Bottom left,* Hypogammaglobulinemia (adult, idiopathic). *Bottom right,* Diffuse hypergammaglobulinemia.

eases, etc., is reflected in a *broad elevation* of gamma globulin. The pattern illustrating a diffuse hypergammaglobulinemia shows an elevation of the slow, major gamma (gamma-2) peak owing to an increase in IgG globulins, and also an increase in the fast gamma (gamma-1) peak, reflecting an increase in IgA and IgM globulins.

The M-type serum and urinary protein abnormalities observed in myeloma, macroglobulinemia, and the other plasma cell dyscrasias are illustrated in Figures 3 and 4. In Figure 3, three sets of serum and urinary patterns from three cases of myeloma illustrate different combinations of abnormalities. Bence Jones proteinuria was present in all three cases of myeloma and was confirmed by the classic precipitation at 55 to 60° C (pH 5.0) and re-solution at 90 to 100° C. Because of their small molecular size, the Bence Jones proteins are rapidly excreted, and their serum concentration is usually too low to be detected by conventional electrophoretic methods. Urine electrophoresis, however, demonstrates the Bence Jones proteins to have the same relative homogeneity as the myeloma serum globulins and electrophoretic mobilities, ranging from slow gamma through beta and into the alpha-2 mobility range. Urine electrophoresis is a more reliable method for the detection of Bence Jones proteins than the usual heat-precipitation procedure. *The finding in the urine of an electrophoretically homogeneous M-type component of gamma, beta, or alpha-2 mobility present in a concentration exceeding that of albumin indicates that the protein*

has a molecular size smaller than albumin (M.W. 70,000). This is strong evidence in favor of Bence Jones proteinuria and can generally be confirmed by precipitation at 55 to 60° C and re-solution at 90 to 100° C *if the pH is carefully adjusted to 4.5 to 5.0.* False negative reactions will be obtained if inadequate attention is given to pH adjustment.

In the case of myeloma illustrated in Figure 3*A* the serum pattern shows a large, electrophoretically homogeneous peak of slow gamma mobility, and the urine pattern shows a large, abnormal M-type peak with a somewhat faster (more anodally positioned) mobility than the serum M-type peak. The lack of correspondence in mobilities of the serum and urinary proteins establishes their *nonidentity.* Immunoelectrophoretically, the serum protein was identified as an IgG globulin and the urinary protein as a Type κ Bence Jones constituent.

In Figure 3*B*, the serum shows a small abnormal peak of slow gamma mobility and an obvious decrease in normal gamma globulin. The urine shows a very large abnormal peak of slow gamma mobility and a minimal amount of albumin. The serum and urinary proteins were both identified immunoelectrophoretically as Type λ Bence Jones protein. Bence Jones protein*emia* is usually not detectable by conventional electrophoresis, although it is almost always demonstrable by the more sensitive technique of immunoelectrophoresis when Bence Jones proteinuria is present.

In Figure 3*C*, the serum pattern shows two overlap-

Figure 3. Serum and urinary protein patterns in three cases of multiple myeloma (*A, B,* and *C*), each with an M-type protein abnormality in the serum and Bence Jones proteinuria. *D,* Macroglobulinemia with nonspecific proteinuria.

ping abnormal peaks of fast gamma (gamma-1) and beta mobility. The urine pattern has an abnormal beta peak along with significant quantities of albumin. In occasional cases of myeloma and other plasma cell dyscrasias, double peaks are found in serum patterns. Most frequently these have been shown to be due to an unusually high concentration of Bence Jones protein in the serum along with an M-type IgG or IgA globulin. Rarely, two distinct globulins such as an IgG *and* an IgA or IgM globulin are found in the serum of a patient with a plasma cell dyscrasia. Although these are commonly referred to as "biclonal gammopathies," detailed structural studies of the two components have shown identity of their V (variable) region sequences, indicating that they are probably derived from a single clone. In Figure 3C, the two serum peaks were immunoelectrophoretically identified, respectively, as IgA globulin and a Type λ Bence Jones protein. The abnormal urinary protein was identified as the same Type λ Bence

Jones constituent present in the serum. There was no detectable IgA globulin in the urine.

In Figure 3D the serum and urinary patterns from a case of primary (Waldenström's) macroglobulinemia are illustrated. The serum has an M-type peak of slow gamma mobility indistinguishable from the IgG abnormality illustrated in Figure 3A. Definitive identification of the abnormal protein as an IgM globulin in this as in all cases of macroglobulinemia was accomplished only by immunoelectrophoretic and ultracentrifugal analyses. The urinary protein pattern revealed nonspecific proteinuria with albumin as the predominant constituent. The virtual absence of the IgM globulin from the urine is noteworthy. Bence Jones proteinuria occurs in a smaller percentage (10 to 20 per cent) of cases of macroglobulinemia than of myeloma (50 to 60 per cent).

Serum and urinary electrophoretic patterns from plasma cell dyscrasias other than typical myeloma and macroglobulinemia are illustrated in Figure 4. The patterns in Figure 4*A* are from a case of generalized amyloidosis with predominant involvement of the tongue, heart, and gastrointestinal tract, classified as "Pattern I amyloidosis." There were no detectable skeletal lesions, but plasma cell dyscrasia was indicated by the finding of Bence Jones proteinuria, and was confirmed by the finding on marrow aspiration of abnormal numbers of plasma cells. The abnormal urinary protein was immunoelectrophoretically identified as a Type λ Bence Jones constituent. The serum pattern shows an elevated alpha-2 globulin and a decreased gamma globulin, without an M-type peak.

In Figure 4*B*, the serum and urinary proteins from a case of γ heavy chain (Fc fragment) disease are shown. The protein elaborated in this condition has been characterized as representing the major portion (Fc fragment) of the IgG H-chain with a molecular weight in the range of 50,000 to 55,000. Because these proteins are larger than Bence Jones proteins, their renal clearance rate is relatively lower, and they are retained in the

serum in sufficiently high concentrations to be detectable by conventional electrophoretic analysis. The abnormal serum and urinary protein peaks are of identical mobility and electrophoretically somewhat more polydispersed than the abnormal peaks in the other plasma cell dyscrasias. The urinary protein pattern, however, is indistinguishable from the patterns observed with Bence Jones proteinuria, and identification of the abnormal protein as related to the IgG heavy chain and unrelated to Bence Jones proteins and light chains must be accomplished by appropriate immunochemical and physicochemical studies.

The serum electrophoretic patterns illustrated in Figures 4*C* and 4*D* are from two cases in which M-type protein abnormalities were discovered in the absence of overt signs or symptoms of myeloma, macroglobulinemia, or any other recognizable disease. These cases are classified as plasma cell dyscrasia of unknown significance (PCDUS). As will be noted subsequently, the clinical and pathologic significance of protein abnor-

Figure 4. Representative electrophoretic patterns in plasma cell dyscrasias. *A,* Plasma cell dyscrasia and amyloidosis of "Pattern I" distribution with a characteristic Bence Jones–type abnormality in the urine pattern. *B,* γ Heavy chain (Fc fragment) disease with corresponding serum and urinary M-type peaks of β mobility. *C* and *D,* Asymptomatic plasma cell dyscrasias with a small (*C*) and a large (*D*) M-type serum peak. *E,* Plasma cell dyscrasia associated with an adenocarcinoma of the rectosigmoid colon. *F,* Plasma cell dyscrasia associated with chronic and recurrent cholecystitis and cholelithiasis.

malities of this type are presently still obscure. In some cases, progression to overt forms of plasma cell dyscrasia, such as myeloma, has been documented, but in many cases the protein abnormality has been found to persist for as long as 20 years without the development of clinically recognizable disease. Rarely, protein abnormalities of this type have been found on subsequent analyses to have disappeared — i.e., transient paraproteinemias — and these almost certainly represent examples of the synthesis of excessively large quantities of functional antibodies.

The M-type gamma globulin abnormalities illustrated in Figures 4*E* and 4*F* were found in association with clinical conditions that may have been related to the development of plasma cell dyscrasias, notably an adenocarcinoma of the rectosigmoid with an intense plasmacytic infiltration surrounding the tumor and in the resected nodes (Fig. 4*E*), and chronic and recurrent cholecystitis and cholelithiasis with extensive plasmacytosis in the gallbladder wall and along the biliary tract (Fig. 4*F*). Until a direct relationship is established between these conditions and the plasma cell dyscrasias, their association must be considered coincidental, but the relative frequency of these associations warrants the search for an occult neoplasm or biliary tract disease in patients found to have asymptomatic M-type gamma globulin abnormalities.

Edelman, G. M.: The antibody problem. Ann. Rev. Biochem., 38:415, 1969.

Farhangi, M., and Osserman, E. F.: Myeloma and xanthoderma due to an IgGλ monoclonal anti-flavin antibody. N. Engl. J. Med., 294:177, 1976.

Haber, E., and Krause, R. M.: Antibodies in Human Diagnosis and Therapy. New York, Raven Press, 1977.

Nisonoff, A., Hopper, J. E., and Spring, S. B.: The Antibody Molecule. New York, Academic Press, 1975.

Osserman, E. F., and Takatsuki, K.: Considerations regarding the pathogenesis of the plasmacytic dyscrasias. Scand. J. Haematol., 4 (Suppl.):28, 1964.

Potter, M.: Antigen binding M-components in man and mouse. In Azar, H. A., and Potter, M. (eds.): Multiple Myeloma and Related Disorders. Vol. I. Hagerstown, Md., Harper & Row, 1973, p. 195.

Potter, M.: The developmental history of the neoplastic plasma cells in mice. Semin. Hematol., 10:19, 1973.

Putnam, F. W.: Immunoglobulin structure: Variability and homology. Science, 163:633, 1969.

Seligmann, M., and Brouet, J. C.: Antibody activity of human myeloma globulins. Semin. Hematol., 10:163, 1973.

Solomon, A.: Bence Jones proteins and light chains of immunoglobulins. N. Engl. J. Med., 294:17, 91, 1976.

510. CLINICAL PATTERNS OF THE PLASMA CELL DYSCRASIAS

510.1. MULTIPLE MYELOMA
(Plasma Cell Myeloma, Myelomatosis)

Multiple myeloma is generally defined as a neoplasm of plasma cells manifested primarily by widespread skeletal destruction and frequently associated with anemia, hypercalcemia, renal functional impairment, and increased susceptibility to infections, Amyloidosis, coagulation defects, and symptoms and signs related to cryoglobulins or increased serum viscosity are less com-

monly associated manifestations. Diagnosis depends upon the roentgenographic demonstration of diffuse osteolytic lesions and/or osteoporosis, documentation of increased numbers of plasma cells in the marrow, and the finding of M-type serum or urinary proteins.

The frequency of myeloma has apparently increased in recent years and now is comparable to that of Hodgkin's disease in many large clinics. Improved diagnostic techniques are unquestionably partly responsible for the apparent increase. Males and females are approximately equally affected. The age of onset of symptoms ranges from young adulthood to advanced years, the peak incidence being in the mid-fifties.

The symptomatic stage of myeloma is preceded by a significant asymptomatic or presymptomatic period in most, and perhaps all, cases. In this presymptomatic period, M-type serum and/or urinary proteins are demonstrable and are usually first suggested by the finding on routine examination of an increased erythrocyte sedimentation rate or unexplained and persistent proteinuria. Because intravenous pyelography may precipitate renal shutdown in the presence of Bence Jones proteinuria, the increased hazard of the procedure should be considered in planning the investigation of a case with unexplained proteinuria. The duration of the presymptomatic period in myeloma is impossible to define, but apparently can range up to 20 years. Repeated bacterial infections, particularly pneumonias, can occur during this period, presumably as a consequence of impaired immunologic mechanisms.

Whey myeloma becomes symptomatic, skeletal pains are the presenting and predominant manifestations in most cases. These may at first be mild and transient, or their onset may be sudden with severe back, rib, or extremity pain after an abrupt movement or effort. The abrupt onset of pain frequently indicates a pathologic fracture. With progression of the disease, more and more areas of bone destruction develop, frequently resulting in marked skeletal deformities, particularly of the sternum and rib cage, and shortening of the spine with as much as 5 or more inches decrease in stature. With earlier diagnosis and more effective chemotherapy and general management, these extreme degrees of skeletal deformity have become less common.

In most cases, multiple osteolytic ("punched-out") lesions are apparent on initial roentgenographic examination (Fig. 5). The skull, spine, ribs, clavicles, sternum, pelvis, and proximal long bones exhibit the greatest destruction, but any part of the skeleton, including the phalanges, may be involved.

In many cases, the initial roentgenographic appearance of the skeleton is that of diffuse osteoporosis without discrete osteolytic lesions. Histologic studies demonstrate a diffuse infiltration of the marrow spaces by myeloma cells, with generalized thinning of trabeculae not detectable by standard roentgenographic techniques. Virtually all patients with this initial pattern of diffuse osteoporosis eventually develop osteolytic lesions as the disease progresses. Possibly the rarest finding in myeloma is an osteoblastic reaction in the absence of a pathologic fracture; there are now several reported examples of this.

In occasional cases, myeloma presents as an *apparently single* skeletal lesion. Although these lesions are commonly designated as solitary plasmacytomas, most patients ultimately develop disseminated disease even if the original lesion is radically excised or irradiated. In

Figure 5.   Characteristic x-ray abnormalities in multiple myeloma. Skull (left) shows multiple osteolytic ("punched-out") lesions. Thoracic spine (right) shows extensive osteoporosis and partial collapse of several vertebral bodies.

cases of apparently solitary plasmacytomas, M-type protein abnormalities are almost invariably demonstrable.

Skeletal destruction results in the release of bone salts, negative calcium balance, and hypercalciuria in virtually all cases. This is generally well tolerated if adequate hydration is maintained. Hypercalcemia ensues, however, if the renal excretory capacity for calcium is exceeded, usually as a consequence of inadequate hydration and diminished urine output. All too frequently, there develops a menacing sequence of hypercalciuria → osmotic diuresis + impairment of renal tubular reabsorption → dehydration → diminished urine output → hypercalcemia + azotemia → anorexia, nausea, vomiting, and further dehydration. This set of circumstances constitutes a major threat requiring prompt therapeutic intervention with rehydration as the primary goal. Prednisone is a useful adjunct in the management of hypercalcemia, but other chemotherapy is contraindicated until hydration is accomplished and renal function restored.

In occasional cases, particularly those with diffuse osteoporosis rather than local skeletal destruction, the initial symptoms are the nonspecific gastrointestinal complaints related to hypercalcemia and the polyuria and polydipsia secondary to hypercalciuria.

Anemia of variable severity is present in virtually all cases, either at the time of diagnosis or developing subsequently as the disease progresses. It may remain moderate (hemoglobin in the range of 7 to 10 grams) and be well tolerated or become severe enough to require repeated transfusions. The anemia is usually normocytic and normochromic, but may be macrocytic. It is characteristically refractory to iron, vitamin B_{12}, folic acid, pyridoxine, and liver therapy. In occasional cases a hypochromic anemia may be related to blood loss from the gastrointestinal tract, to a defect in coagula-

tion, or to plasmacytic or amyloid infiltrates of the intestinal wall. Several factors participate in the production of anemia in myeloma, including marrow replacement, accelerated erythrocyte destruction, blood loss, renal insufficiency, the effects of radiotherapy and chemotherapy, associated infections, and nutritional factors.

Erythrocyte rouleau formation is observed in peripheral blood and marrow films, and in vivo erythrocyte aggregation ("sludged blood") is often demonstrable. This aggregation is probably due to erythrocyte coating by M-type proteins and may contribute to shortened red cell life span. Coombs reactions, however, are usually negative.

Leukocyte and platelet counts are usually within normal limits prior to cytotoxic therapy. Occasionally, however, moderate to severe leukopenia or thrombocytopenia may be observed prior to treatment and, indeed, with therapy, the white cell and platelet counts may rise toward normal. Thrombocytopenia may contribute to a bleeding diathesis and leukopenia to an increased susceptibility to infection. The precise mechanisms responsible for leukopenia and thrombocytopenia in the plasma cell dyscrasias are unknown. The differential white cell count frequently reveals a relative lymphocytosis (40 to 55 per cent) with a variable proportion of immature lymphocytic and plasmacytic forms. Plasma cells in the peripheral blood have been reported in up to 70 per cent of cases. An outpouring of plasma cells into the peripheral blood is occasionally seen in the later stages of disease, and is considered to represent a displacement phenomenon.

A clinical pattern consistent with a diagnosis of plasma cell leukemia, with hepatosplenomegaly and white cell counts in excess of 15,000 and over 50 per cent plasma cells, is occasionally observed, with weakness, anemia, and bleeding manifestations. In the peripheral blood the cells range from typical plasmacytes to immature and atypical forms. Bence Jones proteinuria and abnormal serum globulins occur with the same frequency as in myeloma. The majority of these cases pursue an acute or subacute clinical course. It is of interest that two of the four reported cases of IgE myeloma exhibited the clinical pattern of plasma cell leukemia.

Eosinophilia, with eosinophil counts as high as 15 to 25 per cent, is observed in occasional cases of myeloma and somewhat more commonly in macroglobulinemia and γ heavy chain disease. The significance of eosinophilia in these diseases is unknown.

Marked elevation of the erythrocyte sedimentation rate (ESR) is found in most cases of myeloma. When the M-type serum proteins are cold precipitable (cryoglobulins), the ESR may be markedly temperature dependent, i.e., slower at room termperature or in the cold and accelerated when performed at 37° C.

PATHOLOGIC EFFECTS OF M-TYPE SERUM GLOBULINS AND BENCE JONES PROTEINS. Each M-type protein must be recognized to be individually specific and to possess specific physiochemical properties, such as solubility, intrinsic viscosity, thermostability, and reactivity with other proteins. Certain of these properties can be correlated with specific clinical and pathologic manifestations. Thus coagulation defects are related in certain cases to the interaction (protein:protein complexing) of specific M-type IgG or IgA globulins with specific coagulation factors, including fibrinogen, factors V, VII, prothrombin, and the antihemophilic globulin. Another group of protein-related symptoms are those produced by M-type IgG globulins which are cold precipitable, i.e., cryoglobulins. These include a Raynaud-type phenomenon, circulatory impairment, and, at times, occlusion and gangrene after relatively mild exposure to cold. Circulatory impairment, particularly in the central nervous system and retina, can also be related in certain cases to IgA and IgG globulins with a high intrinsic viscosity. As noted below, these features are relatively more common in Waldenström's macroglobulinemia.

An association between Bence Jones proteinuria and renal functional impairment has long been implied, and is generally ascribed to the tubular precipitation of these proteins and blockage owing to cast formation. More recently, it has been found that Bence Jones proteinuria is occasionally associated with specific defects in renal tubular reabsorption mechanisms, including the adult Fanconi syndrome, indicating that certain Bence Jones proteins have the capacity to interfere with specific tubular transport mechanisms through direct (protein:protein) interaction with tubular cytoplasmic constituents. There is no evident correlation between the antigenic type of a Bence Jones protein and its nephrotoxic potential. The fact that a nephrotoxic potential is *not* common to *all* Bence Jones proteins is indicated by the maintenance of apparently normal renal function in many cases with protracted and profound Bence Jones proteinuria. This is further evidence that several factors in addition to Bence Jones proteinuria, particularly hypercalciuria, hyperuricosuria, and dehydration, contribute to renal dysfunction in myeloma.

Bence Jones proteins have also been implicated in the pathogenesis of amyloidosis. It is postulated that Bence Jones proteins traverse capillary beds because of their small molecular size and polymerize and/or coprecipitate with as yet unidentified tissue proteins or polysaccharides to yield the complex proteinaceous tissue infiltrates designated amyloid (see Ch. 510.3).

ADDITIONAL CLINICAL MANIFESTATIONS. Hyperuricemia and hyperuricosuria are observed in most cases as a result of increased turnover of nucleic acids in the proliferating cell population. Hyperuricosuria is not infrequently associated with renal functional impairment resulting from precipitation of urate crystals or stone formation, or both. The danger of increased urate excretion is particularly great in the initial stages of cytotoxic chemotherapy, and warrants special attention to the maintenance of adequate hydration and possibly therapy with allopurinol. Gouty arthropathy is a rare complication.

Neurologic manifestations may develop from direct pressure on the spinal cord, nerve roots, or cranial or peripheral nerves, or as a result of a pathololologic fracture of a vertebral body or long bone. Spinal cord compression leading to weakness and ultimately paraplegia is an especially serious complication because the osteoporosis and negative calcium balance produced by the myeloma are compounded by the osteoporosis of immobilization. Again, this complication of myeloma has become less common with improved therapeutic management.

Infiltration of peripheral nerves and nerve roots by amyloid can cause peripheral neuropathies or root symptoms that are usually symmetrical and are associated with other evidence of amyloidosis such as macroglossia, cardiac manifestations, and the carpal tunnel syndrome. Rarely, polyneuropathies develop in myeloma and the other plasma cell dyscrasias without demonstrable tumor or amyloid infiltration. The pattern of these polyneuropathies is nonspecific; apparently they are similar to the polyneuropathies of obscure origin occasionally associated with other neoplastic diseases.

Myopathies involving principally proximal muscle groups are also rarely associated with myeloma and other plasma cell dyscrasias and, again, the pathogenic mechanisms are completely unknown.

An apparent increase in the incidence of nonreticular neoplasms, particularly of bowel, breast, and biliary tract carcinomas, has been noted in association with myeloma in one comprehensive postmortem study (19 per cent) and in the author's series (22 per cent).

IMMUNOLOGIC DEFICIENCY. Increased susceptibility to bacterial infections, particularly pneumococcal pneumonia, exists in many cases of myeloma and is at least partially the result of an impaired capacity for antibody formation. This is generally reflected in a decrease in the serum concentration of normal IgG, IgA, and IgM immunoglobulins irrespective of the type of M-protein elaborated. The basis for these deficiencies is presently unknown, but available studies indicate that diminished production is a more significant factor than increased catabolism or loss. Some evidence has been obtained that peripheral blood mononuclear cells from certain myeloma patients suppress in vitro immunoglobulin synthesis by normal lymphocytes. Herpes zoster and generalized varicella infections occur with increased frequency in myeloma and other plasma cell dyscrasias, but apparently no more so than in Hodgkin's disease and lymphosarcoma. Susceptibility to other viral infections apparently is not increased. Studies of the homograft rejection reaction have demonstrated a significant prolongation of rejection time, indicating that the immunologic deficiencies in myeloma may include cell-mediated immune mechanisms.

TREATMENT. Both the comfort and useful life of patients with myeloma can unquestionably be extended by proper management. The importance of *ambulation and adequate hydration* cannot be overemphasized. The constant threats of hypercalcemia, hypercalciuria, and hyperuricemia necessitate continual attention to these cardinal aspects of general care. Many patients are immobilized and bedridden with pain when first seen. In these circumstances, all effort should be made to achieve ambulation by a combination of analgesics, and local radiotherapy, as indicated. In occasional cases orthopedic supports, particularly Taylor-type spine bracing, may facilitate mobilization, but care should be taken to avoid cumbersome braces which may impede ambulation. Plasma cell tumors are characteristically radiosensitive, and x-ray therapy is of established value in the control of localized symptomatic lesions. The field of irradiation and the dosage should be limited in order to spare the marrow as much as possible. A total dose of 1800 to 2200 roentgens is usually adequate for symptomatic control and for the facilitation of ambulation. Pain relief is frequently noted after as little as 200 to 400 r. Salicylates and codeine are usually more effective analgesics for the pain of myeloma than meperidine (Demerol) or propoxyphene (Darvon). Prednisone, as previously indicated, is a useful agent in the management of hypercalcemia, but hydration sufficient to achieve a 24-hour urine output of over 1500 ml is the principal need. Unless mobilization and hydration are accomplished by these measures, it is usually impossible to maintain a patient for the time required to accomplish a remission with chemotherapy.

Of the chemotherapeutic agents presently available, melphalan (1-phenylalanine mustard, Alkeran) and Cytoxan (cyclophosphamide) are the two drugs most useful in the long-term management of myeloma. When properly administered, both agents can achieve significant objective and subjective remissions in approximately 80 per cent of cases. Although both melphalan and Cytoxan are alkylating agents, their precise mechanisms of action must be different, because sensitivity or resistance to one agent does not necessarily imply the corresponding sensitivity or resistance to the other. Thus the two agents can be used sequentially with an increased possibility of achieving a remission. As yet it is not known whether there is a preferential order, but melphalan is generally the first agent employed in the author's clinic. Therapy is usually initiated with an eight- to ten-day course of 8 to 10 mg per day, i.e., an initial course of 64 to 100 mg, depending upon the patient's size, hematologic status, and general condition. After this initial course, continuous maintenance therapy at a dose of 2 mg a day is instituted. It is no longer considered necessary to interrupt therapy between the initial loading dose and institution of maintenance therapy. With this dosage regimen, the peripheral leukocyte count will usually be suppressed to the range of 3000 to 4000 and be maintained in this range with continued therapy. This degree of marrow suppression is tolerated without complications and provides an index of the adequacy of dosage. In some cases, a decrease in white count below 3000 necessitates reducing the maintenance dose to 1 mg per day. With Cytoxan, therapy is

initiated at a dosage level of 200 mg a day for seven to ten days, after which the dose is reduced to 100 mg a day for maintenance. Again, in some cases it is necessary to reduce the maintenance dose to 50 mg a day because of leukopenia or thrombocytopenia, or both. As an alternative to the continuous, low-dose maintenance regimen, melphalan or Cytoxan may be administered intermittently at four- to six-week intervals, alone or in combination with prednisone. The presently available data do not indicate clear superiority of either of these treatment schedules with respect to the frequency, degree, or duration of remission. Accordingly, we generally employ the continuous low-dose regimen in cases with good compliance and use an intermittent (intravenous) regimen for less reliable patients. In a few patients who are refractory to continuous low-dose melphalan or Cytoxan, we have achieved remissions with a combination of Cytoxan, 200 to 400 mg, and daunorubicin (Adriamycin), 40 to 50 mg, administered intravenously every four to six weeks, along with prednisone, 60 mg daily for four to seven days. Adriamycin is discontinued after a total dose of 450 to 500 mg has been administered because of the risk of myocardial toxicity.

With chemotherapy, the objective signs of improvement include a decrease in the concentration of abnormal M-type serum globulins, decreased Bence Jones proteinuria, hematologic improvement, cessation of further skeletal destruction, and occasionally recalcification of osteolytic lesions. In some cases, the concentrations of normal immunoglobulins increase, and this is associated with improved resistance to bacterial infections. It should be recognized, however, that several weeks may elapse between the institution of therapy and the first signs of improvement. Because of the rapid turnover of Bence Jones proteins, a decrease in Bence Jones proteinuria is the earliest objective sign of chemotherapeutic effect, and this has been noted within one week of initiating chemotherapy. A decrease in myeloma serum globulins is usually not observed until the fourth or fifth week. The duration of the remissions which can be achieved with chemotherapy has steadily increased in the past several years; there are now many patients who have been maintained in excellent clinical and functional remission for periods of six years or more. Thus the prognosis in myeloma has greatly improved in the past several years with the introduction of these agents.

An attempt to increase skeletal density by inducing fluorosis with sodium fluoride has been made in some cases with generally equivocal results. At present, this therapy is not recommended. The maintenance of ambulation and the encouragement of exercise are equally as important in the long-term management of myeloma as in the initial phase of therapy. Patients should be encouraged to walk, swim, or engage in other forms of exercise to the extent of their ability, avoiding only those activities which involve excessive lifting and straining.

Azar, H. A., and Potter, M.: Multiple Myeloma and Related Disorders. Vol. I. Hagerstown, Md., Harper & Row, 1973.

Broder, S., Humphrey, R., Durm, M., Blackman, M., Meade, B., Goldman, C., Strober, W., and Waldmann, T.: Impaired synthesis of polyclonal (non-paraprotein) immunoglobulins by circulating lymphocytes from patients with multiple myeloma. N. Engl. J. Med., 293:887, 1975.

Farhangi, M., and Osserman, E. F.: The treatment of multiple myeloma. Semin. Hematol., 10:149, 1973.

Korst, D. R., Clifford, G. O., Fowler, W. M., Louis, J., Will, J., and Wilson, H. E.: Multiple myeloma. II. Analysis of cyclophosphamide therapy in 165 patients. JAMA, 189:758, 1964.

Kyle, R. A., and Bayrd, E. D.: The Monoclonal Gammopathies: Multiple Myeloma and Related Plasma Cell Disorders. Springfield, Ill., Charles C Thomas, 1976.

Osserman, E. F.: Plasma-cell myeloma: II. Clinical aspects. N. Engl. J. Med., 261:952, 1006, 1959.

Waldenström, J.: Diagnosis and Treatment of Multiple Myeloma. New York, Grune & Stratton, 1970.

510.2. MACROGLOBULINEMIA

(Primary or Waldenström's Macroglobulinemia)

Macroglobulinemia is presently classified as a plasma cell dyscrasia involving those cell populations normally responsible for the synthesis of IgM globulins. Recent studies have now established that the monoclonality extends to the B lymphocytes which are the precursors of the IgM-secreting plasma cells. The excessive proliferation of these cells results in the elaboration of large quantities of electrophoretically homogeneous (M-type) IgM globulins and a variable clinical pattern with anemia, bleeding manifestations, and symptoms related to the serum macroglobulins as the predominant features. Males and females are approximately equally affected. Symptoms generally begin in the fifth or sixth decade. As the disease slowly evolves, lymphadenopathy, splenomegaly, and hepatomegaly develop in a variable percentage of cases, producing a clinical pattern resembling a malignant lymphoma or lymphatic leukemia. Skeletal lesions of the type seen in myeloma are exceptionally rare.

Histologic studies of lymph nodes demonstrate a proliferation of lymphocytic-plasmacytic forms often arranged in a pattern of follicular hyperplasia. Immunofluorescent studies have confirmed the synthesis of IgM globulin in these cells, as well as in the corresponding lymphocytic-plasmacytic forms demonstrable in peripheral blood and bone marrow preparations. It is generally impossible to ascertain whether the cellular proliferations observed in macroglobulinemia represent reactive responses or autonomous neoplasia. The possibility that initially benign and reactive proliferations may undergo transformation to neoplastic proliferations is suggested in many cases of macroglobulinemia as in other forms of plasma cell dyscrasia.

When macroglobulinemia becomes symptomatic, anemia is the most common presenting manifestation, and is frequently profound, with hemoglobin levels in the range of 4 to 6 grams per 100 ml. Usually the anemia is due to a combination of factors, including accelerated red cell destruction, blood loss, and decreased erythropoiesis. Coating of erythrocytes with IgM globulin is apparently responsible for the marked rouleaux formation, positive Coombs reactions, and cross-matching difficulties encountered in many cases.

As previously noted, a large percentage of IgM globulins have specific physicochemical properties that are responsible for specific symptom patterns in certain cases. These properties include cold-insolubility (cryoglobulins), high intrinsic viscosity, and the capacity to form complexes with coagulation factors and other plasma proteins. *Cryoglobulin-related symptoms* include Raynaud's phenomenon, cold sensitivity, cold urticaria,

and vascular occlusion with gangrene after exposure to cold. *Viscosity-related manifestations* are most evident in the retinal vasculature, in which a pattern of patchy venous bulging and localized narrowing ("sausage-effect" or "fundus paraproteinemicus") develops, frequently associated with hemorrhages, exudates, and visual impairment. Circulatory impairment in the central nervous system caused by increased plasma viscosity produces changing patterns of neurologic signs and symptoms, e.g., transient paresis, reflex abnormalities, deafness, impairment of consciousness ("coma paraproteinemicum"), frequently terminating with cerebral vascular hemorrhage. Cardiac decompensation and pulmonary symptoms may also develop secondary to increased viscosity in the systemic and pulmonary vascular beds. *Protein:protein interactions* with formation of complexes between IgM globulins and coagulation factors (e.g., fibrinogen, prothrombin, factors V, VII) are an important contributing factor to the bleeding diatheses (particularly epistaxes, oral mucosal bleeding, and purpura) exhibited in many cases. Interference with platelet function (platelet agglutination) and capillary damage secondary to increased serum viscosity are additional factors contributing to bleeding manifestations. It must be recognized that all these symptom patterns are also observed in occasional cases of myeloma with M-type IgG and IgA globulins possessing similar physicochemical properties.

Bence Jones proteinuria is present in approximately 10 per cent of cases of macroglobulinemia, but renal functional impairment is much less common than in myeloma, presumably because of the absence of the contributing factors of hypercalcemia and hypercalciuria. Amyloidosis has been observed in only a few cases of macroglobulinemia, and in all of these, the liver, spleen, and parenchymal organs have been the major areas of involvement (Pattern II) in contrast to the primary, atypical mesenchymal distribution (Pattern I) of amyloid usually observed in myeloma.

Peripheral neuropathies *(Bing-Neel syndrome)* and myelopathy may be progressive and incapacitating. Circulatory impairment in vasa nervorum is a postulated but still unsubstantiated mechanism. Myopathies and rheumatoid-like arthropathies have also been observed.

In the author's series of 57 cases, 15 had clinical or postmortem evidence of an associated nonreticular neoplasm, and an additional 12 had a background of longstanding infection, particularly tuberculosis.

Many of the laboratory findings in macroglobulinemia have already been considered. The presymptomatic cases are usually detected initially as a result of finding an unexplained elevation of erythrocyte sedimentation rate on routine examination, followed by electrophoretic demonstration of an M-type serum protein (Fig. 3) and, finally, its characterization as an IgM globulin by ultracentrifugation or immunoelectrophoresis, or both. The majority of IgM globulins are euglobulins and give a positive Sia water-dilution reaction, but this is not specific for macroglobulins because certain IgG globulins are also Sia-positive euglobulins. Approximately one third of IgM globulins are cryoglobulins, yielding a white precipitate or a thick clear gel on cooling. The temperature and duration of cooling needed for precipitation varies with individual cryoglobulins. With some cryoglobulins, precipitation or gel-formation occurs almost immediately after venipuncture, and a prewarmed syringe is necessary for blood sampling. Others may require up to 24 hours at 10° C for precipitation. Similarly, the increased viscosity of serum containing a viscous M-type macroglobulin may be readily apparent when a tube of serum at room temperature is inverted, or viscosimetric determinations at different temperatures may be required.

Hematologic abnormalities, in addition to anemia, include an absolute lymphocytosis with "atypical, immature, and plasmacytic" forms in many cases, occasionally reaching leukemic proportions. Polymorphonuclear leukopenia, thrombopenia, and eosinophilia are also observed. Bone marrow aspirations characteristically reveal an increase in lymphocytic-plasmacytic forms, accompanied by eosinophils and mast cells in many cases. The small lymphocyte, with a dense pyknotic nucleus, which has been considered most typical for macroglobulinemia, probably represents a degenerating cell undergoing cytoplasmic shedding (so-called "clasmatosis").

Additional laboratory abnormalities in certain cases of macroglobulinemia include positive flocculation reactions, false positive serologic reactions, and positive rheumatoid factors. The latter are occasionally associated with rheumatic symptoms and arthropathy.

TREATMENT. The principal indications for therapy in macroglobulinemia are anemia, bleeding manifestations, and symptoms related to increased plasma viscosity. When the latter symptoms are severe and threaten central nervous system function and vision, plasmapheresis is indicated as a temporary measure. Sufficient plasma should be removed to effect a lowering of viscosity, and the red cells should be returned. In certain cases, a prompt and dramatic improvement in clinical status follows the removal of as little as 500 ml of plasma. Repeated plasmapheresis for a period of several weeks may be required until effective chemotherapy can be instituted.

Chlorambucil (Leukeran) is the chemotherapeutic agent of choice in macroglobulinemia. This should be administered continuously at a dosage level of 4 to 10 mg daily. Although this dosage level is significantly higher than the average employed in most cases of lymphatic leukemia or lymphosarcoma, it is usually well tolerated in macroglobulinemia. A large number of patients have been maintained in objective and subjective remission for periods up to nine years with continuous chlorambucil therapy. More limited studies with melphalan indicate it to be less effective in macroglobulinemia than chlorambucil. Prednisone may be of some value in the control of capillary bleeding.

MacKenzie, M. R., and Fudenberg, H. H.: Macroglobulinemia: An analysis of 40 patients. Blood, 39:874, 1972.
McCallister, B. D., Bayrd, E. D., Harrison E. G., Jr., and McGuckin, W. F.: Primary macroglobulinemia. Review with a report on 31 cases and notes on the value of continuous chlorambucil therapy. Am. J. Med., 43:394, 1967.
Waldenström, J.: Studies on conditions associated with disturbed gamma globulin formation (gammapathies). Harvey Lect., Series 56:211, 1961.

510.3. AMYLOIDOSIS

Amyloidosis is a term applied to a variety of conditions associated with tissue infiltrates composed of insoluble proteins and/or protein-polysaccharide complexes. With the relatively recent development of methods for the isolation and chemical and immunologic analysis of amyloids, it has become evident that there are *at least* two chemical types of amyloid. In one (Ig-type), immunoglobulin light chains appear to be the principal protein component; in the other (protein A–type), an apparently nonimmunoglobulin constituent (protein A) is the major protein. It must be stressed that other chemical types of amyloid have been identified, e.g., calcitonin-related amyloid in certain cases of medullary carcinoma of the thyroid. However, the Ig-type and protein A-type constitute the majority of amyloidosis cases encountered clinically. In both types, the tissue infiltrates apparently represent noncovalently bonded polymers of the basic protein subunit, either alone or in combination with other proteins or polysaccharides. The polymers are sufficiently large to yield a characteristic fibrillar structure which can be visualized by electron microscopy and a distinctive green-yellow dichroic birefringence seen by polarization microscopy after Congo red staining.

As outlined in Table 2, there is some correlation between the chemical type of amyloid and the clinical pattern of amyloid distribution. Thus Ig-type amyloid has been mainly found in cases with either occult plasma cell dyscrasia or overt multiple myeloma. The pattern of distribution of amyloid in these cases is most frequently that previously referred to as primary-type,

TABLE 2. Patterns of Amyloidosis

	Previous Designations	Distribution	Associated Conditions	Type of Amyloid Protein
Pattern I	Primary-type, atypical, para-amyloid, pericollagen, mesenchymal	Tongue, heart, GI tract, muscles, ligaments, skin	Plasma cell dyscrasia, usually with Bence Jones only; overt myeloma	Ig-light chain
Pattern II	Secondary-type, typical, perireticular, parenchymal	Liver, spleen, kidney, adrenal	Chronic infections, rheumatoid arthritis, familial Mediterranean fever	Protein A
Mixed Pattern I and II	—	Various combinations of I and II sites	Plasma cell dyscrasia with complete IgG, A, D, and M globulins	Not known
Localized	Tumor-forming	Lung, GI tract, bladder, eye	Plasma cell dyscrasia	Not known

i.e., principal involvement of the tongue, heart, gastrointestinal tract, skeletal and smooth muscles, carpal ligaments, nerves, and skin. This distribution pattern, referred to as Pattern I, was manifested in 50 per cent of the cases in the author's series.

Protein A–type amyloid has thus far been mainly found in cases of amyloidosis associated with chronic infections (e.g., tuberculosis), rheumatoid arthritis, Hodgkin's disease, and familial Mediterranean fever. The pattern of distribution of amyloid in these cases most frequently is that previously referred to as secondary-type, i.e., principal involvement of the liver, spleen, kidneys, and adrenals. This distribution pattern, now designated Pattern II, was displayed by 17 per cent of the author's cases.

In a significant proportion of cases (30 per cent of the author's series), amyloid involves both Pattern I and II sites to varying degrees, and these cases are now referred to as Mixed Pattern I and II. Monoclonal IgG, A, D, and M globulins, indicative of associated plasma cell dyscrasias, are demonstrable in the majority (82 per cent) of Mixed Pattern I and II cases, but the specific role of these proteins in the amyloid deposits has not been determined. In a small percentage of cases (3 per cent in the author's series) amyloid is apparently localized to one tissue or organ. In all our cases of localized amyloidosis, abnormal collections of plasma cells were found in immediate juxtaposition to the amyloid deposits, and monoclonal immunoglobulins were also demonstrated in all three cases.

Ideally, disease classifications should be based on etiologic factors, and this should eventually be possible with amyloidosis. Until this is achieved, however, the presently suggested classification based on the predominant clinical patterns of amyloid distribution is considered preferable to previously employed designations such as primary, secondary, typical, and atypical. The terms primary and secondary have been particularly confusing, because in usage they have referred either to *presumed* etiologic factors or to particular patterns of amyloid distribution. Because of the prevalence of chronic infections and suppuration in the preantibiotic era, Pattern II amyloid was relatively more common and "typical" than Pattern I ("atypical"). In more recent series, however, Pattern I cases predominate.

The clinical manifestations of amyloidosis are variable and depend on the distribution and extent of the tissue infiltrates. In Pattern I amyloidosis the clinical manifestations may be any one or a combination of the following: cardiac involvement with decompensation (low output failure), often but not invariably refractory to digitalis and associated with decreased pulse pressure, low EKG voltage, conduction defects, and arrhythmias; tongue and salivary gland involvement with progressive macroglossia, change in taste sensation, xerostomia, and dysphagia; gastrointestinal manifestations, particularly anorexia, alternating diarrhea and constipation, abdominal cramps, borborygmi, sprue-like manifestations with malabsorption, and gastrointestinal bleeding; carpal tunnel syndrome with median nerve involvement and arterial insufficiency caused by infiltration of the carpal ligaments; joint and muscle stiffness and limitation of motion, usually not painful or tender and readily distinguishable from rheumatoid arthritis; neuropathies and radiculopathies with varying sensory and motor deficits; or skin and subcutaneous tissue involvement evidenced by subcutaneous hemorrhages and purpura after minimal trauma, particularly in the eyelids and periorbital tissues ("raccoon facies"). Monoclonal immunoglobulins, particularly Bence Jones proteins, and abnormal marrow plasmacytosis can be demonstrated in virtually all Pattern I cases, and overt skeletal lesions consistent with multiple myeloma develop in approximately 50 per cent of these cases.

In Pattern II amyloidosis, the process is usually manifested by the insidious onset of hepatosplenomegaly and progressive hepatic failure, proteinuria, and renal functional impairment, culminating in the nephrotic syndrome. Peripheral edema and anasarca frequently develop as a consequence of the combined effects of hypoalbuminemia (decreased albumin synthesis caused by hepatic dysfunction plus urinary loss) and abnormal arteriolar capillary permeability secondary to amyloid infiltration.

As would be expected, the clinical manifestations in Mixed Pattern I and II amyloidosis also reflect the extent of involvement of specific tissues and organs. Six of 30 cases of Mixed Pattern I and II amyloidosis in our series were associated with overt myeloma.

DIAGNOSIS. The diagnosis of amyloidosis depends on biopsy documentation. If possible, an accessible site with apparent involvement should be biopsied (e.g., skin, muscle), but tongue biopsy should be avoided because of pain and risk of infection. Liver and kidney biopsy are possibly associated with a risk of bleeding, but this has not been a significant problem in most series. Because amyloidosis of Pattern I and Pattern II frequently involves the arterioles of the rectal submucosa, rectal biopsy is a relatively safe and useful diagnostic procedure. All biopsy material should be stained with Congo red and examined by polarization microscopy. This technique not infrequently discloses amyloid deposits not revealed by the usual staining procedures.

In all cases of amyloidosis, detailed examination of the serum and urinary proteins by electrophoresis and immunoelectrophoresis is indicated, along with bone marrow studies, to document a plasma cell dyscrasia. In a case of amyloidosis with proteinuria, the finding of a negative Bence Jones reaction on heat-testing does not exclude the presence of an abnormal constituent of the Bence Jones type, because albumin and other serum proteins in the urine may mask a Bence Jones reaction.

TREATMENT. There is no known method to reverse the deposition of amyloid infiltrates except the identification and control of associated conditions, particularly osteomyelitis, pulmonary abscess, and tuberculosis. Several cases have been reported in which effective antimicrobial therapy or surgery or both for a chronic suppurative process have resulted in cessation of amyloid deposition and reabsorption of existing infiltrates. Unfortunately, this is rare; in most cases the amyloidosis continues despite apparently effective control of associated conditions. A noteworthy exception is the ability of colchicine to block the febrile attacks in familial Mediterranean fever and simultaneously to reduce the incidence of renal amyloidosis.

Experience with melphalan and other cytotoxic therapy in cases of amyloidosis with overt myeloma or occult plasma cell dyscrasia is limited, but results have been generally discouraging. Most patients continue to pursue a downhill course, succumbing to cardiac decompensation or complications related to tongue and gastrointestinal involvement. Corticosteroids occasionally provide slight symptomatic benefit. In cases of macroglossia, careful attention to oral hygiene is important to avoid irritation and ulceration of the tongue.

Cohen, A. S.: Amyloidosis. N. Engl. J. Med., 277:522, 574, 628, 1967.

Franklin, E. C., and Zucker-Franklin, D.: Current concepts of amyloid. *In* Dixon, F. J., and Kunkel, H. G. (eds.): Advances in Immunology. Vol. 15. New York, Academic Press, 1972, p. 249.

Glenner, G. G., Terry, W. D., and Isersky, C.: Amyloidosis: Its nature and pathogenesis. Semin. Hematol., 10:65, 1973.

Isobe, T., and Osserman, E. F.: Patterns of amyloidosis and their associations with plasma cell dyscrasia, monoclonal immunoglobulins and Bence Jones proteins. N. Engl. J. Med., 290:473, 1974.

Osserman, E. F., Takatsuki, K., and Talal, N.: The pathogenesis of "amyloidosis." Studies on the role of abnormal gamma globulins and gamma globulin fragments of the Bence Jones (L-polypeptide) type in the pathogenesis of "primary" and "secondary amyloidosis," and the "amyloidosis" associated with plasma cell myeloma. Semin. Hematol., 1:3, 1964.

Wegelius, O., and Pasternack, A. (eds.): Amyloidosis. London, Academic Press, 1976.

510.4. LICHEN MYXEDEMATOSUS

Lichen myxedematosus (papular mucinosis) is a rare form of plasma cell dyscrasia characterized by the progressive deposition of protein in the dermis of the face, trunk, and extremities (Fig. 6). Recent studies have established that this disorder is apparently consistently associated with the elaboration of unusually basic (cationic) M-type IgG globulins. It has further been demonstrated in one case that the infiltrates of the skin were comprised, at least in part, by this specific protein, presumably deposited in combination with the mucopolysaccharides of the dermis. The possibility that lichen myxedematosus may be an autoimmune disease in which a monoclonal antibody is directed against antigenic constituents of the dermis has been suggested.

510.5. γ HEAVY CHAIN DISEASE

γ heavy chain disease is a relatively rare form of plasma cell dyscrasia characterized by the elaboration of excessive quantities of polypeptide related to the heavy chains and, more specifically, to the Fc fragment of IgG globulin. The clinical pattern resembles a lymphoma with lymphadenopathy, splenomegaly, and hepatomegaly as the predominant manifestations associated with the nonspecific symptoms of weakness, fever, weight loss, and marked susceptibility to bacterial infections. Several patients have exhibited transient palatal erythema and edema resembling that of infectious mononucleosis, and in some there was transient spontaneous regression of the lymphadenopathy after an initially rapid onset. None have had clinical or roentgenographic evidence of skeletal destruction. Most have shown anemia, leukopenia, and thrombopenia, presumably secondary to hypersplenism, and moderate to marked eosinophilia. Bone marrow aspirations and lymph node biopsies demonstrated proliferation of plasmacytic and lymphocytic forms along with eosinophils and large reticulum or reticuloendothelial cells.

Persistent proteinuria (4 to 15 grams per 24 hours) was generally the initial indication of an abnormality of protein metabolism. The characteristic serum and urinary protein electrophoretic patterns are illustrated in Figure 4B and have been described in Ch. 509. Total serum protein concentrations were generally within normal limits. The serum concentration of the abnormal protein ranged from 2 to 4 grams per 100 ml associated with marked decrease in the concentration of normal gamma globulin. Identification of the abnormal protein as related to the γ heavy chain (Fc fragment) and unrelated to Bence Jones and light chain polypeptides must be accomplished by immunochemical and physicochemical analyses.

In contrast to myeloma, erythrocyte sedimentation rates have been normal or only slightly elevated. Additional laboratory findings have included hyperuricemia with normal or only slightly elevated blood urea nitrogen levels and no other evidence of renal functional impairment.

Survival from the time of onset of symptoms has ranged from four months to over five years. Bacterial pneumonia and sepsis caused death in all cases.

Splenic radiation has produced temporary remissions with hematologic improvement. Limited trials of cyclophosphamide, melphalan, and steroids gave little or no benefit.

Figure 6. Lichen myxedematosus (papular mucinosis). A form of tissue proteinosis with extensive involvement of the dermis.

510.6. IgA HEAVY CHAIN (α-CHAIN) DISEASE

IgA heavy chain (α-chain) disease is the most common form of heavy chain disease and over 100 cases have now been reported. As originally described by Seligmann and his associates, the clinical pattern is that previously referred to as "Mediterranean-type abdominal lymphoma." The predominant features are a diffuse lymphoma-like proliferation in the small intestine and mesentery, chronic diarrhea, and malabsorption unresponsive to gluten withdrawal. Although Seligmann's original cases were either non-Ashkenazi Jews or Israeli Arabs, the syndrome, with the specific α-chain abnormality, has subsequently been documented in subjects of diverse ethnic backgrounds. Thus, although genetic factors were considered to be of major importance, the disease is not exclusively restricted to the Mediterranean population.

Chronic diarrhea, malabsorption, and progressive wasting are the major clinical features. Small intestinal biopsies demonstrate a profound infiltration of the lamina propria with abnormal plasma cells. Intestinal absorption studies demonstrate impaired absorption of vitamin B_{12}, glucose, lactose, and fat. Roentgenograms of the small intestines show thickened mucosal folds, segmentation, and dilated intestinal loops. Bone marrow aspiration reveals moderate increases in plasma cells, and skeletal roentgenograms show moderate diffuse osteoporosis but no destructive lesions.

On electrophoretic analysis of serum, the distinctive increase in IgA heavy chains (α chains) has been evidenced by a markedly elevated, broad peak traversing the beta and alpha-2 mobility range. The electrophoretic polydispersity has been shown to be due to polymeric heterogeneity of the alpha chains. This tendency to polymerize also explains the relatively low concentration of alpha chains in the urine as compared with the excretion of gamma chains in IgG heavy chain disease. Confirmation of the identity of the abnormal serum protein as free α-chains is accomplished by demonstrating the absence of associated light chains by appropriate immunologic and chemical analyses.

The association of this particular form of plasma cell dyscrasia with the small intestine is of particular interest in view of the known preponderance of IgA-producing plasma cells in the intestinal tract. Complete regression of the full syndrome of α-chain disease with normalization of the immunoglobulins has now been observed in several patients treated for presumptive intestinal infections with antimicrobial agents, particularly tetracyclines. Thus antecedent chronic infection or irritation of the intestines appears to be an important factor in the pathogenesis of this particular variant of plasma cell cyscrasia.

Frangione, B., and Franklin, E. C.: Heavy chain diseases: Clinical features and molecular significance of the disordered immunoglobulin structure. Semin. Hematol., 10:53, 1973.

Franklin, E. C., Lowenstein, J., Bigelow, B., and Meltzer, M.: Heavy chain disease. A new disorder of serum γ-globulins. Am. J. Med., 37:332, 1964.

Osserman, E. F., and Takatsuki, K.: Clinical and immunochemical studies of four cases of heavy (Hγ₂) chain disease. Am. J. Med., 37:351, 1964.

Seligmann, M.: Alpha chain disease: Immunoglobulin abnormalities, pathogenesis and current concepts. Br. J. Cancer, 31:356, 1975.

510.7. IgM HEAVY CHAIN (μ-CHAIN) DISEASE

IgM heavy chain (μ-chain) disease appears to be a relatively rare variant of plasma cell dyscrasia. The majori-

ty of reported cases have displayed the clinical and hematologic features of chronic lymphatic leukemia with weakness, anemia, peripheral blood lymphocytosis, and hepatosplenomegaly as the predominant manifestations. The specific immunoglobulin abnormality has generally presented as a relatively small monoclonal peak on serum electrophoresis, subsequently shown by immunodiffusion analyses to represent an excess of μ-chains without associated light chains. Because of the relative subtlety of these protein abnormalities, it is likely that the condition may be overlooked in some cases which would otherwise be considered to represent fairly typical chronic lymphatic leukemia. In several cases, Bence Jones proteinuria has been present along with the μ-chain abnormality; in the first reported case, amyloidosis and osteolytic lesions developed in the terminal phase of the illness. Ultrastructural studies of the bone marrow cells in this case demonstrated atypical plasmacytic forms with very large cytoplasmic vacuoles. By immunofluorescence analyses, 70 per cent of cells were found to contain both μ and κ determinants, and it was postulated that a structural defect in the μ-chain interfered with proper assembly of the immunoglobulin molecule.

Ballard, H. S., Hamilton, L. M., Marcus, A. J., and Illes, C. H.: A new variant of heavy chain disease (μ-chain disease). N. Engl. J. Med., 282:1060, 1970.

Dammacco, F., Bonomo, L., and Franklin, E. C.: A new case of Mu heavy chain disease: Clinical and immunological studies. Blood, 43:713, 1974.

Forte, F. A., Prelli, F., Yount, W. J., Jerry, L. M., Kochwa, S., Franklin, E. C., and Kunkel, H. G.: Heavy chain disease of the μ (γ_M) type: Report of the first case. Blood, 36:137, 1970.

510.8. PLASMA CELL DYSCRASIA OF UNKNOWN SIGNIFICANCE AND PLASMA CELL DYSCRASIA ASSOCIATED WITH CHRONIC INFECTIONS, BILIARY DISEASE, AND NONRETICULAR NEOPLASMS

Use of serum electrophoresis as a routine clinical laboratory procedure has resulted in the detection of M-type protein abnormalities, such as are illustrated in Figure 4C and D, in otherwise asymptomatic persons. As previously noted, certain of these later develop signs and symptoms of myeloma, macroglobulinemia, or amyloidosis after many months or years. A fundamental question is whether M-type protein abnormalities are invariably manifestations of plasma cell dyscrasia that will produce clinical symptoms if the patient survives "long enough" (possibly several decades), or whether certain M-type abnormalities are truly benign and "essential." Since this question is presently unanswerable, the term "plasma cell dyscrasia of unknown significance" (PCDUS) is considered preferable to "premyeloma" or "essential or benign monoclonal gammopathy."

In general, asymptomatic M-type protein abnormalities are more commonly observed in older subjects. In many cases there is a background of tuberculosis, syphilis or other chronic infection, chronic biliary tract disease, or a nonreticular neoplasm, particularly large bowel, breast, oropharyngeal, and biliary tract carcinomas. Although a coincidental association cannot be excluded, particularly in older subjects, there is increasing evidence that certain plasma cell dyscrasias in man may be induced by diverse forms of protracted reticuloendothelial stimuli comparable to those described in mice. Because of the frequency of these associations, a careful search for an occult infection or neoplasm should be periodically carried out in all patients with asymptomatic M-type protein abnormalities, with particular attention to the bowel and biliary tracts.

To date, chemotherapy with melphalan or any other agent has not been deemed warranted in asymptomatic subjects, despite the knowledge that a certain percentage of them will later develop overt myeloma. Although there are obvious theoretical advantages to earlier chemotherapy, the unpredictability of the course in any one case and the significant toxicities of presently available agents are strong arguments against the institution of chemotherapy before a distinct clinical pattern is evident.

Hallen, J.: Discrete gamma globulin (M —) components in serum. Clinical study of 150 subjects without myelomatosis. Acta Med. Scand. (suppl.) 462, 127 pp., 1966.

Isobe, T., and Osserman, E. F.: Pathologic conditions associated with plasma cell dyscrasia: A study of 806 cases. Ann. N. Y. Acad. Sci., 190:507, 1971.

Waldenström, J. G.: Benign monoclonal gammapathies. In Azar, H. A., and Potter, M. (eds.): Multiple Myeloma and Related Disorders. Vol. I. Hagerstown, Md., Harper & Row, 1973, p. 247.

Young, V. H.: Transient paraproteins. Proc. R. Soc. Med., 62:778, 1969.

Zawadzki, Z. A., and Edwards, G. A.: Dysimmunoglobulinemia associated with hepatobiliary disorders. Am. J. Med., 48:196, 1970.

510.9. ASSOCIATION BETWEEN PLASMACYTIC AND MONOCYTIC DYSCRASIAS

A close functional relationship is known to exist between the monocyte-histiocyte-macrophage system and plasma cells in the processing of antigens and the synthesis of antibodies. As an apparently related phenomenon, there is a significant association between plasmacytic and monocytic dyscrasias in man. Thus monocytic leukemia develops late in the course of a small but significant number of cases of longstanding plasma cell myeloma, generally after several years of effective chemotherapeutic control of the myeloma. In all cases, the monocytic leukemia is associated with markedly elevated serum and urine lysozyme levels. The onset of monocytic leukemia is usually abrupt, although in some cases transient episodes of peripheral monocytosis and fever precede the development of the terminal leukemic phase.

Additional evidence linking monocytic and plasmacytic dyscrasias has been the finding of M-type gamma globulin abnormalities or diffuse hypergammaglobulinemia, or both, in several cases of monocytic and myelomonocytic leukemia not associated with overt myeloma. Significantly, many of these latter patients have had protracted chronic illnesses, particularly chronic pulmonary infections, tuberculosis, and osteomyelitis, similar to those associated with plasma cell dyscrasia. Thus comparable pathogenic mechanisms may be operative, and may constitute a proliferative stimulus to both plasma cells and monocytes, either simultaneously or sequentially.

Kyle, R. A., Pierre, R. V., and Bayrd, E. D.: Multiple myeloma and acute myelomonocytic leukemia. N. Engl. J. Med., 283:1121, 1970.

Osserman, E. F.: Clinical and biochemical studies of plasmacytic and monocytic dyscrasias and their interrelationships. Trans. Studies, Coll. Physicians, Phila., 36:134, 1969.

Osserman, E. F., and Lawlor, D. P.: Serum and urinary lysozyme (muramidase) in monocytic and mono-myelocytic leukemia. J. Exp. Med., 124:921, 1966.

Rosner, F., and Grunwald, H., for Acute Leukemia Group B: Multiple myeloma terminating in acute leukemia. Am. J. Med., 57:927, 1974.

Section Ten DISEASES OF THE SPLEEN

Richard A. Rifkind

511. INTRODUCTION

Even a brief overview of the functional properties of the spleen provides insight into the confusion which has existed since earliest times over the role of the spleen, Galen's "organ of mystery", with respect to normal physiology and disease. The spleen is responsible for at least four major physiologic functions, calling into play its unique cellular and anatomic characteristics. Of primary importance to the pathophysiology to be discussed in these chapters are the *hemoclastic functions*, concerned with sequestration, pooling, remodeling, and destruction of normal and pathologic blood cells. The spleen is also *an organ of the immune system* — although not an indispensable immunologic organ, because its immunologic functions are shared with the other lymphoreticular organs; nevertheless the spleen serves an important function in protection from blood-borne microorganisms. A third splenic function, of no importance to the healthy adult, but of considerable importance to the embryo and when the bone marrow is pathologically compromised, is the *hemato-poietic function*. During normal embryogenesis and under conditions when the marrow is invaded or is stimulated to expand beyond its capacity to respond, the spleen may become a major site of extramedullary hematopoiesis. In this regard it has been suggested that the spleen may exercise a humoral regulatory function which modulates the hematopoietic activities of the bone marrow. For this hypothetical function there is at present little or no experimental or clinical support. Lastly, the spleen, or the splenic vasculature to be precise, plays a contributory role in the *regulation of portal blood flow* and, by mechanisms not as yet fully established, has an effect on salt and water metabolism and total plasma volume. Although each of these functional properties of the normal spleen is mediated by one or several of the anatomic components of the organ, these structures are so intimately and interdependently disposed in the organ that pathophysiologic mechanisms which, by right, should affect one or another function independently are, in fact, often responsible for major pathophysiologic changes in the behavior of the spleen with respect to many of its functional capabilities. The discussion which follows will attempt to deal with these several functional properties of the spleen in relationship to *hyposplenism*, due most commonly to surgical ablation or vascular accidents; to *splenomegaly*; and to that particular hematologic syndrome termed *hypersplenism*, which sometimes, but by no means invariably, accompanies splenomegaly.

NORMAL ANATOMY AND FUNCTIONS. The principal anatomic components of the spleen are (1) its capsule, composed of a fibrous connective tissue, and extensions of the capsule in the form of trabeculae which course throughout the organ carrying blood vessels, efferent lymphatics, and nerves; (2) a complex and unique branching arterial tree and its venous return; (3) a cordal and sinusoidal system which forms the *red pulp*; and (4) lymphoid tissues, which constitute the *white pulp* (see accompanying figure). The splenic artery divides to form trabecular arteries, which in turn divide to form central arteries, each surrounded by a sheath of thymus-dependent or T lymphocytes, as well as lymph follicles composed principally of non-thymus-dependent B lymphocytes and their plasma cell progeny. Right-angled branches, called follicular arteries, come off each central artery and penetrate the lymphocytic white pulp. The disposition of these small arterial branches creates a skimming effect on the blood, sending a cell-poor, plasma-rich fraction to the white pulp. These follicular arteries serve as the afferent lymphatics for the splenic white pulp; no traditional afferent lymphatic vessels have been detected in this organ. It may be surmised that it is this unique feature of the splenic lymphoid tissues which provides the organ with its special ability with respect to the clearance of and the reaction to blood-borne microorganisms.

Leaving the white pulp, the central arteries divide into small penicillar arteries which deliver a plasma-poor, cell-rich blood to the cords and sinusoids of the red pulp. Although there are, perhaps, direct connections between the terminal penicillar arterioles and the splenic sinusoids, achieving a closed circulation from the arterial to the venous vasculature, there is now incontestable evidence, based upon extensive ultrastructural studies, that a significant portion of this terminal splenic blood flow enters directly into the splenic cords and must navigate this anatomic filtration system in order to reach the splenic sinusoids and the venous circulation. The ultrastructural anatomy of splenic cords and sinusoids is particularly critical to the hemoclastic functions of the spleen.

The splenic (Billroth) cords constitute a true vascular sieve, in the form of a feltwork of loose reticular connective tissue containing macrophages and monocytes as well as the circulating blood cells which are deposited in the red pulp by the terminal splenic arterioles. This sponge-like tissue is separated by a fenestrated basement membrane from the splenic sinusoids, which constitutes the only venous exit for blood in the cordal spaces. The sinusoids themselves are lined by endothelial cells disposed in a longitudinal parallel fashion, much like the staves of a barrel; the sinusoidal basement membrane and endothelial cells together provide a final filtration barrier in the splenic red pulp. Only about 5 per cent of the blood which enters the normal spleen must pass through this vascular filter. Nevertheless, the red pulp is capable of exercising a profound regulatory function with regard to the quality and life span of both normal and injured blood cells. This capability is dependent upon several features. These are the unique anatomic characteristics of the splenic cord-sinusoid complex, the biologic properties of the macrophages which reside there, and the capacity of the spleen to increase blood flow to the cordal circulation and to undergo reticuloendothelial cell hyperplasia in response to a filtration load. The splenic red pulp provides an effective physical filtration system which can retain blood cells, particularly erythrocytes, which have lost their normal deformability. Entrapment in the splenic cords, even transiently, is in itself deleterious to both normal and injured red blood cells. They are subjected to hypoxia, hypoglycemia, and acidosis, which deteriorate their physical properties. This effect, termed *conditioning*, leads to more efficient entrapment on subsequent passages through the spleen and finally to erythrophagocytosis of the senescent cells by the cordal macrophages. Classic examples of the sieving effect of the splenic cords on pathologic red cells are the *Heinz body anemias*. Red cells containing rigid precipitates of

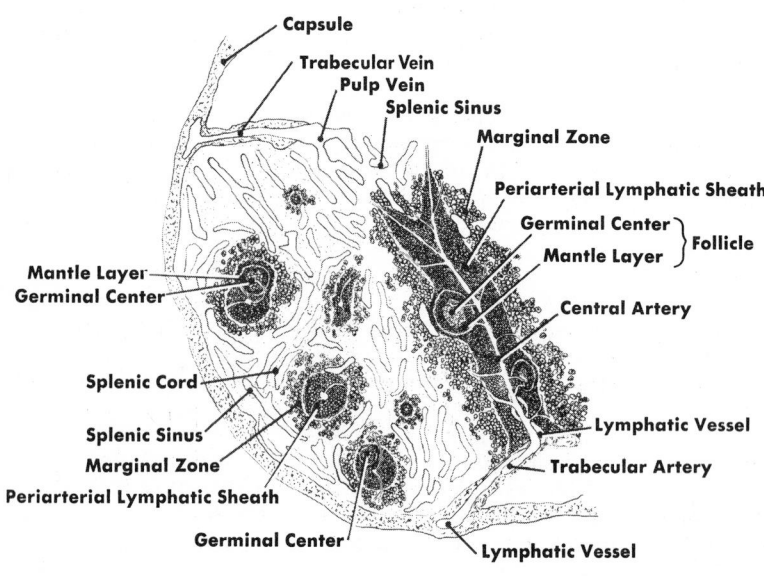

Diagrammatic representation of the structure of the spleen. (From Weiss, L.: Semin. Hematol., October 1970, p. 373.)

denatured hemoglobin (due to enzymatic or globin chain disorders) are trapped in the cordal filter where macrophages ingest them whole (*culling* function) or selectively ingest the inclusions (*pitting* function). Rigid microspherocytes, as in hereditary spherocytosis, are likewise retarded due to their deformity, *conditioned* by the severe cordal environment, and destroyed by macrophages. Cordal sequestration is not only responsive to changes in the physical properties of erythrocytes; red cells sensitized by immunoglobulins or complement may also be retarded within the splenic cords by virtue of specific receptors on cordal macrophages. Although the mechanisms responsible for sequestration of injured red cells are largely understood, at least in their broadest outlines, the role of the spleen in the removal of normal senescent or injured platelets and granulocytes remains less clear. It must be assumed, at least in the case of immunologically injured platelets and granulocytes, that mechanisms similar to those which trap sensitized erythrocytes are effective.

512. HYPOSPLENISM

DEFINITION. Surgical excision, vascular accidents such as the splenic infarctions which occur during the natural history of sickle cell anemia, and congenital asplenia account for most instances of absent or reduced splenic function. Although absence of the spleen is not regularly accompanied by significant signs of disease, there are both laboratory and clinical features which are the consequence of loss or suppression of specific splenic functions and which may, under certain circumstances, be responsible for serious illness.

PATHOPHYSIOLOGY. The consequences of splenectomy relate to each of the specific functional properties of the spleen described in Ch. 511. The spleen is responsible for the sequestration and *pitting* of inclusion-bearing red blood cells. Such inclusions, e.g., *siderosomes* and *Howell-Jolly bodies*, which are intracorpuscular residua of erythroid cell maturation, are removed from intact red blood cells by cordal macrophages. In the absence of the spleen, erythrocytes containing such inclusion bodies may be detected in the peripheral circulation. The presence of Howell-Jolly bodies is a useful criterion for functional or anatomic asplenia. Nucleated red blood cells, which are normally trapped and enucleated in the normal spleen, may be found in small numbers in the peripheral blood following splenectomy or splenic vascular accidents. The splenic cords are also responsible for the normal maturation of the red cell plasma membrane. Young reticulocytes are delivered to the circulation with a relatively high membrane to cytoplasm ratio; during their brief sojourn in the spleen reticulocytes lose membrane and mature to the normal erythrocyte. *Target cells*, displaying a high membrane to cytoplasm ratio, are a common consequence of hyposplenic states.

Although the spleen exerts little or no reservoir function with respect to red blood cells, the normal spleen contains a platelet pool constituting approximately 30 per cent of total circulating platelets. There may, as well, be a small pool of splenic granulocytes. Following splenectomy, a transient modest leukocytosis lasting up to one to two weeks is not uncommon, and should not be mistaken for a sign of infection. A transient thrombocytosis, with platelet counts between 500,000 and 1,000,000 per cubic millimeter, lasting generally for not longer than two to four weeks, is quite regularly observed. Persistent, severe thrombocytosis, which may be associated with thrombotic complications, is particularly apt to occur when hemolytic disease persists following splenectomy. The management of such patients generally dictates the use of anticoagulants. The use of specific platelet functional antagonists, such as aspirin, under these circumstances, is presently the subject of clinical evaluation. Some asplenic patients, the very young and perhaps those whose immune functions are compromised by their primary disease process, appear susceptible to overwhelming septicemia by encapsulated pathogens, most commonly *Diplococcus pneumoniae* and *Hemophilus influenzae*. Depression of a number of immunologic functions, including phagocytosis, serum IgM levels, cell-mediated immune reactivity, and complement-mediated opsonization of microorganisms, may contribute to this predisposition. Although the significance of splenectomy in the etiology of overwhelming septicemia appears established for the very young child, the data are insufficient to evaluate fully the risks of splenectomy to the adult patient. The role of antimicrobial prophylaxis and immunization with pneumococcal polysaccharides in preventing postsplenectomy infection is currently under study.

513. SPLENOMEGALY AND HYPERSPLENISM

DEFINITIONS. Although palpable *splenomegaly* can be detected in small numbers of patients (less than 1 per cent in the Western world) without *apparent* pathophysiologic significance, the presence of a palpably enlarged spleen is best considered a physical finding which demands diagnostic evaluation. Splenomegaly may be accompanied by *hypersplenism*, a term used to describe the blood cytopenia-producing effects of over-activity of the hemoclastic functions of the spleen.

ETIOLOGY AND PATHOGENESIS. The spleen is a functionally complex organ, and the causes of splenomegaly encompass a wide variety of primary illnesses (see accompanying table). The relative incidence of these illnesses associated with splenomegaly depends largely upon geographic and ethnic epidemiologic patterns. Because the spleen is a major reticuloendothelial organ, many *acute and chronic infectious processes* as well as noninfectious *inflammatory disorders* are accompanied by splenomegaly. Septicemia, tuberculosis, typhoid fever, subacute bacterial endocarditis, and infectious mononucleosis may manifest splenomegaly. Splenic abscess is a rare cause of splenomegaly, either due to metastatic infection from another site or to local factors such as infarction, splenic hematoma, localized peritonitis, or other local causes. In non-Western societies, other infectious agents, malaria, leishmaniasis, trypanosomes, and echinococcosis make a significant contribution to the incidence of infectious splenomegaly. Noninfectious inflammatory states such as Felty's syndrome (rheumatoid arthritis with splenomegaly), Boeck's sarcoid, and beryllium disease are also associated with splenomegaly.

Splenomegaly Due to Reticuloendothelial Hyperpla-

Causes of Splenomegaly

Infectious and inflammatory splenomegaly
   Septicemia, typhoid, infectious mononucleosis, subacute bacterial
   endocarditis, disseminated tuberculosis, malaria, leishmaniasis,
   trypanosomes, echinococcosis, Boeck's sarcoid, beryllium, Felty's
   syndrome (rheumatoid arthritis)
Splenomegaly due to reticuloendothelial hyperplasia
   Hemolytic anemias, immune thrombocytopenias, lupus
   erythematosus, thyrotoxicosis
Congestive splenomegaly
   Laennec's and postnecrotic cirrhosis; hepatic schistosomiasis;
   hepatic vein thrombosis; portal vein thrombosis, stenosis, cavernous
   transformation, or occlusion by neoplasm
Infiltrative splenomegaly
   Benign conditions: Gaucher's disease, Niemann-Pick disease,
   amyloidosis, diabetic lipemia, extramedullary hematopoiesis
   Neoplastic conditions: Leukemias, lymphomas, Hodgkin's disease,
   primary tumors, metastatic neoplasm, polycythemia vera,
   myeloid metaplasia

sia. As a reticuloendothelial organ, the spleen is responsible, although not exclusively, for clearance, sequestration, and destruction of injured and senescent blood cells. The volume of splenic tissue is sensitive to the demand for clearance of normal and injured blood cells. Splenomegaly is a frequent finding in hematologic conditions characterized by accelerated clearance of blood cells bearing congenital or acquired defects. Many hemolytic anemias (hereditary spherocytosis, certain hemoglobin disorders, autoimmune hemolytic anemias) as well as other anemias with a significant hemolytic component (the megaloblastic anemias and thalassemias, for example) are associated with splenomegaly. Immune thrombocytopenias (as in lupus erythematosus and, less commonly, idiopathic thrombocytopenia) may also be accompanied by varying degrees of splenomegaly.

Congestive Splenomegaly. An enlarged spleen, with its enlarged vascular bed, may make a significant contribution to increased portal blood flow and portal pressures. More commonly, however, splenomegaly is a consequence of portal hypertension due to any one of a number of obstructive portal vascular diseases, including Laennec's and postnecrotic cirrhosis, hepatic schistosomiasis, and hepatic vein thrombosis, as well as thrombosis, stenosis, cavernous transformation, or tumor compression of the portal vein. Under these circumstances splenomegaly is usually overshadowed by other manifestations of the primary disease such as hepatic failure, ascites, or bleeding esophogeal varices. Hypersplenism, manifested most commonly by granulocytopenia and thrombocytopenia, is a common accompaniment of congestive splenomegaly.

Infiltrative Splenomegaly. Both benign and malignant infiltrative diseases may cause splenomegaly and the hypersplenic syndrome. Metabolic disorders, such as Gaucher's disease, Niemann-Pick disease, and diabetic lipemia, are characterized by accumulation in splenic macrophages of the metabolic product characteristic of each disease. Myelophthisic replacement of the bone marrow by fibrous tissue (myelofibrosis), granulomas or tumor tissue, and chronic medullary stimulation, as in congenital hemolytic anemias, is associated with extramedullary splenic hematopoiesis and splenomegaly due to proliferating blood precursors. Alternatively, splenomegaly may result from involvement of the spleen by truly neoplastic infiltrations such as the acute leukemias, chronic myelogenous leukemia,

and the lymphoproliferative disorders, including chronic lymphocytic leukemia and Hodgkin's and non-Hodgkin's lymphomas. The spleen is an uncommon site for metastasis by nonhematologic malignancies. Primary tumors and cysts of the spleen are also uncommon causes of splenomegaly. These include hemangiomas, lymphangiomas, sarcomas, and hamartomas.

The Hypersplenic Syndrome. The cardinal features of hypersplenism are (1) splenomegaly, (2) some reduction in the number of circulating blood cells, affecting granulocytes, erythrocytes, or platelets in any combination, (3) a compensatory proliferative response in the bone marrow, and (4) the potential for correction of these hematologic abnormalities by splenectomy. Since the functional compartments of the spleen are intimately interconnected, it is not surprising that virtually all causes of splenomegaly may (but certainly need not) be associated with varying degrees of hypersplenism. Both infiltrative and congestive forms of splenomegaly are not uncommonly associated with hypersplenism. The hyperplastic response of splenic reticuloendothelial cells in a hemolytic anemia may initiate nonspecific sequestration of other blood cells, increase the conditioning of both injured and transfused erythrocytes, and accelerate the anemia. The concept of primary or idiopathic hypersplenism, i.e., the hypersplenic syndrome in the absence of a known cause for splenomegaly, is questionable at best. As the relationship between systemic disease, splenomegaly, and the several splenic functions becomes better understood, the number of cases which fall in this wastebasket category is gradually decreasing. It is particularly useful to recall that in this era of world travel the differential diagnosis of splenomegaly and hypersplenism must include worldwide disease patterns.

The mechanisms whereby splenomegaly results in hypersplenism are best understood with respect to erythrocyte sequestration (see Ch. 511). Whether such mechanisms apply to platelets and granulocytes has yet to be determined. It should be recalled, however, that there is normally a large pool of sequestered platelets within the spleen, and with splenomegaly the volume of pooled platelets, transiently withdrawn from the general circulation, increases strikingly. Pooling of otherwise normal platelets may play a significant role in some instances of thrombocytopenia attributable to hypersplenism. Whether such a mechanism is a factor in hypersplenic leukopenia has yet to be documented. Finally, splenomegaly itself makes a contribution, by mechanisms not fully understood, to an expanded total plasma volume. An apparent peripheral blood cytopenia may at times be the result of an expanded plasma volume and be independent of specific splenic sequestration and hemoclastic functions.

DIAGNOSIS. Although the experienced clinician may be reasonably certain that a palpable abdominal left upper quadrant mass represents splenomegaly, additional studies may be required to confirm the physical finding, establish the magnitude of splenomegaly, and evaluate the possibility of hypersplenism. The principal noninvasive technique for determining spleen size is the radionuclide spleen scan. Several techniques are available, including colloidal suspensions of radionuclides such as technetium (^{99m}Tc), as well as the use of mildly heat-injured erythrocytes labeled with ^{51}Cr. Quantitative evaluation of the distribution of chromium-labeled erythrocytes also provides information concerning the relative importance of the spleen, as compared with other reticuloendothelial organs such as the liver, in a hemolytic anemia. Such information may be useful as part of the evidence adduced to determine the advisability of splenectomy. Selective splenic angiography may also be a useful preoperative procedure in the evaluation of splenomegaly.

INDICATIONS FOR SPLENECTOMY. Because there are potential serious risks inherent in splenectomy, including (1) operative and anesthetic morbidity, (2) postsplenectomy thrombosis and thromboembolic complications, and (3) the risk of overwhelming bacterial infection, the indications for splenectomy should be strictly and carefully applied to the individual patient. These include (1) hemolytic syndromes, in which the selective role of the spleen in red cell sequestration and destruction can be documented or is an established aspect of the disease; (2) acute splenic vascular accidents or traumatic rupture requiring immediate surgical intervention; in this context, splenectomy may be indicated prophylactically for massive splenomegaly if there is severe discomfort or a threat of traumatic rupture; (3) immunologically mediated thrombocytopenias (see Ch. 515.1); (4) myeloid metaplasia and other instances of extramedullary hematopoiesis, when clinical evidence suggests that the hematopoietic functions of the enlarged spleen are outweighed by accelerated sequestration and blood cell destruction; and (5) for the staging of Hodgkin's disease or other lymphomas when a therapeutic decision rests upon the presence or absence of splenic disease. In the case of congestive splenomegaly, the factors which determine prognosis are rarely the hypersplenic functions of the enlarged spleen; most commonly these are liver failure and the vascular consequences of portal hypertension. Rectification of these defects must regularly take precedence over hypersplenism. In the face of severe hypersplenism due to infiltrative or hyperplastic splenomegaly (such as Gaucher's disease or severe Felty's syndrome) and when required for the diagnosis of splenomegaly of undetermined etiology, splenectomy may also be entertained after due consideration of the benefits and risks.

Christensen, B. E.: Pathophysiology of "hypersplenism syndrome." Scand J. Haematol., 11:5, 1973.

Frank, M. M.: Pathophysiology of immune hemolytic anemia. Ann. Intern. Med., 87:210, 1977.

Hess, C. E., Ayers, C. R., Sandusky, W. R., Carpenter, M. A., Wetzel, R. A., and Mohler, D. N.: Mechanism of dilutional anemia in massive splenomegaly. Blood, 47:629, 1976.

Jacob, H. S.: Hypersplenism: Mechanics and management. Br. J. Haematol., 27:1, 1974.

Krivit, W.: Overwhelming postsplenectomy infection. Am. J. Hematol., 2:193, 1977.

Nightingale, D., Prankerd, T. H. J., Richards, J. D. M., and Thompson, D.: Splenectomy in anaemia. Quart. J. Med., 41:261, 1972.

Ries, C. A., and Price, D. C.: [⁵¹Cr] platelet kinetics in thrombocytopenia. Correlation between splenic sequestration of platelets and response to splenectomy. Ann. Intern. Med., 80:702, 1974.

Sagoe, A. S.: Tropical splenomegaly syndrome. Long-term proguanil therapy correlated with spleen size, serum IgM, and lymphocyte transformation. Br. Med. J., 3:378, 1970.

Schwartz, S. I., Adams, J. T., and Bauman, A. W.: Splenectomy for hematologic disorders. Curr. Probl. Surg., May 1971, pp. 1–57.

Szur, L., Marsh, G. W., and Pettit, J. E.: Studies of splenic function by means of radioisotope-labeled red cells. Br. J. Haematol., 23:183, 1972.

Section Eleven HEMORRHAGIC DISORDERS: DISORDERS OF PRIMARY HEMOSTASIS

Ralph L. Nachman

514. INTRODUCTION

The major hemorrhagic disorders are associated with malfunction of three physiologic systems either separately or in combination: (1) abnormalities of platelets, (2) abnormalities of blood vessels, and (3) abnormalities of plasma coagulation factors. Clinical disorders associated with qualitative or quantitative platelet defects and/or abnormalities of the blood vessel wall have been referred to as diseases of primary hemostasis or "purpuric syndromes." There are several important clinical and laboratory features which help differentiate this spectrum of diseases from those associated with disorders of coagulation factors (Table 1). Purpuric syndromes are characterized by capillary hemorrhages occurring chiefly in the skin and mucous membranes. Occasionally excessive bleeding may follow trauma; however, the usual lesions encountered are spontaneous petechiae and ecchymoses which result from a breakdown in the anatomic and physiologic integrity of small blood vessel walls. Gastrointestinal and genitourinary bleeding may occur spontaneously with either abnormalities of platelets or coagulation factors. Deep hematomas and hemarthroses are more frequently associated with a coagulation factor abnormality. It is important to note the relationship of excessive bleeding to antecedent trauma or surgery, such as circumcision, tonsillectomy, or tooth extraction. Recurrent bleeding for two to three days or more usually indicates an underlying coagulation disorder. In general, bleeding caused by platelet or blood vessel defects is immediate and responds to direct pressure. A strong familial history of a serious bleeding problem should clearly raise the possibility of a coagulation disorder; however, it is important to note that as many as one third of all hemophilic patients have a negative family history. Several simple bedside procedures are useful for the initial evaluation of a hemorrhagic disorder. The Rumpel-Leede vascular fragility test is usually positive in patients with a purpuric syndrome; however, the procedure is superfluous in patients with spontaneous diffuse petechiae and ecchymoses. The Duke bleeding time is also a valuable bedside test which can help differentiate patients with purpuric disorders from those with underlying coagulation abnormalities. The rebleeding phenomenon should not be confused with the prolonged primary bleeding time. Patients with hemophilia may rebleed one to two hours after an essentially normal Duke or Ivy bleeding time. This results from the forma-

TABLE 1. Differentiation of Purpuric and Coagulation Disorders

Features	Purpuric Syndromes	Coagulation Disorders
Family history	Generally negative	Usually positive
Sex	More common in females	More common in males
Type of bleeding	Skin and mucosal surfaces	Visceral and intramuscular
	Petechiae and ecchymoses	Deep hematomas
	Spontaneous	Usually traumatic
Hemarthroses	Very rare	Frequent
Duration	Recent in onset	Usually lifelong
Bleeding time	Generally prolonged	Normal
Capillary fragility (tourniquet test)	Positive	Negative

tion of a poorly formed friable clot owing to the deficiency of a coagulation factor.

An understanding of the physiology of primary hemostatic mechanisms is important for the interpretation of diagnostic laboratory tests and for the subsequent management of patients with purpuric disorders. The formation of a hemostatic platelet plug can be divided into several separate but interrelated stages. The initial event in the development of the primary plug occurs with great rapidity and involves the adhesion of circulating platelets to exposed subendothelial collagen fibers, microfibrils, or basement membrane at the site of vessel wall injury. The adhesion reaction is mediated by chemical and physical determinants on the collagen molecule and is facilitated by the von Willebrand factor synthesized by endothelial cells. ADP which is stored in platelet granules is released by a process analogous to endocrine gland secretion and leads to platelet aggregation (cohesion). The activation of a platelet membrane phospholipase leads to the generation of arachidonic acid, which is subsequently converted to the prostaglandin derivative thromboxane A_2, which acts as a potent platelet aggregant and vasoconstrictor. A chain reaction of aggregating platelets releasing intracellular ADP which in turn recruits more platelets characterizes the growing plug. Platelet factor 3, a surface lipoprotein complex, and endothelial cell tissue factor become available at the site of the vessel injury probably owing to conformational changes of platelet and endothelial cell membranes. This results in the evolution of thrombin by activation of the intrinsic and extrinsic coagulation pathways. These biochemical events lead to consolidation and contraction of the platelet plug with eventual sealing of the injured vessel wall. The thrombin generated at the local site polymerizes fibrinogen, and the resulting fibrin reinforces the platelet mass at the periphery of the plug.

Marcus, A. J.: Platelet function. N. Engl. J. Med., 280:1213, 1278, 1330, 1968.

Mustard, J. F., and Packham, M. A.: Factors influencing platelet function: Adhesion, release, and aggregation. Pharmacol. Rev., 22:97, 1970.

Nachman, R. L.: Disorders of primary hemostasis. In Mengel, C., Frei, T., and Nachman, R. L. (eds.): Hematology. Chicago, Year Book Medical Publishers, 1972, p. 600.

Weiss, H. J.: Platelet physiology and abnormalities of function. N. Engl. J. Med., 293:531, 580, 1975.

515. QUANTITATIVE PLATELET ABNORMALITIES

515.1. THROMBOCYTOPENIA

Thrombocytopenia is the most common cause of hemorrhagic disease. Thus the peripheral blood of every patient who bleeds should be carefully examined. With experience, it is possible to approximate the platelet count by careful evaluation of a peripheral blood smear. Depending on the individual observer, the microscope, and the technique used in making the smear, there should be approximately three to ten platelets per oil immersion field. Smears prepared from "finger stick" blood samples show platelets which are less evenly distributed than smears from anticoagulated blood. Fewer than 50 platelets per 50 oil immersion fields usually suggests moderate to severe thrombocytopenia. With modern automated counting devices, the average normal platelet count varies from 200,000 to 400,000 per cubic millimeter.

The relationship of the platelet count and clinical bleeding is sometimes obscure. Some patients with severe thrombocytopenia may have little bleeding, but others with only a moderate decrease in platelet number present with a marked hemorrhagic diathesis. It is obvious that a number of contributing variables influence the integrity of the blood vessel wall. Sudden precipitous drops in platelet count, fever, and anemia appear to contribute significantly to petechial hemorrhage. Hormonal influences also can affect vascular integrity, as demonstrated by the beneficial effects of steroids in some patients in the absence of improvement in the platelet count. At very low levels, such as 10,000 platelets per cubic millimeter, major hemorrhagic manifestations such as central nervous system bleeding or massive gastrointestinal hemorrhage are more frequent. It is useful to categorize the many causes of thrombocytopenia in the framework of decreased production, decreased survival or excessive utilization, sequestration, and intravascular dilution (Table 2).

DECREASED PRODUCTION OF PLATELETS

Multiple anatomic as well as biochemical alterations may alter megakaryocyte number and function in the marrow. In such conditions, the erythroid and myeloid cellular elements may also be involved to varying degrees. Megakaryocyte depression from bone marrow infiltration may occur in leukemia, myeloma, carcinoma, lymphoma, granuloma, or myelofibrosis. Drugs, in particular the thiazide derivatives, ionizing radiaiton, and various toxins may cause major injury and megakaryocytic depletion. Familial aplastic anemia (Fanconi's anemia) with thrombocytopenia is a rare fatal childhood illness associated with multiple congenital and skeletal anomalies. A rare syndrome of infancy, congenital amegakaryocytic thrombocytopenia, is associated with bilateral absence of the radii. In congenital rubella, megakaryocytes are decreased in number with an associated

TABLE 2. Thrombocytopenia

I. Decreased production
  A. Reduced marrow megakaryocytes
    Marrow infiltration
    Marrow hypoplasia—radiation, toxins, chemicals, drugs, idiopathic
    Fanconi's anemia
    Congenital amegakaryocytic thrombocytopenia
    Infection—congenital rubella
  B. Normal or increased marrow megakaryocytes
    Megaloblastic anemia
    Paroxysmal nocturnal hemoglobinuria
    Hereditary thrombocytopenia
      Wiskott-Aldrich syndrome
      May-Hegglin anomaly
II. Decreased platelet survival
  A. Increased destruction
    Drug-induced purpura
    Idiopathic thrombocytopenic purpura
    Post-transfusion purpura
    Neonatal purpura
    Secondary immunologic purpura
  B. Increased consumption
    Disseminated intravascular coagulation
    Hemangioma
    Thrombotic thrombocytopenic purpura
    Hemolytic-uremic syndrome
    Acute infections
III. Sequestration (splenomegalic states)
IV. Dilutional

decreased platelet production. In this disease the mega-karyocyte may provide a preferred site for viral replication.

Impaired platelet production may also result from ineffective thrombopoiesis. Under these circumstances, adequate to increased numbers of megakaryocytes are present in the marrow; however, thrombocytopenia results from interference with the functional integrity of the marrow. This is seen in megaloblastic anemias, in paroxysmal nocturnal hemoglobinuria, and in various hereditary thrombocytopenias, including the Wiskott-Aldrich syndrome and the May-Hegglin anomaly.

DECREASED PLATELET SURVIVAL — INCREASED DESTRUCTION

Drug Purpura

Drugs must be considered a possible cause in every adult with thrombocytopenic purpura. Patients with drug purpura may develop hemorrhagic symptoms after weeks or even years of symptom-free use of an agent. Thrombocytopenia may develop within minutes to hours after administration of a drug to a sensitized patient. The bleeding at first is characterized by petechiae, purpura, occasionally hemorrhagic bullae of the oral mucosa, and not infrequently gastrointestinal and/or genitourinary hemorrhage. The petechiae do not itch, are not tender, and are not associated with wheals. In general the skin lesions are distributed over the lower extremities; they are not found on the soles or palms. In the majority of cases, the thrombocytopenic purpura will clear within a few days after removal of the offending drug. Purpura which persists for more than two to three weeks after drug exposure has been terminated should no longer be considered drug induced, and other conditions should be suspected. However, the duration of the purpura may be variable and depends to a large extent on the metabolic fate of

the drug. Thus certain toxic agents such as gold remain in the body for long periods of time after the last injection. Many patients forget that they have been chronically ingesting various common remedies such as aspirin, sedatives, and/or various tranquilizers, which can cause thrombocytopenia.

ETIOLOGY AND PATHOGENESIS. Many agents have been implicated as causes of thrombocytopenia (Table 3). These agents can produce thrombocytopenia by several different mechanisms. Thiazide derivatives, estro-

TABLE 3. Drugs Associated with Thrombocytopenic Purpura

I. Marrow suppression
  Thiazides, alcohol, estrogens
II. Immunologic mechanisms—peripheral destruction
  A. Etiologic relationship established
    Acetazolamide
    Allyl-isopropyl carbamide (Sedormid)
    Arsenical antiluetic drugs
    Carbamazepine
    Cephalothin
    Chlorothiazide
    Digitoxin
    Diphenylhydantoin sodium
    Heparin
    Hydrochlorothiazide
    Hydroxychloroquine
    Methyldopa
    Novobiocin
    Para-aminosalicylic acid
    Quinidine
    Quinine
    Rifampin
    Stibophen
    Sulfathiazole
  B. Etiologic relationship suspected but not confirmed
    Acetaminophen
    Aminopyrine
    Aspirin
    Butabarbitone
    Carbabutamide
    Chloramphenicol
    Chlorpheniramine maleate
    Chlorpromazine
    Chlorpropamide
    Codeine
    Desipramine
    Dextroamphetamine
    Digitalis
    Digoxin
    Disulfiram
    Erythromycin
    Ethyl-allyl-acetylurea
    Furosemide
    Gold
    Iopanoic acid
    Isonicotinic acid hydrazide
    Meperidine
    Meprobamate
    Mercurial diuretics
    Penicillin
    Phenacetin
    Phenylbutazone
    Prednisone
    Prochlorperazine
    Promethazine
    Propylthiouracil
    Reserpine
    Streptomycin
    Sulfadiazine
    Sulfadimidine
    Sulfamethoxypyridazine
    Sulfamerizine
    Sulfisoxazole
    Tetracycline
    Thiouracil
    Tolbutamide

gens, and alcohol may interfere with bone marrow megakaryocyte number and function. Alcohol-related thrombocytopenia is also characterized by a reduced platelet life span. Among the drugs listed in Table 3, *particularly frequent offenders include quinidine, quinine, sulfonamides, and the thiazides.* One should have a high level of suspicion of drug sensitivity when thrombocytopenic purpura develops in a patient receiving any of these drugs. Widely used drugs such as aspirin, penicillin, and phenobarbital have also been reported as offenders. The frequently used drug heparin causes thrombocytopenia by immunologic and nonimmunologic mechanisms. In effect, any drug taken by a patient is a possible cause of purpura.

The most common mechanism implicated in drug purpura is immunologic platelet destruction. In recent years, a convincing body of experimental and clinical evidence has been accumulated that clearly demonstrates the participation of the platelet in immunologic reactions. The external platelet surface is capable of adsorbing certain antibody drug complexes which then lead to platelet damage by an "innocent bystander" effect. According to this theory, the administered drug as hapten binds to a plasma protein or "carrier" to form an antigen. Antibodies stimulated by the immunogen bind to the drug, and these immune complexes secondarily bind with the platelet membrane Fc receptor, leading to cellular damage. Recent evidence also suggests that specific metabolic products of certain drugs rather than the primary agent may act as the offending immunogen.

DIAGNOSIS. A careful history of drug ingestion is an absolute necessity in any patient with thrombocytopenia. In addition to the usual medications, specific questioning is necessary regarding intake of beverages which contain quinine. In general the purpuric lesions with thrombocytopenia develop within hours after exposure to the agent by a sensitized patient. There may be an increased percentage of circulating large young platelets in the peripheral blood which is indicative of increased platelet turnover. A number of laboratory tests have been utilized to demonstrate drug, platelet, and antibody interactions as evidence of drug purpura. Tests involving complement fixation and platelet factor 3 release have proved to be relatively sensitive. Inhibition of clot retraction in the presence of the suspected offending agent is the simplest to perform but only detects high titer antibody. These in vitro tests are based on the premise that the underlying mechanism of the drug purpura is platelet adsorption of immune complexes consisting of drug and antibody with subsequent secondary cell damage. Direct challenge of the patient by a test dose of suspected drug in vivo is potentially hazardous. No single test is capable of detecting all cases of drug purpura. The most sensitive tests are difficult to perform and require expert laboratory assistance.

TREATMENT. All drugs should be discontinued. Medications which are indisputably needed should be replaced with pharmacologically equivalent but chemically different preparations. Adrenal corticosteroids should be given for their beneficial effect on vascular integrity. Platelet transfusions should be used only for life-threatening hemorrhage.

Aster, R. H.: Thrombocytopenia due to enhanced platelet destruction. *In* Williams, W., Beutler, E., Erslev, H., and Rundles, R. W. (eds.): Hematology. New York, McGraw-Hill Book Company, 1977, Chap. 145, p. 1336.

Horowitz, H. I., and Nachman, R. L.: Drug prupura. Semin. Hematol., 2:287, 1965.

Shulman, N. R.: A mechanism of cell destruction in individuals sensitized to foreign antigens and its implications in autoimmunity. Ann. Intern. Med., 60:506, 1964.

Idiopathic Thrombocytopenic Purpura

DEFINITION. Acute. Acute idiopathic thrombocytopenic purpura (ITP) is essentially a disease of young children, affecting both sexes equally. It is characterized by sudden onset of severe thrombocytopenic purpura in an otherwise healthy child, frequently occurring one to two weeks after a sore throat or ordinary cold. Acute ITP is seen most frequently between the ages of two and six years. The manifestations are extensive petechial hemorrhages and purpura with gingival, gastrointestinal, and genitourinary bleeding. There is frequently severe thrombocytopenia (platelet counts below 20,000 per cubic millimeter) with marked hyperplasia of bone marrow megakaryocytes. The spleen is usually not palpable. In over 80 per cent of the patients the disorder is self-limited, clearing spontaneously within two weeks. Patients should be treated with prednisone, 1 to 2 mg per kilogram of body weight, during the period of maximal thrombocytopenia. In some cases the thrombocytopenia may persist for two to six months. Approximately 10 to 15 per cent of affected children will develop chronic ITP, which eventually requires splenectomy.

Chronic. Chronic ITP is predominantly a disease of young adults, affecting females three to four times as often as males. The disorder is characterized by insidious onset with a relatively long history of easy bruising and menorrhagia. Many patients give a history of mild to moderate bleeding after trauma or minor surgery such as dental extractions. The platelet count is usually in the range of 50,000 to 100,000 per cubic millimeter. Bone marrow examination reveals megakaryocytic hyperplasia with predominance of early young forms.

In a typical patient the physical findings are minimal except for petechiae and ecchymoses. There is no characteristic pattern of distribution of the hemorrhagic lesions. The patient is afebrile, and in most cases the spleen is not palpable. The presence of an easily palpable spleen should direct attention away from the diagnosis of ITP. The disease may be present for a number of months to years and may be characterized by remissions and relapses. In most cases, the hemorrhagic complications are not life threatening; however, a rare individual may show central nervous system signs with intracerebral bleeding. In some patients the disorder appears to have cyclical characteristics, with striking exacerbations of systemic hemorrhagic symptoms with menstruation. These patients generally feel quite well except for complaints relating to the four or five days of hemorrhage per month.

ETIOLOGY AND PATHOGENESIS. In approximately 85 per cent of cases, ITP is a disorder produced by a platelet autoantibody that develops in a patient with no evidence of underlying disease or significant exposure to drugs. For this reason, some authors now prefer to define this disease as *autoimmune thrombocytopenic purpura* (ATP).

Although platelet autoantibodies are difficult to demonstrate, a significant body of clinical and experimental evidence has suggested their presence. Thus pregnant women with ITP frequently give birth to thrombocytopenic infants, a situation strongly suggesting the transplacental transfer of antiplatelet antibody. Plasma from patients with ITP produces severe thrombocytopenia when infused into normal individuals. This plasma also produces thrombocytopenia in the donor individual when reinfused at a time of remission. The activity causing thrombocytopenia upon transfusion of ITP plasma has been identified as a 7S gamma globulin which is absorbed by incubation with autologous and homologous platelets.

A number of in vitro test systems have been devised to demonstrate platelet antibodies in ITP. These include platelet agglutination, complement fixation, platelet factor 3 release, anti–gamma globulin consumption tests, and inhibition of labeled serotonin uptake. These tests are generally difficult to perform and are not yet part of routine laboratory studies. With sensitive in vitro systems it has been demonstrated that approximately 85 per cent of chronic ITP patients have antiplatelet antibodies. It is of interest that antibody production has been demonstrated in surgically removed spleens.

DIAGNOSIS. The diagnosis of chronic ITP is in large part an exercise in clinical exclusion. This is because the in vitro tests used to demonstrate circulating antiplatelet antibodies are difficult to perform and are generally not available in most clinical centers. Thus the diagnosis is made by a consideration of the major clinical and laboratory hallmarks as outlined above, paucity of physical findings, absence of underlying systemic disorders, exclusion of other primary immunologic thrombocytopenic conditions, and, finally, response to therapy. In most patients, perhaps the most significant diagnostic differential involves the exclusion of primary drug purpura. It is useful initially to remove or replace all drugs for at least two to three weeks. Thrombocytopenia which persists beyond this period is only rarely associated with previous drug administration, with the possible exception of a gold preparation.

THERAPY AND PROGNOSIS. Adrenal corticosteroids in a fairly high dose range, e.g., 60 mg of prednisone daily, are employed initially in an attempt to promote a significant rise in the platelet count and decrease bleeding. With steroid therapy, reduction in capillary fragility and decreased bleeding are often observed before an appreciable rise in the platelet count occurs. Most patients (approximately 70 per cent) with chronic ITP will respond to this therapy within two to three weeks. Unfortunately most of them will relapse within weeks to months after discontinuation of the steroids. Less than 15 per cent of adults with ITP will make a complete permanent recovery after an initial course of steroid therapy. In general, if significant clinial improvement does not occur within four to eight weeks or can be maintained only with toxic levels of steroids, splenectomy should be considered. For those patients who respond initially to steroids, the drug should be decreased gradually over several weeks so as to maintain the platelet count above 50,000 per cubic millimeter. In practical terms, most patients will require long-term doses of steroids which eventually lead to undesirable side effects. Thus unless the patient represents an unusual surgical risk, splenectomy should be performed.

Approximately 70 per cent of patients will achieve long-term and even permanent remissions after splenectomy. This is due to (1) removal of a major site of platelet destruction and (2) elimination of a major source of synthesis of platelet antibody. Most patients who enter remission after splenectomy show significant rises in the platelet count, often well above normal levels, within a few days. After surgery, up to 10 per cent of patients may require weeks or even months before a significant remission develops. Recent studies suggest that the effectiveness of splenectomy correlates with the response to prior corticosteroid therapy. A good or excellent response to splenectomy may be expected in a high percentage of patients who have shown a significant rise in the platelet count while on steroids.

Postsplenectomy failure with significant bleeding may respond to high-dose steroids even if the patient previously was refractory to the steroid effect. Immunosuppressive agents such as vincristine and cyclophosphamide have proved useful in the treatment of these patients. These agents should also be considered for use in patients with symptomatic chronic ITP in whom splenectomy cannot be performed. As noted previously, a small group of women with ITP who do not respond to splenectomy may develop exacerbations of the hemorrhagic symptoms during the menses. Some of these patients show striking improvement in clinical manifestations after suppression of ovarian function with hormonal agents.

Platelet transfusions should be reserved for life-threatening hemorrhage in chronic ITP. Platelets should not be given prophylactically, because they will be rapidly destroyed by the circulating platelet antibodies.

Aster, R. J., and Keene, R. W.: Sites of platelet destruction in idiopathic thrombocytopenic purpura. Br. J. Haematol., 16:61, 1969.

Baldini, M. G.: Idiopathic thrombocytopenic purpura and the ITP syndrome. Med. Clin. North Am., 56:47, 1972.

Finch, S. C., Castro, O., Cooper, M., Covery, W., Erickson, R., and McPhedran, P.: Immunosuppressive therapy of chronic idiopathic thrombocytopenic purpura. Am. J. Med., 56:4, 1974.

Harrington, W. J., Minnich, V., Hollingsworth, J. W., and Moore, C. V.: Demonstration of a thrombocytopenic factor in the blood of patients with thrombocytopenic purpura. J. Lab. Clin. Med., 38:1, 1951.

Kartapkin, S., and Siskind, G.: In vitro detection of platelet antibody in patients with idiopathic thrombocytopenic purpura and systemic lupus erythematosus. Blood, 33:795, 1969.

Post-Transfusion Purpura

Post-transfusion purpura, occurring almost exclusively in women, is a rare form of immunologic purpura which must be distinguished from ITP and drug purpura. The disease is characterized by sudden explosive onset of thrombocytopenic purpura about five to eight days after transfusion of whole blood. The disease develops because of the mismatching of an inherited platelet antigen with the subsequent development of a complement-fixing antiplatelet isoantibody. The antigen PL^{A1} is found in 98 per cent of the normal population and is absent from the platelets of the patient who develops the disorder. The process is self-limited; however, purpura may last up to six weeks. Conclusive diagnosis rests on the serologic demonstration of platelet antigen mismatching. Post-transfusion purpura should be suspected in any patient who develops sudden purpura in the absence of an overt underlying cause shortly after a blood transfusion. Owing to the danger of intracranial hemorrhage, the therapy consists of exchange transfusion and steroids in high dosage.

Shulman, N. R., Aster, R. J., Leitner, A., and Hiller, M. C.: Immuno-
reactions involving platelets. V. Post-transfusion purpura due to a
complement-fixing antibody against a genetically controlled platelet
antigen: A proposed mechanism for thrombocytopenia and its relevance in "autoimmunity." J. Clin. Invest., 40:1597, 1961.

Neonatal Purpura

Neonatal thrombocytopenia may develop because of
isoimmunization of the mother against fetal platelets
with subsequent transplacental transfer of maternal antibody. The disease is the platelet analogue of erythroblastosis fetalis, with platelets rather than red cells serving as the antigenic stimulus. The infant shows
generalized purpura at delivery, and platelet counts are
usually below 30,000 per cubic millimeter. Intracranial
hemorrhage has occurred in approximately 10 per cent
of cases.

At least four well-defined platelet antigen systems
have been elucidated and appear to be involved in the
development of maternal-fetal incompatibility. These
include the PL^{A1}, PL Gc Ly^{B1}, PL Gc Ly^{C1}, and PL^{E2} antigens. These antigens, which are distinct from erythro-
cyte antigens, are inherited as dominant characteristics.
The B1 and C1 platelet antigens are shared by granulocytes and lymphocytes. Adrenal corticosteroids, transfusion with maternal platelets, and exchange transfusion have been tried in severe cases.

Pearson, H. A., Shulman, N. R., Marder, V. J., and Cove, T. E.: Isoimmune neonatal thrombocytopenic purpura: Clinical and therapeutic
considerations. Blood, 23:154, 1964.

Secondary Immunologic Purpura

Idiopathic thrombocytopenic purpura may be associated with *autoimmune hemolytic anemia (Evans' syndrome)*. Patients with this disorder present with clinical
and laboratory features of Coombs-positive hemolytic
anemia and marked to moderate thrombocytopenia.

Autoimmune thrombocytopenia presenting in a manner identical to that of classic ITP occurs in approximately 10 per cent of patients with *systemic lupus erythematosus*. This entity may present as the only
significant clinical feature of early lupus. For this reason, immunologic tests for lupus erythematosus should
be performed on all patients who present with ITP.
Chronic ITP may present as one of the earliest manifestations of sarcoidosis.

A chronic ITP syndrome can be observed during the
course of *chronic lymphocytic leukemia* and *malignant
lymphoma*. It should be emphasized that the great majority of cases of thrombocytopenia associated with
these diseases are secondary to marrow involvement.
The pathogenesis in these rare cases appears to be the
same as that described in the idiopathic (autoimmune)
disorder. Certain postinfectious thrombocytopenic
states, such as those occasionally seen with *rubella* or
infectious mononucleosis, result from a temporary stimulation of circulating antibody to platelets. The antibody
in some cases of infectious mononucleosis is a cold
agglutinin with "i" specificity which coats platelets
upon exposure to cold. The antibody-coated cells are
sequestered in the spleen.

DECREASED PLATELET SURVIVAL — INCREASED CONSUMPTION

Disseminated Intravascular Coagulation

This group of disorders, which is discussed in Ch.
521.5, is generally associated with significant thrombocytopenia. The platelets are consumed throughout the
vascular tree secondary to the generation of excessive
amounts of thrombin in the circulation.

Cavernous Hemangioma (Kasabach-Merritt Syndrome)

Giant cavernous hemangioma of infancy is generally
detected at birth. Thrombocytopenia, which may be severe, results from excessive consumption of circulating
platelets on the damaged subendothelial surface of the
neoplasm. Intravascular coagulation takes place within
the tumor. Occasionally the tumors are located in visceral sites. In many of these the thrombocytopenia is
the most prominent feature of the generalized coagulation disorder. Surgical excision of the tumor if possible
and radiation have been used successfully in therapy.

Thrombotic Thrombocytopenic Purpura

Thrombotic thrombocytopenic purpura (TTP) is an
acute disease which presents a clinical spectrum, including thrombocytopenic purpura, microangiopathic
hemolytic anemia, transient fluctuating neurologic
symptoms, kidney disease, and fever. Approximately
80 per cent of patients die within one month of onset of
the illness. The most frequently observed symptoms are
related to the fluctuating and, at times, bizarre central
nervous manifestations and the severe hemorrhagic
complications. The anemia is usually brisk, with hematocrits often below 20 per cent on initial examination.
An important diagnostic feature is the striking microangiopathic peripheral blood picture; the blood
smear shows an increased number of schistocytes, burr
cells, and helmet-shaped red cell fragments. Careful
evaluation of the coagulation parameters early in the illness does not support the premise that disseminated
intravascular coagulation (DIC) has a primary role in
this disorder. Later, as the illness becomes more severe
and hepatic failure and sepsis occur, secondary DIC
may be seen. Diagnostic confirmation of TTP requires
histologic demonstration of a characteristic pathologic
lesion: the deposition of hyaline thrombi within the
lumina of arterioles and capillaries in the absence of
vasculitis. These lesions are probably composed of aggregates of degenerating platelets and fibrin. The
relationship of the platelet to the primary process in
this disease remains unclear. Fibrin has been demonstrated in the thrombotic lesions of TTP by immunofluorescence techniques. Since fibrinogen constitutes approximately 10 per cent of the platelet proteins, focal
platelet deposition on blood vessel walls would produce
positive immunofluorescence reactions for fibrin. Radioisotope labeling studies have demonstrated decreased platelet survival but normal fibrinogen survival
in patients with TTP.

The cause of TTP is unknown. The disorder should
be considered a syndrome with multiple etiologic factors producing microcirculatory pathology resulting

from the consumption of circulating platelets throughout the microvasculature at sites of vascular damage. In some cases, the primary lesion may reside in small blood vessels. Electron microscopic studies of capillaries have revealed subendothelial prethrombotic fibrin and accumulations of platelets. TTP has occurred in association with systemic lupus erythematosus and other collagen vascular disorders, supporting the possibility of an immune cause in some cases. *Bartonella*-like bacteria have been isolated from the blood of several patients with TTP. It is possible that other bacterial agents as well as viruses may act as intravascular platelet aggregating agents. Platelet aggregates which are formed in the circulation have been demonstrated to cause microvascular damage by deposition in small vessels and release of vasotoxic factors. Thus under some circumstances, the lesions of TTP could result from insults which primarily affect normal circulating platelets. Whether platelet aggregation is primary or secondary to vessel wall damage, platelet consumption is important in the disease process.

Acute TTP is a medical emergency. Therapy to date has been relatively ineffective, and the current approach is to some extent empirical. Steroids (60 to 100 mg of prednisone daily) and antiplatelet aggregating agents should be started as soon as the diagnosis is made. An effective antiplatelet aggregating combination includes combined dipyridamole and aspirin or sulfinpyrazone. If the clinical situation deteriorates, exchange transfusion with whole blood and/or splenectomy should be performed. Anticoagulant therapy in general has not proved beneficial in this disorder.

Amorosi, E. L., and Ultmann, J. E. L.: Thrombotic thrombocytopenic purpura: Report of 16 cases and review of the literature. Medicine, 45:139, 1966.

Bukowski, R. M., Hewlett, J. S., Harris, J. W., Hoffman, G. C., Battle, J. D., Silverblatt, E., and Yen Yang, I.: Exchange transfusion in the treatment of thrombotic thrombocytopenic purpura. Semin. Hematol., 13:219, 1976.

Jaffe, E., Nachman, R., and Merskey, C. L.: Thrombotic thrombocytopenic purpura. Coagulation parameters in twelve patients. Blood, 42:499, 1973.

Hemolytic-Uremic Syndrome

The hemolytic-uremic syndrome (*Gasser's syndrome*) is a disease of early childhood characterized by acute microangiopathic hemolytic anemia, thrombocytopenia, and renal failure. The explosive onset may follow a minor febrile illness or even prophylactic immunization. Neurologic symptoms are rarely seen, and the patients frequently have hemorrhagic diarrhea. The lesions are usually limited to the kidney and are characteristically focal thromboses of glomerular arterioles and capillaries with renal cortical necrosis. The pathogenesis of the hemolytic-uremic syndrome is unknown. Disseminated intravascular coagulation resulting from circulating immune complexes with deposition of circulating fibrin in the renal microvasculature has been considered as a likely pathogenetic mechanism. Therapy has been primarily directed at management of the acute renal failure. Corticosteroids are probably not helpful. Heparin has appeared to be beneficial in some cases.

The hemolytic-uremic syndrome may also be seen in pregnant or postpartum women or in young women who take oral contraceptive pills. The explosive onset of microangiopathic hemolytic anemia, thrombocytopenia, and acute renal failure may develop in the setting of premature separation of the placenta or toxemia of pregnancy. The pathologic lesions are identical to those seen in young children.

Clarkson, A. R., Lawrence, J. R., Meadows, R., and Seymour, A. E.: The haemolytic-uraemic syndrome in adults. Quart. J. Med., 39:227, 1970.

Acute Infections

Thrombocytopenia may occasionally develop during an acute viral or bacterial infection. Direct platelet damage caused by platelet-bacterium or platelet-virus interaction probably contributes significantly to thrombocytopenia. Extracellular toxins from both staphylococci and streptococci as well as endotoxins from gram-negative organisms lead to platelet damage and aggregation. In cases of severe sepsis, thrombocytopenia may in fact reflect consumption of circulating platelets in association with DIC. In contrast, the thrombocytopenia of some viral infections may be caused by suppression of megakaryocytic function, as is seen in congenital rubella.

SEQUESTRATION THROMBOCYTOPENIA

Thrombocytopenia may occur in any disorder associated with an enlarged spleen. The characteristic clinical picture is prominent splenomegaly with moderate thrombocytopenia (50,000 to 100,000 platelets per cubic millimeter). This entity has also been referred to as *hypersplenic thrombocytopenia*. Under normal circumstances, approximately one third of the total body platelet mass is in the spleen and the splenic platelet pool exchanges with the freely circulating platelets. In splenomegaly of any cause, the splenic platelet pool may be greatly expanded and up to 90 per cent of the platelets can be trapped at any one time. Thus a redistribution of platelets can occur, resulting in thrombocytopenia despite normal platelet production and normal platelet survival. In addition, young platelets tend to accumulate in the spleen to a greater extent than old platelets. The clinical picture will reflect the underlying etiology of the splenomegaly, e.g., cirrhosis with portal hypertension, myelofibrosis, or infiltrative disease such as Gaucher's disease or malignant lymphoma. The thrombocytopenia secondary to splenomegaly is rarely severe enough to produce hemorrhagic disease. Splenectomy, however, will generally restore a normal or even elevated platelet count.

DILUTIONAL THROMBOCYTOPENIA

Massive blood transfusions, extracorporeal circulation, and exchange transfusion may result in moderate thrombocytopenia because of blood volume replacement with platelet-poor banked blood. The severity of the thrombocytopenia is directly related to the number of transfusions.

515.2. THROMBOCYTOSIS

Thrombocytosis refers to clinical situations in which the platelet count is significantly elevated. Benign or secondary thrombocytosis usually occurs as a temporary event in the setting of another condition such as splenectomy, acute or chronic inflammatory disease, hemolytic anemia, acute hemorrhage, or iron deficiency, or as a response to exercise. Asymptomatic secondary thrombocytosis with platelet counts in the range of 700,000 to 1,000,000 per cubic millimeter has been reported in a number of patients with carcinoma, Hodgkin's disease, and other malignant lymphomas. The nature of the reactive thrombocytosis in these conditions is unknown, but it may represent a nonspecific megakaryocytic proliferative response to tissue necrosis. It is of interest that thrombocytosis has been noted after the use of drugs such as vincristine, which interferes with microtubules.

Essential thrombocythemia is characterized by spontaneous bleeding, at times alternating or coinciding with thrombotic episodes accompanied by a sustained elevation in the platelet count. The process may be considered one of the myeloproliferative diseases and can accompany or develop into chronic myelogenous leukemia, polycythemia vera, or myelofibrosis. The platelet count is usually in the range of 1,000,000 per cubic millimeter, and giant irregular forms and aggregates of platelets are seen on the peripheral smear. Platelet function studies such as the bleeding time, platelet factor 3 release, and platelet aggregation in response to epinephrine are frequently abnormal. The platelets are probably qualitatively defective; however, the precise mechanisms underlying the thrombotic and hemorrhagic symptoms are unknown. In some patients essential thrombocythemia has been unmasked after splenectomy for unrelated conditions. *Pseudohyperkalemia* is an interesting laboratory artifact seen in some of these patients. Serum potassium levels may be strikingly elevated in the absence of electrocardiographic evidence of hyperkalemia. In this circumstance the plasma potassium levels are normal, and the elevated serum levels are caused by release of potassium from platelets during blood clotting. Clinically the hemorrhagic and thrombotic symptoms improve as the platelet count is lowered. Busulfan and other myelosuppressive agents have proved useful in the long-term management of these patients. Antiplatelet aggregating agents, such as aspirin and dipyridamole, may prove useful in preventing thrombotic complications.

Gunz, F. W.: Hemorrhagic thrombocythemia: A critical review. Blood, 15:706, 1960.
Levin, J., and Conley, C. L.: Thrombocytosis associated with malignant disease. Arch. Intern. Med., 114:497, 1964.
Silverstein, M. N.: Primary or hemorrhagic thrombocythemia. Arch. Intern. Med., 122:18, 1968.

516. QUALITATIVE PLATELET ABNORMALITIES

Several hemorrhagic disorders have been attributed to abnormalities in platelet function occurring in the presence of adequate numbers of circulating platelets. The abnormalities may result from (1) defects in the primary hemostatic process involving adhesion or cohesion, leading to ineffective platelet plug formation, and/or (2) defects in the procoagulant activity of platelets associated with abnormal platelet factor 3 availability. The bleeding time is probably the most useful in

vivo test for rapid evaluation of platelet function. In addition, a number of in vitro test systems to monitor platelet aggregation and to measure the platelet retention to glass bead columns have helped clarify these different defects. The presence of a qualitative platelet abnormality in a patient is established by the following criteria: (1) hemorrhagic history in the absence of a disorder of the coagulation factors, (2) normal platelet count, and (3) abnormal platelet function.

A large group of qualitative platelet disorders have not yet been satisfactorily characterized. Both morphologic and functional platelet abnormalities have been observed in patients with certain inherited disorders of connective tissue, including *Ehlers-Danlos syndrome, osteogenesis imperfecta,* and *pseudoxanthoma elasticum.* Abnormal platelet function has been reported in the *Wiskott-Aldrich syndrome* and in patients with oculocutaneous albinism (*Hermansky-Pudlak syndrome*). The more important diseases of abnormal platelet function are discussed below.

Weiss, J. J.: Platelet physiology and abnormalities of function. N. Engl. J. Med., 293:531, 580, 1975.

THROMBASTHENIA
(Glanzmann's Disease)

Thrombasthenia is a rare congenital hemorrhagic disease in which there is a profound aberration of the primary hemostatic process. The patients characteristically present with severe bleeding from mucous membranes, usually beginning in childhood. However, some suffer only a minor hemorrhagic problem. There is an autosomal recessive inheritance pattern. The bleeding time is markedly prolonged, and clot retraction is greatly reduced or absent. Platelets from these patients do not aggregate with ADP or thrombin. The basic abnormality is probably due to a defect of one or more of the membrane surface glycoproteins. Defects in platelet size and shape as well as various enzyme abnormalities have been reported. Markedly diminished content of platelet fibrinogen in the presence of normal levels of plasma fibrinogen is a characteristic feature in most patients. The platelets also fail to provide surface platelet factor 3 activity after exposure to activating agents. If clinically significant bleeding occurs, they usually respond to therapy with platelet transfusions.

Caen, J., Castaldi, P. A., Lederc, J. C., Inceman, S., Larrieu, M. J., Probst, M., and Bernard, J.: Congenital bleeding time and normal platelet count. I. Glanzmann's thrombasthenia (report of 15 patients). Am. J. Med., 41:4, 1966.

BERNARD-SOULIER SYNDROME
(Giant Platelet Syndrome)

The Bernard-Soulier syndrome is a rare severe familial bleeding disorder which may be fatal. Cutaneous hemorrhages and deep visceral bleeding are common clinical features. The disorder is characterized by a long bleeding time, a normal or variable degree of thrombocytopenia, and unusually large circulating platelets in the range of lymphocytes or bigger. The patient's platelets in vitro aggregate normally in response to ADP, collagen, or thrombin but fail to aggregate in the presence of the antibiotic ristocetin. Unlike the abnormality in von Willebrand's disease, this defect cannot be corrected by the addition of normal plasma or factor VIII. The basic lesion is presumed to be an abnormality of a membrane surface glycoprotein. Platelet transfusions are the only effective form of therapy.

Howard, M. D., Hutton, R. A., and Hardisty, R. M.: Hereditary giant platelet syndrome: A disorder of a new aspect of platelet function. Br. Med. J., 4:586, 1973.
Nurder, A. T., and Caen, J. P.: Specific roles for platelet surface glycoproteins in platelet function. Nature, 255:720, 1975.

RELEASE REACTION DEFECTS

This involves a group of relatively mild common platelet disorders. Patients present with easy bruising and mild to moderate postoperative bleeding, and the bleeding time may be moderately prolonged. Their platelets when studied in vitro respond normally to high ADP levels but show decreased aggregation with collagen and impaired aggregation with epinephrine. There are several types of abnormality within this group. For example, some patients appear to have decreased intracellular pools of ADP (storage pool deficiency), whereas others have normal storage pools of ADP but are unable to release the nucleotide. The latter category resembles the defect seen after aspirin ingestion by normal subjects.

DRUG-INDUCED PLATELET ABNORMALITIES

Aspirin ingestion results in abnormal platelet function because of inhibition of membrane cyclo-oxygenase, resulting in a failure of the platelets to synthesize cyclic endoperoxides and thromboxane A_2 which mediate the normal release reaction. The bleeding time may be slightly prolonged, and platelet aggregation induced by collagen or epinephrine is abnormal. It is of interest that the effect of a single dose of aspirin may last for several days. In some individuals administration of small amounts of aspirin may prolong the bleeding time and lead to a significant hemorrhagic disorder, particularly if the patient is subjected to a surgical stress. This exaggerated aspirin response may reflect the unmasking of an underlying platelet functional abnormality. Patients with thrombocytopenia or blood coagulation disorders should avoid aspirin.

Other agents also can interfere with normal platelet function. Plasma expanders such as *dextran* and *hydroxyethyl starch* prolong the bleeding time, presumably by interrupting the normal process of adhesion. Numerous other agents currently used in clinical medicine adversely affect normal hemostasis. Included in this group are the anti-inflammatory agents *Butazolidin*, *sulfinpyrazone*, and *indomethacin*, some *antihistamines*, various *local anesthetics*, *clofibrate*, and *dipyridamole*. Some of these pharmacologic agents or structural analogues may be useful as agents to counteract platelet aggregation in thrombotic disorders.

ACQUIRED PLATELET FUNCTIONAL ABNORMALITIES — SYSTEMIC DISEASE

UREMIA. The bleeding time in uremic patients is frequently prolonged out of proportion to that caused by the moderate thrombocytopenia which is commonly present. The most consistent laboratory abnormalities include decreased platelet adhesiveness to glass bead columns and impaired release of the coagulant activity, platelet factor 3. Normal platelets in uremic plasma function abnormally, and the defect in uremia improves significantly after dialysis. It is therefore probable that the platelet functional aberration in uremia results from the accumulation of small molecular weight metabolic waste products.

DYSGLOBULINEMIA. Abnormal platelet function has been observed in patients with macroglobulinemia as well as in multiple myeloma. Macroglobulin probably coats the platelet surface and sterically interferes with the normal hemostatic reactions. Improvement has been noted in patients after plasmapheresis.

Defects in platelet aggregation with prolonged bleeding times have been seen in a number of systemic conditions such as *cirrhosis, systemic lupus erythematosus,* and *pernicious anemia.* The hemorrhagic symptoms in these conditions may be related to the associated qualitative platelet abnormalities.

517. VASCULAR PURPURA

A varied group of clinical syndromes are characterized by intrinsic abnormalities of the blood vessel wall which result in mucosal and skin hemorrhages in the absence of overt defects in platelet function and number or plasma clotting factor defects. These syndromes are listed in Table 4.

Among the most common examples is *purpura simplex*. This is seen in otherwise healthy females who present with frequent but relatively harmless purpuric lesions. The disorder is lifelong, and there is occasionally a positive family history. It is disturbing cosmetically, and there is no effective treatment. It is significant only that this benign condition should be distinguished from the more serious purpuric states.

SENILE PURPURA. This is a relatively harmless, common condition primarily affecting the elderly. Purpuric lesions are mainly localized over the back of the hands and the extensor surfaces of the forearms. Large superficial ecchymotic areas may develop after mild trauma. The lesions occur in thin parchment-like atrophic skin and are presumably related to the regeneration of subcutaneous elastic tissue. They are of little clinical significance.

TABLE 4.   Causes of Vascular Purpura

Senile purpura
Dysproteinemia
   Macroglobulinemia
   Multiple myeloma
   Cryoglobulinemia
   Benign hyperglobulinemic purpura
Nonthrombocytopenic drug purpura
Henoch-Schönlein purpura
Hereditary connective tissue disorders
   Ehlers-Danlos syndrome
   Pseudoxanthoma elasticum
   Marfan's syndrome
   Osteogenesis imperfecta
Cushing's syndrome
Scurvy
Autoerythrocyte sensitivity

DYSPROTEINEMIA. Vascular purpura may be seen in *macroglobulinemia, myeloma,* and *cryoglobulinemia.* As noted previously, the nonthrombocytopenic purpura may develop because of protein coating of the platelet surface as well as coating of endothelial vascular surfaces, leading to impairment in blood vessel integrity. Epistaxis is a common symptom in these patients. It is probable that platelet dysfunction as well as coagulation factor abnormalities contributes to the bleeding diatheses in patients with myeloma, particularly those of the IgA type. Hyperviscosity with sludging of red cells also contributes to capillary anoxia. In cryoglobulinemia, purpuric lesions appear after exposure to cold and are more frequent during the winter months.

Benign hyperglobulinemic purpura primarily affects middle-aged females who present with successive crops of petechiae on the legs occurring at variable intervals, leading to pigmentary changes in the skin. Occasionally local itching or urticaria precedes the petechial eruptions. In half the cases other conditions such as Sjögren's syndrome, disseminated lupus erythematosus, or rheumatoid arthritis are also present. The hypergammaglobulinemia is due to the presence of high titer IgG antiglobulins.

NONTHROMBOCYTOPENIC DRUG PURPURA. Some of the agents listed in Table 3 (Ch. 515.1) may lead to purpura in the absence of thrombocytopenia. The chlorothiazides and chemically related compounds are probably the most common offenders. In these situations, it is probable that the vascular endothelium rather than the circulating platelet serves as a target tissue. Whether this is a true immunologic reaction remains to be determined. The bleeding disorder is usually mild, and the only necessary therapy is removal of the suspected offending agent.

HENOCH-SCHÖNLEIN PURPURA. This allergic vasculitis occurs most frequently in children after a streptococcal infection or, occasionally, after ingestion of a sensitizing food or drug. The skin is invariably involved, usually with extensive elevated purpuric or ecchymotic lesions scattered over the extensor surfaces of the extremities. Initially, the skin lesion is urticarial in nature and gradually becomes hemorrhagic. The rash typically occurs in recurrent crops and may involve the face. Other systems frequently affected include the joints, especially knees and ankles, gastrointestinal tract, and kidneys. Intestinal complications include intramural hematomas and gross mucosal hemorrhage, both of which may be accompanied by severe colicky pain, hematemesis, and melena. Renal involvement with hematuria is seen in approximately 50 per cent of the patients. Chronic nephritis with uremia may also develop (see Ch. 374.4). In the younger patients, the disease is usually self-limited. Steroids have been used, particularly in the more severely ill patients with visceral involvement.

HEREDITARY CONNECTIVE TISSUE DISORDERS. Vascular purpura may be seen in certain inherited disorders of connective tissue, including the *Ehlers-Danlos syndrome, pseudoxanthoma elasticum, osteogenesis imperfecta,* and *Marfan's syndrome.* In some of these disorders abnormal platelet function has also been reported.

CUSHING'S SYNDROME. Nonthrombocytopenic purpura predominantly distributed over the trunk and lower extremities is seen after prolonged administration of exogenous steroids as well as in patients with Cushing's syndrome. The nature of the vascular lesion is unknown; however, some observers believe that chronic exposure of the vasculature to steroids produces a catabolic effect which interferes with vascular integrity.

SCURVY. Chronic vitamin C deficiency is primarily a disease of extremes of age — the very young and the very old. Epistaxis, hematuria, and gastrointestinal bleeding are seen in infants. In adults, deep intramuscular hematomas are frequently encountered. In addition to the vessel wall defect, qualitative platelet defects may also contribute to the bleeding.

AUTOERYTHROCYTE SENSITIVITY. This unusual condition is seen only in women and is characterized by the spontaneous appearance of painful ecchymoses. The lesions occur over the anterior aspects of the upper and lower extremities and spread superficially. Many patients give a history of trauma preceding the onset of the ecchymoses. In general, the lesions appear over areas which are liable to superficial trauma. The etiology of the illness is not known; however, some evidence suggests that certain of these women are sensitive to their own red cells. Many of the patients have significant emotional difficulties, and the lesions at times may be self-inflicted.

Capra, D. J., Winchester, R. J., and Kunkel, H. G.: Hyperglobulinemic purpura. Studies on the unusual anti-α globulins characteristic of the sera of these patients. Medicine, 50:125, 1971.

Gottlieb, A. J.: Disorders of hemostasis — nonthrombocytopenic purpuras. *In* Williams, W., Beutler, E., Erslev, N., and Rundles, R. W. (eds.): Hematology. New York, McGraw-Hill Book Company. 1977, Chap. 151, p. 1385.

Ratnoff, O. D., and Agler, D. P.: Psychogenic purpura: A reevaluation of the syndrome of autoerythrocyte sensitization. Medicine, 47:475, 1968.

518.   HEREDITARY HEMORRHAGIC TELANGIECTASIA
(Osler-Weber-Rendu Disease)

Hereditary hemorrhagic telangiectasia is an inherited disorder associated with intermittent bleeding from vascular abnormalities scattered throughout the body, particularly on mucosal surfaces. Skin lesions appear as small, flattened telangiectases or dilated, raised small vascular nodules which blanch with pressure. The lesions are common on the face and in the mucous membranes of the tongue, lips, and nose. They are also found in the scalp, fingertips, conjunctival surfaces, vagina, and rectum. Visceral lesions are most common in the gastrointestinal tract, but the respiratory and genitourinary systems may also be involved. Approximately 20 per cent of the patients have pulmonary arteriovenous fistulas. Recurrent spontaneous epistaxis is the most common symptom. Severe gastrointestinal bleeding may also be a major clinical problem. The patients invariably have iron deficiency anemia which is sometimes severe. The pathologic lesions involving arterioles, venules, and capillaries are characterized by marked thinning of the vessel wall with ballooning and aneurysm formation. Management consists of symptomatic care of recurrent bleeding. Various plastic surgical procedures have been utilized to diminish the particularly troublesome recurrent episodes of epistaxis. Local pressure with packing is helpful. Systemic estrogen therapy has not proved particularly beneficial. All patients should be maintained on long-term iron administration.

Section Twelve HEMORRHAGIC DISORDERS: COAGULATION DEFECTS

Oscar D. Ratnoff

519. INTRODUCTION

A hemorrhagic disorder often appears when blood coagulation is impaired. Defective hemostasis may be caused by (1) inadequate production of one or more of the procoagulant substances of blood, (2) the synthesis of abnormal forms of these procoagulants, (3) depletion of components required for clotting as a result of increased utilization, (4) the presence in blood of inhibitors of coagulation, or (5) activation of proteolytic mechanisms of plasma. Blood normally contains a relative abundance of each clotting factor, and hemorrhage is rarely the result of deficiency of one of these substances unless its concentration has been reduced to less than 50 per cent of the normal value. Abnormal bleeding may result from a deficiency of the normal form of each of the known clotting factors, with three exceptions. Hageman factor (factor XII), plasma prekallikrein (Fletcher factor), and high molecular weight kininogen (Fitzgerald factor), proteins concerned with the initiation of blood clotting upon contact with foreign surfaces, are apparently not required for normal hemostasis. Depletion of calcium is not a cause of abnormal bleeding, because the cardiovascular and neuromuscular effects of profound hypocalcemia are incompatible with life. Deficiency of a single clotting factor is usually the result of an inherited disorder. Acquired coagulation defects are more likely to involve multiple components of the clotting system. In some clinical situations several mechanisms operate to impair hemostasis, and the extent to which each contributes may be difficult to analyze.

A knowledge of the physiology of blood clotting is essential in interpreting the results of laboratory tests useful in the diagnosis of hemostatic defects. Blood clots when fibrinogen (factor I) is converted to fibrin through the action of a proteolytic enzyme, thrombin (Fig. 1). Fibrinogen is a dimer, each half consisting of three subunits, $A\alpha$, $B\beta$ and γ chains. Thrombin separates two small polypeptides, fibrinopeptides A and B, from the corresponding halves of the fibrinogen molecule. What remains, fibrin monomer, then polymerizes to form insoluble strands of fibrin. The polymerization of fibrin is accelerated by calcium ions at physiologic concentrations. Normally, the molecules of fibrin are chemically bonded to each other by a second enzyme, fibrin-stabilizing factor (factor XIII), a transamidase. These links provide mechanical strength to the fibrin strands.

Thrombin is undetectable in normal blood. When blood is shed, thrombin evolves through one or both of two convergent sequences of chemical reactions, the extrinsic and intrinsic pathways. Presumably, similar mechanisms operate to induce clotting in vivo. Thrombin formation via the *extrinsic pathway* is initiated by components of tissue known as tissue thromboplastin or tissue factor. In the presence of calcium ions, tissue

Figure 1. The formation of fibrin in human plasma.

thromboplastin undergoes what is probably a stoichiometric reaction that allows factor VII to "activate" Stuart factor (factor X). In turn, activated Stuart factor, in concert with proaccelerin (factor V), phospholipid and calcium ions, releases thrombin from prothrombin via an enzymatic process (Fig. 2).

Blood also clots without participation of tissue thromboplastin upon contact with certain negatively charged surfaces such as glass, through sequential steps described as the *intrinsic pathway*: in vivo, collagen and sebum may serve this function. These agents alter Hageman factor (factor XII) so that it can convert plasma thromboplastin antecedent (PTA, factor XI) to an activated state, a process requiring participation of high molecular weight kininogen (Fitzgerald factor) and potentiated in an unknown way by a plasma prekallikrein (Fletcher factor). Hageman factor also participates in other defense reactions of the body, notably conversion of plasma prekallikrein to kallikrein, an enzyme releasing polypeptide "kinins" from plasma kininogens, particularly the high molecular weight kininogens; the kinins increase vascular permeability, dilate small blood vessels, induce pain, contract certain smooth muscles, and probably bring about migration of leukocytes. Additionally, Hageman factor may directly or indirectly augment the action of factor VII, so that the distinction between the extrinsic and intrinsic pathways is not as sharp as was once believed.

Once PTA has been activated, it changes Christmas factor (PTC, factor IX) to an activated state in which it can in turn activate Stuart factor; this reaction requires participation of antihemophilic factor (factor VIII), phospholipids, and calcium ions. Antihemophilic factor is a complex molecule possessing not only procoagulant activity but also the property of supporting aggregation of platelets by the antimicrobial ristocetin, and causing retention of platelets by glass bead columns through

Figure 2. The intrinsic and extrinsic pathways for the formation of thrombin. Omitted from the diagram are inhibitors of the various steps. The phospholipid portion of tissue thromboplastin may function in the activation and action of Stuart factor. The phospholipid for the intrinsic pathway is furnished by platelets and by the plasma itself. An augmentation of the action of factor VII by Hageman factor–mediated reactions is not depicted.

which blood or platelet-rich plasma is filtered. The subsequent steps of the intrinsic pathaway are the same as those of the extrinsic pathway (Fig. 2). Phospholipids for the extrinsic pathway are supplied by tissue thromboplastin, and, for the intrinsic pathway, by platelets and, to a lesser degree, plasma itself. In addition to its action on fibrinogen, thrombin promotes clotting in several ways, liberating phospholipid from platelets, activating fibrin-stabilizing factor from an inert precursor, and altering antihemophilic factor and proaccelerin, a step that potentiates and is probably necessary for their activity.

Plasma contains potent inhibitors of the clotting process, of which those inhibiting thrombin, tissue thromboplastin, and the activated forms of Hageman factor, plasma prekallikrein, PTA, and Stuart factor are most clearly defined. The inhibitors include antithrombin III, α_1-antitrypsin, α_2-macroglobulin, α_2-plasmin inhibitor, and $C\bar{1}$ inactivator, an agent that also inhibits $C\bar{1}$ (C1 esterase), a component of the complement system. The action of antithrombin III is potentiated by heparin, to which it binds, and is directed particularly against thrombin and activated Stuart factor. Plasma also contains plasminogen, the precursor of plasmin, a powerful proteolytic enzyme which can digest fibrinogen, fibrin, and other clotting factors as well as certain other substrates. The sole or principal site of synthesis of several clotting factors — namely, fibrinogen, prothrombin, factor VII, proaccelerin, Stuart factor, and Christmas factor — is the hepatic parenchymal cell. Vascular endothelium has been implicated in the synthesis of at least part of the antihemophilic factor molecule; the locus of synthesis of other factors is not certain, but is probably principally the liver.

The laboratory methods used to differentiate disorders of blood clotting are based upon these physiologic considerations. Thus defects in the extrinsic pathway of coagulation are readily detected by measuring the one-stage prothrombin time, in which tissue thromboplastin and calcium ions are added to decalcified plasma, and the interval of time elapsing until clot-

ting takes place is measured. Defects in the intrinsic pathway are reflected in the test tube by delayed clotting of whole blood, retarded "thromboplastin generation" (a misnomer for the evolution of the activated Stuart factor), deficient conversion of prothrombin to thrombin, i.e., prothrombin consumption, and a prolonged partial thromboplastin time, i.e., the clotting time of recalcified plasma in the presence of phospholipid to which an activator of Hageman factor, such as kaolin or ellagic acid, is often added. The one-stage prothrombin time is normal in persons whose defect is restricted to the early part of the intrinsic pathway, before the participation of Stuart factor, but is prolonged if defects of the later parts of the pathway are present. Defects in the conversion of fibrinogen to fibrin are measured by testing the effect of preformed thrombin on the clotting time of plasma, i.e., the thrombin time, whereas a deficiency of fibrin-stabilizing factor is detected by noting the solubility of fibrin in 5 molar urea or 1 per cent monochloroacetic acid, which cannot dissolve fibrin bonded by this factor. Defects of the platelet-supporting of antihemophilic factor may be recognized by prolongation of the bleeding time, the time elapsing until bleeding stops from a deliberately incised wound of the finger or volar surface of the forearm.

The laboratory procedures available for investigation of defects of coagulation are often crude, nonspecific, and influenced by variations in technique. Accordingly, care is required in selection and performance of the tests and in interpretation of results. Assays are available for each of the known clotting factors. Final identification of a specific deficiency requires mixing of the patients's plasma with that of a patient with a known coagulation defect to determine whether correction occurs. Only fibrinogen can be measured in gravimetric terms, by its conversion to fibrin and by determination of the protein content of the clot.

Biggs, R. (ed.): Human Blood Coagulation, Hemostasis and Thrombosis. 2nd ed. Oxford, Blackwell Scientific Publications, 1976.

Harker, L. A. (ed.): The Hemostasis Manual. 2nd ed. Philadelphia, F. A. Davis Company, 1974.

Ogston, D., and Bennett, B. (ed.): Haemostasis: Biochemistry, Physiology and Pathology. London, John Wiley & Sons, 1977.

Poller, L. (ed.): Recent Advances in Blood Coagulation. Edinburgh, Churchill, Livingstone, 1969 and 1977.

Ratnoff, O. D. (ed.): Treatment of Hemorrhagic Disorders, New York, Harper & Row, 1968.

520. HERITABLE DISORDERS OF BLOOD COAGULATION

520.1. INTRODUCTION

The familial occurrence of a functional deficiency of each of the clotting factors except calcium ions is well established. The cause is either deficient synthesis or the synthesis of functionally defective factors. Transmission of the defect is genetically determined. In most instances, severe functional deficiency of a single clotting factor is encountered in homozygotes in autosomal recessive traits and in male hemizygotes and female homozgotes in X-linked recessive disorders. In some cases, heterozygous carriers can be shown to have a reduced plasma level of the procoagulant, but, except in von Willebrand's disease, the deficiency is rarely sufficient to impair hemostasis. In one anomaly, dysfibrinogenemia, an autosomal dominant gene appears to be responsible for synthesis of a protein that may be normal in quantity but abnormal in structure and function. Rarely, familial deficiency of more than one clotting factor has been encountered. The genetic basis for multiple hemostatic defects is not understood.

Some differential features of hereditary disorders of blood coagulation are listed in Table 1.

520.2. CLASSIC HEMOPHILIA

Classic hemophilia, the best known of the familial disorders of blood coagulation, is the result of functional deficiency of antihemophilic factor (factor VIII). The plasma does not lack antihemophilic factor. Rather, it appears to contain a nonfunctional variant of this clotting factor. The abnormality is attributable to an X-linked recessive gene so that the disorder occurs almost exclusively in males. The sons of a male hemophiliac are unaffected and do not transmit the disease, but all of a hemophiliac's daughters are carriers. Heterozygous females usually do not bleed, but half their sons have hemophilia and half their daughters are carriers. Homozygous females, very rarely encountered, have the typical disease. The clinical manifestations vary from family to family, correlating with the intensity of the functional deficiency of antihemophilic factor, but within a family the degree of the bleeding tendency among affected members is usually about the same; a variant of mild hemophilia, in which the titer of procoagulant antihemophilic factor varies from time to time, has been described by several investigators. A positive family history is obtained in only about two thirds of cases.

CLINICAL MANIFESTATIONS. In severe hemophilia, in which virtually no functional antihemophilic factor is detectable in plasma, serious or lethal hemorrhage may occur in the neonatal period after circumcision, but bleeding from the umbilicus is unusual. In infancy, the bleeding tendency is frequently manifested by the appearance of cutaneous ecchymoses or hematomas in soft tissues, often after injuries so trivial as to be unnoticed. Bleeding from the mouth, in particular from injury to the frenum of the upper lip, is sometimes encountered in young children. After the early years of life, hemorrhages into the joints are characteristic. Increasing deformity, limitation of motion, and destruction of joints result from repeated hemarthroses, commonly the most disabling manifestation of the disease. The ankles, knees, and elbows are particularly likely to be involved, whereas the hands are usually spared. Bleeding is limited by the tension of the joint capsule, and ceases when the synovial space becomes distended. Hemorrhages into soft tissues are not similarly restricted, and may extend widely, dissecting through subcutaneous tissue, along fascial planes, or into muscles. Even enormous hematomas are usually reabsorbed, but sometimes they persist, leaving firm masses that calcify. Pseudotumors can produce symptoms by pressure on other structures, or may erode bone and simulate neoplasms. Hemorrhages into the muscles sometimes cause contractures and deformities such as a claw hand. Bleeding into the lax tissues beneath the tongue, in the pharynx, or in the neck is particularly dangerous, because it may interfere with swallowing or may occlude the respiratory passage. Retroperitoneal hemorrhage can produce symptoms simulating those of appendicitis, or can give rise to other manifestations such as obstructive jaundice owing to occlusion of the common bile duct or fulminant hypertension from compression of the kidneys. Hemorrhage into the mesentery can cause abdominal pain, digestive symptoms, or even avascular necrosis of the bowel. Episodes of hematuria, often accompanied by ureteral colic, are common and tend to persist for weeks if untreated. Hemorrhage into the gastrointestinal tract may occur, sometimes as a complication of peptic ulceration. Epistaxis is relatively uncommon. Excessive bleeding is the rule after dental extraction or minor surgery, and tonsillectomy or major operative procedures may lead to fatal hemorrhage. Subdural hematomas and other hemorrhages into the central nervous system, although uncommon, are an important cause of disability or death, and may result from relatively trivial injury. Hematomas encroaching on nerve trunks may cause sensory loss or paralysis.

Only about half of hemophiliacs present this grim picture. Such individuals have little or no functional antihemophilic factor in their plasma as measured in clotting tests. In others, in whom the titer of this factor may be as high as 40 per cent of the average normal value, the symptoms are proportionately milder, and bleeding may occur only after such challenges as injury, operative procedures, or dental extractions.

DIAGNOSIS. Specific diagnosis can be established only by laboratory tests of blood coagulation, although the character of the bleeding and the family history provide important clues. Tests that detect abnormalities in the intrinsic pathway of coagulation usually give abnormal results, but the clotting time of whole blood may be normal in mildly affected patients. The

TABLE 1. Differentiation of Some Hereditary Coagulation Disorders

Disorder	Usual Hemorrhagic Symptoms	Heredity	Usual Laboratory Findings				Selected Special Tests*
			Thrombin Time	Prothrombin Time	Partial Thromboplastin Time	Bleeding Time	
Disorders of fibrin formation							
Congenital afibrinogenemia	Severe	Autosomal recessive	∞	∞	∞	Normal or ↑	Afibrinogenemia confirmed immunologically
Congenital dysfibrinogenemia	Mild or none	Autosomal dominant	Usually ↑	Usually ↑	Sometimes ↑	Normal	Plasma fibrinogen concentration usually normal; delayed release of fibrinopeptides or/and impaired aggregation of fibrin monomers
Congenital "deficiency" of fibrin-stabilizing factor (factor XIII)	Severe	Unclear†	Normal	Normal	Normal	Normal	Clots soluble in 5 M urea, or 1% monochloroacetic acid
Disorders of the extrinsic pathway of thrombin formation‡							
Hereditary hypoprothrombinemia	Mild to severe	Autosomal recessive†	Normal	↑	↑	Normal	
Parahemophilia (factor V deficiency)	Moderate	Autosomal recessive	Normal	↑	↑	Normal	
Stuart factor (factor X "deficiency")	Severe	Autosomal recessive†	Normal	↑	↑	Normal	Russell's viper venom time usually prolonged
Factor VII "deficiency"	Mild to moderate	Autosomal recessive†	Normal	↑	Normal or ↑	Normal	Russell's viper venom time normal
Disorders of the early intrinsic pathway of thrombin formation							
Classic hemophilia	Mild to severe	X chromosome-linked	Normal	Normal	↑	Normal	Procoagulant titer of antihemophilic factor (factor VIII) decreased; antihemophilic factor–like precipitating antigens normal; ristocetin-induced platelet aggregation normal
von Willebrand's disease	Mild to severe	Autosomal dominant	Normal	Normal	↑	↑	Procoagulant antihemophilic factor and antihemophilic factor–like precipitating antigens usually decreased; ristocetin-induced platelet aggregation decreased.
Christmas disease (factor IX deficiency)	Mild to severe	X chromosome-linked†	Normal	Normal§	↑	Normal	
Plasma thromboplastin antecedent (PTA, factor XI deficiency)	Mild	Autosomal recessive	Normal	Normal	↑	Normal or ↑	
Hageman trait (factor XII deficiency)	None	Autosomal recessive†	Normal	Normal	↑	Normal	
Plasma prekallikrein deficiency (Fletcher trait)	None	Autosomal recessive†	Normal	Normal	↑	Normal	
High molecular weight kininogen deficiency (Fitzgerald trait)	None	Autosomal recessive	Normal	Normal	↑	Normal	

*There are specific assays for each clotting factor.
†In these syndromes cases have been described in which the clotting factor whose activity is decreased in clotting assays is either deficient or is present in a nonfunctional form.
‡And the later steps of intrinsic pathway.
§In some cases of Christmas disease, the prothrombin time is long when bovine thromboplastin is used.

prothrombin time, thrombin time, and bleeding time are normal. Proof of diagnosis requires the use of appropriate clotting tests to demonstrate the functional deficiency of antihemophilic factor, preferably including an assay using the plasma of a known hemophiliac. A normal bleeding time helps differentiate mild cases from von Willebrand's disease; careful analysis of the pattern of inheritance and tests of other relatives may be necessary. Further support for the diagnosis in doubtful cases can be obtained by demonstrating the presence of normal or elevated antigenic material related to antihemophilic factor in the plasma, typical of classic hemophilia, using antiserum raised in rabbits or goats, and normal aggregation of platelets upon addition of the antimicrobial ristocetin to platelet-rich plasma. All patients deficient in antihemophilic factor must be tested for the presence of circulating anticoagulants directed against this substance.

TREATMENT. Patients with hereditary hemorrhagic disease often have difficulty adjusting to the problems inherent in a disorder that poses unexpected threats to normal behavior and to life itself. As soon as the diagnosis is made, the patient or his parents should be instructed concerning the care, prognostic implications, and hereditary nature of his disorder. The parents should be encouraged to rear their afflicted children in as normal a way as is consistent with safety, for emotional crippling is as devastating as that resulting from hemorrhage. While the patient is too young to guard himself, the parents should arrange his environment so that it is as danger free as possible, in order to lessen the need to restrain his behavior. As he grows older, the patient should be advised, within his capacity, to indulge in such sports as swimming, running, tennis, and golf, and to avoid those involving body contact or predisposing to injury. The hemophiliac should prepare for a vocation which is not inherently dangerous; he and his parents should be reminded that hemophilia does not preclude a useful life in business or the professions. The object of therapy is to allow the patient to become a self-supporting adult, capable of caring for himself and living as full a life as possible.

The mainstay of therapy for episodes of bleeding is the transfusion of fractions of plasma rich in antihemophilic factor to correct the specific defect temporarily. The use of whole blood is restricted to the maintenance of blood volume after severe blood loss. Antihemophilic factor–rich fractions must be administered in amounts sufficient to raise the blood level of antihemophilic factor to a degree that permits normal hemostasis. Once transfused, antihemophilic factor disappears rapidly from the circulation, only about half remaining after 10 to 12 hours, so that repeated transfusions must be given until bleeding has been controlled. Therapy with antihemophilic factor–rich fractions carries with it risks of inducing hemolytic anemia from isoantibodies contaminating the preparations, transmitting hepatitis, and bringing about the formation of circulating anticoagulants that specifically inhibit antihemophilic factor. An occasional patient may have allergic reactions manifested by urticaria, headache, backache, chills, fever, and chest distress; antihistaminic agents are helpful both therapeutically and for prophylaxis.

In the event of major injury or in preparation for surgical procedures, the plasma level of antihemophilic factor must be raised to as much as 70 per cent that of a normal individual; lesser amounts may be adequate to control bleeding into joints or minor soft tissue hemorrhage. The use of concentrates of antihemophilic factor that can be administered in a small volume makes it possible to raise the plasma titer of antihemophilic factor adequately without danger of circulatory overload. One preparation in wide use is *cryoprecipitated antihemophilic factor*, separated during the cold thawing of fresh-frozen plasma. A bag of cryoprecipitate separated from 1 unit of blood (450 ml) contains 70 to 100 units of antihemophilic factor, 1 unit being the amount in 1 ml of fresh pooled normal plasma. Plasma levels sufficient for adequate hemostasis in many situations can be achieved by the administration of one bag of cryoprecipitate for each 4 kg of body weight, sustaining the plasma level of antihemophilic factor by administering half this amount every 12 hours. Larger doses may be needed if surgical procedures are undertaken, typically one bag of cryoprecipitate for every 2 kg of body weight initially, the same dose six hours after the first one, and one bag for every 4 kg six hours thereafter, repeated every 12 hours until hemostasis is assured — often as long as several weeks. A similar regimen is suitable when central nervous system bleeding is suspected. Another useful preparation is *lyophilized antihemophilic factor*, separated from plasma either by cryoprecipitation or by addition of glycine or other protein precipitants. Such material can be used under conditions in which frozen cryoprecipitated antihemophilic factor is not available; the dosage is calculated in terms of units of antihemophilic factor.

No rule of thumb can be provided as to how long therapy should be continued. In general, after surgery, dental extraction, or severe bleeding, concentrated antihemophilic factor is administered in the manner described for at least two days after all signs of bleeding have ceased, and the dose is then gradually decreased over the succeeding three or four days. Shorter courses of therapy are used when the danger of renewed bleeding is less threatening, as in most instances of hemarthrosis.

The availability of concentrates of antihemophilic factor has made it possible to abort hemorrhage more readily than was formerly possible without circulatory embarrassment. It has reduced the risk of surgical procedures and dental extractions in hemophiliacs. Indeed, in many patients, elective surgical procedures may be carried out, although surgery should be performed only in hospitals equipped to deal with this special problem.

This optimistic picture must be tempered by the fact that in as many as 20 per cent of severe hemophiliacs a circulating anticoagulant appears in plasma that specifically inactivates antihemophilic factor. The presence of this agent, which is an antibody directed against antihemophilic factor, vitiates the beneficial results of transfusion. Patients in whom this complication is present should under no conditions be subjected to surgery. When bleeding is life threatening and the titer of the anticoagulant is low, hemostasis can sometimes be achieved with large doses of antihemophilic factor. Experimentally, immunosuppressive therapy has been attempted, but the results are usually disappointing. Similarly, therapy with concentrates of the vitamin K–dependent clotting factors that contain "activated" factors has been suggested but is often disappointing.

If the bleeding site is accessible, *hemostasis* may be most effectively achieved by local measures. By appropriate use of local hemostatic agents such as powdered bovine thrombin and the application of cold and gentle pressure, bleeding may often be controlled. These measures must be sustained, for recurrent bleeding is likely over a period of days. Dental extractions in particular require meticulous local measures. Extractions should be carried out only in the hospital and by dental surgeons with special training in the care of hemophiliacs. Except in patients with mild hemophilia, hemostasis should be enhanced by the transfusion of concentrates of antihemophilic factor, e.g., a single dose of one bag of cryoprecipitate or 70 units of AHF for each 4 kg of body weight just before the extraction. The administration of epsilon-aminocaproic acid (4 grams every four hours for ten days in adults) usually obviates the need for further transfusion therapy.

The transfusion of concentrated antihemophilic factor is also useful in aborting *bleeding into joints*. A single dose of cryoprecipitated antihemophilic factor, one and a half bags for every 4 kg of body weight or the equivalent amount of lyophilized antihemophilic factor, combined with a short course of prednisone, 1 mg per kilogram daily for three days, with a maximum of 80 mg per day, has been useful. Acutely swollen joints should be immobilized. Local chilling and application of elastic bandages may be beneficial, but the application of a constricting bandage is contraindicated. Aspiration of the joint is occasionally advantageous, and should be performed only after adequate transfusion therapy. Active motion without weight-bearing is essential after bleeding has stopped in order to prevent persistent limitation of motion. Careful use of physiotherapy may be helpful in preventing and correcting deformities. Traction and splinting is less often used than formerly. Surgical correction of certain deformities has been successfully accomplished, but should be attempted only by experts and under the supervision of someone skilled in the transfusion therapy of hemophiliacs. Increased mobility of joints has sometimes been achieved by synovectomy, and replacement of hip and knee joints has been attempted with some success.

Other forms of bleeding require special types of care. Particularly hazardous is bleeding into the soft tissues of the neck, in which tracheostomy, performed under the cover of transfusion therapy, may be needed. Hemophiliacs should not be given intramuscular or subcutaneous injections, but venipunctures are not hazardous if performed with care. Immunization against tetanus is important, because bleeders are particularly prone to infection with this organism, but this is wisely delayed in severe hemophiliacs until the first course of replacement therapy. Immunization may be carried out without such preparation in mildly affected patients. Regular prophylactic care of the teeth should be provided.

Because bleeding often is painful, analgesics are often needed. Opiates should be used as sparingly as possible because of the possibility of addiction. Moreover, aspirin should be avoided because this agent may impair hemostasis. Acetaminophen, 0.65 gram every four hours in adults and proportionately less in children, combined with codeine if necessary, is a useful substitute but carries the risk of possible hepatic damage.

The availability of concentrates of antihemophilic factor has made possible home transfusion by the patient or a family member. In carefully selected patients, this procedure has reduced hospitalization, increased school attendance, and improved morale.

PROGNOSIS. The outlook for the hemophiliac has been greatly improved by modern methods of treatment. Those with moderately severe or mild hemophilia may seem so little affected that they live virtually normal lives, but even these patients may have exsanguinating hemorrhage after dental extraction, injury, or surgery. Those in whom the defect is more pronounced may require frequent admission to the hospital, and may be crippled by joint deformities. Some meet the challenge and are reasonably productive individuals, although others seem foredoomed to chronic invalidism. The life expectancy of hemophiliacs has lengthened with the availability of transfusion therapy, but death as the result of the complications of hemorrhage still occurs with disturbing frequency.

DETECTION OF CARRIERS. Certain women in hemophilia families are necessarily carriers — the daughters of affected men, the mothers of more than one hemophiliac, and the mother of one hemophiliac who has other affected relatives. The carrier state in other women can be detected with a high degree of certainty by simultaneous measurement of procoagulant antihemophilic factor and antigens related to this agent. In normal women, these two modalities vary from individual to individual, but in proportion. In contrast, in carriers, a relative excess of antigenic material is nearly always present. Because of variations of procoagulant antihemophilic factor titers both in normal women and in known carriers, their measurement alone successfully detects a much smaller proportion of carriers.

Biggs, R. (ed.): Human Blood Coagulation. Hemostasis and Thrombosis. 2nd ed. Oxford, Blackwell Scientific Publications, 1976.

Douglas, A. S. (ed.): Blood coagulation and fibrinolysis in clinical practice. Clin. Haematol., Vol. 2, No. 1, 1973.

Ratnoff, O. D.: Hereditary disorders of hemostasis. *In* Stanbury, J. B., Wyngaarden, J. B., and Fredrickson, D. S. (eds.): The Metabolic Basic of Inherited Disease. 4th ed. New York, McGraw-Hill Book Company, 1978.

Ratnoff, O. D.: Antihemophilic factor. *In* Gordon, A. S., Silber, R., and Lo Bue, J. (eds.): The Year in Hematology. New York, Plenum Book Company, 1977.

Rossi, E. D. (ed.): Symposium on hemorrhagic disorders. Med. Clin. North Am., Vol. 56, No. 1, 1972.

Spaet, T. H. (ed.): Progress in Hemostasis and Thrombosis, Vols. 1–3. New York, Grune & Stratton, 1972–1976.

520.3. OTHER HERITABLE DISORDERS OF BLOOD COAGULATION

Von Willebrand's disease is a hemorrhagic disorder characterized by a long bleeding time and deficiency of antihemophilic factor (factor VIII). Both procoagulant antihemophilic factor and antigens in plasma related to antihemophilic factor are usually reduced, and in proportion. The disease is transmitted by a dominant autosomal mutant gene, but has been detected more often in women than in men. The severity of symptoms varies considerably among affected members of the same family, some of whom may be asymptomatic. Bleeding is particularly severe in homozygotes. Menorrhagia and postpartum bleeding are common. The patient may experience epistaxis and gingival bleeding in severe cases; cutaneous ecchymoses or hematomas may occur. Hemorrhage follows injury or surgical procedures. Hemarthroses are relatively uncommon, but visceral bleeding or severe and even lethal hemorrhage into the gastrointestinal tract has been observed.

A unique feature of von Willebrand's disease is the prolonged bleeding time, an abnormality not usually associated with other hemophilia-like diseases. The coagulation defect can be corrected in vitro by normal but not by hemophilic plasma. In contrast, transfusion of hemophilic as well as of normal plasma or serum is followed by a delayed but pronounced and protracted rise in the patient's plasma level of procoagulant antihemophilic factor. A single unit of normal plasma may lead to the elevation of the antihemophilic activity of the patient's plasma to normal levels for many hours. Paradoxically, usually no corresponding rise in antigens related to antihemophilic factor occurs. These interesting observations are unexplained, although they suggest that the synthesis of antihemophilic factor takes place in at least two steps, one of which is defective in von Willebrand's disease and the second in classic hemophilia. Diagnosis is readily made when a markedly long bleeding time is encountered in a patient with deficiency of antihemophilic factor, as measured in clotting assays. Additionally, certain platelet functions may be disturbed. When normal or hemophilic blood or platelet-rich plasma is filtered through columns of glass beads, a high proportion of platelets is retained within the column; in von Willebrand's disease, platelet retention by the glass bead columns is reduced; this defect may be reflected in nature by impaired adhesion of platelets to expose vascular subendothelial tissue. Aggregation of platelets by the antimicrobial ristocetin, which occurs in normal or hemophilic platelet-rich plasma, is impeded in von Willebrand's disease. These abnormalities of platelet function have been attributed to deficiency of a portion of the antihemophilic factor molecule designated VIII_{VWF}, VWF representing "von Willebrand factor."

Sometimes, within a given family, affected individuals may be found in whom the bleeding time may be prolonged without significant deficiency of antihemophilic factor, or vice versa. Similarly, the deficiency of antigens detected by heterologous antiserum against antihemophilic factor may vary among affected individuals.

Careful study of the patient's relatives may help to differentiate mild classic hemophilia from von Willebrand's disease. When the bleeding time is not significantly prolonged, recognition of the disease is facilitated by demonstration of a concomitant deficiency of antigens related to antihemophilic factor and by impaired ristocetin-induced platelet aggregation.

Treatment of bleeding episodes consists of measures for local control of hemostasis and the administration of fresh plasma, or cryoprecipitates of plasma which contain the agent that induces synthesis of antihemophilic factor in von Willebrand's disease. Rarely, such treatment may be complicated by the appearance of antibodies that can be recognized by their inhibition of ristocetin-induced platelet aggregation. Menorrhagia may be terminated by suppression of menstrual bleeding with hormonal preparations such as norethynodrel. During pregnancy, the titer of antihemophilic factor may rise to levels that would be normal in nonpregnant women, and parturition may occur without hemorrhage, although the bleeding time remains long; postpartum bleeding is frequent.

Christmas disease is attributable to functional deficiency of Christmas factor (factor IX, plasma thromboplastin component), an abnormality transmitted by an X chromosome–linked gene. In most cases patients seem unable to synthesize Christmas factor, whereas in a minority nonfunctional Christmas factor is demonstrable in plasma. The disorder typically occurs in males, and is less common than hemophilia, from which it is clinically indistinguishable. All the clinical manifestations of hemophilia are encountered in patients with Christmas disease. The disorder varies in severity from family to family, manifestations roughly paralleling the degree of the deficiency of Christmas factor measured in the laboratory. In some families, the disorder appears to ameliorate with age. Heterozygous female carriers may have a partial deficiency of Christmas factor, and some have a mild bleeding tendency. A positive family history is obtained in only about two thirds of cases. Diagnosis is established by laboratory tests that demonstrate a defect in the early steps of the intrinsic pathway of thrombin formation, and by specific assay for Christmas factor, using a substrate plasma from a patient with known Christmas disease. The prothrombin time is usually normal, but in one variant of the disease it may be abnormally long when this test is performed with thromboplastin of bovine origin. The treatment of Christmas disease is basically the same as for hemophilia except that cryoprecipitates of plasma and lyophilized preparations of antihemophilic factor lack Christmas factor. Christmas factor is relatively stable, so that the patient can be treated effectively with plasma that has been stored under usual conditions in a blood bank. Large volumes of plasma, for example 1 liter or more, are required to raise the level of Christmas factor sufficiently to provide normal hemostasis; thereafter smaller amounts will sustain the titer of this substance, because its half-disappearance time in the circulation is greater than 20 hours; a typical regimen in an adult is 500 ml of plasma every 12 hours after the initial transfusion of 1000 ml of plasma, until hemostasis is assured. Concentrates of the vitamin K–dependent clotting factors, including Christmas factor, are now available, and can be used to provide large amounts of the missing factor without dangerous expansion of the circulating blood volume. These fractions, however, are often contaminated with hepatitis virus, and after their use for hemostasis during surgery, pulmonary embolism has been reported. In a few cases, the beneficial effects of transfusion are vitiated by the presence in the patient's plasma of a circulating anticoagulant, presumably an antibody directed against Christmas factor.

Plasma thromboplastin antecedent deficiency, a rare familial hemorrhagic disorder encountered in both sexes, is attributable to deficiency of PTA (factor XI). The disorder is inherited in an autosomal recessive manner; in most reported cases, the patients have been Jewish or Japanese. Bleeding episodes may follow trauma or surgical procedures, but spontaneous bleeding is uncommon. Hemorrhage is usually less severe than in hemophilia, and hemarthrosis is rare. Sometimes the disorder is asymptomatic. Laboratory tests demonstrate a defect in the early steps of the intrinsic pathway of clotting, but the specific diagnosis requires matching the plasma with that of a patient known to have PTA deficiency. Rarely, the bleeding time is said to be long. Transfusion of plasma is used in the treatment of bleeding episodes. Since the half-disappearance time of the infused PTA is about three days, correction of the defect is relatively simple.

Hageman trait is the hereditary deficiency of Hageman factor (factor XII). It occurs in both sexes, and is in most instances inherited as an autosomal recessive defect. Hageman trait is usually asymptomatic, although minor bleeding has occasionally been encountered, and families with a propensity for cerebrovascular accidents have been described. The diagnosis may be suspected when the clotting time is prolonged and a defect in the early steps of the intrinsic pathway is detected, but it can be established only by comparison with plasma of patients known to have this disorder. No treatment has been needed in reported cases, but in the event of hemorrhage normal plasma should be efficacious. Both deficiencies of Hageman factor and the presence of an aberrant form of this agent have been observed.

Fletcher trait is a rare, asymptomatic disorder of blood coagulation in which the early steps of the intrinsic pathway of clotting are defective, as demonstrated by prolongation of the partial thromboplastin time. The defect is due to a functional deficiency of Fletcher factor, identical with a plasma prekallikrein, needed for the optimal action of Hageman factor upon PTA. Both deficiency of prekallikrein and the presence of an aberrant form of prekallikrein have been described. No therapy is needed.

Fitzgerald trait (Williams trait, Flaujeac trait) is also an asymptomatic clotting disorder, inherited as an autosomal recessive trait, in which the early stages of the intrinsic pathway are defective, and thus the partial thromboplastin time is abnormally long. The abnormality is associated with a deficiency of high molecular weight kininogen (Fitzgerald factor); variants have been described in which low molecular weight kininogen is also deficient. No therapy is required.

Hageman trait, Fletcher trait, and Fitzgerald trait are distinguished by specific assays for these factors. The patients should be reassured about the benign nature of their laboratory defects.

Parahemophilia, a familial bleeding disorder affecting both sexes, is caused by a functional deficiency of proaccelerin (factor V). The disease is inherited in an autosomal recessive manner. Spontaneous bleeding may occur at numerous sites, but the joints are rarely involved. Menorrhagia and postoperative bleeding may occur, but in some patients the disease is mild or latent. The clue to diagnosis is provided by a prolonged prothrombin time which is not shortened by plasma deficient in proaccelerin. In a few cases the bleeding time is said to be long. A presumptive diagnosis can be made by demonstrating that the prothrombin time is shortened by addition of plasma from which the vitamin K–dependent clotting factors have been removed, but this test does not rule out a deficiency of fibrinogen. During surgical procedures or when abnormal bleeding is sufficiently severe to justify transfusion, fresh blood or plasma should be given in amounts adequate to maintain the plasma level of proaccelerin at about 25 per cent of normal; half the amount of proaccelerin infused disappears from the circulation in 12 to 36 hours. Rarely, patients with parahemophilia may become refractory to the beneficial effects of transfusion because specific antibodies are generated to the proaccelerin in infused plasma.

Hereditary functional deficiency of factor VII is transmitted in an autosomal recessive manner. Homozygous individuals of both sexes display a bleeding tendency of varying severity correlating with the severity of the deficiency. In some patients the plasma contains no material recognizable as nonfunctional factor VII, whereas in others a nonfunctional variant of the protein is present. Numerous hemorrhagic manifestations have been encountered, including umbilical bleeding in the neonatal period, epistaxis, ecchymoses, hemarthroses, menorrhagia, and hemorrhages into the gastrointestinal tract and central nervous system. Nonetheless, in many instances the disorder is clinically mild. Paradoxically, thromboembolism occasionally occurs. The one-stage prothrombin time is prolonged, an abnormality that is not corrected by plasma or serum from patients known to have factor VII deficiency. Factor VII is stable so that stored plasma is of therapeutic value. Large volumes of plasma, infused repeatedly, are required for effective hemostasis because of the rapid disappearance of factor VII from the circulation, half the amount infused being removed in only two to six hours; concentrates of the vitamin K–dependent clotting factors may also be used, with the caveats described in relation to Christmas disease. Menorrhagia may be controlled by the administration of oral contraceptive agents. In a variant form of factor VII deficiency, the partial thromboplastin time is inexplicably slightly prolonged.

Hereditary functional deficiency of Stuart factor, a rare disorder of blood coagulation, is characterized by deficiency of Stuart factor (factor X), and is attributable to an autosomal mutant gene. Only homozygotes have a bleeding tendency, which is similar to that of congenital deficiency of factor VII. In some instances a functionally defective form of Stuart factor is demonstrable in plasma, whereas in others a true deficiency of this agent is apparently present. The prothrombin time is prolonged and is not shortened by plasma from patients with known Stuart factor deficiency. In most instances, the clotting time of recalcified plasma is not shortened to a normal degree by the addition of Russell's viper venom, which requires Stuart factor for its procoagulant effect; in exceptional patients, said to have *Friuli coagulation disorder*, an aberrant form of Stuart factor is present that reacts normally with this venom. Treatment is the same as that for factor VII deficiency, but transfusions have a much more prolonged action, Stuart factor having a half-disappearance time from the blood of about two days, and need not be repeated as frequently.

Hereditary functional deficiency of prothrombin, a rare autosomal recessive trait, is clinically similar to factor VII and Stuart factor deficiencies. Two varieties have been distinguished, a true deficiency of prothrombin and a condition in which one or another nonfunctional prothrombin is detectable in plasma. The prothrombin time is prolonged and is not shortened by the addition of normal serum or of plasma from which the vitamin K–dependent clotting factors have been removed. The treatment of bleeding is the same as that for factor VII deficiency; about half of infused prothrombin disappears from the circulation in three days.

A rare anomaly has been described in which individuals have unusual *resistance to coumarin-like drugs*. As much as 20 times the usual dose is required to achieve a therapeutic effect. The disorder is inherited in an autosomal dominant manner. The mechanism underlying the defect is unknown, but in an analogous disease of rats, the microsomal membranes lack the normal capacity to bind warfarin.

Congenital deficiency of fibrinogen, a rare disorder occurring in both sexes, is apparently transmitted as an autosomal recessive trait. Clinical manifestations may begin at birth with hemorrhage from the umbilicus. In general, bleeding is hemophilia-like, except that permanent joint damage from hemarthroses is uncommon. Some patients have remarkably little bleeding, and even menstrual blood loss may not be excessive, but others have severe hemorrhages that can be fatal in early life. The blood does not clot even after the addition of thrombin, and little or no fibrinogen can be detected in plasma by physical, chemical, or immunologic methods. Bleeding episodes can be satisfactorily treated by intravenous administration of fibrinogen, in the form of cryoprecipitates of plasma, in amounts sufficient to maintain a plasma fibrinogen level in excess of 100 ml. An initial dose of one bag of cryoprecipitate for every 2 kg of body weight should provide hemostasis; subsequent doses should be one bag for every 15 kg daily. Several instances in which therapy has been impeded by the development of antibodies against fibrinogen have been reported. Strangely, death from obstruction of pulmonary circulation by "thrombi" composed of platelets has been described.

Congenital dysfibrinogenemia is a recently described group of familial disorders in which fibrinogen is usually present in normal amounts, but is abnormal in structure and coagulability. The abnormality has occurred in both sexes and in consecutive generations, suggesting autosomal dominant inheritance. The anomaly appears to be different in different families. In some the release of fibrinopeptides is impeded; in others aggregation of fibrin monomers is defective; in still other families, chemical bonding by fibrin-stabilizing factor is impaired. The disorder is usually recognized because the prothrombin time is prolonged, reflecting the presence of the anomalous fibrinogen. The bleeding tendency is usually mild, although severe bleeding has been reported. In some patients wounds have dehisced, whereas in others a paradoxical thrombotic tendency has occurred. Curiously, bleeding appears to be more frequent when the defect is in the release of fibrinopeptides and thrombotic complications or wound dehiscence, when aggregation of fibrin monomers is abnormal. Clots are small and friable and form slowly upon the addition of thrombin to plasma, but fibrinogen concentration as measured immunologically is usually normal. In one family, in which recurrent thrombotic episodes were prevalent, the abnormal fibrinogen clotted unusually rapidly upon the addition of thrombin.

Congenital deficiency of fibrin-stabilizing factor (factor XIII) is a rare disorder in which affected individuals have repeated episodes of serious bleeding after injury. Bleeding from the umbilicus is common. Hematomas, hemarthroses, hematuria, and habitual abortion have been described, and intracranial bleeding is a common cause of death. Sometimes wounds appear to heal slowly, occasionally breaking down repeatedly. The plasma of affected persons usually contains nonfunctional material antigenically similar to fibrin-stabilizing factor. The mode of inheritance of fibrin-stabilizing factor deficiency is not certain. In some families, the disorder is attributable to autosomal recessive mutant genes, whereas in others the syndrome seems limited to males. Diagnosis is established by demonstrating that clots of the patient's plasma are soluble in 5 molar urea or 1 per cent monochloracetic acid, in contrast to normal clots which are insoluble. More sophisticated tests of the transamidation function of fibrin-stabilizing factor have been used. Transfusion of normal plasma transiently corrects the hemorrhagic tendency and facilitates the healing of wounds; the half-disappearance time of infused fibrin-stabilizing factor is three to seven days.

Simultaneous congenital deficiency of several clotting factors has been repeatedly described. The coexistence of *deficiencies of antihemophilic factor and proaccelerin* appears

well established. The defect is probably inherited as an autosomal recessive trait. The bleeding tendency is usually mild, but should treatment of hemorrhage be needed, fresh-frozen plasma should be effective. One authentic case of coexistent deficiency of the vitamin K–dependent factors — prothrombin, factor VII, Stuart factor, and Christmas factor — has been described.

Biggs, R. (ed.): Human Blood Coagulation. Hemostasis and Thrombosis. 2nd ed. Oxford, Blackwell Scientific Publications, 1976.

Ogston, D., and Bennett, B. (ed.): Haemostasis: Biochemistry, Physiology, and Pathology. London, John Wiley & Sons, 1977.

Ratnoff, O. D.: Hereditary disorders of hemostasis. *In* Stanbury, J. B., Wyngaarden, J. B., and Fredrickson, D. S. (eds.): The Metabolic Basis of Inherited Disease. 4th ed. New York, McGraw-Hill Book Company, 1978.

Ratnoff, O. D. (ed.): Treatment of Hemorrhagic Disorders. New York, Harper & Row, 1968.

Rossi. E. D. (ed.): Symposium om hemorrhagic disorders. Med. Clin. North Am., Vol. 56, No. 1, 1972.

Spaet, T. H. (ed.): Progress in Hemostasis and Thrombosis. Vols. 1–3. New York, Grune & Stratton, 1972–1976.

521. ACQUIRED DISORDERS OF BLOOD COAGULATION

521.1. VITAMIN K DEFICIENCY

Vitamin K is required for the synthesis of prothrombin, factor VII, Stuart factor, and Christmas factor. If a deficiency of vitamin K is present, polypeptides are formed and, indeed, released into the plasma, but they lack clot-promoting properties. The role of vitamin K appears to be to transform these polypeptide chains to functional clotting factors through the insertion of a second carboxyl group into certain glutamic acid residues.

If vitamin K is not available in adequate amounts, the plasma levels of the four vitamin K–dependent factors fall and a hemorrhagic disorder ensues. The normal diet contains an abundance of vitamin K; deficiency rarely can be attributed to inadequate diet alone. The bacteria of the intestinal tract synthesize relatively large amounts of the vitamin, which may contribute to the body's supply. Prolonged *oral administration of antibacterial agents* has been associated with depletion of vitamin K and a hemorrhagic disorder reponsive to treatment with this vitamin. This syndrome is most likely to occur in patients undergoing parenteral feeding to whom no vitamin K is provided.

The infant at birth may be deficient in vitamin K and as a result may have *hemorrhagic disease of the newborn*. The disorder is more likely to occur in breast-fed infants; additionally, maternal ingestion of phenobarbital or anti-tuberculous drugs has been incriminated as a precipitating factor. Melena is common, but bleeding may occur from numerous sites. In some cases transfusion is required, and hemorrhage may be fatal. The disorder is self-limited within a few days, because the minute amounts of vitamin K needed by the infant are provided in milk; cow's milk contains more vitamin K than human milk. The establishment of intestinal flora may contribute to the supply, and the administration of antimicrobial drugs to infants requiring correction of congenital gastrointestinal lesions may precipitate hemorrhagic disease of the newborn. The frequency of this disease can be lessened by administration of small amounts of vitamin K to the mother before delivery or to the infant at birth.

Naturally occuring compounds with vitamin K activity are fat soluble and are poorly absorbed from the intestine in the absence of bile salts. Bleeding that accompanies obstructive jaundice or biliary fistula is usually the result of impaired absorption of vitamin K and is promptly responsive to the parenteral injection of the vitamin. Vitamin K should always be given preoperatively in cases of biliary obstruction, for the first evidence of a hemorrhagic disorder often does not appear until the surgical procedure is performed. Administration of cholestyramine, which has an affinity for bile salts needed for absorption of vitamin K, may precipitate deficiency of the factors dependent on its synthesis. Deficiency of the vitamin of a degree sufficient to cause bleeding is encountered in *malabsorption syndromes* such as *sprue* or *celiac disease*, and is readily prevented by parenteral administration of vitamin K.

Derivatives of *coumarin* and *indandione* behave as antagonists of vitamin K. These substances, commonly employed in therapy of thromboembolic disease, impair synthesis of prothrombin and other vitamin K–dependent clotting factors. *Salicylates*, related in chemical structure to coumarin, may produce the same effect when given in large amounts; possibly *propylthiouracil* may have this action in rare instances. Hemorrhage associated with the administration of vitamin K antagonists is usually a complication of therapy. The possibility that hemorrhage complicating anticoagulant therapy is due to potentiation of vitamin K antagonists by other drugs — for example, phenylbutazone, allopurinol, chloral hydrate, salicylates, sulfonamides, glucagon, indomethacin, quinidine, clofibrate, or anabolic steroids — must be kept in mind. Some patients with an obscure hemorrhagic disorder have been discovered to have taken coumarin compounds surreptitiously or because these agents were dispensed in error. A characteristic of the coagulation defects produced by vitamin K antagonists is failure to respond rapidly to injection of large amounts of menadione, a synthetic derivative of naphthoquinone, which ordinarily has potent vitamin K activity; in contrast, vitamin K_1 (phytonadione) is promptly effective. Psychiatric treatment of patients suspected of ingesting coumarin compounds surreptitiously is imperative, because this bizarre behavior may be a manifestation of depression, and the patient may seek more effective means of committing suicide.

Bleeding associated with deficiency of prothrombin and related clotting factors is similar to that occurring with other coagulation defects. Cutaneous ecchymoses, epistaxes, hematuria, gastrointestinal bleeding, and postoperative hemorrhage are common, and intracranial hemorrhage may occur. The hemorrhagic disorder may be fatal.

Diagnosis of vitamin K deficiency is established by the demonstration of a significantly prolonged prothrombin time that is shortened some hours after administration of vitamin K.

Treatment consists of oral or parenteral administration of a preparation of the vitamin. For most deficiency states, including those associated with biliary obstruction and malabsorption syndromes, water-soluble derivatives of menadione (menadiol sodium diphos-

phate or menadione sodium bisulfite) are rapidly and completely effective in correcting the abnormalities of coagulation. An injection of 10 mg of the menadione preparation is adequate, but should be repeated at weekly intervals for patients with a persistent absorption defect. Menadione in moderate amounts can produce serious hemolytic anemia and kernicterus in the newborn, even if given to the mother before delivery. Vitamin K_1 (phytonadione) is preferable, and a single dose of 1 mg, given intramuscularly to the infant at the time of birth, is adequate to prevent hemorrhagic disease of the newborn. To overcome the effects of coumarin derivatives and related drugs, only vitamin K_1 is effective. It is given orally or intramuscularly in doses of 5 to 25 mg. Vitamin K_1 may be administered by slow intravenous injection, but this route should be avoided except in an urgent situation because of the possibility of untoward reactions. Immediate but transient correction of multiple deficiencies of the vitamin K–dependent clotting factors may be provided in life-threatening situations by transfusion of plasma or of concentrates of these factors.

Ansell, J. E., Kumar, R., and Deykin, D.: The spectrum of vitamin K deficiency. JAMA, 238:40, 1977.
Girdwood, R. H. (ed.): Blood Disorders Due to Drugs and Other Agents. Amsterdam, Excerpta Medica, 1973.
Rossi, E. D. (ed.): Symposium on hemorrhagic disorders. Med. Clin. North Am., Vol. 56, No. 1, 1972.

521.2. LIVER DISEASE

Diffuse hepatic disease often produces a hemorrhagic disorder. Ecchymoses and pretibial petechiae are common, and hemorrhage may occur from many sites; bleeding from surgical wounds is frequent. The bleeding tendency may have multiple causes, including vascular abnormalities, thrombocytopenia, and impairment of blood coagulation. Thrombocytopenia is often the result of sequestration within an enlarged spleen, but other causes may be operative. Hypoprothrombinemia and deficiencies of the other vitamin K–dependent clotting factors are common; deficiencies of proaccelerin, PTA, and fibrin-stabilizing factor may contribute to the hemostatic defect. The catabolism of fibrinogen is often accelerated, and rarely, when parenchymal disease is severe, the concentration of plasma fibrinogen may be decreased. In some patients with advanced liver disease, depletion of plasma clotting factors and platelets may reflect diffuse intravascular coagulation. Another rarely encountered disturbance in chronic hepatic disease, particularly primary hepatoma, is the synthesis of a qualitatively abnormal form of fibrinogen which is converted to fibrin by thrombin at an abnormally slow rate. In cirrhosis of the liver, clots prepared from plasma or its euglobulin fraction dissolve abnormally rapidly, but evidence that this test tube phenomenon correlates with a bleeding tendency is insecure, and therapy with inhibitors of fibrinolysis is not recommended. Although the prothrombin time is usually prolonged in patients with hepatic disease who exhibit a bleeding tendency, the administration of vitamin K usually has little or no corrective effect. Transfusion of fresh blood, containing viable platelets, or fresh-frozen plasma may provide transitory correction of the coagulative defect, but is usually not satisfactory in maintaining hemostasis. The use of currently available concentrates of the vitamin K–dependent clotting factors should be avoided, because induction of disseminated intravascular co-agulation has been described and hepatitis is a frequent complication.

An isolated deficiency of factor VII may be found in association with hereditary disorders of bilirubin metabolism, including *Dubin-Johnson syndrome, Gilbert's syndrome,* and the *Rotor syndrome.*

Poller, L.: Coagulation abnormalities in liver disease. *In* Poller, L. (ed.): Recent Advances in Blood Coagulation, Vol. 2. Edinburgh, Churchill Livingstone, 1977, p. 267– 292.

Ratnoff, O. D.: Disordered hemostasis in hepatic disease. *In* Schiff, L. (ed.): Diseases of the Liver. 4th ed. Philadelphia, J. B. Lippincott Company, 1975, pp. 184–203.

521.3.   RENAL DISEASE

Hemorrhagic phenomena, particularly cutaneous bruising, occur with great frequency in patients with renal failure; most disturbing is gastrointestinal bleeding, which occasionally may be severe or lethal. As in the case of hepatic disease, the origin of bleeding manifestations may be complex. Thrombocytopenia is commonplace, but is usually not severe enough to be of much clinical significance. Qualitative defects of platelet function, including impaired aggregation of platelets by adenosine diphosphate or thrombin, impaired retention of platelets by glass bead columns through which blood is filtered, and impaired release of coagulant activity ("platelet factor 3") are often present, and are more likely to be important in the pathogenesis of bleeding; these abnormalities have been attributed to inhibition of platelet function by retained metabolites, particularly guanidosuccinic acid. In some cases the clotting time of whole blood or cell-poor plasma, the prothrombin time and the thrombin time may be abnormally long, perhaps contributing to the bleeding tendency.

Other abnormalities of hemostasis may be present in patients with renal failure. Sometimes plasma fibrinolytic activity may be decreased whereas fibrinogen-related antigens, perhaps the result of fibrinolysis or disseminated intravascular coagulation, may be found in serum, particularly in acute renal failure. Similar antigens are often found in the urine in both acute and chronic renal disease. In nephrotic syndromes, the urine may contain large amounts of one or another clotting factor, e.g., Christmas factor, and the plasma titer of these factors is correspondingly decreased, sometimes resulting in the appearance of a hemorrhagic diathesis.

No specific therapy is available for these various hemostatic abnormalities, but the qualitative defects of platelets may be reversed by hemodialysis or by successful renal transplantation.

Mallick, N. P., and Geary, C. G. Renal disease. *In* Israels, M. C. G., and Delamore, I. W. (eds.): Haematologic Aspects of Systemic Disease. Philadelphia, W. B. Saunders Company, 1976.

521.4.   ACQUIRED DEFICIENCY OF STUART FACTOR

Several cases have now been recorded in which extensive amyloidosis has been associated with severe deficiency of Stuart factor. The pathogenesis of this syndrome is unexplained, although binding to amyloid fibrils has been suggested. A similar transient and un-explained disorder has been described in several individuals without recognized amyloidosis. Therapy with plasma or concentrates of the vitamin K–dependent clotting factors has been suggested, but the half-disappearance time of Stuart factor infused in this way is sharply reduced.

Furie, B., Green, E., and Furie, B. D.: Syndrome of acquired factor X deficiency and systemic amyloidosis. In vitro studies of the metabolic fate of factor X. N. Engl. J. Med., 297:81, 1977.

521.5.   ACQUIRED HYPOFIBRINOGENEMIA AND SYNDROMES OF INTRAVASCULAR COAGULATION AND FIBRINOLYSIS

Deficiency of fibrinogen of a degree sufficient to cause abnormal bleeding is encountered in a number of different clinical syndromes. It occurs only rarely because of retarded production of fibrinogen and more often as a result of rapid utilization. A bleeding tendency encountered in some patients with *cyanotic congenital heart disease* is attributable in part to the very high hematocrit; the fibrinogen concentration of whole blood is so low that an adequate clot cannot form. Whether a similar deficiency of fibrinogen in whole blood contributes to the bleeding tendency of patients with *polycythemia vera* with thrombocythemia is not clear. Although fibrinogen is synthesized in the liver, *hepatic disease* is seldom the cause of profound deficiency.

Normal plasma contains, on the average, about 300 mg of fibrinogen per 100 ml, although individual variation is wide. During pregnancy, infection, inflammation, myocardial infarction, and other stresses, the concentration of fibrinogen in plasma may be much higher, an alteration principally responsible for the elevated erythrocyte sedimentation rate in these conditions. The biologic half-life of fibrinogen is about three to six days, but the nature of its normal catabolism is unknown. Neither consumption by intravascular coagulation, nor deposition at extravascular sites of inflammation, nor fibrinolysis by the proteolytic enzyme, plasmin, seems adequate to explain its continual destruction.

Plasmin is present in circulating plasma in the form of a protein precursor, plasminogen. In the test tube, this proenzyme can be converted to plasmin in many ways, including addition of streptokinase (a product of certain beta-hemolytic streptococci), urokinase (a proteolytic enzyme in normal urine), or a plasminogen activator found in many tissues, most impressively in the endothelium of venules and veins. Under certain conditions, the clotting process itself appears to initiate formation of plasmin, an effect mediated by activated Hageman factor via one or more intermediate agents. The long-recognized activation of plasminogen by incubation of plasma or its euglobulin fraction (that is, the fraction insoluble at low ionic strength and low pH) with chloroform is apparently brought about through this Hageman factor–determined mechanism.

Plasmin can digest a wide variety of substrates, including fibrinogen, fibrin, antihemophilic factor, proaccelerin, gamma globulin, and corticotropin (ACTH). It converts the first component of complement, C1, to its esterolytic form, C$\bar{1}$, changes plasma prekallikrein to kallikrein (an enzyme that releases biologically active kinins, such as bradykinin, from their precursor in plasma, kininogen), and directly severs kinins from kininogen. Additionally, plasmin digests casein, gelatin, and certain synthetic esters and amides of arginine and lysine, all of which have been used for an in vitro assay of plasmin.

Plasma also contains several potent inhibitors of plasmin, notably α1-antitrypsin, α2-macroglobulin, α2-plasmin inhibitor and C1 inactivator, a protein that also inhibits C1, activated Hageman factor, activated PTA, and plasma kallikrein. Platelets, too, possess plasmin-inhibitory properties. Recent evidence also suggests that plasma may inhibit the activation of plasminogen.

Although purified fibrinogen and fibrin appear to be digested by plasmin at comparable rates, this is apparently not true in plasma. For example, fibrin formed in the presence of streptokinase dissolves rapidly, whereas the digestion of fibrinogen in an unclotted mixture of plasma and streptokinase proceeds more slowly. One likely explanation is that plasminogen, adsorbed to fibrin, can be converted to plasmin in situ and then induce fibrinolysis. Presumably, fibrinolysis takes place because the plasmin is physically separated from inhibitors of the activation of plasminogen and of plasmin itself. In unclotted plasma, these inhibitors protect fibrinogen from hydrolysis by plasmin. This phenomenon is of major importance in attempts at therapeutic dissolution of thrombi by the administration of plasminogen activators, with minimal digestion of circulating plasma proteins.

The digestion of fibrinogen by plasmin takes place by steps. The first cleavage of fibrinogen, whose molecular weight is about 340,000, splits this molecule into a fragment with a molecular weight of about 240,000 (fragment X), which can still be clotted by thrombin, and several small fragments. Further digestion of fragment X leads ultimately to the formation of three incoagulable fragments, two with a molecular weight of about 83,000 each (fragments D), and one with a molecular weight of about 50,000 (fragment E). Similar fragments appear during the digestion of fibrin, but in this case fragment X is incoagulable. Fragments X and E are powerful anticoagulants, interfering primarily with polymerization of fibrin, apparently by forming complexes with monomeric units of fibrin, formed by the action of thrombin on fibrinogen. Clots formed in the presence of digestion products of fibrinogen and fibrin are structurally defective. The *degradation products of fibrinogen and fibrin (FDP)* also interfere with earlier stages of clotting, and perhaps with platelet aggregation, but the physiologic significance of these actions is unclear.

EXPERIMENTAL INTRAVASCULAR COAGULATION

When a massive amount of tissue thromboplastin or thrombin is injected intravenously into an animal, its blood clots, presumably because the extrinsic pathway of coagulation has been activated. Death ensues from circulatory obstruction. When, instead, the clot-promoting agent is injected slowly, the animal survives but its blood becomes incoagulable. The slower rate at which thrombin forms under these conditions results in slower, and perhaps incomplete, formation of fibrin, so that plasma may contain intermediates of fibrin formation, such as fibrin monomer, soluble fibrin polymers, or complexes of fibrin monomer and fibrinogen. These products are rapidly removed from the circulation by the reticuloendothelial system, whose cells then contain material recogniz-

able immunologically as related to fibrinogen, whereas the circulating blood is depleted of this protein. Usually thrombi cannot be detected by microscopic examination, although occasionally the smallest blood vessels of the kidneys, adrenals, and other organs contain thrombi. Concomitant with the evolution of afibrinogenemia, the concentration of other clotting factors decreases, particularly prothrombin (presumably utilized in the formation of thrombin), proaccelerin, and antihemophilic factor (the latter two, perhaps, inactivated by thrombin). The platelet count falls, possibly because these cells are clumped by thrombin and removed from the circulation. Animals that have undergone experimental defibrination may undergo hemolysis, and their red blood cells may appear to have been fragmented, as if ruptured by intravascular strands of fibrin. Inconstantly, evidences of intravascular fibrinolysis may be detected, either by demonstration of products of digestion of fibrinogen or fibrin in the animal's serum, or by depletion of plasminogen, the precursor of the fibrinolytic enzyme, plasmin; direct evidence for the presence of fibrinolytic activity in the animal's plasma is more difficult to demonstrate. Nonetheless, fibrinolysis has been invoked as one cause for failure to find thrombi in animals injected with tissue thromboplastin; the plasma often acquires clot-inhibitory properties attributed to the presence either of degradation products of fibrin formed through the action of plasmin, or of complexes of these degradation products, fibrinogen, and dissolved fibrin monomers and polymers, in various combinations.

LABORATORY DIAGNOSIS OF INTRAVASCULAR COAGULATION

When intravascular coagulation has been extensive enough to induce hypofibrinogenemia or afibrinogenemia, rapid diagnosis may be made by observing the appearance of coagulating blood in a test tube. A simple qualitative test for hypofibrinogenemia is the addition of 1 ml of blood to 0.1 ml of bovine thrombin solution containing 1000 NIH units per milliliter. Unless virtually no fibrinogen is present, the blood clots quickly. The size of the clot can then be estimated by tapping the tube and observing the degree to which the clot retracts. The retracted clot may be so small that it is difficult to find among the extruded red blood cells and serum, leading to the misinterpretation that fibrinolysis has occurred. The existence of hypofibrinogenemia is confirmed by additional tests, including quantitative measurement of fibrinogen concentration.

In patients thought to have undergone intravascular coagulation, the thrombin time (that is, the time elapsing until a mixture of plasma and thrombin clots), prothrombin time, and partial thromboplastin time may all be prolonged, both because necessary reactants have been depleted and because of the presence of clot-inhibitory agents. In some cases, intravascular coagulation may be suspected because the concentration of fibrinogen, although within the range found in normal individuals, is decreased below the level anticipated in the light of the patient's clinical condition. In parallel to the changes observed in laboratory animals, the platelet count may be reduced, and deficiencies of prothrombin, proaccelerin, and antihemophilic factor may be observed. Inconstantly, too, rapid dissolution of clots formed from plasma or its euglobulin fraction may suggest that *secondary fibrin-*

olysis has taken place. More frequently, the concentration of plasminogen may be diminished, as if this proenzyme had been converted to plasmin and then inactivated by its inhibitors in plasma, and the plasma may acquire inhibitory properties directed against the clotting process.

Direct evidence that intravascular coagulation has taken place has been provided in several ways. Thus free fibrinopeptide A, separated from fibrinogen through the action of thrombin, can be detected immunologically in the plasma of patients thought to be undergoing intravascular coagulation. Further, the incorporation of radioactive glycine methyl ester into a fraction of plasma rich in fibrinogen has been thought to reflect the presence of dissolved fibrin monomers or polymers; this ester is incorporated into fibrin, but not fibrinogen, through the action of fibrin-stabilizing factor. High molecular weight complexes, seemingly of fibrinogen and fibrin monomer, have been separated from plasma by physical means. And the half-disappearance time of intravenously injected radioactive fibrinogen is dramatically shortened in patients in whom intravascular coagulation is believed to be taking place. These four techniques have not been translated into practical methodology.

Indirect support for the existence of intravascular coagulation can be obtained by demonstrating that the patient's serum, normally devoid of fibrinogen, contains antigenic material related to this protein. Many techniques have been used to demonstrate these fibrinogen-related antigens (FRA), often called by the more restrictive term, fibrinogen degradation products (FDP), which implies that the materials identified are the product of the action of plasmin. Immunodiffusion, immunoelectrophoresis, tanned red blood cell hemagglutination inhibition, and agglutination of latex particles coated with heterologous antifibrin antiserum have all been used to detect fibrinogen-related antigens. Less reliably, gelation of plasma by addition of ethanol or protamine sulfate, or aggregation of certain strains of *Staphylococcus aureus* by the patient's serum may reflect the presence of dissolved polymers, composed particularly of fibrin monomer and fibrinogen but also, perhaps, of fibrin monomer and degradation products of the action of plasmin on fibrinogen or fibrin. Similarly, chilling plasma may induce precipitation of "cryofibrinogen," composed of complexes of fibrinogen and fibrin monomers. And in some patients evidences of intravascular damage to erythrocytes, similar to those seen in experimental animals undergoing defibrination, may be found.

The laboratory abnormalities described have been detected in the blood of patients undergoing disseminated intravascular coagulation. Similar changes, however, are observed in some patients with extensive localized thrombosis, e.g., pulmonary embolism or aortic aneurysm.

HYPOFIBRINOGENEMIC SYNDROMES ASSOCIATED WITH LOCALIZED THROMBOSIS

Rarely, after massive arterial or venous thrombosis or pulmonary embolism, the blood is incoagulable, and marked thrombocytopenia is present. Presumably, the fibrinogen, platelets, and other clotting factors are depleted in the formation of thrombi. A similar coagulation defect may be encountered in *purpura fulminans*, a disease in which acute necrosis of superficial and peripheral parts of the body is associated with thrombosis at the sites of vasculitis in small blood vessels in the affected areas. This rare disorder, which is most prevalent in children and often follows shortly after an apparently banal infection, is usually self-limited, but its course may be aborted by administration of heparin, which inhibits further thrombin formation. Perhaps the rare instances of patchy *cutaneous necrosis during therapy with coumarin-like anticoagulants* have a similar pathogenesis, although hypofibrinogenemia has not been described in this situation. The lesions are most likely to appear at sites rich in fatty tissue, such as the breast, buttocks, and lipomas. The necrotic lesions are preceded by an evanescent, painful erythematous patch, and treatment with vitamin K_1 may abort the episode.

Unusually, hypofibrinogenemia has also been observed with *thrombotic thrombocytopenic purpura*, in which noninflammatory thrombosis of small blood vessels is associated with fever, acute hemolytic anemia, renal failure (see Ch. 515.1). In this disorder, the administration of heparin is usually without benefit. Hypofibrinogenemia may occur in patients with *giant cavernous hemangioma, hemangioepithelioma,* or *cavernomatous transformation of veins*, particularly of the portal system; in these disorders, fibrin thrombi form in the relatively static blood within the vascular lesions. Other syndromes in which widespread thrombosis of relatively large vessels is commonplace, such as *paroxysmal nocturnal hemoglobinuria, Behçet's syndrome, sickle cell disease,* and *homocystinuria*, have not been associated with hypofibrinogenemia.

HYPOFIBRINOGENEMIC SYNDROMES ASSOCIATED WITH DISSEMINATED INTRAVASCULAR CLOTTING

Hypofibrinogenemia or afibrinogenemia may be encountered in other disorders in which thrombosis may be difficult or impossible to demonstrate. In such cases, procoagulant substances are thought to be introduced into the bloodstream sufficiently slowly that massive thrombosis does not ensue. The fate of the fibrin that forms intravascularly is not clear. Perhaps, as is true in laboratory animals, fibrin is removed from the circulating blood by the reticuloendothelial system. Alternatively, soluble fibrin monomers or polymers, perhaps complexed with fibrinogen, are cleared from the bloodstream before insoluble fibrin strands can form, or fibrin is dissolved by plasmin, and the fibrin degradation products, some of which may be complexed with fibrinogen or fibrin monomer, are removed by the reticuloendothelial cells.

Disseminated intravascular coagulation may be suspected in many instances because of the clinical setting, described below. Often suspicion is aroused because of prolonged bleeding from sites of venous or arterial punctures, from surgical or traumatic wounds, or from the uterus. The presence of unexplained ecchymoses, hemorrhagic bullae, and acral cyanosis and gangrene has been emphasized by some authors as suggestive of disseminated intravascular coagulation.

The clearest examples of defibrination by these mechanisms are *amniotic fluid embolism*, in which amniotic fluid and its contaminants enter the maternal bloodstream during parturition, *envenomation* by the bite of snakes whose venom contains procoagulant agents, and the administration of several hundred milliliters of *incom-*

patible blood. In this last circumstance, the products of lysis of the transfused cells may initiate intravascular coagulation and defibrinate the recipient's blood. Envenomation by the bite of the Malayan pit viper, *Agkistrodon rhodostoma,* has been extensively studied; the venom has a thrombin-like action upon fibrinogen, resulting in afibrinogenemia without any of the depletion of other clotting factors or platelets seen in other cases of intravascular clotting. These properties have led to its experimental use in the treatment of thromboembolic disorders.

Similar mechanisms have been evoked to explain hypofibrinogenemia in other disorders, although the evidence is more inferential. For example, hypofibrinogenemia has been encountered in patients with severe *sepsis,* particularly *septic abortion,* and *Waterhouse-Friderichsen syndrome.* In these syndromes, vascular damage may expose the circulating blood to subendothelial tissues which may induce thrombosis through activation of the clotting mechanism or localized aggregation of platelets. A wide variety of both gram-positive and gram-negative organisms have been implicated. The possibility that in some cases intravascular coagulation is part of the human counterpart of the generalized Shwartzman reaction has been advocated. Hypofibrinogenemia has been reported with peculiar frequency in individuals with *pneumococcal sepsis* who have asplenia, usually as the result of splenectomy, or splenic atrophy, such as occurs in sickle cell disease. Vascular damage may also be important in initiating disseminated intravascular coagulation in patients with *viral hemorrhagic fevers* or certain other infectious diseases.

Some cases of *premature separation of the placenta* may be complicated by hypofibrinogenemia; although the introduction of highly thromboplastic placental tissue into the maternal bloodstream has been invoked as an explanation, other mechanisms, such as the formation of a massive retroplacental clot, may be operative. The pathogenesis of hypofibrinogenemia in *prolonged retention of a dead fetus* or *neoplastic diseases* is less clear, although in such cases intravascular coagulation induced by procoagulants derived from the pathologic tissue has been surmised. *Metastatic carcinoma of the prostate* is the most frequent of the many neoplasms that may produce hypofibrinogenemia; this defect has also been encountered in patients with carcinoma of the breast, stomach, gallbladder, pancreas, lung, and colon, disseminated rhabdomyosarcoma, leukemia, most often of the acute promyelocytic type, and other tumors as well.

Hypofibrinogenemia, thrombocytopenia, and other coagulation defects have been encountered during various types of *extracorporeal circulation.* The apparatus may defibrinate the blood if insufficient heparin is employed. *Abnormal bleeding during cardiovascular surgical procedures* may have multiple causes, including the use of too much or too little heparin, as well as the operative procedure itself. Hypofibrinogenemia has also been observed during other surgical procedures, most frequently during pulmonary resection, although this is a rare complication. This syndrome has also been encountered during therapeutic infusion of ascitic fluid, presumably because of its content of thromboplastic substances. Hypofibrinogenemia may accompany *aneurysm of the aorta,* particularly *dissecting aneurysm,* presumably because the exposed subendothelial tissue is clot promoting. Widespread vascular damage may also explain the occurrence of hypofibrinogenemia in patients with *shock* of different origins and *heat stroke.*

Bleeding associated with the defibrinating syndromes is often severe, but the character of the bleeding, as well as the prognosis, is influenced by the nature of the underlying disease. Often, the first indication that defibrination is taking place is bleeding at the sites of arterial or venous puncture. In women with *premature separation of the placenta* or *amniotic fluid embolism,* major hemorrhage is usually from the uterus, although a generalized bleeding tendency may be evident. In patients with more chronic forms of hypofibrinogenemia, ecchymoses, hematoma formation, and bleeding from the gastrointestinal tract may be prominent. Patients with syndromes of disseminated intravascular coagulation may also have symptoms consequent upon the obstruction of the circulation by small thrombi; renal tubular and cortical necrosis caused by thrombosis in the smallest blood vessels are of the greatest moment.

Primary treatment of hypofibrinogenemia or afibrinogenemia caused by intravascular coagulation is that of the basic disease; if this can be eradicated or ameliorated, the coagulation defects are rapidly corrected. Thus the hypofibrinogenemia associated with *amniotic fluid embolism* is self-limited, whereas in patients with *premature separation of the placenta* or *retention of a dead fetus,* recovery follows shortly after the uterus is emptied. Severe bleeding associated with *carcinoma of the prostate* may subside, and the coagulation abnormalities may disappear within days of the institution of estrogen therapy. Similarly, hypofibrinogenemia may subside after specific chemotherapy of *acute myeloid leukemia* or after administration of antivenom after *envenomation by venomous snakes.* Transfusion of fresh blood is often required. Although administration of fibrinogen in the form of cryoprecipitates of plasma (for example, one bag for every 2 kg of body weight) may be of temporary value and tide the patient over an acute episode of bleeding, if the basic pathologic process continues, the transfused fibrinogen is rapidly removed from the circulation and may participate in the formation of new disseminated thrombi. In cases in which the primary disease cannot be treated, intravenous injection of heparin may impede intravascular defibrination by inhibiting the clotting process and raise the levels of depleted clotting factors. A typical course of therapy includes an initial dose of 50 to 100 units of heparin per kilogram of body weight, followed by 10 to 15 units per kilogram per hour, administered by intravenous infusion; more may be needed, and smaller doses may be appropriate if severe thrombocytopenia is present. This seemingly paradoxical approach to treatment is most effective when the disease is self-limited, as in the case of *extensive arterial or venous thrombosis* or *purpura fulminans,* or in cases of chronic defibrination, as in instances of *metastatic disease* or, until surgery is performed, *retention of a dead fetus.* The risks of bleeding from operative wounds or the placental site limit the usefulness of heparin therapy in acute forms of hypofibrinogenemia, but its use has been advocated in such conditions as heat stroke or incompatible blood transfusion in which no overt bleeding site is present.

DISSEMINATED INTRAVASCULAR COAGULATION WITHOUT HYPOFIBRINOGENEMIA

A widely held view is that many pathologic states may induce widespread intravascular coagulation, perhaps insufficient to cause significant hypofibrinogenemia, but adequate to bring about ischemic damage. Under such conditions, the thrombin time, prothrombin time, and partial thromboplastin time may be prolonged; serum may contain agents immunologically resembling fibrinogen; plasma may undergo coagulation upon addition of ethanol or protamine sulfate, and the platelet count may be depressed. In some patients, intravascular hemolysis may be detected, and the erythrocytes may have the morphologic characteristics of those of animals undergoing experimental defibrination, appearing fragmented and often triangular in shape. Such cells, often called *schistocytes*, are characteristic of *microangiopathic hemolytic anemia*, a state seen pre-eminently in *thrombotic thrombocytopenic purpura* and the *hemolytic-uremic syndrome*. In some cases, too, accelerated turnover of fibrinogen and platelets suggests that intravascular coagulation has occurred even though the blood levels of these substances may not be decreased because other compensating mechanisms are operative.

Application of these criteria has led to the assumption that myriad clinical disorders are accompanied by intravascular coagulation. Besides thrombotic thrombocytopenic purpura and the hemolytic-uremic syndrome, these diseases include fulminant *eclampsia* with hemolytic anemia and thrombocytopenia, *malignant hypertension*, *chronic glomerulonephritis, nephrotic syndrome* with proliferative glomerulonephritis, *renal cortical necrosis, cirrhosis of the liver, hyaline membrane disease, sepsis*, especially *meningococcemia* and *rickettsial* and *viral* disorders, *metastatic carcinoma, systemic lupus erythematosus, polyarteritis nodosa,* and *shock* of diverse origins. Intravascular coagulation has also been thought to be important in rejection of *organ grafts*, and may complicate *therapeutic abortion*. This by no means exhausts the disorders in which intravascular coagulation, disseminated or localized to specific organs, is thought to be an important feature (Table 2).

Evidences for the role of intravascular coagulation in the pathogenesis of these various disease states varies in degree of conviction. Particular criticism has been leveled at diagnostic reliance upon hemolysis or changes in red blood cell morphology, because these may occur in the absence of other changes associated with intravascular coagulation, and hemolysis may be the cause rather than the result of defibrination.

The beneficial effects of heparin in some cases of hypofibrinogenemia have led to its use in individuals in whom disseminated intravascular coagulation is suspected in the absence of hypofibrinogenemia. In some cases, a trial of heparin therapy, as outlined for patients with hypofibrinogenemic states, may be justified, and may be followed by clinical and laboratory improvement. In most instances, unfortunately, the results have been disappointing, and skepticism concerning the importance of disseminated intravascular coagulation in pathogenesis seems appropriate.

McKay, D. G.: Disseminated Intravascular Coagulation. An Intermediary Mechanism of Disease. New York, Hoeber Medical Division, Harper & Row. 1965.

Merskey, C.: Defibrination syndromes. *In* Biggs, R. (ed.): Human Blood Coagulation, Haemostasis and Thrombosis. 2nd ed. Oxford, Blackwell Scientific Publications, 1976.

Minna, J. D., Robboy, S. J., and Coleman, R. W. (eds.): Disseminated Intravascular Coagulation in Man. Springfield, Ill., Charles C Thomas, 1974.

Rossi, E. D. (ed.): Symposium on Hemorrhagic Disorders. Med. Clin. North Am., Vol. 56, No. 1, 1972.

TABLE 2.   Disorders Accompanied by Intravascular Coagulation*

A. Hypofibrinogenemic or afibrinogenemic states:
  1. Secondary to the introduction of extrinsic clot-promoting agents
     Amniotic fluid embolism
     Envenomation by snakebite
     Premature separation of the placenta
     Autoadministration of ascitic fluid
  2. Secondary to intravascular elaboration of clot-promoting agents
     Acute hemolytic processes (e.g., mismatched blood transfusion)
     Extracorporeal circulation
     Massive arterial or venous thrombosis; pulmonary embolism
     Near drowning
  3. Secondary to vascular injury, exposing clot-promoting tissues
     Purpura fulminans
     Sepsis with gram-positive or -negative organisms; septic abortion; Waterhouse-Friderichsen syndrome
     Infectious disease (e.g., generalized herpes simplex, dengue, cytomegalic inclusion disease, scrub typhus, Rocky Mountain spotted fever, miliary tuberculosis, subacute bacterial endocarditis, trypanosomiasis)
     Heat stroke
     Aortic aneurysm
     Traumatic shock; burns; head injury; surgical procedures
     Thrombotic thrombocytopenic purpura; hemolytic-uremic syndrome
  4. Secondary to vascular stasis
     Giant hemangioma
     Hemangioendotheliosarcoma
     Cavernomatous transformation of veins
  5. Pathogenesis uncertain (introduction of clot-promoting agents?)
     Malignancy (e.g., carcinoma of prostate, pancreas, etc., neuroblastoma, leukemia)
     Administration of L-asparaginase, cephazolin
     Acute pancreatitis
     Hydatidiform mole
     Relapsing nonsuppurative panniculitis (Weber-Christian disease)
     Hepatitis
B. Conditions in which intravascular coagulation has been implicated in the absence of hypofibrinogenemia:
  1. Secondary to intravascular elaboration of clot-promoting agents
     Hemolytic processes (e.g., paroxysmal nocturnal hemoglobinuria)
     Rejection of organ transplants
  2. Secondary to vascular injury
     Purpura fulminans
     Sepsis with gram-positive or -negative organisms
     Infectious diseases (e.g., exanthematous diseases, viral hemorrhagic fevers, influenza, rickettsial or mycotic disorders, falciparum malaria, bubonic plague, subacute bacterial endocarditis)
     Thrombotic thrombocytopenic purpura, hemolytic-uremic syndrome, eclampsia
     Chronic glomerulonephritis, renal cortical necrosis, lupus erythematosus with renal disease, polyarteritis nodosum, nephrotic syndrome with proliferative glomerulonephritis
     Traumatic, cardiogenic, and anaphylactic shock; burns; surgical procedures
  3. Secondary to vascular stasis
     Malignant hemangioendothelioma
  4. Pathogenesis uncertain
     Malignancy (e.g., metastatic carcinoma of stomach, lung, breast, etc., especially mucin-producing tumors; Wilms' tumor)
     Idiopathic respiratory distress syndrome; hyaline membrane disease
     Cirrhosis of the liver
     Amyloidosis
     Fat embolism
     Poisoning with *Amanita phalloides*, mercuric oxide, alkyl phosphates, dichlorethane
     Cyanotic congenital heart disease
     Cardiogenic shock
     Behçet's syndrome

*This tabulation is not all-inclusive; the classification is tentative, and the evidence supporting the existence of intravascular coagulation as an important component of the disease state varies in its cogency.

521.6. FIBRINOLYTIC STATES

An attractive hypothesis envisions that minor degrees of fibrinolytic activity operate under normal conditions to maintain the fluidity of blood by dissolving thrombi in the microcirculation. Evidence in support of this view is, however, equivocal. As measured in vitro, the fibrinolytic activity of blood or its euglobulin fraction is exaggerated in chronic hepatic disease, under such conditions of stress as traumatic shock, anxiety, electroconvulsive therapy or anoxia, and after the injection of certain vasoactive substances, e.g., epinephrine or nicotinic acid. The enhanced fibrinolytic activity is thought to be due to the presence in plasma of circulating activators of plasminogen, perhaps derived from venous endothelium and, in the case of chronic hepatic disease, inadequately removed from the bloodstream by the liver. The clinical significance of these in vitro observations is uncertain, because the enhanced fibrinolytic activity is not ordinarily reflected in clinical symptomatology, and in vivo the array of inactivators of plasmin in plasma may limit the evolution of significant proteolytic activity. Moreover, demonstration of increased fibrinolytic activity in vitro usually requires the formation or presence of a fibrin clot, to which plasminogen and its activators may be adsorbed. Under these conditions, plasmin may form, physically separated from its inhibitors in plasma, allowing fibrinolysis to take place. In vivo, on the other hand, the array of inactivators of plasmin may limit the evolution of significant proteolytic activity.

Under the stress of intravascular coagulation, local fibrinolysis appears to be an important mechanism in dissolution of small thrombi. Here, as in vitro, plasmin may be capable of digesting clots without reaching effective levels in circulating plasma. Under these conditions, products of fibrinolysis may be found in circulating plasma, where they may inhibit the coagulation process and interfere with the polymerization of fibrin. Usually, direct evidence that fibrinolysis is taking place is meager, but fibrinolysis has been inferred from a fall in the concentration of plasminogen in plasma. The titers of antihemophilic factor and proaccelerin, measured in clotting assays, may also be decreased, and the patient's serum may contain antigenic material related to fibrinogen, possibly products of fibrinolysis but, as has been noted earlier, sometimes the result of incomplete clotting of fibrin. In some patients undergoing intravascular coagulation, fibrinolysis may be so extensive that clotted blood undergoes spontaneous dissolution within minutes or a few hours. This *secondary fibrinolytic state* is most often found in patients in whom defibrination is particularly severe, such as those with *amniotic fluid embolism, premature separation of the placenta, profound hemorrhagic shock,* or *neoplasms,* such as *metastatic carcinoma of the prostate* or *acute leukemia.* In some cases, despite the demonstration of potent fibrinolytic activity in vitro, the concentration of fibrinogen does not fall dramatically, recalling ·the observation noted earlier that fibrinolysis occurs more readily than fibrinogenolysis.

A few patients have been described who, under severe stress, have developed a fulminant hemorrhagic syndrome attributable to excessive fibrinolytic activity. Thus during laparotomy, blood may seem to ooze from every cut tissue; fibrinolysis may be so ·rapid that whole blood appears to be incoagulable, whereas the patient's plasma can be clotted by thrombin, only to redissolve within minutes. Although this rare syndrome has been attributed to a *primary fibrinolytic state,* it is uncertain whether in fact the disorder does not reflect an episode of diffuse intravascular clotting in which fibrinolysis rather than thrombosis dominates the clinical picture. In contrast to the usual case of disseminated intravascular clotting, the platelet count may be normal; other laboratory features, including prolongation of the thrombin time, prothrombin time, and partial thromboplastin time, depletion of clotting factors, and the demonstration of fibrinogen-related antigens in serum, do not distinguish the disorder from diffuse intravascular coagulation. If the diagnosis seems certain, the administration of large amounts of *epsilon-aminocaproic acid,* a drug which inhibits the activation of plasminogen, may be helpful. A typical regimen in an adult is 4 grams every four hours for two or three days. Unfortunately, this agent is strongly contraindicated in individuals undergoing intravascular coagulation, for it may stabilize thrombi which would otherwise dissolve. Thus great circumspection must be used in treating patients with suspected primary fibrinolysis with this agent.

A more certain primary fibrinolytic state may be induced during therapeutic attempts at dissolution of thrombi by administration of streptokinase or urokinase, activators of plasminogen. In such cases, more plasmin forms within the bloodstream than can be effectively neutralized by plasma inhibitors of this enzyme, and fibrinogen and other clotting factors may be depleted, without a concomitant fall in the platelet count. Hemorrhagic symptoms, apparently induced by excessive fibrinolytic activity, are relatively common complications of experimental fibrinolytic therapy. Bleeding has been particularly frequent at sites of venipuncture and cutdown incisions. If bleeding symptoms are alarming, therapy with epsilon-aminocaproic acid in the manner described for primary fibrinolytic states may be indicated, but caution must be exercised in its use, lest the thrombotic state for which therapy was initiated be worsened.

Local fibrinolysis after prostatectomy may lead to protracted and sometimes severe hematuria. The pathogenesis of bleeding under these conditions is uncertain; clots in the operative bed may be dissolved by plasmin, formed through the action either of urinary urokinase or of tissue activators in exposed prostatic tissue. Therapy with epsilon-aminocaproic acid as described above is effective, and is not attended by the dangers inherent in the treatment of thrombotic states. Localized fibrinolysis has also been invoked as an explanation of rebleeding after subarachnoid hemorrhage, and prophylactic administration of epsilon-aminocaproic acid has been advocated by some authorities.

Douglas, A. S. (ed.): Blood coagulation and fibrinolysis in clinical practice. Clin. Haematol. Vol. 2, No. 1, 1973.

Rossi, E. D. (ed.): Symposium on hemorrhagic disorders. Med. Clin. North Am., Vol. 56, No. 1, 1972.

521.7. ANTICOAGULANTS

The presence of an anticoagulant in the circulating blood causes a bleeding tendency that may be severe. This occurrence may follow parenteral administration of heparin, a substance that interferes' with generation of thrombin at several steps as well as with the conversion of fibrinogen to fibrin by potentiating the inhibitory properties of antithrombin III. Heparin rapidly disappears from the circulation so that the hemorrhagic disorder subsides within an hour or two after intravenous injection is terminated. Rarely, inadvertent administration of heparin may be responsible for sudden, unexpected bleeding. A tentative diagnosis can be made by demonstrating that the patient's plasma clots abnormally slowly upon addition of thrombin (whose action is antagonized by heparin) but at a normal rate upon addition of Reptilase, i.e., the venom of *Bothrops atrox* (whose clotting action upon plasma fibrinogen is not blocked by heparin). A number of hemorrhagic disorders have been attributed to the production of heparin in vivo, but there are few if any cases in which this claim is supported by convincing evidence. Antiheparin agents, including protamine sulfate, effectively counteract the action of heparin when given intravenously in precisely calculated amounts; if possible, this titration should be done in vitro, but a rule of thumb is administration of 1 mg of protamine sulfate for every 100 units of heparin. Bishydroxycoumarin (Dicumarol) and related compounds are often referred to as anticoagulants, but they interfere with the synthesis of clotting factors and do not retard coagulation directly.

Endogenously produced anticoagulants are encountered under several circumstances and may produce a hemophilia-like disease. These circulating anticoagulants are usually IgG antibodies, and they most often interfere with the early stages of coagulation. One frequently demonstrable in the plasma of patients with hemophilia specifically inactivates antihemophilic factor and is an antibody against this agent. An anticoagulant of similar nature and specificity sometimes occurs in the plasma of women after pregnancy, producing a hemophilia-like disorder. Hemorrhagic disease attributable to an apparently identical anticoagulant has appeared without obvious cause in persons who were previously healthy, occasionally in those to whom penicillin or related antibiotics or phenytoin has been administered, or in individuals who have a chronic disease. Comparable substances, specifically inactivating other clotting factors, have been encountered in patients with congenital deficiency of the clotting factor in question. A circulating anticoagulant occurring in the plasma of some patients with systemic lupus erythematosus is unusual, because it interferes with the conversion of prothrombin to thrombin; less commonly, patients with this disease have circulating anticoagulants against antihemophilic factor.

The presence of an anticoagulant inhibiting one or another step in the generation of thrombin is detected by demonstrating the retarding action of small proportions of the patient's plasma on the coagulation of normal blood or recalcified plasma. Circulating anticoagulants may disappear spontaneously, sometimes after a period of many months or years, but therapy is difficult. Because of the anticoagulant effect of the patient's plasma, transfusions do not correct the clotting defect. When bleeding is life threatening, exchange transfusion or the injection of massive amounts of the missing factor may be tried. The use of steroids or immunosuppressive agents has been disappointing, and administration of "activated" preparations of the vitamin K–dependent factors to individuals with circulating anticoagulants against antihemophilic factor provides erratic benefit. Patients with myeloma and with other diseases causing dysproteinemia may display impairment of blood coagulation attributable to the presence of the abnormal protein. The bleeding manifestations frequently associated with dysproteinemia are not, however, clearly related to retarded clotting.

Inhibitors of the activation or action of fibrin-stabilizing factor have been described in association with hemorrhagic symptoms that range from mild to none. The inhibitory agents are probably immunoglobulins of the IgG class, and their appearance has been related to isoniazid therapy.

Spaet, T. H. (ed.): Progress in Hemostasis and Thrombosis. Vols. 1–3. New York, Grune & Stratton, 1972–1976.

PART XIX
MEDICAL
ONCOLOGY

522. CANCER AND INTERNAL MEDICINE: AN INTERNIST'S APPROACH TO CANCER AND ITS MEDICAL MANIFESTATIONS

W. P. L. Myers

In some respects oncology is the last bastion of internal medicine. Although an internist is one who is trained to think broadly about medicine and one who should practice his art accordingly, the age of specialization has led to the inescapable tendency for many physicians to view illness from a narrowed perspective. Not so for medical oncologists. The subspecialty of oncology calls for maintaining as broad a perspective as possible if patients are to be evaluated and treated properly. It calls for an appreciation and knowledge of general internal medicine to diagnose and treat the problems which cancer patients present as well as a knowledge of the natural history of cancer and the protean ways in which it can affect patients. In the past, there was a deplorable tendency to dismiss a patient and his problems with the all-inclusive label "cancer" in the belief that it was some mystical, arcane disease entity and, with the label, the light of thought and inquiry in the physician's mind went out. Cancer, although possibly one disease in biologic terms, is many diseases in clinical terms, calling for the broadest understanding and openness of thought.

522.1. INTERNIST'S APPROACH TO THE CANCER PATIENT

All well and good, but still we must have a method, a way of approaching a patient and the neoplastic illness he is suspected of having. The principles of medical analysis discussed below are also employed, in the form of questions, in Ch. 528. They constitute the keystone in the internist's approach to cancer and its medical manifestations.

COMPLETE HISTORY AND PHYSICAL EXAMINATION. A complete history and a physical examination assure that the patient will "pass through" the hands and mind of the physician. Too often, previous examinations are accepted in lieu of a fresh independent look, to the patient's detriment. A detailed chronologic development of all the symptomatology must be undertaken with care, and the patient's observations must not be dismissed because they do not happen to fit the pattern of a disease process the physician is entertaining. What the patient says is to be believed and to be understood to the best of the physician's ability. Thus, if a woman tells her physician that she has noted a breast lump but he is not impressed because of extensive multiple lumps of cystic mastitis, nevertheless, if she has noted one lump above all others, the observation must be believed and acted upon. Too often the physician attempts to reassure prematurely with a pat on the hand and thereby, in effect, to impose his wisdom over the patient's. Patients have their wisdom, too, and it must not be disregarded; as a corollary, a physician should not tell a patient more than he knows. A history relating specifically to the possibility of cancer should emphasize *change* — that is, change in appetite, weight, digestion, bowel habits, voiding, size and color of nevi, or voice — as well as the *appearance of new symptoms*, such as bleeding, pain, or fever. Risk factor analysis is part of this appraisal, and a good cancer history should include facts relating to exposure to carcinogens, drug and hormone use, radiation exposure, immunodeficiency (or suppression), and a family history of cancer. The presence in the history of certain symptoms, not in themselves direct manifestations of cancer, might nevertheless lead to a suspicion of underlying malignancy. Syndromes "guilty by association" with cancer are numerous and include migratory thrombophlebitis, sensorimotor polyneuropathies, cerebellar degeneration, dermatomyositis, and a variety of skin diseases.

As with the history, the physical examination must be complete. The too-frequent incompleteness of physical examinations has led to the facetious definition of a consultant as a physician who does a pelvic and rectal and examines the eyegrounds. The chart entry "Pelvic and rectal: deferred" is all too familiar; completeness of physical examinations in settings where cancer is suspected is a goal which medicine still has not achieved. A brief case history will serve to illustrate this point:

A 45-year-old woman came to the hospital complaining of intermittent lower abdominal discomfort attended by loose watery bowel movements for the previous two to three years. She had noted occasional blood in the stool. There was also a background of intermittent abdominal cramps for the previous ten years. She had experienced no weight loss. The physical examination was noted as showing "nothing really significant," although a pelvic and rectal was not done. The physician then expressed the opinion that he did not think the patient had cancer but rather "some type of colitis. . . ." She was referred for disposition to the gastroenterology clinic (for "long-term management . . ."), where both digital and proctoscopic examination revealed a lesion which proved to be adenocarcinoma of the rectum. The lesion was amenable to anterior resection, and the patient is alive and well without recurrence some three years later.

All of us make mistakes repeatedly, and we hope those we make will not be major ones. One way to keep medical mistakes to a minimum is to begin the analysis of a patient's illness with a thorough physical examination. Special attention must be paid the symptomatic area, and the examining doctor must be honest enough to determine whether his examination was adequate. Thus, if he was able to get only a fleeting view of the vocal cords in a patient complaining of hoarseness, assistance must be sought from someone more skilled in this examination. A flat-of-the-hand palpation of the body is a useful maneuver to detect small subcutaneous lesions, biopsy of which may provide the solution to a problem. Similarly, careful examination of the skin for scars may lead the patient to recall the removal of a nevus, or palpation of the umbilicus may give evidence of a periumbilical cuff of tumor as the only sign of intra-abdominal cancer. The skin must be thoroughly searched for suspicious nevi and for other evidences of skin lesions associated with cancer such as acanthosis nigricans, ichthyosis, and erythema multiforme (see Part XXIII). Anatomic areas deserving of attention, but not commonly examined, include the scalp, alveolar ridges under dentures, perineum, and soles. Palpation and measurement of all suspicious lumps, masses, skin lesions, organ enlargements, and edematous extremities are particularly important. Occasionally primary malignancies remain occult and may be revealed only by the development of an enlarged lymph node; all such nodal enlargements should be noted and measured. Those in the femoral region should not be mistaken for, or dismissed as, femoral hernias. Pelvic and rectal examinations must never be "deferred." If the examination cannot be done at the time of the initial examination, space should be left in the write-up to serve as a reminder that the examination is incomplete.

ESTABLISHMENT OF THE HISTOLOGIC DIAGNOSIS AND PRIMARY SITE. Histologic diagnosis is the cornerstone of cancer treatment. It provides verification that cancer exists and also valuable information as to the stage of the lesion. For example, knowledge whether a surgeon is dealing with a melanoma at Clark's level II or level IV will determine the type of surgical procedure he may employ. With metastatic cancer, the therapeutic implications often vary, depending on the primary site of the tumor. Thus, although the diagnosis of "metastatic cancer" on lymph node biopsy, without definition as to primary site, might suffice in the instance of some cancers (i.e., cancer of the pancreas), with others lack of knowledge of the primary site would be a serious omission (i.e., cancer of the breast or prostate). Accurate definition of the primary site has also led to better understanding of the natural history of certain cancers. Cancers that have been clearly defined as oat-cell cancer of the lung have been found to disseminate so early in their course that nonsurgical treatment has now become the general rule of management. The histopathologic definition of some cancers may be very difficult, and second or third opinions may be necessary. Certainly the oncologist to whom a patient with cancer is referred for treatment should always review the pathologic material. He does this not only for verification purposes but also to stage and classify lesions, as is so necessary in Hodgkin's disease. The grade of a tumor and whether it is well differentiated or not, whether invasive of vessels or not, and whether infiltrated by lymphocytes or not are all additional reasons why histopathology is important. Finally, pathologic examination of adjacent or distant lymph nodes is necessary for staging of cancers. The entire matter of staging by morphologic and clinical criteria has been addressed in the *Manual for Staging of Cancer* (American Joint Committee

for Cancer Staging and End-Results Reporting). In addition to the established standards of histologic examination, histochemistry, electron microscopy, and cell surface marker technology hold promise for vastly increasing the sophistication of the classification of tumors.

CONSIDERATION OF THE POSSIBILITY OF A SECOND PRIMARY CANCER. Although second primary cancers may arise in the same tissue or organ system as the primary lesion or in different organ systems, there remains an irresistible tendency to consider all clinical signs of cancer as manifestations of the original neoplasm, and often inappropriate management is the consequence. Although many reported associations of multiple cancers have been challenged on statistical grounds, from a clinical standpoint the physician would do well to consider a solitary lesion in the lung as a new primary cancer, rather than a metastasis, particularly if the first cancer had originated in the head and neck. Additional associations that have been noted include breast cancer and endometrial cancer, chronic lymphatic leukemia and various solid tumors, and the bilaterality of breast and testicular cancer. In addition to the inherent risk of multiple cancers as a consequence of tumor biology and host response, an added risk of second cancers appears to be developing as a consequence of treatment of the first cancer, by either radiation therapy or chemotherapy or both. These second malignant neoplasms have been described in a variety of clinical settings, among which are included second cancers in children intensively treated with chemotherapy for the first neoplasm and in patients with Hodgkin's disease. Conceivably the widespread current application of adjuvant therapy following the initial surgical treatment of cancer may add further instances of treatment-induced second neoplasms. For all these reasons, an objective approach to the cancer patient must include an evaluation of the possibility of a second primary cancer.

EVALUATION OF THE EXTENT OF DISEASE. A diagnosis of cancer should immediately induce a clinical reflex that asks the extent of the cancer. Chart entries at the end of a history and physical examination that state simply "Hodgkin's disease" or "carcinoma of the lung" are far less informative than those that carry the additional information regarding extent of disease such as "Hodgkin's disease, Stage IIA" or "carcinoma of the lung with metastases to the skeleton and liver." This focus of attention on extent not only concisely summarizes the over-all clinical problem but also sets the stage for treatment. The longstanding generality has been that localized disease is excised, regional nonresectable disease is irradiated, and generalized disease is treated with systemic measures. This generality still holds true, but there are new dimensions to it. This is the age of multimodality therapy in which surgery, radiotherapy, chemotherapy, endocrine therapy, and immunotherapy are interwoven and combined in ways meant to bring about the best possible therapeutic result. Thus regional disease, deemed nonresectable, may be irradiated first and followed by an attempt at surgical removal. Intrapleural BCG (bacille Calmette Guérin) may be instilled following resection of lung cancer. Pulmonary metastases, once thought to be treatable only by nonsurgical means, now may be treated best by surgery combined with chemotherapy, depending upon the type of tumor and other factors. Successes with this approach have been notable particularly in patients whose pulmonary metastases have been secondary to osteosarcoma. The following case report will serve to illustrate the importance of an accurate appraisal of the extent of disease to the selection of treatment:

A 41-year-old man was admitted to the hospital because of suspected recurrent islet cell cancer of the pancreas. He had undergone a subtotal pancreatectomy and splenectomy elsewhere, and although the operation was thought to have been curative, the patient subsequently developed recurrent hypoglycemia. He was referred for chemotherapy. Examination revealed slight hepatomegaly but no intra-abdominal masses. Although a celiac arteriogram and a liver scan suggested that a large metastasis was present in the right lobe of the liver, it was *not* assumed that the patient had nonresectable cancer. At operation, it was established that, contrary to the preoperative laboratory data, no metastasis existed in the liver and it was possible to resect a residual tumor in the head of the pancreas by means of a Whipple procedure. The patient is alive some three years later and is without evidence of recurrent disease.

In this case, an accurate appraisal of the extent of disease, as determined at surgery, led to definitive and possibly curative treatment. Had the disease been *assumed* to be nonresectable, the patient would have been subjected to noncurative forms of treatment.

The detailing of the extent of disease is not only necessary to rational treatment, but it has also led to a better understanding of the clinical behavior of cancer in that certain patterns of extent have emerged. For example, colonic cancer has been observed to recur according to one of four patterns: (1) pelvic recurrence, (2) generalized abdominal metastases, (3) hepatic metastases, and (4) disseminated metastases. These patterns tend to maintain their integrity, and the clinical course of the patient may often be anticipated. Thus in a patient with the pelvic recurrence pattern the physician might anticipate the problems of pain secondary to invasion of the lumbosacral plexus and uremia secondary to ureteral obstruction. The reasons for these patterns, or tropisms, are unknown and pose a major challenge to the clinical investigator.

DEFINITION OF MEDICAL COMPLICATIONS, RELATED AND UNRELATED TO THE CANCER. A remarkable variety of medical complications can be caused by cancer, as the following case history demonstrates:

A 51-year-old woman who had metastatic melanoma was admitted to the hospital for treatment with BCG. Seven months before this an enlarged left axillary node had been excised and found to contain malignant melanoma. Four months later multiple skin metastases developed, and the patient was referred for evaluation and treatment. Physical examination revealed multiple pigmented nodules over the anterior and posterior chest and several pigmented nodules along the suture line of the left axillary biopsy scar. Laboratory studies revealed 4+ proteinuria and 24-hour quantitative urinary protein levels of 17, 24, and 6 grams. The serum albumin was 2.2 grams per deciliter, and the blood urea nitrogen and serum creatinine were normal. The concentration of serum IgG was reported as 290 mg per deciliter (normal, 900 to 1800 mg per deciliter). Studies for urinary tract infection, poststreptococcal infection, and collagen disease were negative. Although a renal biopsy stained by H and E showed only minimal histopathologic change, electron microscopy revealed epimembranous electron-dense deposits, and immunofluorescence studies revealed melanoma antigen immunoglobulin "lumpy-bumpy" deposits. A diagnosis was made of melanoma-induced immune-complex glomerulopathy with the nephrotic syndrome.

This patient demonstrates one of the renal syndromes which may occur as a consequence of cancer. The nephrotic syndrome has been reported also in association with lymphomas and with carcinomas of the lung, colon, and breast. It may be the presenting manifestation of cancer. Of course the nephrotic syndrome may occur in a patient with cancer quite independently of the cancer itself, and antitumor measures might be expected to produce no benefit in these patients. It is this careful delineation of medical problems and complications that forms the basis of good management. At times the medical complication may be more life threatening than the underlying malignancy, constituting an additional reason for the recommended analytical approach.

THOROUGH INVESTIGATION OF PREVIOUS TREATMENT, SPECIFIC AND SUPPORTIVE, AND ITS ADEQUACY; CONSIDERATION OF THE POSSIBLE ETIOLOGIC ROLE OF TREATMENT IN THE PRESENTING CLINICAL PROBLEM. The treatment of all disease depends in part on knowing what the previous treatment has been and whether it can be judged to have been adequate. Effective therapy discarded prematurely because it was *assumed* to have been administered in a proper fashion and in adequate dosage is an avoidable pitfall. If a patient is known to have been treated with a particular chemotherapeutic regimen, exact dosages, duration of treatment, and the patient's response, as well as the response of the tumor, all must be documented. Similarly, if the patient had undergone surgical treatment, its adequacy must be judged. At times "inoperability" is more a consequence of the surgeon's attitude and ability than of the medical and anatomic facts. Supportive treatment should also be judged in these terms; often inadequate supportive measures have been employed and, unless objective data regarding such previous therapy are sought, possible beneficial treatment may be dismissed out of hand. In evaluating previous treatment before initiating a new program, consideration should also be given to the possible etiologic role of previous treatment in the patient's present status. Examples are numerous and would include electrolyte and metabolic disturbances (hyperuricemia, hypercalcemia, steroid diabetes), hematologic disorders (thrombocytopenia, anemia, leukopenia), postsurgical problems (dumping syndrome, diabetes insipidus, adrenal insufficiency), and infectious complications (*Pneumocystis carinii*, gramnegative sepsis).

ASSESSMENT OF THE ACTIVITY OF THE DISEASE PROCESS: ACTIVE AND PROGRESSIVE OR CHRONIC AND STABLE. Judgments concerning cancer and its treatment can be refined when there is some knowledge as to the activity of the disease. Of course, primary operable cancer should be promptly treated surgically whenever it comes to light, regardless of the activity of the cancer, but, in other settings, activity of the process may be a major determinant of treatment. In the surgical treatment of pulmonary metastases, for example, it has been stated that if the doubling time of the pulmonary lesion(s) is less than 20 days, surgical removal should not be attempted because the results are so poor. Although others would dispute this in individual cases, patients with rapidly growing pulmonary lesions in general fare less well with surgical treatment than those whose lesions have a slower doubling time. In other instances patients appear to have established some sort of "truce" with a particular metastatic tumor and the disease process is clearly chronic and stable. Aggressive antitumor measures in such patients, unless the treatment holds remarkable promise, would not be indicated.

522.2. MEDICAL MANIFESTATIONS OF CANCER

Having followed the approach outlined above, the internist is in a position to consider some of the more common medical problems he may encounter in cancer patients. They can be conveniently thought of as (1) those secondary to organ invasion, (2) those secondary to physiologically active tumor products, and (3) those secondary to treatment (Table 1). Medical problems "guilty by association" with cancer have already been alluded to, and many of these undoubtedly constitute examples of syndromes caused by physiologically active tumor products as yet unidentified. For purposes of this discussion, however, problems most likely to be encountered will be discussed. No claim is made for completeness, for the internal medicine of cancer is as vast as internal medicine itself. Neurologic syndromes, pain, cutaneous manifestations of internal malignancy, and syndromes due to the production of ectopic hormones are considered elsewhere and will not be reviewed here.

In considering medical problems in cancer, it is worth remembering that some diseases may simulate cancer. Secondary syphilis with generalized lymphadenopathy has been misdiagnosed as lymphoma, and plasmacytosis incident to subacute bacterial endocarditis has led to the erroneous diagnosis of multiple myeloma. Chronic effusions may cause changes in the mesothelial cells of the pleura or peritoneum that resemble cancer, and care should be taken when basing the diagnosis of cancer solely on cytologic examination of pleural or peritoneal fluid. Awareness of these possibilities, together with the orderly approach outlined above, should make the mistaken diagnosis of cancer highly unlikely.

INFECTIOUS DISEASES. Of all the medical problems encountered in cancer, infections constitute the most important because of the frequency of their occurrence and because so often they may be responsible for the patient's demise. A predisposition to certain infections may occur as a result of cellular defects, as shown in Table 2. Such a classification is useful because it serves to alert the physician to what might reasonably be expected in a given situation of immunodeficiency. As more knowledge is gained, it is likely that we will have other predispositions to infectious agents based on complement deficiency (for example, patients lacking the sixth or eighth components of complement are predisposed to infections with *Neisseria*), but at the moment the immune cell defects noted in Table 2 offer the best working classification. Several general points can be made. The major consideration in treating a given febrile patient is the presence or absence of neutropenia, since it has been observed repeatedly that bacterial infections in such patients can lead to death in 24 to 48 hours, that is, before adequate bacteriologic identification can be made. In neutropenic patients with acute pharyngitis (notably immunosuppressed patients with acute leukemia), the pharyngitis should be regarded as

a medical emergency and the offending organism(s) considered to be gram-negative enteric bacilli pending identification by culture. This means immediate treatment with an antibacterial regimen consisting usually of gentamicin, a cephalosporin, and carbenicillin. The same can be said for neutropenic patients presenting the clinical picture of sepsis. Those organisms most often associated with the picture of sepsis are identified in Table 2. Chloramphenicol or clindamycin (for *Bacteroides fragilis*) might be added to the regimen if an infradiaphragmatic source is suspected, or penicillin in high dosage if clostridial sepsis seems likely. The point is that one should not wait for bacteriologic confirmation before treating the febrile, neutropenic, immunosuppressed patient.

A second general area of concern is pulmonary infection which can range from lobar consolidation to patchy pneumonitis to acute interstitial pneumonia, to fungus balls. Virtually all the organisms listed in Table 2 can be the cause of pulmonary disease in the cancer patient. Pneumonias attended by bacteremia have been cited to have a mortality of 75 per cent, or higher, and prompt treatment, as for sepsis noted above, with carbenicillin added in neutropenic patients, is mandatory while appropriate cultures are pending. Obtaining a good sputum specimen, or, if necessary, tracheal secretions by aspiration, is central to a bacteriologic diagnosis. Unfortunately, in the instance of fungal infections of the lung and in those caused by some parasites and viruses, sputum examination is often not diagnostic, and serologic studies may be necessary, particularly for aspergillosis, cryptococcosis, histoplasmosis, toxoplasmosis, coccidioidomycosis, and cytomegalovirus infection. In anticipation of pulmonary disease, during periods of neutropenia and immunosuppression, collection of serum specimens every two to four weeks, with storage for subsequent analysis, can be an important diagnostic step. In the case of *Pneumocystis carinii* lung biopsy may be the only way in which the diagnosis can be made, and such intervention must be considered after 24 to 48 hours of empirical broad-spectrum antibacterial therapy in a patient who is not responding and in whom no definitive diagnosis has been made. It is useful to remember that a patient infected with *P. carinii* and demonstrating fever, tachypnea, nonproductive cough, and hypoxemia may nevertheless have a normal chest x-ray. The traditional therapy for this organism has been pentamidine, but recent evidence suggests that trimethoprim-sulfamethoxazole is also effective. The possibility of *P. carinii* infection must always be considered in the cancer population, particularly in those patients in whom corticosteroids are being tapered or have recently been discontinued. Since *P. carinii* is the most common infectious cause of interstitial pneumonia in this population, initial empiric therapy might well include trimethoprim-sulfamethoxazole.

With regard to the central nervous system (CNS), the most common infectious causes of meningitis in a cancer population are *Listeria monocytogenes* and *Cryptococcus neoformans*, particularly in patients with impaired cellular immunity. However, neutropenic patients, especially those with leukemias and lymphomas, are still subject to infections with aerobic gram-negative organisms and with *Mucor* species or *Aspergillus*. Patients with meningitis may show few signs of it, and this diagnosis must be considered in any unexplained fever. Definitive bacteriologic examination of the cerebrospi-

TABLE 1. Examples of Common Medical Problems in Cancer

I. Those secondary to involvement of organ systems
    Obstruction and its consequences
        Ureters   Azotemia
        Blood vessels   Superior vena caval obstruction
        Intestine   Perforation; fistulas; pain
        Bronchus   Atelectasis; distal infection
        Biliary excretory ducts   Obstructive jaundice
        Lymph vessels   Lymphedema; malabsorption
    Organ failure secondary to metastases
        Liver   Hepatic coma; hypoglycemia
        Heart   Cardiac arrhythmias; tamponade
        Skeleton   Myelophthisic anemia; fractures; pain
        Lungs   Pneumothorax; respiratory failure
        Endocrine organs   Diabetes insipidus; myxedema
        Anatomic cavities   Ascites; pleural effusion
        Central nervous system   Increased intracranial pressure; cord compression
    Organ failure due to primary neoplasm
        Blood cells   Acute leukemia with infection
        Lymph nodes   Hodgkin's disease with anergy
        Pancreas   Exocrine deficiency with steatorrhea
II. Those secondary to physiologically active tumor products
    Syndromes secondary to ectopic hormone production
        ACTH   Bronchogenic carcinoma with Cushing's syndrome
        PTH   Hypernephroma with ectopic hyperparathyroidism
        ADH   Oat cell carcinoma of the lung with the inappropriate antidiuretic hormone syndrome
        Gastrin   Nonbeta cell carcinoma of the pancreas with the Zollinger-Ellison syndrome
        HCG   Carcinoma of the testis with gynecomastia
        MSH   Carcinoma of the thymus or pancreas with hyperpigmentation
    Syndromes due to excess endogenous hormones
        Cortisol   Carcinoma of the adrenals with Cushing's syndrome
        Insulin   Islet cell cancer of the pancreas with hypoglycemia
        PTH   Carcinoma of the parathyroids with hyperparathyroidism
        Catecholamines   Pheochromocytoma with hypertension
        Erythropoeitin   Hypernephroma with erythrocytosis
    Syndromes due to presumed (but not identified) humoral products
        Cerebellar degeneration
        Sensorimotor polyneuropathies
        Hypertrophic osteoarthropathy
        Migratory thrombophlebitis
        Dermatomyositis
III. Those secondary to treatment
    Infections
        Leukopenia   Chemotherapy
        Immunosuppression   Chemotherapy
        Tuberculosis   Prolonged corticosteroids
        Infections due to invasive procedures   Catheters
        Systemic infection with BCG   Immunotherapy
    Metabolic disorders
        Hypercalcemia   Sex steroids in breast cancer
        Hyperuricemia   Tumor lysis syndrome
        Osteoporosis   Oophorectomy
    Fluid and electolyte disorders
        Edema, hypertension, heart failure   Sex steroids; corticosteroids
        Metabolic alkalosis   Vomiting due to radiotherapy; chemotherapy
        Hyperchloremic acidosis and hypokalemia   Ureterosigmoidostomy
        Hyponatremia, water intoxication   Inappropriate fluid and electrolyte therapy
        Weight loss and anorexia   Chemotherapy; radiotherapy
        B_{12} and folate deficiencies   Gastrectomy and small bowel resections
        Steatorrhea   Vagotomy
    Emotional and behavioral disorders
        Depression   Prolonged corticosteroids
        Psychotic behavior   Amitriptyline (Elavil)
    Hematologic disorders
        Thrombocytopenia, leukopenia, and bleeding   Chemotherapy
        Disseminated intravascular coagulation   Chemotherapy
    Endocrine disorders
        Adrenal insufficiency   Adrenalectomy
        Diabetes insipidus   Hypophysectomy
        Diabetes mellitus   Pancreatectomy
    Cardiorespiratory disorders
        Respiratory insufficiency   Pneumonectomy
        Pneumonitis; pulmonary fibrosis   Radiotherapy, chemotherapy
        Myocardial insufficiency   Doxorubicin (Adriamycin)
        Pericardial effusion   Radiotherapy
    Second primary cancers
        Acute leukemia in Hodgkin's disease   Chemotherapy
        Squamous cancer of the skin   Radiotherapy
IV. Miscellaneous
    Anxiety and depression incident to cancer and its attendant circumstances
    Pain

TABLE 2. Predisposition to Various Infectious Agents According to Cellular Defects*

	Bacteria	Fungi	Protozoa	Viruses
Neutrophil defects	*Streptococcus pyogenes*† *Staphylococcus aureus*† Enteric bacilli†‡	*Candida* species† *Aspergillus* species *Mucor* species		
Monocyte–T cell defects	*Listeria monocytogenes*† *Salmonella* species† *Nocardia asteroides* *Mycobacterium* species	*Cryptococcus neoformans*† *Candida* species *Histoplasma capsulatum* *Coccidioides immitis*	*Pneumocystis carinii* *Toxoplasma gondii*†	Cytomegalovirus† Varicella-zoster Herpes simplex Vaccinia virus
B cell defects	*Streptococcus pneumoniae*† Enteric bacilli†‡ *Hemophilus influenzae*		*Pneumocystis carinii*	Vaccinia virus

*Adapted from Armstrong, D.: Clin. Bull., 6:135, 1976.

†These agents (plus clostridial species) are the most likely causes of clinical sepsis in patients with cancer.

‡Aerobic enteric bacilli: *Escherichia coli, Pseudomonas aeruginosa, Klebsiella* species, and *Proteus* species.

Note: Parasitic infections may also occur in the compromised host, notably *Strongyloides stercoralis* in patients with monocyte–T cell defects and giardiasis, particularly in patients with IgA deficiency.

nal fluid (CSF) depends on the laboratory receiving an adequate amount of fluid, usually about 10 ml. Methods exist for the detection of cryptococcal antigen in the CSF and should be applied routinely in addition to India ink and Gram stain preparations. *Listeria monocytogenes* may be confused with diphtheroids, and such a report in a clinical setting suggesting CNS infection should not be dismissed as being due to a contaminant. Ampicillin is the drug usually recommended to treat *Listeria* meningitis. Infections of the CNS may also give rise to signs and symptoms of a brain abscess (*Toxoplasma, Aspergillus, Mucor* species, *Nocardia*) or encephalitis (varicella-zoster, herpes simplex). Amphotericin B is currently the treatment of choice for fungal infections of the CNS; treatment regimens must be sought that the patient can tolerate, and then continued beyond the return to normal of the various measurements being followed in the CSF, i.e., antigen, cell count, protein, and sugar.

Patients with cancer are especially prone to infection because of the necessity for invasive procedures such as parenteral injections, prolonged infusions, indwelling catheters, endoscopies, blood counts, and marrow aspirations. Reducing these to a minimum, particularly in the neutropenic immunosuppressed patient, together with strict attention to hand washing by all personnel, frequent changing of intravenous catheters, and use of external urinary drainage procedures when possible, will help control such infections.

The use of protected environments has been recommended in certain situations, and although not necessary for management of the majority of patients, their use in severely compromised patients, particularly those in whom marrow transplantation is to be undertaken, appears essential. Transfusion of HLA-compatible white cells is also to be kept in mind in severely neutropenic patients. Efforts to protect susceptible patients against *Pseudomonas aeruginosa* by immunization have not been successful, but more recently polyvalent pneumococcal vaccines have been developed and should be given to patients undergoing splenectomy (Hodgkin's disease, chronic myelogenous leukemia) and to those patients in parts of the world where penicillin-resistant strains of *S. pneumoniae* are being encountered. The use of oral, nonabsorbable antimicrobial agents has been advocated by some to reduce the gut flora in patients undergoing immunosuppressive therapy, but for the most part rigid adherence to hygiene by patients and staff has been the most effective prophylactic measure.

METABOLIC, ELECTROLYTE, AND RENAL DISORDERS. Cancer patients are subject to the same medical and metabolic emergencies as the general population but they are particularly vulnerable to certain of these disorders. *Hypercalcemia* has been variously estimated to occur at some point in the course of neoplastic disease in 15 to 40 per cent of patients, depending upon the type of tumor. It may occur in patients with localized, surgically removable tumors as well as in those with metastases, either skeletal or nonskeletal. In some patients (usually those with bronchogenic or renal carcinoma) the biochemical findings are indistinguishable from primary hyperparathyroidism (hypercalcemia, hypophosphatemia, hypercalciuria, hyperphosphaturia), thereby leading to the designation ectopic hyperparathyroidism. In some of these patients there is evidence by radioimmunoassay to indicate that the tumor can synthesize parathyroid hormone (PTH) or a PTH-like material ectopically, and this is the presumed cause of the hypercalcemia. In others, such evidence is lacking, but other metabolically active tumor products, including prostaglandins (PGE_2) and osteoclast-activating factor (OAF), appear to be of etiologic importance. These patients often present with polydipsia and polyuria — nephrogenic diabetes insipidus — and at times have been erroneously diagnosed as having coincidental idiopathic diabetes insipidus. The symptoms may also cause confusion with diabetes insipidus which can result from metastases to the posterior pituitary, described particularly in patients with breast and lung cancer, or from hypophysectomy. Hypercalcemic patients may experience nausea, vomiting, lethargy, and even coma with rapid elevations of serum calcium, and prompt treatment may be mandatory. Treatment measures include (1) those directed against dehydration, reduced glomerular filtration rate, and enhanced tubular reabsorption of calcium — fluid replacement, intravenous saline, furosemide; (2) those directed against increased bone resorption and/or its causes — oral phosphate, corticosteroids, mithramycin, calcitonin, indomethacin; (3) those directed against the tumor —surgery, endocrine ablation, chemotherapy, radiotherapy; and (4) those directed against coexistent problems such as associated electrolyte abnormalities (e.g., hypokalemic alkalosis), pain, fractures, and myelophthisic anemia.

Hypocalcemia has also been observed in patients with cancer and most often is the consequence of (1) "hungry bones" as seen in patients with osteoblastic metastases, particularly patients with breast cancer after endocrine ablation; (2) hypoparathyroidism secondary to radical neck surgery or tumor replacement of the parathyroids; (3) magnesium deficiency caused, for example, by poor intake, malabsorption, or renal losses; phosphate retention caused by renal failure; (4) hypoalbuminemia with low levels of bound calcium; avitaminosis D induced by malabsorption syndromes; and (5) post-treatment hypocalcemia caused, for example, by mithramycin, chelating agents, or phosphate therapy. The hypocalcemia may be severe enough to cause paresthesias and muscle cramps, and treatment should be directed at the cause.

The *tumor lysis syndrome,* usually marked by azotemia, hyperuricemia, hyperphosphatemia, hyperkalemia and/or hyperkaluria, and hypocalcemia, may occur as a consequence of renal failure secondary to rapid tumor destruction in a patient with a treatment-sensitive tumor. The syndrome is preventable, and patients who are to undergo cytolytic therapy should be well hydrated in advance of treatment and a good urine flow (i.e., about 100 ml per hour) established. Often this requires infusion of mannitol. Allopurinol should also be administered beforehand to block the excess production of uric acid secondary to tumor breakdown.

There are a variety of fluid and electrolyte disorders in cancer. In patients with *hyponatremia* it is often useful to measure a simultaneous urinary sodium; low concentrations of urinary sodium are usually seen with "third space" fluid collections, dilutional states, and hepatic or cardiac insufficiency, whereas high concentrations of urinary sodium usually indicate that adrenal failure, the inappropriate antidiuretic hormone syndrome (SIADH), or diuretics are the cause of the hyponatremia. *Hypernatremia* may indicate pituitary or nephrogenic diabetes insipidus, and variations in serum potassium may be secondary to inadequate intake, gastrointestinal and renal losses, or glucocorticoids (hypokalemia) or to renal failure or tumor lysis (hyperkalemia). Patients with ectopic ACTH-producing tumors are more likely to present with *hypokalemic alkalosis* than with typical Cushing's syndrome, and measurements of serum potassium and bicarbonate are a useful way to screen patients for this syndrome. Disturbances in acid-base balance may be due to either respiratory (see below) or metabolic causes. *Metabolic acidosis* most often reflects renal insufficiency, diarrhea, lactic acidosis, or renal tubular acidosis. *Metabolic alkalosis* is usually associated with chloride, potassium, or magnesium deficiency, alone or in combination, but less common causes, such as protracted treatment with carbenicillin, which may lead to metabolic alkalosis because of its sodium content, must be kept in mind.

The *renal consequences of cancer* include not only obstructive syndromes (ureteral obstruction in carcinoma of the cervix, recurrent carcinoma of the colon, cancer of the prostate) but also renal parenchymal destruction with uremia secondary to invasion and infiltration by the primary neoplasm such as may be seen in malignant lymphoma. Immune complex disease with membranous glomerulopathy and the nephrotic syndrome has been increasingly recognized, and it has been estimated that 6 to 10 per cent of patients with this renal lesion will later be found to have an underlying malignancy. Acute renal failure may result from tumor lysis, as noted above, from hypercalcemia, particularly in patients with multiple myeloma, from acute tubular necrosis, in turn caused by shock, and from drugs such as the combination of the antimicrobials gentamicin and cephalothin with cancer chemotherapeutic agents such as cis-diamminedichloride platinum (II). Excretory urography may result in intrarenal precipitation of paraproteins in multiple myeloma, particularly if the patient is dehydrated, and this diagnostic procedure should be avoided in myeloma whenever possible.

CARDIORESPIRATORY DISEASES. In addition to infectious diseases involving the lungs, as discussed above, pulmonary fibrosis may result from radiation therapy and from chemotherapy (busulfan, bleomycin, methotrexate, cyclophosphamide). Radiation pneumonitis usually precedes fibrosis, and there is characteristically a latent period of about one to three months between the conclusion of radiation treatment and the development of pneumonitis. The pulmonary fibrosis seen with chemotherapeutic agents is variable in its onset and is usually dose related, although hypersensitivity reactions may also be responsible. Decline in vital capacity and other pulmonary function test volumes may be the earliest sign of an adverse effect of chemotherapy, and, accordingly, serial measurements should be made in patients receiving agents known to induce these pulmonary reactions. Cancer may diffusely involve the lungs as in lymphangitic metastases or may appear as coin lesions or mass lesions. For reasons that are not entirely clear but may be related to subpleural localization, sarcomas metastatic to lungs, in contrast to carcinomas, may be accompanied by pneumothorax. In evaluating the extent of disease in bronchogenic carcinoma, it is well to remember the frequent occurrence of brain metastases. A brain scan, or preferably a computerized tomographic scan of the brain, should be done prior to definitive surgery. Small cell (i.e., oat cell) cancers of the lung are best treated by nonsurgical means because of their tendency to early and widespread metastases. Of course, not all central nervous system signs and symptoms are caused by metastases but may represent nonmetastatic syndromes, presumably on a humoral basis, or known metabolic causes such as hypercalcemia or hypoglycemia. Pleural effusions accompanying malignant disease of the lungs, primary or metastatic, often pose difficulties in management. Previously it was thought that effusions need not be treated unless symptomatic, but chronic effusions may lead to fibrothorax and a "trapped lung" with disabling respiratory insufficiency, and it is therefore best that effusions be drained dry and that efforts to prevent their recurrence be applied early. Some will not recur if simultaneous systemic therapy is being applied and is successful. For effusions that do recur, intrapleural chemotherapy — alkylating agents, quinacrine, tetracycline, bleomycin — or pleurectomy may be necessary for control.

All these pulmonary manifestations will cause variable changes in pulmonary function as manifested by symptoms, signs, and changes in blood gases. Respiratory failure may be incident to pulmonary and nonpulmonary causes (drug overdose, cerebrovascular accident), but the common denominator is hypoxemia with or without hypercarbia. Symptoms of severe *hypoxemia* have been likened to ethanol excess — impaired judgment, decreased cognitive function, abnormal behavior (especially agitation and combativeness), incoordination — whereas those of *hypercarbia* have been likened to the effects of an anesthetic — progressive somnolence, depressed consciousness, and, if severe, coma. Patients with cancer are vulnerable to respiratory failure not only because of pulmonary infections and neoplastic infiltrations but also because of the major surgical procedures many of them must undergo, attended, in some instances, by shock and fluid shifts leading to the adult respiratory distress syndrome.

Arterial blood gases are essential to the analysis of respiratory failure, and in making this analysis it is useful to calculate the A-a (alveolar-arterial) gradient in the partial pressure of oxygen. This is best approximated by the formula $PA_{O_2} = 150 - 1.2 \, (Pa_{CO_2})$, where PA_{O_2} is the derived partial pressure of alveolar oxygen and Pa_{CO_2} is the measured partial pressure of arterial carbon dioxide. The simultaneously measured Pa_{O_2} — the partial pressure of arterial oxygen — is then subtracted from the derived PA_{O_2} to obtain the A-a gradient. Normally there is a gradient of about 5 to 10 mm Hg, and it tends to increase with age to about 10 to 20 mm Hg. If the A-a gradient falls outside these normal variations, causes of impaired oxygenation through shunting (adult respiratory distress syndrome), mismatching of ventilation and perfusion (pulmonary embolus), and diffusion impairment (lymphangitic metastases) should be investigated. Simple alveolar hypoventilation, as with narcotic overdosage, will result in hypercarbia with a normal A-a gradient. *Respiratory acid-base changes* may also be seen in the cancer population, and one that deserves special mention is respiratory alkalosis which may herald the onset of septic shock; it may also be seen in association with hepatic failure and early in interstitial pulmonary diseases such as lymphangitic metastases. In one report from a cancer hospital, more than half of the low serum bicarbonate determinations observed were occasioned by respiratory alkalosis, and failure to recognize this as an early sign of septic shock may result in the eventual appearance of metabolic acidosis (resulting from lactic acid accumulation), the occurrence of which is a bad prognostic sign.

Primary neoplastic disease of the heart is rare, but metastatic disease may present several difficult medical problems. Involvement of the pericardium (usually by lung or breast cancer) leading to effusion may cause cardiac tamponade. In some hospitals pericardial effusion has been seen more often among patients with cancer than among those with nonmalignant diseases. Diffuse involvement of myocardium occurs most often with melanoma and acute leukemia, and rhythm disturbances and conduction defects may result. Cor pulmonale has been described as a consequence of lymphangitic disease of the lungs, and patients with mucin-producing adenocarcinomas may have their courses complicated by nonbacterial thrombotic endocarditis (NBTE). The leading cause of stroke in a cancer population has been reported to be embolism secondary to NBTE, a finding consistent with the observation that the lesions almost always involve the aortic or mitral valves or both. A major drug in the chemotherapy of cancer, doxorubicin (Adriamycin), may cause irreversible myocardial toxicity in doses above 500 mg per square meter, so this limit should not be exceeded. *Hypotension and circulatory shock* (cardiogenic, hypovolemic, distributive, obstructive) are commonly encountered among sick cancer patients. Hypovolemia

(external losses of blood or plasma; acute fluid shifts) is usually the most common cause of hypotension, with sepsis being the next. Replacement of intravascular volume in hypovolemia is obvious but the problems of replacement therapy in some patients can become complicated and call for expert management, often in a special unit with techniques available for making critical measurements such as arterial blood gases, blood pH, blood lactate, central venous pressure, urine flow, and cardiac output. In patients in whom left-sided heart failure may be difficult to recognize, the placement of a Swan-Ganz catheter for determination of left atrial pressures may provide lifesaving information. Restoration of tissue perfusion is the basic goal in the therapy of shock, not simply restoration of blood pressure.

GASTROINTESTINAL TRACT. *Gastrointestinal disorders* in cancer are numerous and highly variable. Jaundice presents one of the most challenging problems, there being an almost endless array of possibilities, including disorders leading to extrahepatic obstruction, such as with cancer of the pancreas or bile duct, porta hepatis metastases, or coincidental cholelithiasis; intrahepatic obstruction, such as with the cholestasis of Hodgkin's disease; and hepatic parenchymal damage, as observed with anticancer drugs (methotrexate), viral hepatitis, and extensive replacement of liver parenchyma by tumor. Hemolytic disorders may also be manifested by jaundice, but causes relating to obstruction and parenchymal disease of the liver are more common. Hepatic coma may result from extensive destruction of the liver by tumor or from intercurrent disease such as viral hepatitis or cirrhosis. Precipitating causes include gastrointestinal hemorrhage, rapid removal of ascitic fluid, vigorous diuretic therapy, sepsis, and high protein diets. It had formerly been thought that cirrhotics rarely had liver metastases, but controlled studies have shown that the incidence of hepatic metastases is the same in patients with cirrhosis and those without.

Esophageal varices secondary to cirrhosis are an unusual cause of bleeding in cancer patients, but it should be recognized that cancer metastatic to an otherwise normal liver may also give rise to portal hypertension and esophageal varices. Rarely, gastric varices may arise as a consequence of obstruction of the splenic vein by pancreatic cancer, and hematemesis, congestive splenomegaly, and hypersplenism have been described in this syndrome. Most commonly gastrointestinal bleeding in cancer is the result of gastric mucosal bleeding, whether associated with gastric irritants such as aspirin, aspirin-containing compounds (e.g., Percodan), indomethacin, and adrenal steroids, or with stress ulcers. Stress ulcers have been seen most frequently in the lymphomas and leukemias and in patients with carcinomas of the lung and breast, particularly in those with sepsis, shock and uremia. In all patients with cancer, gastrointestinal bleeding is caused by the cancer in 10 per cent, but this rises to 50 to 75 per cent if the tumor is known to involve the stomach or is a primary gastric cancer or gastric lymphoma. Metastases to the gastrointestinal tract should be considered in the clinical setting of melanoma and cancers of the breast, lung, and testis. Patients with breast cancer under treatment with corticosteroids appear to be prone to the development of gastroduodenal metastases, which may secondarily ulcerate and bleed. Gastrointestinal moniliasis is most common in patients with leukemias and lymphomas, the esophagus constituting a major site of localization. In patients with esophageal moniliasis, bleeding is the most common symptom, followed by dysphagia and substernal pain. Non-beta-cell tumors of the pancreatic islets (gastrinomas) are associated with increased blood levels of gastrin, excess production of gastric acid, and peptic ulcers, involving primarily the duodenum, or duodenitis — the Zollinger-Ellison syndrome — and these, plus those pancreatic tumors (and bronchogenic carcinomas) that secrete vasoactive intestinal peptide (VIP), constitute examples of tumors that produce humoral syndromes, a subject which is addressed further in Ch. 551.

Malabsorption syndromes may result from deficiency of pancreatic enzymes, as will occur with pancreatectomy, from deficient or altered intraluminal bile acids, which may occur with biliary obstruction and jejunal bacterial overgrowth, and from diseases of the small intestine, notably diffuse lymphomatous involvement and ileal resection. The treatment will depend upon the cause: substitution enzyme therapy in pancreatectomy, the use of antimicrobials in bacterial overgrowth, medium-chain triglycerides in ileal resection (more than 100 cm), and antitumor therapy for diffuse involvement by lymphoma.

Other gastrointestinal afflictions in cancer include obstruction and perforation. The possibility of perforation must be kept in mind, not only in patients being treated with corticosteroids, but also in patients in whom lysis of a tumor in the wall of the gastrointestinal tract occurs with treatment, such as may be seen when a lymphomatous tumor, occupying a transmural position in the wall of the gut, shrinks in response to an alkylating agent and leaves a perforation in the wall.

Maintenance of *nutrition* is perhaps the most challenging problem to be faced in caring for cancer patients. Anorexia is common, and not necessarily attributable to parenchymal damage of the liver. It may be marked in patients with carcinoma of the pancreas, but patients whose cancers do not involve the gastrointestinal tract in any way may also experience severe anorexia. Characteristically, and for unknown reasons, breakfast may be the only meal that interests such patients, and physicians can take advantage of this by seeing that ample breakfasts are provided. There have been studies suggesting that the basis of anorexia may be a metabolically active humoral product from the tumor, but confirmation of this has not been forthcoming. In addition to anorexia, the usual causes of malnutrition in cancer patients relate to vomiting, partial or total bowel obstruction or resection, intestinal fistulas, diarrhea, and malabsorption. Losses to the patient include not only calories but also essential nutrients, including vitamins, minerals, and electrolytes. The latter, in particular, may be lost by coexistent renal tubular disorders often associated with nephrotoxic antimicrobials or chemotherapeutic agents. Analysis of nutritional problems, including, most importantly, malnutrition, requires a search for predisposing factors in the history and physical examination, a three-day calorie count, and a 24-hour stool collection for inspection and decision regarding a malabsorption workup. X-ray of the gastrointestinal tract, malabsorption studies (fat absorption, xylose tolerance test, Schilling test), and endoscopy with jejunal biopsy may all be helpful in this analysis. At times anti-cancer treatment measures (surgery, chemotherapy, radiation therapy) are in themselves responsible for an-

orexia, vomiting, diarrhea, or malabsorption. Nutritional therapy includes oral, tube, or intravenous supplementation with individual nutrients and liquid formulations. When oral or tube feeding is contraindicated, total parenteral nutrition (TPN or hyperalimentation) is often useful in improving nutrition during a period of anti-tumor therapy.

HEMATOPOIETIC SYSTEM. Of all the numerous medical manifestations of cancer, disorders of the hematopoietic system are often the most troublesome. Myelophthisic anemia is a consequence of extensive marrow involvement by tumor and, as might be expected, occurs with tumors most notable for their skeletal tropism, such as cancers of the breast and prostate, but may be seen with virtually any cancer. One of the earliest signs of myelophthisis is the appearance of immature leukocytes of the myeloid series in the peripheral blood as well as nucleated red cells out of proportion to the severity of the anemia. The platelet count may be normal or reduced, although at times thrombocytosis may be observed as a consequence of malignancy. Ultimately, anemia, leukopenia, and thrombocytopenia may all be seen. The common problem in differential diagnosis is to distinguish between these effects of myelophthisis and the consequences of chemotherapy. The demonstration of extrinsic cells in the marrow aspirate and biopsy is essential in establishing a cause and effect relationship between myelophthisis and marrow invasion by cancer, as opposed to marrow hypocellularity which is usually the result of therapy. Pre-existing myelosuppression caused by metastases will unfortunately often limit the adequacy of the treatment of cancer by radiation or chemotherapy.

The clinical association between thrombophlebitis and cancer has been recognized for many years, and the spectrum of disorders secondary to abnormal coagulation in cancer varies from this to nonbacterial thrombotic endocarditis (NBTE), disseminated intravascular coagulation (DIC), and hemorrhage. Migratory thrombophlebitis has been most often described in patients with cancer of the pancreas, but this association has been noted also in other carcinomas, particularly carcinoma of the lung. DIC is characterized typically by thrombocytopenia, hypofibrinogenemia, elevated levels of fibrin-fibrinogen degradation products, prolonged prothrombin and thrombin times, variable deficiencies of other coagulation factors, red cell fragmentation, and hemorrhage. It is most characteristically seen in acute promyelocytic anemia, but it may also be a feature of carcinomas, notably metastatic carcinoma of the prostate. Since the level of fibrinogen may be increased in patients with cancer, the finding of a normal level may actually represent a decrease, and serial measurements may be necessary to establish a downward trend. The exact mechanism for the production of DIC is unknown, although some data indicate that products of the neoplastic cells are capable of activating the coagulation and fibrinolytic processes. Malignancies have also been shown to be associated with increased consumption of platelets and fibrinogen within tumor tissues. Cancer treatment may play a role in causing release of active substances with destruction of tumor cells, and sepsis, so often present in these patients, may also be contributory.

Other hematologic phenomena in cancer include classic hemolytic anemias (as distinct from the shortened life span of red cells seen in the "anemia of cancer"), iron deficiency anemias, anemias of chronic infection, coagulation factor deficiencies, leukemoid reactions, and megaloblastic anemias secondary to folate and B_{12} deficiencies, as well as the primary disorders inherent in cancers of the hematopoietic system.

There are many more problems the internist must contend with in the practice of oncology, but the aforementioned examples will serve to illustrate the diversity of these problems and to support the original contention that oncology is the last bastion of internal medicine. The important problem of pain has not been discussed; it is considered in Ch. 260. Likewise, the emotional impact of cancer is often the most serious problem to be dealt with, particularly in the terminally ill. This subject is explored in Ch. 528.

Cancer, then, is many diseases clinically and as broad as the vast scope of internal medicine. Its many faces challenge the internist, but by a careful analytical approach coupled with compassion and a willingness to always try to understand what is happening to his patient, he is in the best position to cause the problems of cancer to yield. In the last analysis the best medical oncologist is first and foremost a good internist.

American Joint Committee for Cancer Staging and End-Results Reporting: Manual for Staging of Cancer, 1977. Chicago, 1977.

Armstrong, D.: Infectious complications of neoplastic disease: Diagnosis and management. Part I. Clin. Bull., 6:135, 1976.

Clarysse, A., Kenis, Y., and Mathé, G. (eds.): Cancer Chemotherapy: Its Role in the Treatment Strategy of Hematological Malignancies and Solid Tumors. New York, Springer-Verlag, 1976.

Hall, T. C. (ed.): Paraneoplastic syndromes. Ann. N. Y. Acad. Sci. 230:1, 1974.

Myers, W. P. L., and Bockman, R.: Studies on the pathogenesis of cancer hypercalcemia. Trans. Am. Clin. Climatol. Assoc., 88:177, 1976.

Sack, G. H., Jr., Levin, J., and Bell, W. R.: Trousseau's syndrome and other manifestations of chronic disseminated coagulopathy in patients with neoplasms: Clincial, pathological, and therapeutic features. Medicine, 56:1, 1977.

Shils, M. E.: Nutrition and neoplasia. In Shils, M. E., and Goodhart, R. S. (ed.): Modern Nutrition in Health and Disease. Philadelphia, Lea & Febiger, 1973, Chap. 37.

523. HUMAN CARCINOGENESIS

Paul A. Marks

INTRODUCTION

Cancer, causing approximately 300,000 deaths per year, is the second leading cause of death in the United States. On the basis of epidemiologic studies, it is estimated that 80 per cent of human cancers are related to environmental, rather than genetic, factors. It follows that a reduction in the incidence of cancer may follow an appropriate alteration of our environment.

A causal relationship between cancer and environmental factors was first suggested in 1775 by Sir Percival Pott, who in his treatise "Chirurgical Observations" noted that chimney sweeps were particularly susceptible to cancer of the skin and scrotum. Pott suggested that "the disease, in these people, seems to derive its origin from a lodgement of soot in the rugae of the scrotum." This remarkably insightful observation went essentially unrecognized for more than 150 years, until Kennaway and his colleagues reported that the

major carcinogenic agents in soot and coal tars were benzo(a)pyrene and related polycyclic aromatic hydrocarbons.

INCIDENCE OF CANCERS

The most common form of cancer of major significance among males in the United States is cancer of the lung; among females, cancer of the breast; and when both sexes are considered together, cancer of the colon and rectum. Cancer of the skin and carcinoma in situ of the uterine cervix are quantitatively the most common types of cancers, but usually do not lead to major clinical problems. The incidence of cancers among children is low when compared with adults, and the age group 1 to 14 years accounts for only 1 per cent of all cancer deaths in the United States. Nevertheless, within this same age group, only accidents exceed cancer as a leading cause of death. In contrast to the type of tumors seen in adults, in children the more frequent types of cancer are leukemias, tumors of the central nervous system, and soft tissue tumors.

Evidence to suggest that environmental factors play an important role in the cause of cancer is derived, in part, from the geographic distribution of different cancer types and the changing patterns of cancer mortality rates over the past several decades. In the United States and western Europe, the mortality rates from cancers of the lung, colon, prostate, and breast are relatively high, whereas rates from cancer of the stomach remain relatively low. By contrast, in Japan, stomach cancer predominates, whereas breast cancer is relatively rare. Cancer of the liver is much more frequent among populations in Africa, southern China, and Japan than in the United States or western Europe. Furthermore, the incidence of various cancers varies with the migration of people from one part of the world to another. For example, the death rates from cancer of the stomach, liver, colon, and prostate among Japanese immigrants to California and their sons tend consistently toward California norms. The change in incidence requires more than one generation. Therefore some of the causative agents could be factors, such as diet, which tend to persist as part of a cultural heritage, rather than factors such as air pollution, which tend to be the same for everyone in a given area. Jewish populations who migrated to Israel from Europe or the United States maintain an incidence of cancer that is typical of their country of origin. But their Israeli-born children have a much lower incidence of almost all kinds of cancer. In this respect, the immigrant children become more like the indigenous Israeli population and the Jewish immigrants from Asia and Africa, among whom the over-all incidence of cancer is relatively lower than in the United States or Europe. Studies of such migrant groups suggest that genetic factors are not usually the principal cause of the most common forms of cancer.

Other striking variations in incidence of different types of cancer suggest environmental factors in causation of these cancers. Skin cancer has a high incidence in Queensland, Australia, but a low one in Bombay, India; cancer of the bronchus is common in the United States and western Europe and rare in Nigeria, Uganda, Israel, and Japan; esophageal and nasopharyngeal cancers are rare in the United States and western Europe, but have a high incidence in northeastern Iran and in southern China, respectively. During the past four decades there has been a marked decrease in deaths from cancer of the stomach in the United States. The cause of this is not known, but it is presumed to be related to alteration in some factor or factors in our environment. A 23-country study of the occurrence of cancer of the colon reveals a strong correlation with per capita meat consumption. The diet in countries with a high incidence of colonic cancer also tends to be higher in refined foods and low in unabsorbed cellulose fiber. Differences in bacterial flora associated with these two types of diet have been documented. Other studies, employing in vitro assays, have identified specific substances in feces and in urine which are mutagenic and possibly carcinogenic.

CERTAIN BIOLOGIC ASPECTS OF CARCINOGENESIS

The group most conspicuously at risk for cancer is the elderly. Various models have been proposed to account for the clustering of cancer in old age. One reasonable theory of carcinogenesis involves a multi-step process, and cancer will not occur until each of these steps (such as mutation of several genes) has occurred. This theory predicts that the log of cancer incidence should be linearly related to the log of age. This rela-

tionship of incidence to age is observed for a number of cancers.

It is a fact that there is a long lag between exposure to potential carcinogens and the appearance of tumors. This lag has been demonstrated for a number of carcinogens, including smoking and radiation, and can vary from 5 to 30 or more years. This lag between exposure and the appearance of cancer has several important implications. First, it suggests that a given cancer may have several factors contributing to its cause. Second, the cancer may be the end result of several events occurring during a lifetime; in other words, we may have to look to environmental factors during the early life of an individual to understand the role of such factors in the causation of cancer. It is critical in taking the history of a patient with cancer to determine possible occupational, social, therapeutic, or other exposures to potentially carcinogenic agents (Table 1). Third, it could take many years before an increased incidence of a particular cancer draws attention to the dangers arising from an environmental factor.

Carcinogenesis appears to be dose dependent. The larger the dose of an environmental carcinogen to which the individual is exposed, the greater the chance of developing a tumor. There is probably no threshold or safe level of exposure to a carcinogen. Information is available for human subjects on cancer incidence in relation to cigarette smoking which suggests that there is

TABLE 1.   Chemicals Recognized as Carcinogens in Human Subjects

Chemical	Site of Cancers
Chemical mixtures	
Soots, coal tars, oils	Skin, lungs, scrotum
Cigarette smoke	Lungs, esophagus, bladder
Industrial chemicals (occupational hazards)	
2-Naphthylamine	Urinary bladder
Benzidine (aniline dye precursors)	Urinary bladder
4-Aminobiphenyl	Urinary bladder
Chloromethyl methyl ether	Lungs
Nickel compounds	Lungs, nasal sinuses
Chromium compounds	Lungs
Asbestos	Lungs, pleura, peritoneum
Arsenic compounds	Skin, lungs
Isopropyl oil	Nasal sinuses
Vinyl chloride	Liver (angiosarcoma)
Benzene	Leukemia
Drugs	
N,N-bis-(2-chloroethyl)-2-naphthylamine	Urinary bladder
Bis-(2-chloroethyl sulfide) (mustard gas)	Lungs
Immunosuppressive drugs	Reticulosarcoma, ? all sites
Diethylstilbestrol	Vagina
Phenacetin	Renal pelvis
Steroid contraceptives	Benign hepatomas
Polycyclic hydrocarbons in ointment	Skin
Naturally occurring compounds	
Betel nuts	Buccal mucosa
Aflatoxins (a mold product)	Liver
Ionizing radiations	
Radar	Bronchus
X-ray, radium	All sites
Ultraviolet	Skin
Thorium, Thorotrast	Bone, reticuloendothelial system
Potent carcinogens in animals to which human populations are exposed	
Sterigmatocystin	Liver
Cycasin	Liver
Safrol	Liver
Pyrrolizidine alkaloids	Liver
Nitroso compounds	Esophagus, liver, kidney, stomach

*Modified from Heidelberger, C.: Ann. Rev. Biochem., 44:79, 1975; and Doll, R.: J. Roy. Coll. Physicians, 11:125, 1977.

no level of consumption which does not elevate the yearly risk of lung cancer. The studies on human subjects exposed to radiation also provide similar data suggesting that there is no so-called safe dose. Although there may be no threshold dose of a carcinogen, a society or an individual may be willing to accept certain risks as trade-offs in life style against the potential costs in avoiding exposure to carcinogenic agents.

SOCIAL FACTORS AND ENVIRONMENTAL CARCINOGENS

One of the most persuasive arguments with regard to environmental factors in the causation of cancer relates to cancer of the lung, essentially a disease of the twentieth century. Initially it predominantly involved men, but recently its incidence has risen sharply in women, reflecting the increase in smoking among women since the late 1940's. One third of all cancer deaths in men in the United States and about one half of such deaths in England are from lung cancer. The incubation period for lung cancer is estimated to be from 10 to 30 years, depending on the quantity an individual smokes, and probably other, as yet unidentified factors. The evidence strongly suggests that the cessation of cigarette smoking would markedly decrease the incidence of lung cancer.

There are other socially related causes of cancer that can be identified in different parts of the world. In Central and Southeast Asia, the chewing of a variety of materials, such as betel, tobacco, and lime, is associated with a high incidence of cancer of the mouth. Aflatoxin, a product of the fungus *Aspergillus flavus*, is a potent carcinogenic agent, causing cancer of the liver. The fungus is a contaminant of certain foods, such as peanuts, particularly in the hot and humid climates of Southeast Asia and Africa. Alcohol consumption has been associated with an increased incidence of a variety of cancers of the upper respiratory and digestive tracts.

In the United States, the black population has a higher incidence of cancer of the prostate, uterine cervix, and oropharynx, while also evidencing a lower incidence of breast cancer than the general population. Over the last ten years, these differences in incidence seem to be diminishing when compared with the previous three to four decades. This emerging pattern suggests that differences in the environment, related possibly to socioeconomic factors, may play a role in accounting for differences in incidences of cancers among the black population and the nonblack population.

CHEMICAL CARCINOGENS

It is apparent from Table 1 that a great many chemicals have been implicated as possible carcinogenic agents. Several represent occupational hazards. Certain drugs and treatments administered for therapeutic purposes can induce cancer in humans. In this regard, it should be recognized that the fetus is very sensitive to the action of carcinogenic agents, including ionizing radiation, and drugs which can cross the placenta. A tumor may not manifest itself in the offspring until adolescence or adulthood, which appears to be the case in

certain instances of vaginal carcinoma associated with fetal exposure to diethylstilbestrol administered to the mother during pregnancy. It is essential to obtain a careful history with respect to medications, exposure to x-ray, and other diagnostic or therapeutic experiences of a patient's mother during pregnancy.

Asbestos, an occupational hazard, has been carried home on workers' clothing, and more than three dozen cases of mesothelioma of the pleura, almost pathognomonic of exposure to asbestos, have been reported from household contacts. Vinyl chloride, used extensively in the plastics industry, places employees making PVC containers at risk for the development of angiosarcoma of the liver. Although it is likely that these occupational hazards account for only a small proportion of all cancers recognized each year, they reflect relatively specific exposures that can be, and in most instances have been, eliminated as health hazards.

A number of environmental carcinogens are not active as such, but require metabolic activation, such as conversion into reactive electrophilic species which form complexes with DNA, RNA, and protein and can alter the function of these macromolecules. For example, a complex with DNA may lead to errors in DNA replication or alter the normal pattern of transcription and cause abnormal cell proliferation and/or function. The body processes have relatively efficient mechanisms that can repair damage to DNA produced by a chemical carcinogen or radiation. This may account for the fact that such damage does not lead to a higher incidence of neoplastic transformation. There is a complex enzyme system which recognizes altered regions of DNA, excises these regions, and then repairs the DNA, restoring it to normal structure and presumably normal function. A genetically determined defect in the DNA repair mechanisms can increase the susceptibility of individuals to cancer. Xeroderma pigmentosum, a genetically determined disorder displaying autosomal recessive inheritance, appears to follow this pattern of susceptibility. Affected individuals are very sensitive to sunlight and develop multiple skin tumors at an early age. Cells in these individuals have a defective ability to repair damaged DNA, suggesting that the increased susceptibility to skin cancer may be due to a failure to repair cellular DNA following exposure to ultraviolet radiation.

GENETIC ASPECTS OF HUMAN CANCER

A complete family history of patients with cancer is of diagnostic importance in identifying the relatively rare genetically determined cancers. Particularly in young individuals and in patients with a history of multiple tumors or bilateral tumors, one should consider the possibility that a hereditary factor contributed to the cause of the cancer. In cataloguing mendelian hereditary disorders in human subjects, McKusick listed 1142 proved single gene traits and 1194 others with suggestive but inconclusive evidence for mendelian inheritance pattern. Among the hereditary disorders, it has been estimated that approximately 200 have genetic factors which predispose the individual to benign or malignant neoplastic disease. In addition, a number of genes might be involved in susceptibility to cancer which do not exhibit a pattern of simple mendelian inheritance. Hereditary tumors may be identified by rec-

TABLE 2. Genetically Determined Cancers

Condition	Preneoplastic Lesions	Cancer
Dominant inheritance pattern		
Polyposis coli	Polyps of colon, osteomas	Colon
Gardner's syndrome	Fibromas, epidermal cysts	
Peutz-Jeghers syndrome	Pigmentation of buccal mucosa, small intestine polyps	Ovarian neoplasms, rare malignant change in polyps
Neurofibromatosis	Neurofibroma, skeletal defects, hamartomas, pheochromocytoma, glioma (brain and optic nerve), acoustic neuroma	Sarcomas
Retinoblastoma	None recognized	Retina
Werner's syndrome	Adenomas of pituitary, thyroid, adrenal, parathyroid, and islet cells	Endocrine gland
Sipple's syndrome	Pheochromocytoma	Medullary thyroid
Von Hippel–Lindau syndrome	Angiomatosis retinae	Pheochromocytoma, hypernephroma, ependymoma
Tylosis palmaris et plantaris	Hyperkeratotic skin lesions	Esophageal
Hereditary multiple exostosis	Exostoses	Chondrosarcoma
Nevoid basal cell syndrome	Osseous developmental anomalies, soft tissue calcification	Basal cell tumors, medulloblastoma, ovarian fibromas
Chemodectomas	None recognized	Paragangliomas of chemoreceptor system
Tuberous sclerosis	Adenoma sebaceum (mental retardation and epilepsy)	Multiple hamartomas, giant cell astrocytomas
Autosomal recessive inheritance pattern		
Bloom's syndrome	Telangiectatic erythema, stunted growth, chromosome breakage and rearrangements	Leukemia and solid tumors
Fanconi's anemia	Pancytopenia, congenital anomalies, chromosome aberrations	Leukemia and solid tumors
Xeroderma pigmentosum	Skin atrophy	Skin
Ataxia telangiectasia	Cerebellar ataxia, oculocutaneous telangiectasia	Lymphoreticular malignancies
X-linked inheritance pattern		
Wiskott-Aldrich syndrome	Eczema, thrombocytopenia, susceptibility to infection	Lymphomas
Bruton type agammaglobulinemia	Humoral antibody deficiency	Lymphocytic leukemia

*Modified from Mulvihill, J. J., et al.: Genetics in Human Cancer. New York, Raven Press, 1977, pp. 138–141.

ognizing other features of the trait or syndrome in the patient or his family (Table 2). Tumors may be the sole manifestation of the gene defects, such as in retinoblastoma and intestinal polyposis, or part of a wider biologic disturbance.

VIRUSES AND CANCER

Viruses are of considerable concern as a possible cause of cancer in man. To date, there is no unambiguous evidence that any class of human cancers is regularly caused by a virus. Some cancers have been shown to be associated with elevated levels of an antibody to certain viruses or viral components. Some cancer cells have been shown to contain viral nucleic acids and certain viral enzymes, and some cancers have been shown to arise in clusters of cases, suggesting an infectious type of transmission, such as Burkitt's lymphoma, which occurs primarily in children in tropical Africa. There is a strong association between Burkitt's lymphoma and human nasopharyngeal carcinoma with the Epstein-Barr virus (EBV) and of cancer of the cervix uteri with herpesvirus type II. However, no direct evidence exists that the viruses and the cancers are causally linked.

DETECTION OF ENVIRONMENTAL CARCINOGENS

With the wide variety of environmental agents which appear to be associated as causal factors in cancer, a critical issue is the development of procedures for detecting carcinogens in our environment before they result in extensive and harmful exposure of human subjects. This is particularly important, because there may be a relatively long lag period between exposure and clinically evident carcinoma.

Among the methods for detecting carcinogens are animal bioassays, usually involving rats and mice. Of the dozen or so organic chemicals known to cause cancer in humans, all cause cancer in animal tests. These animal tests have a number of drawbacks: the number of animals that can be tested is limited; the dose of the carcinogen that must be used in animal tests is generally high; and the cost of the screening procedures is high. Less expensive and quicker approaches to the evaluation of possible carcinogenic agents in our environment have been developed which employ bacteria or animal cells in culture. One such test in relatively wide use is that developed by Bruce Ames, which employs special strains of *Salmonella*. It is based on the concept that since most carcinogens are mutagens, the mutagenic activity of potentially carcinogenic agents is assayed. In these tests, about 90 per cent of the known carcinogens can be detected as mutagens. Although these so-called short-term assays provide important leads to identify potentially carcinogenic agents in our environment, the demonstration of mutagenic agents must be followed up by examination in animal systems of their potential carcinogenic activity. The elimination of potential carcinogenic agents based on these tests presents important issues of public policy. Economic and social factors may place important constraints on the individual or government to act to eliminate exposure to a potential carcinogenic agent. Sir Richard Doll, an authority in this area, has suggested a strategy which would require (1) that no generally mutagenic chemical be released into the environment, or be permitted to be used if there exists a satisfactory nonmutagenic substance; (2) that the extent and rigor of the screening procedure be related to the extent to which man is likely to be exposed to the agent; and, (3) that mutagenic substances be used only if the benefits are judged to be great enough to outweigh the hazards and if appropriate controls are exercised.

Doll, R.: The prevention of cancer. J. Roy. Coll. Physicians, 11:125, 1977.

Hiatt, H. H., Watson, J. D., and Winstein, J. A., (eds.): Origins of Human Cancer, Cold Spring Harbor, N.Y., Cold Spring Harbor Laboratory, 1977.

Marks, P. A.: Nutrition and the cancer problem. *In* Winick, M. (ed.): Nutrition and Cancer. New York, John Wiley & Sons, 1977, p. 7.

Mulvihill, J. J., Miller, R. W., and Fraumeni, J. S., Jr.: Genetics of human cancer. *In* Progress in Cancer Research and Therapy, Vol. 3. New York, Raven Press, 1977.

524. TUMOR MARKERS

Philip S. Schein

524.1. INTRODUCTION

The standard physical examination and diagnostic radiology procedures have been demonstrated to have serious limitations in the early detection and localization of small tumor masses. When a neoplasm is first diagnosed as a lesion of 1 cubic centimeter, a realistic limit of clinical screening, it has already completed approximately 30 doublings or two thirds of its growth. It contains one billion cancer cells, and viable cells are likely to have been shed into the bloodstream or lymphatic system. Despite an "early" diagnosis and surgical removal, the patient may have many established and undetected microscopic metastases. In patients with advanced stages of disease, particularly with intraabdominal malignancy, it is often difficult to assess both disease progression and response to treatment.

In response to this problem, considerable research is now being directed toward the identification of tumor-specific products in body fluids that can serve as indirect evidence of neoplastic growth. These index materials have three potential applications in clinical practice: in early diagnosis of malignancy, in the pre- or postoperative assessment of prognosis, and as a chemical assay of tumor cell burden. An ideal tumor marker should not only be capable of detecting microscopic tumor but should also define the site and morphologic type of the malignancy. Unfortunately the available markers have not attained such a high degree of sensitivity and specificity. The problem of sensitivity has been addressed by the use of radioimmunoassays that can measure nanogram quantities of antigen. The second problem of specificity has been more difficult to resolve. The use of normally occurring hormones, enzymes, proteins, or oncofetal antigens requires that the blood concentration of these materials be present in excess of the established normal range. It is for this reason that attention has been directed toward the placental hormones, which are not normally found in the blood of adult males and nonpregnant females.

524.2. ONCOFETAL ANTIGENS

In the prevailing concept, oncofetal antigens are products of gene expression during the process of fetal tissue differentiation. As the fetal tissues reach full specialization and organization, the same genes are partially or completely repressed and remain inoperative in adult life. However, with the state of dedifferentiation associated with neoplastic transformation there may be a reactivation of dormant genomes and consequently a reappearance of embryonic antigens.

Carcinoembryonic antigen (CEA) was described in 1965 as a specific antigen for adenocarcinoma of the colon and for the digestive organs of the two- to six-month human fetus. It is a glycoprotein, with a molecular weight of 200,000 daltons, which is secreted into the glycocalyx surface of gastrointestinal cells. CEA-like material, measured by radioimmunoassay, has been detected in normal adult colonic mucosae, in the feces of normal volunteers and of patients with colostomies after complete tumor resection, and in the normal secretion of the colon and the pancreaticobiliary system. With invasion of the subepithelial tissues by a malignancy there is a disintegration of the basement membrane. The neoplastic glycocalyx then enters the connective tissue spaces, where it is absorbed into vascular and lymphatic channels. Radioimmunoassays of CEA allow for the quantitative measurement of concentrations less than 1.0 ng per milliliter; CEA levels above 2.5 ng per milliliter are considered abnormal in healthy nonsmoking subjects.

It was initially believed that CEA was specific for colorectal malignancy, and that it would be found in abnormal concentrations in the plasma of virtually all cases. This concept has undergone considerable revision with the demonstration of abnormal serum CEA levels in a wide range of malignancies, particularly the entodermally derived tumors of the gastrointestinal tract and lung. Elevated CEA is also associated with several nonmalignant conditions, including alcoholic cirrhosis and pancreatitis, inflammatory bowel disease, and rectal polyps, in addition to cigarette smoking. Although there is no clear threshold difference in CEA concentration in patients with malignant versus nonmalignant disease, the majority of patients in the latter category have normal levels, and elevations when observed are relatively modest (<20 ng per milliliter). However, patients with early stages of colonic cancer may also have a normal serum CEA concentration. Because of this over-all lack of specificity and sensitivity, the CEA should not be regarded as a diagnostic test for cancer.

Plasma concentrations of CEA in excess of 2.5 ng per milliliter have been reported in 60 to 95 per cent of patients with colonic cancer. The incidence of positive tests is largely dependent upon three factors: (1) the extent of disease: patients with tumor confined to the wall of the colon have an abnormal plasma value in 20 to 40 per cent of cases, compared to 85 to 95 per cent with advanced metastatic disease; (2) the differentiation of the tumor: anaplastic lesions have a lower incidence of positive CEA; (3) the presence or absence of liver metastases: the onset of hepatic involvement with tumor is frequently associated with a marked elevation of CEA resulting from either impaired catabolism or excretion of the glycoprotein. Elevations of plasma CEA have also been associated with advanced stages of pancreatic cancer (90 per cent), gastric cancer (60 per cent), lung cancer (75 per cent), breast cancer (50 per cent), and malignancies of many other organs. The principal clinical importance of the CEA is as a monitor of disease progression and response to treatment. Following the complete resection of a tumor, an elevated preoperative CEA should return to a normal concentration by one month following surgery. A persistent elevation or an increasing concentration on serial testing is strongly correlated with residual or metastatic tumor. In approximately 50 per cent of patients with documented tumor recurrence, a rising CEA will be reported months prior to clinical detection of relapse by physical examination, or radiologic procedures. Conversely, with an objective reduction in tumor mass with either chemotherapy or radiation, a reduction in a previously elevated pretreatment CEA may be anticipated.

Alpha-fetoprotein (AFP) is a 70,000 molecular weight protein with an alpha electrophoretic mobility. It is synthesized by the liver parenchymal cells, yolk sac, and gastrointestinal tract of the human fetus. The peak AFP concentration occurs during the twelfth to fifteenth weeks of gestation, following which it declines to reach the normal adult level (less than 40 ng per milliliter) by the sixth to twelfth month following birth. A similar protein was first demonstrated in the serum of mice bearing a transplantable hepatoma in 1963. In the following year AFP was reported present in the serum of human adults with hepatocellular carcinoma.

The reported incidence of abnormal serum AFP in patients with hepatocellular carcinoma has varied from 30 to 95 per cent. The wide range is partly explained by differences in the sensitivity of the assay systems, immunoprecipitation in agar versus radioimmunoassay, and the patient population studied. A higher incidence of positive AFP has been reported for patients from regions in which hepatoma is endemic, such as the Bantu of South Africa. With the current use of radioimmunoassay, 70 to 95 per cent of all cases have a level in excess of 40 ng per milliliter.

Elevated serum AFP is also found in association with teratocarcinomas and embryonal cell carcinoma of testis, ovary, and extragonadal sites such as the mediastinum and retroperitoneum. In contrast, patients with seminomas, or the corresponding dysgerminoma of the female, have normal blood levels. When measured by radioimmunoassay, an elevated AFP has been found in 75 per cent of men with teratocarcinoma of the testis.

Abnormal levels of AFP have been reported for 23 per cent of patients with pancreatic cancer, 18 per cent of patients with gastric cancer, and 5 to 7 per cent of patients with colonic or lung cancer.

Like CEA, the AFP is not a specific marker for malignancy. The measurement of amniotic fluid AFP is now widely used for the early diagnosis of fetal neural tube defects such as anencephaly and spina bifida. During pregnancy, AFP produced by the fetus crosses the placenta, resulting in an increased maternal concentration. Virtually all patients with ataxia telangiectasia have elevated AFP levels. Patients with hereditary tyrosinemia also have elevated concentrations, attributed to the associated severe liver disease.

The principal sources of "false-positive" elevations of AFP have been benign forms of liver disease. In large series, 15 to 75 per cent of patients with cirrhosis and alcoholic hepatitis have demonstrated abnormal serum levels. Viral hepatitis is also accompanied by a transient elevation in AFP in 16 to 64 per cent of cases.

The serum concentration of AFP in benign disease is usually less than 500 ng per milliliter, whereas the majority of patients with hepatoma have levels greatly in excess of this value. Nevertheless, the AFP should not be considered a diagnostic test for cancer. The principal clinical application is as a monitor of the effectiveness of surgical and chemotherapeutic management of hepatoma and germ cell neoplasms.

Pancreatic oncofetal antigen (POA) is a glycoprotein with a molecular weight of 800,000 that has been found in fetal pancreas and pancreatic cancer tissue, but not in normal adult pancreas. This index substance has now been detected in serum of normal adults, and in elevated concentration in some patients with lung, gastric, colonic, and breast cancer. However, the highest absolute levels and greatest frequency of abnormality have been found for patients with pancreatic cancer. There appears to be no concordance between the POA and CEA.

524.3. PLACENTAL PROTEINS

Human chorionic gonadotropin (hCG) is a glycoprotein hormone which is normally secreted by the trophoblastic epithelium of the placenta villus. It is composed of dissimilar α and β subunits. The alpha subunit shares similarities in primary structure with the comparable alpha subunit of human luteinizing hormone (hLH), whereas there are major differences in their respective beta subunits. Sensitive radioimmunoassays have been developed which utilize antisera produced to the beta subunit, hCG-β, which allow for discrimination between hCG and hLH. hCG can be measured in both fetal and maternal serum during pregnancy and in the immediate postpartum period; however, the presence of hCG in the plasma of a male or nonpregnant female is indicative of underlying neoplasm.

Until recently the principal clinical application of hCG measurements has been for the diagnosis and management of trophoblastic tumors. It enables the chemotherapist to assay chemically for the presence of retained trophoblastic or neoplastic cells, and also furnishes a sensitive guide for follow-up of treated cases.

In the past ectopic production of hCG was suspected in patients presenting with precocious puberty or gynecomastia. It has now been demonstrated that hCG may be secreted by germ cell neoplasms of the testes or ovary, or by extragonadal sites such as the mediastinum or retroperitoneum. In large series hCG has been present in the plasma of 50 to 60 per cent of patients with embryonal and teratocarcinoma of the testis, 40 per cent of patients with seminoma, and virtually all patients with testicular choriocarcinoma. Serial measurements of hCG and AFP increase the accuracy of monitoring the effectiveness of treatment of nonseminomatous testicular cancer. Discordant behavior of the hCG and AFP after treatment suggests that the two markers are synthesized by different clones of cells within the tumor.

Detectable hCG has also been demonstrated in the plasma of patients with adenocarcinoma of the ovary (42 per cent), pancreatic cancer (33 per cent), gastric cancer (22 per cent), and hepatomas (17 per cent).

Human placental lactogen (hPL) is normally found in the serum of pregnant women. Post partum, hPL rapidly disappears and is essentially undetectable within 48 hours. This hormone is secreted by the majority of trophoblastic neoplasms and has been demonstrated in a small percentage of patients with hepatomas, leukemia and lymphomas, endocrine tumors, and lung cancer.

Placental alkaline phosphatase (PAP), or Regan isoenzyme, is synthesized in the trophoblast, where it is located on the macrovilli membranes of the plasma membrane. It is readily distinguished from other isoenzymes of alkaline phosphatase by its heat stability, electrophoretic mobility, and immunochemical specificity. Elevated PAP activity is present in the serum of 5 to 15 per cent of patients with cancer of the female reproductive organs, breast, and lung.

524.4. ECTOPIC POLYPEPTIDES

There are many tumors that produce augmented quantities of hormones or proteins that are normally secreted by the cell of origin. Examples include the hypersecretion of insulin and gastrin by islet cell tumors, the M spike of multiple myeloma, and the elevated serum acid phosphatase activity associated with metastatic cancer of the prostate. The abnormal plasma concentration of these markers must be distinguished from the phenomenon of ectopic secretion.

The concept of ectopic secretion has rested upon the basic assumption that all somatic cells contain a complete genetic complement. In association with malignant transformation there may be selective derepression of a previously dormant genome responsible for the production of a specific polypeptide that can be used as a tumor marker. This theory has been refined in recognition that particular tumors have similarities in embryonic origin, electron microscopic features, and histochemical properties with the normal cell of hormone production. An important example is the APUD system, which describes cells derived from the neural crest. Examples of APUD neoplasms include small cell carcinoma of the lung (ACTH, antidiuretic hormone, calcitonin), islet cell tumors (ACTH, vasoactive intestinal polypeptide, serotonin, hCG, pancreatic polypeptide), carcinoid tumors (ACTH, histamine), and medullary carcinoma of the thyroid (ACTH, serotonin). Recent work has suggested that an elevated plasma hCG or its α subunit can be used to differentiate patients with islet cell carcinoma from those with benign adenomas.

Immunoreactive ACTH has been demonstrated in virtually all tissue extracts of lung cancer, independent of histologic type. In addition, more than half the patients with lung cancer have elevated concentrations of immunoreactive "big" or pro-ACTH in their plasma. This precursor protein has minimal bioactivity, as is evidenced by its failure to produce clinical Cushing's syndrome.

524.5. MISCELLANEOUS

Putrescine, spermidine, and spermine are members of a class of small hydrocarbon polycationic amine substances known as polyamines. They are found in highest concentrations in rapidly proliferating tissues, where they have been linked to the control of RNA metabolism. Elevated urinary excretion of polyamines has been demonstrated in approximately two thirds of patients with metastatic cancer of the large intestine, breast, and lung. Urinary polyamines are not specific

markers for malignancy; increased urinary excretion has also been documented in association with benign prostatic hypertrophy, bronchial adenoma, pernicious anemia, and acromegaly.

Methylated nucleosides and pseudouridine are found in transfer RNA and, to a lesser extent, in ribosomal RNA. Increased transfer RNA methylase activity is a common characteristic of malignancy, and elevated concentrations of methylated bases have been demonstrated in the tRNA of human and animal tumors. Catabolism of these macromolecules results in the excretion of these nucleosides in the urine as free bases, where they can be measured as an index of tRNA methylation and turnover. The methylated nucleoside N^2, N^2-dimethyl guanosine, and pseudouridine have been found in abnormal amounts in the urine of patients with a wide range of hematologic and solid tumors, including 60 per cent of patients with advanced breast cancer.

EDCI is a recently described glycoprotein, molecular weight 27,000, that has been isolated in the urine of patients with acute myelogenous leukemia and adenocarcinoma of the ovary and colon. The cellular origin of this material is not known, but the close correlation between urinary excretion of this antigen and response of the neoplasm to treatment suggests that it is produced by neoplastic cells.

The prostatic acinar epithelium elaborates a specific, tartrate-inhibitable acid phosphatase which has been used as a serum marker for metastatic cancer of the prostate. However, the standard enzymatic assays have not had sufficient sensitivity to diagnose patients with localized tumors. A solid-phase radioimmunoassay for acid phosphatase has recently been developed which combines increased specificity with a high degree of sensitivity. Approximately one third of patients with occult neoplasms and 75 per cent of those with palpable tumors confined within, or locally extending beyond, the prostatic capsule (Stages II and III) can now be detected. A small number of patients with benign prostatic hypertrophy have also been demonstrated to have an elevated serum concentration. This new assay for prostatic acid phosphatase may have a future application for mass screening.

A distinct form of serum galactosyltransferase (GT-II) has been reported to be found in patients with neoplastic disease. This isoenzyme is present in the serum of 75 per cent of patients with gastrointestinal carcinomas and 78 per cent with breast cancer, as well as in prostatic cancer and lymphoproliferative disorders. Although the presence and concentration of GT-II correlates with the extent of disease, the majority of patients with Dukes' B colonic cancer are reported to have detectable levels. False-positive tests are uncommon, but have occurred in association with severe alcoholic hepatitis and celiac disease.

Foti, A. G., Cooper, J. F., Herschman, H., and Malvaez, R. R.: Detection of prostatic cancer by solid-phase radioimmunoassay of serum prostatic acid phosphatase. N. Engl. J. Med., 297:1357, 1977.

Gelder, F. B., Reese, C. J., Moossa, A. R., Hall, T., and Hunter, R.: Purification, partial characterization, and clinical evaluation of a pancreatic oncofetal antigen. Cancer Res., 38:313, 1978.

Gewirtz, G., and Yalow, R. S.: Ectopic ACTH production in carcinoma of the lung. J. Clin. Invest., 53:1022, 1974.

Podolsky, D. K., Weiser, M. M., Isselbacher, K. J., and Cohen, A. M.: A cancer-associated galactosyltransferase isoenzyme. N. Engl. J. Med., 299:703, 1978.

Rosen, S. W., Weintraub, B. D., Vaitukaitis, J. L., Sussman, H. H., Hershman, J. M., and Muggia, F. M.: Placental proteins and their subunits as tumor markers. Ann. Intern. Med., 82:71, 1975.

Rudman, D., Chawla, R. K., Heymsfield, S. B., Bethel, R. E., Shoji, M., Vogler, R., and Nixon, D. W.: Urinary excretion of the cancer-related glycoprotein EDCI: Effect of chemotherapy. Ann. Intern. Med., 86:174, 1977.

Russell, D. H., Levy, C. C., Schimpff, S. C., and Hawk, I. A.: Urinary polyamines in cancer patients. Cancer Res., 31:1555, 1971.

Tormey, D. C., Waalkes, T. P., Ahmann, D., Gehrke, C. W., Zumwatt, R. W., Snyder, J., and Hansen, H.: Biological markers in breast carcinoma: I. Incidence of abnormalities of CEA, HCG, three poly-amines, and three minor nucleosides. Cancer, 35:1095, 1975.

Waldmann, T. A., and McIntire, K. R.: The use of radioimmunoassay for alpha-fetoprotein in the diagnosis of malignancy. Cancer, 34:1510, 1974.

Zamcheck, N.: The present status of carcinoembryonic antigen (CEA) in diagnosis, detection of recurrence, prognosis and evaluation of therapy of colonic and pancreatic cancer. Clin. Gastroenterol., 5:625, 1976.

NONMETASTATIC EFFECTS OF CANCER ON THE NERVOUS SYSTEM

See Ch. 322 to 327.

SKIN MANIFESTATIONS OF MALIGNANT DISEASE

See Ch. 573.9.

525. ENDOCRINE SYNDROMES ASSOCIATED WITH CANCER

Nicholas P. Christy

Neoplasms are often associated with systemic symptoms and signs not explained by local spread or distant metastases. Extreme cachexia in the presence of a small nonmetastatic tumor and glucose intolerance, more often subtle than obvious, are familiar. Many other examples, involving various systems, can be sited. These have been observed in all classes of neoplasms: carcinomas, sacromas, lymphomas, and leukemias. It is not yet possible to ascribe all these effects to humoral agents elaborated by the tumors, although many substances have been postulated, including bradykinin, kallikrein, and others.

There are now humoral explanations for well-defined endocrine syndromes associated with cancer. The weight of evidence is that the tumors themselves, although not arising from glandular tissue, secrete and release substances with the biologic properties of natural hormones. There are also instances of tumors that originate in endocrine tissue but secrete the "wrong" hormone: e.g., rare cancers of the thyroid and adrenal medulla secreting ACTH, testicular tumors secreting gonadotropin. The syndromes are not always obvious. The hyperthyroidism that accompanies choriocarcinoma is more chemical than clinical, and many patients with oat cell carcinoma of the lung have laboratory evidence of hyperadrenocorticism, viz., elevated urinary and plasma 17-hydroxycorticosteroid values, exaggerated re-

sponse of the latter to administered ACTH, and abnormal diurnal variation of plasma corticoids, but do not have clinically detectable Cushing's syndrome. *The point is that there probably are associated with cancer a great many biochemical abnormalities which may turn out to be useful as signals of clinically important problems.* For example, lung carcinoma has been shown to secrete the placental proteins human chorionic somatomammotropin and placental alkaline phosphatase.

The evidence that tumors secrete and release hormones is not perfect, but it is good. What is required for proof is roughly analogous to Koch's postulates as applied to the etiologic significance of a microbe. There must be (1) coexistence of tumor and an endocrine syndrome; (2) a demonstration in blood or urine of the causative hormone; (3) demonstration of large quantities of that hormone in the tumor and evidence that the hormone does not come from its "usual" glandular site; (4) ideally, demonstration in vitro of the tumor's capacity to make large amounts of the hormone; and (5) disappearance of, or definite improvement in, the endocrine syndrome upon removal of the tumor. These five conditions are not always easy to satisfy.

(1) Coexistence of neoplasms and endocrine syndromes is generally accepted; there are now many reported cases, and the syndromes are of at least 11 distinct and recognizable types. (2) Greatly elevated concentrations of hormone activity have been shown by biologic or radioimmunoassay in blood of patients with tumors, e.g., of ACTH in association with Cushing's syndrome, gonadotropins with precocious puberty, and erythropoietin with erythrocytosis. One of the major imperfections in the data is that few of the hormones associated with tumors have been absolutely proved chemically to be identical with the natural product. The ACTH produced by tumors includes an ACTH identical to pituitary ACTH, but also N-terminal and C-terminal fragments. Tumor ADH is identical to the "native" hormone. Tumor MSH sometimes differs in molecular weight from pituitary MSH. PTH (parathyroid hormone) of tumor origin contains a ratio of the various forms of immunoreactive PTH different from that found in hyperparathyroidism. However, the biologic behavior of some of the hormones is so nearly that of the native substance that for clinical purposes there seems no reason to doubt that many of the hormone-like materials elaborated by the tumors are nearly the same as those made by glands. (3) Very high concentrations of these hormones or hormone-like activities have been measured directly in tumors associated with endocrine syndromes, not in most other tumors: ACTH, MSH, gonadotropins, chorionic gonadotropin, prolactin, ADH, parathyroid hormone, glucagon, gastrin, and erythropoietin. In one case of presumed gonadotropin-secreting bronchogenic carcinoma, secretion was proved by showing a higher concentration of FSH in the venous effluent from the tumor than in its arterial supply. With respect to ACTH, high concentrations have been found in plasma and tumor, low concentrations in the pituitary; the inference is that the tumor secretes massive amounts of ACTH, adrenocortical hyperplasia follows, and the induced hypercortisolism suppresses synthesis of ACTH by the pituitary. Similarly, several patients have had tumors containing gonadotropin, gonadotropinuria, and reduced pituitary gonadotropin. (4) In one malignant thymoma associated with Cushing's syndrome, cells propagated in tissue

culture continued to produce ACTH for weeks. (5) There are now many instances of cure or definite remission of endocrine syndromes after successful removal of the associated tumor. For example, Liddle et al. have reported nine surgical cures of Cushing's syndrome by removal of the "ACTH"-producing tumor. Dermal hyperpigmentation has disappeared after tumor removal in several cases of MSH-producing cancer. Radiation to the presumably ADH-secreting lung tumor has brought about temporary remission of inappropriate water retention in at least one case, and there are now several reported remissions of hypercalcemia after removal of a "parathyroid hormone"–secreting tumor. The primary role of the tumor in the secretion of the hormone is further strengthened by return of the hypercalcemia in some of these patients when the tumor recurred.

INCIDENCE. Endocrine and metabolic disturbances associated with cancer and not attributable to metastases are not rare. In a large, unselected series of patients with proved bronchogenic carcinoma, the combined incidence of hypercalcemia, gynecomastia, inappropriate ADH secretion, and Cushing's syndrome was 8.5 per cent.

PATHOGENESIS. The evidence for tumor secretion and release of hormones, mostly polypeptides, is convincing. The mechanisms by which neoplastic tissue manages to synthesize complex molecules with hormonal activity are still conjectural. The prevailing view is that the neoplastic cells in a characteristic process of dedifferentiation lose certain genetic depressor mechanisms so that normally inhibited genetic information is expressed. This hypothesis now appears more tenable than the theory of the "sponge," i.e., the taking up of materials (hormones) from the circulation by the tumor. It is also conceivable that the cancer cell produces a large array of polypeptides, some of which, by chance, have an amino acid sequence capable of bringing about a recognizable biologic activity which can be measured.

The role of APUD cells in "ectopic" production of hormones is discussed in Ch. 540.

TERMINOLOGY. These endocrine manifestations have been termed "ectopic," as in the "ectopic ACTH syndrome" (Liddle). The term is appropriate *only* when the site of the tumor presumably secreting the hormone is clearly not in the organ that ordinarily secretes that hormone, as in an oat cell carcinoma of the lung secreting ACTH, an ovarian tumor secreting parathyroid hormone–like peptide, or a pancreatic tumor secreting serotonin. The term is not appropriate in hyperthyroidism associated with "TSH"-secreting choriocarcinomas, because placental chorionic gonadotropin has thyrotropic properties which account for the thyroid-stimulating effects of these tumors; in erythrocytosis associated with renal carcinoma or renal cyst, because the normal kidney synthesizes an erythropoietin; or in carcinoid tumors associated with argentaffin tumors of the small intestine, because this tissue is a normal site of serotonin production.

CLINICAL MANIFESTATIONS AND TREATMENT. There are practical reasons for recognizing the associations of endocrine syndromes with neoplastic disease. (1) Frequently, the endocrinopathy antedates the appearance of the tumor, and thus may serve as a diagnostic clue to neoplastic disease. (2) The endocrine disorders may be life threatening, as hypoglycemia or hypercalcemia, or severely disabling, as Cushing's syndrome, and yet amenable to palliative treatment. (3) Successful removal

of tumor may cure the endocrine syndrome as well as the cancer. (4) Differences in clinical and biochemical behavior of these tumor-associated endocrinopathies from those associated with the classic glandular hyperfunctional states often make a differential diagnosis possible. The general characteristics of the tumor-associated endocrine syndromes are that the hormone is secreted in *anarchic* fashion, that is, secretion is not regulated by the normal control mechanisms; and, as indicated above, the locus of secretion is *displaced* to a site not ordinarily involved in hormonal synthesis.

The discussion that follows emphasizes comparison of the endocrine syndromes associated with cancer to the classic patterns of hormone overproduction, in order to facilitate differential diagnosis.

Cushing's Syndrome. Clinically evident hypercortisolism has been observed in association with oat cell carcinomas of the lung, thymomas, non-insulin-producing islet cell tumors of the pancreas, pheochromocytomas, and tumors of the thyroid, ovary, prostate, parotid, liver, and neural tissue. A few hundred instances of this association have been reported, and subtle chemical evidence of hypercortisolism has been found in many more, especially with carcinoma of the lung (see above). Large quantities of ACTH have been thoroughly characterized in plasma and in some tumors. In isolated instances of lung and pancreatic cancer, peptides with the properties of corticotropin-releasing factor (CRF) have been detected along with ACTH. That the capacity to synthesize ACTH may be a more general property of tumors can be inferred from the finding of Liddle et al. that about 8 per cent of unselected visceral carcinomas not associated with clinically apparent Cushing's syndrome contained considerable amounts of the hormone.

The most important point to be made about the clinical features of Cushing's syndrome associated with nonendocrine tumors is that they are often *subtle*. Patients may show the classic features, but most do not. The absence of obesity and striae is probably a function of the weight loss accompanying the cancer and the *rapidity* with which the disease progresses. Patients with all forms of Cushing's syndrome have an equal incidence of glucose intolerance and hypertension, about 90 per cent. But in the syndrome associated with tumor, the onset is faster and the sex incidence favors men, whereas the "pituitary" form of Cushing's disease and adrenal adenoma are far more common in women. Patients with the tumor-related form rarely have osteoporosis, probably because the clinical course of the tumor is short. Generalized dermal hyperpigmentation is common in the tumor form, because of the huge quantities of ACTH secreted by the cancer, or of MSH, which may also be produced in large amounts. Severe hypokalemia and weakness, as well as edema, are also more common in this form of the disease, and are best explained by the enormous quantities of cortisol and excessive amounts of deoxycorticosterone secreted by the hyperplastic adrenals. Hypokalemia is not due to aldosteronism; the secretion of aldosterone is normal or low. In the other forms of Cushing's syndrome, the patients die of infection or the effects of hypertension; in the tumor form, the usual cause of death is the cancer. At necropsy, the adrenals are enormously hypertrophied, and the pituitary contains subnormal amounts of ACTH.

The laboratory evidence of hypercortisolism is definite and extreme. Plasma cortisol values (ca. 80 μg per 100 ml) and urinary 17-hydroxycorticosteroid and 17-ketogenic steroids may be ten times normal, all much higher than in the "pituitary" or adrenal adenoma forms of Cushing's syndrome. Provocative tests show autonomous cortisol secretion owing to autonomous ACTH secretion by the tumor; urinary steroids do not rise when metyrapone is given, and do not fall in response to dexamethasone. Differentiation from primary adrenocortical carcinoma, also characterized by very high steroid values, can be made by failure to find a suprarenal mass radiographically, and by measuring plasma ACTH concentration; it is very low in adrenal cancer, very high in the presence of ACTH-secreting tumor (see Ch. 547.7).

To recapitulate: an ACTH-secreting tumor, most likely to be in lung, thymus, or pancreas, should be suspected in any patient with subtle or borderline clinical signs of Cushing's syndrome who has lost, not gained, weight, who has weakness and severe hypokalemia, and whose plasma or urinary corticosteroid values are extremely high.

Management, ideally, is total removal of the tumor, which has been followed by remission of the Cushing's syndrome in several cases. Therefore a vigorous effort should be made to excise tumors completely; some are relatively benign, e.g., bronchial adenomas. If this is not possible, palliative x-radiation or chemotherapy of the cancer is carried out, and chemical palliation of the hyperadrenocorticism can be tried with o,p'-DDD, metyrapone, aminoglutethimide, or combinations of these drugs (see Ch. 547.7). If the effects of hypercortisolism, e.g., hypokalemia, are incapacitating, bilateral total adrenalectomy may be done, and has in some cases provided good relief.

Dermal Hyperpigmentation. Generalized hyperpigmentation of the skin, resembling that of Addison's disease, may occur with oat cell carcinoma of the lung, thymoma, neurogenic tumors, or tumors of the ovary, pancreas, and prostate. Raised concentrations of α-MSH and β-MSH have been measured in plasma by radioimmunoassay; most of the pigmentary effect is due to the β-MSH, which has also been found in the associated cancers. Some tumors of this group have been shown to secrete both excessive MSH and ACTH, with resulting addisonian dermal pigmentation and Cushing's syndrome. Several patients have shown disappearance or diminution of dermal pigment when tumors were successfully removed.

Gynecomastia, Precocious Puberty. About 5 per cent of male patients with lung cancer have gynecomastia, but in only a few have elevated gonadotropin values been detected in blood or urine. Tumor types are "large cell" carcinomas, epidermoid, anaplastic, and oat cell carcinomas, and adenocarcinoma. In some of the patients with gynecomastia, raised levels of urinary estrogens have also been found, possibly a result of adrenal or testicular stimulation by gonadotropin secreted from the tumor; in some cases, striking hypertrophic pulmonary osteoarthropathy has also been present. Its relation to gonadotropin or estrogen excess is not yet clear.

Evidence that the tumor is indeed the site of gonadotropin secretion is convincing (see above). When analyzed by radioimmunoassay, the gonadotropin has been usually LH, on one occasion FSH. There is one report of a patient with galactorrhea whose hypernephroma was shown to secrete prolactin.

Spider angiomas and pulmonary osteoarthropathy may or may not accompany gynecomastia. In such cases, careful search for a pulmonary tumor by roentgenography should be done, and measurements made for urinary estrogens (by bioassay) or plasma LH (by radioimmunoassay). Failure to suppress high urinary or plasma gonadotropin levels by administration of large amounts of estrogen for several days may turn out to be a useful diagnostic test.

Treatment is unsatisfactory. The tumors are very malignant, and most of them have not been surgically curable. Radiation and chemotherapy are ineffective. It remains to be seen whether methotrexate will reduce gonadotropin production, as it does in trophoblastic tumors (see below).

Another group of tumors has been associated with secretion of HCG. In addition to benign or malignant tumors of the placenta, these are choriocarcinomas of the pineal or testis, hepatoblastoma of the liver, and adrenocortical carcinoma. A recent survey has disclosed high levels of plasma HCG, usually without clinical signs, in 12 per cent of a series of patients with cancer. With testicular tumors (by far the most common) excluded, the incidence becomes about 7 per cent, with cancers of the gastrointestinal tract or breast, multiple myeloma, and malignant melanoma the next most frequent. *The interesting point here is the possible value of measurements of HCG as markers in attempts at early detection of cancer* (see above). The advantages and pitfalls of this approach are discussed by Kahn et al. and by Vaitukaitis.

The clinical manifestations, when present, are gynecomastia in the adult male and isosexual precocity in children. In boys, the testes have been enlarged in some, and all show testicular interstitial cell hyperplasia histologically. The gonadotropin has the characteristics of HCG, and has been found in high concentration in the urine, serum, and tumors. In a very few cases, gonadotropin levels have been temporarily lowered by methotrexate which had variable effects on the tumor itself. So far, these tumors have all been fatal.

Hyperthyroidism. In addition to the rare association of hyperthyroidism with tumors of the gastrointestinal tract, hematopoietic system, lung, and other organs, several patients have been identified in whom thyrotoxicosis coexisted with metastatic disease of trophoblastic origin (choriocarcinoma or hydatidiform mole) and, in a few cases, with metastatic embryonal cell carcinoma of the testis. Together with the expected finding of high titer of urinary HCG, these patients have thyrotropic activity in plasma and tumor tissue. The best current evidence indicates that this thyroid-stimulating activity is an intrinsic property of HCG or of a glycoprotein molecule chemically and immunologically similar to HCG. The *clinical manifestations* of hyperthyroidism are usually minimal; many patients have no symptoms, and the rest have only mild symptoms of thyrotoxicosis. All have tachycardia, but other physical signs of the endocrinopathy, e.g., goiter, are generally absent, although laboratory evidence — raised serum PBI and high thyroidal uptake of ^{131}I — is definite. These indices can be controlled with antithyroid drugs or iodides, but most striking is the favorable response of both clinical and laboratory signs of hyperthyroidism to treatment with methotrexate, which is also capable of causing regression of these tumors. The presence of mild thyrotoxicosis, seen in fewer than 10 per cent of women with trophoblastic neoplasms, does not affect prognosis of the tumor.

Inappropriate Antidiuresis. Excessive sodium excretion in patients with lung cancer was first reported in 1938, but not until 1957 did Bartter and Schwartz and their co-workers attribute this abnormality to water retention resulting from abnormally regulated secretion of ADH. Studies done in the last decade have disclosed ADH-like activity in several tumors taken from patients with the syndrome of inappropriate ADH secretion; the tumors have been mostly oat cell carcinomas of the lung, with a few others, e.g., pancreatic and duodenal carcinoma. The ADH-like activity has been completely characterized, and is identical in physical, chemical, and biologic properties with human pituitary ADH, i.e., arginine vasopressin. In some (so far, a minority of) patients, plasma values for arginine vasopressin have been found to be high.

The clinical manifestations of hyponatremia may be minimal or absent, probably because the abnormality has developed slowly. Often, hyponatremia is a chance finding during routine study of a patient with lung cancer. To prove the entity, one has to show a urine hypertonic with respect to plasma, normal GFR, and normal adrenocortical function, i.e., absence of adrenocortical insufficiency. The extracellular space, if measured, is found to be expanded. The pathogenesis of this pattern of abnormalities is discussed in Ch. 530. Treatment with hypertonic salt is useful only as an emergency measure, e.g., for coma or convulsions owing to profound hyponatremia; the only effective medical therapy for long-term use is restriction of water intake to less than 1 liter a day. In a few patients, the water and electrolyte abnormality has undergone temporary remission with successful palliative treatment of the tumor by x-radiation or chemotherapy.

Hypercalcemia. The hypercalcemia of malignant disease may be due to at least four mechanisms: (1) osteolytic lesions of bone associated with widespread metastases, as from carcinoma of the thyroid, prostate, or lung, or lymphoma; (2) osteolysis in the absence of bony metastases, associated with some carcinomas of the breast which presumably elaborate sterols related to vitamin D; (3) osteolysis in the absence of bony metastases, in association with tumors which appear to secrete a parathyroid hormone (PTH)–like substance (a possibility first suggested in 1949 by Fuller Albright and tentatively demonstrated by J. E. Howard in 1953); and (4) osteolysis without bony metastases in the presence of tumors which secrete some humoral substance other than parathyroid hormone or proparathyroid hormone, i.e., a substance or substances not detectable by radioimmunoassays for the various forms of these hormones (see Powell et al.). Tumors have been squamous cell carcinomas of the lung and other organs, and carcinomas of the kidney, ovary, uterus, pancreas, and colon. Evidence for primary secretion of parathyroid hormone by the neoplasm has come from demonstration of immunoreactive PTH in plasma of patients with nonparathyroid tumors and hypercalcemia, from the detection of PTH-like substance in the tumors, disappearance or diminution of hypercalcemia upon tumor removal, and reappearance of the electrolyte abnormality with recurrence of the cancer.

The clinical features of hypercalcemia are presented in detail in Ch. 552.2. The important clinical point is that the hypercalcemia associated with PTH-secreting tumors of nonendocrine tissue is more likely to manifest itself as lethargy, weakness, anorexia, nausea, and vomiting, and less likely to appear as renal stones or bone disease. Patients with the "ectopic PTH syndrome" are more apt to present themselves with general, nonspecific signs, e.g., weight loss or anemia or both.

Separation of these patients from those with hyperparathyroidism by laboratory tests may be difficult. Both may have extreme hypercalcemia, low or normal serum phosphorus, elevated plasma values for PTH, and unresponsiveness of hypercalcemia to corticosteroids; but careful examination, laboratory study, and roentgenographic search, e.g., by chest films and intravenous pyelography, will disclose most of the nonparathyroid tumors. Riggs et al. and Arnaud have discussed the diagnostic difficulties in the use of PTH radioimmunoassays for detection of the immunoheterogeneous substance.

The *treatment* of the hypercalcemia is discussed in Ch. 552.2.

It has been recently postulated that *hypophosphatemic osteomalacia* in the presence of benign hemangiomas may be due to a humoral substance (not PTH) that increases renal clearance of phosphate.

Hypoglycemia. The association of severe fasting hypoglycemia with certain neoplasms, especially very large retroperitoneal or intrathoracic tumors, is well established. Most of the tumors are fibromas or sarcomas, sometimes of huge size — up to 10 kg; others are hepatoma, adrenocortical carcinoma, adenocarcinoma of stomach and colon, undifferentiated bronchial carcinoma, and bronchial carcinoid. As for the mechanism of hypoglycemia, there is some evidence against excessive glucose utilization by the tumor and against stimulation by the tumor of insulin secretion by the pancreas, removal of which does not affect the hypoglycemia. The prevailing view is that the tumor secretes a hypoglycemia-producing substance, which, with only a few exceptions, is not demonstrable as high levels of immunoreactive insulin in plasma or tumor, but only as nonsuppressible "insulin-like" activity. The secretory role of the tumor is affirmed by surgical "cure" of the hypoglycemia in about 20 patients whose tumors have been successfully removed.

The hypoglycemia is indistinguishable clinically and by most of the provocative tests from that associated with islet cell adenoma or carcinoma of the pancreas. However, patients with nonpancreatic tumors lack high plasma immunoassayable insulin values, and the presence of a large tumor is usually apparent.

Treatment is best done by excising the tumor; even incomplete removal may relieve the hypoglycemia temporarily. Failing this, palliative measures must include continuous feeding of carbohydrate and administration of corticosteroids, diazoxide, and possibly glucagon (see Ch. 531.2).

Carcinoid Syndrome. This, the only definite example of an "endocrine" syndrome owing to production of a humoral agent that is not a polypeptide, is discussed in Ch. 551.

Erythrocytosis; Zollinger-Ellison Syndrome. These syndromes, caused by tumor secretion of erythropoietin and gastrin respectively, are discussed in detail in Ch. 478 and 403.

Multiple Hormones Produced by a Single Tumor. Several tumors have been reported which apparently secrete two or even three distinct hormones. The pulmonary and thymic tumors secreting both ACTH and MSH have already been mentioned. A few patients with hepatoma have had both hypoglycemia and polycythemia, and islet cell tumors of the pancreas have been described with coexisting hypoglycemia and carcinoid syndrome, and with Cushing's syndrome and carcinoid syndrome. Three hormones, ACTH, MSH, and gastrin, were found in a single pancreatic tumor, and in one patient with an islet cell carcinoma of the pancreas there was evidence for secretion by the neoplasm of six hormones: glucagon (an "appropriate" hormone for the pancreas), gastrin, ACTH, MSH, ADH, and parathyroid hormone.

Braunstein, G. D., Vaitukaitis, J. L., Carbone, P. P., and Ross, G. T.: Ectopic production of human chorionic gonadotrophin by neoplasms. Ann. Intern. Med., 78:39, 1973.

Kahn, C. R., Rosen, S. W., Weintraub, B. D., Fajans, S. S., and Gorden, P.: Ectopic production of chorionic gonadotropin and its subunits by islet-cell tumors. A specific marker for malignancy. N. Engl. J. Med., 297:565, 1977.

Plimpton, C. H., and Gellhorn, A.: Hypercalcemia in malignant disease without evidence of bone destruction. Am. J. Med., 21:750, 1956.

Powell, D., Singer, F. R., Murray, T. M., Minkin, C., and Potts, J. T.: Nonparathyroid humoral hypercalcemia in patients with neoplastic diseases. N. Engl. J. Med., 289:176, 1973.

Rees, L. H.: The biosynthesis of hormones by non-endocrine tumours — a review. J. Endocrinol., 67:143, 1975.

Riggs, B. L., Arnaud, C. D., Reynolds, J. C., and Smith, L. H.: Immunologic differentiation of primary hyperparathyroidism from hyperparathyroidism due to nonparathyroid cancer. J. Clin. Invest., 50:2079, 1971.

Vaitukaitis, J. L.: Editorial: When is a tumor marker not a tumor marker? N. Engl. J. Med., 293:1370, 1975.

Vaitukaitis, J. L.: Peptide hormones as tumor markers. Cancer, 37:567, 1976.

526. MEDICAL TREATMENT OF HORMONE-DEPENDENT CANCERS

Philip K. Bondy

INTRODUCTION

It is always best, if possible, to cure a malignant tumor by local excision, destruction with radiation, or both. However, if the tumor has already metastasized, local treatment alone is inadequate, and attempts to slow down the growth rate or eradicate the neoplasm require systemic therapy. The factors controlling tumor growth are not clear, but in some instances the endocrine evironment may be important. In general, endocrine manipulations are most useful in tumors of hormone-sensitive organs, e.g., breast and prostate.

The application of endocrine treatment should not be considered as separate from the use of other modalities but should be part of an integrated approach, including surgery, radiotherapy, and chemotherapy as well. Thus the best results are obtained when treatment is planned from the beginning by an experienced team of people who are familiar with current knowledge and are con-

stantly evaluating those results. There is no place for the lone entrepreneur in modern cancer treatment.

CANCER OF THE BREAST

This is a very common disease (incidence about 70 per 100,000 women per year; prevalence about 100 per 100,000 women per year). Incidence is higher in certain families and in childless women. It is increased in obese populations and is reduced by early pregnancy. It is bilateral in 4 to 10 per cent of women when first seen, suggesting a multicentric origin. In spite of this, early diagnosis is desirable and regular examination should be carried out, especially in childless women over 30 years old, when family history is positive, or when a previous breast cancer has occurred. Diagnosis should be confirmed histologically. The prognosis is somewhat better in well-differentiated tumors, or in the presence of lymphocyte infiltration and lymph node histiocytosis.

TREATMENT. The first step in designing treatment is to determine accurately the *distribution* of the tumor. Local disease is usually treated by surgery, supplemented by radiation if local lymph nodes are involved. If the primary tumor is too large for safe surgical treatment, radiation (sometimes followed by local surgery) is proper initial treatment. This local approach cannot be defended (except for palliation of painful or ulcerated masses) if there is evidence of distant dissemination. All patients should therefore have a preoperative work-up, including a chest x-ray and skeletal scintiscan. X-ray survey of the skeleton is much less sensitive and probably not useful in patients without skeletal symptoms or positive scans. Some clinicians also do routine isotopic liver scans, but in my experience this is not very useful. Ultrasonic scans, when available, may be preferable, and elevated plasma alkaline phosphatase activity strongly suggests metastatic spread. High levels of urinary hydroxyproline or plasma carcinoembryonic antigen, chorionic gonadotropin, or chorionic somatomammotropin are also strong indicators of distant spread which should be evaluated preoperatively.

Although discussions of the type of surgery to perform are beyond the scope of this chapter, it is important that an adequate sample of axillary lymph nodes be examined by the pathologist. The presence of any metastatic spread to the nodes seriously impairs prognosis; and if three or more nodes are involved, the probability of surviving five years without clinical recurrence is less than 50 per cent unless some form of successful systemic treatment is undertaken. The design of medical treatment of inoperable or disseminated cancer rests on at least the following four factors:

Status of Ovarian Function. Castration is associated with tumor regression in about one third of premenopausal patients, whereas postmenopausal patients are not helped by removing the ovaries. About a third of them are improved by the administration of estrogen. Cessation of menstrual flow is not by itself a safe guide, however. Many women continue to secrete estrogens for some time after their menses stop, and amenorrhea in younger women is not necessarily associated with depressed ovarian function. Patients whose cancer is first detected within five years of the onset of menopause are therefore a special case, since they are not likely to respond to endocrine manipulations of either type. Chemotherapy is the best method of treatment of metastatic disease in the perimenopausal period.

Sensitivity of the Tumor to Hormones. The only reliable proof of sensitivity is shrinkage of the tumor masses by 50 per cent or more without evidence of progression at any site. Most clinicians also require that the response persist at least two months. Feelings of subjective improvement are treacherous and should not be relied on. Since response is not instantaneous, clinical evaluation may require several months — a very long time in a progressive disease. Endocrine manipulations will benefit only about a third of patients with advanced breast cancer. It would be helpful if a method could be found of minimizing delay in recognizing ineffective treatment and reducing the number of patients subjected to unrewarding endocrine treatment. Early changes in relatively nonspecific indicators such as urinary hydroxyproline or plasma carcinoembryonic antigen may be helpful in minimizing the delay in recognizing lack of response, but they are not entirely reliable.

Attempts have therefore been made to predict whether tumors will respond by evaluating their biologic characteristics. The effective hormonal agents are steroids such as estrogen, androgen, and progestogens. All of these affect cellular metabolism first by binding to a cytoplasmic protein which translocates them to the nucleus, where their metabolic effects take place. Thus the presence of cytoplasmic receptor is essential for their activity. Estrogen receptor (ER) can be measured in samples of the tumor removed at surgery. Whereas the probability of useful clinical response to castration of all premenopausal patients is only about 30 per cent, about 60 per cent of tumors containing ER respond, and only about 5 per cent of tumors lacking ER respond. Comparable data are available for estrogen administration in postmenopausal tumors. Thus it is wasteful to try estrogen manipulations in patients whose tumors lack ER. Unfortunately, ER determinations still fail to identify a large number of nonresponders. Attempts to improve discrimination by measuring receptors for progestogens and androgens are under study. Even when a primary tumor contains ER, in about 25 per cent of cases it will be absent from some of the metastases. The longer the interval between examination of the primary tumor and the metastases, the greater the probability of discrepancy. It appears therefore that nonresponsive forms of the tumor evolve with time.

Disease-Free Interval after Excision. The probability of response is better if this is more than two years.

Distribution of the Metastases. Involvement of soft tissues, for example, tends to respond to estrogens in postmenopausal women, whereas bone involvement is more responsive to androgens. Local skin metastases in postmenopausal women respond to norethisterone more often than to any other endocrine treatment.

Sequence of Treatment. 1. *Adjuvant treatment* refers to treatment given after therapy directed to the primary site has been completed, when a high probability exists of metastatic spread. The common endocrine form is castration at the time of operation in premenopausal women. This is not justified in the absence of disseminated disease, because, although it may defer the onset of clinical metastatic disease, it does not prolong life. Moreover, it deprives the therapist of information

about the sensitivity of the tumor to endocrine manipulations. Some surgeons argue that prolonging the disease-free interval is justified by any means, because of the improved peace of mind it provides. The loss of useful information seems to me to outweigh this consideration, since all future decisions about endocrine treatment will depend on whether the patient responded to estrogen deprivation.

2. The *initial systemic treatment* could be chemotherapy or endocrine. Since the most optimistic expectation, even in ER positive patients, is only about a 50 per cent response, whereas most chemotherapy schedules anticipate a 70 to 80 per cent response, many oncologists now use chemotherapy first (see Ch. 527.3). Endocrine treatment may be preferred because of lesser toxic effects and occasional prolonged remissions. Moreover, chemotherapy is seldom effective in skeletal metastases, whereas endocrine treatment often works well. In premenopausal women, castration is the first endocrine treatment.

The *method of oophorectomy* is unimportant; surgery provides a quicker response than x-ray castration, at the expense of an additional operation. If the patient is desperately ill, surgery is probably preferable. Otherwise, some clinicians prefer irradiation. Abrupt deprivation of estrogen in premenopausal women usually causes severe symptoms, including hot flushes and, in some cases, rapidly progressive osteoporosis. If the tumor has responded to castration, estrogen replacement should not be given; but if no response has occurred, there is nothing to be lost by giving replacement.

In postmenopausal women, administration of estrogens should be tried first. The initial dose may be moderate, but should be increased gradually to a high dose (e.g., diethylstilbestrol, 15 mg daily). A careful watch must be kept for dangerous hypercalcemia, which may occur suddenly and be difficult to control. Many women have nausea and tolerate doses of this magnitude badly.

If the disease responds to the first endocrine treatment, it is worthwhile continuing until relapse; but if no response occurs, chemotherapy should be begun. The probability of responding to other forms of endocrine therapy is low if the first try has been unsuccessful.

3. *Second line endocrine treatment* in premenopausal women is directed toward removing nonovarian sources of estrogen. The adrenal gland can produce both estrogens and precursors such as dehydroepiandrosterone, which are converted to estrogens in body fat, liver, or the tumor. Adrenalectomy is therefore commonly recommended. Surgical extirpation has been used in the past, but pharmacologic blockade has many advantages. Aminoglutethimide, 1 or 2 grams per day in divided doses, together with cortisol, 20 mg twice daily, prevents steroid secretion and also inhibits conversion of precursors to estrogen in the liver and adipose tissue. It also has the virtue of being reversible if unsuccessful. Completeness of blockade is proved if plasma dehydroepiandrosterone concentration falls to undetectable levels. The treatment is more difficult to control if dexamethasone is used rather than cortisol, because its metabolism is altered in an erratic way by aminoglutethimide. Hypophysectomy may be carried out in preference to adrenalectomy. Both treatments are effective in about half the premenopausal women who

have responded to castration. They work best against metastases in bone, local recurrences, and leukoerythroblastic anemia. They are less effective against visceral involvement and are useless in treating brain metastases. Removal of adrenals or pituitary may also be used as a second line of treatment in postmenopausal women, in whom the probability of success and the duration of remission are greater than in premenopausal patients. The explanation of the useful effect in postmenopausal patients is not clear. The postoperative treatment of patients lacking pituitaries or adrenals is discussed in Ch. 543.6 and 547.3.

The success of hypophysectomy depends in some degree on its completeness, but it has not always been possible to demonstrate a good correlation between persistence of ability to secrete growth hormone or prolactin and therapeutic response. The relationship of prolactin to breast cancer has been explored in great detail. At present there is no evidence that this hormone is concerned with growth of the tumor in human beings, and attempts to produce clinical improvement by pharmacologic suppression of prolactin secretion with L-dopa or bromocriptine and other ergot derivatives have been unrewarding.

If hypophysectomy or adrenalectomy is considered inadvisable, another approach is to block the estrogen receptors with an antiestrogen such as tamoxifen, 20 mg daily in divided doses. The drug produces nausea and vomiting in about 10 per cent of patients and hot flushes in 7 per cent. Transient nonprogressive depression of the platelet count occurs in about 10 per cent of patients, but can safely be ignored.

If estrogens have been temporarily beneficial in postmenopausal patients, they should be withdrawn when the disease again becomes active. About 25 per cent of patients who responded to estrogens initially will have a second "rebound" response to their withdrawal, lasting in some instances more than 18 months. As a result, it is inadvisable to institute a new treatment immediately after stopping estrogens, since the effects of the next treatment might be confused by development of a rebound response. It is unlikely that a third response will occur if estrogen treatment is resumed after the beneficial effects of the rebound response have ended. Tamoxifen is often useful when rebound response fails to occur, or after it has ended.

Long-acting preparations of androgens or progestogens are sometimes used as a second line treatment. Androgens produce distressing masculinization, which is minimized by using preparations of low androgenicity such as nandrolone. These hormones have a lower probability of success than the others already mentioned, but may be especially useful in treating skeletal disease. Adrenal corticosteroids are often given (e.g., prednisolone, 10 mg four times daily) but there is no evidence that they are effective specifically against the cancer. They produce euphoria, improve the appetite, and relieve central nervous system symptoms caused by metastases.

4. *Subsequent endocrine treatment* may be justified in patients who have responded to second line therapy. The more endocrine manipulations have succeeded in a given patient, the higher the probability that the next attempt will be successful. It may also be useful to revert to endocrine treatment when chemotherapy has failed. The exact form of endocrine treatment will depend on what has previously been tried and on the nature of the metastatic disease, as discussed previously.

5. *Chemotherapy* is seen in this scheme as a last resort. Usually, *successful* endocrine treatment provides longer remissions than chemotherapy; but the possibility of combining chemotherapy with endocrine treatment has not yet been adequately explored. It has been the writer's practice to combine chemotherapy with the appropriate endocrine manipulation from the very beginning in patients with a bad prognosis, i.e., those with a short disease-free interval or with extensive involvement of the viscera.

PROGNOSIS. In those women who respond, the mean duration of improvement after castration is about a year, and the maximum is several years. Response is more likely after a long disease-free interval and in patients with bone metastases. Patients younger than 35 respond less often.

Most of the information available at present about the rate and duration of response after endocrine treatment is based on observation of patients in whom this was the first treatment for disseminated disease. The recent tendency in some clinics to turn to chemotherapy as the first treatment may affect endocrine responses, since hormonal manipulations will be undertaken at a later stage of the disease and in patients whose tumors may have been subjected to modifications caused by chemotherapy. In addition, chemotherapy, even in small doses used in adjuvant treatment, usually suppresses ovarian function. Thus castration after chemotherapy may sometimes prove redundant. It is impossible at present to predict the effects of early drug treatment on the success of hormonal therapy.

If pregnancy occurs after breast cancer has been diagnosed and treated, the prognosis is not affected, regardless of the outcome of the pregnancy. When the tumor is discovered during pregnancy — especially the third trimester — or during lactation or weaning, the prognosis is much worse. Under these circumstances, termination of the pregnancy does not improve the situation.

COMPLICATIONS OF HORMONAL TREATMENT. Any endocrine treatment may cause a sudden, life-threatening rise of serum calcium, especially in patients with many lytic deposits in bone. This is combated by stopping treatment and by generous hydration; oral prednisolone, 10 mg four times daily, or cortisol, 100 mg intravenously every six hours. Mithramycin, 25 μg per kilogram intravenously at 48-hour intervals for not more than three doses, almost always reduces the serum calcium if these measures fail. The risk of hypercalcemia may be minimized by starting estrogen treatment at low doses (0.1 mg of diethylstilbestrol) for one to two weeks. Even a single course of quadruple chemotherapy usually restores the serum calcium value to normal, even though estrogen treatment is continued. If treatment is successful, rapid healing of osteolytic areas may cause hypocalcemia; this requires treatment with intravenous calcium salts and oral vitamin D until the rate of recalcification slackens off.

Large doses of diethylstilbestrol often cause nausea and vomiting. Conjugated mixed estrogens (Premarin) cause fewer gastrointestinal disturbances if they are given first in oral doses of 2.5 to 5 mg daily. Patients usually tolerate diethylstilbestrol after a week or so in doses of 0.5 mg thrice daily. There is rarely an advantage to larger doses.

Continuous administration of estrogens may cause breakthrough uterine bleeding, but this is unusual. If it occurs, cyclic courses are advisable. Edema may occur during estrogen treatment, and can be managed by diuretics. Increased pigmentation often occurs and is harmless. Thrombophlebitis may be a serious hazard, but whether the danger outweighs the advantage of treatment is not yet known.

In addition to these methods of treatment, radiation should always be available, to toleration, for relief of bone pain or of brain metastases. Proper support of the psyche, nutrition, and bone marrow should be provided.

CANCER OF THE BREAST IN MALES. Malignant breast tumors are very rare in men; but when they occur they are usually much more aggressively malignant than in women. The same principles apply for treating the disease in men as in women, except that castration is generally considered to be an essential part of treatment regardless of age.

CANCER OF THE PROSTATE

This is a very common tumor, affecting between 14 and 46 per cent of all adult males in various autopsy series, but in most instances the tumor is localized and not of clinical significance. About 36 per 100,000 population have clinically significant tumor. In the United States there are about 17,000 deaths and 25,000 new cases per year. About 50 per cent of the clinically important cases can be diagnosed on rectal examination; the remainder are recognized from histologic examination of tissue removed at prostatectomy for benign prostatic hypertrophy. Once the diagnosis is suspected, histologic confirmation is essential, either by prostatectomy or by needle biopsy of suspicious nodules. After the diagnosis is established, the stage of the tumor's growth should be established.

Four stages are generally recognized:

1. Entirely intraprostatic, and too small to be suspected by physical examination or clinical laboratory methods.

2. Apparent on physical examination, but entirely confined to the prostate.

3. Confined to the pelvis. Here the tumor may have spread to other tissues in the pelvis but has not yet metastasized to distant points or bone.

In stages 1, 2, 3, acid and alkaline phosphatase levels are not elevated in the serum, and skeletal x-ray, lymphogram and isotope scanning of bone are negative. In these stages, there is hope of cure by surgery, radiation therapy, or both combined.

4. Distant metastases. Serum acid phosphatase is elevated in about two thirds of these patients. In those with skeletal metastases diagnosed by skeletal x-rays or bone scan, the alkaline phosphatase may also be elevated. These patients can no longer be cured by local treatment.

TREATMENT. The principles applicable to treating cancer of the breast are also appropriate for prostatic carcinoma. So long as the tumor is localized, every rea-sonable effort should be exerted to cure the tumor by surgery, radiation, or both. Chemotherapy or hormonal manipulations should be considered only when local methods are no longer applicable. By the same reasoning, local treatment should not be pushed beyond palliative levels if evidence of distant spread is already available. Careful staging is therefore essential before a decision about appropriate treatment can be made.

Since growth of prostatic cells is dependent on the presence of androgens, it was reasonable for Huggins and his colleagues to try the effects of *castration* on the growth of prostatic tumors (1941). About 80 per cent of cases respond to androgen deprivation by reduced bone pain and size of the tumor masses. In some cases, skeletal metastases may begin to show radiographic evidence of healing. In almost all, the elevated acid phosphatase drops somewhat, but this is an unreliable index of overall response of the tumor, because tumor cells produce less acid phosphatase, even though they may not die, when androgenic stimulation is removed.

Since castration has unpalatable emotional connotations even for aged men, administration of *estrogens* has sometimes been substituted for orchidectomy, with comparable symptomatic results. The dose schedule originally used was much like that for cancer of the breast. In 1967, however, the United States Veterans Administration Cooperative Urological Research Group published the results of a large study demonstrating that administration of high doses of estrogens increased the death rate from cardiovascular causes by about 75 per cent, more than canceling the modest (25 per cent) reduction in mortality from the cancer. A number of studies subsequently have shown that low doses of estrogen are better tolerated. The minimal dose capable of suppressing plasma testosterone concentration to castration levels is 1 mg of diethylstilbestrol three times daily, and this is recommended as the minimal effective dose. Ethinyl estradiol, 0.05 mg twice daily, and Premarin, 2.5 mg thrice daily, work equally well. TACE does not completely suppress plasma testosterone in doses as high as 24 mg daily. The escape of previously responsive patients from estrogen treatment is not associated with a rise of plasma testosterone concentration, but probably reflects development of autonomy of the tumor from hormonal control. In spite of this, a few such patients have a further response to very high doses of estrogens, so it may be justifiable to accept the risks of thromboembolism and try doses of the order of 15 mg or more of diethylstilbestrol daily for a brief period to see whether relief is obtained. Cyproterone, a testosterone-blocking agent, has been tried experimentally in doses of 200 to 300 mg daily, with promising results. It might supplement the effects of estrogen or castration, or prove useful after their effectiveness has worn off.

Since neither estrogens nor castration prolongs life, neither should be used except to relieve pain or urinary tract obstruction; even in these situations, the beneficial effects of radiation to local disease of bone or pelvis should be exploited before hormonal manipulation is tried. If a decision is made to turn to hormone therapy, castration is preferred, because it is not associated with the increased cardiovascular complications seen in estrogen-treated patients. Alternatively, the estrogen program previously described may be tried. *Adrenalec-*

tomy and *hypophysectomy* offer no advantages after castration has failed.

The place of *cytotoxic chemotherapy* is less established in prostatic cancer than in cancer of the breast; but it is the writer's impression that several agents, including cyclophosphamide and methotrexate, sometimes give relief of bone pain, suggesting a response. Objective evidence of reduced tumor size or increased longevity is not at hand. Further studies of chemotherapeutic combinations are needed in this disease.

CANCER OF THE THYROID

Well-differentiated thyroid carcinomas are often under pituitary control, and their growth can be blocked and the metastatic masses may disappear if secretion of thyroid-stimulating hormone (TSH) is suppressed. This is accomplished by giving replacement doses of thyroxine or equivalent hormone combinations of thyroxine and triiodothyronine. Suppression may continue for very long periods with control of the cancer. The matter is discussed in more detail in Ch. 546.8.

OTHER ENDOCRINE CANCERS

There is no evidence that suppressing pituitary ACTH secretion controls the growth or activity of carcinomas of the adrenal cortex, whether functional or not. Endocrine manipulations are ineffective in treating tumors of other endocrine organs. The influence of pituitary growth factors and insulin on tumors of nonendocrine tissues has not yet been established. The cytotoxic effects of *adrenocortical steroids* are used in treating lymphomas, Hodgkin's disease, and other tumors and to ameliorate secondary effects of tumors such as dermatomyositis, neuropathy, and hemolytic disease. They may also relieve pressure by reducing the inflammatory zone surrounding tumor masses, e.g., in cerebral metastases. About 15 per cent of patients with metastases from renal cell carcinoma have objective evidence of regression after treatment with progestogens (e.g., Provera, 100 mg intramuscularly daily for five days of the week, reduced after response to three times a week). The response persists for two months to almost three years. In a few patients it seems clear that life is prolonged by treatment. Subjective improvement is reported by about half the patients. Testosterone has also been tried, but is virtually ineffective.

Band, P. R., Banerjee, T. K., Patwardhan, V. C., and Eid, T. C.: High-dose diethylstilbestrol diphosphate therapy of prostatic cancer after failure of standard doses of estrogens. Can. Med. Assoc. J., 109:697, 1973.

Bloom, H. J. G.: Hormone-induced and spontaneous regression of metastatic renal cancer. Cancer, 32:1066, 1973.

Brown, P. W., Terz, J. J., King, R., and Lawrence, W., Jr.: Bilateral adrenalectomy for metastatic breast carcinoma. Arch. Surg., 110:77, 1975.

Huggins, C., and Hodges, C. V.: Studies on prostatic cancer: Effect of castration, of estrogen, and of androgen injection on serum phosphatase in metastatic carcinoma of the prostate. Cancer Res., 1:293, 1941.

Jensen, E. V., Block, G. E., Smithe, S., Kyser, K., and DeSombre, E.: Estrogen receptors and breast cancer response to adrenalectomy. Natl. Cancer Inst. Monogr., 34:55, 1971.

Legha, S. S., and Carter, S. K.: Antiestrogens in the treatment of breast cancer. Cancer Treat. Rev., 3:205, 1976.

Nestro, R. W., Cady, B., Oberfield, R. A., Pazianos, A. G., and Salzman, F. A.: Rebound response after estrogen therapy for metastatic breast cancer. Cancer, 38:1834, 1976.

Rose, D. P., and Davis, T. E.: Ovarian function in patients receiving adjuvant chemotherapy for breast cancer. Lancet, 1:1174, 1977.

Santen, R. J., Samojlik, E., Lipton, A., Harvey, H., Ruby, E. B., Wells, S. A., and Kendall, J.: Kinetic, hormonal and clinical studies with aminoglutethimide in breast cancer. Cancer, 39:2948, 1977.

Shearer, R. J., Hendry, W. F., Sommerville, I. F., and Fergusson, J. D.: Plasma testosterone: An accurate monitor of hormone treatment in prostatic cancer. Br. J. Urol., 45:668, 1973.

Stoll, B. A.: Endocrine Therapy in Malignant Disease, Philadelphia, W.B. Saunders Company, 1972.

Van Gilder, J. C., and Goldenberg, I. S.: Hypophysectomy in metastatic breast cancer. Arch. Surg., 110:293, 1975.

Veterans Administration Co-operative Urological Research Group: Treatment and survival of patients with cancer of the prostate. Surg. Gynecol. Obstet., 124:1011, 1967.

527. PRINCIPLES OF ONCOLOGIC TREATMENT: IRRADIATION, CYTOTOXIC DRUGS, AND IMMUNOSTIMULATORY PROCEDURES

Paul Calabresi

527.1. GENERAL PRINCIPLES OF ANTINEOPLASTIC THERAPY

INTRODUCTION

With the recognition that medical oncology is an important subspecialty of internal medicine, the internist has accepted a principal responsibility in the care of patients with neoplastic disorders. This concern extends from the role of primary care physician, alert to detect and diagnose cancer in its earliest stages, to that of specialist coordinating a complex multidisciplinary therapeutic plan with appropriate supportive management. Because of this, the internist should be knowledgeable in the principles of neoplasia, its pathophysiology, and related immunologic considerations, and should be aware of genetic conditions, viral agents, occupational risks, and other environmental hazards that may predispose to the development of cancer. In addition to a broad understanding of general internal medicine, the physician must also be familiar with the indications for surgical intervention and the principles of radiotherapy, in order to foster an integrated, combined-modality approach for the care of the patient. Interdisciplinary therapeutic planning conferences, with participation of surgical, radiation, and medical oncologists *before* initiation of individual treatment programs, are highly recommended; one physician, however, must ultimately be responsible for the patient. Before an optimal treatment plan can be designed, it is also necessary to determine the clinical and pathologic extent of a tumor by appropriate staging procedures. This is usually accomplished with the help of surgery, pathology, diagnostic radiology, and nuclear medicine. Although there are several staging classifications, some unique to specific tumors (i.e., lymphomas — Ann Arbor; colonic carcinoma — Duke), the TNM system has broad applicability and is a useful model for understanding the principles of staging. In this system T signifies the primary tumor, N the regional lymph nodes, and M distant metastases; subscripts 1 through 4 indicate increasing degrees of tumor size or involvement, and subscript 0 indicates no evidence of disease in that particular compartment (i.e., T_2, N_1, M_0). T_{is} denotes carcinoma in situ, and N_x is used when the regional lymph node involvement cannot be evaluated clinically. Uniform staging is useful in determining prognosis and in comparing therapeutic results, but it is most valuable as a guide for proper management by defining whether there is *localized, regional,* or *disseminated* neoplastic involvement.

MANAGEMENT OF LOCALIZED OR REGIONAL DISEASE

The preferred treatment of localized cancer is usually surgery and, in some cases, radiotherapy. If a tumor is sufficiently localized and amenable to complete surgical resection, this is the treatment of choice. In tumors that are highly radiosensitive, in patients whose clinical status makes surgery hazardous, or in situations in which surgical resection causes irreparable loss of function and disability (i.e., cancer of the head and neck or uterine cervix), radiotherapy may be preferable. When cancer extends beyond the primary site (T compartment) and invades the regional lymph nodes (N compartment), it may be necessary to supplement surgery with radiotherapy. With some tumors, notably carcinoma of the breast, substantial involvement of regional lymph nodes (four or more) implies a high statistical probability of dissemination of micrometastases in distant organs (M compartment). In other tumors, such as osteogenic sarcoma, approximately 80 per cent of patients already have micrometastases in the lungs at the time of the original surgical amputation. These realizations have led to the use of adjuvant chemotherapy in patients whose clinical disease appears to be limited to the T and N compartments but in whom, despite a clinical M_0 status, there is a high probability of disseminated micrometastatic involvement. This relatively recent use of adjuvant chemotherapy in certain patients with clinically localized or regional disease has resulted in prolonging the duration of complete remission in an increased number of cases and holds promise of achieving a greater percentage of cures than had been possible with surgery and radiotherapy alone. A general concept of strategy using combined modalities for the curative therapy of early cancer would include surgical resection of the primary tumor, irradiation of residual regional disease, and subsequent chemotherapy alone or with immunotherapy for the eradication of disseminated micrometastases when only a relatively small tumor burden remains.

MANAGEMENT OF DISSEMINATED DISEASE

The treatment of choice for disseminated cancer is chemotherapy. In some cases, notably lymphomas, ovarian and testicular tumors, and certain neoplasms of childhood, the use of radiotherapy and surgery may be extremely valuable in reducing tumor bulk. The use of these modalities in combination with chemotherapy has resulted in prolonged disease-free survivals in pa-tients with embryonal rhabdomyosarcoma, Ewing's sarcoma, Wilms' tumor, neuroblastoma, and various lymphomas. Occasionally, surgical resection of solitary and, rarely, multiple metastases has been associated with successful control of disease in patients with carcinomas or sarcomas. More often, the role of surgery or radiotherapy in patients with advanced cancer is to offer palliation for obstruction or compression of vital structures, persistent bleeding, or intractable pain. Although the use of chemotherapy with cytotoxic agents is also predominantly palliative, significant improvements in survival have been obtained in patients with several types of tumors. Indeed, it is now possible to list more than ten disseminated neoplastic diseases in which chemotherapy, alone or in combination with other modalities, has resulted in a normal life expectancy for some patients. In addition to those mentioned above, these include choriocarcinoma in women, acute lymphoblastic leukemia of childhood, testicular carcinomas, Hodgkin's disease, Burkitt's lymphoma, mycosis fungoides, and diffuse histiocytic lymphoma. In most cases these cures have been achieved through the use of combination chemotherapy. The rationale for treatment with multiple cytotoxic agents in combination stems from the concept of achieving total cell-kill without development of drug-resistant tumor cell lines. Since tumors may contain heterogeneous populations of cells with varying sensitivities to different drugs, each of which destroys a constant percentage, rather than a constant number, of tumor cells, successful cytoreductive chemotherapy depends upon effective combination or rational sequences of cytotoxic agents. Because most potent antineoplastic drugs may cause profound suppression of immune responses, intensive cytoreductive therapy may further compromise the ability of the host to withstand both infection by microorganisms and recurrence of the neoplastic process. Accordingly, the role of immunotherapy appears promising in these circumstances and is currently being investigated. The effective management of the patient with disseminated disease depends upon sound clinical judgment and knowledge of the fundamental principles involved in the chemotherapeutic triangle.

THE CHEMOTHERAPEUTIC TRIANGLE

When using cytotoxic agents, the physician should always keep in mind the three principal entities involved in the chemotherapeutic triangle: (1) the host, (2) the drug, and (3) the tumor (Fig. 1). It should be noted that, with the exception of the pharmacologic considerations inherent in the use of *chemical* cytotoxic agents, the same principles apply to the use of irradiation, a *physical* cytotoxic agent.

A series of primary effects and secondary responses involving these factors are illustrated in Figure 1. The relative preponderance or effectiveness of these interactions determines the final outcome for patients receiving chemotherapy. The effect of the tumor on the host is recognized as the "disease." The effects of the drug on the tumor are called "therapy," and those on the host are designated as "toxicity." The tumor may escape from the effects of the drug by one or more mechanisms of resistance. Although the mechanisms for natural and acquired resistance to drugs are not completely established, increased levels of target en-

Figure 1.   The chemotherapeutic triangle.

zyme, deficiency of enzymes required for "lethal synthesis" of the active agent, impaired transport into cells, and increased catabolism of the drug have all been implicated. These and other mechanisms are usually exerted through selection by the drug of resistant cells, as a result of elimination of the susceptible population. The host responds to the toxic effects of the drug by metabolizing and eliminating the compound from the body. It is necessary therefore to be familiar with the mechanisms of detoxification and route of elimination of the drugs administered, as well as with the functional status of the organs involved. This is particularly true for cytotoxic agents, because the therapeutic:toxic ratio is small and the margin for error is slight.

Least understood are the defenses of the host against the tumor, although some degree of natural resistance and considerable variation between different individuals and types of tumors have been recognized for a long time. Recently, specific immunologic mechanisms have received considerable attention, and the importance of cell-mediated immunity through lymphocytes and monocytes has been clearly established. The role of humoral antibodies, on the other hand, may be beneficial to the host when "cytotoxic antibodies" are present, or protective for the tumor when "blocking factors" are involved. Even more nebulous are nonspecific host defense mechanisms, including interferon, local inflammatory responses, phagocytic activity, reticuloendothelial system function, and others yet to be explored. Administration of cytotoxic agents to the host, whether drugs or irradiation, may have profound effects on host defenses, thereby altering a delicate balance that may exist between host and tumor. It is important to remember that these relationships also apply to other parasitic infestations in the body, including viruses, fungi, and bacterial microorganisms. Accordingly, suppression of host defenses may not only facilitate tumor growth, but may render the host more susceptible to infectious complications by pathogenic bacteria or opportunistic organisms. It is of consider-

able importance, therefore, for the medical oncologist to understand the fundamental principles and current applications of tumor immunology, as well as their interaction with antineoplastic therapy.

IMMUNE SURVEILLANCE OF CANCER

The immune surveillance theory first proposed by Burnet and Thomas holds that cancer arises because of a defect in ability of the patient to mount an effective and appropriate defense. The theory further asserts that incipient neoplasms frequently develop in all individuals but never become evident because they are destroyed by the immune system. A corollary of the theory is that cancer cells have antigens that are recognized as foreign by the immune system of the cancer patient. The prototype for the immune response that destroys cancer is the homograft reaction: the ability of the recipient to reject a tissue graft donated by another unrelated member of the same species. Although the mechanisms whereby rejection is accomplished are complex and dependent upon the type of tissue being transplanted, the model for the immune surveillance theory is skin graft rejection, which has been shown to be mediated by T lymphocytes. It has even been suggested that the ability of T lymphocytes to destroy grafts occurred in evolution as a response to the development of neoplasia, an event thought to be of relatively recent occurrence and thus confined to the more advanced species.

Evidence for the immune surveillance theory came from both clinical and experimental observations. It was noted that children with various immunodeficiency diseases have a higher than expected incidence of neoplastic disease, especially of tissues of the immune system. In addition, recipients of kidney transplants, who have been treated with immunosuppressive drugs for long periods of time, also develop cancer at a greater frequency than normal, although these tend to be of either lymphoid or histiocytic origin or else relatively benign, epithelial carcinomas.

Laboratory evidence for the immune surveillance theory was derived from work in animals demonstrating that neonatal thymectomy increases susceptibility to development and growth of certain experimentally induced cancers. This is particularly true for tumors induced by oncogenic DNA viruses.

In recent years, a number of findings have contributed to a decline in popularity of the immune surveillance theory. It is now known that development of T cell immunity and neoplasia are not linked in evolution. Patients who are immunodeficient either by disease or by treatment are not universally more susceptible than normal to development of cancer, but rather to those neoplasms originating in cells of the immune system. It has also been demonstrated that the generalization that patients with cancer, or individuals at high risk of developing cancer, are immunodeficient is incorrect. The concept of immune surveillance has recently been challenged by experimental data. Neonatal thymectomy appears to increase susceptibility to cancer induced by DNA viruses, not to those tumors arising either spontaneously or under the influence of other types of carcinogens. This suggests that depression of antiviral, rather than antitumor, immunity is the basis for the increased incidence. It has also been reported that the incidence of either spontaneous or induced cancer in immunodeficient, athymic, "nude" mice is very low, perhaps lower than that of normal mouse populations.

The complexities that make the simplicity of the immune surveillance theory no longer completely tenable are best illustrated by Prehn's immune stimulation theory. This states that interaction of the immune system with cancer may be bimodal, acting at times, especially early in tumor development or in the presence of "weak" immunity, to stimulate and at other times to inhibit cancer growth. Both lymphocytes and serum antibody have been shown capable of stimulating tumor cell division in experimental systems. Immunization of animals with preparations of experimental tumors may sometimes result in "enhancement," i.e., induction of increased susceptibility to growth of the tumors, as compared to growth in nonstimulated mice. Newer investigations into the interaction of the various components of the immune system have also shown that the action of immune effectors able to inhibit tumor growth can be nullified by other blocking or feedback-interfering immune elements, both humoral and cellular. Thus it is not clear at this time how the immune system influences development or growth of cancer. With some kinds of tumors it may indeed play a pivotal role; in others the immune properties may be incidental or unique to that particular neoplasm and not related to the natural development or growth of the tumor. Nevertheless, it may still be possible to take advantage of the existence of immune properties in a specific cancer for establishing diagnosis, assessing prognosis, or administering therapy. Accordingly, it is important to be familiar with the methods used for measuring immune competence in patients with cancer and to understand their relationship to prognosis and therapy.

IMMUNE COMPETENCE IN PATIENTS WITH CANCER

ASSESSMENT OF GENERAL IMMUNE COMPETENCE. Several different approaches are currently used to measure general immune competence. The most direct is enumeration of either the total number or some subpopulation of peripheral lymphocytes. For example, human T lymphocytes are detected by their ability to form rosettes with sheep red blood cells, and B lymphocytes can be counted as the number of cells with immunoglobulin molecules or complement receptors on their surfaces. Other techniques are being investigated to detect smaller lymphoid cell subpopulations. Total serum immunoglobulin and complement levels can also be determined.

Another type of assay often used is the ability of patients' peripheral lymphocytes to respond by blastogenesis and proliferation to incubation with various mitogens such as phytohemagglutinin (PHA) and concanavalin A (Con A). Typically this reaction is measured by uptake of tritiated thymidine. Both PHA and Con A have been regarded as mitogens for T cells, or subpopulations of T cells, but there is evidence that monocytes may be involved in the response and that B cells can also respond under certain conditions. There is no universally accepted B cell mitogen for humans such as bacterial endotoxin lipopolysaccharide (LPS),

which is used for this purpose in mice. Lymphocyte blastogenesis can also be assessed by reactivity to specific antigens to which nearly all people have been exposed, such as *Candida albicans*.

A third method used to assess general immune competence is the skin test for delayed hypersensitivity, detected by the appearance of erythema and induration 48 hours after intradermal injection or surface application of antigen. Two types of antigens are used: (1) A battery of "recall" antigens to which most people have been exposed in earlier life. These include standard tests to dermatophyton, mumps, tuberculin, streptokinase-streptodornase (Varidase), *Candida albicans,* and, depending upon geographical location, coccidiodin and histoplasmin. (2) An antigen to which very few people have ever been exposed and which can therefore be used to measure primary sensitization. For this purpose 2,4-dinitrochlorobenzene (DNCB) is most often used. Sensitization is achieved by the application of 2000 μg of DNCB dissolved in 0.1 ml acetone to the volar aspect of one arm, previously cleansed with acetone. The extent of exposure is confined by a 2.2-cm diameter plastic ring. The acetone is evaporated and a dressing placed on the site for 48 hours. Simultaneously the patient is tested for previous sensitization by applying doses of 100 and 50 μg of DNCB to the ipsilateral forearm. If no reaction has appeared in 48 to 72 hours, the patient is considered not to have been previously sensitized. Fourteen days after sensitization, challenge doses of 100 and 50 μg are again applied to the ipsilateral forearm, occluded for 24 hours, and observed at 48 and 72 hours for the occurrence of a positive reaction consisting of induration present in an erythematous area involving at least half the size of the test site.

ASSESSMENT OF SPECIFIC ANTITUMOR IMMUNITY. Although tests of general immune competence are frequently used to measure immune function in cancer patients, detection of reactivity to specific tumor antigens might be more useful clinically. Four types of assays have been used in attempts to measure specific antitumor immunity using tumor cells or extracts as antigens: (1) skin tests, (2) cytotoxicity tests, (3) blastogenesis assays, and (4) leukocyte migration and adherence inhibition assays. None of these assays are suitable for routine clinical use. Technical problems inherent in the methods explored to date and difficulties encountered in defining tumor-specific antigens are major obstacles.

RELATIONSHIP OF IMMUNE COMPETENCE TO TYPE OF NEOPLASTIC DISEASE. Patients with cancer are not, as a group, immunologically incompetent. Thus patients with early stage carcinoma of the breast, lung, or colon, melanoma, and sarcoma, or individuals who have been successfully treated for these diseases, show normal range responses to tests of immune competence. An exception to these observations is found in patients with squamous carcinoma of the pelvic or head and neck regions, who often demonstrate depression in cellular immunity independent of disease status. Patients with Hodgkin's disease, especially those with the lymphocyte-depleted type, are frequently deficient in cellular reactivity and hypersensitivity. The depression of reactivity does not correlate, however, with clinical course or survival. Patients with leukemia, myeloma, or lymphoma may exhibit defects in both cellular and humoral immunity. It is often difficult to discriminate between pre-existing defects of immune competence and the results of therapy or secondary effects of neoplasia.

RELATIONSHIP OF IMMUNE COMPETENCE TO PROGNOSIS. The fact that general immunologic incompetence in patients with cancer cannot be demonstrated raises the question of the significance of this finding when it is observed. In particular, it is important to know whether depressed reactivity can be used to identify patients whose prognosis is poor or who may have already developed subclinical recurrence. The many technical difficulties involved in immunologic testing and the wide range in responsiveness of both cancer and normal populations have made this a difficult question to study. Failure to become sensitized to DNCB seems to predict clinical relapse in a variety of neoplasms within six months of testing, whereas sensitization is associated with freedom from disease. Survival in patients with carcinoma of the breast and lung correlates best with PHA-induced blastogenesis. Assessment of reactivity in individual patients, however, is further complicated by the large variability in different studies, and multiple, sequential tests are necessary to obtain the true picture of a given patient's responsiveness. Thus there is no proof that tests of immune competence are clinically useful, regardless of what they may indicate about the biology of neoplasia.

RELATIONSHIP OF IMMUNE COMPETENCE TO CYTOTOXIC THERAPY. The immune competence of a patient with cancer may interact with cytotoxic therapy in several ways. Patients who demonstrate a positive response to various tests of immune function are more likely to respond favorably to chemotherapy than those who are immunologically incompetent. A positive correlation between active immune response and successful results with chemotherapy has been observed in women with choriocarcinoma, a tumor characterized by paternal histocompatibility antigens foreign to the host.

When administering cytotoxic therapy, special attention should be given to dosage schedules. Many experimental studies have shown that cytotoxic drugs at dosage schedules producing only slight immunosuppression are more efficacious than are protocols designed to achieve maximal tumor cell-kill, but which may also produce marked immunosuppression. Thus very high and protracted doses of drug may be less effective than lower doses in controlling disease, although more capable of killing tumor cells. Drug schedules can also be manipulated so that antitumor immune responses are amplified while other immune factors that block effective immunity are suppressed. This phenomenon, called selective immune suppression, is accompanied by an enhanced inhibition of tumor growth. Such effects have been demonstrated for cyclophosphamide, cytarabine, melphalan, and a combination of methotrexate and 5-fluorouracil. Accordingly, the immunosuppressive properties of many antineoplastic agents can be used, paradoxically, to strengthen host immunity.

Clinically, it is known that intermittent administration of high doses of cytotoxic drugs is less immunosuppressive than frequent administration of small doses. Generally speaking, immune function may be severely depressed during the course of treatment, but rapidly rebounds during the next few weeks. Tests of lymphocyte function usually show depressed reactivity within a month or so after major surgery to remove a tumor mass, but the tests return to normal in patients who remain clinically free of disease. This phenomenon may be related to anesthesia, stress, or negative nitrogen balalance. Local radiotherapy for carcinoma of the breast, lung, and laryngopharynx has been reported to result in prolonged lymphopenia and depression of cellular immune function. All three therapeutic modalities are often used aggressively in sequential combinations in an effort to achieve total cell-kill of the neoplastic process. It is particularly unfortunate that these deleterious effects are inflicted upon the immune competence of the host at a time when the total tumor cell burden may be lowest and the possibility of immunologic benefits is highest. Whether immunostimulatory procedures can be helpful at this point is a subject of current investigation.

CONCEPT OF TOTAL CELL-KILL

In order to achieve complete cure of a neoplastic process, every last clonogenic cell, i.e., one capable of giving rise to malignant proliferating daughter cells, must be eradicated. This may be attained surgically when the entire cancer can be excised or it may be accomplished by x-irradiation if sufficient mean lethal doses can be delivered without irreversible damage to normal tissues, so that less than one tumor cell remains. Although the same principles are applicable to chemotherapy, the result has been more difficult to achieve. This is both due to the limitations of currently available cytotoxic agents and because medical oncologists are too often asked to treat patients when the neoplastic process is large, widely disseminated, and not amenable to surgery or radiotherapy.

A number of fundamental principles established by Skipper and his colleagues, using the experimental leukemia L1210 model, offer an excellent basis for understanding the problems involved, and appear to have valid clinical implications. Briefly condensed, they are as follows: (1) A single clonogenic leukemia cell is capable, through its progeny, of producing enough cells eventually to kill the host; (2) the life span of the host is inversely related to either the number of leukemia cells inoculated or the number remaining at the end of therapy; (3) first-order kinetics obtain with respect to leukemic cell-kill by chemotherapy i.e., a given dose of a given drug kills a constant percentage of cells, not a constant number, regardless of the cell numbers present at the time of therapy (fractional kill hypothesis); (4) it is possible to calculate the chances of killing the last cell in populations that are homogeneous with respect to drug sensitivity; and (5) host immune defenses can be augmented, but are detectable only when small numbers of leukemic cells remain. This model has been a major contribution to the rationale of modern antineoplastic therapy and also emphasizes the important need to quantify reliably subclinical numbers of viable clonogenic cells through the use of appropriate tumor cell markers.

TUMOR CELL MARKERS

It is clear that a reliable assay for determining surviving tumor cells would be a highly desirable guide for effective chemotherapy. An important example of a useful marker has been available for trophoblastic tumors of women. In patients with choriocarcinoma and related disorders, it is possible to measure quantitatively human chorionic gonadotropins (hCG) in the urine. This enables assessment of the amount of tumor remaining after each course of treatment and continuation of chemotherapy until the assay indicates that all tumor cells have been killed. Other sensitive markers that may be produced by tumor cells are discussed in Ch. 524. In certain leukemias and lymphomas, rough approximations of cell-kill can be made by counting the number of abnormal cells in the peripheral blood and the marrow or measuring changes in size of visible tumors Some of these neoplasms have responded most successfully to chemotherapy, not only because we are able to monitor the presence of residual tumor cells, but more important, because they are characterized by rapid growth and are more susceptible to cytotoxic drugs. In order to begin to understand the reasons underlying the results obtained with cytotoxic agents, it is essential to have a basic knowledge of cell-cycle kinetics.

CELL-CYCLE KINETICS

The percentage of cells in a tumor or a normal organ undergoing division at any given time represents the *growth fraction* or *proliferating pool*. The larger the growth fraction, the more rapid the growth. Since our most effective cytotoxic agents kill cells that are undergoing DNA synthesis and mitosis, the tumors with larger growth fractions are more susceptible to currently available drugs. These include choriocarcinoma in women, acute lymphocytic leukemia, lymphocytic lymphosarcoma, Burkitt's lymphoma, reticulum cell sarcoma (histiocytic lymphoma), Hodgkin's disease, testicular neoplasms, Wilms' tumor, and Ewing's sarcoma. Other tumors characterized by a small growth fraction, including carcinoma of the lung and various types of adenocarcinomas, are less responsive to, or not inhibited by, cytotoxic drugs. Several normal rapidly proliferating tissues, particularly the bone marrow, the epidermal appendages (hair follicles and nails), and the epithelium of the alimentary tract, are extremely sensitive to cytotoxic drugs, and often constitute the limiting factor to the amount of chemotherapy that can be administered.

The intermitotic time of proliferating cells, i.e., the average time from one mitosis to the next, can be determined by using ^{3}H-thymidine. This interval can be divided into three phases: (1) the presynthetic phase (G_1), (2) the phase of DNA synthesis (S), and (3) the postsynthetic phase (G_2). At this point in the cycle, mitosis (M) transforms one G_2-cell into two G_1-cells, and the cycle may begin again. Implicit in the discussion of growth fraction is the concept that some cells in a tumor, or a normal organ, may be resting and nonproliferating. Some may be permanently incapable of reproduction, and others may be recruited into the proliferating compartment upon receiving an appropriate, but as yet unidentified, stimulus. These recruitable cells are considered to be in a fourth phase, designated as G_0.

Cells that are in cycle are the most vulnerable to cytotoxic drugs, particularly those that are S-phase specific, such as cytarabine (ara-C) and hydroxyurea. Other drugs, including methotrexate (MTX), 5-fluorouracil

(FU), and 6-mercaptopurine (6-MP), exert their major effects during S-phase but, because of their inhibitory effects on RNA and protein synthesis, are self-limiting since they also produce delay of entry into S-phase. The vinca alkaloids are considered cell-cycle specific agents because they interfere with the process of mitosis.

Cells that are not in cycle (G_0) are almost completely insensitive to S-phase specific drugs but may still be affected by cycle-phase nonspecific agents. Alkylating agents, such as cyclophosphamide and 1,3-bis(2-chloroethyl)-1-nitrosourea (BCNU), are called cycle-phase nonspecific, because they react with DNA during any phase of the cell cycle, leading directly to the cell death or to a delayed lethal effect at mitosis. Actinomycin D and the anthracycline antibiotics, daunorubicin and Adriamycin, bind to DNA and interfere with transcription, and are also cycle-phase nonspecific.

Normal tissues with large growth fractions, such as the bone marrow, may have fewer resting cells in G_0 than a slow-growing tumor with a small growth fraction. In this situation, chemotherapy with inhibitors of DNA biosynthesis (S-phase specific drugs) probably would be ineffective, because life-threatening marrow suppression would occur before significant antineoplastic effects. By contrast, the tumors that have responded best to our present generation of cytotoxic agents probably have a larger growth fraction of clonogenic cells than the marrow stem cells of the host. In these patients, judicious administration and scheduling of selected cytotoxic agents can progressively destroy the neoplastic cells while sparing significant numbers of marrow stem cells in G_0, which subsequently could reconstitute the host hematologically.

527.2.   THERAPY BY IRRADIATION

INTRODUCTION

Radiotherapy utilizes the energy of all types of ionizing radiation, which must then be absorbed to act on living systems. The absorbed energy produces excited molecules in the form of free radicals; these interact with macromolecules within the cell to produce molecular changes. The accumulation of these changed molecules, with the resultant irreparable injuries, may produce the death of the cell during the next division. If reproductive integrity is intact, biochemical disturbances may result in defects in cell function or somatic mutations, ultimately manifested by leukemia or other neoplasms some years later. Radiotherapy attempts to impart sufficient absorbed energy within the tumor so that the cells incur such lethal damage that the number of reproducing cells is diminished to less than one.

QUALITY AND QUANTITY OF RADIATION

The short wavelength electromagnetic radiations of x-ray and gamma rays are similar. The former are produced by x-ray generators, Vandergraph generators, linear accelerators, or betatrons. Gamma rays are emitted by the radioactive decay of such elements as ^{60}cobalt, ^{137}cesium, or radium. The quality of the radiation is characterized by the energy of the wavelength.

Gamma rays from radium have a wavelength of 0.01 Å that corresponds to x-rays of 1.2 million volts, which is almost exactly the energy of ^{60}cobalt.

Corpuscular radiations produce their interaction with biologic systems by direct bombardment with electrons. Beta rays are a stream of electrons. Alpha particles are stripped helium nuclei of short range, and protons are hydrogen nuclei having a mass of 1 and carrying a charge of 1. Protons are intermediate between alpha particles and electrons in penetration and ionizing density. Neutrons produce their effect by ejecting a proton from the nucleus of an atom of the absorbing material very much as x-rays produce their effect by ejecting electrons from the atomic shell. The number of ionizations depends upon the media through which the energy passes, with more ionizations in denser material. High energy photon beams (10 MeV or higher) also produce nuclear transformations in the elements through which they pass, and this can be responsible for as much as 5 per cent of the absorbed radiation.

The depth of penetration of a photon beam or gamma ray is dependent upon its initial energy. Initially, the number of ionizations that will occur within its track is low. As the beam slows down, however, more ionizations are produced (linear energy transfer). By contrast, beta rays, which are a stream of electrons, interact heavily initially, giving up their energy within a short distance. Electron beams produced by a betatron or linear accelerator can be specifically energized to impart essentially all their ionizations within a fixed distance within the absorbing media.

The quantity of radiation delivered is expressed in units of roentgens. A roentgen is an exposure of x- or gamma radiation that produces, in 1 gram of air under standard temperature and pressure, 1 electrostatic unit of charge. This is equal to 83 ergs. In biologic systems, however, more important than the exposure dose is the amount of energy that is absorbed. This is calculated in rads, the radiation absorbed dose. One rad is equal to 100 ergs.*

BIOLOGIC EFFECTS OF RADIATION

The radiation biology of the mammalian cell in culture has been the most important tool for understanding the general principles of the relationship of radiation dose to cell survival. Cultured cells that are exposed to radiation show a mitotic delay. This mitotic delay is greatest for cells in G_2, although some delay occurs also in S phase. G_1 cells appear to "catch up" as they move through S phase and G_2 phase to enter mitosis. Some cells will receive a sufficient dose to lose their reproductive integrity. These cells may go through one or two cycles before losing their clonogenic potential. Other cells may never experience a full division but will develop into multinucleated giant cells.

The surviving fraction of cells is a dose- (D) related phenomenon (Fig. 2). There is a shoulder to the curve, which represents the ability of a cell to repair sublethal

*In keeping with an agreement of the International Commission on Radiological Units, the rad is to be replaced with a unit that is consistent with the International System of Units and will be called the Gray, in honor of L. H. Gray, the radiation physicist and radiation biologist. It will be calculated in joules per gram per second.

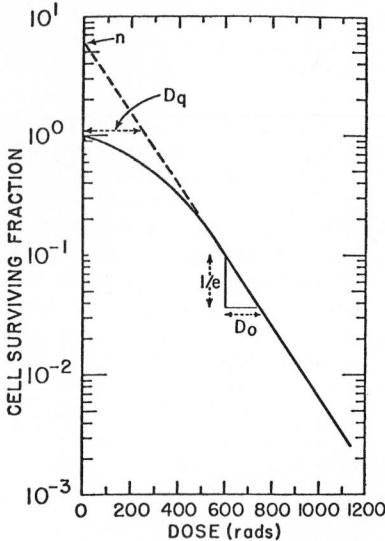

Figure 2.   Radiation dose-response curve.

injury, the so-called D_q (quasi-threshold dose). Beyond this shoulder, there is an exponential relationship between the increase in dose and the decrease in survival. The steeper the slope, the more radiosensitive the cells. In the exponential component of the curve, a dose (D_0) can be determined which reduces the cell population to 37 per cent of the initial population $\left(\dfrac{N_s}{N_0} = 0.37 = e^{-1}\right)$, where N_s = surviving number of cells and N_0 = original number of cells. The D_0 is characteristic of the mammalian cell in the particular culture system and varies between 100 and 200 rads for most cells, malignant or normal. The exponential part of the curve can be extrapolated back to the abscissa to determine the extrapolation number for this system. The extrapolation number also has a rather finite limit of between two and ten. The D_q rarely exceeds 150 to 200 rads under most cell culture conditions. Cells that survive a dose of radiation and maintain their reproductive integrity retain the identical radiation characteristics that they had before the initial dose of irradiation. The D_q, the extrapolation number, and the D_0 remain the same for subsequent doses of irradiation as long as the cell maintains its reproductive capacity.

Several mechanisms may affect the surviving fraction of cells. Synchronous cells in culture show increased radiation sensitivity in G_2 and diminished sensitivity in S. Changes in the dose rate can affect radiation sensitivity. Approximately twice the dose of radiation is required to produce the same decrease in surviving fractions with 10 rads per hour as with 50 rads per hour. Alteration of the physiologic conditions under which the cells are irradiated also affects the surviving fraction. The most important factor that can alter cell survival is the presence or absence of oxygen. The importance of the oxygen effect in radiotherapy is derived from the diminished oxygenation of tumor cells in the center of the tumor. The hypoxic tumor cells may be the critical factor in determining the local curability of a tumor by radiotherapy. While the well oxygenated cells may be destroyed, the protected anoxic cells may survive. A three-fold enhancement of radiation effect can be obtained by going from anoxic to hyperoxic state during irradiation. The more oxygen present, the greater the number of free radicals and therefore the greater the radiation effect. Currently, electrophilic chemical agents such as metronidazole, which contribute free radicals, are being investigated. Alternatively, a physical approach to the problem has been attempted with fast neutrons. Because of the intensity of the local radiation caused by the nuclear change in proton production, neutron irradiation overcomes the tissue's oxygen dependence for radiation effect, eliminating the oxygen enhancement ratio.

CLINICAL APPLICATIONS OF RADIATION

One of the most successful clinical methods of destroying a local tumor by radiation is to fractionate the dose. The dose selected must have high probability of producing at least one log-kill per treatment. Although a proportion of the injury is repaired between treatments, fractionation also allows for reoxygenation of cells within the tumor, so that their sensitivity will improve with each treatment. Using skin erythema, skin tolerance, and cure of cancer as criteria, good correlation can be obtained for a linear relationship between the total dose and the over-all time in which the dose is delivered. In 1944, Strangquest demonstrated that in the higher ranges, there was an increased probability of tissue necrosis, whereas in the lower ranges there was a greater probability of tumor recurrence. As an extension of this concept, Ellis was able to derive a relationship between the total dose (TD), the number of fractions (N) in which the total dose is delivered, the over-all time (T) for this, and an expression of a nominal single dose (NSD) to which this would be equivalent (NSD = TD × $N^{-0.24}$ $T^{-0.11}$). The advantage of the NSD concept is that many alternative fractionation regimens can be considered and assessed with respect to their biologic equivalence. A single dose of 2200 rads might be given to cure a small skin lesion, but 3800 rads in five sessions in a week or 6000 rads in three and one half weeks is biologically equivalent. The advantage of longer fractionation is that normal surrounding tissues are more likely to undergo repair from radiation effects. This results in good function in normal tissue with the same potential for tumor destruction. Another aspect of the selection of time-dose for tumor control is the volume that must be irradiated. Small volumes can be treated with larger fractions for a shorter length of time. Larger volumes require protraction, or the patient's tolerance will be exceeded, limiting the prospect of achieving the desired final dose in the prescribed treatment time. Not infrequently, treatment must be interrupted because of medical reasons such as bone marrow toxicity, severe nausea and vomiting, or tissue intolerance (e.g., mucositis), or as a planned approach to tumor control (i.e., split course). In this situation, the NSD concept cannot be applied directly. The Orton-Ellis modification of the NSD concept, TDF (time-dose fractionation), however, is used to add up the doses in order that a biologic equivalency can be determined for a split course and a continuous course of irradiation (TDF = $NSD^{1.538}$ × 10^{-3}).

Radiotherapy for curative management of tumors is clinically useful alone, or in combination with surgery and chemotherapy, either before or after each of these modalities. In the past, postoperative radiation was frequently used in attempts to enhance the prospect of local control of many tumors, including those involving the head and neck, breast, or gastrointestinal tract. In most instances, postoperative radiotherapy has not been particularly successful in adding to the survival of patients, except perhaps in carcinoma of the head and neck. Of continuing interest has been preoperative radiotherapy, which is being used with some success in carcinoma of the rectum, head and neck, esophagus, and bladder. Radiation alone has produced significant cure rates in early head and neck cancer, cervical cancer, and the lymphomas, especially Stage I and II Hodgkin's disease. Another important role of radiation is in the palliative management of incurable disease. Painful bone metastases, neurologic defects resulting from brain metastases or cord compression, hemoptysis, melena, superior vena cava compression, and other clinical complications of neoplasia can be managed effectively and rapidly by radiotherapy.

TOXIC EFFECTS OF RADIATION

The limiting factor in management of most lesions is the tolerance of the normal surrounding tissue. When compared with tumors, most organs have an increased radiosensitivity. Radiation-induced injury is usually irreversible and may prove catastrophic. Since many patients are currently receiving either concurrent or adjuvant chemotherapy, and interaction of radiotherapy with chemotherapeutic agents may produce increased toxicity, the concepts of radiation and drug sensitivity must be constantly re-evaluated. Although 4000 to 4500 rads in four to five weeks is a tolerable dose on the myocardium, it may be toxic in combination with doxorubicin. A dose of 1200 to 1500 rads on the lung may produce irreversible radiation pneumonitis when administered to patients receiving dactinomycin, cyclophosphamide, or bleomycin. Transient dementia occurs in patients who have received 3000 rads whole brain irradiation and high dose methotrexate.

Another serious long range consequence of radiation is carcinogenesis. In the past, radiation was frequently used for the management of benign conditions such as tonsillitis, enlarged thymus of infancy, acne, bursitis, and arthritis. Radiation-induced neoplasms have included osteogenic sarcoma and carcinomas of the skin and of the breast. Children who received radiation for tonsillitis or enlarged thymus have a thousand-fold increased risk of thyroid carcinoma, and those treated for tinea capitis have an increased incidence of meningiomas.

In the management of neoplastic disease, however, second primaries are less frequent, probably because the higher doses delivered produce lethal injuries to cells and do not allow propagation of a neoplastic somatic mutation. Although there is a four-fold increase in pelvic neoplasms in women who received 2000 rads for the management of metrorrhagia or endometriosis, there is no increase in pelvic neoplasms or leukemia in women who have been successfully treated for carcinoma of the cervix with doses of 6000 rads of external radiotherapy plus intracavitary radium. An appreciable increase in acute myelogenous leukemia has been reported, however, in patients treated for Hodgkin's disease with the combination of total nodal irradiation and chemotherapy with MOPP, as compared with either modality alone.

The increased success of combination treatments in otherwise fatal neoplasms may elicit more examples of combined toxicity in the future. An awareness that this potential hazard exists need not be an absolute deterrent to the use of combined therapy until equally successful alternative modes of treatment have been established.

527.3. THERAPY WITH CYTOTOXIC DRUGS

INTRODUCTION

Although all active drugs exert a certain degree of toxicity on some cells in the body, the term *cytotoxic drugs* usually denotes those compounds that affect the proliferative capacity of cells by their inhibitory action on DNA, RNA, or protein biosynthesis. Accordingly, they are sometimes also called *antiproliferative agents.* The desired result is selective cell death, with destruction of malignant neoplastic cells and relative sparing of viability and function of normal cells. From the large number of compounds studied in experimental systems, only a few have demonstrated sufficient clinical antineoplastic activity, at acceptable levels of toxicity, to deserve the designation of *chemotherapeutic agents.*

Because these drugs inhibit biochemical sites that are not unique to cancer cells, they have also proved valuable in the management of several non-neoplastic disorders. Among these are certain conditions characterized by altered immune reactivity, including those observed in recipients of organ transplantations and in patients afflicted with connective tissue or autoimmune diseases. The term *immunosuppressive agents* has been used properly to describe drugs capable of suppressing

measurable immune responses. It is an oversimplification, however, to attribute all beneficial effects of these drugs to suppression of the immune responses, because this does not take into consideration their anti-inflammatory action or selective enhancement and alterations of complex cellular and humoral immunologic interactions that are probably involved in these disorders.

Other non-neoplastic conditions that have been markedly improved by drugs originally developed for *cancer chemotherapy* include metabolic disorders, such as hyperuricemia and gout, dermatologic diseases, such as psoriasis, and infections caused by DNA viruses and other microorganisms. For these reasons, antiproliferative agents are attracting increasing interest, and their practical importance has expanded beyond the treatment of neoplastic disorders into many other areas of medicine.

SELECTION OF PATIENTS

Proper use of cytotoxic agents requires more than a knowledge of their pharmacology. The physician must be thoroughly familiar with the natural history and pathophysiology of the disease before undertaking therapy. Most important is a careful evaluation of each patient in order to determine the benefit:risk ratio. Special attention must be directed toward factors that may potentiate acute toxicity. Among these, the presence of overt or occult infections, bleeding dyscrasias, poor nutritional status, and severe metabolic disturbances are important considerations. The functional condition of the major organs involved in metabolism and elimination of drugs, usually the liver and kidneys, must be determined. Of cardinal importance is the status of the bone marrow, which may be compromised by the disease process, earlier chemotherapy, or previous irradiation, particularly to the spine or pelvis. Cytotoxic agents have a potential risk for teratogenesis, mutagenesis, and carcinogenesis. Their use during pregnancy or during the reproductive years should be undertaken only after thoughtful consideration and appropriate precautions. In the selection of adjuvant chemotherapy for patients with only moderate risk of tumor recurrence, the possible carcinogenic hazard of some of these compounds is an important consideration. Predictive tests for tumor sensitivity or selective immunosuppression are still research endeavors, but rational selection of patients for chemotherapy is feasible with the judicious application of available clinical and pharmacologic information.

CLASSIFICATION OF DRUGS

Alkylating Agents

Alkylating agents were studied extensively during World War II in programs concerned with chemical warfare research. They became generally available in 1946, when secrecy restrictions were removed. Hundreds of biologically active compounds have been synthesized, using modifications of the basic chemical structure. A number of substances occurring naturally, including certain antimicrobial drugs with antineoplastic activity, such as mitomycin C, porfiromycin, and streptozotocin, probably function as alkylating agents.

Cytotoxic and Immunosuppresive Agents

I. Alkylating agents:	II. Antimetabolites:	III. Natural products:	
Nitrogen mustards	Folic acid analogue	Vinca alkaloids	
Mechlorethamine	Methotrexate	Vinblastine	
Cyclophosphamide		Vincristine	
Melphalan	Pyrimidine analogues		
Uracil mustard	Fluorouracil	Enzyme	
Chlorambucil	Fluorodeoxyuridine	Asparaginase	
	Fluorocytosine		
Ethylenimine	Trifluorothymidine	Antibiotics	
derivatives	Cytaribine	Dactinomycin	
TEM	Azaribine	Daunorubicin	
Thiotepa	Idoxuridine	Doxorubicin	
		Mithramycin	
		Bleomycin	
		Mitomycin C	
Alkyl sulfonate	Purine analogues	IV. Miscellaneous	
Busulfan	Mercaptopurine	agents:	
	Azathioprine	Hydroxyurea	
Nitrosoureas	Thioguanine	Procarbazine	
Carmustine	Adenine	Mitotane	
Lomustine	arabinoside	cis-Platinum	
Semustine			
Streptozotocin			
Triazenes			
Dacarbazine			

Five major types of alkylating agents have established clinical usefulness: (1) the nitrogen mustards, (2) the ethylenimines, (3) the alkyl sulfonates, (4) the nitrosoureas, and (5) the triazenes. The mechanism of cytotoxic action is thought to be similar for most of the agents in this class.

Most alkylating agents, except busulfan, generate highly reactive electrophilic carbonium ions that alkylate, by forming covalent linkages, with various nucleophilic substances. Although many biologically important groups may be targets for the reaction, it is thought that one of the most significant sites is the strongly nucleophilic 7 nitrogen of the purine base, guanine. This could lead to miscoding errors or depurination and, in the case of bifunctional alkylating agents, to cross-linking of adjacent macromolecules, which would interfere with normal mitosis by preventing separation of the strands of DNA. Polyfunctional alkylating agents are more cytotoxic than monofunctional alkylators, although the latter may cause mutagenic and carcinogenic damage that is not lethal to the cell and can therefore be reproduced indefinitely as an inherited mutation. Cells are most susceptible to cytotoxic action of nitrogen mustards or alkyl sulfonates when they are in G_1 or in mitosis (M). Progression from G_1 and S phases to mitosis is impaired after exposure to nitrosoureas, nitrogen mustards, and ethylenimine derivatives. Inhibition of mitosis with double complement of DNA and continuing synthesis of RNA and protein can lead to unbalanced growth, giant cells, and lethal cytotoxicity. Nonproliferating cells in G_0 can also be destroyed by alkylating agents. Cell death may occur during interphase, when many sites, including RNA and protein, are damaged, or may be delayed until mitosis when only cross-linking of DNA has occurred. Lymphocytes appear to be most sensitive to rapid cellular disintegration and lysis by highly reactive nitrogen mustards, whereas busulfan is more toxic to granulocytes. Suppression of the immune response may be pronounced, and depression of erythropoiesis and of platelet production also occur. The intestinal mucosa, the hair follicles, and the reproductive system can be damaged to varying degrees by different drugs in this class.

NITROGEN MUSTARDS. Mechlorethamine (Mustargen, HN₂). The first of the nitrogen mustards to be used clinically, this compound is often abbreviated as HN₂, its chemical warfare code name. Mechlorethamine is a highly reactive agent and a powerful vesicant. For this reason, it is usually administered intravenously (0.4 mg per kilogram)* into the tubing of a rapidly flowing intravenous infusion. Since thrombosis and thrombophlebitis may occur when relatively high concentrations of the drug are in prolonged and direct contact with the intima of the injected vein, its administration into areas of elevated venous pressure, such as superior vena caval obstruction resulting from mediastinal tumors, must be avoided. The use of surgical gloves is advised to protect the hands of the physician preparing and administering the solution. The drug must be dissolved and administered in a few minutes, because it decomposes on standing. Within a few min-

utes after administration, the drug is no longer detectable in active form and is bound to proteins or intracellular macromolecules. Less than 0.01 per cent is excreted in the urine. HN₂ has been administered intraarterially, using techniques involving isolation and perfusion of a tumor-bearing area. The intracavitary use of mechlorethamine (0.2 to 0.4 mg per kilogram) after drainage of malignant pleural effusions can be an effective palliative measure. Intraperitoneal administration is often accompanied by severe gastrointestinal toxicity and is not recommended. Very dilute solutions (0.25 per cent) can be painted on the skin of patients with generalized mycosis fungoides with good results.

The major indications for HN₂ are in the treatment of generalized (Stage III and IV) Hodgkin's disease and other lymphomas, alone or in combination with other agents. The usual dose is 0.4 mg per kilogram administered as a single intravenous dose, because divided consecutive daily doses merely prolong the duration of nausea and vomiting, a direct central nervous system side effect which regularly follows administration of the drug. Premedication with a short-acting barbiturate and an antiemetic is recommended. When extensive neoplastic infiltration of the marrow is suspected, as in malignant lymphoma, lymphocytic type, a reduced dose of 0.2 or 0.3 mg per kilogram is recommended. Beneficial palliative results have also been observed in carcinomas of the lung, breast, and ovary and, occasionally, in less common tumors.

The most serious toxic effect of nitrogen mustard is bone marrow depression, with resultant leukopenia and thrombocytopenia. After four weeks, recovery is usually adequate to permit administration of another course. Dermatologic complications include an idiosyncratic nonrecurring maculopapular skin eruption, overt clinical manifestations of herpes zoster, and local reactions caused by extravasation and vesicant action. The last-named complication may produce a painful, tender, brawny induration, which, in severe cases, may slough. If accidental extravasation occurs, the area should be promptly infiltrated with a sterile isotonic solution of sodium thiosulfate (1/6 molar), or normal saline if this is not immediately available, and an ice compress should be applied intermittently for six to twelve hours.

Cyclophosphamide (Cytoxan, Endoxan). Originally devised as a carrier or transport form of nitrogen mustard, cyclophosphamide is activated by enzymatic cleavage of the phosphorus-nitrogen linkage within the molecule. Although levels of phosphatases and phosphamidases capable of accomplishing this cleavage may be relatively high in some tumors, no evidence for this type of selective activity has been observed and the drug is mainly activated in the liver. Since this occurs through the drug-metabolizing microsomal oxidase system, it is subject to the influence of other compounds that affect these systems. Barbiturates stimulate these enzymes and would increase the activation and toxicity of cyclophosphamide, whereas corticosteroid and sex hormones appear to inhibit the effect. Since cyclophosphamide is frequently used in patients also receiving corticosteroid therapy, special caution is necessary, because a reduction in steroid dosage may increase the toxicity of a previously well-tolerated dose of the alkylating agent. After oral admininistration, maximal plasma levels are achieved in approximately one hour. Disappearance from the plasma is rapid, with a half-life of

*For conversion of milligrams per kilogram of body weight to milligrams per square meter of body surface, a ratio of 1:30 may be used. The conversion factor varies between 1:20 and 1:40, depending on age and body build.

about four hours; urinary recovery of unchanged drug is less than 14 per cent.

The major advantage of cyclophosphamide is its versatility which permits a wide, intermediate range of activity, extending from that of the highly reactive intravenous mechlorethamine to that of the slow-acting oral chlorambucil. It can be administered intravenously at usual initial loading doses of 40 to 50 mg per kilogram, given at the rate of 10 to 20 mg per kilogram daily for two to five days. In patients with compromised bone marrow function, a reduction of one third to one half is recommended. Oral doses usually range between 1 and 5 mg per kilogram daily. The drug can also be administered intramuscularly or into body cavities, and is not associated with vesicant action. A good objective guide for prolonged regulation of maintenance therapy is the total leukocyte count, which should be kept between 2500 and 4000 cells per cubic millimeter.

The major clinical indications for cyclophosphamide are in the lymphoproliferative and myeloproliferative disorders. It is highly effective and has produced cures in Burkitt's lymphoma and is very beneficial in acute lymphoblastic leukemia of childhood, Hodgkin's disease, and other lymphomas. It is active in multiple myeloma, chronic lymphocytic leukemia, ovarian carcinoma, neuroblastoma, and retinoblastoma. Temporary beneficial results have also been observed in carcinoma of the breast, bronchogenic carcinoma, and other neoplasms. Because of its potent immunosuppressive action, it has been used clinically in Wegener's granulomatosis, rheumatoid arthritis, nephrotic syndrome in children, and other conditions associated with altered immune reactivity.

The most important toxic effects are on the bone marrow, but severe thrombocytopenia is probably less common than with other nitrogen mustards. By contrast, alopecia is more frequent and often more severe, though usually reversible. Nausea and vomiting are common, and mucosal ulcerations, hepatic toxicity, increased skin pigmentation, and interstitial pulmonary fibrosis have been reported. Sterile hemorrhagic cystitis, probably caused by accumulation of active metabolites in concentrated urine, has been reported in about 5 per cent of cases. Ample fluid intake and frequent voiding are helpful measures in the prevention of this complication. Because gonadal suppression resulting in sterility has been observed and the mutagenic and carcinogenic potential is high, the use of the drug in patients with reproductive capacity should be carefully considered with respect to possible benefits and risks.

Melphalan (Alkeran). This compound is a phenylalanine derivative of nitrogen mustard. It has the general pharmacologic properties of an alkylating agent of intermediate strength, demonstrating activity in the blood for about six hours. The drug can be administered orally, usually in daily divided doses of 6 mg for two to three weeks; then, after interrupting therapy for four weeks, a daily maintenance dose of 2 to 4 mg is instituted. It is particularly useful in multiple myeloma, alone or in combination with other agents. As with other alkylating agents, the clinical toxicity is mainly hematologic. Nausea and vomiting are infrequent, and alopecia does not occur.

Uracil Mustard. Although synthesized in an attempt to obtain more specificity for the alkylating moiety in pyrimidine biosynthesis, this agent behaves like other nitrogen mustards of intermediate activity. Plasma disappearance is rapid, with no detectable drug after two hours, and less than 1 per cent is recovered intact in the urine. The usual oral daily dose is 1 to 2 mg for three weeks or 3 to 5 mg for one week, with maintenance doses of 1 mg daily. The spectrum of clinical activity is similar to that of other nitrogen mustards. Bone marrow depression is the major toxic manifestation; nausea, vomiting, diarrhea, and dermatitis have been reported, but frank alopecia has not been observed.

Chlorambucil (Leukeran). An aromatic derivative of mechlorethamine, chlorambucil is the slowest-acting and least toxic nitrogen mustard in clinical use. Absorption after oral administration is good, but information on biologic persistence and elimination is inadequate. The usual oral dose is 0.1 to 0.2 mg per kilogram daily for at least three to six weeks. The total daily dose, usually 4 to 10 mg, is given at one time. The dosage is adjusted according to the clinical response, and when maintenance therapy is required, 2 mg daily is recommended. Chlorambucil is the treatment of choice in chronic lymphocytic leukemia. It is effective in Hodgkin's disease, malignant lymphoma, lymphocytic type, polycythemia vera, multiple myeloma, and, particularly, primary macroglobulinemia. It is useful in carcinoma of the ovary, breast, and testes, usually in combination with other agents. Good responses have been reported in the treatment of vasculitis as a complication of rheumatoid arthritis, and in autoimmune hemolytic anemias associated with cold agglutinins. Toxicity to the bone marrow is usually moderate, gradual, and readily reversible. Gastrointestinal and dermatologic toxicity are seldom encountered.

ETHYLENIMINES. Triethylenemelamine (TEM) and triethylenethiophosphoramide (thiotepa) have been largely replaced by the nitrogen mustards, and have similar clinical situations and toxic manifestations.

ALKYL SULFONATE. Busulfan (Myleran). The cytotoxic action of this drug is quite selective, affecting primarily granulocyte production, and, to some extent, platelets. More than 90 per cent disappears from the blood within three minutes and is almost entirely excreted in the urine as methanesulfonic acid and other metabolites. The initial oral dose is 2 to 6 mg daily, and maintenance doses of 1 to 3 mg daily are recommended. It is the treatment of choice in chronic granulocytic leukemia and may be useful in polycythemia vera and myelofibrosis with myeloid metaplasia. It is of no value in acute leukemia or in the "blastic crisis" of chronic granulocytic leukemia. Gastrointestinal toxicity is rare. Occasionally, unusual complications have been reported, including generalized hyperpigmentation of the skin, gynecomastia, cheilosis, glossitis, anhidrosis, and pulmonary fibrosis, but their relation to the drug is poorly understood.

NITROSOUREAS. Carmustine (BCNU). This compound, 1,3-bis(2-chloroethyl)-1-nitrosourea, has activity similar but not identical to that of other alkylating agents. Disappearance of BCNU from the plasma occurs within five minutes. Active metabolites are probably responsible for its cytotoxic actions; entry of these into the cerebrospinal fluid (CSF) is rapid, and levels 15 per cent to 30 per cent of plasma concentrations are achieved. The usual intravenous dose is 100 to 200 mg per square meter monthly. Nausea and vomiting usually occur in two hours. Bone marrow depression is the principal toxicity, with delayed onset and the nadir occurring after four or six weeks. Interstitial pulmonary fibrosis has been reported after long-term administration. Although useful in Hodgkin's disease, lymphomas, and occasionally in malignant melanomas and other solid tumors, the unique property of the nitrosoureas is that they cross the blood-brain barrier, probably because they are are lipid soluble, and have demonstrated some promise in the treatment of primary and metastatic brain tumors.

Lomustine (CCNU). This agent, 1-(2-chlorocthyl)-3-cyclohexyl-1-nitrosourea, is related to BCNU, but is available for oral use. It is also lipid soluble and rapidly metabolized, with prolonged plasma half-life (16 to 48 hours) of its metabolites. These products cross the blood-brain barrier quite effectively, and levels in the CSF reach 50 per cent of the concurrent plasma values. The recommended oral dose of CCNU is 130 mg per square meter, administered as a single dose and repeated every six weeks. Nausea, vomiting, and delayed bone marrow depression occur as with BCNU. Therapeutic indications include brain tumors, Hodgkin's and other lymphomas, as well as some solid tumors.

Semustine (Methyl-CCNU). This methylated analogue of CCNU was selected for clinical studies, along with the parent compound, because of superior activity to BCNU in certain experimental tumors. Semustine is also lipid soluble and so rapidly metabolized that radioactively labeled drug is not detectable in plasma, urine, or CSF, although active metabolites appear in the latter within 30 minutes in significant concentrations. The usual oral dose is 200 mg per square meter once every six weeks. The dose-limiting toxicity is delayed bone marrow depression; nausea and vomiting are frequently noted. The clinical spectrum of activities is similar to BCNU and CCNU, but initial studies indicate more favorable results with Me-CCNU, particularly in adenocarcinoma of the gastrointestinal tract.

Streptozotocin. This naturally occurring glucosamine nitrosourea is diabetogenic in animals and has been effective in patients with islet cell carcinoma of the pancreas and malignant carcinoid tumors. The half-life of the drug in plasma is approximately 15 minutes and only 10 per cent to 20 per cent is excreted unchanged in the urine. The usual dose is 1 gram per square meter intravenously or intra-arterially once a week for four weeks. Nausea and vomiting are frequently noted one to four hours after administration. Hepatic damage has been reported. Bone marrow toxicity occurs in 20 per cent of cases but is usually mild, but nephrotoxicity may be severe and often is the dose-limiting factor.

TRIAZENES. Dacarbazine (Dimethyltriazeno-imidazole Carboxamide, DTIC). Originally considered an antimetabolite, DTIC has demonstrated alkylating activity after metabolic activation in the liver, and is now thought to act by cross-linking DNA. It is not cell-cycle phase specific. After intravenous injection, plasma half-life is about 35 minutes, with 43 per cent excreted intact in the urine in six hours. Elevated urinary levels of 5-aminoimidazole-4-carboxamide (AIC) result from catabolism of DTIC and not inhibition of de novo purine biosynthesis. Intravenous daily doses of 3.5 mg per kilogram for ten days every month are recommended. It is currently the most popular drug in disseminated malignant melanoma, used alone or in combination. Bone marrow depression and gastrointestinal manifestations are the major toxic effects. Fever, myalgias, malaise, alopecia, facial flushing, hepatotoxicity, and paresthesias have been reported.

Antimetabolites

Antimetabolites of nucleic acid biosynthesis are structural analogues of normally occurring substances, metabolites. They interfere with normal biosynthesis by competing with purines, pyrimidines, and their precursors for important enzymatic reactions. They may also be incorporated into nucleic acids in place of the corresponding normal nucleotides. Although the site of action for most of them has been defined, the mechanisms of cell death are incompletely understood. Cytotoxicity may be related to unbalanced growth of cells capable of synthesizing RNA and protein, but not DNA, or to coding, transcription, or translation errors after incorporation of the analogue into DNA or RNA.

The agents with recognized clinical value may be classified as follows: (1) folic acid analogues, (2) pyrimidine analogues, and (3) purine analogues.

FOLIC ACID ANALOGUES. Methotrexate (Amethopterin). The folic acid analogues, aminopterin and subsequently methotrexate, were the first class of antimetabolites to demonstrate effective antineoplastic activity. Other "small-molecule" folate antagonists, pyrimethamine and cycloguanil, have been effective against malaria, and more recently trimethoprim has been useful in bacterial infections of the urinary and respiratory tracts. The primary site of action of methotrexate is the enzyme dihydrofolate reductase which catalyzes the reduction of dihydrofolate to tetrahydrofolate. The kinetics of this inhibition are often referred to as "pseudo-irreversible," because the binding of the inhibitor to the enzyme is tight. This interferes with the transfer of single carbon fragments and blocks the conversion of deoxyuridylate to thymidylate, blocking DNA synthesis. Although RNA and protein synthesis are also inhibited by lack of tetrahydrofolate coenzymes, the thymidylate block is considered to be the most important site of cytotoxic action leading to "thymineless death."

Methotrexate is readily absorbed after oral administration. The mean plasma half-life is approximately two hours, and about 50 per cent of the drug is bound to plasma proteins. Toxicity may be increased through displacement from plasma albumin by a number of drugs, including salicylates, sulfonamides, diphenylhydantoin, tetracycline, and chloramphenicol. Transport across the blood-brain barrier is very poor, and intrathecal administration (0.2 to 0.4 mg per kilogram) is necessary to obtain high concentrations in the cerebrospinal fluid. The major route of elimination is through the kidney, with 50 to 90 per cent of the drug excreted unchanged in the urine, usually within eight hours. Impaired renal function can produce marked increase in toxicity.

The usual daily oral dose is 2.5 to 10.0 mg. Intravenous doses of 25 to 50 mg can be given once or twice weekly. Constant daily infusions of much higher doses have been administered but only when using the technique of leucovorin "rescue."

The rationale for high-dose methotrexate is based on attaining an excess of unbound intracellular drug and thereby inhibiting DNA synthesis almost completely. In order to achieve this, any deficiency of the active, carrier-mediated, transport system must be overcome by extremely high (10^{-3} to 10^{-4} M) extracellular concentrations of methotrexate. After drug infusions ranging from 6 to 30 hours, leucovorin is given as an antidote in order to rescue normal cells and prevent undue host toxicity. When administered by experienced chemotherapists, with laboratories capable of measuring accurate plasma methotrexate concentrations, these investigational regimens are remarkably free of adverse effects. Encouraging results have been observed with these doses, as adjuvant therapy or for treatment of metastatic disease, in osteogenic sarcoma, non-Hodgkin's lymphoma, and carcinomas of the head and neck, breast, and lung. Since methotrexate precipitates in the renal tubules when the urine is acid, impaired excretion may result in life-threatening toxicity. Accordingly, it is imperative to maintain large volume outputs of alkaline urine by appropriate hydration. Because of delayed clearance, high-dose methotrexate is contraindicated in the presence of malignant effusions.

Methotrexate, at standard doses, has produced cures in women with choriocarcinoma and related trophoblastic tumors in approximately 75 per cent of the cases. It is capable of inducing complete remissions in acute lymphoblastic leukemia of childhood, but is of more value for maintenance therapy. It can be useful in Burkitt's lymphoma, mycosis fungoides, and carcinomas of the breast, testes, and oropharynx. It is also effective in severe, recalcitrant psoriasis and as an immunosuppressive agent. In addition to bone marrow depression, it causes ulcerative stomatitis and gastrointestinal toxicity. These adverse reactions can reach serious proportions and even cause death, particularly in the presence of pre-existing folate deficiency or renal insufficiency. Other complications include dermatitis, alopecia, pulmonary interstitial infiltrates, and hepatic dysfunction, sometimes leading to cirrhosis.

PYRIMIDINE ANALOGUES. Fluorouracil (FU) and Fluorodeoxyuridine (FUdR). Both the fluorinated pyrimidine base (5-FU) and its corresponding nucleoside (FUdR) are converted in vivo to 5-fluoro-2'-deoxyuridine-5'-phosphate (F-dUMP). This fraudulent nucleotide has great affinity for thymidylate synthetase, the enzyme involved in transfer of a methyl group from N^5, N^{10}-methylenetetrahydrofolic acid to deoxyuridylic acid (dUMP) in the synthesis of thymidylate. This site of action is responsible for the major cytotoxic effects by blocking DNA synthesis. Inhibition of RNA synthesis and incorporation into RNA also occur and may explain why these compounds are cycle-specific but not phase-specific agents.

These drugs are usually administered intravenously; three hours after injection, no FU can be detected in the plasma. Metabolic degradation occurs primarily in the liver, and special caution must be observed in patients with impaired liver function or extensive hepatic metastases. Approximately 15 per cent of an injected dose of FU appears intact in the urine, most of it within one hour.

The recommended dosage schedule of FU is 12 mg per kilogram intravenously daily for four days and, after toxicity has subsided, 10 to 15 mg per kilogram (not to exceed 1 gram) as a single intravenous weekly maintenance dose. FUdR can be administered either at twice the daily dose of FU intravenously or by continuous intra-arterial infusion at doses of 0.1 to 0.6 mg per kilogram daily.

FU and FUdR have been most useful in the palliative treatment of carcinomas of the breast, colon, and rectum. Occasional responses have been noted in carcinomas of the stomach, pancreas, ovary, urinary bladder, and oropharynx. Topical FU (Efudex) as a 2 or 5 per cent solution of propylene glycol or in a hydrophilic cream base has been successful in eradicating premalignant actinic keratoses, as well as superficial basal cell carcinomas.

The major toxic manifestations are bone marrow depression and ulceration of the epithelium of the alimentary tract, with stomatitis, esophagopharyngitis, nausea, vomiting, and diarrhea. The nadir of the leukopenia is between 9 and 14 days. Dermatitis, hyperpigmentation of the skin, hair loss, and nail changes have been observed.

Other Fluorinated Pyrimidines. 5-Fluorocytosine (FC) is converted to the deoxyribonucleoside (FCdR), an active antimetabolite, by fungi such as *Candida albicans*. It is administered in oral doses of 50 to 150 mg per kilogram daily for one to three months, and is useful in fungal and cryptococcal infections.

Trifluorothymidine (F_3TdR) is beneficial as an antiviral agent when applied topically to the eyes of patients with herpes simplex keratitis. It is active also against vaccinia, another DNA virus.

Cytarabine (Cytosine Arabinoside, Ara-C, Cytosar). This analogue of 2'-deoxycytidine has a structural alteration in the sugar moiety instead of the base. Although the most important site of action has not been completely established, inhibition of DNA polymerase appears to be a primary locus, a concept supported by its cytotoxic effects as an S-phase specific inhibitor. The drug is also incorporated into DNA and RNA, and blocks ribonucleotide reductase. The drug is rapidly deaminated in the blood to an inactive metabolite, uracil arabinoside, which accounts for about 90 per cent of the material in the urine. Ara-C disappears from the blood in approximately 20 minutes, but after intrathecal injection may persist for several hours because of low levels of deaminase in the CSF. The drug is administered intravenously daily for 10 to 20 days at 2 to 4 mg per kilogram, either by rapid injection or by continuous infusion. Ara-C is a potent immunosuppressive agent and, depending on the dosage schedules used, can suppress either humoral or cellular responses, or both. It is effective against DNA viruses and has been used topically with beneficial results in patients with herpes simplex keratitis. In contrast to IUdR, systemic ara-C may have greater immunosuppressive than antiviral action, with detrimental effects in disseminated herpes zoster. Although it has not proved successful against solid tumors, it is the most active drug available in acute myelogenous leukemia, and is particularly effective in combination with thioguanine. Myelosuppressive toxicity can be severe, with leukopenia, thrombocytopenia, and anemia characterized by striking megaloblastic changes. Gastrointestinal disturbances, stomatitis, thrombophlebitis, hepatic dysfunction, dermatitis, and fever have been reported.

Azaribine (Triacetyl-6-Azauridine). This triacetyl derivative of 6-azauridine blocks orotidylate decarboxylase and, thereby, the de novo synthesis of uridylate. Azaribine is well absorbed after oral administration, and provides good levels of 6-azauridine in the blood for approximately six to eight hours, almost 100 per cent of which is recovered intact in the urine. Occasionally, further metabolism to 6-azauracil, probably by gastrointestinal microorganisms, may produce reversible neurologic disturbances. The recommended oral dose is 125 mg per kilogram daily. It is extremely effective in the treatment of psoriasis and psoriatic arthritis. Recent evidence indicates that increased occurrence of thromboembolic disease in psoriasis is reduced by azaribine therapy. Relative absence of toxic manifestations makes it a safe and desirable agent, although at higher doses (270 mg per kilogram daily), it can produce reversible suppression of erythropoiesis. In this dosage it has been beneficial in patients with polycythemia vera and mycosis fungoides.

Idoxuridine (5-Iododeoxyuridine, IUdR, IDU, Stoxil, Herplex, Dendrid). Because the iodine atom in the 5-position of the pyrimidine ring is larger than hydrogen or fluorine and of similar size to the methyl group of thymine, IUdR behaves as an analogue of thymidylate, competitively inhibiting its utilization, and even replacing it in DNA. After parenteral administration, it disappears from the blood within two hours and is metabolized to, and excreted in, the urine as 5-iodouracil, uracil, and iodide. Topical therapy of herpes simplex keratitis is highly effective. Intravenous eight-hour infusions of 60 to 100 mg per kilogram daily for five days are used for systemic DNA virus infections. Beneficial results have been observed in patients with disseminated herpes zoster, vaccinia gangrenosum, and herpes simplex encephalitis. Immunosuppression has not been detected, and, in fact, immunostimulation has been noted. Major toxic manifestations include bone marrow depression, stomatitis, and alopecia. Gastrointestinal toxicity is less frequent than with FU or FUdR. Transverse ridging of the nails and sensitivity to iodine are sometimes encountered.

PURINE ANALOGUES. Mercaptopurine (6-MP, Purinethol). This antimetabolite, after formation of the 5'-phosphate ribonucleotide, blocks by "pseudo-feedback inhibition" the formation of ribosylamine-5-phosphate catalyzed by PRPP-amidotransferase, the first committed step in the de novo pathway of purine biosynthesis. It can also block the synthesis of adenylate and guanylate from the "bridgehead" nucleotide, inosinate. The drug is well absorbed after oral ingestion, and about 50 per cent of the dose is recovered in the urine in 24 hours, largely metabolized to 6-thiouric acid and inorganic sulfate. Attempts to inhibit this degradation led to the development of allopurinol (Zyloprim), a xanthine oxidase inhibitor capable of blocking the catabolism of 6-MP, as well as the formation of uric acid from hypoxanthine and xanthine. Allopurinol has become an important agent in the management of hyperuricemia and gout. The usual oral daily dose of 6-MP is 2.5 mg per kilogram, but *this must be reduced to 25 per cent when allopurinol is being administered concomitantly* at doses of 200 to 600 mg daily to reduce or prevent hyperuricemia. The major clinical indication for 6-MP is acute lymphoblastic leukemia in children. It may be useful in adults with acute leukemia or in chronic granulocytic leukemia. It is not effective in chronic lymphocytic leukemia, Hodgkin's disease, malignant lymphoma, lymphocytic type, or solid tumors. Although active as an immunosuppressive agent, 6-MP has been superseded by its imidazolyl derivative, azathioprine (Imuran). The primary toxic effect is bone marrow depression. Stomatitis and gastrointestinal symptoms are uncommon. Cholestatic jaundice has been reported in

as many as one third of adult patients; this is usually reversible upon discontinuation of therapy.

Azathioprine (Imuran). This imidazolyl derivative of 6-MP is probably the most widely used immunosuppressive agent in organ transplantation and disorders with altered immune reactivity. It is cleaved slowly to 6-MP and has similar actions, catabolism, and toxicity. The usual oral dose is 3 to 5 mg per kilogram daily, but this must also be reduced to 25 per cent if allopurinol is administered simultaneously.

Thioguanine (TG, Tabloid). In addition to being a potent "pseudofeedback inhibitor" and blocking interconversion of purines in a manner analogous to 6-MP, it is more significantly incorporated into DNA and RNA. After oral administration, peak blood levels are reached in six to eight hours, and approximately 40 per cent of the dose is excreted in the urine in 24 hours, mainly as inorganic sulfate and 2-amino-6-methylthiopurine, instead of 6-thiouric acid. Because of this, unlike 6-MP and azathioprine, no reduction in dose of TG is necessary when used together with allopurinol. The usual daily oral dose is 2 mg per kilogram. Clinically, it has a spectrum of antileukemic and immunosuppressive activity similar to that of 6-MP, and similar toxicity. It is particularly useful, together with ara-C, in acute myelogenous leukemia.

Adenine Arabinoside (Ara-A). This investigational compound appears to inhibit DNA polymerase and perhaps ribonucleotide reductase, with little effect on RNA or protein. It has demonstrated activity against several DNA viruses. Recently, beneficial effects have been reported in early herpes simplex encephalitis in humans. Doses of 15 mg per kilogram, administered daily by intravenous 12-hour infusions, are free of clinical toxicity.

Natural Products

An increasing number of naturally occurring substances have attracted attention because of their cytotoxic action. Some are derived from plants that were known for their toxic manifestations many centuries ago, such as the colchicine derivatives of the autumn crocus (*Colchicum autumnale*), and some are of more recent vintage, including the vinca alkaloids from the periwinkle (*Vinca rosea*). The enzyme asparaginase represents an interesting and unique approach to antineoplastic therapy. Finally, countless antimicrobial drugs have been isolated and tested for antitumor activity. Of these, only a few with special clinical pertinence will be discussed.

VINCA ALKALOIDS. The mechanism of action of these compounds is not clearly defined. Inhibition of the cell cycle occurs at metaphase as a result of spindle protein damage. Despite their structural similarity, remarkable differences in cytotoxic action and lack of cross-resistance have been noted among these agents. Oral absorption is unpredictable. Extravasation during intravenous injection may cause considerable irritation and should be treated with local injection of hyaluronidase and heat. The compounds are cleared in less than one hour from the blood and are excreted primarily through the biliary system. Increased toxicity may be encountered in obstructive jaundice. The drugs penetrate the blood-brain barrier poorly.

Vinblastine (Velban, VLB). This drug is administered at weekly intervals, intravenously. The initial recommended dose is 0.1 mg per kilogram, increased by weekly increments of 0.05 mg per kilogram until either moderate leukopenia or the desired beneficial effects are attained, up to a maximum of 0.5 mg per kilogram. Vinblastine is effective in the treatment of lymphomas, particularly Hodgkin's disease. Objective responses have been observed in neuroblastomas, Letterer-Siwe disease, choriocarcinoma, and carcinomas of the breast and testes. The major toxicity is bone marrow depression, usually leukopenia. Gastrointestinal manifestations may be encountered. Neurologic toxicity and alopecia occur less frequently than with vincristine.

Vincristine (Oncovin, VCR). This agent is administered intravenously, at weekly intervals. The initial recommended dose for adults is 0.01 mg per kilogram, increased by weekly increments of 0.01 mg per kilogram until the desired response or toxicity is encountered. Vincristine is particularly effective in the induction of remission in children with acute lymphoblastic leukemia. Vincristine (2 mg per square meter) used together with prednisone (40 to 150 mg per square meter) daily can induce complete remissions in 90 per cent of cases, and with a third drug, such as daunorubicin (25 mg per square meter), this rate approaches 100 per cent. It is also very effective in Hodgkin's disease, other lymphomas, Wilms' tumor, and rhabdomyosarcoma. Responses have been described in choriocarcinoma and carcinomas of the breast, prostate, cervix, and kidney. In contrast to vinblastine, it does not produce bone marrow depression, which makes it particularly useful in combination with other myelosuppressive agents. The combination of nitrogen mustard, Oncovin, procarbazine, and prednisone, the so-called MOPP regimen, is considered the treatment of choice in advanced Hodgkin's disease. The dose-limiting toxicity is neurologic, with paresthesias, loss of deep-tendon reflexes, paresis manifested by footdrop, hoarseness, ptosis, and double vision. Neurogenic constipation may be severe and should be anticipated with an appropriate prophylactic regimen. Alopecia occurs in about 20 per cent of patients. The syndrome of inappropriate antidiuretic hormone (ADH) secretion has been observed in patients treated with vincristine.

ASPARAGINASE. This enzyme, naturally present in guinea pig serum and currently prepared from E. coli as an investigational agent, catalyzes the hydrolysis of plasma asparagine to aspartic acid and ammonia. Because, in contrast to normal cells, certain neoplastic cells lack asparagine synthetase and are dependent on exogenous asparagine, a selective nutritional deficiency is produced. The resulting antineoplastic effect has stimulated considerable hope that exploitable biochemical differences may exist between normal and neoplastic cells. Unfortunately, this expectation has been somewhat tempered by the briefness of the remissions, by rapid development of resistance, and by allergic reactions after repeated administration of foreign protein. Recommended intravenous doses range from 200 IU per kilogram daily for 28 days to 1000 IU per kilogram for periods not exceeding ten days. Asparaginase can produce complete remissions in up to 60 per cent of children with acute lymphoblastic leukemia; it is sometimes beneficial in other leukemias and lymphomas, and occasionally in malignant melanoma. Despite its notable immunosuppressive properties, hypersensitivity reactions occur in 5 to 20 per cent of patients, ranging from urticaria to anaphylactic shock. Inhibition of

protein synthesis often results in mild impairment of hepatic, renal, pancreatic, central nervous, or clotting functions. Although usually expressed only as reversible aberrations of laboratory values, toxicity may occasionally be more severe.

ANTIBIOTICS. Antitumor antibiotics may (1) inhibit DNA synthesis, (2) impair RNA synthesis, or (3) block protein synthesis. Most of those with established clinical usefulness appear to belong to the second category and, after binding with DNA, inhibit DNA-dependent RNA biosynthesis. Bleomycin, however, inhibits DNA synthesis and reacts with DNA, causing strand scission. Most of these agents are rapidly cleared from the blood and are excreted mainly in the bile. They do not penetrate the blood-brain barrier significantly.

Dactinomycin (Actinomycin D, Cosmegen). This agent is administered intravenously in doses of 0.015 mg per kilogram daily for five days, to be repeated after two to four weeks if no toxicity persists. Dactinomycin is highly effective in gestational trophoblastic tumors and, in combination with radiotherapy and surgery, in Wilms' tumor. It is active in testicular tumors and rhabdomyosarcomas. It has an immunosuppressive effect and has been used in renal transplantation. Toxicity includes primarily bone marrow depression, stomatitis, and gastrointestinal reactions. Dermatologic manifestations include alopecia, as well as erythema, desquamation, and hyperpigmentation in areas subjected to radiotherapy. Extravasation can produce severe local injury.

Anthracycline Antibiotics (Daunorubicin and Doxorubicin). These glycosidic anthracycline antibiotics are fermentation products of the fungus Streptomyces peucetius var. caesius. Doxorubicin is the 14-hydroxy-derivative of daunorubicin. In spite of this small difference in chemical structure, doxorubicin possesses, in addition to the antileukemic activity of daunorubicin, a wide spectrum of activity in solid tumors. The mechanism of action of these antibiotics appears to involve a tight binding to DNA with untwisting of the helix to permit intercalation. This distortion impairs the template activity of DNA. Both drugs are administered intravenously and are rapidly cleared from the plasma. The disappearance curves are biphasic, with a short initial half-life of approximately one hour and a long secondary half-life of about 17 hours. Because of this, they are usually administered in large intermittent doses. There is rapid uptake of the drugs in the heart, lungs, kidneys, spleen, and liver, but they do not cross the blood-brain barrier. Metabolic degradation occurs in the liver by an aldehyde reductase and a microsomal reductive glycosidase. Microsomal enzyme inducers enhance this process, and, conversely, severe toxicity may result if the drugs are administered at standard doses in the presence of impaired liver function. Daunorubicin is metabolized primarily to daunorubicinol, whereas doxorubicin appears to have multiple metabolites, the principal one being adriamycinol. Both of these major metabolic products have antineoplastic activity. Although the drugs and their metabolites are primarily excreted in bile, 23 per cent of daunorubicin and its products appear in the urine within five days, in contrast to 6 per cent for doxorubicin. Patients should be advised that these compounds may impart a red color to the urine for one to two days after administration. Myelotoxicity is a major complication, and alopecia, stomatitis, and gastrointestinal manifestations are common. Local vesicant action and tissue necrosis can occur if the drugs are extravasated. A peculiar cardiomyopathy has been observed with these agents.

Two types of cardiotoxicity may occur: an acute type characterized by abnormal electrocardiographic changes, including ST-T wave changes and arrhythmias, which is brief and rarely a serious problem, and a chronic, cumulative, dose-related type manifested by congestive heart failure, unresponsive to digitalis, with a mortality in excess of 50 per cent. Although the frequency of the latter type of cardiomyopathy is negligible at total doses of doxorubicin below 500 mg per square meter, it increases markedly to >20 per cent of patients receiving total doses greater than 550 mg per square meter. With daunorubicin the frequency of congestive heart failure is 1 per cent at cumulative doses of 600 mg per square meter but increases rapidly at higher doses. There is evidence of increased risk of cardiotoxicity in patients previously exposed to irradiation of the cardiac region, cyclophosphamide, or another anthracycline antibiotic. No predictive tests are reliable in the individual patient, and the onset of heart failure is often delayed with 50 per cent of cases occurring after six months from completion of therapy. Although the mechanism of this cardiomyopathy is unclear, the structural similarities of these agents to the cardiac glycosides and their avid binding to cardiac DNA, as well as oxidative damage possibly related to the quinone-hydroquinone locus of the molecule, have been invoked.

DAUNORUBICIN (DAUNOMYCIN, RUBIDOMYCIN, DAUNOBLASTINA). The recommended dose is 30 to 60 mg per square meter intravenously, daily for three days or once weekly. It has also been given at 0.8 to 1.0 mg per kilogram for three to six days. The drug is particularly effective in induction of remission in children with acute lymphoblastic leukemia, usually in combination with vincristine and prednisone; it has some activity in solid tumors in children, and in lymphomas. Daunorubicin is the single most active agent in acute nonlymphocytic leukemias in adults.

DOXORUBICIN (ADRIAMYCIN, ADRIABLASTINA). The recommended dosage is 60 to 75 mg per square meter administered intravenously every three weeks. Doxorubicin is beneficial in acute leukemias and lymphomas but, in contrast to daunorubicin, it has strong activity in a number of solid tumors. It is particularly effective in osteogenic, Ewing's, and soft-tissue sarcomas. The drug is one of the most active single agents against metastatic adenocarcinoma of the breast. It is probably the best available agent in metastatic carcinoma of the thyroid and has shown activity against neuroblastoma, carcinomas of the lung, head and neck, and genitourinary systems in males and females.

Mithramycin (Mithracin). The usual daily dose is 0.025 mg per kilogram, administered during four to six hours intravenously for eight to ten days. Although this drug is useful for the treatment of patients with testicular tumors, it is no longer the treatment of choice, having been surpassed in effectiveness by combinations of other agents, particularly cis-platinum, vinblastine, and bleomycin. The drug has an interesting and unique capacity for lowering the serum calcium level, possibly by interfering with calcium resorption from bone. Prompt reversal of dangerous hypercalcemia and hypercalciuria associated with metastatic disease has been observed with a single intravenous dose of 0.025 mg per kilogram. Sometimes, it is necessary to repeat this for two to three days. The major toxic manifestation is a dangerous hemorrhagic diathesis, usually beginning with epistaxis. This is probably due to a combination of thrombocytopenia, abnormalities in multiple clotting factors, and capillary damage. Other myelo-

suppressive effects, gastrointestinal disturbances, and hepatic and renal abnormalities also occur.

Bleomycin (Blenoxane). The bleomycins are a group of antitumor agents isolated as fermentation products of *Streptomyces verticillus*. The drug in current clinical use is a complex mixture of glycopeptide antibiotics. The recommended dose is 10 to 20 units per square meter, administered intravenously or intramuscularly once or twice weekly. Total courses exceeding 400 units are associated with a marked increase in pulmonary toxicity and should be given with great caution. Renal excretion is the primary route of elimination, and 20 per cent to 40 per cent of the active compound is recovered in the urine. Preferential localization of drug occurs in the skin and the lung; other tissues inactivate the compound by removing 1 mole of ammonia. This probably accounts for the selectivity of therapeutic and toxic effects. It is of palliative value in patients with lymphomas and squamous cell carcinoma of the head, neck, skin, vulva, scrotum, cervix, and penis. It is particularly effective in testicular carcinoma, especially in combination with vinblastine and cis-platinum. Bleomycin alone does not produce bone marrow depression. The most serious toxicity is pulmonary. Although usually age and dose related, occurring more frequently in individuals older than 70 years and at cumulative doses greater than 400 units, it may be encountered in younger subjects at lower doses, particularly when used in combination with other agents. This begins with a picture indistinguishable from pneumonitis and may, in 2 to 15 per cent of cases, progress to pulmonary fibrosis, which has been fatal in about 1 per cent of patients. Stomatitis, alopecia, fever, and marked dermatologic manifestations frequently occur, including hyperkeratosis, ulceration, and hyperpigmentation. Because anaphylactic reactions have been observed in patients with lymphomas, administration of 2 units or less is recommended for the first two doses.

Mitomycin-C (Mutamycin). This water-soluble antibiotic is produced by *Streptomyces caespitosus* and is available as a powder of deep blue-violet crystals. After intracellular enzymatic reduction, it appears to cross-link DNA in a manner similar to the alkylating agents. After intravenous administeration, it disappears rapidly from the blood, with 50 per cent reduction of levels within 6 to 17 minutes. In adults, less than 10 per cent is excreted as active drug in the urine and very little in bile. The currently recommended dose is 50 μg per kilogram daily for five days, repeated for another five days, after a two-day interval. This schedule may be repeated after recovery from hematologic toxicity. Mitomycin is useful in combination with fluorouracil and Adriamycin in palliative therapy of adenocarcinoma of the stomach. It may be temporarily beneficial in carcinomas of the pancreas, colon, rectum, breast, head and neck, lung, cervix, and melanoma. Myelosuppression is a major complication, and gastrointestinal, renal, pulmonary, and mucocutaneous toxicity also occur. Extravasation may produce severe local injury.

Miscellaneous Agents

There are several substances, active as antineoplastic or immunosuppressive agents, that cannot be conveniently categorized under the aforementioned classification of cytotoxic drugs. Some of these are discussed elsewhere, including the steroid hormones — androgens, estrogens, progestins, and adrenocorticosteroids — the nonsteroidal anti-estrogens nafoxidine and tamoxifen, and radioactive isotopes. Four other clinically useful compounds are listed below.

HYDROXYUREA (HYDREA). This structurally simple compound inhibits DNA synthesis, probably by interfering with the enzymatic reduction of ribonucleotides to deoxyribonucleotides. It is an S-phase specific agent and does not block RNA or protein synthesis. It is well absorbed orally, peak plasma concentrations are reached in two hours, and it is undetectable in the blood within 24 hours. About 80 per cent is recovered in the urine; the rest is probably metabolized in the liver. The usual oral dose is 20 to 30 mg per kilogram daily, or 80 mg per kilogram every third day. Hydroxyurea is useful in patients with chronic granulocytic leukemia, who are refractory to busulfan and mercaptopurine. It has recently been demonstrated to be effective in patients with the hypereosinophilic syndrome, including, perhaps, eosinophilic leukemia. It has produced temporary remissions in malignant melanoma and is beneficial in psoriasis. Toxicity includes bone marrow depression, stomatitis, gastrointestinal disturbances, and, more rarely, alopecia, dermatitis, and neurologic manifestations.

PROCARBAZINE (MATULANE). The mechanism of action of this methyl hydrazine derivative is unknown, but it is capable of inhibiting DNA, RNA, and protein synthesis. It is rapidly absorbed from the gastrointestinal tract and readily equilibrates between the plasma and cerebrospinal fluid. Because of rapid metabolism, primarily in the liver, its half-life in the blood is approximately seven minutes, and in 24 hours 25 to 40 per cent is excreted as a metabolite in the urine. The recommended oral daily dose is 50 to 300 mg. It is effective in Hodgkin's disease, particularly in combination with nitrogen mustard, Oncovin, and prednisone (the so-called MOPP regimen), and apparently lacks cross-resistance to other agents. Notable immunosuppressive activity has been reported. Major toxicity includes bone marrow depression and gastrointestinal manifestations. Neurologic, psychic, and dermatologic disturbances have been noted. Augmentation of sedative effects may accompany the concomitant use of CNS depressants. Ethyl alcohol may cause a reaction resembling the acetaldehyde syndrome produced by disulfiram (Antabuse). Because it is a weak monoamine oxidase inhibitor, sympathomimetics, tricyclic antidepressants, and other drugs or foods with high tyramine contents, such as bananas and ripe cheese, should be avoided.

MITOTANE (O,P'-DDD, LYSODREN). This derivative of the insecticides DDD and DDT causes selective destruction of normal or neoplastic adrenocortical cells. It also modifies the peripheral metabolism of corticosteroids. Approximately 40 per cent of the drug is absorbed after oral administration, and about 10 to 25 per cent is recovered as a metabolite in the urine. Blood levels are measurable for six to nine weeks after cessation of therapy. The drug is distributed in all tissues, fat being the primary site of storage. The initial daily dose is 8 to 10 grams, usually given in three or four portions. Maximal tolerated doses vary from 2 to 16 grams per day. Treatment should be continued for at least three months. Beneficial effects have been observed in 35 to 40 per cent of patients with unresectable adrenocortical carcinoma. Gastrointestinal disturbances are common. Somnolence, lethargy, vertigo, and dermatitis also occur. Adverse reactions are usually reversible with reduction in dosage, and do not contraindicate continuation of therapy. Discontinuation of drug

and administration of exogenous corticosteroids are indicated if shock or severe trauma supervenes.

CIS-PLATINUM (CIS-DIAMMINEDICHLOROPLATINUM (II), DDP). A new class of cytotoxic agents, the platinum coordination complexes, was discovered when electrical current delivered between platinum electrodes caused their formation and inhibited replication of *E. coli*. DDP, an inorganic complex containing a central atom of platinum with ammonia and chlorine atoms in the *cis* position on a horizontal plane, was subsequently demonstrated to exert antineoplastic activity. The drug is not cell-cycle phase specific and is capable of cross-linking DNA, although inactivation of DNA also occurs through other mechanisms. After intravenous administration of radioactive platinum, the initial plasma half-life was 25 to 49 minutes and the secondary half-life was 58 to 73 hours. More than 90 per cent of the radioactivity appears to be protein bound, and there is poor penetration into the central nervous system. During the first five days, from 27 to 45 per cent of the radioactivity is excreted in the urine. Various dosage schedules are being studied with this investigational agent. From 50 to 75 mg per square meter can be administered once every three weeks or 15 to 20 mg per square meter daily for five days every three or four weeks. In order to prevent dose-limiting renal toxicity, concomitant administration of intravenous fluids and mannitol, 37.5 to 60 grams, during a period of six to eight hours, with or without 40 mg of furosemide, has been recommended. DDP has shown very promising results in testicular tumors, particularly in combination with vinblastine, bleomycin, and dactinomycin. It is also active in carcinomas of the ovary, head and neck, and bladder. Its major toxic effects are gastrointestinal, renal, and ototoxic. Moderate myelosuppression may occur and anaphylactic reactions, possibly related to DDP, have been reported.

527.4. THERAPY WITH IMMUNOSTIMULATORY PROCEDURES

INTRODUCTION

Attempts to treat cancer by augmenting host defense mechanisms preceded by many years the understanding of these mechanisms. More than 100 years ago, it was appreciated that remarkable improvements, even total regression, occurred in cancers of patients who were recovering from acute bacterial infections. In the early 1900's, Coley showed that bacteria or their products (Coley's toxins) could sometimes be effective in treating cancer.

Modern interest in immunotherapy started in the 1950's and 1960's when Burnet first suggested that the appearance of cancer could be due to a defect in an immune surveillance mechanism and when several workers demonstrated that bacille Calmette-Guérin (BCG) and *Corynebacterium parvum* could inhibit the growth of transplanted tumors in mice. Although the immune surveillance theory has recently been challenged, the rationale for immunotherapy does not really depend upon its basic premise, a state of immune incompetence, but rather on the ability to stimulate host defense mechanisms to levels effective in inhibiting tumor growth. The early work on BCG and *C. parvum* continues to provide impetus for therapeutic studies in man.

THE BASIS FOR IMMUNOTHERAPY

Immunotherapy depends upon the existence of both immunosensitive cancer cells bearing cancer-associated antigens and host immune mechanisms able to mount effective, cytotoxic reactions against them. The definition of cancer-associated antigens in man is still in its infancy. Whether there are antigens associated only with cancer cells, as opposed to those also shared with embryonic, proliferating, or differentiating cells, is unknown. The relationship between cancer antigens and antigens of viruses, associated either etiologically or accidentally with cancer, is not understood. Which antigens, among the myriad of those described, are important in eliciting host defense mechanisms is unclear. Whether antigens unique to each patient's cancer or antigens common to disease from many patients will prove more useful as therapeutic targets remains to be determined. The properties of a cell that render it sensitive to immunologically mediated toxicity are still being studied, although clearly there is more involved than simply bearing the appropriate antigen.

Host defense mechanisms relevant to immunotherapy of cancer are also ill defined. Evidence is accumulating that the T lymphocytes, demonstrated to be important in rejection of histoincompatible skin grafts, may not be of the same type as those reacting against tumor antigens. Other non-T lymphocytes have been detected which are also cytotoxic for cancer cells, but only in the presence of specific antibody, a phenomenon called ADCC, or antibody-dependent cellular cytotoxicity. On the other hand, antibody, antigen-antibody complexes, and soluble tumor antigens have been found, under experimental conditions, to be capable of blocking the ability of cytotoxic lymphocytes to react against cancer cells. Moreover, suppressor cells have also been detected, which are thought to be T cells and other leukocytes able to inhibit both production of antibody and perhaps cytotoxic lymphocytes. Thus the response of an individual patient to cancer is not simply a positive or negative one, but rather a medley of responses, the "balance" of which determines the immunologic picture at any point in time. Simplistic concepts, e.g., cellular immunity is good for the patient and humoral immunity, bad, are no longer tenable. The goal of immunotherapy is to modulate the patient's immune response in his favor, but no direct formula for achieving this is as yet available.

In addition to lymphocytes, the macrophage is capable of killing cancer cells in experimental animals. Ultimately, this component of the host defense mechanism may be most important to immunotherapy; indeed, many of the immunopotentiators currently being tested have significant effects on macrophages. Treatment with BCG can "activate" macrophages, by increasing their phagocytic properties, as well as their capacity to synthesize more digestive enzymes and to undergo mitosis. Activated macrophages can discriminate normal cells from cancer cells growing in culture and destroy the latter by a mechanism apparently unrelated to the tumor-associated antigens recognized by lymphocytes. Macrophages may also be a source of "tumor-necrosis factor," an endogenously released tumor cytoxin that is found circulating in animals given bacterial endotoxin after administration of BCG or *C. parvum*.

SPECIFIC IMMUNOTHERAPY

Another consideration in immunotherapy concerns whether its effects are specifically directed toward enhancing reactivity to cancer antigens, or nonspecifically aimed at increasing either general immune reactivity or host defense mechanisms that do not depend upon the presence of antigens. Macrophages can be involved in specific, as well as nonspecific, reactivity. They may play a vital role in "processing" antigen for effective presentation to lymphocytes and, with the help of cytophilic antibody absorbed to their surface, may also specifically destroy antigen-bearing cells. Our lack of knowledge of the basic mechanisms involved in specific immune reactivity to cancer makes specific immunotherapy not yet clinically practical. Various approaches to this type of therapy are being investigated. One approach involves transfer of passive immunity to patients with cancer either by serum or lymphocytes from sensitized animals, cured patients, or exposed normal individuals. Serum transfer is hazardous because of the possible presence of blocking factors (antigens, antibodies, or antigen-antibody complexes), which could interfere with the development of cytotoxic immunity or lead to enhancement of tumor growth. Recently, however, remarkable benefit in the treatment of leukemia in mice, cats, and other animals has been demonstrated after transfer of serum. The active principles appear to be components of complement that are deficient in the tumor hosts, resulting in a breakdown of antibody-complement–mediated cytotoxicity. Restoration of the complement permits normal activity of the antibody, which was already present at adequate levels. The efficacy of this treatment is now being tested clinically.

Passive transfer of whole viable lymphocytes is also hazardous because of the possibility of graft versus host disease. Attempts are being made to circumvent this by using extracts of immune lymphocytes, such as "immune" RNA and transfer factor, a dialyzable substance capable of transferring skin delayed hypersensitivity reactions in humans. The therapeutic efficacy of both substances is still controversial.

Another approach to specific immunotherapy involves attempts to obtain active immunization of patients by injecting extracted tumor antigens, irradiated tumor cells, and similar preparations. Lack of adequate definition of cancer antigens makes this approach uncertain. One of the most promising uses of active immunization is with cancer cells that have been treated with neuraminidase prior to vaccination. This enzyme removes sialic acid from cell membranes, exposing hidden antigens against which animals and humans may have pre-existing natural immunity. The natural immunity destroys the vaccinated cells, but not before they are able to induce an enhanced response to the tumor antigens.

With better understanding of the etiology of human cancer and more precise knowledge of tumor antigens, prophylactic immunization, or prevention by vaccination, may become a more realistic expectation in the future. Marek's disease, a lymphoproliferative malignancy in chickens, can now be prevented by vaccination with an attenuated form of the causative agent, a herpesvirus.

NONSPECIFIC IMMUNOTHERAPY

The most active area of current research in clinical immunotherapy relates to nonspecific immunostimulators. Such agents have a variety of experimental effects on host immunity to cancer, including stimulation of cellular and humoral immunity and enhancement of macrophage function. In addition, agents such as BCG have been shown to share cross-reacting antigens with tumors, e.g., certain melanomas, suggesting that they may be effecting an active, specific immunization. It remains to be demonstrated whether this laboratory observation is relevant to clinical efficacy. Some of the immunostimulators currently undergoing clinical trial as investigational agents are described below.

BCG. The bacille Calmette-Guérin strain of the tubercle bacillus was first used as a liver vaccine against virulent tuberculosis. BCG is the most widely investigated immune stimulator. It appears to be particularly efficacious when injected directly into the lesions of intradermal melanoma, causing regression of 90 per cent of the injected lesions. Regression of only 10 per cent of the uninjected lesions occurs in the same patients. Injection of subcutaneous lesions is less effective, however, and injection of superficial melanoma lesions has no effect on visceral metastases. BCG and other immunostimulators have not shown clinical activity when given alone against widespread disease. This is in accord with the general observation that immunotherapy is only active in experimental animals against very small numbers of tumor cells, well below clinically detectable levels. To be effective in most patients, it should be given in combination with or after other therapy when the tumor burden is small. Accordingly, BCG has given very encouraging results by increasing survival of patients with Stage I lung cancer, when it was instilled in the pleural cavity after surgical removal of the primary tumor. The same treatment is ineffective against more advanced disease. For many years, BCG or tumor cell vaccines have been claimed to be of benefit in prolonging the disease-free interval and survival of children with acute lymphoblastic leukemia (ALL) who had been previously subjected to intense cytoreductive radiotherapy and chemotherapy. Not all studies have confirmed these findings of efficacy for BCG in ALL, but only a few groups have carried out intensive cytotoxic therapy prior to initiating immunotherapy. Even in patients with widely disseminated disease, however, when it is not possible to reduce the tumor burden to a minimum, BCG has been reported to have some therapeutic effect when given in combination with chemotherapy or tumor cell vaccines. For example, the addition of BCG and irradiated cells to maintenance chemotherapy has been reported to increase survival in patients with acute myelogenous leukemia.

The therapeutic effectiveness of BCG is an area of current controversy. Many studies are marred by poor or inappropriate controls, and several basic parameters, such as optimal BCG strain, dose, time and route of administration, have yet to be determined. Nevertheless, certain principles seem to be emerging that govern the effectiveness of BCG, and probably other immunostimulators: the host must be immunologically competent, and the tumor burden must be small. Effective contact between the agent and the tumor cells appears necessary. Administration of the agent in selected sites, such as the skin in melanoma, yields better results. Successful therapy requires capability of mounting a delayed hypersensitivity response against the organism with a reaction in the tumor mass. There is also experimental evidence that intratumor or adjacent dermal injection of BCG prior to surgical removal of a tumor may prevent development of nodal metastases.

BCG is usually administered intradermally by the multiprong scarification technique or Heaf gun innoculation. One ampule, containing 3×10^8 viable organisms diluted in 0.2 to 0.3 ml of sterile water, is used for each immunization at different sites and various investigational time schedules.

The major clinical problem in administering BCG is the development of severe local, and sometimes systemic, hypersensitivity reactions. A further problem in immunologically deficient patients is development of BCG-osis with septicemia, splenomegaly, and hepatomegaly, although this can be successfully controlled with isoniazid. Ultimately, a more serious concern is the observation in animals, and perhaps humans, that under certain circumstances BCG can accelerate cancer growth. Induction of serum-blocking factors, immune depression consequent to overwhelming infection, or other effects that upset immunologic balance may be responsible.

BCG is a complex agent, containing many different antigens and other substances, which may contribute to the total effect. A nonliving, chemically characterized drug would be obviously easier to control and administer than BCG, and much reasearch effort is being directed to identify such active and nonviable subcomponents.

MER. This methanol-extractable residue of BCG was first shown to have antitumor activity in animals. It is a nonviable, particulate, relatively insoluble powder, which induces local granulomas that may persist for long periods. It is associated with the induction of marked resistance to various experimental neoplasms. Administration is by intradermal injection, divided into five sites, for a total dose of 1.0 mg and repeated on a monthly schedule, with appropriate regulation of dosage depending on response. Initial clinical studies in patients with acute myelogenous leukemia indicate prolongation of remissions after chemotherapy. Its efficacy in other neoplastic disorders is currently also under investigation.

CORYNEBACTERIUM PARVUM. C. parvum is a formalin-fixed, washed suspension of a gram-positive anaerobic bacillus. In some animal tumors its therapeutic ratio is superior to that of BCG, but its modes of action appear similar to those of BCG and MER. It can be administered either systemically or locally into tumors. Although various dosage schedules are used, depending on the investigational protocol, it has been given at 2.5 mg per square meter subcutaneously and intravenously every two to four weeks. Initial clinical results have been encouraging, especially when combined with cytotoxic chemotherapy. Toxic effects include local pain and swelling, as well as chills, fever, changes in blood pressure, and other common reactions observed with injection of crude bacterial preparations. Administration of barbiturates or other anesthetic agents may be hazardous in patients treated with *C. parvum.*

LEVAMISOLE. Levamisole [L-(-)-2,3,5,6-tetrahydro-6-phenylimidazo(2, 1-b)thiazole] is a synthetic agent administered orally and widely used as an anthelmintic drug. The oral dose most commonly used in current clinical trials in adult patients is 150 mg daily for three days, every two weeks. It is capable of augmenting immune reactions, especially in immunodepressed patients. It has also been reported to prolong disease-free interval and survival in women with primary, inoperable breast cancer who have been treated by irradiation to the breast and regional nodes. It is currently being studied in other adjuvant protocols. It has not yet been proved effective by itself against clinically overt disease. Acute toxicity has not been a problem, but, as with other immunostimulators, it is capable of enhancing cancer growth in experimental systems.

The aforementioned represent only some of the "first generation" immunopotentiators undergoing active investigation. As more is learned about their mechanism of action and structure-activity relationships, it is likely that more effective agents will be developed. It is also probable that successful immunotherapy will continue to require the presence of a minimal number of tumor cells and thus will be most effective in combination with the other treatment modalities. The addition of immunostimulators to other therapeutic modalities may help overcome the immunosuppression induced by chemotherapy and radiotherapy, thereby reducing the frequency of infection.

DRUG-IMMUNOPOTENTIATOR INTERACTIONS. As with any other drug combinations, the possibility for interaction between cytotoxic agents and immunostimulators must be considered. Either agent may affect the clinical pharmacology of the other. For example, BCG and *C. parvum* have been reported to interfere with the drug-metabolizing enzymes of the liver, a situation that could modify the therapeutic efficacy of drugs such as cyclophosphamide and dacarbazine, which require activation by these microsomal enzymes, or increase the toxicity of doxorubicin and daunorubicin, which are catabolized by this mechanism.

527.5. SUPPORTIVE CARE

Notwithstanding careful precautions, moderate or severe toxicity may be encountered, with cytotoxic agents, particularly when intensive combination chemotherapy is used, alone or together with irradiation. The physician must be prepared to provide vigorous supportive therapy. Component blood therapy is often required, particularly platelet transfusions. Granulocyte transfusions are more difficult to obtain, unless access to a continuous flow cell separator is available. Accordingly, infectious complications in leukopenic and immunosuppressed patients are common. Although fever may be a manifestation of neoplastic disease, it generally indicates infection. Specific antimicrobial therapy requires prompt identification of the responsible organ-

ism. Bacterial pathogens and opportunistic fungal, viral, or protozoal organisms may be causative agents. Some of these respond to the newer drugs described in Ch. 527.3. Cytotoxic drugs may produce metabolic complications. Hyperuricemia can be prevented by allopurinol; hypercalcemia can be controlled by corticosteroids and mithramycin; and inappropriate ADH secretion can be corrected by fluid deprivation. Other specific measures are discussed above in reference to individual agents. Finally, the importance of psychologic support cannot be overemphasized. Frank discussion of expected but unpleasant complications, such as gastrointestinal disturbances, paresthesias, and alopecia, should include appropriate reassurance of their reversibility. Because palliation is more frequent than cure, the physician's attitude is most important and should combine honesty with optimism and encouragement.

Burnet, M. F.: Immunological Surveillance. Oxford, Pergamon Press, 1970.

Calabresi, P., and Parks, R. E., Jr.: Chemotherapy of neoplastic disease. *In* Goodman, L. S., and Gilman, A. (eds.): The Pharmacological Basis of Therapeutics. 5th ed. New York, The Macmillan Company, 1975.

Chabner, B. A., Myers, C. E., Coleman, C. N., and Johns, D. G.: The clinical pharmacology of antineoplastic agents. N. Engl. J. Med., 292:1159, 1975.

Clark, R. L., and Howe, C. D.: Cancer Patient Care. Chicago, Year Book Medical Publishers, 1976.

del Regato, J. A., and Spjut, H. J.: Cancer. 5th ed. St. Louis, C. V. Mosby Company, 1977.

DeVita, V. T., Young, R. C., and Canellos, G. P.: Combination versus single agent chemotherapy: A review of the basis for selection of drug treatment of cancer. Cancer, 35:98, 1975.

Greenwald, E. S.: Cancer Chemotherapy. Flushing, N.Y., Medical Examination Publishing Company, 1973.

Gutterman, J. U.: Cancer systemic active immunotherapy today — prospects for tomorrow. Cancer Immunol. Immunother., 2:1, 1977.

Heppner, G. H., and Calabresi, P.: Selective suppression of humoral immunity by antineoplastic drugs. Ann. Rev. Pharmacol., 16:367, 1976.

Holland, J. F., and Frei, E.: Cancer Medicine. Philadelphia, Lea & Febiger, 1973.

Kaplan, S. R., and Calabresi, P.: Immunosuppressive agents. N. Eng. J. Med., 289:952, 1234, 1973.

Oettgen, H. F.: Immunotherapy of cancer. N. Engl. J. Med., 297:484, 1977.

Prehn, R. T.: Immunostimulation of the lymphodependent phase of neoplastic growth. J. Natl. Cancer Inst., 59:1043, 1977.

Proceedings of the American Cancer Society's National Conference on Radiation Oncology, Present Status and Future Potential. Cancer, 39:689, 1977.

Sartorelli, A. C., and Johns, D. G.: Antineoplastic and Immunosuppressive Agents. Berlin–Heidelberg–New York, Springer-Verlag, 1974.

Shabel, F. M.: Concepts for systemic treatment of micrometastases. Cancer, 35:15, 1975.

Skinner, M. D., and Schwartz, R. S.: Immunosuppressive therapy. N. Engl. J. Med., 287:221, 281, 1972.

Steinberg, A. D., Plotz, P. H., Wolff, S. M., Wong, V. G., Agus, S. G., and Decker, J. L.: Cytotoxic drugs in treatment of nonmalignant disease. Ann. Inter. Med., 76:619, 1972.

528. THE CARE OF THE PATIENT WITH TERMINAL ILLNESS

W. P. L. Myers

There is perhaps no more controversial medical issue of our time than that dealing with the care of the patient with terminal illness. Endless articles in the lay press dealing with death and dying, death with dignity, a patient's right to die, euthanasia, and so forth are testimony to the enormous interest and concern of the public and to the confusion that abounds. It is not the intent of this chapter to sort out these conflicting attitudes and beliefs, but rather to provide an approach to the problem for the student of medicine. Final answers cannot be written, but the reader will find an approach that is based on long personal experience with terminal illness and on the premise that it is the individual that matters. It is necessary to understand this at the outset, because an entirely different approach could be adopted if one proceeded on the premise that it is the greatest good for the greatest number of people that matters.

The Hippocratic oath demands of each of us that we practice our art for the benefit of our patients. Implicit in this charge is the preservation of life. Nowhere in the original or in its modern version does the word "prolong" appear, with respect to a patient's life. "Prolong" is a word that has come to mean the unnecessary continuation of life in a setting in which, usually in the eyes of a patient's family, recovery is impossible. It is a word most used by the laity because, in general, physicians do not view their efforts in these terms. They are more likely to take the long view and consider that their efforts should be to preserve life, since such efforts are in the main to be equated with what is beneficial for the patient. Therapeutic efforts in a seemingly hopeless situation can be viewed by the patient's family as needless efforts to prolong life, whereas the physician, from his vantage point of seeing a disease in perspective, may regard the same efforts as fully justifiable in terms of his obligation to the patient. The dilemma that arises, however, is that there are those who reasonably question preservation of life as the sole objective of treatment. The physician must always act in his patient's interests, but undoubtedly there are situations in which these are not best served by endless efforts to preserve life. Where does the physician draw the line? How is he to tell when to pursue treatment aggressively and when not to? Are there any guideposts?

MEDICAL ANALYSIS OF THE PATIENT CONSIDERED TO BE TERMINAL

It is important at the outset to define "terminal illness," because an accurate medical analysis of a given situation is the keystone for all future considerations, both medical and humanitarian. How can we tell if a patient is terminally ill? This determination may tax all the skills a physician has, and yet he may end up defining a patient as terminally ill who would not be so regarded by another doctor. We must begin somewhere, however, and there is no better place to begin than to be sure that the medical details have been set forth and have been analyzed in the fullest. It has been said that all problems could be solved if one only knew the right questions to ask. One approach to the matter of determining whether a patient is, in fact, terminally ill is for the physician to ask himself a few brief questions. The seven questions listed below are presented with a cancer patient in mind, but they can serve as a model for this approach to other diseases as well:

1. Has the patient had a complete history and physical examination?

2. Is there histologic evidence of cancer, and where is the primary site?

3. Is the presenting problem caused by a second primary cancer?

4. What is the extent of the disease?

5. What medical complications, both those caused by the tumor and those unrelated to the tumor, exist?

6. What was the previous treatment, and was it adequate?

7. Is the disease process active and progressive or chronic and stable?

The answers to these questions are fundamental to the proper assessment of a patient's illness, as has been discussed in Ch. 522. They have particular applicability in situations in which the patient has been categorized as terminally ill. The questions are considered in greater detail as follows:

Question 1: Has the patient had a complete history and physical examination? It is almost embarrassing to include such a question in a list of this sort, but many patients have been improperly designated as being terminally ill because of what *appears* to be, without the benefit of a complete history and physical examination. Unfortunately the reason for this is that such patients frequently are seen initially by those who lack interest or who are guided by an attitude of hopelessness, especially when it comes to cancer. The following case will serve to emphasize the importance of a complete history and physical examination:

The patient was a 62-year-old white man from Central America who had had mild intermittent diarrhea for several years. Six months before admission he had been treated for malignant lymphoma, histiocytic type, of the stomach. He did well subsequently, but in the week prior to admission he developed anorexia followed by watery diarrhea and rectal bleeding. He had been treated with prednisone, 30 mg daily, for five days before admission. On admission he was found to be febrile and his abdomen was distended and tender, but there was no rebound tenderness. His stool was positive for blood. There was no peripheral lymphadenopathy. It was assumed that he had recurrent intra-abdominal malignant lymphoma, and when he went into shock the day after admission, he was considered to be terminally ill. He responded briefly to medical measures, but shock recurred and he died on the third day after admission. Autopsy disclosed diffuse colonic amebiasis with perforation and peritonitis. There was no evidence of recurrent malignant lymphoma.

In retrospect, further inquiry into the patient's history of intermittent diarrhea should have been made, especially in view of the fact that he came from Central America. The presence of fever, abdominal distention, and rectal bleeding, even without overt signs of perforation at the time of admission, should have led to a more careful examination, in particular a proctoscopic examination, to establish the correct diagnosis. Even so, the patient might not have recovered, but at least he would have had treatment directed against the correct disease, which in this instance was non-neoplastic.

Question 2: Is there histologic evidence of cancer, and where is the primary site? Consignment of patients to the ranks of the "terminally ill" has occurred all too often without histologic evidence of cancer and especially without attempts to define a primary site, if a histologic diagnosis of cancer has been made. The latter does not always have a therapeutic implication, but often it does, notably in those instances in which tumors originate in the breast, prostate, and thyroid. The following is a case in point:

The patient was a 50-year-old man seen in the clinic because of abdominal complaints and back pain. Evidences of tumor were noted intra-abdominally as well as in the lungs and left supraclavicular area. The impression was that he had metastatic carcinoma probably of gastrointestinal tract origin, despite negative gastrointestinal x-rays. A subsequent biopsy of the left supraclavicular lymph node was interpreted as "metastatic carcinoma." The hopeless attitude expressed by one of the patient's attending physicians was brought out by the following note he entered in the patient's record:

"This unfortunate patient has hopeless cancer as evidenced by left supraclavicular nodes. Biopsy shows metastatic adenocarcinoma. The exact site of primary is not apparent. This is now a purely academic question. He has hopeless cancer originating in the upper abdomen and is suitable only for terminal care."

Fortunately, other physicians did not share this opinion, and, in the attempt to discover a primary site, an acid phosphatase was obtained. This proved to be markedly elevated, indicating a diagnosis of metastatic carcinoma of the prostate. After orchiectomy and estrogen therapy, a chest film showed regression of mediastinal disease, and the patient remained alive with his disease in remission for many months. He finally died about three and a half years after having been regarded by one physician as being suitable only for terminal care.

Question 3: Is the presenting problem caused by a second primary cancer? It is difficult for a patient, once treated for cancer, not to have all subsequent clinical disease interpreted as manifestations of the original cancer. A patient previously treated for cancer of the pancreas may now have advanced metastatic disease and correctly be considered terminally ill. But if the metastatic disease is, in fact, caused by a second primary cancer such as carcinoma of the breast, the patient may respond dramatically to hormonal treatment and be anything but terminally ill. This possibility must always be kept in mind, particularly when there has been an appreciable time interval between the diagnosis of the original tumor and the appearance of metastatic disease.

Question 4: What is the extent of the disease? The accurate assessment of the extent of a cancer is the major determinant of treatment. In general, surgery and radiotherapy are utilized for localized and regional disease, whereas systemic treatment is applied to disseminated disease. Patients whose extent of disease is incorrectly evaluated may receive the wrong treatment or may inappropriately be considered to be terminally ill. Obviously, jaundice in a patient with known cancer may or may not represent metastatic disease. Only by judging each manifestation on its own merits can a correct assessment of the extent of disease be made.

Question 5: What medical complications, both those caused by the tumor and those unrelated to the tumor, exist? This question is really a corollary to the last one but deserves special emphasis because a metabolic or infectious complication may be more life-threatening than the underlying cancer, and often if properly identified and treated, the patient may not needlessly lose his life. The following case is illustrative:

A 64-year-old woman was admitted to the hospital with a diagnosis of mammary carcinoma metastatic to the brain. Two

years previously she had undergone a left radical mastectomy for infiltrating duct carcinoma of the breast. She had had positive axillary nodes and received postoperative radiation therapy. She remained well until seven weeks before admission when she developed double vision and dysphagia. On examination she had bilateral ptosis and motor weakness of cranial nerve V bilaterally without sensory impairment. Shortly after admission she underwent emergency tracheostomy for severe stridor, and radiation therapy to the brain was begun. At this point a resident physician, unwilling to assume that everything was caused by metastatic cancer, observed: "This lady really has little evidence for spread of her breast carcinoma. . . . I am hard put to assign her neurologic signs to an anatomic lesion, especially bilateral jaw weakness without any impairment of the sensory component of cranial nerve V. Right now she has marked ptosis bilaterally and paresis of gaze in all directions — without any pupillary abnormalities! The quick fatigue in the jaw muscles brings up myasthenia gravis which could explain all her signs."

A test with edrophonium chloride confirmed the resident's suspicions and a diagnosis of myasthenia gravis was made. The radiation therapy to the brain was stopped and the patient has done very well on medical management of her myasthenia and has had no demonstrable recurrence of breast cancer during these past four years.

Question 6: What was the previous treatment, and was it adequate? Corollary: Was previous treatment in any way responsible for the patient's present problems? At times "terminal" situations arise because patients have not received adequate treatment. No patient should be regarded as terminally ill without a careful review of the type and adequacy of prior treatment, including treatment of coexistent diseases unrelated to the primary one. Of course, previous treatment may also cause problems which can be misinterpreted as manifestations of the underlying malignancy. For example, a rare but remarkable complication of radiotherapy, that of radiation nephritis, is illustrated by the following case:

The patient, a 63-year-old man, was admitted to the hospital for what ultimately proved to be a spindle and giant cell sarcoma of the duodenum which was treated by radiotherapy to the upper abdomen. Two months later, the patient was reexplored and radon seeds were inserted throughout the residual tumor mass. Six months later and during the ensuing 18 months the patient's course was marked by the gradual appearance of recurrent fluid accumulation (peripheral, peritoneal, pleural), hypertension, anemia, thrombopenia, albuminuria, and azotemia. He eventually succumbed to renal failure some 26 months after the initial radiotherapy had been given.

From a clinical viewpoint, the patient had been regarded as having had recurrent intra-abdominal cancer on the basis of a cytologic examination of the peritoneal fluid which was reported to have revealed malignant cells. However, at autopsy none of the organs or tissues showed evidence of residual tumor or metastases. The kidneys presented the classic picture of radiation nephritis, and in retrospect it was apparent that this lesion was responsible for the clinical findings. Had it been recognized that the patient did not have recurrent cancer but rather the renal complications of radiation therapy, it is possible that more aggressive measures directed at his renal failure might have altered the outcome.

Question 7: Is the disease process active and progressive or chronic and stable? There are many so-called terminal diseases, metastatic cancer among them, that pursue a chronic course. A patient may have metastases from a cancer for which we have no specific therapy and he may therefore be "written off" as terminally ill. However, the natural history of the cancer in that patient may not be progressive, and the physician should take this into account when forming his own appraisal of a patient with an incurable illness. In addition, rare but clearly documented, inexplicable remissions of advanced cancer have occurred, and these serve to remind us of the incompleteness of our knowledge and the fallibility of our judgments.

THE TRULY "TERMINAL" PATIENT

If the physician has asked the aforementioned questions and has satisfied himself that, in fact, his patient is nearing death from an illness which is progressive, unrelenting, and disseminated and which cannot be arrested or reversed in our present state of knowledge (or perhaps more accurately, ignorance), how then should he manage the problem? He should, of course, satisfy himself that important general principles, so well summarized in various renditions of a "Bill of Rights for Patients," are being followed, but he should also have a plan or way of thinking about the over-all problem of terminal illness and the specific problems presented by each patient. The technique of asking himself some further critical questions provides such an approach. The principal questions are these:

1. What does the patient know about his situation?
2. What is the patient's attitude regarding the prospect of death?
3. Does he have pain and, if so, is it being relieved?
4. Is the patient being comforted physically, mentally, and spiritually?
5. Is the physician prepared to give of himself to the patient and "go down to the wire" with him? As a corollary, is the physician willing to continue to think about the problems his patient presents until the end?
6. What is the attitude of the patient's family, and how is it being dealt with?
7. Is the patient undergoing experimental study, and, if so, are humanitarian principles being observed or compromised?

There may be other questions one could ask, but these will serve most situations, and they should be considered in some depth.

Question 1: What does the patient know about his situation? Too often the physician fails to ask this question and, if he does, he does not record it on the patient's chart, so there is no general knowledge of this among the various personnel caring for the patient. This, in turn, leads to a lack of coordination in treatment efforts. The care of a patient can be improved substantially if his understanding of his illness is brought to light and recorded in a manner that will permit all medical and nursing personnel involved to know and act accordingly.

By asking a patient what he understands about his illness, the physician provides an opportunity for the patient to tell the physician, directly or indirectly, how much he wants to know. Some patients are quite content to leave it all to the doctor, but usually, if given the opportunity, they will ask questions. There is no standard answer to a given question, but the physician should be truthful insofar as his answer goes. A truthful revelation about a disease should always be supported by a plan of action; an outlook with a grave prognosis can be coupled, in a compassionate manner, with a positive statement regarding what the physician plans to do and how other patients have responded under similar circumstances. Hope should not be false, but it must never be destroyed by a statement of truth thoughtlessly unattended by any words to mollify the implications of that truth. Although this approach is not uniformly followed by the medical profession, it is increasingly so, because doctors have come to know that the erosion of trust between themselves and their patients, created by a failure to tell a patient as much truth as the doctor believes the patient seeks to know, is a more severe blow to the patient than dealing with the truth. There is no need, however, to tell the patient all the details, particularly in view of the fact that our fallibility could lead us to tell a patient more than we know. In addition, by seeking to know what the patient understands, the physician can correct misconceptions which are often the basis of fear and anxiety. Relief of these major burdens of a terminally ill patient should be of primary concern to the physician.

Attempts by a patient's family to persuade the physician to go along with an outright lie regarding the patient's illness should never be acceded to. Good intentions were never more misplaced; the lie creates further problems and is an insult to the patient. In addition, seriously ill patients usually know they are seriously ill, and explanations that do not seem likely create fear that the patient's doctor does not know the real diagnosis. This torment can be worse than the knowledge of the primary illness.

Question 2: What is the patient's attitude regarding the prospect of death? Attitudes toward death and dying are being more openly discussed and analyzed than ever before. The patient stricken with a fatal illness has been noted as going through various stages which have been categorized, progressively, as denial, anger, bargaining, depression, and, ultimately, acceptance (Kübler-Ross). This dissection is useful because it can form a basis for a physician's approach to his patient. For example, understanding that a patient's anger (which may be directed at the physician) is part of the unfolding reaction to his illness permits the physician to deal with this in a helpful rather than defensive manner. Learning about a patient's attitude takes time which a physician may be unwilling or unable to spend. In addition, a physician may be at a loss as to how to broach the subject, although usually this only requires that one give a patient the realization that he will be listened to. This obviously entails choosing a proper time, such as returning to see the patient after regular rounds. The press of time may not always permit this, and under these and other circumstances, the physician would do well to enlist the help of others. The nursing staff usually has considerable insight into the patient's attitudes, and this staff working together as a team with the physician, the clergyman or rabbi, the social worker, and the psychiatrist can often create an atmosphere in which the patient's thoughts can be expressed.

There are times when a patient will feel freer to discuss his or her attitude about death with the spiritual adviser than with anyone else, and the adviser can be of enormous help in these situations. The fear of death is a human emotion widely considered in any discussion of death and dying, but the fear of *not* dying has received little attention. Patients may seek assurances from a clergyman that death is imminent, believing that the physician will not provide such assurances because doing so would be a denial of his role in preserving life.

Those who have had experience in the care of dying patients will not have failed to be impressed with the peace that patients experience when they have become convinced of the inevitability of their own death. Rhoads has written of this penultimate moment: "It was as if tearing away the veil of uncertainty at the same time released him from fear. He became calm, gentle, considerate of those about him, assuming a new dignity, as if he had already partly crossed the threshold."

Question 3: Does the patient have pain, and, if so, is it being relieved? The specter of death being painful is firmly rooted in the lay mind, and there is no doubt that osseous metastases, nerve root compression or infiltration, ischemic neuritis, and so forth can cause great pain. Yet pain as a major feature of terminal illness does not invariably occur, as is so often supposed. When it occurs it is essential that it be relieved; there is no excuse for a terminal illness being marked by uncontrolled pain except that the physician has not fully analyzed the cause of the patient's pain and utilized those measures available to him for control.

The skillful use of narcotics, radiotherapy, nerve blocks, and, rarely, cordotomy can all be applied individually and together to achieve control. Clearly, however, relief of pain will best be achieved by a careful analysis of its cause and by measures directed against the cause. Thus pain in the thigh in a patient with metastatic cancer may be referred pain or it may represent metastases in the femur. Radiotherapy directed to the wrong area will not relieve pain, and it is the primary physician's responsibility to see to it that treatment is directed against the cause.

In a terminal illness narcotics should not be withheld for fear of addiction, assuming the physician has made an accurate determination that the illness is in its terminal stages. Often doctors achieve less than satisfactory results because they fail to adjust the dose of the narcotic to fit the situation. There are no rigid rules of dose and time intervals, but rather these must be adapted to each patient's need. Oral administration of narcotics will usually suffice in all but the most serious pain problems if the dose and time intervals have been carefully adjusted (Saunders). At times, physicians worry too much about the development of tolerance. Of course, the risk of tolerance will increase with increasing doses of a narcotic, but cross-tolerance between narcotics is incomplete and substitution of one narcotic for another may often be helpful if tolerance does become a problem. Also the combination of non-narcotic analgesics with narcotics may permit adequate pain relief with lower doses of narcotics and hence a lower risk of developing tolerance. The guiding principle, then, is to be flexible in adopting a program that is suitable for each individual patient and not to be too concerned with standardized regimens.

The subject of pain and its management is considered in Ch. 260.

Question 4: Is the patient being comforted physically, mentally, and spiritually? There are some who consider that physical, mental, and spiritual comfort for those who are terminally ill can be best accomplished in the home or in a hospice, and adherents to this view are increasing. It is certain that many patients are best cared for under these circumstances, particularly if this is their wish, and families usually feel closer to what is happening to the patient in these settings. It is in the hospital where so often misunderstandings arise because of the vigorous therapeutic stance which, understandably, characterizes our hospitals. In this regard, it is important to draw a distinction between measures undertaken as primary treatment for a disease and those undertaken for the patient's comfort. The latter are often misinterpreted by the laity as needless efforts to prolong life, whereas in the terminally ill patient they are only intended for the relief of discomfort. These measures might include antimicrobial drugs to relieve high fever and drenching sweats caused by infection, oxygen to relieve air hunger, an indwelling catheter to prevent decubitus ulcers secondary to incontinence, and intravenous fluids to relieve thirst and dehydration. These measures do not prolong the life of a dying patient; they, like the relief of pain, merely make more tolerable the period of dying. Yet they have become the targets of those who do not understand and who therefore accuse the medical profession of preventing patients from "dying with dignity." Departing this life in a dignified manner is a noble objective and is often achieved, but in many instances it is not. Dignity is defined in one dictionary as "the presence of poise and self-respect in one's deportment to a degree that inspires respect." This is a reasonable definition; but in those instances in which dignity is lost, it is the illness that is responsible, not the physician, unless through the *injudicious* ordering of drugs, he renders his patient incompetent and robs him of his chance to meet his final hour with courage and character.

Dignity is a quality of human character that is a consequence of what lies within the soul. It is not something that can be taken away by another person. It may lie dormant only to appear under adverse circumstances, such as the prospect of death, or it may be in evidence in all that a person does. Those who have had experience in the treatment of dying patients have often been struck by their fortitude of character and spirit. The medical profession is privileged to go through life with this particular view of humanity, which may only rarely be revealed to people in other walks of life.

Having attended to the patient's physical comfort, the concerned physician will see to it that, to the best of his ability, he brings about mental comfort to the patient. Fear and anxiety are too often left unattended. Narcotics may be useful in allaying both, but even more important is the understanding that physicians can bring to their patients by listening and by giving a patient the realization that his burden is shared by the physician: these, plus a careful interpretation to the patient concerning what is happening to him. Fear can often be counteracted with knowledge and understanding better than with any drug in the pharmacopeia. Lewis Thomas has alluded to the observations of Osler and his own experience that there appears to be no such thing as the agony of death. Regarding the ultimate moment of death he has cited observations that there may be a physiologic mechanism which somehow relieves the patient of all fear and anguish. As we learn more about the pathophysiology of dying, we will undoubtedly come to understand more about such a possible mechanism. The discovery of physiologic substances with pain-relieving properties, the endorphins, is a promising development in this regard.

Finally, is the patient being comforted spiritually? A visit by a clergyman is not necessarily synonymous with spiritual comfort, because some patients do not experience comfort under these circumstances, despite the best efforts of the clergyman. It all depends on the patient's background, and this must be known to his physician. Spiritual comfort can come in many forms, and the doctor who really cares about his patient will see to this aspect of his needs. Usually, however, the clergyman is indispensable in providing spiritual comfort. The physician and clergyman need each other, and the patient needs them both. It has been observed that what a physician can provide a patient in these circumstances will depend upon his own beliefs and his coming to terms with his own mortality. If he views life as simply a biologic accident, one in which consciousness dies with the flesh, and one in which there is no divinity in each person, he will be in no position to help his patient in a spiritual sense. If, on the other hand, he views life as a continuum and divine guidance as something operative in all lives, his manner, compassion, gentleness, and understanding will not be lost on the patient seeking spiritual solace. In considering the question of consciousness and what happens to it, Thomas has written: ". . . there is still that permanent vanishing of consciousness to be accounted for. Are we to be stuck forever with this problem? Where on earth does it go? Is it simply stopped dead in its tracks, lost in humus, wasted? Considering the tendency of nature to find uses for complex and intricate mechanisms, this seems to me unnatural. I prefer to think of it as somehow separated off at the filaments of its attachment and then drawn like an easy breath back into the membrane of its origin, a fresh memory for a biospherical nervous system, but I have no data on the matter."

Question 5: Is the physician prepared to give of himself to the patient and "go down to the wire" with him? As a corollary, is the physician willing to continue to think about the problems his patient presents until the end? The phrase "dying a little with each patient" perhaps sounds trite, but it is a useful way of indicating the eventuality of real commitment to a patient. There is no substitute for making sure that your patient never once worries about being abandoned. Of course, no true physician would ever really abandon his patient, but I am speaking of a greater commitment: one that makes the patient know that you are there at all times, at the very least in spirit. Most people face illness with courage, hope, a willingness to place their trust in others, and a capacity to endure. They do this quietly, not seeking praise but simply because this is the way they are made. For a doctor to abandon a fellow human being at such times, through some well-meant but misguided effort to hurry him out of the world, is breaking the faith that he has pledged to all patients.

Now any position that one takes can be pushed to absurdity, and clearly certain judgments must be taken every day as part of a doctor's life in determining what should or should not be done for a patient. If a patient with far-advanced cancer, whose disease has been resistant to treatment, has a cardiac arrest, he obviously should not be resuscitated. Parenthetically, it is well for hospitals to establish procedures that will ensure that patients who should not be resuscitated are not. Like-

wise, one does not transfuse such a patient to maintain a normal hemoglobin, and so on. Therapeutic intervention need *not* be undertaken just because it *can* be undertaken. Nevertheless, these judgments are thinking judgments, and are made in the context of the earlier remarks. There is often a lot of living that has still to be "lived through" between the diagnosis of a terminal illness and death, and it is the quality of that living which should concern a physician. Helping a patient out of this world usually demands more skill, and certainly more understanding, than helping him into the world. Nevertheless, this can be done without abandoning the principles that guide physicians throughout their lives; if they will but continue to think, they will make decisions as nearly right as they can be.

A. E. Clark-Kennedy has written the following about the moral problem of preserving life: "According to Christian teaching, life is a gift, and the doctor is under a moral obligation to keep his patient alive as long as he can by means put into his hands. . . . A man has been given his life and it is not for him to opt out of it. But even Roman Catholic moralists hold that a doctor is only under an obligation to keep his patient alive as long as life can be reasonably maintained. Further, he need only use ordinary methods. These are those easily available." The key words are "reasonably," "ordinary," and "easily available." Obviously what is reasonable, ordinary, and easily available in a big university hospital will differ from what those terms would mean in a remote hospital in Africa. Further, these terms are also subject to the individual physician's interpretation. In this connection, this same author goes on to identify as "extraordinary" methods of treatment: "palliative surgery such as . . . oophorectomy, adrenalectomy, and even hypophysectomy in carcinoma of the breast." These surgical procedures are certainly available in many countries, but he has chosen to identify them as "extraordinary"; in the United States they would not generally be so regarded. Remissions of metastatic breast cancer have at times been so striking after endocrine surgery (in one recent case report, as long as 25 years after oophorectomy) that there is little doubt as to the value of these procedures in some patients.

One must also consider the thought that physicians may persist in their efforts to preserve life in the realization that they see and know only in part and that some unforeseen event may occur to alter an outcome which the physician, in his fallibility, has come to expect. Further, a patient is less apt to be fearful that his doctor will try to sustain his life than he is that the doctor will give up, notwithstanding the popular idea that healthy persons, contemplating terminal illness, usually express the wish to be allowed to die quickly. Recently, formalized documents have been executed as "living wills," and, although they usually are not legally binding, they are supposed to give some indication as to what a person wants in a terminal illness. These wills state, in part, that the signer "be allowed to die and not be kept alive by artificial means or heroic measures." Some eight state legislatures have passed laws similar to The Natural Death Act of California. This legislation specifies the procedures for executing a refusal of care statement by the patient and obligates the physician to honor this statement when, in his judgment, death is imminent. These pronouncements are generally made by people who are healthy rather than by the sick, who, perhaps because of denial or fear of death, want to live. There is, of course, a middle ground which responsible physicians should take. They should not, on the one hand, aggressively resuscitate a patient who has had prolonged cerebral anoxia after cardiac arrest, or, on the other hand, consign a terminally ill patient to a state of stupor with morphine just to be relieved of the awesome burden of caring for him.

One attempt to articulate the middle ground has been as follows: "When, in the opinion of the attending physicians, measures to prolong life which have no realistic hope of effecting significant improvement will cause further pain and suffering to the patient and the family, we support conservative, passive medical care in place of heroic measures in the management of a patient afflicted with a terminal illness" (New York Academy of Medicine, 1973). Although the word "prolong" appears in this statement, it is qualified by referring to measures which have "no realistic hope of effecting significant improvement," and in this sense it does not conflict with earlier statements about the use, or misuse, of the word "prolong." This statement puts the burden of these decisions squarely on the attending physicians, where it belongs. This burden implies that a doctor will continue to try to analyze what is happening to his patient, but that what action he takes will be dictated by the over-all circumstances. Note also the reference to "physicians," to indicate that decisions to stop active medical care are usually best taken in consultation with one's colleagues. Additional dimensions have been added to these considerations in the matter of discontinuing life-support systems. The principle of the patient's right of privacy and the importance of a return to a "cognitive, sapient state" were central issues in the legal decision permitting withdrawal of these systems in the instance of Karen Ann Quinlan, a 22-year-old woman being so supported but ultimately judged to have no reasonable hope of being restored to such a state of mind from her comatose condition. Ideally, the application of life-sustaining measures should not give rise to such dilemmas, but it is inevitable that at times they will, and the great care, compassion, and scholarliness with which this difficult medical-legal issue was addressed has considerably advanced human understanding.

Question 6: What is the attitude of the patient's family, and how is it being dealt with? Failure of the medical profession to explain to families what is happening to their terminally ill relatives is the cause of many of the articles published in newspapers and magazines about the increasing insensitivity of doctors. One hears repeatedly from families that "no one tells them anything." It is imperative that at least one member of the family, usually the next of kin, be fully informed of the patient's illness by the responsible physician. This should not be a single session but should be reviewed several times during the course of the patient's illness so that members of the family may have as complete an understanding as is possible for laymen to have. This does not mean that the physician has to have individual sessions with every member of the family; his time obligations must be respected. If a number of relatives are involved, it may be useful to meet with them together, because the physician's explanations, relayed by one member to others in the family, are subject to wide distortions.

It is wise to tell the family what you are doing and why, so that they will not harbor misconceptions. If you are giving fluids, antimicrobials, or oxygen, explain that these are designed for the patient's comfort. If members of a family understand, they will be more helpful and supportive to the patient; but if they are kept in the dark, they may sublimate their anxiety into hostility toward everyone and everything connected with their dying relative.

Further, physicians should give families an opportunity to express their own feelings. Guilt, frustration, and fear are all intermingled with grief, and someone must let the family know that their feelings are normal, that such feelings happen to everyone, and that those caring for the patient understand. No one can do this better than the responsible physician, and he should not delegate this to someone else.

The family also needs to have some reasonable projection as to the patient's life expectancy, but it is unwise to be too specific. Only the inexperienced claim such clairvoyance. Also they should know what to expect in terms of new developments in the patient's course. If the natural history of the disease permits some projections, this information should be shared. Finally, it is important not to engage in speculations as to what might have been had this or that been done or not done earlier in the patient's illness. The family likewise should be discouraged from making such speculations themselves, because they serve no useful purpose and may needlessly promote anxiety and bitterness.

Question 7: Is the patient undergoing experimental study, and, if so, are humanitarian principles being observed or compromised? Although this chapter is not concerned primarily with human experimentation, it is necessary to give this important subject some consideration in the context of the care of the terminally ill, because often new procedures or treatments are undertaken for the first time in humans with a limited life expectancy. Under these circumstances the approach of the physician to the terminally ill patient must, of necessity, be modified. In his quest for new knowledge, however, he must be prepared to see to it that the rules under which human experimentation is carried out are strictly observed.

Some have proposed that experiments done not for the immediate good of the patient but for the general welfare of mankind should be carried out by those who do not simultaneously have responsibility for the clinical care of the subject. Thus patients who are the subjects of such experiments would have two physicians: a physician-friend and a physician-investigator. Such a system would avoid the subtle alterations of reasoning that may take place when one physician tries to be both. However, if an investigator is true to himself, to his patient, and to the ethical principles which should guide his professional life, it is quite feasible for the same physician to be both friend and investigator. This relationship between investigator and investigatee has been defined by Guttentag as ". . . a partnership between the two, resulting from the fact of their being fellow human beings. . . ." He characterizes this relationship as one of "mutual trust and confidence, of openness between experimenter and subject." In the last analysis, then, the ethics of human experimentation arise from those of the individual investigator and from his perceptions and integrity in dealing with another human being. The essence of experimentation by one human being on another has been captured in this quotation from Paul Tillich:

Man becomes man in personal encounters. Only by meeting a "thou" does man realize he is an "ego." No natural object within the whole universe can do this to him. Man can transcend himself in all directions in knowledge and control. He can use everything for his purposes. Nobody can say where the final limits of human power lie. In his encounter with the universe, a man is able to transcend any imaginable limit. But there is a limit for man which is definite and which he always encounters, the other man. The other one, the "thou," is like a wall which cannot be removed or penetrated or used. He who tries to do so, destroys himself.

Biomedical research involving human subjects is based upon the integrity of the individual investigator and the obtaining of informed consent, freely given. Various codes have been developed, from the Nuremberg Code (1947) to the revised Declaration of Helsinki (1975), and in one form or another they contain the following provisions:

1. Prior voluntary, informed consent must be obtained from all subjects.

2. The study must hold promise of results for the good of society unprocurable by other means. However, the interest of society must never take precedence over considerations related to the well-being of the subject.

3. The study must be based on animal experimentation and conform to generally accepted scientific principles.

4. It must avoid all unnecessary physical and mental suffering.

5. The degree of risk must never exceed that determined by the humanitarian importance of the problem.

6. It must be conducted only by scientifically qualified and clinically competent persons.

7. The subject must always be at liberty to withdraw.

8. The investigator must be prepared to terminate the study if the subject is seriously endangered.

9. The procedures involved in the study must be formulated in a written protocol which must be reviewed and approved, from a scientific and ethical standpoint, by an independent committee.

Informed consent is still the most difficult thing to achieve, and the physician, in obtaining this, must keep in mind the following additional principles as outlined by the Board of Regents of the University of the State of New York:

(1) . . . it is the patient, and not the physician, who has the right to decide what factors are or are not relevant to his consent, regardless of the rationality of his assessment. . . . A physician has no right to withhold from a prospective volunteer any fact which he knows may influence the decision.

(2) . . . the physician, when he is acting as experimenter, has no claim to the doctor-patient relationship, that, in a therapeutic situation, would give him the generally acknowledged right to withhold information if he judged it in the best interest of the patient.

(3) No person can be said to have volunteered for an experiment unless he had first understood what he was volunteering for. Any matter which might influence him in giving or withholding consent is material. Deliberate nondisclosure of the material fact is no different from deliberate misrepresentation of such a fact.

Physicians dealing with terminal patients who are the subjects of experimentation must assure themselves that all these principles are being observed.

In conclusion, there is no greater test of the qualities of a physician than that imposed by the care of the terminally ill. It calls upon the doctor to exercise medical skill and at the same time to become involved with a fellow human being in the most trying and yet most ennobling of human relationships. How his patient fares will be determined in large part by how the physician meets this test.

Clark-Kennedy, A. E.: Man, Medicine and Morality. Hamden, Conn., Shoe String Press, 1970, pp. 196, 200.

Kübler-Ross, E.: On Death and Dying. New York, The Macmillan Company, 1969.

New York Academy of Medicine: Statement on Measures Employed to Prolong Life in Terminal Illness. Bull. N.Y. Acad. Med., 49 (2nd ser.):349, 1973.

Reiser, S. J., Dyck, A. J., and Curran, W. J. (eds.): Ethics in Medicine. Historical Perspectives and Contemporary Concerns. Cambridge, Mass., and London, The M.I.T. Press, 1977.

Rhoads, P. S.: Management of the patient with terminal illness. JAMA, 192:661, 1965.

Saunders, C. M.: Terminal care. In Bagshawe, K. D. (ed.): Medical Oncology. Oxford, Blackwell Scientific Publications, 1975.

Thomas, L.: The long habit. N. Engl. J. Med., 286:825, 1972.

Tillich, P.: Love, Power and Justice: Ontological Analyses and Ethical Applications. New York, Oxford University Press, 1960, p. 78.

PART XX
DISEASES OF METABOLISM

529. INTRODUCTION

James B. Wyngaarden

The term *metabolism* encompasses the numerous chemical transformations that occur within living organisms. These are often divided into two large categories. Those reactions or processes that are synthetic, and in general result in a larger molecule than any of the reactants, are called *anabolic*. Such reactions are usually energy requiring. Those reactions that are degradative and involve the breakdown of large molecules into smaller products are termed *catabolic*, and are essentially energy yielding processes. The term *intermediary metabolism* refers to all changes which take place between the moment of entry of a nutrient into the organism and the discharge of all of the chemical products into the environment. It is customary to consider separately the intermediary metabolism of carbohydrates, lipids, and proteins, although no sharp lines can be drawn among these three areas of knowledge. The term *basal metabolism* refers to energy requirements for maintenance and conduct of cellular and tissue processes under conditions in which the effects of muscular work and the work of digestion and metabolism of foodstuffs are minimal.

Part XX of this textbook is concerned with Diseases of Metabolism. A disorder is classified as a disease of metabolism when the fundamental pathogenetic mechanism involves a chemical transformation or process. Many diseases of metabolism involve specific enzyme abnormalities, usually deficiencies; a few are consequences of excessive enzyme activities. When these can be attributed to an underlying genetic abnormality, they are termed *inborn errors of metabolism*. Disorders associated with specific enzyme defects have been described for more than 100 individual enzymes. Most of these are described somewhere in this textbook, but not all have been collected into Part XX. For example, hemolytic anemias attributable to specific enzyme defects are included with the other hemolytic anemias in Part XVIII, Hematologic and Hematopoietic Diseases, and adrenal hyperplasia attributable to specific enzyme defects is discussed in Part XXI, Diseases of the Endocrine System. The disorders included in this Part are chiefly those whose manifestations are multisystemic or in which the biochemical and genetic factors dominate the description.

Not all inborn errors of metabolism can be defined at the enzyme level. Some inborn disorders involve transport processes and can at present be characterized only in terms of a functional defect at a membrane level. Examples include cystinuria, Hartnup disease, and renal glycosuria. A relatively new class of inborn errors involves abnormalities of receptor molecules situated within membranes, or within the cytoplasm or nucleus of the cell. Examples include familial hypercholesterolemia, pseudohypoparathyroidism, and nephrogenic dia-

betes insipidus. It is likely that these disorders involve specific structural abnormalities of membrane or receptor proteins. Other inborn errors involve abnormalities of circulating proteins, such as clotting or transport factors. Over 100 abnormalities of structure of both the alpha and beta chains of hemoglobin have been described, and in virtually all of these the specific amino acid replacement, deletion, or addition is known. The term *molecular disease* was introduced by Pauling and coworkers to describe a disorder in which a structural alteration of a macromolecule (sickle cell hemoglobin) caused a specific functional change responsible for the disease state. A molecular abnormality has now been demonstrated for many enzymes in disorders in which the clinical phenotype can be traced to a missing enzyme function, and in which a structurally altered enzyme is present. Thus no sharp distinction should be drawn between molecular diseases of the hemoglobinopathy type and metabolic diseases attributable to altered enzyme function.

There are many examples of metabolic diseases which are acquired rather than hereditary. Gout exists in primary and secondary varieties. The secondary types occur because of excessive nucleic acid turnover in myeloproliferative diseases or chronic hemolytic anemias, or because of impaired renal excretion of uric acid resulting from drug effects upon the kidney or acquired renal disease. Certain varieties of porphyria can be attributed to acquired intoxications. Hyperlipoproteinurias are common accompaniments of other diseases: hypothyroidism, the nephrotic syndrome, acute and chronic alcoholism, biliary obstruction. In many conditions there is a prominent interaction between hereditary and environmental factors: obesity and diabetes mellitus, ingestion of phenylalanine-containing proteins in phenylketonuria, ingestion of milk in galactosemia. Without the environmental stress these conditions would remain silent.

Some of the diseases of metabolism are very common, such as diabetes, with a prevalence in the United States of about 5 per cent, and the hyperlipidemias. Others are quite rare, and a few are perhaps more properly regarded as biochemical anomalies rather than diseases — pentosuria, for example. The study of rare metabolic disorders has provided a better understanding of normal metabolic processes, and in some instances has allowed early recognition of a disorder whose manifestations are preventable simply by adjustment of diet (galactosemia, phenylketonuria). The identification of specific enzyme defects has led to attempts at replacement therapy with inklings of success following enzyme fusion (Gaucher's disease, Fabry's disease) or organ transplantation (bone marrow in immunologic deficiency states; kidney in cystinosis, Fabry's disease, Gaucher's disease).

The chapter on disorders of fluid, electrolyte, and acid-base balance is included in this Part because clinical derangements of acidosis and alkalosis are profoundly metabolic and multisystemic, and an understanding of the composition and disturbances of extra- and intracellular fluids is central to the management of diseases of metabolism as well as many others in this volume.

Bondy, P. K., and Rosenberg, L. E. (eds.): Duncan's Diseases of Metabolism. 7th ed. Philadelphia, W. B. Saunders Company, 1974.

Garrod, A. E.: Inborn errors of metabolism (Croonian Lectures). Lancet, 2:1, 73, 142, 214, 1908.

Stanbury, J. B., Wyngaarden, J. B., and Fredrickson, D. C. (eds.): The Metabolic Basis of Inherited Disease. 4th ed. New York, McGraw-Hill Book Company, 1978.

530. DISORDERS OF FLUID, ELECTROLYTE, AND ACID-BASE BALANCE

William B. Schwartz

Fluid and electrolyte disturbances usually occur as complications of an underlying illness; the disorders considered in this chapter must therefore be viewed not as isolated entities but in the context of the specific clinical settings in which they appear.

As general background, it should be recalled that the water content of the body (approximately 50 to 60 per cent of body weight) is distributed between the intracellular and extracellular compartments. Approximately two thirds of the water is within cells, and the remaining third is divided between the interstitial space and plasma, which together make up the extracellular compartment. Because water moves freely across cell boundaries, changes in tonicity in one compartment induce a transfer of fluid that continues until a new steady state of osmotic equilibrium is established. By contrast, electrolytes are distributed in an asymmetric pattern, most of the ions in the extracellular fluid consisting of sodium, chloride, and bicarbonate and those in the intracellular fluid of potassium and organic anions. Except for the slight deviations attributable to the Donnan effect of the plasma proteins, the electrolyte composition of plasma and interstitial fluid is virtually identical. Thus for clinical purposes plasma composition can be taken as representative of the entire extracellular compartment.

Ch. 369 summarizes the renal regulation of electrolyte and acid-base equilibrium. In the present chapter relevant physiology will be presented entirely within the context of the clinical disorder under consideration.

DEPLETION OF VOLUME

The most common disturbance of fluid and electrolyte equilibrium is volume depletion. Loss of volume may occur from simple dehydration but is seen more frequently in association with a combined loss of water and electrolyte.

CLINICAL MANIFESTATIONS. The symptoms of volume depletion are few and nonspecific. The patient may complain of thirst, but nausea, light-headedness, and weakness are perhaps the most frequent and troublesome manifestations. Volume depletion affects pri-

TABLE 1.   Causes of Volume Depletion

Simple dehydration
  (Loss of water without electrolyte)

Combined depletion of water and sodium
  Gastrointestinal losses
    Vomiting
    Gastric or small bowel drainage
    Diarrhea
    Bowel fistulas (colostomy, ileostomy, etc.)
  Renal losses
    Chronic renal failure
    Diuretic phase of acute tubular necrosis
    Postobstructive nephropathy
    Adrenal insufficiency
    Osmotic diuresis
    Diuretics
  Skin losses
    Sweating
    Burns
  Paracentesis

marily the circulation and renal function. As plasma volume is diminished, blood pressure falls, heart rate rises, and a decrease in renal perfusion leads to oliguria and azotemia. When volume depletion is severe, profound shock becomes an immediate and serious threat to survival. The management of these clinical problems will be discussed after the individual causes of volume depletion have been considered.

PATHOGENESIS. The specific clinical circumstances in which volume depletion is encountered are listed in Table 1 and discussed in the paragraphs that follow.

Simple Dehydration (Loss of Water Without Electrolyte). The fluid requirement of the body is determined by insensible losses through skin and lungs and by the amount of water required to excrete the daily solute load. Ordinarily the minimal intake to maintain water balance is 700 to 1000 ml per day. Thirst ordinarily maintains water intake well above this basal level; if weakness or disability sharply curtails fluid intake, however, dehydration will develop. The magnitude of the fluid deficit will be aggravated when insensible losses are increased by factors such as fever and hyperventilation or when urinary losses are abnormally large — for example, in uncontrolled diabetes insipidus.

Whenever more water than electrolyte is lost, hypernatremia and hypertonicity accompany the depletion of volume. The clinical features and consequences of hypernatremia are discussed later in this chapter.

Combined Depletion of Water and Sodium. Severe volume deficits occur most commonly in patients who have suffered a combined loss of water and sodium, usually from the gastrointestinal tract, the kidneys, or the skin.

GASTROINTESTINAL LOSSES. Volume depletion may occur as the result of losses from any portion of the gastrointestinal tract. Gastrointestinal secretions normally amount to some 8 to 10 liters per day; if the body is deprived of a significant fraction of this total, severe volume depletion will result. Depletion is most commonly the consequence of vomiting, gastric drainage, or diarrhea. It also is seen with small-bowel drainage, ileostomy, colostomy, and pancreatic or biliary fistulas. Most gastrointestinal secretions are either isotonic or slightly hypotonic; thus enteric losses should not by themselves produce a striking change in the sodium concentration of the serum. However, because serum sodium concentration is ultimately determined by overall water balance (as influenced by fluid intake and skin losses, among other factors), either hyponatremia or hypernatremia may be encountered.

RENAL LOSSES. Patients with *chronic renal failure* commonly have a reduced ability to conserve sodium, but the sodium-wasting tendency is seldom severe enough to become apparent if dietary intake of salt is normal. If salt intake is restricted, however, continued excretion of sodium and the associated loss of water may produce severe depletion of extracellular volume. Contraction of volume, in turn, causes a further reduction in glomerular filtration rate and may even precipitate frank uremia. Sodium intake in the azotemic patient should not be curtailed, therefore, without careful sequential observations of body weight and sodium excretion.

Occasionally a patient wastes sodium even while ingesting a normal quantity of salt; most such patients appear to have *medullary cystic disease* as their underlying renal lesion. In such cases of severe salt-wasting, the diet must be supplemented with sodium chloride if volume depletion is to be avoided. It is important to remember that in the patient with renal disease volume depletion should always be considered as a possible explanation for a sudden otherwise unexplained increase in azotemia.

During the *diuretic phase of acute tubular necrosis* the inability of the damaged tubules to reabsorb sodium may lead to a considerable loss of sodium and water. Sodium wasting does not usually persist for more than several days and is not likely to become clinically significant if the salt content of the patient's diet is normal. At times it may be difficult to distinguish between an abnormal diuresis and the physiologic diuresis that occurs when too much fluid and electrolyte have been administered during the oliguric phase of the disease. If the cause is not clear, treatment can ordinarily be delayed for a day or two until the issue is resolved either by the cessation of the diuresis or by the appearance of early signs of volume depletion. In this way an unnecessary and prolonged cycle of saline loading and saline loss can be avoided. A similar period of uncontrolled sodium and fluid loss by the kidney may be observed after renal transplantation.

Postobstructive nephropathy occasionally produces severe sodium and volume depletion in patients in whom complete or nearly complete obstruction has been present for a prolonged period. The defect in sodium reabsorption results from tubular damage and becomes manifest promptly after the relief of obstruction permits the filtered load of sodium to increase. Loss of salt may lead to an obligatory diuresis of as much as 5 or 10 liters per day and thus to an acute contraction of extracellular and plasma volume. Just as with the diuretic phase of acute tubular necrosis, the disorder is usually self-limiting, because the tubules generally recover their capacity to transport sodium within a few days.

Volume depletion following excessive renal losses of fluid and electrolyte may also occur in the absence of structural renal disease. In patients with *adrenal insufficiency* (Addison's disease) a deficiency of salt-retaining steroids reduces the activity of renal transport mechanisms and may allow large quantities of sodium and water to escape into the urine. Continued administration of *diuretics* to the patient who has been but is no

longer edematous will also sometimes produce volume depletion.

Abnormal losses of sodium and water are also induced by the obligatory excretion of a large solute load. Such losses are seen most frequently in association with the glycosuria of *diabetic ketoacidosis* (see Ch. 531.1) and of *nonketotic hyperosmolar coma*. The latter disorder typically occurs in middle-aged or elderly mild diabetics and is characterized by hyperglycemia, hyperosmolality, and profound dehydration. Blood sugar is often in the range of 1000 mg per 100 ml, but the disorder is readily distinguished from diabetic coma by the absence of ketoacidosis. Salt and water depletion caused by osmotic diuresis may also occur with administration of *tube feedings containing large quantities of protein*. Repeated infusions of *mannitol* may have the same effects.

SKIN LOSSES. Large losses of water and electrolyte from the skin may result either from excessive sweating or from burns. *Sweat* is a hypotonic solution normally containing no more than 50 mEq of sodium per liter; sweating will therefore produce a relatively larger deficit of water than of sodium. *Burns* can lead to two types of deficit: isotonic extracellular fluid may be lost by transudation; and water may be lost without electrolyte as the result of increased evaporation through damaged epithelium. An additional factor contributing to a severe depletion of circulating volume is capillary damage, which results in the interstitial accumulation of fluid, particularly during the first days after the burn has occurred. Because it takes place internally, such fluid loss can readily be overlooked.

PARACENTESIS. An occasional patient with cirrhosis and ascites develops circulatory collapse after *paracentesis*. Reduction of pressure within the peritoneal cavity may allow transudation of a large quantity of fluid with consequent contraction of plasma volume. Clinically significant contraction is not likely to occur in patients who have a substantial amount of peripheral edema, apparently because plasma volume can be readily replenished by transfer of fluid from the expanded interstitial space.

DIAGNOSIS. The *history* is frequently of great value in appraising the origin and magnitude of a volume deficit. The patient should be questioned closely about fluid intake and about fluid losses that may have resulted from vomiting, diarrhea, sweating, polyuria, or other disturbances. In many cases, particularly when a reliable history is not available, *physical examination* is the single most valuable diagnostic tool. Reduction in turgor of the skin, particularly over the arms, legs, and face, is the most characteristic finding and is usually accompanied by postural hypotension. The facies are usually pinched, and the tongue is dry. Lowered tension of the eyeballs, a rapid resting pulse, and hypotension in the recumbent position may be observed when dehydration is severe.

Laboratory findings are likely to be less valuable. The concentration of sodium in the serum reflects only the ratio of sodium to water, and whether low, normal, or high, gives no insight into the total volume of extracellular fluid present. Elevated hematocrit and hemoglobin concentrations suggest that plasma volume is contracted, but, unless the values before the acute illness are known, interpretation of these data is likely to be difficult. Measurement of the plasma creatinine concentration is sometimes helpful, because it may provide evidence of volume depletion and impairment of renal function even before the appearance of oliguria. The blood urea nitrogen level is a less useful index of renal dysfunction, because the urea concentration can be elevated by external factors, such as fever or an excess of adrenal corticoids.

Once the diagnosis of a deficit of sodium and water has been made, measurements of sodium excretion may help to identify the source of the losses. If the depletion is of *extrarenal* origin, the contraction in volume will normally lead to relatively prompt and efficient conservation of sodium by the kidney. Increased secretion of aldosterone, a decrease in the rate of glomerular filtration, and other as yet undefined factors augment sodium reabsorption and reduce sodium excretion to less than 5 or 10 mEq per day. If the excretion of sodium exceeds 30 to 40 mEq per day, it can generally be concluded that the losses are of *renal* origin and are the result of primary renal disease, Addison's disease, or osmotic diuresis. If the contraction of volume is sufficiently severe to produce oliguria and a marked reduction in filtration rate, however, sodium excretion will sometimes fall to a low level even in disorders in which the underlying abnormality is defective renal conservation of sodium.

TREATMENT. The most serious threat to the patient with severe volume depletion is circulatory collapse, and the most immediate concern in treatment is restoration of an adequate blood volume and blood pressure. This goal can be accomplished most effectively by the rapid infusion of plasma (if the hematocrit is elevated) or blood. If neither plasma nor blood is available, isotonic saline solution should be given instead; saline is not an entirely satisfactory substitute, however, because a large fraction of administered salt and water is promptly lost from the circulation as it diffuses into the interstitial space.

After shock has been corrected, the remaining fluid and electrolyte abnormalities can be repaired in a more leisurely fashion. Close observation of skin turgor, body weight, blood pressure, and serum creatinine concentration, together with available information about the volume and composition of the losses, will provide a useful guide to replacement therapy. In some cases as much as 4 or 5 liters of fluid will be required to correct the volume deficit. If serum sodium is within normal limits (indicating a virtually equivalent deficit of sodium and water), repair should be carried out largely with isotonic saline solution; water without electrolyte should be given only as needed to replace insensible and renal losses occurring during the period of treatment. Even if serum sodium concentration is moderately abnormal (as low as 130 mEq or as high as 150 mEq per liter), the same approach to therapy can be employed as in the patient with isotonic contraction of extracellular volume. If isotonic saline solution and modest quantities of water are administered, the kidney can be relied on for final adjustment of both volume and tonicity. With gross deviations in sodium concentration, more specific measures will be necessary. Severe hypernatremia will require that considerably more water than salt be given, and, conversely, severe hyponatremia (in the absence of edema) will call for correction, or partial correction, by administration of hypertonic sodium chloride solution. The management of hypernatremia and hyponatremia is discussed in detail later in this chapter.

The composition of the repair solutions must also allow for the presence of other electrolyte abnormalities. If, for example, metabolic acidosis is present, the sodium deficit should be corrected in part with sodium bicarbonate rather than exclusively with sodium chloride.

Treatment of the patient with *nonketotic hyperosmolar coma* requires not only appropriate correction of the fluid and electrolyte deficits but also the administration of adequate amounts of insulin to deal with the hyperglycemia. Some observers have suggested that the amount of insulin required is less than that in the patient with diabetic ketoacidosis, but this question remains to be clarified.

Arieff, A. I., and Carroll, H. J.: Nonketotic hyperosmolar coma with hyperglycemia: Clinical features, pathophysiology, renal function, acid-base balance, plasma–cerebrospinal fluid equilibria and the effects of therapy in 37 cases. Medicine, 51:73, 1972.
Bricker, N. S., and Klahr, S.: Obstructive nephropathy. *In* Strauss, M. B., and Welt, L. G. (eds.): Diseases of the Kidney. 2nd ed. Boston, Little, Brown & Company, 1971, pp. 1018–1020.
Gauer, O. H., Henry, J. P., and Behn, C.: The regulation of extracellular fluid volume. Ann. Rev. Physiol., 32:547, 1970.
Gault, M. H., Dixon, M. E., Doyle, M., and Cohen, W. M.: Hypernatremia, azotemia, and dehydration due to high-protein tube feeding. Ann. Intern. Med., 68:778, 1968.

HYPONATREMIA

Sodium is the ion present in highest concentration in the extracellular fluid, and sodium salts are thus the primary determinant of the osmolality (tonicity) of the extracellular compartment. Changes in sodium concentration therefore have a major influence on the distribution of water between the intracellular and extracellular spaces.

Normally, serum sodium concentration is stabilized at approximately 140 mEq per liter by changes in water balance that occur in response to variations in plasma osmotic pressure. A slight increase in sodium concentration, and thus in osmotic pressure, leads to the release of antidiuretic hormone and to a retention of water that then restores normal tonicity. Conversely, a slight reduction in serum sodium concentration and osmotic pressure inhibits the release of hormone and permits any excess water to be excreted.

A variety of disturbances can lead to an abnormal and sustained reduction in serum sodium concentration. Retention of water without sodium, loss of sodium without a proportional loss of water, or redistribution of water between cells and extracellular fluid may induce hyponatremia. As noted earlier, serum sodium concentration yields no direct information concerning the state of total sodium stores; rather, it indicates only that there has been a disturbance in the ratio of sodium to water.

The specific causes of hyponatremia and the mechanisms that underlie their development are described in detail below. It is convenient, however, to consider first the clinical manifestations and the aspects of treatment that are common to all hypo-osmotic states.

CLINICAL MANIFESTATIONS. The signs and symptoms of the hypo-osmotic state are those of *water intoxication* and are apparently caused by movement of fluid from the extracellular space into the relatively more hypertonic cells. When serum sodium concentration falls to approximately 120 mEq per liter, the patient frequently becomes irritable and confused. More serious disturbances are seen if the sodium concentration falls to 110 mEq or less; the patient often becomes lethargic or comatose, and generalized convulsions develop. Death may result unless appropriate treatment is instituted promptly.

TREATMENT. Severe hyponatremia is best treated by the intravenous administration of hypertonic (3 per cent) sodium chloride. Elevation of serum sodium concentration to a level of 125 or 130 mEq per liter will ordinarily suffice to eliminate all evidence of central nervous system dysfunction. Full correction of hyponatremia need not and should not be carried out over a short time, because the sudden transfer of a large volume of fluid from the intracellular to the extracellular space is sometimes hazardous; an abrupt expansion of plasma volume may elevate central venous pressure and produce symptomatic pulmonary congestion, particularly in the patient with frank or latent heart disease.

Calculation of the amount of salt necessary to produce a given rise in the concentration of sodium must take into consideration the shift of water that will be induced by the increase in extracellular tonicity. As serum sodium concentration is elevated, water moves out of cells along the resulting osmotic gradient; the estimated sodium requirement must therefore be based on the need to restore tonicity throughout the total body water. The following example of this calculation assumes an initial serum sodium concentration of 110 mEq per liter, a final concentration of 125 mEq per liter, and a body weight of 70 kg. Since approximately 50 per cent of the total body weight is water, the amount of sodium necessary to produce the desired change will be 35 liters × 15 mEq per liter, or approximately 500 mEq of sodium. The calculation can be summarized by the following equation:

$$[\text{Desired Na conc.} - \text{initial Na conc.}] \times 0.5 \text{ body weight} = \text{mEq of Na}$$

PATHOGENESIS. Table 2 lists the specific clinical circumstances in which a low sodium concentration is encountered. They are discussed in the following paragraphs.

Functional Disorders Leading to Defective Excretion of Water. DEPLETION OF SODIUM AND EXTRACELLULAR VOLUME. Significant impairment of water excretion often results from severe depletion of sodium and volume, thus making the development of hyponatremia more likely. If water is ingested or infused without electrolyte, the retention of a portion of this water leads to a decreased concentration of sodium in the serum. This sequence of events accounts for the frequent occurrence of hyponatremia in conditions such as vomiting or diarrhea. A reduction in glomerular filtration rate, with a consequent reduced delivery of sodium and water to the distal nephron, probably accounts for the failure to excrete an appropriately dilute urine and for the persistence of hyponatremia.

In most patients with volume depletion, the water intake is not large enough to produce hyponatremia of great severity, and serum sodium concentration decreases by no more than 10 or 15 mEq per liter. In such cases the manifestations of volume depletion rather than of hyponatremia usually dominate the clinical picture; treatment should therefore be aimed primarily at correction of extracellular volume rather than at elevating serum sodium concentration. As discussed earlier, if sodium concentration is only moderately reduced, correction of hyponatremia will occur as a byproduct of expansion with isotonic saline solution; restoration of normal plasma volume will correct the renal defect in water excretion, and an augmented water output will then restore tonicity to normal.

INAPPROPRIATE SECRETION OF ANTIDIURETIC HORMONE. In the syndrome of inappropriate secretion of antidiuretic hormone (SIADH), hypotonicity of the plasma fails to suppress the release of antidiuretic hormone (ADH), with the result that renal excretion of water is impaired. The consequent expansion of extracellular volume not only causes dilution of body fluids, but also induces a sodium diuresis and a negative sodium balance. The increase in sodium excretion in response to expansion of volume is apparently mediated by an increase in the rate of glomerular filtration and other as yet poorly defined factors (for instance, "third factor"). The combination of water retention and salt wasting produces a decrease in serum sodium concentration, with serum levels occasionally falling to as low as 110 or even 100 mEq per liter.

This syndrome has been noted most often in association with bronchogenic carcinoma of the oat cell type but has also been seen in patients with other malignant tumors such as carcinoma of the pancreas. In such patients it appears that the production of vasopressin or a vasopressin-like polypeptide by the tumor is responsible for the abnormal fluid retention. The syndrome is also seen in a variety of other clinical settings, most notably in association with central nervous system disturbances (such as head injuries, brain tumors, and encephalitis) and lung disease (such as cavitating tuberculosis or pneumonia). In each of these conditions, the retention of water apparently results from an aberrant stimulus to ADH release, that is, from a signal which bypasses the osmoreceptors of the hypothalamus.

The following combination of features is virtually diagnostic of SIADH: (1) hyponatremia with renal sodium wasting; (2) normal tissue turgor and normal blood pressure; (3) normal blood urea nitrogen and creatinine concentrations; (4) normal adrenal function; and (5) specific gravity of the urine inappropriately high for a hypotonic subject, that is, in excess of 1.002 or 1.003. Edema is not a usual feature, because water retention does not ordinarily exceed 3 or 4 liters and because some fraction of the retained fluid probably moves into cells.

Although sodium loss is a classic feature of SIADH, the presence of a significant quantity of sodium in the

---

TABLE 2.   Causes of Hyponatremia

1. Functional disorders leading to defective excretion of water
   Depletion of sodium and extracellular fluid volume
   Inappropriate secretion of antidiuretic hormone
   Addison's disease
2. Drug-induced impairment of water excretion
3. Idiopathic hyponatremia
   Congestive heart failure
   Cirrhosis of the liver
4. Excessive water intake in the presence of normal renal function
   Psychogenic polydipsia
5. Renal disease with defective excretion of water
   Acute renal failure with oliguria
   Chronic renal failure
6. Hyponatremia without disturbance in water balance
   Accumulation of solute in the extracellular fluid
   Pseudohyponatremia

urine is not a prerequisite of the diagnosis of the syndrome. As serum sodium concentration falls, a new balance is struck between the reduced filtered load of sodium and the reduced renal capacity for sodium reabsorption. Thus when a new steady state of serum sodium concentration has been achieved, the urine will become virtually sodium free if sodium intake is extremely low. The salt-wasting abnormality can, however, be readily unmasked by the administration of salt either by mouth or by vein.

When the concentration of sodium in the serum is so low that it produces signs of severe water intoxication (such as coma or convulsions), hypertonic sodium chloride solution should immediately be infused to raise the osmotic pressure of plasma. Since the salt so administered will rapidly be excreted if expansion of extracellular volume persists, prompt correction of the state of overhydration should also be undertaken. Diuretic therapy with an agent such as furosemide is an effective means of producing such volume contraction and, when combined with hypertonic salt infusion, will produce a rapid and sustained elevation of serum sodium concentration.

Lithium and demeclocycline, two agents that interfere with the action of vasopressin on the renal tubule, have recently been suggested as yet further means of treating SIADH. The role of these drugs in the management of SIADH is not yet clear, however.

If severe manifestations of water intoxication are not present, appropriate treatment consists simply of restricting fluid intake and allowing insensible and urinary losses of water to contract the volume of extracellular fluid. This program of management not only will restore the capacity for normal renal conservation of sodium but will also correct the component of hyponatremia that has developed as a consequence of dilution. Correction of the element of the hyponatremia caused by renal sodium loss does, of course, require provision of salt either by mouth or by vein. Fluid restriction will not be effective unless it is stringent enough to produce a loss of several kilograms in weight. An intake of 400 to 500 ml per day over three to five days will usually accomplish this goal.

If the patient fails to conserve sodium after a large loss of weight, the diagnosis of SIADH must be questioned seriously, and other disorders, particularly Addison's disease, must be considered. Addison's disease can easily be overlooked unless one recognizes that sodium depletion in adrenal insufficiency need not be accompanied by volume depletion; in some patients the deficiency of cortisol causes an impairment of water excretion of such magnitude that, despite the loss of sodium, hydration remains normal. In such patients the clinical picture can closely mimic SIADH. Thus it is always advisable to carry out studies of adrenal function before concluding that the hyponatremia is due to inappropriate secretion of ADH.

In a disorder such as meningitis or pneumonitis, the water-excreting defect disappears as recovery from the underlying illness takes place. With permanent brain damage, or with carcinoma of the lung, the defect can persist indefinitely, and a moderate degree of water restriction may be necessary to prevent recurrence of severe hyponatremia and salt wasting.

Drug-Induced Hyponatremia. A variety of drugs, notably *chlorpropamide, vincristine, cyclophosphamide,* and *carbamazepine,* interfere with the excretion of a water load by the kidneys and can produce enough retention of water to cause appreciable volume expansion and hyponatremia. These agents stimulate the release of ADH and, at least in the case of chlorpropamide, augment the action of ADH on the renal tubule. The resulting syndrome is indistinguishable from the classic SIADH.

Diuretic agents, such as *furosemide, ethacrynic acid,* and *chlorothiazide,* can also cause water retention and considerable reductions in serum sodium concentration. Such disturbances in water balance are usually seen only if treatment has led to volume contraction of a magnitude which not only stimulates the release of ADH but also lowers the filtration rate and reduces delivery of sodium and water to the diluting segment of the nephron.

In patients ingesting large quantities of fluid, the direct effect of the diuretic in inhibiting sodium reabsorption in the ascending loop of Henle can, in itself, sometimes impair water excretion sufficiently to cause hyponatremia.

Idiopathic Hyponatremia. Hyponatremia frequently appears without warning in the edematous patient entering the late stages of *congestive heart failure* or *cirrhosis of the liver.* In this setting it is an ominous prognostic sign that appears to be the reflection, rather than the cause, of the underlying clinical deterioration.

The factors responsible for this electrolyte disturbance have not been clearly defined. Salt depletion induced by diuretic therapy cannot be held accountable, because the edematous patient has a larger than normal quantity of sodium in his extracellular space. Furthermore, the disorder has been observed in patients who have not received diuretics or in whom diuretics have failed to promote salt excretion. In some cases it can be demonstrated that retention of water is responsible for the hyponatremic state, but in others measurements of body weight give no evidence that fluid was retained during the period that sodium concentration fell. In the latter circumstance it has been proposed that a primary reduction in intracellular osmolality allows water to shift into the extracellular space and that the lowered osmotic pressure of the plasma is simply a passive reflection of the change in cellular tonicity. According to this thesis, failure to increase the excretion of water is explained by the absence of an osmotic gradient between plasma and the osmoreceptors of the hypothalamus.

In some patients with congestive heart failure or cirrhosis, the development of hyponatremia is apparently an indirect consequence of enhanced proximal reabsorption of sodium and water; the delivery of an abnormally small volume of glomerular filtrate from the proximal tubule to the distal nephron prevents the elaboration of a hypotonic urine and leads to pathologic water retention. Inappropriate secretion of antidiuretic hormone has also been invoked as a factor in the genesis of the hyponatremia, but clear support for this hypothesis has yet to be obtained.

As noted above, the appearance of hyponatremia in the edematous patient is usually a grave prognostic sign. Even if the patient does not appear to be critically ill, prolonged survival is uncommon unless treatment directed toward improving the underlying cardiac or liver disease is successful. Elevation of the serum sodium concentration by either water restriction or the administration of hypertonic sodium chloride usually has no beneficial effect. Water restriction usually induces severe thirst before osmolality is restored to normal, and, if the patient is then permitted to increase his fluid intake, he quickly re-establishes the hyponatremic state. The administration of hypertonic saline not only seems to be of little clinical value but appears, in many instances, to hasten rather than retard the downward clinical course.

Hyponatremia of unknown cause is sometimes seen in seriously ill patients with a debilitating disease such as metastatic carcinoma or leukemia. Neither dehydration nor edema is present, and there is no evidence of extrarenal or urinary loss of sodium. The explanation for this disturbance is obscure.

Renal Disease with Defective Excretion of Water. During the oliguric phase of *acute renal failure* dilutional hyponatremia will regularly occur if fluid intake is not adequately restricted. The net loss of water from skin and lungs is normally about 400 to 500 ml per day; if severe oliguria or anuria is present, administration of significantly more than this quantity (for example, 1000 to 1200 ml) will produce overhydration within a relatively short time.

Water intoxication is occasionally seen in *chronic renal failure* and occurs primarily in patients who have been urged to ingest large quantities of fluid in an effort to increase urine volume and thus to promote excretion of urea. Such attempts to force a diuresis not only may be hazardous but also appear to have little beneficial effect on the clinical course, even when they produce a slight reduction in blood urea concentration.

Excessive Water Intake in the Presence of Normal Renal Function (Psychogenic Polydipsia). A syndrome virtually identical to that already described for inappropriate secretion of ADH may be produced by the ingestion of more water than the normal kidney can excrete, that is, more than 1000 or 1200 ml per hour. Intakes in excess of these amounts are unusual, but are occasionally seen in patients with severe psychiatric illness. In such cases the expansion of extracellular volume induced by the positive water balance leads to both hyponatremia and renal wasting of sodium. Characteristically, the urine is maximally dilute (specific gravity of 1.001), and it is this finding that unequivocally demonstrates that the syndrome results from excessive ingestion of water rather than from inappropriate secretion of ADH.

If signs of water intoxication are present, hypertonic saline solution should be given intravenously, but in most cases reduction of water intake and increased ingestion of salt will be the only treatment required.

Hyponatremia Without Disturbance in Water Balance. ACCUMULATION OF SOLUTE IN THE EXTRACELLULAR FLUID. Solutes such as glucose and mannitol, which do not distribute freely throughout the body water, can accumulate in the extracellular space and create an osmotic gradient between cells and interstitial fluid. As a result, water shifts from the intracellular compartment, and the serum sodium concentration falls. Hyponatremia resulting from such a redistribution of fluid is a characteristic feature of the severe hyperglycemia seen in patients with uncontrolled diabetes mellitus; each increment of 100 mg per 100 ml in blood sugar concentration above normal represents the addition of slightly more than 5 milliosmols of solute per kilogram to the extracellular compartment and leads to a reduction in serum sodium concentration of approxi-

mately 1.5 mEq per liter. A blood sugar concentration of 1000 mg per 100 ml can thus be expected to lower sodium concentration from 140 to 125 mEq per liter. Failure to consider the role of hyperglycemia in the genesis of hyponatremia in the diabetic can lead to the administration of an excessive amount of sodium during the treatment of ketoacidosis.

The accumulation of mannitol in the extracellular fluid can also cause a shift of water sufficient to reduce serum sodium concentration. This problem is most likely to be encountered in the patient with acute renal failure in whom an unsuccessful attempt has been made to increase the volume of urine by repeated infusions of mannitol.

Hyperosmolality will not produce hyponatremia if the solute distributes freely across cell membranes and thus increases the osmolality of cells and interstitial fluid to a proportional degree. In uremia, for example, serum sodium concentration is unaffected by the hypertonicity induced by accumulation of urea because it penetrates cells readily and its concentration is elevated throughout body water.

PSEUDOHYPONATREMIA. Pseudohyponatremia is a spurious reduction in sodium concentration resulting from a displacement of some fraction of plasma water by an abnormal accumulation of lipid or protein. Although plasma sodium concentration is usually measured in milliequivalents per liter of plasma, the physiologically significant measurement is the sodium concentration expressed as milliequivalents per kilogram of plasma water. Thus a sodium concentration of 140 mEq per liter measured on whole plasma reflects an actual concentration of 150 mEq per kilogram of water in normal plasma, which contains 93 per cent water. Since the percentage of water in plasma does not vary appreciably under most circumstances, reductions in plasma sodium concentration can generally be taken as reflecting a decrease in the sodium concentration per unit of plasma water and in the tonicity of extracellular fluid. On the other hand, if severe hyperlipemia (or hyperproteinemia) is present, the fraction of plasma made up by water will be lower than normal, and a striking reduction in the sodium concentration per unit volume of plasma will be observed despite the absence of a significant change in the electrolyte concentration per kilogram of plasma water.

Hyperlipemia of sufficient magnitude to produce pseudohyponatremia occurs in a number of diseases, including diabetes mellitus, nephrotic syndrome, and biliary cirrhosis. In nearly all cases in which sodium concentration is reduced by lipidemia the plasma is frankly lactescent. Thus lactescence will often be the first finding that points to the correct diagnosis. *Hyperproteinemia* severe enough to cause pseudohyponatremia is rare and has been seen only in multiple myeloma. In this disease the plasma sodium concentration may be lowered to 125 or 130 mEq per liter.

The contribution of an increased concentration of lipid or protein to a reduced plasma sodium concentration can be readily assessed by determination of plasma osmotic pressure (estimated from freezing-point depression). If osmotic pressure is normal despite the hyponatremia, the concentration of sodium in the aqueous phase of plasma is normal.

Aviram, A., Pfau, A., Czaczkes, J. W., and Ullmann, T. D.: Hyperosmolality with hyponatremia, caused by inappropriate administration of mannitol. Am. J. Med., 42:648, 1967.

Bartter, F., and Schwartz, W. B.: The syndrome of inappropriate secretion of antidiuretic hormone. Am. J. Med., 42:790, 1967.

Harrington, J. T., and Cohen, J. J.: Clinical disorders of urine concentration and dilution. Arch. Intern. Med., 131:810, 1973.

Langgard, H., and Smith, W. O.: Self-induced water intoxication without predisposing illness. N. Engl. J. Med., 266:378, 1962.

Leaf, A.: The clinical and physiologic significance of the serum sodium concentration. N. Engl. J. Med., 267:24, 1962.

Moses, A. M., and Miller, M.: Drug-induced dilutional hyponatremia. N. Engl. J. Med., 291:1234, 1974.

HYPERNATREMIA

Virtually all cases of hypernatremia result from a loss of water that produces a relative excess of sodium in the body fluids. Any hypotonic loss, such as that occurring with sweating or vomiting, will cause a modest degree of hypernatremia that will persist if adequate fluid replacement is not provided. Extreme elevations of plasma sodium concentrations (160 mEq per liter or more) are uncommon and are usually encountered in only one of three clinical settings: decreased or absent fluid intake, diabetes insipidus, or osmotic diuresis. Such extreme increases in tonicity of the extracellular fluid, when they occur, lead to marked cellular dehydration.

The most common cause of hypernatremia is a fluid intake that is inadequate to replace urinary losses and insensible losses of water from skin and lungs. This problem is most frequently encountered in the patient who is stuporous or who has some other disability that prevents him from drinking normally. In the comatose patient in whom *diabetes insipidus* develops after a head injury or a neurosurgical procedure, a large negative water balance is likely to appear with unusual speed. In most cases of diabetes insipidus, polyuria will quickly draw attention to the nature of the problem, but if solute intake is low, the diagnosis can readily be overlooked, because urine volume may not exceed 2 or 3 liters per day.

Osmotic loading can also produce severe hypernatremia. During osmotic diuresis water is lost in excess of sodium; with sustained or repeated diuresis the serum sodium concentration sometimes rises to values greater than 175 mEq per liter. This sequence of events is often observed in comatose patients who are confronted with a massive urea load as the result of being given tube feedings containing large amounts of protein. In such patients maintenance of a normal urine volume by continued solute loading may sometimes obscure the fact that dehydration and hypertonicity are present. Under such circumstances, the progressive loss of weight, the physical signs of volume depletion, and the development of hypernatremia should draw attention to the correct diagnosis.

The specific signs and symptoms produced by a marked elevation of serum sodium concentration have not been clearly defined. Most patients with hypernatremia are already seriously ill; the role of the hypertonicity, as distinguished from that of the underlying disease, is therefore frequently difficult to evaluate. Clinical experience suggests, however, that when hypernatremia is encountered water should be administered (either orally or as 5 per cent glucose intravenously) in quantities sufficient to restore serum sodium concentration to normal. The quantity of water required must be calculated with an appreciation that hypertonicity is present not only in the extracellular fluid but throughout total body water. Thus a 70-kg man with a plasma sodium concentration of 170

mEq per liter will require a 20 per cent expansion of body water, that is, 8 liters of fluid, to restore serum sodium concentration to a normal value of 140 mEq per liter. Observations during the treatment of hypernatremia indicate that full correction should not be carried out over a few hours, because a rapid reduction in tonicity may produce signs of water intoxication.

Gault, M. H., Dixon, E. E., Doyle, M., and Cohen, W. M.: Hypernatremia, azotemia, and dehydration due to high-protein tube feeding. Ann. Intern. Med., 68:778, 1968.

Leaf, A.: The clinical and physiologic significance of the serum sodium concentration. N. Engl. J. Med., 267:24, 1962.

Ross, E. J., and Christie, S. B. M.: Hypernatremia. Medicine, 48:441, 1969.

Weiner, M., and Epstein, F. H.L.: Signs and symptoms of electrolyte disorders. Yale J. Biol. Med., 43:76, 1970.

DISTURBANCES OF POTASSIUM EQUILIBRIUM

Potassium, the major intracellular cation, plays a significant part in control of osmotic pressure and is also an essential activator in a number of enzymatic reactions. In addition, the potassium concentration of body fluids has an important influence on the excitability of both skeletal and cardiac muscle and on the structure and function of the kidneys. Disturbances in potassium equilibrium may therefore produce a wide range of clinical disorders.

The potassium concentraion is normally 3.8 to 5 mEq per liter in extracellular fluid and approximately 150 mEq per liter in intracellular fluid. Since about 20 per cent of body weight is extracellular fluid, only a small fraction of the 2500 to 3000 mEq of potassium within the body is contained in the extracellular space. Changes in plasma potassium concentration often mirror changes in cellular potassium content, however; plasma concentration thus usually provides a useful clinical guide to disturbances in potassium balance. Furthermore, relatively small absolute changes in extracellular concentration, by producing large differences in the ratio of intracellular to extracellular potassium, may have important effects on neuromuscular activity.

Despite the usual wide variations in dietary intake of potassium (40 to 120 mEq per day), plasma potassium concentration is normally stabilized within the narrow range of 4 to 5 mEq per liter by virtue of close renal regulation of potassium balance. Potassium excretion is accomplished largely, if not exclusively, by secretion of potassium in the the distal portion of the nephron; it has been demonstrated that essentially all filtered potassium is reabsorbed in the proximal tubule and that the potassium that appears in the urine is added to the filtrate by a distal process of sodium-cation exchange. Fecal excretion of potassium normally amounts to only a few milliequivalents per day and does not play a significant role in potassium homeostasis.

If a large potassium load is suddenly administered, renal mechanisms do not respond quickly enough to prevent a rise in serum potassium concentration to abnormal levels. Under such circumstances, sequestration of potassium within cells helps prevent a dangerous degree of hyperkalemia. If renal function is normal, the elevation of serum potassium concentration usually persists only briefly.

The clinical aspects of disturbances in potassium metabolism will be considered under two headings, Potassium Deficiency and Potassium Intoxication.

Hypokalemia and Potassium Deficiency

Potassium deficiency may result from either *renal* or *extrarenal losses*. Typically, serum potassium concentration is reduced to a level of 2.5 to 3.5 mEq per liter, but with severe potassium depletion it may fall below 2 mEq per liter. In some circumstances, the reduction in potassium concentration is minimized or prevented by the concomitant presence of acidosis, which shifts the equilibrium between cells and extracellular fluid and tends to make serum potassium concentration high in relation to total body stores.

Hypokalemia can also occur without a loss of potassium from the body in the uncommon disorder known as *hypokalemic familial periodic paralysis*, discussed in Ch. 339.6.

PATHOGENESIS AND DIAGNOSIS. Table 3 lists the common causes of potassium deficiency, both renal and extrarenal in origin. As it shows, a large variety of factors, including adrenal steroids, diuretics, and renal tubular disease, may promote abnormal renal excretion. Nearly all appear to increase sodium-potassium exchange in some fashion. *Adrenal steroids,* whether produced in excessive quantities by the body or given therapeutically, stimulate the sodium-cation exchange mechanism directly and thereby induce a loss of potassuim in the urine. An excess of adrenal steroids resulting from overproduction is seen in *primary aldosteronism, Cushing's syndrome,* and various forms of *secondary aldosteronism* (see Ch. 547.7 to 547.9).

One uncommon cause of secondary aldosteronism and hypokalemia is *Bartter's syndrome*. This disease is characterized by juxtaglomerular hyperplasia, hyperreninemia, hyperaldosteronism, and metabolic alkalosis. Neither hypertension nor edema is present, and there is a subnormal pressor response to the administration of angiotensin. Renal salt wasting and accompanying hyponatremia are frequently striking features of the clinical picture. Bartter's syndrome occurs most commonly in children and in some instances is familial in nature.

Recent studies have raised the possibility that overproduction of prostaglandins by the kidney plays either a primary or an intermediary role in the production of the syndrome. Not only can many of the features of Bartter's syndrome be accounted for in terms of a prostaglandin excess, but it has also been shown that the administration of a potent inhibitor of prostaglandin synthesis, such as indomethacin, partially reverses the clinical picture; during indomethacin therapy, sodium and potassium balance become positive, plasma potassium concentration rises, and both plasma renin and urinary aldosterone levels decrease.

A disorder closely mimicking Bartter's syndrome has recently been observed in states of chronic volume depletion induced by vomiting, diarrhea, or diuretics. Juxtaglomerular hyperplasia, high rates of renin and aldosterone secretion, hypokalemic alkalosis, and a normal blood pressure are present just as in the classic form of Bartter's syndrome. Thus it appears that juxtaglomerular hyperplasia can be produced by a variety of stimuli and that a number of types of Bartter's syndrome will eventually be delineated.

Hypokalemia has also been observed as a cardinal feature of another disorder involving the juxtaglomerular apparatus, namely, *juxtaglomerular cell tumor.* This tumor, as might be expected, produces excessive renin and thereby causes secondary aldosteronism and hypokalemic alkalosis. In striking contrast to Bartter's syndrome, however, blood pressure is markedly elevated rather than normal.

Studies of renal venous renin in the patient with a juxtaglomerular cell tumor will quickly identify one kidney as the source of the excessive renin production. Selective renal angiography will usually demonstrate the tumor, but occasionally the lesion may be so small that it is overlooked; under such circumstances a decision regarding surgery must be made on the basis of the other clinical features. Blood pressure and electrolyte abnormalities usually return to normal shortly after the tumor is removed.

Renal potassium wasting and hypokalemia can also occur as the result of *therapy with diuretics* such as thiazides, ethacrynic acid, and furosemide. These agents affect potassium balance by increasing the delivery of sodium to sodium-avid distal exchange sites and thus accelerating the rate of sodium-potassium exchange. Diuretics that act through inhibition of carbonic anhydrase also cause potassium loss but act directly on the distal exchange mechanism; inhibition of carbonic anhydrase reduces the availability of hydrogen for exchange and thus enhances the exchange of sodium for potassium.

The derangements in function responsible for potassium wasting and hypokalemia in renal tubular diseases such as *renal tubular acidosis* are discussed in Ch. 380.

The only significant extrarenal route of potassium depletion is through the *loss of gastrointestinal secretions.* Gastric juice contains potassium in a concentration somewhat higher than plasma, and diarrheal fluid may have a potassium content as high as 50 to 60 mEq per liter. Thus prolonged vomiting, drainage of the upper gastrointestinal tract, or diarrhea typically produces a considerable deficit of potassium. If intake of potassium is poor, the severity of potassium deficiency will be further aggravated by renal losses; inefficient renal conservation allows considerable quantities of potassium to escape into the urine for as long as ten days or two weeks after potassium intake is lowered sharply. As much as 150 or 200 mEq can be lost before excretion is reduced to a level of less than 10 mEq per day.

In *hypokalemia of unknown origin* the quantity of potassium in the urine frequently provides the clue to the correct diagnosis. If a patient with persistent hypokalemia is excreting considerable quantities of potassium in the

TABLE 3. Causes of Potassium Deficiency

A. Renal
  1. Adrenal steroids
     Primary aldosteronism
     Secondary aldosteronism (including Bartter's syndrome and juxtaglomerular cell tumor)
     Cushing's syndrome
     Adrenal steroid therapy
  2. Diuretics
     Ethacrynic acid
     Thiazides
     Furosemide
     Carbonic anhydrase inhibitors
  3. Renal tubular diseases
B. Extrarenal
  1. Vomiting
  2. Gastric drainage
  3. Diarrhea

urine (30 mEq or more per day), the deficit is clearly of renal origin, and attention can therefore immediately be focused on those disorders listed in Section A of Table 3. Ordinarily the history and other clinical findings will clarify the etiology of such renal losses. There are several exceptions to this statement, however. A common problem, for example, is the evaluation of hypokalemia in the hypertensive patient who has received an agent such as a thiazide as part of his antihypertensive regimen. In such a patient it may be difficult to decide whether potassium deficiency is the result of diuretic therapy or of primary aldosteronism. This question can usually be resolved by observation of the serum potassium level for at least several weeks after the drug has been discontinued.

In the patient with hypokalemia in whom potassium excretion is low (less than 15 mEq per day), the depletion is usually of extrarenal origin (Section B of Table 3). In nearly all such instances a history or other evidence pointing to gastrointestinal losses will easily be obtained, but sometimes the diagnostic problem is more difficult. Ocasionally, a patient with *laxative-induced diarrhea* will deny both laxative ingestion and diarrhea, and it will then be necessary to obtain the relevant history from members of the family. Similarly, some patients with *psychogenic* or *self-induced vomiting* do not admit to their difficulties. Patients with *villous adenomas of the rectum* may also pose a diagnostic problem, because they usually have normally formed stools and, unless asked specifically, may neglect to mention the nearly continuous rectal leakage of mucus-like material that is characteristic of their illness. Accordingly, whenever unexplained chronic hypokalemia is associated with a low urinary potassium excretion, evidence of these uncommon disorders should be sought carefully.

Finally, the patient who has developed potassium depletion as the result of diuretic therapy will sometimes demonstate a low renal excretion of potassium even though the potassium loss was of renal origin. If diuretics are no longer being administered and if metabolic alkalosis is not present, the kidney will promptly begin to conserve potassium, and urinary excretion will remain low until the deficit is fully repaired.

CLINICAL MANIFESTATIONS. The clinical effects of potassium deficiency may be manifested in one or more organ systems, including skeletal muscle, heart, kidneys, and the gastrointestinal tact. Perhaps the most serious disturbances are those affecting the neuromuscular system. At serum potassium concentrations in the range of 2 to 2.5 mEq per liter, muscular weakness is likely to occur; with more severe hypokalemia the patient may develop areflexic paralysis, in which case respiratory insufficiency is an immediate threat to survival. The severity of the neuromuscular disturbance tends to be proportional to the speed with which the potassium level has declined. In an occasional instance, *myoglobinuria* has been noted in association with marked hypokalemia.

Abnormalities in the electrocardiogram that commonly occur in hypokalemia are a sagging of the S-T segment, depression of the T wave, and elevation of the U wave (Fig 1). With marked reductions in serum concentration, the T wave becomes progressively smaller, whereas the U waves show increasing amplitude. In some cases the merging of a flat or positive T wave with a positive U wave may erroneously be interpreted as a prolonged Q-T interval. Ordinarily, there are no serious clinical consequences from the abnormalities in cardiac excitation,

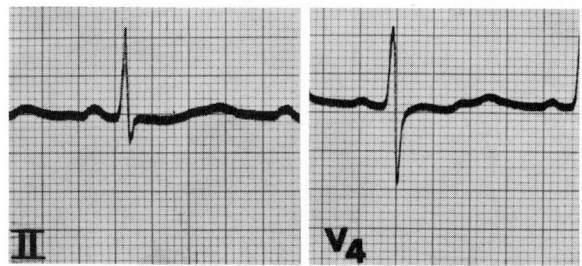

Figure 1. Typical electrocardiographic abnormalities induced by hypokalemia. (Serum potassium concentration 2.8 mEq per liter.) Note in lead II how the merger of the T and U waves might lead to the erroneous interpretation that the Q-T interval is prolonged.

but in digitalized patients the sudden development of hypokalemia may precipitate serious arrhythmias.

Longstanding potassium depletion is apt to produce renal tubular damage, or so-called *hypokalemic nephropathy*; this disorder is discussed in detail in Ch. 380.2. Potassium deficiency is believed to cause dysfunction of the smooth muscle of the gastrointestinal tract and in some patients has been held responsible for the development of *paralytic ileus*.

Potassium deficiency is also a regular concomitant of *metabolic alkalosis*. The role of potassium in the genesis and maintenance of alkalosis is considered later in this chapter.

TREATMENT. Under many circumstances potassium deficiency can be corrected by oral administration of potassium salts. The oral route should be used whenever feasible, because the relatively slow absorption from the gastrointestinal tract prevents a sudden large increase in serum potassium concentration of the sort that can occur during the injudicious administration of potassium intravenously. Correction of a typical deficit of 200 to 500 mEq requires the transfer through the extracellular compartment of a quantity of potassium that has the potential of raising serum concentration to well above lethal levels. When potassium is administered intravenously, therefore, it should ordinarily be given at a rate not exceeding 15 to 20 mEq per hour and at a concentration no higher than 40 to 60 mEq per liter. It is also generally prudent to limit the supplement to 100 or 150 mEq per day and to use the serum potassium concentration as a guide to the need for further replacement. If acidosis is present, the serum potassium concentration may be higher than is appropriate to the degree of potassium deficiency; this discrepancy must be taken into account when treatment is planned. As acidosis is corrected, a more accurate appraisal of further potassium requirements will be possible. Unfortunately, there is no way of directly calculating the quantity of potassium that will be required for full replacement.

The *electrocardiogram* does not provide a reliable guide to the need for replacement therapy but is extremely useful as a convenient and rapid means for determining whether an excessive quantity of potassium has been given. The electrocardiogram in hyperkalemia and potassium intoxication is discussed later.

Potassium chloride, given either intravenously or orally, provides the most reliable means of correcting potassium deficiency. Unfortunately, however, the chloride salt of potassium often produces troublesome upper gastrointestinal symptoms when given orally in a liquid form. To avoid this problem, enteric-coated potassium chloride tablets, which dissolve in the small intestine, were at one time used widely. Clinical experience soon indicated, however, that such preparations sometimes produce severe injury to the small bowel; dissolution of the enteric coating in the small bowel and the resulting high local concentration of potassium on the mucosa occasionally cause ulceration, obstruction, or bleeding. Such preparations have therefore been largely replaced by a new formulation in which a slow release of potassium along the intestine is accomplished by embedding the chloride salt in a wax matrix. Such preparations have rarely been shown to cause any injury to the bowel.

Organic potassium salts can be used as a substitute for the chloride salt if desired. The organic salt can be given as a liquid without producing significant gastric symptoms and without an untoward effect on the mucosa of the small intestine. Potassium gluconate and potassium "triplex" (citrate, acetate, and bicarbonate) are among the agents frequently employed and are effective in patients who are not depleted of chloride. They are, however, relatively ineffective in repairing potassium deficiency when the patient is hypochloremic, alkalotic, and on a low-salt (low-chloride) intake, because in hypochloremic alkalosis a smaller than normal fraction of filtered sodium is reabsorbed with chloride and an increased fraction is reabsorbed by exchange with potassium and hydrogen. As long as hypochloremia and avidity for sodium persist, the accelerated rate of sodium-cation exchange forces a continued high rate of potassium excretion. Thus full repair of potassium deficiency cannot be achieved by administration of an organic potassium salt. Potassium must instead be provided as the chloride salt, or chloride must be made available in some other form, such as ammonium chloride or sodium chloride.

Hyperkalemia and Potassium Intoxication

PATHOGENESIS. Hyperkalemia is most often due to defective renal excretion of potassium. It may arise as the result of primary renal disease, deficiency of adrenal steroids, or the administration of agents that inhibit sodium-potassium exchange by the tubule. Excessively rapid intravenous administration of potassium may also elevate plasma concentration to dangerous levels, as has been mentioned earlier in connection with the treatment of potassium deficiency. Potassium given by mouth rarely causes severe hyperkalemia unless renal function is markedly impaired.

Hyperkalemia secondary to renal damage occurs frequently in *acute tubular necrosis* or in any other form of acute renal failure characterized by oliguria or anuria. In *chronic renal failure* potassium intoxication is usually encountered only in the terminal stages of the disease but is sometimes seen earlier as a sequel to the inadvertent administration of potassium supplements. A deficiency of mineralocorticoid, caused either by *Addison's disease* or by *selective hypoaldosteronism,* a rare disorder, also impairs potassium secretion and may produce hyperkalemia. Selective hypoaldosteronism results, in most instances, from decreased production of renin, caused by damage to the juxtaglomerular apparatus. The disorder is seen most commonly in association with mild to moderate degrees of renal insufficiency. Selective hypoaldosteronism also occurs occasionally as the result of a specific defect in aldosterone synthesis rather than as a consequence of hyporeninemia.

The spironolactones, agents used in diuretic therapy for the purpose of antagonizing the sodium-retaining effects of aldosterone, do not in themselves usually cause a significant elevation in serum potassium concentration. They do, however, impair the ability of the kidney to respond to a potassium load and should not be given in conjunction with potassium supplements. The same caution concerning administration of potassium applies to patients receiving diuretic agents such as *triamterene* and *amiloride,* which also impair the exchange of sodium for potassium by the tubule.

Hyperkalemia also occurs in an uncommon and puzzling disorder known as *familial hyperkalemic periodic paralysis.* In individuals with this disorder, attacks can be induced by the ingestion of potassium. This disease is discussed in detail in Ch. 339.6.

Pseudohyperkalemia has been observed in a few patients with thrombocytosis secondary to a myeloproliferative disorder. The spurious elevation of serum concentration results from release of potassium from platelets during the process of coagulation. Concentrations as high as 9 mEq per liter can be found in the serum at a time when platelet-free plasma has a normal potassium level. Similar spurious elevations in serum potassium concentration resulting from the release of potassium from white blood cells have also been reported in a few patients with chronic myelogenous leukemia. The possibility that one is dealing with pseudohyperkalemia should be considered whenever an elevated serum potassium concentration cannot otherwise be explained.

CLINICAL MANIFESTATIONS. The clinical manifestations of potassium intoxication are related primarily to the heart and the neuromuscular system. *Electrocardiographic abnormalities* are the earliest and most frequent sign of disturbed membrane excitability and are characterized by the development of tall, "tent-shaped" T waves, by decreased amplitude of the P waves, and later by atrial asystole (Fig. 2). Intraventricular block, with widening of the QRS complex, may lead to the development of a sine wave pattern and ultimately to ventricular standstill. Changes in the electrocardiogram usually appear when the serum potassium concentration reaches 7 to 8 mEq per liter, and cardiac standstill is likely to occur at a concentration of 9 to 10 mEq per liter. *Weakness* and *flaccid paralysis* appear only in association with severe hyperkalemia but are not always present even at plasma levels sufficiently high to produce serious deterioration in the electrocardiogram. Indeed, death from cardiac arrest may occur even before muscular weakness is evident. For this reason the electrocardiogram is the single most important guide in appraising the threat posed by hyperkalemia and in determining how aggressive a therapeutic approach is necessary.

Figure 2. Typical electrocardiographic abnormalities induced by a moderate degree of hyperkalemia. (Serum potassium concentration 6.5 mEq per liter.) Note the typical "tent-shaped" T waves.

TREATMENT. The first goal in the treatment of severe potassium intoxication should be to promote the rapid transfer of potassium into cells in order to lower serum potassium concentration and prevent cardiac arrest. Two approaches to this goal are likely to prove effective. Infusion of glucose and insulin induces the cellular deposition of glycogen and at the same time brings about a shift of potassium to the intracellular space; 1 liter of a 10 per cent glucose solution with 30 to 40 units of insulin is generally employed for this purpose. In the acidotic patient further redistribution of potassium can be achieved by the administration of sodium bicarbonate (150 to 300 mEq). In many cases these measures will induce a striking reduction in plasma potassium concentration and prompt improvement in the electrocardiogram. In some instances the administration of calcium (as 2 grams of calcium lactate) is also useful, because calcium, though it has no effect on the plasma potassium concentration, opposes the cardiotoxic effects of potassium. Calcium cannot, incidentally, be given in the same solution with sodium bicarbonate, because precipitation of the calcium ion will result.

Because these techniques do not remove potassium from the body and may be only temporarily effective, longer-term efforts should be directed toward promoting gastrointestinal losses of potassium. A cation-exchange resin in the sodium cycle, such as Kayexelate, will usually achieve this purpose if administered by mouth in a dose of 20 to 30 grams every six hours. Each gram of resin binds approximately 1 mEq of potassium, and within 24 hours a significant effect on plasma potassium concentration should be achieved. To enhance potassium loss and assure the rapid movement of the resin through the gastrointestinal tract, sorbitol, a nonabsorbable polyhydric alcohol, should be given in quantities sufficient to induce a soft or semiliquid bowel movement every few hours. The usual dose for this purpose is 20 ml of a 70 per cent solution three or four times a day. If the patient is unable to take medication by mouth, the resin can be administered by rectum as a retention enema of 100 grams in several hundred milliliters of water.

Hemodialysis is an efficient alternative means of removing excess potassium, but will usually not be required if the program outlined above can be implemented.

Conn, J. W., et al.: Primary reninism. Arch. Intern. Med., 130:682, 1972.

Fleischer, N., Brown, H., Graham, D. Y., and Delena, S.: Chronic laxative-induced hyperaldosteronism and hypokalemia simulating Bartter's syndrome. Ann. Inter. Med., 70:791, 1969.

Gill, J. R., Frolich, J. C., Bowden, R. E., Taylor, A. A., Keiser, H. R., Seyberth, H. W., Oates, J. A., and Bartter, F. C.: Bartter's syndrome: A disorder characterized by high urinary prostaglandins and a dependence of hyperreninemia on prostaglandin synthesis. Am. J. Med., 61:43, 1976.

Ingram, R. H., and Seki, M.: Pseudohyperkalemia with thombocytosis. N. Eng. J. Med., 267:895, 1962.

Michelis, M. F., and Murdaugh, H. V.: Selective hypoaldosteronism. An editorial revisited after 15 years. Am. J. Med., 59:1, 1975.

Schwartz, W. B., and Relman, A. S.: Effects of electrolyte disorders on renal structure and function. N. Eng. J. Med., 276:383, 1967.

DISTURBANCES OF ACID-BASE EQUILIBRIUM

The pH of extracellular fluid normally ranges between 7.35 and 7.45 and is stabilized within these limits despite wide variations in the dietary load of acid or alkali. A large number of body functions are importantly influenced by the pH of body fluids, and disturbances in acid-base regulation often have serious effects on metabolic activity, on the circulation, and on the central nervous system.

As background to a discussion of acid-base disturbances, it is instructive to consider briefly the way in which the body deals with the *normal daily acid load* and thus maintains a steady state of acid-base equilibrium. As food is oxidized, both carbon dioxide (carbonic acid) and nonvolatile acids such as sulfuric and phosphoric acids are added to the extracellular fluid. Immediate buffering within the interstitial fluid, plasma, and red blood cells minimizes the change in pH and permits large quantities of acid to be transferred to the lungs and kidneys for excretion. Because *carbon dioxide* is excreted almost entirely by the lungs, alveolar carbon dioxide tension is the prime determinant of Pco_2 in body fluids. With usual rates of carbon dioxide production, alveolar ventilation maintains the Pco_2 of blood at approximately 40 mm of mercury, that is, 1.2 millimols of dissolved carbon dioxide per liter of plasma.

Nonvolatile acids are excreted solely by the kidney. The process by which this is accomplished is complex, because no significant fraction of the daily hydrogen ion load (some 50 to 100 mEq) can be excreted in an unbuffered form at the minimal urinary pH of 4.0 that the kidney can establish. Virtually all hydrogen must thus be removed as either *titratable acid* or *ammonium*. Acidification of the glomerular filtrate by a process of sodium-hydrogen exchange titrates buffers such as phosphate and also favors the diffusion of ammonia (NH_3) from the tubular cells to the lumen, where it reacts with hydrogen ions to form ammonium (NH_4^+). Bicarbonate generated in tubular cells as the result of acid excretion moves into peritubular blood and replenishes the bicarbonate stores that were previously depleted by the buffering of dietary acid. From all these considerations it is evident that both derangements in either pulmonary or renal function and the imposition of stresses that overwhelm normal regulatory mechanisms can be expected to produce disturbances of acid-base equilibrium.

Because the carbonic acid–bicarbonate buffer pair is the major buffer system in the extracellular fluid, its parameters provide a meaningful and convenient expression of the acid-base status of the organism. The relation between pH and the bicarbonate and carbonic acid concentrations can be expressed in a general fashion according to the familiar Henderson-Hasselbalch equation

$$pH = pK + \log \frac{HCO_3^-}{H_2CO_3} \qquad (1)$$

where pK is the dissociation constant of carbonic acid. In the normal subject this expression will be

$$7.4 = 6.1 + \log \frac{24 \text{ mM/L}}{1.2 \text{ mM/L}} \qquad (2)$$

Traditionally, disturbances in acid-balance equilibrium are considered in terms of a change in the ratio of bicarbonate to carbonic acid, but some believe this approach does not always provide the immediate and intuitive insight that can be derived from the following expression:

$$
\begin{array}{l}
40 \text{ mm Hg} \\
Pco_2 \\
\searrow \quad \searrow \\
H_2CO_3 \;\rightleftarrows\; H^+ \;+\; HCO_3^- \\
1.2 \text{ mM/L} \quad pH\ 7.4 \quad 24 \text{ mM/L}
\end{array}
\qquad (3)
$$

This equation allows ready visualization of the directional changes that can be anticipated in both metabolic and respiratory disturbances of acid-base equilibrium. It is apparent, for example, that a primary reduction in bicarbonate concentration (metabolic acidosis) will cause the reaction to shift to the right, thus increasing hydrogen ion concentration, whereas a primary elevation in bicarbonate concentration (metabolic alkalosis) will cause the reaction to shift to the left, thus decreasing hydrogen ion concentration. Respiratory disorders can be analyzed in the same fashion. A rise in Pco_2 increases the hydrogen ion concentration by shifting the reaction to the right (respiratory acidosis), and a fall has the reverse effect (respiratory alkalosis). In both metabolic and respiratory acid-base disturbances, the widest range of pH values compatible with life is approximately 6.8 to 7.8.

Metabolic Acidosis

Metabolic acidosis results whenever acid is added to the body, alkali is lost from the body, or impaired renal function prevents the excretion of the normal endogenous acid load. In each case the reduction in bicarbonate concentration is accompanied by a rise in hydrogen ion concentration, that is, a decrease in pH.

PHYSIOLOGIC CONSIDERATIONS. The normal organism confronted with a large acid load has a remarkable ability to maintain hydrogen ion concentration within tolerable limits until augmented excretion of acid (and concomitant regeneration of buffer stores) allows restoration of a normal plasma bicarbonate concentration. This resiliency is explained by the magnitude of the total body buffer capacity and the prompt respiratory adjustment of Pco_2.

Body buffers provide a large reservoir of hydrogen ion acceptors distributed through both the extracellular and intracellular compartments. In the extracellular space bicarbonate provides the bulk of the buffer capacity; hemoglobin and plasma proteins, though they make a significant contribution to the buffering ability of blood, are of little quantitative importance when viewed in terms of the entire extracellular compartment. Intracellular buffers, which consist largely of protein and organic anions, provide an additional buffer reserve that is responsible for sequestering half or more of an acid load and that thus serves the important function of protecting against lethal reductions in extracellular pH.

As the price of maintaining electroneutrality during cellular accumulation of hydrogen, both potassium and sodium are forced out of cells. If renal function is normal, the displaced potassium is ultimately lost in the urine. If, on the other hand, renal function is impaired or dehydration has reduced urine volume to oliguric levels, potassium will be retained and potentially dangerous elevations of serum potassium concentration may occur.

Respiratory compensation takes place promptly after the development of metabolic acidosis, an increase in both depth and rate of respiration lowering alveolar and arterial Pco_2. The magnitude of the decrease in Pco_2 becomes larger as the reduction in bicarbonate concentration becomes greater, but respiratory defense is never sufficient to restore pH to normal.

Even with the most severe metabolic acidosis, Pco_2 does not fall below 10 mm of mercury because the physical effort required to produce a further increase in alveolar ventilation increases carbon dioxide production more rapidly than it does pulmonary gas exchange. Thus if bicarbonate concentration is very low and maximal reductions in Pco_2 have already been achieved, a slight further fall in bicarbonate concentration will produce a large decrement in pH.

These comments on respiratory defense have been based, of course, on the assumption that there will be a normal ventilatory response when metabolic acidosis occurs. Indeed, the clinical significance of a given reduction in plasma bicarbonate concentration is judged almost automatically (in the absence of pH measurements) on the basis of experience with the usual degree of respiratory compensation. In some circumstances, however, Pco_2 does not fall in the anticipated manner, and the increase in hydrogen ion concentration is therefore far greater than is customary. This difficulty will be encountered if the respiratory center has been depressed by sedatives or other medications. It is also seen in the patient with pulmonary disease who, though able to maintain a normal Pco_2 under usual conditions, cannot increase alveolar ventilation to a significant degree under stress. In the patient with a plasma bicarbonate concentration of 10 mEq per liter, for example, normal respiratory compensation will usually reduce the Pco_2 to approximately 25 mm of mercury and keep the pH in the range of 7.20 to 7.25, whereas without a reduction in Pco_2 the pH would be 7.00. The measurement of pH or Pco_2 is therefore often important even in circumstances in which the diagnosis of metabolic acidosis is not in question.

Renal compensation is the final step in the defense against metabolic acidosis, but it takes place slowly and does not contribute to the immediate protection of pH. Several days are required before excretion of ammonium and titratable acid rises sufficiently to regenerate bicarbonate and restore plasma concentration to normal. If renal function is impaired, or if underlying renal tubular disease is present, an even longer period may be required for correction to take place.

PATHOGENESIS. Table 4 lists the specific causes of metabolic acidosis, both with and without an increase in unmeasured anions.

Large Acid Loads. Probably the most frequent cause of metabolic acidosis is the addition of a large acid load to the body fluids. Diabetic ketoacidosis is a familiar example of such a disturbance. In diabetic acidosis there is an imbalance between the production and utilization of β-hydroxybutyric and acetoacetic acids, with the result that both acids accumulate in the extracellular fluid. Because these acids are almost completely dissociated at the pH of body fluids, nearly 1 millimol of bicarbonate is dissipated by the addition of each millimol of ketoacid.

Severe ketoacidosis associated with alcoholism has also been noted in nondiabetic patients. This disorder is seen in patients with chronic alcoholism who have been drinking heavily and have eaten little or no food over

TABLE 4. Causes of Metabolic Acidosis

With Increase in Unmeasured Anions	Without Increase in Unmeasured Anions
Diabetic ketoacidosis	Diarrhea
Alcoholic ketoacidosis	Drainage of pancreatic juice
Salicylate poisoning	Obstruction of a ureteroileal
Ethylene glycol poisoning	or ureterosigmoid loop
Methyl alcohol poisoning	Carbonic anhydrase inhibitors
Paraldehyde (rarely)	Ammonium chloride
Lactic acidosis	Renal tubular acidosis
Renal failure	

several days. Typically such patients also have a history of protracted vomiting. The blood sugar level is usually normal or mildly elevated. The acidosis, which is often severe, results from the accumulation of β-hydroxybutyric and acetoacetic acids (and sometimes lactic acid as well), but the severe ketosis can readily be overlooked because the ratio of β-hydroxybutyrate to acetoacetate in the plasma is unusually high; as a result, the nitroprusside test, which detects only acetoacetate, may be negative or only slightly positive. The characteristic history and the findings of a large "anion gap," however, should point strongly to the correct diagnosis.

Accumulation of lactic acid is now recognized as a relatively frequent cause of metabolic acidosis. *Lactic acidosis* is most often encountered in patients with circulatory failure caused by dehydration, hemorrhage, or endotoxic or cardiogenic shock. In these conditions the failure to supply sufficient oxygen to the tissues induces a shift from aerobic metabolism to anaerobic glycolysis and produces a lactic acidosis analogous to that occurring with severe exercise. Lactic acidosis may also occur in the absence of any obvious predisposing cause such as hypotension or hypoxemia. The onset is usually abrupt and without warning, and the acidosis is often very severe. *Spontaneous lactic acidosis* is seen in association with a variety of major illnesses, including diabetes mellitus, hepatic failure, subacute bacterial endocarditis, and leukemia. The etiology of this syndrome remains obscure. Lactic acid may also accumulate in significant quantities during *total fasting in the presence of obesity* and in *glycogen-storage disease*. Severe lactic acidosis has also been seen in association with *phenformin therapy* in diabetics and in association with the ingestion of huge doses of *isoniazid* (15 to 20 grams) taken by accident or in a suicide attempt.

Poisoning caused by the ingestion of *salicylates, methyl alcohol, ethylene glycol,* or occasionally *paraldehyde* leads to the accumulation of relatively strong and highly dissociated organic acids in the body fluids and to marked reductions in plasma bicarbonate concentration. The specific organic acids responsible for the acidosis in these disorders have not been adequately identified.

Metabolic acidosis can also result from the ingestion of mineral acid such as *ammonium chloride*. The release of hydrogen, as ammonium is converted by the liver to urea, makes the administration of ammonium chloride analogous to the administration of an equivalent quantity of hydrochloric acid. *Lysine hydrochloride* and *arginine hydrochloride* have the same effect on acid-base equilibrium, because they too deliver hydrochloric acid to the body fluids. Acidosis resulting from administration of acidifying salts is uncommon, however, because these agents are ordinarily administered only in conjunction with diuretic agents that tend to produce metabolic alkalosis.

Loss of Alkali.   Severe *diarrhea* frequently produces metabolic acidosis, because liquid stools usually contain bicarbonate in concentrations considerably higher than those in extracellular fluid. Loss of *pancreatic juice*, another highly alkaline solution, also leads to a reduction in plasma bicarbonate concentration; such acidosis is encountered almost exclusively in patients who have undergone prolonged drainage of a pancreatic fistula or of the upper portion of the small bowel.

Acidosis can also be seen in patients whose ureters have been transplanted into a loop of ileum or sigmoid colon. The problem of acidosis arises, however, only in patients who develop stasis of urine as the result of obstruction.

Renal Dysfunction.   Inability of the diseased kidney to deal with the normal dietary load of nonvolatile acid will result in a positive acid balance and consequently in a reduction in plasma bicarbonate concentration. In *acute renal failure* the acid-base disturbance is usually transient and mild. In *chronic renal failure* metabolic acidosis is commonly present over an extended period and can be severe. In most patients with chronic renal failure the problem in acid excretion does not arise from any serious difficulty in acidifying the urine or in forming titratable acid but primarily from an inability to excrete normal quantities of ammonium. Defective renal reabsorption of bicarbonate is sometimes an additional contributory factor. Despite these abnormalities, plasma bicarbonate is usually stabilized at a level of 15 to 20 mEq per liter. This new steady state is achieved in part by the enhanced excretion of acid that accompanies the fall in plasma pH and in part by the buffering of some portion of the acid load, probably by alkaline bone salts. The equilibrium is precarious, however, and any factor that increases either the intake or the production of acid (or induces a loss of alkali) is likely to precipitate a dangerous degree of metabolic acidosis.

The foregoing discussion of renal acidosis includes no mention of the traditional view that retention of "acid anions" such as sulfate and phosphate is responsible for the reduction in plasma bicarbonate concentration. This view is inconsistent with modern concepts of physical chemistry that define an acid as any substance that donates hydrogen ions and a base as any substance that accepts hydrogen ions. In these terms substances such as sulfate and dibasic phosphate are actually weak bases rather than acids, and accumulation of these ions could not be expected to have a significant influence on either plasma bicarbonate concentration or pH. The tendency in many patients for bicarbonate to vary more or less reciprocally with the concentration of accumulated anions appears to be the fortuitous consequence of a parallel progression of glomerular and tubular damage, the reduction in filtration rate causing sulfate and phosphate retention, and the damage to tubules impairing acid excretion. Such a parallel change is not inevitable. In some patients, particularly those with chronic pyelonephritis, tubular capacity for acid excretion may be impaired at a time when glomerular filtration rate is only slightly reduced; under these circumstances the decrease in plasma bicarbonate concentration is accompanied by an increase in chloride reabsorption that produces a state of so-called hyperchloremic acidosis.

Hyperchloremic acidosis is also seen in an uncommon form of renal dysfunction known as *renal tubular acidosis*. It is also observed in *Fanconi's syndrome*, a rare disease characterized by a multiplicity of tubular defects. These disorders are discussed in detail in Ch. 380.5 and 534.9, respectively.

Metabolic acidosis accompanied by hyperchloremia also follows the administration of *carbonic anhydrase inhibitors* such as acetazolamide. Carbonic anhydrase has an essential role in making hydrogen available for secretion by renal tubular cells, and inhibition of this enzyme impairs the cation-exchange process and reduces both sodium reabsorption and acid excretion.

DIAGNOSIS.   Hyperventilation is the only clinical finding characteristic of metabolic acidosis, and even this sign is sometimes difficult to detect. For example, patients with acidosis of long duration often appear to be breathing nearly normally at a time when measurements of Pco_2 demonstrate a striking increase in alveolar ventilation. Other clinical disturbances such as lethargy and coma are frequently seen in the patient with severe acidosis, but it is often difficult to decide whether these abnormalities are a manifestation of the acidosis per se or of the underlying disease — for example, diabetic acidosis or uremia.

In most cases, the history, in conjunction with the low plasma bicarbonate concentration and other routine chemical studies, will provide the basis for a tentative diagnosis of metabolic acidosis. However, since plasma bicarbonate concentration can also be reduced by primary hyperventilation (see below), a measurement of pH will be necessary in order to distinguish with certainty between respiratory alkalosis and metabolic acidosis. Subsequent measurements of pH will also serve the important function of providing a guide to effective clinical management.

Once the presence of metabolic acidosis has been documented, it is important to determine the exact cause. In many cases the cause is obvious, but in other instances it is obscure, and some rapid and systematic approach to differential diagnosis is invaluable. Particularly helpful is the calculation of the anion gap, or concentration of unmeasured anions, in plasma. This value, which is estimated by subtraction of the sum of chloride and bicarbonate concentrations from that of sodium, is normally about 8 to 14 mEq per liter (Fig. 3, column I) and represents negative charges contributed to plasma by ions other than chloride and bicarbonate (chiefly phosphate, sulfate, organic anions, and the anionic groups of plasma proteins).

In the patient with metabolic acidosis the reduction in bicarbonate concentration may or may not be accompanied by an increase in the anion gap; this distinction, which can be made on the basis of routine electrolyte measurements, immediately narrows the range of diagnostic possibilities (Table 4). If the concentration of unmeasured anions is increased (Fig. 3, column III), it can be concluded that hydrogen has been added to the body fluids with some anion other than chloride. This finding suggests a diagnosis of diabetic ketoacidosis, drug poisoning, renal failure, or lactic acidosis and gives direction to further studies designed to identify the specific cause of the acid-base disturbance. Lactic acidosis is likely to pose the only special diagnostic problem, because lactate determinations are not yet routinely available in many hospitals. In nearly all cases, however, a tentative diagnosis of lactic acidosis can be made by exclusion of the other disorders characterized by an increased concentration of undetermined anions.

If, on the other hand, the anion gap is not increased (Fig. 3, column II), the reduction in bicarbonate concentration can clearly be attributed either to the accumulation of hydrogen with chloride or to a loss of bicarbonate. With the spectrum thus narrowed, it should again be relatively easy to identify the underlying disorder. A history of diarrhea or of the ingestion of an acidifying agent such as ammonium chloride or acetazolamide will often clarify the problem. The finding of a relatively alkaline urine and of nephrocalcinosis on roentgenographic examination of the abdomen will strongly suggest the diagnosis of renal tubular acidosis.

In some patients, of course, several causes of metabolic acidosis may be present simultaneously, and this possibility should not be overlooked. If, for example, the disappearance of ketonemia during the treatment of diabetic acidosis is not accompanied by restoration of a normal plasma bicarbonate concentration, the presence of a coexistent disorder such as lactic acidosis should be suspected.

In an occasional patient, the anion gap will be reduced below normal levels, to a value of 6 mEq per liter or less. The most common cause of this finding is a random laboratory error in the measurement of sodium, chloride, or bicarbonate. If this possibility is excluded — that is, if a reduced anion gap is seen on repeated examinations —the abnormality will usually be attributable to *bromidism, hypoalbuminemia,* or a *plasma cell dyscrasia.* An elevated plasma bromide concentration causes a spurious increase in the automated analyzer measurement of chloride concentration and thus a false reduction in the anion gap. Hypoalbuminemia exerts its effect by reducing the number of charges contributed by plasma proteins to the moiety of unmeasured anions. The mechanism through which plasma cell dyscrasias exerts its effect on the anion gap is unknown.

TREATMENT. General Principles. Treatment should ordinarily be directed toward any reversible abnormality, such as ketosis or shock, that may be responsible for the acidosis. If the underlying disturbance is not amenable to treatment, however, or if acidosis is life threatening, alkali therapy will be necessary. Calculation of the amount of alkali to be administered must take into account not only the depletion of extracellular bicarbonate stores but also the magnitude of the intracellular acidosis. As mentioned earlier, a large fraction of an acid load is sequestered in cells; restoration of normal acid base equilibrium therefore involves repair of total body buffer stores. Estimates of alkali requirements should thus assume "distribution" of bicarbonate through a volume equivalent to 50 per cent

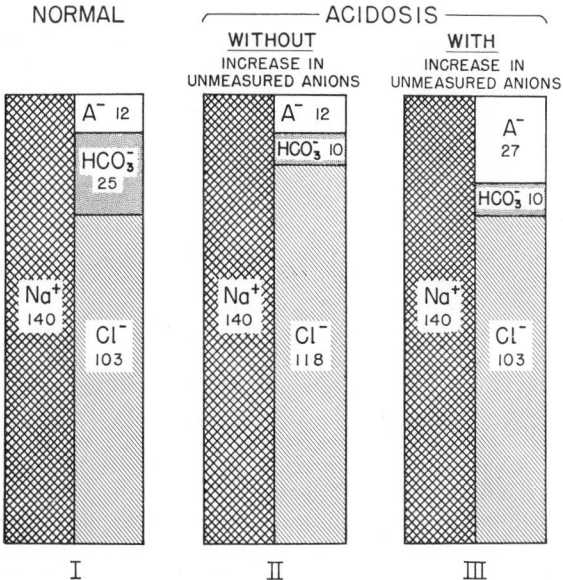

Figure 3. Composition of plasma in various forms of metabolic acidosis, with special reference to the concentration of unmeasured anions ("anion gap"). Column I shows that anions other than chloride and bicarbonate normally make up approximately 12 mEq per liter of the total anion content of plasma. Columns II and III indicate that acidosis can develop with or without an associated increase in concentration of unmeasured anions. The various causes of acidosis that will produce these patterns are listed in Table 4, and the way in which the "anion gap" can be used in differential diagnosis is discussed in the text.

of body weight. The calculation for full repair can be summarized by the following expression:

$$(25 \text{ mEq per liter} - \text{observed plasma HCO}_3 \text{ conc.}) \times 0.5 \text{ body weight (kg)} = \text{mEq of alkali}$$

The figure of 50 per cent for the distribution of bicarbonate is only approximate, but clinical experience has demonstrated that therapy based on this assumption usually induces a rise in plasma bicarbonate concentration close to the predicted level. The only exception to this statement appears to occur in patients in whom plasma bicarbonate concentration is less than 5 mEq per liter. In the presence of such severe degrees of acidosis, the volume of distribution of bicarbonate is of the order of 100 per cent rather than 50 per cent of body weight; larger than usual quantities of alkali will therefore usually be required in order to increase plasma bicarbonate level by the desired amount.

In most patients with severe acidosis immediate correction of the entire alkali deficit is unnecessary; if bicarbonate concentration is increased to 15 or 20 mEq per liter, plasma pH will be returned to a safe level and renal adjustments or continued treatment of the underlying metabolic abnormality can be relied on to complete the corrective process. More rapid correction may, in fact, be undesirable. If bicarbonate concentration is quickly restored to normal or nearly normal levels, blood pH may become frankly alkaline. This apparently paradoxical behavior is the consequence of persistent hyperventilation, which often maintains a state of hypocapnia for as long as one or two days after bicarbonate stores have been replenished.

During the correction of metabolic acidosis, the movement of potassium into cells in exchange for hydrogen tends to lower the concentration of potassium in the serum. In the patient with hyperkalemia and potassium intoxication this reduction serves a useful therapeutic purpose, as discussed earlier. If, however, serum potassium concentration is normal initially, the transfer of potassium from the extracellular fluid may produce hypokalemia and signs of potassium deficiency. This sequence of events has been noted with particular frequency during the correction of diabetic ketoacidosis, but it may also occur during the repair of other acidotic states. Careful clinical observation and occasional measurements of serum potassium concentration should therefore be carried out in the course of treatment to determine the need for the replacement of potassium deficits.

Special Problems in Management. Some of the disorders that cause metabolic acidosis present particular problems in management. This discussion considers such problems as they occur in lactic acidosis, diabetic ketoacidosis, and renal acidosis; salicylate poisoning and methy alcohol poisoning are dealt with in detail in Ch. 23.

In metabolic acidosis resulting from the accumulation of either ketoacids or lactic acid, the bicarbonate deficit may be corrected promptly and fully without administration of exogenous alkali. In both diabetic and lactic acidosis, the anion that has accumulated in the body fluids, if fully oxidized, will regenerate an equivalent quantity of bicarbonate and will restore plasma bicarbonate concentration to normal. A familiar physiologic example of this behavior is seen with the lactic acidosis of exercise; after exertion is discontinued, acidosis is rapidly corrected according to the following reaction:

$$Na^+ + CH_3CH(OH)COO^- + HOH + 3O_2$$

$$\rightarrow \underbrace{Na^+ + OH^- + 3CO_2}_{Na^-HCO_3^- + 2CO_2} + 3H_2O \qquad (4)$$

In *diabetic ketoacidosis* full and rapid oxidation of the organic anion occurs promptly after the administration of adequate quantities of insulin and glucose; thus most patients with ketoacidosis do not require alkali therapy. On the other hand, it is reasonable to administer small quantities of alkali if, at the time of admission, the patient is found to have acidosis of life-threatening severity. Such treatment will have an important influence on pH at a time before insulin can exert a significant effect and will lead to only an inconsequential degree of alkalosis after ketosis has been fully corrected.

In the *ketoacidosis associated with alcoholism*, the only treatment necessary is administration of glucose and isotonic saline solution. Insulin is not required, but small amounts of bicarbonate should probably be given in the early phase of treatment if the metabolic acidosis is of life-threatening proportions.

The ease with which *lactic acidosis* can be corrected depends on the cause of the metabolic abnormality. If shock is responsible for the shift to anaerobic glycolysis, transfusions or other means of restoring blood volume and blood pressure will usually correct the acid-base disturbance. Lactic acidosis of unknown cause (*spontaneous lactic acidosis*) poses a completely different problem. Specific means for remedying the defect in lactate metabolism are not available, and one must therefore rely solely on alkali therapy. Treatment is often further complicated by the unpredictable response to administration of alkali; in some cases bicarbonate concentration rises very little or not at all despite administration of an amount of bicarbonate that, by usual estimates, would be more than sufficient to restore the plasma level to normal. The explanation for this "resistance" to therapy presumably lies in continued addition of lactic acid to the body fluids during the period of treatment. Occasionally, the rate of addition of lactic acid to the body fluids may be so great that as much as 400 to 500 mEq of sodium bicarbonate must be administered over a period of a few hours in order to prevent the development of lethal acidosis.

On the other hand, bicarbonate concentration will sometimes rise spontaneously as a sudden increase in the oxidation of lactate regenerates large quantities of bicarbonate. In the patient who has previously been given alkali, frank metabolic alkalosis may be the result. The acid-base status must therefore be monitored closely during the course of therapy.

Even when the acid-base disorder is well controlled, the majority of patients with spontaneous lactic acidosis do not survive. Any therapeutic approach directed toward the acid-base disturbance alone will obviously be far from satisfactory, because it deals with effect rather than cause. Problems analogous to those seen in spontaneous lactic acidosis were encountered in the management of diabetic acidosis during the preinsulin era; resistance to alkali therapy was common, and death frequently occurred even after plasma bicarbonate concentration was restored to normal.

Chronic *renal acidosis* poses still a different problem. There is no accumulation of organic anion from which bicarbonate can be regenerated, and irreversible renal damage ordinarily precludes correction of the underlying tubular abnormality responsible for the acid-base disturbance. Reliance must therefore be placed on alkali therapy alone. Fortunately, the degree of metabolic acidosis in most patients with renal insufficiency is not great enough to demand treatment; reductions in bicarbonate concentration to 16 to 18 mEq per liter, which occur commonly, do not appear to cause symptoms or to aggravate the uremic syndrome. If, however, acidosis becomes severe, either sodium bicarbonate or sodium citrate should be given by mouth in doses of several grams per day; plasma bicarbonate concentration need not and, in fact, probably should not be raised to normal because of the risk of precipitating tetany if hypocalcemia is present. Sometimes the ingestion of alkali precipitates nausea or vomiting; under these circumstances it may be necessary to discontinue treatment. Sodium bicarbonate is more likely than sodium citrate to produce gastrointestinal symptoms.

If the patient has a sodium-retaining state such as congestive heart failure, it is wise to defer administration of alkali as long as possible and, if treatment must be given, to restrict dietary sodium intake sharply.

The management of *renal tubular acidosis* and that of *Fanconi's syndrome* are discussed in Ch. 380.5 and 534.9, respectively.

Choice of an Alkalinizing Agent. Two agents, *sodium bicarbonate* and *sodium lactate*, have been widely employed in patients requiring the intravenous administration of alkali. Sodium lactate is usually an effective and satisfactory means of treatment, but it has the disadvantage of depending on the intervention of oxidative processes to make bicarbonate available (Equation 4). Thus if there is a defect in lactate metabolism, as in lactic acidosis, the prompt and quantitative conversion of lactate to bicarbonate cannot be relied upon. Bicarbonate, on the other hand, is ideally suited to the treatment of metabolic acidosis because it directly replenishes depleted buffer stores. There thus appears no basis for the continued use of lactate in the treatment of acidotic states.

Metabolic Alkalosis

Metabolic alkalosis results from either an abnormal loss of acid or an excessive retention of alkali. In each case the rise in bicarbonate concentration induces a fall in hydrogen ion concentration, that is, an increase in pH.

PHYSIOLOGIC CONSIDERATIONS. As in metabolic acidosis, pH is defended to a significant extent by *tissue buffering*. In response to alkalinization of the extracellular fluid, hydrogen ions migrate from cells to extracellular space (in exchange for sodium and potassium) and thus mitigate the severity of the acid-base disturbance.

Respiratory compensation may serve as an additional mitigating factor. Diminished ventilation and a resulting rise in Pco_2 tend to restore a more normal ratio between the concentrations of carbonic acid and bicarbonate. Even with severe metabolic alkalosis, Pco_2 does not usually rise above 50 mm of mercury, but values between 50 and 60 mm of mercury are not rare, and Pco_2 may even reach a level of 65 mm Hg of mercury. Respiratory compensation usually becomes significant only when plasma bicarbonate concentration rises to 35 or 40 mEq per liter.

Renal excretion is the route for removal of excess alkali and is thus ultimately responsible for the correction of metabolic alkalosis. Normally, the kidneys reabsorb ap-

proximately 25 mEq of bicarbonate per liter of glomerular filtrate; when plasma concentration is elevated above this level by ingestion or infusion of alkali, the excess bicarbonate is rapidly and quantitatively excreted. Thus even a large alkali load induces only a transient alkalosis. A theoretical example will serve to illustrate this point. If plasma bicarbonate is raised from 25 mEq per liter to 35 mEq per liter by alkali administration, approximately 10mEq of bicarbonate will be excreted each time a liter of glomerular filtrate is formed. With a glomerular filtration rate of 180 liters per day, daily excretion would thus be 1800 mEq. Maintenance of the metabolic alkalosis would therefore require either the daily administration of 150 grams of sodium bicarbonate or the daily loss of 18 liters of gastric juice containing 0.1N HCl. Although such circumstances are rarely encountered clinically, sustained elevations of plasma bicarbonate concentration do occur with considerable frequency. Indeed, plasma concentration of 40 to 50 mEq per liter are seen even in patients who are neither receiving bicarbonate nor losing gastric juice. This finding clearly indicates that renal reabsorption of bicarbonate must be abnormally large, a conclusion borne out by the fact that the urine of the alkalotic patient typically has a pH in the acid range and contains virtually no bicarbonate. The problem confronting the physician is therefore the identification and correction of the cause of the defect in bicarbonate excretion.

Before the causes of metabolic alkalosis are considered, it seems desirable to review briefly the mechanism of bicarbonate reabsorption. Reabsorption of bicarbonate takes place by an indirect process involving the transport of sodium from the glomerular filtrate and the secretion of hydrogen into the lumen in its place. The addition of hydrogen to the filtrate converts bicarbonate to carbonic acid but at the same time generates an equivalent quantity of bicarbonate in the renal tubular cells; the subsequent diffusion of this bicarbonate into the peritubular blood serves as the mode of bicarbonate "reabsorption." Any stimulus that increases the rate of sodium-hydrogen exchange will also increase bicarbonate reabsorption and will sustain a metabolic alkalosis.

PATHOGENESIS. The causes of metabolic alkalosis are outlined in Table 5. A variety of clinical disturbances can produce metabolic alkalosis, but most of these can be grouped under the general headings of *losses from the upper gastrointestinal tract, diuretic therapy,* or *hyperadrenocorticism.* In each instance, as mentioned earlier, the urine is virtually free of bicarbonate, indicating that the rate of sodium-hydrogen exchange is increased. The nature of the mechanisms responsible for the enhanced bicarbonate reabsorption can perhaps best be understood by considering the renal adjustments that occur during vomiting or as the result of gastric drainage. As hydrochloric acid is lost from the stomach, bicarbonate is generated

---

TABLE 5. Causes of Metabolic Alkalosis

Vomiting or gastric drainage
Diuretic therapy
    Ethacrynic acid
    Thiazides
    Furosemide
Cushing's syndrome
Primary aldosteronism
Bartter's syndrome
Adrenal steroid therapy
Relief of chronic hypercapnia

and plasma bicarbonate concentration rises, with the result that sodium formerly filtered with chloride is now filtered with bicarbonate. Because bicarbonate is not as readily reabsorbable as chloride, sodium reabsorption in the proximal tubule cannot proceed normally; much of the newly generated bicarbonate is therefore delivered with sodium to distal exchange sites. Since the distal exchange sites, even when stimulated by a low-sodium diet, cannot fully conserve this additional sodium, some sodium is initially lost into the urine with bicarbonate. A loss of potassium also occurs because a portion of the sodium conserved by the distal nephron is exchanged with potassium.

As sodium loss and contraction of the extracellular volume stimulate sodium reabsorption, and as the depletion of tubular potassium stores reduces the availability of this cation for exchange, sodium-hydrogen exchange is accelerated. As a result, all further sodium and bicarbonate that escapes proximal reabsorption is conserved and there is a sustained elevation of plasma bicarbonate concentration.

The same basic mechanisms account for the metabolic alkalosis seen with diuretic therapy in the edematous patient. Diuretic agents such as furosemide and ethacrynic acid block sodium chloride reabsorption and deliver sodium and chloride to sodium-avid exchange sites where some fraction of the sodium is exchanged with hydrogen and potassium. Hydrogen is therefore lost into the urine with chloride, and an equivalent quantity of bicarbonate is generated. As with gastric alkalosis, two conditions are required for maintenance of the high rate of sodium-hydrogen exchange and of the state of metabolic alkalosis. First, there must be a continued intense stimulus to sodium reabsorption; second, there must be a persistent deficiency of chloride, which maintains the abnormally high ratio of bicarbonate to chloride in the glomerular filtrate.

The exact sequence of events leading to the increase in bicarbonate concentration in both *primary aldosteronism* and *Cushing's syndrome* remains to be determined, but the fundamental renal mechanisms at play are almost certainly the same as those responsible for the alkalosis seen with gastrointestinal losses or diuretic therapy. The syndrome of *posthypercapneic alkalosis* is discussed later in this chapter under Respiratory Acidosis.

The sodium salts of *penicillin, ampicillin,* and *carbenicillin,* when given in large doses, also cause metabolic alkalosis and potassium deficiency. The reason is not clear. Alkalosis can also occur as the result of the *administration of massive amounts of blood* to a patient whose renal function is impaired. Oxidation of the citrate present in banked blood adds alkali to the body fluids and brings about the rise in plasma bicarbonate concentration. If renal function is normal, the alkali should be quickly excreted; if the patient is oliguric or has frank renal insufficiency, however, persistent and severe alkalosis may result.

DIAGNOSIS.   No signs or symptoms are specific for metabolic alkalosis. The diagnosis is usually suspected because there is a history of vomiting, because therapy with diuretics or adrenal steroids has been given, or because the patient has undergone prolonged gastric drainage. Occasionally, an elevation of bicarbonate concentration is discovered accidentally in the course of routine measurements of serum electrolyte values. An unequivocal diagnosis of metabolic alkalosis can be made only after pH is shown to be increased, but, as a practical matter, an elevated bicarbonate concentration in a patient without significant pulmonary disease can be taken as virtually diagnostic.

The finding of unexplained metabolic alkalosis will sometimes lead to the diagnosis of *Cushing's syndrome* even when there are few or no clinical signs of the disease. This sequence of events is most likely to occur with adrenal hyperfunction associated with extra-adrenal neoplasms. The tumor most likely to produce this syndrome is bronchogenic carcinoma.

TREATMENT.   The treatment of metabolic alkalosis (other than that caused by an excess of adrenal steroids) consists of correction of dehydration and of the various ionic deficits. As noted in the discussion of the etiology of metabolic alkalosis, the combination of chloride deficiency and increased avidity for sodium is responsible for the abnormally high rate of bicarbonate reabsorption. Correction can therefore usually be accomplished promptly by administration of sodium chloride and water. Potassium chloride is also effective in the treatment of metabolic alkalosis and is particularly useful in edematous states because sodium administration is usually contraindicated. Organic potassium salts, such as "triplex" and gluconate, will not correct either alkalosis or potassium deficiency unless adequate amounts of chloride are available in the diet.

In cases of metabolic alkalosis of mild or moderate severity, the speed of correction of the acid-base disorder is not a critical factor. Slow correction over several days, achieved by the renal response to repair of the fluid and electrolyte deficit, usually represents optimal management. On occasion, however, an extreme degree of metabolic alkalosis may necessitate a more direct and intensive approach to therapy. In the Zollinger-Ellison syndrome, for example, continuous and massive losses of hydrochloric acid may elevate the plasma bicarbonate concentration to 60 mEq per liter or more. Under such circumstances, direct titration of the excess bicarbonate by the intravenous administration of hydrochloric acid, in the form of ammonium chloride or arginine hydrochloride, may be imperative.

If ammonium chloride is used, it must be given slowly and under close observation, because, if the rate of infusion exceeds the capacity of the liver to convert ammonium to urea, lethal ammonium intoxication may occur. This risk will be greatly increased if there is any element of underlying hepatic disease. Arginine hydrochloride has come into widespread favor as an alternative and safer means of providing hydrochloric acid intravenously.

In treating patients who are receiving diuretics that tend to produce metabolic alkalosis, it may at times be desirable to administer an acidifying salt by mouth. Ammonium chloride, the agent most commonly used for this purpose, can be given without hazard if liver disease is not present. It is usually administered as an enteric-coated form, because it otherwise gives rise to unpleasant gastric symptoms. An amino acid salt such as lysine monohydrochloride is another useful vehicle for the oral provision of acid.

The management of alkalosis in the patient with hyperadrenocorticism (*Cushing's syndrome, primary aldosteronism*) poses a problem different from that encountered in more common clinical states. First, both the elevated plasma bicarbonate concentration and the hypokalemia persist despite a normal dietary intake of potassium, sodium, and chloride. Furthermore, even a large sodium chloride supplement does not correct the electrolyte abnormalities.

Correction of both alkalosis and potassium deficiency can, however, readily be accomplished over several days by administration of potassium chloride either by mouth or by vein. The explanation of this phenomenon remains obscure. Definitive treatment of the electrolyte disturbances associated with hyperadrenalism consists, of course, in the surgical removal of the offending adrenal tissue.

Respiratory Acidosis

Respiratory acidosis results from any disturbance in ventilation that increases arterial P_{CO_2}. An elevation of P_{CO_2} shifts the normal equilibrium of the bicarbonate–carbonic acid buffer system and increases the plasma hydrogen ion concentration (that is, it decreases pH). This effect on pH is mitigated, however, by a secondary increase in plasma bicarbonate concentration that is dependent on two mechanisms. During acute hypercapnia bicarbonate is generated by the titration of body buffers. With more prolonged elevation of P_{CO_2}, additional bicarbonate is added to the extracellular fluid as the result of augmented acid excretion. A concomitant rise in the renal capacity to reabsorb bicarbonate permits conservation of the new bicarbonate and allows plasma concentration to be stabilized at an elevated level (Fig. 4). Experimental studies indicate that the complete process of renal adaptation requires several days or longer. Thus the extent of physiologic adjustment to a given degree of hypercapnia varies as a function of time, and intelligent appraisal of the acid-base changes in respiratory acidosis requires a knowledge of the duration of the ventilatory disturbance.

PATHOGENESIS. *Acute respiratory acidosis* occurs in a variety of clinical settings. Airway obstruction or hypoventilation resulting from central nervous system depression, neuromuscular disorders, or chest wall injuries are perhaps the most frequent causes. Acute hypercapnia may also occur as a result of decreased alveolar ventilation in disorders such as bacterial and viral pneumonias, aspiration pneumonitis, and pulmonary edema. Extreme respiratory acidosis is also often encountered in cardiopulmonary arrest.

Chronic respiratory acidosis is seen with progressive lung diseases such as emphysema or chronic bronchitis. The disturbance in gas exchange results from ventilation-perfusion mismatching and decreased effective alveolar ventilation. Pulmonary diseases characterized primarily by restrictive changes, such as pulmonary fibrosis, do not cause hypercapnia until late in the course of the illness.

DIAGNOSIS. The tentative diagnosis of *acute respiratory acidosis* can often be made on clinical grounds alone if there is obvious impairment of ventilation. The definitive diagnosis depends, however, on demonstration that P_{CO_2} is elevated and that plasma pH is reduced. These measurements are of particular importance when clinical observation cannot be relied on to reveal an impairment of gas exchange, as, for example, in the patient who is being artificially ventilated or who is suffering from intoxication with barbiturates or other central nervous system depressants.

Chronic respiratory acidosis should be suspected in any patient with the symptoms and physical findings of severe lung disease. Although the diagnosis typically rests on the finding of an elevated P_{CO_2} accompanied by a low pH, hypercapnia may occur in some patients with chronic pulmonary disease in conjunction with a normal or even a high pH. Such pH values have sometimes been interpreted as indicating full compensation or even "overcompensation" for the respiratory acidosis, but they are, in fact, almost always attributable to a complicating metabolic alkalosis (see below).

HYPERCAPNIA AND MIXED ACID-BASE DISORDERS. Just as a variety of illnesses, such as vomiting, lactic acidosis, or diabetic ketoacidosis, may produce a metabolic acid-base disturbance in the normal subject, they can do the same in the patient with hypercapnia (Fig. 4). To recognize and assess the magnitude of a complicating metabolic disturbance in pulmonary insufficiency, one must have prior knowledge of the pH and bicarbonate concentration appropriate to the given degree of uncomplicated hypercapnia. Recent observations on changes in plasma composition during exposure of normal subjects to various degrees of acute hypercapnia have provided a background for the appraisal of the acid-base status in *acute respiratory acidosis*. As Figure 5 shows, there is only a slight rise in plasma bicarbonate concentration over a range of carbon dioxide tension up to 90 mm of mercury. From this response curve and other available information, it appears that in uncomplicated acute hypercapnia of mild or moderate severity the bicarbonate concentration should lie between 25 and 30 mEq per liter. Concentrations higher than 30 mEq per liter indicate the presence of a complicating metabolic alkalosis; those below 25 mEq per liter, the presence of a complicating metabolic acidosis.

Unfortunately, physiologic observations on the response to *chronic* hypercapnia are available only in the dog, but data on patients with chronic lung disease suggest that the pattern of response defined experimentally is closely similar to that which occurs clinically. Figure 5 illustrates schematically how data on the adaptation to chronic hypercapnia can be utilized in the analysis of complex acid-base disorders. This figure contains four schematic diagrams depicting, by vectors, the ways in which the acid-base status in pre-existing chronic respiratory acidosis can be deranged. For purposes of discussion, the initial P_{CO_2} is assumed to be 65 mm of mercury.

Figure 5a contains the vector for a superimposed meta-

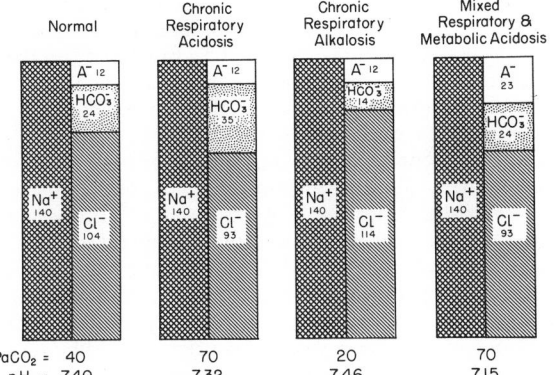

Figure 4. Composition of plasma in representative instances of chronic respiratory acid-base disorders. Note that in *chronic respiratory acidosis* plasma bicarbonate concentration is elevated, whereas in *chronic respiratory alkalosis* it is depressed; in each instance the change in bicarbonate concentration serves to minimize the effect on plasma pH of the abnormality in carbon dioxide tension. The column to the far right depicts a representative example of a *mixed respiratory and metabolic acidosis* in which the "anion gap" is elevated as the result of a disorder such as diabetic ketoacidosis or lactic acidosis.

Figure 5. Schematic diagram of pathways followed by the acid-base disturbances that may complicate chronic respiratory acidosis. The *solid* lines represent the bicarbonate concentrations observed during acute hypercapnia in man, and the *dashed* lines the bicarbonate concentrations seen during chronic hypercapnia in the dog. The origin of each vector has been placed arbitrarily at a point depicting physiologically complete adaptation to a P_{CO_2} of 65 mm of mercury. Each panel is discussed in detail in the text. (Reproduced by permission of the American Journal of Medicine.)

bolic alkalosis. The bicarbonate concentration lies above the level appropriate for chronic adaptation to a P_{CO_2} of 65 mm of mercury and indicates that there has been a pathologic loss of acid or retention of alkali. Such deviations of bicarbonate in the alkaline direction, occurring as a result of diuretics, steroid therapy, or vomiting, could have important clinical consequences, because an inappropriately high pH may diminish respiratory drive and aggravate the pre-existing degree of hypoxemia.

Figure 5b shows the pathway of a superimposed metabolic acidosis. A mild degree of metabolic acidosis, as indicated by the solid portion of the vector, will produce bicarbonate concentrations in the zone lying between the acute and chronic response curves. With a more severe metabolic disturbance, as shown by the dotted extension of the vector, the bicarbonate concentration will be depressed to a level below even the acute response curve.

Figure 5c demonstrates the sequence that will ensue when an acute increase in P_{CO_2} is superimposed on chronic hypercapnia. This disturbance occurs in association with such common complications as pneumonia, heart failure, and excessive sedation, all of which may further compromise alveolar ventilation. As an element of *acute* hypercapnia develops, body buffers can be expected to generate only a small additional amount of bicarbonate; as indicated by the vector, plasma bicarbonate concentration should follow a course roughly parallel to the acute titration curve. For a period of several days — that is, until there is renal compensation appropriate to the new level of hypercapnia — the bicarbonate concentration will remain at a point below the chronic response curve. When either mild metabolic acidosis (Fig. 5b) or acute hypercapnia (Fig. 5c) is superimposed on chronic respiratory acidosis, the bicarbonate values will lie between the acute and chronic response curves. Obviously, the acid-base parameters per se cannot be used to differentiate these two complications, and additional clinical information will be required.

Figure 5d contains the vector resulting from a recent improvement in alveolar ventilation. A sudden fall in P_{CO_2} will titrate body buffers toward normal and induce a

fall in bicarbonate concentration. This titration cannot, however, be expected immediately to erase the renal component of the initial increment in extracellular bicarbonate stores. Plasma bicarbonate concentration will therefore be high in relation to the P_{CO_2}, a condition that has been termed *posthypercapneic alkalosis*. If the diet contains sodium chloride or if the patient is given potassium chloride, the kidney will excrete the excess bicarbonate and the condition will disappear within several days. If chloride intake is low, however, metabolic alkalosis is likely to persist indefinitely. The physiologic mechanisms responsible for this behavior are the same as those already discussed in connection with the metabolic alkalosis resulting from vomiting or from diuretic therapy.

TREATMENT. The treatment of *acute respiratory acidosis* should be directed toward the underlying cause of the impaired ventilation. The measures required will depend on the nature of the clinical problem. If, for example, alveolar gas exchange is impeded by brochospasm, bronchodilators should be used. If inadequate ventilation is the result of a neuromuscular disturbance, artificial ventilation may be necessary.

The treatment of *chronic respiratory acidosis* should be directed primarily toward improving alveolar ventilation, not toward the restoration of a normal pH. Bronchodilators, adrenal steroids, antimicrobials, postural drainage, and artificial ventilation all have a valuable place in therapy at one time or another in the course of the illness. The management of pulmonary insufficiency is dealt with in detail in Ch. 351, but a word of caution should be repeated here concerning the possible hazards of oxygen therapy in worsening chronic respiratory acidosis. In severe hypercapnia the sensitivity of the respiratory center to carbon dioxide may be diminished, and, if this occurs, hypoxemia becomes the major stimulus to respiratory activity. If hypoxemia is then partially or totally corrected, ventilation often undergoes further serious impairment, hypercapnia becomes increasingly severe, and the patient can lapse into coma and die. Thus during oxygen therapy the patient must be watched closely to ensure that improvement in the degree of hypoxemia does not depress ventilation.

Respiratory Alkalosis

Respiratory alkalosis results from any disturbance in ventilation that lowers arterial carbon dioxide tension. A reduction in Pco_2 shifts the normal equilibrium of the bicarbonate–carbonic acid buffer system and decreases the concentration of hydrogen ion in the plasma (that is, it increases pH). This effect on pH is mitigated, however, by a secondary decrease in plasma bicarbonate concentration. During acute hypocapnia bicarbonate is removed from the extracellular fluid by a process of buffering in both blood and tissues; renal excretion of alkali plays only a minor role. During chronic hypocapnia a further reduction in bicarbonate concentration is mediated largely if not entirely by the kidneys. If hyperventilation is sufficiently prolonged (as in persons living at high altitude), these adjustments are sufficient to restore plasma pH to normal or nearly normal levels (Fig. 4).

PATHOGENESIS. Probably the most common cause of respiratory alkalosis is the hyperventilation resulting from extreme anxiety. Other causes are injury to the central nervous system involving the respiratory center, artificial ventilation, fever, hepatic coma, and salicylate intoxication. Hypocapnia is also encountered in the early phase of pulmonary disease if a disturbance in the relation between ventilation and perfusion has produced hypoxemia and hyperventilation.

Finally, as discussed earlier, the persistence of respiratory compensation after the correction of metabolic acidosis may produce a picture chemically indistinguishable from a primary respiratory alkalosis.

DIAGNOSIS. The presence of hyperventilation in a patient suffering from any one of the disorders considered under Pathogenesis should suggest the diagnosis of respiratory alkalosis. In many cases characteristic signs and symptoms provide evidence that one is dealing with primary hyperventilation rather than with respiratory compensation for metabolic acidosis. Respiratory alkalosis produces a typical clinical syndrome in which the cardinal features are lightheadedness, numbness, tingling of the extremities, and circumoral paresthesia. In some patients, frank carpopedal spasm occurs.

The finding of an abnormally low plasma bicarbonate concentration and Pco_2 does not in itself distinguish between metabolic acidosis and respiratory alkalosis; the measurement of plasma pH is often vital to the differentiation. The problem of diagnosis is sometimes further complicated by the presence of a mixed acid-base disorder — that is, one with both respiratory and metabolic components. This combination occurs very often in salicylate poisoning.

TREATMENT. The treatment of respiratory alkalosis should be directed toward correction of the underlying disturbance responsible for the hyperventilation. In the patient with salicylism the goal is to promote removal of the offending drug. One can accomplish this purpose either by augmenting the renal excretion of salicylate (by means of urinary alkalinization and the administration of osmotic diuretics) or by hemodialysis. In the case of injury to the central nervous system or liver failure, the ability to correct respiratory alkalosis will be determined by the effectiveness of therapy directed toward the underlying pathologic process. The hyperventilation syndrome resulting from anxiety can often be effectively controlled if the patient rebreathes into a paper bag. If this method fails, sedation will usually put an end to the acute episode. Recurrences can sometimes be prevented by reassurance and by explanation of the nature of the disorder to the patient, but if these techniques fail, psychotherapy may be indicated.

Arbus, G. S., Herbert, L. A., Levesque, P. R., Etsten, B. E., and Schwartz, W. B.: Characterization and clinical application of the ''significance band'' for acute respiratory alkalosis. N. Engl. J. Med., 280:117, 1969.

Brackett, N. C., Jr., Wingo, C. F., Muren, O., and Solano, J. T.: Acid-base response to chronic hypercapnia in man. N. Engl. J. Med., 280:124, 1969.

Garella, S., Dana, C. L., and Chazan, J. A.: Severity of metabolic acidosis as a determinant of bicarbonate requirements. N. Engl. J. Med., 289:121, 1973.

Levy, L. J., Duga, J., Girgis, M., and Gordon, E. E.: Ketoacidosis associated with alcoholism in nondiabetic subjects. Ann. Intern. Med., 78:213, 1973.

Oliva, P. B.: Lactic acidosis. Am. J. Med., 48:209, 1970.

Relman, A. S.: The acidosis of renal disease. Am. J. Med., 44:706, 1968.

Schnur, M. J., Appel, G. B., Karp, G., and Osserman, E. P.: The anion gap in asymptomatic plasma cell dyscrasias. Ann. Intern. Med., 86:304, 1977.

Schwartz, W. B., and Cohen, J. J.: The nature of the renal response to chronic disorders of acid-base equilibrium. Am. J. Med., 64:417, 1978.

531. DISORDERS OF CARBOHYDRATE METABOLISM

531.1. DIABETES MELLITUS

George F. Cahill, Jr.

GENERAL CONSIDERATIONS. *Diabetes mellitus* is a diagnostic term applied to a constellation of anatomic and biochemical abnormalities which share in common, as part of a syndrome, a disturbance in glucose homeostasis, which is secondary to a deficiency in the beta cells of the endocrine pancreas. This bulky and vague definition cannot be made more specific owing to the marked variability in the disorder. As was once said of syphilis, knowledge of diabetes and its sequelae touches on all areas of medicine.

The syndrome can be completely asymptomatic, or it can appear as an isolated disorder of any organ or system. Fulminant ketoacidosis, fatal unless immediately treated, may be the first sign. Often it is manifested by one of the long-term complications, such as foot ulcer, retinopathy, or proteinuria. Other pathologic states noted to be more frequent in diabetics as compared to the general population may be the clue. For example, the presenting event may be of a myocardial infarction in a young man, an unexpectedly large newborn or pruritus vulvae in the female, recurrent skin infections, or many other phenomena which at first glance appear unrelated. Diabetes mellitus is protean in its manifestations, and this variability is central to its diagnosis and treatment. Furthermore, it tends to be familial.

HISTORY. Descriptions of the disease were made 3000 years ago in Egypt. About 400 B.C., Charak and Susrut in India noted not only the sweetness of the urine, but also the correlation between obesity and diabetes, the tendency of the disease to be passed from one generation to another through the ''seed,'' and even two types of disease, one associated with emaciation, dehydration, polyuria, and lassitude, and the other characterized by "stout build, gluttony, obesity, and sleepiness." Near the beginning of the Christian era, the Romans Aretaeus and Celsus described the disease and gave it the name diabetes (=siphon) mellitus (melli=honey or sweet). Its correlation with gangrene was mentioned by the Arab, Avicenna, 1000 A.D. The sweetness of the urine was again described by Thomas Willis (1675). Dodson, 100 years later, demonstrated that the sweetness was due to sugar and suggested it was not formed de novo by the kidney, but rather that the kidney removed it from the body, a fact scientifically confirmed by the great French physiologist, Claude Bernard, in the mid-1800's.

In 1889 Von Mering and Minkowski first produced experimental diabetes by removing the dog's pancreas. Subsequently Opie (1901) noted changes in the islets of cells in the pancreas (the islets having been described by Langerhans in 1869) in humans dying with the disease. This led to attempts by many to prepare pancreatic extracts which would correct the deficiency. Active fractions were obtained by some, but not until 1921 did Banting and Best in Toronto achieve continuous success, and their discovery was rapidly applied to clinical therapy within six months of their first report. Until then, only a careful semistarvation diet with elimination of excess carbohydrate was even partially effective in prolonging life in the more insulin-deficient juvenile form of the disease, or in ameliorating the symptoms in many patients with the milder maturity-onset variety.

The Banting-Best era changed the outlook of the juvenile diabetic from certain death within two to three years to a nearly normal, albeit shortened, life expectancy. In 1936 the use of long-acting insulin was introduced, simplifying the management of the insulin-requiring diabetic. It became apparent at that time, however, that although insulin therapy prevented many of the acute metabolic problems such as ketoacidosis or those closely correlated with the hyperglycemia, e.g., pruritus vulvae or furunculosis, other sequelae such as retinitis, diabetic neuropathy, or renal glomerulosclerosis appeared in most patients with the juvenile form of the disease for two or more decades in spite of insulin therapy. These complications had been noted prior to the advent of insulin but were relatively unusual, because death from ketoacidosis or infection shortened the life of the patient before these could become manifest. Thus insulin, although a tremendous step forward, did not provide the total solution for the diabetic and his problem. Another development, although less significant than that of insulin, stemmed from the German observation during World War II that certain sulfonamide derivatives lowered blood glucose, and subsequently Loubatières initiated trials in France which established their clinical efficacy. In 1955, oral sulfonylureas began to be generally used as hypoglycemic therapy in diabetics with the milder maturity-onset type of the disease.

PATHOPHYSIOLOGY. Before discussing the etiology, epidemiology, pathology, and clinical aspects of diabetes, the metabolic effects of insulin in normal and abnormal states must be described. Simply, insulin is the animal's "fed" signal. After a large meal, the high circulating levels of insulin tell the body's tissues to take up and store fuel not required for immediate metabolic needs. An intermediate level of insulin resulting from a smaller intake signals the tissues to take up and store fuel less avidly. In contrast, a low level of insulin such as occurs during fasting tells the body that no fuel is entering, and the body's depots should therefore release their stored nutrients back into the blood. Insulin and its normal and abnormal metabolic effects form a continuum of metabolic events (Fig. 1), ranging from those seen when there is a total or near-total lack of insulin's metabolic effects (diabetic ketoacidosis) to those which occur when there are very high levels of insulin (after a large orally ingested mixed meal in a normal individual possessing adequate pancreatic beta cell reserve).

Body Fuels. As shown in Table 1 of Ch. 476.2, average man is about one fifth fat, which stores approximately a two- to three-month supply of calories. Carbohydrate reserves, in contrast, are minimal, about 70 grams (280 kcal) as liver glycogen and 200 to 400 grams (800 to 1600 kcal) in muscle glycogen. Glucose in body fluids is even less, about 15 to 20 grams. Slightly more than 1 kcal per minute is required for basal metabolic needs in a normal resting adult; thus total available carbohydrate in the entire body provides less than one day's supply of fuel. Unlike carbohydrate and fat, there is no depot of protein purely for storage. All is being used for structure, for enzymes, or for other essential purposes. These points emphasize the role of fat as the primary energy storage depot in man and the minimal role of carbohydrate.

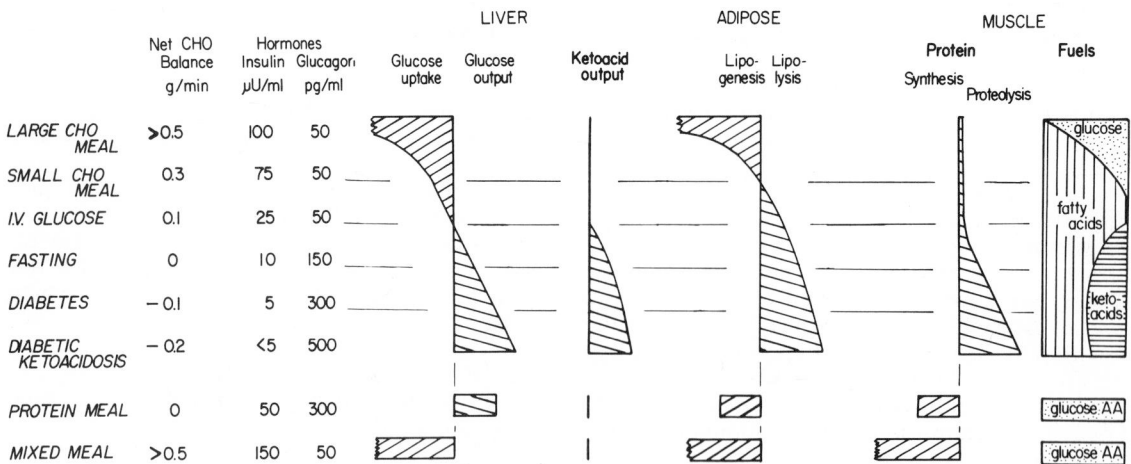

Figure 1. Insulin and glucagon levels and varying rates of organ metabolism as a function of net carbohydrate (CHO) balance in man. The progression from a large positive carbohydrate balance after a large CHO meal to a negative balance as in ketoacidosis forms a continuum of decreasing insulin levels and increasing glucagon levels. Relative metabolic fluxes after protein and mixed meals are also shown. Since the relative contributions of glucose or amino acids (AA) to muscle fuel are not known, these are not differentiated in the scheme with the protein and mixed meals.

Tissue Fuel Utilization. In contrast to storage, in which fat predominates, fuel utilization by brain and, to a lesser degree, by certain other tissues requires a constant supply of glucose. Thus glucose concentration in normal man is confined to a zone between 50 and 150 mg per 100 ml, concentrations above the minimum required by brain and below that saturating the renal reabsorption capacity. Insulin plays the dominant role in maintaining glucose in this range. All other tissues are capable of using glucose and do so when ample amounts are present in the diet, but only if insulin levels are increased. Most of these, particularly fat and muscle, do not utilize glucose when insulin levels are low, and consume instead fat in the form of free fatty acids released from adipose tissue. The capacity of the endocrine pancreas to respond rapidly and adequately to the nutritional state by its rate of insulin release is thus critical to fuel homeostasis.

FED STATE. After eating a mixed meal, gastrointestinal digestion hydrolyzes proteins to single amino acids and carbohydrates to simple sugars, and these enter the portal blood. The liver is easily permeable to all simple sugars and related molecules, and possesses specific enzymes for the phosphorylation and subsequent metabolism of these, particularly of galactose and fructose (see Ch. 531.3 and 531.6). Glucose is phosphorylated and incorporated into glycogen or metabolized by the liver both for its own energy needs and for fat synthesis. These processes require increased insulin levels. After a large carbohydrate-containing meal, much glucose also passes through to the periphery, and the increased insulin levels accelerate the transport of glucose across the muscle and adipose cell wall (Fig. 1).

In muscle, as in liver, glucose is rapidly phosphorylated and used for glycogen synthesis. It is also metabolized to lactate or pyruvate in the cell's cytosol and then, in the presence of adequate oxygen, to carbon dioxide by the cell's mitochondria to provide the bulk of the cell's ATP and, thereby, the muscle's energy needs. In adipose tissue, the augmented glucose uptake in the presence of high insulin levels is metabolized to pyruvate, but instead of the acetyl CoA from the pyruvate being oxidized to CO_2 for energy as in muscle, most is returned to the cytosol and long chain fatty acids are synthesized. In simple terms, the original potential energy available in glucose is converted into potential energy as fatty acid, and the fatty acids are then esterified to glycerol and stored as triglyceride in the oil vacuole in the center of the fat cell. The net effect is transformation of a poor economy type of fuel expressed per unit weight as stored in tissues (carbohydrate) into a much more efficient form (fat).

The amino acids absorbed with the meal are removed by many tissues, particularly by muscle. Insulin augments the transfer of certain amino acids across muscle cell membrane. Insulin also increases the protein-synthetic machinery inside the cell, and the net effect is to increase muscle protein. Thus, as was shown 50 years ago, insulin is anabolic, expanding the body's protein mass.

The third component of the diet, the ingested fat or triglyceride, is partly hydrolyzed in the gut lumen, absorbed by the mucosa where the triglyceride is resynthesized, and incorporated in association with several lipoproteins into a particle, or chylomicron, which is secreted into the lymphatics between the intestinal cells and then, via the thoracic duct, carried into the general circulation (see Ch. 532.2). A major part of these chylomicrons is removed in adipose tissue by an enzyme located at or near the fat-cell membrane, lipoprotein lipase. This enzyme hydrolyzes the triglyceride to yield three free fatty acids, which, in turn, enter into the fat cell, and, like the fatty acid synthesized de novo from glucose, are esterified and incorporated as triglyceride into the central oil droplet. The acceptor for the intracellular re-esterification for fatty acids is glycerol phosphate derived from glucose metabolism. A high insulin level is necessary for the activity of lipoprotein lipase as well as to provide adequate glycerol phosphate for the intracellular esterification of the fatty acids.

In summary, in the "fed" state, a high insulin level is necessary for incorporation of glucose into liver and muscle glycogen, for muscle to consume glucose for energy needs, for both liver and adipose tissue to make fatty acid from glucose, for amino acids to be incorporated into muscle protein, for circulating chylomicrons to discharge their fatty acids into adipose tissue, and for these, in turn, to be re-esterified and incorporated into the triglyceride storage droplet in the middle of the cell.

INTRAVENOUS D AND W. Between the "fed" state, described above, and the fasted state is one in which small amounts of carbohydrate are ingested or administered. This is termed intravenous dextrose and water (IV D and W), because it is frequently employed during partial starvation in patients who cannot or should not be fed by mouth. Glucose, at 100 mg per minute, closely approximates the energy needs of the brain, about one fourth to one fifth the basal caloric need of the body, and thus its administration obviates the need for hepatic glycogenolysis or gluconeogenesis. The body achieves this by the beta cells slightly increasing insulin secretion as a response to the small increase in glucose concentration. This causes circulating insulin levels to rise sufficiently to decrease the release of amino acid from muscle and to prevent hepatic glycogenolysis and gluconeogenesis. It does not increase insulin concentration enough to open up muscle cell and adipose cell membranes to glucose utilization. Thus glucose is yet excluded from most tissues and spared for brain, and, most important, the breakdown of protein to provide precursor for glucose synthesis is no longer necessary. This is the basis for the well-known "nitrogen-sparing effect of carbohydrate." It must again be emphasized that this is probably achieved via levels of insulin slightly above those in simple fasting, and it is the beta cell which increases the insulin level, thanks to its exquisite sensitivity to the minimal but significant increase in blood glucose concentration.

FASTED STATE. As described above, man has minimal carbohydrate reserves, and these are rapidly depleted even during overnight fast. Between meals, glucose levels can be maintained by glycogenolysis, but during more prolonged periods of caloric deprivation, hepatic gluconeogenesis must be initiated to maintain adequate glucose concentrations. This is achieved by a reduction in beta cell release of insulin as glucose falls and thereby in reduced insulin levels, the low levels initiating (1) net muscle proteolysis, (2) the release of amino acids to the liver via the circulation, and (3) gluconeogenesis from these. Subsequently the glucose so produced is consumed by brain. Other tissues, such as renal medulla, red blood cells, peripheral nerve, and, to a limited degree, skeletal muscle, also utilize glucose, but mainly to pyruvate and lactate, and these are returned to the liver for resynthesis to glucose — the so-called Cori cycle. Some of the pyruvate is transaminated to alanine, which also participates in the cycle analogous to lactate and pyruvate. Thus brain is the major tissue metabolizing glucose completely to carbon dioxide and water and requiring gluconeogenesis from amino acids.

For a better understanding of fasting, and particularly of diabetes, more detail is necessary. As insulin level falls, muscle proteolysis outweighs synthesis, certain amino acids are metabolized in the muscle, and those which are glucogenic such as alanine are released. Liver, owing to low insulin and normal or high glucagon levels, is enzymatically poised in the direction of glucose synthesis, and the alanine and glutamine and other glucogenic amino acids are made into glucose. This process requires both energy and hydrogen (reducing equivalent), and these are met by fat oxidation in the liver. The long-chain fatty acids, originally derived from adipose tissue, are partially oxidized to molecules of acetyl CoA, but few of these gain access for terminal combustion via the citric acid cycle to carbon dioxide for reasons incompletely understood. Instead they are condensed and exported from the liver, two at a time, as the *ketone bodies, acetoacetate* and *β-hydroxybutyrate*. Thus during fasting, coupled with gluconeogenesis is the production of ketoacids (ketone bodies).

Acetoacetate and β-hydroxybutyrate are readily utilized by muscle as fuel, and their rate of production by liver in simple fasting closely approximates their utilization, with little "spilling over" into the urine. However, after more than several days of fasting, peripheral tissues diminish their utilization of ketoacids, and their total level in blood rises to approximately 6 to 8 mM. In parallel with this increase is a gradual increase in cerebrospinal fluid ketoacids, sufficient in concentration to provide the major proportion of the brain's energy needs, displacing glucose utilization accordingly. This permits less gluconeogenesis and less mobilization of muscle protein as glucogenic precursor, and survival, thanks to this sparing of body nitrogen, is dramatically prolonged. All these are a result of a continuously low level of insulin, but it must be emphasized that insulin is still playing the central feedback role in the relationship between fuel utilization and mobilization.

Diabetes. With the metabolic state briefly described, it is apparent that abnormalities in insulin secretion must result in altered fuel homeostasis. If insulin secretion cannot be rapidly increased after ingestion of a meal, the rate of intestinal absorption (an insulin-independent process for carbohydrate, amino acid, and fat) will greatly surpass the peripheral uptake of all fuels, resulting in alimentary hyperglycemia, hyperaminoacidemia, and hyperlipemia. This is most easily tested by a simple glucose meal (glucose tolerance), whereby the blood level of glucose given orally or intravenously is followed over time. If insulin release is inadequate, the glucose level is high and remains higher for a longer time owing to failure of the body to receive an adequate "fed" signal. If the insulin deficiency is more marked and is insufficient to facilitate glucose ingress into muscle and adipose cells or glucose incorporation into liver glycogen, but yet enough to depress hepatic ketogenesis and gluconeogenesis, the glucose load will stay in the circulation. Glucose concen-

tration then surpasses the renal threshold and spills into the urine, and dehydration, hypovolemia, and severe hypoglycemia ensue, leading to hyperosmolar coma.

If the insulin deficiency is severe, irrespective of glucose concentration, peripheral amino acid release from muscle protein will provide the liver with more and more glucogenic substrate, and gluconeogenesis and ketogenesis will be rapidly increased. As in prolonged starvation, there is also a decreased peripheral ketoacid utilization, levels of β-hydroxybutyrate and acetoacetate rise quickly in the body, and life-threatening ketoacidosis occurs in addition to the marked hyperglycemia, dehydration, and volume deficiency.

Endocrine Pancreas. The entire carbohydrate, fat, protein, and lipid disorder, as seen in diabetic ketoacidosis, is precisely mimicked by acute pancreatectomy, by chemical destruction of the beta cells with agents such as alloxan or streptozotocin, or by administration of antibody to insulin. Subtotal destruction or removal of beta cells results in less severe degrees of diabetes. Likewise, postmortem examination of human pancreas has shown either total absence of beta cells in juvenile diabetics after several years of the disease or minimal reductions in number with variable nonspecific morphologic changes in the older, maturity-onset type of diabetic, these changes being similar to those associated with aging but occurring prematurely in the diabetic.

Little is known of the natural history of the beta cell. It appears early in the human embryo and continues to divide slowly through life. In states in which there is resistance to insulin's effects, beta cell hyperplasia may be noted. Why the diabetic cannot generate more beta cells to replace his deficiency is unknown, and this deficiency as well as a temporal delay in insulin release by the remaining cells may possibly be the primary underlying defect in the maturity-onset type of diabetes.

The beta cell responds both to the ambient concentration of *glucose* and to changes in glucose concentration by insulin release. This appears to be in two phases, one occurring almost immediately after the increase in glucose concentration and peaking in five to ten minutes, and a later phase occurring 15 to 30 minutes later and persisting as long as the glucose concentration remains elevated. Glucose taken by mouth elicits a greater insulin release than glucose infused parenterally; this is due to a hormonal effect in the gut during carbohydrate absorption which sensitizes the beta cells to release even more insulin in response to changes in glucose concentration. This gut hormone(s) has yet to be identified with certainty, and GIP (gastric inhibitory polypeptide) is a contender. However, GIP and similar intestinal-derived polypeptides share amino acid sequences, and the roles of these components of the gastroenteropancreatic system await characterization (see Ch. 399).

Amino acids also can provoke insulin release. Of particular interest are leucine and arginine, the former being an essential branched-chain amino acid which, in certain children, can induce excessive insulin release, causing symptomatic hypoglycemia (see Ch. 531.2). Arginine, as well as several other amino acids, also induces insulin release, and its administration has been used as one of a battery of research tests for assessing beta cell function. Eating a protein meal results in an apparently greater insulin release than one might expect from the constituent amino acids. This has been explained by the capacity of

Figure 2. Probable sequence of human proinsulin, containing 86 amino acids in a single chain folded back on itself, with closure of 2 sulfhydryl bridges between the beginning and end as well as a bridge between amino acids 71 and 76. When the C-peptide (connecting peptide) is split out in the beta cell as the insulin is being collected into storage granules, the A and B chains are left connected by the sulfhydryl bridges. The eventual human A chain has 21 amino acids and the B chain 30 amino acids. Preproinsulin contains another 23 amino acids before the amino terminus of the B-chain, and the "pre" portion is cleaved as or immediately after the preproinsulin is synthesized on the polysome. The A-B chain insulin differs from pig insulin by a threonine (Thr) instead of an alanine at the end of the B chain. Many more differences exist in the connecting peptides between species; hence the higher antigenicity of the impure insulins. (Illustration courtesy of Dr. D. Steiner.)

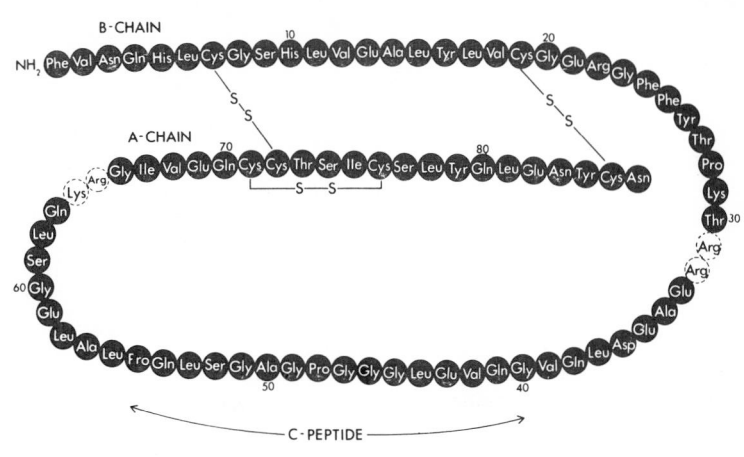

CCK-pancreozymin, the gut hormone released after protein ingestion to stimulate excessive pancreatic secretion, to affect also the endocrine pancreas by promoting insulin release from the beta cells (as well as glucagon from the alpha cells).

Other factors known to stimulate insulin release are the *sulfonylurea class of oral antidiabetic agents,* stimulation of parasympathetic nerves leading to the pancreas, and, to a lesser degree, elevated concentrations of fatty acids, ketoacids, and the potassium ion. The relative importance of innervation and these last-named factors appears to be less than that of glucose and amino acids in man. In other animals, such as the ruminants, ketoacids and related compounds are very active insulin secretagogues.

INSULIN.   Insulin is synthesized inside the beta cell as a single chain preproinsulin of approximately 110 amino acids. The "pre" portion is cleaved as the molecule is being formed. Like other "pre" sequences on proteins synthesized for export from cells, this lead sequence serves to guide the protein into cisternae for transport to the Golgi apparatus. As shown by Steiner in the mid-1960's, this proinsulin molecule folds back on itself, followed by closure of the sulfur bridges (Fig. 2). The connecting peptide is then excised by proteolytic cleavage, residual arginines and lysine are removed, and the insulin molecule is then stored in granules for eventual export along with the remaining C-peptide fragment. The insulin and connecting peptide are packaged together into granules; when the beta cell is stimulated to release insulin, the granules are brought to the surface of the cell, and insulin is discharged with the metabolically inert connecting peptide into the adjacent capillary. Normally a small amount of proinsulin is also released, but this hormone is either inactive or much less active than insulin itself. In abnormal states such as islet cell tumor or in diabetes, the proportion of proinsulin may be increased, a circumstance which has been helpful in diagnosis.

Insulin in blood is unbound. Approximately half is removed as it passes through liver, and most of the remainder is removed by the kidney, being small enough (5734 daltons) to be filtered and catabolized by the tubules on resorption. Thus insulin has a short half-life, approximately three to ten minutes. Most data suggest that changes in its concentration are regulated by alterations in beta cell secretion, not by alterations in removal rates.

Insulin, like other peptide hormones, binds to specific receptors on cell membranes and elicits the release of one or more second messengers, which in turn alter enzyme levels and activities inside the cell. In muscle and adipose tissue, there is also a rapid acceleration of glucose transport across the cell wall after exposure to insulin, as well as augmented transport of certain amino acids and potassium into the cell and changes in the membrane electrical potential. Which of these are primary insulin effects and which are secondary to one or more intracellular messengers remain to be established. In certain tissues, such as liver and adipose, levels of cyclic AMP are reduced by insulin, but the numerous intracellular effects cannot be explained solely by the reduced level of cyclic AMP. Presence of a second messenger is supported by the finding of newly phosphorylated proteins inside cells within minutes after exposure of the intact cell to insulin. No such effect can be found once the cell has been disrupted.

GLUCAGON.   Glucagon is composed of a single strand of 29 amino acids, being synthesized first, like insulin, as a prohormone with the "pro" segment then cleaved prior to storage by the alpha cells in the islets. Its primary effect is to increase the activity of adenyl cyclase in liver by reacting with sites on the liver cell membrane, and thereby to increase hepatic cyclic AMP. This in turn initiates activation of glycogen breakdown, by increasing the activity of the glycogen phosphorylase system and by decreasing the activity of the glycogen synthetase system (see Ch. 531.4). It also increases gluconeogenesis in the liver, again probably because of its effect on adenyl cyclase activity. The precise role of glucagon in man is as yet unclear, but it is probably important in the disposition of the amino acids in a pure protein meal. Its release is prompted by certain amino acids such as arginine and alanine and also by enteric hormones such as CCK-pancreozymin. Its level also increases in many states of stress, such as trauma, hypoglycemia, infection, exercise, and starvation. Unger has shown that at a given glucose concentration it is increased in diabetics as compared to nondiabetics, suggesting either a direct effect of insulin on the alpha cell or a primary alpha cell abnormality. With aggressive insulin therapy of the diabetic, its levels are brought to normal, and the defect is thus probably secondary. Also, destruction of the total pancreas or of beta cells specifically or removal of circulating insulin by administration of antibody in laboratory animals can produce the full-blown diabetic state. Lowering of glucagon levels, using somatostatin, transiently decreases fasting blood glucose levels, and its role is thus probably permissive in maintaining the liver in a glucose-producing mode during fasting or with protein ingestion.

ETIOLOGY. As known to the Hindis centuries ago, diabetes is familial. Environment also plays a large role, particularly overnutrition, as evidenced by the marked decrease in incidence of the disease in Europe during World War II. The geneticist's best tool, a comparison of identical versus fraternal twins, has been used several times, and a much higher concordance rate has been noted in identical twins, indicating an important genetic component. As mentioned before, the disease is a continuum ranging from a total or near total absence of insulin, resulting in death in two to three days in diabetic ketoacidosis, to a slightly elevated glucose level after a glucose load as compared to the disposition of a similar glucose load in a "normal" age-matched population. Terms used for either end of the spectrum include *"juvenile-onset"* or *"ketosis-prone"* for the markedly insulin-deficient, and *maturity-onset "mild"* or *"late-onset"* for the individual whose insulin release after a challenge is insufficient to effect normal glucose tolerance. Although most children exhibit the "juvenile-onset" form of diabetes, they can develop a very mild or "maturity-onset" type of the disease; this latter predisposition, often associated with obesity, appears to be marked in certain families, and dominant inheritance has been suggested for this type of diabetes. Likewise, four fifths or more of all diabetics develop the "maturity-onset" type of the disease in later life and usually are overweight at diagnosis. Ketoacidosis is infrequent in this older-age-onset group, but does occur. A simplified nomenclature has been devised to characterize the diagnosis according to the degree of metabolic abnormality irrespective of age (Table 1). Nonhereditary diabetes, such as that secondary to pancreatitis, should be considered when ketoacidosis develops early in diabetes in this older age group. Curiously, subjects in the eighth or ninth decade of life may also develop the juvenile type of diabetes, but this is infrequent.

Paradoxically, concordance for diabetes is much greater in identical twins developing the disease in middle or later life, approaching 90 to 100 per cent when tested by glucose tolerance. In the juvenile-onset type of diabetes, concordance, which occurs in less than one half of twin pairs, is within one or two years of the diagnosis in the first twin. If the second twin does not develop it within a few years, he frequently never will, suggesting juvenile-type diabetes

TABLE 1.   Classification of Diabetes

Primary diabetes mellitus
A. Insulin-dependent type
B. Not insulin-dependent type
   1. Nonobese
      a. Insulin requiring
      b. Not insulin requiring
   2. Obese
      a. Insulin requiring
      b. Not insulin requiring
Gestational diabetes
Impaired glucose tolerance
Previous abnormality
Potential abnormality
Other conditions with diabetes mellitus or carbohydrate intolerance
A. Hormonal imbalance
B. Drug-induced
C. Pancreatic disease
D. Rare genetic or chromosomal disorders
E. Insulin receptor abnormalities
F. Other rare types

to be less familial than the adult-onset type and possibly more influenced by environment — exactly the reverse of other inherited diseases, in which the more severe form appears to be more transmissible through heredity. Another possibility is that there are different forms of diabetes with a different genetic basis, and this concept of the heterogeneity of diabetes is becoming more accepted.

It has been suggested that juvenile diabetes may be due to viral destruction of beta cells, and British studies have shown juvenile diabetes to occur in clusters associated with certain common viral epidemics (e.g., group B coxsackievirus). Juvenile-onset type diabetes (insulin-dependent in Table 1) correlates strongly with inheritance of genetic factors on chromosome 6. In kindreds with a high prevalence of this disease, over half the affected siblings share an identical chromosome 6 pair. In over 90 per cent of siblings at least one chromosome 6 is shared. In addition, there are significant correlations with certain alleles on the B, C, and D loci of the major histocompatibility complex, in particular B8/DW3 and B15/DW4. Most new cases of juvenile diabetes demonstrate both cell-mediated and antibody-related autoimmunity. In some, these persist for years, and in these there is a greater correlation with B8/DW3. These data suggest a strong pathogenic autoimmune component in some juvenile-type diabetics, and perhaps a viral destruction with secondary autoimmunity, in others. This correlation of diabetes with the histocompatibility antigens on chromosome 6 applies mainly to insulin-dependent (Type I) diabetes (Table 1), or, in other words, the juvenile-onset type of diabetes. In Type II or maturity-onset type diabetes, there is no apparent correlation with factors on chromosome 6.

In diabetes not dependent on insulin, or maturity-onset type diabetes, a progressive age-related diminution of beta cell function appears to be the underlying disorder. This is supported by other suggestions of premature aging, such as accelerated senescence of cells in tissue culture or premature cross-linking of collagen. Little is known of the natural history of the beta cell, and whether the deficiency is accelerated destruction or decreased replacement is not known. In any case, the almost 100 per cent concordance of maturity-onset type diabetes in identical twins suggests a strong hereditary contribution. This accelerated senescence may also contribute to the premature atherosclerosis and other age-related events more prominent in diabetics, such as osteoporosis or senile cataract.

DIAGNOSIS. The sine qua non for diagnosis is demonstration of the inability of a given subject to dispose appropriately of a glucose load, as evidence of a relative or absolute decrease in insulin release and circulating concentration. This legalistic description is, however, markedly qualified. Anxiety, prior carbohydrate deprivation, old age, acute illness, infection, delayed gastric emptying, certain pharmacologic agents, hypokalemia, and many other factors can all result in abnormal glucose tolerance. A normal unstressed subject, having had adequate amounts of dietary carbohydrate (over 200 grams per day for several days), on ingesting 75 or 100 grams of glucose should have a venous whole blood glucose level below 110 mg per 100 ml before glucose ingestion, under 160 mg per 100 ml at one hour, and below 120 mg per 100 ml at two hours (Fig. 3). Capillary levels (mainly arterial) and levels in plasma (caused by the volume occupied by hemoglobin and red cell stroma) will be proportionally higher, and appropriate corrections should be made (i.e., a 10 per cent increase

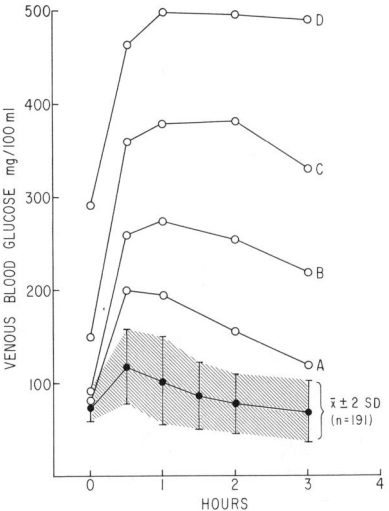

Figure 3. Glucose tolerance tests in four diabetics (A-D) and range of values in 191 healthy controls. Shaded area shows range of two standard deviations in the normal population. Diabetics A and B have sufficient insulin for fasting glucose homeostasis, but an inability to increase insulin release appropriately. Diabetic C has fasting hyperglycemia and marked glucose intolerance. The late fall-off at the end of the curve may be due mainly to glucose loss in urine. Subject D, in whom the tolerance test was clinically unnecessary, is probably almost totally lacking in insulin, and, with this degree of fasting hyperglycemia, is a candidate for the development of ketoacidosis. In such a subject, glucose in the urine may even surpass the load given for the tolerance itself. (Unpublished data of R. Gleason and J. S. Soeldner.)

from the venous blood glucose value). The glucose is given as either pure glucose or commercially available flavored dextrins (i.e., Glucola), which are rapidly hydrolyzed to free glucose in the gut and then absorbed. The glucose may also be given intravenously, 0.5 gram per kilogram, and blood levels determined at several ten-minute intervals up to one hour after its rapid infusion. The per cent disappearance, calculated from half-life (t½) of blood glucose (e.g., the minutes elapsed when glucose levels decrease from 300 to 150 mg per 100 ml, as plotted semilogarithmically) is defined as:

$$K\left(\frac{\text{per cent disappearance}}{\text{minute}}\right) = \frac{0.69}{t\text{½ minutes}} \times 100$$

and should normally be greater than unity. This test has been utilized mainly as a research tool, because it bypasses the gut factor effect elicited by oral glucose. It has been found, however, to be clinically less discriminant than the oral glucose tolerance test.

Rarely, one is presented with a patient with classic diabetic retinopathy or nephropathy but a normal fasting glucose level, and even more rarely the same patient might have a normal glucose tolerance. Is this a diabetic? Probably yes, so the strict adherence fo the legalistic glucose tolerance as being pathognomonic is not warranted. It is highly probable that this subject had had glucose intolerance at one time. This introduces a problem shared by most other diseases of the endocrine system, namely their fluctuating nature and capacity to remit and relapse without known cause.

NATURAL HISTORY AND DEFINITIONS. The disease may present as fulminant diabetic ketoacidosis at any age, but most frequently in childhood or adolescence. It is common for the disease then to remit, little or no insulin being required for several weeks to months, and then to recur as the remission ends. Glucose tolerance through the remission is usually abnormal, but occasionally it may even be normal. Also, the remission may last as long as one or two years, and very rarely the diabetes may not recur. Once the diabetes has recurred in the young individual, it may be relatively easy to manage with a simple morning injection of intermediate-duration insulin, but after several years the glucose levels become more difficult to manage, suggesting termination of all endogenous insulin release. Rubenstein and Steiner have shown connecting peptide (Fig. 2) to be present in plasma, suggesting that some endogenous insulin synthesis and secretion do persist through the early phases of the disease. The diabetes then becomes labile or "brittle" after endogenous insulin secretion ceases and requires more careful matching of diet and insulin, the latter usually necessary twice ("split-dose") instead of once a day.

In the maturity-onset type of diabetic, the insulin deficiency is less severe and may be evidenced only by glucose intolerance of varying degrees. Obesity, for as yet unexplained reasons, requires a higher insulin concentration and therefore a greater rate of insulin release for insulin to exert its metabolic effects (Fig. 4). Binding of insulin to various cells taken from experimentally obese animals has been shown to be decreased, as have the metabolic effects of insulin. Thus obesity unmasks diabetes (as do pregnancy and other endocrine disturbances associated with peripheral resistance to insulin). If the patient loses weight and normal glucose tolerance ensues, the patient was described as a latent diabetic but by the new nomenclature would be classified as "previous abnormality" (Table 1). This same term is applied to a mother with normal glucose tolerance post partum but a diabetic tolerance when pregnant. A "chemical diabetic" was one also asymptomatic at the time but with abnormal glucose tolerance or even an elevated fasting blood glucose value. Depending on the degree of the glucose intolerance, this individual would now be described as diabetic or as having impaired glucose tolerance.

The maturity-onset type of diabetic, as just mentioned, may lose the glucose abnormality with weight loss, or, occasionally, may even lose it without weight loss by dietary therapy alone, meaning carbohydrate restriction. Conversely, the glucose intolerance may progress, with initial worsening of the glucose tolerance itself, followed by insufficient insulin to maintain normal fasting glucose concentrations, with exogenous insulin required to prevent ketoacidosis. Generally, however, the diabetes tends to remain at the severity at which the original diagnosis was made.

INCIDENCE AND PREVALENCE. Surveys in the United States have shown 2 to 4 per cent of the population to have documented diabetes and a similar number to have abnormal glucose tolerance without having been previously diagnosed. The "softness" of this statistic is grossly apparent in view of the "softness" of the criteria for diagnosis. In Michigan, 1 in 600 school children requires insulin; this is probably a good statistic for juvenile diabetes, but there are probably additional children with milder maturity-onset diabetes undiagnosed. In the total diabetic population, the juvenile type of diabetes comprises approximately 10 per cent, but again this is not a firm statistic, because

Figure 4. Glucose and insulin levels in five groups of subjects during 16 hours of the day. The glucose levels are lumped together into nondiabetics and diabetics. The diabetics were specifically selected to be those with a significant degree of fasting hyperglycemia. The obese diabetics show the marked hyperinsulinemia necessary to overcome their generalized resistance to insulin. The estimated peripheral insulin secretion rate in the obese nondiabetic is calculated as 114 units per day, almost four times that of the normal nonobese.

The obese diabetic has also a greater insulin secretion than does the normal, 46 units per day. The thin adult diabetic does less well than the normal, and the juvenile diabetic shows an almost total failure to increase the very meager insulin level after changes in fuel loads. (Data of S. Genuth.)

many patients who have insulin-requiring diabetes do not go into ketoacidosis without insulin but stabilize at a high glucose concentration, thanks to deficient yet significant endogenous insulin production. Thus the disease is a continuum between total insulin lack and the normal, and the characterization of the normal is made arbitrarily. With advanced age, a greater proportion of the population, as high as 40 to 60 per cent in the ninth decade, has abnormal glucose tolerance; so again the definition is arbitrary.

There are diverse cultural and racial differences in incidence and prevalence. Diabetes is rare in the Eskimo; in certain American Indians such as the Pima in Arizona, up to 50 per cent of the population develop diabetes. Similar high rates are observed in Asian Indians who have moved to South Africa and adopted a sedentary, high-caloric style of life. Ketoacidosis is less frequent to absent in these and in blacks in Africa or in the Oriental races, particularly homeland Japanese. The extent to which these differences are genetic on the one hand or environmental or nutritional on the other is under study.

CLINICAL MANIFESTATIONS. The classic juvenile diabetic is a child with one or two weeks or longer of progressive polydipsia and polyuria, weight loss, lassitude, blurred vision, leg cramps, inattentiveness at school, irritability, and frequently a craving for sweet beverages. Such a child, if diabetes is undiagnosed, develops mild and then severe nausea, followed by vomiting, dehydration, stupor, coma, and finally death. The progression may be more rapid, particularly in infants or small children, or it may continue as the three "polys," polydipsia, polyuria, and polyphagia, for from weeks to months, with marked weight loss even to the point of emaciation. These latter subjects apparently still have some endogenous insulin production. Thus the initial presentation of the juvenile diabetic may be due to (1) ketoacidosis; (2) marked hyperglycemia, dehydration, and collapse without ketoacidosis, namely hyperosmolar coma; or (3) an intermediate between these two. Diabetic ketoacidosis always has some degree of hyperosmolarity.

If the insulin deficiency is less marked but fasting hyperglycemia and glucosuria are present, the patient may not be aware of the insidious onset of polydipsia and polyuria and may be brought to the physician's attention

by superimposed infection. Females with glycosuria are particularly susceptible to bacterial and fungal infections of the vulva and vagina, with marked pruritus, excoriation, and bad odor. The hyperglycemia may predispose the subject to other soft tissue infection such as cellulitis, furunculosis, gingival abscess, otitis media, or paronychia. There is also a predisposition to other internal infective processes, such as appendicitis and cholecystitis, and particularly to pulmonary tuberculosis or systemic mycotic infections.

The patient with the milder, maturity-onset type of disease may be asymptomatic, and the diagnosis may be made by finding glycosuria or hyperglycemia or by glucose intolerance. The predisposition of diabetes to premature atherosclerosis frequently provokes medical attention, and the diabetes is then recognized. Myocardial infarction in a young man or, particularly, a woman in the reproductive age, premature peripheral vascular insufficiency, or occasionally diabetic neuropathy or nephropathy may be the first manifestation.

Eye. The ocular manifestations of diabetes are numerous. Hyperglycemia increases glucose concentration in the lens and optic humors, resulting in blurring of vision, weakness of accommodation, and myopia. Very rarely the lens itself may become opacified (the metabolic or *"snowflake" cataract*) presumably owing to sorbitol formation and accumulation; this may disappear after correction of the hyperglycemia. Another manifestation of acute or subacute diabetes is *lipemia retinalis*, the retinal arteries and veins appearing as if they contain cream of tomato soup rather than demonstrating their usual dark red color. Treatment of these conditions is directed to correction of the hyperglycemia (and hyperlipidemia) with appropriate therapy, namely insulin and diet, and other specific agents according to the type of hyperlipidemia.

Most serious and much more prevalent are the *microvascular complications* of the chronic diabetic state. For example, about one sixth of all cases of acquired blindness are due to *diabetic retinopathy*. Approximately two thirds of diabetics with disease for 15 years and over 90 per cent of those with disease for three or four decades have ophthalmoscopically detectable evidence of retinopathy. It most often appears after ten years of known diabetes as an increased tortuosity and widening of the vessels, with scattered, barely visible dots caused by microaneurysms, usually about the macula or about the periphery of the temporal area. With fluorescein angiography, alterations may be noted within the first few years of the disease. Later, small punctate hemorrhages may appear with "waxy" exudates which may either persist or disappear after months to years, leaving a small whitish scar, but with loss of visual elments in that area. Increased capillary permeability leads to extravasation of protein seen as fluffy "cotton-wool" exudates, which also are variable, appearing and disappearing with time.

In the next phase, small vessels may appear over the disc and along the nerves or elsewhere in the retina, and these may then grow into the vitreous. More ominous, they frequently rupture with large hemorrhages and, depending on whether the macular area is involved, with either loss of areas of vision or transient total blindness (Fig. 5). They usually undergo moderate to marked resorption with return of some vision until the next hemorrhage. However, these newly formed vessels, part of the syndrome of retinitis proliferans, usually portend an ominous prognosis unless treated. If there is hemorrhage anteriorly into the vitreous, resorption may be associated with contraction and tearing and detachment of the retina. However, the retinitis may arrest or even regress at any stage without known cause. More commonly, however, proliferating vessels usually lead to legal blindness in the affected eye within four to six years.

The microvascular disease is not limited to the retinal vessels but may also occur in the ciliary body and iris (*rubeosis iridis*), leading to occlusion of the outflow tract, resulting in open-angle neovascular glaucoma, or to hemorrhagic glaucoma after rupture of a vessel.

The pathogenesis of the retinal microangiopathy, as described by Kuwabara and Cogan, is a loss of the pericytes (mural cells) about the capillaries, followed by thickening and weakening of the wall forming the microaneurysm which, in turn, may rupture to cause the visible punctate hemorrhage. In addition shunt vessels, surrounded by areas of capillary closure appear, and it is in these that microaneurysms frequently appear. Another theory postulates small capillary thromboses, vessel distention, rupture, and hemorrhage.

The Joslin Clinic staff and many other specialists have stressed the better visual prognosis in patients who control their diabetes with optimal insulin-carbohydrate homeostasis than in patients taking poorer care of their disease, especially for the first ten years of the disease. Rigid prospective studies on this point are not available, but the rapid acceleration of retinopathy noted in the diabetic decompensation with pregnancy or with infection supports the hypothesis. It is rare to see a patient with normal fundi who has had several episodes of ketoacidosis after 15 to 20 years of the disease; those with normal fundi after many years of the disease usually, but again not always, tend to be the "better controlled."

Treatment of the microangiopathy, if we adhere to the "control" hypothesis, calls for optimal treatment of the diabetes itself through adjustment of insulin and diet from the earliest recognition of the disease. Since many conscientious patients, even with the best effort, still develop retinopathy, numerous therapies, including various vitamins, dietary alterations, and hormones, have been used without effect.

An observation that a patient with diabetic retinopathy underwent remission after spontaneous pituitary necrosis prompted a wave of *pituitary ablative procedures* in the 1960's, including total surgical hypophysectomy, surgical section of the pituitary stalk, proton bombardment of the pituitary, transsphenoidal implantation of yttrium-90, freezing of the pituitary, and others, and a significant delay of the retinopathy or even improvement was observed in many. Many patients with hormonal evidence of total pituitary destruction nevertheless progressed, and a few others, in whom the pituitary was not destroyed, improved. The procedure has since been all but abandoned. It is still not clear why the procedure provided some benefit to the average patient; most authorities attribute its effect to reduction or removal of growth hormone.

Direct therapy of the fundus, using photocoagulation, has been a major advance. Patients with unilateral retinitis pigmentosa and diabetes were observed to have less diabetic retinopathy in the eye with the previous retinitis. This has prompted Aiello and Beetham and others to use laser therapy to apply numerous scattered destructive lesions to the retina as the light is absorbed by the pigment layer, heating and coagulating the adjacent elements. These scattered lesions result in no field defect, and patients with early diabetic neovascularization have had progression of the disease halted or delayed, probably secondary to a diminished vascular need because of diminished tissue in the area treated. Similar results were previously obtained by Wetzig and others, using the polychromatic light of the xenon arc lamp. More recently a green source, the agon laser, has been used to specifically coagulate lesions in the vessels themselves, such as bleeding points, microaneurysms, or the newly forming vessels near or overlying the optic disc; optimal therapy involves treatment of both the specific lesions and the scattered destructive lesions described above.

The eye is occasionally the site of nerve lesions, most frequently the third, resulting in diplopia and strabismus. This disturbing lesion, probably caused by a small vascular infarction, may be preceded by severe pain; it usually reverses itself within several months. The pupil reaction, however, is maintained, because the infarct is usually with the nutrient vessels of the nerve, whereas the pupillary fibers on the outside of the nerve remain nourished by adjacent vessels. Finally, diabetics appear to be more susceptible to the common senile cataract, which appears at an earlier chronologic age and matures more rapidly than usual, and, as mentioned elsewhere, to infections of the eye. Corneal lesions are more pernicious than similar injuries in nondiabetics.

Kidney.   The kidney is also a focal point for diabetes and its complications. The predisposition to infection makes pyelonephritis fairly frequent and serious, and the more severe renal infections may lead to papillary necrosis or perinephric abscess, grave conditions almost unique to the diabetic. For this reason urinary tract instrumentation such as catheterization should be avoided in a diabetic unless absolutely necessary, because subsequent infection is so often observed.

The main problem, however, is the *microangiopathy*. Proteinuria appears in two thirds of patients with diabetes for 20 years and portends progressive renal involvement, with uremia developing in the average patient in five years. Forty per cent of juvenile-type diabetics die from renal failure. Biopsies of kidneys in newly discovered diabetics by Lundbaek's group in Denmark have shown no demonstrable lesion, but after several years there is increased thickness of the capillary basement membrane

and accumulation of material in the mesangial area as seen by the electron microscope, which then may become visible by standard light microscopy after 10 to 15 years. In some unfortunate patients, the nephropathy may be more rapid, occasionally leading to renal failure after only nine to ten years of diabetes. In a very fortunate few, and these appear to be those patients in whom the diabetes has been best controlled by insulin and diet, the signs or symptoms of nephropathy may not develop even after 50 years of the disease. With the progressive thickening and folding of the vascular basement membrane, composed of glycoprotein, as well as the mesangial accumulation of similar material, the lesion is seen as (1) *nodular glomerulosclerosis* as described by Kimmelstiel and Wilson over 30 years ago, (2) a diffuse accumulation of glycoprotein in all areas of the glomerulus, or (3) a mixture of the two. Paradoxically, the thickened basement membrane is more permeable to macromolecules; hence the proteinuria. As the lesion progresses, entire glomeruli may become occluded, with loss of renal function, uremia, and death. Added to these microvascular lesions are the accelerated atherosclerosis and high frequency of hypertension and arteriolar nephrosclerosis in diabetics with nephropathy.

In most diabetics, the severity of retinopathy and nephropathy are similar; however, there are some patients with terminal renal failure secondary to diabetes with only a few scattered microaneurysms and exudates, and, conversely, there are some with retinitis proliferans leading to blindness with minimal proteinuria and normal blood levels of urea and creatinine.

Transplantation of normal kidneys in experimentally diabetic animals has shown similar lesions to appear and to disappear with retransplantation back into nondiabetic animals. A current theory suggests that the abnormality may simply result from glucose molecules reacting with groups on proteins, analogous to the formation of hemoglobin A_{1c}, which results from glucose combining with the amino terminus of the B chain of hemoglobin. Its level increases proportional to the mean glucose level to which the red cell has been exposed.

As with retinopathy, treatment of diabetic nephropathy is directed to the treatment of the diabetes itself. Infection in the genitourinary system in particular, as well as any infection elsewhere with diabetic decompensation, tends to accelerate the nephropathy as well as the retinopathy. With renal failure, chronic dialysis and/or transplantation are the only direct forms of therapy; however, the generalized atherosclerosis makes vascular shunts difficult to create and maintain, and the diabetic's susceptibility to infection creates an even greater problem. Added to this, immunosuppression for transplantation poses such a risk that only subjects with advanced renal failure but otherwise in good condition should be considered as candidates. Basically, therefore, the treatment of diabetic nephropathy is no different from that of renal failure resulting from chronic glomerulonephritis, polycystic kidneys, or other causes; such treatment involves judicious use of diuretics and antihypertensives, a restricted protein diet, and careful adjustment of electrolyte intake.

Nervous System. Diabetes affects the nervous system in many ways as it does other organs and tissues. The marked predilection of the diabetic to atherosclerosis, particularly of medium-sized and small arteries, predisposes him to infarction. If the artery is to the spinal cord, *paraplegia* may result, a very infrequent but disastrous event. Rarely the occlusion may be to a nerve root, resulting in a radiculopathy confined to a dermatome. More frequently, a single peripheral nerve is involved, with sudden loss of sensory and motor function and pain. This may involve the ulnar or peroneal nerve or, more frequently, one of the oculomotor nerves, resulting in acute ophthalmoplegia, or the facial nerve, producing Bell's palsy. Fortunately collateral circulation corrects most or all of the deficit and the mononeuropathy disappears in weeks or months.

By far the most frequent neurologic problem in diabetics is the *peripheral neuropathy* (see Ch. 337.8.) This occurs in over 90 per cent of diabetics who have had the disease for one or more decades. The typical case presents after eight to twelve years of overt diabetes with a grossly symmetrical stocking-type of anesthesia, mainly of the lower extremities, producing decreased vibratory and fine-touch sensation and occasionally progressing after months to years to near-total or total anesthesia. Paradoxically, there may be marked hyperesthesia and pain, frequently nocturnal and occasionally excruciating in character. Fortunately for the patient, the progressive nature of the neuropathy provides relief of the pain after several months or occasionally a year or longer, resulting in hypesthesia to total anesthesia of the area, probably owing to total loss of sensory nerve function. Deep tendon reflexes in the lower extremity are almost always decreased to absent in these subjects. Many elderly subjects may exhibit similar changes; whether these are due to the diabetic syndrome associated with the mild glucose intolerance of the aged can be argued.

Histologic examination reveals segmental demyelinization. Experimental diabetes in animals is associated with

---

Figure 5. *A,* Vitreous and preretinal hemorrhage from the disc area secondary to disc neovascularization.

B, Fibrous band resulting from going into a quiescent stage of retinopathy one year after slide *A* was taken. Patient maintained quiescent stage for eight years until he died a cardiac death.

C, Preretinal hemorrhages in region of macula which also has exudates and superficial hemorrhages. Note boat-shaped dependency type of hemorrhage.

D, Preretinal hemorrhage at site of frond of neovascularization. Note the new vessel fan underneath the boat-shaped preretinal hemorrhage. It is these new vessels which rupture spontaneously or with minimal stress.

E, Extensive fan of new vessels with fibrous network elevated forward into vitreous. Feeding vessels come from multiple arteries and veins at the retinal level, the entire process being analogous to an angioma.

F, Characteristic waxy exudates in macular zone accounting for decrease in vision, apparently due to incompetent capillaries and leaking from central areas of rings of waxy exudates where the red blotches are noted.

G, Fluorescein angiography in a diabetic, showing some very fine microaneurysms and some tiny areas of capillary closure but with good parafoveal network of vessels and 20/20 vision. These are early changes of diabetic retinopathy probably not seen on ophthalmoscopy. (Courtesy of Dr. L. Aiello.)

H, Photograph of retina following laser therapy, showing circumscribed areas of destruction and fibrous replacement. (Courtesy of Dr. M. B. Landers, III.)

an accumulation of sorbitol and fructose in peripheral nerves, probably in the Schwann cells, as well as delayed nerve conduction velocity. Whether this pathogenic sequence explains most instances of diabetic neuropathy is debatable, because the neuropathy occurs with almost equal frequency in diabetics without fasting hyperglycemia, particularly in older people; hence the biochemical basis remains conjectural. A deficiency of another glucose-related product, myoinositol, has also been suggested as related to the neuropathy. The similar findings in elderly subjects without diabetes suggest that the peripheral neuropathy is part of the accelerated senescence of the diabetic as manifested in the nervous system. Occasionally patients with marked hyperglycemia, peripheral pain, and delayed nerve conduction lose their symptoms and signs with reduction of glucose concentration, and this acute diabetic "neuropathy" is more probably related to the direct metabolic disorder of sorbitol and fructose accumulation.

The diabetic neuropathy may progress to total sensory anesthesia, and, as occurs to the hip and knee in syphilis with tabes, the safeguards of the normal foot to protect its structure by afferent signals is lost, and chronic trauma to the joints leads to destruction, the so-called "*Charcot joint.*" Loss of position sense also leads to *ataxia*, the *pseudotabes of diabetes.* Likewise a callus may act as a foreign body, repeatedly injuring the anesthetized foot, leading to ulcer and infection, the "*neuropathic*" *ulcer.* Worse yet, the anesthesia of the foot prevents the patient from recognizing not only the aforementioned problem but also true foreign bodies such as thumb tacks. Daily inspection of the foot, careful and professional management of calluses and bunions, and properly fitted shoes are mandatory to prevent infection, ulcer, and subsequent amputation.

A peculiar syndrome, *diabetic amyotrophy*, usually occurring in middle-aged or older males, involves the anterior thigh muscles, frequently with pain; this may be due to some metabolic aberration at the nerve terminal. Like other mononeuropathy, it may persist without remission, but usually clears in 12 to 24 months.

The *autonomic nervous system* is also affected in the neurologic sequelae, involving both sympathetic and parasympathetic pathways, In the circulatory system this may be manifested as *orthostatic hypotension* caused by involvement of the afferent and efferent autonomic nerves. Decreased angiotensin production resulting from involvement of renal renin production may also contribute to the problem. *Decreased sweating* is also a common observation, although rarely *hyperhidrosis* may occur. *Impotence* in diabetic males is extremely frequent, again resulting from autonomic involvement; retrograde ejaculation is not uncommon. The gastrointestinal system is frequently affected, as evidenced by *delayed gastric emptying* (diabetic gastropathy), with nausea, anorexia, vomiting, and marked weight loss, not unlike that seen in a patient with mental depression or with gastrointestinal malignancy. The bowel itself, both small and large, may be involved, the former leading to a *malabsorption*-like syndrome and the latter to a distressing *diarrhea,* usually nocturnal, or, conversely, to *constipation* and occasionally *megacolon.* Also involved in the autonomic neuropathy is the *bladder,* leading to asymptomatic distention, occasionally with several liters of residual urine. This can be detected by enlargement of the lower abdomen and around-the-clock urination of small overflow volumes.

Obviously, the predilection to urinary tract infection is marked in these subjects. Catheterization, unless essential, is contraindicated.

The treatment of all these disorders is depressingly nonspecific, namely better control of the diabetes. Paradoxically, many patients with peripheral neuropathy who are then placed into better carbohydrate-insulin homeostasis have a worsening of the neuropathy, possibly owing to transient improvement in the afferent nerves. In the specific problems, treatment is at best supportive. The patient with bladder involvement may need chronic catheterization or else genitourinary surgery to revise the outflow tract for better bladder decompression. Various cholinergic agents may be of help to the bladder dysfunction and also for the gastropathy. Occasionally antimicrobial drugs as well as anticholinergics may be palliative to the bowel disorder when diarrhea is severe.

The predisposition of the diabetic to *central nervous system vascular accident*, owing to the accelerated atherosclerosis, has already been mentioned. Of much interest, however, and not correlated with the vascular disease but purportedly associated with peripheral neuropathy is the frequent elevation of cerebrospinal fluid protein, occasionally to levels of 200 to 400 mg per 100 ml. In some patients the protein may be elevated without the neuropathy, and in others neuropathy may be present without the protein. Cellular elements, however, are low to absent, ruling out an infectious or other inflammatory process.

Skin. Dermatologic manifestations of diabetes result from the microvascular and macrovascular abnormalities, from the diabetic's predisposition to infection, and from the secondary lipid disorders in blood.

Necrobiosis lipoidica diabeticorum is a rare but dramatic skin condition, found more frequently in females than in males, which may even antedate the other clinical signs and symptoms of diabetes. Although usually in the pretibial area, it may appear elsewhere, particularly on the dorsum of the foot. The mature lesion is a clearly demarcated painless area of atrophic skin, usually deeply pigmented with small telangiectases about the border. Frequently it follows trauma to the area, but many times its appearance is unprovoked. The lesions, which start as red raised papules that coalesce and expand, may remain stationary or even regress without relation to other problems the patient may have. Many diabetics, particularly those of long standing, have a waxy hue of the skin, and small freckle-like brown spots are frequently seen over the lower extremities. Both these and the necrobiosis are probably due to a microangiopathy similar to that in the renal glomerulus and retinal capillary, although an autoimmune mechanism has also been suggested for the necrobiosis.

Macrovascular disease, or atherosclerosis, often involves the skin in the form of *gangrene* secondary to ischemia. Most commonly one or more toes are affected, but occasionally the entire foot or lower limb may be involved. Rarely the fingers or localized areas of skin anywhere on the body may be affected, probably secondary to occlusion of a small artery, the collaterals have been previously compromised by the same process.

Skin infections are extremely frequent, particularly if the patient is in poor control. The usual staphylococcal and streptococcal infections occur much more frequently than in nondiabetics and may lead to rapid and massive destruction unless antimicrobials are administered and the diabetes is brought under better control. Rectal abscesses, furunculosis, hidradenitis, cellulitis, and intertriginous infections caused by fungi such as dermatophytosis of the feet are all more frequent in the diabetic. Obviously, ischemic areas, especially the feet, are exquisitely susceptible to infection.

Xanthoma diabeticorum (eruptive xanthomatosis): A small percentage of uncontrolled diabetics have a marked elevation in circulating lipids. When triglycerides are chronically elevated, they accumulate not only in macrophages in liver and spleen but also as collections in the skin; these appear as clusters of raised papules, usually on a red base with a pale yellow center, and are referred to as eruptive xanthoma. Most often they are found over the buttocks and extremities, but they may appear anywhere. Diagnosis is made by finding the lipemia in the retinal vessels or by the turbidity or frank creaminess of the serum, and classification is made by electrophoresis into Type I (hyperchylomicronemia), IIb (mixed hypercholesterolemia and hyperchylomicronemia), IV (endogenous hypertriglyceridemia), or V (hyperchylomicronemia and endogenous hypertriglyceridemia) hyperlipidemias. If the diabetes is secondary to Type IV, standard diabetic treatment is indicated with restriction of dietary carbohydrates and, most important if the patient is overweight, a hypocaloric diet. Types IIb, IV, and V are also frequently associated with diabetes, and the hyperlipidemia and diabetes are treated according to the type and severity of each.

Atherosclerosis. Diabetes in all ages is associated with accelerated atherosclerosis. *Coronary insufficiency* in the premenopausal female is twenty times more common than that in the nondiabetic female. A *myocardial infarction* in a male under 40 is almost always associated with either diabetes or a familial lipid disorder. Fifty per cent of all diabetics die prematurely of myocardial infarction. In a diabetic with a myocardial infarction, five-year survival is limited to 30 per cent, whereas 60 per cent of a nondiabetic population would survive this period. *Peripheral arteries* are more severely affected, and gangrene of the feet caused by ischemia is 70-fold more frequent in diabetics. Many explanations have been offered for this accelerated atherosclerosis; one of these implicates defective lipoprotein metabolism. Approximately one fifth of all diabetics have an elevated circulating triglyceride level, mainly in the pre-beta region (endogenous hypertriglyceridemia), and these are diagnosed as Type IV hyperlipoproteinemics. Conversely, over 90 per cent of subjects with Type IV hyperlipoproteinemia have overt diabetes or glucose intolerance. Other lipid disorders, particularly Types IIb, III, and V, have an increased prevalence of diabetes (see Ch. 532.7). However, for the minimal or absent demonstrable circulating lipid abnormality present in most diabetics, their premature atherosclerosis is far out of proportion, unless the recently demonstrated reduction in circulating high density lipoprotein (HDL) in diabetic subjects when inadequately controlled or even in the maturity-onset diabetic with minimal hyperglycemia after meals should play an important role in the atherogenic process. Direct cholesterol synthesis in the vessels has been indicated, as has the basement membrane defect, leading to a microangiopathy of the vasa vasorum and then to atherosclerosis. As in the nondiabetic population, the pathogenic sequence is not clear. Low levels of HDL (high density lipoprotein), which has been associated with atherosclerosis in the nondiabetic population (see Ch. 532.7), are found in poorly controlled diabetics and can be brought back to within the normal range by appropriate diabetic therapy. In addition, a number of platelet abnormalities have also been found in the hyperglycemic diabetic, and, like the levels of HDL, are returned to normal with amelioration of the insulin deficiency and its subsequent abnormal metabolism toward normal.

Treatment poses a quandary, because most diabetic diets are restricted in carbohydrate, calling for a high fat intake which may contribute to the atherosclerosis. A compromise is usually suggested with a diet containing one half the calories as fat, but polyunsaturated in nature. For the specific dyslipidemias, clofibrate or nicotinic acid is used, as is cholestyramine. Interestingly, the waxy exudates in the retinal fundus have been significantly decreased with clofibrate therapy, but visual improvement has not been documented. Most important, the synergistic effect of smoking in augmenting vascular disorders with the diabetic predisposition makes *smoking abstinence* a most important part of therapy in any diabetic. Finally, although there is evidence that optimal diabetic control may mitigate the microvascular complications of diabetes, there is little evidence of any effect of control on the accelerated atherosclerosis, suggesting that this predisposition may be an inherent abnormality closely related to the inheritance of the diabetes itself but independent of the abnormality in insulin-glucose homeostasis.

Infection. At any stage of diabetes, infection is both a diagnostic indicator and a major threat. The reasons are manifold, including a decrease in macrophage mobility, a decrease in the potential of macrophages to phagocytose infectious particles, and the relative substrate richness of hyperglycemia itself for microorganisms. Added to these factors is decreased vascularity, particularly in the lower extremity, which makes infection an even greater threat. Noninvasive organisms, such as various fungi, find the diabetic a unique organism in which to flourish, similar to the patient with immunodeficiency caused by hereditary or acquired disorders. The diabetic is predisposed not only to soft tissue infection such as furunculosis, gingival abscess, or perinephric abscess, but also to meningitis, osteomyelitis, and many others. *Mucormycosis* occurs almost uniquely in the uncontrolled or ketoacidotic diabetic and is evidenced by a rapid invasive and destructive infection of the orbit or nasal sinuses eroding directly into major vessels, into the eye itself, and even into brain substance.

LIPOATROPHIC DIABETES. Patients with this relatively rare syndrome have a peculiar form of diabetes with minimal to absent ketoacidosis, marked resistance to insulin, hypermetabolism, and either congenital or acquired absence of grossly demonstrable adipose tissue. Other prominent features may include marked hyperlipidemia and hepatomegaly, leading to cirrhosis and occasionally to esophageal varices. There are frequently increased musculature, acanthosis nigricans, phlebomegaly, curly hair, thickened skin, and other peculiar anomalies such as cystic angiomatous lesions in bones, genital enlargement, and polycystic ovaries. How these diverse features (Lawrence's syndrome or the *Lawrence-Seip syndrome*) are genetically or metabolically interconnected is obscure. Treatment is symptomatic, and the marked insulin resistance usually makes insulin therapy ineffectual; however, most patients adapt to their marked polydipsia, polyuria, and glucosuria. Histologic examination may demonstrate a diminished number of scattered small adipose cells with minimal lipid. In the congenital variety the paucity of adipose tissue is evident at birth or soon thereafter, but the diabetes and other sequelae may not appear until several years later. In the later or acquired form, the adipose tissue may gradually atrophy through childhood, and again the diabetes occurs several years later. Both forms appear to be inherited as autosomal recessive traits. Hypotheses for this peculiar disorder include a lack of cellular receptors for insulin, a lack of intracellular effects of the insulin response itself, or possibly one or more factors produced in excess by the hypothalamus or pituitary which inhibit insulin's metabolic effects. (See Ch. 539.5.)

SECONDARY DIABETES. Hemochromatosis. Hemochromatosis is a hereditary disease resulting from iron deposition in various tissues such as liver, skin, and pituitary, and including the endocrine pancreas (see Ch. 489). Treatment is directed to the hemochromatosis by iron depletion through phlebotomy or chemotherapy or both, and to the diabetes by standard insulin replacement and diet therapy, depending on the severity of the diabetes. Many patients require more insulin than might be expected from simple destruction of beta cells, and this relative insulin resistance may result from the accompanying liver disease.

Pancreatitis. The endocrine pancreas is also involved in the destruction and scarring that occur with acute and chronic pancreatitis. Thus diabetes occuring with episodic abdominal pain, periumbilical and boring through to the back, particularly in the alcoholic, and associated with elevations of circulating or urinary amylase, makes pancreatitis probable. Treatment of the diabetes is again as indicated by the severity of the disturbed carbohydrate homeostasis; with extensive destruction of the pancreas, total insulin replacement with split doses (two doses daily) of intermediate (with or without rapid-acting insulin) is indicated. The malabsorption resulting fom exocrine deficiency may require oral pancreatic enzyme therapy. In patients with surgical removal of the pancreas because of tumor or, occasionally, pancreatic replacement by tumor or infection, therapy is similar to that for the patient pancreatectomized because of pancreatitis. Many patients in acute diabetic ketoacidosis may have transient elevations of amylase, possibly caused by mild pancreatitis associated with the acute metabolic decompensation, but residual pancreatic exocrine insufficiency is not observed.

Stress Diabetes. During severe stress, sufficient to increase circulating catecholamines and to activate sympathetic innervation of the endocrine pancrease, insulin release is suppressed and glucagon release provoked. The stress-induced hyperglycemia resulting from hepatic glycogenolysis serves to provide emergency fuel for anaerobic metabolism in muscle or in reparative tissue after trauma, without insulin promoting glycogen or fat synthesis from the glucose. Thus there is a true functional diabetes in severe trauma, septicemia, peritonitis, pneumonia, burns, stroke, and myocardial infarction, to name a few. Of course, if the patient had been a mild diabetic previously, the carbohydrate abnormality would be more marked or more easily unmasked. If parenteral glucose is administered, the hyperglycemia resulting from the absolute or relative lack of insulin may become extreme and the patient may progress into hyperglycemic hyperosmolar coma. These patients may have no evidence of diabetes before or after this episode. Should the hyperglycemia be greater than 400 mg per 100 ml, transient insulin therapy is advisable to prevent excess osmolarity. With

lesser degrees of injury, or even with the physical incapacity associated with milder diseases, less severe depression of insulin release may occur, resulting in diabetic glucose tolerance; hence, for diabetes the diagnostic tolerance tests should not be performed until the patient is in good health with adequate nutrition and physical activity.

Acromegaly. Growth hormone administration provokes insulin resistance, and, likewise, excess endogenous growth hormone secretion requires a high concentraion of insulin to maintain glucose homeostasis. In some series, 20 to 50 per cent of patients with acromegaly have been found to have either frank diabetes or glucose intolerance. In all patients there is a decreased sensitivity to administered insulin, as evidenced by a markedly decreased hypoglycemic effect of 0.1 unit of insulin per kilogram of body weight given intravenously. Before growth hormone immunoassays became available, diagnosis was made on clinical grounds and on the findings of enlargement of the sella turcica, elevated serum phosphate, and insulin resistance. Now any patient with suggestive acromegaloid features or evidence of postpubertal growth of extremities and jaw, thickening and coarsening of facial features and of skin, particularly fingers, increased sweating, and the many other signs or symptoms of excess growth hormone should be tested for diabetes and treated accordingly in addition to treatment for the acromegaly (see Ch. 543.7).

Cushing's Syndrome. Excess glucocorticoid, whether administered exogenously or secreted endogenously, may produce either glucose intolerance or frank clinical diabetes in one of five adults. Although there is a slight resistance to the metabolic effects of insulin, the glucose intolerance appears also to be related to increased gluconeogenesis and perhaps to a decrease in beta cell capacity to release insulin. Fajans and Conn have administered small doses of glucocorticoid followed by a glucose tolerance test the next morning as a test for latent diabetes, especially in subjects with strong family histories of diabetes.

Any diabetic, particularly one with early features suggestive of the rounded moon facies, buffalo hump, and truncal obesity, with abdominal striae, osteoporosis, hypertension, or psychosis, must be studied for adrenal hyperactivity. But the clinical challenge is in the less overt or earlier form of the syndrome, and this possibly should always be considered in any newly diagnosed diabetic (see Ch. 547.7). Again, the diabetes is treated according to its signs and symptoms, until the primary cause of the excess glucocorticoid is corrected. It is believed that most of these patients who require insulin have independent diabetes mellitus that has been aggravated by the excess glucocorticoid.

Other Endocrine and Metabolic Disorders. *Pheochromocytoma* is frequently associated with diabetes mellitus because of the suppression of insulin release from beta cells as well as the capacity for adrenal catechols to provoke hepatic glycogen breakdown and peripheral inhibition of glucose uptake. As in patients with major trauma and high levels of catecholamines, this type of diabetes probably may occur in an individual without inherent diabetes, never to return after removal of the tumor. *Thyrotoxicosis*, on the other hand, appears to be able to unmask latent diabetes mellitus, but its direct effect on carbohydrate metabolism is minimal and is possibly related to the relative starvation of the hypermetabolic patient. Also, accelerated gastric emptying and absorption may cause marked hyperglycemia early in an oral glucose tolerance test, similar to that seen in an individual with gastric resection. Other endocrinopathies that are diabetogenic include pregnancy (to be discussed) and the simulated pregnancy found in patients receiving exogenous estrogen. Many latent diabetics can be made overt if given *oral contraceptive agents,* and the estrogen moiety appears more diabetogenic than the progestin. The hypokalemia of *hyperaldosteronism* or during *diuretic therapy* diminishes insulin release from the pancreas and may contribute to diabetes or carbohydrate intolerance. Another factor leading to glucose intolerance is hyperlipidemia, but again many of these patients probably have independent diabetes, and the pathophysiologic relationship is obscure.

Finally, a large number of metabolic and endocrine disorders are associated with a higher incidence of diabetes than one might expect from the general population. These include the Prader-Willi syndrome, sexual ateliotic dwarfism, Schmidt's syndrome, Werner's syndrome, Refsum's syndrome, Friedreich's ataxia, optic atrophy and nerve deafness, Turner's syndrome, and many others. One wonders why the incidence of diabetes is so high in almost all chromosomal aberrations and inborn errors of metabolism. No clear answer is apparent.

TREATMENT. The specific treatment of diabetes depends upon the signs and symptoms of the individual patient presenting with the disease and can be subdivided accordingly. Since the spectrum has at one end fulminant ketoacidosis, which can result in death in coma within several days in the previously well-controlled subject omitting insulin (or in 24 to 48 hours in the child), and at the other end only a slightly abnormal glucose tolerance, the therapy is likewise varied. There is really no fixed regimen for any single patient, even one in ketoacidosis, so only general guidelines will be discussed.

In the terminal ketoacidotic patient in coma, the thready pulse, decreasing blood pressure, rapidly falling arterial pH, and rising P_{CO_2} (signifying inability to achieve compensation of the acidosis by hyperventilation) portend irreversible shock and death, and rapid heroic treatment is mandatory to reverse the fatal outcome. On the other hand, many patients will walk in with mild ketoacidosis, feeling poorly, without nausea or vomiting, but with a glucose level of 500 mg per 100 ml or higher and a total HCO_3^- of 4 to 16 mEq per liter. A liter or two of saline plus 20 to 30 units of crystalline insulin intravenously or intramuscularly may be all that is necessary, as evidenced by correction of the metabolic disorder. This may be followed by the standard insulin dose eight to twelve hours later or, if these patients were not previously on insulin, by a small dose of intermediate-acting insulin (about 20 units) in order to initiate their standard replacement regimen.

The less severe type of diabetic, presenting with polydipsia and polyuria or with any of the sequelae, such as pruritus vulvae, may be handled by diet alone, particularly if over 30 to 40 years of age and overweight. By diet is meant a low calorie, carbohydrate-restricted regimen distributed among meals to avoid excessively large meals at any one time. Should this regimen not be effective in controlling hyperglycemia after one to two months' trial, insulin or one of the oral antidiabetic medications may be indicated in addition to the diet. If insulin is used, it is usually given as a single dose of one of the intermediate types, either NPH or lente, one half hour before breakfast, in order to supplement the endogenously produced insulin. The philosophy, of course, is the reciprocal of the normal physiology wherein the beta cells release insulin proportional to the composition and size of the ingested meal; in the diabetic, the meals are proportioned to match the rate of absorption of the injected intermediate-acting insulin (e.g., a smaller breakfast, a moderate-sized lunch, a mid-afternoon snack, a moderate-sized supper, and a small bedtime snack). Should a larger breakfast be desired, some crystalline insulin may be mixed with the intermediate insulin.

Since ketoacidosis is the most dramatic and life-threatening event, its treatment will be discussed first in greater detail.

Diabetic Ketoacidosis. As in most acute, life-threatening crises, the primary concern is lack of effective circulating volume. The marked hyperglycemia leads to marked glycosuria and an osmotic "washout" of water and electrolyte, mainly sodium and chloride. In addition, as a result of the elevated circulating levels of ketoacids, which are relatively poorly reabsorbed by the renal tubule from the glomerular filtrate, these relatively strong organic acids with pK's below 4 appear in the urine and are coupled with excretion of sodium, potassium, and ammonium, leading to further volume depletion. The ketoacidosis also leads to systemic acidosis, which, in itself, depresses cardiac contractility, as well as the capacity of arterioles to respond to catecholamines, both the circulating epinephrine and the norepinephrine released locally from sympathetic nerve endings. Thus, the thready pulse, hypotension, and poor organ perfusion reflects both hypovolemia and poor physiologic compensation to the decreased volume, the two processes enhancing each other's threat to survival.

Therapy first involves correct diagnosis; the history of polydipsia and polyuria in a patient with marked hyperglycemia and glycosuria together with the demonstration of excess ketoacid in plasma establishes the diagnosis. Usually the patient has omitted insulin because of intercurrent illness, with the mistaken thought that insulin is unnecessary if food is not eaten. Other explanations include the insulin resistance associated with infection or the first trimester of pregnancy, or even emotional stress. In the previously undiagnosed diabetic, the typical history may also include severe abdominal pain, frequently with a rigid, tender abdomen. The marked leukocytosis with immature granulocytes in the blood smear may make an acute surgical abdomen a reasonable diagnosis until the hyperglycemia, glycosuria, ketonemia, and ketonuria provide the correct cause.

In simplest terms, a large indwelling needle is inserted in a vein of the suspect patient, blood is drawn and checked for hyperglycemia by either an approximate bedside procedure. (Testape or Reflectometer) or rapid automatic glucose determination, using glucose oxidase, and plasma or serum ketosis is assessed by a drop placed on one of several commercial preparations (e.g., Acetest, Ketotest, Ketostix). If hyperglycemia and marked ketosis are present, the diagnosis is immediately confirmed and therapy initiated.

The original needle inserted is obviously left in place after drawing the blood, and isotonic saline is run in at a rapid pace, because volume deficit is usually severe. If the patient is critically ill with marked hypotension and barely detectable peripheral pulse, plasma expanders such as plasma itself, albumin, or synthetic colloids can be given in order to improve the circulating hypovolemia. In this case, drawing of arterial gases and pH is mandatory; if the pH is below 7.1, sodium bicarbonate, 1 ampule (44 mEq), should be added to each liter of isotonic saline to help correct myocardial contractility as well as to improve vascular tone. With documentation of the hyperglycemia and the marked increase in ketone bodies, insulin should be given. For many years, large amounts, such as 100 to 200 units, were given initially. This has now been decreased by most physicians, and some have reported what they regard as improved results by giving 5 to 10 units per hour by continuous intravenous infusion or by giving 10 to 20 units hourly intramuscularly during the first hours of treatment. For the present the writer prefers to follow the philosophy that early vigorous reversal of the pathogenic sequence is indicated to spare life, and, once the progression of the metabolic lesion has been reversed, to proceed more slowly in making the final corrections in volume deficit and electrolytes. Thus an initial bolus of 20 units of regular insulin given intravenously or intramuscularly is suggested, with smaller amounts given subsequently on an hourly basis (if needed) according to the blood glucose response. Of importance is the urinary loss of potassium during the development of ketoacidosis, owing partly to the osmotic diuresis and partly to loss of potassium from cells. With volume deficit, aldosterone is also called into play, and distal tubular exchange of potassium for sodium results in an even more marked deficit in body potassium. With the metabolic acidosis there is usually hyperkalemia, approximately 5 to 6.5 mEq per liter in spite of the total body deficit. An initial serum potassium of 4 to 5 mEq per liter or, more striking, of less than 4 mEq per liter signifies severe potassium deficiency. Therefore, potassium, as the phosphate or chloride (preferably the phosphate), should be added to the infusion (40 mEq per liter), particularly after the insulin is injected, because that will accelerate potassium movement into cells, and life-threatening hypokalemia can ensue. Usually potassum administration can be withheld until glucose levels are shown to fall. If bicarbonate is administered because of severe acidosis and hypotension, the fall in potassium may be accentuated and replacement should be more vigorous.

Three or 4 liters of isotonic saline, with bicarbonate in the severely acidotic patient or with potassium in the patient predisposed to hypokalemia, may be given in the first two or three hours of therapy. If there is gastric atony with emesis of a black and frequently benzidine-positive fluid, gastric aspiration helps to return gastric compensation as well as lessening the risk of aspiration pneumonia. These patients may have a demonstrable succussion splash before decompression.

Except in very severe cases, when one may wish to monitor renal perfusion, urinary catheterization is contraindicated. The hyperosmolarity induced by the hyperglycemia exerts a protective effect on the kidney, and acute tubular necrosis after severe diabetic ketoacidosis is extremely rare. Electrocardiographic tracings help monitor the physiologic effects of the potassium levels.

Of prime importance is close observation of the patient, together with the compilation of a detailed bedside flowsheet of all events: insulin administered, chemistries, pulse, blood pressure, and so forth. If blood glucose levels do not fall after the initial insulin injection, the infrequent but serious problem of insulin resistance may be present, requiring intravenous or subcutaneous injection of hundreds to thousands of units. This need to follow the

glucose levels is one of the contraindications to giving exogenous glucose in the initial intravenous therapy until a significant insulin effect is observed, as evidenced by a definite fall in glucose concentration.

Although it appears more logical initially to administer hypotonic saline, since the patient has lost more water than electrolyte, isotonic saline provides a better defense for the maintenance of extracellular fluid volume. As glucose levels fall, thanks to insulin exerting its physiologic effects, the extracellular osmolarity falls and fluid tends to move into cells, decreasing, thereby, extracellular fluid volume; hence the preference for giving isotonic instead of hypotonic solutions initially. Also, the shift of water from the extracellular fluid into cells is shared by the central nervous system, leading tragically, but fortunately rarely, to cerebral edema and death. Hence, again, the principle in the treatment of diabetic ketoacidosis is to initiate treatment rapidly, in order to reverse the process and to correct circulatory fluid volume. Once the patient has begun to improve, the management can proceed more conservatively.

Should bicarbonate and potassium salts be added to the infusate, 0.45 per cent sodium chloride can be used in the basic fluid in order to avoid overly hypertonic solutions.

As blood glucose levels fall, if potassium was not administered initially, it should be added subsequently, 1 ampule per liter (40 mEq) of solution, preferably as the phosphate salt. When the blood glucose level approaches the renal threshold of 180 to 200 mg per 100 ml, glucose as 5 per cent D/W or 2.5 per cent dextrose with 0.45 per cent sodium chloride can be infused in order to prevent hypoglycemia. The patient is returned to long-acting insulin therapy once the threat of hypoglycemia has passed.

Should the initial insulin therapy be ineffective as evidenced by a failure to reduce blood glucose levels in the first or second hour, a second injection must be given, and this is usually twice the first, unless the patient's condition has deteriorated markedly, in which case much larger doses should be given as well as alkali, volume expanders, and all other maneuvers used in the treatment of the patient in shock. If, however, the glucose level is decreased, for example, falling from 600 to 300 mg per 100 ml, a second insulin injection need not be given unless the progressive fall later ceases or glucose levels begin to increase, in which case a small second injection of insulin can be given, perhaps one quarter to one half the initial dose. Thus continuous monitoring and charting of blood glucose concentrations, first at hourly intervals and later at two-hour intervals, are essential. The availability of rapid bedside glucose techniques such as the glucose-oxidase analyzer has greatly simplified this task.

The precipitating event leading to ketoacidosis should always be kept in mind. Usually it is lack of understanding owing to poor education, the patient having omitted insulin when slightly ill from an upper respiratory infection or a gastrointestinal disturbance, believing that the decreased food intake obviated the need for daily insulin. Frequently, an unrecognized infection may provoke sufficient insulin resistance to tip the patient into ketoacidosis. Thus appendicitis, pyelonephritis, meningitis, and other disorders should be considered. The marked leukocytosis with immature forms associated with diabetic ketoacidosis makes exclusion of infection all the more difficult.

Alcohol is metabolized in liver to acetate which is then released for further metabolism by peripheral tissues. Thus alcohol compounds the rate of hepatic acetate production during fasting, particularly in the insulin-deficient diabetic, and severe ketoacidosis may occur with varying degrees of hyperglycemia. In the previously fasting nondiabetic, an alcoholic debauch may even provoke severe ketoacidosis with normal or low blood glucose levels. Thus a careful history is indicated, and in such a subject with severe ketoacidosis, glucose as well as electrolyte may be indicated in the initial therapy.

Hyperosmolar Coma. Coma, usually occurring in an elderly patient, with hyperglycemia caused by dehydration, prerenal azotemia, and marked but not total insulin deficiency, can mimic that of the subject in ketoacidosis. However, the Kussmaul respirations of severe acidosis and the smell of acetone are lacking owing to the low or absent ketonemia. On the other hand, if there are hyperventilation, a low pH, and low bicarbonate without demonstrable ketoacidosis, *lactic acidosis* is a probable diagnosis. The patient in hyperosmolar coma is treated like the patient in diabetic ketoacidosis with an indwelling large needle in a peripheral vein through which isotonic saline is administered rapidly. The usual insulin resistance of ketoacidosis may be absent; if the hyperglycemia is in the range of 500 to 1000 mg per 100 ml or even higher, only 10 units of insulin need be first given intravenously. In these subjects, the requirement for isotonic as opposed to hypotonic fluid replacement is even more strongly indicated, because reduction of glucose levels markedly decreases extracellular osmoles and fluid entry into tissues will markedly compromise extracellular fluid volume as well as producing intracellular fluid overload, especially in the brain. Hence *hypotonic solutions should not be administered* until the patient's circulatory volume is stabilized, and then only slowly and judiciously. Also, as in ketoacidosis, the primary reason for the decompensation should be considered. Bronchopneumonia, myocardial infarction, and local or generalized infections are all included in the differential diagnosis. Again, with the decrease in glucose levels as treatment continues, potassium moves into cells and parenteral potassium replacement may be required. The needed amounts are usually far less than in ketoacidosis, but the same precaution, close observation with frequent monitoring such as precordial electrocardiographic tracings and serum electrolyte levels, is indicated.

Nonketotic or Nonhyperosmolar Patient. In the diabetic with marked fasting and postprandial hyperglycemia, the urgency of the aforementioned two syndromes is not present. In the young individual, particularly under age 20, with polyuria, thirst, and fasting hyperglycemia, insulin therapy is indicated, because deficiency of the hormone, although not as severe as in the patient with ketoacidosis, will eventually be complete or nearly complete. In an adolescent, 20 units of intermediate-duration insulin (lente or NPH) given each morning is a good start, followed by the adjustment of diet and insulin treatment based on urine and blood glucose levels. Since endogenous insulin secretion is moderately compromised, the diet is made to match the rate of insulin absorption within some structure as dictated by social convenience. Many manuals and texts published by the American Diabetes Association and various hospitals and clinics describe this in further detail and should be consulted for specifics. For a more detailed discussion of the diabetic diet, see Ch. 476.4. The patient is taught to test urine for glucose levels and to alter insulin and diet accordingly. If a larger breakfast is desired, or if the present insulin regimen does not cover the breakfast, regular or clear insulin can be added to the intermediate-duration insulin. Likewise, if there is

TABLE 2. Insulin in Clinical Usage*

	Peak Effect (Hours)	Duration of Effect (Hours)
Regular or crystalline	2–3	6–8
Semilente	3–6	10–14
NPH	6–10	16–24
Lente	6–10	16–24
Ultralente	10–16	36+
PZI (protamine zinc insulin)	10–16	36+

*Insulin preparations in the United States and their duration of action. They were formerly available in 40, 80, and 100 units per milliliter, termed U40, U80, and U100 respectively. Standard and disposable syringes calibrated accordingly were also available. The use of the two lower doses is being phased out in view of the simplicity of use of U100. Also available are U500 and U5000 for the rare patient with marked insulin resistance.

glycosuria at bedtime, a short-acting insulin can be given before supper. Since the peak action of intermediate insulin is in the mid-afternoon, hypoglycemia at that time necessitates reduction of the dose (making sure the patient is not omitting the mid-afternoon snack). Conversely, late afternoon hyperglycemia necessitates increasing the morning dose of intermediate-duration insulin. Careful daily records should be kept by the patient of his urine sugar tests as well as hypoglycemic reactions, even if minimal.

If the patient does well through the day but has early morning hyperglycemia and glycosuria, a small injection of intermediate insulin may be necessary before supper or bedtime to carry through the night. This is usually not necessary in the juvenile diabetic in the first years of the disease, thanks to the small endogenous production of insulin. However, after about five years of disease all beta cell function has usually ceased, and the "split" dose of insulin, one in the morning and the other before supper, becomes the rule. In many juvenile-type patients, even the "split" dose with a most careful adherence to diet cannot adequately control the diabetes, and mild hyperglycemia is the compromise to prevent excessive hypoglycemic reactions. In these, occasional collection of a 24-hour urine with quantification of glucose may give an index of overall control, with the hope that excretion is less than 5 to 10 per cent of dietary carbohydrate intake.

In the patient over 20 with marked fasting hyperglycemia, if not overweight but with minimal or mild ketosis, insulin therapy will also probably be necessary. If the patient is overweight, however, the insulin resistance of obesity calls for a trial of rigid dietary restriction and weight reduction, keeping close observation that he does not go into ketoacidosis. Rarely, a fat child without ketosis may fall in this group. Not infrequently, with weight loss, endogenous insulin becomes sufficient to maintain glucose homeostasis for at least several years, occasionally permanently. Too often, unfortunately, weight loss may be minimal because of failure to adhere to a calorically restricted diet; insulin or sulfonylurea therapy is then indicated. The insulin is usually given as a single injection of intermediate acting (NPH or lente) one half hour before breakfast and regulated according to urine and blood tests. Because urine glucose may represent hyperglycemia many hours previously, patients are usually advised to empty the bladder one half hour before the anticipated time of testing, to drink water, and then to void again — the "double-voided" urine specimen.

TABLE 3. Oral Agents

Sulfonylureas	Dosage	Duration of Effect (Hours)
Tolbutamide (Orinase)	0.5–3 grams/day	6–12
Acetohexamide (Dymelor)	0.25–1.5 grams/day	12–24
Chlorpropamide (Diabinese)	0.1–0.5 gram/day	24–48
Tolazamide (Tolinase)	0.1–0.75 gram/day	12–24
Glyburide (Micronase, Diabeta)*	5–35 mg/day	12–24

Biguanides	Dosage	Duration of Effect (Hours)
Phenformin (Meltrol, DBI)†	25–200 mg/day	4–6
Phenformin (Meltrol-50, DBI-TD)†	50–200 mg/day	8–14

*Investigational drug.

†Available only as investigational drug. Removed from market in October 1977 by FDA. Use is restricted to specific, clearly defined situations and requires registration and reporting to FDA.

Oral Hypoglycemic Agents. Although weight reduction by caloric restriction is the ideal approach to the middle-aged overweight diabetic subject, it is almost universally unsuccessful. Thus in these patients, as well as in nonoverweight subjects with maturity-onset type diabetes, addition of the oral hypoglycemic agents is indicated should hyperglycemia persist, although, as discussed below, some controversy exists among experts in the field as to their value and contraindications.

Table 3 lists the oral agents available in the United States. Those of the sulfonylurea type acutely increase insulin release from beta cells in man and in experimental preparations, and their chronic effect is allegedly through this same mechanism, but non-beta-cell effects have also been described, such as inhibition of hepatic glucose output. They differ from each other by their potencies, duration of action, and mechanism of elimination. Tolbutamide, the drug most commonly used, has a relatively shorter duration of action, and its lesser potency requires larger doses to be given as indicated in Table 3. Usually the patient is started on 1 to 2 grams per day, half in the morning and the other half in the evening. Tolbutamide is primarily metabolized to inert products by the liver and then excreted. Should its action not be reflected in lowered glucose levels, a larger dose (3 grams) can be given or else one of the other more potent and longer-acting agents. Acetohexamide is also metabolized by the liver, but its principal product retains hypoglycemic activity. Chlorpropamide, on the other hand, is excreted unchanged by the kidneys and is obviously contraindicated in renal insufficiency. Extremely infrequently these drugs cause skin rashes or other allergic manifestations; an even more rare but serious problem has been protracted hypoglycemia, particularly in elderly individuals, usually from the more potent, long-acting sulfonylureas. Other pharmacologic agents, such as anticoagulants and salicylates, compete with hepatic removal of the sulfonylurea (except chlorpropamide), and drug-drug interactions must always be considered when they are used. If the patient's abnormal glucose tolerance is successfully corrected toward normal or—more easily determined—a one- or two-hour postprandial glucose is less than 160 or 120 mg per 100 ml, respectively, the drug may be continued and later reduced in dosage or perhaps, after a year or so, terminated with the patient observed at quarterly or so intervals to see if glucose intolerance returns.

In a large multicenter study, the University Group Diabetes Project, sponsored by the National Institutes of Health and performed through the 1960's, it was demonstrated that middle-aged subjects on a fixed dose of one of the sulfonylureas, tolbutamide, although showing a small but significant lowering of blood glucose levels, had an increased incidence of sudden death, presumably resulting from myocardial infarction or arrhythmia. This study has limited the indiscriminate use of sulfonylureas, and has placed further emphasis on diet as the primary approach to the maturity-onset type of diabetic. Many experienced students of the disease question the significance of the study and continue to use the agents. Nevertheless, if one adheres to the hypothesis that hyperglycemia is deleterious, in that it leads to the microvascular complications, then the sulfonylureas may be indicated if their benefit outweighs the possible risk of increased myocardial instability. Certainly, in the elderly female with glycosuria, the correction of her discomfort associated with the glycosuria may far outweigh the theoretical increased risk of sudden death as found in the UGDP study. One is obviously hesitant to start older, debilitated individuals on insulin injections unless absolutely necessary, and in these the sulfonylureas may play an important role. With sulfonylurea therapy, many patients may become refractory after several years, and these "secondary failure" patients must be started on insulin therapy.

The biguanides, of which only one, phenformin, was available for general use in the United States, apparently work independently of beta cell insulin release and thus can be used independently of or supplementary to the sulfonylureas. Their mode of action is not yet known, although many experimental metabolic effects have been demonstrated, such as delayed glucose absorption in the gut, augmented peripheral glucose uptake, and inhibition of gluconeogenesis. A predilection to lactic acidosis in patients receiving biguanides, has been described, and these agents are thereby contraindicated in elderly individuals with congestive failure or similar debilitated states. Like the sulfonylurea tolbutamide, an increased number of sudden, supposedly cardiovascular deaths occurred in patients taking phenformin in the UGDP study. In addition, with their correlation with lactic acidosis, the Food and Drug Administration has declared the single biguanide available in the United States unsafe except for the very rare patient who for emotional or religious reasons cannot take insulin and requires a long-acting sulfonylurea plus phenformin to become less symptomatic.

In the milder diabetic with normal fasting glucose and only intermittent or absent glucose in the urine, diet may be all that is necessary. This diet involves reduction or elimination of the easily and rapidly absorbed free sugars: hence no candy, preserves, cookies, or cakes may be eaten, and calories must be distributed throughout the day. Thus a typical diabetic diet of 2200 calories may be composed of 200 to 250 grams of carbohydrate, 100 grams of protein, and the remainder as fat. Again, the standard diabetic texts and handbooks should be used for details such as caloric contents and types of foods as well as exchanges of similar types of foods to provide palatable variability in the diet.

INSULIN PROBLEMS. The most frequent complication of insulin therapy is hypoglycemia, which can generally be prevented by readjustment of insulin type or dose and of diet. A well-controlled juvenile diabetic may experience occasional mild autonomic symptoms indicating a low glucose and respond by eating some carbohydrate, and this is not felt to be deleterious. In fact it may be helpful to demonstrate that ambient glucose levels are in the physiologic range. However, unconsciousness or convulsions are strongly contraindicated, and the insulin therapy is made less stringent in order to prevent these episodes. In many juvenile diabetics, hyperglycemia, as indicated by slightly positive urine tests, may be the compromise to prevent the physiologic and certainly the social consequences of hypoglycemia.

Allergy. Since insulin is a foreign protein, many patients experience slight reddening, discomfort, and occasionally itchiness at the site of injection after the first two or three weeks. These usually disappear in several weeks or months. In rare patients, the insulin may cause generalized hives and itching, requiring antihistamines, or, if more severe, desensitization to insulin according to schedules delineated in the standard diabetes texts. When allergy to insulin occurs, the patient is re-evaluated as to whether insulin per se is mandatory, because a more restricted diet with or without sulfonylureas may suffice. In a juvenile, "ketotic type" diabetic, insulin is mandatory and desensitization must be performed. Also, as discussed under Insulin Resistance, the insulin preparation containing factors least foreign to man should be used.

Insulin Resistance. ANTIBODY-RELATED. Until 1972–73, commercially available insulin preparations contained small amounts of proinsulin and insulin with connecting peptide (C-peptide) still attached to the A or B chains, in addition to other contaminants such as insulin dimers. Thus all patients on daily insulin therapy for several weeks developed antibodies to insulin and these foreign proteins, since beef insulin and pig insulin differ from human insulin by 4 and 1 amino acids respectively. This antibody production, however, did not compromise the effectiveness of insulin except in about 1 in 1000 patients, in whom increasing amounts of insulin were necessary to saturate antibody binding sites in order to permit enough insulin to be physiologically active. By definition, patients receiving 200 units of insulin for two or more days were said to be insulin resistant. Many of these had been on and off insulin therapy on several occasions, an excellent antibody-inducing regimen. Treatment entailed use of the insulin closest in structure to man, pig insulin or pig insulin with the terminal beta-chain alanine removed, making it identical to human insulin minus the terminal beta-chain threonine. In some this decreased the daily insulin dosage, but in others with "resistance" little difference was observed.

In the early 1970's, insulin preparations without contaminants were prepared and found to be much less antigenic than those used formerly. This "single peak" insulin has induced less antibody formation, and the over-all incidence of insulin resistance on this preparation is much less. Thus patients with increasing insulin requirement should be started on "single peak" insulin (or "single component," an electrophoretically pure insulin) and, if available, with the amino acid sequence closest to that of man, namely pig.

Formerly, in those patients with insulin resistance, the insulin doses required for effective therapy frequently fluctuated. The patient might need several thousand units daily for several weeks; then because of unexplained alterations in insulin-antibody interrelationships, he might have frequent hypoglycemic reactions, with daily insulin needs being reduced to 100 or fewer units per day. This instability in management occasionally necessitated treatment with glucocorticoids to reduce antibody formation;

indeed, even immunosuppressive therapy with antimetabolites was used in certain difficult cases in which management became extremely difficult.

ANTIBODY-UNRELATED. A non-antibody-related insulin resistance is seen in many metabolic states and these have been discussed under Secondary Diabetes. Rarely, a patient without prior immunization to insulin may require 100,000 units or more of insulin to correct the metabolic disorder. These patients are frequently young females, and the precise metabolic defect is as yet unknown. It is for these rare patients that the physician must remember that preparations of U500 and U5000 are commercially available and may be lifesaving.

A very rare form of diabetes with antibody to the insulin receptors has been described, mainly in young females who demonstrate marked insulin resistance and (like the lipoatrophic diabetic) acanthosis nigricans. In some older patients with a variant of this disorder, other autoimmune phenomena may be found, such as positive tests for lupus erythematosus or rheumatoid arthritis.

OBESITY. In both laboratory animals and man, obesity is associated with a decreased metabolic response to exogenous and endogenous insulin. Decreased binding sites for insulin have been demonstrated on cell membranes from obese animals and man; Ogilvie, many years ago, found obese man to have true pancreatic hyperplasia at autopsy unless diabetes was present.

The hyperinsulinemia, both basal and postprandial, in obese man is shown in Figure 4. Since insulin degradation rates are equal in normal subjects and in the obese, the pancreas in the latter must secrete five to ten times more insulin to achieve fuel homeostasis. It is thus obvious that a deficient beta cell population is unmasked by obesity, and that, in any diabetic, obesity is a major problem. As discussed previously, the primary therapy in the obese diabetic is the hypocaloric weight-reducing diet. Many middle-aged obese diabetics may require 50 to 100 units of insulin daily, but with weight loss they may not require insulin. Only with weight loss in a given patient can the endogenous insulin secretory reserve be assessed.

SOMOGYI EFFECT. After a hypoglycemic reaction, counterregulatory processes such as increased sympathetic nerve activity and increased circulating catecholamines, glucagon, and cortisol and growth hormone (although the metabolic effects of these latter two are less than those of the first two) all induce peripheral insulin resistance as well as increasing hepatic glucose production from both glycolysis and gluconeogenesis. In addition, overzealous correction by oral intake of carbohydrate adds to the hyperglycemia. Thus as in starvation and diabetic ketoacidosis, the trend is toward hyperglycemia, and a larger than usual dose of insulin is necessary to correct the rebound. Occasionally another hypoglycemic reaction can follow and the sequence be repeated, resulting in marked metabolic swings of hyper- and hypoglycemia. This pattern has been emphasized by Somogyi, and his name is frequently applied to this diabetic instability. Therapy is to reduce the dose of the principal insulin injection and, unless already in use, to administer a second, smaller dose of intermediate-acting insulin before supper in order to "smooth out" the patient's metabolic state. In fact, a true "brittle" diabetic, one in whom glucose levels are highly unstable and unpredictable, is best treated by the "split" or double dose of insulin and occasionally might even do better on a third or, rarely, a fourth injection, judged according to premeal urine tests, the experience of the previous day or two, and anticipated meal size.

Lipoatrophy and Hypertrophy. Not infrequently, and most often in girls in their late teens, lipoatrophy is seen at sites of insulin injection. This disfiguring event, which used to occur in up to one third of all patients, is treated by rotating insulin injections to different sites; however, the new, purer insulin preparations have presumably decreased the incidence of this problem. In many cases, injection of the single peak or single component insulins has even reversed the lesion when given into the same site.

The hypertrophy that occurs at the site of insulin injection of many diabetics, more often in males than in females, is a direct result of insulin's lipogenic action on fat cells. This can also be disfiguring and usually results from repetitive injections into the same site. Treatment is rotation of injection sites, using thighs, buttocks, abdominal wall, and triceps areas as loci, so that no one site is used more than once a week, even in a patient taking two injections daily.

HYPOGLYCEMIA. Any patient on insulin and occasional patients on oral hypoglycemic agents are subject to episodes of hypoglycemia. This is usually evident first as a disturbance in cerebration, such as inability to perform addition or subtraction, or mood changes, followed by parasympathetic signs and symptoms, salivation, hunger, and increased gastric motility. There may then be sympathetic hyperactivity, with sweating, tachycardia, piloerection, and anxiety. The pattern in a given patient may vary, and between patients it varies markedly. Bizarre behavior may arouse suspicion of alcohol or drug intoxication. As hypoglycemia becomes more severe, unconsciousness and convulsions occur which, if prolonged, may lead to severe organic deficit and possibly to an irreversible decorticate or decerebrate state or death. Patient education is most important. Deliberately causing a mild hypoglycemic reaction in a newly discovered and treated diabetic may be advisable so that the patient is aware of the symptoms and signs. Treatment is by administration of carbohydrate as candy or as a sweetened beverage; however, if the patient is stuporous, oral therapy of any sort must not be given because of danger of aspiration. Instead, glucagon, 1 mg given subcutaneously or intramuscularly by a trained family member or friend, or intravenously by a physician, causes sufficient glycogenolysis to elevate glucose transiently to awaken the patient, so further carbohydrate can be given by mouth. Thus glucagon should be in every diabetic kit. Of course, if the hypoglycemia occurs in a hospital or office setting, drawing a blood sample for glucose analysis can be done to document the diagnosis, and glucose (10 to 25 grams) can be given immediately intravenously, usually as a 50 per cent solution.

Symptoms and signs of hypoglycemia may occur literally within minutes and may rapidly progress to total unconsciousness. Thus any diabetic behaving in a bizarre fashion or, particularly, unconscious should be treated as if hypoglycemic until proved otherwise. Ketoacidosis, on the other hand, takes many hours to days to develop; in contrast to hypoglycemia, the patient appears and behaves chronically ill.

Patients on sulfonylureas, particularly the longer-acting agents, may also develop a severe and prolonged hypoglycemia requiring continuous intravenous glucose therapy for as long as two or three days. These are usually elderly patients with mild diabetes or with compromised renal function. As with insulin-induced hypoglycemia, the unconsciousness may be associated with a variable neuro-logic examination, including unilateral or bilateral Babinski reflexes and hyperactive or hypoactive deep tendon reflexes, and may mimic a cerebrovascular accident. A superimposed diabetic neuropathy may make the event all the more confusing, particularly because the deep tendon reflexes in the lower extremity may be decreased to absent.

If a patient taking insulin is found to need a progressive reduction in insulin dosage because of recurrent hypoglycemic episodes, particularly if the daily insulin requirement is less than 15 to 20 units, reasons other than simple fluctuations in insulin responsiveness should be considered. An islet cell tumor, partial hypopituitarism, adrenal insufficiency, hypothyroidism, and pregnancy are all possibilities, particularly pituitary disease, thanks to the diabetic's predilection for vascular infarction secondary to generalized atherosclerosis.

PREGNANCY AND DELIVERY. In the first trimester of pregnancy, a juvenile diabetic receiving insulin frequently needs a reduction in daily dosage owing to recurrent hypoglycemic episodes. In the second trimester, the diabetes tends to become more labile, and more insulin is needed. Ketoacidosis occurs more readily and, if severe, usually results in death of the fetus. Compounded with this lability, particularly in the third trimester, is the increased renal glomerular filtration rate, lowering the threshold and making urine tests less indicative of blood levels. Immediately after delivery there is a dramatic reduction in insulin need, literally within hours, but after one or two weeks the insulin requirement returns to the prepregnancy level.

The pregnant diabetic has a greater tendency to retain sodium and chloride, making her more susceptible to toxemia and to the development of hydramnios. The latter, caused by increased volume, may result in premature labor and delivery before maturation of the infant. Salt restriction and diuretics are indicated. Mothers with juvenile diabetes for less than ten years or with a milder maturity-onset type of diabetes have large babies, especially if permitted to continue hyperglycemic, which may cause obstetric difficulties. In a longstanding juvenile diabetic, particularly with microangiopathic complications or atherosclerosis as evidenced by calcified pelvic vessels, placental function may be decreased and the infant inadequately nourished and "small-for-dates." In both the hypermature or dysmature pregnancy there is a likelihood of sudden intrauterine death, and delivery prior to this catastrophic event is advised. However, the infant is also particularly subject to respiratory distress, and too early delivery is accordingly contraindicated. The thirty-seventh week used to be considered optimal, but fetal movements, maternal hormone excretion (estrogen and estrogen metabolites, placental lactogen), and amniotic fluid concentrations of pulmonary surfactants are all evaluated to select the best time for delivery.

Recent studies have shown that the maintenance of normoglycemia in the pregnant diabetic by frequent blood glucose analyses and insulin administration in a hospital setting corrects all the problems of the infant of the diabetic mother except for the slightly greater predisposition to congenital malformations such as sacral aplasia.

The newborn in the presence of inadequately controlled maternal diabetes may have markedly hyperplastic pancreatic islets and is placed on intravenous dextrose and water to prevent prolonged and severe hypoglycemia. More important, the predisposition to the respiratory distress syndrome makes close supervision mandatory. With better control of the diabetes, more and more pregnancies are being permitted to go to term.

A successful obstetrical outcome results mainly from frequent observation of the pregnant patient and optimal insulin control of her diabetes, with weekly or twice-weekly visits and hospitalization at least for the last two to three weeks. Because diabetic complications such as retinopathy are frequently aggravated by pregnancy, delivery of one or certainly of two viable infants in a juvenile diabetic should raise consideration of measures to prevent further pregnancies.

GENERAL PRINCIPLES IN DIABETIC MANAGEMENT. Since diabetes is a lifelong event, patients must learn to become their own physician. This is accomplished through extensive education. If on insulin therapy, urine testing, with results recorded before each meal and at bedtime, is mandatory, and the insulin dose should be adjusted according to the previous one or two days' records. Patients are taught to reduce insulin or take extra food before strenuous physical activity, or to increase insulin dosage in times of stress, whether it be physical or, occasionally, emotional, particularly as dictated by previous experience. Also if treated with insulin they should be taught about insulin hypoglycemia and should always be in contact with someone who knows of their disease and the therapy of hypoglycemia. If traveling, identification bracelets or cards in the purse or wallet are mandatory. They should also be instructed in foot care, particularly if elderly and with peripheral vascular disease or neuropathy. For educating the young insulin-dependent diabetic, summer camps have been of great help; they have the additional advantage of exposing the child to others with the disease in order to minimize his or her inferiority as being "singled out." Finally, the patient should be especially warned of the threat of infection and of wounds, particularly of the lower extremities. The large number of juvenile and maturity-onset diabetics who have achieved major successes in all walks of life, including athletics, attests to the minimal impact of the disease in many. Unfortunately in many others, particularly with the juvenile-onset form of the disease occurring in childhood, inadequate or improper emotional support and guidance frequently result in gross maladjustment; these patients can become a burden to society as well as a major threat to their own well-being by neglect of their therapy.

American Diabetes Association: Exchange lists for meal planning, New York, 1976; A guide for professionals: The effective application of exchange lists for meal planning, New York, 1977.

Bunn, H. F., Gabbay, K. H., and Gallop, P. M.: The glycosylation of hemoglobin: Relevance to diabetes mellitus. Science, 200:21, 1978.

Creutzfelt, W., Kobberling, J., and Neel, J. V. (eds.): The Genetics of Diabetes Mellitus. New York, Springer-Verlag, 1976.

Crofford, O.: Report of the National Commission of Diabetes. DHEW (NIH) Publication 75–1018. U.S. Government Press, 1975.

Feig, P. U., and McCurdy, D. K.: The hypertonic state. N. Engl. J. Med., 297:1444, 1977.

Fisher, J. N., Shahshahani, M. N., and Kitabchi, A. E.: Diabetic ketoacidosis: Low dose insulin therapy by various routes. N. Engl. J. Med., 297:238, 1977.

Marble, A., White, P., Bradley, R. F., and Krall, L. P.: Joslin's Diabetes Mellitus. 11th ed. Philadelphia, Lea & Febiger, 1971.

Renold, A. E., Mintz, D. H., Müller, W. A., and Cahill, G. F., Jr.: Diabetes mellitus. In Stanbury, J. B., Wyngaarden, J. B., and Fredrickson, D. S. (eds.): Metabolic Basis of Inherited Disease. 4th ed. New York, McGraw-Hill Book Company, 1978, pp. 80–109.

Steiner, D. F.: Insulin today. Diabetes, 26:322, 1977.

Volk, B. W., and Wellman, K. F.: The Diabetic Pancreas. New York, Plenum Publishing Company, 1977.

531.2. HYPOGLYCEMIC DISORDERS

Norbert Freinkel

Homeostatic mechanisms are geared to preserve blood sugar within a narrow range. Fall of blood sugar to a concentration which elicits symptoms caused by glucose deprivation in the central nervous system constitutes hypoglycemia. It is a manifestation of homeostatic failure and can be caused by a variety of diseases. By arbitrary defintion, hypoglycemia in adults has been equated with values for blood sugar below 40 mg per 100 ml (or plasma or serum glucose below 45 to 50 mg per 100 ml).

Because of intermittent eating, all human intermediary metabolism can be subdivided into two categories: the fed state and the fasted state. The fed state begins whenever we eat, and regulation at this time is designed to provide *optimal utilization* of ingested nutrients for oxidative fulfillment, anabolism, and *synchronized* storage. When levels of circulating fuels have returned to pre-eating values, the fasting state is initiated. Regulatory processes are then geared to recall the various foodstuffs from stores in an integrated fashion that is parsimonious and yet adequate for *production* of the endogenous fuels that are required to meet prevailing metabolic needs in the central nervous system and the periphery.

The pathophysiology of hypoglycemia and its attendant symptoms are substantially different in the fed state and in the fasting state. The distinctions justify classification of the hypoglycemic disorders on the basis of their relation to meals (see accompanying table). They also provide a conceptual framework for diagnostic evaluation.

HYPOGLYCEMIA IN THE FED STATE

PATHOPHYSIOLOGY. Increased amounts of insulin can be demonstrated in the peripheral circulation within a few minutes after eating. Concentration of plasma insulin parallels the rise and fall of blood sugar. However, the decrement of insulin lags somewhat behind that of glucose so that normoglycemia is restored before circulating insulin returns to pre-eating levels.

Because of the anatomic location of the pancreas, insulin reaches the liver sooner and in greater amounts than any other structure. During an acute insulin secretory response to eating, net hepatic production of glucose is "turned off" almost immediately. It is "turned on" again when blood sugar returns to normal. However, even in normal subjects, there may be some lag resulting in a transitory hypoglycemic overshoot. The lag is exaggerated in those regulatory disturbances of the fed state which manifest themselves by symptomatic hypoglycemia during the disposition of meals. Such disorders reflect sluggish or thwarted resumption of hepatic glucose output with consequent prolongation of the period of net utilization of alimentary glucose (i.e., "overutilization"). In essence, the acute transition from fed to fasting state is impaired.

CLASSIFICATION. In pediatric practice, hypoglycemia in reaction to eating may be caused by dietary components which produce excessive release of insulin (e.g., leucine sensitivity of infancy or childhood) or metabo-

Pathophysiologic Classification of Hypoglycemic Disorders

I. Hypoglycemia in the fed state ("overutilization" during the dis-
   position of meals; reactive hypoglycemia)
   A. Relative excess of insulin
      1. Alimentary hyperinsulinism
      2. Reactive hypoglycemia of mild maturity-onset diabetes
         mellitus
      3. Leucine hypersensitivity of infancy and childhood
   B. Accumulation of metabolites which inhibit resumption of
      hepatic glucose output
      1. Fructose-1-phosphate aldolase deficiency (hereditary fructose
         intolerance)
      2. Glactose-1-phosphate uridyl transferase deficiency
         (galactosemia)
      3. Familial fructose and galactose intolerance
   C. Mechanism unknown (? glucose-insulin asynchrony)
      1. "Functional" hypoglycemia (idiopathic postprandial
         hypoglycemia)
II. Hypoglycemia in the fasting state ("underproduction" during
    the metabolism of endogenous fuels; spontaneous hypoglycemia)
   A. Absolute production failure (intrinsic limitations in the
      hepatic capacity for glucose output)
      1. Diffuse hepatoparenchymal disease
      2. Defects in liver enzymes for
         a. Final common pathway
            (1) Glucose-6-phosphate deficiency (glycogen storage
                disease, Type I)
         b. Glycogen turnover
            (1) Amylo-1,6-glucosidase deficiency (glycogen storage
                disease, Type III)
            (2) Defects in the phosphorylase enzyme system
                (glycogen storage diseases, Types VI and VIII)
            (3) Glycogen synthetase deficiency (aglycogenosis)
         c. Gluconeogenic formation of glucose-6-phosphate from
            smaller fragments
            (1) Pyruvate carboxylase deficiency
            (2) Fructose-1,6-diphosphatase deficiency
            (3) Phosphoenolpyruvate carboxykinase deficiency
   B. Relative production failure (insufficient glucose output from
      intrinsically normal hepatocytes)
      1. Insulin excess
         a. Functioning pancreatic islet cell tumors
         b. Pancreatic islet cell hyperplasia (rare in adults)

   c. Diffuse islet hyperplasia in infancy and childhood
   d. Nesidioblastosis
   e. Multiple endocrine adenomatosis (MEA I syndrome)
   f. Epithelioid tumors from foregut anlage
   g. Neonatal hypoglycemia in infants of diabetic mothers
   h. Neonatal hypoglycemia in erythroblastosis fetalis
   i. "Autoimmune hypoglycemia": insulin-binding antibodies
      in the absence of prior insulin administration (?)
   2. Excess insulin-like activity
      a. Some nonpancreatic tumors associated with hypoglycemia
         and increased plasma levels of NSILA-s
   3. Deficiency of contrainsulin hormones
      a. Panhypopituitarism
      b. Primary hypoadrenocorticism
      c. Isolated deficiency of growth hormone
      d. Isolated deficiency of ACTH
      e. Hypothyroidism
      f. Isolated deficiency of glucagon?
   4. Limitations in the availability of gluconeogenic substrates
      a. Ketotic hypoglycemia of childhood
      b. Fasting hypoglycemia of late pregnancy
      c. Severe inanition
   5. Insulin independent, supranormal removal of glucose
      a. Severe exercise
      b. Renal glycosuria
   6. Mechanism unknown
      a. Some nonpancreatic tumors associated with hypoglycemia
         but without increased circulating insulin-like activity
      b. Neonatal hypoglycemia in low birth weight infants
      c. "Idiopathic hypoglycemia" of infancy and childhood
III. Hypoglycemia induced in the fasting state (pharmacological
     interruption of mechanisms which preserve normoglycemia in the
     fasting state; e.g., gluconeogenesis, fatty acid oxidation, or both)
   A. Induced insulin excess
      1. Administration of insulin
      2. Administration of oral hypoglycemic agents
   B. Direct inhibition, independent of insulin
      1. Alcohol hypoglycemia
      2. Ingestion of unripe ackee fruit ("Jamaican vomiting
         sickness"; hypoglycin intoxication)
   C. Mechanism unknown
      1. Salicylates

lites inhibitory to resumption of hepatic glucose release which accumulate owing to inherited enzyme defects (e.g., galactose-1-phosphate in galactosemia; fructose-1-phosphate in hereditary fructose intolerance). However, in adults the hypoglycemias in the fed state are usually caused by one of the following three patterns of disturbed interactions between glucose and insulin during alimentation.

When prior *gastrectomy, pyloroplasty* and *vagotomy*, or *surgical bypass of the pylorus* enables ingestion glucose to have more rapid access to absorptive sites in the small bowel, the prompt rise in blood sugar may elicit secretion of insulin that is greater than normal, although appropriate to the hyperglycemia. The accelerated release of insulin may even be abetted by "gut factors" which are elaborated during transduodenal absorption and which prime islet responsiveness to nutrient secretagogues. Rapid utilization of glucose follows as blood sugar falls to pre-eating levels, and the "extra" insulin is not buffered by continuing absorption from a reservoir of carbohydrate within the gastrointestinal tract. Reactive hypoglycemia then occurs during the second or third hour after eating, and the syndrome has been called "alimentary hyperinsulinism." Recently, a group of patients has been described in whom carbohydrate absorption appears to be excessively rapid even without prior surgery. The mechanism has not been clarified, but the glucose-insulin relationships simulate the more classic postsurgery

"alimentary hyperinsulinism." An analogous situation can occur in normal persons when prolonged infusions of glucose sufficient to sustain hyperglycemia are abruptly terminated, or in patients undergoing hemodialysis when dialysates containing large amounts of glucose are suddenly withdrawn.

When *glucose absorption is normal and release of insulin is sluggish,* attenuation of hepatic glucose output and net deposition of glycogen may be retarded, so that blood sugar rises more than normally. This can occur in mild, early maturity-onset diabetes mellitus and lead to another type of reactive hypoglycemia. The continuing stimulus to insulin secretion produces plasma levels of insulin that are high and yet usually still subnormal in relation to the blood sugar. In such a setting of laggard islet cell response, relative hyperinsulinism may prevail once the utilization of glucose exceeds the rate of influx from the intestine. Thus a diabetic pattern of glucose disposition during the first three hours may be followed by reactive hypoglycemia during the fourth or fifth hour after eating. Other factors may be contributory also since some of the early diabetics who become hypoglycemic do not display insulin levels different from those who do not.

More than two thirds of the hypoglycemias that occur in the fed state in adults remain unexplained and have been designated as *"functional hypoglycemia."* Herein, normal or exaggerated "hypoglycemic rebounds" with profound attendant symptoms may occur with seemingly normal rates of glucose absorption, disposition, and insulin release. In some instances, asynchrony of insulin release has been observed with slight delays in the appearance of peak insulin response. The reactive hypoglycemia characteristically occurs during the third or fourth hour after meal eating and following normal prior glucose tolerance. Functional hypoglycemia is particularly frequent in thin, tense, hyperkinetic young women and tends to occur in subjects with vagotonia and compulsive, conscientious, and intense personality patterns. It may also be encountered in patients with peptic ulcer. However, recent studies have disclosed an increased incidence of abnormal Minnesota Multiphasic Personality Inventory tests (MMPI) in patients with *all* types of reactive hypoglycemia.

SIGNS AND SYMPTOMS. Signs and symptoms of the hypoglycemias in the fed state can be readily understood when viewed as "overutilization" during *non-steady-state conditions.* In a sense, the relationships between insulin and glucose simulate those seen when hypoglycemia is induced acutely during an intravenous insulin tolerance test. Thus the symptoms are characterized by precipitous onset and by features of acute epinephrine release, e.g., tachycardia, tremulousness, sweating piloerection, weakness, anxiety, nervousness, and hunger. The temporal sequence of counterregulation to acute insulin-induced hypoglycemia has been documented recently in man. Whereas increases in plasma cortisol and glucagon occurred 30 minutes after intravenous insulin administration and growth hormone rose after 40 minutes, plasma epinephrine was already increased after 20 minutes (coincident with the increase in glucose production after hypoglycemia). Thus adrenergic mechanisms may play the prepotent role in initiating the counter-regulatory response to acute glucopenia. Although the hyperepinephrinemia is triggered by glucose deprivation in the central nervous system, the duration of hypoglycemia is usually too brief to elicit additional signs of central glucopenia other than faintness, inability to concentrate, and sometimes mental confusion or visual disturbance. Consciousness is almost always preserved. The hypoglycemia is evanescent and self-limited, because the extra insulin released in response to alimentation has a finite persistence and glycogen is deposited in the liver during the induction of the hypoglycemia. Thus as soon as sufficient counter-regulation is activated, glycogenolysis can correct the hypoglycemia and activated gluconeogenesis can maintain normoglycemia.

However, such a benign course is not invariable. Hypoglycemic coma can occur in subjects with reactive hypoglycemia, especially when they are receiving therapy with autonomic blocking agents such as propranolol. Thus beta receptor blockade can impair the activated lipolysis and muscle glycogenolysis by which resistance to insulin may be induced and alternate fuels and gluconeogenic precursors mobilized during hypoglycemic rebound. Similarly, in subjects with compromised cardiovascular function, even evanescent hypoglycemia and hyperepinephrinemia may provoke angina, ectopic cardiac rhythms, pulmonary edema, and episodes of transient cerebral ischemia.

DIAGNOSIS. Since blood sugar after overnight or even more prolonged fast is never abnormally low in the aforementioned disorders, diagnosis depends upon eliciting the hypoglycemia during reproduction of the fed state with oral tests of glucose tolerance. Basal con-

ditions should be preserved throughout, and blood samples should be secured from an indwelling venous needle to minimize the trauma of venipuncture. Diagnostic classification depends on the nature of the glucose tolerance curve and the time interval between glucose ingestion and reactive hypoglycemia. To maximize the diagnostic value of the test, blood samples are obtained at least every 30 minutes for five hours. Professional personnel should be in attendance throughout so that vital signs may be monitored at the same time. Symptoms and signs ascribed to hypoglycemia should coincide with nadir values for blood sugar. The evanescent nadir may be missed by adherence to a fixed schedule of blood sampling even with intervals as short as 30 minutes. Increments in plasma cortisol should also be demonstrable 30 to 60 minutes after the symptomatic event and may be used as further evidence that the hypoglycemia threatened homeostasis. Although there has been considerable controversy concerning the limits of normal hypoglycemic rebound that can occur without symptomatology during oral glucose tolerance, recent studies have indicated that decrements in blood glucose to values below 45 mg per 100 ml (that is, plasma glucose less than 50 mg per 100 ml) occur in less than 10 per cent of the population and are associated with symptoms of hypoglycemia in the majority of cases. By definition, patients with reactive hypoglycemia resulting from alimentary hyperinsulinism or functional hypoglycemia should display normal intravenous glucose tolerance. However, data in this regard are sparse.

Rigid diagnostic criteria are imperative because neurasthenic symptoms unrelated to blood sugar, such as those accompanying the hyperepinephrinemia of anxiety attacks, are easily confused with true reactive hypoglycemia. Popular lay misconceptions equating blood sugar with energy have also been responsible for self-diagnosed "hypoglycemia" to explain such symptoms as fatigue, listlessness, diminished mental activity, spasms, and palpitations — i.e., the recently described syndrome of "nonhypoglycemia." Insistence upon precise documentation can spare such subjects unwarranted and frequently ill-advised empiric therapies. However, particularly in functional hypoglycemia, oral glucose tolerance may be normal when tested in the hospital under conditions divorced from daily stresses, and abnormal only in a "real-life" outpatient setting. Hence a single negative glucose tolerance test need not exclude the diagnosis of hypoglycemia in the fed state; more frequent monitoring of blood sugars during symptomatic episodes may be required.

TREATMENT. There are limited prospective studies to define the natural course of the reactive hypoglycemias. In our own hands, some patients with presumed functional hypoglycemia have varyingly displayed oral glucose tolerance compatible with mild maturity-onset diabetes; others have remained remarkably constant during many years of serial testing. The postprandial hypoglycemia of early maturity-onset diabetes may disappear as the diabetes worsens and insulinopenia supervenes. It can also disappear as the diabetes improves in response to weight loss. Thus the duration for which any treatment is to be instituted cannot be defined with certainty.

General objectives of treatment are to dampen the elevations in blood sugar which elicit the subsequent excessive hypoglycemic rebounds. Multiple small feedings have constituted one approach. However, regular meal-eating with diets high in protein (120 to 140 grams), low in carbohydrate (75 to 100 grams), and sufficient in fat to maintain caloric adequacy have been more efficacious. Although long experience has corroborated that high protein, low carbohydrate diets diminish the frequency of all the hypoglycemias in the fed state, their mechanism of action remains unexplained.

Certain more specific therapies may be useful. Anticholinergic drugs in small doses (e.g., 7.5 mg Pro-Banthine 30 minutes before each meal) can be of value by delaying gastic emptying and slowing gastrointestinal motility. Salutary effects have been claimed for weight loss or for sulfonylureas in the reactive hypoglycemia of early diabetics. Reversal of a 10-cm jejunal segment has been reported to ameliorate the reactive hypoglycemia that may follow gastric surgery. Reassurance and judicious use of mild sedatives or tranquilizers may be beneficial in functional hypoglycemia. In the light of existing knowledge, adrenocortical steroids have no place in the treatment of these hypoglycemic disorders.

SPONTANEOUS HYPOGLYCEMIA IN THE FASTING STATE

PATHOPHYSIOLOGY. By the time of waking from overnight sleep, all energy requirements of the body are fulfilled from endogenous resources. Prevailing blood sugar then reflects a balance between the continuing utilization of endogenously derived glucose and the production of additional glucose via gluconeogenesis from smaller fragments to replace the glucose lost. The reliance of the brain on glucose for its oxidative demands determines the major metabolic objective of the fasted state, that is, to produce sufficient glucose for normoglycemia to be preserved. Since net production of glucose requires catabolism of structural protein, the second objective is to restrict utilization of glucose to a minimum. The following adaptations facilitate these objectives: (1) glucose utilization is restrained in most extracerebral tissues, and the more expendable fatty acids are substituted as oxidative fuels; (2) hepatic gluconeogenesis effects essentially complete recovery of lactic acid so that tissues which rely upon glycolysis for energy (e.g., red blood cells, renal medulla) can function without a *net* expenditure of glucose; and (3) hepatic ketogenesis generates lipid products which can cross the blood-brain barrier and replace glucose for *some* of the oxidative needs of the brain once *sufficient ketonemia becomes established.*

The net rate of glucose removal is the physiologic pacesetter for the equilibrium between glucose utilization and production by which normoglycemia is maintained in the fasted state. Hypoglycemia occurs when the liver is unable to "keep up" with rates of glucose removal.

As detailed elsewhere in this text, recent studies permit the relationships in adults to be formulated in quantitative terms. Splanchnic glucose output in normal man after overnight fast approximates 180 grams per day; 80 per cent of that is oxidized completely to carbon dioxide by nervous tissue, chiefly the brain, whereas the remainder undergoes only glycolysis with

the formation of lactate which is recycled to glucose. Since postprandial hepatic glycogen averages only 70 to 75 grams, some de novo formation of glucose is mandatory even after overnight fast. The precursors for the net formation of new glucose have been estimated as originating approximately 50 per cent from amino acids (of which alanine accounts for more than half) and 10 per cent from glycerol derived during lipolysis.

Data are not available concerning the maximal capacity for gluconeogenesis in normal human liver. However, extrapolations from in vitro studies and infusions of gluconeogenic precursors suggest that the biosynthetic ceiling is several-fold greater than the aforementioned values. Thus normal regulation may be delimited by the factors which influence extrahepatic generation of substrates for gluconeogenesis more than by intrahepatic determinants.

CLASSIFICATION. Spontaneous hypoglycemias in the fasting state represent "underproduction" of hepatic glucose and may be classified as "absolute" or "relative" (see table).

The "absolute" production failures are uncommon and arise when intrinsic anatomic or enzymic abnormalities in the liver compromise its capacity to elaborate enough glucose to offset normal rates of glucose utilization in the periphery. Limitations resulting from enzyme deletions are usually confined to pediatric practice. Until recently the recognized entities were limited to enzymes involving the final common pathway for glucose release (i.e., glucose-6-phosphatase deficiency) or glycogen turnover (see table). However, during the past decade, deficiencies in each of the three enzymes which are rate-limiting in the gluconeogenic renewal of glucose-6-phosphate from smaller fragments (i.e., pyruvate carboxylase, phosphoenolpyruvate carboxykinase, and fructose-1,6-diphosphatase) have been implicated in hypoglycemic disorders of infancy. In adults, it used to be held that fasting hypoglycemia via "absolute" production failure occurs only with fulminant necrosis, extensive destruction, or severe congestion of hepatic parenchyma. The recent finding of asymptomatic low blood sugars after overnight fast in patients with viral hepatitis suggests that diffuse involvement of hepatocytes can cause hypoglycemia even without permanent anatomic lesions. In this regard, reduced delivery of gluconeogenic precursors resulting from diminished splanchnic blood flow may contribute to the occasional hypoglycemia of severe congestive heart failure.

"Relative" production failures are far more common. They occur when normal hepatocytes cannot "keep up" with normal or supranormal rates of glucose utilization owing to functional restraints to hepatic glucose output, inadequate generation of alternative fuels of oxidation, of endogenous substrates for gluconeogenesis, or both. In most instances, multiple factors are operative. For example, in the fasting hypoglycemia of insulin excess, direct inhibition of glucose release and ketogenesis in the liver may be combined with restrained lipolysis and protein catabolism and enhanced utilization of glucose in the periphery. Similarly, in the fasting hypoglycemia that may occur when contrainsulin hormones are lacking (e.g., panhypopituitarism, primary hypoadrenocorticism, isolated deficiency of growth hormones; see table), intrahepatic mechanisms for glycogenesis and gluconeogenesis are inadequate, generation of gluconeogenic precursors and mobilization of fat from the periphery are diminished, and the relative effectiveness of circulating insulin is increased due to lack of contrainsulin factors.

In all these disorders, occasional postprandial reactive hypoglycemia may also be encountered. Such episodes arise, presumably, because the factors impairing glucose production during fasting may equally restrain resumption of hepatic glucose output during the hypoglycemic rebound that occurs after eating (see above). They can be readily differentiated from the classic "hypoglycemias in the fed state" described above, because they also have fasting hypoglycemia.

SIGNS AND SYMPTOMS. The fasting hypoglycemias develop slowly, so that manifestations of acute epinephrine discharge are usually not observed. Instead, the clinical picture is dominated by signs and symptoms of more prolonged and severe glucose deprivation in the brain. These may range from confusion, disorientation, and memory lapses to psychotic behavior, paresthesias, transient paralysis, convulsions, and coma. Sclerotic cerebral vessels with selectively compromised blood supply may account for focal abnormalities such as hemiplegias and monoplegias. Vulnerability of different parts of the brain to glucopenia is in reverse order of phylogenetic development. Hence the cerebral cortex is affected first. However, no single constellation of nervous system involvement is diagnostic. Fasting hypoglycemia should be suspected whenever a neuropsychiatric or neurologic complex occurs repeatedly, especially *before breakfast* or after "skipped meals," and is ameliorated almost immediately by food.

DIAGNOSIS. Diagnosis of fasting hypoglycemia presupposes that inadequate delivery of glucose to the brain can be duplicated by simply withholding all food. In well-nourished subjects, normoglycemia and mental acuity are preserved even with several weeks of fasting, although blood sugar stabilizes at somewhat lower levels from the second or third day onward. In rare instances of extreme inanition, hypoglycemia may supervene during shorter periods of fasting, presumably because stores of mobilizable fat and gluconeogenic precursors have been depleted. Some limitation in hepatic gluconeogenic enzymes may be operative also in these situations. However, even in normal subjects, sex differences become manifest after more than 24 hours of withholding food. In a recent report of healthy, nonobese young subjects, the lowest levels of plasma glucose during a 72-hour fast were 55 mg per 100 ml in the males and 36 mg per 100 ml in the females, with mean minimal levels for males and females averaging 61.9 and 52.0 mg per 100 ml and being reached at the sixty-seventh and sixty-second hour, respectively. Feedback relationships between glucose and insulin appear to be equally well preserved in both groups so that levels of plasma glucose and immunoreactive insulin (IRI) decline in parallel with the preservation of constant or slightly falling ratios for IRI/glucose.

Clearly, however, criteria for "fasting hypoglycemia" based solely on arbitrary lower limits for normal blood sugar may require some modification when the fast is extended beyond 24 hours in females. The pregnant woman is particularly vulnerable to fasting hypoglycemia from the second trimester onward because the normal hypoglycemic propensities of being female are exaggerated due to the increased availability of sex hormones of placental origin and the added removal of glucose and amino acids by the conceptus.

Certain findings may occur in all the fasting hypogly-

cemias without regard to etiology. For example, Whipple's triad of (1) symptomatic hypoglycemia, (2) low blood sugar, and (3) alleviation by glucose ingestion is not pathognomonic for any single entity. The blood sugar response to exercise after three days of fasting also has limited specificity. Such exercise may increase blood sugar when the lactic acid derived from the exercised muscles gains access to normal hepatic gluconeogenic mechanisms. On the other hand, the exercise may fail to affect blood sugar or cause further hypoglycemia when the enchancing effects of exercise on glucose utilization cannot be offset because glucose production is impaired for any reason (see table).

Once the general diagnosis of hypoglycemia in the fasting state has been made, procedures should be designed to differentiate between hypoglycemia resulting from absolute insulin excess, lack of contrainsulin factors (e.g., hormonal deficiencies), or limitations in other factors which preserve the normal equilibrium between glucose production and utilization in the fasting state (e.g., organic liver disease, functional liver impairment due to enzyme defects, certain extrapancreatic tumors; see table).

For optimal interpretability, safety, and rigorous exclusion of pharmacologic lowerings of blood sugar by drugs or other *exogenous* agents, diagnostic evaluation should be conducted in the hospital.

FUNCTIONING ISLET CELL TUMORS

Functioning adenomas of the beta cells of the pancreatic islets are the most common cause of fasting hypoglycemia. They are usually single, although multiple adenomas have been reported in 4 to 10 per cent of the cases. Approximately 10 per cent are malignant and 0.5 to 1 per cent are ectopic, usually within the splenic hilum, pancreatic bed, or duodenal wall. A family history of diabetes mellitus is present in approximately 25 per cent of the cases. Peak incidence is encountered between ages 40 and 60; however, cases have been seen in all age groups, although with extreme rarity in infancy and early childhood. Single adenomas are distributed with equal frequency in the head, body, and tail of the pancreas. The incidence of benign adenomas shows no sex difference, whereas malignant functioning islet tumors may be more common in males. In certain instances, functioning islet cell tumors are associated with other endocrine adenomas, particularly in the pituitary, parathyroid, and adrenal (multiple endocrine adenomatosis, Type 1), so that search for multiple endocrinopathy should be instituted whenever disorders of any of these glands occur, especially on a familial basis. Peptic ulcer disease also deserves investigation, because it has been reported in 10 per cent of all islet cell tumor patients, and many believe that the Zollinger-Ellison syndrome (see Ch. 403) and multiple endocrine adenomatosis may represent phenotypic variants of the same mutant gene. A few instances of diffuse microadenomatosis have been described in the adult population; diffuse islet hyperplasia is extraordinarily rare in contrast to the pediatric experience.

DIAGNOSIS. Specific diagnosis of functioning islet cell tumors is made on the basis of secretory properties. Persistence of inappropriately high levels of circulating insulin during hypoglycemia when food is withheld is the single most important diagnostic criterion and often

Plasma glucose and insulin relationships during fasting in a patient with functioning islet cell tumor. Plasma insulin remains within "normal" range despite fall of plasma glucose to hypoglycemic levels; administration of intravenous glucagon at the time of prevailing hypoglycemia elicits a brisk rise in plasma glucose.

suffices. It reflects islet autonomy and disturbed feedback relationships between ambient glucose and basal insulin secretion. Characterization of the prevailing relationships between circulating insulin and proinsulin-like components at this time and the demonstration of other aberrant secretory products may provide further useful documentation, especially when malignancy is suspected (see below). In limited circumstances, additional information may be sought by testing for (1) excessive insulin release in response to certain islet secretagogues or (2) impaired suppressibility of endogenous insulin secretion in response to acute lowering of blood sugar.

Levels of plasma total immunoreactive insulin above the upper limits of normal (25 μU per milliliter) in association with subnormal blood sugar occur in approximately two thirds of patients when blood samples are obtained after overnight fast on at least three separate days. The time relationships are particularly important. We usually do not initiate the fast until 10 P.M. so that the 6 A.M. blood specimen represents ten hours' "overnight fast." For more extended fasting, blood specimens are secured at two-hour intervals until noon and at least every six hours thereafter for a total fast of three days. Close supervision is essential; by simply extending the "overnight fast" from 6 A.M. to noon, abnormal insulin-glucose relationship can be demonstrated in 90 per cent of the insulinoma patients. Termination of the fast by the administration of intravenous glucagon (1 gram dissolved in 20 ml of saline and given intravenously over two minutes) has proved useful in our clinic. In the fasting hypoglycemias that are mediated by excess insulin or "insulin-like" principles, the glucagon elicits a brisk rise in blood sugar despite prevailing hypoglycemia, presumably because hepatic glycogen has been preserved (see accompanying figure). Contrariwise, in patients with fasting hypoglycemias of other causes, or in normal nonobese subjects who have been fasted for three days, glucagon does not elicit meaningful acute increments in blood sugar.

The diagnostic potential of fasting insulin measurements has been expanded considerably by the recogni-

tion that measurable insulin virtually disappears from the circulation at plasma glucose levels of 30 mg per 100 ml. In this context, "normal" insulin levels may be abnormal when associated with fasting hypoglycemia. The relationship may be expressed most conveniently as the "amended" IRI/glucose ratio, i.e.,

$$\frac{\text{plasma IRI in } \mu\text{U/ml} \times 100}{\text{plasma glucose in mg/100 ml} - 30}$$

Values for the ratio above 50 are abnormal when associated with hypoglycemia. The modest elevations of basal insulin that are seen in obesity and other states which are associated with insulin resistance, such as acromegaly or hyperadrenocorticism, are not attended by fasting hypoglycemia.

Plasma "proinsulin-like components" are disproportionately increased (i.e., greater than 20 per cent of the total circulating insulin immunoreactive materials) in more than 80 per cent of patients with islet cell tumors and may provide additional useful characterization of basal insulin secretion, especially when absolute IRI values are borderline. The "proinsulin-like components" exert little hypoglycemic action. In the recently described entity of familial hyperproinsulinemia, fasting blood sugar was normal and consistent with the normal levels of circulating insulin rather than the markedly increased concerntration of plasma proinsulin or proinsulin-like material. The "hyperproinsulinemia" in this autosomal dominant genetic disorder appears to be due to the biosynthesis of an abnormal proinsulin or a deficiency in the enzymes responsible for proinsulin cleavage in the beta cell.

In a study of 76 patients with functioning islet cell tumors, elevated levels of plasma human chorionic gonadotropin (hCG) or one of its subunits (hCG-α or hCG-β) were found in 63 per cent of the 27 patients with islet cell carcinoma and none of the 43 patients with benign disease. Increases in plasma glucagon, gastrin, or both in functioning islet cell tumors may also indicate malignancy as well as microadenomatosis or the multiple endocrine adenomatosis syndrome.

For provocative challenge with islet secretagogues, oral or intravenous glucose has proved unrewarding, and no characteristic patterns have emerged. On the other hand, the insulin secretory response to intravenous tolbutamide (1 gram dissolved in 20 ml of saline and given intravenously over two minutes) is supranormal (i.e., increments greater than 120 μU per milliliter above baseline) in approximately 80 per cent of patients with functioning islet cell tumors; leucine (0.2 gram per kilogram orally or intravenously) elicits greater than normal increases of plasma insulin (i.e., in excess of 30 μU per milliliter) in approximately 70 per cent; and the stimulated release of insulin that follows 1 mg of intravenous glucagon exceeds the peak normal response (i.e., greater than 130 μU per milliliter) in somewhat more than 50 per cent. Since maximal insulin responses occur early, within 3 to 30 minutes after administration of the secretagogue, diagnostic evaluation can be terminated before serious hypoglycemia supervenes. Although equally exuberant releases of insulin may follow tolbutamide or glucagon administration in obesity, acromegaly, late pregnancy, and other states associated with heightened basal insulin secretion, the subsequent hypoglycemia is not commensurate with the hyperinsulinemia under such circumstances. Therefore both blood sugar and insulin values should be monitored during provocative tests for insulinoma.

Although the relationship between insulin and glucose during fasting constitutes a form of suppression test, more acute approaches have been proposed. Endogenous insulin secretion has been monitored by conventional immunoassay during fish insulin–induced hypoglycemia or on the basis of serum connecting peptide (C-peptide) after hypoglycemia induced by the administration of beef or pork insulin. Such tests have confirmed that most islet cell tumors function autonomously and do not attenuate their secretion, like normal islets, in response to acute hypoglycemia.

However, in most circumstances, neither provocative nor acute suppression tests are necessary to diagnose functioning islet cell tumors. Unequivocal diagnoses can usually be established on the basis of the relationships between insulin and glucose during fasting, and concurrent evaluation for other secretory products such as hCG, gastrin, glucagon, and proinsulin may help characterize the nature of the hyperfunctioning tissue.

TREATMENT. *Surgery* constitutes the treatment of choice. Preoperative attenuation of hypoglycemia may be achieved with 100 to 200 mg hydrocortisone per day and appropriate dietary supplementation. The nondiuretic benzothiadiazine, diazoxide, in doses of 200 to 600 mg per day has proved more effective, by inhibiting insulin secretion directly as well as by exerting peripheral actions. Because of its sodium-retaining properties, diazoxide should be combined with a natriuretic thiazide such as trichlormethiazide (2 to 4 mg per day). These medications should be discontinued two days preoperatively.

At surgery, the pancreas should be mobilized and explored carefully for single or multiple lesions that can be "shelled out." Preoperative localization by selective pancreatic arteriography has been successful in approximately half the cases. As yet, no detailed data are available concerning the efficacy of ultrasound or computerized axial tomography, although these modalities also warrant preoperative trial. Quite frequently, however, all efforts at visualization and palpation of the tumor fail. Under such circumstances, the tail and then the body of the pancreas should be excised sequentially, because this will remove a significant proportion of the insulinomas. Failure to find tumor on serial sectioning justifies subsequent excision of most of the head of the pancreas but avoiding duodenal and bile duct resection. Such surgical aggressiveness requires unequivocal preoperative diagnostic confidence — a circumstance that insulin immunoassays have made possible today. Monitoring of blood samples during surgery may also be helpful; a sharp rise in blood sugar within 30 minutes after excision of tumor affords presumptive evidence against residual functioning tumor in situ or additional tumors elsewhere. To facilitate interpretation, intravenous fluids during surgery should be restricted to simple saline if possible.

Successful extirpation of tumor (or tumors) effects complete and prompt cure. However, nonresectable islet cell carcinomas may be functional and accompanied by hypoglycemia. Long-term symptomatic palliation with diazoxide and trichlormethiazide or hormones such as glucocorticoids, long-acting glucagon, or growth hormone has been tried. Streptozotocin, a broad-spectrum antimicrobial with relatively selective cytotoxicity for pancreatic beta cells, has proved more

rewarding. In 52 patients with metastatic pancreatic islet cell carcinoma treated with streptozotocin, measurable response has been observed in 50 and 63 per cent of those with functional and nonfunctional tumors, respectively. Response included tumor regression, rectification of hyperinsulinism, and more than three-fold improvement in survival. The renal and hepatic toxicities of streptozotocin, although appreciable, usually have been reversible.

EXTRAPANCREATIC NEOPLASMS ASSOCIATED WITH HYPOGLYCEMIA

Over 200 instances of massive extrapancreatic neoplasms (ranging from 1.5 to 20 pounds) associated with fasting hypoglycemia have been reported. Four major tumor groups have been involved. Approximately half have been mesothelial tumors (most commonly classified as fibromas, fibrosarcomas, spindle cell sarcomas, and leiomyosarcomas); 20 per cent have been malignant hepatomas; gastrointestinal carcinomas (particularly of the stomach, colon, and bile ducts) and adrenocortical carcinomas have each accounted for about another 10 per cent. The rest have been miscellaneous tumors. About 80 per cent of the tumors have been intra-abdominal.

Although the pathophysiology of this hypoglycemia is not fully understood, it has been associated in a number of cases with heightened glucose utilization by the tumor and restrained hepatic glucose output. Multiple etiologies appear to be implicated. Recent refinements in radioreceptor assay for nonsuppressible insulin-like activity soluble in acid ethanol (NSILA-s) disclosed elevated levels of this peptide in 8 of 15 patients with hypoglycemia in association with nonpancreatic tumors. A number of other workers have elicited insulin-like effects in isolated adipose tissue or rat diaphragms with extracts of some of these tumors. Increased plasma immunoreactive insulin has been observed in one patient with a fibrosarcoma and hypoglycemia. One bronchial carcinoid tumor has been described in which increased immunoreactive insulin was demonstrated in plasma as well as in primary and metastatic tumor tissue.

Massive extrapancreatic tumors associated with fasting hypoglycemia can be readily distinguished from insulinomas. Save for rare exceptions as cited above, plasma immunoreactive insulin is low and usually appropriate to the prevailing hypoglycemia. Responses to tolbutamide and leucine are usually subnormal in terms of glucose as well as insulin, most likely because islet function has been dampened by the antecedent hypoglycemia.

Therapy should be directed toward total surgical excision, or as much tumoricidal ablation as possible. When such therapy is successful, the hypoglycemia has usually disappeared. Glucocorticoids, glucagon, growth hormone, and dietary manipulations have been helpful in managing the hypoglycemia during preparation for surgery and, occasionally, when tumor therapy has been unsuccessful. Diazoxide has been tried also; efficacy has been somewhat less than in other fasting hypoglycemias, perhaps because of the smaller role played by pancreatic insulin.

SPONTANEOUS HYPOGLYCEMIA RELATED TO AUTOIMMUNE MECHANISMS

In 1970, the first case of "autoimmune" insulin hypoglycemia was described, and approximately 13 additional cases have been reported since then. The patients' plasmas contain insulin-binding immunoglobulins, chiefly IgG, capable of reacting avidly with insulins from many species, including human. Prior administration of exogenous insulin has usually been excluded by rigorous history. Despite some continuing controversy, the autoimmune origin of the circulating insulin-binding antibodies appears to have been established by the demonstration that these antibodies do not react to the highly species-specific C-segment of beef or pork proinsulin but are directed to the C-segment of human proinsulin. The patient may exhibit fasting and/or delayed postprandial hypoglycemia.

HYPOGLYCEMIA INDUCED IN THE FASTING STATE

PATHOPHYSIOLOGY. The hypoglycemias which arise *spontaneously* in the fasting state must be differentiated from another group of disorders, the hypoglycemias *induced* in the fasting state. Here, an *exogenous* agent has been introduced which can block the traffic in endogenous fuels by which normoglycemia is preserved when food is withheld. The resulting hypoglycemia may persist for the duration of the biologic effectiveness of the exogenous agent and engender considerable diagnostic confusion in the unwary.

CLASSIFICATION AND MANIFESTATIONS. Two broad groups can be delineated: the hypoglycemias caused by *induced* insulin excess and those caused by drugs which directly impair homeostatic mechanisms, independent of insulin action (see table).

Induced insulin excess should always be suspected when hypoglycemic episodes have no well-defined, recurring pattern and when they involve individuals with ready access to hypoglycemic medications such as diabetics, relatives of diabetics, or medical and paramedical workers. The clinical picture in instances of *surreptitious or accidental administration of insulin* depends on the nature of the insulin involved. Short-acting preparations may elicit the hyperepinephrinemia and the clinical features characteristic of the hypoglycemias in the fed state. Contrariwise, long- or intermediate-acting preparations of insulin may effect a picture indistinguishable from the spontaneous hypoglycemias of the fasting state.

All the *sulfonylureas* have also been associated with life-threatening hypoglycemic comas, presumably owing to stimulation of excessive and/or prolonged insulin release (see table). Vulnerability to this exaggeration of their action is greatest in the elderly, in newborns of diabetic mothers who have received sulfonylureas, and in subjects with reduced hepatic or renal capacities for metabolizing or excreting the drugs. Chlorpropamide has posed the greatest problem. As the longest-acting sulfonylurea, it has been implicated in 120 of the 220 known cases of coma caused by sulfonylurea drugs when used alone. The clinical hypoglycemic syndromes with all these agents have consisted of slowly evolving cerebral dysfunction progressing to coma.

Perhaps the most frequent cause of the hypoglycemias induced in the fasting state in adults is *ethanol* (see table). Although other factors may participate, the principal mechanism is by direct inhibition of gluconeogenesis resulting from the metabolism of alcohol in the cytoplasm of the liver. As each mole of ethanol is oxidized to acetaldehyde and then to acetate (or acetyl CoA) via alcohol and aldehyde dehydrogenase, respectively, two moles of NAD^+ are reduced. The ratio of $NADH/NAD^+$ thereby increases, a reductive environment supervenes, and NAD^+ is diverted from other reactions in the liver. Thus the citric acid cycle is restrained, and there is attenuation of the flux of precursors such as glycerol, lactate, and amino acids which enter the gluconeogenic sequence via NAD^+-dependent reactions. The duration of prior fasting required to lower blood sugar under such circumstances and the latency between imbibition and hypoglycemia depend upon (1) how much glycogen is present for sustaining hepatic glucose output while gluconeogenic renewal is blocked, and (2) how rapidly circulating glucose is being removed and must be replaced in the periphery. In normal adults, more than 24 hours of fasting are usually necessary; infants and children are far more vulnerable, and hypoglycemia may occur shortly after exposure to ethanol and after only minimal dietary deprivation. For reasons which are not yet explained, some chronic alcoholics also appear to be particularly susceptible to ethanol-induced hypoglycemia. Occult liver disease does not seem to be responsible for this sensitivity; acquired limitations in neurohumoral counter-regulatory mechanisms appear more likely.

The clinical signs differ little from other types of hypoglycemia occurring in the fasting state. However, the early mental changes are often mistaken for alcoholic inebriation so that help is not usually sought until patients become comatose. Even then, the transition from alcoholic stupor to hypoglycemic coma may be unsuspected. Hypothermia is common; trismus may be present; and convulsions are particularly prominent in infants and children. The relationship to prior ethanol ingestion need not be obvious. Alcohol metabolism in man usually proceeds at a linear rate (approximately 100 mg per kilogram per hour) until blood alcohol levels decline to 10 to 20 mg per 100 ml and enzyme systems are no longer saturated. Therefore a relatively constant amount of alcohol is oxidized per unit time, and the generation of "reducing equivalents" within the liver may persist for many hours and at low blood alcohol levels, depending upon the initial amount of ethanol ingestion. If there has been no intake of food, hypoglycemia can thus occur 6 to 20 hours after imbibition, and without any clinical signs of alcoholism.

The situation may be particularly complex and dangerous when several agents interact concurrently. For example, irreversible brain damage and even death have occurred from alcohol hypoglycemia in diabetic alcoholics who have received insulin during periods of spree drinking and dietary dereliction.

Salicylates warrant inclusion, because they account for most of the drug-induced hypoglycemias during the first two years of life. Because of the age group involved, salicylates have been associated with the greatest mortality of any hypoglycemic drug (33 per cent in 15 reported cases). The mechanism of hypoglycemic action remains unsettled (see table).

DIAGNOSIS AND TREATMENT. Recognition of hypoglycemia in these comastose patients is imperative. Failure to do so, and to treat accordingly, accounted for fatal terminations in 25 per cent of the children and 11 per cent of the adults with alcohol hypoglycemia reported before 1962. As in all hypoglycemic comas, a high index of suspicion improves prognosis, and response to glucose is usually dramatic unless brain damage has been sustained.

Certain diagnostic aids may be particularly helpful in identifying etiologic agents. Analysis of urine or plasma for C-peptide has proved useful in factitious hyperinsulinism, because the connecting peptide is specific for endogenous islet secretion and therefore will not parallel the circulating levels of administered insulin. Plasma analyses for sulfonylureas or examination of urine for appropriate excretion products may identify sulfonylurea-induced hypoglycemias. In the latter instances, the effect of the drug may be prolonged, and continued administration of glucose, with frequent monitoring of blood sugar, may be necessary for several days. After the patient has been stabilized, it must be established whether the hypoglycemia in the fasting state was *spontaneous* or *induced*. This can only be done in a hospital, because rigorous supervision may be required to exclude *exogenous* agents. After the cause of induced hypoglycemia has been established, no definitive therapy may be required save for dietary instruction, psychiatric help when necessary, and other attempts to modify exposure to the offending agent. However, it must be appreciated that vulnerability to the hypoglycemic potential of drugs like alcohol is far greater in individuals in whom endogenous capacities for gluconeogenesis or lipolysis are already marginal. Therefore diagnostic work-up of the functions that influence blood sugar homeostasis in the fasting state is also indicated. Such evaluations have unmasked occult diseases (e.g., hypopituitarism, hypoadrenocorticism) in several instances of alcohol hypoglycemia in our clinic.

Broder, L. E., and Carter, S. K.: Pancreatic islet cell carcinoma. Ann. Intern. Med., 79:101, 1973.

Couropmitree, C., Freinkel, N., Nagel, T. C., Horwitz, D. L., Metzger, B. E., Rubenstein, A. H., and Hahnel, R.: Plasma C-peptide and diagnosis of factitious hyperinsulinism. Ann. Intern. Med., 82:201, 1975.

Fajans, S. S., and Floyd, J. C., Jr.: Fasting hypoglycemia in adults. N. Engl. J. Med., 294:766, 1976.

Freinkel, N., Singer, D. L., Arky, R. A., Bleicher, S. J., Anderson, J. B., and Silbert, C. K.: Alcohol hypoglycemia. I. Carbohydrate metabolism of patients with clinical alcohol hypoglycemia and the experimental reproduction of the syndrome with pure ethanol. J. Clin. Invest., 42:1112, 1963.

Gabbay, K. H., DeLuca, K., Fisher, J. N., Jr., Mako, M. E., and Rubenstein, A. H.: Familial hyperproinsulinemia: An autosomal dominant defect. N. Engl. J. Med., 294:911, 1976.

Garber, A. J., Cryer, P. E., Santiago, J. V., Haymond, M. W., Pagliara, A. S., and Kipnis, D. M.: The role of adrenergic mechanisms in the substrate and hormonal response to insulin-induced hypoglycemia in man. J. Clin. Invest., 58:7, 1976.

Pagliara, A. S., Karl, I. E., Haymond, M., and Kipnis, D. M.: Hypoglycemia in infancy and childhood, Parts I and II. J. Pediat., 82:365, 558, 1973.

Permutt, M. A.: Postprandial hypoglycemia. Diabetes, 25:719, 1976.

531.3. GALACTOSEMIA

Ernest Beutler

The galactosemias are characterized by inability to metabolize galactose normally. When patients with galactosemia ingest galactose, either in its free form or as the galactose-containing disaccharide lactose, galactose and some of the products of its incomplete metabolism accumulate in the blood, tissues, and usually the urine. Two types of galactosemia exist, each the result of a specific enzyme deficiency. The classic form of the disorder, galactose-l-phosphate uridyl transferase deficiency, is to be distinguished from galactokinase deficiency. Deficiency of epimerase has also been described; although it is associated with increased red cell galactose-l-phosphate levels, there are no clinical consequences, and it is therefore not considered to be a form of galactosemia.

CLASSIC GALACTOSEMIA

ETIOLOGY. Classic galactosemia is an autosomal recessive disorder due to a marked deficiency of the enzyme galactose-1-phosphate uridyl transferase.

INCIDENCE. The incidence of classic galactosemia is approximately 1 per 80,000 births in the white population. It may be somewhat higher in the black population.

PATHOGENESIS. The galactose molecule is identical to the glucose molecule except for the relative position of the hydroxyl and hydrogen groups attached to the fourth carbon. However, the body is unable to utilize this sugar until it has been converted to glucose. The existence of only one pathway for the metabolism of galactose has been established. First, galactose is phosphorylated in the 1-position by ATP through the mediation of the enzyme galactokinase:

$$\text{Galactose} + \text{ATP} \xrightarrow{\text{galactokinase}} \text{galactose-1-P}$$

Next, the galactose-1-P formed exchanges with the glucose-1-P moiety attached to a uridine diphosphate carrier. This reaction is catalyzed by galactose-1-phosphate uridyl transferase (transferase):

$$\text{Galactose-1-P} + \text{UDPG} \xrightleftharpoons{\text{transferase}} \text{glucose-1-P} + \text{UDPGal}$$

Finally, the uridine diphosphogalactose (UDPGal) formed may be converted to uridine diphosphoglucose (UDPG) through the action of epimerase:

$$\text{UDPGal} \xrightleftharpoons{\text{epimerase}} \text{UDPG}$$

In classic galactosemia the absence of galactose-1-phosphate uridyl transferase activity results in accumulation of both galactose and galactose-1-P. Galactose may serve as a substrate for aldose reductase and for L-hexonate dehydrogenase. These enzymes oxidize NADPH, reducing galactose to its polyol derivative, dulcitol, to which cell membranes are relatively impermeable. In the lens of the eye this creates an unbalanced osmotic force resulting in excessive hydration. At the same time it may deplete the lens of its supply of NADPH. The result of these changes is the irreversible precipitation of the lens protein with the formation of cataracts.

Cirrhosis of the liver and mental retardation are also characteristic of classic galactosemia. Since these changes do not occur in galactokinase deficiency (see below), it may be presumed that they are the result of galactose-1-phosphate accumulation.

CLINICAL MANIFESTATIONS. Occasionally infants with galactosemia have cataracts at birth. More typically the symptoms of galactosemia begin within a few days or weeks of birth. The infant takes feedings poorly, vomits frequently, and may have diarrhea. Many galactosemic infants die in the first few weeks of life. Progressive hepatomegaly and ascites may enlarge the abdomen. Jaundice usually appears quite early, and the disorder has at times been mistaken for hemolytic disease of the newborn. Proteinuria and generalized aminoaciduria are constant findings. If cataracts are not present at birth, they may develop within a few weeks, or in some instances not for many months. Mental retardation becomes evident as the infant matures. Administration of large galactose loads, as in the performance of galactose tolerance tests, may produce dangerous hypoglycemia.

DIAGNOSIS. Classic galactosemia is diagnosed by demonstrating that galactose-1-P uridyl transferase activity is absent or nearly absent from the erythrocytes.

TREATMENT. The treatment of galactosemia consists of immediate institution of a diet with a very low galactose content. Because milk contains a high concentration of lactose, a disaccharide of glucose and galactose, a milk substitute such as Nutramigen must be fed during infancy. Although the effectiveness of the low-galactose diet in infants is established, no data are available regarding the necessity for maintaining strict dietary control after the first few years of life. It is likely that the ingestion of small amounts of galactose is relatively harmless after the fifth or sixth year of life. However, until further evidence is available regarding the possible harmful effects of galactose when fed to older galactosemic children and adults, it is probably wise to continue a moderate degree of dietary restriction throughout life.

PROGNOSIS. Untreated infants with classic galactosemia rarely survive more than a few months, and may succumb within a few days. A few cases first diagnosed in later childhood or early adult life are known. With the prompt institution of a low-galactose diet, the development of galactosemic children appears to be normal or nearly so. If treatment is delayed, however, some degree of permanent mental retardation and irreversible cataracts are often present. Signs of liver failure and growth retardation appear to respond promptly to therapy in most instances, and patients who are treated generally survive into adult life.

PREVENTION. Galactosemia can be prevented only through the effects of genetic counseling. Heterozygotes for classic galactosemia have one half normal galactose-1-P uridyl transferase activity in their red cells. However, not all persons with this level of enzyme activity are carriers of galactosemia. Persons homozygous for the gene for the Duarte variant also have one half normal transferase activity, but may be differentiated from those heterozygous for galactosemia on the basis of the electrophoretic properties of the red cell enzyme.

Prevention of the clinical sequelae of galactosemia by early diagnosis and prompt institution of treatment is the most practical means of control. Microbiologic and enzymatic methods for the detection of galactose in the blood or in the urine have been developed and will detect most cases of classic galactosemia in the neonatal period. However, some false positive results are encountered, and false negative results will be found in infants who are so ill as to refuse their feedings. A fluorescent screening test which depends directly upon galactose-1-P uridyl transferase activity will reliably detect classic galactosemia even from cord blood. Prenatal diagnosis can be achieved by assaying cultured amniotic cells for galactose-1-P uridyl transferase.

Segal, S: Disorders of galactose metabolism. In Stanbury, J. B., Wyngaarden, J. B., and Fredrickson, D. S. (eds.): The Metabolic Basis of Inherited Disease. 4th ed. New York, McGraw-Hill Book Company, 1978, pp. 160–181.

GALACTOKINASE DEFICIENCY

ETIOLOGY. Galactokinase deficiency is a hereditary disorder caused by an autosomally inherited enzyme deficiency.

INCIDENCE. Only about 25 families with galactokinase deficiency have been described. Limited data accumulated since 1965 suggest that the incidence may be of the order of 1 in 500,000 births. It is probable that as many as 1 in 100 patients developing cataracts of unknown origin during the first year of life may have this defect.

PATHOGENESIS. Galactokinase catalyzes the first step of galactose metabolism (see above). A deficiency of galactokinase results in the accumulation of galactose in the body, and in the formation of cataracts through the same mechanism outlined under Classic Galactosemia.

It is uncertain whether only galactokinase-deficient individuals with virtually total absence of the enzyme develop cataracts. Since galactokinase is the limiting enzyme in galactose metabolism, it is possible that repeated large galactose loads may result in lenticular damage even in individuals heterozygous for galactokinase deficiency who have one half normal galactokinase activity. An increased incidence of cataracts has been noted among heterozygotes in some families of galactokinase-deficient persons. However, most individuals heterozygous for galactokinase deficiency do not develop cataracts, and the link between partial galactokinase deficiency and cataracts is not firmly established.

CLINICAL MANIFESTATIONS. The only clinical manifestation of galactokinase deficiency is the development of cataracts. Elevated blood galactose levels and galactosuria may be found after ingestion of galactose. A seizure disorder has been described in conjunction with galactokinase deficiency; however, it is not at all clear that a cause-and-effect relationship existed.

DIAGNOSIS. The diagnosis of galactokinase deficiency should be considered in any person developing cataracts of unknown cause during childhood. The diagnosis is established by assaying the galactokinase activity of the red blood cells.

TREATMENT. The treatment of galactokinase deficiency consists of institution of a low-galactose diet (see above).

PROGNOSIS. If a low-galactose diet is initiated at the time of birth or shortly thereafter, cataract formation is prevented. When cataracts are already present, improvement, if any, seems to be very limited.

PREVENTION. The effects of galactokinase deficiency can be prevented by early detection and institution of a low-galactose diet. The heterozygote may be identified by measuring galactokinase activity in red cells. However, one half normal levels of galactokinase are also commonly encountered as an apparently harmless polymorphism in the black population. Genetic counseling can be carried out with families in which a case of galactokinase deficiency has been found. Screening of the blood of neonates by methods which detect increased blood galactose level makes possible early detection so that treatment can be instituted promptly.

Beutler, E., Matsumoto, F., Kuhl, W., Krill, A., Levy, N., Sparkes, R., and Degnan, M.: Galactokinase deficiency as a cause of cataracts. N. Engl. J. Med., 288:1203, 1973.

Gitzelmann, R., Steinmann, B., Mitchell, B., and Haigis, E.: Uridine diphosphate galactose 4'-epimerase deficiency. IV. Report of eight cases in three families. Helv. Paediat. Acta, 31:441, 1976.

Kalckar, H. M., Kinoshita, J. H., and Donnell, G. N.: Galactosemia: Biochemistry, genetics, patho-physiology, and developmental aspects. Biol. Brain Dysfunct., 1:31, 1972.

Segal, S.: Disorders of galactose metabolism. In Stanbury, J. B., Wyngaarden, J. B., and Fredrickson, D. S. (eds.): The Metabolic Basis of Inherited Disease. 4th ed. New York, McGraw-Hill Book Company, 1978, pp. 160–181.

531.4. GLYCOGEN STORAGE DISEASE

J. B. Sidbury, Jr.

DEFINITION. The glycogenoses are a group of heritable disorders of altered glycogen metabolism. Excluded are conditions associated with secondary glycogen accumulation such as Mauriac's syndrome and steroid therapy. A glycogen storage disease was the first inborn error of metabolism to be enzymatically defined. Cori's original classification into four types has been extended progressively to 13. Additions to the original classification have been made in the chronology of the enzymatic definition, except for Type 0 which is so designated because it is characterized by a deficiency of glycogen. Subtypes are designated to reflect different clinical presentation of the same enzymatic defect or when differences in the enzyme can be discerned without a distinguishing phenotypic pattern.

ETIOLOGY. The evidence available is compatible with autosomal recessive transmission except in Type IX which is sex linked. The symptoms associated with Types 0, I, III, IV, IX, XI, and XII can be ascribed to the inadequacy of liver glycogen availability, and the severity of symptoms is related to the degree of impediment in glycogen conversion to blood glucose. In Type IV the symptoms evolve from the resultant cirrhosis. The muscle glycogenoses, Types V, VII, VIII, and X, have symptoms resulting from the inadequacy of glycolysis in the muscle which is usually evident only with vigorous exercise.

CLINICAL MANIFESTATIONS. The enzymatic deficiency of Type 0 results in inadequate rate of glycogen synthesis, and since the rate of degradation is normal, the inadequate glycogen stores are rapidly depleted and hypoglycemia results. Gluconeogenesis alone is inadequate in the infant to sustain the blood glucose. Symptoms are often not manifest until the frequency of feedings is decreased. The other *liver forms* of glycogenosis (see accompanying table) may have symptoms so similar as to be clinically indistinguishable, and the symptoms vary from difficult, symptomatic hypoglycemia and ketoacidosis to essentially asymptomatic hepatomegaly. Types I, III, and VI are more likely to be symptomatic, and the associated findings seen are susceptibility to infections, bleeding tendency, short stature, mild cushingoid features, excessive sweating, and eruptive xanthoma. An occasional patient with Type III may develop a late-onset myopathy severe enough to require differentiation from polymyositis. Gout is unique to Type I, and it is not generally symptomatic until after puberty despite an elevation of uric acid throughout the course. The clinical management of the more symptomatic individuals is most difficult in the first five years of life. As a rule all symptoms and the hepatomegaly resolve with puberty or before in all the classic hepatic types except Type I. In patients with Type IV defect, death almost invariably supervenes as a result of the cirrhosis and portal hypertension before puberty. This is the only glycogen storage disease with splenomegaly.

The *muscle types* of glycogenosis, V, VII, VIII, and X, involve striated muscle. The symptoms may be first noted in early childhood (V, VII, and X) or not until the mature years (VIII). The day-to-day symptoms are unimpressive as are the physical findings, and these individuals are often labeled psychoneurotic for several years before the diagnosis is made. Vigorous exercise is associated with weakness, muscle cramps, and occasionally myoglobinuria. Symptoms tend to be slowly progressive. Seizures associated with myoglobinuria have been reported in individuals with the phosphorylase defect.

Type IIa designates classic *Pompe's disease* or generalized glycogenosis which is seen in infants who appear to be normal for the first two or three months of life and progress to flaccidity, absent reflexes, gross cardiomegaly, and death by one year of age. Patients with Type IIb, with apparently the same enzyme defect, do not have the heart involvement and present simulating relatively severe muscular dystrophy in the first few years of life or as a progressive myopathy in the teen years or later. A variant of Type II with late onset myopathy has been described with low α-glucosidase activity with a reduced enzyme K_m.

DIAGNOSIS. The definite diagnosis of glycogen storage disease is made by enzymatic assay of liver and/or muscle obtained by biopsy. The glycogen is characterized and the content determined. Enzymatic assays of leukocytes can be useful in Types III, IV, VI, and IX. Skin fibroblasts grown in culture have been shown to be useful in diagnosis and in the determination of heterozygosity in Types II and IV, and antenatal diagnosis is possible using these techniques. An antibody to glucose-6-phosphatase has been prepared which will detect the enzyme in the serum of normal individuals and give no precipitin lines with the sera of patients with Type I glycogenosis. The response of blood glucose and lactate to the glucagon tolerance test is useful in that the blood glucose usually does not respond in Types I, III, and VI, and in Type I the lactate

The Enzymatically Defined Glycogenoses

Type	Defect	
0	UDPG-glycogen transferase	(L)
Ia	Glucose-6-phosphatase	(L)
Ib	Glucose-6-phosphatase, functionally	(L)
IIa,b	Lysosomal α-1,4-glucosidase	(M)
IIIa,	Amylo-1,6-glucosidase and/or	
b,c,d	oligo-1,4→1,4-glucantransferase*	(L)
IV	Amylo-1,4→1,6-transglucosylase*	(L)
V	Muscle phosphorylase	(M)
VI	Liver phosphorylase	(L)
VII	Phosphofructokinase	(M)
VIII	Phosphohexosisomerase	(M)
IX	Phosphorylase kinase	(L)
X	Phosphorylase kinase	(M)
XI	Phosphoglucomutase	(L)
XII	Cyclic 3',5'-AMP dependent kinase	(L)

*Glycogen structure abnormal.
(L) Symptoms related to liver.
(M) Symptoms related to muscles.

is high in the fasting state with a further increase in response to the glucagon. The red cell glycogen may be elevated markedly in Type III.

Types V, VII, VIII, and X are characterized by absence of rise in blood lactate consequent to anoxic exercise. This is performed by having the subject exercise the hand with the blood pressure cuff above the elbow inflated above systolic pressure and by obtaining blood from the antecubital vein at intervals for several minutes. The normal individual will have a two- to four-fold rise, whereas the muscle glycogen patients will have none. Type II glycogenosis patients show no abnormality of carbohydrate metabolism that can be approached through blood sampling. Electromyography can be helpful. In the muscle glycogenosis of impaired glycolysis, the signal becomes isoelectric after a period of vigorous exercise. The "dive bomber" effect is characteristically found in Type IIb glycogen storage. Type IIa muscle does not demonstrate a characteristic finding.

TREATMENT. Types I, II, III, IV, and VI are the most likely to be management problems. Individuals with the Type I defect are at risk of severe ketoacidosis in association with infection in the early years. This complication, like the symptomatic hypoglycemia which is frequently seen, is best managed by frequent high carbohydrate feedings. Portacaval shunt has been found to relieve many of the biochemical and physical aberrations. Frequent glucose feedings during the day and constant infusion of glucose of Vivonex at night have been found effective in the therapy of Type I in lieu of the operative shunt. Patients with Type III glycogenosis and the occasional patient with the other forms of hepatic glycogenoses who are symptomatic will respond to a high protein diet with additional carbohydrates when symptomatic. Patients with Type IV glycogenosis are treated symptomatically as one would treat any other child with cirrhosis and portal hypertension. The infant with Type II glycogenosis is managed symptomatically. Digitalis is used for heart failure, but there is little evidence of its efficacy. Patients with glycogen myopathies associated with impaired glycolysis are symptomatic when engaged in vigorous exercise. They must be taught to modulate their activity and seek employment appropriate to their physical capacities. It is reported that fructose administration will help patients with Type VIII glycogen storage disease.

Cori, G. T.: Glycogen structure and enzyme deficiencies in glycogen storage disease. Harvey Lectures, 48:145, 1953.
Moses, S. W., and Gutman, A.: Inborn errors of glycogen metabolism. In Schulman, I. (ed.): Adv. Pediat., 19:95, 1972.

531.5. PENTOSURIA
(Essential Pentosuria)
J. B. Sidbury, Jr.

Pentosuria is a clinically asymptomatic, rare, heritable abnormality of carbohydrate metabolism limited almost exclusively to Jews. It is transmitted as an autosomal recessive condition, with estimated incidence of 1:2000 to 1:5000 of the population at risk. Loading of the glucuronic acid cycle by oral administration of glucuronolactone will cause an increase in urinary 1-xylulose excretion in the homozygote and a lesser response in the heterozygote. Assay of the erythrocytes of affected individuals has demonstrated a deficiency of the specific NADP-linked xylitol dehydrogenase which converts 1-xylulose to xylitol and has further shown that the affinity of the mutant enzyme for NADP is signficantly less than that from normal individuals. As a consequence of the enzyme reduction in the liver, affected individuals excrete 1 to 4 grams of 1-xylulose in the urine daily. The sugar can easily be distinguished from others by paper or thin-layer chromatography. Glucose oxidase, which is the reagent in the dip-stick type of urine test, will not react with this sugar, whereas the reducing methods will. The practical importance of proper identification is in preventing the individual from being labeled a diabetic for treatment and insurance purposes.

Hiatt, H. H.: Pentosuria. In Stanbury, J. B., Wyngaarden, J. B., and Fredrickson, D. S. (eds.): The Metabolic Basis of Inherited Disease. 4th ed. New York, McGraw-Hill Book Company, 1978, p. 110.
Wang, Y. M., and VanEys, J.: The enzymatic defect in essential pentosuria. N. Engl. J. Med., 282:892, 1970.

531.6. FRUCTOSURIA AND HEREDITARY FRUCTOSE INTOLERANCE
J. B. Sidbury, Jr.

FRUCTOSURIA (ESSENTIAL FRUCTOSURIA). Fructosuria is an asymptomatic, rare, autosomal recessive condition resulting from a deficiency of fructokinase, which is the first reaction in the major pathway of fructose metabolism. The incidence of the condition is estimated to be 1:130,000. Fructokinase is normally found only in the liver, kidney, and intestinal mucosa. The diagnosis can be surmised by performing a fructose loading test determining the fructose rise in the blood by difference between total reducing substance and glucose and by identifying the fructose excreted in the urine by chromatography. Normally, under loading conditions the blood fructose will peak at one hour and not exceed 25 mg per 100 ml. No significant fructosuria occurs. Fructose will not react with glucose oxidase but will reduce copper sulfate, even at 80° C. The proper diagnosis is important to the patient in order to prevent his being labeled or treated as a diabetic.

HEREDITY FRUCTOSE INTOLERANCE. This is an autosomal recessive condition associated with a structural alteration of phosphofructoaldolase B. The adult will commonly note dyspepsia and anxiety with fructose ingestion but usually will have learned to avoid offending foods through personal observation. The untreated infant will have vomiting, failure to grow, hypotonia, jaundice, hepatosplenomegaly, ascites, bleeding disorder, hypoglycemia, hypophosphatemia, abnormal liver function tests, aminoacidemia, acidosis, uric acid elevation, proteinuria, mellituria (fructose and sometimes galactose and glucose also), and aminoaciduria. The clinical presentation and findings often make the differential diagnosis between this condition, tyrosinosis, and galactosemia very difficult indeed. Liver biopsy reveals portal and interlobal fibrosis without cellular infiltrate, steatosis, bile retention, and rosette formation. The reported pathology in the kidney is variable. The brain may show diminished neurons. The mechanism of the symptomatology is unclear when the defect is defined in terms of the inability to cleave fructose-1-phosphate to the corresponding trioses. That the symptoms might be similar to those of galactosemia is not surprising, because galactose-1-phosphate accumulates in the cells in galactosemia. In fructose intolerance fructose-1-phosphate accumulates in the liver and kidney, the two primary organs in which fructose is metabolized. Thus symptoms are secondary or tertiary phenomena. The hypoglycemia results from a marked decrease in glucose production by the liver very shortly after fructose loading in these individuals. In spite of the recurrent hypoglycemia in infancy, the affected adults evaluated have had normal intelligence.

The defective enzyme, phosphofructoaldolase B or liver aldolase, has been shown to be decreased in total activity but more specifically to function in a manner analogous to aldolase A or muscle aldolase in that aldolase B normally demonstrates a 1:1 ratio of activity for fructose-1-phosphate and fructose-1,6-diphosphate, whereas aldolase A normally has a ratio of activity for these substrates of approximately 0.1 to 0.2. Kinetic studies of the mutant enzyme have shown a markedly reduced affinity for fructose-1-phosphate. Immunologically the mutant enzyme cross-reacts with the normal and quantitatively correlates with the activity for fructose diphosphate. The enzyme in the liver of parents showed no abnormality.

A presumptive *diagnosis* can be made in an individual whose symptoms are suggstive by an oral or intravenous loading test. Serious hypoglycemia can be induced; hence modified loading doses are recommended, e.g., 0.5 gram per kilogram of body weight orally or 0.25 gram per kilogram intravenously, or 3 grams per square meter of body surface area in children. Demonstrating resultant hypoglycemia, fructosemia, hypophosphatemia, and fructosuria constitutes presumptive evidence for the diagnosis. *Management*, once the diagnosis is made, is simply avoidance of fruits and foods with sucrose.

Froesch, E. R.: Essential fructosuria, hereditary fructose intolerance, and fructose-1,6-diphosphatase deficiency. *In* Stanbury, J. B., Wyngaarden, J. B., and Fredrickson, D. S. (eds.): The Metabolic Basis of Inherited Disease. 4th ed. New York, McGraw-Hill Book Company, 1978, p. 121.

Nordmann, Y., and Schapira, F.: Intolérance au fructose. Biochimie, 54:741, 1972.

Odievre, M., Gantier, M., and Rieu, D.: Intolérance héréditaire au fructose du nourrison. Arch. Franç. Péd., 26:433, 1969.

531.7. PRIMARY HYPEROXALURIA

Lloyd H. Smith, Jr.

Primary hyperoxaluria is a general term for two rare genetic disorders of glyoxylate metabolism productive of excessive synthesis and urinary excretion of oxalic acid. Both disorders are transmitted as autosomal recessive traits. The diseases are characterized by the onset in childhood of recurrent calcium oxalate nephrolithiasis or nephrocalcinosis, or both, usually leading to early death secondary to renal failure. At postmortem examination calcium oxalate may be found widely deposited in extrarenal sites, a condition known as oxalosis. More rarely, milder forms of the disease may be found in adults. Although oxalate is an important constituent in approximately two thirds of all kidney stones, most adult patients with calcium oxalate nephrolithiasis excrete normal amounts of urinary oxalate.

Primary hyperoxaluria Type I (glycolic aciduria) represents a genetic defect in the soluble enzyme α-ketoglutarate: glyoxylate carboligase. The resulting accumulation of glyoxylate leads to its excessive oxidation to oxalate and its reduction to glycolate, both of which are excreted in increased amounts in the urine (more than 60 mg per 1.73 square meters per 24 hours each). In *primary hyperoxaluria Type II* (L-glyceric aciduria) there is a defect in the enzyme D-glyceric dehydrogenase. Hydroxypyruvate accumulates and is reduced by lactic dehydrogenase (LDH) to L-glyceric acid, a compound which is undetectable in normal urine. The reduction of hydroxypyruvate to L-glycerate is probably coupled to the oxidation of glyoxylate to oxalate, both catalyzed by LDH. Each disease can be diagnosed by the characteristic pattern of metabolites in urine: Type I, oxalate and glycolate; Type II, oxalate and L-glycerate. Pyridoxine deficiency in laboratory animals and man also leads to hyperoxaluria and even oxalosis with urinary pattern similar to that of the genetic disease Type I. With the onset of renal failure the clearance of oxalate is reduced (its clearance is normally about 1.2 times that of creatinine) so that its urinary excretion may return to normal. The diagnosis may then be difficult to establish because of the unreliability of current methods for measuring serum oxalate.

No specific methods of treatment are now available. Efforts are directed toward reducing the amount of oxalate excreted and increasing its solubility. Large amounts of pyridoxine (200 to 400 mg per 24 hours) may decrease oxalate excretion in the Type I disease. Dilute urine should be maintained by forcing fluids, and a phosphate or magnesium oxide supplement may offer partial protection against stone formation. Attempts at renal homotransplantation have been disappointing because of rapid deposition of calcium oxalate in the transplanted kidney. Chronic dialysis and pyridoxine are therefore indicated when renal failure is severe. A search for an inhibitor of oxalate synthesis is being conducted.

Increased urinary excretion of oxalate and stone diathesis (in the absence of glycolic aciduria or L-glyceric aciduria) occurs in many patients who have small bowel disease and malabsorption. Normally oxalate and fatty acids of the small intestine compete for available calcium ion, and calcium oxalate is poorly absorbed. This important form of acquired hyperoxaluria results from excessive absorption of dietary oxalate in the presence of significant steatorrhea. It can be controlled by a low oxalate diet.

Boquist, L., Lindquist, B., Östberg, Y., and Steen, L.: Primary oxalosis. Am. J. Med., 54:673, 1973.

Earnest, D. L., Johnson, G., Williams, H. E., and Admirand, W. H.: Hyperoxaluria in patients with ileal resection: An abnormality in dietary oxalate absorption. Gastroenterology, 66:1114, 1974.

Hockaday, T. D. R., Clayton, J. E., Frederick, E. W., and Smith, L. H., Jr.: Primary hyperoxaluria. Medicine, 43:315, 1964.

Williams, H. E., and Smith, L. H., Jr.: Disorders of oxalate metabolism. Am. J. Med., 45:715, 1968.

Williams, H. E., and Smith, L. H., Jr.: Primary hyperoxaluria. *In* Stanbury, J. B. Wyngaarden, J. B., and Fredrickson, D. S. (eds.): The Metabolic Basis of Inherited Disease. 4th ed. New York, McGraw-Hill Book Company, 1978, p. 182.

532. DISORDERS OF LIPID METABOLISM

Richard J. Havel

532.1. INTRODUCTION

Changes in the concentration of lipids in blood plasma occur in a variety of disease states or as a result of inborn errors. In the former, they may provide a clue to diagnosis of the underlying condition. More important, deleterious consequences may occur in both, including premature atherosclerotic vascular disease and recurrent pancreatitis. Taken together, the inborn hyperlipidemias are among the most common metabolic diseases. It is important to recognize them, because reasonably effective treatment is available which may prevent disability and delay death.

532.2. TRANSPORT OF LIPIDS IN THE BLOOD

Because of their insolubility in aqueous environment, essentially all lipids in blood plasma are in complexes (lipoproteins) containing amphiphilic substances which permit the dispersal of the lipids into small particles. The major lipids transported are fatty acids and cholesterol. Fatty acids exist as such in a complex with albumin and as esters of which the main transport form is triglyceride. The former are called free fatty acids (FFA) to indicate that their carboxyl groups are not in ester linkage. Cholesterol is also present in the "free" state (alcohol group not in ester linkage), but it is transported mainly as esters of fatty acids. The normal plasma lipoproteins are spherical particles in which a monolayer of polar lipids (phospholipids and free cholesterol) together with specific apoproteins surround a nonpolar core containing mainly triglycerides and cholesteryl esters (Fig. 1).

EXOGENOUS FAT (TRIGLYCERIDE) TRANSPORT. Dietary fat, after hydrolysis to form partial glycerides and fatty acids, is absorbed from micelles containing conjugated bile acids. From these products, triglycerides are resynthesized in the mucosal cells of the small intestine, appear in particulate form in the Golgi region, and are secreted into the intestinal lacteals. In the lymph, they appear as chylomicrons and are delivered into the blood through the thoracic duct. Normally, chylomicrons are present only during active absorption of fat, because their life span in the blood is only a few minutes. Triglycerides in the core of chylomicrons are removed primarily in tissues other than the liver which contain on the endothelial surface of their capillaries an enzyme, lipoprotein lipase (LPL), which hydrolyzes the triglycerides to FFA and glycerol. These products readily diffuse across the capillary and other cell membranes where they are stored or oxidized.

ENDOGENOUS FAT TRANSPORT. Triglycerides, derived from fat transported in the blood or synthesized from nonlipid precursors, are stored mainly in adipose tissue. Normally, these triglycerides are hydrolyzed to FFA and glycerol at a variable rate controlled by the action of hormones and the adrenergic innervation of the tissue on a "hormone-sensitive" lipase. Catecholamines and growth hormone increase lipase activity, whereas insulin reduces it. The FFA, as albumin complexes, are rapidly transported to various tissues to be oxidized or stored temporarily as lipid esters. They are also the major precursors of endogenous plasma triglycerides, secreted continuously by the liver in particles similar to, but smaller than, chylomicrons (very low density, pre-beta lipoproteins, VLDL; Fig. 1). In the postprandial state, these triglycerides may be derived from dietary fatty acids or from fatty acids synthesized de novo in the liver; in the fasting state, they are derived mainly from plasma FFA. This pathway appears to provide a mechanism for exporting excess fatty acids to sites of storage or oxidation. The metabolism of VLDL-triglycerides resembles that of chylomicrons, but their disposal is less efficient, and they remain in the blood for a considerably longer period.

TRANSPORT OF CHOLESTEROL. Most circulating cholesteryl esters are produced within the blood plasma by transfer of a fatty acid residue from lecithin to cholesterol in a reaction catalyzed by the enzyme lecithin–cholesterol acyltransferase (LCAT) acting upon high density lipoproteins (HDL). "Nascent" HDL are secreted from the liver as discoidal particles composed of a bilayer of phospholipids and free cholesterol stabilized by specific apoproteins. The esters formed by LCAT are stored within the particle to form the normal pseudomicellar plasma HDL or are transferred to other lipo-

PROPERTIES OF PLASMA LIPOPROTEINS

CLASS	HDL	LDL	VLDL			CHYLOMICRONS		
• DIAMETER (Å)	100	200	300	500	800	800	2000	5000
• DENSITY	1.06-1.21	1.006-1.063	0.95 – 1.006			0.94		
• ELECTROPHORETIC MOBILITY	α_1	β	PRE-β			ORIGIN		
PER CENT • COMPOSITION								
• PROTEIN	50	20	15	7	4	4	2	1
• PHOSPHOLIPIDS	25	25	25	18	13	13	8	3
• CHOLESTEROL (FREE + ESTERS)	20	50	45	22	13	13	8	3
• TRIGLYCERIDES	5	5	15	53	70	70	82	93

Figure 1. Properties of plasma lipoproteins. (From Havel, R. J.: Adv. Intern. Med., 15:117, 1969.)

Figure 2. Model for transport of cholesterol in plasma lipoproteins. (From Havel, R. J., Goldstein, J. L., and Brown, M. S., *In* Bondy, P. K., and Rosenberg, L. E. [eds.]: Metabolic Control and Disease. 8th ed. Philadelphia, W. B. Saunders Company, in press.)

proteins. Cholesteryl esters also enter the blood as core components of chylomicrons. These esters, together with esters transferred from HDL, remain in chylomicron "remnants" when triglycerides are removed in various extrahepatic tissues and are subsequently taken up in the liver. The surface cholesterol and lecithin remaining when remnants are formed from chylomicrons or VLDL are transferred in part to HDL as substrates for LCAT. In addition, the same lipids can be transferred to HDL from the surface membranes of cells to provide a pathway for transport of cholesterol from extrahepatic tissues to the liver. In humans, most plasma cholesteryl esters are carried in low density lipoproteins (LDL). LDL are normally formed as an end product of the catabolism of VLDL, presumably through the action of the liver on VLDL-remnants. LDL are removed mainly in extrahepatic tissues by interaction with a specific high-affinity receptor, followed by endocytosis and catabolism in lysosomes. Some LDL are removed by a nonspecific "scavenger" pathway (presumably bulk fluid endocytosis). The cholesteryl esters and free cholesterol in LDL normally supply most of the cholesterol needed by extrahepatic cells for membrane synthesis and synthesis of steroid hormones. The pathways of cholesterol transport in lipoproteins are depicted in Figure 2.

ROLE OF APOLIPOPROTEINS. At least four major groups of apoproteins (termed A, B, and C apoproteins and an arginine-rich apoprotein) have essential roles in lipid transport. The C apoproteins are synthesized in the liver and are transferred from HDL to newly secreted triglyceride-rich lipoproteins. One of them facilitates the hydrolysis of triglycerides by lipoprotein lipase. The A apoproteins are synthesized in both intestine and liver. One of them facilitates the action of lecithin–cholesterol acyl transferase in HDL. The B apoprotein is essential for the formation of VLDL and chylomicrons. In the process of metabolism of triglycerides and cholesterol in chylomicrons and VLDL, this apoprotein appears in LDL. The arginine-rich apoprotein (also called apoprotein E) is synthesized in the liver and is thought to play a role in remnant catabolism.

Dietschy, J. M., Gotto, Jr., A. M., and Ontko, J. A. (eds.): Disturbances in Lipid and Lipoprotein Metabolism. Bethesda, Md., American Physiological Society, 1978, pp. 213–284.
Havel, R. J., Goldstein, J. L., and Brown, M. S.: Lipoproteins and lipid

transport. *In* Bondy, P. K., and Rosenberg, L. E. (eds.): Metabolic Control and Disease. 8th ed. Philadelphia, W. B. Saunders Company, in press.

532.3. CLASSIFICATION OF DISORDERS OF LIPID TRANSPORT

Several classification systems have been devised to distinguish the disorders discussed in these chapters. For the primary disorders, a classification based upon identification of abnormal gene products is ultimately to be preferred, and it will be used when possible. Diagnosis of the common primary hyperlipoproteinemias depends largely upon analysis of blood serum and examination of the familial distribution of abnormal concentrations of lipoproteins. For this purpose, the concentration of total triglycerides and cholesterol in plasma must be determined. These measurements usually permit a fair estimation of the concentration of VLDL and LDL, respectively. The estimate of LDL can be improved by separate measurement of the fraction of total cholesterol associated with HDL. Unlike the direct measurement of LDL-cholesterol, measurement of HDL-cholesterol is simple and does not require special equipment, such as an ultracentrifuge or electrophoretic apparatus. Subtraction of the sum of HDL-cholesterol and the calculated VLDL-cholesterol (estimated from plasma triglyceride concentration) from the total cholesterol gives a good estimate of LDL-cholesterol, provided that the cholesterol:triglyceride ratio in VLDL is normal. Chylomicrons can be evaluated qualitatively by inspection of fasting plasma after storage overnight in a refrigerator. Because of their large size and tendency to aggregate in the cold, these particles rise to form a creamy layer at the surface of the sample.

These four analyses (i.e., total cholesterol, total triglycerides, HDL-cholesterol, and appearance of plasma) permit the concentrations of the major lipoprotein classes to be determined accurately in the great majority of cases. Additional tests that are sometimes needed will be described under the individual disorders. The classification of lipid disorders based upon the concentrations of specific lipoproteins, usually referred to as "phenotyping," is of only limited use in defining the specific primary or secondary disorders of lipid transport. However, phenotypic descriptors are still needed to communicate simply the nature of the lipoprotein abnormality in the many patients for whom a genetic diagnosis is not possible. The accompanying table indicates these descriptors of the hyperlipidemias and lists the disorders with which they are associated.

Havel, R. J.: Classfication of the hyperlipidemias. Ann. Rev. Med., 28:195, 1977.

532.4. NORMAL REGULATION OF PLASMA LIPOPROTEIN CONCENTRATION

Apart from chylomicrons, all lipoprotein classes are present in blood plasma at all times. Among these, the concentration of VLDL, the carrier of endogenous triglycerides, is most variable and is a function of the rate of hepatic triglyceride synthesis. This rate, in turn, depends upon rate of uptake of FFA from the blood or

Hyperlipidemic Disorders*

Generic Designation and Elevated Lipo-protein Class	Synonym	Primary Disorders	Secondary Disorders†
Exogenous hyperlipemia (chylomicrons)	Type I	Familial lipoprotein lipase deficiency Unclassified‡	Dysglobulinemias Systemic lupus erythematosus
Endogenous hyperlipemia (VLDL)	Type IV	Familial hypertriglyceridemia 　(mild form) Familial multiple lipoprotein-type 　hyperlipidemia Sporadic hypertriglyceridemia Tangier disease	Diabetic hyperlipemia§ Glycogenosis, Type I Lipodystrophies Dysglobulinemias Uremia Hypopituitarism Nephrotic syndrome (Diabetes mellitus)¶
Mixed hyperlipemia (VLDL + chylomicrons)	Type V	Familial hypertriglyceridemia 　(severe form) Familial lipoprotein lipase deficiency 　(during pregnancy)	(Alcoholism) (Estrogen use) (Glucocorticoid use) (Stress-induced)
Hypercholesterolemia (LDL)	Type II-a	Familial hypercholesterolemia (LDL 　receptor defects) Familial multiple lipoprotein-type 　hyperlipidemia Polygenic hypercholesterolemia (includes 　exogenous hypercholesterolemia)	Nephrotic syndrome Hypothyroidism Dysglobulinemias Cushing's syndrome Acute intermittent porphyria Hepatoma
Combined hyperlipidemia (LDL + VLDL)	Type II-b	Familial multiple lipoprotein-type 　hyperlipidemia Unclassified	Nephrotic syndrome Hypothyroidism Dysglobulinemias Cushing's syndrome (Glucocorticoid use) (Stress-induced)
Remnant hyperlipidemia (β-VLDL)	Type III	Familial dysbetalipoproteinemia Unclassified	Hypothyroidism Systemic lupus erythematosus
Lamellar hyperlipoproteinemia (vesicular and discoidal lipoproteins)	—	Familial lecithin-cholesterol 　acyltransferase deficiency	Cholestasis (with LP-X) Hepatic failure (with 　lamellar HDL)

*From Havel, R. J., Goldstein, J. L., and Brown, M. S., *In* Bondy, P. K., and Rosenberg, L. E. (eds.): Metabolic Control and Disease. 8th ed. Philadelphia, W. B. Saunders Company, in press.

†Note: all conditions associated with elevated VLDL or β-VLDL are aggravated by hypertrophic obesity.

‡Includes C-II apolipoprotein deficiency.

§Denotes mixed hyperlipemia caused by severe, prolonged insulin deficiency.

¶Parentheses indicate conditions that frequently aggravate a primary hyperlipemia but seldom cause hyperlipemia de novo. These conditions cause some cases of primary hypertriglyceridemia (mild form) to present as mixed hyperlipemia.

synthesis of fatty acids from glucose, and also upon the extent to which the fatty acids are oxidized or converted to triglycerides. Ingestion of glucose initially causes a rapid fall in level of VLDL, presumably related to the accompanying decrease in mobilization of fat from adipose tissue. After one to three days on a high carbohydrate, low fat diet, VLDL level tends to rise. The extent to which this reflects increased hepatic triglyceride synthesis or impaired removal of triglycerides in extrahepatic tissues is uncertain. Ingestion of foodstuffs in excess of need is accompanied by rapid increase in level of VLDL. In addition, in stable obesity, VLDL levels are increased. This has been equated with associated insulin resistance and hyperinsulinism, but the precise mechanism is not clear (see Ch. 474). Increased triglyceride and VLDL levels accompany several other states in which insulin resistance and hyperinsulinism are present.

Plasma levels of LDL and HDL tend to fall as VLDL levels rise. The concentration of HDL is regulated by sex hormones and hence is sex dependent; increases are produced by estrogens and a fall by androgens. The level of LDL is also moderately sensitive to caloric intake, but is influenced more by specific dietary factors. In particular, fats containing saturated fatty acids and cholesterol increase the level of this cholesterol-rich lipoprotein. Substantial differences in lipoprotein levels occur in various population groups throughout the world. The major cause of these differences, which occur predominantly in cholesterol-rich LDL, appears to be dietary (see also Ch. 474).

Conner, W. E., Stone, D. B., and Hodges, R. E.: The interrelated effects of dietary cholesterol and fat upon human serum lipid levels. J. Clin. Invest., 43:1691, 1964.

Dietschy, J. M., Gotto, A. M., Jr., and Ontko, J. A. (eds.): Disturbances in Lipid and Lipoprotein Metabolism. Bethesda, Md., American Physiological Society, 1978, pp. 213–284.

Havel, R. J.: Caloric homeostasis and disorders of fuel transport. N. Engl. J. Med., 287:1186, 1972.

532.5.   INBORN ERRORS OF LIPOPROTEIN METABOLISM

HYPERLIPOPROTEINEMIAS

Whereas characterization of the lipoprotein class or classes responsible for hyperlipoproteinemia in a patient is generally straightforward, establishment of a definitive diagnosis in inherited forms of hyperlipoproteinemia frequently is difficult and may not be possible. There are two major reasons for this. First, lipoprotein concentrations vary with time in an affected individual as well as among affected family members. Second, a given abnormality may represent more than one disorder and pattern of inheritance. Thus both monogenic and polygenic disorders may lead to the same phenotype. Fortunately, treatment usually can be determined simply from quantitative estimation of serum cholesterol and triglycerides, as described earlier, after exclusion of the acquired disorders described below.

Familial Hypercholesterolemia
(Hyperbetalipoproteinemia)

Familial hypercholesterolemia, inherited as a mendelian dominant trait, is characterized by increased concentration of LDL of normal composition. Xanthomas in the tendons, particularly the Achilles, plantar, patellar, and digital extensors of the hands, as well as tuberous xanthomas, xanthelasmas, and early onset of corneal arcus, are frequently encountered. In adults, serum cholesterol concentration usually exceeds 350 mg per 100 ml. In its heterozygous form, the disorder occurs in at least 0.2 per cent of the American population.

ETIOLOGY AND PATHOGENESIS. The disorder results from at least three distinct mutations affecting the function of the high affinity receptor for LDL, leading to a greater use of the less efficient "scavenger" pathway for catabolism of this lipoprotein. In the rare homozygotes, the defect can readily be demonstrated in cultured fibroblasts, which synthesize cholesterol at an abnormally rapid rate when grown in the presence of LDL and fail to take up and catabolize LDL normally.

CLINICAL MANIFESTATIONS. The hyperlipoproteinemia is present from birth or shortly thereafter, and is generally detected as hypercholesterolemia with little or no increase in triglycerides; the xanthomas usually do not appear until after puberty. The patient may not be aware of the presence of large xanthomas in the Achilles or plantar tendons, and the latter may be missed by the physician unless the tendon is put under tension by having the patient extend his toes. Small xanthomas of the extensor tendons of the hands are best detected by observing the tendon while the patient flexes and extends the finger, and small xanthomas in the Achilles tendon are detected by palpation of irregular contour, usually in the central region. Xanthelasmas (raised, yellow plaques about the eyelids near the inner canthus) and corneal arcus are not diagnostic, because they may also be seen in individuals with no discernible abnormality of plasma lipoproteins. The incidence of premature coronary heart disease is several times that of control populations in countries with a "western" culture, and the incidence of peripheral atherosclerotic occlusive disease is also increased. In the homozygous states, the disease is much more severe, with large xanthomas occurring in childhood, together with "malignant" atherosclerotic disease, including calcific aortic stenosis.

DIAGNOSIS. In heterozygotes, the concentration of serum cholesterol is usually about twice normal. However, hypercholesterolemia without hypertriglyceridemia in the absence of known cause, such as hypothyroidism, is not sufficient basis for making a diagnosis unless the cholesterol level exceeds 400 mg per 100 ml. Presence of characteristic xanthomas is diagnostic, and demonstration of familial occurrence (at least one

parent should have hypercholesterolemia) provides strong presumptive evidence. Some individuals or families may have moderate hypertriglyceridemia (combined hyperlipidemia). This must be distinguished from familial dysbetalipoproteinemia, described below. Most normotriglyceridemic individuals whose cholesterol level is 275 to 325 mg per 100 ml (also classified as hypercholesterolemia) have a different disorder, which may be polygenic (see Ch. 532.7).

TREATMENT. No simple method has been devised to reduce lipoprotein levels to normal. Some reduction can be achieved by a diet restricted in saturated fats and cholesterol, with sufficient polyunsaturated fats to provide a total fat intake of 30 to 35 per cent of calories. Nonabsorbable bile acid–binding substances, such as cholestyramine or colestipol (15 to 30 grams daily in divided doses with meals), are more effective. Large doses of nicotinic acid (2 to 8 grams daily in divided doses) may also be effective. When used in combination, these two classes of drugs usually reduce lipoprotein levels to normal. Surgical bypass of the terminal 150 cm of the ileum, which also prevents absorption of bile acids, generally gives good results. Frequent, loose stools are generally produced by this operation. Xanthomatous lesions regress slowly; tendinous lesions seldom disappear. It is reasonable to begin treatment in childhood, although it has not been established that reducing the lipoprotein level will prevent or delay onset of ischemic vascular disease.

Familial Dysbetalipoproteinemia
(Broad-Beta Disease, Type III Hyperlipoproteinemia)

DEFINITION. Familial dysbetalipoproteinemia is an autonormal recessive disorder characterized by accumulation of abnormal beta lipoproteins, which resemble normal pre-beta migrating VLDL in size and flotation characteristics, but differ from them in composition. Planar xanthomas, particularly in the palmar and digital creases, are peculiar to this form of primary hyperlipoproteinemia, but tuberous, tuberoeruptive, and tendinous lesions also occur. It is much rarer than familial hypercholesterolemia; in the older literature, it was frequently called *xanthoma tuberosum*. The mode of inheritance is uncertain.

ETIOLOGY AND PATHOGENESIS. The abnormal lipoprotein contains predominantly the B apoprotein together with an increased amount of the arginine-rich apoprotein, in particles with more cholesteryl ester and less triglyceride than normal VLDL. Its electrophoretic mobility is consequently abnormal, encompassing the beta and extending toward the pre-beta region ("broad beta"). This lipoprotein is thought to represent remnant-VLDL which accumulate because of abnormality in the mechanism responsible for uptake of cholesteryl esters in the liver. The molecular defect appears to reside in the arginine-rich apoprotein. This protein exists normally in three polymorphic forms which differ in their isoelectric points. Patients with familial dysbetalipoproteinemia are homozygous for deficiency of the most basic of these three polymorphic components (apo E-3). Heterozygotes have a reduced amount of apo E-3 but manifest none of the characteristic features of the disease. Population studies indicate that approximately 1 per cent of the population is homozygous and 16 per cent is heterozygous for apo E-3 deficiency. Although abnormal VLDL can virtually always be demonstrated in homozygotes, only a few manifest hyperlipidemia.

Present evidence suggests that other genetic or nongenetic factors are required for expression of hyperlipidemia in homozygotes.

CLINICAL MANIFESTATIONS. The disorder is seldom discovered before early adult life and is usually manifested by appearance of xanthomas when the patient gains weight. The patient may be unaware of the characteristic planar xanthomas which are yellow to orange and tend to fill the palmar and digital creases; they may also appear over the dorsal surfaces of the hands. The tuberous xanthomas tend to be smaller and more numerous than in hyperbetalipoproteinemia and are often confluent and surrounded by an erythematous halo ("tuberoeruptive"). They occur most commonly over the knees and elbows and on the buttocks. Tendinous lesions are usually in the extensors of the hands. Premature coronary and especially peripheral atherosclerotic vascular disease are quite common.

DIAGNOSIS. Hyperlipidemia characteristically involves both cholesterol and triglycerides (combined hyperlipidemia). The levels of these two lipids are often similar, and they change rapidly with alterations in diet. Many hyperlipidemic patients have the characteristic planar xanthomas which, in the absence of obstructive biliary tract disease, are pathognomonic. The serum is usually lactescent. Lipoprotein electrophoresis shows a "broad-beta" pattern with normal or reduced content of alpha lipoproteins. Slight chylomicronemia is often present when hyperlipoproteinemia is severe. Spurious "broad-beta" bands may be seen in other states, particularly in some of the secondary hyperlipemias. Concentration of LDL is characteristically reduced, presumably because of defective remnant catabolism. Hence normolipidemic homozygotes often have low serum cholesterol levels. Definitive laboratory diagnosis requires demonstration of marked apo E-3 deficiency by isoelectric focusing electrophoresis of the apoproteins of VLDL. Because of the high prevalence of the mutant gene for apo E-3 deficiency in the population, vertical transmission of this recessive trait is occasionally observed ("pseudodominance").

TREATMENT. Diet is the mainstay of treatment. In obese subjects, caloric restriction is almost always very effective. The diet should be restricted in simple sugars and in cholesterol, but total fat intake need not be restricted. Concentration of cholesterol and triglycerides will often fall to normal values. For patients who will not adhere to a dietary program and for the few who respond inadequately, clofibrate (the ethyl ester of p-chlorophenoxyisobutyric acid), 500 mg two to four times daily, will almost always produce a good response. Xanthomas invariably regress or disappear with effective reduction in lipid levels. There is some evidence that atheromatous lesions also regress (see Ch. 532.7). This disorder is greatly aggravated by hypothyroidism, in which a similar lipoprotein may accumulate. For this reason, thyroid function should always be carefully evaluated.

Primary Hypertriglyceridemias

Familial Lipoprotein Lipase Deficiency
(Bürger-Grütz Syndrome, Exogenous Hyperlipemia, Fat-Induced Hyperlipemia, Type I Hyperlipoproteinemia)

DEFINITION. This rare disease, inherited as a recessive trait, is characterized by accumulation of chylomicrons proportional to intake of dietary fat and manifested by recurrent acute pancreatitis, usually beginning in childhood.

ETIOLOGY AND PATHOGENESIS. This disorder is caused by deficient activity of lipoprotein lipase with resultant defective removal of triglycerides from the blood. Hydrolytic activity with the characteristic properties of this enzyme on lipoprotein-bound triglycerides is almost absent in blood plasma obtained a few minutes after intravenous injection of heparin, although another lipase, derived from the liver, is present. No lipoprotein lipase activity can be demonstrated in adipose tissue.

CLINICAL MANIFESTATIONS. Chylomicronemia develops as soon as fat is ingested, and the disorder has been diagnosed during the first week of life. Pancreatitis is very common, and many patients diagnosed in adult life have a history of bouts of abdominal pain in childhood. Abdominal pain, not definable as pancreatitis, has been reported frequently, but causes other than pancreatitis have not been established. Other complications, described rarely, include melena and pretibial ulcers. Like the pancreatitis, they may result from ischemia related to agglomeration of chylomicrons in capillaries. Hepatosplenomegaly, presumably the result of phagocytosis of chylomicrons by reticuloendothelial cells, is common, and hypersplenism has been described. Foam cells may be found in the bone marrow. The endogenous hyperlipemia occurring normally during pregnancy is greatly magnified and may lead to repeated attacks of pancreatitis. In infants and children especially, eruptive xanthomas — small yellow papules in the skin, surrounded by an erythematous halo — may occur when lipemia is severe. Lipemia retinalis — whitish reflection from retinal arterioles and venules — can usually be detected when triglyceride levels in plasma exceed 3000 mg per 100 ml and becomes florid with levels above 5000 mg per 100 ml. Other xanthomas do not occur, and premature atherosclerotic vascular disease has not been described. Carbohydrate metabolism is normal.

DIAGNOSIS. Markedly lactescent blood plasma in a young patient with severe midabdominal pain and no history of alcoholism is presumptive evidence for this disorder or one of the other primary hyperlipemias. In exogenous hyperlipemia, the chylomicrons rise to form a creamy layer when the serum is allowed to stand overnight in the refrigerator and the infranatant serum is usually limpid. Triglyceride concentration is increased far more than that of cholesterol. Triglyceride levels fall dramatically when intake of dietary fat is severely restricted for two to three days. Lipolytic activity, measured in blood plasma obtained ten minutes after intravenous injection of 20 USP units of heparin per kilogram of body weight, is reduced, and activity sensitive to inhibition by 0.5 M NaCl and resistant to antiserum to the hepatic postheparin lipase (characteristics of lipoprotein lipase) is virtually undetectable.

TREATMENT. The only established measure is restriction of dietary fat ("saturated" and "polyunsaturated" fats are equivalent) sufficient to reduce fasting triglyceride levels to 500 mg per 100 ml or less. This usually requires an intake of no more than 30 grams per day by adults. On this regimen, xanthomas disappear and pancreatitis is uniformly prevented. Pretibial ulcers have also healed, and hypersplenism has subsided on this regimen. Once pancreatitis occurs, recurrence is very common when large amounts of fat are ingested and may happen within hours. During pregnancy, complete elimination of fat from the diet may be necessary to control hyperlipemia and minimize the possibility of pancreatitis.

Familial Endogenous and Mixed Hypertriglyceridemias
(Types IV and V Hyperlipoproteinemia)

DEFINITION. These apparently dominant disorders are characterized by elevation of VLDL or of VLDL and chylomicrons. The penetrance of the trait in affected families is quite high, but its expression is usually delayed until after age 20. Affected individuals are often obese and manifest glucose intolerance and hyperinsulinism with insulin resistance.

ETIOLOGY AND PATHOGENESIS. Expression of hypertriglyceridemia in affected individuals appears to involve an exaggerated response to the various factors (especially caloric intake and the state of obesity) that normally tend to increase hepatic secretion of VLDL. The disturbance in carbohydrate metabolism, although common, may not be directly linked to the cause of the disorder. It is not known whether the primary disturbance affects the liver (leading to increased secretion of VLDL), extrahepatic tissues (leading to impaired catabolism of VLDL-triglycerides), or both. In most families, affected individuals manifest solely elevations of VLDL (endogenous hypertriglyceridemia). In a few families some affected individuals also regularly have fasting chylomicronemia as well (mixed hypertriglyceridemia). The disorder in these families may be genetically distinct from the usual form of familial endogenous hypertriglyceridemia.

CLINICAL MANIFESTATIONS. Most commonly, individuals with endogenous hypertriglyceridemia are discovered when patients with ischemic vascular disease are screened for metabolic abnormalities. Although endogenous hypertriglyceridemia is commonly found in individuals who develop such disease prematurely, the incidence of vascular complications is uncertain. Obesity and glucose intolerance are common, but fasting hyperglycemia is rare except in the few individuals who have mixed hypertriglyceridemia. In those with mixed hypertriglyceridemia, eruptive xanthomas and pancreatitis may occur, as in familial lipoprotein lipase deficiency. The incidence of hyperuricemia and hypertension seems to be increased in familial hypertriglyceridemias, especially in the severely affected individuals with mixed hypertriglyceridemia.

DIAGNOSIS. Endogenous hypertriglyceridemia is characterized by lactescent serum in the postabsorptive state, with no layering of chylomicrons upon storage in the cold. Serum triglyceride levels seldom exceed 1000 mg per deciliter. Levels of serum LDL remain normal or reduced so that serum cholesterol levels are normal or, if elevated, are less than half the concentration of triglycerides (expressed as milligrams per 100 ml). With mixed hypertriglyceridemia, serum triglyceride levels usually exceed 1000 mg per deciliter and serum stored in the cold separates into a supernatant creamy layer with persisting lactescence in the infranatant serum. Activity of lipoprotein lipase in postheparin plasma is normal or only moderately reduced in these familial hypertriglyceridemias. Both endogenous and mixed hypertriglyceridemias occur as a result of many other diseases (see Ch. 532.6). Endogenous and mixed hypertriglyceridemias also occur sporadically and endogenous hypertriglyceridemias may be aggravated by various factors, including uncontrolled diabetes mellitus, alcohol abuse, and administration of estrogens, producing the phenotype of mixed hypertriglyceridemia. For these reasons, the diagnosis of familial endogenous and mixed hypertriglyceridemia requires careful investigation of first degree relatives of affected individuals.

TREATMENT. For obese patients, caloric restriction (including ethanol) usually reduces levels of both chylomicrons and VLDL effectively. Restriction of simple sugars may contribute to reduction of triglyceride levels in some patients. For patients of normal body weight, avoidance of intermittent excesses of sugar, fat, or ethanol may be helpful. Hyperglycemia, when present, usually responds to the same measures. However, except in the case of accompanying uncontrolled diabetes, oral sulfonylurea drugs and insulin have no specific effect upon the hypertriglyceridemia. Clofibrate (Atromid-S), given as described for familial dysbetalipoproteinemia, is often effective in patients with endogenous hypertriglyceridemia not responding to diet. For those individuals with severe mixed hypertriglyceridemia that does not respond to diet or to p-chlorophenoxyisobutyrate, nicotinic acid, begun at a dose of 100 mg three times daily and increasing gradually as tolerated to as much as 2.5 grams three times daily, is frequently useful. As in exogenous hypertriglyceridemia, recurrent pancreatitis is prevented by effective reduction of lipoprotein levels and eruptive xanthomas disappear. It has not been shown conclusively that atherosclerotic lesions regress or that progression of ischemic vascular disease is slowed by any of the measures that reduce lipoprotein levels.

Familial Multiple Lipoprotein-Type Hyperlipidemia
(Familial Combined Hyperlipidemia)

DEFINITION. This common disorder, only recently recognized, is characterized by a striking variation in the pattern of serum lipid elevation in affected relatives. The hyperlipidemia may be manifested by elevation of either VLDL or LDL, or both. For this reason the term "familial combined hyperlipidemia," which refers only to elevation of both LDL and VLDL, is confusing. The disorder is commonly observed among survivors of myocardial infarction below age 60.

ETIOLOGY AND PATHOGENESIS. In large affected families, hyperlipidemia appears to be transmitted as a dominant trait, but proof of single-gene inheritance is lacking. As in familial hypertriglyceridemia, hyperlipidemia is seldom manifested below age 20. The expression of hyperlipidemia as elevated VLDL, LDL, or both varies not only among individuals in affected families but also with time in the same individual. Because of the close metabolic relationship between the B apoprotein of VLDL and LDL (see Ch. 532.4), it seems likely that the defect involves regulation of the metabolism of this protein, but the nature of this defect and the reasons for the variable expression of the disorder are obscure.

CLINICAL MANIFESTATIONS. Affected individuals are prone to premature atherosclerotic vascular disease, especially myocardial infarction. As in familial hypertriglyceridemia, the prevalence of obesity, hyperinsulinemia, and glucose intolerance seems to be increased. No xanthomas are present.

DIAGNOSIS. Levels of cholesterol, triglycerides, or both tend to be only slightly elevated in the absence of aggravating factors such as uncontrolled diabetes or ethanol abuse. Documentation of the familial nature and character of the hyperlipidemia requires careful study of first degree relatives, as in familial hypertriglyceridemia. In affected families, about 50 per cent of relatives above age 30 will have lipid levels exceeding the ninety-fifth percentile of the general population, but only 10 to 20 per cent of affected children have elevated lipid levels. Hypertriglyceridemia appears earlier in life than hypercholesterolemia.

TREATMENT. Treatment of elevated triglyceride (VLDL) levels is the same as for familial endogenous hypertriglyceridemia. Patients with elevated cholesterol (LDL) levels usually respond to caloric restriction as necessary for obesity and also to restriction of saturated fats and cholesterol. Individuals not responding to diet may benefit from ethyl ester of p-chlorophenoxyisobutyrate, as described for familial dysbetalipoproteinemia. For persisting elevations of LDL, bile acid–binding resins or nicotinic acid are usually effective.

Fredrickson, D. S., Brown, M. S., and Goldstein, J. L.: The familial hyperlipoproteinemias. *In* Stanbury, J. B., Wyngaarden, J. B., and Fredrickson, D. S. (eds.): The Metabolic Basis of Inherited Disease. 4th ed. New York, McGraw-Hill Book Company, 1978, p. 604.

Havel, R. J., Goldstein, J. L., and Brown, M. S.: Lipoproteins and lipid transport. *In* Bondy, P. K., and Rosenberg, L. E. (eds.): Metabolic Control and Disease. 8th ed. Philadelphia, W. B. Saunders Company, in press.

Havel, R. J., and Kane, J. P.: Drugs and lipid metabolism. *In* Elliot, H. W. (ed.): Annual Review of Pharmacology. Vol. 13. Palo Alto, Calif., Annual Review, Inc., 1973, p. 287.

Kane, J. P., Tun, P., Malloy, M. J., and Havel, R. J.: Heterozygous familial hypercholesterolemia: Treatment with combined drug regimens. Clin. Res., 26:529A, 1978.

Leelarthaepin, B., Palmer, A. J., Woodhill, J. M., and Blacket, R. B.: Obesity, diet and Type-II hyperlipidemia. Lancet, 2:1217, 1974.

Miettinen, T. A., and Lempinen, M.: Cholestyramine and ileal by-pass in the treatment of familial hypercholesterolaemia. Eur. J. Clin. Invest., 7:509, 1977.

HYPOLIPOPROTEINEMIAS

These conditions are exceedingly rare, but they have considerable importance for the light that they shed on normal functions of plasma lipoproteins.

Abetalipoproteinemia
(Bassen-Kornzweig Syndrome)

This disease, inherited as an autosomal recessive trait, is characterized by complete absence of LDL, VLDL, and chylomicrons. The absence of the B protein appears to be accompanied by virtually complete loss of ability to transport triglycerides in the blood. It is manifested by severe malabsorption, beginning in infancy, followed by progressive ataxia, nystagmus, distal sensory loss, weakness, and visual impairment with scotomas. These are related, respectively, to inability to deliver triglycerides into the intestinal lymph; demyelination of spinocerebellar tracts, posterior columns, and, occasionally, peripheral nerves; and pigmentary retinal degeneration ("atypical retinitis pigmentosa"). Other findings include peculiar thorny or spiny red cells (acanthocytes) and fatty liver (resulting from failure to export triglycerides in very low density lipoproteins). This disorder is also discussed in Ch. 408.

Diagnosis is established by finding very low cholesterol concentration (about 50 mg per 100 ml) and almost no triglycerides in blood plasma in an individual with one or more of the characteristic symptoms. The disorder should be considered in any patient with hereditary ataxia. On electrophoresis of serum only alpha lipoproteins are present, and blood smears or wet preparations show the characteristic acanthocytes. Treatment is limited to restriction of ordinary fat and supplementation with fat-soluble vitamins. Medium-chain triglycerides are well tolerated. Such measures have not been shown definitively to alter the progressive and disabling course of the disease.

Hypobetalipoproteinemia

A few families have been described in which low concentration of beta lipoproteins is transmitted as an autosomal dominant trait. Some patients have had acanthocytes, but neuromuscular difficulties and retinitis pigmentosa have not been described. No treatment is indicated.

Tangier Disease
(Alpha-Lipoprotein Deficiency)

This disorder, in the homozygous state, leads in childhood to diffuse deposition of cholesterol esters in reticuloendothelial tissues, with enlargement of liver, spleen, and lymph nodes, and especially to grossly enlarged tonsils with a characteristic orange color. Foam cells may be found in the bone marrow. In adults, flocculent corneal infiltrates may occur. Usually, the disorder does not affect growth, nutrition, or general health, but episodic peripheral neuropathy may occur in adults. Electrophoretic or ultracentrifugal examination shows almost no alpha lipoproteins or HDL, and one of the A proteins is reduced to about 1 per cent of the normal level. Heterozygotes have low concentrations of HDL but no other detectable abnormalities. In homozygotes, levels of LDL tend to be reduced, although those of triglycerides and VLDL are high. No treatment is available. There is limited evidence that premature vascular disease may develop.

Lecithin–Cholesterol Acyltransferase Deficiency

This disorder has been reported in only 21 persons. Affected subjects have proteinuria, anemia, and corneal deposits of lipids. HDL are almost absent, levels of VLDL and chylomicrons are variably increased, and abnormal lamellar lipoproteins bearing some resemblance to those found in cholestasis are present (see Biliary Obstruction in Ch. 532.6). Cholesteryl esters comprise less than 10 per cent of total cholesterol in plasma (normal value about 72 per cent) and are found almost entirely in the triglyceride-rich lipoproteins. Their fatty acids are much more saturated than those produced normally by the plasma enzyme lecithin–cholesterol acyltransferase, and this enzyme cannot be detected. Other findings include foam cells in the bone marrow and renal glomeruli and increased concentration of cholesterol and lecithin in the red blood cells. The renal lipid deposition may lead to progressive renal failure in adults. Atherosclerotic disease also occurs, but its incidence and severity are uncertain. Clinicopathologic correlations suggest that the renal disease is related to the concentration of the abnormal lamellar lipoproteins. No definitive treatment is available.

Havel, R. J., Goldstein, J. L., and Brown, M. S.: Lipoproteins and lipid transport. *In* Bondy, P. K., and Rosenberg, L. E. (eds.): Metabolic Control and Disease. 8th ed. Philadelphia, W. B. Saunders Company, in press.

Herbert, P. N., Gotto, A. M., Jr., and Fredrickson, D. S.: Familial lipoprotein deficiency (abetalipoproteinemia, hypobetalipoproteinemia and Tangier disease). *In* Stanbury, J. B., Wyngaarden, J. B., and Fredrickson, D. S. (eds.): The Metabolic Basis of Inherited Disease. 4th ed. New York, McGraw-Hill Book Company, 1978, p. 544.

532.6. ACQUIRED DISORDERS OF LIPOPROTEIN METABOLISM

HYPERLIPOPROTEINEMIAS

These conditions are important as clues to diagnosis or because they may be associated with the premature atherosclerotic vascular disease.

Hypercholesterolemia and Combined Hyperlipidemia

HYPOTHYROIDISM. Hypercholesterolemia is a characteristic finding in myxedema; hypothyroidism must be considered in all patients with this abnormality. Remnant-like lipoproteins of lower density may also accumulate, with accompanying hypertriglyceridemia. All forms of hypercholesterolemia are accompanied by hypercarotenemia, but this is particularly striking in myxedema because of the additional defect in conversion of carotene to vitamin A.

DIETARY. Moderate degrees of hypercholesterolemia occur in some persons who ingest large amounts of cholesterol, usually in eggs and dairy products.

NEPHROTIC SYNDROME. Hypercholesterolemia is frequently observed in nephrotic states when serum albumin concentration falls below 3 grams per 100 ml. As the level of albumin falls below 1.5 grams per 100 ml, the concentration of remnant-like VLDL rises to produce the characteristic nephrotic hyperlipemia. Treatment is that of the underlying disorder.

RESOLVING LIPEMIAS. As levels of chylomicrons or VLDL are reduced in various hyperlipemic states, the concentration of LDL usually rises, presumably reflecting the removal of triglyceride with liberation of component B apoprotein and associated lipids. Such hypercholesterolemia may persist for days to weeks and can lead to confusion if the sequence is not appreciated.

HYPERADRENOCORTICISM. Combined hyperlipidemia of moderate degree is commonly seen in Cushing's disease and subsides with appropriate treatment. Hyperlipidemia also occurs in patients receiving long-term exogenous glucocorticoids, as in patients who have received organ transplants.

OTHER CAUSES. Hypercholesterolemia also occurs commonly in hepatoma and hepatic porphyria.

Endogenous and Mixed Hypertriglyceridemias

DIABETIC HYPERLIPEMIA. Mixed hypertriglyceridemia is characteristic of prolonged insulin deficiency with ketosis. It is generally accompanied by fatty liver and by weight loss and other evidences of a catabolic state. It is not ordinarily seen with acute diabetic ketoacidosis. Defective removal of triglycerides and reduced lipolytic activity in postheparin plasma can be demonstrated. Eruptive xanthomas and lipemia retinalis are commonly seen. With administration of adequate insulin, triglyceride levels fall rapidly and cholesterol levels more slowly. Diabetic hyperlipemia must be differentiated from primary endogenous hyperlipemia and especially mixed hyperlipemia with its frequent associated hyperglycemia. These states are not accompanied by ketosis or wasting and do not respond to insulin. However, uncontrolled diabetes often aggravates an underlying primary hypertriglyceridemia.

ALCOHOLIC HYPERLIPEMIA. This lipemia, usually mixed, is seen in chronic alcoholics with fatty liver and good hepatic function. Diversion of fatty acids entering the liver to triglyceride synthesis accompanies oxidation of ethanol to acetate and appears to be the most important abnormality, but decreased activity of lipoprotein lipase has also been implicated. These patients almost always have underlying primary hypertriglyceridemias, and ingestion of ethanol is an important factor aggravating primary endogenous and mixed hyperlipemias. The association of jaundice and hemolytic anemia with hyperlipemia has been described in patients with alcoholism (Zieve's syndrome), but it has not been shown that the features of this triad are causally interrelated. Pancreatitis and hyperlipemia may also coexist. It is unlikely that pancreatitis causes the hyperlipemia, because the association is confined almost entirely to alcoholics in whom these complications can occur separately. This situation must be clearly distinguished from occurrence of pancreatitis as a complication of one of the primary (usually exogenous or mixed) hyperlipemias.

HYPERLIPEMIA IN GLYCOGEN STORAGE DISEASE TYPE I. Endogenous or mixed hyperlipemia is consistently found in children and adults. It is related both to increased hepatic secretion of triglycerides in VLDL and decreased activity of lipoprotein lipase. Frequent feeding and measures decreasing delivery of absorbed carbohydrate to the liver may be helpful.

HYPERLIPEMIA IN LIPODYSTROPHY. Hyperlipemia is consistently observed in familial and acquired forms of generalized lipodystrophy, and also in familial lipodystrophy of legs and trunk and acquired partial lipodystrophy. The mechanism is not understood; but, as in primary endogenous hyperlipemia, insulin resistance and hyperinsulinism are associated phenomena.

STRESS HYPERLIPEMIA. In a variety of situations, increased secretion of catecholamines, together with growth hormone and ACTH, can lead to hypertriglyceridemia by increasing mobilization of fatty acids from adipose tissue to liver with resultant increased secretion of triglycerides in VLDL. Such hypertriglyceridemia, appearing soon after myocardial infarction, can lead to confusion with primary endogenous hypertriglyceridemia.

ADMINISTRATION OF CONTRACEPTIVE STEROIDS. Mild endogenous hypertriglyceridemia is commonly produced by the estrogenic component of estrogen-progestogen mixtures and is associated with insulin resistance and hyperinsulinism.

OTHER CAUSES. Endogenous hypertriglyceridemia has been described in uremia, hypopituitarism, sphingolipodystrophies, and Werner's syndrome. The prevalence of hypertriglyceridemia is increased in gout.

Dyslipoproteinemias

BILIARY OBSTRUCTION. A low density lipoprotein which has not been detected in health appears in the plasma of patients with extrahepatic or intrahepatic biliary obstruction. It is a spherical vesicle about 400 Å in diameter, the wall of which is a lipid bilayer composed of a 1:1 molar mixture of cholesterol and phospholipids, together with a small amount of C apoproteins. This "cholestasis lipoprotein" or "LP-X" can be detected in virtually all patients with biliary obstruction, but very high levels are most characteristic of the early stages of primary biliary cirrhosis and are frequently accompanied by eruptive and planar xanthomas and xanthelasmas. Bile acid–binding agents, such as cholestyramine, may reduce the concentration of the lipoprotein. Spontaneous subsidence of the hyperlipoproteinemia and disappearance of xanthomas usually signify failing hepatic parenchymal cell function in primary biliary cirrhosis.

PARAPROTEINEMIAS. The abnormal globulins in patients with multiple myeloma and macroglobulinemia may be associated with lipid. In some cases, lipoprotein-globulin complexes have been demonstrated with accompanying hyperlipemia and various xanthomas.

HYPOLIPOPROTEINEMIAS

The secondary states are characterized chiefly by hypobetalipoproteinemia and are the result of malnutrition, malabsorption, or parenchymal liver disease. Presumably they reflect decreased transport of exogenous and endogenous triglycerides, so that formation of LDL is decreased. Reduced concentrations of LDL also occur in healthy individuals when intake of calories and saturated fats is habitually low.

Beck, P.: Contraceptive steroids: Modifications of carbohydrate and lipid metabolism. Metabolism, 22:841, 1973.

Havel, R. J., Balasse, E. O., Kane, J. P., and Segel, N.: Splanchnic metabolism in von Gierke's disease (glycogenosis type I). Trans. Assoc. Am. Physicians, 82:305, 1969.

Havel, R. J., Goldstein, J. L., and Brown, M. S.: Lipoproteins and lipid transport. In Bondy, P. K., and Rosenberg, L. E. (eds.): Metabolic Control and Disease. 8th ed. Philadelphia, W. B. Saunders Company, in press.

McIntyre, N., Harry, D. S., and Pearson, A. J. G.: The hypercholesterolaemia of obstructive jaundice. Gut, 16:379, 1975.

Segura, R., and Gotto, A. M., Jr.: Lipid and lipoprotein abnormalities in renal disease. In Suki, S. N., and Eknoyan, G. (eds.): The Kidney in Systemic Disease. New York, John Wiley & Sons, 1976, pp. 159–200.

Seip, M.: Generalized lipodystrophy. In Frick, P., von Harnack, G.-A., Muller, A.-F., Prader, A., Schoen, R., and Wolff, H. P. (eds.): Ergebnisse der Inneren Medizin und Kinderheilkunde. Berlin, Springer-Verlag, 1971, pp. 59–95.

532.7. HYPERLIPOPROTEINEMIA IN ATHEROSCLEROTIC VASCULAR DISEASE

Although atherosclerosis develops under the influence of a variety of factors, the role of plasma lipoproteins may be decisive in the muscular arteries supplying the heart and lower extremities. Levels of LDL, VLDL, or both tend to be elevated in patients with occlusive atherosclerotic disease in these vessels, particularly before the sixth decade. The level of cholesterol, which closely reflects the level of LDL in large population groups, is a powerful predictor of the incidence of and mortality from coronary heart disease in middle-aged men. Retrospective studies indicate that the level of triglycerides, which closely reflects the level of VLDL, is also associated with premature ischemic vascular disease, but prospective studies suggest that solitary elevation of triglycerides is in any event a less powerful predictor than elevation of serum cholesterol alone.

The cholesterol and cholesteryl esters that accumulate in atherosclerotic plaques are derived predominantly from LDL. It is thought that LDL bind to interstitial glycoaminoglycans and are taken up and catabolized by the proliferating smooth muscle cells that invade the intima under the stimulus of injury to the endothelium.

The level of serum cholesterol is subject to strong familial influence even in the absence of a major gene effect, such as that operating in familial hypercholesterolemia. This influence could be environmental, but available evidence suggests that polygenic inheritance is mainly operative. However, the level of serum cholesterol (and that of LDL) is also influenced by content of cholesterol and saturated fats in the diet. In industrialized countries, where intake of these nutrients is large, cholesterol levels are substantially higher than in underdeveloped countries, where habitual intake of animal fat is low. The much lower incidence of coronary heart disease in underdeveloped countries is consistent with the putative role of LDL-cholesterol in the early development of the atherosclerotic plaque.

In the absence of the major gene effects described in Ch. 532.5, the level of serum triglycerides is less subject to familial influence. The substantial effects of caloric intake and ethanol on serum triglyceride concentration accord with this fact and suggest that sporadic cases of mild to moderate hypertriglyceridemia largely reflect alterations in lipid transport produced by nutritional or other environmental influences.

Studies of survivors of myocardial infarction indicate that hyperlipoproteinemia occurs in about half of those under the age of 50. More than half of the hyperlipoproteinemic survivors, in turn, appear to carry major gene defects. Familial hypercholesterolemia accounts for only about one fifth of these; most of the remainder have familial multiple lipoprotein-type hyperlipidemia or familial hypertriglyceridemia. In addition, polygenic hypercholesterolemia and sporadic cases of hypertriglyceridemia are common among survivors of myocardial infarction.

Recent epidemiologic research suggests that HDL, formerly thought only to be nonatherogenic, may actually be protective against atherosclerotic disease. This is consistent with presumed role of HDL in delivering cholesterol from extrahepatic tissues to the liver for excretion in the bile. High levels of HDL have been linked to longevity.

Whether reduction of lipoprotein levels will prevent progression or cause regression of atherosclerotic lesions has not been clearly established. Experimentally induced atherosclerosis in animals regresses under some circumstances, and recent studies suggest that reduction of dietary cholesterol and saturated fats may delay death from ischemic vascular disease in survivors of myocardial infarction and in elderly men. More direct evidence of regression of occlusive lesions in the femoral artery has recently been obtained. Changes in lesions as determined by quantitative angiography correlated with extent of serum lipid reduction in patients with hyperlipidemia. Thus specific dietary or pharmacologic treatment of hyperlipoproteinemia is probably indicated in coronary heart disease and peripheral atherosclerotic vascular disease as well as for prophylaxis.

Because the risk of developing coronary heart disease is a graded function of the concentration of LDL-cholesterol, the presence of normal levels of cholesterol and triglycerides in survivors of myocardial infarction cannot be taken to exclude a major influence of plasma lipoproteins in the pathogenesis of their disease. Statistical normality of LDL-cholesterol level in industrialized countries should therefore not be confused with the level consistent with maintenance of health. Rather, levels of LDL-cholesterol in the range of 80 to 120 mg per 100 ml serum (equivalent to total cholesterol levels of 140 to 180 mg per 100 ml) may be "normal" in this context. The relative immunity of premenopausal women to complications of atherosclerosis may result from their lower levels of VLDL and higher levels of HDL.

Barndt, R., Jr., Blankenhorn, D. H., Crawford, D. W., and Brooks, S. H.: Regression and progression of early atherosclerosis in treated hyperlipoproteinemic patients. Ann. Intern. Med., 86:139, 1977.

Goldstein, J. L., Hazzard, W. R., Schrott, H. G., Bierman, E. L., and Motulsky, A. G.: Hyperlipidemia in coronary heart disease: I. Lipid levels in 500 survivors of myocardial infarction. II. Genetic analysis of lipid levels in 176 families and delineation of a new inherited disorder, combined hyperlipidemia. III. Evaluation of lipoprotein phenotypes of 156 genetically defined survivors of myocardial infarction. J. Clin. Invest., 52:1533, 1544, 1569, 1973.

Gordon, T., Castelli, W. P., Hjortland, M. C., Kannel, W. B., and Dawber, T. R.: High density lipoprotein as a protective factor against coronary heart disease. Am. J. Med., 62:707, 1977.

Kannel, W. B., Garcia, M. J., McNamara, P. M., and Pearson, G.: Serum lipid precursors of coronary heart disease. Human Pathol., 2:129, 1971.

Small, D. M.: Cellular mechanisms for lipid deposition in atherosclerosis. N. Engl. J. Med., 297:873, 924, 1977.

Turpeinen, O.: Control of atherosclerosis: Progress in primary diet trials. In Jones, R. J. (ed.): Atherosclerosis. Proceedings, Second International Symposium. New York, Springer-Verlag, 1970, p. 572.

533. LIPID STORAGE DISEASES

533.1. FABRY'S DISEASE
(Glycosphingolipidosis)

James B. Wyngaarden

DEFINITION. Fabry's disease is an inborn error of glycosphingolipid metabolism characterized by telangiectatic skin lesions, hypohidrosis, corneal opacities, acral pain and paresthesias, intermittent fevers, renal failure, and cardiovascular, gastrointestinal, and central nervous system disturbance.

INCIDENCE. The disease has an estimated incidence of 1:40,000.

ETIOLOGY AND PATHOGENESIS. Fabry's disease is an X-linked condition, fully manifest in the hemizygous male. Heterozygous females may exhibit the disease in an attenuated form, and usually show corneal clouding; occasionally a female may have most of the features of the full syndrome, including renal failure.

The biochemical defect is a deficiency of the lysosomal enzyme, α-galactosidase-A. The enzymatic defect leads to a progressive deposition of neutral glycosphin-golipids with terminal α-galactosyl moieties in most visceral tissues and fluids of the body. The most prominent of these is a trihexosylceramide called globotriaosylceramide, a product of globoside which is a constituent of membranes. The majority of anatomic and physiologic abnormalities observed in Fabry's disease can be related to the cumulative deposition of glycosphingolipid, particularly in the lysosomes of the cardiovascular-renal system.

PATHOLOGY. Morphologically, Fabry's disease is characterized by widespread tissue deposits of a crystalline glycosphingolipid which shows birefringence with typical Maltese crosses. The glycosphingolipid is deposited in all areas of the body, occurring predominantly in the lysosomes of endothelial, perithelial, and smooth muscle cells of blood vessels, and to a lesser extent in connective tissue. Lipid deposits are also prominent in epithelial cells of the cornea, in glomeruli and tubules of the kidney, in muscle fibers of the heart, and in ganglion cells of the autonomic nervous system. The skin lesions are telangiectases or small superficial angiomas. Capillaries, venules, and arterioles show pathologic lipid storage, and there is marked dilatation of the capillaries of the dermal papillae just below the epidermis. The larger lesions are usually located in the upper dermis, where they may produce elevation, flattening, or hypertrophy of the epithelium, with keratosis; hence the term *angiokeratoma*. On electron microscopy lipid inclusions show a concentrically arranged lamellar structure with alternating light- and dark-staining bands.

CLINICAL MANIFESTATIONS. Telangiectases may occur in childhood and lead to early diagnosis. They increase in size and number with age, and range from barely visible to several millimeters in diameter. The lesions are punctate, dark red to blue-black, and flat or slightly raised. They do not blanch with pressure, and the larger ones may show slight hyperkeratosis. The lesions tend to occur in clusters in the "bathing trunk area," but may occur anywhere, including the oral mucosa. The hips, thighs, buttocks, umbilicus, lower abdomen, scrotum, and glans penis are common sites, and there is a tendency toward bilateral symmetry. In some patients skin lesions are absent and lesions are entirely visceral. Sweating is often decreased, and hair may be sparse; shaving may be required only infrequently. Ocular lesions may be present in all elements of the eye. The most prominent are those of cornea, conjunctiva, and retina. Corneal opacities, observed by slit lamp examination, are present in most heterozygotes. The early lesion is a diffuse haziness of the epithelial layer. Later there may be whorled streaks extending from a central vortex to the periphery. The conjunctival and retinal vessels may show mild to marked tortuosity, with aneurysmal dilatations of thin-walled venules, as well as angulation and segmental, sausage-like dilatation of veins.

Pain is the most debilitating symptom of Fabry's disease. Fabry's crises, lasting from minutes to several days, consist of agonizing, burning pain in palms, soles, and proximal extremities. The pain may become more severe with age, but later may disappear altogether. Pain is usually associated with fever. Attacks of abdominal or flank pain may simulate appendicitis or renal colic. In addition to the intermittent crises, there may be chronic troublesome paresthesias of hands and feet.

With increasing age progressive infiltration of the cardiovascular-renal system with glycosphingolipid gives rise to anginal chest pain, myocardial infarction, cardiomegaly, or congestive heart failure. Involvement of renal parenchymal vessels leads to hypertension. Renal impairment is common with development of azotemia in the second to fourth decade of life. During childhood and adolescence protein, red cells, casts, and desquamated kidney and urinary tract cells appear in the urine. Birefringent lipid globules with characteristic Maltese crosses within and without cells can be observed in the urine sediment by polarized light microscopy. Other features may include chronic bronchitis and dyspnea, lymphedema of the legs without hypoproteinemia, episodic diarrhea, osteoporosis, retarded growth, and delayed puberty. The mean age at death is 41 years, but survival may extend into the sixties.

DIAGNOSIS AND DIFFERENTIAL DIAGNOSIS. The diagnosis in hemizygous males is most readily made from the history of painful paresthesias and episodic crises with fever, and the observation of characteristic skin lesions, corneal opacities, and conjunctival lesions. The disorder is often misdiagnosed as rheumatic fever, erythromelalgia, or neurosis. The skin lesions must be differentiated from the benign angiokeratomas of the scrotum of older men (Fordyce's disease), or from angiokeratoma circumscripta. Angiokeratomas identical to those of Fabry's disease have been reported in alpha-1-fucosidase deficiency. The diagnosis of Fabry's disease is confirmed biochemically by demonstration of markedly deficient α-galactosidase-A activity in plasma or serum, leukocytes, tears, biopsied tissue, or cultured skin fibroblasts. Increased levels of globotriaosylceramide are found in urinary sediment, plasma, or cultured fibroblasts.

Suspect heterozygotes may show corneal opacities, isolated skin lesions, and lipid-laden cells in skin or other tissues or in urinary sediment. Intermediate activities of α-galactosidase A can usually be demonstrated.

Prenatal diagnosis of Fabry's disease may be accomplished by amniocentesis at approximately 14 weeks of gestation and demonstration of deficient α-galactosidase-A activity and XY karyotype in cultured amniotic cells, and accumulated trihexosylceramide in amniotic fluid.

TREATMENT. Relief of pain may be achieved with phenoxybenzamine or diphenylhydantoin in some patients. Diphenylhydantoin combined with carbamazepine and maintenance corticosteroid therapy have also been reported to provide symptomatic relief. Renal insufficiency is treated with chronic hemodialysis or renal transplantation. In some recipients biochemical and clinical regression, with relief of pain, has followed placement of renal allografts, perhaps because of provision of normal α-galactosidase A for substrate metabolism. Transient lowering of serum levels of trihexosylceramide follows administration of normal plasma containing active enzyme. α-Galactosidase-A purified from human placenta has been administered to two hemizygotes. The enzyme was rapidly cleared from plasma and taken up by liver. There was a reduction in level of circulating trihexosylceramide. Current research centers on target delivery of enzyme and methods of protecting it from rapid inactivation.

Desnick, R. J., Klionsky, B., and Sweeley, C. C.: Fabry's disease (α-galactosidase A deficiency). *In* Stanbury, J. B., Wyngaarden, J. B., and Fredrickson, D. S. (eds.): The Metabolic Basis of Inherited Disease. 4th ed. New York, McGraw-Hill Book Company, 1978, p. 810.

533.2. GAUCHER'S DISEASE
(Glucosyl Ceramide Lipidosis)
Donald S. Fredrickson

DEFINITION. Gaucher's disease is a relatively common familial disorder characterized by abnormal accumulation of glucocerebrosides in reticuloendothelial (RE) cells; the accumulation occurs because an enzyme necessary for the degradation of these glycolipids is deficient. The increasing mass of the storage cells accounts for most of the clinical manifestations of the disease, including hepatosplenomegaly, lymph node enlargement, and bone lesions owing to expansion of the involved marrow. At least three syndromes have been recognized: (1) a chronic non-neuronopathic or "adult" form, which is by far the most common, becoming evident at any age and associated with hypersplenism, bone lesions, skin pigmentation and pingueculae, and preponderance among Ashkenazic Jews; (2) an acute neuronopathic form, which is manifest in infancy, is associated with severe neurologic abnormalities, and is usually fatal by three years of age; and (3) a "juvenile" form, which may begin at any time in childhood, combining the features of the chronic form with slowly progressive neurologic dysfunction. At least three different mutations are represented by the different forms of Gaucher's disease. No specific treatment is available.

PATHOLOGIC PHYSIOLOGY AND PATHOGENESIS. Cerebrosides are compounds that contain equimolar amounts of sphingosine, fatty acid, and hexose. In the brain the hexose component is galactose, and the galactocerebrosides form an essential part of the myelin in the white matter. In tissues outside the brain, except for the kidney, practically all the small amounts of cerebroside present contain only glucose. These glucocerebrosides arise mainly from the degradation of more complex sphingoglycolipids, the most important source probably being the normal breakdown of both white and red blood cells. In Gaucher's disease there is a specific deficiency in the activity of glucosylceramide-β-glucosidase (glucocerebrosidase), one of the acid hydrolases found in the lysosomes. Glucocerebroside, a *relatively* insoluble compound, then accumulates in RE cells.

The morphologic hallmark of Gaucher's disease is the *Gaucher cell*, a round or polyhedral pale reticulum cell 20 to 80 μ in diameter, with a small eccentrically placed nucleus and a wrinkled ("crumpled silk") cytoplasm that contains an irregular network of fibrils. With electron microscopy the fibrils are shown to represent tubules or strands of glucocerebroside contained within secondary lysosomes having a single limiting membrane. Evidence of active phagocytosis or pinocytosis is present at the cell border, and fragments of erythrocytes are often visible. A few cells may have two or more nuclei. The cytoplasm does not stain with fat stains, but numerous wavy fibrillae are stained deeply with the periodic acid–Schiff reaction or with Mallory's trichrome connective tissue stain. The cytoplasm also demonstrates strong acid phosphatase activity. Examination of unstained smears of aspirated bone marrow by phase microscopy affords the best visualization of the cells (see accompanying figure, part *A*).

Proliferation and expansion of the Gaucher cells are responsible for the enlargement of spleen, liver, and intrathoracic and intra-abdominal lymph nodes. The concentration of glucocerebrosides may be increased 50 to 100 times normal in these organs. The spleen may become tremendous in size. Hemosiderin may be increased in the skin and other organs. Gaucher cells are also scattered diffusely throughout the marrow, and in some areas form tumor-like accumulations that may expand, erode the cortex, and lead to pathologic fractures. Infiltration of the lungs, kidneys, thymus, tonsils, thyroid, adrenals, and lymphatic tissue of the intestinal tract also occurs. Functional impairment of these organs is unusual, except for the lungs. Serious pulmonary infections are common in children, and pulmonary hypertension may occur in adults. Pathologic changes in the brains of adults are restricted to the presence of perivascular adventitial cells swollen in the typical Gaucher configuration. In children with the acute neuronopathic type of disease, such "perivascular cuffing" is accompanied by acute nerve cell degeneration with active phagocytosis of the cellular remains by histiocytes and microglia, and cytoplasmic storage of periodic acid–Schiff positive lipid in either neurons or glial cells. These changes are distributed focally in the cerebrum, cerebellum, brainstem, and spinal cord. In the juvenile form the ballooning of neurons is accentuated. An accumulation of both glucocerebrosides and gangliosides has been reported in the brains of infants with the acute neuronopathic type. It is not known why the severity of the effect on the brain is so different in the several forms of the disease.

Acid phosphatase activity, not inhibited by L-tartrate (in contrast to the prostatic enzyme), is characteristically elevated in plasma and has diagnostic value. The enzyme is apparently spilled into plasma from the Gaucher cells. Plasma cerebroside concentrations are elevated after splenectomy.

CLINICAL MANIFESTATIONS. Chronic Non-neuronopathic Type. The disease affects both sexes equally. It has been reported in Caucasians, Negroes, and Orientals; but a very high proportion of cases occurs among Ashkenazic Jews. Manifestations may appear at any age; the diagnosis has been made in the first month of life and past the age of 80 years. The course is extremely variable and tends to be more severe in affected children. Often, particularly in adults, the patient has no symptoms for a long time except awareness of a progressively enlarging mass in the left upper abdomen. The spleen may become very large; the liver is usually palpable. The second most common presenting abnormality is related to bone lesions. From 50 to 75 per cent of patients have roentgenographic changes, mostly asymptomatic. A common change is expansion of the cortex of of the lower end of the femur, producing a characteristic radiolucent area with the configuration of an Erlenmeyer flask. The phalanges, long bones, vertebrae, ribs, and pelvis are more commonly involved than the skull. Bone pain or aching and pathologic fractures may appear at sites of skeletal lesions. With destruction of the head and neck of the femur, walking may become progressively more difficult. The hip abnormalities are sometimes confused with Legg-Perthes disease. In younger patients episodic attacks of bone pain simulating acute osteomyelitis are common. The long bones are usually affected; fever, joint tenderness, and redness occur, and draining sinus tracts may form. The cause is believed to be interference with the blood supply of the highly vascular metaphysis. Attacks usually last several weeks and no longer recur when growth is complete.

A high percentage of patients with Gaucher's disease develop hematologic changes of hypersplenism at some time during the course of their disease: hemolytic anemia, leukopenia, thrombocytopenia, or any combination of the three. The peripheral cytopenia is accompanied by a normal or increased number of the progenitors of the involved formed element in the bone marrow. Chronic Gaucher's disease usually involves only a single generation, but it has been observed in two generations. Otherwise normal parents, siblings, and other close relatives of patients sometimes have slight splenomegaly or small Gaucher cells in the marrow. Although the disease sometimes appears to behave like a dominant trait, most patients probably are homozygous for an autosomal recessive allele or alleles.

Acute Neuronopathic Type. This "infantile" form of the disease is usually evident by three months of age but may become so any time between birth and 18

Appearance of the typical Gaucher cell (*A*) and a foam cell seen in Niemann-Pick disease (*B*). Both are viewed under phase microscopy in unstained smears of aspirated bone marrow. Magnification can be estimated from adjacent red cells.

months. Among the earliest signs are splenomegaly, chronic cough, and psychomotor retardation. Other neurologic signs indicative of brainstem and cranial nerve involvement usually appear by the age of six months. The children have a stereotyped appearance: hepatosplenomegaly, strabismus, head retroflexed, lips retracted, and often spastic extremities held in flexion. The disease is fatal within three years; the average life span is about one year, respiratory infection and distress being the principal cause of death. Sex distribution is about equal. If one child in a family is afflicted, all other affected sibs will have the same form of disease. The disease appears to be transmitted as an autosomal recessive gene and is expressed only in the homozygote. The mutant gene is present in low frequency in many ethnic groups. Four of about 70 reported cases have occurred in Jews.

Juvenile Type. About 25 examples of subacute neuronopathic Gaucher's disease have been described. Hepatosplenomegaly, hypersplenism, bone lesions, and other features of the chronic type appear from infancy onward. These are combined with mental retardation, behavioral problems, seizures, choreoathetoid movements, and sometimes strabismus, trismus, and other evidence of brainstem involvement. In several related Swedish families, glucocerebrosidase deficiency was demonstrated. Glycolipids other than glucocerebrosides may be stored in the spleen and liver, and a clear-cut phenotype has not been established.

DIAGNOSIS. Gaucher's disease should be ruled out in any patient with unexplained splenomegaly, especially with elevated plasma acid phosphatase activity (not inhibited by L-tartrate). A presumptive diagnosis is made from detection of Gaucher cells, usually in marrow aspirates. Diagnosis should be confirmed by demonstration of absence or severe deficiency in activity of glucosylceramide β-glucosidase. The enzyme activity can be measured most accurately in circulating leukocytes or fibroblasts cultured from skin, bone marrow, or amniotic fluid (for prenatal diagnosis). If there is any doubt, liver biopsy will permit confirmation of both specific enzyme deficiency and accumulation of glucocerebrosides, provided that the tissue is stored in the absence of fixatives. Heterozygotes are detectable by enzyme assay.

TREATMENT AND PROGNOSIS. No specific therapy exists; enzyme replacement remains experimental. X-ray therapy to bone lesions may alleviate pain, but usually does not arrest the destructive process. Bone pain may also respond well to corticosteroid therapy. Splenectomy corrects the manifestations of hypersplenism but does not otherwise influence the course of the disease. Because of the possibility that bone involvement may be accelerated by splenectomy, the indication for the procedure should be clear cut. The course is protracted, often extending over many years. Most older patients die of intercurrent diseases rather than Gaucher's disease per se.

Brady, R. O.: Glucosylceramide lipidosis: Gaucher's disease. *In* Stanbury, J. B., Wyngaarden, J. B., and Fredrickson, D. S. (eds.): The Metabolic Basis of Inherited Disease. 4th ed. New York, McGraw-Hill Book Company, 1978, pp. 731–746.

Matoth, Y., and Fried, K.: Chronic Gaucher's disease: Clinical observations in 34 patients. Isr. J. Med. Sci., 1:521, 1965.

Miller, J. D., McCluer, R., and Kanfer, J. N.: Gaucher's disease: Neurologic disorders in adult siblings. Ann. Intern. Med., 78:833, 1973.

533.3.   NIEMANN-PICK DISEASE
(Sphingomyelin Lipidosis)
Donald S. Fredrickson

DEFINITION. The eponym Niemann-Pick disease refers to several rare disorders characterized by extensive tissue storage of sphingomyelin. All patients have hepatosplenomegaly and large macrophages filled with lipid droplets in the bone marrow (see figure in Ch. 533.2, part B); some also have severe neurologic abnormalities. The "sphingomyelin lipidoses" fall into two major groups. In the first, there is clear-cut inheritable deficiency of activity of sphingomyelinase, a lysosomal enzyme that catalyzes the hydrolysis of phosphorylcholine from sphingomyelin. Sphingomyelin concentrations in tissues are 10 to 100 times normal. The second includes a heterogeneous group of disorders with clinical manifestations similar to the first. The tissue activity of sphingomyelinase is normal or only slightly deficient, however, and increases in sphingomyelin concentrations of liver or spleen are relatively small.

The sphingomyelinase-deficient disorders usually occur in either an acute neuronopathic form (type A) or a chronic, non-neuronopathic form (type B). All affected members of the same family are phenotypically the same, and the two disorders are presumably "allelic," i.e., they represent different mutations at or near the same locus governing the activity of sphingomyelinase.

CLINICAL MANIFESTATIONS.   Type A. Type A is usually manifested by six months of age by abdominal enlargement and evidence of physical and mental retardation. Hepatosplenomegaly and roentgenographic evidence of diffuse pulmonary infiltration may be present as early as one month of age. Throughout the nervous system the neurons and glial cells are ballooned with lipid, the nuclei are pushed to one side, and Nissl substance disappears. Neuronal loss, gliosis, and demyelination are severe. Retinal degeneration in the macular area usually causes a cherry-red spot to appear. The disease progresses to a vegetative state, and death nearly always occurs by the fourth year of life. There are a few exceptional patients, perhaps representing different mutations, who early have retinal changes and other central nervous system signs and who have a much more prolonged course. Both sexes are affected. The disease occurs in all races; it is disproportionately frequent in Ashkenazic Jews.

Type B. Children with type B may develop evidence of visceral involvement as severe and as early as those with type A, but the central nervous system apparently is spared, and mental development is normal. Chronic pulmonary infections and hypersplenism are sometimes life-threatening, but a reasonably normal life span may be possible. Types A and B are inherited as autosomal recessives.

DIAGNOSIS. The typical presentation of Niemann-Pick disease is a very young child with hepatosplenomegaly in whose bone marrow foam cells (see figure in Ch. 533.2, part B) are present. From the appearance of the cells Gaucher's disease can be excluded but the diagnosis of Niemann-Pick disease cannot be made. Indistinguishable foam cells occur with severe hyperglyceridemia and many other lysosomal enzyme deficiencies. The next diagnostic step should be assay of sphingomyelinase in cultured skin fibroblasts or leukocyte preparations. When the assay is appropriately controlled, sphingomyelinase activity between 0 and 20 per cent of normal permits a presumptive diagnosis. Distinction between type A and type B rests on frequent observation for development of neurologic abnormalities. Niemann-Pick disease is also detectable prenatally by enzyme assays of fetal cells grown from amniotic fluid. Separation of types A and B in utero can only be presumed from phenotype of a previously affected sib. Heterozygotes have intermediate levels of enzyme activity, best measured in cultured fibroblasts.

Indeterminate Forms of Sphingomyelin Storage. When the patient has unexplained hepatosplenomegaly and marrow foam cells and the tissue assay for sphingomyelinase is normal or slightly deficient, open liver biopsy is advisable. Tissue must be kept frozen without fixatives for chemical and enzymatic analyses. Careful morphologic examination is also advisable, but neither light nor electron microscopy is capable of distinguishing between most of the lipid storage diseases. Exhaustive analyses of the concentrations of phospholipids, neutral lipids, and glycolipids, in combination with assay of various lysosomal hydrolases and other appropriate enzymes, must be carried out.

In a number of patients an increase of only one- to two-fold in sphingomyelin and cholesterol has been detected. These are usually children who have appeared normal for one or more years before moderate hepatosplenomegaly is noted. Later neurologic abnormalities appear; these may include seizures, behavioral disorders, and mental retardation. Frequently such abnormalities are familial and have been referred to as chronic neuronopathic forms of Niemann-Pick disease. If the sphingomyelinase activity is modestly decreased, such patients have been referred to as Niemann-Pick disease, Type C, or as Type D for a similar disorder occurring in related patients of Nova Scotian ancestry. They may possibly represent other mutations affecting sphingomyelinase, but probably they and other similar phenotypes in which the enzyme activity is unequivocally normal represent other undetermined lysosomal enzyme deficiencies in which sphingomyelin metabolism is only incidentally affected.

TREATMENT. There is no specific treatment for any of the sphingomyelin storage disorders. Chronic administration of sphingomyelinase has not been attempted. Because phospholipid storage leads to excessive lipid peroxidation and ceroid pigment deposition in tissue, long-term administration of an antioxidant, such as vitamin E, has been empirically recommended.

Brady, R. O.: Sphingomyelin lipidosis: Niemann-Pick disease. *In* Stanbury, J. B., Wyngaarden, J. B., and Fredrickson, D. S. (eds.): The Metabolic Basis of Inherited Disease. 4th ed. New York, McGraw-Hill Book Company, 1978, pp. 718–730.

534. INBORN ERRORS OF AMINO ACID METABOLISM

534.1. HYPERAMINOACIDURIA

Charles R. Scriver

GENERAL COMMENTS. A certain amount of L-aminoaciduria, representing less than 2 to 3 per cent of the total urinary nitrogen, is a normal phenomenon. A small fraction, usually less than 5 per cent, of the filtered load of the amino acids in plasma is not absorbed completely by the proximal portion of the renal tubule and is excreted in the urine. In the healthy person, the efficiency of renal tubular transport for the individual amino acids is related to their chemical and steric structure, the amount in the glomerular filtrate, and the sex, age, and physiologic state of the subject. Data for normal range and mean values of endogenous renal clearance rates, plasma levels, and urinary excretion rates of approximately 20 L-amino acids exist for infants, children, and adults, both male and female, in fasting and nonfasting states. Advances in the knowledge of aminoaciduria have come primarily from the development of chromatographic methods, which allow rapid qualitative screening and reliable quantitative estimation of the complex amino acid composition of physiologic fluids.

Renal tubular absorption of amino acids is mediated by reactive sites which are believed to be membrane proteins. The transport process is saturable (equivalent to the T_m) and is susceptible to competitive and noncompetitive inhibition. The specificity of the site is genetically controlled.

Transfer of the amino acid across the membrane (a directional process) is by a mechanism which either is coupled to metabolic reactions which produce energy (nondirectional reactions) or elicits coupled fluxes in the same or opposite direction of other solutes.

Abnormal aminoaciduria will result when there is an acquired or hereditary disturbance of cellular metabolism or transport of amino acids. The known hyperaminoacidurias (Table 1) can be classified according to four basic mechanisms:

1. *Saturation:* Substrate is at elevated concentration and approaches or exceeds the capacity of the system ("overflow" aminoaciduria).

2. *Competition:* One substrate itself at elevated concentration competes with other members for access to the system ("combined" aminoaciduria).

3. *Modification of reactive site(s):* Substrate(s) not transported efficiently because access to the system is modified ("renal" aminoaciduria).

4. *Inhibition of substrate transfer:* Impaired energy-dependent processes, coupled to the transfer of substrates across membrane ("renal" aminoaciduria).

In some diseases, e.g., in Group III of Table 1, gene mutation affects amino acid transport in both the renal tubule and the intestine. Furthermore, it appears that the individual mechanisms required for transport of each amino acid can be grouped into at least five major gene-controlled and nonoverlapping systems, each having a particular *preference for a group of amino acids* normally found in plasma and usually elucidated in a particular aminoacidopathy. Another series of reactive sites *recognizes individual amino acids,* one site for each of the protein amino acids. Yet *another series permits transepithelial absorption of oligopeptides* in the intestine, with hydrolysis following uptake of the peptides. The *group-specific sites* used by free amino acids, and particularly evident through the inborn errors of amino acid metabolism, are classified as follows:

1. *The β-amino system:* β-alanine, β-aminoisobutyric acid, and taurine (viz., hyper-β-alaninemia).

2. *The α-amino systems:*

Text continued on page 2021

TABLE 1. Hereditary and Acquired Aminoacidopathies

The aminoacidurias presented in this table are divided into acquired and inherited types. Disturbances related to perinatal adaptive phenomena of multifactorial origin are included. The classification recognizes physiologic factors affecting amino acid distribution between plasma and urine, and whether the disorder primarily affects catabolism or membrane transport of the amino acid(s). Thus the disorders are grouped according to mechanism and preferred fluid for detection. The data refer to those conditions associated with perturbation of the normal content of ninhydrin-reactive metabolites in plasma or urine; some exceptions have been made to include ninhydrin-negative metabolites.

GROUP IA

The primary defect is in catabolism. There is a low renal clearance of amino acid but a hyperaminoaciduria by saturation of transepithelial transport. Detection in the plasma is preferable unless otherwise indicated, but the use of urine for screening (or diagnosis) is not precluded; assignment to this group implies primarily that diagnosis (or screening) of the condition is feasible by virtue of significant metabolite accumulation in blood (or plasma). *Amino Acid Affected:* ↓ = decreased; ↑ = increased. Source of enzyme number is *Enzyme Commission. IP:* Apparent inheritance pattern; AR = autosomal recessive; (AR) = probably autosomal recessive; XL = X-linked. *Remarks:* CNS = central nervous system; CoA = coenzyme A; CSF = cerebrospinal fluid. Data in brackets refer to the column heading in brackets.

Condition or Disease	Amino Acid Affected	Enzyme Affected (Synonym) [Enzyme Commission No.]	IP	Remarks
		*Common Perinatal (Adaptive) Traits**		
1. Neonatal hyperphenyl-alaninemia	Phenylalanine	Phenylalanine 4-monooxygenase (phenylalanine-hydroxylating system) [1.14.16.1]	—	Benign; may respond to folic acid; often occurs with tyrosinemia
2. Neonatal tyrosinemia	Tyrosine	4-Hydroxyphenylpyruvate dioxygenase (*p*-hydroxyphenyl pyruvic acid hydroxylase) [1.13.11.27]	—	Benign; responds to ascorbic acid and reduced protein intake
3. Hypermethioninemia	Methionine	? Methionine adenosyltransferase (ATP:L-methionine S-adenosyltransferase) [2.5.1.6]	—	Benign; usually found with high protein intake
4. Hyperhistidinemia	Histidine	? L-Histidine ammonia-lyase [4.3.1.3]	—	Benign; related to high protein intake
		Inherited Traits		
Hyperphenylalaninemias				
5. Classic phenylketonuria	Phenylalanine	Phenylalanine 4-monooxygenase (L-phenylalanine, tetrahydropteridine:oxygen oxidoreductase [4-hydroxylating]) [1.14.16.1]	AR	Plasma phenylalanine >16 mg/100 ml; causes mental retardation; when treated, L-phenylalanine tolerance in diet is 250–500 mg/deciliter
6. Atypical phenylketonuria	Phenylalanine	Same as for entry 5	(AR)	Plasma phenylalanine >16 mg/100 ml; similar to entry 5, but dietary tolerance for L-phenylalanine is >500 mg/deciliter
7. Transient phenylketonuria	Phenylalanine	Same as for entry 5	(AR)	Plasma phenylalanine >16 mg/100 ml; change in status to that for entry 8, or normal, several months or years after birth
8. Benign hyperphenyl-alaninemia	Phenylalanine	Same as for entry 5	AR	Plasma phenylalanine <16 mg/100 ml on normal diet; benign trait
9. Phenylketonuria (dihydropteridine reductase deficiency)	Phenylalanine	Dihydropteridine reductase [1.6.99.7]	—	Resembles classic phenylketonuria, but no CNS response to diet; enzyme can be assayed in cultured skin fibroblasts
Hypertyrosinemias				
10. Tyrosinosis (Medes)	Tyrosine	? Tyrosine aminotransferase (L-tyrosine:α-ketoglutarate aminotransferase) [2.6.1.5]	(AR)	One case known; myasthenia gravis probably incidental finding
11. Hypertyrosinemia	Tyrosine	Soluble (cytosol) tyrosine aminotransferase [2.6.1.5]	(AR)	Associated with developmental retardation; Richner-Hanhart syndrome in some patients
12. Hereditary tyrosinemia	Tyrosine (and methionine in acute stage)	4-Hydroxyphenylpyruvate dioxygenase† [1.13.11.27]	AR	Hepatic cirrhosis and renal tubular failure; usually fatal in absence of tyrosine restriction
Hyperhistidinemias‡				
13. Classic form	Histidine (alanine in some cases)	L-Histidine ammonia-lyase§ [4.3.1.3]	AR	Occasionally associated with mental retardation and speech defect
14. Variant form	Histidine	L-Histidine ammonia-lyase¶ [4.3.1.3]	(AR)	Same as for entry 13
*Branched-chain hyperaminoacidemia** *				
15. Classic "maple syrup urine disease"	Leucine, isoleucine, valine, alloisoleucine	Branched-chain α-ketoacid oxidase(s) (probably decarboxylase component)	AR	Postnatal collapse; mental retardation in survivors; diet therapy can be effective

TABLE 1. Hereditary and Acquired Aminoacidopathies (Continued)

Condition or Disease	Amino Acid Affected	Enzyme Affected (Synonym) [Enzyme Commission No.]	IP	Remarks
16. Intermittent form	Leucine, isoleucine, valine, alloisoleucine	Branch-chain α-ketoacid oxidase(s)††	(AR)	Intermittent symptoms; development may be otherwise normal
17. Mild form	Same as for entry 16	Same as for entry 16	(AR)	Unremittent; milder than for entry 15
18. Thiamin-responsive form	Same as for entry 16	Same as for entry 16	(AR)	Mild form; responsive to thiamin (vitamin B_1)
19. Hypervalinemia	Valine	Branched-chain-amino-acid aminotransferase (valine aminotransferase) [2.6.1.42]	AR	Retarded development and vomiting; responds to diet
20. Hyperleucinemia	Leucine or isoleucine	Branched-chain-amino-acid aminotransferase (leucine/isoleucine aminotransferase) [2.6.1.42]	(AR)	Retarded development
Sulfur aminoacidemias				
21. Homocyst(e)inuria‡ (cystathionine β-synthase deficiency)	Methionine and homocyst(e)ine	Cystathionine β-synthase (L-serine hydro-lyase [adding homocysteine]) [4.2.1.22]	AR	Usually associated with thromboembolic disease, mental retardation, and Marfan-like phenotype
22. Homocyst(e)inuria (methylene THF reductase deficiency)	Methionine (low) and homocyst(e)ine (high)	5,10-Methylenetetrahydrofolate reductase [1.1.1.68]	AR	Defective remethylation of homocysteine to methionine; Neurologic and behavioral symptoms associated
23. Homocyst(e)inuria (with methylmalonic aciduria)	Homocyst(e)ine (high), methionine (low); plus methylmalonate	Defective cobalamin coenzyme biosynthesis	(AR)	Defective remethylation of homocysteine and methylmalonyl-CoA mutase (MMA mutase) activity; severe neurologic signs and acidosis after birth
24. Cystathioninuria‡	Cystathionine	Cystathionine γ-lyase [4.4.1.1]	AR	Probably benign trait; vitamin B_6 corrects biochemical trait in most patients
Hyperglycinemias				
25. Ketotic form	Glycine and other glucogenic amino acids	Propionyl-CoA carboxylase (ATP-hydrolyzing) (propionyl-CoA:carbon-dioxide ligase [ADP-forming]) [6.4.1.3]	AR	Ketosis, neutropenia, mental retardation; often fatal; detectable in skin fibroblasts
26. Ibid.		Methylmalonyl-CoA racemase [5.1.99.1] or methylmalonyl-CoA mutase [5.4.99.2]	(AR)	Symptoms are those of methylmalonic aciduria with acidosis (some mutase-affected patients are responsive to vitamin B_{12})
27. Ibid.		Acetyl-CoA acyltransferase (β-ketothiolase) [2.3.1.16] deficiency‡‡	(AR)	Symptoms are those of α-methyl-β-hydroxybutyric aciduria (with or without tiglic aciduria) and acidosis
28. Nonketotic form	Glycine	Glycine cleavage reaction (CO_2, NH_3, and hydroxymethyltetrahydrofolate formed)	AR	Severe CNS depression soon after birth; high CSF:plasma glycine ratio; benzoate decreases plasma glycine; no effect on CNS prognosis; strychnine improves seizures
29. Sarcosinemia‡	Sarcosine	Sarcosine oxidase (sarcosine:oxygen oxidoreductase [demethylating]) [1.5.3.1]	AR	Benign trait (probably)
Hyperprolinemias				
30. Type I	Proline	Pyrroline-5-carboxylate reductase (L-proline:NAD(P)$^+$ 5-oxidoreductase; proline oxidase) [1.5.1.2]	AR	Benign trait, sometimes associated with hereditary nephritis
31. Type II	Proline	1-Pyrroline dehydrogenase (Δ^1-pyrroline-5-carboxylate:NAD$^+$ oxidoreductase) [1.5.1.12]	AR	Possibly benign trait, sometimes associated with CNS disease; Δ^1-pyrroline-5-carboxylate and 3-hydroxy-1-pyrroline-5-carboxylate excreted in urine; proline concentration > type I
32. Hydroxyprolinemia	Hydroxyproline	4-Oxoproline reductase (4-hydroxy-L-proline:NAD$^+$ oxidoreductase) [1.1.1.104]	AR	Sometimes associated with CNS disease; probably benign
Hyperlysinemias				
33. Type I	Lysine (and glutamine)	Saccharopine dehydrogenase (NADP$^+$, lysine-forming) [1.5.1.8]	AR	Associated with mental retardation and hypotonia
34. Type II	Lysine, arginine (sometimes NH_3)	? Partial defect of enzyme in entry 33 or different enzyme	(AR)	Hyperammonemia symptoms, related to protein intake
35. Saccharopinuria‡	Lysine, saccharopine, citrulline	? Saccharopine dehydrogenase (NADP$^+$, L-glutamate-forming) (saccharopine dehydrogenase) [1.5.1.10]	(AR)	Two cases; associated with mental retardation
36. Hydroxylysinemia	Free hydroxylysine	? Hydroxylysine kinase [2.7.1.81]	(AR)	Mental retardation

Table continues on following page. See bottom of following page for footnotes.

TABLE 1. Hereditary and Acquired Aminoacidopathies (Continued)

Condition or Disease	Amino Acid Affected	Enzyme Affected (Synonym) [Enzyme Commission No.]	IP	Remarks
37. α-Aminoadipic aciduria	α-Aminoadipic acid (and α-ketoadipic acid)	? "α-Ketoadipate dehydrogenase"	(AR)	Mental retardation
38. Pipecolic acidemia‡	Pipecolic acid	? L-Pipecolate dehydrogenase (pipecolate oxidase) [1.5.99.3]	(AR)	Hepatomegaly and mental retardation
Hyperammonemias§§				
39. Carbamyl phosphate synthetase (CPS) deficiency	Glycine, glutamine	Carbamate kinase (ATP:carbamate phosphotransferase) [2.7.2.2]	AR	Group of diseases with ammonia intoxication, protein intolerance, hepatomegaly, vomiting, etc.; argininosuccinic aciduria also has trichorrhexis nodosa
40. Ornithine transcarbamylase (OTC) deficiency	Glutamine	Ornithine carbamoyltransferase (carbamoylphosphate:L-ornithine carbamoyltransferase) [2.1.3.3]	XL	Same as above
41. Hyperornithinemia	Ornithine	a. L-Ornithine; 2-oxoacid aminotransferase [2.6.1.13]	—	a. Associated with gyrate atrophy of choroid and retina but no hyperammonemia (HOGA syndrome)
		b. Unknown; mitochondrial ornithine transport system	—	b. Associated with hyperammonemia and homocitrullinemia (HHH syndrome)
42. Citrullinemia	Citrulline	Argininosuccinate synthetase (L-citrulline:L-aspartate ligase [AMP-forming]) [6.3.4.5]	AR	See entry 39
43. Argininosuccinic-aciduria‡	Argininosuccinic acid	Argininosuccinate lyase (L-argininosuccinate arginine-lyase) [4.3.2.1]	AR	See entry 39
44. Hyperargininemia	Arginine	Arginase (L-arginine amidinohydrolase) [3.5.3.1]	(AR)	Deterioration of CNS function and I.Q. in childhood; hyperammonemia (inconstant) aggravated by protein
45. Hyperalaninemias	Alanine	Pyruvate dehydrogenase (lipoate) (pyruvate dehydrogenase) [1.2.4.1] deficiency	(AR)	Lactic acidosis, intermittent ataxia, mental retardation
46. Ibid.		Pyruvate carboxylase [6.4.1.1] deficiency	(AR)	Intermittent lactic acidosis, intermittent hypoglycemia
47. Aspartylglucosaminuria	Glycoasparagines	Aspartylglucosylaminase (2-acetamido-1-[β¹-L-aspartamido]-1,2-dideoxyglucose amidohydrolase) [3.5.1.26]	AR	? Lysosomal disease; mental retardation
48. "Glutathionemia"	Glutathione or related peptide	γ-Glutamyltransferase (γ-glutamyl-transpeptidase) [2.3.2.2]	(AR)	Mental retardation associated with finding

Other Conditions Which May Affect Amino Acids in Plasma

Condition or Disease	Amino Acid Affected		IP	Remarks
49. Protein-calorie malnutrition	Tryptophan/leucine/isoleucine/valine ↓; tyrosine/glycine/proline ↑	—	—	Severity of change related to severity of malnutrition
50. Prolonged fasting	Alanine ↓; threonine, glycine ↑	—	—	Early fasting does not show same pattern
51. Obesity	Leucine/isoleucine/valine/phenylalanine/tyrosine ↑; glycine ↓	—	—	Reflects insulin insensitivity
52. Hepatitis	Methionine/tyrosine ↑	—	—	Reflects severity of liver disease

*These conditions have been detected by screening methods applied in the newborn period of life. They should not be misdiagnosed as permanent disorders of amino acid metabolism also identifiable by screening.

†Probably secondary defect; primary unknown.

‡Urine screening is as efficient as, or even more reliable than, blood screening in these conditions.

§Liver and epidermis.

¶Liver only.

**A number of disorders of branched-chain amino acid catabolism cause accumulation of substances which are ninhydrin negative. These compounds can usually be detected by gas-lipid chromatographic methods.

††Partial activity less than 2 per cent of normal.

‡‡Hyperglycemia observed only in some patients with this enzyme deficiency.

§§See also entry 34.

TABLE 1. Hereditary and Acquired Aminoacidopathies (Continued)

GROUP IB

The primary defect is in catabolism. There is a high renal clearance of amino acid and a hyperaminoaciduria by saturation of transepithelial transport. Detection in the urine is preferable. See also entries 21, 24, and 43 in Group IA.

Source of enzyme number is *Enzyme Commission. IP:* Apparent inheritance pattern; AR = autosomal recessive; (AR) = probably autosomal recessive; AD = autosomal dominant. Data in brackets refer to the column heading in brackets.

Condition or Disease	Substance Affected (Synonym)	Enzyme Affected (Synonym) [Enzyme Commission No.]	IP	Remarks
1. Hypophosphatasia	Phosphoethanolamine	? Deficiency of ethanolaminephosphate phospho-lyase (*O*-phosphorylethanol-amine phospho-lyase) [4.2.99.7]	AR	"Rickets" unresponsive to vitamin D; craniosynostosis; hypercalcemia
2. Pseudohypophosphatasia	Phosphoethanolamine	"Alkaline phosphatase" activity present but altered (K_m mutant)	(AR)	Same as for entry 1
3. β-Aminoisobutyric-aciduria	β-Aminoisobutyric acid	?	AD/AR	Benign polymorphic trait
4. Hyper-β-alaninemia	β-Alanine	? β-Alanine–pyruvate aminotransferase (β-alanine transaminase) [2.6.1.18]	(AR)	Seizures; somnolence; mental retardation
5. Carnosinemia	Carnosine	Aminoacyl-histidine dipeptidase (carnosinase) [3.4.13.3]	AR	Seizure and mental retardation; or benign possibly
6. Pyroglutamic aciduria*	L-Pyroglutamic acid (5-oxo-L-proline; pyrrolidone-2-carboxylic acid)	Glutathione synthetase [6.3.2.3]	(AR)	L-Pyroglutamic acid (5-oxo-L-proline) results from overproduction via modified γ-glutamyl cycle

*Urine screening is as efficient as, or even more reliable than, blood screening in these conditions.

GROUP II

There is a primary defect in catabolism and a secondary defect in transport. Hyperaminoaciduria is of combined origin—saturation and competition. Detection is possible in both plasma and urine.

Disease	Amino Acids		Remarks
	Affected in Plasma	Present in Urine	
1. Hyperprolinemia, types I and II	Proline	Proline, + hydroxyproline and glycine	See entries 30 and 31 in Group IA; competition occurs on iminoglycine transport system (see Group III)
2. Hyper-β-alaninemia	β-Alanine	β-Alanine, + β-aminoisobutyric acid and taurine	See entry 4 in Group IB; competition occurs on β-amino transport system
3. Hyperlysinemia	Lysine	Lysine, + ornithine and arginine	See entries 33–36 in Group IA; competition occurs on "dibasic" transport system (see Group III)
4. Hyperargininemia	Arginine	Ornithine and lysine, and sometimes generalized hyperaminoaciduria	See entry 44 in Group IA; competition occurs on "dibasic" transport system (see Group III); pathogenesis of generalized aminoaciduria unknown

GROUP III

The primary defect is in the membrane transport site. There is a high renal clearance of amino acid, and detection is possible only in the urine. *Activity Affected:* Presumed gene product activity affected by mutant gene. *IP:* Apparent inheritance pattern; AD = autosomal dominant; (AD) = probably

autosomal dominant; AR = autosomal recessive; (AR) = probably autosomal recessive; XL = X-linked. *Remarks:* hetz = heteroxygote; homoz = homozygote. PTH = parathyroid hormone.

Trait	Substance Affected	Activity Affected	Other Tissues Affected	IP	Remarks
Common Perinatal (Adaptive) Trait					
1. Neonatal imino-glycinuria	Proline, hydroxy-proline, glycine	Specific proline and specific glycine transport (probably)	—	—	Benign adaptive trait; prolinuria subsides at ~100 days, glycinuria at ~200 days after full-term birth
2. Neonatal cystine-lysinuria	Cystine and dibasic amino acids (lysine, ornithine, and arginine)	Specific dibasic transport system	—	—	Transient; evident in newborn period in some but not all infants

Table continues on following page

TABLE 1.　Hereditary and Acquired Aminoacidopathies (Continued)

GROUP III (Continued)

Trait	Substance Affected	Activity Affected	Other Tissues Affected	IP	Remarks
	Inherited Hyperaminoacidurias				

Selective

Trait	Substance Affected	Activity Affected	Other Tissues Affected	IP	Remarks
3. Hyperdibasic aminoaciduria	Lysine, ornithine, arginine ("dibasic" group)	Shared "dibasic" amino acid transport system	Intestine; ? liver; ? brain	AD/AR	Two alleles (? different loci); type I associated with protein intolerance, failure to thrive, hyperammonemia (? mitochondrial defect); hetz silent; type II associated with mental retardation in recently discovered homoz; hetz have modest dibasic aminoaciduria
4. Cystinuria	Lysine, ornithine, arginine, and cyst(e)ine	Shared membrane system (? for efflux)	Intestine; ? brain (skin fibroblasts are normal)	AR	"Negative" reabsorption of affected amino acid can occur; three alleles (? same locus), each causing different phenotypes: in type I hetz, no amino acids in urine ("silent"); in type III homoz, intestinal transport intact (or partial defect)
5. Hypercystinuria	Cystine	Specific system for cyst(e)ine	?	(AR)	One pedigree only
6. Iminoglycinuria	Proline; hydroxyproline; glycine	Shared system for imino acids, glycine (and sarcosine)	Intestine	AR	Four alleles (? same locus); I and II are silent hetz; III and IV are hyperglycinuric hetz; I associated with intestinal defect; IV with K_m mutant
7. Hartnup syndrome	Neutral amino acids (excluding imino acids and glycine)	Shared system for large neutral amino acid group (luminal membrane)	Intestine (skin fibroblasts are normal)	AR	Two alleles (? same locus); I, intestine affected; II, intestine normal; hetz "silent" in both
8. Histidinuria	Histidine	? Specific histidine system	Intestine	(AR)	Associated with mental retardation in siblings
9. Dicarboxylic aminoaciduria (glutamate-aspartate transport defect)	Glutamic acid, aspartic acid	? Shared dicarboxylic acid transport system	? Intestine	(AR)	Hypoglycemia

Generalized

Trait	Substance Affected	Activity Affected	Other Tissues Affected	IP	Remarks
10. Idiopathic Fanconi's syndrome	Generalized effect on all solutes and water	? Coupling of energy; ? tight junction integrity	Secondary to renal phenotype	AR (and ?AD)	Adult onset and infantile-childhood forms are differentiated; basic defect unknown; probably several alleles

Symptomatic forms of Fanconi syndromes

Trait	Substance Affected	Activity Affected	Other Tissues Affected	IP	Remarks
11. Cystinosis: type I, type II, and type III	Same as for entry 10 (secondary response)	Cystine storage (lysosomal defect), with secondary damage to tubule and glomerulus (later)	Secondary to renal phenotype	AR*	Several alleles; infantile (type I) and adolescent (type II) forms have differing rates for onset of nephropathy; "adult" form (type III) has no nephropathy
12. Hereditary fructose intolerance	Same as for entry 10, + fructose	Fructose-1-phosphate aldolase (fructose bisphosphate aldolase) (with secondary effects on cellular ATP)	Secondary to renal phenotype (hepatic cirrhosis)	AR	Nephropathy dependent on intact PTH-cAMP axis in kidney; responds to fructose withdrawal
13. Galactosemia	Same as for entry 10, + galactose	Galactose-1-phosphate uridylyltransferase (with secondary effects on cellular ATP)	Secondary to renal phenotype (cataracts, CNS effects)	AR	"Galactosemia" due to galactokinase deficiency does *not* have Fanconi's syndrome; Fanconi's syndrome responds to galactose withdrawal
14. Hereditary tyrosinemia	Same as for entry 10, + tyrosine metabolites	Unknown (with secondary effects on cellular ATP)	Secondary to renal phenotype (hepatic cirrhosis)	(AR)	Fanconi's syndrome responds to tyrosine restriction
15. Wilson's disease	Same as for entry 10, with proximal and distal renal tubular acidosis	Unknown (? secondary effects on cytochrome oxidase system)	Hepatolenticular degeneration	(AR)	Fanconi's syndrome responds to depletion of copper storage

TABLE 1.   Hereditary and Acquired Aminoacidopathies (Continued)

GROUP III (Continued)

Trait	Substance Affected	Activity Affected	Other Tissues Affected	IP	Remarks
16. Lowe's oculocere-brorenal syndrome	Generalized dysfunction with defective urinary NH_3 production	Unknown	An oculocerebro-intestinal-renal syndrome (? involving tissues with high γ-glutamyl cycle activity)	XL†	Basic defect still unknown; treatment for tubular reclamation defects does not improve mental retardation or the cataracts and hydrophthalmia
17. Vitamin D dependency (pseudodeficiency rickets)	Generalized defect (secondary response)	Type I: 25-Hydroxy-vitamin D-1-α-hydroxylase Type II: Defective binding of hormone	Vitamin D hormone synthesis occurs in kidney mitochondria; deficiency of synthesis or binding affects intestinal absorption of calcium and initiates PTH response	AR	Nephropathy dependent on PTH excess and hypocalcemia (phenocopy occurs in vitamin D deficiency)
Miscellaneous 18. Glucoglycinuria	Glucose and glycine	Unknown (the two solutes do *not* share a common carrier)	—	(AD)	Asymptomatic; normal-Tm (type B) glucosuria; possibility that this is a heterozygous manifestation of a Fanconi-like tubulopathy merits consideration
19. Luder-Sheldon syndrome	Generalized amino acids, glucose, and phosphate	Unknown	—	(AD)	Same as for entry 18; symptoms of Fanconi's syndrome have occurred in probands
20. Rowley-Rosenberg syndrome	Generalized aminoaciduria	Unknown	—	(AR)	Associated components of syndrome: growth retardation, muscular hypoplasia, pulmonary involvement, and right ventricular hypertrophy

*For each type.
†Recessive.

General References:
1. Scriver, C. R., and Rosenberg, L. E.: Amino Acid Metabolism and Its Disorders. Philadelphia, W. B. Saunders Company, 1973.
2. Scriver, C. R., et al.: Kidney Int., 9:149, 1976.
3. Scriver, C. R.: Table 75, Biological Handbook II: Human Health and Disease. Bethesda, Md., FASEB, 1977.

a. "Basic" system: lysine, arginine, ornithine (and cystine, although not as a "basic" amino acid, viz., cystinuria).
b. "Acidic" system: aspartic, glutamic (viz., dicarboxylic aminoaciduria).
c. Neutral-I system: prolone, hydroxyproline, and glycine (viz., hyperprolinemia and renal iminoglycinuria).
d. Neutral-II system: the remaining neutral α-amino acids (viz., Hartnup disease).

It is usually possible to classify the aminoaciduria by analyzing the amino acid content of plasma and urine collected conjointly (Table 1). Chromatographic techniques will reveal the details of hyperaminoaciduria more accurately than any other method. The recognition of a specific aminoaciduria can provide an accurate clinical diagnosis for which there may be appropriate therapy.

Scriver, C. R., and Rosenberg, L. E.: Amino Acid Metabolism and Its Disorders. Philadelphia, W. B. Saunders Company, 1973.

534.2.   BRANCHED-CHAIN AMINOACIDURIA

Charles R. Scriver

MAPLE SYRUP URINE DISEASE. The colloquial term describes a characteristic odor of patients with *branched-chain ketoaciduria and aminoacidopathy*. The disease is autosomal recessive, and its apparent rarity may reflect, in part, missed diagnoses in patients dying in infancy. Severe hypotonia, apnea, feeding difficulty, and hypoglycemia appear in the first week of life, progressing to seizures, decorticate rigidity, severe mental retardation, and death. At least three variants with episodic illness or mild mental retardation presenting in later infancy have been reported.

The primary enzymatic defect is a block in decarboxylation of branched-chain α-keto acids; consequently leucine, isoleucine, alloisoleucine, and valine and their equivalent α-keto acids and α-hydroxyacids accumulate after birth; symptoms are primarily related to abnormal leucine metabolism. The aminoacidopathy can be detected in blood and urine within the first week of life; the enzyme defect can be assayed in leukocytes and in cultured skin fibroblasts.

The disease reponds to dietary control of leucine, isoleucine, and valine intake, the best results following the earliest possible treatment. One variant is responsive to thiamin at ten times the normal daily intake.

HYPERVALINEMIA. Symptoms of vomiting, blindness, and retardation of physical and mental development in a singe Japanese infant were reported, which improved abruptly with a valine-restricted diet. Valine transaminase is the defective enzyme; hence only valine accumulates in body fluids.

534.3. HYPERHISTIDINEMIA

Charles R. Scriver

Many cases of this autosomal recessively inherited disease are now known. Inactivity of the enzyme histidase (L-histidine, ammonia lyase) which nonoxidatively deaminates histidine to uraconic acid, can be detected in epidermis and liver. Accumulation of histidine (and sometimes of alanine) above normal levels and depressed serotonin levels are found in blood; increased excretion of imidazolepyruvic acid and a positive ferric chloride test are found in urine. The risk of mild mental retardation is believed to be higher than normal (>5 per cent). Histidinemic sibs of reported probands had 40 per cent frequency of mental retardation. The frequency is not more than 20 per cent in probands followed prospectively after detection by newborn screening and without treatment. Low-histidine therapy is feasible and, in view of the risk of delayed mental development, is probably indicated.

534.4. THE HYPERPROLINEMIAS AND HYDROXYPROLINEMIA

(Iminoacidopathies)

Charles R. Scriver

HYPERPROLINEMIAS. *Type I* (L-proline oxidase deficiency) is a recessively inherited condition. Proline is the only amino acid elevated in plasma, but a "combined" aminoaciduria involving proline, hydroxyproline, and glycine is found. In *Type II* hyperprolinemia the block is apparently at the second step in proline degradation (Δ-pyrroline-5-carboxylate dehydrogenase); the pyrroline derivative is also excreted in urine. Type I hyperprolinemia is sometimes associated with familial hematuric nephropathy, but pedigree studies show that prolinemia and nephropathy are not the consequences of a single gene effect; seizures also occur in both types of hyperprolinemia.

HYDROXYPROLINEMIA. The first enzyme for free hydroxy-L-proline catabolism is distinct from that for L-proline, and the deficient enzyme in hydroxyprolinemia is a hydroxyproline-specific "oxidase." The condition is probably benign.

534.5. DISEASES OF THE UREA CYCLE

Charles R. Scriver

A number of enzymes are involved in the incorportaion of ammonia and its delivery as urea. Differences in their relative activity (Table 2) and their location in the cell may account for some of the differences in clinical severity of the inborn errors of the urea cycle. In addition to the catalytic steps, two transport steps across the mitochrondrial membranes are involved, one of which delivers citrulline to the cytoplasm from the mitochondria, the other returning ornithine to the mitochondrion. *Carbamyl phosphate synthetase deficiency* is an intramitochondrial disease with severe hyperammonemia and a rapidly fatal course after birth; inheri-

TABLE 2. Enzymes in Urea Cycle and Relative Activities*

Carbamyl phosphate synthetase	4.5
Ornithine transcarbamylase	163.0
Argininosuccinic acid synthetase	1.0
Argininosuccinic acid lyase	3.3
Arginase	149.0

*From Scriver, C. R., and Rosenberg, L. E.: Amino Acid Metabolism and Its Disorders. Philadelphia, W. B. Saunders Company, 1973.

tance is probably autosomal recessive. *Ornithine transcarbamylase deficiency* is an X-linked disease, with males severely, even fatally, affected and females exhibiting a variable range of clinical symptoms as expected in an X-linked trait. *Citrullinemia* and *argininosuccinicaciduria* are each autosomal recessive, their names identifying the substrate which accumulates in the presence of their respective enzyme deficiencies. *Argininemia* is an autosomal recessive disorder of the last step of the cycle.

Ornithinemia (HOGA) is apparently an autosomal recessive disease in which the defective enzyme is L-ornithine: 2-oxo-acid aminotransferase (EC 2.6.1.13). The deficiency state has no ammonia accumulation and is associated with a characteristic gyrate atrophy of choroid and retina and reduced whole blood glutamate levels. A second form of hyperornithemia (HHH), also autosomal recessive, is associated with hyperammonemia and homocitrullinemia; the catalytic defect is unknown in this second condition.

Each disease of the urea cycle is accompanied by a set of similar findings which include hyperammonemia, metabolic alkalosis, failure to thrive, convulsions, hepatomegaly, and mental retardation. A fatal outcome is common.

The severity of symptoms and biochemical imbalance varies with the site of the defect and with its completeness. Some patients maintain normal or nearly normal urea synthesis, presumably reflecting only a partial block in the urea cycle compensated for by marked substrate accumulation. Symptomatic treatment with low protein diet and prevention of ammonia intoxication is sometimes feasible. More often it is necessary to restrict nitrogen intake drastically and to utilize a mixture of "essential" keto acids as a source of carbon chains which can incorporate endogenous ammonia to form essential amino acids and thus sustain protein synthesis. Careful genetic counseling, coupled with the option for prenatal diagnosis in some of the diseases, is recommended.

534.6. β-AMINOISOBUTYRICACIDURIA

Charles R. Scriver

β-Aminoisobutyric acid (βAIB) is a derivative of thymine and valine metabolism. High urinary excretion (more than 100 μmoles per gram total N) occurs in some humans who are probably homozygous for a gene controlling βAIB metabolism. In these subjects, plasma levels of βAIB are elevated; the renal clearance rate of the natural isomer, D-(-), βAIB, exceeds that for inulin, indicating net renal "secretion" of βAIB; probenecid can suppress excretion. Hyperexcretors are common in the Mongolian race but infrequent (approximately 5 per cent) in Caucasians; the adaptive significance for the mutation is unknown. Increased βAIB excretion can also be acquired under catabolic stress.

534.7. THE HYPERGLYCINURIAS

Charles R. Scriver

Six forms of isolated hyperglycinuria are known:
1. Hyperglycinemia with "overflow" hyperglycinuria.
   a. Type I (ketotic): Vomiting, acetonuria, neutropenia, thrombocytopenia, and leucine intolerance occur in the neonatal period; retardation of growth and mental development follow if the infant survives. The findings to a lesser or greater degree are found in propionicacidemia (propionyl CoA carboxylase deficiency), methylmalonicacidemia (methylmalonyl CoA mutase deficiency), and a disorder of isoleucine catabolism (β-ketothiolase deficiency). Restriction of dietary protein intake may be helpful.
   b. Type II (nonketotic): There is severe developmental and mental retardation. Conversion of glycine to carbon dioxide, methylenetetrahydrofolate, and ammonia is apparently impaired.
2. Renal glycinurias.
   a. Impaired renal conservation of glycine occurs as the heterozygous phenotype in one form of familial iminoglycinuria.
   b. Resistant rickets and renal hyperglycinuria occur in association with (i) hyperphosphaturia, (ii) hyperphosphaturia and glucosuria (both renal).
   c. Dominantly inherited, asymptomatic renal glycinuria with renal glucosuria has been reported from Switzerland.

534.8. RENAL HYPERAMINOACIDURIAS

Charles R. Scriver

Certain hyperaminoacidurias reflect impairment of specific transport systems; the transport lesion is frequently demonstrable in the gut as well as in the kidney. The renal clearance rates of affected amino acids are high, and their plasma levels are low or normal, rather than elevated.

CYSTINURIA. Three homozygous cystinuric phenotypes are now recognized; in all, there is elevated urinary excretion of cystine, lysine, ornithine, and arginine. In Type I, gut transport of the four amino acids is also abnormal; the heterozygote has normal aminoaciduria (complete recessive). Type II has defective gut transport of the basic amino acids but not of cystine; the heterozygote has elevated urinary lysine and cystine (incomplete recessive.) Type III has normal gut transport; the heterozygote phenotype is "incomplete." The exact mechanism of the hyperaminoaciduria is unclear.

Genetic classification of patients now extends to include "genetic compounds," that is, individuals who resemble homozygotes in their findings but who have inherited two *different* mutant alleles (e.g., I-III, I-II, or II-III). Further details appear in Ch. 534.12.

HARTNUP DISEASE. Episodic clinical features include pellagra-like symptoms with photosensitive dermatitis, cerebellar ataxia, and psychosis. Biochemical findings include reduced blood levels of tryptophan metabolites, e.g., nicotinic acid and serotonin, and a fluctuant increase in urinary excretion of indolic acids and derivatives. A constant transport defect for certain neutral α-amino acids is demonstrable in kidney. The abnormal "indoluria" is dependent on intestinal flora degrading unabsorbed L-tryptophan, with absorption and renal excretion of the products. Defective intracellular transport of tryptophan may account for the deficiency of its endogenous metabolites. Good protein nutrition, normal general intestinal health, and nicotinamide supplements (40 to 200 mg per day) can maintain good general health of the patient.

PROLINE-HYDROXYPROLINE-GLYCINURIA (IMINOGLYCINURIA). This finding is normal in early infancy. Failure of the group-specific transport system to develop has been observed as a benign autosomal recessive trait. Presence or absence of an associated intestinal transport defect indicates at least two mutant genotypes.

534.9. FANCONI'S SYNDROME

Charles R. Scriver

The term "Fanconi's syndrome" describes a disturbance of proximal renal tubular function of multiple causation and comprising generalized hyperaminoaciduria, renal glucosuria, and hyperphosphaturia, as well as renal loss of potassium, bicarbonate and water, and other substances conserved by the proximal tubule. Fanconi's syndrome should be considered as the final result of any one of many possible primary insults to proximal tubular function (see Group III aminoacidurias, Table 1). The patient's symptoms reflect the disturbance of tubular function, in addition to the primary cause of the syndrome. Osteomalacia is a particularly prominent clinical finding primarily reflecting phosphate wasting. Acidosis accompanies the bicarbonate loss, whereas muscular weakness may be a prominent manifestation of hypokalemia.

Fanconi's syndrome may be inherited or acquired. The various hereditary forms are predominantly recessive, different alleles being responsible for the different diseases causing the syndrome. For example, cystinosis is a recessive, inherited disease, with cystine accumulation occurring in tissues and accompanied by the syndrome that first appears about six months after birth. The idiopathic Fanconi syndrome in adults is a recessively inherited disorder of early middle age. Acquired causes are numerous; deteriorated tetracycline (epianhydrotetracycline) is an interesting example of a toxic cause of the syndrome.

The syndrome appears to follow inhibition of cellular mechanisms sustaining transport function in the proximal tubule. As a result, the tubular capacity for transport is impaired. In severe cases, morphologic changes also occur, with reduction in cell organelles and cell mass of the proximal portion of the proximal convoluted tubule (swan-neck lesion). There is considerable experimental evidence that solutes enter urine in excess not only because of impaired absorption but also by back-flux from renal cells after entry into kidney tissue from peritubular capillaries.

The disturbance of proximal tubular function results in the alterations in urine and plasma composition referred to above. The final levels of expression of the syndrome are more peripheral, and are related to both the disturbances in renal physiology and the primary causes of the syndrome. Evidence for the primary cause of the syndrome, e.g., cystine crystals in the cornea, Kayser-Fleischer rings of Wilson's disease, a history of exposure to antimicrobial drugs or toxins, or other affected family members should always be pursued.

TREATMENT. Attempt to eliminate the primary cause, e.g., removal of exogenous toxic agents or deficiency states. Other primary conditions may be ameliorated, e.g., removal of milk in galactosemia or removal of copper in Wilson's disease.

Offset the disturbance in tubular physiology. Osteomalacia is readily treated, and prevented, with oral phosphate supplements (1.0 to 2.0 grams phosphorus per day, equivalent to 20 grams of "neutral" phosphate salt); supplemental vitamin D as $1,25-(OH)_2D_3$ may also be required in doses adjusted to the patient's need. Shohl's solution, 30 ml three times daily for adults, usually controls the acidemia. Hypokalemia may be corrected with potassium salts (as phosphate or citrate). Adequate fluid intake is indicated to prevent dehydration.

Nyhan, W. L. (ed.): Amino Acid Metabolism and Genetic Variation. New York, McGraw-Hill Book Company, 1967.

Scriver, C. R., and Rosenberg, L. F.: Amino Acid Metabolism and Its Disorders. Philadelphia, W. B. Saunders Company, 1973.

534.10. THE HYPERPHENYLALANINEMIAS

Charles R. Scriver

Mass screening of newborn infants in recent years has shown that all that is hyperphenylalaninemia is not necessarily phenylketonuria. Hence this chapter includes several hyperphenylalaninemic phenotypes evident in the human race.

METABOLISM OF PHENYLALANINE. L-Phenylalanine is an essential amino acid for man. In infancy half or more of its dietary intake is used for protein synthesis, and the remainder is oxidized to tyrosine by hydroxylation in the liver. As body size increases, the phenylalanine intake increases from 1/2 gram per day at birth to as much as 4 grams daily in the older child and adult; at the same time that the rate of growth slows, a larger fraction of phenylalanine is catabolized to tyrosine, and the amount required for anabolism decreases proportionately. Any impairment of oxidation, without change in the other parameters, will cause the free phenylalanine pool to enlarge and its plasma concentration to rise above the normal maximum (1.2 mg per 100 ml). When this happens, other minor pathways of phenylalanine catabolism are called upon, and increased amounts of normal minor metabolites will appear in body fluids.

The key step in L-phenylalanine catabolism, namely, hydroxylation to tyrosine, has received much attention. This complex reaction involves several genes which control various components (Table 3). Not surprisingly, several types of hyperphenylalaninemias are known; further variants will undoubtedly be discovered in the future.

TABLE 3. The Mammalian Phenylalanine Hydroxylating System*

	Gene Locus†	Mutant Alleles Identified
1. Apoenzyme		
Phenylalanine hydroxylase (EC 1.14.16.1)	1	+ (Several)
Dihydropteridine reductase (EC 1.6.99.7)	2	+
Dihydrofolate reductase (EC 1.5.1.4)	(3)§	
2. Cofactor or coenzyme		
Tetrahydrobiopterin (cofactor for apohydroxylase)	Several for biosynthesis pathway	+
NADPH + H⁺		
3. Additional factor¶		
Phenylalanine hydroxylase–stimulating protein	4	
Lysolecithin	Several for biosynthesis	

*Adapted from Kaufman (1976).
†Loci are arbitrarily numbered.
‡Clinical, biochemical, and genetic evidence indicates mendelian inheritance of variants.
§Probably of little importance in maintaining cofactor (tetrahydrobiopterin) for apohydroxylase.
¶Factors active only in presence of tetrahydrobiopterin.

CLASSIC PHENYLKETONURIA

DEFINITION. The disease was first described by Følling in 1934. In its fully expressed form, there is persistent hyperphenylalaninemia in excess of 1 mM (16.5 mg per 100 ml), mental retardation (in most cases), and excessive urinary excretion of phenylpyruvic acid and other phenylalanine derivatives. The condition is autosomal recessive, being the result of complete or near-complete absence of phenylalanine hydroxylase activity. Mass screening of newborn infants for this trait and genetic counseling is effective, so that the patient with classic untreated phenylketonuria has become an oddity, often mentioned but rarely seen.

PREVALENCE. The homozygote occurs once in about 12,000 live births in Caucasians, with significant variation in frequency among ethnic groups. The disease is rare in the black and in the Ashkenazic Jew; in the latter cases, the mutation may not be allelic with the gene causing Caucasian phenylketonuria.

CLINICAL MANIFESTATIONS. The most important and consistent feature is mental retardation. This becomes evident by mid-infancy and in later childhood 98 per cent of untreated patients have an I.Q. below 70. Phenylketonuric patients are clinically normal at birth, distinguishable only by hyperphenylalaninemia, which is established in the first postnatal week. Other manifestations, such as seizures (often with the hypsarrhythmic EEG pattern), psychotic behavior, eczema, dermatographia, "mousy" odor (owing to excretion of phenylacetic acid), and pigment dilution, are found in untreated patients. None of these signs are seen in patients who benefit from early diagnosis and proper treatment.

THE METABOLIC ERROR. Homozygotes are almost completely lacking in phenylalanine hydroxylase activity; heterozygotes have partial activity, sufficient to maintain normal phenylalanine metabolism under ordinary circumstances.

Phenylalanine accumulates when the catabolic pathway is blocked, and is found in excessive amounts in blood, urine, and cerebrospinal fluid. Minor pathways are then overutilized, and, characteristically, phenylpyruvic acid is formed and excreted in urine. Additional compounds such as the lactic and acetic derivatives and the glutamine conjugate are also formed and excreted. Orthohydroxylation can occur and the corresponding ortho series of metabolites may be present.

Excessive amounts of phenylalanine and its derivatives can inhibit other enzymes. As a result disturbances of tyrosine and tryptophan metabolism occur. Diminished formation of catecholamines, melanin, and serotonin is observed in untreated phenylketonuria.

The cause of mental retardation in phenylketonuria is still unknown. It is probably due to many abnormalities which occur as a consequence of the disturbed chemical environment during the critical early postnatal stage of brain development.

DIAGNOSIS. Recognition of the trait should result from early postnatal detection of hyperphenylalaninemia. Subsequent studies to assess the degree of hyperphenylalaninemia, the dietary phenylalanine tolerance, and the persistence of the trait will help to distinguish it from other genetic variants affecting phenylalanine metabolism. Testing of the urine with ferric chloride (a few drops of 5 per cent solution in 0.1N HCl added to 1 to 2 ml urine) is not recommended for diagnosis in the newborn, because this test requires the excretion of phenylpyruvic acid, whose formation is dependent on transamination of phenylalanine; the latter function may not mature for at least three weeks after birth, even in full-term babies. All current newborn screening programs employ a specific microbiologic assay, fluorometric assay, or partition chromatography to detect excess phenylalanine in a few microliters of capillary blood collected from the heel of the infant.

TREATMENT. Replacement of phenylalanine hydroxylase is not feasible. Partial liver transplantation from a normal homozygote or heterozygote would give the patient a stable source of enzyme, and perhaps this mode of treatment will be possible in the future. At present dietary restriction of phenylalanine is the only practical therapy. By means of semisynthetic diets containing a low-phenylalanine hydrolysate, it is possible to restrict L-phenylalanine intake to about 250 to 500 mg daily while providing the recommended amounts of other essential amino acids and of calories and other nutritional factors. Close supervision of this treatment is important, and is best performed at centers experienced with such regimens.

Reduction of hyperphenylalaninemia to about 4 to 12 mg per 100 ml (relaxed regimen) when begun within 60 days of birth, allows normal physical and mental development. Delayed or inadequate treatment impairs normal mental development. There is an emerging impression that dietary treatment should be continued throughout the first decade at least. Female homozygous phenylketonurics should be treated during pregnancy to prevent harm to the fetus from intrauterine hyperphenylalaninemia.

HYPERPHENYLALANINEMIC VARIANTS

The following phenotypes behave as independent autosomal recessives. Their description is almost certainly a minimal report, since there are probably many mutant alleles which in like pairs (homozygotes) or combinations (genetic compounds) will yield all manner of phenotypic variation. Their recognition is important in order to avoid inappropriate treatment and counseling.

ATYPICAL PHENYLKETONURIA (MILD VARIANT). This variant is characterized by its high dietary tolerance for phenylalanine, which allows the patient to ingest between 700 and 2000 mg of the amino acid in the diet. Phenylalanine hydroxylase deficiency in the liver is probably incomplete; impaired intestinal absorption or excessive renal or fecal loss of phenylalanine does not account for this variant.

TRANSIENT PHENYLKETONURIA. Several sibships are known in which disappearance of the phenylketonuric phenotype and restoration of normal or nearly normal dieatry phenylalanine tolerance occur spontaneously during infancy or childhood. The precise enzymatic basis for the phenotype has not been established.

BENIGN PERSISTENT HYPERPHENYLALANINEMIA. The concentration of phenylalanine in plasma of homozygotes consuming normal diets is usually less than 1 mM (16.5 mg per 100 ml). Mental and physical development is normal without treatment in these subjects.

"LETHAL" PHENYLKETONURIA. As screening programs have retrieved more and more patients, it has become apparent that some phenylketonuric patients treated from the postnatal period in the accepted manner have not developed normally. In these patients, mental retardation appeared despite good control of phenylalanine levels, and these have also developed a seizure disorder; most are dead by the fifth year. They constitute perhaps 3 per cent of all "phenylketonuria" patients.

Their enzyme defect involves the natural cofactor (tetrahydrobiopterin) regenerating system; dihydropteridine reductase activity (Table 3) is deficient. Phenylalanine hydroxylase activity is normal in the presence of an adequate supply of tetrahydropterin in vitro, but with deficient reductase activity in vivo hydroxylation activity cannot be maintained; accordingly the conversion of phenylalanine to tyrosine is impaired. At the same time hydroxylation of L-tryptophan to 5 hydroxytryptophan and of tyrosine to L-dopa is compromised in brain, since the dihydropteridine reductase enzyme maintains these hydroxylation reactions as well. Therefore mutation at the dihydropteridine reductase locus affects one hepatic and two brain hydroxylation reactions. The neurologic complications are believed to reflect the disorder of brain enzymes in this variant.

Treatment of the condition requires phenylalanine restriction and replacement of 5-OH tryptophan and L-dopa at levels sufficient to repair the cerebral deficits. Replacement of tetrahydrobiopterin is not feasible, since it cannot penetrate cells (or brain) effectively, and the rate of replacement would have to be equimolar with the amount of phenylalanine oxidized per unit time.

A further variant of the "lethal" type has recently been discovered. In this form of "phenylketonuria," phenylalanine hydroxylase and dihydropteridine reductase enzymes are both normal but the cellular (hepatic) tetrahydrobiopterin level is greatly diminished. The deficit in this instance is believed to involve a step —as yet unspecified — in the biosynthesis pathway that yields tetrahydrobiopterin.

Diagnosis of "lethal" variants is of practical importance. Accurate counseling as to expected outcome and the anticipated efficacy of (low phenylalanine) dietary therapy is not possible until it is known whether the patient has a primary phenylalanine hydroxylase deficiency or a disorder of the cofactor system. Because the reductase enzyme can be assayed in skin fibroblasts, specific diagnosis of "phenylketonuria" patients will now require evaluation of this component of the system. Another option under investigation is the analysis of cofactor byproducts in body fluids, including urine; they should be increased in the reductase deficiency and diminished in the cofactor biosynthesis disorder.

Kaufman, S.: The phenylalanine hydroxylating system in phenylketonuria and its variants. Biochem. Med., 15:42, 1976.

Scriver, C. R., and Rosenberg, L. E.: Amino Acid Metabolism and Its Disorders. Philadelphia, W. B. Saunders Company, 1973, pp. 290–337.

534.11. ALCAPTONURIA

James B. Wyngaarden

DEFINITION. Alcaptonuria is a rare hereditary disease in which the enzyme homogentisic acid oxidase is missing. Because of this defect homogentisic acid produced during the metabolism of phenylalanine and tyrosine cannot be further metabolized. It therefore accumulates and is excreted in the urine. It causes pigmentation of cartilage and other connective tissue (ochronosis) and in later years a degenerative arthritis of the spine and the larger peripheral joints. The disease has great historic significance, for it was chiefly on the basis of study of families with alcaptonuria that Sir Archibald Garrod developed the concept of inborn errors of metabolism.

INCIDENCE. At least 600 cases have been reported. An incidence of 3 to 5 per million individuals was found in a population study in Northern Ireland.

ETIOLOGY. The disease is inherited as an autosomal recessive trait. In a family in which alcaptonuria in five successive generations at first suggested a dominant form of the disease, further study disclosed at least three instances of consanguinity and pedigree analysis confirmed a recessive pattern of inheritance. No method of detection of heterozygotes has been found.

PATHOGENESIS. The activity of homogentisic acid oxidase in the normal adult human liver is sufficient to metabolize over 1600 grams of homogentisic acid per day. Normally, no homogentisic acid can be detected in plasma or urine. In alcaptonuric individuals there is no detectable activity of this enzyme in liver or kidney tissue obtained by biopsy. Plasma levels of homogentisic acid rise to about 3 mg per deciliter, and the urinary excretion ranges from 4 to 8 grams per day. Mammalian tissue contains an enzyme called homogentisic acid polyphenol oxidase which catalyzes the oxidation of homogentisic acid to an ochronotic pigment, but pigment can also be produced nonenzymatically in the presence of oxygen and alkali, as for example in urine. The homogentisic acid polymer has a high affinity for cartilage and connective tissue macromolecules. The stained tissue is fragile and eventually may break down, leading to degenerative intervertebral disc or joint disease. Homogentisic acid may also have a direct effect upon collagen synthesis through inhibition of lysyl hydroxylase. In organ culture of embryonic chick calvariae, hydroxylation of lysine as well as subsequent hydroxylysine-derived cross-link formation was significantly inhibited by homogentisic acid administration. There is no spontaneously occurring animal model of alcaptonuria or ochronosis.

PATHOLOGY. In an elderly alcaptonuric patient cartilage in many areas, particularly the costal, laryngeal, and tracheal cartilage, is densely pigmented, sometimes being coal-black in appearance. Pigmentation is also present throughout the body in fibrous tissue, fibrocartilage, tendons, and ligaments. To a lesser degree it is also found in the endocardium, in the intima of larger vessels, in various organs such as kidney and lung, and in the epidermis. The pigment is deposited both intracellularly and intercellularly, and may be granular or homogeneous.

CLINICAL MANIFESTATIONS. Homogentisic acid is present in urine from birth, but urine is colorless when passed. Before the days of disposable napkins the diagnosis was sometimes made when diapers turned brown in alkaline soaps. Homogentisic acid reduces Benedict's reagent to give a yellow-orange-brown precipitate, and this reaction has given rise to false-positive diagnoses for diabetes. Pigment may appear in perspiration and stain clothing in the axillary region. Generally, the earliest change that can be detected externally is a slight pigmentation of the sclerae or the ears, beginning at 20 or 30 years of age. The cartilage of the ears may be slate blue or gray and feel irregular and thickened. Sometimes dusky discolorations of underlying tendons can be seen through the skin over the hands. In many patients, however, pigment is scarcely evident at all. The arthritis usually presents with some degree of limitation of motion of the hips, knee joints, or shoulders. There may be periods of acute inflammation, and later there is usually rather marked limitation of motion and ankylosis in the lumbosacral region. The arthritic complications are often severe and painful and may lead to extensive crippling. In addition, alcaptonuric patients appear to have a high incidence of cardiovascular disease, including generalized arteriosclerosis and chronic mitral and aortic valvulitis, with calcification of valves and annulus. Myocardial infarction is a common cause of death. Other reported complications include ruptured intervertebral discs, prostatitis, or renal stones.

X-RAY CHANGES. These may be almost pathognomonic of alcaptonuria. The vertebral bodies of the lumbar spine show degeneration of the intervertebral discs with narrowing of the space and dense calcification of remaining disc material. There is a variable degree of fusion of vertebral bodies, but little osteophytic formation and minimal calcification of intervertebral ligaments are present. The degenerative changes of ochronotic arthritis are most severe in the hip, shoulder, and knee, and there may be calcific deposits in the muscle tendons. The sacroiliac joints and smaller joints of the extremities usually show little or no abnormality. Ear cartilage may be calcified.

DIAGNOSIS AND DIFFERENTIAL DIAGNOSIS. The diagnosis is suggested by the history of pigmentary changes of urine, the presence of nonglucose reducing substance, the pigmentation of sclerae or cartilage, the arthritic episodes, and especially the typical x-ray changes of the lumbar spine. Specific identification of homogentisic acid in urine can be accomplished by chromotographic or enzymatic assays.

The ochronotic changes of skin and cartilage may possibly be confused with pigmentary changes resulting from prolonged use of Atabrine, or use of carbolic acid dressings for chronic cutaneous ulcers. The arthritis must be differentiated chiefly from rheumatoid arthritis, osteoarthritis, and gout.

TREATMENT. There is no effective treatment. Dietary restriction of phenylalanine and tyrosine of the degree necessary to reduce homogentisic aciduria is impractical and potentially deleterious. Large amounts of ascorbic acid have been given in an effort to reduce pigment formation. Ascorbic acid protects lysyl hydroxylase from inhibition by homogentisic acid in vitro. It does not alter the metabolic defect.

La Du, B. N.: Alcaptonuria. In Stanbury, J. B., Wyngaarden, J. B., and Fredrickson, D. S. (eds.): The Metabolic Basis of Inherited Disease. 4th ed. New York, McGraw-Hill Book Company, 1978, p. 268.

Pinnell, S. R.: Disorders of collagen. In Stanbury, J. B., Wyngaarden, J. B., and Fredrickson, D. S. (eds.): The Metabolic Basis of Inherited Disease. 4th ed. New York, McGraw-Hill Book Company, 1978, p. 1366.

534.12. CYSTINURIA

James B. Wyngaarden

DEFINITION. Cystinuria is an inherited disorder of amino acid transport affecting the epithelial cells of the renal tubules and gastrointestinal tract. The disease is characterized clinically by precipitation of cystine in the urine with formation of crystals and calculi, and a potential for obstruction, infection, and ultimately renal insufficiency.

INCIDENCE. The over-all incidence of the disease is about 1 in 7000, which makes cystinuria one of the more common inherited disorders. Screening programs in newborn babies show an incidence in England of 1 in 2000, in Australia of 1 in 4000, and in the United States of 1 in 15,000.

ETIOLOGY AND PATHOGENESIS. The disease is characterized by deficient transport of dibasic amino acids, cystine, lysine, ornithine, and arginine. Since this aminoaciduria occurs with a normal or reduced filtered load of cystine and other dibasic amino acids, it was postulated earlier that cystinuria is a disorder of tubular transport in the kidney. Subsequent demonstration of comparably defective transport in the intestine established the present view that this disorder is an inherited defect of a special transepithelial transport mechanism, which is expressed in two areas, the kidney and the intestine.

Three homozygous cystinuric phenotypes are recognized. In Type I, gut transport of the four amino acids is also abnormal. The heterozygote shows no abnormal urinary amino acid excretion. Thus Type I behaves as a completely recessive trait. Type II has defective gut transport of the basic amino acids but not of cystine; the heterozygote has elevated urinary lysine and cystine (incomplete recessive). Type III has normal gut transport. Cystinuria also presents as genetic compounds, that is, in individuals who resemble homozygotes in their findings but who have inherited two different mutant alleles (for example, I-III, I-II, or II-III).

Urinary cystine values in homozygotes range from 250 to 1000 mg per gram of creatinine per day. Cystine is poorly soluble in acid or neutral urine, where the limit is 300 to 400 mg per liter.

CLINICAL MANIFESTATIONS AND DIAGNOSIS. The disease occurs equally in both sexes, but males are more severely affected and have a higher mortality rate. The greater severity in the male may be related to urinary tract anatomy. The peak times for expression of cystinuria are the second and third decades of life, but the disease may appear during the first year or as late as the ninth decade. The most common presenting symptom is renal colic, and this may be associated with urinary tract obstruction. Recurring calculi lead to infection and eventual loss of renal function. Hypertension and renal failure may occur. Cystine stones are radiopaque. On roentgenograms they appear smooth but are less dense than calcium stones. They may occur singly, as multiple recurrent stones, or as staghorn calculi filling the entire renal pelvis. Patients with infection may form mixed stones containing cystine and calcium.

The diagnosis of cystinuria should be considered in every patient with urinary calculi. The first morning specimen or other concentrated urine may show typical cystine crystals. Patients with a positive nitroprusside test result should be studied further for identification of urinary amino acids by such methods as thin layer chromatography or high voltage electrophoresis. These tests will disclose increased quantities of cystine, lysine, arginine, and ornithine. Cystinuria has been associated with hyperuricemia, hemophilia, retinitis pigmentosa, muscular dystrophy, and mongolism. As a group cystinuric subjects are slightly shorter than the general population, perhaps because of malabsorption of essential amino acids.

TREATMENT. The aims of treatment are to reduce excretion and increase the solubility of cystine. Therapeutic approaches include (1) dietary restriction aimed at reducing cystine production and excretion, (2) attempts to increase cystine solubility by physical means, and (3) attempts to convert cystine to a more soluble compound.

Results of dietary restriction of methionine have been variable. It is possible to design a nutritionally adequate diet low in methionine. Avoidance of excess methionine intake is reasonable, but discomforting diets are not indicated.

Cystine solubility can be enhanced by providing liberal fluid intakes. However, a subject who excretes 1 gram of cystine per day will require fluid intake of 4 or more liters per day. Solubility can be increased by alkalinization of urine above 7.5, but the risks of persistently excessive alkaline loads must be considered. A major problem in stone formers is the supersaturation of urine which occurs at night when urine flow is low. The intake of 2 glasses of water at bedtime repeated at 2 or 3 A.M. has been recommended in cystinuria. Hydration therapy was successful in preventing stone formation in about two thirds of patients who adhered to it during a 10-year study conducted by Dent and associates. For those who are apparently not helped by diet, fluid, and alkalinization, the introduction of D-penicillamine for use in cystinuria represented a great advance. On penicillamine therapy, usually 1 to 2 grams per day in divided doses, cystine excretion may be kept below 200 mg per gram of creatinine, a level at which stone formation is minimal. Penicillamine has certain undesirable side effects. As many as 50 per cent of patients receiving the drug will develop allergic reactions, usually fever and rash, sometimes including arthralgias. More severe reactions include the nephrotic syndrome and pancytopenia. These are usually rapidly reversible when the drug is discontinued. Epidermolysis, thrombocytosis, loss of taste, and a fatal Goodpasture-like syndrome have also been reported. In view of the drawbacks of D-penicillamine therapy, its use should be restricted to patients in whom more conservative therapy has failed, or who have lost one kidney from cystine stone disease. Therapy should be started in the hospital in order to monitor reactions of hypersensitivity. In those patients initially sensitive to the drug, adequate results have been obtained by readministering the medication in gradually increasing dosages over one to two months. A related compound, N-acetyl-D-penicillamine, appears to have fewer side effects. Cystine crystalluria has been reported to be reduced in patients receiving diazepoxide, but this is unexplained. Mercaptopropionylglycine has recently been used orally, reportedly preventing stones without side effects.

Dent, C. E., Friedmann, M., Green, H., and Watson, L. C. A.: Treatment of cystinuria. Br. Med. J., 1:403, 1965.

Thier, S. O., and Segal, S.: Cystinuria. In Stanbury, J. B., Wyngaarden, J. B., and Fredrickson, D. S. (eds.): The Metabolic Basis of Inherited Disease. 4th ed. New York, McGraw-Hill Book Company, 1978, p. 1578.

534.13.   HOMOCYSTINURIA

James B. Wyngaarden

DEFINITION. The term homocystinuria designates a biochemical abnormality, not a specific disease entity. There are several genetic disorders leading to homocystinuria. The most common condition, and the one of greatest importance in the adult, is that due to cystathionine β-synthase deficiency. In this condition ectopia lentis, mental retardation, lax ligaments, lengthened extremities, malar flush, and sparse fine hair are present. Death from thromboembolic phenomena is frequent.

INCIDENCE. More than 300 adequately documented cases have been reported. Screening of newborn infants has led to an apparent frequency of 1 in 200,000 in the United States, Europe, Australia, and New Zealand.

ETIOLOGY AND PATHOGENESIS. Cystathionine β-synthase deficiency is inherited as an autosomal recessive trait. The disease occurs in the homozygote, and the heterozygote is without known risk. Deficient enzyme activity has been demonstrated in liver extracts from at least 28 homocystinuric patients. Activity is also deficient in brain, skin fibroblasts, and lymphocytes. The enzyme deficiency results in a failure of homocysteine to react with serine to form cystathionine on the pathway to cysteine. Homocystine is the disulfide oxidation product formed from two molecules of homocysteine. Normally, homocystine is not detected in human plasma by methods of the usual sensitivity. In cystathionine β-synthase–deficient patients fasting plasma concentrations of up to 0.2 μmol per milliliter of homocystine have been reported. The urine may contain up to 1 mmol of homocystine per day. Many of the manifestations of homocystinuria are related to abnormal connective tissue. Outwardly these patients may resemble those with Marfan's syndrome, but the joints are not hyperextensible. Skin collagen from patients with homocystinuria is more soluble in acid solutions, and cross-links are diminished compared with normal collagen. The stability of insoluble collagen is reduced. The pathogenesis of the thrombotic tendency is not clearly understood. Some evidence exists for specific abnormalities of each of the following, but the generali-

ty and reproducibility of these abnormalities have not been established: structural abnormality of collagen leading to abnormal hemostasis, abnormal platelet adhesiveness, abnormal aggregation of platelets, activation of Hageman factor by homocystine, platelet vacuolization, and endothelial damage leading to increased platelet consumption.

PATHOLOGY. There is fraying and disruption of the zonular fibers of the lens, with resulting subluxation. The skeleton is markedly osteoporotic, and the vertebrae show rarefaction of spongy bone with biconcave (codfish) compression. Thrombi and emboli have been reported in almost every artery or vein, even in many smaller vessels. These result in brain infarcts, coronary occlusion and myocardial infarction, pulmonary infarcts, renal infarcts, and thrombophlebitis with pulmonary emboli. The liver shows fat accumulation, largely in the centrilobular hepatocytes.

CLINICAL MANIFESTATIONS. The clinical abnormalities in this disorder develop after birth. Probably the most consistent finding is ectopia lentis, rarely occurring before age three, but generally noted by age ten years. The dislocation is usually downward, although it may occur in any direction. The osteoporosis has rarely been noted in early childhood, but may be present by ages six to eleven. The spine is the most common site, followed by the long bones. Scoliosis occurs in many individuals, although kyphosis is infrequent. Vertebral collapse and pathologic factors of long bones may occur. The long bones are generally thin and excessively lengthened. Pectus carinatum or excavatum is common. Mental retardation is frequent, and may be obvious as a developmental delay within the first weeks of life, but more commonly becomes manifest in the first or second year. However, at least 20 per cent of patients have average or above average intelligence. Convulsions occur in 10 to 15 per cent of patients, and the electroencephalogram may show excessive slow wave activity. The life-threatening complication of cystathionine β-synthase deficiency is thromboembolism. Large and small arteries and veins may be affected. Vascular occlusions may occur at any age. Major cerebral vascular thrombosis may occur in infancy. Sudden death from coronary occlusion may occur in young adult or early childhood years. Thrombi are particularly likely to occur following surgery. Venous thrombosis with pulmonary emboli is common. There are some data suggesting that cystinuric women have difficulty in carrying a fetus to term, perhaps because of a tendency for placental thrombosis. The number and severity of clinical complications vary markedly. At the mild end of the spectrum are those with only ectopia lentis and virtually no other discernible clinical complications.

DIAGNOSIS AND DIFFERENTIAL DIAGNOSIS. The diagnosis is suggested by ectopia lentis and thromboembolic phenomena, together with other features mentioned above. The urinary cyanide-nitroprusside test reaction is positive. Homocystine is identified by paper or thin layer chromatography or high voltage electrophoresis. Cystathionine β-synthase deficiency is confirmed by demonstration of markedly reduced enzyme activity in a liver biopsy specimen, or with cultured phytohemagglutinin-stimulated lymphocytes, or with cultured skin fibroblasts.

Heterozygotes may be tentatively identified by assay of cystathionine β-synthase activity in liver biopsy tissue, cultured fibroblasts, or phytohemagglutinstimulated lymphocytes. In most instances values on obligate heterozygotes fall below the control range, but there is some overlap.

Homocystinuria may also occur in patients with lesions leading to decreases in 5-methyltetrahydrofolate–dependent homocysteine methylation, owing to (1) inability to form or accumulate methylcobalamin; (2) decreased 5,10-methylenetetrahydrofolate reductase activity; or (3) Imerslund's syndrome (familial pernicious anemia and proteinuria, due to defective absorption of vitamin B_{12} in the presence of intrinsic factor). Homocystinuria also occurs following 6-azauridine triacetate administration, because of inhibition of cystathionine β-synthase.

TREATMENT. Management is concerned with the control or elimination of the biochemical abnormality with the aim of preventing or ameliorating clinical manifestations, and with the clinical treatment of complications.

A low methionine diet (with cystine supplementation) begun in infancy results in some degree of control of biochemical abnormalities, but no reversal of major clinical abnormalities. There have been suggestions that thromboembolic episodes may have been prevented, but this is uncertain. The diet is unpalatable. Pyridoxine administered in relatively large amounts effectively reduces or eliminates the biochemical abnormalities in more than 50 per cent of patients with cystathionine β-synthase deficiency. An occasional patient will respond to doses as low as 25 mg per day. According to Perry, a patient should not be considered unresponsive to pyridoxine until a dose of 500 to 1000 mg per day has been given for a period of several weeks. For patients incompletely responsive to pyridoxine, methionine restriction is also recommended. The biochemical basis for vitamin B_6 responsiveness is not clear. Some patients show small increases in synthase activity in vitro, whereas others do not. No patients have been treated from birth on, so that the long-term efficacy of such intervention is not yet established.

Mudd, S. H., and Levy, H. L.: Disorders of transsulfuration. *In* Stanbury, J. B., Wyngaarden, J. B., and Fredrickson, D. S. (eds.): The Metabolic Basis of Inherited Disease. 4th ed. New York, McGraw-Hill Book Company, 1978, pp. 458–488.
Perry, T. L., Dunn, H. G., Hansen, S., MacDougall, L., and Warrington, P.D.: Early diagnosis and therapy of homocystinuria. Pediatrics, 37:502, 1966.

534.14. ALBINISM
(Oculocutaneous Albinism)
Alexander G. Bearn

The term albinism has come to refer to a genetically heterogeneous group of disorders in which there is an inherited defect in melanin metabolism. It is characterized by a decrease of melanin in the skin, hair, and eyes, and is due to a failure of melanocytes to produce normal melanin. The metabolic defect may involve melanocytes in more than one system (oculocutaneous albinism) or be restricted to one system (ocular albinism). Several independent genetic defects in tyrosine metabolism lead to the same phenotypic effect. Oculocutaneous albinism occurs in two distinct autosomal recessively inherited forms. In one form, the melanocytes lack the enzyme tyrosinase, leading to "tyrosinase-negative" albinism; in the second, the enzyme is present and the defect is probably due to a limitation in the availability of tyrosine, the melanogenic substrate for the enzyme.

"Tyrosinase-negative" albinism is the classic form of albinism; it occurs with a frequency of about 1 in 34,000 and is equally common in whites and blacks. The skin and hair color are strikingly white and do not darken with age. The skin is particularly susceptible to sunlight and often appears wrinkled. Precancerous keratoses in the areas exposed to sunlight are common, and there is a marked increase in the frequency of basal cell and squamous cell carcinomas of the skin. Photophobia, astigmatism, horizontal nystagmus, and severe defects in visual acuity are common. Strabismus is almost invariable. The ocular fundus of albinos is unpigmented and appears bright red.

"Tyrosinase-positive" albinism is more frequently found among blacks than among whites. In the black population the phenotypic frequency is 1 in 15,000, whereas in the white population the frequency is approximately 1 in 40,000. In contrast with "tyrosinase-negative" albinism, the pigmentation of the skin and eyes increases with advancing age. Blacks with "tyrosinase-positive" albinism may be darker than many blonde Caucasoids. Freckles and pigmented nevi are common. Photophobia is less pronounced, and not all patients exhibit nystagmus.

Ocular albinism is a very rare variety in which the defect in pigmentation is restricted to the iris and fundus of the eye. Nystagmus, head-nodding, and defective vision also occur. It is inherited as an X-linked recessive trait and is closely linked to the Xg blood group (recombination fraction 0.15).

Cutaneous albinism (partial albinism, piebald trait) is limited to the skin and hair. In almost all patients a triangular white forelock is present. The trait is inherited in a dominant fashion.

Albinism with hemorrhagic diathesis (Hermansky-Pudlak syndrome) is an exceedingly rare autosomal recessively inherited syndrome. It consists of tyrosinase-positive albinism, a bleeding diathesis caused by storage pool–deficient platelets, and an accumulation of ceroid-like material in the reticuloendothelial system.

DIFFERENTIAL DIAGNOSIS. Circumscribed areas of cutaneous depigmentation may occur in vitiligo. Idiopathic vitiligo is inherited in a dominant fashion and is characterized by an absence of melanocytes. Vitiligo may also occur in a variety of diseases, such as Addison's disease, hyperparathyroidism, hyperthyroidism, and pernicious anemia. White macules, particularly on the buttocks and back, may be seen in tuberous sclerosis.

Witkop, C. J., Jr., Quevedo, W. C., Jr., and Fitzpatrick, T. B.: Albinism. *In* Stanbury, J. B., Wyngaarden, J. B., and Fredrickson, D. S. (eds.): The Metabolic Basis of Inherited Disease. 4th ed. New York, McGraw-Hill Book Company, 1978.

535. DISORDERS OF PURINE AND PYRIMIDINE METABOLISM

535.1. GOUT
Lloyd H. Smith, Jr.

DEFINITION. Gout represents a group of *genetic* diseases and acquired disorders of purine metabolism or

TABLE 1.   Classification of Hyperuricemia and Gout

I. Metabolic gout—excessive synthesis of urate
  A. Genetic (primary)
    1. Unknown defects of rate control—most frequent cause of
       excessive synthesis
    2. Hypoxanthine–guanine phosphoribosyltransferase
       deficiency—Lesch-Nyhan syndrome or incomplete forms
    3. PP-ribose-P synthetase variants with increased activity
    4. Glycogen storage disease Type I (partial explanation,
       see below)
  B. Aquired (secondary to excessive tissue turnover)
II. Renal gout—reduced clearance of urate, presumed to be
  secondary to reduced renal tubular secretion
  A. Genetic (primary)
    1. Idiopathic—most frequent cause of underexcretion gout
    2. Lactic acidosis—glycogen storage disease Type I
  B. Acquired
    1. Renal failure—especially that of lead nephropathy
    2. Inhibition of urate transport—drugs and certain
       metabolites (lactic acid, β-hydroxybutyric acid)

excretion ordinarily identifiable by *hyperuricemia*. When clinically manifest, gout presents as an acute inflammatory *arthritis*, the accumulation of sodium urate deposits as *tophi, uric acid nephrolithiasis,* or *renal failure*. These manifestations can occur in any combination. This definition, which must remain arbitrary until the pathogenesis of each gouty syndrome has been more firmly established, has several points of emphasis which will be discussed more fully later in this chapter. First, it emphasizes the genetic or familial origin of most forms of clinical gout. This attribute has long been recognized. Galen attributed gout to "debauchery, intemperance, and an hereditary trait," and Sydenham emphasized its early occurrence in patients "when they have received the ill seeds of this disease from their parents by inheritance." Second, gout is defined here in terms of its chemical derangement, essential hyperuricemia. This is analogous to the diagnosis of diabetes mellitus as essential hyperglucosemia. The clinical manifestations are complications of hyperuricemia (or hyperuricaciduria) which may or may not occur in the individual patient. It has been estimated that these complications in some combination occur in only 10 to 20 per cent of individuals with hyperuricemia, the incidence increasing in rough proportion to the level of serum uric acid. Finally, the definition emphasizes the heterogeneity of gout. Several different diseases lead to the common feature of persistent hyperuricemia (see Pathogenesis and Table 1).

In a sense all of us have inappropriate hyperuricemia because of two errors in evolution. Uricase catalyzes the conversion of relatively insoluble urate to soluble allantoin, which would be a much more appropriate end product for the mammalian kidney. The evolutionary retention of this enzyme would have obviated both gout and uric acid nephrolithiasis. A second error compounds the first. The mechanism by which the human kidney excretes uric acid is complex, including glomerular filtration, tubular reabsorption, and tubular secretion. The net result is renal retention of more than 90 per cent of that filtered. At equilibrium, the same amount of uric acid is presumably excreted but at the cost of relative hyperuricemia. Renal tubular reabsorption of filtered uric acid is not present in other primates, which therefore have serum uric acid levels of less than 0.05 mg per deciliter. The suggestion has been made that renal retention might help to modulate

bursts of uric acid excretion owing to purine ingestion, and also might shunt more urate into the gut for bacterial destruction. Whether this is true or not, it seems clear that gout represents an exaggeration of a genetic legacy of hyperuricemia common to all.

HISTORY. Gout has figured largely in history, perhaps rivaled only by pandemics of infectious diseases and mental illness. Its classic manifestations were noted in classical times, and the occurrence of osseous tophi and uric acid stones has allowed archeologic diagnoses to be made with confidence. Hippocrates, who recognized and described podagra, devoted three of his aphorisms to the disease, saying in effect: 28, Eunuchs do not take the gout, nor become bald; 29, Women do not take the gout until their menses be stopped; 30, Young men do not take the gout until they indulge in coition. Galen described tophaceous gout and commented upon the familial occurrence of the disease. The term gout, derived from the Latin word *gutta,* came into usage during the Middle Ages to reflect a theory of pathogenesis that this form of arthritis resulted from the "dropping" of a poisonous "*noxa*" into the joint. It is interesting to see the recent confirmation of this theory and the identification of sodium urate microcrystals as the *noxa*. In the seventeenth century, Thomas Sydenham (1683), sometimes called the Shakespeare of gout, wrote clinical descriptions of the disease which have yet to be improved on. He wrote with an authority based on intense personal experience with gouty arthritis and stones. Uric acid was first discovered as a component of stones by Scheele in 1776 (designated lithic acid), followed two decades later by its identification in tophi by Wallaston (1797). In the middle of the nineteenth century the elder (A. B.) Garrod developed a crude but ingenious method for estimating uric acid in serum (crystallization on a linen fiber), and found it to be elevated in patients with gout, demonstrating for the first time the chemical hallmark of the disease. His postulate that acute gouty arthritis was due to deposits of sodium urate was convincingly supported by the work of Freudweiler (1899), who demonstrated the inflammatory potential of sodium urate microcrystals and leukocytic phagocytosis of such crystals in acute gout. This contribution was lost in the sediment of subsequent investigations, the phenomenon of *microcrystalline synovitis* being independently rediscovered approximately 18 years ago. In 1931, the younger (A. E.) Garrod proposed that gout should be classified as one of the inborn errors of metabolism. Over the past two decades studies in many laboratories, notably those of Buchanan, Greenberg, Seegmiller, and Wyngaarden, have elucidated the pathways of purine biosynthesis and degradation and the controlling mechanisms for modulating the appropriate rate of control of purine metabolism. It is against this background that current studies of pathogenesis, to be reviewed below, are being conducted.

The history of gout has been intermingled with sociologic and cultural variables as well as the march of medical and biochemical progress. From earliest observations the disease has been associated with dissipation and venery. Even gouty Sydenham wrote, "the gout generally attacks those aged persons who have spent most of their lives in ease, voluptuousness, high living, and too free use of wine and other spirituous liquors." It gradually became a disease in caricature in the eighteenth and nineteenth centuries, used by novelist, satirist, and political cartoonist alike as symbolic of medical retribution for excessive indulgence of natural appetites. Ambrose Bierce defined gout as "a physician's name for the rheumatism of a rich patient." The disease gradually won grudging respect ("disease of kings and king of diseases") because of its remarkable association with men of genius and exceptional achievement. An incomplete list of those alleged to have suffered from the gout includes Alexander the Great, Louis XIV, Isaac Newton, William Harvey, Martin Luther, John Calvin, Leonardo da Vinci, Samuel Johnson, and Benjamin Franklin. It is an amusing sequel that several recent studies have confirmed positive statistical correlations of serum uric acid levels and intelligence or social status.

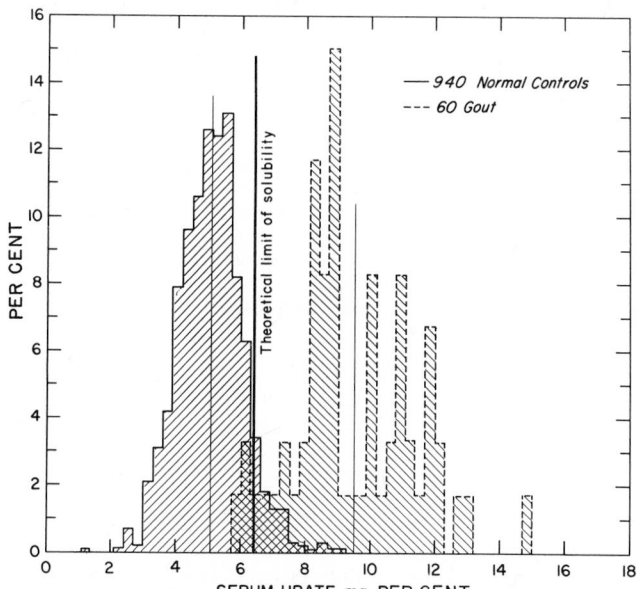

Figure 1. Distribution of serum urate concentrations in normal and gouty male subjects and calculated limit of solubility of sodium urate in serum. (From Seegmiller, J. E.: Diseases of purine and pyrimidine metabolism. *In* Bondy, P. K., and Rosenberg, L. E. [eds.]: Duncan's Diseases of Metabolism. 7th ed. Philadelphia, W. B. Saunders Company, 1974.)

GENETICS OF GOUT. Family aggregation of clinical gout has been observed since the first clinical descriptions of the disease in antiquity. Gout has appeared in an irregular pattern both in successive generations and in sibships. A positive family history for clinical gout is found in about 10 to 20 per cent of patients with the primary disorder. Attempts have been made to use hyperuricemia as a more precise marker for the presence of the gouty trait. Within the restrictions imposed by the statistical uncertainties of the boundary between normal and abnormal serum urate levels (Fig. 1), hyperuricemia has been found in 15 to 25 per cent of close relatives of patients with clinical gout. It is sometimes stated that primary gout is transmitted as an autosomal dominant with incomplete penetrance. The pattern of inheritance of hyperuricemia has varied so widely that it may be polygenic in origin. Many variables affect the phenotypic expression of the gouty trait: age, sex, diet, and renal function. It is noteworthy that in the two forms of gout in which a specific enzyme defect of purine metabolism has been most clearly established, the syndrome of hypoxanthine–guanine phosphoribosyltransferase deficiency and the syndrome of PP-ribose-P synthetase variants with excessive activity, the genetic transmissions have been established as sex-linked recessive traits. Glycogen storage disease Type I, which is associated with a specific form of secondary gout, is transmitted as an autosomal recessive trait. It seems probable that the mode of inheritance of other forms of gout will not be clearly established until genetic markers more specific than hyperuricemia are available. This must await clarification of the pathogenesis of the various gouty syndromes in more specific phenotypic terms.

PATHOGENESIS. It has been established for over 100 years (A. B. Garrod) that the hallmark of gout is hyperuricemia. All the clinical manifestations of gout, with the single exception of uric acid nephrolithiasis,

derive from the crystallization of sodium urate from extracellular fluids where it has accumulated in a supersaturated concentration. No one has shown that sodium urate in solution is toxic. There are several questions which relate to the pathogenesis of gout: What leads to the accumulation of urate in extracellular fluid? What are the variables in its precipitation? How do sodium urate crystals lead to inflammatory arthritis?

The Cause of Hyperuricemia. The accumulation of any metabolite in excess must result from one (or a combination) of four variables: increased absorption, decreased metabolism, decreased excretion, or increased biosynthesis. There is no evidence that gouty patients habitually ingest excessive purines or have an increased avidity for purine absorption. Elimination of purine ingestion usually results in a reduction of serum urate of about 0.6 mg per deciliter in normal subjects and about 1.0 mg per deciliter in gouty patients. Under experimental conditions, ingestion of a diet very high in nucleic acids may lead to hyperuricemia in normal subjects comparable to gouty levels. In summary, absorption of preformed purines from dietary sources may modify extracellular urate levels, but does not represent a primary cause of gout.

Uric acid is the end product of purine metabolism, most of it being excreted as free urinary urate. There are at least two mechanisms by which it is partially destroyed in man. Leukocytes contain verdoperoxidases capable of degrading uric acid to allantoin and carbon dioxide. Of much greater importance quantitatively, uric acid is secreted into the gut where uricolysis is carried out by bacterial enzymes. Approximately one third of that synthesized daily is degraded through these mechanisms. Studies in gout have not supported decreased uricolysis as a mechanism for hyperuricemia. In fact, with high urate concentrations, especially after the onset of renal insufficiency, excretion into the gut, and uricolysis there, may be enhanced as an important second line of defense. Particular attention has therefore been directed toward increased synthesis or decreased excretion as primary mechanisms for hyperuricemia in gout.

Uric acid is synthesized from xanthine and from hypoxanthine (via xanthine), these successive oxidations being catalyzed by xanthine oxidase (Fig. 2). The free purine bases bear complex metabolic relationships to various pools of purine nucleotides. In part the free bases are reutilized to form functioning nucleotides; in part they are converted to uric acid for excretion. Be-

Figure 2. Pathway of uric acid synthesis catalyzed by xanthine oxidase and the site of action of allopurinol.

Figure 3. De novo pathway of purine nucleotide biosynthesis and the feedback control mechanisms ($\longrightarrow$). E_1, Amidophosphoribosyltransferase; E_2, inosine 5'-phosphate dehydrogenase; E_3, adenylsuccinic acid (AMP-S) synthetase; XMP, xanthosine 5'-phosphate.

cause of this reutilization, sometimes called "salvage synthesis," uric acid synthesis represents only a part of the purine nucleotide turnover rate. At equilibrium, however, that part should approximate the de novo synthetic rate of purine nucleotides. Small amounts of hypoxanthine, xanthine, and other trace purines are normally excreted in the urine as well. Several methods have been widely applied in an attempt to determine whether there is excessive purine synthesis in gout: measurement of urate excreted on a low purine diet, use of isotopic urate to determine its pool size and turnover rate, and study of the time course of incorporation of a purine precursor, usually glycine, into urate (Fig. 3). Each of these methods is subject to limitations which cannot be detailed here. The following information has emerged from such studies. In normal man the daily rate of production of uric acid on a low purine diet averages about 750 mg. The miscible pool of uric acid is about 1.0 to 1.3 grams, so that two thirds to three fourths of the body pool turns over daily. Urinary excretion of urate varies widely even during dietary regulation, averaging in men 426 ± 81 mg per 24 hours. The difference between the estimated production rate of urate and that excreted in the urine represents uricolysis, mostly by bacterial action in the gut.

By use of these methods, evidence for excessive synthesis of uric acid has been obtained in about two thirds of patients with primary gout. Overproduction is readily understood in patients with diseases resulting in increased tissue breakdown, e.g., myeloid metaplasia, polycythemia vera, and leukemia. The hypoxanthine–guanine phosphoribosyltransferase deficiency syndrome is discussed in Ch. 535.3 as the biochemical basis for excessive purine synthesis in one form of gout. The first step unique to purine nucleotide biosynthesis and the major site of metabolic regulation is that of the synthesis of phosphoribosylamine, catalyzed by the amidophosphoribosyltransferase.

$$\text{Glutamine} + \text{PP-ribose-P} + H_2O \xrightarrow{Mg^{++}} \text{glutamic acid} +$$
$$\text{5-phosphoribosylamine} + \text{pyrophosphate}$$

There are several possibilities for loss of normal rate control at this regulatory site; these include (1) excessive concentrations of the substrates glutamine, PP-ribose-P, or both; (2) a structural alteration in the enzyme, rendering it more active or less sensitive to normal feedback control by purine nucleotides; or (3) a partial deficiency of one of the nucleotides (adenylic, guanylic, and inosinic acids), which, in concert, exert allosteric modulation of the enzyme (Fig. 3). In several families, gout has been found to be secondary to altered kinetic properties of PP-ribose-P synthetase. The resulting increased concentration of PP-ribose-P drives purine production by furnishing a key substrate and by allosteric activation of amidophosphoribosyltransferase. Increased availability of PP-ribose-P may also contribute to the hyperuricemia of glycogen storage disease type I. It can be anticipated that future studies will document further heterogeneity in the mechanisms by which purine synthesis is enhanced in various types of overproduction gout.

In about one third of patients with primary gout there is no evidence for overproduction of uric acid by any of the methods now available. Evidence suggests that these patients have an inherited disorder (or group of disorders) of the renal tubule resulting in decreased urate clearance as the cause of hyperuricemia. Renal clearance of urate is a complex function of filtration, tubular reabsorption, and tubular secretion. There is partial binding of urate to plasma proteins, but this does not seem to represent a significant fraction under physiologic conditions at 37° C. Using the assumption that urate is completely filterable at the glomerulus, there is net tubular reabsorption of 90 to 95 per cent. Urate which is excreted is in part and perhaps in toto that secreted by the tubule. Patients with "renal gout" exhibit reduced clearances of urate, the differences being most evident when compared to normal controls with dietary induction of comparable plasma levels of uric acid. The differences have not always been striking, and in some cases may be difficult to interpret because of early impairment of renal function by gout. In renal gout reduced net clearance of urate probably results from a defect in its tubular secretion, although enhanced tubular reabsorption of urate has not been excluded. In theory, an increase in the bound fraction of urate would also reduce clearance by reducing that filtered. An impaired tubular secretion of urate might be an intrinsic defect of the transport mechanism which has not yet been clarified biochemically. It might also result from a genetic or acquired metabolic disorder in some other pathway which leads to the accumulation of a metabolite which secondarily interferes with tubular urate secretion. An example of this latter mechanism is the hyperuricemia associated with the lactic acidosis of

Type I glycogen storage disease (see Ch. 531.4). Idiopathic renal gout might similarly result from the accumulation of other uric acid transport inhibitors not yet identified. When over-all reduction of renal function occurs, as happens not infrequently in gout, hyperuricemia is further exacerbated, and an increased percentage of urate is excreted into the gut for uricolysis.

In summary, the important causes of persistent hyperuricemia are those of excessive synthesis and decreased renal clearance. This allows for a rational classification of gout as shown in Table 1. Such a classification reflects only a progress report. Although hypoxanthine–guanine phosphoribosyltransferase deficiency and PP-ribose-P synthetase excess represent the only types of metabolic gout for which specific enzymatic defects have been established, new defects in the rate control mechanisms will almost certainly be established in the future, possibly as abnormalities of excessive synthesis of pentose phosphate compounds. Similarly, the genetic types of renal gout will probably prove to be more heterogeneous in future studies. A variety of drugs (notably the chlorothiazide diuretics) and metabolites (lactate, β-hydroxybutyrate) diminish urate clearance in the normal kidney, and may precipitate clinical gout.

Precipitation of Urate. Uric acid is not toxic to man in its soluble state. Although hyperuricemia has been associated epidemiologically with a number of conditions, e. g., coronary artery heart disease and hypertension, there is no evidence that it has any pathogenic relationship to those disorders. Uric acid seems to produce disease "physically" rather than "chemically" when precipitated as sodium urate at pH 7.40, or as uric acid in acidic urine. Its precipitation as amorphous sodium urate, which may occur in virtually any tissue in the body except for the central nervous system, results in tophi with tissue disruption and destruction but with minimal inflammatory response. Its precipitation as microcrystals of critical size in certain tissues, especially in synovial tissues and spaces, leads to an acute inflammatory reaction to be described below. Its precipitation in the renal distal collecting tubules as uric acid may rarely lead to acute renal failure. The precipitation of uric acid in a protein matrix in the renal pelvis, or more rarely in the ureter or bladder, leads to uric acid nephrolithiasis.

Sodium urate is soluble in human plasma to a concentration of only about 7 mg of urate per deciliter. Values above this denote supersaturated solutions, although sodium urate may remain in supersaturated solution with considerable stability. Why do some patients with serum uric acid levels of 9 mg per deciliter have severe tophaceous gout or acute gouty arthritis or both, whereas others may maintain similar levels for years or even for life with no evidence of precipitation, i.e., of clinical gout? The reasons for these differences in threshold of precipitation are not known. One variable is that of protein binding of urate in plasma to a specific α_1-α_2 globulin (Alvsaker) and to albumin. The report that some patients with tophaceous gout have reduced protein-binding of urate is provocative but has not been confirmed. Furthermore, the importance of protein-binding of urate, which probably does not exceed 4 or 5 per cent in normal plasma, remains to be established.

The solubility of urate in urine decreases with increasing acidity because of the shift to free uric acid.

The titration curve is such that the undissociated uric acid increases to 85 per cent at pH 5.0. At this pH only 15 mg of urate is soluble per deciliter of urine so that supersaturation is required to excrete an average uric acid load in a normal urine volume. The solubility increases more than 10-fold at pH 7.0 over that at pH 5.0. Three factors are therefore important in the urinary precipitation of uric acid: urine volume, the amount of urate excreted per 24 hours, and urine pH. It is possible that the availability of stone matrix and the level of stabilizing substances in urine may also play important roles.

Cause of Acute Gouty Arthritis. There are four cardinal clinical manifestations of gout: acute gouty arthritis, tophaceous gout, uric acid nephrolithiasis, and gouty kidney with varying degrees of impairment of renal function. Of these clinical manifestations or complications associated with hyperuricemia, acute inflammatory arthritis is that which has been most obscure in its pathogenesis. Garrod the elder, in the second of his ten propositions on "the true nature or essence of gout" (1859), wrote: "Investigations recently made in the morbid anatomy of gout prove incontestably that true gouty inflammation is always accompanied with a deposition of urate of soda in the inflamed part." This proposition was strongly supported by the experimental work of Freudweiler (1899), who was able to produce inflammation with sodium urate crystals and observe their subsequent presence in leukocytes. For many years, however, this work was ignored because of evidence which seemed to indicate that retention of uric acid, the seemingly obvious basis of tophi, was unrelated to the sudden acute attacks of inflammatory arthritis. Several pieces of evidence supported that view. The onset of acute attacks bore no relation to changes in serum urate levels. Joints severely involved with tophaceous deposits were often free from acute attacks. Despite its almost specific therapeutic effectiveness, colchicine had no demonstrable effect on urate metabolism. During reductions of serum urate levels with uricosuric drugs, attacks of acute gouty arthritis were fairly often exacerbated. Because of these and other observations, major attention was directed toward alternative explanations, such as abnormalities in the metabolism of trace purines.

Acute gouty arthritis represents an inflammatory reaction to microcrystals of sodium urate, mediated by a series of chemical changes accompanying phagocytosis of the crystals by leukocytes. This basic pathogenetic mechanism has been firmly established. In fact, the presence of sodium urate microcrystals in synovial fluid from gouty joints during acute inflammation, both free and in leukocytes, is so constant as to be of diagnostic value (Fig. 4). This was the key observation that led to the experiments supporting the early Garrod-Freudweiler concept. The injection of sodium urate microcrystals into joints of normal controls or gouty patients produces typical gout responsive to colchicine. Aspiration of these joints demonstrates phagocytosis of some of the injected crystals. No experimental gouty arthritis can be produced in laboratory animals in the absence of leukocytes. The inflammatory reaction of microcrystalline synovitis is a nonspecific one, being produced by injection of other crystals of appropriate size and shape, such as sodium orotate or calcium pyrophosphate dihydrate.

The exact mechanism by which sodium urate crystals

Figure 4. Sodium urate monohydrate crystals phagocytized by leukocytes in synovial fluid from acute gouty arthritis examined by polarized light. (Reproduced with permission of Daniel J. McCarty, Jr.)

initiate inflammation has not been established. The crystals can activate Hageman factor, and in this way initiate the chain of events resulting in bradykinin synthesis. Bradykinin levels are raised in synovial fluid from gouty joints, but injection of carboxypeptidase B, which destroys bradykinin, does not prevent experimental gout. The requirement for leukocyte-crystal interaction was noted above. Uric acid has been found to be leukotactic. Phagocytosis of the crystals leads to increased metabolic activity of the leukocyte, release of lysosomal enzymes, and increased lactic acid production. Interesting studies on the molecular basis of crystal-induced inflammation have been carried out (Weissmann, McCarty). Phagocytosis of sodium urate crystals leads to rapid destruction of the phagolysosome membrane, releasing its hydrolytic enzymes into the cell cytoplasm. This results in cell lysis. The original crystal, the hydrolytic enzymes, and the cytoplasmic enzymes from the destroyed leukocyte are released into the surrounding tissue. This crystal-membrane interaction, which can be simulated with artificial lipid membranes ("liposomes") as well, is thought to result from hydrogen bonding between the rigid crystal and elements in the lipid membrane surface, leading to breaks in its continuity. The attack of the leukocyte on the sodium urate crystal is therefore both suicidal and counterproductive, setting in motion an inappropriate inflammatory response which is injurious to the host.

Although the biochemical events of inflammation are poorly understood, the establishment of the general mechanism of microcrystalline synovitis has allowed a rational explanation of acute gouty arthritis. Still unexplained are the mechanisms by which the acute attack is initiated, i.e., what leads to the presumed burst of microcrystallization at a given time. How are the known precipitating events of acute gouty arthritis, which may be roughly grouped together as stresses, translated into microcrystallization?

The model of leukocyte-crystal interaction may offer an explanation for the action of colchicine. As stated, in the therapeutic range colchicine has no effect on net purine metabolism as reflected in levels of extracellular uric acid or in its excretion. On the other hand, colchicine diminishes leukocyte migration and modifies many of the metabolic concomitants of phagocytosis in the leukocyte, possibly through combining with microtubular elements of the internal cytoskeleton. The use of such an in vitro model may allow the rational development of other therapeutic agents in the future.

CLINICAL MANIFESTATIONS. As previously stated, the clinical manifestations of gout can be arbitrarily divided into four categories: acute gouty arthritis, tophaceous gout, uric acid nephrolithiasis, and gouty kidney. Although the basic metabolic abnormalities of genetic gout must be presumed to have been present since conception, clinical gout is extraordinarily rare before the rise in extracellular uric acid levels which accompanies puberty in the male. Exceptions to this are seen in the juvenile gout of the Lesch-Nyhan syndrome and in glycogen storage disease Type I. Clinical gout usually makes its appearance in middle life in men, although the majority of patients with hyperuricemia never exhibit these complications. As observed by Hippocrates, clinical gout in women rarely occurs before the menopause, at which time there is a further rise in uric acid levels. In most series, gout in women accounts for only 5 to 10 per cent of cases.

The epidemiology of gout and hyperuricemia has received increasing attention beyond the genetic studies of families. The positive statistical correlation of uric acid levels with education, intelligence, and social status was pointed out above. Exceptionally high frequencies of hyperuricemia have been found in Filipinos (in the United States but not in the Philippines), in Maoris, and in the natives of the Marianas Islands. The over-all incidence of clinical gout in the United States has been estimated as 3 patients per 1000 population. As a generality it has been stated that gout makes up about 5 per cent of arthritis.

Acute Gouty Arthritis. Acute gouty arthritis is the most frequent first clinical manifestation of the disease. It has been eloquently described by many who have endured it, but by none more effectively than Sydenham, who wrote, "it [the affected part] is not able to bear the weight of the cloths upon it, nor hard walking in the chamber." He further alluded to the pain as being "like the gnawing of a dog." Acute gouty arthritis often follows a precipitating event: surgery, injury, alcohol ingestion, dietary excess, emotional stress, or even the minor stress of excessive walking. In view of the current concept of the pathogenesis as that of microcrystalline synovitis, such stress must somehow be translated into localized sodium urate crystallization, or must alter the tissue reaction to such crystals. Since sodium urate usually exists in a supersaturated solution in the gouty patient, the initiating event need introduce only a single crystal focus for seeding a cascade of precipitation. Some of the precipitating events, such as starvation and alcohol ingestion, increase urate levels by inhibition of renal urate excretion through the accompanying ketosis and lactic acidosis, respectively. The particular association of gout with spirituous liquors, legendary in medieval history ("in the young wine goes to the head; in the aged it goes to the feet"), therefore finds some scientific basis at the level of the renal tubule. A particularly puzzling and important kind of exacerbation of acute gouty arthritis is that which frequently occurs during early stages of treatment designed to lower extracellular urate levels. This may complicate the use of uricosuric agents or of allopurinol, to the great distress of both patient and physician. It has been difficult to explain the exacerbation of gout in the face of a falling urate concentration. It is possible that mobilization of amorphous tophaceous deposits may allow for local precipitation of the microcrystals conducive to inflammation. The frequent occurrence of this complication may occasionally obviate or delay effective treatment.

Gout usually presents as a sudden, exquisitely painful arthritis. After a few premonitory twinges the onset of inflammation may occur within minutes with severe arthritis within a few hours. Typically a patient may retire for the night in good health, yet be awakened a few hours later with excruciating pain in the affected joint. He may develop podagra (gouty arthritis of the first metatarsophalangeal joint) with such rapidity that he is unable to remove his shoe in time. More rarely the warning signals of impending arthritis develop into a crescendo pattern ending in the acute attack.

Gouty arthritis exhibits a marked predilection for the larger joints, particularly in the feet and ankles. Hippocrates described podagra, which still represents the most frequent site of involvement (Fig. 5). This may reflect the trauma of weight-bearing which in the normal foot produces the greatest force per unit area (pressure) there. Other frequent sites of early attacks are the ankle, the instep, or occasionally the knee. Less frequently the elbow, wrist, or metacarpophalangeal joints are the sites of gouty arthritis. The hips, shoulders, and spine are very rarely the sites of microcrystalline synovitis, and almost never the sites of initial involvement. Gouty arthritis is usually monoarticular, especially in the earliest attacks. Some patients may have marked to-

phaceous gout with bone and articular destruction and few if any attacks of acute gout. Involvement of a joint by tophi does not seem to predispose that area to acute attacks, and some clinicians have even suggested that tophaceous areas enjoy relative immunity from acute inflammation.

Acute gouty arthritis is characterized by severe inflammation, not only in the joint itself but typically in the periarticular tissues and skin. The presence of heat, marked swelling, exquisite tenderness, and rubor extending well beyond the immediate vicinity of the joint capsule has often led to the erroneous diagnosis of septic arthritis or cellulitis. Occasionally lymphangitis may be evident. The skin over the area of inflammation is usually tense and shiny, and after subsidence of the attack undergoes superficial desquamation as is seen in erysipelas. Systemic signs of inflammation may include fever, leukocytosis, and elevation of the sedimentation rate which may further suggest an infectious etiology. The severity of the associated pain has been referred to above, and commands respect and attention rather than the traditional jocularity. When untreated, an attack of acute gouty arthritis usually subsides gradually over a period of one to two weeks. Generally there are no residual signs or symptoms; more rarely, stiffness persists, or a second flareup supervenes before there is complete recovery.

As stated, only about one of six patients with hyperuricemia will eventually have one or more of the complications of clinical gout. Moreover, the clinical course of gout after an initial attack of acute arthritis is highly variable. Some patients have only a single attack of monoarticular arthritis and then remain free of symptoms despite the persistence of hyperuricemia. More often, after a symptom-free interval, but usually within the first year, there is recurrence of an attack. In Gutman's series, 62 per cent had recurrences within the first year, 16 per cent in one to two years, 11 per cent in two to five years, 4 per cent in ten years, and 7 per cent, no recurrence during prolonged follow-up. In the usual pattern, subsequent attacks come with increasing frequency over the years unless prophylactic measures are taken, with gradual reduction in the duration of the

Figure 5. Acute gouty arthritis of great toe.

Figure 6.   Chronic gouty arthritis with tophaceous destruction of bone and joints.

Figure 7.   Advanced tophaceous gout, with ulcerations.

symptom-free intervals (sometimes called intercritical gout). In about one third of patients, the number of attacks occurring each year remains constant, and rarely, there is a spontaneous decline in frequency with increasing age of the patient. When attacks become more frequent they also tend to become more severe, both in the extent and duration of the inflammation and in the number of joints affected. The patient may reach a state at which he is rarely free of gouty inflammation, and at which even with subsidence of an acute attack there is enough residual swelling, stiffness, and pain in the involved joints to give permanent disability not responsive to the measures usually effective in acute attacks.

Tophaceous Gout. Sodium urate may accumulate in virtually any tissue in the body with the exception of the central nervous system, where the concentration is reduced by the blood-brain barrier. Tophi occur most often in and around joints in cartilage, bone, bursae, and subcutaneous tissue. As foreign bodies, these deposits elicit a low-grade chronic inflammatory process with disruption of tissues and fibrosis. Destruction of tissue is particularly evident in cartilage and bone, leading to radiolucent "punched-out" lesions of bone and gross deformities of joints (Figs. 6 and 7). Deposits of sodium urate may be massive, particularly in the hands and feet and around the olecranon bursa. Subcutaneous deposits may be easily visible as yellowish-white excrescences, which on occasion may erode through the skin and discharge a pale paste composed largely of crystalline needles of sodium urate. In advanced cases, deposits of several hundred grams may lead to grotesquely deformed extremities. Rarely, involvement of the heart has been observed with tophi causing conduction disturbances. A frequent site of tophaceous deposits is the external ear, especially in the helix and antihelix. The local factors that control the sites of crystallization are not known. Massive tophi may be found in the hands, feet, and elbows with none of the typical auricular deposits. Conversely, the external ear may be the only site of visible tophi over many years of gouty diathesis. As stated above, reports that patients most susceptible to tophi may have reduced protein binding of urate have not been generally confirmed.

About one half of all patients with clinical gout have visible tophi at some stage of their disease. Other patients may have more diffuse deposition of sodium urate without local nodules or infiltrates demonstrable by physical or radiologic examination. The destruction and gross distortion of articular structures (cartilage, bone, capsule, synovial membranes) by tophi leads to a form of chronic gouty arthritis which compounds the stiffness, pain, and fibrosis that may follow repeated attacks of acute gouty arthritis. Although symptomatic and objective improvement may occur with proper therapy, this late stage of destructive gout cannot be completely reversed. One of the objectives of modern management is to prevent the excessive accumulation of urate that results in tophaceous destruction and connective tissue reaction.

Uric Acid Nephrolithiasis. Kidney stones are very common. It has been estimated that 1 in every 1000 inhabitants of the United States is hospitalized annually because of a kidney stone. This figure does not include those whose stones remain in situ or are passed without hospitalization. In large series it has been found that 5 to 10 per cent of all kidney stones in adults are composed mainly of uric acid deposits within a protein matrix. Uric acid may serve as the nidus for a stone of mixed composition, in particular in association with calcium oxalate. Pure uric acid stones are radiolucent, being demonstrable only by the use of contrast media. Other radiolucent stones, so-called matrix stones which are predominantly proteinaceous, xanthine stones, and 2,8-dihydroxyadenine stones are extremely rare.

Most patients with uric acid stones do not have clinical gout. On the other hand, patients with gout are much more likely to have stones. The frequency of stones in primary or genetic gout has been estimated at 15 to 20 per cent, and in secondary overproduction gout (e.g., myeloid metaplasia, polycythemia vera) at 35 to 40 per cent. Stone formation may occur at any stage in the disease, as the first manifestation of gout or as a late complication in the course of crippling arthritis. Stones may be infrequent or, rarely, they may be the main problem, with almost constant uric acid gravel and superimposed episodes of acute renal colic from passage of larger stones.

As noted earlier, the absolute amount of uric acid excreted per 24 hours is only one of the factors conducive to stone formation. A concentrated acidic urine increases the likelihood of stones at any level of uricaciduria. Some investigators have reported that patients with gout, and certain other patients with uric acid stone diathesis, habitually excrete more acid urine. It is postulated that this reflects a shift toward increased titratable acidity rather than ammonia excretion because of a relative defect in renal ammonia production. These data have been both confirmed and denied, perhaps an indication in part of the difficulty in choosing proper controls.

Gouty Renal Disease. A selective defect in urate excretion may be the basic defect in possibly one third of all patients with gout. Extracellular urate rises nonspecifically in all patients with renal insufficiency, uric acid representing one component of nonprotein nitrogen. The onset of renal failure in gout tends to exacerbate the disease, especially the frequency and severity of tophaceous deposits. More generally, renal tubular reabsorption of urate in man, as opposed to other primates, leads to inappropriate urate retention without which there would be no gout. The kidney therefore plays a significant role in the pathogenesis and progression of gout.

Conversely, gout may impair renal function and lead to death in uremia. The so-called gouty kidney represents a variable mixture of factors. Sodium urate may crystallize in the renal interstitial tissue, especially in the pyramids, with tissue destruction and distortion and a low-grade inflammatory reaction leading to fibrosis. In addition to this primary lesion, uric acid stones lead to obstruction with hydronephrosis and increased susceptibility to chronic pyelonephritis, a complication quite often found in late-stage gouty kidney. A distinctive form of glomerulosclerosis has been described with thickening of the glomerular capillary basement membranes and increased cellularity in capillary loops. Finally, gout, or at least hyperuricemia, carries a statistical association with accelerated vascular disease and hypertension, so that nephrosclerosis may contribute in some measure to impairment of renal function. There are no characteristic clinical or laboratory findings to distinguish gouty kidney from chronic glomerulonephritis except for the association of the former with clinical gout. The question whether gout (i.e., hyperuricemia) ever leads to renal failure in the absence of the other three manifestations of the disease, i.e., arthritis, tophi, and stones, is pertinent to the prophylactic treatment of patients discovered to have essential hyperuricemia (considered here to be gout without complications). Gouty kidney in the absence of these manifestations of clinical gout is extraordinarily rare, and even then the entity may be open to question because of variable interpretations of renal pathology.

A particular form of uric acid nephropathy may be found in the absence of clinical gout. With sudden exceptionally high levels of uric acid excretion, seen almost exclusively after chemotherapeutic or radiation therapy of certain malignant myeloproliferative disorders, crystals may occlude the distal collecting tubules, leading to acute renal failure. These intraluminal crystals are uric acid rather than sodium urate, precipitate in the distal tubule in which maximal concentration and acidification occur, and lead to intranephronic hydronephrosis. This complication is easy to prevent with fluids, alkalinization of the urine, and allopurinol inhibition of urate synthesis. Oliguria, once established, usually follows a course similar to that seen with acute renal failure secondary to shock or to an incompatible blood transfusion.

Diseases Associated with Gout (Table 2). Several diseases have been described in association with gout. In some cases, the relationship seems to be clear pathogenically, as outlined in the classification of gout in Table 1. Some associations have not yet been so explained. Many diseases which lead to continued tissue synthesis and breakdown may produce hyperuricemia and clinical gout because of the resulting increased turnover of nucleic acids and functional nucleotides. This form of secondary or acquired metabolic gout is that seen with polycythemia vera, myeloid metaplasia, chronic leukemia, mast cell disease, extensive psoriasis, and sarcoidosis. The triad of sarcoidosis-psoriasis-gout has been described in a small number of patients, although this may represent the fortuitous coincidence of common diseases, both of which may be productive of secondary gout. Severe gout may be a major complication in surviving patients with glycogen storage disease Type I because of the constant lactic acidosis which inhibits renal tubular urate secretion. Studies with isotopic glycine also suggest excessive synthesis of urate in this disease. As noted above, this may result from excessive synthesis of PP-ribose-P, one of the substrates for the rate-limiting initial step in purine synthesis. The hyperuricemia of starvation results largely from inhibition of renal tubular urate secretion by the accumulated β-hydroxybutyrate. The association of gout and diabetes mellitus is not a strong one. Three to 5 per cent of patients with gout have diabetes, but this figure is not far from that of the incidence of diabetes in the general population when adjusted for age. Some diabetic patients considered to have atypical gout in the past in fact have pseudogout, as described in Ch. 60. Over the last decade several clinics have documented a high incidence of hyperuricemia and clinical gout in patients with primary hyperparathyroid-

TABLE 2.   Diseases Associated with Gout

---

1. Myeloproliferative disorders and hemolytic anemias
2. Chronic renal disease—glomerulonephritis, pyelonephritis, hereditary nephropathy
3. Hyperparathyroidism
4. Sarcoidosis and chronic beryllium disease
5. Psoriasis
6. Lead poisoning
7. Glycogen storage disease Type I (glucose-6-phosphatase deficiency)
8. Down's syndrome
9. Nephrogenic diabetes insipidus

---

ism even in the absence of overt renal failure. The hyperuricemia has usually not responded to successful surgical treatment of hyperparathyroidism, so may be secondary to early calcium nephropathy. Hyperuricemia may also be found in hypothyroidism. Renal insufficiency is a common cause of hyperuricemia. It is surprising how rarely this results in clinical gout in view of the high concentrations of uric acid which may be found. It may be that hyperuricemia in uremia does not have sufficient duration, i.e., time at risk, to result in a high incidence of sodium urate precipitation. Uremia may also interfere in some way with the crystallization potential of sodium urate, as it does for bone salts in osteoid, or diminish the inflammatory response to such crystals when they occur. Garrod commented upon the association of lead poisoning and gout in his treatise of 1876, and this has been repeatedly confirmed in subsequent reports. Saturnine gout, as it has been called, is particularly prevalent in the southeastern region of the United States, where it is usually a byproduct of ingesting large amounts of illicitly distilled ("moonshine") whiskey of high lead content. Hyperuricemia induced by chronic lead poisoning appears to be secondary to lead nephropathy rather than to enhanced catabolism of tissue. Hyperuricemia has also been described in Down's syndrome and in nephrogenic diabetes insipidus.

Pseudogout. The syndrome of pseudogout, also called *chondrocalcinosis articularis*, is considered as a separate entity in Ch. 60.

Hypoxanthine–Guanine   Phosphoribosyltransferase (HGPRT) Deficiency. The X-linked genetic disease HG-PRT deficiency is associated with overproduction of urate in which a specific enzymatic defect has been clearly established. A virtually complete deficiency of activity of HGPRT results in a devastating neurologic disorder of male children, called the Lesch-Nyhan syndrome. It is described in Ch. 535.3. A partial deficiency of HGPRT activity results in articular gout, associated with renal stones and renal damage. Partial HGPRT deficiency may be suspected in a young adult male patient with severe gout, possibly with minor neurologic abnormalities, who excretes uric acid in an amount greater than 0.75 times that of creatinine. The final diagnosis can best be made by enzymatic assay of a hemolysate preparation, preferably sent to one of the laboratories engaged in research on purine metabolism. Therapy is ineffective in preventing or reversing neurologic damage, but may reduce the complications directly related to urate accumulation and excretion, as described below.

DIAGNOSIS. The diagnosis of acute gouty arthritis rarely offers difficulties when there is sudden onset of typical inflammatory involvement of a susceptible joint in a patient with hyperuricemia. Rarely, the serum uric acid concentration may be within the upper range of normal at the time of measurement (Fig. 1), or the arthritis may be atypical in its location or persistence. Rapid response of the pain and inflammation after administration of colchicine is so characteristic as to be of diagnostic usefulness. Some response of rheumatoid arthritis or sarcoid arthritis has been described with colchicine, but the effects are not so dramatic as those in gout. Demonstration of the typical needle-shaped birefringent crystals of sodium urate in leukocytes of synovial fluid is diagnostic of gout. With proper technique, intraleukocytic sodium urate crystals are found in over 95 per cent of aspirates from joints affected by acute gout (Fig. 4). Although use of a polarizing microscope is preferable, sodium urate crystals can also be demonstrated in centrifuged, heparinized joint fluid by examining the sediment with an ordinary microscope. Positive identification of the crystals may be achieved by incubation of the synovial fluid preparation with uricase. The particular characteristics of pseudogout or *chondrocalcinosis articularis* are described in Ch. 60. Occasionally, gout may simulate infectious arthritis or be confused with monarticular rheumatoid arthritis. Examination of the joint fluid, measurement of serum uric acid, and response to colchicine should suffice to establish the diagnosis.

A classification of types of gout according to pathogenesis has been outlined in Table 1. It is clearly important to determine whether gout is secondary to a myeloproliferative disorder, renal failure, or drug or metabolite interference with renal tubular secretion of urate. In the study of the average patient with idiopathic gout, in the absence of the aforementioned disorders, it is not necessary to establish whether the disease is metabolic (overproduction) gout or renal (underexcretion) gout in order to institute proper treatment. In the absence of clear-cut hyperuricaciduria on a low purine diet, this further classification is still a laborious procedure requiring isotopic studies.

TREATMENT. Genetic gout cannot be cured, but its phenotypic expression can usually be modified and progression of its clinical complications controlled or reversed. The therapeutic program differs according to the complications present. Generally, in the majority of patients, the treatment of gout is now quite adequate with the introduction of potent uricosuric drugs and allopurinol, and more skilled use of colchicine as a prophylactic agent. The purpose of every therapeutic program is to prevent the complications of gout or, failing complete prophylaxis, to treat each complication specifically when it occurs.

Acute Gouty Arthritis. Although acute gouty arthritis is self-limited in duration, the severity of the pain and the persistence of the untreated inflammatory process over one to two weeks call for early intervention. The earlier the onset of treatment, the more likely a rapid response. The affected joint should be placed at rest. Usually the degree of pain will demand this, and on occasion specific medication, i.e., a narcotic, for pain may be required. Four types of drugs have been utilized with repeated success in the treatment of acute gout: colchicine; phenylbutazone, indomethacin, and glucocorticoids (or ACTH).

Colchicine is still widely used and is a relatively specific agent for the treatment of acute gout. A number of regimens can be used. It is recommended that an initial dose of 1.0 or 1.2 mg (2 tablets) be given orally, followed by 0.5 or 0.6 mg (1 tablet) every hour until the relief of pain or the onset of gastrointestinal symptoms (nausea, vomiting, abdominal pain, and, especially, diarrhea). The therapeutic response and the gastrointestinal symptoms often occur more or less simultaneously. No more than 6.0 to 8.0 mg of colchicine should be given orally for an acute attack; no more than that should be given over a 72-hour period. Colchicine may preferably be given intravenously (1.0 to 3.0 mg given in 20 ml of saline over a ten-minute period) instead of orally, with less gastrointestinal reaction, and repeated if necessary after an interval of four to six hours. Not more than 4.0 mg should be administered intravenously within a 24-hour period. Diarrhea is the most frequent complication of oral colchicine therapy and often requires treatment, e.g., paregoric, for rapid relief. Colchicine is excreted by the kidney and should be used

cautiously in uremia. Large amounts of colchicine may cause transient leukopenia. The probable mechanism of action of colchicine has been discussed earlier. Because of the frequent occurrence of gastrointestinal symptoms during its use, colchicine has been replaced by the anti-inflammatory agents phenylbutazone or indomethacin as the first drug of choice in the treatment of acute gouty arthritis in the ambulatory patient in many if not most clinics.

Phenylbutazone (Butazolidin) or *oxyphenbutazone* (Tandearil) is given in a dose of 200 mg four times a day for two days, with rapid tapering to discontinuation over the following two days. With such brief therapeutic periods, toxicity is minimized. *Indomethacin* (Indocin) may be given in doses of 50 mg three to four times daily for two days with early resolution of acute attack and subsequent tapering of dosage over two days. Some but not all physicians have described a higher incidence of side effects with indomethacin (largely headache and gastrointestinal symptoms) than with phenylbutazone in the treatment of acute gouty arthritis. Glucocorticoid (or ACTH) therapy is not recommended for routine use in acute gouty arthritis because of variability in response and the high incidence of rebound arthritis after its discontinuation. ACTH has proved to be useful in postoperative gout when parenteral therapy is mandatory. Here it may be given as 40 units by slow intravenous drip on the first day, combined with 40 units of ACTH gel intramuscularly on each of the first three days.

When effective treatment has been given, improvement in symptoms usually begins within 6 to 12 hours, with virtually complete remission within 24 to 48 hours. In about 5 to 10 per cent of patients, no rapid relief is obtained, especially if treatment is begun late in the course, and the resolution of the inflammatory arthritis is more gradual. The use of uricosuric agents is not indicated in the management of acute gout.

One of the purposes of therapy is to prevent acute attacks of arthritis. By experience, patients may become aware of stressful experiences or dietary or alcoholic excesses which precipitate attacks, and in this way be able to avoid them. The proper use of uricosuric agents or allopurinol will lower urate levels below the saturation concentration over time, and in this way help to prevent the crystallization which precedes attacks. The short-term effect of such treatment, however, usually leads to exacerbation of gouty arthritis during periods of mobilization of urate deposits. Daily colchicine (0.5 or 0.6 mg once or twice a day) reduces the number of acute attacks in patients subject to recurrent gouty arthritis. Colchicine prophylaxis is not recommended for patients with a single attack (which may never recur) but should be instituted for all patients with frequent attacks of arthritis. Finally, the importance of aborting acute attacks by the use of colchicine or phenylbutazone during the earliest premonitory symptoms should be stressed. This will be the responsibility of the patient himself.

Tophaceous Gout. There are two ways to remove or reduce the size of tophi: surgical removal or redissolving sodium urate crystals. In extracellular fluid, sodium urate crystals can be dissolved only by lowering urate below the saturation level (approximately 7 mg per deciliter, assuming normal protein binding). The rate of redissolving sodium urate bears a direct relationship to the degree of unsaturation achieved, although it may be modified by blood supply, fibrosis, and the area of crystal surface exposed. Two methods are in general use to lower urate levels: the use of uricosuric drugs to increase renal clearance, and the use of allopurinol to inhibit urate synthesis. Dietary restriction may help reduce urate synthesis from preformed purines, but with the advent of the aforementioned methods of treatment it has become less important. In theory an ideal approach to treatment would be to increase urate excretion into the gut (normally one fourth to one third of that synthesized) for bacterial uricolysis. No agent has yet been found which selectively increases gut excretion of urate.

Two uricosuric agents are most often employed, *probenecid* (Benemid) or *sulfinpyrazone* (Anturane). Either of these drugs should be started in small amounts with forced fluids and mild alkalinization of the urine (if no contraindications exist), in order to prevent uric acid stone formation. If the patient has been subject to acute arthritis, prophylactic colchicine should be administered simultaneously to anticipate the exacerbation of gouty arthritis during the early phases of uricosuric therapy. Probenecid should be started at a dose of 0.25 gram twice daily, gradually increasing over a two-week period to a maintenance dose of 0.5 gram two or three times daily. A few patients, particularly those with reduction in renal function, may require 2.5 to 3.0 grams daily in order to reduce serum urate to satisfactory levels, preferably lower than 6.0 mg per deciliter. Sulfinpyrazone may be used as an alternate in beginning doses of 50 mg twice daily, gradually increasing to a maintenance dose of 100 mg three to four times daily. Exceptionally, sulfinpyrazone may be required in doses of 200 mg four times daily for effective uricosuria. In general, both drugs are well tolerated. The most frequently reported reactions are those of gastrointestinal intolerance and drug-induced dermatitis. Very rarely, marrow suppression and hepatic necrosis have been reported. Although uricosuric in large doses, salicylates should not be used in the treatment of gout. At usual therapeutic levels they may primarily inhibit renal tubular secretion of urate and therefore be uricoretentive.

The availability of *allopurinol* (Zyloprim) has introduced a new approach to the treatment of gout. This analogue of hypoxanthine and its oxidation product oxypurinol competitively inhibit xanthine oxidase, and in this way reduce the oxidation of hypoxanthine to xanthine and of xanthine to uric acid (Fig. 2). The human kidney clears hypoxanthine and xanthine much more efficiently than uric acid, so that their extracellular fluid concentrations do not rise commensurately with the fall in urate. The total amount of purine bases excreted is generally somewhat reduced, owing probably to increased reutilization of the oxypurines for salvage synthesis of nucleotides. De novo purine synthesis may also be reduced by feedback inhibition of amidophosphoribosyltransferase by purine ribonucleotides and by depletion of PP-ribose-P. Furthermore, the more equitable distribution of purines excreted among the three metabolites reduces the tendency toward urinary saturation by either xanthine or uric acid (hypoxanthine being highly soluble). Allopurinol is usually given in a single dose of 300 to 600 mg per day. As in the case of uricosuric drugs, its use may initially increase the number of acute attacks of gouty arthritis unless colchicine prophylaxis is used. The pharmacologic production of xanthinuria, an analogue of the genetic disorder, has rarely resulted in difficulties from xanthine stone formation, notably in two patients with the Lesch-Nyhan syndrome and in a few patients being treated with antineoplastic agents. The nucleotide of allopurinol is formed in vivo, and inhibits the enzyme orotidylic decarboxylase with secondary orotic aciduria and orotidinuria. This partial inhibition of pyrimidine synthesis has not been shown to be adverse, and no incorporation of allopurinol nucleotide into nucleic acid as a possible mutagenic agent has been found. Toxic effects of allopurinol are rare (3 to 5 per cent of patients), and consist of dermatitis, fever, headache, diarrhea, transitory leukopenia, and elevation of serum transaminase enzymes of hepatic origin. Intramuscular crystals of xanthine and oxypurinol have been described in patients receiving allopurinol. The significance of this observation in terms of ultimate toxicity is not clear.

The availability of two general methods of treatment allows choice in the management of tophaceous gout or marked hyperuricemia productive of acute gout. In general, it is recommended that uricosuric agents be given an initial trial in the treatment of milder forms of gout in the absence of renal failure, allopurinol being withheld for more specific indications. Probenecid has been widely used for almost 30 years, whereas the use of allopurinol, although the known toxic effects are few and rarely severe, represents the introduction of a foreign purine base and nucleotide widely used therapeutically for perhaps a dozen years. This expression of some therapeutic restraint in the use of allopurinol is a conservative position, for there is a definite trend toward using this agent in the initial treatment of hyperuricemia. Allopurinol is definitely indicated for certain patients: when uricosuric treatment proves ineffective in lowering the extracellular urate level sufficiently (to less than 6 mg per deciliter); when there are toxic reactions to uricosuric drugs; when tophaceous gout is particularly severe (which often accompanies some degree of renal functional impairment and poor response to uricosuric agents); or when there have been recurrent uric acid stones. In general, the allopurinol regimen is more effective in rapidly lowering urate levels without the added hazard of passing extra uric acid through the kidney and urinary tract. A uricosuric drug may be used in conjunction with allopurinol with more rapid reduction in serum urate, but higher doses of allopurinol may be required, because probenecid increases the renal excretion of oxypurinol as well as that of uric acid. Combined treatment has been used successfully for patients with severe tophaceous gout with good renal function when neither drug alone has sufficed to lower urate levels adequately.

With prolonged treatment, remarkable reversal of tophaceous gout may be obtained. Treatment should then be continued for life to prevent recurrence of hyperuricemia and its complications.

Gouty Kidney. There is no specific way to treat gouty kidney when renal failure has occurred. There is rarely any evidence of improvement in renal function when urate values are reduced enough to mobilize tophaceous deposits. Treatment is limited to control of pyelonephritis if it exists, prevention of further stone formation, lowering extracellular urate levels by the methods previously described in order to prevent further injury, treatment of hypertension to modify the progress of nephrosclerosis, and the general metabolic measures used to treat any patient with diminished renal function. With early diagnosis and treatment, renal failure is becoming a much rarer complication of gout. With uremia, the dose of allopurinol used should be lower.

A particular form of gouty kidney, acute tubular blockade by uric acid with oliguria or anuria, can be prevented in patients being treated with cytotoxic agents by the use of fluids, alkalinization of the urine, and, in particular, full doses of allopurinol *before* the treatment of the myeloproliferative disorder. If anuria occurs, the usual measures for the treatment of acute renal failure should be instituted in anticipation of tubular regeneration over a 10- to 14-day period.

Uric Acid Stones. As previously described, the tendency to form uric acid stones is a function of the concentration of free uric acid, as opposed to sodium urate, in urine. Preventive measures attempt to reduce uric acid concentration by increasing urine volume (forcing of fluids, particularly at night), increasing urine pH (administration of sodium citrate or bicarbonate to maintain urine pH greater than 6), or reducing urate excretion (allopurinol). In most patients, fluids and mild alkalinization suffice to prevent uric acid stones. When uricaciduria is marked, when excess sodium is contraindicated, or when these measures are not successful, the use of allopurinol offers a specific method for the prevention of uric acid stones. As stated, the theoretical possibility of substituting xanthine stones for uric acid stones exists, but this complication has so far occurred only in the Lesch-Nyhan syndrome.

Essential Hyperuricemia. In this chapter, essential hyperuricemia is considered to be gout without complications. The incidental discovery of elevated serum urate values in the absence of any of the clinical manifestations of gout has increased with the broader use of screening laboratory determinations. One of the most vexing problems facing the physician is whether asymptomatic hyperuricemia should be treated. There are few firm data on which to base a decision. Although hyperuricemia has been associated epidemiologically with hyperlipidemia, hypertension, obesity, glucose intolerance, and accelerated vascular disease, there is no evidence that it is primary in any of these derangements, or that lowering uric acid levels affects their course. Similarly, gout may lead to renal failure, but documentation of gouty kidney in the absence of other clinical manifestations is exceedingly rare. Finally, only a minority of patients develop complications of gout despite a lifetime of hyperuricemia in the postpubertal period, although the incidence of complications is roughly proportional to the degree of sodium urate supersaturation in extracellular fluid. Because of these uncertainties, it does not seem justified to start therapy for life in essential hyperuricemia. On the other hand, when serum uric acid values are consistently above 9.0 mg per deciliter, the degree of supersaturation is such that the incidence of complications is perhaps 90 per cent. It would seen reasonable to treat such patients with uricosuric agents, or allopurinol, in order to maintain safer uric acid levels.

Gutman, A. B., and Yü, T.-F.: Uric acid nephrolithiasis. Am. J. Med., 45:756, 1968.

McCarty, D. J., Jr.: Mechanisms of the crystal deposition diseases — gout and pseudogout. Ann. Intern. Med., 78:767, 1973.

Rieselbach, R. E., and Steele, T. H.: Influence of the kidney upon urate homeostasis in health and disease. Am. J. Med., 56:665, 1974.

Spillberg, I.: Current concepts of the mechanism of acute inflammation in gouty arthritis. Arthritis Rheum., 18:129, 1975.

Weissman, G.: Crystals, lysosomes, and gout. Adv. Intern. Med., 19:239, 1974.

Wyngaarden, J. B., and Kelley, W. N.: Gout. *In* Stanbury, J. B., Wyngaarden, J. B., and Fredrickson, D. S. (eds.): The Metabolic Basis of Inherited Disease. 4th ed. New York, McGraw-Hill Book Company, 1978, p. 916.

Wyngaarden, J. B., and Kelley, W. N.: Gout and Hyperuricemia. New York, Grune & Stratton, 1976.

Yü, T.-F.: Milestones in the treatment of gout. Am. J. Med., 56:676, 1974.

535.2. XANTHINURIA

Lloyd H. Smith, Jr.

Xanthinuria is a rare genetic disorder secondary to deficiency of xanthine oxidase. Approximately 24 cases have been described, and some of these have not been fully investigated. It is probably transmitted as an autosomal recessive trait, although this has not been firmly established and there is no method now available for detection of heterozygotes. Deficient activity of xanthine oxidase has been demonstrated in liver and gut mucosa in xanthinuria. The normal function of this enzyme is to catalyze the oxidation of hypoxanthine to xanthine and of xanthine to uric acid.

Most patients with xanthinuria have been asymptomatic, being discovered in the investigation of hypouricemia (serum urate less than 1 mg per deciliter). Three patients had xanthine kidney stones, which resemble uric acid stones in their radiolucency. Two of the patients had muscle cramps, made worse by exercise, and were found on muscle biopsy to have intracellular crystals of xanthine and hypoxanthine. Although one patient with xanthinuria had hemochromatosis, no other patients have shown abnormal avidity for iron absorption.

The diagnosis is established by the demonstration of hypouricemia and hypouricaciduria with increased excretion of hypoxanthine and xanthine. In xanthinuria these oxypurines are usually excreted in amounts somewhat less than the normal value for uric acid. Hypoxanthine is partially reutilized to form inosine-5'-phosphate, a reaction catalyzed by hypoxanthine guanine phosphoribosyltransferase, the enzyme which is deficient in the Lesch-Nyhan syndrome. Xanthinuria is simulated pharmacologically by the use of the allopurinol which is a competitive inhibitor of, as well as a substrate for, xanthine oxidase. (See Ch. 535.1.) Hypouricemia may also occur in proximal renal tubular disease (Fanconi's syndrome, Wilson's disease) and during treatment with uricosuric agents. Uricosuric agents include aspirin, x-ray contrast agents, and glyceryl guaiacolate. Hypouricemia has been described repeatedly in association with neoplastic diseases. It has also been described in several healthy individuals who had an isolated defect in renal tubular reabsorption of urate (clearance of urate 1.3 times creatinine clearance), similar to that found in the Dalmatian coach hound and in primates other than man. Probably a few patients have had xanthine stones or mixed stones containing xanthine as one component in the absence of the genetic disease. The solubility of hypoxanthine prevents its precipitation in the urinary tract.

Treatment is usually not required. A program for the prevent of xanthine stones would be similar to that for uric acid stones, i.e., forcing fluids, alkalinization of the urine (although the enhancement of solubility of xanthine by alkalinization is not as great as that of urate), and possibly a low purine diet if the above does not suffice. Despite the very low levels of xanthine oxidase, studies on a single patient suggest that allopurinol might increase the amount of oxypurine excreted as the more soluble hypoxanthine.

Seegmiller, J. E.: Xanthine stone formation. Am. J. Med., 45:780, 1968.

Seegmiller, J. E.: Hereditary xanthinuria. *In* Bondy, P. K., and Rosenberg, L. E. (eds.): Duncan's Disease of Metabolism. 7th ed. Philadelphia, W. B. Saunders Company, 1974, p. 739

Wyngaarden, J. B.: Xanthinuria. *In* Stanbury, J. B., Wyngaarden, J. B., and Fredrickson, D. S. (eds.): The Metabolic Basis of Inherited Disease. 4th ed. New York. McGraw-Hill Book Company, 1978, p. 1037.

535.3.   THE LESCH-NYHAN SYNDROME

(HGPRT Deficiency)

James B. Wyngaarden

DEFINITION. The Lesch-Nyhan syndrome is an inherited disorder characterized clinically by choreoathetosis, spasticity, mental retardation, self-mutilation, hyperuricemia, excessive production of uric acid, hyperuricaciduria, renal stones, and renal failure. Death usually occurs in the second or third decade from infection or renal failure. The disease affects males only.

INCIDENCE. The disease is rare. About 100 cases have been reported.

ETIOLOGY AND PATHOGENESIS. The Lesch-Nyhan syndrome is an X-linked condition, fully manifest in the hemizygous male. The biochemical defect is a deficiency of an enzyme of purine metabolism, hypoxanthine–guanine phosphoribosyltransferase. The enzymatic defect leads to a failure of salvage of the purine bases hypoxanthine and guanine as they are produced in the turnover and degradation of nucleic acids and purine nucleotides. Guanine is deaminated to xanthine by guanase; hypoxanthine is oxidized to xanthine, and xanthine is oxidized to uric acid by the enzyme xanthine oxidase. As a consequence of the enzymatic defect there is gross overproduction of uric acid, with marked hyperuricemia and hyperuricaciduria. These observations provide an understanding of the features of the syndrome associated with raised concentrations of uric acid, such as urinary stones, and hyperuricemic and uric acid nephropathies. The neurologic and behavior aberrations have not been satisfactorily explained. It is thought likely that critical abnormalities of neurologic development may be secondary to regulation of intracellular nucleotide levels at key stages of neural growth, but this has not been proved.

PATHOLOGY. At autopsy there is evidence of growth retardation and self-mutilation, and of bilaterally shrunken kidneys with striking deposits of monosodium urate and uric acid. Routine histologic examination of the nervous system does not reveal any significant changes, except in patients dying of renal failure in which the findings can probably be attributed to severe uremia preceding death.

CLINICAL MANIFESTATIONS. Patients with the Lesch-Nyhan syndrome generally appear normal at birth. The earliest consistent abnormality is a delay in motor development which appears by three to four months of age. Between eight months and one year extrapyramidal signs develop. These are characterized by fine athetoid movements of the hands and feet, dystonia, and chorea. The athetosis, which is similar to that associated with asphyxia, birth injury, and hyperbilirubinemia, accounts at least in part for the dysarthria which appears later in life. At about one year signs of pyramidal tract involvement such as hyperreflexia, sustained ankle clonus, extensor plantar responses, and scissoring of the legs also develop. These developments preclude ambulation in the older patient.

The most striking neurologic feature is compulsive self-destructive behavior. Between 2 and 16 years of age affected children begin to bite their fingers, lips, and buccal mucosa. This compulsion for self-mutilation becomes so extreme that it may be necessary to keep the elbows in extension with splints, or to wrap the hands with gauze or restrain them in some other manner. In some patients mutilation of lips can only be controlled by extraction of teeth. The compulsive urge to inflict painful wounds appears to grip the patient irresistibly. Often he will be content until one begins to remove an arm splint. At this point a communicative patient will plead that the restraints be left alone. If the arm is freed, the patient will become agitated and extremely upset. Finally, when completely unrestrained he will begin to put his fingers into his mouth. An older patient will plead for help, and if one takes hold of the arm, the patient will show obvious relief. If help is not forthcoming, a painful and often severe injury may be inflicted. Lesch-Nyhan patients also attempt to injure themselves in other ways, by hitting their heads against objects, or by placing their extremities in dangerous places such as the spokes of a wheelchair. Lesch-Nyhan patients may exhibit unusual aggressiveness toward others, and may strike at visitors, relatives, or medical personnel.

Most patients with the Lesch-Nyhan syndrome appear to be mentally deficient. I.Q. testing by routine methods usually gives values ranging from 39 to 65. The poor performance in formal testing may in part be related to dysarthria and choreoathetosis. Approximately 50 per cent of patients have had seizures.

All patients with the Lesch-Nyhan syndrome exhibit excessive production of uric acid. Excretion of uric acid ranges from 25 to 143 mg per kilogram per day, compared with an upper limit in normal children of 18 mg per kilogram per day. The ratio of excretion of uric acid to creatinine is raised. The increased quantity of uric acid in the urine leads to uric acid crystalluria. Orange crystals may be noted on the diaper during the first few weeks of life. Many patients develop uric acid nephrolithiasis, and this may lead to obstructive uropathy with severe and unrelenting uremia. Serum urate concentrations usually range from 7 to 18 mg per deciliter. An occasional patient develops classic gouty arthritis and tophaceous deposits of monosodium urate, although these are rare before the age of 12 or 13. Some patients have exhibited a megaloblastic anemia which responds to adenine but not to folic acid. Lesch-Nyhan children may have an increased susceptibility to infections, and some appear to have a B-lymphocyte immunologic dysfunction.

DIAGNOSIS AND DIFFERENTIAL DIAGNOSIS. The diagnosis should be suspected in a male child with the clinical features described, associated with hyperuricemia, and with self-destructive mutilation. The diagnosis is established by demonstration of immeasurably low levels of activity of hypoxanthine–guanine phosphoribosyltransferase in erythrocytes. The syndrome must be distinguished from cerebral palsy and other instances of delayed motor development and self-mutilation in patients who are not hyperuricemic and have normal HGPRT activity.

Suspect heterozygotes usually show normal plasma levels of uric acid, and normal erythrocyte activity values of HGPRT. They can be identified as heterozygotes by growth of fibroblasts in tissue culture, and demonstration of mosaicism with respect to HGPRT activity. HGPRT$^+$ and HGPRT$^-$ cells can be distinguished by radiographic techniques, and the two types of cells can be grown selectively in specific media. Heterozygotes can also be identified by analysis of enzyme activity of hair follicles which exhibit a degree of clonal differentiation. Prenatal diagnosis of the Lesch-Nyhan syndrome can be made with cultured cells obtained from amniotic fluid. In at least two instances the diagnosis of HGPRT deficiency has been made in utero and the pregnancy has been interrupted.

TREATMENT. There is no definitive treatment. Allopurinol effectively lowers the serum urate concentration and the uric acid content of urine. This drug can be used to prevent uric acid stone formation, uric acid and urate nephropathy, gouty arthritis, and tophi. A few patients with the Lesch-Nyhan syndrome have developed xanthine stones during allopurinol treatment. No agents have been found which alleviate the central nervous system dysfunction. Improvement on the metabolic ward that has occasionally been attributed to an experimental therapy probably reflects the positive response of patients to supportive measures and protection from self-mutilation.

Kelley, W. N., and Wyngaarden, J. B.: The Lesch-Nyhan syndrome. *In* Stanbury, J. B., Wyngaarden, J. B., and Fredrickson, D. S. (eds.): The Metabolic Basis of Inherited Disease. 4th ed. New York, McGraw-Hill Book Company, 1978, p. 1011.

535.4. 2,8-DIHYDROXYADENINE RENAL STONES
(APRT Deficiency)
James B. Wyngaarden

Several children have been described with 2,8-dihydroxyadenine crystalluria and renal stones, associated with complete deficiency of adenine phosphoribosyltransferase (APRT) activity. This enzyme normally catalyzes reconversion of adenine to adenylic acid. When its activity is absent, adenine, 8-hydroxyadenine, and 2,8-dihydroxyadenine appear in urine, and together may represent one fourth of urinary purines. The last two compounds are derived from adenine by action of xanthine oxidase. 2,8-Dihydroxyadenine is 50 times less soluble in water than uric acid, and forms crystals and stones as the urine is concentrated. The nephrotoxicity of 2,8-dihydroxyadenine is well known from experiments after adenine administration in man and animals.

The disease is inherited as an autosomal recessive trait, and parents have half or less of the normal activity of APRT in erythrocytes. The carrier state is not rare, one estimate being 1 per cent of the population. If this estimate is correct, the homozygous state should occur once in 40,000 births. The ultraviolet spectral characteristics of 2,8-dihydroxyadenine are similar to those of uric acid; it has been suggested that 2,8-dihydroxyadenine crystalluria and stones may be more frequent than presently recognized, especially among "uric acid" stone formers in the pediatric age group. Partial APRT deficiency has been associated with gout in at least ten patients, but this may represent bias of ascertainment as several surveys were conducted in gout clinics. When the propositus was excluded, only 2 of 26 carriers were hyperuricemic, and none had gout. In addition, APRT and hyperuricemia were discordant in the families.

Treatment with a low purine diet and allopurinol reduces 2,8-dihydroxyadenine excretion and averts further stone formation.

Fox, I. H., Lacroix, S., Planet, G., and Moore, M.: Partial deficiency of adenine phosphoribosyltransferase in man. Medicine, 56:515, 1977.
Van Acker, K. J., Simmonds, A., Potter, C., and Cameron, J. S.: Complete deficiency of adenine phosphoribosyltransferase. Report of a family. N. Engl. J. Med., 297:127, 1977.

535.5. MISCELLANEOUS DISEASES OF PURINE METABOLISM
James B. Wyngaarden

About 50 per cent of patients with severe combined immunodeficiency disease have an associated *adenosine deaminase (ADA) deficiency*. A few cases have been associated with *purine nucleoside phosphorylase (PNP) deficiency*. These disorders are discussed in Ch. 40.5. The mechanisms of T and B lymphocyte dysfunction resulting from these enzyme deficiencies are not known with certainty, but two classes of potentially toxic mediators have been proposed. Erythrocytes of ADA-deficient patients contain 50- to 100-fold elevations of deoxyadenosine triphosphate. Some patients respond immunologically to periodic infusions of irradiated erythrocytes containing ADA. The excess erythrocyte deoxyATP disappears after infusion of normal erythrocytes. Cells of PNP-deficient patients accumulate 10-fold elevations of deoxyGTP. DeoxyATP and deoxyGTP inhibit ribonucleotide reductase, an enzyme involved in DNA synthesis. ADA-deficient cells also accumulate elevated levels of S-adenosyl-homocysteine. This metabolite inhibits many S-adenosyl-methionine–dependent methylases with resulting impairment of methylation reactions.

A deficiency of *ecto-5'-nucleotidase* has been described in several different types of hypogammaglobulinemia.

Myoadenylate deaminase deficiency is associated with a generalized nonprogressive myopathy of children and young adults. The disease presents with muscular weakness or cramping after exercise. In patients with this disorder muscle exercise results in elevations of plasma lactic acid, but not of plasma ammonia concentrations. In the normal individual concentrations of these metabolites rise in parallel during exercise. These relationships provide the basis for a presumptive diagnostic test. Muscle biopsy specimens are histologically normal but lack myoadenylate deaminase activity by histochemical stain and solution essays.

Cohen, A., Hirschhorn, R., Horowitz, S. D., Rubinstein, A., Polmar, S. H., Hong, R., and Martin, D. W., Jr.: Deoxyadenosine triphosphate as a potentially toxic metabolite in adenosine deaminase deficiency. Proc. Natl. Acad. Sci., 75:472, 1978.
Fishbein, W. N., Armbrustmacher, V. W., and Griffin, J. L.: Myoadenylate deaminase deficiency: A new disease of muscle. Science, 200:545, 1978.
Kredich, N. M., and Martin, D. W., Jr.: Role of S-adenosyl homocysteine in adenosine mediated toxicity in cultured mouse T lymphoma cells. Cell, 12:931, 1977.

535.6. DISORDERS OF PYRIMIDINE METABOLISM
Lloyd H. Smith, Jr.

Pyrimidine nucleotides share equally with purine nucleotides the chemical chore of transmitting genetic information for reproduction or for phenotypic expression within the cell. They also function in the intermediary metabolism of lipids and carbohydrates. Only a few disorders of pyrimidine metabolism have been recognized.

Hereditary orotic aciduria is a rare genetic disorder of pyrimidine metabolism characterized by megaloblastic anemia resistant to the usual hematinic agents, leukopenia, failure of normal growth and development, and the continued excessive urinary excretion of orotic acid. Orotic acid is highly insoluble and often forms a heavy sediment of urinary crystals which may on occasion result in ureteral or urethral obstruction. The disorder, which is transmitted as an autosomal recessive trait, is usually characterized by reduced activities of two consecutive enzymes in pyrimidine biosynthesis, orotate phosphoribosyltransferase (OPRT) and orotidine 5'-phosphate decarboxylase (ODC). A single patient has been described with isolated deficiency of ODC. There is a prompt and sustained hematologic and general clinical response to oral uridine (2 to 4 grams per day), which must be continued indefinitely as replacement therapy. The disease has attracted special attention because it represents a block in the de novo pathway of pyrimidine synthesis, is an example of a double enzyme defect, and produces a requirement for replacement of a normal metabolic intermediate, uridine.

Orotic aciduria, without the characteristic hematologic abnormalities, also occurs in *ornithine transcarbamylase deficiency*. It is presumed that this results from the overflow of carbamyl phosphate from urea synthesis (partially blocked in this disease) to pyrimidine synthesis.

Excessive urinary excretion of orotic acid and orotidine occurs during treatment with *allopurinol* or *6-azauridine*. Metabolic products of both compounds inhibit orotidine 5'-decarboxylase activity.

Beta-aminoisobutyricaciduria is a benign hereditary disorder of thymine catabolism which occurs in 5 to 10 per cent of Caucasians and in a much higher percentage of Asians. The defect presumably lies in the transamination of beta-aminoisobutyric acid to methylmalonic acid semialdehyde. The aminoaciduria which results, representing the only known disorder of pyrimidine catabolism, has no known biologic disadvantage.

Pyrimidine 5'-nucleotidase deficiency is a rare form of hereditary hemolytic anemia, transmitted as an autosomal recessive trait. The erythrocytes exhibit prominent basophilic stippling due to aggregates of undegraded ribosomes and on analysis contain very high concentrations of cytidine and uridine nucleotides. The mechanism by which the nucleotidase deficiency leads to hemolysis is unclear.

Kelley, W. N., and Smith, L. H., Jr.: Hereditary orotic aciduria. *In* Stanbury, J. B., Wyngaarden, J. B., and Fredrickson, D. S. (eds.): The Metabolic Basis of Inherited Disease. 4th ed. New York, McGraw-Hill Book Company, 1978, p. 1045.

Smith, L. H., Jr.: Pyrimidine metabolism in man. N. Engl. J. Med., 288:764, 1973.

Valentine, W. N., Fink, K., Paglia, D. E., et al.: Hereditary hemolytic anemia with human erythrocyte pyrimidine 5'-nucleotidase deficiency. J. Clin. Invest., 54:866, 1974.

536. PORPHYRIA

Rudi Schmid

536.1. INTRODUCTION

Porphyrins are tetrapyrrole pigments in which four monopyrroles are linked by four carbon bridges to form a planar ring structure. Each of the pyrroles has two substituent side chains, and the various porphyrins such as uro-, copro-, and protoporphyrin differ only in the nature of these side chains. Their sequential arrangement in specific porphyrins determines the structural isomer type, numbered I to IV. In nature, only porphyrins of the isomer types I and III have been identified. With the exception of protoporphyrin IX (belonging to the isomer type III series), which in the form of ferroprotoporphyrin (heme) serves as the prosthetic group of hemoglobin and other essential heme proteins, porphyrins apparently neither possess physiologic functions nor act as metabolic intermediates. Rather, they are metabolic byproducts that have escaped from the biosynthetic path to heme by irreversible oxidation of the corresponding reduced porphyrinogens (see accompanying figure). The latter are intermediates in heme biosynthesis and are formed from the monopyrrole porphobilinogen (PBG), which in turn is synthesized by condensation of 2 moles of δ-aminolevulinic acid (ALA). The over-all rate of heme and porphyrin biosynthesis is regulated primarily by the activity of ALA synthetase, which condenses glycine and succinyl-CoA to ALA. This mitochondrial enzyme is reversibly repressed and inhibited by the final product, heme, and it is likely that this and other regulatory mechanisms are responsible for preventing both overproduction of heme and accumulation of metabolic intermediates. In porphyria, the increased excretion of ALA, PBG, or porphyrins results from inherited defects or acquired dysfunction of individual enzyme systems or control mechanisms of heme biosynthesis. Catabolism of hemoglobin and other heme proteins does not lead to formation of porphyrins; instead, the ferroprotoporphyrin ring is cleaved to biliverdin and bilirubin which are linear tetrapyrroles.

Although all aerobic cells can synthesize heme-containing chromoproteins, heme formation is particularly active in the erythroid elements of bone marrow and in liver. The small quantities of porphyrins and porphyrin precursors excreted normally in urine and bile are derived primarily from these sources. Similarly, the metabolic defects in porphyria that result in the accumulation and consequent increased excretion of porphyrins or their precursors usually can be traced to the erythroid cells of the bone marrow or to the liver, or to both. This distinction serves as a convenient basis for the classification of the porphyrias on page 2045.

The metabolic pathway from glycine and succinate to heme. Abbreviations: ALA, δ-aminolevulinic acid; PBG, porphobilinogen; UROgen, uroporphyrinogen; COPROgen, coproporphyrinogen; PROTOgen, protoporphyrinogen; URO, uroporphyrin; COPRO, coproporphyrin; PROTO, protoporphyrin; I, III, isomer types I and III.

A. Congenital erythropoietic porphyria
B. Hepatic porphyrias
   1. Genetic forms
      a. Acute intermittent porphyria
      b. Hereditary coproporphyria
      c. Variegate porphyria
      d. Porphyria cutanea tarda
   2. Acquired (toxic) porphyria
C. Protoporphyria

This classification indicates the major anatomic site of the metabolic disturbance and distinguishes the hereditary forms of porphyria from the instances in which porphyria appears to be acquired.

Increased urinary excretion of porphyrins or precursors, including ALA and PBG, occurs in a variety of conditions other than porphyria. Chronic lead poisoning is commonly associated with increased ALA, and elevated PBG occasionally has been observed in carcinomatosis, Hodgkin's disease, cirrhosis, and affections of the nervous system. Normal urine contains only traces of uroporphyrin, but increased concentrations may be present in heavy metal poisoning and occasionally in parenchymal liver disease; gross uroporphyrinuria has been reported in patients with benign or malignant tumors of the liver. Coproporphyrin frequently is increased in lead poisoning, hemolytic or refractory anemia, hepatitis, cirrhosis, infectious mononucleosis, and alcoholism. In liver disease, coproporphyrinuria may not indicate increased formation of the pigment, but rather its diversion from bile to urine. Protoporphyrin, which has only 2 carboxyl groups and consequently is poorly soluble in water, does not appear in urine, but is excreted exclusively in the bile. The feces regularly contain copro-, proto-, and deuteroporphyrin, but these pigments may be derived in part from food, intestinal hemorrhage, and colonic microflora. Because of the wide range in fecal porphyrin concentration, values up to 200 μg per gram dry weight may not be indicative of porphyria without other diagnostic evidence.

536.2. CONGENITAL ERYTHROPOIETIC PORPHYRIA

(Congenital Photosensitive Porphyria, Günther's Disease)

This very rare disease is due to a hereditary defect of porphyrin metabolism in the erythroid cells that leads to chronic photosensitivity, hemolytic anemia, and increased urinary excretion of uroporphyrin. Only about 80 cases in both sexes have been reported. Inheritance is by autosomal recessive transmission; heterozygous individuals appear clinically normal.

Excretion of pinkish urine usually begins shortly after birth, whereas cutaneous lesions on exposed parts, increased hemolysis, and splenomegaly may not be detected until later. Hypertrichosis and erythrodontia are virtually always present. Urine contains high concentrations of uroporphyrin I and coproporphyrin I, but excretion of ALA and PBG is normal. Hemoglobin frequently is decreased, and reticulocytes and fecal urobilinogen are increased. Erythrocytes contain much uroporphyrin I, and normoblasts and reticulocytes exhibit intense red fluorescence. The metabolic defect involves faulty conversion of PBG to uroporphyrinogen

III in the maturing erythroid cells of the bone marrow. Death may occur in childhood, but if patients live to maturity, they usually exhibit severe scarring and mutilation of hands and face. Successful pregnancy with delivery of phenotypically normal children has been reported. Treatment is symptomatic and prophylactic, consisting essentially of rigorous protection from sunlight. In some instances hemolytic anemia, photosensitivity, and porphyrin excretion have been improved by splenectomy.

536.3. HEPATIC PORPHYRIAS

ACUTE INTERMITTENT PORPHYRIA

DEFINITION, INCIDENCE, AND GENETICS. Acute intermittent porphyria (synonyms: *acute porphyria, porphyria hepatica, pyrroloporphyria, Swedish type*) is an abnormality of pyrrole metabolism inherited as a dominant trait. It is associated with recurrent attacks of abdominal pain, gastrointestinal dysfunction, and neurologic manifestations. It is probably the most common form of porphyria, with an over-all incidence of approximately 1 per 100,000 population, but, because of its occurrence in large families, regional incidence may be much higher. The total number of reported cases suggests that people of Scandinavian, Anglo-Saxon, and German ancestry are affected more frequently, whereas the disease is very rare in blacks.

Acute attacks are rarely seen before puberty; they most often begin in the third or fourth decade, and occur more frequently in women. Manifestations may appear only in later life, or recurrent symptoms may be so vague and protean as to escape recognition. Indeed, persons carrying the genetic abnormality may remain free of clinical manifestations throughout life; such latent porphyria tends to be more frequent in men. This probably accounts for the alleged preponderance of porphyria in women of child-bearing age.

CLINICAL MANIFESTATIONS. Moderate to severe abdominal pain, often colicky, is frequently the initial or most prominent symptom. The pain may be localized, generalized, or radiating to the back or loins, but the abdomen usually is soft. Abdominal tenderness and distention may exist, but are much less striking than would be expected from the intensity of the pain. Leukocytosis and mild fever may be present. Diarrhea occasionally occurs. Severe vomiting and persistent constipation are frequent and may be accompanied by lack of bowel sounds and dilatation of the stomach. Roentgenograms of the abdomen may reveal distended intestinal loops proximal to areas of spasm; volvulus and gangrene have been reported. Gastrointestinal complications commonly lead to weight loss and occasionally to severe emaciation. Prolonged vomiting may cause dehydration, oliguria, and azotemia.

Neurologic disturbances frequently, though not always, are associated with abdominal manifestations and may involve the peripheral, central, or autonomic nervous system. Peripheral neuropathy usually is predominantly motor, may be asymmetrical, and may vary from mild weakness in one extremity to complete flaccid quadriplegia. These motor disturbances may be preceded or accompanied by severe pain, particularly in the legs. Deep tendon reflexes are usually diminished or absent and, although subjective sensory symptoms are frequent, objective sensory loss is less common. Cranial nerve involvement leads to optic atrophy, ophthalmoplegia, facial palsy, dysphagia, and vocal cord paresis. Weakness of abdominal, intercostal, or diaphragmatic musculature may progress to respiratory paralysis, which has a poor prognosis and ranks as the chief cause of death. Wasting and contracture of affected muscles frequently occur but are reversible to a surprising degree during prolonged remissions.

Many patients have a long history of nervousness, emotional instability, and functional disturbances that may remain unexplained until an acute attack occurs. Striking psychiatric abnormalities include personality changes, hysteria, psychoses, and confusional states. With more severe central nervous system involvement, delirium, coma, and epileptic seizures may occur; on occasion they have followed ingestion of barbiturates or maladvised surgical exploration of the abdomen.

Sinus tachycardia frequently accompanies acute attacks, and the pulse rate has been found to be a good index of the activity of the disease. This is believed to be due to vagal neuropathy, which also may account for nonspecific electrocardiographic abnormalities. Transient hypertension is often present, and on occasion spasm of retinal arteries has been observed. Frank photosensitivy does not occur in acute intermittent porphyria, but mild and apparently reversible pigmentation, particularly of exposed parts of the body, may accompany acute phases of the disease.

Acute episodes vary widely in duration and frequency. Some patients complain merely of occasional and intermittent abdominal pain, whereas in others the initial attack may begin almost explosively and may terminate fatally within days to several weeks. In the majority of cases, distinct attacks recur at irregular intervals over months or years, but tend to decrease in frequency and severity with age. There is strong evidence that attacks frequently are precipitated by a variety of drugs, including barbiturates, sulfonamides, griseofulvin, estrogens, and contraceptives, all of which are metabolized by microsomal enzyme systems of the liver, that contain hemoproteins. Occasionally, periodic exacerbations are correlated with the menstrual cycle, or latent porphyria may become clinically manifest late in pregnancy, shortly after delivery, or during fasting.

LABORATORY FINDINGS AND PATHOGENESIS. The most characteristic laboratory finding is excessive ALA and PBG in the urine. PBG is a colorless chromogen giving a red complex with Ehrlich aldehyde (p-dimethylaminobenzaldehyde in HCl) which after neutralization cannot be extracted with chloroform or butanol (*Watson-Schwartz test*). By contrast the red color produced by Ehrlich aldehyde with urobilinogen or indoles is readily extractable with chloroform or butanol. Ingestion of antipyrine or admixture of methyl red (Zephiran) results in urine that turns red on acidification alone, whereas compounds of the phenolphthalein group show red only in alkaline urine. During acute episodes of porphyria, the Watson-Schwartz test is almost always strongly positive; if the reaction is faintly pink or negative, the diagnosis remains doubtful. In latent porphyria or in patients recovered from an acute attack, urinary excretion of PBG frequently is less pronounced or may be normal so that the Watson-Schwartz test may be negative. In these instances, urinary ALA and PBG should be quantitated by chromatographic methods, which commonly but not invariably reveal increased excretion of these porphyrin precursors. Freshly passed urine may be normal in color and usually contains relatively little preformed uro- and coproporphyrin. It darkens on standing because of conversion of PBG and other precursors to porphyrins and porphobilin, a dark brown pigment of unknown structure. Fecal porphyrins are within normal limits, except in rare instances when urine porphyrins are markedly elevated; under these circumstances fecal porphyrins may exceed normal values.

Except for a moderate reduction in the circulating red cell volume, hematologic abnormalities usually are absent. Conventional liver function tests frequently yield normal results except for increased BSP retention. The urine may contain increased concentrations of amino acids and indoles; the latter sometimes give an atypical Ehrlich reaction. Elevated protein-bound iodine, cholesterol, and β-lipoprotein levels have been reported. During acute attacks hyponatremia may become an alarming complication; although this often can be ascribed to prolonged vomiting or excessive intravenous fluid replacement, inappropriate secretion of antidiuretic hormone has been demonstrated. The liver is microscopically normal or shows mild focal or centrilobular necrosis and fatty changes. It usually does not exhibit porphyrin fluorescence, but contains much PBG. Inconstant neuropathologic changes include patchy demyelination of the peripheral or central nervous system and chromatolysis of anterior horn cells.

The inherited biochemical defect consists of a partial deficiency of the enzyme *uroporphyrinogen synthetase* which converts PBG to uroporphyrinogen. The ensuing impairment of heme synthesis secondarily leads to derepression of ALA synthetase, which results in increased formation and urinary excretion of ALA and its condensation product, PBG. Although this enzymatic defect is demonstrable in a variety of tissues, including circulating erythrocytes, its functional expression appears to be limited to the liver. Drugs and hormones known to aggravate the disease have been shown to induce the activity of hepatic ALA synthetase. The pathogenesis of the abdominal and nervous manifestations remains obscure; a direct toxic effect of ALA or PBG now seems unlikely.

DIAGNOSIS AND DIFFERENTIAL DIAGNOSIS. The diagnosis rests primarily on the determination of increased urinary excretion of ALA and PBG. As a screening procedure, the qualitative Watson-Schwartz test usually is adequate, but for a definitive diagnosis, quantitative determination with chromatographic methods is essential. In prepubertal children and in asymptomatic adults suspected of having latent porphyria, urinary ALA and PBG may be normal; in these instances detection of the inherited defect requires demonstration of reduced uroporphyrinogen synthetase activity in erythrocytes or other tissues. Lead intoxication may produce severe abdominal pain and neuropathy, but the urine rarely contains sufficient PBG to give a positive Watson-Schwartz test, although ALA excretion frequently is increased.

The possibility of porphyria should always be considered in the presence of unexplained abdominal pain, because the disease has been mistaken for cholelithiasis, renal colic, peptic ulcer, appendicitis, bowel obstruction, pancreatitis, and pelvic disorders. Some patients have undergone several surgical procedures before the correct diagnosis was established. Acute attacks seldom last less than 48 hours, and very brief episodes of pain followed by complete remission rarely occur. Obscure neurologic disturbances, especially unexplained peripheral neuropathy, regional muscle weakness, flaccid paralysis, or bulbar palsy, should suggest the possibility of porphyria. Similarly, if hysterical behavior, psychoneurosis, psychosis, or unexplained epilepsy is aggravated by barbiturates, coincides with the menstrual cycle, or is noted in patients under treatment with contraceptives, porphyria should be suspected.

Persistent tachycardia, muscle weakness, and elevated protein-bound iodine may lead to confusion with hyperthyroidism. Occasionally weakness, abdominal pain, pigmentation, and hyponatremia may suggest Addison's disease. During the last trimester of pregnancy, hypertension, vomiting, and oliguria suggestive of eclampsia may in reality be due to porphyria. Provocative diagnostic tests, such as deliberate fasting or administration of barbiturates, carry a definite risk, and with the availability of reliable assay methods for erythrocyte uroporphyrinogen I activity are neither desirable nor necessary.

TREATMENT AND PROGNOSIS. There is no specific treatment for acute intermittent porphyria, and therapy remains symptomatic and prophylactic. Acute pain and psychic manifestations usually can be alleviated or controlled with phenothiazines, reserpine, or merperidine. Oral phenothiazines, such as chlorpromazine (25 to 100 mg four times daily), are the preferred treatment for abdominal and muscle pain. Neuropsychiatric manifestations frequently respond to relatively small doses of reserpine. Meperidine (Demerol) by intramuscular injection in doses of 50 to 100 mg may give prompt though transient relief; but, in general, use of opiates should be limited, because the severity and chronicity of the pain render porphyric patients particularly susceptible to addiction. When recurrent manifestations are clearly related to the menstrual cycle, ovarian suppression with either estrogens (oral contraceptives) or androgens has been helpful in a few patients.

Acute attacks often can be aborted by prompt administration of carbohydrate ("glucose effect"). Intravenous infusion of glucose at a rate of 10 to 20 grams per hour for 24 hours frequently results in remarkable and rapid remission, particularly in patients whose attack has been precipitated aggravated by anorexia, nausea, and vomiting. If the attack does not abate within 24 hours of continued glucose infusion or if neuropsychiatric manifestations progress, rapid improvement usually is achieved by intravenous infusion of hematin (4 mg per kilogram of body weight, dissolved in 50 ml 0.1 M sodium carbonate solution, adjusted with hydrochloric acid to pH 8.0, infused into a large vein over 10 to 15 minutes, and repeated after 12 hours). In addition, supportive treatment is of great importance. Dehydration and hyponatremia should be prevented. If bulbar signs are present, respiratory paralysis should be anticipated and a mechanical respirator made available. Fever and leukocytosis are suggestive of occult infection, most often of the respiratory or urinary tract. Penicillin and aminoglycoside antibiotics and cephalosporins have not been implicated in precipitating porphyric attacks and can be used in this situation. On the other hand, sulfonamides, rifamycin, and related compounds, as well as drugs in general, should be avoided.

In the earlier literature, the prognosis of acute intermittent porphyria was considered grave, with a mortality of 80 per cent within five years of the first attack. This figure undoubtedly is too high; indeed, more recent reports set it around 25 per cent. With the judicious use of intravenous glucose and, if indicated, hematin infusion, most acute attacks now are reversible and fatality appears to be substantially reduced. Death occurs most frequently during the second and third decades, whereas beyond this age manifestations tend to be less severe and the prognosis distinctly improves. In latent porphyria, a high carbohydrate diet is of no apparent prophylactic benefit.

HEREDITARY COPROPORPHYRIA

Hereditary coproporphyria was recognized only recently as a distinct entity. Clinically it resembles variegate porphyria except that a larger percentage of affected individuals remain asymptomatic, or phostosensitivity may be the only symptom. As in acute intermittent and variegate porphyria, drugs may precipitate acute attacks which are associated with increased urinary excretion of ALA and PBG. The unique biochemical abnormality is the striking increase in fecal coproporphyrin excretion, whereas fecal protoporphyrin concentration usually is low. During acute attacks, urinary coproporphyrin excretion also may be very high. The disease is caused by a dominantly inherited partial deficiency of the enzyme coproporphyrinogen oxidase which converts coproporphyrinogen III to protoporphyrinogen IX. Both sexes are equally affected. Treatment is the same as for acute intermittent porphyria.

VARIEGATE PORPHYRIA

DEFINITION, INCIDENCE, AND GENETICS. Variegate porphyria (synonyms: *porphyria cutanea tarda, protocoproporphyria hereditaria, mixed hepatic porphyria, South African genetic porphyria*) is a hereditary abnormality of porphyrin metabolism associated with chronic cutaneous manifestations alone or in conjunction with acute, transient attacks of abdominal pain and neuropathy. The disease is inherited as a dominant trait and the sexes are equally affected. Because of its occurrence in large family groups, the incidence varies widely in different parts of the world. Among white settlers of South Africa it is estimated at 3 per 1000. It undoubtedly is very much less elsewhere, although reliable figures are not available.

CLINICAL MANIFESTATIONS. Cutaneous symptoms consist of dermal abrasions, superficial erosions, and blister formation after trivial trauma, and commonly are first noted during the second or third decade. The excessive mechanical fragility is usually limited to exposed parts of the skin. The lesions tend to heal slowly, often leave pigmented or slightly depressed scars, and are subject to secondary infection. Direct sensitivity to sunlight is infrequent, but the distribution of the cutaneous lesions leaves little doubt that light exposure is an important pathogenic factor. Hyperpigmentation of the face and hands is common, and women often exhibit hypertrichosis, particularly of the temporal margins. The extent of these manifestations varies considerably, but after increased fragility of the skin has developed, it rarely disappears completely. In some instances the abnormality is minimal and remains unnoticed, whereas in others chronicity and secondary infection lead to severe scarring and disfigurement. Cutaneous lesions are uncommon before puberty; they are usually milder in women, but during pregnancy become more pronounced.

Although in many patients manifestations remain limited to the skin, acute episodes of abdominal pain, neuropathy, and encephalopathy, similar in all aspects to those in acute intermittent porphyria, are not uncommon. Barbiturates, sulfonamides, general anesthetics, and excessive amounts of ethanol or estrogens frequently appear to be precipitating or aggravating factors. During acute episodes mortality is approximately 25 per cent, but since many patients never develop acute manifestations, the over-all mortality of variegate porphyria is much lower. Genetic studies from South Africa suggest that before the widespread use of barbiturates and sulfonamides, kinships with porphyria survived and propagated as well as the unaffected population. Unless they terminate fatally, acute attacks commonly resolve completely, although neuropathy and muscle weakness may persist for several months. Evidence of hepatic dysfunction and histologic abnormality, including steatosis, fibrosis, or cirrhosis, is not uncommon, and biopsy material from the liver frequently shows extensive porphyrin fluorescence.

LABORATORY FINDINGS AND PATHOGENESIS. The characteristic finding in variegate porphyria is the large amount of copro- and particularly protoporphyrin in the bile and feces. Fecal excretion of these pigments is continuous throughout the course of the disease, and takes place even in those patients with minimal cutaneous manifestations and in asymptomatic children with the genetic trait. PBG and porphyrin levels in the urine are usually slightly elevated, but the qualitative test for PBG is frequently negative. During acute attacks urinary excretion of ALA, PBG, and, at times, uro- and coproporphyrin is greatly increased, and may reach values comparable to those in acute intermittent porphyria in relapse. Azotemia, hypochloremia, hyponatremia, and jaundice may be present, but readily resolve as the acute attack subsides and the disease converts to its cutaneous form.

The exact nature of the inherited biochemical defect is unclear; the pattern of porphyrin overproduction suggests that conversion of protoporphyrin IX to heme is defective. Exposure to sunlight is important in the pathogenesis of the cutaneous lesions, but the mechanism underlying the abnormal mechanical fragility of the skin is unclear.

DIAGNOSIS AND DIFFERENTIAL DIAGNOSIS. The diagnosis can best be established by demonstrating increased porphyrin in the feces. The following qualitative test frequently suffices. A small piece of stool is thoroughly mixed with four parts of ethyl ether and one part of glacial acetic acid, the mixture is filtered, and the filtrate is extracted with 5 per cent hydrochloric acid. Under ultraviolet light with a Wood filter, extracts of porphyric feces exhibit intense red fluorescence, which is faint or absent with normal stool. In quantitative determinations, values in excess of 120 μg of protoporphyrin per gram of dry feces are suggestive of porphyria. During acute attacks the diagnosis can be ascertained by demonstrating increased ALA and PBG excretion in the urine.

Chronic cutaneous lesions limited to exposed parts, abnormal skin fragility, a positive family history, and increased fecal porphyrin excretion usually permit differentiation of variegate porphyria from most other skin diseases. Protoporphyria is the only other light-sensitive dermatosis associated with increased fecal porphyrins, but in this condition erythrocyte or plasma protoporphyrin is usually increased, and the reaction to light is prompt and transient. During acute attacks it may be difficult to distinguish between variegate and acute intermittent porphyria, except that the former diagnosis is suggested by concomitant skin involvement or a positive personal or family history of cutaneous manifestations.

TREATMENT. Treatment is symptomatic and prophylactic. Management of acute attacks is the same as for acute intermittent porphyria. Exposure to direct sunlight should be minimized and the hands protected from mechanical trauma by gloves. Of paramount importance is avoidance of drugs known to precipitate porphyria.

PORPHYRIA CUTANEA TARDA

Porphyria cutanea tarda (synonyms: *porphyria cutanea tarda symptomatica; constitutional or idiosyncratic porphyria; symptomatic porphyria*) is a relatively frequent sporadically occurring form of cutaneous porphyria, characterized by chronic skin lesions, hepatic dysfunction, and uroporphyrinuria. Abdominal and neurologic manifestations are absent. The disease is more common in males and usually begins insidiously, most often in the fourth to sixth decade. It occurs in all parts of the world, but is most frequent in the Bantus of South Africa. Exposed skin shows abnormalities similar to those of variegate porphyria, ranging from slight dermal fragility to severe chronic scarring and disfiguration. The lesions often are more active in summer and tend to heal in winter. Hyperpigmentation and hirsutism are frequent and may be the presenting symptoms. Hepatomegaly with chemical and histologic evidence of liver disease, often caused by chronic alcoholism, is present in the great majority of patients. Disseminated lupus erythematosus appears to occur in porphyria cutanea tarda more frequently than can be accounted for by coincidence.

In addition to large amounts of porphyrin, variable degrees of hemosiderosis are frequently found in the liver. Urinary excretion of uro-type porphyrins and, to a lesser extent, coproporphyrin is greatly increased, and urine may be pink or brownish. Fecal porphyrins are normal or only slightly increased, and excretion of ALA or PBG is almost never elevated. The excessive formation of uro-type porphyrins in the liver appears to be caused by hereditary partial deficiency of uroporphyrinogen decarboxylase associated with a superimposed form of acquired liver injury, most often hepatic siderosis, or alcoholic liver disease. The mode of genetic transmission of the enzyme defect is controversial. In the absence of acquired liver disease, the enzymatic deficiency alone does not appear to produce recognizable clinical manifestations, which may explain the frequent lack of a positive family history. Porphyria cutanea tarda frequently is strikingly improved by removal of hepatic iron by repeated venesection or chelation therapy. Abstinence in alcoholic patients commonly results in significant improvement or disappearance of the porphyric manifestations. Chloroquine, which purges the liver of uroporphyrin, is not recommended as treatment because in the presence of excessive hepatic porphyrin it produces hepatic necrosis.

In rare instances, intoxications may lead to a form of hepatic porphyria that is *acquired*. Porphyria characterized by cutaneous manifestations, hepatic dysfunction, and uroporphyrinuria has been reported in population groups accidentally exposed to hexachlorobenzene or biphenyls.

536.4. PROTOPORPHYRIA
(Erythropoietic Protoporphyria)

In this form of porphyria, high concentrations of protoporphyrin in erythrocytes, plasma, and feces are associated with solar urticaria or solar eczema. Short exposure to sunlight results in intense pruritus, erythema, and edema of exposed skin. These lesions appear during or immediately after exposure, subside in 12 to 24 hours, and usually heal without significant scarring, atrophy, or pigmentation. Occasionally cutaneous manifestations develop only after prolonged exposure to sunlight, or the initial acute skin lesions may progress to a chronic eczematous stage, persisting for weeks and healing with superficial scar formation. Skin manifestations commonly begin during childhood or adolescence, are more severe in summer, and recur throughout life. Affected skin shows neither abnormal mechanical fragility nor blister formation characteristic of the other forms of photosensitive porphyria. Erythrodontia, hirsutism, hyperpigmentation, and neurologic manifestations are lacking. Photosensitivity is mediated by protoporphyrin in plasma and skin and is evoked by near-ultraviolet light in the 400 nm range, in which porphyrins absorb maximally. The excessive protoporphyrin in plasma and feces is derived primarily from young erythroid cells and probably also from the liver. Fasting increases the plasma protoporphyrin level, whereas carbohydrate administration reduces both protoporphyrin formation and photosensitivity. Urinary porphyrin excretion is normal.

The metabolic defect is due to a dominantly inherited partial deficiency of ferrochelatase which inserts the iron into protoporphyrin IX to form heme. Although this mitochondrial enzyme defect is demonstrable in maturing erythroid cells, liver, and cultured fibroblasts, a significant percentage of persons carrying the genetic abnormality remain clinically asymptomatic, and detection may be possible only by repeated determination of erythrocyte and fecal protoporphyrin concentration. The disease generally has a good prognosis, and neither results in permanent disability nor influences normal life expectancy. However, the incidence of protoporphyrin cholelithiasis is distinctly increased, and chronic intrahepatic cholestasis progressing to fatal cirrhosis has been reported. Treatment is prophylactic and consists largely in protection from direct sunlight. Substantial improvement in photosensitivity has been achieved by treatment with β-carotene. The therapeutic usefulness of cholestyramine which binds protoporphyrin in the intestine remains to be evaluated.

Dean, G.: The Porphyrias. 2nd ed. London, Pitman Medical Publishing Company, 1971.

Dhar, G. J., Bossemaier, I., Petryka, Z. J., Cardinal, R., and Watson, C. J.: Effects of hematin in hepatic porphyria. Further studies. Ann. Intern. Med., 83:20, 1975.

Eales, L., Grosser, Y., and Sears, W. G.: The clinical biochemistry of the human hepatocutaneous porphyrias in the light of recent studies of newly identified intermediates and porphyrin derivatives. Ann. N.Y. Acad. Sci., 244:441, 1975.

Elder, G. H., Gray, C. H., and Nicholson, D. C.: The porphyrias: A review. J. Clin. Pathol., 25:1013, 1972.

Goldberg, A.: Porphyrins and porphyrias. In Goldberg, A., and Brain, M. C. (eds.): Recent Advances in Haematology. Edinburgh and London, Churchill Livingstone, 1971.

Meyer, U. A., and Schmid, R.: The porphyrias. In Stanbury, J. B., Wyngaarden, J. B., and Fredrickson, D. S. (eds.): The Metabolic Basis of Inherited Disease. 4th ed. New York, McGraw-Hill Book Company, 1978.

Meyer, U. A., and Schmid, R.: Hereditary hepatic porphyrias. Fed. Proc., 32:1649, 1973.

Tshudy, D. P.: Porphyrin metabolism and the porphyrias. In Bondy, P. K., and Rosenberg, L. E. (eds.): Duncan's Diseases of Metabolism. 7th ed. Philadelphia, W. B. Saunders Company, 1974.

Waldenström, J., and Haeger-Aronsen, B.: The porphyrias: A genetic problem. Prog. Med. Genet., 5:58, 1967.

537. WILSON'S DISEASE
(Hepatolenticular Degeneration)

Alexander G. Bearn

Wilson's disease is a rare, autosomal recessively inherited disease characterized by degenerative changes in the brain, particularly in the basal ganglia, and cirrhosis of the liver. A brownish pigmented ring at the corneal margin, the Kayser-Fleischer ring, is pathognomonic of the disease.

CLINICAL MANIFESTATIONS. The disease is frequently insidious in onset, manifesting itself as tremor and incoordination in the second or third decade of life. Deteriorating handwriting and difficulty in speech may be common early symptoms. While the patient is at rest, the tremor is often minimal and can be alleviated by resting the hands on a table or placing them in a pocket. Attempts to perform purposive movements are less successful, and a wild ataxia frequently develops. Rarely, symptoms occur as early as four years of age or may be delayed until the fourth decade of life. In late childhood and early adolescence, the disease is more likely to be rapidly progressive; rigidity, dysarthria, and dysphagia occur more frequently than tremor. Uncontrollable choreoathetotic movements and staggering may be particularly distressing. The sensory system is unaffected, and pyramidal signs are usually absent. In the terminal stages of the disease the patient is frequently febrile and emaciated. Muscular rigidity, contractures, and mental deterioration dominate the clinical picture, and the patient becomes completely bedridden.

In adults, clinical signs of severe hepatic insufficiency are uncommon, although slight abnormalities in liver function can be detected, and cirrhosis can be recognized by liver biopsy. In childhood, however, the disease commonly presents as atypical or prolonged hepatitis, which may be indistinguishable from juvenile cirrhosis. Signs of central nervous system dysfunction are minimal or absent. Portal hypertension can frequently be demonstrated, and ascites and hepatic coma may supervene. Rarely, massive bleeding from esophageal varices may be the first manifestation of the disease. Jaundice may be an early symptom, and is frequently followed by several years of normal health.

Behavioral and personality changes, acute schizophrenic episodes, transient hemiparesis, and unexplained Coombs-negative hemolytic anemia may also herald the onset of the disease. Unusual pigmentation of the lower extremities, azure lunulae of the nails, and bone lesions may be found.

GENETICS. The disease is ubiquitous and occurs in approximately 1 in 200,000 persons. It is particularly common in populations with a high inbreeding coefficient. As anticipated in a rare autosomal recessive disease, an increased consanguinity in the parents of affected persons is extremely common; in one series the frequency of marriages among first cousins was 36 per cent. Clinically normal heterozygous carriers of the gene have been estimated to occur with a frequency of approximately 1 in 200.

PATHOGENESIS. A decrease in the biliary excretion of copper is the primary disturbance in Wilson's disease; this results in an accumulation of copper in the brain, liver, kidney, and other tissues, including Descemet's membrane of the cornea, where it gives rise to the characteristic *Kayser-Fleischer ring.* The copper first accumulates in the liver and is stored initially in the hepatocytes, and later in the lysosomes. As the disease progresses, the accumulation of copper causes hepatocellular damage with release of copper from within the hepatocyte. The copper released from the liver is distributed and deposited in various tissues of the body, giving rise to cellular and organ damage.

In normal persons, approximately 95 per cent of the copper in serum is bound to ceruloplasmin, whereas the remaining 5 per cent is loosely bound to serum albumin. In patients with Wilson's disease, there is a decrease in the concentration of serum ceruloplasmin and total serum copper and an increase in the easily dissociable albumin-bound copper. The excretion of copper in the urine is usually considerably increased. Exceptionally, and particularly in girls with chronic active hepatitis or cirrhosis, the serum copper and ceruloplasmin levels may be normal. Accumulation of copper in the kidneys selectively damages the proximal renal tubules. Aminoaciduria, glycosuria, phosphaturia, uricosuria, and calciuria may be present. The serum phosphate and serum uric acid concentrations also may be decreased.

PATHOLOGY. Although it is assumed that accumulation of copper in the tissues is responsible for the symptoms, the brain may appear surprisingly normal at autopsy. Slight generalized atrophy is common, particularly of the basal ganglia. An accumulation of large astrocytes is found throughout the central nervous system and is more marked in the basal ganglia and cerebral cortex. In the rare acute form of the disease, cavitation of the putamen, globus pallidus, caudate nucleus, and cerebral cortex may be evident. In the asymptomatic stage of the disease, the liver is grossly and histologically normal despite an increase in the hepatic concentration of copper. As the disease progresses, liver damage occurs and the characteristic pathologic changes of chronic active hepatitis or postnecrotic cirrhosis become evident. Glycogen degeneration of hepatic cell nuclei, with the accumulation of cytoplasmic fat droplets, is frequently observed.

DIAGNOSIS. The disease should be suspected in all cases of unexplained tremor and rigidity, particularly in early adult life. The differential diagnosis includes Parkinson's syndrome, cerebellar ataxia, chorea, and choreoathetosis. In children and young adults, the disease frequently presents with symptoms resulting from chronic active hepatitis, and the disease should be suspected in all cases of juvenile cirrhosis. The presence of *Kayser-Fleischer rings* is pathognomonic of the disease, but these may be absent in children under the age of ten. They are golden brown or green-brown, and are located at the limbus and may encircle the entire cornea. In the early stages of the disease, a careful slit-lamp examination may be needed to demonstrate their presence with certainty. Needle biopsy of the liver and determination of the hepatic copper concentration should be undertaken in all patients in whom the diagnosis is suspected. In most patients with Wilson's disease the copper content of the liver is usually greater than 250 μg per gram dry weight (normal, less than 50 μg per gram dry weight); in some patients the copper content may reach a level of 2000 μg per gram. In the absence of prolonged cholestasis this finding is pathognomonic for the disease. A decrease in serum ceruloplasmin (less than 20 mg per 100 ml) can nearly always be observed and, in the absence of malnutrition, sprue, or the nephrotic syndrome, is virtually diagnostic. The disease is difficult to diagnose unequivocally in the first six months of life, because decreased ceruloplasmin and increased hepatic copper are common in normal children.

TREATMENT. The aim is to decrease the total body copper and prevent its reaccumulation. A high-protein, low-copper diet with the addition of sulfurated potash, technical (20 mg three times daily, with meals), is often recommended, although it is not as important as intensive and continued drug therapy. The administration of D-penicillamine (β, β-dimethylcysteine), 1 to 2 grams a day, depending on body weight, is the treatment of choice and should be continued indefinitely. A "sensitivity" reaction associated with fever, arthralgia, and leukopenia may occur. Desensitization with steroids should be undertaken and penicillamine therapy cautiously reinstituted. Except for the occasional occurrence of skin reactions, toxic reactions are seldom seen. The nephrotic syndrome has been reported in a few patients, and the urine should be monitored regularly for proteinuria. Pyridoxine deficiency, as a result of treatment with penicillamine, may give rise to optic neuritis but can be prevented by administration of pyridoxine, 50 mg daily. A new oral decoppering agent, triethylene tetramine dihydrochloride,* 1.0 gram a day, has been recently introduced by Walshe and may play a useful role in those exceptional patients who cannot tolerate penicillamine.

Persistent decrease in serum ceruloplasmin accompanied by elevated hepatic copper in an asymptomatic sib of a patient with Wilson's disease is an indication to begin therapy. In newborn infants treatment should be delayed until it is apparent that the decreased serum ceruloplasmin and increased hepatic copper have persisted beyond the normal physiologic period of three to six months. When penicillamine treatment is started early and continued indefinitely, symptomatic improvement is usually dramatic and long continued. In the absence of treatment the disease is invariably fatal.

Sass-Kortsak, A., and Bearn, A. G.: Wilson's disease. *In* Stanbury, J. B., Wyngaarden, J. B., and Fredrickson, D. S. (eds.): The Metabolic

---

*Investigational drug.

Basis of Inherited Disease. 4th ed. New York, McGraw-Hill Book Company, 1978.

Sass-Kortsak, A.: Hepatolenticular degeneration (Kinnear-Wilson's disease). *In* von Schwiegk, H. (ed.): Handbuch der Inneren Medizin. 5th ed. Berlin, Springer-Verlag, 1974.

Sternlieb, I.: Evolution of the hepatic lesion in Wilson's disease (hepatolenticular degeneration). *In* Popper, H., and Schaffner, F. (eds.): Progress in Liver Diseases. Vol. IV. New York, Grune & Stratton, 1972.

Walshe, J. M.: Copper chelation in patients with Wilson's disease; a comparison of penicillamine and triethylene tetramine dihydrochloride. Quart. J. Med., N. S., 42:441, 1973.

538. INHERITED DISORDERS OF CONNECTIVE TISSUE

538.1. THE MUCOPOLYSACCHARIDOSES

Alexander G. Bearn

HURLER'S SYNDROME
(Mucopolysaccharidosis I H, MPS I H)

DEFINITION. Hurler's syndrome is an autosomal recessively inherited abnormality of mucopolysaccharide metabolism characterized by skeletal abnormalities, hepatosplenomegaly, corneal clouding, mental retardation, and increased mucopolysaccharide excretion in the urine.

ETIOLOGY. The disease, which has an incidence of 1 in 100,000 births, is caused by excessive intracellular accumulation of the mucopolysaccharides dermatan sulfate (chondroitin sulfate B) and heparan sulfate (heparatin sulfate). These substances are preferentially deposited in those tissues and organs in which they normally occur. An increased intracellular deposition of mucopolysaccharides can be demonstrated in cultured fibroblasts of patients and their heterozygous relatives. Prenatal diagnosis using cultured amniotic cells is reliable. The primary inherited defect in Hurler's syndrome is a deficiency of the lysosomal enzyme α-L-iduronidase which is responsible for the degradation of the polysaccharide side chains of dermatan sulfate and heparan sulfate. Particularly noteworthy is the discovery that the same enzymatic defect, which can be detected in cultured fibroblasts, occurs in *Scheie's syndrome* (see below). This biochemical finding indicates that Hurler's syndrome and Scheie's syndrome, long thought to be closely related, are caused by allelic genes.

PATHOLOGY. The most characteristic pathologic feature of the disease is the excessive accumulation of intracellular mucopolysaccharides. Cells of the nervous system, liver, reticuloendothelial system, endocrine glands, cartilage, bone, and heart muscle are involved. Abnormal deposits are also present in the cornea, meninges, epicardium, pericardium, chordae tendineae, heart valves, tracheobronchial cartilages, upper air passages, and coronary and larger peripheral arteries. Distention of fibroblasts with this material causes the appearance of "clear" or "gargoyle" cells.

CLINICAL MANIFESTATIONS. Although the patient may appear normal at birth, the disease becomes evident during the first year or two of life and progresses during childhood and adolescence. In the full-blown disorder, the head is large and there is hyperostosis of the sagittal suture that sometimes extends onto the forehead. The facial features are usually coarse and ugly. A broad saddle nose, wide nostrils, thick lips, large tongue, open mouth, and noisy breathing are characteristic. Skeletal abnormalities include short neck, dorsal and lumbar kyphosis with gibbus, short stature, and flaring of the costal margins. The hands are broad with stubby fingers, and there is a tendency for the fifth finger to bend radially. There may be a deformity of joints such as genu valgus, coxa valga, pes planus, or talipes equinovarus. The skin, especially over the upper extremities and thorax, is ridged and grooved, and may present nodular thickenings. Fine lanugo hairs are prominent over much of the cutaneous surface, and the extremities are likely to show profuse growth of large coarse hair. The heart is enlarged, and valvular involvement produces murmurs that may simulate those of rheumatic heart disease. Disease of coronary arteries may give rise to angina or other evidence of occlusive disease. The abdomen is large and protuberant, and the liver and spleen are commonly enlarged. Umbilical and inguinal hernias are frequent. Clouding of the cornea is extremely common; slit-lamp examination of the eyes may be needed to detect the corneal opacification in the early stages of the disease. Mental deterioration is severe and progressive.

Abnormalities demonstrable by roentgenogram include a large skull with frontal and occipital hyperostosis, hypertelorism, long shallow sella turcica with anterior pocketing, and deformities of the facial bones. Gibbus is associated with wedge-shaped deformities and anterior hooklike projections of the vertebral bodies. The ribs are broad, spatulate, and saber shaped. The terminal phalanges of the hands are broad and short, and the long bones, especially of the arms, show swollen shafts from expansion of medullary cavities. The heart is often enlarged, and pulmonary congestion may be present.

DIAGNOSIS. Diagnosis depends upon recognition of the characteristic clinical manifestations, biopsy, blood and bone marrow studies, and examination of the urine for increased mucopolysaccharide content. A simple screening test for this consists of adding acidified bovine serum albumin to the urine. A positive result is indicated by a dense white precipitate owing to the reaction of albumin and acid mucopolysaccharide at low pH. A more specific screening test can be performed by allowing urine to dry on filter paper and adding acetic acid and toluidine blue O. A purple color develops in the urine of patients with Hurler's syndrome. Metachromatic granules in the cytoplasm of circulating lymphocytes (*Reilly bodies*) are usually demonstrable and are useful diagnostic adjuncts. Since the primary inherited defect, a decrease in α-L-iduronidase, occurs in both Hurler's syndrome (MPS I H) and Scheie's syndrome (MPS I S), the distinction between the two syndromes must still be made on clinical grounds (see accompanying table). That Hurler's and Scheie's syndromes should be so different clinically yet have the same enzymatic defect is compatible with genetic allelism. The same gene undergoes mutation in both diseases but at different points on the same

The Common Inherited Mucopolysaccharidoses

Disease	Clinical Features	Inheritance	Enzyme Defect
Hurler's syndrome (MPS I H)	Mental retardation, early corneal clouding; death before age 10	Recessive	α-L-Iduronidase
Scheie's syndrome (MPS I S)	Normal intelligence, corneal clouding, stiff joints; normal life span	Recessive	α-L-Iduronidase
Hunter's syndrome (MPS II)	Mental retardation, no corneal clouding; milder course; death before 15	X-linked	Iduronate sulfatase
Sanfillipo's syndrome A (MPS III A) Sanfillipo's syndrome B (MPS III B)	Mental retardation, no corneal clouding; skeletal changes mild; death before 20	Recessive	Heparan-N-sulfatase N-acetyl-α-glucosaminidase
Morquio's syndrome (MPS IV)	Normal intelligence, cloudy cornea, cervical myelopathy; skeletal changes; death before 55	Recessive	Hexosamine-6-sulfatase
Maroteaux-Lamy syndrome (MPS VI)	Normal intelligence, corneal clouding; death by 30	Recessive	N-acetyl-galactosamine-4-sulfatase (aryl sulfatase B)
MPS VII	Mental deficiency, hepatospleno-megaly, leukocyte inclusions very rare	Recessive	β-Glucuronidase

Notes:
1. Hurler-Scheie compounds (1H/1S) of intermediate phenotypes have been described.
2. Two forms of Hunter's syndrome have been described, a mild and a severe form.
3. Morquio's syndrome may be genetically very heterogeneous.
4. Three forms of Maroteaux-Lamy syndrome have been described, all varying in severity.

codon or in different codons of the same cistron. An analogous situation exists in hemoglobin SC disease.

Hurler's syndrome has features of cretinism but differs in that bone age is normal, tests of thyroid function are normal, and the patient is active.

TREATMENT. Although enzyme replacement with α-L-iduronidase may provide a new therapeutic approach to this disease, further work is needed to establish its clinical usefulness.

SCHEIE'S SYNDROME
(Mucopolysaccharidosis I S, MPS I S)

This rare autosomal variant of Hurler's syndrome is characterized by stiff joints, particularly of the hands and feet, near normal intelligence, marked clouding of the cornea, and an increased urinary excretion of dermatan sulfate and heparan sulfate. The frequency of the disease is approximately 1 in 500,000 births. Aortic regurgitation and the carpal tunnel syndrome are common features of this mucopolysaccharidosis. Survival into adult life is not uncommon. The primary inherited defect is deficiency of α-L-iduronidase. A deficiency of α-L-iduronidase also occurs in Hurler's syndrome (see above).

HUNTER'S SYNDROME
(Mucopolysaccharidosis II, MPS II)

This is the only mucopolysaccharidosis known to be inherited in an X-linked recessive fashion. In rather less than a third of cases the disease is the result of a new mutation. The disease may vary in severity, and this is probably due to genetic heterogeneity. The disease is similar to but clinically less severe than classic Hurler's syndrome. Grotesque features, stiff joints, and slow mental deterioration are prominent features. Clouding of the cornea is absent. Nodular thickening of the skin, particularly in the scapular region, and deafness are common. Cardiac enlargement and pulmonary hypertension have been reported. An increased urinary

excretion of dermatan sulfate and heparan sulfate occurs; in some instances heparan sulfate may be the only mucopolysaccharide excreted in excess. A deficiency of the enzyme iduronate sulfatase can be demonstrated in serum and cultured fibroblasts, as well as in cultured amniotic fluid cells, the latter enabling the disease to be diagnosed prenatally. Since the disease is X-linked, cloning of the amniotic cells, an expensive procedure, is necessary for unequivocal prenatal diagnosis.

SANFILIPPO'S SYNDROME
(Mucopolysaccharidosis III, MPS III)

Sanfilippo's syndrome is rare and is characterized by severe progressive mental retardation with relatively minor somatic changes. Corneal clouding is extremely uncommon, and dwarfism and hepatosplenomegaly are only moderately severe. The disease is inherited as an autosomal recessive and occurs in approximately 1 in 100,000 to 1 in 200,000 individuals. Many patients languish in mental institutions undiagnosed. As in the other mucopolysaccharidoses, cultured fibroblasts from affected individuals and heterozygous carriers demonstrate increased mucopolysaccharides. An increased urinary excretion of heparan sulfate, but not of dermatan sulfate, is virtually diagnostic. Two clinically indistinguishable forms of Sanfilippo's syndrome have been found to have different enzymatic deficiencies. In one type, Sanfilippo A, the enzyme heparan-N-sulfatase is deficient, whereas in Sanfilippo B, the enzyme N-acetyl-α-glucosaminidase is lacking.

MORQUIO'S SYNDROME
(Morquio-Brailsford Syndrome, Chondro-osteodystrophy, Mucopolysaccharidosis IV, MPS IV)

Patients with this recessively inherited syndrome are strikingly dwarfed, and growth beyond the age of eight years is rare. The characteristic radiologic features of the disease become evident after the age of two and consist of marked osteoporosis, platyspondyly, abnormalities of the femoral heads, and knock knees. The odontoid process of the second cervical vertebra is absent. Severe skeletal changes may lead to symptoms of spinal cord or medullary compression. Intelligence is unimpaired or trivially decreased. Aortic regurgitation is common. The disease has an estimated frequency of 1 in 40,000 births. Although not invariably present, an increased excretion of keratan sulfate in the urine is diagnostic. The urinary excretion of dermatan sulfate and heparan sulfate is normal. A deficiency of hexosamine-6-sulfatase has been reported. The syndrome is probably genetically heterogeneous.

MAROTEAUX-LAMY SYNDROME
(Mucopolysaccharidosis VI, MPS VI)

Normal intelligence and early corneal clouding are the distinguishing features of this rare autosomal recessively inherited syndrome. An increased excretion of dermatan sulfate can be demonstrated. Unlike Scheie's syndrome, the skeletal abnormalities are severe and aortic disease is absent. A deficiency of aryl sulfatase B is characteristic of this syndrome.

The comparative clinical and biochemical features of the various mucopolysaccharidoses discussed in this chapter are summarized in the table.

McKusick, V. A.: Heritable Disorders of Connective Tissue. 4th ed. St. Louis, C. V. Mosby Company, 1972, pp. 521–686.

McKusick, V. A., Neufeld, E. F., and Kelly, T. E.: The mucopolysaccharide storage diseases. In Stanbury, J. B., Wyngaarden, J. B., and Fredrickson, D. S.: The Metabolic Basis of Inherited Disease. 4th ed. New York, McGraw-Hill Book Company, 1978, pp. 1282–1307.

Neufeld, E. F.: The biochemical bases for mucopolysaccharidoses and mucolipidoses. In Steinberg, A. G., and Bearn, A. G. (eds.): Progress in Medical Genetics. Vol. X. New York, Grune & Stratton, 1974.

538.2. MARFAN'S SYNDROME
(Arachnodactyly, Dolichostenomelia)

Alexander G. Bearn

Marfan's syndrome is a generalized disorder of connective tissue with skeletal, ocular, and cardiovascular manifestations. The molecular nature of the defect is not precisely known, and abnormalities of collagen as well as elastin have been implicated. The condition occurs equally in the sexes, and is inherited as a dominant trait with variable expression. Its prevalence has been estimated to be 1.5 per 100,000 of the population, and approximately 15 per cent of all cases are due to new mutations. The average age of fathers of patients with Marfan's syndrome resulting from "new mutations" is about seven years in excess of the mean age of fathers generally.

MANIFESTATIONS. Skeleton. The extremities are characteristically long and thin. The arm span is greater than the height, and the lower segment measurement (pubis-to-sole) is in excess of the upper segment (pubis-to-vertex). Excessive longitudinal growth gives rise to arachnodactyly, pectus excavatum or pigeon breast, dolichocephaly, long narrow face, and high arched palate. This last feature, contrary to common opinion, is not specific for Marfan's syndrome, because it may be seen in congenital myopathy and myotonic dystrophy. Weakness and reduplication of ligaments and joint capsules lead to "double-jointedness," backward curvature of the knees, flat feet, and recurrent dislocation of the hips, patella, and other joints. Cutaneous striae may be present, and probably reflect the abnormal elastic fibers. An unexplained sparsity of subcutaneous fat is a feature in many patients. Femoral hernias are not uncommon.

Eyes. The eyes show subluxation of the lens (ectopia lentis). Although this is usually severe and bilateral, minor degrees of subluxation require careful slit-lamp examination for their detection. Diagnosis of Marfan's syndrome in the absence of subluxation or redundancy of the suspensory ligament and without affected family members should be made with extreme caution. Other ocular signs include tremor of the iris and glaucoma. Severe myopia and spontaneous retinal detachment are common and often lead to gross impairment of vision.

Cardiovascular Defects. Disruption and loss of the elastic fibers of the media, associated with an increase in collagen and smooth muscle, is the primary basic defect. The lack of elasticity results in progressive diffuse dilatation of the proximal segment of the ascending aorta and severe aortic regurgitation. The aorta is widest at the sinuses of Valsalva. Aortic regurgitation, owing to dilatation and stretching of the aortic cusps, may occur in the absence of roentgenographic evidence of aortic dilatation. An early systolic click is commonly heard at the apex as well as at the aortic area. *Mitral regurgitation* is being observed with increasing frequency, and appears to be due to stretching of the chordae tendineae. Myxomatous transformation of the mitral ring may occur. Heart failure and rupture of the aorta resulting from *dissecting aneurysm* are the most common causes of death. Prominence of the pulmonary artery is frequently seen, and is due to displacement of the dilated aortic ring as well as to dilatation of the pulmonary artery. Bacterial endocarditis may be superimposed on the cardiac lesion. Cystic disease of the lung may occur as an integral part of Marfan's syndrome.

DIFFERENTIAL DIAGNOSIS. Marfan's syndrome exhibits wide variation in clinical severity. It must be distinguished from *homocystinuria*, which clinically it may closely resemble. It has been estimated that 5 per cent of patients with nontraumatic ectopia lentis, one of the cardinal signs of classic Marfan's syndrome, have homocystinuria. Ectopia lentis, pectus excavatum, and pigeon breast are common to both syndromes. The lens is more likely to be dislocated upward in Marfan's syndrome but downward in homocystinuria. The presence of a malar flush, generalized osteoporosis, and moderate to severe mental retardation are characteristic of homocystinuria and are not found in Marfan's syndrome; patients with homocystinuria do not develop dissecting aneurysm. Homocystinuria is inherited as a recessive trait. The diagnosis can be made by a positive urinary nitroprusside test result or, definitively, by paper electrophoresis of the urine. The primary defect in homocystinuria is a deficiency of cystathionine synthetase in the liver. This deficiency can also be revealed in cultured skin fibroblasts. Rats given β-aminoproprionitrile (or seeds of *Lathyrus odoratus*) develop skeletal changes and dissecting aortic aneurysm reminiscent of some of the features of Marfan's syndrome.

TREATMENT. In patients with clinical or radiologic evidence of aortic dilatation, propranolol may be used to reduce the force of ventricular contraction. Surgical repair of the aortic dilatation is difficult but is becoming increasingly successful in selected cases.

McKusick, V. A.: Heritable Disorders of Connective Tissue. 4th ed. St. Louis, C. V. Mosby Company, 1972, pp. 61–200.

538.3. EHLERS-DANLOS SYNDROME

Sheldon R. Pinnell

DEFINITION. The Ehlers-Danlos syndrome is a group of inherited disorders of connective tissue sharing phenotypic expressions, including hyperextensible skin and joints, easy bruisability, and friability of tissues with poor wound healing. Seven forms of the condition are recognized on the basis of clinical, genetic, and biochemical evidence. Life-threatening complications, including spontaneous arterial rupture and gastrointestinal perforation, occur especially in the ecchymotic form (type IV).

ETIOLOGY. Biochemical abnormalities in collagen biosynthesis have been described in four of the varieties of the syndrome. Fragility and hyperelasticity of tissues would seem to be consistent with altered collagen structure, since strength and limited extensibility are characteristics of normal collagen. Deficiency of α_1-antitrypsin has been reported in patients with chronic emphysema and Ehlers-Danlos syndrome.

INCIDENCE. Ehlers-Danlos syndrome has been reported most often in persons of European ancestry, but dark-skinned races may be involved. Incidence is estimated at 1:200,000, although mild forms of the disease are undoubtedly common and unrecognized.

PATHOLOGY. No diagnostic abnormality is ordinarily apparent in skin and connective tissues by routine histologic techniques. Reports of increased elastic tissue in skin may actually represent diminished collagen content, and fragmentation of elastic tissue may occur as a result of recurrent damage to fragile tissue. Electron microscopic studies have revealed diminished collagen fiber diameters. Molluscoid pseudotumors represent herniations of fat into dermis with connective tissue proliferation and calcification.

PATHOGENESIS. Of the seven recognized types of Ehlers-Danlos syndrome, abnormalities in collagen biosynthesis have been described in four. Patients with type IV (ecchymotic) have been reported with diminished levels of type III collagen. This species of collagen molecule is present in most tissues of the body, but is predominant in blood vessels and the gastrointestinal tract — tissues most severely involved in this form of the disease. The normal absence of type III collagen in bone helps explain a lack of bony abnormalities in this form of the syndrome. Lysyl oxidase, an enzyme necessary for collagen and elastin cross-linking, has been reported to be diminished in type V (X-linked) Ehlers-Danlos syndrome. Type VI (hydroxylysine-deficient collagen disease) is associated with diminished hydroxylysine levels in tissue collagens resulting from a deficiency of lysyl hydroxylase. Hydroxylysine is necessary for collagen cross-linking, and its lack results in

structural weakness. In type VII (procollagen peptidase deficiency) an enlarged form of collagen accumulates. Collagen is synthesized in precursor form (procollagen), which is converted to collagen by an enzyme(s) (procollagen peptidase), which cleaves polypeptide chains from both ends of the molecule. Deficiency of this enzyme results in an enlarged, incompletely processed collagen molecule which is incapable of entering into normal collagen fibril formation and subsequent cross-linking.

CLINICAL MANIFESTATIONS. Clinical features are variable and many are shared among the different forms of the disorder. Common facial features include epicanthal folds, a flat nasal bridge, and ears which stick out from the side of the head and point downward.

The skin is unusually soft and feels like chamois. It may be thin and is often strikingly hyperextensible; its response to stretching is usually rubber-like, although with aging, skin may sag, particularly over the elbows. In contrast to the rest of the body, skin over the palms and soles is often wrinkly and redundant. Fragile skin may split with blunt trauma, and gaping wounds may result which often require taping to repair because the tissue is too friable to hold stitches. Wound healing is prolonged and scar tissue is of poor quality. Wide "fish mouth" scars result from poor retraction of the atrophic scar tissue. So-called molluscoid pseudotumors are common over elbows and knees and apparently result from repeated trauma, hemorrhage, connective tissue organization, fatty degeneration, and calcification. Pea-sized, freely movable calcified spherules can often be palpated subcutaneously over the arms and legs.

Easy bruisability may be the most striking clinical manifestation of the disease and may result in extensive hematologic evaluation. Since clotting parameters are ordinarily normal, ecchymoses are thought to be related to friable blood vessels and dissection of blood through planes of tissue which are poorly held together. Varicosities are often prominent under the thin skin.

Joints may be remarkably hyperextensible, and some persons with the disorder have made their living as contortionists. Chronic dislocations of patellae, shoulders, hips, clavicles, and temporomandibular joints are particularly common and may require surgical intervention. Hypermobile joints make motor control difficult during early life. Repeated falls during this time, coupled with friable skin and poor wound healing often result in appreciable cosmetic disfigurement. In time, joint hypermobility may lead to "wear and tear" arthritis and joint effusion. Although there is notable lack of bony fragility in Ehlers-Danlos syndrome, kyphoscoliosis is frequent; joint looseness and hypotonic musculature may contribute to this complication. Pes planus is common. Teeth may be carious, and periodontitis is occasionally severe.

Ophthalmologic involvement, including blue sclerae, microcornea, and myopia, is common. Ocular fragility may occur, and keratoconus, keratoglobus, dislocated lens and retinal detachment have been described.

Rupture of large arteries is a dramatic and often catastrophic manifestation of type IV (ecchymotic). Angiography is risky and should ordinarily be avoided. Mitral valve prolapse can regularly be demonstrated by echocardiography, but functional insufficiency is unusual. Many congenital cardiac defects, including atrial septal defect, tetralogy of Fallot, heart block, and aortic arch anomalies, have been described. Emphysema, as well as lung rupture and pneumothorax, can occur.

Inguinal, hiatal, and umbilical hernias occur at all ages, and recurrence after repair is frequent. Diverticula of the gastrointestinal and genitourinary tract are common. Visceral perforation may be life threatening and is most often associated with type IV (ecchymotic). Surgery must be undertaken with caution; serious bleeding as well as persistent oozing, hematoma formation, difficulty in working with friable tissue, and poor healing leading to wound dehiscence may prove disastrous.

Pregnancy is likewise risky; perinatal lacerations and hemorrhage regularly occur. Forceps delivery should be avoided so that fragile tissues are not unnecessarily torn. Prematurity is common and is often associated with premature rupture of fetal membranes. Since the membranes are mostly derived from the fetus, they share its poorly made connective tissue.

Type I (gravis) is characterized by striking hyperextensibility of skin and joints, fragile skin which bruises easily, poor wound healing, hernias, and prematurity associated with premature rupture of fetal membranes. The inheritance is autosomal dominant.

Type II (mitis) has only mild manifestations and often goes undiagnosed. Joint hypermobility is usually limited to hands and feet; skin hyperextensibility and bruisability are mild. Inheritance is autosomal dominant.

Type III (benign hypermobile) has as its major manifestation marked hyperextensibility of joints which occasionally become arthritic. Skin hyperextensibility is variable, and inheritance is autosomal dominant.

Type IV (ecchymotic) is associated with impressive bruising. Joint and skin hyperextensibility are minimal. Serious internal manifestations, including arterial rupture and intestinal perforation, are often life threatening. Both autosomal dominant and autosomal recessive forms occur.

Type V (X-linked) has only moderate involvement of skin and joints. Inheritance is sex-linked recessive.

In Type VI (hydroxylysine-deficient collagen disease) joint hypermobility is extreme, and dislocated joints and kyphoscoliosis are common. Skin hyperextensibility, easy bruisability, and poor wound healing are usual, and ocular fragility has been described. Inheritance is autosomal recessive.

Type VII (procollagen peptidase deficiency) patients have short stature; their joints are lax, and hip dislocation is frequent. Inheritance is autosomal recessive.

DIAGNOSIS. The combination of hyperextensible skin and hypermobile joints usually suggests the diagnosis. Involvement of other family members helps establish the genetic type. Biochemical studies to document abnormalities in collagen biosynthesis are research procedures of limited availability.

In *cutis laxa*, the skin may be hyperextensible, but in contrast to Ehlers-Danlos syndrome it is loose and inelastic and hangs in folds. Joint hypermobility is not usually present. Joint hypermobility without other manifestations of Ehlers-Danlos syndrome has been described as a familial tendency. Hypermobile joints and blue sclerae are associated with *osteogenesis imperfecta,* but prominent bony fragility and lack of skin hyperelasticity usually suggest this diagnosis. Hypermobile joints and skeletal deformities are found in *Marfan's syndrome,* but prominence of lens dislocation and disproportionate long bone growth usually make this diagnosis apparent. Hyperelastic joints and skin may be found in *Bonnevie-Ullrich-Turner syndrome,* but other features of this disorder, including dwarfism, webbing of the neck, gonadal dysgenesis, and XO chromosome pattern, establish this diagnosis.

TREATMENT. Ascorbic acid, 4 grams per day, was reported to be helpful in a patient with hydroxylysine-deficient collagen disease. Protection from trauma to skin and joints is helpful. As children learn to walk on unstable joints, environmental protection is particularly important. Proper repair of lacerations is necessary to prevent cosmetic disfigurement. Taping is often helpful, and because wound healing is delayed, support from sutures and tape must remain for as long as needed. An exercise program to strengthen muscles around hypermobile joints may improve function. Surgical procedures are risky, as fragile tissues may unexpectedly tear, suturing may be difficult or impossible, and massive bleeding is often impossible to control. Genetic counseling can be expected to become more precise as the biochemical nature of the different forms of the disease is better understood.

PROGNOSIS. Prognosis for life is good except in the ecchymotic form of the disease, in which arterial rupture or visceral perforation may be catastrophic. Connective tissue strength improves with age, and most clinical problems lessen as the patient gets older.

Beighton, P.: The Ehlers-Danlos Syndrome. London, William Heinemann Medical Books Limited, 1970.

McKusick, V. A.: Heritable Disorders of Connective Tissue. 4th ed. St. Louis, C. V. Mosby Company, 1972.

Pinnell, S. R.: Disorders of collagen. *In* Stanbury, J. B., Wyngaarden, J. B., and Fredrickson, D. S. (eds.): The Metabolic Basis of Inherited Disease. 4th ed. New York, McGraw-Hill Book Company, 1978, pp. 1366–1394.

539. MISCELLANEOUS DISORDERS

539.1. FAMILIAL MEDITERRANEAN FEVER

(Paroxysmal Polyserositis, Familial Recurrent Polyserositis, Periodic Fever)

Anthony S. Fauci

DEFINITION. Familial Mediterranean fever is an inherited disease characterized by acute self-limited attacks of fever accompanied by signs of peritonitis, pleuritis, and arthritis. The attacks recur at irregular, unpredictable intervals.

ETIOLOGY. Although numerous pathogenic mechanisms have been proposed, the etiology of familial Mediterranean fever remains unknown. There is no solid or consistent evidence that the disease is related to an underlying infection, hypersensitivity or autoimmune disease, inborn error of metabolism, or elevated levels of circulating hormones such as etiocholanolone. Because psychologic stress may precipitate attacks and because many patients with this disease have secondary psychologic abnormalities, it has been suggested that psychologic factors may play a primary role in the etiology of the disease. There is no good evidence to support this concept.

This disorder is often referred to as a periodic disease, but there is no true periodicity to attacks in most cases. They are irregular, sporadic, and unpredictable.

INCIDENCE, PREVALENCE, AND GENETICS. The disease occurs predominantly in patients of Mediterranean or Middle East origin, particularly Sephardic or non-Ashkenazic Jews, Armenians, Arabs, and Turks. However, it is also seen less commonly in other parts of the world and in Italians, Greeks, Anglo-Saxons, and others.

The disease appears to be inherited as a single autosomal recessive trait. In Israel, the gene frequency is 0.22 and the homozygote incidence is 1:2000. There is a male:female predominance of 3:2.

PATHOLOGY. The pathologic findings related to the acute attack are nonspecific. Serosal exudates from peritoneum, pleura, and joint spaces contain predominantly polymorphonuclear leukocytes. In addition, biopsy specimens of serosal surfaces such as peritoneum show acute inflammation. Inflammatory changes are transient and reversible. However, repeated attacks may result in secondary adhesions. In particular, intra-abdominal adhesions may result in mechanical obstruction of bowel.

The most striking and serious histopathologic findings relate to the amyloidosis which accompanies certain cases of familial Mediterranean fever. Amyloid is deposited in the intima and media of arterioles, as well as the subendothelial region of venules in all organs. In addition, there is a characteristic pattern of parenchymal distribution of amyloid, including extensive involvement of renal glomeruli, adrenals, spleen, and pulmonary alveolar septa, with remarkable sparing of the liver sinusoids and heart muscle.

CLINICAL MANIFESTATIONS. Characteristically, patients appear and feel quite normal until their first attack, which in most cases is during the first or second decade. Rarely, onset may be in infancy or as late as the fifth or sixth decade. The acute attacks are of short duration, usually lasting from 24 to 48 hours but occasionally as long as several days. Between attacks, patients look and feel quite normal. The duration and particularly the frequency of attacks vary considerably among patients and in the same patient. On the whole, attacks usually occur once or twice a month. However, some patients have attacks as frequently as one to two per week or as infrequently as one per year. Rarely, some patients go without attacks for years and then resume the more frequent pattern. Freedom from attacks is characteristic during pregnancy, with resumption of episodes postpartum.

The acute attack is characterized in most cases by fever, which may reach as high as 39 to 40° C. Rarely, the fever may occur without symptoms of serositis, but it usually occurs together with the other classic findings of peritonitis, pleuritis, or arthritis. The peritoneal attack is the most common, occurring in more than 95 per cent of patients. The intensity of symptoms is quite variable, but in its severe form the attack is characterized by pain which begins locally and then spreads over the entire abdomen, gaining in intensity. It may be associated with abdominal distention, rigidity, rebound tenderness, and evidence of ileus. Abdominal x-rays may reveal small fluid levels and bowel wall edema. Nausea and vomiting sometimes occur. Because this pattern is indistinguishable from an acute abdomi-

nal catastrophe, many patients with familial Mediterranean fever have undergone laparotomy, some more than once.

Approximately 75 to 85 per cent of patients develop pleuritic attacks which resemble acute febrile pleuritis with pleuritic pain (usually unilateral), diminished breath sounds, and small pleural effusions.

Acute arthritis during one or more attacks is seen in up to 75 per cent of Israeli patients. However, frank arthritis is seen much less commonly in the United States. When arthritis occurs, it usually involves a single large joint, particularly the knee, although this is variable. Arthritic attacks usually last a few days but may assume a protracted course of weeks or, rarely, months. Radiologic findings are nonspecific, including reversible soft tissue swelling, mild osteoporosis, and occasionally osteoarthritic changes (in chronic attacks).

Erysipelas-like skin lesions occur in approximately 25 per cent of patients. They are characterized by painful, rather sharply circumscribed, patchy areas of erythema and swelling, usually on the lower extremity below the knee.

The most serious and dreaded complication of this disease is amyloidosis which is progressive and usually leads to death in renal failure. In Israel, this complication occurs in a high proportion of cases and may cause death in adolescence or even earlier. Patients in Israel have been classified according to phenotypes. More than 90 per cent of patients are of phenotype I in which the acute attacks precede the development of amyloidosis. In phenotype II, amyloidosis precedes the onset of acute attacks, negating the concept that recurrent febrile or inflammatory episodes lead to amyloidosis in this disease.

Amyloidosis is only very rarely seen in the United States as a complication of familial Mediterranean fever, although there are many Jews of different ethnic subgroups, Armenians, and others with the disease in the United States. The explanation for this difference is unknown, but it strongly suggests the interrelationship of environmental or other factors with the known genetic factors in the development of amyloidosis in this disease.

American patients with familial Mediterranean fever but without amyloidosis live much longer than their Middle East counterparts, but are subjected to another serious complication of the disease, namely, drug addiction resulting from inappropriate administration of narcotics during repeated acute attacks.

Laboratory findings are nonspecific. During acute attacks, these include an elevated erythrocyte sedimentation rate, leukocytosis (up to 30,000 per cubic millimeter), and elevated acute phase reactants such as C-reactive protein, plasma fibrinogen, serum haptoglobin, and ceruloplasmin. Laboratory findings with amyloidosis reflect the resulting nephrotic syndrome and renal failure.

DIAGNOSIS. When the characteristic clinical presentation of recurrent self-limited attacks is present in a person of appropriate ethnic background with or without a positive family history, the diagnosis is not difficult. However, because of frequent failure to think of the disease as a possible diagnosis, patients still go undiagnosed for substantial periods of time, and may be subjected to one or more laparotomies.

Any given abdominal attack must be differentiated from the spectrum of acute abdominal disorders, particularly appendicitis, pancreatitis, cholecystitis, and intestinal obstruction. Porphyria and hyperlipidemias with acute abominal symptoms must also be considered.

Pleural attacks may closely mimic acute infections or pulmonary emboli with infarction, whereas joint manifestations may resemble the acute infectious and noninfectious arthritides, including the connective tissue diseases.

Patients with this disease who present with fever alone are quite rare, and all ultimately manifest serositis. When encountering a rare familial Mediterranean fever patient who presents with fever alone, an orderly approach to a fever of unknown origin should be undertaken.

TREATMENT. Up until recently, many forms of therapy, including corticosteroids, have been tried with no effect. During acute attacks symptomatic and supportive measures are indicated. Because of the recurrent nature of the disease, narcotics should be avoided except in unusual circumstances.

Recently, it has been shown in controlled trials that the prophylactic use of colchicine* will reduce the number of acute attacks in most but not all patients with familial Mediterranean fever. A dose of 0.6 mg of colchicine three times a day by mouth is most effective. If patients develop gastrointestinal symptoms on this dose, it may be reduced to 0.6 mg twice a day. Since familial Mediterranean fever is a lifelong disease and since chronic colchicine therapy may cause azoospermia and chromosomal abnormalities, patients who require therapy should be tried on a course of intermittent colchicine consisting of 0.6 mg every hour for four hours, then every two hours for four hours, and then every twelve hours for two days. The colchicine should be started at the first prodromal indication of an attack. Such a regimen has been shown to abort attacks in some patients. The mechanism of colchicine effect in this disease is uncertain, although it is speculated that the drug interferes with the cellular phase of the inflammatory response.

PROGNOSIS. The prognosis for normal longevity with this disease in the United States is excellent. Patients are usually normal between attacks without residua or debilitation. However, psychologic difficulties related to the chronic and recurrent nature of the disease may occur. In addition, drug addiction may result from the inappropriate administration of narcotics.

The prognosis in patients in the Middle East who develop amyloidosis is quite poor. Death, usually from renal failure, almost always occurs.

Dinarello, C. A., Wolff, S. M., Goldfinger, S. E., Dale, D. C., and Alling, D. W.: Colchicine therapy for familial Mediterranean fever. A double-blind trial. N. Engl. J. Med., 291:934, 1974.

Schwabe, A. D., and Peters, R. S.: Familial Mediterranean fever in Armenians. Analysis of 100 cases. Medicine, 53:453, 1974.

Siegal, S.: Familial paroxysmal polyserositis: Analysis of fifty cases. Am. J. Med., 36:893, 1964.

Sohar, E., Gafni, J., Pras, M., and Heller, H.: Familial Mediterranean fever. A survey of 470 cases and review of the literature. Am. J. Med., 43:227, 1967.

Wright, D. G., Wolff, S. M., Fauci, A. S., and Alling, D. W.: Efficacy of intermittent colchicine therapy in familial Mediterranean fever. Ann. Intern. Med., 86:162, 1977.

Zemer, D., Revach, M., Pras, M., Modan, B., Schor, S., Sohar, E., and Gafni, J.: A controlled trial of colchicine in preventing attacks of familial Mediterranean fever. N. Engl. J. Med., 291:932, 1974.

*Investigational drug for this purpose.

539.2. ACATALASIA
(Acatalasemia, Takahara's Disease)
Alexander G. Bearn

Acatalasia is a rare, autosomal, recessively inherited trait characterized by a deficiency of catalase in many tissues of the body, including the erythrocytes, bone marrow, liver, and skin. The disease is particularly common among Japanese, Koreans, and Chinese, but has also been reported from Germany, Switzerland, and Israel. Manifestations are usually restricted to the oral cavity and are related to the increased susceptibility to tissue damage caused by the H_2O_2 produced by normal microbial flora. Oral sepsis may lead to severe gangrenous lesions, including alveolar bone destruction. Approximately 50 per cent of acatalasic subjects are asymptomatic; after puberty gangrenous lesions in the oral cavity are rare. An absence of catalase in individuals homozygous for the trait and intermediate values for the clinically normal heterozygous carriers are characteristic of the families reported from Japan. Homozygotes from Germany, Switzerland, and Israel commonly show residual catalase activity and are symptomatically normal. When hydrogen peroxide is added to acatalasic blood, it turns a brownish black color owing to the formation of methemoglobin; by contrast normal blood bubbles vigorously and remains pink. At least two forms of acatalasia exist in Japan where more than 50 patients with the disease have been reported. Genetic heterogeneity is suggested both from variations in the clinical expression of the disease and in the level and stability of residual catalase activity in different populations. The estimated frequency of homozygotes in Japan is approximately 4×10^{-6} and the heterozygote frequency is approximately 1.7×10^{-3}. Considerable variations in the gene frequency within Japan have been reported. Local surgical excision, extraction of teeth, and antimicrobial therapy have been employed. A similar disease occurs in mice, guinea pigs, dogs, and the domestic fowl.

Aebi, H. E., and Wyss, S. R.: Acatalasemia. *In* Stanbury, J. B., Wyngaarden, J. B., and Fredrickson, D. S. (eds.): The Metabolic Basis of Inherited Disease. 4th ed. New York, McGraw-Hill Book Company, 1978.

539.3. FAMILIAL DYSAUTONOMIA
(Riley-Day Syndrome)
Alexander G. Bearn

Dysautonomia is a rare, recessively inherited disease of childhood, occurring almost exclusively in Ashkenazi Jews. The disease is characterized by a small-fiber peripheral neuropathy, associated with a decrease in the number of neurons in the dorsal roots of sympathetic ganglia. Nerve conduction is decreased. Hypersensitivity of the pupil to instillation of methylcholine is common. Features include defective lacrimation, emotional instability, absence of the fungiform papillae of the tongue, blotching of the skin, relative indifference to pain, poor motor coordination, disturbed esophageal motility, and absent deep tendon reflexes. Dysphagia in childhood may be the presenting symptom. Many patients die in childhood from secondary pneumonia. In certain dysautonomic patients an increase in nerve growth stimulating factor is present in the serum. This factor is antigenetically similar to, but functionally unlike, that found in control serum.

Diagnostic confirmation of autonomic disturbance should include an absence of a skin flare after histamine injection, an increase in urinary vanillylmandelic acid, and a decrease in homovanillic acid. A deficiency in serum dopamine beta-hydroxylase has been reported but awaits confirmation.

The differential diagnosis includes amyloidosis and the congenital and hereditary sensory neuropathies which may present with insensitivity to pain.

Brunt, P. W., and McKusick, V. A.: Familial dysautonomia. A report of genetic and clinical studies, with a review of the literature. Medicine, 49:343, 1970.

Mobley, W. C., Server, A. C., Ishii, D. N., Riopelle, R. J., and Shooter, E. M.: Nerve growth factor. N. Engl. J. Med., 297:1211, 1977.

539.4. LAURENCE-MOON SYNDROME

(Laurence-Moon-Biedl Syndrome)

Alexander G. Bearn

The salient features of this recessively inherited syndrome are mental retardation, retinitis pigmentosa, hypogonadism, obesity, and polydactyly. There is a high parental consanguinity rate, and in Switzerland, where the disease appears to be particularly common, consanguinity has been established in more than 50 per cent of the affected sibships. Rigid classification is not possible, and the limits of the syndrome are poorly defined. Although retinitis pigmentosa appears relatively late, it is a common and well-defined feature. Other ocular signs include atypical retinal changes and retinitis without pigmentation. Mental retardation is only moderately severe and is usually noted soon after entering school. Unexplained obesity before the age of ten, associated with polydactyly and hypogonadism, should arouse suspicion of the disease. This condition must be distinguished from Fröhlich's syndrome, in which more convincing disturbances in hypothalamic-pituitary dysfunction have been described.

Warkany, J.: Congenital Malformations. Chicago, Year Book Medical Publishers, 1971.

539.5. LIPOATROPHIC DIABETES

Alexander G. Bearn

The features of this disfiguring and invariably fatal disease include a loss of subcutaneous and body fat, hyperlipemia, hepatomegaly caused by fatty infiltration, phallic enlargement, hyperpigmentation and hypertrichosis with acanthosis nigricans, and insulin-resistant hyperglycemia. In all patients, the binding of insulin to insulin receptors on circulating monocytes is greatly reduced (1 to 50 per cent).

The pathogenesis of this disease, which is usually inherited in a recessive fashion, is obscure. It has been

suggested that the disease may be due to hypothalamic-pituitary dysfunction which affects dopamine-β-hydroxylase. Since this enzyme is rate limiting in the conversion of dopamine to norepinephrine, dopamine accumulates in the brain and is accompanied by a relative decrease in the quantity of norepinephrine. The excess dopamine and decreased norepinephrine may in turn cause an increase in the hypothalamic releasing factors (corticotropin-releasing hormone, luteinizing-releasing hormone, and melanocyte-stimulating hormone) which can then be detected in the peripheral blood. The possibility that dopamine receptor blockers might influence the course of the disease has been raised and requires further investigation. Rarely, this disease has been reported to follow nonspecific viral infections.

Bar, R. S., and Roth, J.: Insulin receptor status in disease states of man. Arch. Intern. Med., 137:474, 1977.

Mabry, C. C., Hollingsworth, D. R., Upton, G. V., and Corbin, A.: Pituitary-hypothalamic dysfunction in generalized lipodystrophy. J. Pediat., 82:625, 1973.

Rossini, A. A., and Cahill, G. F., Jr.: Lipoatrophic diabetes. *In* de Groot, L. J., et al. (eds.): Metabolic Basis of Endocrine Disease. New York, Grune & Stratton, 1979.

539.6. LIPOID PROTEINOSIS

(Cutaneous-Mucosal Hyalinosis)

Alexander G. Bearn

This rare, autosomal recessively inherited disease, particularly common in South Africa, is characterized by the combination of a husky voice from birth and scarring maculopapular eruptions around the face, arms, and trunk. The mucous membranes of the mouth, tongue, and larynx are diffusely infiltrated with hyaline-like material. The extracellular deposits resemble those seen in histiocytosis X. Recurrent painful parotitis may occur. Calcification of the hippocampal gyri is an inconstant but pathognomonic sign of the disease. No consistent biochemical abnormalities have been reported. The disease must not be confused with porphyria. Although there is no clear-cut evidence for their effectiveness, corticosteroids have been employed in the treatment of this disorder. The disease is compatible with a normal life expectancy.

Gordon, H., Gordon, W., and Botha, V.: Lipoid proteinosis in an inbred Namaqualand community. Lancet, 1:1032, 1969.

539.7. WERNER'S SYNDROME

Alexander G. Bearn

This rare, autosomal recessively inherited syndrome is characterized by scleroderma-like changes in the skin, especially in the extremities where ulceration of the ankles is common, symmetrical growth retardation with absence of the adolescent growth spurt resulting in shortness of stature, and premature graying of the hair. Early cataracts, soft tissue and vascular calcifications, generalized arteriosclerosis, osteoporosis, and premature loss of teeth are common. Diabetes mellitus occurs in 50 per cent of patients and is of the insulin-resistant type. Ten per cent of patients develop malignancies, with an unusually high incidence of sarcoma; an evaluation for occult neoplasms in such patients is advisable. Certain features of Werner's syndrome resemble premature aging. Werner's syndrome and the pediatric syndrome progeria have been considered possible models for aging.

DeBusk, F. L.: The Hutchinson-Guilford syndrome. J. Pediat., 80:697, 1972.

Epstein, C. J., Martin, G. M., Schultz, A. L., and Motulsky, A. G.: Werner's syndrome. A review of its symptomatology, natural history, pathological features, genetics and relationship to the natural aging process. Medicine, 45:177, 1966.

PART XXI
DISEASES OF THE ENDOCRINE SYSTEM

540. INTRODUCTION

Nicholas P. Christy

FUNCTIONS OF THE ENDOCRINE SYSTEM

Like the nervous system, the endocrine "system" provides mechanisms by which the mammalian organism adapts to an environment that is always changing. Parts of the endocrine system may indeed be regarded as extensions of the nervous system: the *adrenal medulla,* which secretes epinephrine in response to environmental change, is of ectodermal origin, arising from the neural crest; many environmental stimuli cause cells in the *hypothalamus* to secrete neurohumoral peptides which are carried in the hypothalamic-hypophysial portal venous system to cells in the anterior pituitary, which then secrete growth hormone, adrenocorticotropin, or gonadotropins (see Ch. 542). These two glands, the adrenal medulla and the anterior pituitary, are particularly clear examples of endocrine organs whose secretions mediate between the external and internal environments. No less important examples are the neurohypophysial response to rises and falls in hydration and the fluctuations of adrenocortical secretion of aldosterone with changes in dietary Na^+. These and the other endocrine glands, by steady, oscillating, or waxing and waning secretion of hormones, wield an important *regulatory* influence on cellular metabolism.

Again like the nervous system, the endocrine system has both *vegetative* and *adaptive* functions. The essential roles of pituitary growth hormone and thyroxine in normal growth and the effects of the sex steroids, testosterone and estradiol, on the gradual and orderly maturation of the secondary sex characters are examples of *vegetative* activity. Rapid *adaptive* functions are numerous: insulin secretion in response to hyperglycemia; epinephrine secretion during profound hypoglycemia; antidiuretic hormone secretion in the presence of increased osmolarity of the plasma; and the instantaneous hypersecretion of pituitary adrenocorticotropic hormone (ACTH) in response to many noxious stimuli, of growth hormone to severe muscular exercise, and of aldosterone to hemorrhage-induced hypovolemia. It is apparent that both the vegetative and adaptive, that is, the slowly acting and rapidly acting functions are in effect homeostatic.

But "homeostasis" must not be defined too rigidly. It is usually taken to mean "a tendency to stability in the normal body states (internal environment) of the organism . . . achieved by a system of control mechanisms activated by negative feedback . . ." (Dorland's Medical Dictionary). The word "homeostasis," in its radical sense, has a rigid cast about it. The Greek words from which it is derived are *homeo:* always the same, un-

changing; and *stasis:* a standing still. Yet, in the definition quoted above, there is the word "metabolism," meaning "change," so that in sameness there is also in that modified definition the suggestion of alterability. And indeed homeostasis itself must be changeable. The internal environment is only *relatively* constant. In his famous and much quoted generalization, Claude Bernard said: "All the vital mechanisms, varied as they are, have only one object: that of preserving constant the conditions of life in the *milieu intérieur.*" But, as the American physiologist L. J. Henderson wrote in 1926, "This should not be thought of as absolute constancy, and it should be understood that variations in the properties of the internal environment may be both cyclical and adaptive, that is, functional. . . ." Normal metabolism thus operates to keep the cellular environment in a state appropriate to constantly changing conditions: growth, reproduction, and aging; and changes in body temperature, hydration, and nutrition. It is a mistake to think of the constancy of the *milieu intérieur* as simply a ceaseless struggle of the cells to return to some fixed and immutable baseline. The baseline is always changing, at least slightly. It should not be thought of schematically as a horizontal straight line, but rather as slanting a bit up or down, moving in either direction stepwise, or describing any sort of family of curves, large or small.

It is a mistake to think of the endocrine system as a system in a rigid sense (see below). It is true that the endocrine organs are all by definition ductless structures that secrete hormones which have many actions at sites remote from those structures. It is also true that several hormones may conspire to affect single, well-defined functions or substances. For example, it can be shown that all the following hormones have the capacity to influence the concentration of blood glucose: pituitary growth hormone, ACTH, thyroxine, cortisol, epinephrine, insulin, and glucagon. Pituitary growth hormone, ACTH, cortisol, aldosterone, and antidiuretic hormone all affect serum Na^+ concentration. But in either of these groupings, it is difficult to know in a given set of circumstances which hormone is quantitatively the most important, and to calculate accurately how the several hormones, with their complementary, supplementary, synergistic, or opposing actions, operate together to regulate the serum concentration of glucose or Na^+. Further, it is hard to see, for example, how epinephrine secretion by the adrenal medulla relates to the secretion of parathyroid hormone, how growth hormone secretion bears on thyroxine secretion, and how aldosterone and gonadotropins inter-relate. *There are at least as many examples of independent as of interdependent functions among the endocrine glands.*

Therefore it seems most reasonable not to regard the endocrine glands as such a tightly integrated system as the anatomically distinct nervous system, but rather as a loose group of secretory organs, arising from different embryologic layers, having made their appearance at different stages in evolution, and possessing a broad range of functions, some separate and distinct and some interdigitated. These regulatory functions are exerted by circulating chemical substances upon biochemical processes of all cells and tissues.

It is possible to construct plausible schemata for describing the operation of the endocrine system: how it is itself controlled and how it exerts its regulatory actions upon cellular processes. In such diagrams, the entire endocrine armamentarium, numerous and variegated as it is, is held to bear on a kind of "ionic net" or conceptual membrane in a concerted and orderly way. It is even possible to draw fairly convincing parallels between the ways in which hormones regulate physiologic events in the whole organism on one hand and minute intracellular events on the other (Rasmussen). Such parallels and such patterns have the *virtues* of penetrating scholarship, ingenuity, and a degree of coherence. Also, they may be heuristic. They have the *defects*, chiefly those of oversimplification and teleology, inherent in all scientific hypotheses constructed prematurely on the basis of very incomplete information. The question always is: Are such inventions in tune with biologic truth or not? In the present state of endocrinology I think not. It seems proper to warn the student to examine such schematic representations with cautious skepticism, bearing in mind T. S. Eliot's injunction that experience ". . . imposes a pattern, and falsifies," or at least harbors within it the seeds of falsification.

The difficulty in accepting schemes of endocrine "system" organization and control may be illustrated in many ways. One series of questions may suffice: What are the limits of the endocrine "system"? What is a gland? What is not a gland? When is a gland not a gland? When is a nongland a gland? We are used to thinking of the endocrine organs as the hypothalamus–anterior pituitary unit and its dependents: the gonads, the thyroid, and the adrenal cortex; the supraoptic nuclei–posterior pituitary unit; the parathyroids; and the adrenal medulla. This is the conventional textbook arrangement. But investigations dating from as long ago as Bayliss and Starling's work of 1902 suggest that the definition of a *hormone* (from a Greek verb meaning "to set in motion," "to spur on") should probably be more inclusive than our present narrow and arbitrary view permits. The following examples illustrate some of the conceptual and practical problems:

1. *The pineal* (see Ch. 545): This organ, often included among the endocrine glands, perhaps should not be. The pineal synthesizes several peptides and amines, including one unique substance, melatonin, which has vivid hormonal effects in lower animals, but none so far demonstrated in man.

2. *The thymus:* The thymus used to be referred to as a gland before its importance in the immune system was understood. Now that its place there is firmly established, it is also known to secrete a number of humoral substances, including thymin and thymosin. Should these be considered hormones or not? They exert effects at remote sites and therefore qualify as "chemical messengers" in the Bayliss-Starling sense of the term.

3. *The kidney:* The kidneys synthesize erythropoietin and renin which also, directly or indirectly, have hematopoietic and vascular actions distant from their site of origin. Should the kidney therefore be regarded as an endocrine gland?

4. *The gut:* The alimentary tract has been referred to as the biggest manufacturer of endocrine substances in the body, largely through the secretory activity of its so-called APUD cells (APUD is an acronym for cells with these cytochemical properties: high *A*mine content, a capacity for amine *P*recursor *U*ptake from the surrounding medium, and the presence of the enzyme amino acid *D*ecarboxylase. These cells are located not only in the gut but also in the *CNS* — hypothalamus, anterior and posterior pituitary, and pineal body; and *"generally"* distributed — in the thyroid [C cells], adrenal medulla, carotid body, lungs, urinary tract, and skin) (Welbourn). A partial list of gastrointestinal hormones of APUD cell origin is given in Table 1. Should the gut and its appendages be regarded as an endocrine gland? Is the APUD system a kind of endocrine subsystem, neoplasms of which are perhaps easier to explain as they appear in the patterns observed in the various forms of multiple endocrine adenomatosis (MEA I and MEA II) and in "ectopic" secretion of hormones by cancers (see below)?

5. *The lung:* Many workers now look upon the lung as a "paraendocrine organ." The lungs have the capacity to process in a selective manner hormones, prohormones, and other "excitatory substances": some are inactivated (serotonin, bradykinin), some are unaltered (angiotensin II), some are activated (angiotensin I), and some are synthesized (certain prostaglandin-related compounds) (Ryan and Ryan, 1977). Pulmonary diseases, mostly but not all neoplastic, are often associated with the secretion of hormonal compounds (Table 2). The lung would seem to qualify reasonably well as a gland of internal secretion under both normal and pathologic conditions.

TABLE 1. APUD Cells of the Gut and Their Products*

| Organs | Cell Type | Products | |
		Polypeptides	Amines
Stomach	G	Gastrin	
	D	Somatostatin	
	EC	Substance P	5-HT
			?5-HTP
Pancreas			
Islet cells	B (β)	Insulin	
	A (α)	Glucagon	
	D ($\delta_1\alpha_1$)	Somatostatin	
Inter-acinar cells	D₁	Pancreatic polypeptide	
	EC	?	5-HT
			?5-HTP
Duodenum and	S	Secretin	
small intestine	EC	Motilin	5-HT
		?Substance P	
	I	CCK	
	K	GIP	
	?	Gastrin	
	D	Somatostatin	
	?H	VIP	
	?	Bombesin	
Large intestine	?H	VIP	
	EG	Enteroglucagon	

5-HTP = 5-Hydroxytryptophan; CCK = cholecystokinin-pancreozymin; GIP = gastric inhibitory polypeptide; VIP = vasoactive intestinal polypeptide; EC = enterochromaffin.

*Reprinted with permission from Welbourn, R. B.: Am. J. Surg., 133:13, 1977.

TABLE 2.   Hormonal Secretion by Pulmonary Tumors: Paraneoplastic Syndromes*

Hormone	Syndrome	Lesion
ACTH	Hypokalemic alkalosis, edema, Cushing's syndrome	Oat cell carcinoma, adenoma
ADH (arginine vasopressin)	Hyponatremia (SIADH)	Oat cell carcinoma, adenoma; also, tuberculosis, pneumonia, aspergillosis
PTH or related peptide, PGs	Hypercalcemia	Squamous cell carcinoma, adenocarcinoma and large-cell undifferentiated carcinoma
Gonadotropins	Gynecomastia (adults), precocious puberty (children)	Large-cell anaplastic carcinoma
Calcitonin	No clinical findings	Adenocarcinoma, squamous and oat cell carcinoma
VIP or related peptide	Watery diarrhea or no symptoms	Squamous, oat or large-cell carcinoma
Growth hormone(?)	Hypertrophic osteoarthropathy	Squamous cell carcinoma
Serotonin, kinins (and PGs)	"Carcinoid"	Bronchial adenoma, oat cell carcinoma
Insulin-like peptide	Hypoglycemia	Mesenchymal cell tumors
Glucagon or related peptide	Diabetes	Fibrosarcoma
Prolactin	Galactorrhea (or no symptoms)	Anaplastic cell carcinoma
Combination of above	Multiple syndromes	Anaplastic cell carcinoma

ACTH, Adrenocorticotropic hormone; SIADH, syndrome of inappropriate secretion of antidiuretic hormone; PTH, parathyroid hormone; PGs, prostaglandins; VIP, vasoactive intestinal polypeptide.

*Reprinted with permission from Said, S. I., *In* Kendig, E. L., Jr., and Chernick, V. (eds.): Disorders of the Respiratory Tract in Children. 3rd ed. Philadelphia, W. B. Saunders Company, 1977, p. 62.

6. *Cancers that secrete hormones* (see Ch. 525): Whether tumors of APUD cells ("apudomas," see above) or not, neoplasms of about every organ in the body have been reported to secrete one or more hormones, which, in many instances, have chemical structures identical with those of the "native" hormones (e.g., ACTH, ADH). It would seem not unreasonable to regard many if not most cancers as autonomous, that is, uncontrolled glands.*

Given the difficulty, set forth above, in determining what are the dimensions of the endocrine system and which circulating substances are hormones and which are not (cf., for example, prostaglandins; the enkephalins and endorphins "secreted" by the brain), it becomes clear that no presently available construct is comprehensive or flexible enough to account in a precise way for the manner in which "hormones" act in concert, or independently, or both, to help maintain a reasonable degree of homeostasis within the body.

The *disorders of what we conventionally regard as the endocrine glands* become clinically apparent through excessive, deficient, or untimely secretion of a hormone, owing either to primary disease of the endocrine gland or to an abnormal secretion by that gland in response to disease of some other organ (see Categories of Endocrine Disease, below). *All endocrine diseases have this property in common: the secretion of the hormone is not regulated or is improperly regulated by the control mechanisms that operate under normal conditions; that is, the production of the hormone is autonomous, anarchic, or inappropriate, a state of affairs that leads to disordered homeostasis.* (See Principles of Endocrine Diagnosis, below.)

*In reading articles on the APUD cell, the APUD "system," and "apudomas," the student should again be on guard against a tendency toward overschematization. The questions of whether the APUD concept explains adequately the patterns of multiple endocrine adenomatosis and accounts satisfactorily for the types and patterns of "ectopic" secretion of hormones by neoplasms of "nonendocrine" organs and tissues remain matters of active controversy.

BIOCHEMISTRY AND MODE OF ACTION OF HORMONES

The *chemical nature* of human hormones is now well known. The substances are amines (epinephrine), amino acids (thyroxine), peptides (vasopressin or antidiuretic hormone), proteins (pituitary growth hormone, parathyroid hormone), and steroids (aldosterone). Despite intensive study by many workers, the mode of action of hormones at the cellular level, the importance of "second messengers," and the role of cellular receptors are still not completely understood. The subject is discussed in detail in Ch. 541.

UBIQUITY OF HORMONAL EFFECTS

Since all hormones circulate in the blood, their actions are to be found everywhere. The effects of disordered endocrine function impinge upon most organs and systems. Some examples are the characteristic changes in the skin, central nervous system, muscles, gastrointestinal tract, heart, and blood vessels in severe *hypothyroidism;* the changes in the psyche, the eyes, the regulation of blood glucose, the blood pressure, water metabolism, and the structure and function of the sexual apparatus in fully developed *pituitary insufficiency;* and the changes in the personality, central nervous system, muscles, gastrointestinal tract, kidneys, and skeleton that are characteristic of *hyperparathyroidism.*

Many acute and chronic diseases impinge on the endocrine glands. Examples are such changes as increased adrenocortical and adrenal medullary secretion of cortisol and epinephrine during *acute myocardial infarction,* increased aldosterone secretion in the accelerated phase of *hypertension,* decreased pituitary gonadotropin secretion with hypogonadism accompanying *anorexia nervosa* (see Ch. 475), and the secondary hyperparathyroidism of *renal insufficiency* (see Ch. 371 and 552). "Simple" obesity is often accompanied by well-marked abnormalities in the metabolism of cortisol and of sex hormones.

Looking at endocrine disease from another point of view, many common symptoms and signs may be parts of endocrine syndromes. *Hypertension* is common in acromegaly and *Cushing's syndrome;* not all patients with these diseases can be diagnosed on inspection. Fixed hypertension is also present in *pheochromocytoma,* in *aldosteronism,* and in some patients with *congenital adrenal hyperplasia.* In the differential diagnosis of *coma,* one must consider the hypercalcemia of *hyperparathyroidism,* the hypoglycemia associated with *islet cell tumors* or *panhypopituitarism,* and the severe water intoxication sometimes associated with the syndrome of *inappropriate secretion of antidiuretic hormone.* Serious *psychologic disturbance,* including psychosis, may be an important feature of *pituitary insufficiency, hypothyroidism, hyperthyroidism, hyperparathyroidism,* any of the *hypoglycemias, Addison's disease,* and *Cushing's syndrome.*

The aim here is to sensitize the reader to the systemic but less obvious signs of endocrine disease; one does not need to be reminded that the patient with clear signs of thyrotoxicosis may have disease of an endocrine gland.

CATEGORIES OF ENDOCRINE DISEASE

In the light of the discoveries made during the past two decades, it is no longer enough to think of endocrine disease simply as too much or too little hormone. For clinical purposes, the following may be a helpful classification:

PRIMARY HYPERFUNCTION OF ENDOCRINE GLANDS. Most diseases in this group are due to *benign tumors* of endocrine glands, such as the pituitary adenoma of acromegaly, the "toxic adenoma" which produces hyperthyroidism, the parathyroid adenoma of hyperparathyroidism, the insulin-secreting islet cell adenoma of the pancreas, benign pheochromocytoma, and the adrenal cortical adenoma of Cushing's syndrome.

Malignant hormone-secreting tumors of the anterior pituitary and thyroid are extremely rare, but cancers of the parathyroids, islet cells, adrenal medulla, and adrenal cortex are occasional causes of severe and intractable endocrine disease. No more is known about the etiology of these endocrine cancers than about that of any other cancer.

There are hyperfunctional states *not associated with endocrine tumors.* An example is Graves' disease or toxic diffuse goiter, which was formerly believed to be due to pituitary oversecretion of TSH. It is not; plasma TSH concentrations are low (see Ch. 546.2).

SECONDARY HYPERFUNCTION OF ENDOCRINE GLANDS. This term defines overactivity of a "target" gland owing to *hyperfunction of the anterior pituitary.* Cushing's syndrome not associated with adrenal tumor is caused by excessive and unremitting ACTH secretion; there are very rare instances of hyperthyroidism associated with TSH overproduction by pituitary tumors.

PRIMARY HYPOFUNCTION OF ENDOCRINE GLANDS. Primary glandular failure is the usual cause of endocrine deficiency syndromes. The etiology is often obscure. Fibrosis or even absence of the anterior pituitary has been discovered at autopsy *without anatomic evidence of any cause.* Destruction of a gland by formation of *autoantibodies* to that gland has been postulated as a cause of the hypothyroidism of Hashimoto's thyroiditis, and

also as a cause of hypoparathyroidism and of "idiopathic" Addison's disease. Autoantibodies to thyroid, parathyroid, and adrenals have indeed been demonstrated in many patients with these disorders, but it is not clear whether the antibodies are the primary cause of the glandular destruction or are secondary consequences, arising from damage to the glands by unknown agents. Autoimmune mechanisms may play a role in the pathogenesis of *juvenile diabetes mellitus.* There has been recent interest in the possibility that delayed or cellular hypersensitivity related to abnormal "lymphoid recognition" may play a part, especially in cases of polyglandular insufficiency. The possible role of genetic defects in immune surveillance, that is, defects in suppressor "T" lymphocytes, as bases for both hypoendocrine and hyperendocrine function have been presented by Volpé; some examples are given in Table 3.

Tumors may destroy a gland. Breast cancer and lymphomas may metastasize or spread to invade the neurohypophysis or supraoptic nuclei, giving rise to diabetes insipidus; chromophobe adenoma is the most common cause of anterior pituitary insufficiency (see Ch. 543). Several cancers, especially lung cancer, very often metastasize to the adrenals, but rarely cause enough destruction to produce clinically recognizable adrenocortical insufficiency.

Infections are not very common causes of glandular failure: tuberculosis and syphilitic gummas used to be occasional causes of pituitary destruction, but are now museum pieces; tuberculosis, histoplasmosis, and blastomycosis may destroy the adrenals with ensuing Addison's disease. *Chromosomal disorders,* such as Klinefelter's syndrome and gonadal dysgenesis (Turner's syndrome), are not rare as causes of primary gonadal deficiency in phenotypic males and females (see Ch. 548.4 and 549.2).

SECONDARY AND TERTIARY FAILURE OF ENDOCRINE GLANDS. *Secondary* glandular deficiency means failure of the gonads, thyroid, or adrenals owing to *pituitary insufficiency.* Although it is true that the growth hormone–secreting and gonadotropic functions of the pituitary are usually the first to drop out during the course of destructive pituitary disease, and, as a corollary, if only one function is affected, it is likely to be either growth (hypopituitary dwarfism) or gonadal function, the other functions, i.e., thyrotropic or adrenocortico-

TABLE 3. Human Endocrine Disorders Considered to Be of an Autoimmune Nature, and Other Associated Autoimmune Diseases*

Endocrine Disorders	Other Nonendocrine, Organ-Specific Autoimmune Associations
Hashimoto's thyroiditis	Pernicious anaemia
Graves' disease	Vitiligo
Diabetes mellitus (insulinopenic group)	Rheumatoid arthritis
	Idiopathic thrombocytopenic
Idiopathic Addison's disease	purpura
Autoimmune oophoritis or orchitis	Myaesthenia gravis
Idiopathic hypoparathyroidism	Sjögren's syndrome
Possibly some cases of infertility	Chronic active hepatitis
Possibly some cases of hypophysitis	

*Reproduced with permission from Volpé, R.: Ann. Intern. Med., 87:86, 1977.

tropic, may fail singly or in any combination (see Ch. 543.6). The key to diagnosis is to study the patient carefully for the presence of pituitary disease in every instance of growth failure, hypogonadism, hypothyroidism, or hypoadrenocorticism. There may be good clinical evidence to implicate or rule out pituitary involvement, but, if not, assessment of thyroid or adrenal response to TSH or ACTH or direct measurement by radioimmunoassay of the tropic hormones in plasma or urine will clarify the diagnosis.

When the anterior pituitary insufficiency is the result of hypothalamic disease, the target gland failure is defined as tertiary, e.g., "tertiary hypothyroidism" (see Ch. 542 and 543).

"FUNCTIONAL" DISORDERS OF THE ENDOCRINE GLANDS. The response of endocrine glands to certain disease states may be clinically important or clinically trivial. Important endocrine responses are the secondary hyperparathyroidism of renal failure, leading to renal osteodystrophy, and the secondary aldosteronism of portal cirrhosis and of the nephrotic syndrome with ascites and edema — aldosterone is an important contributing factor in edema formation.

Responses which are not yet of proved clinical significance are altered metabolism of thyroxine in liver disease and in patients acutely ill from a variety of causes; the altered metabolism of cortisol in portal cirrhosis; the abnormal metabolic disposition of androgens in acute intermittent porphyria; and many others.

FAILURE OF AN END-ORGAN TO RESPOND TO A HORMONE. There are several examples of this in human medicine. One is *nephrogenic diabetes insipidus,* a heritable defect in which the kidney fails to respond to vasopressin in the face of adequate secretion of vasopressin by the supraoptic nuclei. Another is *pseudohypoparathyroidism,* a hereditary disease characterized by renal and osseous resistance to measurable effects of parathyroid hormone (PTH), which is secreted in normal or greater than normal amounts by normal or hyperplastic parathyroids. In both these diseases, the respective hormones, vasopressin and PTH, fail to activate the adenylate cyclase system of the appropriate renal tubular cells; there is no rise in cyclic AMP and no metabolic effect of the hormone. Still another type of failure of end-organ response, the so-called *pseudohypoparathyroidism type II,* is characterized by adequate cyclic AMP response to PTH but absence of phosphaturia or rise in serum calcium concentration. The inference is that there is a failure to receive the intracellular cyclic AMP "message." A third example is the syndrome of *testicular feminization,* a developmental defect in which "target tissues" are unresponsive to endogenous or administered androgen. In some patients with this disorder the mechanism of end-organ failure to respond appears to be related to absent or inadequate conversion of testosterone to dihydrotestosterone, presumably the "active" form of the androgen.

PRODUCTION BY AN ENDOCRINE GLAND OF AN ABNORMAL OR UNUSUAL HORMONE. Such lesions are characteristic of the inborn errors of metabolism. In *congenital adrenocortical hyperplasia,* deficiencies of C-21 and C-11 hydroxylases cause metabolic blocks in the synthesis of cortisol, with the additional result that several cortisol precursors, e.g., pregnanetriol and 17α-hydroxyprogesterone, normally present in very small amounts, are secreted in amounts much greater than normal, as are

C_{19} androgens (see Ch. 547.10). In *goitrous cretinism* enzymic blocks in the synthesis of thyroxine give rise to thyroidal secretion into the bloodstream of large quantities of mono- and diiodotyrosines. In "T_3 thyrotoxicosis" hyperthyroidism is present and serum PBI and thyroxine concentrations are normal; for unknown reasons the goiter or thyroid nodule apparently synthesizes excessive quantities of the normally less abundant hormone, triiodothyronine (T_3) (see Ch. 546.2). A form of hypoparathyroidism ("*pseudoidiopathic hypoparathyroidism*") has been described in which the glands secrete a biologically ineffective PTH, possibly because of a defect in conversion of proparathyroid hormone to an active form.

PRODUCTION OF A HORMONE BY A NONENDOCRINE ORGAN. Cancers of many organs (lung, thymus, pancreas) may produce substances that cannot be chemically or immunologically distinguished from normal endocrine products, usually proteins, such as ACTH, MSH, gonadotropins, erythropoietin, and others. The clinical features and hypotheses concerning the mechanisms by which these "hormones" are secreted are discussed in Ch. 525.

PROSTAGLANDINS. Unlike the classic hormones, which must be carried considerable distances from their sites of formation to their sites of action, prostaglandins in general act locally upon target cells in the immediate vicinity of their site of biosynthesis. Among the most potent pharmacologic agents known, prostaglandins exert their biologic effects at exceedingly low concentrations, and because they need not be transported in large volumes of plasma, they are formed in correspondingly minute quantities.

Few compounds have excited so much interest over the past decade, and few exhibit such a bewildering array of biologic effects. They are virtually ubiquitous in body tissues and fluids, and the list of their recognized pharmacologic properties continues to expand. All prostaglandins are 20-carbon unsaturated fatty acids containing an internal cyclopentane ring from C_8 to C_{12}, and even subtle modifications such as the substitution of hydroxyl groups or the introduction of double bonds at different sites in the parent structure may result in enormous differences in biologic activity, and at times even reversals in biologic effects. A partial list of prostaglandin activities includes effects on vasomotor tone, capillary permeability, extravascular smooth muscle tone, platelet aggregation, and exocrine and endocrine secretion, as well as diverse effects on autonomic and central nervous system function. Although there is evidence that at least certain of these effects are mediated by a stimulation or inhibition of cyclic AMP accumulation in target cells, it appears likely that additional mechanisms are also involved.

The role of the prostaglandins in both normal physiology and a variety of pathologic conditions is only beginning to be understood. It is of interest that both aspirin and indomethacin have been shown to be potent inhibitors of the enzyme responsible for the formation of the internal cyclopentane ring essential in prostaglandin structure. Prostaglandins have now found limited pharmacologic or experimental use in a number of conditions. These include their employment in the induction of abortion or labor, in the treatment of refractory asthma, and in the reduction of hydrochloric acid secretion by the stomach.

IATROGENIC ENDOCRINE DISEASE. By far the most

common of these is iatrogenic Cushing's syndrome caused by administration of ACTH or cortisol and its derivatives in pharmacologic doses for many allergic, inflammatory, and neoplastic diseases. In the United States, there are hundreds of thousands of patients receiving long-term steroid therapy. An unknown number of these are getting very large doses (more than 50 mg per day of cortisol, or equivalent), and an unknown proportion of them have overt hyperadrenocorticism. The features of this entity are the physical signs of spontaneously occurring Cushing's syndrome, but with a lesser incidence in the iatrogenic form of diabetes, hypertension, and psychosis, and perhaps a higher incidence of peptic ulcer and certain rarer untoward effects, e.g., pseudotumor cerebri, glaucoma, pancreatitis, and "aseptic necrosis" of the hip joint. In addition, an unpredictable and probably small number have enough suppression of pituitary-adrenal function to be important in times of intercurrent acute illness or surgical emergency. The writer has developed elsewhere the idea that these patients are addicted to corticosteroids (see References; also Ch. 547.6). The point is that one should be as restrained as possible in the dosage of corticosteroids.

Prescription of sex hormones and thyroid hormone to patients without gonadal or thyroidal deficiency rarely produces iatrogenic disease, but there have been instances of surreptitious thyroxine ingestion leading to thyrotoxicosis. Overenthusiastic use of estrogen may induce endometrial hyperplasia and breakthrough bleeding; some patients are apparently hypersensitive to methyl testosterone, which may cause cholestatic jaundice. The unfavorable changes in glucose tolerance, serum triglycerides, and liver function tests and the increased incidence of structural abnormalities in the liver and of thromboembolic disease associated with administration of oral contrceptives have all become familiar.

The protein hormones are sometimes troublesome. Various kinds of hypersensitivity to administered insulin are common. There are more than 80 reported instances of anaphylaxis owing to ACTH. For further details about the toxicity of hormonal products, the reader is referred to textbooks of pharmacology. The keys to successful hormonal therapy are accurate diagnosis and great restraint in dosage.

PRINCIPLES OF ENDOCRINE DIAGNOSIS

Although it is a cliché, it is nevertheless necessary to emphasize that endocrine disease, like all other disease, is best detected by the alert and careful physician who carries out an attentive and thorough *history* and *physical examination*. As suggested above (Ubiquity of Hormonal Effects), the examiner should be alert to the straightforward symptoms and signs of endocrine disease. These include, among others, decline in sexual function (patients rarely complain of the opposite), infrequency of shaving, amenorrhea, virilism or hirsutism in women, unilateral or bilateral exophthalmos, and gross changes in dermal pigmentation. It is easier to overlook the subtler or more general signs of endocrine disease (again, see above). They must be carefully evaluated in areas as different as hypertension, altered states of consciousness, and psychiatric illnesses.

The multiplicity and subtlety of endocrine manifestations are easy to illustrate. For example, *anterior pituitary diseases* should be suspected and looked for under at least these 11 sets of circumstances: hypertrophy of acral structures, growth acceleration, growth retardation, precocious puberty, delayed puberty, postpubertal gonadal failure (e.g., infertility, impotence), adrenocortical insufficiency, hypothyroidism, galactorrhea, neurologic signs and symptoms pointing to mechanical involvement of juxtasellar structures, and diabetes insipidus or other symptom complexes which suggest disease of the hypothalamus (see Ch. 543). Lethargy or otherwise unexplained congestive heart failure may be the only evidence for *hyperthyroidism* (the so-called "apathetic hyperthyroidism") in elderly patients. One must keep in mind the facts that asthenia or exaggerated sensitivity to minor illness (coryza, minor gastrointestinal upsets) may be the only clues to the presence of *Addison's disease.* Many patients with primary adrenocortical insufficiency are assumed by the unwary physician to be "merely" psychoneurotic, a problem which is further compounded by the substantially greater prevalence of severe emotional disturbances, including frank psychosis, in authentic addisonians (Knowlton, 1971). Impotence in the male and frigidity in the female indeed occur in *hypopituitarism, hypoleydigism,* and *primary ovarian failure,* but these two symptoms are far more commonly due to primary emotional causes. Finally, the physician must be alert to the "hyperendocrine syndromes" which have come to be regarded as markers of "ectopic" secretion of hormones by cancers of "nonendocrine" organs (see Ch. 525).

As to *physical examination,* a few examples will serve. Moniliasis and abnormal dentition may occur in association with *primary hypoparathyroidism.* Dermal hyperpigmentation is a sign of *Addison's disease,* but is found in only 60 per cent of the patients (Knowlton, 1971). Obesity is a common sign in *Cushing's syndrome* of any etiology, but most obese patients, although they may show certain biochemical features of hypercortisolism (e.g., raised cortisol secretory rate) do not have Cushing's syndrome. On the other hand, *hypothyroidism* is not a cause of true obesity, even though many obese patients are mistakenly treated for overweight by the administration of thyroid hormone. Menstrual disturbances are observed in women with *hyperthyroidism* and *myxedema,* but the great majority of patients with amenorrhea, hypomenorrhea, oligomenorrhea, and menorrhagia do not have thyroid disease of any kind.

It follows from the above that the task of the internist or endocrinologist is just as often to *exclude* endocrine disease in the causation of systemic or local changes as it is to *ferret out* some obscure endocrine lesion.

LABORATORY DIAGNOSIS. The laboratory diagnosis or confirmation of endocrine disease depends upon two exercises: first, the accurate *measurement* of the hormone suspected to be present in deficient or excessive quantity; and second, the *detection of an altered state of control of the secretion of that hormone.*

Quantification. Many good methods now exist for the satisfactory measurement of virtually all hormones in blood, urine, or cerebrospinal fluid. Precise chemical techniques have replaced the cumbersome biologic assays that endocrinologists formerly relied upon. By far the most revolutionary and useful of these new techniques is the *radioimmunoassay* developed over the

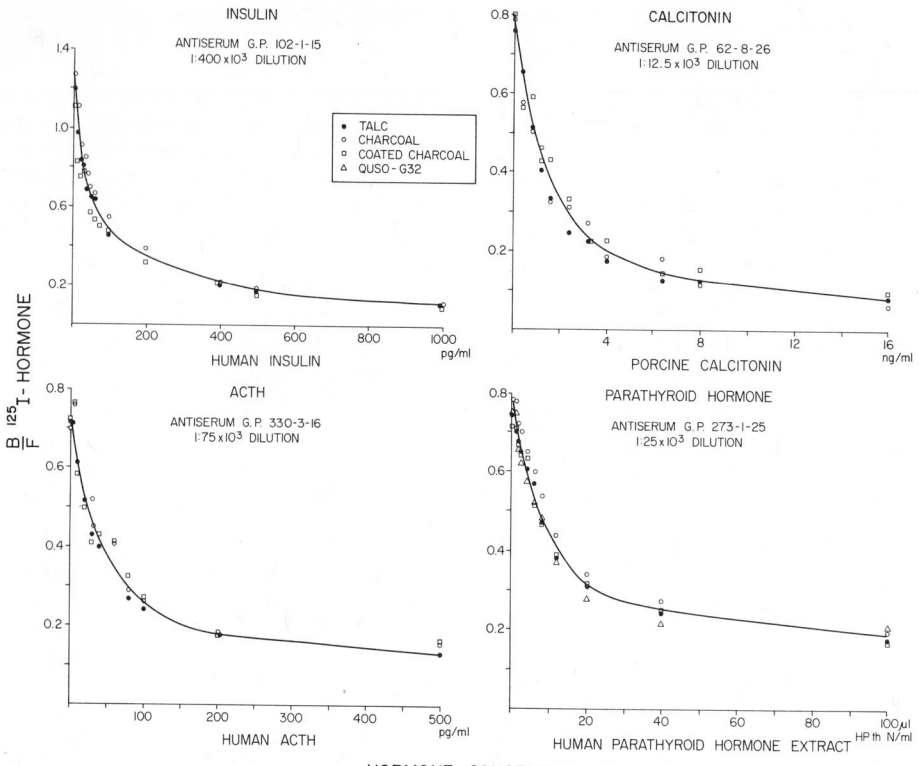

HORMONE CONCENTRATIONS

Standard curves obtained by separation of bound and free labeled hormone. Four different hormones are illustrated. If the B/F ratio for labeled ACTH (lower left panel) in an unknown sample were measured as 0.3, the concentration of ACTH in that sample (plasma) would be about 90 pg per ml. (Reprinted by permission from Yalow, R. S., and Berson, S. A., *In* Odell, W. D., and Daughaday, W. H. [eds.]: Principles of Competitive Protein-Binding Assays. Philadelphia, J. B. Lippincott Company, 1971, p. 1. [Also from Palmieri, G. M. A., Yalow, R. S., and Berson, S. A.: Horm. Metab. Res., 3:301, 1971.])

last two decades by S. A. Berson and R. S. Yalow. This method depends upon the principle of competitive protein binding, as shown at the bottom of this page. In a heterologous species (rabbit, guinea pig) antibody is raised against the antigen, i.e., the hormone one wishes to measure. Most of the polypeptide hormones are adequate antigens. Steroid hormones and small molecules which are not themselves significantly antigenic are used as haptenes, that is, they are covalently linked to proteins. The resulting antigen is then injected into the animal with satisfactory antibody formation. Antigen (hormone) labeled with ^{131}I or ^{125}I is then reacted with the specific antibody in the presence of unlabeled antigen (hormone) in the unknown, the sample of blood or urine to be tested. The higher the concentration of unlabeled antigen (hormone) in the unknown sample, the greater will be the amount of labeled antigen (hormone) displaced from the antibody,

that is, the greater will be the detectable amount of free, unbound labeled hormone (F). This can be measured directly, or after separation the ratio of bound to free hormone (B/F ratio) can be determined when the reaction has come to or near equilibrium. As may be seen in the accompanying figure, the lower the B/F ration, the higher is the concentration of unknown (unlabeled hormone) in the sample. This concentration is simply read off a standard curve constructed for each laboratory run by measuring with the same technique the quantities of unlabeled hormone in graded samples of known hormone concentration.

The method enables the detection of hormones in the physiologic range 10^{-12} to 10^{-7} molar, has permitted the estimation of daily turnover rates of peptide hormones, has led to the discovery that the anterior pituitary hormones undergo complex oscillatory rhythms throughout the day and night (HGH, prolactin, ACTH), and has

---

Labeled* antigen		Specific antibody		Labeled* antigen-antibody complex
Ag* (F) (Free)	+	Ab + Ag Unlabeled antigen ⇅ Ag-Ab Unlabeled antigen-antibody complex	⇌	Ag*-Ab (B) (Bound)

defined precisely the slower rhythms of the gonadotropins throughout the month and over the longer seasons of life: the gradual rise of FSH and LH from infancy through adolescence into maturity and old age.

Radioimmunoassay has been applied to nearly every branch of medicine. It is now possible to measure in plasma more than 40 hormones, including polypeptides, thyroid hormones, steroids, and prostaglandins. In addition, the method is capable of detecting and quantifying many nonhormonal substances as diverse as intrinsic factor, various enzymes, Australia antigen, folic acid, drugs (digoxin, morphine), and small molecules like cyclic AMP. The applications to metabolic and pharmacokinetic problems and to the prevention, diagnosis, and treatment of disease are apparent.

A second group of methods has brought about major advances in the understanding of the secretion and metabolism of all classes of hormones. These techniques, many of which are also applicable to the diagnosis of endocrine diseases, are based upon the *principle of isotope dilution*, as used, for example, in classic studies of cholesterol turnover rate and purine metabolism. The radical relationship is the dilution law as applied to solutions:

$$(\text{Concentration})_{\text{initial}} \times (\text{Volume})_{\text{initial}} = \\ (\text{Concentration})_{\text{final}} \times (\text{Volume})_{\text{final}}$$

As presented in its clearest form by P. K. Siiteri (see References), further relationships may be derived from this simple equation with the use of several assumptions. The derivations are not obvious, and the interested reader should consult the literature. In simplified form, the procedures may be summarized in this way. One starts with an isotopically labeled (tracer) substance whose weight is trivial in comparison with that of the "native" substance existing in a body or body compartment. One then develops methods for measuring the specific activity (the ratio of counts per minute or cpm to the weight of the compound) of that substance detected in blood or urine, after injection of a minute amount of the labeled material. Then these assumptions are made: the isotope has no important chemical effect on the behavior of the substance in vitro; dilution per se has no effect; the labeled substance is handled by the body in a manner identical to that by which the unlabeled native substance is metabolized; and, at least in certain circumstances, a unique metabolite of the administered labeled substance can be isolated, that is, a metabolite to whose production no other precursor can contribute. It then becomes possible to write this equation for the urinary production rate of a hormone:

$$PR_u = \frac{R}{SA_m \times t}$$

where PR_u is the production rate, e.g., micrograms of aldosterone per 24 hours, R is the amount of radioactivity injected, SA_m is the specific activity of such a unique urinary metabolite (tetrahydroaldosterone), and t is the time of urinary collection, usually 24 hours for most steroid hormones. As can readily be seen, the units in the equation work out in this way:

$$PR_u = \frac{\text{cpm}}{\text{cpm}/\mu g \times 24 \text{ hrs}} \text{ or, dividing, } \frac{\mu g}{24 \text{ hrs.}}$$

Further derivations permit the estimation of the "blood production rate" of a hormone, particularly its metabolic clearance rate (MCR), which is defined by J. F. Tait (1963) as the volume of blood or plasma "totally and irreversibly cleared of a hormone per unit time" (Siiteri). The MCR is important because it directly relates the blood production rate of a hormone to its peripheral concentration in blood.

The isotope dilution methods allow the estimation of interconversions and rates of interconversion of hormones. These techniques have also made it possible to determine which hormonal secretory rates can be measured (certain polypeptide hormones, thyroxine, cortisol, aldosterone) and which cannot (estradiol) (Siiteri).

This sort of method has the great advantage of not requiring complete recovery of hormones for chemical measurement, since, as can be seen from the equations above, one is always estimating ratios, not absolute quantities. The resulting investigations have yielded important quantitative data concerning hormone production and metabolic fate, have enabled estimates of how various physiologic and pathologic perturbations influence hormone secretion and metabolism, and have shown in several instances (growth hormone [HGH] and cortisol) that the daily production rate of a hormone is strikingly close to the daily replacement dosages given in glandular deficiency states (hypopituitary dwarfism, Addison's disease), dosages previously arrived at by empirical clinical means. The predictive value of having at hand some prior estimate of the production rate of a hormone is thus obvious.

Detection of Altered Control of Hormonal Secretion. As stated at the beginning of this chapter, endocrine disease is characterized by altered or *anarchic states of the control of hormonal secretion*. These states can be presented in order of increasing complexity. Included is a discussion of certain imperfections and pitfalls.

1. *First level — excessive or deficient secretion of a hormone by a single gland with minimal involvement of other hormones or chemical substances.* In this category, detection of excess or deficiency suffices. Control of hormone secretion is not an issue. Examples are "simple" overproduction of *prolactin* by a pituitary microadenoma in association with galactorrhea, and "simple" deficit in the secretion of *parathyroid hormone* (PTH) in idiopathic primary hypoparathyroidism. Diagnosis of both conditions can be firmly established by finding raised plasma prolactin levels and low or absent plasma PTH values, respectively. Another example might be virilism in women; here, raised plasma testosterone definitely indicates excessive androgen secretion but tells nothing about its source (ovary vs. adrenal cortex). The difficulties in differential diagnosis are discussed in Ch. 549.2.

It can also be readily understood that detection of a reduced plasma concentration of a hormone will not always allow definitive diagnosis. In authentic *diabetes insipidus* basal plasma arginine vasopressin (AVP) should of course be low or undetectable, but will also be reduced or absent in *psychogenic polydipsia,* owing to suppression of AVP secretion by a chronic hypo-osmolar state (see Ch. 544.2).

2. *Second level — deficient secretion of a hormone by a single pituitary-dependent gland.* Application of what is known about negative feedback inhibition systems in endocrinology permits intelligent evaluation of gonadal, thyroidal, and adrenocortical deficiency states. Plasma

gonadotropin (FSH/LH) values are raised in the primary ovarian failure of the *menopause* and *Turner's syndrome,* the blood TSH levels are high in *primary myxedema,* and plasma ACTH is elevated in *Addison's disease* and the *adrenalectomized subject.* In each instance, the pituitary tropic hormone is secreted in excess because of *disordered endocrine control;* the normal inhibitory influence upon pituitary hormone release is absent because the controlling hormone of the defective "target" gland is lacking.

3. *Third level — hierarchy of secretory control (example, hypothalamic vs. anterior pituitary disease).* In theory, these two classes of disease should be distinguishable. Administration of a synthetic hypophysiotropic hormone (gonadotropin-releasing hormone [LHRH] and thyrotropin-releasing hormone [TRH]) should induce augmented secretion of pituitary hormone (LH, TSH) if the primary lesion is in the hypothalamus. If the anterior pituitary is primarily affected, as in a destructive lesion like chromophobe adenoma, there should be no hormonal response to administered hypophysiotropic hormone (see Ch. 543). Unfortunately, there is considerable overlap in response between the two categories, so that this approach does not provide a definitive differential diagnostic tool (Edwards and Besser, 1974) (see Ch. 543).

4. *Fourth level — "takeover" by an abnormal control mechanism.* Plasma TSH values are low or undetectable in *toxic diffuse goiter* (hyperthyroidism associated with Graves' disease) because an abnormal, one might say "ectopic" thyroid stimulator (LATS or some other) has induced hypersecretion of thyroid hormone, which in turn suppresses pituitary secretion of thyrotropin (see Ch. 546.2). Another obvious example is that class of hyperendocrine syndromes accompanying hormone secretion by *cancers of nonendocrine organs* (see Ch. 525). Disturbances of the normal plasma ACTH–plasma cortisol relationship can usually be demonstrated in patients with the hypercortisolism that characterizes the "ectopic ACTH syndrome" observed in oat cell carcinoma of the lung and certain neoplasms of the thymus and pancreas (see Ch. 547.7).

5. *Fifth level — disorders of complex negative feedback inhibition systems.* In *pituitary-dependent Cushing's syndrome,* small doses of corticosteroids (e.g., dexamethasone) do not suppress endogenous pituitary secretion of ACTH as they do in normal subjects. This abnormality is due to *disordered control* of ACTH secretion, in which the plasma ACTH–plasma cortisol ratio is *inappropriate* because of a pathologic "driving force" to corticotropin secretion, emanating either from the hypothalamus or from the anterior pituitary itself (Liddle, 1965) (see Ch. 547.7).

In some patients with *acromegaly,* or overproduction of HGH by a pituitary tumor, infusion of glucose does not lower plasma HGH values as is the case in normal people. *A normal control mechanism is defective.*

The plasma PTH–plasma calcium relationship is *inappropriate* in *primary hyperparathyroidism.* As set out in Ch. 552, infusion of calcium should fail to suppress the plasma PTH values in *autonomous* primary parathyroid disease (e.g., a parathyroid adenoma), but this maneuver should lower hormonal levels in a normal fashion when the primary disease is located elsewhere, as in chronic renal insufficiency. Difficulties in differential diagnosis may, however, arise in the so-called "tertiary

hyperparathyroidism," when, as a consequence of protracted renal failure and protracted parathyroid gland stimulation by hypocalcemia, the function of the parathyroids appears to become *autonomous.* The problems, methodologic and other, are spelled out in Ch. 552.

6. *Sixth level — disturbances in the oscillatory rhythms of hormones.* Such abnormalities are only beginning to be recognized. Their origin may be in the hypothalamus or located elsewhere in the cerebrum. Further studies will be required to determine whether, for example, one may be able to clarify problems of *delayed* or *precocious puberty* by discovering altered rhythms in, rather than simply abnormal single values of, plasma FSH and LH. Analogous studies of plasma HGH oscillations may yet elucidate disorders of *accelerated* or *retarded* growth in children, but sufficient data are not now at hand.

As with the other forms of endocrine disease set forth above, the answers to the clinical problems (including earlier detection of disorder) are likely to come from investigations of *subtle disturbances in the control of hormonal secretion.*

HORMONES AS MEDICINES

Hormones are legitimately given to patients in three sets of circumstances: (1) for replacement of lost functions. (2) as tests of endocrine function, and (3) to achieve a pharmacologic purpose.

REPLACEMENT THERAPY. This is probably the most gratifying use of hormones to both patient and physician, and is the easiest to defend. So long as an endocrine deficiency is clearly and definitely demonstrated, in most instances a realistic goal owing to the availability of good chemical tests for most hormonal diseases, the physician can achieve brilliant clinical results with small doses of hormones. Cortisol for adrenal insufficiency, thyroid hormone USP or thyroxine for hypothyroidism, and human growth hormone for hypopituitary dwarfism are all given in amounts very close to the estimated daily production rates of the respective hormones. It is common practice to give too much cortisone to patients with primary or secondary adrenal insufficiency, i.e., enough to induce signs of mild Cushing's syndrome; daily doses of not more than 10 to 25 mg per day are usually quite sufficient. With thyroid hormone replacement, restraint is also necessary, especially in older people with coronary artery disease, in whom the maintenance dose should be attained gradually. The writer believes that triiodothyronine is never indicated for treatment of longstanding myxedema; too many elderly patients with atherosclerosis have had bouts of severe coronary insufficiency or even myocardial infarction when this rapidly acting hormone is given. Triiodothyronine may have a place in the treatment of myxedema coma (see Ch. 546.4).

Replacement dosages of sex hormones have been arrived at by "clinical experience." In the writer's experience, treatment to promote the development of deficient secondary sex characters is best given just before or at the expected time of puberty. If replacement therapy with estrogen or testosterone is delayed until late in the second or well into the third decade, the induced sexual development is suboptimal. This puts a premium on early diagnosis as the basis for early treatment.

Few protein hormones are used routinely in treatment. Although it would be theoretically most correct, say in hypopituitarism, to replace absent tropic hormones by giving gonadotropins, TSH or ACTH, this is not practical, owing to antibody formation, short supply, and the need for parenteral administration. Gonadotropins are given only in short courses to induce ovulation in women (see Ch. 549.2); to stimulate ovarian or testicular function over a long period of time is cumbersome, so sex hormones, which can be administered orally, are used instead. Treatment of secondary hypothyroidism and hypoadrenalism is much more easily done with thyroid hormone and cortisone than with TSH or ACTH; allergic reactions to ACTH have been alluded to above. Parathyroid hormone from human sources is not available; vitamin D and calcium salts are simpler to give. The only protein hormone other than insulin that is generally used as replacement therapy is human growth hormone because there is still no satisfactory substitute for it.

TESTING. TSH and ACTH are still useful for assessing thyroidal and adrenal response in differentiating between primary and secondary deficiencies of these glands, and the triiodothyronine suppression test of thyroidal ^{131}I uptake is a useful adjunct in diagnosis of some patients with hyperthyroidism. These testing procedures entail the direct chemical or physical measurement of a hormone or of a glandular function. Such methods, together with radioimmunoassay measurement of TSH, ACTH, and other peptide hormones, have largely superseded indirect methods of estimating endocrine activity (e.g., the BMR and the eosinophil count). Some of the older techniques, being provocative tests, were potentially dangerous, e.g., the water-loading and salt withdrawal tests for Addison's disease. These should now be abandoned.

By testing, the writer does not mean the administration of a hormone as a *therapeutic trial*, that is, to determine by the patient's response whether he has or does not have an endocrine deficiency. This approach may be tolerable in an emergency, as for a patient in acute shock when there seems to be some possibility of adrenocortical insufficiency and there is no time for careful chemical study. *Under any other conditions, failure to establish a diagnosis is an inexcusable basis for giving hormonal therapy.*

HORMONES GIVEN TO ACHIEVE A PHARMACOLOGIC END. Hormones customarily are given to patients in high doses to achieve some pharmacologic, not physiologic, goal in three sets of circumstances: treatment of diseases in which large doses of hormones are *often beneficial*; treatment of diseases for which large doses of hormones are *possibly* or *sometimes beneficial*; and treatment of diseases for which large doses of hormones are *never beneficial* or of very doubtful value.

Beneficial Uses. The obvious examples are of course ACTH and cortisol and its congeners. Although ACTH is usually associated with fewer serious untoward effects and with less danger of a "withdrawal syndrome" when treatment is stopped, the corticosteroids are preferred because of the convenience of the oral route of administration, more flexibility in spacing of doses, shorter action, the larger doses attainable, and the absence of serious allergic reactions. *The ideal use of high-dosage corticosteroids is in acute, self-limited diseases such as serum sickness owing to penicillin allergy or bouts of status asthmaticus.* In serious inflammatory diseases such as pemphigus, ulcerative colitis, acute rheumatic fever, and lupus erythematosus, in hematologic disorders such as acute lymphoblastic leukemia of childhood, and in bronchial asthma of allergic origin, among other conditions, there is good evidence that corticosteroids often alter the course of the disease in a favorable direction. As in giving any other medicinal agent, the physician has to balance the probability of benefit from corticosteroid therapy against the disability or danger incurred by giving the patient corticosteroids, with the attendant risk of iatrogenic Cushing's syndrome. To make this semiquantitative judgment, the doctor has to have the fullest possible knowledge of the *natural history* of what he proposes to treat, that is, the natural course of the disease untreated (Feinstein, 1967).

Possibly or Sometimes Beneficial Uses. The efficacy of corticosteroids in such disorders as scleroderma and endotoxin shock remains arguable. The same statement applies to the use of testosterone or estrogen, or both, in the treatment of postmenopausal osteoporosis (q.v.); the use of vasopressin or mineralocorticoids in the management of idiopathic postural hypotension; administration of small doses of corticosteroids to women with "acquired adrenal virilism," an entity which may or may not exist; and many others. In this group of diseases, further work is needed toward an understanding of pathogenesis; only this will provide a rational basis for giving or withholding treatment.

Uses That Are Never Beneficial. These uses are derived by the trial and error method, with emphasis on the latter. Examples are numerous; outstanding ones are the widespread administration of thyroid hormone for obesity, for fatigability, and for infertility and menstrual disturbances, the use of estrogens to treat frigidity in the female, and the use of testosterone for impotence in the male. *The major objection to such therapies is that they are ineffective.* Further, they are often expensive and raise false hopes. The physician must resist the temptation to keep trying one hormonal remedy after another in the hope that something will work. "The empiricist," said Claude Bernard, "is never at a loss." It is the patient who loses.

Drezner, M., Neelon, F. A., and Lebovitz, H. E.: Pseudohypoparathyroidism, Type II: A possible defect in the reception of the cyclic AMP signal. N. Engl. J. Med., 289:1056, 1973.

Nusynowitz, M. L., and Klein, M. H.: Pseudoidiopathic hypoparathyroidism. Hypoparathyroidism with ineffective parathyroid hormone. Am. J. Med., 55:677, 1973.

Odell, W. D., and Daughaday, W. H. (eds.): Principles of Competitive Protein-Binding Assays. Philadelphia, J. B. Lippincott Company, 1971.

Rassmussen, H.: Organization and control of endocrine systems. *In* Williams, R. H. (ed.): Textbook of Endocrinology. 5th ed. Philadelphia, W. B. Saunders Company, 1974, p. 1.

Rimoin, D. L., and Schimke, R. N.: Genetic Disorders of the Endocrine Glands. St. Louis, C. V. Mosby Company, 1971.

Siiteri, P. K.: Qualitative and quantitative aspects of adrenal secretion of steroids. *In* Christy, N. P. (ed.): The Human Adrenal Cortex. New York, Harper & Row, 1971, p. 1.

Sterling, K., Refetoff, S., and Selenkow, H. A.: T_3 thyrotoxicosis. Thyrotoxicosis due to elevated serum triiodothyronine levels. JAMA, 213:571, 1970.

Volpé, R.: The role of autoimmunity in hypoendocrine and hyperendocrine function. Ann. Intern. Med., 87:86, 1977.

Welbourn, R. B.: Current status of the apudomas. Ann. Surg., 185:1, 1977.

Werner, S. C., and Ingbar, S. H. (eds.): The Thyroid. 4th ed. Hagerstown, Md., Harper & Row, 1978.

541. MODE OF ACTION OF HORMONES

John N. Loeb

The physiologic effects of the endocrine secretions have long been recognized as among the most dramatic in clinical medicine. The conspicuous consequences of castration in the male have been known since ancient times, and by the mid-nineteenth century the results of ablation of various other endocrine tissues had begun to be appreciated. By the end of the first quarter of the present century most of the currently recognized syndromes of endocrine hypersecretion had been described as well, and at the present time it is recognized that an enormous diversity of metabolic processes, exerting profound effects on growth, differentiation, and homeostasis, are under endocrine control.

In recent years there has been a concerted effort to understand the biochemical mechanisms by which these processes are regulated, and in particular to account, in molecular terms, for the diverse and dramatic effects of the endocrine secretions on structure and function. The development of sensitive biochemical techniques has permitted a shift in focus from simple observations of hormonal effects to efforts at defining mechanisms by which such effects are mediated. It is becoming increasingly clear that, despite the variety of their physiologic effects, the fundamental modes of action of many hormones are similar. This chapter outlines some of the patterns which are beginning to emerge and discusses some of their implications.

PROPERTIES COMMON TO ALL HORMONES

As non-neuronal carriers of information between different organs, hormones must interact specifically and reversibly with target cells, and this interaction must have the capacity to result in widespread cellular effects. The fact that hormones are normally present in extraordinarily low concentrations (e.g., 10^{-11} to 10^{-8} molar) moreover requires that target tissues be sensitive to even minute changes in hormone concentration. It follows that hormone–target cell interactions must have at least two characteristics: *specificity*, and the capacity for *amplification* of an initial hormone signal in terms of subsequent biochemical events. These two characteristics will be discussed in some detail below for different classes of hormones.

STEROID HORMONES

A general model for the mode of action of a steroid hormone is shown in Table 1. After secretion, the hormone, either alone or complexed to a specific plasma-binding protein, circulates to its target cell. The free hormone then diffuses into the cytoplasm, where it becomes attached to another specific binding protein called a "receptor" protein. This attachment results in a change in the three-dimensional configuration of the protein and the formation of steroid-receptor complexes which have a high affinity for specific regions of the nuclear chromatin (DNA-histone complex). These steroid-receptor complexes then enter the nucleus, be-

come attached to these regions of the chromatin, and, through mechanisms still unknown, interact with the chromatin to bring about an increased rate of transcription (synthesis) of specific messenger RNA (mRNA) molecules. The resulting mRNA molecules leave the nucleus and enter the cytoplasm, where they are "translated" into molecules of corresponding specific proteins (see Part V). These latter proteins, at least some of which are enzymes, then influence specific intracellular biochemical pathways and account for the ultimate "biologic effects" of the hormone. In recent years a number of steroid hormones have been studied, and in all instances their mechanism of action, insofar as it has been elucidated, appears to conform to this model.

THYROID HORMONES

Despite the relative simplicity of their chemical structures, the thyroid hormones exert their biologic effects by mechanisms that have only recently begun to be understood. It is now clear that, at least in outline, the mode of action of thyroxine and triiodothyronine resembles that of the steroid hormones in that interaction of nuclear hormone-receptor complexes with chromatin brings about the transcription of specific mRNA, which in turn leads to the synthesis of specific proteins which mediate the biologic effects (see Table 1). In contrast to the steroid hormones, however, receptors for the thyroid hormones appear to be largely if not entirely restricted to the nucleus. The possibility that additional, extranuclear receptors may mediate certain other actions of the thyroid hormones is nevertheless currently being explored.

The *calorigenic* effect of the thyroid hormones is now known to be due to increased activity of a "sodium pump" whose primary function is to maintain normal sodium and potassium ion gradients across the limiting membranes of virtually all mammalian cells. Active sodium transport (extrusion of sodium ions against an electrochemical gradient from the interior of cells, where their concentration is low, to the extracellular fluid environment, where it is considerably higher) is accomplished by the hydrolysis of ATP in the presence of a sodium-potassium–activated ATPase and may account for a third or more of the energy requirement of resting cells. One of the nuclear effects of thyroid hormone may be the synthesis of mRNA which leads to increased synthesis of these "pumps."

CATECHOLAMINE, POLYPEPTIDE, AND PROTEIN HORMONES

In contrast to the steroid and thyroid hormones, which must reach the cell *nucleus* before influencing cellular events, many other hormones exert their biochemical effects by interacting directly with the external cell surface. These latter hormones include many polypeptide and protein hormones as well as the catecholamines, and in these instances the hormone receptors, instead of being located in the cytoplasm of the target cell, appear to be located in the external cell membrane ("plasma membrane") itself. As shown in Table 1, the result of the interaction of one of these hormones with its receptor in the cell membrane depends upon the nature of the hormone. As first shown by the brilliant work of Sutherland, a large number of membrane-

TABLE 1. Outline of Modes of Action of Some Different Classes of Hormones

Hormone Class	Location of Receptor	Primary Result of Interaction with Receptor	Consequences	
Steroids	Target cell cytoplasm	Steroid-receptor complexes in cytoplasm migrate to nucleus, bind to specific region(s) of chromatin, and result in increased rate of synthesis ("transcription") of specific mRNA molecules	mRNA molecules migrate to cytoplasm, where they are "translated" into molecules of protein (e.g., specific enzymes) →	Changes in enzyme concentrations, which can then influence the rates of specific biochemical events within the cell
Thyroid hormones	Target cell nucleus	Hormone-receptor complexes formed in nucleus bind to specific region(s) of chromatin and result in increased rate of synthesis ("transcription") of specific mRNA molecules	Same →	Same
Catecholamines Polypeptides Most proteins	Target cell outer membrane	1. Modification of adenyl cyclase activity: a. Stimulation of cAMP synthesis (e.g., catecholamines, majority of polypeptide and protein hormones—see Table 2)	Increased intracellular concentration of cAMP →	Changes in enzyme activities, changes in cell permeability, etc. (effects of cAMP dependent upon nature of particular target cell—see Table 2)
		b. ? Inhibition of cAMP synthesis (e.g., to account for effects of insulin on liver and fat cell cAMP levels)	Decreased intracellular concentration of cAMP →	Increased rate of liver glycogen synthesis; decreased rate of gluconeogenesis, glycogenolysis, and lipolysis
		2. ? Direct effect on membrane transport processes (e.g., effects of insulin on glucose uptake by adipose tissue and skeletal muscle)	Increased rate of glucose entry →	Increased rate of glucose utilization and glycogen synthesis

active hormones exert their effects by interacting specifically with the enveloping cell membrane to activate *adenyl cyclase,* an enzyme present in the membranes of a great variety of cells. Activation of adenyl cyclase causes an increased rate of synthesis of 3',5'–cyclic adenosine monophosphate ("cAMP") from ATP. This mechanism leads to an increase in the intracellular concentration of cAMP and accounts for the action of the catecholamines and of most polypeptide and protein hormones for which mechanisms are currently known. An increase in cAMP concentration in a target organ can have diverse and important biochemical consequences which depend upon the cell type and which account for the physiologic effects of the hormone on its target tissue. The diversity of these effects is illustrated in Table 2. In contrast to the steroid hormones, the effects of which require new RNA and protein synthesis (see above), the catecholamine and most of the polypeptide hormones act directly to influence the activity of pre-existing enzyme systems. Many of their physiologic effects can thus be observed almost instantaneously (e.g., those of epinephrine), in contrast to those of the steroid hormones, which often require many minutes or longer to become clinically apparent (e.g., the effects of hydrocortisone).

Insulin, in contrast to the hormones discussed in the preceding paragraph, is known to produce a *decrease* in the cyclic AMP content of several tissues. Although it is possible that a fall in intracellular cAMP accounts for some of the effects of insulin in liver and adipose tissue, it is by no means clear that it explains *all* the biologic effects of the hormones. Other important effects of insulin, such as the stimulation of glucose uptake by skeletal muscle, appear thus far to take place in the absence of any demonstrable change in adenyl cyclase activity or total intracellular cAMP concentration and may instead reflect direct and independent effects of the hormone on membrane transport processes.

The action of *growth hormone* appears to be mediated at least in part by *somatomedins,* a family of serum proteins of low molecular weight generated (probably by the liver) in response to growth hormone. Somatomedins stimulate sulfate incorporation into cartilage and possess an insulin-like activity that can markedly stimulate the proliferation of a variety of other cells in vitro.

TABLE 2. Some Hormonal Responses Dependent Upon an Activation of Adenyl Cyclase

Hormone	Target Tissue	Response
Catecholamines	Liver	Activation of phosphorylase
		Inactivation of glycogen synthetase
	Skeletal muscle	Activation of phosphorylase
		Inactivation of glycogen synthetase
	Heart	Activation of phosphorylase
		Positive inotropic response
	Adipose tissue	Lipolysis
	Salivary gland	Amylase secretion
	Kidney	Renin production
	Pineal gland	Melatonin synthesis
Glucagon	Liver	Activation of phosphorylase
	Pancreatic beta cell	Insulin release
	Adipose tissue	Lipolysis
ACTH*	Adrenal cortex	Steroidogenesis
	Adipose tissue	Lipolysis
LH (ICSH)*	Corpus luteum	Steroidogenesis
	Testis	Steroidogenesis
Vasopressin	Renal collecting tubule	Increase in permeability to water
GnRH*	Anterior pituitary	FSH* and LH release
?TRH*	Anterior pituitary	TSH and prolactin release
TSH*	Thyroid	Thyroid hormone release
Gastrin	Gastric parietal cell	Production of HCl
Parathormone	Renal tubule	Excretion of phosphate
	Bone	Calcium mobilization
Calcitonin	Bone	Inhibition of calcium mobilization
	Kidney	Calcium and sodium excretion

*ACTH, adrenocorticotropic hormone; FSH, follicle-stimulating hormone; GnRH, gonadotropin-releasing hormone; LH (ICSH), luteinizing hormone (interstitial cell-stimulating hormone); TRH, thyrotropin-releasing hormone; TSH, thyroid-stimulating hormone (thyrotropin). (Modified after Sutherland, E. W., et al.: Circulation, 37:279, 1968.)

To what extent somatomedin production can account for the multiple and diverse biologic effects of growth hormone still remains unclear.

SPECIFICITY OF HORMONAL EFFECTS; "AMPLIFICATION" OF HORMONAL SIGNALS

Two characteristics of hormonal effects have already been mentioned: their *specificity*, and the fact that hormones exert their biochemical effects at extremely low molecular concentrations. Both characteristics will be considered briefly as they apply to the different models for hormone action described above. In the models presented for *steroid hormone* and *thyroid hormone* action, specificity resides in the affinities of these hormones for appropriate receptor proteins inside their target cells. Thus tissues which are estrogen-sensitive contain an estrogen-binding receptor protein in their cytoplasm, whereas those which are unresponsive to estrogen do not. "Amplification" of the initial hormonal signal can occur at several subsequent steps: interaction of the hormone-receptor complex with the nuclear chromatin can bring about the transcription of more than one molecule of mRNA from a given DNA gene; each of these can then be translated into many enzyme molecules, each of which in turn can catalyze the transformation of many molecules of intracellular substrate into product.

The model presented for *those hormones which operate through cAMP* provides a similar opportunity for both specificity of hormone effect and amplification of the hormonal signal. The mechanisms, however, are different. In the case of the polypeptide and catecholamine hormones, specificity is determined not only by the presence or absence of specific hormone receptors in a cell membrane, but also by the response of that cell to an increased level of cAMP once adenyl cyclase has been activated (see, e.g., Table 2 and References). Mechanisms by which the adenyl cyclase system can amplify an initial hormonal signal are described under the following heading.

Cyclic AMP

BIOLOGIC EFFECTS. The effects of changes in the intracellular concentration of cAMP depend upon the nature of the cell in which these changes occur. Thus in various cells an increase in intracellular cAMP may affect enzyme activities (for example, that of phosphorylase in liver or muscle), may affect permeability of the external cell membrane (as in the renal collecting tubule), may influence gene transcription, or, in certain tissues, may actually stimulate the production or release of certain hormones (see Table 2). The generation of cAMP in response to a hormonal signal at the surface of the cell permits the conversion of an external hormonal signal into a new kind of (*intracellular*) signal, referred to by Sutherland as a "second messenger," and can greatly amplify the original hormonal signal; by stimulating adenyl cyclase activity, a single hormone molecule can potentially cause the synthesis of many molecules of cAMP, which in turn can produce a whole cascade of events within the cell. Both the complexity of these events and their extraordinary rapidity, despite this complexity, are illustrated by the familiar example of hepatic glycogenolysis in response to epinephrine. The steps involved are illustrated in Figure 1; the many steps which intervene between the binding of epinephrine to receptor sites in liver cell membranes and the clinical "result" (an elevation of the blood sugar) are evident.

REGULATION OF INTRACELLULAR CYCLIC AMP CONCENTRATION. The intracellular concentration of cAMP is controlled both by regulation of its rate of synthesis and by regulation of its rate of degradation. Degradation of cAMP occurs via a phosphodiesterase which rapidly hydrolyzes cAMP (3',5'-cyclic AMP) to the noncyclic monoester 5'-AMP. It has been found that many substances not conventionally considered hormones are capable of affecting intracellular cAMP levels and hence of mimicking the effects of certain hormones (Fig. 2). Epinephrine and theophylline, for example, have very different primary biochemical actions, yet through entirely different mechanisms they both cause an increased concentration of cAMP in many cells. In view of this "final common path" it is not surprising that

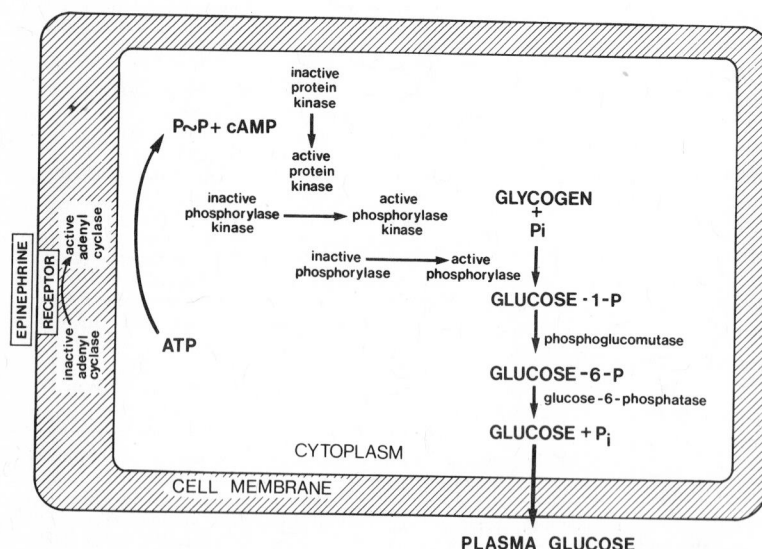

Figure 1. Steps required in the activation of liver phosphorylase by epinephrine resulting in glycogenolysis and hyperglycemia. The activation of phosphorylase is only one of the consequences of an increased level of cAMP in the liver; the mechanism by which this is accomplished has recently been shown in all probability to conform closely to that established earlier for skeletal muscle. (P $\sim$ P, pyrophosphate; P_i, inorganic phosphate; enzymes are indicated in small type.)

Figure 2. Influence of various physiologic and pharmacologic substances on the formation and degradation of cyclic AMP. → ⊕ implies stimulation; → ⊖ implies inhibition. Prostaglandins can also affect adenyl cyclase activity, but whether they induce an increase or a decrease in the level of cyclic AMP depends upon target cell type. (Modified after Sutherland, E. W., et al.: Circulation, 37:279, 1968.)

many of the familiar physiologic effects of theophylline and epinephrine (e.g., tachycardia, positive inotropic effect, dilatation of the coronary arteries, bronchodilatation, nervousness, sweating, glycogenolysis, lipolysis) are so similar.

ONSET AND DURATION OF BIOLOGIC EFFECT(S)

The time that must elapse between the administration of a hormone and the *appearance of a particular biologic effect* is determined by the time required for the accomplishment of the necessary intervening biochemical steps following initial attachment of the hormone to its receptor. Thus, as indicated earlier, effects produced by the steroid and thyroid hormones, most or all of which are mediated by new RNA and protein synthesis, are generally slower to appear than effects mediated through the influence of changes in cAMP concentration on pre-existing enzyme systems. The *duration of a hormonal effect* is similarly dependent upon the mechanism by which the effect is biochemically mediated. In general, effects mediated through changes in intracellular cAMP concentration are short lived, since cAMP turns over rapidly and intracellular levels consequently return promptly to their basal values upon disappearance of an adenyl cyclase–active hormone from the plasma. In contrast, the effects of a steroid or thyroid hormone may persist long after the hormone itself has disappeared from the plasma, for these latter effects are largely if not entirely mediated by newly synthesized enzymes, many of which are degraded relatively slowly. Since, moreover, not all enzymes induced by a given hormone necessarily turn over at the same rate, it is evident that certain effects may last longer than others, and hence that, even for a single hormone, "duration of biologic effect" is an ambiguous expression unless a particular effect is specified. The term "biologic half-life," occasionally employed to describe the duration of action of a hormone in contrast to its decay rate from plasma, is conceptually unsound and should be avoided.

REGULATION OF RECEPTOR OCCUPANCY

Implicit in the discussion thus far is the assumption that the initial determinant of the magnitude of a given hormonal response is the number of hormone-receptor complexes formed in the presence of hormone. Although the concentration of such occupied receptors, and hence the magnitude of the response, might thus be expected to be determined largely by the concentration of the hormone itself, it is at least theoretically possible that the number of such complexes, and hence the magnitude of the response *to a given concentration of hormone* might also be influenced by variations in the initial concentration of available receptors or by changes in the affinities of these receptors for hormone. Recent evidence suggests that a number of "spontaneous" as well as pharmacologically induced pathologic conditions resulting in partial hormonal "resistance" may indeed be associated with a decrease in total receptor concentration.

HORMONE STRUCTURE AND SPECIFICITY

The relation between hormone structure and specificity is imperfectly understood, but studies of the relation between molecular structure and function in simpler systems suggest concepts that may apply to hormones and their target-cell receptors. In most of the systems studied so far it appears that the number of indispensable functional groups per molecule is small. For steroid hormones, for example, it is probable that the steroid nucleus itself functions little more than as a rigid spacer to hold essential functional groups in fixed relation to each other. Thus the stilbestrol molecule, a potent but nonsteroidal synthetic estrogen, bears only superficial resemblance to estradiol except in the relative (and fixed) positions of its phenolic hydroxy groups.

In the more complex polypeptide hormones it is possible that one portion of the molecule is responsible for specific binding to a membrane receptor, while another portion interacts with adenyl cyclase to stimulate the synthesis of cAMP. Thyroid-stimulating hormone (TSH) and luteinizing hormone (LH), for example, both exert their biologic effects by stimulating adenyl cyclase in their respective target tissues. Both hormone molecules consist of subunits made up of two different proteins, and one of these two subunits is identical in both hormones. It is tempting to speculate that the subunit which is shared in common contains the site that interacts with adenyl cyclase, whereas the other subunit, which is different in the two hormones, contains the determinants for their tissue specificity.

It now seems likely that those hormone molecules which act by influencing cAMP synthesis and which have tissue specificity contain not only functional groups capable of interacting with adenyl cyclase, but also functional groups which confer an affinity for specific receptors in their target cell membranes. An ingenious and attractive, though still unproved, hypothesis has been advanced by Beers and Reich. They have suggested that certain essential tyrosinyl, histadyl, and tryptophanyl residues in the polypeptide hormones may represent the evolutionary descendents of three "primeval" adenyl cyclase–stimulating amines, epinephrine, histamine, and serotonin, and that these amino acids may play an analogous role in the stimulation of adenyl cyclase in target tissues. The rest of the polypeptide molecule is regarded as an elaborate appendage which has been acquired in the course of evolution to confer necessary tissue specificity and to maintain the amino acid at the adenyl cyclase–active site in an appropriate three-dimensional orientation. Epinephrine, for example, is a simple amine and stimulates adenyl cyclase in a great variety of target cells (see, e.g., Table 2); in contrast, the specificity of a substance like parathormone may, by this hypothesis, be attributed to the acquisition of a portion of the molecule which is capable of binding to a more restricted range of target tissues, and which may in fact be at some distance from the site which interacts with adenyl cyclase.

"PHYSIOLOGIC" VS. "PHARMACOLOGIC" EFFECTS

The diversity of the human hormones and their striking tissue specificity are apparent. With the ready availability of many of these hormones in pure form, and with the present ability of the biochemist to detect even subtle effects, an ever-increasing number of hormonal "effects" are being described. One must be cautious in interpreting some of these observations, particularly those made at hormone concentrations which greatly exceed those present in the normal organism. At high concentrations of hormone it is possible that certain exquisite end-organ specificities are simply overcome; under such conditions occasional "anomalous effects" on "surprising" target organs may have little *physiologic* significance.

Archer, J. A., Gorden, P., and Roth, J.: Defect in insulin binding to receptors in obese man: Amelioration with calorie restriction. J. Clin. Invest., 55:166, 1975.

Baxter, J. D.: Glucocorticoid hormone action. Pharmacol. Therapeutics, B–2:605, 1976.

Czech, M. P.: Molecular basis of insulin action. Ann. Rev. Biochem., 46:359, 1977.

Edelman, I. S.: Thyroid thermogenesis. N. Engl. J. Med., 290:1303, 1974.

Lefkowitz, R. J., Limbird, L. E., Mukherjee, C., and Caron, M. G.: The β-adrenergic receptor and adenylate cyclase. Biochem. Biophys. Acta, 457:1, 1976.

Lesniac, M. A., and Roth, J.: Regulation of receptor concentration by homologous hormone: Effect of human growth hormone on its receptors in IM-9 lymphocytes. J. Biol. Chem., 251:3720, 1976.

Loeb, J. N.: Models for hormone action, In Christy, N. P. (ed.): The Human Adrenal Cortex. New York, Harper & Row, 1971, pp. 191–203.

Maddaiah, V. T.: A model for hormone specific activation of adenyl cyclase. J. Theor. Biol., 25:495, 1969.

O'Malley, B. W.: Mechanisms of action of steroid hormones. N. Engl. J. Med., 284:370, 1971.

Oppenheimer, J. H., Silva, E., Schwartz, H. L., and Surks, M. I.: Stimulation of hepatic mitochondrial α-glycerophosphate dehydrogenase and malic enzyme by L-triiodothyronine: Characteristics of the response with specific nuclear thyroid hormone binding sites fully saturated. J. Clin. Invest., 59:517, 1977.

Rall, J. E.: Mechanism of action of T₄. In Werner, S. C., and Ingbar, S. H. (eds.): The Thyroid: A Fundamental and Clinical Text. 4th ed. New York, Harper & Row, 1978, pp. 138–148.

Robison, G. A., Butcher, R. W., and Sutherland, E. W.: Cyclic AMP. New York, Academic Press, 1971.

Roth, J.: Peptide hormone binding to receptors: A review of direct studies in vitro. Metabolism, 22:1059, 1973.

Sutherland, E. W.: Studies on the mechanism of hormone action. Science, 177:401, 1972.

Thompson, E. B., and Lippman, M. W.: Mechanism of action of glucocorticoids. Metabolism, 23:159, 1974.

Van Wyk, J. J., Underwood, L. E., Hintz, R. L., Clemmons, D. R., Voina, S. J., and Weaver, R. P.: The somatomedins: A family of insulinlike hormones under growth hormone control. Recent Prog. Horm. Res., 30:259, 1974.

542. THE CONTROL OF ANTERIOR PITUITARY SECRETION

Seymour Reichlin

Although the anterior pituitary gland lacks a direct nerve supply, the secretion of each of its hormones is under the control of the central nervous system. Through specialized secretory neurons localized in the ventral hypothalamus, the function of the pituitary and, in turn, of its target glands becomes responsive to changes in the external and internal environment. In addition, the neurohumoral connections of the anterior pituitary are important in the "feedback" regulation of a number of hormones such as cortisol, the gonadal steroids, thyroxine, and prolactin, and serve as part of the integrated mechanism by which behavioral and metabolic adaptation to the external enviroment is accomplished.

During the last few years, as the importance of neural factors in the control of pituitary secretion has become increasingly apparent, a division of study of endocrinology has developed which is termed *neuroendocrinology*. This area deals mainly with the interaction of neural and hormonal factors in endocrine and metabolic control systems.

HYPOTHALAMIC NEUROSECRETION: HYPOPHYSIOTROPIC NEURONS

The pituitary gland and hypothalamus are closely related anatomically, as may be seen in Figure 1. This relationship has both embryologic and functional significance. The neural lobe develops as a downgrowth of axons from the diencephalon, whose cells of origin are located in the paraventricular and supraoptic nuclei of the hypothalamus. These nerve fibers pass as unmyelinated axons through the neural stalk and terminate in the neural lobe. Like neurons elsewhere, supraopticohypophysial and paraventriculohypophysial neurons are electrically excitable, conduct action potentials, and are responsive to neurotransmitters. Unlike most other neurons, these cells are neurosecretory, that is, they synthesize hormonal substances which are released into blood vessels for action at a remote site rather than locally at synapses, as is characteristic of most neurons. Hormones of the neurohypophysis are synthesized mainly in cell bodies located in the hypothalamus and pass in granule form (associated with a protein carrier substance, neurophysin) to the nerve endings in the neural lobe, where they are stored. Neurosecretory neurons thus manifest the properties of both nerve and gland. This kind of nerve cell of which the neurohypophysial neurons are the classic example, have been termed by Wurtman and Axelrod "*neuroendocrine transducers.*" Neurosecretory cells are the major effector links between the nervous system and the endocrine gland.

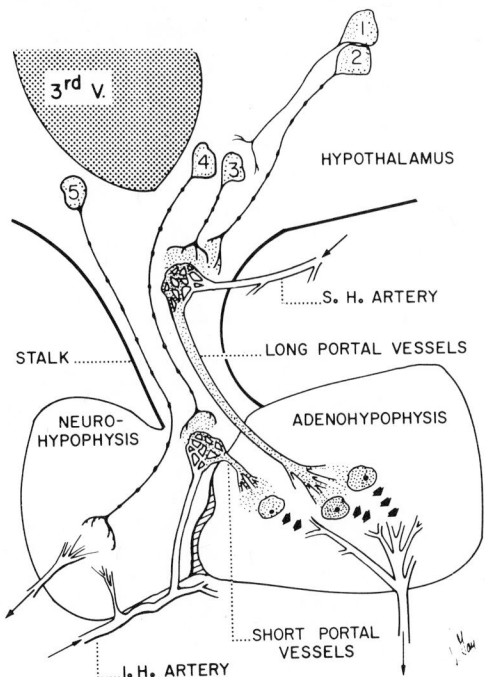

Figure 1. The functional elements of control of the hypothalamic-pituitary unit. Two general types of neurons are involved in anterior pituitary regulation. One type, the peptidergic neuron, forms the releasing hormones (shown here as No. 3, ending in the median eminence, and No. 4, ending in the pituitary stalk), both in relation to the capillary plexus of the hypophysial-portal vessels. These neurons (corresponding to the designation "tuberohypophysial" neurons) are neurosecretory. That is, they combine the function of excitable electrical tissue and secretory function and serve as "neuroendocrine transducers" (Wurtman, 1971) to convert neural information to hormonal information. Their function is analogous to the function of the classic supraopticohypophysial neuron (No. 5), the structure responsible for secretion of vasopressin. The second type of neuron is the link between the rest of the brain and the peptidergic neuron. These are largely monaminergic and are believed to end on the cell body of the peptidergic neuron in a conventional manner (No. 1), or to end on the axon terminus of the peptidergic neuron (No. 2) in a manner termed by Schneider and McCann "axo-axonic." Some tuberohypophysial neurons are dopaminergic. Abbreviations: S.H., superior hypophysial; I.H., inferior hypophysial; 3rd V., third ventricle. (From Gay, V.: Fertility and Sterility, 23:50, 1972.)

Although the neural lobe lies close to the anterior lobe of the pituitary and neurohypophysial secretory products are identifiable in blood reaching the pituitary, the secretions of the neurohypophysis (oxytocin, vasopressin, neurophysin) have no established regulatory action in the anterior lobe but are released into the systemic circulation to affect remote tissues such as the kidney, breast, and uterus.

Neuroendocrine cells that regulate the anterior pituitary are distributed relatively widely throughout the hypothalamus, as shown by immunohistochemical methods that utilize antisera to the hypothalamic hormones. Their axons project to the median eminence of the hypothalamus. From the median eminence, the hypophysiotropic secretions of the hypothalamus (also called *releasing factors*) reach the anterior pituitary through a specialized system of capillaries and veins, the hypophysial-portal circulation. Hypophysiotropic

neurons resemble neurohypophysial neurons in being electrically active, pharmacologically excitable, and responsive to a wide variety of nerve impulses arising from other sites in the brain. They also respond to feedback hormonal stimuli. Neuron endings of the stalk–median eminence region (tuberohypophysial neurons) and the associated blood vessels have been likened to the posterior lobe and can be looked upon as a "median eminence gland"; taken together, these structures constitute the "final common pathway" for neural control of the anterior pituitary gland.

This outline of anterior pituitary regulation is the *portal vessel chemotransmitter hypothesis.* According to this view, lesions of the hypothalamus (and of the portal vessel complex of the stalk) reduce most anterior pituitary functions by causing a deficiency of releasing factors. Direct electrical stimulation of the tuberohypophysial neurons, or reflex activation of these neurons, caused, for example, by emotional stress, activates the anterior pituitary by the release of hypophysiotropic hormones.

Initially based on indirect physiologic experiments, this hypothesis has been established by demonstration of hypothalamic substances which selectively affect each of the known pituitary hormones. These are CRF (corticotropin-releasing factor), TRH (thyrotropin-releasing hormone), GHRF (growth hormone–releasing factor), LHRH, GnRH (luteinizing hormone–releasing hormone, gonadotropin-releasing hormone), and PRF (prolactin-releasing factor). Inhibitory hypophysiotropic hormones have also been identified. These are PIF (prolactin inhibitory factor) and somatostatin (SRIF, somatotropin release–inhibiting factor).

The chemical nature of TRF, now termed thyrotropin-releasing hormone (TRH), was identified in 1969 as a tripeptide amide, pyroglutamyl histidyl prolineamide (Fig. 2). The chemical nature of LRF (LHRH) was identified in 1971 as a decapeptide (Fig. 2), the amino terminal of which (like TRH) is pyroglutamic acid and the carboxyl terminal an amide. A substance with powerful growth hormone release inhibitory activity, chemically identified in 1973 as a linear peptide composed of 14 amino acids (Fig. 2), was named by its discoverers *somatostatin.* The Nobel prize in Medicine or Physiology was awarded in 1977 to Roger Guillemin and Andrew Schally for their work in isolating and identifying these three factors. TRH also possesses intrinsic prolactin-releasing activity, but other peptides of the hypothalamus, including one or more as yet uncharacterized factors are active as a PRF. The principal PIF is dopamine.

---

pyroGlu-His-Pro–NH$_2$

TRH, Thyrotropin-releasing hormone

pyroGlu-His-Trp-Ser-Tyr-Gly-Leu-Arg-Pro-Gly–NH$_2$

LHRH, Luteinizing hormone–releasing hormone, gonadotropin-releasing hormone, GnRH

$$\overset{\text{S-S}}{\overline{\hspace{3cm}}}$$
H-Ala-Gly-Cys-Lys-Asn-Phe-Phe-Trp-Lys-Thr-Phe-Thr-Ser-Cys-OH

Somatostatin, SRIF

Figure 2. Structural formulas of the established hypophysiotropic hormones.

Figure 3. Monaminergic pathways in mammalian brain. The principal localization of the neurons containing norepinephrine, dopamine, and serotonin is in the mesencephalon and pons. Axons of these cells are distributed to widespread areas of cortex, limbic system, and striatum. The dopaminergic system of the arcuate is an exception to this general scheme of distribution. *Abbreviations:* MFB, medial forebrain bundle; AN, arcuate nucleus; OC, optic chiasm. (From Martin, J. B., Reichlin, S., and Brown, G. M.: Clinical Neuroendocrinology. Philadelphia, F. A. Davis Company, 1977.)

Other peptides or neurotransmitters may also act as PIF. Neither CRF nor GHRF has been chemically characterized. Although the primary activity of the aforementioned chemically identified releasing hormones is related to the original bioassay properties used in purification and identification, it is now apparent that there are certain crossover effects of these hormones. Thus TRH is a potent releaser of prolactin in man and certain other species and releases GH in some acromegalics. LHRH releases FSH as well as LH and is the only gonadotropin-releasing hormone (GnRH) for regulation of both of these gonadotropins. Somatostatin inhibits TSH secretion as well as somatotropic hormone secretion.

In the human subject, TRH and LHRH have been widely used for physiologic and diagnostic studies of pituitary function. These are considered later in this chapter.

One of the important consequences of these discoveries is that means have now been provided for selective manipulation of the secretion of TSH, LH-FSH, prolactin, and GH.

BIOGENIC AMINE CONTROL OF HYPOPHYSIOTROPIC FUNCTIONS

The hypophysiotropic peptide–secreting neurons of the hypothalamus are in turn innervated by specialized monoaminergic neurotransmitter neurons that arise in characteristic midbrain or brainstem nuclei. The principal bioaminergic pathways, dopaminergic, noradrenergic, and serotonergic, arise respectively in the substantia nigra, locus ceruleus, and raphe nuclei (Fig. 3). In addition to the nigral-hypothalamic input, there is another independent set of dopamine aminergic neurons, those of the arcuate nucleus (a nucleus found in the base of the hypothalamus), which are distributed to the median eminence and may be directly involved in the regulation of prolactin secretion. Drugs that act as dopamine agonists (for example, L-dopa or apomorphine) stimulate the release of growth hormone, and inhibit the release of prolactin. Noradrenergic agonists also stimulate GH release and, in addition, gonadotropins and TSH. Serotonin agonists (for example, tryptophan, a precursor of brain serotonin) release GH and prolactin, and suppress TSH release. Specificity of control derives both from neuropharmacologic coding and anatomic coding of these bioaminergic pathways. In turn, the functions of the central biogenic system are under the domination of inputs from various parts of the so-called visceral brain and hence are responsive to stress and emotional disturbance. Certain of the hormonal systems have rather complex control inputs. For example, each of the neurotransmitters capable of stimulating GH release (presumably through GHRH) respond to a certain class of physiologic stimuli. Sleep-induced GH is serotonin mediated, whereas hypoglycemia-induced GH release is an alpha-adrenergic dependent function. Each of the other anterior pituitary hormones is also controlled by a complex neuropharmacologic array of signals.

The central bioaminergic system serves other important functions in addition to its role in anterior pituitary regulation. The best known is the function of the dopaminergic pathway in control of extrapyramidal motor activity, disturbance of which gives rise to parkinsonism. Bioaminergic systems are also involved in determination of affective state, sleep and wakefulness, appetite and drinking behavior, and temperature regulation. Neuroleptic agents, widely used in psychiatry to modify mood or thought processes, act, at least in part, by stimulating or suppressing central bioaminergic pathways and may thereby interfere with or modify anterior pituitary function. Common examples are the administration of chlorpromazine, which inhibits GH secretion and stimulates prolactin, or reserpine, which inhibits TSH release and stimulates prolactin secretion. The serotonin antagonist cyproheptidine, used clinically as an antipruritic agent, will under certain circumstances inhibit nocturnal release of both GH and ACTH. Such agents are being used on an experimental basis to treat some forms of pituitary hypersecretion.

The hypophysiotropic neurons and the pituitary itself are involved in hormone feedback control of pituitary secretions. The relative importance of hypothalamic and pituitary feedback appears to differ to some degree from one system to another. The pituitary-thyroid axis is the best worked out of these control systems. Thyroid hormone regulates TSH secretion through a direct inhibitory effect on the anterior pituitary. These inhibitory effects are opposed by the stimulatory effect of hypothalamic drive brought about by TRH secretion. TRH secretion, a neurogenic function, is responsive to a variety of neural signals, including those involved in temperature regulation. Recent work indicates that somatostatin tonically inhibits TSH secretion.

Gonadotropic hormone secretion is regulated by a complex interaction of ovarian or testicular hormone feedback on both the pituitary and hypothalamus. Testosterone inhibits LH and FSH secretion through its action on the hypothalamus. Estrogens inhibit LH and FSH secretion in men at least in part by a direct inhibitory action on the pituitary, whereas in normal women, estrogens transiently inhibit and later sensitize the pituitary to LHRH. In fact, it is the sensitizing effect that may be responsible for mid-cycle ovulatory "surge" of LH. In addition to this hormonal interaction, gonadotropin secretion is subject to "open-loop" effects such as emotional stress (which in the human can inhibit ovulation) and in animals such as the rabbit copulation can trigger reflex ovulation.

Growth hormone secretion is almost exclusively controlled by the central nervous system. Estrogenic hormones appear to sensitize the pituitary to the growth hormone–releasing factor, and metabolic (as well as stress related) events are mediated at the level of the hypothalamus. An important aspect of GH regulation is so-called short-loop feedback control. Plasma GH itself is capable of inhibiting the secretion of GHRF, either directly or through the intervention of somatostatin.

Prolactin secretion, like GH secretion, is largely regulated by the nervous system; there is a short-loop feedback control, and estrogen also appears to sensitize the pituitary to the effects of PRF.

Cortisol feedback inhibition of the pituitary-adrenal axis appears to act both on the hypothalamus and the pituitary; cortisol may also act on suprahypothalamic neural structures. Some workers believe that all feedback control is directed at the pituitary and that results of experiments in which intrahypothalamic injection of cortisol was effective in inhibiting ACTH were due to transport of the cortisol via the median eminence to the pituitary.

An important recent insight is that pituitary secretion of growth hormone, prolactin, and ACTH is regulated by intrinsic brain rhythms related to the sleep-wake cycle or to changes in lighting, rather than by specific homeostatic requirements. Nocturnal GH secretion (largely related to early deep sleep) accounts for more than half of total daily GH secretion, values at night approaching the levels found in acromegaly. Nocturnal prolactin secretion begins about the same time that GH secretion does but appears to last longer. The secretion of ACTH with a peak in the early morning hours is linked to the day-night lighting cycle. Nocturnal rhythms for TSH and (under certain circumstances) gonadotropins have also been shown. Disturbances in sleep-related hormonal secretion may be the earliest indication of incipient or mild hypothalamic-pituitary disturbance. Proper evaluation of total endocrine function under physiologic or pathologic states must take into account these diurnal rhythms.

CENTRAL PEPTIDERGIC NEURON SYSTEMS

One of the most dramatic advances in neurobiology in the last decade has been the discovery of extensive peptidergic neuron systems analogous to the hypophysiotropic neuron system but with a broader distribution and wider physiologic importance. Two of the peptidergic pathways involve hypothalamic hormones, namely, the TRH and the somatostatinergic peptidergic pathways. TRH-containing nerves are distributed throughout the brain and spinal cord, and in the latter position appear to innervate the motor ventral horn cell. Somatostatinergic cells are widely distributed throughout the brain except for the cerebellum. They are found in the dorsal root ganglia as bipolar nerve cells, the central axon of which is directed to the dorsal horn of the spinal cord. Other important central peptidergic neuron systems include those containing angiotensin II, the endorphins, substance P, neurotensin, and cholecystokinin (Table 1). Cells containing certain of these peptides are distributed outside the brain, where they exert important regulatory functions. For example, somatostatin-containing cells are found in the gut and pancreatic islets, and in these locations regulate gastric acid, gastrin, insulin, and glucagon secretion. Enzyme systems for formation of angiotensin II in situ are found in the brain; angiotensinergic systems in the brain are involved in regulation of drinking behavior, ADH release, and blood pressure regulation. Substance P is found in dorsal root ganglia, in bipolar cells whose axons are distributed to skin, and in dorsal horn. These neurons are responsible for the flare component of the triple reaction observed upon skin injury, and may also be part of the pain perception pathway.

The endorphin system has important neuroendocrinologic implications. Endorphins are a class of endogenous brain constituents that bind to opiate receptors. They were discovered during efforts to identify substances in brain extracts that act like morphine. Several endorphins have been identified chemically, including two pentapeptides, leucine and methionine enkephalin, and three endorphins, termed alpha, beta, and gamma. The beta compound is the most powerful of all endorphins, and on a molar basis is more potent than morphine. There is evidence that methionine enkephalin and beta endorphin are found in neurons and in nerve endings within the brain. All the endorphins and meth-enkephalin appear to be parts of a larger molecule identical to the pituitary hormone β-lipotropin. The large linear peptide molecule (91 amino acids) also contains a segment identical to β-MSH and itself is part of a still larger prohormone which includes a segment identical with ACTH. The endorphins arise in the brain in situ (since they are demonstrable even in hypophysectomized rats), but may also arise by degradation from β-lipotropin.

The endorphins exert numerous physiologic effects on brain function as well as on endocrine function. They are involved in pain perception (raise pain threshold, cause addiction and tolerance to morphine, change motor function), and when injected into animals act on the hypothalamus to bring about the release of GH, prolactin, and ACTH. The endorphinergic system may be part of a "stress pathway."

On the basis of embryologic and histologic study, it has been proposed that all peptidergic neural systems, including those distributed both within and without the brain, are derived from embryonic neuroectoderm where they make up part of the APUD (amine precursor uptake decarboxylase) system, cell lines which also include melanocytes, sympathetic ganglia, pituitary basophils, thyroid C cells, and argentaffin cells of the gut from which carcinoid tumors arise. Because so many secretory and neurosecretory cells appear to arise from neural ectoderm, it has been proposed by Pearse and Guillemin that the endocrine system is in fact a division of the nervous system, although not all endocrinologists would agree with this assertion.

TABLE 1.   Several Hypothalamic Peptides Whose Structure and Action Are Known but Whose Physiologic Function Is Not Fully Understood*

Name	Structure
Substance P†	Arg-Pro-Lys-Pro-Gln-Gln-Phe-Phe-Gly-Leu-Met-NH₂
Neurotensin‡	<Glu-Leu-Tyr-Glu-Asn-Lys-Pro-Arg-Arg-Pro-Tyr-Ile-Leu-CoOH
Angiotensin II§	Asp-Arg-Val-Tyr-Ile-His-Pro-Phe
Leu-enkephalin¶	Tyr-Gly-Gly-Phe-Leu-OH
Meth-enkephalin¶	Tyr-Gly-Gly-Phe-Met-OH
α-Endorphin¶	Tyr-Gly-Gly-Phe-Met-Thr-Ser-Glx-Lys-Ser-Gln-Thr-Pro-Leu-Val-Thr-OH
β-Endorphin¶	Tyr-Gly-Gly-Phe-Met-Thr-Ser-Glu-Lys-Ser-Gln-Thr-Pro-Leu-Val-Thr-Leu-Phe-Lys-Asn-Ala-Ile-Val-Lys-Asn-Ala-His-Lys-Gly-Gln-OH
γ-Endorphin¶	Tyr-Gly-Gly-Phe-Met-Thr-Ser-Glu-Lys-Ser-Gln-Thr-Pro-Leu-Val-Thr-Leu-OH
Vasoactive inhibitory peptide**	His-Ser-Asp-Ala-Val-Phe-Thr-Asp-Asn-Tyr-Thr-Arg-Leu-Arg-Lys-Gln-Met-Ala-Val-Lys-Lys-Tyr-Leu-Asn-Ser-Ile-Leu-Asn-NH₂

*From Reichlin, S., *In* Reichlin, S., Baldessarini, R. J., and Martin, J. B. (eds.): The Hypothalamus. New York, Raven Press, 1978.

†Substance P (permeability factor) was originally found in dorsal root ganglia and now has been shown to be distributed in both peripheral and central axon projections of sensory ganglia. This peptide is probably responsible for the wheal reaction in the triple response to skin damage. Its function in brain and sensation is unknown, but it is believed to interact with the endorphins. In large doses it has an intense sialagogic effect.

‡Neurotensin is widely distributed in brain, and its identification in synaptosomes indicates a role as a neurotransmitter regulator of brain function. It causes a lowering of blood pressure and widespread increased capillary permeability and vasodilation.

§In the periphery, angiotensin II, a potent pressor agent, is formed from angiotensin I. Angiotensin II formed in situ in the hypothalamus, as in the periphery by converting enzyme, is believed to be involved in central regulation of blood pressure, drinking behavior, and ADH secretion.

¶The endorphins and enkephalins make up a class of compounds that react with endogenous opiate receptors in various brain sites, including hypothalamus, amygdala, dorsal root entry zone, and areas in ascending pain pathways. Their special function in the hypothalamus (as distinct from a role in pain perception) is unknown.

**VIP is found in the small intestine and in pancreatic islet cell tumors and more recently in hypothalamic extracts and in axonal endings in brain neurons. Although this peptide has many actions (produces hyperglycemia, acts as a hypotensive, stimulates water excretion by gut), its physiologic role in either the brain or the extraneural tissues is unknown.

NEUROENDOCRINE DISEASES OF THE PITUITARY GLAND

Any consideration of the neuroendocrine diseases of the pituitary overlaps the descriptions of diseases of the pituitary itself (see Ch. 543.5 to 543.7). The following paragraphs emphasize, primarily, neuroendocrine disorders of the anterior pituitary.

In the context of the foregoing description of the hypothalamic-pituitary unit, disorders of pituitary secretion can be viewed as occurring at many "levels" of function. Defects may arise resulting from destruction of the pituitary itself (as by a tumor), or from genetically determined deficiency of a particular type of pituitary cell. At a higher level, disorders may arise through disruption of the stalk–median eminence neurons or of their essential vascular channels to the anterior pituitary gland. Such destruction of the "final common path" of anterior pituitary regulation occurs after surgical stalk section, in tumors of the stalk region, e.g., craniopharyngioma, infundibuloma, or teratomas, and in such inflammations as sarcoidosis. In precocious puberty, the tonically active inhibitory system which determines the time at which the hypophysiotropic neurons will become active may be destroyed or inactivated too soon. Disease may also arise from abnormal stimulation of the hypophysiotropic neurons. The major endocrine syndromes of hypothalamic origin are listed in Table 2. The causes of hypothalamic disease are shown in Table 3.

Hypophysiotropic Hormone Deficiency

Introduction of TRH and LHRH into clinical medicine has made it possible to identify several syndromes of hypophysiotropic neuron failure. Deficiency of TSH secondary to TRH deficiency has been identified as a cause of thyroid failure. This disorder has been termed "*hypothalamic hypothyroidism*" or "*tertiary*" hypothyroidism. Isolated LHRH deficiency accounts for the endocrine deficiency in many patients with isolated gonadotropin deficiency, as in Kallmann's syndrome (hypogonadotropic hypogonadism with hyposmia). Isolated GHRF deficiency appears to underlie the growth hormone secretory failure in the bulk of patients with idiopathic dwarfism. There also appears to be a disorder of "panhypophysiotropic failure" in which all pituitary functions are lost. Most children with idiopathic panhypopituitarism fall into this category. The association of hypophysiotropic deficiency with abnormal EEG's, and a history of birth trauma in some cases, or its occurrence as a congenital loss of hypophysiotropic secretion, suggests an analogy with other forms of birth injury.

Hypophysiotropic deficiency can be induced by destruction of the hypophysiotropic area of the hypothalamus, of the stalk, or of the vascular supply to the anterior pituitary. Under most circumstances, acquired hypophysiotropic deficiency (as in surgical stalk section) results in a moderate to severe degree of pituitary failure, but the extent of endocrine deficit is not as extreme as that seen after hypophysectomy. This residuum of func-

TABLE 2. Endocrine Syndromes of
Hypothalamic Origin

Hypophysiotropic hormone deficiency:
 Surgical pituitary stalk section
 Basilar meningitis and granuloma, sarcoidosis, tuberculosis,
  sphenoid osteomyelitis, eosinophilic granuloma
 Craniopharyngioma
 Hypothalamic tumor
  Infundibuloma
  Teratoma (ectopic pinealoma)
  Neuroglial tumors, particularly astrocytoma
 Maternal deprivation syndrome
 Isolated GHRF deficiency
 Hypothalamic hypothyroidism
 Panhypophysiotropic failure
Disorders of regulation of LHRH:
 Female
  Precocious puberty
  Delayed puberty
  Neurogenic amenorrhea
   Pseudocyesis
   Anorexia nervosa
   "Functional amenorrhea"
   "Functional oligomenorrhea"
   Drug-induced amenorrhea
 Male
  Precocious puberty
  Fröhlich's syndrome
  Olfactory-genital dysplasia (Kallmann's syndrome)
Disorders of regulation of prolactin-inhibiting hormone (nonpuerperal galactorrhea):
 Tumor
 Sarcoid
 Drug-induced
 Reflex
  Herpes zoster of chest wall
  Post-thoracotomy
  Nipple manipulation
  Spinal cord tumor
 "Psychogenic"
 Chiari-Frommel syndrome
 Hypothyroidism
 CO_2 narcosis
Disorders of regulation of CRF:
 Paroxysmal ACTH discharge (Wolff's syndrome)
 Loss of circadian variation
 Depression

TABLE 3. Etiology of Hypothalamic Disease (by Age)*

I. Premature infants and neonates:
  Intraventricular hemorrhage
  Meningitis: bacterial
  Tumors: glioma, hemangioma
  Trauma
  Hydrocephalus, hydranencephaly, kernicterus
II. 1 month–2 years:
  Tumors:
   Glioma, especially optic glioma
   Histiocytosis X
   Hemangiomas
  Hydrocephalus, meningitis
  "Familial" disorders: Laurence-Moon-Biedl, Prader-Labhart-Willi
III. 2–10 years:
  Tumors:
   Craniopharyngioma
   Glioma, dysgerminoma, hamartoma, histiocytosis X, leukemia
   Ganglioneuroma, ependymoma, medulloblastoma
  Meningitis
   Bacterial
   Tuberculous
  Encephalitis
   Viral and demyelinating
   Various viral encephalitides and exanthematous
    demyelinating encephalitides
   Disseminated encephalomyelitis
  "Familial" disorders: diabetes insipidus, etc.
IV. 10–25 years:
  Tumors
   Craniopharyngioma
   Glioma, hamartoma, dysgerminoma
   Histiocytosis X, leukemia
   Dermoid, lipoma, neuroblastoma
  Trauma
  Subarachnoid hemorrhage, vascular aneurysm, arteriovenous
   malformation
  Inflammatory diseases, meningitis, encephalitis, sarcoid,
   tuberculosis
  Associated with midline brain defects: agenesis of corpus callosum
  Chronic hydrocephalus or increased intracranial pressure
V. 25–50 years:
  Nutritional: Wernicke's disease
  Tumors
   Glioma, lymphoma, menigioma
   Craniopharyngioma, pituitary tumors
   Angioma, plasmacytoma, colloid cysts
   Ependymoma, sarcoma, histiocytosis X
  Inflammatory
   Sarcoid
   Tuberculosis, viral encephalitis
  Subarachnoid hemorrhage, vascular aneurysm, arteriovenous
   malformation
  Damage from pituitary radiation therapy
VI. >50 years:
  Nutritional: Wernicke's disease
  Tumors
   Sarcoma, glioblastoma, lymphoma
   Meningioma, colloid cysts, ependymoma, pituitary tumors
  Vascular
   Infarct, subarachnoid hemorrhage
   Pituitary apoplexy
  Infectious: encephalitis, sarcoid, meningitis

*From Plum, F., and Van Uitert, R., *In* Reichlin, S., Baldessarini,
R. J., and Martin, J. B. (eds.): The Hypothalamus. New York, Raven
Press, 1978.

tion (which is readily duplicated in laboratory animals) has been thought in the past to represent the "autonomous" capacity of the pituitary to function independent of the hypothalamus. With the identification of syndromes of hypophysiotropic failure, as in "hypothalamic hypothyroidism" and panhypophysiotropic failure, has come the recognition that pituitary deficiency as severe as that observed after hypophysectomy can at times follow loss of hypothalamic function. It is probable that most of the so-called pituitary autonomy after stalk section is the result of residual hypothalamic hypophysiotropic function.

The main endocrine manifestations of hypothalamic failure are variable loss of TSH secretion, abolition of gonadotropin secretion, loss of normal GH secretory responses to hypoglycemia and other stimuli, and loss of normal sleep pattern. Circadian and tonic baseline corticotropin secretion is abolished, as is feedback control by circulating cortisol levels, but the response to certain kinds of stress, such as pyrogens, may be retained, suggesting that there are extrahypothalamic sites of formation of CRF. In sharp contrast to the hypophysectomized patient, individuals with hypothalamic disease usually have high circulating levels of prolactin owing to loss of PIF influence. Galactorrhea develops in about one fourth of women after section of the pituitary stalk,

although all have elevated prolactin levels in plasma. The most sensitive signs of hypothalamic damage appear to be loss of diurnal GH rhythms, loss of GH secretory responses to stress, and the capacity to have an ovulatory surge of LH secretion.

Disorders of Regulation of GHRF

In addition to idiopathic hypophysiotropic failure and specific damage to the hypothalamus or stalk, growth hormone deficiency may arise on a psychogenic basis in the so-called maternal deprivation syndrome (MDS). Such patients, generally children from grossly disturbed homes, may fail to grow despite adequate food intake. When they are brought into the hospital and given loving care, growth rate returns to normal. GH secretion is impaired or absent in such children, and they do not respond to the usual stimuli such as hypoglycemia or arginine infusion. Since this disturbance is reversible after psychologic management, it has been concluded that a functional inhibition of the hypophysiotropic GH-regulating neurons has taken place in these children. Deprivation in infants can cause marasmus. In contrast to purely psychosomatic interpretations of GH inhibition, some pediatricians believe that most such cases are attributable to food restriction rather than to bad mothering. Others attribute the poor growth to disordered sleep with consequent loss of characteristic sleep-induced GH release.

In adults a somewhat analogous situation is seen in severe "monopolar" depression. Failure to release GH in response to hypoglycemia or to L-dopa administration suggests that in such patients there is an abnormality in central hypophysiotropic function. In the light of modern ideas about the role of biogenic amines in determination of affective states, it is believed that the GH unresponsiveness in depression may be a reflection of abnormalities in central noradrenergic pathways in the hypothalamus.

In additon to GH unresponsiveness, some children with MDS may have unresponsive pituitary-adrenal function with loss of the circadian rhythm and of the response to the metyrapone test of ACTH reserve.

Excessive GHRF secretion has been proposed to be the cause of some cases of acromegaly.

Disorders of Regulation of GnRH

The concept of "levels" of neurogenic disruption of pituitary control is best illustrated in abnormalities of secretion of the gonadotropins. Deficiency of both LH and FSH occurs after destruction of the hypophysiotropic neurons. But disturbances also occur if the hypophysiotropic neurons are themselves abnormally stimulated. The characteristic pattern of male gonadotropin regulation is one of tonic low-level secretion of LH and FSH which leads to growth, development, and maturation of the spermatozoa, a process taking place over a 70-day period. The characteristic pattern of human female regulation is that of the recurring menstrual cycle, dependent upon a recurring surge of LH secretion, which is in turn dependent upon cyclic secretion of estrogens by the ovary. In certain forms of hypothalamic disease, the characteristic normally recurring cyclic pattern of LH secretion may be lost. Because this often occurs transiently in a setting of severe psychologic stress, as after incarceration in concentration camps, in bombing attacks, or after minor stress such as going away to school, and develops in the absence of evident structural disease of the pituitary or hypothalamus, it is probable that loss of LH cycling may be an acquired psychologic disorder. The terms "functional amenorrhea," "functional oligomenorrhea," and "hypothalamic amenorrhea" have been applied to such cases. These probably represent a neural inhibition of estrogen-induced LHRH secretion. A similar correlation appears likely in pseudocyesis, most often a manifestation

of hysteria, and in anorexia nervosa. In about half the cases of anorexia nervosa, amenorrhea begins coincident with the disturbance in eating, and for this reason must be regarded as a concomitant rather than a consequence of inanition. Resumpton of menstrual cycling does not occur until the patient has returned to a "critical weight," thus supporting the role of nutritional factors in this disease. Amenorrheic anorexia nervosa patients may show nocturnal LH secretory patterns appropriate to those seen in prepubertal girls.

Besides these more obvious psychogenic changes in menstrual function, many women with "secondary" amenorrhea are encountered who have no apparent psychologic distress, but in whom the pattern of menstrual irregularity, amenorrhea, and oligomenorrhea is similar to that seen in the neurogenic syndromes. In one series, fully one fourth of the women in this category who were placed into a research study after one year or more of anovulation developed normal cycles within a month of their entry into the research project.

Next to pregnancy, "functional" amenorrhea is the most common cause of a secondary failure to menstruate. A clear-cut differential diagnosis between functional amenorrhea and disease of the anterior pituitary or hypothalamus can now be made in most cases. The patient with pituitary or hypothalamic disease most often has more than one trophic hormone deficiency, may have evidence of local pituitary damage, e.g., enlarged sella by x-ray, visual field defects, and behavioral or other neurologic abnormalities of the hypothalamus. Sixty to 80 per cent of patients with "functional" amenorrhea release luteinizing hormone after treatment with the drug clomiphene. An important cause of amenorrhea is hyperprolactinemia, caused by a prolactinoma (whether roentgenographically apparent or occult) or attributable to no specific etiology. It has been suggested that idiopathic prolactinemia, like idiopathic gonadotropin failure, is in some women a psychosomatic disease. The use of LHRH as a diagnostic aid is outlined below.

Drug-induced anovulation should be borne in mind as a cause of amenorrhea. Reserpine and the phenothiazines are particularly common causes. Many patients who fail to resume normal menses after discontinuance of contraceptive pills ("post-pill amenorrhea") are suffering from hyperprolactinemia. Prolactin causes amenorrhea by a "short loop feedback" suppression of LHRH secretion at the hypothalamic level.

Gonadotropin regulatory difficulties may arise from loss of hypophysiotropic function, from failure of the intrinsic cycling mechanism, and, at a higher functional level, from precocious or delayed development of sexual maturation. The timing of the onset of puberty is a neural function, and involves a patterned development of brain analogous to the patterns of development of other brain functions such as crawling, sitting, or walking and the development of abstract ability. Both delayed and accelerated puberty can be observed. When sexual function is normal in other respects, the term *precocious puberty* is applied, in contradistinction to the condition arising from primary secretory abnormalities of the gonads, properly termed *pseudoprecocious puberty*. All true precocious puberty is neurogenic in origin. In males, more than half the cases are due to brain lesions which directly or indirectly impinge upon the hypothalamus. In girls, fewer than 10 per cent have demonstrable lesions, although a high proportion have EEG abnormalities and may be regarded as suffering from mild degrees of brain damage.

In the male, primary isolated gonadotropin failure is a well recognized cause of delayed puberty. In one type, there is an association with failure to develop rhinencephalic brain structures, manifested clinically by hyposmia. Such cases have been termed olfactory-genital dysplasia (Kallmann's syndrome), and appear to be due to failure to develop hypophysiotropic function, because the patients usually respond to injections of LHRH, albeit sluggishly. Cases of isolated gonadotropic failure resulting from intrinsic pituitary disease have also been identified.

Disorders of Regulation of PIF

Many conditions cause lactation unrelated to pregnancy (nonpuerperal galactorrhea). Certain chromophobe pituitary tumors may secrete prolactin and induce lactation (see Ch. 543.5). Hypothalamic disturbance or "psychogenic" factors are important causes of galactorrhea. Causes listed in Table 2 have in common a presumed deficiency of prolactin inhibitory hormone, whether caused by irritation of the neural pathways involved in normal suckling reflexes (herpes zoster, nipple stimulation, post-thoracotomy) or by drugs, encephalopathy, hypothyroidism, or direct damage to the hypothalamus or stalk. Still uncertain is the relative frequency of small chromophobe adenomas as a cause of prolactin hypersecretion.

USE OF THE HYPOTHALAMIC HORMONES IN DIAGNOSIS OF ANTERIOR PITUITARY DISEASE

Synthetic TRH and LHRH have been widely used for diagnostic purposes. The intravenous injection of TRH (15 to 800 μg; usual dose, 500 μg) is followed within five minutes by a rise in TSH which peaks between 15 and 45 minutes (Fig. 4). Changes in TSH secretion lead to a detectable increase in T_3 and a slight and less consistent increase in T_4. Mean responses in normal men are slightly less than in normal women, presumably owing to the estrogen sensitization of the anterior pituitary. In one series of normal subjects, mean maximal increment, $\pm$S.D. after 400 μg was 16.0 μU per ml$\pm$2.5; in another, mean response to 500 μg was 25 μU$\pm$10 of TSH. In normal people, prolactin levels also rise, and in many acromegalics (unlike the normal) GH levels may also rise. Pituitary failure causes a loss of the response to TRH or a reduction in response, and in patients with TRH hypophysiotropic failure the response may be

Figure 4. TSH and prolactin secretory response to TRH infusion (500 μg intravenously) in patient with hypothalamic hypothyroidism secondary to eosinophilic granuloma.

slightly delayed in onset, but may rise higher, presumably owing to the associated hypothyroidism. Thus, in theory, this test permits the differentiation between pituitary and hypothalamic forms of secondary hypothyroidism. However, in practice the TRH test has been somewhat disappointing in distinguishing sharply between pituitary and hypothalamic causes of TSH failure. Some patients with unquestionable hypothyroidism secondary to pituitary disease may respond normally to TRH, whereas some patients with hypothalamic disease may show poor responses. It is possible that the misleading cases with pituitary disease may have intrapituitary blockade of normal transmission of endogenous TRH from the hypothalamus. Normal older men particularly have relatively poor response to TRH (as low as 2 mU per 100 ml increment), and for this reason it is especially difficult to identify a pituitary abnormality with this test. (For a summary of normal values in the TRH test, see Table 4.) Because of the fact that thyroid hormone inhibits the pituitary, the response to TRH is also abolished in patients being treated with thyroid hormone, or in individuals with hyperthyroidism which may be so mild as to be barely detectable. This response, in fact, is a very sensitive test for mild degrees of hyperthyroidism. Recovery of TSH responsiveness may be very much delayed (as long as six weeks) after a course of thyroxine treatment.

LHRH has been used as a diagnostic aid in patients with hypogonadism caused by pituitary disease. The

TABLE 4.   Normal TSH Responses to TRH*

Sex	Dose (μg IV)	Response (μU/ml)
Women	500	>6
Men		
Age <30	500	>6
Age 40–79	500	>2
Men and women	500	Mean 15 (8.5–27.0)†
Children (1-10/12 to 14-3/12	500	23.3 ± 3.3 SEM

*Adapted from Martin, J. B., Reichlin, S., and Brown, G. M.: Clinical Neuroendocrinology. Philadelphia, F. A. Davis Company, 1977.

†Range of responses.

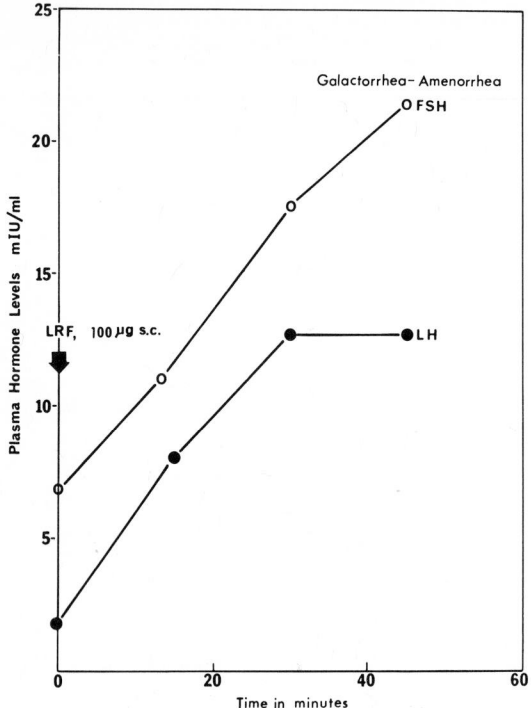

Figure 5. Changes in plasma LH and FSH after injection of LHRH. This patient with a chromophobe adenoma of the pituitary had been amenorrheic for 15 years. Plasma prolactin levels (not shown) were 365 ng per ml. The prompt and striking response to LHRH indicates that the amenorrhea was secondary to hypophysiotropic failure, in this case owing to prolactin-induced inhibition of LHRH secretion.

administration of 20 to 500 μg (usual dose, 100 μg) intravenously is followed by a prompt rise in serum LH and a somewhat less marked and later rise in serum FSH concentration (Fig. 5). Many patients show only the rise in serum LH. These responses vary with prior hormonal status. Patients with primary gonadal failure, i.e., menopause, have increased secretion rates of LH

and FSH, and show increased responses to LHRH. On the other hand, brief treatment with estrogenic hormones (one to three days) causes inhibition of responsiveness in women, whereas longer periods of treatment usually sensitize the pituitary response. In men, estrogenic hormones uniformly suppress pituitary responses to LHRH. In prepuberal boys there may be a relatively larger secretion of FSH than LH owing to the absence of inhibin, a peptide hormone secreted by the testis which selectively inhibits FSH release. It is important to recognize that the initial responses to LHRH may be markedly reduced, even in patients whose hypogonadism is secondary to hypothalamic disease. This is due to the fact that pituitary responsiveness to LHRH depends upon prior LHRH exposure. LHRH sensitizes the pituitary to LHRH. In patients with intrinsic pituitary failure sufficient to cause hypogonadism, LHRH may nevertheless be capable of stimulating release of LH and FSH. Because of these seemingly paradoxical responses, the use of LHRH as a diagnostic tool has not thus far permitted clear differentiation of hypothalamic from pituitary disorder, but is complementary to other studies. The role of LHRH as a diagnostic agent is still under investigation. Standard values are shown in Table 5. LHRH may prove to be of greatest clinical value in the *treatment* of hypogonadotropic hypogonadism rather than in its diagnosis.

Side effects after TRH include mild nausea, a transient lowering of blood pressure, and a sense of urinary urgency. "Allergic" symptoms have occasionally been observed, but no serious reactions have been reported, and even these mild symptoms are prevented if the material is injected over a two-minute period instead of a single rapid "bolus." No side effects have been observed after LHRH injection.

Guillemin, R., and Gerich, J.: Somatostatin: Physiologic and clinical significance. Ann. Rev. Med., 27:379, 1976.

Hayward, J. N.: Functional and morphological aspects of hypothalamic neurons. Physiol. Rev., 57:574, 1977.

Martin, J. B., Reichlin, S., and Brown, G. M.: Clinical Neuroendocrinology. Philadelphia, F. A. Davis Company, 1977.

Martini, L., and Ganong, W. F. (eds): Neuroendocrinology. New York, Academic Press, Vol. 1, 1966; Vol. 2, 1967.

TABLE 5.   Normal Responses to LHRH*

	Mean Max. Δ LH (mIU ± S.D.)	Mean Max. Δ FSH (mIU ± S.D.)
Men		
50 μg IV		
Age 21–30	37.7 ± 9.6	2.0 ± 0.3
250 μg IV		
Age 20–39	53.7 ± 31.7	3.0 ± 2.8
Age 40–49	54.3 ± 29.0	2.9 ± 2.3
Age 60–79	37.9 ± 18.5	1.1 ± 2.7
100 μg IV		
Age 18–40	32.2 ± 6.2	3.0 ± 1.4
Age >65	22.6 ± 3.8	3.2 ± 0.8
25 μg IV		
Infants 8–35 months	10.28 ± 2.01 (3.75–19.8)†	18.47 ± 6.43 (9.25–67.50)†
Women		
100 μg IV		
Follicular phase	17.5 ± 2.7	3.1 ± 0.6
Around LH peak	162.0 ± 49.0	7.6 ± 2.6
Luteal phase	49.6 ± 8.2	2.5 ± 0.4

*Adapted from Martin, J. B., Reichlin, S., and Brown, G. M.: Clinical Neuroendocrinology. Philadelphia, F. A. Davis Company, 1977.

†Range of responses.

Martini, L., and Ganong, W. F. (ed.): Frontiers in Neuroendocrinology. New York, Oxford University Press and Raven Press, Vol. 1, 1969; Vol. 2, 1971; Vol. 3, 1973; Vol. 4, 1975; Vol. 6, 1978.

Martini, L., and Besser, G. M.: Clinical Neuroendocrinology. New York, Academic Press, 1977.

Mortimer, C. H., et al.: The luteinizing hormone and follicle stimulating hormone–releasing hormone test in patients with hypothalamic-pituitary-gonadal dysfunction. Br. Med. J., 4:73, 1974.

Reichlin, S., Baldessarini, R. J., and Martin, J. B. (eds.): The Hypothalamus. New York, Raven Press, 1978.

Snyder, P. J. et al.: Diagnostic value of thyrotropin-releasing hormone in pituitary and hypothalamic diseases; assessment of thyrotrophin and prolactin secretion in 100 patients. Ann. Intern. Med., 81:751, 1974.

543. THE ANTERIOR PITUITARY

(Adenohypophysis)

Nicholas P. Christy

543.1. INTRODUCTION

Diseases of the anterior pituitary manifest themselves in two ways: mechanically, when space-occupying pituitary tumors impinge upon adjacent structures; and functionally, when there is deficient, excessive, or untimely secretion of some or all of the several hormones secreted by the gland.

HISTORY. The pituitary gland was first described by Vesalius in 1543. The earliest known artistic representation of pituitary disease is found in a sculptured figure on the Rheims Cathedral (thirteenth century): one of the gargoyles has distinctly acromegalic features. Good clinical and pathologic descriptions of acromegaly were provided by Verga (1864) and Fritzsche and Klebs (1884). Pierre Marie (1886) named the disease "acromegaly" because of the hypertrophy of the extremities. The pituitary tumor was recognized by Minkowski (1887) and by Broca (1888). In 1900, Benda ascribed the disorder to eosinophilic adenoma of the hypophysis.

Hypofunction of the pituitary was suspected by Lorain (1871), who associated dwarfism with pituitary destruction in man. Simmonds (1914) described the necropsy findings in an emaciated woman who proved to have extreme atrophy of the anterior pituitary and ovarian fibrosis and splanchnomicria. He correctly attributed the clinical picture to pituitary destruction, which he later showed could also result from tuberculosis or tumor (1916). Many later authors described clinical features now interpreted as those of pituitary insufficiency in patients with tumors of the infundibulum and chromophobe adenomas of the anterior lobe (Cushing and others, 1923–1938). The association of pituitary destruction with the puerperium was definitely established by H. L. Sheehan (1937–1949). He demonstrated acute pituitary necrosis in women dying shortly after difficult labor and traced the syndrome of chronic hypopituitarism and pituitary atrophy to episodes of postpartum hemorrhage.

Experimental elucidation of the functions of the pituitary began with Aschner's demonstration (1909) that hypophysectomy caused arrest of growth in young dogs. P. E. Smith observed failure of growth after hypophysectomy in the frog and the rat (1916–1926). In 1921, Evans and Long made the important observation that administration of pituitary extracts restored normal growth in the hypophysectomized animal and that large amounts of such growth-promoting extracts produced gigantism in the rat. Smith (1927–1930) described the

repair by hypophysial extracts of the gonadal, thyroidal, and adrenocortical atrophy that follows hypophysectomy. He also showed the distinctive effects of destruction of the pituitary (hypopituitarism) as opposed to the hypothalamus (obesity).

The last four decades have witnessed rapid progress in knowledge of the physiologic and biochemical effects of pituitary ablation in animals and man. The work of many investigators has led to methods for the extraction of progressively purer pituitary hormones for physiologic study and clinical use, to knowledge of the chemical structure of several, and to the measurement of all in plasma by radioimmunoassay (Berson and Yalow). Current experimental and clinical interest centers around the central nervous system control of anterior pituitary function (Harris and others), especially the role of the hypothalamic "releasing hormones" (see Ch. 542). Recent developments (1975–1978) have uncovered a new class of peptides isolated from brain (enkephalins) and from brain and pituitary (endorphins or "endogenous opiates"). These substances are structurally related to pituitary β-lipotropin, ACTH, and MSH. All those peptide hormones react to appropriate stimuli in a parallel manner. The potent opioid and behavioral properties of enkephalins and endorphins have suggested their possible importance in brain-pituitary interactions, pain mechanisms, affective disorders, and narcotic addiction (Goldstein, Guillemin).

For their methodologic and conceptual contributions to the detection and measurement of cerebral, hypothalamic (see Ch. 542), and pituitary peptides, the Americans R. S. Yalow, R. Guillemin, and A. V. Schally were awarded the Nobel Prize for Medicine or Physiology in 1977.

ANATOMY. The adult pituitary gland weighs 0.4 to 0.9 gram, averaging about 0.6 gram. It enlarges during pregnancy, and after repeated pregnancies may attain a weight of 1.0 to 1.5 grams; the weight tends to decrease in old age. The gland rests in the bony sella turcica and is bounded superiorly by the tough diaphragma sellae, a lamina of the dura mater. The pituitary stalk perforates the diaphragma and connects the pituitary to the hypothalamus; it contains the neurosecretory fibers, which pass from the supraoptic and paraventricular nuclei to the posterior pituitary (neurohypophysis) and the complex arterial and hypothalamic-hypophysial portal venous system, which serves as the functional connection between the nuclei of the hypothalamus and the anterior pituitary (see Ch. 542). For clinical purposes, the *gross anatomy* of the pituitary is the anatomy of the sella turcica; roentgenographic changes in that structure provide evidence of pituitary enlargement in the form of increase in the linear measurements of the sella and erosion, demineralization, or displacement of its bony borders. The normal sella can be oval, round, or flat. In normal adults, the anteroposterior diameter (sagittal plane) should not exceed 17 mm, the vertical diameter 14 mm, and the normal width (frontal projection) about 19 mm. Measured roentgenographically, the calculated area of the normal adult pituitary fossa (sagittal plane) does not exceed 130 sq mm; the volume is about 1100 cu mm. Even when sellar measurements are normal, pituitary tumor is suspected if there is suprasellar calcification, elevation or destruction of the anterior or posterior clinoids, demineralization or depression of the floor of the sella (Fig. 1), or "ballooning" of the fossa.

The pituitary fossa is enlarged in many but not all instances of intrasellar tumor; intrasellar calcification may be present. The fossa is also large in some suprasellar tumors with intrasellar extension, e.g., craniopharyngioma, metastases to the sella (as from carcinoma of the breast or prostate), longstanding increase of

Figure 1. Craniopharyngioma in a 69-year-old woman. The lateral (sagittal) film of the skull shows suprasellar calcification and a normal-sized sella with depression of the sellar floor and some flattening of the dorsum sellae. Craniopharyngioma more commonly has its clinical onset in late childhood.

pic'' or ''mammotropic'') can be distinguished from the growth hormone–secreting acidophil by special stains. Increased numbers of these cells, now accepted as *prolactin*-secreting, are found in the pituitaries of pregnant and lactating women and patients with galactorrhea. A recognizable type of basophil secretes gonadotropins; there is some evidence that two distinct subtypes of basophils produce FSH and LH. Gonadotropin-secreting basophils are few or absent in childhood, but increase in number at puberty; there are subtle changes during the menstrual cycle; marked changes are observed after castration and menopause. The thyrotropin-secreting cell is another identifiable type of basophil. The number of these cells increases, and the morphology changes with thyroprivic states. The corticotropin- (ACTH-) secreting basophil, known as the (R) basophil, probably also secretes MSH in man; the human pituitary lacks a definite intermediate lobe, the source of MSH secretion in lower animals. ACTH, β-lipotropin, and endorphins occur in the same pituitary cells and within the same secretory granules.

The pituitary tumors described by Cushing in hyperadrenocorticism are basophilic. In the absence of pituitary tumor, the most notable feature of pituitary cytology in patients with Cushing's syndrome is in the basophils; the cytoplasm becomes hyalinized (''Crooke's change''), an abnormality also found in patients with hyperadrenocorticism due to large doses of administered adrenocortical steroids. In the aggressive pituitary tumors that occur after bilateral adrenalectomy in 10 to 15 per cent of patients with Cushing's syndrome with bilateral adrenal cortical hyperfunction (owing to oversecretion of ACTH by the pituitary), the cell type is a distinctive kind of chromophobe which often has the capacity to secrete MSH as well as ACTH (see Ch. 547.7).

Abrams, H. L., and McNeil, B. J.: Medical implications of computed tomography (''CAT scanning''). N. Engl. J. Med., 298:255, 310, 1978.

Adams, J. H., Daniel, P. M., and Prichard, M. M. L.: Observations on the portal circulation of the pituitary gland. Neuroendocrinology, 1:193, 1965/66.

Baker, B. L.: Functional cytology of the hypophysial pars distalis and pars intermedia. *In* Knobil, E., and Sawyer, W. H. (eds.): Handbook of Physiology, Section 7, Endocrinology, Vol. IV: The Pituitary Gland and Its Neuroendocrine Control, Part I. Washington, D.C., American Physiological Society, 1974, p. 45.

Berglund, R. M., Ray, B. S., and Torack, R. M.: Anatomical variations in the pituitary gland and adjacent structures in 225 human autopsy cases. J. Neurosurg., 28:93, 1968.

Guillemin, R.: Editorial: Endorphins, brain peptides that act like opiates. N. Engl. J. Med., 296:226, 1977.

Harris, G. W., and Donovan, B. T. (eds.): The Pituitary Gland, 3 vols. Berkeley, University of California Press, 1966.

New, P. F. J.: The sella turcica as a mirror of disease. Radiol. Clin. North Am., 4:75, 1966.

Russfield, A. B.: Adenohypophysis. *In* Bloodworth, J. M. B. (ed.): Endocrine Pathology, Baltimore, Williams & Wilkins Company, 1968, p. 75.

intracranial pressure from any cause, the so-called ''empty sella syndrome,'' and hypothyroidism (see Ch. 543.5). The fossa is often small in patients with postpartum pituitary necrosis (Sheehan's syndrome), hypopituitary dwarfism without pituitary tumor, and myotonic muscular dystrophy. Rarely observed in presumably normal people, the significance of the small sella is not clear. Roentgenographic changes in the base of the skull may involve the sella in several disorders, e.g., osteoporosis, Paget's disease, Hand-Schüller-Christian disease, and Hurler's syndrome.

When pituitary tumors extend upward through the diaphragma sellae they encroach upon the optic chiasm to produce bitemporal hemianopia. When such tumors impinge on the pituitary stalk or the diencephalon there may be symptoms of hypothalamic involvement (diabetes insipidus, galactorrhea). Such upward extensions can often be seen roentgenographically with the use of pneumoencephalography, carotid artery angiography, or computerized axial tomography (''CAT scanning'').

The *microscopic anatomy* of the anterior pituitary is complex. The classic concept of secretory acidophilic (eosinophilic) and basophilic cells and functionless chromophobes has to be modified in the light of recent data. There appear to be at least five or six distinct kinds of cells; it is probable that each pituitary hormone is secreted by one of the distinct cell types. Somatotropic cells are acidophils which secrete growth hormone. The pituitary tumors associated with acromegaly (excessive secretion of growth hormone) are usually composed of acidophils; sometimes the tumors consist of acidophils mixed with chromophobes, chromophobes alone, or cells which have features of both types of cell (''amphophils''). Another kind of acidophil has been identified in the primate and human pituitary. This larger acidophil (known as ''lactotro-

543.2. ANTERIOR PITUITARY FUNCTION IN NORMAL SUBJECTS AND IN PATIENTS WITH SYSTEMIC DISEASES

By means of the ten or more peptide hormones it secretes, the anterior pituitary helps to regulate orderly growth, timely maturation, reproduction, and many aspects of metabolism.

The role of the maternal pituitary in governing the normal growth and development of the *fetus* is not clear. Hypopituitary dwarfs nearly always have normal birth weight and length, yet maternal growth hormone does not pass across the placental barrier. The operative growth factor may be placental lactogen. In anencephalic infants whose pituitary tissue is often diminished in amount or abnormal, the *"target glands"* — thyroid, fetal adrenal cortex, gonads — tend to be partly atrophied. In *childhood* the anterior pituitary influence on *growth* is profound. Deficiencies in HGH secretion announce themselves early in the first year of life. Anterior pituitary insufficiency, stemming from either hypothalamic or intrinsic hypophyseal disease, often is manifest in *delayed puberty*. Exactly what mechanisms trigger the onset of *normal puberty* (i.e., the onset of increased pituitary secretion of gonadotropins) are not clear. Factors that are probably important include changes in the positive feedback relationships between gonadal steroids and pituitary FSH/LH release, changes in the sensitivity of gonadotropin response to hypothalamic LHRH, and the emergence of episodic secretory patterns of gonadotropins and of gonadal steroids. The integrity of anterior pituitary function is essential in the *adult* for most of the proper functions of the gonads, thyroid, and adrenal cortex. Normal maintenance of *early pregnancy* and of *lactation* depends upon an intact pituitary. The adenohypophysis usually undergoes progressive fibrous replacement and sometimes deposition of iron with *aging*. The functional significance of these findings is not known.

Abnormalities of pituitary hormonal secretion have been demonstrated in many *nonendocrine systemic diseases*. Some of these changes may be merely laboratory curiosities and not of much clinical importance, but several may turn out to be of concern to the patient and physician. Further studies will be needed to permit evaluation of the significance of these altered pituitary functions in systemic disorders. A list of representative abnormalities is given in Table 1.

Christy, N. P., and Warren, M. P.: Disease syndromes of the hypothalamus and anterior pituitary. *In* DeGroot, L. J., et al. (eds.): The Metabolic Basis of Endocrinology. New York, Grune & Stratton, 1979, in press.

Grumbach, M. M., Grave, G. D., and Mayer, F. E (eds.): Control of the Onset of Puberty. 4th ed. New York, John Wiley & Sons, 1974.

Schönberg, D. K.: Dynamics of hypothalamic-pituitary function during puberty. J. Clin. Endocrinol. Metab., 41:57, 1975.

543.3. THE HORMONES OF THE ANTERIOR PITUITARY

Many *protein* or *peptide hormones* have been isolated from human pituitary tissue. These include growth hormone, prolactin, follicle-stimulating hormone, luteinizing hormone, thyrotropin, adrenocorticotropin, melanocyte-stimulating hormone, β-lipotropin, and endorphins. Each is regulated by the *releasing hormones of the hypothalamus* which stimulate the secretion of pituitary peptides; it is not yet certain that the releasing factors act to increase the synthesis of all the pituitary hormones. *Hypothalamic inhibitory factors* also exert an important regulatory influence. The tonic control of prolactin secretion is exerted by prolactin-inhibiting factor (PIF), and there are inhibitory peptides for growth hormone ("somatostatin") and MSH.

Pituitary hormones act directly (prolactin) or through "second messengers." The growth-promoting activity of growth hormone is possibly via an intermediary protein, "somatomedin" (see below); the gonadotropins, TSH and ACTH, stimulate hormone synthesis in their corresponding target glands via cyclic AMP.

TABLE 1. Abnormalities of Anterior Pituitary Function in Various Systemic Conditions*

Disorder	Pathologic Manifestation	Frequency	Clinical or Chemical Manifestation
Carcinomatosis	Pituitary metastases	Rare (0.1%)	Hypopituitarism (rarely)
Histiocytosis X	Hypothalamic-pituitary infiltration	Uncommon	HGH deficiency
Radiotherapy of extrasellar tumors	Hypothalamic injury	Common	Altered HGH secretion
Severe acute illness (e.g., cardiac surgery)	Pituitary necrosis	Unknown	?Fatal outcome
Myocardial infarction	Unknown	Unknown	Altered TSH secretion
Generalized sepsis, meningitis, pneumonia	Unknown (?pituitary abscess)	Rare	Varying degrees of hypopituitarism
Starvation (anorexia nervosa, maternal deprivation syndrome)	Hypothalamic injury (presumed)	Common	HGH secretion raised or reduced; altered TSH values
Chronic renal failure	Unknown	Not rare	Decreased somatomedin Hyporesponse of TSH to TRH
Myotonic muscular dystrophy	Small pituitary fossa	Common	Altered FSH levels Altered HGH response Low testosterone values
Thalassemia major	?Iron deposits in pituitary	Unknown	Raised plasma HGH
Fanconi's anemia	Unknown	Unknown	Low HGH values (sometimes)
Parkinsonians treated with L-dopa	"Poisoning" of the hypothalamus (presumed)	Unknown	"Abnormal function"
Carcinoid syndrome	Unknown	Unknown	Altered LH secretion
Emotional disorders			
Homosexuality (male)	None known	Common	FSH and LH values normal
Hebephrenic schizophrenia	None known	Unknown	HGH response to hypoglycemia sometimes low
Drug administration			
Alcoholism (chronic)	Unknown	Unknown	Raised LH response to LHRH Testosterone sometimes raised TSH hyporesponse to TRH
Lithium carbonate (chronic)	Unknown	Unknown	TSH hyper-response to TRH
Morphine (acute)	Unknown	Unknown	Raised plasma prolactin values

*Data abstracted from Christy, N. P., and Warren, M. P., *In* DeGroot, L. J., et al. (eds.): The Metabolic Basis of Endocrinology. New York, Grune & Stratton, 1979, in press.

Largely controlled by the central nervous system (see Ch. 540 and 542), the anterior pituitary hormones profoundly affect growth, maturation, reproduction, and metabolism. The paragraphs immediately following deal with the chemistry, physiology, and regulation of these hormones under normal conditions; pathologic states are discussed in Ch. 543.4.

Berson, S. A., and Yalow, R. S.: Methods in Investigative and Diagnostic Endocrinology. Vol. 2A, Peptide Hormones. New York, American Elsevier Publishing Company, 1973.

Knobil, E., and Sawyer, W. H. (eds.): Handbook of Physiology, Section 7, Endocrinology, Vol. IV: The Pituitary Gland and Its Neuroendocrine Control, Part 2. Washington, D.C., American Physiological Society, 1974.

Reichlin, S.: Neuroendocrinology. In Williams, R. H. (ed.): Textbook of Endocrinology. 5th ed. Philadelphia, W. B. Saunders Company, 1974, p. 774.

GROWTH HORMONE
(Somatotropin)

Pituitary growth hormone is the substance that, secreted or given in excessive amount, induces gigantism and acromegaly in animals and man; its absence results in failure to grow. The hormone exerts a major influence on somatic growth in man from an early stage of infancy. It also has widespread metabolic effects in both young and adult subjects.

Chemically, human growth hormone (HGH) is a single-chain peptide containing 190 amino acids whose sequence is now known; the molecular weight is 21,500.

Within the substance of the gland and in the plasma, HGH is heterogeneous, existing in at least two forms. "Orthodox" HGH (the 21,500 peptide) has in common with prolactin and placental lactogen several segments of identical amino acid sequence; all three hormones may be phylogenetically descended from a single primordial peptide. The production rate is about 500 μg per day.

The physiologic effects of HGH are many. The salient action is anabolic. In the hypophysectomized, dwarfed animal, GH administration induces symmetrical growth of the skeleton (chondrogenesis and osteogenesis), the musculature, and viscera. Several effects of HGH on cartilage appear to operate through the obligatory intermediate, *"sulfation factor"* or *"somatomedin,"* a protein of molecular weight 8000 whose site of origin is the liver. Somatomedin is thought to play a vital role in HGH-induced skeletal growth. Optimal growth response also requires the presence of thyroid hormone and insulin. HGH causes both cellular hypertrophy and hyperplasia; there is an increased rate of cellular mitosis, as well as an increase in tissue and organ weight. The hormone induces accelerated transport of specific amino acids into cells, stimulates synthesis of messenger and ribosomal RNA, and influences the activity of several enzymes.

HGH augments protein anabolism in hypophysectomized or hypopituitary human subjects. Nitrogen retention occurs within 24 to 48 hours; BUN concentration falls even earlier, within 12 to 24 hours. Nitrogen storage is great (3 to 4 grams per day) for the first several days of treatment, then falls to an amount compatible with growth requirements, about 0.3 gram of nitrogen retained per day in children 9 to 13 years of age. Linear growth can be induced in hypopituitary dwarfs (see Pituitary Insufficiency in Childhood, in Ch. 543.6).

HGH evokes changes in electrolyte and water metabolism. Tissue protein and water are increased. Phosphorus and potassium are stored, the latter in amounts larger than can be accounted for by the estimated quantity of new tissue formed. Moderate sodium retention occurs. Hypercalciuria is the rule, but most studies of calcium metabolism indicate an over-all positive calcium balance.

The increase in tissue mass induced by administration of HGH is not accompanied by fat deposition. The hormone is in fact adipokinetic. Although many other pituitary hormones have fat-mobilizing properties, e.g., prolactin, thyrotropin, corticotropin, MSH, and several other peptides, HGH appears to be the major adipokinetic principle of the human anterior pituitary. Administration of this hormone to hypophysectomized man rapidly stimulates the release of fat from adipose tissue, with a rise in plasma free fatty acids. This HGH effect on fat metabolism may operate in the anabolic response by ensuring a supply of calories, yet sparing protein breakdown through gluconeogenesis. In acromegalic patients, fat deposition is notably absent; obesity is extremely rare.

HGH also affects carbohydrate metabolism. The hormone is well known to be diabetogenic; many acromegalics have diabetes. The diabetic state is characterized by fasting hyperglycemia, impaired glucose tolerance, insulin resistance, lipemia, and ketosis. HGH given to normal subjects produces only minor changes; in diabetics the diabetes is often substantially exacerbated. Nondiabetic and diabetic subjects are much more sensitive to this effect of growth hormone after hypophysectomy.

The closely interrelated effects of HGH on fat and carbohydrate metabolism may be of great importance in concert with insulin, not only in promoting growth but also in maintaining homeostasis during feast or famine.

Most important observations have followed the recent development of accurate methods for the measurement of HGH in serum by radioimmunoassay (see Ch. 543.4). The findings have provided new insights into the role of the hormone in the growth of children. Basal serum concentrations and secretion rates are slightly higher in young children and adolescents than in older children or adults.

The serum concentration of HGH in *adults* is extremely labile, responding to many stimuli, and being spontaneously secreted in periodic bursts under the influence of the CNS. Serum values rise at the onset of deep sleep. Rapid rises in the serum levels of HGH are induced by hypoglycemia, fasting, and exercise; in some obese subjects these responses are blunted. HGH response to hypoglycemia is inhibited by corticosteroids. Hypoglycemia-induced rises in HGH level are quickly suppressed when glucose is given. Ambulation raises the serum levels of HGH in women, not in men; estrogen administration reproduces this increase. Increases in ambulatory (not basal) serum levels of growth hormone occur during the luteal phase of the menstrual cycle. Growth hormone also participates in the response to *stress*, e.g., surgery, but the pattern of response differs from that of ACTH; this suggests that the neural pathways influencing the two hormones are different. Infusion of amino acids, ACTH, glucagon, and large amounts of catecholamines and oral administration of L-dopa also stimulate HGH secretion. Chlorpromazine and the hypothalamic hormone somatostatin inhibit pituitary release of HGH. The production rate of HGH is subnormal in hypothyroidism, raised in hyperthyroidism.

Apart from the obvious value of measuring serum levels of HGH for the diagnosis of hypopituitarism and acromegaly, the aforementioned findings have clearly shown that HGH is not secreted at a uniform rate in adults. The lability of response to many metabolic events indicates that the hormone is not functionless in adults, as formerly thought, but participates in the day-to-day regulation of organic metabolism.

The use of the hormone in treatment of HGH deficiency is discussed in Ch. 543.6 under Pituitary Insufficiency in Childhood.

Berson, S. A., and Yalow, R. S.: Radioimmunoassay of peptide hormones in plasma. N. Engl. J. Med., 277:640, 1967.
Guillemin, R., and Gerich, J.: Somatostatin: Physiologic and clinical significance. Ann. Rev. Med., 27:379, 1976.
Li, C. H.: Hormones of the adenohypophysis. Proc. Am. Philosoph. Soc., 116:365, 1972.
Martin, J. B.: Neural regulation of growth hormone secretion. N. Engl. J. Med., 288:1384, 1973.
Van Wyk, J. J., and Underwood, L. E.: Relation between growth hormone and somatomedin: Definition of somatomedin. Ann. Rev. Med., 26:427, 1975.

PROLACTIN
(Lactogenic Hormone)

Because of many chemical and biologic similarities to HGH, prolactin was not recognized as a separate hormone in man until recently. Human prolactin is now definitely established as a distinct hormone, distinguishable from HGH. The evidence is this: the human pituitary during pregnancy and lactation and in galactorrhea contains many acidophils that are unlike HGH-secreting acidophils; patients with galactorrhea do not have high plasma HGH concentrations; plasma HGH is not raised in lactating women; normal postpartum lactation occurs in mothers with isolated HGH deficiency; pituitary tumors from women with galactorrhea have been shown to contain large amounts of prolactin activity not neutralizable with anti-HGH antiserum; bioassay experiments have indicated high prolactin activity in the presence of low immunoassayable HGH in normal and pathologic lactation; and prolactin has been found to be immunologically distinct from HGH.

In women, prolactin governs growth, development, and milk formation in the breast. These effects require the presence of estrogens, progestogens, adrenocortical steroids, insulin, and perhaps HGH. The physiologic role of prolactin in men is not yet clear.

The hormone is a single polypeptide chain (molecular weight about 23,000) containing 198 amino acids; its chemical similarity to HGH and human placental lactogen (HPL) has been described above.

Prolactin has more than 20 physiologic and behavioral actions in animals and man, most of them related to reproduction. Apart from its effect on the primate breast, prolactin controls cutaneous "milk" secretion in certain teleost fish, the renal osmoregulatory adaptation of salmon migrating to fresh water, hormone secretion by the corpus luteum in some rodents, and broodpatch formation in birds. In man, prolactin has growth-promoting (and nitrogen-retaining) effects similar to but much weaker than those of HGH; the hormone may also induce renal sodium, potassium, and water retention. The role of prolactin in human breast cancer is now under intense study.

Prolactin is secreted throughout the day in *periodic bursts* temporally unrelated to those of HGH. Plasma levels are lowest during the waking hours, rising 60 to 90 minutes after the onset of sleep and reaching highest concentrations at 5 to 7 A.M. Plasma levels do not vary from day to day throughout the normal *menstrual cycle*, but rise progressively during *pregnancy*; there are sharp rises during *breast feeding*.

Many *physiologic stimuli* elicit increased secretion of prolactin. These include suckling in postpartum women, stimulation of the nonlactating breast (women show a greater response than men), strenuous physical exercise, sexual intercourse in women (most striking when orgasm occurs), profound hypoglycemia, and surgical stress; plasma prolactin values fall with prolonged fasting. Several *pharmacologic agents* alter plasma prolactin levels. Rises follow the administration of TRH, estrogens (but not progesterone), arginine, phenothiazines and other tranquilizing drugs (which sometimes cause galactorrhea), and reserpine. L-Dopa, nicotine, and ergot alkaloids induce falls in plasma prolactin concentration. Chlorpromazine and L-dopa appear to exert their effects by respectively inhibiting and stimulating the hypothalamic secretion of PIF.

Frantz, A. G.: Prolactin, N. Engl. J. Med., 298:201, 1978.
Friesen, H. G., Guyda, H., Hwang, P., Tyson, J. E., and Barbeau, A.: Functional evaluation of prolactin secretion: A guide to therapy. J. Clin. Invest., 51:706, 1972.
Smithline, F., Sherman, L., and Kolodny, H. D.: Prolactin and breast carcinoma. N. Engl. J. Med., 292:784, 1975.
Tyson, J. E., Friesen, H. G., and Anderson, M. S.: Human lactational and ovarian response to endogenous prolactin release. Science, 177:897, 1972.

FOLLICLE-STIMULATING HORMONE
(FSH)

Follicle-stimulating hormone is the pituitary hormone essential for the normal cyclic growth of the ovarian follicle and for restoration of follicular growth in the hypophysectomized female; it stimulates spermatogenesis in the male without significant influence on the androgen-secreting interstitial cells of the testis. For optimal effect upon both ovary and testis, FSH seems to require the presence of luteinizing hormone (LH).

The molecular weight of human FSH is not finally established; estimates vary between 24,000 and 35,000. It is a glycoprotein, containing 7 per cent carbohydrate. Sialic acid is an integral part of the molecule; biologic activity is lost on exposure to neuraminidase. The purest preparations contain slight LH activity. FSH comprises two subunits: an α subunit which resembles the α subunits of LH and human chorionic gonadotropin (HCG), and a unique β subunit in which the specific biologic activity of FSH probably resides.

Administration of purified human FSH to amenorrheic women elicits increased secretion of estrogens and may stimulate the ovary to polycystic enlargement; given together with HCG, FSH sometimes provokes spermatogenesis. Discussion of the use of human gonadotropins in the treatment of infertility in men and women is found in Ch. 548.4 and 549.2.

Gonadotropin concentrations are low in the pituitaries and in the plasma and urine of infants and young children. The hormones rise to reach detectable levels

SECRETION OF PITUITARY AND OVARIAN HORMONES
IN THE NORMAL MENSTRUAL CYCLE

and negative feedback control of gonadotropin release by estrogens and progesterone is dealt with in Ch. 549.1. This chapter sets out the pattern of hormone secretion during the normal menstrual cycle. Figure 2 shows the cyclic secretion of FSH, LH, estradiol, and progesterone. During the early *follicular phase,* plasma FSH rises from its nadir during menstruation, and then, while estrogen secretion is rising, falls toward mid-cycle. In this phase, plasma LH progressively rises toward mid-cycle. Just after the peak level of estrogen, now thought to stimulate gonadotropin (LH) release, both FSH and LH reach their maximal secretion rate (day 0 in Fig. 2); the average daily production rates of FSH and LH are 15 and 30 μg per day, respectively, increasing 10- to 15-fold at *mid-cycle,* when *ovulation* occurs. Values for plasma FSH and LH then decline through the *luteal phase* (FSH being lowest when progesterone levels are high), LH rising slightly as estrogen and progesterone values fall just before menses.

Unopposed by the negative feedback action of gonadal hormones, plasma and urinary FSH values are high, as in ovariectomized and postmenopausal women. In females, the negative feedback is in part due to estrogen inhibition of hypothalamic gonadotropin-releasing hormone (LHRH); in the male, the inhibiting testicular hormone may be elaborated by the seminiferous tubule, testosterone being a weak suppressor of FSH secretion.

Baghdassarian, A., Guyda, H., Johnson, A., Migeon, C. J., and Blizzard, R. M.: Urinary excretion of radioimmunoassayable luteinizing hormone (LH) in normal male children and adults, according to age and stage of sexual development. J. Clin. Endocrinol. Metab., 31:428, 1970.

Odell, W. D., and Moyer, D. L.: Physiology of Reproduction. St. Louis, C. V. Mosby Company, 1971.

Rifkind, A. B., Kulin, H. E., and Ross, G. T.: Follicle stimulating hormone (FSH) and luteinizing hormone in the urine of prepubertal children. J. Clin. Invest., 46:1925, 1967.

Ross, G. T., Cargille, C. M., Lipsett, M. B., Rayford, P. L., Marshall, J. R., Strott, C. A., and Rodbard, D.: Pituitary and gonadal hormones in women during spontaneous and induced ovulatory cycles. Recent Prog. Horm. Res., 26:1, 1970.

Schally, A. V., Nair, R. M. G., Redding, T. W., and Arimura, A.: Isolation of the luteinizing and follicle-stimulating hormone-releasing hormone from porcine hypothalami. J. Biol. Chem., 246:7230, 1971.

Vande Wiele, R. L., Bogumil, J., Dyrenfurth, I., Ferin, M., Jewelewicz, R., Warren, M., Rizkallah, T., and Mikhail, G.: Mechanisms regulating the menstrual cycle in women. Recent Prog. Horm. Res., 26:63, 1970.

Figure 2. Notice the fall of plasma estradiol values on the day before the midcycle peak of FSH and LH. Plasma estradiol and progesterone concentrations both rise during the luteal phase after the midcycle "surge" of gonadotropin. The luteal rise in progesterone is reflected by a rise in basal body temperature (BBT) and increased urinary excretion of pregnanediol. The black bar denotes menses. (Adapted from Yen, S. C. C., Vela, P., Rankin, J., and Littell, A. S.: JAMA, 211:1513, 1970; and Catt, K. J.: Lancet, 1:1097, 1970.)

well before puberty. In adult women, the values are about the same as those for men during the preovulatory (follicular) and postovulatory (luteal) phases of the menstrual cycle. In adult men, FSH and LH are secreted in arrhythmic, pulsatile bursts (like ACTH [q.v.]), during sleep, but without temporal relation to the phasic peaks of HGH and prolactin secretion.

SECRETION OF GONADOTROPINS DURING THE NORMAL MENSTRUAL CYCLE. Hypothalamic control of FSH and LH secretion by one or more hypothalamic releasing factors is discussed in Ch. 542, and the role of positive

LUTEINIZING HORMONE OR INTERSTITIAL CELL–STIMULATING HORMONE
(LH or ICSH)

Luteinizing hormone is essential for ovulation, for the formation of the corpus luteum, and for stimulation of steroid hormone secretion by that structure. Acting alone, it does not produce follicular growth; to be effective, LH requires the prior action of FSH on the follicle. Human LH is assumed to be the luteotropic hormone; there is evidence that the corpus luteum has an intrinsic life span that is not much influenced by pituitary hormones. LH also stimulates the growth and secretory activity of the testicular interstitial cells. This interstitial cell–stimulating activity is sufficient to correct the testicular endocrine defect of hypophysectomy, producing androgen secretion and maintenance of the secondary sex organs. The steroidogenic action of LH on the corpus luteum and the Leydig cells is mediated by cyclic AMP. Spermatogenesis in man requires the synergism of FSH.

Like FSH, LH is a glycoprotein. Human LH (ICSH) has a molecular weight estimated at about 28,000. It is composed of two subunits, designated α and β; the α subunit is chemically similar to that of FSH and TSH, so that the hormonal specificity of LH probably resides in the β subunit. The hormone has been little used therapeutically; the more readily available human chorionic gonadotropin (HCG), which also contains an α subunit similar to that of human LH, has predominantly LH properties and is used instead.

The circadian and cyclic secretion of LH is described above (see FSH and Fig. 1). Partly through their action on the elaboration of hypothalamic FSH/LH-releasing hormone (LHRH), testosterone, estrogen, and progestogens inhibit the secretion of LH. In men testosterone lowers plasma LH levels; in women estrogen-progestin combinations (as in antiovulatory drugs) suppress the mid-cycle "surge" of LH and reduce LH secretion in the postmenopausal state (*negative* feedback inhibition). Conversely, LH values are high in castrate men and postmenopausal women. It appears that the concentration of circulating estrogen in the late follicular phase of the menstrual cycle *stimulates* LH release, an example of *positive* hormonal feedback.

Lipsett, M. B., Cargille, C. M., and Ross, G. T.: Reproductive endocrinology: Methodologic advances and clinical studies. Ann. Intern. Med., 72:933, 1970.

Marsh, J. M., Butcher, R. W., Savard, K., and Sutherland, E. W.: The stimulating effect of luteinizing hormone on adenosine-3',5'-monophosphate accumulation in corpus luteum slices. J. Biol. Chem.; 241:5436, 1966.

Santen, R. J., and Bardin, C. W.: Episodic luteinizing hormone secretion in man. Pulse analysis, clinical interpretation, physiologic mechanisms. J. Clin. Invest., 52:2617, 1973.

Saxena, B. B., Beling, C. G., and Gandy, H. M. (eds.): Gonadotropins. New York, Wiley-Interscience, 1972.

Schalch, D. S., Parlow, A. F., Boon, R. C., and Reichlin, S.: Measurement of human luteinizing hormone in plasma by radioimmunoassay. J. Clin. Invest., 47:665, 1968.

THYROTROPIN
(Thyrotropic or Thyroid-Stimulating Hormone, TSH)

Thyrotropin repairs the atrophy of the thyroid gland that follows hypophysectomy. The hormone also restores the ability of the thyroid to synthesize and secrete thyroxine and triiodothyronine. If given in large doses to normal or hypophysectomized animals or man, thyrotropin evokes the morphologic and secretory changes of hyperthyroidism. TSH elicits a rapid release of thyroxine and triiodothyronine from the gland; the content of colloid is reduced, and the quantity of organic iodine is decreased.

Thyrotropin is a glycoprotein, containing hexose and glucosamine. The molecular weight is about 28,000; there are two subunits, the α subunit being essentially identical to the α subunit of LH and similar to those of FSH and HCG, and the β subunit comprising the hormone-specific properties. The linear amino acid sequences of the two subunits are known. There is evidence that the TSH molecule is heterogeneous. The hormone stimulates many metabolic processes in the thyroid, e.g., the uptake and oxidation of glucose, the production of TPNH, and many others. The rapid discharge of thyroxine from the thyroid follicles is in part due to the action of TSH upon a proteolytic enzyme that accelerates the release of the hormone from the intrafollicular thyroglobulin. Within 24 hours after the administration of TSH, hypertrophy and hyperplasia of the thyroid epithelium occur. The weight of the thyroid increases. TSH augments the capacity of the thyroid to take up iodide, to convert iodide to organic iodine, and to synthesize thyroxine. These effects can be reproduced by cyclic AMP; this and other evidence indicates that the nucleotide is an important mediator of TSH action on the thyroid.

Hypothalamic TRH appears to be the most important regulator of TSH secretion; the daily production rate of TSH is about $100\mu U$. Circadian rhythm of plasma TSH levels in man is slight, and, in contrast to other anterior pituitary hormones, TSH secretion remains remarkably constant in the face of many kinds of stimuli. Except for a transitory increase in early neonatal life, there is no age-related change in plasma TSH values; they are the same in both sexes and do not change in response to exercise, the stress of surgery, or the administration of vasopressin, glucagon, arginine, or, surprisingly, antithyroid drugs. Corticosteroids cause transitory suppression of TSH secretion, and prolonged exposure to cold slightly increases it. Thyroxine and triiodothyronine also exert important effects on the hypothalamic and pituitary control of TSH secretion; values are high in primary hypothyroidism and low in naturally occurring and iatrogenic hyperthyroidism (see Ch. 546.2).

Bovine thyrotropin and synthetic TRH are available for medical use; diagnostic tests of pituitary-thyroid function are discussed in Ch. 543.4.

Anderson, M. S., Bowers, C. Y., Kastin, A. J., Schalch, D. S., Schally, A. V., Snyder, P. J., Utiger, R. D., Wilber, J. F., and Wise, A. J.: Synthetic thyrotropin-releasing hormone. N. Engl. J. Med., 285:1279, 1971.

Hershman, J. M., and Pittman, J. A.: Control of thyrotropin secretion in man. N. Engl. J. Med., 285:997, 1971.

Pierce, J. G., Liao, T., Howard, S. M., Shome, B., and Cornell, J. S.: Studies on the structure of thyrotropin: Its relationship to luteinizing hormone. Recent Prog. Horm. Res., 27:165, 1971.

Utiger, R. D.: Assay and secretory physiology in man. In Werner, S. C., and Ingbar, S. H. (eds): The Thyroid, a Fundamental and Clinical Text. 4th ed. Hagerstown, Md., Harper & Row, 1978, p. 196.

ADRENOCORTICOTROPIN
(ACTH, Corticotropin)

Adrenocorticotropin repairs the adrenocortical atrophy and failure to synthesize steroid hormones that follow hypophysectomy. In most species, ACTH administration causes hypertrophy and hyperplasia of the adrenal. The main effect appears to be upon the fascicular and reticular zones. The hormone stimulates the synthesis and release of cortisol, corticosterone, and androgens; it also elicits a moderate increase in the secretory rate of aldosterone, but this increase is not sustained. Large amounts of exogenous corticotropin cause enlargement and hyperemia of the adrenal, and hemorrhagic infarction has occurred rarely.

The chemical nature of adrenocorticotropin is known. It is a single polypeptide made up of 39 amino acids. Smaller fragments of the ACTH peptide, e.g., that containing amino acids 1 to 20, have full biologic potency. The complete hormone has been synthesized; its molecular weight is 4567, its potency 100 to 140 units per milligram. ACTH exists in at least two forms in the pituitary; "big ACTH" may serve as a prohormone, whereas "little" ACTH (molecular weight 4500) is the circulating, biologically active hormone. One international unit, equal to 1 USP unit, is the biologic activity of 1 mg of international standard. The daily production rate of ACTH in man is small, about 10 μg per day.

The action of the hormone upon the adrenal cortex is complex. It stimulates increased mitotic activity. The increase in steroidogenesis is the result of an increase in the rate of steroid biosynthesis, not simply of accelerated release of steroid into the bloodstream. The precise point in the biosynthetic pathway at which corticotropin acts is debatable; the increased steroid production may be mediated by ACTH stimulation of a particular messenger RNA. An important mechanism by which ACTH induces increased steroid synthesis is its capacity to stimulate the synthesis of active adrenocortical phosphorylase by raising the concentration of cyclic AMP in the gland. The increased phosphorylase activity makes available more glucose-6-phosphate from the hexose monophosphate shunt, thus providing larger quantities of NADH (TPNH), a compound essential for the synthesis and hydroxylation of steroids.

Corticotropin has extra-adrenal actions. It stimulates the release of free fatty acids from adipose tissue; the importance of this effect is unknown. In large doses it causes darkening of the skin.

In man, the short-term administration of adrenocorticotropin causes a rapid increase in the secretion of cortisol, reflected by an abrupt rise in plasma cortisol concentration. This effect has proved useful in the diagnostic assessment of adrenocortical response, as has the biologic and immunologic assay of ACTH in human serum. Radioimmunoassay measurements of plasma ACTH concentration have confirmed earlier ideas about the extraordinary lability of this hormone in response to physiologic and pathologic stimuli. Plasma ACTH undergoes a free-running circadian cycle under CNS (hypothalamic CRF) influence. The hormone is secreted in episodic bursts, with highest levels tending to be in the early morning; a nadir is reached by late evening. Plasma cortisol levels roughly reflect this circadian rhythm. Hospitalized patients not acutely ill often have ACTH concentrations higher than normal, and severely ill patients occasionally show extremely elevated levels. Plasma ACTH rises in addisonian and adrenalectomized patients and in response to metyrapone, and falls when suppressive doses of adrenocortical steroids, e.g., dexamethasone, are given (see Ch. 547.2). Stressful stimuli, such as surgery under general anesthesia, electroshock, and hypoglycemia, and the administration of histamine and vasopressin are usually followed by raised plasma ACTH concentrations.

The long-term effects of adrenocorticotropin in human subjects are the same as those produced by cortisone, cortisol, and their synthetic analogues. In contrast to the adrenocortical steroids, corticotropin evokes sensitivity reactions, but antihormone formation does not occur. ACTH brings about a greater degree of sodium and water retention, more androgenicity, and a more constant elevation in serum cholesterol than do steroids. Large doses elicit the stigmata of Cushing's syndrome (e.g., osteoporosis, hyperglycemia, psychosis). The unpleasant symptoms associated with abrupt withdrawal of steroid therapy are said to occur rarely after a course of ACTH therapy.

The hormone regulates the growth, structural integ-

rity, and steroid secretion of the adrenal cortex. This constantly changing regulatory influence is exerted by central nervous system control of the anterior pituitary and by a reciprocal relation between the amounts of circulating cortisol and ACTH. In man, noxious stimuli such as acute illness or severe and prolonged emotional disturbance provoke an increased or abnormally regulated output of adrenocortical steroids, mediated via an increased rate of endogenous corticotropin release.

ACTH is available for diagnostic purposes in lyophilized and repository (with gelatin or zinc) forms. Two synthetic ACTH preparations are also available in unmodified and repository forms: $\alpha^{1\text{-}24}$ ACTH (Synacthen, Cortrosyn), and $\alpha^{1\text{-}18}$ ACTH (see Ch. 543.4 and 547.3). ACTH has also been used *therapeutically*, but most clinicians think that the diseases which respond to hyperadrenal therapy are more simply managed with corticosteroids than with ACTH.

Berson, S. A., and Yalow, R. S.: Radioimmunoassay of ACTH in plasma. J. Clin. Invest., 47:2725, 1968.

Gill, G. N.: Mechanism of ACTH action. Metabolism, 21:571, 1972.

Kendall, J. W.: Feedback control of adrenocorticotrophic hormone secretion. In Martini, L., and Ganong, W. F. (eds.): Neuroendocrinology, Vol. 2. New York, Oxford University Press, 1971, p. 177.

Weitzman, E. D., Fukushima, D., Nogiere, C., Roffwarg, H., Gallagher, T. F., and Hellman, L.: Twenty-four hour pattern of the episodic secretion of cortisol in normal subjects. J. Clin. Endocrinol. Metab., 33:14, 1971.

MELANOCYTE-STIMULATING HORMONE
(MSH)

MSH produces darkening (addisonian pigmentation) in human skin. Two MSH peptides have been identified in pituitary tissue. One of the pituitary lipotropins (β-LPH or γ-LPH) may be the prohormone for the MSH peptides. The smaller and more potent molecule, α-MSH, is made up of 13 amino acids and has a molecular weight of 1823; it is found in the pituitaries of pigs, cows, and monkeys, and may be present in the neurohypophysis of man. The characteristic human peptide, β-MSH, contains 22 amino acids and has a molecular weight of 2734. α-MSH has a common 13-amino acid sequence with ACTH; β-MSH a 7-amino acid sequence. These partial identities of structure may account for common physiologic properties among the three molecules: ACTH has a slight pigmentary effect on skin; both MSH molecules and ACTH are adipokinetic; both MSH's have weak adrenal-stimulating activity. Studies of plasma β-MSH concentration in man have shown that the hormone undergoes a circadian rhythm in normal subjects and that its secretion is regulated by the same factors that control ACTH. Metyrapone raises and adrenocortical steroids depress plasma β-MSH levels.

The functional significance of human β-MSH is not known; nor is it certain that MSH should be regarded as a separate hormone in man. Plasma values are the same in pigmented and nonpigmented races, and are normal in albinism and in several diseases characterized by increased dermal pigmentation.

Abe, K., Nicholson, W. E., Liddle, G. W., Orth, D. N., and Island, D. P.: Normal and abnormal regulation of β-MSH in man. J. Clin. Invest., 48:1580, 1969.

Bloomfield, G. A., Scott, A. P., Lowry, P. J., Gilkes, J. J. H., and Rees, L. H.: A reappraisal of human beta-MSH. Nature, 252:692, 1974.

Lerner, A. B., and McGuire, J. S.: Effect of alpha- and beta-melanocyte stimulating hormones on skin colour of man. Nature (London), 189:176, 1971.

LIPOTROPINS AND ENDORPHINS

The anterior pituitary is known to contain several substances with lipolytic properties. In addition to HGH, ACTH, and MSH, there are at least two other lipotropic peptides: β-lipotropin (β-LPH) and γ-lipotropin (γ-LPH) (Li, 1976). Their molecular weights are 9500 and 5810, respectively; they share a common sequence of 58 amino acids, and have an 18-amino acid sequence in common with β-MSH. β-LPH and γ-LPH are lipotropic, melanotropic, and weakly adrenocorticotropic, and fragments of β-LPH have strong opiate activity. There is evidence that the lipotropins may be the prohormones of MSH. Both lipotropins are detectable in the human circulation, but their peripheral function in man is not yet known (see Ch. 543.4).

A new class of small anterior pituitary peptides, the endorphins, has aroused intense investigative and clinical interest. These compounds are structurally related to ACTH, β-MSH, and β-LPH. A close *functional* relationship among those three hormones and endorphins is suggested by several lines of evidence. Antigenic determinants for ACTH and LPH may reside in the same molecule. ACTH, β-LPH, and endorphins are found in the same type of pituitary basophil and within the same secretory granules. Under most physiologic and pathologic conditions, stimuli that augment or reduce ACTH release from the pituitary affect β-LPH and β-MSH in a parallel way. "Ectopic" ACTH-producing cancers usually secrete β-MSH-like peptides also. Endorphins and ACTH appear to share a common precursor molecule.

The endorphins, which are found not only in the pituitary but also in the brain, chemically resemble the cerebral enkephalins. Enkephalins and endorphins both have potent opiate ("opioid") properties and attach to the "specific" brain receptors for morphine. Endorphins exert profound neuropsychologic effects in animals, and, in some studies, affect human behavior. Active work is now being done to detect endorphins in human circulation, to elucidate their possible role in "stress" as "natural" or endogenous opiates, to determine whether they are of any importance in human psychoses or in narcotic addiction, and to clarify further the biochemical and functional interrelationships between the anterior pituitary and the brain.

Bloom, F., Segal, D., Ling, N., and Guillemin, R.: Endorphins: Profound behavioral effects in rats suggest new etiological factors in mental illness. Science, 194:630, 1976.
Goldstein, A.: Opioid peptides (endorphins) in pituitary and brain. Science, 193:1081, 1976.
Goldstein, A., and Cox, B. M.: Opioid peptides (endorphins) in pituitary and brain. Psychoneuroendocrinology, 2:11, 1977.
Guillemin, R., Vargo, T., Rossier, J., Minick, S., Ling, N., Fivier, C., Vale, W., and Bloom, F.: β-Endorphin and adrenocorticotropin are secreted concomitantly by the pituitary gland. Science, 197:1367, 1977.
Mains, R. E., Eipper, B. E., and Ling, N.: Common precursor to corticotropins and endorphins. Proc. Natl. Acad. Sci. U.S.A., 74:3014, 1977.

543.4. ASSESSMENT OF ANTERIOR PITUITARY FUNCTION

CLINICAL DETECTION OF PITUITARY DISEASE. Clinical suspicion of hypopituitarism must be entertained in patients with short stature, delayed puberty, primary and secondary amenorrhea, sterility, and hypothyroidism. Typical ocular findings or the incidental discovery of an enlarged pituitary fossa (as in a skull film taken for head injury) also require diagnostic study of pituitary function (see below).

STRUCTURAL DETECTION OF PITUITARY DISEASE. This is discussed in Ch. 543.1 under Anatomy and in Ch. 543.5.

FUNCTIONAL DETECTION OF PITUITARY DISEASE. This is based on measurement of hormones in plasma or urine. In addition to detection of abnormally high or low levels of pituitary hormones, such measurements permit an evaluation of abnormal *regulation* of pituitary hormone secretion (see Ch. 542). *Direct* measurement of pituitary hormones is made when possible, as for growth hormone and gonadotropins; *indirect* evaluation of TSH and ACTH is done by measuring the hormones of glands that are under their tropic control if immunoassay methods are not available, e.g., thyroidal response to TSH, adrenocortical response to ACTH (see below).

GROWTH HORMONE

Radioimmunoassay of plasma growth hormones is now a routine procedure, and can be done at most medical centers and commercial laboratories. This is the most direct method for detecting hypopituitary states and acromegaly. In *hypopituitary dwarfism*, radioimmunoassay for growth hormone has superseded the crude indirect indices that clinicians have had to rely on, e.g., measurements of body proportions, chromosomal analysis, roentgenographic estimate of bone age, and laborious exclusion of all other causes of short stature. In pituitary dwarfism, basal plasma HGH values of less than 1.0 ng per milliliter may be found; these low values are not diagnostic, because the normal range is 0 to 5 ng per milliliter. One must demonstrate failure of growth hormone to respond to a stimulus, e.g., hypoglycemia. When suspicion is strong, the starting dose of insulin should be 0.05 unit per kilogram, given intravenously; if the hypoglycemia is inadequate, the dose can be increased to 0.1 or even 0.15 unit per kilogram, given under careful supervision to avoid prolonged hypoglycemia. Adequate stimulus requires a lowering of blood glucose to one half the basal value or to 40 mg per 100 ml for at least ten minutes; if this condition is satisfied, patients without growth hormone deficiency show a rise in HGH value of at least 7 ng per milliliter above the basal level 60 minutes after injection. *Failure of growth hormone response to hypoglycemia is the most common laboratory abnormality in adult hypopituitarism, and is characteristic only of the dwarfism associated with growth hormone deficiency.* Certain amino acids also have the property of inducing growth hormone release; intravenous administration of neutralized arginine hydrochloride, 0.5 gram per kilogram, is preferred by some workers, because one avoids possibly dangerous hypoglycemia. The rise in growth hormone value is again 7 ng per milliliter above the resting levels.

In *acromegaly* also, HGH radioimmunoassay has begun to replace the highly unsatisfactory indirect methods clinicians have struggled with for years: histologic changes in the cartilage of the costochondral junction, measurement of serum phosphorus, PBI, urinary calcium, urinary hydroxyproline excretion, and so forth. Basal plasma HGH may be in the range of 50 to more than 100 ng per milliliter. Many patients with untreated acromegaly fail to show the normal sharp drop in plasma HGH concentration after administration of glucose (given as for a standard glucose tolerance test, blood samples being taken for glucose and growth hormone determinations at 30-minute intervals for at least three hours). It will require protracted follow-up studies of acromegalic patients before and after treatment and careful correlation with clinical findings, e.g., acral growth, to assess the usefulness of this nonresponse to hyperglycemia as an index of "acromegalic activity." In some acromegalics, plasma HGH paradoxically *rises* in response to glucose.

Glucagon and L-*dopa* have been recently introduced as provocative tests of HGH adequacy. Both have the virtue of simplicity. One mg of glucagon is given subcutaneously or intramuscularly; in normal subjects plasma HGH rises to 8 ng per milliliter or more within two to three hours. L-Dopa, 0.5 gram, is given orally; normal subjects raise HGH levels more than 5 ng per milliliter with a peak rise at 90 minutes. Response is said to be subnormal or absent in pituitary disease. These two maneuvers are promising but require further trial.

Beck, P., Parker, M. L., and Daughaday, W. H.: Paradoxical hypersecretion of growth hormone in response to glucose. J. Clin. Endocrinol. Metab., 26:463, 1966.
Eddy, R. L., Gilliland, P. F., Ibarra, J. D., Jr., McMurry, J. F., Jr., and Thompson, J. Q.: Human growth hormone release: Comparison of provocative test procedures. Am. J. Med., 56:179, 1974.
Mitchell, M. L., Byrne, M. J., Sanchez, Y., and Sawin, C. T.: Detection of growth hormone deficiency: The glucagon stimulation test. N. Engl. J. Med., 282:539, 1970.
Pecile, A., and Muller, E. E. (eds.): Growth and Growth Hormone. Amsterdam, Excerpta Medica, 1972.
Rabkin, M. T., and Frantz, A. G.: Hypopituitarism: A study of growth hormone and other endocrine functions. Ann. Intern. Med., 64:1197, 1966.

PROLACTIN

The development of sensitive radioimmunoassay measurements for plasma prolactin has introduced a new and useful method for evaluating pituitary disease and *galactorrheic states*. Normal values are the same for adult men and women, usually less than 15 ng per milliliter, with an extreme upper limit of 25 ng per milliliter. Plasma prolactin is usually elevated in patients who have had *pituitary stalk section*, owing to interference with the action of hypothalamic PIF (see Ch. 542). A finding of major importance is detection of high plasma prolactin levels in patients with various kinds of *pituitary tumors*, often in the absence of clinical or structural evidence of pituitary enlargement, often in the absence of galactorrhea, and sometimes when all other pituitary hormones are low and there is clinical panhypopituitarism. Raised prolactin levels may on occasion constitute the *only* chemical evidence of pituitary disease with or without tumor. The mechanism is either mechanical interference with PIF action or actual oversecretion of prolactin by a pituitary tumor. Plasma prolactin measurement may turn out to be valuable as an early hormonal sign of "nonfunctional" chromophobe adenoma. Raised prolactin levels are usually but not always found in patients with *galactorrhea*: e.g., in the *Chiari-Frommel syndrome* (postpartum amenorrhea and low gonadotropin levels), the *Argonz-Del Castillo syndrome* (amenorrhea and low gonadotropin levels but not in relation to parturition), the *Forbes-Albright syndrome* (amenorrhea and low FSH/LH values but associated with chromophobe adenoma), and the *"oversuppression" syndrome* (amenorrhea and low FSH/LH values after cessation of antiovulatory medication, occasionally in *acromegaly*, and rarely in *primary hypothyroidism* (especially when the pituitary is enlarged) and injury to the chest wall. Prolactin levels are often high in renal failure but are usually normal in gynecomastia (see Hypersecretion of pituitary hormones other than HGH, in Ch. 543.7).

Provocative tests have been devised to distinguish between hypothalamic and pituitary disorders of prolactin secretion: stimulation with TRH and chlorpromazine and suppression with L-dopa. Panhypopituitary patients have low plasma prolactin levels which fail to respond to all three tests; patients with hypothalamic involvement respond abnormally to one or more of the three agents. Details of protocols and interpretation are given by Tolis et al.

Boyer, R. M., Kapew, S., Finkelstein, J. W., Sassani, J. F., Fukushima, D. K., Wertzman, E. D., and Hellman, L.: Hypothalamic-pituitary function in diverse hyperprolactinemic states. J. Clin. Invest., 53:1588, 1974.
Forsyth, I. A., Besser, G. M., Edwards, C. R. W., Francis, L., and Myres, R. P.: Plasma prolactin activity in inappropriate lactation. Brit. Med. J., 2:225, 1971.
Kleinberg, D. L., Noel, G. L., and Frantz, A. G.: Galactorrhea: 235 cases including 48 with pituitary tumors. N. Engl. J. Med., 296:589, 1977.
L'Hermite, P., Copinschi, G., Golstein, J., Vanhaelst, L., Leclercq, R., Bruno, O. D., and Robyn, C.: Prolactin release after injection of thyrotropin-releasing hormone in man. Lancet, 1:763, 1972.
Tolis, G., Goldstein, M., and Friesen, H. G.: Functional evaluation of prolactin secretion in patients with hypothalamic-pituitary disorders. J. Clin. Invest., 52:783, 1972.

GONADOTROPINS
(FSH and LH)

Biologic assay of urinary gonadotropin is useful in distinguishing primary from secondary gonadal failure after the expected age of puberty. In the former, urinary gonadotropin titers are elevated; in the latter (resulting from pituitary deficiency), levels are not detectable. Results of urinary gonadotropin (human pituitary gonadotropin) assays, done by the mouse uterine weight or rat ovarian weight method, are expressed in mouse uterine units (muu) or rat units (RU). In the mouse assay, a reported value of "positive at 20 muu" means that one twentieth of the extract of a 24-hour urine just induces a definite response in the injected mice. If one twentieth of a 24-hour urinary extract produces a definite response in the rat assay, results are reported as "20 RU per 24 hours." The rat assay is the more sensitive; normal people occasionally have undetectable values in the mouse assay. There is no official reference standard for this bioassay. Representative mean values for the rat assay are as follows: adult men, 10; women in the follicular and luteal phases, 7; women at midcycle, 15; postmenopausal women, 75 — all values being expressed in RU per 24 hours. Corresponding figures for the mouse assay are 35, 20, 55, and 200 — all expressed in muu per 24 hours. In pituitary insufficiency, urinary gonadotropins are usually undetectable; this abnormality is one of the earliest laboratory signs to appear in the course of the disease.

TABLE 2. Plasma Gonadotropin Values as Measured by Radioimmunoassay in Normal People (with the "2nd IRP–Human Menopausal Gonadotropin" as Standard)

	FSH, mIU/ml	LH, mIU/ml
Children	3–19	5–15
Adult males	3–42	3–32
Adult females		
Follicular phase	10–18	7–27
Mid-cycle	20–30	70–100
Luteal phase	6–18	7–22
Postmenopausal	35–215	0–90

The highly sensitive radioimmunoassays for plasma FSH and LH are now available for routine clinical use, and have largely supplanted the bioassay methods. As expected, values are low or undetectable in pituitary insufficiency and high in primary gonadal failure. The normal ranges for various stages of the reproductive cycle are set out in Table 2.

Use of FSH and LH radioimmunoassay measurements has permitted sharper diagnostic accuracy in *delayed puberty* and the identification of patients with *hypogonadotropic hypogonadism*, e.g., isolated FSH deficiency and gonadotropin deficiency associated with *anosmia* or *hyposmia (Kallmann's syndrome)*, in some of whom the defect may be in the synthesis or release of gonadotropin-releasing factor (FSH-LH/RF or LHRH). *Provocative tests* which entail administration of LHRH or clomiphene have been used in attempts to distinguish hypothalamic from pituitary hypogonadotropism. In theory, patients with intrinsic anterior pituitary disease should show no FSH or LH response to administered LHRH, and in people with hypothalamic lesions the response should be present but subnormal or delayed. Unfortunately, there is enough overlap in results so that clear differentiation between pituitary and hypothalamus as the primary site of disease cannot always be made, and other evidence must be used. Clomiphene may be therapeutically effective in some patients with gonadotropin deficiency. (For detailed protocols, see references.)

Edwards, C. R., and Besser, G. M.: Diseases of the hypothalamus and pituitary gland. Clin. Endocrinol. Metab., 3:475, 1974.

Hamilton, C. R., Henkin, R. I., Weir, G., and Kliman, B.: Olfactory status and response to clomiphene in male gonadotrophin deficiency. Ann. Intern. Med., 78:47, 1973.

Newton, J., Ramsay, I., and Marsden, P.: Clomiphene as a test of pituitary function. Lancet, 2:190, 1971.

Rabin, D., Spitz, I., Bercovici, B., Bell, J., Laufer, A., Benveniste, R., and Polishuk, W.: Isolated deficiency of follicle-stimulating hormone: Clinical and laboratory features. N. Engl. J. Med., 287:1313, 1972.

Vaitukaitis, J., Becker, R., Hansen, J., and Mecklenberg, R.: Altered LRF responsiveness in amenorrheic women. J. Clin. Endocrinol., Metab., 39:1005, 1974.

Yohimota, R., Moridera, K., and Imura, H.: Plasma luteinizing hormone and follicle-stimulating hormone responses to luteinizing hormone releasing hormone in patients with hypogonadism. Endocrinol. Japon., 21:191, 1974.

THYROTROPIN
(TSH)

Radioimmunoassay for serum thyrotropin is available for general clinical use; normal values are 0.5 to 10 μU per milliliter. Serum TSH values are undetectable in Graves' disease (see Ch. 546.2). The values in primary myxedema, as expected, are high, falling to normal when thyroid hormone is given. A *provocative test*, in which 200 to 500 μg of TRH is given intravenously and plasma TSH rise is measured 30 to 60 minutes later, has been used in an attempt to differentiate between "hypothalamic" and pituitary hypothyroidism. TSH rise may be normal in the former and absent in the latter, but there is enough overlap of TSH response in the two entities so that this is by no means a perfect discriminatory test (Edwards and Besser, 1974). In intrinisc pituitary disease, the basal TSH level is low; if this measurement cannot be obtained, an acceptable method for distinguishing primary myxedema from secondary thyroid deficiency is the thyrotropin stimulation test. The most reliable technique seems to be measurement of 24-hour ^{131}I uptake by the thyroid before and after intramuscular administration of bovine TSH, 10 USP units per day intramuscularly for three days. In primary myxedema, there is no response; normal subjects respond briskly; patients with myxedema secondary to pituitary failure respond, but subnormally. Exceptions are some patients with Sheehan's disease of long duration, who may be unresponsive.

Costom, B. H., Grumbach, M. M., and Kaplan, S. L.: Effect of thyrotropin-releasing factor on serum thyroid-stimulating hormone. J. Clin. Invest., 50:2219, 1971.

Foley, T. P., Jr., Owings, J., Hayford, J. T., and Blizzard, R. M.: Serum thyrotropin responses to synthetic thyrotropin-releasing hormone in normal children and hypopituitary patients. J. Clin. Invest., 51:431, 1972.

Pittman, J. A., Haigler, E. D., Hershman, J. M., and Pittman, C. S.: Hypothalamic hypothyroidism. N. Engl. J. Med., 285:844, 1971.

Reichlin, S.: Neuroendocrine Control. *In* Werner, S. C., and Ingbar, S. H. (eds.): The Thyroid, a Fundamental and Clinical Text. 4th ed. Hagerstown, Md., Harper & Row, 1978, p. 151.

Shenkman, L., Mitsuma, T., Suphavai, A., and Hollander, C. S.: Triiodothyronine and thyroid-stimulating hormone response to thyrotropin-releasing hormone. Lancet, 1:111, 1972.

ADRENOCORTICOTROPIN
(ACTH)

Measurement of the ACTH secretion of the pituitary is usually done *indirectly* by testing adrenocortical response. A safe and specific method is intravenous administration of 25 units of lyophilized ACTH in 500 ml of 0.9 per cent saline over a four-hour period. Five per cent glucose in water should not be used as a diluent, because it may aggravate pre-existing hyponatremia. In primary adrenocortical failure (Addison's disease) there is no response of plasma corticosteroids; in pituitary deficiency with secondary adrenal failure, response is present but subnormal. Equally useful is intravenous infusion of ACTH over several days with measurement of urinary steroid excretion; some workers think this is a more certain method for differentiating primary and secondary adrenal insufficiency. It is prudent to give 0.5 to 1.0 mg of dexamethasone orally to obviate untoward reactions to ACTH. Use of the synthetic corticotropins avoids these reactions, but results are not yet widely standardized. The nonspecific methods, insulin tolerance test and water loading, can be dangerous and are not recommended.

Four other methods have been used to assess pituitary ACTH release; like the ACTH-response test described above, the index is rise or failure to rise of plasma or urinary corticosteroid values. Three of the methods entail stimulation of ACTH release by giving a more or less noxious stimulus: insulin-induced hypoglycemia, vasopressin, and bacterial pyrogen. Although it is true that patients with hypopituitarism show absent or subnormal rises in plasma cortisol concentration after all three of these, there is no agreement about which is the most discriminating or the most sensitive; but Edwards and Besser (1974) present convincing evidence that the insulin-hypoglycemia test with simultaneous measurement of HGH and cortisol response is a reliable index of anterior pituitary reserve. The insulin, vasopressin, and pyrogen tests have not found favor as clinical methods in this country. The fourth method, the metyrapone test, a measure of pituitary ACTH reserve, is described in Ch. 547.2 and 547.5. To make certain that the adrenal has the capacity to respond to ACTH, a standard ACTH response test should be done before metyrapone is given. In a few patients with severe hypopituitarism, metyrapone blockade of adrenocortical biosynthesis coupled with poor or absent ACTH reserve has resulted in clinically significant adrenal insufficiency. In patients with possibly advanced hypopituitarism, "coverage" with 0.5 to 1.0 mg of dexamethasone is therefore a reasonable safeguard during a metyrapone test.

Biologic assay and radioimmunoassay of plasma ACTH, although not yet generally available for clinical purposes, are *direct* techniques which have yielded valuable information about the fluctuations of this hormone. Normal values are a mean of about 0.3 mU per 100 ml by bioassay and a mean of 22 pg per milliliter by radioimmunoassay (normal range, 12 to 80 pg per milliliter). Values are occasionally ten times higher in severely ill patients; as expected, levels are low or not detected in hypopituitarism. The changes in plasma ACTH concentration that occur in the various forms of Cushing's syndrome are discussed in Ch. 547.7.

Jasani, M. K., Freeman, P. A., Boyle, J. A., Reid, A. M., Diver, M. J., and Buchanan, W. W.: Studies of the rise in plasma 11-OH-CS in corticosteroid-treated patients with rheumatoid arthritis during surgery: Correlations with the functional integrity of the hypothalamo-pituitary-adrenal axis. Quart. J. Med., 37:407, 1968.
Wood, J. B., Frankland, A. W., James, V. H. T., and Landon, J.: A rapid test of adrenocortical function. Lancet, 1:243, 1965.

MELANOCYTE-STIMULATING HORMONE (MSH)

A radioimmunoassay for plasma β-MSH has been developed but is not used for clinical purposes. Normal levels are 20 to 110 pg per milliliter. The values are raised in untreated Addison's disease and congenital adrenal hyperplasia, and fall during corticosteroid administration. Plasma β-MSH is slightly raised, as is plasma ACTH, in the "pituitary" form of Cushing's syndrome (see Ch. 547.7), and very much elevated in patients who develop pituitary tumors and dermal hyperpigmentation after bilateral adrenalectomy for this disease. Elevations of plasma β-MSH tend to parallel those of plasma ACTH, and large amounts of each peptide have been found in extracts of hormone-secreting tumors (see Ch. 525). That the parallelism of rise and fall of MSH and ACTH together is not always perfect is seen in patients with "isolated" pituitary ACTH deficiency, some of whom have normal or excessive dermal pigmentation. A finding of great interest is the detection of raised plasma β-MSH levels in patients with parkinsonism; this raises the possibility that β-MSH functions as a neuroregulatory hormone. However,

since "MSH" may not be a distinct entity in man (see above) but a "split product" of pituitary β- or γ-LPH, there is some question about the significance of circulating β-MSH in human plasma.

Abe, K., Nicholson, W. E., Liddle, G. W., Island, D. P., and Orth, D. N.: Radioimmunoassay of β-MSH in human plasma and tissues. J. Clin. Invest., 46:1609, 1967.
Editorial: Melanocyte-stimulating hormone? Br. Med. J., 1:533, 1977.
Shuster, S., Thody, A. J., Goolamali, S. K., Burton, J. L., Plummer, N., and Bates, D.: Melanocyte-stimulating hormone and parkinsonism. Lancet, 1:463. 1973.

LIPOTROPINS AND ENDORPHINS

No clinical syndromes of lipotropin or endorphin excess or deficiency have yet been identified, but radioimmunoassay measurement of the lipotropins in blood has found some diagnostic use. In the "pituitary" form of Cushing's syndrome, plasma ACTH concentration is said to be higher than that of LPH; the opposite is true when the hormonal source is "ectopic", i.e., a nonendocrine tumor (see Ch. 525 and 547.7). It may also turn out that one can distinguish between pituitary and ectopic sources of hormone hypersecretion by measuring the ratio of plasma γ-LPH to β-LPH in plasma.

Gilkes, J. J. H., Rees, L. H., and Besser, G. M.: Plasma immunoreactive corticotrophin and lipotrophin in Cushing's syndrome and Addison's disease. Br. Med. J., 1:996, 1977.

543.5. DIAGNOSIS AND TREATMENT OF PITUITARY TUMORS

Epidemiologic studies indicate that there are about 2500 newly diagnosed pituitary tumors per year in the United States. Tumors of the pituitary may be *asymptomatic.* In an autopsy study of 1000 "normal" pituitaries, adenomas were found in nearly 25 per cent, over half being chromophobic, more than a quarter basophilic, and the rest (7.5 per cent) acidophilic. Although some pathologists believe, on the basis of special stains, that most pituitary tumors are chromophilic and contain stainable, possibly hormone-secreting granules, the majority of tumors are chromophobic by conventional light microscopy, whatever implication this may have for their secretory capacities. Thus in a recent collection of nearly 1000 cases of known pituitary adenoma, 98 per cent were chromophobic, the remaining 2 per cent being acidophilic. Malignant chromophobe adenomas are rare. Extrasellar and suprasellar cysts and tumors, especially gliomas of the optic chiasm and craniopharyngiomas, are less common tumors that may involve the pituitary, either by direct extension into the pituitary fossa or by impingement upon the adjacent hypothalamus or pituitary stalk.

Patients with pituitary tumor are more likely to seek medical aid because of visual or neurologic symptoms than for complaints of endocrine dysfunction. However, careful questioning will almost always disclose the fact that *some endocrine symptom long antedated the appearance of the neurologic change;* but it is still true that the neurologic symptom is what brings the patient to the doctor. In a recent series, about three quarters of the patients had headaches (not by themselves sufficiently typical to be diagnostic of a pituitary lesion), two thirds had impair-

Figure 3. Chromophobe adenoma in a 36-year-old man. Roentgenogram of the skull shows moderate enlargement of the sella (24 mm in the anterior-posterior diameter, 16 mm in depth on the original film). The sellar floor shows a double contour, indicating uneven downward growth of the tumor, which depresses one side of the sella more than the other. The dorsum sellae is thin; the posterior clinoids are intact. The texture and appearance of the skull and facial bones are normal (cf. acromegaly, Fig. 4).

ment of visual fields, and the same proportion had impairment of visual activity; about 40 per cent complained of decreased libido, and one third had diplopia, decrease in potency, dizziness (postural hypotension), change in amount of sexual hair, or intolerance to cold. By far the most common visual field defect is *bitemporal hemianopia*, occurring in 70 to 80 per cent of patients; it is noteworthy that about 15 per cent of patients with this defect are unaware of it. Sometimes, in rapidly growing pituitary tumors, the visual field defects are scotomatous. Paralysis of the extraocular muscles innervated by cranial nerves III, IV, and VI usually denotes a large tumor extending outside the sella turcica. Among *endocrine symptoms*, about 90 per cent of patients give a history of some degree of gonadal insufficiency on careful questioning, about 80 per cent have symptoms of thyroid failure, and perhaps half report evidence of what appears to be adrenocortical deficiency. Even when pituitary tumors rise up out of the sella turcica and exert pressure on the diencephalon, they rarely cause *hypothalamic symptoms;* diabetes insipidus and disorders of sleep or temperature regulation are rare and do not occur unless the diencephalon is grossly damaged. About one eighth of patients may have symptoms caused by *"pituitary apoplexy"* (abrupt hemorrhage into the tumor) (see below).

Physical findings in pituitary tumor are also more commonly related to the eyes than to the endocrine system. In addition to bitemporal hemianopia, up to 85 per cent of patients can be shown to have reduced visual acuity, more than half have optic atrophy, and one third have cranial nerve palsies. About two fifths of patients are found to have loss of body hair, and a third or fewer have changes in the skin or genital atrophy.

Roentgenographic detection (see Anatomy in Ch. 543.1) should be based on frontal as well as sagittal views of the skull and sella. In addition to changes in the length and depth of the pituitary fossa, the examiner looks for erosion or destruction of the anterior and posterior clinoids and of the tuberculum sellae, suprasellar calcification (Fig. 1) (chromophobe adenoma, craniopharyngioma), and "double floor" of the sella, seen when a tumor extends downward unevenly (Fig. 3). Laminagraphy may show intrasellar calcification or extension of a tumor into the sphenoid sinus. Carotid artery angiography and particularly pneumoencephalography or CAT scanning may show quite accurately the degree of upward extension of an intrasellar tumor; these procedures should always be done before craniotomy for pituitary tumor, and are also necessary guides in the design of a radiotherapeutic program. Many neurosurgeons insist upon pneumoencepha-

Figure 4. Skull roentgenogram typical of acromegaly; 66-year-old woman with acromegaly of 43 years' duration. Radiotherapy to sella within five years of onset. Intermittent increases in the acral parts. No symptoms of endocrine deficiency (serum protein-bound iodine normal, normal blood glucose two hours after a meal). The film shows thickening and hyperostosis of the cranial vault and occipital protuberance, and very large size of the frontal and maxillary sinuses. As is not uncommonly true in acromegaly, the sella is only slightly enlarged (18 mm in the sagittal plane). The dorsum sellae is pneumatized. Prognathism is indicated by the overlapping lower teeth.

lography before undertaking pituitary surgery, especially transsphenoidal adenomectomy, in order to ascertain precisely the anatomic relation between the pituitary and the subarachnoid space. In *acromegaly*, plain films of the skull show not only enlargement of the sella turcica in 80 to 90 per cent of patients, but also thickening of the calvarium, enlargement of the paranasal sinuses, and widening of the mandibular angle with prognathism (Fig. 4). Films of the hands disclose gross increase in the mass of soft tissue, a more characteristic finding than tufting of the distal phalanges (Fig. 5). Spinal films may reveal anterior lipping of vertebral bodies; lateral films of the os calcis often show thickening of the heel pad.

CHROMOPHOBE ADENOMA. Natural History. These tumors may occur in adolescence but are most common between the ages of 30 and 60, with equal distribution between men and women. They are the largest of pituitary tumors, having a tendency to extend upward for a considerable distance. The clinical picture is variable. The tumors may be asymptomatic; the symptoms may be predominantly ocular or neurologic; or *endocrine symptoms* and signs may predominate, the most common being secondary gonadal failure (amenorrhea, decreased

frequency of shaving, impotence), with evidence of secondary thyroidal and adrenocortical failure being less common and occurring later in the course. *Galactorrhea* may be the only endocrine symptom (Forbes-Albright syndrome) or may coexist with elements of hypopituitarism. Recent studies have called attention to the possibility that longstanding *primary hypogonadism* or *hypothyroidism* may give rise to pituitary enlargement, owing to chromophobe adenoma in most cases (Bower; Lawrence et al.). In contrast, there are rare instances of *oversecretion* of a *pituitary* hormone, e.g., TSH, by a chromophobe adenoma.

Treatment. It is now clear that chromophobe adenoma must be treated; it is not safe to manage "expectantly" a patient suspected to have this lesion. A recent study has shown that of 16 such patients left untreated, 14 eventually required treatment, and during the observation period (6 months to 15 years) growth of the adenoma produced further and irreversible damage in 8. The best treatment appears to be *surgery*, followed by *conventional radiotherapy* (4000 to 5000 rads over five to six weeks); this method yields a control rate of about 75 per cent. Surgery (mortality rate 5 per cent or less) is mandatory if there is

Figure 5. X-ray of the hands in acromegaly. There is tufting of the distal phalanges, but the most characteristic finding is increase in soft tissue mass.

evidence of recent or rapid growth of the adenoma or if there is a major threat to vision. Since surgery alone is followed by an appreciable recurrence rate, radiotherapy should be added. The long-term remission rate after surgery alone is about 65 per cent. This can be raised to 85 per cent with postoperative radiation. In selected cases, radiotherapy alone may suffice. Preliminary results suggest that treatment with *heavy particles* (protons, α-particles) may be as effective as conventional radiotherapy for this tumor; the method is available only at those few centers that have cyclotrons.

Treatment of *galactorrhea* is either *surgical* or *pharmacologic.* If the pituitary tumor is large and threatens vision, surgery must be done. Hardy has had considerable success with *transsphenoidal* removal of laterally located prolactin-secreting microadenomas without producing hypopituitarism (Kohler and Ross). With or without pituitary tumor, treatment of galactorrhea with L-*dopa* and *ergot alkaloids* has shown promise, eliciting falls in plasma prolactin levels and, after several weeks, suppressing the inappropriate lactation.

ACIDOPHILIC ADENOMA WITH ACROMEGALY. Natural History and Pathogenesis. There is some evidence that acidophilic tumors may arise through an abnormality in HGHRH (growth hormone–releasing hormone) secretion by the hypothalamus. The course and prognosis of this lesion are more unfavorable than used to be thought. Life expectancy is reduced; in one series half the patients were dead before age 50 and nearly 90 per cent by age 60; among 194 patients followed for up to 30 years in London, the death rate was almost twice that in a matched group of patients without acromegaly (see Ch. 543.7). Treatment is therefore mandatory, even in "mild" cases without ocular or neurologic symptoms.

Treatment. Several modes of therapy are available; each is more or less effective and more or less hazardous.

As Gorden and Roth have put it (Kohler and Ross): "At the present time patients are treated largely on the basis of regional expertise or preference. No single mode of therapy has emerged as ideal or clearly preferable. All therapeutic modalities to date leave some patients with distinctly elevated growth hormone concentrations." *Conventional pituitary radiation* (4000 to 5000 rads over five weeks) probably controls tumor growth in over 70 per cent of patients; if one is willing to wait, plasma HGH values will fall somewhat by one to two years after radiation and will be reduced by nearly 80 per cent after three to six years, with some values in the normal range; untoward effects are not common. Treatment with *heavy particles* (4500 to 6500 rads over 11 days) sometimes produces dramatic results; there are more untoward effects than with conventional external radiation. The method works best where there is no major extrasellar extension of the tumor. Plasma HGH falls to levels below 10 ng per milliliter within two years after radiation in about three fourths of patients; at these levels metabolic improvement is almost always seen.

More in Europe than in the United States, *transsphenoidal implantation of radioactive isotopes* (^{90}Y, ^{198}Au) into the pituitary has found favor. There are many reports of beneficial effect, with resolution of soft tissue and osseous abnormalities and reduction of plasma HGH levels, but there is an appreciable rate of complications (meningitis, CSF rhinorrhea), and a still higher rate may be expected during the developmental phase at a given institution.

Many *surgical approaches* have been tried. *Transfrontal hypophysectomy* is effective and has a mortality rate of well under 5 per cent in experienced hands; the difficulty is in achieving total removal of the tumor, for short of that plasma HGH values remain elevated. *Transsphenoidal* removal, especially of small adenomas, may be highly successful in skilled hands; in a recent series of 40 patients treated by this method, 25 had clinical "cure" with return of plasma HGH to normal levels, and 10 showed improvement with substantial falls of plasma HGH: there was one late postoperative death. Both *stereotaxic* and *transsphenoidal cryohypophysectomy* have also been used in small numbers of patients.

Several *pharmacologic agents* have been tried: *estrogens, chlorpromazine, progestins,* and *somatostatin* (HGH-inhibiting hormone). These drugs may prove to be suitable in selected "mild" cases; further trials over long periods will be required for full evaluation of efficacy.

BASOPHILIC ADENOMA WITH CUSHING'S SYNDROME. Natural History. These tumors are *small,* being rarely visible by routine radiographic methods. They can sometimes be seen by microtomography of the pituitary fossa. If the sella is enlarged, the lesion is most likely a chromophobe adenoma; those pituitary tumors occurring after bilateral total adrenalectomy for Cushing's syndrome have chromophilic granulations, are aggressive, and may secrete ACTH and β-MSH with dermal pigmentation (Nelson's syndrome).

Treatment. *Conventional external pituitary radiation* (up to 4000 rads) in the "pituitary" type of Cushing's syndrome may yield results better than the 30 to 40 per cent of incomplete or temporary remissions that could be achieved in the past (Orth and Liddle, 1971). In *Nelson's syndrome,* tumors may be aggressive or malignant, and require more radiation; with *heavy particles,* doses of 12,000 to 16,000 rads have been given with control of most tumors. In the faster-growing adenomas, particularly those with large extrasellar extension, *surgery* is required.

Transsphenoidal surgery for removal of these tumors, especially when small (microadenomas), has, in many patients, corrected the ACTH and β-MSH oversecretion and controlled the tumor without producing hypopituitarism. When there is a large suprasellar component, the *transfrontal* approach is preferable.

CRANIOPHARYNGIOMA (RATHKE'S POUCH TUMOR, ADAMANTINOMA). Although they may first appear in adult life, most of these tumors become manifest in childhood. Signs of increased intracranial pressure, changes in visual fields and acuity, and slowing or cessation of growth in late childhood are typical; because of the suprasellar location of the major portion of the tumor mass, *hypothalamic symptoms,* especially *diabetes insipidus,* occur occasionally. About 80 per cent of craniopharyngiomas display suprasellar calcification on x-ray (Fig. 1); the sella may be normal, eroded, or enlarged. Since these tumors are cystic (lined with squamous or columnar epithelium not resembling pituitary cells), they are not very radiosensitive; *transfrontal surgery* is usually indicated.

MULTIPLE ENDOCRINE ADENOMATOSIS. Clinical Characteristics. Acidophilic or chromophobic adenomas of the pituitary are occasionally accompanied by functioning islet cell tumors of the pancreas and adenomas of the parathyroids and adrenal cortex. Intractable peptic ulcer (hypergastrinemia, Zollinger-Ellison syndrome; q.v.) is often associated. The disorder is familial in many instances. Presenting symptoms may be those of pituitary tumor (ocular, neurologic, acromegaly), hypoglycemia, hyperparathyroidism (e.g., renal colic) or gastrointestinal hemorrhage. Acromegaly with hypertension has been associated with surgically proved primary *aldosterone-secreting adrenal adenoma.* It is probably more correct to regard multiple endocrine adenomatosis (also known as Wermer's syndrome) as a complex of separate genetic abnormalities than as a series of consequences of a single primary disease. This syndrome (known as multiple endocrine adenomatosis Type I or MEA I) should not be confused with MEA Type II: medullary carcinoma of the thyroid, pheochromocytoma and parathyroid hyperplasia (also known as Sipple's syndrome), which is a familial disease transmitted as an autosomal dominant trait with a high degree of penetrance (see Ch. 546.2, 546.8, and 552.2).*

Treatment. This syndrome may present the physician with a nice problem in deciding which tumor to treat first. Generally, the pituitary tumors are not so threatening as the others; unless there is a major or rapidly progressive impairment of vision, treatment of the pituitary adenoma or of acromegaly can wait. Obviously, the gastrointestinal problem, the hypoglycemia, or the hypercalcemia will have to be attacked first, depending upon which is the most acute or the most incapacitating.

PITUITARY APOPLEXY. This acute event, literally "pituitary stroke," means infarction or necrosis of or hemorrhage into a pituitary tumor. It was first described in 1905 and is said to occur in 5 to 10 per cent of patients with pituitary tumor. Sheehan's syndrome (see Ch. 543.6) may perhaps be thought of as a kind of pituitary apoplexy, which can also be seen in association with any type of pituitary tumor and now and again in diabetic patients without pituitary neoplasms. Precipitating causes cited have been anticoagulation therapy, radiotherapy to the pituitary region, pneumoencephalography, and fractures of the base of the skull. There have been very few studies of anterior pituitary function before and after pituitary apoplexy. In acromegaly, the plasma HGH value may fall, but the endocrine symptoms have been variously reported as remitting or staying the same. Pituitary responses to administered TRH and LHRH have also been variable. The early literature on pituitary apoplexy depicts a catastrophic clinical picture with a high mortality rate. More recently, there have appeared a number of reports of spontaneous recovery without neurosurgical intervention and without significant worsening of ocular or neurologic deficits. Pituitary apoplexy can on occasion destroy enough adenohypophysial tissue to produce an "empty" sella (see below). In summary, the importance of pituitary apoplexy is this: it should be considered in any patient with a known pituitary tumor who sustains a bout of acute unconsciousness, blindness, or headache; fortunately, many and perhaps most patients recover spontaneously and do not necessarily require surgery. If further endocrine deficiency supervenes after the event, appropriate changes in hormonal replacement therapy are of course indicated.

PITUITARY TUMORS DURING PREGNANCY. This paragraph deals with pre-existing tumors, not with the normal "physiologic" swelling of the adenohypophysis that occurs during gestation (see Anatomy in Ch. 543.1). Destruction of the anterior pituitary by tumor is not a rare cause of infertility in women. Now that artificial (hormonal) induction of ovulation with the successful carrying of pregnancy to term has become possible (see Ch. 549), many women have sustained gestation and delivery in the presence of *treated* pituitary tumors. Apparently, the usual pregnancy-induced pituitary swelling is not sufficient to create an important clinical problem in such

---

*These syndromes are sometimes referred to as "multiple endocrine neoplasia," Type I or II, or as MEN I or MEN II. For the relation of these adenomatoses to "apudomas," see Ch. 525.

Figure 6. "Empty" sella in a 56-year-old woman. Pneumoencephalogram, lateral (sagittal) view of the sella which shows depression of the sellar floor (1). The striking abnormality is downward extension of air (2) into the sella; the pituitary is flattened downward and posteriorly (3). Normally, no air should enter the sella. If an intrasellar tumor were present, one would expect it to elevate the air column above the sella and encroach upward upon the third ventricle (4).

patients. If ocular signs (hemianopia) occur during gestation, they are generally reversible. In the very few reported patients who have undergone successful pregnancies in the face of *untreated* pituitary tumors, there seems to be a 5 per cent likelihood of blindness owing to swelling of the hypophysial tumor, but this frightening sign disappears post partum.

THE "EMPTY" SELLA SYNDROMES. Pathogenesis and Clinical Characteristics. In an unknown proportion of cases, enlargement of the pituitary fossa as seen on lateral x-rays of the skull is not due to pituitary tumor. In recent studies of patients with enlarged pituitary fossae, a quarter to a third of enlarged sellae were found on pneumoencephalography to contain not too much but too little pituitary tissue (Fig. 6). One autopsy series has revealed a 5.8 per cent incidence of this lesion in nearly 800 presumably normal people, the space above the pituitary remnant being replaced by a subarachnoid sac filled with cerebrospinal fluid. "Empty" sella may occur as a consequence of Sheehan's syndrome or of necrosis of a pituitary adenoma, either spontaneous (secondary to pituitary apoplexy) or after x-irradiation. The sella may be radiologically enlarged or normal. The pathogenesis is debated. Possible mechanisms include pseudotumor cerebri (benign intracranial hypertension), a defective diaphragma sellae through which an outpouching of subarachnoid membrane may descend, and medial kinking of the internal carotids compressing the "waist" of the dorsum sellae, with consequent expansion ("ballooning") of the pituitary. The *clinical picture* may show *no endocrine abnormality* or *frank hypopituitarism*. Usually symptoms of pituitary deficiency are not prominent, but one or more defects in anterior pituitary hormone secretion can be shown by test. There seems to be a curious predisposition to empty sella in obese middle-aged women who have had many children.

Diagnosis and Treatment. This lesion emphasizes the need for *pneumoencephalography* in all cases of enlarged sella (Fig. 6) in which radiotherapy or pituitary surgery might be contemplated; such treatment, directed to an unsuspected empty sella, is likely to produce a permanent CSF fistula. CAT scanning is not yet regarded as a foolproof method in the detection of "empty" sella. If an empty sella is found, the only therapy required is replacement of lost hormonal functions if any are shown to exist.

GUIDELINES FOR THE DIAGNOSIS AND TREATMENT OF PITUITARY TUMORS. The following "rules" will be helpful in the management of patients suspected of having pituitary tumors.

1. Sellar x-rays should be done in any patient with persistent headache. There is *nothing* specific about the headache of pituitary tumor.

2. Optic atrophy or visual field defect demands diagnostic study of the pituitary.

3. Juxtasellar calcification (by x-ray) requires careful study of pituitary structure and function.

4. Any hypogonadal, hypothyroid, or hypoadrenocortical patient must have a hypophysial cause excluded.

5. Galactorrhea is or can be a signal of pituitary disease.

6. If a pituitary tumor is definitely present, it has to be treated because (a) if associated with acromegaly, the mortality rate is about double that of the age-matched population at large; (b) if associated with a "functionless," presumably chromophobic adenoma, 80 to 90 per cent of patients will come to a bad end neurologically; if treated (e.g., by simple external radiotherapy), 80 to 90 per cent of patients will have their pituitary tumor arrested, at least from the mechanical if not from the endocrine point of view.

7. Raised serum prolactin levels may turn out to be a valuable early clue to detecting the presence of an otherwise invisible chromophobe adenoma.

8. Not all enlarged sellas contain pituitary tumors. A significant portion (25 to 33 per cent) are "empty" sellas.

9. Treatment is still controversial. The choices are conventional (up to 5000 rads) external x-radiation, proton beam therapy, transfrontal and transsphenoidal hypophysectomy, or adenomectomy. Each method has advocates and detractors.

To summarize, the practice of this writer is as follows. Any patient with acromegaly has to be treated, either by conventional external radiotherapy (which works pretty well over the long pull and is quite innocuous) or transsphenoidal adenomectomy, depending on which method is the more readily available. For "functionless" and presumably chromophobic adenomas, those that are associated with no ocular, neurologic, or endocrine symptoms or signs can be managed by close observation alone, i.e., physical examination and skull films every six months. For "presumed" chromophobe adenomas that are associated with symptoms in any of the aforementional three categories, "conventional" sellar radiotherapy will suffice in most cases, with minimal morbidity. Large tumors which have produced significant impairment of vision may be successfully treated by radiation; if this is not effective, adenomectomy should be done by the most reasonable means: transsphenoidal if the tumor is small, transfrontal if there is considerable upward or anterior extension of the tumor. For prolactin-secreting tumors, transsphenoidal surgery and radiotherapy may well be equally efficacious. "Basophilic" adenomas associated with Cushing's syndrome seem to be treated as well by the proton beam method as by transethmoidal removal of the microadenoma.

Bower, B. F.: Pituitary enlargement secondary to untreated primary hypogonadism. Ann. Intern. Med., 69:107, 1968.

Fürst, E.: On chromophobe pituitary adenoma. Acta Med. Scand. (Suppl. 452), 1966.

Jordan, R. M., Kendall, J. W., and Kerber, C. W.: The primary empty sella syndrome. Analysis of the clinical characteristics, radiographic features, pituitary function and cerebrospinal fluid adenohypophysial hormone concentrations. Am. J. Med., 62:569, 1977.

Kohler, P. O., and Ross, G. T. (eds.): Diagnosis and Treatment of Pituitary Tumors, New York, American Elsevier Publishing Company, 1973.

Lawrence, A. M., Wilber, J. F., and Hagen, T. C.: The pituitary and primary hypothyroidism: Enlargement and unusual growth hormone secretory responses. Arch. Intern. Med., 132:327, 1973.

LeMay, M.: The radiologic diagnosis of pituitary disease. Radiol. Clin. North Am, 5:303, 1967.

Reich, N. E., Zelch, J. V., Alfidi, R. J., Meany, T. F., Duchesnau, P. M., and Weinstein, M. A.: Computed tomography in the detection of juxtasellar lesions. Radiology, 118:333, 1976.

Schimke, R. N.: Multiple endocrine adenomatosis syndromes. Adv. Intern. Med., 21:349, 1976.

Weisberg, L. A.: Pituitary apoplexy: Association of degenerative change in pituitary adenoma with radiotherapy and detection by cerebral computed tomography. Am. J. Med., 63:109, 1977.

Weisberg, L. A., Zimmerman, E. A., and Frantz, A. G.: Diagnosis and evaluation of patients with an enlarged sella turcica. Am. J. Med., 61:590, 1976.

543.6. HYPOPITUITARISM

PITUITARY INSUFFICIENCY IN THE ADULT

DEFINITIONS. Hypopituitarism is the clinical condition resulting from destruction of the anterior pituitary; it is accompanied by secondary atrophy of the gonads, thyroid, and adrenal cortex. The term *panhypopituitarism* has been used to designate total absence of all the known pituitary secretions. *Simmonds' disease* is used synonymously. The term *Sheehan's disease* describes hypopituitarism resulting from postpartum necrosis of the gland. The designation *pituitary insufficiency* is inclusive.

ETIOLOGY, PATHOLOGY, AND PATHOGENESIS. The most common cause of pituitary insufficiency in adult life is *pituitary tumor,* particularly chromophobe adenoma; the most common cause of *very severe* adult hypopituitarism is probably postpartum necrosis of the gland. This lesion occurs rarely in the western world but is frequent as a cause of hypopituitarism in developing nations, e.g., in South America and Africa. The pathogenesis is debated. The common denominator is obstetric accident. According to Sheehan, peripheral vascular collapse is followed by spasm of local vessels, then thrombosis, and then infarction. McKay holds that the primary event is not arteriolar spasm but thrombosis of pituitary vessels as part of generalized intravascular coagulation. Neither view accounts for the peculiar susceptibility of the swollen pituitary to damage in the postpartum period The well-demarcated infarctions are small or nearly total. Sheehan and Summers have shown that pituitary insufficiency does not occur unless the lesion is very large. The late lesion is fibrosis with residual small nests of normal chromophils.

Lesions other than tumors (see Ch. 543.5) are fibrosis of unknown cause, granulomas, which may be nonspecific, syphilitic, or tuberculous, and aneurysms of the *internal carotid artery.* Ischemic necrosis has occasionally followed acute infection (usually associated with diabetes mellitus), meningitis, basal skull fracture, and septic cavernous sinus thrombosis. Other rare causes are abscesses, metastatic carcinoma or lymphoma, and various juxtasellar cysts and tumors. In some patients the primary defect may be in the hypothalamus (e.g., sarcoidosis, Hand-Schüller-Christian disease, histiocytosis X, idiopathic).

General pathologic findings in pituitary insufficiency include widespread *splanchnomicria* with particularly striking atrophy of the gonads, thyroid, and adrenal cortex.

CLINICAL MANIFESTATIONS AND NATURAL HISTORY. The speed of onset of pituitary insufficiency depends upon the nature and size of the lesion. When *postpartum necrosis* of the pituitary is extensive and severe, acute symptoms such as *diabetes insipidus* and *hypoglycemia* occur during the puerperium and may be only transitory; the patient may suddenly die within weeks, probably as a consequence of acute adrenocortical insufficiency. More commonly, the onset after obstetric accident is slow, occurring over months to years. The first symptom is usually failure to lactate; pubic and axillary hair fails to grow; menses do not return owing to gonadal failure, or the periods are scanty and transitory; amenorrhea follows. Libido is lost. Symptoms of *thyroid and adrenocortical failure* occur later as a rule than do those of ovarian deficiency, but *there is no set pattern.* General deterioration ensues. Patients become weak, easily fatigued, indifferent to their surroundings, slothful, and negligent of household duties. *Personality changes* range from mild idiosyncrasies to frank psychosis. Intolerance of cold, as in primary hypothyroidism, may be exteme. *Hypopituitary coma* with hypotension and hypothermia, probably in most instances resulting from *hypoglycemia,* may have its onset gradually with no apparent cause, or rapidly in response to minor illness. At times collapse is preceded

Fig. 7   **Fig. 8**

Figure 7. A patient with documented hypopituitarism 21 years after postpartum necrosis of the pituitary. Pubic and axillary hair is gone. Notice the absence of cachexia. Compare with Figure 8. (Reproduced by permission from Sheehan, H. L., and Summers, V. K.: Quart J. Med., 42:319, 1949.)

Figure 8. The patient is a 30-year-old unmarried woman with anorexia nervosa who had lost 55 pounds (compare with the good nutritional state of the patient with hypopituitarism, Fig. 7). Pubic hair was present and menses continued but were scanty and irregular. (Reproduced by permission from Bliss, E. L., and Branch, C. H. H.: Anorexia Nervosa, New York, Paul B. Hoeber, Inc., 1960.)

by clinical manifestations of *adrenal crisis* with nausea, vomiting, high fever, and hypotension. Although *anorexia* is a prominent feature in some patients, cachexia is uncommon and is a terminal event in the neglected patient. Pre-existing diabetes is on rare occasions ameliorated abruptly, with sudden lowering of the insulin requirement after pituitary destruction ("Houssay phenomenon").

The *physical examination* discloses a fair state of nutrition as a rule (Fig. 7). The skin is thin, smooth, cool and pale, with fine wrinkling about the eyes (geroderma). The dry, scaly skin and puffy face of primary myxedema are unusual but occur on occasion. Pubic and axillary hair is absent or sparse. The pulse is slow and thin, the blood pressure low. Symptomatic hypotension on orthostasis is common. The breasts may appear well preserved, but genital atrophy is the rule.

General *laboratory examination* shows a moderate normochromic anemia that is less striking than the pallid appearance suggests. Roentgenogram of the skull is normal (there is no expanding intrasellar lesion). Blood glucose concentration is often low. The serum sodium concentration may be 120 mEq per liter or lower without symptoms of adrenal insufficiency. Hyponatremia is probably related to hemodilution owing to inadequate excretion of water, which in turn is due to deficient cortisol secretion. Episodic hyponatremia in patients with pituitary insufficiency is correlated with measurable water retention (increased total body water), not with sodium depletion. The level of serum potassium is normal or low (not high, as in classic primary adrenocortical insufficiency [Addison's disease, see Ch. 547.3]). As in the hypophysectomized animal or man, the aldosterone function of the adrenal cortex is fairly well preserved; the hypopituitary patient responds to salt withdrawal by a slow but adequate increase in aldosterone secretion and consequent retention of sodium. In very severe hypopituitarism with complete adrenal destruction, this capacity may be lost. The urinary 17-ketosteroids and corticosteroids are decreased. The serum T_4 and T_3 RU are depressed, but thyroidal uptake of ^{131}I is often inexplicably normal even when the patient is clinically hypothyroid.

The typical clinical picture becomes obvious as late as 15 to 20 years after the obstetric accident. Acute adrenocortical failure with or without superimposed infection is the chief cause of death in untreated patients.

Expanding intrasellar tumors — e.g., chromophobe adenoma — may have a similar insidious onset. The clinical picture and natural history are discussed in Ch. 543.5. In patients with intrasellar tumor, both the chief complaint and the ultimate cause of death are more commonly mechanical results of the adenoma than of pituitary failure.

DIAGNOSIS. A history of postpartum hemorrhage, symptoms and signs of an intracranial tumor with chiasmal pressure, or evidence of multiple glandular deficiencies should raise the question of hypopituitarism. Diagnosis is difficult early in the course of the disease, before symptoms and signs of deficiency of more than one target gland are definite. Hypopituitarism should be suspected in patients with onset of gonadal failure in adult life. Amenorrhea occuring in a fertile woman before the expected age of menopause requires inquiry about obstetric hemorrhage in the past. Loss of axillary and pubic hair and atrophy of the external genitalia make hypopituitarism likely in a relatively young woman with amenorrhea. In men, loss of previously normal libido and potency and loss of body hair with or without genital atrophy are suggestive; roentgenogram of the skull shows sagittal stretching or ballooning of the sella if a pituitary tumor is present (Fig. 3). Reduced visual acuity, optic atrophy, and bitemporal hemianopia provide evidence of suprasellar expansion of an intrasellar mass (see Ch. 543.5). Failure of sexual development late in the second decade raises the question of hypopituitarism in either sex.

In the *differential diagnosis,* primary gonadal failure and primary hypothyroidism must be considered. *Primary gonadal failure,* in the *male* especially, may resemble pituitary insufficiency. The degree of eunuchoidism (disproportionately long arms and legs owing to late closure of the epiphyses of the long bones) depends on the age of onset of hypoleydigism, being extreme if early, absent if late. Many males with gonadal failure have fine, pale, wrinkled skin like that seen in hypopituitarism, but thyroid and adrenal function is normal. *Anorexia nervosa* is not difficult to differentiate, because only gonadotropic deficiency is present and the degree of emaciation is extreme (Fig. 8; see Ch. 475).

Levels of urinary gonadotropin are elevated in testicular deficiency, undetectable in pituitary failure. Klinefelter's syndrome (seminiferous tubule dysgenesis) is easily distinguished. In the female the same principles apply: The level of urinary gonadotropin is undetectable in hypopituitarism, high in natural menopause. *Primary myxedema* is generally characterized by more noticeable dryness and puffiness of the skin, and the serum cholesterol tends to be higher. In hypothyroidism resulting from pituitary failure, other glandular deficiencies (e.g., gonadal) are often present and should be sought. Measurement of plasma immunoassayable TSH or of thyroidal response to thyrotropin is helpful (see Ch. 543.4). *Primary adrenocortical failure* (Addison's disease) is not hard to differentiate. The skin is darkly tanned (MSH) rather than pale, gonadal function is often normal, and thyroidal function is unimpaired, unless Hashimoto's thyroiditis is associated (Schmidt's syndrome). Diagnosis of this entity is discussed in Ch. 547.3. Primary adrenal failure is ruled out, and subtle adrenal insufficiency caused by pituitary failure is diagnosed by measuring the response of plasma or urinary corticosteroids to intravenous corticotropin. This constitutes more specific evidence of adrenal deficiency than do low urinary steroid values, which are reduced in a great variety of chronic, debilitating diseases. Measurement of plasma ACTH levels by radioimmunoassay (if available) should yield low values in hypopituitary patients.

TREATMENT. *Long-term medical management* of the patient with hypopituitarism consists of careful replacement of lost functions. (Management of intrasellar mass lesions is discussed in Ch. 543.5.) Tropic hormones are not used because of expense and the bother of daily injections. By far the most important defect is that of the *adrenal cortex;* acute adrenal crisis may come on abruptly and without warning, and may lead to death.

Under ordinary conditions, cortisone or hydrocortisone (10 to 25 mg per day in two divided doses, by mouth) provides a sense of well-being and adequate protection against hypotension, hypoglycemia, and water and electrolyte imbalance. Small doses are preferred, because patients with hypopituitarism have a peculiar susceptibility to the effects of larger doses of corticosteroids (peptic ulcer, facial rounding, psychosis) possibly because of coexisting secondary hypothyroidism in which metabolism of corticosteroids is much delayed. Added salt and a mineralocorticoid are only occasionally required. In the female, diethylstilbestrol, 0.5 to 1.0 mg per day or Premarin, 1.25 mg daily, for 20 days of each month, provides good maintenance of developed secondary sex characters and, in time, leads to an artificial menstrual cycle. Induction of ovulation in women with hypopituitarism is discussed in Ch. 549.2. In the male, a fair degree of libido and potency can be conferred by androgens (methyltestosterone, 20 to 30 mg per day orally; testosterone propionate, 25 to 100 mg two to three times per week by intramuscular injection; or a long-acting ester, e.g., testosterone enanthate, 100 to 200 mg once per month intramuscularly). Thyroid replacement should be started with small doses (8 to 15 mg per day of USP thyroid orally), which are gradually

increased over a period of several weeks; for optimal effect a dose as large as 0.180 gram may be needed. Roughly equivalent doses of L-thyroxine are 0.1 to 0.2 mg per day. Triiodothyronine should not be used. Its onset of action is too fast and its duration of activity too short. It is probably wise to begin corticosteroid therapy first, because adrenal crisis has allegedly been precipitated by vigorous treatment with thyroid hormone alone.

Treatment of an acute illness or management during a surgical procedure, e.g., craniotomy for intrasellar tumor, is that of adrenal crisis. Thyroid hormone is not necessary. *Corticotropin should never be relied upon,* because the degree of endogenous adrenal response is unpredictable. Correct treatment is hydrocortisone (100 to 300 mg per day of a water-soluble ester in isotonic saline intravenously). It is better to err on the side of *moderately* excessive doses, because untoward reactions are not likely to occur during the few days of vigorous treatment generally required; the dose should be reduced as quickly as possible to the maintenance level. If in an emergency there is doubt concerning the presence of secondary hypoadrenalism, one should assume that it exists rather than attempt a time-consuming laboratory evaluation of adrenal status. If *diabetes insipidus* occurs postoperatively, treatment is as set out in Ch. 544.2.

Martin, L. G., Martul, P., Connor, T. B., and Wiswell, J. G.: Hypothalamic origin of idiopathic hypopituitarism. Metabolism, 21:143, 1972.

McKay, D. G.: Pituitary. *In* Disseminated Intravascular Coagulation. New York, Hoeber Medical Division, Harper & Row, 1965, pp. 405, 460.

Naidich, T. P., Pinto, R. S., Kushner, M. J., Lin, J. P., Kricheff, I. I., Leeds, N. E., and Chase, N. E.: Evaluation of sellar and parasellar masses by computed tomography. Radiology, 120:91, 1976.

Pittman, J. A., Jr: Hypopituitarism. *In* Werner, S. C., and Ingbar, S. H. (eds.): The Thyroid: A Fundamental and Clinical Text. 4th ed. Hagerstown, Md. Harper & Row, 1978, p. 936.

Sheehan, H. L., and Davis, J. C.: Pituitary necrosis. Br. Med. Bull., 24:59, 1968.

Sheehan, H. L., and Summers, V. K.: The syndrome of hypopituitarism. Quart, J. Med., 42:319, 1949.

Sheehan, H. L., and Stanfield, J. P.: The pathogenesis of post-partum necrosis of the anterior lobe of the pituitary gland. Acta Endocrinol., 37:479, 1961.

Warren, M. P., and Vande Wiele, R. L.: Clinical and metabolic features of anorexia nervosa. Am. J. Obstet. Gynecol., 117:435, 1973.

DEFICIENCY OF SINGLE ANTERIOR PITUITARY HORMONES

It is hard to determine in an individual case whether there is isolated deficiency of a pituitary hormone or whether one is observing an early stage of what will turn out to be panhypopituitarism. Whereas some *pituitary dwarfs* are panhypopituitary, others have *isolated HGH deficiency,* either of pituitary or hypothalamic origin (see below). Patients who have Hand-Schüller-Christian disease with short stature have also been shown to have isolated HGH deficiency. It is not yet known whether women who have failure of postpartum lactation are deficient in *prolactin* secretion and deficient in the secretion of that hormone *alone.* Idiopathic isolated FSH and LH failure exists in several forms, with or without anosmia, in men and women. *Isolated deficiencies of TSH and ACTH* have been reported; in one instance of the latter, pituitary basophils were virtually absent. Isolated corticotropin deficiency has been found as part of the hypothalamic disorder of acute intermittent porphyria. As indicated previously, it is not always possible to distinguish between a hypothalamic and a pituitary cause of isolated pituitary hormone deficiency (Edwards and Besser, 1974).

The most common form of isolated ACTH deficiency occurs in patients receiving *long-term corticosteroid therapy*, which is discussed in Ch. 547.6. Prolonged treatment with thyroid hormone and antiovulatory drugs usually induces *self-limited* TSH and gonadotropin deficiency; rarely, the latter persists ("oversuppression syndrome," see Ch. 549.2).

TREATMENT. Thyrotropin and adrenocorticotropin deficiencies are usually treated with thyroid hormone (or thyroxine) and corticosteroids, respectively. Administration of purified human FSH and HCG is effective in the induction of ovulation in hypopituitary women and sometimes of spermatogenesis in men (see Ch. 548.2 and 549.2).

Braunstein, G. D., and Kohler, P. O.: Pituitary function in Hand-Schüller-Christian disease. Evidence for deficient growth-hormone release in patients with short stature. N. Engl. J. Med., 286:1225, 1972.

Carlson, H. E., and Hershman, J. M.: The hypothalamic-pituitary-thyroid axis. Med. Clin. North Am., 59:1045, 1975.

Christy, N. P.: Iatrogenic Cushing's syndrome. *In* Christy, N. P. (ed): The Human Adrenal Cortex, New York, Harper & Row, 1971, p. 395.

Christy, N. P.: Editorial: The clinical significance of pituitary-adrenal suppression by exogenous corticosteroids. J. Chron. Dis., 26:261, 1973.

Males, J. L., Townsend, J. L., and Schneider, R. A.: Hypogonadotropic hypogonadism with anosmia — Kallmann's syndrome. Arch. Intern. Med., 131:501, 1973.

Mejer, J.: Isolated adrenocorticotrophic hormone deficiency: A case report. Danish Med. Bull. 23:45, 1976.

Melby, J. C.: Systemic corticosteroid therapy: Pharmacology and endocrinologic considerations. Ann. Intern. Med., 81:505, 1974.

Rabin, D.: The syndromes of isolated gonadotropin deficiency. Birth Defects, 11:73, 1975.

HYPOPHYSECTOMY-INDUCED HYPOPITUITARISM

Since 1952, pituitary ablation has been used as a palliative treatment for metastatic cancer and for diabetic retinopathy. The mortality rate of the operation is 1 to 2 per cent, higher in diabetic patients.

The metabolic consequences of hypophysectomy in man are familiar. They are repaired by hormonal replacement therapy. If *diabetes insipidus* is a sequela, it is treated with vasopressin as set forth in Ch. 544.2. The postoperative incidence of diabetes insipidus is 10 to 15 per cent, with about 5 per cent being permanent; the lesion is much more common (50 per cent) in patients subjected to electrocoagulation of the pituitary stalk. Diabetes insipidus almost never follows any form of pituitary radiotherapy. Loss of gonadotropic function, observed as disappearance of detectable urinary gonadotropin, occurs within a week after hypophysectomy. Gonadal steroids are not given to patients with cancer, because the induced hypogonadism may be an important part of the palliative therapy. Loss of thyrotropic function is apparent from fall of serum T_4 values to myxedematous levels at one week and of thyroidal uptake of ^{131}I at two weeks after pituitary ablation. If hypophysectomy is incomplete, these indices decline, only to return to normal within a month after surgery. Loss of adrenocorticotropic function is notable only if hypophysectomy has been virtually total. Some investigators believe that the metyrapone test and measurement of plasma prolactin concentration are the most sensitive indices of completeness of hypophysectomy. In the completely hypophysectomized patient, withdrawal of replacement therapy precipitates symptoms and signs of secondary adrenocortical failure within five to ten days.

Conventional medical treatment consists of thyroid USP in daily doses of 0.120 gram (or L-thyroxine, 0.1 to 0.2 mg) and cortisone acetate, 25 mg or less, both given by mouth.

Methods for pituitary ablation are numerous: transfrontal and transsphenoidal hypophysectomy, cryosurgery, stereotaxic radiofrequency surgery, pituitary stalk section, implantation of radioactive gold or yttrium (^{198}Au, ^{90}Y), and external delivery of heavy particles (proton beam) from the cyclotron. It is not yet possible to decide which of these techniques is the safest or the most effective for all patients. It is also not clear why pituitary ablation is effective at all; there is evidence that adequate palliation may not be closely or uniquely related to the degree of reduction in growth hormone or prolactin secretion.

The present position can be summarized in this way. Methods for predicting the efficacy of hypophysectomy are not yet satisfactory. Carefully selected patients with advanced, widespread metastases from cancer of the breast have objective remissions in bony, cutaneous, and pulmonary metastases in about 40 per cent of cases treated with surgical hypophysectomy. The best results are achieved in women with osseous metastases only. In metastatic prostatic cancer, remissions occur in fewer than half the patients. The methods which bring about less complete ablation of the pituitary tend to be associated with lower remission rates (see Ch. 526), but it is now generally agreed that *total* hypophysectomy is not an absolute requirement.

In patients with diabetic retinopathy, surgical hypophysectomy is rarely done now. Most ophthalmologists now favor retinal photocoagulation. Hypophysectomy is ineffective in proliferative retinopathy, and in several series the remission rate of hemorrhages and exudates is about the same in hypophysectomized as in untreated groups of patients. Some recent studies have yielded good results (70 per cent remission rate) in hypophysectomized patients with florid retinopathy but without fibrosis. There appears to be a positive correlation between ocular response and completeness of hypophysectomy. If one can establish a close relationship between retinal improvement and suppression of HGH secretion, *somatostatin* might turn out to be a useful therapeutic tool.

Brendler, H.: Adrenalectomy and hypophysectomy for prostatic cancer. Urology, 2:99, 1973.

Howitz, P. R.: Hypophysectomy and thyroid function. Danish Med. Bull., 27:308, 1975.

Luft, R., and Olivecrona, H.: Hypophysectomy in treatment of malignant tumors. Cancer, 10:789, 1957.

VanGilder, J. C., and Goldenberg, I. S.: Hypophysectomy in metastatic breast cancer. Arch. Surg., 110:293, 1975.

Zimmerman, B. R., and Molnar, G. D.: Prolonged follow-up in diabetic retinopathy treated by sectioning the pituitary stalk. Mayo Clin. Proc. 52:233, 1977.

PITUITARY INSUFFICIENCY IN CHILDHOOD

Lesions involving the pituitary in childhood cause *dwarfism*; like that of gonadotropin, secretion of HGH appears to be more sensitive to impairment than the thyrotropic or adrenocorticotropic functions of the pituitary. Pituitary insufficiency is an uncommon cause of short stature, accounting for fewer than 10 per cent of instances, and having an incidence no greater than 1 to 30,000 live births. About two thirds of pituitary dwarfs have no evidence of pituitary tumor; usually there is no evidence of an anatomic lesion. The lesion may in some cases be hypothalamic. Idiopathic hypophysial *fibrosis* has been occasionally observed. Of the tumors, *craniopharyngioma* (adamantinoma) is the most common. This neoplasm arises from fragments of oral epithelium remaining from the embryologic invagination (see Ch. 543.5). Other causes are *suprasellar cysts* and *Hand-Schüller-Christian disease*. Reversible isolated HGH deficiency has been documented in children with the maternal deprivation syndrome (MDS).

Diagnosis of pituitary dwarfism is often difficult early in life. The infant's size may be normal at birth. Growth does not stop entirely, but is obviously retarded in early infancy. Evidence of thyroid and adrenocortical insufficiency, e.g., hypoglycemic attacks, is strongly suggestive, but may be subtle or absent. If, however, the patient reaches the early years of the second decade with continued retardation of growth and complete failure of sexual development, suspicion of pituitary dwarfism is raised. The physical examination discloses relatively normal proportions. The facies is childish, but the skin may become wrinkled early, imparting an incongruous aspect of aging. Laboratory study shows absence of urinary gonadotropin, reduced concentration of serum protein-bound iodine, and subnormal response of plasma corticosteroids to intravenous adrenocorticotropin. Idiopathic hypopituitary dwarfism may occur either as an isolated, recessively inherited deficiency of growth hormone, or sporadically. When sporadic, the deficiency may involve growth hormone alone or several pituitary hormones.

The *differential diagnosis* of pituitary dwarfism includes constitutional retardation of growth and constitutional delay in the onset of puberty (see Ch. 548.2 and 549.2); in the latter condition, the family history is often positive, evidence of thyroidal and adrenocortical insufficiency is lacking, and in time normal growth and maturation take place. *Systemic and other endocrine diseases* may cause dwarfism; among these are chondrodystrophy, rickets, Hurler's syndrome, intestinal malabsorption, chronic renal disease, hypoxia associated with congenital cardiac malformations, hypothyroidism, and sexual precocity with premature fusion of the epiphyses. These conditions are distinguished by the inappropriately short extremities, osseous deformities, overt malnutrition and evidence of fat intolerance, gross proteinuria and nitrogen retention, cyanosis and heart murmur, mental deficiency and other stigmata of cretinism, or precocious development of the genitalia. D. W. Smith has presented a list of 52 conditions associated with short stature, some of which are recognized at a glance by seasoned pediatricians; Smith also lists the numerous systemic diseases in which growth retardation is observed.

Special mention should be made of those patients, known as sexual ateliotic (incomplete) dwarfs, who become miniature adults often capable of producing normal offspring. During childhood, physical examination cannot distinguish these patients from patients with other varieties of hypopituitary dwarfism. McKusick and his coworkers have shown that in some of these patients the failure to grow in association with normal gonadal and secondary sexual development and normal thyroid and

adrenal cortical function is due to a deficiency of end-organ response to growth hormone. With radioimmuno-assay measurements of serum growth hormone, it is possible to define four subgroups of ateliotic dwarfs, some of whom fail to raise sulfation factor (somatomedin) activity when HGH is administered. It is interesting that the African pygmy also has subresponsiveness to administered growth hormone, whereas endogenous growth hormone release is apparently normal (Table 3). The differentiation of pituitary dwarfism in the female and *gonadal dysgenesis (Turner's syndrome)* may be difficult before puberty; patients with this disorder are phenotypic females who often have associated congenital anomalies (webbed neck, coarctation of the aorta) and short stature; the distinguishing features are less immature facies, less delay in epiphysial closure, slight but definite growth of pubic hair at puberty, a frequently negative (male) chromatin pattern on buccal smear, and, after the age of 9 to 13, an elevated rather than absent titer of urinary gonadotropin (see Ch. 549.2). Recognition of *progeria* is easy; this rare idiopathic condition is characterized by retardation of growth, baldness, loss of subcutaneous fat, premature fusion of epiphyses, and atherosclerosis or arterial calcification, all occurring within the first few years of life. The life span is short; there is no evidence of endocrine disease.

As indicated in Ch. 543.4, the best way to detect growth hormone deficiency is to test the response of serum growth hormone values to insulin-induced hypoglycemia. If a metabolic ward is available, demonstration of a sharp increase in nitrogen retention in response to administered growth hormone is diagnostic of classic idiopathic HGH deficiency (see also Table 3). Analysis of the growth curve determines whether or not to subject the patient to elaborate testing procedures.

As to *treatment*, a moderate degree of linear growth can be achieved in hypopituitary dwarfs through the administration of thyroid hormone in combination with gonadal steroids. Impressive skeletal growth can be induced, with the administration of purified human growth hormone.

TABLE 3.   Classification of Pituitary Dwarfism*

I. *HGH undetectable:*
  A. Idiopathic hypopituitarism (primary disorder of pituitary or secondary to deficiency of hypothalamic HGHRF)
    1. Panhypopituitarism
    2. Isolated HGH deficiency (may be familial)
  B. Organic hypopituitarism
    1. Tumors
    2. Trauma
    3. Infection
    4. Hand-Schüller-Christian disease
  C. HGH unreactive immunologically, partially active biologically (Merimee's Type II ateliotic dwarf)
    1. Absent HGH response to provocative tests
    2. Evidence that endogenous HGH has some activity
    3. Resistance to exogenous HGH (including no rise in somatomedin)
    4. Autosomal dominant inheritance in some cases

II. *HGH detectable but ineffective:*
  A. Laron dwarf
    1. Normal plasma HGH response to provocative tests
    2. Plasma HGH normal or high
    3. Deficient generation of somatomedin when HGH is given
  B. African pygmy
    1. Normal plasma HGH response to provocative tests
    2. Plasma HGH normal
    3. Somatomedin low and showing no rise when HGH is given

*Compiled from many sources by Dr. C. A. L. Abrams.

The optimal dose is about 20 to 45 mg per month (see Tanner et al.). This therapy is limited by the short supply of the hormone; if it is used, gonadal steroids should not be given until maximal linear growth is attained so that epiphysial closure will not occur; thyroid hormone augments the somatotropic effects. Detailed criteria for diagnosis and treatment of pituitary dwarfism and descriptions of appropriate responses to growth hormone are readily available. The hormone causes only minimal if any increase in linear growth rate in children whose short stature is not due to deficiency of HGH. Since growth hormone should therefore be reserved for patients with growth hormone deficiency, a high premium is placed upon accurate diagnosis.

Laron, Z.: Syndrome of familial dwarfism and high plasma immunoreactive hormone. Israel J. Med. Sci., 10:1247, 1974.

Maclaren, N. K., Cornblath, M., and Raiti, S.: Human growth hormone. A symposium. Am. J. Dis. Child., 127:906, 1974.

Merimee, T. J.: Isolated growth hormone deficiency and related disorders. Ann. Rev. Med., 25:137, 1974.

Pertzelan, A., Kauli, R., Assa, S., Greenberg, D., and Laron, Z.: Intermittent treatment with human growth hormone (GH) in isolated GH deficiency and in multiple pituitary hormone deficiency. Clin. Endocrinol., 5:15, 1976.

Rabinowitz, D., and Merimee, T. J.: Isolated human growth hormone deficiency and related disorders. Israel J. Med. Sci., 9:1598, 1973.

Rimoin, D. L.: Genetic forms of pituitary dwarfism. Birth Defects, 7:12, 1971.

Smith, D. W.: Compendium on shortness of stature. J. Pediat., 70:463, 1967.

Tanner, J. M., Whitehouse, R. H., Hughes, P. C. R., and Vince, F. P.: Effect of human growth hormone treatment of 1 to 7 years on growth of 100 children with growth hormone deficiency, low birthweight, inherited smallness, Turner's syndrome, and other complaints. Arch. Dis. Child., 46:745, 1971.

543.7. HYPERPITUITARISM

ACROMEGALY

DEFINITION. Acromegaly is a chronic disease of middle life characterized by overgrowth of bone, connective tissue, and viscera in response to prolonged and excessive secretion of adenohypophysial growth hormone. The term "acromegaly" denotes the typical enlargement of acral or distal parts of the body — the hands, feet, face, and head.

ETIOLOGY. The increased secretion of growth hormone results from overactivity of the acidophil cells of the pituitary. The evidence for excessive growth hormone is that (1) similar pathologic changes are produced in animals by administration of the hormone, and (2) increased concentrations of growth hormone have been detected in plasma of patients with acromegaly. Hyperactivity of the anterior pituitary is deduced from (1) the almost invariable necropsy finding of pituitary enlargement, (2) histologic observation of overgrowth of the acidophilic cells, and (3) the clinical improvement that frequently follows destruction of the gland.

INCIDENCE AND PREVALENCE. Acromegaly is a rare disorder with about 300 new cases per year being discovered in the United States. The sexes are affected equally. Acromegaly starts most commonly in the third and fourth decades; a few patients trace the start of acromegaly to adolescence. Some 30 acromegalic children have been reported.

PATHOLOGY AND PATHOGENESIS. Acidophilic or mixed acidophilic and chromophobe adenoma is found in 75 per cent or more of autopsied patients with acromegaly. Rarely, acidophil cell hyperplasia is observed, malignancy almost never. The growth of the tumor may obliterate normal cells. The assumption is that if hypopituitarism occurs, it is a result of atrophy of normal pituitary tissue owing to the pressure of the tumor. Over 90 per cent of adenomas cause sufficient enlargement of the sella turcica to be visible in roentgenograms of the skull. Sellar enlargement may be minimal or gross (Fig. 4). Upward extension rarely produces clinical evidence of hypothalamic involvement, e.g., diabetes insipidus, but invasion of the optic tracts of chiasm is of clinical significance (visual field changes, optic atrophy) in about 60 per cent of patients.

The excessive secretion of growth hormone affects virtually all organs and tissues. The response of cartilage and bone is obvious and distinctive. The histologic appearance of chondrogenesis and osteogenesis is somewhat disorderly. The cartilaginous and bony response occurs at points of special sensitivity, e.g., mandible, zygoma, ribs, and clavicles. The uneven growth is thought to be due to the effect of pressure or of muscular traction. Increased *chondrogenesis* is most obvious in hypertrophy of the costal cartilages, which contributs to the increased circumference of the thorax. *Acromegalic arthritis*, affecting chiefly the large joints and the spine, resembles osteoarthritis and results from proliferation of deep layers of joint cartilage with thinning of articular cartilages. Hypertrophy of nasal and aural cartilage accounts for part of the enlargement of nose and ears. *Osteogenesis* from the thickened periosteum is accelerated; absorption of bone is also rapid; late in the disease *osteoporosis* may be striking. There is overgrowth of the supraorbital ridge. The anterior temporal ridge advances with forward growth of the lateral portions of the orbit, expansion of the frontal sinuses, and forward displacement of the zygoma. Overgrowth of the maxilla (Fig. 4) lengthens the face, and the teeth are separated by heaping up of alveolar bone. The ramus of the mandible grows longer; the angle between ramus and body opens out to produce mandibular prognathism (Fig. 4). The ribs and clavicles widen and reach a length 2 to 3 inches greater than normal. The *long bones* thicken and become massive. The humerus and femur may be lengthened, and the latter may be deformed by bowing. The vertebral bodies are increased in the anteroposterior diameter; the greatest changes occur in the thoracic spine with deposit of new bone upon diaphyses, particularly anteriorly; this change makes forward flexion of the spine difficult.

The visible *enlargement of distal parts* is chiefly due to proliferation of soft tissue, not bone (Fig. 5). Subcutaneous connective tissue is grossly increased, giving the characteristic thick and fleshy appearance of the *hands* and *feet*, enlargement of the *lips*, and *accentuation of skin folds*. The skin itself is greatly thickened; there are increased sweating and seborrhea; hirsutism occurs in a few female patients. The *tongue* may be so large as to protrude from the mouth. Widespread splanchnomegaly is the rule. The heart, lungs, liver, spleen, and intestines are variously enlarged two- to five-fold. There may be gross cardiomegaly (up to 1300 grams); there is still debate about the relative importance of coexistent hypertension, coronary artery atherosclerosis, or simply raised HGH levels in the pathogenesis of *acromegalic heart disease*. The kidneys are enlarged by the growth of individual nephrons; studies of renal function indicate increased glomerular filtration rate and proximal tubular activity. The endocrine glands participate in the splanchnomegaly. A possible role of accompanying oversecretion of tropic hormones is not proved. The gonads, although often functioning subnormally and showing histologic evidence of failure, may be large. The *adrenal cortex* is hypertrophied, nodules are often found, and the secretory rate of cortisol is occasionally elevated but without accompanying signs of hyperadrenocorticism. The *thyroid* may be eight to nine times the normal size; goiters are diffuse or nodular. True hyperthyroidism is uncommon. The *parathyroids* are usually enlarged, and adenomas occur, often as a part of the syndrome of multiple endocrine adenomatosis (MEA I) (see Ch. 543.5). Although there is generalized enlargement of tissues and organs and a considerable gain in weight, obesity is almost unknown, possibly because of the adipokinetic effect of growth hormone. The weight of the *brain* is increased, and there is a more or less specific peripheral hypertrophic *neuropathy*. The muscles enlarge somewhat but without conspicuous hypertrophy; edema and deposition of mucopolysaccharide in muscle have been reported; weakness and atrophy are late findings.

CLINICAL MANIFESTATIONS AND NATURAL HISTORY. The onset of acromegaly is usually so insidious and so subtle that it escapes detection by the patient and his intimate associates. The gradualness and subtlety of onset are such that a third of the patients seek medical help for unrelated diseases, being unaware of their acromegaly. In Davidoff's series of 100 patients, the mean age of onset was estimated as 27 years, but the mean age at which the patients presented themselves was over 40; this average lapse of 13 or 14 years implies chronicity and a generally slow course. Careful analysis of the history reveals that early symptoms are related to peripheral effects of growth hormone or, much less commonly, to the mechanical pressure of the intrasellar tumor. Even before the obvious changes in appearance are noticed patients may complain of excessive sweating, paresthesias of the hands and feet, and pain and stiffness of the slowly expanding fingers and toes. Arthralgias are common. Accounts of hypersexuality and greatly increased muscular strength early in the course of the disease are rare and of doubtful authenticity. Complaints of hypogonadism (amenorrhea, loss of libido) are common. Headache may be extremely severe; the mechanism is not clear, because, in many instances, there is little clinically detectable enlargement of the pituitary tumor. Impairment of visual acuity or symptomatic encroachment upon visual fields occurs in over 60 per cent of patients at one time or another.

The *clinical picture* of advanced acromegaly is easily recognized on physical examination, but the changes are occasionally subtle. The typical acromegalic is large and burly; in late stages the forward carriage of the head, prognathism, kyphosis, bowing of the legs, and rolling gait are distinctive. The features are blunt and coarse, the nose and ears large; the brow is prominent and the jaw prognathous; the facial wrinkles are exaggerated; the lips are full. The skin is thick and hairy, the voice husky and cavernous. The hands and feet are enlarged; shaking hands with an acromegalic patient gives the startling impression of losing one's hand in a mass of dough. The superficial veins of the extremities are thick and prominent. The thoracic cage is widened

and deepened and thoracic kyphosis is present. Galactorrhea is an occasional finding in both men and women.

Most routine *laboratory data* are within normal limits. The basal metabolic rate is elevated in more than half the patients, but other evidence of hyperthyroidism (increased thyroidal uptake of ^{131}I or level of serum T_4) is usually lacking even when the thyroid is palpably enlarged. Appraisal of adrenocortical function reveals normal plasma cortisol values, normal response to ACTH, occasionally increased excretion of urinary 17-ketosteroids or corticosteroids, and sometimes raised cortisol secretory rate and a degree of adrenal refractoriness to suppression by dexamethasone. Urinary gonadotropin titer is normal or reduced; semen analysis generally shows oligospermia. Despite the reported increased insulin activity of acromegalic plasma, glycosuria or glucose intolerance is found in about a third of acromegalic subjects and frank diabetes in about one fifth. The diabetes is usually mild and somewhat resistant to insulin, but management of the diabetes presents no unusually difficult problems, and ketoacidosis is rare. Hypercalciuria is a common finding, and hypercalcemia occurs in a few patients; in some this abnormality is apparently due to hypersecretion of growth hormone, because it disappears with successful treatment of the acromegaly. However, in others the hypercalcemia persists and can be shown to be due to associated hyperparathyroidism as part of the syndrome of *multiple endocrine adenomatosis*.

As the disease progresses, muscular weakness (predominantly of proximal muscle groups) supervenes; kyphosis increases, partly because of osteoporosis. Visual impairment may become aggravated to the point of blindness. Partial or total pituitary insufficiency may ensue. The course is extremely variable; it is hard to know with accuracy the natural history, because the onset is usually so insidious and because most patients have received some sort of treatment. Life expectancy is reduced (see Ch. 543.5). The course may be fulminant, resulting in death within three years (usually because of tumor growth in younger patients) or benign and intermittent, lasting 50 years or longer. Death comes from the tumor (expansion, hemorrhage into its substance, "pituitary apoplexy"), cardiac failure (owing to "acromegalic heart disease"), or the effects of hypertension (found in 20 to 50 per cent of patients) or degenerative vascular disease. The causes of death in years past were diabetes and hypopituitarism; these are now rarely lethal because of the availability of adequate treatment.

DIAGNOSIS. The typical acromegalic is recognized at a glance. *The great need is a means of early diagnosis.* If acromegaly is suspected, a history of increasing size of gloves and shoes and of increasingly poor fit of dentures provides useful clues. Tightness of old rings is suggestive; comparison of the patient's features with old photographs is helpful. Roentgenogram of the skull and tests of the visual fields usually give confirmatory evidence.

The differential diagnosis rarely presents difficulties. The large tongue, hoarse voice, and periorbital edema may suggest myxedema, but the other physical and laboratory abnormalities of hypothyroidism are absent. Patients with pachydermoperiostosis, some of whom look quite acromegalic, do not have involvement of the pituitary, and plasma HGH values are normal. Some patients receiving anticonvulsants for long periods may develop "acromegaloid" coarsening of the features. The articular pains of acromegaly are usually distinguishable from those associated with other forms of arthritis by the typical acromegalic aspect.

There is no generally satisfactory method for the *indirect* assessment of the *secretory activity* of the adenoma. History of recent acral enlargement is the best evidence of active secretion, and some clinicians believe that excessive sweating and seborrhea are good guides. Laboratory data are disappointing. Elevation of serum phosphorus follows administration of human growth hormone, but is an unreliable index of "activity" of the disease in acromegaly. The same may be said of the glucose tolerance test and serum T_4 level. Some investigators consider the insulin tolerance test useful. Biopsy of costal cartilage may show active endochondral bone formation. Urinary excretion of hydroxyproline is increased. None of these laboratory indices has been conclusively proved to correlate closely with the clinical course of the disease. If plasma growth hormone measurements cannot be made, one must rely on a synthesis of historical, physical, and laboratory findings. Without

documentary evidence of recent acral growth, judgment of secretory activity is highly subjective.

The use of *radioimmunoassay of plasma growth hormone* is the method of choice for *direct* assessment of the secretory activity of the acidophilic tumor. It is known that most untreated acromegalics have high concentrations. After hypophysectomy these fall, often to normal, but sometimes they remain elevated, presumably when hypophysectomy is not complete. After pituitary radiation, levels often do not fall. Not enough data are yet available to allow a complete appraisal of growth hormone response to physiologic stimuli (hypoglycemia, glucose administration) as a measure of "activity" in acromegaly. What is needed is careful correlation (over a period of years) of plasma growth hormone levels with objective studies of acral growth. Such studies will reveal the value of plasma growth hormone measurements as indices of secretory activity. At the moment, it appears that sharp falls in basal plasma growth hormone value, or recovery of growth hormone responsiveness to administered glucose, are closely related to clinically arrested disease.

Figure 9. Evolution of acromegaly. *A,* Age 38, within a year after onset of the disease. *B,* Age 55, after two courses of radiation therapy to sella; disease has progressed with moderate coarsening of features: thickening of lips, enlargement of nose and ears. *C, D,* Age 64, 26 years after onset, after a third series of x-ray treatments to sella (total dose of radiation to the pituitary, 10,000 rads); nose and ears have enlarged further, supraorbital ridge and zygoma have become more prominent, and jaw is more prognathous; frontal view shows deepening of skin wrinkles (temporal atrophy is a result of x-irradiation). *E, F,* Age 64, volar and dorsal aspects of hand, showing broadened fingers and characteristically "meaty" appearance owing to gross increase in soft tissue, not bone. The patient died 12 years later at age 76 of cardiac and respiratory failure. By that time diabetes mellitus and hypopituitarism (thyroid and adrenocortical deficiency) had developed and were treated, but the last plasma HGH measurement, six years before death, was still elevated—27 ng per milliliter.

TREATMENT. Treatment is discussed in detail in Ch. 543.5. No single method has been shown to be ideal (Fig. 9). Most endocrinologists believe that *external pituitary radiation* will in time control the majority of cases of acromegaly. As stated above, one may have to wait two years for visible results. *Proton beam radiotherapy* and *transsphenoidal adenomectomy* carry a higher rate of morbidity, but the therapeutic results are usually more dramatic and appear sooner. *Transfrontal surgery* should probably be reserved for patients with major visual impairment or radiographic evidence of large-scale extension of the tumor upward or anteriorly. *Medical management* of pituitary tumors associated with acromegaly must be restricted to patients whose neoplasms are not mechanically threatening and whose metabolic disease is mild. Somatostatin, chlorpromazine, and progestational agents (e.g., medroxyprogesterone), all of which suppress HGH secretion, must still be regarded as experimental therapeutic agents.

Cryer, P. E., Daughaday, W. H., Coxe, W. S., and Avioli, L. V.: Diagnosis and therapy of acromegaly. Arch. Intern. Med., 135:338, 1975.

Davidoff, L. M.: Studies in acromegaly: III. The anamnesis and symptomatology in one hundred cases. Endocrinology, 10:461, 1926.

Hardy, J.: Transsphenoidal hypophysectomy. J. Neurosurg., 34:582, 1971.

Lawrence, A. M., Pinsky, S. M., and Goldfine, I. D.: Conventional radiation therapy in acromegaly: A review and reassessment. Arch. Intern. Med., 128:369, 1971.

Lawrence, J. H., Tobias, C. A., Linfoot, J. A., Born, J. L., Lyman, J. T., Chang, C. Y., Manougian, E., and Wei, W. C.: Successful treatment of acromegaly: Metabolic and clinical studies in 145 patients. J. Clin. Endocrinol. Metab., 31:180, 1970.

Roth, J., Gorden, P., and Brace, K.: Efficacy of conventional pituitary irradiation in acromegaly. N. Engl. J. Med., 282:1385, 1970.

Wright, A. D., Hill, D. M., and Lowy, C.: Mortality in acromegaly. Quart. J. Med., 39:1, 1970.

GIGANTISM

Gigantism is arbitrarily defined as height exceeding 80 inches or, in children, exceeding a height three standard deviations above the mean for age. This rare disorder has been conventionally regarded as the childhood counterpart of acromegaly, i.e., as oversecretion of growth hormone by a pituitary adenoma in a growing organism *before closure of the epiphyses.* However, acromegaly occurs in young children. It is reasonable to doubt a pituitary cause when (1) there is no evidence of acromegaly, (2) the sella is not enlarged, or (3) there is a strong familial history of unusually tall stature suggesting constitutional gigantism. Several forms of "cerebral gigantism" are described in children: associated features of one form are macrocrania, large extremities, large hands and feet, evidence of cerebral dysfunction, and normal values and normal response of plasma growth hormone. An additional cause of abnormally tall stature is hypogonadism or late puberty, resulting in prolongation of the period of linear growth because of delayed epiphysial closure. In such patients, the bodily proportions are eunuchoidal, with a lower segment greater than the upper segment and arm span greater than height.

In those giants who are acromegalic, management is that of acromegaly. Treatment of the pituitary adenoma must be *vigorous.* The radioimmunoassay for growth hormone provides more accurate assignment of cause in gigantism and a more objective criterion as a guide to management.

Baumann, G., Cain, J. P., and Dingman, J. F.: Gigantism with hypopituitarism: A re-evaluation. Am. J. Med., 53:805, 1972.

Haigler, E. D., Jr., Hershman, J. M., and Meador, C. K.: Pituitary gigantism: A case report and review. Arch. Intern. Med., 132:589, 1973.

Hook, E. B., and Reynolds, J. W.: Cerebral gigantism. Endocrinological and clinical observations of six patients, including a congenital giant, concordant monozygotic twins, and a child who achieved adult gigantic size. J. Pediat., 70:900, 1967.

Stock, J. M., Glatak, N. R., and Oppenheimer, J. H.: Unsuspected meningioma in a patient with pituitary gigantism. Case report with autopsy findings. Metabolism, 24:767, 1975.

Wu, N. F. T., and Kushnick, T.: The Beckwith-Wiedemann syndrome: The exophthalmos-macroglossia-gigantism syndrome. Clin. Pediat. 13:452, 1974.

HYPERSECRETION OF PITUITARY HORMONES OTHER THAN HGH

Excessive secretion of each of the anterior pituitary hormones occurs and is associated with a clinical syndrome. Hypersomatotropism, the cause of acromegaly and of pituitary gigantism, has been discussed above. Hyperprolactinemia with or without a pituitary tumor is often but not always observed in patients with *nonpuerperal galactorrhea.* Generally, the plasma prolactin levels are higher when a pituitary tumor is present. It must be emphasized that *prolactin-secreting tumors* tend to be laterally located, small, and visible radiographically only with the most careful microtomography. The most popular method of treatment at the moment is transsphenoidal adenomectomy, but some workers believe that conventional external radiotherapy to the sellar region is equally effective.

Pituitary adenomas, usually chromophobic, may rarely secrete excessive quantities of *TSH, gonadotropins, ACTH,* and *"MSH."* As indicated above, ablation of the "target" glands, the thyroid, gonads, and adrenals, may once in a great while give rise to pituitary overgrowth (see Ch. 543.5). More rarely still, what appear to be *primary* hypersecreting pituitary adenomas occur, causing thyrotoxicosis, hypergonadotropic hypogonadism, the "pituitary" form of Cushing's syndrome, and hyperpigmentation of the skin.

The clinical syndromes associated with oversecretion of pituitary peptides by cancers of nonendocrine organs are discussed in Ch. 525.

Hamilton, C. R., Jr., Adams, L. C., and Maloof, F.: Hyperthyroidism due to thyrotropin-producing pituitary chromophobe adenoma. N. Engl. J. Med., 283:1077, 1970.

Kleinberg, D. L., Noel, G. L., and Frantz, A. G.: Galactorrhea: 235 cases including 48 with pituitary tumors. N. Engl. J. Med., 296:589, 1977.

Nelson, J. C., Kollar, D. J., and Lewis, J. E.: Growth hormone secretion in pituitary disease. Arch. Intern. Med., 133:459, 1974.

Snyder, P. J., and Sterling, S. H.: Hypersecretion of LH and FSH by a pituitary adenoma. J. Clin. Endocrinol. Metab., 42:544, 1976.

544. POSTERIOR PITUITARY

Alexander Leaf

544.1. ANTIDIURETIC HORMONE

NORMAL PHYSIOLOGY. Antidiuretic hormone is produced in nuclei of the anterior hypothalamus. The major source of this hormone is the supraoptic nuclei, but contributions from the paraventricular and filiform nuclei are thought to be added. The hormone produced in these neural centers is transported by a process of neural secretion down the supraopticohypophysial tract to the neurohypophysis or posterior pituitary where the hormone is stored until released into the blood according to the state of hydration of the subject.

The antidiuretic hormone in man was identified by du Vigneaud as the octapeptide arginine vasopressin. The hormone is released normally in response to osmotic stimuli; a rise in concentration of solute, largely the salts of sodium, in the plasma or extracellular fluid, serves as the stimulus for release of vasopressin from the neurohypophysis. The hormone circulates to the kidney where its major action is on the epithelium lining the collecting ducts. In the presence of vasopressin this epithelium becomes more permeable to water so that water is transported from the tubular lumen to the more concentrated peritubular fluids. This serves to reduce urine volume and increase its concentration, thereby conserving body water. Dilution of plasma or extracellular fluids, as occurs after water ingestion, inhibits release of antidiuretic hormone. The dilute luminal fluid entering the distal convoluted tubule is excreted with little modification in concentration, with the result that a copious flow of dilute urine characterizes the absence of antidiuretic hormone. This rids the body of any excess of water.

Studies by G. Robertson, using a specific radioimmunoassay to determine concentrations of vasopressin in the plasma, have provided quantitative information regarding the sensitivity of this system in man. Increase in plasma osmolality within the physiologic range from 280 to 295 mOsm produces a five-fold increase in plasma vasopressin, from 1.0 to 5 pg per milliliter. This increase in plasma concentration of the hormone is associated with a rise of urine concentration from 100 mOsm during water diuresis to 1000 mOsm during water restriction. A 2 mOsm increase in plasma causes a 1.0 pg per milliliter rise in hormone concentration in plasma, and this in turn is associated with a 200 mOsm elevation of urine concentration. Thus a change in plasma concentration of 1.0 mOsm alters urine concentration by 100 mOsm; the multiplication factor via vasopressin levels accounts for the remarkable homeostatic sensitivity of this system.

The thirst center is functionally and anatomically closely related to the antidiuretic mechanism. Andersson has shown that osmotic or electrical stimulation creates a sensation of thirst; dilution of plasma inhibits thirst. The responsive sensor in the anterior hypothalamus for both release of antidiuretic hormone and thirst now seems to be cells in the anterior wall of the third ventricle which can sense changes in their ambient sodium concentration. The integrated activity of thirst and antidiuretic mechanism serves to regulate the concentration of body fluids as follows:

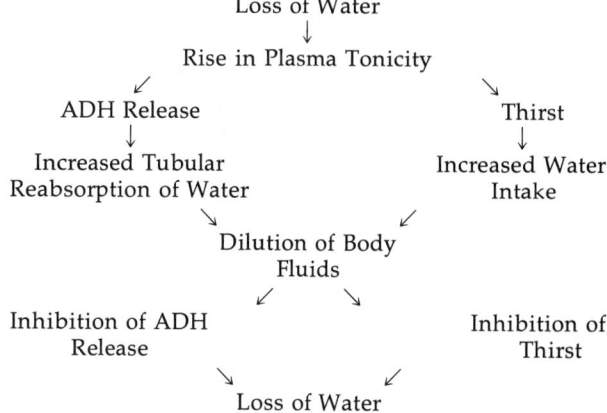

This double negative feedback system works with remarkable effectiveness to preserve the concentration of sodium in the serum between some 136 and 143 mEq per liter. Since intracellular fluids are in osmotic equilibrium with the extracellular fluids, this mechanism regulates the tonicity of the body fluid compartments.

In addition to the usual osmotic stimuli regulating release of vasopressin, other factors may affect this process. Pain and emotional states have been associated with antidiuresis, as have a number of pharmacologic agents which act to release the hormone. These include cinchoninic acid, acetylcholine, nicotine, morphine, barbiturates, ferritin, and bradykinin. Alcohol may inhibit release of antidiuretic hormone, but the effect is weak and is often obscured. Physiologically, reduction in the effective plasma volume is also a stimulus for secretion of antidiuretic hormone. The afferent limb appears to be parasympathetic via stretch receptors in the left atrium, carotid sinus, and aortic arch. An increase in tension on these receptors inhibits and a reduced tension enhances impulses via the glossopharyngeal and vagus nerves to the hypothalamus to affect hormone secretion. Thus antidiuretic hormone release responds to both concentration and volume changes in the plasma. Generally concentration regulation appears dominant, but when volume is seriously compromised antidiuretic hormone will be regulated so as to prevent further impairment in volume even at the expense of aggravating abnormality of concentration.

It is now appreciated that in a considerable number of clinical conditions there is an apparent inappropriate secretion of substances possessing antidiuretic activity. The adjective "inappropriate" is used to indicate that neither osmotic nor circulatory (volume) stimuli are responsible for the excessive, persistent antidiuretic activity. Furthermore, the antidiuretic substances may not arise in all instances from the neurohypophysis but may be secretory products of the tumors or inflammatory tissue which give rise to the syndrome of inappropriate antidiuretic hormone secretion (see Ch. 530).

Andersson, B.: Regulation of body fluids. Ann. Rev. Physiol., 39:185, 1977.

Gauer, O. H., and Henry, J. P.: Neurohormonal control of plasma volume. Int. Rev. Physiol., 9:146, 1976.

Leaf, A.: The clinical and physiologic significance of the serum sodium concentration. N. Engl. J. Med., 267:24, 77, 1962.

Leaf, A., Bartter, F. C., Santos, R. F., and Wrong, O.: Evidence in man that urinary electrolyte loss induced by pitressin is a function of water retention. J. Clin. Invest., 32:868, 1953.

Robertson, G. L., Sheldon, R. L., and Athar, S.: The osmoregulation of vasopressin. Kidney Int., 10:25, 1976.

Schrier, R. W., and Berl, T.: Nonosmolar factors affecting renal water excretion. N. Engl. J. Med., 292:81, 141, 1975.

Schwartz, W. B., Bennett, W., Curelop, S., and Bartter, F. C.: A syndrome of renal sodium loss and hyponatremia, probably resulting from inappropriate secretion of antidiuretic hormone. Am. J. Med., 23:529, 1957.

Verney, W. B.: The absorption and excretion of water: The antidiuretic hormone. Lancet, 2:739, 781, 1946.

544.2. DIABETES INSIPIDUS

ETIOLOGY. Diabetes insipidus is an uncommon disturbance resulting from any condition which damages the neurohypophysial system. Idiopathic cases constitute the major group, comprising approximately 45 per cent. The idiopathic condition may become manifest at any age and affect either sex. It is unusual in infancy, but may commence in early childhood. Familial diabetes insipidus is very uncommon, but may occur in infancy or childhood and affect either sex. The condition has been noted in seven generations of one family. Familial diabetes insipidus is to be distinguished from nephrogenic diabetes insipidus, which is a renal tubular defect, inherited largely by males, in whom the affected tubules are unresponsive to antidiuretic hormone.

Head trauma (accidental or neurosurgical) and neoplasms (primary or metastatic) are the major causes of acquired diabetes insipidus. Of the metastatic tumors, breast cancer seems to have a special predilection for the hypothalamic area. Other rarer etiologic factors include sarcoidosis, birth injuries, eosinophilic granuloma, and a variety of local infections. Even with lesions directly in the hypothalamus, diabetes insipidus is rare, because a small fraction of normal tissue suffices to protect against manifest dysfunction. Since the posterior and anterior pituitary have separate blood supplies, infarction of the latter need not be associated with failure of the former; a space-occupying lesion is suspect when insufficiency of both occurs.

CLINICAL MANIFESTATIONS. The polyuria and polydipsia can be so dramatic that adult patients may remember an exact date or even hour when symptoms started. The fluid exchanges may reach the distressing proportions of 5 to 10 liters or more per 24 hours. The specific gravity of the urine is usually 1.001 to 1.005; corresponding concentrations will be about 100 to 200 mOsm per liter. With restriction of fluid intake the specific gravity may reach 1.010, or even slightly higher with severe water lack, and urine concentration may increase to 300 mOsm per liter. Urine slightly hypertonic to serum has been produced experimentally in the complete absence of antidiuretic hormone by greatly reducing the glomerular filtration rate. The elaboration of a hypertonic urine by a patient with diabetes insipidus during severe dehydration or with acute reduction of the glomerular filtration rate from any cause need not therefore indicate the presence of residual neurohypophysial function.

Other than the annoyance of polyuria and polydipsia, there may be no evidence of ill health or of other physiologic disturbance associated with the condition, unless the patient suffers from the underlying local or systemic disease which has destroyed the neurohypophysial system. The assumption that patients with diabetes insipidus suffer from severe dehydration is not supported by measurements of serum sodium or total solute concentrations. A slight elevation of sodium and total solute concentrations of serum has been demonstrated statistically, but the overlap in individual cases is such as to make these determinations of little assistance diagnostically: 297 ± 12 mOsm per liter (S.D.) for diabetes insipidus and 285 ± 4 mOsm per liter (S.D.) for normal persons. As long as the patient's thirst center remains intact, the total solute concentration of the body fluids will be preserved close to normal values, but at the expense of polydipsia and the large fluid exchange characteristic of the condition. After a period of water restriction, these differences may be accentuated and have greater diagnostic value.

With unconsciousness resulting from trauma or anesthesia, the inability of the patient to demand water may be fatal. This situation may occur at the onset of diabetes insipidus secondary to head injury or intracranial surgery, and is one of the causes of hypernatremia after trauma to the head. A careful record of urine volumes and urine and serum concentrations in patients with acute head trauma and coma will prevent the occurrence of severe dehydration.

DIFFERENTIAL DIAGNOSIS. A patient with persistent polyuria and urine of low concentration may have one or more of three basic disturbances: (1) inability of the kidney to elaborate a concentrated urine despite adequate vasopressin, (2) deficient vasopressin, or (3) persistent excessive water intake. Any condition which disturbs the renal concentrating mechanism, rendering it unresponsive to vasopressin, may produce polyuria. Hypercalcemia, potassium depletion, or renal failure (both chronic and acute) may impair maximal concentrating ability, but none of these conditions cause the urine to be persistently hypotonic, and in only a few patients does the resulting polyuria suggest diabetes insipidus. These conditions are readily excluded in establishing the diagnosis of diabetes insipidus. The rare nephrogenic diabetes insipidus results from a failure of the renal tubule to respond to vasopressin. Patients with uncontrolled diabetes mellitus may exhibit extreme polyuria and polydipsia, but the specific gravity of the urine is high, although its osmolality may not be over 300 mOsm per liter; the large contribution which glucose makes to the specific gravity accounts for this seeming discrepancy.

Although it is evident that polyuria in diabetes insipidus is primary to polydipsia, compulsive water drinking may give rise to a condition which closely mimics diabetes insipidus. Chronic ingestion of large volumes of water impairs the renal concentrating mechanism, making it sometimes quite difficult to distinguish this psychogenic disturbance from true diabetes insipidus.

Several special procedures have been devised to assist in establishing the diagnosis of diabetes insipidus in patients with polyuria and polydipsia. They all test ability to respond to osmotic stimuli by elaboration of a concentrated urine, whether failure to do so is the consequence of a lack of endogenous vasopressin or of an inability of the renal tubules to respond to the hormone.

Water restriction with observation of urine volume and concentration constitutes the simplest test. Weight should be followed to avoid the hazards of incurring loss of more than 3 to 5 per cent of body weight. Small children and infants are especially liable to serious circulatory disturbances if dehydration is allowed beyond this limit. A normal subject may be expected to reduce urine flow to less than 0.5 ml per minute and increase urine concentration to greater than 800 mOsm per liter (corresponding to a specific gravity of 1.020 or above). In patients with diabetes insipidus, urine volumes well above this limit persist, and urine concentration remains below 200 mOsm per liter (specific gravities of 1.001 to 1.005) until advanced states of dehydration are present. Unfortunately, the differences are often not so clear, and patients with neurohypophysial insufficiency may concentrate their urine to 300 to 400 mOsm per liter (specific gravities of 1.008 to 1.014) with marked dehydration.

Another means of increasing plasma osmolarity to test the release of antidiuretic hormone is by the infusion of hypertonic solutions. After an initial hydrated state is established, 2.5 per cent sodium chloride is infused intravenously at a rate of 0.25 ml per minute per kilogram of body weight for 45 minutes. Urine flow is measured at 15-minute intervals. If neurohypophysial and renal functions are normal, urine flow will drop promptly to 25 per cent or less of control.

If either the water deprivation test or the infusion of hypertonic saline fails to reduce urine flow or to increase urine concentration as expected, the ability of the patient's kidneys to respond to exogenous vasopressin must be demonstrated, in order to separate nephrogenic causes from hormone deficiency. For this purpose 5mU per minute of aqueous vasopressin (vasopressin injection, USP) may be administered intravenously for at least one hour by a slow drip, or 5 units of the long-acting vasopressin tannate in oil may be administered intramuscularly. An injection of the latter material in the evening, with urine samples collected on arising the following morning and hourly for three successive hours thereafter, should induce maximal concentration.

These simple measures will readily distinguish diabetes insipidus from nephrogenic causes of diminished response to vasopressin. To distinguish true diabetes insipidus from compulsive water drinking may be more difficult, because continued polydipsia lowers the maximal urinary concentrations achievable after dehydration, infusions of hypertonic saline, or exogenous vasopressin. Barlow and de Wardener have pointed out that a normal subject with intact neurohypophysis will achieve a higher urinary concentration after water deprivation than after administration of vasopressin without water restriction. The patient with diabetes insipidus has just the opposite response, i.e., higher urine concentration after vasopressin than after water restriction. Patients with psychogenic polydipsia respond in this regard normally; whatever the absolute value of urine concentration they achieve, concentrations during dehydration will exceed those attained after injections of vasopressin. In addition to the laboratory studies, it should be remembered that compulsive water drinking to a degree which is confused with diabetes insipidus constitutes a severe psychogenic disorder. Clinical evaluation is usually rewarding in revealing other neurotic symptoms supporting the suspicion of a serious personality or behavioral disturbance.

TREATMENT. If symptoms are mild, no therapy may be warranted, although a thorough search for underlying causative factors should be conducted. When symptoms interfere with sleep or interrupt work, treatment is indicated. Replacement therapy intramuscularly with long-acting vasopressin in oil (1.0 ml ampule contains 5 units per milliliter; 0.5 to 1.0 ml injected every 24 to 72 hours, as necessary to control polyuria) is generally reserved for the more severe cases, whereas an aqueous nasal spray of lysine-vasopressin will usually provide symptomatic relief for two to four hours. The longer-acting 1-desamino-8-D-arginine vasopressin, dDAVP, which also can be self-administered intranasally, will control symptoms in doses of 5 to 10 μg two or three times daily. Although expensive at present, dDAVP affords the best symptomatic control. The oral hypoglycemic agent chlorpropamide has been found to enhance the antidiuretic activity of residual endogenous antidiuretic hormone; 100 to 500 mg once daily will usually relieve polyuria and polydipsia in patients with incomplete neurohypophysial failure. Thiazide diuretics — 250 mg of chlorothiazide two or three times daily — presumably by sustaining a condition of persistent mild salt depletion, will blunt a water diuresis, and in patients with diabetes insipidus may reduce urine flow by some 50 per cent. In patients with nephrogenic diabetes insipidus this form of antidiuretic agent is also effective.

Barlow, E. D., and de Wardener, H. E.: Compulsive water drinking. Quart. J. Med., 28:235, 1959.

Coggins, C. H., and Leaf, A.: Diabetes insipidus. Am. J. Med., 42:807, 1967.

Dashe, A. M., Cramm, R. E., Crist, C. A., Habener, J. F., and Solomon, D. H.: A water deprivation test for the differential diagnosis of polyuria. JAMA, 185:71, 1963.

Leaf, A.: Diabetes insipidus. In Astwood, E. B. (ed.): Clinical Endocrinology, I. New York, Grune & Stratton, 1960.

Williams, R. H., and Henry, C.: Nephrogenic diabetes insipidus: Transmitted by females and appearing during infancy in males. Ann. Intern. Med., 27:84, 1947.

545. THE PINEAL

Seymour Reichlin

The pineal gland was discovered more than 20 centuries ago, and its function has long been a matter of scientific and philosophic speculation. Arising embryologically from ependyma lining the roof of the third ventricle, the pineal consists of parenchymal cells supported by a meshwork of neuroglia. In the adult, the gland weighs between 100 and 180 mg and is a cone-shaped organ lying in the groove formed by the superior colliculi. Although connected to the epithalamus by a peduncle, the pineal does not receive a direct nerve supply from this source. Instead, it is innervated by postganglionic nerve fibers which arise in the cervical sympathetic ganglia and travel along the great vein of Galen. The sympathetic inflow to the pineal is in turn regulated by impulses arising in the suprachiasmatic nuclei, paired structures lying just above the optic chiasm (Fig. 1). This nucleus is innervated by a direct nerve pathway from the retina termed the retinohypothalamic tract. Changes in external lighting influence pineal activity (and other endocrine functions) via this pathway even when pathways mediating conscious light perception have been severed. The suprachiasmatic nucleus is also believed to serve as an internal "clock" (or biologic oscillator), regulating a number of endogenous endocrine rhythms. Circadian changes can occur even in the absence of external sensory cues, including light changes, thus indicating that there is a mechanism for determination of intrinsic rhythms. The rhythm of the endogenous oscillator can be modified by external signals such as normal light-dark cycles which have been termed "zeitgebers" (time givers). The pineal contains an incredible variety of neurotransmitter substances, including norepinephrine, serotonin, histamine, melatonin, dopamine, octopamine, and gamma-aminobutyric acid. It also contains the hypothalamic peptides somatostatin and TRH, and a peptide, vasotocin, an analogue of vasopressin and oxytocin. Of all these biologically active substances, only melatonin has been shown to be secreted into the blood and can be looked upon as a true hormonal secretion of the pineal. There is also evidence that some important pineal functions are mediated by a peptide of undetermined nature. Melatonin has been demonstrated by highly specific methods to be present in blood, cerebrospinal fluid, and urine of many species of animals, including man. Hormone levels show a marked diurnal rhythm, with night values up to ten times higher than day values. In the sheep, high nighttime melatonin levels in the blood drop dramatically upon exposure to light. Melatonin is believed to exert suppressive effects on a number of endocrine functions in experimental animals, the most important of which is on the release of gonadotropic hormones. When given to man in high dosage, melatonin was shown to suppress plasma LH levels and stress-induced growth hormone secretion. It also lightened the skin pigmentation in one of five patients. Important effects of melatonin injection in man are the production of sleepiness and changes in the electroencephalogram, mainly an increase of alpha waves. Since melatonin is secreted in response to darkness, it is an attractive hypothesis (as yet unproved)

that melatonin release contributes to nocturnal drowsiness. Melatonin is formed by a series of enzymatic steps from tryptophan (Fig. 1). One of the intermediates is serotonin, which in turn is converted to N-acetylserotonin by the enzyme N-acetyl transferase; the conversion of N-acetylserotonin to melatonin is accomplished by the enzyme hydroxy-o-methyl transferase (HIOMT). Measurement of the activities of these enzymes has been used to study the factors controlling melatonin synthesis and, by inference, melatonin secretion. Both enzyme activities are influenced by alterations in the light-dark cycle. It was initially believed that the HIOMT enzyme was the rate-limiting step for melatonin synthesis. More recent work indicates that the acetyltransferase system is more important, but both enzymes may be involved in final control of pineal secretion. Enzymic activity of the pineal gland and its secretory function are regulated by noradrenergic nerve endings on pinealocytes (Fig. 2). Beta catecholamine receptors activate adenyl cyclase with the formation of cyclic AMP through the classic second messenger mechanism. The activated ATP-protein kinase is believed to promote the formation of the melatonin-synthesizing enzymes. Norepinephrine also stimulates pineal uptake of the precursor tryptophan.

The pineal gland has no known function in man but becomes of clinical significance because of the occurrence of calcification and of tumor formation. Calcific nodules termed *acervuli* form in a matrix of ground substance secreted by pinealocytes. This process begins in early childhood and becomes increasingly evident by roentgenography beginning in the second decade of life. Calcification has no known effect on pineal function, as inferred from the fact that the characteristic enzymes of the pineal (HIOMT, monoamine oxidase, and histamine N-methyl transferase) maintain normal concentrations throughout life.

Diseases of the pineal are rare. A few cases of hypo-

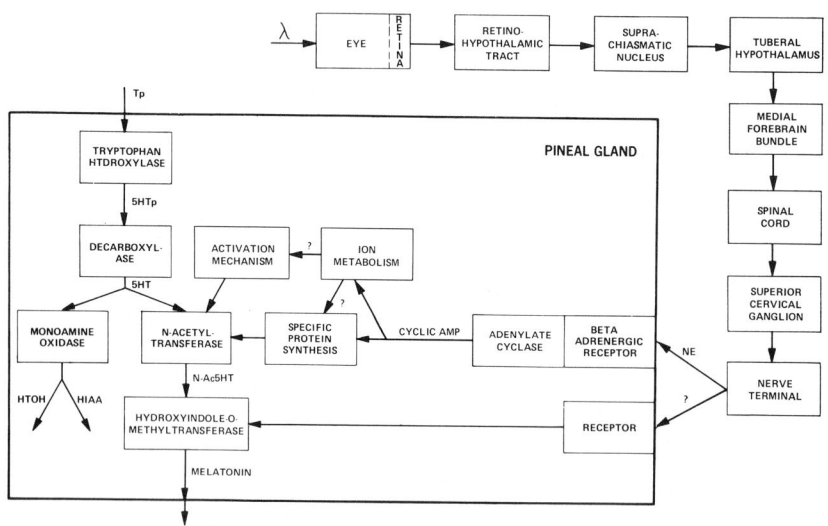

Figure 1.   Control system for pineal regulation. Environmental lighting impinging on the retina is transduced into a neural signal, which projects to one suprachiasmatic nucleus of the hypothalamus. Thence, descending pathways via the medial forebrain bundle impinge upon the cervical outflow of the sympathetic nervous system, which reaches the pineal via the superior cervical ganglia. Norepinephrine released at nerve endings within the pineal interact with beta receptors on pineal cells. Through second messenger and sequential changes in protein synthesis, the formation of melatonin from tryptophan precursors is regulated. Detailed pathways are shown in Figure 2. (From Klein, D. C., *In* Reichlin, S., Baldessarini, R. J., and Martin, J. B. [eds.]: The Hypothalamus. New York, Raven Press, 1978, p. 303.)

Figure 2. Biosynthesis of melatonin from tryptophan in the pineal gland. Step 1 is catalyzed by tryptophan hydroxylase; Step 2 by L-aromatic amino acid decarboxylase; Step 3 by N-acetylating enzyme; and Step 4 by HIOMT. (From Wurtman, R. J., Axelrod, J., and Kelly, D.: The Pineal. New York, Academic Press, 1968, p. 60.)

plasia and aplasia have been reported, and these have been associated in a relatively high proportion with genital precocity. Less than 1 per cent of intracranial neoplasms are tumors of the pineal gland, and they are seen almost exclusively in young males. The term pinealoma refers to a tumor of the pineal parenchymal cell, called pineoblastoma or pineocytoma according to its degree of differentiation. In one series of pineal tumor cases, only 9 of 53 fitted this category and there were 13 glial tumors, including astrocytomas and glioblastomas. The most common tumor, according to DeGirolami and Schmidek, is best termed germinoma because it apparently arises from germ cells. Approximately half the cases studied by these authors were so classified. In the literature of pathology germinomas are also called ectopic pinealomas (germinoma-like lesions arising away from the pineal), or seminomatous pinealomas (from their resemblance to testicular tubules). Although the pineal gland is often the site of origin of germinomas, they do not arise from pineal parenchymal cells. They are believed to be due to embryologic rests of germ cells. Identical tumors are found in the testis and anterior mediastinum. Approximately 10 per cent of intracranial germinomas metastasize to the spinal cord. Germinomas arising in the pineal gland may infiltrate the third ventricle and the floor of the hypothalamus, producing a characteristic triad: diabetes insipidus, hypogonadism, and optic atrophy. It is likely that an identical clinical presentation can be due to germinomas arising from midline tissues at the base of the brain. X-ray of the skull rarely shows abnormality even when hypothalamic functions are grossly deranged. Teratomas may also arise in the pineal region, and rarely give rise to choriocarcinomas. Several cases of precocious puberty have been reported to be caused by gonadotropin-secreting choriocarcinomas of the pineal, an abnormality associated with detectable HCG in the spinal fluid.

Pineal tumors also cause sexual precocity by hypothalamic damage which destroys structures normally inhibitory to the development of puberty. Pinealomas cause precocious puberty almost exclusively in males. The most important local manifestations of pineal neoplasms are due to pressure on the quadrigeminal plate of the midbrain. An enlarging mass in the pineal region compresses the aqueduct of Sylvius and distorts the upper brainstem. Internal hydrocephalus gives rise to characteristic headache, vomiting, papilledema, and disturbed consciousness. Pressure of the superior colliculi causes paralysis of conjugate upward gaze (Parinaud's syndrome). The characteristic wide-based gait may be due to pressure on the cerebellum or brainstem.

Although a number of surgical cures have been reported, pineal tumors are rarely resectable by the time that clinical signs appear. Fortunately, the germinoma type is radiosensitive, and prolonged survival has been observed. Most workers recommend that craniotomy be carried out for diagnostic purposes, but that removal be attempted only if the lesion is favorably localized, or if it is a radioresistant lesion. Supervoltage roentgen therapy is usually given. There is little experience with chemotherapy of these tumors. In emergency situations presenting with hydrocephalus, it is usually necessary to carry out a shunt procedure.

DeGirolami, U., and Schmidek, K.: Clinicopathological study of 53 tumors of the pineal region. J. Neurosurg., 39:455, 1973.

Klein, D. C.: The pineal gland: A model of neuroendocrine regulation. In Reichlin, S., Baldessarini, R. J., and Martin, J. B. (eds.): The Hypothalamus. New York, Raven Press, 1978, p. 303.

Martin, J. B., Reichlin, S., and Brown, G. M.: The pineal gland and periventricular organs. In Clinical Neuroendocrinology. Philadelphia, F. A. Davis Company, 1977, pp. 229–246.

Nordlund, J. J., and Lerner, A. B.: The effects of oral melatonin on skin color and on the release of pituitary hormones. J. Clin. Endocrinol. Metab., 45:768, 1977.

Stein, B. M.: The infratentorial supracerebellar approach to pineal lesions. J. Neurosurg., 35:197, 1971.

Wolstenholme, G. E. W., and Knight, J. (eds.): The Pineal Gland. Ciba Foundation Symposium. Edinburgh and London, Churchill Livingstone, 1971.

Wurtman, R. J., Axelrod, J., and Kelly, D. E.: The Pineals. New York, Academic Press, 1968.

Wurtman, R. J., and Moskowitz, M. A.: The pineal organ. N. Engl. J. Med., 296:1329, 1383, 1977.

546. THE THYROID

Leslie J. DeGroot

546:1. INTRODUCTION

Thyroid hormone serves as a metabolic thermostat, regulating the level of biochemical activity of most tissues. In general, malfunction of the thyroid gland leads to two sets of symptoms: those related to the local effects of a mass in the neck, and the generalized effects of an excess or deficiency of hormone. Illnesses involving this gland are relatively common medical disorders and, excluding diabetes, account for nearly four fifths of endocrine disease.

DEVELOPMENT AND ANATOMY

The embryonic thyroid gland develops from segments of the fourth pharyngeal pouches, joined by a midline anlage from the base of the tongue. During the first three months of growth, the thyroid gland is unable to synthesize and release thyroid hormone. Accordingly, if hormone is needed in this period, the fetus must depend upon the maternal supply of thyroid hormone. By the end of the first trimester, the gland has assumed its adult shape and position, concentrates iodide, synthesizes thyroglobulin, and functions under the control of the fetal pituitary. During the remainder of intrauterine life, the gland produces the hormone required for the developing fetus. If necessary because of malfunction of the fetal gland, the fetus derives some hormone from the maternal circulation. However, the placenta is poorly permeable to thyroid hormone, and serum hormone levels in the athyreotic fetus are typically much below the normal range. During the first 18 or 20 years after birth, the gland doubles in size three to four times to attain a weight of 15 to 20 grams. In the absence of disease or changes in iodine supply, the size and function of the gland remain relatively constant throughout life until advanced age, when hormone production gradually diminishes.

The normal thyroid gland is butterfly shaped, firm, smooth, and red-brown. It consists of two elongated lobes on either side of the trachea connected by a thin isthmus of tissue at or below the level of the cricoid cartilage. (Often, a remnant of the lingual anlage, the pyramidal lobe, extends superiorly from one side of the isthmus. Under normal circumstances, this is too small to be detected by external palpation.) The fine structure consists of numerous follicles, each approximately 300 μ in diameter and made up of clusters of cells surrounding a colloid-filled luminal space. The colloid is a mixture of proteins, of which thyroglobulin comprises about 80 per cent.

The thyroid cells are 15 μ high; the borders facing the lumen have microvilli and pseudopods thought to be involved in secretory and resorptive activities. In hyperplastic glands the cells are taller, and colloid space is reduced. Certain cells do not contact the luminal surface and have slightly different staining properties; these perifollicular or "C-cells" secrete the hormone calcitonin and are involved in regulation of calcium metabolism. The parathyroid glands occur as two pairs, one posterior to the upper poles of the thyroid and the other below or embedded in the substance of the lower poles. The recurrent laryngeal nerves pass immediately beneath the lower poles of the thyroid, or are sometimes embedded in the substance of the thyroid gland. Occasionally bits of normal-appearing thyroid tissue are present adjacent to the gland.

PHYSIOLOGY OF THE THYROID

It is best to view the thyroid gland as part of a system designed to provide a constant supply of hormone to somatic cells. Thyroid hormone is transported from blood to the peripheral tissues, where it produces its characteristic metabolic stimulation, and is in turn degraded. The thyroid gland replenishes this supply by secreting about 90 μg of tetraiodothyronine (thyroxine, T_4) and 10 μg of triiodothyronine (T_3) daily. If the hormone supply to tissue is depleted, the change is sensed by the pituitary (and possibly the hypothalamus), which increases the secretion of thyroid-stimulating hormone (TSH). TSH increases secretion of hormone by the thyroid gland in a feedback control system until the circulating level of hormone returns to the original level and suppresses TSH to its control level.

IODIDE METABOLISM (Fig. 1). Iodine bears a unique relation to thyroid physiology, because the element is a major and characteristic constituent of the hormones. The average daily American diet contains 150 to 600 μg of iodide, depending in part on the consumption of certain varieties of bread, which may contain much iodate, and milk, which may contain considerable iodide. Another major source is iodized salt. Most forms of ingested iodine are reduced to iodide in the gastrointestinal tract before absorption. Absorption is usually complete in one hour. Iodide is cleared from plasma by the salivary glands and gastric parietal cells into their secretions, but normally this iodide is recycled to plasma. Iodide is cleared unidirectionally by the kidney from plasma at a rate of about 30 ml per minute. The normal

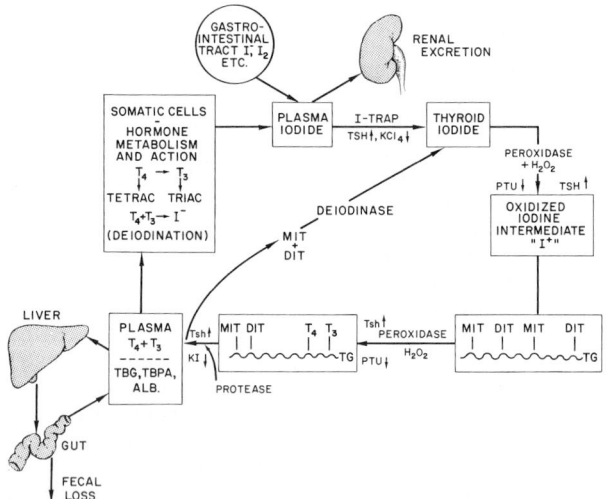

Figure 1. The iodide cycle and thyroid hormone metabolism. The pathway includes iodide absorption, thyroid trapping, oxidation by peroxidase, iodination of tyrosine and intramolecular coupling, proteolysis, plasma hormone transport, and finally hormone action and metabolism with recirculation of iodide.

thyroid clears plasma iodide at a rate of 4 to 12 ml per minute. The TSH feedback control system regulates the clearance rate to provide the gland with enough iodide for hormone production, and this control point is probably the prime determinant of thyroid hormone production. If iodide intake is low and thyroid uptake of iodide is diminished, thyroxine production is reduced and the level of hormone in plasma falls. TSH secretion is then increased and augments iodide clearance by the thyroid gland. Under the influence of TSH or in thyroid hyperactivity of the thyrotoxicosis, clearance may be elevated 5 to 20 times the normal range. With augmented levels of iodide ion in the body, e.g., during therapy with Lugol's solution, thyroid clearance falls to a fraction of a milliliter per minute. The thyroid cells actively transport iodide and maintain a concentration gradient of 20 to 1 over the level in plasma. The iodide concentration process is blocked competitively by perchlorate or thiocyanate ions. These drugs can thus interfere with formation of thyroid hormone. They are also used to establish the presence of elevated amounts of free iodide in the gland (see below).

HORMONOGENESIS. As rapidly as iodide is transported into the normal thyroid cell it is oxidized by a peroxidase and bound to tyrosine residues present in thyroglobulin. This iodination process takes place near the apical cell border, either in secretory vesicles before liberation of thyroglobulin to colloid or inside the colloid space. The iodine acceptor protein, thyroglobulin, is a huge glycoprotein of 670,000 molecular weight. Each thyroglobulin molecule contains about 120 tyrosine residues and, after iodination, 26 atoms of iodine. The iodination of the tyrosyl residues in thyroglobulin leads to the production of monoiodotyrosine (MIT) and diiodotyrosine (DIT) in the peptide chain. Then two iodotyrosyl groups couple to form an iodothyronine (T_3 or T_4), still within the peptide chain of thyroglobulin. In the iodine-replete gland, each thyroglobulin molecule contains about one iodothyronine molecule (T_3 or T_4). The ratio of T_4 to T_3 molecules is about 10 to 1.

HORMONE SECRETION. As thyroglobulin is iodinated and coupling of iodotyrosines occurs, some molecules are hydrolyzed to release hormone and others are stored in the colloid for days or weeks. Resorption from colloid occurs as pseudopods on the surface of the thyroid cell surround a small fragment of colloid, and a droplet is thus formed within the cell. The colloid droplet then fuses with a lysosome, producing a phagosome within which thyroid protease hydrolyzes thyroglobulin to its component amino acids. MIT and DIT are released and deiodinated by a dehalogenase present in the microsomal fraction of the cell; the liberated iodide is reincorporated into new MIT and DIT in thyroglobulin. The thyroxine and triiodothyronine released from thyroglobulin are secreted into blood, along with some unhydrolyzed thyroglobulin, small amounts of iodotyrosines, and small amounts of iodide. The thyroid also iodinates other proteins, including a protein very similar to serum albumin, and secretes this iodinated protein into the circulation. Other particulate and soluble iodoproteins are formed in the gland, but their metabolic role is unknown. Some T_4 may be monodeiodinated to form T_3 within the thyroid cell.

HORMONE TRANSPORT. The T_4 and T_3 secreted by the gland are transported in plasma largely bound by noncovalent bonds to plasma proteins. Of these, the main and most specific hormone-binding protein is thyroxine-binding inter-alpha-globulin, or TBG. Approximately 80 per cent of T_4 in the blood is carried by this protein. Perhaps 5 per cent of thyroxine is bound to thyroxine-binding prealbumin (TBPA), and the remainder is bound to albumin. Triiodothyronine is less tightly bound to TBG, and insignificant amounts bind to TBPA. T_4 binds firmly to the proteins; only 0.04 per cent of the hormone exists free in solution at any one time. The plasma protein–hormone interaction is reversible. The binding proteins control distribution of hormone between serum and cells, serve as a reservoir constantly replenishing free hormone, and also prevent the iodinated thyronines from being excreted in urine. Free hormone gains access to cells and appears to be the metabolically important fraction. The level of TBG is raised by estrogen treatment and lowered by testosterone. TBG is rarely absent or present in excess on a congenital basis, and its formation is depressed in serious malnutrition or liver disease. In these conditions there may be wide variations in the total thyroid hormone content of plasma, but since the absolute level of free hormone remains constant, the patients remain metabolically normal (Fig. 2).

Free hormone also penetrates cells and controls the feedback mechanism in the pituitary. Approximately one third of the extrathyroidal hormone is loosely bound in the liver. The hormone slowly penetrates most other tissues, reaching an equilibrium within tissue (e.g., muscle) in two or three days.

T_4 leaves the blood with a disappearance half-time of about six days, and T_3 with a half-life of approximately

Figure 2. Variations in plasma hormone level. Plasma T_4 (and T_3) is largely bound to protein, whose capacity for holding the hormone is partially saturated. The small fraction of free hormone regulates metabolism. Variations in total hormone primarily reflect the protein-bound fraction, and must be combined with analysis of the fraction that is free in order to assess properly that hormone which is active on body tissues.

one day. The usual ratio of T_4 to T_3 secreted by the thyroid is 10 to 1. Because of the difference in T_4 and T_3 binding to plasma proteins and metabolism, the ratio of T_4 to T_3 in plasma is about 40 to 1. About 30 per cent of T_4 is converted to T_3 by monodeiodination in peripheral tissues. A significant fraction of this T_3 returns to plasma. T_4 may be considered to be a plasma hormone, or pro-hormone, and T_3 the main tissue hormone. T_3 is less firmly bound to plasma proteins, and enters the cells much more rapidly. T_3 is somewhat selectively taken up and bound by receptor molecules in the cell nuclei. Because of extensive conversion of T_4 to T_3, and the threefold greater metabolic potency of T_3 in comparison to T_4, a large proportion of the metabolic stimulation caused by the hormones may be due to T_3.

METABOLIC ACTION. The exact metabolic action of the hormone is unclear. In animals made hypothyroid by ablation of the gland, administration of thyroid hormone is followed by stimulation of liver nuclear protein synthesis in about five hours, increased nucleic acid synthesis in eight to ten hours, and increased mitochondrial oxidative phosphorylation, reaching a peak within two to seven days. Coincident with this increased synthetic and oxidative activity in the cell, the activity of many enzymes, including alpha-ketoglutarate dehydrogenase, malic enzyme, and phosphokinases, is stimulated.

Usually several hours elapse before any action of the hormone is observed after administration to animals or man. After a single dose, peak action is seen within two to five days, and gradually decays over a period of two to three weeks. T_3 has a slightly more rapid onset of action than T_4, and its action is more rapidly dissipated. It is of interest that some tissues (brain, spleen, and testes) do not appear to respond to thyroxine.

Treatment of animals with large doses of thyroid hormone or addition of thyroid hormone is vitro induces uncoupling of mitochondrial oxidative phosphorylation. For years one theory of the primary action of thyroid hormone action has centered on this phenomenon. There are two objections to this theory. (1) The change from the sluggish metabolic activity of the hypothyroid state to the normal or mildly hyperactive state induced by administration of physiologic doses of thyroid hormone to animals is accompanied by an increased rate of oxidative phosphorylation *without* loss of efficiency. (2) Studies of mitochondria taken by biopsy from patients with severe hyperthyroidism have shown increased metabolic activity but normally coupled oxidative phosphorylation.

Many other actions of thyroid hormone have been observed, including stimulation of protein synthesis in isolated mitochondria and microsomes, inhibition of pyridine nucleotide–linked dehydrogenases, and swelling of mitochondria.

Recent studies indicate that T_3 and, to a lesser extent, T_4 are accumulated rapidly in the nuclei of responsive tissues and are found tightly but noncovalently linked to a protein associated with chromatin. Although no specific effects of this T_3-protein complex are known, it is postulated that the complex may modulate nuclear RNA synthesis, leading to subsequent increases in protein synthesis and enzyme actions. The importance of these putative receptors is supported by four sets of data: (1) their affinity for analogues of T_3 corresponds in general with metabolic potency; (2) capacity of receptor corresponds to tissue responsiveness to T_3; (3)

saturation of receptor parallels hormone response; and (4) receptors are abnormal in certain children resistant to thyroid hormone.

Thyroid hormone seems to differ in its mechanism of action from the peptide hormones which act on the adenyl cyclase system at the cell membrane, or the steroid hormones which cause an almost immediate stimulation of nuclear RNA synthesis.

THYROID HORMONE METABOLISM. A major portion of T_4 is metabolized by monodeiodination in peripheral tissues to form T_3. In fact T_4 is considered by some as only a pro-hormone, but evidence indicates that T_4 can independently affect tissue metabolism. In adult man T_4 is also metabolized by deiodination of the inner phenolic ring to form "reverse T_3" (rT_3) which has minimal (1 per cent) of the metabolic effect of L-T_3. Conversion of T_4 to L-T_3 or rT_3 is affected by different enzymes, is under metabolic control, and is in many instances reciprocally related. Thus during fetal life, acute and chronic illness, and starvation, rT_3 production is augmented and little L-T_3 is formed. This may be viewed teleologically (and correctly or incorrectly?) as a homeostatic defense mechanism used by the body to lower levels of the catabolic hormone L-T_3 during times of stress. In any event, T_4 to T_3 conversion must be considered a very important aspect of normal hormone metabolism. In a few instances (in the fetus, in severe illness), low serum and tissue T_3 levels occur in the absence of clinical hypothyroidism. The significance of these findings is not clear, although it is postulated that, under some circumstances, serum T_3 may not validly reflect the saturation of nuclear T_3 receptors.

T_4 and T_3 are metabolized to form butanol-insoluble iodoprotein, some of which may be covalently bound hormone. This material is formed in the microsomal fraction of cells, and some in plasma. Most likely it is a degradative product of thyroid hormone. The alanine side chain of the molecule is metabolized to the acetic acid and pyruvic acid derivatives, analogues which are significantly less active than the parent compound. The hormone is also metabolized extensively by deiodination without rupture of the ether linkage. In some tissues the ether linkage is broken with formation of a hydroquinone and protein-bound DIT. As a final result of metabolism, the hormone is deiodinated and the iodide is returned to plasma to follow the same fate as newly absorbed dietary iodine.

Approximately 10 to 20 per cent of hormone is lost in the feces after secretion by the liver as glucuronide and in other conjugates. A small amount of hormone derived from free T_4 and T_3 in plasma is cleared by the kidneys to urine.

FEEDBACK CONTROL. Each day the thyroid releases approximately 60 to 100 μg of hormonal iodide, of which 90 per cent is thyroxine and 10 per cent is triiodothyronine. If production falls because of inefficiency in the gland or diminished iodide supply, the level of free hormone in blood decreases, and this alteration is detected by the pituicytes which synthesize increased TSH. The signal recognized by the pituicyte requires RNA and protein synthesis. It is presumed that T_3 and T_4 exert the same sort of metabolic activity on the tissues involved in feedback control as they do in other cells and that this metabolic process constitutes the feedback signal.

In turn, the feedback control of T_4 on the pituitary is modulated by the hypothalamus. Neural centers in the hypothalamus synthesize and secrete the tripeptide pyro-glutamyl-histidyl-proline amide known as thyrotropin-releasing hormone (TRH). This hormone travels down the hypophysial-portal vessels and stimulates TSH release. There is a delicate balance between the TRH stimulation and T_3-T_4 feedback inhibition of the pituicyte; excess of either can overcome the effect of the other. TRH probably acts by binding to membrane receptors and augmenting adenyl cyclase activity. This leads to increased synthesis and secretion of TSH. T_4 opposes the action of TRH by a mechanism which requires increased protein synthesis.

TRH is needed for normal tonic control of TSH secretion, as evidenced by the hypothyroidism occurring when the hypothalamus is damaged and TRH is no longer formed. However, the physiologic control of TRH is unclear. Secretion may be altered in response to neural stimuli or cold, but there is no evidence that an excess or deficiency of thyroid hormone alters secretion of TRH. TRH is also a potent stimulant of pituitary prolactin release, but its exact role in the physiologic control of prolactin synthesis and secretion is unknown.

TSH ACTION ON THE THYROID. TSH released by the pituitary binds to a receptor on the thyroid cell membrane and initiates a sequence of reactions, including stimulation of adenyl cyclase and formation of increased intracellular cyclic adenosine monophosphate (cAMP). It is believed that this cAMP "second messenger" somehow mediates all the metabolic stimulatory actions of TSH, including increased uptake and binding of iodide, increased thyroglobulin synthesis, increased colloid resorption, proteolysis, and hormone release.

OTHER CONTROLS OF THYROID FUNCTION. As described above, pituitary TSH is the main regulator of thyroid function. The adrenal gland exerts some control; excess cortisol depresses pituitary production of TSH by blunting the pituitary sensitivity to TRH. Cortisol also directly depresses the level of TBG, in plasma, and augments urinary excretion of iodide. Pregnancy, associated with its increased estrogen production, augments the level of circulating TBG, and increases the concentration of circulating T_4 and T_3. However, the turnover rate of the hormone in blood is proportionately decelerated, so that net hormone utilization remains unchanged. Androgens have an effect on TBG and thyroxine turnover that is the converse of the action of estrogen. Severe illness and stress inhibit T_4 conversion to T_3, and cause a rapid lowering of serum T_3 levels. Thyroid hormone utilization is accelerated in animals by exposure to cold and in man by conditioning to strenuous exercise.

In a very real sense, the average daily intake of iodide controls thyroid function. The feedback control system is designed to maintain a constant level of serum T_4 and T_3. To achieve this the gland must accumulate a constant amount of iodide each day. Thus variations in iodide intake are countered by reciprocal changes in thyroid activity (uptake and binding of iodide, for example) which achieve homeostasis.

THYROID FUNCTION TESTS

In examining a patient with thyroid disease, one seeks to determine the level of tissue metabolic activity and the nature of the thyroid disease. The most direct measure of metabolic activity is the basal metabolic rate (BMR), but the wide range of normal values and the changes in the BMR caused by nonthyroidal factors make the determination of limited diagnostic value. There is no other good approach to assaying the peripheral action of thyroid hormone, although numerous measurements can be made. The serum cholesterol concentration is elevated in hypothyroidism and depressed in hyperthyroidism. The relaxation half-time of the deep tendon reflexes is sometimes shortened below 240 msec in hyperthyroidism, and characteristically prolonged beyond 360 msec in hypothyroidism. Plasma tyrosine levels are elevated in hyperthyroidism, urinary hydroxyproline excretion is depressed in hypothyroidism, and CPK, SGOT, and LDH activities are elevated in hypothyroidism. None of these tests are useful for definitive diagnosis, because they are nonspecific and similar alterations can be caused by other disease processes.

MEASUREMENT OF SERUM HORMONES. Lacking a good measure of hormone action in the tissues, most physicians turn to a measure of thyroid hormone in blood. The standard determination for years was the serum protein-bound iodine (PBI) or butanol-extractable iodine (BEI). Direct measurements of serum T_4 and T_3 by competitive displacement (T_4D and T_3D) or radioimmunoassay (T_3-RIA and T_4-RIA) have now largely replaced PBI and BEI. When combined with a measure of saturation of TBG by hormone, such as thyroxine dialyzable fraction (per cent DT_4) or resin uptake (T_3RU), a measure of serum free thyroxine (FT_4) or triiodothyronine (FT_3) is obtained. The latter values are the most precise measures of thyroid hormone supply to tissues currently available.

The PBI measures all iodine in serum precipitable by protein-denaturing agents. Ordinarily this consists mainly of thyroid hormone, but if large quantities of iodide are present, or if any of the roentgenographic contrast medium used for gallbladder examinations, intravenous pyelograms, or arteriograms is present in plasma, the level is falsely elevated. Iodoproteins, formed by the thyroid in augmented amounts in some conditions, e.g., thyroiditis, are also precipitated. The normal range is 4 to 8 μg of iodine per 100 ml. It is wise to determine total plasma iodine as well; if the level is no more than 2 or 3 μg per 100 ml above the PBI, it can be assumed that contamination with excess quantities of free iodide is not present. The butanol-extractable iodine (BEI) procedure is technically more sophisticated and is more specific for thyroid hormone because it excludes iodoproteins. If the PBI exceeds the BEI by more than 20 per cent, abnormal amounts of iodoprotein are present. Neither of these tests is widely used for diagnosis at present since specific measurement of T_4 or T_3 eliminates problems of "contamination" of serum by iodide.

SERUM THYROXINE AND TRIIODOTHYRONINE. A competitive protein-binding assay for thyroxine, similar in principle to the radioimmunoassay of peptide hormones, is widely available. The technique is in practice like the resin uptake test. T_4 is extracted from a serum sample. The T_4 of the plasma sample is then mixed with isotope-labeled T_4 in a standard TBG-containing solution, and its capacity to displace some of the radioactive-labeled hormone from the TBG to a resin is quantitated by comparison to a standard curve made with known amounts of T_4. The test is technically demanding, but is extremely useful because it is specific for tetraiodothyronine and triiodothyronine. In practice it measures mainly T_4, because so little T_3 is present in plasma. Serum T_4 by displacement analysis (T_4D) is usually 4 to 10 μg per 100 ml, expressed as quantity of thyroxine, not iodide. The normal range varies depending upon the methodology used in a particular laboratory. Serum T_3 can also be measured specifically by this technique if the T_3 is first extracted from serum and separated chromatographically from T_4, but this is rarely done.

Specific antibodies to T_4 and T_3 have been generated, allowing radioimmunoassay of T_4 (T_4-RIA) and T_3 (T_3-RIA). These techniques are gradually becoming available in most medical centers and commercial laboratories. T_4 (RIA) results are similar to T_4(D). The levels of T_3 reported from various laboratories have varied widely, but most results suggest that normal T_3 (RIA) is about 140 (100 to 200) ng per 100 ml. Usually T_4 and T_3 vary concordantly. Under some circumstances (limited availability of iodine, diminished peroxidase, thyroid hyperplasia), excess T_3 may be produced relative to T_4. More commonly seen is a decrease in serum L-T_3 in comparison to L-T_4, associated with reduced L T_3 5'-deiodination in severe illness, starvation, and fetal life. Measurement of L-T_4 (or better, free thyroxine index; see FTI, below) is the best current index of metabolic function. Occasionally serum T_3 must also be determined to assess hyperthyroidism correctly. Serum T_3 is not a useful diagnostic measure in hypothyroidism.

Variation in total T_4 or T_3 in serum may occur because of excess or diminution of hormone supply, or because of increase or decrease in serum TBG. Changes in hormone supply represent chemical thyrotoxicosis or hypothyroidism. Increased TBG results from pregnancy, estrogen administration, or heredity. Decreased TBG or TBPA results from liver disease, severe malnutrition, severe illness, steroids, or testosterone. These changes are accompanied by concordant alterations in T_4 and T_3 but reciprocal alterations in per cent free T_4 and T_3, resulting in normal quantities of FT_4 and FT_3. To differentiate between these two possible causes of high or low serum thyroid hormone concentrations, one must assess the level of TBG, or measure per cent DT_4 (Fig. 2).

T_3 **RESIN UPTAKE (T_3RU).** Serum is incubated with a trace amount of labeled T_3 and a resin. Uptake of the tracer by the resin varies directly with total serum T_4 and T_3 and per cent FT_4 if TBG levels are normal, and inversely with serum TBG if it is altered. Resin uptake is *inversely* proportional to, and can be used as an estimate of, unoccupied TBG and varies *directly* with free hormone fraction. For example, T_3RU is elevated in hyperthyroidism, low in hypothyroidism, elevated in severe liver disease, and low in normal pregnancy.

PER CENT FT_4. Serum plus a labeled T_4 tracer is dialyzed to equilibrium against a buffer. The dialyzable fraction, normally $\pm$ 0.04 per cent of the total T_4, represents the free hormone fraction.

FREE THYROID HORMONE. Multiplication of the total serum T_4 × per cent FT_4 yields FT_4, the actual concentration of free — non-protein-bound — T_4. The usual range is 1.5 to 3.5 ng per 100 ml. The same measure can be derived for T_3 (FT_3) if T_3 concentration and per cent FT_3 are available.

In most laboratories advantage is taken of the relationship of the resin uptake to per cent FT_4 in order to calculate an "index," as first suggested by Clark and Horn. Total $T_4 \times \dfrac{\text{Patient's } T_3RU}{\text{Standard } T_3RU}$ equals the free thyroxine index (FTI), which is a very good approximation of free T_4 and correlates exactly with FT_4.

FT_4 or FTI constitutes the best available contemporary measure of hormone supply to tissues, is independent of variations in plasma thyroid hormone binding proteins, and is not affected by excess iodide or iodide-containing compounds. However, the FTI is not foolproof. Extreme alterations in TBG may produce apparently abnormal FTI values unless the standard test is modified. Certain drugs (Dilantin, ASA) may produce false depressions of the FTI.

Certain problems must be remembered when performing function tests. Excess iodine in any form may elevate the PBI and BEI and depress the radioactive iodide uptake test. Roentgenographic contrast dyes may for a short time depress the radioactive uptake test, and for periods of weeks or months falsely elevate the PBI and BEI. Alterations in binding proteins caused by heredity, hormones, illness, liver disease, or malnutrition can cause increases or decreases in the PBI, BEI, serum thyroxine, and T_3 values without altering the level of free thyroid hormone. In most circumstances (with the few exceptions noted above), determination of the FTI provides a reliable assessment of free hormone despite changes in binding proteins.

RADIOACTIVE IODINE UPTAKE. Another commonly used measure of thyroid activity is the thyroidal radioactive iodide uptake (RAIU). The patient is given a trace dose of radioactive iodide, and the fraction accumulated in the gland is determined at 2, 6, or 24 hours, the last of these being the most widely used end-point. The normal uptake is inversely dependent upon available iodide supply. In areas where the iodide intake is 150 to 200 μg per day, it ranges from 20 to 50 per cent. In most of the United States, an increase in iodide in the diet up to 400 to 600 μg per day has reduced the normal range to 10 to 25 per cent. This procedure measures the activity of the thyroid trapping and binding process, which can be augmented owing to excess TSH stimulation or because of inherent thyroid hyperactivity. The RAIU is characteristically elevated in areas of iodide deficiency.

PERCHLORATE DISCHARGE TEST. The presence of trapped but unbound iodide in the thyroid gland can be ascertained by administering 1 gram of $KClO_4$ orally two hours after a ^{131}I tracer. Discharge of more than 10 per cent is characteristic of thyroid organification defects of congenital (e.g., Pendred's syndrome) or acquired (e.g., Hashimoto's thyroiditis) types (Fig. 3).

SERUM TSH ASSAY. Measurement of serum TSH by RIA is now a standard and useful determination. Normal TSH varies from undetectable to 8 μU per milliliter. TSH is characteristically suppressed by exogenous or endogenous excess of thyroid hormone. Elevations of 20 to 40 μU per milliliter occur in primary thyroid failure of any cause. Mild elevations (10 to 20 μU) are of less certain significance and may represent mild hypothyroidism or euthyroidism (compensated hypothyroidism) achieved by the elevated TSH. Undetectable or normal TSH levels are found in pituitary hypothyroidism, hypothalamic damage, and in almost all patients with thyrotoxicosis.

TESTS FOR SPECIFIC CONDITIONS. The nature of the disease process affecting the thyroid can be evaluated by a number of other procedures.

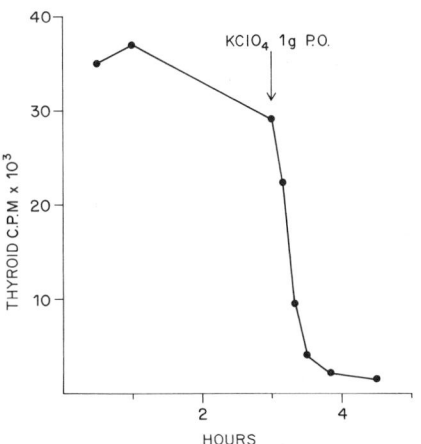

Figure 3. KClO$_4$ discharge test. In the usual test thyroid RAIU is measured sequentially over two to three hours after a tracer dose of ^{131}I. One gram of KClO$_4$ is given orally, and thyroid uptake determinations are continued. In this patient with organification defect resulting from complete lack of peroxidase, KClO$_4$ caused nearly complete release of accumulated iodide, indicating that the tracer existed in the gland as iodide and had not been bound in the normal manner to thyroglobulin.

T$_3$ Suppression Test. A high thyroid ^{131}I uptake caused by endogenous TSH can be reduced in most circumstances to or below the normal range by administration of 100 μg of triiodothyronine daily for one week. Serum T$_4$ will also be lowered, and its determination is useful when administration of radioiodine is contraindicated (e.g., pregnancy). Thyroid activity is not suppressible in most patients with active Graves' disease (see Ch. 546.2). This response is seen whether the basal RAIU is elevated or normal and is accepted as the most characteristic abnormality in this illness. However, nonsuppressibility also occurs in the closely related syndrome of Hashimoto's thyroiditis and if autonomous functioning thyroid nodules are present.

TSH Stimulation Test. The presence of functioning thyroid tissue can be evaluated by administration of 5 units of TSH subcutaneously daily for three days, with a radioactive iodide uptake test (and sometimes a scan) before and after. TSH should raise the radioactive iodide uptake to a normal level or at least double it in a patient whose basal function is low because of deficient TSH. The test is also useful for demonstrating normal tissue which has been suppressed by a functioning "hot" nodule.

TRH Test (Fig. 4). The ability of the pituitary to secrete TSH can be elevated by administration of 400 μg of TRH intravenously and measuring serum TSH during the subsequent 90 minutes. Hypothalamic hypothyroidism is associated with normal basal TSH, responding to the administration of exogenous TRH. Primary thyroid failure is associated with a high basal level of TSH hyperresponsive to TRH. Hypothyroidism resulting from pituitary failure causes low serum TSH and absent TRH response. Administration of replacement doses of T$_4$ or T$_3$ or excess endogenous or exogenous T$_4$ or T$_3$ obliterates the response to TRH. Thus TRH nonresponsiveness can serve as a measure of normal or excessive thyroid hormone supply, derived from an administered pill or autonomous thyroid function.

Antibodies and LATS. Autoimmunity against thyroid antigens can be demonstrated by measuring antithyroglobulin antibodies by the tanned red cell agglutination procedure, or antithyroid microsomal antibodies by the

immunofluorescent, complement fixation, or tanned red cell agglutination methods. Positive test results are found in Hashimoto's thyroiditis, primary thyroid failure, and Graves' disease. Thyroid stimulatory immunoglobulins measured by several methods, including the LATS bioassay, are described in Ch. 546.2.

Thyroid Scans. A scintiscan performed after administration of ^{199m}TcO$_4$ or radioactive iodide provides anatomic localization of functioning thyroid tissue. Adenomas may appear inactive ("cold") or hyperactive ("hot"). Graves' disease shows diffuse uptake, and Hashimoto's thyroiditis gives a diffuse or mottled uptake, whereas multinodular goiter gives a mottled picture. Uptake outside the thyroid identifies aberrant thyroid tissue, metastatic thyroid cancer, and struma ovarii.

Recently, fluorescent scanning with a ^{241}Am source has been developed. This technique identifies concentration and distribution of the stable ^{127}I present in the gland (Fig. 5). It is a useful technique when radioisotopes should be avoided (children, pregnant women, lactation). In addition, it provides another independent index of thyroid function. The Hashimoto's gland is characteristically and diagnostically found to be devoid of stored iodine. Also, the thyroid can be shown by fluorescent scanning to have a normal appearance and iodine content in pituitary hypothyroidism and when uptake of a tracer is suppressed by administration of exogenous hormone or iodide.

Needle Biopsy. Needle biopsy of the thyroid is a useful procedure in properly selected cases and can provide a histologic diagnosis when all other techniques fail. Recently, fine-needle aspiration for cytologic examination has gained favor for the same purpose.

INITIAL SELECTION OF FUNCTION TESTS. In most thyroid diseases careful history and physical examination lead to the diagnosis, and laboratory procedures serve to confirm the clinical impression. In the initial evaluation of most patients, it is useful to measure the serum thyroxine, the free thyroxine index, and occasionally the radioactive iodine uptake. A scan can be done at the same time if there is a question of nonuniformity of gland function raised by history or examination of the neck. The TSH level should be checked if hypothyroidism is suggested. The test for antithyroglobulin antibodies is also useful in the initial evaluation of many patients. To follow the progress of

Figure 4. TSH responses to intravenous TRH. The normal rapid elevation of plasma TSH after TRH is obliterated in thyrotoxicosis, by thyroid hormone administration, or in pituitary destruction. An excessive response occurs in primary thyroid failure.

NORMAL   **THYROIDITIS**

Figure 5. Fluorescent thyroid scan. Fluorescence by ^{241}Am indicates distribution and concentrations of stable ^{127}I in the normal gland. By contrast, the gland affected by Hashimoto's thyroiditis is nearly devoid of iodine.

therapy, the most useful procedure is serial determination of FTI. Frequent measurement of the patient's weight also constitutes an excellent measure of whole body metabolism.

Further tests are dictated by the progress of the evaluation. Many specialized assays are available if needed to define unusual congenital or acquired diseases.

Bernal, J., and Refetoff, S.: The action of thyroid hormone. Clin. Endocrinol., 6:277, 1977.

Burrows, A. W., Cooper, E., Shakespear, R. A., Aickin, C. M., Fraser, S., Hesch, R. D., and Burke, C. W.: Low serum L-T$_3$ levels in the elderly sick: Protein binding, thyroid and pituitary responsiveness, and reverse T$_3$ concentrations. Clin. Endocrinol., 7:289, 1977.

Chopra, I. J.: An assessment of daily production and significance of thyroidal secretion of 3,3',5'-triiodothyronine (reverse T$_3$) in man. J. Clin. Invest., 58:32, 1976.

DeGroot, L. J., and Niepomniszcze, H.: Biosynthesis of thyroid hormone: Basic and clinical aspects. Metabolism, 26:665, 1977.

Faglia, G., Ferrari, C., Paracchi, A., Spada, A., and Beck-Peccoz, P.: Triiodothyronine response to thyrotrophin-releasing hormone in patients with hypothalamic-pituitary disorders. Clin. Endocrinol., 4:585, 1975.

Hershman, J. M., and Pittman, J. A.: Utility of the radioimmunoassay of serum thyrotrophin in man. Ann. Intern. Med., 74:481, 1971.

Refetoff, S.: Tests of thyroid function. In Gottschalk, A., and Potcher, E. J. (eds.) Diagnostic Nuclear Medicine. Baltimore, Williams & Wilkins Company, 1976, p. 237.

Taurog, A.: The mechanism of action of the thioureylene antithyroid drugs. Endocrinology, 98:1031, 1976.

546.2.   GRAVES' DISEASE AND HYPERTHYROIDISM

Hyperthyroidism refers to a state of heightened thyroid gland activity associated with the production of excess quantities of thyroid hormone. The clinical state is also referred to as *thyrotoxicosis.* Most commonly hyperthyroidism is a part of a syndrome which may include goiter, exophthalmos, and pretibial myxedema, known as *Graves' disease* or *Basedow's* disease. Thyrotoxicosis can also be caused by excessive production of hormone by a *single "toxic" nodule,* by a *toxic multinodular goiter,* by occasional *functioning thyroid carcinomas,* or by *medication.* Rarely, it is caused by a TSH-secreting pituitary adenoma, is asso-

ciated with acromegaly, occurs because of production of TSH-like material in trophoblastic tumors or embryonal cell carcinomas, or is due to hyperfunctioning teratoma (struma ovarii).

INCIDENCE.   Hyperthyroidism is not a reportable condition, so exact data on incidence are unavailable. Incidence is probably in excess of 3 per 10,000 adults per year. It is largely a disease of adult women, with a sex ratio of approximately 5 to 1. Peak incidence is between 30 and 50 years of age.

ETIOLOGY AND PATHOGENESIS.   The manifestations of Graves' disease fall into two categories: (1) the primary disease involving the thyroid (plus eyes and skin), and (2) the circulatory, neurologic, and metabolic abnormalities, described below, which are secondarily caused by excess thyroid hormone produced by the thyroid gland impinging on tissues.

There are two recurring themes in discussions of the etiology of Graves' disease: (1) it often seems related to emotional trauma, or (2) it may be an "autoimmune." disease. The previous impression that the thyroid in Graves' disease was responding to excess TSH is erroneous, because TSH in plasma of patients with this disorder is characteristically reduced or absent, apparently suppressed by increased circulating thyroid hormone.

For decades it has been suggested that Graves' disease is induced by emotional stress, because of the frequency with which physicians obtain a history of emotional trauma occurring before the onset of hyperthyroidism. Characteristically the event is a marital problem or death of a loved one. Although such testimonials are frequent, the meager factual data available are inconclusive. Psychiatric evaluations indicate that there is nothing special about the individual who becomes a victim of Graves' disease, and that the incidence of emotional stress in these patients is comparable to that in a control population. Perhaps, in the individuals who report a stressful circumstance, Graves' disease was already present and made the emotional reaction more dramatic. Also, the patient suffering from Graves' disease has anxiety and tremulousness as a result of the illness; these symptoms may be misinterpreted as causal.

Autoimmunity directed against thyroid antigens is currently thought to be the most probable cause. Antibodies directed against endogenous thyroid antigens were detected in patients with Hashimoto's thyroiditis in 1956, and several thyroid antibody-antigen systems have since been found in patients with thyroiditis, idiopathic myxedema, and Graves' disease (see Ch. 546.3). Sixty to 80 per cent of patients with Graves' disease have antibodies directed against thyroglobulin or against thyroid microsomes. In addition, Adams and Purves described in 1956 a factor (long-acting thyroid stimulator, LATS), present in the serum of about half the patients with Graves' disease, which stimulated the release of hormone from the prelabeled thyroid of a test animal. LATS is now known to be a polyclonal gamma globulin, probably an autoantibody directed against a component of the thyroid cell membrane. LATS can be neutralized by reacting with antibodies prepared against 7S human IgG. LATS adsorbs to thyroid microsomes, but the reaction is not entirely specific and does not require complement. In addition to causing release of hormone, LATS stimulates increased synthesis of nucleic acids and proteins, increases incorporation of phosphate into phospholipids, stimulates glucose metabolism, and causes thyroid growth.

LATS is, however, found in at most 80 per cent of patients with Graves' disease, and its presence or level does not correlate uniformly with thyroid hyperactivity. Recent data suggest that there are several thyroid stimulatory immunoglobulins present which can be detected in different assays. One of these is the "human thyroid stimulator" (HTS) of Onaya et al.; another possible factor is the "LATS protector" (LATS-P) of Adams. Others are detected by their ability to displace TSH from human thyroid plasma membrane receptors for TSH. It is probable that all these immunoglobulins have the ability to interact with the TSH receptor site and stimulate it as does TSH. They are probably IgG's of variable structure, having different affinities for human and animal TSH receptors. Whether they are truly antibodies, formed in response to some aberrant stimulus by the thyroid cell TSH receptor, is the key question waiting to be answered.

A contemporary interpretation is that LATS, LATS-P, and other thyroid stimulatory immunoglobulins (TSI) mimic the action of TSH and stimulate the synthesis and release of thyroid hormone. In patients whose thyroids are capable of responding to such a trophic stimulus, TSI may be the mediator of hyperthyroxinemia. TSI cross the placenta and cause transient hyperthyroidism in some neonates born to mothers who have high circulating levels of the antibody.

In addition to circulating antibodies (humoral immune response), there is much evidence for cell-mediated immunity (CMI) in Graves' disease, as well as in Hashimoto's thyroiditis and primary myxedema. The CMI is probably involved in a cell-destructive response. Our theory is that the manifestations of Graves' disease represent a balance between the stimulatory or blocking effect of circulating antibodies such as LATS and HTS and the cell-destructive effects of CMI.

Exophthalmos has also been related to autoimmunity. In serum of patients with exophthalmos, a factor causing experimental exophthalmos in animals is found. Various reports also indicate an abnormality in binding of gamma globulin from exophthalmic patients to orbital antigens, and other studies indicate that patients with exophthal-

mos have CMI against these antigens. Other theories indicate that thyroglobulin binds to extraocular eye muscles and causes secondary binding of antithyroglobulin antibodies, and that these complexes initiate the eye disease.

Why the body should develop a humoral antibody and CMI response active against its own tissues remains unknown. There is no evidence for an abnormal antigen in these conditions, or for an abnormal sequestration or release of antigen. Because of the association of thyroid autoimmunity with immunity against several other organs of the body, it seems possible that Graves' disease is basically a manifestation of deranged immune homeostasis.

Much evidence indicates that *a strong hereditary factor is involved in Graves' disease, Hashimoto's thyroiditis, and myxedema*, and that the three diseases are intimately related. Patients with Graves' disease and thyroiditis usually have a family history positive for the same condition. Thyroid autoantibodies, including LATS, are found in relatives of patients with these diseases. The incidence of any one of the other two diseases is increased in relatives of patients who have one of the three. Some patients appear to have a combination of thyroiditis and Graves' disease that has been called "Hashitoxicosis." Two studies report that the frequency of HLA-B8 transplantation antigen is increased in patients with Graves' disease. This suggests the occurrence of Graves' disease may be conditioned by inheritance of particular immune response genes.

Another intriguing bit of circumstantial evidence related to etiology is the occasionally reported occurrence of Graves' disease after consumption of desiccated thyroid for weight reduction. It is as if the ingestion of thyroid hormone somehow conditioned the body to a high level of the substance and "demanded" continued thyroid hyperfunction after the exogenous hormone was withdrawn.

Iodine administration occasionally induces hyperthyroidism. This "Jod-Basedow" phenomenon typically occurs in areas of endemic goiter when iodinization of salt is introduced, but can occur after administration of iodine to patients in nonendemic areas. Apparently the thyroid was functioning autonomously at a hyperactive level before the introduction of iodine, but was unable to manifest hyperthyroidism owing to the limitation of hormone synthesis imposed by the low iodide intake. Supplemental iodide then allows excess production of hormone.

Little is known about other causes of hyperthyroidism. The etiology of the toxic nodular goiter, the toxic solitary nodule, or the hyperfunctioning thyroid carcinoma is related to the problem of tumor formation. Hyperthyroidism found in association with acromegaly may be due to increased TSH production, although this has not been established. Hyperthyroidism associated with trophoblastic tumors is due to the production of a trophic substance by the tumor. A placental thyrotropin is believed to be a normal placental product; a different protein is formed in excess in patients with hydatidiform mole and in choriocarcinoma. It is immunologically related to bovine thyrotropin, but does not cross-react with antibodies to human thyrotropin. The most widely accepted view at present is that this protein is in fact human chorionic gonadotropin (hCG), or a closely related aberrant protein. hCG appears in several studies to have about 1/4000 the ability of TSH to stimulate the thyroid gland.

PATHOLOGY. The main pathologic abnormality in Graves' disease is in the size of the thyroid cells. The cells are tall, and the size of the average follicle is reduced. Small amounts of colloid are present in the lumen. The picture is analogous to a gland under intense TSH stimulation. In addition there is characteristically an infiltration of mononuclear cells, mainly small lymphocytes and some plasma cells, and lymphoid germinal centers may be apparent. Sometimes the process shades into a picture characteristic of Hashimoto's thyroiditis. There is generalized lymph node hyperplasia, the thymus is enlarged, and the proportion of active thymic tissue is increased. Active germinal centers are also found in the thymus, and the histology is similar to that of myasthenia gravis or lupus erythematosus. The muscles are usually microscopically normal, but occasionally the cells are atrophic, multiple nuclei are present, striations are indistinct, and a lymphocyte infiltrate is apparent. Hepatic changes include cellular edema, focal necrosis, and lymphocyte infiltrates. The epidermis and dermis are thinned. Bones may show osteoporosis or osteomalacia. Pathology of the eye and "localized myxedema" are described below.

CLINICAL MANIFESTATIONS. In many patients the changes are so obvious as to be inescapable; in others the subtlety of the disease defines anything except a laboratory diagnosis. The patient may notice weakness, increased fatigue, insomnia, weight loss, or tremulousness. The skin becomes fine and moist, and there is excess perspiration. The hair thins, and the nails become thin and brittle. Increased tolerance to cold or decreased tolerance to moderate heat is noted. Friends observe that the eyes are prominent, and the patient appears to be staring. Double vision, blurred vision, burning, tearing, and decreased visual acuity may occur. Often the patient finds a mass in the neck, although this produces few local symptoms. A hyperactive heart, palpitations, dyspnea on exertion, and ankle edema may be evident, usually in the absence of congestive failure. Weight loss occurs despite increase in appetite. There may occasionally be abdominal pain reminiscent of an ulcer and frequent loose bowel movements. Subdeltoid bursitis may occur. Menstrual periods become scanty, the cycle is shortened, some periods may be missed, and fertility is reduced. Usually libido is not altered. Thirst and polyuria are sometimes noted. Weakness of the muscles is prominent; it may be the primary symptom in older persons who have had chronic low-grade thyroid hyperfunction for months or years. Such patients report that they cannot climb stairs or get up easily from a chair. Pruritus is frequently noticed, and occasionally hives occur.

On examination the patient appears anxious, tremulous, and restless, and is typically quick to cooperate. The hair is fine and thin, and females may show some temporal recession of the hairline. The skin feels moist, hot, thin, or even silky, and pigmentation may be increased. Vitiligo, especially of the hands and feet, is present in about 7 per cent of cases. The nails are thin, and the hyponychium is often seen to have receded, forming an irregular concave erosion under the distal portion of the nail. This change (onycholysis or Plummer's nails) is most typically found bilaterally on the fourth digit. The elbows are sometimes red, as are the palms.

The eyes may appear prominent, and the sclera is visible above the iris on upward or downward gaze (lid lag). The lids may be grossly puffy. Proptosis (forward displacement of the globes in the orbits) may be evident, and if severe the lids may not close adequately. Edema of the scleral conjunctiva may form loose pockets filled with clear liquid (chemosis). Extraocular muscle function may be diminished, often first with a loss of upward gaze, and

later with a fixed strabismus caused by contracture of a damaged muscle. In severe cases total loss of ocular motility and convergence are present. With proptosis the edge of the lacrimal gland may be felt bulging below the supraorbital ridge. The beefy red insertion of the lateral rectus can sometimes be seen. Depending on the severity of the process, there may be papilledema or hemorrhages and exudates in the retina. Visual acuity may be severely reduced.

The thyroid typically is enlarged, usually three to four times the normal size, although rarely the gland may be of normal dimensions. Usually the gland is symmetrically involved and may be lobulated. It characteristically feels rather firm and beefy, and often the pyramidal lobe is palpable. Lymph nodes are often present in the supraclavicular fossae and may be tender. A systolic bruit may be heard over the thyroid or palpated ("thrill") in very vascular glands.

The precordium is hyperactive, and the heart sounds are intensified. A systolic murmur is usually audible, and sometimes a scratching systolic sound (Lerman's sound) is heard in the second or third left intercostal space. Murmurs present before the onset of thyroid disease are intensified. Occasionally murmurs suggestive of mitral insufficiency or stenosis are audible; they disappear after hyperthyroidism is controlled. Recent studies prove that mitral regurgitation can be induced by thyrotoxicosis in individuals with an otherwise apparently normal heart. Tachycardia is usually present, and there is an increased propensity to atrial fibrillation. Axillary lymph nodes are frequently palpable; on examination of the abdomen, the spleen or liver or both may be minimally enlarged. Muscle strength and bulk may be reduced. Reflexes are exaggerated in speed and strength.

Rarely, typical attacks of hypokalemic periodic paralysis occur during severe hyperthyroidism, especially in young men of Oriental extraction.

Occasionally patients develop severe hyperthyroidism but present few classic manifestations. In this picture, termed *masked hyperthyroidism,* to which older people are most prone, the tremor, anxiety, and hyperkinesis may be lacking. Instead, the patient is apathetic, sometimes mentally confused, or obtunded. There may be extreme weakness and muscle atrophy. The skin may not be thinned, and the sweating and eye signs may also be lacking. Usually, however, tachycardia, goiter, and low-grade fever are present. Coincidental atrial fibrillation and weight loss should suggest this diagnosis.

DIAGNOSIS. The flagrant case with all the characteristic manifestations is usually recognized by laymen who refer the patient to the physician for therapy. Other patients do not present with more than a few of the signs and symptoms of Graves' disease, and in these patients laboratory studies become critical. Diagnosis begins with the history and physical examination. Serial weights should be recorded, because progressive loss of weight is a strong clue to the diagnosis. To prove the diagnosis, the serum thyroxine (or better, the free thyroxine index), serum T_3, and RAIU are probably the most useful tests. The BMR, cholesterol, T_3RU, and reflex time may occasionally be helpful. The antithyroglobulin or antimicrosomal antibody tests are useful, because a positive test result indicates that the patient has some variety of thyroid autoimmune disease. Often patients develop a normochromic and normocytic anemia with 9 to 11 grams of hemoglobin per 100 ml. Alkaline phosphatase may be elevated because of increased rate of bone turnover, and serum calcium, urinary calcium, and hydroxyproline excretion may be increased. Bilirubin is occasionally elevated. Roentgenograms of the skull and views of the orbits should be obtained if there is a question of an intracerebral or orbital space-occupying lesion, especially if unilateral exophthalmos occurs before the onset of hyperthyroidism. All the tests must be carefully evaluated in the light of the patient's known iodide intake, exposure to radiographic contrast media, and medications. If there is doubt about the diagnosis, a T_3 suppression test may be useful. *Nonsuppressibility of the thyroid is considered the most characteristic feature of Graves' disease.* A TRH test, giving evidence of pituitary nonresponsiveness, provides similar (but not identical) information and is safer to perform in elderly or ill patients, since it does not cause significant elevation of thyroid hormone.

T_3 Toxicosis. In some patients who have clinical symptoms suggestive of hyperthyroidism, but in whom the radioactive iodide uptake and serum thyroxine are normal, measurement of elevated plasma triiodothyronine may confirm the condition known as "T_3 toxicosis." This condition can be the presenting feature of Graves' disease, but is more frequently found in patients with an autonomous nodule or residual tissue after radioiodide (RAI) or surgical therapy, or in areas of iodine deficiency. Some reports indicate that as many as one tenth of patients have T_3 toxicosis without elevated T_4 levels. This has not been the author's experience. Although it is imperative to remember that T_3 toxicosis can explain the unusual case, the great majority of patients present with both high T_4 and high T_3, and cause no difficulty in diagnosis by the more commonly available serum T_4 measurement.

It is especially important to consider this diagnosis in elderly patients who have atrial fibrillation or congestive heart failure. Other diagnostic hints are unexplained diarrhea, severe muscle weakness, bursitis, and vitiligo of the hands and feet.

Severe pulmonary disease, anxiety, carcinoma, malabsorption, cirrhosis, and myasthenia can have features similar to thyrotoxicosis, and must be considered in the differential diagnosis.

In this age of dependence upon chemistry, it is not rare to be faced with a patient who has negligible signs and symptoms but in whom an elevated T_4 or T_3 has been detected by chance. In such patients it is wise to establish as carefully as possible the presence or absence of disease by RAIU, T_3 suppression test, and FT_4 or FT_3 levels, and then to observe events for a period of time. In some ill patients T_4 is transiently elevated for reasons that are yet obscure. The process may subside, show evidence of damage to cardiac, hepatic, or osseous tissues, indicating need for treatment, show no change, or progress gradually into overt thyrotoxicosis.

In fact, major reliance is placed on the laboratory tests. A significant elevation of FT_4 or FT_3 can alone be the determining feature of Graves' disease and demand therapy.

The RAIU, formerly a very useful test, is now of less value because elevated intake of iodide has depressed the normal and thyrotoxic values and confused the area of overlap between them. It is not necessarily required for diagnosis, but is useful when planning RAI therapy and with a scan when defining autonomous thyroid function caused by an adenoma or multinodular goiter.

Differentiation from Other Mitochondrial Diseases. The symptoms and signs of thyrotoxicosis are due to hypermetabolism, and theoretically could be mimicked by any cause of uncontrolled mitochondrial function. In fact few conditions have been reported in which mitochondrial oxidative phosphorylation is disturbed, and only one syndrome has caused confusion in diagnosis. A unique illness suggestive of thyrotoxicosis was reported by Luft. Weakness, excessive perspiration, marked hypermetabolism, and weight loss led to thyroidectomy, but induction of overt hypothyroidism failed to control the illness. Muscle mitochondria from this patient were unusually abundant and large, and had excessive crista formation. Respiration was not controlled as in normal tissues, and uncoupled oxidative phosphorylation was demonstrated. The cause of this illness is unknown.

Other cases that less clearly represent mitochondrial disease have been described, but none resemble thyrotoxicosis. Distorted mitochondria in hepatocytes and a defect in electron transport between dehydrogenases and the cytochromes have been observed in the fatal congenital "cerebro-hepato-renal syndrome." Abnormal increased, diminished, and absent muscle mitochondria have been detected in various idiopathic myopathies, in steroid-induced myopathy, and in cardiac muscle in experimental left ventricular failure. Experimental iron deficiency can lower tissue cytochrome content, and copper deficiency may be associated with diminished cytochrome oxidase. The clinical correlates of these observations are unknown. Considering the importance of mitochondria in cell homeostasis, they so far appear to be remarkably immune from disease-related pathology.

THERAPY. The choice of therapy for hyperthyroidism resulting from Graves' disease has been debated for decades, and final resolution is not yet in sight. During the period from 1950 to 1970, sentiment gradually swung to the use of RAI in most adults because of its simplicity and absence of surgical complications or hospitalization. When hypothyroidism was observed to occur in 40 to 70 per cent of patients in the five- to ten-year period after treatment with "conventional" doses of RAI, many clinics adopted a "low dose" ^{131}I treatment program. This clearly reduced the incidence of early hypothyroidism, but is associated with a need for multiple doses and continued treatment of many patients with various other agents over one to five years. Dissatisfaction with ^{131}I has swung the pendulum, to some extent, back toward surgery. Recognition that short-term (four to six months) antithyroid drug therapy gains most of the drug-induced remissions that might come from more prolonged therapy has also altered one's approach. Recognizing that no rules are hard and fast, the author's current therapeutic approach is, by age group, as follows:

0 to 25 — antithyroid drug, prolonged if necessary, followed by surgery if needed.

25 to ±40 — short-term trial of antithyroid drug, followed, if necessary, by surgery.

40 + — usually RAI ^{131}I.

The reasons for this approach are discussed below.

Although the three common treatments for hyperthyroidism are excellent, each has its built-in disadvantages and none of the therapies can be considered ideal.

Antithyroid Drugs. Children and young adults are best treated initially by a course of antithyroid drug. Patients with small goiters, recent onset of disease, and mild symptoms respond most frequently to this therapy. Usually propylthiouracil, 100 mg every eight hours, or methimazole, 10 mg every eight hours, is given orally. If this is not effective within two to four weeks, the dose may be doubled. Rarely, 1 gram of propylthiouracil or 100 mg of methimazole will be needed daily. It is imperative that the patient be instructed to take the medication at the scheduled times. Antithyroid drugs have a short duration of action, and one of the main causes of treatment failure is that patients do not adhere to a rigorous time schedule. As a response is obtained, the dose is progressively lowered to 50 or 100 mg of propylthiouracil every 12 hours, or a comparable dose of methimazole. Many patients can be maintained on a single daily dose of medication. Some physicians prefer to maintain a higher dose of the antithyroid drug and to add replacement doses of thyroid hormone in order to avoid hypothyroidism. Overtreatment with antithyroid drugs will of course block formation of thyroid hormone, lower the T_4, and cause a TSH response. This is usually evident in rapid enlargement of the thyroid.

Symptoms of thyrotoxicosis usually abate within two to six weeks, and the patient should be metabolically normal after this period of time. The thyroid gland, in the absence of induced hypothyroidism, either remains at the original size or gets smaller. The latter is a favorable prognostic sign. Another favorable prognostic sign is return of thyroid suppressibility after administration of T_3 (T_3 suppression test), which has been documented to occur in some patients as early as eight weeks after the start of antithyroid drug treatment. The appropriate duration of therapy is a matter of current discussion. Traditionally patients have been treated for a year, on the belief that this provided an optimal chance for a prolonged remission. Recent studies have contested this view, and suggest that therapy until euthyroidism is reached, or for four to six months, is long enough to achieve a remission in most cases. The medication is continued for the desired time and then is gradually discontinued. One third to half the treated patients will enter a prolonged remission. Others will relapse within 1 to 12 months, and are either retreated with the same drug or given an alternative form of therapy. The incidence of remission is higher after the first year of therapy, and decreases among patients who have failed to remit with each subsequent year of treatment.

During antithyroid drug administration, patients must be carefully monitored for occurrence of side effects such as pruritus, rash, and epigastric pain, and for the more serious but less frequent occurrence of neutropenia or even agranulocytosis. A mild skin rash may disappear spontaneously. Pruritus can be treated by the addition of an antihistaminic drug. A severe rash calls for discontinuation of the antithyroid drug. It is possible to reinstitute therapy with an alternative antithyroid medication, because cross-reactions do not always occur. The leukocyte count should be checked at each visit during administration of antithyroid drugs. Occasionally, a count as low as 3500 cells per cubic millimeter may be observed spontaneously in patients with thyrotoxicosis. If, however, the blood count falls from a normal range down to a level of 3500 or lower during therapy, the antithyroid drug should be discontinued. Occasionally agranulocytosis develops, requiring intensive care in a hospital, but is usually reversible.

Radioactive Iodide. For adults older than 25, administration of radioactive iodide appears to be a satisfactory form of treatment. So far there is no evidence that this therapy causes an increased incidence of leukemia or significant somatic damage. Hypothyroidism, attributable to an "overeffective" treatment, is a disadvantage and will be discussed below. The radiation dose delivered to the gonads during treatment is similar to that given during an intravenous pyelogram or barium enema and is probably inconsequential. Patients have now been treated with this agent for nearly three decades, and there is still no evidence of ^{131}I-induced tumor formation. Evidence on this point must continually be accumulated, but for the moment it does not appear that radiation of the adult thyroid with ^{131}I leads to subsequent thyroid malignancy.

A major difficulty with radioactive iodine treatment has been the onset of hypothyroidism, either immediately or long after the treatment. The incidence of hypothyroidism may approach 40 to 70 per cent after ten years. Most patients are now treated with a dose of radioactive iodide approximately half that used five or ten years ago, in an effort to diminish the incidence of hypothyroidism.

Therapy is planned to deliver a retained dose of 40 to 100 μC per estimated gram of weight at 24 hours, the dose per gram increasing with thyroid size from 20 to 100 grams. The formula by which the author treats patients is as follows:

$$\text{uCi given} = \frac{\text{Est. thyroid weight} \times \text{uCi/gram}}{\text{Fractional RAIU at 24 hours}}$$

Thyroid weight, grams	^{131}I dose, μCi/gram
10-20	40
21-30	45
31-40	50
41-50	60
51-60	70
61-70	75
71-80	80
81-90	85
91-100	90
100+	100

This approach corrects for variation in RAIU, attempts to compensate for gland size, and obviously depends on estimates of gland weights, but in practice has been proved effective in the author's clinic. With this dose, many patients do not achieve immediate euthyroidism, and require ancillary therapy such as administration of potassium iodide solution or an antithyroid drug if hyperthyroidism is not controlled within two or three months. These agents should be continued for 6 to 12 months, because the full effect of radiation is not obtained until then. At the end of 6 or 12 months, the potassium iodide or the antithyroid drug or both are discontinued, and if hyperthyroidism recurs, a second treatment of radioactive iodide is given. Thirty to 50 per cent of the patients need a second treatment, and occasionally a third dose is required (Fig. 6). In selected individuals, in whom it is imperative that hyperthyroidism be rapidly controlled, a two- to three-fold larger dose is administered, and re-treatment is given at three months if required. If prompt control is necessary, antithyroid drug and then KI can be instituted within one day of administration of the therapeutic ^{131}I dose, with loss of about one fifth of the radiation effect. Control of the disease with this combined treatment is usually achieved in one to four weeks. Patients with coincident heart disease are usually given fractionated doses (one third to one half the full dose every three to six months, until controlled) or pretreated with antithyroid drugs to deplete endogenous hormone stores.

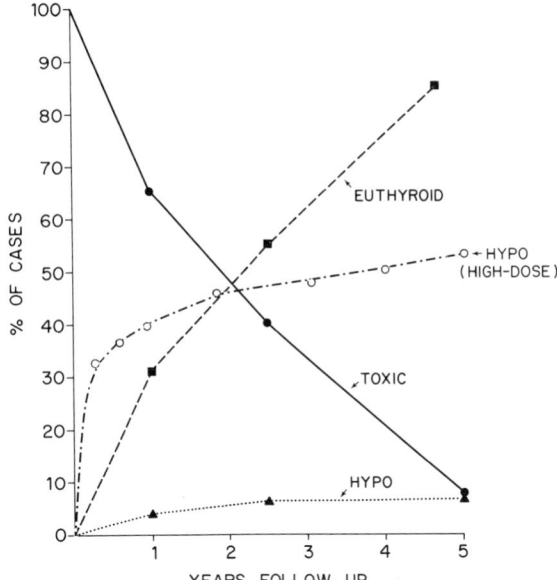

Figure 6. Graphic representation of current therapeutic results achieved with "low-dose" [131]I therapy of thyrotoxicosis. Although hypothyroidism is infrequent in the first five years, many patients remain toxic for a prolonged period after initial therapy. The high and progressively increasing incidence of hypothyroidism after "high-dose" therapy is also indicated.

All women in the reproductive age who are to receive radioactive iodide must be questioned for possible pregnancy or lactation, which are contraindications to this treatment. It is best to give the radioactive iodide shortly after a menstrual period. Women should be advised to avoid pregnancy for a period of at least one year, because the possible need for re-treatment will not be eliminated before this time has elapsed.

There was a recent wave of interest in the use of ^{125}I for therapy, on the basis that it would be less likely to produce hypothyroidism. The few reported trials do not establish any improved efficacy of ^{125}I over [131]I.

Surgery. Subtotal thyroidectomy performed by a skilled surgeon is also very effective. It is the preferred therapy in children who fail to respond to antithyroid drugs or have had adverse reaction to the drug, in young adults who do not wish to pursue a prolonged course of treatment, in patients who are apprehensive about the possible adverse effects of radioactive iodide, in patients who have huge thyroids, and in patients whose glands are believed to harbor a carcinoma. Although the author now treats many adults up to age 40 with a course of antithyroid drug in an attempt to secure a medical remission, surgery is an equally acceptable form of therapy and probably offers the most prompt return to normal function. Although no hard data can be offered, it also seems preferable to RAI therapy in patients with marked exophthalmos. The procedure is accompanied by a mortality rate of less than 1 in 1000, an incidence of permanent hypothyroidism in from 5 to 40 per cent, recurrence of thyrotoxicosis in 5 per cent or more (depending on the extent of the initial resection), occasional instances of damage to the recurrent laryngeal nerves and parathyroids, need for hospitalization, and considerable expense. Patients should be rendered euthyroid with an antithyroid drug in preparation for surgery, and should be given potassium iodide (saturated solution of potassium iodide, 2 drops twice daily) or Lugol's solution (10 drops twice daily) for a period of one to two weeks before the operation. Iodide decreases vascularity of the gland and makes the surgical procedure less difficult. Induction of euthyroidism before surgery is desirable, because cardiac arrhythmias during surgery are frequent in patients with thyrotoxicosis. Recently patients have been prepared for surgery by the administration of propranolol, 20 to 40 mg every six hours, for one to two weeks, and continued in the immediate postoperative period. Although numerous reports attest to the safety of this technique, it does not seem logical as yet to discard the time-tested approach, especially in patients with severe thyrotoxicosis. Propranolol does certainly provide a useful alternative in patients who must go to surgery and are allergic to antithyroid drugs and/or iodides.

Iodine. Iodine was introduced for control of hyperthyroidism 50 years ago but is rarely used today as the sole treatment. When given in doses of greater than 6 mg per day, iodide blocks further formation of iodotyrosines (Wolff-Chaikoff effect), and diminishes release of thyroid hormone by inhibiting proteolysis of thyroglobulin. Most patients are benefited initially by iodide, although some respond only partially, and some have an exacerbation of their illness despite continuation of iodine. Iodine treatment may induce hypothyroidism, especially in patients who have previously been treated with surgery or radioactive iodide. Addition of antithyroid drugs to the regimen of patients who are already receiving iodide has been known to induce a severe exacerbation of hyperthyroidism. At present the three more certain and well defined modes of treatment described above seem preferable to the use of potassium iodide, but it is probable that further study of this treatment will be forthcoming in future years, especially in treatment of mild hyperthyroidism.

Potassium perchlorate is rarely used at present for control of hyperthyroidism because of its reported association with fatal aplastic anemia.

Cortisone and immunosuppressive treatments have been tried experimentally, but no data indicate that they are appropriate for routine use. However, glucocorticoids such as prednisone, in doses of 10 to 20 mg every six hours, promptly lower serum T_4 and T_3 by inhibiting gland secretion and peripheral T_4 conversion. This effect may be desirable in therapy of thyroid storm.

Ancillary Treatments. Most patients benefit from a period of rest, a good diet, and added vitamins and calcium. The response to a few days in a hospital bed is often remarkable even before specific therapy is instituted. Phenobarbital and diazepam are useful for sedation.

Much recent interest has been given to propranolol as a specific therapy because of its ability to counteract the alleged beta-adrenergic mediated features of thyrotoxicosis. Although the mechanism may be uncertain, in doses of 10 to 40 mg by mouth four times daily, propranolol will reduce tachycardia and provide a beneficial calming effect in some patients. The author believes it is a useful drug, but does not find it to be more than an adjunct to usual therapy. Its role in preparation for surgery is discussed above.

Therapy in Pregnancy. The choice of therapy in pregnancy is between antithyroid drug and surgery during the middle trimester. At present most patients are probably treated by administration of antithyroid drugs, although there is no certain superiority of one method. It is advisable to use the smallest dose necessary to bring the FTI into the high normal range, that is, between 9 and 13, if this coincides with a remission of symptoms. This precaution is taken because induction of fetal hypothyroidism by the antithyroid drug could result in mental damage. Therapy is followed by measurement of the FTI, or FT_4. These tests avoid the problem of interpreting the effect of pregnancy on T_4 and T_3 (high TBG). An alternative (although not preferred) program is to continue the antithyroid drug and to institute coincident therapy with thyroid hormone. Since this method exposes the fetus to a higher level of antithyroid drug than is needed in the absence of added hormone, and since there is no evidence that the added hormone has any protective effect, it is not recommended. Surgery can be safely performed during the middle trimester after antithyroid drug preparation. KI is used only briefly, since there is evidence that the fetus is especially sensitive to KI-induced block of hormone synthesis.

Some patients with Graves' disease have an amelioration of their symptoms during pregnancy, requiring progressively smaller doses of drug or even none.

Since the immunoglobulins that cause Graves' disease pass the placenta, infants of mothers with active or treated Graves' disease may have neonatal thyrotoxicosis and should be observed carefully for this complication.

Therapy in Children. Thyrotoxicosis in children is usually less severe than in adults. Restlessness, inability to concentrate, weight gain or loss, emotional lability, and poor performance at school may be the presenting signs. Exophthalmos is rarely severe, and pretibial myxedema does not occur.

After surgery, there is a pronounced tendency for the disease to recur, unless an extensive subtotal resection is done; this increases the likelihood of postoperative hypothyroidism. RAI is avoided in individuals under the age of 25, if possible, because of the belief that children are most susceptible to induction of tumors. Thus individuals under age 25 are typically given a one- to two-year trial of antithyroid drugs before considering an alternative approach. Sometimes the drugs are continued for four to seven years if a remission does not occur after one year, in an attempt to delay a more drastic form of therapy until the child is older. Subtotal resection is an appropriate alternative therapy if a one- to two-year trial of drug treatment fails to induce remission or if the child is unable for some reason to maintain a drug regimen satisfactorily over the required months or years. RAI has been used only rarely, when some problem such as a severe reaction to both propylthiouracil and methimazole occurred, preventing adequate preparation for surgery and making the radiation hazard the least of the several evils.

PROGNOSIS. Untreated hyperthyroidism can result in death from inanition, congestive heart failure, and other causes. All three major forms of therapy should result in prompt control of hyperthyroidism, and most patients subsequently lead a normal life. It is interesting to observe that none of the treatments are directed toward the cause of the illness. There is a tendency for a patient who responds to antithyroid drugs (less so to surgery) to have recurrence of the illness years later. This rarely if ever occurs in patients who have been adequately treated with radioactive iodide. *Delayed onset of hypothyroidism must always be watched for,* and therefore patients who have been treated with surgery, RAI, or antithyroid drugs should be followed indefinitely at yearly intervals. The prognosis for the ophthalmologic and dermatologic complications of Graves' disease is not so sanguine. Often these complications persist for years or even decades and may be incapacitating. As set out below, their course

seems to be little influenced by the course of hyperthyroidism.

COMPLICATIONS OF GRAVES' DISEASE

OPHTHALMOPATHY. Mild lid retraction and stare are probably effects of hyperthyroxinemia and in themselves are inconsequential. The remaining abnormalities of Graves' ophthalmopathy (described previously) appear to be due to infiltration of the retro-orbital tissues, extraocular muscles, and lacrimal gland by lymphocytes, plasma cells, and polymorphonuclear leukocytes, as well as an increase in tissue water, mucopolysaccharides, and mucoproteins. The extraocular muscles are often swollen to five or ten times their normal diameter, and the muscle fibers may be largely destroyed, leading in time to contractures. The lacrimal gland may likewise be severely swollen and damaged, although keratitis sicca does not appear. The initial presentation is as a cosmetic defect owing to proptosis and lid edema, often with tearing, burning, or retrobulbar pain. As the condition increases, the patient's difficulties include diplopia, susceptibility to infection, and the more severe complications such as loss of visual acuity, corneal ulceration, and panophthalmitis. Occasionally the process presents essentially as retrobulbar neuritis with loss of vision and few other signs. Infiltrative ophthalmopathy may occur at any time in relationship to the hyperthyroidism of Graves' disease. Most typically it develops with the onset of hyperthyroidism and subsides coincident with therapy. Changes of infiltrative ophthalmopathy are present in 10 to 20 per cent of patients with Graves' disease, and severe progressive ("malignant") exophthalmos occurs in 2 to 3 per cent.

The cause of this complication is unknown. Plasma of patients with progressive exophthalmos has been found to contain a factor which stimulates exophthalmos in certain test animals; the material is known as exophthalmos-producing substance (EPS). Some data suggest that EPS may be a fragment of TSH. Although LATS is present more frequently in patients with exophthalmos and typically in higher titers than in the average patient with Graves' disease, there is no evidence that LATS itself causes exophthalmos. No localization of gamma globulin orbital tissue has been recognized, and retro-orbital tissue does not bind and neutralize LATS. Gamma globulin from exophthalmic patients is reported to bind to retrobulbar antigens in what may be a pseudoimmunologic reaction. These patients also have cell-mediated immunity against orbital antigens. Recent studies suggest that thyroglobulin may bind to extraocular muscle and then bind antithyroglobulin antibodies, thus setting up an immunologic reaction. Thus the belief exists that exophthalmos is an autoimmune phenomenon, but the cause and nature of the antigens are not known with certainty. Although there is usually little diagnostic confusion, some degree of exophthalmos may occur in Cushing's syndrome, Turner's syndrome, and cirrhosis. Orbital tumor, sphenoid ridge meningioma, and thrombosis of the cavernous sinus must also be considered in reaching a diagnosis, especially when the exophthalmos is unilateral, and differentiation from other causes of optic neuritis must be considered. Evaluation is not complicated if the process is bilateral and associated with thyrotoxicosis. Unilateral eye signs may be difficult to relate to Graves' disease. In this instance anatomic evaluation by orbital x-rays, CAT scanning, or orbital echo scanning is in order, along with a search for any evidence of Graves' disease, such as family history, antibodies, LATS assay, T_3 suppression or TRH test, serum T_3, or RIA.

Treatment. Patients with any degree of exophthalmos should be reassured that the process is almost invariably self-limiting. The eyes usually return to an essentially normal condition, although some degree of proptosis may persist. Useful local measures include shielding the eyes from excessive light and dust, avoidance of smoke and other irritants, and instillation of artificial tears. Patients may find it useful to sleep with the head of the bed elevated, and to cover the eyes at night with cold saline compresses. If proptosis is severe, the lids may be taped together with cellophane tape which holds a piece of wet gauze and Saran Wrap over the eyelids. Diuresis (chlorothiazide, 500 mg every day) may be useful. Diplopia can be alleviated in part by covering one eye with a patch or obscuring one lens of the patient's glasses. Any sign of infection should be treated by appropriate antimicrobial ointments or, if necessary, by parenteral administration of antimicrobial drugs. If proptosis is severe, muscle function is progressively lost, and especially if vision deteriorates, glucocorticoids may be helpful. Most patients who have progressive exophthalmos respond, whereas those who have stable changes do not. A common starting dose is 20 to 40 mg of prednisone daily in divided doses, although occasionally, and especially in patients with retrobulbar neuritis, doses up to 120 mg daily may be required. This medication induces Cushing's syndrome. It should be given in effective doses until improvement occurs or it is clear that no response will be obtained, after which an attempt should be made to reduce the dose gradually. Sometimes improvement can be maintained with 10 to 20 mg of prednisone daily or every other day. The response is variable, ranging from none at all to a complete remission of muscle paresis, papilledema, improvement in visual acuity, and recession of exophthalmos.

In recent years the use of radiotherapy to the postlenticular orbital contents (2000 r to each side) has been revived. Many patients appear to benefit, and side effects are believed minimal. This therapy may be especially useful when irritative symptoms are prominent and vision is not threatened.

In patients resistant to steroids but requiring therapy, a Kronlein lateral decompression or other operative procedures such as the Naffziger supraorbital decompression or decompression into the antrum and ethmoids may be performed. The results are unpredictable, but often improvement is gained, and a few patients respond dramatically. In more chronic cases, operations on the muscles may restore binocular vision, and recession of the levator palpebrae superioris can help alleviate a disturbing stare. Muscle surgery, however, should not be done during the stage of progression but should be reserved for a time when fibrosis has occurred and diplopia is stable.

Lateral tarsorrhaphy is useful in patients whose eyes become damaged because the lids do not close during sleep. It provides some protection against corneal abrasions and infection and, sometimes, cosmetic benefits but has little effect on the basic process.

When these procedures have been exhausted, one sometimes resorts to methods whose basis is speculative. Some patients have been treated with azathioprine. Total surgical ablation of the thyroid followed by radioactive iodide has been proposed as being universally effective, but reports from several clinics indicate that it has no predictable effect on exophthalmos. Hypophysectomy, hypophysial stalk section, and x-ray treatment of the pituitary have all been espoused, but none is of proved value.

The *course and prognosis* of this illness are difficult to predict. In general, patients whose thyroid disease is successfully controlled will in time do well, although they may go through a period of severe discomfort. Typically, in 6 to 18 months, the activity of the process appears to abate, and there is subsequent slow but progressive evolution toward normality. Rarely sight is severely impaired or even lost, despite the administration of steroids and use of local x-ray and decompressive surgery. In general it is best to treat coincident hyperthyroidism by the most logical means irrespective of the ophthalmologic complication, and to maintain the patient in a *euthyroid* state after the initial control of the thyrotoxicosis. It is possible that RAI therapy, perhaps by inducing release of antigens and an augmented immune response, may exacerbate exophthalmos. With considerable reservation about the scientific basis for the recommendation, surgery is preferred over RAI by the author for patients who have evidence of possibly dangerous exophthalmos.

PRETIBIAL MYXEDEMA (Fig. 7). In the simplest form, pretibial or localized myxedema presents as a firm bulging over the lateral aspect of the lower leg, just above the lateral malleolus. Often the skin is shiny and has an orange-peel appearance. The deposits may extend from an area of a few centimeters to involve multiple areas or even the entire anterior leg and foot. Occasionally, similar deposits can be found on the abdomen, hands, or face. Histologically there is an infiltration of mucopolysaccharide and mucoprotein material in the dermis, an increase in fluid, fraying of connective tissue fibers, and increase in collagen. The pattern is very similar to that observed in thyroid hormone deficiency, although there is no evidence that local thyroid hormone deficiency is present. There is a characteristic increase in hyaluronic acid in the lesions and also in uninvolved skin. The process almost invariably occurs in patients who have exophthalmos. It typically is first noted during the onset of hyperthyroidism, but may occur without associated hyperthyroidism and even in some patients whose thyroid appears to have been destroyed by thyroiditis and who are euthyroid or hypothyroid. Usually the process is not incapacitating, and except for its cosmetic disadvantage it requires no therapy. Topical application of triamcinolone ointment under Saran Wrap may be temporarily useful. It is striking that patients with this lesion characteristically have high and sometimes remarkable levels of serum LATS. If LATS disappears, so does the pretibial myxedema. Nevertheless, no etiologic relationship with LATS or other autoimmunity has been shown.

THYROID STORM. Sudden severe exacerbation of hyperthyroidism may occur as a feature of the basic disease process or because of coincident infection, trauma, or surgery. Without treatment, and even with therapy, the illness carries a *high mortality*. The patients develop severe hyperkinesis; tachycardia, hyperpyrexia, vomiting, and shock, and may drift into coma. Dehydration may be prominent.

If the diagnosis seems reasonable, treatment of the hyperthyroidism should begin at once, pending laboratory confirmation. Oral or parenteral blocking doses of propylthiouracil should be given, followed in one hour with potassium iodide. The latter agent should cause a rapid remission in the symptoms of hyperthyroidism, and it is

Figure 7. *A,* An example of severe "localized myxedema" involving the entire legs, feet, and hands, and coincident exophthalmos. *B,* Deposits of localized myxedema on the dorsum of the second, third and fourth digits, which are unusual manifestations of this condition.

active in the presence of an antithyroid drug block. Saturated solution of KI, 2 drops, or Lugol's solution, 8 drops, may be given orally twice daily. Intravenous sodium iodide 100 to 200 mg daily, is also effective. The prior introduction of an antithyroid drug block ensures that the gland will not be flooded with iodide and guards against a subsequent flare of the illness. If the patient is not obtunded, sedatives such as phenobarbital (60 mg intramuscularly every four to six hours) or reserpine (1 to 3 mg every eight hours) should be given. Propranolol, 10 to 40 mg every six hours orally, or 2 to 10 mg every four hours intravenously, has been introduced for therapy of this condition and is useful. This drug should be given with caution in the presence of congestive heart failure. Dehydration should be treated by appropriate fluid supplementation. Cultures should be taken to exclude infection, and antimicrobial therapy given as indicated. Adrenocortical steroids (50 to 100 mg of hydrocortisone intramuscularly every six hours) can cause a prompt reduction of serum T_4 and especially T_3. Occasionally plasma, blood, or norepinephrine is required to support the circulation. Hyperthermia can be treated by cooling. Digitalis may be needed to control congestive heart failure.

TREATMENT IN THE PRESENCE OF HEART DIS-EASE. Usually this complication occurs in older patients who would typically receive RAI. The FTI usually decreases progressively after RAI therapy, and no exacerbation of the heart disease (angina, congestive heart failure, myocardial infarction, arrhythmia) is seen. But if there is concern about therapy because of the gravity of the heart disease, several not very certain approaches can be suggested. RAI, followed in 24 hours by methimazole and then Lugol's solution, is probably safe and effective. Multiple low doses of RAI can be used, but therapeutic response is delayed. A safe but slow method is to pretreat the patient with antithyroid drugs in order to deplete the gland of stored hormone, and give RAI when the FTI has reached the normal range. Discontinuation of antithyroid drug for 48 hours before the required RAIU is sufficient.

Adams, D. D., Fastier, F. N., Howie, J. B., Kennedy, T. H., Kilpatrick J. A., and Stewart, R. H. D.: Stimulation of the human thyroid by infusions of plasma containing LATS protector. J. Clin. Endocrinol. Metab., 39:826, 1974.

Birkhäuser, M., Busset, R., Burer, T., and Burger, A.: Diagnosis of hyperthyroidism when serum-thyroxine alone is raised. Lancet, 2:76, 1977.

Dorfman, S. G., Cooperman, M. T., Nelson, R. L., Depuy, H. Peake, R. L., and Young, R. L.: Painless thyroiditis and transient hyperthyroidism without goiter. Ann. Intern. Med., 86:24, 1977.

Georges, L. P., Santangelo, R. P., Mackin, J. F., and Canary, J. J.: Metabolic effects of propranolol in thyrotoxicosis. I. Nitrogen, calcium, and hydroxyproline. Metabolism, 24:11, 1975.

Hollingsworth, D. R., and Mabry, C. C.: Congenital Graves' disease. Am. J. Dis. Child., 130:148, 1976.

Mullin, B. R., Levinson, R. E., Friedman, A., Henson, D. R., Winand, R. J., and Kohn, L. D.: Delayed hypersensitivity in Graves' disease and exophthalmos: Identification of thyroglobulin in normal human orbital muscle. Endocrinology, 100:351, 1977.

Orgiazzi, J., Williams, D. E., Chopra, I. J., and Solomon, D. H.: Human thyroid adenyl cyclase–stimulating activity in immunoglobulin G of patients with Graves' disease. J. Clin. Endocrinol. Metab., 42:341, 1976.

Roudebush, C. P., Hoye, K. E., and DeGroot, L. J.: Compensated low-dose ^{131}I therapy of Graves' disease. Ann. Intern. Med., 87:441, 1977.

Solomon, D. H., and Kleeman, K. E.: Concepts of pathogenesis of Graves' disease. Adv. Intern. Med., 22:273, 1976.

546.3. THYROIDITIS

Three types of thyroiditis are recognized: chronic, acute, and subacute. Chronic thyroiditis is not an infection or, in the usual sense, an inflammation, and therefore the name may be inappropriate. Two varieties are defined by pathologists: lymphocytic thyroiditis and Riedel's struma. In lymphocytic thyroiditis (Hashimoto's thyroiditis, struma lymphomatosa), the thyroid is replaced to a varying degree by lymphocytes forming germinal centers and fibrous tissue, leading to goiter, parenchymal destruction, and thyroid hormone insufficiency. Riedel's thyroiditis (ligneous thyroiditis) is a possibly related, slowly progressive fibrosis of the thyroid, of great rarity. These two processes will be considered separately, with the main emphasis on Hashimoto's thyroiditis.

HASHIMOTO'S THYROIDITIS

ETIOLOGY AND PATHOGENESIS. Hashimoto's thyroiditis is thought to be an autoimmune disease. In 1956, Doniach and Roitt, and Witebsky, coincidentally discovered antibodies to thyroid antigens in patients with this illness. The thyroid antigen-antibody systems that are now known include (1) antibodies reacting with thyroglobulin, usually detected by the tanned red cell agglutination test; (2) antibodies reacting with a component of thyroid cytoplasm, detected by the immunofluorescent technique, by a complement-fixing reaction with thyroid microsomes, or by a variation of the tanned red cell technique; and (3) antibodies reacting with a colloidal antigen which is distinct from thyroglobulin. When antibodies against thyroglobulin and thyroid cell cytoplasm are both measured, about 95 per cent of patients with Hashimoto's thyroiditis have a positive titer in one or both tests, and frequently the titers are very high.

Thyroiditis with a similar histologic pattern can be induced by immunization of animals with thyroid tissue. The experimentally induced disease cannot in general be transferred from animal to animal by serum, but can be transferred in inbred guinea pigs by transfer of lymphocytes. This observation, as well as the poor correlation of circulating antibody titers with the course of the disease, suggested that *cell-mediated immunity* (CMI) was important in the destruction of thyroid cells. This has been abundantly confirmed in the past few years by studies demonstrating CMI by in vitro techniques such as leukocyte migration inhibition assay and lymphotoxin assay. Patients with thyroiditis, primary thyroid failure, and Graves' disease are found to have lymphocytes presensitized to thyroid antigens. The antigens are associated with particulate fragments of the cell. CMI is most obvious in patients with primary myxedema, and is less intense in patients with thyroiditis or Graves' disease. Probably both circulating antibodies and CMI contribute to thyroid cell dysfunction and/or death.

Why individuals should produce antibodies against thyroid antigens remains a mystery. It might be supposed that an abnormal antigen exists in the cells, but none has been found. It has been suggested that thyroglobulin or other thyroid antigens are normally hidden from the organism during fetal life when immune tolerance is established, and that subsequent escape of the thyroglobulin from the thyroid follicle could induce immunity in the adult. This seems unlikely, because thyroglobulin normally circulates in the blood. Possibly viral infection or other injury could alter thyroid tissue and produce neoantigens. There is a strong hereditary pattern for the illness, and the propensity to produce antibodies is transmitted as a dominant trait. Further, thyroiditis is associated with a number of other possibly autoimmune diseases, including pernicious anemia, idiopathic adrenal insufficiency, rheumatoid arthritis, Sjögren's syndrome, ulcerative colitis, lupoid hepatitis, disseminated lupus erythematosus, and hemolytic anemia. The relationship to pernicious anemia is especially prominent. Fifty per cent of patients with pernicious anemia have antibodies against thyroid tissue antigens, and the converse is also true. There is also an associated increased incidence of antibodies against parathyroid tissue and antibodies against the pancreas and ovary. These observations suggest that some ill-understood hereditarily defined abnormality in immune homeostasis occurs in these patients, predisposing them to develop reactivity to self-antigens.

In the author's view, Graves' disease, Hashimoto's thyroiditis, and myxedema are variants of a common process. Among the relatives of patients with one of these three diseases, it is typical to find examples of the other two. The histology of Graves' disease shades into that of Hashimoto's thyroiditis, and the histology of idiopathic thyroid failure is interpreted by some as the end-stage of lymphocytic and fibrotic replacement of the thyroid. Antibody titers against thyroid cell antigens are high in each condition. It is as if an abnormality in immune homeostasis were at the root of each illness, possibly triggered by some environmental factor. Perhaps with the development of antithyroglobulin and anticytoplasmic antibodies, plus a cell-mediated response, Hashimoto's thyroiditis occurs. If the destructive cell-mediated response is severe, the process may go on to thyroid failure. If, in addition to or in the absence of the other antibodies, LATS or other thyroid-stimulating antibodies are formed, and if the thyroid is capable of responding, thyroid hyperplasia and hypersecretion occur with the picture of Graves' disease. Although this formulation is by no means universally accepted, it embodies the thinking of many workers in the field.

PATHOLOGY (Fig. 8). On gross inspection the thyroid appears pale yellow-tan and has a lumpy surface. The normal thyroid structure is replaced with dense infiltration by lymphocytes, and lymphoid germinal centers are evident. The remaining thyroid tissue often shows hyperplasia, with small empty follicles. The cells frequently are enlarged and eosinophilic. In many specimens, fibrosis is prominent. The thymus is characteristically enlarged, and germinal centers are seen. There may be lymph nodes showing reactive hyperplasia in the area surrounding the thyroid.

CLINICAL MANIFESTATIONS. This illness occurs with an incidence roughly similar to that of Graves' disease. There is good evidence that it has tripled in frequency in the past three decades. Hashimoto's thyroiditis may present with thyroid enlargement or symptoms of hypothyroidism. The disease is 20 times as frequent in women as in men. It can occur even in young children, but is most common between ages 30 and 50. In children the process is occasionally seen to subside spontaneously. In other instances, extensive destruction of the gland can lead to thyroid failure and growth retardation (Fig. 8). Most characteristic is the thyroid enlargement, which varies from two to five times normal, averaging 30 to 50 grams. The gland may be soft, normal, or firm, and there is no thrill or bruit. The surface may feel lobulated, but distinct nodules are usually not found. Their presence suggests that a mass of lymph nodes is present or that a thyroid adenoma or malignancy is present. Typically the pyramidal lobe is palpable. Sometimes patients complain of choking or difficulty in swallowing or of a sensation of local pressure, but usually the goiter is asymptomatic. Rarely, the illness proceeds more rapidly, and there are pain and tenderness in the thyroid gland. The trachea is characteristically in the midline. The remainder of the physical examination is unremarkable unless there are signs of hypothyroidism.

The presence of an asymptomatic diffuse thyroid enlargement (with a palpable pyramidal lobe) in a middle-aged woman who appears to be euthyroid is indicative of Hashimoto's thyroiditis. The serum thyroxine may be normal or depressed, depending on the stage of development of the process. The PBI may be low, normal, or elevated owing to butanol-insoluble iodinated albumin in plasma. This can be detected by simultaneous determination of the PBI and BEI, or the PBI and serum T_4. The RAIU test may be elevated, normal, or low, but usually is normal unless the patient has developed hypothyroidism. Other tests of thyroid function reflect the ability of the thyroid to

Figure 8. *A,* Identical twins, age 12, both of whom developed Hashimoto's thyroiditis. One boy ceased growing at age 8 and was hypothyroid. *B,* Biopsy specimen from one twin, showing small hyperplastic residual follicles, fibrosis, and lymphocytic infiltration. (Photographs provided by Dr. Frank Milgram.)

produce hormone. Characteristically, the scintiscan shows an enlarged thyroid with a smooth outline and diffuse or mottled distribution of the isotope. Fluorescent scans show a diminution or virtual absence of thyroid-stable iodine. The diagnosis can be made with certainty in this setting if the hemagglutination test for thyroglobulin and/or microsomal antigens is positive. However, only 60 per cent of the patients have a positive tanned red cell agglutination test result, and only 95 per cent are positive if both tests are performed. If it seems imperative that the diagnosis be established and the antibody response is not in the diagnostic range, needle biopsy is both safe and effective. A diagnostic piece of tissue will be obtained in perhaps 80 per cent of the biopsies. Failure of radioactive iodide uptake to rise after administration of TSH is also suggestive, indicating the syndrome of low thyroid reserve. Further, some patients will show a positive perchlorate discharge test. Occasionally there are striking elevations of the serum gamma globulin.

THERAPY.   In patients with thyroid deficiency, therapy with thyroid hormone is indicated. It is also useful to give replacement therapy to euthyroid individuals who have developed a goiter causing a cosmetic defect or local symptoms, or to prevent further thyroid enlargement. In young patients, treatment results in disappearance of the goiter, but in older persons whose thyroid enlargement has been present for a prolonged period, it may have little effect. When the thyroid is minimally enlarged, it is debatable whether therapy is indicated. Serial biopsies have shown that the histologic picture may not change over a decade.

Further, there is no evidence that the process tends to spread to other organs.

Usually therapy is with thyroid hormone, although there are reports of other approaches. In children steroid therapy causes diminution of goiter and suppresses antibody titers, but the entire process recurs when therapy is withdrawn. This approach does not appear to have merit.

PROGNOSIS.   There is a tendency for the involved thyroid to enlarge slowly and for hypothyroidism to develop. Spontaneous thyroid atrophy may occur, and it is hypothesized that this sequence may be the cause of "idiopathic" myxedema.

RIEDEL'S THYROIDITIS

In Riedel's thyroiditis, a very uncommon condition, the gland is replaced by a mass of dense, infiltrative fibrotic tissue which extends into the capsule of the thyroid, the trachea, and the surrounding strap muscles. Patients seek attention because of local symptoms such as choking or difficult swallowing, because a small goiter is observed, or because of hypothyroidism. The disease is more frequent in women than in men and characteristically occurs after age 40. Some circumstantial evidence suggests that it is a variant of Hashimoto's thyroiditis. Patients have been observed who first had typical lymphocytic thyroiditis but later had the histology of Riedel's struma. On examination, the thyroid is found to be of normal size, reduced in bulk, or moderately enlarged, and is usually firm and densely adherent to the trachea. Thyroid function tests reveal normal function or hypothyroidism. There is no specific diagnostic test, and antibody titers to thyroid antigen are not elevated in this condition as in Hashimoto's thyroiditis.

Diagnosis is usually made at operation, when the surgeon finds fibrotic thyroid tissue bound to the trachea. Often the process suggests a sclerosing carcinoma, and the diagnosis is made on frozen sections. The only known therapy is surgery if pressure symptoms are sufficient to warrant this approach. The gland may be resected or the isthmus may be exposed and divided, allowing the two halves of the gland to fall laterally, thus avoiding tracheal constriction. Since resection may cause loss of the parathyroids or recurrent laryngeal nerve, simple division of the isthmus and mobilization of the lateral lobes is the preferred approach. Thyroid hormone therapy may be required.

An association has been suggested between this process and sclerosing cholangitis, mediastinal fibrosis, and periureteral fibrosis (see Ch. 71). Since some of these processes may respond to steroid administration, it is possible that this would be a useful therapy in Riedel's thyroiditis; information on this therapeutic approach is not available.

ACUTE THYROIDITIS

Acute and subacute thyroiditis are etiologically unrelated. Both are transient inflammatory reactions involving the thyroid, and they are clinically distinct from chronic thyroiditis. "Acute thyroiditis" (acute infectious thyroiditis, suppurative thyroiditis) means an uncommon condition in which the thyroid gland is invaded by pathogenic bacteria. This occurs as part of a cellulitis in the neck or because of infection of a cyst in a multinodular goiter. Usually the patient presents with fever, pain in the neck, and a mass involving the thyroid area. The area is erythematous and tender to palpation. Often only one portion of the thyroid is involved, and contiguous infection is evident. The leukocyte count is elevated. The serum thyroxine is normal. On scintiscan there may be some depression of radioiodine uptake in a portion of the thyroid, but RAIU is usually normal.

Cultures should be taken and appropriate antimicrobials administered. With suitable therapy, the process subsides rapidly. Occasionally resection of a portion of the thyroid is indicated or drainage of an abscess may be required.

SUBACUTE THYROIDITIS

Subacute thyroiditis (granulomatous thyroiditis, acute thyroiditis, de Quervain's thyroiditis) is an inflammatory condition of the thyroid causing painful enlargement, lasting over a period of weeks or months, with a prominent tendency to relapse. Its incidence is not known, but it appears to be about one tenth as common as Graves' disease.

ETIOLOGY. Subacute thyroiditis frequently occurs two to three weeks after viral upper respiratory infection. This association suggests that the thyroiditis represents an immunologic response to the viral infection. Other data imply that direct viral invasion of the thyroid may be

the cause. Thyroiditis has occurred in outbreaks of mumps, and the mumps virus has been cultured from the thyroid. Numerous other attempts at viral culture have been negative. Volpé finds that most patients have antiviral antibody titers which are high at the time of diagnosis, and tend to fall progressively over subsequent weeks. Antibodies are frequently found against common pathogens such as echovirus, coxsackievirus, and adenovirus, and often one finds significant changes in titers against two or even three viral antigens. The reported occurrence with mumps virus or in mumps epidemics may represent one possible etiology, but is not the most common. The causation remains obscure.

PATHOLOGY. The thyroid may be enlarged with dense infiltration by polymorphonuclear cells, lymphocytes, and plasma cells. Fibrosis is prominent. Many pyknotic thyroid follicular cells are apparent. The follicular structure is often destroyed, and in its place are found small granulomas with giant cells. There is poor correlation between the histologic abnormalities, which may be extreme, and the clinical picture.

CLINICAL MANIFESTATIONS. Subacute thyroiditis may be painful and disabling, but it does not last long. The patient usually notices gradual onset of severe pain and tenderness involving one or both sides of the lower neck, sometimes localized to the thyroid. The process may begin in one lobe and travel over several days to the other. There may be fullness and the sensation of pressure. Pain typically radiates up the lateral aspects of the neck and into the jaw and ear. Swallowing may be uncomfortable, causing the patient to choke over saliva. There is often mild fever, sore throat, malaise, and fatigue. Sometimes the process is entirely asymptomatic.

On examination the thyroid is enlarged and often extremely tender. The process may be restricted to one portion of a lobe or may involve the entire gland. Lymph nodes are usually not enlarged. Sometimes the patient develops symptoms and signs of mild hyperthyroidism, but usually the clinical status is that of euthyroidism or rarely hypothyroidism. The disease tends to remit spontaneously or because of therapy, only to recur after a period of two to three weeks, and this cycle may recur several times. Over the course of one to twelve months the process finally subsides.

DIAGNOSIS. The typical history of pain and the tender enlargement of the thyroid are highly suggestive of subacute thyroiditis. The leukocyte count may be elevated to 15,000 to 20,000, or may be normal. The sedimentation rate is characteristically high, and may reach 100 mm per hour (Westergren). Anemia is said to accompany the illness, although the cause is unknown. On scan, RAIU is suppressed in the involved portion of the gland, which may be one lobe or the entire thyroid, and the RAIU is often zero. Fluorescent scanning shows the involved thyroid tissue to have lost all iodine stores. The PBI, T_4, and FTI may be elevated because of iodoprotein or excess thyroid hormone released during the acute phase of the illness, making the patient thyrotoxic. Serum thyroglobulin is also elevated. During recovery, the TSH and RAIU may be transiently elevated while T_4 is depressed, and then over a period of two to three months all test results return to normal. Antibody titers against thyroid antigens may be transiently demonstrable, but they rarely if ever reach the levels found in Hashimoto's thyroiditis, and the responses are not sustained.

This process can usually be differentiated from acute thyroiditis because of the localization to the thyroid, absence of signs of infection, characteristically high sedimentation rate, and depressed radioactive iodide uptake. Occasionally, aspiration biopsy may be necessary to prove the diagnosis. Rarely, Hashimoto's thyroiditis presents with a rather acute and painful onset, and it may be difficult to make the distinction short of biopsy. Sometimes the diagnosis of Graves' disease is suggested by a painless goiter and thyrotoxicosis, but in these cases the patient fails to have the appropriate history or physical evidence of long-term thyrotoxicosis. Exogenous iodine can depress RAIU in Graves' disease to near zero, offering another source of confusion. Serial observations over a few weeks will identify the proper diagnosis.

THERAPY. In mild cases the inflammatory process subsides spontaneously, and all that is needed is mild analgesia. Aspirin, up to 6 grams daily, is useful in suppressing the pain. It is probably advantageous to give thyroid hormone if the disease has gone on for more than a few days (and the patient is not thyrotoxic), because TSH stimulation may exacerbate the process. If the illness does not subside with these simple measures, corticosteroids are useful; 20 to 40 mg of prednisone is given daily for a period of one to four weeks, with progressive diminution of the dose as symptoms are controlled. Often withdrawal of steroids is followed by exacerbation of the process, and such a cycle may recur several times before the illness eventually subsides. Rarely, a chronic, tender enlargement of the thyroid persists despite therapy and requires surgical resection.

PROGNOSIS. In the author's experience, all patients with subacute thyroiditis, with the exception of one who required surgery, have eventually returned to normal thyroid function and become asymptomatic. It is reported that up to 10 per cent of the patients develop permanent hypothyroidism.

Amino, M., and DeGroot, L. J.: Insoluble particulate antigen(s) is cell-mediated immunity of autoimmune thyroid disease. Metabolism, 24:45, 1975.

Appel, G. B., and Holub., D. A.: The syndrome of multiple endocrine gland insufficiency. Am. J. Med., 61:129, 1976.

Gordin, A., and Lamberg, B. A.: Natural course of symptomless autoimmune thyroiditis. Lancet. 2:1234, 1975.

Greene, J. N.: Subacute thyroiditis. Am. J. Med., 51:97, 1971.

Kalderon, A. R., and Bogaars, H. A.: Immune complex deposits in Graves' disease and Hashimoto's thyroiditis. Am. J. Med., 63:729, 1977.

Ling, S. M., Kaplan, S. A., Weitzman, J. V., Reed, G. B., Costin, G., and Larding, B. H.: Euthyroid goiter in children: Correlation of needle biopsy with other clinical laboratory findings in chronic lymphocytic thyroiditis and simple goiter. Pediatrics, 44:695, 1969.

Rapoport, B., Block, M. B., Hoffer, P. B., and DeGroot, L. J.: Depletion of thyroid iodine during subacute thyroiditis. J. Clin. Endocrinol. Metab., 36:610, 1973.

Tunbridge, W. M. G., Evered, D. C., Hall, R., Appleton, D., Brewis, M., Clark, F., Evans, J. G., Young, E., Bird, T., and Smith, P. A.: The spectrum of thyroid disease in a community: The Wickham survey. Clin. Endocrinol., 7:481, 1977.

546.4.   HYPOTHYROIDISM AND MYXEDEMA

Hypothyroidism (Gull's disease) refers to the morbid state characterized by progressive slowing of all bodily activities owing to deficiency in thyroid hormone. The severest form is known as myxedema because of the characteristic infiltration of the skin by nonpitting, mucinous edema.

ETIOLOGY. Probably most cases of "idiopathic" hypothyroidism and myxedema develop as the end-stage of Hashimoto's thyroiditis. The histologic pattern confirms this suggestion; antithyroglobulin and antimicrosomal antibody are frequently present in high titers, and progression from Hashimoto's thyroiditis to hypothyroidism can be observed. More commonly, thyroid failure occurs because of administration of RAI to control the thyrotoxicosis in Graves' disease or after subtotal thyroidectomy for Graves' disease, multinodular goiter, or Hashimoto's thyroiditis. Hypothyroidism sometimes occurs as part of the presentation of Graves' syndrome, with coincident exophthalmos and pretibial myxedema. Less frequently, hypothyroidism occurs as the only feature of hypopituitarism because of isolated failure of the pituitary to produce TSH or because of damage in the hypothalamus inhibiting TRH secretion. Hypothyroidism is reported to occur in 10 per cent of patients who have had subacute thyroiditis (see Ch. 546.3). Some patients with multinodular goiter are hypothyroid. Hypothyroidism is also found in patients with congenital metabolic defects of thyroid hormone synthesis, is sometimes caused by severe iodine deficiency in areas of endemic goiter, and can be induced by medications such as the antithyroid drugs, resorcinol, lithium chloride, or para-aminosalicylic acid. In some individuals, administration of iodine (more than 6 mg per day) induces inhibition of thyroid hormone synthesis and release, with the development of goiter and hypothyroidism.

PATHOGENESIS AND PATHOLOGY. Whatever the cause of thyroid hormone deprivation, the effects are similar. Over a period of months and years, there is progressive infiltration of the skin by mucoprotein and mucopolysaccharides, giving a puffy appearance. Similar deposits of mucopolysaccharide are reported to occur under the sarcolemma of striated muscle. Muscle fibers become frayed, and the cells may become necrotic. Effusion can occur in any serosal space. Thickening of joint capsules and joint effusion also occur. There is a generalized decreased rate of nucleic acid and protein synthesis, and almost all enzyme systems are reported to be underactive.

In idiopathic myxedema the thyroid is replaced by scar tissue containing a few scattered thyroid cells and many lymphocytes. In secondary hypothyroidism resulting from pituitary failure, the thyroid is small, with flattened, cuboidal epithelium and acini filled with colloid. In other conditions the pathology is that of the primary process. In goiter resulting from metabolic defects in hormone formation or the action of thyroid blocking drugs or iodide, the characteristic picture is extreme hyperplasia, which may look much like papillary adenocarcinoma.

CLINICAL MANIFESTATIONS. Quite typically the patient has no complaints. He or, more commonly, she may be brought to the doctor because someone else recognized unusual sluggishness, weight gain, or sleepiness. Sometimes the presenting symptom is edema or menorrhagia. We have seen several women whose menorrhagia, caused by myxedema, was treated first by hysterectomy and only later by thyroid hormone. The symptoms and signs are in proportion of the severity and duration of the illness. In advanced cases the diagnosis is obvious. The patient notices fatigue and somnolence, often falling asleep at inopportune times. There is marked increase in sensitivity to cold. Hearing may be diminished. The eyes are puffy or watery. The hair is brittle, sparse, and coarse; curl tends to be lost. The eyebrows are sparse, and the outer third may be missing. The skin is thickened and dry, and sweating rarely occurs. There is generalized thickening and puffiness of the face and extremities; pitting is not characteristic, but may occur in the presence of fluid retention or congestive heart failure. True obesity is not characteristic. The patients have a jocular air about them, their answers to questions often being delayed and seemingly humorous but inappropriate. As a group they tend to be uncomplaining and hardly recognize the marked change that may have occurred in their appearance and behavior. The tongue is thick, and papillae may be atrophic, especially if there is coincident pernicious anemia, which occurs in 12 per cent of patients with idiopathic thyroid failure. The thyroid may be absent or palpable, depending on the etiology. The heart is quiet, the pulse is slow, and diastolic blood pressure may be elevated. Although pericardial effusion is frequently present, physical signs of tamponade are rarely if ever found. Pleural effusion may occur, and the abdomen may be distended by ascites. These fluids may have a high specific gravity. The patient complains of severe constipation, and ileus and megacolon have been reported. Irregular menstrual pattern and severe menorrhagia frequently occur in younger women. Deep tendon reflex relaxation time is markedly prolonged. Other neurologic signs include diminished hearing, paresthesias, vertigo, and ataxia with lateral column signs. Often the skin shows perifollicular keratoses. The nails may be thickened. Joint stiffness, thickening of the joint capsules, joint effusion, arthritis, and bursitis are occasionally seen.

Overt *psychosis* may develop as a manifestation of prolonged and severe myxedema. Hallucinations, disorientation, paranoia, and attempted suicide have been reported. With substitution therapy, the psychosis usually clears, although some patients never regain sanity. Occasionally patients develop overt psychosis as therapy is introduced. The name "myxedema madness" has been applied to these conditions.

The degree of abnormality is by no means always as great as that described. In mild hypothyroidism it may be impossible to make a clinical distinction from the normal state.

DIAGNOSIS. In the classic case the diagnosis can be confirmed at the bedside by evaluation of the slow relaxation time of the Achilles tendon reflexes. Other tendon jerks are less reliable. The serum T_4 is characteristically low, as is the RAIU, except in individuals who have a block in thyroid hormone formation as a cause of their thyroprivia. Both the T_4 and the RAIU tend to be less severely depressed in patients with hypothyroidism of pituitary origin, and in these subjects the values tend to overlap the normal range. The RAIU is not a very useful test now, because normal values (down to 10 per cent) overlap the values found in hypothyroid patients. The BMR is depressed, the serum cholesterol and carotene are elevated, and there may be marked elevation of the enzymes GOT, LDH, and CPK. Uric acid is sometimes elevated. The EKG shows slow rate and low voltage. Most patients have anemia. This may be due to menorrhagia causing iron deficiency or to coincident pernicious anemia, or may be normocytic or macrocytic and be related solely to hypothyroidism. Pernicious anemia, nephritis, uremia, and mongolism are occasional causes for confusion in differential diagnosis.

When the conclusion is reached that the patient is hypothyroid, it is imperative that the cause be evaluated. If there is atrophy of thyroid tissue, the presence of thyroiditis may be ascertained by tests for antithyroglobulin and antimicrosomal antibodies. Goiter and a positive $KClO_4$ discharge test may be found in hypothyroidism caused by congenital metabolic defects, including Pendred's syndrome, and Hashimoto's thyroiditis. Pituitary dysfunction should be considered unless there is strong evidence incriminating primary thyroid failure. In primary thyroid failure, the sella turcica is usually normal, but it may be enlarged in cretins and in some adults with longstanding myxedema. Plasma cortisol is normal, although ketosteroid and hydroxycorticoid excretion is depressed, and the adrenal response to metyrapone may be delayed and low. Follicle-stimulating hormone is characteristically elevated in postmenopausal women with primary thyroid failure, but is occasionally low, returning to an elevated level after therapy with thyroid hormone has been started. Growth hormone should be present in primary thyroid failure, but the response to insulin hypoglycemia is often depressed. TSH is characteristically very high in primary thyroid failure, often 20 to 1000 μU per milliliter. Absent or normal TSH and a failure to respond to exogenous TRH indicate pituitary damage. Hypothyroidism and a normal TSH which responds to exogenous TRH identify "hypothalamic hypothyroidism." This condition may be the cause of most instances of secondary hypothyroidism in children, and can be acquired by trauma or neoplastic lesions.

THERAPY. Treatment with desiccated thyroid is a remarkably satisfactory therapeutic maneuver. Usually it is advantageous to initiate treatment with a low dose of hormone, such as 15 or 30 mg of USP desiccated thyroid daily or the equivalent dose of one of the synthetic mixtures of T_4 and T_3 (liotrix). Subsequent increments of 15 or 30 mg are made at intervals of 7 to 14 days, until a full replacement dosage is reached in two to three months. Marked improvement should be seen with 30 mg. The usual replacement dosage is 90 to 120 mg of desiccated thyroid daily given in one dose, although a range of 60 to 200 mg per day is found, with some dependence upon patient's size. Equivalent doses of L-thyroxine (100 μg = 60 mg UPS desiccated thyroid) or L-triiodothyronine (37.5 μg = 60 mg USP desiccated thyroid), may be used for replacement therapy. If desiccated thyroid or liotrix is used to achieve replacement therapy, the FTI should be in the normal range when the patient is optimally replaced. Using thyroxine alone, the T_4 or FTI will be in the upper range of normal or slightly elevated. When T_3 is given, the T_4 or FTI will be near zero even when replacement is quite adequate.

In patients who have congestive heart failure, previous myocardial infarction, or angina pectoris, it is best to initiate therapy very gradually. Often such conditions are exacerbated by therapy, although some patients cease to have angina pectoris on replacement of the hormone. Triiodothyronine is theoretically useful because of the more rapid disappearance of its effect should toxicity be encountered, but in most patients, replacement with desiccated thyroid or liotrix is preferred, because with these medications the T_4 is within the normal range during adequate therapy and is a useful guide.

The best guide to treatment is the patient's and the physician's progressive re-evaluation of the clinical status. There should be a return to a normal and steady weight, a disappearance of all symptoms, and a feeling of well-being. Severe myalgias and arthralgias may occur during therapy, but disappear gradually if therapy is continued. It is sometimes useful to increase the dose until symptoms of thyroid hormone excess appear and then return to a slightly lower dose, in order to be certain that sufficient medication is administered. Once the dosage is established, the patient may take exogenous hormone for years or decades without change. Patients must be cautioned to continue taking the medication indefinitely, for some will feel that treatment is no longer needed once well-being has been restored. It is especially important that women be urged to continue the medication without interruption and at the same dosage level throughout pregnancy. Dosage need not be changed in preparation for or during surgery.

PROGNOSIS. The prognosis for treatment of hypothyroidism in the ambulatory patient is excellent; usually there is a complete return to normal health.

SPECIAL PROBLEMS IN HYPOTHYROIDISM

MYXEDEMA COMA. As myxedema worsens, the affected individual becomes more and more lethargic, and episodes of apparent sleep may become frequent, culminating in severe obtundation or even coma from which the patient cannot be aroused. In other instances coma develops abruptly during an intercurrent illness such as pyelonephritis, pneumonia, or cellulitis. Patients with severe myxedema may develop sepsis with minimal symptoms, no fever, and little leukocytosis.

Typically, if a history is available, it is that the patient had previous surgery or radioactive iodine therapy for hyperthyroidism, did well for a number of years afterward, but then over five or ten years gradually lapsed into hypothyroidism, finally developing coma. Often such people have received replacement therapy with thyroid hormone, but have for some reason discontinued it.

The mechanism of myxedema coma is unknown. Blood flow to the brain is diminished, but oxygen consumption is allegedly not diminished. Altered cortical activity is apparent in sluggish mentation and slowing of the alpha rhythm of the EEG. The pathologic correlates of these changes are not well known. Progressive hypothermia, hypoglycemia, and carbon dioxide retention may be specific causes of coma in some patients.

The clinical manifestations are fundamentally those of severe myxedema, as described before. Localizing neurologic signs are characteristically absent. The reflexes are symmetrical and depressed, and the relaxation time is delayed. Babinski reflex may be evident. Often the patients are severely obtunded rather than comatose, and they are typically disoriented. It may be possible to arouse the patient from his stupor, only to have him immediately slip back into a depressed state. The temperature should be carefully recorded, and may be as low as 29.5 to 30.5° C.

The diagnosis is usually suggested by physical examination which reveals signs of advanced hypothyroidism and cutaneous myxedema. The scar of a thyroidectomy, a history of previous thyroid surgery or radioactive iodide treatment, and a history of thyroid therapy are important diagnostic clues. The thyroid is impalpable or replaced by fibrous tissue. Careful search should be made for precipitating causes such as infection of the lungs or urinary tract, as well as other causes of coma, e.g., cerebrovascular accidents, renal and hepatic failure, and drug ingestion. The last-named cause is important, because hypothyroid patients are excessively sensitive to the usual doses of barbiturates and opiates. Diagnosis rests on finding abnormally low blood levels of thyroid hor-

mone, but usually these tests are not immediately available. Clinical judgment is called for in the interim; this can sometimes be supplemented by measurement of the deep tendon reflex relaxation time. Severe hyponatremia and hypoglycemia may occur as a manifestation of primary or secondary thyroid failure. The usual measures needed for differential diagnosis of primary and secondary thyroid failure, including FTI, antibody tests, TSH levels, measurement of plasma cortisol, skull films, and measurement of plasma LH and FSH, should be carried out. Carbon dioxide retention should be excluded, if necessary, by arterial gas determination, because hypoventilation may induce coma in some patients. If the diagnosis seems probable but cannot be established at the time the patient is admitted, it is best to institute treatment without a diagnosis because of the urgency of the condition.

The appropriate treatment remains a matter of debate. Failure has consistently been reported in patients treated with very slow supplementation of thyroid hormone, and an impressive series of successes has been reported in patients given a massive intravenous dose of T_4 or T_3 in an attempt to return the circulating thyroid hormone to normal levels without delay. Approximately 300 μg of thyroxine is administered intravenously and 100 to 200 μg is given daily thereafter with monitoring of the plasma thyroid hormone blood levels. If possible, it is probably wise to give L-T_3 intravenously in doses of 100 μg initially and 25 to 50 μg per day as well. Hypothermia is best treated by covering the patient with warm blankets and allowing endogenous body heat to bring up the temperature gradually. Rapid warming by means of electrical blankets or hot baths has resulted in shock and death. Appropriate antimicrobial therapy should be given if there is evidence of infection. If there is carbon dioxide retention, the patient should be placed on a respirator to provide an adequate ventilatory exchange. If there is any suggestion of pituitary failure, shock, or hyponatremia suggestive of adrenal steroid insufficiency, the patient should be given 100 to 200 mg of hydrocortisone intravenously. Occasionally blood pressure must be supported by transfusions or by use of norepinephrine. Fluid and electrolyte therapy should be given with caution, since cutaneous and respiratory losses are extremely small; 600 to 1000 ml of fluid per day, of which one third to one half is a balanced electrolyte solution, is sufficient. Overhydration is the major problem in therapy and may lead to congestive failure, cerebral edema, and death. Hyponatremia should be treated preferably by fluid restriction rather than by administration of hypertonic saline, because with thyroid hormone therapy excess stored salt in myxedema tissue is mobilized and may precipitate congestive failure.

If the patient survives the critical first few days and is able to take medication orally, replacement therapy can be switched to any standard preparation of thyroid hormone. The blood thyroxine level should be checked to assay adequacy of replacement.

Despite some advances in understanding of the precipitating causes of this illness, therapy remains unsatisfactory, and mortality rates of 50 to 90 per cent are reported.

MYXEDEMA HEART. Cardiomegaly and congestive failure often accompany myxedema. The ECG shows low voltage, flattened T waves, and occasionally first degree AV block. Is there a specific variety of heart disease associated with thyroid hormone deficiency? Obviously patients who develop myxedema may be in the older age groups expected to have a high incidence of hypertension and coronary artery disease. The coexistence of mild hypertension, which may be alleviated by therapy with thyroid hormone, has previously been noted. Another and probably more common cause of presumptive cardiomegaly is the frequent pericardial effusion found in this illness. The pericardial effusion is usually functionally insignificant, but rare instances of cardiac tamponade have been reported.

Atherosclerosis was for many years thought not to be accelerated by hypothyroidism, but present evidence indicates that there is an association between these two conditions.

In addition, it appears that severe myxedema can be associated with a specific cardiac lesion, evident pathologically as an edema of the myocardium, deposition of mucopolysaccharides and mucoproteins between the cells, fraying of cardiac myofibrils, and death and necrosis of cells. Probably this represents a very advanced stage of myxedema, and these changes are not found in most patients dying of myxedema coma.

Although the effusion, decreased cardiac output, and ECG changes are manifestations of hypothyroidism per se, most instances of heart failure associated with myxedema are probably due to coexistent organic heart disease. Occasionally the problem may not be overt before institution of therapy because of the lesser cardiac output required in the hypothyroid patient. With therapy increased demands are put upon the heart, and congestive failure, angina, and even myocardial infarction may occur.

Bland, J. H., and Frymoyer, J. W.: Rheumatic syndromes of myxedema. N. Engl. J. Med., 282:1171, 1970.

Fisher, D. A., and Burrow, G. N. (eds.): Perinatal Thyroid Physiology and Disease. New York, Raven Press, 1975.

Holvey, D. N., Goodner, C. J., Nicoloff, J. T., and Dowling, J. T.: Treatment of myxedema coma with intravenous thyroxine. Arch. Intern. Med., 113:89, 1964.

Lawrence, A. M., Wilber, J. F., and Hagen, T. C.: The pituitary and primary hypothyroidism. Arch. Intern. Med., 132:327, 1973.

Sanders, V.: Neurologic manifestations of myxedema. N. Engl. J. Med., 266:547, 1962.

Stock, J. M., Surks, M. I., and Oppenheimer, J. H.: Replacement dosage of L-thyroxine in hypothyroidism. N. Engl. J. Med., 290:529, 1974.

Walfish, P. G.: Evaluation of three thyroid-function screening tests for detecting neonatal hypothyroidism. Lancet, 1:1208, 1976.

546.5. MULTINODULAR GOITER

Multinodular goiter refers to an enlargement of the thyroid associated with more than one identifiable nodule. In fact the condition more specifically refers to a replacement of the normal homogeneous cytostructure of the thyroid by a collection of nodules of variegated histologic pattern, ranging from colloid-filled cysts and colloid adenomas to follicular and fetal adenomas. There may be some residue of histologically normal thyroid between the lumps, but more typically the structure between the more discrete adenomatous nodules consists of follicles with distended colloid-filled lumina. Often there is considerable associated fibrosis, sometimes there is calcification in the fibrous tissue or in the nodules, and hemorrhage into the nodules may be evident. Sometimes there is lymphocytic infiltration.

ETIOLOGY. The cause of this condition is not known with certainty, but there is evidence that mild deficiency in thyroid hormone production with consequent long-term stimulation of the gland (by TSH?) is one etiology. In areas of iodide deficiency, children under age 10 typically have diffuse enlargement of the thyroid, which on histologic examination shows a pattern of follicles distended with colloid and low cuboidal epithelium. Between ages 10 and 20, there is a gradual transformation of the process into the multinodular structure. Alternate periods of iodide deficiency with thyroid hyperplasia, and iodide sufficiency with involution, may lead first to colloid goiter and later to the typical multinodular goiter. Experimental proof of this theory in man is lacking. Presumably the hypertrophy of the thyroid in the iodide-deficient areas is due to TSH stimulation, but why this should lead to a colloid goiter rather than to hyperplasia is uncertain. For some reason the iodide-deficient gland forms excessive poorly iodinated thyroglobulin which is resistant to hydrolysis by intrathyroidal proteases, and thus accumulates.

Another possible cause is an inherited partial defect in hormone synthesis. Some patients with typical multinodular goiter secrete a large proportion of the iodide from the thyroid in a butanol-insoluble form, apparently an iodinated protein. These patients are usually euthyroid. Multinodular goiter tends to occur with high incidence in some kindreds. It has been generalized from this evidence that mild forms of metabolic defects in hormone synthesis, or perhaps the heterozygous carrier state for such a defect, may lead to the development of sporadic multinodular goiter.

PREVALENCE. The prevalence of multinodular goiter is related to geography, age, and heredity, among other factors. In iodide-deficient areas, multinodular goiter may occur in most individuals. In the United States a conservative estimate of the prevalence of palpable multinodular goiter among adults is 2 per cent, but this is probably low. Identical pathologic changes in the thyroid which do not produce gross enlargement of the gland are present in a much higher proportion of individuals at autopsy. It is evident, however, that multinodular goiter is a disappearing disease in the United States. Large goiters are rarely seen except in adults. This probably is due to increased dietary iodide.

CLINICAL PRESENTATION. Most commonly the condition exists throughout life and is not detected. In some patients enlargement and nodularity of the thyroid are found on routine physical examination. Since the incidence is 10 to 20 times as great in women as in men, and since it develops and progressively increases in size during life, it is often found in females of 50 to 70. Usually the condition is asymptomatic, but with progressive growth there may be a visible enlargement in the neck; tracheal compression, producing a sensation of choking or coughing; and occasionally pressure on the recurrent laryngeal nerve or edema, causing hoarseness. Sometimes there is hemorrhage into a cyst, producing sudden enlargement and tenderness in one area of the goiter. The problems of thyrotoxicosis and malignancy are discussed below.

DIAGNOSIS. The diagnosis of multinodular goiter is usually made on the basis of physical examination. In its most typical form, the goiter feels like a bunch of grapes. The nodules vary in size from 0.5 to several centimeters in diameter and are of variable consistency. The patients are usually euthyroid on clinical examination, and this is confirmed by measuring the serum T_4 or FTI and the RAIU. Single nodules and Hashimoto's thyroiditis are the most common sources of confusion with multinodular goiter. Extensive development of one portion of the gland may lead to the impression of a single nodule; some thyroid enlargements thought to be single nodules turn out at operation to be multinodular goiters. The gland of Hashimoto's thyroiditis may have a lobulated texture, making it impossible to distinguish from multinodular goiter. Thyroid scintiscan may be useful if it shows a mottled distribution of radiosotope in the gland with definite "hot" and "cold" areas. Fluorescent thyroid scans show the same mottled distribution of stable iodine, in contrast to the uniform and diminished stable iodine in the gland of thyroiditis. Roentgenographic examination of the neck may give evidence of broad septate calcification or ringlike calcification in nodules. Often the trachea is deviated because of pressure by the goiter; this is rare in Hashimoto's thyroiditis. If diagnosis is imperative and cannot be made on the basis of the examinations already mentioned, needle biopsy is useful, but obviously gives information relevant to only one tiny area of the gland.

THERAPY. Small nodular goiters in euthyroid subjects require no therapy. However, the natural history is progressive enlargement, and therefore it is appropriate to place patients on permanent therapy with desiccated thyroid in the hope that this will suppress TSH and prevent further enlargement of the gland. This should be done with careful observation, because some of the glands become autonomous, and the additional metabolic effect of exogenous hormone occasionally causes thyrotoxicosis. If the gland is grossly enlarged and causes a cosmetic defect or tracheal compression, resection may be indicated. Subsequently such patients should be placed on replacement therapy, because there is a pronounced tendency for regrowth. Sudden swelling and pain in the gland owing to hemorrhage into a cyst usually subside spontaneously over several weeks, and can be treated with analgesics. Nodular goiters that have progressively enlarged and have become displaced below the clavicles (substernal goiter) may cause tracheal compression and should be resected. Such lesions can usually be removed through a cervical incision. Long-term pressure on the trachea occasionally produces tracheomalacia. The cartilaginous rings of the trachea are destroyed with a loss of normal rigidity. In such patients it is imperative that the function of the trachea be examined during inspiration and expiration at operation. Occasionally it is necessary that a tracheostomy be performed. The tracheostomy tube is left in place for 10 to 14 days to induce a fibrous reaction in the trachea and give it some rigidity.

PROGNOSIS. The prognosis in untreated multinodular goiter is for slow enlargement of the gland. Administration of thyroid hormone may prevent progressive growth. It is also typical for longstanding multinodular goiter to develop autonomy and produce clinical hyperthyroidism.

COMPLICATIONS OF MULTINODULAR GOITER

TOXIC NODULAR GOITER. Many years ago Plummer observed that after nodular goiters had been present for an average of 17 years, thyrotoxicosis tended to develop. This may be due to the coincident occurrence of Graves' disease in the normal tissue between the nodules, but more often it is due to the uncontrolled hyperfunction of one or more nodules in the multinodular gland. In areas of endemic goiter this is the most common cause of hyperthyroidism, especially when iodine supplementation is first introduced into a previously deficient area. It is presumed that nodules developing because of TSH stimulation eventually become autonomous. Also, some autonomously functioning nodules in which hormone production has been limited by restricted iodine supplies are, in the presence of iodide supplementation, able to augment greatly the production of thyroid hormone. Patients with toxic nodular goiter are typically elderly, and symptoms are often minimal. Although the pathophysiology does not differ from that of other forms of thyrotoxicosis, congestive heart failure, atrial fibrillation, and muscle weakness tend to be prominent. The diagnosis should be suspected in any individual with a multinodular goiter and symptoms suggestive of hyperthyroidism, especially if heart failure or atrial fibrillation is present. The RAIU and FTI may be in the high normal range or elevated. The diagnosis is further substantiated by a thyroid scan which localizes radioactivity to one or more of the nodules of the gland. In some of these patients it has been shown that there is a preferential secretion of T_3, leading to an increased ratio of T_3 to T_4 in blood. If the thyrotoxicosis is caused primarily by the excess T_3, the serum T_4 level may be normal. This diagnosis can be partially corroborated by observing failure of suppressibility of the gland, but must be confirmed by direct measurement of T_3. Nonsuppressibility by exogenous T_3 defines autonomy, but does not prove thyrotoxicosis. Nonresponsiveness to TRH is also typically present in toxic multinodular goiter, but it must be remembered that failure to respond to TRH is compatible with either normal or excess hormone production by an autonomous gland.

Toxic multinodular goiter may be treated either by thyroidectomy after appropriate preparation with antithyroid drugs and potassium iodide or by administration of larger doses of radioiodine than are used in the treatment of Graves' disease, typically 10 to 15 mCi. Hypothyroidism is rarely produced because the isotope is distributed unevenly throughout the gland, and some portions are spared from radiation. The gland usually shrinks, but does not disappear. If the patient has significant heart disease, it is best to pretreat with antithyroid drugs before giving RAI, or to use multiple small doses of isotope (5 mCi every two to three months) until euthyroidism is achieved. Release of stored hormone after vigorous RAI therapy can otherwise precipitate congestive failure or infarction.

Administration of small dose of iodine (1 to 4 mg per day) occasionally induces thyrotoxicosis in previously euthyroid individuals with multinodular goiter. The thyrotoxicosis may be transient or may require treatment.

THE CANCER PROBLEM. Although the vast proportion of patients with multinodular goiter are never referred for evaluation or for surgery, the occurrence of sudden growth of one area of a multinodular gland, the palpation of an unusually firm area, or the development of hoarseness may raise the question of malignancy. Patients who come to surgery are obviously highly selected because they have developed symptoms that brought them to a physician and that were considered significant enough for referral to a surgeon. Among those who are operated upon, the incidence of verified carcinoma, usually papillary adenocarcinoma, varies from 2 to 20 per cent. Because of this frequency, some physicians view the presence of multinodular goiter as sufficient indication for thyroidectomy. The gross illogic of this reasoning can be seen by some simple calculations. If 2 per cent of the population have multinodular goiter and 10 per cent of these have thyroid malignancy, at least 400,000 papillary cancers would be present in the United States. In fact it is known that the prevalence of multinodular goiter is much greater than the figure used. In contrast, only 8100 thyroid cancers are detected annually, and the majority of these are found in patients whose thyroids are normal except for the malignancy. Because of this, it seems more logical to accept multinodular goiter as a measure of assurance that malignancy is not present. Multinodular goiter should not be resected because of a general fear of malignancy, but thyroidectomy is logical in the presence of signs that in themselves are suggestive of malignant change. In contrast, glands harboring a single nodule carry a real increase in risk of thyroid carcinoma.

Gemsenjäger, E., Staub, J. J., Girard, J., and Heitz, P. H.: Preclinical hyperthyroidism in multinodular goiter. J. Clin. Endocrinol. Metab., 43:810, 1976.

Mortensen, J. C., Woolner, L. D., and Bennett, W. A.: Gross and microscopic findings in clinically normal thyroid glands. J. Clin. Endocrinol. Metab., 15:1270, 1955.

Rapport, B., Niepomniszcze, H., Bigazzi, M., Hati, R., and DeGroot, L. J.: Studies on the pathogenesis of poor thyroglobulin iodination in non-toxic multinodular goiter. J. Clin. Endocrinol. Metab., 34:822, 1972.

Shimaoka, K., and Sokal, J. E.: Suppressive therapy of nontoxic goiter. Am. J. Med., 57:576, 1974.

Vagenakis, A. G., Wang, C. A., Burger, A., Maloof, F., Braverman, L. E., and Ingbar, S. H.: Iodide-induced thyrotoxicosis in Boston. N. Engl. J. Med., 287:523, 1973.

Vander, J. B., Gaston, E. A., and Dawber, T. R.: The significance of nontoxic thyroid nodules. Ann. Intern. Med., 69:537, 1968.

546.6. ENDEMIC GOITER

In the United States the average iodide intake is 200 to 600 μg or more per day, and detectable thyroid enlargement occurs in 2 to 4 per cent of adults. In contrast, in areas where iodide deficiency is present, as shown by urinary iodine excretion below 50 μg per day, the incidence of palpable enlargement of the thyroid increases in inverse relation to the average urinary iodide excretion. Endemic goiter exists in many mountainous areas of the world, including the Andes, central New Guinea, and Switzerland, as well as in many lowland areas such as the Baltic Plains and Zaïre. In almost all well-studied endemics, the cause is deficient iodide in the soil and water, leading to deficient iodide intake. Presumably, iodide privation leads to diminished production of thyroid hormone, which is sensed by the pituitary, resulting in augmented secretion of TSH, and thus to increased thyroidal clearance of plasma iodide. With this there is also growth (both hyperplasia and hypertrophy) of the thyroid. The thyroid strives to gain the necessary 60 to 100 μg of iodide needed daily for hormonogenesis, and does so by accumulating almost all the iodide ion entering the vascular compartment, either from the diet or from degradation of hormone within the body. The uptake of a radioactive tracer is 90 to 98 per cent in some endemic areas. Initially the gland is diffusely enlarged, and the histologic picture in adolescence is a "colloid goiter" with large follicles and flat cuboidal epithelium. In time the picture changes into the multinodular goiter described previously; the histology is identical with that of sporadic multinodular goiter found in other regions. Usually diffuse goiter predominates in youth, and multinodular goiter in older persons. The incidence is higher in women than in men unless the endemic is unusually severe. In some areas, practically all adults have thyroid enlargement.

PATHOGENESIS. The biochemical abnormalities that lead to the formation of multinodular goiters in response to iodide deficiency are not known. Alternate periods of iodide deficiency and repletion may lead to hyperplasia and involution and produce the picture of endemic goiter.

TSH is elevated in some severe endemics, but in Argentina adults have been found to have endemic goiter in the presence of normal levels of plasma TSH. Possibly these people had elevated TSH levels earlier in their lives, or perhaps owing to iodide deficiency the gland is more sensitive to TSH. The thyroglobulin of endemic goiters is iodine poor and characteristically has an excess of MIT over DIT, and the content of T_4 and T_3 tends to be low. Possibly these alterations of iodide content or distribution in the amino acids of thyroglobulin lead to abnormalities in degradation of thyroglobulin and produce the picture of a colloid-filled goiter.

Goitrogens. In a few instances factors other than iodide deficiency operate to cause endemic goiter. Thus a factor present in water appears to be associated with an endemic in Colombia. Thiocyanates are derived from some plants, e.g., cassava eaten in Central Africa. Potent goitrogens related in action to the thioureas are found in some plant species and are transmitted through cow's milk to humans in Tasmania and Finland. As fascinating as these examples are, they account for only a minute fraction of endemic goiter, a condition that involves many millions of people throughout the world.

CLINICAL MANIFESTATIONS. Patients with goiter in endemic zones present with thyroid enlargements that may be diffuse or nodular and that vary in size from barely detectable to as large as the head (Fig. 9). In some places monstrous enlargement of the thyroid is accepted as normal. Usually such individuals, when adult, are euthyroid, and thus appear to have adapted to iodide deficiency by growth of the goiter. All the problems related to thyroid enlargement, such as dysphagia, respiratory difficulty, tracheal deviation and compression, and cosmetic problems may of course be associated with the thyroid enlargement. Occasionally, in severe endemics, some people are hypothyroid clinically and by laboratory examination. In contrast to the condition known as endemic cretinism, described below, patients with endemic goiter do not have neurologic signs or gross mental retardation. Aside from what might be considered by foreigners a cosmetic blemish, endemic goiter itself is inconsequential to most adults with this condition. However, there is evidence, discussed below, that the neural complications of iodide privation may be important.

DIAGNOSIS. The diagnosis of endemic goiter is best made by study of a population group. The characteristic feature is reduced excretion of iodide in the urine. Iodide excretion is often 30 to 50 μg per day, although values as low as 5μg per day have been recorded. RAIU values are elevated to the 70 to 95 per cent range. Thyroid hormone in blood, as measured by the PBI or T_4, is normal, or rarely is depressed, and the patients are hypothyroid. The T_4 may be low in the presence of euthyroidism; these patients maintain normal metabolism by producing relatively more T_3. The findings of diminished urinary iodide, augmented thyroid uptake, and high incidence of goiter are sufficient to incriminate iodide as the cause of the endemic. If iodide intake is sufficient, i.e., above 100 μg per day in the presence of endemic goiter, some other cause must be sought, such as a goitrogenic agent in foodstuffs.

TREATMENT. The best treatment for endemic goiter is iodine prophylaxis applied to the entire population group. The most convenient approach is salt iodinization, adding about 50 μg of iodide per gram of salt as iodate or as potassium iodide. Another approach is to inject population groups with iodinated poppyseed oil. This provides a

Figure 9. A young woman from the Nepalese village of Wapsa which has severe iodine deficiency and a high incidence of endemic goiter. (Photograph kindly provided by Professor Kaye Ibbertson of the University of Auckland, Private Bag, New Zealand.)

depot of 1 to 2 grams of potential iodide, and is sufficient to supply iodide for one to four years. Treatment with desiccated thyroid should prevent further enlargement of the goiters and suppress diffuse goiters in children. It usually has little effect on the multinodular goiters of adults. Local symptoms caused by massive enlargement of the thyroid may require thyroidectomy.

Thyrotoxicosis is rarely seen in areas of severe endemic goiter, apparently because the limitation of iodide supply prevents its development. Occasionally it does occur, and may be difficult to recognize because RAIU values are elevated even in "normal" subjects. The FTI or serum T_4 may be elevated, or may be normal if the patient secretes an excess of T_3. After administration of iodine in salt or by injection, some patients develop thyrotoxicosis. Sometimes this process (Jod-Basedow) is self-limiting, but therapy with antithyroid drugs, radioactive iodine, or surgery may be required.

There is no convincing evidence that carcinoma occurs with increased frequency in areas of endemic goiter, but there is a strong suggestion that a higher proportion of the tumors that do occur are poorly differentiated or sarcomatous.

ENDEMIC CRETINISM

This term refers to defective individuals having a typical constellation of signs and symptoms found with increased frequency in areas of severe endemic goiter. If recognized shortly after birth and if the children are hypothyroid, there is a typical appearance with increased hair, low forehead, puffy features, umbilical hernia, enlarged tongue, and sluggish behavior. Other abnormalities may be detected: deaf-mutism, mental retardation, and evidence of spastic paraplegia. These may occur with or without overt hypothyroidism, or as individual entities. If there is continued hypothyroidism, retarded growth and retarded bone age and epiphysial stippling occur. The individual may be goitrous, or no thyroid tissue may be present. In childhood, most endemic cretins achieve a euthyroid metabolic state, but stunted growth, deaf-mutism, mental subnormality, and diplegia give evidence of the syndrome. Endemic cretinism is probably caused by severe iodide deficiency leading to hypothyroidism in both mother and child during fetal development. Athyreotic individuals born to normal mothers in nonendemic zones rarely if ever develop the full-blown syndrome, apparently because significant quantities of thyroid hormone are transported from the mother to the fetus across the placenta. When investigated during childhood or adult life, endemic cretins may be hypothyroid or euthyroid. Treatment of euthyroid adult cretins with thyroid hormone has had no beneficial effect on mental function, deafness, or neurologic damage. The only known therapy is iodine prophylaxis, as described above for endemic goiter. Studies by Fierro in Ecuador suggest that in severe endemics associated with cretinism, mental subnormality may afflict a much larger portion of the population. Thus the effects of endemic iodide deficiency, goiter, and cretinism appear to be even more devastating than was previously known, making iodine prophylaxis of crucial importance in these areas.

Bray, G. A.: Increased sensitivity of the thyroid in iodine-depleted rats to goitrogenic effects of thyrotropin. J. Clin. Invest., 47:1640, 1968.

Chopra, I. J., Hershman, J. M., and Hornabrook, R. W.: Serum thyroid hormone and thyrotropin levels in subjects from endemic goiter regions of New Guinea. J. Clin. Endocrinol. Metab., 40:326, 1975.

Delange, F., Thilly, C., and Ermans, A. M.: Iodine deficiency, a permissive condition in the development of endemic goiter. J. Clin. Endocrinol. Metab., 28:114, 1968.

Dumont, J. E., Ermans, A. M., and Bastenie, P. A.: Thyroidal function in a goiter endemic. IV. Hypothyroidism and endemic cretinism. J. Clin. Endocrinol. Metab., 23:325, 1963.

Ermans, A. M., Bastenie, P. A., Galperin, H., Beckers, C., Van Den Schrieck, H. G., and DeVisscher, M.: Endemic goiter in the Uele region. II. Synthesis and secretion of thyroid hormones. J. Clin. Endocrinol. Metab., 21:996, 1961.

Fierro-Benitez, R., Penafiel, W., DeGroot, L. J., and Ramirez, I: Endemic goiter and endemic cretinism and in the Andean region. N. Engl. J. Med., 280:296, 1969.

Stanbury, J. B., and Kroc, R. L. (eds.): Human Development and the Thyroid Gland. Relation to Endemic Cretinism. New York, Plenum Press, 1972.

Thilly, C. H., Delange, F., Goldstein-Golaire, J., and Ermans, A. M.: Endemic goiter prevention by iodized oil: A reassessment. J. Clin. Endocrinol Metab., 36:1196, 1973.

546.7. METABOLIC DEFECTS IN THYROID HORMONE FORMATION, TRANSPORT, AND ACTION

CONGENITAL METABOLIC DEFECTS IN THYROID HORMONE FORMATION
(Sporadic Goitrous Hypothyroidism or Goitrous Cretinism)

The biosynthesis of thyroid hormone proceeds via transport of iodide into the thyroid, binding of iodide to tyrosine in thyroglobulin, coupling of iodotyrosines, subsequent proteolysis of thyroglobulin with release of iodotyrosines and thyronines, intrathyroidal deiodination of iodotyrosines and reutilization of their iodide, and release of thyroid hormone to the blood. Specific enzymatic defects causing diminished efficiency in the formation of thyroid hormone have been identified at several of these steps. The various genotypes usually produce a common phenotype, characterized by the presence of a hyperplastic thyroid plus hypothyroidism or euthyroidism.

Defect in Iodide Trapping. A few patients have been recognized with hyperplastic thyroid glands and congenital hypothyroidism associated with inability to transport iodide into the thyroid and thyroidal uptake of tracer isotope near zero. Thyroid tissue from such patients, studied in vitro, is unable to establish an iodide concentration gradient. The patients also fail to transport iodide into saliva and gastric juice; this observation forms the basis of a simple test for the defect. The concentration of iodide in saliva is compared with that in plasma two hours after administration of a radioactive iodide tracer. In affected individuals the ratio is 1, whereas in normal individuals and in presumed heterozygotes it is from 10 to 100. Thyroid tissue of these patients contains the other enzymes needed for hormone synthesis. It should be remembered that the usual cause for failure of iodide uptake during a tracer test is that the gland is saturated by exogenous iodine rather than a faulty iodide-concentrating mechanism.

Iodide Organification Defect. The most common defect in hormone synthesis is at the iodide-binding step. The patients are able to transport and concentrate iodide in the thyroid, but the iodide is not bound to tyrosine in thyroglobulin. Iodide in the thyroid remains in equilibrium with that in plasma, and as iodide in plasma is cleared to the urine, the free thyroidal iodide gradually returns to plasma. Such patients have an elevated thyroid uptake shortly after administration of a tracer and a low uptake at 24 hours. The iodide content of the gland is greated reduced. Reduced amounts of iodinated compounds are formed or released to plasma. T_4 is low.

A defect in binding can be identified by administration of potassium perchlorate two hours after administration of a radioactive iodide tracer. The potassium perchlorate will effectively block the iodide transport mechanism. If there is a large pool of free intrathyroidal iodide, potassium perchlorate will cause a release of this material to plasma, with a dramatic drop in the thyroid iodide content. A release of 10 per cent or more of the iodide present at two hours is considered a positive test result.

A variant of this condition is found in association with congenital nerve deafness (Pendred's syndrome). This condition is transmitted as a mendelian dominant, but is expressed to varying degrees. Deafness ranges from complete through nearly normal hearing, and hypothyroidism may be severe or thyroid function may be normal.

The biochemical basis of the organification defect syndromes has been identified in patients studied in the author's laboratory. Some patients have diminished or absent iodide peroxidase. Others have an abnormal peroxidase apo-protein which fails to bind the hematin prosthetic group firmly; thus the enzyme is not fully active. In other patients, an abnormality of thyroglobulin synthesis results in a diminished quantity of iodide acceptor. Other proteins are iodinated, but apparently inefficiently, resulting in a buildup of free intrathyroidal iodide and failure to produce iodothyronines.

"Coupling" Defect. Some individuals with congenital goiter have large, hyperactive thyroids and low thyroid hormone in plasma. Large amounts of MIT and DIT are found in their thyroglobulin. An abnormality of the coupling process is implied by these observations, but it is by no means certain what this abnormality is. It could, for example, be an abnormality in energy supply, an abnormality in the structure of the thyroglobulin, or perhaps lack of peroxidase enzyme related to the coupling process. It is currently believed that there is no "coupling enzyme," rather that peroxidase mediates this process as well as initial iodination of thyroglobulin. Although patients with congenital thyroid disease, hypothyroidism, low plasma T_4, and plentiful iodotyrosines in the thyroid must have a defect of the coupling process, a more exact definition will require new information about the normal synthetic process.

Iodotyrosine Dehalogenase Defect. Thyroglobulin is degraded in the thyroid by a combination of protease and peptidases, and each amino acid of the thyroglobulin peptide chain is thus separated. Normally the iodotyrosines are deiodinated by a dehalogenase present in the microsomes. The liberated iodide is reutilized for the iodination of tyrosine to form more MIT and DIT. Each day about four times as much iodide goes through this cycle as enters the thyroid from the blood. Some patients have a specific defect of the dehalogenase. In the most carefully studied cases, the enzyme defect also exists in other tissues. Because of the defect in the thyroid, iodotyrosine is liberated from the gland into the blood. Because of lack of the enzyme in other tissues, iodotyrosines are not deodinated, but are excreted in the urine. This iodide loss causes marked hypothyroidism and thyroid enlargement. The disease can be diagnosed by the identification of labeled iodotyrosines in plasma or urine after administration of a radioactive iodide tracer. Also, infused iodotyrosine is not deiodinated, but is excreted unchanged in the urine. Parents of affected individuals, who are presumed to be heterozygous, often show a minor abnormality in their ability to deiodinate iodotyrosine.

Serum Iodoprotein Defect. Many patients with congenital or familial thyroid enlargement and hypothyroidism have in their plasma iodine insoluble in acidified butanol, and thus not T_4 or T_3. This material is formed in the thyroid, and is of heterogeneous nature. Some glands secrete large amounts of iodinated albumin, prealbumin, or both. Others seem to secrete iodinated proteins that do not react with antihuman albumin serum, and do react in part with antithyroglobulin antibodies. Possibly these are abnormal subunits or fragments of thyroglobulin. The iodoproteins usually contain mainly MIT and DIT and no T_4 or T_3.

This inefficient utilization of glandular iodide restricts the formation of T_4 and causes thyroid hyperplasia. The basic abnormality is poorly understood, but is probably related to inadequate production of normal thyroglobulin. Other proteins may then gain access to the gland and be iodinated. Another possibility is an abnormality in the proteolytic enzymes of the thyroid so that iodinated subunits of thyroglobulin are released to plasma. Attempts to identify defective protease activity have been inconclusive.

EPIDEMIOLOGY. The metabolic defects in hormone synthesis occur sporadically or in family groupings. Affected siblings may be identifiable, and occasionally parents are found to have a minor metabolic abnormality. Typically there is inbreeding in the family. The metabolic defects usually represent the expression of a homozygous recessive genetic abnormality. An exception to this is in Pendred's syndrome, which may be inherited as a mendelian dominant.

PATHOLOGY. Typically there is marked hyperplasia of the thyroid. The gland is beefy, the cells are columnar, there is little or no colloid, and hypervascularity is marked. The extreme hyperplasia may take on the appearance of a papillary carcinoma. In other instances the longstanding thyrotropin stimulation of the gland results in change into a carcinoma, metastases, and death. Disease, other than in the thyroid, depends upon the degree of hypothyroidism. In Pendred's syndrome there is in addition nerve deafness, but information on the nature of the lesion is lacking.

CLINICAL PRESENTATION. Patients present a common phenotype. Usually the illness is not suspected at birth but becomes apparent within the first few months or, more frequently, during childhood. If the illness is severe, the child will develop evidence of hypothyroidism. There is symmetrical enlargement of the thyroid from two to ten times normal size. The gland is usually very vascular, and typically a bruit and thrill are present. The signs and symptoms of hypothyroidism are those described previously. The presence of metastases, including pulmonary infiltrates, indicates malignant change in the goiter.

DIAGNOSIS. The diagnosis is suggested by observation of a hyperplastic thyroid in an individual who is apparently euthyroid or hypothyroid. The iodide-trapping defect can be demonstrated by the inability of the gland to accumulate iodide during a tracer uptake study. A corroborative finding is lack of concentration of iodide in the saliva. An iodide organification defect can be shown by a positive perchlorate discharge test and hypothyroxinemia. The iodotyrosine dehalogenase defect can be identified by chromatography revealing iodotyrosine in plasma and urine after administration of a tracer. The butanol-insoluble iodoprotein defect is detected by an abnormal difference between the PBI and BEI or between the PBI and serum T_4 iodine. Normally the difference is no more than 20 per cent. In patients with the syndrome, the BEI or T_4 iodine may be only 30 to 40 per cent of the PBI. Identification of the labeled protein can be made by electrophoresis of plasma or thyroid proteins obtained at biopsy after administration of a radioiodide tracer.

THERAPY. Since the patients have a goitrogenic response to TSH caused by deficiency of thyroid hormone, the obvious therapy is to replace thyroid hormone. This corrects existing hypothyroidism and in children usually results in complete regression of the goiter. In older people in whom multinodular goiter has developed, there may be little change in size. In patients with the iodide trapping or dehalogenase defects, administration of a few drops of Lugol's solution daily will compensate for the defect. Development of thyrotoxicosis during iodide therapy for dehalogenase defect has been reported.

PROGNOSIS. It is imperative that individuals with these syndromes be treated with suppressive doses of thyroid hormone or potassium iodide, as indicated, for the duration of their lives. Inadequate therapy will allow continued TSH stimulation of the gland, and malignant degeneration may occur. In general the patients and parents can be reassured that if the defect has been detected early so that there is no neurologic abnormality, treatment will result in normal health and longevity. Further, it is highly unlikely that progeny will be affected if there is no inbreeding.

DEFECTS IN HORMONE TRANSPORT

Occasionally patients have a great elevation or depression of blood thyroid hormone in the absence of corresponding clinical symptoms, owing to the presence of abnormal quantities of thyroxine-binding globulin (TBG). In well-studied kinships, the abnormalities have been shown to be transmitted as X-linked traits. Thus the affected or "carrier" females are typically heterozygous, and affected males are homozygous. In families with hypo-TBG-emia, the males have extremely low or undetectable levels of TBG, with PBI or T_4 values in the range of 1 to 2 μg per 100 ml. Affected females usually have about half-normal TBG and PBI or serum T_4 values. The abnormality is the altered production of a normal protein, because no protein immunologically related to TBG is found in the serum of TBG-deficient subjects and turnover of labeled normal TBG injected into these subjects is similar to turnover in unaffected individuals. The decrease in total bound hormone in the plasma of such patients is counterbalanced by an increased fraction of free hormone. The absolute free hormone concentration is therefore normal, and the patients are eumetabolic. Aside from the confusion caused in the interpretation of laboratory tests, there is no known physiologic abnormality associated with this defect.

A few individuals have been reported with elevations of TBG to approximately two times normal and gross elevation of serum T_4. Again this appears to be genetically X-linked, with affected males exhibiting TBG elevation about twice that of affected (carrier) females. The patients are euthyroid, and no change in the availability of thyroid hormone to tissues can be shown.

The possibility of genetically induced decreased or (rarely) increased TBG should always be kept in mind when a thyroid hormone test reveals a level that appears to be discordant with the observed clinical state and no hormonal or disease-related cause exists. Measurement of absolute free T_4 content, or of the FTI, will indicate that the amount of functioning thyroid hormone in the plasma is normal. Another way to show the nature of the condition is by measurement of the T_4 carrying capacity of TBG. Evaluation of other members of the family will help verify the diagnosis.

HEREDITARY RESISTANCE TO THE ACTION OF THYROID HORMONE

Three of eight children in one reported sibship have apparent resistance to the action of thyroid hormone. The children have a characteristic facial appearance, retarded growth, delayed bone age, stippled epiphyses, deaf-mutism, and elevated thyroid hormone concentration in blood. The hormone in blood is T_3 and T_4, and there is no abnormality of binding proteins. Their thyroids produce about five times the normal amount of hormone daily, and this quantity is likewise degraded in the peripheral tissues. They appear to be euthyroid. A large body of laboratory data supports the conclusion that these children are resistant to the action of thyroid hormone. In compensation, an increased quantity of hormone is made available to the peripheral tissues. Even with this, some organs (e.g., the ears and bones) receive an insufficient supply of hormone. It is hypothesized that the hypothalamus shares in the decreased sensitivity. Lymphocytes from one of these children lack the normal "receptor" molecule for thyroid hormone. It is believed that the receptor abnormality causes thyroid hormone resistance, which is partially compensated for by high plasma hormone levels. A few similar sporadic or familial cases have been reported.

Bernal, J., DeGroot, L. J., Refetoff, S., Fang, V. S., and Barsano, C.: Absent nuclear thyroid hormone receptors and failure of T_3-induced TRH suppression in the syndrome of peripheral resistance to thyroid hormone. Thyroid Research; Proceedings, Seventh International Thyroid Conference, Boston, June 1975.

DeGroot, L. J., and Stanbury, J. B.: The syndrome of congenital goiter with butanol insoluble serum iodine. Am. J. Med., 27:586, 1959.

Lissitzky, S., Bismuth, J., Codaccioni, J. L., and Cartouzou, G.: Congenital goiter with iodoalbumin replacing thyroglobulin and defect of deiodination of iodotyrosines. Serum origin of the thyroid iodoalbumin. J. Clin. Endocrinol. Metab., 28:1797, 1968.

Lissitzky, S., Torresani, J., Burrow, G. N., Bouchilloux, S., and Chabaud, O.: Defective thyroglobulin export as a cause of congenital goitre. Clin. Endocrinol., 4:363, 1975.

Niepomniszcze, H., Castells, S., DeGroot, L. J., Refetoff, S., Kim, O. S., Rapoport, B., and Hati, R.: Peroxidase defect in congenital goiter with complete organification block. J. Clin. Endocrinol. Metab., 34:607, 1972.

Refetoff, S., DeGroot, L. J., Benard, B., and DeWind, L. T.: Studies of a sibship with apparent hereditary resistance to the intracellular action of thyroid hormone. Metabolism, 21:723, 1972.

Stanbury, J. B., and Chapman, E. M.: Congenital hypothyroidism with goiter. Absence of an iodide-concentrating mechanism. Lancet, 1:1162, 1960.

Stanbury, J. B., Kassenaar, A. A. H., Meijer, J. W. A., and Terpstra, J.: The occurrence of mono- and di-iodotyrosine in the blood of a patient with congenital goiter. J. Clin. Endocrinol. Metab., 15:1216, 1955.

546.8. THYROID NEOPLASMS

Thyroid neoplasms are adenomas and malignant tumors. Pathologically, adenomas are classified into fetal, follicular, Hürthle cell, and papillary forms. Carcinomas are usually grouped into papillary, follicular, mixed, Hürthle cell, medullary, and anaplastic varieties. Lymphoma and lymphosarcoma are also found in the thyroid.

ETIOLOGY. As in all other neoplasms, the exact etiology is unknown. In the case of thyroid cells, it is certain that both radiation and TSH stimulation are involved. After the original observation by Duffy and Fitzgerald, a relation between x-ray to the pharyngeal or thymic area in early childhood and subsequent development of thyroid carcinoma (usually papillary) was well documented. In children who develop thyroid carcinoma under the age of 20, this association is characteristically present. Although the tumors are presumed to occur because of x-ray damage to the thyroid, it is possible that the pathogenesis involves damage to the immunologic surveillance system of the thymus, or that the response is fundamentally due to x-ray damage to the thyroid with subsequent TSH hypersecretion.

Thyroid carcinoma is now known to follow radiation given for thymic enlargement, tonsillar-adenoid hypertrophy, acne, and tumors in the neck area. The relationship between dose and incidence shows no significant threshold effect, and is probably linear through 700 to 1000 rads, with an incidence of about 3 cases per 10^6 persons per rad per year. The effect is not restricted to radiation given in childhood. Radiation induces both benign and malignant tumors (ratio of 3:1), with a latency usually of 10 to 20 years. The lesions are almost always the well differentiated slow-growing tumors typically found in young people. It is believed that several hundred thousand people may have been exposed to this radiation. It is recommended that such individuals should receive a careful physical examination and other tests as described below if an abnormality is found. Discovery of a clear cut nodule(s) (usually over 1 cm in diameter) constitutes reason for explorative surgery.

Another known relationship is between chronic TSH stimulation and the formation of invasive thyroid carcinoma, best identified in patients with congenital metabolic defects. A third relationship is to a variety of the multiple endocrine adenomatosis syndrome (Type 2), involving pheochromocytoma and medullary thyroid carcinoma, which is transmitted as a dominant genetic trait. Multiple cutaneous neuromas are also seen in association with this syndrome, and occasionally parathyroid adenomas. Many thyroid tumors are known to be TSH dependent, in that administration of suppressive doses of thyroid hormone leads to decrease in or regression of the malignancy. The exact relation of x-ray or TSH to induction of autonomous growth is unclear, although it is presumed to involve a mutational change with deletion of genes that restrict growth of the thyroid cells.

Little is known about the development of thyroid adenomas, although it may be presumed that the same sort of change that causes thyroid carcinoma is involved in the pathogenesis of adenomas. Thyroid adenomas, or at least nodularity, are present with increased frequency in patients who have received x-ray therapy to the thymus, and adenomas are produced in laboratory animals subjected to long-term TSH stimulation. Multiple follicular adenomas are occasionally found in family groups. Although adenomas may develop into thyroid carcinomas, this is not a common process.

A high incidence of thyroid carcinoma has been found in patients coming to surgery with multinodular goiter. The reasons for this have been discussed in Ch. 546.5. It has been stated for years that the incidence of thyroid cancer in Graves' disease is diminished, but this is not certain. In a recently reported large series, 0.5 per cent of patients undergoing thyroidectomy for Graves' disease were found to have papillary thyroid carcinoma.

"Minimal" Papillary Cancer. Evidence exists that if thyroids of individuals coming to autopsy are examined with great care, up to 7 per cent may have tiny foci of papillary cancer, often surrounded by a fibrotic reaction. The incidence of these lesions is best described in individuals over age 40. Ninety per cent of these are under 4 mm in size, and thus they are not detectable by any current clinical examination and often would be missed by observation or palpation at surgery. Although it is certain that most of these lesions will not be associated with a clinically significant problem, the exact relationship to the cancers found in patients who have received prior neck irradiation, and to the much smaller number of clinically evident cancers, is yet unknown. For the moment, such lesions under 1 cm in size are labeled "minimal" papillary thyroid cancers, and it is believed that the incidental discovery of such a lesion at surgery is not an indication for radical surgery.

THYROID ADENOMAS

PATHOLOGY. Adenomas are new growths of thyroid tissue having a homogeneous histologic pattern, surrounded by a capsule composed of fibrous tissue or compressed normal cells. They may present as single structures in otherwise normal glands or, less frequently, as two or three discrete adenomas, or they may be a feature of the multinodular goiter. The most common variety is the follicular adenoma, composed of large colloid-filled follicles with flattened cuboidal epithelium. A common variety of this growth has large colloid-filled follicles and an ill-defined capsule, leading to its designation as a "colloid nodule." Whether or not these are true adenomas is debated. Occasionally there may be degeneration, and the adenoma is then cystic and filled with a gelatinous material. Evidence of old or recent hemorrhage into a degenerating adenoma is common. Some adenomas have the histologic appearance of normal thyroid tissue. Adenomas with smaller follicles and more cellularity are termed fetal or embryonal and are occasionally transitional forms between adenomatous and carcinomatous growths. In the Hürthle cell adenoma the cells are eosinophilic and have the appearance of liver cells. All of these are variants of the follicular adenoma. Papillary "adenomas" have characteristic fronds of cells projecting into a sparsely filled lumen; these may in fact be carcinomas.

CLINICAL PRESENTATION. *The clinical problem most often presented by the thyroid adenoma is management of a solitary thyroid nodule.* This may be asymptomatic, or, less commonly, may be brought to attention because of hoarseness, pain, or difficulty in swallowing. Single nodules are present in 2 per cent of the adult population. They are much less frequent in men than in women. It is certain that most remain without significant danger for long periods of time.

The problem is in differentiation of such lesions from thyroid cancer. In the vast majority of persons, the clinical finding is limited to a nodule in an otherwise normal gland. Nodules in individuals under age 30 and in males are considered more suspicious because benign nodules are less frequent in these groups. Contrariwise, lesions in women over 60 to 65 are more often benign. The presence of recent growth, pain fixation, and lymph nodes suggests possible malignancy. A history of prior radiation exposure is especially important, since at least 30 per cent of individuals with a nodule and prior radiation will have a cancer at operation.

The main problem comes in deciding what to do about the majority of the patients who do not fit into any of the aforementioned categories. These are typically women between ages 30 and 60. On clinical and laboratory examination, most patients are euthyroid, although some are clinically toxic. RAIU and scanning studies may show that the nodule is "cold" (most commonly), that it is equal in uptake of radioactive iodide to that of the normal tissue, or that it concentrates radioactive iodide selectively. Some of the "hot" nodules produce excessive hormone and suppress the normal gland or produce clinical thyrotoxicosis. Nodules may be "cold" because they are biochemically unable to transport radioactive iodide into the thyroid or are unable to bind it, but most frequently they are "cold" because they are cystic. If the nodule is "cold," is unusually firm, is fixed to the trachea or surrounding structures, is irregular in contour, or is known to have recently grown, or if cervical nodes are felt, the likelihood of malignancy is increased. However, it is certain that clinical examination and isotope scanning cannot segregate carcinomas from benign adenomas. Carcinoma may occur in nodules that are functioning on scanning; from 3 to 10 per cent of carcinomas are warm or hot by this technique. However, the possibility of malignancy is reduced in warm nodules (as compared to cold), and is low in hot nodules that suppress the remainder of the gland. Solitary nodules in the thyroids of children and men are particularly dangerous. It cannot be taken for granted that a nodule known to have been present for a few years is benign. Further, it is probably not advantageous to treat such lesions for a long time with desiccated thyroid in an attempt to suppress their growth, because this rarely causes disappearance of the nodule. Short-term therapy before surgery may be of value since it makes the lesion more discrete and facilitates a localized resection. Positive diagnosis of cancer can be made in the infrequent medullary carcinomas by detection of elevated thyrocalcitonin levels, if this assay is available.

The author's current approach to single nodules is as follows. Nodules in individuals who have received significant radiation exposure are resected, as are most nodules with signs or symptoms suggestive of malignancy, including growth, nodes, unusual fixation or firmness, pain, and hoarseness. Most single nodules in men and women under 30 are likewise resected. In females between 30 and 60 to 65 years, an attempt is made to classify nodules on the basis of scanning, symptoms, needle biopsy, or aspiration cytology into those with a high or low probability of malignancy. Cysts can be aspirated one or more times, but often recur. Nodules with strong support for a benign diagnosis can be followed with thyroid hormone suppressive therapy; this plan can always be altered in the light of a changing clinical course. Lesions with suggestive findings on history or physical examination, those with biopsy or cytologic studies suggestive of malignancy, those that are cosmetically a problem, or nodules causing a real degree of anxiety are best resected by a competent surgeon. In women over 60 to 65 the proportion of benign nodules is high and complicating medical illness is more common; in these circumstances medical therapy is usually advised. The operative procedure is usually subtotal lobectomy if the lesion appears to be benign and if there are no observable lymph nodes. Frozen sections are made; if the diagnosis of adenoma is confirmed, no further procedure is done. If the lesion is malignant, a more extensive procedure is carried out, as discussed below. Patients who have a subtotal resection for a benign adenoma should be placed on permanent thyroid hormone replacement therapy. *Some of the "single nodules" subjected to surgery are found to be multinodular goiters, and from 10 to 20 per cent are diagnosed by the surgical pathologist as thyroid carcinoma.*

Hyperfunctioning nodules can be ablated by large doses of ^{131}I (30 to 60 mCi). An alternative and preferable approach in the author's mind is surgical resection, except in older individuals.

THYROID CARCINOMAS

Papillary Carcinoma. Nearly 80 per cent of thyroid carcinomas are papillary tumors, and there is debate over whether a benign papillary adenoma actually exists. The tumors have fronds of cellular tissue projecting into slit-like lumina containing scant or no colloid. Other portions of the lesion may show differentiation into a relatively normal follicular structure. The lesions are frequently very small and often are found as incidentally observed microscopic tumors in glands removed for some other lesion. Papillary tumors tend to metastasize early to lymph nodes in the neck, often when the primary tumor cannot be detected by physical examination or by scanning. The tumor remains confined to cervical lymph nodes for a long time, but may invade locally into strap muscles and the larynx, and metastasize to lungs. The histologic patterns of the primary and metastatic disease may be quite different, with follicular elements in either area. Growth tends to be partially dependent on TSH. The disease is less aggressive in individuals under age 40. Ten-year survival with various forms of therapy is 80 to 90 per cent.

Up to two thirds of the thyroid tumors in the differentiated papillary group cannot be categorized as either purely papillary or follicular, but are mixed. These tumors behave more or less like pure papillary lesions. It is impossible to tell which element has metastasized, and there may be major discrepancies in architecture and function between the primary and the metastatic deposits.

Follicular Carcinoma. Follicular thyroid carcinoma varies in appearance from relatively normal-looking thyroid tissue, to microfollicular structures, large follicles, or areas of solid, rather anaplastic-appearing tumor. Often some areas have Hürthle cell changes. These tumors metastasize early via the bloodstream to lung and bones. The tumors are TSH responsive and tend to pick up and metabolize iodide and to form thyroid hormone. Occasionally the unchecked biosynthetic activity of the tumor results in clinical thyrotoxicosis. The ten-year survival in patients with this illness is approximately 50 per cent.

Hürthle cell carcinoma tends to invade and metastasize locally in the neck. It has a morbidity approximately like that of follicular carcinoma.

Medullary Carcinoma. Medullary cell carcinoma is derived from the "C" cells, or calcitonin-secreting parafollicular cells of the thyroid. These tumors form sheets of cells with large nuclei. There is usually extensive deposition of amyloid and considerable fibrosis; lymphocyte infiltration may also be prominent. The tumors tend to metastasize locally to the neck and finally to the lungs and soft tissues. Their course is like that of follicular carcinoma, despite their undifferentiated "solid tumor" appearance. The tumors may occur sporadically or be associated with two familial syndromes. In multiple endocrine neoplasia syndrome Type I, there are associated islet cell adenomas (2E syndrome), parathyroid adenoma, and occasionally pituitary, thyroid, and adrenal adenoma. In MEN Type II, the association is with pheochromocytoma and parathyroid hyperplasia–adenoma (II-A), or with the mucosal neuroma–pheochromocytoma syndrome (II-B). It is clear that they produce calcitonin and rarely cause hypocalcemia. In response to this they may induce parathyroid adenomas. The tumors may also secrete "hormonal" polypeptides and, through this mechanism, may cause Cushing's syndrome and may produce excess serotonin. A history of familial cancer, pheochromocytoma, or hypocalcemia should suggest this diagnosis, and assay for calcitonin should be done.

Anaplastic Carcinomas. Anaplastic thyroid cancer ranges from small cell tumors through carcinosarcomas, giant cell tumors, and epidermoid tumors. These tend to invade locally and behave much as malignant neoplasms in any other portion of the body. Survival is usually less than 10 to 20 per cent after one year.

Lymphoma and lymphosarcoma may also involve the thyroid. It is doubtful that this is related to the occurrence of Hashimoto's thyroiditis. The mortality rate depends upon the histologic nature of the lesion.

TREATMENT OF THYROID CANCER. The selection of patients for operation has been discussed above. Patients with a neck mass thought to be due to thyroid cancer, or those with a thyroid mass plus cervical nodes, should have *thyroidectomy* unless some contraindication to surgery is present. At surgery diagnosis is made on the basis of examination of the primary lesion by the physician, resection of lymph nodes, and examination of frozen sections. If the lesion is differentiated papillary cancer under 1 cm in size and is confined to the thyroid, a total lobectomy is done on the involved side, resection of the lymph nodes in the tracheoesophageal groove is carried out, and a subtotal resection is performed on the opposite side. If there is evidence of multicentricity, if the tumor is over 1 cm in size, if there is a history of radiation, or if it has metastasized to the neck, a near-total thyroidectomy is done, with preservation of the parathyroids by careful dissection or transplantation, and a homolateral limited neck dissection is performed. The extent of dissection is dictated by clinical findings and biopsies obtained at operation. In most instances a modified radical neck technique is employed. Occasionally patients will present with metastatic disease. If there is proved thyroid cancer with a solitary metastasis, it may be profitable to extract both the thyroid and the metastasis, because some patients will survive for a long time. In preparation for surgery and after surgery, patients with thyroid cancer should be on thyroid hormone therapy in order to suppress endogenous TSH. Many tumors are TSH dependent, and this therapy will prevent growth or actually cause tumor involution over years or decades.

If there is definite evidence of lymph node involvement or metastases, the patients are given one or more doses of 50 mCi ^{131}I to ablate residual thyroid tissue. If uptake in the metastasis can be demonstrated by scanning techniques after stimulation by endogenous or exogenous TSH, then patients are given courses of approximately 150 mCi of radioactive iodide-131 at intervals of 3 to 12 months (Fig. 10). Except when receiving ^{131}I therapy, all should receive thyroid hormone. Some spectacular cures of metastatic thyroid cancer are obtained by ^{131}I, but all too frequently tumor uptake is low or declines with treatment, and there is a gradual overgrowth of tumor which does not concentrate isotope. Invasive and metastatic papillary and follicular cancer may respond to radiotherapy. Chemotherapy is probably useful, but indications are not well defined.

Medullary thyroid cancer is treated by surgery followed by x-ray therapy to the neck, because this tumor rarely concentrates radioactive iodide.

Anaplastic thyroid cancer is treated by local dissection to the extent possible. A radioactive iodide scan should be performed, but it is most unlikely that these tumors will concentrate radioactive iodide. Roentgen therapy is

Figure 10. *A,* Chest roentgenogram demonstrating pulmonary and mediastinal deposits of functioning follicular thyroid cancer in a 43-year-old woman. *B,* Two years and 450 mCi ^{131}I later, the original nodules are invisible. However, nonfunctioning osseous metastasis has destroyed the body of D2, requiring a steel brace to alleviate spinal cord compression.

useful. After surgery, patients are placed on suppressive doses of thyroid hormone. Patients with lymphoma or lymphosarcoma are usually treated by surgery combined with postsurgical radiotherapy. The long-term survival is excellent in the lymphomas, and is perhaps 50 per cent at ten years in lymphosarcoma.

Recent reports indicate that the antitumor agents bleomycin and Adriamycin may be useful in treating thyroid cancer unresponsive to surgery, ^{131}I, or x-ray therapy.

Block, M. B., Roberts, J. P., Kadair, R. G., Seyfer, A. E., Hull, S. F., and Hofeldt, F. D.: Multiple endocrine adenomatosis type IIb. Diagnosis and treatment. JAMA, 234:710, 1975.

DeGroot, L. J., Frohman, L. A., Kaplan, E. L., and Refetoff, S. (eds.): Radiation-associated thyroid carcinoma. New York, Grune & Stratton, 1977.

Keiser, H. R., Beaven, M. A., Doppman, J., Wells, S., Jr., and Buja, L. M.: Sipple's syndrome: Medullary thyroid carcinoma, pheochromocytoma, and parathyroid disease. Ann. Intern. Med., 78:561, 1973.

Leeper, R. D.: The effect of ^{131}I therapy on survival of patients with metastatic papillary or follicular thyroid carcinoma. J. Clin. Endocrinol. Metab., 36:1143, 1973.

Mazzaferri, E., Young, R. L., Oertel, J. E., Kemmerer, W. T., and Page, C. P.: Papillary thyroid carcinoma: The impact of therapy in 576 patients. Medicine, 56:171, 1977.

Sampson, R. J., Woolner, L. B., Bahn, R. C., and Kurland, L. T.: Occult thyroid carcinoma in Olmsted County, Minnesota: Prevalence at autopsy compared with that in Hiroshima and Nagasaki, Japan. Cancer, 34:2072, 1974.

Simpson, W. J. K.: Radiotherapy in thyroid cancer. Can. Med. Assoc. J., 113:115, 1975.

Walfish, P. G., Hazani, E., Strawbridge, H. T. G., Miskin, M., and Rosen, I. B.: Combined ultrasound and needle aspiration cytology in the assessment and management of hypofunctioning thyroid nodule. Ann. Intern. Med., 87:270, 1977.

547. ADRENAL CORTEX

Grant W. Liddle

547.1. THE ADRENAL STEROIDS AND THEIR FUNCTIONS

The function of the adrenal cortex is to secrete hormonal steroids, and the major disorders of the adrenal cortex arise from deficiencies or excesses of one or another of the adrenal steroids.

Table 1 lists the major adrenal steroids, their most abundant metabolites, their functions, and the clinical consequences of steroid deficiencies or excesses.

It has been known since the publication of Thomas Addison's classic monograph in 1855 that the adrenal cortex is essential for life. The two essential hormones are cortisol and aldosterone. The former provides resistance to a variety of stresses and maintains the activity of a number of enzyme systems; the latter enables the organism to withstand salt deprivation. In the quantities normally secreted, all the other adrenal steroids may be regarded as relatively weak or inactive precursors, metabolites, or byproducts of cortisol and aldosterone. Cortisol and aldosterone are, indirectly, self-regulating, because each one is capable of initiating a series of physiologic events that result in the suppression of their respective stimulators.

TABLE 1. Properties of the Major Adrenal Steroids

Steroid	Regulated by	Major Metabolites	Methods of Measurement*	Major Actions	Clinical Consequences of Deficiency	Clinical Consequences of Excess
Cortisol	ACTH	Tetrahydro-cortisol Tetrahydro-cortisone	17-OHCS (Porter-Silber) Fluorogenic 17-KGS	Suppression of ACTH Protein catabolism Impairs glucose utilization Stabilizes lysosomes Suppresses inflammation Na retention K excretion	Hyperpigmentation (high ACTH) Fasting hypoglycemia Anorexia and vomiting Weight loss Apathy Impaired water excretion	Impaired glucose tolerance Thinning of skin Ecchymoses Poor wound healing Osteoporosis Weakness Hypertension Impaired growth Central obesity
Aldosterone	Angiotensin K, Na, ACTH Volume	Tetrahydro-aldosterone Aldosterone-18-glucuronide	Isotopic Radioimmunoassay	Na retention K excretion	Hypotension Hyponatremia Hyperkalemia	Hypertension Hypokalemia
Deoxycorticosterone (DOC)	ACTH	Tetrahydro-DOC	Isotopic Radioimmunoassay	Na retention K excretion		Hypertension Hypokalemia
Dehydroisoandrosterone	ACTH	Androsterone Etiocholanolone	17-KS	Weekly androgenic and anabolic	Lack of axillary hair in women	Virilization of women and children
Unidentified androgens	ACTH			Androgenic	Lack of axillary hair in women	Virilization of women and children
Unidentified estrogens	ACTH			Estrogenic		Feminization in men and children
11-Deoxycortisol (S)	ACTH	Tetrahydro-S	17-OHCS 17-KGS			
17α-OH-progesterone	ACTH	Pregnanetriol	17-KGS			
Corticosterone	ACTH	Tetrahydro-corticosterone	Fluorogenic			

*Methods such as 17-OHCS, 17-KS, fluorogenic, and 17-KGS are not specific; isotopic and chromatographic methods are used in specific identification of individual steroids.

Although cortisol and aldosterone are essential for life, when secreted in excessive quantities they can be life threatening. Beyond the scope of this chapter is the fact that supraphysiologic doses of cortisol and certain of its synthetic analogues can be used to modify the courses of a wide variety of nonendocrinologic disorders, particularly inflammatory and allergic processes.

Cortisol is the most important product of the human adrenal cortex in the sense that it is the one steroid that corrects most of the pathophysiologic effects of adrenalectomy when given in doses comparable to the amounts normally secreted. Cortisol is synonymous with hydrocortisone (the official pharmaceutical term) and, chemically, is 11β,17α,21-trihydroxy-pregn-4-ene-3,20-dione. It is closely related to *cortisone,* the glucocorticoid first produced synthetically on a large enough scale for widespread use as a therapeutic agent. Chemically, cortisone differs from cortisol in only one small detail: it has an 11-keto group instead of an 11β-hydroxyl group. This small chemical difference is extremely important biologically, however, for cortisone itself is lacking in biologic activity. It becomes effective in the body only because it can be converted to cortisol.

Cortisol is secreted by the zona fasciculata in response to adrenocorticotropic hormone (ACTH). A specific biosynthetic step that is catalyzed by ACTH is the conversion of cholesterol to pregnenolone (3β-hydroxy-pregn-5-ene-20-one). Pregnenolone is then transformed by a series of adrenal enzymes to progesterone → 17α-hydroxyprogesterone → 11-deoxycortisol → cortisol. An inborn error in one of these enzymes or pharmacologic inhibition of one of them diminishes the efficiency of cortisol production and results in hypersecretion of the precursor occurring immediately before the inhibited step.

Upon entering the circulation, cortisol is reversibly bound to an α₂-globulin, transcortin. The major process of metabolic inactivation is carried out in the liver and involves reduction of ring A: Cortisol → dihydrocortisol → tetrahydrocortisol → tetrahydrocortisol glucuronide. The glucuronide is rapidly excreted by the kidneys. Some of the cortisol is oxidized to cortisone and then reduced and excreted as tetrahydrocortisone glucuronide. Tetrahydrocortisol and tetrahydrocortisone are the two most abundant end-products of cortisol metabolism; together, they account for almost 50 per cent of the total disposition of cortisol.

A widely used method for measuring cortisol in biologic fluids is the Porter-Silber reaction, utilizing the chromogenicity of the product resulting from the combination of phenylhydrazine with steroids having 17,21-dihydroxy-20-keto side chains (17-hydroxycorticosteroids, 17-OHCS). Normally, cortisol is the only major 17-OHCS in plasma, and tetrahydrocortisol and tetrahydrocortisone are the only major 17-OHCS in urine.

Another simple method for estimating plasma cortisol is based on the fact that it fluoresces; the fluorogenic steroid method is not applicable to the measurement of tetrahydrosteroids. Urinary tetrahydrocortisol and tetrahydrocortisone can be oxidized to 17-ketosteroids by bismuthate and are, therefore, 17-keto*genic* steroids (17-KGS). This method is somewhat less specific than the Porter-Silber reaction; nevertheless, it is widely used for estimating cortisol metabolites.

Cortisol is ubiquitous as a physiologic regulator; hardly a tissue in the body is unaffected by this hormone. Cortisol influences the level of activity of certain enzymes. It restrains the secretion of ACTH by the pituitary. It accelerates the catabolism of protein and the hepatic metabolism of amino acids. It increases the appetite and promotes the deposition of fat in the facial, cervical, and truncal portions of the body. It retards the uptake of glucose by muscle cells and promotes hepatic gluconeogenesis from amino acids, pyruvate, lactate, and bicarbonate. It stabilizes lysosomes and suppresses a variety of inflammatory processes. It stimulates a number of electrolyte transport systems. As will become apparent in the discussions of Addison's disease and Cushing's syndrome, most of the manifestations of these clinical disorders can be understood in terms of inadequacies or exaggerations of the physiologic actions of cortisol.

Aldosterone is secreted by the zona glomerulosa in response to angiotensin, potassium, and ACTH. Like cortisol, it is metabolized by the liver to an inactive tetrahydro derivative; but, in addition, about 10 per cent is conjugated by the liver and kidneys to aldosterone-18-glucuronide. This is an acid hydrolyzable conjugate which recovers its identity as biologically active aldosterone when exposed to acid, a fact which has been exploited in the measurement of urinary aldosterone. Aldosterone is extremely potent, and the concentrations encountered in clinical situations are so low that they can be measured precisely only with highly sophisticated isotopic methods or radioimmunoassays.

The physiologic effects of aldosterone stem from its property of stimulating transport of electrolytes by epithelial cells of the sweat glands, gastrointestinal tract, and, of greatest importance, the nephron. In response to aldosterone all these tissues tend to conserve sodium and lose potassium. Aldosterone deficiency leads to sodium depletion, loss of extracellular fluid, hypovolemia, and hypotension. An excess of aldosterone leads to sodium retention, expansion of extracellular volume, and hypertension.

11-Deoxycorticosterone (DOC) is normally secreted at about the same rate as aldosterone (of the order of 0.1 mg per day), but since it has only about one thirtieth the mineralocorticoid potency of aldosterone it is usually of little physiologic importance. DOC normally occurs in the biosynthetic pathway as a precursor of corticosterone and aldosterone, but in certain varieties of congenital adrenal hyperplasia it may be secreted in quantities sufficient to cause hypertension. It is metabolized to tetrahydro-DOC, but the quantities of either DOC or its metabolite that appear in biologic fluids are so small that isotopic techniques are usually required to measure them.

Dehydroisoandrosterone, a weakly androgenic 17-ketosteroid, is the most abundant steroid secreted in response to ACTH. A small portion is excreted as such; some is excreted in the form of androsterone and etiocholanolone; a minute portion is converted to testosterone. Dehydroisoandrosterone is the major precursor of the urinary 17-ketosteroids. Except in states in which it is secreted in grossly excessive quantities, such as virilizing congenital adrenal hyperplasia, it is of little physiologic importance.

11-Deoxycortisol (Reichstein's substance S) is the immediate precursor of cortisol and is, therefore, produced in response to ACTH. Normally, it is retained by the adrenal long enough to undergo 11β-hydroxylation, resulting in formation of cortisol. Inefficiency of 11β-hydroxylase can occur as an inborn error of metabolism (hypertensive congenital adrenal hyperplasia), in carcinomatous adrenals, and as a consequence of treatment with an 11β-hydroxylase inhibitor (metyrapone). It has little biologic activity. Like cortisol it has a 17,21-dihydroxy-20-ketone side chain and is, therefore, measurable either as a 17-OHCS or as a 17-KGS.

17α-Hydroxyprogesterone is the cortisol precursor preceding the formation of 11-deoxycortisol and is under the regulatory control of ACTH. It has little biologic activity, and probably has no important role in the clinical manifestations of virilizing congenital adrenal hyperplasia. It is normally secreted in trivial quantities, but in the most common variety of congenital adrenal hyperplasia (21-hydroxylase deficiency) it is secreted in large amounts. This steroid is metabolized to a tetrahydro derivative, pregnanetriol, which is excreted in the urine and is of diagnostic value: a large excess of urinary pregnanetriol is practically pathognomonic of virilizing congenital adrenal hyperplasia owing to 21-hydroxylase deficiency. Although pregnanetriol is not a 17-OHCS by the Porter-Silber reaction, it is a 17-KGS and thus contributes to the nonspecificity of the latter as an index of cortisol production.

547.2. REGULATION OF ADRENAL STEROID SECRETION

The adrenal cortex may be regarded as two related but distinct organs. The inner portion of the cortex (zona fasciculata and zona reticularis) is under the control of ACTH and secretes all the adrenal steroids except aldosterone. The outer portion of the cortex (zona glomerulosa) secretes aldosterone in response to angiotensin, potassium, and ACTH.

ACTH activates adrenal adenyl cyclase, stimulating the formation of adenosine-3',5'-monophosphate (cyclic AMP). Cyclic AMP is thought to activate an enzyme system that catalyzes the conversion of cholesterol to 20α-hydroxy-cholesterol, which in turn is converted to pregnenolone. The latter serves as a precursor for all hormonal steroids. The pattern of steroids secreted depends upon the enzymatic makeup of the adrenal cortex. Under normal circumstances the most abundant secretory products of the human adrenal cortex are cortisol and dehydroisoandrosterone, but a deficiency of one of the enzymes involved in the conversion of pregnenolone to its normal derivatives results in increased secretion of the biosynthetic intermediates occurring before the impaired step. Such distortions of adrenal secretory patterns are observed in congenital adrenal hyperplasia, in certain adrenal neoplasms, and during treatment with pharmacologic inhibitors of adrenal enzymes.

Since the secretory activity of the adrenal cortex is directly controlled by ACTH, many questions concerning the regulation of adrenal steroid secretion can be transformed into questions of what controls the secretion of ACTH. In brief, there are three major determinants of ACTH secretion in man. The *first* of these is the level of cortisol. Of all the products of the human adrenal cortex, only cortisol has significant ACTH-regulating potency. The higher the cortisol level, the greater is its restraining influence on ACTH secretion; the lower the cortisol level, the less the restraint on ACTH secretion. A *second* factor governing the secretion of ACTH is the sleep schedule. In people in the habit of sleeping at night, plasma ACTH (and cortisol secretion) begins to rise at about 2 A.M. It crests at about the time of awakening; then during the day it falls irregularly to low values during the evening. Thus there is a "diurnal rhythm" in the secretion of ACTH. The *third* factor governing the secretion of ACTH has been referred to as stress. Such experiences as pyrogenic reactions, acute hypoglycemia, electroconvulsive treatments, and major surgical operations bring about increases in ACTH secretion. Corticotropin-releasing factor (CRF), of hypothalamic origin, is thought to stimulate ACTH secretion (thus mediating the diurnal rhythm and the response to stress). The action of CRF on the pituitary is thought to be counteracted by cortisol.

For practical purposes, in people with normal adrenal responsiveness, the plasma cortisol concentration can be used as an indirect index of ACTH secretion. Within the physiologic range of ACTH concentrations the adrenal response is directly proportional to the amount of ACTH reaching it. The cortisol secretory response to ACTH begins within minutes and continues as long as the plasma ACTH concentration is maintained. Once ACTH secretion has ceased, the plasma ACTH concentration falls with a half-time of about ten minutes; and once cortisol secretion has ceased, the plasma cortisol concentration falls with a half-time of one to two hours.

The secretion of aldosterone is only partially under the control of ACTH. Large amounts of ACTH induce increases in aldosterone transiently; but if ACTH is administered for more than two or three days, aldosterone secretion diminishes to pretreatment levels. Aldosterone is also influenced by potassium; depletion of bodily potassium diminishes aldosterone secretion. Impressive increases in aldosterone secretion can be brought about simply by depletion of bodily sodium, thus inducing hypovolemia. Hypovolemia of any cause induces renal production of renin, which catalyzes the generation of angiotensin; and angiotensin stimulates adrenocortical secretion of aldosterone. It is currently thought that the renin-angiotensin system is the principal regulator of aldosterone secretion in most of the conditions grouped under the heading Secondary Aldosteronism (see Ch. 547.9).

547.3. ADDISON'S DISEASE
(Primary Adrenal Cortical Insufficiency)

INCIDENCE AND ETIOLOGY. Addison's disease has been estimated to occur with an incidence of 1 case per 100,000 population. It is usually caused by granulomatous destruction or idiopathic atrophy of the adrenal cortex. Clinical adrenal insufficiency usually does not occur unless at least 90 per cent of the adrenal cortex has been destroyed. The most common granulomatous disease destroying the adrenal cortex is tuberculosis, but, in certain regions, disseminated fungal infections are almost equally common. Idiopathic atrophy of the adrenal cortex is thought by some to be a consequence of an autoimmune process. All other causes of Addison's disease are decidedly rare. They include amyloidosis,

adrenal apoplexy, and destruction of the adrenal cortex by metastatic tumor.

PATHOGENESIS. From the foregoing comments, it should be apparent that Addison's disease commonly arises in association with other significant disease processes. Thus the patient with Addison's disease resulting from granulomatous destruction of his adrenal glands should be considered to have had hematogenous spread of a tuberculous or fungal infection, and should be carefully surveyed for evidence of an active infection of other organs, particularly the genitourinary and respiratory systems. Patients with "autoimmune" atrophy of their adrenals have an increased probability of having other diseases such as diabetes mellitus, hypothyroidism, and hypoparathyroidism. Patients with Addison's disease preceded by the nephrotic syndrome should be suspected of having amyloidosis.

The pathology of the granulomatous adrenal was described in masterful detail in a monograph written in 1931 by Rowntree and Snell. Of interest to physiologists in later years was the fact that the few remaining adrenal cells were often "arranged in adenoma-like nodules . . . suggesting . . . compensatory hypertrophy." All the pathophysiologic consequences of Addison's disease can now be understood in terms of deficiencies of cortisol, aldosterone, and adrenal androgen.

Cortisol deficiency results in increased pituitary secretion of ACTH and melanocyte-stimulating hormone (MSH), and these pituitary hormones are responsible for the mucocutaneous accumulation of melanin in classic Addison's disease. Cortisol deficiency also results in loss of appetite, loss of vigor, inability to maintain adequate blood glucose levels during prolonged fasting, inability to excrete a load of free water with normal rapidity, and inability to withstand severe or even rather minor stresses without going into shock.

Aldosterone deficiency renders the distal convoluted tubule of the nephron unable to carry out cation exchange at a normal rate. Consequently, there is failure to conserve sodium and excrete potassium normally. As a result of sodium wastage, there is depletion of extracellular fluid volume, blood volume decreases, blood pressure falls, cardiac output falls, and heart size diminishes. This process may culminate in peripheral vascular collapse, and is a prominent feature of addisonian crisis. Hyponatremia results from failure to conserve sodium and, as noted before, impaired ability to excrete a water load. Impaired ability to excrete potassium causes serum potassium concentrations to rise. If serum potassium concentrations exceed about 7 mEq per liter, disturbances of cardiac electrophysiology occur, manifested by sharp peaking of the T waves of the electrocardiogram and cardiac standstill in diastole.

Adrenal androgen deficiency is of no consequence in the male, because testicular androgen production suffices to induce adequate virilization. In women, however, the adrenal is responsible for a major portion of the total production of androgen, and loss of adrenal function results in a decreased growth of axillary and pubic hair.

The clinical manifestations of Addison's disease are usually insidious, and often exist in mild form, for several weeks or months before correct diagnosis leads to proper treatment. Throughout this time, however, the patient with severely compromised adrenal function is in jeopardy of fatal addisonian crisis, either through progression of the chronic abnormalities or through superimposition of some acute stress such as fasting (vomiting), injury (surgical operation), or infection.

The mechanisms of death are peripheral vascular collapse (shock) and hyperkalemic cardiac standstill; perhaps hypoglycemia plays a role in some cases.

CLINICAL MANIFESTATIONS. One can hardly do better than to quote or paraphrase the clinical descriptions in the monographs by Addison and by Rowntree and Snell, written before synthetic steroids became available to alter the natural course of Addison's disease. Addison wrote:

The patient, in most of the cases I have seen, has been observed gradually to fall off in general health; he becomes languid and weak, indisposed to either bodily or mental exertion; the appetite is impaired or entirely lost; . . . the pulse small and feeble . . . excessively soft and compressible; the body wastes . . . slight pain or uneasiness is from time to time referred to the region of the stomach, and there is occasionally actual vomiting . . . it is by no means uncommon for the patient to manifest indications of disturbed cerebral circulation. . . . We discover a most remarkable, and, so far as I know, characteristic discoloration taking place in the skin, — sufficiently marked indeed as generally to have attracted the attention of the patient himself, or of the patient's friends. . . . It may be said to present a dingy or smoky appearance, or various tints or shades of deep amber or chestnut-brown. . . . The body wastes . . . the pulse becomes smaller and weaker, and . . . the patient at length gradually sinks and expires.

In their experience with 108 cases of Addison's disease, Rowntree and Snell noted that asthenia, weight loss, gastrointestinal symptoms (anorexia, nausea, vomiting, and abdominal pain), and hypotension were almost always part of the syndrome. Hyperpigmentation was present in most cases and was described in such terms as "a suntan which does not wear off . . . tinged somewhat with blue or gray . . . dirty in appearance." The exposed portions of the body (hands, face, neck, and arms), points of pressure and friction, nipples, freckles, recently formed scars, genitalia, and creases of the palms often showed exaggerated pigmentation. Brown, blue, or gray spots on the lips and buccal mucous membranes were common.

Nowadays, earlier diagnosis and specific therapy make it possible to correct the compensatory hypersecretion of ACTH and MSH before development of prominent mucocutaneous hyperpigmentation, so that this manifestation may disappear in the patient who has been treated for a long time. Hyperpigmentation is not present in all untreated patients, so one should not take the position that the absence of characteristic hyperpigmentation rules out the diagnosis of Addison's disease.

The mental state of the untreated addisonian patient was frequently characterized as "asthenia, languor, exhaustion, or disinclination to physical or mental effort." Less frequently, irritability, confusion, and delusions were noted. Almost invariably the patients lacked the vigor to carry on productive lives.

Fever was not found in "uncomplicated" cases of Addison's disease. When it did occur it was attributable to coexisting infection.

It is of historical interest that the laboratory abnormalities of Addison's disease as listed by Rowntree and Snell were limited to such items as gastric achlorhydria, elevated serum urea, and delayed excretion of phenolsulfonphthalein and water. It was only later that hyponatremia and hyperkalemia were recognized as being commonplace abnormalities in the chemical profile of Addison's disease.

It is important to remember that Addison's disease often occurs in association with other diseases. Since the clinical manifestations of Addison's disease are shared by many other debilitating disorders, it is easy to overlook the possible presence of Addison's disease while attributing all the manifestations to some coexisting condition. Fortunately, it is now possible to establish with certainty whether a patient has Addison's disease with a specific test for adrenocortical reserve, and this should be carefully performed without hesitation whenever the possibility of Addison's disease seems realistic, for example, in any patient with a syndrome of hypotension, weakness, anorexia, and weight loss.

DIAGNOSIS AND DIFFERENTIAL DIAGNOSIS. To establish the diagnosis of Addison's disease one should measure the steroid secretory response to a standard dose of ACTH. A standard test, which has a number of modifications, all valid in experienced hands, is to give 50 units of ACTH as a constant intravenous infusion for eight hours and measure the resulting rise in plasma cortisol. Individuals with normal adrenal glands should respond with increases in plasma cortisol to at least 30 μg per 100 ml. Addisonian patients show little or no increase in plasma cortisol, which is usually less than 15 μg per 100 ml both before and during the infusion of ACTH. Intermediate (subnormal) responses are observed in patients with adrenocortical insufficiency secondary to hypopituitarism or prolonged corticosteroid therapy; these conditions can be distinguished from Addison's disease by demonstrating that repetitive treatment with ACTH, over several successive days, induces a stepwise increase in adrenal steroids until normal values are attained. Among the acceptable modifications of this standard test are procedures employing intramuscular injection of a good quality of depot ACTH and measurement of urinary 17-OHCS, 17-KGS, or 17-ketosteroids. The crucial point is that the patient with Addison's disease has little or no adrenocortical capacity to respond to ACTH (Fig. 1).

TREATMENT. The most important principles to observe

Figure 1. Urinary 17-OHCS: (1) during a control day and (2) during a day on which 50 units of ACTH was administered intravenously over a period of eight hours. In contrast to normal subjects and patients with Cushing's disease, patients with Addison's disease have low steroid values on both days.

in the management of Addison's disease are (1) that only two adrenal hormones, cortisol and aldosterone, are vitally important; (2) that the physiologic requirements for these two hormones fluctuate; (3) that cortisol substitution therapy should never be totally withdrawn unless it can first be demonstrated that the diagnosis of Addison's disease was erroneous; and (4) that sodium chloride must be administered in liberal quantities in order to correct extracellular fluid depletion.

Treatment of Addisonian Crisis. The patient in addisonian crisis is in immediate danger of losing his life because of glucocorticoid deficiency, extracellular fluid depletion, and hyperkalemia. Without delay, he should be treated with an intravenous infusion of physiologic sodium chloride; the infusion should be given rapidly, on the assumption that the patient probably has a deficit of at least 20 per cent of his extracellular volume (at least 3 liters in the adult). A water-soluble glucocorticoid such as hydrocortisone phosphate, 100 mg, should be added to the infusion. Within a few hours, if the electrolyte imbalance is corrected, the endocrinologic crisis may be considered to be over, and therapy should be adapted to meet the patient's current needs; if there is no stressful complication, the dose of glucocorticoid may be reduced to the physiologic range of approximately 20 mg of hydrocortisone daily; but if the patient is stressed, larger doses will be required. An attempt should be made to determine whether the crisis might have been precipitated by some stress such as an infection, and if so, this should be treated specifically.

If the diagnosis of Addison's disease has not previously been established and the patient's illness is suggestive of addisonian crisis, one should without delay initiate therapy and, at the same time, carry out a definitive diagnostic test for Addison's disease. Physiologic sodium chloride solution should be administered as outlined above. Instead of adding hydrocortisone phosphate to the saline infusion, one should add the potent water-soluble glucocorticoid dexamethasone phosphate, 4 mg. This will be equivalent to 100 mg of hydrocortisone in biologic potency, but will not obscure the adrenal response to an infusion of ACTH. To the intravenous infusion one may add ACTH in a dose sufficient to asure that the patient receives at least 5 units each hour for eight hours. Plasma cortisol should be measured prior to the addition of ACTH and again toward the end of the ACTH infusion. An adequate rise in plasma cortisol in response to ACTH excludes the diagnosis of Addison's disease; a negligible adrenal response confirms the diagnosis. As an alternative to giving ACTH intravenously, one may give a good preparation of depot ACTH; and as an alternative to measuring plasma cortisol, one may measure urinary 17-OHCS in evaluating adrenal responsiveness, as outlined under Diagnosis and Differential Diagnosis, above.

Chronic Treatment of Intercritical Addison's Disease. Therapeutic strategy in Addison's disease aims at simulating normal rates of secretion of cortisol and mineralocorticoid. Normal adults secrete about 20 mg of cortisol per day, and adults with Addison's disease usually require approximately 20 mg of cortisol (hydrocortisone) daily in the form of medication; it may be administered orally or parenterally in single or divided doses. Various synthetic glucocorticoids may be substituted for hydrocortisone, provided that proper adjustment is made for their differences in biologic potency.

Normal adults receiving unrestricted diets usually consume 100 to 300 mEq of sodium daily, and while on such diets they secrete approximately 0.1 mg of aldosterone daily. Aldosterone is not available for therapeutic use, but a synthetic mineralocorticoid, fludrocortisone (9α-fluorohydrocortisone), is available, and a tablet containing 0.1 mg taken once daily usually suffices as aldosterone substitute. Another useful preparation is *desoxycorticosterone pivalate*, a slowly absorbed suspension given intramuscularly in doses of about 50 mg (2 ml) per month. A patient who has a history of hypertension prior to the onset of Addison's disease may not require mineralocorticoid replacement therapy as long as he receives glucocorticoids and ordinary amounts of dietary sodium. No addisonian patient will do well, however, without an ample intake of sodium chloride.

Children with Addison's disease require smaller doses of steroids than adults. The daily cortisol dose should be about 12 mg per square meter of body surface. If the child's linear growth does not proceed normally, it should be assumed that the dose of cortisol might be excessive, and the dose should be adjusted downward. The dose of mineralocorticoid should be adjusted as necessary to maintain normal blood pressure.

Treatment During Stresses. The maximal response of the normal pituitary-adrenal system to extreme stress results in the secretion of 200 to 500 mg of cortisol per day. This is the dosage range of hydrocortisone phosphate to be administered parenterally to patients undergoing bilateral adrenalectomy or to addisonian patients undergoing extensive surgical procedures. Hydrocortisone phosphate administered parenterally in doses of 100 mg every four to six hours should suffice as glucocorticoid replacement therapy in any severely stressed addisonian patient. As the stress subsides, the dose of hydrocortisone should be diminished accordingly. For example, after a major surgical operation, the daily dose of hydrocortisone can usually be decreased by decrements of 50 per cent each day until the usual dosage employed in chronic substitution therapy is reached.

For one reason or another, severely stressed patients usually do not consume adequate diets. It is important that addisonian patients be given at least 1 liter of physiologic sodium chloride solution daily until they resume their normal diets; a particularly hazardous period in convalescence is that during which orders are ordinarily given for the patient to take a "soft diet" or "surgical liquids." During this period the patient often does not even take all that is offered and may become depleted of extracellular fluid.

Mild stresses such as minor surgical operations and injuries require only minor increases in corticosteroid therapy. Usually a two- to four-fold increase in glucocorticoid treatment on the day of the stress will suffice. Oral medications may be used if they can be retained. Again, it is important that the addisonian patient who is fasting or vomiting be given parenteral sodium chloride solution.

Treatment in the Presence of Infection. In the presence of infection, it is particularly important that glucocorticoid dosage should simulate the cortisol secretion rate of the similarly infected but endocrinologically normal person. Overtreatment might impair the patient's mechanisms for defending against invading microorganisms, whereas undertreatment might predispose the infection-stressed patient to addisonian crisis. As a rule, an endocrinologically normal person secretes no more than 20 to 100 mg of cortisol per day in response to infection. This then is the hydrocortisone dosage range that is appropriate for the addisonian with an intercurrent infectious illness. A practical rule is to be guided by the patient's body temperature. If it is in excess of 39° C, the dose of hydrocortisone should be increased to whatever amount is needed to reduce the temperature to less than this level. If the temperature is normal, the hydrocortisone dosage should be lowered until maintenance doses are reached. If the temperature is between 38 and 39° C, it may be assumed that the dose of hydrocortisone is appropriate (presumably between 20 and 100 mg per day). It is of utmost importance that infections be specifically diagnosed and specifically treated as quickly as possible.

Mineralocorticoid vs. Sodium Chloride Therapy. Mineralocorticoids are used in treating intercritical adrenal insufficiency in order to assist the well-fed patient in maintaining adequate sodium stores without taking supplemental sodium chloride. Ordinary doses of mineralocorticoids do not adequately protect the addisonian patient from sodium and extracellular fluid depletion during periods of fasting or vomiting. Once sodium depletion has occurred, it must be corrected by the administration of sodium chloride; if adequate attention is given to this matter, upward adjustment of mineralocorticoid dosage (simulating the normal aldosterone secretory response to sodium depletion) will be unnecessary. Patients who sustain losses of sodium chloride but who are still capable of retaining oral medication, e.g., patients who sweat excessively, may be given supplemental sodium chloride tablets in doses of 2 grams two to four times daily.

Identification Bracelet and Injectable Hydrocortisone. The patient with Addison's disease should wear an identification bracelet stating his name, nearest kin's name and telephone number, and physician's name and telephone number. It should also state: "I have adrenal insufficiency. In any emergency involving injury, vomiting, or loss of consciousness, the hydrocortisone in my possession should be injected under my skin, and my physician should be notified." The patient should carry a small, clearly labeled kit containing 100 mg of hydrocortisone phosphate solution in a sterile syringe ready for injection. Even if never used, the bracelet and kit are of educational value to the addisonian patient, who must understand that his survival depends upon the timely use of steroids.

PROGNOSIS. With the advent of synthetic corticosteroids the prognosis of Addison's disease became radically altered from one of almost certain fatal termination within months (rarely years) to one of normal activity and life expectancy. The well-treated addisonian patient should have essentially normal steroid and electrolyte values under all circumstances; therefore he should not be incapacitated or have his life expectancy shortened by the fact that he has Addison's disease. All of the author's addisonian patients are productively employed unless they suffer from some additional disorder which is in some way incapacitating. Addisonians must, however, face the perils of emergencies in which they are incapable of caring for themselves and in which they might depend upon the assistance of others to assure that the essential steroids and electrolytes are administered. Their prognosis might also be limited by other diseases sometimes associated with Addison's disease, such as tuberculosis, histoplasmosis, diabetes mellitus, or amyloidosis. Most of the addisonian patients who have been discovered since synthetic cortisone became generally available are still living, and there are no accurate data to indicate whether Addison's disease per se, when adequately treated, alters life expectancy.

ADRENAL INSUFFICIENCY SECONDARY TO BILATERAL ADRENALECTOMY

Adrenal insufficiency secondary to bilateral adrenalectomy is one variant of Addison's disease which should never present any diagnostic difficulty inasmuch as it is iatrogenic. Treatment is the same as that outlined under Addison's Disease.

547.4. ADRENAL APOPLEXY

Hemorrhagic infarction of the adrenal glands can occur in the course of meningococcal septicemia (Waterhouse-Friderichsen syndrome) or as a complication of anticoagulant therapy. The occurrence of hypotension in either of these clinical settings should alert the physician to the possibility of adrenal apoplexy, and treatment similar to that outlined under the heading Treatment During Stresses (Ch. 547.3) should be undertaken on an emergency basis. Specific treatment for the underlying disorder (meningococcemia or coagulation defects) should also be carried out without delay. If the patient survives, he may at some later date undergo a standard test for adrenocortical reserve in order to determine whether steroid replacement therapy can be withdrawn safely.

Although the adrenal glands are hemorrhagic in the Waterhouse-Friderichsen syndrome, hypotension, shock, and death in this condition are usually not attributable to adrenal insufficiency. Cortisol should be given in large doses, because it is impossible to rule out adrenal insufficiency within the time that is available to initiate decisive therapy; the patient who might have true adrenal insufficiency in association with adrenal apoplexy should not be denied the benefits of adequate cortisol therapy.

547.5. ADRENAL INSUFFICIENCY SECONDARY TO HYPOPITUITARISM

DEFINITION AND INCIDENCE. Since normal adrenal function is dependent upon the stimulatory action of ACTH secreted by the pituitary, it follows that any disorder in which the pituitary is damaged in such a way as to reduce ACTH secretion to subnormal values leads to secondary adrenocortical hypofunction. This situation is encountered in approximately 1 of 1000 patients admitted to hospitals. (See Ch. 543.6.)

PATHOGENESIS. Whether associated with tumor, infarction, infection, histiocytosis, surgical resection, or intensive irradiation, loss of pituitary function is attributable to loss of pituitary tissue or to interruption of the connections between the hypothalamus and the pituitary. The degree of hypopituitarism is variable from patient to patient, ranging from such profound deficiencies as to be incompatible with survival to such mild deficiencies that special tests of pituitary reserve are required to demonstrate an abnormality.

Absence of ACTH results in decreased secretion of cortisol and adrenal androgen, but aldosterone secretion remains relatively intact. Cortisol deficiency results in loss of appetite, loss of vigor, inability to maintain adequate blood glucose levels during prolonged fasting, inability to excrete free water with normal rapidity, and inability to withstand severe stresses without going into shock. Hyponatremia is commonly encountered in patients with hypopituitarism who have been given liberal amounts of fluid, and it is directly attributable to the difficulty these individuals have in excreting free water. If they are given glucocorticoid so that they can excrete water adequately, they can be shown to have the capacity to adapt to simple sodium chloride deprivation by increasing their aldosterone secretion sufficiently to enable them to excrete urine that is virtually sodium free.

Absence of adrenal androgen is itself of little consequence; but when adrenal insufficiency is secondary to hypopituitarism, it is usually accompanied by a deficiency of gonadotropins with secondary hypogonadism and a consequent decrease in testicular secretion of testosterone. Therefore, in contrast to Addison's disease, in which only the adult female shows evidence of androgen deficiency, in hypopituitarism patients of either sex are likely to exhibit manifestations of androgen deficiency.

CLINICAL MANIFESTATIONS. There are several similarities and a few important differences between hypopituitarism and Addison's disease with regard to their clinical manifestations. Like the addisonian, the patient with hypopituitarism "falls off in general health; he becomes languid and weak, indisposed to either bodily or mental exertion; the appetite is impaired. . .and there is occasionally actual vomiting." Fasting may lead to hypoglycemia, and hypoglycemic symptoms (including loss of consciousness) are probably more common in untreated hypopituitarism than in Addison's disease. A liberal intake of water may lead to severe hyponatremia and manifestations of water intoxication such as confusion, incoordination, stupor, and convulsions. Severe stress may precipitate peripheral vascular collapse.

In contrast to the addisonian, the patient with hypopituitarism does not show mucocutaneous hyperpigmentation (this abnormality, in Addison's disease, is a consequence of *excessive* secretion of the pituitary hormones ACTH and MSH). Unlike the addisonian, the patient with hypopituitarism can tolerate simple sodium deprivation without developing shock or hyponatremia. In addition to the manifestations of adrenal insufficiency, the patient with hypopituitarism usually exhibits manifestations of hypogonadism and hypothyroidism, and may show other evidence of pituitary or intracranial disease, e.g., erosion of the sella turcica and temporal visual field defects.

DIAGNOSIS AND DIFFERENTIAL DIAGNOSIS. The diagnosis of secondary adrenal insufficiency is established by the demonstration that cortisol levels in blood and cortisol metabolite levels in urine are subnormal and that they can be induced to rise to normal or above normal by repetitive treatment with ACTH over a period of one to three days. Urinary 17-ketosteroids are also subnormal, but rise in response to ACTH.

Primary adrenal insufficiency (Addison's disease) is easily differentiated from secondary adrenal insufficiency by the failure of steroids to rise substantially regardless of the dosage or duration of treatment with ACTH.

It is advisable to measure both plasma and urinary steroids in order to avoid pitfalls in differentiating secondary adrenal insufficiency from certain disorders of cortisol metabolism in which a normal relationship between plasma and urinary corticosteroids is lacking. Thus in primary hypothyroidism, hepatic insufficiency, and severe renal insufficiency, and during treatment with drugs that alter the extra-adrenal metabolism of cortisol (diphenylhydantoin, aminoglutethimide, amphotericin, o,p'-DDD, triparanol), the urinary 17-OHCS do not adequately reflect cortisol secretion rates and are falsely low in relation to plasma cortisol levels. In these situations, plasma cortisol concentrations accurately reflect cortisol secretion under basal conditions and in response to ACTH, whereas urinary 17-OHCS might falsely suggest the presence of secondary adrenal insufficiency. In contrast, there is a familial disorder in which plasma transcortin concentrations are subnormal, even though cortisol secretion rates, plasma free cortisol concentrations, and urinary 17-OHCS are all normal. In this situation, plasma cortisol concentrations alone might erroneously suggest the presence of secondary adrenal insufficiency.

Various clinical clues are also helpful in arriving at a correct diagnosis of secondary adrenal insufficiency, e.g., hypothyroidism with normal responsiveness to thyrotropin, hypogonadism with subnormal gonadotropin levels in plasma or urine, or growth failure with consistently negligible levels of growth hormone in serum (even after provocative maneuvers such as arginine infusion or insulin-induced hypoglycemia). Other evidence of pituitary disease, such as erosion of the sella turcica or a history of postpartum hemorrhage, should also alert the physician to the possibility that the patient might have hypopituitarism, subnormal ACTH production, and secondary adrenocortical deficiency.

A mild degree of ACTH deficiency can exist with normal or slightly subnormal plasma and urinary corticosteroids and normal or slightly subnormal responses to ACTH. Such mild degrees of ACTH deficiency are referred to as limited pituitary reserve, and are characterized by failure of the pituitary to secrete normal quantities of ACTH (and therefore a failure of the adrenal glands to secrete normal quantities of corticosteroids) in response to stress or to standard test doses of metyrapone.

TREATMENT. Secondary adrenocortical insufficiency requires cortisol replacement therapy in the same doses and under the same conditions as outlined for Addison's disease (see Ch. 547.3). Mineralocorticoid therapy is unnecessary. An identification card and hydrocortisone phosphate for emergency use should be employed as in Addison's disease.

If the patient suffers from hypogonadism, hypothyroidism, or diabetes insipidus, these conditions should be treated with androgens or estrogens, thyroid, or Pitressin, as outlined in Ch. 548.4, 546.4, and 544.2, respectively.

PROGNOSIS. As in the case of Addison's disease, the prognosis in secondary adrenal insufficiency is excellent if intelligent use is made of hormones for replacement therapy and if the primary basis for the hypopituitarism is not otherwise incapacitating or life threatening (see Ch. 543.6).

547.6. ADRENAL INSUFFICIENCY SECONDARY TO PITUITARY-ADRENAL SUPPRESSION BY CORTICOSTEROIDS

Prolonged administration of glucocorticoids or prolonged secretion of cortisol by an adrenal tumor in quantities sufficient to cause Cushing's syndrome consistently causes suppression of ACTH secretion and consequent adrenocortical atrophy. Withdrawal of steroid therapy or removal of the adrenal tumor results in adrenal insufficiency. Diagnosis should not be difficult in view of the physician's or surgeon's role in bringing about the condition. If the hypercortisolism has been severe and has existed continuously for at least one year, the course of pituitary-adrenal recovery may be slow, requiring several months for completion. Early in the course the basal corticosteroid levels, the adrenal response to ACTH, and the pituitary-adrenal response to metyrapone are all subnormal, simulating adrenal insufficiency secondary to hypopituitarism. Treatment consists of giving a physiologic dose of hydrocortisone, 20 mg once daily, to prevent symptoms of adrenal insufficiency. Over a period of months this dose can gradually be reduced to 5 mg daily and finally withdrawn altogether as pituitary-adrenal function gradually returns to normal. Until pituitary-adrenal recovery is complete, one should treat the patient as if he had hypopituitarism during periods of stress or infection (see Ch. 543.6).

547.7. CUSHING'S SYNDROME

DEFINITION. Cushing's syndrome is the clinical and metabolic disorder resulting from a chronic excess of glucocorticoids. *Cushing's syndrome medicamentosus* is a common iatrogenic disorder caused by any of several synthetic glucocorticoids. Spontaneous Cushing's syndrome, on the other hand, is caused solely by cortisol, the only glucocorticoid produced in significant quantities by the human adrenal cortex.

ETIOLOGY. Normally, cortisol is not secreted except in response to ACTH, and ACTH is not secreted in the presence of supraphysiologic levels of cortisol. Therefore the very occurrence of Cushing's syndrome implies a disorder in the regulation of cortisol or ACTH secretion: either the adrenal gland has acquired the capability of secreting cortisol in the absence of ACTH, or ACTH secretion is not normally suppressible by cortisol. There are three well-established causes of Cushing's syndrome. *First,* adrenocortical tumors can secrete cortisol autonomously, that is to say, in the virtual absence of ACTH. The tumors may be carcinomas, solitary adenomas, or (rarely) multiple adenomas. *Second,* certain nonpituitary neoplasms secrete ACTH, which stimulates the adrenal cortices to secrete supraphysiologic quantities of cortisol. This clinical entity is sometimes referred to as the ectopic ACTH syndrome (see Ch. 525). *Third,* pituitary function can become disordered so that ACTH is secreted in excessive quantities, thus stimulating excessive secretion of cortisol by the adrenals. This condition is referred to by the specific term Cushing's disease. The pituitary can be normal in appearance, contain a small basophil adenoma, or contain a chromophobe adenoma; regardless of the morphologic appearance of the pituitary, virtually all patients with excessive pituitary ACTH show similar patterns of ACTH secretion. There is loss of normal diurnal rhythmicity, relative but not absolute resistance to suppression by glucocorticoids, and increased secretion of ACTH in response to a reduction of cortisol levels to normal.

INCIDENCE: Cushing's syndrome resulting from adrenal tumor occurs in approximately 1 of every 10,000 hospital admissions. Cushing's disease occurs in approximately 1 of every 4000 admissions. The incidence of the ectopic ACTH syndrome is difficult to estimate, because it is frequently overlooked. There is evidence that ectopic ACTH might be produced by as many as 8 per cent of

visceral carcinomas. Careful screening of patients with nonpituitary tumors might reveal the production of ectopic ACTH to be the most common cause of hypercortisolism.

PATHOGENESIS. The major features of Cushing's syndrome are understandable in terms of the known actions of cortisol. When present in excessive quantities, this hormone accelerates the catabolism of protein and stimulates the hepatic uptake and deamination of amino acids. It also inhibits the transport of amino acids into extrahepatic tissues. As a consequence of these actions, prolonged high concentrations of cortisol cause clinical manifestations of protein wasting. Children show retardation of linear growth. Wasting of the integument and increasing capillary fragility result in ecchymoses. Cutaneous striae form in areas where the skin is stretched by an accumulation of adipose tissue. In extreme cases, wasting of muscle results in pronounced weakness. Wasting of bone matrix results in osteoporosis.

Abnormally high levels of cortisol alter the body's responses to injury and infection. Cortisol stabilizes lysosomal membranes, thus diminishing the tendency of injured tissues to perpetuate their own damage. It suppresses the sticking of leukocytes to endothelial surfaces, and diminishes the accumulation of leukocytes at sites of tissue injury. It inhibits the diapedesis of white blood cells and impairs their migration through tissues. In high concentrations over long periods of time, cortisol impairs antibody production and inhibits the proliferation of lymphocytes. Thus almost every aspect of the normal cellular response to injury or infection is suppressed by high concentrations of cortisol, leaving the patient with impaired capacity to limit the spread of invading organisms.

Cortisol promotes potassium excretion and sodium retention by stimulating cation exchange by the distal convoluted tubules. A severe excess of cortisol can result in depletion of bodily potassium to such a degree that hypokalemia, electrocardiographic abnormalities, muscular weakness, and impairment of renal concentrating capacity develop. Retention of sodium and elevated blood pressure occur. Steroid hypertension, like other varieties of hypertension, leads to left ventricular hypertrophy and predisposes the patient to congestive heart failure and strokes. Even without frank congestive heart failure, some patients experience expansion of their extracellular fluid volumes to the point of edema.

In addition to stimulating the formation of new glucose from amino acids, lactate, pyruvate, and bicarbonate, cortisol impairs the action of insulin in transporting glucose across cell membranes. Consequently, abnormally high amounts of cortisol tend to raise the level of blood glucose; this is most readily apparent in the prolongation of hyperglycemia after a glucose load; a minority of patients with hypercortisolism have abnormally high fasting blood glucose levels. Frank diabetes mellitus with glycosuria occurs in fewer than 20 per cent of patients with Cushing's syndrome (see Ch. 531.1).

Adrenal carcinomas that secrete cortisol usually secrete significant quantities of adrenal androgen as well. In men this is of no clinical consequence, but in women and children it gives rise to virilism. Benign adenomas that cause Cushing's syndrome are somewhat less likely to produce excessive quantities of androgen. Mild virilism, usually amounting to nothing more than acne, thinning of scalp hair, and some degree of facial hirsutism, is common in women with Cushing's disease or the ectopic ACTH syndrome. In these disorders the increased levels of ACTH result in increased production of adrenal androgens as well as cortisol.

Although Cushing's syndrome is due entirely to an excess of corticosteroids, one must realize that the clinical illness of the patient may be affected by other factors as well. This is readily apparent in the ectopic ACTH syndrome when the clinical picture is usually dominated by other effects of the ACTH-secreting tumor. These patients often have a degree of weakness out of proportion to the severity of their hypercortisolism, and they often lose weight, in contrast to patients with classic features of Cushing's syndrome. Many patients with severe hypercortisolism associated with cancer have no signs of obesity, cutaneous striae, or osteoporosis, but may have persistent hypokalemia as the initial clue leading to a diagnosis of Cushing's syndrome.

CLINICAL MANIFESTATIONS. The clinical manifestations of Cushing's syndrome are familiar to every physician who has seen a patient treated with large doses of a cortisol-like steroid for several weeks or longer. In addition to the picture of cortisol excess, there will, in some patients, be features of virilism and mineralocorticoid excess as well. The frequencies of various clinical manifestations in Cushing's syndrome are listed in Table 2.

General Appearance and Physiognomy. The typical patient with Cushing's syndrome has central obesity, with rounding of the face, thickening of the fat pads in the supraclavicular fossae, and thickening of the thoracico-abdominal panniculus (Fig. 2). In longstanding cases, the abdominal obesity can progress to grotesque proportions while the extremities remain remarkably slender. People with pre-existing obesity from other causes can, of course, develop Cushing's syndrome; under such circumstances it is difficult to decide on clinical grounds alone whether the patient has Cushing's syndrome and, if so, to what extent his obesity is attributable to the steroid excess. Patients with malignant tumors often show little or no obesity, even though their steroid levels are high and other features of Cushing's syndrome are fully expressed.

Cutaneous Manifestations. The face and neck often have a ruddy hyperemic appearance. Trivial trauma often results in ecchymosis. In advanced cases, the skin over the forearms and legs becomes thin, having the appearance of parchment. Slight injury to the skin can result in purpuric extravasation of blood; the sites of venipunctures sometimes show extensive subcutaneous hemorrhage. Removal of adhesive tape sometimes denudes the delicate skin of the patient with the advanced protein-wasting of Cushing's syndrome. Wounds heal slowly

Figure 2. The appearance of a patient with Cushing's syndrome (A) before and (B) one year after removal of an adrenal adenoma. (C) Profile, before treatment.

and often become the sites of indolent infections. In areas where the weakened skin is stretched by the underlying accumulation of fat (particularly the abdomen, shoulders, and hips), wide purplish striae may form.

The reaction to infection is attenuated in Cushing's syndrome. Superficial fungal infections, e.g., tinea versicolor, occur in about 20 per cent of cases. In more severe cases, bacterial infections are not well confined in the form of discrete abscesses of short duration, but are more likely to be chronic and to give rise to cellulitis and bacteremia. This is a dangerous situation which may escape notice, because the patient with Cushing's syndrome often has less discomfort and experiences less of a febrile reaction than would ordinarily be expected with a given degree of infection.

Largely as a function of an associated excess of androgens, acne and hirsutism commonly occur in patients with Cushing's syndrome. The hirsutism is usually slight, downy, and distributed over the cheeks and shoulders, but coarse hairs may appear in the beard area and on the chest and abdomen. In men, of course, this aspect of hyperadrenocorticism is unnoticed.

Reproductive Functions. Most women with Cushing's syndrome have oligomenorrhea. Although it is difficult to evaluate with certainty, many of them may have diminished fertility; however, this is by no means uni-

TABLE 2. Frequency of Clinical Manifestations in Cushing's Syndrome

	Per Cent
Impaired glucose tolerance	94
Central obesity	88
Hypertension	82
Oligomenorrhea	72
Osteoporosis	58
Purpura and striae	42
Muscle atrophy	36
Hirsutism	30
Edema	20
Hypokalemia (unprovoked)	18
Kidney stones	12
Psychotic mentation	6

form. Men with Cushing's syndrome are sometimes said to be troubled with impotence; this is certainly not always so, and might not be related to the hyperadrenocorticism when it does occur. Most men with Cushing's syndrome have subnormal serum testosterone levels, which rise to normal following correction of the hypercortisolism.

Musculoskeletal Manifestations. Children with Cushing's syndrome experience arrest of linear growth. If obesity in a child is associated with growth arrest, the possibility of Cushing's syndrome should receive strong consideration; continued normal linear growth is strong evidence that the child's obesity is not due to Cushing's syndrome. Insidious atrophy of the skeleton results in mild hypercalciuria and, in time, in frank osteoporosis. Severe osteoporosis of the vertebral bodies may result in bulging of intervertebral discs, giving the appearance of codfish vertebrae in lateral roentgenographic views. Compression fractures with anterior wedging of the vertebral bodies result in kyphosis and loss of height. Pathologic fractures of ribs and hips occasionally occur.

In severe Cushing's syndrome, muscular atrophy may progress to such an extent that the patient is too weak to rise from a squatting position without assistance. Muscular weakness is usually not noticeable in milder cases.

Cardiovascular and Renal Manifestations. Most patients with Cushing's syndrome have hypertension, the course and complications of which are similar to those of essential hypertension. Edema can occur as a manifestation of congestive heart failure, but in 10 to 20 per cent of cases, mild edema occurs in the absence of congestive failure.

Hypokalemia with hypochloremic alkalosis occurs spontaneously in about 10 to 20 per cent of the cases (usually those with the most severe excesses of steroid secretion), and may occur in others as a complication of diuretic therapy.

Renal lithiasis can occur in chronic cases of Cushing's syndrome.

Hematologic Features. Some patients with Cushing's syndrome have erythrocytosis, granulocytosis, lymphopenia, and eosinopenia.

Carbohydrate Tolerance. Impaired carbohydrate tolerance occurs in more than 90 per cent of cases of Cushing's syndrome. In the majority it is manifested merely by a failure of the blood glucose to return to normal fasting levels during the first three hours after a glucose load. In about 20 per cent it is manifested as clinical diabetes mellitus.

Psychologic Abnormalities. Alterations of mood are common in Cushing's syndrome. Many patients feel irritable and weep with little provocation. A few experience psychotic mentation with delusional content. A few patients are depressed, and some attempt suicide. Manic and hypomanic behavior may also occur.

DIAGNOSIS AND DIFFERENTIAL DIAGNOSIS. It is important for the physician to know when to suspect Cushing's syndrome and then how to prove or disprove the diagnosis, keeping in mind the need for economy and precision. Taken singly, the various clinical manifestations of Cushing's syndrome are not very specific. Thus only a minute percentage of all hypertensive patients have Cushing's syndrome; only a minute percentage of diabetic patients have Cushing's syndrome; only a minute percentage of patients with renal lithiasis have Cushing's syndrome, and so forth. The coexistence of multiple clinical manifestations greatly increases the probability that a given patient might have hypercortisolism. If one encounters a patient with a single manifestation of Cushing's syndrome, he should always ask himself if hypercortisolism could be present; but if no other symptoms or signs of the syndrome can be found in the course of a complete medical evaluation, it will usually be unrewarding to pursue this line of investigation. Here we are discussing only probabilities, and should recognize that rare examples of hypercortisolism have been unequivocally diagnosed in the virtual absence of clinical manifestations.

Under certain conditions, one can make a clinical diagnosis quite confidently. For example, a patient with protein wasting (osteoporosis, easily denuded skin) and centripetal obesity probably has hypercortisolism. A child who simultaneously develops central obesity and experiences arrest of linear growth probably has Cushing's syndrome. Osteoporosis occurs commonly in patients beyond the age of 50 and is of limited value in diagnosis in this group; but osteoporosis in children and young adults should make one alert to the possibility of Cushing's syndrome. Although impaired glucose tolerance, taken by itself, is not especially suggestive of Cushing's syndrome, *normal* glucose tolerance is rare in Cushing's syndrome (about 10 per cent) and is therefore useful in discounting the probability of hypercortisolism. Patients with tumors of any organ and unprovoked hypokalemia should be suspected of having hypercortisolism, regardless of lack of obesity or signs of protein wasting.

Whenever the suspicion of Cushing's syndrome cannot be dismissed confidently, one should proceed with assays of plasma cortisol or urinary 17-hydroxycorticosteroids under basal conditions and during treatment with standard small doses of dexamethasone. At this point, a reliable laboratory with well-established ranges of normal values is indispensable. Equally important is close supervision of the patient so that specimens are collected properly, so that stresses or medications which might lead to high steroid values are avoided, and so that the physician knows that the dexamethasone is taken as prescribed.

Normal subjects have plasma cortisol concentrations of 8 to 25 μg per 100 ml in the morning and less than 8 μg per 100 ml in the evening. Patients with untreated Cushing's syndrome almost always have plasma cortisol concentrations in excess of 15 μg per 100 ml at all times. Normal subjects have urinary 17-OHCS of 3 to 7 mg per gram of urinary creatinine. Patients with untreated Cushing's syndrome almost always have urinary 17-OHCS in excess of 10 mg per gram of creatinine.

In response to small doses of dexamethasone (0.5 mg every six hours for two days), normal subjects show decreases in plasma cortisol to less than 5 μg per 100 ml and excrete less than 2 mg of 17-OHCS per gram of creatinine. Under similar conditions, patients with Cushing's syndrome almost always maintain plasma cortisol concentrations above 8 μg per 100 ml and excrete more than 3 mg of 17-OHCS per gram of creatinine.

Having established the fact that a patient has hypercortisolism, the physician must then determine whether it is caused by autonomous adrenal function, ectopic secretion of ACTH, or inappropriate secretion of pituitary ACTH. There are many useful guides in making this differential diagnosis, but the most reliable approach is to perform a large-dose dexamethasone suppression test and then, if pituitary-adrenal suppressibility cannot be demonstrated, to perform an assay for plasma ACTH if this measurement is available. The purpose of the large dose of dexamethasone is to determine whether adrenal function is under pituitary control. In almost all cases of Cushing's syndrome caused by inappropriate secretion of ACTH by the pituitary, it is possible to suppress adrenal function distinctly and reproducibly (through not necessarily profoundly) by administering dexamethasone in doses of 2 mg every six hours for two days. If a distinct, reproducible decrease in adrenal function does not occur, one should assume that adrenal function is autonomous or that it is under the control of ectopic ACTH. The distinction between these two disorders can be made by assaying plasma ACTH. In patients with autonomous adrenal function, plasma ACTH concentrations should be subnormal; but in patients with the ectopic ACTH syndrome plasma ACTH is high-normal or distinctly elevated (Fig. 3). The reason for emphasizing the importance of reproducibility in the large-dose dexamethasone suppression test is to avoid diagnostic errors that might result if spontaneous decreases in tumor activity should occur or if inadequate urine collections happen to be made at the same time as the administration of dexamethasone. Such coincidences should not be reproducible, but suppression of pituitary ACTH secretion should be. Frequently it is unnecessary to carry out the large-dose dexamethasone test, because all the information one requires can be derived from an analysis of the results of the small-dose test. Many patients with an excess of pituitary ACTH show partial suppression of their steroid output in response to 0.5 mg of dexamethasone every six hours. Definite, reproducible suppression of adrenal function with any dose of dexamethasone implies that adrenal function is under the control of the pituitary.

Blind reliance upon a single set of laboratory values is not to be recommended; for example, high levels of estrogen, such as those encountered in pregnancy or during treatment with oral contraceptives, lead to elevations of plasma cortisol by raising the concentration of cortisol-binding globulin, but there is no increase in cortisol secretion rate or in urinary 17-OHCS. Hyperthyroidism can lead to accelerated removal of cortisol from the circulation and a compensatory increase in cortisol secretion rate, accompanied by an increase in urinary 17-OHCS, but plasma 17-OHCS values are not elevated. Awareness of the total clinical condition and use of more than one dimension in evaluating adrenal function should protect one from making diagnostic errors.

Although the approach described above is the most economical and reliable method of establishing a definitive diagnosis of Cushing's syndrome, the following points may often offer additional help (Fig. 4):

	NORMAL	ADRENAL TUMOR	"CUSHING'S DISEASE"	ECTOPIC ACTH SYNDROME
PLASMA CORTISOL	10-25 μg% RHYTHMIC	HIGH, NO RHYTHM	HIGH, NO RHYTHM	HIGH, NO RHYTHM
PLASMA ACTH	0.1-0.4 mU%	LOW	HIGH	HIGH
17-OHCS RESPONSE TO ACTH	3-5 FOLD RISE	+,0	+	+,0
RESPONSE TO METYRAPONE	2-4 FOLD RISE	0	+	+,0
RESPONSE TO DEXAMETHASONE	0-3 mg/d	NO FALL	PARTIAL FALL	NO FALL
PLASMA ACTH AFTER ADRENALECTOMY, ON NORMAL CORTISOL	NORMAL	LOW	HIGH	HIGH

Figure 4. Typical cortisol, ACTH, and urinary 17-OHCS values in normal subjects and in the hypercortisolism associated with (a) adrenal tumor, (b) Cushing's disease (pituitary ACTH excess), and (c) the ectopic ACTH syndrome. (From Liddle, G. W.: Am. J. Med., 53:638, 1972. By permission.)

1. Patients with Cushing's disease almost invariably respond to metyrapone with increased secretion of ACTH and total 17-OHCS (the increase in 17-OHCS is attributable to a large increase in 11-deoxycortisol). Patients with Cushing's syndrome caused by adrenal tumor do not respond to metyrapone with increased 17-OHCS production. Patients with the ectopic ACTH syndrome vary in their responses; some show increases in 17-OHCS and others do not.

2. In patients with hypercortisolism, a grossly disproportionate elevation of urinary 17-ketosteroids is highly suggestive of adrenal carcinoma. The same may be said if more than 30 per cent of the urinary 17-OHCS are made up of 11-deoxycortisol and its tetrahydrometabolite.

3. Virtually all patients with Cushing's disease respond to exogenous ACTH with large increases in cortisol secretion; this is also true of patients with the ectopic ACTH syndrome unless their basal levels of cortisol are very high. Patients with Cushing's syndrome resulting from adrenal carcinoma almost never respond to brief infusions of ACTH. Patients with cortisol-secreting adenomas vary in their responses; about half of them respond and half do not.

4. Adrenal carcinomas are usually so inefficient in producing steroids that they do not cause Cushing's syndrome until they have become large enough to be readily demonstrated by intravenous urography or arteriography; some are so large that they can be palpated through the anterior abdominal wall by the time the patient exhibits Cushing's syndrome.

TREATMENT. The prime therapeutic objectives in Cushing's syndrome are to reduce cortisol levels to normal and to eradicate any associated tumors. Secondary objectives are to avoid producing hormonal deficiencies and to avoid making the patient chronically dependent upon medication. All these objectives can be achieved in some patients in each of the three categories of Cushing's syndrome. In many cases, however, compromises must be made. Sound therapeutic strategy begins with precision in diagnosis.

In Cushing's disease, ideal therapeutic results can be achieved in up to 80 per cent of adults by transsphenoidal resection of a pituitary microadenoma. In children, comparable results can be achieved by irradiation of the pituitary with about 4500 r. Microadenomectomy has not been extensively tried in children. In adults with Cushing's

SUSPECTED CUSHING'S SYNDROME

| NORMAL 17-OHCS PROFOUND SUPPRESSION OF 17-OHCS WITH DEXAMETHASONE 0.5 mg q̄ 6 h | ELEVATED 17-OHCS RESISTANCE TO SUPPRESSION WITH DEXAMETHASONE 0.5 mg q̄ 6 h |

NO CUSHING'S SYNDROME / CUSHING'S SYNDROME

NO SUPPRESSION WITH DEXAMETHASONE 2 mg q̄ 6 h / DISTINCT SUPPRESSION WITH DEXAMETHASONE 2 mg q̄ 6 h

HIGH PLASMA ACTH / LOW PLASMA ACTH / PITUITARY ACTH EXCESS

ECTOPIC ACTH SYNDROME / ADRENAL NEOPLASM

Figure 3. Diagnostic flow sheet for Cushing's syndrome.

disease, the "cure rate" in response to 4500 r has been only about 15 per cent. Why there should be a difference between adults and children with respect to radiosensitivity of ACTH-secreting microadenomas remains obscure. In either children or adults, failure to respond to the aforementioned modes of therapy usually calls for more aggressive therapy unless the hypercortisolism and its manifestations are so mild that they do not constitute a problem for the patient.

A technical advance in pituitary irradiation has been achieved recently through careful use of a cyclotron to deliver intensive irradiation to a sharply localized region. Through this means, it is possible to deliver 10,000 r to the pituitary gland with little risk of injury to neighboring structures. Information thus far available indicates that this form of therapy might cure at least two thirds of the patients with Cushing's disease; however, there is at least a small risk of producing hypopituitarism, a problem that did not arise in connection with conventional irradiation with less than 5000 r.

Only three other modes of therapy have been consistently effective in Cushing's disease. With each of them, normalization of cortisol is usually achieved, but the patient incurs life-threatening hormonal deficiencies which require lifelong substitution therapy. Bilateral adrenalectomy is most widely practiced. Substitution therapy with a glucocorticoid (and usually a mineralocorticoid) must begin at the time of adrenalectomy and continue for the duration of the patient's life. The principles of substitution therapy are outlined in Ch. 547.3. Subtotal adrenalectomy is not to be recommended because of the likelihood of recurrence of hyperadrenocorticism and the frequent impossibility of finding and removing all the regenerative remnant from a scarred mass of perinephric fat at a second operation.

Hypophysectomy and subtotal ablation of the pituitary by means of transsphenoidal microdissection, cryosurgery, or the implantation of radioactive gold or yttrium have been mastered in several medical centers. These forms of therapy carry the risk of producing hypopituitarism and are therefore not to be recommended for the young patient to whom reproductive capacity and normal growth are, obviously, important matters. When, in the course of an attempted microadenomectomy, it is impossible to identify a microadenoma, it would be reasonable to perform an anterior hypophysectomy if it has previously been ascertained that the patient does not wish to preserve reproductive capacity.

Selective destruction of the zona fasciculata and zona reticularis without the induction of aldosterone deficiency can be achieved with prolonged administration of the adrenocorticolytic drug mitotane (o,p'-DDD). This mode of therapy is attended by at least minor gastrointestinal side effects and entails the risk of producing virtually complete loss of glucocorticoid secretory capacity unless the physician is able to follow the patient closely enough to adjust the dose of o,p'-DDD so that plasma cortisol concentrations remain within the optimal range. The advantage of this form of treatment, apart from the avoidance of operative risks, is the preservation of the aldosterone secretory mechanism so that the patient is not so vulnerable to sodium depletion as is the totally adrenalectomized patient.

In the ectopic ACTH syndrome, ideal therapeutic results can be achieved only if the ACTH-secreting tumor can be completely removed. Thus far this has been possible in fewer than a hundred cases. In those cases in which the ACTH-secreting tumor cannot be removed, it is still possible to curtail the hypercortisolism by treatment with metyrapone.* This drug inhibits the final step in cortisol synthesis and leads to secretion of the biologically weak precursor, 11-deoxycortisol. One can start with small doses of 250 mg every eight hours and increase them if necessary to achieve the desired reduction of cortisol production (under these circumstances the simplest way to estimate cortisol levels is to measure plasma fluorogenic steroids). Doses in excess of 500 mg every six hours are rarely required. Bilateral adrenalectomy or o,p'-DDD therapy might be employed in selected patients in whom the hypercortisolism offers a more immediate threat to life than does the ACTH-secreting tumor. It should be borne in mind that o,p'-DDD so alters the extra-adrenal metabolism of cortisol that the measurement of urinary 17-OHCS is unreliable in evaluating cortisol secretion; the patient's progress should be followed by measurements of plasma cortisol.

The only completely satisfactory treatment of Cushing's syndrome resulting from adrenal tumor is the surgical removal of the tumor. Most tumors are benign and unilateral, and removal of the tumor-bearing gland is curative. It is essential that the patient be supported with glucocorticoids during and for several days after the operation, because chronic suppression of ACTH production will have resulted in atrophy of the nontumorous adrenal. A regimen similar to that employed during bilateral adrenalectomy is appropriate. Postoperatively, glucocorticoid therapy should be progressively reduced so that within a week or so the patient receives only 20 to 30 mg of cortisol per day. This supportive therapy should be withdrawn gradually over the ensuing year. It is possible during this period to give the entire daily steroid supplement as a single dose in the morning, thus permitting the pituitary-adrenal system to escape from the suppressive influence of cortisol for a portion of each day. On this schedule the daily dose of cortisol can gradually be reduced from 30 mg to 5 mg and then discontinued altogether. Throughout this first year the physician and patient should be alert to the possible need for increased cortisol dosage in the event of an acute stress. The principles of therapy in this situation are the same as those described for patients with adrenal insufficiency. After steroids have been withdrawn for a time, the patient's recovery of normal pituitary-adrenal function can be verified by a metyrapone test. A normal response should indicate that the patient no longer needs to be concerned about pituitary-adrenal insufficiency.

Approximately 5 to 10 per cent of patients with Cushing's syndrome resulting from benign adrenal adenomas have bilateral tumors. These patients require bilateral adrenalectomy followed by lifelong treatment, as for Addison's disease.

Although adrenal surgery is curative in some patients with adrenal carcinoma, a majority have either apparent or occult metastases by the time they seek medical attention. In about two thirds of these patients, the adrenocorticolytic drug o,p'-DDD will induce a temporary remission of hyperadrenocorticism, and about one half of these experience regression of tumor mass for several months to a few years. The dose ranges from 3 to 10 grams per day, depending upon the severity of gastrointestinal side effects. If measures to control growth of the tumor are unsuccessful, it is still possible to control hypercortisolism with metyrapone given in divided doses totaling 1 to 2 grams

---

*Experimental drug for this purpose.

daily. In patients with adrenal tumors, overtreatment with adrenal inhibitors can result in adrenal insufficiency; this can be avoided by erring on the side of undertreatment or by giving 0.5 mg of dexamethasone daily as a supportive measure.

SIGNIFICANCE OF VIRILISM IN ASSOCIATION WITH CUSHING'S SYNDROME. Clinical and chemical evidences of androgen hypersecretion are not uncommon in Cushing's syndrome. Although not a highly reliable rule, it is usually true that when a patient with Cushing's syndrome exhibits marked evidence of androgen excess, the cause is likely to be adrenocortical carcinoma. In other varieties of Cushing's syndrome, virilism is usually mild or inapparent.

The most important question to be settled early in the evaluation of any patient with virilism is whether or not this is associated with hypercortisolism, for virilism associated with hypercortisolism should be managed according to the principles outlined above for Cushing's syndrome, but virilism without hypercortisolism represents an entirely different group of disorders requiring drastically different treatment (see Ch. 547.10, 547.11, 548.3, and 549.2).

547.8. PRIMARY ALDOSTERONISM

DEFINITION, ETIOLOGY, AND INCIDENCE. Narrowly defined, "primary aldosteronism" is the constellation of chemical and clinical abnormalities resulting from the "autonomous" hypersecretion of aldosterone. The words "primary" and "autonomous" are employed to set this condition apart from "secondary aldosteronism," which refers to hypersecretion of aldosterone in response to a known stimulus such as angiotensin. Usually primary aldosteronism is due to an aldosterone-secreting adenoma (Conn's syndrome), but occasionally it is associated with adrenal hyperplasia or with morphologically normal adrenals (idiopathic hyperaldosteronism).

The incidence of primary aldosteronism is perhaps 1 per cent of the hypertensive population. It has been reported in about twice as many females as males.

PATHOGENESIS. Virtually all the features of primary aldosteronism are attributable to the fact that aldosterone promotes the conservation of sodium and the excretion of potassium.

Excessive conservation of sodium leads to expansion of extracellular volume, elevation of the blood pressure, and suppression of renin production. In the absence of circulatory insufficiency, modest expansion of extracellular volume leads to physiologic adjustments which enable the excretory system to come into equilibrium with the sodium intake; progressive expansion of extracellular volume is thus avoided, and overt edema is absent or only slight. (These adjustments are sometimes referred to as the "escape phenomenon.")

Excessive excretion of potassium can result in potassium depletion, hypokalemic alkalosis, muscular weakness, areflexia, tetany, paresthesias, electrocardiographic abnormalities (S-T depression, flattening of T waves, and appearance of U waves), idioventricular arrhythmias, and kaliopenic nephropathy, with impaired renal concentrating capacity that cannot be corrected by vasopressin. Despite the hypokalemia, urinary potassium excretion usually exceeds 30 mEq per day. Since potassium secretion in the distal nephron is, in part, a function of the quantity

of fluid reaching that portion of the nephron, a high sodium intake tends to exaggerate the potassium-wasting process, and a low sodium intake tends to mask it.

The action of aldosterone in promoting the conservation of sodium and the rejection of potassium is observable not only in the kidney but in all epithelialized organ systems which carry on cation exchange. Thus in hyperaldosteronism one can often demonstrate depression of the sodium:potassium ratio in sweat, saliva, and gastrointestinal secretions.

Apart from the relatively rare patients who develop alarming ventricular arrhythmias or incapacitating muscular weakness as a result of potassium depletion, the great dangers of primary aldosteronism are the common complications of hypertensive cardiovascular disease: cardiac hypertrophy, congestive heart failure, strokes, and progressive impairment of renal function. Although uncommon, malignant hypertension can occur as a complication of primary aldosteronism and can be associated with either elevated or suppressed plasma renin activity.

CLINICAL MANIFESTATIONS. All patients who have been proved to have primary aldosteronism have had hypertension. This is somewhat tautologic because physicians do not usually consider the diagnosis in the absence of hypertension. Nevertheless, the clinical importance of primary aldosteronism is in the main related to hypertension and its sequelae. There are no characteristics of the hypertension of primary aldosteronism that are helpful in distinguishing it from "essential" hypertension.

The coexistence of hypertension and *unprovoked* hypokalemia is highly suggestive of primary aldosteronism. Indeed, in some studies as many as 50 per cent of patients with this combination of abnormalities have ultimately been shown to have primary aldosteronism. In a large percentage of patients the hypokalemia is asymptomatic. In an uncertain but probably small percentage it is not demonstrable at all. The clinical manifestations of potassium depletion have been summarized under Pathogenesis. Another possible consequence of potassium depletion in primary aldosteronism is impairment of carbohydrate tolerance.

DIAGNOSIS AND DIFFERENTIAL DIAGNOSIS. In practice, the diagnosis of primary aldosteronism usually begins with the recognition that the patient has hypertension. Serum potassium should be determined on several occasions while the patient is on a liberal sodium intake and is not receiving kaliuretic drugs (diuretics) or experiencing diarrhea or vomiting. The finding of unprovoked hypokalemia in association with hypertension calls for measurements of aldosterone and renin. If the aldosterone secretion rate, urinary aldosterone excretion rate, and plasma aldosterone concentration are elevated, it may be assumed that the patient has either primary or secondary aldosteronism. If plasma renin activity is suppressed while aldosterone remains elevated, one may assume that the patient has primary rather than secondary aldosteronism. Anecdotal evidence indicates that some patients have coexistent primary and secondary aldosteronism, but it is impossible to diagnose primary aldosteronism with certainty until the secondary aldosteronism has been corrected and it can be demonstrated that the hypersecretion of aldosterone persists in spite of subnormal plasma renin activity.

Hypokalemia is not an essential feature of primary aldosteronism but the diagnosis is not easy to establish in its absence, when total reliance must be placed on the aldosterone and renin determinations. There is no substitute for a sophisticated and reliable laboratory if one is to practice competently in this area of medicine.

Conditions that can lead to concomitant hypertension and hypokalemia include malignant hypertension, Cushing's syndrome (especially the ectopic ACTH syndrome), congenital adrenal hyperplasia caused by 17-hydroxylase deficiency or 11-hydroxylase deficiency (see below), ingestion of large quantities of licorice, and a familial renal disorder simulating primary aldosteronism but with negligible aldosterone secretion (Liddle, Bledsoe, and Coppage). Except for the last condition, all these disorders should be recognizable in the course of a routine evaluation, which includes a determination of 17-OHCS.

Once the diagnosis of primary aldosteronism has been established by demonstrating that, under carefully standardized conditions, the patient has an abnormally high aldosterone secretion rate, plasma aldosterone, and urinary aldosterone, in combination with an abnormally low plasma renin activity, one would like to know whether the hypersecretion of aldosterone is unilateral or bilateral. If the source of aldosterone is a unilateral adenoma, the condition can usually be cured by unilateral adrenalectomy with the expectation that the contralateral adrenal gland will then function normally. If the source of aldosterone is bilateral (with or without adenomas), the disorder usually cannot be surgically corrected short of bilateral adrenalectomy, and this is too high a price to pay in view of the fact that medical therapy with the mineralocorticoid antagonist spironolactone will generally correct both the hypokalemia and the hypertension of primary aldosteronism.

The art of distinguishing between unilateral and bilateral hypersecretion of aldosterone is still under development. Kahn and Melby have found it possible to determine which of the two adrenal glands contains an aldosterone-secreting adenoma by catheterizing the adrenal veins (via a femoral vein) and measuring aldosterone concentrations in the adrenal effluents before and after brief injection of angiotensin. This procedure is not generally useful owing to the extraordinary expertise that is required in placing the adrenal venous catheters properly. Adrenal venography has been used to demonstrate the location of aldosterone-secreting tumors, but this procedure carries the danger of rupturing the adrenal vein. Scanning of adrenals with radioactive iodocholesterol has been used to demonstrate the location of a small number of adenomas, but this procedure is not highly reliable and is still limited to a few centers where active investigative programs are in progress. Robertson has developed a computer program for distinguishing between unilateral adenoma and bilateral hypersecretion, combining a large variety of clinical and laboratory data, but the applicability of the program to patients in other medical centers does not yield distinctions having the reliability that Robertson found in his original study in Scotland, presumably because other medical centers employ somewhat different standard conditions for collecting and reporting their data. In summary, many medical centers still find it necessary to explore both adrenals surgically in order to determine whether primary aldosteronism is attributable to unilateral or bilateral hypersecretion of aldosterone.

TREATMENT. Unless the patient is a poor surgical risk, the treatment of choice in primary aldosteronism is surgical excision of an adenomatous adrenal gland. During the weeks prior to operation the patient's hypertension and potassium depletion should be corrected by treatment with the aldosterone antagonist spironolactone in doses of 200 to 400 mg daily. Unless preoperative studies have provided conclusive evidence as to the location of the aldosterone-secreting adenoma, both glands are exposed, inspected, and palpated before a decision is made as to what should be resected. If one gland is found to contain an adenoma, it should be removed, and the contralateral gland should be left intact. If no adenoma can be found, one gland may be removed and sectioned carefully in search of a small tumor; if one is found, nothing further is required. If a tumor is not found in the first gland to be removed, half of the second gland may be resected in search of an adenoma. Even if an adenoma is not encountered, the operation should be terminated at this point rather than risk permanent adrenal insufficiency.

Patients who are poor surgical risks, those who are unwilling to undergo adrenal exploration, and those whose hyperaldosteronism persists after subtotal adrenalectomy should be treated chronically with spironolactone in doses of 100 to 200 mg daily.

PROGNOSIS. Without treatment, patients with primary aldosteronism will sooner or later have the disabling and fatal complications common to hypertensive cardiovascular disease in general; they have been known to die of strokes, congestive heart failure, and renal insufficiency. Within several days to several months after the successful removal of an aldosterone-secreting tumor, 70 per cent of the patients become normotensive, 25 per cent exhibit significant lowering of blood pressure but not to normal levels, and only 5 per cent are unimproved. Correction of the electrolyte disturbance is uniformly observed after correction of the aldosterone excess. Adequate treatment with spironolactone is almost equally effective in correcting the hypertension and potassium depletion of primary aldosteronism, but not infrequently it leads to gynecomastia, impotence, or menstrual irregularity.

547.9.   SECONDARY ALDOSTERONISM

The normal response of the adrenal cortex to increased stimulation by the renin-angiotensin system is to secrete increasing quantities of aldosterone. The aldosterone, in turn, promotes sodium conservation and potassium excretion. The retention of sodium results in expansion of extracellular volume and tends to restrain further production of renin. Physiologically the sympathetic nervous system and the renin–angiotensin–aldosterone–sodium-volume sequence can be viewed teleologically as a compensatory mechanism designed to support blood flow by expanding extracellular volume. Thus severe dehydration, sodium depletion, hemorrhage, hypoalbuminemic states, and sequestration of blood on the venous side of circulation are all conditions in which venous return is diminished, calling forth increased production of catecholamines, renin, and aldosterone. Secondary aldosteronism, then, is not a disease but, rather, is a response of the normal adrenal to physiologic demands arising in the course of a variety of disease processes, notably the nephrotic syndrome and hepatic cirrhosis.

547.10.   CONGENITAL ADRENAL HYPERPLASIA

GENERAL   CONSIDERATIONS,   DEFINITION,   ETIOLOGY. Steroidal hormones are derived from cholesterol through a long series of enzymatically controlled steps. Each enzyme system carries the biosynthetic process one step along the pathway from ultimate precursor through an orderly series of intermediates to the final, biologically potent derivative. Many of these enzyme systems are common to both the zona fasciculata and zona glomerulosa, and some are important in the biosynthesis of gonadal androgens and estrogens as well as corticosteroids.

An inborn error in an adrenal enzyme system which impairs the efficiency of any step in the biosynthesis of cortisol or aldosterone can lead to congenital adrenal hyperplasia. Impairment of cortisol synthesis leads to a compensatory increase in ACTH secretion by the pituitary, and impairment of aldosterone synthesis leads to a compensatory increase in the production of renin and angiotensin. These tropic hormones stimulate the production of cortisol and aldosterone precursors and induce hyperplasia of the adrenal cortex. If the block in cortisol or aldosterone biosynthesis is not complete, and if the compensatory increase in ACTH or renin secretion is adequate, the resultant production of cortisol and aldosterone may be within the normal range. However, the chemical hallmark of an intra-adrenal enzyme deficiency would still be evident: a distortion of steroid secretory pattern with conspicuous overproduction of the intermediates that occur in the biosynthetic pathway immediately prior to the blocked step. The clinical manifestations of congenital adrenal hyperplasia are determined in part by the biologic properties of the biosynthetic intermediates which are excessively secreted and in part by the degree of deficiency of cortisol, aldosterone, or gonadal steroids.

Beyond the fact that the enzymatic defects that lead to congenital adrenal hyperplasia are genetically determined, little is known about their etiology. The pattern of familial occurrence is usually consistent with the view that congenital adrenal hyperplasia is inherited as a recessive trait. Within any one family, the same enzyme appears to be defective in all affected members.

VARIETIES OF CONGENITAL ADRENAL HYPERPLASIA. Thus far, six varieties of congenital adrenal hyperplasia have been described, each resulting from impaired function of a different enzyme (Fig. 5).

Deficiency of 20α-Hydroxylase. The first step in the conversion of cholesterol into hormonal steroids is 20α-hydroxylation. Impairment of this process results in clinical adrenal insufficiency and, in the male fetus, incomplete differentiation of the external genitalia. The adrenal glands are hyperplastic and contain high concentrations of cholesterol. This is an extremely rare disorder.

Deficiency of 3β-Hydroxysteroid Dehydrogenase. This too is a rare disorder; it is characterized by genital ambiguity in infants of either sex. The explanation for this is that these patients have impaired capacity to transform Δ⁵ steroids into Δ⁴ steroids. Cortisol, aldosterone, and the potent androgens are all Δ⁴ compounds; therefore these hormones are subnormal in this disorder, and affected patients have clinical adrenal insufficiency. Males have inadequate genital differentiation owing to lack of testicular androgen during fetal life. In response to increased levels of ACTH, both males and females secrete superabundant amounts of the Δ⁵ steroids, pregnenolone and dehydroisoandrosterone. Although the latter is not a very strong androgen, it is secreted in large enough quantities to cause partial masculinization of the external genitalia of the female fetus. Both males and females therefore have adrenal insufficiency, ambiguous genitalia, and ele-

GLAND	ENZYME	ENZYME DEFICIENCY RESULTS IN:	
		UNDERPRODUCTION OF:	OVERPRODUCTION OF:
Adrenal and Gonad	20-Hydroxylase	Cortisol, Aldosterone, 17-KS, Testosterone, Estrogen	Cholesterol
Adrenal and Gonad	3-OH-Dehydrogenase	Cortisol, Aldosterone, Testosterone, Estrogen	Pregnenolones, 17-KS
Adrenal and Gonad	17-Hydroxylase	Cortisol, 17-KS, Testosterone, Estrogen	DOC and Corticosterone
Adrenal	21-Hydroxylase	Cortisol, Aldosterone	17-OH-Progesterone, 17-KS
Adrenal	11-Hydroxylase	Cortisol, Aldosterone	DOC, Substance S, 17-KS
Adrenal	18-Hydroxylase	Aldosterone	Corticosterone

Figure 5. Summary of the enzymatically regulated reactions through which cholesterol is converted to hormonal steroids. A deficiency of each enzyme results in underproduction of certain important adrenal or gonadal hormones and overproduction of their precursors and byproducts.

Reaction Group 1
20-Hydroxylase
22-Hydroxylase
20,22-Desmolase

Reaction Group 2
3β-OH-Dehydrogenase
Δ⁵—Δ⁴ Isomerase

Reaction Group 3
17α-Hydroxylase
17,20-Desmolase
17-Reductase

Reaction 4
21-Hydroxylase

Reaction 5
11β-Hydroxylase

Reaction 6
18-Hydroxylase
18-OH-Dehydrogenase

vated urinary 17-ketosteroids (derived from dehydro-isoandrosterone).

Deficiency of 17α-Hydroxylase. Congenital adrenal hyperplasia resulting from a deficiency of 17α-hydroxylase has only recently been described; it is undoubtedly a very rare disorder but is nevertheless important because it represents a curable cause of hypertension. Cortisol synthesis is impaired at the step where progesterone is converted to 17α-hydroxyprogesterone. Androgen and estrogen synthesis, whether by the adrenal, ovary, or testis, also depend on hydroxylation at the 17α-position prior to cleavage of the 17-20 carbon-carbon bond. Thus impairment of 17α-hydroxylation leads to a deficiency of estrogen and androgen. The patient with 17-hydroxylase deficiency has subnormal cortisol production, a compensatory increase in ACTH, and a consequent increase in the secretion of 17-deoxycorticosteroids, the most prominent of which are DOC and corticosterone. The excessive mineralocorticoid results in hypertension and suppression of renin production; aldosterone production is subnormal. Estrogen and androgen deficiencies result in sexual infantilism and compensatory increases in gonadotropin secretion.

Deficiency of 21-Hydroxylase. The most common variety of congenital adrenal hyperplasia is attributable to a deficiency of 21-hydroxylase activity. This condition affects approximately one person in 10,000 of our general population. Cortisol synthesis is impaired at the step at which 17-hydroxyprogesterone should be converted to 11-deoxycortisol, and aldosterone synthesis is impaired at the step where progesterone is normally converted to 11-deoxycorticosterone. If the defect is severe, the patient during the first weeks of life may show signs of adrenocortical insufficiency such as salt-wasting, dehydration, hypotension, shock, prerenal azotemia, hyponatremia, hyperkalemia, vomiting, hypoglycemia, and poor tolerance to stress. Plasma ACTH and renin levels are high. Hypersecretion of 17-hydroxyprogesterone is of no clinical consequence, but it results in the excretion of a diagnostically specific urinary metabolite, *pregnanetriol*.

Adrenal androgens do not require 21-hydroxylation for their synthesis, and as part of the adrenal response to high levels of ACTH they are produced in excessive quantities. Chemically, this is reflected in excessive levels of urinary 17-ketosteroids. The clinical consequence is virilization. The precise clinical manifestations of virilism depend upon the sex of the patient, the age at which the androgen excess occurs, and the severity of the androgen excess. In the male fetus, testicular production of androgen is sufficient to bring about completely masculine differentiation of the genitalia, and even a large excess of adrenal androgen has no obvious effect on genital differentiation or growth. The female fetus, though lacking gonadal androgen, is nevertheless very sensitive to androgens. In females with virilizing congenital adrenal hyperplasia, an excess of adrenal androgen results in partial masculinization of those portions of the genitourinary system that are the last to undergo differentiation. The abnormalities include the development of a urogenital sinus, fusion of labioscrotal folds, and hypertrophy of the clitoris. In extreme cases the external genitalia may be so ambiguous that on superficial examination the patient appears to be a male with hypospadias and bilateral cryptorchidism. In general, female infants with the most profound deficiencies of cortisol and aldosterone (the so-called salt-wasters) are likely to have conspicuous genital abnormalities, and the diagnosis should be suspected at birth, well in ad-

vance of any clinical difficulty from adrenal insufficiency. Salt-wasting males, on the other hand, lacking abnormalities of genital differentiation, are unlikely to attract special attention until they are in trouble with vomiting, dehydration, and other consequences of adrenal insufficiency. A positive family history, however, sometimes assists the pediatrician in considering the diagnosis before clinical complications arise.

Unless he or she succumbs or is treated, the patient with 21-hydroxylase deficiency grows rapidly and becomes quite muscular; at some time between two and ten years of age, pubic and axillary hair appear; this is followed by facial hirsutism and deepening of the voice. Investigation at this time reveals that the bone age is advanced beyond the height age, which, in turn, is advanced beyond the chronologic age. Early epiphysial closure foredooms the patient to short stature during adult life.

Clinically, the male patient may appear normal except for precocious puberty. The untreated female patient, however, does not undergo true pubertal changes but simply shows slowly progressive virilization; she lacks the feminization, mammary development, uterine development, and menstrual cycles that are a part of true puberty in the female.

The definitive diagnosis of 21-hydroxylase deficiency is based upon the demonstration of excessive quantities of pregnanetriol in the urine together with *easy* suppressibility of pregnanetriol and 17-ketosteroids by administration of glucocorticoids. This maneuver aids in distinguishing patients with congenital adrenal hyperplasia from those with Cushing's syndrome and those with adrenal tumors.

Deficiency of 11β-Hydroxylase. The second most common variety of congenital adrenal hyperplasia is attributable to a deficiency of 11β-hydroxylase. Fewer than 100 cases have been recognized thus far. The final step in cortisol synthesis is impaired so that cortisol secretion is subnormal, ACTH secretion is excessive, and the biologically inactive precursor of cortisol, 11-*deoxycortisol*, is secreted in large quantities. Normally, corticosterone is secreted by the zona fasciculata in quantities of the order of 2 mg daily, but in patients with 11β-hydroxylase deficiency the final step in corticosterone synthesis is impaired, and large quantities of 11-*deoxycorticosterone (DOC)* are secreted. DOC is a mineralocorticoid having about one thirtieth the potency of aldosterone. When secreted in quantities of several milligrams daily, DOC induces hypertension. Renin and aldosterone levels are low.

Adrenal androgens do not require 11β-hydroxylation for synthesis, and they are produced in excessive quantities as part of the adrenal response to high levels of ACTH. The consequent virilization is similar in its pathogenesis to that observed in patients with 21-hydroxylase deficiency.

The clinical manifestations of 11β-hydroxylase deficiency are simply those of hypertension and virilism. Plasma and urinary 17-OHCS are elevated because 11-deoxycortisol and its tetrahydro derivative behave like cortisol and its tetrahydro derivatives in chemical tests based on the presence of the 17,21-dihydroxy-20-keto configuration. Despite the elevation of 17-OHCS, this condition should not be confused with Cushing's syndrome, because plasma fluorogenic steroids should be normal or low in 11β-hydroxylase deficiency, the elevated steroids should be *readily* suppressible by the administration of glucocorticoids, and the clinical features of central obesity, protein wasting, and impaired carbohydrate tolerance are absent. The history of lifelong abnormalities together with *easy* suppressibility of the high steroid levels should distinguish 11β-hydroxylase deficiency from an adrenal tumor.

Deficiency of 18-Hydroxysteroid Dehydrogenase. This rare disorder results in a selective impairment of the final step in aldosterone biosynthesis. As a consequence the patient suffers excessive sodium loss, dehydration, and hypotension; there is a compensatory increase in formation of the aldosterone precursor 18-hydroxycorticosterone.

TREATMENT OF CONGENITAL ADRENAL HYPERPLASIA. The major abnormalities in congenital adrenal hyperplasia stem from deficiencies of cortisol or aldosterone or both. Compensatory increases in secretion of ACTH or renin or both then stimulate overproduction of the precursors or byproducts of these important steroids. The rationale of therapy is to provide physiologic quantities of glucocorticoid and mineralocorticoid, thus correcting the deficiency state, suppressing the tropic hormones, and curtailing the secretion of steroid precursors and byproducts.

The technique of treatment is similar to that employed in adrenal insufficiency. For the first several days it is advisable to employ slightly greater than physiologic doses of glucocorticoid in order to hasten the involution of the hyperplastic, very responsive adrenal cortex. Thereafter only physiologic doses are required, and overtreatment must be assiduously avoided so that growth will not be inhibited.

In those varieties of congenital adrenal hyperplasia that are characterized by the excessive excretion of 17-ketosteroids, glucocorticoid dosage should be adjusted from time to time so as to bring daily 17-ketosteroid excretion to approximately 1 mg for each year of chronologic age, up to 12 years. More profound suppression of 17-ketosteroids is not necessary to prevent progression of virilism, but would be indicative of excessive glucocorticoid dosage. During intercurrent stressful illnesses, corticosteroid doses should be adjusted upward in the same manner and for the same reason as in treating adrenal insufficiency.

Several steroid preparations are available, and with proper consideration of relative potencies, effective routes of administration, and duration of effect, one can substitute one glucocorticoid for another and one mineralocorticoid for another at will. Many patients do well on approximately 12 mg of hydrocortisone and 0.06 mg of 9α-fluorohydrocortisone per square meter of body surface per day. In any case, the dosage must be adjusted to suit individual requirements; the objectives of therapy are to avoid adrenal insufficiency, to normalize 17-ketosteroid excretion, and to maintain normal blood pressure.

Certain therapeutic considerations are peculiar to the specific varieties of congenital adrenal hyperplasia. Mineralocorticoid therapy is required only for patients with salt-wasting varieties of congenital adrenal hyperplasia and not for those with the hypertensive varieties. Glucocorticoid therapy is not required in treating 18-hydroxysteroid dehydrogenase deficiency. Estrogen and androgen therapy may be needed to induce secondary sex characteristics in patients with 17α-hydroxylase deficiency, those with 20α-hydroxylase deficiency, or those with 3β-hydroxysteroid dehydrogenase deficiency.

Plastic surgery to correct gross abnormalities of the external genitalia should be carried out before the age of two years, by which time the child's psychosexual identity should be unambiguously established.

PROGNOSIS. Without treatment, patients with various salt-wasting forms of congenital adrenal hyperplasia are unlikely to survive infancy. Patients with the hypertensive varieties also have decreased life expectancy. Many experience psychosexual problems arising from pseudohermaphroditism in the females and precocious puberty in the males.

If recognized early and treated properly, patients with any variety of congenital adrenal hyperplasia should theoretically be able to live normal lives. This is true for the patients with 21-hydroxylase and 11β-hydroxylase deficiency, except that they have usually not attained normal height. It appears that reproductive functions can sometimes be normal if proper treatment is started before adulthood. It is of interest that a child whose bone age has advanced beyond about 13 years before suppressive treatment with glucocorticoids is instituted will exhibit adult pituitary-gonadal relationships (females will undergo breast development and establish their menstrual cycles) when glucocorticoid treatment is finally begun; this is true even if the chronologic age is only seven or eight years.

The other varieties of congenital adrenal hyperplasia have less favorable prognoses. In 17α-hydroxylase deficiency, reproduction will probably not be possible even though the hypertension can be controlled and all other clinical manifestations of steroid deficiency corrected. The survival of patients with deficiencies of 20α-hydroxylase or 3β-hydroxysteroid dehydrogenase has been unaccountably poor up to the present time.

547.11. VIRILIZING TUMORS

Adrenal tumors that produce a clinically significant excess of androgen along with cortisol have been discussed in Ch. 547.7. Somewhat less common are adrenal tumors that secrete androgen without significant quantities of cortisol. Most of these tumors are malignant, and the majority are large and have metastasized by the time they are clinically apparent. The clinical hallmark of such tumors is virilization; this manifestation, of course, is limited to children and women; adult males usually recognize no increased virilization as a result of even large excesses of the relatively weak adrenal androgens. The common chemical hallmark of a purely virilizing tumor is the excessive excretion of 17-ketosteroids. This is a remarkably uniform characteristic of adrenal carcinomas. Several adrenal carcinomas have, probably erroneously, been reported as being nonfunctioning simply because they did not give rise to clinical virilization. Evidence was inadequate to support this conclusion, however, whenever 17-ketosteroid excretion was not measured.

It is not sufficient just to measure urinary 17-ketosteroids; under basal conditions one should also carry out dexamethasone suppression tests and demonstrate that urinary 17-ketosteroids can reproducibly be reduced to less than 6 mg per day within three days before concluding that an adrenocortical carcinoma is nonfunctioning. Nonsuppressibility of plasma pregnenolone and 17-hydroxypregnenolone (with dexamethasone) may also serve as useful clues to the presence of adrenocortical neoplasms.

Suprarenal "masses" that are discovered accidentally during roentgenographic examinations almost never prove to be adrenal cortical tumors if basal 17-OHCS and

17-ketosteroids are normal and normally suppressible, and they almost never prove to be adrenal medullary tumors if catecholamines are consistently normal.

Virilizing adrenal tumor must be differentiated from congenital adrenal hyperplasia, Cushing's syndrome with virilism, ovarian tumor, idiopathic hirsutism, and precocious puberty. This can be accomplished by a history of late onset of first clinical manifestations, absence of Cushing's syndrome, presence of a palpable abdominal mass, abnormal resistance to suppression of 17-ketosteroids with dexamethasone, absence of ovarian mass, and presence of an adrenal mass on urography or arteriography.

Treatment is with surgical resection and with o,p'-DDD. A sizable minority responds favorably to each mode of therapy, at least temporarily.

547.12. FEMINIZING ADRENAL TUMORS

Feminization as a clinical manifestation of adrenal tumor is exceedingly rare. The most common sign is gynecomastia, and this is one of the least common causes of gynecomastia. The diagnosis is made by the observation of other signs of adrenal overactivity, e.g., hypertension, demonstration of excessive estrogen in the urine, and demonstration of a suprarenal mass by intravenous urography or arteriography. If positively diagnosed, the tumor may be treated by surgical resection, and, if this fails, with o,p'-DDD. Experience is too limited to support a generalization as to prognosis.

Addison, T.: On the constitutional and local effects of diseases of the suprarenal capsules. London, Samuel Highley, 1855.

Bartter, F. C., Albright, F., Forbes, A. P., Leaf, A., Dempsey, E., and Carroll, E.: The effects of adrenocorticotropic hormone and cortisone in adrenogenital syndrome associated with congenital adrenal hyperplasia: An attempt to explain and correct its disordered hormonal pattern. J. Clin. Invest., 30:237, 1951.

Baulieu, E. E., and Robel, P. (eds.): Aldosterone: Prague Symposium. Oxford, Blackwell Scientific Publications, 1964.

Blizzard, R. M., and Kyle, M.: Studies of the adrenal antigens and antibodies in Addison's disease. J. Clin. Invest., 42:1653, 1963.

Bongiovanni, A. M., Eberlein, W. R., Goldman, A. S., and New, M.: Disorders of adrenal steroid biogenesis. Recent Prog. Horm. Res., 23:375, 1967.

Christy, N. P. (ed.): The Human Adrenal Cortex. New York, Harper & Row, 1971.

Conn, J. W., Knopf, R. F., and Nesbit, R. M.: Clinical characteristics of primary aldosteronism from an analysis of 145 cases. Am. J. Surg., 107:159, 1964.

Cope, C. L.: Adrenal Steroids and Disease. 2nd ed. Philadelphia, J. B. Lippincott Company, 1972.

Cushing, H.: The basophil adenomas of the pituitary body and their clinical manifestations (pituitary basophilism). Bull. Johns Hopkins Hosp., 50:137, 1932.

Eisenstein, A. B. (ed.): The Adrenal Cortex. London, J. & A. Churchill, Ltd., 1967.

Gabrilove, J. L., Sharma, D. C., Wotiz, H. H., and Dorfman, R. I.: Feminizing adrenocortical tumors in the male: A review of 52 cases including a case report. Medicine, 44:37, 1965.

Glaz, E., and Vecsei, P.: Aldosterone: International Series of Monographs in Pure and Applied Biology. New York, Pergamon Press, 1971.

Graber, A. L., Ney, R. L., Nicholson, W. E., Island, D. P., and Liddle, G. W.: Natural history of pituitary-adrenal recovery following long-term suppression with corticosteroids. J. Clin. Endocrinol. Metab., 25:11, 1965.

Jennings, A. S., Liddle, G. W., and Orth, D. N.: Results of treating childhood Cushing's disease with pituitary irradiation. N. Engl. J. Med., 297:957, 1977.

Krieger, D. T., and Ganong, W. F. (eds.): ACTH and related peptides: Structure, regulation, and action. Ann. N.Y. Acad. Sci., Vol. 297, 1977.

Lee, P. E., Plotnick, G. D., Kowarski, A. A., and Migeon, C. J. (eds.):

Congenital Adrenal Hyperplasia, Baltimore, University Park Press, 1977.

Liddle, G. W.: Adrenal cortex. In Williams, R. (ed.): Textbook of Endocrinology, 5th ed. Philadelphia, W. B. Saunders Company, 1974, pp. 233-284.

Liddle, G. W.: Tests of pituitary-adrenal suppressibility in the diagnosis of Cushing's syndrome. J. Clin. Endocrinol. Metab., 20:1539, 1960.

Liddle, G. W., Bledsoe, T., and Coppage, W. S., Jr.: A familial renal disorder simulating primary aldosteronism but with negligible aldosterone secretion. Trans. Assoc. Am. Physicians, 76:199, 1963.

Liddle, G. W., Island D., and Meador, C. K.: Normal and abnormal regulation of corticotropin secretion in man. Recent Prog. Horm. Res., 18:125, 1962.

Orth, D. N., and Liddle, G. W.: Results of treatment in 108 patients with Cushing's syndrome. N. Engl. J. Med., 285:243, 1971.

Rowntree, L. G., and Snell, A. M.: A Clinical Study of Addison's Disease. Mayo Clinic Monographs. Philadelphia, W. B. Saunders Company, 1931.

Temple, T. E., and Liddle, G. W.: Inhibitors of adrenal steroid biosynthesis. Ann. Rev. Pharmacol., 10:199, 1970.

Thorn, G. E. (ed.): Symposium on the adrenal cortex. Am. J. Med., 53:No. 5, 1972.

Tyrrell, J. B., Brooks, R. M., Fitzgerald, P. A., Cofoid, P. B., Forsham, P. H., and Wilson, C. B.: Cushing's disease: Selective trans-sphenoidal resection of pituitary microadenomas. N. Engl. J. Med., 298:753, 1978.

548.   THE TESTIS

Mortimer B. Lipsett

548.1.   INTRODUCTION

FETAL DEVELOPMENT

The primordial gonad arises in the urogenital ridge from intermediate mesoderm during the fifth week of gestation. Early in its development, the bipotential primitive gonad (Fig. 1) is composed of two unipotential mesodermal primordia, each with a distinct physiologic as well as morphologic capacity: (1) a cortical component, consisting of the germinal epithelium; and (2) a medullary component, made up of the primary sex cords derived from the germinal epithelium, and mesonephric and blastemal elements. A third constituent, the primordial germ cell, which appears to be bipotential, arises in an extragonadal site and migrates to the gonads. Under the influence of the Y organizer, a surface protein of cells carrying the Y chromosome, the medullary component differentiates as a testis (Fig. 1). The cortical component can differentiate as an ovary only in the absence of Y organizer.

When the gonad destined to become a testis begins to differentiate in a male direction during the seventh to eighth week of embryonic life, the cortical component involutes. Within the medulla, seminiferous tubules form from the primary sex cords and anastomose with the rete testis and testicular ducts, and Leydig cells develop. Leydig cells proliferate predominantly during the first half of gestation, but then gradually decrease in number and involute after birth. Leydig cells acquire the capacity to synthesize testosterone, and this steroid hormone has been found in the fetal testis. At the time of pubescence morphologic differentiation of Leydig cells occurs, and testosterone production is greatly increased.

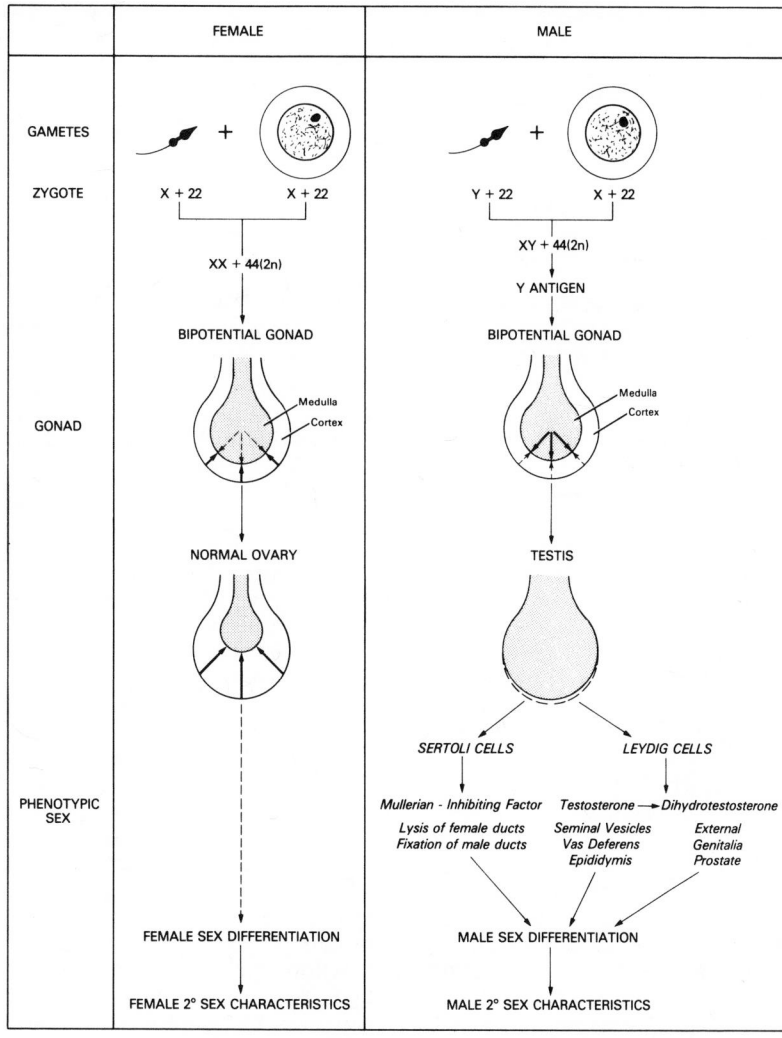

Figuré 1. Diagrammatic scheme of human sex determination and differentiation.

ACCESSORY SEX STRUCTURES

Recent experimental results and observation of fetal sex anomalies have now clarified the roles of fetal hormone. A fetal testicular morphogenetic substance, probably a peptide secreted by Sertoli cells, acts locally to cause regression of the müllerian ducts. Testosterone induces development of wolffian duct structures, the epididymis, vas deferens, and seminal vesicles, and dihydrotestosterone causes development of the prostate and external genitalia. Most disorders of sexual differentiation can be understood by reference to the separate actions of each hormone. These disorders will be discussed more fully in Ch. 548.4 and 548.5.

CHEMISTRY AND PHYSIOLOGY OF THE TESTICULAR HORMONES

The testicular hormone *testosterone*, secreted from the Leydig cell, has the primary role in the development and maintenance of the male accessory sex organs, prostate, and seminal vesicles, in the elaboration of semen, and in the development of masculine secondary sexual characteristics. These properties define a class of substances, the androgens; the important androgen secreted by the testis is testosterone. The 5α-reduced derivative of testosterone, 5α-dihydrotestosterone, is the active form of the hormone at the nuclear receptor within the male accessory sex structures, and is responsible for inducing growth of these organs.

The adrenal cortex secretes little testosterone. The weak androgenic potency of adrenocortical steroids such as androstenedione and dehydroepiandrosterone can be attributed to their conversion to testosterone in small yield.

The contention that testosterone is the principal testicular androgen has been confirmed by the measurement of this steroid in human spermatic vein blood. Healthy young men secrete about 7 mg of testosterone per day. From animal experiments in which the seminiferous tubules were destroyed without affecting the Leydig cells, it has been concluded that testosterone originates in the Leydig cells, although the seminiferous tubule has a weak capacity for testosterone synthesis. Clinical signs of androgen deficiency are absent in certain testicular disorders in man associated with defective seminiferous tubules but with intact Leydig cells.

Pathways for the biosynthesis of testosterone by the Leydig cell resemble those in other steroid-synthesizing glands. Precursors such as acetate and cholesterol are converted enzymatically to testosterone via 17-hydroxypregnenolone and 17-hydroxyprogesterone. The testis can also aromatize testosterone to estradiol. In adult man 10 to 15 μg of estradiol is secreted daily; an additional 25 to 30 μg is produced peripherally by aromatization of blood testosterone in other tissues. The Leydig cells and the tubules synthesize estradiol. Aromatization of testosterone to estradiol by the tubules is increased by FSH. Estrone, however, is predominantly a product of adrenal cortical secretions.

The liver is the main site of catabolism of testosterone and of the conjugation of its known metabolites with glucuronic or sulfuric acid; other tissues play a less important role in its metabolism. The major identifiable urinary metabolites are the 17-ketosteroids androsterone and etiocholanolone, which are excreted principally as glucuronides and account for 20 to 40 per cent of the testosterone secreted. A small amount of testosterone (0.2 to 2 per cent) is excreted as testosterone glucuronide.

The two functions of the testis, the synthesis of testosterone and sperm production, are under the control of the hypothalamic-pituitary unit. Luteinizing hormone (LH) acts on the Leydig cell to induce testosterone synthesis, although FSH may synergize to a limited extent. FSH is necessary to initiate spermatogenesis, but it is uncertain whether it has any other role in the process. An androgen-binding protein, similar to plasma sex-steroid-binding globulin, is secreted by the Sertoli cell and regulated by FSH in the rat. The function of this protein in the rat and its occurrence in man are problematic.

The Sertoli cell is a target tissue for androgen, and there are many data showing that the high concentration of testosterone in the fluid bathing the tubule is functionally important. In hypophysectomized man or monkey spermatogenesis continues if intratesticular testosterone concentration is maintained by human chorionic gonadotropin (HCG) administration or testosterone implants, respectively.

Testosterone exerts a negative feedback on LH secretion, although it is not clear whether the steroid combining at the pituitary and hypothalamic receptor sites is testosterone or one of its metabolites, dihydrotestosterone or estradiol. It seems likely that both androgen and estrogen receptors modulate LH secretion. The hypothalamus and the pituitary have the capacity to metabolize testosterone to dihydrotestosterone and estradiol. Plasma FSH also is suppressed by testosterone, but an additional factor, inhibin, a polypeptide derived from the Sertoli cell, also modulates FSH secretion. Thus plasma FSH and LH are high in the absence of Leydig cell secretions, but FSH alone is increased when there is severe seminiferous tubule disease. These relationships are shown diagrammatically in Figure 2. Prolactin, at normal levels, may promote Leydig cell function. At high levels, it apparently inhibits testosterone biosynthesis.

EVALUATION OF TESTICULAR FUNCTION

CLINICAL ASSESSMENT. Adequacy of androgen production can be estimated from the degree of develop-

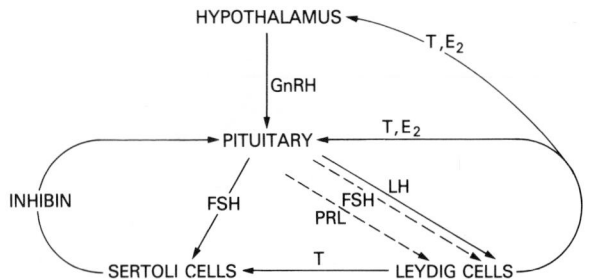

Figure 2. Diagram of hypothalamic-pituitary-testis interactions. Dashed arrows indicate probable action.

ment of the penis and scrotum, size of the prostate, general maturity and status of male secondary sex characteristics, habitus and skeletal proportions, muscular development, and sexual potency. This assessment has limitations in the mature adult, however, because regression of secondary sexual characteristics is slow even after complete loss of Leydig cell function. Furthermore, distribution of facial and body hair can be highly variable owing to differences in responsiveness of these skin appendages to hormonal stimulation. The American Indian, the black African, and some Orientals have sparse or absent facial and body hair despite normal testicular function and plasma testosterone concentration.

URINARY 17-KETOSTEROIDS. About 80 per cent of the urinary 17-ketosteroids (17-KS) is derived from adrenocortical steroids that have little intrinsic androgenic activity. Less than 3 mg daily is derived from Leydig cell secretions. Androsterone and etiocholanolone, the principal urinary metabolites of testosterone, are also metabolites of adrenocortical 11-deoxysteroids. Thus, since urinary 17-KS are an index chiefly of adrenal cortical function, they cannot be used to assess testicular function. Testosterone, which has a hydroxyl group at carbon atom 17, is not a 17-ketosteroid.

The normal range of 17-KS excretion in men is 8 to 20 mg per day (mean, 15 mg). Before puberty only small amounts are detectable in urine. In adult men and women after the third decade, urinary 17-KS decrease gradually owing to lessening adrenal secretion of dehydroepiandrosterone. The excretion of 17-KS may be reduced in eunuchoidism, although the values obtained in such patients are often within the normal range. In panhypopituitarism the function of both the testis and the adrenal cortex is impaired, and the excretion of urinary 17-KS is greatly decreased. Low values are also frequently found in chronic debilitating disease and renal insufficiency. Measurement of urinary 17-KS has little clinical value in diseases of the testis or adrenal cortex except as a screening test for congenital adrenal hyperplasia and adrenal tumors (see Ch. 547.10 to 547.12).

PLASMA AND URINARY ESTROGENS. Maddock and Nelson suggested that the increase in urinary estrogen after the administration of chorionic gonadotropin (a placental gonadotropin with LH-like activity) could be a useful index of Leydig cell function. Although the Leydig cell is the important source of almost all of the plasma estradiol in men, neither measurement of plasma estradiol concentration nor that of urinary estrogen excretion is a practical index of Leydig cell function.

PLASMA AND URINARY TESTOSTERONE. Measurement of plasma or urinary testosterone, the latter as the glucuronide conjugate, provides reliable indices of Leydig cell function. The production rate of testosterone can be estimated, but the method is too cumbersome for routine use. Young adult males excrete 40 to 100 μg per day of testosterone glucuronide; women excrete less than 6 μg, and boys before puberty less than 0.5 μg. The concentration of testosterone in plasma of young adult men ranges from 0.3 to 1.2 μg per 100 ml (mean 0.65 μg per 100 ml), and the concentration in women varies from 0.034 to 0.06 μg per 100 ml (mean, 0.054 μg per 100 ml). More than 98 per cent of testosterone in plasma is bound to a specific β-globulin, sex-steroid binding globulin, and thus only 1 to 2 per cent is available for diffusion into cells. The administration of HCG to adult men induces a rise in plasma and urinary testosterone; this procedure has been used to assess the responsiveness of the Leydig cell and to distinguish between primary and secondary testicular disease.

PLASMA AND URINARY GONADOTROPINS. Only a small proportion of the FSH and LH secreted daily appears in the urine in a biologically active form. The normal range of gonadotropin excretion assayed by the mouse uterine weight method is 10 to 100 mouse uterine units per day, and by the rat ovarian weight method 5 to 20 rat units per day. The common bioassays of urinary gonadotropins measure the combined excretion of LH and FSH and do not give meaningful information about variations in individual hormones. Further, the imprecision of the measurements is such that only successive determinations will permit a statement about low or normal levels. For these reasons and because of the availability of radioimmunoassays, routine bioassay of urinary gonadotropins is no longer a recommended diagnostic procedure.

The advent of radioimmunoassays has led to the development of sensitive, accurate, practical methods for measurement of these glycoproteins in serum and urine. The values obtained by immunoassay are expressed in terms of International Units of the Second International Reference Preparation (2nd IRP) of human menopausal gonadotropin or in ng of a human pituitary FSH and LH standard. The mean plasma FSH concentration in adult men is 11.7 mIU per milliliter (range 4 to 27 mIU per milliliter) and the mean plasma LH concentration is 9.1 mIU per milliliter (range 4 to 18.9 mIU per milliliter). Plasma FSH levels remain fairly constant throughout the day; nonsystematic pulsatile fluctuations of LH are commonly noted. Increased excretion or plasma concentration of these hormones indicates primary testicular disease; isolated increases of FSH point to severe seminiferous tubular disease (see below).

ASSESSMENT OF HYPOTHALAMIC-PITUITARY GONADOTROPIN RELEASE. Clomiphene citrate, an analogue of the nonsteroidal estrogen chlorotrianisene, is an estrogen antagonist and competes with estrogen at hypothalamic receptor sites. When administered to normal men by mouth, 100 to 200 mg per day for five to seven days, it evokes a mean increase in the concentration of plasma FSH of 130 per cent and of plasma LH of 160 per cent. It also induces a rise in urinary FSH and LH and of plasma testosterone. Little or no increase in FSH or LH secretion is elicited in men with pituitary disease.

The recent identification and synthesis of the hypothalamic decapeptide LH-releasing hormone (LHRH) has enabled the physician to establish pituitary responsiveness directly (see Ch. 543.4). It has been valuable in distinguishing between pituitary and hypothalamic disease.

TESTICULAR BIOPSY. This procedure can be of great value in the diagnosis and prognosis of testicular disorders. It provides information concerning primarily the gametogenic function of the testis — the status of the seminiferous tubules and the stages of spermatogenesis. Biopsy examination of the testis is of use in diagnosis of tubular disease, in assessing processes of sperm maturation, and in distinguishing azoospermia resulting from obstruction to the passage of sperm from azoospermia of other causes.

EXAMINATION OF SEMEN. Specimens of semen for analysis should be obtained two to three days after the last ejaculation. The volume of the specimen, the total number of sperm, and the motility and morphology of the sperm are determined. The minimal number of sperm necessary for normal fertility is unknown, but a total sperm count of 60 million may be considered normal. Less than this in general means decreased fertility. Because of the wide variations in sperm count among several specimens from the same patient, evaluation of therapy requires long control periods. Assessment of motility and morphology may require examination of many specimens to establish an accurate baseline.

SEX CHROMATIN PATTERN. The number of X chromosomes in the sex chromosome complex can be assessed indirectly by cytologic methods because of sexual dimorphism in the nuclear structure of somatic cells. Preparations suitable for examination can be obtained from smears of buccal mucosa, skin biopsy specimens, or blood (see Ch. 18.1). This test is widely used in the investigation of abnormalities of sex differentiation, particularly of males with defective testes and azoospermia or severe oligospermia. When a chromatin-positive (female-type) nuclear sex chromatin pattern is detected in a phenotypic male with bilateral testes, it suggests that an associated congenital primary testicular disorder may be present (see Ch. 548.4).

Instances have been described in which some of the nuclei from phenotypic males or females contained two or more sex chromatin bodies. The maximal number of sex chromatin bodies in somatic nuclei is equivalent to one less than the number of X chromosomes in the sex chromosome complex. For example, XO and XY individuals have chromatin-negative (male-type) somatic nuclei (no chromatin bodies), whereas a high proportion of diploid nuclei in individuals with XX or XXY sex chromosome constitution contain a maximum of one sex chromatin body. Similarly, in XXX females and XXXY males a maximum of two bodies is found in somatic nuclei.

Quinacrine hydrochloride, an acridine derivative, when utilized as a stain, produces intense fluorescence of the Y chromosome in interphase nuclei, in metaphase preparations, and in sperm. This discovery makes it possible to detect XYY, XXYY, and other double Y syndromes by the simple buccal smear technique. Recent studies using an immunologic assay for Y antigen have shown that Y chromosomal material is present whenever there is a testis.

Clermont, Y.: Kinetics of spermatogenesis in mammals: Seminiferous epithelium cycle and spermatogonial renewal. Physiol. Rev., 52:198, 1972.

Lipsett, M. B.: Regulation of testicular functions. Andrologia, 8:43, 1976.

Steinberger, E.: Hormonal control of mammalian spermatogenesis. Physiol. Rev., 51:1, 1971.

Troen, P., and Nankin, H. R. (eds.): The Testis in Normal and Infertile Men. New York, Raven Press, 1977.

Van Thiel, D. H., Sherins, R. J., and DeVita, V. T., Jr.: Evidence for a specific seminiferous tubular factor affecting follicle-stimulating hormone secretion in man. J. Clin. Invest., 51:1009, 1972.

Wilson, J. D., and Gloya, R. E.: The intra-nuclear metabolism of testosterone in the accessory organs of reproduction. Recent Prog. Horm. Res., 26:309, 1970.

548.2. PUBERTAL DEVELOPMENT IN THE MALE

There are wide variations in the age of onset, duration, and sequence of events that characterize the biologic pattern of male puberty. In normal boys signs of puberty may appear at any age between 10 and 17 years; the average age of onset is 12 to 13 years. Once initiated, the major changes are usually completed or well advanced in three to four years; in a small percentage of normal persons, maturity is not attained until the age of 21, and rarely thereafter.

A substantial body of evidence suggests that the stimulus for release of pituitary gonadotropin at puberty originates in the hypothalamus and is mediated by a neurohormonal secretion, LHRH. It seems likely that a certain level of physiologic maturation, presumably including the central nervous system, is necessary before this complex and incompletely understood mechanism is activated. This level of development can be best correlated with the degree of osseous and epiphyseal development (bone age) rather than with the chronologic age. Small amounts of FSH and LH are secreted by prepubertal children. There is good evidence in animals as well as some data in man showing that the hypothalamic-pituitary-testicular negative feedback mechanism is operative and set at a low level before pubescence.

The sequence of events that marks the pubertal period starts with an acceleration in the growth of the testes and scrotum. The initial increase in testicular size, occurring between 11 and 12 years, is largely attributable to changes in the seminiferous tubules, which occupy about 90 per cent of the volume of the testis. After initial acceleration of testicular growth, there is an increase in the size of the penis, the appearance of pubic hair, which has at first a transverse growth, and gradual enlargement of the prostate and other accessory organs and glands. It should be noted that the increase in testis size precedes the first appearance of pubic hair by approximately two years and peak height velocity by three years, and is an important clinical feature in ascertaining onset of early puberty. With pubescence, pulsatile and increased release of LH is observed, first at night and then throughout the 24 hours. Similarly, plasma testosterone concentration is first increased only during the night, reaching its normal adult levels as LH secretion increases.

The physician should be cognizant of the wide range of normality of the pubertal process in time of onset, intensity, and duration, and also of normal variations in the degree of development of the secondary sex characteristics. In normal men, the pitch of the voice, the size of the external genitalia, the amount of body hair, and the body habitus vary from individual to individual, and are largely attributable to genetic factors and not to differences in the secretion of testosterone.

DELAYED ADOLESCENCE. Delayed adolescence, although a normal variant and benign, is often a severe psychologic handicap to the patient and a cause of parental anxiety. Many of these boys are short, and a delay of several years in osseous development is not uncommon. There may be a history of late onset of puberty in other members of the family. Retardation of puberty can be due to inadequate dietary intake or to chronic illness, because these may be associated with either diminished secretion of pituitary gonadotropin or Leydig cell dysfunction.

Pubertal failure or arrest in pubertal development secondary to pituitary-hypothalamic dysfunction or gonadal disease must be excluded in cases of delayed puberty. To exclude pituitary tumor, roentgenographic examination of the skull and careful examination of the fundi and visual fields are required, as well as search for other signs of neurologic involvement in boys who are significantly delayed in their sexual development, particularly when this is accompanied by stunting of growth. It is advisable to assess other pituitary functions, especially if the delayed maturation is accompanied by short stature or a decreased rate of growth. A buccal smear for sex chromatin and determination of urinary or plasma gonadotropins may clarify the clinical situation. The response to clomiphene will not differentiate between delayed puberty and hypogonadotropic hypogonadism, because both groups are clomiphene unresponsive. LHRH causes a similar pattern of LH and FSH release in both groups so that the response to this agent also is not diagnostic.

Treatment. Treatment should be directed toward correction of the basic disturbance, e.g., measures to improve nutrition or surgical removal or irradiation of a pituitary neoplasm. Substitution therapy with male sex hormone should be started at about 13 or 14 years of age so that the onset of the patient's maturation coincides with that of his contemporaries. The use of this regimen does not preclude subsequent induction of spermatogenesis with FSH and HCG in those individuals with hypogonadotropic hypogonadism.

Less well defined is the treatment of boys in whom no apparent etiologic factor is found. Many will mature spontaneously before 17 years of age and merely represent an extreme of the normal range. Although indiscriminate use of hormonal treatment in this group is unwise, sociopsychologic considerations may make it expedient to treat such boys. A therapeutic trial with human chorionic gonadotropin, 500 to 1000 IU three times weekly injected intramuscularly, or with a testosterone preparation for three to six months will cause virilization, and often maturation will progress after treatment is discontinued.

Marshal, W. A., and Tanner, J. M.: Variations in the pattern of pubertal changes in boys. Arch. Dis. Child., 45:13, 1970.

548.3. SEXUAL PRECOCITY

Isosexual precocity in boys is defined as the occurrence of signs of masculinization before the age of ten years. Skeletal maturation is accelerated and the epiphyses fuse at a premature age, leading to short stature in adult life. On the other hand, mental and dental development are not precocious. Sexual precocity occurs about three times more frequently in girls than in boys. There are four main causes of isosexual precocity in boys: *cerebral, adrenocortical, testicular,* and *tumors secreting HCG.*

The cerebral causes of sexual precocity may be functional or organic. They are associated with premature activation of the hypothalamic-pituitary mechanism and the release of pituitary gonadotropins. This form, designated true precocious puberty or complete isosexual precocity, is manifested by maturation of the Leydig cells, spermatogenesis, and enlargement of the testis.

True precocious puberty may be caused by organic lesions of the brain either directly or indirectly involving the posterior hypothalamus, such as hypothalamic and pineal tumors, hamartoma of the tuber cinereum, craniopharyngioma, hydrocephalus, postencephalitic lesions, congenital defects, tuberous sclerosis, and neurofibromatosis. The *McCune-Albright syndrome* of sexual precocity, polyostotic fibrous dysplasia, and pigmented areas of skin is rare in boys. The mechanism whereby such lesions activate the hypothalamic-pituitary secretion of gonadotropins is unknown. Cerebral lesions, particularly tumors, accompanied by precocious puberty may affect other hypothalamic functions, causing diabetes insipidus, bulimia, obesity, somnolence, emotional lability, or disturbances in temperature regulation. The syndrome of diabetes insipidus and precocious puberty suggests aberrant pinealoma. Signs of puberty may precede the onset of detectable neurologic involvement, and prolonged observation with repeated careful neurologic examinations, roentgenograms of the skull, and determinations of the visual fields is necessary before it is possible to exclude cerebral neoplasm. When no organic cause is found, the condition is described as *idiopathic precocious puberty;* in some instances, it is transmitted as a sex-limited autosomal dominant trait. In the idiopathic cases, seizure disorders and abnormal electroencephalographic patterns are appreciably more frequent than in normal children.

In all varieties of precocious puberty, plasma and urinary testosterone values are increased, because either Leydig cell secretion is stimulated or testosterone is produced elsewhere. In contrast to precocious pseudopuberty, pituitary gonadotropin is excreted in the urine; frequently, however, this is not detectable early except by the more sensitive radioimmunoassay procedures for FSH and LH. The pulsatile secretion of LH that normally occurs with pubescence has been noted in precocious puberty. Medroxyprogesterone acetate, a synthetic long-acting progestin, administered intramuscularly, is occasionally of value in the management of patients with idiopathic precocious puberty by virtue of its capacity to inhibit pituitary LH secretion. Rarely secretion of HCG by extrapituitary neoplasms, such as hepatoblastoma, causes isosexual precocity.

In other forms of isosexual precocity not related to intracranial causes, the testes remain immature, in contrast to the enlarged phallus, and true puberty does not occur. Accordingly, this type has been called *incomplete sexual precocity* or *precocious pseudopuberty.*

The most common cause of incomplete sexual precocity in boys is adrenocortical hyperfunction resulting from congenital virilizing adrenal hyperplasia or a virilizing adrenocortical tumor. With few exceptions the testes remain prepubertal in size despite enlargement of the penis and scrotum and development of other secondary sexual characteristics. In congenital adrenal hyperplasia ectopic nodules of hyperplastic adrenal tissue are occasionally palpable in the testis, and may be confused with Leydig cell tumor, especially in rare instances in which striking enlargement of the testis is found. The excretion of 17-KS is increased in relation to chronologic age, and urinary pregnanetriol is high in congenital adrenal hyperplasia.

Interstitial cell tumor of the testis is a rare cause of isosexual precocity. In almost all reported cases the tumor has been unilateral, and the contralateral testis is immature. Gynecomastia is occasionally present. The excretion of 17-KS is usually normal, although occasional high values have been reported. Plasma testosterone concentration has generally been in the normal adult male range. Spermatogenesis has been observed in the tubules surrounding the tumor only, thereby confirming the importance of high intratesticular androgen concentrations for spermatogenesis.

Iatrogenic sexual precocity has been produced by the administration of male sex hormone, but is seen most frequently in boys who have been treated with large doses of HCG for cryptorchidism.

548.4. HYPOGONADISM

Hypogonadism may refer to a decrease in either the endocrine or the gametogenic function of the testis or to both. Primary hypogonadism is due to testicular disease, whereas secondary hypogonadism is a result of hypothalamic-pituitary disease. The excretion or blood level of gonadotropins is normal or high in primary hypogonadism, and is decreased in secondary hypogonadism. Of common occurrence are primary lesions of the testis involving only spermatogenesis, resulting in infertility. On the other hand, whenever testosterone secretion is deficient, spermatogenesis is impaired.

ANDROGEN DEFICIENCY. The clinical signs of androgen deficiency depend upon the age of onset and upon severity and duration of the deficiency. Total loss of testicular androgenic function, usually secondary to surgical castration or congenital defects of the testes, before or during early puberty results in eunuchoidism in adulthood. Eunuchoidism causes disproportionate growth of the long bones owing to delay in epiphysial closure. The span exceeds the height by several inches, and the distance between the symphysis pubis and the sole (lower segment) measures more than 55 per cent of the height. Tall stature is common, but not invariable. (The characteristic skeletal proportions of the eunuch are not pathognomonic and may be found in otherwise normal men.) The shoulders tend to be narrow and, although the habitus may be lean or obese, excessive fat deposition often occurs about the pectoral region, hips, thighs, and lower abdomen. Muscular development is poor. Except for the appearance of sparse pubic hair, secondary sex characteristics fail to appear, and the voice remains juvenile. Gynecomastia occurs in association with Klinefelter's syndrome and with male pseudohermaphroditism. Acne and baldness do not occur. Sex drive and potentia are absent or greatly reduced. The hematocrit and hemoglobin levels are characteristic of those for women and increase with administration of androgen.

The effects on somatic and sexual development of partial loss of testicular androgenic function are less striking and vary greatly in degree. Characteristic of the milder forms of eunuchoidism are the scant growth of facial hair and a female distribution of pubic hair. In men who have attained sexual maturity, castration does not result in complete regression of secondary sexual characteristics, and the signs of androgen deficiency are less conspicuous. The most common signs are reduction in prostatic size, diminished rate of growth of the beard and body hair, the appearance of fine wrinkles around the eyes, and a pasty, sallow complexion. Semen volume is reduced. Potentia and libido, although usually diminished, occasionally persist. There may be vasomotor phenomena, including hot flushes.

The most useful substances for the treatment of androgen deficiency are the preparations of testosterone that are available in forms suitable for intramuscular, oral, and buccal or sublingual administration. The mode of administration depends, for the most part, on the preference of the patient and the cost.

Esterification of testosterone with organic acids potentiates its activity when injected as an oily solution. Testosterone propionate in doses of 25 to 50 mg by intramuscular injection two or three times weekly is adequate for replacement therapy. However, longer-acting esters are available that can be administered less frequently. One dose of 200 to 400 mg of testosterone cyclopentylpropionate or testosterone enanthate is highly effective when injected at two- to four-week intervals.

Methyltestosterone is an effective preparation for oral and buccal or sublingual use. It is usually administered in doses of 50 mg (30 to 75 mg) orally or about 25 mg per day by sublingual absorption. It is not metabolized to 17-KS as is testosterone. No potent protein anabolic steroid lacking androgenic properties in man is available at present, although intensive efforts have been made to obtain one.

Undesirable effects of androgens include edema caused by retention of extracellular electrolyte (a rare effect except with use of large doses or in elderly persons with diminished cardiac reserve), polycythemia, acne, gynecomastia, and premature closure of the epiphyses. Rarely, methyltestosterone causes intrahepatic cholestatic jaundice. Androgen therapy may be contraindicated in patients with carcinoma of the prostate. The use of androgens by normal men to increase athletic performance remains controversial; it is certain, though, that the androgens will markedly decrease spermatogenesis.

PRIMARY HYPOGONADISM
(Primary Failure of the Testis)

The problem of classification of primary hypogonadism has not been entirely resolved, because the etiology of many of the disorders in this group is uncertain. Primary hypogonadism may result from genetic and developmental defects, such as seminiferous tubule dysgenesis and Laurence-Moon-Biedl syndrome, or from other causes: trauma, destruction of spermatogonia after orchitis, exposure to ionizing radiation, chemotherapy, and surgical castration. Disorders in this group may or may not be accompanied by androgen deficiency, although in some eunuchoidism is a constant or frequent feature. Disorders of spermatogenesis characterized only by oligospermia and infertility are likewise examples of primary hypogonadism. Plasma LH is increased with hypofunction of the Leydig cells as in old age or myotonic dystrophy. Plasma FSH is increased whenever tubular damage is severe enough to compromise Sertoli cell function. A high plasma FSH concentration signifies infertility, the ultimate prognosis depending on the cause.

Klinefelter's Syndrome; Seminiferous Tubule Dysgenesis

This syndrome was described in 1942 by Klinefelter, Reinfenstein, and Albright and is characterized classically by small, firm testes, azoospermia, gynecomastia, and elevated urinary gonadotropins. The features become apparent during early puberty, and may include eunuchoidism. Histologically there are atrophy and hyalinization of the seminiferous tubules; Leydig cells tend to occur in large clumps and are apparently increased in number, but total Leydig cell volume is probably normal. The few remaining tubules are lined by Sertoli cells; rarely, germ cells are present. Elastic fibers in the tunica propria are absent, indicating failure of pubertal maturation. The cause of the syndrome is a developmental defect of the gonad associated with and probably resulting from a sex chromosome abnormality. Klinefelter's syndrome and its variants are now defined by the single constant finding of an increase in the number of X chromosomes in at least one cell line.

The discovery in 1956 that most persons with the classic features of Klinefelter's syndrome are chromatin positive, followed by the detection of sex chromosome abnormalities, served to identify an especially well-defined disorder caused by a nonfamilial, genetically determined gonadal defect. In accord with this observation and the histopathologic characteristics of the testicular lesion the term "seminiferous tubule dysgenesis" has been suggested. This disorder, which occurs sporadically, is an important cause of male infertility and a common type of sexual anomaly. The results of several large surveys of newborns in nurseries indicate that the frequency of chromatin-positive seminiferous tubule dysgenesis is of the order of 1 in 500 newborn males.

The most frequent clinical feature of Klinefelter's syndrome is the small size of the testes, the long diameter usually being less than 2 cm. The testes are firmer than normal owing to hyalinization of the tubules. Gynecomastia is present in fewer than 50 per cent of cases, and eunuchoidism is variable. Patients with this disorder are often tall, and the skeletal proportions frequently are eunuchoid as a consequence of the disproportionately long lower extremities, even though epiphysial fusion is not delayed and skeletal maturation usually follows the normal male pattern (Fig. 3). Cryptorchidism and hypospadias are infrequent. Mental retardation and psychopathic behavior are not uncommon, and there is often evidence of poor social adaptation. This disorder has been reported in association with mongolism and with leukemia. It has been suggested that chronic pulmonary disease and varicose veins are more prevalent in affected adults. The frequency of impaired glucose tolerance and of mild diabetes is increased.

In the classic form of the disease plasma FSH is increased as a result of the extensive tubular destruction. Plasma LH may be either high or normal, depending on whether Leydig cell function is normal. The plasma concentration of testosterone is often low, and may increase only slowly with the daily administration of human chorionic gonadotropin for four to five days.

Figure 3. *A* and *B*, Typical 19-year-old phenotypic male with chromatin-positive seminiferous tubule dysgenesis (Klinefelter's syndrome). This patient had a positive sex chromatin pattern and an XXY karyotype. His 17-ketosteroid excretion was 11.2 mg per 24 hours, and his urinary gonadotropin excretion was more than 100 mu. These patients vary widely in their habitus and degree of virilization. This patient is well virilized, but had long extremities with eunuchoidal proportions and exhibited gynecomastia. The testes measured 1.8 × 0.9 cm and were small and firm. Testicular biopsy, *C*, revealed a severe degree of hyalinization of his seminiferous tubules and Leydig cell hyperplasia. *D*, Forty-eight-year-old man with chromatin-positive Klinefelter's syndrome who came to medical attention only because his severe leg varicosities were thought to reveal a "female trait." (From Van Wyk, J. J., and Grumbach, M. M.: Disorders of sex differentiation. *In* Williams, R. H. [ed.]: Textbook of Endocrinology. 4th ed. Philadelphia, W. B. Saunders Company, 1968.)

The common abnormality of the sex chromosomes in Klinefelter's syndrome is a 47,XXY karyotype. Less common types of sex chromosome abnormalities in this disorder include phenotypic males with the genotypes 48,XXYY, 48,XXXY, or 49,XXXXY that have been found so far only in mentally retarded persons. Unusually tall stature has been found in the XXYY group, along with a tendency to more aggressive and delinquent behavior. The 48,XXXY sex chromosome complex is associated with two sex chromatin bodies in a proportion of diploid somatic nuclei, and the 49,XXXXY constitution with three sex chromatin bodies. In addition to mental retardation, the XXXXY men have had severe congenital malformations, including very small, usually undescended testes; hypoplastic external genitalia; minor skeletal deformities, including radioulnar synostosis; and other congenital anomalies. It seems that with increasing numbers of X chromosomes, the severity of the abnormalities increases.

Instances of sex chromosome mosaicism have also been described in which at least two populations of cells with different cell chromosome complexes were found in the same individual, e.g., XY/XXY (one cell line with an XY sex chromosome complex and another with an XXY sex chromosome complex), XY/XXXY, XX/XXY, and XXXY/XXXXY. Sex chromosome mosaics arise from a mitotic error in an early division after fertilization in a zygote that originally had either a normal or an abnormal sex chromosome constitution. The detection of a chromatin-positive sex chromatin pattern on buccal smear should not by itself be used as incontrovertible evidence of sterility. Active spermatogenesis was found in the testes of an XY/XXXXY mosaic, and additional examples of potential fertility may be found in chromatin-positive males with other forms of sex chromosome mosaicism, especially XY/XXY. In several carefully studied men with Klinefelter's syndrome, only an XX sex chromosome constitution was found. The maternal origin of the two X chromosomes suggests that a Y chromosome was present early in ontogeny and was lost or more likely translocated to an X chromosome or autosome, or that these men were mosaics and the Y-bearing cell line has escaped detection.

The typical XXY sex chromosome constitution of seminiferous tubule dysgenesis may arise from an abnormality of meiosis during gametogenesis or from a mitotic error in the fertilized zygote (see Ch. 18). The positive association of this disorder with advanced maternal age and the results of surveys of color blindness (a sex-linked recessive trait) and of the Xg blood group suggest a maternal origin with nondisjunction occurring during oogenesis. Using X-linked markers, a paternal origin of one X has been established in several informative pedigrees, nondisjunction during spermatogenesis giving rise to an XY-bearing sperm and fertilization yielding an XXY zygote. More complex sex chromosome anomalies may arise from meiotic or mitotic errors, or from a combination of both.

The gonadal defect is a consequence of the abnormal sex chromosome constitution. The single Y chromosome is a sufficiently powerful male determiner to suppress the cortical component (ovarian anlage) of the primordial gonad despite the presence of two (or even four) X chromosomes. The fetal testes that develop may have either an adequate number or a deficiency of germ cells, but bring about normal male differentiation of the genital tract. At puberty, if the function of the Leydig cells is adequate, male secondary sexual characteristics develop, but the seminiferous tubules lack or are severely deficient in germ cells. Tubular hyalinization usually does not begin until the later prepubertal period. It seems likely that the characteristic appearance of the testes in adolescent and adult cases depends on the direct or indirect action of pituitary gonadotropins from the onset of puberty on an inherently defective testis, which, before this time, shows only subtle signs of an abnormal histologic structure.

TREATMENT. If there is evidence of androgen deficiency, testosterone replacement is indicated. Testosterone treatment may produce transient increase in gynecomastia and nipple tenderness. Mastectomy may be necessary in some patients, primarily for cosmetic reasons.

Chromatin-Negative Klinefelter's Syndrome

This term is a misnomer and was bestowed before the fundamental distinction was made on the basis of karyotype. The small testes and azoospermia suggest the Klinefelter phenotype. The testicular lesion resembles that of Klinefelter's syndrome, but the testis can react to injury in only a limited number of ways. The patients have none of the associated anomalies seen in Klinefelter's syndrome, but hypogonadism is sometimes present. It is probable that so-called chromatin-negative Klinefelter's syndrome is the end-stage of several different disease processes, the final result being hyalinization of the tubules with loss of spermatogonia. Some of these patients may be unrecognized mosaics with one cell line bearing an XXY karyotype and would thus be classified as Klinefelter's syndrome. Plasma testosterone levels have varied from normal to low.

XYY Syndrome

Although the XYY syndrome is discussed under the topic of primary hypogonadism, in fact primary hypogonadism is unusual in XYY subjects. The XYY syndrome is characterized by a chromosome complement of 47 with an extra Y chromosome and a sex chromatin–negative buccal smear that contains nuclei with two small fluorescent Y chromatin masses, and is estimated to occur in 1 per 500 to 1 per 1000 male births. Newborn males and young boys with this syndrome have a normal phenotype. A number of associated characteristics have been reported in the adolescent and adult XYY male. These include tall stature (often over 6 feet), severe acne, and skeletal abnormalities, e.g., radioulnar synostosis. In studies of criminals with a history of aggressive crimes, an increased frequency of the XYY genotype has been noted. On the other hand, many adult XYY males are physically and mentally normal, and the genotype is present with greater frequency in tall men.

Although the extra Y apparently confers the potential for increased stature, Leydig cell function and plasma and urinary testosterone concentrations have been normal.

Germinal Aplasia
(Sertoli-Cell-Only Syndrome)

This condition is characterized by seminiferous tubules lined with Sertoli cells, little or no tubular fibrosis, and absent germinal cells. The patients are first seen by the physician because of sterility. Leydig cell function is normal. Azoospermia is an invariable finding. The testes are normal or slightly reduced in size. Plasma FSH levels are increased four- to five-fold, whereas LH levels are within normal limits. The karyotype is 46,XY. Germinal aplasia is probably a congenital disease of the Sertoli cell, and these cells are abnormal by electron microscopy. The lesion has also been described after exposure of the testes to ionizing radiation and after extensive chemotherapy with cytotoxic agents. There is no treatment for the spontaneous form, but the lesion after damage to the spermatogenic epithelium may be reversible.

Myotonic Muscular Dystrophy

Testicular atrophy, occurring in middle age, is found in about 80 per cent of affected men with myotonic dystrophy. This syndrome is characterized by myotonia, muscle wasting, frontal baldness, and lenticular opacities. Signs of androgen deficiency occur in 18 per cent of the patients and gynecomastia in 12 per cent. As the disease progresses, increasing tubular fibrosis results in high plasma FSH levels and Leydig cell failure increases LH levels. The histology of the testis shows tubular fibrosis, hyalinization, and disordered spermatogenesis. There are other metabolic abnormalities which, in association with the testicular findings, have been described as accelerated aging.

Anorchia

Absence of both testes in phenotypic males has been described but is exceedingly rare. Careful surgical exploration is required to establish the diagnosis. In a few cases, catheterization of the spermatic vein revealed a testosterone gradient, suggesting that a nidus of Leydig cells in the expected position of the testis remained functional. Unilateral anorchia is more common, and may result from testicular atrophy after herniorrhaphy, from attempted orchiopexy, or from a developmental disturbance, in which case there may be associated anomalies of the genitourinary tract.

Infertility

In many testicular lesions, the defect involves only spermatogenic function and results in infertility. Endocrine manifestations are absent. Either the semen lacks sperm or the number or quality of sperm is diminished. Testicular biopsy has a major role in differentiating the various disturbances in spermatogenic activity and in determining prognosis. Azoospermia is usually associated with severe tubular fibrosis, germinal aplasia, or spermatogenic arrest, and oligospermia with germinal cell desquamation, hypospermatogenesis, incomplete spermatogenic arrest, and less severe forms of tubular fibrosis. In general, only azoospermia or severe oligospermia is associated with increased plasma FSH concentrations. In most cases the cause is unknown. Azoospermia may also result from obstruction in the afferent ducts secondary to gonorrhea, tuberculosis, or a nonspecific infection. Absence or atresia of the vas deferens and a rudimentary epididymis are common bilateral lesions in boys with cystic fibrosis, but may occur spontaneously. Azoospermia in the presence of a normal FSH suggests obstructive disease and warrants biopsy and urologic consultation.

OLIGOSPERMIA. This condition is composed of many variants. There may be partial arrest of spermatogenesis at the primary or secondary spermatocyte stage or at the spermatid stage. Abnormalities of the meiotic chromosomes and reduction in chiasma formation have been noted in men with oligospermia. Sperm morphology may be abnormal. Of interest are the nonmobile sperm seen in Kartagener's syndrome (sinusitis, bronchiectasis, and situs inversus). The cause of immobility is the absence of the dynein arms of the microtubular elements of the sperm tail, and this defect is related to the immobility of the cilia in the bronchi.

VARICOCELE. This condition is associated with decreased sperm count in 25 to 65 per cent of men, and there are varying abnormalities of sperm morphology. In general, measures of endocrine function have been normal. Results of varicocelectomy have been uneven, the incidence of restored fertility varying from 25 to 75 per cent. The role of the varicocele in producing infertility remains obscure.

OTHER CAUSES. Sterility is a common sequel of bilateral cryptorchidism and may occur in association with unilateral cryptorchidism. Sterility may follow orchitis caused by mumps, gonorrhea, brucellosis, leprosy, or occasionally other systemic infection; it may result from radiation of the testes or treatment with chemotherapeutic agents; it may be of developmental origin, as in seminiferous tubule dysgenesis. Even relatively minor illnesses may cause profound depression in sperm count. Starvation and chronic debilitating diseases associated with inanition adversely affect spermatic function. Estrogen and androgen administration also inhibit spermatogenesis by suppression of gonadotropins with concomitant decrease in intratesticular testosterone concentration. Chemotherapeutic agents, alcohol, and other drugs may cause reversible damage to the spermatogenic epithelium.

TREATMENT OF INFERTILITY IN THE MALE. Although important advances have been made in the evaluation of spermatogenic function, treatment of infertility caused by primary testicular disease is unsatisfactory. The results of therapy of hormonally normal men with oligospermia by the use of large doses of androgenic steroids, gonadotropins, pregnenolone, thyroid hormone, clomiphene, and vitamin preparations have been generally unsuccessful. The intermittent use of large doses of testosterone to take advantage of the "rebound effect" on spermatogenesis has not been established as efficacious, although occasional men seem to benefit.

SECONDARY HYPOGONADISM

Secondary hypogonadism is due to decreased secretion of gonadotropins, and may result from neoplastic, inflammatory, traumatic, vascular, and degenerative lesions involving the pituitary or hypothalamus. These lesions include such entities as pituitary adenoma, craniopharyngioma, astrocytoma, infarction, carotid aneurysm, granulomas such as tuberculosis, histiocytosis X, and hemochromatosis. In many instances, the nature of the underlying lesion is not known. A functional and reversible depression of gonadotropin secretion occurs in malnutrition, in chronic disease states associated with inanition and nutritional deficiencies, and in some patients with myxedema. High concentrations of androgen and estrogen, as in the adrenogenital syndrome, may cause secondary hypogonadism by suppression of gonadotropin secretion. Excessive estrogen, either from ingestion or endogenous, as from a feminizing adrenal tumor, depresses the secretion of pituitary gonadotropin. The testicular atrophy that occurs in some patients with severe liver disease is due in part to increased levels of estrogen. Decreased gonadotropin secretion may also result from the nutritional and metabolic disturbances accompanying hepatic cirrhosis.

Decreased secretion of pituitary gonadotropins occurs either as an isolated defect, *hypogonadotropic hypogonadism*, or, more commonly, in association with a deficiency of growth hormone and other anterior pituitary hormones. On the other hand, hypoadrenocorticism or hypothyroidism secondary to pituitary failure is rarely found without concurrent involvement of gonadotropic function and secondary hypogonadism. Secondary hypogonadism is usually characterized by both inadequate androgenic function and, with rare exceptions (see below), absent or deficient spermatogenesis.

The clinical manifestations vary with age of onset, degree of the deficiency, and whether there is coexistent deficiency of other anterior pituitary hormones. Hypopituitarism occurring during childhood, commonly designated "pituitary dwarfism," results in proportionate dwarfism and complete sexual infantilism. The characteristic features of prepubertal or pubertal gonadotropic failure are eunuchoid habitus, small testes, lack of development of secondary sexual characteristics, an increased frequency of anosmia or hyposmia, low or absent gonadotropins, and low plasma testosterone concentration. The absence of gynecomastia, regarded by some as a salient feature, is of no clinical value in differentiating primary from secondary hypogonadism. It is important to detect organic disease of the pituitary region. Such evaluation should include study of the visual fields, roentgenography of the sella turcica, and, when indicated, such procedures as tomography of the sella, pneumoencephalography, and carotid and venous angiography.

A familial form of isolated hypogonadotropic hypogonadism limited to males occurs in association with anosmia or hyposmia *(Kallmann's syndrome)* and is transmitted as either an X-linked or a sex-linked dominant trait. Aplasia of the olfactory lobes has been found in autopsied cases. Leydig cell responsiveness to HCG in some of these patients may be decreased. Both familial and sporadic forms of isolated FSH and LH deficiency are known, and these may be associated with a variety of somatic anomalies and neurologic defects. Although the initial response to LHRH has been variable, with continued administration the response becomes normal. These data suggest that hypothalamic synthesis or release of LHRH is impaired in these patients and in most patients with hypogonadotropic hypogonadism.

The testis in patients with hypogonadotropic hypogonadism remains infantile, the tubular diameter being the same as that of the fetal testis. When pituitary function is decreased in adult life, tubular collapse, fibrosis, and hyalinization occur at variable times after the onset of gonadotropic failure.

Isolated LH Deficiency. Pasqualini and Bur described a group of eunuchoidal men with relatively normal-sized testes and some spermatogenic function. Later, McCullagh applied the term "fertile eunuch" to patients with this syndrome. The patients are not fertile, however, because spermatogenesis is decreased, and libido and potentia are absent. Leydig cells are absent or few in number, and androgen deficiency is always present. The concentration of plasma LH and the excretion of urinary LH are low or undetectable, whereas the secretion of FSH is normal. Chorionic gonadotropin stimulates Leydig cell function, ameliorates the androgen deficiency and increases spermatogenesis. These patients have an isolated deficiency of LH, which may arise from an abnormality in the hypothalamus (and the synthesis or release of LHRH) or in the pituitary gland. A kindred with two affected brothers has been reported. Rarely, a pituitary tumor or idiopathic delayed adolescence may manifest itself as isolated LH deficiency.

TREATMENT. A physiologic approach to the treatment of secondary hypogonadism characterized by decreased spermatogenesis requires the use of gonadotropins. FSH preparations derived from animal sources are not consistently effective and, when injected repeatedly, stimulate antibody formation that reduces the effect of the hormones. However, gonadotropins prepared from menopausal urine have been used successfully in combination with HCG to induce spermatogenesis in patients with hypogonadotropic hypogonadism. As little as 25 IU of FSH three times a week in combination with 1000 IU of HCG three times a week has induced spermatogenesis. It is of interest that impregnation often occurs with total sperm counts below 20 million. This suggests that the infertility seen in men with oligospermia whose sperm counts may be higher is due to factors other than sperm number. Testosterone cannot be used in place of HCG, because intratesticular testosterone concentrations do not reach the levels attained when the Leydig cells are stimulated by HCG. HCG does not have a direct effect on the seminiferous tubules, although in a few instances of partial gonadotropic failure spermatogenic as well as Leydig cell function improved after its use. HCG has been effective in maintaining spermatogenesis after hypophysectomy for diabetic retinopathy. When only androgen substitution therapy is needed, one of the long-acting testosterone preparations is preferred.

Bardin, C. W., Ross, G. T., Rifkind, A. B., Cargille, C. M., and Lipsett, M. B.: Studies of the pituitary–Leydig cell axis in young men with hypogonadotropic hypogonadism and hyposomia: Comparison with normal men, prepubertal boys, and hypopituitary patients. J. Clin. Invest., 48:2046, 1969.

Brasel, J. A., Wright, J. C., Wilkins, L., and Blizzard, R. M.: An evaluation of seventy-five patients with hypopituitarism beginning in childhood. Am. J. Med., 38:484, 1965.

Kelch, R. P., Jenner, M. R., Weinstein, R., Kaplan, S. L., and Grumbach, M. M.: Estradiol and testosterone secretion by human, simian, and canine testes, in males with hypogonadism and in male pseudohermaphrodites with the feminizing testes syndrome. J. Clin. Invest., 51:824, 1972.

Mancini, R. E., Seiguer, A. C., and Perez Lloret, A.: Effect of gonadotropins on the recovery of spermatogenesis in hypophysectomized patients. J. Clin. Endocrinol., 29:467, 1969.

Paulsen, C. A., Gordon, D. L., Carpenter, R. W., Gandy, H. M., and Drucker, W. D.: Klinefelter's syndrome and its variants: A hormonal and chromosomal study. Recent Prog. Horm. Res., 24:321, 1968.

Santen, R. J., and Paulsen, C. A.: Hypogonadotropic eunuchoidism. I. Clinical study of mode of inheritance. J. Clin. Endocrinol. Metab., 36:47, 1973.

548.5. MALE PSEUDOHERMAPHRODITISM

Male pseudohermaphroditism may be considered a form of fetal hypogonadism, because those fetal structures normally responsive to androgen develop incompletely or not at all. Depending on the degree of androgen deficiency, the adult phenotype may range from almost normal female to male with minimal abnormalities. Male pseudohermaphroditism is most often familial and is transmitted either as a sex-linked autosomal dominant or as a sex-limited recessive trait manifest in the male.

SYNDROME OF TESTICULAR FEMINIZATION

This form of familial male pseudohermaphroditism deserves detailed consideration because the pathophysiology illuminates areas of hormone action and fetal regulation. The patients have primary amenorrhea, absent or sparse axillary and pubic hair, female external genitalia, a short blind vaginal pouch, absence of uterus and usually of the male genital ducts, and undescended or labial testes. The phenotypic women are usually tall, have good breast development, and show cornification of the vaginal mucosa. The karyotype is 46 XY.

The cause of the syndrome is a congenital resistance to androgens. Exogenous androgens have been shown to be ineffective in causing axillary or pubic hair growth, virilization, or nitrogen retention. From studies of rat and mouse models of this syndrome and of man, it is probable that the androgen resistance is usually due to absence of the cytosol androgen-binding protein receptor present in androgen-responsive tissues. This receptor is also present normally in the male gonaducts. In its absence, the male fetus receives no effective androgenic stimulus, resulting in failure of fusion of the genital folds and swellings to form penis and scrotum, respectively, and a lack of posterior migration of the labioscrotal folds. The fetal testicular inducer of müllerian duct regression is not an androgen and continues to be secreted by the fetal testis in this syndrome. Thus, since the upper third of the vagina is a müllerian duct derivative, it regresses and the vagina remains short. Wolffian duct derivatives such as the vas deferens, however, are induced by androgen and therefore are usually absent in this syndrome.

The hormonal relationships in the adult are likewise of interest. Plasma testosterone concentrations are within the normal range for men, and plasma estradiol levels are in the high normal range. Plasma LH is increased, presumably because of end-organ resistance of hypothalamic receptors. Plasma FSH is normal, however, suggesting that feedback is normal owing to a combination of normal estradiol concentration and "tubular factor" originating in the Sertoli cell.

The testes in these patients have tubules containing only Sertoli cells and showing variable peritubular fibrosis. Spermatogenesis is rare. The Leydig cells appear hyperplastic.

A phenotypic variant of testicular feminization has been identified in which androgen receptors are present in normal amounts. The cause of the androgen insensitivity then must lie at some subsequent step in androgen action.

Treatment consists of orchiectomy, because the risk of cancer in these gonads is several times that in the normal individual. The patients should receive replacement doses of an estrogen such as 0.5 mg of diethylstilbestrol or 0.05 mg of ethinyl estradiol daily to prevent the vasomotor instability characteristic of castration and to maintain normal female secondary sexual characteristics.

THE SPECTRUM OF MALE PSEUDOHERMAPHRODITISM

A variable decrease of cytosol androgen receptors can produce inadequate androgen stimulation during fetal life and consequent incomplete masculinization of internal and external genitalia. With a severe defect, the phenotype may be female; lesser defects are expressed as failure of posterior migration of the labioscrotal folds with incomplete midline fusion, microphallus, bifid scrotum, or only hypospadias. Gynecomastia is usually present due to incomplete suppression by androgen of the breast anlage. These disorders have been termed "incomplete testicular feminization."

Another and newly described type of male pseudohermaphroditism is due to a deficiency of 5α-reductase, the enzyme converting testosterone to dihydrotestosterone. These boys have a small phallus and a urogenital sinus. Internally, differentiation of the wolffian duct structures is complete and müllerian duct inhibition occurs. The ambiguity of the external genitalia indicates the role of dihydrotestosterone in promoting their growth during fetal life, whereas the wolffian duct responds to testosterone. Penile enlargement occurs at puberty, but there is no prostate growth, no acne, and absence of facial and male pattern hair — all these being dihydrotestosterone-mediated phenomena. Complete spermatogenesis is present, so that one may conclude that testosterone is the proximate androgenic hormone at the tubule.

Other types of male pseudohermaphroditism resulting from variants of congenital adrenal hyperplasia are discussed in Ch. 547.10.

Imperato-McGinley, J., and Peterson, R. E.: Male pseudohermaphroditism: The complexities of male phenotypic development. Am. J. Med., 61:251, 1976.

548.6.   CRYPTORCHIDISM

The terms "cryptorchidism" and "undescended testes" are used synonymously to designate testes that have never descended into the scrotum. Unilateral cryptorchidism is approximately four times as common as bilaterally undescended testes. A cryptorchid testis may be situated in the abdomen, within the inguinal canal, or in an ectopic position outside the scrotum and the normal pathway of descent. The majority of undescended testes are inguinal. To avoid needless treatment,

it is essential to distinguish this condition from retractile testes, which lie in the lower or upper scrotum and are withdrawn into the inguinal region and occasionally into the abdomen by slight stimulus.

The testes usually descend into the scrotum about the eighth fetal month; but occasionally descent is delayed until shortly after birth. Incomplete descent is common in premature male infants. Scorer found undescended testes at birth in 3.4 per cent of 1500 full-term male infants; during the first month of life 50 per cent of undescended testes reached the scrotum. In a prospective study of the incidence of congenital anomalies only 0.5 per cent of 2793 liveborn male infants had undescended testes at 12 months of age. The incidence of unilateral and bilateral cryptorchidism in large series of adult males has been variously estimated at 0.2 to 0.4 per cent. Spontaneous descent occurs frequently during the first year of life and is less common after this age.

The etiology is not understood. Not infrequently a normal testis resides in the superficial inguinal pouch, its descent arrested by Scarpa's fascia. However, the cryptorchid testis is often dysgenetic. In rare instances, unilateral or bilateral cryptorchidism is the only overt anatomic abnormality of the external genitalia in individuals with fetal testicular dysfunction.

DIAGNOSIS. The most difficult aspect of diagnosis is distinguishing the true undescended testis from the more common retractile testis of childhood; repeated examinations may be necessary, especially in obese boys. It is important to ascertain by careful inquiry whether the testes have at any time been observed in the scrotum. In cryptorchidism the ipsilateral side of the scrotum is empty and poorly developed. The patient should be carefully examined while standing, squatting, and in a recumbent position, in a warm room and with warm hands. Bimanual examination and palpation while the patient performs a Valsalva maneuver or while the examiner applies pressure to the lower abdomen are also useful procedures. In boys with retractile testes, elicitation of the cremasteric reflex often results in a localized puckering of the scrotal skin. If the testis is palpated in the normal pathway of descent, gentle manipulation should be used in an attempt to displace it into the scrotum. Such mobile testes do not require therapy and will remain in the scotum with the advent of puberty. Failure to palpate a testis on multiple occasions suggests that the testis is intra-abdominal, atrophic, or absent. An increase in plasma FSH and an augmented response to LHRH indicates Sertoli cell dysfunction in some patients with cryptorchidism.

TREATMENT. The treatment of undescended testes is a vexing and controversial subject; experienced observers differ in their approach to the problem. Major considerations are (1) the potential fertility of the undescended testis, (2) the likelihood of spontaneous descent, and (3) the propensity of the undescended testis to undergo malignant change.

It is well established that during or after puberty the undescended testis shows degenerative changes that eventually proceed to atrophy. With good reason these changes have been ascribed to the deleterious effect of the higher temperature of an extrascrotal environment on the testes, especially on the germinal epithelium. The tubules gradually undergo progressive fibrosis and loss of germinal elements, although androgenic function may persist for many years. These degenerative changes may also be manifestations of a dysgenetic testis. This distinction is important, because the risk of cancer in the dysgenetic gonad is considerably greater than in the normal gonad.

Men with bilateral undescended testes are sterile. However, general agreement is lacking as to the age at which the fertility potential of the cryptorchid testis is impaired. A lag in development of the seminiferous tubules and, in some instances, a mild degree of fibrosis in testes retained after the age of six to ten years have been observed. The significance of these changes is uncertain, but after puberty irreversible degenerative changes frequently occur.

The incidence of cancer in undescended testes is considerably greater than in scrotal testes, and more so in abdominal than in inguinal testes. Although precise statistics are not available, the over-all risk appears to be small, with the exception of the dysgenetic, frequently undescended gonads of intersexes, which are especially prone to malignant degeneration.

The most important problem in the treatment of patients with cryptorchidism is the age at which it is advisable to attempt correction. Treatment consists of orchiopexy or of the administration of HCG followed by orchiopexy when necessary. It is generally agreed that therapy must be started before pubescence if irreparable testicular damage is to be prevented, but opinions differ about the optimal age for treatment. In the more common unilateral cryptorchid, the scrotal testis, if normal, is adequate for fertility. Treatment is recommended for cosmetic reasons, to facilitate examination for neoplasm, and as additional insurance against infertility in the event that the scotal testis is defective or impaired at a later age.

In bilateral cryptorchidism preservation of fertility is the major consideration, but the results of treatment are disappointing. Bilateral orchiopexy is generally followed by tubular fibrosis and atrophy. Since many undescended testes descend before puberty, it is justifiable to delay treatment until nine years of age unless the testis is ectopic or associated with a hernia.

When hormonal therapy is effective it is probable that the testis would have descended spontaneously at puberty under the stimulus of endogenous gonadotropin. To minimize a theoretical risk of damage to the tubule, short intensive courses of 4000 units of HCG administered intramuscularly daily for three days or 4000 units three times a week for three weeks may be used. Hormonal treatment is contraindicated when the testis lies outside the normal pathway of descent.

If the undescended testis is atrophic and biopsy examination at the time of surgery shows irreversible changes, it is generally advisable to perform orchiectomy, provided that the contralateral testis is in the scrotum. This also applies to a testis that, despite all attempts at mobilization, cannot be brought into the scrotum.

548.7. IMPOTENCE

Impotence is a complicated problem that may be either relative or complete and may involve any phase of the sexual act. Although it is a symptom of androgen deficiency and of genitourinary or neurologic disease, in most instances it is psychic in origin. Multiple sclerosis, tabes dorsalis, and diabetic neuropathy are com-

monly associated with impotence. Impotence without apparent impairment of libido has been described in patients with temporal lobe lesions. Many agents used in the therapy of hypertension can cause impotence. When impotence is the principal complaint of a patient, it is usually the result of an emotional disturbance, and in this case androgen therapy is valueless. Several recent studies show clearly that, in men as well as in women, stress can decrease gonadotropic secretion and thereby affect androgen secretion and spermatogenesis (see Ch. 549.2). Increased prolactin, resulting from tumor or drugs, may produce impotence by directly suppressing LH and by interfering with Leydig cell function.

548.8. "MALE CLIMACTERIC"

The spontaneous occurrence of a male climacteric is still controversial. Although in women during the fifth or sixth decade ovarian failure with a consequent rise in gonadotropin excretion is an anticipated and physiologic accompaniment of the aging process, spontaneous testicular deficiency of sufficient degree to produce symptoms is rare. Many of the symptoms ascribed to this syndrome are common in psychoneurotic syndromes in middle-aged and elderly men. The diagnosis should be documented by finding an increased excretion of gonadotropin and a low concentration of plasma testosterone, and should be confirmed by obtaining a therapeutic response to androgen therapy but not to placebos. Plasma testosterone concentrations show little change until after 70 years of age. However, increasing concentrations of testosterone-binding globulin (TeBG) are associated with the gradually decreasing concentration of plasma-free testosterone that has been noted after the age of 50. A progressive increase in plasma LH levels after age 50 has been described. The frequency of alterations in tubular histology increases progressively after age 30, prominent changes being thickening of the basement membrane, intratubular fibrosis, and loss of germ cells. Plasma FSH increases after age 70 in response to this seminiferous tubule damage.

548.9. ORCHITIS

Acute orchitis, a common complication of mumps, is a rare occurrence in the course of other specific infectious diseases (see Ch. 88).

Chronic orchitis is associated with painless, hard, sometimes nodular enlargement of the testis. *Syphilis*, the most common cause, may produce an interstitial orchitis in which the testis is characteristically smooth and wooden in consistency ("billiard ball" testis); involvement is frequently bilateral. Other causes include *tuberculosis, leprosy, brucellosis, glanders*, and certain parasitic infections such as *filariasis* and *bilharziasis*. In these disease, Leydig cell function almost always remains intact, but severe tubular destruction may result.

548.10. TUMORS OF THE TESTIS

Tumors of the testis are uncommon, comprising about 0.7 per cent of all forms of cancer in the male. They occur in about 0.002 per cent of men, and frequently are malignant. The greatest incidence occurs in the third and fourth decades. Testicular tumors may arise from any of the cellular components of the testis or their embryonal precursors.

Considerable uncertainty applies to classification, especially of those neoplasms whose origin has been ascribed to the totipotent germ cell. Melicow has suggested the classification shown in the accompanying table.

GERMINAL TUMORS

Most common are germinal tumors, and, of these, seminoma exceeds in frequency all other testicular tumors. *Seminoma,* although usually fairly uniform in cellular architecture, may contain embryonal elements such as chorionic syncytium in the primary growth or in metastatic lesions. In contrast to the embryonal tumors, which tend to invade the spermatic cord and to metastasize early, especially to lung, seminomas in general are relatively slow growing and commonly invade the iliac and periaortic lymph nodes before generalized dissemination is demonstrable. In addition, seminomas are frequently highly radiosensitive, whereas embryonal tumors are usually resistant to radiotherapy. The significantly increased incidence of germinal tumors, particularly seminoma, in undescended testes and in the dysgenetic gonads of intersexes has been discussed above.

Many patients with germinal tumors excrete increased amounts of chorionic gonadotropin. This may almost always be attributed to the presence of trophoblastic elements in the tumor. Response to therapy or evidence of recurrence may be monitored by measurement of plasma HCG levels. Other fetal protein markers such as carcinoembryonic antigens may also be secreted by these cancers.

The germ cell tumors of the testis are responsive to therapy. Removal or radiation of regional and paraortic lymph nodes has produced survival rates of 80 to 95 per cent in men with seminoma. Choriocarcinoma and embryonal cell carcinoma have responded to multiagent chemotherapeutic regimens. With the addition of cis-diamminedichloroplatinum to combinations of methotrexate, dactinomycin, and chlorambucil, response rates of 40 to 70 per cent have been achieved in men with

Tumors of Testis: Classification

I. Primary tumors
  A. Germinal
    1. Seminoma
    2. Embryonal tumors
      a. Embryoma
      b. Choriocarcinoma
      c. Embryonal carcinoma
      d. Teratocarcinoma
      e. Adult teratoma
    3. Combinations of seminoma and embryonal tumor and of the various types of embryonal tumors
    4. Gonadal tumors in intersexes (gonadoblastomas)
  B. Nongerminal tumors
    1. Interstitial cell tumor
    2. Sertoli cell tumor
    3. Tumors of testicular stroma: fibroma, lipoma, etc.
II. Secondary tumors
  A. Lymphoma, plasmacytoma, leukemia, etc.
  B. Metastatic carcinoma

metastatic disease. About 20 per cent of these patients are apparently in long-term remission.

INTERSTITIAL CELL TUMORS

Tumors of this type are rare, occur at any age, and are usually but not invariably benign. The tumors are small and often difficult to palpate. In boys interstitial cell tumors cause sexual precocity but not true puberty, because spermatogenesis is absent in the contralateral testis. The only recognizable endocrine manifestation in the adult is gynecomastia, which has been observed in about 10 per cent of cases. Malignant interstitial cell tumors that retain their steroid-synthesizing capacities have been reported.

Melicow, M. M.: Classification of tumors of the testis. J. Urol., 73:547, 1955.

549. THE OVARIES
Nathan Kase

549.1. OVARIAN STRUCTURE AND FUNCTION

The human ovary has a dual physiologic responsibility: (1) development and release of ova and (2) elaboration of estrogen and progesterone. From menarche to menopause both these activities are bound to the cycle of follicle development, ovulation, corpus luteum formation, and regression. In reality each ovary is a heterogeneous, cyclically changing tissue containing subunits with differing properties. During its brief interval of dominance each subunit defines the function of the total organ. The sequential appearance of each unit and their respective gametogenic and endocrine performances are directed by pituitary secretion of varying quantities of gonadotropins: follicle-stimulating hormone (FSH) and luteinizing hormone (LH). Release of these factors is controlled by a specific neurosecretory substance (gonadotropin-releasing hormone [GnRH or LRH]) originating in hypothalamic nuclei that are sensitive to "feedback" levels of circulating ovarian hormones. The ranges of peptide and steroid hormone concentrations in a normal ovulatory cycle are shown in Figure 1.

The ovary contains specialized cells in the cortical and medullary areas that may contribute to abnormal ovarian function in certain pathologic conditions, but its major elements are the follicle and corpus luteum. The follicle consists of the ovum and two layers of tissue surrounding it: an inner band of granulosa cells without blood vessels, and an outer vascularized mantle of theca cells. At any given time in the preovulatory phase a number of follicles display varying degrees of developmental maturity: cystic changes, hormonal activity, and atresia. The factors responsible for the selection of one to attain full maturity and ovulation while others atrophy are unknown. Morphologic clues indicating development of a follicle are the degree of thecal proliferation and vascularity and the ratio of granulosa layer thickening to cystic distention of the antrum. The formation of a true corpus luteum is a direct consequence of final maturation and ovulation of the follicle.

Figure 1. Steroid and peptide hormone concentrations during an ovulatory menstrual cycle. (From Speroff, L., Glass, R. H., and Kase, N. G.: Clinical Gynecologic Endocrinology and Infertility. Baltimore, Williams and Wilkins Company, 1978.)

In a variety of animal experiments the physical expulsion of the oocyte appears to be dependent on a preovulatory surge in prostaglandin synthesis within the follicle. Inhibition of this prostaglandin synthesis produces a corpus luteum with an entrapped oocyte.

As uncertain as the factors which "choose" the follicles for maturity in any particular cycle is the mechanism by which, in most cases, only a single unit is selected for the final burst of maturity expressed as ovulation. Recent evidence has implicated local concentrations of estradiol within a follicle unit as an important organizational factor. As FSH quantities diminish prior to ovulation, it appears that the most mature follicle, and thus the most efficient estrogen producer, selectively binds available FSH better than less differentiated units. As a result the limited FSH supplies are directed to the single maturing follicle.

The ruptured follicle is transformed by proliferation, vascularization, and luteinization of the granulosa into the yellow body that characterizes the last two weeks of an ovulatory cycle. Contrary to evidence obtained in other mammals, the human corpus luteum appears to possess an inherent life span of two weeks, during which it is sustained by modest postovulatory pituitary secretion of LH. After this period, the corpus luteum recedes unless renewed major tropic stimulation appears in the form of human chorionic gonadotropin (HCG) originating in a flourishing mass of syncytiotrophoblasts associated with an implanted conceptus.

OVARIAN HORMONE FUNCTION: GONADOTROPIN-STEROID INTERACTIONS; GONADOTROPIN SECRETION THROUGH FETAL LIFE, CHILDHOOD, AND PUBERTY

Gonadotropin production has now been documented throughout fetal life, during childhood, and into the adult years. Remarkable levels of FSH and LH, similar to postmenopausal levels, can be measured in the fetus. The peak concentrations of FSH and LH occur at approximately midgestation, at about 20 weeks of intrauterine life (Fig. 2).

The production of gonadotropins until midgestation reflects the growing ability of the hypothalamic-pituitary axis to perform at full capacity. Beginning at midgestation, there is an increasing sensitivity to inhibition by steroids, i.e., a maturation of the negative feedback system. Full sensitivity to steroids is not reached until late in infancy. The rise in gonadotropins after birth reflects loss of the high levels of placental steroids.

Testicular function in the fetus can be correlated with the fetal hormonal patterns. Initial testosterone production and sexual differentiation are in response to the high fetal levels of HCG, whereas further testosterone production and differentiation appear to be maintained by the fetal pituitary gonadotropins. Decreased testosterone levels in late gestation despite continued significant gonadotropin levels may be due to heterogeneity of the gonadotropins (and thus decreased biologic activity), the decrease in gonadotropins being due to placental steroids, interference with steroidogenesis by prolactin, or interference with Leydig cell function by the placental steroids, particularly estrogen. In the female, the peak of oogenesis and the onset of atresia appear to coincide with peak production of pituitary gonadotropins in the fetus.

There is a sex difference in gonadotropin levels. In fetal life, there are higher FSH and LH levels in female fetuses. The lower male levels may be due to elevated testosterone levels. In infancy the postnatal FSH rise is more marked and more sustained in females, whereas LH values are not as high.

The precise signal which initiates the events of puberty is unknown. In girls, the very first steroid to rise in the blood is dehydroepiandrosterone (DHA), beginning at six to eight years. This is followed by a rise in androstenedione at eight to ten years of age, and the estrogens do not begin to rise until ten to twelve years of age. A positive correlation can be demonstrated between bone age and the rise in the adrenal steroids.

Puberty is associated with the development of episodic LH secretion associated with sleep. At the time of the appearance of secondary sex characteristics, the mean LH levels are two to four times higher during sleep than during wakefulness, and the number of LH spurts correspond to the number of sleep cycles of rapid and nonrapid eye movements (REM and NREM). This pattern is not present before or after puberty, and is an early sign of changes taking place in the hypothalamus. FSH levels plateau by mid-puberty, whereas LH and estradiol levels continue to rise until late puberty.

ADULT FEMALE CYCLIC STEROID-PEPTIDE INTERACTIONS

The human menstrual cycle is a recycling system dependent upon changes in estradiol levels at key times. The interplay between the follicle, the hypothalamus, and the anterior pituitary depends upon estradiol functioning as a classic hormone, i.e., to reflect the status of the differentiating follicle, to transmit messages of negative and positive feedback to the hypothalamus, to enhance pituitary sensitivity to GnRH, and to work locally within the follicle of origin to ensure gonadotropin sensitivity.

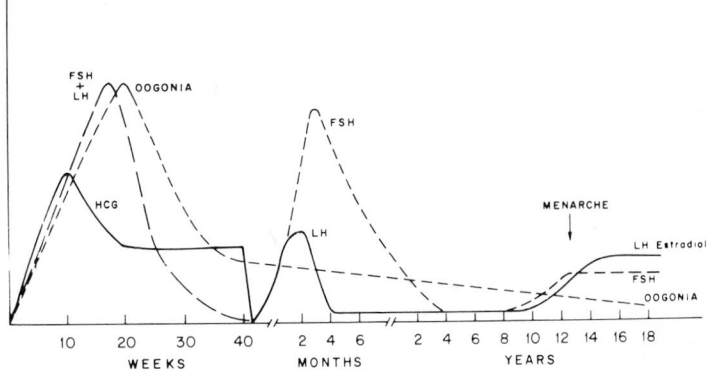

Figure 2. Steroid-peptide hormone interactions in fetal, neonatal, prepubertal, and pubertal periods. (After Winter et al.)

THE FEEDBACK SYSTEMS

The interaction between estrogen and FSH and between estrogen and LH is complex, and is best understood by attention to the following theoretical model. As one increases estradiol in the hypergonadotropic state (postmenopause), the effect of graded increments of estradiol is first seen as suppression of LH, followed at higher levels of estradiol by a suppression of FSH. At still higher doses of estradiol, FSH remains low, but LH secretion is now stimulated. The changes in hormonal levels are regulated therefore by feedback mechanisms. In the case of FSH there is a negative inhibitory feedback relationship with estradiol (the most potent and effective estrogen in the human), whereas in the case of LH there is a negative inhibitory feedback at low levels of estradiol and a positive stimulatory feedback at high levels of estradiol. Thus in the early part of the cycle as estrogens rise, one would expect a decrease in FSH caused by a negative feedback effect. A concomitant decrease in LH does not occur, since the positive hypothalamic center is responding to the rising levels of estrogen and overriding the negative feedback center. The negative feedback of estrogens upon LH secretion therefore operates at a very low level and is probably maximal throughout the cycle. Accordingly, fluctuations in LH reflect the positive feedback of estradiol during the follicular and ovulatory phases. During the luteal phase LH secretion is suppressed by the negative feedback of progesterone. In contrast, FSH levels are regulated throughout the cycle by the negative feedback of estrogen.

The positive feedback system is activated by an increase in circulating estradiol. There are two critical features in this mechanism: (1) the concentration of estradiol and (2) the length of time during which the estradiol elevation is sustained. In women the estradiol concentration necessary to achieve a positive feedback is over 200 pg per milliliter, and this concentration must be sustained for approximately 50 hours. In contrast, a change in circulating estradiol (in the Rhesus monkey) of only 20 pg per milliliter will activate the negative feedback system within minutes.

The negative feedback system may consist of two components: (1) a major system within the hypothalamus involving the tonic center, and (2) a modulating system governing the response of the pituitary to GnRH. A rapid increase in circulating estradiol results in a direct inhibitory effect of the pituitary response to GnRH. In the monkey physiologic doses of estradiol which depressed circulating levels of LH did not decrease levels of GnRH in blood collected from the pituitary stalk. The increasing concentration of estradiol at midcycle augments the pituitary response to GnRH in women, whereas, as noted, acute increases in estradiol inhibit the response to GnRH. Thus the nature of the steroid present in the circulation (estradiol, progesterone, androgens), the steroid concentration, and the time course all influence behavior of the hypothalamic pituitary system.

OVARIAN HORMONE FUNCTION — THE ENDOMETRIAL CYCLE

It is helpful to consider the function of ovarian hormones relative to their ability to provide an appropriate milieu for fertilization, implantation, and nutrition of the early embryo. Before menstruation has ceased, preparation for a more successful ovum is resumed. FSH and small quantities of LH renew follicle growth and augment estrogen secretion. Under the influence of estradiol and estrone, endothelial and mucosal repair takes place. In the ensuing fortnight continued estrogen stimulation produces growth of glands and spiral arterioles. These vessels remain unbranched to the periphery where a terminal capillary network is formed. Accompanying this proliferation, endometrial expansion is accomplished by accumulation of ground substance and modest edema of the stroma. This estrogen-induced phenomenon unfolds the collapsed stromal reticulum. In this way follicle estrogen produces an endometrium with sufficient height, vascularity, and concentrations of glycogen and protein to satisfy the early requirements of the anticipated embryo. Furthermore, estrogen-dependent changes in cervical mucus aid sperm migration.

The midcycle preovulatory peak of estrogen probably signals the release of pituitary LH. The brief surge of this gonadotropin induces acute follicle distention. By unknown mechanisms necrosis of the thinned follicle wall occurs, leading to capsular rupture and permitting extrusion of the ovum. The corpus luteum is formed, and secretion of progesterone rapidly increases. This hormone and sustained levels of estrogen combine to inhibit further LH secretion.

In the absence of a conceptus, at day 12 post ovulation, the corpus luteum recedes and hormone levels wane. With stromal cell shrinkage and loss of ground substance, the endometrium thins. The vessels buckle, and diminished peripheral blood flow is reduced further by tonic vasoconstriction of spiral arterioles. Localized peripheral ischemia and fragmentation occur, with progressive hemorrhage and disruption of superficial zones of the endometrium. With the loss of the peripheral binding epithelium, menstruation begins.

OVARIAN STEROID BIOSYNTHESIS

Appropriate target organ processes are dependent on periodic variations in the quantity and type of hormone emanating from the ovary. How does the ovary accomplish the initial production of microgram quantities of estrogen and then milligram secretion of progesterone? The analyses in vitro of Ryan, using isolated follicles and corpora lutea and radioactive steroid precursors, contributed significantly to the understanding of these processes. This work confirmed the accumulated evidence bearing on the dominance of two biosynthetic pathways leading to estrogen production in the ovary. These routes (A and B) are depicted in Figure 3. Route A provides for conversion of pregnenolone to estrogen via a pathway in which the 3β-ol,Δ^5 characteristic is maintained to the C_{19} stage. Route B projects immediate conversion of pregnenolone to progesterone (change from Δ^5-3β-ol to Δ^4-3 ketone in ring A) prior to loss of sidechain and estrogen generation. Ryan's data suggest that whereas the corpus luteum utilizes the pathway

via progesterone (B), the follicle employs route A, bypassing formation of this biologically active intermediate. Individual cell studies have shown that granulosa and theca cells have similar biosynthetic capabilities and that only quantitative differences exist between these tissues. Apparently both granulosa and theca cells are necessary for adequate steroid production in biologic studies.

The understanding of the biosynthetic processes by which the *combination* of theca and granulosa cells produced estradiol has been extended by recent investigations (Fig. 4). Theca cells provide the C_{19} androgen precursors, i.e., testosterone for the granulosa cell aromatase systems necessary for estrogen synthesis. This biosynthetic conversion may be a crucial factor determining the maturational potential of the follicle. As the local concentrations of estradiol *enhance* differentiation of the follicle, androgen effect will *inhibit* this process.

SITE OF ACTION OF FSH

In small follicles (such as those found at the beginning of the cycle) FSH, not LH, is found in follicle fluid. Although it is useful to consider FSH as the gonadotropin responsible for follicle growth and LH the stimulation of steroidogenesis, such a distinction is not completely accurate. FSH receptors are probably confined to the granulosa cells. Thus FSH may contribute to steroidogenesis by specifically stimulating the steroid aromatizing system within the granulosa. However, such a direct effect on steroidogenic capability of the follicle is not the major role for FSH. In terms of steroidogenesis, the principal contribution of FSH is to increase the activity or the number of LH receptors, this representing but one aspect of the total anabolic and differentiating stimuli FSH brings to the follicle.

LOCAL STEROID EFFECTS

Many of the most important advances in the understanding of ovarian physiology concern the interrelationships of steroids (estradiol and testosterone) and peptides (FSH and LH) on follicle growth and function.

Once initial follicle growth is achieved, continued maturation is dependent on gonadotropins and is correlated with increasing production of estradiol. As the follicle matures, the number of gonadotropin receptors increases. This continued growth is not an expression of an increased affinity for the peptides but of an increase in receptors. The increased FSH receptor number is stimulated by estradiol. Estradiol is necessary for continued response to FSH by increasing the ovarian uptake of FSH and the stimulation of granulosa cell proliferation and aromatase activity. Thus the interaction of FSH and estradiol is mutually enhancing. Estradiol increases FSH receptors, and FSH allows a greater estradiol availability by also indirectly increasing steroidogenesis through the induction of LH receptors. Estradiol alone does not increase LH receptors, but the FSH action is enhanced by estradiol. This sequence of events may be summarized as follows: (1) initial follicle growth → (2) FSH stimulation of further follicle growth → (3) estradiol production, increasing sensitivity to FSH by increasing FSH receptors → (4) FSH induction of LH receptors (enhanced by estra-

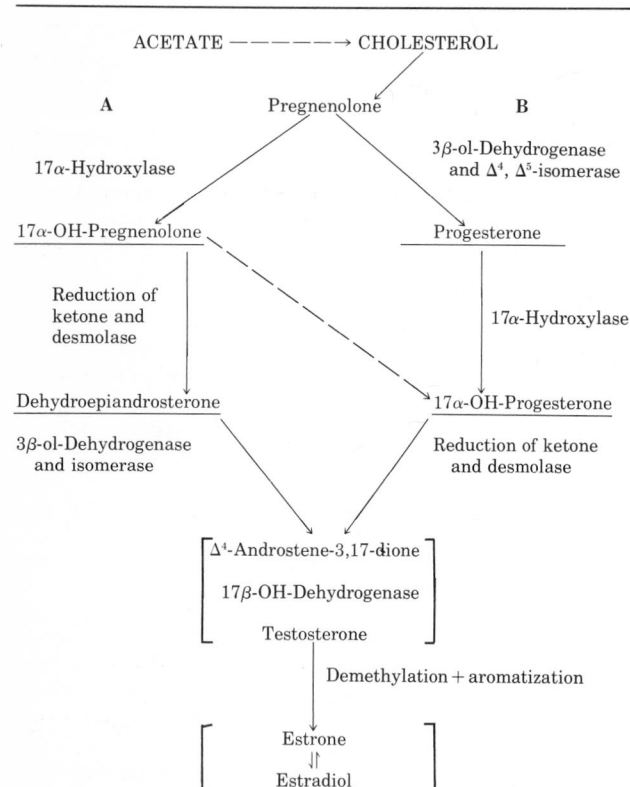

Figure 3.   Pathways of ovarian steroid biosynthesis.

THECA INTERNA

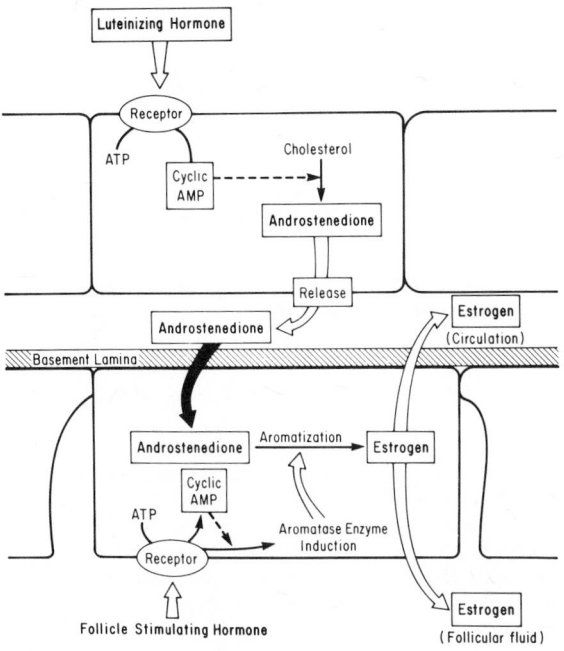

GRANULOSA CELLS

Figure 4. Combined theca–granulosa cell participation in follicle biosynthesis of estrogen. (From Erickson, G. F.: Clin. Gynecol., 21:46, 1978.)

diol) → (5) theca cell differentiation and stimulation with greater estradiol production.

The local ovarian role of androgens in suppressing follicle maturation and inducing atresia has also been explored. Intraovarian androgens accelerate granulosa cell death and follicle atresia. The mechanism for this action may be suppression of granulosa cell receptors for estradiol.

Catt, K. J., and Dufau, M. L.: Basic concepts of the mechanism of action of peptide hormones. Biol. Reprod., 14:1, 1976.

Chan, L., and O'Malley, B. W.: Mechanism of action of the sex steroid hormones. Parts I-III. N. Engl. J. Med., 294:1322, 1372, 1430, 1976.

Faiman, C., Winter, J. S. D., and Reyes, F. I.: Patterns of gonadotrophins and gonadal steroids throughout life. Clin. Obstet. Gynecol., 3:467, 1976.

Louvet, J. P., Harman, S. M., Schrieber, J. R., and Ross G. T.: Evidence for a role of androgens in follicular maturation. Endocrinology, 97:366, 1975.

McNatty, K. P., Hunter, W. M., McNeilly, A. S., and Sawers, R. S.: Changes in the concentration of pituitary and steroid hormones in the follicular fluid of human graafian follicles throughout the menstrual cycle. J. Endocrinology, 64:555, 1975.

Richards, J. S., and Midgley, A. R., Jr.: Protein hormone action: A key to understanding ovarian follicular and luteal cell development. Biol. Reprod., 14:82, 1976.

Ross, G. T., et al.: Pituitary and gonadal hormones in women during spontaneous and induced ovulation cycles. Recent Prog. Horm. Res., 26:1, 1970.

Schally, A. V., et al.: Gonadotropin-releasing hormone: One polypeptide regulates secretion of luteinizing and follicle stimulating hormones. Science, 173:1036, 1971.

549.2. OVARIAN DISORDERS PERTINENT TO GENERAL MEDICINE

EVALUATION OF OVARIAN FUNCTION

The simple existence of ovarian function may be inferred from the development and maintenance of the breasts and the internal and external genitalia. However, a range of ovarian secretion essential to the full activity of these organs is more critically expressed by the periodic phenomenon of ovulatory menstruation. With the corpus luteum's inherent life span of two weeks, an implicit termination point for each cycle is provided in the menstruation resulting from estrogen and progesterone withdrawal and the recycling surge of FSH.

It is helpful to group disorders of ovarian function within the following descriptive categories:

Sexual precocity: the onset of menses before the age of ten years or development of breasts or pubic (not vulvar) hair growth before the age of eight years. Although these elements may appear as isolated manifestations, this general term usually applies to premature appearance of all three aspects of sexual maturation.

Primary amenorrhea: the delay of menarche beyond the age of 18. Statistically 5 per cent of girls initiate menses after 16 and 1 per cent after age 18. In the presence of breast development, pubic hair growth, and a normal adolescent growth spurt, diagnostic evaluation of delayed menarche may be postponed until 18.

Secondary amenorrhea: the cessation of uterine bleeding at any age in women who have previously menstruated. The elapsed interval of amenorrhea necessary for the diagnosis cannot be rigidly defined, and is often dictated by other clinical factors. However, if the patient has not bled within a length of time equivalent to three or four of her normal cycles, then investigation is warranted.

Oligomenorrhea: a recurrent prolongation of intermenstrual intervals leading to a decreased frequency of menses (three to six per year). This irregularity is commonly seen in postmenarchal and premenopausal women. In the absence of other signs and symptoms, intensive workup is not required at these times. Evaluation is in order in other age groups because anovulatory infertility is frequently associated with this menstrual anomaly.

Hypomenorrhea: a diminution in the quantity of menstrual flow based on tampon or napkin requirement. It is of little diagnostic significance if found as a solitary problem. Investigation beyond a physical examination, which includes a pelvic examination and cytologic smear, is unnecessary.

Hypermenorrhea: a definite relative increase in duration or quantity (or both) of menstrual flow that occurs at normal cycle intervals. A subgrouping called *polymenorrhea* designates menstrual flow close to normal in quantity and duration but which occurs too frequently (less than 21 days apart). Each group requires immediate gynecologic assessment. Because each is frequently associated with anovulation, endocrine evaluation may also be in order.

AIDS TO DIAGNOSIS

The clinical categories just described represent a spectrum of abnormal ovarian function which appears clinically as changes in sexual development, menstrual regularity, and ovulation. Such malfunction may be caused by primary ovarian disease, abnormal stimulation of the ovary by other glands, disease of target organs, or systemic disease. Steps to appropriate diagnosis begin with a complete history and physical examination, including careful examination of the pelvic

TABLE 1.   Values for Gonadotropins in Serum

Clinical State	Serum FSH	Serum LH
Normal adult female	5–30 mIU/ml, with ovulatory midcycle peak two times baseline	5–20 mIU/ml, with ovulatory midcycle peak three times baseline
Hypogonadotropism (prepubertal, hypothalamic and pituitary dysfunction)	Less than 5 mIU/ml	Less than 5 mIU/ml
Hypergonadotropism (postmenopause, castrate, ovarian failure)	Greater than 40 mIU/ml	Greater than 25 mIU/ml

organs and external genitalia. When properly selected, certain procedures and laboratory tests can be of great diagnostic assistance.

PITUITARY GONADOTROPIN FUNCTION. Pituitary gonadotropins may be measured by bioassay or by radioimmunoassay. The bioassay requires a 24-hour urine collection from which gonadotropins are extracted by a process including acidification, kaolin absorption and elution, followed by acetone precipitation. The extract is diluted and injected into immature female mice, and the increase in the weight of the mouse uterus is measured. The assay depends on the FSH and LH in the extract to stimulate the immature mouse ovaries to produce estrogen. The greatest dilution of the urine extract which causes a 100 per cent increase in uterine weight is the titer of gonadotropins, and the result is expressed in mouse uterine weight units (muu) per 24 hours. Less than 6 muu per 24 hours indicates normal prepubertal levels or adult hypogonadotropism. A castrate or postmenopausal level is greater than 200 muu per 24 hours.

This assay is notoriously unreliable and has been entirely replaced by specific radioimmunoassays for FSH and LH in serum. It must be remembered (Fig. 1) that wide swings in gonadotropin levels are typical of ovulatory cycles. Table 1 depicts the ranges of gonadotropins in various clinical circumstances.

OVARIAN FUNCTION. Tests that are based on biologic effects of ovarian hormones are simply performed, providing immediate and valuable data at little cost to the patient. Therefore more costly laboratory evaluations of hormone excretion or blood concentrations are rarely required for clinical purposes.

Gonadal Hormone Effects. CORNIFICATION OF VAGINAL EPITHELIUM. The percentage of fully cornified cells is related to ovarian estrogen production. Because cytologic criteria and staining methods vary from center to center, no normal values can be given. However, because other factors affect this evaluation (progesterone, cortisone, and androgen diminish, although digitalis increases cornification), the stage of the cycle as well as current therapy must be considered in evaluation of test results.

Endometrial biopsy tests endometrial responsiveness as well as the existence of appropriate ovarian hormone secretion during the cycle. Evaluation must take into consideration the stage of the cycle when the biopsy specimen is taken.

In addition to the quantity and clarity of *cervical mucus,* the development of an arborization pattern in a dried specimen *(the "fern" test)* indicates the presence of estrogen. Correlation with cycle dates is essential, for secretion of progesterone inhibits this phenomenon.

The *basal body temperature* will demonstrate the occurrence of ovulation if serial readings are taken throughout a cycle. Based on the mild thermogenic properties of progesterone, a sustained postovulatory rise of temperature (0.3° C or more) of two weeks' duration indicates corpus luteum function. Retrospectively, the timing of ovulation in the cycle can be estimated from the date when the effect of progesterone first appeared.

PROGESTERONE WITHDRAWAL BLEEDING. If menses can be induced after administration of progesterone or a nonestrogenic derivative, this event indicates prior ovarian estrogen secretion and its proliferative or "priming" effect on the endometrium.

Gonadal Hormone Plasma Concentrations. The normal levels for total plasma estrogens or estradiol and plasma progesterone vary with the time in the menstrual cycle when the blood sample is drawn. (For the pattern of these variations, see Fig. 2.) The normal ranges of plasma gonadal steroids as measured by radioimmunoassay are depicted in Table 2.

Gonadal Hormone Excretion. TOTAL URINARY ESTROGENS PER 24 HOURS. The measurement of estrogen ina a 24-hour urine sample is useful in guiding replacement FSH-LH therapy for the induction of ovulation. The range of estrogen excretion during various clinical states is shown in Table 3.

URINARY PREGNANEDIOL EXCRETION. Pregnanediol is the main urinary metabolite of progesterone but accounts for only 7 to 20 per cent of total progesterone production. Measurement of this metabolite in urine has been used to document ovulation and the presence and well-being of early pregnancy. The range of excretion of pregnanediol is seen in Table 4.

URINARY PREGNANETRIOL EXCRETION. Although not exclusively a metabolite of gonadal hormone production, the concentration of this metabolite of 17α-OH-progesterone in a 24-hour urine specimen is useful in the diagnosis of adrenocortical hyperplasia. In normal circumstances urinary pregnanetriol excretions in children and adults are within the ranges shown in Table 5.

Other Tests. Other tests of importance include those that estimate *adrenal cortex and thyroid activity.* Specific details concerning interpretation of results and the diagnostic manipulations involved are given in other

TABLE 2.   Values for Plasma Estrogens and Progesterone

Cycle Phase	Total Estrogen or Estradiol	Progesterone
Follicle phase	25– 75 pg/ml	Less than 1 ng/ml
Midcycle peak	200–600 pg/ml	
Luteal phase	100–300 pg/ml	5– 20 ng/ml
Pregnancy, first trimester	1– 5 ng/ml	20– 30 ng/ml
Pregnancy, second trimester	5– 15 ng/ml	50–100 ng/ml
Pregnancy, third trimester	10– 40 ng/ml	100–400 ng/ml

TABLE 3. Values for Urinary Estrogen

Clinical Circumstance	Total Urinary Estrogen/24 Hours
Prepubertal	0– 5 μg/24 hr
Follicle phase	10– 25 μg/24 hr
Midcycle peak	35–100 μg/24 hr
Luteal phase	25– 75 μg/24 hr
Postmenopausal	5– 15 μg/24 hr

sections of this text. Dysfunction of either organ may have pronounced effects on ovarian and target organ physiology.

HUMAN CHORIONIC GONADOTROPIN. Secretion of human chorionic gonadotropin (HCG) by the synctiotrophoblast cells of the placenta is directed predominantly into the maternal circulation. The assay of HCG in maternal urine has been the basis of many pregnancy tests since the original Aschheim-Zondek test.

These bioassays depend upon the response of ovaries or testes in immature animals to the gonadotropic properties of HCG when present in urine. The endpoints were increased gonadal weight, hyperemia, or response in sex organs to increased gonadal steroidogenesis induced by HCG. The expulsion of ova or sperm in amphibia was also a widely used clinical assay. These biologic tests have been entirely replaced by the clinical application of immunoassays for HCG in urine — the urinary chorionic gonadotropin (UCG) test.

Three types of immunologic assays are used: hemagglutination-inhibition, complement-fixation, and radioimmunoassay. In the hemagglutination-inhibition reaction, the presence of HCG in maternal urine inhibits an agglutination reaction between HCG-coated red cells and the antisera. In some commercial methods latex particles are used in place of red cells. A rapid although less sensitive slide test using latex particles is available, but the two-hour red cell test is more reliable. A first morning voided urine specimen is preferred.

HCG and LH are similar in structure and considerable immunologic cross-reaction exists. The sensitivity of most commercial HCG assays is limited to 1000 IU per liter of urine to avoid false positive cross-reactions with LH. Because of the limitations in sensitivity, a positive test result does not appear until ten days to two weeks after the missed menstrual period. From that point the levels of HCG rise to an average peak of 100,000 IU per liter at 10 weeks' gestation, and then declines over the next four weeks to 20,000 IU per liter, at which point excretion levels are sustained for the remainder of the pregnancy.

Patients with *hydatidiform moles* generally display urinary HCG levels around 300,000 IU per liter. *Choriocarcinoma* may be associated with levels in the millions of

TABLE 4. Values for Urinary Pregnanediol

	Urinary Pregnanediol/24 Hours
Follicle phase	Less than 1 mg
Luteal phase	2–5 mg
Pregnancy, 20 weeks	40 mg
Pregnancy, 30 weeks	80 mg
Pregnancy, 40 weeks	100 mg

TABLE 5. Values for Urinary Pregnanetriol

	Urinary Pregnanetriol/24 Hours
Children	Less than 0.5 mg
Adults	0.2 to 2–4 mg (upper limits vary with laboratory)

IU. Although absolute levels are helpful, they are not absolutely diagnostic of disease. Multiple gestations may also show high levels of UCG excretion.

A semiquantitative estimation of HCG in a 24-hour urine may be useful in evaluating threatened abortion of ectopic gestation. A low or declining level of UCG indicates a poor prognosis for an intrauterine pregnancy, whereas a low level of HCG (below 5000 IU per liter of urine) is commonly seen when the pregnancy test is positive in ectopic pregnancy.

Three weeks after a spontaneous or therapeutic abortion, the urinary pregnancy test result should reverse to negative. Before that time positive test results may still be encountered.

Development of specific assays for the β subunit of HCG has increased diagnostic sensitivity and precision in three clinical areas: early pregnancy, monitoring patients with HCG-secreting tumors, and diagnosing ectopic pregnancies.

With specific HCG radioimmunoassay, pregnancy can be detected as early as ten days after fertilization. This represents a 100-fold increase in sensitivity compared with conventional pregnancy tests.

Clinical assays. *In* Speroff, L., Glass, R. H., and Kase, N. G.: Clinical Gynecologic Endocrinology and Infertility. Baltimore, Williams & Wilkins Company, 1978, Chap. 20.

PUBERTY

The initiation of menstrual function in humans occurs with greatest frequency at age 12 or 13, but there is a considerable "normal" variation in the time of its onset. When menstruation begins before the age of 10 or after 16, a decision must be made whether the precocious or delayed menarche is a physiologic variant or whether it is due to some abnormality. Furthermore, since menarche is but one of several important changes associated with puberty and a variation in its timing is by no means the only feature of disease, it is useful to review the characteristic sequence of female puberty.

The *first sign of puberty* is generally the appearance of the *breast bud*. Pubic hair quickly follows breast development, but appearance of axillary hair is normally delayed as much as two years. At about the time of breast development the adolescent growth in linear height begins, and over the next year of peak growth a girl will grow 6 to 11 cm. In the typical pubescence, within two years of initiating this growth spurt, the first menstruation, i.e., the menarche, occurs.

Because the growth of pubic and axillary hair is almost certainly due to an increased production of adrenal androgens at puberty, this event is often referred to as *adrenarche* as well as pubarche. Premature thelarche (premature breast development) as an isolated biologic event is less common. The etiology of these events is not understood at present; gonadotropin and estrogen levels are not elevated.

Although pubescence has been described in terms of

the two-year sequence — increased linear growth rate, breast development, pubarche, and menarche — varying patterns occur frequently and are not necessarily indicative of dysfunction or disease.

Certain aspects of the neuroendocrine mechanism involved in normal puberty have been uncovered. It has been shown that the anterior pituitary of infants contains adequate quantities of gonadotropins and that an intact pituitary is essential for the prepubertal development and maintenance of the gonads. Removal of the ovaries in this age group is associated with increased gonadotropin excretion, the formation of castration cells in the pituitary, and enlargement of the gland. These changes can be prevented by estrogen therapy in very low doses. Therefore the small quantity of estrogen secreted prepubertally is sufficient to inhibit all but a small clinically undetectable quantity of gonadotropin release. Further indirect evidence that this central inhibition is the critical mechanism in the *normal* delay of sexual maturation can be seen in the fully responsive competence of the premenarchal ovary to exogenous gonadotropin therapy. Certain areas in the hypothalamus are believed to be responsible for this temporary extreme sensitivity to inhibiting levels of circulating steroids. It has been suggested that neoplastic and vascular disorders that alter hypothalamic function probably reverse this low threshold inhibition and lead to precocious puberty.

SEXUAL PRECOCITY

Precocity may be due to organic or constitutional (idiopathic) causes. Ninety per cent of patients with this symptom will fall in the latter category despite thorough evaluation. However, it is essential that these cases be distinguished from those with lesions of the brain or the rare diseases of ovary and adrenal that produce premature development.

CONSTITUTIONAL SEXUAL PRECOCITY. This is due to the premature release of the adult sequence and levels of gonadotropin, which are sufficient to initiate prematurely the normal physiologic and endocrine processes of breast development, appearance of pubic and axillary hair, and menstruation. Although it is assumed that hypothalamic inhibitory influences have been diminished, the precise inciting factor is unknown. Diminished secretion of inhibitory quantities of melatonin by the pineal gland is suggested as one possible etiologic factor. Generally the normal, orderly, albeit more rapid appearance of breast development, pubic hair growth, and then menarche is found in the five- to eight-year age group. However, menarche may be the first symptom noted and may occur as early as three months of age. The usual sequential maturation pattern may be altered or only partially displayed. Although not all patients will ovulate, biologic manifestations of ovulation rule out precocity based on gonadotropin-independent estrogen production by ovarian or adrenal disease. Estrogen production from any source is likely to induce accelerated linear growth and advancement of bone age, which is seen best in roentgenograms of carpal bones, knee, and elbow. Although these children are temporarily taller than their normal counterparts, premature closure of epiphyses produces a final height that is less than normal. Thus the diagnostic criteria for a constitutional etiology of precocity include the sequence of secondary sex characteristics, advanced bone age, adult levels of estrogen and gonadotropin, nor-

mal urinary adrenal metabolites, and normal neurologic examination and skull films. Optimal therapy (reversible suppression of gonadotropins without peripheral target organ stimulation) may be achievable with long-acting nonestrogenic depomedroxyprogesterone acetate.* This potent progestational agent, when administered in large doses (400 mg) intramuscularly monthly for three months and then once every three months, provides long-term inhibition of gonadotropin secretion. Pubic hair does not disappear, but further menstruation, breast development, and growth may be inhibited. The response to progestins is not uniformly positive; it is not possible to determine which child will respond favorably in advance of therapy.

These children present a serious emotional and social problem not only because they are distinctly different from their contemporaries, but also because they are insufficiently mature emotionally to cope with the sexual interest they provoke in others. That they are capable of reproduction has been demonstrated many times, but most dramatically in the case of a Peruvian girl, Lena Medina, who was delivered of a normal child by cesarean section at five and a half years of age.

PRECOCITY DUE TO ORGANIC CAUSES. Cerebral Lesions. A variety of brain disorders produce sexual precocity secondary to premature gonadotropin release, presumably by the abolition of the inhibitory effects of the hypothalamus. Although the anatomic location of these inhibitory centers is uncertain, three general groups of tumors may cause precocity: lesions in the tuber cinereum, lesions in the posterior hypothalamic mammillary body area, and lesions destroying the pineal. In addition, disorders indirectly affecting hypothalamic function (internal hydrocephalus, encephalitis, meningitis, and cranial trauma) may be associated with precocity. Differential diagnosis of this type of precocity from the constitutional variety cannot be achieved by endocrine survey. Only after intensive neurologic, roentgenographic, and pediatric evaluation and follow-up reappraisal will proper diagnosis be made.

Organic Precocious Pseudopuberty Due to Adrenal and Ovarian Hyperfunction. The term pseudopuberty defines the basic difference between precocity resulting from premature gonadotropic activity (constitutional, central types) and those lesions in which adrenal and ovarian estrogen stimulates target organs. In the latter, gonadotropin is absent, and therefore ovulation does not occur.

Although certain elements of premature maturation (pubic hair, bone age advancement) appear in adrenal disorders, the masculinization and rarity of vaginal bleeding (delayed menarche is usual) make the diagnosis relatively simple. Isosexual pseudopuberty is more commonly associated with estrogen-producing ovarian tumors. Although the diagnosis of tumor is always considered, it is rarely confirmed. Only 5 per cent of *granulosa tumors* occur before true puberty. The presence of a palpable adnexal mass and the absence of urinary gonadotropin, ovulation, and regular cyclic bleeding support the diagnosis. In addition, the exceedingly rare *choriocarcinoma, teratoma, or dysgerminoma* of the ovary may be associated with pseudopuberty. However, these will sometimes pose a diagnostic complication. The production of chorionic gonadotropin by these tumors will give falsely elevated adult levels of "FSH" in mouse uterine

---

*Investigational drug for this purpose.

weight tests and elevated serum LH values in routine radioimmunoassay, in addition to positive pregnancy tests. The finding of an ovarian mass calls for laparotomy.

Albright's syndrome, consisting of cystic bone lesions, patchy skin pigmentation, and sexual precocity, is grouped with pseudopuberty in that gonadotropin excretion and ovulation are absent. Normal puberty and ovulation follow and fertility is not decreased.

Bidlingmaier, F., Butenandt, O., and Knorr, D.: Plasma gonadotropins and estrogens in girls with idiopathic precocious puberty. Pediat. Res., 11:91, 1977.

Di George, A. M.: Albright syndrome: Is it coming of age? J. Pediat. 87:1018, 1970.

Greulich, W. W., and Pyle, S. L.: Radiographic Atlas of Skeletal Development of the Hand and Wrist. Stanford, Stanford University Press, 1950.

Jones, K. L.: Feminization, virilization and precocious sexual development that results from neoplastic processes. Ann. N.Y. Acad. Sci., 230:195, 1974.

Korth-Schutz, S., Levine, L. S., and New, M. I.: Serum androgens in normal prepubertal and pubertal children and in children with precocious adrenarche. J. Clin. Endocrinol. Metab., 42:117, 1976.

Marshall, W. A., and Tanner, J. M.: Variations in the pattern of pubertal changes in girls. Arch. Dis. Child., 42:291, 1969.

Money, J., and Clopper, R. R., Jr.: Psychosocial and psychosexual aspects of errors of pubertal onset and development. Hum. Biol., 46:173, 1974.

Tanner, J. M.: Growth at Adolescence. 2nd ed. Oxford, Blackwell, 1962.

THE AMENORRHEAS

DEFINITION OF AMENORRHEA. Any patient fulfilling the following criteria should be evaluated for clinical amenorrhea: (1) No period by age 14 in the absence of growth or development of secondary sexual characteristics. (2) No period by age 16 regardless of the presence of normal growth and development with the appearance of secondary sexual characteristics. (3) In a woman who has been menstruating, the absence of periods for a length of time equivalent to a total of at least three of the previous cycle intervals or six months of amenorrhea.

DIAGNOSTIC EVALUATION OF AMENORRHEA. It is useful to employ a diagnostic evaluation system (Fig. 5) which segregates causes of amenorrhea into the following categories: (1) disorders of outflow tract or uterine target organ; (2) disorders of the ovary; (3) disorders of the anterior pituitary; and (4) disorders of central nervous system (hypothalamic) factors and functions.

All patients with amenorrhea are exposed to the following combined therapeutic and laboratory steps:

Step One. The initial step is to assess the level of endogenous estrogen and the competence of the outflow tract, and to measure the serum prolactin level. In order to test the pituitary-ovarian system, a course of a pure progestational agent totally devoid of estrogenic activity is administered. There are only two choices: progesterone in oil (100 mg intramuscularly) or the orally active compound, medroxyprogesterone acetate (Provera), 10 mg daily for 5 days.

The patient will either bleed or not bleed within two to seven days after the conclusion of progestational medication. If the patient bleeds, a diagnosis of *anovulation* is made. The presence of a functional outflow tract and a uterus lined by reactive endometrium sufficiently prepared by endogenous estrogen is confirmed. With this demonstration of the presence of estrogen, at least minimal function of the ovary, pituitary, and central nervous system is established. Obviously, perfect integration of these systems has not been achieved, the dysfunction resulting in anovulation.

In the absence of galactorrhea, and if the serum prolactin level is normal (less than 20 ng per milliliter), evaluation for a pituitary tumor is not necessary. If the serum prolactin level is elevated, polytomography of the sella turcica (discussed below) is essential. The presence of galactorrhea, regardless of the bleeding pattern or the prolactin level, dictates pituitary evaluation. Only a rare patient with a pituitary or nearby tumor will bleed following progestational medication, and prolactin level serves as an effective screen for these patients.

Step Two. If the course of progestational medication does not produce withdrawal flow, either the target organ outflow tract is inoperative or preliminary estrogen preparation of the endometrium has not occurred. Orally active estrogen is administered in quantity and duration certain to stimulate endometrial proliferation and withdrawal bleeding, provided that a completely reactive uterus with patent outflow tract exists. An appropriate dose is 2.5 mg conjugated estrogens daily for 21 days.

As a result of this pharmacologic test, the patient with amenorrhea will either bleed or not bleed. If there is no withdrawal flow, the diagnosis of a *defect in the endometrium or outflow tract is made.* If withdrawal bleeding does occur, these systems have normal functional abilities if properly stimulated by estrogen.

Step Three. With the elucidation of the amenorrheic patient's inability to provide adequate stimulatory amounts of estrogen, the physiologic mechanisms responsible for the elaboration of this steroid must be tested. In order to produce estrogen, gonads containing a normal follicular apparatus and sufficient pituitary gonadotropin as the hormonal means to stimulate the apparatus are required. Step three determines which of these two components (gonadotropins or follicular activity) is functioning improperly.

This step involves an assay of the level of gonadotropins. The normal range for LH in serum is 5 to 20 mIU per milliliter; under 5 mIU per milliliter is abnormally low, and over 25 mIU is abnormally high. One should keep in mind that the midcycle surge of LH is approximately three times the baseline level. Therefore if the patient does not bleed two weeks after the blood sample was

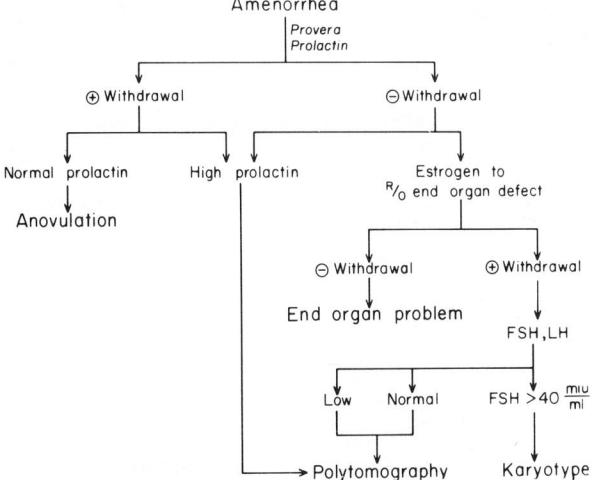

Figure 5. "Flow" diagram of standard diagnostic workup of amenorrhea.

obtained, the high level can be safely interpreted as abnormal. An FSH level below 5 mIU is abnormally low and over 40 mIU is abnormally high.

Step three is designed to determine whether the lack of estrogen is due to a fault in the follicle or in the CNS-pituitary axis. The result of the gonadotropin assay in the amenorrheic woman who does not bleed following a progestational agent will be abnormally high, abnormally low, or in the normal range. If the FSH is over 40 mIU per milliliter, the cause of the amenorrhea is *gonadal failure*. If gonadotropins are abnormally low or in the normal range, *pituitary failure or inactivity is diagnosed*. In practice, a low LH (less than 5 mIU per milliliter) has been found to be a more reliable indicator of hypogonadotropism, whereas a high FSH (over 40 mIU per milliliter) has proved to be a reliable indicator of ovarian failure. FSH values within the normal range (5 to 30 mIU per milliliter) indicate the presence of ovarian follicles, whereas values over 40 mIU per milliliter are found only when the supply of ovarian follicles has been exhausted.

HIGH GONADOTROPINS.   Patients with FSH levels over 40 mIU per milliliter will not respond to ovulatory drugs and should be considered sterile. The association between a high FSH and ovarian failure is so reliable that further attempts to document the state of the ovaries are unnecessary. Because the result of a high FSH has such an immense bearing on the future fertility of the patient, repeat sampling is a wise precaution. Rarely a condition is encountered in which there is a single gonadotropin deficiency. A patient with an isolated deficiency of FSH would have primary amenorrhea, a high LH level, and undetectable FSH.

LOW GONADOTROPINS.   If the gonadotropin assay is abnormally low or in the normal range, one final localization is required to distinguish between a pituitary or CNS-hypothalamic cause for the amenorrhea. Special skull x-rays (polytomography) should be obtained to examine the sella turcica for signs of abnormal change.

Polytomography consists of tomographic sections (at approximately 1 mm increments) of the sella turcica in the lateral and anteroposterior projections with a hypocycloidal movement which blurs structures not in the plane of section and gives excellent focal resolution. This technique will detect a microadenoma of 5 to 10 mm in size. With a tumor of this size, a routine skull film will indicate a normal sella turcica. Typical polytomographic findings consistent with a pituitary tumor are localized bulging of the anteroinferior wall on one side (lateralization is a significant characteristic) and erosion (demineralization) of the anterior or posterior floor of the sella. When the adenoma grows above 10 mm, the diameters of the sella are increased. Visual field examination is reserved for the evaluation of the patient with an abnormal polytomogram.

If amenorrhea is the only presenting symptom in an otherwise normal individual, sella turcica evaluation should be obtained annually as a precaution to rule out an emerging tumor. The patient with an insidiously evolving pituitary tumor may present with amenorrhea years before the tumor becomes evident by sella turcica x-rays. A spectrum beginning with a mildly compromised ovulatory capacity and extending to panhypopituitarism can be encountered. Usually, over the course of time, deterioration in tropic activity is seen, with withdrawal of activity following a fairly predictable pattern: first growth hormone, then FSH and LH, and finally TSH and ACTH. Less commonly, peculiar isolated loss of specific tropic hormones may be found. Only rare cases have been reported of gonadotropin-producing pituitary tumors.

EVALUATION OF THE ABNORMAL SELLA TURCICA.   Expectations for the utilization of gonadotropin-releasing hormone (GnRH) to discriminate between disorders of the hypothalamus and the anterior pituitary have not been realized. Tremendous variability in response is the rule, even to the degree that the patient with a pituitary tumor may or may not respond to GnRH stimulation. Likewise, maneuvers designed to alter prolactin secretion (L-dopa, phenothiazine, and ergot alkaloid administration) cannot identify the patient with a pituitary tumor. Therefore the serum prolactin level and polytomography are the two major screening procedures.

There is a positive correlation between prolactin levels and the size of the sella turcica. However, significant tumors may be found in amenorrheic women with normal or slightly elevated prolactin levels. Further sampling is not useful, since a random single blood sample appears to be reliable in detecting elevated levels of prolactin.

If the x-ray of the sella and neurologic scrutiny raise the suspicion of tumor, further evaluation requires an inpatient program along with consultation with an expert neurosurgeon. Inpatient evaluation of an abnormal sella turcica includes dynamic testing of tropic hormones, computerized axial tomography, pneumoencephalography, and visual field examination.

Specific Disorders Leading to Amenorrhea

Disorders of Outflow or Uterine End-Organ

ASHERMAN'S SYNDROME.   Secondary amenorrhea follows destruction of the endometrium (Asherman's syndrome). This condition generally is the result of an over-zealous postpartum curettage resulting in intrauterine scarification and showing a typical pattern of multiple synechiae on a hysterogram. In the presence of normal ovarian function, the basal body temperature over one month's time will be biphasic. Asherman's syndrome is treated with dilatation and curettage (D and C) to break up the synechiae and an on-the-table hysterogram to ensure a free uterine cavity. Current clinical investigation indicates that hysteroscopy with direct lysis of adhesions is a preferred alternative to the "blind" dilatation and curettage.

At operation, a method should be utilized to prevent the sides of the uterine cavity from readhering. Previously an intrauterine device was used for this purpose; however, a pediatric Foley catheter appears to be a better method. The bag is filled with 3 ml of fluid, and the catheter is removed after seven days. A broad-spectrum antimicrobial agent is started preoperatively and maintained for ten days. The patient is treated for six months with high stimulatory doses of estrogen (e.g., conjugated estrogens, 10 mg daily, three weeks out of four, with Provera, 10 mg daily, added during the third week).

Infectious impairment of the endometrium resulting in amenorrhea is usually attributed to tuberculosis, a rare but still present condition in the United States. Diagnosis is made by culture of the menstrual discharge or endometrial biopsy. Uterine schistosomiasis may be another rare cause of end-organ failure, and eggs may be found in urine, feces, rectal scrapings, menstrual discharge, or endometrium.

MÜLLERIAN ANOMALIES.   In primary amenorrheas, discontinuity by segmental disruptions of the müllerian tube should be ruled out. Good clinical practice demands a survey which begins distally and works proximally. Thus imperforate hymen, obliteration of the vaginal orifice, and lapses in continuity of the vaginal canal must be ruled out by direct observation. The cervix or the entire uterus may be absent. Far less commonly the uterus may be present but the cavity absent, or in the presence of a cavity the endometrium may be congenitally lacking. With the exception of these latter items, the clinical problem of amenorrhea is compounded by the painful distention of hematocolpos, hematometra, or hematoperitoneum. In all instances an effort must be made to incise and drain from below at the points of closure of the müllerian tube. In complicated circumstances re-establishment of müllerian duct continuity can be achieved surgically. Depending on the type of anomaly, associated lesions of lower genitourinary and gastrointestinal tracts should be ruled out.

MÜLLERIAN AGENESIS. Lack of müllerian development (Mayer-Rokitansky-Küster-Hauser syndrome) is the diagnosis for the individual with primary amenorrhea and no apparent vagina. This is a relatively common cause of primary amenorrhea, more frequent than testicular feminization, and second only to gonadal dysgenesis. These patients have an absence or hypoplasia of the vagina. The uterus may be normal, but lacking a conduit to the introitus, or there may only be rudimentary bicornuate cords present. If a partial endometrial cavity is present, cyclic abdominal pain may be a complaint. Because of the similarity to some types of male pseudohermaphroditism, it is worthwhile to demonstrate the normal female karyotype. Ovarian function is normal, and can be documented with basal body temperatures or peripheral levels of progesterone. Growth and development are normal. Although usually sporadic, occasional occurrence may be noted within a family.

Further evaluation should include radiologic studies. Approximately one third have abnormal kidneys and 12 per cent or more have skeletal anomalies, mostly involving the spine. When the presence of a uterine structure is suspected on examination, ultrasound may be utilized to depict the size and symmetry of the structure.

Therapy includes surgery or the vaginal pressure technique of Frank and Wabrek to establish a coitally functional vagina.

TESTICULAR FEMINIZATION. When a blind vaginal canal is encountered and the uterus is absent, the possibility of testicular feminization must be excluded. The patient with testicular feminization is a male pseudohermaphrodite. The adjective *male* refers to the gonadal sex; thus the individual has testes and an XY karyotype. *Pseudohermaphrodite* means that the genitalia are opposite of the gonads; thus the individual is phenotypically female, but with absent or meager pubic and axillary hair.

The male pseudohermaphrodite is a genetic and gonadal male with failure of virilization. Failures in male development can be considered as a spectrum, with incomplete forms of testicular feminization being represented by some androgen response. Transmission of this disorder is by means of an X-linked recessive gene responsible for the dihydrotestosterone receptor. Clinically the diagnosis should be considered in (1) a female child with inguinal hernias, since the testes are frequently partially descended; (2) a patient with primary amenorrhea and an absent uterus; and (3) a patient with absent body hair.

These patients appear normal at birth, except for the possible presence of an inguinal hernia, and most patients are not seen by a physician until puberty. Growth and development are normal, although over-all height is usually greater than average and there may be a eunuchoidal tendency (long arms, big hands and feet). The breasts, although large, are abnormal; actual glandular tissue is not abundant, and the nipples are small and areolae are pale. More than 50 per cent have an inguinal hernia; the labia minora are usually underdeveloped, and the blind vagina is less than normal. Rudimentary fallopian tubes are composed of fibromuscular tissue with only occasional epithelial lining.

The testes may be intra-abdominal, but often are in the hernia. They are similar to any cryptorchid testis except that they may be nodular. After puberty, the testis has immature tubular development and is lined by immature germ cells and Sertoli cells. There is no spermatogenesis. The incidence of neoplasia in these gonads is high. In 50 reported patients 30 years old or more, there were 11 malignancies, 15 adenomas, and 10 benign cysts — a 22 per cent incidence of malignancy and a 52 per cent incidence of neoplasia. Therefore once full development is attained after puberty, the gonads should be removed and the patient placed on hormonal replacement therapy. This is the only exception to the rule that gonads with a Y chromosome should be removed prior to puberty. The reason is that development achieved with hormonal replacement does not seem to match the smooth pubertal changes caused by endogenous hormones.

When first studied, it was found that the urinary 17-ketosteroids were normal, and it was suggested that there might be a resistance to androgen action rather than an absence of androgens — a congenital androgen insensitivity. Indeed, the plasma levels of testosterone are in the normal to high male range, and the plasma clearance and metabolism of testosterone are normal. Thus these patients produce testosterone, but they do not respond to androgens, either their own or those given locally or systemically. Therefore the critical steps in sexual differentiation which require androgens fail to take place, and development is totally female.

Cases of incomplete testicular feminization represent individuals with some androgen effect. Such patients may have clitoral enlargement, or a phallus may even be present. Axillary and pubic hair develop, along with breast growth. Gonadectomy should not be deferred in such cases, but would in fact obviate unwanted further virilization. Patients with a deficit in testicular 17-dehydrogenase activity will have impaired testosterone production, and present clinically as incomplete testicular feminization. Since treatment is the same, precise diagnosis is not essential.

Disorders of the Ovary

Gonadal failure is best classified in two large groups: gonadal dysgenesis and gonadal agenesis.

TURNER'S SYNDROME (Fig. 6). Gonadal dysgenesis (Turner's syndrome) is a well-known entity. The characteristics of short stature, webbed neck, shield chest, and increased carrying angle, combined with hypergonadotropic hypoestrogenic amenorrhea, usually make a correct diagnosis possible on the most superficial evaluation. However, special attention must be given to the less common variations of this syndrome. Coarctation of the aorta and various renal collecting system anomalies must

Figure 6. Turner's syndrome.

be ruled out. A karyotype should be performed on all patients with elevated gonadotropins, despite the appearance of a typical case of Turner's syndrome. The presence of the syndrome, 45,X chromosome single cell line, should be confirmed.

MOSAICISM. The presence of mosaicism (multiple cell lines of varying sex chromosome composition) must be ruled out for a very important reason. The presence of a Y chromosome in the karyotype requires laparotomy and excision of the gonadal areas, on the basis that the presence of any medullary (testicular) component within the gonad is a predisposing factor to tumor formation and to heterosexual development (virilization). Only in the patient with the complete form of testicular feminization can laparotomy be deferred until after puberty, since the individual is resistant to androgens. In all other patients with a Y chromosome, gonadectomy should be performed before puberty to avoid virilization. One should be aware that approximately 30 per cent of patients with a Y chromosome will not develop any signs of virilization. Therefore even the normal-appearing adult patient with elevated serum levels of gonadotropins must be karyotyped to detect a silent Y chromosome, so that prophylactic gonadectomy may be performed before neoplastic changes occur.

The impact of mosaicism, even in the absence of a

Y-containing line, is significant. With an XX component (e.g., XX/XO), functional cortical (ovarian) tissue can be anticipated to exist within the gonad, leading to a variety of responses, including some degree of female development, and on occasion even menses and reproduction. These individuals may appear normal, attaining normal stature before premature menopause is experienced. The menopause is early, presumably because the number of functioning follicles was limited by an abnormal chromosomal constitution.

This complex array of gonadal dysgenesis variations, from the typical form to an otherwise normal-appearing and functioning woman with premature menopause, is the result of mosaicism which produces a complex mixture of cortical and medullary gonadal tissue. The clinical importance of this information justifies obtaining karyotypes in all cases of elevated gonadotropins.

GONADAL AGENESIS. No complicated clinical problems accompany the gonadal failure caused by agenesis. Without precise information, only conjecture as to the causes of absent development can be made. Thus viral and metabolic influences in early gestation are suspected events. Nevertheless, the final result is irretrievable — hypergonadotropic hypogonadism.

THE RESISTANT OVARY SYNDROME. Rare patients with amenorrhea have elevated gonadotropins despite the presence of ovarian follicles. These patients require large amounts of exogenous gonadotropins in order to produce follicular growth and estrogen production. In order to arrive at a correct diagnosis, laparotomy is necessary to achieve adequate histologic evaluation of the ovaries (since laparoscopic biopsy is not representative). Because of the rarity of this condition, and the very low chance of achieving pregnancy even with high doses of exogenous gonadotropins, performing a laparotomy for the purpose of ovarian biopsy on every patient with amenorrhea, high gonadotropins, and a normal karyotype is not productive clinically.

A situation similar to the resistant ovary syndrome may be encountered in the perimenopausal period. In the perimenopausal period (whether it be premature at age 30 to 38, or at the expected time) the remaining few follicles may fail to respond until a high level of gonadotropin is reached. Hence a period of amenorrhea with postmenopausal levels of FSH and LH may be followed by a pregnancy.

Premature ovarian failure caused by antibodies to steroid-producing cells is almost always associated with idiopathic Addison's disease.

Disorders of the Anterior Pituitary

Disorders of the hypothalamic-pituitary axis pose the most exacting diagnostic challenge. Through the appearance of amenorrhea, the patient with a slowly growing pituitary tumor may present years before the tumor becomes evident by radiologic techniques. Sometimes the suspicion of tumor is increased because of clinical signs of acromegaly, Cushing's syndrome resulting from excessive secretion of ACTH, or inappropriate lactation, although nonfunctioning tumors must also be considered. Prolactin-secreting tumors may be seen in preadolescent and adolescent children, and may thus be a cause of failure of growth and development.

Not all intrasellar masses are neoplastic. Gummas, tuberculomas, and fat deposits have been reported as causes of pituitary compression leading to hypogonadotropic amenorrhea. Nearby lesions such as internal carotid artery aneurysms and obstruction of the aqueduct of Sylvius may also cause amenorrhea. Pituitary insufficiency may be secondary to ischemia and infarction and appear as a late sequela to obstetric hemorrhage — Sheehan's syndrome.

PITUITARY TUMORS. With the utilization of the serum prolactin assay and the increased sensitivity of the polytomographic technique, the association of amenorrhea and small pituitary tumors (microadenomas of 5 to 10 mm in diameter) is being recognized more frequently. At this time the exact incidence of this clinical problem is unknown. In autopsy series, the number of pituitary glands found to contain adenomas ranged from 9 to 22.5 per cent. The age distribution ranged from 2 to 86, with the greatest incidence in the sixth decade of life. The sex distribution was equal.

Exact statements regarding incidence and frequency will require further accumulation of clinical experience. Preliminary information suggests the following:

1. A high prolactin level may be encountered in 20 per cent of women with no obvious cause of amenorrhea. (It is not surprising that prolactin levels are not elevated in women with obvious causes of amenorrhea, such as genetic problems, anorexia nervosa, and ovarian failure.)

2. Only one third of patients with high prolactin levels will have galactorrhea, probably because the low estrogen environment associated with the amenorrhea prevents a normal response of the breast to prolactin.

3. Possibly as many as one third of patients with secondary amenorrhea will have a pituitary adenoma; if galactorrhea is present, perhaps one half will have an abnormal sella turcica.

4. In patients with pituitary tumors, the association of amenorrhea and elevated prolactin levels is high. In one series of 62 patients with pituitary tumors (without acromegaly or Cushing's syndrome), 75 per cent of the patients with amenorrhea had elevated prolactin levels.

An important consideration of this problem is the behavior of the adenoma during pregnancy. In the latter half of pregnancy, pituitary and parasellar tumors can expand and lead to optic chiasmal compression, which usually regresses after delivery. This sequence may return in successive pregnancies, eventually leading to complete blindness. In addition to visual disturbances, persistent or worsening headaches are usual symptoms of an enlarging tumor.

Fortunately the increased ability to detect pituitary tumors has been accompanied by the development of a surgical technique which very effectively removes the small tumors with a high margin of safety. This technique is the transsphenoidal approach to the sella turcica, utilizing the operating microscope. The transsphenoidal approach is via a sublabial incision, with dissection under the nasal mucosa, removal of the nasal septum to expose the sphenoidal sinus, and resection of the floor of the sphenoidal sinus to expose sella turcica. The operating microscope adds magnification to allow direct visualization. Tumor tissue is usually distinguishable from the yellow-orange, firm tissue of the normal anterior pituitary. However, since pituitary adenomas do not have a capsule, the borderline between tumor and normal tissue is often doubtful. The ideal time for excision is when the adenoma is a small nodule. When enlarged, it becomes difficult to distinguish normal from pathologic tissue. Once the adenoma leaves the sella, total removal by this method is impossible. The need for postoperative irradiation is determined by histologic examination of the edges of the resected tissue and postoperative prolactin levels. Visual impairment caused by suprasellar extension improves immediately with operative relief of pressure on the optic nerves.

The reason for the amenorrhea associated with elevated prolactin levels is not exactly clear. Prolactin may interfere with ovarian response to gonadotropins as well as pituitary response to GnRH. Regardless of the mechanism, treatment which lowers the circulating levels of prolactin restores ovarian responsiveness and menstrual function. This is true whether the treatment consists of removal of a prolactin-secreting tumor or suppression of prolactin secretion. Because ergot alkaloids inhibit both prolactin secretion and growth of tumor cells, surgical treatment may not be necessary for all patients, especially those with only minimal radiologic evidence for a tumor.

THE EMPTY SELLA SYNDROME (see Ch. 543.5). A patient may have an abnormal sella turcica, but rather than a tumor, she may have the empty sella syndrome. This is a condition in which there is a congenital incompleteness of the sellar diaphragm, allowing an extension of the subarachnoid space into the pituitary fossa.

An empty sella is found in approximately 5 per cent of autopsies, and approximately 85 per cent are in women, mostly middle-aged and obese. In approximately one third of cases gonadotropins are decreased and there is a reduced response of growth hormone to hypoglycemia. Adrenal and thyroid function are rarely affected. Occasionally, rhinorrhea may develop. This condition is benign; it rarely progresses to pituitary failure.

Disorders of the Central Nervous System

HYPOTHALAMIC AMENORRHEA. Hypothalamic problems are usually diagnosed by exclusion of pituitary lesions, but are the most common category of hypogonadotropic amenorrheas. Frequently there is an association with a stressful situation. In a study of the total female population aged 18 to 35 years of Uppsala, Sweden, pronounced psychologic stress was more frequent in women with secondary amenorrhea than in their age-matched controls. There was also a higher proportion of underweight women and a higher occurrence of previous menstrual irregularity. Nevertheless, the physician is obliged to go through the process of excluding other causes of amenorrhea prior to prescribing hormone replacement therapy or attempting induction of ovulation in order to achieve pregnancy.

ANOREXIA. A special example of hypothalamic amenorrhea is that associated with weight loss. It is true that obesity may be associated with amenorrhea, but amenorrhea in an obese patient is usually due to anovulation, and a hypogonadotropic state is not encountered unless the patient also has a severe emotional disorder. Acute weight loss, on the other hand, in some unknown way may lead to the hypogonadotropic state. Again the physician must exclude the presence of a tumor, and the diagnosis is made by exclusion.

Clinically, a spectrum is encountered from a limited period of amenorrhea associated with a crash diet to the severely ill patient with the life-threatening attrition of anorexia nervosa. It is a common experience for the gynecologist to be the first to recognize anorexia nervosa in a patient presenting with the complaint of amenorrhea. It is important that attention be directed to this syndrome, which is associated with a mortality rate of approximately 7 per cent.

The borderline anorexic frequently presents as a teenager characterized by low body weight, amenorrhea, and hyperactivity (excellent grades and many extracurricular activities). The amenorrhea can precede, follow, or appear coincidentally with the weight loss. Endocrine studies can be summarized as follows: The FSH level is normal. The LH level is low. 17-Ketosteroids and 17-hydroxysteroids may be low, and plasma cortisol may lose its diurnal variation. Thyroid studies are normal, except for low T_3 levels, suggesting an impaired peripheral conversion of T_4 to T_3. Prolactin levels are normal.

The central origin for the amenorrhea is suggested by the demonstration that the response to GnRH is regained at approximately 15 per cent below the ideal weight, and this return to normal responsiveness occurs before the resumption of menses. This change in pituitary responsiveness is not seen in women with secondary amenorrhea which is not associated with self-imposed weight loss.

AMENORRHEA AND ANOSMIA. A rare condition in females is the syndrome of hypogonadotropic hypogonadism associated with anosmia. A similar syndrome in the male is hereditary and is known as Kallmann's syndrome. In the female, this problem is characterized by primary amenorrhea, infantile sexual development, low gonadotropins, a normal female karyotype, and the inability to perceive odors, e.g., coffee ground or perfume. The gonads can respond to gonadotropins; therefore induction of ovulation with exogenous gonadotropins has been successful. However, clomiphene is ineffective.

POSTPILL AMENORRHEA. It has been assumed that amenorrhea may reflect persistent suppressive effects of oral contraceptive medication or the use of the intramuscular depot form of medroxyprogesterone acetate. Recently it has been appreciated that the fertility rate is normal following discontinuance of either of these forms of contraception. Therefore amenorrhea following the use of steroids for contraception requires investigation as described in order to avoid missing a pituitary tumor.

The Polycystic Ovary

In contrast to the characteristic picture of fluctuating estradiol levels in the normal cycle, a "steady state" of tonic gonadotropin and estrogen function, associated with persistent anovulation, can be depicted. This steady state is only relative, and is being exaggerated here to present a concept of this clinical syndrome (Fig. 7).

In patients with chronic anovulation, the average daily production of estrogen and androgens is increased. This is reflected in higher circulating levels of testosterone and androstenedione and higher levels of estrogen, largely estrone derived from the peripheral conversion of androstenedione. When compared to levels found in normal women, patients with this syndrome have higher mean concentrations of LH, but low or low-normal levels of FSH. The elevated levels of LH may be in the range of the midcycle surge or even equivalent to postmenopausal values. Evidence suggests that the elevated LH levels are due to an increased sensitivity of the pituitary to releasing hormone stimulation. This increased sensitivity is probably the effect of the increased estrone levels, since a correlation exists between estrogen and LH levels. It is possible that the elevated androgens contribute to the increased LH in another fashion. The hypothalamus aromatizes androgens to estrogens, and this local change may raise estrogen levels in the anterior hypothalamus to sensitize and stimulate the positive feedback mechanism. The lower FSH levels probably represent the sensitivity of the FSH negative feedback system to the elevated levels of estrogen.

Because the FSH levels are not totally depressed, new follicular growth is continuously stimulated, but not to the point of full maturation and ovulation. Despite the fact that full growth potential is not realized, follicular life span may extend several months in the form of multiple follicular cysts, 2 to 6 mm in diameter. These follicles are surrounded by hyperplastic theca cells, often luteinized in response to the high LH levels. The accumulation of follicular tissue in various stages of development allows an increased and relatively constant production of

Figure 7. Comparison of steroid and gonadotropin concentrations and patterns in an ovulatory cycle and the steady state of persistent anovulation. (From Speroff, L., Glass, R. H., and Kase, N. G.: Clinical Gynecologic Endocrinology and Infertility. Baltimore, Williams and Wilkins Company, 1978.)

steroids in response to the gonadotropin stimulation. This condition is self-sustaining. Because of the low levels and limited excursion of FSH levels, as arrested follicles undergo atresia, they can only be replaced by new follicles of similar limited growth potential.

The tissue derived from follicular atresia is also sustained by the steady state, and now contributes to the stromal compartment of the ovary. This functioning stromal tissue secretes significant amounts of androstenedione and testosterone. In response to the elevated LH levels, the androgen production in this gonadal compartment is increased. In turn, the elevated androgen levels, through the process of extraglandular conversion, result in elevated estrogen levels and are a major factor in sustaining this condition by depressing FSH levels and elevating LH secretion by augmenting the pituitary response to GnRH. The elevated androgens may also contribute to the morphologic effect within the ovary by blocking the actions of estradiol on the granulosa cells and inducing premature atresia. Indeed, the ovulatory response to wedge resection appears to follow a sustained reduction in testosterone levels, suggesting that the intraovarian androgen effects are the major obstacles to complete follicular maturation and normal cycling.

In this manner the classic picture of the polycystic ovary is attained, displaying numerous follicles in all stages of development and atresia, and dense stromal tissue. The loss of recycling has resulted in a hormonal steady state causing persistent anovulation which may be associated with the increased production of androgens. This condition has been referred to by many names, most commonly the Stein-Leventhal syndrome, polycystic ovary disease, or sclerocystic ovaries.

The polycystic ovary is palpably enlarged (up to two times) and is characterized by a smooth pearly white capsule. For years, it was erroneously believed that the thick sclerotic capsule acted as a mechanical barrier to ovulation. Rather, one should have the concept that the polycystic ovary is a consequence of the loss of ovulation and the achievement of a steady state of persistent anovulation. The histologic characteristics reflect this dysfunctional state. An accumulation of atretic tissue along with the constant and elevated LH stimulation results in stromal hyperplasia called hyperthecosis. It is doubtful that hyperthecosis represents a separate syndrome. Hyperthecosis refers to patches of luteinized theca-like cells scattered throughout the ovarian stroma, and it is characterized by the same clinical, histologic, and endocrine findings as are seen with polycystic ovaries. It is likely that both are morphologic manifestations of the same process, anovulation with hyperthecosis representing the more prolonged and clinically profound end of a continuous spectrum of this syndrome.

One group of investigators has indicated that high LH levels in anovulatory patients are associated with big ovaries, whereas low LH levels are found in association with small ovaries. Another group has failed to find a relationship between the size of polycystic ovaries and the levels of LH. There is a spectrum of time involved in the development of this clinical syndrome, and it is useful to view the attainment of high LH levels and large ovaries as a stage of maximal effect of persistent anovulation. However, the key to understanding this clinical problem is an appreciation of the disruption in ovulatory recycling function. The size of the ovaries is not a critical feature, nor is it necessary to assign a specific etiology. The polycystic ovary may be associated with a variety of disorders in the hypothalamic-pituitary-ovarian axis, as well as with extragonadal sources of androgens or with androgen-producing tumors.

It appears that at least one group of patients with this condition inherits the disorder, possibly by means of an X-linked dominant or autosomal dominant transmission. Studies of families have indicated that there is a two-fold higher incidence of hirsutism and oligomenorrhea, with paternal transmission, but with marked variability of phenotypic expression.

The adrenal gland becomes involved in this syndrome. Higher circulating levels of dehydroepiandrosterone sulfate (DS), almost exclusively an adrenal product, testify to adrenal participation.

CLINICAL EFFECTS AND TREATMENT OF THE POLYCYSTIC OVARY SYNDROME. Anovulation is the key feature of this syndrome, presenting as amenorrhea in approximately 55 per cent of cases and with irregular, heavy bleeding in 28 per cent. True virilization is rare, but 70 per cent of anovulatory patients complain of cosmetically disturbing hirsutism.

Obesity has been classically regarded as a common feature, but its presence is extremely variable and has no diagnostic value.

Although an elevated LH value in the presence of a low or low-normal FSH may be diagnostic, the diagnosis is easily made by the clinical presentation alone. The symptoms are a consequence of the loss of ovulation: dysfunctional bleeding, amenorrhea, hirsutism, and infertility. The presentations each require a specific diagnostic and therapeutic approach.

There are potentially severe clinical consequences of the steady state of hormone secretion. Besides the problems of infertility, hirsutism, amenorrhea, and bleeding, the effect of the unopposed and uninterrupted estrogen is to place the patient at risk for cancer of the breast and endometrium. If left unattended, patients with persistent anovulation develop clinical problems, and therefore appropriate therapeutic management is essential for all anovulatory patients.

The typical patient presents with anovulation and irregular menses. If there is no hirsutism or virilism, evaluation of androgen production is not necessary. There is no need for urinary 17-ketosteroids, plasma testosterone, or any other laboratory procedures. In the patient whose only problem is longstanding anovulation, especially if she is over 35, an endometrial biopsy is a wise precaution. The well-known association between this syndrome and abnormal endometrial changes must be kept in mind. Documentation of anovulation is usually unnecessary, especially in view of menstrual irregularity with periods of amenorrhea.

Therapy of most anovulatory patients can be planned at the first visit. If the patient desires pregnancy, she is a candidate for the medical induction of ovulation. If the patient presents with amenorrhea, an investigation must be pursued. The management of significant dysfunctional uterine bleeding may also be required.

For the patient who does not wish to become pregnant and does not complain of hirsutism but is anovulatory and has irregular bleeding, therapy is directed toward interruption of steady state effect on the endometrium. The use of Provera is favored to ensure complete withdrawal bleeding and to prevent endometrial hyperplasia and atypia. Spacing of the progestational medication in this fashion will allow the patient to be aware of spontaneous bleeding caused by the onset of ovulatory cycles.

The use of oral contraceptive medication for therapy in these patients requires individual patient judgment. When reliable contraception is essential, the use of low dose combination oral contraception in the usual cyclic fashion is appropriate.

Chang, R. J., Keye, W. R., Jr., Young, J. R., Wilson, C. B., and Jaffee, R. B.: Detection, evaluation, and treatment of pituitary microadenomas in patients with galactorrhea and amenorrhea. Am. J. Obstet. Gynecol., 128:356, 1977.

Fries, H., Nillius, S. J., and Pettersson, F.: Epidemiology of secondary amenorrhea. Am. J. Obstet. Gynecol., 118:473, 1974.

Griffin, J. E., Edwards, C., Madden, J. D., Harrod, M. J., and Wilson, J. D.: Congenital absence of the vagina. Ann. Intern. Med. 85:224, 1976.

Judd, H. L., Rigg, L. A., Anderson, D. C., and Yen, S. S. C.: The effects of ovarian wedge resection on circulating gonadotropin and ovarian steroid levels in patients with polycystic ovary syndrome. J. Clin. Endocrinol. Metab., 43:347, 1976.

Klein, S. M., and Garcia, C. R.: Asherman's syndrome: A critique and current review. Fertil. Steril., 23:72, 1973.

Neelon, F. A., Goree, J. A., and Lebovitz, H. E.: The primary empty sella: Clinical and radiographic characteristics and endocrine function. Medicine, 52:73, 1973.

Sheehan, H. L., and Stanfield, J. P.: The pathogenesis of postpartum necrosis of the anterior lobe of the pituitary gland. Acta Endocrinol., 37:479, 1972.

Vigersky, R. A., Anderson, A. E., Thompson, R. H., and Loriaux, D. L.: Hypothalamic dysfunction in secondary amenorrhea associated with simple weight loss. N. Engl. J. Med., 297:1141, 1977.

Treatment of Amenorrhea

The therapy of inadequate ovarian hormone function depends not only on the degree of hormonal failure, but also on the therapeutic objectives. Certainly menstruation is not a necessity, for its absence does not represent a threat to the life expectancy of the patient. Therefore except in the treatment of infertility, and possibly in rare psychologic situations, a patient need not be treated solely for the purpose of recreating menstrual cycles. On the other hand, certain patients who show other evidence of estrogen deficiency, such as loss of secondary sex characteristics, deserve substitutive therapy. At no time should artificial cycles be instituted without preliminary investigation to uncover serious underlying lesions.

HYPERGONADOTROPIC HYPOGONADISM. The patient with gonadal dysgenesis should be given cyclic exogenous estrogen therapy indefinitely for development and maintenance of adequate secondary sexual characteristics. The transformation induced by cyclic estrogen therapy in these otherwise anatomically, biologically, and cosmetically handicapped patients is particularly gratifying. Among the oral regimens available, 1.25 mg of conjugated equine estrogens daily for 21 days is satisfactory; during the last seven days of treatment, the addition of 10 mg daily of medroxyprogesterone acetate orally provides endometrial stability and controlled withdrawal flow.

The woman with premature ovarian failure (before the age of 40 years) presents a somewhat different therapeutic problem. In this situation replacement medication is required to sustain systems already developed and dependent upon ovarian hormone secretion. Patients of this type are concerned not only about secondary amenorrhea and the termination of their reproductive capabilities but also about the usual severe vasomotor symptoms that attend this type of ovarian failure. These *hot flashes* are not seen in primary hypogonadism, although gonadotropins are elevated in both conditions. Probably as a consequence of these disabilities and the fear of further restrictions, there are various subjective symptoms such as depression, anxiety, and loss of libido. No satisfactory

treatment of this condition exists at present except substitution therapy with estrogen. Control of vasomotor instability, preservation of a serviceable vagina, and maintenance of other feminine aspects, including menses, are possible with cyclic conjugated equine estrogens (Premarin, 1.25 mg every day), or ethinyl estradiol (Estinyl, 0.02 mg every day). Again, the terminal addition of a progestin after 21 days of estrogen is advantageous. It should be noted that these doses of estrogen stimulate menstrual function and are higher than necessary for nonmenstrual metabolic requirements. This point comes into active consideration when determining what, if any, therapy should be given for ovarian failure occurring after the age of 40.

Menopause. The menopause is a physiologic and not a pathologic phenomenon. Menstruation ceases for a variety of reasons at other times of life, but after 40 the ovary becomes atrophic and ceases to respond to gonadotropic stimulation. No amount of gonadotropic stimulation can produce activity in the menopausal ovary. It becomes small, pale, and more wrinkled. The few remaining follicles undergo atresia so that none are found within a few years after cessation of menses. Diminution of all ovarian elements proceeds, resulting in a firm structure one third the size of the active organ.

Vasomotor instability and genital atrophy are the only clinical symptoms definitely associated with ovarian aging that occurs when otherwise the woman may be active, healthy, and vital physically, emotionally, and mentally. However, because of improved general health, women can expect to live for 20 to 25 years beyond the menopause, and interest has increased in the possible amelioration of certain disease states associated with the menopause by administration of exogenous estrogen therapy. Whether actual causal relationships exist between certain disorders and diminished estrogen secretion has not been established. Nevertheless, beneficial effects on extragenital organs and prevention of atherosclerosis and osteoporosis have been claimed.

A statistical rise in coronary atherosclerosis in postmenopausal women has been ascribed to estrogen deficiency. Castration performed before natural menopause also has been associated with increased coronary and peripheral vascular disease. The ability of estrogen to reverse abnormal serum lipids in laboratory animals as well as in human subjects is a possible mechanism by which treated castrates may have a lower incidence of abnormal electrocardiograms and hypertension than untreated women.

However, *excessive therapy* has been observed to pose increased risks. Studies of the preventive effects of estrogens for heart attacks have yielded variable results. Administration of 10 mg of conjugated estrogens per day appeared to be associated with beneficial survival statistics but revealed a disturbing incidence of early vascular accidents. In the Coronary Drug Project, 5 mg conjugated estrogen therapy was associated with an excess of nonfatal myocardial infarctions over controls. In the Stroke Study, estrogens were associated with increased recurrent cerebral accidents and myocardial infarctions rather than protection against these two insults.

Postmenopausal osteoporosis is also believed to be related to estrogen deficiency. Estrogen induces positive calcium balance and reduces bone resorption, but bone formation also drops within three to nine months after initiation of therapy. Although there is no net increase in bone mass in the osteoporotic woman, estrogen would seem to stabilize bone turnover at a new and slower rate. However, there is no *prospective* evidence that estrogen can prevent osteoporosis-induced mechanical fragility leading to fracture. Appropriate diet and exercise are certainly also involved in bone matrix biology. Conclusive proof is lacking that diminished estrogen is a factor in this and other age-related disorders such as arthritis, muscular weakness, migraine headache, and stomatitis. On the other hand, atrophic changes in the distal urinary tract, particularly in the urethra, which result in urinary frequency, burning, and occasionally stress incontinence, are reversible by the administration of local or systemic estrogen. Finally, estrogen controls the often embarrassing and sometimes disabling irritations of atrophic vaginitis and vulvitis.

In the postmenopausal situation, in which menstrual function is not required, only small doses of cyclic estrogen are necessary for appropriate therapy. Conjugated estrogen, 0.625 mg daily for three weeks of every four, is sufficient. Despite the ease of administration and its obvious physiologic and clinical value, estrogen therapy has often been limited in duration or actively avoided. The reason for this restraint is the concern that protracted estrogen treatment will induce neoplastic changes in estrogen-sensitive aging tissues. The contribution of endogenous estrogen to the pathogenesis of uterine and breast carcinoma is still speculative, but suspicion has been aroused, particularly as to the effects of unopposed estrogen in the stimulation of endometrial disease. Several retrospective studies have appeared in which the use of estrogen was linked to the appearance of endometrial cancer. Duration of use, dosage, constant versus cyclic application, and the absence of periodic progestin-induced withdrawal bleeding were all shown to increase risk of endometrial disease. Clearly, indiscriminate use of this hormone in high doses without periodic evaluation is condemned. On the other hand, if therapy is given within the restrictions stated, there is more evidence in favor of than against its use.

In this regard the importance of frequent medical evaluations in this age group should not be understated. In addition to the opportunities such interviews present for continual psychologic support of the apprehensive patient, the full physical examination performed on these occasions may uncover basic organic disease, the symptoms of which have been incorrectly minimized by the woman as further evidence of "a change of life."

HYPOGONADOTROPIC HYPOGONADISM. Before embarking on a therapeutic program in this form of amenorrhea, the physician must have assured himself of the absence of various intracranial diseases that inhibit or destroy gonadotropin secretion.

In the absence of neoplastic, vascular, or congenital anomaly to account for disruption in pituitary function, there is usually a history of some stressful circumstance as the precipitating event. Improved dietary habits or psychotherapy may result in return of ovulatory cycles. In fact, the frequency of spontaneous remission is so high that simple observation is often satisfactory. However, when amenorrhea is prolonged and is associated with incipient atrophy of dependent organs and infertility, or is accompanied by lactation, more active therapeutic measures must be undertaken.

Inappropriate Lactation — Galactorrheic Syndromes. Galactorrhea refers to the inappropriate mammary secretion of milky fluid that is not immediately related to pregnancy or the needs of a neonate. The quantity of secretion is not an important criterion. Galactorrhea may involve both breasts, or one or the other breast consecutively or alternately. Amenorrhea does not necessarily accompany galactorrhea, even in the most serious disorders.

A variety of eponymic designations have been applied to variants of the lactation syndromes. These are based on the association of galactorrhea with intrasellar tumor (Forbes, Henneman, Griswold, and Albright, 1954), antecedent pregnancy with inappropriate persistence of galactorrhea (independently reported by Chiari and Frommel in 1852), and the absence of previous pregnancy (Argonz and Del Castillo, 1953). In all these types, the association of galactorrhea with eventual amenorrhea was observed. On the basis of currently available information, categorization of individual cases according to these eponymic guidelines neither is helpful nor permits discrimination of patients who will eventually develop serious intrasellar lesions.

The differential diagnosis of galactorrhea syndromes is a difficult and complex clinical challenge. The difficulty arises from the multiple factors involved in the control of prolactin release. In most pathophysiologic systems, the final common pathway leading to galactorrhea is an inappropriate augmentation of prolactin release.

Prolactin is a polypeptide secreted from the anterior pituitary and has a half-life of 15 to 30 minutes. Prolactin is apparently under a chronic, tonic inhibition owing to hypothalamic secretion into the pituitary portal system of prolactin-inhibiting factor (PIF). The following considerations are important in differentiation of causes of excess prolactin:

1. *Excessive estrogen* (as may be administered in birth control pills) can lead to milk secretion via hypothalamic suppression, causing inhibition of PIF and consequent release of pituitary prolactin. Progesterone, on the other hand, seems to have a restraining effect, perhaps by a stimulatory effect on the hypothalamus leading to production of PIF.

2. Prolonged intensive *suckling* can also release prolactin, via hypothalamic reduction of PIF control of prolactin. Similarly, thoracotomy scars, cervical spinal lesions, and herpes zoster can induce prolactin release by activating the afferent sensory neural arc.

3. A variety of *drugs* can also inhibit hypothalamic PIF. There are nearly 100 phenothiazine derivatives with indirect mammotropic activity. In addition, many phenothiazine-like compounds, reserpine derivatives, amphetamines, and a variety of other drugs can initiate galactorrhea via hypothalamic suppression (thioxanthenes, diazepines, butyrophenones, α-methyldopa).

4. *Emotional stresses* (presumably capable of increasing hypothalamic PIF and diminishing prolactin secretion) can also inhibit hypothalamic PIF and induce the secretion of prolactin and galactorrhea. Severe anxiety and trauma often occur in temporal relation to the onset of galactorrhea. The posthysterectomy or menopausal onset of this symptom is a rare but known entity.

5. *Hypothalamic lesions,* stalk lesions, or compression — events that physically reduce production or delivery of PIF to the pituitary — can release excess prolactin, leading to galactorrhea.

6. *Hypothyroidism* (juvenile or adult) can be associated with galactorrhea. The mechanism of this relationship requires the introduction of a positive hypothalamic material (prolactin-releasing factor, PRF) that can release, not inhibit, pituitary secretion of prolactin. PRF exists in

various fowl (e.g., pigeon, chicken, duck, turkey, and the tricolored blackbird). Although the identity of this material has not been elucidated or its function substantiated in normal human physiology, in pathologic situations such as hypothyroidism, thyrotropin-releasing hormone (TRH) may be active as a PRF. Synthetic TRH is a potent stimulant of prolactin secretion in man. With diminished circulating levels of thyroid hormone, hypothalamic TRH is produced in excess and as such may act as a PRF to release prolactin from the pituitary. Adult hypothyroidism associated with galactorrhea is well known. In juvenile hypothyroidism, prepubertal breast development and galactorrhea may be seen. Reversal with thyroid hormone therapy is strong circumstantial evidence in support of this thesis.

7. Also acknowledged as a rare cause of galactorrhea is *Cushing's disease*. It is not known whether the direct effect of excessive free cortisol enhances otherwise nonstimulating levels of prolactin secretion to cause galactorrhea, or whether hypothalamic-pituitary dysfunction involves not only increased corticotropin-releasing hormones but also excess PRF or reduced PIF.

8. Increased prolactin release may be the consequence of prolactin elaboration and secretion from *pituitary tumors* which function independently of the otherwise appropriate restraints exerted by PIF from a normally functioning hypothalamus. This dangerous tumor with endocrine, neurologic, and ophthalmologic liabilities makes the differential diagnosis of persistent galactorrhea a major clinical challenge. Beyond prolactin production, the tumor may also suppress pituitary parenchyma by expansion and compression interfering with other tropic hormones.

9. *Ectopic production of prolactin* has been reported in one patient without galactorrhea and with a bronchogenic carcinoma, and in one patient with galactorrhea and a hypernephroma. An occult carcinoma, although a remote possibility, should be considered.

Symptoms of galactorrhea may antedate the recognition of intrasellar tumors by many years. It is recognized that a mean duration of 10 to 12 years of galactorrhea and amenorrhea may precede the radiologic demonstration of a pituitary adenoma. As a result, follow-up must be prolonged and zealous. Furthermore, the criterion of antecedent pregnancy does not necessarily suggest that a different pathophysiologic process is involved in the galactorrhea. Cases of pituitary adenoma which did not alter competent gonadotropin secretion are known, and conception has occurred in some of these patients.

Galactorrheic women with pituitary tumors shown by x-ray can demonstrate withdrawal from progesterone and even have menses and ovulate, as stated above. Obviously, the presence of galactorrhea is not incompatible with gonadotropin release. However, in the majority of patients a single lesion is sufficiently extensive or critically placed to impair both mechanisms and, on rare occasions, other tropic hormones (TSH, ACTH).

Therefore regardless of the clinical circumstances, in galactorrhea of six months' to one year's duration, a pituitary tumor must be considered. The longer the follow-up, with the progressive exclusion of other benign causes, the higher the incidence of tumor diagnosis in persistent galactorrhea. The diagnosis of pituitary tumor has been dealt with earlier in this chapter.

Gonadotropin Therapy. HUMAN PITUITARY FOLLICLE-STIMULATING HORMONE (HPFSH) AND HUMAN CHORIONIC GONADOTROPIN (HCG) THERAPY. In 1958 Gemzell reported the use of a human pituitary preparation that stimulated follicular growth and estrogen production in amenorrheic women. The material was extracted from pituitary tissue collected at autopsy and partially purified by ammonium sulfate fractionation. When assayed against relatively specific standards, it revealed combined FSH and LH potencies, but with the former dominating the biologic activity. Ovulation occurs during HCG administration. Dose size and duration are adjusted according to the ovarian response noted. In limited trials it has been found that more than 90 per cent of patients ovulated once or several times, and more than 50 per cent became pregnant. The limited availability of material (requiring approximately 10 pituitaries to produce an ovulation with this system) has been its major disadvantage.

HUMAN MENOPAUSAL URINARY GONADOTROPIN (HMG-FSH, PERGONAL). Although menopausal urine has been recognized as a potential source of gonadotropins (FSH activity by animal studies) since 1930, toxic reactions precluded utilization in human investigations. Acceptable material is now available clinically as Pergonal, which contains 75 units of FSH and 75 units of LH potency per ampule. Toxic and allergic reactions have been eliminated. At least 90 per cent of appropriately selected patients ovulate, and 50 to 70 per cent achieve pregnancy. The usual dose required is 8 to 12 days of 2 ampules of human menopausal gonadotropin (HMG) per day, followed by 10,000 units of HCG. However, variable ovarian reactivity has been encountered. In addition to monitoring HMG-induced ovarian stimulation by biologic expressions of estrogen (cervical mucus changes), urinary estrogen excretion or plasma estradiol concentrations have proved to be useful. An excretion range between 100 and 200 μg total estrogen or plasma level of E_2 about 1000 pg per milliliter is the goal of HMG therapy, at which time the ovulatory dose of exogenous HCG can be applied. In this range, an optimal ratio between induced pregnancy rate and incidence of serious side effects (hyperstimulation and multiple pregnancy) is expected.

The results of species-specific FSH (as HMG) therapy (two to five courses) are 90 per cent ovulation, 50 to 70 per cent pregnancies, 20 per cent abortion, 20 per cent multiple gestation (15 per cent twins, 5 per cent three or more), and 1 per cent serious side effects (hyperstimulation).

SIDE EFFECTS OF GONADOTROPIN THERAPY. Certain side effects have been noted that may limit general application of these agents. The reactions encountered are attributable to the effects of ovarian enlargement and production of unusual quantities of ovarian hormones. These consist of abdominal pain, bloating, pressure, nausea, and general malaise. Acute distention can even cause ovarian rupture and hemorrhage. Because many of the reactions are self-limiting, nonsurgical supportive therapy is advised, laparotomy and conservative surgery short of castration being reserved for the deteriorating circumstance. In this regard hypovolemic shock resulting from a syndrome of severe ascites and hydrothorax has been recognized. Additional expressions of ovarian hyperstimulation are the frequency of abortion and multiple pregnancy and the consequent diminution in fetal salvage noted in all series. Finally, it has become clear that gonadotropin therapy is effective only during the treatment interval. Regardless of frequency of ovulation or the occurrence of pregnancy, patients revert to pretreatment hypogonadal status upon cessation of therapy or conclusion of pregnancy. For this reason gonadotropin induction of ovulation is currently withheld until other modes of treatment have failed.

NORMOGONADOTROPIC NORMOESTROGENIC ANOVULATION. In this type of amenorrhea, the chain of events leading to normal ovulation and menstruation is upset by the absence of the midcycle surge of LH. Lacking progesterone secretion, continued unopposed estrogen stimulation leads to hyperplasia of the endometrium. For this reason amenorrhea may be punctuated by prolonged, sometimes severe uterine hemorrhages (*metropathia hemorrhagica*) that require special attention. In addition, infertility further complicates this syndrome. Clearly the correction of both these circumstances is found in the return of recurrent ovulation.

Correction of Menstrual Pattern. There may be no specific requirement for reproductive function, but the inconvenience and uncertainty of the menstrual pattern prompt the patient to seek hormonal regulation of her cycle. In the absence of serious underlying disease, this may be accomplished by inducing progesterone withdrawal flow with an oral progestin such as 10 mg of medroxyprogesterone acetate for five days after an interval of endogenous estrogen stimulation. Two to five days after progestin withdrawal, menses will appear. Retreatment with progestin should be delayed for sufficient time (six weeks) to determine whether spontaneous ovulation will return. Only in cases of too frequent menstruation (polymenorrhea) is the disadvantage of complete cycle coverage by combined estrogen and progestin (as in the birth control medications) acceptable. Medication should be withdrawn periodically, because spontaneous correction may have occurred during therapy.

When severe dysfunctional bleeding occurs, an effort must be made to obtain an endometrial biopsy, but curettage is not essential. Regardless of the duration or severity of flow, anovulatory bleeding of this type is treated by converting the proliferative endometrium to a secretory endometrium from which limited withdrawal flow will occur. Three to four times the contraceptive doses of oral 19-nor steroids will rapidly diminish dysfunctional bleeding with complete cessation within 12 hours. Therapy is then continued, and is gradually tapered to allow an interval for blood replacement as well as general, gynecologic, and hematologic evaluation. The possibility of underlying disorders of coagulation must always be considered. After withdrawal flow, contraceptive doses of 19-nor steroids must be resumed for two to three cycles. The initial use of high doses of estrogen intravenously (Premarin, 25 mg) before progestin conversion is limited to those cases in which bleeding has been prolonged or severe and immediate cessation is required. On the other hand, if agents such as 19-nor steroids do *not* control abnormal flow, then pathologic bleeding is diagnosed and curettage is mandatory.

Reversal of Anovulation. Correction of proved adrenocortical and thyroid disease will reverse associated anovulation. The drug Clomid (a synthetic nonsteroidal analogue of chlorotrianisene) has proved useful in the treatment of diagnostically nonspecific anovulation. It has almost entirely replaced the low-dose corticosteroid regimens and has virtually eliminated the need for operative wedge resection of the ovaries to achieve resumption of ovulation. With 50 to 100 mg daily for five days of each cycle, induction of ovulation is achieved in patients with intermediate follicle maturation arrest but with sufficient function to secrete some estrogen. The drug appears to enhance endogenous gonadotropin secretion. In properly

selected patients, 80 per cent can be expected to ovulate and approximately 50 per cent become pregnant. The percentage of pregnancies per number of induced ovulatory cycles is 15 per cent. The multiple pregnancy rate in accumulated national statistics is approximately 8 per cent, almost entirely twins. The abortion rate is 20 per cent. The incidence of congenital anomalies is not increased as a result of Clomid-induced ovulation. There is no evidence that the effect of Clomid is long lasting; it is considered to be limited to the cycle in which the drug is used. The side effects are similar to those of the gonadotropins and are related to increased ovarian size, hormone production, and multiple pregnancies. In the event that Clomid (after gradually increased doses over four to six months) is unsuccessful, then bilateral wedge resection of the ovaries or HMG plus HCG therapy is advised. Because all the therapies cited present some risk to the patient and none guarantee lasting results, other aspects of the fertility potential of the involved couple must be fully evaluated before ovulation induction is undertaken.

Baird, D. T., Corhen, C. S., Davidson, D. W., Hunter, W., Michie, E. A., and Van Look, P. A.: Pituitary ovarian relationships in polycystic ovary syndrome. J. Clin. Endocrinol. Metab., 45:798, 1977.

Givens, J. R.: Hirsutism and hyperandrogenism. Adv. Intern. Med., 1:221, 1976.

Jones, G. S.: Luteal phase defects. *In* Berhrman, J. S., and Kistner, R. W. (eds.): Progress in Infertility. Boston, Little, Brown & Company, 1975, p. 299.

Judd, H. L., Rigg, L. A., Anderson, D. C., and Yen, S. S. C.: The effects of ovarian wedge resection on circulating gonadotropin and ovarian steroid levels in patients with polycystic ovary syndrome. J. Clin. Endocrin. Metab., 43:347, 1976.

Kase, N., Mroueh, A., and Olson, L. E.; Clomid therapy for anovulatory infertility. Am. J. Obstet. Gynecol., 98:1037, 1967.

Kistner, R. W.: Induction of ovulation with clomiphene citrate. *In* Behrman, S. J., and Kistner, R. W. (eds): Progress in Infertility. Boston, Little, Brown & Company, 1975, p. 509.

Naftolin, F., and Ryan, K. J.: The metabolism of androgens in central neuroendocrine tissues. J. Steroid Biochem., 6:993, 1975.

Siiteri, P. K., and MacDonald, P. C.: Role of extraglandular estrogen in human endocrinology. *In* Geyer, S. R., Astwood, E. B., and Greep, R. O. (eds): Handbook of Physiology, Section 7, Endocrinology. Washington, D.C., American Physiology Society, 1973, p. 615.

INVESTIGATION OF INFERTILITY

Approximately 10 per cent of married couples in the United States are unable to conceive. The cause of infertility varies with geographic and socioeconomic factors, but some general statements can be made regarding the frequency of certain etiologic factors. Of 100 couples in whom a definite disorder is identified, approximately 40 will show a male factor deficiency, 20 a female hormonal defect, 30 a female tubal disorder, and 10 a cervical defect. Ten to 20 per cent of couples with infertility remain undiagnosed as to the cause of their problem. Because investigation of infertility in the female is time consuming and expensive, evaluation of the male factor is carried out first.

MALE FACTOR. The most important procedure is the analysis of the semen. Although some estimate of sperm can be made from postcoital cervical examinations, before any final conclusion of deficiency is made, three separate masturbatory specimens should be examined for volume, sperm count, motility, morphology, and viability. A normal ejaculate is considered to have a volume not less than 1 ml and not more than 6 ml, 60 per cent active forms after two hours, 60 per cent normal morphology, and at least 20 million sperm per milliliter. If counts are below 20 million, full urologic and medical investigation is warranted. Regardless of count, the male partner should be questioned and instructed when necessary in the development of appropriate sexual and social habits.

FEMALE FACTOR. Once it is established that ovulation regularly occurs (by means of basal body temperature curves, appropriately timed examination of cervical mucus, endometrial biopsy, and pregnanediol excretion), investigation of the female attempts to certify functional and anatomic competence of the reproductive tract to permit union of sperm and ovum in the ampulla of the oviduct.

The postcoital test is performed at the expected date of ovulation, not less than 2 and not more than 16 hours after intercourse. A specimen of endocervical mucus is inspected for clarity, ferning, elasticity, and the number and activity of spermatozoa. In this way the adequacy of coital position, intromission, and ejaculate content, as well as the cervical environment, can be evaluated. Sperm survive in mucus that is abundant, clear, and elastic. The presence of this type of mucus is indicative of adequate local cervical and ovarian function. Repeatedly poor postcoital examinations, despite documented ovulation, make examination of the male factor and coital habits imperative. Furthermore, anatomic abnormalities of the cervix or hostile mucus resulting from erosions, infections, and other local disorders of the cervix should be investigated and specifically treated.

Tubal competence is evaluated by tubal insufflation with carbon dioxide (the Rubin test), by roentgenographic demonstration of patency by hysterosalpingography, or by direct visualization by laparoscopy or culdoscopy. Each serves distinct functions and should be included in the definitive infertility work-up.

The *Rubin test* is best performed before ovulation. It involves transcervical introduction of carbon dioxide under a carefully monitored flow rate and pressures and insufflation of gas through the uterus and the ostia of the tubes into the peritoneal cavity. A positive test result (indicating tubal patency) involves demonstration of gas under the diaphragm by the appearance of referred shoulder pain. The insufflation occurs at a gas pressure usually less than 120 mm of mercury. If tubal blackade exists, escape of gas is prevented and the pressure readings rise continuously to above 200 mm of mercury. At this point the test should be discontinued. It must be remembered that a single negative test result is not diagnostic, because functional occlusion (tubospasm) is frequently encountered. Multiple studies are essential and may be undertaken with paracervical block local anesthesia. On the other hand, a positive Rubin test does not rule out the presence of distortions of the tube or tubal-ovarian junction secondary to pelvic adhesions. For this reason if infertility persists in the face of positive tubal insufflation, then ancillary tests of tubal competence are required.

Hysterosalpingography is ordinarily performed by instillation of 3 to 6 ml of radiopaque oil into the uterine cavity and oviducts under fluoroscopic observation. In this way defects in the uterine cavity that may interfere with implantation and alteration in tubal architecture can be visualized and permanently recorded. The presence of peritubal adhesions may be diagnosed by the dye diffusion pattern about the tubal ostia at the time of examination and 24 hours later.

Laparoscopy (which has virtually replaced culdoscopy) accompanied by tubal insufflation with methylene blue is probably the most effective means of diagnosing peritubal and pelvic adhesions producing infertility. Combined with salpingography, these procedures offer detailed information as to the feasibility and type of corrective adnexal surgery to be undertaken.

Uterine factors were once considered important elements in infertility. However, current views no longer give significance to the multiple anatomic variations in uterine displacement from the usual anterior position. However, abnormalities of the uterine cavity, such as congenital anomalies and submucous myomas, deserve surgical repair if associated with otherwise unexplained infertility.

FERTILITY CONTROL
(Population Control)

Discussion of the need for population control is beyond the scope of this text. Obviously, once the public health issues of the demographic gap and its consequences are put aside, the basic issue remains the acceptability of the form of fertility control offered to the individual couples. If 100 women of proved fertility are exposed to pregnancy for one year, approximately 80 pregnancies will result. Clearly, then, *any* method of contraception is more effective than none. It must be remembered that significant discrepancies always exist between the theoretical and practical effectiveness of any contraceptive method, as is illustrated by experience with the "rhythm" method. The fertile phase (requiring sexual continence) is estimated as extending from the eighteenth day before the onset of the earliest likely menstruation up to and including the eleventh day before the onset of the latest likely menstruation. The method assumes that ovulation occurs about 14 days before menstruation, that spermatozoa can fertilize for 48 hours after intercourse, and that the ovum can be fertilized for about 24 hours after it emerges from the ovary. The method depends on motivation to accumulate menstrual records for one year before use and to remain continent during the fertile period. Studies of the effectiveness of this method reveal pregnancy rates of about 15 conceptions per 100 years of exposure. Although this is about double the conception rates with mechanical devices (condom, diaphragm), it represents an important reduction compared with the projected rate of 80 which would have been expected. All physicians must be prepared to teach this method as long as a substantial proportion of the population is limited by religious belief to this method alone.

When considering the other available contraceptive modalities, it is apparent that with advancing scientific knowledge and public awareness the traditional, folklore-based methods (douche, withdrawal, household spermicides) have given way to proved methods of prevention. Vaginal jellies, foams, diaphragms, and condoms are all safe and fairly reliable. Their relative acceptability varies geographically and according to social class. Their application and use are described in Calderone's manual.

Two modern methods of contraception have altered worldwide concepts of conception control. These are the oral ovulation-inhibiting steroid "pill" and the intrauterine device (IUD).

Steroid Contraception

The ovulation inhibition noted during pregnancy had been recognized, but it was not until the 1950's that orally active progestins became available and applied in women seeking contraception. Currently over 50 million women are using the oral contraceptives. Although these drugs offer practically 100 per cent use effectiveness, various side effects occur related to the biochemical characteristics and doses of the steroid utilized.

THE ESTROGEN COMPONENT. There are two estrogens used in the over 25 oral contraceptives available (see Fig. 8): ethinyl estradiol and mestranol. The addition of an ethinyl group at carbon 17 yields an orally active compound. Mestranol (ME) is the 3-methyl ether of ethinyl estradiol (EE) and must be converted to EE in vivo to achieve estrogenic potency. Although much has been written concerning potency of the two estrogens, it is best to consider EE and ME as equipotent with respect to blood levels, endometrial histology, ovulatory inhibition, and gonadotropin inhibition.

THE PROGESTIN COMPONENT. The addition of the ethinyl group to the 17 portion of testosterone yields oral activity (ethisterone). Removal of the 19 carbon from ethisterone converts an androgen into a 19-norprogestin. There are five of these steroids used in birth control pills (Fig. 9): norethindrone, norethynodrel, norethindrone acetate, ethynodiol diacetate, and norgestrel. Some anabolic and estrogen qualities are retained in these steroids, but they are not clinically important factors.

MECHANISM OF ACTION. The combined (E & P) birth control pill inhibits ovulation at the hypothalamic centers by suppressing LH by negative feedback. In addition, the estrogen component inhibits FSH-suppressing follicle development, and progestin alters endometrium and cervical mucus to reduce implantation of the fertilized egg and inhibit sperm migration. This formation is so effective that major reductions in steroid content have occurred — estrogen 50 μg and lower, progestin 1 mg and lower — without loss of efficacy. However, major and minor side effects have been noted.

SIDE EFFECTS. Birth control pills have been studied in large retrospective and prospective studies. The reader is directed to several of these studies, such as those of the Royal College of General Practitioners, the Boston Collaborative Drug Surveillance Program, and the British Family Planning Council. A summary of critical issues is presented here.

Figure 9. Progestogens in the birth control pill.

Deep Thrombosis of the Leg. In the English prospective study the risk of deep thrombosis of the leg was 5.7 times that of controls. Furthermore the attributable risk of deep thrombosis on 50 μg estrogen pills was 80 per 100,000 users per year, whereas on higher doses it was 112 per 100,000 per year, a decrease of 28 per cent.

Neurovascular Accidents. Pill use increases the risk of thrombotic stroke by three times and hemorrhagic stroke by two times, with an over-all risk of 1 per 200,000 users per year. The onset of visual symptoms or severe headaches is regarded as a warning signal requiring discontinuation of therapy.

Myocardial Infarction. Oral contraceptives act synergistically with risk factors associated with myocardial infarction (hypercholesterolemia, hypertension, and cigarette smoking). There is also an increased incidence with age (over 35) (see Fig. 10).

Carbohydrate Metabolism. Both the estrogen and progestin components of the pill produce an increase in the peripheral resistance to insulin action. Individuals who cannot respond with a compensatory increase in insulin have an abnormal glucose tolerance. This is seen in 15 to 40 per cent of pill users. The clinical significance of the elevated blood sugar (aside from monilial vaginitis) remains uncertain. In the English prospective study there was no evidence that users had an increased development of clinical diabetes or its complications. Furthermore, overt diabetics did not experience a worsening of disease while on the pill. Only gestational diabetes may become overt diabetes as a consequence of birth control steroids.

Liver Adenomas. This rare development is produced by steroids of both estrogen and androgen type. Two different lesions can be seen: peliosis (dilated vascular spaces without endothelial lining) and adenomatous changes (nodular hyperplasia or adenomas). These tumors are not malignant, and they may regress after the pill is stopped. Their significance lies in sudden hemorrhagic complications.

Gallbladder Disease. A two-fold increase in risk of cholelithiasis and/or cholecystitis has been noted. The mechanism appears to be an estrogen-induced rise in bile concentration of cholesterol.

Hypertension. In the English prospective study 5 per cent of pill users developed hypertension after five years of use. The mechanism is thought to be related to the increased plasma angiotensinogen (8×) seen in recipients. In the majority of women vasoconstriction by excess

Figure 8. Estrogens in the birth control pill.

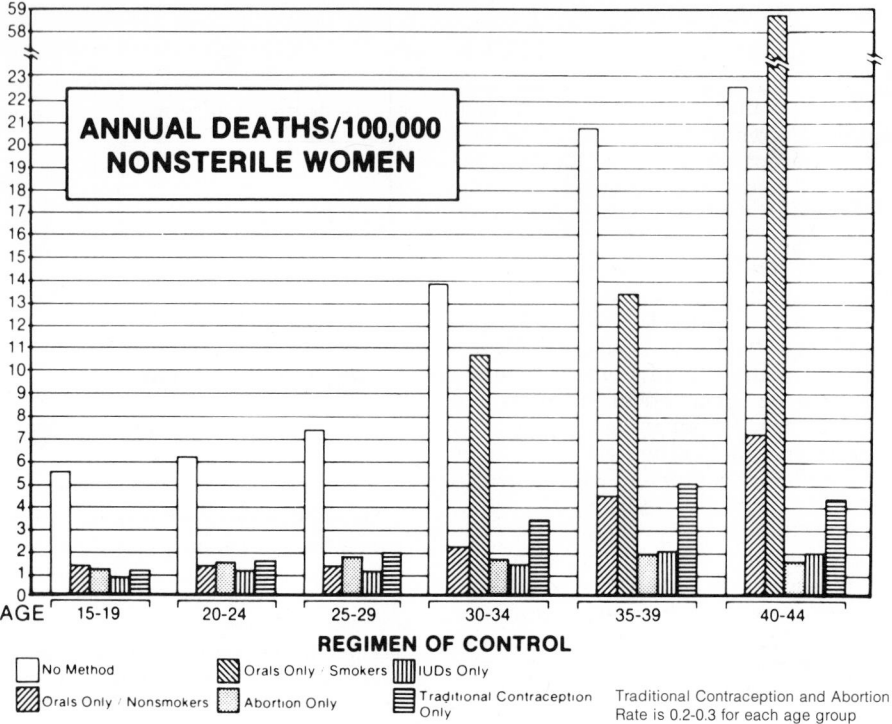

Figure 10.   Mortality estimates in various fertility control measures.

angiotensin II production is avoided by decreased renin concentration. A failure in this response has been suggested as responsible for clinical hypertension. Other sodium retention related factors (volume changes, vessel wall sensitivity to vasoconstrictors) are also considered. The incidence of hypertension increases with duration of use of the pill; but hypertension recedes following discontinuation of pills and renin-angiotensin changes return to normal in three to six months. At this time there is no method of detecting the susceptible patients.

Cancer.   There is no evidence that birth control pill use increases the risk of uterine or cervical cancer. Both prospective and retrospective studies show no evidence of an association of breast cancer and the pill.

Lipid Metabolism.   Progestins have no apparent effect on lipids, whereas estrogens increase plasma triglycerides and phospholipids. Because these changes can be seen in subjects on fat-free diets, estrogen either increases hepatic lipogenesis or impairs removal into adipose tissue by inhibiting heparin action on lipase activity. The clinical significance of these changes is not known. In women with strong family histories of coronary disease, periodic measurement of triglyceride levels while on contraceptive pills seems a wise precaution.

Liver.   Estrogen influences the synthesis of hepatic DNA and RNA, hepatic cell enzymes, serum enzymes formed in the liver, and plasma proteins. Estrogenic hormones also affect hepatic lipid and lipoprotein formation, the intermediary metabolism of carbohydrates, and intracellular enzyme activity. The active transport of biliary components is impaired by a large number of estrogens and some progestins. Cholestatic jaundice and pruritus are occasional complications of the pill and are similar to the recurrent jaundice of pregnancy. BSP retention is abnormal in 20 per cent of users, and serum alkaline phosphatase is elevated in 2 per cent; but SGOT eleva-

tion, if persistent, is not caused by the pill. Pre-existing acute and chronic cholestatic hepatic disease is a contraindication to the use of steroidal contraception. Cirrhosis and previous hepatitis do not seem to be aggravated.

Adrenal Cortex.   For some time it has been known that estrogen increases the cortisol-binding globulin transcortin. It has been thought that the increase in plasma cortisol while taking birth control medication was due to increased binding by the globulin without increase in the concentration of free cortisol. Recently, free cortisol has also been shown to be elevated in people taking these steroids. The prolonged effects of this elevation are unknown. The pituitary-adrenal reaction to stress is unimpaired, although the adrenal reaction to metyrapone may be subnormal (owing to estrogen-influenced conjugation of metyrapone).

Other Metabolic Effects.   Gastrointestinal effects, breast discomfort, and weight gain remain common disturbing effects of birth control pills. Fortunately, these are most intense in the early months of use and usually disappear thereafter. Weight gain on medication is very common but responds to caloric restriction. For some patients, weight gain is a particularly discouraging symptom because of the additional burden of periodic fluid retention.

Chloasma, an increase in facial pigment, was at one time found in as many as 5 per cent of users, but is less commonly seen with the current reduction of the steroid content of pills. Once chloasma does appear, it fades slowly and incompletely. Skin-blanching medications may be useful in cosmetically burdened women.

Oral contraception may inhibit the absorption of folate polyglutamates, and prolonged use may lead to megaloblastic anemia in patients with folic acid–deficient diets. Pyridoxine deficiences may also be seen.

Hematologic effects reported include increased fibrinogen, increased sedimentation rates, increased serum total iron-binding capacity, and a decrease in prothrombin time.

In some women mental depression or reduction in libido, or both, may require search for an alternative contraceptive method.

ABSOLUTE CONTRAINDICATIONS TO THE USE OF THE PILL. As a result of these observations, the following list of absolute contraindications to use of birth control pills has been developed: (1) Thrombophlebitis, thromboembolic disorders, cerebral vascular disease, coronary occlusion, a past history of these conditions, or conditions predisposing to these problems. (2) Markedly impaired liver function; steroids are contraindicated in patients with acute hepatitis until liver function tests return to normal. (3) Known or suspected carcinoma of the breast. (4) Known or suspected estrogen-dependent neoplasia, specifically carcinoma of the endometrium. (5) Undiagnosed abnormal genital bleeding. (6) Cholestatic jaundice in pregnancy. (7) Congenital hyperlipidemia.

Further, certain contraindications apply in which clinical judgment will define the benefit-risk ratio of pill use: (1) Migraine headaches. (2) Hypertension. (3) Uterine fibroids. (4) Epilepsy. (5) Varicose veins. (6) Gestational diabetes. (7) Vaginal adenosis secondary to diethylstilbestrol. (8) Elective surgery; the pill should be discontinued one month prior to elective surgery to avoid an increased risk for postoperative thrombosis.

Intrauterine Devices for Contraception

With increased use and experience, pregnancy rates in users of various intrauterine spiral or loop devices (IUD's) vary from 2 to 5 per 100 woman years, and therefore tend to be similar to rates observed for other mechanical contraceptives. Obviously the advantage of this mode of contraception is that it minimizes the factor of patient error and is therefore suited to large-scale application in the lower socioeconomic groups. A complicating factor is the often unnoticed expulsion of the device, with consequent loss of contraceptive protection. Pregnancy has occurred with the device in place. The disturbing incidence of intermenstrual spotting, menorrhagia, reproductive tract infection, and perforation of the uterus detracts from the acceptability of these devices. Furthermore, contraindications to their application include distorting fibromyomas and adnexal disease.

The mechanism of action is not understood. In rats the devices affect ovum transport, in rabbits implantation and postimplantation stages are affected, and in monkeys tubal ova are lost. Objective studies of associated alterations in human physiology have not appeared. Their usefulness to date has been in large-scale programs requiring minimal patient cooperation.

IUD's are now divided into two groups: *Medicated* IUD's are those that carry a biologically active contraceptive into the uterine cavity; the *nonmedicated* IUD's do not contain a drug in their matrix. With medicated types the IUD need only be the carrier or platform for the medication, thereby reducing the properties of shape, size, or volume which may be related to pain, expulsion, bleeding, and infection but maximize contraceptive efficacy. Because the drug duration is limited, these IUD's have the limitation of requiring repeated reinsertions (one- to three-year frequencies) and depend on a reliable follow-up. Although theoretically expected to have greater contraceptive success, medicated IUD's as yet have not been shown to improve efficacy in formal prospective studies.

A worrisome aspect of IUD use is the problem of infection — pelvic infection with subsequent infertility resulting from salpingitis, and the risk of septic abortion in pregnancies existing with an IUD in utero. Various studies have implicated a rise (two to eight times) in pelvic infection in users of IUD's versus women employing other methods. This rise is most striking in nulliparous women. Although this infection rate is almost certainly due to a high rate of multiple partners and venereal disease exposure in the population most likely to rely on IUD's, the case is persuasively made to avoid this procedure in nulliparas except in situations in which other methods cannot be utilized.

Although the septic abortion problem was observed in IUD's such as the Dalkon Shield with multifilament tails, good practice dictates removal of all IUD's in pregnancy and abortion counseling when appropriate. Finally, if the patient conceives with the IUD in place, the threads are not visible (with enlargement of the uterus these markers are drawn up into the cavity), and she wishes to continue the pregnancy, she should be advised that her chance of having a spontaneous abortion is increased approximately three-fold, and her chance of ectopic pregnancy is increased ten-fold (although the IUD prevents intrauterine pregnancy, ectopic gestational protection is nil). Any bleeding, fever, or chills must be reported and treated as potential evidence of septic abortion.

Beral, V., and Kay, R. K.: Mortality among oral contraceptive users. Lancet, 2:727, 1977.

Boston Collaborative Drug Surveillance Program: Oral contraceptives and venous thromboembolic disease, gall bladder disease, and breast tumors. Lancet, 1:1399, 1973.

Johansson, B. W., Kaij, L., Kullander, S., Lenner, H. C., Svanberg, L., and Astedt, B.: On some late effects of bilateral oophorectomy in the age range 15–30 years. Acta Obstet. Gynecol. Scand., 54:449, 1975.

Klatskin, G.: Hepatic tumors: Possible relationship to use of oral contraceptives. Gastroenterology, 73:386, 1977.

Lindsay, R., Hart, D. M., Artken, J. M., MacDonald, E. B., Anderson, J. B., and Clarke, A. C.: Longterm prevention of postmenopause osteoporosis by estrogen. Lancet, 1:1038, 1976.

Lipsett, M. B.: Estrogen use and cancer risk. JAMA, 237:1112, 1977.

Speroff, L., Glass, R. H., and Kase, N. G.: Clinical Gynecologic Endocrinology and Infertility. Baltimore, Williams & Wilkins Company, 1978.

Weiss, N. S., Szekely, D., and Austin, D. F.: Increasing incidence of endometrial carcinoma in the United States. N. Engl. J. Med., 294:1259, 1976.

COUNSELING IN GYNECOLOGY

The emphasis in the preceding discussions has been directed to analysis of changes in the primary ovarian function of ovulation. In these concluding paragraphs some mention of the physician's role in sexual counseling must be made.

Whereas deep-seated sexual problems are usually discussed in psychiatry teaching programs in the medical curriculum, ordinarily no instruction is given the medical student in the normal aspects of sexual life or in its commonly occurring abnormalities. The physician therefore enters practice without benefit of the usual guidelines of diagnosis and management that he has developed for most of the other disorders he will be called upon to see. However, because of his professional status he is often asked for advice in sexual matters and, owing to the uncertainty of applying his own intuitive perception to these matters, the physician usually avoids comment. Unfortunately, this attitude compounds the official silence with which these subjects are treated by schools, religious groups, and families.

As a result of the important observations and clinical activities of Masters and Johnson, recorded in two widely read volumes, a factual description of the biophysical progression of male and female sexual response associated with orgasm as well as an approach to diagnosis and therapy of sexual dysfunction is available. Using rapid (two-week) therapeutic methods involving instructional and interpretive interactions between the dysfunctional couple and a male and female co-therapy team, an overall treatment success rate of 80 per cent has been achieved in the four main categories of human sexual inadequacy: premature ejaculation, male impotence, female orgasmic deficiency, and vaginismus.

In general, the direction of therapy, regardless of the type of presenting distress, is based upon the premise that subjective appreciation of sexual responsivity derives from positive pleasure in sensory experience. For the sexually dysfunctional individual the sensory deprivation originates in one of several possibilities: fear and apprehension of sexual situations, denial of personal sexual identity, rejection of partner or the circumstance of sexual encounter, and lack of sexual awareness through either emotional or physical fatigue or preoccupation. It is not known what special susceptibility causes only a fraction of individuals exposed to these traumas to undergo protracted sexual dysfunction.

The therapist's role is to provide an accurate "mirror" of professional objectivity and knowledge to the troubled couple. In doing this, myths and misconceptions are dismissed, and fear of poor performance, lack of goal orientation, and the notion of the patient as a "spectator" in sexual activity are eliminated. Furthermore, since there appears never to be a purely unilaterally dysfunctional partner, the couple must be trained to communicate needs and exchange sexual vulnerabilities. Thus a nonverbal and verbal signal system is established to maximize pleasure, excitation, mutual satisfaction, and avoidance of stereotyped performance. In this process of reorientation, education, and physical direction, exploration without performance pressures, development of "sensate focus," and carefully graded escalation of sexual involvement compose the therapeutic sequence.

ORGASMIC DYSFUNCTION—MALE. *Premature ejaculation* exists if the male cannot control the onset of his ejaculation for a sufficient length of time during intravaginal containment to satisfy his partner in at least 50 per cent of coital opportunities. Obviously, this problem also affects female function. It limits her ability to express sexual reactions and to achieve satisfactory relief of mounting sexual tensions, inevitably leading to frustration at "just being used." On the other hand, the rapid conclusion of sexual contact is a welcome relief from involvement in unpleasant and unrewarding service. The derivations of this self-centered male expression of need appear to be initial teenage exposures to prostitutes, exclusive reliance on "heavy petting" and coital simulation, and dependence on withdrawal as a contraceptive technique. Under all these circumstances there was no need either to learn ejaculatory control or to undertake responsibility for the partner's reactions and responses. Apparently, masturbation practices do not play an etiologic role.

Therapy by "squeeze technique" and gradual resumption of coital contact has led to almost complete therapeutic success (98 per cent).

Male impotence is classified as *primary* when a male has never been able to achieve and/or maintain an erection qualitatively sufficient to accomplish coital connection. His erection may be achieved but then dissipated without ejaculation. This male may masturbate successfully. Masters and Johnson assign certain events in adolescence as factors influencing the formation of primary impotence. These include untoward maternal influences, the psychosocial restrictions of religious orthodoxy, homosexual functioning, and personal devaluations from experiences with prostitutes. These events lead in a very few men to a longstanding and deep concern about subsequent sexual performance. Therapy has been successful along the general lines outlined above with the augmenting use of replacement partners or partner surrogates.

Secondary impotence is said to exist if at least one successful coital intromission has occurred; as many as several hundred may have been experienced before the onset of secondary impotence. Inability to obtain or maintain a satisfactory erection for coitus normally occurs as an accompaniment to fatigue or distraction. However, if 25 per cent of opportunities are not achieved, then secondary impotence exists. Among the etiologic factors involved are premature ejaculation, alcoholism, excessive dominance of either parent, homosexuality, and religious orthodoxy. Only rarely are physiologic causes (diabetes, neurologic disease, drug intake, genitourinary problems) found as responsible for impotence. All too often the effect of inadequate counseling is a precipitating or prolonging factor.

The treatment of impotence is directed at combating the male's personal insecurity and his feelings that "nothing can be done," that the problem is unique to the patient, that the partner is viewed as a liability leading to disability, and that the problem must be kept secret even from the therapist. In therapy, the patient must be convinced that he can never "will" an erection. As fears of sexual performance are reduced, the patient's concept of being a spectator of his own dysfunction is diminished. The female partner must also be supported and instructed. Thorough discussion, discovery of sensate focus (the opportunity to think and feel sexually without orientation to performance), sharing mutual genital manipulation and masturbation pleasures with verbal and nonverbal communication, and a "tease" technique in graded resumption of coital opportunities lead to repair of sexual dysfunction in 60 to 70 per cent of cases.

ORGASMIC DYSFUNCTION — FEMALE. The physician may incorrectly assume that the "modern" girl is well versed in genital anatomy and physiology and the technique of the sexual act. Practical experience indicates that in many instances the young woman approaching marriage knows too little and has the disturbing notion, perhaps by conditioning from her mother's experience, that marital sex for the female is overrated, exploitative, and sinful. In such instances, without adequate counseling for both partners, repeated dissatisfaction may confirm these attitudes and set the pattern for a lifetime of maladjusted performance of a "wifely duty." Although it may appear too simple a solution for a problem of such magnitude, the physician can help the couple to avoid this situation by tactful and sympathetic review of basic facts during premarital examinations or any other occasion requiring medical consultation.

The fear of genital injury or expectation of pain and

hemorrhage owing to rupture of the hymen during sexual intercourse poses a threat to achievement of vaginal-oriented orgasm. Such preconceived attitudes can be dispelled by the assurance of the physician that the pelvic examination just performed reveals anatomically adequate external and internal genitalia. Some pain is usually experienced on entry into the vagina, but lubrication, a considerate partner, and repeated experience favor prompt resolution of this difficulty.

Because mutual precoital sexual excitement is imperative, varying patterns of stimulation as well as coital techniques must be encouraged and instruction given. Every effort must be made to motivate both partners to seek this result by experimentation and frank discussion. In this situation affectation of false modesty or "man of the world" all-knowing attitudes should be discouraged. In 223 dysfunctional couples, 107 had bilateral impairment in which an anorgasmic female was paired with a male who was a premature ejaculator.

It must be made clear that, no matter how satisfactory the circumstances, few women experience orgasm regularly. Often this misunderstanding, if uncorrected, provokes undue concern and tension that may produce further diminution in satisfaction, a change in coital frequency, substitution of clitoral orgasm, or pretending satisfaction when none occurs. Once these patterns are set, reconditioning for vaginal orgasm is possible but only after a long and difficult period of adjustment. Some of the factors leading to the initial lack of coital orgasm are fear of pregnancy, the possibility of discovery by parents or children, economic and social pressures, poor health, and fatigue. All these profoundly influence both partners' interest in and response to intercourse. Possibly the most common factor in the development of aversion to sexual intimacy in the somewhat older married woman is that over the years these intimacies have tended to follow a monotonous, routine sameness of time, place, and practice. Reluctance to discuss the matter with her husband or with her physician abets the situation. The alert physician can usually suspect this problem from the patient's response during history taking and the nature of her physical complaints. Again sympathetic but informative discussions will bring a more open and intelligent outlook on the part of the patient, and whereas no quick cure exists, reorientation of sexual practice and renewed motivation can occur, with an increasing degree of satisfaction derived. Coaching the couple in the recognition of the female indicators of sexual arousal and the sequence leading to achievement of orgasm is particularly helpful. Delay of coitus until extragenital and genital responses in the female (generalized skin flush, retraction of the clitoris, ballooning of the vagina, color changes in the labia) will increase the frequency of coital orgasm, release female sexual tension, and make the anxious, uncertain couple more confident and eager for sexual contact. The therapeutic use of testosterone and alcohol in the sexually frigid woman is not recommended. The effects are temporary and only serve to postpone the necessary personal examination that must be carried out. *Cantharis vesicatoria* (Spanish fly) is a severe irritant to the clitoris and has no place in therapeutics.

Sometimes problems appear to be so complicated and deep seated that psychiatric help is worthwhile. Fortunately these are rare. However, if sexual frigidity appears to have the malicious motivation of deprivation, if sexual intercourse and practice are revolting prospects, or if the

woman displays pronounced aggressive or homosexual tendencies, psychiatric evaluation is in order.

Vaginismus is a constriction of the outer third of the vagina by spastic involuntary contractions of the muscles of the pelvic floor. This occurs in reaction to imagined, anticipated, or real attempts at vaginal penetration. As a result, penile penetration is exceedingly difficult or impossible and coitus is rare or the marriage is unconsummated. It is not infrequently found in association with a male partner who suffers from primary impotence or other male dysfunction. In addition, religious orthodoxy, early psychosexual trauma (e.g., rape), recurrent vaginitis or dyspareunia caused by endometriosis, pelvic inflammatory disease, postoperative adhesions, or homosexual preferences are seen as contributory factors. Therapy of the primary pathologic problem and vaginal dilators lead to nearly 100 per cent therapeutic success.

Masters, W. H., and Johnson, V. E.: Human Sexual Response. Boston, Little, Brown & Company, 1966.

Masters, W. H., and Johnson, V. E.: Human Sexual Inadequacy. Boston, Little, Brown & Company, 1970.

550. THE ADRENAL MEDULLA AND SYMPATHETIC NERVOUS SYSTEM

Karl Engelman

The sympathetic nervous system is made up of cellular elements distinguished by their embryologic derivation from neural crest cells and by their distinct chemistry and pharmacology relating to the synthesis and release of the postsynaptic neurotransmitter catecholamine compounds. The cells are found widely distributed throughout the body with major foci located in the central nervous system as well as in ganglia associated with the thoracolumbar segments of the spinal cord. Peripheral sites of localization include the innervation of the heart, blood vessels, smooth muscle of the gastrointestinal tract, sweat and salivary glands, adipose tissue, and adrenal medulla.

Alterations of sympathetic nervous system activity may lead to a wide variety of clinical manifestations. Within the central nervous system, abnormalities result in changes of mood and emotional status as well as movement and tremor disorders. Peripheral manifestations include deficits in vasomotor control with resultant hypo- or hypertension, and altered motility and secretory activity of other visceral organs. In addition, tumors may develop from sympathetic neural tissue, producing clinical syndromes dependent upon the biochemical and pharmacologic activity of the hormones synthesized and released from these cells.

HORMONES OF THE ADRENAL MEDULLA AND SYMPATHETIC NERVOUS SYSTEM

The hormones of the sympathetic nervous system are dopamine, norepinephrine, and epinephrine; the last-named is primarily synthesized and released by the ad-

Figure 1. Biosynthetic pathway of the catecholamines.

renal medulla. These compounds are classified chemically as *catecholamines,* because they are amine derivatives of the catechol (dihydroxybenzine) nucleus. In common usage the term is usually applied only to norepinephrine and epinephrine. The accepted pathway for synthesis of these hormones was first postulated by Blaschko in 1939, and the intermediate steps with the related enzymes are shown in Figure 1. The rate-limiting step in the pathway is hydroxylation of tyrosine to form dihydroxyphenylalanine (dopa), a reaction under feedback control by end-product (norepinephrine) inhibition.

Synthesis of the catecholamines is a unique capability of sympathetic nervous tissue; except for the enzyme aromatic-L-amino acid decarboxylase, the biosynthetic enzymes are found only within sympathetic nervous cells. The enzyme required for the conversion of norepinephrine to epinephrine is found solely within the adrenal medulla. Tyrosine hydroxylase and dopamine beta-hydroxylase (DβH) are found almost universally in sympathetic neural cells where synthesis normally terminates with norepinephrine. The adrenal medulla contains very large quantities of both norepinephrine and epinephrine, the latter comprising 70 to 80 per cent of the total. These catecholamines are normally stored within sympathetic nerve terminals in intracellular granules which migrate to the cell membrane at the time of neural activity and discharge the amines.

When catecholamines are released from sympathetic tissues other than the adrenal medulla, the primary route of physiologic inactivation is effected by an active transport mechanism which returns the unaltered catecholamine into the nerve ending. Either the residual

hormone is metabolized locally, or a small portion may diffuse away to appear in the circulation where it may be further metabolized (liver and lung) or excreted unchanged by the kidney. In contrast, catecholamines released from either the adrenal medulla or hormone-producing tumors appear directly in the circulation and manifest their peripheral effects as a result of their concentration in plasma. The primary routes of catecholamine metabolism are shown in Figure 2. For circulating catecholamines, the major route is O-methylation by the enzyme catechol-O-methyltransferase, followed by oxidative deamination via aldehyde dehydrogenase and monoamine oxidase. In contrast, catecholamines metabolized either within the sympathetic nerve cells or in sympathetic tumors are in large part initially converted by oxidative deamination, followed by O-methylation. In either case, the initial metabolic product is pharmacologically inactive, and the major end-product is vanillylmandelic acid (VMA).

The catecholamines and their metabolites are primarily excreted in the urine, and VMA makes up 75 to 80 per cent of the total. The methoxyamines (metanephrines) comprise 10 to 15 per cent, and free catecholamines in the urine usually represent less than 1 per cent of the quantity released. Quantitatively, norepinephrine and its metabolites make up 80 per cent of the total, with epinephrine and its metabolites comprising the balance. Under usual circumstances and with normal activity, humans excrete from 10 to 70 μg of norepinephrine and from 5 to 30 μg of epinephrine per 24 hours. After adrenalectomy the excretion of epinephrine decreases to minimal values, whereas norepinephrine excretion is little changed. Normal excretion of the methoxyamines (normetanephrine plus metanephrine) ranges from 0.3 to 1.3 mg per 24 hours and that of VMA from 2.0 to 6.8 mg per 24 hours.

PHARMACOLOGY. Important quantitative differences between epinephrine and norephinephrine, relating to the proportionately greater beta-adrenergic potency of epinephrine, are observed when small doses (5 to 10 μg per minute) are administered intravenously to humans. Although a potent direct vasoconstrictor in some vascular beds, epinephrine produces over-all vasodilatation and a decrease in peripheral resistance as well as striking increases in cardiac output and heart rate. Systolic blood pressure is increased, but diastolic pressure remains unchanged or falls, and there is little change in

Figure 2. Major routes of catecholamine metabolism.

the mean arterial pressure. In contrast, norepinephrine causes an increase of both systolic and diastolic pressure owing to generalized vasoconstriction. Although norepinephrine also has potent beta-sympathomimetic activity, the predominating rise in pressure leads to reflex slowing of the heart, resulting in little change or decrease in cardiac output. When very large doses of norepinephrine or epinephrine are infused into humans or are released from catechol-producing tumors, these differences in physiologic activities of the hormones are usually muted.

Both norepinephrine and epinephrine produce profound metabolic effects, including increased lipolysis and oxygen consumption, elevation of body temperature, and hyperglycemia caused by increased glycogenolysis, as well as inhibition of insulin release from the pancreas. Many of the varying alpha- and beta-sympathetic effects of these hormones have been shown to be mediated through changes in the adenyl cyclase system. Current theory holds that beta-sympathomimetic effects are primarily induced by stimulation of adenyl cyclase and increased cyclic-AMP generation, whereas alpha-adrenergic effects inhibit adenyl cyclase activity.

Under normal conditions secretion of epinephrine and norepinephrine by the adrenal medulla is probably not of great physiologic significance. Although hormone production from this sympathetic tissue achieves greater importance during conditions of stress, as in insulin hypoglycemia, the role of the adrenal medulla in normal physiology appears to be mainly supportive in nature. Deficiency states are not generally noted in patients who have had total adrenalectomy with adequate adrenocortical replacement. On the other hand, neuropathic or pharmacologic interruption of the nonadrenal sympathetic tissues appears to produce profound effects most notable in vasomotor control and propulsive activity of the hollow viscera. Among the more commonly encountered clinical conditions in which there is disorder in the sympathetic nervous system are idiopathic orthostatic hypotension and the Riley-Day syndrome (familial dysautonomia), conditions in which both sympathetic and parasympathetic functions are abnormal. In addition, results of recent investigations tend to implicate an increase in sympathetic nervous system activity as a causative factor in a significant number of patients with what has previously been called essential hypertension.

PHEOCHROMOCYTOMA

Pheochromocytoma is a catecholamine-producing tumor arising from cells of the sympathetic nervous system. The first clinical description of the syndrome is credited to Labbé and his associates in 1922, and successful surgery for this condition was first performed in 1927 by Dr. Charles H. Mayo.

The most distinctive feature is hypertension, although pheochromocytoma is responsible for far less than 1 per cent of all patients with hypertension. Although potentially lethal if undiagnosed and untreated, it is curable in about 90 per cent of cases.

In general, patients with pheochromocytoma are between 5 and 25 years of age. In young women the diagnosis is frequently made during pregnancy, in part because the blood pressure is taken more frequently then

and in some measure because the enlarging uterus may produce pressure on the tumor, inducing more frequent attacks. The tendency to develop pheochromocytoma may be inherited in association with certain other neuroectodermal disorders. Patients with von Recklinghausen's disease and associated disorders have a high incidence of pheochromocytoma within the family. Furthermore, pheochromocytomas can be inherited in association with medullary carcinoma of the thyroid and a tendency to parathyroid hyperfunction resulting from hyperplasia or multiple parathyroid adenomas (*Sipple's syndrome*). In some instances these patients also manifest multiple mucocutaneous neuromas as well as generalized ganglioneuromatosis of visceral organs (Fig. 3). These conditions are inherited as autosomal dominant traits, and the pheochromocytomas are almost always multiple, including bilateral adrenal tumors.

PATHOLOGY. More than 95 per cent of pheochromocytomas arise within the abdominal and pelvic cavities. The majority are found in one or both adrenal glands, but other sites of origin include embryologic rests of neural crest tissue found usually in association with major arteries. Areas of predilection for extra-adrenal tumors include the paravertebral sympathetic ganglia, and in particular those at the bifurcation of the aorta which make up the organ of Zuckerkandl. Very rarely, tumors arise from sympathetic ganglia within the wall of the urinary bladder, producing distinctive symptoms which should strongly suggest this diagnosis. The majority of those arising in the chest are in paravertebral sympathetic ganglia. Other chemodectomas, especially of the carotid body, may produce increased amounts of catecholamines and the clinical syndrome of pheochromocytoma, but the majority of these do not appear to produce hormone syndromes. Extremely rarely, cate-

Figure 3. Multiple neuromas of the tongue and lips in a patient with bilateral multiple adrenal pheochromocytomas, medullary carcinoma of the thyroid, exstrophy of the bladder, and multiple visceral ganglioneuromas.

Figure 4. Bilateral adrenal medullary pheochromocytomas from a patient with Sipple's syndrome. The five largest tumors have been extirpated from the specimens, and an additional five tumors, each measuring approximately 2 mm in diameter, are depicted by the arrows on the specimens.

cholamine-producing tumors may arise from sympathetic tissue in association with intracranial branches of the vagus nerve. Collectively, these tumors, known as glomus jugulare tumors, are found along the base of the skull in the jugular foramen, within the mastoid and temporal bones and the middle ear. Most glomus jugulare tumors are nonfunctional. An increasing number of patients, especially in families with Sipple's syndrome, have been described with typical symptoms of pheochromocytoma in association with *adrenal medullary hyperplasia*. In most instances, anatomic enlargement is bilateral and histologic changes suggest nodular hypertrophy of the medulla with atypical medullary cells.

Most tumors are benign. They may be multiple in up to 20 per cent of patients, usually of the adrenal medulla (Fig. 4). An occasional patient may present with both an adrenal medullary and ectopic tumor. Malignant tumors are found in fewer than 10 per cent of patients. The definition of malignancy is difficult, since benign tumors may present with bizarre nuclear and cellular patterns. The diagnosis of malignancy rests on the finding of metastatic tissue, e.g., in the liver, bone, lymph nodes, lung, and marrow.

Benign tumors may vary from less than a gram to almost a kilogram in weight; most are in the range of 15 to 100 grams. The smallest tumors are usually found in association with other large tumors, especially in the hereditary cases (Fig. 4). Solitary tumors less than 10 grams in weight rarely produce symptoms. They are highly vascular and usually well encapsulated. In the larger tumors there may be central areas of necrosis and fibrosis. The cells are polygonal or spheroidal with granular cytoplasm and are often arranged in masses separated by connective tissue. Multinucleate and bizarre-looking cells are frequent. When unfixed sections are exposed to chromium salts, the tissue may take on a brown color, thus giving rise to the term "chromaffin cells." The catecholamine content is generally greater than that of the adrenal medulla, usually in the range of 1 to 10 mg per gram of tumor. All tumors contain increased quantities of norepinephrine, but fewer than 50 per cent appear to synthesize epinephrine as well. The ma-

jority of those containing epinephrine arise from the adrenal medulla and intrathoracic ganglia. This is in contrast to the catecholamine content of densely sympathetically innervated tissues such as heart and brain, which contain 5 to 10 μg of norepinephrine per gram of tissue.

CLINICAL MANIFESTATIONS. The most common finding is *hypertension* which is usually paroxysmal in character, occurring in association with palpitations, tachycardia, a feeling of malaise and apprehension, and excessive sweating. Many patients are persistently hypertensive, having superimposed paroxysmal rises in blood pressure. An approximately equal number have fluctuating blood pressures, normal at times and hypertensive at others (Fig. 5). Most patients with pheochromocytoma will be hypertensive on at least 50 per cent of readings. Patients who have attacks only at intervals of several days to several weeks are extremely rare, and probably comprise less than 1 per cent of the total group. Symptoms usually occur spontaneously and vary considerably in frequency, severity, and duration in different patients. They often occur while the patient is at rest, or may be precipitated by emotional upset, postural changes or bending, physical exertion, and eating. Attacks coincidental with micturition suggest that the patient has a primary bladder tumor. Before an attack patients may experience apprehension, frequently associated with abdominal or low back pain, which evolves with palpitations, pounding headache, and even angina pectoris. Occasional patients will describe a peculiar, poorly defined sensation of tightness beginning in the lower abdomen and rising through the thorax into the neck and through the head at the onset of attacks. Because of the frequency with which these patients are manifestly anxious or tremulous, it is not uncommon for them to be labeled as having functional disorders. Observers will frequently note tremulousness and pallor or flushing of the face and extremities as well as dilatation of the pupils and marked diaphoresis. Blood pressures during severe attacks may exceed 300 mm Hg, and after the attack the patient may complain of prostration, lassitude, or fatigue. In some instances a "shocklike" state has been recorded in which peripher-

Figure 5. Pattern of blood pressure in a patient with pheochromocytoma. Note variability of blood pressure and presence of orthostatic hypotension prior to therapy and surgery.

al blood pressure has not been obtainable. Although shock and myocardial infarction may occur as a result of a severe attack, frequently the inability to obtain a peripheral blood pressure is due to severe peripheral vasoconstriction. Under these circumstances central blood pressures are usually very high, and very strong central pulses are usually palpable in the axillary or carotid arteries. In rare instances when intense vasoconstriction persists for long periods of time, necrosis and ulceration of tissue may occur. The most serious complications of severe attacks are myocardial infarction, intracerebral hemorrhage, cardiac failure, or hyperpyrexia, all of which may result in death.

In rare instances only special manifestations will suggest this diagnosis in a patient who might otherwise be thought to have essential hypertension. Of prime importance are *excessive sweating* or *hypermetabolism with weight loss* unexplained by overactive thyroid function and the presence of *orthostatic hypotension* in a hypertensive patient not receiving antihypertensive drugs (Fig. 4). This manifestation is found in approximately 70 per cent of patients and reflects a paradoxical impairment of autonomic reflex responses to standing. *Polycythemia* has been noted in several patients and is explained by high plasma and tumor concentrations of erythropoietin. Other important features include *impaired glucose tolerance, paradoxical pressor responses* to autonomic blocking agents such as guanethidine, and *enhanced pressor responses* to sympathomimetic agents such as the amphetamines and commonly used nasal and bronchial decongestants. Severe *constipation* is found in some individuals — presumably because of the marked inhibitory effect of the catecholamines on bowel motility and enhanced sphincter tone. For unknown reasons the incidence of *cholelithiasis* is markedly increased in patients with pheochromocytoma.

Additional clinical features relate to the *inherited disorders which may be found in association with pheochromocytoma.* Most prominent among these are *von Recklinghausen's disease* and *Sipple's syndrome.* In the latter, diarrhea and remarkable flushing resulting from prostaglandin and serotonin production by the tumor may simulate certain aspects of the carcinoid syndrome, and biochemical evidence for hyperparathyroidism exists when secondary parathyroid hyperplasia or tumor induction occurs.

Untreated, the disease may progress in a manner similar to other forms of hypertension, although it is relatively unusual for patients to present with advanced atherosclerotic changes or renal impairment. The primary mode of death in the untreated patient is a cardiovascular or cerebral catastrophe associated with a severe rise in blood pressure. In some instances chronic congestive heart failure caused by a metabolic cardiomyopathy (*"catecholamine cardiomyopathy"*) may be the most serious manifestation.

DIAGNOSIS. Recognition of the variety of clinical features associated with pheochromocytoma should provide the most important asset in suspecting this diagnosis. Often included in the differential diagnosis are essential hypertension, hyperthyroidism, diabetes mellitus, and a variety of psychoneurotic conditions. Once the diagnosis is suspected, it can usually readily be confirmed.

Pharmacologic Tests. Historically, pharmacologic tests were the primary means of confirming or excluding the diagnosis of pheochromocytoma. With the general availability of good biochemical assays for catecholamines and metabolites, the use of pharmacologic tests has been relegated to a secondary or even lesser role in the evaluation of this condition.

Pharmacologic tests may be divided into two categories: *provocative* (producing a rise in blood pressure) and *blocking* (producing a vasodepressor response). Drugs in the former group include histamine, glucagon, and tyramine. Regitine (phentolamine) is the only commonly used vasodepressor agent. Both categories of tests result in as high as a 30 per cent incidence of *false-positive* and *false-negative* responses. In addition, they may produce serious or life-threatening responses in occasional patients. Details as to the dose of drug and positive response will be omitted, since these tests are considered primarily of historical interest. Their use is now discouraged, with preference given to chemical analyses to demonstrate excessive catecholamine production.

Chemical Tests. Reliable assays are now universally available for the measurement of urinary catecholamines (either as total content or fractionated into norepinephrine and epinephrine components), metanephrines (combined normetanephrine plus metanephrine), and VMA. Increased quantities of one (and usually all) of these substances can be documented in any 24-hour urine collection of almost all patients with pheochromocytoma (Fig. 6). In most instances, two-fold or greater increases will be found. However, in rare patients who truly have intermittent symptoms or spells at intervals of many hours or days, and who are otherwise asymptomatic and normotensive, it may be possible only to document significant increases in catecholamine excretion over relatively short, carefully timed periods in association with documented changes in blood pressure and symptoms. Close observation of vital signs, hydration of the patient, and separate collection of each sequential voided urine specimen with determina-

URINARY EXCRETION OF CATECHOLAMINES AND METABOLITES IN PHEOCHROMOCYTOMA

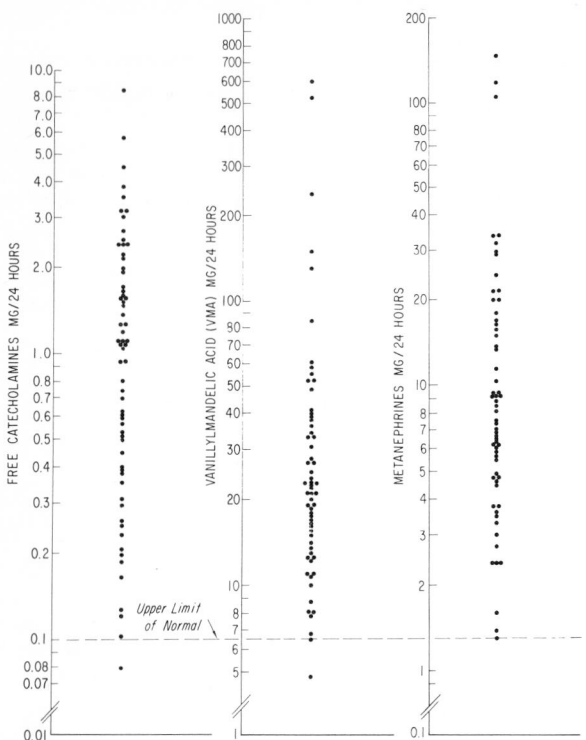

Figure 6. Distribution of excretion values for catecholamines and metabolites determined on single 24-hour urine collections in 64 patients with pheochromocytoma. The vertical axis depicts values on a logarithmic scale.

tion of norepinephrine and epinephrine content in selected samples are usually required to document the episodic nature of two-fold or more increases in catecholamine excretion. In patients manifesting this syndrome more dramatic rises are usually found in epinephrine excretion, and when such patients have been subjected to surgery they have usually been found to have either very small adrenal tumors or adrenal medullary hyperplasia. VMA and metanephrine excretions in these same samples do not usually show significant changes. Determination of plasma catecholamine content (a very difficult assay performed well in only a few laboratories) is not a suitable screening test for pheochromocytoma, since plasma catecholamine values may vary widely under a variety of circumstances even in patients without the tumor.

Certain drugs in common use may interfere with the analyses and interpretation of catecholamines and metabolites in plasma or urine (see accompanying table). It is usually not necessary to discontinue all therapy, provided

that the appropriate choice of tests is made. Dietary restriction, especially prior to determination of VMA, was advocated in the past because crude, nonspecific screening tests were used, which relied upon color reactions with phenolic acids that might be derived from a wide variety of food flavorings, beverages, fruits, and vegetables. Generally available more specific tests for VMA do not necessitate strict diets. As a general rule, laboratory procedures which accept as normal VMA excretion values exceeding 6.5 to 7 mg per 24 hours are prone to this type of dietary interference and *should not be used.*

Tumor Localization. Since almost all pheochromocytomas are found within the abdominal and pelvic cavities, the major preoperative diagnostic attempts to localize the tumor should be directed at *excluding* the presence of an intrathoracic pheochromocytoma or one arising from the neck or in the skull. Such conditions are readily determined by palpating the area of the carotid bifurcations for the presence of a hard mass. Functioning intracranial glomus jugulare tumors should be suspected by the presence of deficits in cranial nerves VII to XII or by the appearance of tumor tissue in the outer or middle ear which can readily be seen by otoscopic examination. In almost all instances in which chest x-rays were obtained in patients having intrathoracic pheochromocytomas, the tumor was readily seen as a posterior mediastinal paravertebral mass. To exclude the presence of such tumors, all patients with pheochromocytoma should have chest fluoroscopy as well as routine and oblique x-rays of the chest. Intra-abdominal pheochromocytomas present no problem of localization at the time of operation (see Treatment, below), and large tumors can usually be demonstrated by the relatively noninvasive technique of intravenous pyelography with laminagrams of the renal and retroperitoneal areas. If the tumor is not seen, evidence of its presence by distortion of the renal contour or shift in the position or axis of the kidney or ureter gives strong indication of its position. Arteriography may readily define large tumors, but small or ectopic tumors may be missed, and the hazard and cost of the procedure do not seem to justify its routine use. Computerized axial tomography of tumor-bearing areas is undergoing evaluation and may prove safe and helpful, although expensive. Precise anatomic location is rarely necessary other than to rule out the presence of extra-abdominal tumors.

In exceptional cases, routine preoperative evaluation and thorough surgical exploration will fail to identify tumor tissue, and in such circumstances it may be necessary to perform venous catheterization of the superior and inferior vena cava as well as their major tributaries to collect blood samples for catecholamine determination. These assays are extremely difficult and can be performed accurately in only a few laboratories, so such problem patients are best handled by experts. Demonstration of a

Urinary Values and Interfering Drugs

Metabolite	Normal Excretion Rate (mg/24 hr)	Usual Range in Pheochromocytoma (mg/24 hr)	Drug	Drug Effect on Excretion Rate
1. Free catecholamines	< 0.1	0.2–4.0	Methyldopa	False increase
			L-Dopa	False increase
2. Metanephrines (normetanephrine plus metanephrine)	< 1.3	2.5–40	MAO inhibitors	Increase
3. Vanillylmandelic acid (VMA)	< 6.8	10–250	MAO inhibitors	Decrease
			Clofibrate (Atromid–S)	False decrease
			Nalidixic acid (NegGram)	False increase

step-up in plasma catecholamine concentrations at any particular level indicates the probable area in which the venous drainage of the tumor enters the major veins. It is noteworthy that falsely elevated values may be produced inadvertently by the person performing the catheterization if radiopaque dye is instilled into the adrenal veins under sufficient pressure to cause local tissue damage. This will result in sufficient catecholamine release from normal adrenals to simulate tumor secretion. Values obtained from the hepatic vein may be most helpful in evaluating the patient for possible hepatic metastases. Under normal circumstances, hepatic venous effluent should have a very low catecholamine concentration because of metabolism of these compounds in the liver. Values from this source as high as or higher than those obtained from other systemic veins indicate hepatic metastases.

TREATMENT. The objective of therapy of pheochromocytoma is prevention of the physiologic and metabolic effects of the catecholamines secreted by the tumor. The preferred therapy is complete surgical excision of the single or multiple tumors, and this can be achieved successfully in approximately 90 per cent of patients. In the remainder, who either have metastatic disease or are not operative candidates for reasons of serious medical complications, pharmacologic therapy can prove very effective in reversing the symptoms of the disease and markedly prolonging life. Regardless of the ultimate form of therapy, pharmacologic therapy will have to be instituted in almost every patient. Adequate control of the effects of catecholamines is necessary before surgery, because the greatest danger to the patient exists during induction of anesthesia and intraoperative manipulations, when life-threatening or lethal rises in blood pressure and arrhythmias may occur as a result of tumor stimulation. Two categories of adrenergic blocking drugs are useful in such cases: those which competitively block the peripheral effects of circulating catecholamines, and a still experimental drug which has proved useful in competitively inhibiting the synthesis of the catecholamines by the tumor. The competitive peripheral sympathetic blocking drugs may be further divided into two groups: the alpha- and beta-sympathetic blockers. The *alpha-blockers* (Dibenzyline and phentolamine) compete primarily with the peripheral vasoconstrictor effects of the catecholamines, thus reducing blood pressure, and they also are effective in blocking the alpha-mediated inhibition of insulin release. Dibenzyline (phenoxybenzamine) is a very long-acting drug which may be administered orally once or twice daily. The usual dose range necessary for the control of most patients is from 20 to 60 mg per day. Occasional patients may require larger doses. The onset of action is rapid, and maximal effect from a single dose is usually achieved in one to two hours. Phentolamine, although also available in an oral dose form, is primarily used intravenously because of its short duration of action, as acute adjunctive therapy to control severe hypertensive crises during surgery. Again, it should be noted that patients whose tumors produce significant amounts of epinephrine alpha-blockers may produce exaggerated hypotensive responses.

The only *beta-sympathetic blockers* available for use in the United States at this time are propranolol and metoprolol. The primary salutary effect is as a specific antagonist of the catecholamine-induced arrhythmias and tachycardia, although it is not usually suggested for use for the latter condition unless the pulse rate is above the range of 110 to 120 beats per minute. Propranolol may be administered either orally or intravenously; metoprolol is currently available only in an oral form. Patients with pheochromocytoma are extremely sensitive to their effects, because use in this condition is specifically related to the causative agent (excess catecholamine stimulation), unlike other instances in which the drugs may be used. Oral doses of 5 to 10 mg every six hours are frequently sufficient to reduce heart rate and abolish arrhythmias. During surgery, doses of propranolol in the range of 0.5 to 2.0 mg may be used intravenously to control arrhythmias when they present a danger. Because of the negative inotropic effects of these drugs, they must be used with caution, especially in patients who have catecholamine cardiomyopathy and who may be thrown into severe congestive failure by very small doses. Paradoxical rises in blood pressure are usually produced when beta-blockers, such as propranolol, are administered to patients whose tumors produce epinephrine. Under these cirucmstances, the drug blocks beta-mediated vasodilatation, thus producing a net increase in peripheral resistance by converting epinephrine pharmacologically into norepinephrine ("epinephrine reversal"). This type of effect should not be produced by metoprolol since it is a β_1-selective blocker, and it should not block the β_2-vasodilating effects of epinephrine. Both types of adrenergic blockers are effective in reducing the sweating and hypermetabolism associated with this condition.

In contrast to the selective effects produced by the adrenergic blocking drugs, experimental competitive inhibitors of the rate-limiting step in catecholamine synthesis, the conversion of tyrosine to dopa (catalyzed by the enzyme tyrosine hydroxylase), produce a panoramic effect, because all catecholamine actions are reduced in proportion to the inhibition of hormone synthesis. The most effective of these experimental drugs is the tyrosine analogue alpha-methyl-para-tyrosine. In doses of 2.0 to 4.0 grams per day, this drug inhibits catecholamine synthesis by as much as 85 to 90 per cent. Sedation and diarrhea have limited its use in some patients and the very low solubility of the drug has produced crystalluria in patients receiving large doses and inadequate hydration. Despite these shortcomings this drug appears to be the pharmacologic treatment of choice for pheochromocytoma.

After control of the physiologic abnormality produced by the pheochromocytoma, the patient may be explored. Successful surgery depends on a concerted and prearranged team effort, involving the surgeon, anesthetist, and internist-pharmacologist. The procedure is greatly facilitated by constant electronic monitoring of blood pressure and electrocardiogram so that appropriate use of blocking drugs may be made to counter any sudden changes in pressure or rhythm. Drugs to control catecholamine effects in the preoperative management of the patient should not be discontinued prior to the day of surgery, and the fear that they may produce untoward effects during surgery appears to be unsubstantiated. Preanesthetic medications should be limited to sedation the evening before surgery, but the use of atropine or other anticholinergic drugs as a routine may present problems because of the tachycardia produced by these compounds. Satisfactory anesthesia has been achieved with combinations of nitrous oxide and ether, as well as with the use of the newer halogenated hydrocarbon gases. Halothane and ethrane have proved especially useful because they possess potent alpha-blocking properties. In common with other halogenated hydrocarbons, the effects do seem to enhance the development of cardiac arrhythmias in the presence of excessive catecholamine secretion. Cyclopropane is contraindicated for anesthesia in these patients because of its marked arrhythmic effects. Propranolol should be available for rapid intravenous administration in case serious disturbances of cardiac rhythm occur. Doses in the range of 0.5 to 2.0 mg usually suppress dangerous rhythm disturbances for sufficient periods of time to permit the tumor to be removed and the surgery to be completed. Lidocaine is also useful in this regard, but its duration of effectiveness is very short compared to that of propranolol. If hypertensive crises occur during surgery despite preoperative preparation, small doses of phentolamine (1 to 5 mg) should be given rapidly intravenously for blood pressure control.

When the tumor is thought to be within the abdominal cavity, exploration should be done through an anterior transabdominal approach because of the likelihood of multiple tumors being found at the time of surgery, some of which might not be suspected after preoperative testing. This approach permits direct visualization and palpation of both adrenal glands as well as all the other common sites from which these tumors may arise between the floor of the pelvis and the diaphragm. Even when tumors have not been located by diagnostic procedures before surgery, it is usually not difficult for the surgeon to locate small ectopic masses. Direct digital stimulation of tumor tissue, even when the mass is inapparent to the surgeon, usually results in significant changes in cardiac rate and rhythm or blood pressure. When these occur, careful selective palpation with monitoring of vital signs will readily lead the surgeon to the tumor. Multiple and bilateral adrenal pheochromocytomas occur almost universally in patients with Sipple's syndrome, and in most instances total bilateral adrenalectomy must be performed or residual tumor tissue will be left behind (Fig. 4). However, multiple ectopic tumors must be suspected in *all* patients, and despite the removal of a large tumor, patients must be thoroughly explored to exclude other foci. Great care must be taken in the dissection of these tumor masses, because they bleed profusely when incised. In a number of instances, it appears that metastases have spread as a result of incision or rupture of a tumor and implantation of otherwise benign cells throughout the field of surgery.

After removal of all tumors, blood pressure almost invariably falls to hypotensive levels. The mechanism of this hypotension is thought to relate to persistent impairment of autonomic reflexes and not to hypovolemia. Nonetheless, all blood loss should be replaced quantitatively during the course of surgery. In anticipation of final severance of the tumor blood supply, rapid expansion of intravascular volume by the administration of plasma or plasma substitute (5 per cent albumin in normal saline) has been found most effective in sustaining a normal blood pressure at this time. This maneuver has proved much more effective than pressor drug infusions which are frequently difficult to discontinue for hours to days after surgery and have sometimes led to the demise of the patient in what was called "intractable shock."

During the first postoperative day, most patients will become hypertensive, especially in the period in which they are experiencing pain as they emerge from the effect of anesthesia. The usual cause of this hypertension is a combination of the cardiovascular responses to stress and iatrogenic hypervolemia induced in the course of treat-

ment of the hypotensive reaction. This rise in blood pressure is usually unresponsive to intravenous phentolamine; although it usually diminishes rapidly over the period of the ensuing day, it may be treated parenterally with rapidly acting diuretics such as furosemide or ethacrynic acid. Other causes of postoperative hypertension include inadvertent damage to a kidney or ligation of a renal artery or one of its branches during the course of surgery, or the presence of residual pheochromocytoma tissue, persisting either as additional undiscovered benign primary tumors or as metastases. When residual pheochromocytoma is suspected, postoperative urine collections should be obtained for catecholamine or metabolite assays in an attempt to determine whether the previously elevated values have returned to normal. Since most patients normally excrete increased quantities of these compounds for four to five days after surgery, the collection should be delayed until the end of the first postoperative week so that the results of the tests are interpretable. Before discharge from the hospital, all patients who have undergone surgery for pheochromocytoma should have repeat analyses to determine the adequacy of surgery. Follow-up determinations, initially at six-month and then at yearly intervals, seem adequate to exclude development of new tumors or metastases unless clinical symptoms dictate an earlier reevaluation. When the patient has associated evidence of von Recklinghausen's disease or Sipple's syndrome, it is mandatory to extend the investigation to members of the family, especially those who are hypertensive, in an attempt to discover other cases. Even in apparent sporadic cases, hypertensive members of the family should be evaluated to exclude this potentially curable form of hypertension.

In patients who cannot undergo surgery or who are not cured by surgery, prolonged therapy with either adrenergic blocking agents or alpha-methyl-tyrosine has proved successful in controlling the signs and symptoms of the disease. This is especially important because most patients with malignant pheochromocytoma die as a result of cardiovascular catastrophes rather than because of the directly aggressive nature of the cancer. Indeed, most patients with this condition have exceedingly slow-growing tumors, and patients with documented metastases have been treated successfully for more than ten years, often without evident progression. These tumors have uniformly proved unresponsive to treatment with either high-voltage radiation or chemotherapeutic agents.

OTHER TUMORS ARISING FROM SYMPATHETIC TISSUES

Depending upon the state of differentiation of primitive neural crest cells, sympathetic tissues may contain either immature pluripotential cells or cells which have differentiated into mature ganglion cells or adrenal medullary pheochromocytes. Tumors may arise from cell types which run the whole gamut of this differentiation. The most common are classified as ganglioneuromas or neuroblastomas, the latter originating from more primitive cell types. It is not unusual to encounter multiple cell types within any particular tumor, and the pathologic classification usually is based upon the predominant cell morphology. Although certain clinical features have been associated with the presence of these tumors (evidence of vasomotor instability, flushing, fever, and diarrhea), they generally have been considered to be nonfunctional. However, these tumors not only produce catecholamines, their precursors, and metabolites, but are also capable of producing other hormones which may contribute to clinical syndromes. There appears to be some correlation between the degree of differentiation of the primary cell types of the tumor and the pattern of catechol excretion. Those which are primarily composed of immature cells tend to excrete relatively larger quantities of dopa, dopamine, and their primary metabolites, whereas the most mature tumors tend to excrete relatively greater quantities of norepinephrine and its metabolites. Regardless of the nature of the tumor, VMA and metanephrine values are almost universally increased and serve as excellent screening and diagnostic tests in confirming the diagnosis preoperatively.

Ganglioneuromas are usually well encapsulated and rarely malignant. They may arise from any of the sympathetic ganglia, and they are frequently found in childhood as prominent posterior mediastinal paravertebral masses. Less commonly, they arise in the adrenal medulla or para-aortic sympathetic ganglia in the abdomen, and they also may be found in association with sympathetic ganglia in the bowel wall. This latter occurrence is especially notable among those patients with Sipple's syndrome in association with multiple cutaneous neuromas and multiple visceral ganglioneuromas. The tumor is composed of mature ganglion cells which are surrounded by connective tissue containing nerve fibers.

Neuroblastomas are highly malignant tumors occurring during infancy and early childhood; except for Wilms' tumor, they are the most common retroperitoneal tumors in children. They arise most commonly in the adrenal medulla, but they may also develop in other sympathetic ganglia within the thorax or abdomen. They metastasize early with widespread involvement of lymph nodes, liver, bone, lung, and marrow. When the tumor is diagnosed prior to obvious metastases, the prognosis is often good, but with metastases prognosis is poor despite the extensive use of radical surgery, deep x-ray therapy, and chemotherapeutic agents. As with patients with ganglioneuroma, these patients may demonstrate marked diarrhea in addition to other systemic effects The demonstration of very high concentrations of prostaglandins within both tumor tissue and plasma lends considerable support to the hypothesis that the gastrointestinal manifestations and flushing may be related to tumor production of these hormones. Recent experimental evidence relating to the elaboration of increased quantities of a hormone stimulating nerve growth (nerve growth factor, NGF) has raised questions about the role of this tropic hormone in this disease.

Catalona, W.J., Engelman, K., Ketcham, A.S., and Hammond, W.G.: Familial medullary thyroid carcinoma, pheochromocytoma, and parathyroid adenoma (Sipple's syndrome), study of a kindred. Cancer, 28:1245, 1971.

Cooperman, L.H., Engelman, K., and Mann, P.E.G.: Anesthetic management of pheochromocytoma employing halothane and beta-adrenergic blockade. A report of 14 cases. Anesthesiology, 28:575, 1967.

Engelman, K.: Assay of plasma catecholamines; an approach to evaluating altered sympathetic activity in essential hypertension. In Laragh, J.H. (ed.): Hypertension Manual, New York, Yorke Medical Books, 1973, p. 605.

Engelman, K., Horwitz, D., Jéquier, E., and Sjoerdsma, A.: Biochemical and pharmacologic effects of alpha-methyl-tyrosine in man. J. Clin. Invest., 47:577, 1968.

Gifford, F.W., Kvale, W.F., Maher, F. T., Roth, G.M., and Priestley, J. T.: Clinical features, diagnosis, and treatment of pheochromocytoma: A review of 76 cases. Mayo Clin. Proc., 39:281, 1964.

Landsberg, L.(ed.): Catecholamines. Clin. Endocrinol. Metab., Vol. 6, November 1977.

Regulation of catecholamine metabolism in the sympathetic nervous system (New York Heart Association Symposium). Pharmacol. Rev., 24:161, 1972.

Sandler, M., Kari, S.M., and Williams, E.D.: Prostaglandins in amine-peptide-secreting tumours. Lancet, 2:1053, 1968.

551. THE CARCINOID SYNDROME

Karl Engelman

DEFINITION. Tumors of the gastrointestinal tract composed of cell types now associated with carcinoid tumors have been known since the early 1800's. In 1907, Oberndorfer postulated that these tumors were a morphologic entity, and although he thought them to be malignant on the basis of their cellular appearance, they behaved in a very indolent and benign manner. For this reason he coined the name "karzinoid" (carcinoma-like). At various times they were thought to be derivates of autonomic nerve tissue, as well as of several types of intestinal mucosal cells. Masson advanced the hypothesis in 1928 that carcinoid tumors arose from argentaffin cells (Schmidt's cells, Kulchitsky's cells) which are normal constituents of the intestinal mucosa near the base of the crypts of Lieberkühn. The term argentaffin derives from the fact that many of these cells reduce and fix certain silver salts. In the early 1950's, Thorson, Waldenström, and others suggested that the constellation of signs and symptoms in patients harboring this tumor might be related to production of hormones. Initially, both serotonin and histamine were found in large quantities in most carcinoid tissues. Subsequently, tumor production of vasoactive kinin peptides and prostaglandins provided additional bases for the clinical syndrome. It is now possible to define several subsets of the syndrome, based on specific variants of clinical features, anatomic site of the primary tumor, and biochemical differences in secretion products.

PATHOLOGY. The *carcinoid syndrome* occurs only in relation to malignant tumors which have metastasized, usually with extensive hepatic implants. The most common primary tumor arises from the terminal third of the ileum; other sites include other areas of the small and large bowel, the bronchi, gastric mucosa, pancreas, common bile ducts, and ovaries. Carcinoid tumors of the appendix are rarely malignant and almost never cause the carcinoid syndrome; carcinoids of the rectum are frequently multicentric in origin, usually nonfunctional, and rarely malignant. Several patients with ovarian carcinoids have been described as having the systemic findings in the absence of metastases.

Diarrhea and intestinal obstruction are the most common gastrointestinal symptoms but these symptoms are rarely produced by the primary tumor itself. The primary tumor is often a very small, innocuous-looking lesion which can rarely be found by radiographic procedures. When the disease is diagnosed on the basis of the typical syndrome, it is unusual for the primary tumor to constitute more than 1 per cent of the tumor mass in the body. Mechanical impairment of gastrointestinal tract continuity and function is usually attributable either to local sclerosing metastases in the bowel wall or to extensive mesenteric lymph node metastases which sclerose and coalesce to shorten the mesentery and impair the blood supply. At its end-stages, the bowel often has the appearance of a parachute in which the shrouds have been pulled tightly toward the center so that the loops of small bowel are kinked, narrowed, and relatively fixed in position to a central retroperitoneal point. Contributing to this process is an unusual proliferation of fibrous tissue. Other areas in which dense fibrosis may occur — entirely without evidence of local tumor growth — include peritoneal and pleural surfaces and the endocardium of the heart chambers and valves. When there is extensive involvement of the peritoneal surfaces, retroperitoneal and pelvic fibrosis may result in obstruction of urinary drainage and simulate retroperitoneal fibrosis (see Ch. 71.2).

In the heart minimal to massive fibrotic proliferation occurs mainly on the right side and involves the valvular surfaces as well as the endocardium. Pulmonic stenosis and tricuspid stenosis and insufficiency are the most common lesions. Lesser degrees of involvement on the left side of the heart occur under circumstances of longstanding carcinoid syndrome, but they occur earlier in patients who have primary bronchial lesions or when there is an atrial septal defect with a right-to-left shunt. Pathologically, the distribution of the fibrosis is distinctive and readily differentiated from endomyocardial fibroelastosis and generalized myocardial fibrosis. The fibrotic lesion of this syndrome does not disrupt the internal elastic lamina of the myocardial and heart valves and the fibrosis appears in apposition to the endocardial surface. There is a predilection for fibrosis on the underside of the heart valves, upstream from the direction of blood flow (i.e., on the ventricular surface of the tricuspid valve and the pulmonary arterial surface of the pulmonic valve).

The extensive fibrosis observed in the carcinoid syndrome remains unexplained. Several lines of evidence indicate that serotonin may be implicated. When introduced into fibroblast tissue culture, serotonin results in marked stimulation of cellular growth and fiber production. Furthermore, the serotonin antagonist methysergide, used in treatment of migraine headache, occasionally causes extensive retroperitoneal fibrosis with ureteral obstruction. Chronic methysergide therapy may also produce endocardial and valvular lesions indistinguishable from that of the carcinoid disease, lending further support to the hypothesis that these lesions may be related in some way to serotonin metabolism.

CLINICAL MANIFESTATIONS. The carcinoid syndrome, because of its variable clinical features, is frequently misdiagnosed for many years.

Vasomotor. A cardinal feature of the carcinoid syndrome is *flushing*, chiefly occurring over the face and neck and in sun-exposed areas. Its onset may be sudden and it may range from a bright red to a violaceous hue. Facial and periorbital edema, tachycardia, hypotension, and pulmonary and gastrointestinal symptoms frequently accompany a flush. Black patients, in whom the change in color may be less apparent, frequently report a feeling of warmth or intense heat, and vascular dilatation may be apparent only in the bulbar conjunctivae. Certain distinctive features of the flush, including anatomic distribution, temporal relationships, and color, vary with the anatomic site of the primary tumor (see Variant Syndromes, below). Precipitating stimuli include ingestion of food and especially alcohol, pain, physical activity, and emotional upset. Small doses of intravenous catecholamines are potent flush-provoking agents. Both alpha and beta agents cause the flushing. Although this phenomenon has been proposed as a diagnostic test for the carcinoid syndrome, the associated hypotension or shock produced by the massive flushing reaction may be life threatening, and the use of this pharmacologic test is not encouraged. When patients have experienced flushing for several years, they usually develop fixed cutaneous changes in the areas in which flushing occurs. These include multiple fine telangiectasias and a fixed purple hue, usually over the malar areas, the nose, the upper lip, and the chin.

Gastrointestinal. Recurrent attacks of mild to explosive diarrhea, abdominal pain, bloating, and severe tenesmus are common. Frequently, the loose bowel movements are misdiagnosed for .years as functional bowel disease. Nausea and vomiting may also develop, especially in association with small bowel obstruction. When hepatic metastases grow to massive size, patients may experience episodic severe right upper quadrant pain, fever, right shoulder pain, leukocytosis, and all the features of an acute abdomen. Most commonly these features represent hemorrhage and necrosis within a hepatic metastasis which has outgrown its blood supply. With small bowel suction and other conservative measures, the entire syndrome may evolve and disappear in a week to ten days. Surgery for this condition is rarely necessary. *Peptic ulcer disease* also appears more commonly in patients with carcinoid syndrome than in the general population.

Cardiopulmonary. Blood pressure is usually normal or low. During flushing attacks severe *hypotension* and even life-threatening shock may occur. *Hypertension* has rarely been found in association with the carcinoid syndrome, despite the widely held clinical impression that this is a feature of the disease. However, hypertension and severe headache tend to occur more commonly in patients with metastatic bronchial primary tumors.

Cardiac involvement (see Pathology, above) is a progressive complication which occurs late in the disease. Right-sided congestive heart failure is a serious problem and a common cause of death. Edema may be enhanced by hypoproteinemia which commonly results from severe diarrhea, protein loss, and replacement of liver by tumor. Auscultatory evidence of pulmonic stenosis and tricuspid stenosis and insufficiency can usually be demonstrated in patients with longstanding carcinoid disease. Murmurs indicating left-sided heart involvement are less common. Pulmonary symptoms caused by primary heart failure are rare except in those with predominantly left-sided lesions, but bronchospasm and wheezing in association with flushing attacks occur in 20 to 30 per cent of the patients. This may be indistinguishable from bronchial asthma, and the use of glyceryl guaiacolate–containing expectorants may further complicate diagnosis by yielding false-positive results for urinary serotonin metabolites (see Diagnosis, below).

Nutritional. Chronic weight loss, often leading to cachexia, may be attributed not only to the catabolic effects of the tumor but also to severe diarrhea. Satisfactory control of the diarrhea is beneficial with regard to sense of well-being and the development of positive nitrogen balance. Patients with far-advanced carcinoid disease may develop the signs and symptoms of pellagra, including dementia and typical skin lesions in sun-exposed areas. Niacin deficiency has a dual etiology. First, patients with poor nutrition have a decreased intake of niacin and its amino acid precursor, tryptophan. Second, the carcinoid tumor diverts dietary tryptophan from the kynurenine–nicotinic acid pathway to production of serotonin and its metabolites (see Chemistry, below).

Malignant carcinoid tumors have also been associated with ectopic hormone production. The bronchogenic tumors have been more commonly associated with peptide hormone synthesis than have the ileal or other tumors. In addition to the production of prostaglandins and 5-hydroxyindole compounds, excessive ectopic production of parathyroid hormone, gonadotropins, ACTH, insulin, and probably growth hormone have all been documented.

CHEMISTRY. The biochemical hallmark of malignant carcinoid tumors is excessive production of *5-hydroxyindole compounds* (Fig. 7). The essential amino acid tryptophan is hydroxylated to 5-hydroxytryptophan (5-HTP) by the enzyme tryptophan hydroxylase, the rate-limiting step in serotonin synthesis. With the tumor (except in gastric carcinoid — see below) the 5-HTP is further metabolized to serotonin (5-HT), its pharmacologically active metabolite. Small quantities of serotonin are normally produced in the body, major depots being the gastrointestinal mucosa, the brain, and the platelets. Normally, less than 1 per cent of total dietary tryptophan (1000 to 1500 mg per day) is converted to 5-hydroxyindole compounds, but

when very large masses of malignant carcinoid tissue are found in the body, as much as 600 to 1000 mg of 5-HIAA may be excreted in the urine daily. This may represent almost all the dietary tryptophan available to the patient; this accounts for the development of niacin deficiency and pellagra (see above). When the clinical condition results in the inability to eat, the urinary 5-HIAA values fall to low values only to rise after dietary tryptophan ingestion increases, thus demonstrating the limiting relationships of dietary tryptophan on niacin and serotonin synthesis. Excessive quantities of histamine may also be synthesized by carcinoid tumors, especially those of gastric origin.

PHYSIOLOGY. The pharmacologic effect of serotonin as a smooth muscle agonist has long been considered responsible for the hyperperistalsis, diarrhea, and bronchial constriction of the carcinoid syndrome. Although serotonin was also thought to be related to the severe flushing, this hypothesis does not fit with the known effects of serotonin as a peripheral vasoconstrictor and the observations that infusions of serotonin do not reproduce these features of the syndrome. Peart and coworkers demonstrated that the flushing is indirectly mediated by sympathetic stimulation. Subsequently, Oates and others showed that the kinin peptide bradykinin appeared in the circulation after catecholamine stimulation of the tumor. The catecholamines were shown to activate a tumor enzyme — kallikrein — which in its active form is capable of cleaving the decapeptide lysyl-bradykinin from a circulating α_2-globulin precursor, kininogen. After its release into the hepatic vein, the decapeptide is converted to the potent vasoactive nonapeptide bradykinin, primarily by a converting enzyme found in the endothelium of the pulmonary capillary vasculature; the same enzyme also converts angiotensin I to angiotensin II. Although infusions of bradykinin reproduce the carcinoid flush, it was not possible to demonstrate increased kinin levels in some patients with severe flushing. Carcinoid tumors also produce large quantities of prostaglandins, which could explain some of the flushing.

DIAGNOSIS. The diagnosis of carcinoid syndrome should be suspected on the basis of distinctive clinical features. Confirmation can be achieved preoperatively by demonstration of increased 5-hydroxyindole production. Since approximately 99 per cent of serotonin infused intravenously is converted to 5-HIAA, this metabolite rather than the hormone should be measured in the urine of patients suspected of this disease. Both qualitative and quantitative tests are available for the assay of 5-HIAA in urine.

The *qualitative screening test* is a simple procedure requiring only 0.2 ml of urine from any random voiding. Indole compounds in the urine are converted to colored derivatives by the addition of nitrosonaphthol reagent. After extraction with an organic solvent, the color in the aqueous layer is compared with that of a blank sample to which water was added instead of the urine sample. A positive test result is indicated by the presence of a faint to deep purple color, depending upon the quantity of indole compounds present in the urine sample. Assuming a normal daily urine volume of 1000 to 1500 ml, this qualitative screening test will not be positive unless the patient is excreting 30 to 50 mg of 5-HIAA per 24 hours (Fig. 8). Thus since the upper limit of normal for 5-HIAA excretion is 9 mg per 24 hours, some patients with this disease may have a

Figure 7. Synthesis and metabolism of serotonin.

false-negative screening test when their urinary 5-HIAA excretion is less than 50 mg per day total.

A simple modification of the screening tests yields a specific *quantitative test* for 5-HIAA. Prior to and during the collection of the 24-hour urine specimen, certain dietary precautions must be taken because of the presence of significant quantities of serotonin in certain foods (bananas, pineapples, walnuts, red plums, avocados) so that 5-HIAA excretion will not be increased spuriously. In addition, drugs such as mephenesin and especially cough preparations containing glyceryl guaiacolate (see Cardiopulmonary, above) produce metabolites which are excreted in the urine and which produce *false-positive test results* by both the qualitative and quantitative assays. Phenothiazines, often used for the prevention or treatment of flushing, reduce the color yield of the test reaction and produce false-negative results. Patients with malignant carcinoid usually excrete 50 to 500 mg of 5-HIAA daily, but some patients excrete values closer to the upper limit of normal. They must be distinguished from patients with nontropical sprue who have been reported to have moderately elevated (10 to 15 mg per 24 hours) 5-HIAA excretion.

Except in the carcinoid syndrome associated with gastric tumor (see below), urinary serotonin is rarely increased significantly because it is so readily converted to 5-HIAA. Thus in the vast majority of patients with carcinoid, determinations of serotonin in urine are of little value. In most patients with carcinoid syndrome total blood or platelet serotonin is high, but these determinations are not diagnostic and should not be part of the general workup.

Histologic confirmation of the diagnosis may be obtained by biopsy of the primary tumor or metastases. However, the constellation of the typical clinical features, increased 5-HIAA excretion in the urine, and demonstration of metastases, especially to the liver, is usually sufficient to confirm the diagnosis without invasive procedures such as exploration or liver biopsy.

VARIANT SYNDROMES. Ileal Tumor ("Classic Carcinoid Syndrome"). The majority of patients with carcinoid syndrome have a primary tumor in the terminal portion of the ileum metastatic to the liver, producing typical symptoms of flushing, diarrhea, valvular heart disease, and, in a significant minority of patients, asthmatic attacks. Flushing is usually episodic with a red to cyanotic coloration (Fig. 9). Duration of flushing varies from 1 to 30 minutes, and in patients with more advanced disease it may be relatively constant. Right-sided heart lesions and right-sided heart failure predominate. 5-Hydroxyindoles in the urine appear almost exclusively as 5-HIAA. Metastases to regional mesenteric lymph nodes with massive involvement of the liver always occur prior to the onset of typical clinical symptoms; metastases to bone or other peripheral tissues are rare. Abdominal pain, especially in association with intestinal obstruction, is common, and irremediable intra-abdominal mechanical obstruction or resistant right-sided heart failure is the usual cause of death.

Bronchial Tumor. Carcinoid tumors of the bronchial tree are generally nonfunctioning and are removed after incidental finding of a solitary pulmonary lesion. Rarely, when systemic signs and symptoms are produced by this tumor, there are a number of unique clinical features which distinguish it from the ileal tumor syndrome. The most important is the nature of the flushing episodes. With functioning bronchial carcinoids, the flushes are a livid red, and they are of devastating severity, frequently lasting for hours to days. Hypotension is common during severe flushes, often resulting in oliguria or anuria, and patients may have to be treated acutely with intravenous volume-expanding fluids and large doses of glucocorticoids in an attempt to abort the attack and to sustain the circulation. Marked chemosis, tearing, nasal discharge, and excessive salivation are fairly constant concomitants. During the intense flushes patients frequently develop swelling of the entire face, and, unlike other carcinoid flushes, this flush may involve most of the body. Left-sided cardiac lesions may develop, along with or before right-sided lesions. As with the ileal variant, systemic symptoms rarely occur without distant metastases, especially in the liver. In common with other carcinoids derived from embryologic foregut areas (stomach, bile duct, and pancreas), metastases to bone are common, and they are frequently osteoblastic in nature. Biochemically, these tumors may produce both serotonin and 5-HTP, so the pattern of urinary 5-hydroxyindole excretion products may more closely resemble that of the gastric carcinoid variant (see below). In addition, other endocrine syndromes may be produced, most notably Cushing's syndrome resulting from ACTH production by the tumor. In contrast to other forms of the carcinoid syndrome, between flushing attacks these patients have a tendency to be hypertensive. Headaches are also prominent, and marked enlargement of lacrimal, parotid, submaxillary, and submandibular salivary glands may develop with time. Patients who survive the disease for several years tend to develop thickening and creasing of the skin about the face and forehead. Rhinophyma is prominent, and the fixed, thickened, hard skin folds of the upper face and forehead lend the semblance of "leonine facies" (Fig. 10). Graham has observed that patients with longstanding migraine headaches, a disease postulated to be related to an abnormality of serotonin metabolism, develop the same peculiar facial features.

Gastric Tumor. The syndrome associated with primary tumors of gastric origin is distinctive from other carcinoid syndromes in both clinical and biochemical features. The flush is characterized by raised, wheal-like lesions of a reddish-brown coloration with variegated borders (Fig. 11). These lesions may occur on any part of the body and frequently are migratory, sometimes involving the palms and soles, where they may become intensely pruritic. Metabolic products of these tumors also differ from the other varieties. Oates and Sjoerdsma, acting on the previous suggestions by Sandler and Waldenström, were able to demonstrate in a patient with gastric carcinoid that although the major 5-hydroxyindole excretion product was 5-HIAA, this constituted only about 60 per cent of the total 5-hydroxyindoles in the urine as opposed to more than 99 per cent in the usual carcinoid patient. Studies by bidirectional paper chromatography of small samples of the urine revealed excretion of large quantities of serotonin and 5-HTP. Quantitatively, the serotonin comprised 25 per cent of the total and the 5-HTP, 17 per cent. It was suggested that the tumor hydroxylated tryptophan to 5-HTP but was incapable of the further conversion to serotonin. After release from the tumor, the 5-HTP was subsequently decarboxylated in other

Fig. 8

Fig. 9

Fig. 10

Fig. 11

Figure 8. Qualitative screening test for carcinoid (tubes, left to right): carcinoid patient excreting approximately 200 mg 5-HIAA per day; color reaction in normal subject taking 15 ml cough preparation containing glyceryl guaiacolate on the previous day; normal urine; and the same urine to which had been added 5-HIAA to give the final concentration noted on each tube. The color of a positive test is first detected visually at a 5-HIAA concentration of approximately 50 mg per liter.

Figure 9. Classic or ileal carcinoid flush.

Figure 10. Bronchial carcinoid flush.

Figure 11. Gastric carcinoid flush.

tissues, especially kidney, leading to the urinary excretion of both serotonin and 5-HIAA. Infusion of 5-HTP into normal subjects resulted in the same excretion pattern observed in patients with the gastric carcinoid syndrome. Subsequent analysis of a gastric carcinoid tumor revealed the absence of aromatic-L-amino acid decarboxylase, confirming this hypothesis. Markedly increased urinary excretion of histamine has also been observed in patients with gastric carcinoid. The unique pruritic, wheal-like flushing which occurs with this carcinoid variant may be related to histamine production.

"Noncarcinoid" Tumor. Typical features of the carcinoid syndrome may occur with what are considered to be noncarcinoid tumors. Most common among these is *medullary carcinoma of the thyroid* (see Pheochromocytoma in Ch. 550, and Ch. 546.8), which, in addition to producing calcitonin, has also been shown to produce increased quantities of prostaglandins and serotonin. Carcinoid-like flushing and multiple watery bowel movements may be common features in patients with these tumors, especially when the primary thyroid tumors are very large or when there are multiple metastases. Urinary 5-HIAA values as high as 300 to 600 mg per 24 hours have been recorded, although usually the values are little, if at all, increased. As yet, there have been no reports of extensive fibrotic lesions in the endocardium and other tissues in association with the medullary thyroid carcinoma. *Tumors of ovarian origin* have also been implicated in this syndrome. Usually these arise from ovarian teratomas and differ from other carcinoid variants in that all the typical symptoms of ileal carcinoid as well as fibrotic thickening of endocardium and mesothelial cavity linings may occur, but notably without metastases in the liver or other organs. This is probably related to the fact that the venous drainage of the tumors is not via the portal system; thereby tumor products are introduced directly into the general circulation. This could explain the otherwise universal finding that abdominal carcinoids do not produce systemic symptoms until extensive hepatic metastases have developed.

Tumors of the common bile duct or pancreatic islets may produce biochemical and clinical features of the carcinoid syndrome. In common with other carcinoid tumors of embryologic foregut origin (bronchial and gastric), these tend to produce both 5-HTP and serotonin.

PROGNOSIS AND THERAPY. Patients with malignant carcinoid syndrome frequently have symptoms for several years before the diagnosis is made, and it is not unusual for them to survive for 10 to 15 years after the initial diagnosis. The course is frequently characterized by spontaneous remissions and exacerbations, although the over-all status progresses slowly and inexorably. With proper nutritional and pharmacologic therapy, and with *surgical restraint,* these patients can usually be carried for long periods of time before they succumb to cardiac or hepatic failure or to complications of mechanical obstruction in the gastrointestinal tract. Above all, it must be understood by physician, patient, and family that this is a chronic disease, and the diagnosis of malignancy, even with widespread hepatic metastases, does not carry with it the dire immediate implications of other bowel tumors with similar distribution. Patients frequently suffer periods of severe pain, often requiring hospitalization for days to weeks. In view of the expected protracted course and its inevitable outcome, the psychologic aspects of patient care are extremely important and may prove most taxing for the physician and family.

Except in rare instances in which a primary bronchial or ovarian tumor may cause symptoms of the carcinoid syndrome in the absence of metastases, patients cannot be cured by surgery. Indeed, in the usual ileal case the eventual clinical course of the patient may be seriously prejudiced by an attempt to remove large segments of small bowel. Not uncommonly in such instances, patients who have had tolerable or controllable diarrhea prior to surgery develop malnutrition and fluid and electrolyte loss postoperatively owing to marked increase in the number and magnitude of watery bowel movements. This change in the course of the disease may be attributable to decreased bowel area for absorption of nutrients, fluid, and electrolytes. Resection of the distal ileum also compromises the enterohepatic circulation of bile salts which in themselves may constitute a potent cathartic. If a patient is explored for diagnostic reasons or to attempt to remedy an area of small bowel obstruction, the surgeon should carry out the minimal resection necessary to restore continuity. Frequently, the most effective measures are to create one or several enteroenterostomies to bypass areas of obstruction while retaining as much absorptive surface of small bowel as is possible. Hypotension, especially during surgery, is a serious problem and requires special consideration of the pharmacology of vasopressor substances. Most sympathomimetic pressor drugs produce *paradoxical hypotension* in patients with carcinoid syndrome because they induce flushing and severe peripheral vasodilatation via the activation of tumor kallikrein and bradykinin synthesis. Only two vasopressor compounds — methoxamine (Vasoxyl) and angiotensin II (Hypertensin) — may be used safely. Prophylactic treatment with corticosteroids may prevent flushes by endogenous sympathetic mechanisms, and thus hypotensive episodes may be minimized during the operation.

The results of chemotherapy and irradiation have generally been unrewarding regardless of the site of origin. Temporary responses to *cyclophosphamide* (Cytoxan), *methotrexate, phenylalanine mustard*, or oral administration or hepatic artery perfusion with *5-fluorouracil* or *cytosine arabinoside* (Cytosar) have been reported. More recent enthusiasm for the use of *streptozotocin* has appeared to be ill substantiated when examined critically. In many instances the death of patients has been hastened by use of cytotoxic drugs.

Nonetheless, significant control of some of the clinical complications of the carcinoid syndrome may be achieved by other pharmacologic agents which do not directly affect tumor growth. Basic to all therapy is the maintenance of adequate nutrition with vitamin supplementation, especially of niacin (see Chemistry, above) and other vitamins. Modification of food intake does not uniformly provide relief for patients with the carcinoid syndrome. The patient should be permitted to select foods which seem not to exacerbate symptoms.

Flushing attacks may be controlled or diminished by the use of *antiadrenergic drugs* and those which have antikinin properties. Phenothiazine compounds which have alpha-adrenergic blocking activity, such as prochlorperazine (Compazine), 5 to 10 mg, or chlorpromazine (Thorazine), 25 to 50 mg, orally every six hours, may be helpful in reducing the incidence of flushing; the alpha-adrenergic blocker phenoxybenzamine (Dibenzyline), 10 to 50 mg daily, may prove very effective. Beta-sympathetic blocking drugs have no effect on the flushing. Reducing the intake of alcohol and other known stimulants to flushing may reduce the need for drugs. The use of glucocorticoids (10 to 40 mg of prednisone per day) should be reserved for unusually severe and protracted periods of flushing. In patients with bronchial carcinoids whose continuous flushing may be life threatening it is frequently necessary to use suppressive doses of steroids chronically.

Diarrhea and tenesmus are best treated with the use of conventional antidiarrheal drugs, sometimes in association with specific serotonin antagonists. Belladonna alkaloids, camphorated tincture of opium (paregoric), or kaolin- and pectin-containing compounds may prove useful. In severe diarrhea opium alkaloids such as diphenoxylate (Lomotil), 1 or 2 tablets every three or four hours, or tincture of opium, 6 to 12 drops every three to four hours, may be required. If diarrhea does not respond to these more conservative measures, the specific serotonin antagonists cyproheptadine (Periactin), 4 to 8 mg every six hours, or methysergide (Sansert), 2 to 4 mg three to four times daily, may be tried. Use of the latter, even though often successful, is to be discouraged because of the severe complications relating to both fluid retention and the development of fibrotic lesions of the retroperitoneal area, heart valves, and other tissues which would be presumed to be accelerated in a patient with the carcinoid syndrome. For patients whose diarrhea is exacerbated by resection of small bowel with resultant bile salt–enhanced diarrhea, oral cholestyramine (Questran), 4 to 8 grams every six hours, may prove useful by its ability to bind and inactivate the bile salts.

Discovery of a specific inhibitor of the enzyme tryptophan hydroxylase, the rate-limiting step in serotonin synthesis, has provided the opportunity to test the hypothesis that serotonin is one cause of diarrhea. Parachlorophenylalanine, when administered in doses of up to 3 grams daily, has proved uniquely successful in reducing 5-hydroxyindole production by as much as 90 per cent while concomitantly producing reduction or complete remission of diarrhea. Other manifestations of the syndrome do not seem to have been affected by this experimental therapy. Unfortunately, a majority of patients using the drug for more than six weeks develop allergic reactions. Nonetheless, it offers the hope that a compound with similar mechanism of action may be discovered which will prove effective in symptomatic treatment.

A recent publication describes an ingenious approach to infarcting large masses of tumor by selectively thrombosing the hepatic artery. Significant clinical remission occurred following this therapy, although it should be considered only in experienced centers where the massive release of kinin peptide resulting from tumor infarctions can be handled appropriately.

Adamson, A. R., Peart, W. S., Grahame-Smith, D. G., and Starr, M.: Pharmacological blockage of carcinoid flushing provoked by catecholamines and alcohol. Lancet, 2:293, 1969.

Allison, D. J., Modlin, I. M., and Jenkins, W. J.: Treatment of carcinoid liver metastases by hepatic artery embolization. Lancet, 2:1323, 1977.

Engelman, K., Lovenberg, W., and Sjoerdsma, A.: Inhibition of serotonin synthesis by parachlorophenylalanine in patients with the carcinoid syndrome. N. Engl. J. Med., 277:1103, 1967.

Graham, J. R.: Cardiac and pulmonary fibrosis during methysergide therapy for headache. Am. J. Med. Sci., 254:23, 1967.

Melmon, K. L., Sjoerdsma, A., and Mason, D. T.: Distinctive clinical and therapeutic aspects of syndromes associated with bronchial carcinoid tumors. Am. J. Med., 39:568, 1965.

Oates, J. A., and Sjoerdsma, A.: A unique syndrome associated with secretion of 5-hydroxytryptophan by metastatic gastric carcinoid. Am. J. Med., 32:333, 1962.

Peart, W. S., Robertson, J. I. S., and Andrews, T. M.: Facial flushing produced in patients with carcinoid syndrome by intravenous adrenaline and noradrenaline. Lancet, 2:715, 1959.

Sandler, M., Karim, S. M. M., and Williams, E. D.: Prostaglandins in amine-peptide–secreting tumors. Lancet, 2:1053, 1968.

552. PARATHYROID

G. D. Aurbach

552.1. PARATHYROID HORMONE AND CALCITONIN

Parathyroid hormone, the principal peptide hormone controlling calcium metabolism in man, has been characterized definitively as a polypeptide 84 amino acids in length. The complete structure of the bovine and porcine hormones and part of the sequence of human parathyroid hormone are known, and active analogues of the hormones have been synthesized. Biosynthesis of the hormone proceeds through a ribosome-bound prehormone (approximately 110 amino acids) that is converted immediately to a prohormone molecule 90 amino acids in length. The prohormone is rapidly cleaved within the gland to the 84 amino acid hormone for storage and subsequent secretion. Calcium is the major known factor controlling secretions of the hormone clinically. A fall in blood calcium concentration provokes secretion of the hormone, which in turn causes an increased rate of transfer of calcium from bone and glomerular filtrate to the extracellular fluids. The same peptide hormone also causes increased urinary excretion of phosphate by direct action on the kidney (possibly by inhibition of the reabsorption of phosphate) and increases activity of the renal 25-OH-D-1-alpha hydroxylase. By regulating this enzyme activity, parathyroid hormone controls the concentration of the most potent endogenous calciferol metabolite, which in turn controls intestinal absorption of calcium. The action of parathyroid hormone is mediated by cyclic 3',5'-adenosine monophosphate (3',5'-AMP) produced through direct specific hormonal activation of the enzyme adenylate cyclase in bone and kidney. The consequent increase in concentration of 3',5'-AMP in the renal cortex and bone activates other intracellular processes which account for the physiologic actions of the hormone. The increase in concentration of 3',5'-AMP effected by parathyroid hormone in the renal parenchyma is manifested also by increased urinary excretion of 3',5'-AMP.

Calcitonin is another polypeptide hormone involved in regulation of calcium and bone metabolism. The structures of the calcitonins from many species are known, syntheses have been completed, and radioimmunoassays have been developed, but the physiologic significance of calcitonin for normal man is still uncertain. Calcitonin is secreted from the parafollicular cells found in the mammalian thyroid but related embryologically to the ultimobranchial body of lower vertebrate species. The rate of secretion of calcitonin is a direct function of the concentration of calcium in plasma, whereas parathyroid hormone is secreted at a rate inversely proportional to calcium concentration. The hypocalcemic action of calcitonin is effected through an inhibition of resorption of mineral from bone, and the physiologic actions of this hormone seem to be mediated through the adenylate cyclase–cyclic AMP system.

Diseases of the parathyroid gland include hyperparathyroidism and hypoparathyroidism. Pseudohypoparathyroidism encompasses the general clinical and laboratory features of hypoparathyroidism but is an abnormality not of parathyroid gland function but of the receptor tissue for parathyroid hormone. Medullary carcinoma of the thyroid is a tumor that secretes excessive amounts of calcitonin into plasma. Primary hyperparathyroidism, pheochromocytoma, Cushing's syndrome, and multiple neuromas are found associated in some cases.

Aurbach, G. D., and Chase, L. R.: Biochemical actions of parathyroid hormone and calcitonin: Cyclic nucleotides in the hormonal control of calcium metabolism. In Aurbach, G. D. (ed.): Parathyroid Gland. Washington, D. C., American Physiological Society, 1976, pp. 353–381. (Handbook of Physiology, Endocrinology Section, R. O. Greep and E. B. Astwood [eds.], Section 7, Vol. VII.)

Chase, L. R., and Aurbach, G. D.: Renal adenyl cyclase: Anatomically separate sites for parathyroid hormone and vasopressin. Science, 159:545, 1968.

Copp, D. H., Cockcroft, D. W., and Kueh, Y.: Calcitonin from ultimobranchial glands of dogfish and chickens. Science, 158:924, 1957.

DeLuca, H. F.: Metabolism and function of vitamin D. In Aurbach, G. D. (ed.): Parathyroid Gland. Washington, D.C., American Physiological Society, 1976, pp. 265–280. (Handbook of Physiology, Endocrinology Section, R. O. Greep and E. B. Astwood [eds.], Section 7, Vol. VII.)

Habener, J. F., Kemper, B. W., Rich, A., and Potts, J. T.: Biosynthesis of parathyroid hormone. Recent Prog. Horm. Res., 33:249, 1977.

Hirsch, P. F., Gauthier, G. F., and Munson, P. L.: Thyroid hypocalcemic prinicple and recurrent laryngeal nerve injury as factors affecting the response to parathyroidectomy in rats. Endocrinology, 73:244, 1963.

Munson, P. L.: Physiology and pharmacology of thyrocalcitonin. In Aurbach, G. D. (ed.): Parathyroid Gland. Washington, D.C., American Physiological Society, 1976, pp. 443–464. (Handbook of Physiology, Endocrinology Section, R. O. Greep and E. B. Astwood [eds.], Section 7, Vol. VII.)

Potts, J. T., Jr., and Aurbach, G. D.: Chemistry of calcitonins. In Aurbach, G. D. (ed.): Parathyroid Gland. Washington, D.C., American Physiological Society, 1976, pp. 423–430. (Handbook of Physiology, Endocrinology Section, R. O. Greep and E. B. Astwood [eds.], Section 7, Vol. VII.)

552.2.   HYPERPARATHYROIDISM

DEFINITION. Primary hyperparathyroidism is the clinical condition caused by excessive and incompletely regulated secretion of hormone from the parathyroid glands. The manifestations, which may include hypercalcemia, tissue calcification, and osteitis fibrosa cystica, represent the result of excessive parathyroid hormone action on bone and kidney.

ETIOLOGY. The etiology of primary hyperparathyroidism is unknown. *Secondary hyperparathyroidism* develops as a compensatory mechanism in any state tending to produce true hypocalcemia; this may occur in hypovitaminosis D, vitamin D dependent rickets, malabsorption of calcium, chronic renal disease, hyperphosphatemia, or renal tubular acidosis. There is a suggestion that prolonged, progressive secondary hyperparathyroidism may evolve into autonomous hy-

perparathyroidism in some cases. Parathyrotropic substances have not so far been implicated in the development of primary or secondary hyperparathyroidism. Recent studies on parathyroid cells in vitro suggest that in parathyroid adenomas there is abnormally low affinity (or high K_i, inhibitor constant) for calcium as an inhibitor of parathyroid secretion. Several families with autosomal dominant hyperparathyroidism have been reported; thus a genetic factor is involved in some cases. Recently an association between past irradiation of the neck and primary hyperparathyroidism has been suggested.

INCIDENCE. Modern diagnostic methods and wide clinical awareness have facilitated recognition of the disease. Automated laboratory facilities now make possible routine analysis of serum calcium for all clinic subjects and foster thereby ready discovery of new cases. In one clinic, routine analyses yielded an incidence of hyperparathyroidism as high as one case per thousand.

PATHOLOGY. Hypersecretion of parathyroid hormone as a manifestation of primary parathyroid disease may be caused by a single adenoma, primary chief cell or clear cell hyperplasia of all parathyroid glands, or carcinoma. Differentiation between hyperplasia and adenoma on the basis of histology alone is difficult. If more than one parathyroid gland is pathologically involved, the diagnosis of hyperplasia is warranted. In 60 to 80 per cent of the cases primary hyperparathyroidism is attributable to a single parathyroid adenoma, and in less than 2 per cent carcinoma of the parathyroid gland is the cause. Other cases are caused by chief cell or clear cell hyperplasia. Hyperparathyroidism in families or in the MEN I (multiple endocrine neoplasia I) syndrome is due virtually invariably to hyperplasia of all glands. A syndrome analogous to primary hyperparathyroidism can result from ectopic production of parathyroid hormone by nonparathyroid tissue. Usually parathyroid adenomas vary in size from 1 to 5 grams, but occasionally very large tumors, 50 grams or more, may develop. In general, large tumors are more likely to be associated with clinically evident bone disease, marked hypercalcemia, very high concentrations of parathyroid hormone in plasma, and relatively short interval between development of symptoms and establishment of diagnosis. Histologic examination usually shows chief cells and some water-clear cells; sometimes the latter are predominant. Rarely adenomas are composed of oxyphil cells. Occasionally adenomas of other endocrine glands are found in hyperparathyroidism (multiple endocrine neoplasia; see Clinical Manifestations, below). The pathologic manifestation of the disease in bone is osteitis fibrosa cystica generalisata. When the kidneys are affected, nephrolithiasis or nephrocalcinosis is apparent; pyelonephritis often complicates the course of the kidney disease.

Muscle biopsy often shows neuropathic (not myopathic) atrophy of type II and, later, type I muscle fibers. This denervation-type structural change (probably secondary to a metabolic lesion in the nerve itself) parallels the severity of muscle weakness in hyperparathyroidism.

Pancreatitis, acute or chronic, is recognized as a possible complication of hyperparathyroidism. About half of the patients with advanced hyperparathyroidism examined at autopsy show calcification in the pancreas. It is possible that chronic hypercalcemia contributes to the development of pancreatitis, but the actual mechanism of this association has not been established.

PATHOLOGIC PHYSIOLOGY AND CHEMISTRY. Hypersecretion of parathyroid hormone from adenomatous or hyperplastic glands is expressed in acceleration of the normal physiologic actions of the hormone on bone and kidney. The effect on bone leads to an increase in rate of resorption of calcium from bone and, in more severe cases, to pathologic development of macroscopic cystic areas of bone resorption (osteitis fibrosa cystica). The effect on the kidney causes an increase in rate of resorption of calcium from the renal tubular lumen as well as increased renal clearance of phosphate from plasma with consequent hypophosphatemia. The renal concentrating ability may decrease, resulting in polyuria and polydipsia. Hypercalcemia results from the actions of the hormone on bone and kidneys. Parathyroid hormone and hypophosphatemia synergize in increasing the activity of renal 25-OH-D 1-alpha-hydroxylase. This leads to increased amounts in plasma of $1,25(OH)_2D$ that acts directly on the intestine to increase absorption of calcium. The urinary excretion of 3',5'-AMP is greater than normal.

Most new cases of hyperparathyroidism discovered in the clinic show little or no detectable bone disease. This might be attributable to technology (widespread precise determinations of serum calcium allowing discovery of early and mild forms of the disease) and general recognition of the problem. Some early or mild cases become clinically apparent chiefly by nephrolithiasis and hypophosphatemia, with little or no hypercalcemia or skeletal abnormality. Ten to 20 per cent of all cases of nephrolithiasis are associated with primary hyperparathyroidism.

The classic laboratory manifestations of primary hyperparathyroidism are low serum phosphate and high serum calcium concentrations. Frequently 24-hour urinary excretion of calcium is high because of significant hypercalcemia and, consequently, high renal filtered load of calcium, even though the renal clearance of calcium is relatively reduced. Hypercalciuria, with calcium excretion in excess of intake, is particularly apparent when diets low in calcium are given. The alkaline phosphatase activity in plasma may be high in hyperparathyroidism when there is significant bone disease. This is probably attributable to release of skeletal alkaline phosphatase isoenzyme from osteoblasts, a manifestation of increased bone formation compensating for the high rate of bone resorption induced by excessive parathyroid hormone secretion. Another manifestation of increased bone resorption is increased urinary excretion of hydroxyproline. Kinetic studies utilizing radioactive calcium frequently show evidence of increased bone formation and resorption rates.

CLINICAL MANIFESTATIONS. The disease tends to segregate into three categories in terms of clinical presentation. In the mildest form there may be no symptoms or signs, and discovery is made only through routine determination of serum calcium concentration. The second category develops insidiously, sometimes over a period of years, and presents predominantly as renal colic. In the third group the interval between development of symptoms and diagnosis may be much shorter, and there may be marked hypercalcemia, weight loss, debility, and bone pain, sometimes with pathologic fracture. Debility,

weight loss, anemia, and elevated sedimentation rate may be so prominent in the severe form of the disease as to suggest malignancy. The most frequent symptoms of the disease in general are weakness, fatigability, and renal colic. Epigastric pain, neurologic abnormalities, and constipation are also common. Hypercalcemia may cause polydipsia, polyuria, anorexia, nausea, and vomiting. Neurologic abnormalities include impaired mentation, loss of memory for recent events, depression, emotional lability, hyperactive deep tendon reflexes, sensory loss for pain and vibration, and proximal muscle weakness, particularly in the lower extremities. There may also be abnormal movements (resembling fasciculations) of the tongue, glossal atrophy, ataxic gait, hoarseness, dysphagia, anosmia, and abnormal flexor reflex. Careful clinical examination sometimes elicits neurologic abnormalities even in patients who are seemingly asymptomatic.

Still other symptoms cannot be clearly related to distinct pathophysiologic mechanisms. There may be burning in the throat or abdomen, vague malaise, back or coccygeal pain, or dry skin. Occasionally headache or pruritus is the sole presenting complaint. It is of interest in this regard that the pruritus of uremia may be dramatically relieved after removal of parathyroid glands showing secondary hyperplasia. Anemia, elevated erythrocyte sedimentation rate, and hypertension also are each observed in 25 per cent or more of some series.

Hypercalcemia may depress sensitivity to electrical stimuli of ganglia and peripheral nerves (Erb's sign). Shortening of the Q-T interval (between the onset of the Q wave and the beginning of the T wave) in the electrocardiogram is found in some patients with hypercalcemia. Prolonged hypercalcemia may lead to calcification in the eye displayed as *"band keratopathy,"* opaque material appearing in vertical lines parallel to and within the limbus, or as conjunctival crystals without the limbus or under the eyelids. Detection of these may require examination by slit lamp.

Bone disease in hyperparathyroidism, osteitis fibrosa cystica, may be recognized by roentgenographic examination (Fig. 1); it sometimes causes bone pain or pathologic fracture. Roentgenographically, bone disease may appear as generalized osteopenia, loss of the lamina dura about the teeth, erosion of the distal ends of the clavicles, bone cysts (Fig. 1B), "brown tumors" of bone, epulis of the jaw, or subcortical bone resorption, most readily observed in the phalanges (Fig.1A) or distal clavicles. Calcifications in soft tissues, kidneys (nephrocalcinosis), blood vessels, or cartilage (chrondrocalcinosis, Fig. 1B) may be found by roentgenography.

Hypercalciuria may lead to *nephrolithiasis* and passage of calcium oxalate or calcium phosphate stones with or without renal colic. In other instances *nephrocalcinosis* may develop, sometimes causing progressive renal failure. Infection may complicate either type of renal disorder.

Peptic ulcer is common in hyperparathyroidism and can reflect coexisting Zollinger-Ellison syndrome. It also may reflect a potentiating effect of hypercalcemia on acid secretion. An association between acute or chronic *pancreatitis* and hyperparathyroidism is recognized more and more frequently. Hyperparathyroidism may exist in any case of pancreatitis, and may be masked by the acute lowering of serum calcium concentration in pancreatitis.

In addition to pancreatitis and peptic ulcer, several other diseases may be associated with primary hyperparathyroidism. Hypertension occurs in up to 50 per cent of

Figure 1. Roentgenographic signs in hyperparathyroidism. *A,* Bone resorption. There is severe bone resorption with general loss of mineral, thinning of the cortices, marked subperiosteal resorption along the cortical surfaces of the proximal and distal phalanges, and gross resorption of the distal phalangeal tufts. *B,* Cysts (osteitis fibrosa cystica) in femur and tibia in subject with severe hyperparathyroidism. Also note intra-articular chrondrocalcinosis (thin line of calcification in knee joint indicated by arrow).

cases. It cannot be clearly related to any particular factor (e.g., associated renal disease) and does not often regress after surgical cure. There is an increased incidence of ill-defined arthralgia as well as of gout and pseudogout. The latter is associated with intra-articular deposition of calcium pyrophosphate crystals. Discovery of pseudogout should suggest possible coexistence of primary hyperparathyroidism. Primary hyperparathyroidism may exist as part of the multiple endocrine neoplasia syndromes type I or type IIa. In MEN I, tumors may produce associated endocrinopathies. These include acromegaly or hypopituitarism (pituitary tumors), peptic ulceration with excessive gastrin secretion (Zollinger-Ellison syndrome), or hypoglycemia resulting from secretion of insulin (pancreatic islet cell tumors). Hyperparathyroidism may also occur in MEN IIa in association with medullary carcinoma of the thyroid (see Ch. 552.6), and sometimes pheochromocytoma as well. Each of the two types of multiple endocrine neoplasia syndromes may be familial with autosomal dominant transmission. Sporadic cases of hyperparathyroidism have also been observed in association with hyperthyroidism, sarcoidosis, Albright's fibrous dysplasia of bone, Paget's disease, Cushing's syndrome, and malignancy.

Metabolic acidosis occurs in about one fourth of patients, with hyperchloridemia and low serum bicarbonate concentration. The acidosis can be attributed to impaired tubular reabsorption of bicarbonate and parallels the increase in phosphate clearance. It may become worse in the immediate postparathyroidectomy period when hypophosphatemia is accentuated. A similar defect in proximal tubular reabsorption of bicarbonate may occur in a number of metabolic disorders characterized by secondary hyperparathyroidism or cellular depletion of phosphate, or both. The abnormality can be documented by carrying out a test for T_m of bicarbonate reabsorption. Eventually metabolism returns to normal after surgical removal of hyperplastic or adenomatous parathyroid glands. Hypokalemia and hypomagnesemia also are occasionally observed in hyperparathyroidism. The hypokalemia is attributed to decreased distal tubular reabsorption of potassium and may be made worse by treating subjects with high doses of phosphate by mouth. Phosphate depletion may also account for decreased magnesium reabsorption.

DIFFERENTIAL DIAGNOSIS. Hypercalcemia, demineralizing disease of bone, and nephrolithiasis are clinical problems that commonly suggest the diagnosis of hyperparathyroidism. *Hypercalcemia* may be expressed in diverse metabolic, endocrine, or malignant diseases, including hyperparathyroidism, several types of cancer, sarcoidosis, milk-alkali syndrome, vitamin D intoxication, hyperthyroidism, acute adrenal insufficiency, and a rare disease, hypophosphatasia. Thiazides can produce a slight increase in serum calcium concentration and are currently one of the most common causes of hypercalcemia. In Paget's disease or osteoporosis, hypercalcemia may develop upon prolonged bed rest. Familial hypercalcemia occurs in MEN I and in *familial hypocalciuric hypercalcemia,* an autosomal dominant disorder characterized by high penetrance for hypercalcemia, disproportionately low urinary calcium clearance, and low cure rate with parathyroidectomy. Hypercalcemia may occur in malignancy as a consequence of one or more etiologic factors: osteolytic metastases causing hypercalcemia through local resorptive influence of the lesions in bone; production by the tumor of substances (e.g., prostaglandins or osteoclast-activating factors) capable of inducing bone resorption and hypercalcemia; production of an abnormal blood protein capable of binding calcium, the increase in serum calcium being attributable simply to a higher concentration of bound calcium in the plasma compartment (some cases of multiple myeloma); or "ectopic" hyperparathyroidism, in which a nonparathyroid tumor produces parathyroid hormone itself. The last-named may be particularly difficult to diagnose, because the laboratory findings do not differ from those of hyperparathyroidism caused by parathyroid adenoma or hyperplasia; blood calcium is high, blood phosphate is low, and the alkaline phosphatase may be elevated. A "pseudohyperparathyroid" syndrome (production of a unique bone-resorbing humoral substance unrelated to parathyroid hormone) may occur with associated hypophosphatemia. There is no detectable parathyroid hormone by immunoassay either in the tumor or in plasma. Hypercalcemia caused by malignancy and unrelated to parathyroid hormone tends to be associated with metabolic alkalosis, in contradistinction to the metabolic acidosis (decreased proximal renal tubular reabsorption of bicarbonate) sometimes associated with primary hyperparathyroidism (see above). The question of malignancy with hypercalcemia requires extensive studies to ascertain the true nature of the disease. Severe cases of true primary hyperparathyroidism may present particular diagnostic problems, because the disease itself can cause anemia, weight loss, debility, and increased erythrocyte sedimentation rate suggestive of malignant disease. Moreover, there are several reports of primary hyperparathyroidism coexisting with unrelated malignancies.

Paget's disease of bone, osteoporosis, osteomalacia, multiple myeloma, and malignancies metastatic to bone show varying degrees of skeletal demineralization. The roentgenographic appearance in each of these disorders, though, is more or less characteristic. In osteoporosis, the serum calcium, phosphate, and alkaline phosphatase values are normal. Extensive Paget's disease is attended by an increase in serum alkaline phosphatase activity, but phosphate and calcium concentrations in blood are normal except during periods of immobilization, when hypercalcemia may develop. Examination of bone marrow is helpful in excluding multiple myeloma, and is occasionally of value in diagnosing lymphoma or metastatic malignancy. Analysis of plasma and urine for myeloma proteins should be routine in suspected cases. Osteomalacia may be caused by hypovitaminosis D, resistance to vitamin D, intestinal malabsorption syndromes, or renal tubular acidosis. In these conditions, serum calcium concentration is normal or low, sometimes with tetany; blood phosphate concentration is low; and the alkaline phosphatase activity is elevated. The differential diagnoses of hyperparathyroid bone disease (osteitis fibrosa cystica), osteomalacia, fibrous dysplasia of bone, Paget's disease, and osteoporosis are discussed also in Part XXII.

Secondary hyperparathyroidism in chronic renal disease

may produce the histologic picture of osteitis fibrosa cystica. In general, serum phosphate concentration is high and there is a tendency to hypocalcemia. Occasionally, however, primary hyperparathyroidism may become superimposed upon chronic renal failure. This complication (sometimes called "tertiary hyperparathyroidism") becomes evident by an increase in serum calcium content to the high normal or hypercalcemic range. In this event hyperplastic or adenomatous parathyroid glands should be removed surgically.

Development of nephrolithiasis with calcium phosphate or calcium oxalate stones, particularly when associated with hypercalciuria, requires clinical testing to rule out primary hyperparathyroidism. "Idiopathic hypercalciuria" with recurrent nephrolithiasis may be associated with hypophosphatemia, making the distinction more difficult. This category may still include some patients with bona fide hyperparathyroidism. Repeated tests of serum calcium concentration are essential in reaching the correct conclusion. In some cases in which the diagnosis has been doubtful, hyperparathyroidism is obvious at the follow-up examination 6 to 12 months later.

DIAGNOSTIC INVESTIGATIONS. Hypercalcemia is almost always present in primary hyperparathyroidism. Indeed, hypercalcemia per se, detected in a general clinic population, can be attributed on chance alone to primary hyperparathyroidism in almost half the cases. Although malignancy is an equally common cause of hypercalcemia in the general population, hypercalcemia associated with hypophosphatemia and a long relatively benign clinical history makes the diagnosis of primary hyperparathyroidism more likely. In any one patient, though, particularly with an early or mild case, serial analyses may show fluctuations of serum calcium concentrations into the normal range. In rare instances hypomagnesemia or vitamin D deficiency may mask hyperparathyroidism. Correction of the magnesium or vitamin D deficiency in these cases allows the hypercalcemia to be expressed. In general, though, the finding of high serum calcium concentration is the laboratory test most likely to lead to the diagnosis. Several further investigations based on assessing the secretion or actions of parathyroid hormone help establish the diagnosis.

Several tests have been based on the known physiologic action of parathyroid hormone in causing increased phosphate clearance (and decreased tubular reabsorption of phosphate, TRP). Although these procedures are constantly modified in attempts to obtain greater diagnostic accuracy, none offer sufficient specificity to be of regular clinical value.

Prednisone Suppression Test. Hypercalcemia in sarcoidosis, vitamin D intoxication, or certain lymphoproliferative syndromes is particularly amenable to correction with corticosteroid therapy; subjects with the milk-alkali syndrome may respond also. These observations form the basis of a test that is helpful in differentiating among several types of hypercalcemia. Either prednisone, 60 mg daily, or hydrocortisone, 120 mg daily, is given in divided doses for ten days. The hypercalcemia of hyperparathyroidism, ectopic or primary, almost invariably is resistant to the effects of this treatment. The response in other types of hypercalcemia is more variable. The milk-alkali syndrome and hypervitaminosis D both respond to withdrawal of the offending agents. Hypercalcemia in sarcoidosis may respond to therapy with chloroquine. In general, the clinical, laboratory, and roentgenographic features cited under diagnosis of the particular disease should lead one to the proper diagnosis in the other disorders listed. Hypercalcemia in hyperthyroidism is best treated by correcting the hyperthyroid state. Hypercalcemia that persists in the euthyroid state indicates the existence of a second disease.

Urinary Excretion of Cyclic AMP. Parathyroid hormone exerts its effects on target tissues by activating adenylate cyclase and causing thereby an increase in tissue concentration of cyclic $3',5'$-AMP. Part of the cyclic $3',5'$-AMP accumulating within renal cells in response to parathyroid hormone is excreted in the urine; this nephrogenous contribution to the urinary excretion of cyclic $3',5'$-AMP in man is approximately 40 to 50 per cent of the total excreted. In primary hyperparathyroidism the mean urinary excretion of $3',5'$-AMP is elevated, and conversely in hypoparathyroidism the rate of excretion is low. After surgical correction of hyperparathyroidism, the rate of excretion falls to normal; this is a reliable index of successful surgery. The ratio of cyclic AMP to creatinine in the urine in normal subjects is 1.3 to 4.2 (average 2.7) μmoles per gram of creatinine. In hyperparathyroid patients cyclic AMP excretion averages 5.2 (standard deviation 2.2) μmoles per gram of creatinine. Expression of cyclic AMP per 100 ml of glomerular filtrate ([μmoles of cAMP per milligram of urine creatinine] $\times$ serum creatinine) provides a much better index (3.2 $\pm$ 0.68 for normal subjects; 6.3 $\pm$ 2.1 for hyperparathyroidism). Urinary cAMP per 100 ml of glomerular filtrate is abnormally high in most cases of proved hyperparathyroidism and is almost as useful in discriminating between normal subjects and primary hyperparathyroidism as is determination of nephrogenous cAMP (urinary cAMP per 100 ml of glomerular filtrate minus plasma cyclic AMP). The latter test requires plasma cAMP determination, which is not yet generally available. A high cyclic AMP excretion per 100 ml of glomerular filtrate in association with clinical hypercalcemia is very highly suggestive of hyperparathyroidism, primary or ectopic. Certain nonparathyroid cancers producing hypercalcemia are associated with low rates of cyclic AMP excretion, reflecting suppressed parathyroid hormone secretion, and thus can be distinguished from hyperparathyroidism.

Radioimmunoassay for Parathyroid Hormone. Radioimmunoassays for parathyroid hormone have been developed in several laboratories, but radioimmunoassay alone, particularly in random peripheral plasma samples, is not a uniformly reliable diagnostic index for primary hyperparathyroidism. After the hormone is secreted from the gland, it undergoes degradation to fragments in the periphery. One of the principal fragments remaining is immunologically reactive but biologically inert. This fragment (derived from the carboxyl two thirds of the molecule) disappears relatively slowly from the circulation and accumulates to an even greater extent in chronic renal disease. Moreover, some antisera are relatively more reactive than others with the carboxyl terminus of the molecule. Thus results for radioimmunoassays in peripheral plasma samples vary from one laboratory to another on the basis of differences in antisera and standards employed in the assay as well as differences in renal function in any particular patient. Nevertheless, in hyperparathyroidism, use of the assay usually shows abnormally high concentrations (particularly relative to calcium content of plasma) of hormone in the plasma. Hypercalcemia from causes unrelated to parathyroid hormone is usually associated with

undetectable hormone in plasma. Moreover, the immunoassay is particularly applicable to studies on samples obtained by selective venous catheterization. Blood drawn directly from the thyroid veins contains hormone immediately as it is secreted and before it has undergone degradation in the periphery. Such sampling allows preoperative localization of abnormal parathyroid tissue, helps establish the exact diagnosis, and should be utilized before further surgery in patients having persistent or recurrent hyperparathyroidism subsequent to prior parathyroid operations.

High concentrations of hormone in peripheral plasma have been found also in cases of hyperparathyroidism resulting from ectopic production of hormone by nonparathyroid tumors as well as in secondary hyperparathyroidism and pseudohypoparathyroidism. The difficulty of precise analysis for parathyroid hormone in peripheral plasma will undoubtedly be lessened by developing assays more specific for the active form. Radioimmunoassay (or possibly a radioreceptor assay) for parathyroid hormone coupled with an index of nephrogenous cAMP will undoubtedly become the principal diagnostic tests for hyperparathyroidism, as well as several other hypercalcemic or hypocalcemic disorders.

Preoperative Localization of Abnormal Parathyroid Tissue. Several methods have been proposed for identification of parathyroid adenomas before surgery. Occasionally large glands have been identified simply on esophagography; other procedures that have been used include scanning with [75]selenium-labeled methionine, intraoperative vital staining with toluidine blue, thermography, and arteriography (Fig. 2). None of these methods have been highly successful. The advent of the radioimmunoassay for parathyroid hormone, coupled with selective arterial and venous catheterization, has provided a means for more specific localization. Before undertaking further parathyroid surgery for persistent or recurrent hyperparathyroidism, it is advantageous to carry out selective arteriography of thyroid and mediastinal arteries and selective venous catheterization of vessels in the same distribution. Localization of adenomas is possible when each of the thyroid veins can be selectively catheterized with radioimmunoassays for parathyroid hormone in samples obtained. Arteriography should be carried out first in an attempt to delineate the thyroid venous anatomy as well as to uncover lesions representing potential parathyroid tissue. Computerized axial tomography has allowed identification of adenomas in some cases.

PROGNOSIS. Untreated, hyperparathyroidism with significant hypercalcemia may cause progressive renal impairment and ultimately death. Occasionally severe hypercalcemia develops rapidly ("hyperparathyroid crisis") and causes an immediate threat to life. On the other hand, the disease may exist in mild form without symptoms, and it is probable that some patients in apparently excellent health harbor hyperfunctioning parathyroid tissue for decades and die of unrelated causes.

Uncomplicated primary hyperparathyroidism is correctable definitively by surgery. Occasionally a second adenoma becomes apparent after initial resection was apparently successful. When primary hyperplasia of the parathyroid glands is the cause and insufficient tissue has been resected, recurrence of the disease will show itself by return of preoperative symptoms and signs.

TREATMENT. *Hypercalcemia* (from whatever cause) that is neither severe nor progressive requires treatment

Figure 2. Arteriographic localization of large parathyroid adenoma. *A,* Arrows outline large parathyroid adenoma filled by radiographic dye injected into right inferior thyroid artery. This phase of the arteriographic study shows also a rich arterial vascular plexus within the gland. *B,* Late phase of arteriographic study, showing vein (delineated by arrows) draining the adenoma. Subsequent selective venous sampling showed a very high gradient for parathyroid hormone concentration at the point marked by the large arrow.

directed only toward correction of the underlying disease state. On the other hand, progressive and severe hypercalcemia ("*hypercalcemic crisis*") leads to marked weakness, mental deterioration, coma, progressive uremia, and death within a short period. Several methods have been proposed for control of progressive hypercalcemia which may be so severe as to require emergency attention. Intravenous infusions of EDTA, sodium sulfate, or phosphate salts have been recommended, but each of these may produce hazardous side effects. Phosphate by mouth is effective in doses equal to those given intravenously, and there is probably less danger in this approach. Dehydration is often an important contributory factor in the development of progressive hypercalcemia and uremia. It is therefore important to restore extracellular fluids parenterally. Intravenous saline and furosemide are highly effective in reducing hypercalcemia but may lead to massive electrolyte losses. This treatment should only be employed with intensive monitoring and appropriate replacement of electrolytes. Treatment with phosphate by mouth for the first few days should consist of the equivalent of 2 grams of elemental phosphorus given in divided doses four times daily. After three to five days when control of hypercalcemia has begun to be effective, the dosage of phosphorus should be reduced to 1 to 1.5 grams daily. Calcium, phosphate, and urea nitrogen in plasma should be analyzed daily to assure that the desired effect is obtained. It is best not to allow the blood phosphorus concentration to exceed 6 mg per 100 ml because of possible soft tissue calcification. Some patients with primary hyperparathyroidism have been maintained with nearly normal blood calcium concentrations for periods up to six months, pending clarification of other complications before parathyroidectomy. However, this form of treatment should be regarded

as temporary; at the earliest possible moment, definitive therapy for the underlying disease should be instituted. Phosphate therapy may cause hypokalemia in these patients, requiring administration of potassium supplements. Calcitonin has not proved to be generally efficacious in controlling hypercalcemia. Mithramycin, which inhibits skeletal resorption, is the most potent agent available for the pharmacologic treatment of refractory hypercalcemic crisis. It should not be used in uncomplicated cases, however, because of its potential toxicity.

Surgery is the only definitive treatment yet devised for primary hyperparathyroidism. In very mild cases it may be deferred, but only if frequent and regular observation of the patient is possible. It is the author's view that treatment should be deferred only so long as the patient is completely asymptomatic, can return for frequent evaluation, shows no clinical symptom or sign of the disease, and maintains a serum calcium concentration under 11.5 mg per 100 ml. Otherwise parathyroidectomy should be performed by a surgeon qualified by extensive experience. It is essential that the highest possible rate of success be obtained at the *initial* surgical procedure. As would be expected, multiple explorations for parathyroid adenomas carry increased risk and expense, as well as greater difficulty for the surgeon, particularly when scarring from earlier surgery is significant. One side of the neck should be searched meticulously first. If an adenoma and a normal gland on that side are each proved by biopsy (frozen section), the adenoma should be removed and the wound closed. This leaves the contralateral side undisturbed and suitable for accurate exploration at a future time in the unlikely event this becomes necessary.

If the lesion is not found initially, the surgeon should extend the procedure to the contralateral side and attempt to identify all four parathyroid glands. Biopsy identification of all glands (results of frozen section at surgery should be confirmed by analysis of permanent sections) is then essential for subsequent surgical exploration if needed and also facilitates diagnosis of hyperplasia, which is an indication for removal of seven eighths of all parathyroid tissue found. Familial hyperparathyroidism or MEN I with hyperparathyroidism virtually always reflects multiple gland hyperplasia. In rare instances there are more than four hyperplastic glands.

If neither hyperplastic nor adenomatous glands are found in the neck, a mediastinal exploration should be considered at a later date. Mediastinal tumors account for approximately 20 per cent of parathyroid adenomas; 95 per cent of them lie superiorly embedded in or attached to the mediastinal fat pad. As such, they are readily removable along with the fat pad through the routine neck incision. Thus only 1 per cent of all parathyroid adenomas should require a sternal splitting procedure. This conclusion is borne out by the observation that virtually all missed adenomas, discovered at subsequent surgical explorations, prove to be in the neck. Arteriography and selective venous catheterization (see Preoperative Localization, above) should be carried out before a second surgical procedure. The results of surgery can be assessed readily with serial analyses of serum calcium concentrations. Determination of urinary cyclic 3′,5′-AMP will show a decrease to normal after successful parathyroidectomy.

Postoperatively, tetany may be expected in patients who show significant bony demineralization. Treatment at intervals with 10 per cent calcium gluconate (10 to 30 ml in 500 to 1500 ml of saline) intravenously and administration of vitamin D, 50,000 units or more daily by mouth is required until severe hypocalcemia shows signs of control. Adequate dietary intake of calcium (at least 1 gram daily) should be assured; if necessary, calcium lactate should be given by mouth. Therapy should be withdrawn as rapidly as clinical progress allows. Almost invariably, remaining parathyroid tissue recovers normal function; definite signs of recovery are usual within seven to ten days. Hyperphosphatemia greater than 6 mg per deciliter in the postoperative period suggests permanent hypoparathyroidism. The latter can be differentiated from the hypocalcemia of remineralization by monitoring urinary cAMP. It is best to allow some degree of hypocalcemia during the recovery period as long as symptoms are controlled, because hypercalcemia would tend to inhibit recovery of remaining parathyroid tissue. Excessive therapy with calcium by vein or vitamin D by mouth is neither necessary nor desirable.

Other complications in the postoperative period include temporary worsening of renal function or metabolic acidosis (see above), hypomagnesemia, pancreatitis, and gout or pseudogout. The physician should be particularly alert to the potential for the last two of these in subjects with intra-articular calcification or history of prior attacks.

Aurbach, G. D., Mallette, L. E., Patten, B. M., Heath, D. A., Doppman, J. L., and Bilezikian, J. P.: Hyperparathyroidism: Recent studies. Ann. Intern. Med., 79:566, 1973.

Broadus, A. E., Mahaffey, J. E., Bartter, F. C., and Neer, R. M.: Nephrogenous cyclic adenosine monophosphate as a parathyroid function test. J. Clin. Invest., 60:771, 1977.

Brown, E. M., Brennan, M. F., Hurwitz, S., Windeck, R., Marx, S. J., Spiegel, A. M., Koehler, J. O., Gardner, D. G., and Aurbach, G. D.: Dispersed cells prepared from human parathyroid glands: Distinct calcium sensitivity of adenomas versus primary hyperplasia. J. Clin. Endocrinol., 46:267, 1978.

Goldsmith, R. S., and Ingbar, S. H.: Inorganic phosphate treatment of hypercalcemia of diverse etiologies. N. Engl. J. Med., 274:1, 1966.

Mallette, L. E., Bilezikian, J. P., Heath, D. A., and Aurbach, G. D.: Primary hyperparathyroidism: Clinical and biochemical features. Medicine, 53:127, 1974.

Marx, S. J., Spiegel, A. M., Brown, E. M., and Aurbach, G. D.: Family studies in patients with primary parathyroid hyperplasia. Am. J. Med., 62:698, 1977.

Mundy, G. R., Luben, R. A., Raisz, L. G., Oppenheim, J. J., and Buell, D. N.: Bone-resorbing activity in supernatants from lymphoid cell lines. N. Engl. J. Med., 290:867, 1974.

Seyberth, H. W., Segre, G. V., Morgan, J. L., Sweetman, B. J., Potts, J. T., Jr., and Oates, J. A.: Prostaglandins as mediators of hypercalcemia associated with certain types of cancer. N. Engl. J. Med., 293:1278, 1975.

Sherwood, L. M., O'Riordan, J. L. H., Aurbach, G. D., and Potts, J. T., Jr.: Production of parathyroid hormone by nonparathyroid tumors. J. Clin. Endocrinol., 27:140, 1967.

552.3.   HYPOPARATHYROIDISM

DEFINITION. Hypoparathyroidism is the syndrome characterized by deficient secretion of parathyroid hormone, with consequent hypocalcemia.

ETIOLOGY. In most instances hypoparathyroidism is the consequence of mechanical injury to or removal of parathyroid glands during surgery for primary thyroid disorders or occasionally parathyroid disorders. Idiopathic hypoparathyroidism is rare; approximately 100 cases are known. It is usually recognized in childhood or adolescence and, in distinction to pseudohypoparathyroidism, it may be associated with pernicious anemia, ovarian failure, moniliasis, or Addison's disease; it occurs with equal incidence in males and females, and occasionally is familial.

PATHOLOGY. In postsurgical and most cases of idiopathic hypoparathyroidism there is complete absence of the parathyroid glands. There may be calcification in the basal ganglia and cataracts. The bones may be abnormally dense, and the calvarium may be thickened. Idiopathic hypoparathyroidism may reflect autoimmune disease or in other instances an organ maldevelopment associated with abnormalities of adjacent bronchial structures.

PATHOLOGIC PHYSIOLOGY AND CHEMISTRY. The physiologic consequences of insufficient secretion of parathyroid hormone are low blood calcium and high blood phosphate concentrations and a low rate of phosphate clearance into the urine. Attendant upon hypocalcemia is a very low concentration of calcium in the urine. As a general rule, the clearance of calcium into the urine approaches zero as its concentration in blood falls below 7 mg per deciliter.

Hypocalcemia in hypoparathyroidism is a manifestation of the reduced rate of bone resorption in the absence of sufficient parathyroid hormone. The diminished concentration of calcium in extracellular fluid leads to increased neuromuscular excitability and tetany. Hyperphosphatemia in this disorder is primarily attributable to lack of the effect of both PTH and calcium itself on phosphate clearance by the kidney. The rate of urinary excretion of 3′,5′-AMP is reduced, but in distinction to pseudohypoparathyroidism there is a normal renal response to exogenous parathyroid hormone.

CLINICAL MANIFESTATIONS. The principal symptoms of hypoparathyroidism are due to a low concentration of calcium in the extracellular fluid. Hypocalcemic tetany is manifested by numbness and tingling in the fingers and toes and around the lips, and sometimes by laryngeal stridor with "crowing" inspiration, dyspnea, and cyanosis. In severe tetany, cramps of individual muscle groups occur in the hands and feet as carpopedal and tarsopedal spasms. The differential diagnosis of tetany is discussed below. There may also be convulsions or abdominal pain, nausea, and vomiting. Epileptiform attacks are a striking symptom of hypoparathyroidism. Usually the seizures are of a grand mal type, but they are not always preceded by aura, loss of consciousness, involuntary trauma, or incontinence. The electroencephalogram may show abnormalities typical of idiopathic epilepsy. The seizures and usually the abnormal electroencephalographic pattern associated with tetany respond to treatment with calcium, whereas the latter is without effect in idiopathic epilepsy. Sometimes seizures of the petit mal type are expressed. Other cases may display choreiform movements, and in general there is increased sensitivity in hypoparathyroidism to the dystonic reactions of phenothiazine drugs.

Mental abnormalities may occur in hypoparathyroidism. Irritability, emotional lability, moroseness, impairment of memory, mental confusion, lethargy, depression, and mental deficiency have been described.

Papilledema, sometimes associated with increased intracranial pressure, may also accompany the hypocalcemia of hypoparathyroidism. These manifestations as well as the electroencephalograms return to normal when hypocalcemia is corrected. Cataracts are a characteristic consequence of chronic hypoparathyroidism. Other forms of ectopic calcification may be exhibited in the basal ganglia or subcutaneous tissues. The calvarium may be thickened.

Patients with idiopathic hypoparathyroidism may display abnormalities of the ectodermal structures, including the teeth, skin, nails, and hair. A characteristic feature of hypoparathyroidism early in life is blunting of the roots of the teeth and dysplasia of the enamel. The nails may be malformed and brittle and show transverse grooves. In addition, there is a significant incidence of moniliasis in idiopathic hypoparathyroidism, and when this involves the nails they become pitted and flaky in appearance. The transverse grooves, but not moniliasis, disappear when the serum calcium concentration is corrected toward normal. The hair is thin, there may be patchy alopecia, and the skin is sometimes coarse and dry and may show vitiligo.

DIAGNOSIS. Complaints of numbness and tingling in the extremities and around the mouth should suggest tetany. "Latent" tetany may be detected by eliciting Chvostek's sign by tapping over the facial nerve. A positive response consists of twitching of the muscles about the mouth and sometimes the nose and eyelids. Trousseau's sign is sought by producing ischemia with a cuff inflated above systolic pressure for three minutes. Characteristically, carpal spasm becomes evident during the course of the test. In latent tetany one may find increased sensitivity to galvanic current in producing muscle contraction (Erb's sign). The electrocardiogram may show a Q-T interval that is prolonged in proportion to the degree of hypocalcemia.

Patients with atypical epilepsy, other manifestations of increased neuromuscular irritability, or bizarre mental symptoms should be investigated for possible hypoparathyroidism. Obviously a history of prior thyroid surgery should alert one to this possibility. Tetany associated with Addison's disease, pernicious anemia, or moniliasis should immediately suggest a diagnosis of idiopathic hypoparathyroidism. Each of these diseases may be caused by or associated with autoimmunity, and autoantibodies to these endocrine tissues have been detected.

PROGNOSIS. Hypoparathyroidism that follows thyroid or parathyroid surgery may often be transient. One should try withdrawing therapy several months postoperatively in such cases before it is concluded that permanent hypoparathyroidism exists. The prognosis is excellent with full life expectancy in established cases adequately treated. Untreated, the subject with hypoparathyroidism may suffer the discomfort and morbidity of muscular spasms, convulsions, cataracts, and mental impairment. It is not certain that cataracts can be prevented in hypoparathyroidism by correction of hypocalcemia early in the course of the disease. Epileptiform seizures are generally alleviated as hypocalcemia is corrected.

TREATMENT. Acute hypocalcemic tetany requires treatment with intravenous calcium, for example, 1 to 2 mg per kilogram acutely or 10 to 15 mg per kilogram over 6 to 12 hours given as necessary to control the symptoms. At the same time 40,000 to 80,000 IU daily of ergocalciferol (vitamin D_2) should be given by mouth. Adequate intake of at least 1 to 2 grams of calcium by mouth should be assured, and sometimes further supplementation with 15 grams of calcium lactate (equivalent to 2 grams of calcium) in divided doses is necessary. The amount of vitamin D and calcium should be gradually reduced as serum calcium approaches normal. Crystalline dihydrotachysterol or new synthetic biologically active calciferol analogues may be used instead of vitamin D and are advantageous should withdrawal be required in cases of toxicity because their biologic half-lives are shorter than that of vitamin D itself. In the absence of parathyroid hormone, vitamin D may cause an inordinately high rate of excretion of urinary calcium with the danger of nephrolithiasis. Sulkowitch's test is not of value in the management of these patients; quantitative analyses for 24-hour excretion of calcium are required.

552.4. PSEUDOHYPOPARA-THYROIDISM AND PSEUDO-PSEUDOHYPOPARATHYROIDISM

DEFINITION. *Pseudohypoparathyroidism* is a clinical state of hypoparathyroidism characterized by appropriate secretion of hormone from the parathyroid glands, but with a genetic defect in the renal receptor tissue so that there is little or no response in the action of the hormone. The defect is transmitted as a sex-linked dominant trait, and is associated with characteristic abnormalities of physiognomy and growth. The genetically related disorder *pseudopseudohypoparathyroidism* (see below) represents an incomplete form of the syndrome, shows the constitutional features without the chemical findings of hypoparathyroidism, and may occur in the same families with pseudohypoparathyroidism.

ETIOLOGY AND GENETICS. Recent clinical investigations in this disorder as well as current studies on the mechanism of action of parathyroid hormone have shed light on the pathophysiology of this syndrome. The original hypothesis of Albright and his associates that the receptor tissues, bone, and kidney are unresponsive to parathyroid hormone accounts for the endocrinopathology of this disorder. Other hypotheses such as secretion of a biologically inactive form of parathyroid hormone, circulating antibodies to the hormone, or secretion of excessive amounts of calcitonin have been tested without substantiation. The direct action of parathyroid hormone on the kidney is reflected in the urinary excretion of cyclic 3',5'-AMP. Normal subjects show a marked increased in excretion of the nucleotide after injection of parathyroid hormone. Pseudohypoparathyroidism is characterized by a defective response to exogenous parathyroid hormone assessed by urinary excretion of 3',5'-AMP. The most reasonable interpretation of this finding, and the probable explanation for the disorder, is the genetic transmission of defective or deficient receptor–adenylate cyclase complex in the renal cortex and perhaps other tissues of those affected.* These subjects, when hypocalcemic, secrete parathyroid hormone at increased rates reflected in high concentrations of the hormone in peripheral plasma. The secretory rate responds normally, though, to blood calcium levels.

The genetics of the disorder is currently best explained by a sex-linked dominant mode of inheritance. The sex incidence ratio is female to male 2:1; no instances of male-to-male transmission of the complete syndrome have been documented with biochemical testing. Possibly the short stature characteristic of the syndrome is also attributable to an abnormal X chromosome. Genetic studies of sex-linked disorders indicate that in order to achieve normal height two functional sex chromosomes are required; that is, both the X chromosomes in females or both X and Y in males must be normal in the segments controlling growth. Pseudopseudohypoparathyroidism, in females at least, may reflect genetic mosaicism with a relatively greater degree of inactivation of the abnormal X chromosome. Several patients with hypocalcemia, reactive hyperparathyroidism, increased urinary cyclic AMP, but low phosphate clearance have been recently classified as pseudohypoparathyroidism type II. They appear to manifest a defective renal response to generated cAMP, possibly a defect in the cAMP receptor–protein kinase complex.

INCIDENCE. Pseudohypoparathyroidism and its incomplete variant pseudopseudohypoparathyroidism are rare. The average case is recognized earlier in life than is idiopathic hypoparathyroidism. Approximately 100 cases of pseudohypoparathyroidism and still fewer cases of the variant have been reported.

PATHOLOGY. The parathyroid glands are normal or hyperplastic. Shortening of the carpal and metatarsal bones and metastatic calcification, including calcification of the basal ganglia, occur. Also, there may be thickening of the calvarium, defective enamel of the teeth, dental aplasia, coxa vara, coxa valga, and bowing of the long bones. Cataracts are common.

PATHOLOGIC PHYSIOLOGY AND CHEMISTRY. The clinical chemical findings, hypocalcemia, hyperphosphatemia, and a low urinary calcium, are qualitatively similar but sometimes milder than those found in idiopathic or postoperative hypoparathyroidism. However, in pseudo-

hypoparathyroidsm, biologically active hormone under normal secretory control is elaborated from the parathyroid glands, but the target tissues do not respond. Exogenously administered parathyroid hormone causes little or no effect. The calcemic (skeletal) but not the renal response to PTH is restored after vitamin D therapy, indicating that the skeletal unresponsiveness is a manifestation secondary to inadequate renal production of active vitamin D metabolites in response to parathyroid hormone. Other endocrinopathies may coexist. Hypothyroidism (nongoitrous primary hypothyroidism or that caused by selective pituitary TSH deficiency), diabetes mellitus, hypomenorrhea, prolactin deficiency, or gonadal dysgenesis may be found associated with pseudohypoparathyroidism. Conversely, moniliasis, Addison's disease, and pernicious anemia, which may be associated with idiopathic hypoparathyroidism, have not been found in cases of pseudohypoparathyroidism.

CLINICAL MANIFESTATIONS. The symptoms and signs of pseudohypoparathyroidism encompass those of hypoparathyroidism plus certain unique abnormalities of physiognomy and growth. Mental retardation, short, stocky, obese stature, and round facies are characteristic. The hands and feet are usually disproportionately short, resulting in about 75 per cent of cases from shortening of one or more metacarpal and metatarsal bones. This is readily recognized when the first is clenched, thereby causing a dimple over the head of the affected bone. Less frequently, shortening of the phalanges or uniform brachydactyly may occur. The calvarium is thickened in over one third of the patients. There may be delayed dentition, defective enamel, or complete dental aplasia. Less common defects include normally dense or lucent bones, exostoses, coxa vara, coxa valga, bowing of the ulna, radius, tibia, and fibula, and loss of "tubulation" of the long bones. Calcification occurs in the basal ganglia and in the dentate nucleus, and there may be actual ossification as well as calcification in the skin, subcutaneous tissue, and deep connective tissues. Cataracts are also common. Most cases of true pseudohypoparathyroidism show the abnormalities of physiognomy and growth originally described by Albright and his associates.

DIAGNOSIS. The diagnosis is established by the characteristic constitutional changes, by the clinical and laboratory abnormalities of hypoparathyroidism, and by testing the response to purified parathyroid hormone or parathyroid extract given intravenously. The earlier test for pseudohypoparathyroidism based on measurement of urinary phosphate excretion did not allow clear-cut separation of pseudohypoparathyroidism from normal subjects who vary widely in response; determination of 3',5'-AMP in the urine in response to parathyroid hormone affords virtually complete differentiation between the two groups. Normal subjects, but not those with pseudohypoparathyroidism, show a marked rise (to give 3'5'-AMP–to–creatinine ratios greater than 15 μmoles per gram) in the rate of excretion of urinary 3',5'-AMP within 15 to 45 minutes after injection of 200 USP units of parathyroid hormone intravenously. There is no overlap of results between normal subjects and those with the disease. Baseline excretion of cyclic AMP is lower than normal in patients with idiopathic, postsurgical, and pseudohypoparathyroidism, but higher than normal in pseudopseudohypoparathyroidism. The last-named group comprises patients with the physiognomy of pseudohypoparathyroidism but a normal response to

---

*It is possible that the defect does not involve the receptor itself or the enzyme adenylate cyclase. In one instance, the only case in which adenylate cyclase from renal tissue was tested directly, there appeared to be a normal in vitro response to parathyroid hormone. Other biochemical abnormalities, such as defective nucleotide or phospholipid regulatory site on the enzyme or a defect distal to generation of cyclic nucleotide, have not been excluded. However, these patients respond normally to exogenous dibutyryl cyclic 3',5'-AMP, and thus it seems that the metabolic defect must be at a site prior to formation of cyclic 3',5'-AMP.

parathyroid hormone. Parathyroid hormone in peripheral plasma is high (as long as hypocalcemia is not corrected) in pseudohypoparathyroidism, in contrast to other forms of hypoparathyroidism in which it is undetectable. Some patients previously categorized as having pseudohypoparathyroidism associated with intestinal malabsorption syndromes, osteitis fibrosa cystica, or both, should be re-examined with the newer diagnostic procedures. It is the author's view that opinions should be deferred pending further tests before accepting a patient with atypical family history or clinical findings as a true example of pseudohypoparathyroidism.

TREATMENT. In general the treatment of pseudohypoparathyroidism is the same as that of hypoparathyroidism. Usually hypocalcemia is easier to control in pseudohypoparathyroidism, although occasional patients seem relatively resistant to vitamin D and require unusually high doses to achieve normal calcium concentration in blood. The disease may fluctuate in severity, and sometimes affected subjects show normal serum calcium and phosphorus concentrations for long periods of time without treatment.

552.5. TETANY

Tetany may develop in hypocalcemia, alkalosis, potassium deficiency, and occasionally hypomagnesemia. The symptoms and signs of tetany are discussed in Ch. 552.3. In addition to the information obtained by clinical examination, the laboratory findings are particularly important in diagnosing the cause of tetany. In hypoparathyroidism the serum phosphate concentration is high, whereas in the hypocalcemic states of rickets or osteomalacia serum phosphate values may be below normal. Urinary calcium is low in hypocalcemic tetany. Tetany caused by alkalosis is associated with normal serum phosphate and calcium values and normal urinary excretion of calcium, but the blood pH is high. Alkalotic tetany may occur in hyperventilation, usually a manifestation of psychoneurosis, and can be corrected by inducing the patient to reduce the respiratory rate or breathe into a paper bag to increase carbon dioxide retention.

Metabolic alkalosis, caused by persistent vomiting, hypokalemic alkalosis, or excessive treatment with alkali, may also produce tetany. In excessive treatment with alkali, the serum calcium and phosphate concentrations are normal as long as there is no renal impairment, but the serum pH is high. Tetany is produced by overcorrection of acidosis in chronic renal disease. In such a condition, there is a tendency to hypocalcemia as well as hyperphosphatemia. In respiratory alkalosis plasma bicarbonate concentration is low or normal, whereas in metabolic alkalosis plasma bicarbonate concentration is high. The history should suggest the appropriate diagnosis in cases of excessive intake of alkali or excessive loss of gastric acid. The diagnosis is supported by finding a high concentration of bicarbonate in the serum and an alkaline urine. Treatment is directed at checking the cause. Hypokalemic alkalosis may appear in primary aldosteronism or treatment with corticosteroid analogues, and calls for correction of hormone excess and repletion of body potassium. Neonatal hypocalcemia may occur after asphyxia in premature infants, or in the progeny of diabetic or hyperparathyroid mothers. This last is a transient phenomenon secondary to hypercalcemia attendant upon primary hy-

Differential Diagnosis of Tetany

Cause	Serum			Urine	
	Ca	P_i	pH	Ca	pH
Hypocalcemia					
Hypovitaminosis D		↓	↓	N	—
Resistance to vitamin D	N or ↓	↓	N	—
Intestinal malabsorption		↓	↓	N	—
Hypoparathyroidism		↓	↑	N	—
Hypomagnesemia	N or ↓	N or ↑	N	N or ↓	—
Alkalosis					
Respiratory	N	N	↑	N	
Metabolic	N	N	↑	N	

Ca = Calcium. P_i = Phosphate. N = Normal. (−) = Indeterminate. ↑ = High. ↓ = Low.

perparathyroidism in the mother. Hypomagnesemia is a rare cause of tetany refractory to treatment with calcium; magnesium deficiency in those instances should be corrected.

Albright, F., Burnett, C. H., Smith, P. H., and Parson, W.: Pseudohypoparathyroidism — an example of the "Seabright-Bantam syndrome." Endocrinology, 30:922, 1942.

Blizzard, R. M., Chee, D., and Davis, W.: The incidence of parathyroid and other antibodies in the sera of patients with idiopathic hypoparathyroidism. Clin. Exp. Immunol., 1:119, 1968.

Bronsky, D., Kushner, D. S., Dubin, A., and Snapper, I.: Idiopathic hypoparathyroidism and pseudohypoparathyroidism: Case reports and review of the literature. Medicine, 37:317, 1958.

Carlson, H. E., Brickman, A. S., and Bottazzo, G. F.: Prolactin deficiency in pseudohypoparathyroidism. N. Engl. J. Med., 296:140, 1977.

Chase, L. R., Melson, G. L., and Aurbach, G. D.: Pseudohypoparathyroidism: Defective excretion of 3′,5′-AMP in response to parathyroid hormone. J. Clin. Invest., 48:1832, 1969.

Drezner, M. K., Neelon, F. A., Haussler, M., et al.: 1,25-Dihydroxycholecalciferol deficiency: The probable cause of hypocalcemia and metabolic bone disease in pseudohypoparathyroidism. J. Clin. Endocrinol., 42:621, 1976.

Harrison, H. E., Lifshitz, F., and Blizzard, R. M.: Comparison between crystalline dihydrotachysterol and calciferol in patients requiring pharmacologic vitamin D therapy. N. Engl. J. Med., 276:894, 1967.

Marx, S. J., Hershman, J. M., and Aurbach, G. D.: Thyroid dysfunction in pseudohypoparathyroidism. J. Clin. Endocrinol., 33:822, 1971.

552.6. CALCITONIN AND MEDULLARY CARCINOMA OF THE THYROID

Medullary carcinoma of the thyroid (see also Ch. 546.8) arises from the parafollicular cells of the thyroid which derive embryologically from the final or ultimobranchial cleft. These particular cells of the ultimobranchial cleft may, like chromaffin tissue, take origin initially in the neural crest. In submammalian vertebrates the ultimobranchial cells remain separate as the ultimobranchial gland, whereas in mammals the anlage merges with the embryologic thyroid. In either instance, the cells derived from the ultimobranchial cells constitute the gland that synthesizes and secretes calcitonin. Medullary carcinoma may be sporadic or familial and is part of a syndrome (the so-called "multiple endocrine neoplasia type II") encompassing hyperplasia or adenoma of the parathyroid glands, sometimes expressed as primary hyperparathyroidism, pheochromocytoma, multiple neuromas, and Cushing's syndrome. Abnormally high concentrations of calcitonin are found in medullary thyroid tumors as well as in plasma taken from these patients. The variant familial medullary thyroid carcinoma (MEN IIb or MEN III) shows an unusually high incidence of mucosal neuromas and a very low incidence of primary hyperparathyroidism.

INCIDENCE. Medullary carcinoma of the thyroid accounts for 5 to 10 per cent of the cases of thyroid cancer. In the familial form it follows the autosomal dominant form of inheritance.

PATHOLOGY. Histologically this tumor differs from other cancers of the thyroid in that the cells resemble parafollicular cells, there is often amyloid infiltration, and there are no papillary folds, follicles, or polymorphonuclear infiltrates in the tissue. (Sometimes artifacts of fixation look like papillary folds in sections.) The tumor usually does not appear to be encapsulated, and may show areas of calcification. The tissue does not take up radioactive iodine. As noted above, pheochromocytoma or parathyroid hyperplasia or adenoma may be associated with medullary carcinoma of the thyroid.

PATHOLOGIC PHYSIOLOGY. Although these tumors elaborate calcitonin at a high rate, hypocalcemia is unusual. Moreover, as stated above, there may be frequent occurrence of primary hyperparathyroidism in the syndrome. Calcitonin, at least under experimental conditions, can directly stimulate secretion of parathyroid hormone; hyperparathyroidism might thus arise as a consequence of prolonged effects of calcitonin acting directly as a secretagogue or (less likely in adults) indirectly by inhibiting skeletal resorption and provoking secondary hyperparathyroidism. The concentration of histaminase in serum frequently is increased in metastatic medullary carcinoma.

Measurements by radioimmunoassay or bioassay show that hypercalcemia induces secretion of calcitonin from normal parafollicular cells as well as from medullary carcinoma tissue. In addition, glucagon or gastrin, injected intravenously in pharmacologic doses, causes secretion of calcitonin in certain animals as well as in patients with medullary carcinoma. These responses to calcium, glucagon, or gastrin are valuable in conjunction with radioimmunoassay as diagnostic tests for the syndrome. Completely asymptomatic cases in the familial syndrome have been detected by this means. Indeed, thyroid C-cell "hyperplasia" has been discovered in some family members showing abnormal secretory responses to calcium.

CLINICAL MANIFESTATIONS, PROGNOSIS, AND TREATMENT. Medullary carcinoma may become evident simply as a mass in the thyroid or by the clinical expression of the associated endocrinopathies, pheochromocytoma, primary hyperparathyroidism, or Cushing's syndrome.

The tumor, local or metastatic, may be hard or tender, and sometimes is calcified to a degree detectable by x-ray. Severe diarrhea may occur, possibly related to elaboration by the tumor of prostaglandins, serotonin, or calcitonin, any of which can stimulate intestinal secretion. Intestinal motility problems may also result from ganglioneuromas of the autonomic nervous system. Other conditions occasionally associated with the syndrome include orbital, lingual, or buccal neuromas or extensive ganglioneuromas anywhere in the gastrointestinal tract, peculiar facies, megacolon or Marfan's syndrome–like habitus. Medullated nerves in the cornea are detected in some cases on slit lamp examination. The tumor often spreads locally, and metastases may grow to huge size. Hypertension from adrenal medullary disease (hyperplasia or pheochromocytoma) is another cause of serious morbidity. Surgery represents the best treatment and should consist of bilateral thyroidectomy, avoiding local seeding with tumor fragments. Isolated metastases may also be amenable to surgery. Chemotherapy in this disorder generally has not been valuable. Persistent high concentrations (basally or after provocative tests) of calcitonin in plasma reflect residual unresected tumor or metastases. Spread of tumor to nodes carries a poorer prognosis than when nodes are free of disease.

Carney, J. A., Go, V. L. W., Sizemore, G. W., and Hayles, A. B.: Alimentary-tract ganglioneuromatosis: A major component of the syndrome of multiple endocrine neoplasia, type 2b. N. Engl. J. Med., 295:1287, 1976.

Hazard, J. B., Hawk, W. A., and Crile, G., Jr.: Medullary (solid) carcinoma of the thyroid — a clinicopathologic entity. J. Clin. Endocrinol., 19:152, 1959.

Hennessy, J. F., Gray, T. K., Cooper, C. W., and Ontjes, D. A.: Stimulation of thyrocalcitonin secretion by pentagastrin and calcium in two patients with medullary carcinoma of the thyroid. J. Clin. Endocrinol., 36:200, 1973.

Keiser, H. R., Beaven, M. A., Doppman, J., Wells, S., Jr., and Buja, M.: Sipple's syndrome: Medullary thyroid carcinoma, pheochromocytoma and parathyroid disease: Studies in a large family. Ann. Intern. Med., 78:561, 1973.

Khairi, M. R. A., Dexter, R. N., Burzynski, N. J., and Johnston, C. C., Jr.: Mucosal neuroma, pheochromocytoma and medullary thyroid carcinoma: Multiple endocrine neoplasia type 3. Medicine, 54:89, 1975.

Melvin, K. E. W., Tashjian, A. H., Jr., and Miller, H. H.: Studies in familial (medullary) thyroid carcinoma. Recent Prog. Horm. Res., 28:399, 1972.

Steiner, A. L., Goodman, A. D., and Powers, S. R.: Study of a kindred with pheochromocytoma, medullary thyroid carcinoma, hyperparathyroidism and Cushing's disease: Multiple endocrine neoplasia, type 2. Medicine, 47:371, 1968.

Wolfe, H. J., Melvin, K. E. W., Cervi-Skinner, S. J., Saadi, A. A. A., Juliar, J. F., Jackson, C. E., and Tashjian, A. H., Jr.: C-cell hyperplasia preceding medullary thyroid carcinoma. N. Engl. J. Med., 289:437, 1973.

PART XXII
DISEASES OF BONE

Louis V. Avioli

553. CALCIUM, PHOSPHORUS, AND BONE METABOLISM

553.1. CALCIUM

Calcium is the most abundant cation and fifth most common inorganic element of the human body. It not only serves as the principal component of the skeletal tissue, imparting to it the structural integrity essential to support the increasing body size of the individual during growth, but also plays a vital role in a variety of essential physiologic and biochemical processes. The functions of the calcium ion include its influence on blood coagulation, neuromuscular excitability, cellular adhesiveness, transmission of nerve impulses, maintenance and function of cell membranes, and activation of enzyme reactions and hormone secretion. The skeleton, a huge reservoir of insoluble complexed forms of calcium, is in dynamic equilibrium with physiochemically soluble forms of circulating calcium. These are maintained at a remarkably constant level, with a diurnal plasma variation of ±3 per cent. This fluctuation in circulating calcium is comparable to that of plasma sodium (± 3 per cent) and is lower than the range of variation for the potassium (± 12 per cent) or the hydrogen ion (± 10 per cent). Although the primary homeostatic mechanism that controls the plasma calcium concentration is a function of the parathyroid glands, a variety of other hormones, vitamins, inhibitors of biologic calcification such as inorganic pyrophosphate, and other less well understood factors prevent the fluctuation of calcium over a wide range despite the enormous insoluble skeletal reservoir and great variations in intake and output. Primary disruption of this exquisite control system leads ultimately to derangements in skeletal and extraosseous mineral metabolism. These, in turn, often result in characteristic clinical manifestations and alterations in both chemical and roentgenographic findings which serve to define the pathologic state.

CALCIUM IN BONE

The average adult human contains 1000 to 1200 grams of calcium or 20.7 to 24.8 grams per kilogram of fat-free body tissue. Whereas quantitatively 30 per cent of body sodium and 50 per cent of magnesium are stored in bone, over 99 per cent of the body calcium resides in the skeleton. Calcium in the solid mineral phase of bone is usually considered to be a variant of poorly crystalline hydroxyapatite, $Ca_{10}(PO_4)_6(OH)_2$, the unit cell of the crystal lattice containing all 18 ions of the formula. It has been suggested from studies on synthet-

ic and biologic hydroxyapatites that the apatite portion of bone mineral does not have the ideal stoichiometry, $Ca_{10}(PO_4)_6(OH)_2$, but is approximately 10 per cent deficient in calcium, with the structure remaining generally intact. A noncrystalline amorphous phase combined with phosphate, $Ca_3(PO_4)_2$, has also been identified in osseous tissue. The hydroxyapatite crystals are tubular hexagons, with average dimensions of $40 \times 50 \times 600$ Å. Although calcium and phosphate are the principal ions in hydroxyapatite, the crystal contains significant amounts of Na+, Mg++, CO_3^{-2} and citrate^{-3} ions, which, with the exception of Mg++, can substitute for either calcium or phosphate in the apatitic lattice, as well as being adsorbed on its surface or incorporated into its hydration shell. Other so-called "bone seeking" ions such as strontium (Sr), radium (Ra), plutonium, lead, and fluorine are also incorporated into or adsorbed onto the crystal. This assumes importance when their radioactive isotopes (e.g., Sr^{90} from fallout or Ra from luminous paints) are ingested, since their accumulation may lead to radiation damage and malignant degeneration of bone cells. The release of mineral from bone during resorption buffers hydrogen ions, whereas the formation of bone mineral generates hydrogen ions, eight H$^+$ released per unit cell of the crystalline lattice. This may assume significant proportions in the growing skeleton wherein, during the process of skeletal mineralization and hydroxyapatite synthesis, approximately 20 mEq of H$^+$ is released by the deposition of 1 gram of calcium. Bone, therefore, not only represents a calcium depot for the miscible calcium pool but also assumes an important role as a reservoir for electrolytes and buffers. The presence of the amorphous calcium phase accounts for a Ca:P ratio in bone (1.5) lower than that found in synthetic hydroxyapatite. This metastable noncrystalline calcium phase is characteristic of newly deposited bone mineral and spontaneously changes to the poorly crystallized hydroxyapatite after it is deposited. The relative concentration of the amorphous phase in bone decreases with increasing biologic age of the skeleton.

CALCIUM IN PLASMA

The total calcium concentration of blood plasma or serum of man is remarkably constant, ranging between 2.25 and 2.75 mM, with 2.5 mM (10 mg per 100 ml or 5.0 mEq per liter) the average value. In men, the serum calcium decreases with age, paralleling a decrease in both total serum protein and albumin, whereas in women, despite similar decrements in total serum proteins, serum calcium remains rather constant with advancing years. Serum total calcium also decreases 5 to 10 per cent from the normal average during pregnancy until the end of the third trimester, when it tends to rise. The values begin to fall in the second or third month, attaining the lowest values in the seventh or eighth month. The "free" ionized calcium concentration is not significantly altered during pregnancy, so the reduction in total calcium can best be explained by the lower amount of protein-bound calcium. The latter may reflect the 20 to 30 per cent fall in circulating albumin which normally obtains during the third trimester.

Calcium exists in three forms in the blood and body fluids: (1) protein-bound calcium, (2) ionized calcium, and (3) diffusible calcium complexed with organic acids like citrate or inorganic acids like sulfate or phosphate. The free and complexed calciums are often referred to as the non-protein-bound or ultrafilterable fraction. The physiologic properties of calcium are all functions of the free ionic calcium. In view of the compartmentalization of plasma calcium, total calcium may often fail to reflect the free ionic calcium levels, particularly in subjects with acidosis, alkalosis, or abnormal plasma protein concentrations. In normal plasma the protein-bound calcium accounts for about 46 to 50 per cent of the total. Albumins and globulins are the principal plasma proteins to which calcium is bound, with the prealbumin fraction accounting for the highest degree of binding affinity. About 81 per cent of the protein-bound calcium is bound to albumin, the globulins accounting for the remainder. A nomogram for estimating protein-bound calcium has been established and can be applied when the serum albumin and arterial pH values are known. The calcium binding by serum proteins obeys the mass-law equation for a monoligand association and is not specific, since other cations compete with calcium for the binding proteins. For example, magnesium and calcium complexes with protein in serum are similar and are probably formed at the same protein sites. A knowledge of the protein binding of plasma calcium is of practical significance clinically, since low plasma albumin concentrations which occur commonly in hepatic cirrhosis or nephrosis are accompanied by low values for total calcium while the ionized calcium is normal. Hyperglobulinemia may also contribute to the elevated total calcium values occasionally noted in myelomatosis and sarcoidosis. The normal protein affinity for calcium is such that 1 gram of albumin binds approximately 0.0350 mEq (0.7 mg) of calcium. For comparison, the magnesium binding affinity of albumin is 0.0128 mEq per gram. A formula devised for the calculation of the plasma protein-bound calcium based on the differential binding affinities of albumin and globulin is as follows:

Per cent protein bound Ca = 8 albumin (grams per 100 ml) + 2 globulin (grams per 100 ml) + 3

For the protein-poor fluids of the body, such as the cerebrospinal and extracellular fluids, the calcium concentration is generally about 1.25 mM per liter (5 mg per 100 ml) and is virtually all in the ultrafilterable form. A small fraction of this is also in the form of unionized diffusible complexes which have no known physiologic significance. Since the ionized calcium fraction is the physiologically active form, alterations in its concentration are critical for the regulation of neuromuscular excitability.

Plasma ionized calcium concentrations normally range between 0.94 and 1.33 mM per liter (mean, 1.14 mM per liter). When this plasma concentration is reduced, increased neuromuscular irritability results. Although increases in total serum calcium are usually associated with increases in the level of ionized calcium, there is no apparent correlation between serum ionized and total calcium concentrations. Thus neither serum total calcium nor ultrafilterable calcium provides a reliable index of serum ionized calcium. A variety of factors control the continuous dynamic exchange of calcium between the compartmental subsystems. The binding of calcium to serum proteins increases with increasing pH, and a systemic alkalosis may thus precipitate hypocalcemic tetany. Consistent pH effects on ionized calcium do obtain at physiologic pH values between 6.8 and 7.5, with ionized calcium concentrations varying inversely with pH. Despite this relationship between plasma pH and ionized calcium, the so-called protective effect of acidosis against hypocalcemic tetany may not result entirely from an increased concentration of ionized calcium, since the hydrogen (or hydroxyl) ion exerts a depressive effect on neuromuscular irritability even though it does not affect the inotropic response of the heart to calcium ions. Furthermore, the relative lack of tetany in uremic patients with metabolic acidosis and low plasma ionized calcium levels may also be ascribed to associated elevations in ionized magnesium, since hypermagnesemia can also lead to depressed neuromuscular activity.

In normal subjects, a relation exists between plasma calcium and inorganic phosphate. When expressed in terms of total calcium (mg per cent) and inorganic phosphate (mg per cent), the ion product or Ca × P solubility product described clinically normally averages 35. Although useful, this calculated circulating ion product has no theoretical significance, and its values are extremely variable in normal man. In molar untis, the ion product calculated by this method is 0.2 to 0.3 times the actual plasma ion product, $(Ca^{2+}) \times (HPO_4^{2-})$, which in human plasma averages $0.72 \times 10^{-6}M$. A solubility product constant can be defined as the ion product at concentrations of the ions at which the rates of solution and precipitation of the salt are equal. A solubility product constant thus physicochemically defines conditions present at equilibrium. Despite many uncertainties concerning the mineralizing propensity of plasma and the exact chemical nature of either the earliest form of bone mineral or the fluids in direct contact with bone mineral in vivo, it has been suggested that ionic interchange between bone and tissue fluids exhibits a solubility relationship. The ion product of hydroxyapatite $(1 \times 10^{-25}M)$ is considerably lower than that of $(Ca^{2+}) \times (HPO_4^{2-})$ in extracellular fluid. At normal plasma pH the body fluids are in effect supersaturated with respect to the final mineral bone phase of bone. These facts have been interpreted as meaning that mineral can be extracted from the surrounding fluids with great efficiency during bone formation. Moreover, it has been suggested that a fall in the Ca × P ion product in the extracellular fluid leads to a dissolution of the exchangeable bone mineral and, conversely, that an increase leads to increased transition of these elements into bone. Presently, it seems more than likely that the formation of inorganic crystals in bone must occur by a process of heterogeneous phase transformation which does not occur within the lumen of blood vessels and soft tissue. This implies that calcium and phosphate from the fluids bathing bone are rendered "mineralizable" by the interaction of ions in the bathing fluids with a unique "nucleating center" in bone (most probably collagen fibrils). In order for heterogeneous nucleation to occur, the tissue fluid in contact with the nucleation center in bone must be in metastable equilibrium. To date, this hypothesis has not been verified, since it cannot be determined a priori from the chemical composition and the properties of the fluids bathing bone whether it is in metastable equilibrium with the mineral phase of bone. Therefore, until the determination of the plasma Ca × P ion product can be correlated in vivo with the mineralizing propensity of plasma, and until the effective ion product which governs mineralization in vivo is known, it appears unwise to consider the plasma Ca × P ion product a precise physiologic determinant of new bone formation and skeletal turnover.

CALCIUM HOMEOSTASIS

Calcium Absorption

The homeostasis of calcium in blood and extracellular fluid represents one of the most exquisite biologic control systems in man. The level of circulating calcium depends on a balance between the amount added by the resorption of bone and intestinal absorption and renal reabsorption on one hand and the calcium lost by skeletal formation or "accretion" and by renal and intestinal excretion on the other. It should be stressed that measurements of "calcium balance" in man are likely to be poor estimates of actual calcium retention. Since the "balance" is in essence the calculated difference between a large intake and a large excretion, the difference between these is inherently inaccurate. The usual errors, namely, failure of the subject to consume all the diet and failure to collect all the excreta, may lead to false-positive balances The extent to which such errors have influenced prevailing concepts of calcium homeostasis in health and disease is presently unknown.

The average diet consumed daily by human subjects contains approximately 400 to 800 mg of calcium. The recommended dietary intake for adults approximates 10 mg per kilogram of body weight per day. Whereas up to 75 per cent of ingested calcium may be absorbed by children during periods of rapid skeletal growth and remodeling, 30 to 50 per cent of the dietary intake is absorbed in adults. The division of calcium intake into multiple feedings rather than a single feeding is less likely to saturate intestinal absorptive mechanisms and will increase calcium absorption. An intestinal adaptation demonstrated by individuals ingesting low calcium diets is achieved by more efficient absorption of dietary calcium than in people accustomed to higher intakes. Calcium is absorbed primarily in the duodenum and upper jejunum. All the mechanisms which condition or regulate the absorptive process are still incompletely defined, although vitamin D is most effective in this regard. It appears well established, however, that net calcium absorption depends on both simple passive or facilitated diffusional and active transport processes (i.e., a net movement against a concentration gradient). The latter requires metabolic energy in the form of oxidative phosphorylation, intact mitochondria, a specific ATP-ase, and a soluble intestinal calcium-binding protein. The efficiency of calcium absorption is increased by vitamin D, parathyroid hormone, lactose, systemic alkalosis, an acid environment in the intestinal lumen, growth hormone, and certain amino acids such as ar-

ginine, lysine, and tryptophan. Its absorption is decreased by cortisol or synthetic glucocorticoids such as prednisone, by excess unabsorbed fatty acids in the intestinal contents, by thyroid hormones, by diets rich in oxalate and undigestible organic phosphates (such as hexaphosphoinositol in bran), by the ingestion of alkali, in chronic debilitating diseases, after gastric surgery, and in clinical disorders characterized by increased gastrointestinal transit time. Although alleged to interfere with calcium absorption as the result of formation of poorly soluble calcium phosphate, high phosphate intakes probably exert minimal effects on calcium absorption in humans. In man, as in animals, calcium absorption also decreases with advancing age. Fecal calcium consists not only of unabsorbed ingested calcium but also of that calcium endogenously secreted into the gastrointestinal tract which is not absorbed. About 85 per cent of the calcium entering the intestine in this manner is secreted proximal to the site of absorption, presented to the absorptive sites, and assumed to be handled with the same efficiency as the calcium of dietary origin. Total intestinal calcium excretion in man averages 0.194±0.073 grams per day, whereas the secreted calcium which is not absorbed, or *endogenous fecal calcium,* averages 0.130±0.047 grams per day. Thus approximately 15 per cent of the total intestinal calcium secretion is assumed to be nonabsorbable, even under conditions when dietary calcium is completely absorbed. These values are based on the assumption that dietary calcium mixes homogeneously with endogenously secreted calcium, that the absorptive efficiencies for both are identical, and that a portion of the endogenous calcium is unabsorbed because it enters the gut distal to the absorptive site(s). There is general agreement that this endogenous fecal fraction, like the daily losses of calcium in sweat, exerts little control on the day-to-day regulation of calcium balance. It should be noted, however, that in certain clinical situations such as thyrotoxicosis, the calcium losses in sweat, which normally range between 20 and 350 mg per day, may be considerable because of the increased concentrations of calcium in the sweat as well as the increased volume of sweat. In addition, calcium losses in sweat may approximate 1 gram per day in individuals working at high temperatures.

Following alterations in dietary calcium intake, a consistent pattern of changes obtains in calcium homeostasis. Whereas bone formation rates are unaffected by dietary perturbations, calcium excretion and bone resorption rates respond homeostatically to alterations in calcium intake. Calcium can be administered orally in the form of its lactose, gluconate, carbonate, or sulfate salts. There seems to be little difference in the intestinal utilization of calcium from the gluconate, carbonate, sulfate, or lactate salts.

Calcium Excretion

Once absorbed, the calcium enters the extracellular fluid and rapidly exchanges with the calcium in the exchangeable moiety of bone mineral and that in the glomerular filtrate. The daily urinary excretion of calcium in normal human subjects on diets containing 400 to 800 mg per day ranges between 80 and 250 mg. An exponential relationship exists between dietary and urinary calcium so that wide variations in intake are accompanied by parallel but only slight alterations in excretion. The urinary excretion of calcium is determined more by the absorption of calcium from the intestine than by the dietary intake. The more efficient the intestinal absorption, the greater will be the absolute change in urinary calcium for a given change in calcium intake. Since the efficiency of absorption decreases in man with advancing age, the variation of urine calcium with calcium intake is greater in young than in older individuals. Variations in urinary calcium excretion normally play an insignificant role in modifying the effect of wide swings in calcium intake in calcium homeostasis. There is a diurnal variation in the rate of calcium excretion, the greatest excretion occurring during the day and a nadir during the evening hours.

The amount of non-protein-bound calcium filtered by the glomeruli in man averages 10,000 mg per 24 hours. Normally, approximately 99 per cent of the filtered load is reabsorbed by the renal tubules so that, on the average, 100 mg of calcium is excreted per day. In hypocalcemic states (i.e., serum calcium concentrations below 7.5 mg per 100 ml), renal tubular reabsorption of calcium is so complete that it virtually disappears from the urine. The major part of calcium reabsorption, like that of sodium, occurs in the proximal convoluted tubules and in the ascending limb of Henle's loop, the remainder presumably absorbed in more distal parts of the nephron. Whereas the distal tubular reabsorption of calcium appears independent of sodium, calcium and sodium ions appear to share a common transport pathway in the proximal tubule. To this extent, calcium excretion is dependent upon sodium intake and excretion. Calcium excretion is increased not only by saline diuresis but also by diets rich in carbohydrate, protein, or magnesium, by phosphate deprivation, by metabolic acidosis, by cortisol or any of the synthetic glucocorticoids, or by thyroid and growth hormones. Hypercalciuria is often seen in metabolic or metastatic bone disease characterized by rapid bone destruction with or without simultaneously occurring hypercalcemia. The renal tubular reabsorption of calcium is increased by parathyroid hormone, a fall in plasma calcium, metabolic alkalosis, and benzothiazine diuretics.

553.2. PHOSPHORUS

Of the 11 to 14 grams of phosphorus per kilogram of fat-free tissue in the normal adult, 85 per cent is in the skeleton. The remainder is distributed between tissue and membrane components of skeletal muscle, skin, nervous tissue, and other organs. Whereas most of the phosphorus in soft tissue and cell membranes is in the form of organic esters, almost all the phosphorus in bone is contained in the mineral phase as inorganic orthophosphate and small amounts of inorganic phosphate. The regulation of plasma phosphate is not as readily explained as that of plasma calcium, since the circulating phosphate is in equilibrium not only with skeletal and cellular inorganic phosphate but also with a large number of organic compounds resulting from cellular metabolism. The phosphate ion is essential for the metabolism of carbohydrate, lipids, and protein, functioning as a cofactor in a multitude of enzyme systems and contributing to the metabolic potential in the form of "high energy phosphate" compounds. Phos-

phate functions to modify acid-base equilibrium in plasma and within cells and plays fundamental roles in modifying the development and maturation of bone, in the renal excretion of hydrogen ions, and in modifying the effects of the B vitamins.

Although the sequence of events which obtains during the nucleation of bone collagen is still imperfectly understood, collagen fibrils exhibit a remarkable faculty to form covalent bonds with phosphate. The phosphorylation of collagen has been considered the initiating event in the nucleation of bone. In addition to this conditioning role played by phosphate in the formation of the apatitic structure, it also affects bone resorption, mineralization, and collagen synthesis and thus plays an integral role in calcium homeostasis. The available evidence is consistent with the interpretation that these effects are due to a direct effect of phosphate upon the metabolic functions of bone cells.

PLASMA PHOSPHATE

In the human adult, plasma inorganic phosphate ranges between 2.5 and 4.4 mg per deciliter, with a mean of 3.5 mg per deciliter. Dietary phosphate, stage of growth and age, time of day, hormonal interplay, and renal function all contribute to the variability of the fasting serum phosphate concentration. Eighty-eight per cent of the plasma phosphate is unfilterable; some of this is complexed with mono- or divalent cations, such as $Na+$, $Ca++$, and $Mg++$. At normal blood pH, 85 per cent of the ultrafilterable phosphate is in the form of HPO_4^{-2}, the remainder existing mainly as $H_2PO_4^-$.

As noted earlier for calcium, the concentration of plasma phosphate varies with age. In prepubertal children the mean value for circulating phosphate approximates 5 mg per 100 ml with an upper normal limit approaching 6 mg per 100 ml. Normal adult values are gradually approached by the third decade, after which, in men, plasma phosphate decreases progressively with advancing age. The trend of values for plasma phosphate in females represents a unique circumstance; they decline gradually between ages 20 and 35 and rise after age 40. The higher levels of phosphate in the female over 40 years of age seem to be related to the menopause. This assumes more significance, since not only are postmenopausal females deficient in estrogen (a phosphaturic substance) but a positive correlation reportedly exists between serum inorganic phosphate and the extent of bone resorption in middle-aged and elderly women. Total serum phosphate may also normally fluctuate by as much as 1 to 2 mg per 100 ml. These variations generally reflect abrupt shifts of inorganic phosphate between extracellular fluid and intracellular compartments, rather than a net gain or loss of phosphate from the body. The administration of hexoses or hormones, such as insulin, glucagon, or epinephrine, results in a reduction in serum phosphate, presumably by stimulating the cellular utilization of glucose and accelerating the formation of intracellular phosphate esters. A systemic alkalosis has been associated with a fall in circulating phosphate and attributed to a shift of phosphate out of the extracellular fluid compartment. The fall in plasma phosphate concentration is apparently greater in respiratory than in comparable levels of metabolic alkalosis. Thus the evaluation of hypophosphatemia should always include measurements of the pH and total CO_2 content of plasma.

Whereas starvation is occasionally associated with a decrease in plasma inorganic phosphate, acidosis and excessive catabolism of body tissue associated with starvation or lysis of neoplastic lymphoid cells during therapy may lead to cellular release of phosphate, hyperphosphatemia, and reciprocal hypocalcemia. Severe hypophosphatemia has also been reported in hypokalemic states, independent of the attendant metabolic alkalosis. Variations in the plasma level of inorganic phosphate most probably contribute to the regulation of bone turnover and to bioactivation of the vitamin D metabolite 25-hydroxycholecalciferol to 1,25-dihydroxycholecalciferol. It is noteworthy in this regard that severe dietary phosphate deprivation results in hypophosphatemia and increased circulating 1,25-dihydrocholecalciferol in women, whereas insignificant changes in the plasma levels of either substance obtain in phosphate-depleted males.

PHOSPHATE ABSORPTION

Most or all of the dietary phosphorus is absorbed as free phosphate. The efficiency of phosphate absorption is a function of both the dietary intake and the food source. Sixty to 70 per cent is absorbed on a normal intake, and maximal absorption (up to 90 per cent) is achieved on very low intakes. Various dietary forms of organic phosphate esters, such as the phytic acid of cereals and seeds, are not readily available to man, since the human intestine is relatively deficient in the enzyme phytase, essential for hydrolysis of the organic esters. Organic phosphate ester compounds may also interfere with calcium absorption, since they form insoluble calcium salts within the intestinal lumen. In animals, unsaturated fatty acids, iron, and aluminum interfere with intestinal phosphate absorption. Vitamin D increases intestinal phosphate absorption in certain animal species; however, a direct effect of vitamin D (or its biologically active metabolites) on phosphate absorption in man is yet to be adequately demonstrated. There is no known effective physiologic mechanism regulating the intestinal absorption of phosphate in man, the control of the phosphate economy being achieved primarily by variations in dietary intake and renal excretion. Fecal phosphorus represents both unabsorbed phosphate and that secreted into the gastrointestinal tract. In man with phosphorus intakes of approximately 1 to 1.50 grams per day, the secretion of endogenous phosphate into the intestinal lumen averages 3 mg per kilogram per day. Dietary phosphorus is absorbed to a greater extent than is calcium, and consequently the renal excretion of phosphate is much greater than that of calcium.

PHOSPHATE EXCRETION

Urinary phosphorus is largely inorganic phosphate, the amount depending primarily upon how much is absorbed from the intestinal tract. Phosphate exists in the forms of $HPO_4^{2-}/H_2PO_4^-$ in the glomerular filtrate in the ratio of 4 to 1. With normal renal function, urinary phosphorus usually amounts to approximately two thirds of the dietary phosphorus. Normally, a diurnal variation in phosphate clearance occurs with the usual pattern, that of a matutinal increase in urinary phosphorus:creatinine ratios. This circadian rhythm is related to physical activity, with the nadir appearing a few hours after the end of sleep. The loss of diurnal variation in adrenal-insufficient states and the documented inverse correlation between phosphate excretion and plasma cortisol levels suggest that this rhythm is controlled by the adrenal glands.

In man, the tubular reabsorption of phosphate cleared by the glomeruli is normally 85 to 95 per cent. This process is age related and rate limited, with a maximal tubular reabsorptive capacity in adults of 4 to 8 mg per minute. The tubular reabsorption of phosphate is increased by short-term cortisol therapy and growth hormone, and is decreased by digoxin, estrogen, thyroid hormone, parathyroid hormone, long-term cortisol therapy, and elevations in circulating calcium.

PHOSPHORUS REQUIREMENTS

The average daily phosphorus requirement of adults in the United States is estimated at 0.8 to 1.5 grams per day. The primary source of calcium in the American diet is milk; other major sources of phosphorus are poultry, fish, and meat. Non-nutritious soft drinks containing excess phosphorus in the form of phosphoric acid also serve as sources for children and adults alike. The relatively greater availability of phosphate-containing foodstuffs in Western diets has resulted in a calcium:phosphate dietary ratio much lower than that recommended to maintain the integrity of skeletal tissue. This matter is of some concern, since diets with a low Ca:P ratio have led to progressive bone loss in rats, dogs, and horses and may stimulate secondary hyperparathyroidism in man.

With the exception of young infants, the recommended allowance of phosphorus per day is the same as that of calcium, although the Ca:P ratio of diets ingested throughout the world today is reportedly less than 0.75. The Ca:P ratio of cow's milk of 1.3:1, compared with a Ca:P ratio of 2:1 in breast milk, may contribute to the syndrome of idiopathic hypocalcemia and tetany of infants on formula feedings. Phosphate depletion in man, a syndrome characterized by weakness, anorexia, malaise, and skeletal aches, can obtain during prolonged and excessive intake of nonabsorbable antacids. Specific abnormalities, such as hemolytic anemia, granulocyte dysfunction, erythrocyte glycolysis, hypercalciuria, and renal calculi, may also result from phosphate depletion. The syndrome has been experimentally produced in man and is readily reversed when the medication is discontinued and sufficient amounts of dietary phosphorus are consumed. Its frequency in the very large population of individuals ingesting antacids is unknown, but it is probably rare, based on the infrequency of published reports of this complication. Recognition and appropriate therapy require medical supervision, particularly when adjustments in drug therapy for peptic ulcer are involved.

Since the kidney is capable of excreting 600 to 900 mg of phosphorus daily, hyperphosphatemia is rare in the absence of chronic renal disease, and then only when the glomerular filtration rate falls below 20 ml per minute. Hyperphosphatemia is also characteristic of disorders of parathyroid secretion and metabolism, such as hypoparathyroidism and pseudohypoparathyroidism, and can be accentuated by phosphate feeding. There are no specific signs or symptoms of hyperphosphatemia per se, although the hypocalcemia often associated with hyperphosphatemia (and exacerbated by phosphate feeding) can cause enhanced neuroexcitability, tetany, and convulsions.

553.3. THE STRUCTURE OF BONE AND ITS RELATION TO CALCIUM HOMEOSTASIS

Bone functions not only as a supporting organ for the body but also as a well organized dynamic system consisting of mineral, a matrix of collagen fibers, and cells. The cells include osteocytes, osteoblasts, and osteoclasts and occupy 3 to 4 per cent of the total volume. The collagen fibers are spatially oriented, highly organized in interlacing bundles and layers, and embedded in a gelatinous mucopolysaccharide ground substance which accounts for 4 to 5 per cent of the organic bone matrix. The mucopolysaccharides (or glycosaminoglycans), covalently linked to specific noncollagenous proteins in combination with collagen, form the matrix of connective tissue. They are composed of a polypeptide or "core protein," to which side chains of polysaccharides are attached. The polysaccharide chain consists of repeating disaccharide units composed of alternating hexosamine and uronic moieties. Although the dermatan sulfate, heparan sulfate, and keratan sulfate are quantitatively minor components of skeletal tissue, they appear to contribute significantly to bone matrix maturation and mineralization and bone remodeling. Inherited lysomal storage diseases in which mucopolysaccharides accumulate as a result of deficiency of specific degradative enzymes (i.e., mucopolysaccharidoses such as Hurler's or Hunter's syndrome) result in the accumulation of skeletal mucopolysaccharides and a spectrum of skeletal dysplasias (see Ch. 538.1).

In fully mineralized mature bone, the protein matrix accounts for approximately 35 per cent of the volume of the intercellular material, with mineral occupying most of the remainder. The molecular architecture of collagen demonstrates a characteristic x-ray diffraction pattern, with a wide-angle line of 2.86 Å and a low-angle diffraction diagram of 640 to 700 Å repeated along the individual fibril. The collagen fiber in bone is actually an aggregate of rod-shaped fundamental tropocollagen subunits. Individual units are made up of three polypeptide chains, each coiled in a left-handed helix and wound about each other in right-handed fashion. Each polypeptide unit has a molecular weight of approximately 120,000 and is composed of four subunits overlapping one another by one quarter of their length and joined by an ester linkage. This spatial orientation of the individual units is essential to the process of phase transformation and heterogeneous nucleation which initiates the deposition of microcrystalline material within and upon the fibrils. The specific orientation of collagen fibrils in the bone matrix and their spatial relationship to the crystalline phase also impart to the skeleton the mechanical properties of a two-phase system

and condition the so-called "breaking strength" and "elasticity" of bone. Cross-linkages between individual collagen polypeptide units and between tropocollagen subunits appear as collagen matures and, to a large extent, determine its physicochemical properties.

Collagen is chemically distinguished by its amino acid composition, with one third of its amino acid residues being glycine and another third proline, hydroxyproline, and alanine. The remaining third contains a variety of amino acids, the most important of which are lysine and hydroxylysine. Hydroxylysine is found almost exclusively in collagen and participates in the intermolecular cross-linkage between collagen subunits. In addition, the carbohydrates glucose and galactose are linked to collagen through the hydroxylysine residues. Although the relative amounts of the glycosylated hydroxylysines are quite constant for collagen-containing organs such as skin and bone, galactosylhydroxylysine predominates in bone, whereas glucosylgalactosylhydroxylysine predominates in skin. Recent studies indicate that the excretion of glycosylated hydroxylysines reflects the rate of bone collagen turnover, since patients with diseases of increased bone turnover, e.g., Paget's disease of bone and hyperparathyroidism, excrete increased amounts of galalactosylhydroxylysine. Hydroxyproline constitutes some 14 per cent of the collagen molecule and is derived not from dietary sources but from the hydroxylation of proline during the early stages of collagen biosynthesis by osteoblasts. Since the destruction of bone collagen involves the liberation of hydroxyproline which cannot be reutilized in the biosynthetic process, the urinary excretion of hydroxyproline-containing peptides is also commonly used as an indicator of bone turnover and collagen metabolism.

The maturation of bone matrix is dependent upon osteoblastic activity and certain bioelectrical fields in bone which are constantly produced by external mechanical stress. This latter electrical phenomenon, known as piezoelectricity, has been shown to influence the spatial orientation of collagen fibrils and to play an important role in directing the architecture and structural development of bone. As bone matrix is deposited on a bone-forming surface, an "osteoid seam" is formed which, following a complex sequence of biochemical changes, is normally mineralized. During this bone maturation and mineralization process, the enzyme alkaline phosphatase can be detected by appropriate staining techniques within osteoblasts and in the surrounding layers of newly deposited matrix. Although an elevation in plasma "bone" alkaline phosphatase (characteristically heat labile when compared to other isoenzymes such as placental or hepatic alkaline phosphatases) is often seen in actively growing children and in patients with disorders characterized by increased bone turnover, the role of this enzyme in active bone formation is still entirely conjectural. The bone alkaline phosphatase appears to be intrinsically related to the formation of collagen and may actually prepare the matrix for calcification by hydrolyzing inorganic pyrophosphate, a known inhibitor of biologic calcification. In favor of this hypothesis is the observation that there is a marked or total deficiency in bone alkaline phosphatase in hypophosphatasia, a disease characterized by increased pyrophosphate excretion and defective bone matrix calcification.

Bone resorption is characterized by concomitant dissolutions of both bone matrix and mineral and is histologically associated with large multinucleated cells known as osteoclasts. The mechanisms by which bone solids are solubilized are largely unknown. Collagenase and a variety of lysosomal proteases are involved in matrix hydrolysis, and large quantities of H^+ are consumed in solubilization of the mineral (approximately one proton for each calcium ion). The H^+ production derives from both organic acids and carbonic anhydrase, and is both dependent upon and stimulated by O_2 levels in the bathing fluids. Carbonic anhydrase has been specifically localized to osteoclasts, and its inhibitors can directly reduce bone resorption. Like the osteoblasts, the osteoclasts have been shown to arise from bone mesenchymal cells, although extraskeletal sites of production have also been demonstrated. When compared to the rate of bone formation, osteoclastic resorption of bone is an extremely fast and efficient process. Consequently, stimulation of osteoclastic activity may result in the immediate release of large quantities of mineral from bone. Although the resorption of the mineral phase of bone and the arrested synthesis and degradation of organic matrix can be adequately explained by histochemical evidence demonstrating local accumulation of citrate and lactate, the exact mechanism by which osteoclasts resorb bone is still unknown. The osteocyte is another cellular element which regulates bone resorption. Osteocytes are localized within the substance of densely mineralized compact cortical bone. These cells release alkaline phosphatase, proteases, and lysosomal acid hydrolases. Histologic evidence of osteolytic resorption of compact bone in pregnancy, hyperparathyroidism, osteomalacia, and thyrotoxicosis suggest that osteocyte-mediated resorption may play a significant role in the rapid mobilization of calcium from bone. In contrast, the role of the osteoclast may be more important in regulating the normal remodeling process of skeletal tissue and in the chronic resorptive response to hormones.

Bone affords an enormous depot of calcium which, when appropriately stimulated by a variety of hormones and metabolic agents, serves as the guardian of the circulating calcium pool. Unlike the mineral of tooth enamel, which is relatively inert, bone undergoes constant remodeling and turnover. The dynamic process of bone turnover normally releases into blood and then reaccumulates from 250 mg to 1 gram of calcium per day. Little calcium is deposited in the fetus during the first trimester of pregnancy, but the concentration rises rapidly during the early gestation until a body weight of 0.5 kg is attained. Gradual increments are observed thereafter until term. During the final trimester, the human fetus acquires approximately 20 grams of calcium from maternal sources. The total calcium content of a full-term neonate weighing 3500 grams approaches 30 grams, or about 1 per cent of the body weight. The turnover of skeletal calcium varies with age. It has been estimated to be 100 per cent per annum in infants up to one year and decreases with age to a turnover rate of 10 per cent in older children. The skeleton weighs approximately 100 grams at birth and actually doubles in weight during the first year of life. Skeletal growth during childhood involves calcium retention of not more than 150 mg per day until after the first decade. During peak adolescent growth, bone development is at its maximum, and calcium retained

as bone may range between 275 and 500 mg per day. The rate of turnover is higher in cancellous or trabecular bones (e.g., vertebrae and ribs) than in compact bones such as the skull and mandible. In adults, after epiphyseal closure and longitudinal growth have ceased, the turnover rate is approximately 2 to 4 per cent per annum. During adult life, skeletal growth does not entirely cease, since there is both continuing subperiosteal bone formation and a continuation of the later adolescent shift to endosteal bone formation or apposition. At this time skeletal maintenance requires the deposition of approximately 180 grams of calcium per annum, or 18 per cent of the total skeletal content. The skeleton is in a relative steady state, since bone formation equals bone resorption with no net change in skeletal mass. Between the fourth and fifth decades, there is a shift in this equilibrium and bone resorption dominates. Skeletal mass then begins to decline with advancing age at a rate approximating 0.7 per cent of the total mass per annum. This inevitable decrease in bone mass with advancing years obtains independent of wide variations in calcium intake and dietary habits. The significant features of this universal loss of skeletal mass are as follows: (1) among young adults, the skeletal mass is greater in males than females and greater in blacks than whites; (2) the loss begins earlier in females than in males; (3) taller subjects of both sexes lose bone less rapidly; and (4) although the onset of loss in females antedates the menopause, the rate of skeletal loss in some females is distinctly accelerated after the menopause. Thus since the maximal skeletal maturity is less for the white female than for the male or for blacks of either sex, and since the loss begins earlier in the female and proceeds at a more rapid rate after the menopause, net skeletal mass is lowest in the postmenopausal white female.

The exchange of calcium between bone and circulating fluids is still ill defined and poorly understood. It appears to be divisible into the slow processes of bone formation and resorption and the far more rapid processes of ion exchange with accessible crystal surfaces. The extensive osteon surface (or haversian units of compact bone) plus that afforded by trabecular bone provides an enormous surface area for interchange between extracellular fluids and bone mineral. Normally, less than 1 per cent of the skeletal calcium is available for free ionic exchange with the extracellular fluid. The calcium in blood, extracellular fluid, and extraosseous cellular compartments accounts for 1 per cent of whole body calcium and, together with the exchangeable calcium of bone, comprises the miscible, or readily exchangeable, calcium pool. Since most of the skeletal calcium is not in a form readily diffusible to combat hypocalcemia and maintain homeostasis, calcium must be mobilized by active resorptive processes.

Bone lability is maintained by the concurrent activities of bone formation and resorption. Osseous tissue is continually being deposited and resorbed, mainly as a result of the activity of the connective tissue cells covering its surfaces. Changes in bone resorption are not simply a consequence of changes in the activity of existing cell machinery, but depend on the continuous transformation of resting undifferentiated cells to osteocytic cells, osteoblasts, and osteoclasts. Osteoclastic and osteocytic response to parathyroid hormone represents one of the most effective control mechanisms available to homeostatic control of bone turnover. This regulating action of parathyroid hormone is normally accomplished through continuous secretion, which, as detailed in Ch. 552.1, is inversely related to the extracellular fluid calcium ion concentration. In contrast to the action of parathyroid hormone on bone, the inhibition of bone resorption is the principal, or perhaps sole, function of calcitonin (see Ch. 552.1). In addition, vitamin D, through its biologically active metabolites, alters the responsiveness of bone to both parathyroid hormone and calcitonin so that alterations in bone resorption serve the needs of skeletal growth and remodeling, as well as calcium homeostasis. Although the roles of parathyroid hormone, calcitonin, and vitamin D metabolites in maintaining calcium homeostasis are of paramount importance, it should also be appreciated that insulin, growth hormone, somatomedin, thyroxine, androgens, estrogens, adrenal glucocorticoids, and circulating inorganic phosphate may also be contributory.

Bourne, G. H. (ed.): The Biochemistry and Physiology of Bone. Vol. IV, Calcification and Physiology. New York, Academic Press, 1976.

Keating, P. R., Jones, J. D., Elveback, L. R., and Randall, R. V.: The relation of age and sex to distribution of values in healthy adults of serum calcium, inorganic phosphorus, magnesium, alkaline phosphatase, total proteins, albumin, and blood urea. J. Lab. Clin. Med., 73:825, 1969.

Moore, E. W.: Ionized calcium in normal serum, ultrafiltrates and whole blood determined by ion-exchange electrodes. J. Clin. Invest., 49:318, 1970.

Raisz, L. G.: Bone metabolism and calcium regulation, In Avioli, L. V., and Krane, S. M. (eds.): Metabolic Bone Disease, Vol I. New York, Academic Press, 1977, pp. 1–42.

Vaughn, J.: The Physiology of Bone. 2nd ed. New York, Oxford, University Press, 1975.

554.   VITAMIN D

Vitamin D_3 is normally produced in the epidermal layer of skin when ultraviolet irradiation is absorbed by the provitamin 7-dehydrocholesterol. Although the manner in which 7-dehydrocholesterol is normally converted to vitamin D_3 in skin has not been established, it is assumed that the chemistry is similar to that observed in vitro wherein an unstable form of 7-dehydrocholesterol is produced during irradiation and converted to a vitamin D precursor (previtamin D). Previtamin D is then converted to a vitamin D_3 slowly without additional ultraviolet activation. To date, the endogenous production rate of vitamin D_3 in man is unknown, but it must be at least equivalent to the minimal vitamin D dietary dose of 200 to 400 IU daily essential to cure vitamin D–lack rickets, since it has been observed that ultraviolet skin irradiation alone is curative in this regard.

Following the photochemical conversion of 7-dehydrocholesterol to vitamin D_3, the preformed vitamin D_3 is absorbed into the subepidermal microcirculation and transported in plasma to the liver and target organs bound to a specific globulin with a molecular weight of 50,000 to 60,000. Dietary vitamin D_3 (cholecalciferol) or vitamin D_2 (ergocalciferol) is absorbed primarily from the duodenum and jejunum into lymphatic channels, with both bile salts and intraluminal lipids permissive in this regard. Although lipoproteins do not appear to be quantitatively important for the transport of vitamin D_3 in plasma, most of the vitamin absorbed from the intestine of animals and man is transported in lymph by chylomicrons. Presently, the site of transfer of vitamin D_3 from chylomicrons to its specific plasma globular transport protein has not been established, although it appears likely that the liver is fundamental for this transformation. The absorbed vitamin D_2 or vitamin D_3 then admixes with endogenously synthesized vitamin D_3 and is either sequestered into storage depots such as adipose tissue and muscle by specific tissue-binding proteins or metabolically transferred by the liver. It seems likely that these tissue-binding proteins also play a role in the regulation of the metabolism of vitamin D and its metabolites. In man, circulating vitamin D (vitamin D_3 + vitamin D_2) levels normally range between 8 and 45 ng per milliliter. Whereas at normal plasma concentrations vitamin D disappears with a biologic half-time of 19 to 25 hours, its metabolic disposal is conditioned by the state of vitamin D nutrition and plasma concentrations with high and low circulating levels, resulting in a decrease and increase, respectively, in the plasma disappearance rate.

Endogenously synthesized and dietary vitamin D_3 and presumably dietary vitamin D_2 are subsequently metabolized to their respective 25-hydroxylated derivatives, i.e., 25-hydroxycholecalciferol ($25OHD_3$) and 25-hydroxyergocalciferol ($25OHD_2$), by a hepatic microsomal enzyme system that requires reduced pyridine nucleotide and molecular oxygen. Although it has been demonstrated that the hepatic 25-hydroxylation of vitamin D is substrate specific and to some extent feedback regulated by the reaction product, the exact nature of this servocontrol mechanism is still in doubt, as is its function in preventing the toxic effects of vitamin D overdosage. The hydroxylated vitamin D metabolites $25OHD_2$ and $25OHD_3$ also circulate bound to a globular protein, indistinguishable from that which binds the parent vitamin D, with a biologic half-time of 12 days. Circulating levels of 25OHD ($25OHD_2$ + $25OHD_3$) in normal subjects living in the United States, as measured by competitive protein-binding radio-ligand assays, range between 15 and 30 ng per milliliter. Reported lower mean circulating 25OHD levels of adults from the British Isles presumably reflect both the higher dietary intake of vitamin D and the greater sunshine exposure in the United States because of its more southerly latitudes. A direct correlation does appear to exist between circulating and fetal 25OHD, as well as between plasma 25OHD and age, sunlight exposure, and diet. Not only do $25OHD_2$ and $25OHD_3$ represent the major circulating forms of vitamin D; they have also been shown to concentrate in bone, to stimulate calcium absorption, and to increase bone resorption without further structural modification. $25OHD_3$ increases the proximal renal tubular reabsorption of calcium, sodium, and phosphate in certain mammals (rats) with the control of phosphate excretion antagonistic to the phosphaturic effect of parathyroid hormone.

Whereas the metabolic fate of $25OHD_3$ in intestine, bone, and storage depot sites such as adipose tissue and muscle is presently ill defined, it is further hydroxylated by the kidney to either 1,25-dihydroxycholecalciferol ($1,25(OH)_2D_3$) or 24,25-dihydroxycholecalciferol ($24,25(OH)_2D_3$) by a carbon monoxide–sensitive mitochondrial system requiring reduced pyridine nucleotide and molecular oxygen for maximal activity. A number of observations made either in intact animals or from renal homogenates, isolated renal mitochondria, or proximal tubular preparations are consistent with the view that the control of $1,25(OH)_2D_3$ production by the kidney is indeed complex, with potassium, calcium, inorganic phosphate, estrogen, prolactin, and cyclic AMP as well as parathyroid hormone, calcitonin, and pH all implicated as controlling factors. However, the conversion of $25OHD_3$ to $1,25(OH)_2D_3$ is regulated primarily by a sensitive servo-control mechanism modulated by circulating calcium and $1,25(OH)_2D_3$ levels, as well as by parathyroid hormone and the inorganic phosphate content of renal cortical cells. Whereas $1,25(OH)_2D_3$ once synthesized by the kidney is metabolized to a substance with unknown biologic activity, $24,25(OH)_2D_3$, which circulates at a concentration of 1.68 ± 0.82 ng per milliliter, is further metabolized by the kidney to 1,24,25 trihydroxyvitamin D_3 $(1,24,25(OH)_3D_3)$. Both $25OHD_3$ and $1,25(OH)_2D_3$ can also be converted to $1,24,25(OH)_3D_3$. $1,24,25(OH)_3D_3$ is reportedly 60 per cent as active as vitamin D_3 in curing rickets in animals and is less active on a weight basis than $1,25(OH)_2D_3$ in stimulating and sustaining the intestinal absorption of calcium and bone resorption. Presently, $1,24,25(OH)_3D_3$ is considered to exert its biologic activity preferentially by promoting the intestinal absorption of calcium, with the kidney essential for its formation.

$1,25(OH)_2D_3$, i.e., $1,25(OH)_2D_2 + 1,25(OH)_2D_3$, circulates with a biologic half-life of 24 hours at concentrations of 25 to 33 pg per milliliter in adults. Preliminary studies suggest that young adolescents have higher plasma levels, i.e., 49 to 66 pg per milliliter. It seems well established that the 1,25-hydroxylated vitamin D_3 derivative is *the* metabolic or hormonal form of vitamin D_3 which controls the intestinal transport of calcium (and perhaps the remodeling of bone), since it is some 4 to 13 times as effective as vitamin D_3 and over twice as effective as $25(OH)D_3$ in this regard. Unlike $25-OHD_3$, $1,25(OH)_2D_3$ has a minimal effect on the renal tubular reabsorption of phosphate. $1,25(OH)_2D_3$ does, however, possess significant bone resorptive properties, with an in vitro effectiveness some one hundred times that of the parent $25(OH)D_3$. The isolation of molecular receptors for $1,25(OH)_2D_3$ in bone and the preferential accumulation of $1,25(OH)_2D_3$ in the nucleus of bone cells suggest a mechanism of $1,25(OH)_2D_3$ action in bone similar to that proposed for the control of calcium translocation across the intestinal cell. Finally, although another vitamin D_3 diol metabolite, 25,26-dihydroxycholecalciferol, with weak biologic activity has been isolated from plasma and structurally identified, its tissue of origin and metabolic fate are still unknown. There is rather substantial evidence that this dihydroxy vitamin D metabolite is not a byproduct of the renal tubular or intestinal cellular metabolism of $25(OH)D_3$, $1,25(OH)_2D_3$, $24,25(OH)_2D_3$, or $1,24,25-(OH)_3D_3$. Thus on the basis of experimental evidence obtained in man and a variety of animal species, the current working hypothesis depicts vitamin D_3 primarily as an inert reservoir substance; $25(OH)D_3$ as the major circulating biologically active metabolite; and $1,25(OH)_2D_3$ as the metabolite with maximal biologic activity, which, together with parathyroid hormone and calcitonin, regulates the intestinal absorption of calcium and remodeling of bone.

The manner in which the vitamin D metabolites exert control over the molecular events that precede and condition the intestinal absorption of calcium and bone turnover is still uncertain. Preliminary observations suggest that the diol or triol metabolites are initially bound to specific cytosol proteins in bone and intestine prior to their incorporation onto nuclear receptor sites, where they ultimately affect the transcriptional processes directly or regulate the release or transport of nuclear-derived RNA. Vitamin D metabolites may also be considered tropic substances for the intestinal mucosa, since the administration of vitamin D_3 stimulates mucosal growth as well as protein synthesis.

Gray, R. W., Caldas, A. E., Wilz, D. R., Lemann, J., Jr., Smith, G. A., and DeLuca, H.: Metabolism and excretion of ^3H-1,25-(OH)$_2$–vitamin D_3 in healthy adults. J. Clin. Endocrinol. Metab., 46:756, 1978.

Haussler, M. R., and McCain, T. A.: Basic and clinical concepts related to vitamin D metabolism and action. N. Engl. J. Med., 297:947, 1041, 1977.

555. HYPERCALCEMIA

Although hypercalcemia has been traditionally associated with primary hyperparathyroidism (see Ch. 552.2), it has been well established that metastatic malignancy and a variety of clinical syndromes may be associated with this laboratory finding. Regardless of etiology, the syndrome of hypercalcemia should be considered a potentially lethal one. Moreover, since automated multiple screening laboratory procedures have documented a 2 per cent incidence of hypercalcemia during routine screening maneuvers and because of the protean clinical manifestations of hypercalcemia states, the physician is now more than ever confronted with the differential diagnostic spectrum of this disorder. Familiarity with the syndrome and its causes and complications, as well as with modern acceptable modes of therapy, can be lifesaving.

Hypercalcemia may result from a variety of nonrelated pathologic states as well as from inappropriate blood sampling and laboratory error. The latter can be effectively eliminated as a cause of spurious hypercalcemia by avoiding the use of cork stoppers and by utilizing acid-washed glassware and calcium-free disposable syringes.

MALIGNANCY

The most common cause of hypercalcemia is cancer. The spectrum is wide, ranging from solid tumors, predominantly breast, lung, and kidney, to hematologic malignancies such as multiple myeloma, lymphoma, and leukemia. Breast carcinoma accounts for over half the reported malignancies with hypercalcemia, followed in frequency by carcinoma of the lung, kidney, and cervix. The hypercalcemia of malignancy commonly results from widespread destruction of bone by metastasis and is characterized by a normal or elevated serum phosphate level. On occasion, because of inadequate food intake, patients with hypercalcemia and metastatic skeletal lesions may actually present with abnormally low serum phosphate values. The hypercalcemia is believed to result from accelerated osteolysis and a release of calcium and phosphorus from the bone into the vascular compartment at rates greater than those at which these substances are cleared by the kidney and gastrointestinal tract. In this regard, it should be noted that approximately 100 mg of calcium is ordinarily released by the replacement of 1 gram of bone. The relative insensitivity of conventional skeletal roentgenograms and the fact that only 50 per cent of patients with histologically documented skeletal metastasis have radiographic findings indicative of invasive carcinoma often make it difficult to document metastatic bone disease. Often hypercalcemia occurs in previously normocalcemic patients with breast carcinoma following initiation of therapy with estrogens, androgens, or progestational agents. In this instance, the offending agent is discontinued and glucocorticoids administered. This sequence of events may seem paradoxical, since estrogen and/or androgens have also been used effectively to combat the hypercalcemia that develops in untreated patients with metastatic breast carcinoma.

Less often, the hypercalcemia of malignancy is caused by increased bone resorption secondary to the action of a substance(s) produced and secreted by the neoplasm. This syndrome has often been known as "pseudohyperparathyroidism," since immunochemical and physicochemical data indicate a close similarity to or identity of this ectopic humoral substance with native parathyroid hormone. The parathyroid glands are invariably normal in this syndrome, surgical removal of the neoplasm is followed by an abrupt fall in serum calcium toward normal, and recurrent hypercalcemia accompanies recurrent tumor growth. This sequence of events, although documented for ovarian, endometrial, and hepatic carcinomas, lymphomas, and a variety of other neoplasms, occurs with much greater frequency in renal cell carcinoma and carcinoma of the lung. The symptoms of hypercalcemia accompanying malignant disease are generally more conspicuous, appear abruptly, and often demonstrate rapid and relentless progression. They tend to be associated with a rapidly progressive illness with morbidly elevated serum calcium levels. In bedridden patients, the increased bone resorption attending immobilization may further contribute to the hypercalcemia. Although patients with the ectopic-hormone-producing neoplasms and hypercalciuria are less likely to present with clinical or radiographic evidence of bone disease or a history of recurrent renal calculi and tend to have serum chloride levels less than 102 mEq per liter, the clinical and laboratory expressions of this syndrome are quite often indistinguishable from those of patients with primary hyperparathyroidism. Hyperprostaglandinemia has also been implicated in the pathogenesis of hypercalcemia in some patients with solid tumor neoplasia and normal circulating immunoreactive parathyroid hormone. In this instance specific inhibitors of fatty acid cyclo-oxygenase such as indomethacin and aspirin may decrease prostaglandin synthesis and reverse the hypercalcemia. Elevations in serum calcium observed in patients with islet cell carcinoma and pancreatitic cholera have been attributed to the hypercalcemic effect of secretin.

Hypercalcemia is generally considered to be a rare complication of lymphoma and chronic leukemia. The frequency of hypercalcemia in acute (usually lymphatic) leukemia, which is approximated at 5 per cent, presumably develops as a result of extensive infiltration of bone and subsequent osteolysis. The relatively greater incidence of hypercalcemia in acute leukemic processes is probably related to the observation that skeletal lesions in adults with chronic leukemia are relatively uncommon, whereas the frequency of bone lesions in acute leukemia ranges between 50 and 90 per cent. Hypercalcemia complicating the acute leukemia state may precede other signs and symptoms of acute leukemia and become clinically manifest with gastrointestinal or central nervous system symptoms and/or the appearance of bone pain in a manner mimicking that resulting from local tissue invasion with leukemia cells. Thus serum calcium determinations are mandatory for the correct diagnosis and the institution of proper therapy. In reported instances of leukemia with hypercalcemia, common features include leukopenia, azotemia, and extensive infiltration of bone and other tissue. Hypercalcemia associated with Hodgkin's disease, lymphosarcoma, or reticulum cell sarcoma presumably also develops as a result of extensive malignant invasion of bone. Although reports of ectopic parathyroid hormone production have been recorded for acute myeloblastic and "undifferentiated" leukemia, there appears to be a greater tendency for solid tumors to be associated with an ectopic-PTH hypercalcemia. In this regard, it may be noteworthy that lymphomas are more often associated with hypo- than with hyperphosphatemia.

Although plasma alkaline phosphatase activity is usually normal in patients with multiple myeloma, the incidence of hypercalcemia in this disorder ranges between 20 and 50 per cent. In some but not in all instances, the hypercalcemia is attended by hypercalciuria. In some patients with multiple myeloma the hypercalcemia results from excessive osteoclastic bone resorption owing to the secretion of an osteoclastic-activating-factor (OAF) by the tumor cells. Dysproteinemia and specific gammopathies are also common and outstanding features of multiple myeloma and not infrequently result in elevations in total serum calcium. In these circumstances the total protein-bound calcium is high but ultrafilterable, and ionized calcium fractions are either normal or disproportionately low. Thus hypercalcemia in myeloma patients should not be categorically interpreted as a reflection of skeletal osteolysis. In fact, not infrequently patients with typical "punched out" x-ray lesions present with normal serum calcium levels. When associated with hypercalciuria and hyperphosphatasia, bone dissolution is probably much more likely. Serum inorganic phosphate may be normal, low, or slightly elevated in this disorder. Since renal function may be impaired by the deposition of calcium in renal tubules in the presence of longstanding renal disease and uremia, serum phosphate may also be markedly elevated.

VITAMIN D TOXICITY

Hypercalcemia results from vitamin D overdosage primarily because of an increase in intestinal calcium absorption. The documented osteolytic activity of the vitamin D metabolites, 25-hydroxycholecalciferol and 1,25-dihydroxycholecalciferol suggests that a stimulated skeletal resorption may also contribute to the hypercalcemia.

Vitamin D toxicity is a rare occurrence in adults and usually appears after treatment with 100,000 to 300,000 units daily for many months to years. There is wide variation in individual susceptibility, however, with hypercalcemia observed in some patients taking as little as 50,000 units per day for a few weeks. It should be stressed that the first sign of vitamin D intoxication is hypercalciuria (i.e., urinary calcium > 4 mg per kg per 24 hours) and not hypercalcemia. A high dietary calcium and pre-existing renal disease predispose to an early appearance and enhanced severity of intoxication. In some instances, calcification of soft tissues has been described mainly in the kidneys, bronchi, arteries, and periarticular tissue. Renal calcification is primarily arterial, with tubules and glomeruli involved less often. The syndrome has been observed with decreasing frequency in recent years, probably because the use of vitamin D in the treatment of rheumatoid arthritis has been virtually discontinued, and because the numerous reports of serious complications during high dose vitamin D therapy have caused certain restrictions with regard to dosage and duration of treatment. Serum phosphorus is usually normal or slightly elevated in this disorder, and alkaline phosphatase normal. Plasma 25OHD may increase five- to ten-fold, although 1,25(OH)$_2$D levels are normal. Treatment usually consists of adrenocortical steroids, hydration, oral sodium phytate, and cellulose phosphate. Regression of soft tissue calcification and improvement in renal function occur when therapy is initiated at an early stage.

VITAMIN A TOXICITY

Although not confined to bone, the effects of chronic excessive vitamin A intake may be most apparent in the skeleton. Such intoxication is rare; it has occurred most frequently in young children and elderly females who receive doses on the order of 100 times the normal daily vitamin requirement and in hunters who have ingested large quantities of polar bear liver. The initial bony change is painful periosteal proliferation, particularly of the ulnae, clavicles, and metatarsals. These are readily apparent on roentgenographic examination. Higher doses in small animals produce severe osteoporosis and multiple fractures. The diagnosis is suggested by a history of excessive vitamin intake and by finding high vitamin A levels in the plasma. Bone healing is usually complete when vitamin exposure ceases. The hypercalcemia results from direct action of vitamin A in bone and, indirectly, via vitamin A–induced elevations in parathyroid hormone secretion. The dangers of vitamin A intoxication will continue as long as over-the-counter multivitamin preparations containing more than the recommended daily requirements (3000 IU in children and 5000 IU in adults) exist. For this reason vitamin A preparations containing more than 5000 IU per dose should be dispensed only by prescription.

SARCOIDOSIS

The reported frequency of hypercalcemia in sarcoidosis varies widely, with reported incidences ranging from 2 to 60 per cent. In a recent review of over 4000 patients with this disease, the incidence of hypercalcemia approximated 12 per cent. The hypercalcemia of sarcoidosis occurs twice as frequently in males as in females and predominantly in patients with chronic or generalized disease. Although most patients have minimal elevation of serum calcium that either reverts to normal spontaneously or responds rapidly to therapy, occasionally the hypercalcemia is life threatening or causes progressive metastatic calcification with eventual death from uremia. In the latter instance, the hypercalcemia may be characterized by wide spontaneous fluctuations, by elevations persisting or recurring for as long as ten years, and by calcium levels as high as 20 mg per 100 ml.

The frequency of skeletal lesions in sarcoidosis is variably estimated at 5 to 26 per cent. The changes usually fall into one of three categories: (1) single or multiple rounded radiolucencies in the epiphyses, often referred to as punched-out lesions; (2) diffuse cortical thinning and widening of medulla, and a reticular pattern of the trabeculae producing a honeycombed configuration; or (3) coalescing lesions, producing bone destruction. The hands and feet are usually involved with greater frequency. Although the hypercalcemia has often been attributed to granulomatous invasion of bone, there is no apparent correlation with the hypercalcemia, serum phosphate, alkaline phosphatase, or radiographically evident bone disease. In fact, most patients with demonstrable bone involvement have not had hypercalcemia. Since circulating α_2 and β-globulin may also be increased in sarcoidosis, in some instances elevations in total calcium concentration may be secondary to increased calcium binding by these protein fractions. Hypercalciuria is at least twice as common as hypercalcemia in sarcoidosis. Persistent hypercalcemia may be present without hypercalciuria if the glomerular filtration rate is sufficiently reduced by renal disease and even, on occasion, when renal function is normal. In some patients, both the hypercalcemia and hypercalciuria are due to an excessive sensitivity to vitamin D and an enhanced intestinal absorption of calcium. This "sensitivity" is presently undefined, since plasma levels of 25OHD$_3$, the major circulating form of vitamin D, are normal in sarcoidosis, as is the conversion of 25OHD$_3$ to 1,25(OH)$_2$D$_3$, the vitamin D metabolite which primarily regulates the intestinal absorption of calcium. This hyperabsorptive state responds dramatically to glucocorticoid therapy. Until the exact cause of hypercalcemia in this disease is established, the mechanism by which cortisol or its structurally related synthetic analogues correct the hypercalcemia is still in doubt. The most provocative theory is one which invokes complete or partial metabolic antagonism between glucocorticoids and vitamin D metabolism. In this regard, it has been demonstrated that cortisone interferes with the metabolic conversion of vitamin D to its biologically active metabolite(s), increases the rate of degradation of 1,25(OH)$_2$D$_3$, and also directly inhibits the action of vitamin D on the intestinal absorption of calcium. The hypothesis which attributes the hypercalcemia and hypercalciuria of sarcoidosis to vitamin D$_3$ hypersensitivity is compatible with the observation that the hypercalcemia is more common in the summer months when the production of vitamin D$_3$ in the skin by sunlight is enhanced and that hypercalcemia can be induced in some patients by ultraviolet irradiation.

Although hyperparathyroidism may rarely simulate sarcoidosis, the major source of diagnostic confusion has been the frequency with which sarcoidosis has mimicked the biochemical abnormalities of hyperparathyroidism, since hypercalcemic patients with sarcoidosis frequently demonstrate elevations in serum alkaline phosphatase and hypophosphatemia. Although normal or low serum phosphorus levels may occur with either disorder, hypercalcemia and normal or elevated phosphate levels in a patient with good renal function should suggest sarcoidosis. In doubtful circumstances the so-called "cortisone suppression" test may be used to differentiate hyperparathyroidism from hypercalcemic sarcoidosis. One administers 50 mg of cortisone or 5 to 10 mg of prednisone orally every eight hours for 10 to 12 days. The hypercalcemia of sarcoidosis, vitamin D intoxication, and adrenal insufficiency is characteristically corrected by the tenth day, whereas that of hyperparathyroidism is usually unaffected. Glucocorticoids still remain the drugs of choice for the short-term treatment of hypercalcemia caused by sarcoidosis. In view of the potential hazards of long-term steroid therapy, dietary restriction of calcium, sodium phytate, and cellulose phosphate and avoidance of sunlight are considered more acceptable alternatives for treating the prolonged hypercalcemic states.

IDIOPATHIC HYPERCALCEMIA

Idiopathic hypercalcemia of infancy is a disorder characterized by a peculiar elfin facies, retardation of growth and mentality, osteosclerosis, and renal dysfunction associated with hypercalcemia, hypercalciuria, and azotemia. Nonspecific cardiac murmurs, cardiac failure, hypertension, and metastatic calcifications have also been observed in this disorder. Bone changes often considered diagnostic for this disease consist of sclerotic changes on the frontal and basal region of the skull and in the long bones where dense rings and bands of bone are noted near the epiphyseal margins. Idiopathic hypercalcemia is considered to represent an inborn error of calcium metabolism and has been known to be exacerbated by vitamin D administration. As in vitamin D intoxication and sarcoidosis, the intestinal absorption of calcium is increased and is antagonized by adrenal steroids. In fact, these steroids presently represent the only efficacious therapy for the hypercalcemia in this disorder.

HYPERTHYROIDISM

The serum calcium of hyperthyroid patients is frequently higher than normal when matched for age and sex. Serum ionized calcium also tends to be elevated, possibly because of the tendency these patients have to hypoalbuminemia. The extent of the hypercalcemia can be extremely variable and bears no relation to the severity of the thyrotoxicosis. Although the hypercalcemia in this disorder is generally not severe enough to warrant emergency therapeutic measures, symptoms of thyrotoxic hypercalcemia, such as nausea, vomiting, abdominal pain, and constipation, may be dramatic and mask the accompanying thyrotoxic state. Despite the documented hypercalciuria of thyrotoxic patients, renal calculi and metastatic calcification are quite rare, although urine calcium may approach 1.0 gram per day, and both nephrocalcinosis and renal tubular acidosis have been described. Although reported elevations of alkaline phosphatase in hypercalcemic thyrotoxic patients have been slight and inconsistent, the elevation in serum calcium is presumed to result from the direct metabolic effect of thyroid hormone on bone. The skeletal disorder is an osteopenia characterized by increased bone resorption and normal or increased bone formation. Thyrotoxic bone disease (osteoporosis or osteomalacia) is infrequently documented clinically, probably because the underlying disorder is usually corrected before the demineralization proceeds to a level which can be detected with conventional radiographic techniques. The mechanisms responsible for thyrotoxic hypercalcemia appear to be independent of the parathyroid glands. This is supported by the tendency toward hyperphosphatemia and an increased tubular resorption of phosphate (per cent TRP), which reverts to normal when the hyperthyroidism is treated. These observations are consistent with the interpretation that endogenous parathyroid hormone secretion is already sup-

pressed by the hypercalcemia imposed by the thyrotoxic state. However, the coexistence of hyperparathyroidism and hyperthyroidism is greater than that attributable to chance alone. Thus parathyroid exploration may be mandatory if the hyperalcemia of thyrotoxic states does not respond to treatment of the hyperthyroidism. Paradoxically, hypercalcemia may also occur in hypothyroid states. In this case, decreased bone turnover and retarded bone formation result in inadequate transfer of calcium from blood to bone. The mild hypercalcemia responds appropriately to thyroid medication.

ADRENAL INSUFFICIENCY

Although Addison's disease may be a relatively rare cause of hypercalcemia, it must be emphasized that the clinical presentation of adrenal insufficiency and hypercalcemia may be identical. The mechanism for production of the hypercalcemia is still conjectural. Hypercalcemia with serum calcium values as high as 15 mg per cent has also been noted in patients during the postoperative course of subtotal adrenalectomy, and hypercalciuria has been documented during reduction of high-dose, long-term glucocorticoid therapy. In contrast, hypercalcemia is not associated with adrenalectomy for disorders other than hyperadrenocorticism. These observations suggest that an abrupt lowering of high circulating levels of glucocorticoids is necessary to produce the hypercalcemia. Corticosteroids inhibit organic matrix formation and decrease both bone formation and resorption, the former much more than the latter. Corticosteroids have also been shown to impair the intestinal absorption of calcium. Since there is mounting evidence that cortisone and vitamin D are biochemical antagonists in intestinal and bone tissue, it has been speculated that a rapid lowering of steroid hormone levels results in a "functional hypervitaminosis D" with unabated bone resorption and intestinal calcium absorption. Whatever the mechanism, one should always consider the possibility of hypercalcemia in symptomatic patients suddenly deprived of high levels of endogenous or exogenous adrenal steroids. The dose of steroids required to decrease the serum calcium levels may be considerably higher than that required for maintenance in patients with adrenal insufficiency.

IMMOBILIZATION

Immobilization results in a loss of bone mineral, and so-called "disuse osteopenia" occurs locally in patients with isolated fractures or hemiplegia and is generalized in quadriplegia. Immobilization for the treatment of simple fractures does not produce hypercalciuria in the great majority of patients. Yet rapid demineralization and hypercalciuria have been demonstrated in patients immobilized for multiple fractures and also in normal individuals whose activity is markedly reduced by bed rest. When normal subjects are subjected to complete bed rest for up to seven weeks, the rate of calcium loss is significant and approximates 0.4 to 0.6 per cent of total body calcium per month. The hypercalcemia of immobilization is found most commonly in children or adolescents immobilized because of fractures or osteomyelitis, or in adults with metabolic or metastatic skeletal disease or Paget's disease of bone. Classically, disuse osteopenia is associated with a relative increase in bone resorption attributed to mechanical factors: either to absence of pressure transmitted to bone or to absence of tension applied to bone by muscle, or both. Evidence has accumulated that the absence of pressure forces on bone is primarily responsible for tissue osteopenia, possibly by altering piezoelectric forces within bone. This potentially serious complication in immobilized subjects can be dramatically relieved by quiet standing maneuvers, simple ambulation, or the use of oscillating mattresses. The last-named approach is apparently useful only when skeletal or muscle mass has not been significantly compromised by the primary disorder requiring immobilization, as might obtain in hemi- or paraplegic immobilized patients or in individuals immobilized in whole body plaster casts.

DIURETICS AND HYPERCALCEMIA

It has been well established that diuretics can appreciably influence calcium metabolism in man. The oral administration of thiazides and chlorthalidone to normal subjects and patients with disuse osteopenia, idiopathic hypercalciuria, congestive failure, and metabolic bone disease has consistently resulted in a decrease in urinary calcium. Hypercalcemia during thiazide administration has also been observed transiently in normal subjects as well as in patients with osteoporosis and metabolic bone disease. With the exception of patients with underlying hyperparathyroidism (see Ch. 552.2), restoration of previous plasma calcium levels and disappearance of symptoms caused by the hypercalcemia rapidly follow the discontinuation of the drug. Since elevations in plasma calcium caused by thiazides do not correlate with the magnitude of the attendant fall in urinary calcium, effects of thiazides other than hypocalciuria may contribute to the hypercalcemia. These accumulated observations dictate the cautious administration of thiazide diuretics to hypercalcemic patients, to those with potentially hypercalcemic disorders (i.e., immobilization), and to normocalcemic patients with diseases characterized by an accelerated bone resorption. In these instances, the associated hypercalciuria may actually be preventing or delaying the onset of hypercalcemia.

DISORDERS IN RENAL FUNCTION

Hypercalcemia has been also observed in the diuretic phase of acute renal failure and following renal transplantation. The former syndrome is initially characterized by oliguria and a history of antecedent severe muscle or soft tissue damage, or both. In this syndrome, hypercalcemia usually develops with the first or second week of diuresis and may persist from one to three weeks, with normocalcemia achieved only when the blood urea nitrogen is normal or nearly so. An acute form of secondary hyperparathyroidism and immobilization appear to contribute to the hypercalcemia. Various forms of therapy include ambulation, peritoneal dialysis, hemodialysis solutions containing calcium in a concentration of 2.5 per cent, hydration, and glucocorticoids. In each instance, the elevated serum calcium characteristically falls as both renal function and plasma parathyroid hormone levels approach normal.

The hypercalcemia reported to occur following renal transplantation probably results from a combination of autonomous parathyroid function, a resistance to the action of parathyroid hormone and vitamin D, and hyper-

phosphatemia, all of which characterize the pretransplant period. When such patients receive functioning homografts, renal function is restored and phosphate levels decrease because of depleted reserves conditioned by preoperative therapy with phosphate-binding antacids. In addition, the resistance to vitamin D and to supernormal levels of circulating parathyroid hormone is removed. In some individuals, these rapid changes lead to a syndrome of hypercalcemia and hypophosphatemia. Since hypomagnesemia may also stimulate parathyroid hormone release, the fall in plasma magnesium often noted following successful transplantation may also trigger an exaggerated release of parathyroid hormone from large hyperplastic glands and perpetuate the hypercalcemia. Hypercalcemia observed for the first time in the post-transplantation period appears self-limited and will usually disappear within three to six months. Post-transplantation hypercalcemia can usually be reversed with a combination of oral phosphate and steroid therapy. If hypercalcemia persists for months despite medical therapy, one should anticipate the development of metastatic calcification and nephrocalcinosis. Such complications may warrant surgical intervention and subtotal parathyroidectomy.

Hypercalcemia has also been observed when calcium resins are administered to hyperkalemic uremic patients during dialysis. The mechanisms responsible for this are not well understood. It appears extremely unlikely, however, that the hypercalcemia is due solely to the absorption of free calcium ion from the gut, since the maximum amount of free calcium ion liberated in the gut from 15 to 45 grams of calcium resin is 0.6 to 1.8 grams per day, an amount unlikely to result in hypercalcemia in patients with advanced renal failure, even if it were all available for absorption.

MILK-ALKALI SYNDROME

The oral ingestion of calcium salts alone may rarely induce elevations in serum calcium. If absorbable alkali containing calcium salts is ingested, hypercalcemia frequently ensues. The so-called milk-alkali syndrome is observed in individuals with a history of chronic ingestion of milk and absorbable alkali. Typical blood chemical findings include hypercalcemia, normal or elevated phosphorus, normal alkaline phosphatase, azotemia, and mild alkalosis. Since chronic renal insufficiency with "secondary hyperparathyroidism" is normally attended by acidosis, the combination of alkalosis and azotemia may be a valuable clue to the correct diagnosis. Urinary calcium may be high, normal, or low in this syndrome, reflecting glomerular filtration rates. Patients usually demonstrate band keratopathy and conjunctival deposition of calcium, and the hypercalciuria characteristically responds to the withdrawal of milk and alkali and maximal hydration. The fall in serum calcium, although prompt in the majority of circumstances, may be delayed for months. If therapy is not instituted early, permanent renal damage may occur despite the correction of hypercalcemia by dietary restriction and cessation of alkali therapy.

MISCELLANEOUS CAUSES

Hypercalcemia has been noted in patients with *pheochromocytoma* and attributed to catecholamine-stimulated parathyroid hormone release. Following remedial surgery, the serum calcium returns to normal. If serum calcium is still elevated following surgical excision of the pheochromocytoma(s), the possibility of an existing parathyroid adenoma should be considered. *Multiple endocrine adenomatosis syndromes* (i.e., MEA types I and II) may include medullary carcinoma, bilateral pheochromocytomas, and parathyroid adenomas (see Ch. 543.5). A benign form of familial hypercalcemia has also been observed in children and young adolescents. This disorder, inherited in an autosomal dominant mode, presents with elevations in total and ionized blood calcium and normal immunoassayable parathyroid hormone.

Fungal and mycobacterial infections have also been attended by hypercalcemia and/or hypercalciuria. Characteristically the serum calcium is normalized when the underlying disease is treated. Hypercalcemia occurring in patients with active tuberculosis may be due to an abnormal sensitivity to vitamin D similar to that observed in sarcoidosis. For this reason, the administration of vitamin D and calcium supplements to tuberculosis patients should be carefully monitored.

SIGNS AND SYMPTOMS OF HYPERCALCEMIA

Although the varied causes for hypercalcemia are usually readily distinguished from one another on clinical grounds alone, there is often considerable diagnostic difficulty when one or several of the clinical manifestations of hypercalcemia, rather than those of the underlying condition, predominate. For purposes of analysis, the symptoms arising from hypercalcemia can be placed in two general categories: in the first instance, the hypercalcemia is but one of a variety of mechanisms responsible for the symptoms. Sarcoidosis, hyperthyroidism, myxedema, steroid withdrawal states, and malignancies serve as adequate examples of this group. The second category includes situations in which the hypercalcemia alone is responsible for the clinical picture. Vitamin D intoxication, hyperparathyroidism, immobilization hypercalcemia, thiazide ingestion, and idiopathic hypercalcemia are considered representative of this group.

Clinical manifestations of patients with hypercalcemia are protean, since gastric secretion, contractility of skeletal, smooth, and cardiac muscle, excitability of nervous tissue, renal and cerebral function, and vascular tone are all altered by elevations in extracellular calcium ion concentration. Thus hypercalcemia may result in anorexia, apathy, nausea, vomiting, generalized fatigue, hypertension, constipation, subjective proximal muscular weakness and myopathy, stupor, and coma. Unlike the majority of symptoms attributed to hypercalcemia, the degree of elevation of the serum calcium does not appear to correlate with the severity of the myopathy. Hypercalcemia has been associated with reversible hypertension and is known to produce spasm in renal vessels as well as actual renal vascular damage. There is substantial experimental and clinical evidence that the calcium ion has a direct effect on vascular tonicity and that significant renal disease is not a prerequisite to the association of hypercalcemia and hypertension. Blood pressure elevation may be a clue to the diagnosis of hypercalcemia and may contribute to the management of patients with an inherent predisposition to hypertension. The effects of hypercalcemia on renal function include defective water conservation leading to polyuria, polydipsia, and noc-

turia and a clinical picture which resembles a vasopressin-resistant diabetes insipidus. The polyuria, when accompanied by prolonged vomiting, leads to dehydration and decreased glomerular filtration. Hypercalcemia also appears to have an inhibitory effect on sodium transport by the renal tubules and consequently results in decreased free-water reabsorption and formation and increased sodium excretion. With progressive hypercalciuria, deposition of calcium in the renal parenchyma may result in potassium wasting and hypokalemia, nephrocalcinosis, albuminuria, and persistent hyposthenuria. The polyuria is thereby aggravated, and eventually azotemia and renal failure may occur. The combination of nausea, constipation, and weakness, together with a diabetes insipidus–like state with ensuing dehydration and severe weight loss, may mimic terminal malignant cachexia.

The serum calcium level is essential for the regulation of cardiac excitability and contraction and, as such, functions to regulate the contraction-relaxation cycle. In humans, infusions of calcium lead to shortening of the systolic time intervals resulting from a positive inotropic action of calcium on the myocardium. Sinus bradycardia, sinus arrhythmia, shifting pacemaker, and varying degrees of atrioventricular block have also been induced by hypercalcemia. The bradycardiac effect of calcium has been considered vagotonic in action, since it is abolished by atropinization or vagotomy. In addition to bradycardia, hypercalcemia shortens mechanical ventricular systole, increases myocardial contractility, and decreases myocardial automaticity. Responses in the systolic time intervals and electrical systole correlate quite well with the level of serum calcium. Electrocardiographic manifestations of hypercalcemia include slight P-R interval and QRS complex prolongation and S-T segment shortening which produces a short Q-T interval. The T wave is usually normal, although on occasion it may be slightly depressed. Shortening of the Q-T interval is almost invariable with a serum calcium greater than 13 mg per 100 ml. The decreased conduction velocity and shorter refractory period of hypercalcemia predispose to cardiac arrhythmias. The fact that synergism exists between digitalis and calcium with respect to their myocardial effects has long been known. Hypercalcemia mimics digitalis both in shortening the Q-T interval and in its toxic effects. Since the inotropic and toxic manifestations of digitalis may be potentiated by hypercalcemia, measurements of serum calcium should be made in any individual who develops arrhythmias or cardiographic patterns characteristic of digitalis intoxication.

Hypercalcemia is associated with a depression of cerebral function and nonspecific (see also with hypokalemia) electroencephalographic (EEG) patterns. These are characterized by a diffusely slow record with paroxysms of frontal dominance and 2 to 4 cycle per second bursts of moderately high voltage. Reversal of the hypercalcemia leads to a gradual disappearance of the abnormal EEG pattern. Drowsiness and lethargy are usually the earliest signs of altered cerebration in hypercalcemic states. There may be generalized muscular weakness, hypotonia, and hypoactive or absent deep tendon reflexes. Although thick speech and transient aphasia have been observed, neurologic signs are usually generalized rather than localized. Elevations in serum calcium can also produce visual hallucinations, ataxia, and hemianopia. When these symptoms are coupled with the more common ones of nausea, vomiting, and weakness, a syndrome resembling basilar artery insufficiency may result. Convulsions are not a symptom of hypercalcemia per se, although hyperexcitability has often been observed. The documented synergistic action of elevated calcium and decreased magnesium concentrations in facilitating acetylcholine release may account for the hyperexcitability and nonrhythmic twitchings reported in situations when the hypercalcemia is attended by hypomagnesemia.

Mental disturbances attributed to hypercalcemia range from simple functional behavioral disorders, confusion, and depression to severe neurasthenic personality changes, organic psychosis, and catatonic stupor. There also appears to be a definite quantitative correlation between the degree of psychosocial disturbance and serum calcium, since the higher the serum calcium, the more severe the mental disturbances. Moreover, the disturbed behavioral patterns are completely reversed when the serum calcium is returned to normal. Relatively small variations in the extracellular calcium concentration appear to have significant influence on brain function. The deleterious effect of hypercalcemia on the central nervous system needs specific emphasis, since in a hypercalcemic crisis the vague symptoms of lassitude, weakness, fatigability, and anorexia, if untreated, may gradually progress to nausea and vomiting, polyuria, dehydration, somnolence, confusion, disorientation, stupor (or delirium), coma, and death.

Rarely hypercalcemia may be associated with clinical evidence of bone destruction such as severe kyphosis or pseudoclubbing of the fingers caused by telescoping of the distal phalanges. Not infrequently, patients also present with "red eyes" and complain of pruritus and conjunctival irritation. These symptoms are due to subconjunctival calcium phosphate deposits, variously described as white flecks or glasslike crystals and identified with the aid of a slit lamp. The deposits tend to localize within the conjunctiva of the palpebral fissure region. Another distinct type of ocular abnormality associated with hypercalcemia, often referred to as band keratopathy, consists of diffuse, hazy gray granular epithelial and subepithelial corneal opacities running concentrically with the limbus on either the nasal or the temporal side, or both. The limbic margin is usually abrupt, and the calcification is characteristically separated from the limbus by a clear margin. This keratopathy is usually inconspicuous and asymptomatic. Although the conjunctival opacities might be confused with calcification, which occurs commonly in the absence of local or systemic disease, the band corneal opacities are usually readily distinguished from arcus senilis, which may normally accompany senescence. Rarely, hypercalcemia may also produce a diffuse generalized corneal calcification. The corneal lesions and ectopic conjunctival calcifications are commonly noted in situations wherein *both* serum calcium and phosphate levels are elevated, as may obtain in sarcoidosis, malignancy, the milk alkali syndrome, vitamin D overdosage, and the secondary hyperparathyroid state accompanying chronic renal disease. Despite assertions to the contrary, these lesions are not necessarily related to the extent or duration of the hypercalcemia.

TREATMENT OF HYPERCALCEMIA

When the serum calcium is moderately raised (i.e., less than 12 mg per cent), therapy directed against the un-

derlying causes is usually quite effective in reversing the hypercalcemia. In this regard, oral glucocorticoid therapy has ameliorated the hypercalcemia of sarcoidosis, vitamin D intoxication, idiopathic hypercalcemia of infancy, lymphomas, multiple myeloma, and breast carcinoma; propranolol decreases the hypercalcemia of thyrotoxic individuals; alkalating agents such as melphalan and cyclophosphamide have also normalized the hypercalcemia of patients with multiple myeloma, as has definitive ablative endocrine surgery for the hypercalcemia of hyperparathyroidism, hyperthyroidism, and breast carcinoma. A moderate hypercalcemia is also corrected by long-term, nonspecific therapy directed toward either a reduction in calcium absorption or a decrease in bone turnover, or both. Oral chelating agents such as cellulose phosphate, sodium phytate (the sodium salt of inositol hexaphosphoric acid), and sodium phosphate have been advocated for the control of hypercalcemia. Although cellulose phosphate in a dose of 15 grams per day is reportedly quite effective in controlling hypercalcemia, symptomatic hypomagnesemia may occasionally complicate its use. However, the lack of relatively serious side effects and effective inhibition of intestinal calcium absorption make this agent particularly useful in the long-term therapy of hypercalcemia associated with renal impairment and hyperabsorption of calcium. Ethylenediamine tetra-acetate (EDTA) is often tolerated poorly and should be avoided because of the propensity to nephrotoxicity. The hypocalcemic action of sodium phytate has been attributed both to the formation of nonabsorbable calcium compounds in the gut and to the hydrolysis of as much as two thirds of the ingested phosphate, with subsequent absorption of the liberated inorganic phosphorus. Sodium phytate in daily doses of 6 to 9 grams has been used effectively in sarcoidosis and hyperparathyroidism. Symptomatic complications of continuous treatment with sodium phytate for as long as 18 months have included diarrhea, anorexia, nausea, and vomiting. The absorption of liberated phosphate may also impose limitations on its long-term administration similar to those attending long-term sodium phosphate therapy. The long-term administration of sodium phosphate in recommended doses equivalent to 2 grams of elemental phosphorus per day, although also repeatedly effective in the control of hypercalcemia as well as hypercalciuria, may produce extraskeletal calcification, secondary hyperparathyroidism, acute pancreatitis, and depressed renal function. Mithramycin, a cytotoxic antibiotic used mainly in the therapy of embryonal testicular tumors and Paget's disease of bone, does lower serum calcium levels in normocalcemic as well as hypercalcemic subjects. Its toxic side effects, which include bleeding due to thrombocytopenia and hepatocellular and renal damage, have restricted its use primarily to patients with malignancy and hypercalcemia. When given as a direct single intravenous injection of 25 to 50 μg per kilogram of body weight, it appears to be effective in lowering the serum calcium within 24 to 48 hours. Although the duration of the effect is variable, repeated injections have successfully controlled the hypercalcemia of patients with metastatic carcinoma. The drug works primarily by decreasing skeleton resorption and may be a valuable therapeutic agent in patients with cancer and intractable hypercalcemia in whom the potential benefits outweigh the risks of toxicity. Calcitonin, the calcium-lowering hormone secreted by the thyroid which inhibits bone resorption (see Ch. 552.1) has been administered to hypercalcemic patients with varied effectiveness. Doses of 4 MRC units per kilogram of body weight induce modest falls in serum calcium of 1 to 2 mg per cent in hypercalcemic patients. The calcium-lowering effect is maximal at six to nine hours, and characteristically wears off within 24 hours. The efficacy of calcitonin in the regulation of plasma calcium homeostasis appears to depend on the prevailing rate of bone resorption, with maximal effectiveness noted in patients with hypercalcemia and rapid skeletal turnover rates.

Glucocorticoids have also been widely used in the treatment of hypercalcemia. High doses (30 to 100 mg per day of prednisone or equivalent doses of other steroids) may result in the lowering of serum calcium in a variety of hypercalcemic disorders. Satisfactory results have been recorded in hypercalcemia associated with sarcoidosis, malignant tumors, and hypervitaminosis D. In some instances (e.g., multiple myeloma), the response may be quite dramatic, with falls in serum calcium from 16 to 18 mg per cent to near normal values a day or two after treatment is initiated. In most cases, however, normocalcemic levels are gradually approached over a period of seven to ten days. The hypercalcemia of hyperparathyroidism is characteristically resistant to glucocorticoid therapy. Although glucocorticoids decrease intestinal calcium absorption, increase renal calcium excretion, and cause alterations in vitamin D metabolism, their effect on serum calcium in hypercalcemic states is in most cases due to suppression of the underlying disease.

With very high concentrations of serum calcium, the danger of cardiac arrest and obtundation demands more rapid treatment than that offered by adrenal steroids, oral chelating agents, sodium phosphate, mithramycin, or calcitonin, since the response to these agents is relatively slow. The measures presently available for emergency treatment of hypercalcemia include the infusion of sodium salts of chloride, sulfate, and phosphate. Although the intravenous administration of EDTA has been recommended in the past for emergent therapy of hypercalcemia, the subjective discomfort observed during its administration, its short-lived action of 12 to 24 hours, and renal toxicity limit its usefulness. The initial and most important therapeutic approach to the patient with life-threatening hypercalcemia is hydration with isotonic sodium chloride. A water diuresis, as opposed to a diuresis produced by a sodium chloride solution, is relatively ineffective in this regard. Rehydration with isotonic sodium chloride often leads to volume repletion, increased glomerular filtration, and enhanced renal calcium clearance. In addition, the resulting natriuresis is accompanied by an increase in calcium excretion independent of changes in filtration rate due probably to a combination of volume expansion and the competitive inhibition of calcium reabsorption by the proximal renal tubular cells. Infusion of solutions of isotonic sodium sulfate (38.9 grams of sodium sulfate decahydrate per liter) has also been advocated for the immediate therapy of hypercalcemia. In this instance, 3 liters of isotonic sodium sulfate is administered over a period of eight to nine hours. Sodium sulfate has been effective in the treatment of hypercalcemia, mainly by virtue of increasing the urinary excretion of calcium. There is also evidence that the sulfate ion inhibits the effect of calcium on cardiac contractility. One should proceed cautiously with this agent in patients with renal or cardiovascular disease, since an isotonic solution of sodium sulfate is hypertonic with respect to sodium (i.e., 242 mEq/Na per liter) and hypernatremia with marked hypertonicity of the body fluids

may obtain during the treatment period. Since hypertonicity per se may produce marked alterations in the sensorium with hyperactivity, confusion, stupor, and even coma, the clinical responsiveness of the hypercalcemic patient may be severely compromised. One might avoid these complications if serum sodium is monitored during sodium sulfate infusion and appropriate amounts of dextrose in water administered. Finally, since hypokalemia and hypomagnesemia frequently accompany intravenous sulfate therapy, it is also advisable to monitor potassium and magnesium levels and to administer $MgSo_4$ and/or KCl as needed.

Unlike the response to isotonic sodium chloride or sodium sulfate infusion, intravenous phosphate therapy leads to a fall in serum calcium and a *reduction* in urinary calcium. Although this form of therapy is quite effective, its mechanism of action is still not completely understood. Unlike intravenous therapy with sodium chloride or sodium sulfate solutions, intravenous (or oral) phosphate causes a decreased rather than an increased renal calcium clearance. The prevailing opinion is one which attributes the induced fall in serum calcium to a combination of skeletal and ectopic soft tissue calcification. One usually administers a solution containing 50 mmoles of phosphorus, 80 mEq of sodium, and 10 mEq of potassium diluted in 500 to 1000 ml 5 per cent dextrose in water over six to eight hours if renal function is normal. If renal impairment coexists, profound hypocalcemia may develop. A total of 60 to 90 mmoles of phosphate can effect a dramatic fall in serum calcium which is directly proportional to both the increment in plasma phosphate and the initial height of the plasma calcium. Not infrequently, however, this form of treatment is temporary and calcium levels return to preinfusion values within 24 hours after terminating the infusion. In patients with extreme hypercalcemia, attempts to reduce serum calcium precipitously to normal or subnormal levels are hazardous and unwise, since severe hypotension and acute renal failure may develop. Although phosphate therapy may be more advantageous in patients with congestive heart failure, since a reduction in serum calcium is accomplished with minimal fluid (i.e., 0.5 to 1 liter of phosphate compared to 3 liters of sulfate), phosphate should be reserved for extreme degrees of intractable hypercalcemia and is contraindicated in the presence of renal dysfunction. The hazards of either sodium sulfate or sodium phosphate therapy are quite real. Once the life-threatening hypercalcemia episode has been effectively treated with either of these agents, a concerted effort should be made to maintain a normal serum calcium level by other means and to treat the underlying disease.

Since calcium is reabsorbed both in the proximal convoluted tubules and in the more distal segments of the nephron, a variety of diuretic agents which exert their effect at these sites have also proved quite successful in the management of "hypercalcemic crises." Although experience with these agents is somewhat limited, furosemide, a potent natriuretic agent which increases calcium excretion in direct proportion to sodium excretion, appears to have effective therapeutic potential, especially in patients with compromised cardiac reserve and moderate renal insufficiency. This agent is administered intravenously in doses of 80 to 100 mg, and its circulating concentration is sustained by the injection of similar amounts at intervals of one to two hours. The resultant diuresis is brisk and the fall in serum calcium is usually quite significant, ranging from 2 to 4 mg per 100 ml. Since the forced diuresis is also accompanied by a considerable loss of potassium and magnesium, and since the contraction of the extracellular fluid volume may result from the large losses of sodium and water in the urine, furosemide therapy of hypercalcemia should be attended by measurements of plasma potassium and magnesium and the administration of electrolyte solution with a concentration of sodium and potassium closely approximating the urine composition at a rate equaling that of urine flow. Since mental obtundation may result from hypomagnesemia, supplemental magnesium therapy may also be required.

Successful dialysis treatment of intractable hypercalcemia is also an easily accessible measure against life-threatening hypercalcemia when all other methods fail. The transient effect of dialysis can, however, be of special value if an underlying disease state such as hyperparathyroidism can be immediately corrected after the calcium level has been brought to normal.

Christensson, T., Hellstrom, K., and Wengle, B.: Clinical and laboratory findings in subjects with hypercalcemia. Acta Med. Scand., 200:355, 1976.

Heilbron, D. C., Eastman, J. W., and Kelly, D.: Warning methods for quality control in determinations of serum calcium. Clin. Chem., 20:1416, 1974.

Rodman, J. S., and Sherwood, L. M.: Disorders of mineral metabolism in malignancy. In Avioli, L. V., and Krane, S. M. (eds.): Metabolic Bone Disease, Vol. II. New York, Academic Press, 1978, pp. 577–631.

Schneider, A. B., and Sherwood, L. M.: Calcium homeostasis and the pathogenesis and management of hypercalcemic disorders. Metabolism, 23:975, 1974.

Shai, F., Baker, R. K., Addrizzo, J. R., and Wallach, S.: Hypercalcemia in mycobacterial infection. J. Clin. Endocrinol., 34:251, 1972.

Shaw, J. W., Oldham, S. B., Rosoff, L., Bethune, J. E., and Fichman, M. P.: Urinary cyclic AMP analyzed as a function of the serum calcium and parathyroid hormone in the differential diagnosis of hypercalcemia. J. Clin. Invest., 59:14, 1977.

556. HYPOCALCEMIA

In addition to clinical syndromes characterized by either a deficiency of or an inherited end-organ refractoriness to parathyroid hormone (see Ch. 552.3), hypocalcemia is also observed in intestinal malabsorption syndromes, uremia, acute pancreatitis, osteoblastic metastatic bone disease, and hypoalbuminemic states such as cirrhosis and nephrosis. The hypocalcemia of cirrhotic or nephrotic patients is characteristically not attended by clinical tetany. Although on an absolute scale the ionized calcium may be slightly reduced in cirrhosis, the fraction of total calcium which is ionized is actually increased. In cirrhotics, the change in serum total calcium is almost quantitatively accounted for by a corresponding change in serum albumin, since, in contrast to normal subjects, there is no detectable binding of calcium to serum globulins. The presence of overt tetany or irritability in patients with uremia and hypocalcemia depends on the circulating levels of potassium and magnesium as well as the severity of the acidosis of hydrogen ion concentration. In acute pancreatitis with fat necrosis, blood calcium levels may fall within the first four days and remain depressed for seven to ten days. The drop in serum calcium and muscle irritability usually parallels the severity of the pancreatitis. The fall in serum calcium may also be accompanied by hypomagnesemia, so that tetany which persists after restoration of calcium to normal may require magnesium therapy. The fall in serum calcium (and to a limited extent, magnesium) in acute pancreatitis probably results from a combination of precipitation of calcium soaps, fatty acids liberated by lipolytic destruction of abdominal and retroperitoneal fat, and the attendant elevations in circulating glucagon and other enteric hormones which are potent secretagogues for calcitonin. Occasionally, the tetany observed in hypocalcemic subjects with intestinal malabsorption is refractory to intravenous calcium therapy, whereas it responds promptly to infusions of magnesium salts. This sequence of events stems from a malabsorption of magnesium and subsequent hypomagnesemia, and has been ascribed to both a "permissive" action of magnesium on parathyroid hormone–induced bone resorption and decreased parathyroid hormone secretion.

Hypocalcemia with marked irritability and frank convulsions has also been observed in the neonate. Neonatal hypocalcemia, like neonatal convulsions, has two peaks of incidence: one in the first 48 hours of life, and one between the fourth and tenth days of life. The cause of the hypocalcemia appears to be quite distinct for each group. Those infants who develop hypocalcemia within the first 48 hours of life are typically the product of an operative delivery, are often of low birth weight for gestational age, usually have an associated hypoglycemia and elevated blood calcitonin levels, and may be magnesium deficient. Following premature or traumatic delivery, calcium levels fall in the first 48 hours below the levels for infants delivered spontaneously at term. Hypocalcemia occurring within the first 48 hours of birth has been noted in children born of mothers with hyperparathyroidism and may also be complicated by hypomagnesemia. Those newborn infants who develop hypocalcemia after the first two days of life are usually full-term babies of average weight who have been artificially fed. In this case, the infant is faced with a large phosphate intake as a result of early cow's milk feeding. Hyperphosphatemia probably results because the immature kidney cannot adequately handle a phosphate load caused by a combination of low glomerular filtration rates and a blunted response to parathyroid hormone. Although hypocalcemic hypomagnesemic convulsions refractory to calcium infusions have also been documented in this second group of children, breast feeding or use of low phosphate milk products is often curative and substantially reduces the incidence of convulsions.

Neuromuscular irritability and tetany accompanying the hyperventilation syndrome have been variably ascribed to a systemic respiratory alkalosis and/or hypocalcemia. In this instance, the symptoms most probably result directly from a decreased hydrogen ion concentration and increased neuromuscular irritability, since hyperventilation per se induces a rise in serum calcium.

It has been well established that diphenylhydantoin, phenobarbital, and structurally related compounds stimulate the hepatic microsomal conversion of vitamin D_3 and $25OHD_3$ to biologically inactive metabolites, resulting ultimately in decreased circulating concentrations of $25OHD_3$, intestinal malabsorption of calcium, hypocalcemia, and osteomalacia. The observation that anticonvulsant-induced hypocalcemia and osteomalacia respond favorably to vitamin D therapy suggests that exogenous supplementation is the treatment of choice for correcting the drug-induced alteration in calcium homeostasis. Patients on high doses of anticonvulsant drugs known to stimulate hepatic drug–metabolizing enzymes, especially those with marginal dietary intakes and decreased sunlight exposure, or patients with diseases predisposing to vitamin D malabsorption should be carefully screened for evidence of vitamin D deficiency.

SIGNS AND SYMPTOMS OF HYPOCALCEMIA

Tetany, when apparent, may be characterized by carpopedal spasm, muscle twitching, laryngeal stridor, hyperreflexia, choreiform movements, muscle cramps, and changes in electrical excitability of peripheral nerves. The presence of subclinical or latent tetany may be demonstrated by Chvostek's sign (unilateral contraction of the facial musculature and nasal alae on percussion of the ipsilateral facial nerve anterior to the ear) or Trousseau's sign (hyperextension and close adduction of the fingers induced by tourniquet-induced ischemia of the arm). Chvostek's sign is usually elicited in untreated hypocalcemic states but may also be positive in 10 per cent of normal adults. It has been repeatedly emphasized that these signs are only crude indications of increased neuromuscular excitability. Quite often, the only symptomatic manifestations of the hypocalcemia are perioral or distal extremity paresthesias. These sensations have been interpreted as signs of activation of peripheral sensory nerve receptors by hypocalcemia. Not uncommonly, the tetany is latent in hypocalcemic patients for years, the only symptoms being muscular weakness, fatigue, palpitations, and paresthesias of the upper extremities.

The increased neural excitability occasioned by hypocalcemia also results in seizures and EEG abnormalities, which include a paucity of alpha rhythm, increased fast activity, sporadic spike activity, and slow waves (6 to 7 per second) with frontal preponderance. In general, the abnormal EEG pattern will disappear following calcium infusions; but since chronic hypocalcemia may also induce organic brain deterioration, calcium infusion may prove ineffective in this regard. Hypocalcemia is also believed to result in increased intracranial pressure. On occasion, convulsions or unilateral neurologic manifestations may be accompanied by papilledema, stimulating an expanding intracranial mass. Patients with hypocalcemia may also present with nausea, vomiting, and abdominal pain. These gastrointestinal symptoms may be related in part to the effect of the hypocalcemia on the sympathetic ganglia of the gastrointestinal tract, since the response to different stimuli may be increased in hypocalcemic states and the efferent discharge may be increased in the presence of a constant amount of perfusing acetylcholine.

The most common electrocardiographic manifestation of hypocalcemia is S-T interval prolongation with a normal T wave. This pattern contrasts with the Q-T interval prolongation of hypokalemia. With combined hypocalcemia and hypokalemia, the electrocardiographic abnormalities are those of *hypokalemia* and are normalized by potassium, rather than by calcium administration. Hypocalcemia with a serum calcium level below 6 per 100 ml may also lead to prolongation of the Q-T interval. This effect is proportional to the degree of hypocalcemia and reversed by calcium infusion. Hypocalcemia may attentuate digitalis effect on the myocardium and potentiate the electrocardiographic changes of hyperkalemia. In fact, the associated calcium concentration in hyperkalemia may actually determine the severity of atrioventricular and intraventricular conduction defects and determine the vulnerability to ventricular fibrillation.

Hillman, L. S., Rojanasathit, S., Slatopolsky, E., and Haddad, J. G.: Serial measurement of serum calcium, magnesium, parathyroid hormone, calcitonin and 25-hydroxyvitamin D in premature and term infants during the first week of life. Pediat. Res., 11:739, 1977.

Robertson, N. R. C., and Smith, M. A.: Early neonatal hypocalcemia. Arch. Dis. Child., 50:604, 1975.

Schneider, A. B., and Sherwood, L. M.: Pathogenesis and management of hypoparathyroidism and other hypocalcemic disorders. Metabolism, 24:871, 1975.

557. THE OSTEOPOROTIC SYNDROMES

Osteoporosis is a form of osteopenia leading to decreased radiographic density because of a decrease in the total mass of bone below the levels required for mechanical support. This disorder must be differentiated histologically from other forms of osteopenia such as osteomalacia, which is characterized by decreased mineralization rates and wide osteoid seams. In osteoporosis, a deficiency of bone tissue per unit volume of bone as an organ exists. According to both chemical and ordinary histologic criteria, the bone that remains in the osteoporotic skeleton has a normal mineral-osteoid ratio. Microscopically the fibrous and fatty marrow that fills the void once occupied by mineralized trabeculae is also normal. Occasionally increased osteoclastic activity and increased marrow mast cell counts are noted. Since approximately 30 to 50 per cent of bone mineral must be lost before bone rarefaction becomes radiologically evident, so-called "early" radiographic changes actually represent a large diminution in skeletal mass. The amount of bone loss essential for detection of the osteopenic process actually varies considerably in different bones and in different parts of the same bone, depending on the structural composition of the skeletal segment. It may take years before appreciably radiographic abnormalities can be noted in osteoporotic subjects. By the same token, it may also require years before therapeutically induced improvement in the mineral content of the skeleton would be appreciated by routine radiographs. However, the availability of more sophisticated analyses of bone content such as radiogrammetry of short tubular bones and forearm mass quantitation by photon densitometry offers promise for the early detection of bone loss.

The net loss of bone which characterizes osteoporosis is reflected histologically by an imbalance between the rate of bone formation and the rate of bone destruction. This imbalance could be the result of a primary decrease in the rate of bone formation, a primary increase in the rate of bone destruction, or various combinations thereof. Osteoporosis may develop at either low or high rates of bone turnover, but in each instance bone resorption must be higher than formation. Small increments in resorption may suffice to perpetuate the osteopenic process, since it appears from detailed histologic studies that osteoclastic bone resorption is much more effective than osteoblastic bone formation.

The amount of tissue removed by one osteoclast is replaced by approximately 150 osteoblasts. High rates of bone turnover with disproportionate increments in bone resorption characterize the osteoporosis of hyperthyroidism, acromegaly, and immobilization, whereas the osteoporosis seen in Cushing's syndrome or in patients on prolonged adrenocortical steroid therapy develops at low rates of bone formation with an increase in bone resorption accompanied by a decrease in bone formation. Glucocorticoid-induced osteoporosis differs from that of senile or postmenopausal osteoporosis, since in the latter instance the increased bone resorption is in general accompanied by a normal rate of bone formation.

Osteoporosis represents a generalized decrease in bone mass which may often appear subtle. The radiographic changes, when apparent, include cortical thinning of long bones with irregularity of endosteal surfaces and diffuse demineralization and thinning of the tables of the calvarium. Occasionally the demineralization is spotty and resembles multiple myeloma or metastatic carcinoma. These changes are often associated with decreased density of the floor and dorsum of the sella turcica. Pelvic and femoral involvement is characterized by a thin rim of well mineralized cortex and a decreased amount of trabeculae or spongiosa. The remaining trabecular pattern in the pelvis and femoral necks reflects the lines of stress applied to the skeleton and may actually appear more dense. Identical changes occur in the vertebrae; the cortex becomes thin and may impart the false appearance of increased density because of the loss of trabeculae in the main body. In postmenopausal or senile osteoporosis, the cortex, although thin, is uninterrupted. Erosion of the cortex is rare and should lead one to suspect malignant disease. The superior and inferior vertebral cortices are usually thickened or eburnated in glucocorticoid-induced osteoporosis. As the disease progresses, the trabecular pattern is accentuated because of the loss of horizontal trabecular structure and maintenance of vertical trabeculae, according to the structural lines of stress. Further progression of the osteoporotic process results in a variety of vertebral deformities. These include biconcave compression of the end-plates by the pressure of the intervertebral discs, resulting in "codfish" vertebrae and localized herniations of the nucleus pulposus into the vertebral body, producing Schmorl's nodes. These pathologic changes lead subsequently to wedge or compression fractures. In osteoporosis, the apex of the wedge fracture is anterior. Posterior wedging strongly suggests a different disease such as Paget's disease, trauma, or metastatic malignancy. Progressive waves of vertebral fractures finally terminate in dorsal kyphosis and loss of stature. The vertebral collapse is asymptomatic (except during acute fracture) in over 50 per cent of patients, but spinal tenderness is characteristically noted when percussion or pressure is applied to the involved vertebra. The backache of osteoporosis is classically situated in the lumbar of lower thoracic vertebrae, is nonradiating and longstanding, and is usually exacerbated by bending forward or lifting heavy objects. Progressive vertebral collapse leads finally to kyphosis and associated downward angulation of the ribs which, in thin subjects, produce prominent horizontal folds over the chest and abdomen and a variety of constitutional gastrointestinal symptoms.

PRIMARY OSTEOPOROSIS

The term osteoporosis actually defines a heterogeneous group of disorders, with varied etiologies and pathophysiologic features, each of which requires different forms of therapy. Primary (involutional, postmenopausal, or senile) osteoporosis is the most common form of the disorder. This form of the disease becomes increasingly common with age in women after the menopause and in men after 60 years; hence the derivation of the terms postmenopausal and senile osteoporosis. It most probably is a consequence of the universal loss of bone with age, which begins earlier and progresses more rapidly in women than in men. In general, biochemical hallmarks are lacking, since plasma calcium, phosphate, and alkaline phosphatase are usually normal. In some instances, severe osteopenia with structural alterations pathognomonic of primary osteoporosis is associated with a modest elevation in circulating alkaline phosphatase and parathyroid hormone. The relative hyperphosphatasia probably results from the simultaneous presence of osteomalacia. Osteoporosis is probably the most common bone disorder which confronts the average clinician. It has been estimated that 16 to 18 million women in the United States have a significant degree of vertebral atrophy and that approximately 1.5 to 2.0 million have asymptomatic fractures of the dorsolumbar vertebrae. Epidemiologic studies also suggest that approximately 25 to 30 per cent of all white females in the United States develop symptomatic osteoporosis. A direct relationship obtains between osteoporosis and the incidence of hip, femoral, neck, and trochanteric fractures in women age 45 and older, with the fracture rates twice as high in women with radiographically detectable osteopenia when compared to age-matched women with greater skeletal density. Based on these findings, it is estimated that of the approximately 1 million fractures experienced each year by women 45 years or older in the United States, about 700,000 are incurred by women with osteoporosis. Although elderly males develop symptomatic osteoporosis between ages 50 and 70, it is predominantly a disease of females. Evidence has accumulated that the disease is rare among black males of any age and that black females and females of southern European ancestry are much less vulnerable than their Anglo-Saxon sisters.

The cause of postmenopausal and senile osteoporosis is unknown. The sexual and racial differences appear to be related primarily to differences in the amount of skeletal mass accumulated at maturity, rather than to any inherited, dietary, or environmental protection against bone loss. Although many attempts have been made to ascribe gonadal hormonal deficiency following the menopause as the primary cause for an accelerated decrease in bone mass, this relationship has yet to be clearly established. Surgically castrated females do not routinely develop osteoporosis sooner than noncastrated women; moreover, poor correlation exists between the age at menopause and the onset of symptomatic osteoporosis. The fact that osteoporosis is frequently observed in young prepubescent girls with congenital absence of functioning ovaries (gonadal dysgenesis) probably represents a skeletal manifestation of the genetic defect rather than a premature lack of ovarian steroids. Moreover, patients with congenital 17-

hydroxylase deficiencies who are estrogen deficient do not develop osteoporosis prematurely, and circulating estradiol and estrone are comparable in postmenopausal females with or without vertebral compression fractures and symptomatic osteoporosis. At best, the course of the disease may be slowed by short-term estrogen therapy in some females, with relief of the associated spasm of paravertebral muscles. This seemingly paradoxical response has been attributed to estrogen-induced suppression of the skeletal response to parathyroid hormone, which may be elevated in approximately 15 to 20 per cent of females with this disorder.

A second prevailing concept expanded to define the cause of postmenopausal or senile osteoporosis is that calcium consumption is inadequate to permit a positive mineral balance. This hypothesis has been expanded to include the concept that a chronically negative calcium balance could also result from impaired intestinal calcium absorption or from a failure of renal calcium conservation in the presence of seemingly adequate amounts of dietary calcium. The hypothesis is an intriguing one, since a net calcium loss of as little as 50 mg per day could reduce the skeletal mass by 15 to 20 per cent per decade. However, it has been well established by international epidemiologic studies that this disorder occurs in patients with higher than average calcium intakes and that structural changes such as vertebral wedging and compression are unrelated to the level of dietary calcium over a wide range of estimated values. In addition, similar changes in calcium conservation and decreased intestinal calcium absorption have been observed in normal men and women 20 to 30 years older than osteoporotic patients. If alterations in calcium intake and retention are in any way related to osteoporosis, they most probably represent a contributory rather than a primary cause. Until more definitive interpretations are available, one must assume that the cause of postmenopausal or senile osteoporosis is multifactorial and related to (1) a failure to generate a normal bone mass during adolescence; (2) a variety of dietary or environmental indiscretions; (3) the decreased intestinal absorptive efficiency for elements and nutrient fuels which normally accompanies senescence; and (4) an alteration in the hormonal milieu, another necessary concomitant of the aging process.

ENDOCRINE OSTEOPOROSIS

Patients with a variety of endocrinopathies may present with radiographic signs which are indistinguishable from those of postmenopausal or senile osteoporosis. *Hyperthyroidism, hyperparathyroidism, Cushing's syndrome,* and *acromegaly* are usual offenders. Currently available diagnostic hormone assays for growth, thyroid, and parathyroid hormones and for plasma and urinary free cortisol afford an easy solution to the differential diagnosis. Acromegaly with its classic clinical stigmata is usually associated with a normal skeletal radiograph. The most characteristic abnormality is increased concavity of the posterior surfaces of the vertebral bodies. The skeletal response to elevated circulating growth hormone levels is unique for high-turnover bone disease in that cortical bone seems to be principally affected. This is reflected in an increased amount of periosteal new bone, overtubulation of pe-

ripheral bones, and increased posterior concavity of the lumbar vertebrae. Although a sparse trabecular pattern in pelvic and peripheral bones has been observed in this disorder, osteoporosis is a rare finding despite assertions to the contrary.

In contrast, osteoporosis is rather common in Cushing's syndrome and in patients on long-term adrenocorticoid therapy. Cortical bone may be a relatively insensitive indicator of bone disease in the presence of excess adrenal steroids. Osteoporosis is observed in the spine and pelvis, where the proportion of trabecular bone is high, before it is recognized in the long bones, in which the proportion of cortical bone is high. The contrast between "deossified" trabecular bone and unaffected cortical bone may be striking. The vertebral cortical plates may become thick and fuzzy during the active phase of Cushing's disease (or with adrenocortical steroid excess). This is peculiar to glucocorticoid excess and may be considered pathognomonic of the disease. With healing the cortical plates become thin and less dense. Severe bone loss may also obtain in patients (usually young adults) with micronodular adrenal disease with minimal clinical manifestations of hypercortisolism.

Both cortical and trabecular bone are involved in hyperthyroidism; patients may present with extensive skeletal demineralization, hypercalcemia, hypercalciuria, and bone fractures. The osteopenia and high rate of bone turnover in this disease are not due to osteoporosis alone, since osteitis fibrosa and wide osteoid seams are also frequently observed histologically. Occasionally the only radiographic evidence of bone disease in thyrotoxic patients is generalized demineralization. The bones may have a ground glass appearance caused by indistinct trabeculae and distortion of the normal trabecular architecture. Granular deossification ("salt and pepper sign") may be seen in the skull, with blurring of the inner and outer tables. Since the incidence of hyperparathyroidism in thyrotoxic patients is greater than that observed in the general population, osteopenia and hypercalcemia which are not reversed following cure of the thyrotoxic state should be investigated further.

MISCELLANEOUS CAUSES OF OSTEOPOROSIS

Patients treated with large amounts of *heparin* (15,000 to 30,000 units for six months or longer) develop symptomatic osteoporosis which regresses after withdrawal of heparin therapy. The mechanism whereby this phenomenon occurs is unknown, but it has been postulated that heparin, via lysosomal activation, directly stimulates bone resorption. This view is supported by the observations that heparin stimulates bone resorption in tissue culture and that osteoporosis occurs in mastocytosis, a clinical disorder characterized by an overproduction of heparin-producing mast cells.

Immobilization or "disuse" osteoporosis is usually a localized disorder confined to extremities which have been artificially immobilized following a traumatic insult. In traumatic or paralytic lower motor neuron disease, the entire skeleton may be involved. The osteopenia stems from a massive increase in bone resorption because of the absence of the normal mechanical stress imposed by functioning musculature. Radiographically, one initially sees a decrease in the cancellous portions of bone, since it is more easily mobilized than compact cortical bone. Ultimately, the cortex thins and a patchy increase in density occurs throughout the immobilized bone. These changes progress and result in a homogeneous deossification. Although disuse osteoporosis often aggravates pre-existing osteoporosis of other causes, the most serious complication of disuse bone atrophy is that of hypercalciuria and the formation of renal calculi. Patients should be well hydrated and all attempts directed toward rapid and efficient mobilization with appropriate physical therapeutic manipulations.

Osteogenesis imperfecta is an inherited disorder characterized by a variety of phenotypic abnormalities, the most significant being osseous fragility and fractures. It is usually inherited as an autosomal dominant, although autosomal recessive patterns have been documented. Clinically, patients are usually divided into two groups: congenita and tarda — the former defined by the presence of fractures at birth, blue sclerae, wormian bones, and severe skeletal deformities, and the latter by the absence of fractures at birth, with deformities resulting from recurrent fractures in later life. Although the disease has been described in the medical literature for almost 200 years, the pathogenesis is still ill defined. Abnormalities in the molecular organization of skin and bone collagen have been documented, as well as changes in the metabolism of noncollagenous bone proteins. The skeletal lesion is characterized by an accumulation of stainable glycosoaminoglycans, an abnormal orientation of collagen fibers, and an increase in bone resorption. Alterations in bone metabolism in osteogenesis imperfecta often result in elevations in plasma alkaline and acid phosphatases, and in urinary hydroxyproline, pyrophosphate, and glycosoaminoglycans. The congenital form of the disease is often complicated by recurrent fractures and prolonged periods of immobilization, the latter often contributing most dramatically to the osteoporosis and increased bone fragility. Proposed regimens for the management of the progressive osteopenia that invariably occurs in the majority of young adults with this disorder include therapy with sodium fluoride, vitamin D, androgens, and magnesium oxide, but the clinical response to these agents has been less than adequate. Favorable responses in the tarda variety have been reported with calcitonin. In this form of the disease, a decreased incidence of fractures is also observed after puberty, whereas increased incidence occurs after menopause. The disease may be confused with idiopathic juvenile osteoporosis. However, in that skeletal disorder, the sclerae are normal in color, the osteoporosis is typically localized to the vertebral column, and the family history for fractures and resulting deformities is negative. Osteogenesis imperfecta in children may also mimic the juvenile form of hypophosphatasia, although the low circulating alkaline phosphatase, rachitic skeletal changes, and phosphorylethanolaminuria which accompany the hypophosphatasia syndrome should make the disorder readily identifiable. Because of an exceedingly wide range of phenotypic expressivity of the inherited connective tissue defect in osteogenesis imperfecta, the disease may often be misdiagnosed in the adult as a routine case of postmenopausal or idiopathic osteoporosis. A detailed family history and bone biopsy evaluation may prove helpful in establishing the correct diagnosis.

Homocystinuria, a metabolic disease with an autosomal recessive inheritance pattern, is characterized clinically by mental retardation, chronic back pain, kyphoscoliosis, anterior chest deformities in adults (either pectus carinatum or pectus excavatum), genu valgum, joint laxity, ectopia lentis, vascular dilatation, and thrombotic diatheses, and radiographically by osteopenia. Fractures occur with relatively minor trauma, with severe vertebral osteopenia and concavity of the vertebral end-plates, contributing to the associated kyphoscoliotic deformities. Other skeletal findings include punctate or linear longitudinal radiologic densities in the distal ulna and radius, microencephaly, and large paranasal sinuses with abnormally thick calvaria. The basic defect in homocystinuria is a deficiency in the enzyme cystathionine synthetase, resulting in elevations in plasma homocysteine, homocystine, and methionine and an "overflow" homocystinuria. Homocysteine interferes with the formation of intermolecular cross-links, which normally stabilize the collagen macromolecular network by binding to the aldehydic functional groups of the collagen molecule. Since the administration of lathyrogens such as β-aminopropionitrile to animals leads to disturbances in collagen cross-linking and to connective tissue and bone abnormalities not unlike those seen in homocystinuria, the osteoporosis of homocystinuria is presently attributed to the homocysteine effect on bone collagen maturation. Vitamin B_6 (a cofactor for cystathionine synthetase) deficiency also leads to osteoporosis in the rat. When vitamin B_6 is administered to homocystinuric patients in pharmacologic doses of 50 to 300 mg per day, the level of urinary homocystine, an oxidation product of homocysteine, falls. Since the reported homocysteine effect on the collagen molecule is also reversible, continued high dose vitamin B_6 therapy may ultimately prove therapeutic for the osteopenia seen in patients with homocystinuria.

Although the incidence is much less than that seen with homocystinuria, increased radiolucency of the vertebrae and exaggeration of the normal concavity of the dorsal aspect of the vertebral bodies have also been reported in *Marfan's syndrome* and *Ehlers-Danlos syndrome*. Although the fundamental defect in Marfan's syndrome is still unknown, the connective tissue and bone defects of Ehlers-Danlos syndrome may be related to the faulty bone collagen maturation.

Osteoporosis is also observed in children with *Menkes' syndrome,* an X-linked recessive inherited disorder of connective tissue characterized by an intestinal malabsorption of copper, low serum copper ceruloplasmin concentration, severe copper deficiency, growth retardation, and kinky or "steely" hair. The skeletal pathology may also result from maturational defects in bone collagen, since the lysine oxidase enzyme essential for collagen cross-link formation is copper dependent. Cultured human fibroblasts may ultimately prove valuable in establishing this diagnosis, since they exhibit elevated copper concentrations in patients with this disorder.

Decreased bone density and radiologically detectable osteoporosis has also been reported in an inherited disorder characterized by hypercalciuria, hypouricemia, and increased uric acid clearance and in the *Riley-Day syndrome* (familial dysautonomia), a rare autosomal recessive disorder found mostly in Jewish children of Eastern European extraction. Other distinctive features of the Riley-Day syndrome include scoliosis, hyperhidrosis, disordered swallowing, dysarthria, motor incoordination, relative insensitivity to pain, episodic hypertension, postural hypotension, and transient blotching of the skin. Although inherited forms of vitamin D resistant rickets classically present with rachitic deformities (children) or pseudofractures (adults), severe osteopenia without distinct alterations in epiphyseal bone maturation may also occur.

Juvenile (idiopathic) osteoporosis is a rare disorder of prepubertal children between the ages of 8 and 14 years, characterized by an abrupt onset of bone pains (usually close to the metaphyses of long bones), fractures following minimal trauma, and osteoporosis of the entire skeleton, including the hands and feet. When uncomplicated by the sequelae of recurrent fractures, the disease is self-limited, most patients recovering completely within four or five years. As noted in children successfully treated for Cushing's syndrome, endochondral new bone is deposited around less dense permanently altered bone during the recovery phase. Histologically, haversian bone remodeling is severely impaired, osteoid content is decreased, bone formation rates are either normal or low, and bone resorption is strikingly increased. Serum calcium and phosphate are usually at the upper limits; serum alkaline phosphatase and urinary hydroxyproline may be abnormally high for the patient's age. Transient hypercalciuria and calcium malabsorption have also been observed. A detailed family history and iliac crest bone biopsy may be essential to differentiate juvenile osteoporosis from osteogenesis imperfecta, since both disorders may present with a history of fractures and slender bones with thin cortices. The juvenile form of osteoporosis may also mimic the bone disease associated with childhood leukemic syndromes. Because of the self-limited course, therapy other than minimizing immobilization and avoiding excessive weight gain is unwarranted.

Sudeck's atrophy is a form of regional osteoporosis seen in patients with reflex sympathetic dystrophy and commonly localized to the hands and feet. The disorder, often recurrent and episodic, may terminate in permanent skeletal injury. This form of localized osteopenia is characterized clinically by atrophic, glossy, tight skin with swelling, tenderness, and sweating over the affected area. Abnormal autonomic vasomotor regulation has been implicated as the cause. Paravertebral lumbar or stellate ganglion sympathetic block may produce dramatic relief. Although frequently disabling, the disease is usually self-limited and in most instances heals spontaneously over a period of several months to a few years. Corticosteroids in a dosage equivalent to 30 to 40 mg of prednisone per day may prove effective in alleviating the pain which often precludes programmed ambulation and skeletal mobilization. In particularly severe or protracted cases, regional sympathectomy may be indicated. Reports of beneficial response to chronic calcitonin therapy, although promising, require further confirmation.

TREATMENT OF OSTEOPOROSIS

In the majority of instances, the therapy of osteoporosis depends upon reversing the underlying disease. Thus mobilization results in a rapid cure of disuse osteoporosis, as does appropriate surgery in the osteoporosis seen in a variety of endocrinopathies. Since the cause(s) of postmenopausal or senile osteoporosis is still unknown, the therapy is largely empirical. Bed rest is contraindicated and physical therapy desirable. An adequate calcium intake of 1.5 to 2.0 grams per day is essential, as is exposure to sunlight and vitamin D ingestion (e.g., 500 to 1000 IU daily). Since oral neutral sodium and potassium phosphates of 1.0 to 1.5 gram per day actually increase the rate of bone loss, this approach is contraindicated. Since fluorapatite is more stable and less soluble than hydroxyapatite, it has been reasoned that the skeleton of fluoride-treated subjects should be less susceptible to the enhanced skeletal resorption which perpetuates the osteopenia. Therapy with sodium fluoride in doses of 40 to 60 mg per day should, however, be tempered by the knowledge that arthralgia and joint effusions may develop and that excessive fluoride ingestion leads to *more* brittle bones. Since women reared in endemic areas where the fluoride content of water is greater than average (e.g., 3 to 4 ppm) have a decreased incidence of vertebral collapse, *low-dose* prophylactic fluoride therapy may actually retard the accelerated postmenopausal bone loss observed in some individuals. Since hormones may possibly play a role in preventing the accelerated bone loss of postmenopausal females, prophylactic estrogen therapy in ordinary replacement doses of 1.0 mg 17β estradiol per day or its equivalent in *nonconjugated* estrogens may also be administered for short periods to the young castrated female or to women in the early menopausal state with emphasis on the additional need for adequate dietary intake and physical activity. The injudicious use of long-term conjugated estrogens in elderly women with severely compromised bone mass cannot be presently sanctioned as an effective mode of therapy, since such agents increase the incidence of endometrial carcinoma and have not yet proved of significant therapeutic value in this aged population. Finally, the clinician must always be cognizant of the fact that thyrotoxicosis, multiple myeloma, and osteomalacia may be occult in the aged. In the absence of pseudofractures, osteomalacia cannot be diagnosed by routine radiographic techniques. Thus before any form of empirical therapy is instituted for senile or postmenopausal osteoporosis, attempts should be made to rule out occult endocrine and malignant disorders and osteomalacia by functional testing and bone biopsy procedures if the latter prove nondiagnostic.

Avioli, L. V.: Osteoporosis, pathogenesis and therapy. *In* Avioli, L. V., and Krane, S. M. (eds.): Metabolic Bone Disease, Vol. I. New York, Academic Press, 1977, p. 307.

Bassan, J., Frame, B., and Frost, H.: Osteoporosis: A review of pathogenesis and treatment. Ann. Intern. Med., 58:539, 1963.

De Takats, G.: Sympathetic reflex dystrophy. Med. Clin. North Am., 39:117, 1965.

Gallagher, J. C., Aaron, J., Horsman, A., Marshall, D. H., Wilkinson, R., and Nordin, B. E. C.: The crush fracture syndrome in postmenopausal women. *In* Clinics in Endocrinology and Metabolism. London, W. B. Saunders Company, 1973, p. 293.

Hahn, T. J., and Hahn, B. H.: Osteopenia in patients with rheumatic diseases: Principles of diagnosis and therapy. Semin. Arthritis Rheum., 6:165, 1976.

Heaney, R. P.: A unified concept of osteoporosis. Am. J. Med., 39: 877, 1965.

Rosenberg, E., Lang, R., Boisseau, V., Rojanasathit, S., and Avioli, L. V.: Effect of long-term calcitonin therapy on the clinical course of osteogenesis imperfecta. J. Clin. Endocrinol. Metab., 44:346, 1977.

Steinbach, H. L.: The roentgen appearance of osteoporosis. Radiol. Clin. North Am., 2:191, 1964.

558. OSTEOMALACIA AND RICKETS

The two major types of bone in man are fibrous and lamellar. Fibrous bone (often called "woven" or "fetal" bone) is elaborated rapidly, and its formation is governed by phenomena which differ from those which initiate and control lamellar bone formation. The adult human skeleton is composed almost exclusively of lamellar bone, and osteomalacia represents a skeletal disorder characterized by a disturbance in lamellar bone metabolism. As detailed earlier, the organic phase of lamellar bone is formed by osteoblasts. Normal lamellar bone is formed by cellular activity which deposits an osteoid layer on pre-existing bone at the rate of 1 μ per day, and is characterized by the presence of osteoid seams. A lamellar "osteoid seam" is defined as a layer of new bone matrix that is not as yet mineralized. An osteoid seam therefore exists in temporal limbo between its formation by osteoblasts and the onset of mineralization. Osteoid seams are normally less than 12 μ in width (average, 10 μ) and accompany lamellar bone formation at all ages and in both sexes. The number of osteoid seams per unit volume of bone is maximum at birth; it decreases gradually until age 30, after which an increase in number obtains with increasing age.

Osteoid seams normally occur in actively forming haversian systems, in actively forming endosteal bone sites, and in actively forming new trabeculae or portions of new trabeculae in cancellous bone. Tetracyclines have a special affinity for bone tissue, and when administered orally or parenterally they deposit in skeletal areas at the "calcification front" when new bone matrix or hyaline cartilage is actively mineralizing. The pattern of tetracycline deposition is the same as the patterns of new mineralization and the deposition of calcium. In essence, the tetracycline "labels" new bone mineralization, being taken up only during periods of active osteoid mineralization. There is no apparent diffusion of the bone-fixed tetracycline molecules and no apparent permanent absorption of the drug in the resting skeletal mineral mass. Tetracycline deposited in the skeleton at sites of new mineralization is permanently fixed in situ as long as subsequent osteoid mineralization is not interrupted. It is conventional to term tetracycline deposited and fixed in this manner as a "label." When the labeled skeletal tissue is reabsorbed during the remodeling process, the tetracycline is released to and diluted by the bloodstream and lost to subsequent optical detection. In normal adults, tetracycline will deposit in a band 4 to 5 μ wide at the mineralization front within two hours of administration. With continued tetracycline administration, 1 μ per day of formed osteoid will be labeled, and at the end of a 10 day course the tetracycline-labeled zone should therefore be approximately 15 μ wide. If, for example, the width of the tetracycline band was distinctly less than 15 μ after a ten-day labeling period, one could conclude that the bone mineralization, or "appositional," rates were decreased if newly formed matrix mineralizes as soon as elaborated, tetracycline-labeled bone should appear in the histologic section without a bordering osteoid seam. If, however, mineralization of new matrix occurs a few days after formation, an osteoid seam bordering tetracycline-labeled bone should appear. The time required for osteoid mineralization can then be quantitated with appropriate measurements of the distance between the calcifying point and the fluorescent-tetracycline band obtained following a single tetracycline dose, or by quantitating the amount of osteoid calcified between two labels given at predetermined intervals before the biopsy. In the latter instance, the mean distance between the centers of the tetracycline bands approximates the appositional rate, in microns per day, of new bone mineralized in the time interval between labels. These measurements of bone formation or osteoid content can be made only on undecalcified sections, since decalcification often distorts the distinction between osteoid seams and recently mineralized bone and interferes with the location and quantitation of osteoid content. In addition, estimates of bone appositional or formation rates using the calcification front and a single tetracycline label are fraught with interpretive difficulties on routine decalcified specimens stained with hematoxylin and eosin.

Although the optimal concentrations of calcium and inorganic phosphate essential for osteoid mineralization are unknown, mineralization does not proceed optimally when their plasma and extracellular fluid concentrations are decreased. Other conditions required for normal mineralization include an adequate collagen matrix, low concentrations of calcification "inhibitors" such as specific protein polysaccharide moieties and inorganic pyrophosphate, and intact metabolic and transport functions of osteoblasts and chondrocytes.

Osteomalacia, a term which means bone softening, is characterized by the accumulation of increased amounts of osteoid in bone matrix that either fails to calcify or does so very slowly. The term *rickets* refers to an identical syndrome in children with distinct epiphyseal abnormalities, since, unlike the adult skeleton, endochondral skeletal growth is still incomplete in growing children. In rickets, mineralization is defective in both bone and cartilage, since in endochondral bone formation cartilage is normally remodeled and organic matrix replaced as ossification of the cartilage model proceeds. In both osteomalacia and rickets, the distinguishing histologic features observed on trabecular surfaces or newly forming haversian systems are wide osteoid seams and an increased number of osteoid seams per unit area of bone. In addition to these changes, one classically finds, with tetracycline labeling techniques, a decreased rate of osteoid mineralization, or a low appositional rate. These combined diagnostic criteria are essential to the diagnosis of true osteomalacia, since other disorders of bone metabolism characterized by *elevated* appositional rates (e.g., Paget's disease, hyperthyroidism, or primary hyperparathyroidism) may also lead to an increased number of osteoid seams.

CLINICAL AND RADIOGRAPHIC FINDINGS. Osteomalacia complicates a variety of clinical disorders and, although clinically quite obvious in the child, often presents in the adult with vague symptoms of skeletal pain and tenderness which, although characteristically diffuse, may be limited to the spine, pelvis, and lower extremities. When it occurs, pain may be especially prominent about the hips, resulting in an ataxic gait. Weakness, usually proximal in distribution, may become severe enough to mimic primary muscle disorders. In children, growth is retarded, the skeleton becomes fragile, and fractures may occur repeatedly with minimal trauma. Thickened and irregular epiphyseal plates, curvature and flaring of the metaphyses of long bones, and prominent smooth beading of the costochondral junctions (rachitic rosary) develop as a result of distorted skeletal remodeling and defective mineralization. Indentation of the lower ribs at the site of attachment of the diaphragm ("Harrison's groove") may also be evident. Characteristically, swelling of wrists and ankles becomes apparent. In advanced rickets, calvarial sutures are open and soft (craniotabes), and frontal and parietal bossing gives the head a boxlike appearance. Defects in dentition with delay in eruption and extensive caries may also occur.

In the adult, osteomalacia may occur without radiologic abnormalities, and the features of the underlying disorder may dominate. Although a generalized decrease in bone density or osteopenia may be seen in adults with this disorder, it stems most probably from an associated osteoporosis. In patients in whom the osteomalacia is not attended by osteoporosis, the bone mass is normal and the skeleton may actually appear *more* dense roentgenographically. The cause for this "hyperostosis" is unknown. Microscopically the trabeculae are covered with abnormally thickened osteoid seams, and the bone is still subject to fracture with relatively little trauma. Cortices of long bones may be thin; the skull may be mottled and resemble the appearance found in hyperparathyroidism. On occasion, stimulated parathyroid activity (secondary hyperparathyroidism) may lead to subperiosteal bone resorption along the radial margin of middle phalanges. The x-ray changes of secondary hyperparathyroidism are usually seen in the more severe forms of osteomalacia which accompany renal osteodystrophy and intestinal malabsorption. The only characteristic roentgenographic changes in adults with osteomalacia are pseudofractures (Milkman's lines, Looser's zones). Pseudofractures (which are rare in children) are ribbon-like zones of decalcification extending into bones at approximately right angles to the margin and are often bilateral and symmetrical. They usually occur at the axillary margin of the scapula, metatarsals, femoral neck, pubic and ischial rami, and ribs and correspond anatomically to the location of major blood vessels or nutrient arteries. In children, the roentgenographic features of rickets are seen most readily in the fastest growing portion of bones such as the proximal ends of tibia and humerus, distal ends of radius and ulna, and sternal ends of ribs. If growth ceases because of an intercurrent illness, the skeletal lesion may actually heal even though the underlying disorder is still uncorrected.

LABORATORY FINDINGS. Changes in plasma concentrations of calcium, inorganic phosphorus, and alkaline phosphatase vary with the different disorders. In vitamin D deficiency states, whether resulting from dietary lack, inadequate sunlight exposure, or intestinal malabsorption, serum calcium levels are normal or low, whereas phosphorus levels are characteristically low. The osteomalacia reported in patients with benign soft tissue tumors is also attended by strikingly low serum phosphorus values. In adults, phosphorus concentrations less than 3.0 mg per deciliter are abnormal; in children, the lower limit of normal is closer to 4.0 or 4.5 per deciliter. In *severe* states of vitamin D depletion hypocalcemia may also be seen, occasionally sufficient to produce tetany. Mild acidosis and generalized aminoaciduria may also be found as a result of secondary hyperparathyroidism or intrinsic renal tubular disease. As a rule, patients with renal tubular disorders maintain normal serum calcium levels, while hypophosphatemia is characteristic. Other laboratory findings, such as glycosuria, aminoaciduria, acidosis, and hypouricemia, reflect variable degrees of disturbance of proximal tubular function, secondary hyperparathyroidism, or features of the underlying disease (e.g., low plasma ceruloplasmin in Wilson's disease or abnormalities of immunoglobulins in multiple myeloma). In chronic renal failure, hyperphosphatemia and either normal or low plasma calcium are usually seen, and circulating alkaline phosphatase may be normal or elevated. Serum phosphorus levels are also normal or elevated in hypophosphatasia, an inherited disorder characterized by abnormally low circulating and alkaline phosphatase levels. Increased excretion of hydroxyproline peptide and cyclic AMP are noted in those conditions in which secondary hyperparathyroidism and excessive bone resorption are associated with the defect in mineralization.

Levels of alkaline phosphatase in plasma are usually elevated in rickets or osteomalacia but typical and even severe osteomalacia, especially that due to renal tubular disorders, may be accompanied by normal or only borderline elevations. Alkaline phosphatase and hydroxyproline excretion may increase during the early phases of therapy. Occasionally the source of the elevations in circulating alkaline phosphatase may be misleading. Patients with osteomalacia or malabsorption may present with elevations in either the intestinal or skeletal isoenzyme, and a predominance of the intestinal isoenzyme may occur in patients with severe hepatic insufficiency and osteomalacia. Moreover, a variety of drugs also result in elevations in circulating alkaline phosphatase during routine laboratory testing. In this regard, measurements of 5'-nucleotidase and/or gamma glutamyl transpeptidase (GGTP) activities may prove diagnostically significant. Elevations in GGTP and 5'-nucleotidase indicate that the hepatic isoenzyme is the main cause of the associated elevations in circulating alkaline phosphatase. If the rise in plasma alkaline phosphatase results from disturbances in the hepatobiliary system, circulating leucine aminopeptidase (LAP), an enzyme not elevated in simple rickets or osteomalacia, may also be high. Elevations in alkaline phosphatase (the Regan enzyme) may also result from carcinoma without evidence of metastatic lesions in the liver or bone.

Circulating levels of 25-hydroxycholecalciferol and 1,25-dihydroxycholecalciferol, normal in a variety of osteomalacic or rachitic disorders, may be decreased in patients with hepatic dysfunction, small bowel or gastric resections, or renal insufficiency, and in those on anticonvulsant medications or with nutritional deficiencies. Hypomagnesemia, noted in patients with hepatic insufficiency and/or intestinal malabsorption, may be attended by hypocalcemia and severe neuroirritability. As noted earlier, a state of "functional hypoparathyroidism" obtains in this situation; clinical symptoms and hypocalcemia are characteristically reversed only after the hypomagnesemia has been corrected.

VITAMIN D DEFICIENCY

Vitamin D deficiency rickets in children, often termed classic, infantile, or nutritional rickets, is almost always the result of inadequate exposure to the ultraviolet irradiation of sunlight and/or dietary deficiency. Although rickets is more common in premature and fat infants, it may appear even in association with protein-calorie malnutrition, making diagnostic confirmation difficult. Nutritional childhood rickets or osteomalacia is virtually unheard of in modern developed communities, since foods fortified with vitamin D contain amounts sufficient to prevent rickets in growing children or adults living in temperate zones. These disorders are still diagnosed in their most florid forms in underdeveloped regions of the world and in urban areas where pigmented populations have migrated from sunny to cloudy climates and ignored prescribed preventive measures. Although the disease may present at birth as a result of maternal vitamin deficiency or later in the neonatal period, it is classically seen in infants between six months and two years of age. Irritability is usually seen; tetany and convulsions, although infrequent, can occur when skeletal mineralization is initiated by phosphate feeding or when phosphate is liberated from intracellular stores during periods of prolonged fasting or increased metabolic requirements of acute febrile illnesses. Since initiation of healing by very small doses of vitamin D or exposure to sunlight may also precipitate neuromuscular irritability and tetany, it is advisable to treat with doses of vitamin D in excess of prophylactic requirements (i.e., 1000 to 10,000 IU daily) for a period of several months. Healing becomes evident within weeks, with a rapid return of the serum calcium and inorganic phosphate to normal and a more gradual decline in serum alkaline phosphatase. Occasionally, healing is heralded by a brief increase or "flare" in the circulating alkaline phosphatase level and urinary hydroxyproline. Subsequent therapy is primarily the ensuring of an adequate dietary supply of vitamin D.

Nutritional osteomalacia is rare in adults, since the mature skeleton with its relatively slow turnover rate is able to withstand short periods of vitamin D deficiency without deleterious effects, and body adipose tissue vitamin D stores are often more than sufficient to maintain normal mineral homeostasis. It has been estimated, however, that osteomalacia may develop in adults of any age when the diet contains less than 70 to 100 IU of vitamin D per day. The usual dietary history obtained is of avoidance of fatty foods or of strict vegetarianism. Certain immigrants and elderly females appear to be most susceptible to the nutritional form of osteomalacia, which characteristically responds to therapy with vitamin D and 25-hydroxycholecalciferol.

GASTROINTESTINAL MALABSORPTION AND HEPATIC DISEASE

Osteopenia (osteomalacia and/or osteoporosis) is relatively common after gastric surgery, in disorders of the small and large intestine, and in chronic hepatic diseases. Estimates of the incidence of bone disease following gastrectomy vary between 1 and 42 per cent and depend on the type of surgery and the interval after surgery, as well as appropriate diagnostic testing and the diagnostic criteria used. Bone disease appears with greater frequency after the Polya or the Billroth II types of gastric resection and gastroenterostomy, less often after the Billroth I procedure. The pathogenesis of the bone disease following gastrectomy is still virtually unknown. The incidence of osteopenia increases with time after surgery. Postoperative steatorrhea is probably a predisposing factor. Since intestinal absorption of calcium and vitamin D is found to be normal in gastrectomized patients, their poor appetite may cause inadequate intake of calcium, protein, and vitamin D, thus contributing to the progressive loss in skeletal mass and demineralization.

Characteristically, patients present with variable degrees of muscle weakness and diffuse tenderness and aching of the bones. Bone tenderness is usually elicited by tibial pressure or by compression of the rib cage. The tenderness may be localized to pseudofracture areas. Whereas serum calcium and inorganic phosphate values may seldom lead to detection of postoperative bone disease, the serum alkaline phosphatase levels may be used as a reliable index. Although normal in patients with small bowel resection and early bone disease, this enzyme serves reasonably well as a screening test for osteomalacic bone disease after gastrectomy procedures. In the absence of Paget's disease of bone or hepatic dysfunction, a raised serum alkaline phosphatase after gastrectomy is usually indicative of either overt or subclinical osteomalacia. Subclinical osteomalacia can only be diagnosed with certainty by bone biopsy, and as a rule a decalcified section will not suffice. Low circulating levels of vitamin D_3 and 25-hydroxycholecalciferol, wide osteoid seams, and the absence of calcification fronts in biopsied bone strongly support a diagnosis of osteomalacia, and the response to appropriate vitamin D therapy offers further confirmation.

Osteomalacia is not uncommon as a complication of intestinal malabsorption; it often accompanies idiopathic steatorrhea, nontropical sprue, regional enteritis, prolonged biliary obstruction, and chronic pancreatic insufficiency. Dietary vitamin D and 25-hydroxycholecalciferol, which is produced by the liver and normally secreted into the intestine, are absorbed in the form of chylomicron complexes. This process is impaired in diseases with steatorrhea, such as chronic biliary obstruction in which emulsification of fat is disturbed. Factors other than failure to absorb vitamin D may contribute to the osteomalacia in patients with small bowel disease, such as inadequate absorbing surfaces and/or failure of intestinal cells to respond to the active vitamin D metabolite, as may obtain in gluten-sensitive enteropathy syndromes and tropical sprue with folate deficiency. Osteomalacia may also complicate the course of obese patients treated with jejunocolic or jejunoileal anastomoses. When associated with recurrent calcium oxalate stones (also noted in these patients), the bone pain of osteomalacia may be misinterpreted and inappropriately ascribed to hyperparathyroidism. Although steatorrhea and calcium malabsorption contribute to the osteomalacic bone disease in patients with small bowel disease, it appears most likely that the defective absorption of vitamin D and of 25-hydroxycholecalciferol are major factors in its pathogenesis. As noted earlier for gastrectomized patients, hypophosphatemia and/or hyperphosphatasia are often the only chemical hallmarks of the bone disease. Treatment with vitamin D in disorders of intestinal malabsorption is usually combined with that of calcium supplements (1 to 2 grams of elemental calcium per day) and gluten-free diets. In cases of nontropical sprue, gluten-free diets are continued indefinitely whereas the vitamin D (10,000 to 50,000 IU daily) may be discontinued once the osteomalacia has been cured. In treatment of the osteomalacia resulting from obstructive jaundice, large parenteral doses of vitamin D (200,000 to 500,000 IU every two to four weeks) may be essential. The observed "resistance" to vitamin D therapy in these disorders stems from malabsorption and/or the failure of the diseased liver to convert vitamin D to 25-hydroxycholecalciferol, since much smaller doses of the latter compound (10,000 IU per day) are quite effective in reversing the bone lesions.

Chronic pancreatitis, intestinal malabsorption, and steatorrhea frequently complicate the course of anicteric patients with liver disease. Moreover, since adipose tissue serves as a large storage depot for vitamin D, prolonged malnutrition, decreased sunlight exposure, and decreased fat stores which frequently characterized the clinical course of patients with chronic hepatic dysfunction may also contribute to a decrease in the available body stores of vitamin D. Patients with chronic liver disease and osteomalacia may also demonstrate unequivocal histologic evidence of osteoporosis. This form of bone disease is probably a result of cachexia and prolonged inactivity.

VITAMIN D RESISTANT RICKETS
(VDRR)

VDRR is predominantly a familial disorder and is almost always transmitted by an X-linked dominant gene. The disorder should not be confused with pseudo–vitamin D deficiency rickets, a separate disorder characterized by an autosomal recessive inheritance pattern. Using *fasting* hypophosphatemia as a genetic determinant, the frequency of VDRR has been estimated as 1:25,000. Asymptomatic hypophosphatemic adult carriers (i.e., individuals with affected children but with no past history of clinical or radiographically demonstrable bone disease) are almost always females. These VDRR individuals should be contrasted with those adults presenting with sporadic hypophosphatemia and osteomalacia, who differ from patients with the inherited form of VDRR by the onset of symptoms during adolescence or adult life, severe myopathy, and glycinuria.

Clinically, VDRR is characterized by reduced growth rate and short stature, fractures (more often in adults), and varus and valgus knee deformities in growing children secondary to the presence of epiphyseal rachitic lesions. These changes are not specific for VDRR and may be seen in other acquired or vitamin D deficient forms of rickets. In untreated or poorly managed patients (i.e., those treated with vitamin D alone) the secondary deformities which present after epiphyseal closure such as coxa vara and "saber shins" may be quite severe. Trunk length is normal in children with VDRR, and leg length shortening accounts for most of the statural defect in these patients. Retardation of bone maturation is not ordinarily attended by striking delay in bone age.

Although hypophosphatemia is the hallmark of the disorder and supplemental phosphate administration is therapeutic with more rapid healing and acceleration of growth of children initially treated with vitamin D alone, there is no relationship between the observed height deficits and the degree of hypophosphatemia. Clinical signs of rickets, such as growth failure, genu varum, or genu valgum, are usually less obvious in affected females than in affected males despite comparable degrees of hypophosphatemia. On the average, heterozygous females manifest a mild degree of hypophosphatemia and less severe skeletal deformities. When bone disease is present, however, objective measurements such as skeletal radiograms and growth rates do not demonstrate differences in severity between males and females. Patients with VDRR may initially present to dental consultation because of tooth fracture or attrition. Moreover, loose abscessed teeth with gingival fistulas, with or without gross evidence of pulp exposure from caries, and enamel hypomineralization and hypoplasia have been observed before changes in growth rates or rachitiform deformities were clinically apparent. Radiologically these changes are associated with varying degrees of facial-osseous abnormalities, delayed tooth eruption, obscure lamina dura, and enlarged pulp chambers.

Patients with VDRR may present with either rachitic (children) or osteomalacic (adult) lesions, although in severe cases diffuse osteopenia may be observed. Histologically, the skeletal lesion is generalized and characterized by an abundance of unmineralized osteoid (collagen) and mineralization defects, specifically around the osteocytes. In some skeletal areas failure of osteoclastic resorption results in osteomalacic osteosclerosis. Evidence of bone cell population dynamics in VDRR also reveals major dynamic disturbances in bone turnover, osteoprogenitor cell activity, and osteoblastic function. The osteomalacic lesion observed in adults with VDRR may be either undetected radiologically or limited to pseudofractures. Accessory ossicles, skeletal proliferation in the areas of ligamentous or tendinous insertion (particularly the intervertebral spaces and neural arches of the lower thoracic and lumbar vertebrae) and a coarsened trabecular osteosclerotic pattern may be observed. In adults with fused epiphysis, VDRR may be confused with the tarda form of achondroplasia, since short stature and disproportionate length of the extremities and spine, thick and dense long bones, wedging of the pelvis, and well developed musculature are common to both disorders. Adults with VDRR may also present with either dome-shaped or narrow and long cranial contours. These changes have been ascribed to premature closure of the cranial sutures (most commonly the sagittal suture), a phenomenon observed in one third to one half of individuals with active rickets.

Fasting hypophosphatemia, elevations in circulating alkaline phosphatase, phosphaturia, and hydroxyprolinuria have all been well documented in this disorder. In contrast to the general finding of elevated values in simple vitamin D deficiency rickets, circulating levels of immunoreactive parathyroid hormone (iPTH) have been variably reported as normal, elevated, or lower than normal in VDRR. Part of this disparity may be due to differences between antisera with regard to the recognition of the heterogeneous circulating fragments of parathyroid hormone and/or differing basal phosphate and vitamin D intake patterns of the patients. Although hypomagnesemia has been reported, serum magnesium is usually normal. Slight elevations in urinary amino acids and glycosuria have also been observed.

Earlier isotopic studies of vitamin D metabolism in VDRR revealed a delayed plasma disappearance of intravenously injected radioactive vitamin D_3 with decreased formation of lipid-soluble metabolites and increased formation of polar water-soluble metabolites. These changes were consistent with a decreased conversion of vitamin D to one or more of its biologically active metabolites. Subsequently it was demonstrated that circulating levels of 25OHD were normally maintained in patients with VDRR, with an appropriate increase in 25OHD following vitamin D administration, and that serum 1,25(OH)$_2$D levels in untreated VDRR patients were low and inappropriate for the marked hypophosphatemia. This defective response of renal 1α-hydroxylase to hypophosphatemia is consistent with alterations in phosphate transport in the renal tubule.

Since parathyroid hyperplasia and elevations in circulating iPTH have been documented in VDRR, it has been proposed that patients with this syndrome inherit either a basic defect in intestinal calcium transport or a blunted response to vitamin D. This theory assumes that the propensity to malabsorb calcium results in parathyroid overactivity, the latter leading to an exaggerated phosphaturia and chronic hypophosphatemia. The skeletal lesions of rickets or osteomalacia are attributed to a persistently low Ca × P product. The hypothesis is consistent with reports of calcium malabsorption and alterations in the morphology of the intestinal cell, the reversal of the phosphaturia during calcium infusion, and the development of parathyroid hyperplasia and parathyroid adenoma in patients with longstanding VDRR.

It has also been proposed that the skeletal lesions and hypophosphatemia which characterize VDRR result from primary defects in intestinal and renal tubular phosphate transport systems. Phosphate transport defects in patients with VDRR have been localized to the intestine and kidney, with red cell and salivary phosphate transport systems apparently intact. This hypothesis is consistent with the blunted 1α-hydroxylase response to hypophosphatemia, reports of defective phosphate absorption by patients with this disorder and in the C57/Hyp mouse laboratory model for VDRR, and observations that ^{32}P uptake by small bowel mucosal biopsies obtained from VDRR males and heterozygous females is decreased. It also accounts for the observations that some males who carry the gene for VDRR lack a parathyroid hormone–sensitive renal phosphate transport system, and other reports of net tubular *secretion* of phosphate in individuals with VDRR.

The ideal response to vitamin D therapy of any rachitic or osteomalacic disorder is seen in patients with classic vitamin D lack rickets due to nutritional inadequacy or poor sunlight exposure, or both. In simple D lack rickets, serum calcium, phosphorus, alkaline phosphatase, and PTH return to values which are normal for the age of the patient, the skeletal lesions heal completely, and, in children, skeletal maturity and growth rate are once again normalized. This response is to be contrasted with the effect of vitamin D therapy on children with VDRR, which is characterized primarily by healing of the rachitic lesions and a decrease in circulating alkaline phosphatase. The hypophosphatemia and growth retardation are relatively unaffected even during long-term therapy with doses as high as 500,000 IU per day. Not infrequently, the rachitic VDRR child treated only with high dose vitamin D regimens, which fail to correct the hypophosphatemia (i.e., serum phosphorus <3.0 mg per deciliter), is "healed" at the expense of short stature and skeletal deformities. The need for careful monitoring of serum and urinary calcium must be emphasized, since, as noted previously, long-term high dose vitamin D therapy may result in hypercalcemic crises, hypercalciuria, and nephrocalcinosis. Although it has been assumed that an increase in

the serum calcium level above the upper limit of normal provides a reliable sign of vitamin intoxication, it would be more appropriate to monitor calcium excretion at frequent intervals, since prolonged hypercalciuria (i.e., 24-hour urinary calcium greater than 4 mg per kilogram of body weight) should be avoided. Moreover, in many instances hypercalciuria actually antedates the hypercalciuria in VDRR subjects on high dose vitamin D regimens.

Although the ideal therapeutic dose of vitamin D is difficult to establish, the concomitant administration of oral phosphate supplements in doses of 1 to 4 grams per day results in more rapid healing of the skeletal lesions, amelioration of the hypophosphatemia, and acceleration of growth not attainable when vitamin D is administered alone. The recommended phosphate preparation for children with VDRR consists of dibasic sodium phosphate, 136 grams per volume; phosphoric acid (NF 85 per cent), 58.5 grams per volume; and 1 liter of water. One ml of this solution provides 30 mg of elemental phosphorus. Treatment is usually initiated with 5-ml doses, with stepwise increments in multiples of 5 until an average intake of 15 ml every four hours five times daily is achieved. When phosphate is added to the therapeutic regimen, the rachitic skeletal lesions heal with vitamin D doses of 25,000 to 75,000 IU daily, a range which rarely proves toxic. The main disadvantages of phosphate therapy are the frequency (five to six doses per day) with which the medication must be administered and the diarrhea which usually occurs during the first one to two weeks of therapy. These problems should not preclude attempts to initiate phosphate therapy in growing children with VDRR, with emphasis on maintaining circulating phosphate levels >3.0 mg per deciliter. It should be emphasized that the administration of phosphate alone cannot heal or prevent the recurrence of rickets, so that vitamin D therapy must be continued, albeit at lower dose schedules. During the initial stages of either vitamin D or phosphate therapy, or a combination thereof, urinary hydroxyproline and serum alkaline phosphatase may actually rise. This seemingly paradoxical response is only temporary and is actually associated with and followed by clinical, biochemical, and radiologic healing. Some patients with VDRR also present with mild glycosuria, decrease in the tubular reabsorption of glucose, and a further decrease in the maximal tubular reabsorption of phosphate following oral glucose loading. High carbohydrate feeding should be avoided in them because the induced phosphaturia often renders the hypophosphatemia more resistant to phosphate supplementation.

In the past, once the active rickets was controlled, surgery was usually considered appropriate for correction of the severe leg deformities. Operative intervention, necessitating immobilization before radiographic and biochemical evidence of skeletal healing was achieved, was frequently unsuccessful and deformities recurred. Moreover, spasmodic or inadequate therapy also resulted in recurrence of the deformities, although leg abnormalities which were surgically corrected in patients older than 12 years did not tend to recur. Since the incidence of leg deformities and short stature should be considerably reduced if VDRR is diagnosed early in childhood and phosphate added to vitamin D therapy, the need for ultimate corrective surgical intervention would be minimized. If surgery necessitating strict immobilization is ultimately required, vitamin D and phosphorus supplementation should be drastically reduced until an active mobilization program is reinstituted.

PSEUDO–VITAMIN D DEFICIENCY RICKETS
(PDR)

PDR, also called vitamin D dependent rickets, hereditary pseudo–vitamin D deficiency rickets or pseudodeficiency rickets, is often mistakenly confused with VDRR. PDR, inherited as a simple autosomal recessive trait, is characterized by signs and symptoms usually appearing in the first year of life which may mimic those seen in simple nutritional vitamin D deficiency. The rachitic skeletal lesions are similar to those of VDRR, but convulsions and severe muscular weakness, notably present in VDRR, are characteristic for PDR. Biochemically, PDR is characterized by hyponatremia, mild hypophosphatemia (in some cases the serum phosphate is actually normal), marked elevations in alkaline phosphatase, a metabolic renal tubular acidosis, and generalized amino aciduria. Circulating parathyroid hormone levels are usually elevated, although normal values have been reported in a pedigree with PDR and relative hypoparathyroidism. Whereas controversy still exists regarding the malabsorption of calcium in VDRR, calcium malabsorption is the rule in PDR. The term "dependency" arises from the observation that the skeletal and biochemical derangements in PDR respond dramatically to vitamin D in doses approximately 100 times the normal daily requirement of 400 IU per day. Unlike VDRR, in which phosphorus supplementation is mandatory for normal growth and skeletal maturation and normalization of circulating phosphate, vitamin D *alone* is therapeutic for children with PDR.

In contrast to the VDRR syndrome, which has been attributed (either directly or indirectly) to renal and intestinal phosphate transport defects independent of vitamin D, the pathogenesis of PDR has been ascribed to defective or absent 1-hydroxylation of 25OHD to $1,25(OH)_2D_3$. This in turn supposedly results in decreased calcium absorption, hypocalcemia, and stimulated release of parathyroid hormone. The associated mild renal tubular acidosis, aminoaciduria, phosphaturia, and elevations in urinary cyclic AMP are all assumed to represent the normal renal tubular response to high circulating parathyroid hormone levels. As such, PDR may be considered a mendelian trait affecting the bioactivation of vitamin D. Whereas $25OHD_3$ and $1,25(OH)_2D_3$ are relatively ineffective in VDRR, healing of the rachitic lesions and reversal of the biochemical defects have been observed with "physiologic" (1 μg per day) doses of $1,25(OH)_2D$, or the synthetic analogue, 1α-hydroxycholecalciferol in PDR. This therapeutic response is consistent with the hypothesis that PDR (unlike VDRR) is due to a specific inborn error of vitamin D metabolism caused by a recessively inherited defect in the renal enzyme 25-hydroxycholecalciferol 1-hydroxylase. More definitive confirmation and direct evidence of 1-hydroxylase deficiency in this disorder are essential before this assumption can be accepted, however, since long-term administration of either $1,25(OH)_2D$ or 1α-hydroxyvitamin D_3 in smaller doses (0.5 μg per day), which are therapeutic for patients

with simple nutritional rickets, have limited biologic effectiveness in patients with PDR.

RENAL TUBULAR DISORDERS AND DE TONI-DEBRÉ-FANCONI SYNDROME

Other tubular defects which lead to rickets or osteomalacia belong to a heterogeneous group of disorders usually categorized as renal tubular acidosis and the De Toni-Debré-Fanconi syndrome(s). The pathogenesis of rickets and osteomalacia in renal tubular acidosis is not well delineated; hypophosphatemia and hyperphosphaturia, systemic acidosis, decreased intestinal absorption of calcium, and a mild but persistent hypercalciuria all probably contribute to the alterations in skeletal mineralization. In the pure form of renal tubular acidosis, the phosphaturia seems to be a secondary phenomenon, related to the acidosis since the osteomalacia and hypophosphatemia are corrected by alkali. The acidosis of proximal tubular defects also plays a role in the development of osteomalacia in rickets, possibly by altering the metabolism of vitamin D and the renal handling of calcium of phosphorus. Individuals with renal tubular acidosis may also have a mild degree of azotemia, which may further compromise normal skeletal growth and remodeling. When the osteomalacia or rickets is minimal (as is the usual case in renal tubular acidosis), it is likely that supplemental vitamin D–calcium therapy will result in bone healing. When the skeletal lesions are severe, the combination of moderately large vitamin D doses (i.e., 50,000 to 100,000 IU daily) and alkali (i.e., Shohl's solution) is recommended, the vitamin D to be discontinued as soon as skeletal repair occurs. In most circumstances, high-dose vitamin D therapy is not essential and often contraindicated because it may increase the hazard of nephrocalcinosis and renal calculi formation.

The De Toni-Debré-Fanconi syndrome represents a heterogeneous group of disorders characterized by hypophosphatemia, glycosuria, and aminoaciduria. Accompanying features may include systemic acidosis, hypokalemia, hypouricemia, and proteinuria. Children with this syndrome may also have an inherited cystine storage disease or cystinosis characterized by widespread tissue disposition of cystine crystals and an early demise in hepatic and/or renal failure. The De Toni-Debré-Fanconi syndrome in the older child or the adult is most often idiopathic or acquired (i.e., Wilson's disease, multiple myeloma, lead or cadmium intoxication), not associated with cystinosis, and frequently complicated by osteomalacia or rickets. The skeletal lesions are presumably due to the chronic hypophosphatemia and mild acidosis. Effective therapy of the skeletal lesions in these multifactorial renal tubular disorders usually requires large doses of vitamin D (up to 250,000 IU daily), indicating a resistance to vitamin D exceeding that observed in renal tubular acidosis. The potential nephrotoxicity of high-dose vitamin D therapy may be circumvented by treatment with a combination of oral phosphate supplements and correction of the systemic acidosis with alkali. These observations further emphasize the importance of extracellular phosphate levels in the genesis of osteomalacia in this as well as the hypophosphatemic disorders cited earlier.

Hypophosphatemic osteomalacia and high renal phosphate clearance have also been associated with either benign of malignant giant cell tumors or reparative granulomas and soft tissue hemangiomas. In some of these instances removal of the tumor has resulted in normalization of renal phosphate clearance, rise in serum phosphorus, and remission of the rickets or osteomalacia. The mechanism of this response has not yet been elucidated, although an acquired defect in vitamin D metabolism has been incriminated by some.

ANTICONVULSANT RICKETS AND OSTEOMALACIA

Rickets or osteomalacia has been reported in treated epileptic populations throughout the world, with the incidence of hypocalcemia and clinical evidence of osteomalacia or rickets varying from 4 to 75 per cent depending on the population studied and the level of sensitivity of the diagnostic techniques employed. The clinical severity of drug-induced osteomalacia varies considerably, ranging from subclinical decreases in bone mass detectable only by the most sensitive techniques to marked hypocalcemia and severe osteopenia with multiple, recurrent bone fractures.

It has been established that virtually all the common anticonvulsants and many of the major and minor tranquilizers are capable of inducing liver microsomal mixed oxidase enzyme activity. Since steroids share the hepatic microsomal degradation pathways with foreign substances, induction of these enzyme systems leads to an increased catabolism of a variety of steroid hormones. This, in turn, results in accelerated production of polar, hydroxylated biologically inactive products which are eliminated in the bile and urine, effects previously demonstrated in the case of estrogens, progesterone, and corticosteroids. Since vitamin D and its biologically active metabolites are structurally similar to the steroid hormones, chronic anticonvulsant drug therapy also results in an increase in their biodegradation rates. Significant reductions in serum levels of 25OHD have been repeatedly demonstrated in patients receiving long-term anticonvulsant drug therapy, although levels of $1,25(OH)_2D$ are normal. Serum calcium levels in these patients usually demonstrate a direct correlation with serum 25OHD levels. Moreover, concomitant with the decrease in serum calcium there is an appropriate secondary increase in serum parathyroid hormone levels.

Anticonvulsant drugs also exert direct effects on mineral and bone metabolism independent of their effects on vitamin D metabolism. This is particularly true in the case of diphenylhydantoin, which has been demonstrated to alter ion transport across cell membranes by virtue of its effect on membrane bound ATP-ase transport systems. When diphenylhydantoin is administered to animals in doses that do not appear to alter vitamin metabolism, there is significant inhibition of intestinal calcium absorption; phenobarbital does not produce this effect. Additionally, both diphenylhydantoin and phenobarbital have been shown to have direct effects on bone calcium mobilization and the skeletal response to parathyroid hormone, calcitonin, and $1,25 (OH)_2D_3$. Patients with anticonvulsant-induced bone disease may give a history of repeated fractures, and present with bone deformities (in children), hypocalcemia, hypo-phosphatemia, and radiologic signs of rickets (in children) or severe osteopenia with pseudofractures (in adults). Even more rarely, a patient may experience a significant increase in seizure frequency with the institution of higher doses of anticonvulsant drugs, presumably owing to increased neuromuscular instability resulting from progressive hypocalcemia. Occasionally proximal myopathy similar to that seen in other forms of severe vitamin D deficiency may occur. The basis for the myopathy is unclear, but may be related to the fact that vitamin D metabolites appear to play an important role in the maintenance of intracellular phosphate concentrations required to maintain normal ATP levels in muscle. On the other hand, the usual patient is likely to have a much more subtle presentation. Bone symptoms may be minimal or absent; serum calcium, phosphate, and alkaline phosphatase levels obtained on a random blood specimen may be within the normal range; and routine x-rays may fail to detect any bone abnormalities. In most large series, the *mean* reduction in serum calcium in groups of anticonvulsant-treated patients as compared to control subjects averages between 0.3 and 0.8 mg per deciliter, with the incidence of frank hypocalcemia varying from 4 to 30 per cent and the incidence of elevated serum alkaline phosphatase levels ranging between 24 and 40 per cent. Inorganic phosphate levels are occasionally reduced but are usually within the normal range. The risk factors predisposing to increased severity of anticonvulsant-induced osteomalacia include multiple anticonvulsant drug regimens, decreased vitamin D intake or sunlight exposure, physical exercise, coexisting diseases such as malabsorption or renal insufficiency, and drugs such as acetazolamide which induce calciuria.

In patients on anticonvulsants with clinically obvious bone disease, several strategies have been employed. Vitamin D in doses of 2000 to 4000 units per day in combination with 500 mg of calcium per day for three months produces a 3 to 5 per cent increase in bone mass as measured by photon absorption densitometry in both pediatric and adult patients with drug-induced osteomalacia. Alternatively, it has been suggested that vitamin D in a dose of 4000 units per day can significantly reduce seizure incidence in patients with drug-induced mineral disorders, presumably by normalizing serum ionized calcium levels. In adults with clinically or radiologically apparent bone disease and/or definite hypocalcemia, an initial dose of 50,000 to 75,000 units of vitamin D (50,000 units per square meter of body surface area) per *week* in divided doses, plus 500 mg of supplemental calcium per day, should be maintained for a period of four to six months. In children, doses are reduced according to body area. After normalization of biochemical and radiologic parameters, patients can then be maintained on approximately 10,000 units of vitamin D per week. When this regimen is employed, it is essential to follow serum and urine calcium levels carefully so that vitamin D and calcium supplementation can be adjusted to individual requirements and inadvertent vitamin D overdosage avoided.

MISCELLANEOUS CAUSES

Fibrogenesis imperfecta ossium is another rare disorder which leads to osteomalacia and generalized and progressive skeletal pain and tenderness. The disease appears limited to middle-aged males and is characterized by normal plasma values for calcium and inorganic phosphate but substantial elevations in circulating alkaline phosphatase. Radiographically, the pathology involves both axial and appendicular bone with thickened and amorphous trabeculae, leading to an over-all impression of *increased* skeletal density; pseudofractures have also been observed. Histologically, one finds increased numbers of osteoid seams, impaired mineralization of matrix, and altered polarization of collagen fibers. Whereas this form of osteomalacia is resistant to vitamin D therapy, it is remarkably sensitive to dihydrotachysterol. Although similar in many respects to fibrogenesis imperfecta ossium, the syndrome of *axial osteomalacia* appears to represent a separate disorder in skeletal metabolism leading to osteomalacia. In this instance, patients are relatively asymptomatic, skeletal pathology is limited to the axial skeleton, and circulating alkaline phosphatase values and collagen polarization are normal.

Hypophosphatasia is a hereditary, generalized skeletal disorder that follows on autosomal recessive pattern and has been categorized into four types according to the age of onset and the severity of the clinical and radiologic manifestations. Childhood forms of the disease resemble rickets radiologically. The adult form, although relatively rare, should be considered in individuals who present with fractures following minimal trauma or localized arthropathy. Adults with the mild form of the disease characteristically give a history of renal stones, dentition difficulties, delayed growth, and/or childhood "rickets." Radiologically, the disorder is characterized by radiolucent bones and pseudofractures. The biochemical hallmarks of the disease are abnormally low tissue and circulating levels of alkaline phosphatase activity and increased excretion of phosphoethanolamine. Increased urinary phosphoethanolamine is also found in vitamin C deficiency, hypothyroidism, celiac disease, and magnesium deficiency. Elevations in urinary phosphocholine and phosphoserine have also been noted. When the diagnosis is clinically suspected in a patient with elevations in urinary phosphoethanolamine, a "normal" alkaline phosphatase need not be considered inappropriate. In certain nutritional states the intestinal isoenzyme alkaline phosphatase may prove to be the primary circulating form of alkaline phosphatase in contrast to the pattern identified in normal individuals. Attempts to reverse the skeletal calcification defect of hypophosphatasia with vitamin D, cortisone or structurally related synthetic analogues, and phosphate supplements have been unsuccessful; fractures usually heal normally with conventional forms of orthopedic management.

Byers, P. D.: The diagnostic value of bone biopsies. *In* Avioli, L. V., and Krane, S. M. (eds.): Metabolic Bone Disease, Vol. I. New York, Academic Press, 1977, p. 184.

Dent, C. E., and Stamp, T. C. B.: Vitamin D, rickets and osteomalacia. *In* Avioli, L. V., and Krane, S. M. (eds.): Metabolic Bone Disease, Vol. I. New York, Academic Press, 1977, p. 237.

Drezner, M. K., and Feinglos, M. N.: Osteomalacia due to $1\alpha25$-dihydroxycholecalciferol deficiency. Association with a giant cell tumor of bone. J. Clin. Invest., 60:1046, 1977.

Hahn, T. J., Hendin, B. A., Scharp, C. R., Boisseau, V. C., and Haddad, J. G., Jr.: Serum 25-hydroxycalciferol levels and bone mass in children on chronic anticonvulsant therapy. N. Engl. J. Med., 292:550, 1975.

Hahn, T. J., Hendin, B. A., Scharp, C. R., and Haddad, J. G., Jr.: Effect of chronic anticonvulsant therapy on serum 25-hydroxycalciferol levels in adults. N. Engl. J. Med., 287:900, 1972.

Stanbury, S. W.: Osteomalacia. *In* Clinics in Endocrinology and Metabolism. London, W. B. Saunders Company, 1972, p. 239.

559. RENAL OSTEODYSTROPHY

Chronic renal insufficiency is attended by derangements in skeletal metabolism and in the homeostatic control of calcium, phosphate, magnesium, and a variety of other minerals. These include impaired absorption of calcium and magnesium from the gastrointestinal tract; parathyroid hyperactivity; resistance to the biologic effects of vitamin D, metastatic soft tissue, and vascular calcification; and a steadily progressive form of bone disease (renal osteodystrophy), which presents both histologically and radiographically as a mixture of osteosclerosis, osteomalacia, osteoporosis, and osteitis fibrosa cystica.

THE NATURE OF THE DEFECT IN BONE

Osteomalacia or rickets is also observed in the chronic uremic state. In young adults prior to epiphyseal closure, the fundamental histologic and radiographic findings are indistinguishable from those of nutritional rickets. In older patients, osteomalacia occurs with wide osteoid seams in the trabeculae of the diaphyseal spongiosa, and pseudofractures may be observed. Tetracycline labeling studies reveal an increase in the relative and absolute amounts of osteoid seams per unit amount of bone and decreased bone mineralization or appositional "rates." Radiographically, excessive osteoid tissue in the form of "woven bone" imparts the so-called "rugger-jersey sign." (The phrase "rugger-jersey" refers to the alternating striped shirts commonly worn by British rugby teams.) The expression has been used to describe the increased density of the upper and lower margins of the vertebral body separated by a central horizontal zone of decreased density. This localized form of osteosclerosis, commonly seen in young adults with severe osteodystrophy, may progress and involve the entire spine, as well as the pelvis and long bones. Although the pathogenetic mechanism(s) responsible for the osteosclerosis of chronic uremia is still ill defined, it is most probably the result of excess production of woven bone secondary to excessive levels of circulating parathyroid hormone, the latter leading to osteoblastic hyperactivity and increased matrix production. The abnormal mineral composition of the bone of uremic subjects (i.e., reduction in bone carbonate content and increase in less crystalline moieties), combined with the observation that the dissolution of the apatitic crystal proceeds more slowly than normal in uremia, may also contribute to the osteosclerosis.

Azotemic rickets and osteomalacia are usually accompanied by parathyroid hyperplasia (secondary hyperparathyroidism) and elevations in immunoassayable parathyroid hormone, using the carboxyterminal antibody assay. At times, in the early stages of renal insufficiency, the secondary hyperparathyroidism is mild and undetectable radiographically. In children with end-stage renal disease, however, osteitis fibrosa cystica may be the prominent process both radiographically and histologically. The skeletal changes with secondary hyperparathyroidism, often indistinguishable from those of primary hyperparathyroidism, include a moth-eaten, granular appearance of the skull, cyst-like lytic lesions in the long bones, and subperiosteal resorption of bone seen best in the digital phalanges, medial aspect of the proximal tibia, outer third of the clavicle, sacroiliac joints, and symphysis pubis.

There is substantial evidence to suggest that the metabolic acidosis of uremia also contributes to the skeletal abnormalities. As the patient with chronic renal failure progressively loses nephrons and retains hydrogen ions, the accumulation of unexcretable protons in the extracellular fluids is buffered by the solubilization of skeletal carbonate and anionic exchange. This chronic acidotic state also contributes to the decrease in intestinal calcium absorption and skeletal wasting of calcium. The full-blown osteodystrophy of chronic renal insufficiency can be considered an extreme of a continuous spectrum of bone demineralization caused primarily by the need for day-to-day homeostatic adjustments in calcium, phosphate, and acid-base balance. Renal osteodystrophy thus represents a varied radiographic and histologic picture, with the predominant lesion in a given instance dependent on age, individual nutritional state, duration and severity of the renal failure, and type of therapy imposed.

SECONDARY HYPERPARATHYROIDISM

Normally, the rate of parathyroid hormone secretion is controlled by the plasma-ionized calcium levels (see Ch. 552.1). Since, to date, parathyroid-tropic factors have not been identified in chronic renal failure, hypocalcemia, which results from a combination of defective renal biodegradation of parathyroid hormone, calcium malabsorption, progressive hyperphosphatemia, abnormal vitamin D metabolism, and a relative resistance to the skeletal response to parathyroid hormone, prompts the development of secondary hyperparathyroidism. In general, the hyperparathyroidism of renal insufficiency can be reversed somewhat by calcium infusions, as well as by elevating the serum calcium by large doses of vitamin D and calcium-containing salts (usually calcium carbonate) and the oral administration of phosphate-binding gels. In patients with more advanced and prolonged renal failure, the calcium-parathyroid negative feedback control mechanisms no longer function, and hypercalcemia, hyperphosphatasia, progressive osteitis fibrosa, and severe bone pain characterize their clinical course. This apparent failure of the negative feedback mechanism may be a function of an autonomous adenoma formed in chronically overstimulated glands or of an extraordinarily large mass of hyperplastic parathyroid tissue which, though partially suppressed, continues to secrete an excessive amount of hormone.

Despite increased parathyroid hormone secretion to 50 to 100 times the normal rate and defective renal degradation of the hormone, the hypocalcemia observed in patients with chronic renal disease is only partially compensated. The nature of this apparent end-organ resistance to the skeletal response to parathyroid hormone is still uncertain. It may result from a relative deficiency of $1,25(OH)_2D_3$ or $25OHD_3$, since these normally play a permissive role for the action of parathyroid hormone on bone. Long-term hemodialysis therapy, although effectively ameliorating many of the clinical manifestations and biochemical derangements of chronic renal failure and extending the life span of the uremic patient, is comparatively ineffective in reversing either the calcium malabsorption or the associated skeletal lesions. In fact, overt skeletal lesions with progressive osteitis fibrosa and osteomalacia occur with increasing frequency as the period of dialysis is prolonged.

CALCIUM MALABSORPTION AND VITAMIN D "RESISTANCE"

The impaired intestinal absorption of calcium in uremic subjects is resistant to both oral and parenteral vitamin D therapy and has been observed in patients without manifest azotemia. Although not all the pathophysiologic factors contributing to the intestinal defect in calcium transport and absorption are known, it is evident that abnormal protein synthesis and mitochondrial activity of the mucosal cell, increased intraluminal concentrations of potassium, the systemic acidosis, and defective production of $1,25(OH)_2D_3$ play a role in the development and progression of the intestinal defect. In view of the homeostatic necessity to maintain a normal level of plasma-ionized calcium, the decreased input of calcium into plasma invariably contributes to the insidious development of secondary hyperparathyroidism and skeletal osteitis fibrosa. The gradual emergence of hyperphosphatemia in the chronic uremic state also contributes to the fall in ionized calcium. In this regard, the advancing uremic state with progressive reduction in nephron population and resultant decreased phosphate clearance, acquired cellular intolerance to insulin action, and autonomous growth hormone secretion probably all contribute to the observed abnormalities in phosphate homeostasis.

Although acknowledged for years, the exact nature of the vitamin D resistance of azotemic man has only recently been clarified. A failure in end-organ (intestinal) responsiveness has been suggested by the clinical observation that raising plasma vitamin D levels to ten times the normal value fails to influence the intestinal malabsorption of calcium. Demonstrated low values of vitamin D activity in some untreated uremic subjects who absorb vitamin D normally also suggest nutritional deficiencies and/or alterations in its metabolism. Studies on the metabolism of vitamin D in uremic subjects reveal a low plasma $25OHD_3$ in some and low $1,25(OH)_2D_3$ in almost all patients. Whereas the defect in the generation of $1,25(OH)_2D_3$ can be adequately explained by a decrease in renal functioning mass, the nature of the abnormality which results in decreased circulating $25OHD_3$ levels is still uncertain. The disturbances in vitamin D metabolism may explain, at least in part, the clinically observed resistance to vitamin D therapy and the intestinal malabsorption of calcium. The altered metabolic sequence may also account for the resistance to parathyroid hormone, the observed depression of the skeletal "appositional" or bone formation rate, and the delay in the maturation period of bone matrix, all of which are seen in the chronic uremic state. The disorders in vitamin D metabolism, although unaffected by long-term intermittent dialysis, are completely reversed by homotransplantation. These observations are consistent with others which demonstrate that chronic dialysis fails to correct the resistance to large doses of vitamin D and the defect in calcium absorption which accompany renal failure. They are also in accord with the observation that low levels of circulating vitamin D activity are unchanged after chronic dialysis, whereas they return to normal after successful renal homotransplantation.

TERTIARY HYPERPARATHYROIDISM

The development of an autonomous parathyroid adenoma in chronically overstimulated hyperplastic parathyroid glands has been designated by some as tertiary hyperparathyroidism. Continued and accelerated interest in renal transplantation as the definitive therapeutic procedure for patients with chronic renal disease has uncovered a new constellation of biochemical abnormalities characterized by hypercalcemia, hypophosphatemia, and hyperphosphatasia in previously hypocalcemic, hyperphosphatemic patients. With rare exceptions, these findings are coupled with diffuse hyperplasia of all parathyroid glands. In most instances, tertiary hyperparathyroidism does not in fact persist, since the biochemical abnormalities uncovered by the renal homograft are of transient nature, reverting to normal within three to six months following surgery. The prevailing opinion regarding the mechanism(s) which underlie this post-transplantation syndrome is one wherein the hypercalcemia and hypophosphatemia are attributed to the secondary hyperparathyroidism established during the interval which preceded surgery. The observed alterations in serum calcium and phosphate are considered as sequelae of the persistent excessive rates of parathyroid hormone secretion by a large mass of hyperplastic tissue. The return of normal renal function corrects the abnormality in vitamin D metabolism acquired in the uremic state and reverses the tendency toward hyperphosphatemia and hypocalcemia that masks the effects of parathyroid hormone in the pretransplantation period. Accentuation of the hypercalcemia and hypophosphatemia also occurs in the post-transplantation period because of the use of phosphate-binding antacids frequently administered with immunosuppressive agents such as prednisone, and the mobilization of metastatic calcified deposits. In general, involution of the hyperplastic parathyroid glands and reduction in circulating immunoassayable parathyroid hormone ultimately follow transplantation surgery. Since autonomous "tertiary hyperparathyroidism" rarely occurs following renal transplantation, when suspected, it should be carefully documented by serial measurements of parathyroid hormone and failure of calcium infusion to suppress parathyroid hormone secretion. The longer the patient can be managed conservatively following transplantation, the greater the likelihood that surgical intervention can be avoided.

TREATMENT

Choice of therapy for derangements in calcium and skeletal metabolism seen in chronic uremic patients should be based on (1) adequate appraisal of the bone disease radiographically and measurements of circulating calcium, phosphate, alkaline phosphatase, parathyroid hormone, $25OHD_3$, and $1,25(OH)_2D_3$ levels; (2) the degree of clinical disability such as nausea, vomiting, intractable pruritus, bone pain, or pathologic fractures; (3) the presence or absence of soft tissue and/or vascular calcifications; and (4) evaluation of the over-all therapeutic approach to the chronic uremic state in each instance, including the plans for either long-term dialysis without renal transplantation or intermittent dialysis in preparation for transplantation surgery. It must be emphasized that in each instance therapy of the derangements in mineral metabolism must be considered an adjunct to the over-all management of the chronic renal insufficiency.

Although chronic uremia may be attached by hypocalcemia, it is rarely symptomatic, since both ultrafilterable and ionic calcium concentrations are usually normal despite significant depressions in total plasma calcium. In the occasional uremic patient with signs and symptoms of tetany the parenteral administration of calcium-containing preparations is justified. There is not substantial evidence that alkali (sodium bicarbonate) administration per se plays a beneficial role in management of the hypocalcemia and osteodystrophy of chronic renal failure. In fact, the long-term administration of alkali salts can result in irritability and tetany. Bicarbonate administration to patients undergoing intermittent dialysis also may augment a previously existing tendency to alkalemia secondary to respiratory alkalosis and accentuate soft tissue calcification. Symptomatic improvement in anorexia, vomiting, and neuromuscular irritability occurs in azotemic patients receiving oral chronic calcium therapy with concomitant increments in serum calcium, carbon dioxide combining power and the circulating calcium-phosphate products. Since the tendency for metastatic tissue calcification correlates directly with the calcium-phosphate products, this parameter should be evaluated periodically during oral calcium therapy. Hypocalcemia in the patient on long-term dialysis may also be corrected by maintaining a positive gradient of calcium from dialysate to plasma-diffusible calcium with dialysate calcium concentrations of 6.0 to 6.5 mg per 100 ml. Since chronic intermittent dialysis is often inadequate to "normalize" the serum phosphate level, attempts should also be made in the dialyzed patient to bind dietary inorganic phosphate in the gastrointestinal tract with aluminum hydroxide gel preparations. These phosphate-binding gel preparations should not be used indiscriminately, since they may prove toxic to the uremic patient as a result of central nervous system accumulation of the aluminum ion.

The judicious use of vitamin D and oral calcium preparations has also been advocated to maintain the serum calcium at a level which effectively suppresses the excessive parathyroid hormone secretion, thereby reducing the tendency toward skeletal demineralization. Frequent monitoring of serum calcium and phosphate levels is also considered mandatory when vitamin D, $25OHD_3$, or $1,25(OH)_2D_3$ is used in hemodialyzed patients to avoid life-threatening hypercalcemia and extensive soft tissue calcification.

Therapy with either vitamin D or $25OHD_3$ is perhaps most advantageous to those patients with osteomalacia dominating the osteodystrophic skeletal pattern, whereas $1,25(OH)_2D_3$ or its synthetic analogue $1\alpha OHD_3$ is more effective for those with predominant osteitis fibrosa. The response to therapy with either of these agents can be effectively established in undialyzed or dialyzed subjects by analyzing undecalcified bone biopsy sections. The prevailing plasma levels of calcium and phosphate may provide a valid clue to the primary nature of the bone disease in the undialyzed patient. Serum calcium phosphate products (in milligrams per 100 ml) below 60 in patients with radiographic evidence of osteopenia without associated osteitis fibrosa are consistent with a significant degree of osteomalacia, which may respond favorably to vitamin D or $25OHD_3$. If no apparent change occurs in 6 to 12 weeks, as reflected in clinical improvement, progressive rise in plasma calcium, or fall in plasma alkaline phosphatase, the daily dose of the vitamin D preparations should be gradually and cautiously increased. It should be noted that a maximal response to vitamin D therapy is achieved with a dietary calcium-phosphate ratio of 1:1. Excessive use of oral phosphate binding gels may be harmful if persistent hypophosphatemia results. The latter may actually cause progression of the osteomalacic component of the skeletal lesion.

Although the osteomalacic manifestations of uremic osteodystrophy may improve with oral calcium, limited phosphate restriction, and treatment with one of the biologically active metabolites of vitamin D, patients with osteitis fibrosa may not be helped by this regimen.

Long-term dialysis therapy inevitably results in a greater incidence of recognizable osteodystrophy. Recent evidence suggests that the use of fluoridated water in the dialysate may enhance the rate at which osteodystrophy develops. There is, however, convincing evidence that secondary hyperparathyroidism plays a significant or perhaps a major role in the progressive skeletal demineralization seen in the undialyzed patient with longstanding uremia, or in the subject on intermittent dialysis. Attempts to suppress parathyroid activity by establishing a mild hypercalcemia either with combinations of vitamin D, oral antacids, and calcium salts or by increasing dialysate calcium concentrations have been moderately effective. However, the combination of an acquired disturbance in vitamin D metabolism which is not reversed by chronic dialysis, persistent hyperphosphatemia, and the inability to maintain suppressive levels of plasma calcium without accelerating metastatic calcification often leaves much to be desired of this form of treatment. In carefully selected cases, elective parathyroidectomy may offer a therapeutic advantage over conservative medical attempts to suppress parathyroid activity. The exact indications and ideal time for parathyroid surgery are uncertain. Circumstances in which immediate parathyroidectomy appears mandatory include rapidly progressive vascular calcification, intractable pruritus, or progressive debilitating bone disease either in patients awaiting renal transplantation or in those destined to remain in long-term intermittent dialysis programs. In the former group vascular calcification may complicate the surgical procedures, while the vascular integrity required for effective cannulation may be severely compromised. Parathyroidectomy should not be injudiciously used to ameliorate the osteodystrophic syndrome without careful consideration of each case and the plans for the patient's subsequent management. This surgical procedure is not without risk in severely ill uremic patients and should not be undertaken except in those instances in which adequate attempts at medical management have failed, and when symptoms of metastatic calcification, bone pain, and pathologic fractures are incapacitating. It is maintained by some that total, rather than subtotal, parathyroidectomy is the operation of choice, particularly for those patients who are not candidates for transplantation, since rapid growth of the remaining parathyroid tissue may occur, necessitating repeat surgical intervention. The clinical response to parathyroidectomy is often striking, particularly regarding soft tissue calcification and pruritus. This often disabling complication of chronic uremia may disappear within one week of surgery. Vascular complications may be slow to resolve, although ischemic symptoms may be relieved by parathyroid excision. More important, however, elective parathyroid surgery may often result in remineralization of skeletal defects. Patients with metastatic calcification also appear to heal more quickly than those without detectable extraskeletal mineralization. X-ray evidence of skeletal healing may occur within three months of parathyroidectomy, although it is often the last pathologic parameter to demonstrate evidence of improvement. Some dialyzed patients, particularly those with severe osteomalacia, may, however, continue to sustain fractures without evidence of improvement of their osteodystrophy.

It must be emphasized that parathyroidectomy may be followed by severe hypocalcemia and tetany in a uremic patient. This sequence is most often noted in patients subjected to total parathyroidectomy with transplantation of some homologous parathyroid tissue to a muscle bed in the arm. Moreover, in uremic individuals with severe osteodystrophy, the "hungry-bone syndrome," rapid decrease in circulating parathyroid hormone results in acute fall in bone resorption, with accelerated entry of calcium and magnesium into bone.

Avioli, L. V.: Renal osteodystrophy. *In* Avioli, L. V., and Krane, S. M. (eds.): Metabolic Bone Disease, Vol. II. New York, Academic Press, 1978, p. 214.

Kleeman, C. R. (ed.): Divalent ion metabolism and osteodystrophy in chronic renal failure. Arch. Intern. Med., 124:261, 389, 519, 619, 1969.

Stanbury, S. W.: Azotemic renal osteodystrophy. *In* Clinics in Endocrinology and Metabolism. London, W. B. Saunders Company, 1972, p. 267.

560. PAGET'S DISEASE (Osteitis Deformans)

INCIDENCE. Paget's disease is a relatively common form of localized bone disease with an incidence of 3 per cent of the population over the age of 40 and 10 per cent over the age of 70 when the frequency is determined by systematic pathologic examination of the skeleton. With the advent of radiographic bone scanning techniques and routine measurements of plasma alkaline phosphatase, the recognition of asymptomatic lesions is much greater. The disease is relatively rare in Scandinavia, Japan, China, India, Africa, and the Middle East, with the majority of cases observed in the United States, United Kingdom, Australia, France, and Germany. A significant male predominance exists and, although the disorder is rarely detected *clinically* before the age of 40 years, it may involve multiple skeletal sites (polyostotic) by the second decade and progress rapidly. A rare inherited childhood disorder (hyperostosis corticalis deformans juvenilis), characterized by hyperphosphatasia and bone deformities which superficially resemble those of adult Paget's disease, is often mistakenly referred to as juvenile Paget's disease. Histologically, however, the lesions are quite distinct. Despite isolated reports of familial clustering of Paget's disease, a specific genetic vertical transmission pattern has not yet been uncovered.

PATHOGENESIS. Histologically, this disorder is characterized by extensive vascularity, increased marrow fibrosis, and intense cellular activity with irregular areas of lamellar bone interspaced by poorly stained "cement" lines, the latter simulating a mosaic pattern. At times an osteolytic phase predominates; bone resorption resulting from multinucleated osteoclastic activity is so rapid and extensive that new lamellar bone formation lags and the original bone is replaced by fibrous tissue. At other times, an increase in irregular mosaic lamellar bone dominates and, combined with waning osteoclastic activity, results in a "sclerotic" or "osteoblastic" lesion. These phases are "coupled" to a considerable extent and may vary in intensity at the same time in different skeletal sites or during the progressive course of the disease in any one individual. The etiology of Paget's disease is unknown despite claims for an inborn error of connective tissue metabolism, a disorder of hormone secretion, and either an acquired vascular disorder or an autoimmune state. Recently, a viral etiology has been proposed and osteoclastic intranuclear inclusions which resemble the nucleocapsids of measles-like viruses demonstrated.

CLINICAL MANIFESTATIONS. The clinical expressions of this disorder may be protean and dependent on the specific area of skeletal involvement. Many patients with Paget's disease are totally asymptomatic during the course of their disease. In fact, the disorder may prove to be an incidental finding 20 per cent of the time. Lesions in weight-bearing bones tend to be the most symptomatic. Involvement of the skull results in headaches, intermittent tinnitus and vertigo, and hearing loss, usually of the sensorineural type. Although the hearing loss has been attributed by many to compression of the eighth cranial nerve as it traverses the canal in the temporal bone, this appears unlikely, since the facial nerve which parallels the course of the eighth nerve is rarely affected. In patients with severe skull involvement, the increased blood flow through the external carotid artery and its branches may contribute to an increased incidence of vascular and migraine headaches, as well as the "pagetic steal syndrome," with symptoms analogous to the subclavian steal syndrome. With severe involvement of the occipital region of the skull, basilar impression and cervical herniation may cause pressure on the pons and cerebellum, spinal cord compression, and loss of coordination, muscle strength, and central control of respiration, as well as slurred speech, diplopia, impaired gait, and urinary incontinence. Maxillary or mandibular involvement may result in a variety of sinus headaches, facial deformities, and leontiasis ossea. This abnormality, although much more typical of fibrous dysplasia, can be easily distinguished by the age of onset. Paget's disease rarely results in facial deformity before the sixth decade, whereas in fibrous dysplasia the deformities invariably occur before age 30.

Vertebral involvement, although occasionally asymptomatic (especially with cervical involvement), may prove symptomatic due to a sudden compression fracture, compression of a sensory nerve root or spinal cord by a displaced vertebra, or progressive vertebral enlargement. Stiffness of the back, chronic intermittent dull aching back pain, and limitation in spinal flexion may mimic ankylosing spondylitis. Pain associated with pelvic involvement may be severe when both acetabulum and femoral head are affected, or mild when the disease is restricted to either of these sites. Since degenerative arthritis of the hip and occasionally the knee joints is a complicating factor in pagetic patients, decreased mobility and "arthritic" pains, which are often severe and incapacitating, may occur. Unlike lesions in the appendicular skeleton (especially the lower limbs), it is occasionally impossible to explain the source of pain in patients with axial skeletal involvement. When it is limited to a specific area in a long

bone, careful radiographic evaluation may reveal small hairline cortical fractures. Lesions in the upper extremity may also present as nerve palsy syndromes. Osteogenic sarcoma in adults, which most often arises in pagetic lesions, may result in persistent pain because of sarcomatous elevation of the periosteum. Angioid streaks, which are detected funduscopically in 10 to 15 per cent of patients with polyostotic Paget's disease, may rarely result in blindness. The increase in cardiac output observed when Paget's disease involves more than 30 to 40 per cent of the skeleton may cause cardiac enlargement and congestive failure. The increased cardiac output has been ascribed in the past to the hypervascularity of active osteolytic bone lesions, with resting skeletal blood flow ranging from 5 to 19 per cent of blood volume per minute. Elevations in skin temperature noted over an affected extremity are probably caused by associated increments in cutaneous blood flow.

RADIOGRAPHIC AND LABORATORY FINDINGS. As noted earlier, Paget's disease is primarily an osteolytic destructive process, usually followed by an osteoblastic, sclerotic phase. The destructive phase is best seen in the skull and long bones. The active destructive phase is characterized by a wave of osteolysis which, when seen on skull films, is classically defined as "osteoporosis circumscripta." Well demarcated osteolysis usually begins in the occipital or frontal area, extending to the rest of the calvaria with time. This initial osteolytic state is eventually followed by a second osteoblastic or reparative phase with early sclerosis of the inner surface of the outer table of the skull extending gradually throughout the calvaria, resulting in a "cotton ball" appearance and a thickened sclerotic outer table. At this juncture, the disease becomes relatively quiescent. Concomitant involvement of the facial bones may result in skeletal sclerosis and overgrowth and the clinical features of leontiasis ossea mentioned earlier.

Thickening of the pelvic brim or ileopectineal line is a frequent, and often the earliest, sign of Paget's disease of the pelvis. Although noted also in osteopetrosis, this "brim sign" is often considered pathognomonic for Paget's disease. Other features of pelvic disease are thickened and prominent trabeculae, asymmetrical diffuse sclerosis, widening of pubic and ischial bones, and acetabular protrusion. Although some of these features are occasionally confused with the osteoblastic metastatic disease of prostatic carcinoma, ileopectineal sclerosis and widening of the pubic and ischial bones, frequently present in Paget's disease, are rarely noted in patients with osteoblastic metastases.

The early lytic phase of Paget's disease in long bones is usually manifested by a well defined V-shaped or "blade of grass" area of osteolysis. Occasionally bubble-like lesions can be demonstrated which also precede the sclerotic phase. The latter usually results in cortical thickening and new bone formation within the medullary cavity, with trabeculae eventually fusing with the cortex to form the characteristic deforming long bone curvatures. Weight bearing often leads to small cortical fractures which tend to heal only at their periosteal and endosteal surfaces, leaving a permanent linear cortical defect. Pathologic true fractures of the tibia or femur, which are usually transverse and heal readily, may be seen during the active phase of the disease.

Vertebral, specifically lumbosacral, involvement is

also quite frequent. The most common presenting features are thickened margins and coarse vertical striations imparting a "box-like" or "frame" configuration. Diffuse sclerosis of a single vertebra, with or without activity, as confirmed by scintigraphic imaging, is also noted. The short tubular bones of the hands and feet may also be involved by the pagetic process, although the lesions are usually asymptomatic.

Serum alkaline phosphatase and urinary hydroxyproline, elevated in patients with Paget's disease, can usually be correlated with the extent and activity of the disease. Normal alkaline phosphate values have been noted in 15 per cent and normal hydroxyproline excretion observed in more than 50 per cent of patients with early active disease detected by radioisotopic scintigraphic imaging. Since heat fractionation can distinguish the heat labile bone alkaline phosphatase isoenzyme from the more stable isoenzymes produced by other tissue, heat sensitivity studies may ultimately confirm disease activity detected by scintigraphic imaging despite normal total alkaline phosphatase and normal radiographs. Wide fluctuations in alkaline phosphatase levels do occur in the same patient without therapy; intercurrent infections and immobilization may result in a decrease in alkaline phosphatase and a rise in serum calcium and hydroxyproline excretion. When osteosarcoma develops, a striking and rapid increase in alkaline phosphatase (phosphatase flare) may be observed, with minimal if any change in urinary hydroxyproline and a negative bone scan.

Serum calcium and phosphorus concentrations in the mobilized patient are usually normal but may be increased or decreased. Urinary calcium concentration is variable, although an abrupt rise paralleling the hydroxyprolinuria is seen in immobilized subjects. Hyperuricemia with clinical gout, elevations in serum and urinary citrate, and high erythrocyte sedimentation rates have also been noted in some patients.

THERAPY. Until the last decade, the treatment of Paget's disease was unsatisfactory. Although symptomatic, clinical and histologic improvements were observed with glucocorticoid, aspirin, or sodium fluoride therapy, adverse side effects minimized their effectiveness. Within recent years calcitonin, mithramycin, and disodium ethane-1-hydroxy-1,1-diphosphonate (EHDP) have proved to be more effective. Calcitonin treatment results in symptomatic and biochemical improvement as well as a decrease in bone blood flow after the first few months of therapy. It has also been beneficial to patients with deafness and neurologic complications such as cranial nerve palsies and nerve compression syndromes. Symptomatic improvement has been maintained as long as one year after long-term therapy is discontinued (e.g., for two years at doses of 50 to 100 MRC units thrice weekly). However, the serum alkaline phosphatase may increase toward pretreatment values six months after treatment has been discontinued despite maintained depression of the urinary hydroxyproline. Since readily available forms of calcitonin are obtained only from salmon or pig, as many as 40 per cent of patients develop circulating antibodies to these foreign calcitonins. Some patients become resistant to therapy, as judged by a rebound of both biochemical changes and clinical symptoms to pretreatment levels. The "resistance" can be effectively reversed with human calcitonin preparations. To date, antibodies to human calcitonin have not been detected in patients subjected to long-term therapy with this preparation.

Disodium ethane-1-hydroxy-1,1-diphosphonate (EHDP) has also proved effective in reducing the serum alkaline phosphatase and urinary hydroxyproline excretion in Paget's disease. However, in doses of 10 to 20 mg per kilogram per day, this agent paradoxically results in a lower rate of symptomatic improvement (with increased fracture incidence) and a relatively greater rate of deterioration than that observed on lower dose regimens (e.g., 2.5 to 5.0 mg per kilogram per day). It appears that long-term therapeutic EHDP regimens with doses of 5 mg per kilogram per day maximize the benefits while minimizing the adverse effects. Unlike preparations of calcitonin which, because of the peptide structures, must be administered parenterally, EHDP is available for oral ingestion.

Dramatic symptomatic improvement has also been reported following mithramycin therapy. This agent, an inhibitor of DNA-directed RNA synthesis, has been administered intravenously in doses of 10 to 15 μg per kilogram once or twice weekly with prompt amelioration of pain and reversal of the biochemical abnormalities. Although those favorable responses have been associated with radiologic improvements, reports of nephrotoxicity, thrombocytopenia, and hepatotoxicity suggest that intravenous mithramycin therapy should be administered with reluctance and caution.

Barry, H.: Paget's Disease of Bone. Baltimore, Williams & Wilkins Company, 1969.
De Deuxchaisnes, C. N., and Krane, S. M.: Paget's disease of bone; clinical and metabolic observations. Medicine, 43:233, 1944.
Haddad, J. G., Jr., Birge, S. J. and Avioli, L. V.: Effects of prolonged thyrocalcitonin administration of Paget's disease of bone. N. Engl. J. Med., 283:549, 1970.
Singer, F. R.: Paget's Disease of Bone. New York, Plenum Press, 1977.

561. OSTEONECROSIS*

Osteonecrosis denotes the clinical syndrome associated with death of bone cells in a localized volume of bone. The term osteonecrosis is used here interchangeably for aseptic necrosis of bone or avascular necrosis of bone.

ETIOLOGY. Osteonecrosis may result from traumatic disruption of the blood supply of bone and is usually noted in the femoral head after a subcapital fracture of the hip or traumatic dislocation of the hip; the semilunar, navicular, and scaphoid bones in the wrist; the tibial tuberosity; and the epiphysis of the os calcis before closure. Nontraumatic necrosis is believed to be due to obstruction of bony end-arteries by sludged red cells, gas bubbles, lipid droplets, uric acid crystals, or vasculitis. These may arise in Gaucher's disease, in sickle cell anemia, in caisson disease, in systemic lupus erythematosus, in hyperlipemia associated with chronic alcoholism or pancreatitis, and with chronic corticosteroid therapy, as may obtain in patients following renal transplantation. Perthes' disease is an osteonecrosis of the femoral head occurring for uncertain reasons, large-

---

*Portions of this chapter and the following short chapters on other bone diseases are unchanged from those in the previous edition by Dr. Paul D. Saville.

ly in males between four and ten years of age. Osteochondritis dissecans of the medial femoral condyle of children is a similar condition, as is osteonecrosis of the weight-bearing portion of the medial femoral condyle seen in older adults. The disease also occurs in the talus, the capitellum, and the humeral head.

INCIDENCE. Osteonecrosis of the femoral head occurs in about 50 per cent of cases of subcapital fracture of the hip and in 50 per cent of patients on immunosuppressive therapy for kidney homograft. Perthes' disease of the hip occurs in one of 820 boys and one of 4500 girls.

CLINICAL MANIFESTATIONS AND DIAGNOSIS. In adults, pain may occur up to three years after the original subcapital fracture. The disease, which occurs in alcoholics and immunosuppressed patients as well as in an idiopathic variety, usually manifests itself with sudden bone pain. At first, there are no radiographic changes, but after two months there may be a small radiolucent zone in bone under the articular cartilage. High resolution bone scans with agents such as ^{99m}Tc diphosphonate invariably reveal a focus of intense isotope uptake before radiographic changes become apparent. Later, increased bone density indicates attempted healing of the lesion. Before healing can occur, the resorptive phase leads to weakened bone, which may collapse on weight bearing and result in bone deformity. This often results in secondary osteoarthrosis.

TREATMENT. Treatment consists of discontinuing weight bearing until healing has occurred. This may take up to three years. Occasionally bone grafts are inserted through the femoral neck into the head to speed up the healing process in the hip. When osteonecrosis affects bones in the wrist, severe osteoarthrosis of the joint is common, and wrist fusion may be required to relieve pain. Prostheses may be used with success when deformity of bone and secondary osteoarthritis occur in weight-bearing joints.

Glimcher, M. J., and Kenzora, J. E.: The biology of osteonecrosis of the human femoral head and its clinical implications. Clin. Orthop. Rel. Res., 130:47, 1978.

Zinn, W. M.: Idiopathic Ischemic Necrosis of the Femoral Head in Adults. Baltimore, University Park Press, 1971.

562.   OSTEOMYELITIS

Osteomyelitis is an infectious lesion in bone produced by a microorganism. Before puberty, infection starts in the metaphyseal sinusoidal veins. Because bone tissue is inelastic, local edema accumulates under pressure and leads to necrosis of tissue, breakdown of bone trabeculae, and removal of both matrix and calcium. Infection extends along haversian canals, through the marrow cavity, and beneath the periosteum, damaging the vascular channels and causing death of osteocytes. This leads to the formation of a sequestrum. The periosteal new bone formation which takes place on top of already dead bone is known as an involucrum.

ETIOLOGY. Patients can often be shown to have infection elsewhere, particularly in the skin, where *S. aureus* is probably the most common causative organism; but its prevalence has dropped in the United States from 80 per cent in the past to about 50 per cent at present. In infants and children, nonhemolytic streptococci and *H. influenzae* are also offending agents, with septic arthritis compli-

cating the osteomyelitis. Gram-negative bacilli are important etiologic agents in adults with vertebral osteomyelitis. *M. tuberculosis* occurs mainly in the spine, especially among economically deprived individuals. Tuberculous and fungal infections of bone can usually be traced to pulmonary disease. Persons with sickle cell disease have a special susceptibility to *Salmonella* osteomyelitis. Osteomyelitis may follow colorectal surgery or infection of the genital, urinary, or biliary tracts. Osteomyelitis, predominantly spondylitis, is also an important sequel of drug abuse. The affected areas are usually in the axial skeleton, mainly the lumbar vertebrae or sacroiliac joints. The organisms causing the infection are unusual, e.g., *Pseudomonas aeruginosa* or *Klebsiella aerobacter*, although *Staphylococcus* and *Candida* may also be causative in this regard.

CLINICAL MANIFESTATIONS. In the past, over 85 per cent of cases occurred in children under 16. Recently there has been a shift of the disease to older age groups. Infection usually occurs in the metaphyseal region, particularly of the femur and tibia, and multiple bone involvement is not rare. In patients over age 50, the most common site of osteomyelitis is the spine.

In children, onset is sudden, with high fever, chills, and pain in a limb. Increasing numbers of patients are seen with atypical features, including low-grade temperature elevation and even no fever at all. There is usually leukocytosis. Acute local tenderness and swelling may occur because of elevation of the periosteum by pus. In adults, pyogenic spondylitis is seldom heralded by an acute febrile episode. Usually there is simply insidious onset of deep boring pain in the back, aggravated by movement, coughing, sneezing, or straining. Symptoms gradually increase. The drug abuse patient who presents with spontaneous onset of localized musculoskeletal pain should be promptly investigated for gram-negative osteomyelitis to permit specific antimicrobial therapy. Patients may complain of abdominal pain when the lumbar vertebrae are involved. Paravertebral or psoas abscesses were once thought to be indicative of tuberculous spondylitis, but today such abscesses in the United States or Western Europe are more likely to be associated with staphylococcal infection than with tuberculosis. In the adult, no changes are visible radiographically, often for many weeks after onset of infection. The delay in radiographic diagnosis is due to the interval required for either the bone matrix to be fully mineralized and thus become apparent, or for more than 50 per cent of the bone mineral to be removed before a lytic process can be visualized. Periosteal elevation or reaction or irregularities in the cortex may be noted from two to four weeks after the onset of symptoms. The radiographic changes include destruction of a disc space and the adjacent vertebral end-plates above and below. Later sclerosis of bone occurs and new bone forms, often with fusion of two vertebrae and obliteration of the intervertebral space. In childhood disease, blood cultures are frequently positive for the causative organism, but this is infrequent in adult pyogenic spondylitis.

Subacute pyogenic osteomyelitis, known as *Brodie's abscess*, is usually located in a metaphysis and appears as a lucent lesion sometimes surrounded by slight sclerosis. Its onset is insidious; pain is a prominent symptom, but fever is rare. It is usually due to the presence of *S. aureus*, occasionally *S. albus*, or even more occasionally gram-negative organisms.

Chronic osteitis in the hands or feet is usually due to

tuberculosis or syphilis. Asymmetric osteitis in the hands or feet is more likely to be due to group A *Streptococcus* and *S. aureus*.

Radiographic changes develop late in osteomyelitis, but scintigraphy, using ^{99m}Tc diphosphonate, will point to a lesion early in the disease, either in the spine or in the long bones. This is particularly helpful in the adult, in whom there is little clinical evidence to indicate spinal disease.

TREATMENT. It is important to identify the organism responsible for the infection and to determine the antimicrobial sensitivity. In vertebral osteomyelitis, needle biopsy with aspiration of tissue is necessary. For sensitive organisms, penicillin G is the best antimicrobial and should be used in large doses, preferably 20,000,000 units per day intravenously. Alternatively, oxacillin, methicillin, nafcillin, or cloxacillin may be given in daily doses of 8 to 16 grams intravenously in an adult. Treatment should be maintained for at least four to six weeks. There is no place for bacteriostatic drugs in the initial stages of treatment. Most cases of hematogenous osteomyelitis in children should be surgically drained even when the organism is known and the appropriate antimicrobial is given in large doses.

When osteomyelitis has been clinically cured, it can be assumed that viable organisms remain in haversian and Volkmann canals. It may recur up to four decades later because of the same organisms. These recurrences are often precipitated by trauma.

OSTEOMYELITIS DUE TO CONTIGUOUS INFECTION

Osteomyelitis may be caused by infection gaining entrance to a bone from a compound fracture or through surgical operation, especially with internal fixation. Infection of the phalanges of the hands and feet may occur from soft tissue infections, especially in the hands. Infection of the jaws occurs from dental abscesses and radiation. Infection from the frontal or ethmoid sinuses causes osteomyelitis of the frontal bone by spread from the blood vessels of the mucosal lining of the sinuses. When the frontal bone is infected, pus collects under the periosteum, causing swelling and edema over the forehead known as Pott's puffy tumor. With frontal osteomyelitis, epidural and even subdural abscesses may occur, with severe headache and signs of increased intracranial pressure.

A local infection occurring after a compound fracture or internal fixation is usually associated with pain, pus, and fever. When infection occurs after introduction of a prosthetic device, there is frequently an insidious onset of pain, which may take months or even years after the surgical procedure to become manifest. Extensive bone destruction may occur without clear-cut signs of infection or fever. The existence of infection may be obscured by the use of prophylactic antimicrobials given at the time of surgery. The diagnosis may be helped by needling of the suspected lesion or by open surgery. When a prosthetic device has been used, it is often necessary to remove this before the infection can be controlled.

Infections of the bones of the feet or toes occur frequently in patients with diabetes mellitus or with severe peripheral vascular disease. The patients frequently have pain and swelling in the affected limb and may have painless ulcers due to peripheral neuropathy. More often than not they have no systemic manifestations such as fever. Response to treatment with antimicrobials is usually unsatisfactory, and amputation is often necessary.

Holzman, R. S., and Bishko, F.: Osteomyelitis in heroin addicts. Ann. Intern. Med., 75:693, 1971.

Vu Quoc Dich, Nelson, J. D., and Haltalin, K. C.: Osteomyelitis in infants and children. Am. J. Dis. Child., 129:1273, 1975.

Waldvogel, F. A., Medoff, G., and Swartz, M. M.: Osteomyelitis: A review of clinical features, therapeutic considerations and unusual aspects. N. Engl. J. Med., 282:198, 260, 316, 1970.

Waxman, A. D., Bryan, D. and Siemsen, J. K.: Bone scanning in the drug abuse patient: Early detection of hematogenous osteomyelitis. J. Nucl. Med., 14:647, 1973.

563. RADIONUCLIDE BONE TOXICITY

Many radioactive isotopes accumulate in the skeleton and, although ingested in doses too small to produce acute systemic effects, may lead years later to severe bone disease. Skeletal damage consists of (1) growth retardation if exposure occurred prior to epiphyseal closure; (2) osteonecrosis, osteomyelitis, and bone abscess; (3) brittleness and tendency to fracture; and (4) osteogenic sarcoma. There are three categories of exposure: (1) strontium-90 and yttrium-91 from radioactive fallout of atom bomb fission products (2) radium and thorium from industrial and medical exposure, and (3) uranium and transuranic elements from processing of nuclear reactor fuel and wastes. Strontium and radium, like calcium, are alkaline earth elements and readily form phosphate salts. They are trapped in newly forming bone at the time of its mineralization. The localization of thorium, uranium, and the transuranic elements is less well understood, but appears to be predominantly on bone surfaces adjacent to the innumerable small vessels of bone. Radiation damage in each case is produced by the α and β particles, rather than by the γ radiation. Because of the extremely short range of these particles in bone, the damage is thus confined microscopically to the areas of isotope deposition. Cell death is the usual result, cell sensitivity varying with cell type, as follows: chondroblasts > osteoblasts > osteocytes > osteoclasts. The surrounding bony material, deprived of continuing cellular influence, becomes hard and brittle. Ultimately it is subject to slow resorptive removal. The mechanism of sarcoma production is not known but is presumably the same as for radiation carcinogenesis elsewhere.

Clinical features are variable and not distinctive. Bone pain may be present, and spontaneous fractures may occur through bone that appears roentgenographically normal. Occasionally the long bones may present a punched-out appearance reminiscent of multiple myeloma. Radium dial painters frequently developed necrosis and osteomyelitis of the jaw, related to localization of radium in the periodontal tissues. Radiation damage, once it has occurred, is irrevocable, and no treatment is beneficial. Bone localization after acute accidental ingestion of radium and strontium can be minimized by calcium infusion and deliberate production of sustained hypercalciuria.

Hasterlik, R. J., and Finkel, A. J.: Diseases of bones and joints associated with intoxication by radioactive substances, principally radium. Med. Clin. North Am., 49:285, 1965.

Vaughn, J. M.: The effects of radiation on bone. *In* Bourne, G. H. (ed.): Biochemistry and Physiology of Bone, Vol. 3. 2nd ed. New York, Academic Press, 1971.

564. FLUOROSIS

Fluoride is one of the more common constituents of the earth's crust, occurring particularly in association with phosphates, silicates, and calcium. It is abundant in sea water and in many fresh water supplies, and was undoubtedly a component of the environment in which life evolved. It probably functions as an important trace element in human nutrition, though a fluoride deficiency syndrome is not recognized. In optimal concentrations fluoride stabilizes the crystal structure of tooth enamel and probably also that of bone. In high concentrations fluoride acts as a general protoplasmic poison, resulting in death; but between toxic intake levels (>100 mg) and probably optimal intakes (about 1 mg daily), chronic intake produces changes confined largely to the skeleton. Intoxication occurs because of accidental ingestion of fluoride-containing insecticides, chronic inhalation of industrial dusts (particularly in the aluminum mining and phosphate fertilizer industries), or prolonged drinking of certain fresh waters containing large amounts of fluorides. The skeletal lesions in man vary with the intake but consist of a combination of osteosclerosis and osteomalacia. The malacic lesions are more prominent at higher intake levels and represent interference with matrix maturation or crystal nucleation. Sclerosis consists of coarsening of trabeculae, periosteal new bone deposition, osteophyte formation, and ossification of tendons and ligaments. Severely fluorotic bone is chalky white in appearance and exhibits a crumbly consistency, cutting easily with a knife.

Early there are no specific complaints. As the skeletal disease advances, there may be vague pains in the small joints of hands and feet. As osteophyte formation and periosteal bone growth progress, kyphosis, restriction of spine motion, genu valgum flexion contractures of hips and knees, and ultimately nerve root and spinal cord compression develop. The neurologic involvement produces paresthesias, weakness, and ultimately paralysis. Early the neurologic involvement may simulate peripheral neuropathy, spinal cord tumor, or syringomyelia. Affected children may develop genu valgum and secondary hyperparathyroidism. Although serum calcium is normal in patients with skeletal fluorosis, parathyroid gland hyperactivity and increased circulating parathyroid hormone become manifest because of the decreased solubility of the bone fluoroapatite and the compensatory need to maintain normal extracellular ionized calcium equilibrium.

No municipal water supply in the United States has yet been identified with more than 6 to 8 parts per million of fluoride. This concentration, although sufficient to produce mottled tooth enamel, almost never produces bone disease. In certain regions of India and Arabia, water-related fluoride intake reaches sufficient levels to produce fluoride intoxication. In the Punjab, for example, osteofluorosis with genu valgum is the most common form of bone disease. Deliberate osteofluorosis has sometimes been induced to halt the explosive skeletal demineralization of diseases such as multiple myeloma.

There is no effective treatment for the advanced syndrome except for orthopedic and supportive measures. Effort should be directed at prevention, particularly in the context of industrial exposure. Excess body burdens of fluoride are retained for years after exposure has terminated. Fluoride trapped in bone crystals is released only when bone resorption occurs, and some of the liberated ions are redeposited at sites of new bone formation. If the intake is low, however, urinary excretion will gradually lower the total body content.

Editorial: Genu valgum due to fluoride toxicity. Nutr. Rev., 33:76, 1975.
Epker, B. N.: A quantitative microscopic study of bone-remodeling and balance in a human with skeletal fluorosis. Clin. Orthop. Rel. Res., 55:87, 1967.
Singh, A., Jolly, S. S., Bansal, B. C., and Mathur, C. C.: Endemic fluorosis: Epidemiological, clinical and biochemical study of chronic fluorine intoxication in Punjab (India). Medicine, 42:229, 1963.
Sivakumar, B., and Krishnamachari, D. A. V. R.: Circulating levels of immunoreactive parathyroid hormone in endemic genu valgum. Horm. Metab. Res., 8:317, 1976.
Srikantia, S. G., and Siddiqui, A. H.: Metabolic studies in skeletal fluorosis. Clin. Sci., 28:477, 1965.
Teotia, S. P. S., and Teotia, M.: Hyperactivity of the parathyroid glands in endemic osteofluoroses. Fluoride, 5:115, 1972.

565. FIBROUS DYSPLASIA

Fibrous dysplasia, a developmental disorder of the bone mesenchyme, is characterized by replacement of bone by large masses of cellular fibrous tissue containing immature bone spicules and islands of cartilage. Except for the cartilage component, the histologic features are very similar to those of osteitis fibrosa, as is the roentgenographic appearance, but the two diseases differ in many respects. Fibrous dysplasia is a local disorder, and although lesions may be widespread, there is always normal, uninvolved bone somewhere; furthermore, the disease is relatively slowly progressive and lacks the rapid bone resorption and formation of osteitis fibrosa. When the disease occurs in young girls, it is sometimes associated with precocious puberty and patchy brownish skin pigmentation. This triad is known as Albright's syndrome. Since large doses of estrogens produce a similar metaphyseal lesion in very young animals, it is not clear whether the precocious puberty of Albright's syndrome is simply a part of the picture or a contributing cause of the bone disease. The sexual precocity noted in some females is not associated with ovulation or with demonstrable follicle-stimulating hormone. Moreover, short stature is not a constant finding at the end of the growth surge in females. In some individuals the adrenarche occurs prematurely, and sexual precocity may be found in female patients without the cutaneous pigmentation characteristic of the syndrome or fibrous dysplasia of the skull. The syndrome may be comparable to other pluriglandular adenomatosis syndromes (see Ch. 543.5), since the disorder may be associated with hyperparathyroidism, hyperthyroidism, or gigantism.

The actual age of onset with bone involvement is usually unknown, and the disease first becomes apparent between ages 5 and 15, commonly because of deformity or pathologic fracture. Typical roentgenographic changes are cystlike lesions of metaphyseal or shaft bone, with expansion of the cortex and sometimes severe destruction of bony architecture. Areas of increased density are frequently seen; as the patient ages, the lesions gradually acquire a uniform, ground-glass type of opacity. Plasma calcium and phosphorus are normal; the alkaline phosphatase is usually normal, but may be elevated when the disease is extensive.

Bone involvement is commonly unilateral. The femur and pelvis are frequently involved, as is the skull. Repeated fractures through involved areas of the upper femur lead to the characteristic "shepherd's crook" deformity. In the skull, however, lesions are osteomatoid rather than fibrous, and roentgenograms reveal dense, featureless opacification and distortion of the facial bones and base of the skull. Encroachment on cranial nerves may produce neurologic symptoms. Osteomalacia, vitamin D resistant rickets, and myositis ossificans may also be present in some individuals. Growth is slow throughout childhood and usually ceases entirely in adolescence. The principal significance of the disorder lies in the production of fractures and deformity, but occasionally osteogenic fibro- or chondrosarcoma may occur. Except for indicated orthopedic procedures, treatment is generally supportive. In isolated instances rapidly progressive skeletal lesions have responded favorably to human calcitonin treatment.

Benedict, P. H.: Endocrine features in Albright's syndrome (fibrous dysplasia of bone). Metabolism, 11:30, 1962.
Falconer, M. A., and Cope, C. L.: Fibrous dysplasia of bone with endocrine disorders and cutaneous pigmentation (Albright's disease). Quart. J. Med., 4:121, 1942.
Firat, D., and Stutzman, L.: Fibrous dysplasia of the bone. Am. J. Med., 44:421, 1968.
Huvos, A. G., Higinbotham, N. L., and Miller, T. R.: Bone sarcomas arising in fibrous dysplasia. J. Bone Joint Surg., 54A:1047, 1972.

566. HYPERTROPHIC OSTEOARTHROPATHY

Hypertrophic osteoarthropathy is a syndrome consisting of clubbing of the fingers, painful swelling, and periosteal new bone deposition in the long bones of the extremities, and sometimes moderate joint swelling and tenderness, particularly at the wrists, ankles, and knees. The disorder is almost always associated with disease elsewhere in the body. It occurs in association with intrathoracic malignancies, usually a lung cancer or mesothelioma, but also with metastatic malignancies and mediastinal tumors, as well as bronchiectasis. Clubbing is common with chronic intestinal diseases; true osteoarthropathy is rare but has been described with ulcerative colitis, portal cirrhosis, and juvenile biliary cirrhosis. Very rarely it exists without apparent predisposing disease, and there is also a distinct hereditary form of the disorder, *pachydermoperiostosis*, associated with thickening of the skin of the scalp, face, and hands. In pachydermoperiostosis onset is usually at puberty. A family history of the disorder can be obtained in about one fourth of the cases.

In the fingertips the predominant changes are edema, hyperemia, and soft tissue fibrous proliferation; bony changes are variable and usually not prominent. Grossly the fingertips appear bulbous, and there is increased curvature of the nails in all directions. The most typical bony lesions are found in the distal shafts of the bones of the forearm and leg, where there is distinct periosteal new bone deposition. Overlying tissues may be edematous, and the entire region is painful and tender to pressure. More advanced disease may involve the entire forearm and leg bones, and later the femur and humerus are affected.

The cause is unknown. The changes are probably mediated by alterations in periosteal blood flow. There is reason to suspect abnormal visceral reflex patterns, triggered by centrally located disease. Innominate artery aneurysms have been reported in association with osteoarthropathy confined to the involved extremity. In any case, surgical correction of lung lesions responsible for the disorder frequently produces dramatic relief of pain and swelling and prompt healing on roentgenographic examination.

Early in the course of the disorder the arthritic complaints may be misdiagnosed as rheumatoid arthritis. The later periosteal manifestations must be differentiated from disorders such as scurvy, syphilitic periostitis, polyarteritis nodosa, and progressive diaphyseal dysplasia. The skin changes of pachydermoperiostosis may suggest a diagnosis of acromegaly; however, absence of sinus enlargement and presence of periosteal reaction allow differentiation by roentgenography.

The disorder is important for two reasons. First, it usually serves as an indicator of serious disease elsewhere in the body and sometimes, particularly with pulmonary neoplasia, may be the first manifestation. Second, it is usually painful and may contribute significantly to the over-all disability of the primary disease.

Treatment must be directed at the underlying disease. Analgesics, and sometimes narcotics, are required for symptomatic relief. Vagotomy has also been reported to provide relief.

Fischer, D. S., Singer, D. H., and Feldman, S. M.: Clubbing, a review, with emphasis on hereditary acropachy. Medicine, 43:459, 1964.
Herman, M. A., Massaro, D., Katz, S., and Sachs, M.: Pachydermoperiostosis — clinical spectrum. Arch. Intern. Med., 116:918, 1965.
Pugh, D. G.: Roentgenologic Diagnosis of Diseases of Bone. New York, Thomas Nelson & Sons, 1951.

567. OTHER CONGENITAL AND/OR HEREDITARY DISORDERS INVOLVING BONE

Osteopetrosis (Albers-Schönberg's disease, marble bone disease) is a rare familial disorder of the skeleton characterized by an increase in density of all bones owing to failure of bone resorption and bone remodeling.

There are probably dominant as well as recessive types of inheritance. The severe variety presents in infancy with anemia and hepatosplenomegaly. These children have little or no bone marrow and require blood transfusions. Failure to resorb bone results in optic atrophy, deafness, and hydrocephalus. Osteomyelitis of the jaws from dental infection may require antimicrobials. Early death is frequent. Milder cases may come to medical attention later in childhood or in adult life because of retarded growth or increased bone fragility.

Hypersplenism may require splenectomy for improvement of anemia. There is no specific treatment for the bone disease. Bone resorption can be restored in mice with inherited osteopetrosis by transplants or normal bone marrow and spleen cells. Additional studies are essential to determine whether the migratory cells are precursors of osteoclasts or the source of humoral substances such as the osteoclast activity factor (OAF) or prostaglandins which may regulate activities of bone-resorbing cells.

Melorheostosis is a rare disorder of bone resulting in massive endosteal thickening, affecting one or more long bones, which begins proximally and proceeds distally like the flow of wax down a candle. The condition is painful. The cause is unknown, and there is no specific treatment.

Osteopoikilosis is inherited as an autosomal dominant trait. It consists of multiple dense zones or streaks occurring throughout the skeleton and frequently is associated with local patches of elastic fiber hyperplasia in the skin. It is of little clinical importance.

Hereditary hyperphosphatasia (hyperostosis corticalis deformans juvenilis) is a rare disease inherited as an autosomal recessive trait. It is characterized by multiple fractures and bone deformity in childhood, presenting radiologically some of the features of Paget's disease of bone. Plasma alkaline phosphatase is extremely high. Bone turnover is rapid, and there is increased urinary hydroxyproline. There may be mental retardation. As in Paget's disease, the skeletal lesions respond to calcitonin therapy, with healing of the lytic component and gradual development of normal bone contours.

Ellis–van Creveld syndrome (chondroectodermal dysplasia) is characterized by polydactyly of the hands and, rarely, of the feet, dwarfism, and dysplasia of the fingernails. It is inherited as an autosomal recessive trait. In contrast to classic achondroplasia, the shortening of the extremities is more marked distally than proximally. Fusion of the capitate and hamate bones of the wrist and a defect in the lateral aspect of the proximal part of the tibia, producing knock knees, are consistent features. Congenital heart disease is frequently present; atrial septal defect is the most common cardiac malformation. An abnormally short upper lip, bound down by multiple frenula, and premature eruption of the teeth are frequent features. The disease is rare, but occurs as the main cause of dwarfism in the inbred socioreligious group known as the Old Order Amish in Lancaster County, Pennsylvania, where it occurs with a frequency of 5 per 1000 births. One third of those affected die before two weeks of age. The condition must be distinguished from familial polydactyly and classic achondroplasia.

Achondroplasia is a form of inherited dwarfism caused by retardation of endochondral bone formation. This relatively common disorder is inherited as an autosomal dominant trait. The abnormality is confined to cartilage and consists of failure or retardation of interstitial cellular proliferation and growth. As a result bones formed in cartilage are shortened. This is most apparent in the long bones of the extremities and in the base of the skull, and to a much lesser extent in the vertebrae. Membrane bone formation is normal; thus the bones of the cranial vault are able to grow normally and even accommodate themselves to the restricted growth of the base of the skull. Similarly, bone shafts enlarge normally. Microscopically there is a lack of normal cartilage cell columns at the epiphyseal growth plates, so that formation of the primary spongiosa proceeds very slowly and irregularly. Clinically, there is dwarfism, with disproportionate shortening of the extremities. Final height is usually less than 1.4 meters. The bridge of the nose is flattened and depressed, and the forehead may appear prominent and bulging. The hands and feet are short, and the fingers tend to be nearly equal in length. The vertebrae are slightly and symmetrically flatter than normal. There is usually a dorsal kyphosis, along with compensatory posterior rotation of the sacrum and pelvis. The hip joints may thus be displaced backward and the pelvic inlet narrowed by the sacral promontory. Achondroplastic dwarfs exhibit entirely normal intelligence, endocrine function, and calcium metabolism, and, apart from their characteristic dwarfing and the problems it imposes, are able to live normal, useful lives. Achondroplasia presents such a typical picture that it is not usually confused with other causes of dwarfism except vitamin D resistant rickets (VDRR). Occasionally patients with osteogenesis imperfecta may have very short extremities because of multiple fractures, but the true nature of the disease is immediately apparent roentgenographically. When diagnosis is difficult, measurement of the interpeduncular distance in the lumbar spine may be helpful. In normal people, interpeduncular distance increases (as one goes down) from T12 to L5, but in patients with achondroplasia T11 or 12 is the widest vertebra, while the lumbar interpeduncular distance either does not increase or actually decreases. Because of this restricted bony canal in the lumbar region, prolapsed intervertebral discs cause extremely severe symptoms.

Ollier's dyschondroplasia (multiple enchondromatosis) is a rare disorder in which projections or islands of epiphyseal cartilage proliferate down into the metaphysis. These cartilage remnants fail to undergo the changes required for mineralization but retain the growth potential of the epiphyseal plate, and under continued stimulation by growth hormone may expand slowly until much of the normal metaphyseal architecture is destroyed. There may be gross enlargement of the metaphysis. On the roentgenogram the lesions vary from elongated radiolucent patches to a fragmented, expanded picture that conveys the impression of a violent internal explosion within the metaphysis. Growth may cease and calcification may take place after puberty, but the inclusions may continue to enlarge throughout life, sometimes developing into chondrosarcomas. One side of the body is usually more severely involved than the other, but the lesions are fundamentally bilateral. The long bones and the ilia are most commonly involved, and when severe the disease may result in crippling and invalidism. The only treatment available consists of orthopedic procedures for correction of deformities and pathologic fractures.

Probably the most common of the osteodyschondroplasias, the syndrome of *hereditary multiple exostoses*, consists of irregular bony protuberances with a cartilage growth cap that projects out from the subepiphyseal metaphyseal cortex and backward along the shaft. Lesions are bilateral, although not truly symmetrical, and represent more an abnormality of development of bony contour than a true exostosis. The metaphyseal cortex extends out around the periphery of the protuberances, and their trabecular structure and marrow spaces are continuous with that of the adjacent metaphysis. The disease occurs in families, but the mode of transmission is not known. Although the lesions begin to develop early in childhood, they rarely become apparent for several years. The basic abnormality is not known, but the disorder behaves as if portions of the zone of proliferating cartilage extended down the side of the metaphysis and in the process of growing split off from the growth plate and migrated back along the shaft, leaving a wake of normal endochondral bone behind them. The lesions are confined to the metaphyses of bones with active growth plates, and when severe may limit joint motion. Growth usually ceases when the epiphyses fuse. Very rarely the cartilaginous cap of an exostosis may develop into a chondrosarcoma.

Bargman, G. J., Langer, L. O., Jr., and Opitz, J. M.: Achondroplasia and thanatophoric dwarfism: With a review of several forms of short-limb dwarfism. In Gardner, L. I., (ed.): Endocrine and Genetic Diseases of Childhood and Adolescence. Philadelphia, W. B. Saunders Company, 1975, p. 870.

McKusick, V. A.: Heritable Disorders of Connective Tissue. 4th ed. St. Louis, C. V. Mosby Company, 1972.

Nyhan, W. L., and Sakati, N. D.: Genetic and Malformation Syndromes in Clinical Medicine. Chicago, Year Book Medical Publishers, 1976.

Rubin, P.: Dynamic Classification of Bone Dysplasias. Chicago, Year Book Medical Publishers, 1964.

PART XXIII
CERTAIN CUTANEOUS DISEASES WITH SIGNIFICANT SYSTEMIC MANIFESTATIONS

Marie-Louise Johnson

568.   INTRODUCTION

The skin is our interface with the world, and more. It is the glassine bag through which physiologic and chemical changes are perceived; the self-substance that is invaded and traumatized from within and without; an organ that responds and repairs; and one that shares the burdens of growing up and growing old, of environmental insults, and of systemic disease.

As an organ system it is unique. It stretches before the examiner patently obvious with significant data waiting to be read. The student attuned to palpating and auscultating forgets to look. He misses basic physiologic facts about his patient, perhaps significant signals of serious disease, even gross pathology. Further, when the patient draws attention to a skin change, the student is chagrined at his uncertainty as to what it may be or its importance. If the patient is sufficiently persistent, or the examiner sufficiently compulsive, a consultation can be obtained, usually with dispatch during medical school and house staff training. But later, when the examiner is removed from the medical center and the logistics and economics of the consultation must be reckoned, decisions are made on shaky foundations. The risk of ignoring the mortal and promoting morbidity is increased as much as is the cost of care through unnecessary referral. Such decisions are not infrequent; some 30 per cent of Americans have a dermatologic problem that should be seen by a physician; further, 52 per cent of all problems related to the skin present to internists, pediatricians, and generalists.

This is not to say that every practicing physician needs to be a dermatologist; he could not, in the limited time for training. It does suggest that every doctor involved in patient care should be comfortable recognizing and treating *common* skin problems, ten of which constitute 76 per cent of the burden of skin disease as established by population survey (Table 1).

In Part XXIII it is our intention to review pathophysiologic mechanisms that will prepare the observer for an informed assessment of the skin. Once there is confidence in identifying the morbid processes observed, the facts can be interpreted and the diagnosis elaborated. Without awaiting a confirmed impression, however, the patient can be made more comfortable; thus Ch. 571 will emphasize principles of therapy as well as precautions and proscriptions. Finally, the more common

TABLE 1.   Prevalence of Common Dermatologic Disease in the United States*

	Rate per 1000	Numbers (in 1000's)
Fungus infections	81.1	15,733
Tinea pedis	38.7	7509
Tinea unguium	21.8	4232
Tinea versicolor	8.4	1623
Tinea cruris	6.7	1301
Acne vulgaris	68.1	13,217
Cystic acne	1.9	375
Acne scars	1.7	321
Seborrheic dermatitis	28.2	5476
Verruca vulgaris	8.5	1684
Folliculitis	8.0	1553
Atopic dermatitis	6.9	1332
Lichen simplex chronicus	4.5	882
Hand eczema	1.6	311
Dyshidrotic eczema	2.1	405
Psoriasis	5.5	1070
Vitiligo	4.9	957
Herpes simplex	4.2	824

*Persons 1 to 74 years of age—noninstitutionalized.

dermatologic conditions will be reviewed, as well as those that have implications for systemic illness, and those which in their management utilize medications and modalities of therapy uncommon to other disciplines. Our aim is to ensure an ease of recognition and management for the common dermatoses; to provide a useful guide to the identification and assessment of cutaneous signs of systemic disease; and, finally, to sharpen suspicion and enhance understanding of the risk and challenge of the more significant dermatologic diagnoses as judged by morbidity and mortality. In no way are the following chapters an attempt to substitute for a text in dermatology; hence frequent reference will be made to the literature, especially to selected texts and review articles, where the reader can further his knowledge.

Johnson, M. L., and Roberts, J.: Prevalence of dermatological diseases among persons 1 to 74 years of age, United States. *In* Advance Data, National Center for Health Statistics, No. 4, 1977.

Stern, R. S., Johnson, M-L., and DeLozier, J.: Utilization of physician services for dermatologic complaints. Arch. Dermatol., 113:1062, 1977.

General Dermatology Reference Texts

Braverman, I. M.: Skin Signs of Systemic Disease. Philadelphia, W. B. Saunders Company, 1970.

Fitzpatrick, T. B., Eisen, A. Z., Wolff, K., Freedberg, I. M., and Austen, K. F. (eds.): Dermatology in General Medicine. 2nd ed. New York, McGraw-Hill Book Company, in press.

Moschella, S. L., Pillsbury, D. M., and Hurley, H. J., Jr.: Dermatology, 2 vols. Philadelphia, W. B. Saunders Company, 1975.

Rook, A., Wilkinson, D. S., and Ebling, F. J. G.: Textbook of Dermatology, 2 vols. Oxford, Blackwell Scientific Publications, 1968.

569. PATHOPHYSIOLOGY

The skin is an essential organ. Deprived of significant amounts, as by burn and trauma, we cannot survive. Excessive losses of fluid and electrolytes are difficult to replace, and without the natural barrier to organisms infection is hard to contain.

But the disruptions of the integument are not always so gross. To understand challenges that have targeted effects, to interpret disease processes that show characteristic anatomic change or deposits of immune proteins at selected sites, some detailed information about the structure and function of the skin is required.

ANATOMIC CONSIDERATIONS

The living envelope which enfolds us contributes 16 per cent or so to the body weight of the average adult. It is composed of two mutually dependent layers of distinct developmental origin: the outer *epidermis* from the ectoderm and the inner *dermis* from the mesoderm, both cushioned on the fat-containing subcutaneous tissue, the *panniculus adiposus* (Fig. 1). Mesenchymal structures such as collagen, blood vessels, and fat originate from the mesoderm.

The stratified cellular epidermis is derived by a division of a basal layer of cells which forms successive sheets moving outward as keratinocytes synthesizing the insoluble protein keratin. From the *stratum germanitivum* the columnar basal cell resting on a basement membrane generates, by mitosis, daughter cells, one or both of which progress to the surface, becoming more polyhedral as they go; still nucleate, they are bound at the tufts called desmosomes, to which are fixed cytoplasmic filaments constituting by their quill-like appearance the *stratum spinosum* (Fig. 2). In the course of 14 days the matured daughter cell will have flattened from a polyhedral form to a pancake, acquiring keratohyaline granules that in the aggregate suggest the label *stratum granulosum*. Eventually it will lose its nucleus to become part of the *stratum corneum*. In another 14 days, by wear and programmed replacement from beneath, it will be shed completely; this slough of skin is continuous and imperceptible in the normal individual, with a turnover time of four weeks from basal cell to extinction. Anatomically there is some variation. The stratum corneum has its greatest thickness on the palms and soles, for example, and in these areas epidermal turnover is prolonged.

The differentiation of the migratory epidermal cells involves the formation of one or more fibrous proteins known collectively as keratin. The process, complete in the stratum corneum, yields mature keratin, a system of filaments embedded in a continuous matrix within a thickened cell membrane. As the stratum corneum, keratin serves as a rate-limiting membrane affecting the passage of ions and molecules. It is the protective layer against harmful chemicals; it also admits selected substances, including topical allergens as well as topical therapy. It freely admits water, up to four times its weight, and it freely yields water to the environment as insensible perspiration. Transport across the membrane is enhanced by increased temperature, by the lipid solubility of the solute, and by increased hydration of the stratum corneum itself.

Pathologic processes that disorder the differentiation of epidermal cells toward keratin may manifest themselves as blocking the transport of insensible water, the admission of topical therapy, or even the clinical appearance of casings or scale, be it retained or overproduced keratin. Further, in the loss of the spinous adherence of cells at desmosomes, the intercellular spaces trap fluid to the consequent development of blisters.

Although the pathogenesis may vary, the disrupted cell is the keratinocyte—that general name for the epidermal cell derived from the basal layer. In the epidermis, however, there are also *melanocytes* which originate in the neural crest of the embryo and retain migratory capabilities in the adult. They transfer pigment to the epidermal cells through their dendritic processes. Malfunction can mean absence of pigment or pigment production to the extreme, both potential cosmetic disasters. Also present in the epidermis are Langerhans' cells, of long recognition, of obscure origin and function, and of recent focus for their suspected role in contact dermatitis and delayed hypersensitivity.

Figure 1. Structure of the skin.

SWEAT DUCT
STRATUM CORNEUM
S. LUCIDUM
S. GRANULOSUM
S. SPINOSUM
DERMO-EPIDERMAL JUNCTION
SUB-PAPILLARY PLEXUS
ECCRINE GLAND
DERMO-EPIDERMAL JUNCTION
ARRECTOR PILI
SEBACEOUS GLAND
ECCRINE GLAND
DERMAL PAPILLA OF HAIR FOLLICLE
FAT OF SUB-CUTIS

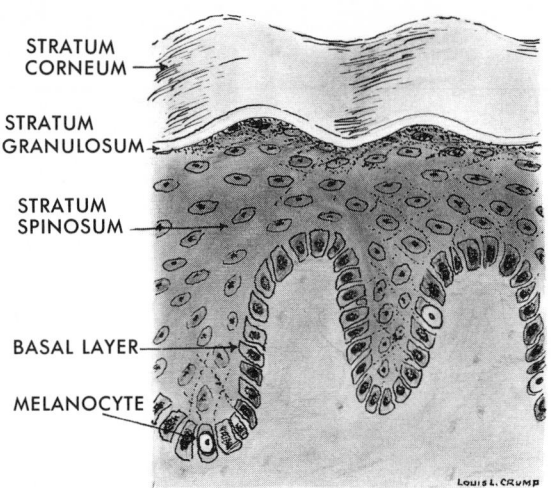

STRATUM CORNEUM

STRATUM GRANULOSUM

STRATUM SPINOSUM

BASAL LAYER

MELANOCYTE

LOUIS L. CRUMP

Figure 2. The stratified cellular epidermis.

Beneath the epidermis is the principal mass of skin, the dermis, a mixture of fibrous protein and collagen embedded in mucopolysaccharide along with water, elastic fibers, nerves, blood vessels, lymph channels, glands, appendages, and a few cells, largely fibroblasts, mast cells, and histiocytes. Actually eccrine sweat glands and the pilosebaceous apparatus, although dermal in location, are of ectodermal origin and formed from embryonic invaginations into the mesoderm. Because the stratum corneum covers only the most superficial part, transport through these structures is more rapid. Undoubtedly the pilosebaceous and sweat glands contribute heavily to the transport of molecular substances through the skin.

MECHANICAL CONSIDERATIONS

The mechanical properties of skin are important from the standpoint of toughness and resistance to forces of disruption, to shearing, but also as they relate to wound healing, to the aging process, or to inherited disorders in which structural elements are defective. Strength and flexibility are signficant attributes, and the extracellular components of the dermis are important contributors. *Collagen* fibers, for example, give high tensile strength, and their loose mesh permits the mobility of joints. The return of collagen to the unstressed state depends on the elastic restoring forces of *elastin.* In old age the degradation of the elastic fiber network leaves the collagen mesh without the support to restore fully its original configuration, and wrinkled skin is the surface evidence. The ground substance, which is less well understood, through its viscous and elastic properties, resists compression and accepts molding, thus serving to reduce point pressure on more sensitive skin structures.

PHYSIOLOGIC CONSIDERATIONS

The individual cannot survive without skin, and skin cannot survive without oxygen and nutrients. Although the prime provider role of blood vessels is dramatically underscored in its disruption, as with gangrenous toes

and stubborn leg ulcers, the skin compared to other organs is low in metabolic requirements. Like the kidney, its blood flow is far in excess of nutritional need, and its vascular system is adapted to mechanisms that meet other demands such as the regulation of body heat. In normal and warm environments blood flow is greater in the digits and other acral skin areas, achieved in part through the arteriovenous shunt of the glomus body, a dermal vessel peculiar to the acral areas. At normal environmental temperatures and low work levels, dermal blood flow is the only thermoregulatory mechanism required to maintain a constant body temperature. Increase in the metabolic rate of the body will increase skin blood flow. Posterior hypothalamic centers in the brain control dermal blood flow through deep vasoconstrictor mechanisms of the sympathetic nervous system.

Apart from nutrition and thermal regulation, dermal blood vessels participate in the inflammatory response and demonstrate recognizable pathologic changes in specific diseases. Reacting to a noxious stimulus, transient vasoconstriction will be followed by dilatation with a ten-fold increase in blood flow, an increase in vessel permeability, and a consequent escape of fluid into the interstitial space. There is a relaxing of precapillary sphincters which become refractory to vasoconstrictor stimuli, and finally, initiation of the cellular response. With certain traumatic stimuli to normal skin in disease states, the dermal response may be a vascular proliferation or constriction, or even development of the complete lesion of the disease, the isomorphic response as seen in collagen diseases, psoriasis, and lichen planus.

SWEAT GLANDS

Eccrine

The thermoregulatory mechanism depends significantly on the eccrine sweat gland, which produces and transports to the skin surface a hypotonic solution for evaporation and cooling. Given sufficient thermal stimulation, an individual through his 2 to 3 million sweat glands can produce 2 to 3 liters of sweat per hour for a short interval. Each gland is a simple tubule with a coiled secretory segment deep in the dermis and a straight duct extending up to become spiraled terminally before it pierces the stratum corneum. It is well supplied with blood vessels, and, in its secretory part, with unmyelinated nerve endings, anatomically sympathetic but functionally parasympathetic.

Lesions develop with anatomic blockage of the sweat duct. A rupture in the mid-dermis nearer the secretory part stimulates little dermal response, although the trapped sweat may be visible in the skin. Like a deep millet seed, it is called descriptively *miliaria profunda.* Rupture more distally near the papillary plexus ensures proximity to blood vessels and nerve endings, which provokes redness and itching because of reactive dilatation of the capillaries and stimulation of the *c* fibers of the nerves. Clinically it is known as *miliaria rubra* or, more commonly, *prickly heat.* Inability of sweat to escape at the surface leaves a superficial drop of sweat with few symptoms, scattered dew drops in transparent casings; it is important only to be recognized for what it is — *miliaria crystallina.* In all physiologic entrap-ments of sweat the therapy is to reduce the activity of the gland, remove blockage at the duct orifice, and counteract the local irritant effects of escaped intradermal sweat. Cooling will reduce the need to sweat; mild keratolytics will free the eccrine sweat pores of retained keratin and lipid, and anti-inflammatory agents such as topical steroids will reduce erythema and pruritus.

Sweat is formed not by passive filtration but by active metabolic processes, with lactate produced in the secretory segment and sodium resorbed in the ductal segment. Sweat appearing on the skin is usually lower in sodium and chloride and higher in lactate than interstitial fluid from which it is derived. The maximal capacity to resorb sodium is only one quarter the capacity to secrete. Hence at times of profuse sweating, significant amounts of sodium can be lost. True adaptation can be seen with repeated intense thermal stress, leading to a conservation of sodium through a mechanism that may involve increased adrenal aldosterone secretion and enhanced reabsorption in the ductal segment.

An increase in body heat arouses temperature-sensitive centers in the hypothalamus and serves as a potent stimulus for generalized sweating. Pyrogens raise the hypothalamic temperature threshold for inducing sweating, and fever is the consequence, the heat produced through shivering if the ambient temperature is low. When the receptor function returns to normal levels and body temperature is then perceived as too high, profuse sweating ensues.

It is of interest and an aggravation to certain dermatologic problems that the palms and soles have large eccrine sweat gland populations. Although they respond poorly to thermal stimulation, they do respond immediately and profusely to psychogenic stimuli. Palmar sweat as an index of emotional stress is used in the polygraph or lie-detector test.

The physical aspects of heat loss and retention have their obvious dramatic roles in the desert and polar regions, but they also have an important and certainly more extensive role in prophylactic skin care and management of dermal pathology. Heat may be lost or gained relative to environmental temperature by radiation, conduction, or convection. Ordinary metabolic heat from organs and muscle is transported by the blood to the skin, where it is lost through radiation and convection by adjustments in cutaneous circulation effecting perhaps small changes in skin surface temperature. The balance is maintained readily and without sweat. With excessive metabolic heat the regulated blood flow through skin is accelerated; the increased vascular surface area permits heat to be lost to the lower ambient temperature of the air, to colder solid or liquid surfaces as to rocks or lake water, and through the evaporation of water or sweat from the skin, which reduces the available heat by the 2260 joules needed to convert each gram of water to water vapor.

At rest in a 35° C, windy dry environment, an elevated body temperature will lose heat not by radiation or convection but through evaporation calculated as 150 grams of sweat per hour to remain stable. With exercise and consequent increase in metabolic heat, and with an extreme environmental temperature to 46° C, 830 grams of sweat per hour would be needed for stabilization. In a hot humid environment with evaporation restricted, profuse sweat drips rather than evaporating and the heat load is difficult to dissipate, with risk of severe hyperthermia, dehydration, and sodium depletion,

which may be followed by collapse, failure of the eccrine apparatus, and fatal heat stroke; the victim's skin is flushed, warm, and dry. In hot environments it is vital to replace salt and water losses continuously and to promote cooling by evaporation with air currents, nonrestrictive clothing, and cool water immersion.

The conservation of body heat, less dramatic physiologically, is a more common phenomenon, since there is greater risk to life from unexpected or prolonged exposure to cold. Survival in water of 0° C unprotected is no more than 30 minutes. Actually one primary physiologic defense to cold, to shut down the cutaneous circulation, thus increasing the distance heat must be conducted to be lost at the surface, is inadequate for most environmental cold. We rely heavily on shelter and clothing. In pathologic conditions with inflammation, body heat loss can be impressive even with common protection at average temperatures, and the comfort of patients is compromised by their constant sense of chill. It is recognizing heat loss as it manifests the pathologic process and modifies the therapeutic management that is most important for our consideration in dermatology.

The Pilosebaceous-Apocrine Apparatus

The hair unit, including sebaceous and apocrine glands, develops in utero over the entire skin surface except the palms and soles. One would never see a furuncle, for example, an abscess of a hair follicle, on the palm, sole, or glans penis, unless the patient had had a skin graft from a hairy site. Before birth the apocrine portion of the hair-gland apparatus atrophies in most complexes, but persists as a full pilosebaceous-apocrine apparatus in the axillae and genital area, occasionally at the areolae of the breast, and about the umbilicus. The breast is actually a modified apocrine gland, as are the ceruminous glands of the ear and Moll's glands of the eyelid. At puberty apocrine glands enlarge to produce an oily, colorless substance, which remains odorless until bacterial decomposition results in a characteristic body odor. Individuals vary in the intensity of odor related to apocrine gland size and personal hygiene. Short chain fatty acids and ammonia are the major odorogenic products of bacterial degradation, but other unidentified substances in the sweat or on the skin could contribute to individual variations in the malodorous emanations.

A rare individual may have colored apocrine sweat, apocrine chromhidrosis, which can be axillary or exceptionally facial or, even more rarely, of the scalp, according to where vestigial apocrine glands are functional. Apart from concern and the need for reassurance, the nuisance of stained underclothing is a common complaint in those with axillary chromhidrosis. Most frequently yellow, the pigment can be green, blue, or blue-black and is attributed to one or more lipofuscins produced, for reasons unknown, within the apocrine gland. The staining must be distinguished from that resulting from surface pigments of corynebacteria or piedra, which thrive in the axilla and lend their pigment to colorless sweat after it leaves the sweat duct. The latter staining can be controlled with shaving and topical antimicrobial agents; true chromhidrosis cannot. As a side note, patients with ochronosis may stain axillary secretions or skin brown but would have a positive urine test result for homogentisic acid.

As with eccrine sweat, apocrine secretions can be plugged, disrupting the duct, breaking into the dermis, and triggering intense pruritus with erythema. The problem, often provoked by emotional stimuli to apocrine excretion through adrenergic sympathetic discharge, is really an apocrine miliaria and is known as *Fox-Fordyce disease.* Usually involving the axillae, often the genital area, and occasionally the periareolar glands, the trapped apocrine sweat raises small discrete rounded lesions with a consequent relative apocrine anhidrosis. Therapy of variable success is aimed at reducing stimuli to apocrine sweating, limiting maceration from eccrine sweat, and counteracting the inflammatory response with topical and injectable steroids.

As distressing and persistent as apocrine miliaria may be, the severe disease of apocrine glands is the chronic, suppurative, and cicatricial problem known as *hidradenitis suppurativa.* It may involve the axillae exclusively, as it often does in women, or the anogenital area, or both; in some affected individuals it is associated with severe scarring acne, occasionally with cicatrizing perifolliculitis of the scalp, or a pilonidal cyst. Although an isolated axillary or inguinal lesion might be mistaken for an abscess, multiple lesions or recurrences, especially an associated acne or scalp problem, should suggest the diagnosis. Once made, vigorous antimicrobial therapy with topical preparations and systemic antibiotics is indicated to reduce smoldering infection and minimize sinus tract formation. Early surgery may reduce the number of glands at risk and abort a potentially devastating disease (Fig. 3).

The *sebaceous gland* specialized for lipid synthesis is widely distributed over the body but concentrated in the scalp, face, upper back, and chest. Each hair follicle is associated with sebaceous glands, but the converse is not true. Some sebaceous glands without associated hairs open directly into the surface and are known as sebaceous follicles; others, by reason of anatomic localization and modification, are singled out for special identification. In the buccal mucosa and at the vermilion border of the lip, for example, they are known as

Fordyce's spots; around the female areola, as Montgomery's tubercles; at the prepuce, as Tyson's glands; and on the eyelids, as meibomian glands. As sebaceous glands they share in the pathophysiologic mechanisms to be considered; as normal anatomic structures they should not be confused with skin pathology.

The sebaceous gland depends upon and is extremely receptive to androgenic hormones. Maternal androgens ensure full development and function at birth. The vernix caseosa covering the neonate is mostly sebum. Normally the gland then atrophies until the child's pubertal hormones stimulate it once more. Sebaceous gland activity in children can result from congenital adrenal hyperplasia or anabolic hormone therapy as given in aplastic anemia. Disorders of androgen excess in adult women are associated with increased sebaceous gland activity. Androgen insufficiency in either sex such as primary or secondary hypogonadism or adrenal insufficiency is associated with decreased activity. Androgens increase the sebaceous gland size, increase the secretion of sebum, and increase sebaceous gland mitotic rate. Estrogens decrease the gland in size and secretion but do not decrease the mitotic rate. Their effect may be from the suppression of androgens primarily at sites of androgen synthesis rather than at the glandular level. It is noteworthy that in women, adrenal androgens in addition to gonadal androgens are a source of sebaceous stimulation. Progesterone in physiologic amounts has no effect, and the role of the pituitary is most likely indirect through tropic hormones. With severe caloric deprivation sebum secretion levels decrease.

The function of sebaceous gland lipid is in question. Although variously touted as a barrier to microbes or other hostile environment, as a regulator of percutaneous absorption, and as a vitamin D precursor, all these roles have been challenged. Further, skin conditions characterized by dry skin, such as ichthyosis or asteatosis, are allegedly associated with decreased sebum production, but without supporting data.

What is known is that sebaceous gland maturation, which begins at age eight to ten and continues through adolescence, remains fairly unchanged through adult life until it decreases after the climacteric, some time past the fifth decade in women and the seventh decade in men. Patients with Parkinson's disease and postmenopausal women with breast cancer have statistically higher rates of sebum secretion than the average. Because the distribution of sebum levels overlaps with normal values, an individual reading has limited diagnostic importance. Although the reason for the higher sebum levels is not known, it is not likely to be androgenic, since circulating androgens are not increased in such patients.

The final portion of the pilosebaceous apparatus to be considered is the hair, and any understanding of hair implies some knowledge of its *growth cycle* and *pattern.* *Hair growth* can be reckoned in three phases: *telogen* when it is resting in its cornified sac, *anagen* when it is actively growing, and *catagen* when it is involuting. Throughout telogen, the resting hair is high in the follicle at the level of the arrector pili muscle, a stubby hair bulb resembling a club, and is inactive mitotically. When anagen begins, there is a burst of mitosis and downward growth. The newly formed hair shaft dislodges the old resting hair bulb, the club hair. With a hand lens a fallen or plucked hair can be determined from root inspection as having been resting or actively

Figure 3.   Hidradenitis suppurativa, axilla.

growing. Catagen is the brief respite when mitosis ceases and the hair pulls upward in the dermis and hair shaft to become a club hair. In the adult most hairs, 85 per cent, are in anagen at any given time, 14 per cent in telogen, and 1 per cent in catagen.

Hair growth cycles vary with *hair type,* of which there are several in man. Vellus hair is fine, soft, short, nonpigmented, and common to "nonhairy" areas of the body. Its anagen phase is short and telogen long. A terminal hair is coarse, long, pigmented, and located in "hairy" areas — scalp, beard, eyebrow, eyelash, axilla, and pubes. The ratio of the duration of anagen to telogen in terminal hairs varies. It is short and equal for eyebrows, but for scalp hair anagen is long, two to six years, and telogen short, about three months. Hair length depends upon duration of active growth compared to that of resting.

Acute disease, high fever, and gross metabolic illness can all markedly affect the hair cycle. Classic postfebrile hair loss tends to be diffuse, with the loss first noted two to three months after the fever. The suggested mechanism is that the altered physiologic state stuns the actively growing follicles into a resting state. Following the ordinary physiologic pattern, the hair rests for three months, then is shed at the time new growth begins, a phenomenon called *telogen effluvium.* Excessive hair fall may continue over a month or more. Stress as from anesthesia, normal delivery, or psychic shock may do the same. Malabsorption or the serious malnutrition of kwashiorkor often has an associated severe hair loss. Debilitated chronically ill patients may lose hair, too, but more often they merely note change in texture. Depletion of dietary protein, anemia, and iron deficiency can be correlated with damaged hair shafts, suggesting insults insufficient to trigger the resting phase but enough to deform the hair. Complete disruption can follow more severe deprivation.

Interference with essential amino acid incorporation, as suggested for the effect of thallium ingestion, leads to a fracture of the hair shaft within the follicle. Once used for depilation in the therapy of scalp fungus, hair shedding occurs about one week after treatment. In an unsuspected (or intended) ingestion of rat poison containing thallium, hair loss should be anticipated, a so-called *anagen effluvium,* since the fall occurs during the active phase of the follicle cycle. Similar alopecias are seen with the antimitotic agents used in chemotherapy. The damage can be dose related, for if mitosis is merely impaired, not halted, the hair shaft may not be disrupted but merely narrowed, as with methotrexate therapy for psoriasis or colchicine for gout. Heparin and coumarin, although they, too, show some mitotic inhibition, have their full effect through shunting anagen follicles into telogen until occasionally as many as half the follicles are at rest. At two to three months after the initiation of anticoagulant therapy, hair will fall; the cosmetic significance of the alopecia will depend upon the original density of hair growth and the percentage of follicles in telogen.

In many instances hair loss may be anticipated or its cause immediately identified. Even with the sparse or absent scalp hair of congenital ectodermal defects, the diagnosis is apparent from the history, perhaps reinforced by pedigree, and the physician feels no compulsion to justify the defect. With alopecia areata, however, there is a difference. Of obscure etiology, it is a problem of increased incidence in patients with autoimmune disease, Addison's disease, diabetes mellitus, or vitiligo. It commonly presents as one or two small circumscribed bald areas, usually of the scalp, which may not progress but in some few patients will increase in size, coalesce, and extend until all scalp hair is lost (alopecia totalis) or all body hair (alopecia universalis). Most patients with alopecia areata will do well; four out of five will get full regrowth of hair. Initially the course is unpredictable but deserves guarded optimism. However, when the alopecia is extensive, recurs, is associated with nail dystrophy, or lasts more than a year, the prognosis for recovery is not good.

In the instances of hair loss cited thus far, the scalp, on inspection, would appear as normal skin devoid of some or all hair. There would be no scarring. When inflammatory and infiltrative diseases affect the scalp so as to produce hair loss, the basic lesion is grossly evident. The hair is lost because of the pathologic process disrupting and perhaps destroying the hair follicle. This is true even with traction alopecia when the pull of hair styles or the self-plucking of hairs, consciously or unconsciously as in trichotillomania, leads to the permanent damage of the hair follicles and occasionally their destruction.

As to *growth pattern,* the hair follicles common to both sexes that produce the same type of hair in pre- and postpubertal individuals are not hormone dependent. Others, common to both sexes, are androgen dependent, such as the conversion of vellus to terminal hair in the axillae, the lower pubic triangle, and the temporal area of the scalp. In males responding to higher concentration of androgens there is a conversion from vellus to terminal hair in the follicles of the beard, ears, nasal tip, sternum, and upper pubic triangle. At the same time on a genetic basis some terminal hair may change to vellus in the vertex and frontal regions of the scalp, with slow recession of the anterior hair line to produce male pattern baldness. Similar pattern loss occurs in women but rarely progresses to the total bare crown seen in men. In both, hereditary factors influence the time of onset, pattern, and severity, with androgen playing an undisputed role. Castration interrupts pattern baldness in males, and masculinizing diseases of women produce baldness subject to genetic predisposition.

Hypertrichosis and Hirsutism

Excessive hair growth may be genetically determined, as in a nevus, or from repeated local trauma, as with weights carried on the shoulders. It may be generalized and appear after encephalitis or with the onset of multiple sclerosis. It is seen in dermatomyositis and is induced by drugs such as diphenylhydantoin. Although the reason for the increased hair may be obscure, an association can be made with a genetic determinant or recognized problem.

Hirsutism, however, a term used mainly for the excessive growth of coarse terminal hair occurring in women in the adult male distribution, is more of a diagnostic challenge. In most, the hair growth is idiopathic without underlying pathology. Genetic and racial differences are considerable, and their recognition may help differentiate a familial problem from an underlying masculinizing process. If there is no menstrual abnormality, no male pattern balding, no increase in muscle mass or deepening of the voice, and a normal pelvic examination, the problem should probably not be pursued further. On the other hand, diffuse vellus hairs occuring suddenly over the face of women past 40 should arouse suspicion of underlying malignancy.

Aging and Actinic Damage

With age, the epidermis thins and the skin appendages atrophy. Hair becomes sparse and sebaceous secretions decrease, with consequent susceptibility to dryness, chapping, and fissuring. The dermis diminishes with loss of elastic and collagen fibers — hence loss of elasticity and support for dermal vessels easily visualized and readily ruptured (senile purpura).

Sunlight exposure wreaks far greater destruction on the skin than time itself, however, as the contrast between covered and exposed skin clearly shows, even in the skin of the elderly. It intensifies and augments the aging process. Sun-damaged skin is thin, wrinkled, and variably hyperpigmented with fine thread-like telangiectatic vessels and small erythematous scaling spots of actinic keratoses. Yellow papules in a reticulated pattern may occur on the nose and forehead. Comedones and follicular cysts appear in the periorbital region. The back of the neck becomes thickened in the rhomboidal pattern of sailor's skin. Histologically collagen is replaced by amorphous or granular material of slightly basophilic stain on hematoxylin and eosin preparation. Called elastotic, it gives its name to the clinical observation of thinning and sagging, senile elastosis.

570. THE EXAMINATION OF THE SKIN

The traditional approach to the medical patient is to elicit the chief complaint and elaborate the history before seeking supportive clinical findings. The dermatologist on the contrary looks first, with an eye trained to see and recognize, his hand lens being more important than his stethoscope. He has the advantages of concurrent review — the history of the present illness often being written for him in the skin — markers of genetic predisposition, and even something of the patient's physiologic age and exposure to the elements and to actinic radiation. It is all there: the ectoderm and the mesoderm; the blood vessels and the nerves; the collagen, the elastin, the ground substance. It is there and sharing, perhaps, in an inflammatory, metabolic, or even neoplastic change that is widespread in the body but comes to focus first in the skin. Dermatology is a visual specialty, and its excitement derives from the direct and patent entry into general medicine that the skin provides, and from the clarity with which pathologic processes can be assessed and followed. It is a showcase for reaction patterns and for responses to therapy.

For the examination of the skin, to see *what* is there and *all* that is there is the only cardinal rule. Good lighting is essential. Nonglaring north light is best for both lesion configuration and true color, but a mix of fluorescent bulbs to simulate daylight is acceptable. It can never be too bright, but the capability of side lighting in a darkened room is also useful for detecting minimally raised and depressed lesions.

The skin should be observed from head to toe in a routine repetitive way so that no orifice or appendage is overlooked. For the writer, the horizontal patient completely disrobed and covered with a sheet is easiest to examine in a systematic way. In the *supine* position the frontal scalp is examined first, then the face, with special attention to the eyes (conjunctiva, iris and pupil, eyelids), followed by the ears, nose, lips, mouth (observing mucosa and dentition), pharynx, neck, thorax, abdomen, genital area, anterior legs, and then the fingernails, forearms, and arms, anterior and posterior. With the patient changed to the *prone* position and the knees flexed, the feet, toenails, and webs can be examined easily, next the posterior aspect of the legs, the perianal and sacral area, the back, lower and upper, nuchal area, and then the full scalp to complete the round. By uncovering only limited areas of the body at a time the patient is mostly covered and comfortable throughout the examination. If the presenting complaint has been only a finger wart, the surprised patient is usually reassured that his integument has been assessed for present or potential pathology and good preventive medicine has been practiced.

After having surveyed the entire skin surface, *generalized observation* warrants first notation. A blue man with argyria, the result of silver deposits in sweat glands and elastic fibers, may present with a fungus infection. Although the pigmentation may be untreatable and permanent, it nonetheless is an important part of his dermatologic assessment. So, too, is the *pattern of a problem*. Skin change following a dermatome distribution is significant. At a distance a segmental color change over the thorax might suggest a diagnostic differential between herpes zoster and nevus, but on close inspection viral vesicles would resolve the diagnosis. The limitation of the specific viral lesions to a dermatome makes the presumptive diagnosis. It underscores the importance of the pattern of appearance — important for description and the diagnostic process, as well as for the record for others to interpret.

The examiner, then, must be aware of the whole skin and the pattern of the problem before focusing on specific lesions. He will have noted signs of aging, trauma, pigment response, general turgor, nutrition, and hygiene. He will attempt to assess the pathology he notes with reference to configuration and anatomic location. Distribution may follow innervation, as in the dermatome, or vascular patterns, as in the reticulated changes in mottled skin of chilled swimmers, cutis marmorata. The pathology may be localized or generalized, perhaps universal, involving the entire integument, including hair and nails. Most important, the examiner will try to assess what physical change has occurred in the skin. Is it flushed or blanched? If red, is it the hot bright red of infection or the cool blue red of a connective tissue disorder? He will attempt to make a microscopic judgment and decide whether the skin surface is normal or thickened, raised or flat, infiltrated with cells and at what level, filled with fluid, filled with pus, freely movable, bound down, atrophic, excoriated, or ulcerated.

Often the consultation request proffers dermatologic terms that bear no relation to the lesion described. It is far better to call an urticarial lesion a hive, or a lesion resembling a mosquito bite, than to define it as an erythematous papule, which is interpreted differently by the indoctrinated. Terms are useful in descriptive interchange, but if they defeat the honest analysis of the pathophysiologic process, their value is lost.

Despite this conviction, it is necessary to provide some

guide to the description of pathologic changes in skin. A defined lesion that leaves the epidermis and dermis unchanged except in color is a *macule*. Stroking the lesion and adjacent normal skin with eyes closed resolves any doubt; the macule cannot be distinguished. If the surface is raised in a circumscribed way by an infiltrate of cells or change in anatomic thickness, the lesion is a *papule* and should be further described as rounded or flat-topped, perhaps as angular, smooth, or verrucous (the roughness of a wart), and by color. If penetration of the process into the dermis gives greater substance and depth, the lesion is *nodular* rather than papular. Either may be a sac for entrapped cellular debris and secretions, a *cyst*, suspected by the palpation of a soft center.

For wheals or hives, edema in the upper dermis produces raised rounded or plateau-like evanescent lesions known as *urticaria*, which, according to size, may be ordinary or giant. Trapped fluid in the skin produces a *vesicle* if the blister is less than 0.5 cm, a *bulla* if larger. The anatomic level of the fluid and its cellular content will affect translucency and stability. Significant vesicles may be so numerous as to become confluent and indistinguishable as vesicles, presenting instead as a weeping denuded area. Superficial bullae also rupture easily and in the mouth are rarely seen intact. Ones that occur more deeply, such as friction blisters, can persist, and some may be so overlayered with skin that it is difficult to distinguish them from a papule. When the fluid-filled sac contains abundant neutrophils, with or without bacteria, it is considered a *pustule*. If it occurs anatomically related to a pilosebaceous apparatus, it is a follicular pustule, usually conical, and with a protruding hair.

When skin is abnormal and raised over a relatively large but circumscribed area, the term *plaque* is used. If the skin surface is denuded, it may just be a superficial *erosion*; if the defect penetrates into the dermis, it is an *ulcer*. Coagulated blood elements can provide a *crust* for such lesions. When the deeper ones heal, there will be scar, pink and vascularized at first, then *atrophic*, i.e., white and avascular. Healing could occur with an exuberant pink raised hypertrophic scar that subsequently flattens or perhaps persists as a fibrous, rubbery cicatrix, a *keloid*. Even without recognized injury the skin may become depressed, with the normal skin markings and appendages diminished or effaced. Such *atrophy* can be part of a pathologic process or may result from such topical therapy as steroids.

In contrast to atrophic change, the skin in certain conditions may be thickened with accentuation of the normal epidermal pattern, as is caused by rubbing, *lichenification*; or the thickness may be from *scale*, flaking keratin, that may be loose or adherent, thick as an oyster shell (ostracious), or fine as cigarette paper; scale may be dry or greasy and slough in a localized desquamation or generalized exfoliation.

Finally, the descriptive process will reflect pigment, its presence or absence, and the vascular changes that affect skin color, not only physiologically because of blood flow, but because of anatomic considerations. Lips, red or blue, are transparent to blood color because of a thin to absent stratum corneum. New vessel growth or suffusion can produce hemangiomas. Superficial wispy dilated vessels, *fine telangiectasia*, one of the stigmata of solar damage, may, without the hand lens, be mistaken for erythema; coarse telangiectasia would not, but should be identified for its association with acrosclerosis, for example, and roentgen damage where it is found with atrophy

and pigmentary change. The trick is to see what is present in the skin without prejudice and to tabulate the data without premature interpretation.

With the distribution of lesions noted and their pattern of arrangement determined, whether in a dermatome (zosteriform) or linear (/), annular (o), arciform ($\cap$), polycyclic (∞), or serpiginous ($\sim$), the individual lesion can be assessed according to the broad description given. The eye may detect different kinds of lesions which in fact may be the same at different stages of development, or a primary lesion that has been subjected to the trauma of scratching or secondary infection or perhaps to an adverse reaction to therapy. The search for the representative lesion should yield the most typical and the most recent.

SUPPORTING TESTS

TZANCK SMEAR. If the primary lesion is a vesicle or bulla, a rapid cytologic examination known as the Tzanck test can be helpful. The vesicle or bulla is unroofed with a sterile scissors and the base curetted lightly with the blunt side of a scalpel. A smear is made and stained with Wright's or Giemsa's stain to reveal the multinucleated epidermal giant cells of a viral infection or the rounded acantholytic cells devoid of their intercellular bridges, a phenomenon present in certain blistering diseases and in viral vesicles as well, but not in friction blisters or burns or in the vesicles of contact dermatitis.

THE KOH TEST AND CULTURE. Should the primary problem be a circumscribed scaling dermatitis of the sort that suggests a diagnosis of fungus, a very simple examination for the presence of mycelia should be done. Heating a sample of scale with 10 per cent potassium hydroxide to dissolve the keratin (and a drop of methylene blue to improve visualization), the fungal elements, if present, can be observed by direct microscopic examination. At the same time the scale should be cultured in Sabouraud's medium to establish the identity of the fungus involved. If repeated attempts to visualize hyphae and grow fungus are negative, the diagnosis of mycotic infection is certainly in question.

WOOD'S LIGHT. Examination under long wave ultraviolet light will be helpful in detecting hair and skin infected with fungi that fluoresce at 360 nm; it is important for diagnosis and for plucking infected hairs for culture.

The Wood filter, made of nickel oxide and silica fitted to a high pressure mercury lamp, is opaque to all light under 320 nm and above 400 nm. Inspection under Wood's light is also useful in differentiating between hypo- and depigmented areas of skin, an important diagnostic clue, and in detecting porphyrins in the urine of patients suspected of having porphyria.

BACTERIOLOGIC CULTURES. When the primary lesion is a pustule, bacteriologic cultures should be taken, especially if it is suspected that a micrococcus may be the etiologic agent. The nephritogenic strains of the *Streptococcus* are associated with glomerulonephritis, and certain strains of *Staphylococcus pyogenes* as well as the *streptococcus* can produce a severe infection with bright erythema and extensive desquamation.

BIOPSY. Of all that may be done to aid the assessment of the primary lesion, the very best is to re-examine it with the clinical eye, using magnification greater than the hand lens, and to see it in cross-section. The biopsy has no magic other than the wonderment of seeing precisely

Figure 4.   Punch biopsy of the skin.

what is going on at every level of the skin. For this to be pertinent, we must be looking at the right lesion, the representative one, and for best comparisons we should see it against the patient's normal skin for that area. A remarkably thickened keratin layer means nothing if the biopsy is from the palm unless it is seen against normal palm with less keratin.

For the most complete histopathologic assessment,

especially if for reasons of concern or cosmetics the lesion is to be removed, an elliptical excision is best. One procedure removes the lesion, secures tissue for diagnosis, and leaves a defect easily sutured. Of greater speed and ease, and of quite useful yield, is the punch biopsy, which at 2 mm is hardly more than a venipuncture but permits adequate tissue to be removed and examined. After anesthetizing the site with deep rather than superficial infiltra-

4

tion to avoid histologic distortion, a tubular blade bears through the skin by slight rotary motion, clockwise and back, to the depth of the subcutis. By light external pressure with a curved iris scissors astride the plug, the specimen lifts without the distorting pressure of forceps and can be easily clipped at its base through the loose subcutaneous tissue. The plug gently lifted to absorbent paper attaches upright, the fat adherent to the paper, the epidermis on top. Such orientation and some detailed instruction for fixing and sectioning is needed by even the most experienced technician who is unaccustomed to handling small specimens.

To enhance the value of the biopsy by contrast with normal tissue, the excision should, if possible, cut through normal and abnormal tissue, but here the laboratory will need a diagram (Fig. 4), and in addition a pre-biopsy directional scratch on the skin sample made with a scalpel to establish the direction for histopathologic sectioning. Rotating the sections 90 degrees could provide all lesion or, most distressing, all normal skin.

For the punch biopsy suturing is not necessary for hemostasis; a Gelfoam plug to fill the defect or Monsel's solution on an applicator stick will suffice, but the cosmetic result will not be as fine as with a suture. Anatomic location and convenience of suture removal will influence the choice.

571. PRINCIPLES OF THERAPY

Before considering more detailed diagnostic formulations, it is possible to look at therapy as it seeks to correct the pathologic situation observed. Specific metabolic changes and cell infiltrates, as with lymphomas, will require a particular treatment regimen for management, but, apart from these, there is a broad group of pathologic changes that can be reversed and symptoms alleviated by therapeutic maneuvers directed toward restoration to the normal state.

The skin that is undergoing an *inflammatory* response with coalescent allergic or viral vesicles, so that it quite figuratively "weeps," requires a reduction of heat and a drying of the serous ooze through evaporation and coagulation of serum proteins. Superimposed infection will require antimicrobial therapy; debridement may be indicated. All of this can be accomplished with the wet dressing.

WET DRESSINGS

OPEN WET DRESSINGS. The prototype is a piece of undyed finely woven cloth, cotton or linen, thoroughly wet with clear water, wrung out so as not to drip, and then applied to the skin. Considered solely for its physical effects, the water evaporates, cooling and drying the underlying skin. As the cloth dries and is removed to be reimmersed, it cleanses. To get maximal benefit from evaporation, the dressing should not be more than a layer or two thick and should be changed every 15 to 30 minutes, depending on the ambient temperature and humidity. If permitted to dry completely and become adherent, the debriding effect will be greater, perhaps damaging. Remoistening the dressing in place may be needed to facilitate removal.

The wet dressing described can be initiated anywhere, even on a camping trip. In ordinary practice, however, the effectiveness of the wet dressing can be enhanced by medications added to the water. A mild protein precipitant, aluminum acetate, serves to coagulate bacterial and serum protein. As a 5 per cent preparation it is known as Burow's solution, and it must be further diluted for use. Appropriate concentrations, indications, and modes of prescribing various medications are shown for convenience in Table 2. If infection is a complication, potassium permanganate or silver nitrate should be in the wet dressing, but with precautions; potassium permanganate is a poison and must be kept from children's reach. Both preparations stain the skin and everything else they touch. Patient compliance will be improved by forewarnings. To use rubber gloves to protect nails from becoming brown, for example, and to use disposable containers for mixing solutions and plastic liners for sinks and tubs if porcelain is old or porous will reduce the burden of therapy. One further caution concerns the maneuver of removing the wet dressing to reimmerse the cloth rather than basting on new solution. Although important to enhance the cleansing effect, it is absolutely essential with potassium permanganate and silver nitrate, in which evaporation can permit the solute to increase in the dressing to concentrations sufficient to cause irritation or chemical burn.

The question is often raised about the use of antimicrobial agents in wet dressings. Apart from the risk of sensitization which limits the topical use of penicillin and neomycin, the quantities needed for adequate concentration in the dressing would make their use exceedingly inefficient and wasteful. The same might be said for enzymic preparations for debridement. Although the physical effects of the wet dressing would be helpful to reduce erythema and free tissue, the manipulations of the wet dressings would deactivate the enzymes prematurely. When required, they are best used separately as creams or gels.

Wet dressings, if needed at all, are needed three to four hours a day divided according to the patient's schedule. Although best split into four to five treatments of equal duration, two or three ten-minute dressings with the

TABLE 2. Use of Wet Dressings

Condition	Ingredient	Effect	Prescribed	Prepared Preparation H₂O	Approximate Final Concentration
Eczematous	A1Ac (Burow's Solution)	Protein coagulation	Tablets or powder packets	1 tab/packet 500 ml / 1 tab/packet 1000 ml	1:20 / 1:40
Mild infection	AgNO₃	Antimicrobial (especially gram-negative)	10% stock solution / 25% stock solution	10 ml 1000 ml / 5 ml 1000 ml	1:1000 / 1:800
Infection	KMnO₄	Antimicrobial	Tab 300 mg	1 tab 1500 ml / 1 tab 3000 ml	1:5000 / 1:10,000

balance in the evening or whenever the patient is free are preferable to one solid four-hour bloc in the evening. Use of long narrow wrappers the length of a forearm or whole leg, just wide enough to circumvent it once, pinned top, bottom, and in between, obviates winding as with an Ace bandage, and hence is fast. Knowing that the dressing can be secured and ordinary work continued gives the patient a sense of release from an imprisoning routine. Dermatologic treatments can be time consuming and a nuisance; patients would much rather swallow a pill. The physican's attention to convenience and realistic scheduling may mean the difference between treatment and no treatment.

BATHS AND SOAKS. Should the need for wet dressings be extensive — head to toe or even half that — it requires little imagination to sense the chilling experience of lying naked under a wet sheet. It matters little that the initial temperature of the wet dressing was warm. Actually the solution need be of no set temperature. It should neither chill nor scald and is best at a temperature that the patient finds comfortable. However, evaporation from a wet dressing over an extensive surface of inflamed skin will soon cause chill. The useful alternative is to immerse the total body in water of selected temperature which permits regulated cooling; if starch powders are added to the bath, there will be an after-film and a drying effect. With infections potassium permanganate can be added to the tub. To protect against undissolved crystals burning the skin, tablets crushed with a hammer in fibrous paper should be dissolved in a small container and the solution decanted into the bath. When infection or necrotic debris is a problem in a limited area, such as the draining sinus tracts of a diabetic toe, foot immersion in appropriate medication serves as a limited therapeutic bath. Because there is the mechanical need to force the solution to the depths of the tract, such irrigation is difficult to achieve except with immersion. The same can be said for the treatment of pilonidal cysts and for many anogenital problems.

CLOSED WET DRESSINGS. The need for the open wet dressing or immersion soak will diminish as inflammation subsides, lesions dry, and draining infection is controlled. Further, not all lesions are benefited by cooling and drying. A patient with much retained keratin of the palms or soles or even generalized scaling may need maceration rather than drying. Another with an early abscess may need heat to focalize the infection. For these problems the *open* wet dressing can be covered with an impervious material to induce maceration and heat retention and to enhance penetration of a specific medication; it thereby becomes known as a *closed* wet dressing, prescribed because of need for its physical effects. Compared to the open dressing, its use is infrequent. However, it can be inadvertently created when a fastidious nurse or patient covers the open wet dressing with plastic to protect the bedclothing or furniture. The routine instructions for open wet dressings should include a warning about covering with plastic. Although it is unlikely that any significant harm has come from the extended or untimely use of open wet dressings, the inadvertent or injudicious use of occlusion can lead to a phenomenon in which a pruritic papular eruption occurs at the site of active dermatitis and then distally in body folds, and may even progress to become generalized. Unfortunately termed "autosensitization," the phenomenon is nonetheless very real.

TOPICAL THERAPY

In the general approach to therapy, wet dressings are but the beginning. Topical medications are the mainstay. Their array can be bewildering if some basic principles of selection are overlooked. They must be sorted out by active ingredients, but equal importance must be given to the vehicle that contains the active preparation.

BASES. Topicals vary in their base from lotions, through creams, to ointments. Beginning at one side of the spectrum with the simplest shake lotion, talc in water, there is a progression of relative concentrations of oil and water bases in the first of which water is the continuous phase with dispersed oil droplets. These are the water-washable bases, easy to apply and easy to wash away. They are nongreasy and vanish into the skin. As the oil-water ratio reverses and oil becomes the continuous phase with water dispersed, the preparation is more lubricating, leaves a film on the skin, and is cosmetically less elegant. At the far end of this spectrum is 100 per cent inert oil such as mineral oil or petrolatum.

Confusion about bases derives from mislabeling as lotions preparations that are other than powder and water, and from forgetting that the fluid state has little to do with the composition of the base. Water in oil and oil in water bases may pour or not. The same is true with inert oil. Mineral oil pours; petrolatum does not. A cream may be either an oil in water (water-washable) or water in oil; an ointment may be water in oil or inert oil. Both cream and ointment must be further defined if a prescription is to be compounded. Writing for the right medication in an unspecified inert oil base may result in having a preparation in mineral oil streaming down the patient's face.

BASE SELECTION. The selection of the base depends on the need for its physical properties. A powder in water such as the classic calamine lotion permits evaporation and cooling with some drying from the powder, suggestive surely of an open wet dressing. Petrolatum by contrast conserves heat, promotes maceration, and recalls completely the closed wet dressing. The inert oil has one additional role that may be overlooked, that of protection. One would not swim the English Channel without a covering of grease.

In between these two extremes there is a spectrum of possibilities permitting some cooling but adding lubrication. Choice will weigh need and cosmetic acceptance. When a medication is to be applied to the face or scalp, a greasy base would be unsightly and underutilized. If it is an antimicrobial, for example, known to penetrate better in an ointment base, the physician will nonetheless opt for a vanishing cream, recognizing the value of compliance and preferring therapy with less penetration over no therapy at all.

Having made a judgment about the base required, a separate selection is made for the active ingredients. Some compromises may be required. Steroids, for example, may be needed and a lotion base indicated, but because lotions are easily spilled and too lavishly applied, the same steroid in a nonpouring water-washable base may prove as effective and more economical. Similarly, when lubrication is needed, the ointment base of a steroid may serve just as well without the steroid and at a fraction of the cost. In such a situation a steroid cream used sparingly and rubbed well into the skin can be overlayered with a lubricating ointment for better utilization of both.

TOPICAL STEROIDS. Although specific medications will be included under consideration of the specific diseases, some of broad use across the specialty are more conveniently considered together — for example, the steroids. It is difficult to imagine dermatology without them. As topical therapy their local anti-inflammatory action is a major stroke toward restoration of the skin to normal. By vasoconstriction they halt the edema and cellular infiltrates that contribute to pruritus and local discomfort. By breaking the itch-scratch cycle with its consequent tissue damage, they permit healing. By modifying the full effect of the antigen-antibody complexes in delayed hypersensitivity reactions, they abort the intensity of the inflammatory response and permit the situation to defuse over time with the erosion of the antigen. Here, they are curative in the sense that they erase the effects of the reaction until the reaction no longer occurs. When steroids alleviate the symptoms of a specific infection, as with some yeasts and fungi, they are not curative and infection will persist unless overcome by the host's defenses. The same is true with certain opportunistic organisms that overtake an area of active dermatitis. The response of the dermatitis to steroids with consequent restoration of the skin may discourage the invader. With more aggressive organisms and in the immunocompromised patient eradication will depend on specific antimicrobial therapy.

Hydrocortisone is the "Model A" of topical steroids. In a 1 per cent concentration it is still a useful preparation and continues to serve as a norm for comparing potency of the subsequently synthesized fluorinated corticosteroids, powerful anti-inflammatory agents at concentrations as low as 0.01 per cent. Less potent than the fluorinated steroids, prednisolone and methylprednisone are also less frequently used; concentration for concentration, they are more effective than hydrocortisone.

The adverse effects reported with steroids relate almost exclusively to the fluorinated compounds, no doubt because of their high potency and because of their frequent use under occlusion (an impervious dressing analogous to the closed wet dressing which enhances absorption). Epidermal and dermal atrophy can be a pronounced adverse effect; decreased collagen synthesis and reduced stromal support for blood vessels lead to telangiectasia, purpura, and striae. A perioral dermatitis has also been reported with the fluorinated steroids, as well as aggravation of facial erythema, restricting absolutely the extended use of these compounds for the face. Further, the provoking of elevated intraocular pressure warrants a strong proscription against the prolonged application of any topical steroids near the eyes.

The reality of systemic absorption of topical steroids presents an additional hazard. Lowering of the plasma cortisol level is seen with as little as 20 per cent of the body under occlusion. The risk of rebound after discontinuing steroids in those skin diseases characterized by the phenomenon cannot be overlooked. Despite all side effects, steroids, systemically and topically, are supremely useful therapy, saving life and the quality of life.

$$\begin{array}{c} \text{C} \qquad\qquad \text{R}' \\ \text{or} \qquad\qquad \diagup \\ \text{R}-\text{N}-\text{CH}_2\,\text{CH}_2\text{N} \\ \text{or} \qquad\qquad \diagdown \\ \text{O} \qquad\qquad \text{R}'' \end{array}$$

Figure 5. The three antihistamine linkages.

With the hesitation and full medical precautions accorded any initiation of steroid therapy, plus the close monitoring on treatment, systemic steroids are used for three major groups of dermatologic patients. First are the severely ill with a life-threatening disease known to be responsive to corticosteroids. Initial doses will be high, 80 to 100 mg of daily prednisone or equivalent; if response is poor, the dose may be doubled. In the second group are those with an acute but severe self-limiting problem which the steroids will control or suppress during a predicted activity. Intermediate doses of 40 to 60 mg of prednisone will be initiated, and a planned but *supervised* taper would be extended over one to two weeks. Last are the patients with chronic problems who because of exacerbation or other stresses need a respite. For them the doses will be low, no more than 15 to 20 mg of prednisone, with a concurrent focus on increased supportive topical therapy so that the systemic treatment can be phased out.

ANTIHISTAMINES. Before leaving the general considerations of dermatologic therapy, antihistamines deserve mention. Used often for their soporific and tranquilizing effect, they are still helpful in blocking one or more of the effects of histamine. No one antihistamine blocks all the effects. They are biochemically arranged in three major groups according to the linkage of their side arm through a C or N or O (Fig. 5). The selection of an effective agent for a given patient may be from any one group (Table 3) or from a combination of groups, but is unlikely to be enhanced by combining antihistamines within the group. If response to one antihistamine is minimal or poor, another from another group should be added or substituted.

572. THE DIFFERENTIAL DIAGNOSIS

With the primary lesion assessed, a representative site biopsied, and perhaps general therapy initiated to reduce discomfort, the dermatologic diagnosis, if not immediately obvious, can be elaborated. There are broad classifi-

TABLE 3. Selected Antihistamines Grouped by Molecular Linkage

Carbon	Nitrogen	Oxygen
Chlorpheniramine (DL mixture) (Chlor-Trimeton)	Tripelennamine (Pyribenzamine)	Diphenhydramine (Benadryl)
Chlorpheniramine (D form) (Polaramine)	Pyrilamine (Neo-Antergan)	Bromodiphenhydramine (Ambodryl)
Parabromdylamine (Dimetane)	Promethazine (Phenergan)	Dimenhydrinate (Dramamine)
Pyrrobutamine (Pyronil)		
Meclizine (Bonamine)		

cations and wide-ranging considerations which help frame a diagnostic grid so that a reasonable differential can be narrowed. The skin has only a finite number of ways to respond, and many diagnoses have predilections for selected anatomic areas, suggesting their identity by their location. Further, the bulk of dermatologic problems is distributed among no more than a dozen diagnoses, so the framework need not be too cumbersome.

In the examination of the skin, noting the pattern of lesions has been stressed, but the value of the pattern has not been exploited. With a look to commonly encountered problems by anatomic region it is possible to check the supporting evidence that might be expected in a given diagnosis.

572.1.   THE HEAD AND NECK

SEBORRHEIC DERMATITIS

In the scalp if there is scale and erythema but no evidence of atrophy or hair follicle disruption, the most likely diagnosis is that of seborrheic dermatitis. There may be pattern baldness and the complaint of hair thinning, but the observed pathology is a greasy scale, covering a yellow-red marginated base. The problem is common; it is shared by 12 million Americans, of whom 5.5 million have it severely enough to warrant medical consultation. Although usually a problem limited to the scalp or perhaps by extension to the retroauricular fold, it can in some patients involve the eyebrows and skin between, the eyelids in blepharitis, or the pinna in otitis externa, as well as the alae nasi, axillae, anterior thorax, periumbilical area, and genital area with focus in the crural and intergluteal folds. Obese patients with a predisposition to seborrheic dermatitis can have severe erythema and maceration in all intertriginous areas. An occasional individual can progress to a generalized exfoliative dermatitis.

The differential diagnosis in the adult is fairly limited. If scalp scaling is severe, laminated, and adherent, psoriasis must be considered. In fact, seborrheic dermatitis of such severity may be a forme fruste of psoriasis. Axillary and genital erythema raise the question of infection of the body folds with *Candida albicans* or *Corynebacterium*, but the presence of scalp lesions and the inability to demonstrate causative organisms support the diagnosis of seborrheic dermatitis. Even with positive routine cultures as for *Candida*, characteristic scalp lesions and other stigmata of seborrheic dermatitis (periumbilical erythema and scale) may suggest the diagnosis. It should be noted further that the high prevalence of seborrheic diathesis may extend features of seborrheic dermatitis to an associated eruption. Lupus erythematosus has been observed in a seborrheic distribution with a greasiness to the lupus scale. Present, too, however, were atrophy, telangiectasia, and follicular plugging, classic for lupus erythematosus but not part of seborrheic dermatitis. In Parkinson's disease in which sebaceous glands are enlarged and sebum production is increased, seborrheic dermatitis is frequently a problem. Although treatment with L-dopa lowers sebum production, there is not always correlation of the degree of sebum suppression and neurologic improvement. Seborrheic dermatitis has been noted unilaterally in association with neurologic lesions, and

with sympathetic nerve regeneration it has disappeared.

The tendency to develop seborrheic dermatitis in those genetically predisposed cannot be altered, but its manifestations can be suppressed, often by a simple acceptable routine. To reduce risk of progression and to delay hair fall, active treatment ought to be encouraged. Therapy should control inflammation and scaling, thereby reducing pruritus and oiliness. Medicated shampoos containing antimicrobial agents and salicylic acid may be all that is needed. Frequent shampooing is important, daily at first, although it need not always be with the medicated preparation. Topical steroid in lotion bases applied to the scalp two or three times daily will reduce erythema. If scale is marked, however, no medication will penetrate; warm oil soaks under plastic occlusion with or without salicylic acid will loosen the scale.

Once control has been achieved and the scalp appears normal, therapy may be reduced gradually until a minimal maintenance is determined: topical steroids every other day or less often; medicated shampoos alternating with regular shampoos in a determined repetitive pattern. As a rule, maintenance requirements will increase in winter.

For seborrheic dermatitis of areas other than the scalp, a similar routine is effective. The maceration of scale in body folds obviates the need for oil occlusion. In fact, warmth and erythema may suggest wet dressings as an initial therapy. These, combined with topical steroid, will usually control the problem, but ultraviolet light, cautiously administered, often hastens resolution.

Recognizing the anatomic distribution of seborrheic dermatitis, it is also important to recognize associated conditions. Severe *acne vulgaris*, for example, is always found with some seborrheic dermatitis and so is *acne rosacea*.

ACNE

Diagnostically, acne will not be a problem. Its stigmata have become a hallmark of adolescence, and the advertising media have brought into sharp focus the characteristic erythematous papules and pustules of the pilosebaceous apparatus, the comedones open and closed (blackheads and whiteheads). When acne appears suddenly and for the first time in the 30-year-old or menopausal woman, everyone is surprised, the diagnosis is doubted, and there is uneasiness about underlying pathology. Unless there are other clinical indications of virilization or endocrine dysfunction, the diagnosis of acne should merely be a challenge to active and adequate therapy, not to hormonal evaluation.

This is not to take acne lightly as a diagnosis. So prevalent in the second decade as to be considered almost a normal physiologic phenomenon, acne vulgaris defaces youth at a most vulnerable and insecure time. Further, it can persist throughout life and be severe and disfiguring, as in the conglobate form, causing marked morbidity and debility. Even severe cases that resolve can leave such destructive scarring that the psychologic burden never lifts.

There is other acne that is aggravated or perhaps frankly caused by oil, such as mechanics experience in their work, and by medications such as halogens and systemic steroids. Industrial exposure to the chlorinated hydrocarbons will almost invariably produce acne in exposed workers (chloracne). For these, improving the environment, removing the oil, discontinuing the bromides or iodides, or reducing the steroid dosage will be therapeutically advantageous. However, in most instances treating acne successfully relies on patient compliance derived mostly from an understanding of the pathophysiologic process. The patient should know that the aim of therapy is to foster the free drainage of the pilosebaceous unit, to avoid rupture, and to limit bacterial growth. The hydrolysis of the triglycerides of sebum by cutaneous bacteria yields fatty acids which have an inflammatory effect on the follicle, and which then, with its disruption, pass into the surrounding tissue as a primary irritant. The abnormality in acne is at the follicular dyskeratosis that plugs the duct. Comedones, open and closed, must be dislodged, and surface bacteria, especially *Corynebacterium acnes,* suppressed.

The patient should be instructed in the need for simple cleansing every four to six hours to stun bacteria and discourage their logarithmic growth. Washing with soap will do, or a mild alcohol preparation carried or kept in a locker may be used. A topical antimicrobial preparation should be applied twice daily, benzoyl peroxide 5 or 10 per cent, for example, or the antimicrobial clindamycin, tetracycline, or erythromycin 1 or 2 per cent in an alcohol base. Plugged follicles will respond to topical retinoic acid, presumably through the labilization of lysosomes in the keratinizing cells of the follicles. A brisk erythematous response is often induced that may necessitate a reduction in the concentration or frequency of application of the vitamin A acid. Further, the concern for enhanced damage from solar radiation, or the possibility of a co-carcinogenic effect as suggested by experiments in hairless albino mice, contraindicates its use in summer or in light-complexioned individuals. For these as for all patients with acne, the mechanical removal of comedones and the incision and drainage of pustules and cysts foster resolution.

Systemic broad-spectrum antimicrobials in low to moderate doses given over long periods have proved a useful management for more severe acne, and, contrary to the expectations of some, have not been complicated by microbial resistance or superinfections. The tetracyclines, although commonly used, carry risk of dental discoloration and photosensitivity. They should not be prescribed from the fourth fetal month through age 12; hence all patients of the childbearing age should be cautioned if prolonged therapy is anticipated. Photosensitivity, impossible to predict, must be considered in the event of untoward reaction. More severe acne may require more extensive surgical procedures, higher doses of antimicrobials, intralesional steroid, or even systemic steroid. Estrogens have been used in selected women with stubborn severe acne with good results, but used as cyclic estrogen progestin therapy they have all the attendant risk of anovulatory preparations given for contraception. X-ray has no part in the management of acne. The question of diet is invariably raised, but there is no evidence to support a role for diet as either cause or aggravation.

ACNE ROSACEA

Characteristically appearing in the central one third of the face, acne rosacea occurs more commonly in women of 30 to 50 years, but more severely in men; it can be seen in

Figure 6. Rhinophyma.

both sexes at any age. Comedones are lacking, and the acne pustules are associated with telangiectasia and persistent flush; spices, alcohol, hot drinks, and temperature extremes that foster flushing aggravate the condition. Rhinophyma (Fig. 6) is associated with longstanding rosacea, but ocular involvement (blepharitis, conjunctivitis, episcleritis, and keratitis) can be by far the more serious complication. Therapy as outlined for acne vulgaris can be helpful for the pustular component of rosacea, but the flush and telangiectasia remain. Foods and situations that provoke flushing should be avoided. For both acne vulgaris and acne rosacea, control of the seborrheic dermatitis is important for management.

572.2.   THE THORAX

In the course of the regional examination, note is constantly made of the isolated pigmentary lesions (see Ch. 573) and the stigmata of aging and actinic exposure (see Ch. 569). The present larger focus is the pattern of appearance of eruptions.

DRUG ERUPTION

Symmetrical, scaling, erythematous macules or papules on the thorax, if of sudden onset, would suggest a drug eruption (Fig. 7). Itching need not be present but would support the impression.

PITYRIASIS ROSEA

Should the lesions be oval with a collarette of fine scale and follow skin cleavage lines (Fig. 8), the diagnosis of pityriasis rosea is likely. In this self-limited eruption, which is not uncommon and is often seen in young adults,

Figure 7. Drug eruption.

there is occasionally recognition of a larger antecedent lesion, the herald patch. Usually on the trunk it can be several centimeters in size, erythematous, and scaling. It is often mistaken for fungus; the negative KOH test result would correct that error. When the generalized eruption appears, the immediate reflex of the knowing examiner is to look again at the pharynx and palms lest luetic lesions be overlooked. Secondary syphilis is always in the differential diagnosis, and a serological test should be obtained; but without systemic symptoms, coryza, or palmar and plantar lesions, syphilis is an unlikely cause of the eruption.

LICHEN PLANUS

Lichen planus must be included in the differential diagnosis of scattered scaling lesions of the thorax, especially if there are lesions on the flexor aspect of the wrists, lower legs, or genitalia. Most often the typical polygonal flat-topped papule with a lilac hue and, on close inspection, the delicate whitish lines of Wickham's striae can be found. The classic lesion is diagnostic, and the histology supports the diagnosis. Mouth lesions are seen in half the patients, a lacy white network involving the buccal mucosa and lips. Ulcerative, erosive, hypertrophic, and atrophic variants have been described, and lichen planus–like eruptions have been induced by certain drugs, heavy metals, and color photo developers. The drugs include streptomycin, methyldopa, gold, phenothiazine, and the antimalarials chloroquine and quinacrine.

The etiology remains obscure, but the known association with drugs and chemicals and the observation of deficiency of glucose-6-phosphate dehydrogenase in lichen planus skin support a hypothesis that certain susceptible enzyme-deficient individuals respond to various chemicals and other environmental factors with lichen planus–like lesions. Eruptions resembling lichen planus

have also been observed with polymyositis and lymphoma.

PSORIASIS

Psoriasis, too, although classically presenting with plaques over the elbows and knees, can appear suddenly over the thorax as small, scattered papulosquamous lesions described as guttate. If these are the first manifestation of the disease, the finding of supporting stigmata may be essential. Characteristic silvery micaceous scale would be a helpful clue, and so, too, would be severe scaling of the scalp. Pitting of the fingernails with lifting and flaring is supportive, and a change suggestive of an oil droplet underneath the nail is pathognomonic. Historical or current evidence of scaling plaques of the elbows or knees, erythema or fissuring of the intergluteal fold, and associated arthritis of the distal interphalangeal joints all leave the diagnosis hard to challenge. In severe cases much of the skin may be involved (Fig. 9).

In the United States more than one million people have psoriasis, and of these more than 11 per cent have experienced disability of such severity as to compromise employment and effectiveness. The disease can begin at any age and has its peak appearance in the third decade. Its severity, course, and remissions are unpredictable. It is inherited in a pattern still unclear. There are studies relating two HL-A antigens and psoriasis. One, W17, is a useful genetic marker for that group of psoriatic patients with a high rate of affected relatives and a mean age of onset under 20 years (18.2 years). Those with HL-A$_{13}$ have little heritable tendency and milder disease.

Patients whose psoriasis requires therapy, or patients who demand it, are usually referred to a dermatologist, for, in general, physicians do not appreciate the discomfort and disfigurement of the disease and the potential for severity, arthritis, generalized exfoliation, or even death. Lesions are often dismissed as untreatable, or sometimes are subjected to an overkill with systemic therapy and attendant significant side effects. Systemic corticosteroids, for example, can induce prompt resolution of psoriatic lesions, but suppression requires ever-increasing doses. When therapy is tapered, there is a

Figure 8. Pityriasis rosea.

Figure 9. Psoriasis.

therapy in a significant percentage. Treatment requires traveling to a center and risk of burn or eye damage from normal sunlight before and after therapy until the psoralen is metabolized. The importance of long-term assessment is recognized because of the laboratory inducement of skin malignancies and cataracts in albino mice on high dose psoralens and intense exposure to UVA.

The effect of the topical modalities utilizing ultraviolet light is believed to be through mitotic arrest and the consequent return toward normal of the psoriatic cell turnover time, which is at an accelerated three to four days rather than the normal 27 to 28 days. Surely the antimetabolites have this effect on mitosis and thereby induce involution of psoriatic lesions. Arsenic used as Fowler's solution was an early cellular poison for psoriasis, and its previous use in a given patient is an important historical fact to alert the examiner to search for sequelae of arsenic ingestion. Aminopterin, amethopterin or methotrexate, and azaribine have also been used for therapy, methotrexate being the most widely used and the only one still accepted. Its prescription in psoriasis is limited to grave situations and to rigid guidelines set by the Psoriasis Task Force, National Program for Dermatology.

Because patient care is so often fragmented among specialists and because not all patients appreciate the gravity of therapy, it is important for any physician to inquire about every treatment regimen prescribed for his patient. The psoriasis in a patient with clear skin on methotrexate may escape detection. In the same way the dermatologist should know if the patient whose skin cancer he is about to curette and electrodesiccate is on anticoagulation and has a pacemaker.

Isolated psoriatic lesions, especially if circinate, and psoriasis limited to the seborrheic areas such as axillae or groin may suggest the differential diagnosis of fungus infection. For that matter, so would the "herald patch" of pityriasis rosea. If there is any question, scrapings should be taken for KOH examination and culture. Not uncommonly, ubiquitous organisms are opportunistic. Patients *can* have two diagnoses, but the KOH test result and cultures sooner or later must support the clinical impression of fungus.

rebound phenomenon, with extension of lesions possibly to exfoliation. If systemic steroids are used for other valid reasons in patients with psoriasis, the risk of aggravated psoriasis should be recognized and weighed in the decision for initiating therapy.

Psoriasis is without cure but is responsive to treatments which can induce remission of many months to years and maintenance therapy that can help sustain the remission. Corticosteroids applied topically under occlusion or given intralesionally promote blanching and flattening of lesions. If the impetus to remit is enhanced by the use of tar and ultraviolet light through the Goeckerman regimen, the chance of steroid rebound will lessen and a true remission may be realized. Black coal tars are applied directly to the skin in sufficient amounts to penetrate, and then are wiped clean so as not to filter out the light to which they have sensitized the skin. Increasing exposures to ultraviolet light are given on a set schedule — as often as twice daily for inpatients, perhaps once or twice weekly for outpatients. The duration of exposure is pushed to tolerance of erythema but not burn, lest the Koebner phenomenon, the isomorphic response by which tissue injury induces new lesions, activate a psoriatic flare. Within three to four weeks the most extensive psoriasis is usually resolved. Continuing the use of light and tar, alone or together if possible, at reduced intervals helps preserve the favorable response. Variations of the Goeckerman method have included the use of anthralin paste with dressings after the baths and light.

Long wave ultraviolet light (UVA) has also been used from a high intensity source through photosensitization with oral psoralens which potentiate the effect of the light. Experience with PUVA (psoralens plus UVA) suggests good resolution of the psoriatic lesions in most patients with 20 treatments, but with a need for maintenance

FUNGUS INFECTIONS

Scaling lesions of the thorax, with macular patches of all sizes and shapes, varying in color from white to tan to brown, represent *tinea versicolor* (Fig. 10). Extending sometimes to the neck, face, and arms, it is asymptomatic and is usually just a cosmetic bother. Wood's light examination aids visualization because of skin pigment change and because of the brick-red fluorescence of the causative organism, *Malassezia furfur (Pityrosporon orbiculare)*, which is not readily cultured. Scraping of the lesion removes scale and leaves normal skin beneath. Direct microscopic examination of the scale shows short hyphal filaments and grape-like clusters of budding forms. The therapy prescribed is usually the common fungicides. Any preparation with sodium thiosulfate, haloprogin, or tolnaftate, for example, is useful, as is clotrimazole or miconazole. The problem tends to recur, but can be prevented by daily scrubs with a keratolytic antimicrobial soap. No systemic therapy is indicated.

In general, if scaling lesions show hyphal elements and the appropriate cultures are positive but if another diagnosis is still suspected, the basic problem may not be

Figure 10.   Tinea versicolor.

fungus. A course of antifungal therapy should resolve the question; if it is a secondary invader, it will disappear, leaving the underlying pathology.

Traditionally, fungus is considered anatomically, from head to foot. Tinea capitis, so common to children, is hardly ever seen in adults except for a rare *Trichophyton tonsurans* infection. Occasionally parents of children with infected scalps can have glabrous or smooth, nonhairy skin involvement, having come in contact with the child's infection, but such anthropophilic fungi provoke little in tissue reaction. Animal fungi by contrast can stimulate a brisk reaction. From the broken hair "black dot" infection of *T. tonsurans* the spectrum extends through the red scaling dermatophytosis of groin and foot characteristic of *Trichophyton* and *Epidermophyton* infections to the boggy, bumpy tumefaction, raised, red, and tender, of a *Microsporum* infection such as *M. gypseum, M. canis,* or even *M. audouini.* These kerions resemble bacterial abscesses and initially can be misdiagnosed and mistreated. The importance of the direct and immediate examination for fungus by the KOH preparation cannot be overemphasized.

Scaling lesions of the trunk or body folds, if KOH-positive for hyphal elements, are tinea until proved otherwise. In areas where fungus has been associated with the continued maceration of wet clothing, as from occupation or wet swim trunks, plaques and nodules may develop; the history of maceration is important. Therapy which can be specific topically and systemically is less effective when good local care is neglected. Tub baths for adequate cleansing, removal of wet garments promptly, and use of drying powders can all be helpful.

Scaling lesions of the hands and feet offer a wider differential, since contact and chronic irritant dermatitis

are so common. The differential diagnosis will be considered below. Persistent inflammation of nail beds and the presence of psoriatic lesions in the nail plate can deform nails without fungal infection. However, the opportunities for fungi to infect macerated keratin further the confusion. Scrapings for fungal study should be taken from glabrous skin and nails as well as finger and toe webs. Too often oral griseofulvin is prescribed for scaling lesions without benefit of confirmatory KOH examination and culture. Rarely it may be considered for a therapeutic trial despite negative test results but never without them. It is useful against most dermatophytes but inactive against deep fungi and *Candida* species. It works best for fungal infection of the scalp, trunk, or groin.

When griseofulvin is given as 1 gram per day after a fatty meal to enhance absorption, pruritus, if a symptom, should disappear in 24 to 48 hours. Glabrous skin involvement should clear in 7 to 14 days. Dystrophic, infected nails, however, will require continuing therapy for as long as the pregriseofulvin keratin is retained, i.e., as long as it takes for replacement — three to four months for fingernails, six months or longer for toenails. Interrupting therapy will permit reinfection from retained infected keratin. Even throughout constant therapy and thereafter, a topical antifungal agent should be used.

The lengthy duration of required treatment should give the physician pause about committing a patient to a half year or more of a medication that can have unpleasant neurologic, hematologic, and gastrointestinal side effects. Further, once cleared, the chance of reinfection is considerable because of the ubiquitous organisms and the selected inability of some individuals to resist such infections.

A useful alternative to prolonged treatment is to clear glabrous skin with a short oral course of griseofulvin while instituting a vigorous topical program that ideally will contain the infection in the nails and keep the skin free of disease. Should there be a relapse at a future date, the oral course can be repeated. Most mild to moderate tinea infections require only topical medication such as tolnaftate or haloprogin.

YEAST INFECTIONS

Yeast infections of the skin mimic fungal infections as in the groin, but most often the erythema is a bit brighter, the scale is more macerated, and there will be telltale satellite lesions at the periphery of the patch. When *Candida* infects webs or paronychia — a common hazard of the prolonged water immersion experienced by bartenders and janitors — or when it involves the mouth or vagina as a sequela of systemic antimicrobial therapy — perhaps a signal of the diabetic diathesis — the lesions are more characteristic. The erythematous base is often raw with a cheesy exudate, and there may be pruritus, but more often tenderness and pain occur.

Therapy to reduce erythema and itching is helpful in initiating symptomatic relief, and eradication of the underlying predisposing factors is mandatory, but specific topical anticandidal medications, such as nystatin, amphotericin, or clotrimazole, are also indicated and would be prescribed, as might be expected, in a water-washable or lotion base, never occlusive. The sexual partner of a patient with balanitis or vulvovaginitis should be alerted to the possibility of infection and treated if the patient's problem is slow to clear or recurrent. Vaginal suppositories of nystatin are available, as well as oral suspension for direct application to mouth lesions.

Candida albicans is usually the infecting species, but several others of the same genus, *Candida tropicalis*, for example, may be the agent under predisposing conditions, especially with paronychial infections. Since they are common organisms of the gastrointestinal tract, the chance for reinfection with *Candida* organisms is ever present. Precautions should include adequate cleansing and drying of the body folds routinely but especially after defecation, and the adding of an anticandidal preparation to any topical antibacterial medication that is to be used in the anogenital area. Neither nystatin nor amphotericin B is sufficiently absorbed from the gastrointestinal tract to be of value as systemic therapy; but taken orally, either agent will reduce the *Candida* population of the intestine. This may be indicated if topical control fails in the vulvovaginitis of *Candida*-induced pruritus among those on contraceptives or long-term antimicrobial therapy.

Despite the tendency to chronicity and recurrence, and despite the acute discomfort of the active infection, most candidiasis is responsive to therapy. Occasionally severe infection can have quite generalized erythematous crusting and be associated with horny excrescences on granulomatous bases. Labeled chronic mucocutaneous candidiasis, this intractable infection may appear at birth or early childhood and may be associated with endocrinopathy such as hypoparathyroidism, hypoadrenalism, and diabetes, or with congenital thymic disorders affecting lymphocyte function and cell-mediated immunity. There are data to suggest that chronic mucocutaneous candidiasis results from a deficiency of migration inhibitory factor or from the presence of an inhibitor to this factor or other mediator of delayed hypersensitivity. Despite endocrinopathy and the compromised immune status in the presence of severe extensive mucocutaneous infection, systemic candidiasis develops rarely — all the more surprising because in general medicine systemic manifestations of *Candida* infection are not that unusual.

In systemic infection, bronchopulmonary and pulmonary candidiasis are the most common manifestations seen as complications of chronic primary pulmonary disease, especially in the diabetic or those on systemic corticosteroids or antimicrobial agents. Candidemia, with or without seeding, is a complication of surgery associated with prolonged use of indwelling catheters, and of those conditions requiring long-term therapy with immunosuppressive agents and antimetabolites.

Because of the frequent finding of *Candida* in and on the body, establishing *Candida* as a cause of a particular problem requires the demonstration of budding yeasts and filaments in the scraping or biopsy from the lesion in question, a generous and repeated growth of the organism or culture, and a fit of the lesions to what might be anticipated for a *Candida* infection.

572.3. DERMATITIS OF THE HANDS AND FEET

The problem of redness and scaling of the hands and feet can be exasperating to clinician and patient alike. Hands and feet have similar and sympathetic reaction patterns. A dermatitis on one may produce an "id" on the other. Both are subjected to trauma and both are exposed to abundant contactants, greater in variety on the hands perhaps, but greater in intensity on the feet in their enclosed pressure casings.

Thus far, a consideration of psoriasis and of fungus has included hands and feet, but the differential has not been extended for those from whom no fungus could be isolated and no stigmata of psoriasis identified. Erythema and scale of long standing, a chronic dermatitis, might mean a continuing contact dermatitis or the late manifestations of atopic dermatitis, or perhaps might be part of an ill-defined group of reaction patterns that are quite characteristic in their manifestations but of obscure etiology.

CONTACT DERMATITIS

Of all the dermatitides of the hands and feet, contact dermatitis is perhaps the most important. Irritants and allergic sensitizers commonly involve hands and feet. If the offending substance can be identified, avoidance or protection can restore a patient to normal. If the problem is ignored or the offender escapes detection and the dermatitis smolders, a chronicity is established that may totally disable the patient.

Any dermatitis that presents acutely with erythema and vesicles warrants intense restorative therapy and an undaunted search for the cause. Plants and airborne contactants can leave their linear vesicles or exposure pattern as a clue; the distribution in a hand or foot problem may not be that revealing. Nonetheless, history taking and patch testing may narrow the field. Screening trays are available to test to common allergens, to medications, to the components of shoes, and to cosmetics, and for every patient it is possible to test with the part of his own environment that is suspect, a part of the lining of a shoe, as an example. For hands rather than feet, photosensitivity may be checked to establish if the minimal erythema dose for the individual is lowered or if a photo-contact reaction can be demonstrated in association with medications or soaps.

If the offending irritant or allergen is identified, the source of the patient's exposure and other occult and unsuspected sources can be established to ensure protection. Fisher's text is the definitive reference for elaborating a suspected contact dermatitis and then sorting out the cross-reactions and tabulating where the allergen is to be found. Contact dermatitis placed first in prevalence among 75,000 consecutive visits to the Skin and Cancer Clinic of New York University. There were 11,100 visits for contact and an additional 4600 for chronic dermatitis of obscure etiology. The importance of recognition and identification cannot be overstated.

ATOPIC DERMATITIS

In that same pool of diagnoses atopic dermatitis placed seventh, a disease determined by heredity and characterized by a lower threshold to pruritus. With scratching, the skin becomes spongiotic and weeps, the eczematous form seen more often in the young. At any age rubbing can produce lichenification with accentuation of skin markings. Across the United States, 0.7 per cent of the population has this inherited diathesis of sufficient severity that a physician's consultation is warranted. Most cases contributing to the burden of the problem occur in infancy or childhood. After a period of quiescence from age two or three, it can recur in late childhood, in adolescence, or in early adult life, tending to localize in flexural areas of the neck, antecubital and popliteal folds, often about the eyelids, behind the ears, and at the wrists. Of those who are afflicted in adulthood, occasionally to the fifth decade, chronic hand and foot eczema is a common expression of the problem. At any age, a pruritic dermatitis in the "atopic distribution" should raise the possibility of the diagnosis. Such patients will have a personal history of atopic dermatitis and a personal or family history of atopy, asthma, hay fever, or perhaps urticaria, which is part of the complex but of more obscure relationship.

The atopic diathesis is manifest in the skin by a blanching response to injections of acetylcholine or methacholine, in contrast to normal skin in which vasodilatation results in erythema. The skin of the atopic has been shown to contain up to 60 times the concentration of acetylcholine of skin in nonatopic rashes, as well as an excess of cholinesterase. Sweat glands in the atopic have an increased sensitivity to acetylcholine rather like that produced by a partial beta receptor blockade. Atopic skin also differs from normal in its exquisite sensitivity to epinephrine and norepinephrine. In fact the "grainy" skin of patients with atopic dermatitis has been ascribed to a permanent state of piloerection mediated by norepinephrine.

The role of allergy in atopic dermatitis is not completely elaborated. Immediate urticarial reactions to skin tests with common antigens are frequently observed. The skin-sensitizing antibody can be transferred by serum to another subject and has been identified as a distinct immunoglobulin, IgE. Some patients with atopic dermatitis will have excessive serum levels of IgE but with little correlation between the serum level and the severity of the dermatitis. Further, high levels of IgE have been reported in nonatopic conditions. T-cell function is said to be deficient in atopic dermatitis, whether depressed by elevated IgE levels or de novo with the IgE rise in response to reacting B cells.

The major implications of these documented facts are that atopic skin responds to slight trauma with vasoconstriction and pruritus, leading to a weeping vesicular dermatitis acutely, and then more chronically to dry lichenified skin. Wet dressings, if indicated, will physically reduce erythema and weeping, and topical steroids and systemic antihistamines will alter the pruritus and inflammatory response. Dry or lichenified skin may suggest lubrication, but the inability to sweat may be aggravated by occlusive lubricants which, with retained heat, may increase pruritus. Should secondary pyogenic or fungal infection be present, specific therapy may be needed to control it. Restoring the integrity of the skin will thwart opportunistic organisms.

One major risk of atopic dermatitis derives from the depression of T-cell function which makes the patient more susceptible to widespread viral infection with vaccinia, herpes simplex, and of less concern, molluscum contagiosum and verruca vulgaris. Even without active dermatitis, infection with herpes simplex can lead to a generalized vesicular eruption with high fever and significant mortality. With the control of variola and the need for vaccinia almost obviated, there is no longer a public health requirement for vaccination, which is absolutely contraindicated in the atopic patient and all his close contacts. Protection from latent herpes simplex virus is not so easy to achieve.

Any acute flare in the dermatitis of an atopic should be inspected closely for vesicles. If they are present, to differentiate viral vesicles from the eczematous process of atopy, a Tzanck smear should be done in search of multinucleated giant cells indicative of viral infection. If such cells are found, the patient warrants close assessment and continued expectant observation. Widespread infection can occur; its severity will dictate therapy. Corticosteroids, topically and systemically, would be contraindicated because of the risk of viral dissemination, but all other topical therapy to promote resolution of the atopic dermatitis should be undertaken. Specific therapy with idoxuridine should be used as a last measure and monitored closely. Because contained viral infections can also occur in the atopic, all that may be needed is good supportive care.

Infection with the virus of verruca vulgaris or with molluscum contagiosum, even though generalized, merely requires a good topical regimen. Although some physicians would anesthetize and curette all lesions from the start, a trial of salicylic acid in flexible collodion or plaster, with self-peeling or paring by the patient, is less traumatic with less risk of scar. Destroying the epidermal cells in which the virus lives is all that is needed, but repetition and persistence are required to ensure extinction. The diagnosis of both these viral problems is usually obvious once one has seen a common verruca or an umbilicated shiny flesh-colored papule from which a core can be easily shelled. Both verruca vulgaris and molluscum contagiosum are seen most commonly in children, and both can be seen as venereal problems in young adults, but they are of greatest challenge and concern when widespread in the immunosuppressed patient or the atopic individual.

One further risk borne by the severe atopic is that of developing cataracts, which may be minimal or blinding. Occurring most frequently in the second and third decades, they are a serious complication of the atopic diathesis and may be further aggravated by corticosteroid therapy.

Canales, L., Middlemas, R. O., III, Louro, J. M., and South, M. A.: Immunological observations in chronic mucocutaneous candidiasis. Lancet, 2:567, 1969.

Chilgren, R. A., Quie, P. G., Meuwissen, H. J., and Hong, R.: Chronic mucocutaneous candidiasis: Deficiency of delayed hypersensitivity, and selective local antibody defect. Lancet, 2:688, 1977.

Farber, E. M., and Cox, A. J. (eds.): Psoriasis: Proceedings of the Second International Symposium. New York, Yorke Medical Books, 1977.

Fisher, A.: Contact Dermatitis. 2nd ed. Philadelphia, Lea & Febiger, 1973.

Montes, L. F., Pittman, C. S., Moore, W. J., Taylor, C. G., and Cooper, M. D.: Chronic mucocutaneous candidiasis. JAMA, 221:156, 1972.

573. SIGNIFICANT DERMATOLOGIC SIGNS OF DISEASE

573.1. INTRODUCTION

In assessing the skin for pathology the diagnostic range extends to systemic implications of cutaneous signs. The integument nourished by blood with a markedly elevated bilirubin is a dramatic indicator of pathology. Because serologic tests can detect preclinical icterus, the clinical fact of jaundice loses its edge. However, there is an array of metabolic substances, abnormal or in excess of normal, that settle in the skin and await recognition. Lipids and amyloid are good examples. Pathologic processes such as vasculitis can affect

Figure 11. Acanthosis nigricans.

enocarcinoma, the acanthosis nigricans has been labeled "malignant," a poor choice of terminology, for the skin change is in no way malignant. Its appearance may precede the malignancy (20 per cent), follow it (20 per cent), or be noted simultaneously (60 per cent). Regression of the skin sign has been observed following therapy for the malignancy, and reappearance with reactivation of the tumor. The stomach is the most common site of malignancy (70 per cent), but it may appear elsewhere in the gastrointestinal tract — colon, esophagus, liver, gallbladder, pancreas — and less often in the ovaries, prostate, breast, or lung. There are rare reports of association with lymphomas and squamous cell carcinoma.

Acanthosis nigricans unassociated with malignancy is found with developmental, hormonal, and metabolic pathology, and after the administration of certain drugs and hormonal agents. In the inherited form benign cutaneous changes are considered nevoid genodermatoses present from birth or childhood with the possibility of spread or intensification at puberty. In the juvenile idiopathic type with cushingoid obesity, the onset is frequently at puberty. Acanthosis nigricans is found with adrenal insufficiency, Cushing's syndrome, acromegaly, Stein-Leventhal syndrome, and various pituitary and hypothalamic tumors or other lesions involving the base of the brain. It has been postulated that a pituitary peptide hormone secreted under hypothalamic control may stimulate papillary dermal hypertrophy. Crude preparations of MSH have been shown to induce acanthosis nigricans in a patient with melanoma, with MSH-like peptides the most likely agent. Diethylstilbestrol, corticosteroids, and nicotinic acid have also been implicated in the cutaneous phenomenon, and there are reports of appearance and disappearance correlated with the use of oral contraceptives. In insulin-resistant diabetes associated acanthosis nigricans tends to remit as the glucose intolerance lessens. Correlation is made with the antibody titer to insulin receptors.

Although there is no local therapy for acanthosis nigricans, the early recognition of the cutaneous sign, especially in the adult, warrants an immediate and thorough search for underlying pathology, especially tumor. The associated malignancies tend to be aggressive and rapidly fatal. Extension of the acanthosis nigricans is an ominous sign.

Banuchi, S. R., Cohen, L., Lorinca, A. L., and Morgan, J.: Acanthosis nigricans following diethylstilbestrol therapy: Occurrence in patients with childhood muscular dystrophy. Arch. Dermatol., 109:545, 1974.

Curth, H. O., Hilberg, A. W., and Machacek, G. F.: The site and histology of the cancer associated with acanthosis nigricans. Cancer, 15:364, 1962.

Givens, J. R., Kerber, I. J., Wiser, W. L., Andersen, R. N., Coleman, S. A., and Fish, S. A.: Remission of acanthosis nigricans associated with polycystic ovarian disease and a stromal luteoma. J. Clin. Endocrinol. Metab., 38:347, 1974.

Kahn, C. R., Flier, J. S., Bar, R. S., Archer, J. A., Gorden, P., Martin, M. M., and Roth, J.: Syndromes of insulin resistance and acanthosis nigricans: Insulin receptor disorders in man. N. Engl. J. Med., 294:739, 1976.

Lerner, A. B.: On the cause of acanthosis nigricans. N. Engl. J. Med., 281:706, 1969.

Nordlund, J. J., and Lerner, A. B.: Cause of acanthosis nigricans (letter). N. Engl. J. Med., 293:200, 1975.

both viscera and skin, and malignancy can extend or metastasize to both. There are also physiologic symptoms of pruritus or weakness and skin changes of ichthyosis or weeping dermatitis that relate to occult malignancy and respond to therapy directed at the malignancy. But most curious of all, there are congenital aberrations and pigmentary hallmarks that are associated with specific systemic disease in an established but obscure relationship.

The purpose of the present chapter is to review these various skin stigmata so that they may be identified by the examiner, providing him with some broad indications of the kinds of problems with which they may be associated. Then, grouped with a specific organ system as the key, selected skin signs are tabulated and ranked for potential value in suspecting or establishing a diagnosis (see Tables 6 to 9).

573.2. ACANTHOSIS NIGRICANS

A brown-black velvety skin change, verrucous and creased, and localized in the axillae, nuchal folds, or groin is readily recognized as acanthosis nigricans (Fig. 11). Blending into normal adjacent skin, it is characteristically bilateral and symmetrical. Affecting any body fold and favoring flexural surfaces, it may rarely be generalized. Histologically there is epidermal thickening and folding over a hypertrophic papillary layer. Because acanthosis nigricans can occur with malignancy, with hormonal dysfunction, or as an inherited disorder, it is a clinical sign of note; yet neither the clinical nor the histologic appearance helps in the differential diagnosis of associated pathology.

When found with visceral malignancy, usually an ad-

573.3. ICHTHYOSIS

An integument that is rough and dry with retained scale but free of erythema suggests a "fish skin" desig-

Figure 12. Ichthyosis.

may have a yellow cast because of carotenemia; it will appear with the disease and be supported by laboratory evidence of decreased thyroid function.

MALIGNANCY. The onset of ichthyosis in an adult without drug inducement or metabolic disorder is of grave significance, suggesting an underlying malignant process. Hodgkin's disease is found most frequently, but also other lymphomas, multiple myeloma, and carcinoma of the breast. As with *acanthosis nigricans*, the regression and recurrence of the tumor may be reflected in the activity of the dermatosis.

For those attuned to this significant cutaneous sign, the question of possible malignancy is often raised when the observation is of minimal dryness and polyhedral scale over the legs, arms, or abdomen of the older patient. Winter dryness at any age, but especially in the lipid-deprived skin of the elderly, is prone to pruritus and ichthyosiform change. If the problem is mild, limited, and historically of long standing or winter occurrence, the dermatosis observed is probably not a sign of tumor and should respond to simple lubrication. More intensive therapy would be to increase environmental moisture and free retained keratin with special lubricants, especially those containing urea, 15 to 30 per cent.

Frost, P., and Van Scott, E. J.: The ichthyosiform dermatoses. Classification based on anatomical and cellular kinetic observations. Arch. Dermatol., 94:113, 1966.

Steinberg, D., Vroom, F. Q., Engel, W. K., Cammermeyer, J., Mize, C. E., and Avigan, J.: Refsum's disease — a recently characterized lipoidosis involving the nervous system. Combined Clinical Staff Conference at the NIH. Ann. Intern. Med., 66:365, 1967.

573.4. ACQUIRED ERYTHRODERMAS

ICHTHYOSIFORM

Generalized dryness and scaling with erythema in a universal distribution may be total body psoriasis. The plaque-like quality of the lesions is no longer discerned, but nail stigmata and severe scalp involvement, as well as an antecedent diagnosis of psoriasis, may aid the differential. An explosive ichthyosiform erythroderma may be a manifestation of mycosis fungoides (see Ch. 574.5).

Localized ichthyosiform or psoriasiform erythroderma may be of equal significance. *Bowen's disease*, a sharply demarcated red-brown plaque moderately thickened with scale, loose or adherent, is sometimes misdiagnosed as psoriasis. It commonly occurs on covered areas of the body, and since it can be a sequela of arsenic ingestion, patients treated in the past with Fowler's solution for psoriasis may have both psoriasis and Bowen's disease. They may also have the stigmata of

nation (Fig. 12). On close inspection there may be fine scale with keratin-plugged follicles, or large polyhedral scales loosely adherent. The palms and soles may be normal, or may be thickened with accentuation of normal creases.

INHERITED. If the condition has been present from birth or childhood, perhaps only clinically apparent in dry winter months, the diagnosis is likely to be one of the *ichthyosiform dermatoses*, an inherited disorder in which excessive amounts of keratin are retained at the skin surface. Through an analysis of clinical and anatomic findings as well as a consideration of the cellular kinetics and genetic aspects, distinctions are made among the four more common types (Table 4). These ichthyoses are important to be recognized for what they are and to be differentiated from the ichthyosis-like dermatoses of abnormal lipid metabolism and the acquired ichthyosis of malignancy.

METABOLIC. Except for an inherited metabolic disorder as in Refsum's disease, the ichthyosis of abnormal lipid metabolism will appear later in life and be associated temporally with a drug which inhibits lipid synthesis, such as the butyrophenones or triparanol. So too, the dryness and scale of hypothyroidism, which

TABLE 4.   Common Ichthyosiform Dermatoses

	Inheritance	Onset	Distribution	Clinical Associations	Kinetics
Lamellar ichthyosis	Autosomal recessive	Birth	Body, palms, soles	Ectropion	Increased
Epidermolytic hyperkeratosis	Autosomal dominant	Birth	Predominant flexural involvement	Blisters	Increased
X-linked ichthyosis	X-linked	Birth	Trunk	Corneal opacities	Normal
Ichthyosis vulgaris	Autosomal dominant	Childhood	Spares flexural areas	Atopy	Normal

arseniasis: arsenical keratoses, discrete hyperkeratotic papules of the palms and soles, plus the raindrop hyperpigmentation over the thorax. Bowen's disease is a cutaneous premalignancy, and the diagnosis can be established by biopsy. Any unremitting erythematous scaling lesion of long duration, especially if slowly enlarging, should be regarded with suspicion.

PAGET'S DISEASE

Paget's disease is another example. A sharply defined plaque of erythema, often eczematous with crusting or even erosion, it can be psoriasiform. Classically of the breast, it involves the nipple and areola unilaterally, perhaps only a portion, and is associated with underlying malignancy, most often a ductal adenocarcinoma. It appears usually, but not exclusively, in women; the mean age is 55 years. Extramammary Paget's disease, frequently of the anogenital area, occurs in both sexes at about the same age, but more often in women. It is without the invariable association of malignancy, which is found in less than half the patients. The malignancies that do occur derive most often from cutaneous apocrine structures.

Histologically Paget cells lie within the epidermis. Large round cells with large nuclei and abundant cytoplasm, they can be confused with nevus cells and those of Bowen's disease, although mucin stains are helpful in the differential. The histopathology is definitive and underscores the importance of biopsy for any persistent psoriasiform or eczematous lesion anywhere, but especially of the breast. In the patient with skin that is otherwise normal, the lesion of Paget's disease is obvious and the course clear. It is the patient with other psoriasiform and eczematous dermatitis who is at risk of having Paget's disease overlooked. Any suspicious lesion of the areola should be treated intensively for a week or two; if the skin does not return to normal, the lesion should be biopsied.

ACRODERMATITIS ENTEROPATHICA

This condition is occasionally misdiagnosed as psoriasis, and more often as candidiasis because of periorificial dermatitis, but it can present with reddened ichthyosiform plaques. It is a persistent dermatitis about the mouth, with acral involvement that begins as vesicles but is soon crusted, thickened, and perhaps superinfected with bacteria or *Candida,* and may be associated with diarrhea. Because of its onset in childhood and poor prognosis without therapy, the adult form, even if not controlled, will have been identified. Two thirds of patients have a family history of the disease, and an autosomal recessive inheritance is suggested. The affected children tend to be slow in growth and development, and to have a deficiency in cell-mediated immunity. They are reported to have increased IgA and deficient or "absent" thymus, and to lack germinal centers and plasmacytosis of lymph nodes and spleen. In the bowel, in the fasting state, jejunal cytoplasmic inclusions are found by electron microscopy. Plasma zinc levels are low, but also decreased are serum lipids and arachidonic acid. Prostaglandin synthesis is defective. Zinc supplements will dramatically reverse all clinical manifestations of the disease within a few days, even in adult patients plagued with the disease from childhood. Abnormalities of the intestinal mucosa were noted to revert to normal on oral zinc therapy.

Although it is not clear that the defect in zinc uptake is the primary lesion, prostaglandin "zinc-binding ligand" is necessary for zinc absorption. Aspirin, which inhibits prostaglandins, impairs zinc absorption in rats. Arachidonic acid, decreased in acrodermatitis enteropathica, is known to be a prostaglandin precursor. There is the further evidence of clinical benefit from a dietary supplement of zinc or prostaglandin. Curiously, human milk has PGE_2 as a zinc ligand; cow's milk has none, fitting the frequently observed onset of the disease at weaning. Because calcium ingestion can impede zinc absorption in the gastrointestinal tract, as can soy milk protein, the prescribing of zinc supplements should include precautions about calcium, soy proteins, and aspirin.

Evans, G. W., and Johnson, P. E.: Defective prostaglandin synthesis in acrodermatitis enteropathica (letter). Lancet, 1:52, 1977.
Hirsch, F. S., Michel, B., and Strain, W. H.: Gluconate zinc in acrodermatitis enteropathica. Arch. Dermatol., 112:475, 1976.
Kelly, R., Davidson, G. P., Townley, R. R. W., and Campbell, P. E.: Reversible intestinal mucosal abnormality in acrodermatitis enteropathica. Arch. Dis. Child., 51:219, 1976.
Michaelson, G.: Zinc therapy in acrodermatitis enteropathica. Acta Derm. Venereol., 54:377, 1974.

EXFOLIATIVE ERYTHRODERMA

When the skin is normal rather than thickened but generally red with fine scale, the term exfoliative erythroderma (Fig. 13) is used. It can be the eventuality of any extensive eruption; when seen, of itself, it gives few clues to the etiology. Drug allergy, contact dermatitis, an eczematous process, seborrheic dermatitis or psoriasis, the lymphomas and leukemias, or any extensive inflammatory insult to the skin may be the cause. Older patients are more predisposed to the phenomenon, and it is most difficult to clear in them; it may smolder for months or years.

The best treatment is prevention. Any acute dermatitis of whatever etiology should be quieted with wet dressings and topical steroids, with antihistamines or other sedation, and with rest. The specific cause should

Figure 13. Exfoliative erythroderma.

be sought, although it may remain obscure. If the eruption continues to progress, systemic steroids or immune suppression should be considered. If generalized exfoliation has occurred, initial efforts should be conservative and supportive, but systemic therapy will probably be needed.

PHOTOSENSITIVITY

The skin of the normal individual will react to sunlight in a range of responses that are modified by pigmentary protection, geographic location, solar and solstice time, and duration of exposure. The data derived would be a base line of normal and predictable responses, however varied or unpleasant, from no reaction through erythema to blistering; cumulatively one could anticipate actinic damage (see Ch. 569) and malignancy (see Ch. 574.5). Here, however, consideration is given only to responses that deviate from the normal as modified by genetic, chemical, allergic, or nutritional factors.

The patient with an abnormal light reaction could present with an exaggerated sunburn in a patterned exposure with the outline of protective clothing, but more often there is merely the subtle sparing of the submental area of the chin or the eyelids, perhaps with accentuation at the "V" of the neck. Frequently the lesions are not as diffuse as a burn but are characterized by papules or urticaria, or even an eczematous response.

To sort out the etiology, light must be suspected from historical or physical evidence and from any recognized predisposition to sun sensitivity. Seasonal recurrences, especially in the spring or early summer, would arouse suspicion. The evoked reaction may be to light alone, to light in association with abnormal metabolites as in the porphyrias, or to light plus chemicals and medications applied to the skin or ingested.

Light Alone

Adverse reactions to light alone are rare and may all have a genetic predisposition. *Xeroderma pigmentosum*, for example, inherited as an autosomal recessive problem has a defect in DNA repair replication. The light-exposed skin undergoes severe early solar damage with erythema, spotty pigmentation, atrophy, and neoplasm. From infancy there is photophobia and a prolonged erythematous response to sun. In albinism, too, there is photophobia and increased sun sensitivity, but the skin, except for lacking the protective shield of pigment, is normal. Repair is normal. The defect in the tyrosinase function of the melanocyte leaves the albino with a sunburn susceptibility comparable to that of the lightest-complexioned Celt.

But more than an exaggerated response to sun damage, light alone can evoke a polymorphous light eruption. Common among certain North American Indians, and reported in families and identical twins, it is without indication of genetic factors in most patients. As the name polymorphous photodermatitis implies, the eruption .is a mixture of papules and vesicles which may become confluent. It occurs at any age but usually has its onset in young adulthood with no evidence of sex predisposition or protection from melanin; it is seen in a range of patients of all races from the lightly to the heavily pigmented. Pursuing a chronic course, it

flares each spring until some sun tolerance develops in summer. Selected sun protection and topical steroids are the mainstay of therapy.

Light Plus

METABOLITES.   With the porphyrias as an example, the onset of photosensitivity in childhood and the associated severe scarring, hair loss, and discolored teeth readily suggest the diagnosis of congenital erythropoietic porphyria. The manifestations of photosensitivity in the adult onset porphyrias are more subtle, however. The appearance of skin fragility with bullae and erosions localized to the dorsa of the hands, possibly involving the forehead or scalp of the balding older patient, is frequently missed as a sign of porphyria cutanea tarda (Fig. 14). Such patients excrete urinary uroporphyrins and some coproporphyrins and can be shown to be photosensitive to those wavelengths of light which the porphyrin molecule absorbs best: 400 to 410 nm in the blue-violet region, and 500 to 600 nm in the orange. Their sun-exposed skin becomes prematurely aged, with associated hypertrichosis characteristically found at the outer canthus of the eyes. Therapy by phlebotomy to reduce the circulating porphyrins and the use of sun screens to filter out the damaging light rays give most patients with acquired porphyria sustained remissions from the dermatologic manifestations of the disease.

Photosensitivity is also observed with the aminoacidurias. In Hartnup disease, for example, in which there is a transport defect of tryptophan, with hydroxykynureninuria and tryptophanuria, minimal exposure to sun can lead to erythema, edema, and even vesicula-

Figure 14.   Porphyria cutanea tarda.

tion. At least for Hartnup disease, the eruption is associated with a cellular deficiency of nicotinamide. As in nutritional pellagra, high doses of nicotinamide improve the dermatitis. Recognizing that patients deficient in nicotinamide excrete increased amounts of certain porphyrins and indican, it is suggested for all these photosensitivity responses that sunlight induces photochemical reactions in the skin that lead to tissue destruction and antigen formation.

EXOGENOUS AGENTS. Of even greater diagnostic challenge are the many phototoxic and photoallergic reactions encountered. *Phototoxicity* occurs without recognized immune mechanisms. It is the kind of reaction seen in patients receiving systemic antimicrobial therapy such as declomycin or sulfonamides; dyes such as acridine, methyl violet, or eosin; psychotherapeutic drugs such as phenothiazine; the sulfonylurea hypoglycemic agents; the thiazide diuretics; and the antifungal agent griseofulvin. Upon exposure to light there is burning, followed by prompt erythema and edema reaching a maximum intensity in 12 to 24 hours, and then by desquamation and hyperpigmentation. The initial reaction is common to a large number of people upon first exposure. The sensitivity will not persist, and future exposure to ultraviolet light will be normal.

Photoallergy differs in that reactions, although occasionally prompt and urticarial, can appear after 24 hours or more. They occur in only a small number of exposed individuals, are often persistent, and show cross-photosensitization; with photo patch testing there may be flares at previous reaction sites. Few oral ingestants contribute to the phenomenon, although sulfanilamide, sulfadiazine, and sulfisoxazole have been implicated as being both phototoxic and photoallergic. The bulk of photoallergy is through topical exposure, whether airborne or applied, and such reactions should be known as *photoallergic contact dermatitis*. It is postulated that light acts upon the offending chemical to form a haptene that binds protein, accounting for persistence and recurrence.

Therapy for all photodermatitis is the treatment for burn and contact dermatitis. With phototoxicity, if there is merely marked erythema, or if the reaction is noted early, topical steroids with occlusion will encourage vasoconstriction and reduce the over-all intensity of the reaction. With photoallergy antihistamine may be helpful. Whether phototoxic or photoallergic, the offending agent must be sought to be identified and avoided, along with its cross-reactants.

Brodthager, H.: Polymorphous light eruption. *In* Urbach, F. (ed.): The Biologic Effects of Ultraviolet Radiation. Oxford, Pergamon Press, 1969.

Cleaver, J. E.: Defective repair replication of DNA in xeroderma pigmentosum. Nature, 218:652, 1968.

Cleaver, J. E.: Xeroderma pigmentosum: Variants with normal DNA repair and normal sensitivity to ultraviolet light. J. Invest. Dermatol., 58:124, 1972.

Urbach, F., Davies, R. E., and Forbes, P. D.: Ultraviolet radiation and skin cancer in man. *In* Montagna, W. (ed.): Advances in Biology of Skin Carcinogenesis. Oxford, Pergamon Press, 1966.

Light-Sensitive Diseases

Lupus erythematosus known for its photosensitivity is characterized by the isomorphic response whereby exposure to sunlight will evoke lesions of lupus erythematosus in the skin. In the patient with recognized disease the untoward response will be accepted and skin lesions, however mildly erythematous or urticarial, will be clinically identified as the disease. In a patient without antecedent diagnosis, however, an urticarial response to sunlight may be overlooked as a first manifestation of a collagen disease. Persistence of the hive, bluing of the erythema, development of scale, and follicular plugging should suggest the diagnosis, and histopathologic evidence should support it.

573.5. PIGMENTARY DISTURBANCES

Color changes in the skin and mucous membrane are common and occasionally important. The wide range of normal hues and markings that racial diversity extends makes it necessary to review continuously the full array of normal possibilities through attention to the multiple banal lesions in every patient examined.

Melanin contributes significantly to the color of eyes, hair, and skin. It is most conspicuous in its heavy concentration or total absence. Brown to black eumelanin is a high molecular weight, relatively insoluble polymer, a polyquinone. In man it is derived from the phenolic precursors tyrosine and 3,4-dihydroxyphenylalanine (dopa). Tyrosinase, a copper-containing enzyme, catalyzes the oxidation of tyrosine in the cytoplasm of the melanocyte. Formed melanin is then transferred to keratinocytes; thus skin color derives from pigment in the epidermal cells as well as the melanocytes. When deep in the skin, melanin can appear blue or slate colored because of light scatter of the Tyndall effect.

Although melanocyte distribution is varied throughout the body, with twice higher concentrations in the skin of the head and forearms than in the rest of the skin (excepting the scrotum and foreskin), there are no differences in distribution or total numbers among races. Genotypic variations that underlie racial differences are within the ultrastructure of the melanocyte relating to the production and distribution of melanosomes following ultraviolet light irradiation or other stimulation. In situations in which generalized pigmentation is induced, the pigment pattern will reflect the melanocyte concentration.

HYPERPIGMENTATION

Ephelides

Increased concentrations of melanin may be localized or diffuse. The circumscribed melanoses commonly observed include *ephelides* or freckles, the small flat macules of less than 0.5 cm that first appear on sun-exposed areas at about age four and tend to fade in later life. Long wave ultraviolet light, 300 to 400 nm, will darken them. The melanocytes of ephelides are not increased in number but are more arborized and more active in melanin production.

Lentigines

These small flat macular lesions resemble ephelides clinically but are histologically distinct because of increased numbers of normal-appearing melanocytes. Evoked by aging and solar damage, they come in later life — so-called "liver spots," the *senile lentigo*.

A separate group unrelated to light, in fact occasionally involving mucous membranes, appearing at any age and genetically determined, is the *nevoid lentigines*. Associated with inherited syndromes such as the "leopard" syndrome and Moynihan's syndrome, they are present from birth and are found with a wide range of defects and mental retardation. In Peutz-Jeghers syndrome, the perioral mucous membrane and digital lentigines are associated with small bowel polyps, especially of the jejunum. These histologically distinct hamartomas arising from the muscularis mucosae have little malignant propensity in the small bowel, but when also present in the colon the risk of malignancy is increased.

Freckles of the axillae, especially when seen with irregular hyperpigmented mottling of the skin elsewhere, are known as Crowe's sign of neurofibromatosis. The pigment changes are believed to be a variant of café-au-lait spots, the large tan uniformly pigmented macules that may be present at birth anywhere on the skin or may appear later. Café-au-lait spots larger than 1.5 cm and more numerous than six are suggested as presumptive evidence of neurofibromatosis. They are also seen in other neurocutaneous syndromes such as tuberous sclerosis. In Albright's syndrome the circumscribed hypermelanotic macules may appear in a linear, rarely segmental, pattern on one side or the other without crossing the midline. They occur on the forehead, nuchal and sacral areas, and buttocks. Their distribution rather than their clinical appearance or histology distinguishes them from the café-au-lait lesions of neurofibromatosis.

Pigmented Nevi

Pigmented nevi, often called moles, are formed of clusters of melanocytes and are rarely present from birth. They are divided clinically and histologically into four groups: the nevus spilus, and junctional, com-

Figure 16.   Junctional nevus.

pound, and dermal nevi or moles. The nevus spilus (Fig. 15) is a small oval macule from tan to dark brown or black, usually of uniform color. Hyperpigmentation of the keratinocyte is intense, and there may be elongation of the rete ridges. The melanocytes are normal, not nested. Histologic differentiation is also used for the further classification of the moles or nevi, often called nevus cell nevi to distinguish them from the epidermal and connective tissue nevi. Junctional nevi have nevus cell nests above the basement membrane, compound nevi have them in both the epidermis and dermis, and intradermal nevi have them in the dermis alone. Junctional nevi tend to be flat and pigmented, dark brown to

Figure 15.   Nevus spilus.

Figure 17.   Intradermal nevus.

Figure 18. Incontinentia pigmenti.

terned pigmentation should warn the examiner of the possibility of ectodermal defects and the need for genetic counseling. Although incontinentia pigmenti is of unknown etiology, the evidence suggests genetic transmission of the disease as an autosomal dominant with expression mainly in females or as an X-linked trait lethal for males. It presents with an inflammatory vesicobullous phase with little or no pigment change, and evolves either through a verrucous papillomatous phase or directly to the distinctive pigmentation. One or more of the stages may be present at birth or may begin in the first weeks of life. Despite the extent of the inflammatory lesion, the patient is afebrile. There may be pronounced eosinophilia of the blood and vesicle fluid.

The importance of recognizing the pigmentary stigma is the identification of a significant genodermatosis and the association of the diagnosis with other ectodermal abnormalities in 60 per cent of patients. Eyes, teeth, central nervous system, and cutaneous appendages are affected. Eye problems include strabismus, nystagmus, blue sclerae, optic atrophy, exudative chorioretinitis, papillitis, congenital retinal folds, and retrobulbar glioma. With the dental abnormalities, permanent dentition is compromised. There are impacted and missing teeth, pegged teeth, and malformed crowns. Neurologically, seizures and spastic paralysis are seen, and there may be mental retardation, deafness, and homonymous hemianopsia. Occasionally there are cardiac abnormalities and skeletal deformities, including syndactyly and shortened extremities.

Other Hyperpigmentations

Blotchy pigmentation of the skin without discrete lesions may be seen following inflammation, especially if the individual pigments easily. Thus it may follow trauma such as cuts and burns, generalized eruptions, or exposure to photosensitizers. It can also occur without antecedent erythema in a mask-like distribution known as *melasma* (Fig. 19). Aggravated by sunlight, the patterned pigmentation can be seen in pregnancy and with the taking of oral contraceptives, but it is also seen in men without laboratory evidence of abnormal hormonal levels.

Generalized hyperpigmentation is often associated with abnormalities of the endocrine system but can also be related to nutritional, metabolic, or chemical factors and to drugs. In primary adrenocortical insufficiency the pituitary activity increases in response to the decreased cortisol. With melanocyte-stimulating hormone (MSH) elaborated in excess by the pituitary along with the corticotropin (ACTH), there is consequent darkening of the skin. An MSH-producing tumor of the pituitary would have the same effect. If increased ACTH were also produced, the stimulation of the adrenal might make the initial clinical impression that of Cushing's syndrome. Without appreciation for the central lesions the adrenals might be removed.

Diffuse melanosis is seen in the cachectic and with metabolic problems such as hemochromatosis and biliary cirrhosis. It has been noted with inorganic arsenical poisoning and with a number of drugs, including busulfan and long-term high dose chlorpromazine. In malignancies such as melanoma, melanin may be deposited directly in the dermis. With certain tumors, as of the lung, MSH-like peptides have been identified which stimulate generalized darkening.

black, with the pigment orderly and the skin markings preserved (Fig. 16). Compound and intradermal nevi (Fig. 17) may be dome shaped, polypoid, or even verrucoid. They may be deeply pigmented but mostly are light or even skin colored.

Occasionally a depigmented area may develop around a nevus cell nevus, sometimes with eventual obliteration of the nevus. Occurring primarily in children and young adults, the *"halo nevus"* has been associated with vitiligo and noted in melanoma.

Not nevi but sometimes confused with them are *seborrheic keratoses*, the benign keratotic tumor of aging. Their distribution, growth, and depth of pigment are sunlight related, and their numbers can be legion. Beginning as yellow to light brown flat lesions with a verrucous or velvety surface, they can develop from less than 1 cm to several centimeters, become dark brown with a greasy keratotic scale, and assume a "tacked on" appearance.

Their importance is in differentiating them from nevi or not overlooking a changing nevus among them; also, they have been reported in their explosive appearance or sudden enlargement to be associated with underlying malignancy (the sign of Leser-Trélat).

Pigment in Patterns

Whorls of pigmentation, zebra stripes, and angular flecks and sprays, occurring in no known neural or anatomic configuration and crossing the midline, should suggest *incontinentia pigmenti* (Fig. 18). The macules are dark brown or slate colored and intensely pigmented in childhood. With gradual fading they leave few dermatologic residua in later adult life. However, the pat-

Figure 19.   Melasma.

DEPIGMENTATION

Partial Albinism

Areas of depigmentation in otherwise normal skin have a limited differential diagnosis. In partial albinism or piebaldism, the depigmentation is unchanged from birth, with melanocytes absent in the white areas. It is inherited as a simple autosomal dominant; there is often an associated white forelock. When it occurs with Waardenburg's syndrome, there is perceptual deafness and heterochromia iridis.

Vitiligo

Vitiligo can be present from infancy but usually is not. Half the patients note the onset before the third decade. Pigment is lost in exposed areas, about body orifices, over pressure points, and from the axillae, genitalia, hair, and nevi (halo nevus). Occurring in 0.5 per cent of the population of the United States, vitiligo is inherited as a dominant trait. Familial early graying is frequently found. Melanocytes, present from birth, persist in the vitiliginous areas for a time but eventually disappear. Autoimmune mechanisms have been suggested for the melanocyte destruction, and also the converse, the failure to protect against toxic intermediates generated during melanogenesis.

Individuals with vitiligo are usually healthy, but the prevalence of vitiligo is higher than expected among patients with diseases suspected of autoimmune pathogenesis: pernicious anemia, thyroid dysfunction, Addison's disease, and alopecia areata. Circulating antibody for gastric parietal cell antigens, thyroglobulin,

HYPOPIGMENTATION

Localized

In assessing a circumscribed area of leukoderma the distinction between hypopigmentation and depigmentation is crucial, and should be confirmed by Wood's light examination, which shows the depigmented lesion as ivory white.

Tuberous Sclerosis

A polygonal hypomelanosis, an ovoid lesion rounded at one end and tapered at the other like the leaf of a mountain ash, is seen from birth in 85 per cent of patients with tuberous sclerosis. Found in the skin over trunk and limbs, the lesions range in size from a few millimeters to several centimeters. They appear before the other skin signs and can be of signal value in the differential diagnosis of seizures. By age four, 90 per cent of patients will have developed *adenoma sebaceum* (Fig. 20) — actually angiofibromas without sebaceous gland involvement. Clinically these are red-pink nodules with a smooth surface found at the nasolabial folds, over the cheeks and chin, and occasionally on the forehead and scalp. In the lumbosacral area the shagreen patch, a circumscribed area of subepidermal fibrosis, is almost always found. Skin-colored and slightly raised, it resembles studded leather. The ungual fibromas, soft pink papules growing out from the nail bed, are the fourth skin sign of tuberous sclerosis and appear first at puberty.

Figure 20.   Tuberous sclerosis angiofibromas.

Figure 21. Neurofibromatosis—von Recklinghausen's disease.

the same ocular features, but no deficiency of cutaneous pigment, is inherited as a sex-linked recessive.

Fitzpatrick, T. B., Quevedo, W. C., and Witkop, C. J.: Albinism. *In* Stanbury, J. B., Wyngaarden, J. B., and Fredrickson, D. S. (eds.): The Metabolic Basis of Inherited Disease. 4th ed. New York, McGraw-Hill Book Company, 1978, pp. 283–316.

Gorlin, R. J., Anderson, R. C., and Blaw, M.: Multiple lentigines syndrome. Am. J. Dis. Child., 117:652, 1969.

Lerner, A. B.: Vitiligo. Prog. Dermatol., 6:1, 1972.

573.6.   NEUROFIBROMAS

Clinical neurofibromatosis of the skin (Fig. 21) is no diagnostic challenge. With its multiple skin-colored pedunculated tumors and subcutaneous nodules along nerve sheaths, the cosmetic disfigurement is vivid and remembered. If the disease is early, or not fully expressed, or even without the disease at all, an individual may have a solitary neurofibroma, an organoid overgrowth of Schwann cells and endoneurium that presents clinically as a smooth, flesh-colored, dome-shaped papule, soft to firm, looking rather like an intradermal nevus. A doughy feel and the ability to invaginate the lesion could aid the differential diagnosis. When seen in association with the café-au-lait spots (Fig. 22) and axillary freckles as described above, the diagnosis should be made.

Neurofibromatosis of von Recklinghausen is a dominantly inherited disorder with systemic manifestations in the nervous system, bone, and soft tissues as well as skin. Half the cases are sporadic, presumably representing new mutations, but once expressed they will transmit the disease as a mendelian dominant. It occurs in one of 3000 births and has a prevalence of 0.04 per cent.

and adrenal antigens has been demonstrated in patients with vitiligo, with and without endocrine pathology or pernicious anemia. In adult onset diabetes, vitiligo is encountered five times more frequently than in controls. Further, a number of ocular syndromes with uveitis, as well as gastritis, gastric cancer, IgA deficiency, and melanoma, are reported with vitiligo.

When vitiligo is *universal* and includes the hair, eye color remains. Even without a history of pigment loss, such a totally depigmented patient is readily distinguished from the albino. There is no photophobia. Biopsy would also differentiate between the two, for melanocytes are present in normal numbers in the albino; the pathology is in the enzyme tyrosinase which is defective or absent.

Albinism

Albinism may be oculocutaneous or may involve only the eyes. In the oculocutaneous group there are various degrees of expression relating to the completeness of the defect in the tyrosinase. Two types are distinguished: tyrosinase positive and tyrosinase negative, according to plucked hair darkening upon incubation with tyrosine. The deficiency of pigment in hair and skin is thus variable, as it is in the ocular fundi and irides. Horizontal nystagmus is observed, along with photophobia and refractive errors, especially myopia. With time and sunlight there is severe actinic damage to the skin. The prevalence of oculocutaneous albinism in the general population is given as between 0.004 and 0.02 per cent; among the Cuna Indians off the Panama coast it is between 1 and 7 per cent. It is inherited as an autosomal recessive; ocular albinism which shows

Figure 22.   Café-au-lait spot.

The pigmentary stigmata of neurofibromatosis can be present at birth, and 90 per cent of patients with the disease will have them. The tumors, with rare exceptions, begin to develop after birth but before puberty, becoming constantly more numerous throughout life. They may arise in all tissues, including bone and lung, in which they cause cystic lesions. Bone lesions, occurring in half the patients, are quite variable, and may represent growth disturbances as well as erosion by tumor. Scoliosis, severe kyphoscoliosis with gibbus formation, lordosis, and pseudoarthrosis are seen. Of greater significance are the neurofibromas in the brain or cranial nerves, eye, or bowel. Full mental capacity may be diminished by the disease, and mental deficiency is not unusual. Bilateral acoustic neuromas lead to deafness; gliomas of the optic nerve present with exophthalmia and decreased visual acuity. There may be nodules of the iris and hamartomas of the retina.

In patients with pheochromocytoma, 5 to 10 per cent have neurofibromatosis; bilateral pheochromocytomas occur. The presenting sign is usually hypertension, but this might also be the result of renal vascular anomalies such as atresia associated with the disease. In a syndrome of familial amyloid-producing medullary carcinoma of the thyroid and pheochromocytoma, one patient with bilateral pheochromocytoma had neurofibromatosis. Malignant pheochromocytoma with metastases has been reported.

Although the quality of life is severely compromised in von Recklinghausen's disease, the prognosis for survival is fairly good. Mesenteric and colonic neurofibroma may cause obstruction or result in bleeding. There is risk of malignancy — 5 to 16 per cent in various series. The malignant tumors seen are not always neurofibrosarcomas or histologically malignant nonmetastasizing brain tumors, but may be liposarcomas, rhabdomyosarcomas, or undifferentiated sarcomas. The dangers for patients with neurofibromatosis are hypertension and sudden enlargement of a tumor. Blood pressure should be checked regularly and tumors with growth spurts biopsied. In younger patients, or those with limited numbers of lesions, continuing excisions of neurofibromas of the head and arms may contain the cosmetic disfigurement.

Crowe, F. W.: Axillary freckling as a diagnostic aid in neurofibromatosis. Ann. Intern. Med., 61:1142, 1964.
Fienman, N. L., and Yakovac, W. C.: Neurofibromatosis in childhood. J. Pediat., 76:339, 1970.
Person, J. R., and Perry, H. O.: Recent advances in phakomatoses. Int. J. Dermatol., 17:1, 1978.
Schenkein, I., Beuker, E. D., Helson, L., Axelrod, F., and Dancis, J.: Increased nerve-growth-stimulating activity in disseminated neurofibromatosis. N. Engl. J. Med., 290:613, 1974.
Snyder, S. H.: Nerve growth in neurofibromatosis (editorial). N. Engl. J. Med., 290:626, 1974.

573.7.   PSEUDOXANTHOMA ELASTICUM

A change in the skin of the neck and axilla that is reticular and sometimes telangiectatic, with small 1- to 3-mm tan-yellow papules resembling chicken skin, should bring pseudoxanthoma elasticum to mind. Although actinic damage might be considered in the differential diagnosis, especially of early cases, the occurrence of lesions in covered areas of the body would distinguish it from sun-induced change. The problem is an inherited disorder of elastic tissue, transmitted as an autosomal recessive trait, that involves the skin, eyes, and vascular system. Prevalence rates are estimated at 0.001 to 0.006 per thousand, and females are affected more frequently than males.

The skin lesions develop in the second decade or later and are progressive. Characteristically seen at the sides of the neck, in axilla, and in groin, they may be found in the flexural areas of arms and legs or about the umbilicus, and may involve the breast and penis or even the mucosal surfaces of the mouth, vagina, rectum, and stomach. Initially, and in mild cases, the small papules are best seen in stretched skin. Eventually, there will be thickening of the skin and redundancy with exaggerated folds. The earliest histologic change evident is deposits of calcium on elastic fibers that seem otherwise normal. Fibrils with the histochemical characteristics of elastin show autofluorescence. Although the epidermis and upper corium remain normal, large aggregates of granular material with the properties of elastic fibers form in the mid-dermis. Collagen is decreased.

The full expression of the defect, known as Grönblad-Strandberg syndrome, consists of the distinctive and diagnostic skin lesions, angioid streaks of the retina, and vascular abnormalities. The combination of skin and eye changes is found most often (60 per cent); eye changes only are found in 30 per cent; skin changes only are found least frequently (10 per cent). Nearly all patients (80 per cent) have some cardiovascular abnormality.

The angioid streaks, which underlie the retinal vessels, cross the fundus radially from the optic disc. Flat red to brown or gray lines, several times wider than the retinal vessels, they represent breaks in the elastic tissue of Bruch's membrane. Although the angioid streaks do not limit vision unless the macula is involved, retinal hemorrhage from damaged vessels and chorioretinitis may lead to severe visual difficulties. Angioid streaks are also seen with Paget's disease of the bone, Ehlers-Danlos syndrome, and sickle cell anemia.

The vascular lesions can present as internal hemorrhage. Gastrointestinal bleeding, occurring in 10 per cent of patients, may be the initial event in an unsuspected case. Although there may be a peptic ulcer or hiatal hernia aggravated by the vascular defect, often no specific cause of the bleeding is found. Hematuria is seen, and hypertension is found in half the patients secondary to renal artery involvement, beginning as early as the second decade. By age 30 radiographic demonstration of arterial calcification is found in many patients, along with diminished or absent peripheral pulses and associated intermittent claudication. These premature and advanced arterial changes lead to angina, arrhythmias, and cerebrovascular occlusion and hemorrhage.

The prognosis for an individual patient with pseudoxanthoma elasticum is uncertain. Many have a normal life span, some may have visual impairment, and a few may become blind. The skin lesions of signal importance in labeling the defect are of questioned correlative value for the intensity and scope of the defect, and ultimately are only of cosmetic consequence often helped by plastic repair. The hypertension must be managed, but risk from hemorrhage in viscera or brain, or from coronary occlusion, persists.

Altman, L. K., Fialkow, P. J., Parker, F., and Sagebiel, R. W.: Pseudo-xanthoma elasticum, an underdiagnosed genetically heterogenous disorder with protean manifestations. Arch. Intern. Med., 134:1048, 1974.

McKee, P. H., Cameron, C. H. S., Archer, D. B., and Logan, W. C.: A study of four cases of pseudoxanthoma elasticum. J. Cut. Pathol., 4:146, 1977.

McKusick, V. A.: Heritable Disorders of Connective Tissue. 4th ed. St. Louis, C. V. Mosby Company, 1972.

573.8. NODOSE LESIONS OF THE LEG

The differential diagnosis of tender erythematous nodules of the lower legs is not so much of the lesion itself, which is a reaction pattern, but of the number of significant diagnoses which are characterized by such lesions. The cutaneous nodules vary in size, number, and location, appear suddenly or gradually, and disappear over weeks or months with or without scar or ulceration. They are sorted out according to their onset, course, distribution, and associations.

ERYTHEMA NODOSUM

Appearing acutely is the classic erythema nodosum, recognized as a clinical entity since 1798 and associated with a variety of infections and drug reactions. It is considered a hypersensitivity vasculitis; the ordinary presentation is of bilateral pretibial red nodules, occasionally with lesions of the extensor aspect of the arms. Rare in children and the elderly, it is seen most commonly between 15 and 23 years and is found in females three times more often than in males. According to the country and prevailing infections, it will be reported with tuberculosis, leprosy, sarcoid, streptococcal pharyngitis, pertussis, measles, primary atypical pneumonia, lymphogranuloma venereum, gonorrhea, syphilis, and also the superficial and deep fungus infections. It is seen in chronic ulcerative colitis and, less frequently, in regional enteritis or as a reaction to drugs such as iodides, bromides, sulfonamides, arsphenamine, contraceptives, and others.

The onset is often associated with fever and arthralgia, and occasionally with gastrointestinal upsets. It is a self-limited disease with a three- to five-week course and resolution without scarring. Recurrences and relapses occur in fewer than 10 per cent of patients. Any hematologic or roentgenographic abnormalities observed would be those of the underlying disease, to which the therapy should be directed. In more than a quarter of the cases, however, no etiology can be determined.

The histopathologic changes in the skin are nonspecific and are completely reversible. The venous walls can be edematous and the fat lobules show disintegration, but there is no leukocytoclastic or lymphocytic angiitis.

ACUTE FEBRILE NEUTROPHILIC DERMATOSIS

The same is true of the rare, self-limiting acute febrile neutrophilic dermatosis of Sweet. Characterized by high persistent fever with painful nodules and plaques occurring asymmetrically over the extremities, face, and neck, it is often noted to follow an upper respiratory infection and is considered a probable hypersensitivity reaction. The disease is reported most in middle-aged women, in whom it is associated with leukocytosis and an elevated sedimentation rate. Histopathologic examination of the skin lesions shows vasodilatation and endothelial swelling, with infiltration of polymorphonuclear leukocytes in the upper and mid-dermis. There is no suppuration and no scarring.

NODULAR LIQUEFYING PANNICULITIS

In this condition, by contrast, there are foci of fat necrosis with preservation of cell membranes but with basophilic granular changes of the cytoplasm, as well as loss of nuclear staining in the fat septum to produce characteristic ghost-like cells. The recurrent crops of red painful nodules 0.5 to 5 cm, which appear on the legs but occasionally elsewhere, can be noted to soften and drain a viscous aseptic material as evidence of fat liquefaction. Associated with pancreatitis or occasionally with acinous adenocarcinoma of the pancreas, the fat necrosis has been attributed to the action of the pancreatic enzyme lipase on the subcutaneous fat. Occurrences may be associated with episodes of abdominal pain, polyarthritis, and fever. The problem is rare. The differential diagnosis is that of other nodular lesions of the leg rather than Weber-Christian disease, a nonsuppurative panniculitis in which the nodular lesions are primarily on the trunk and thighs, and are associated with fever and recurrence.

ERYTHEMA INDURATUM

This chronic recurring nodular vasculitis of the lower legs is not rare, at least in Europe or Japan. It is found predominantly in women from the teens to old age; there are peak appearances in adolescence and at the menopause. Histologically panniculitis and vasculitis are seen, along with a granulomatous reaction that may be nonspecific or tuberculoid.

The lesions occur mostly on the posterior rather than anterior aspect of the lower legs and, rarely, on the thighs. The nodules, painful to pressure, may ulcerate with subsequent scarring, or resorb, leaving an atrophic depressed surface. Traditionally associated with tuberculosis, active disease is hardly ever found. Most observers now designate a group of nodose lesions as nodular vasculitis and distinguish between those associated with tuberculous infection (erythema induratum of Bazin) and those not.

The usual course of the problem is protracted and subject to remission and exacerbations. If there is antecedent or current evidence of tuberculosis infection, antituberculous therapy may be beneficial.

573.9. CUTANEOUS MANIFESTATIONS OF INTERNAL MALIGNANCY

Of the many dermatologic signs described thus far, many have been noted to be associated with malignancy as well as with other pathologic processes. This chapter focuses on noncutaneous malignancy as it relates to the skin, and reviews the symptoms and signs that make one think first of tumor, either with assurance or with grave suspicion.

TUMOR

Internal malignancy may extend or metastasize to the skin. Primary lesions in lung or bone can appear by direct lymphatic extension but usually not until the primary is of considerable size. Metastatic lesions, however, may be the first sign of tumor; solitary papules or nodules, firm or hard, and often of innocent appearance, they are found freely movable in the skin or just beneath it. One notable exception is the inflammatory sclerosing breastplate of cutaneous metastases, the carcinoma en cuirasse that occurs with malignancy of the breast. In order of decreasing frequency, metastatic tumors to the skin will originate from breast, (50 per cent), stomach (15 to 30 per cent), lung (12 per cent), uterus (9 per cent), kidney (9 per cent), and, less often, colon, prostate, ovary, or testicle. Any nodule or plaque of obscure origin and uncertain diagnosis should be biopsied, especially if there are reasons to suspect malignancy. The anaplastic cells may or may not define the origin of the tumor, but they will identify it clearly as noncutaneous.

NONTUMOR

Without the stamp of malignant tumor cells, there are certain ominous cutaneous signs that indicate malignancy. *Intense pruritus* is one. The malignant itching of lymphoma or Hodgkin's disease is often refractory to all therapy except the successful treatment, at least to remission, of the underlying pathology. The pruritus can be intolerable and unremitting, and can lead to suicide. It may begin with the feet or legs, often associated with burning sensations, and then become generalized. Initially the skin may appear normal except for excoriations and the occasional papules or nodules that are the cutaneous response to the trauma of scratching. With leukemia, the normal-appearing skin may become erythematous until there is a generalized erythroderma or even exfoliation.

It is the intensity and persistence of the pruritus that is such a powerful indicator of malignancy. This is not so with milder, intermittent itching. Although it, too, can occur with tumor, or herald it, as for example with gastrointestinal malignancies and those of the bronchus, ovaries, and prostate, the variability in severity and localization of the itching makes it a weaker signal. In the older patient the most common cause of pruritus is dry skin. If the skin appears normal, however, and there is no underlying thyroid disease or diabetes, and if the symp-

TABLE 5. Cutaneous Lesions Associated with Malignancy

Lesion or Syndrome	Description and Distribution	Malignancy
Frequent association:		
Dermatomyositis (>40 yrs)	Heliotrope erythema on eyelids, upper cheeks, forehead, temples; edema of hands and arms; scaly bluish-red plaques over knuckles; erythema of scalp and alopecia; cutaneous calcification	Breast, lung, gastrointestinal tract, genitourinary system, lymphoma
Gardner's syndrome	Epidermal inclusion cysts and sebaceous cysts on scalp and face (trunk)	Colon
Acquired hypertrichosis lanuginosa	Long, fine, silky hair on face and other sites normally clinically hairless (does not involve palms and soles)	Bronchus, gallbladder, rectum, bladder
Ataxia telangiectasia	Telangiectasia on bulbar conjunctiva → ears, eyelids, cheeks, limbs; hair may be prematurely gray	Reticulum cell sarcoma, lymphosarcoma, Hodgkin's disease, gastric
Stewart-Treves syndrome	Edematous upper extremity following radical mastectomy; livid or dusky red blebs exuding fluid with lymph chemistries	Lymphangiosarcoma
Paget's disease	Marginated scaling of the nipple and areola	Breast
Leser-Trélat sign	Sudden development of a large number of seborrheic keratoses	Carcinoma of stomach
Extramammary Paget's disease	Erythematous to gray-white plaque which may be scaly, crusted, ulcerated, or papillary in appearance on vulva or perianal area	Rectum, cutaneous adnexal tumors
Systemic mastocytosis	Multiple reddish-brown or yellow macules, papules, or nodules; heavily pigmented macules or erythroderma	Mast cell leukemia
Sipple's syndrome	Multiple neuromas of lips, eyelids, nares, and anterior two thirds of tongue (pink nodules)	Thyroid, pheochromocytoma
Acquired pachydermoperiostosis	Skin of forehead and scalp thickened and thrown into folds; skin of hands and feet thickened; increased sebaceous activity on face and scalp	Bronchus, stomach, esophagus, thymus, mesothelioma
Wiskott-Aldrich syndrome	Eczematous lesions on scalp, face, flexures, and buttocks; purpura on skin and mucous membranes	Reticuloendothelial
Carcinoid	Telangiectasias on face and upper trunk; hyperpigmentation (gray-black) on legs, forearms, trunk with hyperkeratosis; yellow-brown pigmentation on forehead, back, wrists, and thighs	Metastatic carcinoids
von Hippel–Lindau syndrome	Angiomas	Hypernephroma, pheochromocytoma
Cowden's syndrome	Warty papules and nodules on central face, oral mucosa, hands, and dorsal forearms	Breast, thyroid, female reproductive
Necrolytic migratory erythema	Dermatitis of two forms: (1) generalized symmetrical dermatitis initially eczematous over perineum, buttocks, and extremities; (2) erythematous areas with central blister formation progressing to central crusting and healing, followed by hyperpigmentation of perineum, buttocks, groin, lower abdomen, and lower extremities	Glucagonoma
Erythema gyratum repens	Irregular wavy bands with peculiar gyrate or serpiginous outline, with marginal desquamation on trunk, neck, and extremities	Breast, lung, tongue
Acanthosis nigricans	Confluent hyperpigmented, hyperkeratotic verrucosities in body folds, especially axillae, nipples, and umbilicus; diffuse keratoderma of palms and soles	Adenocarcinoma of stomach, pancreas, colon, lung, breast, uterus, ovary, rectum, cystic and hepatic ducts

TABLE 5. Cutaneous Lesions Associated with Malignancy (*Continued*)

Lesion or Syndrome	Description and Distribution	Malignancy
Occasional association: Tylosis	Late onset keratosis palmaris et plantaris; diffuse palmar and plantar hyperkeratoses with hyperhidrosis	Esophageal
Systemic amyloidosis (secondary)	Small, glistening papules on eyelids, central area of face, lips, and tongue; macroglossia; nodules in auditory meatus and body flexures; small hemorrhages induced by stroking skin; may have leonine facies due to plaques	Multiple myeloma
Reticulohistiocytoma	Small, firm, pink, moderately pruritic papules or nodules on dorsa of hands, forearms, scalp, face, ears, trunk, and mucosa of lip; fluctuates in severity	Sarcoma, gastric, colon, lung
Neurofibromatosis (von Recklinghausen)	Café-au-lait spots; axillary freckles; white macular areas; multiple tumors which may be small to large, soft to firm, most numerous on trunk and limbs—rare (elephantiasis neuromatosa—wrinkled and pendulous skin with overgrowth of subcutaneous tissue along nerve trunk with diffuse neurofibromatosis)	Sarcomas pheochromocytomas, astrocytomas, gliomas
Congenital nevi	Sebaceous nevus—circumscribed, slightly raised hairless plaques of orange-yellow which become verrucous and nodular in puberty; bathing trunk nevus or other; congenital pigmented nevus—dark brown and raised surface which is irregular with small mammillary projections (may have hair, well defined margins); nevus verrucosus and nevus unius lateris—skin colored or yellow-brown with rough warty surface, more often on limbs and trunk	Melanoma, basal cell epithelioma, squamous cell carcinoma
Alopecia mucinosa	Well demarcated, slightly raised plaque which is erythematous and indurated; may have fine scale—face, neck, head	Mycosis fungoides, lymphomas
Nodular liquefying panniculitis (with pancreatitis)	Tender subcutaneous erythematous nodules, lower legs and thighs occasionally	Pancreatic carcinoma
Erythroderma	Generalized erythematous skin with scaling	Lymphoma, lung, rectum, leukemia Variable; skin lesions reported to disappear with excision of malignancy and to reappear with recurrence or metastases
Erythema annulare centrifugum	Small pink papule slowly enlarges to form a ring; as the central area flattens and fades, may attain diameter of 6 to 8 cm; buttocks, thighs, upper arms	
Thrombophlebitis migrans	Successive crops of tender, linear, and oval nodules affecting large and small vessels throughout the body	Lung, pancreas, breast, colon, stomach
Peutz-Jeghers-Touraine syndrome	Discrete mucocutaneous pigmentation, including lips, face, buccal mucosa, and hands; brown-black, discrete macular lesion 2 to 5 mm	Malignancy proximal to ligament of Treitz
Bloom's syndrome	Erythema of face most pronounced in butterfly area—may involve margins of eyelids, forehead, and ears; sunlight may provoke bullae, bleeding, and crusting	Leukemia
Cushing's syndrome	Redistribution of subcutaneous fat, vascular fragility, moon face, striae, hirsutism, obese trunk and slender limbs	Oat cell of lung, pituitary, hypothalamus, adrenal
Acquired ichthyosis	Usually starts at the legs; generalized dry, cracking skin; hyperkeratotic palms and soles; alopecia	Hodgkin's disease
Tuberous sclerosis	Adenoma sebaceum—firm discrete, yellow or telangiectatic papules 1 to 10 mm to extend from nasolabial fold, occasionally in the ear; periungual fibroma and smooth firm, flesh-colored excrescences emerging from nailbeds (5 to 10 mm); shagreen patch—irregular soft, elevated plaque in lumbosacral area; ash leaf spots; poliosis	Brain, rhabdomyoma
Dyskeratosis congenita	Dystrophic nails, suppurative paronychia, fine reticulate gray-brown pigment on neck, thighs, and involving greater part of trunk with telangiectasias; face is red and atrophic with irregular macular pigmentation; mucous membranes—bullae, erosions, and leukoplakia; hands and feet—atrophic shiny skin; palms and soles may be hypohidrotic and form bullae with trauma	Carcinoma develops in area of leukoplakia (squamous cell)

tom of pruritus is new and unresponsive to simple measures, then malignancy is suspect.

Other strong signals of malignancy include *Paget's disease of the breast* (see Ch. 573.4), which is almost invariably associated with underlying breast carcinoma. Dusky papules arising on a persistently edematous upper extremity following radical mastectomy indicate a lymphangiosarcoma until proved otherwise (Stewart-Treves syndrome). Nodules arising in a giant pigmented hairy nevus are almost certainly indicative of melanoma (see Ch. 574.5).

Lesser signals, but those still with frequent association of malignancy, may be grouped as the systemic and/or cutaneous signs which appear in previously normal individuals, as distinct from those cutaneous markers which identify an antecedent syndrome or inherited diathesis that places an individual at greater risk of malignancy.

The onset of weakness and the heliotrope erythema of *dermatomyositis* are frequently associated with malignancy in those over 40 years of age. It precedes the appearance of the tumor by six months in most cases (80 per cent), but they may appear together. At least two patients, one with a malignancy of the breast, the other of the lung, have been shown to have an immediate intradermal reaction to tumor extracts and also positive passive transfer reactions.

Color changes of the skin are far less specific; the pallor of anemia, the flush of carcinoid, the dusky erythema of polycythemia, and the hyperpigmentation secondary to excessive MSH or MSH-like peptides all can be associated with malignancy, but they may not be. The same holds true for the altered keratinization limited to the palms and soles or generalized, and the erythemas: generalized exfoliative erythroderma, erythema nodosum, and urti-

TABLE 6. Cutaneous Lesions Associated with Gastrointestinal Disease

Diseases	Lesion and Description	Gastrointestinal Disorders and Symptoms	Other
Disorders Associated with Gastrointestinal Bleeding			
Degos' disease	Pink papules → small white scar with peripheral telangiectasias; spares palms, soles, and face	Cramps, vomiting, enteritis, bowel perforation, hemorrhage	CNS involvement
Osler-Weber-Rendu syndrome	Telangiectasias (multiple), especially upper half of body	Hemorrhage, hepatic arteriovenous anastomoses, hepatomegaly, cirrhosis	Epistaxis
Syndrome of phlebectasia of jejunum, oral cavity, and scrotum	Fordyce lesions (scrotum), caviar spots (tongue), phlebectasia (buccal mucosa and lips)	Hemorrhage and ulcer symptoms	
Blue rubber bleb disease	Cutaneous hemangiomas (predominantly on trunk and arms)	Hemorrhage; lesions involve liver and spleen	Lesions in CNS, lung, kidney, adrenal
Ehlers-Danlos syndrome	Easy bruising, fragile skin, pseudotumors at pressure points, stretchability of skin	Hiatal hernia, diverticula, rupture of bowel, hemorrhage	Pneumothorax, CNS bleeding, hyperextensible joints
Pseudoxanthoma elasticum	1- to 3-mm yellowish papules in plaques associated with telangiectasia, especially on neck and flexures; soft lax skin in folds at neck, axilla, umbilicus, face, antecubital fossa, groin	Hemorrhages	Angioid streaks of retina; vascular abnormalities, hypertension
Kaposi's sarcoma	Dark blue–purple macules → nodules initially on extremities; also hands, ears, nose	10% visceral involvement, hemorrhage, perforation, intestinal obstruction	
Henoch-Schönlein purpura	Erythematous macules which become papules, urticarial, purpuric, or necrotic (external aspects of limbs, buttocks, and occasionally face)	75% of patients >2 years old have abdominal complaints: colic, vomiting, diarrhea, melena, hematemesis	Arthritis; renal involvement; fever
Polyarteritis nodosa	Tender nodules in groups along superficial arteries—may be cutaneous or subcutaneous; purpuric plaques, gangrene, Osler's nodes, and splinter hemorrhages have been noted	Pain, peritonitis; infarcts in bowel, liver, spleen; hemorrhage, pancreatitis, steatorrhea, gangrene of bowel	Multisystem: hypertension, myocardial infarction, renal thrombosis; neurologic —encephalopathy, convulsions, neuritis; arthralgia; myopathy
Disorders Associated with Gastrointestinal Polyposis			
Gardner's syndrome	Epidermal and sebaceous cysts, inclusion cysts; primarily on face and scalp	45% incidence of malignancy of colonic polyps	Osteomas, desmoid tumors
Peutz-Jeghers-Touraine syndrome	2- to 5-mm brown-black macules on lips, face, buccal mucosa, hands	Polyps with predilection for jejunum and ileum (malignancy proximal to ligament of Treitz)	
Cronkhite-Canada syndrome	Diffuse hyperpigmentation affecting palms, volar surface of fingers, face, and neck; alopecia (patchy → complete); dystrophic nails	Diarrhea, acquired polyps of gastrointestinal tract	
Disorders Associated with Dysphagia			
Scleroderma	Raynaud's, tense, smooth, hardened, and bound-down skin, starting with hands → upper extremities, face, trunk; cutaneous calcification; resorption of terminal phalanges	Dysphagia, malabsorption	Pulmonary fibrosis, arthritis
Plummer-Vinson syndrome	Angular stomatitis, brittle nails, koilonychia, atrophic tongue	Dysphagia due to strictures in esophagus	Anemia, iron deficiency
Epidermolysis bullosa	Trauma results in blisters which heal with scarring	Dysphagia due to strictures in esophagus	
Behçet's disease	Recurrent oral and genital ulcerations; pyoderma of groin and genitalia; sterile pustules at puncture sites	Dysphagia	Photophobia, uveitis, CNS abnormality
Disorders Associated with Diarrhea or Malabsorption			
Carcinoid	Flushing and patchy cyanosis and telangiectasia on face and upper trunk; hyperpigmented, hyperkeratotic lesions on legs, trunk, forearms, without hyperkeratosis on forehead, back, wrists, thighs	Diarrhea, metastatic lesions of carcinoid	Asthma, valvular heart disease, arthritis
Ulcerative colitis	3 to 34% have skin lesions: pyoderma gangrenosum (1 to 10%), purpura, aphthae, erythema nodosum, erythema multiforme, perianal fistula, and abscess (10 to 20%), pyostomatitis vegetans	Diarrhea, hemorrhage	Arthritis (46 of 555)
Systemic mastocytosis	Flushing (secondary histamine release); generalized multiple reddish-brown or yellow macules, papules or nodules, or erythroderma	Symptoms in 23%—abdominal pain, cramps, diarrhea	(Mast cell leukemia is a possible complication)
Hartnup disease	Dry, scaly, well-marginated, affecting light-exposed area; stomatitis and glossitis	Diarrhea	Cerebral ataxia; renal aminoaciduria
Acrodermatitis enteropathica	Alopecia, pustular eruption around orifices and and bullous or verrucous on extremities	Diarrhea	Zinc deficiency

TABLE 6. Cutaneous Lesions Associated with Gastrointestinal Disease (Continued)

Diseases	Lesion and Description	Gastrointestinal Disorders and Symptoms	Other
Dermatitis herpetiformis	Papular and vesicular lesions with severe pruritus over extensor surfaces; symmetrical, chronic with recurrences; mucous membranes clear	Gluten enteropathy	
Reiter's syndrome	Mucocutaneous lesions, 80% keratosis blennorrhagica of palms and soles; hyperkeratosis of scalp; onycholysis, shedding and dystrophies of nails; scrotal and penile erosions; balanitis circinata sicca	Dysentery may precede other symptoms	Nonspecific urethritis, conjunctivitis, asymmetric arthritis
Crohn's disease	20% (15 to 50%) perineal ulceration with fistula formation; occasional pyoderma gangrenosum; 20% abdominal wall sinuses	Diarrhea, obstruction, perforation	Arthritis, iritis
Dermatogenic enteropathy	Erythroderma due to psoriasis, eczema or other etiology	Steatorrhea (malabsorption)	
Malabsorption syndrome	90% stomatitis; 50% angular stomatitis, purpura, petechiae; 10 to 20% have dermatitis, either erythematous or scaling like seborrheic dermatitis or psoriasis; in others, eczema, ichthyosis, asteatosis; alopecia, Beau's lines in nails, koilonychia; hyperpigmentation: melasmic, addisonian, or pellagroid	Diarrhea	
Pellagra	Hard, rough, cracked blackish and brittle epidermis of fingers, face, neck (Casal's necklace), dorsa of hands, arms, feet; fissures on palms and soles; earlier, may have blisters	Diarrhea; 50% achlorhydria	Dementia

Disorders Associated with Liver Disease

Laennec's cirrhosis	Spider angiomas in 75%; palmar erythema; men—sparse axillary, pubic, and pectoral hair; Dupuytren's contracture; purpura; opaque white nails in 25%	Cirrhosis, hemorrhage from esophageal varices	Ascites, varices, testicular atrophy
Biliary cirrhosis	Jaundice, melanotic hyperpigmentation generalized but more prominent on exposed areas; xanthelasma; tuberous xanthomas over extensor and pressure areas; flat xanthomas in palmar creases and scars	Biliary cirrhosis	Pruritus
Total lipoatrophy	Loss of subcutaneous fat; hypertrichosis, xanthomas, axillary and inguinal folds, associated with hyperpigmentation and linear epidermal thickenings (in congenital form)	Hepatic failure hematemesis, hepatomegaly	↑ Bone growth; diabetes; hyperlipemia; enlarged genitalia; renal, neurologic, and cardiac disorders
Hemochromatosis	15 to 20% gingival, palatal, buccal, and conjunctival hyperpigmentation—pigment most noticeable on flexures; loss of pubic and axillary hair	Cirrhosis	Diabetes, hypogonadism
Symptomatic porphyria	Bullous lesions on exposed parts of body; milia; hypertrichosis; onycholysis; conjunctival injection	Chronic liver dysfunction	

Disorders Associated with Pancreatic Disease

Necrolytic migratory erythema	Symmetrical dermatitis initially eczematous over perineum, buttocks, and extremities → central blister with crusting, followed by hyperpigmentation, stomatitis	Glucagon-secreting tumor of pancreas	Weight loss, depression, anemia
Weber-Christian disease	Tender subcutaneous nodules on upper thighs and buttocks which resolve with depressed atrophic areas	Ileus, perforation	Fever, malaise
Nodular fat necrosis	Recurrent crops of red painful, inflammatory subcutaneous nodules 0.5 to 5 cm initially on legs, especially lower; in 2 to 3% of patients with pancreatic disease, heal without atrophy	Pancreatitis or pancreatic neoplasm	Fever, eosinophilia, synovitis
Grey Turner's sign	Bruise-like discoloration of skin of left flank	Pancreatitis or other abdominal hemorrhage	
Cullen's sign	Bruise around umbilicus	Acute pancreatitis or ruptured common bile duct or perforated duodenal ulcer	

Miscellaneous Disorders

Familial angioedema	Recurrent swelling of skin and mucous membranes	Nausea, vomiting, colic	Urinary symptoms, deficient in C1 esterase inhibitor
Familial Mediterranean fever	40% (8 to 45%) have erysipelas-like erythema on feet or lower legs	95 to 98% have abdominal pain	Fever, chest pain, arthralgia, renal amyloidosis
Acanthosis nigricans	Gray-brown to black pigmentation with thickened skin covered by small papillomas over axilla, sides of neck, groin, anogenital region; thickened palms; nails may be brittle or ridged	Gastric adenocarcinoma	Endocrinopathy

caria. Discussed in previous chapters, they are included where appropriate in Table 5.*

Tabulated, too, are the various syndromes and dermatologic markers that are associated with malignancy. Gardner's syndrome, for example, of dominant inheritance, characterized by cutaneous cysts, fibromas, lipomas, and osteomas, is associated with colonic polyps which undergo malignant change before the age of 40 years in more than half the patients. The syndrome, although uncommon, is important to identify in an affected individual because of his high attendant risk of bowel malignancy and need for close surveillance. The purpose of Table 5 is to assemble in a readily retrievable form the many cutaneous signs and syndromes that have an association with internal malignancy. Distinction is made between those of frequent association and those less frequent.

573.10. CUTANEOUS CORRELATIONS WITH SPECIFIC ORGAN SYSTEMS

Throughout Ch. 573, the focus has been on the lesion observed to identify and differentiate it from similar clinical presentations. Since multiple etiologies can generate the same lesion, a further focus was directed to the manifestations of internal malignancy. Here, we will redistribute the dermatologic manifestations according to disorders of specific systems.

In Table 6* are the gastrointestinal problems associated with dermatologic diagnoses and lesions that may have as a complication gastrointestinal bleeding or polyposis,

*Tables 5 and 6 were compiled with Dr. Virginia Fallon-Pellicci.

TABLE 7.   Diseases with Renal and Cutaneous Manifestations

Diseases	Cutaneous Manifestations	Renal Manifestations	Other
Tumors			
Hypernephroma	Solitary vascular lesions — tend to be pedunculated	Hypernephroma	
Tuberous sclerosis	60 to 70% skin lesions; adenoma sebaceum; periungual fibroma, shagreen patch, ash leaf spots, poliosis	Benign renal hamartomas, hematuria	Mental retardation (60 to 70%), epilepsy (70%), eye lesions (8 to 40%), rhabdomyoma
von Hippel–Lindau syndrome	Angiomas of skin	20% hypernephromas	Angiomas of retina, brain, epididymis; pheochromocytoma
Anomalies of Development			
Oral-facial-digital syndrome	Short upper lip; hypertrophied frenula of lips and tongue; multilobed tongue; clefts of hard and soft palate; sparse hair; numerous milia	Polycystic kidneys	Polycystic liver; 50% mentally retarded; dental caries; brachydactyly and syndactyly
Neurofibromatosis	Neurofibromas, nodules in relation to peripheral nerves; 5 to 15% sarcomatous change in neurofibroma; café-au-lait spots; axillary freckles; oral tumors	60% oligophrenia; defect of renal tubules; osteomalacia	Spinal deformities, endocrine and neurologic abnormalities
Metabolic Disorders			
Sarcoidosis	Lupus pernio, plaques, maculopapular eruptions, erythema nodosum	25% hypercalciuria; nephrocalcinosis; polyuria, nocturnal polydipsia; 1 to 3% renal failure	Anemia, joint pain, adenopathy, CNS involvement, pulmonary fibrosis
Metastatic calcinosis	Nodules or plaques from 0.5 to 5 cm symmetrically on extremities and trunk — discharge of chalk-like material from lesions	Deposits in kidney of Ca^{++}	Blood vessels of muscles, stomach, lungs, and large blood vessels have deposits of Ca^{++}
Systemic amyloidosis, urticaria, and deafness syndrome	Urticaria	Nephropathy secondary to amyloid	Chills, malaise, deafness
Gout	Subcutaneous nodules, pink and most common on helix of ear, bursae of elbow, digits of hands and feet; chalky drainage	Renal calculi	
Cold agglutinins	Acrocyanosis	Hematuria	Anemia; may be associated with *Mycoplasma* pneumonia, reticulosarcoma, or lymphoma
Multiple myeloma	Plasmacytoma, petechial bleeding at perianal and periocular sites	Proteinuria, nephrolithiasis	Anemia; 10 to 20% amyloid; bone destruction; frequent infection; neuropathy
Diabetes mellitus	Necrobiosis lipoidica diabeticorum, granuloma annulare, carotenemia, lipodystrophy, frequent cutaneous infections	Kimmelstiel-Wilson disease; papillary necrosis	Heart, vascular, neurologic disease
Fabry's disease	Dry skin, dark red or black macule or papule in groups, especially on thighs, scrotum, and periumbilical	Hypertension, albuminuria, hematuria, uremia	Coronary artery disease, cerebrovascular attacks, eye lesions
Alcaptonuria	Skin discoloration (bluish-black) of nose tip, ear, extensor tendons, and costochondral junctions	Renal disease accelerates other abnormal findings; homogentisic acid in urine	Arthropathy
Hartnup disease	Stomatitis, glossitis; dry scaly eruption in light-exposed areas.	Aminoaciduria	Diarrhea, cerebellar ataxia, psychiatric problems
Familial Mediterranean fever	40% erysipelas-like erythema	Death from renal amyloidosis	Fever, abdominal and chest pain, arthralgia, synovitis

TABLE 7.   Diseases with Renal and Cutaneous Manifestations (*Continued*)

Diseases	Cutaneous Manifestations	Renal Manifestations	Other
Glomerulitis			
Hypersensitivity angiitis	Palpable purpura, urticaria, ulcerations	Necrotizing glomerular nephritis	Cardiac, neurologic, pulmonary, and joint involvement
Henoch-Schönlein purpura	Erythematous macules → papular and urticarial → purpuric lesions on external aspects of limbs, buttocks, face	40% microscopic hematuria (worse in adults)	Edema of feet and hands; polyarthritis; abdominal pain; fever, headache, anorexia
Scleroderma	Raynaud's, tense smooth, hardened, and bound-down skin; initially of distal extremities, spreads proximally; cutaneous calcification	Hypertension; 60% have abnormal BUN and creatinine	Arthritis, edema of hands; dysphagia; pulmonary fibrosis; malabsorption
Systemic lupus erythematosus	70 to 85% cutaneous lesions—butterfly erythema; maculopapular rash primarily above waist; chronic discoid lesions; alopecia; mucosal ulcers; periungual erythema; bullae; ecchymoses	50% renal disease (proteinuria-hematuria); 10% have nephrotic syndrome	Fever, fatigue, arthritis, pericarditis, neurologic involvement, pleural involvement
Polyarteritis nodosa	Tender nodules in group along arteries; purpuric plaques, splinter hemorrhages, Osler's nodes	Cortical infarction, glomerulosclerosis, thrombosis	Malaise, fever, weight loss, abdominal pain, neurologic and cardiac involvement, arthralgia, myopathy
Nail-patella syndrome	Nails absent or hypotrophic	Chronic glomerulonephritis, renal dysplasia	Skeletal abnormalities; decrease in size or absence of patella
Wegener's granulomatosis	50% cutaneous lesions—other 61/118 (51%); early (32/118), have papulonecrotic or vesicular lesion symmetrical on elbows, knees, buttocks; later (29/118), erythematous, purpuric, or vesicular lesions generalized; oral ulceration	Facial necrotizing glomerulitis, renal failure	CNS involvement; destruction of paranasal sinus, nasopharynx, and lung
Miscellaneous Disorders			
Osler-Weber-Rendu syndrome	Telangiectasias on upper half of body	Hematuria	Hemorrhages, epistaxis; cirrhosis, liver, atriovenous anastomoses
Pseudoxanthoma elasticum	Yellow papules 1 to 3 mm in confluent plaques on neck and flexures; skin soft and lax	Hypertension from involvement of renal arteries	Gastrointestinal hemorrhage, circulatory abnormalities, arterial degeneration
Partial lipodystrophy	Loss of subcutaneous fat from face spreading downward	Nonspecific renal abnormalities; ↑ incidence	
Erythema multiforme	Erythematous macules, bullae, and target lesions symmetrical on distal extremities	Transient albuminuria	Infections or allergies possibly related
Sickle cell disease	Leg ulcers at early age; increased pigment in lower leg	Acute pyelonephritis, hematuria	Fever, abdominal pain, osteomyelitis, bone pain
Congenital ichthyosis, mental retardation, dwarfism, and renal impairment	Nonbullous congenital ichthyosiform erythroderma, most marked on back and extensor surfaces	Elevated BUN and creatinine, 50% of glomerular filtration rate	Mental retardation, dwarfism

or that may be associated with dysphagia or diarrhea, or with hepatic or pancreatic disease. In the same way renal, hematologic, and rheumatic disorders are presented, with a synopsis of the skin pathology, in Tables 7 to 9,* respectively. The data given are not all discussed in the text, for space does not permit this, but the standard general dermatologic references cited in Ch. 568 will provide depth of detail.

574.   SELECTED SIGNIFICANT DERMATOLOGIC DIAGNOSES

574.1.   THE BLISTERING DISEASES

The concentrated accumulation of fluid in the skin sufficient to replace the pre-existent tissue structure and produce a visible vesicle or bulla can be the result of

forces as divergent as friction and infection, or may be from causes completely obscure. For blisters of unknown etiology categorization yields to microscopic morphologic grouping and to further sorting according to the clinical expression of disease. It is among these, the blisters known to be other than infectious, chemical, or traumatic, that the searchlight of immunofluorescence has been disclosing immune complexes to correlate with clinical disease and its course. Antibodies, circulating and tissue-fixed, whether cause or effect of the observed pathology, are important indicators that must be fully assessed.

In this chapter we shall assume that historical information and close observation will have enabled the examiner to identify blisters associated with solar and thermal burn, with infections such as herpes simplex, or with vesicants such as cantharidin used in the treatment of warts but found in certain stinging insects and flies. It is the differential diagnosis of the one or several blisters on a fairly normal base that is to be considered. In the physical examination, the distribution of the lesions and any extension to mucous membranes or eyes would have been noted. The tenseness of the bulla would have been assessed to estimate the morphologic depth of cleavage and whether this split is easily re-

---

*Tables 7 to 9 were compiled with Dr. Virginia Fallon-Pellicci.

TABLE 8.   Cutaneous Lesions in Disorders with a Hematologic Component

Diseases	Cutaneous Lesions	Hematologic Component	Other
Fanconi's syndrome	85% generalized olive-brown pigmentation most prominent on lower trunk, in flexures, and on neck with macules of hyper- and hypopigmentation	Hypoplastic anemia, neutropenia, thrombocytopenia, increased incidence of leukemia	Short broad hands, microcephaly, mental retardation, hypogonadism, aplasia of radii
Dyskeratosis congenita	Nail dystrophy; reticulate gray-brown pigmentation of neck, thighs, trunk; face and hands, atrophic skin; bullae on hands and feet secondary to trauma; leukoplakia on mucous membranes	Myeloid aplasia, refractory anemia, pancytopenia, blood dyscrasias, possible Fanconi's anemia	Dental abnormalities; mental and physical growth retarded
Sickle cell anemia	Leg ulcers at early age; increased pigment of lower leg	Anemia with typical red cells	Fever, abdominal pain, bone osteomyelitis
Cold agglutinin syndrome	Acrocyanosis, ulceration, gangrene	Anemia (hemolytic)	Hematuria, may be associated with *Mycoplasma* pneumonia, lymphoma, or reticulosarcoma
Gardner-Diamond syndrome	Recurrent painful erythematous and purpuric lesions	Autoerythrocyte sensitization	Psychiatric disturbances may be present
Chédiak-Higashi syndrome	Light color hair, skin, retinas, and translucent irides	Lethal defect in leukocytes	Frequent infections
Job's syndrome	Red, scaly, crusted lesions over scalp, ears, periorbital, skin, groin	Defect in polymorphonuclear neutrophil function	Recurrent pneumonia; liver, spleen, and lymph nodes enlarged
Leukemia cutis	Erythroderma, papules, nodules, nonspecific infection, purpura, urticaria	Chronic lymphocytic leukemia most common type to develop lesions (11% of patients with acute myeloblastic or monocytic leukemia, as compared to 1.3% of acute lymphoblastic leukemia, developed leukemia cutis)	
Sézary's syndrome	Pruritus and generalized erythroderma, dystrophic nails, alopecia; thickening and convolution of skin, especially on face	Variant of mycosis fungoides or leukemia form of it	Adenopathy
Systemic mastocytosis	Urticaria pigmentosa, erythroderma	Mast cell leukemia	23% flushing, diarrhea, abdominal pain
Pernicious anemia	Glossitis, vitiligo, cheilitis (pallor, hyperpigmentation, jaundice)	Anemia, B_{12} deficiency	
Plummer-Vinson syndrome	Koilonychia, glossitis, cheilitis	Microcytic hypochromic anemia	Dysphagia, cancer of upper gastrointestinal tract
Methemoglobinemia	Violet or brownish skin color	Intrinsic defect in red cell enzyme of altered structure of hemoglobin	Inherited, acquired from medications
von Willebrand's disease	Albinism; ecchymoses or hematomas	Deficiency of factor VIII (long bleeding time)	
Polycythemia	Ruddy cyanosis; erythralgia; acne urticata; polycythemia; favors face and extensor surfaces of extremities; pruritus	May be primary or secondary; primary associated with ↑ red blood cells, white blood cells, platelets; secondary with ↑ red blood cells	Splenomegaly in primary form
Congenital erythropoietic porphyria	Photosensitivity and vesiculobullous eruption in light-exposed areas; hypertrichosis, alopecia; scarring marked	Hemolytic anemia; fluorescence of red blood cells	Splenomegaly; erythrodontia; nausea and vomiting on exposure to sunlight
Erythropoietic protoporphyria	Photosensitivity resulting in swelling and erythema and burning sensation; may have vesicular eruption in center of face with small scars; skin over knuckles thickened	High concentration of protoporphyrin in red blood cells—may have fluorescence of red blood cells	Cholecystitis, cholelithiasis
Paroxysmal cold hemoglobinuria	Pain and acrocyanosis; urticaria	Hemolysis on warming	Seen in syphilis, viral infections; chills, fever, aching, asthma
Multiple myeloma	Plasmacytoma; petechial bleeding at perianal, periocular areas	Plasma cell leukemia (eventual anemia, thrombocytopenia)	Proteinuria, nephrolithiasis, amyloidosis, bone destruction, neuropathies, frequent infections
Strawberry hemangioma (multiple)	Most common on head; superficial lesions red; deeper components dark blue or purple; grow rapidly after birth; ulceration and spontaneous involution	May have thrombocytopenia	Cardiac hypertrophy due to high output; neurologic manifestations of lesions in CNS
Systemic lupus erythematosus	70 to 85% cutaneous lesions; butterfly erythema; maculopapular rash above waistline, chronic discoid lesions, alopecia; mucosal ulcers; bullae and ecchymoses occasionally; photosensitivity	Anemia, thrombocytopenia	Fever, fatigue, arthritis, renal disease, serositis, neurologic disease

TABLE 9. Diseases with Both Cutaneous and Rheumatic Components

Diseases	Cutaneous Lesions	Rheumatic Component	Other
Stevens-Johnson syndrome	Vesiculobullous and urticarial lesions; target lesions on mucous membranes and distal extremities	Arthralgias	Fever, malaise, nausea, vomiting, myalgias, chest pain, sore throat, eye involvement
Reiter's syndrome	80% have mucocutaneous lesions (macules, papules, erosions); keratoderma blennorrhagicum of palms and soles, hyperkeratosis of scalp and umbilicus, onycholysis, dystrophy of nails, balanitis circinata sicca, scrotal and penile erosions	Asymmetric arthritis of weight-bearing joints; tendinitis, fasciitis, ankylosing spondylitis	Urethritis, conjunctivitis (dysentery)
Behçet's disease	Superficial grayish erosions or deeply punched-out erosions on oral and genital mucosa; pyoderma; pustule at puncture sites	Arthralgia, noninflammatory joint effusions	Iritis or uveitis, fever, malaise, phlebitis, gastrointestinal ulcers, pericarditis, neurologic involvement

vealed or extended by light pressure or rubbing as one would skin a ripe peach (Nikolsky's sign).

Bullae that are flaccid on normal-appearing skin which is easily denuded, favoring a truncal location with associated mouth erosions, should suggest pemphigus. If few bullae are unroofed, there will still be a history of blisters. The presence of an erythematous base or of other nonbullous papular to urticarial lesions might mean erythema multiforme. Taut preserved bullae are found in pemphigoid and dermatitis herpetiformis, although in the latter the more common presentation is vesicular with marked pruritus and a characteristic distribution over the extensor aspect of the limbs, the shoulders, and the buttocks. The further diagnostic assessment and the support from biopsy and immunofluorescence studies are shown in Table 10, which is best perused after a review of the specific diseases.

PEMPHIGUS

Pemphigus is a cluster of blistering entities characterized histologically by acantholysis (see Ch. 570) with resultant fluid accumulation within bullae, and immunologically by the unexplained presence of circulating autoantibodies to an intercellular epidermal antigen. Of unknown etiology, it is found throughout the world, in both sexes, and in all races, with a reported higher incidence in Jews. The onset commonly occurs between 40 and 60 years. It has been seen in children and in families as fogo selvagem, or Brazilian wildfire. Broadly, and according to the intraepidermal level of the acantholytic blister, pemphigus is divided into suprabasilar pemphigus vulgaris and, if more superficial and just under the corneum, subcorneal pemphigus foliaceous.

Pemphigus vulgaris, which had a 95 per cent mortality before the advent of steroids, can still present acutely and run a swiftly fatal course despite therapy. More often it is a controlled but chronic problem of varying severity. Occasionally it remains localized for months with lesions of the mouth or scalp, perhaps axilla or groin; within a year or so it can be predicted to become generalized. Those presenting with mouth lesions tend to have a poorer prognosis, and some 30 to 40 per cent of all those diagnosed will succumb to the disease or side effects of therapy. The Nikolsky sign is present in uninvolved as well as involved skin, and areas readily traumatized become sloughed. When this extends to the pharynx and larynx, hoarseness is a clinical sign. In general, lesions tend to favor the seborrheic areas—the scalp; the periocular, paranasal, and perioral areas;

TABLE 10. The Blistering Diseases: Correlations with Histology and Immunofluorescence

	Pemphigus	Pemphigoid	Erythema Multiforme	Dermatitis Herpetiformis
Histology				
Blister	Intraepidermal	Subepidermal	At basal layer	Subepidermal
Special	Acantholysis	Eosinophils predominate in papillary dermis	Vacuolar alteration at basal layer, necrotic keratinocytes	Neutrophils at tips of dermal papillae
Tzanck test	Acantholytic cells	Negative	Negative	Negative
Immunofluorescence				
Indirect	Positive—intercellular*	Positive—basement membrane	Negative	Negative
Direct	Positive—intercellular	Positive—basement membrane	Negative	Positive—granular deposits in papillary dermis, less often along basement membrane
Treatment	Corticosteroids Immunosuppressives Cyclophosphamide Azathioprine Gold	Corticosteroids ?Immunosuppressives	Supportive ?Corticosteroids	Sulfones Gluten-free diet

*Antibody levels correlate with disease activity.

the presternum; the mid-back; the area around the umbilicus; and the groin. Denuded intertriginous lesions may tend to become vegetative through heaped peripheral collarettes of epidermis and crust, lending a descriptive name to the clinical subdivision of *pemphigus vegetans*. It is further classified into Neumann and Hallopeau types; the former affects younger patients, and the latter tends to follow a more benign course. Noted for pustules extending peripherally, both these pemphigus variants are characterized by vegetative lesions containing eosinophilic abscesses. Both variants can be fatal.

Pemphigus foliaceus is a milder disease, with finer, smaller lesions and more crust and scale; it almost always spares the mouth. It affects mainly the older patient, occasionally children, and is believed to occur in a localized variant as pemphigus erythematosus and as an endemic problem in Brazil, where it affects immigrants as well as Brazilians. In the era before steroids some 40 per cent succumbed.

Therapy for pemphigus includes corticosteroids, immunosuppressives, and gold in combinations which will vary according to the form and severity of the disease and the current persuasion of the practitioner. For active widespread disease, most will treat initially with high dose steroids (100 to 150 mg of prednisone or equivalent) to suppress the disease; if there is failure to respond, the dosage will be increased, perhaps doubled. When no new bullae form for several days, a slow taper is begun by first gradually reducing to zero the dosage for alternate days. If it is clear that prolonged or high dose corticosteroid therapy will be required, many elect to begin immunosuppressive therapy from the start: methotrexate,* azathioprine,* or cyclophosphamide.* Gold therapy,* too, is being used with new interest, and in some patients is reported to be effective even without initial corticosteroid control. Of note is the unexplained but beneficial effect of ACTH infusion on those whose disease is uncontrolled by more than 200 mg of prednisone or equivalent. The management of pemphigus also includes therapeutic baths, protective ointments and powders, and intralesional injection of corticosteroids when bullae are few. Disease activity can be correlated with the titer of indirect immunofluorescent intercellular antibody.

A benign suprabasalar acantholytic disease is Hailey-Hailey disease; an incompletely penetrating autosomal dominant genodermatosis also known as *benign familial chronic pemphigus*. Small flaccid vesicles are noted about the neck and in body folds where they are aggravated by heat and humidity. The disease is rarely widespread and rarely involves the mouth. Two of three patients will have a family history of the problem. All can expect prolonged spontaneous remission.

PEMPHIGOID

Pemphigoid is a chronic and comparatively benign blistering disease in which subepidermal bullae *without* acantholysis present clinically as large, tense, irregular blisters frequently on an erythematous base. It is often associated with or preceded by pruritus and an urticarial, perhaps eczematous eruption. Serum IgG antibody to basement membrane of skin, capable of fixing complement, occurs at the site of pathologic change and suggests an autoimmune pathogenesis. However, the disease cannot be transferred passively and, unlike pemphigus vulgaris, antibody levels do not correlate with disease activity.

Pemphigoid is a problem of the elderly; it is chronic and subject to exacerbations and remissions. Lesions, which may occur anywhere, favor the abdomen, groin, inner aspect of the thighs, and flexor aspect of the forearms. Mucosal lesions occur but are small; they heal readily with minor discomfort and, unlike pemphigus vulgaris, are no threat to nutrition.

In *benign mucosal pemphigoid* subepidermal bullae without acantholysis form on the mucous membranes, less often the skin, with the possibility of severe residual scarring. Women are afflicted twice as often as men, but both may have involvement of the conjunctivae as well as the oral cavity, pharynx, larynx, esophagus, genitalia, and anus. Secondary fibrous bands may lead to dysphagia, hoarseness, blindness, and stenotic anogenital orifices. Response to steroid therapy — topical, intralesional, and systemic — is poor.

Lever, W. F., and Schaumburg-Lever, G.: Immunosuppressants and prednisone in pemphigus vulgaris. Therapeutic results obtained in 63 patients between 1961 and 1975. Arch. Dermatol., 113:1236, 1977.

Penneys, N. S., Eaglstein, W. H., and Frost, P.: Management of pemphigus with gold compounds: A long-term follow-up report. Arch. Dermatol., 112:185, 1976.

Rosenberg, F. R., Sanders, S., and Nelson, C. T.: Pemphigus: A 20-year review of 107 patients treated with corticosteroids. Arch. Dermatol., 112:962, 1976.

DERMATITIS HERPETIFORMIS

Dermatitis herpetiformis is grouped with the blistering diseases. It can occasionally have bullae, but presents most often with intense pruritus and with excoriated papules or grouped vesicles in classic distribution over buttocks, shoulders, elbows and knees, and sometimes scalp, face, and ears. Histologically papillary microabscesses occur with aggregates of neutrophils leading to dermoepidermal separation and widespread destruction of the basement membrane. Direct immunofluorescent staining of uninvolved paralesional skin is positive at the dermoepidermal junction. Although IgG and IgM may be identified, as well as complement at the tips of the dermal papillae, IgA is the immunoglobulin most predominant; in fact, without it the diagnosis of dermatitis herpetiformis is in question. Since IgA does not fix complement by the direct pathway beginning with C1q, some other mechanism is necessary to implicate IgA. There is rather convincing evidence to suggest activation of the alternate pathway of complement through IgA aggregates, not unlike that which is known to occur in myeloma. Conventional complexes have been demonstrated, but circulating immunoglobulin and significant serum complement levels have not been detected.

Dermatitis herpetiformis appears between the second and fifth decades. It occurs in men twice as often as women. Of special interest, however, is its association with malabsorptive enteropathy. As in celiac disease, enzymatic disaccharidase and dipeptidase activities are decreased, and there is villous atrophy of the small intestine most apparent in the proximal jejunum. In patients diagnosed as having dermatitis herpetiformis

---

*Investigational drugs for this purpose.

with IgA deposits at the dermoepidermal junction of the skin, 19 of 23 had total or partial villous atrophy. As in the celiac syndrome they had autoantibodies to thyroid, reticulin, and parietal cells, as well as atrophic gastritis and overt pernicious anemia. Comparisons of histocompatibility indicate that HLA1, A8, and 4b have a high frequency in dermatitis herpetiformis when contrasted to normals, and even higher in adult celiac disease. No correlation can presently be made with HLA type and the presence or absence of intestinal involvement from the data at hand, but to identify villous atrophy may take more than one biopsy.

Whether dermatitis herpetiformis is a reaction pattern and whether the activity and extent of skin lesions can be correlated with observed enteropathy are not yet known. Three reports in as many years which document jejunal lymphoma complicating a clinical dermatitis herpetiformis, characterized by IgA skin deposits and intestinal villous atrophy, warrant careful consideration. Further, the riddle of antireticulin antibody titers and the degree of villous atrophy must be solved. There is a cross-reactivity reported between fraction III of gluten and reticulin. However, the anticipated favorable response to the gluten-free diet, important in the management of celiac disease, has not been noted consistently in dermatitis herpetiformis and is challenged. In a match of diet, HLA type, and mucosal abnormality in a series of 44 patients, 22 with celiac disease and 22 with dermatitis herpetiformis, milk antibody titer was used as an index of mucosal abnormality. It was similar in both groups, but antigluten antibody was consistently higher in celiac disease, suggesting that the antigluten response may not be part of the enteropathy of dermatitis herpetiformis. One patient with both diseases finds that her dermatitis herpetiformis is not benefited by the gluten-free diet that controls her celiac disease.

The classic case of dermatitis herpetiformis is not difficult to diagnose, and at its onset the severe pruritus and paucity of lesions might be confused only with scabies, which the telltale burrow and mite would differentiate. Halogens have been known to aggravate the disease or even to provoke it, and thus may provide a clue. A skin patch test with 20 per cent KI is frequently positive and has been known to induce characteristic lesions with IgA deposition. One last and perhaps definitive test is the therapeutic response to sulfapyridine or diaminodiphenylsulfone, each of which has a dramatic beneficial effect that suppresses pruritus and lesions in 12 to 24 hours. The individual dose required to maintain the patient must be titrated. The end-point is surprisingly sharp. Because the medications must be continued for long periods, there is considerable risk of hematologic or perhaps carcinogenic effects (sulfone), or hepatic and renal side effects (sulfa); hence treatment must be monitored closely.

Baker, P. G., and Palmer, R. K.: Autoantibodies in patients with coeliac disease and dermatitis herpetiformis. Lancet, 1:750, 1976.

Charlesworth, E. N., Backe, J. T., and Garcia, R. L.: Iodide-induced immunofluorescence in dermatitis herpetiformis. Arch. Dermatol., 112:555, 1976.

Fausa, O., Larsen, T. E., Husby, G., and Thune, P.: Gastro-intestinal investigations in dermatitis herpetiformis. Acta Derm. Venereol., 55:203, 1975.

O'Donoghue, D. P., Lancaster-Smith, M., Johnson, G. D., and Kumar, P. J.: Gastric lesion in dermatitis herpetiformis, Gut, 17:185, 1976.

Scott, B. B., and Losowsky, M. D.: Gluten antibodies in coeliac disease and dermatitis herpetiformis. Gut, 17:398, 1976.

Silk, D. B. A., Mowat, N. A. C., Riddell, R. H., and Kirby, J. D.: Intestinal lymphoma complicating dermatitis herpetiformis. Br. J. Dermatol., 96:555, 1977.

HERPES GESTATIONIS

Should an extremely pruritic vesiculobullous disease occur in pregnancy, the most likely diagnosis is herpes gestationis. If the pregnancy is early and unsuspected, the grouped vesicles and intense pruritus might suggest dermatitis herpetiformis, but the lesions lack symmetry and pigmentation, are frequently bullous and occasionally urticarial, and resemble erythema multiforme more than any other diagnosis. Histopathologically they are subepidermal bullae with abundant eosinophils indistinguishable from those of bullous pemphigoid. The possibility of a toxic or allergic reaction to fetal or placental protein or their metabolites, or to hormones, has been considered but remains unproved. With exacerbations and remission the disease is likely to persist throughout the pregnancy and perhaps into the puerperium, especially if the onset is just ante partum. It can recur with the menses for a year or more after delivery and is likely to recur with subsequent pregnancies.

The problem for the mother is only one of discomfort, but for the fetus it is significant, with threat of abnormalities or death. Recent experience with successful outcome using systemic steroids would give a more optimistic, although guarded, prognosis.

Pruritus in pregnancy with erythematous papules in the absence of blisters may represent the rare papular dermatitis of Spangler that is generalized, intensely pruritic, difficult to control, and also associated with fetal risk. In the more benign prurigo gestationis of Besnier, without threat to the fetus, the pruritic papules occur mostly over the extremities in the last trimester and are usually amenable to topical therapy. In the differential diagnosis both conditions suggest drug eruptions and excoriations from other causes of pruritus, rather than any of the blistering diseases.

ERYTHEMA MULTIFORME

Erythema multiforme is a reaction pattern in the skin and mucous membranes, an angiitis which in the upper corium leads to symptomless erythematous lesions, perhaps edematous or bullous, that darken with age, leaving the concentric rings of an "iris" or "target" lesion. Acute appearances and recurrences have been associated with recognized infections such as herpes simplex and, more recently, *Mycoplasma pneumoniae*, as well as with vaccinations, drugs, melignancy, deep x-ray therapy, and even infectious mononucleosis, but a third of the cases defy explanation. The expression of erythema multiforme may range from minor disease with a few scattered lesions to major illness with extensive bullous erosions, life-threatening fever, and prostration. The syndrome described and named erythema exsudativum multiforme by Hebra in 1866 was not familiar to Stevens and Johnson, who reported "a new eruptive fever with stomatitis and ophthalmia" in 1922, giving their names to the extreme expression of the disease.

In the severe form, erythema multiforme can be associated with mild prodromal symptoms suggestive of an upper respiratory infection that would be unremarkable except for the very sudden and dramatic eruption that ensues. The eyes are involved almost as often as the mouth and vagina. Endoscopy reveals erosions of the esophagus and colon, leading to gastrointestinal symptoms. Nephritis and uremia may be a further complication. Its course lasts two to four weeks or longer, and is prone to recur. Although systemic steroids are usually used in severe cases, the improvement is not as prompt as expected in steroid-responsive blistering diseases and can be questioned. An underlying cause of erythema multiforme must always be sought, particularly with recurrent disease. Although most patients are between 10 and 30, in those over 50 years old a search for malignancy is warranted.

TOXIC EPIDERMAL NECROLYSIS

This eruption resembles scalded skin and may not be in the clinical differential of classic erythema multiforme, but the reaction pattern is analogous. Both diseases probably represent part of a continuous disease spectrum. Toxic epidermal necrolysis has a prodrome followed by the appearance of erythema and the loss of skin in sheets, with a threat of death and liability of recurrence. Two forms are recognized: one occurring mainly in young children with associated staphylococcal infections of phage Type 71, and the other affecting adults or older children and associated with drugs or other infections and conditions. When toxic epidermal necrolysis is induced by staphylococcal toxins, the epidermal cleavage is in the malpighian or granular layer, in contrast to the subepidermal split of toxic epidermal necrolysis from other causes. The prognosis is good. It is now separately labeled the staphylococcal scalded skin syndrome (SSSS), the histology reflecting the effect of toxin on the intercellular region of the lower granular layer without significant cytotoxic change in adjacent cells. The usefulness of corticosteroids and antimicrobial agents in the course of the epidermal change has not been demonstrated; but with the delay in developing a humoral response to staphylococcal toxin, and risk of contagion, specific prompt antimicrobial therapy is indicated. In toxic epidermal necrolysis of other causes, the epidermal cleavage occurs just above or at the basal layer as a result of basal cell disintegration. Although non-staphylococcal infections, immunizations, and vaccinations have been implicated, the reaction is more often precipitated by drugs such as the sulfonamides, phenylbutazone, penicillin, hexametaphosphate, tetracycline, mithramycin, barbiturates, aspirin, amidopyrine, procaine, phenolphthalein, allopurinol, dapsone, gold salts, and hydantoin. Even a gin and tonic has caused toxic epidermal necrolysis, presumably from the quinine, and it has been reported following inhalation of acrylonitrile, a pesticide. Since the full thickness of the epidermis is separated in toxic epidermal necrolysis, the serum loss is greater and the prognosis is more guarded. Unlike staphylococcal scalded skin syndrome the mucous membranes are often involved, and associated membranoproliferative glomerulonephritis has been noted.

The clear histologic distinction between staphylococcal scalded skin syndrome and toxic epidermal necrolysis of other causes makes the biopsy an important diagnostic tool for differentiation and prognosis. By using the Nikolsky sign to advantage, skin peeled from a fresh wound of staphylococcal scalded skin syndrome shows, on frozen section, the stratum corneum with focally adherent granular cells. The Tzanck smear from the denuded base has broad cells with a low nucleus-to-cytoplasm ratio. In toxic epidermal necrolysis the full thickness of the epithelium is found on the frozen peeled specimen and the Tzanck preparation shows inflammatory cells, basal cells, and a high nucleus-to-cytoplasm ratio. Further, direct immunofluorescent staining in toxic epidermal necrolysis has shown intercellular fixation of immunoglobulins and complement at the basal cell layer, suggesting that drugs bind to intercellular epidermal protein and that the basal cells are the site of damage. Therapy is supportive with close attention to fluid balance, but corticosteroids or even renal dialysis may be required.

574.2. MUCOCUTANEOUS LYMPH NODE SYNDROME

A recently recognized entity, presently observed only in children, the mucocutaneous lymph node syndrome is included with the blistering diseases and erythema multiforme because of the ocular and conjunctival involvement, the mucous membrane erythema and erosions, and the severe prostration with fever, rash, and lymphadenopathy. Of obscure etiology and unresponsive to recognized therapy, it can be associated with myocardial involvement and death from coronary artery occlusion.

First reported in Japan in 1967 and observed there in epidemic proportions, it has also been documented in Caucasian children. It presents with ulcerative gingivitis, rhinitis, and fever which can last one to two weeks. On the third day or so of illness, a generalized macular eruption appears with intense bright erythema and edema of the palms and soles, followed by desquamation of the skin of fingers and toes. Proteinuria, pyuria, diarrhea, and mild icterus may be observed, with leukocytosis and a shift to the left, slight anemia, and perhaps an elevated transaminase. There are complaints of photophobia and arthralgia.

Although the course is usually benign and self-limited, sudden death has been reported in 1 to 2 per cent of patients; electrocardiograms have suggested myocarditis or pericarditis in 70 per cent of cases. Further, abnormal coronary angiograms were noted in more than half of 20 patients studied three weeks to four years after their illness.

Darby, C. P., and Kyong, C. U.: Mucocutaneous lymph node syndrome. JAMA, 236:2295, 1976.
Kato, H., Koike, S. , Yamamoto, M., Ito, Y., and Yano, E.: Coronary aneurysms in infants and young children with acute febrile mucocutaneous lymph node syndrome. J. Pediat., 86:892, 1975.
Kawasaki, T., Kosaki, F., Okawa, S., Shigematsu, I., and Yanagawa, H. L.: A new infantile acute febrile mucocutaneous lymph node syndrome (MLNS) prevailing in Japan. Pediatrics, 54:271, 1974.

574.3. BEHÇET'S DISEASE

So often considered in the differential diagnosis of erythema multiforme because of oral and genital erosions with inflammatory ocular disease, Behçet's disease is best considered here. A chronic and frequently multisystem disease, it is characterized by the triad cited and often by joint and bowel disease, with vasculitis important to the pathogenesis.

Most patients have arthralgias and arthropathy with polyarthritis and hydrarthrosis. Thrombophlebitis occurs in a third of patients; although usually superficial, perhaps migratory, it can occasionally be deep and may rarely involve the retinal veins, the dural sinus, or the superior and inferior vena cava. Arterial thrombosis has been reported, as well as aneurysms of the aorta and popliteal artery. When the central nervous system is involved, headache and fever can herald or accompany symptoms of cerebellar ataxia, paresis, and cranial nerve palsies. Meningomyelitis, meningoencephalitis, encephalopathies, seizures, multiple sclerosis—like disorders, and organic confusional states are recognized; although they occur in a small percentage of all cases, they portend a grave prognosis, with a 50 per cent mortality within one year.

Originally reported from the Middle East, Behçet's disease is seen worldwide. It occurs most often in males between 15 and 45 years of age; however, women can be affected, and familial occurrences have been documented. HLA typing, although inconclusive, suggests some mode of genetic inheritance or predisposition involving genetic information in the vicinity of HLA coding. Circulating antibodies to mucous membranes and esophagus have been described in the disease, and characteristic symptoms have been induced in rabbits through inoculations of patient isolates, but there is no conclusive support for the autoimmune and viral factors postulated. The disease is of uncommon occurrence despite alleged underreporting. It appears regularly in the differential diagnosis of aphthae, recurrent severe herpes simplex, and Reiter's syndrome, but the variability in expression of the entity and the lack of minimal criteria or specific diagnostic tests for irrefutable identification leave clinical considerations unconfirmed.

Oral and genital ulcerations are usually the first symptoms, followed within days, months, or years by the uveitis and other clinicial signs that may express an associated thrombophlebitis or vasculitis. Fever, malaise, and arthralgia are usually present during periods of active disease.

The mucosal lesions may be superficial erosions or deep punched-out ulcers, with necrosis leading to pain, with dysphagia and fetor if of the mouth, and to perforation of the labia minora in the genital area. If the colon is involved, discrete mucosal ulcers can be observed, with intervening normal bowel; thus it is differentiated from the continuous inflammatory change of ulcerative colitis. Of all lesions, however, the ocular pathology produces the most disability. Iridocyclitis and uveitis with hypopyon, chronic recurring inflammations, are the most serious complications, leading to blindness, partial or total. Only one eye may be involved at first, and then eventually both. Other ocular changes can occur, such as keratitis, retinitis, choroiditis, optic neuritis, and atrophy, as well as the thrombotic occlusion of retinal vessels previously noted.

Cutaneous lesions occur in some 80 per cent of cases: follicular pustules, furuncles, inflammatory dermal nodules, acneiform lesions, cellulitis, and other forms of pyoderma. Of interest, and perhaps of diagnostic significance, sterile pustules occur after intradermal injection of normal saline or even a needle prick. The histology of induced sterile pustules shows mild to intense perivascular round cell infiltrates at 24 hours, with an occasional cluster of polymorphonuclear leukocytes. On immunofluorescent study, no deposits of immunoglobulins, complement, fibrinogen, or albumin are noted, although circulating alpha$_2$ globulin, gamma globulin, IgA, IgG, and IgM have been elevated.

The range of organ involvement and the spectrum of symptomatology without conclusive diagnostic criteria leaves Behçet's disease frequently mentioned and rarely confirmed. For diagnosis some insist upon the classic triad of uveitis and oral and genital ulcers. Others feel that any two of these with skin lesions, thrombophlebitis, or bowel or joint disease should be sufficient. For the records and for estimates of prevalence, unanimity would be an advantage.

Therapy for the basic disease process is probably not helpful. Corticosteroids systemically and topically may reverse some of the inflammatory processes, but the condition is known for its natural clinical fluctuations. Immunosuppressive therapy, azathioprine and cyclophosphamide, is used to reduce the need for corticosteroids.

Chavatzas, D.: Popliteal artery thrombosis in Behçet's syndrome: A new manifestation of a very little known condition. Angiology, 25:773, 1974.

Haim, S., Sobel, J. D., and Friedman-Birnbaum, R.: Thrombophlebitis: A cardinal symptom of Behçet's syndrome. Acta Derm. Venereol., 54:299, 1974.

Haim, S., Sobel, J. D., Friedman-Birnbaum, R., and Lichtig, C.: Histological and direct immunofluorescence study of cutaneous hyperreactivity in Behçet's disease. Br. J. Dermatol., 95:631, 1976.

O'Duffy, J. D., and Golstein, N. P.: Neurologic involvement in seven patients with Behçet's disease. Am. J. Med., 61:170, 1976.

Pallis, D. B.: Behçet's disease and the nervous system. Transcript, St. John's Hospital Dermatol. Soc., 52:201, 1966.

Stanley, R. J., Tedesco, F. J., Melson, G. L., Geisse, G., and Herold, S. L.: The colitis of Behçet's disease, a clinical radiographic correlation. Radiology, 114:603, 1975.

574.4. MAST CELL DISEASE

Mast cell disease is a group of entities of which the common denominator is the spindle-shaped, dendritic connective tissue mast cell which aggregates in excessive numbers in the skin and occasionally in other organs. Symptoms relate to the pharmacologic effect of the histamine released by the degranulated mast cell and to the disruption of the organ structure and strength, as in bones, by mast cell infiltrates.

Several schemata distinguish among the clinical manifestations of mastocytosis. The cells may appear in the skin alone, or with systemic involvement, rarely as systemic infiltrates without skin lesions. The classic mast cell infiltrate appears as a small, discrete, reddish brown pigmented macule that becomes hive-like when stroked (Darier's sign), the released histamine having provoked a wheal. Such *urticaria pigmentosa* is the most common form of mastocytosis, occurring primarily in children, with half the patients clearing and almost all improving before adult life. Occasionally in infants there may be a single nodular lesion, a larger aggregate of cells known as a *mastocytoma*. Stroking for urtication can induce systemic effects of flushing and colic, with sufficient local edema to produce vesicles and bullae. Rarely is there *diffuse mastocytosis* with the skin so widely infiltrated as to become thickened, doughy, and lichenified. When the diffuse form is seen in children or when the urticaria pigmentosa has its onset in adulthood, noncutaneous organ involvement must be suspected. Any tissue where the mast cell is found can be affected. The central nervous system is thus excluded, leaving bone, liver, spleen, and gastrointestinal tract as sites of predilection in *systemic mastocytosis*. Here the associated mascular lesions of the skin may acquire persistent telangiectasia, or may become more papular, suggestive of leukemia cutis. A small percentage of patients with systemic mastocytosis actually develop leukemia, which can be mast cell leukemia but is usually not.

Urticaria pigmentosa without systemic involvement accounts for 90 per cent of persons affected with mast cell disease. These and the balance of patients with systemic mastocytosis demonstrating cutaneous involvement all have skin lesions readily recognized by the trained eye and provable by biopsy. The nests of mast cells are diagnostic. When selecting a lesion for histology, however, care must be taken lest the granules be discharged and thus rendered invisible by stroking or other manipulation prior to biopsy. Brisk skin cleansing must be avoided, and anesthesia should be injected at a distance and deeply. After fixation in 10 per cent formalin or absolute alcohol and staining with Giemsa, toluidine blue, or methylene blue, the characteristic basophilic metachromatic granules will be seen in the cytoplasm of the mast cell.

It is the rare systemic case without cutaneous involvement that is the diagnostic challenge. Bone films may be of help, since cystic lesions are found in 10 to 30 per cent of patients with systemic disease. The pelvis, spine, ribs, and skull are the most common sites of involvement. Areas of decreased density alternate with small areas of sclerosis. The radiolucencies have been attributed to granulomatous aggregates of mast cells in the marrow which release histamine, inducing fibrotic change in the adjacent marrow, with subsequent conversion to osteoid tissue and the deposition of calcium salts to produce dense foci. The striking bone pattern that results on the x-ray although not pathognomonic of osseous mast cell disease, is strongly suggestive.

The symptomatology of mast cell disease varies with the site and extent of organ involvement. If it is confined to the skin, more than half the patients are asymptomatic. A third or so complain of pruritus, flushing, and headache often induced by the mechanical degranulation of the mast cell, as with hot baths and exercise, or by the pharmacologic degranulation, as with codeine and aspirin. In more extensive involvement patients may experience diarrhea and peptic ulcer, usually without acid hypersecretion. Patients with systemic mastocytosis can have bone pain and can even sustain pathologic fractures. Hepatic infiltrates may lead to hepatomegaly and portal fibrosis with impaired hepatic function. Splenomegaly can be marked. Mast cell proliferation in the bone marrow can result in anemia, leukopenia, and thrombocytopenia. The latter, in association with heparin released from cutaneous mast cells, may account for the purpuric lesions that have been discussed and may have a role in the gastrointestinal bleeding seen in 10 per cent of patients. A malabsorption syndrome may develop, as well as diarrhea, with or without steatorrhea.

Those mast cell lesions present at birth or appearing in childhood and limited to the skin have an excellent prognosis. In fact mast cell disease confined to skin and bone is compatible with life and minimal morbidity. Solitary lesions can be excised. Therapy otherwise relates to symptomatology, the avoidance of maneuvers and situations that lead to mast cell degranulation, or the selection of time for such discharge when it interferes least with the patient's life style and can be anticipated with antihistamine coverage. There is also claim for the control of the associated diarrhea with cromolyn. If the mechanism of action is to block the activation of the mast cell at the degranulation level of antigenic stimulation, it would seem a potentially useful drug to control many of the symptoms of mast cell disease. Since it is short acting, the required high blood levels cannot be sustained, and planned intermittent therapy would be necessary. Further, there are other data which suggest that the diarrhea may not always be the result of histamine release but of lymphatic obstruction by mast cells in the lamina propria. An H_2-receptor antagonist such as cimetidine has been shown to abolish acid hypersecretion in a patient with mast cell disease without altering the steatorrhea or diarrhea. Systemic mastocytosis, although it can be a static and fairly benign disease, may progress with extensive reticuloendotheliosis and with consequent weakness, weight loss, nausea, vomiting, and cachexia. The presence of mast cells in the peripheral blood is an ominous sign. Anaplasia indicates malignant transformation. Patients may develop pancytopenia and succumb to infection, hemorrhage and leukemia.

Clinicopathologic Conference: Systemic mastocytosis. Am. J. Med., 61:671, 1976.

Feldman, E. J., and Isenberg, J. I.: Effects of Metiamide on gastric acid hypersecretion, steatorrhea and bone-marrow function in a patient with systemic mastocytosis. N. Eng. J. Med., 295:1178, 1976.

Gagnon, J. H., Kalz, F., Kadri, A. M., and Von Graefe, I.: Mastocytosis: Unusual manifestations, clinical and radiologic changes. Can. Med. Assoc. J., 112:1329, 1975.

Keller, R. T., and Roth, H. P.: Hyperchlorhydria and hyperhistaminemia in a patient with systemic mastocytosis. N. Eng. J. Med., 283:1449, 1970.

574.5.   MALIGNANCY

Skin can undergo malignant change, and it can support the metastatic malignant growth of other organs. Even more, as elaborated in Ch. 573.9, it can respond to the systemic presence of malignancy in ways that challenge the implication of the malignant cell and process. Considered here are the common *cutaneous malignancies,* often radiation induced; then *mycosis fungoides,* an uncommon neoplastic disease but a distinct histopathologic and clinical entity first manifested in the skin; and finally *melanoma.*

THE COMMON CUTANEOUS MALIGNANCIES

The individual at highest risk for developing skin cancer is the light complexioned, blue-eyed freckler who has had considerable ultraviolet light exposure, whether geographically determined or influenced by occupation and avocation. The effect of such natural radiation will be augmented by any x-irradiation every received, or by any exposure to carcinogens such as the oral inorganic arsenicals or to chronic cutaneous infection, ulceration, or burn.

Basal Cell Epithelioma

The most common cancer of the skin by far is the basal cell epithelioma, which affects the white population but rarely blacks or Orientals. The prevalence in the United States is 3.9 per 1000, or 757,000 cases. The average patient is over 40 years of age, but basal cell epithelioma can be seen in young adults or even children. Men are more often affected than women (2.2:1.7). The clinical lesion is a raised nodule with a pearly translucent border showing telangiectatic vessels (Fig. 23). It may be ulcerated and, more rarely, pigmented. Some lesions remain unchanged for years; others can, be ulcerated and invasive from the first clinical observation. When removed completely by any destructive measure — excision, desiccation and curettage, even x-ray — the subsequent morbidity of the enlarging eroding lesion is thwarted. Proximity to sensitive structures and the capacity to burrow compel early recognition. The clinical diagnosis is readily confirmed by biopsy. Therapy should be selected to ensure removal with minimal cosmetic compromise and without increasing risk through long-term radiation effects. X-ray therapy, for example, which induces cutaneous malignancy in 15 to 20 years and augments all other radiation effects, should be reserved for the feeble and elderly. Recurrent lesions, or those proximal to the eye, at the inner canthus, for example, where neither should normal tissue be sacrificed nor risk of recurrence permitted, are best treated by the microscopically monitored removal of the last malignant cell through the tedious staging of Mohs' chemosurgery; fixed or frozen tissue is charted, and each shaved specimen is checked for the persistence of the readily recognized basophilic cell.

Basal cell epitheliomas usually appear singly, but may not, and the individual who has developed one is prone to develop others. The areas most struck by sunlight in the erect individual are the surfaces prone to actinic damage and consequent cutaneous malignancy: cheeks, forehead, and nasolabial fold. Certain basal cell lesions, such as the sclerosing waxy morphea type occurring on the head and neck or the superficial spreading type seen on the trunk, may confound the inexperienced, but biopsy will usually be definitive. Nevoid tumors such as trichoepithelioma can occasionally be confused with keratotic basal cell epithelioma, especially if solitary. Multiple basal cell tumors appearing in childhood should alert the observer to the basal cell nevus syndrome and its associated abnormalities of skin, bone, central nervous system, eye, and gonads.

Squamous Cell Carcinoma

Induced by the same factors as basal cell epithelioma but with a fraction of the prevalence, squamous cell carcinoma arises in the light-exposed areas from keratinizing epidermal cells. The typical patient is more than 60 years old and male with a history of considerable sun exposure. The tumors arising on sun damaged skin are, when compared to other squamous cell carcinoma, less aggressive, and less likely to metastasize, except perhaps for those of the ear and lip which, even when small, can metastasize to local lymph nodes. Squamous cell tumors induced by x-ray or arsenicals, or arising in burn scars, or in chronic granulomas such as lupus vulgaris, are of greater concern and have a poorer prognosis. Commencing in chronic ectodermal change as they do, they may go unnoticed or unappreciated until extensive and metastatic. Ordinarily squamous cell carcinoma appears as a slowly enlarging nodule with an inflamed, indurated base growing more rapidly than a basal cell tumor. Therapy is urgent complete removal. The prognosis is guarded for lesions of the lip, especially of the vermilion border, and for all lesions with metastases. Patients treated for cutaneous malignancy must be assessed periodically for recurrence and for new tumor. Those who have had one skin cancer are at risk of developing others even when the initiating factors are not apparent. They should be cautioned about this and about the need for surveillance, as well as the harmful effects of continued sun exposure.

MYCOSIS FUNGOIDES

Mycosis fungoides is a chronic fatal disease of the reticuloendothelial system, a T-cell lymphoma which initially and primarily involves skin but can involve lymph nodes and viscera. It is distinguishable from Hodgkin's disease and other malignant lymphomas. Clinically there is an erythematous pretumor stage which progresses to thickened, indurated, plaque-like lesions, and ultimately tumor. The early premycotic stage may last from months to years, with scaling and erythema persisting to the end; uncommonly, the presenting complaint can be a tumefaction. The disease is not rare, accounting for perhaps 1 per cent of deaths from lymphoma; it occurs in all races, usually in those from 40 to 60 years, but has been seen in teenagers.

A psoriasiform or eczematous dermatitis, chronic, persistent, and pruritic, that is not caused by drug or contactant should bring mycosis fungoides into the differential diagnosis. Fixed giant hive-like lesions or plaques are further clinical indicators, as is lymphadenopathy. Often, histopathologic confirmation of the diagnosis is delayed for years past the clinical impression of mycosis fungoides. Biopsies from plaques or tumors, however, provide the histologic features that establish the diagnosis: Pautrier's microabscesses, atypical cells nested within the

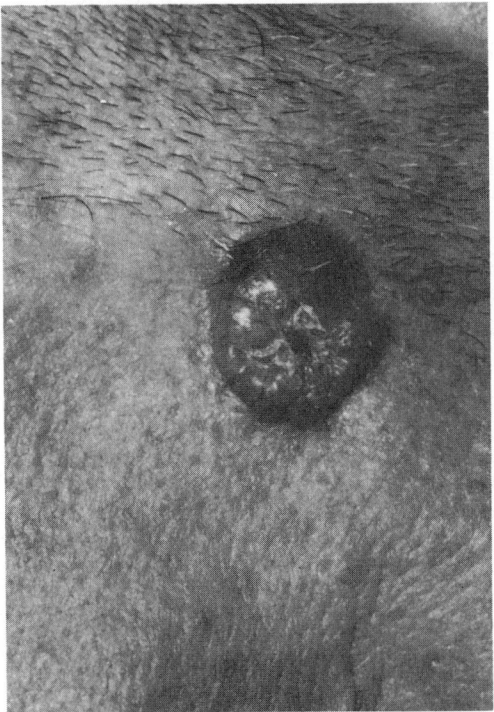

Figure 23. Basal cell epithelioma.

epidermis; an infiltrate of atypical mononuclear cells; and hyperchromatic larger cells with irregular nuclei, the "mycosis cells." After the appearance of tumor, lymphadenopathy, or ulceration, the median survival is less than two to five years; with the appearance of all three, the median survival is less than one year.

Extracutaneous dissemination of mycosis fungoides, once thought rare, is no longer considered uncommon; visceral involvement is noted in two thirds of patients (61 to 82 per cent) at autopsy. Lung, liver, and spleen are the more common sites, but nearly every organ or tissue may be involved with atypical cells. Any lymph node involvement indicates the likelihood of spread to other extracutaneous sites. Staging for prognosis will have impetus as treatment protocols are developed. It must not be forgotten that one third of patients who succumb to mycosis fungoides have disease limited to the skin.

Therapy for this uniformly fatal disease has been palliative. Pruritus, dermatitis, and tumor are treated at each stage as they appear. Corticosteroids have been used, as well as chemotherapeutic agents such as cyclophosphamide and chlorambucil, and also the antimetabolites azaribine and methotrexate. Bleomycin is a promising cytotoxic antibiotic because of its concentration in the skin (and lung). Electron beam therapy is of advantage for the remission of lesions if not the disease, as is conventional x-ray. More recently, skin painting with nitrogen mustard or by intralesional injection has given favorable results, as have psoralens with high intesity ultraviolet light. To date, however, no protocol or series has been adequate to provide the definitive data for the proper treatment of this devastating disease.

No consideration of mycosis fungoides is complete without mention of Sézary's syndrome. Probably a variant of mycosis fungoides, it is characterized by an extensive exfoliative erythroderma with intense pruritus, lymphadenopathy, and large mononuclear cells in the skin and blood. Elevated leukocyte counts are found in most patients; all have a lymphocytosis, with atypical cells varying in size from 10 to 20 μ recognized as Sézary cells by their folded, lobulated nucleus and rim of PAS-positive, diastase-resistant cytoplasm. A "small cell" variant has been described. Studies of the ultrastructure of these abnormal lymphocytes have identified them in cutaneous infiltrates of mycosis fungoides. In Sézary's syndrome these abnormal thymus-derived cells constitute more than 40 per cent of purified lymphocyte fractions from the peripheral blood. In patients affected, immune mechanisms are generally not impaired.

Although Sézary's syndrome might be looked upon as the erythrodermatous phase of mycosis fungoides, it does not respond well to palliative therapy, even electron beam irradiation. Reduction of the intravascular neoplastic T cells by leukapheresis to effect a mobilization and reduction of tissue infiltrates gives a new and innovative but not yet fully assessed approach to the management.

Edelson, R. L., Kirkpatrick, C. H., Shenock, E. M., Schein, P. S., Smith, R. W., Green, I., and Lutzner, M.: Preferential cutaneous infiltration by neoplastic thymus derived lymphocytes: Morphological and functional studies. Ann. Intern. Med., 80:685, 1974.

Epstein, E. H., Levin, D. L., Croft, J. D., and Lutzner, M. A.: Mycosis fungoides. Survival, prognostic features, response to therapy and autopsy findings. Medicine, 51:61, 1972.

Thomas, L. E., and Rappaport, H.: Mycosis fungoides and its relationship to other malignant lymphomas. In Rebuck, J. W., et al. (eds.): The Reticuloendothelial System. Baltimore, Williams & Wilkins Company, 1975.

Van Scott, E. J., and Haynes, H. A.: Cutaneous lymphoma. In Fitzpatrick, T. B. (ed.): Dermatology in General Medicine. New York, McGraw-Hill Book Company, 1971, pp. 556–573.

MELANOMA

Melanoma is a neoplasm of melanocytes that has the potential for invasion and metastasis. It contributes little to the burden of cutaneous malignancy by case load (fewer than 3 per cent of new skin cancers), but by mortality it accounts for two thirds of the deaths from skin cancer, and at an appreciably young age. In fact, those who develop any malignancy between ages 35 and 40 are at greater risk only for cancer of the lung, breast, or cervix.

Along with other skin cancer, melanoma shows a currently increasing incidence, highest in Caucasians, and influenced adversely by ultraviolet light exposure as judged by the anatomic distribution of lesions and by occupational and geographical factors. As with other skin cancers, patients who develop melanoma are apt to have a light complexion and light-colored eyes, and to sunburn readily. They may have a family predisposition to the development of melanoma, or they may have had one primary melanoma which places them at greater risk of having a second primary.

Three out of four melanomas that develop in the skin undergo progressive change over an extended period from not less than six months to many years, thereby providing the informed examiner with a prolonged opportunity to recognize and remove surgically the potentially lethal lesion for probable cure. Change in texture, color, or size of a pre-existing nevus arouses suspicion of melanoma, but even without such signs there are clinical characteristics that make a pigmented lesion suspect. Any brown-black spot with areas of red or red-purple, plus white, whether gray-white or pink-white, and blue, should be examined histopathologically. There is further suspicion of melanoma if the borders of the lesion are irregular, appear notched or smudged, and have pigment streaming from the pigmented edge. Of grave concern is the lesion with a surface that is elevated or ulcerated and devoid of skin markings.

Regarding all melanotic lesions with red, white, and blue as possible melanoma and hence in need of definitive histopathologic diagnosis, one may gather a few vascular lesions and a rare pigmented basal cell epithelioma, but would also net a significant number of early melanomas when most are at a curative stage. This underscores the importance of examining the entire integument carefully, in good light, and with hand lens magnification, for all suspicious pigmented lesions. It presumes confidence in recognizing the common benign pigmented lesions of the skin reviewed in Ch. 573.5.

Primary cutaneous melanoma can be classified according to clinicohistologic type, the level of invasion, the thickness of the lesion, and the density of the inflammatory response. With the establishment of criteria for sorting among the various clinical presentations, realistic comparisons can be made, prognoses given, and the value of therapeutic measures assessed. Clinically, several types are recognized and the histology correlated.

Lentigo maligna (Fig. 24) begins as a small tan macular lesion, a circumscribed precancerous melanosis, the melanotic freckle of Hutchinson. Usually a lesion of the el-

Figure 24. Lentigo maligna.

Figure 25. Superficial spreading melanoma.

derly, it can occur in the 20's. Over years, or even decades, it may enlarge by lateral growth, with the margins becoming irregular and the color modified to brown-black and pink-white. Eventually there will be dermal invasion, the vertical growth phase, associated with a papular on nodular surface. Melanotic freckles are mostly seen on the face but may occur anywhere on the skin where there has been significant sunlight exposure. The radial growth phase of 5 to 7 cm and measured in years provides the long lead time for therapy before active malignant invasion. Unfortunately, the benignity of appearance and the confusion of the smaller early lesion with a solar lentigo often delay definitive treatment until size alone precludes simple excision.

Superficial spreading melanoma occurs in younger individuals; it may appear anywhere in the body, characteristically on the upper back in both sexes and on the legs of women (Fig. 25). Fairly regular in outline, sometimes notched, lesions range in color from tan to black, with the telltale combination of red, white, and blue. Initially barely palpable, these, too, become papular or nodular with the vertical growth phase.

Nodular melanoma, as might be suspected from the terminology, does not have a discernible radial growth phase but, from the first, is observed as a nodule or plaque, dark brown or black, with a gray or blue cast (Fig. 26). It is invasive from the start, and the prognosis is never as good as with other melanomas. Further, the nodular variety can occasionally be amelanotic and extremely difficult to diagnose clinically.

The clinicohistologic grouping recognizes an *acral lentiginous melanoma* of the palms, soles, and terminal phalanges, which is similar in its benign clinical appearance to *lentigo maligna melanoma,* but which, like it and like *superficial spreading melanoma,* can develop a vertical growth phase. It also distinguishes nodular melanoma of the mucous membranes, occurring more frequently in blacks and Orientals, and a miscellaneous group of melanomas that arise in various nevi, the central nervous system, and the viscera.

In all melanomas there is correlation between the depth of the histologic invasion and the prognosis. Clark and his coworkers have designated intraepidermal malignancy as Level I, invasion of the papillary dermis as Level II, filling the papillary dermis and impinging upon but not invading the reticular dermis as Level III, reaching into the reticular dermis as Level IV, and reaching into the subcutaneous tissue as Level V. Correlated with these levels is an increasing mortality: 8.3 per cent for Level II; 35.2 per cent for Level III; 46.1 per cent for Level IV; and 52 per cent for Level V. There is also a difference in survival according to the clinical type of melanoma, with lentigo maligna melanoma having the longest survival, followed by superficial spreading melanoma, and, poorest, nodular melanoma. Further correlations have been made between survival and depth of invasion as measured with an ocular micrometer.

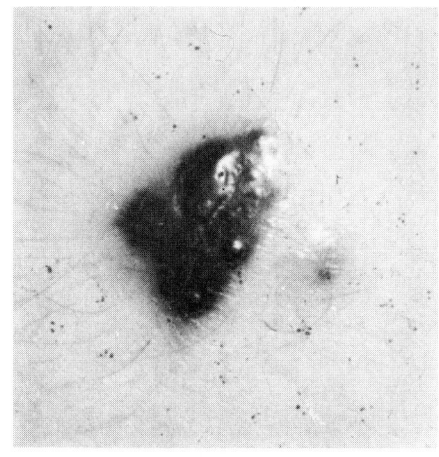

Figure 26. Nodular melanoma.

Prognosis, in addition to a consideration of the type of melanoma, its size, and depth of invasion, is also dependent on the age and sex of the patient, the anatomic location of the tumor, and the presence or absence of metastases and of pigment. With similar lesions women fare better than men, and lesions of the leg or of the head or neck permit longer survival than those of the trunk. Absence of pigment portends a poor prognosis. So may pregnancy, although this is not certain for a given patient. In a study of women with melanoma there was no indication of benefit to the melanoma patient from termination of the pregnancy, oophorectomy, adrenalectomy, or hypophysectomy. Survival of those with localized disease was unchanged when compared to nonpregnant melanoma patients at the same stage. Those with nodal disease and pregnant did less well. They and those whose lesions had been activated during gestation should be cautioned against subsequent pregnancies.

The question of melanoma arising in pre-existing nevi is always posed. Congenital nevi account for fewer than 0.1 per cent of the nevi of the average young adult, but they are usually larger than acquired nevi and, since present from birth, are likely to be identifiable by the patient or his family. The risk of malignant change in such nevi is probably proportional to the numbers of aggregated melanocytes — hence the size of the lesion. Giant pigmented congenital nevi (the giant hairy or bathing trunk nevi) have an incidence of malignant change variously reported from 15 to 42 per cent. Although melanoma is rare before puberty, almost half of those occurring in childhood arise in such giant congenital nevi. However, of all patients who develop melanoma, only one in four will recall a pre-existing pigmented lesion present from childhood, a figure supported by the 20 per cent of melanoma lesions that have histologic evidence of associated nevus.

The removal of giant congenital nevi is indicated for malignant risk as well as cosmetic disfigurement, but often it is not surgically feasible. For small congenital nevi there are no data to support significant risk. If one accepts the relationship of size to risk, such aggregates of melanocytes must pose greater risk per unit area than normal skin. There is probably value in considering the removal of all congenital nevi larger than 1 cm after weighing the possibility of cosmetic disfigurement and such factors as complexion, eye color, and anatomic location.

Melanoma, capable of persisting for years before active metastatic spread, can signal its presence by metastases with the primary lesion undiscoverable. In such cases (15 per cent in two large series) the occult primary melanoma may have undergone spontaneous regression, since melanoma, even visceral metastatic disease, has been known to disappear without therapy.

Perhaps parts of this phenomenon are the areas of depigmentation observed around nevi, and occasionally around the primary or metastatic cutaneous lesions of patients with melanoma. Such leukoderma is clinically indistinguishable from that present in halo nevi of the individual *without* melanoma, in whom the depigmentation can progress to the obliteration of the pigmented nevus clinically and histopathologically. In such individuals, free of malignancy, circulating anti-melanoma antibodies have been reported.

With suspected melanoma, an unequivocal diagnosis is mandatory. Clinical diagnoses can be quite wrong, and histopathologically certain pigmented lesions such as the Spitz nevus (benign juvenile melanoma) can be misread or confused with melanoma. A biopsy must be done and the histology reviewed.

The suspected lesion should be excised with a 5- to 10-mm border and penetration to the subcutaneous fat. If the size of the lesion precludes simple excision, an incisional biopsy is probably justified despite concern over dissemination of tumor.

With confident histologic confirmation, a wide surgical excision is indicated. Depending upon the type and level of the tumor, further surgery or therapy may be suggested. Systemic and regional chemotherapy have been used and, more recently, immunotherapy with vaccinia and BCG. The staging of melanoma which guides therapy varies according to several classifications presently in use. None upon which there is agreement includes characteristics of the tumor and the level of penetration of the malignant cells — important parameters for prognosis.

In sum, melanoma is a capricious and intriguing tumor, evident but inactive for years, or metastatic from an occult primary. It may appear with pigment or without, and may disappear before treatment. It can express itself in pedigrees in comparable anatomic locations, or as multiple primary tumors, and in families with a higher incidence of malignancy of all types. Its cells are tagged with a pigment marker. Melanoma is a challenge and model for the study of all malignancy.

Kopf, A. W., Bart, R. S., and Rodriguez-Sains, B. A.: Malignant melanoma: A review. J. Dermatol. Surg. Oncol., 3:41, 1977.

Mihm, M. C., Jr., Fitzpatrick, T. B., Brown, M. M. L., Raker, J. W., Malt, R. A., and Kaiser, J. S.: Early detection of primary cutaneous malignant melanoma. A color atlas. N. Eng. J. Med., 289:989, 1973.

Shiu, M. H., Schottenfeld, D. , Maclean, B., and Fortner, J. G.: Adverse Effect of pregnancy on melanoma: A reappraisal. Cancer, 37:181, 1976.

PART XXIV
DISEASES OF THE EYE

Maurice B. Landers, III

575. INTRODUCTION

The eye presents a unique opportunity to study systemic disease processes and, indeed, has been referred to as a microcosm of the entire body. Within Part XXIV, material is presented on the ocular manifestations of several of the more common systemic diseases. Some of the eye disorders likely to be seen initially by the general physician are also discussed.

576. THE DIFFERENTIAL DIAGNOSES OF THE ACUTE RED EYE

INTRODUCTION. The main differential diagnoses of an acute red eye include conjunctivitis, anterior uveitis, acute closed angle glaucoma, and corneal trauma or infection. A composite of the main differential diagnostic signs and symptoms of the inflamed eye is given in Table 1.

THE RED EYE. The red eye is caused by congestion or hemorrhage of the conjunctival vasculature. Subconjunctival hemorrhage occurs suddenly and produces a characteristic bright red area with no other signs or symptoms. These hemorrhages can be the result of trauma, hypertension, blood dyscrasias, straining, or violent fits of sneezing or coughing, but often no cause is apparent. The subconjunctival hemorrhage requires no treatment and gradually resorbs over a few weeks with the characteristic color changes of hemoglobin degradation products.

Vascular congestion, on the other hand, is a cardinal sign of intraocular inflammation or conjunctival irritation. A differentiation between ciliary injection and conjunctival injection should be made if possible.

Ciliary injection is seen in inflammations of the cornea and anterior uvea and in angle closure glaucoma. It appears as dull red to violet colored vessels that do not move with the conjunctiva. The vessels are most evident encircling the limbus and fade away toward the fornices. They are not affected by topical instillation of 1:1000 epinephrine drops.

Conjunctival injection is a sign of conjunctivitis. It appears as superficial, bright red or pink tortuous vessels that move with the conjunctiva. The vessels tend to be more numerous in the fornix and fade away toward the limbus. When occluded by pressure through the lids, the vessels may be seen refilling from the periphery. Epinephrine drops constrict these superficial vessels and whiten the conjunctiva.

CONJUNCTIVITIS. Conjunctivitis is the most common cause of the acute red eye. The most useful classification of the myriad types of conjunctivitis is by etiology, which includes bacterial, viral, chlamydial, rickettsial, fungal, allergic, traumatic, parasitic, and inflammatory conjunctivitis of unknown etiology (or in association with systemic disease).

Although the conjunctiva is rich in blood vessels and lymphoid tissue, it has relatively few pain fibers. Therefore symptoms of vague ocular discomfort, scratchiness, or burning are characteristic of conjunctivitis. (Severe pain is suggestive of corneal inflammation.) Itching, tearing, and mild photophobia are exhibited by many patients, especially those with allergic conjunctivitis. An exudate is usually present and can be purulent (primarily in bacterial disease), thin and watery (viral disease), or white and stringy (allergic disease). Vision may be blurred periodically by copious secretions floating over the cornea, but in most patients the visual axis is unaffected and vision when tested carefully is normal. The characteristic conjunctival injection outlined above is present to various degrees. Pupillary size and reflexes are normal. Palpable preauricular nodes may or may not be present, depending on

TABLE 1. Differential Diagnoses of the Acute Red Eye

	Conjunctivitis	Anterior Uveitis	Acute Closed-Angle Glaucoma	Corneal Trauma or Keratitis
Incidence	Very common	Common	Uncommon	Common
Onset	Gradual	Usually gradual	Sudden	Sudden (trauma) or gradual
Pain	Mild discomfort, ± itching	Moderate ocular pain	Severe with facial radiation	Moderate to severe, superficial
Vision	Normal	Slight blurring	Marked blurring	Usually blurred
Injection	Conjunctival	Ciliary	Ciliary	Ciliary or diffuse
Discharge	Moderate to copious, clear to mucopurulent	None	None	Mild to moderate, watery to purulent
Media	Clear	Cells, flare, keratitic precipitates	Steamy cornea	Corneal ulcers, erosions, and opacities, related to cause
Pupil	Normal	Small, irregular	Large	Normal
Pupillary reflex	Normal	Sluggish	Absent	Normal
Intraocular pressure	Normal	Usually low to normal	Elevated	Normal
Smear	± organisms	Negative	Negative	± organisms
Systemic complaints	Occasionally upper respiratory infection	Few	Prostration, nausea, and vomiting	None

the etiologic agent. Localized conjunctival lesions such as follicles, papillary nodules, phylctenules, and granulomas, as well as conjunctival membranes, when present, aid in the etiologic classification of the conjunctivitis. Associated constitutional symptoms may be present in viral syndromes but are seldom seen in primary bacterial, chlamydial, or other infectious processes.

The diagnosis is made by history and examination, Gram's and Giemsa stains, and culture of conjunctival scrapings. Keratitis, uveitis, and glaucoma should be ruled out early in the workup. Treatment is directed toward the etiologic agent.

ACUTE ANTERIOR UVEITIS. The uveal tract is the vascular middle layer of the globe and includes the iris, the ciliary body, and the choroid. Any or all three structures can be involved in an inflammatory process. Inflammations of the iris or ciliary body go under the preferred general term of "anterior uveitis," whereas choroiditis or chorioretinitis usually is called "posterior uveitis." Although some conditions can cause an isolated iritis, or more rarely an isolated cyclitis, many inflammations involve both structures simultaneously. Acute anterior uveitis is a common disorder in young and middle-aged individuals and is one of the main differential diagnostic etiologies of the acute red eye.

Iritis or iridocyclitis is characterized by a deep, aching pain unlike the discomforting foreign body sensation of conjunctivitis. Photophobia, mild tearing, and slight blurring of vision are usual symptoms. Typically, a ciliary injection (circumcorneal flush) is seen, although there may be an associated conjunctival injection due to a concurrent conjunctivitis. The pupil in anterior uveitis is usually miotic due to engorgement of iris vessels and a third nerve reflex response to irritation. In chronic cases, posterior synechiae can form, producing pupil irregularities and diminishing the light reflex. Exudation of protein into the normally protein-poor aqueous humor results in clouding, which is visible on slit lamp examination. Protein aggregates can form on the posterior corneal surface (keratitic precipitates). Inflammatory cells may be present in the anterior chamber and may gravitate along with cellular debris and protein aggregates to the inferior portion of the anterior chamber. Intraocular pressure is initially normal and helps differentiate uveitis from acute glaucoma. With chronicity, however, the pressure may be elevated due to blockage of the angle, inflammation of the outflow channels, or posterior synechiae with adhesions of the iris to the lens. Inflammation of the ciliary body may cause a deficiency in aqueous secretion and result in ocular hypotension.

The most difficult differential diagnosis is between angle closure glaucoma and uveitis with synechiae and a secondary rise in ocular pressure. This distinction is important because atropine-induced dilation of the pupil is indicated in anterior uveitis to lessen the chance of synechiae formation. The same drug can precipitate or worsen closed angle glaucoma. Systemic analgesics, dark glasses, and topical steroid drops are also used to treat anterior uveitis. When the disease is complicated by a secondary glaucoma, it is still very important to dilate the pupil and treat the elevated intraocular pressure with other agents such as carbonic anhydrase inhibitors or topical epinephrine.

ACUTE ANGLE CLOSURE GLAUCOMA. Angle closure glaucoma is a sudden increase in intraocular pressure due to mechanical blockage of the outflow channels in the angle. The blockage is caused by the iris coming in contact with the trabecular meshwork. Although angle closure glaucoma is the least frequent cause of an acute red eye, it represents an ophthalmologic emergency. Permanent optic nerve damage can be caused within 24 to 48 hours following a rise of ocular pressure above 50 mm Hg.

Angle closure glaucoma is heralded by a sudden attack of severe ocular, orbital, or facial pain with a blurring of vision. Associated nausea and vomiting can occur and falsely suggest abdominal disease. The intraocular pressure is markedly elevated during an attack. A shallow anterior chamber is usually evident on oblique illumination of the iris. The cornea becomes edematous and has a "steamy" appearance. The pupil is moderately dilated, and the reflexes are diminished or absent. The deep ciliary injection pattern is usually seen.

Medical attempts at lowering intraocular tension should begin with oral or intravenous osmotic agents combined with miotics. If the pressure is not relieved within four to six hours by medical therapy, surgical correction (usually a peripheral iridectomy) is indicated.

KERATITIS AND CORNEAL TRAUMA. Infectious agents are the most frequent cause of keratitis or keratoconjunctivitis. Corneal trauma and infection are common causes of an acute red eye. Since the conjunctival and corneal epithelium are continuous structures, inflammations frequently involve both structures. Corneal inflammation also can result from hypersensitivity reactions, ischemic vascular disease, nutritional deficiency, lacrimal disorders, exposure, or denervating disease. The cornea is rich in pain fibers and produces more pain, photophobia, and reflex blepharospasm than the inflamed conjunctiva. Blurring of vision is common but varies with location and type of corneal defect. There is usually no discharge unless a purulent bacterial ulcer is present. A ciliary injection is seen characteristically in corneal inflammation.

Newell, F. W., and Ernest, J. T.: Ophthalmology Principles and Concepts. 3rd ed. St. Louis, C. V. Mosby Company, 1974.
Scheie, H. G., and Albert, D. M.: Textbook of Ophthalmology, 9th ed. Philadelphia, W. B. Saunders Company, 1977.
Vaughan, D., and Asbury, T.: General Ophthalmology. 8th ed. Los Altos, Calif., Lange Medical Publications, 1977.

577. ARTHRITIC DISEASES

RHEUMATOID ARTHRITIS. Rheumatoid arthritis (RA) may affect the conjunctiva, cornea, sclera, aqueous outflow channels, and lacrimation apparatus. Ocular involvement is primarily seen in severe cases of RA and in those patients with extra-articular manifestations. Remissions and exacerbations of ocular disease usually parallel the activity of the systemic disease.

The most common ocular complication of RA is keratoconjunctivitis sicca, which appears in 10 to 35 per cent of cases. When these two entities are present, the diagnostic criteria for Sjögren's syndrome are met.

Four scleral and episcleral lesions may be identified: (1) episcleral rheumatoid nodules, (2) necrotizing nodular scleritis, (3) scleromalacia perforans, and (4) massive granuloma of the sclera (brawny scleritis).

Episcleral rheumatoid nodules are yellow-white, raised lesions several millimeters in diameter which are usually surrounded by dilated vascular channels.

Though uncommon, these lesions can be painful and hyperemic, although they may be asymptomatic and clinically overlooked. These lesions usually resolve spontaneously without serious sequelae.

Rheumatoid nodules within the sclera produce two clinically different lesions. The first, necrotizing nodular scleritis, is an acutely painful, hyperemic lesion that may or may not be bilateral, occurs equally in both sexes, and may rarely be seen preceding all other manifestations of RA. The second form of scleritis, scleromalacia perforans, is a more "benign" lesion with much less inflammation. It is usually bilateral and more commonly seen in females with at least ten years of rheumatoid disease. Both forms of scleritis result in devitalization and sloughing of scleral tissue, leaving permanent scleral defects and exposing the pigmented uvea beneath it. Approximately 6 per cent of patients with rheumatoid arthritis will develop either of the two forms of scleritis.

The fourth type of scleral lesion is a massive granuloma known as brawny scleritis. This infrequent complication is characterized by a severely painful, diffuse scleral thickening beneath an inflamed, swollen conjunctiva. All portions of the globe, including the cornea, can be involved in this process.

Corneal infiltrates and vascularization frequently occur subsequent to any of the latter three scleral lesions when they are located near the corneoscleral junction, or limbus. Primary corneal involvement is rare. Non-nodular ulcerative sclerokeratitis may produce a marginal, furrowed ulcer around the limbus. This process is usually bilateral and not associated with marked inflammation or vascularization but can progress to corneal perforation. In other cases, a small ulcer is seen in a relatively quiet eye. This may progress rapidly to perforation.

Scleral inflammation can lead to a variety of secondary complications. These include glaucoma resulting from aqueous outflow channel inflammation, cataract, chorioretinitis, retinal detachment, and perforation of the globe. The incidence of uveitis in adults with RA is the same as that of the general population.

Many serious ocular complications result from drug therapy for RA and the other arthritides. Steroids, antimalarials, gold salts, and other various anti-inflammatory agents may have significant ocular side effects.

Topical steroids are often beneficial for episcleritis, although these lesions usually are self-limiting. Steroids can suppress the inflammatory component of scleritis but do not apparently affect the pathologic process. Immunosuppressive therapy has been successful in some patients with rheumatoid scleritis when steroids were of no benefit. Retrobulbar alcohol injection is occasionally needed for relief of the pain associated with scleritis. Corneoscleral patch grafts can be used when perforation is imminent, but soft contact lenses may be of benefit earlier.

JUVENILE RHEUMATOID ARTHRITIS. Although juvenile rheumatoid arthritis (JRA) has many features in common with the adult form of the disease, the ocular involvement is quite different in the two forms. Although adults with RA tend to get keratoscleritis after severe longstanding disease, children with JRA are affected with severe uveitis early in their disease, and scleritis is almost unknown.

Anterior uveitis is primarily seen in children with the monoarticular or oligoarticular form of JRA. Ocular disease is relatively uncommon in the two other forms of JRA — the acute systemic disease with fever, rash, lymphadenopathy, hepatosplenomegaly, and leukocytosis (Still's disease), and the symmetrical polyarticular disease. The incidence of iritis in mono- and oligoarticular disease ranges from 19 to 42 per cent, but is seen in only 2 to 5 per cent of polyarticular cases. The iritis usually occurs after the onset of arthritis but may precede it by many years. It is more frequent in children with a negative test for rheumatoid factor and positive tests for antinuclear antibodies.

The iritis may cause redness, pain, photophobia, and tearing in the affected eye, but is most often asymptomatic. In these cases, extensive ocular damage and visual impairment can occur before the process is recognized. Therefore it is recommended that children with JRA, especially the monoarticular form, be examined by an ophthalmologist at three- to six-month intervals until adulthood.

The characteristic uveitis is a bilateral, chronic, or recurring anterior uveitis. Chronic uveitis is more common in younger females, and carries a worse visual prognosis than acute, isolated iritis which is seen more often in older male children. The acute form responds better to topical steroids and cycloplegic-mydriatic drops and may resolve without sequelae.

The most common sequela of the uveitis of JRA is band keratopathy. Other sequelae of chronic uveitis include cataract, anterior or posterior synechiae, and secondary glaucoma. The ocular triad of JRA consists of iritis, band keratopathy, and cataract. Other ocular manifestations such as macular edema, papillitis, and keratoconjunctivitis sicca have been described, but are rare.

SJÖGREN'S SYNDROME. Sjögren's syndrome is described as a combination of any two of the following entities: keratoconjunctivitis sicca, xerostomia, and rheumatoid arthritis or other connective tissue disease. Ocular involvement is a feature in an estimated 80 per cent of cases, particularly when RA is the systemic component of the syndrome. It usually begins in the fourth to sixth decade and has a 9:1 female predominance. It is estimated that 10 to 35 per cent of patients with RA develop this syndrome.

Keratoconjunctivitis sicca (KCS) is a nonspecific condition due to deficient tear film production. In addition to Sjögren's syndrome, KCS can be caused by congenital absence or hypoplasia of the lacrimal glands, by abnormalities in lacrimal gland innervation (e.g., familial dysautonomia), or in association with certain systemic diseases such as sarcoidosis, leukemia, or lymphoma.

Sjögren's syndrome is almost always a bilateral disease, although involvement may be asymmetric. Clinical symptoms of redness, itching, burning, dryness, photophobia, and foreign-body sensation evolve insidiously. Often these symptoms appear only in times of increased tear demand such as crying or environmental irritation. The conjunctiva usually appears normal but may be lusterless and gray. Lacrimal glands are rarely enlarged. The most characteristic ocular sign is the presence of accumulations of thick mucus near the palpebral fissures. The tear film is thin and viscous with epithelial and mucous debris on slit lamp examination. Occasionally, small focal areas of wrinkling, superficial corneal pits, or epithelial filaments can be discerned on the corneal surface. Corneal and conjunctival signs are highlighted by instillation of ophthalmic dyes such as rose bengal or fluorescein.

The most common diagnostic test for KCS is the Schirmer tear test. This test gives a crude approximation of lacrimal gland secretion. A 5 × 35 mm strip of filter paper is hooked over the lower lid margin in an anesthetized eye. After five minutes, the length of paper moistened is measured. Less than 5 mm of wetting is considered a positive (abnormal) test. Another consistent finding in KCS is a decreased lysozyme concentration in tears measured by lysis of bacteria on an agar plate.

Symptomatic treatment of the KCS of Sjögren's syndrome involves instillation of artificial tears and lubricants as often as necessary. Occlusion of the lacrimal puncta to retard drainage may be necessary in severe cases of xerosis. Soft contact lenses have been helpful to some patients.

ANKYLOSING SPONDYLITIS. Ankylosing spondylitis (Marie-Strümpell disease) is associated with an acute, recurrent anterior uveitis. In general, one third of the patients with ankylosing spondylitis will have this ocular complication. The uveitis is unrelated to the severity of the systemic complaints and usually follows the onset of arthritis symptoms, although it has been the initial complaint of some patients. In a study of young adult males with anterior uveitis, 41 per cent showed x-ray evidence of ankylosing spondylitis. Over-all, 12 to 17 per cent of cases of uveitis have such x-ray changes.

The anterior uveitis is heralded by acute pain, redness, photophobia, constricted pupil, sluggish pupillary reflex, and a circumcorneal conjunctival injection. It often resolves without complications but may result in anterior or posterior synechiae, or cataracts.

Treatment of the uveitis consists of topical or subconjunctival corticosteroids and cycloplegic drugs. Systemic steroids may be necessary in severe cases.

REITER'S SYNDROME. In 1916, Reiter described the classic triad of nongonococcal urethritis, arthritis, and conjunctivitis. The diagnosis of Reiter's syndrome is often made in the absence of the ocular symptom, however. Although conjunctivitis is occasionally the presenting symptom, it usually follows the onset of urethritis and arthritis by several days. The association of the HLA-27 antigen in 76 per cent of patients with urethritis and arthritis alone rises to 90 to 92 per cent in patients who also have the ocular component.

The most common eye disorder is a bilateral, mucopurulent conjunctivitis. This is associated with chemosis, lid edema, papillary hypertrophy, conjunctival hemorrhage, follicles, and preauricular lymphadenopathy. The conjunctivitis usually resolves spontaneously in seven to ten days.

Corneal lesions in Reiter's disease are usually associated with conjunctivitis. The most common disorder is a superficial punctate keratitis with underlying subepithelial opacities. This may subsequently involve the central stroma and finally the peripheral cornea. These lesions tend to regress spontaneously after several weeks without scarring; however, the stromal opacities may persist for months.

An anterior uveitis develops in up to 40 per cent of patients with Reiter's syndrome. It is especially common in recurrent attacks and may be the only feature of such recurrences. Although initial attacks tend to be unilateral, recurrences usually are bilateral.

Other ocular complications such as nodular scleritis,

episcleritis, retinal edema, and optic neuritis have been reported, but are rare.

Therapy of the eye disease consists of topical steroids and cycloplegics.

INFLAMMATORY BOWEL DISEASE. Both ulcerative colitis and regional enteritis (Crohn's disease) may cause ocular complications such as a recurrent nongranulomatous anterior uveitis, conjunctivitis, episcleritis, scleritis, and marginal keratitis. Ocular complications are usually limited to those patients with other nonintestinal manifestations. It is estimated that uveitis is more common in cases of granulomatous colitis than in ulcerative colitis.

The ocular inflammations respond to topical steroids and cycloplegics, although the uveitis tends to spontaneously resolve in four to six weeks.

RELAPSING POLYCHONDRITIS. The most common eye lesion seen in relapsing polychondritis is episcleritis, which develops in 40 per cent of the cases and is the initial presenting sign in 8 per cent of the cases. Conjunctivitis is seen in 24 per cent of patients with this disorder. Anterior uveitis affects 20 per cent of all patients. Other less common ocular complications have been reported. These include scleritis, keratoconjunctivitis sicca, retinal edema, retinal detachment, chorioretinal scarring, optic neuritis, exophthalmos, lateral rectus palsy, and Horner's syndrome.

As in other rheumatic diseases, the ocular complications tend to respond to topical or systemic corticosteroid therapy.

BEHÇET'S DISEASE. The classic triad of Behçet's disease includes recurrent aphthous stomatitis, genital ulcerations, and anterior uveitis, although many other manifestations such as arthritis, inflammatory bowel disease, CNS disease, and thrombophlebitis are often seen. The ocular complications, however, are the most frequent cause of disability seen with this disease. The most common complication is a severe recurrent anterior uveitis with hypopyon formation. It is occasionally unilateral during the initial attack; however, bilateral involvement is the rule during recurrences. Other infrequent ocular manifestations include conjunctivitis, keratitis, retinitis, choroiditis, optic neuritis, optic atrophy, and retinal vein occlusion. Corticosteroids and immunosuppressive drugs are used to control ocular complications.

Gold, D. H.: Ocular manifestations of connective tissue (collagen) diseases. In Duane, T. D. (ed.): Clinical Ophthalmology, Vol. 5. Hagerstown Md., Harper & Row, 1976, pp. 1–24.

Michels, R. G.: Ocular manifestations in arthritis. In Ryan, S. J., and Smith, R. E. (eds.): Selected Topics on the Eye in Systemic Disease. New York, Grune & Stratton, 1974, p. 363.

Rodnan, G. P. (ed.): Primer on the rheumatic diseases. JAMA, 224(5) (suppl.), 1973.

Schlaegel, Jr., T. F.: Uveitis of the suspected viral origin. In Duane, T. D. (ed.): Clinical Ophthalmology, Vol. 4. Hagerstown, Md. Harper & Row, 1976, pp. 1–11.

Shearn, M. A.: Sjögren's syndrome. In Smith, L. H. (ed.): Major Problems in Internal Medicine, Vol. 2. Philadelphia, W. B. Saunders Company, 1971, pp. 21–37.

Van Bijsterveld, O. P.: Diagnostic tests in the sicca syndrome. Arch. Ophthalmol., 82:10, 1969.

578. CONNECTIVE TISSUE DISEASES

INTRODUCTION. This chapter presents the pathophysiology, clinical features, and treatment of the ocular manifestations of systemic sclerosis, periarteritis nodosa, giant cell arteritis, Wegener's granulomatosis, polymyositis-dermatomyositis, and systemic lupus erythematosus. The ophthalmic features of other related disorders that primarily affect the joints (e.g., rheumatoid arthritis, Sjögren's syndrome, Reiter's syndrome) are discussed in Ch. 577.

SYSTEMIC LUPUS ERYTHEMATOSUS. Ocular manifestations of systemic lupus erythematosus (SLE) are usually seen during the acute flare-ups of severe systemic disease. SLE can involve the lids, conjunctiva, cornea, uveal tract, retina, optic nerve, and CNS visual pathway.

The eyelids, as with skin elsewhere, may have an erythematous rash, telangiectases, purpura, and pigmentary changes. A line of telangiectatic vessels just superior to the cilia on the upper lids can occasionally be seen.

The anterior segment may show a number of nonspecific signs. Conjunctivitis, injection, and scarring, as well as episcleritis, scleritis, and anterior uveitis, have all been reported in SLE patients. Keratoconjunctivitis sicca is occasionally seen. The cornea may show epithelial keratitis, band-like stromal infiltration, ulceration, and vascularization. These nonspecific signs are usually very mild but evident on careful slit lamp examination.

The most commonly observed ophthalmic sign of SLE is the cotton wool spot (Fig. 1E). This is caused by microinfarcts of the nerve fiber layer of the retina and is also a nonspecific sign seen in diabetic and hypertensive retinopathy. These lesions are usually found in the posterior pole. Superficial retinal hemorrhages, retinal edema, disc edema, fatty exudates, and perivasculitis have also been reported in SLE patients.

CNS complications of SLE can produce field defects (especially homonymous hemianopsia), optic atrophy, nystagmus, gaze palsies, and internuclear ophthalmoplegia. Diplopia, ptosis, and pupillary defects caused by third and sixth nerve lesions are also seen.

Many of the ocular complications of SLE and other connective tissue disorders are secondary to systemic steroid or antimalarial therapy. Posterior subcapsular cataracts from steroids, epithelial keratopathy, accommodation disorders, and degenerative retinopathies from chloroquine or hydroxychloroquine therapy are frequently encountered.

Ocular manifestations of SLE usually correlate to active systemic disease and are best treated by control of the systemic disease.

PROGRESSIVE SYSTEMIC SCLEROSIS. Progressive systemic sclerosis (scleroderma) may affect the lids, conjunctiva, cornea, retina, and extraocular muscles. One of the most common manifestations found is the skin of eyelids becoming indurated and tight, which can be minimal or cause severe restriction of eyelid movement. The other common ocular manifestation is decreased lacrimation, which can be found in 30 to 50 per cent of patients with scleroderma. The changes of keratoconjunctivitis sicca may be seen and are discussed in Ch. 577. Shallowing of the conjunctival fornices and mild chemosis may occasionally occur. Ocular motility may be involved in rare instances. Restriction of movements and heterotropias have been reported with laboratory and histologic evidence of inflammatory ocular myopathy.

Retinal changes resulting from scleroderma are uncommon. Many reports describe the changes of hypertensive retinopathy or anemia that may be superimposed and are not specifically signs of scleroderma. Ophthalmoscopic findings of uncomplicated scleroderma are limited to cotton wool spots and, less frequently, superficial retinal hemorrhages, retinal edema, and optic disc edema.

PERIARTERITIS NODOSA. The characteristic vasculitis of periarteritis nodosa can involve almost every ocular tissue. Conjunctival injection, edema, and subconjunctival hemorrhages are commonly seen. As in any of the connective tissue disorders, keratoconjunctivitis sicca can develop.

Necrotizing sclerokeratitis, similar to that seen in rheumatoid arthritis or Wegener's granulomatosis, may be present. A furrowed ulceration develops at the limbus of the cornea which may spread around and form a ring ulcer. This can progress anteriorly to involve the central cornea and produce scarring, vascularization, or perforation. This process may extend to the sclera and cause scleritis or episcleritis. Scleral nodules may also occur. An anterior uveitis (iridocyclitis) can accompany the sclerokeratitis. Posterior uveitis is rarely detectable clinically but is often present as choroidal arteritis on histologic examination. Choroidal arteritis is thought to produce retinal edema, flat detachment, and patchy atrophy in the overlying retina.

Visible fundus changes resulting from vasculitis have been estimated to occur in 10 to 20 per cent of patients with periarteritis. The nonspecific retinal changes include hemorrhages, edema, fatty exudates, cotton wool patches, vascular narrowing, retinal detachments, and branch or central retinal artery occlusions (Fig. 1C). The nephrogenic hypertension seen in periarteritis frequently causes retinopathy. Involvement of the optic nerve takes the form of disc edema (10 per cent of patients) or papillitis. Exophthalmos caused by orbital involvement is seen rarely.

CNS effects of periarteritis can produce field defects, an Argyll Robertson pupil, amaurosis fugax, Horner's syndrome, nystagmus, tropias, and cranial nerve palsies.

There is no satisfactory treatment of the ocular complications of periarteritis. The side effects of steroid or antimalarial therapy often add to the ocular problems.

WEGENER'S GRANULOMATOSIS. Of the classic triad of necrotizing granulomas of the respiratory tract, focal vasculitis, and renal glomerulitis, the first two can give rise to ocular manifestations in approximately 40 per cent of patients with Wegener's granulomatosis. Orbital invasion by granulomas of the upper respiratory tract often results in proptosis. A spectrum of ophthalmic signs similar to those of periarteritis nodosa may be present due to the necrotizing vasculitis. These signs include chemosis, uveitis, scleritis, episcleritis, corneal ring ulcer, retinal venous congestion, extraocular muscle disorders, cotton wool patches, and optic disc edema. Ophthalmic manifestations of CNS disease and hypertensive retinopathy are more common in periarteritis, whereas direct orbital involvement (proptosis) is suggestive of Wegener's granulomatosis.

GIANT CELL ARTERITIS. Giant cell arteritis, also known as temporal arteritis, cranial arteritis, and Horton's arteritis, has many features in common with periarteritis nodosa and Wegener's granulomatosis. A differential diagnosis on ophthalmic examination is not always possible. Ocular manifestations of giant cell arteritis are often more severe, more common, and more

Figure 1. *See facing page for legend.*

detrimental to vision than the other forms of vasculitis. Therefore a greater emphasis should be placed on the ophthalmic examination as an aid in early treatment of giant cell arteritis.

The incidence of ocular involvement in giant cell arteritis is approximately 50 per cent. The eye disease is frequently the most serious aspect of the disease and results in blindness in approximately 27 per cent of patients. Bilateral involvement occurs in 35 per cent of the cases. Ocular findings usually occur within weeks or months after the onset of systemic involvement, but may be delayed for several years. Acute visual loss can be seen in the absence of other systemic signs or symptoms and is known as occult temporal arteritis. This is due to arteritis of the ophthalmic, central retinal, or ciliary arteries.

The most frequent cause of visual loss is ischemic optic neuropathy. This presents as sudden visual loss with a pale, edematous disc and small peripapillary hemorrhages. Visual loss is usually complete, but various field defects have been described. The consensual pupillary reflex is normal, but the direct response is sluggish or absent, indicating an afferent pupillary defect. Disc edema resolves in a few days, leaving a waxy pallor to the disc. Ischemic optic neuropathy is also seen as a consequence of arteriosclerosis. Occlusion of the central retinal artery resulting from giant cell arteritis is a less common cause of sudden visual loss. This appears ophthalmoscopically as a gray-white ischemic retina with blood sludging in the vessels and a cherry red macula.

Other ocular manifestations of giant cell arteritis include transient diplopia caused by third or sixth nerve palsies, ptosis, episcleritis, scleritis, iritis, branch artery occlusion, rubeosis iridis, ocular hypotony, scintillating scotomas, photophobia, and periorbital pain. All of these may be present during the acute phase of the arteritis but are generally infrequent complications.

Although the nonspecificity of the erythrocyte sedimentation rate (ESR) is stressed, an elevated ESR is a characteristic feature of the disease, even in the absence of other signs or symptoms. A temporal artery biopsy is the most reliable diagnostic test, however. The histologic appearance is that of granulomatous arteritis with giant cells within the vessel walls, fragmentation of the internal elastic lamina, and intimal thickening or fibrosis. False-negative biopsies can occur, as can the positive histologic findings when there is no other clinical evidence of disease. A temporal arteriogram may also aid in the diagnosis and increase the biopsy yield by locating involved areas. Polymyalgia rheumatica is associated with giant cell arteritis and may represent different manifestations of the same disease. Therefore the characteristic proximal muscle symptoms of pain and stiffness despite normal muscle enzymes, biopsy, and electromyogram should aid in the diagnosis of giant cell arteritis.

The only effective therapy is systemic corticosteroids. Early treatment is indicated following diagnosis to prevent occurrence of the eye signs. Prednisone is administered until clinical and laboratory evidence (e.g., ESR) of disease activity is under control. Although visual loss is usually permanent, a few patients may regain some visual acuity after early steroid therapy. The essence of therapy therefore is early diagnosis and treatment.

POLYMYOSITIS, DERMATOMYOSITIS. Ocular manifestations of dermatomyositis and polymyositis are uncommon. They are all nonspecific changes that are seen in any of the connective tissue diseases. These include keratoconjunctivitis sicca, cotton wool spots, hemorrhages, edema, and vessel tortuosity in the retina. The ophthalmoscopic signs generally parallel the systemic disease and are improved with steroids. The most serious ocular complications are those of systemic steroid or antimalarial therapy.

Cullen, J. F., and Colerio, J. A.: Ophthalmic complications of giant cell arteritis. Surv. Ophthalmol., 20:247, 1976.

Gold, D. H.: Ocular manifestations of connective tissue (collagen) diseases. In Duane, T. D. (ed.): Clinical Ophthalmology, Vol. 5. Hagerstown, Md., Harper & Row, 1976, pp. 1–24.

Jaeger, E. A.: Retinopathy in the connective tissue diseases. In Duane, T. D. (ed.): Clinical Ophthalmology, Vol. 3. Hagerstown, Md., Harper & Row, 1976, pp. 1–8.

Michels, R. G.: Ocular manifestations in connective tissue disorders (CTD). In Ryan, S. J., Jr., and Smith, R. E. (eds.): Selected Topics on the Eye in Systemic Disease. New York, Grune & Stratton, 1974, pp. 301–313.

Figure 1. *A,* Papilledema secondary to increased intracranial pressure. The disc shows loss of normal contour with edema fluid in the peripapillary layers. There is associated loss of nerve fiber layer pattern, small flame hemorrhages and exudates, and marked dilatation of the venous system.

B, End-stage glaucoma. The disc shows marked pallor with loss of normal disc architecture. The nasal vessels curl behind the enlarged cup of the disc, which is suggestive but not pathognomonic of a glaucomatous process. Notice the temporal border of the disc which shows minimal to absent nerve fiber layer rim.

C, Central retinal artery occlusion. The fundus shows a milky retinal reflex secondary to edema of the retinal layers. The disc is hazy secondary to ischemia. The macular region shows a "cherry red spot" which is seen as a dark area in the photograph. This corresponds to active choroidal circulation seen through the thin retina at the fovea in the face of a markedly malfunctioning ischemic retinal circulation.

D, Central retinal vein occlusion. This fundus finding is known as the "squashed tomato" fundus in which the central retinal vessels become obstructed. The vascular insult causes capillary and surface hemorrhage with exudation and swelling at the disc.

E, Cotton wool spots. The fundus shows fluffy "cotton wool spots" which are indicative of nerve fiber layer ischemia and infarction. Note that the cotton wool spots overlying the retinal vessels indicate their anatomic location at the innermost retinal layer.

F, Grade 4 hypertensive retinopathy. Note the swelling at the disc with the engorged vessels and disc edema. Multiple areas of retinal exudate and hemorrhage are present. In the macular area accumulation of fluid in the outer plexiform layer of the retina gives the appearance of a partial macular "star."

G, Ocular toxoplasmosis. Note the large atropic pigmented macular scar from an ocular toxoplasmosis lesion. Approximately one half disc diameter nasally is a small area of acute toxoplasmic retinal inflammation.

H, Presumed ocular histoplasmosis syndrome (POHS). This fundus reveals the classic triad of presumed ocular histoplasmosis. Note (1) peripapillary scarring and atrophy at the disc margin, (2) a macular histoplasmosis "spot," and (3) punched-out "spots" elsewhere and in the periphery (seen in this photograph to be inferior to the macular lesion).

579. DIABETES MELLITUS

INCIDENCE. The most common and potentially serious ocular complication of diabetes is diabetic retinopathy. The development of retinal lesions caused by diabetic microangiopathy is related to the duration of diabetes in most patients. Therefore the incidence of diabetic retinopathy and other ocular lesions has been steadily increasing over the last two generations as advances in medical management have increased the average life span of patients with this disease.

Approximately 1.5 per cent of the population of Europe and the Americas has diabetes mellitus. Of the patients with juvenile-onset diabetes, 10 per cent have retinopathy 5 to 9 years after onset of diabetes, 50 per cent after 15 years, and 80 to 90 per cent after 25 years of disease. Patients with maturity-onset diabetes develop retinopathy sooner in their disease, but the manifestations are milder than those of juvenile-onset diabetics. In patients developing diabetes between the ages of 30 and 60, 30 per cent of these have retinopathy after 5 years, 40 to 50 per cent after 10 years, 60 per cent after 15 years, and 70 to 80 per cent after 25 years of disease. Similarly, after 10 years of diabetes, 0.1 to 2.1 per cent of patients will be blinded by their disease, whereas 1.6 to 7.1 per cent of diabetics will be blind after 30 years of disease. In the United States, between 10 and 15 per cent of all cases of acquired blindness are due to diabetic retinopathy.

PATHOLOGY. The characteristic small vessel disease seen elsewhere in the body also occurs in the retinal vasculature. In the capillaries and venules, there is thickening and vacuolization of the basement membrane with deposits of PAS-positive material. In addition, capillary mural cells (pericytes) are lost, and endothelial cells proliferate with hyalinization. Finally, focal closure of capillaries occurs, with subsequent redirection of blood flow through arteriovenule shunts or anastomoses.

Venous dilatation is one of the earliest retinal signs of diabetic retinopathy. This change may be due to arterial insufficiency or may be in response to some alteration (e.g., hypoxia) of local retinal tissues.

Microaneurysm formation is a characteristic early lesion of diabetic retinopathy, although microaneurysms are seen in other disorders such as sickle cell anemia, macroglobulinemia, arteritis, and hypertension. The microaneurysms are 50 to 200 μ saccular dilatations of capillaries and venules. These may originate at bends of shunt vessels where the hydrostatic pressure is greatest and where the vessel wall is weakened by loss of mural cells.

With advancing retinopathy, the retinal veins become more tortuous and dilated. Rupture of these abnormal vessels leads to large retinal or vitreous hemorrhages. Mesenchymal proliferation from within the ruptured vessels causes a neovascularization of poorly differentiated vessels and connective tissue. These new vessel tufts frequently invade the vitreous body and also may lead to vitreal hemorrhage. Vitreous shrinkage or contraction, caused by the fibrotic response to hemorrhage resorption, leads to retinal traction, rupture of retinal surface vessels (preretinal hemorrhage), or retinal detachment.

The exact pathophysiologic alteration that leads to these changes is still under speculation. The theory currently receiving the most attention centers on inadequate retinal oxygenation because of either microcirculatory insufficiency or disordered oxygen transplant by erythrocytes.

CLINICAL MANIFESTATIONS. Extraocular. The lids, conjunctiva, extraocular muscles, and orbital tissue can be involved in diabetes. The lids of diabetics have xanthelasma more frequently than nondiabetic patients. These elevated yellowish plaques have only cosmetic significance and can be surgically excised if desired. Conjunctival vessels can show venular and arteriolar dilatation, vasoconstriction, and microaneurysms.

Extraocular muscle palsies are commonly seen in diabetics. They often develop suddenly, are associated with periorbital pain, and regress spontaneously after four to six weeks. The lateral rectus is the most commonly involved muscle. Characteristically, the pupillary response is preserved when the third nerve is involved. Third and sixth nerve palsies may be due to vascular insufficiency to the neurons rather than to a primary neuropathy.

A rare but serious complication of diabetes is orbital mucormycosis. About 50 per cent of all cases occur in diabetic patients whose disease is in poor control. The diagnosis is suggested by rapidly developing rhinitis, headaches, unilateral ptosis, lid edema, and ophthalmoplegia. Although it may be fatal, it is usually responsive to local and systemic amphotericin B therapy.

Cornea. Wrinkling of Descemet's membrane is common in diabetics. This finding, which is only detectable on slit lamp examination, may be an early clinical sign that precedes most other ocular manifestations. Similar but less well defined wrinkles are seen occasionally in elderly nondiabetics. Corneal sensation may be decreased in diabetics. The corneal epithelium may heal poorly following a corneal abrasion.

Iris. Rubeosis iridis is the characteristic iris lesion in diabetes. This is a fibrovascular membrane which proliferates from the iris stroma and is almost always secondary to proliferative retinopathy. This membrane covers the anterior surface of the iris and can produce a neovascular glaucoma by obliteration of the aqueous outflow channels. These cells are fragile and may rupture and release iris pigment into the anterior chamber during pupillary dilation or anterior chamber surgery.

Lens. Hyperglycemia causes an increased refractive power of the lens. Therefore transient refractive errors are seen when the blood glucose level fluctuates. The lens changes in hyperglycemia may be due to an increased glucose concentration and water content of the lens. The lens becomes thicker and thus increases its refractive power. Nearsightedness is the initial symptom of diabetes in approximately 33 per cent of all cases. Since this change is reversible, corrective lenses should not be prescribed when the glucose level is uncontrolled.

The incidence of senile cataracts is increased in diabetics; they also tend to develop earlier than in nondiabetics. Less frequently seen is the characteristic "snowflake" opacity or "true" diabetic cataract seen in juvenile diabetics. These bilateral cataracts may produce complete opacity of the lens within several weeks. They appear as white subcapsular bands and uniform needle-shaped opacities which progress to total opacity in many cases. Surgical extraction is the only therapy.

Ciliary Body. The basement membrane of the ciliary process is thickened in diabetics. The clinical significance of this histologic finding is unknown.

Retina and Vitreous. The most common and potentially serious ocular complications of diabetes occur in the retina. Diabetic retinopathy is usually always bilateral, and of approximately equal severity in both eyes. Profound asymmetry suggests unilateral carotid artery disease, previous chorioretinal or optic nerve disease, unilateral high myopia, or increased intraocular pressure.

Diabetic retinopathy generally occurs in two phases: a nonproliferative phase and a proliferative phase. The earliest ophthalmoscopic changes of diabetes are those of nonproliferative or background retinopathy. In this phase the retinal veins become more dilated and tortuous. Numerous microaneurysms appear. These are barely perceptible, tiny red dots which may be impossible to differentiate from tiny retinal hemorrhages. Retinal hemorrhages and exudates are also characteristic of background retinopathy. Dot hemorrhages are small round hemorrhages in the compact inner nuclear layer of the retina. Flame-shaped hemorrhages, similar to those seen in hypertensive retinopathy, blood dyscrasias, papilledema, or central vein obstruction (Fig. 1D), represent more superficial bleeding into the nerve fiber layer. Hemorrhage into the preretinal space produces a characteristic "blot" appearance. Most hemorrhages resolve spontaneously. Exudates in the retina have been described classically as "hard" or "soft." Hard exudates are small, glistening, yellow-white spots that tend to gradually enlarge and coalesce. These represent serum lipid and protein exudates into areas of ischemic retina. Soft exudates or cotton wool patches, as previously mentioned, represent microinfarcts of the nerve fiber layer which are seen commonly in patients with hypertension and connective tissue disease.

The development of neovascular tufts heralds the proliferative diabetic retinopathy phase and is a poor prognostic sign. Between 6 and 20 per cent of all patients with background retinopathy progress to the proliferative phase. Neovascularization occurs primarily at arteriovenous crossings or over the optic disc. The superior temporal vein is involved most frequently, followed by the inferior temporal, superior nasal, and inferior nasal veins. These new vessels frequently extend beyond the internal limiting membrane or protrude from the disc and may become adherent to or even penetrate the posterior vitreous face. Vitreous hemorrhage, vitreous contraction with retinal traction, and retinal detachment represent the most serious complications of the neovascularization.

An additional ophthalmoscopic feature occasionally encountered in diabetics is lipemia retinalis. Usually seen during ketoacidosis, lipemia retinalis is due to a gross hyperlipemia in the range of 3.0 to 3.5 grams per 100 ml. The retinal vessels become engorged, and the blood column assumes a salmon pink to creamy white color because of the higher lipid content. Vision is not affected, however. This sign is occasionally helpful in the rapid evaluation of a comatose patient in suspected diabetic ketoacidosis. When the ketosis is corrected, serum lipids normalize and lipemia retinalis disappears.

DIAGNOSIS. The characteristic retinopathy, along with laboratory evidence of disordered carbohydrate metabolism, usually establishes the diagnosis. The ophthalmoscopic features rarely can precede chemical abnormalities but have been reported in patients who never develop an abnormal glucose tolerance curve. The differentiation between background and proliferative retinopathy is an important task because it alters prognosis and therapeutic regimens. Fundus photography and fluorescein angiography, which demonstrate the vascular abnormalities, are invaluable tools for detection and observation of subtle changes such as microaneurysms, venous dilatation, arteriovenular shunts, and neovascular tufts.

TREATMENT. The goal of treatment is to delay or retard visual impairment caused by retinopathy. Many different approaches to therapy have been tried or are being tested, and considerable debate remains concerning the various efficacies of each.

Medical Therapy. Much disagreement exists over the value of rigid control of the biochemical parameters of diabetes. The consensus is that optimal control of blood glucose levels decreases the risk of microvascular complications. Many other medical therapies such as vitamins, anticoagulants, anabolic steroids, lipotropic agents, and salicylates have been tried but without encouraging results.

Pituitary Ablation. Pituitary ablation has been advocated for the management of diabetic retinopathy. Most favorable reports, however, are of small and uncontrolled clinical trials. Considering the morbidity and mortality of the surgery and the resulting panhypopituitarism, this form of therapy seems to create considerable risks for questionable benefits.

Photocoagulation. Xenon arc and laser photocoagulation can be used for direct application to neovascular tissue, for obliteration of microaneurysms and leaking retinal vessels, or for widespread ablation of retinal tissue. This scattered, panretinal photocoagulation in eyes with proliferative retinopathy is of benefit in reducing the amount of visual loss from the retinopathy. Panretinal photocoagulation should be considered in all patients with early signs of proliferative complications of diabetes. There is still questionable benefit for photocoagulation of background retinopathy alone, however.

Vitrectomy. Vitreous hemorrhages occasionally fail to reabsorb spontaneously. Recent advances in vitreous surgery have made it possible to remove the blood-stained vitreous from the eye while leaving the other ocular structures intact.

Neovascular Glaucoma. Glaucoma secondary to rubeosis iridis is refractory to most medical and surgical treatment. A few patients have been helped with partial freezing of the ciliary body to decrease aqueous production, but treatment for this complication is generally unsatisfactory.

PROGNOSIS. Diabetic retinopathy primarily affects the posterior pole and spares the periphery, which is the reverse of the pattern seen in sickle cell anemia and the dysproteinemias. Its natural history is to fluctuate in severity and to progress. There is a 10 to 30 per cent rate of spontaneous regression or improvement of neovascular retinopathy. An additional 10 to 70 per cent of patients have a stable, nonprogressive disease over an observation period of one to four years. Visual deterioration is more rapid in older diabetics. In patients with diabetic retinopathy, legal blindness (best corrected vision of less than 20/200) occurs in 3 per cent of those less than 60 years old and 20 per cent of those over 60. Photocoagulation significantly improves the prognosis for patients with proliferative retinopathy.

Cahill, G. F., Etzwiler, D. D., and Freinkel, N.: Control and diabetes. N. Engl. J. Med., 294:1004, 1976.

Diabetic Retinopathy Study Research Group: Preliminary report on effects of photocoagulation therapy. Am. J. Ophthalmol., 81:383, 1976.

Duane, T. D.: Diabetic retinopathy. *In* Duane, T. D. (ed.): Clinical Ophthalmology, Vol. 3. Hagerstown, Md., Harper & Row, 1976, pp. 1–19.

Frank, R. N.: Diabetic retinopathy. *In* Ryan, S. J., Jr., and Smith, R. E. (eds.): Selected Topics on the Eye in Systemic Disease. New York, Grune & Stratton, 1976, pp. 65–118.

Goldberg, M. F., and Fine, S. L. (eds.): Symposium on the Treatment of Diabetic Retinopathy. Washington, D.C., U.S. Department of Public Health Publication No. 1890, 1968.

Henkind, P.: The eye in diabetes mellitus: Signs, symptoms, and their pathogenesis. *In* Mausolf, F. A. (ed.): The Eye and Systemic Disease. St. Louis, C. V. Mosby Company, 1976, pp. 195–204.

Mandelcorn, M. S., Blankenship, G., and Machemer, R.: Pars plana vitrectomy for the management of severe diabetic retinopathy. Am. J. Ophthalmol., 81:561, 1976.

Wise, G. N., Dollery, C. T., and Henkind, P.: The Retinal Circulation. New York, Harper & Row, 1971.

580.   GLAUCOMA

DEFINITION. The glaucomas are a collection of ophthalmic disorders in which the intraocular pressure is sufficiently elevated to cause excavation and degeneration of the optic disc and typical visual field defects due to nerve fiber bundle damage. An estimated 2 per cent of all people over 40 years of age have glaucoma. As one of the leading causes of acquired blindness, glaucoma accounts for 12 to 30 per cent of the total cases (Fig. 1*B*).

The glaucomas are generally classified as primary, secondary, or congenital disorders. Primary glaucoma is a genetically determined, bilateral disease which is further subdivided into angle-closure and open-angle forms. Secondary glaucoma is characterized by increased intraocular pressure caused by some antecedent or concomitant ocular disorder such as tumor, inflammation, trauma, or neovascularization. These also may be divided into angle-closure and open-angle forms. Congenital glaucoma occurs as a result of anterior segment anomalies developed during gestation or at birth, although the classic signs and symptoms may not emerge until adult life.

Measurement of Intraocular Pressure. The two most common methods for estimating intraocular pressure are Schiøtz and applanation tonometry. The Schiøtz tonometer is a portable hand-held device which is the most practical, cheapest, and easiest method for routine screening. This tonometer measures the amount of corneal indentation produced by a standardized pressure. Applanation tonometry gives a more reliable and accurate reading but requires more complex equipment. This method measures the force required to flatten a standard area of cornea.

The intraocular pressures of a normal population approximate a normal distribution with a mean value of approximately 16 mm Hg. Pressure readings between 10 and 21 mm Hg are generally considered normal. The pressure varies 1 to 2 mm Hg with each heartbeat, and there may be a 2 to 5 mm Hg diurnal fluctuation in intraocular tension. Many other factors such as venous hypertension or marked variation in plasma osmolarity may have temporary effects on the intraocular pressure as well.

An intraocular pressure of greater than 21 mm Hg is not diagnostic of glaucoma, just as a pressure of less than that does not strictly rule it out. Glaucoma is present with any pressure sufficient to produce optic nerve damage. Although some patients normally run pressures above 21 mm Hg without any evidence of optic nerve degeneration, others show progressive visual impairment with pressures of less than 21 mm Hg.

PRIMARY OPEN-ANGLE GLAUCOMA. Open-angle glaucoma, also known as simple or chronic glaucoma, is a slowly progressive bilateral disease of insidious onset. There are usually no symptoms until significant irreversible field losses have occurred.

Primary open-angle glaucoma has been demonstrated to be a familial and hereditary disorder. It is predominantly inherited as a multifactorial trait, although variations in penetrance or expressivity of the gene in certain individuals can account for those patients who develop open-angle glaucoma despite a negative family history. The disease occurs predominantly in people 40 years or older. It is the most common form of all the glaucomas and accounts for over 90 per cent of primary adult disease cases.

In over 99 per cent of cases of open-angle glaucoma, the elevation of intraocular pressures is due to an outflow obstruction resulting from degenerative changes in the trabecular meshwork, Schlemm's canal, or adjacent efferent channels.

The patient with open-angle glaucoma rarely has any symptoms, and visual field loss is so gradual that subjective complaints are not made until late in the disease. Characteristically, the elevated intraocular pressure gradually destroys bundles of optic nerve fibers at the nervehead. This results in a specific arcuate-shaped scotoma arising from the blind spot, curving around the fovea, and ending abruptly at the horizontal meridian. Peripheral field loss, especially in nasal and superior fields, also commonly occurs later in the course of the disease. The fibers from the central fixation area are usually spared until late in the disease process, so that central visual acuity may be normal despite extensive field defects. Visual acuity therefore is a poor index of the degree of glaucomatous damage. Although the disease is invariably bilateral, asymmetric involvement is frequently seen.

Another important sign of glaucoma is optic disc excavation and degeneration. Early changes may be indistinguishable from normal variations in the size of the physiologic cup. The cup in glaucoma gradually enlarges and deepens, often asymmetrically toward the temporal (macular) side. The cup/disc ratio is thus increased from an average normal value of 0.3. The large retinal vessels become nasally displaced and seem to disappear over the rim of a deep, bean pot–shaped depression. The affected area of the disc becomes atrophic and appears grayish white rather than the normal pink.

The diagnosis of open-angle glaucoma is made when an increased intraocular pressure is combined with the characteristic field defects and optic disc degeneration. The elevated pressure usually precedes the neural damage by many years. Pressures over 21 mm Hg without other signs are suggestive of early open-angle glaucoma and warrant the need for frequent follow-up or referral to an ophthalmologist for special diagnostic procedures.

Treatment of open-angle glaucoma is usually medical, although surgery may be required in some refractory individuals. Initial therapy usually begins with miotic drops to facilitate the aqueous outflow. Parasympathomimetics such as pilocarpine (1 to 4 per cent) or anticholinesterases such as echothiophate iodide (0.03 to 0.25 per cent) are the usual drugs of choice for open-angle glaucoma. Epinephrine (0.5 to 2 per cent) is often added to one of the aforementioned miotics to decrease aqueous production and further enhance outflow. Other agents such as carbonic anhydrase inhibitors (acetazolamide) also are used if miotics and epinephrine do not adequately lower the intraocular pressure.

Response to medical therapy is usually good. However, despite adequate control of ocular pressure, some patients' field defects continue to progress. A variety of surgical techniques are available for medically uncontrollable cases. If left untreated, the disease will slowly progress to complete blindness.

ANGLE-CLOSURE GLAUCOMA. Acute angle-closure glaucoma is a sudden increase in intraocular pressure due to a mechanical blockade of the outflow channels in the angle. The blockage is caused by the iris coming in contact with the trabecular meshwork. Affected individuals genetically predisposed to the development of an acute glaucomatous attack have some anatomic variation that results in a shallow anterior chamber and a narrow angle. Although it is relatively uncommon and constitutes less than 5 per cent of all cases of primary glaucoma, angle-closure glaucoma is an important disease to recognize and treat quickly. The severe pain associated with an acute attack and the rapidity with which visual impairment ensues make angle-closure glaucoma a true ophthalmic emergency.

An acute attack of angle-closure glaucoma produces dramatic ocular and systemic symptoms. There is a sudden onset of excruciating pain which often produces prostration, nausea, and vomiting. The pain may be localized in or around the eye or may be distributed over the fifth cranial nerve area. Vision becomes blurred or foggy, and colored halos are seen around lights as the cornea obtains a steamy appearance.

Paralysis of the pupillary sphincter muscle by a markedly increased intraocular pressure results in a fixed, mid-dilated pupil. Ciliary injection is seen, as well as varying degrees of iris and conjunctival venous engorgement and aqueous flare. The optic disc may become swollen within 24 hours, and complete visual loss can occur in just a few days. Glaucomatous cupping and specific field defects are seldom seen. The main differential diagnostic conditions which also produce an acutely painful red eye include anterior uveitis, conjunctivitis, and corneal trauma.

A number of factors which can precipitate an acute attack of angle-closure glaucoma have been identified. Dilation of the pupil can thicken the peripheral iris sufficiently to obstruct the angle and produce an attack. Therefore the depth of the anterior chamber should be estimated in all patients prior to dilation for funduscopy by oblique illumination (Fig. 2). Long-acting or irreversible mydriatics such as atropine should not be used in patients with shallow anterior chambers or narrow angles. Increased

thickness of the lens can also encroach upon the angle and precipitate an attack of acute glaucoma. The lens normally thickens with age and further increases in width during accommodation. Fibrous adhesion of the pupil to the lens is also a cause of angle-closure glaucoma and can follow any of a number of intraocular inflammations.

Prior to considering surgery, lowering intraocular pressure with miotics and intravenous or oral hyperosmotic agents should be tried. Oral glycerin and pilocarpine drops are the initial drugs of choice. If glycerin treatment is unsuccessful, intravenous hypertonic mannitol or urea can be effective. Systemic analgesics such as meperidine are also indicated for relief of pain and sedation. A peripheral iridectomy is indicated within four to six hours after initiating treatment if the pressure is not lowered sufficiently. The iridectomy also acts as a prophylactic measure against future episodes of angle-closure glaucoma.

Kolker, A. E., and Hetherington, J.: Becker-Shaffer's Diagnosis and Therapy of the Glaucomas. 4th ed. St. Louis, C. V. Mosby Company, 1976.
Newell, F. W., and Ernest, J. T.: Ophthalmology Principles and Concepts. 3rd ed. St. Louis, C. V. Mosby Company, 1974.
Scheie, H. G., and Albert, D. M.: Textbook of Ophthalmology. 9th ed. Philadelphia, W. B. Saunders Company, 1977.
Vaughan, D., and Asbury, T.: General Ophthalmology. 8th ed. Los Altos, Calif., Lange Medical Publications, 1977.

581. OCULAR HISTOPLASMOSIS

DEFINITION. Ocular histoplasmosis consists of disseminated choroiditis which results in scars in the periphery of the fundus and near the optic nerve, and characteristic disciform macular lesions. Epidemiologic, experimental, and clinical evidence strongly suggests *Histoplasma capsulatum* as the causative agent. However, organisms have only rarely been recovered from eyes of patients having this clinical syndrome. This has prompted many writers to refer to the presumed ocular histoplasmosis syndrome (POHS) (Fig. 1H).

INCIDENCE. Characteristic atrophic chorioretinal scars ("histo spots") are seen in 1 to 2 per cent of the population

NORMAL (DEEP) CHAMBER   SHALLOW CHAMBER

SIDE VIEW   SIDE VIEW

Figure 2. Estimating anterior chamber depth.

ANTERIOR VIEW
(NOTE SMALL NASAL SHADOW)   ANTERIOR VIEW
(NOTE LARGE NASAL SHADOW)

in the Midwest. Ocular histoplasmosis is seen in patients of all ages from 7 to 70 years, with the highest incidence between 30 and 39 years of age. Although skin sensitivity to histoplasmosis is equal between blacks and whites, ocular histoplasmosis is seen 20 times more often in whites. Ocular histoplasmosis has the same geographic distribution and endemic areas as systemic histoplasmosis.

ETIOLOGY.   Since ocular histoplasmosis has never been proved to be associated with systemic disease and since few organisms have ever been recovered from these eyes, the term presumed ocular histoplasmosis is often used. However, there is evidence supporting this association: (1) the ocular syndrome is rarely seen outside the areas endemic for histoplasmosis; (2) histoplasmin skin tests are positive in 93 per cent of the patients with the characteristic eye findings, and they differ significantly from a control group of the same area; and (3) there is usually an absence of other causes of uveitis in these patients.

PATHOLOGY AND PATHOPHYSIOLOGY.   Although there are few histopathologic studies of ocular histoplasmosis in humans, the eyes studied to date have shown focal areas of disruption of the outer retinal layers, loss of the pigment epithelium, loss of the choriocapillaris, chorioretinal adhesion, and minimal inflammation. Macular lesions show focal granulomatous choroiditis, disruption of Bruch's membrane, hemorrhagic retinal detachment, disruption of the pigment epithelium, and abnormal vessel formation in fibrovascular scars.

CLINICAL MANIFESTATIONS.   The three classic lesions of presumed ocular histoplasmosis are (1) peripheral chorioretinal scars ("histo spots"), (2) scars surrounding the optic nerve, and (3) macular scars.

Histo Spots.   Early lesions of ocular histoplasmosis appear as subtle, yellow nodules in the choroid without pigment changes or hemorrhage. Histo spots are atrophic chorioretinal scars that appear as discrete round or oval punched-out lesions about 0.5 to 1.0 mm in diameter. They usually have a pale atrophic center with a surrounding pigmented margin. These spots vary in number from 1 to 70, with a mean of 8 per eye. Scars are bilateral in over 60 per cent of the cases, and in 90 per cent they are posterior to the equator. Histo spots do not produce overlying haze in the vitreous. They should be differentiated from tuberculosis, sarcoidosis, nocardiosis, coccidioidomycosis, and cryptococcosis.

Circumpapillary Choroiditis.   Circumpapillary choroiditis refers to chorioretinal scars surrounding the papilla, or optic nerve, that are usually separated from the disc by a rim of pigment. Hemorrhage under the retina may occur from these scars and lead to secondary detachment of the retina in 50 per cent of these cases, which results in significant visual impairment.

Circumpapillary choroiditis is seen in 70 to 85 per cent of patients with macular disciform disease and in 30 per cent of patients with histo spots alone. The most important aspect of this ocular sign is to help recognize the characteristic ocular findings of histoplasmosis. The differential diagnosis of these lesions includes myopic crescents, senile halos, inferior crescents, atypical colobomas, and drusen.

Macular Disciform Lesions.   Macular disciform lesions are important observations in histoplasmosis because of their potential adverse effects on vision. These lesions occur equally in both sexes primarily between the ages of 20 and 50, with a peak incidence in the fourth decade. Macular disease usually occurs 10 to 20 years after the onset of peripheral atrophic scars (histo spots) and almost never during acute systemic histoplasmosis. Perhaps 5 per cent of all patients with histo spots will eventually develop symptomatic macular lesions.

Symptoms usually begin with metamorphopsia, which progresses slowly to paracentral and central scotoma with blurred vision.

The earliest ophthalmoscopic signs are subretinal fluid accumulation adjacent to old parafoveal scars or a gray-white thickening of the choroid with blurred margins under a normal retina and vitreous.

Macular lesions usually progress through the several stages resulting in gliotic scarring and severe visual impairment. The lesions become hemorrhagic in 63 per cent of cases. Hemorrhages tend to recur and active lesions persist for about two years. Hemorrhage and serous transudation follow choroidal neovascularization with extensions through Bruch's membrane into the subretinal space. This may lead to serous detachment of the pigment epithelium with yellow circinate exudates surrounding the detachment. The areas of disciform retinal detachment can be larger than the area of choroidal disease and obscure the funduscopic view. Late lesions are inactive, white, elevated scars due to chronic disciform detachment with microcystic degeneration and fibrosis secondary to recurrent hemorrhage. Rarely, blood may leak into the vitreous body, usually in anticoagulated patients. Otherwise, the eye findings are limited to the posterior uvea and retina. The anterior segment and the vitreous are characteristically free of disease.

Macular lesions can occur in the second eye in about 10 per cent of the affected population. Symptomatic macular lesions in the second eye occur from one month to one or two decades after first eye involvement, with an average lag of five to seven years.

DIAGNOSIS.   The characteristic posterior lesions provide the basis for the diagnosis of presumed ocular histoplasmosis. There is no specific laboratory test to establish the diagnosis. The most valuable test is the histoplasmin skin test, although false negatives may occur in up to 11 per cent of the population with characteristic ocular lesions. Complement fixation tests are positive in only one third of patients with eye findings, but this test may be useful if skin tests are negative. The chest x-ray shows fibrocalcific changes consistent with pulmonary histoplasmosis more frequently in people with macular lesions than a control group. The diagnosis may be made in people with suggestive fundus lesions, a history of residence in an endemic area, and some evidence of previous infection, i.e., immunologic, serologic, or radiographic.

TREATMENT.   Disseminated atrophic choroidal scars (histo spots) are usually asymptomatic and require no therapy. Treatment of macular lesions is directed toward prevention of progression to blinding fibrovascular scarring. Amphotericin B, the mainstay of systemic histoplasmosis therapy, is contraindicated in ocular histoplasmosis.

Corticosteroids and photocoagulation are the two major modes of therapy. Some authors feel that high dose corticosteroids (100 mg of prednisone daily) given at first indication of macular disease may prevent early disciform lesions. Periocular injections beneath Tenon's capsule can be used in patients who do not tolerate systemic steroids or who require long-term therapy for control of their disease. Others feel that corticosteroids do not favorably influence the long-term prognosis.

If medical therapy produces no improvement or if hemorrhage occurs during therapy, photocoagulation has been recommended for extrafoveal lesions.

The goal of steroids and photocoagulation is to decrease transudation of fluid from the choroid beneath the retina and to prevent or inhibit bleeding from subretinal neovascular membranes.

PROGNOSIS. Almost 60 per cent of untreated eyes with macular involvement will have 20/200 vision or worse following ocular histoplasmosis. The effect on vision is dependent on the location of the lesions and the occurrence and severity of hemorrhage and detachment. Disciform lesions outside the fovea may result only in paracentral scotoma with preservation of central acuity. Hemorrhage is associated with a 50 to 60 per cent chance of permanent central visual loss. Prognosis rapidly declines with increasing severity of the macular lesions. With minimal involvement over 80 per cent may retain normal vision. Most patients with advanced, central lesions have vision worse than 20/200 despite optimal therapy.

Histo spots usually do not affect vision unless located in the fovea but should be observed for early signs of development of potentially blinding macular disciform lesions.

Campinchi, R., Faure, J. P., Bloch-Michel, E., and Haut, J. (translated by Golden, B., and Givoiset, M. M.): Uveitis: Immunologic and Allergic Phenomena. Springfield, Ill., Charles C Thomas, 1973.

Francois, J., and Rysselaere, M.: Oculomycoses. Springfield, Ill., Charles C Thomas, 1972.

Klintworth, G. K., Hollingsworth, A. S., Lusman, P. A., and Bradford, W. D.: Granulomatous choroiditis in a case of disseminated histoplasmosis. Histologic demonstration of *Histoplasma capsulatum* in choroidal lesions. Arch. Ophthalmol., 90:45, 1973.

Roth, A. M.: *Histoplasma capsulatum* in the presumed ocular histoplasmosis syndrome. Am. J. Ophthalmol., 84:293, 1977.

Smith, R. E.: Ocular histoplasmosis. *In* Ryan, S. J., and Smith, R. E.: Selected Topics on the Eye in Systemic Disease. New York, Grune & Stratton, 1974, pp. 135–165.

Schlaegel, Jr., T. F.: Presumed ocular histoplasmosis. *In* Duane, T. D.: Clinical Ophthalmology, Vol. 4. Hagerstown, Md., Harper & Row, 1976, pp. 1–19.

582. SYSTEMIC HYPERTENSION AND ARTERIOLOSCLEROSIS

INTRODUCTION. Ophthalmoscopy provides the clinician with a unique opportunity to directly visualize a patient's small retinal arteries, arterioles, and accompanying veins. Although the much discussed vascular changes and retinopathy of systemic hypertension and arteriolosclerosis seldom produce significant visual complications, they do provide a clue to the condition of small vessels elsewhere in the body.

ARTERIOLOSCLEROSIS. Terminology of arteriosclerotic vascular disease is often misunderstood. Arteriosclerosis is a general term referring to all processes which cause hardening and thickening of arteries. Subgroups of this include internal atherosclerosis, medial sclerosis, and arteriolosclerosis. Atherosclerosis and arteriolosclerosis are the two forms commonly evident in retinal vessels.

Atherosclerosis primarily affects large and medium-sized arteries and can involve the central retinal artery and its branches immediately adjacent to the optic disc. Atheromatous plaques in the central retinal artery can cause narrowing of the lumen with diminished retinal blood flow. Total occlusion of the central retinal artery or large branch arteries can also occur. Occasionally one notices atheromatous or thrombotic emboli within retinal arterioles with a boxcar effect of the blood column distal to the obstruction.

Arteriolosclerosis is an arteriole response to systemic hypertension. Subinternal deposition of hyalin, fibrinoid necrosis, and replacement fibrosis in response to hypertension produce changes in arterioles visible on ophthalmoscopy.

The retinal vascular changes of arteriosclerosis are outlined as follows:

1. *Alteration of caliber:* Arteriolar attenuation may be the most consistent sign of hypertension but also the one most difficult to interpret consistently. Narrowing may be generalized or segmental; although it is reversible in early disease, narrowing becomes permanent as the hypertensive disease progresses. Attenuated vessels are best appreciated at least two bifurcations beyond the optic disc. The often heard alteration of arteriovenous ratio (AV ratio) from the normal 2:3 to 1:2 or 1:3 can be a meaningless observation because of a number of factors: arteriolar narrowing is often focal; ratios are subjective and vary over different areas of the retina; venous engorgement is often superimposed; age and refractive error of the patient change the apparent size of the vessels; and comparable anatomic divisions of both artery and vein are not always seen in the same ophthalmoscopic field.

2. *Alteration of central light reflex:* The "vessels" visualized in ophthalmoscopy are actually the intraluminal blood columns. The vessels themselves are transparent under normal conditions. As the arteriolar wall is infiltrated with lipid and cholesterol and becomes hyalinized and sclerotic, the vessels become more opaque. First, a broadening of the light reflex is noted. As the disease progresses, a grayish yellow appearance of the vessels gives the blood column a "copper wire" appearance. Severe arteriolosclerosis produces a narrow, white "silver wire" arteriole which completely hides the blood column owing to its opacity. In the final stage, the vessels appear as thin threads or are invisible.

3. *Arteriolar sheathing:* Arteriolar sheathing is a sign of advanced sclerosis as well as of leukemia, periarteritis nodosa, and other forms of vasculitis. It appears as two thin white lines paralleling the blood column and representing vessel wall opacities (seen in cross section). The parallel sheathing can progress until the entire vessel is seen as a broad white ribbon that obscures the blood column — a condition called pipe-stem sheathing.

4. *Arteriolovenous crossing changes (AV nicking):* AV nicking is a significant sign of arteriolosclerosis when it is observed more than one disc diameter from the disc. The earliest change is arteriolar concealment of underlying venules, which obscures the venous blood column passing beneath it. As a vein crosses a thickened arteriole, it may be deflected more deeply into the retina or "hump" over the arteriole. Venous banking is seen when the vein distal to the AV crossing is more curved and engorged than normal and suggests venous compression at the crossing. Venous deviation at the AV crossing is also seen. The vessels tend to assume a perpendicular orientation at the crossing which produces an S-shaped deviation of the venule.

HYPERTENSION. Arterial hypertension, regardless of etiology, produces vasoconstriction, hemorrhages, and exudates in the retina. The ophthalmoscopic signs of hypertension generally precede those of arteriolosclerosis but are less specific. The earliest changes are focal or generalized arteriolar narrowing. In hypertension alone, this narrowing is thought to represent reversible arteriole spasm and differs from the attenuation caused by arteriolosclerosis. As mentioned above, however, arteriolar narrowing is a very difficult sign to quantify, and has led many to abandon this finding as a "hard" sign of hypertension.

The retinopathy of hypertension is most likely a result of capillary insufficiency or ischemia and is composed of hemorrhages, microaneurysms, cotton wool patches, exudates, edema, and papilledema. The characteristic hemorrhages of hypertensive retinopathy are streaked, flame-shaped hemorrhages of extravasated blood in the nerve fiber layer. These usually are seen paralleling the blood vessels. Deeper, round blot hemorrhages can be seen, but not as frequently. Unless they involve the macula, hemorrhages produce few symptoms and are of no great significance. They resolve spontaneously in a few weeks.

Microaneurysms are more common in hypertensive eyes than in normal ones but less common than in diabetic eyes. A more detailed description of microaneurysms is included in Ch. 579.

Cotton wool patches are fluffy, white, "soft" exudates characteristic of diabetes, connective tissue diseases, papilledema, and other conditions as well as hypertension. They usually are located in the posterior pole near the optic disc. The appearance of cotton wool patches in hypertensive patients, without other diseases such as diabetes or a connective tissue disorder, is an indication for immediate blood pressure reduction. In the absence of other causes, it represents necrotizing arteriolitis or microangiopathic hemolytic anemia, which, if left untreated, can result in irreversible renal damage within days.

Hard exudates are smaller, round, yellowish-white deposits in the retina. The exudates of hypertensive patients tend to be of lower fat content and appear grayer than the waxy exudates of diabetics. Hard exudates represent edema residues from leaking capillaries or arterioles or degenerating nerve tissue. Occasionally, the edema residue collects in the outer plexiform layer in the posterior pole and produces a "macular star" appearance. Although nonmacular hard exudates spontaneously resorb in a few weeks, the exudates in the macular star may persist for months or years. They usually disappear more quickly, however, if the blood pressure is successfully lowered.

Various degrees of retinal edema are seen in hypertensive patients. Small focal areas of edema can obscure vascular detail and produce mild visual disturbances if located near the fovea. The development of optic disc swelling is an ominous sign, however. Optic disc edema is an indication that the hypertensive disease is in a "malignant" phase and that renal function is in severe jeopardy. Although it can be caused by arterial hypertension alone, other causes of optic disc edema must be ruled out. Unlike the changes associated with arteriolosclerosis, the retinopathy of hypertension is usually reversible. (The one specific treatment is control of the systemic hypertension.) Serial ophthalmoscopic examinations are often good indications of the efficacy of the antihypertensive therapy. However, exudates and optic disc edema may take weeks or months to resolve. At any level of diastolic blood pressure, the prognosis declines with increasing severity of the retinopathy.

CLASSIFICATION OF HYPERTENSIVE AND ARTERIOLOSCLEROTIC RETINOPATHY. Over the years, a number of classification systems have been proposed for grading the severity of hypertensive retinal changes (Fig. 1F). The system most commonly used by internists is the four-grade Keith-Wagener-Barker classification. This grouping is frowned on by many ophthalmologists, as it lumps hypertensive and arteriolosclerotic changes together. The Scheie classification is preferred by many who feel that hypertensive and arteriolosclerotic retinal changes have different prognostic significance and should be grouped separately.

The Scheie classification defines four grades of hypertensive changes based on arteriolar narrowing, vasospasm, hemorrhages, exudates, and disc edema. Four grades of arteriolosclerotic changes are also defined according to alterations of the central light reflex and arteriolovenous crossing abnormalities (Table 2).

Becker, R. A.: Hypertension and arteriolosclerosis. *In* Duane, T. D. (ed.): Clinical Ophthalmology, Vol. 3. Hagerstown, Md., Harper & Row, 1976, pp. 1–21.

Breshin, D. J., Gifford, F. W., Fairbairn, J. F., and Kearns, T. P.: Prognostic importance of ophthalmoscopic findings in essential hypertension. JAMA, 195:91, 1966.

Chester, E. M.: The Ocular Fundus in Systemic Disease. Chicago, Year Book Medical Publishers, 1973.

Keith, N. M., Wagener, H. P., and Barker, N. W.: Some different types of essential hypertension: Their course and prognosis. Am. J. Med. Sci., 197:332, 1939.

Kirkendall, W. M.: Retinal changes of hypertension. *In* Mausolf, F. A. (ed.): The Eye and Systemic Disease. St. Louis, C. V. Mosby Company, 1975.

Newell, F. W., and Ernest, J. T.: Ophthalmology Principles and Concepts. 3rd ed. St. Louis, C. V. Mosby Company, 1974.

Scheie, H. G.: Evaluation of ophthalmoscopic changes of hypertension and arteriolar sclerosis. Arch. Ophthalmol., 49:117, 1953.

Scheie, H. G., and Albert, D. M.: Textbook of Ophthalmology. 9th ed. Philadelphia, W. B. Saunders Company, 1977.

Vaughn, D., and Asbury, T.: General Ophthalmology. 8th ed. Los Altos, Calif., Lange Medical Publications, 1977.

TABLE 2. Scheie Classification*

Hypertension	Arteriolosclerosis
Normal – Mild hypertension without ophthalmoscopic retinal changes	Normal – Some patients with hypertension have no evidence of sclerosis
Grade 1 – Arteriolar narrowing, particularly in the smaller secondary branches; no irregularity in the caliber	Grade 1 – An early, recognizable increase in the light reflex or a broadening of the reflex, associated with a minimal amount of arteriolovenous compression
Grade 2 – Arteriolar narrowing is more pronounced, with some localized or focal irregularities and constrictions	Grade 2 – More severe or more marked changes than in grade 1
Grade 3 – Narrowing and irregularity of the arterioles, usually more severe and usually accompanied by edema residues and retinal hemorrhages	Grade 3 – Arteriolosclerosis is represented by copper wire arterioles and more marked arteriolovenous compression
Grade 4 – All of those described in grade 3 plus neuroretinal edema and papilledema	Grade 4 – This is represented by silver wire arterioles and marked arteriolovenous crossing changes

*Adapted from Becker, R. A.: Hypertension and arteriolosclerosis. *In* Duane, T. D. (ed.): Clinical Ophthalmology, Vol. 3. Hagerstown, Md., Harper & Row, 1976.

583. THE OPTIC NERVE

PAPILLEDEMA. Definition. Papilledema refers to all forms of passive disc swelling that result from increased intracranial pressure (Fig. 1*A*). It does not include the many forms of disc edema or swelling of other local or systemic etiology.

Incidence and Etiology. Papilledema is usually bilateral, although some degree of asymmetry is common. It can take from 4 to 48 hours for the earliest ophthalmoscopic signs of papilledema to develop after the acute elevation of intracranial pressure (ICP). It is estimated that 60 per cent of all patients with papilledema have expanding intracranial lesions caused by neoplasms. Papilledema is more common in patients with infratentorial tumors than in those with supratentorial lesions. Approximately 70 per cent of infratentorial and 50 per cent of supratentorial tumors produce papilledema. Unilateral papilledema may occur in patients with pre-existing contralateral optic atrophy, congenital abnormalities of the optic nerve sheath, or abnormalities of the orbit.

Pathogenesis. The mechanism that produces the prelaminar edema, vascular changes, hemorrhages, and exudates of papilledema, in response to increased ICP, is subject to debate. Some clinical and experimental observations concerning the pathogenesis of papilledema are as follows: (1) Chronically increased ICP does not alter pressure in the ophthalmic vein. (2) Increased ICP tends to increase both pressure and blood flow in the posterior ciliary branch of the ophthalmic artery which supplies arterial blood to the prelaminar portion of the optic nerve. (3) Elevated ICP is transmitted to the intravaginal sheath about the optic nerve and may impede venous return from the retina and capillary circulation of the nervehead. Occlusion of the central retinal vein, however, does not produce papilledema. (4) Optic atrophy prevents the development of papilledema. (5) Rapid increases in subarachnoid fluid pressure produce papilledema more rapidly than an insidious elevation.

The majority of currently accepted theories on pathogenesis suggest a mechanical blockage of fluid flow (e.g., blood, lymph, cerebrospinal fluid) from the eye, resulting in fluid accumulation in the nervehead. Currently the most accepted theory relates to deficiencies in axoplasmic flow.

Recent electron microscopic studies have shown that the axon itself swells early in the development of papilledema. Autoradiographic studies have also shown that there is blockage of axoplasmic flow at the level of the lamina cribrosa. It is therefore felt that the earliest ophthalmoscopic signs of papilledema may be related to swelling of the axons with accumulation of intra-axon organelles. Following this stage, there will be abnormalities in venous return, resulting in a vascular component to the optic disc edema.

Pathology. Edema of varying degrees is the primary characteristic. It can be mushroom shaped and limited to the nervehead, but usually spreads into the adjacent retina. Compression, lateral displacement, detachment, or degeneration of retinal tissue can ensue. The lamina cribrosa bows forward, and varicosities separating the nerve fibers appear. The neurofibrils can subsequently degenerate into cytoid bodies. Phagocytic microglia and fibrous astrocytes proliferate. Inflammatory cells are rare, but hemorrhages are usually present on the disc and in the neighboring retina.

Clinical Signs and Symptoms. Symptoms of nausea, headache, diplopia, loss of consciousness, and bradycardia are associated with increased ICP and the pathologic entity which caused it. Visual symptoms related to papilledema include transient blurring of vision, enlargement of the blind spot, and constriction of the peripheral fields. Pupillary reflexes and acuity are ordinarily normal. Visual field and acuity alterations usually are seen only in well-developed papilledema unless retinal hemorrhages invade the macular region.

The ophthalmoscopic signs of papilledema are classified into four stages: early, fully developed, chronic, and atrophic.

Stage 1 — Early incipient papilledema. Subtle funduscopic changes prior to disc swelling can be seen on careful examination. Pupil dilation, a bright source, and red-free light are used to accentuate these signs: (1) hyperemia of the disc due to dilated capillaries and venous stasis; (2) loss of the spontaneous venous pulsations which are normally present in 90 per cent of patients; (3) blurring of the superior and inferior poles of the disc margin; (4) blurring of the fine parallel linear striated pattern of light reflexes from the nerve fiber layer; (5) loss of perivenous highlights and fine vessel background; and (6) dulling of vessel light reflex.

Stage 2 — Fully developed papilledema. Accentuation of all the aforementioned signs is seen as well as (1) splinter hemorrhage in the nerve fiber layer; (2) ischemic infarcts of the nerve fiber layer — "cotton wool spots"; (3) exudates; and (4) disc elevation.

Stage 3—Chronic papilledema. Neuronal degeneration and gliosis in chronic papilledema produce the following changes: (1) hyperemia giving way to a boggy, milk-gray appearance, and (2) resolution of hemorrhages and exudates.

Stage 4 — Atrophic papilledema. Chronic papilledema can result in optic nerve atrophy, decreased vision, and visual field losses. Ophthalmoscopic features are (1) decreased prominence and size of the optic disc, (2) gray-white gliosis of the entire disc, and (3) narrowing of retinal vessels.

After lowering intracranial pressure, venous distention and capillary dilatation immediately disappear. Distinct disc margins and nerve fibers may not be evident for several weeks. Resolution of fully developed papilledema is usually complete by six to eight weeks. Retinal hemorrhages may occur during resolution but are of no consequence and regress spontaneously. There is no residual visual impairment unless chronic swelling results in nerve fiber loss and optic nerve atrophy occurs.

Diagnosis. The diagnosis of papilledema is made by ophthalmoscopy in association with other systemic signs and symptoms of the etiologic disease. Observation of subtle progressive features is important in detecting the earliest signs of papilledema and differentiating these from congenitally blurred disc and other forms of disc swelling listed in Table 3.

Treatment. Papilledema is a reliable sign of intracranial hypertension. The goal of therapy is to reduce the pressure by appropriate therapy of the underlying pathologic process. Optic nerve sheath decompression can be attempted when vision is threatened and when no treatable underlying process is found.

PSEUDOPAPILLEDEMA. Definition. Pseudopapilledema is any condition resulting in an optic disc configuration that may be confused with papilledema.

TABLE 3.   Etiology of the "Swollen" Disc*

Congenital
  Anomalous elevation
  Hyaline bodies (drusen)
  Gliotic dysplasia
Ocular disease
  Uveitis
  Hypotony
  Vein occlusion
Metabolic
  Dysthyroidism
  Juvenile diabetes
  Proliferative retinopathies
Inflammatory
  Papillitis
  Neuroretinitis
  ?Papillophlebitis
Infiltrative
  Lymphoma
  Reticuloendothelial
Systemic disease
  Anemia
  Hypoxemia
  Hypertension
Disc tumors
  Hemangioma
  Glioma
  Metastatic
Vascular
  Ischemic neuropathy
  Arteritis, cranial
  Arteritis, collagen
Orbital tumors
  Perioptic meningioma
  Glioma
  Sheath "cysts"
  Retrobulbar mass
Elevated intracranial pressure (papilledema)
  Mass lesion
  Pseudotumor cerebri
  Hypertension

*From Glaser, J. S.: Topical diagnosis: Prechiasmal visual pathways. In Duane, T. D. (ed.): Clinical Ophthalmology, Vol. 2. Hagerstown, Md., Harper & Row, 1976.

Etiology.   The most commonly seen condition simulating papilledema is drusen of the optic nervehead. Other causes include hyperopia, gliotic hyaloid remnants, myelinated nerve fibers, and other congenital abnormalities of the disc.

DRUSEN.   Intrapapillary drusen (or hyaline bodies or colloid bodies) are masses of hyaline material that are often calcified. Drusen are bilateral in 72 per cent of cases and are clinically evident in 3.4 per 1000 individuals. They are primarily seen in blond Caucasians and are extremely rare in other races. There is equal sex distribution. These lesions usually progress slowly over many years but almost never affect macular vision. Field defects, principally concentric constriction, baring of the blind spots, and nerve fiber bundle defects are found in 87 per cent of the cases. These are due to compression of nerve fibers in the papilla. Occasionally drusen have been known to produce splinter hemorrhages on the disc, papillary hemorrhages extending into the vitreous, and peripapillary subretinal hemorrhages. Drusen are thought to be inherited as an irregular dominant trait.

The appearance of disc drusen depends on their location on the disc. Superficial drusen, more characteristic in adults, are refractive white or yellow globular masses that appear to have glowing edges. Deep-seated drusen are more common in children and lack sharp margins if they are visible at all. They tend to emerge later in adult life but

may remain undetected. Features of papillary drusen that help differentiate them from papilledema are (1) normal appearance of nerve fiber layer entering the disc; (2) increased number of large vessels on the disc with abnormal pattern; (3) elevation confined to the disc seldom affecting the retina; (4) absence of hyperemic disc, dilated vasculature, and exudates; and (5) an irregular, scalloped border to the disc.

SEVERE HYPEROPIA.   Some individuals with severe hyperopia develop a raised, hyperemic disc which can be confused with papilledema. Venous changes, edema of the nerve fiber layer, hemorrhages, and exudates are not associated with this condition, however. Some feel that the elevated disc of hyperopia represents a normal variant, as it is also occasionally seen in patients with normal vision.

PERSISTENT HYALOID REMNANTS.   Persistent embryonic glial tissue can produce fibrous membranes that obscure the disc margins and retinal vasculature in the nervehead. Anomalous branching or tortuosity of the retinal arteries and veins is commonly associated with this condition. The other characteristic findings of papilledema are absent, allowing for easy differentiation.

MYELINATED NERVE FIBERS.   Myelinated (medullated) nerve fibers can obscure disc margins but are easily differentiated by their white color, flame-shaped appearance, and location in the superficial nerve fiber layer, which partially obscures the underlying retinal vessels. This condition occurs in 1 per cent of the patients, has equal sex distribution, and is bilateral in 8 per cent of the cases.

Diagnosis.   Despite good ophthalmoscopic skill and knowledge of the characteristics listed above, physicians may still find some discs that remain a diagnostic enigma. For physicians with this uncommon dilemma, the following rules have been suggested by Savino and Glaser: (1) Examine family members, as congenital anomalies of the disc are often familial. (2) Consider the general condition of the patient. A questionable disc in an asymptomatic patient is probably not papilledema. (3) If a firm diagnosis of the optic disc is not made, management of the patient is dictated by other signs and symptoms — as if the fundi were not visualized. (4) The presence of congenitally anomalous optic discs does not exclude the possibility of an additional superimposed pathologic process.

Treatment.   Pseudopapilledema rarely produces symptoms requiring treatment. Recognition of the symptoms as an interesting physical finding and not as an ominous sign of intracranial hypertension should exempt the patient from extensive neurologic workup.

PAPILLITIS.   Definition.   Papillitis, or intraocular optic neuritis, is an inflammatory disorder of the nervehead which causes disc swelling.

Incidence.   Papillitis and disc swelling are evident in perhaps 20 per cent of adults with optic neuritis. It is a much more common form of neuritis in children, in whom 80 per cent will show disc swelling.

Etiology.   A variety of systemic and local diseases have been implicated, including (1) demyelinating diseases such as multiple sclerosis and postinfectious encephalomyelitis; (2) systemic infections such as poliomyelitis and the viral diseases of children; (3) metabolic disorders such as diabetes, dysthyroidism, vitamin deficiencies, and neuropathy of pregnancy; (4) local inflammatory disorders such as sinusitis, meningitis, and orbital or intraocular inflammation; (5) toxic neuropathies such as tobacco, methanol, lead, quinine, and arsenic; and (6) ischemic neuropathy such as atherosclerotic vascular disease and any form of arteritis.

Pathology. The optic nerve is infiltrated with white blood cells and fat-laden macrophages. With chronicity, a predominant polymorphonuclear infiltrate gives way to lymphocytes and plasma cells. Nerve fibers become swollen and fragmented. The medullary sheaths undergo fatty degeneration prior to axonal degeneration. Later microglial phagocytes and astrocytes herald the scarring stage.

Clinical Appearance. The onset of papillitis is usually acute and almost invariably associated with profound visual symptoms. Vision is rapidly reduced, and large central scotomas are usually present. Pupillary reaction is diminished. The patient often complains of retrobulbar pain, especially on movement of the eye.

Ophthalmoscopically, the disc becomes hyperemic. There is venous engorgement, blurring of the disc margins, and obliteration of the physiologic cup. Retinal edema, exudates, and hemorrhages in the nerve fiber layer can occur.

Diagnosis. The following manifestations of papillitis help differentiate it from papilledema: (1) visual loss and field defects, (2) ocular pain, (3) pupillary reflex defect, (4) cells in the vitreous over the papilla, (5) loss of central cup, and (6) deep retinal exudates.

Prognosis. Loss of vision is rapid after onset of the disease and then returns to near normal acuity in two to three weeks (although wide variation exists). Progressive atrophy occasionally develops with permanent visual impairment.

Treatment. Treatment is directed toward the underlying etiology, if known. Systemic corticosteroids can be used, but efficacy is questionable.

Brodrick, J. D.: Drusen of the disc and retinal hemorrhages. Br. J. Ophthalmol., 57:299, 1973.

Glaser, J. S.: Topical diagnosis: Prechiasmal visual pathways. In Duane, T. D. (ed.): Clinical Ophthalmology, Vol. 2. Hagerstown, Md., Harper & Row, 1976, pp. 1–70.

Hayreh, S. S.: Pathogenesis of oedema of the optic disc. Doc. Ophthalmol., 24:289, 1968.

Hedges, T. R.: Papilledema: Its recognition and relation to increased intracranial pressure. Surv. Ophthalmol., 19:201, 1975.

Hoyt, W. F., and Knight, C. L.: Comparison of congenital disc blurring and incipient papilledema in red-free light — a photographic study. Invest. Ophthalmol., 12:241, 1973.

Savino, P. J., and Glaser, J. S.: Pseudopapilledema versus papilledema. Int. Ophthalmol. Clin., 17:115, 1977.

Walsh, F. B., and Hoyt, W. F.: Clinical Neuro-ophthalmology, Vol. 1. 3rd ed. Baltimore, Williams & Wilkins Company, 1969.

Wirtschafter, J. D., Rizzo, F. J., and Smiley, B. C.: Optic nerve axoplasm and papilledema. Surv. Ophthalmol., 20:157, 1975.

584. OCULAR SARCOIDOSIS

Ocular involvement is present in 20 to 50 per cent of all patients with sarcoidosis and is the reason for initial presentation in 7 to 15 per cent of all cases. The disease shows a predilection for blacks in the 20- to 40-year age group, and ocular involvement is seen equally in males and females.

The most common ocular manifestation is iridocyclitis. It is seen in 70 to 80 per cent of the patients with ocular sarcoidosis and represents approximately 3 per cent of all cases of uveitis. Other tissues vulnerable to disease include the lacrimal glands, posterior uveal tract, conjunctiva, cornea, retina and the optic nerve.

ETIOLOGY. The cause of sarcoid remains speculative and is discussed fully in Ch. 65.

PATHOLOGY AND PATHOPHYSIOLOGY. The granulomatous inflammation associated with sarcoidosis can occur in and around the ocular tissues. Discrete granulomas are found in the anterior and posterior uvea, lids, conjunctiva, lacrimal glands, retina, and optic nerve. Retinal neovascularization can also occur.

CLINICAL MANIFESTATIONS. Anterior Uveitis. Iridocyclitis is the most frequent ocular involvement in sarcoidosis. Acute iridocyclitis is frequently bilateral and associated with pain, decreased visual acuity, perilimbal injection, and aqueous flare and cells in the anterior chamber. It may be associated with fever, erythema nodosum, and transient lymphadenopathy. Acute iridocyclitis can resolve without sequelae and has a better prognosis than the chronic inflammatory type.

Chronic iridocyclitis, in contrast, is slowly progressive with little pain. Large "mutton fat" keratitic precipitates on the posterior surface of the cornea and iris granulomas (Koeppe and Busacca nodules) are occasionally present.

Posterior Uveitis. Sarcoid involves the posterior uvea as chorioretinitis, periphlebitis retinae, chorioretinal granulomas, optic nerve granulomas, edema, atrophy, preretinal infiltrates, and vitreous opacities. Posterior uveitis is much less common than anterior involvement, is equal in sex distribution, and is often associated with anterior uveitis, which obscures the fundus examination.

Retinal lesions may be exudative or inflammatory in character. Small, waxy grayish or yellow-white masses ("candlewax drippings") along the retinal veins are characteristic of sarcoidosis. They vary in number and may sometimes disappear spontaneously in a few months but usually last for years. Small self-limiting hemorrhages may occur but are infrequent. Large granulomatous masses arising from the retina have also been reported. Thrombosis, macular edema, and irregular macular pigmentation have been noted rarely.

Retinal periphlebitis is the most frequent funduscopic lesion seen in sarcoidosis. These are scattered, gray-white exudates found around the retinal veins with candlewax drippings. A nonspecific form of chorioretinitis may present with a hazy, inflamed area which later shows chorioretinal atrophy, scarring, and pigment clumping.

Uveoparotid fever (Heerfordt's disease) is uveitis, fever, salivary gland enlargement, and cranial nerve involvement (usually facial palsy). It can be seen with gastrointestinal and cerebral symptoms and skin eruptions.

Vitreous Body. The vitreous body in sarcoidosis may show many discrete fluffy "snowball" opacities in the inferior regions. This "string of pearls" is not specific to sarcoidosis, however, and may be seen in peripheral uveitis, toxoplasmosis, and Behçet's disease. Vitreous hemorrhage may also be seen following massive retinal hemorrhage or retinal neovascularization extending into the vitreous.

Optic Nerve. Involvement of the optic nerve can be due to direct granuloma infiltration or to edema secondary to intracranial disease. Sarcoid granulomas of the nervehead are present in 1 to 5 per cent of patients with sarcoidosis, and occur without regard to anterior segment involvement. Central nervous system manifestations, usually seen in 10 to 15 per cent of cases, are twice as common when fundus lesions are found.

Glaucoma. Secondary glaucoma can result from anterior or posterior synechiae, in response to steroid administration, or from inflammation of the aqueous outflow channels.

Cataract. The lens may become cataractous secondary to anterior chamber inflammation or in response to steroid administration.

Cornea. "Mutton fat" keratitic precipitates may sometimes be found on the posterior surface of the cornea when iridocyclitis is present. The most common corneal lesion, however, is band keratopathy. Hypercalcemia and chronic anterior chamber inflammation may be causative factors, although band keratopathy is seen in sarcoid patients with normal calcium levels. Corneal anesthesia and ulceration are rare sequelae of sarcoidosis.

Conjunctiva. Conjunctival granulomas can be seen on the palpebral surfaces. Conjunctival biopsy has been suggested for histologic confirmation of sarcoidosis, but various authors have reported only 2 to 33 per cent positive findings.

Sclera. Yellow sarcoid nodules appear in the episclera and have a predilection for areas near the insertions of the rectus muscles. These lesions mimic chalazia and episcleritis.

Periorbital. The lacrimal glands contain sarcoid granulomas in 7 to 10 per cent of sarcoid patients. Using rose bengal staining and slit lamp examination, some investigators have found keratoconjunctivitis in 70 per cent of their sarcoid patients. Sarcoid granulomas may also be found in the lacrimal sac. Orbital involvement other than the lacrimal glands is exceedingly rare.

The eyelids, like skin elsewhere, can have small "millet seed" nodules which are rare but can be very important clinically. Muscle palsies and other neurologic manifestations can be rare presenting signs of sarcoidosis and may complicate the differential diagnosis.

DIAGNOSIS. The diagnosis of sarcoidosis is often suggested by characteristic although not pathognomonic ocular signs. Ocular signs may be the first clinical evidence of the disease or may help confirm suspicions arising from other clinical clues. Chest x-ray, the Kveim-Siltzbach test, negative tuberculin skin test, and certain biochemical parameters combined with the characteristic clinical presentation are the basis for diagnosis. Inspection, ophthalmoscopy, and slit lamp examination are essential for the diagnosis of ocular sarcoidosis. Special procedures such as conjunctival biopsy, fluorescein angiography, visual fields, and lacrimation tests may be helpful in selected cases.

TREATMENT. Early lesions respond to steroid therapy more readily than late, fibrotic, hyalinized lesions. Topical steroids are effective in some patients. Systemic corticosteroids are indicated for severe anterior uveitis, optic neuritis, and posterior uveitis of any degree; large doses may be required over a six- to nine-month period. Ocular side effects of steroid administration should be periodically checked for. Other pharmacologic agents have been tried but without clear benefit in the management of ocular lesions. Photocoagulation to areas of retinal neovascularization may be required occasionally.

PROGNOSIS. Ocular symptoms usually coincide with the severity of systemic complaints. Some patients have an acute self-limiting form of the disease, whereas others have a slowly progressive or chronic form that ultimately results in blindness.

Campinchi, R., Faure, J. P., Bloch-Michel, E., and Haut, J. (translated by Golden B. and Givoiset, M. M.): Uveitis: Immunologic and Allergic Phenomena. Springfield, Ill., Charles C Thomas, 1973.

Klintworth, G. K., and Landers, M. B.: The Eye: Structure and Function in Disease. Baltimore, Williams & Wilkins Company, 1976.

Mausolf, F. A. (ed.): The Eye and Systemic Disease. St. Louis, C. V. Mosby Company, 1975.

Newell, F. W., and Ernest, J. T.: Ophthalmology Principles and Concepts. 3rd ed. St. Louis, C. V. Mosby Company, 1974.

Ryan, S. J., Jr., and Maumenee, A. E.: Ocular sarcoidosis. In Ryan, S. J., Jr., and Smith, R. E. (eds.): Selected Topics on the Eye in Systemic Disease. New York, Grune & Stratton, 1974.

Schlaegel, T. F., Jr., and Coles, R. S.: Uveitis and miscellaneous general diseases. In Duane, T. D. (ed.): Clinical Ophthalmology, Vol. 5. Hagerstown, Md., Harper & Row, 1976, pp. 6–13.

585. SICKLE CELL DISEASES

DEFINITION. The inherited sickle cell hemoglobinopathies produce a variety of intraocular lesions primarily confined to the retina. Two patterns of retinopathy are observed: proliferative sickle retinopathy and nonproliferative sickle retinopathy.

INCIDENCE. Ocular abnormalities can occur in all types of sickle cell disease. Proliferative sickle retinopathy is far more common in adults with hemoglobin SC and SThal (60 to 70 per cent) than in those with SS disease (10 per cent). Proliferative sickle retinopathy is seen primarily in the third and fourth decades of life, although it can occur earlier. Both sexes are equally affected. The particular incidences of nonproliferative sickle retinopathy are discussed later in this chapter.

ETIOLOGY. The sickling disorders are inherited and are discussed fully in Ch. 485.4.

PATHOPHYSIOLOGY. Most or perhaps all of the ocular abnormalities are related to vascular occlusion. Under conditions of decreased oxygen tension, red blood cells (RBC) containing sickle hemoglobin assume the characteristic sickle shape and become less pliable than normal RBC. These sickle cells impede blood flow in small vessels, creating ischemia, hypoxia, and necrosis of the surrounding tissues. Vaso-occlusion can be secondary to arterial emboli of sickled RBC, hemolyzed RBC debris, blood coagulants, or bone marrow, or it can be secondary to capillary or venous stasis.

Following vascular occlusion either of two pathophysiologic mechanisms can ensue, leading to proliferative or nonproliferative retinopathy (Fig. 3). In proliferative sickle retinopathy, arteriolar occlusion is followed by arteriolar-venular anastomosis at the junction of the normal and ischemic retina. Vascular proliferation can later be observed on funduscopic examination over these same areas. This neovascularization is not specific for sickle hemoglobinopathies and can occur in any disease causing local retinal ischemia such as diabetic retinopathy, retinal branch vein occlusion, retrolental fibroplasia, pulseless disease, sarcoidosis, chronic myelogenous leukemia, and Eales' disease. Retinal atrophy caused by ischemia or chronic vitreous traction often ensues.

Chronic capillary transudation or hemorrhage into the vitreous body can result in liquefaction, fibrosis, and shrinkage of the vitreous, which leads to retinal tears and detachments.

The changes associated with nonproliferative sickle retinopathy are seen following sub-, intra-, or preretinal hemorrhage due to arteriolar obstruction and vascular rupture. Salmon-patch hemorrhages less than two disc diameters in size have a pink-red coloration, prob-

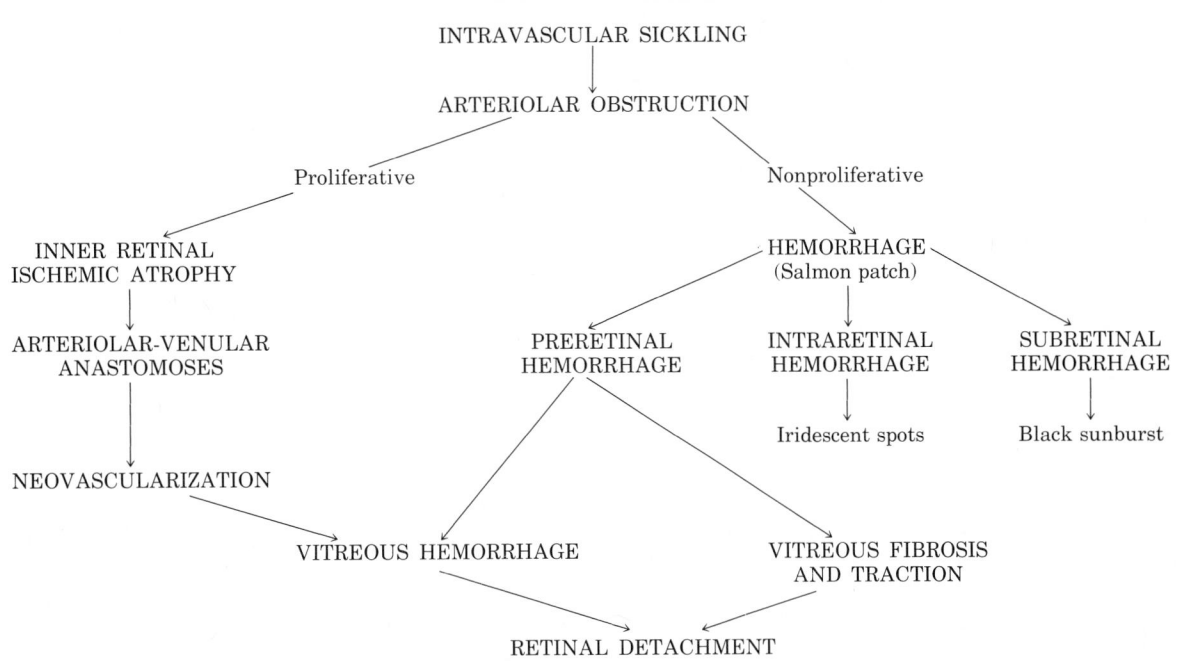

Figure 3. Presumed pathogenesis of sickle retinopathy. (Derived from Romayananda et al. and Goldberg.)

ably caused by hemoglobin degradation products. Refractile iridescent spots are also characteristically seen. These are thought to represent resorbed intraretinal hemorrhage. Black sunburst spots are typically seen in sickling disorders. These represent old subretinal or deep retinal hemorrhages. Histologic examination of these lesions has shown hypertrophy, hyperplasia, and migration of the retinal pigment epithelium, hemosiderin-laden macrophages, and deposition of hemosiderin.

PATHOLOGY. Histologic examination of enucleated eyes reveals vascular occlusions by sickled RBC and fibrin, cytoid bodies, ischemic atrophy, vascular necrosis, and capillary acellularity distal to arterial occlusions.

CLINICAL MANIFESTATIONS. Conjunctiva. Characteristic dilatation of the conjunctival blood vessels can be a pathognomonic sign of sickle cell disease. Serjeant et al. found these abnormal vessels in 64 of 66 cases of homozygous sickle cell disease. No false positives have been reported. The approximate incidence of false negatives (1 per cent) may occur after transfusion or in young children with hemoglobin F levels. Other nonspecific conjunctival signs of sickle cell disease include scleral icterus, telangiectasias, and vascular stasis.

Uvea. Uveal manifestations of sickle cell disease are rare. Iris atrophy, both spontaneous and following retinal detachment operations, has been reported in a few patients with SC hemoglobin.

Optic Nerve. Capillary and precapillary occlusion and dilatation are seen infrequently on the optic nerve-head. Vision usually is not altered.

Retina. NONPROLIFERATIVE SICKLE RETINOPATHY. *Asymptomatic Lesions.* (1) Venous tortuosity may be seen in 47 per cent of patients with SS disease and in 32 per cent of patients with SC disease. It is uncommon in AS or SThal individuals. This nonspecific sign also is seen as a normal variant, as an inherited trait, and in such diseases as cystic fibrosis, familial dysautonomia, and some mucopolysaccharidoses. (2)

Black sunbursts are dark, ovoid lesions approximately 0.5 to 2 disc diameters in size with stellate or spiculate borders and frequent clumps of yellowish refractile granules within them. They are usually located in the peripheral fundus and therefore rarely affect vision. They may be seen in 35 per cent of SS patients, in 41 per cent of SC patients, in 20 per cent of SThal patients, and rarely in sickle cell trait. These lesions represent the end-stage of subretinal hemorrhages. The intermediate lesions have an uneven mottled brown surface with a narrow halo of paler retina. (3) Salmon patches are small (0.25 to 1.0 disc diameter) intraretinal hemorrhages. They are usually round to oval and can be flat or dome shaped. Initially, they are bright red, but over a course of weeks to months they turn salmon pink, then orange, and finally yellowish-white as the hemorrhage is resorbed. The lesions may result in areas of thin, atrophic retina, pigmented patches resembling black sunbursts, or small cystic, hemosiderin-stained retinoschisis cavities that appear as glistening, refractile areas containing iridescent spots. These lesions are seen in 13 per cent of SS patients and 18 per cent of SThal patients. (4) Silver wire arterioles are chalky white peripheral arteriolar occlusions. These lesions can be nonprogressive or precede the phase of neovascular proliferation. (5) Whitening of the peripheral retina has been called a sign of sickle cell disease and is present in 82 to 93 per cent of patients with SS, SC, or SThal disease. This sign is also seen in the general population and is not specific to sickle cell disease. (6) Asymptomatic retinal holes can develop in the peripheral fundus and are often obscured by vitreal fibrovascular membranes or traction bands. They should be treated early to prevent retinal detachment.

Symptomatic Lesions. Symptomatic lesions of nonproliferative sickle retinopathy are infrequent and are primarily due to vascular occlusion. Central retinal artery occlusion is the most devastating and results in permanent blindness. Although it is more often seen in elderly patients, it has been reported in children and infants with sickling disorders. Arteriolar lesions at the macula include occlusion, tortuosity, dilatation, and microaneurysm formation. These are seen in 40 per cent of SS patients and 10 per cent of SThal patients. Retinal venous occlusions and choroidal vascular occlusion are rare manifestations seen in any age group. Angioid streaks have been reported in all types of sickle cell disease and sickle cell trait. These are seen in about 2 per cent of sickle patients under 40 years of age and in as many as 22 per cent in patients over 40.

PROLIFERATIVE SICKLE RETINOPATHY. Five stages of proliferative sickle retinopathy have been classified. These stages reflect the increasing severity and presumed pathogenesis of each lesion.

Stage I: Peripheral Arteriolar Occlusions. The earliest abnormality seen in proliferative sickle retinopathy is peripheral arteriolar occlusion at the equator. Normally bright red arterioles become dark, beefy red owing to the clumped, deoxygenated sickled RBC. Most frequently, the occlusions occur at arteriolar branching points. The obstructions are frequently broken down with subsequent sclerosing of the vessels. The demarcation of normal orange-brown peripheral retina and ischemic grayish-brown retina is usually sharp. Silver wire arterioles are frequently seen within the blurred nonperfused zone.

Stage II: Peripheral Arteriolar Venular Anastomosis. Arteriolar-venular anastomoses occur at the interface of normal and ischemic retina. Nonleakage of dye on fluorescein angiography indicates that these channels are dilated capillary connections and not neovascularization. The arteriolar occlusions and anastomoses are difficult to detect by ophthalmoscopy. Therefore fluorescein angiography is frequently required to detect the changes of Stage I and II proliferative sickle retinopathy.

Stage III: Neovascular Proliferation. Neovascularization begins at the same site as the occlusions and anastomoses. Patches of neovascularization assume a "sea fan" configuration and almost always grow in the direction of the ischemic retina. These small vascular buds blend easily with the adjacent fundus and can be easily overlooked. They resemble telangiectases or microaneurysms. Spontaneous regression of sea fans may be observed in up to 20 per cent of patients with PSR.

Neovascularization most frequently affects the superotemporal quadrant, followed by the inferonasal quadrant. This is a pattern also seen in other neovascular disorders such as proliferative diabetic retinopathy and retrolental fibroplasia.

Stage IV: Vitreous Hemorrhage. Vitreous hemorrhage from neovascularization frequently occurs in SC and SThal patients and only occasionally in SS or AS patients. Forty-four per cent of patients with Stage I to Stage III proliferative sickle retinopathy will suffer vitreous hemorrhage at some time during their disease.

Hemorrhages occur after ocular trauma or as a result of vitreous traction on adherent neovascular tissue. They usually are asymptomatic and remain localized over the neovascular tufts but can spread into the visual axis, causing a decrease in vision, visual field defects, or vitreous floaters.

Stage V: Retinal Detachment. Retinal detachment results from vitreous traction and is usually confined to patients with SC disease and has only rarely been observed in AS and SS patients.

DIAGNOSIS. The conjunctival sign and characteristic retinopathy are highly suggestive of sickle cell retinop-

athy. Unequivocal laboratory diagnosis is discussed in Ch. 485.4.

TREATMENT. The goal of therapy in sickle cell retinopathy is to prevent transudation and hemorrhage into the vitreous and to prevent or repair retinal detachments. Therefore therapy is not indicated for Stage I or II disease. Patients at high risk (i.e., patients with SC or SThal disease or patients with AS and SS hemoglobin with retinal signs of proliferative sickle retinopathy) should be examined by ophthalmoscopy every 6 to 12 months.

Treatment includes diathermy, xenon arc or argon laser photocoagulation, and cryocoagulation for neovascularization, surgery for retinal detachment, and vitrectomy for persistent vitreous hemorrhage. Photocoagulation of sea fan neovascularization results in a 90 per cent eradication of neovascular tissue, although the risk of induced hemorrhage is somewhat greater. Repeated treatments are usually needed.

Barnhart, M. J., Henry, R. L., and Lusher, J. M.: Sickle Cell. A Scope Publication. Kalamazoo, Upjohn Company, 1974, p. 62.

Goldberg, M. F.: Sickle cell retinopathy. In Duane, T. D. (ed.): Clinical Ophthalmology, Vol. 3. Hagerstown, Md., Harper & Row, 1976, pp. 1–45.

Nagpal, K. C., Goldberg, M. F., and Rabb, M. F.: Ocular manifestations of sickle hemoglobinopathy. Surv. Ophthalmol., 21:391, 1977.

Romayananda, N., Goldberg, M. F., and Green, W. R.: Histopathology of sickle cell retinopathy. Trans. Am. Acad. Ophthalmol., Otolaryngol., 77:652, 1973.

Serjeant, G. R., Serjeant, B. E., and Condon, P. I.: The conjunctival sign in sickle cell anemia. A relationship with *irreversibly* sickled cells. JAMA, 219:1428, 1972.

586. THYROID EYE DISEASE

DEFINITION. Graves' disease is characterized by goiter, hyperthyroidism, infiltrative dermopathy, infiltrative ophthalmopathy, and exophthalmos. The eye findings were well described by Graves in 1835, and they were further elucidated by von Basedow in 1840. The characteristic infiltrative ophthalmopathy of Graves' disease may also occur in euthyroid or hypothyroid patients, and in patients with Hashimoto's disease. Thyroid ophthalmopathy may progress .in euthryoid or hypothyroid patients following treatment for hyperthyroidism.

INCIDENCE. Thyroid ophthalmopathy is the most common single cause of both unilateral and bilateral exophthalmos in adults. Ocular signs occur in 50 per cent of patients with toxic diffuse goiter, but are only rarely associated with toxic nodular goiter. Ocular signs occur much more frequently in women than in men, but both sexes are equally affected by the severe, infiltrative ophthalmopathy. All age groups are affected.

ETIOLOGY. The etiology of thyroid infiltrative ophthalmopathy is unknown. Many patients with thyroid ophthalmopathy have antibodies, and it is hypothesized that an ag-ab interaction takes place in the orbit, which in turn causes breakdown of the extraocular muscle membrane and an autoimmune reaction against muscle antigen, producing an orbital inflammatory infiltrate.

PATHOLOGY. Abnormalities are present throughout the orbit and are usually most marked in the extraocular muscles. The eye becomes proptotic, and there is edema of the orbital tissues. The extraocular muscles are markedly enlarged and have a firm, rubbery consistency. Macrophages and extensive lymphocytic infiltration of the extraocular muscles and surrounding structures are present. Plasma cells and mast cells may also be seen. Other prominent features include a marked increase of glycosaminoglycan, collagen, and glycoproteins in the orbit. Fibrosis of extraocular muscles occurs late in the disease.

CLINICAL MANIFESTATIONS. Thyroid ophthalmopathy is clinically best divided into two categories: (1) dysthyroid ocular signs and (2) infiltrative ophthalmopathy.

Dysthyroid ocular signs include the prominent stare of Graves' disease, which is secondary to lid retraction. This sign is present in up to 90 per cent of patients with Graves' disease. Lid lag, in which the sclera superior to the cornea becomes visible on downgaze as the upper lid "lags" behind the downward-moving globe, occurs in 50 per cent of patients with Graves' disease. These signs are related to the metabolic abnormality of Graves' disease and do not necessarily indicate infiltrative eye disease. They do not produce serious abnormalities of vision and do not require treatment.

Infiltrative ophthalmopathy is a serious disorder that can progress to significant loss of vision. The characteristic findings of infiltrative ophthalmopathy are as follows: (1) True exophthalmos: Exophthalmometer readings of >20 mm in Caucasians and >22 mm in blacks, or a >2 mm difference between the two eyes. (2) Lid edema. (3) Conjunctival edema and engorged conjunctival vessels (chemosis). (4) Enlarged extraocular muscles, which may even be palpable. (5) Limitation of extraocular movements secondary to extraocular muscle fibrosis, often associated with diplopia. (6) Lagophthalmos (inability to close lids over the cornea) secondary to exophthalmos, often associated with corneal exposure. (7) Optic neuropathy secondary to compression of the optic nerve by markedly enlarged extraocular muscles in the posterior aspect of the orbit and loss of vision.

Exophthalmos occurs in over 20 per cent of patients with Graves' disease. It may be cosmetically unsatisfactory for the patient, but by itself it does not produce visual symptoms unless lagophthalmos and exposure keratopathy occur. Corneal ulcers, perforation of the globe, and endophthalmitis are the sequelae of lagophthalmos.

Symptoms of conjunctival and corneal irritation are common. Patients will complain of a burning or gritty sensation, photophobia, tearing, and red eyes. Ocular signs include lid fullness, palpable extraocular muscles, chemosis, and dilatation of bulbar vessels.

Diplopia results from swelling and fibrosis of the extraocular muscles. The inferior rectus muscle is most frequently involved, producing diplopia and limitation of upgaze. The medial rectus muscle is the next most frequently involved muscle. The important clinical signs associated with fibrosis of the extraocular muscles are limitation of passive motion and inability to elicit the full range of motion on forced duction testing, in which direct traction is applied to the involved muscle.

Enlargement of the extraocular muscles and orbital edema and inflammation may produce a compressive optic neuropathy. Optic nerve involvement is manifested by any combination of the following: (1) decreased visual acuity, (2) visual field defects, and (3) optical atrophy or optic disc edema. These are serious signs that require prompt treatment.

DIAGNOSIS. The differential diagnosis of unilateral or bilateral exophthalmos should always include thyroid ophthalmopathy. Evaluation of the systemic disorder includes T_4 level, RT3U, and thyroid index. A T_3 suppression test result is positive in 75 per cent of patients with Graves' ophthalmopathy, and a thyroid suppression test generally shows nonsuppressibility in 75 per cent of the cases.

The differential diagnosis of exophthalmos includes tumor, orbital cellulitis, carotid–cavernous sinus fistula, orbital pseudotumor, high myopia, and unilateral enophthalmos, which produces pseudoexophthalmos on the opposite side. Unilateral ptosis may also produce pseudoexophthalmos on the opposite side.

Evaluation of the orbits should include an examination by an ophthalmologist, including visual acuity, visual fields, extraocular motility evaluation, and a funduscopic examination with pupils dilated. X-rays of the orbits and skull should be obtained to help rule out a mass lesion. Orbital ultrasound and orbital computerized axial tomography are extremely valuable, as they will generally show marked enlargement of the extraocular muscles in thyroid infiltrative ophthalmopathy.

TREATMENT. Thyroid ophthalmopathy is an unpredictable disease characterized by spontaneous remission. The course of the disease is independent of the level of thyroid activity, and the eye signs may even show progression following treatment of the underlying thyroid disease. Therefore evaluation of treatment can be quite difficult.

Prominent stare and lid lag require no treatment, and may resolve over a period of months to years following treatment of the thyroid disorder. Progressive exophthalmos, diplopia, exposure keratopathy, and optic nerve damage are indications for vigorous therapy. Initial treatment usually consists of high doses of prednisone (60 to 80 mg per day). If exposure keratopathy is present, artificial tears, topical antimicrobial agents, and a surgical lid adhesion may be used in addition to the steroids. Supervoltage x-ray treatment has also been reported as successful in the treatment of infiltrative ophthalmopathy.

Indications for surgery include (1) diplopia, (2) exposure keratopathy, and (3) optic nerve damage. The most frequently used surgical procedure is an orbital decompression performed by removing the floor of the orbit. This procedure is usually done only after medical attempts at controlling the disease have failed.

Bloch, R. S., and Henkind, P.: Ocular manifestations of endocrine and metabolic diseases. In Duane, T. D. (ed.): Clinical Ophthalmology, Vol. 5. Hagerstown, Md., Harper & Row, 1976.

Dardenne, M. U.: Endocrine diseases (excluding diabetes): Ophthalmic aspects. In Mausolf, F. A. (ed.): The Eye and Systemic Disease. St. Louis, C. V. Mosby Company, 1975.

Donaldson, S. S., Bagshaw, M. A., and Kriss, J. P.: Supervoltage orbital radiotherapy for Graves' ophthalmopathy. J. Clin. Endocrinol. Metab., 37:276, 1973.

Duke-Elder, S., and MacFaul, P. A.: System of Ophthalmology, Vol. XIII. St. Louis, C. V. Mosby Company, 1974.

Solomon, D. H.: The eye in endocrine diseases, especially Graves' ophthalmopathy. In Mausolf, F. A. (ed.): The Eye and Systemic Disease. St. Louis, C. V. Mosby Company, 1975, pp. 155–168.

Symposium on Graves' disease. Mayo Clin. Proc., 47:801, 1972.

Werner, S. C., and Day, R. M.: Ocular manifestations. In Werner, S. C., and Ingbar, S. H. (eds.): The Thyroid. New York, Harper & Row, 1971.

587. OCULAR TOXOPLASMOSIS

INCIDENCE. This disease has a prevalence of 20 to 60 per cent in various parts of the world (Fig. 1G). In the United States the infection is acquired at a rate of 1 per cent of the population per year. Congenital toxoplasmosis is detected in about 1 in 10,000 births in the United States, 1 in 1000 births in France, and 1 in 500 births in Norway. Transplacental transmission occurs from mothers who acquired the infection during pregnancy. Approximately 40 per cent of infants of mothers infected during pregnancy acquire toxoplasmosis, although only one third to one half show clinical evidence of the disease at birth.

It remains unclear whether late-onset ocular disease is due to an acquired infection or to reactivation of clinically silent congenital toxoplasmosis.

PATHOLOGY AND PATHOPHYSIOLOGY. *Toxoplasma gondii* travels easily through most tissue and multiplies in any nucleated cell. Transmission to the eye is probably via circulating leukocytes. The intraocular protozoa have a predilection for the nerve fiber layer of the retina and so far have been found only within the retina in the eye. Intracellular multiplication of *T. gondii* has no apparent adverse effects on host cell function until the cell wall bursts, releasing the organisms and inducing an intense inflammatory reaction. A pseudogranuloma is formed, consisting of a central area of necrosis and polymorphonuclear leukocytes surrounded by a zone of plasma cells, lymphocytes, and giant cells. Local retinal tissue is completely destroyed. The released protozoa then spread by direct extension into neighboring healthy retinal cells. Adjacent choroidal, scleral, and vitreous structures show secondary inflammatory effects resulting from the retinitis. A giant cell reaction is seen in the choroid. Although retinal pigment is seen within these choroidal giant cells, *Toxoplasma* organisms are rarely or never seen outside the retina. Cellular debris and inflammatory exudates are released into the vitreous body and create a characteristic vitreal haze. Frequently, there is an intense granulomatous iritis accompanying the chorioretinitis.

Occasionally, in a resistant host, or in one with less virulent *Toxoplasma* organisms, some cells are not lysed and form a membrane around the intracellular parasites. These cysts are seen more commonly in chronic infections and may be up to 70 μ in size. The cysts seem inert but may release viable organisms up to 25 years later. Recurrent posterior lesions may be caused by the release of organisms from these dormant cysts as the result of unknown stimuli. There is less destruction in recurrent contiguous or satellite lesions due to local immunologic reactions and delayed hypersensitivity. Widespread dissemination is seen in the immunocompromised host, however.

CLINICAL MANIFESTATIONS. Toxoplasmosis is seen in acquired and congenital forms. Differentiation between the two by ophthalmoscopy may be impossible, although acquired toxoplasmosis often is unilateral, whereas the congenital form is usually bilateral. This disease may have systemic involvement but is more commonly limited to the eyes. Ocular features of each form are discussed separately.

Acquired Systemic Toxoplasmosis. Ocular disease (retinitis) is a very rare manifestation of acquired systemic toxoplasmosis. Most cases of ocular toxoplasmosis result from congenital infections or acquired ocular toxoplasmosis alone, which many authors believe to be a recurrence of a clinically silent congenital form of the disease.

Congenital Systemic Toxoplasmosis. The diagnosis of congenital toxoplasmosis is suggested by the three C's: convulsions, intracranial calcifications and chorioretinitis. Microphthalmia, microcephaly, mental retardation, hepatosplenomegaly, pneumonitis (exanthem), and fever may also be part of the clinical spectrum. Eighty per cent of children with congenital toxoplasmosis have chorioretinitis, and 85 per cent of these have bilateral disease. Lesions are usually limited to the posterior part of the retina. Early severe intrauterine infection often causes nystagmus, cataract, pupillary membrane, vitreous organization, and microphthalmos, usually in association with generalized central nervous systemic disease and developmental anomalies. Infections occurring around parturition or in the neonatal period are less severe. In these patients, the chorioretinitis is limited to the posterior part of the retina and results in chorioretinal scarring and varying degrees of visual impairment, depending upon the location of the lesions. Frequently, congenital toxoplasmosis is diagnosed for the first time after the development of crossed eyes or amblyopia due to macular scarring or after the discovery of decreased vision during a routine preschool examination.

Acquired and Congenital Ocular Toxoplasmosis. Ocular toxoplasmosis, whether acquired or congenital, begins with an acute focal retinochoroiditis with exudation of cells and inflammatory debris into the vitreous cavity. This vitreal haze decreases vision and fundus visualization, producing a "headlight in the fog" appearance. In congenital cases, this appearance helps differentiate toxoplasmosis from the retinal lesions of cytomegalovirus infection which have fewer vitreal exudates. In the acquired form the lesions are usually single and unilateral, and posterior to the equator in persons 11 to 40 years of age. In contrast to congenital disease, the acquired form has no macular predilection.

A severe granulomatous anterior uveitis with keratic precipitates, anterior chamber flare and cells, and posterior synechiae is usually seen along with acquired toxoplasmic retinochoroiditis. Occasionally recurrent iridocyclitis is seen in patients with no visualized active retinal lesions.

Papillitis and papilledema can be seen in ocular toxoplasmosis. Papillitis is diagnosed when vitreous cells are found concentrated in front of the optic disc and when no other apparent source of cells is observed. Papilledema of both involved and uninvolved eyes is seen secondary to increased intracranial pressure which can follow the spontaneous rupture of intracerebral toxoplasmic cysts and the subsequent inflammatory reaction.

Posterior detachment of the vitreous with precipitates on the detached surface is common in ocular toxoplasmosis. Occasionally vitreal lesions described as "grapevines covered with wet snow" are seen.

Recurrent Toxoplasmic Retinitis. Seventy-five per cent of recurrent retinitis occurs between the ages of 10 and 35 years. It is rarely seen after 50. Recurrences are usually satellite lesions of old pigmented scars and appear as yellow-white, ill-defined lesions frequently with a vitreous haze and a posterior detachment. They may also be seen as focal peripheral lesions, as peripapillary lesions, or as focal perivascular lesions. Recurrent retinitis is classed in three categories. The mild form (smaller than one disc diameter) is seen as typical satellite lesions or as punctate inner or punctate outer retinal lesions. Punctate lesions consist of small single or multiple gray areas of retinitis with minimal edema and vitreous reaction. These forms heal in 1 to 12 weeks. They may mimic the lesions of histoplasmosis. Moderate recurrent retinal lesions from one to three disc diameters in size are the most common. Severe recurrent lesions have intense inflammation, edema, vitreal exudate, and anterior chamber reaction. The average healing time is several months, and 40 per cent will have a significant decrease in vision. Complications of retinal detachment, glaucoma, cataract, vitreal hemorrhage, cystic macular edema, and chronic iridocyclitis are usually limited to this latter group.

DIAGNOSIS. The diagnosis of ocular toxoplasmosis may be presumed by observing the typical clinical features and confirmed by laboratory evidence. Main differential possibilities in the adult include tuberculosis, syphilis, and fungal chorioretinitis, and, in the neonate, cytomegalovirus, herpes simplex, neonatal hemolysis, torulosis, cerebral trauma, focal retinoblastoma, and macular coloboma.

Serologic testing is the most common laboratory test for ocular toxoplasmosis. With the Sabin-Feldman methylene blue dye test, any positive antibody titer (1:8 or greater) is significant. However, three cases of confirmed toxoplasmosis in patients with false-negative dye tests have been documented. Ninety-five percent of patients with ocular toxoplasmosis have positive skin tests to toxoplasmin. Because of the ubiquitous occurrence of toxoplasmosis, however, 35 to 50 per cent of clinically normal individuals will have positive skin and serologic tests. Comparison of aqueous humor and serum toxoplasma antibody levels and fluorescent antibody tests have been used by some authors when the Sabin dye test is equivocal. The mainstay of diagnosis, however, is the characteristic clinical presentation of this exudative retinochoroiditis.

TREATMENT. Chemotherapy for any type of active toxoplasmic retinochoroiditis is indicated for macular lesions or large lesions with massive vitreous inflammation. Small peripheral lesions usually resolve spontaneously and require only topical mydriatics and corticosteroids to check anterior chamber inflammation. No known therapy has proved effective for eradicating *T. gondii* in the cyst stage. It is suggested that active congenital toxoplasmosis, regardless of the degree of ocular or systemic involvement, be treated pharmacologically.

The treatment of choice for ocular toxoplasmosis is a combination of oral sulfonamides, pyrimethamine (Daraprim), and corticosteroids. There is considerable debate over the particular drugs and dosage schedules, but the following are recommended:

1. Sulfadiazine, 4 grams (orally) loading dose, followed by 1.0 gram four times daily.

2. Pyrimethamine, 100 mg loading dose, followed by 25 mg twice daily.

3. Prednisone, 40 to 60 mg daily, tapered rapidly to 20 mg daily.

4. In pyrimethamine-intolerant patients, chlortetracycline, 2-gram (orally) loading dose, followed by 250 mg four times daily, may be used. Subconjunctival clindamycin has also been used.

Weekly urinalyses and complete blood counts are indicated to check for early toxicities to these therapeutic agents.

Photocoagulation and cryotherapy also have been used in an effort to destroy cysts or to check "creeping" chorioretinitis, but the results have not been encouraging.

Klintworth, G. K., and Landers, M. B.: The Eye: Structure and Function in Disease. Baltimore, Williams & Wilkins Company, 1976.

Newell, F. W., and Ernest, J. T.: Ophthalmology Principles and Concepts. 3rd ed. St. Louis, C. V. Mosby, 1974.

Schlaegel, T. F., Jr.: Toxoplasmosis. *In* Duane, T. D. (ed.): Clinical Ophthalmology, Vol. 4. Hagerstown, Md., Harper & Row, 1976, pp. 1–16.

Smith, R. E.: Ocular toxoplasmosis. *In* Ryan, S. J., and Smith, R. E. (eds.): Selected Topics on the Eye in Systemic Diseases. New York, Grune & Stratton, 1974, pp. 259–273.

PART XXV
DRUG-DRUG INTERACTIONS

Rubin Bressler

588. INTRODUCTION

Drug-drug interactions are modifications of the effect of a drug when used in association with another drug. These interactions can result in either an augmentation or diminution of pharmacologic activity and may account for a significant proportion of all adverse drug reactions. It has been reported that hypersensitivity (the signs and symptoms resulting from an immune response to a standard dose of drug), idiosyncrasy (the inordinate response to a usual dose), and the predictable response (toxicity expected from overdose) account for less than 50 per cent of drug reactions.

The treatment of a number of pathologic states such as hypertension, arthritis, congestive heart failure, depression, neoplastic disease, infectious disease, and inflammatory disease involves the use of multiple drug therapy. The trend toward simultaneous use of increasing numbers of pharmacologic agents over long periods of time raises new considerations and concerns. Since the efficacy and toxicity of any new pharmacologic agent is ascertained by tests in which the drug is the sole agent used, the testing results may not be valid in the clinical arena of actual drug use. It is unrealistic to assume that drugs do not interact and that a drug will produce the same effect when used with another drug as when used alone. Each chemical agent has its separate and distinct side effects which occur at a characteristic frequency. The concomitant use of two or more drugs, however, may result in unexpected increases or decreases in potencies of the several drugs being used simultaneously. It has been found that there is a 7 per cent adverse drug reaction rate in patients using six to ten drugs, whereas the reaction rate is 40 per cent in patients using 16 to 20 drugs. At all numbers of multiple drugs taken, adverse drug reactions to antihypertensive and anticoagulant drugs lead the list by a considerable margin, followed by antimicrobial, antiarrhythmic, and diuretic agents.

Tissue levels of physiologically or pharmacologically active substances are limited by their rates of appearance (synthesis or absorption) and their rates of removal (enzymatic inactivation, binding, or excretion). Since drugs may directly or indirectly alter enzymatic activity, binding capacity, and transport processes, it might be expected that the presence of one drug might markedly influence the efficacy of another drug either by affecting the rate of appearance or removal of the drug itself or of an endogenous compound necessary for the action of the second drug. The course of such interactions may enhance drug efficacy, lead to undesirable side effects, or even result in marked toxicity.

The time course of drug activity is determined by pharmacokinetic characteristics. These include (1) absorption, (2) distribution, (3) metabolism, and (4) excretion. Since most drugs are orally administered, absorption is usually from the gastrointestinal tract. Distribution is of importance in delivery of drugs to target tissues. Distribution is also important in the termination of action of those drugs with high extraction coefficients which are removed by hepatic uptake. Metabolism occurs to the greatest extent in the liver, but also to some extent in the gastrointestinal tract, kidney, and lung. Excretion is primarily by the kidney, but also occurs via the biliary system.

589. PHYSICAL-CHEMICAL PROCESSES

CHEMICAL REACTIONS IN VITRO. The drug-drug interactions that occur prior to administration usually represent physical-chemical incompatibilities. For example, the delayed hypoglycemia that follows the mixture of regular with protamine zinc insulin is due to the binding of the regular insulin by the excess of protamine present in the sustained action insulin preparation. Other instances of drug inactivation prior to administration include the diminution of penicillin and semisynthetic penicillin activity caused by carbohydrate solutions at alkaline pH, and the decrease in gentamicin activity caused by chemical alteration of the aminoglycoside when given in solutions containing carbenicillin.

ABSORPTION. Clinical responses to orally administered drugs can be modified by changes in the rate of drug absorption or the total quantity of drug absorbed. Since nonionized drugs are better absorbed, acidic drugs are more readily absorbed in the stomach (salicylates, sulfonamides, phenytoin, barbiturates, warfarin) and basic drugs in the small intestine (phenothiazines, tricylic antidepressants, antihistamines, quinidine, erythromycin). However, the small intestine, because of its greater surface area, accounts for the majority of absorption of both acidic and basic drugs.

Drugs which alter gastric and small intestinal motility can affect the rate or quantity of drug absorption. Drugs such as anticholinergics and opiates increase gastric retention time and decrease intestinal motility. This serves to increase transit time in the small intestine, where most drug absorption occurs, because of the large mucosal absorption surface. Digoxin, a drug whose absorption is normally incomplete, has its plasma levels increased by simultaneously administered anticholinergic agents. This effect presumably occurs as a result of increased intestinal transit time. Decreased digoxin absorption would be anticipated with simultaneous use of drugs which decrease intestinal transit time such as cathartics and cholinomimetics.

Impairment of drug absorption may result from binding of drugs to other interacting drugs or to foods. This is exemplified by the binding of iron and penicillin to food and the precipitation of tetracyclines as insoluble complexes with magnesium, calcium, and aluminum commonly found in antacid preparations and with iron.

Drug absorption can be affected by the concomitant use of antacid and kaolin products. The large surface area of these preparations favors nonspecific absorption of drugs. Simultaneous use of acidic drugs with antacid preparations may further promote the ionization of the acidic drugs in the small intestine where they are already ionized to some extent. The ionized drug state favors nonspecific drug adsorption to the antacid preparation and decreases and/or delays absorption. The absorption of lincomycin is impaired by ingestion of kaolins. Phenothiazines, which are bound by antacid preparations, lose their effects with long-term use of antacids.

Therapeutic use of these nonspecific surface adsorption phenomona has led to the use of charcoal and kaolin for treatment of drug overdoses. These preparations diminish drug absorption and permit removal of the drug from the gastrointestinal tract.

Cholestyramine and polystyrene sulfonate are insoluble exchange resins which have been used to prevent intestinal absorption and facilitate elimination of certain substances (bile acids, potassium). Cholestyramine is an anion exchanger which has been found to alter the absorption of warfarin. Interactions of the exchange resins and acidic and basic drugs are probable, but the extent and clinical significance are not known.

DRUG BINDING TO PLASMA PROTEINS. Most drugs are reversibly bound to plasma albumin to varying degrees. The drug-albumin complex serves as a circulating reservoir of drug. Only the unbound form of the drug is active — free to diffuse through capillary walls and reach tissue sites of drug action. The availability of drugs to sites of drug action is directly related to the quantity of free drug present. The quantity of free drug is related to the total concentration of drug, the amount of albumin present, and the binding affinity of the drug for albumin. Albumin is capable of binding anionic and cationic drug species. These ionic interactions are not strong, and other forces play important roles in binding. These include hydrogen bonding, hydrophobic bonding, and van der Waals' forces.

When two or more drugs are simultaneously administered, the binding of one may be affected by the other(s). Displacement of a drug initially results in a greater quantity of free drug and a resultant intensification of pharmacologic action. However, since the free drug is more rapidly eliminated via glomerular filtration and hepatic metabolism, the half-life may be shortened.

Most displacing drugs are acidic. The displacement is more marked with high concentrations of drugs which have high affinities for albumin-binding sites relative to the bound drug. A list of highly bound drugs is shown. The bound-free percentage of drug is shown at therapeutic plasma levels.

Diazepam	99–1
Phenylbutazone	99–1
Tolbutamide	99–1
Indomethacin	97–3
Warfarin	97–3
Chlorpromazine	96–4
Amitriptyline	96–4
Propranolol	94–6
Methotrexate	94–6
Phenytoin	91–9
Clofibrate	90–10
Digitoxin	90–10
Acetylsalicylic acid	84–16

Even a small displacement of a highly bound drug can result in a large increase in the free (active) species. For highly bound drugs, the free form can be doubled by as little as a 1 per cent displacement of the bound drug. A 1 per cent displacement of phenylbutazone doubles the free drug concentration, whereas a 3 per cent displacement will do so for warfarin.

The pharmacologic effects of drug displacement are most marked if the displaced drug is highly bound (greater than 90 per cent at therapeutic plasma levels) and has a narrow therapeutic index and a small apparent volume of distribution. If the volume of distribution of the drug is large, then displacement results only in a small rise in plasma concentration of free drug, and the pharmacologic effect will be small. If the volume of distribution is small, then displacement will result in a significant rise in plasma concentration of the free drug, resulting in a more marked pharmacologic effect. Many drugs bound to plasma albumin can be displaced with little discernible clinical effect because they do not fulfill these criteria for intensification of drug action. Examples are penicillin, which has a very large therapeutic index, and amitriptyline, which has a large volume of distribution.

A number of clinically significant displacement reactions have been reported with oral anticoagulants and tolbutamide. These drugs have been displaced from their binding to albumin by acidic drugs such as sulfonamides, phenylbutazone, ethacrynic acid, nalidixic acid, and acetylsalicylic acid, resulting in bleeding or hypoglycemia.

Displacement can occur both competitively and noncompetitively. Acetylsalicylic acid influences the binding of other drugs to albumin by acetylating a lysine residue of albumin which modifies the binding of anionic drugs.

Hepatic and renal disease are associated with decreased drug binding to plasma albumin. This is due to decreased levels of plasma albumin and to qualitative changes in the albumin which diminish binding.

Drug Interactions at Receptor Sites and Cell Membranes. The actions of some drugs and endogenous compounds are associated with their binding to cell surface receptors. Alterations of this binding by other drugs can modify the usual receptor response.

Antagonism is based on inhibition of drug binding to receptor, and it may be competitive or noncompetitive. These types of inhibitions are the basis of the actions of a number of drugs. These include inhibition of the cardiac accelerator actions of norepinephrine by propranolol, a β-adrenergic receptor blocking agent; reduction of the respiratory depression effects of morphine by naloxone; and inhibition of the bradycardiac effect of acetylcholine by atropine, a cholinergic receptor blocking agent. These are all examples of competitive inhibitions. Thyroxine has been reported to potentiate the anticoagulant effects of warfarin without altering the warfarin plasma half-life. This is probably a noncompetitive effect.

Drugs may influence the actions of other drugs by blocking their uptake into or facilitating their release from cells. The monoamine oxidase (MAO) inhibitors deter the intracellular inactivation of active catecholamines which accumulate in adrenergic neurons. These vasoactive catecholamines can be released from the cell by a number of drugs, including amphetamines. A variety of foods contain tyramine, which is normally metabolized in the gastrointestinal tract by MAO. Because of the MAO inhibition, the tyramine gains access to the circulation and acts like amphetamines to release the increased stores of catecholamines and causes marked adrenergic effects (tachycardia, hypertension, headache).

Tricyclic antidepressants (TCA) block the amine uptake system(s) in neural tissues. They inhibit the uptake of norepinephrine and serotonin, which is considered to be at least in part the basis of their actions. They also inhibit the uptake of guanethidine, which cannot gain access to its site of action; its antihypertensive effect is reversed by simultaneous use of TCA.

DRUG INTERACTIONS AND RENAL CLEARANCE. Renal clearance of drugs may occur by means of glomerular filtration or tubular secretion. Drug-drug interactions can influence drug clearance by either of these mechanisms.

Non-protein-bound drugs are filtered through the glomerulus. The free drug in the glomerular filtrate is reabsorbed by the renal tubules by a passive diffusion process. The reabsorption occurs in varying degree, depending in part on the polar nature of the drug, and on the pH of the urine. Because less polar (uncharged) drugs are more readily reabsorbed, the pH of the urine can determine the extent of drug clearance. Weakly acidic drugs such as salicylic acid and phenylbutazone are rapidly excreted in alkaline urine, whereas weakly basic drugs such as amphetamine and quinidine are readily excreted in acid urine. The renal clearance of quinidine at a urine pH of 7.5 is only 10 per cent of that at a urine pH of 6.0. Drugs can alter the pH of urine and influence the half-lives of other drugs which are significantly excreted by the kidney (>20 per cent). Drugs such as sodium bicarbonate and acetazolamide alkalinize the urine, whereas drugs such as mandelic acid and ascorbic acid acidify urine. These principles are the basis for alkalinization of the urine in the treatment of aspirin and phenobarbital overdoses, and for acidification of the urine in amphetamine overdoses.

Drug-drug interactions may occur if a drug which is cleared by the kidney is used in conjunction with a drug which is nephrotoxic. The aminoglycoside antimicrobials such as gentamicin and kanamycin decrease glomerular filtration. Digoxin and quinidine toxicity may occur when these drugs are used in association with gentamicin because they are significantly cleared by glomerular filtration.

Many acidic drugs such as penicillins, thiazides, salicylic acid, and indomethacin are eliminated by renal tubular secretion, an active process. Drug-drug interactions occur when two drugs, both of which are cleared by renal tubular secretion, are used simultaneously. The elimination of methotrexate is slowed by acetylsalicylic acid, and phenylbutazone inhibits the elimination

of hydroxyhexamide, a hypoglycemic metabolite of acetohexamide. The inhibitions result in increased half-lives of active drugs and overdose toxicities. This type of interaction has been used beneficially in the case of simultaneous use of penicillin and probenecid. Probenecid blocks the tubular secretion of penicillin, resulting in higher blood levels for longer periods of time.

590. DRUG DISPOSITION

STIMULATION OF DRUG METABOLISM. Drugs and other xenobiotics are in the main metabolized in the liver, but also to a lesser extent in the kidney, gastrointestinal tract, and lungs. These compounds undergo a variety of structural modifications which tend to produce products which are more polar and water soluble. The biotransformations in general create drug metabolites which are less capable of permeating cells. The more polar metabolites are generally more readily eliminated by means of renal or biliary excretion.

The enzymes of drug metabolism are both nonpotent and nonspecific. The number of these enzymes is not known, and isolation and purification studies are ongoing. Many but not all of these enzymatic reactions are oxidative, and they are often followed by additional conjugation reactions.

Biotransformation of drugs usually implies loss of pharmacologic activity, but this is not always so. There are instances in which metabolism results in the conversion of an inactive precursor to an active metabolite, and in which both the precursor and metabolite are pharmacologically active. Some examples of these reactions are as follows:

Cytoxan (inactive)	→ Cytoxyl alcohol (active)
Parathion (inactive)	→ Paraoxon (active)
Acetohexamide (active)	→ Hydroxyhexamide (more active)
Phenylbutazone (active)	→ Oxyphenylbutazone (active)
Imipramine (active)	→ Desipramine (active)

The enzymes of drug metabolism are sensitive to a variety of chemical influences which can increase their activity. The increased activity may be engendered by prior exposure in vivo to drugs, insecticides, or environmental chemicals and by smoking cigarettes (see Ch. 21). The augmentation of drug-metabolizing enzyme activity is termed induction and is thought to be due to enhanced synthesis of enzymes in the liver.

It has been established that induction is a nonspecific phenomenon. For example, phenobarbital and warfarin are both capable of accelerating the metabolic disposition of a number of other drugs.

In general, drugs are capable of inducing the metabolism of other drugs, depending on their lipid solubility at physiologic pH (nonpolar), their concentration, and their duration of exposure.

The effects of enzyme induction can be clinically important when a drug is either added to or withdrawn from a therapeutic regimen employing multiple drug therapy. In the case of the addition of a second drug there may be an acceleration of metabolic disposition of the first drug, resulting in decreased plasma concentrations and a diminished therapeutic effect. In the case of withdrawal of a drug from a multiple drug therapy regimen, the opposite effect may occur. Drug withdrawal results in the concentration of the drug whose metabolism had been accelerated rising to higher and perhaps toxic levels.

Induction of drug-metabolizing enzymes by xenobiotics has produced a variety of unexpected clinical responses to drugs. An often-cited example is the drug-metabolizing enzyme stimulation induced by phenobarbital. Under conditions of phenobarbital administration, both warfarin and bishydroxycoumarin are metabolized more rapidly. An anticoagulated patient given a barbiturate will require larger doses of anticoagulants than are usually required to maintain a suitable state of anticoagulation. On the other hand, if the barbiturate is discontinued and the dose of anticoagulants is not readjusted, bleeding may occur. Similar effects have been seen in other conditions of multiple drug use. Adjustments of drug regimens must be considered upon the institution or discontinuation of an enzyme-inducing drug. A clue to the occurrence of drug interactions resulting from altered drug metabolism is the development of unexpected sensitivity to a drug under conditions in which a drug has been discontinued from a therapeutic regimen or the development of drug resistance after the addition of a drug to a therapeutic regimen.

Environmental exposure to chlorinated hydrocarbon insecticides such as lindane and DDT has been found to accelerate the metabolism of antipyrine in subjects chronically exposed to these agents. A loss of the anticoagulant effects of warfarin has also been reported after occupational exposure to insecticides. This exposure required an increase in the warfarin maintenance dose from 7.5 to 17.5 mg a day.

An effect of cigarette smoking on the plasma clearance of phenacetin has been described. The accelerated disposition of phenacetin from the plasma of cigarette smokers was probably due to increased phenacetin metabolism resulting from induction of drug metabolizing enzymes by xenobiotics contained in the inhaled cigarette smoke.

It has been found that long-term therapy of epilepsy with phenobarbital, phenytoin, or both may result in hypocalcemia, osteomalacia, and depressed plasma levels of 25-hydroxycholecalciferol in some patients. It is believed that these drugs accelerate the metabolism of vitamin D_3 (cholecalciferol) to hydroxylated metabolites which are biologically inactive.

Rifampin, a drug used in the treatment of tuberculosis, has been suspected of modifying the effects of the steroidal oral contraceptives because of a number of pregnancies which have occurred while subjects were simultaneously being treated with both agents. This drug interaction is thought to result from an acceleration of the metabolism of the oral contraceptive drugs.

Phenobarbital caused a 44 per cent reduction in the plasma half-life of dexamethasone when the two drugs were used together. Simultaneous use of these drugs resulted in clinical deterioration in asthmatic patients who had previously been satisfactorily maintained on dexamethasone. These effects are probably a result of enzyme induction and acceleration of dexamethasone metabolism by phenobarbital.

Ethanol also may play a role in drug interactions because of its capacity to induce microsomal enzymes of drug metabolism and accelerate the biotransformation of such drugs as tolbutamide and warfarin. The role of ethanol as an inhibitor of drug metabolism is discussed below.

INHIBITION OF DRUG METABOLISM. Drug inhibition of drug metabolism is not uncommon and may be clinically more important than stimulation interactions. Because of the nonpotent and nonspecific nature of the drug-metabolizing enzymes, inhibition of drug metabolism may be nonspecific and the metabolism of a drug may be inhibited by chemically and pharmacologically unrelated drugs. The inhibition is thought to be due to saturation of the drug-metabolizing enzymes. Drug inhibition of drug metabolism usually results in both an intensification of drug action and an increase in its duration. If drug metabolism results in an increase of pharmacologic activity, then an inhibition would cause a decrease in drug activity. A number of human studies have shown that inhibition of drug metabolism by other drugs increases the half-life of the primary drug and elevates its steady-state plasma concentration. Tolbutamide metabolism is inhibited by bishydroxycoumarin, chloramphenicol, clofibrate, and sulfaphenazole, which increase its half-life from a range of 4.5 to 6 hours to 11 to 18 hours. The metabolism of phenytoin is inhibited by simultaneous administration of bishydroxycoumarin, disulfiram, isonicotinic acid, chloramphenicol, and sulfaphenazole. The metabolism of bishydroxycoumarin is inhibited by allopurinol, chloramphenicol, and clofibrate. These inhibitions are probably competitive and produce toxic effects at therapeutic doses of the drugs: tolbutamide (hypoglycemia), phenytoin (ataxia), bishydroxycoumarin (bleeding).

Although inhibition of drug metabolism by other drugs is generally a nonspecific phenomenon, there are interesting exceptions. Simultaneous use of warfarin and metronidazole has resulted in increased steady-state plasma levels of warfarin and increased prothrombin times. This is probably due to metronidazole inhibition of warfarin metabolism. The inhibitory effect was found when either S (−) warfarin or the racemic mixture was used. No inhibition of the metabolism of R (+) warfarin was found. The stereoselective inhibition of S (−) warfarin metabolism by metronidazole could be lessened or avoided by chronic therapy with R (+) warfarin.

A number of drugs exhibit dose-dependent pharmacokinetics. The plasma levels of these drugs decline more slowly after a large than after a small dose of drug. This phenomenon has been well studied in the case of bishydroxycoumarin, phenytoin, acetylsalicylic acid, and probenecid. The plasma half-life of bishydroxycoumarin at an oral dose of 2 mg per kilogram is around 24 hours, whereas at a dose of 4 mg per kilogram the half-life is 48 hours. Dose-dependent kinetics is a special case of inhibition. It is self-inhibition of drug metabolism secondary to saturation of the metabolizing enzymes. It has important implications for therapy of drug overdoses. Larger drug intakes can lengthen the clearance time of drugs from plasma.

Clofibrate inhibits the metabolism of Cytoxan to cytoxyl alcohol. Because the metabolite is the active pharmacologic species, the inhibition diminishes drug action.

Drug-drug interactions may also occur by means of drug inhibition of specific enzymes. These inhibitions may provide therapeutic advantage, as in the case of allopurinol and dihydroxyphenylalanine hydrazide.

Allopurinol is an inhibitor of xanthine oxidase. Since both azathioprine and mercaptopurine are metabolized to inactive compounds via xanthine oxidase, its inhibition by allopurinol serves to prolong the duration and increase the intensity of action of these two drugs.

L-Dihydroxyphenylalanine (L-dopa) is converted to dopamine (DA), a central nervous system (CNS) transmitter, by the nonspecific L-aromatic amino acid decarboxylase, which is ubiquitous in tissues. Normally 90 per cent or more of orally administered L-dopa is decarboxylated outside the CNS, and the DA does not penetrate into the CNS where it can relieve the signs and symptoms of Parkinson's disease. Because of this, the L-dopa doses used have to be high, in the 4 to 12 grams per day range. These doses of L-dopa cause nausea, vomiting, tachycardia, hypotension, and cardiac arrhythmias secondary to the DA formed extracerebrally. Combinations of L-dopa and an L-dopa decarboxylase inhibitor (dopa hydrazide), which does not penetrate into the CNS, have been used. The inhibition of DA formation in extracerebral tissues increases the quantity of L-dopa available for decarboxylation to DA in the CNS and reduces the deleterious side effects of peripheral DA. The inhibition of the dopa decarboxylase is a beneficial one which has permitted a reduction in the quantity of L-dopa used in the therapy of Parkinson's disease by two- to three-fold.

Ethanol has been found to play a complex role in drug metabolism. Ethanol is a poor substrate for the hepatic drug metabolizing enzyme systems, and ethanol metabolism is not significantly influenced by these enzymes (induction or inhibition), because most ethanol metabolism proceeds via the alcohol dehydrogenase–aldehyde dehydrogenase systems. However, ethanol at blood concentration of 200 to 300 mg per 100 ml does influence drug metabolism in spite of its behavior as a poor substrate for these enzymes. It can (1) induce microsomal enzymes of drug metabolism, as discussed above, and (2) act as a competitive inhibitor of the metabolism of other drugs. In the chronic alcoholic who is acutely intoxicated, ethanol may potentiate the action of other drugs by decreasing their metabolism (competitive inhibition due to high blood levels). On the other hand, in the sober chronic alcoholic, ethanol is an inducer of drug metabolism, and the patient may be less responsive to other drugs (due to an increased rate of drug metabolism).

The metabolism of a number of drugs, including bishydroxycoumarin, phenytoin, and meprobamate, has been found to be inhibited by ethanol.

HEPATIC BLOOD FLOW. Orally administered drugs pass through the liver before entering the systemic circulation. Those drugs which are highly extracted by the liver have a low order of bioavailability. This is termed a "first pass effect." Drugs known or suspected to show first pass effect pharmacokinetics include lidocaine, nortriptyline, morphine, pentazocine, and propranolol. Lidocaine has been extensively studied in man because of its intravenous use in cardiac arrhythmias. It undergoes rapid intravenous clearance and has a very low oral availability. Its hepatic extraction ratio is approximately 0.7. Pathologic decreases in hepatic blood flow secondary to congestive heart failure or portacaval shunting significantly affect lidocaine's clearance from plasma.

A number of drugs have been shown to either increase or decrease hepatic blood flow, and therefore influence the clearance from plasma of drugs with high hepatic extraction ratios.

Drugs which increase hepatic blood flow include glucagon, isoproterenol, and phenobarbital. Halothane and propranolol decrease hepatic blood flow by 33 per cent, and simultaneous administration of lidocaine and propranolol results in a 50 per cent reduction in lidocaine clearance.

Significant reductions in hepatic blood flow have a potential for increasing the activity and duration of action of drugs handled by first pass kinetics. The use of drugs which decrease hepatic blood flow simultaneously with drugs having high hepatic extraction ratios holds a potential for adverse effects resulting from unexpectedly high levels of bioavailability. Little information is as yet available from human studies in regard to these drug interactions, but there is good probability of their existence.

A number of significant drug interactions have been validated and their mechanisms elucidated. Several of these are presented in the accompanying table. Because of the multiple mechanisms available for drug interactions, these phenomena may be complex, involving more than one mechanism. Such an interaction occurs with simultaneous use of tolbutamide and warfarin. Warfarin inhibits tolbutamide metabolism, causing hypoglycemia, and tolbutamide displaces warfarin from its binding to albumin, causing bleeding.

Some Clinically Important Drug Interactions

Primary Drug	Interacting Drug	Adverse Effect	Mechanism
Quinidine	Phenytoin	Decreased antiarrhythmic effect	Induction of drug metabolism
Warfarin	Barbiturates	Decreased anticoagulant effect	Induction of drug metabolism
Tolbutamide	Rifampin	Decreased hypoglycemic effect	Induction of drug metabolism
Phenytoin	Isoniazid	Cerebellar ataxia	Inhibition of drug metabolism
Warfarin	Chloramphenicol	Increased anticoagulant effect	Inhibition of drug metabolism
Tolbutamide	Warfarin	Increased hypoglycemic effect	Inhibition of drug metabolism
Warfarin	Nalidixic acid	Increased anticoagulant effect	Displacement from binding
Tolbutamide	Salicylates	Increased hypoglycemic effect	Displacement from binding
Salicylates	Probenecid	Salicylate toxicity	Inhibition of renal excretion
Lincomycin	Kaolin-pectin	Decreased lincomycin effect	Decreased absorption
Tetracyclines	Antacids	Decreased tetracycline effect	Decreased absorption
Guanethidine	Tricyclic antidepressants	Decreased antihypertensive effect	Blockade of uptake at target site
Dopa	Phenothiazines	Decreased dopa effects	Blockade of uptake at target site

591. ADVERSE DRUG REACTIONS

A great deal of attention has been given to the incidence, nature, and cost of adverse drug reactions. Karch and Lasagna have defined an adverse drug reaction as "any response to a drug that is noxious and unintended and that occurs at doses used in man for prophylaxis, diagnosis or therapy, excluding failure to accomplish the intended purpose." Claims have been made for adverse drug reactions as a major cause of patient hospitalization, increased duration of hospital stay, and death. The adverse drug reaction problem is complex, and the available data do not allow strict quantification of the size of the problem. A number of drugs in current use are potent, efficacious pharmacologic agents which are not expected to be completely devoid of adverse effects even when appropriately and properly used. Warranted drug use has a recognized benefit-risk ratio. Firmly establishing the nature of adverse drug reaction may itself be a formidable problem. Drugs are used in a setting of disease, and adverse drug reactions may be difficult to discern from the manifestations of the disease. Moreover, many ill patients are treated with multiple drug therapy and may be expected to experience drug-drug interactions as well as placebo effects of drug ingestion, which are common. Cause-effect relationships are made more difficult by the absence of standardized procedures for defining adverse drug reactions. Even when adverse drug reaction surveillance has been undertaken, use of controls is not possible, since most illnesses have recognized drug therapy. Most data on adverse drug reactions have been derived from acute medical inpatient services at university hospitals, and it is not known whether these data are truly representative of other types of patients and settings.

The Boston Collaborative Drug Surveillance Program found a 5 per cent incidence of adverse drug reactions in inpatient medical services. Most of these were self-limited and of little consequence in the course of the primary illness. Serious adverse drug reactions were found to occur mostly in severely ill patients. The reactions tended to occur with standard drugs which are considered worthwhile in light of their generally accepted risk-benefit ratios. These drugs included digital-is, diuretics, antimicrobials, tranquilizers, antihypertensives, anticoagulants, and steroids.

Data relating to the effects of adverse drug reactions on increasing the length and cost of hospital stay, and on admission to the hospital, are few. Estimates of adverse drug reactions causing admission to the hosptial range from 0.3 to 5.0 per cent. The data are derived without operational criteria and do not define the drug-illness setting. These estimates must be considered arbitrary, as must the cost estimates derived from the admission and length of stay data.

Deaths resulting from adverse drug reactions have been estimated at 0.24 to 2.9 per cent in hospitalized patients. Deaths were generally associated with severe illness and soon-to-be-fatal diseases and with use of drugs considered to be of potential value in the disease setting. The drugs included digitalis, insulin, morphine, KCl, and heparin. One third of these events were instances of fluid overload and KCl excess. In the Boston Collaborative Drug Surveillance Program experience, about two thirds of the adverse drug reactions which terminated fatally occurred in patients with advanced cancer or liver disease.

Because of the large population treated with efficacious drugs, adverse drug reactions are probably not completely preventable in the course of warranted drug use. The data are incomplete, uncontrolled, unrepresentative, and nonrigorously obtained. Thus the quantitative nature of the problem and the possibility of ameliorating it are still unanswered.

Brown, D. D., and Juhl, R. P.: Decreased bioavailability of digoxin due to antacids and kaolin-pectin. N. Engl. J. Med., 295:1034, 1976.

Karch, F. E., and Lasagna, L.: Adverse drug reactions. A critical review. JAMA, 234:1236, 1975.

Koch-Weser, J.: Drug interactions in cardiovascular therapy. Am. Heart J., 90:93, 1975.

Koch-Weser, J., and Sellers, E. M.: Binding of drugs to serum albumin. N. Engl. J. Med., 294:311, 326, 1976.

Kolmodin-Hedman, R.: Decreased plasma levels of antipyrine and phenylbutazone in workers occupationally exposed to lindane and DDT. In Morselli, P. L., Garrattini, L., and Cohen, S. H. (eds.): Drug Interactions. New York, Raven Press, 1974, p. 249.

Pantuck, E. J., Kuntzman, R., and Conney, A. H.: Decreased concentration of phenacetin in plasma of cigarette smokers. Science, 175:1248, 1972.

Perel, J., Dayton, P., Snell, M. M., Yu, T. F., and Gutman, A. B.: Studies of interactions among drugs at the renal level: Probenecid and sulfinpyrazone. Clin. Pharm. Therap., 10:834, 1969.

Wilkinson, G. R., and Shand, D. G.: A physiologic approach to hepatic drug clearance. Clin. Pharmacol. Ther., 18:377, 1975.

NORMAL LABORATORY VALUES OF CLINICAL IMPORTANCE

James B. Wyngaarden

592. THE USE AND INTERPRETATION OF LABORATORY-DERIVED DATA

When you can measure what you are speaking about, and express it in numbers, you know something about it. Lord Kelvin, 1889

The basic workup of a patient begins with the acquisition of data. The experienced clinician will insist upon a discerning and sensitive history, a thorough physical examination, and such laboratory tests as are necessary to evaluate the general health of the patient, to arrive at a specific diagnosis, to assess the functional status of involved organs, and to provide a basis for monitoring effectiveness of therapy.

The inclusion of a panel of chemical tests or enzyme assays of blood (or urine) as a part of a basic medical evaluation is now routine practice. A decade ago many physicians would have ordered a fasting blood sugar and blood urea nitrogen determination as a part of the general workup, and other tests only if suggested by a differential diagnosis constructed from the clinical evaluation.

In 1966 Thiers published a provocative study comparing the results of a screening battery of eleven tests run by an automated multichannel analyzer with those of tests specifically ordered on the same patients by physicians as part of the admission workup. The screening battery detected twice as many abnormal test results of significance to the patient as were uncovered by selective ordering. The most common findings were elevated glucose or uric acid concentration values. Ensuing developments were rapid. Ingenious automated analyzers have brought an increasing number and variety of tests of diagnostic utility within the reach of all practitioners. The cost of such a screening battery is now no greater than that of three or four selected tests run manually a decade ago.

This new practice has profound implications in the teaching of medical students and house officers. One can no longer evaluate the reasoning process which led the house officer to order a serum calcium determination. Some of the intellectual discipline of the construction of a logical differential diagnosis is now gone. The information comes automatically by a computer printout. Attention has shifted from the selective acquisition of data to the interpretation and use of it, including the evaluation of significance of test results and (perhaps)

the selection of a second round of tests and studies. The gains surely outweigh the losses. Since many diseases present initially with rather nonspecific constitutional symptoms, the clinical approach may not suggest the most appropriate laboratory tests, and the initial laboratory screen may disclose unexpected hypercalcemia, acidosis, azotemia, or evidence of liver disease.

In order to utilize the results of laboratory tests intelligently (and economically), the physician must be able to evaluate the validity of the test result, must understand principles of variation and distribution of values, and must be able to integrate the data received from the laboratory with the information acquired from the patient. If the test result deviates from values found in a healthy control population, is the difference trivial, or is it indicative of important dysfunction? Should the test be repeated? How often need a particular measurement be followed? What additional tests or studies are indicated on the basis of these leads?

The more information the physician has, the more effective the physician should be in caring for the patient. To ensure that this is the result requires a sophisticated knowledge of medical science, excellent clinical judgment, and a profound respect for the limitations of the laboratory. One of the best ways of acquiring the constructively critical attitude so essential to the proper evaluation of laboratory test results is for the student or house officer to work in a laboratory for a while. There is a paradox in the present pattern of medical education: at a time of increasing reliance upon an expanding universe of laboratory tests in the practice of medicine, first-hand learning experiences in the laboratory are being progressively eliminated from the medical curriculum.

SOME LIMITATIONS OF THE LABORATORY

CRITERIA FOR EVALUATION OF LABORATORY METHODS. A trustworthy laboratory test must pass critical evaluations of specificity, sensitivity, accuracy, and precision.

Specificity refers to the detection of the substance in question and no other. It is doubtful that any test is absolutely specific for the substance being measured. There is always some other substance around that is capable of reacting. In biochemical analyses this limitation is most serious in tests dependent upon color development, less in the case of assays dependent upon degradation by purified enzymes, and perhaps least in such procedures as atomic absorption spectroscopy.

Sensitivity refers to the ability of the test to detect the substance in question at the required concentrations, namely, those at which the compound exists in body fluids.

Accuracy refers to the quantitative detection of the correct amount of the substance being measured. This property rests upon both specificity and sensitivity. A test may be accurate in the absence of certain interfering drugs, and only in a certain range of values. It may fail this criterion under other conditions.

Precision embodies *repeatability*, the obtaining of the same result on samples analyzed in replicate fashion, and *reproducibility*, representing quality control over time. Precision rests upon the specificity, sensitivity, and accuracy of the method, and characterizes the procedure under conditions of actual use in the diagnostic laboratory.

THE "LAW OF ERRORS." Early in the nineteenth century, the German mathematician and physicist, Johann C. F. Gauss, introduced the "law of errors." This law states that in repeated measurements of the *same* object or substance, the random component on the errors will be distributed about the mean as a frequency function. This distribution, which is bell shaped, is often called "normal" or "gaussian." Note that the law applies to repeated measurements of the same item. Its extension to a population of those items is justifiable only under certain circumstances, for not all distributions are bell shaped, and not all bell-shaped distributions are gaussian. The matter of distributions will be discussed further below, when we consider the topic of "normal range" of a biological variable. First, however, it may be pertinent to emphasize the topic of error, for every laboratory measurement is subject to it.

SOURCES OF ERROR

These are legion, and include some factors under the control of the clinician, such as the dietary preparation of the patient, and the techniques of collection and handling of samples. Reduction of the error factor to an acceptable minimum requires continuous compulsive attention to every detail of the process.

LABORATORY ERRORS. There is imprecision in every measurement. In tests run by hand, pipetting, timing, reading, and recording errors occur. They are more frequent when technicians are overworked or fatigued. It is common to find greater scatter of results of replicate tests at the end of the day than at the beginning. Technician fatigue can be largely eliminated by automation, but there will always remain the technical limitations of machines and the human error in the preparation of reagents in the standardization of instruments, and in the copying of test results. The last is not totally avoided by the computer print-out, as even typewriters make misteaks. Quality control of laboratory performance is both a science and an art. Control criteria vary widely from laboratory to laboratory. Split samples submitted to different laboratories may show surprising disparities in results.

DRUG INTERFERENCE. According to Osler, man is distinguished from all other members of the Animal Kingdom by his desire to take drugs. Since many patients do not regard proprietary pain remedies or vitamins as drugs, the physician may obtain a negative drug history unless questions are appropriately phrased. Drugs have great potential for interference

with laboratory tests. High resolution chromatography of urine yields about 300 peaks of ultraviolet absorbing materials. Two hundred and fifty of these disappear if the "normal subject" abstains from salicylates and vitamins for a few days. Salicylates and vitamins also produce chromogens which interfere with certain analytic methods employed in automated tests, particularly of the urine.

DISTRIBUTIONS OF VALUES

There is widespread belief among medical students and graduate physicians that if the sample of test results from a healthy population is large enough, the distribution will be "normal" (gaussian); that on this assumption one may justifiably determine a mean value ($\bar{x}$) and its standard deviation (δ); that the value, $\bar{x} \pm 2\delta$, will include the central 95 per cent of all measurements; that this segment of the distribution is the "normal range;" and that values which fall outside this range are by definition "abnormal." All these beliefs are erroneous in most instances. The experimental fact is that for most physiological variables the distribution is smooth, unimodal, and skewed, and that $\bar{x} \pm 2\delta$ does not cut off the desired central 95 per cent. Among the distributions of serum calcium, inorganic phosphorus, magnesium, alkaline phosphatase, total proteins, albumin, uric acid, and blood urea, only that of albumin is gaussian. All others are skewed, leptokurtic, or both. The value $\bar{x} \pm 2\delta$ will cut off many more measurements in one tail of the distribution than the other. The uncritical application of principles of normal distributions in situations in which variables are not normally distributed leads occasionally to values of $\bar{x} - 2\delta$ which are negative, surely a biological absurdity.

Once we discard the notion that the distribution of values in healthy persons is gaussian, the question of estimating the mean and standard deviation does not arise. One is then spared the awkward exercise of fitting skewed distributions to bell-shaped curves by constructing histograms of logarithms of the data (a technique which has the effect of compressing the skewed tail to create a "log-gaussian distribution"), or by constructing plots of cumulative frequencies of values (or log-values) on probability paper in search of the linear relationship indicative of a normal distribution (see accompanying figure).

These pitfalls can be circumvented by use of *nonparametric* methods for estimating the normal range, that is, methods which do not involve any a priori assumption regarding the parental distribution shape except that it is continuous. Two nonparametric methods of normal range estimation are the method of *percentile estimates* with associated nonparametric confidence intervals, and the method of nonparametric *tolerance intervals* which include a specified proportion of the population with a specified probability. The required sample sizes of healthy persons for the normal value studies are large, just as they are with parametric methods.

The percentile method of expressing interindividual variation in many kinds of data has been in use for a long time. Physicians are familiar with its use in pediatric growth charts of height and weight. The method avoids the arbitrary distinction of normal and abnormal. It also removes the aura of precision of the standard deviation, expressed to two or more decimal places.

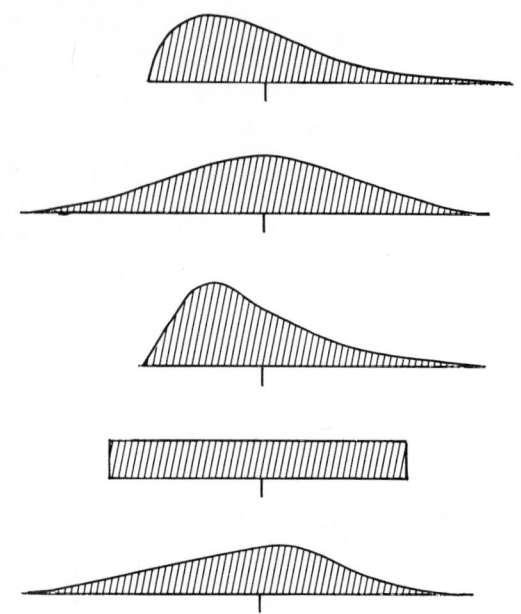

Five distributions with the same mean and standard deviation ($\bar{x} = 4$, $\delta = 2.83$). From top to bottom: χ_4^2 normal, lognormal, rectangular, and mixture of two normals. (From Elveback, L. R.: Mayo Clinic Proc., 47:93, 1972; with permission.)

The percentile method appropriately fits the real world of nongaussian distributions.

From every laboratory test for which a good normal-value study has been done, the laboratory can report not only the result but also the percentile corresponding to that result and appropriate to the age and sex of the patient under study. With this information the clinician can know how common or how unusual the test result is. This information obviates the necessity of remembering a large number of complicated relationships. The percentile method is superior to an arbitrary definition of a normal range, such as $\bar{x} \pm 2\delta$, even in those few cases in which a distribution is gaussian, for it indicates for each test result the relationship of that result to the healthy population. The percentile method is also superior to the definition of the normal range as the range of all observed values in a healthy sample population, for this method seriously underestimates any selected segment, e.g., the central 95 per cent, in small samples, and overestimates it in large samples.

The percentile method does not systematically over- or underestimate any selected range, regardless of sample size. If one wishes to cut off the lowest and highest 2.5 per cent, or 5 per cent, one simply orders all values and finds the value that cuts off the desired percentage of observations at either tail of the distribution. The complete percentile range is readily defined. No assumptions are required about distribution shape except that it is continuous. From the size of the healthy population represented in the distribution, the confidence limits of a given percentile may be ascertained, with known probability, by reference to standard tables. The method should particularly appeal to clinicians who utilize local norms, which are often based on small samples.

THE "NORMAL RANGE." From this discussion, it is clear that "normal range" is an arbitrary and potentially misleading term. By whatever method it is defined, the normal range will exclude observations of the parental distribution of healthy subjects and will very likely include some values of other distributions. What is desired by the clinician is an expression of cut-off points at either end of a distribution, such that by far the largest number of values of healthy individuals is included in the central segment, and as few values as possible are included that are part of another distribution, i.e., that the number of false positives and false negatives are both minimized. Ingrained habits, perhaps now indelible, will probably lead us to continue to select the central 95 per cent of the parental distribution as "clinical limits," even though there is no magic in this number. Some clinical investigators have advocated use of the central 90 per cent.

Influence of Age. The distributions of values of many plasma constituents vary with age in the healthy population. For example, plasma cholesterol concentrations, mean and 90 per cent limits, are 180 (120 to 240) mg per deciliter in the "normal" 20- to 29-year age group, and 245 (160 to 330) mg per deciliter in the "normal" 50- to 59-year age group.

Influence of Sex. Distributions in men may differ from those in women. For example, plasma urate concentration values, mean and 90 per cent limits, are 4.9 (2.7 to 7.2) mg per deciliter in men, and 4.0 (2.5 to 6.3) mg per deciliter in premenopausal women. Mean serum calcium values in normal men decline 0.0068 mg per deciliter per year from age 20 to age 80. Those of women show no regression against age. This is an important point in the diagnosis of hyperparathyroidism which is chiefly a disease of the older age group.

BIOLOGICAL RATHER THAN STATISTICAL NORMS. Whether values of serum cholesterol of 325 mg per deciliter in the 50- to 59-year age group are biologically "normal" simply because they fall in the 90 to 95 percentile range could be debated. Epidemiological studies show that the more serum cholesterol values exceed about 180 mg per deciliter the shorter is the life expectancy.

Clinical norms of serum cholesterol concentrations should perhaps be defined in terms of age-related values that are noninjurious, rather than as a 90 percentile range. Such an approach requires a biological rather than statistical definition. Data are not yet available to set reliable limits in this manner for more than a few substances.

One secure example concerns urate concentration values. An electrolyte solution with the sodium concentration of plasma is saturated with urate at 6.4 to 6.8 mg per deciliter. In addition, proteins of plasma bind urate equivalent to about 4 per cent of the amount in solution. Values above 7.0 (perhaps 7.2) mg per deciliter represent supersaturation and are "abnormal" in that they are associated with increased risk of renal stone and clinical gout. The risk factors increase as urate concentration values increase above 7.0 mg per deciliter. The 95 per cent limits of serum urate values in "healthy" male New Zealand Maoris are 4 to 10 mg per deciliter and 10 per cent of adult males develop gout. Surely the central 95 per cent of the distribution of the general male population cannot be considered "normal," even though the reference sample is appropriately selected by the usual criteria.

DISCONTINUOUS DISTRIBUTIONS. Some traits may be distributed bimodally, or trimodally. Such relationships are most likely to emerge from studies of families in which there is a monogenetic disease characterized by a chemical abnormality. For example, measurements of galactose-1-phosphate uridyltransferase activity in the families of patients with transferase deficiency galactosemia are distributed trimodally. The effects of two and of one mutant allele are clearly distinguishable from the normal and from each other. Assay values in the three modes are zero, 7.5 to 13.5 units, and 19.5 to 32 units. The intermediate enzyme assay values are found in subjects who are presumed heterozygotes by pedigree analysis. It is common to hear the term "heterozygote value" applied to an enzyme activity value approximately one half of normal. This practice is justifiable only when assay data are combined with pedigree data, for there may be other reasons for a reduced enzyme assay value that have nothing to do with genetics.

An apparent continuous distribution with marked skewing may at times be dissected into two or even three distribution modes by appropriate clinical and pedigree studies. For example, the distribution of plasma cholesterol concentrations in familial hypercholesterolemia displays marked overlap between subjects who are clinically normal and those who are heterozygotes by pedigree analysis. Similarly, there is considerable overlap between heterozygotes and abnormal homozygotes. Only a complete family pedigree permits adequate definition of the range of values in each distribution mode.

THE PHYSICIAN AND THE LABORATORY TEST RESULT

The tables in Ch. 593 contain values which define the limits of the clinical norms. They represent the best data currently available, but are subject to all the uncertainties discussed above. In some instances more selective data of an age- and sex-matched control population will need to be consulted by the physician.

Clinical judgment rather than exclusive reliance on published normal ranges will always be required. For example, a serum BUN concentration of 22 mg per deciliter is not a normal value for a patient on a rice diet. Also electrolyte test results of sodium 145 mEq per liter, potassium 3.5 mEq per liter, chloride 96 mEq per liter, and CO_2 30 mEq per liter may indicate metabolic alkalosis even though all individual values fall within published normal ranges.

Laboratory tests are critical to the diagnosis of disease and management of patients. They have both great value and inherent imprecision. The doctor must know the limits of reliability and usefulness of each test result in the clinical setting of the individual patient. This is particularly true when all deviant test results have returned to normal but the patient is not improving. It is especially when laboratory data provide little or no help that the patient needs a doctor.

Bryan, D. J., Wearne, J. J., Viau, A., Musser, A. W., Schoonmaker, F. W., and Thiers, R. E.: Profile of admission chemical data by multichannel automation: An evaluative experiment. Clin. Chem., 12:137, 1966.

Elveback, L. R., Guillier, C. L., and Keating, F. R.: Health, normality, and the ghost of Gauss. JAMA, 211:69, 1970.

Keating, F. R., Jones, J. D., Elveback, L. R., and Randall, R. V.: The relation of age and sex to distribution of values in healthy adults of serum calcium, inorganic phosphorus, magnesium, alkaline phosphatase, total proteins, albumin, and blood urea. J. Lab. Clin. Med., 73:825, 1969.

Mainland, D.: Remarks on clinical "norms." Clin. Chem., 17:267, 1971.

593. COMMON LABORATORY VALUES OF CLINICAL IMPORTANCE

HEMATOLOGIC VALUES

"Complete blood count"	*Mean*	*Mean ± 2 standard deviations*
Hematocrit		
Males	46	40–52 ml/dl (%)
Females	41	35–47 ml/dl (%)
Newborn		49–54 ml/dl (%)
Children (varies with age)		35–49 ml/dl (%)
Hemoglobin		
Males	15.5	13.3–17.7 grams/dl
Females	13.7	11.7–15.7 grams/dl
Newborn		16.5–19.5 grams/dl
Children (varies with age)		11.2–16.5 grams/dl
Cell counts		
Erythrocytes: Males	5.1	4.4–5.9 million/cu mm
Females	4.5	3.8–5.2 million/cu mm
Children		4.5–5.1 million/cu mm
Leukocytes		
Total	7250	3500– 11,000/cu mm

Differential	*Percentage*	*Absolute*
Myelocytes	0	0/cu mm
Juvenile neutrophils	3–5	150–400/cu mm
Segmented neutrophils	54–62	3000–5800/cu mm
Lymphocytes	25–33	1500–3000/cu mm
Monocytes	3–7	285–500/cu mm
Eosinophils	1–3	50–250/cu mm
Basophils	0–0.75	15– 50/cu mm

(Infants and children have greater relative numbers of lymphocytes and monocytes)

Platelets	150,000–350,000/cu mm
Reticulocytes: Adults	25,000–75,000/cu mm
	0.5–1.5% of erythrocytes
Newborns	4.6% of erythrocytes
Hemoglobin, special studies	
Hemoglobin, plasma	0–5.0 mg/dl
Hemoglobin, fetal	Less than 1% of total
Hemoglobin A_2	1.5–3.0% of total
Hemoglobin A_{1c}	5% of total
Hemoglobin heat stability	No precipitation
Hemoglobin oxygen affinity (p50)	26–28 mm Hg
Carboxyhemoglobin	Up to 5% of total
Methemoglobin	0.03–0.13 grams/dl
Erythrocytes, special studies	
Corpuscular values of erythrocytes	
(Values are for adults; in children, values vary with age)	
MCH (mean corpuscular hemoglobin)	27–31 pg
MCV (mean corpuscular volume)	80–105 cu micra
MCHC (mean corpuscular hemoglobin concentration)	32–36%
Hemolysis	
Acid hemolysis test (Ham)	No hemolysis
Cold hemolysis test (Donath-Landsteiner)	No hemolysis
Osmotic fragility of erythrocytes	
Immediate	10% lysis in 0.45–0.50% NaCl
	50% lysis in 0.40–0.45% NaCl
	90% lysis in 0.35–0.42% NaCl
After 24 hours incubation	10% lysis in 0.57–0.66% NaCl
	50% lysis in 0.47–0.60% NaCl
	90% lysis in 0.28–0.50% NaCl
Sedimentation rate	
Wintrobe: Males	0–5 mm in 1 hr
Females	0–15 mm in 1 hr
Westergren: Males	0–15 mm in 1 hr
Females	0–20 mm in 1 hr

(May be slightly higher in children and during pregnancy)

HEMATOLOGIC VALUES (*Continued*)

Coagulation studies
    Coagulation screening tests
        Bleeding time
            Ivy   Less than 7 min
            Duke   1–7 min
        Coagulation time (Lee-White) (room temperature)   5–15 min (glass tubes)
                         19–60 min (siliconized tubes)
                         Begins in 30–60 min
        Clot retraction, qualitative   24–38 sec
        Partial thromboplastin time (cephalin activated)   Over 80% consumed in 1 hr
        Prothrombin consumption   12.0–14.0 sec (ratio to control
        Prothrombin time (one stage)   0.90–1.15)
                         10–15 sec
        Thrombin clotting time   Compared to normal control
        Thromboplastin generation test   Ten or fewer additional
        Tourniquet test   petechiae in a 2.5 cm circle
                         after 5 min with cuff at
                         100 mm Hg
        Whole blood clot lysis   No clot lysis in 24 hrs
    Coagulation factors
        Factor I (fibrinogen)   200–400 mg/dl
        Factor II (prothrombin)   60–140% of reference control
        Factor V (accelerator globulin)   60–140% of reference control
        Factor VII-X (proconvertin-Stuart)   70–130% of reference control
        Factor VIII (antihemophilic globulin)   50–200% of reference control
        Factor IX (plasma thromboplastic cofactor)   60–140% of reference control
        Factor X (Stuart factor)   70–130% of reference control
        Factor XI (plasma thromboplastic antecedent)   60–140% of reference control
        Factor XII (Hageman factor)   60–140% of reference control
        Cryofibrinogen   Negative
        Cryoglobulin   Negative
    Fibrinolytic studies
        Euglobulin lysis time   120–240 minutes
        Fibrinogen split products: 16 mg
            Method I   Negative reaction at greater
            latex agglutination (Thrombo-Wellcotest)   than 1:4 dilution
            Method II   Positive reaction at greater
            (staphylococcal clumping)   than 1:16 dilution
        Thrombin time   Less than 5-sec deviation
                         from control

	Average	Range
Bone marrow, differential cell count		
Myeloblasts	2.0%	0.3– 5.0%
Promyelocytes	5.0%	1.0– 8.0%
Myelocytes: Neutrophilic	12.0%	5.0–19.0%
Eosinophilic	1.5%	0.5– 3.0%
Basophilic	0.3%	0.0– 0.5%
Metamyelocytes ("juvenile" forms)	22.0%	13.0–32.0%
Polymorphonuclear neutrophils	20.0%	7.0–30.0%
Polymorphonuclear eosinophils	2.0%	0.5– 4.0%
Polymorphonuclear basophils	0.2%	0.0– 0.7%
Lymphocytes	10.0%	3.0–17.0%
Plasma cells	0.4%	0.0– 2.0%
Monocytes	2.0%	0.5– 5.0%
Reticulum cells	0.2%	0.1– 2.0%
Megakaryocytes	0.1%	0.03– 3.0%
Pronormoblasts	4.0%	1.0– 8.0%
Normoblasts	18.0%	7.0–32.0%

	Mean	Range
Volume		
Blood		
Male	67.8 ml/kg	52–83 ml/kg
Female	62.3 ml/kg	50–75 ml/kg
Plasma		
Male	34.2 ml/kg	25–43 ml/kg
Female	36.6 ml/kg	28–45 ml/kg
Red cell		
Male	28.9 ml/kg	20–36 ml/kg
Female	24.7 ml/kg	19–31 ml/kg

Electrolytes, fluid-acid-base factors, blood gases

Acetoacetate plus acetone	0.3–2.0 mg/dl
"Anion gap" $(Na^+ - [Cl^- + HCO_3^-])$	6– 18 mEq/liter
Base, total, serum	145–160 mEq/liter
Bicarbonate	23– 28 mEq/liter
Carbon dioxide content, serum	24– 30 mEq/liter Infants: 20–28 mEq/liter
Carbon dioxide tension (Pco_2), blood	34– 45 mm Hg
Chloride, serum	96–106 mEq/liter
Lactic acid, blood	6– 16 mg/dl 0.6–1.8 mEq/liter
Magnesium, serum	1.5–2.5 mEq/liter
Osmolality, serum	285–295 mOsm/kg H_2O
Oxygen, blood	
Capacity	16– 24 ml/dl (varies with Hb)
Content: Arterial	15– 23 ml/dl
Venous	10– 16 ml/dl
Saturation: Arterial	94–100% of capacity
Venous	60– 85% of capacity
Tension, Po_2 Arterial	75–100 mm Hg
pH, arterial, blood	7.35–7.45
Potassium, serum	3.5–5.0 mEq/liter
Sodium, serum	136–145 mEq/liter

Other chemical values, serum

Alpha amino nitrogen	4–6 mg/dl
Ammonia nitrogen, blood	75–196 μg/dl
plasma	56–122 μg/dl
Ascorbic acid	See Vitamin C, below
Bilirubin, serum	
Direct	0.1–0.4 mg/dl
Indirect	0.2–0.7 mg/dl
Total	0.3–1.1 mg/dl
Calcium, serum	4.3–5.2 mEq/liter (8.5–10.5 mg/dl) (Slightly higher in children) (Varies with protein concentration)
Calcium, serum ionized	2.1–2.6 mEq/liter (4.25–5.25 mg/dl)
Carotenes, serum	50–300 μg/dl
Cholesterol, serum	
Total	150–250 mg/dl
Esters	68–76% of total cholesterol
Copper, serum	
Male	70–140 μg/dl
Female	85–155 μg/dl
Creatine, serum	0.2–0.8 mg/dl
Creatinine, serum	0.7–1.5 mg/dl
Delta-aminolevulinic acid	Less than 200 μg/dl
Fatty acids, total, serum	190–420 mg/dl
Ferritin	20–700 ng/ml
Folic acid, serum	7–16 ng/ml

Glucose (fasting)

Blood, true (hexokinase)	60–100 mg/dl
Neocuproine	70–110 mg/dl
Plasma or serum (hexokinase)	70–115 mg/dl

Iron

Iron, serum	75–175 μg/dl
Iron binding capacity, total serum	250–410 μg/dl
% saturation	20–55%
Lipids, total, serum	450–850 mg/dl
Nitrogen, nonprotein, serum	15–35 mg/dl
Osmolality, serum	285–295 mOsm/kg serum water
Phenylalanine, serum	Less than 3 mg/dl
Phosphate, inorganic, serum (expressed as phosphorus)	3.0–4.5 mg/dl (Children: 4.0–7.0 mg/dl)
Phospholipids, serum (expressed as lipid phosphorus)	6–12 mg/dl

Proteins, plasma

Albumin and globulins	
Total	6.0–8.0 grams/dl
Albumin	3.5–5.5 grams/dl
Globulin	2.5–3.5 grams/dl
Electrophoresis	
Albumin	3.5–5.5 grams/dl 52–68% of total
Globulin	
Alpha$_1$	0.2–0.4 grams/dl 2–5% of total
Alpha$_2$	0.5–0.9 grams/dl 7–14% of total
Beta	0.6–1.1 grams/dl 9–15% of total
Gamma	0.7–1.7 grams/dl 11–21% of total
Alpha-1-antitrypsin	200–400 mg/dl
Ceruloplasmin, serum	23–44 mg/dl
Fibrinogen, plasma	200–400 mg/dl
Haptoglobin, serum	40–170 mg/dl
Pyruvic acid, plasma	0.4–0.9 mg/dl 0.5–1.2 mEq/liter
Sulfates, inorganic, serum (expressed as sulfur)	0.8–1.2 mg/dl
Triglycerides, serum	0–150 mg/dl
Urea, blood	21–43 mg/dl
plasma or serum	24–49 mg/dl
Urea nitrogen, blood (BUN)	10–20 mg/dl
plasma or serum	11–23 mg/dl
Uric acid, serum	
Male	2.5–7.7 mg/dl
Female	2.1–6.6 mg/dl
Vitamin A, serum	20–80 μg/dl
Vitamin B, serum	200–800 pg/ml
Vitamin C, blood	0.4–1.5 mg/dl

ENZYME ASSAYS

Serums

Aldolase, serum	0.8–3.0 milliunits/ml (IU) (30°) (Sibley-Lehninger)
Amylase, serum	80–160 Somogyi units/dl
Cholinesterase, serum	0.5–1.3 pH units/hr
Creatine phosphokinase, serum	
Male	0–50 milliunits/ml (IU) (30°)
Female	0–30 milliunits/ml (IU) (30°) (Oliver-Rosalki)
Hydroxybutyric dehydrogenase, serum	0–180 milliunits/ml (IU) (30°) (Rosalki-Wilkinson) 114–290 units/ml (Wroblewski)
Lactic dehydrogenase, serum	0–300 milliunits/ml (IU) (30°) (Wroblewski modified) 150–450 units/ml (Wroblewski) 80–120 units/ml (Wacker)

Lipase, serum	0–1.5 units (Cherry-Crandall)
5'-Nucleotidase	0.3–2.6 units/dl (Bodansky) 1.6–17 milliunits/ml (IU) (Wootton)
Phosphatase, acid, serum	1.0–5.0 units (King-Armstrong) 0.5–2.0 units (Bodansky) 0.5–2.0 units (Gutman) 0.0–1.1 units (Shinowara) 0.1–0.63 unit (Bessey-Lowry)
Phosphatase, alkaline, serum	5.0–13.0 units (King-Armstrong) 2.0–4.5 units (Bodansky) 3.0–10.0 units (Gutman) 2.2–8.6 units (Shinowara) 0.8–2.3 units (Bessey-Lowry) 30–85 milliunits/ml (IU) (Values are higher in children)

ENZYME ASSAYS (*Continued*)

Transaminase, serum	
Glutamic oxalacetic transaminase (SGOT) (Aspartate aminotransferase)	0–19 milliunits/ml (IU) (30°) (Karmen modified) 15–40 units/ml (Karmen) 18–40 units/ml (Reitman-Frankel)
Glutamic pyruvic transaminase (Alanine aminotransferase)	0–17 milliunits/ml (IU) (30°) (Karmen modified) 6–35 units/ml (Karmen) 5–35 units/ml (Reitman-Frankel)
Leukocyte	
Alkaline phosphatase	Total score 14–100% positive
Erythrocyte	
Cholinesterase	5.5–1.0 pH units/hr
Glucose-6-phosphate dehydrogenase	12.1±2.1 IU/gram Hb
Glutathione reductase	10.4±1.5 IU/gram Hb
6-Phosphogluconate dehydrogenase	8.8±0.8 IU/gram Hb
Pyruvate kinase	15.0±2.0 IU/gram Hb

NORMAL URINE VALUES

Acetone and acetoacetate	0
Alpha amino nitrogen	50–200 mg/24 hrs (not over 1.5% of total nitrogen)
Amino acids	200–400 mg/24 hrs
Ammonia nitrogen	20–70 mEq/24 hrs
Amylase	35–260 Somogyi units/hr
Bence Jones protein	Negative
Bilirubin (bile)	Negative
Calcium	
Low Ca diet (Bauer-Aub)	Less than 150 mg/24 hrs
Usual diet	Less than 250 mg/24 hrs
Chloride	110–250 mEq/24 hrs (varies with intake)
Copper	0–30 μg/24 hrs
Creatine	
Male	0–40 mg/24 hrs
Female	0–100 mg/24 hrs (Higher in children and during pregnancy)
Creatinine	15–25 mg/kg of body weight/24 hrs
Cystine or cysteine, qualitative	Negative
Delta-aminolevulinic acid	1.3–7.0 mg/24 hrs
Glucose (reducing substances)	0
Hemoglobin and myoglobin	Negative
Homogentisic acid, qualitative	Negative
Iron	500 mg/24 hrs
Osmolality	38–1400 mOsm/kg water
Oxalate	12–40 mg/24 hrs
pH	4.6–8.0, average 6.0 (depends on diet)
Phenylpyruvic acid, qualitative	Negative
Phosphorus	0.9–1.3 grams/24 hrs (varies with intake)
Porphobilinogen	
Qualitative	Negative
Quantitative	Less than 2.0 mg/24 hrs
Porphyrins	
Coproporphyrin	50–250 μg/24 hrs
Uroporphyrin	10–30 μg/24 hrs
Potassium	25–100 mEq/24 hrs (varies with intake)

NORMAL URINE VALUES (*Continued*)

Protein
    Qualitative   0

    Quantitative — 10–150 mg/24 hrs

Sodium — 130–260 mEq/24 hrs (varies with intake)

Solids, total — 30–70 grams/liter, average 50 grams/liter (to estimate total solids per liter, multiply last two figures of specific gravity by 2.66, Long's coefficient)

Specific gravity — 1.003–1.030

Titratable acidity — 20–40 mEq/24 hrs

Uric acid — 250–800 mg/24 hrs (varies with purine intake)

Urobilinogen — Up to 1.0 Ehrlich unit/2 hrs (1–3 P.M.) 0–4.0 mg/24 hrs

NORMAL VALUES FOR CEREBROSPINAL FLUID

Bilirubin — 0

Cells — Fewer than 5 cu mm, all mononuclear

Chloride — 120–130 mEq/liter (20 mEq/liter higher than serum)

Colloidal gold test — Not more than 1 in any tube

Glucose — 50–75 mg/dl (20 mg/dl less than blood)

Pressure — 70–180 mm water

Protein, total (lumbar) — 15–45 mg/dl
    Albumin — 52%
    Alpha$_1$ globulin — 5%
    Alpha$_2$ globulin — 14%
    Beta globulin — 10%
    Gamma globulin — 19% (IgG 2.0–5.9 mg/dl)

Protein, total (cisternal) — 15–25 mg/dl

Protein, total (ventricular) — 5–15 mg/dl

HORMONE AND HORMONE PRODUCTS

	Plasma	*Urine*
Steroids		
Aldosterone	210 mEq sodium diet:	
	Supine (fasting, at rest)	
	48±29 pg/ml	3–20 µg/24 hrs
	Upright (2 hr)	
	65±23 pg/ml	
	110 mEq sodium diet:	
	Supine (fasting, at rest)	
	107±45 pg/ml	
	Upright (2 hr)	
	239±123 pg/ml	
	10 mEq sodium diet:	
	Supine (fasting, at rest)	
	175±75 pg/ml	
	Upright (2 hr)	
	532±228 pg/ml	

HORMONE AND HORMONE PRODUCTS (*Continued*)

Cortisol, plasma
  Cortisol
      8 A.M. (Fasting)
        5–25 μg/dl   20–70 μg/24 hrs
      8 P.M. (at rest)
        Below 10 μg/dl
      4 hr ACTH test (20 U ACTH,
        IV per 4 hrs)
        30–45 μg/dl
      Overnight suppression test
        (8 A.M. sample after
        dexamethasone at midnight)
        Below 5 μg/dl

11-Deoxycortisol
      Basal
        Below 1 μg/dl
      After metyrapone
        Above 10 μg/dl

Estrogens	*Male*	*Female*
Estrone	3–8 μg/24 hrs	4–31 μg/24 hrs
Estradiol	0–6 μg/24 hrs	0–14 μg/24 hrs
Estriol	1–11 μg/24 hrs	0–72 μg/24 hrs
Total	4–25 μg/24 hrs	5–100 μg/24 hrs
		(Markedly high during pregnancy)

Etiocholanolone   Below 1.2 μg/dl

17-Hydroxycorticosteroids
    Male   2–12 mg/24 hrs (3–7 mg/gram creatinine)
    Female   2–8 mg/24 hrs (varies with method used)
17-Ketogenic steroids   5–15 mg/24 hrs
17-Ketosteroids

Age	Males (mg/24 hrs)	Females (mg/24 hrs)
10	1–4	1–4
20	6–21	4–16
30	8–26	4–14
50	5–18	3–9
70	2–10	1–7

Pregnanediol (females)   Below 1 mg/24 hrs (follicular)
      5–12 mg/24 hrs (luteal)

Pregnanetriol   Less than 2.5 mg/24 hrs in adults

Testosterone
      Adult male
        300–1100 ng/dl
      Adolescent male
        Over 100 ng/dl
      Female
        25–90 ng/dl

Unbound testosterone
      Adult male
        3.06–24.0 ng/dl
      Adult female
        0.09–1.28 ng/dl

Polypeptide hormones
  Adrenocorticotropin (ACTH)   15–70 pg/ml
  Calcitonin   Undetectable in normals; >100
      pg/ml in medullary carcinoma
  Follicle-stimulating hormone (FSH)   6–18 mIU/ml (males)
      5–50 mIU/ml (females)
      >50 mIU/ml (postmenopausal)
  Gastrin, serum   30–200 pg/ml
  Gonadotropin, chorionic   0
  Gonadotropins, pituitary   Less than 250 mg/24 hrs
      5–10 rat units/24 hrs
      10–50 mouse units/24 hrs

  Growth hormone
      Fasting, at rest
        Below 5 ng/ml
      After exercise
        Children: Over 10 ng/ml
      After glucose load
        Adult male: Below 5 ng/ml
        Adult female: Below 10 ng/ml

  Insulin
      Fasting
        Below 20 mU/ml
      Hypoglycemia, blood sugar <50 mg/dl
        Below 5 mU/ml

HORMONE AND HORMONE PRODUCTS (*Continued*)

Luteinizing hormone	6–18 mIU/ml (male)
	5–22 mIU/ml (female)
	30–250 mIU/ml (female, mid-cycle)
Parathyroid hormone	150–300 pg/ml
Renin (angiotensin-I RIA)	150–300 pg/ml
Peripheral plasma	Normal diet:
	Supine: 0.3–1.9 ng/ml/hr
	Upright: 0.2–3.6 ng/ml/hr
	Low sodium diet:
	Supine: 0.9–4.5 ng/ml/hr
	Upright: 4.1–9.1 ng/ml/hr
	Diuretics + low sodium diet:
	6.3–13.7 ng/ml/hr
Renal vein concentration	Normal ratio (high: low):
	less than 1.5
Thyroid-stimulating hormone (TSH)	Up to 10 μU/ml

Miscellaneous
   Catecholamines

Epinephrine	Less than 20 μg/24 hrs
Norepinephrine	Less than 100 μg/24 hrs
Vanillylmandelic acid (VMA)	1–8 mg/24 hrs

Serotonin, platelet suspension	0.1–0.3 μg/ml blood
serum	0.10–0.32 μg/ml
5-Hydroxyindoleacetic acid (5-HIAA)	
Qualitative	Negative
Quantitative	1.7–8.0 mg/24 hrs

NORMAL VALUES FOR SEROLOGIC PROCEDURES

Alpha-fetoglobulin	Abnormal if present
Anti-DNA antibodies, plasma	Less than 20% DNA bound (Farr)
	Not more than 5 μg DNA bound/ml plasma (Ginsberg/Keiser)
	Not more than 8 μg DNA bound/ml plasma (Kredich)
Anti-hyaluronidase	Less than 1:200; significant if rising titer can be demonstrated at weekly intervals
Antimitochondrial antibodies, serum	Negative at 1:5 dilution
Antinuclear antibodies (ANA), serum	Negative at 1:32 dilution of serum; if positive, titer and fluorescent pattern (peripheral, shaggy, or ring; homogeneous; speckled; nucleolar) are important
Anti-streptolysin O titer	Less than 166 Todd U/ml; single test usually has little significance; rise in titer or persistently elevated titer is significant
Bacterial agglutinins	Significant only if rise in titer is demonstrated or if antibodies are absent
Bence Jones protein (urine)	Abnormal if present
Carcinoembryonic antigen (CEA)	Less than 2.5 ng/dl

Complement
   Whole hemolytic activity, serum   37– 55 CH50 units/ml

   Classic pathway components

C1q	100– 200 μg/ml
C1r	100 μg/ml
C1s (C1 esterase)	110– 120 μg/ml
C2	25– 30 μg/ml
C3 (β-1-C globulin) Males	880–2520 μg/ml
Females	880–2060 μg/ml
C4 (β-1-E globulin)	120– 750 μg/ml
C5 (β-1-F globulin)	75– 80 μg/ml
C6	60– 75 μg/ml
C7	55– 75 μg/ml
C8	80 μg/ml
C9	1– 230 μg/ml

   Alternative pathway components

Properdin	25 μg/ml
Properdin factor B	200– 225 μg/ml

   Inhibitors

C1 esterase inhibitor (C1 inactivator)	180 μg/ml
C3b inactivator (KAF)	25 μg/ml

NORMAL VALUES FOR SEROLOGIC PROCEDURES (*Continued*)

Complement fixation tests	Titers of 1:8 or less are usually not significant. Paired sera showing rise in titer of more than two tubes are usually considered significant.
C reactive protein (CRP)	Negative
Heterophile titer	Low titers may be present normally, but these antibodies are absorbed by Forssman antigen (guinea pig kidney). In infectious mononucleosis an elevated heterophile titer is present. The titer is only minimally reduced after incubation with guinea pig kidney but is significantly reduced after incubation with beef red cell stroma.

Immunoglobulins, serum, adults
    (Values vary with age, sex and
    race — see Buckley and Dorsey)   (95% range)

IgG	640–1430 mg/dl (70–176 IU/ml)
IgA	30– 300 mg/dl (16–164 IU/ml)
IgM	20– 140 mg/dl (19–134 IU/ml)
IgD	Less than 20 mg/dl
IgE	6– 780 ng/ml

Lupus erythematosus (LE) cell test	Abnormal if LE cells present	
Proteus OX-19 agglutinins	1:80	Negative
	1:160	Doubtful
	1:320	Positive
Rheumatoid factor test (Latex)	1:40	Negative
	1:80	Weakly positive
	1:160	Positive
Sensitized sheep cell agglutination (SCAT) (Rose-Waaler test)	1:4	Negative
	1:8	Doubtful
	1:16	Positive
Tularemia agglutinins	1:80	Negative
	1:160	Doubtful
	1:320	Positive

NORMAL VALUES FOR GASTRIC ANALYSIS

Basal gastric secretion (one hour)

	Concentration Mean ± 1 S.D.	Output Mean ± 1 S.D.
Male	25.8 ± 1.8 mEq/liter	2.57 ± 0.16 mEq/liter
Female	20.3 ± 3.0 mEq/liter	1.61 ± 0.18 mEq/liter

After histamine stimulation

Normal	Mean output = 11.8 mEq/hr
Duodenal ulcer	Mean output = 15.2 mEq/hr

After maximal histamine stimulation

Normal	Mean output 22.6 mEq/hr
Duodenal ulcer	Mean output 44.6 mEq/hr

Diagnex blue (Squibb):	Anacidity	0–0.3 mg in 2 hrs
	Doubtful	0.3–0.6 mg in 2 hrs
	Normal	Greater than 0.6 mg in 2 hrs

Volume, fasting stomach content	50–100 ml
Emptying time	3–6 hrs
Color	Opalescent or colorless
Specific gravity	1.006–1.009
pH (adults)	0.9–1.5

NORMAL VALUES FOR DUODENAL DRAINAGE

pH	5.5–7.5
Amylase	Over 1200 U per total sample
Trypsin	Values from 35 to 160 per cent "normal"
Viscosity	3 min or less

GASTROINTESTINAL ABSORPTION TESTS

d-Xylose absorption test	After an 8-hour fast, 25 grams in 500 ml water is given by mouth. Nothing further by mouth is given until the test has been completed. All urine voided during the following 5 hours is pooled. Normal value is 5–8 gm excreted over a 5-hr period.
Schilling test (oral administration of ^{60}Co-labeled vitamin B_{12})	8.5–28% excreted in urine/24 hrs

NORMAL VALUES FOR FECES

Bulk	100–200 grams/24 hrs
Dry matter	32–32 grams/24 hrs
Fat, total	Less than 6.0 grams/24 hrs
Nitrogen, total	Less than 2.0 grams/24 hrs
Urobilinogen	40–280 mg/24 hrs
Water	Approximately 65%

LIVER FUNCTION TESTS

Cardiogreen	Less than 5% remaining in serum 45 minutes after injection of 5 mg/kg of body weight
Cephalin cholesterol flocculation	0–1+ in 24 hrs, 2+ or less in 48 hrs
Galactose tolerance	Excretion of not more than 3.0 grams of galactose in the urine 5 hours after ingestion of 40 grams of galactose
Glycogen storage	Increase of blood glucose 45 mg/dl over fasting level 45 minutes after subcutaneous injection of 0.01 mg/kg body weight of epinephrine
Hippuric acid	Excretion of 3.0–3.5 grams hippuric acid in urine within 4 hours after ingestion of 6.0 grams of sodium benzoate

or

Excretion of 0.7 gram of hippuric acid in urine within 1 hour after intravenous injection of 1.77 grams of sodium benzoate

Thymol turbidity	0–5 units
Zinc turbidity	2–12 units

PANCREATIC (ISLET) FUNCTION TESTS

Glucose tolerance tests	Patient should be on a diet containing 300 grams of carbohydrate per day for 3 days prior to test
Oral	After ingestion of 100 grams of glucose or 1.75 grams of glucose/kg body weight, blood glucose is not more than 160 mg/dl after 60 minutes, 140 mg/dl after 90 minutes, and 120 mg/dl after 120 minutes. Values are for blood; serum measurements are approximately 15% higher.
Intravenous	Blood glucose does not exceed 200 mg/dl infusion of 0.5 gram of glucose/kg body weight over 30 minutes. Glucose concentration falls below initial level at 2 hours and returns to preinfusion levels in 3 or 4 hours. Values are for blood; serum measurements are approximately 15% higher.
Cortisone-glucose tolerance test	The patient should be on a diet containing 300 grams of carbohydrate per day for 3 days prior to test. At 8½ and again 2 hours prior to glucose load, patient is given cortisone acetate by mouth (50 mg if patient's ideal weight is less than 160 lb, 62.5 mg if ideal weight is greater than 160 lb). An oral dose of glucose, 1.75 grams/kg body weight, is given and blood samples are taken at 0, 30, 60, 90, and 120 minutes. Test result is considered positive if true blood glucose exceeds 160 mg/dl at 60 minutes, 140 mg/dl at 90 minutes, and 120 mg/dl at 120 minutes. Values are for blood; serum measurements are approximately 15% higher.

RENAL FUNCTION TESTS

Clearance tests (corrected to 1.73 square meters of body surface area)
    Glomerular filtration rate (GFR)
        Inulin clearance,
        mannitol clearance, or
        endogenous creatinine clearance

	Males	110–150 ml/min
	Females	105–132 ml/min

    Renal plasma flow (RPF)
        p-Aminohippurate (PAH) or Diodrast

	Males	560–830 ml/min
	Females	490–700 ml/min

    Filtration fraction (FI)

$$FF = \frac{GFR}{RPF}$$

	Males	17–21%
	Females	17–23%

Urea clearance (C_u)

Standard	40–65 ml/min
Maximal	60–100 ml/min

Concentration and dilution

Specific gravity >1.025 on dry day
Specific gravity <1.003 on water day

Maximal Diodrast excretory capacity T_{MD}

Males	43–59 mg/min
Females	33–51 mg/min

Maximal glucose reabsorptive capacity T_{MG}

Males	300–450 mg/min
Females	250–350 mg/min

Maximal PAH exretory capacity $T_{M_{PAH}}$ 80–90 mg/min

Phenolsulfonphthalein excretion (PSP)
    (After injection of 1 ml PSP intravenously)

25% or more in 15 min
40% or more in 30 min
55% or more in 2 hrs

NORMAL VALUES FOR SEMEN

Volume	2–5 ml, usually 3–4 ml
Liquefaction	Complete in 15 min
pH	7.2–8.0; average 7.8
Leukocytes	Occasional or absent
Count	60–150 million/ml
	Below 60 million/ml is abnormal
Motility	80% or more motile
Morphology	80–90% normal forms

NORMAL SYNOVIAL FLUID

	Mean	*Range*
Volume (knee joint)	1.1 ml	0.13–4.0 ml
pH		7.3–7.6
Relative viscosity, 37°		High
Cells	63/cu mm	13–180/cu mm
Differential		
Polymorphonuclear cells	6.5%	0–25%
Monocytes	47.9%	0–71%
Lymphocytes	24.6%	0–78%
Clasmatocytes	10.1%	0–26%
Unclassified	4.9%	0–21%
Synovial cells	4.3%	0–12%
Complement activity, whole hemolytic		12–22 CH50 units/ml
Protein	1.7 grams/dl	0.45–2.7 grams/dl
Albumin	63%	
α-1 globulin	7%	
α-2 globulin	7%	
β-globulin	9%	
γ-globulin	14%	
Fibrinogen	0	
Crystals	0	
Fibrin dot	Absent	
Mucin dot	Type 1 or 2	Grades as: Type 1-tight clump Type 2-soft clump Type 3-soft clump that breaks up Type 4-cloudy, no clump

Hyaluronic acid	2.45–3.97 grams/liter
Glucose, uric acid	Approximately the same as in serum
Sodium, potassium, calcium concentrations	Slightly lower than serum, as determined by Donnan equilibrium

THYROID FUNCTION TESTS

Protein bound iodine (PBI)	3.5–8.0 μg/dl
Butanol extractable iodine (BEI)	3.2–6.4 μg/dl
Thyroxine, serum	
Total T_4	4.0–11.0 μg/dl
T_4-iodine	2.6–7.2 μg/dl
Free T_4	0.8–2.4 ng/dl
Free thyroxine index (FT$_4$I)	1 – 4 ng/dl
Thyroxine-binding globulin, serum	10–26 μg T_4/dl
Triiodothyronine, serum	70–190 ng/dl
T_3 uptake	
RBC	11–19%
Resin (T$_3$RU)	25–35%
Thyroid-stimulating hormone (TSH)	0–10 milliunits/ml
Radioactive iodine (^{131}I) uptake (RAI)	10–25% administered dose in 24 hrs. in U.S. with dietary iodine intake of 400–600 μg/day
Radioactive iodine (^{131}I) excretion	30–70% of administered dose in 24 hrs
Radioactive iodine, protein bound (PB^{131}I)	Less than 0.3% of administered dose per liter of plasma at 72 hrs

DRUGS AND TOXIC SUBSTANCES

	Therapeutic or Usual Range	Toxic or Excessive Levels
Amitriptyline	180 ng/ml	
Arsenic, blood	Less than 6 μg/dl	
Arsenic, urine	Less than 25 μg/24 hrs	More than 100 μg/24 hrs
Barbiturates, serum		
Phenobarbitol	1.5–4.0 mg/dl	Above 5.5 mg/dl; Coma: 8–12 mg/dl
"Short-acting"		Coma: 2.5–3.5 mg/dl
Bromide, serum		Above 100 mg/dl (12.5 mEq/liter)
Cadmium, blood	Less than 10 ng/ml	
Cadmium, urine	Less than 15 ng/24 hrs	
Carbamazepine (Tegretol), serum	2–10 μg/ml	
Carbon monoxide, blood	Less than 3% of Hgb (heavy smokers up to 15%)	Over 20% of Hgb
Chlordiazepoxide (Librium), serum	Up to 1 μg/ml	Over 5 μg/ml
Chromium, serum	Less than 25 ng/ml	
Chromium, urine	Less than 8 μg/24 hrs	
Cobalt, serum	0.4–1.0 μg/dl	
Desipramine, serum	120 ng/ml	
Diazepam (Valium), serum	1 μg/ml	Over 1 μg/ml
Digoxin, serum	0.5–1.5 ng/ml	Over 2 ng/ml
Digitoxin, serum	5–40 ng/ml	
Diphenylhydantoin (Dilantin), serum	10–20 μg/ml	
Doxepin, serum	120 ng/ml	
Ethanol, blood		Marked intoxication, 0.3–0.4% Stupor, 0.4–0.5% Coma, above 0.5%
Ethchlorvynol (Placidyl), serum	10–20 μg/ml	Over 25 μg/ml
Ethosuximide (Zarontin), serum	40–80 μg/ml	
Glutethimide (Doriden), serum	Less than 7 μ/ml	Over 7 μg/ml
Ipramine, serum	180 ng/ml	
Lead, blood	Less than 40 μg/dl	
Lead, urine	Less than 80 μg/24 hrs	More than 100–125 μg/24 hrs
Lithium, serum	0.6–1.2 mEq/liter	Over 1.5 mEq/liter
Mercury, blood	Less than 50 μg/dl	
Mercury, urine	Less than 20 μg/24 hrs	
Methaqualone (Parest), serum	20–30 μg/ml	
Methyprylon (Noludar), serum	Up to 10 μg/ml	Over 30 μg/ml
Nortriptyline, serum	5–150 ng/ml	
Phenothiazines, serum		
Compazine	Less than 0.5 μg/ml	More than 1 μg/ml
Mellaril	1.0–1.5 μg/ml	More than 10 μg/ml
Stelazine	Less than 0.5 μg/ml	More than 1 μg/ml
Thorazine	Less than 0.5 μg/ml	More than 1 μg/ml
Primidone (Mysoline), serum	7–11 μg/ml	
Procainamide (Pronestyl), serum	4–8 μg/ml	Over 12 μg/ml
Quinidine, plasma	1.5–3.0 μg/ml	About 10 μg/ml
Salicylate, serum	15–25 mg/dl (adult) 20–30 mg/dl (children)	Tinnitus, 19–49 mg/dl Hyperventilation, over 35 mg/dl Death, 45–75 mg/dl
Sulfonamides, blood	100–200 μg/ml	
Theophylline, serum	10–20 μg/ml	

Buckley, C. E., and Dorsey, F. C.: Serum immunoglobulin levels throughout the life-span of healthy man. Ann. Intern. Med., 75:673, 1971.

Halsted, J. A.: The Laboratory in Clinical Medicine. Philadelphia, W. B. Saunders Company, 1976.

Lynch, M. J., Raphael, S. S., Mellor, L. D., Spare, P. D., and Inwood, M. J. H.: Medical Laboratory Technology and Clinical Pathology. 2nd ed. Philadelphia, W. B. Saunders Company, 1969.

Müller-Eberhard, H. J.: Complement. Ann. Rev. Biochem., 44:697, 1975.

Normal reference laboratory values. N. Engl. J. Med., 298:34, 1978.

Owen, C. A., Jr.: Mayo Medical Laboratories Handbook. Rochester, Minn., Mayo Medical Laboratories, 1977.

Williams, W. J., Beutler, E., Erslev, A. J., and Rundles, R. W.: Hematology. 2nd ed. New York, McGraw-Hill Book Company, 1977.

Note: In this index the expression "vs." has been used to denote "differential diagnosis." Thus "Amebiasis, vs. malaria" is the equivalent of "Amebiasis, differential diagnosis from malaria." **Boldface entries and folios** in the index indicate main discussions in the text. *Italic folios* indicate illustrations and tables.

Abdomen
actinomycosis of, 474
acute, 1578–1582
distention of, in pneumococcal
pneumonia, 352, 356
injury to, in electric injury, 93
pyogenic infections of, enteric
bacteria in, 454
Abdominal angina, 1587, 1588
Abdominal aorta
aneurysms of, 1293, 1590
ultrasonography in, *1466*
coarctation of, 1290
Abdominal pain, 1476–1477
referred, 1477
Abdominal ultrasonography, 1465–1466,
1465, 1466
Abducens nerve, disorders of, 899
Abetalipoproteinemia, *42,* 1539, **2008**
Abiotrophies, 764
Abortion
physician counseling in, 690
septic, hypofibrinogenemia in, 1894
Abscess(es)
anorectal, 1617
appendiceal, vs. regional enteritis,
1565
at subcutaneous injection sites,
enteric bacteria causing, 455
brain, 804–807
amebic, 592
cerebrospinal fluid findings in, *803,*
806, 807
enteric bacteria causing, 454
epilepsy associated with, 852
in nocardiosis, 475
presenting as "acute meningitis,"
806
vs. brain tumor, 868, 869
vs. cerebral infarction, 790
vs. herpes simplex encephalitis, 823
vs. viral meningitis or encephalitis,
820
Brodie's, 2260
Candida, 548
cerebellar, 806
cerebral epidural, 808
cerebrospinal fluid findings in,
803
frontal lobe, 806
"gas," 434
hepatic, acute, 1656–1657
amebic, 590, 591, 592, 593
computerized tomography in, *1467*

Abscess(es) (*Continued*)
hepatic, pyogenic, vs. hepatic
amebiasis, 592
vs. pneumococcal pneumonia, 354
in infective endocarditis, 388, 389
in staphylococcal infection, 397
injection, "atypical" mycobacteria
causing, 500
ischiorectal fossa, 1617
lung, 979–982
amebic, 591, 980, 981
cavitary, vs. pulmonary
tuberculosis, 486
vs. pulmonary paragonimiasis, 620
parietal lobe, 806
pelvic, tuberculous, 492
pelvirectal, 1617
perianal, 1617
perinephric, 1410
perirectal, enteric bacteria causing,
455
tuberculous, 492
peritonsillar, in streptococcal
tonsillitis, 373
skin, in heroin addiction, 696
spinal epidural, 810, 811
cerebrospinal fluid findings in, *803*
primary, 404
vs. transverse myelitis, 812
subdiaphragmatic, pleural effusion
in, 1018
vs. pneumococcal pneumonia, 354
submucous, 1617
subphrenic, 1594
radionuclide imaging in, *1469*
vs. hepatic amebiasis, 592
temporal lobe, 806
"Welch," 434
Absence attack, 854
Absolute polycythemia, 1793–1800
Absorption
amino acid, 1525
calcium, 1526, 2227
carbohydrate, 1525
abnormal, manifestations of,
1529
disorders of, 1523–1550. See also
Malabsorption syndrome.
drug, rate of, changes in, 2336, 2337
electrolyte, 1525
diminished, in malabsorption
syndrome, 1529
fat, 1524
folic acid, 1525

Absorption (*Continued*)
gastrointestinal, tests for, 2353
iron, 1526, 1744, *1745*
impaired, in malabsorption
syndrome, 1529
normal, mechanism of, 1523–1526
phosphate, 2229
protein, 1525
tests for, 2353
vitamin B_{12}, 1525
tests of, in malabsorption
syndrome, 1532
water, 1525
diminished, in malabsorption
syndrome, 1529
Abstinence syndrome
in alcohol abuse, 668, 709, 710
in central nervous system depressant
abuse, 699, 700
in opiate abuse, 695, 696
Acalculia, 658
Acalculous cholecystitis, 1626
Acanthamoeba castellani, 603
Acanthamoeba polyphaga, 604
Acanthocytosis, 1539. See also
Abetalipoproteinemia.
Acanthosis nigricans, 2285, *2285, 2296,*
2299
Acariasis, sarcoptic, 110–111
Acatalasia, *43,* 2057
Accelerated hypertension, 1204
prognosis in, 1217
retinopathy in, 1205
Accelerated idioventricular rhythms,
1254, *1254*
Accidental poisoning, common, 71–76
Accommodation, visual, anomalies of,
headache from, 733
Acebutolol, in hypertension of chronic
renal failure, 1362
Acervuli, 2112
Acetaminophen
in migraine syndrome, 732
in pain, 723, 724, *724*
in pain of classic hemophilia, 1886
liver injury caused by, 1658
Acetazolamide
in acute mountain sickness, 101
in epilepsy, *859,* 860
in familial periodic paralysis, 922
in heart failure, *1104,* 1105
metabolic acidosis from, 1962
Acetohexamide, in diabetes mellitus,
1986, *1986*

Acetophenetidin, in pain, *724*
Acetylcholine, 751
   in regulation of gastric secretion,
      1505, 1506
   in regulation of pepsin secretion, 1506
Acetylcholine receptor, antibodies to, in
   myasthenia gravis, 925, 927
Acetylsalicylic acid. See *Aspirin.*
Acetylstrophanthidin, as diagnostic test
   for adequacy of digitalization, 1097
Achalasia, 1486–1488, *1487*
   cricopharyngeal, 1483
   esophageal carcinoma and, 1597, 1598
Acholuric jaundice, 1638
Achondroplasia, 2264
Acid(s). See names of specific acids.
Acid perfusion test, in esophagitis, 1484
Acid phosphatase, prostatic, as tumor
   marker, 1913
Acid-base balance
   disorders of, 1950, **1960–1969**
      in shock, 1046
      respiratory, in cancer patient, 1905
   kidney in, 1322–1323
Acidemia
   alpha-methyl-beta-hydroxybutyric, *41*
   isovaleric, *41*
   pipecolic, *2018*
Acidophilic adenoma with acromegaly,
   2097, 2098
Acidosis
   hyperchloremic, 1962
      in chronic renal failure, 1354
      in total parenteral nutrition, 1708
   hypokalemic, in cancer patient, 1904
      in chronic renal failure, 1357, 1358
   in shock, 1110
      correction of, 1118
   lactic, in louse-borne relapsing fever,
      528
      metabolic acidosis from, 1962, 1964
   metabolic, 1322, **1961–1965**
      causes of, *1961*
      complicating chronic respiratory
         acidosis, 1968, *1968*
      in acute renal failure, 1372
      in cancer patient, 1904
      in hyperparathyroidism, 2216
      in shock, 1046
   renal, 1962, 1964, 1965
      in interstitial nephritis, 1417, 1418
   renal tubular, 43, **1441–1442**
      rickets and osteomalacia in, 2252
   respiratory, 1961, **1967–1969**
      chronic, acid-base disturbances
         complicating, 1967, *1968*
      plasma composition in, *1967*
Aciduria
   alpha-aminoadipic, *2018*
   beta-hydroxyisovaleric, *41*
   L-glyceric, 2001
   glycolic, 2001
   methylmalonic, homocystinuria with,
      2017
      prevention and management of, 55
      vitamin B₁₂ responsive, *41*
      vitamin B₁₂ unresponsive, *41*
   orotic, *42,* 2044
      prevention and management of, 55
   proglutamic, *2019*
   xanthurenic, *42*
Acinar cell carcinoma of pancreas, vs.
   Weber-Christian disease, 222

Acne rosacea, 2279
Acne vulgaris, 2278–2279
   pustular, 400
Acoustic neuroma, 868
   hearing loss from, 736
Acral lentiginous melanoma, 2311
Acrocentric chromosomes, 50, *50*
Acrocyanosis, 1307
   vs. ergotism and methysergide
      toxicity, 1308
   vs. Raynaud's disease and
      phenomenon, 1306
Acrodermatitis enteropathica, 2287, *2298*
Acrodynia, 80
Acromegaly, 2105–2108, *2107*
   acidophilic adenoma with, 2097, 2098
   arthritis in, 199, 2105
   diabetes mellitus in, 1982, 2106
   growth hormone radioimmunoassay
      in, 2091, 2092
   neuropathy of, 909
   osteoporosis in, 2244
   prolactin levels in, 2092
   roentgenography in, 2096, *2096, 2097*
Acrosclerosis, 171. See also *Scleroderma.*
Acrylamide, neuropathy from, 911
Actamer. See *Bithionol.*
ACTH, 2089–2090. See also
   Adrenocorticotropin and
   Corticotropin.
   in multiple sclerosis, 847
Actinomyces bovis, 474
Actinomyces israelii, 474
Actinomycin D, in oncologic treatment,
   1936
Actinomycosis, 473–474
   vs. nocardiosis, 475
Activated charcoal, in accidental
   poisoning, 74
Active transport, in normal absorption,
   1524
Acupuncture analgesia, 726
Acute abdomen, 1578–1582
Acyanotic Fallot's tetralogy, 1164
ADA deficiency, 2043
Adamantinoma, 2098
Adams-Stokes syndrome, 743
Adaptive colitis, 1493
Addisonian crisis, 2147
   treatment of, 2149
Addison's disease, 2147–2150
   diagnosis of, principles of, 2065
   eosinophilia in, 226
   HLA system and, 39
   hyperkalemia in, 1959
   volume depletion in, 1951
   vs. acute intermittent porphyria, 2047
   vs. adrenal insufficiency secondary to
      hypopituitarism, 2151
   vs. hypopituitarism, 2102
   vs. malabsorption syndrome, 1535
Adenine arabinoside, *556,* 1935
   in herpes simplex encephalitis, 824
**Adenine phosphoribosyltransferase
   deficiency, 2043**
Adenitis
   cervical, "atypical" mycobacteria
      causing, 500
   suppurative, in streptococcal
      pharyngitis, 373
   mesenteric, acute, vs. acute
      appendicitis, 1581

Adenitis (*Continued*)
   tuberculous, vs.
      paracoccidioidomycosis, 541
Adenocarcinoma
   colonic, vs. chronic cholecystitis, 1625
   colorectal, 1607
   gallbladder, in chronic cholecystitis,
      1625
   small intestinal, 1604, 1605, *1605*
Adenohypophysis, 2083–2108. See also
   Anterior pituitary.
Adenoid cystic carcinoma, 1012
Adenoma(s)
   acidophilic, with acromegaly, 2097,
      2098
   basophil, 863
      with Cushing's syndrome, 2098
   bile duct, 1635
   bronchial, 1011
   chromophobe, 863, *2095,* 2096, 2097
   eosinophilic, 863
   **functioning, islet cell, fasting
      hypoglycemia caused by, 1993–1995**
   gallbladder, 1634
   gastric, 1604
   hepatic, 1667
      oral contraceptive use and, 2195
   parathyroid, 2214
      preoperative localization of, 2218,
         2219
   pituitary, excessive hormone
      secretion in, 2108
   polypoid, colorectal carcinoma risk
      and, 1607, *1607*
   renal, 1461, 1462
   small intestinal, 1605
   thyroid, 2141, **2142**
   villous, 1610
      rectal, hypokalemia in, 1958
Adenoma sebaceum, in tuberous
   sclerosis, 770, 2292, *2292*
Adenomatosis, multiple endocrine, 2098
   detection of, in relatives, *58*
   hypercalcemia in, 2238
   in acromegaly, 2106
Adenomatous hyperplasia of
   gallbladder, 1634
Adenomyomatosis of gallbladder,
   1634
Adenomyomatous hyperplasia of
   gallbladder, 1634
Adenopathy
   hilar, in pulmonary tuberculosis, 484,
      485
   inguinal, vs. lymphogranuloma
      venereum, 335
Adenosine deaminase
   deficiency of, 2043
   **severe combined immunode-
      ficiencies with,** *139,* **141–142**
   excessive, hemolytic anemia in, 1761
Adenosine monophosphate, cyclic,
   2071, **2072–2073,** *2072, 2073*
   urinary excretion of, in
      hyperparathyroidism, 2218
Adenoviral infections, 236–238
   vs. influenza, 245
   vs. ocular chlamydial infections, 334
Adenoviral pharyngitis
   vs. diphtheria, 431
   vs. streptococcal pharyngitis, 372
Adenoviral pneumonia, 237
   vs. mycoplasmal pneumonia, 345

Adenoviruses, 236, 237
  associated with common cold, *230*
Adenyl cyclase, activation of, hormonal responses dependent upon, 2071, *2071*
Adhesive capsulitis, 207
Adie's myotonic pupil, 900
Adnexal tumors, 864
Adolescence, 17–22. See also *Puberty.*
  delayed, 1756
  psychosocial development in, 20–22
Adrenal(s)
  congenital hyperplasia of, 2158–2161
    hypertension from, 1211
    vs. primary aldosteronism, 2158
  hyperfunction of, organic precocious pseudopuberty due to, 2182, 2183
  insufficiency of
    hypercalcemia in, 2236
    secondary to hypopituitarism, 2150–2151
    secondary to pituitary-adrenal suppression by corticosteroids, 2151–2152
  tuberculosis of, 498
  tumor of
    Cushing's syndrome resulting from, 2152
      treatment of, 2156
    feminizing, 2162
    virilizing, 2161–2162
Adrenal apoplexy, 2150
Adrenal cortex, 2144–2162
  effects of oral contraceptives on, 2196
  in acromegaly, 2106
  insufficiency of, primary, 2147–2150. See also *Addison's disease.*
Adrenal medulla, 2199–2207
  hormones of, 2199–2201
Adrenal steroids
  functions of, 2144–2146, *2145*
  secretion of, regulation of, 2146–2147
Adrenarche, 2181
Adrenergic neuron–blocking drugs, in arterial hypertension, *1212,* 1215
Adrenocortical hyperplasia, congenital, 2064
Adrenocorticotropin, 2089–2090
  in diagnosis of Addison's disease, 2148, *2148*
  in regulation of adrenal steroid secretion, 2146
  secretion of
    control of, 2146, 2147
    measurement of, 2093–2094
Adrenogenital syndrome, *43*
Adrenoleukodystrophy, 849, 850
Adriablastina, 1937
Adriamycin, 1937
  cardiotoxicity from, 1287
  in Hodgkin's disease, 1846
  in multiple myeloma, 1861
  in non-Hodgkin's lymphomas, *1836*
Adult respiratory distress syndrome, 1024, **1033–1045**
  conditions associated with, *1024*
Adulthood, 22–24
  crises of, 23–24
  development to, 17–22
    psychosocial, 20–22
    pubertal changes and, 17–20, *18*
  stages of, 22–23

Adynamic ileus, 1490, 1491
Aedes aegypti
  Chikungunya virus transmitted by, 279
  dengue hemorrhagic fever transmitted by, 297
  dengue transmitted by, 277
  yellow fever transmitted by, 293, 294
Aedes africanus, 294
Aedes albopictus, 277
Aedes dorsalis, 288
Aedes luteocephalus, 294
Aedes scutellaris, 277
Aedes simpsoni, 294
Aedes sollicitans, 286
Aedes triseriatus, 288
Aedes vexans, 286
Aeration, lung, abnormalities of, 965–966
Aerobic gram-negative bacilli, pneumonia and nosocomial respiratory infections caused by, 361–365
Aerophagia, 1479, 1489
  psychogenic, 1489
Aerosol sprays, inhalation of, 705
Aerotitis media, 96
Afibrinogenemia, *43, 1884*
Aflatoxins
  food contamination by, 69, 70
  hepatoma and, 1668
African hemorrhagic fever, 300–301
African tick typhus, 324–325
African trypanosomiasis, 575, 576–579
Afterload, cardiac, 1065, 1083, 1084
  reduction of, in heart failure, 1100, *1100,* 1101, *1101*
  in shock, 1121
Agammaglobulinemia, infantile, X-linked, *43,* **139–140,** *139, 140*
  Bruton type of, 139, 150, *1910*
Aganglionic megacolon, 1495–1496, *1495*
Aganglionosis, 1495
Age
  blood pressure and, 1200
  renal transplantation and, 1382
  selection of antimicrobial agents and, 553
Agglutination test(s)
  in brucellosis, 477, 478
  in rickettsial diseases, *314,* 315
Agglutinin(s)
  cold, syndrome of, 1764–1765
    autosensitization in, 132
  sheep cell, in infectious mononucleosis, 266
Aging, 25–30
  as risk factor for atherosclerosis, 1219
  effects of, on aorta, 1292
  management of, special problems of, 29–30
  physician's responsibility in, 30
  psychosocial problems of, 29
  skin changes with, 27, *2272*
  structural and functional changes with, 25–27
  theories of, 28–29
Agnogenic myeloid metaplasia, 1827–1829
  portal hypertension in, 1639
  vs. myelophthisic anemia, 1742

Agnosia, 658
  finger, 658
Agranulocytosis
  angina of, vs. diphtheria, 431
  drugs causing, 156
Agraphia
  alexia with, 657
  alexia without, 657
  in Gerstmann's syndrome, 658
  pure, 657
Air
  chemical contamination of, 60–64
  swallowing of, 1479, 1489
Air conditioner lung, *971*
Air embolism
  hyperbaric oxygen therapy in, 104
  transfusion reaction caused by, *1785, 1786*
Air encephalography, in head injury, 881
Air travel, problems of, 95–97
Airway(s)
  acute reactions in, to organic particles, 996–997
  chemical agents affecting, 1000
  continuity of, interruption of, nosocomial pneumonia and, 362
  control of, in acute respiratory failure, 1039, 1040
  esophageal obturator, in cardiopulmonary resuscitation, 1055
  establishment of, in acute respiratory failure, 1025–1026
    in cardiopulmonary arrest, 1054
  function of, tests of, 934, *934*
  in coma from sedative overdose, 713
  in head injury, 882
  in tetanus, 439
  narrowing of, 934
  obstruction of, diseases associated with, 951–964
    respiratory failure in, 1022–1023, *1023*
    due to organic particles, 997–998, *997*
    in bullous disease, 1003
    localized, 964
    pathophysiology of, 952–953, *952*
  small, disease of, 951
  upper, neoplasms of, vs. midline granuloma, 221
Airways resistance, 933, 934, *934*
  tests of, in ventilatory disorders, 936, *936*
Ajellomyces dermatitidis, 540
Akinesia, in paralysis agitans, 753
Akinetic mutism, in midbrain infarctions, 787
Akinetic seizure, 854
Akodon arenicola, 299
Alastrim, 257
Albers-Schönberg's disease, 2263
Albinism, *41,* **2029**
  oculocutaneous, 2029, 2293
  partial, 2292
  photophobia in, 2288
Albright's syndrome, 2183, 2262
  lentigines in, 2290
Albumin
  in shock, 1118
  salt-free, in pseudomembranous enterocolitis, 1585

Albumin (*Continued*)
  salt-poor, in ascites complicating
    cirrhosis, 1666
  in malabsorption syndrome, *1536*
  synthesis of, measurement of, 1646
Alcaptonuria, *41,* **2026–2027,** *2300*
Alcohol
  abuse of, 705–711
    cirrhosis in, 1663–1665
  acute intoxication with, 707, *712*
    vs. hypoglycemias induced in
      fasting state, 1996
  acute pancreatitis and, 1551, 1552
  addiction to, 706, 708
  chronic pancreatitis and, 1555
  excessive ingestion of, withdrawal
    symptoms after, 668, 709, 710
  hypoglycemia induced by, 1705
  hypomagnesemia induced by, 1705
  liver disorders due to, 709, 1658,
    1663, 1664. See also names of
    specific diseases.
  methyl, poisoning by, 75
    metabolic acidosis from, 1962
Alcoholic cardiomyopathy, 1284, 1285
Alcoholic cerebellar degeneration, 775
Alcoholic hepatitis, acute, 1664
  vs. acute cholecystitis, 1627
  vs. acute viral hepatitis, 1654
  vs. hepatic amebiasis, 592
Alcoholic hyperlipemia, 2009
Alcoholic ketoacidosis, 1705
  metabolic acidosis from, 1961, 1962,
    1964
Alcoholic myopathy, 924
Alcoholic neuropathy, 772–773
  esophagus in, 1488
Alcohol-related illness, 705–711
Aldomet. See *Methyldopa.*
Aldosterone
  circulating level of, effect of, on
    potassium excretion, 1323
  deficiency of, *43*
    in Addison's disease, 2147
  properties of, 2144, *2145,* 2146
  secretion of, control of, 1321, 2147
Aldosterone antagonists, in heart
  failure, 1105
Aldosteronism
  primary, 2157–2158
    metabolic alkalosis in, 1966
  secondary, 2158
    vs. primary aldosteronism, 2157
Aleppo evil, 587
Aleukemic leukemia
  acute, vs. rheumatic fever, 383
  vs. visceral leishmaniasis, 586
Aleukia, alimentary toxic,
  trichothecenes causing, 70
Alexia with or without agraphia, 657
Algid malaria, 572
Alimentary form of lead poisoning, 78
Alimentary hyperinsulinism, 1990
Alkali
  in treatment of renal calculi, 1446
  in treatment of renal tubular acidosis,
    1441, 1442
  loss of, metabolic acidosis from, 1962
Alkaline phosphatase
  placental, as tumor marker, 1913
  plasma levels of, in osteomalacia,
    2248
  serum levels of, in Paget's disease,
    2259

Alkalòsis
  metabolic, *1322, 1961,* **1965–1967**
    causes of, *1965*
    complicating chronic respiratory
      acidosis, 1967, 1968, *1968*
    in cancer patient, 1904
    potassium deficiency and, 1958
    tetany from, 2223
  respiratory, *1961,* **1969**
    plasma composition in, *1967*
Alkeran. See *Melphalan.*
Alkyl sulfonate, in oncologic treatment,
  1932
Alkylating agents. See also names of
  specific agents.
  in oncologic treatment, 1930–1933
Allelic genes, 40
Allergens, injected, in allergic rhinitis,
  159, 160
Allergic alveolitis
  extrinsic, 970–972, *971*
    vs. Goodpasture's syndrome, 976
Allergic angiitis, granulomatosis and,
  166, 182
  treatment of, 183
  vs. classic periarteritis nodosa, 183
  vs. Wegener's granulomatosis, 183
Allergic aspergillosis, 956
Allergic asthma, 956
Allergic encephalomyelitis,
  experimental, 844
Allergic gastroenteritis, 1542–1543
Allergic rhinitis, 157–160
  perennial, 157
  sensitization to external antigens in,
    131
Allergy(ies). See also *Hypersensitivity.*
  drug, 154–157
    vs. malaria, 573
  epilepsy associated with, 853
  food, 1498, 1499
    sensitization to external antigens
      in, 131
    urticaria caused by, 161
  gastrointestinal, 1498–1499
    in children, 1499
  in insulin therapy of diabetes
    mellitus, 1987
  sarcoidosis caused by, 210
  to arthropod products, 112–113
  to house-dust mites, 118
  to insect stings, 113, 114, 163
  transfusion reaction from, *1785,* 1787
Allescheria boydii, 542
Alloantibodies, high-titer, in group O
  donor blood, transfusion reaction
  from, 1787, 1788
Allopurinol
  as nephrotoxin, 1432
  in agnogenic myeloid metaplasia,
    1828
  in renal calculi, 1446
  in renal complications of chronic
    granulocytic leukemia, 1823
  in tophaceous gout, 2040
  in uric acid synthesis, *2031*
  urinary orotic acid excretion and,
    2044
  xanthine oxidase inhibition by, 2340
Alopecia, 2271
Alopecia mucinosa, *2297*
Alpha thalassemia, 1779
Alpha-adrenergic receptor–blocking
  drugs, in arterial hypertension, 1215

Ālpha-aminoadipic aciduria, *2018*
Alpha₁-antitrypsin deficiency, *43,* 962
Alpha-chain disease, 1866
  lymphoma in, 1545
Alpha-fetoprotein, as tumor marker,
  1912
Alpha-1-fucosidase deficiency, vs.
  Fabry's disease, 2012
Alpha-lipoprotein deficiency, 2008
Alpha-methyl-para-tyrosine, in
  pheochromocytoma, 2205
Alport's syndrome, 1329, **1402**
Altitude(s)
  high, at birth, congenital heart
    disease and, 1150
    disorders associated with, 100, 101,
      102
    pulmonary arterial pressure at, 1137
    secondary polycythemia and, 1798,
      1799
    varying, pressure changes at, 97,
      98, *98*
Aluminosis, 990
Aluminum, accumulation of, in chronic
  renal failure, 1360
Aluminum hydroxide
  in hyperphosphatemia of acute renal
    failure, 1373
  in peptic ulcer, 1513
Alveolar hydatid cysts, 609
Alveolar hypoventilation
  pulmonary hypertension in, 1146,
    1147, 1148
  secondary polycythemia in, 1799
Alveolar lipoproteinosis, in silicosis,
  989
  management of, 993
Alveolar macrophages
  bacterial ingestion by, 339, 340
  in immunocompromised patient,
    nosocomial pneumonia and, 363
Alveolar proteinosis, pulmonary, 978
Alveolar surfactant, 932
Alveolar ventilation, maintenance of, in
  acute respiratory failure, 1027
Alveolar-capillary block syndrome, 937
Alveolar-capillary membrane, in
  diffusion, 936, 937, 938
Alveolitis, allergic
  extrinsic, 970–972, *971*
    vs. Goodpasture's syndrome, 976
Alveolus(i)
  bacteria in, inactivation of, 339
  fluid in, pneumococcal pneumonia
    and, 348
  phagocytosis in, 340, 341
Alzheimer's disease, 661–662
  vs. hereditary chorea, 759
  vs. Pick's disease, 661, 662
Amanita species, poisoning by, 69
Amantadine hydrochloride, *556*
  in parkinsonism, 755
Amatoxins, 69
Amaurosis fugax
  in benign intracranial hypertension,
    870
  in intracranial tumors, 865
Amaurotic idiocy, 850
Ambilhar. See *Niridazole.*
Amblyomma americanum, 322
Amblyomma cajennense, 322
Amblyopia
  nutritional, 774–775
  tobacco-alcohol, 774–775

Amebiasis, 566, **589–594**
  antimicrobial agents for, *558*
  cutaneous, 591
  hepatic, 590, 591, 592, 593
    vs. clonorchiasis, 618
  immunodiagnostic tests for, *565*
  intestinal, 590, 591, 592, 593
  vs. actinomycosis, 474
  vs. malaria, 573
Amebic brain abscess, 592
Amebic colitis, vs. ulcerative colitis, 1572
Amebic dysentery, 589–594
  Trichuris and, 629
  vs. balantidiasis, 603
Amebic encephalitis, vs. viral encephalitis, 820
Amebic liver abscess, 590, 591, 592, 593
Amebic lung abscess, 591, 980, 981
Amebic meningoencephalitis, primary, 603–604
Amebic pericarditis, 592
Amebic peritonitis, 590, 591, 592
Amebic ulceration, 590, 591
Amebomas, 590, 591, 592
Amenorrhea(s), 2183–2193
  anosmia and, 2188
  diagnostic evaluation of, 2183, *2183*
  disorders leading to, 2184–2188
  functional, 2080
  hypothalamic, 2080, 2187
  in anorexia nervosa, 1700, 1703, 2080, 2187
  "post-pill," 2080, 2188
  primary, 2179
  secondary, 2179
  treatment of, 2190–2193
American mucocutaneous leishmaniasis, *588, 589*
American trypanosomiasis, 579–583. See also *Chagas' disease.*
Amethopterin, 1933, 1934. See also *Methotrexate.*
Amidopyrine, neutropenia induced by, 1809
Amikacin, *556,* 561
  adverse reactions to, 562
  as nephrotoxin, 1426
Amiloride, hyperkalemia and, 1959
Amino acid(s)
  absorption of, 1525
  in chronic renal failure, 1361
  insulin release provoked by, 1972
  isotonic, in intravenous nutrition, 1708
  metabolism of, inborn errors of, 41, **2015–2029**
Amino acid sequence of immunoglobulins, 127
Aminoacidemias, sulfur, *2017*
Aminoacidopathies, hereditary and acquired, classification of, *2016–2021*
Aminoaciduria(s)
  branched-chain, 2021
  dicarboxylic, *2020*
  hyperdibasic, *41, 2020*
  photosensitivity in, 2288
Aminoacyl-tRNA synthetases, 32
α-Aminoadipic aciduria, *2018*
γ-Aminobutyric acid, 751
  deficiency of, in hereditary chorea, 758, 759
Aminocaproic acid, in bleeding of chronic renal failure, 1364

Aminoglutethimide, in breast cancer, 1919
Aminoglycosides, *556–557,* 561. See also names of specific agents.
  adverse reactions to, 561, 562
  as nephrotoxins, 1425, 1426
  neuromuscular block caused by, 929
β-**Aminoisobutyricaciduria,** *2019,* **2022–2023,** 2044
δ-Aminolevulinic acid, in porphyria, 2044
Aminophylline
  in asthma, 958, 959
  in chronic respiratory failure, 1029
  in pulmonary embolism, 1133
  in status asthmaticus, 959
Aminosalicylic acid, *556*
Amitriptyline
  abuse of, 698
  in muscle-contraction headaches, 732
  in pain, 724, 725
  in parkinsonism, 755
  in postherpetic neuralgia, 728
  poisoning by, *712*
Ammonia
  exposure to, respiratory effects of, 1000
  formation of, in urinary tract infection, 1410
  in chronic renal failure, 1360
Ammonium chloride, ingestion of, metabolic acidosis from, 1962
Amnesia
  after head injury, 659
  anterograde, 658
  functional, 659
  retrograde, 658
Amniocentesis
  in chromosome analysis, 49, 50
  in genetic counseling, 58, 59
Amniotic fluid embolism, hypofibrinogenemia in, 1893, 1894
Amoxicillin, *557,* 558
  in typhoid fever, 448
AMP, cyclic, 2071, **2072–2073,** *2072, 2073*
  urinary excretion of, in hyperparathyroidism, 2218
Amphetamine(s)
  abuse of, 701–702
  poisoning by, 75, 702, *712*
    schizophrenia-like syndrome in, 668
Amphetamine psychosis, 702
Amphiphils, in fat absorption, 1524
Amphoric breath sounds, in pulmonary tuberculosis, 486
Amphotericin B, *556*
  as nephrotoxin, 1427, 1428
  in blastomycosis, 541
  in candidiasis, 549
    in compromised host with leukopenia, 152
  in chromomycosis, 543
  in coccidioidomycosis, 539
  in cryptococcosis, 544
  in cutaneous leishmaniasis of new world, 589
  in fungal endocarditis, 394
  in histoplasmosis, 537
  in maduromycosis, 542
  in mucormycosis, 546
  in paracoccidioidomycosis, 541, 542
  in sporotrichosis, 545

Amphotericin B (*Continued*)
  in visceral leishmaniasis, 586, 587
Ampicillin, *557,* 558
  adverse reactions to, 559
  in bacterial meningitis, 415, 416
  in bacterial overgrowth causing malabsorption, 1538
  in chronic respiratory failure, 1029
  in gonococcal disease, 409, 410
  in granuloma inguinale, 429
  in infective endocarditis, 394
  in infective endocarditis prophylaxis, 396
  in malabsorption syndrome, *1536*
    postgastrectomy, 1546
  in meningococcal disease, 421
  in nocardiosis, 475
  in regional enteritis, 1566
  in shigellosis, 459
  in simple chronic bronchitis, 954
  in toxic megacolon, 1575
  in typhoid carriers, 448
  in typhoid fever, 448
  in Whipple's disease, 1542
Ampullary stenosis, 1636
Amyl nitrite, inhalation of, 705
Amylase, blood, determination of, in acute pancreatitis, 1553
Amyloidosis, 1863–1865
  cardiac, 1285–1286
  electrophoretic patterns in, 1857, *1857*
  in familial Mediterranean fever, 2056
  malabsorption in, 1543
  neuropathy in, 910
    vs. idiopathic autonomic insufficiency, 763
  patterns of, *1863*
  renal changes in, 1405–1406
  systemic, internal malignancy and, *2297*
Amyotrophic lateral sclerosis, 765–766
  vs. multiple sclerosis, 847
  vs. muscular dystrophies, 918
  vs. myasthenia gravis, 927
Amyotrophy, diabetic, 902, 909, 1980
Anaerobic bacteremia, 443
Anaerobic bacteria, nonsporeforming, disease due to, 441–445
Anaerobic cellulitis, 434, 443
  treatment of, 435
  vs. clostridial myonecrosis, *435*
Anaerobic cocci, 441
  susceptibility of, to antimicrobial agents, *445*
Anaerobic endocarditis, 443
Anaerobic gram-negative bacilli, 441
Anaerobic streptococcal myonecrosis, 434
Anaerobic streptococci, 367
Anagen, 2270
Anagen effluvium, 2271
Anal diseases, 1616–1618
Anal fissure, 1617
Anal sensory receptors, 1482, 1483
Anal sphincters, 1482
Analbuminemia, *43*
Analgesic agents, 723–725, *724*
  narcotic, 694–698, 723, 724, *724*
Analgesic nephropathy, 1409, 1412, 1419–1420
  chronic renal failure and, 1352
Anaphylactic reaction, complicating therapy of serum sickness, 154

Anaphylactoid purpura, renal involvement in, 1400, 1401
Anaphylaxis, generalized, in drug allergy, 156
Anasarca, in right ventricular failure, 1093
Ancylostoma braziliense, 625
Ancylostoma caninum, 625
Ancylostoma ceylonicum, 624
Ancylostoma duodenale, 559, 624
Ancylostomiasis, 624–625
Androgen deficiency, 2167, 2168
in Addison's disease, 2147
Anemia(s), 1714–1751
  aplastic, 1733–1740
    drugs causing, 156, 1734
    etiologic classification of, *1733*
    idiopathic, acute leukemia in, 1814
    neutropenia in, 1810
    therapeutic principles in, 1719
  associated with infection and chronic systemic diseases, 1731–1733
  classification of, 1717–1718, *1718*
  Cooley's, 1778
  Fanconi's, 1733, 1737, *1910*
    unrepaired chromosomal breakage in, 54
  hemolytic, *42*, 1751
    acquired, 1762–1770
    autoimmune, idiopathic thrombocytopenic purpura associated with, 1867
    cause of, diagnosis of, 1753
    compensated, 1752
    congenital, 1755–1762
    drugs associated with, 156
    immune, Coombs-negative, 1763
    in chronic lymphocytic leukemia, 1825
    in cold agglutinin syndrome, 1765
    in glucose-6-phosphate dehydrogenase deficiency, 45
    microangiopathic, 1766–1767, *1767*
    therapy of, 1754
    traumatic, cardiac, 1767
    uncompensated, 1752
    unstable hemoglobins causing, 1776–1777, *1777*
  hemorrhagic, acute, 1729–1730
  hookworm, 624, 625
  hypochromic, 1743–1751
    not caused by iron deficiency, 1751
  hypoplastic, 1733. See also *Anemia(s), aplastic.*
  in acute leukemia, 1816, 1817, 1820
  in acute tubular necrosis, 1372
  in analgesic nephropathy, 1419, 1420
  in cancer, 1732
  in cerebral infarction, 781
  in chloramphenicol therapy, 562
  in chronic renal failure, 1363, *1363*, 1364, 1731
  in dialysis patients, 1381, 1731, 1732
  in endocrine disorders, 1732
  in gastric carcinoma, 1601
  in Hodgkin's disease, 1842
  in infective endocarditis, 391
  in liver disease, 1643, 1732
  in macroglobulinemia, 1862
  in malabsorption syndrome, 1529
  in malaria, 569, 571
  in multiple myeloma, 1859
  in non-Hodgkin's lymphomas, 1834

Anemia(s) (*Continued*)
  in regional enteritis, 1566
  in rheumatic fever, 381
  in rheumatoid arthritis, 189, 1732
  in scurvy, 1691
  in systemic lupus erythematosus, 178
  iron deficiency, 1743–1751
    benign intracranial hypertension with, 872
    in hookworm disease, 625
    vs. anemia of chronic disorders, 1732
    vs. other hypochromic anemias, 1751
    vs. sideroblastic anemia, 1741
  leukoerythroblastic, 1742, 1827
  Mediterranean, 1778
  megaloblastic, 1719–1729
    clinical manifestations of, 1724
    differential diagnosis of, 1725, *1725*
    etiologic classification of, 1719, *1720–1721*
    incidence and prevalence of, 1722
    laboratory findings in, 1725
    pathogenesis of, 1719
    pathology of, 1723
    therapeutic principles in, 1719
    therapy of, 1726
  miner's, 624–625
  myelophthisic, 1742
    in cancer patient, 1906
    therapeutic principles in, 1719
    vs. aplastic anemia, 1738
  normochromic normocytic, 1729–1742
  of chronic disorders, 1731–1733
  pernicious, 1719
    adult, gastric carcinoma and, 1600
    clinical manifestations of, 1725
    cutaneous lesions in, *2302*
    eosinophilia in, 226
    immunologic aspects of, 133
    incidence and prevalence of, 1723
  severe, vs. arteriosclerosis obliterans, 1301
  sickle cell, 1773–1775
    air travel and, 97
    cutaneous lesions in, *2302*
    genetic screening for, 59
    heterozygote detection in, *58*
    pneumococcal infections in, 348, 349
    Salmonella infections in, 451
    vs. rheumatic fever, 383
  sideroblastic, 1740–1741, *1741*, 1751
    therapeutic principles in, 1719
  simple chronic, 1731–1733
  target cell, 1778
  therapy of, principles of, 1718–1719
Anencephaly, frequency and sex ratio of, *48*
Anesthetics
  flurane, as nephrotoxins, 1433
  malignant hyperthermia from, genetic basis of, 46
Anesthetized patient, hemolytic transfusion reaction in, 1787
Aneurysm(s)
  aortic, 1292
    abdominal, 1293, 1590
      ultrasonography in, *1466*
    arteriosclerotic, 1292, 1293
    classification of, 1292
    congenital, 1291

Aneurysm(s) (*Continued*)
  aortic, dissecting, 1295–1297, *1296*
    vs. acute pericarditis, 1273
    vs. myocardial infarction, 1233
    in syphilis, 511, 1294, 1295
    "students'," 1293
  arterial, intracranial hemorrhage from, 794–795, *795*
    arteriography in, 798, 799
    prognosis in, 799
    treatment of, 800
  berry, intracranial hemorrhage from, 794, 795, *795*
  congenital, of sinuses of Valsalva, 1169–1170
  fusiform, intracranial hemorrhage from, 795
  mycotic, in infective endocarditis, 389, 390
    intracranial hemorrhage from, 795
  Rasmussen's, in pulmonary tuberculosis, 486
  renal artery, 1457
  ventricular, after myocardial infarction, 1237
"Angel dust," 704
Angiitis
  allergic, granulomatosis and, 166, 182
    treatment of, 183
    vs. classic periarteritis nodosa, 183
    vs. Wegener's granulomatosis, 183
  historical review of, 165–166
  hypersensitivity, 166, 167, *2301*
    drug-induced, vs. periarteritis nodosa, 183
  necrotizing, 165
    classification of, 166–167, *166*
    generalized, vs. classic periarteritis nodosa, 183
    hepatitis B antigenemia and, 181
    incidence of, at necropsy, *181*
Angina
  abdominal, 1587, 1588
  Ludwig's, 443
    vs. actinomycosis, 474
  Vincent's, 443
    vs. diphtheria, 431
    vs. infectious mononucleosis, 266
Angina decubitus, 1225
Angina pectoris, 1223–1229
  in aortic regurgitation, 1195
  in aortic stenosis, 1191
  preinfarction, 1228
  Prinzmetal's, 1228, 1229
  surgical treatment of, 1238, 1239, 1241
  unstable, 1228, 1229
    vs. myocardial infarction, 1232
  variant, 1229
  vs. esophagitis, 1484
Angiocardiography
  in asymmetric septal hypertrophy, 1279
  in congenital valvular aortic stenosis, 1157
  in endocardial cushion defect, 1171
Angioedema, 162–163
  hereditary, *43*, 162, 163, *2299*
Angiofibromas, in tuberous sclerosis, 2292, *2292*
Angiography
  in cerebral infarction, 790

Angiography (*Continued*)
  in colonic diverticulum, 1471, *1471*
  in head injury, 881
  in hepatic tumors, *1470*, 1471
  in intracranial hemorrhage, 798, 799
  in intraspinal compression, 892
  in nephrocarcinoma, 1459
  in pancreatic carcinoma, *1470*, 1471
  in primary pulmonary hypertension, 1141
  in pulmonary disease, 943, 944
  in splenic and hepatic rupture, 1471, *1471*
  visceral, 1470–1471, *1470, 1471*
Angioimmunoblastic lymphadenopathy, 1832
Angiokeratoma circumscripta, vs. Fabry's disease, 2012
Angiokeratoma corporis diffusum, 912
Angiolymphoid hyperplasia with eosinophilia, 226
Angioma(s), 863
  cavernous, intracranial hemorrhage from, 795
    of spinal cord, 898
  spider, in liver disease, 1645
Angiomyolipoma, renal, 1461
Angioneurotic edema, 162–163. See also *Angioedema.*
Angiopathy, necrotizing, neuropathy associated with, 908
Angiosarcoma, hepatic, 1668
Angiostrongyliasis, 631–632
Angiostrongylus cantonensis, 631, 632
Angiotensin
  circulatory effects of, 1111
  in control of aldosterone secretion, 1321
  renin and, in blood pressure regulation, 1207, 1208
Angiotensin-converting enzyme, serum, assay of, in sarcoidosis, 214
Angle closure glaucoma, 2323, *2323*
  acute, *2313*, 2314
Anhedonia, sexual, 689
Anicteric hepatitis, 1652
Animals
  marine, venomous, 123–125
  poisonous, 68–69
Anion gap, calculation of, in metabolic acidosis, 1962, *1962*
Anisakiasis, 628
Anisakis marina, 628
Ankles, swelling of, during air travel, 96
Ankylosing spondylitis, 194–195
  aortic regurgitation in, 1194
  eyes in, 2316
  genetic factors in, 39, 194
  pulmonary disability with, 1020
  regional enteritis and, 198, 1561
  ulcerative colitis and, 198, 1568
  vs. degenerative joint disease, 205
  vs. psoriatic arthritis, 196
Anomic aphasia, 657
Anopheles mosquitoes, in malaria, 566, 567, 568
Anorchia, 2170
Anorectal abscess, 1617
Anorexia
  amenorrhea in, 2187, 2188
  in cancer patient, 1906
Anorexia nervosa, 1699–1703, *1700, 1702*
  amenorrhea in, 1700, 1703, 2080, 2187

Anorexia nervosa (*Continued*)
  in male, 1701
  vomiting in, 1477, 1700, 1701
  vs. hypopituitarism, *2101*, 2102
Anoscopy, in diagnosis of constipation, 1481
Anosmia, 899
  amenorrhea and, 2188
Anosognosia, 658
  in cerebral infarction, 786
Anovulation, normogonadotropic normoestrogenic, 2193
Ant stings, 113–114
Antacids, in peptic ulcer, 1513, 1514
Antegrade pyelography, 1343
Anterior pituitary, 2083–2108
  anatomy of, 2083
  disorders of, amenorrhea due to, 2186–2187
    diagnosis of, hypothalamic hormones in, 2081–2082, *2081, 2082*
    diagnostic principles in, 2065
    vs. functional amenorrhea, 2080
  function of, 2084–2085, *2085*
    assessment of, 2091–2094
  hormones of, 2085–2091
    deficiency of, 2102, 2103
  secretion of, control of, 2074–2083
Anterior poliomyelitis, acute, 829–833
Anterior tibial compartment syndromes, 1305
Anterior uveitis
  acute, *2313*, 2314
  in ankylosing spondylitis, 2316
  in Behçet's disease, 2316
  in juvenile rheumatoid arthritis, 2315
  in sarcoidosis, 2329
Anterocollis, 761
Anterograde amnesia, 658
Anthracosilicosis, host response to tuberculosis in, 483
Anthracycline antibiotics, in oncologic treatment, 1936, 1937
Anthrax, 470–471
Antiarrhythmic drugs, 1264–1266. See also names of specific agents.
Antibiotics, antitumor, 1936, 1937
Antibody(ies), 96
  administration of, measles modified by, 249
  antinuclear, in systemic lupus erythematosus, 178
  autoimmune, hemolysis due to, 1763–1764
  cold agglutinin, classification of, *1765*
  cold-reacting, hemolysis due to, 1764–1766
  drug-induced, hemolysis due to, 1766
  formation of, in malnutrition, 1679
  heterophil, in infectious mononucleosis, 266
  isoimmune, hemolysis due to, 1763
  skin-sensitizing, 128
  types and properties of, 96–98, *97*
  warm-reacting, hemolysis due to, 1763–1764
Antibody tests, in malaria, 572
Anticapsular opsonins, in pneumococcal pneumonia, 349
Anticholinergics. See also names of specific agents.
  excessive ingestion of, 705
  in hypoglycemia in fed state, 1992

Anticholinergics (*Continued*)
  in parkinsonism, 755
  in peptic ulcer, 1515
Anticoagulant(s). See also names of specific agents.
  adrenal apoplexy in, 2150
  hemorrhagic complications from, 793, 795
  in cerebral infarction prevention, 792, 793
  in circulating blood, 1896–1897
  in completed stroke, 793
  in myocardial infarction, 1234, 1235
  in progressive stroke, 793
  in pulmonary embolism, 1133, 1134
  in stroke-in-evolution, 793
  in transient ischemic attacks, 792
  resistance to, genetic basis of, 46
Anticonvulsants. See also names of specific agents.
  as nephrotoxins, 1432
  rickets and osteomalacia induced by, 2253
Antidepressants. See also names of specific agents.
  in pain, *724*
  poisoning by, 712
  tricyclic, in depression of manic-depressive psychosis, 671
Antidiuretic hormone, 2109–2110
  function of, 1321, 1322, 2109
  inappropriate secretion of, 1953, 1954, 2109
    associated with cancer, 1917
    in bronchogenic carcinoma, 1006
    in head injury, 882
Antidote(s)
  specific, in accidental poisoning, 75
  "universal," 74
Antigen(s)
  autologous, sensitivity to, 132–133
  carcinoembryonic, as tumor marker, 1911, 1912
  foreign, sensitivity to, 131–132
  HLA, in sarcoidosis, 209
  oncofetal, as tumor markers, 1911–1912
  rickettsial, demonstration of, in acute phase urine, 312
Antigen-antibody complexes, in systemic lupus erythematosus, 175
Antigenemia, hepatitis B, in periarteritis nodosa, 181
Anti-glomerular basement membrane antibody disease, 1324, *1324*
Antihemophilic factor, 1881
  cryoprecipitated or lyophilized, in classic hemophilia, 1885, 1886
  deficiency of, coexistent proaccelerin deficiency and, 1889
  in classic hemophilia, 1883, *1884*
  in von Willebrand's disease, *1884*, 1886
Antihistamines
  excessive use of, 705
  in dermatologic therapy, 2277, *2277*
  in Hymenoptera stings, 114
Antihypertensive drugs, 1212–1217, *1212, 1215.* See also names of specific agents.
Antimetabolites. See also names of specific agents.
  in oncologic treatment, 1933–1935

Antimicrobial agents, 553–564. See also names of specific agents.
adverse reactions to, 556
as nephrotoxins, 1425–1428
broad-spectrum, in malabsorption syndrome, *1536*
combination therapy with, 555
failure of, 564
in bacterial, fungal, and viral infections, *556–557*
in chronic respiratory failure, 1029
in regional enteritis, 1566
pairings of, 552
prophylaxis with, 564, *564*
resistance to, forms of, 551, 552
selection of, 552, **553–556**
absorption and distribution in, 555
excretion in, 555
host determinants in, 553
Antimony, poisoning by, 81
Antimony sodium gluconate, in leishmaniasis, *558*
Antineoplastic therapy, principles of, 1922–1927
Antinuclear antibodies, in systemic lupus erythematosus, 178
Antirabies vaccination, neuroparalytic accidents following, 838–839
Antisera, in T cell detection, 130
Antistreptolysin O determination, in rheumatic fever, 382
Antithyroid compounds in plants, goiter caused by, 69
Anti-tissue antibody–mediated renal diseases, 1324, *1324*, 1325
Antitoxin
in clostridial myonecrosis, 434, 435
in diphtheria, 432
tetanus, 437, 438
trivalent, in botulism, 68
Anti-tubular basement membrane antibody disease, *1324*, 1325
Antitumor antibiotics, 1936, 1937
Antivenin(s)
in jellyfish sting, 123
in scorpion sting, 116, 117
in snakebite, 122
in spider bite, 115
in stonefish sting, 125
Anton's syndrome, in posterior cerebral artery occlusion, 787
Antrectomy, truncal vagotomy and, in duodenal ulcer, 1519, *1519*
Anturane. See *Sulfinpyrazone.*
Anus. See also *Anal.*
diseases of, 1616–1618
Anxiety, 672, **673–675**
atherosclerosis and, 1221
chronic, 675
in dementia, 660
in heart failure, 1093
WAIS scores in, 682
Anxiety neurosis, vs. angina pectoris, 1227
Aorta
abdominal, aneurysms of, 1293, 1590
ultrasonography in, *1466*
coarctation of, 1290
aneurysms of, 1292
arteriosclerotic, 1292, 1293
classification of, 1292
congenital, 1291

Aorta (*Continued*)
aneurysms of, dissecting, 1295–1297, *1296*
vs. acute pericarditis, 1273
vs. myocardial infarction, 1233
in syphilis, 511, 1294, 1295
"students'," 1293
atresia of, 1291
coarctation of, 1157–1158, 1209, 1289, 1290
at aortic isthmus, 1289, 1290
murmurs in, 1158, 1290
roentgenography in, 1158, 1290
surgical treatment of, 1290
diseases of, 1288–1299
congenital, 1289–1291
heredofamilial, 1291–1292
traumatic, 1293, *1294*
effects of aging on, 1292
enlarged, 1292–1293
in ankylosing spondylitis, 194, 195
in polychondritis with arthritis, 199
in relapsing polychondritis, 218
insufficiency of, in syphilis, 511
pseudocoarctation of, 1290
Aortic arch
absence of, 1290
right-sided, 1290, 1291
Aortic arch syndrome, 1288, **1297**
Aortic isthmus, coarctation of aorta at, 1289, 1290
Aortic occlusion syndromes, 1298–1299
Aortic regurgitation, 1194–1197
Austin Flint murmur in, 1196
vs. mitral stenosis, 1183
general physiologic effects of, 1174, 1175, *1175*
ventricular septal defect with, 1171
Aortic stenosis, 1190–1194
calcific, underlying infective endocarditis, 387
differential diagnosis of, *1192*, 1193
general physiologic effects of, 1174, 1175, *1175*
subvalvular, discrete, 1167
supravalvular, 1167, 1289
valvular, congenital, 1156–1157
vs. mitral regurgitation, 1187
Aortic valve
bicuspid, functionally normal, 1155–1156
replacement of, in aortic stenosis, 1193, 1194
Aortitis
miscellaneous forms of, 1297–1298, *1298*
syphilitic, 511, **1294–1295,** *1295*
Aortocoronary bypass grafts, 1238–1241
Aortography, in pulmonary disease, 944
Aortoiliac disease, isolated, in arteriosclerosis obliterans, 1300
"Apathetic hyperthyroidism," 923, 2065
Aperistalsis, esophageal, 1486–1488, *1487*
Aphasia, 656–657
anomic, 657
Broca's, 657
apraxia in, 658
conduction, 657
fluent, 656, 657
in intracranial tumor, 865
in left handers, 657

Aphasia (*Continued*)
nonfluent, 656
vs. dementia, 660, 661
Wernicke's, 657
Aphasic syndromes in children, 657
Aphemia, 657
Aphthous fever, 261
Aphthous ulcers, 149
Aplasia
germinal, 2170
pure red cell, 1735
Aplastic anemia, 1733–1740
drugs causing, 156, 1734
etiologic classification of, *1733*
idiopathic, acute leukemia in, 1814
neutropenia in, 1810
therapeutic principles in, 1719
Aplastic crises
in hereditary spherocytosis, 1756
in sickle cell anemia, 1774
Apnea, sleep, 654, 655
Apocrine chromhidrosis, 2269
Apodemus agrarius, 301
Apolipoproteins, in lipid transport, 2003
Apoplexy, 794–801. See also *Intracranial hemorrhage.*
adrenal, 2150
pituitary, 2098
Appendectomy, 1582
Appendiceal abscess, vs. regional enteritis, 1565
Appendicitis, acute, 1578–1582
vs. acute cholecystitis, 1627
vs. gonococcal salpingitis, 408
vs. pleurisy of pneumococcal pneumonia, 354
vs. regional enteritis, 1565
Apraxia, 658
of gait, 741
Apresoline. See *Hydralazine.*
APRT deficiency, 2043
APUD cells, hormone products of, 2061, *2061*
APUD system, 1913
Ara-A. See *Adenine arabinoside.*
Ara-C. See *Cystosine arabinoside.*
Arachnodactyly, 2053–2054. See also *Marfan's syndrome.*
Arachnoiditis
in amphotericin B treatment of coccidioidomycosis, 539
spinal, 897
vs. spinal epidural infections, 811
Arboviral encephalitis, 283–291
Arboviruses, 276–302
group A, 276
fevers caused by, 279–280, *279*
group B, 276
tick-borne diseases caused by, 290–291
meningitis and encephalitis from, 818, *818*, 819
Arc burns, 93
Arc of Riolan, 1587, *1587*
Arches, high, 903
Arenaviruses, 276
hemorrhagic diseases caused by, 298–300
Arfonad. See *Trimethaphan.*

Argentine hemorrhagic fever, *293,* **298–300**

Arginine, insulin release provoked by, 1972

Arginine hydrochloride, ingestion of, metabolic acidosis from, 1962

Argininemia, 2022

Argininosuccinicaciduria, *41, 2018,* 2022
dietary restriction in, 55

Argonz–Del Castillo syndrome, 2191
prolactin levels in, 2092

Argyll Robertson pupil, 900
in neurosyphilis, 512, 814, 815

Ariboflavinosis, 1686–1687

Armadillo disease, 930

Armillifer armillatus, 119

Arnold-Chiari malformation, 875
syringomyelia and, 769

Aromatic hydrocarbons, exposure to, aplastic anemia after, 1735

Arousal, sleep and, hypothalamus in, 715

Arrhythmia(s), 1242–1268. See also names of specific arrhythmias.
cardioversion of, by DC electroshock, 1266–1267
drugs for, 1264–1266
faintness in, 740
in acute pericarditis, 1272
in atrial septal defect, 1161
in cardiac amyloidosis, 1285
in digitalis toxicity, 1098
in myocardial infarction, 1230, 1235
in shock, treatment of, 1118
sinus, 1243

Arsenic
nephrotoxicity from, 1431
peripheral neuropathy from, 910, 911
poisoning by, 76–77

Arsenic trioxide, poisoning by, 76

Arsenous oxide, poisoning by, 76

Arsine, poisoning by, 76

Arterial aneurysms, intracranial hemorrhage from, 794–795, *795*
arteriography in, 798, 799
prognosis in, 799
treatment of, 800

Arterial baroreflex, in blood pressure regulation, 1206, 1207

Arterial blood gas values, significance of, 940–941

Arterial blood volume, effective, in control of sodium excretion, 1321

Arterial emboli, renal infarction from, 1407

Arterial embolism, 1303–1304
prevention of, 1134
vs. arteriosclerosis obliterans, 1301

Arterial hypertension, 1199–1218
cardiovascular disease risk factors in, 1201, 1202, *1202*
evaluation of, 1204
reduction of, 1212
causes of death in, 1203
clinical manifestations of, 1203
clinical syndromes of, 1204
epidemiology of, 1200
etiology of, 1209
headaches associated with, 732, 1203
mechanisms of, 1206
prognosis in, 1217
treatment of, 1211
drugs for, 1212–1217, *1212, 1215*
cessation of, 1216

Arterial hypertension (*Continued*)
treatment of, drugs for, choices of, 1216, 1217
combinations of, 1215, *1215*

Arterial hypoxia, causes of, in acute respiratory failure, 1036, *1037*

Arterial obstruction, organic, peripheral vascular diseases due to, 1299–1305

Arterial pressure
factors regulating, 1069
maintenance of, control systems for, 1206–1208
measurement of, 1074, 1200
monitoring of, in shock, 1047, 1116, 1117

Arterial pulses, examination of, 1074
in congenital heart disease, 1155

Arterial system, 1066, 1067

Arterial thrombi, renal infarction from, 1407

Arteriography
bronchial, 944
cerebral, 749
in brain tumor, 867
in cerebral infarction, 790
in epilepsy, 857
in herpes simplex encephalitis, 823
in intracranial hemorrhage, 798, 799
coronary, in angina pectoris, 1226
in selection of patients for myocardial revascularization, 1239
in arteriosclerosis obliterans, 1301
in ergotism and methysergide toxicity, 1308
in thromboangiitis obliterans, 1303
renal, 1343, *1343*

Arteriolosclerosis, eyes in, 2325–2326, *2326*

Arteriosclerosis, 1218

Arteriosclerosis obliterans, 1299–1302
vs. ergotism and methysergide toxicity, 1308
vs. erythromelalgia, 1308
vs. thromboangiitis obliterans, 1303

Arteriosclerotic aortic aneurysm, 1292, 1293

Arteriosclerotic pseudoparkinsonism, 753–754

Arteriovenous anomalies
rupture of, intracranial hemorrhage from, 795
arteriography in, 799
clinical manifestations of, 797
prognosis in, 799
treatment of, 801
spinal cord, 897–898

Arteriovenous fistula, 1312–1313
coronary, congenital, 1169
portal hypertension in, 1639
pulmonary, congenital, 1168–1169

Arteritis
cranial, 216–218
neuropathy in, 908
giant cell, 166, 216–218
eyes in, 2317, 2319
vs. periarteritis nodosa, 183
in rheumatic fever, 166
necrotizing, in rheumatoid arthritis, 187
peripheral, in systemic infections, 1305
temporal, 216–218

Artery(ies). See also names of specific arteries.
structural changes in, in hypertension, 1208
veins and, abnormal communications between, peripheral vascular diseases due to, 1312–1313

Arthralgia(s)
in fevers caused by group A arboviruses, 279
in periarteritis nodosa, 182
in rat-bite fever, 531
in systemic lupus erythematosus, 176

Arthritic diseases, eyes in, 2314–2316

Arthritis, 184
bacterial, 185–186
vs. rheumatic fever, 383
diseases associated with, 198–200
gonococcal, 185, 407, 408
vs. Reiter's syndrome, 197
gouty, acute, 2030
cause of, 2033, 2034, *2034*
clinical manifestations of, 2034, 2035, *2035*
treatment of, 2039
in obesity, 1696
in acromegaly, 199, 2105
in Behçet's syndrome, 199
in familial Mediterranean fever, 2056
in hemochromatosis, 199
in hyperparathyroidism, 200
in hypogammaglobulinemia, 199
in obesity, 1696
in polychondritis, 199
in rat-bite fever, 531
in regional enteritis, 198
in rheumatic fever, 379, 380
in sarcoidosis, 199
in sickle cell disease, 200
in ulcerative colitis, 198, 1575
in Whipple's disease, 199
infectious, 185–186
vs. gout, 2039
Lyme, 202
meningococcal, 417
miscellaneous forms of, 200–202
mycotic, 186
psoriatic, 196–197, *197*
vs. rheumatoid arthritis, 190
purulent, anaerobic, 444
pyogenic, gonococcal, 407
in bacterial meningitis, 414
rheumatoid, 186–193
adrenocorticosteroid therapy in, 192
anemia in, 189, 1732
aortic regurgitation in, 1194
Caplan's syndrome in, 187, 992, 993
clinical course of, 189
clinical manifestations of, 188
differential diagnosis of, 190
eosinophilia in, 226
epidemiology of, 186
extra-articular manifestations of, 187, 188, 189
eyes in, 2314, 2315
gastric ulcer and, 1504
HLA system and, 39
immune mechanisms in, 133, 134
immunosuppressive therapy in, 193
incidence of, 186
juvenile, 195–196
eyes in, 2315
laboratory findings in, 189
management of, 190

Arthritis (*Continued*)
  rheumatoid, mode of onset of, 188
    neuropathy in, 908
    neutropenia in, 1809
    orthopedic surgery in, 193
    pathogenesis of, 187
    pathology of, 187
    pericarditis caused by, 1271
    physical measures in, 191
    physical signs of, 188
    pleura in, 1017
    prognosis in, 189
    pulmonary involvement in, 974
    rest in, 191
    roentgenographic findings in, 189
    salicylates in, 191
    skeletal manifestations of, 188, *188,*
      189
    splenomegaly in, 193
    symptoms of, 188
    variants of, 193–194
    vs. degenerative joint disease, *203,*
      204
    vs. gonococcal arthritis, 408
    vs. gout, 2039
    vs. periarteritis nodosa, 183
    vs. polymyalgia rheumatica, 217
    vs. rheumatic fever, 383
    vs. tuberculous arthritis, 186
  syphilitic, 186
  tuberculous, 185–186, 497
  viral, 186
  vs. arteriosclerosis obliterans, 1301
Arthritis-dermatitis syndrome, 409
Arthrogryposis multiplex, 920
Arthropod-borne viral encephalitides,
  283–291
Arthropod-borne viral fevers,
  undifferentiated, 277–282, *279*
Arthropod-borne viruses, 276–302. See
  also *Arboviruses.*
Arthropods
  as environmental agents of disease,
    108–119
  products of, allergy to, 112–113
Arthus reaction
  in drug allergy, 155, 157
  in serum sickness, 131
"Asbestos bodies," in primary
  mesothelioma, 1595
Asbestosis, *987,* **990–992**
  neoplasia associated with, 994, 995
  pleura in, 990, 991, 1017
  pulmonary hypertension in, 1147
Ascariasis, 626–627
  bile duct obstruction by, 1632, 1633
  immunodiagnostic tests for, *565*
  vs. hepatic amebiasis, 592
Ascaris lumbricoides, 559, 605, 626
  life cycle of, *621*
Ascaris suum, 626
Ascites, 1592–1593, *1592, 1593*
  bile, 1593
  chylous, 1593
  cirrhosis and, 1640, 1665, 1666
    renal failure in, 1644
    spontaneous peritonitis in, 1594
  differential diagnosis of, 1592
  fluid of, evaluation of, 1592
  in chronic renal failure, 1366
  in portal hypertension, 1640
  in right ventricular failure, 1093
  "pseudochylous," 1593
  urine, 1593

Ascorbic acid
  deficiency of, 1689–1691, *1690*
    clinical signs of, *1677*
    perifolliculitis of, *1675*
  in clinical medicine, 1691
  in Ehlers-Danlos syndrome, 2055
  in scurvy, 1691
  nutrient value of, 1672
  recommended allowances of, *1671*
Aseptic meningitis, 817, 818, 820
  in Colorado tick fever, 280
  in epidemic pleurodynia, 272
  in leptospirosis, 533
  in mumps, 262
  vs. infectious mononucleosis, 267
Aseptic necrosis of bone, after renal
  transplantation, 1385
Asherman's syndrome, 2184
Asiatic cholera, 460–462
Asinocytosis, 1718
Asparaginase, in oncologic treatment,
  1936
Aspartylglucosaminuria, *43, 2018*
Aspergilloma, 547
Aspergillosis, 546–547
  allergic, 956
  in neutropenic patients on
    corticosteroid therapy, 149
  serologic tests for, 947
  vs. pneumocystosis, 599
Aspergillus flavus, 546
Aspergillus fumigatus, 546
Aspergillus-induced endocarditis, 387
Aspiration
  hepatic, in amebiasis, 592, 593, 594
  nasogastric, in hemorrhage of peptic
    ulcer, 1516
  percutaneous transtracheal,
    microbiologic diagnosis by, 342
Aspiration liver biopsy, in sarcoidosis,
  214
Aspiration pneumonitis, 1478
Aspirin
  in common cold, 233
  in degenerative joint disease, 205
  in erythromelalgia, 1309
  in headache with brain tumor, 730
  in influenza, 245
  in measles, 250
  in migraine syndrome, 732
  in pain, 723, 724, *724*
  in rheumatic fever, 383, 384
  in rheumatoid arthritis, 191
    juvenile, 196
  in subacute thyroiditis, 2132
  in thrombophlebitis, 1127
  in transient ischemic attacks, 792
  nephropathy from, 1419
  platelet dysfunction caused by,
    1879
  poisoning by, 75, 76
  ulcerogenesis and, 1504
Asplenia, 1869
Association, genetic, 37, 38
Astasia-abasia, 741
Asterixis
  in hepatic encephalopathy, 1641
  in metabolic brain disease, 648
Asthenia
  neurocirculatory, vs. angina pectoris,
    1227
  postinfluenzal, 243
Asthma, 951, 955–959
  allergic, 956

Asthma (*Continued*)
  as reaction to organic particles, 996,
    997
  intrinsic, 956
  nonallergic, 956
  pulmonary eosinophilia with, *969,*
    970
  vs. pulmonary embolism, 1133
  vs. simple chronic bronchitis, 954
Asthma-like reactions to chemical
  agents, 999–1000
Astigmatism, headache from, 733
Astrocytoma, 863
Asymmetric septal hypertrophy,
  1278–1279, 1280
Asymptomatic bacteriuria, 1409
Atabrine. See *Quinacrine hydrochloride.*
Ataxia
  Friedreich's, 767–768
    cardiomyopathy in, 1281
    vs. leprosy, 504
  in intracranial tumor, 865
  locomotor, 814–815. See also *Tabes*
    dorsalis.
Ataxia telangiectasia, 771, *1910*
  immunodeficiency with, *139,* **143–144**
  internal malignancy and, *2296*
  unrepaired chromosomal breakage in,
    54
Ataxic neuropathy, in diabetes mellitus,
  908
Atelectasis, 965
  obstructive, 964, 965
  roentgenographic appearance of, 941
  vs. pneumococcal pneumonia, 354
  vs. pulmonary embolism, 1133
Atenolol
  in arterial hypertension, *1212,* 1213
  in hypertension of chronic renal
    failure, 1362
Atheromas, 1218, 1219
Atherosclerosis, 1218–1222
  angina pectoris from, 1223
  diabetes mellitus and, 1981
  hyperlipoproteinemia in, 2010–2011
  in cerebral infarction, 779, *779*
  postmenopausal, 2190
  syncope in, 744, 745
Atherosclerotic plaques, 1218, 1219
Athetosis, 751, 760
  vs. dystonia musculorum deformans,
    761
Athetosis simplex, 760
Atlas, fractures of, 885
Atmospheric pressure, alterations in,
  97–103
  direct effects of, 98–99
  indirect effects of, 99–103
Atonic constipation, 1480
Atopic dermatitis, 2283–2284
Atransferrinemia, *43*
Atresia
  aortic, 1291
  pulmonary, Fallot's tetralogy with,
    1164, 1165
  tricuspid, 1171–1172
Atrial contractions, premature, 1246
Atrial extrasystoles, 1246–1247, *1246*
Atrial fibrillation, 1247–1248, *1247*
  DC electroshock in, 1267
  in aortic stenosis, 1191
  in mitral stenosis, 1180, 1181
  in myocardial infarction, 1230, 1235
  in pericardial constriction, 1275

Atrial flutter, 1248–1249, *1248*
 DC electroshock in, 1266
Atrial myxoma
 left, vs. mitral stenosis, 1183
 vs. infective endocarditis, 392
Atrial septal defect, 1160–1162
 ostium primum, 1171
 ostium secundum, 1160, 1161, 1162
 pulmonary vascular disease in, 1142,
  1143
 vs. mitral stenosis, 1183
Atrial tachycardia
 in myocardial infarction, 1235
 paroxysmal, 1249–1251, *1249, 1251*
"Atrialized right ventricle," 1168
Atrioventricular block
 first degree, 1260, *1260, 1261*
 functional or physiologic, 1263–1264
 second degree, 1260–1262, *1261, 1262*
 third degree, 1263, *1263, 1264*
 2:1, 1263, *1263*
Atrioventricular conduction, 1242, 1243,
 1243
 disorders of, 1260–1264
  in myocardial infarction, 1230
Atrioventricular dissociation, 1255–1256,
 1256
Atrioventricular junction, 1242
Atrioventricular junctional rhythms,
 1256
Atrioventricular valves, functional
 anatomy of, 1063
Atrium(a)
 common, 1169
 functional anatomy of, 1063
 left, vena caval drainage into, 1170
Atropa belladonna, poisoning by, 70
Atrophic gastritis, gastric carcinoma
 and, 1600
Atrophy
 muscular, peroneal, dominantly
   inherited hypertrophic
   neuropathy type of, 912
  neuronal type of, 913
  vs. muscular dystrophies, 918
 progressive, 765
 optic, 813, 815
  hereditary motor and sensory
   neuropathy with, 913
 Sudeck's, 206, 727, 2246
 yellow, acute, in fulminant hepatitis,
  1655
  in viral hepatitis, 1652
Atropine
 in diagnosis of myasthenia gravis,
  927
 in myocardial infarction, 1235
 in poisoning by phosphate ester
  insecticides, 75
 in sinus bradycardia complicating
  shock, 1118
 in ventricular fibrillation, 1057
 in vertigo, 739
 ingestion of, 705
 poisoning by, 75, *712*
Atypical facial neuralgia, 731
Atypical pneumonia, primary, vs.
 influenza, 245
Auchmeromyia luteola, 112
Audiometry
 in evaluation of dizziness, 738
 in hearing loss, 735

Auer bodies, in acute leukemia, 1815
Aura, in epilepsy, 853
Aurothioglucose, in rheumatoid
 arthritis, 192
Auscultation, cardiac, 1075
Austin Flint murmur, in aortic
 regurgitation, 1196
 vs. mitral stenosis, 1183
Australian X disease, 290
Autoantibodies, 126
 in systemic lupus erythematosus, 178,
  179
Autoerythrocyte sensitivity, 1880
Autoimmune antibodies, hemolysis due
 to, 1763–1764
Autoimmune diseases, silicosis and, 990
"Autoimmune" drug-induced
 hemolysis, 1766
Autoimmune hemolytic anemia,
 idiopathic thrombocytopenic purpura
 associated with, 1876
Autoimmune mechanisms, spontaneous
 hypoglycemia related to, 1996
Autoimmune phenomena, in systemic
 lupus erythematosus, 175
Autoimmune thrombocytopenic
 purpura, 1874
Autoimmunity, 126
 exophthalmos and, 2121
 Graves' disease and, 2121
 rheumatic fever and, 378, 379
 sarcoidosis and, 210
Autologous antigens, sensitivity to,
 132–133
Automated data management, in
 intensive care unit, 1032
Autonomic activity, in metabolic brain
 disease, 648
Autonomic insufficiency, idiopathic,
 762–763
Autonomic nervous system
 in diabetes mellitus, 1980
 in heart failure, 1088
 in tetanus, 439
Autonomic neuropathy, 909
 inflammatory, acute, 907
Autonomic seizures, 855
Autosensitization in human disease,
 132, 133
Autosomal dominant traits, 34, 35, *35*
Autosomal genes, 34
Autosomal inheritance, 34
Autosomal linkage of genes, 38
Autosomal recessive traits, 35, *35,* 36
AV. See *Atrioventricular.*
Avascular osteonecrosis, in
 adrenocorticosteroid therapy of
 rheumatoid arthritis, 192
Axial osteomalacia, 2254
Axis, fractures of, 885
Azaribine, in oncologic treatment, 1934,
 1935
Azathioprine, 1935
 in autoimmune hemolytic anemia,
  1764
 in chronic active hepatitis, 1662
 in regional enteritis, 1567
6-Azauridine, urinary orotic acid
 excretion in, 2044
Azotemia
 complicating diuresis for ascites in
  cirrhosis, 1665

Azotemia (*Continued*)
 in leptospirosis, 534
 prerenal, 1369
  vs. acute tubular necrosis, 1373
Azulfidine. See *Salicylazosulfapyridine.*
Azygography, in pulmonary disease,
 944

B cells, 126, 128
 alterations of, in disease states, 130
 characteristics and estimation of,
  129–130, *129*
 deficiency of, infections in, *148,* 150
 development of, *128*
 in host defense, 146
  diagnostic evaluation of, 150, 151,
   151
 primary immunodeficiency diseases
  and, 138–143
Babesia species, 600, 601
Babesiasis, 600–602
Babesiosis, 600–602
Bacillary dysentery, 457, 458
 vs. amebic dysentery, 592
Bacille Calmette Guérin
 in oncologic treatment, 1940
 in prevention of tuberculosis, 483
Bacillus(i)
 Battey, 480, 498, 499
 dysentery, 457, 458
 gram-negative, aerobic, pneumonia
  and nosocomial respiratory
  infections caused by, 361–365
 anaerobic, 441
 bacteremia caused by, 455, 456
  treatment of, 456, 457
 meningitis caused by, 411
  treatment of, 416
 gram-positive nonsporeforming
  anaerobic, 442
 Shiga, 457, 458
 tubercle, 481
  disappearance rate of, after drug
   therapy, 489
Bacillus anthracis, 470
Bacillus cereus food poisoning, 66
Bacillus mallei, 468
Bacillus whitmori, 469
Bacitracin, *556,* 561
 in bacterial meningitis, 416
 malabsorption from, 1548
Back-diffusion of acid, peptic ulcer and,
 1505
Backwash ileitis, vs. regional enteritis,
 1566
Baclofen, in multiple sclerosis, 847
Bacteremia
 anaerobic, 443
 gonococcal, 407
 gram-negative, 455–456
  treatment of, 456, 457
 in bacterial meningitis, 413
 in brucellosis, 476
 in hepatic cirrhosis, 455
 in infective endocarditis, 387, 388, 391
 in pneumococcal pneumonia, 349
 Klebsiella, 358
 "placental," 455
 preallergic, in tuberculosis, 481, 482

Bacteremia (*Continued*)
  Salmonella, 449, 450
    clinical manifestations of, 451
    diagnosis of, 452
    treatment of, 452
  staphylococcal, 403–404
**Bacteria, nonsporeforming anaerobic,
  disease due to, 441–445**
Bacterial arthritis, 185–186
  vs. rheumatic fever, 383
Bacterial bronchopneumonia, vs.
  pneumocystosis, 599
"Bacterial encephalitis," 806, 807
Bacterial endocarditis, 386–396. See also
  Endocarditis, infective.
Bacterial food poisoning, 64–66
Bacterial infection(s), 307–535
  antimicrobial agents for, *556–557*
  enteric, 453–457
    treatment of, 456, 457
  in chronic renal failure, 1364
  liver disease associated with, 1656
Bacterial lysis, complement-mediated,
  137
Bacterial meningitis, 411–416
  cerebrospinal fluid findings in, 413,
    414, *803*
  recurrent, 415
  vs. arboviral encephalitis, 284
  vs. poliomyelitis, 831
  vs. viral meningitis, 820
Bacterial myocarditis, 1282
Bacterial overgrowth
  malabsorption in, 1537, 1538
    treatment of, 1538
  tests for, 1531, 1532
Bacterial pneumonia(s). See also names
    of specific pneumonias.
  in influenza, 245
  recurrent, 340
  vs. coccidioidomycosis, 539
  vs. Goodpasture's syndrome, 976
  vs. malaria, 573
  vs. psittacosis, 338
  vs. pulmonary tuberculosis, 487
Bacterial sepsis, vs. congenital
  cytomegalovirus infection, 828
Bacterial toxins, destruction of, in
  malnutrition, 1680
Bactericidal drugs, 555
Bacteriostatic drugs, 555
Bacteriuria
  asymptomatic, 1409 .
  bacteriologic findings in, 1411
  epidemiology and natural history in,
    1412
  significant, concept of, 1411
Bacteroides fragilis, 441, 442, 445
  susceptibility of, to antimicrobial
    agents, *445*
Bacteroides melaninogenicus, 441, 442
  susceptibility of, to antimicrobial
    agents, *445*
Bacteroides oralis, 441
Bacteroides species, in tropical
  phagedenic ulcer, 530
Bagassosis, *971*
Bagdad boil, 587
Bag-valve-mask units, in
  cardiopulmonary arrest, 1055
BAL. See *Dimercaprol.*
Balance, impaired, 737, 741
Balantidiasis, 603

Balantidium coli, 603
Balkan nephropathy, 1421–1422
Ballism, 751
Bamboo spine, in ankylosing
  spondylitis, 195
Bancroftian filariasis, 633–634
Band keratopathy
  in hypercalcemia of
    hyperparathyroidism, 2215
  in juvenile rheumatoid arthritis, 2315
Banocide. See *Diethylcarbamazine.*
Bantu hypokinetic heart disease, 1283
Bárány rotation, in evaluation of
  dizziness, 738
Barbiturates. See also names of specific
    agents.
  abuse of, 698, 699, 700
  poisoning by, *712*
  sensitivity to, in porphyria, 46
Baritosis, 987
Barium, poisoning by, 76
Barlow's disease, 1691
Barometric pressure, alterations of, at
  differing altitudes, 98, *98*
Baroreflex, arterial, in blood pressure
  regulation, 1206, 1207
Barosinusitis, 99
Barotitis media, 98
Barr body, 37, 51
Barrett's esophagus, 1484
Barrett's ulcer, 1484
Bartonella bacilliformis, 331
Bartonellosis, 331–332
  Salmonella infections in, 451
Bartter's syndrome, 1957
Basal body temperature, in evaluation
  of ovarian function, 2180
Basal cell epithelioma, 2308–2309, *2309*
Basal ganglia, diseases of, 750–763
Basal metabolism, 1949
Base, selection of, in dermatologic
  therapy, 2276
Basedow's disease, 2120
Basilar artery, 782, 783, *783*
  ischemia of, 784, 785
  occlusion of, 788
Basilar impression, 875
Basilar skull fracture, 883
Basophil adenomas, 863
  with Cushing's syndrome, 2098
Basophilia, punctate, 1718
Bassen-Kornzweig syndrome, 767, 2008
  vs. Friedreich's ataxia, 768
Baths, in dermatologic therapy, 2276
Batten Spielmeyer-Vogt disease, 850,
  851
Battey bacillus, 480, 498, 499
"Battle fatigue," 674
Battle's sign, in stupor or coma, 643
Bay sore, *588*
Bazin's disease, 498
BCG
  in oncologic treatment, 1940
  in prevention of tuberculosis, 483
BCNU, in oncologic treatment, 1932,
  1933
Bechterew's syndrome, 194–195. See
  also *Ankylosing spondylitis.*
Becker dystrophy, 917
Beclomethasone, in asthma, 959
Bedsores. See *Decubitus ulcers.*
Bedwetting, 655
Bee stings, 113–114, 163

Beef tapeworm, 607–608
  antimicrobial agents for, *559*
  treatment of, 608–609
Beer drinker's hyponatremia, 719
Beetles, blister, 114
**Behavior, nervous system and,
  disorders of, 639–930**
Behavior modification, in obesity, 1698
Behçet's disease, *2298, 2303,* **2306–2307**
  arthritis in, 199
  eyes in, 2316
  neurologic involvement in, 842
  vs. bacterial meningitis, 415
Bejel, 522–523
Bejel treponeme, 522
Belching, 1479
Belesh, 522–523
Bell's palsy, 900
Benadryl. See *Diphenhydramine.*
Bence Jones protein, in cardiac
  amyloidosis, 1286
Bence Jones proteinuria, in multiple
  myeloma, 1858, 1860
Bendrofluazide, in arterial
  hypertension, *1212*
Bends, in decompression sickness, *103*
Benemid. See *Probenecid.*
Benserazide, in parkinsonism, 755
Bentonite flocculation test
  in protozoan and helminthic diseases,
    565
  in rheumatoid arthritis, 190
  in trichinosis, 631
Bentyl. See *Dicyclomine hydrochloride.*
Benzathine penicillin
  in cardiovascular syphilis, 1295
  in diphtheria prevention, 433
  in group A streptococcal infection,
    375
  in prevention of rheumatic fever, 385
  in rheumatic fever, 383
  in yaws, 521
Benzathine penicillin G, 557, *557*
  in bejel, 523
  in congenital syphilis, 517
  in erysipeloid of Rosenbach, 473
  in neurosyphilis, 816
  in pinta, 525
  in prophylaxis of streptococcal
    infection, 377
  in streptococcal pharyngitis, 376
  in syphilis, *515, 516*
Benzene, chronic exposure to, acute
  leukemia and, 1814
Benzene hexachloride, in Chagas'
  disease prophylaxis, 583
Benznidazole, in Chagas' disease, 583
Benzol, exposure to, aplastic anemia
  after, 1735
Benzoyl peroxide, in acne, 2279
Benztropine, in parkinsonism, 755
Benzyl penicillin G, aqueous, in
  syphilis, *515*
Bephenium, in malabsorption
  syndrome, *1536*
Bephenium hydroxynaphthoate, in
  fasciolopsiasis, 620
Berberine sulfate, in cutaneous
  leishmaniasis of old world, 588
Beriberi, 1688–1689
  cerebral, 773
  dry, 772–773
Beriberi heart disease, 1284, 1689

Bernard-Soulier syndrome, 1878–1879
Berry aneurysms, intracranial
  hemorrhage from, 794, 795, *795*
Berylliosis, pulmonary hypertension in,
  1147
Beryllium, sarcoidosis and, 210
Beryllium disease of lung, chronic, 990,
  991
Besnier, prurigo gestationis of, 2305
Beta cells, in diabetes mellitus, 1972,
  1973
Beta thalassemia
  heterozygous, 1778–1779
  homozygous, 1778
Beta-adrenergic blocking drugs
  in angina pectoris, 1228
  in arterial hypertension, *1212*, 1213,
    1214
Beta-aminoisobutyricaciduria, *2019*,
  2022–2023, 2044
Beta-glucuronidase deficiency, *41*
Beta-hydroxyisovaleric aciduria, *41*
Beta-lactamase, in drug resistance, 551
Betamethasone, in rheumatoid arthritis,
  192
Bethanidine, in hypertension
  complicating tetanus, 440
Bhang, 702
Bicarbonate, pancreatic secretion of, in
  chronic pancreatitis, 1556
Bicarbonate threshold concentration,
  1322
Bicillin. See *Benzathine penicillin G.*
Bicipital tendinitis, 206
Bicuspid aortic valve, functionally
  normal, 1155–1156
Bidirectional tachycardia, 1254, *1255*
Bielschowsky's disease, 850
Bifidobacterium eriksonii, 442
Bigeminy, ventricular, 1252, *1252*
Biguanides, in diabetes mellitus, 1986,
  1986
Bile, 1618
  average composition of, *1619*
  bilirubin secretion in, 1636, 1637
Bile acid breath test, in malabsorption
  syndrome, 1531
Bile acids
  conjugated, deficiency of, 1536, 1537
    treatment of, 1538
  in fat absorption, 1524
  deconjugation of, decreased,
    treatment of, 1538
    increased, 1537
  metabolism of, in liver disease, 1642,
    1643
  serum, measurement of, 1646
Bile ascites, 1593
Bile duct(s)
  common, tumors of, carcinoid
    features of, 2212
  diseases of, 1618–1636
    roentgenologic examination in,
      1622–1623, *1623*
  obstruction of
    extrahepatic, vs. biliary cirrhosis,
      1666
    uncommon causes of, 1632–1633
  tumors of, benign, 1635
    malignant, 1634–1635
Bile peritonitis, in needle biopsy of
  liver, 1648
Bile pigments, fecal and urinary
  excretion of, 1638–1639

Bile pigments (*Continued*)
  fecal and urinary excretion of,
    measurement of, 1646
Bile salts, 1619
  intestinal reabsorption of, 1619
Bilharziasis, 611–617. See also
  Schistosomiasis.
Biliary cirrhosis, 1666–1667, *2299*
  conjugated bile acid deficiency in,
    1537
  vs. chronic active hepatitis, 1662
  vs. malignant bile duct tumors, 1635
Biliary colic, 1624–1625
  vs. myocardial infarction, 1233
Biliary obstruction, dyslipoproteinemia
  in, 2010
Biliary stricture, 1631–1632
  vs. choledocholithiasis, 1630
  vs. malignant bile duct tumors, 1635
Biliary tract
  diseases of, 1618–1636
    acute pancreatitis and, 1551
    diagnosis of, procedures for, 1648
    endoscopic retrograde
      cholangiopancreatography in,
      1472–1473, *1472*, *1473*
    plasma cell dyscrasia associated
      with, 1866–1867
    roentgenologic examination in,
      1622–1623, *1623*
    neoplasm of, vs. choledocholithiasis,
      1630
Bilious typhoid, 526–529
Bilious vomiting, after peptic ulcer
  surgery, 1520
Bilirubin
  conjugated, excretion of, 1637
    reduced, 1638
  conjugation of, hepatic, reduced, 1638
    impaired, neonatal, 1649
  hepatic uptake of, 1637
    reduced, 1638
  in hemolytic disorders, 1753
  intestinal degradation of, 1638
  metabolism of, 1637–1638
    disorders of, 1648, 1649, 1650
  production of, 1637
    excessive, 1638
  serum, measurement of, 1645
  transport and distribution of, 1637
Bilirubin encephalopathy, 1649
Bing-Neel syndrome, in
  macroglobulinemia, 1862
Bioaminergic pathways in brain, 2076,
  2076
Biochemical processes, renal injury
  from, 1329–1330
Biologic aspects of carcinogenesis,
  1908–1909, *1908*
Biologic factors, role of, in disease, 13, 14
Biologic processes in puberty, 17–20, *18*
Biological science, medical practice
  and, 6–8
Biopsy
  bone marrow, in agnogenic myeloid
    metaplasia, 1828
    in aplastic anemia, 1738
    in Hodgkin's disease, 1842, *1843*
    in myelophthisic anemia, 1742
  brain, 750
    in intracranial inflammatory
      disease, 804
  cerebral, in herpes simplex
    encephalitis, 823

Biopsy (*Continued*)
  endometrial, 2180
  hepatic
    in chronic active hepatitis, 1662
    in hemochromatosis, 1791
    in sarcoidosis, 214
    needle, 1647–1648
  jejunal, in malabsorption syndrome,
    1532, *1533*, *1534*, *1535*
    in protein-losing enteropathy, *1549*
  lung, 950
  lymph node, in pulmonary disease,
    949, 950
  meningeal, in intracranial
    inflammatory disease, 804
  muscle, in differentiation of
    neurogenic and myopathic
    disease, 915
    in polymyositis and
      dermatomyositis, 172
    in trichinosis, 630, 631
  nerve, in peripheral neuropathy, 905
  peritoneal, 1592
  pleural, 950, 1014
  rectal, in congenital megacolon, 1495
    in schistosomiasis, 615
    in ulcerative colitis, 1569
  renal, 1345, 1346
    in interstitial nephritis, 1418
    in nephrotic syndrome, 1389
  skin, 2273, 2274, *2274*
    in systemic lupus erythematosus,
      176
  techniques of, in pulmonary disease,
    949–950
  temporal artery, in polymyalgia
    rheumatica, 217
  testicular, in evaluation of testicular
    function, 2165
  thyroid, needle, 2119
Biotin, nutrient value of, 1672
Bird breeder's lung, *971*
Bird spiders, bites of, 114
Birth control, 2194–2197
Biskra button, 587
Bismuth
  colloidal, in peptic ulcer, 1515
  nephrotoxicity from, *1428*, 1431
Bite(s)
  centipede, 117
  flea, 110
  snake-, 121–123
  spider, 114–115
Bithionol
  in fascioliasis, 619
  in paragonimiasis, *559*, 620
Biton. See *Bithionol.*
Bitot spots, in hypovitaminosis A, 1675,
  1684, *1685*
Bittersweet, poisoning by, 70
Black widow spider bites, 115
Blackfat tobacco smokers' lung, 998, 999
Blackout, weightlifter's, 746
Blackwater fever, 569, 572, 1770
Bladder
  anomalies of, 1458
  function of, after myocardial
    infarction, 1234
  in diabetes mellitus, 1980
  inflammation of, 1409, 1410
  lining of, candidiasis in ͫ
Blast crisis, in chronic gͥ
  leukemia, 1822, 1823
Blastoma, pulmonary, 101.

Blastomyces dermatitidis, 540
Blastomycosis, 540–541
  European, 543–544
  North American, 540–541
  South American, 541–542
  vs. chromomycosis, 543
  vs. coccidioidomycosis, 539
  vs. cutaneous leishmaniasis of new
    world, 589
Bleeding. See also *Hemorrhage(s).*
  **capillary, infiltrative diseases
    associated with, 976**
  gastrointestinal, 1520–1523
    angiography in, 1471, *1471*
    disorders associated with,
      cutaneous signs of, *2298*
    in cancer patient, 1905
    in hypothalamic dysfunction, 717
    in peptic ulcer, 1516, 1517
    iron deficiency from, 1748
    portal hypertension and, in
      cirrhosis, 1665
  in anticoagulant therapy of
    thrombophlebitis, 1127, 1128
  in liver disease, 1643
  in louse-borne relapsing fever, 527
  tendency to, in chronic renal failure,
    1364
Bleeding diathesis(es), 1523
  albinism with, 2029
  in malabsorption syndrome, 1529
  intracranial hemorrhage from, 795
Bleeding esophageal varices, 1523
  in cancer patient, 1905
  in schistosomiasis, 614
Bleeding time
  in hereditary coagulation disorders,
    1884
  in von Willebrand's disease, 1887
Blenoxane. See *Bleomycin.*
Bleomycin, 1937
  in esophageal carcinoma, 1599
  in Hodgkin's disease, 1846
  in non-Hodgkin's lymphomas, *1836*
"Blind boil," 400
Blind loops, malabsorption from, 1537
"Blind staggers," 745
Blindness
  air travel and, 96
  as hysterical symptom, 679
  river, 635–636
    antimicrobial agents for, *559*
Blister beetles, 114
Blistering diseases, 2301, 2303–2306,
  2303
Blood
  banked, contaminated, transfusion
    reaction from, *1785,* 1786
  changes in, cerebral infarction from,
    781
    with aging, 26
  **circulating, anticoagulants in,
    1896–1897**
  coagulation of. See also *Coagulation.*
    defects of, 1881–1897
  culture of, in pneumococcal
    pneumonia, 352
  diseases of, 1713–1897
    cutaneous lesions in, *2302*
    in cancer patients, 1906
  group O donor, high-titer
    alloantibodies in, transfusion
    reaction from, 1787, 1788
    bacterial meningitis, 413

Blood (*Continued*)
  in cerebral metabolism, 646
  in visceral leishmaniasis, 586
  laboratory values for, 2346–2347
  lipid transport in, 2002–2003
  loss of, acute, clinical manifestations
    of, 1729, *1729*
    exceptional, hyperbaric oxygen
      therapy in, 104
    iron deficiency from, 1747, 1748
  **purification of, by dialysis,
    1376–1382.** See also *Hemodialysis.*
  replacement of, in head injury, 882
  transfusion of. See *Transfusion(s).*
  viscosity of, increased, in cerebral
    infarction, 781
Blood amylase, determination of, in
  acute pancreatitis, 1553
Blood cells. See names of specific blood
  cells and diseases affecting them.
Blood chemical values, 2348
Blood cultures
  in infective endocarditis, 391
  sterile, endocarditis with, treatment
    of, 394
Blood flow
  cutaneous, 2268
  hepatic, 1639
  mechanical obstruction to, in shock,
    1110
  pulmonary, 1136
    distribution of, 938
  redistribution of, in heart failure,
    1088
  renal, 1316
    impaired, renal injury from, 1330
    in shock, 1112
    measurement of, 1340, 1341
Blood gas exchange, assessment of, in
  acute respiratory failure, 1036
Blood gas values, arterial, significance
  of, 940–941
Blood glucose, as cardiovascular risk
  factor, 1062
Blood lipids, circulating, elevated, as
  risk factor for atherosclerosis, 1220
Blood pressure
  arterial, factors regulating, 1069
    maintenance of, control systems
      for, 1206–1208
    measurement of, 1074, 1200
    monitoring of, in shock, 1047, 1116,
      1117
  as risk factor for atherosclerosis, 1219,
    1220
  emergency reduction of, 1215, 1216
  high. See *Hypertension.*
  in obesity, 1695
  sustenance of, peripheral mechanisms
    for, in heart failure, 1088, 1089
"Blood sludging," in shock, 1112, 1113
Blood smears, in malaria diagnosis, 572
Blood transfusion. See *Transfusion(s).*
Blood vessels
  autoregulatory adjustment of, local,
    1111, 1112
  changes in, with aging, 26
  in electric injury, 93
Blood volume, 1070, 1071
  arterial, effective, in control of
    sodium excretion, 1321
  in shock, 1109
  maintenance of, in gastrointestinal
    bleeding, 1522

Blood volume (*Continued*)
  pulmonary, 1136
  pulmonary capillary, in diffusion,
    937, 938
Bloom's syndrome, *1910,* 2297
  acute leukemia in, 1814
  unrepaired chromosomal breakage in,
    54
"Blue bloaters," in chronic obstructive
  pulmonary disease, 961
Blue bottle, infestation by, 112
Blue rubber bleb disease, *2298*
Bochdalek, foramen of, herniation
  through, 1019
Bodily posture, disturbances in, 752
  in paralysis agitans, 753
Body louse, 108, 109
  in epidemic typhus, 318
Body plethysmography, 933
Body proportions, pubertal changes in,
  18, 19
Body temperature, basal, in evaluation
  of ovarian function, 2180
Boerhaave's syndrome, 1478
Boils, 399, 400
  Bagdad, 587
  "blind," 400
  Delhi, 587
Bolivian hemorrhagic fever, *293,*
  298–300
Bone
  anaerobic infection of, 444
  aseptic necrosis of, after renal
    transplantation, 1385
  calcium in, 2225
  calcium storage and exchange by,
    2231
  changes in, with aging, 267
  **congenital or hereditary diseases
    involving, 2263–2265**
  destruction of, in multiple myeloma,
    1858, *1859*
  diseases of, 2225–2265. See also
    names of specific diseases.
    in chronic renal failure, 1359, 1360
    in hyperparathyroidism, 2215, *2216*
  eosinophilic granuoma of, 1848
  fibrous dysplasia of, 2262–2263
  hydatid cyst of, 609, 610
  in acromegaly, 2105
  in bejel, 523
  in cryptococcosis, 544
  in Gaucher's disease, 2013
  in homocystinuria, 2028
  in sarcoidosis, 213, 214, 2235
  in tophaceous gout, *2036,* 2037
  lamellar, 2247
  lesions of, "atypical" mycobacteria
    causing, 500
  Paget's disease of, 2257–2259
    vs. hyperparathyroidism, 2217
  protein matrix of, 2230
  radionuclide toxicity of, 2261
  remodeling of, 2231
  resorption of, 2231
  **structure of, calcium homeostasis
    and, 2230–2232**
  tuberculosis of, 496–497
    cystic, 497
  turnover of, 2231
Bone marrow
  biopsy of, in agnogenic myeloid
    metaplasia, 1828
  in aplastic anemia, 1738

Bone marrow (*Continued*)
  biopsy of, in Hodgkin's disease, 1842, *1843*
    in myelophthisic anemia, 1742
  examination of, in acute leukemia, 1817
    in anemia of chronic disorders, 1731
    in aplastic anemia, 1733, 1736
    in chronic granulocytic leukemia, 1821
    in chronic lymphocytic leukemia, 1824
    in hereditary spherocytosis, 1756
    in Hodgkin's disease, 1841, *1843*
    in myeloproliferative disorders, 1826
    in non-Hodgkin's lymphomas, 1834
    in polycythemia vera, 1794, *1794*, 1795, 1796
    in sideroblastic anemia, 1740
    in visceral leishmaniasis, 585
  neutrophil development in, 1800, *1801*, 1807
  production of, diagnostic evaluation of, 150, *151*
  transplantation of, in aplastic anemia, 1738, 1739
    in hematologic form of acute radiation syndrome, 90
Bone scanning, in intraspinal compression, 892
Bonine. See *Meclizine*.
Bonnevie-Ulrich-Turner syndrome, vs. Ehlers-Danlos syndrome, 2055
Bordetella bronchiseptica, 426
Bordetella parapertussis, 426
Bordetella pertussis, 426, 427
Bornholm disease, 271–272
Borrelia duttonii, 526, 529
Borrelia recurrentis, 526, 528
Borrelia vincentii, 530
Boston exanthem, 274
Botflies, infestation by, 112
Botulism, 67–68
  neuromuscular block caused by, 929
  vs. myasthenia gravis, 927
Bouba, 518–522, *520.* See also *Yaws.*
Bouchard's nodes
  in degenerative joint disease, 203, *203*, 204
  vs. rheumatoid arthritis, 190
Bourneville's disease, 770–771
Bouton de Crete, 587
Boutonneuse fever, 325
  clinical features of, *313*
  epidemiologic features of, *310*
Bowel. See *Intestine(s)* and names of specific intestinal components.
Bowen's disease, 2286, 2287
Brachial plexus, neuropathy of, 902
Bradycardia
  in intracranial tumors, 864
  in shock, 1109
  sinus, 1243
    in myocardial infarction, 1230, 1235
    in shock, 1118
    in sick sinus syndrome, 1244
Bradycardia-tachycardia syndrome, 1244, *1244*
Bradykinin, circulatory effects of, 1111
Brain
  abscess of, 804–807
    amebic, 592
    cerebrospinal fluid findings in, *803*, 806, 807

Brain (*Continued*)
  abscess of, enteric bacteria causing, 454
    epilepsy associated with, 852
    in nocardiosis, 475
    presenting as "acute meningitis," 806
    vs. brain tumor, 868, 869
    vs. cerebral infarction, 790
    vs. herpes simplex encephalitis, 823
    vs. viral meningitis or encephalitis, 820
  bioaminergic pathways, in, 2076, *2076*
  biopsy of, 750
    in intracranial inflammatory diseases, 804
  disorders of, respiratory failure in, *1023*, 1024
    sexual precocity due to, 2182
    WAIS scores in, 682
  function of, in intracranial tumors, 864
  fungal infections of, vs. dementia in cancer, 877
  in acromegaly, 2106
  in arboviral encephalitis, 283
  in decompression sickness, *103*
  in Reye's syndrome, 839
  in right ventricular failure, 1093
  "interstitial" edema of, in benign intracranial hypertension, 871
  metabolic disease of, 644–651
    autonomic activity in, 648
    causes of, *644*
    causing coma, 642
    clinical features of, 647–649
    diagnosis of, 649–651
    electroencephalography in, 649
    laboratory evaluation of, 649, *649*
    mental changes in, 647, 648
    motor activity in, 648
    pathophysiologic aspects of, 645–647
    prognosis and treatment of, 651, *651*
    suspected, physical examination in, *647*
    ventilation in, 649
  metastatic disease of, vs. dementia in cancer, 877
  nonmetastatic effects of cancer on, 876–878
  structural and vascular anatomy of, 781–784, *781–784*
  structural lesions of, vs. narcolepsy, 654
  swelling of, in bacterial meningitis, 412, 416
  tumors of, 863–869
    epilepsy associated with, 853
    headache in, 730, 864, 865
    intracranial hemorrhage in, 795
      arteriography in, 799
    metastatic, 864, 868
    primary, 863
    vs. benign intracranial hypertension, 872
    vs. cerebral infarction, 790
  vasogenic edema of, 864
Brain death, criteria for, 1031
Brain scan, radionuclide, 748–749
  in brain abscess, 806
  in cerebral infarction, 790
  in herpes simplex encephalitis, 823

Brainstem
  hemorrhage into, clinical manifestations of, 798
  in acute head injury, 881
  infarctions in, 786, 787
  ischemia of, 784
  tumors of, 868
Branched-chain aminoaciduria, 2021
Branched-chain hyperaminoacidemia, *2016–2017*
Branched-chain ketoaciduria, intermittent, *41*
Branham's sign, in arteriovenous fistula, 1312
Brawny scleritis, 2315
Breast(s)
  cancer of
    in males, 1921
    medical treatment of, 1918–1921
  development of, *18, 19*
  Paget's disease of, 2287
    anal involvement in, 1618
    breast carcinoma and, *2296,* 2297
    pigeon, 1020, 1021
    tuberculosis of, 498
Breathing. See also *Respiration*.
  assisted, in cardiopulmonary arrest, 1054, 1055
  control of, 932, 938–939
    abnormalities of, 939
Bridegroom's palsy, 902
Brill-Zinsser disease, 320
  clinical features of, *313*
  epidemiologic features of, *310*
  serologic responses in, *314*
Briquet's syndrome, 679
Broad Street pneumonia, 359
Broad-beta disease, 2005–2006
Broca's aphasia, 657
  apraxia in, 658
Brodie's abscess, 2260
Bromide intoxication, 700, 701, 714
Bromocriptine, in parkinsonism, 756
Bromophenol blue test for proteinuria, 1337
Brompheniramine
  in allergic rhinitis, 160
  in angioedema, 163
  in drug allergy, 157
  in serum sickness, 154
  in urticaria, 162
  in vasomotor rhinitis, 160
Bromsulphalein clearance, 1646
Bronchial adenoma, 1011
Bronchial arteries, 1135
Bronchial arteriography, 944
Bronchial carcinoid tumors, 1011, 2210, *2211*
Bronchial hygiene, in simple chronic bronchitis, 955
Bronchial type of chronic obstructive pulmonary disease, 961, *961*
Bronchiectasis, 982–983
  pulmonary hypertension in, 1147
  respiratory failure from, 1023
  vs. mucopurulent bronchitis, 954
  vs. pulmonary paragonimiasis, 620
  vs. pulmonary tuberculosis, 486
  vs. simple chronic bronchitis, 954
Bronchiolitis fibrosa obliterans, 1001
Bronchitis, 235–236, *235*
  chemical, acute, 1000
  chronic, 952
    antimicrobial prophylaxis in, *564*

Bronchitis (*Continued*)
  chronic, simple, 951, **953–955**
    mucopurulent, 954
    mycoplasmal, 343, 345
    obstructive, chronic, 951, 960
    occupational, 995–996
    respiratory failure from, 1023
Bronchodilators
  in chronic respiratory failure, 1029
  in simple chronic bronchitis, 955
Bronchogenic carcinoma, 1005–1010
  dust exposure and, 994, 995
  hepatic metastases in, scanning in, *1469*
  staging of, 1008, *1009*
  vs. lung abscess, 981
Bronchogenic cysts, 1002
Bronchography, in pulmonary disease, 943
Bronchopneumonia
  bacterial, vs. pneumocystosis, 599
  in nocardiosis, 475
Bronchopulmonary sequestration, 1003
Bronchoscopy
  fiberoptic, in sarcoidosis, 214
    microbiologic diagnosis by, 342
  in bronchogenic carcinoma, 1008
  in pulmonary disease, 949
Bronchospasm, in asthma, 955
Brown-Séquard's syndrome, 890
  in meningovascular syphilis, 814
Brucella abortus, 475, 476
Brucella agglutination test, 477, 478
Brucella canis, 476
Brucella melitensis, 475, 476
Brucella skin test, 477, 478
Brucella suis, 475, 476
Brucellosis, 475–479
  vs. Chagas' disease, 582
  vs. psittacosis, 338
  vs. toxoplasmosis, 597
  vs. visceral leishmaniasis, 586
Brugia malayi, 605, 632, 634
Bruton type of agammaglobulinemia, 139, 150, *1910*
BSP clearance, 1646
Bubonic plague, 463, 464, 465
Budd-Chiari syndrome, 1661
Buerger's disease, 1302
Buffalo leeches, as agents of disease, 120
Bulbar encephalitis, in cancer, 877
Bulbar myasthenia gravis, vs. hysteria, 679
Bulbar palsy, progressive, 765
Bulbar paralysis, in botulism, 67, 68
Bulbar poliomyelitis, 831
Bulk-forming agents, in constipation, 1482
Bullae, 2273, 2301, 2302
Bullous disease of lung, 1003–1004
Bullous impetigo, 400
Bullous myringitis, in mycoplasmal pneumonia, 345, 346
Bundle branch block, in myocardial infarction, 1236
Bundle of His, 1242
Bürger-Grütz syndrome, 2006–2007
Burkitt's lymphoma, 1838–1839
  malaria and, 567
Burning feet syndrome, 773
Burns
  antimicrobial prophylaxis in, *564*
  arc, 93

Burns (*Continued*)
  ascorbic acid deficiency in, 1691
  surfaces of, enteric bacteria in, 455
  thermal, hyperbaric oxygen therapy in, 105
  volume depletion in, 1951
Burr holes, in diagnosis of head injury, 881
Bursae
  synovial, extension or rupture of, in rheumatoid arthritis, 188
  tuberculosis of, 497
Bursitis, 207
  calcific tendinitis and, 206
Buruli ulcer(s), 500
  vs. tropical phagedenic ulcer, 530
Buschke, scleredema adultorum of, vs. scleroderma, 170
Busulfan, 1932
  in agnogenic myeloid metaplasia, 1828
  in chronic granulocytic leukemia, 1823
  in polycythemia vera, 1797
  pulmonary hypersensitivity reactions from, 975
  toxicity of, 1823
Busulfan lung, 1823
Butanol-extractable iodine, determination of, 2117
Butazolidin. See *Phenylbutazone*.
Butterfly cod, envenomation by, 124
Butterfly rash, in systemic lupus erythematosus, 174, 175, 176
Bypass grafts, aortocoronary, 1238–1241
Byssinosis, 997–998

C1 deficiency, 137
C'1 esterase inhibitor, deficiency of, in angioedema, 162, 163
C1q deficiency, *43*
C1r deficiency, *43*, 144
C2 deficiency, *43*, 137, 144
C3 deficiency, *43*, 138, 144, 1804
  infections in, *148*
C3b inactivator deficiency, 136, 138
C4 deficiency, 137
C5 deficiency, 144
C5 dysfunction, 1804
  infections in, *148*
C5-C8 deficiency, 138
C6 deficiency, 144
C7 deficiency, 144
Cachexia, in right ventricular failure, 1093
Caddis flies, allergic response to, 112
Cadmium
  nephrotoxicity from, *1428*, 1429
  poisoning by, 81–82
Cadmium oxide, exposure to, respiratory effects of, 1000
Café-au-lait spots, 2290
  in neurofibromatosis, 2293, *2293*
Caisson disease, 102–103
Calabar swellings, in loiasis, 635
Calcific tendinitis, bursitis and, 206
Calcification
  gallbladder, in chronic cholecystitis, 1625
  pineal, 2112
Calcinosis, metastatic, *2300*

Calcitonin, 2213–2214
  in hypercalcemia, 2239, 2240
  in Paget's disease, 2259
  medullary carcinoma of thyroid and, 2223–2224
Calcium, 2225–2228
  absorption of, 1526, 2227
  elemental, in osteomalacia of malabsorption, 2249
  excretion of, 2227–2228
    in chronic renal failure, 1359, *1359*
  homeostasis of, 2227–2228
    bone structure and, 2230–2232
  in bone, 2225
  in hypoparathyroidism, 2221
  in plasma, 2225–2227
  in shock, 1048
  malabsorption of, in maintenance hemodialysis, 1381
    in uremia, 2255
  metabolism of, in sarcoidosis, 215
    renal disease secondary to, 1402
  parathyroid hormone in, 2213
  nutrient value of, 1673
  plasma concentrations of, in osteomalacia, 2248
  recommended allowances of, *1671*
Calcium carbonate
  in peptic ulcer, 1513
  in renal calculi, 1446
Calcium chloride, in ventricular fibrillation, 1057
Calcium disodium edetate, in lead poisoning, 79
Calcium ethylenediamine-tetraacetate, in lead nephropathy, 1429
Calcium gluconate
  in colic of lead poisoning, 79
  in malabsorption syndrome, *1536*
  in postoperative tetany complicating hyperparathyroidism, 2220
  in puss-caterpillar dermatitis, 119
  in renal calculi, 1446
Calcium lactate
  in hyperkalemia, 1960
  in hypoparathyroidism, 2221
Calculi, renal, 1443–1446
  2,8-dihydroxyadenine, 2043
  in gout, 2037
    treatment of, 2041
  in paraplegia, 888
  in regional enteritis, 1564
California arbovirus complex, 288
California encephalitis, 288
Callosal syndromes, 658
Calluses, painful, 903
Calomel, hypersensitivity to, 80
Calomys callosus, 299
Calomys laucha, 299
Calomys musculinus, 299
Caloric balance, feeding behavior and, 717–718
Caloric supplementation, in malabsorption syndrome, *1536*
Caloric test, in evaluation of dizziness, 738
Calories, nutrient value of, 1670
Calymmatobacterium granulomatis, 429
Camp fever, 318–320
Canavan's disease, 850
Cancer(s), 1898–1948. See also *Carcinoma* and names and sites of specific malignancies.
  anemia in, 1732

Cancer(s) (*Continued*)
 Cushing's syndrome and, 1914, 1915, 1916, *2297*
 dermatomyositis in, 879, *2296, 2297*
 disseminated, management of, 1923
 endocrine syndromes associated with, 1914–1918
 environmental factors in, 1907–1911
 extent of, evaluation of, 1899, 1900
 genetic factors in, 1909–1910, *1910*
 histologic diagnosis of, 1899
 hormone-dependent, medical treatment of, 1918–1922
 hypercalcemia associated with, 1903, 1917, 2233–2234
 immune surveillance of, 1924–1925
 in renal transplant recipient, 1385, 1386
 incidence of, 1907–1908
 internal medicine and, 1898–1907
 localized, management of, 1923
 medical complications of, definition of, 1900
 medical manifestations of, 1901–1907, *1902*
 multinodular goiter and, 2136, 2137
 nonmetastatic effects of, on nervous system, 876–879, *877*
 patient history in, 1898
 patient with
  immune competence in, 1925–1926
  internist's approach to, 1898–1901
 physical examination in, 1898
 previous treatment of, investigation of, 1900
 primary site of, establishment of, 1899
 second, possibility of, 1899
 process of, activity of, assessment of, 1900
 regionalized, management of, 1923
 terminal, patient care in, 1941–1948
 treatment of, principles of, 1922–1941
  supportive care in, 1941
 viruses and, 1910
Cancer family syndrome, 1606
Candida abscesses, 548
Candida albicans, 547, 548
Candida denture stomatitis, 548
Candida endocarditis, 387
Candida granuloma, 548
Candida infections of skin, 2282, 2283
Candida meningitis, 548
Candida parapsilosis, 547
Candida tropicalis, 547
Candida vaginitis, 548
Candidiasis, 547–549
 systemic, in neutropenia, 149
Candidosis, 547–549
Canicola fever, 532
Cannabis, 702–703
Cannulas, nasal, for oxygenation in acute respiratory failure, 1027
Cantharidin, 114
Capillaria hepatica, 623
Capillaria philippinensis, 623
Capillariasis, 623
Capillary(ies)
 blood flow through, shock and, 1112, 1113
 pulmonary, 1135
Capillary bleeding, infiltrative diseases associated with, 976
Capillary system, 1067

Caplan's syndrome, 992, 993
 in rheumatoid arthritis, 187, 992, 993
Capreomycin, *556*
 in pulmonary tuberculosis, 488, 490
Capsular hemorrhage, clinical manifestations of, 797, 798
Capsulitis, adhesive, 207
Caput medusae, in portal hypertension, 1640
Carate, *520,* 524–525
Carbamazepine
 hyponatremia induced by, 1954
 in dystonia musculorum deformans, 761
 in epilepsy, *859,* 860
 in tabes dorsalis, 512
 in trigeminal neuralgia, 727
Carbamyl phosphate synthetase deficiency, *2018,* 2022
Carbenicillin, *557,* 558, 559
 adverse reactions to, 559, 560
 in bacterial meningitis, 416
 in infective endocarditis, 394
Carbenoxolone sodium, in peptic ulcer, 1515
Carbohydrate(s)
 absorption of, 1525
 abnormal, manifestations of, 1529
 in chronic renal failure, 1361
 in kwashiorkor, 1682
 metabolism of, disorders of, 1969–2001
  in liver disease, 1642
  inborn errors of, *41*
  oral contraceptive use and, 2195
 nutrient value of, 1670
 tolerance to, in Cushing's syndrome, 2154
 unabsorbed, tests for, 1530, 1531
Carbon dioxide, diffusion of, 936
Carbon monoxide poisoning, 82–84
 acute, hyperbaric oxygen therapy in, 104
 chronic, secondary polycythemia in, 1799
Carbon monoxide–diffusing capacity, 937
 abnormalities of, 937–938
Carbon tetrachloride
 as hepatotoxin, 1658
 as nephrotoxin, 1434
 poisoning by, 75
Carbonic anhydrase inhibitors
 in heart failure, *1103, 1104,* 1105
 metabolic acidosis from, 1962
Carboxyhemoglobin concentrations, in carbon monoxide poisoning, 82, 83
Carbuncles, 400
Carcinoembryonic antigen
 as tumor marker, 1911, 1912
 in colorectal carcinoma, 1609
Carcinogenesis, human, 1907–1911
Carcinogens
 biologic aspects of, 1908–1909, *1908*
 chemical, 1908, *1908,* 1909
 environmental, detection of, 1910–1911
Carcinoid flush, 2208, *2211*
 treatment of, 2212, 2213
Carcinoid syndrome, 2207–2213, *2298*
 classic, 2210, *2211*
 malignant, metastatic, malabsorption in, 1547

Carcinoid tumors, 2207
 bronchial, 1011, 2210, *2211*
 gastric, 2210, *2211,* 2212
 ileal, 2210, *2211*
 vs. regional enteritis, 1565
Carcinoma. See also *Cancer(s)* and names and sites of specific malignancies.
 adenoid cystic, 1012
 anal, 1618
 bronchogenic, 1005–1010
  dust exposure and, 994, 995
  hepatic metastases in, scanning in, *1469*
  staging of, 1008, *1009*
  vs. lung abscess, 981
 colonic, 1606–1610
  in ulcerative colitis, 1574
  vs. amebiasis, 592
  vs. diverticulitis, 1583
 cutaneous, squamous cell, 2309
 eosinophilia in, 226
 esophageal, 1597–1599
 gallbladder, 1633–1634
 gastric, 1599–1603
 hepatic, primary, 1668
  secondary, 1667
 neuropathy associated with, 910
 pancreatic, 1557–1559
  acinar cell, vs. Weber-Christian disease, 222
  acute pancreatitis and, 1551
  angiography in, *1470,* 1471
  percutaneous transhepatic cholangiography in, *1473*
 polymyositis and, 172
 prostatic
  hypofibrinogenemia in, 1894
  medical treatment of, 1921–1922
 rectal, 1606–1610
 renal, 1458–1460
  embryonal, 1460
 small intestinal, in adult celiac disease, 1541
 thyroid, 2141, 2143–2144, *2144*
  medical treatment of, 1922
  medullary, 2143, 2223–2224
   carcinoid features of, 2212
Carcinomatosis, lymphangitic, pulmonary hypertension in, 1147
Carcinomatous meningitis, 867
Carcinomatous myopathy, 923
Carcinosarcoma(s)
 esophageal, 1599
 pulmonary, 1012
Cardiac. See also *Heart.*
Cardiac amyloidosis, 1285–1286
Cardiac arrest
 causes of, 1053, *1053*
 ventricular fibrillation causing, 1056, 1057
Cardiac arrhythmia, 1242–1268. See also *Arrhythmia(s)* and names of specific arrhythmias.
Cardiac auscultation, 1075
Cardiac catheterization, 1078–1079
 in acquired valvular heart disease, 1178
 in aortic regurgitation, 1196
 in aortic stenosis, 1193
 in asymmetric septal hypertrophy, 1279
 in atrial septal defect, 1162
 in congenital valvular aortic stenosis, 1157

Cardiac catheterization (*Continued*)
  in mitral regurgitation, 1187
  in mitral stenosis, 1183
  in mitral valve prolapse syndrome,
    1189
  in pericardial constriction, 1275
  in primary pulmonary hypertension,
    1141
  in selection of patients for myocardial
    revascularization, 1239
Cardiac cirrhosis, 1092, **1667**
Cardiac compression, external, in
  cardiopulmonary resuscitation, 1055
Cardiac contractility, 1066, *1066*, 1083,
  1084, 1085
**Cardiac hemolytic anemia, traumatic,
  1767**
Cardiac murmur. See *Murmur(s).*
Cardiac myxoma, 1288
Cardiac output, 1083, 1084, *1084*
  during exercise, 1070
  factors determining, 1068, 1069
  in arterial hypertension, 1208
  in liver disease, 1644
  in shock, 1109
    monitoring of, 1117
  increase of, in management of heart
    failure, 1093
  regional distribution of, 1067
  serial determinations of, 1032, 1083
  sustenance of, peripheral mechanisms
    for, in heart failure, 1088, 1089
Cardiac pacemakers, 1267–1268, *1267,
  1268*
  in cardiopulmonary resuscitation, 1057
Cardiac rupture, in myocardial
  infarction, 1231
Cardiac standstill, reflex, syncope in,
  743
Cardiac tamponade, 1273
Cardiac tumors, 1288
Cardiac valve, prosthetic, underlying
  infective endocarditis, 387
Cardiogenic shock, surgical treatment
  in, 1121, 1122
Cardiomyopathy(ies), 1276–1288
  alcoholic, 1284, 1285
  catecholamine, 2203
  cobalt-beer, 1285
  congestive, 1277
  familial, 1280–1281
  in Chagas' disease, 581, 582, 583, 1283
  infective, 1281–1283
  inflammatory, 1281–1283
  miscellaneous, 1286–1287
  nutritional, 1283–1285
  obstructive, hypertrophic, 1278
  peripartum, 1287
  restrictive, 1277
**Cardiopulmonary arrest, resuscitation
  in, 1053–1058,** *1054*
Cardiospasm, 1486–1488, *1487*
Cardiotoxicity, digitalis, 1098
  treatment of, 1099
Cardiovascular syphilis, 511, **1294–1295,**
  1295
  treatment of, 516, 1295
Cardiovascular system
  changes in, in arterial hypertension,
    1208
  **circulatory function and control in,
    1063–1072**
  diseases of, 1059–1315

Cardiovascular system (*Continued*)
  diseases of, data collection in, 1072
    death rates for, *1060, 1061*
    history in, 1072, 1073
    **patient with, approach to,
      1072–1079**
    physical examination in, 1073–1075
    **prevalence and epidemiology of,
      1059–1063,** *1060, 1061, 1062*
    risk factors for, 1061, 1062, *1062,*
      1063, 1201, 1202, *1202*
  in acute radiation syndrome, 88, 90
  in acute renal failure, 1372
  in cancer patient, 1905
  in carcinoid syndrome, 2208
  in chronic renal failure, 1365
  in Cushing's syndrome, 2154
  in electric injury, 93
  in hypothalamic dysfunction, 717
  in liver disease, 1644
  in maintenance hemodialysis, 1381,
    1382
  in Marfan's syndrome, 2053
  in obesity, 1695
  in paraplegia, 887
  in rickettsial diseases, 316
  in systemic lupus erythematosus, 177
  in tetanus, 440
  integrated function of, 1068–1072
  response of, to stress, 1070, *1070*
Carditis, in rheumatic fever, 380
Carey-Coombs murmur, in carditis of
  rheumatic fever, 380
Caries
  dental, pathogenesis of, 367
  tuberculous, 497
Carmustine, in oncologic treatment,
  1932, 1933
Carnosinemia, *41, 2019*
Caroli's disease, 1632
Carotid artery, internal
  occlusion of, 786–787
  stenosis of, ischemia from, 784, 785
  thrombosis of, in head injury, 884
Carotid sinus
  hypersensitivity of, dizziness in, 740
  stimulation of, in evaluation of
    dizziness, 737
Carotid sinus syncope, 743, 744
Carotid–cavernous sinus fistula, in head
  injury, 884
Carotene, serum, measurement of, in
  malabsorption syndrome, 1530
Carpal tunnel syndrome, 207, 901
Carrier state
  after *Salmonella* infection, 449, 451
  in acute viral hepatitis type B, 1654
  in alpha thalassemia, 1771
  in chronic granulomatous disease,
    1805
  in classic hemophilia, 1886
  in diphtheria, 433
  in meningococcal disease, 422
  in pneumococcal pneumonia, 348
  in typhoid fever, 447
    treatment of, 448
Carrión's disease, 331–332
Carvallo's sign
  in staphylococcal endocarditis, 403
  in tricuspid regurgitation, 1198
Carybdea species, envenomation by, 123
Casal's necklace, in pellagra, 1688
Castor bean, poisoning by, 70

Casts, urinary, 1338, 1339
  in chronic renal failure, 1353, 1354
CAT. See *Computerized tomography.*
Cat scratch disease, 302–305, *303, 304*
  vs. toxoplasmosis, 597
  vs. tularemia, 467
Cat scratch skin test, 303, 304
Catabolic states, energy requirements
  in, 1704, 1705
Catagen, 2270, 2271
Cataplexy, 653, 654
Cataract(s)
  extraction of, dizziness after, 741
  in classic galactosemia, 1997, 1998
  in galactokinase deficiency, 1998
  in radiation injury, 89
  in sarcoidosis, 2330
  "snowflake," in diabetes mellitus,
    1976, 2320
Catatonia, periodic, 668
Catatonic symptoms, in schizophrenia,
  666
Catecholamine(s), 2200
  excess of, hypertension associated
    with, 1209, 1210
  metabolism of, routes of, 2200, *2200*
  mode of action of, 2070, 2071, *2071*
  pharmacology of, 2200, 2201
  synthesis of, 2200, *2200*
  urinary measurement of, in
    pheochromocytoma, 2203, 2204,
    2204
Catecholamine cardiomyopathy, 2203
**Caterpillars, dermatitis caused by,
  118–119**
Catfishes, envenomation by, 124, 125
Cathartic colon, 1614
Cathartic medication, 1482
  abuse of, 1481
  systemic effects of, 1614
Catheterization
  cardiac, 1078–1079
    in acquired valvular heart disease,
      1178
    in aortic regurgitation, 1196
    in aortic stenosis, 1193
    in asymmetric septal hypertrophy,
      1279
    in atrial septal defect, 1162
    in congenital valvular aortic
      stenosis, 1157
    in mitral regurgitation, 1187
    in mitral stenosis, 1183
    in mitral valve prolapse syndrome,
      1189
    in pericardial constriction, 1275
    in primary pulmonary
      hypertension, 1141
    in selection of patients for
      myocardial revascularization,
      1239
  central venous, in shock, 1116
  Swan-Ganz, in acute respiratory
    failure, 1043
    in shock, 1116
  urinary, in paraplegia, 888
    in shock, 1116
Cattle grub, infestation by, 112
Cauda equina
  compressive lesions of, 891, 892
  disease of, vs. arteriosclerosis
    obliterans, 1301
  in ankylosing spondylitis, 195

Cauda equina (*Continued*)
   intermittent claudication of, 895
   tumors of, anal pain from, 1618
      vs. hysteria, 679
Causalgia, 727
Caustics, poisoning by, 75
Cavernous angiomas
   intracranial hemorrhage from, 795
   of spinal cord, 898
Cavernous hemangioma, 1876
Cavernous sinus
   occlusion of, 789
   thrombosis of, 780, 808
      vs. Romaña's sign in Chagas'
        disease, 582
Cavitary *Klebsiella* disease, chronic, 358
Cavity formation
   in coccidioidomycosis, 538
   in pulmonary tuberculosis, 482
CCNU, in oncologic treatment, 1933
Cecal diverticulum, solitary, 1502
Cecum, vascular abnormalities of, 1590
Cefazolin, *556*, 560
   in gonococcal disease, 410
      in pregnancy, 409
   in infective endocarditis, 392, 393, 394
   in pneumococcal pneumonia, 356
   in staphylococcal pneumonia, 402
Cefoxitin, 560
Celiac axis, 1586, *1586*
Celiac compression syndrome, 1588
Celiac disease, adult, 1539–1541, *1541*
   clinical manifestations of, 1527
   jejunal histology in, 1533, *1533,*
      1534
   roentgenography in, 1532, *1533,*
      1540
   vs. chronic pancreatitis, 1557
   vs. eosinophilic gastroenteritis,
      1543
   vs. tropical sprue, 1545, 1546
Celiac sprue, 1539. See also *Celiac
disease, adult.*
Cell(s)
   APUD, hormone products of, 2061,
      2061
   B, 126, 128
      alterations of, in disease states, 130
      characteristics and estimation of,
        129–130, *129*
      deficiency of, infections in, *148,* 150
      development of, *128*
      in host defense, 146
        diagnostic evaluation of, 150, 151,
          151
      primary immunodeficiency diseases
        and, 138–143
   beta, in diabetes mellitus, 1972, 1973
   blood. See names of specific blood
      cells and diseases affecting them.
   Downey, in infectious
      mononucleosis, 266
   epithelioid, in sarcoidosis, 211
   foam, in Niemann-Pick disease, *2013,*
      2014
   Gaucher, 2012, 2013, *2013*
   "giant," in radiation injury, 87
      in sarcoidosis, 211
   in aging process, 26
   K, 129
   killer, 129
   Leydig, 2162
   "Pick," 661

Cell(s) (*Continued*)
   preparation of, for chromosomal
      analysis, 49
   Reed-Sternberg, in Hodgkin's
      disease, 1839, 1840
   stem, dysfunction of, in polycythemia
      vera, 1794, 1795
   T, 126, 128
      alterations of, in disease states, 130
      characteristics and estimation of,
        129–130, *129*
      deficiency of, treatment of, 152
      deficiency or dysfunction of,
        infections in, *148,* 150
      development of, *128*
      in host defense, 146
        diagnostic evaluation of, 150, 151,
          151
      in sarcoidosis, 210, *210,* 211
      primary immunodeficiency diseases
        and, 138–143
Cell count, in bacterial meningitis, 413
Cell membranes, drug interactions at,
   2337, 2338
Cell-cycle kinetics, cytotoxic agents and,
   1927
Cell-kill, total, concept of, in neoplastic
   therapy, 1926
Cell-mediated immunity
   impairment of, in sarcoidosis, 210
   in Graves' disease, 2121
   in Hashimoto's thyroiditis, 2129
   in malnutrition, 1679
   in measles, 247
Cell-mediated renal injury, 1327
Cellular defects, infections resulting
   from, in cancer, 1901, *1903*
Cellular membranes, in shock, 1114
Cellulitis
   anaerobic, 434, 443
      treatment of, 435
      vs. clostridial myonecrosis, *435*
   clostridial, 434
   crepitant, nonclostridial, 434
   in heroin addiction, 696
   orbital, vs. cavernous sinus
      thrombosis, 808
      vs. Romaña's sign in Chagas'
        disease, 582
   streptococcal, vs. erysipeloid of
      Rosenbach, 473
   vs. glanders, 469
Cellulose phosphate, in hypercalcemia,
   2239
Centipede bites, 117
Central core disease, 919
Central hearing loss, 734, 736
Central nervous system
   acute leukemia in, treatment of, 1818
   depressants of, abuse of, 698–701
      poisoning by, *712*
   **disorders of, amenorrhea due to,
      2187–2188**
   in acute radiation syndrome, 88, 90
   in acute renal failure, 1371, 1372
   in alcohol abuse, 709
   in arboviral encephalitis, 283
   in cat scratch disease, 303, 304
   in Colorado tick fever, 280
   in meningococcal infections, 420
   in periarteritis nodosa, 182
   in Rocky Mountain spotted fever, 323
   in schistosomiasis, 615

Central nervous system (*Continued*)
   in systemic lupus erythematosus, 180
   in western equine encephalitis, 285
   **infections and inflammatory diseases
      of, 802–816**
      in cancer patient, 1901, 1903
   lipidoses of, 850–851
   stimulants of, abuse of, 701–702
      poisoning by, *712*
   suppurative diseases of, cerebrospinal
      fluid findings in, *803*
   surgery of, in pain relief, 726, 727
   syphilis of, 812–816. See also
      Neurosyphilis.
   vascular accident to, in diabetes
      mellitus, 1980
Central peptidergic neuron systems,
   2077, *2078*
Central pontine myelinolysis, 775–776
Central venous catheterization, in
   shock, 1116
Central venous pressure, in acute
   respiratory failure, 1039
Centric fusion translocations, 53, *53*
Centrilobular emphysema, 960
Centromere, 50, *50,* 51
Centronuclear myopathy, 919
Centruroides sculpturatus, 116, 117
Cephalexin, *556,* 560
Cephaloridine, *556,* 560
   adverse reactions to, 560
Cephalosporins, *556,* 560
   adverse reactions to, 560
   as nephrotoxins, 1426
Cephalothin, *556,* 560
   adverse reactions to, 560
   as nephrotoxin, 1426
   in infective endocarditis, 392, 393, 394
   in infective endocarditis prophylaxis,
      396
   in pneumococcal pneumonia, 356
   in staphylococcal pneumonia, 402
Cephamandole, 560
Cephapirin, *556,* 560
   adverse reactions to, 560
Cephradine, *556,* 560
Ceramide lactoside lipidosis, 42
Cercopithecus aethiops, 300
Cerebellar abscess, 806
Cerebellar artery occlusion, posterior
   inferior, 788
Cerebellar cortical degeneration, 775
Cerebellar degeneration
   alcoholic, 775
   parenchymatous, 775
   subacute, in cancer, 877
Cerebellar hemorrhage, clinical
   manifestations of, 798
Cerebellar herniation, in intracranial
   tumors, 864
Cerebellar lesions, dysequilibrium in,
   741
Cerebellopontine angle tumor, 868
   vertigo caused by, 740
Cerebellum
   nonmetastatic effects of cancer on, 877
   tumors of, 867
Cerebral angiography
   in cerebral infarction, 790
   in head injury, 881
   in intracranial hemorrhage, 798, 799
Cerebral arterial occlusive disease,
   syncope in, 744, 745

Cerebral arteriography, 749
 in brain tumor, 867
 in cerebral infarction, 790
 in epilepsy, 857
 in herpes simplex encephalitis, 823
 in intracranial hemorrhage, 798, 799
Cerebral artery(ies)
 anterior, 781, *781*, *782*
  occlusion of, 787
 inflammatory states involving,
   cerebral infarction and, 779
 middle, 782, *782*
  occlusion of, 787
  thrombosis of, in head injury, 884
 posterior, *781*, 782, *782*, *784*
  occlusion of, 787
Cerebral beriberi, 773
Cerebral biopsy, in herpes simplex
  encephalitis, 823
Cerebral collateral circulation, cerebral
  infarction and, 779
Cerebral degenerative diseases, epilepsy
  associated with, 853
Cerebral edema
 following cardiopulmonary
   resuscitation, 1058
 in bacterial meningitis, 412
 in cerebral infarction, 778, 791
 in head injury, 881, 882, 883, 885
 in intracranial tumors, 864
 in louse-borne relapsing fever, 528
 in Reye's syndrome, 839
Cerebral emboli, 778
 anticoagulant drugs in, 793
 cerebral infarction from, 779–780
 vs. cerebral transient ischemic
   attacks, 785
Cerebral embolism, 788
 in head injury, 885
Cerebral epidural abscess, 808
 cerebrospinal fluid findings in, *803*
Cerebral gnathostomiasis, vs.
  angiostrongyliasis, 631
Cerebral hematoma, 794
 surgical removal of, 801
Cerebral hemispheres, tumors of, 867
Cerebral hemorrhage, 1205
Cerebral infarction, 778–794
 course of, 790–791
 differential diagnosis of, 790
 etiology of, 778
 incidence of, 778
 mechanisms of, 778–781
 neuropathology of, 778
 physical and laboratory findings in,
   789–790
 prevention of, 792–793
 prognosis in, 791
 signs and symptoms of, 785–786
 treatment of, 791–792
 vs. intracerebral hemorrhage, 797
Cerebral ischemia, 778–794. See also
 Cerebral infarction.
Cerebral malaria, 574
Cerebral metabolism, 646
Cerebral palsy, 760
Cerebral paragonimiasis, 620
Cerebral schistosomiasis, 615
Cerebral transient ischemic attacks,
  784–785
 anticoagulant drugs or surgery in, 792
Cerebral vascular. See *Cerebrovascular.*
Cerebral venous inflammation, cerebral
  infarction from, 780

Cerebral venous thrombosis, 788–789
 cerebral infarction from, 780
Cerebrospinal fever, 417
**Cerebrospinal fluid examination,
  747–748, 802–804,** *803*
 in acute disseminated
   encephalomyelitis, 837
 in acute hemorrhagic encephalitis,
   803
 in African trypanosomiasis, 578
 in bacterial meningitis, 413, 414, *803*
 in benign intracranial hypertension,
   870
 in brain abscess, *803*, 806, 807
 in cerebral epidural abscess, *803*
 in cerebral infarction, 789
 in coccidioidomycosis, 539
 in cryptococcal meningitis, *803*
 in cryptococcosis, 544
 in diffuse meningeal neoplasia, 867
 in epilepsy, 857
 in general paresis, 814
 in herpes simplex encephalitis, 823
 in hydrocephalus, 873
 in infective endocarditis with
   embolism, *803*
 in intracranial hemorrhage, 798
 in intracranial tumor, 866, 867
 in intraspinal compression, 892, 893
 in malaria, 571, 572
 in meningococcal meningitis, 420, 421
 in meningovascular syphilis, 814
 in multiple sclerosis, 844, 846
 in neoplastic meningitis, *803*
 in neurosyphilis, 511
 in nonsuppurative meningitis, *803*
 in poliomyelitis, 830
 in sarcoid meningitis, *803*
 in spinal epidural abscess, *803*
 in spinal epidural infections, 811
 in subdural empyema, *803*, 807
 in suppurative diseases of central
   nervous system and meninges, *803*
 in syphilitic meningitis, *803*, 813
 in tabes dorsalis, 815
 in thrombophlebitis, *803*
 in transverse myelitis, 812
 in tuberculous meningitis, *803*
 in ventricular empyema, *803*
 in viral encephalitis, 820
 in viral meningitis, *803*, 820
 normal values for, 2350
Cerebrospinal fluid fistula, in head
  injury, 883
Cerebrospinal meningitis, epidemic,
  417
Cerebrotendinous xanthomatosis, *42*
Cerebrovascular disease(s), 777–801
 epilepsy associated with, 853
 prevalence and epidemiology of, 1059
 signs and symptoms in, 784–789
  pathogenesis of, 781–784
 vertigo from, 739
Cerebrovascular insufficiency, vs.
  epilepsy, 858
Cerebrum, nonmetastatic effects of
  cancer on, 876
Cerumen, impacted, hearing loss from,
  735
Cervical adenitis
 "atypical" mycobacteria causing, 500
 suppurative, in streptococcal
   pharyngitis, 373
Cervical discs, herniated, 894

Cervical mucus, examination of, 2180
 in infertility, 2194
Cervical myelopathy, 895
Cervical radiculopathy, 895
Cervical spine
 compressive lesions of, 891
 degenerative disease of, 204
 hypertrophic spurs of, dysphagia
   from, 1483
 injuries of, 885, 886
Cervical spondylosis, 895
 pain of, vs. angina pectoris, 1227
 vs. multiple sclerosis, 847
 vs. vitamin B$_{12}$ deficiency, 776, 777
Cervical tuberculous lymphadenitis, 495
**Cervical vertebrae, congenital fusion of,
  875**
 syringomyelia and, 769
Cervicitis
 in chlamydial infection, 334
 mycoplasmal, 347
Cervicofacial actinomycosis, 474
Cervicogenic vertigo, 739
Cervix, tuberculosis of, 496
Cestodes, 606–611, *606*
 antimicrobial agents for, *559*
 prevalence of, *605*
Chagas' disease, 566, 575, 576, **579–583**
 immunodiagnostic tests for, *565*
 megacolon in, 582, 583, 1496
 myocarditis in, 581, 582, 583, 1283
Chagoma, 581
α-Chain disease, 1866
 lymphoma in, 1545
μ-Chain disease, 1866
Chains, polypeptide, in
  immunoglobulin structure, 126, *127*
Chancre
 in sleeping sickness, 577, 578
 in syphilis, 508, *509*
Chancroid, 425
 ulcers of, vs. syphilitic ulcer, 508
 vs. lymphogranuloma venereum, 335
Charas, 702
Charbon, 470
Charcoal, activated, in accidental
  poisoning, 74
Charcot joints, 200, 512
 in diabetes mellitus, 1980
Charcot-Marie-Tooth disease, 913
 vs. muscular dystrophies, 918
Charcot's triad, in intermittent
  cholangitis, 1629
Chédiak-Higashi syndrome, *43*, 144,
  1806–1807, *2302*
 host defense defects in, 149
Cheese worker's lung, *971*
Cheilosis, in malabsorption syndrome,
  1530
Chemical agents
 asthma-like reactions to, 999–1000
 carcinogenic, 1908, *1908*, 1909
 pericarditis caused by, 1272
 pulmonary effects of, *984*
 **pulmonary infiltrative disease caused
   by, 979**
 sarcoidosis caused by, 210
**Chemical and physical irritants to
  lungs, 983–1002,** *984*
Chemical bronchitis, acute, 1000
**Chemical contamination of water and
  air, 60–64**
Chemical factors in disease, 13
Chemical food poisoning, 70

"Chemical" meningitis, vs. bacterial meningitis, 414
Chemical pneumonitis, acute, 1000
Chemical pulmonary edema, 1001
in acute chemical bronchitis or pneumonitis, 1000
Chemodectomas, *1910*
Chemotaxis, 1801, *1801*
defects of, 1803
infections in, *148, 149, 150*
in host defense, 146
Chenodeoxycholate, 1619
in gallstones, 1620–1621
Chest
examination of, in pneumococcal pneumonia, 352
in stupor or coma, 643
funnel, 1020
pain in, in bronchogenic carcinoma, 1006
in diffuse collagenous pneumoconioses, 991
in pneumococcal pneumonia, 351
in pulmonary tuberculosis, 486
roentgenography of
in acquired valvular heart disease, 1177
in angina pectoris, 1226
in cardiovascular disease, 1075, 1076
in pulmonary disease, 941–944
wall of, disorders of, 1019–1021
respiratory failure in, *1023*, 1024
dynamic properties of, 933–935
static properties of, 932–933, *932*
volume-pressure relationships of, 932, *932*
Cheyne-Stokes respiration, in left ventricular failure, 1090
CHF-Congo virus, 298
Chiari-Frommel syndrome, 2191
prolactin levels in, 2092
Chickenpox, 253–255, 824, 825
acute disseminated encephalomyelitis after, 836, 837
vs. mild smallpox, 257
vs. rickettsialpox, 326
Chicle ulcer, *588*
Chigger-borne rickettsiosis, 327–328
Chiggers, 113
Chigoe bites, 110
Chikungunya fever, 279–280, *279*
Chikungunya virus, 279
Chilblain, 1310–1311
Chill(s)
in bronchogenic carcinoma, 1006
in louse-borne relapsing fever, 527, 528
in malaria, 571
in pneumococcal pneumonia, 351
Chilomastix mesnili, 602
China clay miners, pneumoconiosis in, 987
Chinese restaurant syndrome, 70
Chiropsalmus species, envenomation by, 123
Chlamydia psittaci, 336
Chlamydia trachomatis, 332
Chlamydiae
diseases caused by, 332–338
properties of, 332
Chloasma
oral contraceptive use and, 2196
vs. pinta, 525

Chloracne, 2279
Chloral hydrate
in heart failure, 1094
in insomnia, 653
in sleep disturbances complicating dementia, 663
Chlorambucil, 1932
in chronic lymphocytic leukemia, 1825
in macroglobulinemia, 1863
in polycythemia vera, 1797
Chloramphenicol, *556,* 562
aplastic anemia caused by, 1734, 1735
contraindications to, 553
in anaerobic infections, 445, *445*
in bacterial meningitis, 415, 416
in bartonellosis, 332
in lung abscess, 982
in malabsorption syndrome, *1536*
in plague, 465
in rickettsial diseases, 315
in tularemia, 468
in typhoid fever, 448
neuropathy from, 910
Chlordiazepoxide
abuse of, 698
in alcohol withdrawal syndrome, 710
in anxiety, 675
in depression, 678
poisoning by, *712*
Chlorinated hydrocarbon insecticides, poisoning by, 75
Chlorine, exposure to, respiratory effects of, 1000
Chloroguanide hydrochloride, in malaria prophylaxis, 575
Chloromas, 1822
Chlorophenothane, poisoning by, 75
Chloroquine
in amebiasis, *558*
in hepatic amebiasis, 593
in malaria, *558,* 573
in malaria prevention, 575
in Weber-Christian disease, 222
Chloroquine diphosphate, in clonorchiasis, 618
Chloroquine phosphate, in babesiosis, 601
Chloroquine susceptibility test, in malaria, 572
Chloroquine-resistant malaria, 573, 574, 575
Chlorosis, in iron deficiency anemia, 1748
Chlorothalidone, in arterial hypertension, *1212*
Chlorothiazide
hyponatremia induced by, 1954
in diabetes insipidus, 2111
in exophthalmos complicating Graves' disease, 2127
in heart failure, 1104, *1104*
Chlorpheniramine, in allergic rhinitis, 160
Chlorpromazine
in acute intermittent porphyria, 2047
in amphetamine poisoning, 75
in anorexia nervosa, 1702
in carcinoid flush, 2212
in dystonia musculorum deformans, 761
in mania of manic-depressive psychosis, 671
in pain, *724*

Chlorpromazine (*Continued*)
in schizophrenia, 669
in vertigo, 739
neutropenia induced by, 1808, 1809
Chlorpromazine jaundice, 1659
Chlorpropamide
hypoglycemic coma induced by, 1996
hyponatremia induced by, 1954
in diabetes insipidus, 2111
in diabetes mellitus, 1986, *1986*
Chlortetracycline, *557,* 562
in ocular toxoplasmosis, 2335
Chlor-Trimeton. See *Chlorpheniramine.*
Chokes, in decompression sickness, *103*
Cholangiography
in chronic pancreatitis, 1556
intravenous, 1622, 1623
in acute cholecystitis, 1626
transhepatic, 1622, 1623
percutaneous, 1473–1474, *1473, 1474*
Cholangiohepatitis, Oriental, 1633
Cholangiopancreatography, endoscopic retrograde, 1472–1473, *1472, 1473*
in biliary disease, 1622, 1623, *1623*
in chronic pancreatitis, 1556
Cholangitis, 1629–1631
destructive, chronic nonsuppurative, 1666
intermittent, 1629
obstructive, 1631
sclerosing, 224, 1633
stenosing, vs. biliary cirrhosis, 1666
suppurative, 1631
liver abscess in, 1657
Cholecalciferol, 2232
Cholecystectomy
abdominal symptoms after, 1635–1636
in acute cholecystitis, 1627
in chronic cholecystitis, 1625
Cholecystenteric fistula, in acute cholecystitis, 1626, 1628
Cholecystitis
acalculous, 1626
acute, 1625–1628, *1627*
complicating chronic cholecystitis, 1625
vs. acute appendicitis, 1580
vs. acute pericarditis, 1273
vs. peptic ulcer, 1508
cholelithiasis and, plasma cell dyscrasia with, electrophoretic patterns in, *1857,* 1858
chronic, 1624–1625
emphysematous, 1628
vs. angina pectoris, 1227
vs. pleurisy of pneumococcal pneumonia, 354
Cholecystitis cystica, 1634
Cholecystitis glandularis proliferans, 1634
Cholecystography
nephrotoxicity in, 1433, 1434
oral, 1622, *1623*
in chronic cholecystitis, 1625
Cholecystokinin
in colonic motility, 1493
in gallbladder function, 1619
in gastroduodenal motility, 1476, 1489
Cholecystostomy, in acute cholecystitis, 1628
Choledochal cysts, 1632
Choledocholithiasis, 1629–1631, *1629*
in chronic cholecystitis, 1625
vs. biliary stricture, 1631, 1632

Choledocholithiasis (*Continued*)
  vs. malignant bile duct tumors, 1635
Cholelithiasis
  cholecystitis and, plasma cell
    dyscrasia with, electrophoretic
    patterns in, *1857, 1858*
  vs. angina pectoris, 1227
Cholera, 460–462
Cholera vaccine, 462
Choleretic diarrhea, 1479
Cholestasis, 1638
  intrahepatic, chlorpromazine-
    induced, 1659
    sex hormones causing, 1658
    vs. choledocholithiasis, 1630
Cholestatic hepatitis, 1652, 1653
Cholesterol
  absorption of, 1524
  elevated, as cardiovascular risk factor,
    1062, 1220
  serum, measurement of, 1646, 1647
  synthesis of, in liver disease, 1642
  transport of, 2002, 2003, *2003*
Cholesterol flocculation test, in
  protozoan and helminthic disease,
  565
Cholesterol gallstones, 1619, 1620, *1620*
Cholesterol pericarditis, 1276
Cholesterol polyps, 1634
Cholesterolosis, 1624
Cholesterylester storage disease, *42*
Cholestyramine
  in biliary cirrhosis, 1667
  in chlorpromazine jaundice, 1659
  in diarrhea after ileal resection, 1567
  in diarrhea of carcinoid syndrome,
    2213
  in esophagitis, 1485
  in familial hypercholesterolemia, 2005
  in malabsorption syndrome, *1536*
  malabsorption caused by, 1548
Choline, nutrient value of, 1672
Choline chloride, in hereditary chorea,
  759
Cholinergic drugs. See also names of
  specific agents.
  in myasthenia gravis, 928
Cholinergic urticaria, 161
Chondrocalcinosis, 201–202
  in hyperparathyroidism, 2215, *2216*
  vs. rheumatoid arthritis, 190
Chondrodystrophy, vs. pituitary
  dwarfism, 2104
Chondroectodermal dysplasia, 2264
Chondromalacia patellae, 204
Chondromatosis, synovial, 202
Chondro-osteodystrophy, 2052–2053,
2052
Chondrosarcoma, synovial, 202
Chordomas, 864
Chorea(s), 751, 757–759
  acute, 757–758
  hereditary, 758–759
  Huntington's, 758–759
    dementia in, 663, 758, 759
    screening for, 44
    vs. acute chorea, 758
    vs. striatonigral degeneration, 765
  infectious, 757–758
  progressive, chronic, 758–759
  senile, 759
    vs. hereditary chorea, 759

Chorea(s) (*Continued*)
  Sydenham's, 757–758
    in rheumatic fever, 381
    vs. African trypanosomiasis, 578
    vs. dystonia musculorum deformans,
      761
Choreoathetosis, 760
Choriocarcinoma, pulmonary
  embolization by, 1143
Chorioepithelioma, pulmonary
  embolization by, 1143
Choriomeningitis, lymphocytic, 818, *818*
  vs. arboviral encephalitis, 284
Chorionic gonadotropin, human
  as tumor marker, 1912
  in amenorrhea, 2192
  in cryptorchidism, 2174
  in delayed adolescence, 2166
  in evaluation of ovarian function,
    2181
  in secondary hypogonadism, 2172
Choroid papillomas, 864
Choroidal tubercles, in disseminated
  tuberculosis, 498
Choroiditis, circumpapillary, in ocular
  histoplasmosis, 2324
Christmas disease, *1884,* **1887**
Christmas factor, 1881
Chromatids, 50, *50*
Chromatin-negative Klinefelter's
syndrome, 2170
Chromhidrosis, apocrine, 2269
Chromite miners, pneumoconiosis in,
  987
Chromium, nutrient value of, 1674
Chromomycosis, 542–543
Chromophobe adenoma, 863, *2095,*
  2096, 2097
Chromosome(s)
  acrocentric, 50, *50*
  analysis of, amniocentesis for, 49, 50
    preparation of cells for, 49
  bands of, nomenclature for, 51, *51*
  breakage of, 53
    in LSD users, 704
    unrepaired, diseases associated
      with, 54
  deletions of, 54
  disorders of, 49–54
    congenital heart disease and, 1150
    frequency of, 49
    from changes in chromosomal
      structure, 53–54, *53*
    from changes in chromosome
      number, *52,* **53**
    in radiation injury, 88
    nomenclature for, 51
  endoreduplication of, 54
  identification of, methods of, 50, *50*
  karyotypic arrangement of, *50,* 51
  metacentric, 50, *50*
  Philadelphia, in chronic granulocytic
    leukemia, 1822
  rearrangements of, 53, *53,* 54
  reciprocal translocations of, 53, *53*
    transmission of, 53, 54
    submetacentric, 50, *50*
Chvostek's sign, in hypocalcemia, 2242
Chylomicronemia, in familial
  lipoprotein lipase deficiency, 2006
Chylothorax, 1014
Chylous ascites, 1593

Chylous pericardial effusion, 1276
Chyluria, 1442
  in bancroftian filariasis, 634
Chymotrypsin, in protein absorption,
  1525
Cicuta species, poisoning by, 70
Cigarette smoking
  after myocardial infarction, 1234
  as cardiovascular risk factor, 1062,
    1220
  dust exposure and, neoplasia
    associated with, 994, 995
  in bronchogenic carcinoma, 1005
  in chronic obstructive pulmonary
    disease, 960
  in peptic ulcer, 1503, 1516
  in simple chronic bronchitis, 953, 954
  in "stress polycythemia," 1793
  in thromboangiitis obliterans, 1302
  occupational bronchitis and, 995, 996
Ciguatera poisoning, 69
Ciliary body, in diabetes mellitus, 2320
Cimetidine
  in chronic pancreatitis, 1557
  in peptic ulcer, 1514, *1514,* 1515
Circle of Willis, anomalies of, cerebral
  infarction and, 779
Circulating immune complex–mediated
  renal diseases, 1325, *1325,* 1326
Circulation
  cerebral collateral, cerebral infarction
    and, 779
  function and control of, 1063–1072
    in shock, 1108–1113, *1109*
  hormonal effects on, 1111
  in etiology of acute pancreatitis, 1551
  in sedative overdose, 714
  mesenteric, anatomy, physiology and
    pathophysiology of, 1586–1587,
    1586, 1587
  neurogenic control of, 1110
  peripheral, 1066–1067
  pulmonary
    functions of, 938
    in mitral stenosis, 1145–1146
    normal, 1135–1137
  renal, lesions of, renal injury from,
    1330
  variations in, 1457
  slowed, in heart failure, 1088
Circulatory overload, transfusion
  reaction from, *1785,* 1786
Circulatory shock, hypotension and, in
  cancer patient, 1905
Circumpapillary choroiditis, in ocular
  histoplasmosis, 2324
Cirrhosis, 1663–1667
  ascites and, 1640, 1665, 1666
    renal failure in, 1644
    spontaneous peritonitis, 1594
  bacteremia in, 455
  biliary, 1666–1667, *2299*
    conjugated bile acid deficiency in,
      1537
    vs. chronic active hepatitis, 1662
    vs. malignant bile duct tumors,
      1635
  cardiac, 1092, 1667
  complications of, treatment of,
    1665–1666
  diabetes mellitus and, 1642
  hypocalcemia in, 2241

Cirrhosis (*Continued*)
hyponatremia in, 1954
idiopathic, 1663
in alcoholic, 1663–1665
Laennec's, *2299*
macronodular, 1663
portal hypertension and, 1144, 1665
posthepatitic, 1663
postnecrotic, 1663
vs. visceral leishmaniasis, 586
Cis-platinum, in oncologic treatment, 1938
Cisternography, radioisotope, 749
Citrullinemia, *41, 2018,* 2022
dietary restriction in, 55
Cladosporium carrioni, 542
Claudication, intermittent
in arteriosclerosis obliterans, 1300
of cauda equina, 895
Claw hand, 903
Cleft lip and cleft palate, frequency and sex ratio of, *48*
Clethrionomys glareolus, 301
Click-murmur syndrome, 1187, 1188–1190
Climacteric, male, 2174
Clindamycin, *556,* 560, 561
in acne, 2279
in anaerobic infections, 445, *445*
in lung abscess, 982
in staphylococcal pneumonia, 402
Clinical medicine
biological science and, 6–8
laboratory investigation and, 4, 6, 7
psychologic testing in, 681–683
science, spectrum of disease and, 3–6
study of, 1–3
Clioquinol, neuropathy from, 910
Clofazimine, in leprosy, 504
Clofibrate, in familial dysbetalipoproteinemia, 2006
Clomiphene, in amenorrhea complicating anorexia nervosa, 1703
Clomiphene citrate, in assessment of hypothalamic-pituitary gonadotropin release, 2165
Clomipramine, in cataplexy, 654
Clonazepam
in dystonia musculorum deformans, 761
in epilepsy, *859*
in spasmodic torticollis, 762
Clonidine
in arterial hypertension, *1212,* 1214
in hypertension of chronic renal failure, 1363
withdrawal of, catecholamine excess following, 1209
Clonopin. See *Clonazepam.*
Clonorchiasis, 617–618
Clonorchis sinensis, 605, 617, 618
bile duct obstruction caused by, 1633
Clostridial cellulitis, 434
Clostridial contamination of wounds, 434
Clostridial diseases, 433–441
histotoxic, classification of, *434*
uterine, 435
Clostridial food poisoning, 65–66, 436
Clostridial gastroenteritis, 436
Clostridial myonecrosis, 433–435
differential diagnosis of, *435*
hyperbaric oxygen therapy in, 104
Clostridial septicemia, 436

Clostridium bifermentans, 433
Clostridium botulinum, 67
Clostridium difficile, 405
Clostridium fallax, 433
Clostridium histolyticum, 433
Clostridium novyi, 433
Clostridium oedematiens, 433
Clostridium perfringens, 433
type A, food poisoning caused by, 65
type C, intestinal disease associated with, 66
Clostridium septicum, 433
in septicemia, 436
Clostridium sordelli, 433
Clostridium tetani, 436, 437
Clotting. See *Coagulation.*
Cloxacillin, *557,* 559
in osteomyelitis, 2261
Clubbing, digital
in bronchogenic carcinoma, 1007
in hypertrophic osteoarthropathy, 201
in infective endocarditis, 390
Cluster headache, 729, 731
treatment of, 732
Clutton's joints, in congenital syphilis, 186, 513
Coagulation
alterations in, in cerebral infarction, 781
complement system and, 137
defects of, 1881–1897
acquired, 1889–1897
heritable, 1883–1889
differentiation of, *1884*
in bacterial meningitis, 414
in critically ill patient, 1052–1053
in liver disease, 1643, 1644
vs. purpuric disorders, 1871, *1872*
intravascular
disorders accompanied by, *1895*
disseminated, hypofibrinogenemic syndromes associated with, 1893–1894
in cancer patient, 1906
in critically ill patient, 1052
in shock, 1113
without hypofibrinogenemia, 1894–1895
experimental, 1892
laboratory diagnosis of, 1892–1893
syndromes of, 1891–1895
renal injury induced by, 1327–1328
tests of, as measurement of hepatic function, 1646
Coal workers, progressive massive fibrosis of, 992, 993
Coal workers' pneumoconiosis, 987
pulmonary hypertension in, 1147
Coarctation of abdominal aorta, 1290
Coarctation of aorta, 1157–1158, 1209, 1289, 1290
at aortic isthmus, 1289, 1290
murmurs in, 1158, 1290
roentgenography in, 1158, 1290
surgical treatment of, 1290
Cobalt
nutrient value of, 1674
poisoning by, 76
secondary polycythemia caused by, 1799
Cobalt-beer cardiomyopathy, 1285
Cocaine
abuse of, 701–702

Cocaine (*Continued*)
poisoning by, 702, *712*
"Cocaine bugs," 702
Cocaine psychosis, 702
Cocci, anaerobic, 441
susceptibility of, to antimicrobial agents, *445*
Coccidioides immitis, 537, 538
Coccidioidin skin test, 539
Coccidioidomas, 538
Coccidioidomycosis, 537–540
serologic tests in, 946
skin test in, 539, 946
vs. tularemia, 467
Coccidiosis, 604
Coccygodynia, 1618
vs. proctalgia fugax, 1497
Cochin-China diarrhea, 622–623
Cochliomyia hominivorax, 112
Code, genetic, 33
population genetics and, 47
Codeine, 694–698
in pain, *724,* 725
terpin hydrate with, in common cold, 233
Codeine phosphate, in headache of intracranial hemorrhage, 800
Codeine sulfate
in diarrhea, 1480
in headache of intracranial hemorrhage, 800
in influenza, 245
in measles, 249, 250
in pleural pain of pneumococcal pneumonia, 356
Co-dominance, genetic, 34
Codons, 31, 32, 33, 34
chain-terminating, 33, *33*
Coelenterates, envenomation by, 123
Coenurus infections, 611
Cogan's syndrome, 740
Cogentin. See *Benztropine.*
Cognition, disturbances in, in metabolic brain disease, 647
Cognitive function, tests of, in dementia, 660, 661
Coitus, 686, 687
premarital, 690
Colace. See *Dioctyl sodium sulfosuccinate.*
Colchicine
in acute gouty arthritis, 2039
in familial Mediterranean fever, 2057
malabsorption caused by, 1548
Cold
common, 230–234, *230, 232*
vs. influenza, 245
disorders due to, 84, 85–86
exposure to, peripheral vascular diseases due to, 1309–1312
sensitivity to, 1309
Cold agglutinin antibodies, classification of, *1765*
Cold agglutinin disease, chronic, of elderly, 1765
Cold agglutinin syndrome, 1764–1765, *2302*
autosensitization in, 132
Cold hemagglutinin test, in mycoplasmal pneumonia, 345, 346
Cold hemoglobinuria, paroxysmal, 1765–1766, *2302*
immune mechanisms in, 132
in syphilis, 507
Cold urticaria, 161, 162

Cold water immersion foot, 1309, 1310
**Cold-reacting antibodies, hemolysis
due to, 1764–1766**
Colectomy, in ulcerative colitis, 1575
Colestipol, in familial
hypercholesterolemia, 2005
Colic
biliary, 1624–1625
vs. myocardial infarction, 1233
lead, 78
painter's 78
renal, in renal calculi, 1444
ureteral, in analgesic nephropathy,
1420
Colistimethate sodium, *557*, 562
as nephrotoxin, 1426
Colistin, neuromuscular block caused
by, 929
Colistin sulfate, *557*, 562
Colitis
adaptive, 1493
amebic, vs. ulcerative colitis, 1572
granulomatous, 1576–1578
vs. amebiasis, 592
vs. diverticulitis, 1583
ischemic, 1589
vs. Crohn's disease of colon, 1578
vs. diverticulitis, 1583, 1584
vs. ulcerative colitis, 1572
mucous, 1493
postdysenteric, 591
radiation, 1584–1585
vs. ulcerative colitis, 1572
soap, 1614
ulcerative, 1568–1576
ankylosing spondylitis in, 198, 1568
arthritis in, 198, 1575
clinical manifestations of, 1570
colorectal carcinoma and, 1607
complications of, 1574
cutaneous signs of, *2298*
diagnosis of, 1571
differential diagnosis of, 1572
disease manifestations of,
mechanisms of, 1571
eosinophilia in, 226
epidemiology of, 1568
etiology of, 1568
eyes in, 2316
genetics in, 1568
incidence and prevalence of, 1568
laboratory studies in, 1571
pathology and pathogenesis of,
1569
physical examination in, 1570
regional enteritis and, 1561, 1562
sclerosing cholangitis and, 1633
toxic megacolon in, 1569, *1570*,
1570, 1574–1575
treatment of, 1572
surgical, 1575
vs. amebic dysentery, 592
vs. balantidiasis, 603
vs. Crohn's disease of colon, 1576
vs. shigellosis, 459
Colitis cystica profunda, 1611
Colitis cystica superficialis, 1611
Collagen, 164, 165, 2230
formation of, in malnutrition, 1680
synthesis of, in scleroderma, 168
"Collagen disease," 164–183
eosinophilic, 226
myopathy in, 923

Collagenosis, mediastinal, pulmonary
venous hypertension from, 1145
Collagenous pneumoconioses, 984
diffuse, 990–992
nodular, 988–990
Collagenous sprue, 1541
Collateral vessels, portal-systemic, in
portal hypertension, 1640
Colloidal bismuth, in peptic ulcer, 1515
Colloids, hydrophilic
in constipation, 1482
in diarrhea, 1480
in irritable bowel syndrome, 1494
Colon
adenocarcinoma of, vs. chronic
cholecystitis, 1625
arterial supply to, 1587, *1587*
ascending, tuberculosis of, 492
carcinoma of, 1606–1610
in ulcerative colitis, 1574
vs. amebiasis, 592
vs. diverticulitis, 1583
cathartic, 1614
Crohn's disease of, 1576–1578
vs. amebiasis, 592
vs. diverticulitis, 1583
diverticula of, 1501–1502
angiography in, 1471, *1471*
gastrointestinal bleeding in, 1522
diverticulitis of, 1582–1584. See also
Diverticulitis.
diverticulosis of, 1501–1502
familial polyposis of, colorectal
carcinoma and, 1606
detection of, in relatives, *58*, *59*
fibrous strictures of, in amebiasis,
591
ileus of, 1497–1498
in scleroderma, 169
infarction of, vs. ulcerative colitis,
1572
irrigations of, in accidental
poisoning, 74
irritable, 1493. See also *Irritable bowel
syndrome.*
left, small, 1498
malakoplakia of, 1613
motility in, disorders of, 1492–1498
in ulcerative colitis, 1571
normal, 1492, *1492*, 1493
nervous, 1493
pain originating in, 1476
perforation of, in amebiasis, 591
in ulcerative colitis, 1575
pseudo-obstruction of, 1497–1498
segmentation in, 1492, *1492*
sigmoid, diverticulitis of, vs. Crohn's
disease of colon, 1578
vs. ulcerative colitis, 1572
tuberculosis of, 492
spastic, 1493
strictures of, in ulcerative colitis, 1574
transverse, tuberculosis of, 492
**ulcer of, nonspecific or solitary,
1615–1616**
unstable, 1493
vascular ectasias of, 1590
villous adenomas of, 1610
Colonoscopy, in colorectal carcinoma,
1608, 1609, *1609*
Colorado tick fever, *279*, 280–281
Colorado tick fever virus, 280
Colorectal carcinoma, 1606–1610

Coma
acute hepatitis with, 1655, 1656
common causes of, *640*
hepatic, 1640–1641
in cirrhosis, 1666
hyperosmolar, in diabetes mellitus,
treatment of, 1985
nonketotic, volume depletion in,
1951
hypoglycemic, in reactive
hypoglycemia, 1991
sulfonylureas inducing, 1996
hypopituitary, in hypopituitarism,
2100
"hysterical," vs. metabolic brain
disease, 649, 650
in acute drug poisoning, 713
in intracranial hemorrhage, 796, 797
treatment of, 799, 800
in malaria, 571
in Reye's syndrome, 839
in viral encephalitis, 821
laboratory examination in, 643
myxedema, 2134
pathogenesis of, 640–643
patient in, approach to, 642–643
Coma vigil, in midbrain infarctions, 787
Combined hyperlipidemia, *42, 2004*
acquired, 2009
familial, 2007–2008
**Combined immunodeficiencies, severe,
139, 141**
**with adenosine deaminase
deficiency, *139*, 141–142**
Combined system disease
vitamin B_{12} deficiency with, 776
vs. multiple sclerosis, 847
Commissural syndrome, 890
Common atrium, 1169
Common bile duct, tumors of, carcinoid
features of, 2212
Common cold, 230–234, *230*, *232*
vs. influenza, 245
Common cold vaccines, 233
Common cold viruses, 230, *230*, 231
Common faint, 743
Common nightshade, poisoning by, 70
**Common variable immunodeficiency,
142–143**
Communicating hydrocephalus, 873
Compazine. See *Prochlorperazine.*
Complement, 135–138
activation of, glomerulonephritis
associated with, 1327
in shock, 1115
modulation and control of, 136
pathways of, 135, *135*, 136
bacterial inactivation by, 339
biologic function of, 136, 137
clinical assays for, 137
components and cleavage products of,
biologic functions of, *135*
components of, selective deficiencies
of, 144
disease and, 137–138
in B cell determination, 129
in drug reactions, 131
in rheumatoid arthritis, 187
in systemic lupus erythematosus, 178,
179
interaction of, with coagulation,
fibrinolytic and kinin systems, 137
metabolism of, 137

Complement deficiency disease, hereditary, 137, 138
Complement fixation test
in Chagas' disease, 582
in coccidioidomycosis, 539
in lymphogranuloma venereum, 336
in protozoan and helminthic diseases, 565
in rickettsial diseases, 313, *314*
in toxoplasmosis, 597
Complete heart block, congenital, 1166
Compliance, in acute respiratory failure, 1036
Compromised host, 145–152. See also *Host defense(s).*
Computerized tomography
in brain abscess, 806
in brain tumor, 867
in cerebral infarction, 789, 790
in chronic pancreatitis, 1556
in epilepsy, 857
in evaluation of jaundice, 1622
in fatty infiltration of liver, *1467*
in gastrointestinal disease, 1466–1468, *1467*
in head injury, 881
in hepatic abscess, *1467*
in herpes simplex encephalitis, 823
in intracranial hemorrhage, 798
in intracranial inflammatory disease, 804
in intraspinal compression, 892
in nephrocarcinoma, 1459
in neurologic diagnosis, 747
in obstructive jaundice, *1467*
in peritoneal disease, 1592
in pulmonary disease, 944
in renal investigation, 1344
Concanavalin A
in assessment of immune competence in cancer, 1925
in T cell competence assay, 130
Concussion, 880
inner ear, hearing loss from, 736
Conduction, defects of, in myocardial infarction, 1230, 1235, 1236
Conduction aphasia, 657
Conductive hearing loss, 734, 735
Condylomata acuminata, vs. condylomata lata, 509
Condylomata lata, in syphilis, 509, *509*
Cone shell stings, 123, 124
Confabulation, in Korsakoff's syndrome, 659
Confusional state, acute or subacute, 645
Congenital adrenal hyperplasia, 2158–2161
hypertension from, 1211
vs. primary aldosteronism, 2158
Congenital adrenocortical hyperplasia, 2064
Congenital afibrinogenemia, *43, 1884*
Congenital aneurysms of sinuses of Valsalva, 1169–1170
Congenital aortic diseases, 1289–1291
Congenital complete heart block, 1166
Congenital coronary arteriovenous fistula, 1169
Congenital cytomegalovirus infection, 827, 828, 829
Congenital dysfibrinogenemia, *1884,* 1889

Congenital ectopia of kidney, 1457
Congenital erythropoietic porphyria, 42, 2045, *2302*
hemolytic anemia in, 1761
Congenital fibrinogen deficiency, 1888, 1889
Congenital fusion of cervical vertebrae, 875
Congenital glucose-galactose malabsorption, 1539
Congenital heart disease, 1149–1174
clinical classification of, *1152*
death rates for, *1060*
diagnosis of, 1151, *1153,* 1154, 1155
etiology of, 1149, 1150
frequency and sex ratio of, *48*
incidence of, 1149
physiologic adaptation to, after birth, 1150
pulmonary vascular disease in, 1141–1143
underlying infective endocarditis, 387
vs. neonatal myocarditis, 273
Congenital hemolytic anemias, 1755–1762
Congenital hepatic fibrosis, 1667
Congenital hydronephrosis, 1457
Congenital hypertrophic pyloric stenosis, 1490
Congenital lymphedema, 1314
Congenital malformations, 48–49. See also names of specific congenital disorders.
eosinophilia in, 226
epilepsy associated with, 852
Congenital megacolon, 1495–1496, *1495*
Congenital mesoblastic nephroma, 1460
Congenital multicystic kidney, 1450, 1451, 1452
vs. childhood polycystic kidney disease, 1453
Congenital myasthenia gravis, 927
Congenital myopathies, 919–920
Congenital neurosyphilis, 815–816
Congenital neutropenia, 1809, 1810
Congenital nevi, 2312
internal malignancy and, *2297*
Congenital ocular toxoplasmosis, 2334
Congenital pericardial lesions, 1276
Congenital photosensitive porphyria, 2045
Congenital pulmonary arteriovenous fistula, 1168–1169
Congenital pulmonary valve regurgitation, 1168
Congenital rubella, 251, 252
hearing loss from, 735
vs. congenital cytomegalovirus infection, 828
Congenital syndromes, obesity in, 1697
Congenital syphilis, 512, 513
follow-up examinations in, 517
IgM FTA-ABS test for, 515
treatment of, *515,* 516, 517
Congenital toxoplasmosis, 595, 596, 597, 598
Congenital valvular aortic stenosis, 1156–1157
Congestive cardiomyopathies, 1277
Congestive heart failure, 1081, 1082. See also *Heart failure.*
hyponatremia in, 1954
in infective endocarditis, 390

Congestive heart failure (*Continued*)
in pneumococcal pneumonia, 354
vs. asthma, 957
vs. congested state, 1081, 1082
Congestive splenomegaly, 1870
neutropenia in, 1809
Conglomerate silicosis, 989
Conium maculatum, poisoning by, 70
Conjugated hyperbilirubinemia, 1638
Conjunctiva
in sarcoidosis, 2330
in sickle cell diseases, 2331
Conjunctival myiasis, 112
Conjunctivitis, 2313, *2313,* 2314
adenoviral, 237
follicular, chronic, vs. ocular chlamydial infections, 334
gonococcal, 406
Hemophilus aegyptius causing, 425
hemorrhagic, acute, 274–275
poliomyelitis-like syndrome in, 270, 275
in Reiter's syndrome, 2316
inclusion, trachoma and, 332–335
vs. Romaña's sign in Chagas' disease, 582
Connective tissue
diseases of, 164–183. See also *Rheumatoid arthritis.*
eyes in, 2316–2317, 2319
inherited, 2051–2055
vascular purpura in, 1880
"mixed," 171, 179
pericarditis caused by, 1271, 1272
pulmonary manifestations of, 973–974
renal involvement in, 1400–1401
increased synthesis of, atherosclerosis and, 1222
structure and function of, 164–165
Conn's syndrome, 2157
Consanguinity, 37
Consciousness, 640
disturbances of, 640–655
in cerebral infarction, 786
in hepatic encephalopathy, 1641
state of, in metabolic brain disease, 647
Constipation, 1480–1482
after myocardial infarction, 1234
atonic, 1480
causes of, 1480, 1481
colonic motility in, 1492
diagnosis of, 1481
imaginary, 1481
in intracranial hemorrhage, 800
in irritable bowel syndrome, 1493
spastic, 1480
treatment of, 1481, 1482
Constrictive pericarditis, 1274–1275
protein-losing enteropathy and, 1549
Contact dermatitis, 2283
photoallergic, 2289
Contact sensitivity, 130
Contamination
chemical, of water and air, 60–64
radionuclide, diagnosis of, 89
treatment of, 91
Continence, fecal, maintenance of, mechanisms for, 1482
Continuous positive pressure ventilation, in acute respiratory failure, 1027

Contraception, 2194–2197
Contraceptives
　intrauterine, 2197
　oral, 2195–2197
　　cerebral infarction and, 781
　　contraindications to, 2197
　　hypertension and, 1211
　　side effects of, 2195, 2196
Contractility, cardiac, 1066, 1066, 1083, 1084, 1085
Contractions, premature
　atrial, 1246
　ventricular, 1251
Contracture(s), 930
　aging patient and, 30
Contrast media, radiographic, as nephrotoxins, 1433–1434
Convulsions. See also Seizures.
　febrile, in epilepsy, 852
　generalized, in delirium, 650
　in subarachnoid hemorrhage, 797
　major, 853
Cooley's anemia, 1778
Coombs-negative immune hemolytic anemia, 1763
COPD, 960–964, 961. See also Obstructive pulmonary disease, chronic.
Copper
　hemolysis caused by, 1770
　in Wilson's disease, 2050
　nephrotoxicity from, 1428, 1430, 1431
　nutrient value of, 1673
Copper acetoarsenite, poisoning by, 76
Coproporphyria, hereditary, 42, 2047
Cor pulmonale
　in acute respiratory failure, 1022
　in chronic obstructive pulmonary disease, 961, 963
　in chronic respiratory failure, 1022
　treatment of, 1029–1030
Cor triatriatum, 1145, 1172
　vs. mitral stenosis, 1183
Coral snake, bite of, 122
Corals, envenomation by, 123
Cordotomy, in pain relief, 726
Corkscrew esophagus, 1485–1486, 1486
Cornea
　in diabetes mellitus, 2320
　in Reiter's syndrome, 2316
　in sarcoidosis, 2330
　trauma to, 2313, 2314
Corns, painful, 903
Coronary arteriography
　in angina pectoris, 1226
　in selection of patients for myocardial revascularization, 1239
Coronary arteriovenous fistula, congenital, 1169
Coronary artery(ies)
　disorders of, 1223–1241
　　surgical treatment of, 1238–1241
　left, anomalous origin of, 1172
　left main, stenosis of, surgical treatment of, 1239, 1239
Coronary care unit, 1236
Coronary heart disease. See also names of specific disorders.
　death rates for, 1060
　prevalence and epidemiology of, 1059
Coronaviruses, associated with common cold, 230
Corrigan pulse, in aortic regurgitation, 1195

Cortical degeneration, cerebellar, 775
Cortical thrombophlebitis, 808
　in bacterial meningitis, 412
Corticocerebellar degeneration, in bronchogenic carcinoma, 1007
Corticosteroids. See also names of specific agents.
　pituitary-adrenal suppression by, adrenal insufficiency secondary to, 2151–2152
Corticosterone, properties of, 2145
Corticotropin, 2089–2090
　in adult celiac disease, 1540
　in malabsorption syndrome, 1536
　in nongranulomatous ileojejunitis, 1542
　in regional enteritis, 1567
　in toxic megacolon, 1575
　in ulcerative colitis, 1573
　in Whipple's disease, 1542
　myopathy induced by, vs. polymyositis, 174
Corticotropin-releasing factor, 2075
Cortisol
　as index of ACTH secretion, 2147
　deficiency of, in Addison's disease, 2147
　in breast cancer, 1919
　in hypercalcemia complicating hormonal treatment of breast cancer, 1920
　plasma concentrations of, in Cushing's syndrome, 2154
　properties of, 2144, 2145, 2145, 2146
　secretion of, in Cushing's syndrome, 2152
Cortisone
　immunosuppressive doses of, varicella and, 254
　in hypopituitarism, 2102
　in rheumatoid arthritis, 192
Corynebacterium diphtheriae, 429, 430
Corynebacterium parvum, in oncologic treatment, 1940, 1941
Coryza, acute, 230–234, 230, 232
Cosmegen. See Dactinomycin.
Costochondral junction, tuberculosis of, 497
Co-trimoxazole, 556, 563
　in gonococcal disease, 410
　in pneumocystosis, 558, 600
Cotton, processing of, byssinosis in, 997, 998
Cotton wool spots
　in retinopathy of arterial hypertension, 1203, 1205
　in systemic lupus erythematosus, 177, 2317, 2318
Cough
　in bronchiectasis, 983
　in bronchogenic carcinoma, 1006
　in chronic obstructive pulmonary disease, 961
　in diffuse collagenous pneumoconioses, 991
　in influenza, 243
　in left heart failure, 1089
　in mycoplasmal pneumonia, 344
　in pneumococcal pneumonia, 351
　in pulmonary tuberculosis, 486
　in simple chronic bronchitis, 953, 954
　in whooping cough, 426, 427
　smoker's, 953, 954

Cough syncope, 740, 744
Coumarin compounds
　as vitamin K antagonists, 1890
　in thrombophlebitis, 1126, 1127, 1128
Coumarin-like drugs, resistance to, 1888
Councilman bodies
　in dengue hemorrhagic fever, 297
　in yellow fever, 294
Countercurrent immunoelectrophoresis, in diagnosis of bacterial meningitis, 413
Counterimmunoelectrophoresis, in pneumococcal pneumonia, 353
"Coupling" defect, in thyroid hormone synthesis, 2139
Cowden's syndrome, 2296
Cowpox virus, 255
Cow's milk, allergy to, 1499
Coxarthrosis, 203
Coxiella burnetii, 309, 309, 310, 329
Coxsackievirus(es)
　diarrhea associated with, 275
　distinctive features of, 268
　group A, 268, 269, 269
　group B, 268, 269, 269
　infection with, general aspects of, 269–270, 269
　paralysis and other neurologic complications due to, 270
　pericarditis and myocarditis caused by, 272, 273
Coxsackievirus B heart disease, 1281, 1282
Crab louse, 108, 109
"Crab yaws," 519
Cramps, 930
　in chronic renal failure, 1365
　in maintenance hemodialysis, 1381
Cranial arteritis, 216–218
　neuropathy in, 908
Cranial mucormycosis, 546
Cranial nerves
　disorders of, 899–900
　in bacterial meningitis, 412
　in head injury, 883
　nonmetastatic effects of cancer on, 876–878
Craniopharyngioma(s), 863, 2098
　pituitary dwarfism caused by, 2104
　roentgenography in, 2084
Craniovertebral junction, anomalies of, 874–876
Craw-craw, in onchocerciasis, 636
C-reactive protein, complement activation by, 136
Creatine phosphokinase activity, in myocardial infarction, 1232
Creatinine clearance
　in estimation of glomerular filtration rate, 1339, 1340, 1340
　with peritoneal dialysis, 1378
Creatinine urine/plasma ratio, in acute renal failure, 1373, 1373, 1374
Creeping eruption, 625
Creeping myiasis, 112
Crepitant cellulitis, nonclostridial, 434
CREST syndrome, 169
Cretinism
　endemic, 2138
　goitrous, 2064, 2138–2140
Creutzfeldt-Jakob disease, 840–841
　dementia in, 663
Cricopharyngeal achalasia, 1483

Cricopharyngeal sphincter, normal physiology of, 1475
Crigler-Najjar syndrome, *42*, 1638, 1649
  prevention and management of, 55
Crimean hemorrhagic fever, 293, 298
Critical care medicine, 1031–1058
  acute respiratory failure in, 1033–1045
  coagulation disorders in, 1052–1053
  instrumentation for, 1032–1033
  massive blood transfusions in, 1051–1052
  renal function in, 1050–1051
  shock in, 1045–1050
Crocodile skin, in onchocerciasis, 636
Crohn's disease
  cutaneous signs of, *2299*
  eosinophilia in, 226
  of colon, 1576–1578
    vs. amebiasis, 592
    vs. diverticulitis, 1583
  of small intestine, 1560–1567. See also *Enteritis, regional.*
    vs. eosinophilic gastroenteritis, 1543
Cromolyn, in asthma, 958
Cronkhite-Canada syndrome, *2298*
  colorectal carcinoma and, 1606, 1607
Crooke's change, in Cushing's syndrome, 2084
Croup, 235–236, *235*, 239–240
Crowe's sign of neurofibromatosis, 2290
Crusted itch, 111
Cruveilhier-Baumgarten syndrome, 1640
Cryoglobulinemia
  essential, renal changes in, 1406
  mixed, vs. periarteritis nodosa, 183
  vascular purpura in, 1880
Cryptococcal meningitis, 543, 544
  cerebrospinal fluid findings in, *803*
Cryptococcosis, 543–544
  serologic tests for, 947
Cryptococcus neoformans, 543
Cryptogenic tularemia, 466
Cryptorchidism, 2173–2174
Crystalloids in urine, 1443, 1444
CT scan. See *Computerized tomography.*
Culex annulirostris
  in Japanese B encephalitis, 290
  in Murray Valley encephalitis, 290
Culex gelidus, 290
Culex melanoconion, 286
Culex melanura, 285
Culex nigripalpus, 289
Culex pipiens
  in St. Louis encephalitis, 289
  in West Nile fever, 278
Culex quinquefasciatus, 289
Culex tarsalis
  in California encephalitis, 288
  in St. Louis encephalitis, 289
  in western equine encephalitis, 284
Culex tritaeniorhyncus, 289
Culex univittatus, 278
Cullen's sign, *2299*
Curling, esophageal, 1485–1486, *1486*
Cushing reflex, 1136
Cushing's disease, 2152
  diagnosis of, 2155
  galactorrhea caused by, 2192
  treatment of, 2155, 2156
Cushing's syndrome, 2152–2157
  anterior pituitary in, 2084
  associated with cancer, 1914, 1915, 1916, *2297*

Cushing's syndrome *(Continued)*
  basophilic adenoma with, 2098
  bronchogenic carcinoma and, 1006
  clinical manifestations of, 2153, *2153*
  diabetes mellitus in, 1982
  hypertension from, 1211
  iatrogenic, 2065
  metabolic alkalosis in, 1966
  obesity in, 1697
  osteoporosis in, 2244
  vascular purpura in, 1880
  vs. 11β-hydroxylase deficiency, 2160
  vs. primary aldosteronism, 2158
Cushing's syndrome medicamentosus, 2152
Cushing's ulcer, in intracranial tumors, 866
Cutaneous. See also *Skin.*
Cutaneous amebiasis, 591
Cutaneous anthrax, 471
Cutaneous blastomycosis, 540
Cutaneous candidiasis, 548
Cutaneous diphtheria, 431
  vs. tropical phagedenic ulcer, 530
Cutaneous diseases, 2266–2312. See also *Skin, diseases of,* and names of specific diseases.
Cutaneous larva migrans, 625
  vs. gnathostomiasis, 626
Cutaneous leishmaniasis, 583
  of new world, *588*, *589*
    diffuse, *588,* 589
  of old world, 587–589, *588*
    diffuse, 588
  vs. yaws, 521
Cutaneous lesions, viral diseases characterized by, 246–264
Cutaneous lymphatic form of sporotrichosis, 545
Cutaneous manifestations of internal malignancy, 2295–2297, 2300, *2296–2297*
Cutaneous melanoma, primary, 2310
Cutaneous myiasis, 112
Cutaneous staphylococcal infections, 399–401
  in diabetes mellitus, 398
  prevention of, 401
  treatment of, 400–401
Cutaneous stimulation, in pain relief, 725
Cutaneous tuberculosis, 498
  vs. lupoid leishmaniasis, 588
Cutaneous-mucosal hyalinosis, 2058
Cutis laxa, vs. Ehlers-Danlos syndrome, 2055
Cyanide poisoning, 75
  acute, hyperbaric oxygen therapy in, 104
  chronic, from cyanogenic glycosides, 69
Cyanocobalamin, 1673
  in vitamin B₁₂ deficiency, 777
Cyanogenic glycosides, chronic cyanide poisoning caused by, 69
Cyanosis
  abnormal hemoglobins producing, 1777, 1778, *1778*
  in congenital heart disease, *1153*, 1154, *1154*
  in liver disease, 1644
  in methemoglobinemia, 1781
  in pneumococcal pneumonia, 352
  in right ventricular failure, 1091

Cyanotic Fallot's tetralogy
  classic, 1164, 1165
  vs. right ventricular origin of both great arteries, 1173
Cyclazocine, 698
Cyclic AMP, 2071, 2072–2073, *2072, 2073*
  urinary excretion of, in hyperparathyroidism, 2218
Cyclic neutropenia, 1810
Cyclizine, in motion sickness, 95
Cyclophosphamide, 1931, 1932
  hyponatremia induced by, 1954
  in aplastic anemia, 1740
  in autoimmune hemolytic anemia, 1764
  in Hodgkin's disease, 1845
  in multiple myeloma, 1861
  in non-Hodgkin's lymphomas, *1836*
  in rheumatoid arthritis, 193
  in Wegener's granulomatosis, 219
  pulmonary hypersensitivity reactions from, 975
Cycloserine, *556*
  in pulmonary tuberculosis, 488, 490
Cycrimine, in parkinsonism, 755
Cylindromas, 1012
Cylindruria, in asymptomatic individual, 1333
Cyproheptadine
  in cold sensitivity, 1309
  in diarrhea of carcinoid syndrome, 2213
  in malabsorption of metastatic malignant carcinoid syndrome, 1547
Cyproterone, in cancer of prostate, 1921
Cyst(s)
  bone, in sarcoidosis, 213, 214
  choledochal, 1632
  hydatid, 609, 610
    vs. hepatic amebiasis, 592
  lung, 1002
    vs. lung abscess, 981
  mesenteric, 1596
  ovarian, twisted, vs. acute appendicitis, 1581
  pancreatic, in chronic pancreatitis, 1556, *1556*
  pericardial, congenital, 1276
  popliteal, rupture of, in rheumatoid arthritis, 188
  renal
    benign, 1461
    simple, 1451
Cystathionine β-synthase deficiency, *2017,* 2028
Cystathioninuria, *41, 2017*
Cystic carcinomas, adenoid, 1012
Cystic diseases of kidney, 1450–1456
  classification of, 1450–1451, *1451*
  medullary, adult-onset, 1454
    volume depletion in, 1951
  symptoms and signs of, *1450*
Cystic fibrosis, 43, 1559–1560
Cystic renal medulla, nephronophthisis and, 1454–1455
Cystic tuberculosis of bone, 497
Cysticercosis, 608
  granulomas of, 864
  vs. brain tumor, 868, 869
  immunodiagnostic tests for, *565*
  vs. angiostrongyliasis, 631
Cysticercus cellulosae, 608
Cysticercus racemosus, 608

Cystine-lysinuria, neonatal, *2019*
Cystinosis, *41, 2020*
  renal transplantation in, 55
Cystinuria, *41,* 1539, *2020, 2023,*
  2027–2028
  renal calculi and, 1445, 1446
Cystitis, 1409, 1410
  honeymoon, 1412
Cytarabine, *556,* 1934. See also *Cytosine arabinoside.*
Cytogenetics, human, 49–54
Cytology, exfoliative
  in colorectal carcinoma, 1609
  in gastric carcinoma, 1602
Cytomegalic inclusion disease, 827–829
  vs. Chagas' disease, 582
Cytomegalovirus infections, 827–829
  vs. congenital toxoplasmosis, 597
  vs. pneumocystosis, 599
Cytomegalovirus mononucleosis, 828
  vs. infectious mononucleosis, 267
Cytomegaly, 827–829
Cytosar. See *Cytosine arabinoside.*
Cytosine arabinoside, *556,* 1934
  in acute myelocytic leukemia, 1819
  in herpes simplex encephalitis, 824
  in non-Hodgkin's lymphomas, *1836*
Cytotoxic agents, 1930–1938. See also
  names of specific agents.
  cell-cycle kinetics and, 1927
  classification of, 1930
  immune competence and,
    relationship of, 1926
  nosocomial pneumonia and, 362, 363
  patient selection for, 1930
  use of, therapy vs. toxicity in,
    1923–1924, *1924*
Cytoxan. See *Cyclophosphamide.*

Dacarbazine, in oncologic treatment,
  1933
Dactinomycin, in oncologic treatment,
  1936
Dactylometra species, envenomation by,
  123
Dactylopterus species, envenomation by,
  124
Dagga, 702
Danazol, in hereditary angioedema, 163
Dangerous universal donor, transfusion
  reaction from, 1787, 1788
Dapsone
  in leprosy, 504
  in malaria prophylaxis, 575
  in relapsing polychondritis, 218
Daraprim. See *Pyrimethamine.*
Darkfield examination
  in pinta, 525
  in syphilis, 513
Darvon. See *Dextropropoxyphene.*
Data management, automated, in
  intensive care unit, 1032
Datura stramonium, poisoning by, 70
Daunorubicin, 1936, 1937
  in multiple myeloma, 1861
Dawson's encephalitis, 841
DC electroshock, cardioversion of
  arrhythmias by, 1266–1267
dDAVP, in diabetes insipidus, 2111
DDS. See *Dapsone.*

DDT
  human health and, 61, 62
  poisoning by, 75
de Quervain's syndrome, 207
de Quervain's thyroiditis, 2131
De Toni-Debré-Fanconi syndrome, 2252
Deadly nightshade, poisoning by, 70
Deafness, 734–737
  air travel and, 96
  as hysterical symptom, 679
  hereditary, 735
  word-, pure, 657
Death
  brain, criteria for, 1031
  causes of, in hypertension, 1203
  dying and, 1941–1948
    in aged patient, 30
  risk of, Gompertz concept and, 27–28,
    27
  sudden, 1237–1238
    in aortic stenosis, 1191
Decadron. See *Dexamethasone.*
Decompensation, hemodynamic, in
  acute respiratory failure, 1034
Decompression, surgical, in spinal
  injuries, 886
Decompression sickness, 99, **102–103,**
  103
  hyperbaric oxygen therapy in, 103,
    104
Decubitus ulcers
  enteric bacteria in, 455
  in aging patient, 30
  in paraplegia, 887
Degeneration(s)
  cerebellar
    alcoholic, 775
    parenchymatous, 775
  cerebellar cortical, 775
    subacute, in cancer, 877
  cerebral, epilepsy associated with, 853
  corticocerebellar, in bronchogenic
    carcinoma, 1007
  hepatolenticular, 2049–2051
    vs. dystonia musculorum
      deformans, 761
  nigrospinodentatal, 765
  olivopontocerebellar, 768
  spinocerebellar, 766–768
    in bronchogenic carcinoma, 1007
    vs. multiple sclerosis, 847
  spongy, of white matter, 850
  striatonigral, 764–765
Degenerative diseases of nervous
  system, inherited, 764–772
Degenerative heart disease, underlying
  infective endocarditis, 387
Degenerative joint disease, 202–205, *203*
  in acromegaly, 199
  vs. ankylosing spondylitis, 195
  vs. polymyalgia rheumatica, 217
  vs. rheumatoid arthritis, 190
Deglutition. See also *Swallowing.*
  disorders of, 1478–1479
Degos' disease, *2298*
  malabsorption in, 1543
  vs. periarteritis nodosa, 183
Dehydration
  in malabsorption syndrome, 1529
  volume depletion from, 1950
7-Dehydrocholesterol, 2232
Dehydroemetine dihydrochloride, in
  amebiasis, 593

Dehydroisoandrosterone, properties of,
  2145, 2146
Deletions, chromosomal, 54
Delhi boil, 587
Delirium, 644–651
  differential diagnosis in, 650
  in intracranial hemorrhage, 800
  ventilation in, 649
Delirium tremens, 709
  in pneumococcal pneumonia, 356
Delta-aminolevulinic acid, in porphyria,
  2044
Delusions
  in manic-depressive psychosis, 670
  in schizophrenia, 666
Demeclocycline, as nephrotoxin, 1427
Dementia, 645, 660–663
  clinical manifestations of, 660
  diagnosis of, 660
  diagnostic issues in, 661
  "dialysis," 1381
  in Alzheimer's disease, 661, 662
  in cancer, 876, 877
  in Creutzfeldt-Jakob disease, 663
  in Huntington's chorea, 663, 758, 759
  in Pick's disease, 662
  multi-infarct, 661
  "presenile," 662
    vs. brain tumor, 868
  senile, 30
  treatment of, 663
  vs. delirium, 650
Dementia paralytica, 814
Demerol. See *Meperidine.*
Demethylchlortetracycline, *557,* 562
  as nephrotoxin, 1427
Demyelinating diseases, 843–851
  epilepsy associated with, 853
  vs. brain tumor, 868
Demyelination, status, 760
Dendrid. See *Idoxuridine.*
Dengue, 277–278, *279*
  vs. malaria, 573
  vs. rat-bite fever, 531
  vs. smallpox, 257
  vs. West Nile fever, 278
Dengue hemorrhagic fever, *293,* **296–298**
Dengue shock syndrome, 296, 297
Dengue virus, 277
  hemorrhagic fever caused by, 296
Dental. See *Teeth.*
Denture stomatitis, *Candida,* 548
11-Deoxycorticosterone
  properties of, *2145,* 2146
  secretion of, in 11β-hydroyxylase
    deficiency, 2160
11-Deoxycortisol
  properties of, *2145,* 2146
  secretion of, in 11β-hydroxylase
    deficiency, 2160
Deoxyribonucleic acid, 31
  replication of, 31
  synthesis of, slowed, megaloblastic
    anemia from, 1723, 1724
  Watson-Crick model for, 31
Depakene. See *Valproic acid.*
Depersonalization, in phobic anxiety
  syndrome, 674
Depigmentation, 2292–2293
Depomedroxyprogesterone acetate,
  nonestrogenic, in constitutional
  sexual precocity, 2182
Deprenyl, in parkinsonism, 756

Depressants, central nervous system
abuse of, 698–701
poisoning by, *712*
Depressed fractures, in head injury,
883
Depression, 675–678
in aged patients, 29
in anxious patient, 675
in dementia, 660
in maintenance hemodialysis, 1381
in manic-depressive psychosis, 669,
670
treatment of, 671
in paraplegia, 887
in rheumatoid arthritis, 190
mid-life, memory impairment in, 659
"monopolar," growth hormone
release failure in, 2080
vs. schizophrenia, 666, 667
WAIS scores in, 682
Dermacentor andersoni
in Colorado tick fever, 280
in Rocky Mountain spotted fever, 322
in tick paralysis, 117
in tularemia, 466
Dermacentor variabilis
in Rocky Mountain spotted fever, 322
in tick paralysis, 117
in tularemia, 466
Dermal leishmaniasis
post-kala-azar, 585, 587, *588*
vs. leprosy, 504
Dermatitis
atopic, **2283–2284**
**caterpillars and moths causing,
118–119**
contact, 2283
photoallergic, 2289
exfoliative, generalized, 400
gold-induced, complicating therapy of
rheumatoid arthritis, 192
in local radiation injury, 89
in malabsorption syndrome, 1530
in pellagra, 1688
millipedes causing, 117
of hands and feet, 2283–2284
papular, of Spangler, 2305
schistosome, 613
seborrheic, 2278
trombiculid mites causing, 113
"whip-lash," 114
Dermatitis herpetiformis, *2299, 2303,*
2304–2305
hemolytic anemia in, 1761
in adult celiac disease, 1541
Dermatoarthritis, lipoid, 201
Dermatobia hominis, 112
Dermatogenic enteropathy, *2299*
Dermatomyositis, 171–174, 923
as sign of internal malignancy, 879,
2296, 2297
childhood form of, 172, 173
eyes in, 2319
pulmonary involvement in, 974
Dermatophagoides farinae, 118
Dermatophagoides pteronyssinus, 118
Dermatosis(es)
febrile neutrophilic, acute, 2295
ichthyosiform, 2286, *2286*
Dermis, 2267, 2268
reticular, in slceroderma, 168
Dermoids, 864
Dermotypho, 318–320

Desferrioxamine
in hemochromatosis, 1791
in poisoning by iron salts, 75
Desferrioxamine test, in
hemochromatosis, 1791
Desiccocytosis, 1757
Deslanoside, in heart failure, *1096, 1097*
Desoxycorticosterone pivalate, in
Addison's disease, 2149
**Desquamative interstitial pneumonitis,
978**
DET, 704
Detergents, manufacture of, asthma-like
reactions in, 996, 997
**Development, human, growth and,
11–30**
Devic's disease, 849
Devil's grip, 271–272
Dexamethasone
in allergic rhinitis, 160
in bacterial meningitis, 416
in decompression sickness, 103
in diagnosis of Cushing's syndrome,
2154, 2155
in intracranial tumors, 869
in post-traumatic cerebral edema, 883
in rheumatoid arthritis, 192
phenobarbital and, simultaneous use
of, effects of, 2339
Dexamethasone phosphate, in
addisonian crisis, 2149
Dexamethasone sodium, in lead
encephalopathy, 79
Dexamethasone spray, in vasomotor
rhinitis, 160
Dextran(s)
in acute hemorrhagic anemia, 1730
in prevention of postoperative
thrombophlebitis, 1126
in shock, 1117, 1118
low molecular weight, as
nephrotoxins, 1434, 1435
Dextroamphetamine
abuse of, 701
in pain, *724, 725*
Dextroamphetamine sulfate, in
narcolepsy, 654
Dextropropoxyphene, in pain, *724, 725*
Dextroversion of heart, 1166
Diabetes insipidus, 2110–2111
hypernatremia in, 1956
in eosinophilic granuloma, 1849
in head injury, 882
nephrogenic, 1435–1437, 2064, 2110,
2111
posthypophysectomy, 2103
renal, *43*
X-linked, prevention and
management of, 55
Diabetes mellitus, 1969–1989
acromegaly and, 1982, 2106
air travel and, 96
arteriosclerosis obliterans in, 1299
atherosclerosis and, 1981
cerebral infarction and, 779
cirrhosis and, 1642
classification of, *1974*
clinical manifestations of, 1976
Cushing's syndrome and, 1982
cutaneous staphylococcal infections
in, 398
diagnosis of, 1974
diet in, 1709, 1710

Diabetes mellitus (*Continued*)
etiology of, 1974
eyes in, 1976, 1977, *1978,* **2320–2322**
hemochromatosis and, 1791, 1982
hyperosmolar coma in, treatment of,
1985
incidence and prevalence of, 1975
infection in, 1981
insulin in, 1985, *1985*
complications of, 1986, 1987, 1988
resistance to, 1987
juvenile-onset, 1974
HLA system and, 39
ketosis-prone, 1974
lipoatrophic, 1981, 1982, **2058**
malabsorption in, 1547, 1548
maturity-onset, 1974
mucormycosis in, 545
mumps and, 263
natural history of, 1975
obesity and, 1696, 1975, *1976*
oral hypoglycemic agents in, 1986,
1986
pancreatitis and, 1982
pathophysiology of, 1970
patient education in, 1989
peripheral neuropathy with, 908–909,
1979, 1980
vs. idiopathic autonomic
insufficiency, 763
pheochromocytoma and, 1982
pregnancy and, 1988, 1989
recurrence risks for, 57
renal changes in, 1403, 1977, 1979
secondary, 1982
skin in, 1980, 1981, *2300*
Somogyi effect in, 1987
stress, 1982
thyrotoxicosis and, 1982
treatment of, 1983
tuberculosis in, 483
vs. diabetes insipidus, 2110
Diabetic amyotrophy, 902, 909, 1980
Diabetic coma, hyperosmolar, treatment
of, 1985
Diabetic diarrhea, 1496–1497
Diabetic hyperlipemia, 2009
Diabetic ketoacidosis, 1975
fatty liver in, 1660
metabolic acidosis from, 1961, 1964
treatment of, 1983, 1984
volume depletion in, 1951
Diabetic lumbosacral plexus
neuropathy, 909
Diabetic nephropathy, 1403, 1977, 1979
acute renal failure in, 1369
Diabetic neuropathy, 908–909, 1979,
1980
Charcot joints in, 200
esophagus in, 1488
vs. acute abdomen, 1581
Diabetic retinopathy, 1976, 1977, *1978,*
2320, 2321
hypophysectomy and, 2103
Diabinese. See *Chlorpropamide.*
Dialysis, 1375, **1376–1382.** See also
Hemodialysis.
anemia in, 1381, 1731, 1732
fluid for, composition of, *1377, 1377*
in acute tubular necrosis, 1372
pericarditis and, 1272
peritoneal, 1377–1378
in accidental poisoning, 74

Dialysis (*Continued*)
  rapid, disequilibrium syndrome
    precipitated by, 1366
  ''Dialysis dementia,'' 1381
Dialysis encephalopathy, in chronic
    renal failure, 1366
Diamox. See *Acetazolamide.*
Diaphragm, diseases of, 1019
Diaphragmatic hernias, 1019, 1485,
  1485
Diarrhea, 1479–1480
  after extensive small intestinal
    resection, 1544
    for regional enteritis, 1567
  associated with coxsackie- and
    echoviruses, 275
  choleretic, 1479
  Cochin-China, 622–623
  colonic motility in, 1492
  diabetic, 1496–1497
  differential diagnosis in, 1480
  disorders associated with, cutaneous
    signs of, *2298–2299*
  epidemic, 305–306
  etiology of, 1479, 1480
  in bacterial food poisoning, 65
  in carcinoid syndrome, 2208
    treatment of, 2213
  in cholera, 461
  in chronic renal failure, 1365
  in clostridial food poisoning, 65
  in irritable bowel syndrome, 1493
  in regional enteritis, 1563
  in *Salmonella* gastroenteritis, 451
  in shigellosis, 458
  in typhoid fever, 447
  in Zollinger-Ellison syndrome, 1508
  large volume, 1479
  laxative-induced, hypokalemia in,
    1958
  metabolic acidosis from, 1962
  osmotic, 1479
  painless, 1493
  postvagotomy, 1520
  small volume, 1479, 1480
  treatment of, 1480
''Diarrhea treatment solution,'' in
    cholera, 462
Diathesis(es), bleeding, 1523
    albinism with, 2029
    in malabsorption syndrome, 1529
    intracranial hemorrhage from, 795
Diazepam
  abuse of, 698
  in bacterial meningitis, 416
  in convulsions of chronic renal
    failure, 1366
  in delirium tremens complicating
    pneumococcal pneumonia, 356
  in dystonia musculorum deformans,
    761
  in heart failure, 1094
  in hyperactive labyrinths, 740
  in hyperventilation-induced
    dizziness, 741
  in metabolic brain disease, 651
  in pain, *724*
  in spasmodic torticollis, 762
  in status epilepticus, *859*, 861
  in tetanus, 439
  poisoning by, *712*
Diazoxide
  in arterial hypertension, 1215
  in emergency reduction of blood
    pressure, 1216

Diazoxide (*Continued*)
  in hypertension of chronic renal
    failure, 1363
  in hypoglycemia caused by
    functioning islet cell tumors, 1995
  in toxemia of pregnancy, 1415
Dibenzyline. See *Phenoxybenzamine.*
Dicarboxylic aminoaciduria, *2020*
Dichuchwa, 522–523
Dicloxacillin, *557*, 559
Dicrocoeliasis, 618
Dicrocoelium dendriticum, 618
Dicyclomine hydrochloride
  in colonic diverticulosis, 1501
  in irritable bowel syndrome, 1494
Dientamoeba fragilis, 602
Diet(s), 1708–1712. See also *Nutrition.*
  after myocardial infarction, 1234
  aging patient and, 29
  high protein, in nephrotic syndrome,
    1389
  in acute renal failure, 1372
  in acute viral hepatitis, 1654
  in adult celiac disease, 1540
  in anorexia nervosa, 1702
  in chronic renal failure, 1711
  in classic galactosemia, 1998
  in colonic diverticulosis, 1501
  in constipation, 1481, 1482
  in diabetes mellitus, 1709, 1710
  in epilepsy, 861
  in irritable bowel syndrome, 1494
  in obesity, 1697, 1710
  in peptic ulcer, 1515
  in pneumococcal pneumonia, 356
  in rheumatoid arthritis, 190
  in ulcerative colitis, 1572
  normal, 1709
  protein-restricted, 1711
  sodium-restricted, 1711, 1712
Diethylcarbamazine
  in bancroftian filariasis, 634
  in bancroftian filariasis prevention,
    634
  in filariasis, *559*
  in loiasis, 635
  in onchocerciasis, 636
  in pulmonary tropical eosinophilia,
    637
  in river blindness, *559*
  in toxocariasis, 628
Diethylpropion, abuse of, 701
Diethylstilbestrol
  in cancer of prostate, 1921
  in hypopituitarism, 2102
  in prevention of hypercalcemia
    during hormonal treatment of
    breast cancer, 1920, 1921
  in testicular feminization, 2173
Diethyltryptamine, 704
Dietl's crisis, in nephroptosis, 1457
Diffuse collagenous pneumoconioses,
  990–992
Diffuse cutaneous leishmaniasis
  of new world, *588, 589*
  of old world, 588
Diffuse esophageal spasm, 1485–1486,
  1486
Diffuse mastocytosis, 2307
Diffuse meningeal neoplasia, 867
Diffuse sclerosis, 849–850
Diffusing capacity of lung for gases,
  936–937
Diffusion, 932, 936–938
  impaired, 940, 1022

DiGeorge's syndrome, 140–141
Digestive system, diseases of,
  1463–1669
Digital clubbing
  in bronchogenic carcinoma, 1007
  in hypertrophic osteoarthropathy, 201
  in infective endocarditis, 390
Digitalis
  blood levels of, determination of,
    1099
  effects and mechanisms of, 1095
  in acute myocardial infarction, 1099,
    1100
  in acute pulmonary edema of heart
    failure, 1094
  in heart failure, 1094–1100
  in shock, 1121
  preparations of, choice of, 1095, 1096,
    1096, 1097
    diagnostic, 1097
    intravenous, 1097
    oral, 1096
  proper dosage of, guides to, 1097,
    1098
  prophylactic use of, 1098
  toxicity of, 1098
    ectopic atrial tachycardias from,
      1250, 1251, *1251*
    treatment of, 1099
Digitoxin. See also *Digitalis.*
  in heart failure, 1095, *1096*, 1097
Digoxin. See also *Digitalis.*
  in acute tubular necrosis, 1373
  in atrial fibrillation, 1248
  in heart failure, 1095, 1096, *1096*, 1097
  in myocardial failure complicating
    relapsing fever, 528
  in shock, 1121
Dihydrocodeine, in pain, 725
Dihydropteridine reductase deficiency,
  2016
2,8-Dihydroxyadenine renal stones,
  2043
1,25-Dihydroxycholecalciferol, calcium
  absorption by, 1526
Diiodohydroxyquin, in amebiasis, *558,*
  593
Di-isocyanato diphenyl methane,
  asthma-like reactions to, 999
Dilantin. See *Diphenylhydantoin.*
Dilutional thrombocytopenia, 1877
Dimenhydrinate, in motion sickness,
  95
Dimercaprol
  in antimony poisoning, 81
  in arsenic poisoning, 76
  in gold-induced complications of
    rheumatoid arthritis, 192
  in lead poisoning, 79
Dimetane. See *Brompheniramine.*
2,5-Dimethoxy-4-methylamphetamine,
  704
Dimethyltriazeno-imidazole
  carboxamide, in oncologic treatment,
  1933
Dimethyltryptamine, 704
2,4-Dinitrochlorobenzene, in
  assessment of immune competence in
  cancer, 1925
Dinobdella species, as agents of disease,
  120
Dioctyl sodium sulfosuccinate
  after myocardial infarction, 1234
  in acquired megacolon, 1496
  in constipation, 1482

Dipetalonema perstans, 605, 632, **635**
Dipetalonema streptocerca, 632, 637
Diphenhydramine
  in anaphylactic reaction complicating
    therapy of serum sickness, 154
  in angioedema, 163
  in drug allergy, 157
  in insect stings, 163
  in parkinsonism, 755
  in senile tremor, 757
Diphenoxylate
  in diarrhea, 1480
  in diarrhea of carcinoid syndrome,
    2213
Diphenoxylate hydrochloride
  in diarrhea after extensive small
    intestinal resection, 1544
  in malabsorption syndrome, *1536*
Diphenylhydantoin, 1265–1266
  as nephrotoxin, 1432
  hypocalcemia induced by, 2241
  in cramps, 930
  in digitalis toxicity, 1099
  in epilepsy, *859,* 860
  in intracranial tumors, 869
  in myotonia congenita, 920
  in myotonic dystrophy, 918
  in status epilepticus, 861
  in tabes dorsalis, 815
  rickets or osteomalacia induced by,
    2253
2,3-Diphosphoglycerate, in oxygen
  dissociation, 1771
2,3-Diphosphoglyceric acid, levels of, in
  shock, 1113
Diphtheria, 429–433
  cutaneous, 431
    vs. tropical phagedenic ulcer, 530
  peripheral neuropathy with, 905
  vs. infectious mononucleosis, 266
  vs. streptococcal pharyngitis, 372
Diphtheria antitoxin, 432
Diphtheritic myocarditis, 431, 432, 1282
Diphyllobothrium latum, 559, 605, 606,
  607
Diphyllobothrium mansonoides, 607
Diphyllobothrium pacificum, 607
Diplacusis, in sensorineural hearing
  loss, 734
Diplopia, 899
  in brain tumors, 865
  in myasthenia gravis, 926
  in thyroid eye disease, 2333
Dipylidium caninum, 611
Dirofilaria conjunctivae, 637
Dirofilaria immitis, 637
Dirofilaria repens, 637
Dirofilaria tenuis, 637
Dirofilariasis, 637
Disaccharidase deficiency, 1529, **1539**
Disc(s)
  cervical, herniated, 894
  intervertebral, protrusion of, 893–894
    staphylococcal infections of, 402
  lumbar, diseases of, vs.
    arteriosclerosis obliterans, 1301
  herniated, 894
Discoid lupus erythematosus, 176
Disease. See names of specific diseases.
Disequilibrium, linkage, 39
Disequilibrium syndrome
  after dialysis in chronic renal failure,
    1366
  complicating maintenance
    hemodialysis, 1381

Disodium cromoglycate, in asthma,
  958
Disodium ethane-1-hydroxy-1,1-diphos-
  phonate, in Paget's disease, 2259
Disopyramide, 1266
Dissecting aortic aneurysm, 1295–1297,
  1296
  vs. acute pericarditis, 1273
  vs. myocardial infarction, 1233
Disseminated encephalomyelitis, acute,
  836–838, 849
Disseminated infection, "atypical"
  mycobacteria causing, 500
Disseminated intravascular coagulation
  hypofibrinogenemic syndromes
    associated with, 1893–1894
  in cancer patient, 1906
  in critically ill patient, 1052
  in shock, 1113
  without hypofibrinogenemia,
    1894–1895
Disseminated listeriosis in infants, 472
Disseminated tuberculosis, vs. glanders,
  469
Dissociation, atrioventricular,
  1255–1256, *1256*
Distal myopathy, 918
Disuse osteopenia, 2236, 2237
"Disuse" osteoporosis, 2244, 2245
Diuresis, forced, in acute drug
  poisoning, 714
Diuretics. See also names of specific
  agents.
  as nephrotoxins, 1432
  hypercalcemia and, 2237
  hypokalemia from, 1957, 1958
  in arterial hypertension, 1212, *1212,*
    1213
  in heart failure, 1102–1106, *1102, 1103,*
    1104
  in nephrotic syndrome, 1389
  metabolic alkalosis from, 1966
  osmotic, in accidental poisoning, 74
  in head injury, 882
Diuril. See *Chlorothiazide.*
Diverticulitis, 1582–1584
  Meckel's, 1500, 1501
  sigmoid, vs. Crohn's disease of colon,
    1578
  vs. ulcerative colitis, 1572
  vs. acute appendicitis, 1581
  vs. amebiasis, 592
Diverticulosis
  colonic, 1501–1502
  gallbladder, 1634
  vs. diverticulitis, 1583
Diverticulum(a)
  cecal, solitary, 1502
  colonic, 1501–1502
    angiography in, 1471, *1471*
    gastrointestinal bleeding in,
      1522
  duodenal, 1500
    bile duct obstruction by, 1632
  epiphrenic, 1500
  esophageal, 1499–1500
  gastric, 1500
  hypopharyngeal, 1499
  ileal, 1500–1501
  jejunal, 1500–1501
    malabsorption in, 1537
  Meckel's, 1500–1501
    radionuclide imaging in, 1470
  mid-esophageal, 1499
    pericardial, 1276

Diverticulum(a) (*Continued*)
  urethral, 1458
  Zenker's 1499
Diving
  atmospheric pressure changes with,
    98, *98*
  deep-sea, accidents during, vertigo
    caused by, 740
  hazards of, 98, 99, 102, 103
  scuba, air travel after, 96
Dizziness, 737–742
  conditions producing, 738–742
  epileptic, 741
  evaluation of, 737–738, *738*
  hyperventilation-induced, 741
  in cerebral transient ischemic attacks,
    785
  multisensory, 741, 742
  psychiatric disease producing, 742
  types of, 737
Dizziness simulation battery, 737, 738
DNA, 31
  replication of, 31
  synthesis of, slowed, megaloblastic
    anemia from, 1723, 1724
  Watson-Crick model for, 31
DNA–anti-DNA complexes, in systemic
  lupus erythematosus, 134
Dog tapeworm, 611
Dolichostenomelia, 2053–2054
Dolophine. See *Methadone.*
DOM, 704
Dominance, functional, 656
Donovan body, in granuloma inguinale,
  429
Donovania granulomatis, 429
L-Dopa, in assessment of growth hor-
  mone, 2092
Dopamine, 751, 2199, 2200
  cerebral, functional excess of, schizo-
    phrenia and, 668
  in shock, 1048, 1120
Doriden. See *Glutethimide.*
Dorsal root ganglionitis, in cancer, 878
Double outlet right ventricle, 1173
Downey cells, in infectious
  mononucleosis, 266
Down's syndrome
  acute leukemia in, 1814
  clinical and cytogenetic characteristics
    of, *52*
  frequency and sex ratio of, *48*
  heterozygote detection in, *58*
  intrauterine diagnosis of, 59
Doxinate. See *Dioctyl sodium sulfo-*
  succinate.
Doxorubicin. See also *Adriamycin.*
  in oncologic treatment, 1936, 1937
Doxycycline, 557, 562
  in epidemic louse-borne typhus, 319
  in louse-borne relapsing fever, 528
  in rickettsial diseases, 316
  in trachoma and inclusion conjunc-
    tivitis, 334
dp/dt, indices of, 1085
Dracontiasis, 633
Dracunculus medinensis, 605, 633
Dramamine. See *Dimenhydrinate.*
Dressings, wet, in dermatologic therapy, 2275, *2275,* 2276
Dressler's syndrome, 1237, 1271
Drop attacks, in brainstem ischemia,
  784, 785
Droplet nuclei, tuberculosis infection
  by, 480

Drowning, 105–108
Drug(s). See also names of specific
    agents.
  absorption of, rate of, changes in,
    2336, 2337
  abuse of, 692–714
    infective endocarditis in, 390
  acute poisoning with, 711–714, *712*
  aging patient and, 29, 30
  antiarrhythmic, 1264–1266. See also
    names of specific agents.
  bactericidal and bacteriostatic, 555
  binding of, to plasma proteins, 2337
  cytotoxic, 1930–1938. See also
    Cytotoxic agents and names of spe-
    cific agents.
  dependence upon, 692–714
  genetically determined responses to,
    45–46
  hypersensitivity reactions to, 154–157
  in obesity, 1698
  interactions of, 2336–2341. See also
    Drug-drug interactions.
  intoxication with, 692–714
  metabolism of, drug interactions and,
    2338–2340
    in liver disease, 1641
    inhibition of, 2339, 2340
    stimulation of, 2338, 2339
  microbes and, 549–553
  oral contraceptive, cerebral infarction
    and, 781
  ototoxic, hearing loss from, 736
    vertigo from, 739
  pairing of, 552
  peripheral neuropathy associated
    with, 910
  reactions to, adverse, 2341
    hypersensitivity, 154–157
      liver disease due to, 1659–1660
    immune mechanisms in, 131
  therapeutic and toxic levels of, 2356
Drug allergy, 154–157
  vs. malaria, 573
Drug eruption, 2279, *2280*
  vs. secondary syphilis, 510
Drug fever, 155, 156
  vs. infective endocarditis, 392
Drug idiosyncrasy, vs. drug allergy, 155
Drug intolerance, vs. drug allergy, 155
Drug purpura, 1873–1874, *1873*
  nonthrombocytopenic, 1880
Drug rash, vs. measles, *249*
Drug resistance
  forms of, 551, 552
  in pulmonary tuberculosis, 488, 489
Drug susceptibility, in antimicrobial
  agent selection, 554
Drug-drug interactions, 2336–2341
  adverse reactions from, 2341
    at receptor sites and cell membranes,
      2337, 2338
    in management of heart failure, 1094,
      1095
  physical-chemical processes in,
    2336–2338
  renal clearance and, 2338
Drug-induced acute pancreatitis, 1551
Drug-induced antibodies, hemolysis
  due to, 1766
Drug-induced aplastic anemia, 156, 1734
Drug-induced benign intracranial
  hypertension, 871
Drug-induced embryopathy, 48, 49

Drug-induced fasting hypoglycemia,
  1996
Drug-induced galactorrhea, 2191
Drug-induced hemolysis, 1769
Drug-induced hepatitis, vs. acute viral
  hepatitis, 1653
Drug-induced hypersensitivity angiitis,
  vs. periarteritis nodosa, 183
Drug-induced hyponatremia, 1954
Drug-induced malabsorption, 1548
Drug-induced myocarditis, 1287
Drug-induced myopathy, 924
Drug-induced neutropenia, 1808,
  1809
Drug-induced parkinsonism, 753
Drug-induced peptic ulcer, 1504
Drug-induced pericarditis, 1272
Drug-induced platelet abnormalities,
  1879
Drug-induced polycythemia, 1799
Drug-induced pulmonary hyper-
  sensitivity reactions, 974–976
Drug-induced systemic lupus erythe-
  matosus, 156, 179, 975, *975*
Drug-induced urticaria, 161
Drusen, intrapapillary, 2328
Dry beriberi, 772–773
Dry pleurisy, 491
  in pulmonary tuberculosis, 486
DTIC, in oncologic treatment, 1933
dU suppression test, in megaloblastic
  anemias, *1725, 1726*
Dubin-Johnson syndrome, *42,* 1638,
  1649, 1650
Duchenne dystrophy, 915, 916, *916,* 917,
  918
  cardiomyopathy in, 1280, 1281
  heterozygote detection in, 57, 58, *58*
Ductus arteriosus, patent, 1162–1164
  pulmonary hypertension in, 1141,
    1142
Dumping syndrome, 1520
Duodenal drainage, normal values for,
  2353
Duodenal ulcer. See also *Peptic ulcer.*
  duodenitis and, 1508
  hyperparathyroidism and, 1504
  pain in, radiation of, 1477
  pathogenesis of, 1503, 1504
  pathophysiology of, 1504, 1505, 1506,
    1507
  radiographic appearance of, 1511,
    1511, 1512
  surgical treatment of, indications for,
    1519
  types of, 1519, *1519*
Duodenitis, duodenal ulcer and, 1508
Duodenogastric reflux, peptic ulcer and,
  1507
Duodenoscopy, in peptic ulcer, 1511
Duodenum
  adenocarcinoma of, *1605*
  arterial supply to, 1586, *1586*
  diverticula of, 1500
    bile duct obstruction by, 1632
  in scleroderma, 169
  motility in, disorders of, 1488–1490
    normal, 1488, 1489
  pain originating in, 1476
  tuberculosis of, 492
Dural sinuses, major, thrombosis of,
  808–809
Duroziez' sign, in aortic regurgitation,
  1195

Dust(s)
  "angel," 704
  exposure to, neoplasia associated
    with, 994–995
    occupational bronchitis and, 995,
      996
  inorganic, cellular reaction to, 985
    pneumoconioses due to, diagnosis
      of, 986
    treatment and prevention of,
      993–994
    pulmonary effects of, *984*
  organic. See *Organic particles.*
Dwarf tapeworm, 609
Dwarfism
  achondroplastic, 2264
  hypopituitary, growth hormone
    radioimmunoassay in, 2091
  pituitary, 2103, 2104, 2105
    classification of, *2104*
    management of, 55
Dye dilution, cardiac output
  determination by, 1032
Dysautonomia, familial, 912, 2057–2058
  osteoporosis in, 2245, 2246
Dysbaric osteonecrosis of divers and
  caisson workers, 102
Dysbetalipoproteinemia, familial,
  2005–2006
Dyschondroplasia, Ollier's, 2264
Dyscrasia(s)
  plasma cell, 1852–1867, *1852*
    clinical patterns of, 1858–1867
    of unknown significance, 1852,
      1866–1867
      electrophoretic patterns in, 1857,
        1857
    paraproteins of, 1853, *1853*
    pathogenesis of, 1852
    serum and urinary proteins in,
      electrophoretic patterns of, 1854,
      1855, 1856, 1857
  plasmacytic and monocytic,
    association between, 1867
Dysentery
  amebic, 589–594
    Trichuris and, 629
    vs. balantidiasis, 603
  bacillary, 457, 458
    vs. amebic dysentery, 592
Dysequilibrium, 737, 741
Dysfibrinogenemia, congenital, *1884,*
  1889
Dysglobulinemia, platelet abnormalities
  in, 1879
Dyskeratosis congenita, 2297, *2302*
Dyskinesia, tardive, 669, 753
Dyslipoproteinemias, 2010
Dyspareunia, 689
Dyspepsia, functional, vs. peptic ulcer,
  1508
Dysphagia, 1479
  cervical spine spurs producing, 1483
  disorders associated with, cutaneous
    signs of, *2298*
  in achalasia, 1487
  in bronchogenic carcinoma, 1006
  in diffuse esophageal spasm, 1486
  in esophageal carcinoma, 1597
  in iron deficiency anemia, 1748
  in myasthenia gravis, 926
  in polymyositis and dermatomyositis,
    173
  in tetanus, 439

Dysphagia (*Continued*)
neurologic disorders causing, 1483
sideropenic, 1483
esophageal carcinoma and, 1597
Dysphagia lusoria, 1483
Dysphasia, in cerebral infarction, 786
Dysplasia
chondroectodermal, 2264
fibrous, 2262–2263
Dyspnea
in angina pectoris, 1225
in aortic regurgitation, 1195
in asthma, 956, 957
in bronchogenic carcinoma, 1006
in chronic obstructive pulmonary
disease, 960
in complicated pneumoconiosis, 993
in diffuse collagenous
pneumoconioses, 991
in inorganic dust pneumoconioses,
986
in left ventricular failure, 1089
in mitral stenosis, 1180
in primary pulmonary hypertension,
1139
in scleroderma, 169
Monday morning, in byssinosis, 997,
997
paroxysmal nocturnal, in left
ventricular failure, 1090
Dysproteinemia(s)
renal changes in, 1406
vascular purpura in, 1880
Dyssebacea, 1675
Dyssynergia cerebellaris myoclonica,
768
Dystonia, 751
torsion, 760–761
Dystonia musculorum deformans,
760–761
vs. striatonigral degeneration, 765
Dystrophy(ies)
muscular, 915–918
Becker, 917
Duchenne, 915, 916, *916*, 917, 918
cardiomyopathy in, 1280, 1281
heterozygote detection in, 57, 58,
58
fascioscapulohumeral, 915, *916*, 917
limb-girdle, 915, *916*, 917
myotonic, 915, *916*, 917, 918
cardiomyopathy in, 1281
testicular atrophy in, 2170
ocular, 918
respiratory failure in, 1024
vs. polymyositis, 173, 923
reflex neurovascular, 206
"reflex sympathetic," 727
Dysuria, in diverticulitis, 1583

Ear(s)
disease of, head pain and, 733
in mycoplasmal pneumonia, 346
in mycoplasmal respiratory diseases,
344, 345
in relapsing polychondritis, 218
middle, infection of, brain abscess
from, 805
inflammation of. See *Otitis media.*
tuberculosis of, 492
East African sleeping sickness, 576
Eastern equine encephalitis, 285–286

Eastern equine encephalitis virus, 285
Eastern Hemisphere, tick-borne
rickettsioses of, 324–325
Eaton-Lambert syndrome, 929
Ebola virus, 300
Ebstein's anomaly of tricuspid valve,
1168
Ecchymoses, in scurvy, 1690, *1690*
Echidnophaga gallinacea, 110
Echinococcosis, 609–610
bile duct obstruction by, 1632
immunodiagnostic tests for, *565*
Echinococcus granulosus, 605, 606, 606,
609, 610
Echinococcus granulosus var. canadensis,
609, 610
Echinococcus multilocularis, 606, 609, 610
Echinoderms, envenomation by, 124
Echinostoma species, infection by, 621
Echocardiography
in acquired valvular heart disease,
1178, *1179*
in acute pericarditis, 1273
in aortic regurgitation, 1196
in aortic stenosis, 1192
in atrial septal defect, 1162
in cardiovascular disease, 1076, *1077*
in congenital pulmonary valve
regurgitation, 1168
in discrete subvalvular aortic stenosis,
1167
in Ebstein's anomaly, 1168
in endocardial cushion defect, 1171
in Fallot's tetralogy, 1165, 1166
in idiopathic hypertrophic subaortic
stenosis, 1278, *1278*
in mitral regurgitation, 1187
in mitral stenosis, *1179*, 1182
in mitral valve prolapse syndrome,
1189
in pericardial constriction, 1275
in pericardial effusion, 1274
in scleroderma, 170
in tricuspid regurgitation, 1198
in tricuspid stenosis, 1198
Echoencephalography, 749, 750
in head injury, 881
Echography, abdominal, 1465–1466,
1465, 1466
Echothiophate iodide, in glaucoma,
2322
Echoviruses
diarrhea associated with, 275
distinctive features of, 268
infection with, general aspects of,
269–270, *269*
pericarditis and myocarditis caused
by, 272
Eclampsia, 1414
vs. acute intermittent porphyria, 2047
Economo's disease, parkinsonism
secondary to, 753
Ecthyma, vs. tularemia, 467
Ecto-5'-nucleotidase deficiency, 2043
Ectopia, renal, congenital, 1457
Ectopia lentis, in homocystinuria, 2028
Ectopic ACTH syndrome, 2152, 2153
diagnosis of, 2155
treatment of, 2156
Ectopic atrial tachycardia, 1250–1251,
1251
Ectopic beats, ventricular, in myocardial
infarction, 1230, 1235
"Ectopic" hyperparathyroidism, 2217

Ectopic polypeptides, as tumor
markers, 1913
Eczema vaccinatum, 260
EDCI, as tumor marker, 1913
Edecrin. See *Ethacrynic acid.*
Edema
angioneurotic, 162–163. See also
Angioedema.
brain, "interstitial," in benign
intracranial hypertension, 871
cerebral, following cardiopulmonary
resuscitation, 1058
in bacterial meningitis, 412
in cerebral infarction, 778, 791
in head injury, 881, 882, 883, 885
in intracranial tumors, 864
in louse-borne relapsing fever, 528
in Reye's syndrome, 839
hunger, 1684
in acute poststreptococcal
glomerulonephritis, 1395, 1396
in chronic obstructive pulmonary
disease, 963
in chronic renal failure, 1363
in kwashiorkor, 1681, *1682*
in malabsorption, 1528
in minimal change glomerular
disease, 1392
in nephrotic syndrome, 1388, *1388*
in nutritional deficiency, 1676
in toxemia of pregnancy, 1414, 1415
pulmonary
acute, in left ventricular failure,
1090
management of, 1094
chemical, 1001
in acute chemical bronchitis or
pneumonitis, 1000
diseases causing, respiratory failure
in, 1023–1024, *1023*
high altitude, 101
in chronic renal failure, 1363
in malaria, 571, 572, 574
"neurogenic," 717
vs. Goodpasture's syndrome, 976
vs. pulmonary embolism, 1133
refractory, in heart failure, 1106
subcutaneous, in right ventricular
failure, 1092
vasogenic brain, 864
Edrophonium
in diagnosis of myasthenia gravis,
927
in myasthenia gravis, 928
Edwards' syndrome, clinical and
cytogenetic characteristics of, *52*
EEG, 749. See also
Electroencephalography.
Effective arterial blood volume, in
control of sodium excretion, 1321
Effort syncope, 744
Effort syndrome, vs. angina pectoris,
1227
Effusion(s)
pericardial, 1273–1274
chylous, 1276
in right ventricular failure, 1093
pleural
in cancer patient, 1904
in pneumococcal pneumonia, 353
in pulmonary infarction, 1130
in systemic diseases, 1017, 1018
with pneumonia, 1015
pleurisy and, tuberculous, 485

Effusion(s) (*Continued*)
serofibrinous pleurisy with, 482, 491
subdural, in bacterial meningitis, 412
EHDP, in Paget's disease, 2259
Ehlers-Danlos syndrome, 2054–2055, *2298*
aortic complications of, 1291
osteoporosis in, 2245
Eisenmenger's complex, 1170
Ejaculation, 687
premature, 688, 2198
Ejection fraction, 1085
Elapidae, bites by, 121, 122
Elastase, in protein absorption, 1525
Elastin, 164, 165
Elavil. See *Amitriptyline.*
Elbow, tennis, 207
Electric shock and electric injury, 92–94, *93*
Electrical control mechanisms for intestinal motility, 1475
Electrocardiography, 1075
in accelerated idioventricular rhythms, 1254, *1254*
in acquired valvular heart disease, 1177, 1178
in acute pericarditis, 1272
in acute renal failure, 1372
in alcoholic cardiomyopathy, 1284
in angina pectoris, 1225, 1226
in anomalous origin of left coronary artery, 1172
in aortic regurgitation, 1196
in aortic stenosis, 1192
in arterial hypertension, 1204
in asymmetric septal hypertrophy, 1278, 1279
in atrial extrasystoles, 1246, *1246*
in atrial fibrillation, 1247, *1247*
in atrial flutter, 1248, *1248*
in atrial septal defect, 1161
in atrioventricular dissociation, 1255, *1256*
in bradycardia-tachycardia syndrome, 1244, *1244*
in cardiac amyloidosis, 1285
in cerebral infarction, 789
in Chagas' disease, 582
in chagasic myocarditis, 1283
in chronic obstructive pulmonary disease, 961, 962
in common atrium, 1169
in congenital aneurysms of sinuses of Valsalva, 1170
in congenital complete heart block, 1166
in congenital coronary arteriovenous fistula, 1169
in congenital pulmonary valve regurgitation, 1168
in congenital valvular aortic stenosis, 1157
in dextroversion of heart, 1166
in dissecting aortic aneurysm, 1296
in Ebstein's anomaly, 1168
in ectopic atrial tachycardia, 1250, *1251*
in Fallot's tetralogy, 1165
in hypercalcemia, 2238
in hyperkalemia, 1959, *1959*
in hypocalcemia, 2242
in hypokalemia, 1958, *1958*
in Lutembacher's syndrome, 1169
in mitral regurgitation, 1187

Electrocardiography (*Continued*)
in mitral stenosis, 1182
in mitral valve prolapse syndrome, 1189
in myocardial infarction, 1231, 1232
in paroxysmal atrial tachycardia, *1249,* 1250, 1251, *1251*
in patent ductus arteriosus, 1163
in pericardial constriction, 1275
in pericardial effusion, 1274
in primary pulmonary hypertension, 1140
in pulmonary disease, 950
in pulmonary embolism, 1132
in pulmonic stenosis, 1159
in rheumatic carditis, 380, 381
in right ventricular origin of both great arteries, 1173
in scleroderma, 170
in shock, 1116
in sinoatrial block, 1245, *1245*
in situs inversus, 1166
in tricuspid atresia, 1171–1172
in tricuspid regurgitation, 1198
in tricuspid stenosis, 1198
in ventricular extrasystoles, 1252, *1252*
in ventricular fibrillation, 1255, *1255*
in ventricular septal defect, 1170
in ventricular tachycardia, 1253, *1253*
in Wolff-Parkinson-White syndrome, 1257, *1257, 1258, 1259*
Electroconvulsive treatment, in depression of manic-depressive psychosis, 671
Electroencephalography, 749
in akinetic seizure, 854
in brain tumor, 866
in epilepsy, 854, 855, 857, 858
in focal seizures, 855
in generalized seizures, 854
in head injury, 881
in herpes simplex encephalitis, 823
in hypercalcemia, 2238
in hypocalcemia, 2242
in hypoparathyroidism, 2221
in mental disturbances accompanying chronic renal failure, 1366
in metabolic brain disease, 649
in myoclonic seizures, 854
in petit mal, 854
in syncope, 742
in viral meningitis and encephalitis, 820
Electrolytes
absorption of, 1525
diminished, in malabsorption syndrome, 1529
disorders of, 1950–1969
in cancer patient, 1904
in cholera, 461, 462
in impaired gastric emptying complicating peptic ulcer, 1517
in intestinal obstruction, 1491
in kwashiorkor, 1683
in myxedema coma, 2134
in pneumococcal pneumonia, 356
in rickettsial diseases, 316
in shigellosis, 458, 459
Electromyography, 749
in differential diagnosis of neuropathy, 904
in differentiation of neurogenic and myopathic disease, 915
in intraspinal compression, 892

Electromyography (*Continued*)
in polymyositis and dermatomyositis, 173
single-fiber, in myasthenia gravis, 926, 927
Electronystagmography, in evaluation of dizziness, 738
Elephantiasis
in bancroftian filariasis, 634
in lymphogranuloma venereum, 335
vs. maduromycosis, 542
Elephantiasis neuromatosa, 770
ELISA test
in protozoan and helminthic diseases, *565*
in sleeping sickness, 578
Elliptocytosis, hereditary, 1757
Ellis–van Creveld syndrome, 2264
Embden-Meyerhof pathway enzymes, defects in, 1758–1759
Embolectomy
in arterial embolism, 1304
in pulmonary embolism, 1134
Embolism
air, hyperbaric oxygen therapy in, 104
transfusion reaction from, *1785,* 1786
amniotic fluid, hypofibrinogenemia in, 1893, 1894
arterial, 1303–1304
prevention of, 1134
vs. arteriosclerosis obliterans, 1301
cerebral, 788
in head injury, 885
gas, in diving, 99
infective endocarditis with, cerebrospinal fluid findings in, *803*
mesenteric artery, 1589
pulmonary, 1015, 1129–1134
in myocardial infarction, 1231
massive, vs. myocardial infarction, 1232, 1233
Embolization, pulmonary, vs. acute pericarditis, 1273
Embolus(i), 1122
arterial, renal infarction from, 1407
cerebral, 778
anticoagulant drugs in, 793
cerebral infarction from, 779–780
vs. cerebral transient ischemic attacks, 785
in arterial embolism, 1303
in infective endocarditis, 389, 390
in mitral stenosis, 1181
pulmonary, pulmonary vascular disease in, 1143
Embryonal carcinoma of kidney, 1460
Embryopathy, drug-induced, 48, 49
Emesis, induced, in accidental poisoning, 74
Emetine hydrochloride
in amebiasis, 593
in stonefish sting, 125
Emotion
angina pectoris provoked by, 1225
hypothalamic dysfunction and, 716
irritable bowel syndrome and, 1493
Emotional expression, in schizophrenia, 666
Emphysema, 951, 960, 961, 962
air travel and, 96
mediastinal, 1018
respiratory failure from, 1023
roentgenographic appearance of, 942

Emphysematous cholecystitis, 1628
Emphysematous type of chronic
  obstructive pulmonary disease, 961,
  961
"Empty nest" crisis, 24
Empty sella syndrome, 870, 2099, *2099*
  amenorrhea due to, 2187
Empyema, 1015
  in acute cholecystitis, 1626, 1628
  in hemolytic streptococcal
    pneumonia, 375
  in pneumococcal pneumonia, 353
    treatment of, 356
  subdural, 807–808
    cerebrospinal fluid examination in,
      803, 807
  ventricular, cerebrospinal fluid
    findings in, *803*
Empyema necessitatis, in pneumococcal
  pneumonia, 353
Encephalitic complications of viral
  infections and vaccines, 836–839
Encephalitis(des)
  amebic, vs. viral encephalitis, 820
  "bacterial," 806, 807
  bulbar, in cancer, 877
  California, 288
  Dawson's, 841
  epidemic, vs. dystonia musculorum
    deformans, 761
  epilepsy associated with, 852
  equine, eastern, 285–286
    Venezuelan, 286–288
    western, 284–285
  hemorrhagic, acute, cerebrospinal
    fluid findings in, *803*
    drugs causing, 156
  herpes simplex, 821–824
    vs. arboviral encephalitis, 284
  in Colorado tick fever, 280
  in fulminating meningococcemia, 419
  in influenza, 243
  in mumps, 262
  in nonpolio enteroviral infections, 270
  in varicella, 254
  inclusion body, subacute, 841
  infectious, vs. acute disseminated
    encephalomyelitis, 838
  Japanese B, 289–290
  Murray Valley, 290
  postinfectious, vs. arboviral
    encephalitis, 284
  postvaccinal, vs. arboviral
    encephalitis, 284
  postvaccinial, 260
  Russian spring-summer, 290–291
  St. Louis, 288–289
  viral, 817–821
    arthropod-borne, 283–291
    vs. malaria, 573
    vs. poliomyelitis, 831
  viruses associated with, 817, *817*, 818,
    818
Encephalitis lethargica, parkinsonism
  secondary to, 753
Encephalitis periaxialis diffusa, 849
Encephalography
  air, in head injury, 881
  isotope, in brain tumor, 867
Encephalomyelitis, 817
  allergic, experimental, 844
  disseminated, acute, 836–838, 849
  following antirabies vaccination,
    838–839

Encephalomyelitis (*Continued*)
  in measles, 248
  myalgic, benign, 307
    vs. poliomyelitis, 831
  necrotizing hemorrhagic, acute, 849
  postinfectious, 836
  postvaccinal, 836, 837
  postvaccination, 836
Encephalopathy(ies)
  bilirubin, 1649
  dialysis, in chronic renal failure, 1366
  hepatic, 1640–1641
    in cirrhosis, 1665, 1666
  hypertensive, 793–794, 1205
  lead, 78, 79
  metabolic, 645. See also *Brain,*
    metabolic disease of.
    causes of, *644*
    coma caused by, 642
    diagnosis of, 649–651
    endogenous, 645
    exogenous, 645
    in chronic liver disease, 1640, 1641
    vs. dementia in cancer, 877
  portal-systemic, 1640–1641
  progressive subcortical, 794
  pulmonary, benign intracranial
    hypertension in, 872
  toxic, vs. arboviral encephalitis, 284
Enchondromatosis, multiple, 2264
Encopresis, in acquired megacolon,
  1496
End-diastolic pressure, ventricular, 1084
Endemic cretinism, 2138
Endemic goiter, 2137–2138, *2138*
Endemic hemoptysis, in
  paragonimiasis, 619
Endemic syphilis, 522–523
End-expiratory pressure, in acute
  respiratory failure, 1027, 1041, 1042
Endobronchial tuberculosis, 491
Endocardial cushion defect, 1171
Endocardial fibroelastosis, 1280
Endocarditis
  anaerobic, 443
  Aspergillus, 387
  bacterial, 386–395. See also
    Endocarditis, infective.
  Candida, 387
  enterococcal, 386, 390
    treatment of, 393
  fibroplastic, Löffler's, 1286
  fungal, 387
    treatment of, 394
  gonococcal, 387, 407, 408, 410
    treatment of, 394
  infective, 386–396
    acute, clinical manifestations of, 389
      vs. subacute endocarditis, 386,
        386
    antimicrobial prophylaxis in, *564*
    aortic regurgitation in, 1194
    bacteremia in, 387, 388, 391
    cerebral manifestations of, 809
    classification of, 386, *386*
    clinical manifestations of, 389
    differential diagnosis of, 391
    embolism and, cerebrospinal fluid
      findings in, *803*
    epidemiology of, 387
    fungi in, 387
    glomerulonephritis in, 1397–1398
    in aortic stenosis, 1191
    in drug abusers, 390, 696, 697

Endocarditis (*Continued*)
  infective, laboratory findings in, 391
    laboratory findings in, 391
    lesions of, mechanisms in
      production of, 388, 389
    microbiology of, 386
    neurologic disorders in, 390, 809
    pathogenesis and pathology of, 387
    portal of entry in, 388
    prognosis in, 395
    prophylaxis of, 395
    special syndromes of, 390, 391
    subacute, clinical manifestations of,
      389
    in heroin addiction, 696, 697
    vs. acute endocarditis, 386, *386*
    vs. rheumatic fever, 383
    vs. viral meningitis or
      encephalitis, 820
    treatment of, 392
      antimicrobial, 392
        untoward effects of, 394
      response to, 395
      surgical, 395
    vs. bacterial meningitis, 414
    vs. malaria, 573
  marantic, 387
  meningococcal, 394
  nonbacterial, verrucous, in systemic
    lupus erythematosus, 176, 177
  nonbacterial thrombotic, 387
    in cancer patient, 1905
    vs. infective endocarditis, 392
  pneumococcal, 353, 386
    treatment of, 394
  prosthetic valve, 391
  Q fever, 330
  staphylococcal, 386, 403–404
    treatment of, 393, 404
  streptococcal, 386
    treatment of, 392, 393
  with sterile blood cultures, treatment
    of, 394
Endocardium, candidiasis of, 548
Endocrine adenomatosis, multiple, 2098
    detection of, in relatives, *58*
    hypercalcemia in, 2238
    in acromegaly, 2106
Endocrine neoplasia, multiple,
    inherited, neuropathy with, 909
Endocrine osteoporosis, 2244
Endocrine system
  changes in, in liver disease, 1641,
    1642
  with aging, 26
  diseases of, 2060–2224
    anemia in, 1732
    associated with cancer, 1914–1918
    benign intracranial hypertension
      with, 871
    categories of, 2063–2065
    diagnosis of
      laboratory, 2065, 2066, *2066*, 2067
      principles of, 2065–2068
    "functional," 2064
    iatrogenic, 2064, 2065
    in bronchogenic carcinoma, 1006,
      1007
    in etiology of acute pancreatitis,
      1551
    myopathy in, 923, 924
    of hypothalamic origin, *2079*
    peripheral neuropathy with, 909
    physical examination in, 2065

Endocrine system (*Continued*)
failure of, secondary and tertiary, 2063, 2064
functions of, 2060–2062
hyperfunction of, peptic ulcer and, 1508–1509
primary, 2063
secondary, 2063
hypofunction of, primary, 2063
in anorexia nervosa, 1701
in chronic renal failure, 1361, 1362
in kwashiorkor, 1683
in malnutrition, 1680
in systemic lupus erythematosus, 175
Endolimax nana, 602
Endometrial cycle, 2177–2178
Endometriosis, 1612–1613
pelvic, vs. colorectal carcinoma, 1610
Endometrium
biopsy of, 2180
destruction of, amenorrhea from, 2184
tuberculosis of, 496
Endomyocardial fibrosis, 1286
Endomyocarditis, eosinophilic, Löffler's, 225
Endophthalmitis, in toxocariasis, 628
Endoreduplication, chromosomal, 54
Endorphins, 2077, *2078*, 2083, **2091**
measurement of, 2094
Endosalpinx, tuberculosis of, 496
Endoscopic retrograde cholangio-pancreatography, 1472–1473, *1472, 1473*
in biliary disease, 1622, 1623, *1623*
in chronic pancreatitis, 1556
Endoscopy
in achalasia, 1487
in diagnosis of constipation, 1481
in gastric carcinoma, 1601, 1602, *1602*
in gastrointestinal bleeding, 1522
in peptic ulcer, 1511, 1512
Endothelial glomerulonephritis, 1399, 1400
Endotoxemia, tests for, 454
Endotoxin, in enteric bacterial infections, 453
Endotracheal intubation
in acute respiratory failure, 1026, 1039, 1040
in cardiopulmonary arrest, 1055
Endoxan. See *Cyclophosphamide*.
Enemas, in constipation, 1482
Enkephalins, 2077, *2078*, 2083
Entamide furoate, in intestinal amebiasis, 593
Entamoeba coli, 592, 602
Entamoeba hartmanni, 592
Entamoeba histolytica, 558, 570, 589, 590, 592
Entamoeba polecki, 592
Enteric bacterial infections, 453–457
treatment of, 456, 457
Enteric fever, 449
clinical manifestations of, 451
diagnosis of, 452
treatment of, 452
Enteric form of tularemia, 466
Enteritis
granulomatous, vs. eosinophilic gastroenteritis, 1543
infectious, acute, malabsorption in, 1546
radiation, 1584–1585
malabsorption syndrome in, 1547

Enteritis (*Continued*)
regional, 1560–1567
ankylosing spondylitis in, 198, 1561
arthritis in, 198
clinical complications of, 1564
clinical manifestations of, 1562, 1563
diagnosis of, 1564
differential diagnosis of, 1565
epidemiology of, 1561
etiology of, 1561
eyes in, 2316
genetics in, 1561
laboratory studies in, 1563
malabsorption in, 1543, 1564
pathogenesis of, 1562
pathology of, 1562, *1562*
physical examination in, 1563
prognosis in, 1567
sclerosing cholangitis and, 1633
treatment of, 1566
Enteritis necroticans, 66
Enterobiasis, 629–630
Enterobius vermicularis, 559, 605, 629
life cycle of, *621*
Enterococcal endocarditis, 386, 390
treatment of, 393
Enterococcal meningitis, 416
Enterococci, 366, 367
Enterocolitis
pseudomembranous, 1585
necrotizing, acute, 405
radiation, 1584–1585
staphylococcal, 404–405
Enteropathy
dermatogenic, *2299*
exudative, in X-linked infantile agammaglobulinemia, 140
gluten, 1539
HLA system and, 39
protein-losing, 1528, **1548–1549,** *1548, 1549*
Enterotoxin
in cholera, 461
in shigellosis, 458
Enteroviral diseases, 268–275
vs. arboviral encephalitis, 284
vs. measles, *249*
vs. smallpox, 257
Enteroviruses, 268, *268*
exanthems caused by, 274
meningitis and encephalitis from, 818, *818,* 819
newer, 269
nonpolio
distinctive features of, 268–269
infection with
general aspects of, 269–270, *269*
paralysis and other neurologic complications of, 270
pericarditis and myocarditis caused by, 272–273
respiratory illness due to, 275
Enthrane, as nephrotoxin, 1433
Entomophobia, 108
Entrapment neuropathies, 901, 902
Enuresis, 655
Environment, 12–15
heredity and, in disease development, 11, 12
Environmental factors
blood pressure and, 1200, 1201
classification of, 13–14
in cancer, 1907–1911
colorectal, 1606

Environmental factors (*Continued*)
in congenital malformations, *48*
in development of alcohol abuse, 706
in disease, 12, 13–14, **60–125**
behavioral change and, 15
in health improvement, 14, *14*
in host defense compromise, 146
in pathogenesis of peptic ulcer, 1503
response to, determinants of, 12–13
Environmental pressure, physics of, 97, 98, *98*
Enzyme(s)
amplification of activity of, in management of genetic disease, 55
deficiencies of, hemolysis from, 1758–1761
in kwashiorkor, 1682
replacement of, in management of genetic disease, 55
serum, concentrations of, in myocardial infarction, 1232
in acute pericarditis, 1272
in differentiation of neurogenic and myopathic disease, 915
in liver disease, 1647
Enzyme assays, 2348–2349
Eosinophilia
diffuse fasciitis associated with, vs. dermatomyositis, 174
diseases associated with, 225–226
helminthic infections and, 638
in multiple myeloma, 1860
in neoplastic disorders, 226
in scarlet fever, 371
in strongyloidiasis, 623
in toxocariasis, 628
in trichinosis, 630
pulmonary, prolonged, 969–970, *969*
simple, 969, *969*
tropical, 225, 637, 969, 970
with asthma, *969,* 970
with periarteritis nodosa, *969,* **970**
pulmonary infiltration with, 225, **968–970,** *969*
drugs causing, 156
radiation-related, 226
Eosinophilic adenomas, 863
Eosinophilic collagen disease, 226
Eosinophilic endomyocarditis, Löffler's, 225
Eosinophilic gastroenteritis, 1542–1543
vs. regional enteritis, 1566
Eosinophilic granuloma, 978, 1543, **1848–1850,** *1849*
treatment of, 1850–1851
Eosinophilic leukemia, 226
Eosinophilic leukemoid reactions, 1813
Eosinophilic lung, 637
Eosinophilic meningoencephalitis, *Angiostrongylus cantonensis* causing, 631
Eosinophilic syndromes, 225–226
pulmonary, 225
Ependymoma, 863
spinal cord, 897
Ephedrine
in asthma, 958
in erythromelalgia, 1309
Ephelides, 2289
Epicondylitis, 207
Epidemic cerebrospinal meningitis, 417
Epidemic diarrhea, 305–306
Epidemic encephalitis, vs. dystonia musculorum deformans, 761

Epidemic hemorrhagic fever, *293,*
301–302
Epidemic louse-borne typhus fever,
318–320
clinical features of, *313*
epidemiologic features of, *310*
Epidemic myalgia, 271–272
Epidemic neuromyasthenia, 307
vs. poliomyelitis, 831
Epidemic pleurodynia, 271–272
Epidermal necrolysis, toxic, 2306
staphylococcal, 400
Epidermis, 2267
stratified cellular, *2267, 2267, 2268*
Epidermolysis bullosa, *2298*
Epidermolytic hyperkeratosis, *2286*
Epididymides, tuberculosis of, 496
Epididymitis, gonococcal, 407, 409
Epidural abscess
cerebral, 808
cerebrospinal fluid findings in, *803*
spinal, 810, 811
cerebrospinal fluid findings in, *803*
primary, 404
vs. transverse myelitis, 812
Epidural granulomas of spinal cord, 494
Epidural hematoma
in head injury, 883, 884
spinal, 898
Epidural infections, spinal, 810–811
Epidural tumors, in Hodgkin's disease,
1844
Epiglottitis, *Hemophilus influenzae* type
b, 424
Epilation, in local radiation injury, 89
Epilepsia partialis continua, 842, 856
Epilepsy(ies), 851–862. See also
Seizure(s).
acquired, 852, 853
after head injury, 852, 883
clinical examination in, 857
clinical manifestations of, 853
diagnosis of, 856
differential diagnosis of, 858
etiology of, 852
focal, chronic, 842
grand mal, 853, 854
history in, 856
idiopathic, 852
in tuberous sclerosis, 770
interseizure state in, 856
Kozhevnikov's, 842
laboratory investigations in, 857
myoclonus, 854
pathogenesis of, 851, 852
petit mal, 854
prevalence of, 851
psychomotor, 855
schizophrenia-like syndrome in, 668
vs. syncope, 745
"reflex," 852
sensory-induced, 852
symptomatic, 852
treatment of, 858
dietary, 861
medical, *857, 858*
psychologic, 861
surgical, 862
vestibulogenic, 741
vs. brain tumor, 869
"Epileptic cry," 853
Epileptic discharge, basic mechanisms
of, 851

Epileptic dizziness, 741
Epiloia, 770–771
Epimembranous nephritis, 1393
Epimerase deficiency, 1997
Epinephrine, 2199, 2200, *2200*
in anaphylactic reaction complicating
therapy of serum sickness, 154
in angioedema, 163
in asthma, 959
in drug allergy, 157
in food allergy, 1499
in glaucoma, 2322
in insect stings, 163
in reaction to injected allergen in
allergic rhinitis, 160
in shock, 1120
in urticaria, 162
in ventricular fibrillation, 1056, 1057
metabolic effects of, 2201
pharmacology of, 2200, 2201
secretion of, 2201
Epinephrine hydrochloride, in
Hymenoptera stings, 114
Epiphrenic diverticulum, 1500
Episcleral rheumatoid nodules, 2314,
2315
Episcleritis, in relapsing polychondritis,
2316
Episomal transfer, drug resistance
characterized by, 551
Epispadias, 1458
Epithelioid cells, in sarcoidosis, 211
Epithelioma, basal cell, 2308–2309,
2309
Epstein-Barr virus
in Burkitt's lymphoma, 1838
in infectious mononucleosis, 264
Equanil. See *Meprobamate.*
Equine encephalitis
eastern, 285–286
Venezuelan, 286–288
western, 284–285
Erethism, in mercury poisoning, 80
Ergocalciferol, 2232
in hypoparathyroidism, 2221
Ergot, toxicity of, 1308
Ergotamine, toxicity of, 1308
Ergotamine tartrate, in migraine
syndrome, 731, 732
Ergotism, 1308
Eristalis tenax, 112
Erosive osteoarthritis, 204
Eructation, 1479
Eruption(s)
creeping, 625
drug, *2279, 2280*
vs. secondary syphilis, 510
Eruptive xanthomatosis, in diabetes
mellitus, 1981
Erysipelas, 374–375
Erysipeloid of Rosenbach, 473
Erysipelothrix rhuziopathia, 473
Erythema
in local radiation injury, 89
migratory, necrolytic, *2296, 2299*
palmar, in liver disease, 1645
Erythema annulare centrifugum, *2297*
Erythema circinatum, in rheumatic
fever, 381
Erythema gyratum repens, *2296*
Erythema induratum, 498, **2295**
Erythema marginatum, in rheumatic
fever, 381

Erythema multiforme, *2301, 2303,*
2305–2306
in coccidioidomycosis, 538
Erythema nodosum, 2295
in coccidioidomycosis, 538
in enteritis with arthritis, 198
in pulmonary tuberculosis, 484
in sarcoidosis, 213
Erythema nodosum leprosum, 503, 504
Erythermalgia, 1308–1309
Erythrocyanosis, 1310–1311
Erythrocyanosis frigida crurum, 1311
Erythrocyte(s)
acquired hypersusceptibility of, to
oxidative stress, 1761
distribution of, in circulation, 1717
enzyme deficiencies of, hemolysis in,
1755, **1758–1761,** *1758*
formation of, 1716
glycolysis in, pathways of, 1758, *1758*
in congenital hemolytic anemias,
1755, 1756
life span of, measurement of, 1753
membrane of, abnormalities of,
hemolysis in, 1755, **1756–1758**
acquired dysplastic alteration of,
hemolysis due to, 1768–1769
chemical alteration of, hemolysis
due to, 1769–1770
immunologic alteration of,
hemolysis from, 1762–1766
traumatic alteration of, hemolysis
due to, 1766–1768
metabolism of, inborn errors of, 42
oxygen affinity of, 1771
sheep, in T cell detection, 129, 130
structure and function of, 1715
survival of, 1717
shortening of, in anemia of chronic
disorders, 1731
values of, normal range of, *1717*
Erythrocyte incompatibility, transfusion
reaction from, *1785,* 1787
Erythrocyte sedimentation rate
in multiple myeloma, 1860
in rheumatoid arthritis, 189
Erythrocytosis
abnormal hemoglobins causing, 1778,
1779
in nephrocarcinoma, 1459
primary, vs. polycythemia vera, 1796
Erythroderma(s), *2297*
acquired, 2286–2289
exfoliative, 2287–2288, *2288*
ichthyosiform, 2286, 2287
Erythroleukemia, 1814, 1816
Erythromelalgia, 1308–1309
Erythromycin(s), *556,* 560, 561
in acne, 2279
in diphtheria, 432
in diphtheria carriers, 433
in gonorrhea in pregnancy, 409, 410
in infective endocarditis prophylaxis,
396
in legionnaires' disease, 360
in malabsorption of scleroderma, 171
in mycoplasmal pneumonia, 346
in mycoplasmal urethritis, 347
in pneumococcal pneumonia, 356
in pseudomembranous enterocolitis,
1585
in rheumatic fever, 383
in rheumatic fever prophylaxis, 376

Erythromycin(s) (*Continued*)
 in syphilis, 516
 in whooping cough, 428
Erythropoiesis, 1716
 in anemia of chronic disorders, 1731
 ineffective, 1716
  excessive bilirubin production
   from, 1638
Erythropoietic porphyria, congenital,
 42, **2045**, *2302*
 hemolytic anemia in, 1761
Erythropoietic protoporphyria, 2049,
 2302
Erythropoietin, 1716
 plasma, in chronic renal failure, 1361
 polycythemia caused by, 1798, 1799,
  1800
Eschar, in rickettsial diseases, 310, *313*
 in rickettsialpox, 326
Escherichia coli
 gastroenteritis caused by, 454
 pneumonia due to, 361, 365
Esophageal curling, 1485–1486, *1486*
Esophageal motility
 disorders of, 1483–1488
 tests of, in achalasia, 1487
Esophageal obturator airway, in
 cardiopulmonary arrest, 1055
Esophageal reflux, vs. angina pectoris,
 1227
Esophageal ring, lower, 1488, *1488*
Esophageal spasm, diffuse, 1485–1486,
 1486
Esophageal sphincter(s)
 in swallowing, 1478, *1478*, 1479
 lower, hypertensive, 1488
 normal physiology of, 1475
Esophageal tamponade, in portal
 hypertension with gastrointestinal
 bleeding, 1523
Esophageal varices
 bleeding, 1523
  in cancer patient, 1905
  in schistosomiasis, 614
 in portal hypertension, 1640
Esophagitis, 1483–1485
 peptic, vs. peptic ulcer, 1507
  with stricture, vs. esophageal
   carcinoma, 1598
 reflux, 1484
  hiatal hernia and, 1485
Esophagogastric trauma from retching,
 1478
Esophagus
 Barrett's, 1484
 candidiasis of, 548
 carcinoma of, 1597–1599
 carcinosarcomas of, 1599
 corkscrew, 1485–1486, *1486*
 diverticula of, 1499–1500
 in alcoholic neuropathy, 1488
 in diabetic neuropathy, 1488
 in scleroderma, 169, 1488
 in swallowing act, 1478, *1478*
 inflammation of, 1483–1485. See also
  Esophagitis.
 leiomyomas of, 1599
 malignant lymphomas of, 1599
 motility of, disorders of, 1483–1488
  tests of, in achalasia, 1487
 neoplasms of, 1597–1599
 obstruction of, in esophageal
  carcinoma, 1597, 1598

Esophagus (*Continued*)
 pain originating in, 1476
  radiation of, 1477
 peristalsis in, 1478
 rupture of, vs. myocardial infarction,
  1233
 tuberculosis of, 492
 ulcer of, radiographic appearance of,
  1509, *1510*
Espundia, *588*, *589*
Essential cryoglobulinemia, renal
 changes in, 1406
Essential fructosuria, 2000
Essential hematuria, 1398–1399
Essential hypernatremia, 718, 719
Essential hypertension
 "benign," 1206
 catecholamine excess in, 1209
Essential pentosuria, 2000
Essential thrombocythemia, 1878
Essential tremor, 756–757
Estradiol
 in ovarian function, 2177, 2178
 plasma, values for, 2180, *2180*
Estrogen(s)
 excessive, galactorrhea and, 2191
 in oral contraceptives, 2195, *2195*
 in ovarian function, 2177
 plasma, values for, 2180, *2180*
 plasma and urinary, in evaluation of
  testicular function, 2164
 urinary, values for, 2180, *2181*
Ethacrynic acid
 hyponatremia induced by, 1954
 in heart failure, *1103*, 1104, *1104*, 1105
 metabolic alkalosis from, 1966
Ethambutol, *556*
 as nephrotoxin, 1427
 in pulmonary disease caused by *M.
  kansasii*, 499
 in pulmonary tuberculosis, 488, 489,
  490
 neuropathy from, 910
Ethanol
 acute poisoning with, 710
 effects of, on liver, 1663, 1664
 hypoglycemia induced by, 1996
 in drug interactions, 2339, 2340
 metabolism of, 707
Ethinyl estradiol
 in cancer of prostate, 1921
 in testicular feminization, 2173
Ethionamide, *556*
 in pulmonary tuberculosis, 488, 490
Ethosuximide, in epilepsy, *859*
Ethyl mercury, poisoning by, 80
Ethyl stibamine, in visceral
 leishmaniasis, 586
Ethylene glycol
 as nephrotoxin, 1434
 poisoning by, metabolic acidosis
  from, 1962
Ethylenimines, in oncologic treatment,
 1932
Ethylphenylhydantoin, in epilepsy, *859*
Eualleles, 40
Eubacterium alactolyticum, 442
Eubacterium lentum, 442
Eubacterium limosum, 442
Eubacterium species, susceptibility of, to
 antimicrobial agents, *445*
Euproctis flava, 119
European blastomycosis, 543–544

European typhus, 318–320
Eutonyl. See *Pargyline.*
Evans' syndrome, 1876
Eventration of diaphragm, 1019
Ewart's sign, in pericardial effusion,
 1274
Exanthem(s)
 enteroviruses causing, 274
 febrile, vs. secondary syphilis, 510
Exanthema subitum, vs. measles, *249*
Exchange transfusion, in accidental
 poisoning, 74
Excretory system, changes in, with
 aging, 26
Exercise
 angina pectoris provoked by, 1224
 cardiac output in, 1070
 in ankylosing spondylitis, 195
 in constipation, 1481
 in obesity, 1698
 in parkinsonism, 754
 in rheumatoid arthritis, 191
 in shoulder-hand syndrome, 206
 isotonic, 1070
 lack of, as risk factor for
  atherosclerosis, 1221
 myoglobinuria from, 924
Exercise tests, in angina pectoris, 1225,
 1226
Exfoliative cytology
 in colorectal carcinoma, 1609
 in gastric carcinoma, 1602
Exfoliative dermatitis, generalized, 400
Exfoliative erythroderma, 2287–2288,
 2288
Exhaustion, heat, 85
 vs. heat stroke, 84
Exogenous hyperlipemia, *2004*,
 2006–2007
Exophthalmos
 autoimmunity and, 2121
 in Graves' disease, 2126, 2127, 2332,
  2333
Exostosis, multiple, hereditary, *1910*,
 2264, 2265
Experimental allergic encephalomyelitis,
 844
Expiratory flow rate, maximal, 934, *934*
Expiratory flow–volume curve, maximal,
 934
Expiratory volume, forced, 934, *934*
Expressivity, genetic, 37
Extracapillary glomerulonephritis, with
 epithelial crescents, 1399, *1399*
Extracellular fluid, solute accumulation
 in, 1955
Extracellular fluid compartments, in
 right ventricular failure, 1092, 1093
Extracranial headache, 729, 730–733
Extradural spinal cord tumors, 896
Extramedullary hematopoiesis,
 myelofibrosis with, 1827
Extramedullary spinal cord tumors,
 intradural, 896–897
Extraneural cryptococcosis, 544
Extraocular myalgia, in influenza, 243
Extraocular palsy, pupillary
 disturbances and, 899, 900
Extrapulmonary tuberculosis, 491–498
 drug therapy in, 491
Extrapyramidal disorders, 750–763
Extrasystoles
 atrial, 1246–1247, *1246*

Extrasystoles (*Continued*)
junctional, 1256
ventricular, 1251–1252, *1252*
Extrinsic allergic alveolitis, 970–972, *971*
Exudative enteropathy, in X-linked
infantile agammaglobulinemia, 140
Exudative pharyngitis, nonstreptococcal,
237
vs. streptococcal pharyngitis, 372
Exudative tonsillitis, 443
Eye(s)
as source of headache, 733
changes in, with aging, 27
diseases of, 2313–2335
examination of, in stupor or coma,
643
in acute hemorrhagic conjunctivitis,
275
in albinism, 2029, 2293
in ankylosing spondylitis, 2316
in ariboflavinosis, 1686
in arterial hypertension, 1203, 1205,
1206
in arthritic diseases, 2314–2316
in Behçet's disease, 2316
in benign intracranial hypertension,
870
in brain tumors, 865
in cavernous sinus thrombosis, 808
in chronic renal failure, 1366
in congenital rubella, 252
**in connective tissue diseases,
2316–2317,** *2318*
in cranial arteritis, 217, 218
in dermatomyositis, 2319
in diabetes mellitus, 1976, 1977, *1978,*
2320–2322
in Ehlers-Danlos syndrome, 2054
in giant cell arteritis, 2317, 2319
in Graves' disease, 2126, 2127, 2332,
2333
in herpes zoster, 826
in histoplasmosis, *2318,* **2323–2325**
in hypercalcemia, 2239
in hyperthyroidism, 2122, 2332, 2333
in juvenile rheumatoid arthritis, 2315
in loiasis, 635
in Marfan's syndrome, 2053
in measles, 247
in myasthenia gravis, 926
in neurosyphilis, 815
in nutritional amblyopia, 774, 775
in nutritional deficiency, 1675
in onchocerciasis, 636
in periarteritis nodosa, 2317
in polymyositis, 2319
in radiation injury, 89
in regional enteritis, 2316
in Reiter's syndrome, 2316
in relapsing polychondritis, 2316
in rheumatoid arthritis, 2314, 2315
in sarcoidosis, 213, **2329–2330**
in scleroderma, 2317
in sickle cell diseases, 2330–2332,
2331
in Sjögren's syndrome, 2315, 2316
**in systemic hypertension and
arteriolosclerosis, 2325–2326**
in systemic lupus erythematosus, 177,
2317, *2318*
in tabes dorsalis, 512
in thyroid disease, 2332–2333
in toxoplasmosis, 596, 597, 598, *2318,*
2334–2335

Eye(s) (*Continued*)
in ulcerative colitis, 2316
in Wegener's granulomatosis, 219,
2317
motor nerves to, disorders of, 899
**red, acute, differential diagnoses of,
2313–2314,** *2313*
trachomatous infection of, 332, 333
tuberculous infections of, 498
Eyelids
in diabetes mellitus, 2320
in sarcoidosis, 2330
in scleroderma, 2317
in systemic lupus erythematosus,
2317

F body, 51
Fabry's disease, *42,* **912,** 1280, 1329,
2011–2012, *2300*
renal transplantation in, 55
Face
in paralysis agitans, 752
infections of, brain abscess from, 805
Facial hemispasm, chronic, 900
Facial myokymia, 900
Facial nerve, disorders of, 900
Facial neuralgia, atypical, 731
Factor I, 1881
Factor V, 1881
deficiency of, *1884,* 1888
Factor VII, 1881
deficiency of, *43, 1884,* 1888
Factor VIII, 1881
deficiency of, in classic hemophilia,
1883, *1884*
in von Willebrand's disease, *1884,*
1886
Factor IX, 1881
deficiency of, *1884,* 1887
Factor X, 1881
deficiency of, *43, 1884,* 1888
acquired, 1891
Factor XI, 1881
deficiency of, *1884,* 1887
Factor XII, 1881
deficiency of, 1887, 1888
Factor XIII, 1881
congenital deficiency of, *1884,* 1889
Faget's sign, in yellow fever, 295
Faint. See also *Syncope.*
common, 743
due to heat, 85
hysterical, 744
impending, 737
"Fainting lark," 746
Faintness, 740–741
Falciparum malaria, 567, 569
clinical manifestations of, 571
complications of, 571
drug-resistant, 573
erythrocyte forms of, *570*
recrudescent, prevention of, 574
supportive therapy in, 574
vs. louse-borne typhus, 312
Fallot's tetralogy, 1164–1166
cyanotic, classic, 1164, 1165
vs. right ventricular origin of both
great arteries, 1173
Familial cardiomyopathy, 1280–1281
Familial chronic pemphigus, benign,
2304

Familial colonic cancer without polyps,
1606
**Familial combined hyperlipidemia,
2007–2008**
Familial dysautonomia, 912, **2057–2058**
osteoporosis in, 2245, 2246
**Familial dysbetalipoproteinemia,
2005–2006**
**Familial endogenous
hypertriglyceridemias, 2007**
Familial goiter, *43*
prevention of, 55
Familial hyperbradykinism, vs.
idiopathic autonomic insufficiency,
763
Familial hypercholesterolemia, 2005
detection of, in relatives, *58*
Familial hyperkalemic periodic
paralysis, 1959
Familial hyperparathyroidism, detection
of, in relatives, *58*
Familial juvenile nephronophthisis,
1454
Familial lipochrome histiocytosis, 1806
**Familial lipoprotein lipase deficiency,
2006–2007**
Familial Mediterranean fever, 2055–2057
arthritis in, 199
cutaneous signs of, *2299, 2300*
pericardial involvement by, 1276
**Familial mixed hypertriglyceridemias,
2007**
**Familial multiple lipoprotein–type
hyperlipidemia, 2007–2008**
Familial myoglobinuria, 920–921
Familial periodic paralysis, 921–922
Familial polyposis
colorectal carcinoma and, 1606
detection of, in relatives, *58, 59*
**Familial recurrent polyserositis,
2055–2057**
Familial tremor, 756–757
Family-planning counseling, 690
Famine fever, yellow, 526–529
Fanconi's anemia, 1733, 1737, *1910*
unrepaired chromosomal breakage in,
54
Fanconi's syndrome, 2023–2024
acute leukemia in, 1814
cutaneous lesions in, *2302*
idiopathic, *2020*
symptomatic forms of, *2020–2021*
toxic nephropathy with, 1425
Farcy, 468–469
Farmer's lung, *971*
Fasciitis
diffuse, associated with eosinophilia,
vs. dermatomyositis, 174
gas-forming, 434
Fasciola hepatica, 618, 619
Fascioliasis, 618–619
vs. angiostrongyliasis, 631
vs. toxocariasis, 628
Fasciolopsiasis, 620
Fasciolopsis buski, 605, 620
Fascioscapulohumeral dystrophy, 915,
916, 917
Fasting, prolonged, effect of, on plasma
amino acids, *2018*
Fasting hypoglycemia
**functioning islet cell tumors causing,
1993–1995**
induced, *1990,* **1996–1997**
spontaneous, *1990,* **1992–1993**

Fat(s). See also *Lipid(s)*.
  absorption of, 1524
  nutrient value of, 1670
  stool, measurement of, in
    malabsorption syndrome, 1530
  transport of, 2002
Fat embolism, cerebral, in head injury, 885
Fat emulsions for intravenous nutrition, 1708
Fat necrosis, nodular, *2299*
Fatigue, in chronic renal failure, 1366
Fat-induced hyperlipemia, 2006–2007
Fat-soluble vitamins
  nutrient value of, 1670, 1672
  recommended allowances of, *1671*
Fatty acids
  deficiency of, essential, in total
    parenteral nutrition, 1708
  free, 2002
Fatty liver, 1660–1661
  computerized tomography in, *1467*
Fatty streaks, in atherosclerosis, 1219
Fauces, in herpangina, 270
Faucial diphtheria, 431
Favism, 1760, 1761
  genetic basis of, 45
Febre maculosa, 322–324
Febrile convulsions, in epilepsy, 852
Febrile neutrophilic dermatosis, acute, 2295
Febrile nodular nonsuppurative panniculitis, relapsing, 221–222
Febrile pharyngitis
  acute, 237
  in listeriosis, 472
Febrile transfusion reactions, unexplained, *1785*, 1788
Fecal excretion of bile pigments, 1638–1639
  measurement of, 1646
Fecal impaction, 1615
  in paraplegia, 887
Fecal incontinence, 1482–1483
  in acquired megacolon, 1496
Feces, normal values for, 2354
Feeding behavior, caloric balance and, 717–718
Feet. See *Foot (feet)*.
Felty's syndrome, 193, 1809
Female genital tuberculosis, 496
Female infertility, 2193–2194
Female mid-life crises, 24
Female orgasm, 687
  dysfunction of, 688, 2198, 2199
Female pubertal development, *18, 19*, **2181–2182**
Female sexual precocity, 2179, 2182–2183
Feminization, testicular, 2064, 2172–2173
  amenorrhea in, 2185
  incomplete, 2173
Feminizing adrenal tumors, 2162
Femoral neuropathy, 902, 909
Fenoprofen, in rheumatoid arthritis, 191
Fern test, in evaluation of ovarian function, 2180
Ferritin, 1743
  plasma, measurement of, 1745
  serum, estimation of, in
    hemochromatosis, 1791
Ferrokinetics, 1745, 1746

Ferrous fumarate, in iron deficiency
  anemia, 1749
Ferrous gluconate
  in iron deficiency anemia, 1749
  in malabsorption syndrome, *1536*
Ferrous sulfate
  for iron needs in pregnancy, 1750
  in acute alcoholic hepatitis, 1664
in fragmentation hemolysis, 1767
in hookworm anemia, 625
in iron deficiency anemia, 1749
Fertility, impairment in, in radiation
  injury, 89
Fertility control, 2194–2197
Fetal gonadotropin secretion, 2176
Fetal hamartoma, renal, 1460
Fetal hemoglobin, hereditary
  persistence of, 1772
Fetor hepaticus, 1641
Fetus
  maternal smallpox and, 257
  pulmonary arteries in, 1135
  radiation injury to, 89
Fever. See also names of specific
    diseases, e.g., *Q fever, Scarlet fever.*
  agitated delirium with, 650
  in arboviral encephalitis, 284
  in bacterial meningitis, 414
  in bronchogenic carcinoma, 1006
  in brucellosis, 476
  in Colorado tick fever, 280
  in dengue, 277
  in diverticulitis, 1582, 1583
  in drug allergy, 155
  in epidemic hemorrhagic fever, 301
  in epidemic pleurodynia, 272
  in familial Mediterranean fever, 2056, 2057
  in Hodgkin's disease, 1841
  in infectious mononucleosis, 265
  in infective endocarditis, 389, 395
  in influenza, 243
  in intracranial tumors, 866
  in legionnaires' disease, 360
  in leptospirosis, 533
  in liver disease, 1645
  in louse-borne relapsing fever, 527, 528
  in malaria, 571
  in measles, 248
  in mumps, 262
  in mycoplasmal pneumonia, 344
  in plague, 464
  in pneumococcal pneumonia, 351, 353
  in Q fever, 330
  in rat-bite fever, 531
  in renal malignancy, 1459
  in respiratory syncytial viral disease, 238
  in rheumatoid arthritis, 188
  in rickettsialpox, 326
  in Rift Valley fever, 281
  in Rocky Mountain spotted fever, 322
  in shigellosis, 458
  in subarachnoid hemorrhage, 797
  in systemic lupus erythematosus, 180
  in trench fever, 329
  in tularemia, 466, 467
  in typhoid fever, 447
  in varicella, 254
  in visceral leishmaniasis, 585
  in West Nile fever, 278
  in western equine encephalitis, 285
  in yellow fever, 295

Fiberoptic bronchoscopy
  in sarcoidosis, 214
  microbiologic diagnosis by, 342
Fibrillation
  atrial, 1247–1248, *1247*
    DC electroshock in, 1267
    in aortic stenosis, 1191
    in mitral stenosis, 1180, 1181
    in myocardial infarction, 1230, 1235
    in pericardial constriction, 1275
  ventricular, 1255, *1255*
    cardiac arrest from, 1056, 1057
    DC electroshock in, 1267
    in digitalis toxicity, 1098, 1099
    in myocardial infarction, 1230, 1235
    sudden death due to, 1237, 1238
Fibrin, formation of, 1881, *1881*
  disorders of, differentiation of, *1884*
Fibrinogen, 1881
  deficiency of, acquired, 1891
    congenital, 1888, 1889
  digestion of, by plasmin, 1891, 1892
Fibrinoid, 164
  in systemic lupus erythematosus, 176
Fibrinolysis, complement system and, 137
Fibrinolytic states, 1896
Fibrin-stabilizing factor, 1881
  congenital deficiency of, *43*, *1884*, 1889
Fibroelastosis, endocardial, 1280
Fibrogenesis imperfecta
  ossium, 2253, 2254
Fibromas, small intestinal, 1605
Fibroplastic endocarditis, Löffler's, 1286
Fibrosclerosis, multifocal, 222–224
Fibrosing syndromes, 222–224
Fibrosis
  cystic, *43*, **1559–1560**
  endomyocardial, 1286
  hepatic, congenital, 1667
  interstitial, drug-induced, vs.
    pneumocystosis, 599
  mediastinal, 224
  periureteral, 223–224
  pleural, in asbestosis, 1017
  progressive massive, of coal workers, 992, 993
  pulmonary, complicating cancer
    therapy, 1904
    in collagenous pneumoconioses, 990, 991
    in paraquat ingestion, 1001
    radiation, 1002
    pulmonary hypertension in, 1147
  retroperitoneal, 223–224
    sclerosing cholangitis and, 1633
Fibrositis, 208
Fibrothorax, in empyema, 1015
Fibrous dysplasia, 2262–2263
Fibrous strictures, colonic, in
  amebiasis, 591
Fiebre manchada, 322–324
Fiebre petequial, 322–324
Filariasis, 632–637
  antimicrobial agents for, *559*
  bancroftian, 633–634
  immunodiagnostic tests for, *565*
  Malayan, 634
  occult, 637
Filarioidea, common, *632*
Filling pressure, decrease in, in shock, 1109

Filtration fraction, renal, 1317
Finger agnosia, 658
Fingers
  clubbing of, in bronchogenic
      carcinoma, 1007
    in hypertrophic osteoarthropathy,
        201
    in infective endocarditis, 390
    in Raynaud's phenomenon, 1306
Fire ants, stings of, 113, 114
Fire medusae, envenomation by, 123
Fish(es)
  poisoning by, 69
  venomous, 124
Fish tapeworm, 607
  antimicrobial agents for, *559*
  treatment of, 608–609
Fissure, anal, 1617
Fistula(s)
  arteriovenous, 1312–1313
    coronary, congenital, 1169
      portal hypertension in, 1639
    pulmonary, congenital, 1168–1169
  carotid–cavernous sinus, in head
      injury, 884
  cerebrospinal fluid, in head injury,
      883
  cholecystenteric, in acute
      cholecystitis, 1626, 1628
  malabsorption in, 1537
  paraprosthetic-enteric, 1590
  perirectal, in regional enteritis, 1562
  rectovaginal, in ulcerative colitis,
      1574
Fistula in ano, 1617
  tuberculous, 492
Fitzgerald factor, 1881
Fitzgerald trait, *1884, 1888*
Fitz-Hugh–Curtis syndrome, 408
  vs. acute cholecystitis, 1627
Five-day fever, 329
Flaccid paralysis, in hyperkalemia, 1959
Flagyl. See *Metronidazole.*
"Flashback" phenomena, after LSD use,
    704, 705
Flatulence, 1489
Flaujeac trait, 1888
Flea-bite, 110
Flea-borne typhus fever, 320–321
Fleckfieber, 318–320
Flesh flies, infestation by, 112
Fletcher factor, 1881
Fletcher trait, *1884, 1888*
Flies. See *Fly(ies).*
**Floppy mitral valve syndrome,
    1188–1190**
Flowering plants, poisoning by, 70
Flucytosine, *556*
  in fungal endocarditis, 394
Fludrocortisone, in Addison's disease,
    2149
Fluent aphasia, 656, 657
Fluid(s). See also *Water.*
  ascites, evaluation of, 1592
  **cerebrospinal, examination of,
      747–748, 802–804,** *803.* See also
      Cerebrospinal fluid examination.
  dialysis, composition of, 1377, *1377*
  disorders of, 1950–1969
    in cancer patient, 1904
  extracellular, solute accumulation in,
      1955
  in acute renal failure, 1372
  in acute respiratory failure, 1044

Fluid(s) *(Continued)*
  in bacterial meningitis, 416
  in cholera, 461, 462
  in head injury, 882
  in impaired gastric emptying
      complicating peptic ulcer, 1517
  in intestinal obstruction, 1491
  in myxedema coma, 2134
  in pneumococcal pneumonia, 356
  in pseudomembranous enterocolitis,
      1585
  in pulmonary embolism, 1133
  in rickettsial diseases, 316
  in shigellosis, 458, 459
  in shock, 1047, 1048, 1117, 1118
  in tetanus, 440
  in volume depletion, 1952
Fluid compartments, extracellular, in
    right ventricular failure, 1092,
    1093
Fluid volume, regulation of, 1207
Flukes
  antimicrobial agents for, *559*
  diseases caused by, 611–621
    hermaphroditic, 617–621
      hepatic, 617–619
      intestinal, 620–621
      lung, 619–620
  prevalence of, *605*
Fluorescent antibody technique, surface
    Ig staining by, 129, *129*
Fluorescent antibody test(s)
  in protozoan and helminthic diseases,
      565
  indirect, in rickettsial diseases, *314,*
      315
  in toxoplasmosis, 596, 597
Fluorescent treponemal antibody
    absorption test, in syphilis, 514
Fluoride
  accumulation of, in chronic renal
      failure, 1360
  nutrient value of, 1673, 1674
Fluorinated agents, anesthesia with,
    hepatitis after, 1659–1660
5-Fluorocytosine
  in candidiasis, 549
  in cryptococcosis, 544
  in oncologic treatment, 1934
Fluorodeoxyuridine, in oncologic
    treatment, 1934
90α-Fluorohydrocortisone, in congenital
    adrenal hyperplasia, 2161
Fluoromebendazole, in echinococcosis,
    610
Fluoroscopic image intensifiers, in
    critical care medicine, 1032
Fluoroscopy
  in pericardial constriction, 1275
  in pulmonary disease, 942
Fluorosis, 1676, *1677,* **2262**
Fluorouracil, in oncologic
    treatment, 1934
Fluoxymesterone
  in anemia of chronic lymphocytic
      leukemia, 1825
  in paroxysmal nocturnal
      hemoglobinuria, 1769
Fluphenazine, in pain, *724*
Flurane anesthetics, as nephrotoxins,
    1433
Flurazepam, in insomnia, 653
Flurazepam hydrochloride, in
    depression, 678

Flushing, in carcinoid syndrome, 2208,
    2211
  treatment of, 2212, 2213
Flutter, atrial, 1248–1249, *1248*
  DC electroshock in, 1266
Fly(ies)
  flesh, infestation by, 112
  tsetse, 576
Fly agaric, poisoning by, 69
Fly larvae, infestation by, 111–112
Foam cells, in Niemann-Pick disease,
    2013, 2014
**Focal disturbances of higher nervous
    function, 656–659**
Focal epilepsy, chronic, 842
**Focal glomerulonephritis with recurrent
    hematuria, 1398–1399**
Focal glomerulosclerosis, 1393
Focal seizures, 851, 854
Focal sensory seizures, 855
Focal siderosis, 1790
Fog, urban, human health and, 62, 63
Foix-Alajouanine syndrome, 849
Folacin
  nutrient value of, 1672
  recommended allowances of, *1671*
Folate
  deficiency of, biochemical and
      hematologic sequence in, 1723,
      1723
    in pregnancy, 1723
    vs. vitamin B$_{12}$ deficiency, 1725,
        1725
  metabolism of, 1722, *1722*
Folic acid
  absorption of, 1525
  deficiency of, causes of, *1721*
    in liver disease, 1643
    in malabsorption syndrome, 1529
    neutropenia in, 1809
  in acute alcoholic hepatitis, 1664
  in hereditary spherocytosis, 1757
  in homozygous beta thalassemia, 1778
  in malabsorption syndrome, *1536*
  in megaloblastic anemia, 1726, 1727
  in sickle cell anemia, 1775
  in tropical sprue, 1546
Folic acid analogues, in oncologic
    treatment, 1933, 1934
Folinic acid, in toxoplasmosis, *558,* 598
Follicle-stimulating hormone, 2087–2088
  human pituitary, in amenorrhea, 2192
  in ovarian function, 2175, 2176
  in secondary hypogonadism, 2172
  measurement of, 2092–2093, *2093*
  site of action of, 2178
Follicular conjunctivitis, chronic, vs.
    ocular chlamydial infections, 334
Follicular hyperkeratosis, 1675
Folliculitis, 399, 400
Food, antigen entrance into body
    through, 131
Food allergy, 1498, 1499
  sensitization to external antigens in,
      131
  urticaria caused by, 161
Food intolerance, 1498–1499
Food poisoning, 64–70
  Bacillus cereus, 66
  bacterial, 64–66
  chemical, 70
  clostridial, 65–66, 436
  staphylococcal, 64–65, 404
    vs. *Salmonella* gastroenteritis, 452

Food poisoning (*Continued*)
Vibrio parahaemolyticus, 66
vs. motion sickness, 95
Foot (feet)
"burning," syndrome of, 773
dermatitis of, 2283–2284
immersion, 1309–1310
insensitive, treatment of, 912
Madura, 542
paddy-field, 1309
swelling of, during air travel, 96
trench, 1309–1310
Foot-and-mouth disease, 261
Foramen magnum, compressive lesions of, 891
Forbes-Albright syndrome, 2191
prolactin levels in, 2092
Forced expiratory volume, 934, *934*
Forced vital capacity, 934, *934*
Fordyce's disease, vs. Fabry's disease, 2012
Forebrain, herniation of, 641
Foreign antigens, sensitivity to, 131–132
"Forest yaws," *588*
Forestier's syndrome, 1483
Forgetfulness, benign, syndrome of, 659
Formiminotransferase deficiency, *43*
Fort Bragg fever, 534
Foville's syndrome, 788
Fowler's solution, poisoning by, 76
Fox-Fordyce disease, 2270
Fracture(s)
depressed, in head injury, 883
rib, vs. angina pectoris, 1227
skull, basilar, 883
spinal, 885, 886
Fragmentary seizure, 854
Fragmentation hemolysis, 1766, 1767
in abnormalities of heart and great vessels, 1767
Frambesia tropica, 518–522, *520*. See also *Yaws*.
Francisella tularensis, 465, 466
Frank-Starling mechanism, 1083, 1084, *1084*
Freckle(s), 2289
melanotic, of Hutchinson, 2310, 2311
Free fatty acids, 2002
Free thyroid hormone, determination of, 2118
Frei test, in lymphogranuloma venereum, 336
Friction rub, pericardial, in acute pericarditis, 1272
Friedländer's bacillus, pneumonia caused by, 357–358
vs. pneumococcal pneumonia, 354
Friedreich's ataxia, 767–768
cardiomyopathy in, 1281
vs. leprosy, 504
Frequency, gene, 46, 47
Frigidity, 687, 688
Friuli coagulation disorder, 1888
Frontal lobe abscess, 806
Frostbite, 1311–1312
Frozen shoulder, 206–207
Fructose, hereditary intolerance to, *41*, 2000–2001, *2020*
Fructose-1,6-diphosphatase deficiency, *41*
Fructosuria, *41*, 2000
FSH, 2087–2088. See also *Follicle-stimulating hormone*.
FTA-ABS test, in syphilis, 514

Fucosidosis, *41*
Fuel homeostasis in health and disease, 1703–1705
Fuller's earth workers, pneumoconiosis in, 987
Fulminant hepatitis, 1655–1656
hepatic encephalopathy in, 1641
Fulminating meningococcemia, 419, *419*
treatment of, 421
Functional amenorrhea, 2080
Functional amnesia, 659
Functional dyspepsia, vs. peptic ulcer, 1508
Functional psychoses, 665–672
Functional residual capacity, 932, *932*
in acute respiratory failure, 1035, *1035*, 1036
Fungal diseases, 535–549. See also *Mycoses* and names of specific diseases.
dermatologic, 2281–2282, *2282*
of brain, vs. dementia in cancer, 877
Fungal endocarditis, 387
treatment of, 394
Fungal granulomas, vs. lupoid leishmaniasis, 588
Fungal meningitis
vs. arboviral encephalitis, 284
vs. poliomyelitis, 831
vs. viral meningitis, 820
Fungemia, in infective endocarditis, 391
Fungizone. See *Amphotericin B*.
Funnel chest, 1020
Furosemide
hyponatremia induced by, 1954
in acute mountain sickness, 101
in differential diagnosis of acute renal failure, 1374
in edema of acute poststreptococcal glomerulonephritis, 1396
in heart failure, 1104, 1105
in hypercalcemic crisis, 2240
in hypertension of chronic renal failure, 1362
in oliguric renal failure, 1051
in pulmonary edema of chronic renal failure, 1363
in renal complications of transfusion, 1789
metabolic alkalosis from, 1966
Furuncles, 399–400
prevention of, 401
treatment of, 400, 401
vs. tularemia, 467
Furuncular myiasis, 112
Furunculosis, 400
Fusiform aneurysms, intracranial hemorrhage from, 795
"Fusion figures," 54
Fusobacterium mortiferum, 441
Fusobacterium necrophorum, 441
exudative tonsillitis caused by, 443
Fusobacterium nucleatum, 441
Fusobacterium species, susceptibility of, to antimicrobial agents, 445
Fusobacterium varium, 441, 445
susceptibility of, to antimicrobial agents, *445*

Gait
apraxia of, 741
in Alzheimer's disease, 662
Galactokinase deficiency, *41*, 1998

Galactorrhea, 2191–2192
nonpuerperal, 2108
prolactin radioimmunoassay in, 2092
Galactose, absorption of, 1525
Galactosemia, *41*, 1997–1999, *2020*
classic, 1997–1998
dietary restriction in, 55
Galatose-1-phosphate uridyl transferase deficiency, 1997, 1998
Galactosyltransferase, serum, as tumor marker, 1913
Gallbladder
adenocarcinoma of, in chronic cholecystitis, 1625
benign tumors and pseudotumors of, 1634, *1634*
calcification of, in chronic cholecystitis, 1625
carcinoma of, 1633–1634
diseases of, 1618–1636
oral contraceptive use and, 2195
roentgenologic examination in, 1622–1623, *1623*
in typhoid fever, 446, 447
pain originating in, 1476
radiation of, 1477
perforation of, in acute cholecystitis, 1626, 1628
strawberry, 1624
Gallop rhythm, in left ventricular failure, 1090
Gallstone ileus, 1626, 1628–1629
Gallstones, 1619–1620. See also *Cholecystitis*.
acute pancreatitis and, 1551, 1553, 1554
asymptomatic, 1623–1624, *1624*
cholesterol, 1619, 1620, *1620*
dissolution of, by chenodeoxycholic acid, 1620–1621
pathophysiology of, 1621, *1621*
pigment, 1619, 1620
roentgenologic examination in, 1622–1623, *1623*
ultrasonography in, *1466*
vs. pancreatic carcinoma, 1559
Gambian sleeping sickness, 576
clinical features of, 577
diagnosis of, 578
epidemiology of, 576
treatment of, 578, 579
vs. Rhodesian sleeping sickness, *577*
Gamma camera scanning, renal, 1345, *1345*
Gamma globulin
in common variable immunode-ficiency, 142
in whooping cough, 428
in X-linked infantile agammaglobu-linemia, 140
Gamma glutamyl transpeptidase, measurement of, in osteomalacia, 2248
Gamma heavy chain disease, 1865
electrophoretic patterns in, 1857, *1857*
Gamma-aminobutyric acid, 751
deficiency of, in hereditary chorea, 758, 759
Gammopathy, monoclonal, benign, renal changes in, 1406
Ganga, 702
Ganglia, basal, diseases of, 750–763

Ganglioneuromas, 2206, 2207
Ganglionitis, dorsal root, in cancer, 878
Gangliosidoses, *42*
Gangosa, in yaws, 521
Gangrene
  bilateral, of digits, 1306
  gas, 433–435
    hemolysis in, 1770
    postoperative, 435
  in arteriosclerosis obliterans, 1302
  in diabetes mellitus, 1980
  Meleney's synergistic, 367
  of extremities, in systemic infections, 1305
Gardner-Diamond syndrome, *2302*
Gardner's syndrome, *1910, 2296, 2298*
  colorectal carcinoma and, 1606
  detection of, in relatives, *58*, 59
Gas(es)
  diffusing capacity of lung for, 936–937
  in lungs, measurement of, 933
"Gas abscess," 434
Gas dilution or washout, lung gas measurement by, 933
Gas embolism, in diving, 99
Gas exchange, 931, 939–941
  abnormal, 939–940, 1021–1022
  normal, 939, 1021
Gas gangrene, 433–435
  hemolysis in, 1770
  postoperative, 435
Gas-forming fasciitis, 434
Gas-forming soft tissue infections, differential diagnosis of, *435*
Gasoline, poisoning by, 75
Gasser's syndrome, 1877
Gasterophilus intestinalis, 112
Gastrectomy
  malabsorption after, 1538
  subtotal, in duodenal ulcer, 1519, *1519*
    malabsorption after, 1546, 1547
Gastric. See also *Gastro-* and *Stomach*.
Gastric acid, secretion of, 1505, 1506
  in peptic ulcer, 1506
  in Zollinger-Ellison syndrome, 1509
Gastric analysis, normal values for, 2353
Gastric carcinoid tumor, 2210, *2211*, 2212
Gastric carcinoma, 1599–1603
Gastric crises, in tabes dorsalis, 814
Gastric dilatation, acute, 1489
Gastric drainage, metabolic alkalosis from, 1965, 1966
Gastric irradiation, in peptic ulcer, 1516
Gastric lavage
  in accidental poisoning, 74
  in acute drug poisoning, 714
Gastric mucosa, peptic ulcer and, 1504, 1505
Gastric outlet obstruction, 1490
  in peptic ulcer, 1507, 1517, 1518
  vs. acute appendicitis, 1580
Gastric secretory tests, in peptic ulcer, 1512
Gastric ulcer. See also *Peptic ulcer*.
  malignant, 1508
  pathogenesis of, 1503, 1504
  pathophysiology of, 1504, 1505, 1506, 1507
  radiographic appearance of, 1510, *1510*
  rheumatoid arthritis and, 1504

Gastric ulcer (*Continued*)
  surgical treatment of, indications for, 1519
  types of, 1520
Gastric vagotomy, proximal, in duodenal ulcer, 1519, *1519*
Gastric varices, in portal hypertension, 1640
Gastric volvulus, 1489–1490
Gastrin
  in colonic motility, 1492, 1493
  in gastric secretion, 1505, 1506
  in gastrointestinal motility, 1476, 1489
  in pepsin secretion, 1506
Gastrinomas, in Zollinger-Ellison syndrome, 1508, 1509
Gastrin-secreting tumor, in Zollinger-Ellison syndrome, 1508, 1509
Gastritis
  atrophic, gastric carcinoma and, 1600
  in peptic ulcer, 1502, 1503
  ulcer-like symptoms in, 1508
Gastro-. See also *Gastric* and *Stomach*.
Gastrodiscoides hominis, 621
Gastroduodenal motility
  disorders of, 1488–1490
  normal, 1488, 1489
Gastroenteritis
  allergic, 1542–1543
  clostridial, 436
  enteric bacteria causing, 454
  eosinophilic, 1542–1543
    vs. regional enteritis, 1566
  infectious, acute, vs. acute appendicitis, 1581
  infectious nonbacterial, acute, 305–306
  Salmonella, 449
    clinical manifestations of, 451
    diagnosis of, 452
    pathogenesis of, 450
    treatment of, 452
  staphylococcal, 404–405
  Vibrio parahaemolyticus causing, 66
  viral, Norwalk-like agents and rotaviruses causing, 305–306
Gastrointestinal absorption, tests for, 2353
Gastrointestinal allergy, 1498–1499
  in children, 1499
Gastrointestinal bleeding, 1520–1523
  angiography in, 1471, *1471*
  disorders associated with, cutaneous signs of, *2298*
  in cancer patient, 1905
  in hypothalamic dysfunction, 717
  in peptic ulcer, 1516, 1517
  iron deficiency from, 1748
  portal hypertension and, in cirrhosis, 1665
Gastrointestinal motility
  disorders of, 1475–1502
    pathophysiology and cardinal symptoms of, 1476–1483
    relation of symptoms to, 1476
  hormonal control of, 1476
  normal, 1475–1476
Gastrointestinal myiasis, 112
Gastrointestinal sphincters, normal physiology of, 1475
Gastrointestinal tract
  changes in, with aging, 26

Gastrointestinal tract (*Continued*)
  diagnostic imaging procedures for, 1464–1474
  diseases of, 1463–1669
    cutaneous lesions associated with, *2298–2299*
    neoplastic, 1596–1610
  diverticula of, 1499–1502
  endocrine functions of, 2061, *2061*
  in acute radiation syndrome, 88
    management of, 90
  in acute renal failure, 1371
  in analgesic nephropathy, 1419
  in cancer patient, 1905, 1906
  in carcinoid syndrome, 2208
  in Chagas' disease, 581, 582
  in chronic renal failure, 1364, 1365
  in hypothalamic dysfunction, 717
  in iron deficiency anemia, 1748
  in mucormycosis, 546
  in non-Hodgkin's lymphomas, 1832
  in obesity, 1696
  in paraplegia, 887
  in periarteritis nodosa, 181
  in right ventricular failure, 1093
  in scleroderma, 169
  in systemic lupus erythematosus, 177
  procedures or surgery on, infective endocarditis prophylaxis in, 396
  secretions of, loss of, potassium depletion from, 1957
  upper, losses from, metabolic alkalosis caused by, 1965, 1966
  water and sodium loss from, 1950, 1951
Gastrointestinal tuberculosis, 492
Gastroscopy, in gastric carcinoma, 1601, 1602, *1602*
"Gate control" theory of pain, 721, 725, 726
Gaucher cell, 2012, 2013, *2013*
Gaucher's disease, *41*, **2012–2014,** *2013*
Gegenhalten, in arteriosclerotic pseudoparkinsonism, 754
Gender role behavior, 686
Gene(s), 31
  allelic, 40
  autosomal, 34
  autosomal linkage of, 38
  expression of, modification of, 37
  frequency of, 46, 47
  nonallelic, 40, *44*
  pleiotropic effect of, 38
  protein synthesis and, 31
  regulatory, 34
  "risk," 45
  structural, 34
General paresis, 512, 813, 814
  treatment of, 516
Generalized exfoliative dermatitis, 400
Generalized hypertrophic osteoarthritis, primary, 204
    vs. rheumatoid arthritis, 190
Generalized salivary gland virus disease, 827–829
Generalized seizures, 851, 853, 854
Genetic code, 33
  population genetics and, 47
Genetic compounds, 36
Genetic control of protein synthesis, 32, *32*, 33
  regulatory mechanisms of, 34
Genetic counseling, 56–59, *57, 58*

Genetic disease
  detection of, in relatives, *58, 59*
  prevention and management of, 54–56
Genetic factors
  in aging, 28
  in alcohol abuse, 706
  in ankylosing spondylitis, 39, 194
  in antimicrobial agent selection, 554
  in atherosclerosis, 1221
  in cancer, 1909–1910, *1910*
  in colorectal carcinoma, 1606
  in complement system, 137
  in congenital malformations, *48*
  in diabetes mellitus, 1974
  in disease, 11, 12
  in familial Mediterranean fever, 2056
  in gastric carcinoma, 1599, 1600
  in gastrointestinal neoplasms, 1597
  in gout, 2031
  in manic-depressive psychosis, 671
  in pathogenesis of peptic ulcer, 1503
  in pseudohypoparathyroidism, 2222
  in regional enteritis, 1561
  in sarcoidosis, 209
  in schizophrenia, 667
  in systemic lupus erythematosus, 175
  in ulcerative colitis, 1568
  in Wilson's disease, 2050
Genetic heterogeneity, 40, *44*
Genetic load, 47
Genetic principles, 31–59
Genetic risks, in genetic counseling, 56, 57, *57*
Genetic screening, 59
  in inborn errors of metabolism, 44
Genetics
  internal medicine and, 31
  pharmaco-, 45–46
  population, 46–48
Genital tuberculosis, 496
Genitourinary blastomycosis, 540
Genitourinary disease, mycoplasmas in, 346–347
Genitourinary myiasis, 112
Genitourinary tract
  anaerobic infection of, 443
  anomalies of, 1456–1458
  in periarteritis nodosa, 182
  procedures or surgery on, infective
    endocarditis prophylaxis in, 396
Genitourinary tuberculosis, 496
Gentamicin, *556*, 561
  adverse reactions to, 562
  as nephrotoxin, 1426
  in bacterial meningitis, 416
  in infective endocarditis, 393, 394
  in infective endocarditis prophylaxis, 396
Geriatric medicine, aging and, 25–30
Geriatrics, 25
German measles, 250–252. See also *Rubella.*
Germinal aplasia, 2170
Germinal tumors, testicular, 2175
Germinomas, pineal, 2113
Gerontology, 25
Gerstmann's syndrome, 658
  in anomic aphasia, 657
  in parietal lobe abscess, 806
Ghon complex, 481
Giant cell arteritis, 166, 216–218
  eyes in, 2317, 2319
  vs. periarteritis nodosa, 183
Giant cell myocarditis, 1283

Giant cell pneumonia, in measles, 249
"Giant cells"
  in radiation injury, 87
  in sarcoidosis, 211
Giant platelet syndrome, 1878–1879
Giardia lamblia, 558, 602
Giardiasis, 602
  antimicrobial agents for, *558*
  malabsorption in, 1546
Gid, 611
Gigantism, 2108
Gilbert's syndrome, *42*, 1638, 1649
Gilles de la Tourette's disease, 759
Gingivae, in nutritional deficiency, 1676
Gingivostomatitis, herpetic, primary,
  vs. herpangina, 271
Giordano-Giovannetti diet, in chronic
  renal failure, 1711
Glabrous skin, trichophytosis of, vs.
  pinta, 525
Glanders, 468–469
Glanzmann's disease, 1878
Glaucoma, *2318*, 2322–2323
  angle closure, 2323, *2323*
    acute, *2313*, 2314
  following glucocorticoid instillation,
    genetic basis of, 46
  headache from, 733
  in sarcoidosis, 2329, 2330
  neovascular, in diabetes mellitus,
    2321
  open-angle, 2322
Glioblastoma multiforme, 863
Glioma(s), optic nerve, 868
Globoid cell leukodystrophy, *41*, 850
Globulin(s)
  serum, measurement of, 1646
  thyroxine-binding, abnormal
    quantities of, thyroid hormone
    transport defect from, 2140
Globus hystericus, vs. true dysphagia,
  1479
Glomangioma, 1313
Glomerular disease, 1386–1406
  cell-mediated immunity in, 1327
  circulating immune
    complex-mediated, 1325, 1326
  membranous, idiopathic, 1393
  minimal change, 1391–1393
    vs. nephrotic syndrome, 1389
  **Glomerular filtrate, processing of, by
    renal tubules, 1317–1320, *1320***
  Glomerular filtration, 1317
  **Glomerular filtration rate, 1317,
    1339–1340, *1340***
    in acute renal failure, 1370, 1371
    in chronic renal disease, 1347, 1348,
      1349, 1354
    in obstructive nephropathy, 1448
  **Glomerular function, elements of,
    1316–1317**
Glomerular proteinuria, 1337
Glomerulitis
  acute, vs. acute tubular necrosis, 1373
  acute renal failure from, 1368
  cutaneous signs in, *2301*
  in periarteritis nodosa, 181
  in systemic lupus erythematosus, 180
Glomerulonephritis, 1390–1400
  acute, epidemiology of, 370, *370*
    vs. Goodpasture's syndrome, 976
  anti-glomerular basement membrane
    antibody–mediated, 1324, *1324*
  biopsy in, 1346

Glomerulonephritis (*Continued*)
  classification of, *1391*
  complement activation–associated,
    1327
  endothelial, 1399, 1400
  etiology of, 1390
  extracapillary, with epithelial
    crescents, 1399, *1399*
  **focal, with recurrent hematuria,
    1398–1399**
  immune complexes in, 134
  in infective endocarditis, 1397–1398
  in pregnancy, 1414
  in sarcoidosis, 1403
  in systemic lupus erythematosus, 176,
    177, 180
  membranoproliferative, 1327, 1398
  mesangiocapillary, 1398
  poststreptococcal, acute, 1394–1397
  prevention of, 376
  proliferative, 1394–1400
    in staphylococcal bacteremia and
      endocarditis, 403
  recurrent, after renal transplantation,
    1385
  subacute or chronic, exacerbations of,
    vs. acute poststreptococcal
    glomerulonephritis, 1396
  vs. Chagas' disease, 582
Glomerulosclerosis, focal, 1393
Glomerulotubular balance
  homogeneity of, 1348
  in unilateral renal disease, 1347,
    1348
Glomus jugulare, tumors of, 867
Glomus tumor, 1313
Glossina morsitans, 577
Glossina palpalis, 577
Glossina tachinoides, 577
Glossitis, peripheral neuropathy and, in
  malabsorption syndrome, 1529
Glossopharyngeal neuralgia, 727
Glucagon, 1973
  in assessment of growth hormone,
    2092
  in heart failure, 1100
  metabolism of, in chronic renal
    failure, 1361
Glucantime. See *Meglumine antimoniate.*
Glucocorticoids, risk of glaucoma with,
  genetic basis of, 46
Glucoglycinuria, *2021*
Glucose
  absorption of, 1525
  accumulation of, in extracellular fluid,
    1955
  blood, as cardiovascular risk factor,
    1062
  in acute intermittent porphyria, 2047
  in cerebral metabolism, 646
  in cerebrospinal fluid, in bacterial
    meningitis, 413
  in coma of doubtful cause, 642
  in coma of metabolic brain disease,
    651
  in diabetic ketoacidosis, 1984
  in hyperkalemia, 1960
  in tissue fuel utilization, 1971
  insulin release provoked by, 1972
  intolerance to, as risk factor for
    atherosclerosis, 1221
  in chronic renal failure, 1361
  plasma, in functioning islet cell tumor
    during fasting, 1994, *1994*

Glucose tolerance, decreased, in obesity, 1694, 1695
Glucose tolerance test, in diabetes mellitus, 1974, 1975, *1975*
Glucose-galactose malabsorption, *41*, 1539
Glucose-6-phosphate dehydrogenase deficiency, 1759–1761
hemolytic reactions in, after drug administration, 45
leukocytic, severe, 1806
Glucosuria, in chronic renal failure, 1353
Glucosyl ceramide lipidosis, 2012–2014, *2013*
β-Glucuronidase deficiency, *41*
Glue, toluene in, inhalation of, 705
Glutamate-aspartate transport defect, 2020
Glutamic oxaloacetic transaminase, in myocardial infarction, 1232
Glutathione peroxidase deficiency, 1761
Glutathione reductase deficiency, 1761
"Glutathionemia," *2018*
Gluten enteropathy, 1539
HLA system and, 39
Gluten-free diet, in adult celiac disease, 1540
Glutethimide
abuse of, 698
poisoning by, *712*, *713*
Glyburide, in diabetes mellitus, *1986*
L-Glyceric aciduria, 2001
Glycerin suppositories, in constipation, 1482
Glyceryl trinitrate, in angina pectoris, 1228
Glycogen storage disease, 919, 1999–2000, *1999*
type I, hyperlipemia in, 2009
Glycogenoses, *41*, 1999–2000, *1999*
Glycolic aciduria, 2001
Glycolysis, pathways of, in mature erythrocyte, 1758, *1758*
Glycolytic enzymes, Embden-Meyerhof pathway, defects in, 1758–1759
Glycosides, cyanogenic, chronic cyanide poisoning caused by, 69
Glycosphingolipidosis, 2011–2012
Glycosuria, renal, *41*
Gnathostoma spinigerum, 626
Gnathostomiasis, 626
cerebral, vs. angiostrongyliasis, 631
Goiter
endemic, 2137–2138, *2138*
familial, *43*
prevention of, 55
multinodular, 2135–2137
complications of, 2136–2137
nodular, toxic, 2136
Goitrous cretinism, 2064, 2138–2140
Goitrous hypothyroidism, sporadic, 2138–2140
Gold, as nephrotoxin, *1428*, 1430
Gold compounds
in rheumatoid arthritis, 191, 192
neuropathy from, 910
Gompertz concept, 27–28, *27*
Gonadal agenesis, 2186
Gonadal deficiency, obesity in, 1697
Gonadal dysgenesis, 2185, 2186, *2186*
vs. pituitary dwarfism, 2104
Gonadal failure, primary, vs. hypopituitarism, 2101

Gonadal hormones
excretion of, values for, 2180, *2181*
plasma concentrations of, 2180, *2180*
Gonadotropin(s)
assay of, in amenorrhea, 2183, 2184
chorionic, human, as tumor marker, 1912
in amenorrhea, 2192
in cryptorchidism, 2174
in delayed adolescence, 2166
in evaluation of ovarian function, 2181
in secondary hypogonadism, 2172
function of, assessment of, 2092–2093, *2093*
hypothalamic-pituitary release of, assessment of, 2165
menopausal urinary, human, in amenorrhea, 2192
pituitary, measurement of, 2180
plasma and urinary, in evaluation of testicular function, 2165
secretion of, 2176
during menstrual cycle, 2088, *2088*
serum, values for, *2180*
therapy with, side effects of, 2192
Gonadotropin-releasing hormone, 2075
regulation of, disorders of, 2080–2081
Gonococcal arthritis, 185, 407, 408
vs. Reiter's syndrome, 197
Gonococcal bacteremia, 407
Gonococcal conjunctivitis, 406
Gonococcal disease, 404–410
Gonococcal endocarditis, 387, 407, 408, 410
treatment of, 394
Gonococcal epididymitis, 407, 409
Gonococcal meningitis, 410
Gonococcal ophthalmia neonatorum, 410
Gonococcal perihepatitis, 408, 409
vs. acute cholecystitis, 1627
Gonococcal pharyngitis, 406, 407
Gonococcal proctitis, 407
Gonococcal prostatitis, 407, 409
Gonococcal salpingitis, 406, 407, 408, 410
vs. acute appendicitis, 1581
Gonococcal seminal vesiculitis, 407, 409
Gonococcal urethritis, 406, 407
Gonococcal vulvovaginitis, 406
Gonorrhea, 404–410
vs. bancroftian filariasis, 634
Gonyaulax catanella, 68
Gonyaulax tamarensis, 68
Goodpasture's syndrome, 976
autosensitization in, 132
immune injury in, 1390, *1390*
renal involvement in, 1401
vs. idiopathic pulmonary hemosiderosis, 976
vs. periarteritis nodosa, 183
vs. Wegener's granulomatosis, 219
Goundou, in yaws, 521
Gout, *42*, 2029–2041
chronic renal failure in, 1352
classification of, *2030*
clinical manifestations of, 2034
cutaneous manifestations of, *2300*
diagnosis of, 2038
diseases associated with, 2038, *2038*
genetics of, 2031
pathogenesis of, 2031
pseudo-, 201–202

Gout *(Continued)*
saturnine, in lead poisoning, 78
tophaceous, 2030, *2036*, 2037
treatment of, 2039, 2040
treatment of, 2039
vs. gonococcal arthritis, 408
vs. rheumatoid arthritis, 190
vs. sarcoidosis, 215
Gouty arthritis
acute, 2030
cause of, 2033, 2034, *2034*
clinical manifestations of, 2034, 2035, *2035*
treatment of, 2039
in obesity, 1696
Gouty kidney, 1420–1421, 2037, 2038
treatment of, 1421, 2040, 2041
Gowers' sign, in muscular dystrophy, 917
Graafian follicles, ruptured vs. acute appendicitis, 1581
Gradenigo's syndrome, 808
Graft vs. host reaction, 130
Grafts, skin, impaired, hyperbaric oxygen therapy in, 105
Graham Steell murmur
in atrial septal defect, 1161
in mitral stenosis, 1182
Gram-negative bacilli
aerobic, pneumonia and nosocomial respiratory infections caused by, 361–365
anaerobic, 441
bacteremia caused by, 455, 456
treatment of, 456, 457
meningitis caused by, 411
treatment of, 416
Gram-negative septicemia, liver disease in, 1656
Gram-positive nonsporeforming anaerobic bacilli, 442
Grand mal, 853, 854
Granular casts, 1339
Granular cell myoblastomas of lung, 1013
Granulocytes, overproduction of, in polycythemia vera, 1794, 1795
Granulocytic leukemia
acute, vs. leukemoid reaction, 1813
chronic, 1821–1824
vs. neutrophilic leukemoid reaction, 1813
Granulocytic sarcomas, 1822
Granulocytopenia
in acute leukemia, 1821
in aplastic anemia, 1736, 1737
in liver disease, 1643
nosocomial pneumonia and, 362
Granuloma(s)
affecting nervous system, 864
Candida, 548
eosinophilic, 978, 1543, 1848–1850, *1849*
treatment of, 1850–1851
epidural, of spinal cord, 494
fungal, vs. lupoid leishmaniasis, 588
hepatic, 1667
in cysticercosis, 864
vs. brain tumor, 868, 869
in sarcoidosis, 211, *211*, 864, 1667
midline, 220–221
vs. Wegener's granulomatosis, 219
Granuloma inguinale, 429
ulcer of, vs. syphilitic ulcer, 508
vs. lymphogranuloma venereum, 335

Granulomatosis
allergic angiitis and, 166, 182
treatment of, 183
vs. classic periarteritis nodosa, 183
vs. Wegener's granulomatosis, 183
lipophagic intestinal, 1541
lymphomatoid, vs. Wegener's
granulomatosis, 219
Wegener's, 166, **218–220,** 972–973
cutaneous signs in, *2301*
eyes in, 219, 2317
neuropathy in, 908
renal involvement in, 219, 1400
vs. allergic angiitis and
granulomatosis, 183
vs. Goodpasture's syndrome, 976
vs. midline granuloma, 221
Granulomatous colitis, 1576–1578
vs. amebiasis, 592
vs. diverticulitis, 1583
Granulomatous disease(s)
chronic, *43*, **1804–1806**
variants of, 1806
of childhood, chronic septic, 144
of unproved etiology, 209–226
Granulomatous enteritis, vs.
eosinophilic gastroenteritis, 1543
Granulomatous inflammation, in
chronic schistosomiasis, 614
Granulomatous intraocular infection,
498
Granulomatous thyroiditis, 2131
Granulomatous vasculitis, 972–973
Grass pollen, allergic rhinitis from, 157
Graves' disease, 2120–2128
complications of, **2126–2128**
eyes in, 2126, 2127, 2332, 2333
hereditary factor in, 2121
HLA system and, 39
vs. subacute thyroiditis, 2132
Gray baby syndrome, 553, 562
Great arteries
both, right ventricular origin of, 1173
transposition of, complete, 1172
congenitally corrected, 1166–1167
Great vessels, abnormality of,
hemolysis due to, 1767
Green bottle, infestation by, 112
Green monkeys, in African hemorrhagic
fever, 300
Grey Turner's sign, *2299*
Grief, 676
Grippe, summer, 275
Griseofulvin, in fungus infections of
skin, 2282
Grönblad-Strandberg syndrome, 2294
Ground itch, 624
Growth
development and, human, 11–30
pubertal spurt of, 17, 18
rate of, in chronic renal failure, 1365
Growth hormone, 2086–2087
function of, assessment of, 2091–2092
mode of action of, 2071
purified, in pituitary dwarfism, 2104,
2105
radioimmunoassay of, in acromegaly,
2107
secretion of, regulation of, 2077
Growth hormone–releasing factor, 2075
regulation of, disorders of, 2079–2080
Grub, cattle, human infestation by, 112
GT-II, as tumor marker, 1913

Guanethidine
in arterial hypertension, *1212*, 1215
in Raynaud's disease, 1307
Guanidine
in botulism, 68
in Eaton-Lambert syndrome, 929
Guanidine hydrochloride, in
myasthenic syndrome complicating
cancer, 879
Guillain-Barré syndrome, 906–907
associated with swine influenza
vaccination, 246
during enteroviral infections, 270
vs. hysteria, 679
vs. idiopathic autonomic
insufficiency, 763
vs. polymyositis, 174
Guinea worm, infection with, 633
Gull's disease, 2132
Gumma(s)
in syphilis, 510, 511, 813, 815, 864
in yaws, 519, 521
Gums, in nutritional deficiency, 1676
Günther's disease, 2045
Gymnodinium breve, 68
Gynecology, counseling in, 2197–2199
Gynecomastia
as manifestation of cancer, 1916
in bronchogenic carcinoma, 1006

H chains, 126, 127, *127*
Habit spasms, 759–760
vs. acute chorea, 758
Haemadipsa species, as agents of
disease, 120
Haemagogus mosquitoes, in yellow
fever, 294
Hageman factor, 1881
Hageman trait, *43*, 1887, 1888
Hailey-Hailey disease, 2304
Hair, 2269
changes in, with aging, 27
growth cycle of, 2270, 2271
disease and, 2271
growth of, excessive, 2271, 2272
in kwashiorkor, 1681
in nutritional deficiency, 1675
kinky, Menkes' syndrome of, *43*
osteoporosis in, 2245
loss of, 2271
in local radiation injury, 89
pubic, development of, *18*, 19
types of, 2271
Haldol. See *Haloperidol.*
Hallucinations
hypnagogic, 654
in alcohol addiction, 709
in metabolic brain disease, 648
in schizophrenia, 666
Halo nevus, 2291
Haloperidol
in dementia, 663
in dystonia musculorum deformans,
761
in Gilles de la Tourette's disease, 759
in mania of manic-depressive
psychosis, 671
in spasmodic torticollis, 762
Halothane
anesthesia with, hepatitis after,
1659–1660
inhalation of, 705

Halzoun, 120
Hamartoma
of lung, 1013
renal, 1461
fetal, 1460
Hamman-Rich syndrome, 967
pulmonary hypertension in, 1147
Hamman's sign, in mediastinal
emphysema, 1018
Ham's test, in paroxysmal nocturnal
hemoglobinuria, 1768, 1769
Hand(s)
care of, in scleroderma, 171
claw, 903
dermatitis of, 2283–2284
in degenerative joint disease, 203, *203*
in psoriatic arthritis, 196, *197*
in Raynaud's phenomenon, 1306
in rheumatoid arthritis, 188, *188*, *189*
insensitive, treatment of, 912
Hand-foot syndrome, in sickle cell
anemia, 1774
Hand-foot-and-mouth disease, 274
vs. herpangina, 271
Hand-Schüller-Christian syndrome,
1848
"Hangman's fracture," 885
Hangover, 708
Hansen's disease, 501–505. See also
Leprosy.
Haplotype, 39
Hardy-Weinberg law, population
genetics and, 46
Hartnup disease, *41*, 1539, *2020, 2023,*
2300
cutaneous signs of, *2298*
photosensitivity in, *2288, 2289*
Harvest mites, 113
Hashimoto's thyroiditis, 2128–2130,
2130
autosensitization in, 132
hereditary factor in, 2121
hypothyroidism developing from,
2132
vs. multinodular goiter, 2135, 2136
Hashish, 702–703
Hashitoxicosis, 2121
Haverhill fever, 531
Hawaii agents, acute infection with,
305, 306
Hay fever, 157–160. See also *Allergic*
rhinitis.
Head
dermatologic diseases of, 2278–2279
injuries of, 879–885
acute, evaluation of, 881–882
management of, 882–883
prognosis in, 885
complications of, 883–885
epilepsy associated with, 852, 883
hearing loss from, 736
memory disorder following, 659
vertigo from, 739
vs. cerebral infarction, 790
Head bobbing, in aortic regurgitation,
1195
Head louse, 108, 109
in epidemic typhus, 318
Headache(s), 728–733
classification of, 729
cluster, 729, 731
treatment of, 732
ear disease and, 733

Headache(s) (*Continued*)
  extracranial, 729, 730–733
  eyes as source of, 733
  hot dog, 70
  in arterial hypertension, 732, 1203
  in benign intracranial hypertension, 870
  in brain abscess, 805
  in brain tumor, 730, 864, 865
  in carbon monoxide poisoning, 83
  in cerebral infarction, 786
  in influenza, 243
  in intracranial hemorrhage, treatment of, 800
  in intracranial hypotension, 873
  in meningitis, 729, 730
  in Paget's disease, 2258
  in subarachnoid hemorrhage, 796
  in subdural empyema, 807
  intracranial, 729–730
  lumbar puncture, 730
  migraine, 729, 731–732
    vertiginous, 740
    vs. cerebral transient ischemic attacks, 785
  muscle-contraction, 732
  nasal and paranasal structures as source of, 733
  pathogenesis of, 729
  post-traumatic, recurrent, 732
  sinus, 733
  tooth disease and, 733
  vascular, 730–731
Hearing
  examination of, 734–735
  loss of, 734–737. See also *Deafness.*
Hearing aids, 736
Heart. See also *Cardiac.*
  abnormality of, hemolysis due to, 1767
  as component of circulation, 1087–1089
  as muscle, 1087
  as pump, 1083–1085, *1083*
  changes in, with age, 26
  contractile process of, subcellular bases for, 1082
  dextroversion of, 1166
  diastolic properties of, 1064, *1064*
  dilatation of, in heart failure, 1086, *1086*
  disease of. See *Heart disease* and names of specific cardiac disorders.
  failure of. See *Heart failure.*
  functional anatomy of, 1063, 1064
  herniation of, through pericardial defect, 1276
  in arterial hypertension, 1203, 1208
  in cancer patient, 1905
  in carcinoid syndrome, 2208
  in Chagas' disease, 581
  in chronic renal failure, 1365
  in Cushing's syndrome, 2154
  in hyperthyroidism, 2122
  in left ventricular failure, 1090
  in liver disease, 1644
  in louse-borne relapsing fever, 527
  in Marfan's syndrome, 2053
  in periarteritis nodosa, 182
  in pericardial constriction, 1275
  in pneumococcal pneumonia, 352
  in primary pulmonary hypertension, 1140
  in rheumatoid arthritis, 187

Heart (*Continued*)
  in rickettsial diseases, 311
  in right ventricular failure, 1091
  in sarcoidosis, 213
  in scleroderma, 169, 170
  in shock, 1109, 1110
  in sickle cell anemia, 1774
  inotropic characteristics of, 1083, 1085
  myxedema, 2134, 2135
  myxoma of, 1288
  oxygen consumption of, 1087
  performance of, assessment of, 1083–1088
    factors altering, 1064–1066, *1065, 1066*
  pressures and volumes in, *1067*
  soldier's, vs. angina pectoris, 1227
  surgery of, infective endocarditis prophylaxis in, 396
  tumors of, 1288
  work of, decrease of, in management of heart failure, 1093, 1094
Heart attack. See *Infarction, myocardial.*
Heart block. See also *Atrioventricular block.*
  complete, congenital, 1166
  in myocardial infarction, 1230, 1235, 1236
Heart disease
  Bantu hypokinetic, 1283
  beriberi, 1284
  congenital, 1149–1174
    clinical classification of, *1152*
    death rates for, *1060*
    diagnosis of, 1151, *1153,* 1154, 1155
    etiology of, 1149, 1150
    frequency and sex ratio of, *48*
    incidence of, 1149
    physiologic adaptation to, after birth, 1150
    pulmonary vascular disease in, 1141–1143
    underlying infective endocarditis, 387
    vs. neonatal myocarditis, 273
  coronary. See also names of specific disorders.
    death rates for, *1060*
    prevalence and epidemiology of, 1059
  degenerative, underlying infective endocarditis, 387
  hyperthyroidism and, treatment of, 2128
  in cerebral infarction, 780
  ischemic, 1223
  organic, syncope in, 744
  rheumatic, death rates for, *1060*
    prevalence and epidemiology of, 1059
    underlying infective endocarditis, 387
  scleroderma, 170
  secondary polycythemia in, 1799
  syphilitic, 1294–1295
  valvular, acquired, 1174–1199
    cardiac catheterization and operation in, 1178–1179
    evaluation of, 1176–1178
    physiologic effects of, 1174–1176, *1175*
Heart failure, 1071, **1080–1107**
  acute, 1080, 1081
    liver in, 1661

Heart failure (*Continued*)
  acute, vs. idiopathic autonomic insufficiency, 763
  acute pulmonary edema in, 1090
    management of, 1094
  anasarca in, 1093
  anxiety in, 1093
  ascites in, 1093
  autonomic nervous system in, 1088
  backward, 1081
  blood pressure in, sustenance of, peripheral mechanisms for, 1088, 1089
  brain in, 1093
  cardiac output in, sustenance of, peripheral mechanisms for, 1088, 1089
  categories of, 1080–1082
  Cheyne-Stokes respiration in, 1090
  chronic, 1080, 1081
    compensatory mechanisms in, 1085–1087
  clinical manifestations of, 1089–1093
  congestive, hyponatremia in, 1954
    in infective endocarditis, 390
    in pneumococcal pneumonia, 354
    vs. asthma, 957
    vs. congested state, 1081, 1082
  cyanosis in, 1091
  dyspnea in, 1089
    paroxysmal nocturnal, 1090
  extracellular fluid compartments in, 1092
  forward, 1081
  gallop rhythm in, 1090
  gastrointestinal tract in, 1093
  heart in, 1090, 1091
  hemoptysis in, 1090
  high output, 1081
  hydrothorax in, 1092
  in hemochromatosis, 1791
  in infective endocarditis, 395
  in myocardial infarction, 1236
  initiating mechanisms of, 1081
  kidney in, 1093
  left, 1081, 1089–1091
    acute pulmonary edema in, 1090
      management of, 1094
    hypertensive, 1206
    in myocardial infarction, 1231
  liver in, 1092
  low output, 1081
  lungs in, 1091
  management of, 1093–1107
    digitalis in, 1094–1100
    diuretics in, 1102–1106, *1102, 1103, 1104*
    general measures in, 1093–1094
    inotropic agents in, 1094–1102
    sympathomimetic amines in, 1100
    vasodilator therapy in, 1100–1102, *1100, 1101*
  orthopnea in, 1089
  pericardial effusion in, 1093
  pulmonary function tests in, 1090
  pulsus alternans in, 1090
  radiologic findings in, 1090
  refractory, surgical therapy of, 1106–1107
  refractory edema in, 1106
  right, 1081, 1091–1093
    in acute respiratory failure, 1022
    in chronic respiratory failure, treatment of, 1029–1030

Heart failure (*Continued*)
right, in primary pulmonary
hypertension, 1140
pulmonary hypertension and, in
pulmonary disease, 1147, 1148
salt restriction in, 1102
salt retention in, 1089
slowed circulation in, 1088
subcutaneous edema in, 1092
systemic venous congestion in, 1092
venous hypertension in, 1087, 1088
water restriction in, 1102
water retention in, 1089
Heart rate, 1066
factors determining, 1068
in myocardial infarction, 1235
in shock, 1109
increased, in heart failure, 1086
Heartburn, 1479
in esophagitis, 1484
Heat
body, conservation of, 2269
loss of, through skin, 2269
disorders due to, 84–85
prickly, 2268
regulation of, hypothalamic
dysfunction and, 716–717
Heat exhaustion, 85
vs. heat stroke, 84
Heat stroke, 84–85
vs. malaria, 573
Heat syncope, 85
vs. heat stroke, 84
Heat-labile opsonins, in pneumococcal
pneumonia, 349
Heavy chain disease
IgA, 1866
IgM, 1866
γ **Heavy chain disease, 1865**
electrophoretic patterns in, 1857, *1857*
Heavy metal poisoning, 76–82
vs. acute abdomen, 1581
Heberden's nodes, in degenerative joint
disease, 203, *203*, 204
Heerfordt's syndrome, 213, 2329
Height, pubertal spurt of, 17, 18
Heinz bodies, 1718
in glucose-6-phosphate
dehydrogenase deficiency, 1759,
1760
in hemolytic anemia, 1754
Helminthic diseases, 565, 605–638
antimicrobial agents for, *558*
eosinophilia and, 638
hepatic, 1657
immunodiagnostic tests for, *565*
malabsorption in, 1546
prevalence of, *605*
Hemagglutination, intravascular, in
shock, 1112, 1113
Hemagglutination test(s)
in protozoan and helminthic disease,
565
in rheumatoid arthritis, 190
in streptococcal pharyngitis, 372
Hemangioblastomas, 863
Hemangioma(s)
cavernous, 1876
cutaneous, in Sturge-Weber disease,
771
hepatic, 1667
small intestinal, 1590, 1605
strawberry, *2302*
Hemangiopericytoma, renal, 1462

Hemarthrosis, 200
in hemophilia, 200, 1883, 1886
Hematemesis, 1520, 1521
in schistosomiasis, 614
Hematin, in acute intermittent
porphyria, 2047
Hematite miners, pneumoconiosis in,
987
Hematochezia, 1520
Hematogenous staphylococcal
osteomyelitis, 402
Hematogenous tuberculosis
chronic, 492
generalized acute, 481
Hematologic abnormalities in liver
disease, 1643–1644
Hematologic and hematopoietic
diseases, 1713–1897
Hematologic form of acute radiation
syndrome, 88
treatment of, 90
Hematologic laboratory values,
2346–2347
Hematoma(s)
aortic, dissecting, 1295–1297, *1296*.
See also *Dissecting aortic aneurysm.*
cerebral, 794
surgical removal of, 801
epidural, in head injury, 883, 884
in hemophilia, 1883
intracerebral, in head injury, 884
intracranial, in head injury, 883, 884
spinal epidural, 898
subdural, complicating maintenance
hemodialysis, 1381
in head injury, 884
vs. benign intracranial
hypertension, 872
vs. brain tumor, 868
vs. California encephalitis, 288
vs. cerebral infarction, 790
Hematopoiesis, extramedullary,
myelofibrosis with, 1827
Hematopoietic system, in cancer
patient, 1906
Hematoside sphingolipodystrophy, *42*
Hematuria
essential or benign, 1398–1399
in acute poststreptococcal
glomerulonephritis, 1395
in asymptomatic individual, 1332,
1333
in chronic renal failure, 1353
in renal calculi, 1444
in sickle cell hemoglobinopathy, 1404
recurrent, focal glomerulonephritis
with, 1398–1399
Heme
absorption of, 1744
biosynthesis of, 2044
catabolism of, in hemolytic disorders,
1753
metabolism of, inborn errors of, *42*
Hemianopia
in brain tumors, 865
in subarachnoid hemorrhage, 797
Hemiballism, 762
in midbrain infarctions, 787
Hemiparesis, in subarachnoid
hemorrhage, 797
Hemiplegia
in intracranial tumor, 865
in subarachnoid hemorrhage, 797
Hemispasm, facial, chronic, 900

Hemlock, poisoning by, 70
Hemobilia, 1632
Hemochromatosis, 43, 1790–1792
arthritis in, 199
cutaneous signs of, *2299*
detection of, in relatives, *58*
diabetes mellitus and, 1791, 1982
prevention and management of, 55
Hemodialysis, 1376–1382
anemia in, 1381, 1731, 1732
ascites in, 1593
extracorporeal, 1378–1380, *1378, 1379*
in accidental poisoning, 74
in acute drug poisoning, 714
in scleroderma, 171
maintenance, 1380–1381
medical complications of, 1381–1382
Hemodynamic decompensation, in
acute respiratory failure, 1034
Hemoglobin(s), 1714, 1715, 1743, **1771**
abnormal, hereditary
methemoglobinemia due to, 1780,
1781
abnormalities of, 1771–1778
defective, secondary polycythemia in,
1799
fetal, hereditary persistence of, 1772
oxygen affinity of, 1771
sickle cell, screening for, 44
synthesis of, disorders of, 1751
in lead poisoning, 78
unstable
drug sensitivity of, 46
hemolytic anemias caused by,
1776–1777, *1777*
with abnormal oxygen affinity,
disorders caused by, 1777–1778,
1778
Hemoglobin A, 1715, 1716, 1771
Hemoglobin Bart's, hydrops fetalis
with, 1779
Hemoglobin C disease, homozygous,
1776
Hemoglobin C trait, 1776
Hemoglobin C–thalassemia, 1776
Hemoglobin D Punjab disease,
homozygous, 1776
Hemoglobin E disease, homozygous,
1776
Hemoglobin F, 1715, 1716, 1771
Hemoglobin H bodies, 1718
Hemoglobin H disease, 1779
Hemoglobin M, hereditary
methemoglobinemia due to, 1780,
1781
Hemoglobin mutants, effect of, on
terminator codons, 33, *33*
Hemoglobinemia
hemoglobinuria and, 1783
in hemolytic disorders, 1753
Hemoglobinopathies, 1771–1778
clinical syndromes associated with,
1773–1776
heritable, 1772
Hemoglobinuria, 1782–1784
as transfusion reaction, 1787
in hemolytic disorders, 1753
march, 924, 1767–1768, 1783
paroxysmal cold, 1765–1766, *2302*
immune mechanisms in, 132
in syphilis, 507
paroxysmal nocturnal, 1768–1769
acute leukemia in, 1814
aplastic anemia and, 1734, 1737

Hemolysis
  causes of, 1751, 1752
    classification of, *1752*
  due to abnormalities of
    microcirculation, 1766–1767, *1767*
  due to abnormality of heart and great
    vessels, 1767
  due to acquired abnormalities,
    1762–1770
  due to acquired dysplastic alteration
    of membrane, 1768–1769
  due to autoimmune antibodies,
    1763–1764
  due to chemical alteration of
    membrane, 1769–1770
  due to cold-reacting antibodies,
    1764–1766
  due to drug-induced antibodies, 1766
  due to intracorpuscular
    abnormalities, 1755–1762
  due to isoimmune antibodies, 1763
  due to overactivity of
    reticuloendothelial system, 1770
  due to traumatic alteration of red cell
    membrane, 1766–1768
  due to warm-reacting antibodies,
    1763–1764
  excessive bilirubin production by,
    1638
  fragmentation, 1766, 1767
    in abnormalities of heart and great
      vessels, 1767
  in glucose-6-phosphate
    dehydrogenase deficiency, 1759
    prevention of, 1761
  intravascular, as transfusion reaction,
    1787
    hemoglobinuria following, 1783
    massive, in malaria, 572
  laboratory signs of, 1752, 1753
  uncompensated, in liver disease, 1643
Hemolytic anemia(s), *42,* 1751
  acquired, 1762–1770
  autoimmune, idiopathic
    thrombocytopenic purpura
    associated with, 1867
  cause of, diagnosis of, 1753
  compensated, 1752
  congenital, 1755–1762
  drugs associated with, 156
  immune, Coombs-negative, 1763
  in chronic lymphocytic leukemia,
    1825
  in cold agglutinin syndrome, 1765
  in glucose-6-phosphate
    dehydrogenase deficiency, 45
  microangiopathic, 1766–1767, *1767*
  therapy of, 1754
  traumatic cardiac, 1767
  uncompensated, 1752
  unstable hemoglobins causing,
    1776–1777, *1777*
Hemolytic disorders, 1751–1784
  classification of, *1752*
  of newborn, 131, **1763**
    kernicterus in, 1754
Hemolytic jaundice, 1638
Hemolytic streptococcal pneumonia, 375
Hemolytic transfusion reactions, 1787
Hemolytic-uremic syndrome, 1877
  renal involvement in, 1401
Hemophilia
  carriers of, detection of, 1886

Hemophilia (*Continued*)
  classic, 1883–1886, *1884*
    vs. von Willebrand's disease, 1887
  hemarthrosis in, 200, 1883, 1886
  heterozygote detection in, 57, 58, *58*
Hemophilia A, *43*
Hemophilia B, *43*
Hemophilia-like disease, circulating
  anticoagulants producing, 1897
Hemophilus aegyptius, 423, 425
Hemophilus aphrophilus, 425
Hemophilus ducreyi, 423, 425
Hemophilus hemolyticus, 423, 425
Hemophilus influenzae infections, 423,
  423
  bacterial meningitis caused by, 411
    treatment of, 415
  type b, 424, 425
  pneumonia caused by, vs.
    pneumococcal pneumonia, 354
  type b, 423–425
Hemophilus parahemolyticus, 423
Hemophilus parainfluenzae, 423, 425
Hemophilus species, clinical
  differentiation of, *423*
Hemoptysis
  endemic, in paragonimiasis, 619
  in bronchogenic carcinoma, 1006
  in left ventricular failure, 1090
  in mitral stenosis, 1180
  in pulmonary tuberculosis, 486
Hemorrhage(s). See also *Bleeding.*
  brainstem, clinical manifestations of,
    798
  capsular, clinical manifestations of,
    797, 798
  cerebellar, clinical manifestations of,
    798
  cerebral, 1205
  complicating massive blood
    transfusions, 1052
  complicating needle biopsy of liver,
    1648
  complicating tracheostomy, in acute
    respiratory failure, 1040
  gastrointestinal, 1520–1523. See also
    Gastrointestinal bleeding.
  in acute leukemia, 1817
  in anticoagulant therapy, 793
  in hemophilia, 1883
  in peptic ulcer, 1516, 1517
  in regional enteritis, 1564
  in retinopathy of accelerated
    hypertension, 1205
  in ulcerative colitis, 1574
  intestinal, in typhoid fever, 447
    intramural, 1590
  intracerebral, 794
    arteriography in, 799
    clinical manifestations of, 797, 798
    pathology and pathogenesis of, 796
    treatment of, 801
  intracranial, 794–801
    clinical manifestations of, 796–798
    etiology of, 794–796, *794, 795*
    laboratory findings in, 798–799
    pathology and pathogenesis of, 796
    prognosis in, 799
    treatment of, 799–801
    vs. cerebral infarction, 790
  putamen, clinical manifestations of,
    797, 798
  splinter, in infective endocarditis, 389

Hemorrhage(s) (*Continued*)
  subarachnoid, 794
    clinical manifestations of, 796, 797
    pathology and pathogenesis of, 796
    with intracerebral extension, 794
  subhyaloid, 797
  subperiosteal, in scurvy, 1690
  tendency to, in chronic renal failure,
    1364
  thalamic, clinical manifestations of,
    798
  vitreous, in sickle cell diseases, 2332
Hemorrhagic anemia, acute, 1729–1730
Hemorrhagic conjunctivitis, acute,
  274–275
  poliomyelitis-like syndrome in, 270,
    275
Hemorrhagic disorder(s), 1871–1897
  arenaviruses causing, 298–300
  in kidney disease, 1891
  in liver disease, 1890, 1891
  in vitamin K deficiency, 1889, 1890
  of newborn, 1889
Hemorrhagic encephalitis
  acute, cerebrospinal fluid findings in,
    803
  drugs causing, 156
Hemorrhagic encephalomyelitis,
  necrotizing, acute, 849
Hemorrhagic fever(s)
  African, 300–301
  Argentine, *293,* **298–300**
  Bolivian, *293,* **298–300**
  Crimean, *293,* **298**
  dengue, *293,* **296–298**
  epidemic, *293,* **301–302**
  Korean, *293,* 301
  Omsk, 290–291, *293*
  viral, 292–302, *293*
Hemorrhagic hypotension, in shock,
  1117
Hemorrhagic leukoencephalitis, acute,
  836
Hemorrhagic mediastinitis, in anthrax,
  470, 471
Hemorrhagic meningitis, in anthrax,
  470, 471
Hemorrhagic nephrosonephritis, *293,*
  301–302
Hemorrhagic telangiectasia, hereditary,
  1880
Hemorrhoids, 1617
  vs. amebiasis, 592
Hemosiderin, 1743
Hemosiderosis, 1790
  pulmonary, idiopathic, 976
    pulmonary hypertension in, 1147
  transfusion, 1785
Hemostasis, primary, disorders of,
  1871–1880
Henbane, poisoning by, 70
Henderson-Hasselbalch equation, 1960
Henle, loops of, 1316, 1317
  function of, 1318, 1319, *1320*
Henoch-Schönlein purpura, 1880, *2298,*
  2301
  arthritis in, 201
  renal involvement in, 1400, 1401
  vs. periarteritis nodosa, 183
He-O$_2$ curve, 934, 935
Heparin
  administration of, bleeding tendency
    after, 1896, 1897

Heparin (*Continued*)
  in disseminated intravascular
    coagulation, 1052
  in pulmonary embolism, 1133
  in thrombophlebitis, 1126, 1127
  in thrombosis, 1124
  osteoporosis induced by, 2244
Hepatic. See also *Liver*.
Hepatic abscess
  acute, 1656–1657
  amebic, 590, 591, 592, 593
  computerized tomography in, *1467*
  pyogenic, vs. hepatic amebiasis, 592
  vs. pneumococcal pneumonia, 354
Hepatic amebiasis, 590, 591, 592, 593
  vs. clonorchiasis, 618
Hepatic coma, 1640–1641
  in cirrhosis, 1666
Hepatic diseases, 1637–1669. See also
  Liver, diseases of.
Hepatic encephalopathy, 1640–1641
  in cirrhosis, 1665, 1666
Hepatic fibrosis, congenital, 1667
Hepatic granulomas, 1667
Hepatic hermaphroditic flukes, 617–619
Hepatic porphyria(s), 2045–2049
  mixed, 2047
Hepatic precoma, 1640–1641
Hepatic schistosomiasis, 614, 1657
Hepatic tuberculosis, primary, 493
Hepatic vein occlusion, 1661
Hepatitis
  acute, with coma, 1655, 1656
  after anesthesia with fluorinated
    agents, 1659–1660
  alcoholic, acute, 1664
    vs. acute cholecystitis, 1627
    vs. acute viral hepatitis, 1654
    vs. hepatic amebiasis, 592
  anicteric, 1652
  aplastic anemia in, 1735
  cholestatic, 1652, 1653
  chronic active, 1661–1663
    cirrhosis in, 1663
    eosinophilia in, 226
    HLA system and, 39
    vs. acute viral hepatitis, 1654
  chronic persisting, 1652, 1653
    vs. chronic active hepatitis, 1662
  cirrhosis after, 1663
  drug-induced, vs. acute viral
    hepatitis, 1653
  effect of, on plasma amino acids, *2018*
  fulminant, 1655–1656
    hepatic encephalopathy in, 1641
  icteric, 1652, 1653
  in syphilis, 510
  infectious, 1650
    vs. psittacosis, 338
    vs. secondary syphilis, 510
  isoniazid, 484, 487, 489, 1658–1659
  lupoid, vs. systemic lupus
    erythematosus, 177
  methyldopa, 1660
  toxic, 1657–1659
    cirrhosis in, 1663
    vs. acute viral hepatitis, 1653
  viral, acute, 1650–1655
    cirrhosis in, 1663
    vs. acute cholecystitis, 1627
    complicating maintenance
      hemodialysis, 1382
    in opiate addiction, 697

Hepatitis (*Continued*)
  viral, non-A, non-B, 1656
    non-A, non-B, 1656
    polyarthritis associated with, 186
    type A, 1650, 1651
      prophylaxis of, 1654, 1655
      vs. cytomegalovirus
        mononucleosis, 828
    type B, 1650, 1651
      in chronic renal failure, 1366
      prophylaxis of, 1655
      vs. cytomegalovirus
        mononucleosis, 828, 829
    types A and B, differentiation of,
      1654
    vs. hepatic amebiasis, 592
    vs. jaundice of malaria, 573
    vs. leptospirosis, 534
    vs. louse-borne relapsing fever, 528
    vs. rat-bite fever, 531
Hepatitis A virus, 1650, 1651
Hepatitis B antigenemia, in periarteritis
  nodosa, 181
Hepatitis B virus, 1650, 1651
Hepatocellular jaundice, 1638
Hepatolenticular degeneration,
  2049–2051
  vs. dystonia musculorum deformans,
    761
Hepatoma, 1668
  angiography in, *1470, 1471*
  liver scanning in, *1469*
Hepatomegaly, 1639
  in malaria, 571
Hepatorenal syndrome, 1644, 1645
  acute renal failure in, 1369
  vs. acute tubular necrosis, 1373
Hepatosplenic schistosomiasis, 614
Hepatotoxins, 1657
Hereditary angioedema, *43*, 162, 163,
  2299
Hereditary chorea, 758–759
Hereditary coagulation disorders,
  1883–1889
Hereditary complement deficiency
  diseases, 137, 138
Hereditary coproporphyria, *42,* 2047
Hereditary deafness, 735
Hereditary elliptocytosis, 1757
Hereditary fructose intolerance, *41*
  2000–2001, *2020*
Hereditary hemorrhagic telangiectasia,
  1880
Hereditary hyperphosphatasia, 2264
Hereditary hypoprothrombinemia, *1884*
Hereditary methemoglobinemia, 1780,
  1781
Hereditary motor and sensory
  neuropathies, 912–913
Hereditary multiple exostosis(es), *1910,*
  2264, 2265
Hereditary myeloperoxidase deficiency,
  1806
Hereditary nephritis, 1402
Hereditary orotic aciduria, 2044
Hereditary pseudo–vitamin D
  deficiency rickets, 2252
Hereditary pyropoikilocytosis, 1758
Hereditary sensory neuropathies,
  911–912
  vs. leprosy, 504
Hereditary spastic paraplegia, 768
  vs. vitamin B_{12} deficiency, 777

Hereditary spherocytosis, 1756–1757
  detection of, in relatives, *58*
  vs. pyruvate kinase deficiency, 1758,
    1759
Hereditary stomatocytosis, 1757
Hereditary tyrosinemia, *2016, 2020*
Heredity, 11–12
  environment and, in disease
    development, 11, 12
Heredofamilial aortic diseases,
  1291–1292
Heredofamilial diseases, renal injury
  from, 1329–1330
Hermansky-Pudlak syndrome, 2029
Hermaphroditic flukes, 617–621
  hepatic, 617–619
  intestinal, 620–621
  lung, 619–620
Hernia(s)
  diaphragmatic, 1019, **1485,** *1485*
  hiatal, 1485, *1485*
    esophageal reflux with, vs. angina
      pectoris, 1227
Herniated disc syndromes, 204
Herniation
  cardiac, through pericardial defect,
    1276
  cerebellar, in intracranial tumors, 864
  intervertebral disc, 893, 894
  of forebrain, 641
  uncal, in intracranial tumors, 864
Heroin, 694–698
  acute reactions to, 696
  poisoning by, *712*
Herpangina, 270–271
  vs. hand-foot-and-mouth disease,
    274
Herpes gestationis, 2305
Herpes labialis, in pneumococcal
  pneumonia, 354
Herpes simplex
  vs. congenital cytomegalovirus
    infection, 828
  vs. herpes zoster, 826
Herpes simplex encephalitis, 821–824
  vs. arboviral encephalitis, 284
Herpes simplex virus
  encephalitis from, 818, *818,* 821, 822
  meningitis from, 818, *818*
Herpes zoster, 253, 824–827
  facial paralysis in, 900
  neuralgia after, 728
  peripheral neuropathy with, 905
  vertigo caused by, 740
Herpetic gingivostomatitis, primary, vs.
  herpangina, 271
Herpetic keratoconjunctivitis, vs. ocular
  chlamydial infections, 334
Herpetic ulcer, vs. syphilitic chancre,
  508
Hetastarch, in shock, 1118
Heteroalleles, 40
Heterogeneity, genetic, 40, 44
Heterophil antibodies, in infectious
  mononucleosis, 266
Heterophyes heterophyes, 621
Heterozygosity, 34
Heterozygote detection, in genetic
  counseling, 57, 58, *58*
Heterozygous beta thalassemia,
  1778–1779
Hetrazan. See *Diethylcarbamazine*.
Hexokinase deficiency, 1759

Hexose monophosphate shunt pathway, enzyme activity related to, deficiency in, 1759–1761
Hexylresorcinol, in fasciolopsiasis, 620
HGPRT deficiency, 2038, **2042–2043**
Hiatal hernia, 1485, *1485*
 esophageal reflux with, vs. angina pectoris, 1227
Hiccup, 1019
 in chronic renal failure, 1366
Hidradenitis suppurativa, 400, 2270, *2270*
Hilar adenopathy, in pulmonary tuberculosis, 484, 485
Hines' ulcers, vs. ischemic ulcers of arteriosclerosis obliterans, 1301
Hip
 congenital dislocated, frequency and sex ratio of, *48*
 degenerative disease of, primary, 203
Hippel-Lindau disease, 771, *1910*
 cutaneous manifestations of, *2300*
 internal malignancy and, *2296*
Hirschsprung's disease, 1495–1496, *1495*
Hirsutism, 2271–2272
Hirudiniasis, 120–121
His, bundle of, 1242
His-Purkinje conduction delay, 1260, *1261*
His-Purkinje system, 1242
Histamine
 circulatory effects of, 1111
 in regulation of gastric secretion, 1505, 1506
Histamine H_2-receptor antagonists, in peptic ulcer, 1514, *1514,* 1515
Histidinemia, *41*
Histidinuria, *2020*
Histiocytic lymphoma(s), 1830, *1830,* 1831, *1833*
Histiocytic-lymphocytic lymphomas, mixed, 1830, *1830,* 1831, 1832, *1833*
Histiocytosis, lipochrome, familial, 1806
"Histiocytosis X," 1848
Histo spots, in ocular histoplasmosis, *2318,* 2324
Histocompatibility locus
 disease associations of, mechanisms of, 39
 disease susceptibility and, 38, 39, *39*
Histocompatibility testing, in renal transplantation, 1383–1384
Histoplasma capsulatum, 536
Histoplasma duboisii, 536
Histoplasmosis, 536–537
 ocular, *2318,* **2323–2325**
 serologic tests for, 946
 skin test in, 537, 946
 vs. coccidioidomycosis, 539
 vs. pulmonary tuberculosis, 486
 vs. tularemia, 467
Historic typhus, 318–320
Histotoxic hypoxia, 100
Histones, 34
Hitzig zones, in tabes dorsalis, 815
Hives, 160–162. See also *Urticaria.*
HLA antigens, in sarcoidosis, 209
HLA system
 disease associations of, mechanisms of, 39
 disease susceptibility and, 38, 39, *39*
Hoarseness, in bronchogenic carcinoma, 1006

Hodgkin's disease, 1839–1848
 clinical manifestations of, 1840
 clinical problems in, 1844
 diagnostic evaluation in, 1844
 eosinophilia in, 226
 epidemiology of, 1839
 etiology and pathogenesis of, 1839
 histopathologic classification of, *1840*
 lungs as primary site of, 1011, 1012
 pathology of, 1839
 prognosis in, 1847
 staging in, 1845
 treatment of, 1845
  complications of, *1847*
 tuberculosis complicating, 483, 1844
 vs. histoplasmosis, 537
Hoechst-BUDR technique, 51
Hoffman's syndrome, 923
Holt-Oram syndrome, 1160
Homans' sign, in thrombophlebitis, 1125
Homocystinuria, *2017,* **2028–2029**
 aorta in, 1291, 1292
 osteoporosis of, 2245
 prevention and management of, 55
 pyridoxine responsive, *41*
 pyridoxine unresponsive, *41*
 vs. Marfan's syndrome, 2053
Homogentisic acid, in alcaptonuria, 2026
"Homologous disease," 130
Homosexuality, 691
Homozygosity, 34
Homozygous beta thalassemia, 1778
Homozygous hemoglobin C disease, 1776
Homozygous hemoglobin D Punjab disease, 1776
Homozygous hemoglobin E disease, 1776
Honeybee stings, 113
"Honeycomb" lung, 991, **1003**
Honeymoon cystitis, 1412
Hookworm anemia, 624, 625
Hookworm disease, 624–625
 antimicrobial agents for, *559*
 prevalence of, *605*
Hookworm infection, 624
Hormone(s). See also names of specific substances.
 abnormal or unusual, production of, 2064
 anterior pituitary, 2085–2091
  deficiency of, 2102, 2103
 antidiuretic, 2109–2110
  function of, 1321, 1322, 2109
  inappropriate secretion of, 1953, 1954, 2109
   associated with cancer, 1917
   in bronchogenic carcinoma, 1006
   in head injury, 882
 as medicines, 2068–2069
 biochemistry of, 2062
 effects of, circulatory, 1111
  onset and duration of, 2073
  "physiologic" vs. "pharmacologic," 2074
  specificity of, 2072
  ubiquity of, 2062–2063
 end-organ response to, failure of, 2064
 follicle-stimulating, 2087–2088
  human pituitary, in amenorrhea, 2192

Hormone(s) (*Continued*)
 follicle-stimulating, in ovarian function, 2175, 2176
  in secondary hypogonadism, 2172
  measurement of, 2092–2093, *2093*
  site of action of, 2178
 gonadal, excretion of, values for, 2180, *2181*
  plasma concentrations of, 2180, *2180*
 gonadotropin-releasing, 2075
  regulation of, disorders of, 2080–2181
 growth, 2086–2087
  function of, assessment of, 2091–2092
  mode of action of, 2071
  purified, in pituitary dwarfism, 2104, 2105
  radioimmunoassay of, in acromegaly, 2107
  secretion of, regulation of, 2077
 hypophysiotropic, deficiency of, 2078–2079, *2079*
  structural formulas of, *2075*
 hypothalamic, in diagnosis of anterior pituitary disease, 2081–2082, *2081, 2082*
 in control of gastrointestinal motility, 1476
 interstitial cell–stimulating, 2088–2089
 laboratory values for, 2351, 2353
 lactogenic, 2087. See also *Prolactin.*
 luteinizing, 2088–2089
  deficiency of, isolated, 2172
  in ovarian function, 2175, 2176
  measurement of, 2092–2093, *2093*
 luteinizing hormone–releasing, in diagnosis of anterior pituitary disease, 2081, 2082, *2082*
 melanocyte-stimulating, 2090
  function of, measurement of, 2094
 metabolism of, inborn errors of, *43*
 mode of action of, 2062, 2070–2074
 multiple, produced by single tumor, 1918
 ovarian, function of, 2176, *2177,* 2177–2178
 parathyroid, 2213–2214
  immunoreactive, circulating levels of, in vitamin D resistant rickets, 2250, 2251
  radioimmunoassay for, in hyperparathyroidism, 2218
  secretion of, in chronic renal failure, 1355, 1358
 pharmacologic uses of, 2069
 polypeptide, mode of action of, 2070, 2071, *2071*
 production of, by nonendocrine organ, 2064
 products of, laboratory values for, 2350–2352
 properties common to, 2070
 protein, mode of action of, 2070, 2071, *2071*
 replacement therapy with, 2068, 2069
 secretion of, altered control of, detection of, 2067, 2068
  by pulmonary tumors, 2061, *2062*
 steroid, mode of action of, 2070, *2071*
 structure and specificity of, relation between, 2073–2074

Hormone(s) (*Continued*)
testicular, chemistry and physiology of, 2163–2164
thyroid, action of, hereditary resistance to, 2140–2141
formation of, congenital metabolic defects in, 2138–2140
free, determination of, 2118
metabolic action of, 2116
metabolism of, 2114, *2114*, 2116
mode of action of, 2070, *2071*
secretion of, 2115
synthesis of, defects of, 2138, 2139
transport of, 2115, *2115*
defects in, 2140
thyroid-stimulating, 2089
action of, on thyroid, 2117
function of, assessment of, 2093
serum, assay of, 2118
thyrotropic, 2089
thyrotropin-releasing, 2075, 2117
synthetic, in diagnosis of anterior pituitary disease, 2081, *2081*
Hormone-dependent cancers, medical treatment of, 1918–1922
Horner's syndrome
in cluster headache, 731
in internal carotid artery occlusion, 787
in midbrain infarctions, 788
in syringomyelia, 769
Hornet stings, 113–114, 163
Horseshoe kidney, 1457
Hospital-acquired pneumonia, 361–364
factors predisposing to, 362
mechanisms and prevalence of, 361
possible future management of, 363
Hospital-acquired staphylococcal infections, 398
Host defenses
components of, 145, *145*, 146
compromised, 145–152
antimicrobial agent selection in, 553
clinical manifestations of, 147
diagnosis of, 150, 151, *151*
etiology of, 146
infections in, *148–149*
management of, 151, 152
pathogenesis and pathology of, 146
toxoplasmosis in, 596
cytotoxic agents and, 1923–1924, *1924*
mediation of, complement in, 136
Hot dog headache, 70
House-dust mites, allergy to, 118
Houssay phenomenon, in hypopituitarism, 2101
Howell-Jolly bodies, 1718
in hemolytic anemia, 1754
Human growth and development, 11–30
Humidification, in acute respiratory failure, 1026
Humidifier lung, *971*
Humoral mediators in host defense, 146
Hunger edema, 1684
Hunter's syndrome, *41*, **2052,** *2052*
cardiomyopathy with, 1280
Huntington's chorea, 758–759
dementia in, 663, 758, 759
screening for, 44
vs. acute chorea, 758
vs. striatonigral degeneration, 765
Hurler's syndrome, *41*, **2051–2052,** *2052*
aortic regurgitation in, 1194
cardiomyopathy with, 1280

Hurler's syndrome (*Continued*)
vs. pituitary dwarfism, 2104
Hutchinson, melanotic freckle of, 2310, 2311
Hutchinson-Gilford syndrome, vs. scleroderma, 170
Hutchinson's teeth, in congenital syphilis, 513
Hyaline casts, 1338
Hyalinosis
cutaneous-mucosal, 2058
segmental, 1393
Hydatid cyst(s), 609, 610
vs. hepatic amebiasis, 592
Hydatid disease, 609–610
Hydatidiform moles, human chorionic gonadotropin levels in, 2181
Hydralazine
in arterial hypertension, *1212*, 1214, 1215
in heart failure, 1101
in hypertension of chronic renal failure, 1362, 1363
in toxemia of pregnancy, 1415
neuropathy associated with, 910
Hydrarthrosis, intermittent, 198
Hydrocarbons
aromatic, exposure to, aplastic anemia after, 1735
as nephrotoxins, 1434
ingestion of, poisoning by, 75
Hydrocephalus, 873–874
communicating, 873
frequency and sex ratio of, *48*
in bacterial meningitis, 412
in neurofibromatosis, 770
noncommunicating, 873
occult "normal pressure," 874
ototic, 871
Hydrochlorothiazide
in arterial hypertension, *1212*
in ascites complicating cirrhosis, 1665
in renal calculi, 1446
Hydrocortisone
in Addison's disease, 2149, 2150
in adrenal insufficiency secondary to pituitary-adrenal suppression by corticosteroids, 2152
in chronic respiratory failure, 1029
in congenital adrenal hyperplasia, 2161
in Hymenoptera stings, 114
in hypoglycemia caused by functioning islet cell tumors, 1995
in hypopituitarism, 2102
in louse-borne relapsing fever, 528
in myxedema coma, 2134
in orchitis complicating mumps, 263
in rheumatoid arthritis, 192
in rickettsial diseases, 316
in status asthmaticus, 959
in thyroid storm, 2128
in toxic megacolon, 1575
in ulcerative colitis, 1573
Hydrocortisone phosphate, in addisonian crisis, 2149
Hydrocytosis, 1757
Hydrogen fluoride, exposure to, respiratory effects of, 1000
Hydrogen ion, excretion of, in chronic renal failure, 1357
Hydrolysis, intraluminal, defective, malabsorption syndrome caused by, 1535–1539

Hydromyelia, 768
Hydronephrosis
congenital, 1457
in paraplegia, 888
vs. adult polycystic kidney disease, 1454
vs. nephroblastoma, 1460
Hydropericardium, 1276
Hydrophilic colloids
in constipation, 1482
in diarrhea, 1480
in irritable bowel syndrome, 1494
Hydrophobia, 833–836, *833, 835*. See also *Rabies*.
Hydrops
in acute cholecystitis, 1626
in chronic cholecystitis, 1625
Hydrops fetalis, with Hemoglobin Bart's, 1779
Hydrothorax
in right ventricular failure, 1092
simple, 1014–1015
Hydroxychlorobenzamide, in tapeworm infections, 608, 609
Hydroxychloroquine, in solar urticaria, 162
25-Hydroxycholecalciferol, 2232, 2233
25-Hydroxyergocalciferol, 2232, 2233
Hydroxyethyl starch, in shock, 1118
5-Hydroxyindolacetic acid, measurement of, in malabsorption syndrome, 1531
5-Hydroxyindole compounds, excessive production of, in carcinoid syndrome, 2209, 2210
11β-Hydroxylase, deficiency of, *2159*, 2160, 2161
17α-Hydroxylase, deficiency of, *2159*, 2160, 2161
20α-Hydroxylase, deficiency of, 2159, *2159*, 2161
21-Hydroxylase, deficiency of, *2159*, 2160, 2161
Hydroxylysinemia, *2017*
Hydroxy-o-methyl transferase, 2112
17α-Hydroxyprogesterone, properties of, *2145*, 2146
Hydroxyprolinemia, *41*, *2017*, 2022
Hydroxyprolinuria, in sarcoidosis, 215
3β-Hydroxysteroid dehydrogenase, deficiency of, 2159, *2159*, 2161
18-Hydroxysteroid dehydrogenase, deficiency of, 2161
2-Hydroxystilbamidine, in blastomycosis, 541
Hydroxyurea, in oncologic treatment, 1938
Hydroxyzine, in chronic urticaria, 162
Hymenolepis diminuta, 611
Hymenolepis nana, 606, *606*, **609**
Hymenoptera, stings of, 113–114, 163
Hyoscine, in motion sickness, 95
Hyoscyamine, ingestion of, 705
Hyoscyamus niger, poisoning by, 70
Hypemic hypoxia, 100
Hyperadrenocorticism
combined hyperlipidemia in, 2009
myopathy in, 924
obesity in, 1697
Hyperaeration, localized, 966
Hyperalaninemias, *2018*
Hyperaldosteronism
idiopathic, 2157
primary, hypertension from, 1211

Hyperaldosteronism (*Continued*)
  selective, hyperkalemia in, 1959
  vs. familial periodic paralysis, 922
Hyperalgesic neuropathy, 908, 909
Hyperalimentation
  intravenous, after extensive small
    intestinal resection, 1544, *1544*
  parenteral, 1706, 1707, 1708
Hyperaminoacidemia, branched-chain,
  2016–2017
Hyperaminoaciduria(s), 2015, 2021
  renal, 2023
Hyperammonemia, *41, 2018*
  dietary restriction in, 55
  in total parenteral nutrition, 1708
Hyperargininemia, *41, 2018, 2019*
Hyperbaric oxygen, therapeutic
  application of, 103–105
  in clostridial myonecrosis, 435
Hyperbeta-alaninemia, *41, 2019*
Hyperbetalipoproteinemia, 2005
Hyperbilirubinemia
  conjugated, 1638
  shunt, 1649
  unconjugated, 1638, 1648, 1649
    idiopathic, 1649
Hyperbradykinism, 743
  familial, vs. idiopathic autonomic
    insufficiency, 763
Hypercalcemia, 2233–2241
  complicating hormonal treatment of
    breast cancer, 1920
  diuretics and, 2237
  idiopathic, 2236
  in acute renal failure, 1369, 2237
  in adrenal insufficiency, 2236
  in bronchogenic carcinoma, 1007
  in cancer patient, 1903, 1917,
    2233–2234
  in chronic renal failure, 1354
  in fungal and mycobacterial
    infections, 2238
  in hyperparathyroidism, 2215, 2216,
    2217
    treatment of, 2218, 2219
  in hyperthyroidism, 2236
  in milk-alkali syndrome, 2237
  in multiple endocrine adenomatosis,
    2238
  in pheochromocytoma, 2237, 2238
  in renal function disorders, 2237
  in sarcoidosis, 215, 2235–2236
  in vitamin D toxicity, 2234–2235
  mental disturbances with, 2239
  of immobilization, 2236–2237
  signs and symptoms of, 2238–2239
  treatment of, 2239–2241
  vs. diabetes insipidus, 2110
Hypercalcemic crisis(es)
  in hyperparathyroidism, 2219
  treatment of, 2240
Hypercalcemic nephropathy, 1438–1440
Hypercalciuria, in sarcoidosis, 215
Hypercapnia, 1022
  acid-base disturbances in, 1967, *1967*
  clinical manifestations of, 1025
  in chronic obstructive pulmonary
    disease, 963
Hypercarbia, in cancer patient, 1904,
  1905
Hyperchloremic acidosis, 1962
  in chronic renal failure, 1354
  in total parenteral nutrition, 1708
Hypercholesterolemia, *42, 2004*
  acquired, 2009

Hypercholesterolemia (*Continued*)
  familial, 2005
    detection of, in relatives, *58*
Hypercoagulability, in cerebral
  infarction, 781
Hypercortisolism, 2152, 2154, 2155
Hypercystinuria, *2020*
Hyperdibasic aminoaciduria, *41, 2020*
Hyperdipsia, primary, 719
Hyperemia, reactive, in Raynaud's
  phenomenon, 1306
Hypereosinophilic syndrome, 226
Hypergammaglobulinemia
  electrophoretic patterns in, 1854,
    1855, *1855*
  immunodeficiency with, *139*
  in chronic active hepatitis, 1662
  in liver disease, 1662
Hypergastrinemia, 1508, 1509
Hyperglobulinemic purpura, benign,
  1880
Hyperglycemia
  in acute pancreatitis, 1553
  in total parenteral nutrition, 1707
Hyperglycinemias, *41, 2017*
Hyperglycinurias, 2023
Hypergonadotropic hypogonadism,
  treatment of, 2190
Hyperhistidinemia, *2016*, 2022
Hyperinfective syndrome, in
  strongyloidiasis, 622
Hyperinsulinemia, in obesity, 1694
Hyperinsulinism
  alimentary, 1990
  vs. polymyositis, 174
Hyperkalemia, 1959–1960
  complicating diuresis for ascites in
    cirrhosis, 1665
  complicating massive blood
    transfusions, 1051, 1052
  in acute renal failure, 1372
  in chronic interstitial nephritis, 1418
  in chronic renal failure, 1356, *1357*
  in familial periodic paralysis, 921,
    1959
Hyperkeratosis
  epidermolytic, *2286*
  follicular, 1675
  of soles, in yaws, 521
Hyperleucinemia, *2017*
Hyperlipemia
  alcoholic, 2009
  diabetic, 2009
  endogenous, *2004*
  exogenous, *2004*, 2006–2007
  fat-induced, 2006–2007
  in glycogen storage disease type I,
    2009
  in lipodystrophy, 2009
  mixed, *2004*
  pseudohyponatremia produced by,
    1955
  stress, 2009
Hyperlipidemia
  as risk factor for atherosclerosis,
    1220
  combined, *42, 2004*
    acquired, 2009
    familial, 2007–2008
  in acute pancreatitis, 1553
  in chronic renal failure, 1361
  in nephrotic syndrome, 1388, 1389
  multiple lipoprotein–type, familial,
    2007–2008
  remnant, *2004*

Hyperlipidemic disorders, classification
  of, 2003, *2004*
Hyperlipoproteinemia(s)
  acquired, 2009–2010
  in atherosclerotic vascular disease,
    2010–2011
  inherited, 2004–2008
    type I, 2006–2007
    type III, 2005–2006
    type IV, 2007
    type V, 2007
  lamellar, *2004*
Hyperlucent lung, unilateral, 1004
Hyperlysinemia(s), *41, 2017–2018, 2019*
Hypermenorrhea, 2179
Hypermethioninemia, *2016*
Hypermetropia, headache from, 733
Hypernatremia, 1956
  essential, 718, 719
  in cancer patient, 1904
Hypernephroma, cutaneous
  manifestations of, *2300*
Hyperopia, severe, elevated disc of,
  2328
Hyperornithinemia, *2018*, 2022
Hyperosmolar coma
  in diabetes mellitus, treatment of,
    1985
  nonketotic, volume depletion in, 1951
Hyperostosis corticalis deformans
  juvenilis, 2257, 2264
Hyperoxaluria, *41*
  primary, 2001
Hyperparathyroid crisis, in
  hyperparathyroidism, 2218
Hyperparathyroidism, 2214–2220
  arthritis in, 200
  complicating maintenance
    hemodialysis, 1381
  duodenal ulcer and, 1504
  "ectopic," 2217
  familial, detection of, in relatives, *58*
  hypercalcemia in, 2215, 2216, 2217
    treatment of, 2218, 2219
  myopathy in, 924
  osteoporosis in, 2244
  secondary, 2214
    in chronic renal failure, 2217, 2255
  tertiary, 2256
  vs. hypercalcemia of sarcoidosis, 2235
  vs. medullary sponge kidney, 1456
  vs. polymyositis, 174
  Zollinger-Ellison syndrome and, 1509,
    2215, 2216
Hyperphenylalaninemia(s), *2016*,
  2024–2026, *2024*
  benign, *2016*
  benign persistent, 2025
  neonatal, *2016*
Hyperphosphatasia, hereditary, 2264
Hyperphosphatemia, 2229, 2230
  in acute renal failure, 1372, 1373
  in hypoparathyroidism, 2220
Hyperpigmentation, 2289–2291
  associated with cancer, 1916, 2297
  generalized, 2291
  in Addison's disease, 2148
Hyperpituitarism, 2105–2108
Hyperpnea, 939
Hyperprolactinemia, 2108
Hyperprolinemia(s), *41, 2017, 2019,*
  2022
Hyperproteinemia, pseudohyponatremia
  produced by, 1955
Hypersarcosinemia, *41*

Hypersensitivity. See also *Allergy(ies)*.
  carotid sinus, dizziness in, 740
  delayed type of, 130
  in mercury poisoning, 80
  penicillin, in treatment of infective
    endocarditis, 394
  to Hymenoptera stings, 113, 114
  tuberculin, 481
Hypersensitivity angiitis, 166, 167, *2301*
  drug-induced, vs. periarteritis
    nodosa, 183
**Hypersensitivity drug reactions,
  154–157**
  liver disease due to, 1659–1660
  pulmonary disorders due to, 974–976
**Hypersensitivity pneumonitis, 970–972,
  *971***
Hypersomnia, 653–655
Hypersplenic syndrome, 1870
Hypersplenic thrombocytopenia, 1877
Hypersplenism, 1869–1871
Hypertension
  accelerated, 1204
    prognosis in, 1217
    retinopathy in, 1205
  after renal transplantation, 1385
  arterial, 1199–1218
    cardiovascular disease risk factors
      in, 1201, 1202, *1202*
      evaluation of, 1204
      reduction of, 1212
    causes of death in, 1203
    clinical manifestations of, 1203
    clinical syndromes of, 1204
    epidemiology of, 1200
    etiology of, 1209
    headaches associated with, 732,
      1203
    mechanisms of, 1206
    prognosis in, 1217
    treatment of, 1211
      drugs for, 1212–1217, *1212, 1215*
        cessation of, 1216
        choices of, 1216, 1217
        combinations of, 1215, *1215*
  as risk factor for atherosclerosis, 1062,
    1219, 1220
  associated with catecholamine excess,
    1209, 1210
  cerebral infarction and, 779
  complicating maintenance
    hemodialysis, 1382
  death rates for, *1060*
  essential, "benign," 1206
    catecholamine excess in, 1209
  in acute poststreptococcal
    glomerulonephritis, 1395, 1396
  in acute renal arterial occlusive
    disease, 1407
  in analgesic nephropathy, 1420
  in carcinoid syndrome, 2208
  in cerebral infarction, 780
  in chronic renal failure, 1356, *1356*
    management of, 1362, 1363
  in glomerular disease, 1386, 1387
  in hyperparathyroidism, 2215,
    2216
  in interstitial nephritis, 1417
  in nephronophthisis–cystic renal
    medulla complex, 1455
  in obesity, 1695
  in pheochromocytoma, 2201, 2202,
    2203, *2203*
  in pregnancy, 1205, 1206, 1414, 1415,
    1416

Hypertension (*Continued*)
  in primary aldosteronism, 2157
  in tetanus, 440
  intracranial, benign, 870–872, *871*
  intracranial hemorrhage from, 795
    prognosis in, 799
  left atrial, 1144–1146
  malignant, 1204, 1205
    vs. primary aldosteronism, 2158
  mineralocorticoid excess, 1211
  oral contraceptive use and, 2195, 2196
  portal, 1639–1640
    ascites in, 1593
    cirrhosis and, 1144, 1665
    diagnostic procedures in, 1648
    gastrointestinal bleeding and, 1523
      in cirrhosis, 1665
    manifestations of, 1639, 1640
  postoperative, in pheochromocytoma,
    2206
  prevalence of, 1059
  pulmonary, 1135–1149
    **disorders of respiration and,
      1146–1149**
    in atrial septal defect, 1161
    **in cirrhosis with portal
      hypertension, 1144**
    in coarctation of aorta, 1289
    **in congenital heart disease,
      1141–1143**
    in mitral stenosis, 1180, 1181
      vs. atrial septal defect, 1162
    primary, 1137–1141
      vs. mitral stenosis, 1183
  pulmonary venous, 1144–1146
  renal, 1210–1211
  renin-dependent, 1210
  renoprival, 1207
  retinopathy in, 1206, *2318, 2325, 2326,
    2326*
    in chronic renal failure, 1366
  salt and water overload, 1210
  systemic, eyes in, 2325–2326, *2326*
    in intracranial tumors, 864
    severe, aortic regurgitation in, 1194
  systolic, 1209
  ulcers of, vs. ischemic ulcers of
    arteriosclerosis obliterans, 1301
  venous, in heart failure, 1087, 1088
Hypertensive encephalopathy, 793–794,
  1205
Hypertensive left ventricular failure,
  1206
**Hypertensive lower esophageal
  sphincter, 1488**
Hyperthermia
  hypothalamic dysfunction and, 716,
    717
  in metabolic brain disease, 648
  malignant, anesthetic agents causing,
    genetic basis of, 46
    myoglobinuria in, 924, 925
Hyperthyroidism, 2120–2128
  "apathetic," 923, 2065
  associated with cancer, 1916, 1917
  eyes in, 2122, 2332, 2333
  hypercalcemia in, 2236
  in pregnancy, 2125, 2126
  malabsorption in, 1548
  masked, 2122
  osteoporosis in, 2244
  vs. acute intermittent porphyria, 2047
Hypertrichosis, 2271–2272
Hypertrichosis lanuginosa, acquired,
  2296

Hypertriglyceridemia(s), *42*
  endogenous, acquired, 2009
    familial, 2007
    in obesity, 1695
  mixed, acquired, 2009
    familial, 2007
  primary, 2006–2008
Hypertrophic neuropathy
  dominantly inherited, 912
  recessively inherited, 913
Hypertrophic obstructive
  cardiomyopathy, 1278
Hypertrophic osteoarthritis, primary,
  generalized, 204
    vs. rheumatoid arthritis, 190
**Hypertrophic osteoarthropathy, 201,
  2263**
  in bronchogenic carcinoma, 1007
Hypertrophic pachymeningitis, 813
Hypertrophic subaortic stenosis,
  idiopathic, 1278, *1278,* 1279
    vs. aortic stenosis, *1192,* 1193
    vs. mitral regurgitation, 1187
    vs. mitral valve prolapse syndrome,
      1189
Hypertyrosinemias, *2016*
Hyperuricemia, *42*
  acute renal failure in, 1369
  in gout, 2030
    cause of, 2031
    classification of, *2030*
    treatment of, 2041
  in multiple myeloma, 1860
  in sarcoidosis, 215
Hyperuricosuria, in multiple myeloma,
  1860
Hypervalinemia, *41, 2017,* 2021
Hyperventilation, 745–746, 939
  dizziness from, 741
  in acute respiratory failure, 1033
  in metabolic acidosis, 1962
  in metabolic brain disease, 649
  in shock, 1046
  respiratory alkalosis from, 1969
  Valsalva maneuver with, 746
Hyperventilation syndrome, 674, 745,
  746
  hypocalcemia in, 2241
  vs. asthma, 957
  vs. hysterical fainting, 744
Hypervitaminosis A and D, 1691–1692
Hypesthesia, in radicular syndromes,
  889
Hypnagogic hallucinations, 654
Hypoaeration, localized, 965
Hypoalbuminemia, in portal
  hypertension, 1640
Hypobetalipoproteinemia, *42,* 2008
Hypocalcemia, 2241–2242
  in acute pancreatitis, 1553, 2241
  in cancer patient, 1904
  in hypoparathyroidism, 2220, 2221
  in malabsorption syndrome, 1528, 2241
  in newborn, 2241
  signs and symptoms of, 2242
Hypochromic anemias, 1743–1751
  not caused by iron deficiency, 1751
Hypoderma lineatum, 112
**Hypofibrinogenemia, acquired,
  1891–1895**
Hypofibrinogenemic syndromes
  associated with disseminated
    intravascular clotting, 1893–1894
  associated with localized thrombosis,
    1893

Hypogammaglobulinemia
arthritis in, 199
electrophoretic patterns in, 1854, *1855*
immunodeficiency and thymoma
associated with, 142
in chronic lymphocytic leukemia,
1825
malabsorption in, 1547
transient, of infancy, *139*
Hypoglossal nerve, disorders of, 900
Hypoglycemia, 1989–1997
alcohol-induced, 1705
associated with cancer, 1917
**extrapancreatic neoplasms associated
with, 1995**
**fasting, functioning islet cell tumors
causing, 1993–1995**
induced, *1990*, **1996–1997**
spontaneous, *1990*, **1992–1993**
functional, 1990, 1991
in fed state, 1989–1992, *1990*
in insulin therapy of diabetes
mellitus, 1986, 1988
in liver disease, 1642
in Reye's syndrome, 839
pathophysiologic classification of,
1990
postinfusion, in total parenteral
nutrition, 1707
reactive, 1990
hypoglycemic coma in, 1991
spontaneous, related to autoimmune
mechanisms, 1996
syncope in, 745
Hypoglycemic agents, oral, in diabetes
mellitus, 1986, *1986*
Hypoglycemic coma
in reactive hypoglycemia, 1991
sulfonylureas inducing, 1996
Hypoglycemic disorders, 1989–1997
Hypogonadism
female, hypergonadotropic, treatment
of, 2190
hypogonadotropic, treatment of,
2191, 2192
male, 2167–2172
hypogonadotropic, 2171
primary, 2168–2171
secondary, 2171–2172
Hypokalemia, 1957–1959
after thiazide therapy in heart failure,
1104
hypocalcemia and, 2242
in familial periodic paralysis, 921
in primary aldosteronism, 2157
of unknown origin, 1957, 1958
Hypokalemic acidosis, in cancer
patient, 1904
Hypokalemic nephropathy, 1437–1438
Hypokinetic heart disease, Bantu, 1283
**Hypolipoproteinemias
acquired, 2010
inherited, 2008–2009**
Hypomagnesemia
alcohol-induced, 1705
in chronic renal failure, 1356, *1357*
in malabsorption syndrome, 1528,
1529
tetany caused by, 2223
Hypomenorrhea, 2179
Hyponatremia, 1952–1956
beer drinker's, 719
causes of, *1953*
complicating diuresis for ascites in
cirrhosis, 1665

Hyponatremia (*Continued*)
drug-induced, 1954
idiopathic, 1954
in acute renal failure, 1372
in cancer patient, 1904
in hypopituitarism, 2101
in malabsorption syndrome, 1529
without disturbance in water balance,
1955
Hypoparathyroidism, 2220–2221
malabsorption in, 1547
pseudoidiopathic, 2064
Hypopharyngeal diverticulum, 1499
Hypophosphatasia, *43*, 2019, 2254
juvenile form of, vs. osteogenesis
imperfecta, 2245
Hypophosphatemia
in total parenteral nutrition, 1707,
1708
in vitamin D resistant rickets, 2250
Hypophosphatemic rickets, X-linked,
dietary treatment of, 55
Hypophysectomy-induced
hypopituitarism, 2103
**Hypophysiotropic hormones
deficiency of, 2078–2079,** *2079*
structural formulas of, *2075*
Hypophysiotropic neurons, 2074–2076
biogenic amine control of, 2076–2077
Hypopigmentation, 2292
Hypopituitarism, 2100–2105
**adrenal insufficiency secondary to,
2150–2151**
adrenocortical insufficiency secondary
to, vs. Addison's disease, 2148, *2148*
hypophysectomy-induced, 2103
in childhood, 2103–2105
Hypopituitary coma, in
hypopituitarism, 2100
Hypopituitary dwarfism, growth
hormone radioimmunoassay in, 2091
Hypoplastic anemia, 1733. See also
Aplastic anemia.
Hypoplastic kidney, 1457
Hypoproteinemia, in chronic renal
failure, 1353
Hypoprothrombinemia, *43*
hereditary, *1884*
Hyposensitization, in allergic rhinitis,
159, 160
Hypospadias, 1458
Hyposplenism, 1869
in adult celiac disease, 1541
Hypotension
after tumor removal in
pheochromocytoma, 2206
compensated, in shock, 1107
hemorrhagic, in shock, 1117
in cancer patient, 1905
in cerebral infarction, 780
in malabsorption syndrome, 1529
in myocardial infarction, 1230
in sedative overdose, 714
intracranial, 873
orthostatic, 742, 743
faintness in, 740
idiopathic, 762–763
in diabetes mellitus, 1980
Hypothalamic amenorrhea, 2080, 2187
**Hypothalamic hormones, in diagnosis
of anterior pituitary disease,
2081–2082,** *2081, 2082*
Hypothalamic hypothyroidism, 2078
**Hypothalamic neurosecretion,
2074–2076**

Hypothalamic obesity, 718, 1697
Hypothalamus
diseases of, causes of, *716, 2079*
vs. functional amenorrhea, 2080
functional anatomy of, 715, *715*
lesions of, galactorrhea in, 2191
neurologic disorders and, 715–719
pituitary and, 2074, *2075*
Hypothermia, 84, **85–86**
complicating massive blood
transfusions, 1051
hypothalamic dysfunction and, 716
in heat stroke, 85
paroxysmal, 716
Hypothyroidism, 2132–2135
cardiomegaly in, 1272
galactorrhea in, 2191, 2192
goitrous, sporadic, 2138–2140
hypercholesterolemia in, 2009
hypothalamic, 2078
in radiation injury, 89
in radioactive iodide therapy of
hyperthyroidism, 2124
myxedema coma in, 2134
myxedema heart in, 2134, 2135
obesity and, 1697
peripheral neuropathy with, 909
primary, prolactin levels in, 2092
tertiary, 2078
vs. adrenal insufficiency secondary to
hypopituitarism, 2151
vs. pituitary dwarfism, 2104
Hypoventilation, 939, 940, 1021
alveolar, pulmonary hypertension in,
1146, 1147, 1148
secondary polycythemia in, 1799
in metabolic brain disease, 649
in sedative overdose, 713
Hypovitaminosis A, 1684–1686
Hypovolemia
correction of, in shock, 1117, 1118
in cancer patient, 1905
intravascular, vs. idiopathic
autonomic insufficiency, 763
**Hypoxanthine–guanine
phosphoribosyltransferase deficiency,**
2038, **2042–2043**
Hypoxemia, in cancer patient, 1904
Hypoxia, 100–101, *100*
arterial, causes of, in acute respiratory
failure, 1036, *1037*
clinical manifestations of, 1025
effects of, on cerebral metabolism, 646
in shock, 1109, 1110
correction of, 1118
polycythemia and, 1798
pulmonary circulation in, 1137
terminal, in acute respiratory failure,
1034
Hypoxic hypoxia, 100
Hypsarrhythmia, infantile massive
spasms associated with, 854
Hysteria, 678–680
vs. dystonia musculorum deformans,
761
vs. poliomyelitis, 832
"Hysterical coma," vs. metabolic brain
disease, 649, 650
Hysterical fainting, 744
Hysterical pain, 678
"Hysterical personality," 678, 679
Hysterical seizures, vs. epilepsy, 679,
858
Hysterical weakness, vs. myasthenia
gravis, 927

"Hysteroepilepsy," 858
Hysterosalpingography, in infertility, 2194

Ibuprofen, in rheumatoid arthritis, 191
Iceland disease, 307
vs. poliomyelitis, 831
I-cell disease, *41*
Ichthyosiform dermatoses, 2286, *2286*
Ichthyosiform erythrodermas, 2286, 2287
Ichthyosis, 2285–2286, *2286*
acquired, internal malignancy and, *2297*
Ichthyosis vulgaris, *2286*
ICSH, 2088–2089
Icteric hepatitis, 1652, 1653
Icterus, 1637. See also *Jaundice.*
Idiocy, amaurotic, 850
Idioventricular rhythms, accelerated, 1254, *1254*
Idoxuridine, *556,* 1935
Ig, surface, on B cell, detection of, 129, *129*
Ig chain structure, 127, *127*
Ig deficiency, selective, *139*
IgA, 126
biologic properties of, *127*
deficiency of, selective, *43, 139,* **143**
serum, in sarcoidosis, 215
structure of, 127, *127*
IgA heavy chain disease, 1866
IgD, 126
biologic properties of, *127*
serum, in sarcoidosis, 215
structure of, 127, *127*
IgE, 126
biologic properties of, *127*
serum, in sarcoidosis, 215
skin-sensitizing antibodies and, 128
structure of, 127, *127*
IgG, 126
complement activation by, 135, 136
deficiency of, recurrent bacterial infections and, management of, 152
Fc portion of, in B cell determination, 129
serum, in sarcoidosis, 215
structure of, 127, *127*
IgG1, 126
biologic properties of, *127*
IgG2, 126
biologic properties of, *127*
IgG3, 126
biologic properties of, *127*
IgG4, 126
biologic properties of, *127*
IgG–anti-IgG complexes, 128
in renal disease, 134
IgG-IgM cryoglobulinemia, mixed, renal changes in, 1406
IgM, 126
biologic properties of, *127*
complement activation by, 135, 136
increased, X-linked immunodeficiency with, *43, 139*
serum, in sarcoidosis, 215
structure of, 127, *127*
IgM FTA-ABS test, in congenital syphilis, 515
IgM heavy chain disease, 1866
Ileal bypass operation
in obesity, 1698

Ileal bypass operation (*Continued*)
malabsorption after, 1547
Ileal carcinoid tumor, 2210, *2211*
vs. regional enteritis, 1565
Ileal resection, malabsorption after, 1547
Ileitis
backwash, vs. regional enteritis, 1566
regional. See *Enteritis, regional.*
Ileocecal sphincter, 1492
Ileocecal tuberculosis, 492
vs. regional enteritis, 1565
Ileojejunitis, nongranulomatous, 1542
vs. eosinophilic gastroenteritis, 1543
Ileum
disease of, malabsorption in, 1547
diverticula of, 1500–1501
perforation of, in regional enteritis, 1564
Ileus, 1490–1492
adynamic, 1490, 1491
colonic, 1497–1498
gallstone, 1626, **1628–1629**
paralytic, in pneumococcal pneumonia, 354
in spinal cord dysfunction, 887
potassium deficiency inducing, 1958
Iliofemoral thrombophlebitis, acute, vs. arterial embolism, 1304
Image intensifiers, fluoroscopic, in critical care medicine, 1032
Imerslund's syndrome, 2029
Imferon. See *Iron dextran.*
Iminoacidopathies, 2022
Iminoglycinuria, *41, 2020,* 2023
neonatal, *2019*
Imipramine
in depression, 675, 678
in depression of manic-depressive psychosis, 671
in depressive symptoms complicating dementia, 663
in pain, *724*
in parkinsonism, 755
poisoning by, *712*
Immersion foot, 1309–1310
Immobilization
hypercalcemia of, 2236–2237
osteoporosis of, 2244, 2245
Immune competence in cancer patients, 1925–1926
Immune complex disease, 133–134
Immune complexes
circulating, in sarcoidosis, 210
in rheumatoid arthritis, 187
Immune deficiency syndromes, eosinophilia in, 226
Immune disease, 126–163
Immune hemolytic anemia, Coombs-negative, 1763
Immune mechanisms
in chronic active hepatitis, 1661
in Hodgkin's disease, 1843
in liver disease, 1644
in multiple myeloma, 1860
in pneumococcal pneumonia, 347, 348
in rheumatoid arthritis, 187
in toxic nephropathy, 1423, 1424
in ulcerative colitis, 1569
in Wegener's granulomatosis, 219
Immune response(s), 146
abnormal, in systemic lupus erythematosus, 174, 175, 178, 179

Immune response(s) (*Continued*)
cellular basis of, *138*
defects of, infections in, *148, 150*
management of, 152
diagnostic evaluation of, 150, 151, *151*
to infection, in malnutrition, 1679
Immune response gene hypothesis, 39
Immune surveillance of cancer, 1924–1925
Immune system, cellular, in scleroderma, 168
Immune-mediated renal disease, 1324–1327, *1324, 1325*
Immunity
after viral infections, 229
altered, presumed, neuropathy associated with, 906
cell-mediated, in Graves' disease, 2121
in Hashimoto's thyroiditis, 2129
in malnutrition, 1679
in measles, 247
cellular, impairment of, in sarcoidosis, 210
mechanisms of, in common cold, 231, 232
Immunoblastic lymphadenopathy, eosinophilia in, 226
Immunocompromised patient, nosocomial pneumonia and, 362
Immunodeficiency(ies)
combined, severe, *43, 139,* **141**
common variable, 142–143
primary, 138–145, *139*
Swiss type, 141
thymoma with, *139,* **142**
varicella and, 254
with ataxia telangiectasia and Wiskott-Aldrich syndrome, *139,* **143–144**
X-linked, with increased IgM, *43, 139*
Immunoelectrophoresis, countercurrent, in diagnosis of bacterial meningitis, 413
Immunoglobulins, 126. See also names of specific immunoglobulins: *IgG, IgM,* etc.
amino acid sequence of, 127
bacterial inactivation by, 339
isolated absence of, 143
properties of, 126–128, *127*
serum, in sarcoidosis, 215
structure of, 127, *127*
Immunologic purpura, secondary, 1876
Immunologic reactions, hemolysis effected by, 1762–1766
Immunology, 126
aging and, 28
microbial diseases and, 228
Immunosuppressive agents, 1930, *1930.* See also names of specific agents.
in regional enteritis, 1567
in rheumatoid arthritis, 193
in ulcerative colitis, 1574
Immunotherapy
in acute leukemia, 1818
in bronchogenic carcinoma, 1010
in cancer, 1938–1941
Impaction, fecal, 1615
in paraplegia, 887
Impetigo, 374, 400
bullous, 400
in streptococcal pharyngitis, 373
treatment of, 401

Impetigo (*Continued*)
  vs. yaws, 521
Impetigo contagiosa, 374
Impotence, 687, **2174,** 2198
  in diabetes mellitus, 1980
Imuran. See *Azathioprine.*
Inborn errors of metabolism, 40–44,
  41–44, 1949
  amino acid, 2015–2029
  lipoprotein, 2004–2009
  screening for, 44
Inclusion body encephalitis, subacute,
  841
Inclusion conjunctivitis, trachoma and,
  331–335
Inclusion disease, 827–829
Incontinence, fecal, 1482–1483
  in acquired megacolon, 1496
Incontinentia pigmenti, 2291, *2291*
  vs. pinta, 525
Indian tick typhus, 324
Indiana type of inherited amyloidosis,
  910
Indican, measurement of, in
  malabsorption syndrome, 1531
Indicator dilution techniques, cardiac
  output determination by, 1032, 1083
Indocin. See *Indomethacin.*
Indomethacin
  in acute gouty arthritis, 2039
  in ankylosing spondylitis, 195
  in degenerative joint disease, 205
  in pain, *724*
  in Reiter's syndrome, 198
  in rheumatoid arthritis, 191
Infant(s)
  athetosis in, 760
  beriberi in, 1689
  botulism in, 67
  disseminated listeriosis in, 472
  newborn. See *Newborn(s).*
  polycystic kidney disease in, 1453
  premature, congenital heart disease
    and, 1150
  recommended dietary allowances for,
    1671
  scurvy in, 1691
  streptococcal pharyngitis in, 372
  transient hypogammaglobulinemia of,
    139
Infantile agammaglobulinemia,
  X-linked, *43,* **139–140,** *139, 140*
  Bruton type of, 139, 150, *1910*
Infantile massive spasms, 854
Infarction
  brainstem, 786, 787
  cerebral, 778–794
    course of, 790–791
    differential diagnosis of, 790
    etiology of, 778
    incidence of, 778
    mechanisms of, 778–781
    neuropathology of, 778
    physical and laboratory findings in,
      789–790
    prevention of, 792–793
    prognosis in, 791
    signs and symptoms of, 785–786
    treatment of, 791–792
    vs. intracerebral hemorrhage, 797
  colonic, vs. ulcerative colitis, 1572
  intestinal, acute, 1588, 1589
    nonocclusive, 1589
  medullary, 788

Infarction (*Continued*)
  midbrain, 787–788
  myocardial, 1223, **1229–1237**
    after myocardial revascularization
      procedures, 1240, 1241
    air travel after, 96
    clinical course of, 1230
    clinical features of, 1229
    complicating maintenance
      hemodialysis, 1381, 1382
    complications of, early, 1230
      late, 1237
      surgical intervention in, 1239,
        1240
    diabetes mellitus and, 1981
    diagnosis of, 1231
    differential diagnosis of, 1232
    digitalis in, 1099, 1100
    Dressler's syndrome after, 1237,
      1271
    etiology and pathology of, 1229
    oral contraceptive use and, 2195
    pathophysiology of, 1229
    pericarditis associated with, 1231,
      1270, 1271
    physical examination in, 1230
    prognosis in, 1233
    recurrent, prevention of, 1236
    treatment of, 1233
    unstable angina preceding, 1228
    vs. acute appendicitis, 1581
    vs. acute pericarditis, 1273
    vs. angina pectoris, 1227
    vs. dissecting aortic aneurysm, 1296
    vs. peptic ulcer, 1507
    vs. pulmonary embolism, 1133
  pontine, 788
  pulmonary, 1015, **1129–1134**
    vs. acute appendicitis, 1581
    vs. pneumococcal pneumonia, 354
  renal, from arterial thrombi and
    emboli, 1407
  splenic, vs. acute pericarditis, 1273
Infection(s). See also names of specific
  infectious diseases.
  adenoviral, 236–238
    vs. influenza, 245
    vs. ocular chlamydial infections,
      334
  anemia associated with, 1731–1733
  arthritis associated with, 185–186
  bacterial, 307–535. See also names of
    specific bacterial diseases.
    antimicrobial agents for, *556–557*
    enteric, 453–457
      treatment of, 456, 457
      in chronic renal failure, 1364
    liver disease associated with, 1656
  chronic, plasma cell dyscrasia
    associated with, 1866–1867
  complicating maintenance
    hemodialysis, 1382
  cutaneous, in diabetes mellitus, 1980,
    1981
  cytomegalovirus, 827–829
    vs. congenital toxoplasmosis, 597
    vs. pneumocystosis, 599
  delayed hypersensitivity induced by,
    130
  disseminated, "atypical"
    mycobacteria causing, 500
  effect of malnutrition on, 1679–1680
  fungal, 535–549. See also *Mycoses* and
    names of specific diseases.

Infection(s) (*Continued*)
  fungal, of skin, 2281–2282, *2282*
  hemolysis in, 1770
  in acute leukemia, 1817, 1820, 1821
  in acute respiratory failure, 1044
  in Addison's disease, treatment of,
    2149, 2150
  in cancer, 1901, 1903, *1903*
  in diabetes mellitus, 1981
  in head injury, 885
  in paroxysmal nocturnal
    hemoglobinuria, 1768
  in pathogenesis of rheumatoid
    arthritis, 187
  in patients with host defense defects,
    148–149
  in X-linked infantile
    agammaglobulinemia, 140
  lung, in cancer patient, 1901
    routes of, 339
  malabsorption syndrome from,
    1545–1546
  mechanisms of, in common cold, 231,
    232
  mediastinal, 1018
  meningococcal, 417–423
    antimicrobial prophylaxis for, *564*
    myopathy in, 924
  neuropathy associated with,
    905–906
  neutropenia in, 1809, 1810
  nutrition and, 1678–1680
  of central nervous system and
    coverings, 802–816
  parameningeal, 804–809
    vs. bacterial meningitis, 414
    vs. viral meningitis, 820
  parasitic, 565–638. See also names of
    specific parasitic diseases.
    immunodiagnostic tests for, *565*
    of brain, vs. dementia in cancer, 877
  pelvic, intrauterine device use and,
    2197
  peritoneal, 1593–1595
  renal calculi caused by, 1446
  renal injury from, 1329
  Salmonella, **449–452**
  sarcoidosis caused by, 209
  site of, as factor in antimicrobial
    agent selection, 553
  slow, of nervous system, 839–843
  spinal epidural, 810–811
  staphylococcal, 396–405. See also
    Staphylococcal infections and names
    of specific diseases.
  streptococcal, 366–385. See also
    Streptococcal infections and names of
    specific diseases.
  systemic, peripheral arteritis and
    gangrene in, 1305
  thrombocytopenia in, 1877
  urinary tract, 1335, 1409–1413
    after renal transplantation, 1385
    in chronic renal failure, 1354
    urinary tract obstruction from, 1447,
      1448
  viral, 229–307. See also *Viral diseases*
    and names of specific infections.
  yeast, of skin, 2282–2283
Infectious arthritis, 185–186
  vs. gout, 2039
Infectious chorea, 757–758
Infectious encephalitis, vs. acute
  disseminated encephalomyelitis, 838

Infectious enteritis, acute,
  malabsorption in, 1546
Infectious gastroenteritis, acute, vs.
  acute appendicitis, 1581
Infectious hepatitis, 1650
  vs. psittacosis, 338
  vs. secondary syphilis, 510
Infectious lymphocytosis, vs. infectious
  mononucleosis, 267
Infectious mononucleosis, 264–268, *267*
  acute disseminated encephalomyelitis
    after, 836, 837
  cold agglutinin syndrome following,
    1765
  liver disease and, 265, 1656
  vs. acute viral hepatitis, 1653, 1656
  vs. Chagas' disease, 582
  vs. cytomegalovirus mononucleosis,
    828
  vs. diphtheria, 431
  vs. listeriosis, 472, 473
  vs. measles, *249*
  vs. psittacosis, 338
  vs. rubella, 252
  vs. secondary syphilis, 510
  vs. streptococcal pharyngitis, 372
  vs. toxoplasmosis, 597
  vs. tularemia, 467
**Infectious nonbacterial gastroenteritis,
  acute, 305–306**
Infectious pericarditis, 1269–1270
Infective cardiomyopathy, 1281–1283
Infective endocarditis, 386–396
  acute, clinical manifestations of, 389
    vs. subacute endocarditis, 386, *386*
  antimicrobial prophylaxis in, *564*
  aortic regurgitation in, 1194
  bacteremia in, 387, 388, 391
  cerebral manifestations of, 809
  classification of, 386, *386*
  clinical manifestations of, 389
  differential diagnosis of, 391
  embolism and, cerebrospinal fluid
    findings in, *803*
  epidemiology of, 387
  fungi in, 387
  glomerulonephritis in, 1397–1398
  in aortic stenosis, 1191
  in drug abusers, 390, 696, 697
  laboratory findings in, 391
  lesions of, mechanisms in production
    of, 388, 389
  microbiology of, 386
  neurologic disorders in, 390, 809
  pathogenesis and pathology of, 387
  portal of entry in, 388
  prognosis in, 395
  prophylaxis of, 395
  special syndromes of, 390, 391
  subacute, clinical manifestations of,
    389
    in heroin addiction, 696, 697
    vs. acute endocarditis, 386, *386*
    vs. rheumatic fever, 383
    vs. viral meningitis or encephalitis,
      820
  treatment of, 392
    antimicrobial, 392
      untoward effects of, 394
      response to, 395
    surgical, 395
  vs. bacterial meningitis, 414
  vs. malaria, 573
Inferior mesenteric artery, 1587, *1587*

Infertility
  female, **2193–2194**
  male, **2170–2171,** 2193, 2194
Infiltration, pulmonary
  diseases of, 966–979
    respiratory failure in, 1023, *1023*
    with eosinophilia, 225, **968–970,** *969*
    drugs causing, 156
Infiltrative disease of liver, 1667–1668
Infiltrative splenomegaly, 1870
Inflammation
  energy requirements in, 1704, 1705
  granulomatous, in chronic
    schistosomiasis, 614
  in rheumatoid arthritis, 187
  neuropathy associated with, 906
**Inflammatory autonomic neuropathy,
  acute, 907**
**Inflammatory cardiomyopathy,
  1281–1283**
Inflammatory disease(s)
  **intracranial and intraspinal, aids to
    diagnosis in, 802–804,** *803*
  **of central nervous system and
    coverings, 802–816**
  of intestines, 1560–1586
**Inflammatory polyradiculo-
  neuropathy(ies)**
  acute, 906–907
  chronic, 908
Inflammatory response, 145, 146
  defects of, infections in, *148,* 149, 150
  diagnostic evaluation of, 150, *151*
  disorders of, management of, 152
  mediation of, complement in, 136
Influenza, 240–246
  acute disseminated encephalomyelitis
    after, 836, 837
  clinical manifestations of, 243
  complications of, 243, 244, *244,* 245
  course of, 243, *244*
  diagnosis of, 245
  endemic, 242, 243
  "epidemic," interpandemic, 242
  epidemiology of, 241
  etiology of, 241
  pandemic, *241,* 242
  pathology and pathogenesis of, 243
  prevention of, 245
  prognosis in, 245
  swine, 241, 242, 246
  treatment of, 245
  vs. coccidioidomycosis, 539
  vs. listeriosis, 473
  vs. malaria, 573
  vs. psittacosis, 338
Influenza vaccine, 245, 246
Influenza virus pneumonia
  bacterial pneumonia and, combined,
    245
  primary, 243, 244, *244*
  vs. mycoplasmal pneumonia, 345
Influenza viruses, 241, *241,* 242
Inguinal adenopathy, vs.
  lymphogranuloma venereum, 335
Inhalants, abuse of, 705
Inheritance
  autosomal, 34
  polygenic and multifactorial, 44–45,
    45
  X-linked, 36, *36*
  Y-linked, 37
**Inherited degenerative diseases of
  nervous system, 764–772**

Inherited disease
  discovery or precipitation of, by drug
    use, 45, 46
  pedigree analysis in, 34–40
Inherited polymorphisms, *44*
Injection abscesses, "atypical"
  mycobacteria causing, 500
"Innocent bystander" reaction, in
  drug-induced hemolysis, 1766
Inoculation lymphoreticulosis, 302–305,
  303, 304
Inorganic dusts
  cellular reaction to, 985
  **pneumoconioses due to, diagnosis of,
    986**
    **treatment and prevention of,
      993–994**
  pulmonary effects of, *984*
Inotropic agents. See also names of
  specific agents.
  in heart failure, 1095–1102
Insane, general paralysis of, 814
Insecticides
  aplastic anemia associated with, 1735
  chlorinated hydrocarbon, poisoning
    by, 75
  phosphate ester, poisoning by, 75
Insects. See also names of specific
  insects.
  stings of, 113–114, 163
Insomnia, 652–653
  hypothalamic, 715
  in chronic renal failure, 1366
Insulin
  decreased sensitivity to, in obesity,
    1694
  in diabetes mellitus, 1985, *1985*
    complications of, 1986, 1987, 1988
    resistance to, 1987
  in diabetic ketoacidosis, 1984
  in hyperkalemia, 1960
  in hyperosmolar coma, 1985
  induced excess of, hypoglycemia due
    to, 1996
  metabolic effects of, 1970, *1970*
  mode of action of, 2071
  plasma, in functioning islet cell tumor
    during fasting, 1994, *1994*
  release of, stimulation of, 1972, 1973
  synthesis of, 1973, *1973*
Insulinomas, vs. extrapancreatic
  neoplasms associated with
  hypoglycemia, 1995
Integument, changes in, with aging, 27
Intelligence, 681–682
Intelligence quotient, 682
Intensive care unit, 1031
  instrumentation for, 1032–1033
Interferon, 229
"Intermediate syndrome," 1223
Intermittent branched-chain
  ketoaciduria, *41*
Intermittent cholangitis, 1629
Intermittent claudication
  in arteriosclerosis obliterans, 1300
  of cauda equina, 895
Intermittent hydrarthrosis, 198
Intermittent porphyria, acute, *42,*
  2045–2047
    vs. acute abdomen, 1581
    vs. acute inflammatory
      polyneuropathy, 907
    vs. hysteria, 679
    vs. lead poisoning, 78

Intermittent porphyria (*Continued*)
acute, vs. variegate porphyria, 2048
Intermittent positive pressure
ventilation, in acute respiratory
failure, 1027
**Internal medicine, cancer and,
1898–1907**
**Interstitial cell–stimulating hormone,
2088–2089**
Interstitial fibrosis, drug-induced, vs.
pneumocystosis, 599
Interstitial nephritis, 1416–1422
chronic, etiologic types of, 1418–1422
idiopathic, 1422
penicillin-induced, 1426, 1427
Interstitial nephropathy(ies), 1416–1422
etiologic classification of, *1416*
Interstitial pneumonia, 998–999
Interstitial pneumonitis
desquamative, 978
lymphocytic, 1011, 1012
lymphoid, 979
usual, 978–979
Intervertebral disc(s)
protrusion of, 893–894
staphylococcal infections of, 402
Intestinal amebiasis, 590, 591, 592, 593
Intestinal flora, changes in, in
malnutrition, 1680
Intestinal granulomatosis, lipophagic,
1541
**Intestinal hermaphroditic flukes,
620–621**
Intestinal infarction
acute, 1588, 1589
nonocclusive, 1589
Intestinal ischemic syndromes
acute, 1588–1590
chronic, 1587–1588
Intestinal lipodystrophy, 1541
Intestinal lymphoma, primary, 1545
Intestinal nematodes, 622–630
antimicrobial agents for, *559*
life cycle of, *621*
prevalence of, *605*
Intestine(s). See also names of specific
intestinal components, e.g., *Colon,
Jejunum.*
blind loop of, malabsorption from,
1537
hemorrhage of, in typhoid fever, 447
intramural, 1590
inflammatory diseases of, 1560–1586
chronic, 1560–1578
microcirculation of, 1587
motility of, electrical control
mechanisms for, 1475
neural regulatory mechanisms for,
1475, 1476
obstruction of, 1490–1492
Ascaris causing, 627
in congenital megacolon, 1495
perforation of, in typhoid fever, 447,
448
pseudo-obstruction of, 1497
malabsorption in, 1538
small
adenocarcinoma of, 1604, 1605, *1605*
arterial supply to, 1586, 1587, *1587*
carcinoma of, in adult celiac
disease, 1541
Crohn's disease of, 1560–1567. See
also *Regional enteritis.*
disease of, intraluminal, 1539–1543

Intestine(s) (*Continued*)
small, hemangiomas of, 1590, 1605
in scleroderma, 169
ischemia of, malabsorption in, 1543
leiomyosarcoma of, 1604, 1605
lymphomas of, 1604, 1605
in adult celiac disease, 1541
malabsorption secondary to,
1544, 1545
neoplasms of, 1604–1605
obstruction of, vs. acute
appendicitis, 1580
pain originating in, 1476
resection of, malabsorption after,
1543, 1544, *1544*
tuberculosis of, 492
ulceration of
in adult celiac disease, 1541
primary nonspecific, 1585–1586
tuberculosis of, malabsorption in,
1545
vascular diseases of, 1586–1591
Intra-abdominal infection, anaerobic,
443
Intracerebral hematoma, in head injury,
884
Intracerebral hemorrhage, 794
arteriography in, 799
clinical manifestations of, 797, 798
pathology and pathogenesis of, 796
treatment of, 801
**Intracorpuscular abnormalities,
hemolysis due to, 1755–1762**
Intracranial headache, 729–730
Intracranial hematomas, in head injury,
883, 884
Intracranial hemorrhage, 794–801
clinical manifestations of, 796–798
etiology of, 794–796, *794, 795*
laboratory findings in, 798–799
pathology and pathogenesis of, 796
prognosis in, 799
treatment of, 799–801
vs. cerebral infarction, 790
**Intracranial hypertension, benign,
870–872,** *871*
Intracranial hypotension, 873
**Intracranial inflammatory disease, aids
to diagnosis in, 802–804,** *803*
Intracranial pressure
increased
in hydrocephalus, 873
in intracranial tumors, 864
in papilledema, 2327
states causing, 863–876
without localizing signs, 868
monitoring of, in head injury, 883
Intracranial tumors, 863–869
classification of, 863
clinical manifestations of, 864
congenital, 864
diagnosis of, 866
differential diagnosis of, 868
headache in, 730, 864, 865
pathology of, 863
pathophysiology of, 864
treatment of, 869
Intradermal nevus, *2290,* 2291
Intradural extramedullary spinal cord
tumors, 896–897
Intrahepatic cholestasis
chlorpromazine-induced, 1659
sex hormones causing, 1658
vs. choledocholithiasis, 1630

Intraluminal hydrolysis, defective,
malabsorption syndrome caused by,
1535–1539
**Intraluminal small bowel disease,
1539–1543**
Intramedullary spinal cord tumors, 897
Intramural intestinal hemorrhage, 1590
Intraocular infection, granulomatous,
498
Intraocular neuritis, 848
Intrapulmonary shunts, in acute
respiratory failure, 1037
Intraspinal compression, 889–898
**Intraspinal inflammatory disease, aids
to diagnosis in, 802–804,** *803*
Intrathoracic sarcoidosis, 212, 213, *213*
**Intrauterine devices for contraception,
2197**
Intrauterine diagnosis of genetic
disease, 58
Intravascular coagulation
disorders accompanied by, *1895*
disseminated, hypofibrinogenemic
syndromes associated with,
1893–1894
in cancer patient, 1906
in critically ill patient, 1052
in shock, 1113
without hypofibrinogenemia,
1894–1895
experimental, 1892
laboratory diagnosis of, 1892–1893
syndromes of, 1891–1895
Intravascular hemagglutination, in
shock, 1112, 1113
Intravascular hemolysis
as transfusion reaction, 1787
hemoglobinuria following, 1783
massive, in malaria, 572
Intravascular hypovolemia, vs.
idiopathic autonomic insufficiency,
763
Intravenous cholangiography, 1622, 1623
in acute cholecystitis, 1626
Intravenous nutrition
long-term, 1706, 1707, 1708
short-term, 1706
Intravenous pyelography, in
nephrocarcinoma, 1459
Intravenous urography, 1342, *1342,* 1343
in analgesic nephropathy, 1420
Intraventricular pressure, increase in,
rate of, 1085
Intrinsic factor, in vitamin B_{12}
absorption, 1525
Intubation, endotracheal
in acute respiratory failure, 1039,
1040
in cardiopulmonary arrest, 1055
Intubation-assisted ventilation, in
chronic respiratory failure, 1028–1029
Involuntary movements, abnormal, 751
Iodamoeba butschlii, 602
Iodide
metabolism of, 2114, *2114*
radioactive, in hyperthyroidism, 2123,
2124, *2125*
trapping of, defect in, in thyroid
hormone synthesis, 2139
Iodide organification defect, in thyroid
hormone synthesis, 2139
Iodine
butanol-extractable, determination of,
2117

Iodine (*Continued*)
deficiency of, 1676, *1677*
in hyperthyroidism, 2125
nutrient value of, 1674
protein-bound, determination of, 2117
radioactive, uptake of, determination of, 2118
recommended allowances of, *1671*
5-Iododeoxyuridine, 1935
Iodotyrosine dehalogenase defect, 2139
Iopanoic acid, hepatic excretion of, 1648
Ipecac, syrup of, in accidental poisoning, 74
Iridocyclitis, 2314
in ankylosing spondylitis, 194, 195
in juvenile rheumatoid arthritis, 196
in sarcoidosis, 2329
in tick-borne relapsing fever, 529
Iris, in diabetes mellitus, 2320
Iritis, 2314
in juvenile rheumatoid arthritis, 2315
Iron
absorption of, 1526, 1744, *1745*
impaired, in malabsorption syndrome, 1529
deficiency of, clinical signs of, *1677*
megaloblastic anemia and, 1723
distribution of, in body, 1743, *1743*
excretion of, 1747
impaired release of, in anemia of chronic disorders, 1731
metabolism of, 1743
nutrient value of, 1674
plasma, concentration of, in hemochromatosis, 1791
recommended allowances of, *1671*
requirements for, dietary, 1747, *1747*
storage of, 1746
transport of, 1745
turnover of, in body, 1745, 1746
Iron deficiency anemia, 1743–1751
benign intracranial hypertension with, 872
in hookworm disease, 625
vs. anemia of chronic disorders, 1732
vs. other hypochromic anemias, 1751
vs. sideroblastic anemia, 1741
Iron dextran, in iron deficiency anemia, 1749, 1750
Iron overload, 1790
Iron salts, poisoning by, 75
Iron sorbitex, in iron deficiency anemia, 1749, 1750
Iron storage disease, 1790–1792. See also *Hemochromatosis.*
Iron-binding capacity, measurement of, 1745, *1745*
Irradiation therapy, 1927–1930. See also *Radiotherapy.*
Irritable bowel syndrome, 1480, 1493–1494
vs. amebiasis, 592
vs. chronic cholecystitis, 1625
vs. ulcerative colitis, 1572
Irritants, physical and chemical, to lungs, 983–1002, *984*
Ischemia
brainstem, 784
cerebral, 778–794. See also *Infarction, cerebral.*
myocardial, in shock, 1110
small intestinal, malabsorption in, 1543

Ischemic attacks, transient, 784–785
anticoagulant drugs or surgery in, 792
Ischemic colitis, 1589
vs. Crohn's disease of colon, 1578
vs. diverticulitis, 1583, 1584
vs. ulcerative colitis, 1572
Ischemic heart disease, 1223
Ischemic optic neuropathy, in giant cell arteritis, 2319
Ischemic syndromes, intestinal
acute, 1588–1590
chronic, 1587–1588
Ischemic ulcers, in arteriosclerosis obliterans, vs. Hines' ulcers, 1301
Ischiorectal fossa abscess, 1617
Islet cells, tumors of
carcinoid features of, 2212
functioning, fasting hypoglycemia caused by, 1993–1995
Isocyanates, asthma-like reactions to, 999
Isoimmune antibodies, hemolysis due to, 1763
Isoniazid, *556*
in miliary tuberculosis, 493
in pulmonary disease caused by *M. kansasii*, 499
in pulmonary tuberculosis, 485, 487, 488, 489, 490
in tuberculosis chemoprophylaxis, 484
in tuberculous meningitis, 494
in tuberculous pericarditis, 494
neuropathy from, 910
overdose of, lactic acidosis from, 1962
pyridoxal phosphate deficiency caused by, 773
slow inactivation of, genetic basis of, 46
Isoniazid form of drug resistance, 551
Isoniazid hepatitis, 484, 487, 489, 1658–1659
Isoproterenol
in asthma, 958
in conduction disorders complicating myocardial infarction, 1236
in Hymenoptera stings, 114
in pulmonary embolism, 1133
in shock, 1048, 1120
in ventricular fibrillation, 1057
Isosorbide dinitrate, in angina pectoris, 1228
Isospora belli, 604
Isosporiasis, 604
Isosthenuria, in chronic renal failure, 1355
Isotonic exercise, 1070
Isotope dilution methods, in diagnosis of endocrine disease, 2067
Isotope encephalography, in brain tumor, 867
Isovaleric acidemia, *41*
Itai-itai byo, 82, 1429
Itch
crusted, 111
ground, 624
perianal, 1617, 1618
"seven-year," 110
swimmer's, 613
IUdR, 1935
Ixodes holocyclus, 118
Ixodes muris, 601
Ixodes scapularis, 601

Jackknife seizures, 854
Jacksonian motor seizure, 855
Jail fever, 318–320
Janeway's lesions, in infective endocarditis, 390
Japanese B encephalitis, 289–290
Japanese B virus, 289
Japanese flood fever, 327–328
Japanese river fever, 327–328
Jarisch-Herxheimer reaction
in leptospirosis, 535
in louse-borne relapsing fever, 528
in syphilis, 517
Jaundice, 1637–1639
acholuric, 1638
chlorpromazine, 1659
classification of, 1638
clinical evaluation of, 1621–1622, *1621*
hemolytic, 1638
hepatocellular, 1638
in acute viral hepatitis, 1652, 1653
in cancer patient, 1905
in malaria, 571
in non-Hodgkin's lymphomas, 1832
in pancreatic carcinoma, 1558
in pneumococcal pneumonia, 354
in sclerosing cholangitis, 1633
neonatal, 1638
obstructive, 1638
computerized tomography in, *1467*
cutaneous manifestations of, 1645
ultrasonography in, *1465*
pathophysiology of, 1638
recurrent, of pregnancy, 1658
JC virus, 842
Jectofer. See *Iron sorbitex.*
Jefferson's fracture, 885
Jejunal aspirates, culture of, in malabsorption syndrome, 1532
Jejunoileal bypass, malabsorption after, 1543, 1544
Jejunum
biopsy of, in malabsorption syndrome, 1532, *1533, 1534, 1535*
in protein-losing enteropathy, *1549*
diverticula of, 1500–1501
malabsorption in, 1537
fat absorption in, 1524
Jellyfish, envenomation by, 123
"Jet lag," 96
"Jigger flea" bites, 110
Jimson weed, poisoning by, 70, 75
Job's syndrome, 1803, *2302*
host defense defects in, 149
Jod-Basedow phenomenon, 2121
Joints
anaerobic infection of, 444
Charcot, 200, 512
in diabetes mellitus, 1980
Clutton's, in congenital syphilis, 186, 513
diseases of, 184–208
degenerative, 202–205, *203*
in acromegaly, 199
vs. ankylosing spondylitis, 195
vs. polymyalgia rheumatica, 217
vs. rheumatoid arthritis, 190
neuropathic, 200
hemorrhages into, in hemophilia, 200, 1883, 1886
in Ehlers-Danlos syndrome, 2054
in gonococcal arthritis, 407
in relapsing polychondritis, 218
in rheumatic fever, 380

Joints (*Continued*)
in rheumatoid arthritis, 188, *189*
in scleroderma, 169
in systemic lupus erythematosus, 176
in tophaceous gout, *2036*, 2037
lesions of, "atypical" mycobacteria causing, 500
of Luschka, degenerative changes in, 204
tuberculosis of, 496–497
tumors affecting, 202
Joseph's disease, 764–765
Junctional extrasystoles, 1256
Junctional nevi, 2290, *2290*
Junctional rhythms, atrioventricular, 1256
Jungle yellow fever, 293, *293*, 294
Junin virus, 298, 299
Juvenile melanoma, benign, 2312
Juvenile nephronophthisis, familial, 1454
Juvenile osteoporosis, 2246
vs. osteogenesis imperfecta, 2245
Juvenile polycystic kidney disease, 1453
Juvenile rheumatoid arthritis, 195–196
eyes in, 2315
Juvenile-onset diabetes mellitus, 1974
HLA system and, 39
Juxtaglomerular apparatus, 1321
Juxtaglomerular cell tumor, hypokalemia in, 1957

K cell, 129
Kala-azar, 584–587
vs. Chagas' disease, 582
Kallmann's syndrome, 2078, 2081, 2171, 2188
Kanamycin, *556*, 561
adverse reactions to, 562
as nephrotoxin, 1426
in malabsorption syndrome, *1536*
in pulmonary tuberculosis, 488, 490
malabsorption caused by, 1548
neuromuscular block caused by, 929
Kaposi's sarcoma, *2298*
Kartagener's syndrome, mucociliary movement in, 146
Karyotype, *50*, 51
polymorphic variations in, 51
Kasabach-Merritt syndrome, 1876
Katayama fever, 613
Kato technique, in nematode infections, 622
Kayexelate, in hyperkalemia, 1960
Kayser-Fleischer ring, in Wilson's disease, 2049, 2050
Kearns-Sayre syndrome, 918
Keloid, 2273
Keratin, 2267
Keratitis, *2313*, 2314
punctate, in onchocerciasis, 636
in Reiter's syndrome, 2316
Keratonconjunctivitis, 2314
adenoviral, 237
herpetic, vs. ocular chlamydial infections, 334
phlyctenular, 498
in pulmonary tuberculosis, 484
Keratoconjunctivitis sicca, 2314
in Sjögren's syndrome, 2315, 2316
Keratoma plantare sulcatum, vs. yaws, 521

Keratomalacia, 1684–1686, *1685*
Keratopathy, band
in hypercalcemia of hyperparathyroidism, 2215
in juvenile rheumatoid arthritis, 2315
Keratoses, seborrheic, 2291
Kerley B lines, in mitral stenosis, 1145
Kernicterus, 1649
in hemolytic disease of newborn, 1754
Kerosene, poisoning by, 75
Ketoacidosis
alcoholic, 1705
metabolic acidosis from, 1961, 1962, 1964
diabetic, 1975
fatty liver in, 1660
metabolic acidosis from, 1961, 1964
treatment of, 1983, 1984
volume depletion in, 1951
Ketoaciduria, branched-chain, intermittent, 41
Ketogenic diet, in epilepsy, 861
Ketosis-prone diabetes mellitus, 1974
17-Ketosteroids, urinary, in evaluation of testicular function, 2164
Ketotic hyperglycemia, *41, 2017*
Kidney(s). See also *Renal.*
adenoma of, 1461, 1462
agenesis of, bilateral, 1457
angiomyolipoma of, 1461
anomalies of, 1457
antimicrobial agent clearance from, 555
artificial, 1378
components of, 1379, *1379*
solute clearance by, 1379, *1379*
biopsy of, 1345, 1346
in interstitial nephritis, 1418
in nephrotic syndrome, 1389
blood flow through, 1316
impaired, renal injury from, 1330
in shock, 1112
measurement of, 1340, 1341
calculi of, 1443–1446
2,8-dihydroxyadenine, 2043
in gout, 2037
treatment of, 2041
in paraplegia, 888
in regional enteritis, 1564
carcinoma of, 1458–1460
embryonal, 1460
circulation of, variations in, 1457
concentrating capacity of, in interstitial nephritis, 1417
congenital ectopia of, 1457
cyst(s) of
benign, 1461
simple, 1451
diseases of, 1316–1462
chronic, pathophysiology of, 1346–1351
chronic progressive, acute renal failure in, 1369
cutaneous manifestations of, *2300–2301*
cystic, 1450–1456
classification of, 1450–1451, *1451*
medullary, adult-onset, 1454
volume depletion in, 1951
symptoms and signs of, *1450*
hemorrhagic phenomena in, 1891

Kidney(s) (*Continued*)
diseases of, hypertension in, 1210, 1211
hypertension in, 1210, 1211
immune complexes in, 133, 134
in cancer patient, 1904
in hyperparathyroidism, 2215
in pregnancy, 1414–1416
metabolic acidosis in, 1962
secondary polycythemia in, 1800
syndromes caused by, 1331–1336
volume depletion in, 1951
with defective water excretion, hyponatremia in, 1955
double, 1457
drug clearance by, drug-drug interactions and, 2338
dysplasia of, 1452
endocrine functions of, 2061
failure of, acute, 1334, 1367–1375. See also *Renal failure, acute.*
chronic, 1334, 1351–1367. See also *Renal failure, chronic.*
irreversible, transplantation and dialysis in, 1375–1386
function of, 1316–1323
abnormalities of, in interstitial nephritis and interstitial nephropathy, 1417, 1418
changes in, in liver disease, 1644–1645
disorders of, hypercalcemia in, 2237
in chronic renal failure, 1355
in critically ill patient, 1050–1051
in head injury, 882
in louse-borne relapsing fever, 527
in unilateral renal disease, 1347
investigation of, 1336–1341
normal, excessive water intake with, 1955
regional, investigation of, 1341–1346
tests of, 2354
gouty, 1420–1421, 2037, 2038
treatment of, 1421, 2040, 2041
hamartoma of, 1461
horseshoe, 1457
hypoplastic, 1457
in acid-base homeostasis, 1322–1323
in amyloidosis, 1405–1406
in anaphylactoid purpura, 1400, 1401
in cadmium poisoning, 82
in connective tissue diseases, 1400–1401
in Cushing's syndrome, 2154
in diabetes mellitus, 1403, 1977, 1979
in electric injury, 93
in Goodpasture's syndrome, 1401
in hemolytic-uremic syndrome, 1401
in infective endocarditis, 389, 390
in leptospirosis, 532, 533
in malaria, 569, 571, 572, 574
in non-Hodgkin's lymphomas, 1832
in periarteritis nodosa, 181, 1400
in periarteritis nodosa caused by drugs, 156
in potassium homeostasis, 1323
in regional enteritis, 1564
in rickettsial diseases, 311, 316
in right ventricular failure, 1093
in sarcoidosis, 1402–1403
in schistosomiasis, 615
in scleroderma, 169, 170, 171, 1401
in sickle cell anemia, 1774
in sickle cell disease, 1404

Kidney(s) (*Continued*)
 in systemic lupus erythematosus, 175, 176, 177, 178, 1400
 in visceral leishmaniasis, 585
 in Wegener's granulomatosis, 219, 1400
 inflammation of, 1409–1413
 injury of
  coagulation-induced, 1327–1328
  immune-mediated, 1324–1327, *1324, 1325*
  infection-mediated, 1329
  mechanisms of, 1323–1331
  toxin-mediated, 1328–1329, *1328*
 malrotation of, 1457
 medullary sponge, 1455–1456
  vs. adult polycystic kidney disease, 1454
 metastatic disease to, 1462
 multicystic, congenital, 1450, 1451, 1452
  vs. childhood polycystic kidney disease, 1453
 neoplasms of, vs. adult polycystic kidney disease, 1454
 pancake, 1457
 polycystic, 1450, 1451, **1452–1454**
  in adults, 1453–1454
  in children, 1452–1453
   vs. medullary sponge kidney, 1456
 ptotic, 1457
 salt and water excretion by, factors controlling, 1321–1322
 scanning of, 1344, *1344*
  gamma camera, 1345, *1345*
 size of, in chronic renal failure, 1354
 solitary, 1457
 structure of, 1316–1323
  investigation of, 1341–1346
 susceptibility of, to toxins, 1423
 toxic damage to, 1422–1435. See also *Nephropathy, toxic.*
 transplantation of, 1375, *1375,* **1376,** *1376,* **1382–1386**
  biopsy after, 1346
  hypercalcemia after, 2237
  in cystinosis, 55
  in Fabry's disease, 55
  in scleroderma, 171
  rejected, acute renal failure in, 1369
   pathologic features of, 1384
  rejection crisis in, 1384
 tuberculosis of, 496
 tumors of, 1458–1462
  benign, 1461, 1462
  classification of, 1458, *1458*
 vascular disorders of, 1407–1409
Kif, 702
Killer cell, 129
Kimura test, 656
Kinins, circulatory effects of, 1111
Kinky hair syndrome, Menkes', *43*
 osteoporosis in, 2245
Klatskin tumor, 1634, 1635
Klebsiella disease, chronic cavitary, 358
Klebsiella **pneumonia, 357–358**
 vs. pneumococcal pneumonia, 354
Kleine-Levin syndrome, 655
Klinefelter's syndrome, 2168–2170, *2169*
 chromatin-negative, 2170
 clinical and cytogenetic characteristics of, *52*
 frequency and sex ratio of, *48*

Klippel-Feil syndrome, 875
 syringomyelia and, 769
KMIF test, in sarcoidosis, 214
Knee, degenerative disease of, 203, 204
KOH test, 2273
Koilonychia, in iron deficiency anemia, 1748
Koplik's spots, in measles, 247, *248*
Korean hemorrhagic fever, *293,* 301
Korsakoff's syndrome, 659, 774
 vs. dementia, 660, 661
 Wernicke's disease and, 773–774
Kozhevnikov's epilepsy, 842
Krabbe's disease, 850
Kufs' disease, 851
Kuru, 840
Kveim test, in sarcoidosis, 214, 946, 977
Kwashiorkor, 1283, 1284, 1680, **1681–1683,** *1682*
 fatty liver in, 1660
Kyasanur Forest disease, 290–291, *293*
Kyasanur Forest disease virus, 290, 291
Kyphoscoliosis, 1020
 alveolar hypoventilation in, 1147
 in syringomyelia, 769
Kyphosis, 1020
 in paraplegia, 887, 888

L chains, 126, 127, *127*
La Crosse virus, 288
Laboratory investigation, clinical medicine and, 4, 6, 7
Laboratory values of clinical importance, 2346–2357
Laboratory-derived data, use and interpretation of, 2342–2345
Laburnum, poisoning by, 70
Labyrinth(s)
 hypo- and hyperactivity of, 740
 toxic damage to, vertigo from, 739
Labyrinthitis
 acute, 738
 hearing loss from, 735, 736
Laceration, scalp, 881, 882
Lacrimal glands, in sarcoidosis, 2330
Lactase deficiency, *41,* 1539
Lactate dehydrogenase, in myocardial infarction, 1232
Lactation
 inappropriate, 2191, 2192. See also *Galactorrhea.*
 recommended dietary allowances during, *1671*
Lactic acidosis
 in louse-borne relapsing fever, 528
 metabolic acidosis from, 1962, 1964
Lactoferrin, 1743
Lactogen, placental, human, as tumor marker, 1912, 1913
Lactogenic hormone, 2087. See also *Prolactin.*
Lactosylceramidosis, *42*
Laennec's cirrhosis, *2299*
Lamellar bone, 2247
Lamellar hyperlipoproteinemia, *2004*
Lamellar ichthyosis, *2286*
Land leeches, as agents of disease, 120
Landry-Guillain-Barré-Strohl syndrome, 906–907. See also *Guillain-Barré* syndrome.
Langerhans granules, in eosinophilic granuloma, 1849, *1849*

Language
 abnormal, in schizophrenia, 666
 disorders of, 656–657
  in dementia, 660
Laparoscopy, in infertility, 2194
Laparotomy, exploratory
 in Hodgkin's disease, *1842, 1844*
 in non-Hodgkin's lymphomas, 1835
Laplace relationship, 1086, *1086*
Larva migrans
 cutaneous, 625
  vs. gnathostomiasis, 626
 visceral, 627–628
  vs. clonorchiasis, 618
Larvae, fly, infestation by, 111–112
Laryngeal diphtheria, 431
Laryngitis
 in measles, 248
 viral, 235–236
Larynx, tuberculosis of, 491
Lassa fever, *293,* **298–300**
Lassa virus, 298, 299
Lateral rectus palsy, in intracranial tumors, 866
Lateral sclerosis, amyotrophic, 765–766
 vs. multiple sclerosis, 847
 vs. muscular dystrophies, 918
 vs. myasthenia gravis, 927
Lateral sinus thrombosis, 789, 808, 809
Latex agglutination test, in protozoan and helminthic disease, *565*
Latex fixation text, in rheumatoid arthritis, 190
Lathyrism, 69
Lathyrus sativus, 69
Latrodectus mactans, 115
LATS, in Graves' disease, 2121
Laurence-Moon syndrome, 2058
Lavage, gastric
 in accidental poisoning, 74
 in acute drug poisoning, 714
Lawrence-Seip syndrome, 1981
Laxative(s), 1482
 abuse of, 1481
Laxative-induced diarrhea, hypokalemia in, 1958
Lazy leukocyte syndrome, 1803
LE cell, in systemic lupus erythematosus, 178
Lead
 exposure to, normal and abnormal values in, 79
 nephrotoxicity from, 1428, *1428,* 1429
 poisoning by, 77–80
  chronic, hypochromic anemia from, 1751
  neuropathy from, 911
  vs. arsenic poisoning, 77
Lead colic, 78
Lead encephalopathy, 78, 79
"Lead line," in lead poisoning, 78
Lecithin-cholesterol acyltransferase, 2002, 2003
 deficiency of, 2008–2009
Leeches as agents of disease, 120–121
Left atrial hypertension, 1144–1146
Left atrial myxoma, vs. mitral stenosis, 1183
Left colon, small, syndrome of, 1498
Left coronary artery, anomalous origin of, 1172
Left handers
 aphasias in, 657
 pathologic, 656

Left heart failure, 1081, 1089–1091
    acute pulmonary edema in, 1090
        management of, 1094
    hypertensive, 1206
    in myocardial infarction, 1231
Leg
    deep thrombosis of, oral
        contraceptives and, 2195
    milk, in thrombophlebitis, 1126
    nodose lesions of, 2295
Leg vein thrombi, 1124, 1125
Legionnaires' disease, 359–360
    vs. pneumococcal pneumonia, 354
Leiner's syndrome, 144, 1804
Leiomyoma(s)
    esophageal, 1599
    gastric, 1604
    small intestinal, 1605
Leiomyosarcoma(s)
    gastric, 1603
    small intestinal, 1604, 1605
Leishmania aethiopica, 587
Leishmania brasiliensis, 558, 583, 588, 589
Leishmania chagasi, 584
Leishmania donovani, 558, 570, 583, 584
Leishmania infantum, 584
Leishmania mexicana, 583, *588,* 589
Leishmania tropica, 558, 583
Leishmania tropica major, 587
Leishmania tropica minor, 587
Leishmaniasis, 566, 583–589
    antimicrobial agents for, *558*
    cutaneous, 583
        of new world, *588,* **589**
            diffuse, *588,* 589
        of old world, 587–589, *588*
            diffuse, 588
            vs. yaws, 521
    dermal, post-kala-azar, 585, 587, *588*
        vs. leprosy, 504
    immunodiagnostic tests for, *565*
    lupoid, 587, 588
    mucocutaneous, American, *588,* **589**
    "rural," 587
    "urban," 587
    visceral, 583, **584–587**
        vs. malaria, 573
        vs. paracoccidioidomycosis, 541
Leishmaniasis recidiva, 587
Leishmanin test, 584
    in cutaneous leishmaniasis of old
        world, 588
Lennert's lymphoma, 1832
Lenses, in diabetes mellitus, 2320
Lentigines, 2289–2290
    nevoid, 2290
    senile, 2289
Lentiginous melanoma, acral, 2311
Lentigo maligna, 2310, 2311, *2311*
Lepra reactions
    lepromatous, 503
    nonlepromatous, 503
    treatment of, 504, 505
Lepromatous leprosy, *502,* 503
Lepromatous neuropathy, vs.
    syringomyelia, 769
Lepromin test, in leprosy, 501, *502*
Leprosy, 501–505
    classification of, 502, *502*
    peripheral neuropathy with, 905
    vs. chromomycosis, 543
    vs. yaws, 521
Leptospira interrogans, 532
**Leptospiral and spirillary diseases,
    526–535**

Leptospirosis, 532–535
    hepatic involvement in, 533, 1656
    vs. acute viral hepatitis, 1653
    vs. hemorrhagic diseases caused by
        arenaviruses, 299
    vs. louse-borne relapsing fever, 528
    vs. malaria, 573
    vs. rat-bite fever, 531
Leptotrombidium deliense group, 327
Leriche's syndrome, 1299
    in arteriosclerosis obliterans, 1300
Lerman's sound, in hyperthyroidism,
    2122
Lesbianism, 691
Lesch-Nyhan syndrome, *42,* **2038,
    2042–2043**
    heterozygote detection in, *58*
Letterer-Siwe syndrome, 1850
Leucine, insulin release provoked by,
    1972
Leucovorin. See *Folinic acid.*
Leukemia(s)
    acute, 1813–1821
        clinical manifestations of, 1816
        epidemiology of, 1816
        etiology of, 1814
        neutropenia in, 1809
        pathogenesis of, 1815
        therapy of, 1817
    aleukemic, acute, vs. rheumatic fever,
        383
        vs. visceral leishmaniasis, 586
    as delayed effects of radiation injury,
        89
    central nervous system, treatment of,
        1818
    chronic, 1821–1826
    eosinophilic, 226
    granulocytic
        acute, vs. leukemoid reaction, 1813
        chronic, 1821–1824
            vs. neutrophilic leukemoid
                reaction, 1813
    intracranial hemorrhage from, 795
    lymphatic, chronic, 1824–1826
    lymphocytic
        acute, 1814
            epidemiology of, 1816
            pathogenesis of, 1816
            therapy of, 1817, 1818, 1819, 1820
            vs. leukemoid reaction, 1813
        chronic, 1824–1826
            idiopathic thrombocytopenic
                purpura in, 1876
    "lymphosarcoma-cell," 1824
    monocytic, acute, 1814
        in multiple myeloma, 1867
    myeloblastic, 1814
    myelocytic
        acute, 1814
            epidemiology of, 1816
            pathogenesis of, 1816
            treatment of, 1819, 1820
        chronic, 1821–1824
            subacute, vs. aplastic anemia, 1738
    myelogenous, chronic, 1821–1824
    myeloid, chronic, 1821–1824
    myelomonocytic, 1814
        acute, in Hodgkin's disease, 1842,
            1843
    neuropathy with, vs. acute
        inflammatory polyneuropathy, 907
    plasma cell, in multiple myeloma,
        1859, 1860
    portal hypertension in, 1639

Leukemia(s) (*Continued*)
    promyelocytic, 1814
        hemorrhage in, 1817
    subacute, vs. aplastic anemia, 1738
    tuberculosis complicating, 483
    varicella and, 254
    vs. histoplasmosis, 537
    vs. infectious mononucleosis, 266
    vs. leukemoid reaction, 1813
Leukemia cutis, *2302*
Leukemogenesis, radiation, 1814
Leukemoid reactions, 1812–1813
    vs. chronic granulocytic leukemia,
        1822
Leukeran. See *Chlorambucil.*
Leukocyte(s)
    donor, sensitivity to, transfusion
        reaction from, *1785,* 1788
    in host defenses, 147
    "lazy," syndrome of, 1803
    metabolism of, inborn errors of, *43*
    polymorphonuclear, neutrophilic
        antibacterial activity of, 340
        dysfunction of, syndromes of,
            1803–1807, *1803*
        function of, **1800–1802,** 1801
Leukocyte alkaline phosphatase score
    in chronic granulocytic leukemia,
        1822
    in leukemoid reactions, 1813
Leukocyte sensitization, complicating
    massive blood transfusions, 1051
Leukocytic glucose-6-phosphate
    dehydrogenase deficiency, severe,
    1806
Leukodystrophy(ies), 850–851
    globoid cell, *41,* **850**
    metachromatic, *42*
    sudanophilic, 850
Leukoencephalitis, hemorrhagic, acute,
    836
Leukoencephalopathy
    metachromatic, 850
    multifocal, progressive, 841–842
        vs. brain tumor, 868
        vs. dementia in cancer, 877
Leukoerythroblastic anemia, 1742, 1827
Leukonychia, in nephrotic syndrome,
    1388
Leukopenia(s), 1807–1812
    host defense compromise in, 147, 149
        management of, 152
    in multiple myeloma, 1859
Levallorphan, in opiate poisoning, *712*
Levamisole, in ascariasis, 627
Levodopa, in parkinsonism, 754, 755
Levorphanol, in pain, 723, *724,* 725
Leydig cells, 2162
LH, 2088–2089. See also *Luteinizing
    hormone.*
Lhermitte's sign, in radiation injury,
    870
Libman-Sacks verrucous nonbacterial
    endocarditis, in systemic lupus
    erythematosus, 176, 177
Librium. See *Chlordiazepoxide.*
Lice. See under *Louse.*
Lichen myxedematosus, 1865, *1865*
Lichen planus, 2280
    vs. secondary syphilis, 510
Lidocaine, 1264
    in digitalis toxicity, 1099
    in myofascial pain syndromes, 728
    in reflex sympathetic dystrophies,
        728

Lidocaine (*Continued*)
  in ventricular ectopic beats
    complicating myocardial
    infarction, 1235
  in ventricular fibrillation, 1057
  in ventricular tachycardia, 1253
  in ventricular tachycardia
    complicating shock, 1118
Life cycle, phases of, 23
Life span, life expectation and, 25
Life support, termination of, legal
  aspects of, 1031
**Life-cycle perspective in medicine,
  16–17**
Light, pupillary reactions to, in
  metabolic brain disease, 648
Lighter fluid, poisoning by, 75
Lightheadedness, 737, 741–742
Limb-girdle dystrophy, 915, *916*, 917
Limnatis species, as agents of disease,
  120
Lincomycin, *556, 560, 561*
  in granuloma inguinale, 429
  in malabsorption syndrome, *1536*
  in postgastrectomy malabsorption,
    1546
Linguatula serrata, 119
Linguatuliasis, 119–120
Linkage disequilibrium, 39
Lion fishes, envenomation by, 124
Liotrix, in hypothyroidism, 2133
Lip(s)
  cleft, frequency and sex ratio of, *48*
  in ariboflavinosis, 1686
Lipase, pancreatic, in fat absorption,
  1524
Lipemia retinalis
  in diabetes mellitus, 1976
  in familial lipoprotein lipase
    deficiency, 2006
Lipemias, resolving, 2009
Lipid(s). See also *Fat(s).*
  circulating, elevated, as risk factor for
    atherosclerosis, 1220
  deposition of, in atherosclerosis,
    1218, 1219
  in chronic renal failure, 1361
  in kwashiorkor, 1682
  **metabolism of, disorders of,
    2002–2011**
    inborn errors of, 42
    oral contraceptive use and, 2196
  storage of, diseases of, 919, **2011–2015**
  transport of, 2002–2003
    **disorders of, classification of, 2003,
      *2004***
Lipid A, 453
Lipidosis(es)
  ceramide lactoside, *42*
  glucosyl ceramide, 2012–2014, *2013*
  of central nervous system, 850–851
  sphingomyelin, *2013,* **2014–2015**
  sulfatide, 850
Lipiduria, 1442
Lipoatrophic diabetes, 1981, 1982, **2058**
Lipoatrophy
  at site of insulin injection, 1988
  total, *2299*
Lipochrome histiocytosis, familial, 1806
Lipodystrophy
  hyperlipemia in, 2009
  intestinal, 1541
  mesenteric, 222
  partial, 1697, *2301*
Lipoid dermatoarthritis, 201

Lipoid nephrosis, 1327, 1391–1393
Lipoid pneumonia, 998–999
Lipoid proteinosis, 2058
Lipomas, small intestinal, 1605
Lipomatosis, multiple, 1697
Lipophagic intestinal granulomatosis,
  1541
Lipoprotein(s)
  high density, 2002, *2002,* 2003
  low density, *2002,* 2003
  **metabolism of, acquired disorders of,
    2009–2010**
    inborn errors of, 2004–2009
  **plasma, concentration of, normal
    regulation of, 2003–2004**
    properties of, 2002, *2002*
  very low density, 2002, *2002,* 2003
Lipoprotein lipase
  deficiency of, familial, *42,* **2006–2007**
  in obesity, 1695
Lipoproteinosis, alveolar, in silicosis,
  989
    management of, 993
Lipoteichoic acid, in streptococcal
  infections, 368
Lipotropins, 2091
  measurement of, 2094
Liquefying panniculitis, nodular, 2295,
  2297
Listeria monocytogenes, 471
Listeriosis, 471–473
Literal paraphasias, 656
Lithium, nephrotoxicity from, 1431
Lithium carbonate, in mania of
  manic-depressive psychosis, 671
Little sister, 587
Liver. See also *Hepatic.*
  abscess of, acute, 1656–1657
    amebic, 590, 591, 592, 593
    computerized tomography in, *1467*
    pyogenic, vs. hepatic amebiasis,
      592
    vs. pneumococcal pneumonia, 354
  acetaminophen-induced injury to,
    1658
  acute yellow atrophy of, 1652, 1655
  adenomas of, 1667
    oral contraceptive use and, 2195
  alcohol metabolism in, 707
  amebiasis of, 590, 591, 592, 593
    vs. clonorchiasis, 618
  angiosarcoma of, 1668
  antimicrobial agent clearance from,
    555
  aspiration of, in amebiasis, 592, 593,
    594
  bilirubin conjugation of, reduced,
    1638
  bilirubin uptake by, 1637
    reduced, 1638
  biopsy of
    in chronic active hepatitis, 1662
    in hemochromatosis, 1791
    in sarcoidosis, 214
    needle, 1647–1648
  blood flow through, 1639
  carbon tetrachloride injury to, 1658
  carcinoma of, primary, 1668
    secondary, 1667
  cirrhosis of, 1663–1667. See also
    Cirrhosis.
  diseased, physical changes of, 1639
  diseases of, 1637–1669
    alcohol-related, 709, 1658. See also
      names of specific diseases.

Liver (*Continued*)
  diseases of, altered hepatic function
    in, patterns of, 1647
    anemia in, 1643, 1732
    bacterial infections and, 1656
    cardiovascular changes in, 1644
    chronic, 1661–1667
    cutaneous manifestations of, 1645,
      2299
    diagnostic procedures in, 1645–1648
    drug metabolism changes in, 1641
    drug-induced, 1657–1660
    **hematologic abnormalities in,
      1643–1644**
    hemorrhagic disorder in, 1890–1891
    **hypersensitivity drug reactions
      causing, 1659–1660**
    immune mechanisms in, 1644
    in polycystic kidney disease, in
      adults, 1454
    in children, 1453
    infectious mononucleosis and, 265,
      1656
    infiltrative, 1667–1668
    mechanisms in, 1637–1645
    **metabolic disorders causing,
      1648–1650**
    metabolic encephalopathy in, 1640,
      1641
    **neuropsychiatric abnormalities
      associated with, 1640–1641**
    nonspecific symptoms in, 1645
    **nutritional and metabolic
      abnormalities in, 1642–1643**
    osteomalacia in, 2249, 2250
    peripheral neuropathy with, 909
    protozoan or helminthic, 1657
    **renal function changes in,
      1644–1645**
    secondary polycythemia in, 1800
    toxic, 1657–1660
  drug allergy and, 156
  drug metabolism in, 2338, 2340
  effects of alcohol on, 1663, 1664
  effects of oral contraceptives on, 2196
  enlargement of, 1639. See also
    Hepatomegaly.
  failure of, hemolysis in, 1770
  fatty, 1660–1661
    computerized tomography in, *1467*
  function of, tests of, 1645–1647, 2354
    in cirrhosis, 1664
  granulomas of, 1667
  hemangiomas of, 1667
  **impaired detoxification by, clinical
    manifestations resulting from,
    1641–1642**
  in acute heart failure, 1661
  in drug therapy of pulmonary
    tuberculosis, 488
  in hemochromatosis, 1790, 1791
  in Hodgkin's disease, 1841
  in hydatid cyst, 610
  in leptospirosis, 533, 1656
  in louse-borne relapsing fever, 527
  in malaria, 569, 571
  in non-Hodgkin's lymphomas, 1832
  in Reye's syndrome, 839
  in rickettsial diseases, 311, 316
  in right ventricular failure, 1092
  in schistosomiasis, 614, 1657
  in shock, 1661
  in sickle cell anemia, 1774
  in systemic lupus erythematosus, 177
  in toxocariasis, 628

Liver (*Continued*)
in typhoid fever, 446, 447, 1656
in visceral leishmaniasis, 585
in Wilson's disease, 2049, 2050
insufficiency of, vs. adrenal
insufficiency secondary to
hypopituitarism, 2151
metastases to, from lung carcinoma,
scanning in, *1469*
polycystic disease of, 1667
rupture of, angiography in, 1471
sarcomas of, 1667–1668
scanning of, 1468, *1468, 1469,* 1470,
1648
sex hormones and, 1658
tuberculosis of, primary, 493
tumors of
angiography in, *1470, 1471*
benign, 1667
malignant, 1667–1668
"Liver spots," 2289
Loa loa, 559, 605, 632, 635
Loboa loboi, 541
Lobo's disease, 541
Lockjaw, 436–441
Locomotor ataxia, 814–815. See also
Tabes dorsalis.
Löffler's eosinophilic endomyocarditis,
225
Löffler's fibroplastic endocarditis, 1286
Löffler's syndrome, 225, **969,** *969*
Löfgren's syndrome, 213
Loiasis, 635
Lomidine. See *Pentamidine isethionate.*
Lomotil. See *Diphenoxylate.*
Lomustine, in oncologic treatment, 1933
Long-acting thyroid stimulator, in
Graves' disease, 2121
Longitudinal sinus, superior, occlusion
of, in head injury, 884, 885
Loops of Henle, 1316, 1317
function of, 1318, 1319, *1320*
Lordosis, in paraplegia, 887, 888
Louping ill, 290–291
Louping ill virus, 291
Louse infestation, 108–110
Louse-borne relapsing fever, 526–529
**Louse-borne typhus fever, epidemic,
318–320**
clinical features of, *313*
epidemiologic features of, *310*
Lowenberg, sphygmomanometer cuff
pain test of, in thrombophlebitis,
1125
Lowe's oculocerebrorenal syndrome,
2021
**Lown-Ganong-Levine syndrome,
1256–1257**
Loxosceles reclusa, 115
LSD, 703–705
poisoning by, *712*
Luder-Sheldon syndrome, *2021*
Ludwig's angina, 443
vs. actinomycosis, 474
Luft's syndrome, vs. thyrotoxicosis,
2123
Lugol's solution
in preparation for thyroidectomy,
2125
in thyroid storm, 2128
Lumbar disc(s)
disease of, vs. arteriosclerosis
obliterans, 1301
herniated, 894

Lumbar plexus neuropathy, 902, 903
diabetic, 909
Lumbar puncture, 747–748. See also
Cerebrospinal fluid examination.
in coma, 643
in dementia, 661
in head injury, 881
in meningococcal meningitis, 421
intracranial hypotension after, 873
Lumbar puncture headache, 730
Lumbar spine
degenerative disease of, 204
stenosis of, 895
Lumbar spondylosis, 895
Lumbar sympathectomy, preganglionic,
in arteriosclerosis obliterans, 1301
Lumbosacral region, compressive
lesions of, 891
Lung(s). See also *Pulmonary.*
abscess of, 979–982
amebic, 591, 980, 981
cavitary, vs. pulmonary
tuberculosis, 486
vs. pulmonary paragonimiasis, 620
aeration of, abnormalities of, 965–966
air conditioner, *971*
beryllium disease of, chronic, 990, 991
biopsy of, 950
bird breeder's, *971*
blackfat tobacco smokers', 998, 999
busulfan, 1823
carcinoma of, 1005–1010. See also
Bronchogenic carcinoma.
cavitary disease of, chronic, *Klebsiella*
causing, 358
changes in, with age, 26
cheese worker's, *971*
circulation of, normal, 1135–1137
compliance of, 932, *932*
cysts of, 1002
vs. lung abscess, 981
diffusing capacity of, 936–937
disease of
"atypical" mycobacteria causing,
499–500
bullous, 1003–1004
chronic, *H. influenzae* organisms
and, 425
hormones secreted in, 2061, *2062*
infiltrative, 966–979
respiratory failure in, 1023, *1023*
**pulmonary hypertension in,
1146–1149**
dynamic properties of, 933–935
effects of atmospheric pressure
changes on, 99
elastic properties of, 932, *932*
endocrine functions of, 2061
eosinophilic, 637
farmer's, *971*
function of, in diffuse collagenous
pneumoconioses, 991
gas in, measurement of, 933
"honeycomb," 991, 1003
host defense system of, 339, 340, 348
humidifier, *971*
hyperlucent, unilateral, 1004
in Hodgkin's disease, 1844
in hydatid cyst, 610
in left ventricular failure, 1090
in nocardiosis, 475
in rickettsial diseases, 311
in right ventricular failure, 1091
in scleroderma, 168, 169

Lung(s) (*Continued*)
in strongyloidiasis, 623
infections of, in cancer patient, 1901
routes of, 339
lymphoma of, primary, 1011–1012
maple bark stripper's, *971*
mushroom worker's, *971*
neoplasms of, 1005–1013, *1005*
metastatic, 1012
paprika splitter's, *971*
**physical and chemical irritants to,
983–1002,** *984*
pituitary snuff, *971*
pseudolymphoma of, 1011, 1012
radiation injury to, *984,* **1001–1002**
shock, 1113
static properties of, 932–933, *932*
tissue response of, to organic dusts,
985
tumors of, benign, 1013
hormonal secretion by, 2061, *2062*
volume-pressure relationships of,
932, *932*
Lung capacity, total, 932, *932*
Lung hermaphroditic flukes, 619–620
Lung perfusion scan, 944
Lung purpura, nephritis and, 1401
Lung tissue, examination and culture
of, microbiologic diagnosis by, 342
Lung volumes, changes in, in
ventilatory disorders, 936, *936*
Lupoid hepatitis, vs. systemic lupus
erythematosus, 177
Lupoid leishmaniasis, 587, 588
Lupus erythematosus
discoid, 176
systemic, 174–180
autoantibodies in, 178, *179*
autoimmune thrombocytopenia in,
1876
clinical symptoms in, frequency of,
176
cutaneous signs in, *2301, 2302*
drug-induced, 156, 179, 975, *975*
eyes in, 177, 2317, *2318*
immune complexes in, 134
immune mechanisms in, 132
laboratory abnormalities in, 178, *178*
malabsorption in, 1543
pericarditis caused by, 1271
photosensitivity in, 2289
pleura in, 1017
pregnancy and, 177, 1414
pulmonary hypertension in, 1141,
1143
pulmonary involvement in, 974
renal involvement in, 175, 176, 177,
178, 1400
vs. infective endocarditis, 392
vs. leprosy, 503
vs. periarteritis nodosa, 183
vs. rheumatic fever, 383
vs. rheumatoid arthritis, 190
Lupus pernio, upper respiratory tract
sarcoidosis and, 212
Lupus vulgaris, 498
Luschka, joints of, degenerative
changes in, 204
Luteinizing hormone, 2088–2089
deficiency of, isolated, 2172
in ovarian function, 2175, 2176
measurement of, 2092–2093, *2093*
Luteinizing hormone–releasing factor,
2075

Luteinizing hormone–releasing hormone, in diagnosis of anterior pituitary disease, 2081, 2082, *2082*
Lutembacher's syndrome, 1169
Lutzomyia longipalpis, in visceral leishmaniasis, 584
Lutzomyia species, in cutaneous leishmaniasis of new world, *588*
Lycosa species, bites of, 115
Lye, poisoning by, 75
Lye damage, esophageal, carcinoma after, 1597
Lye stricture, esophageal, vs. carcinoma, 1598
Lyme arthritis, 202
Lymph nodes
  biopsy of, in pulmonary disease, 949, 950
  in infectious mononucleosis, 265
  in leprosy, *502*
  in listeriosis, 472
  in systemic lupus erythematosus, 177
  in toxoplasmosis, 595, 596
  in visceral leishmaniasis, 585
  mucocutaneous, syndrome of, 534, 2306
Lymphadenitis
  "atypical" mycobacteria causing, 500
  nonbacterial regional, benign, 302–305, *303, 304*
  tuberculous, 495
    malabsorption in, 1545
    vs. bancroftian filariasis, 634
Lymphadenopathy
  angioimmunoblastic, 1832
  immunoblastic, eosinophilis in, 226
  in acute leukemia, 1817
  in bancroftian filariasis, 634
  in bronchogenic carcinoma, 1006
  in Hodgkin's disease, 1840, *1840,* 1841
Lymphangiectasia, malabsorption in, 1545
Lymphangiography, retroperitoneal, in non-Hodgkin's lymphomas, 1834, 1835
Lymphangitic carcinomatosis, pulmonary hypertension in, 1147
Lymphangitis, 1315
  in paracoccidioidomycosis, 541
Lymphatic leukemia, chronic, 1824–1826
Lymphatic obstruction, malabsorption in, 1544, 1545
Lymphatic tissue, pharyngeal, tuberculosis of, 492
Lymphatic vessels, peripheral, diseases of, 1314–1315
Lymphedema, 1314–1315
  in bancroftian filariasis, 634
Lymphocele, after renal transplantation, 1385
Lymphocyte culture reaction, mixed, in T cell function assay, 130
Lymphocytes, 126, 128–129, *128*
  abnormal function of, nosocomial pneumonia and, 363
  B. See *B cells.*
  leukemoid reactions involving, 1813
  T. See *T cells.*
Lymphocytic choriomeningitis, 818, *818*
  vs. arboviral encephalitis, 284
Lymphocytic interstitial pneumonitis, 1011, 1012
Lymphocytic leukemia
  acute, 1814

Lymphocytic leukemia (*Continued*)
  acute, epidemiology of, 1816
    pathogenesis of, 1816
    therapy of, 1817, 1818, 1819, 1820
    vs. leukemoid reaction, 1813
  chronic, 1824–1826
    idiopathic thrombocytopenic purpura in, 1876
Lymphocytic lymphoma(s), 1830, *1830*
  poorly differentiated, 1831, *1833*
  well differentiated, 1831, *1833*
Lymphocytosis, infectious, vs. infectious mononucleosis, 267
Lymphogranuloma venereum, 335–336
  lesion of, vs. syphilitic ulcers, 508
  vs. amebomas, 592
  vs. plague, 464
  vs. ulcerative proctitis, 1572
Lymphoid interstitial pneumonitis, 979
Lymphoma(s)
  Burkitt's, 1838–1839
    malaria and, 567
  esophageal, malignant, 1599
  gastric, 1603
  histiocytic, 1830, *1830,* 1831, *1833*
  histiocytic-lymphocytic, mixed, 1830, *1830,* 1831, 1832, 1833
  intestinal, primary, 1545
  Lennert's, 1832
  lung, primary, 1011–1012
  lymphocytic, 1830, *1830*
    poorly differentiated, 1831, *1833*
    well differentiated, 1831, *1833*
  malignant, idiopathic thrombocytopenic purpura in, 1876
    with high content of epithelioid histiocytes, 1832
  neuropathy with, vs. acute inflammatory polyneuropathy, 907
  non-Hodgkin's, 1830–1838
    clinical manifestations of, 1832
    epidemiology of, 1831
    etiology of, 1830
    lungs as primary site of, 1011, 1012
    pathology of, 1831
    prognosis in, 1837
    staging in, 1834, *1834*
    treatment of, 1835
  pleomorphic, 1830, *1830,* 1832, *1833*
  portal hypertension in, 1639
  small intestinal, 1604, 1605
    in adult celiac disease, 1541
    malabsorption secondary to, 1544, 1545
  varicella and, 254
  vs. eosinophilic gastroenteritis, 1543
  vs. malaria, 573
  vs. toxoplasmosis, 597
  vs. visceral leishmaniasis, 586
  vs. Whipple's disease, 1541
Lymphomatoid granulomatosis, vs. Wegener's granulomatosis, 219
Lymphonodular pharyngitis, acute, 271
Lymphopenia, 1807, 1812
Lymphoproliferation, in sarcoidosis, 210
Lymphoreticular neoplasms, 1829–1848
  classification of, *1830*
Lymphoreticulosis, inoculation, 302–305, *303, 304*
Lymphosarcoma, vs. regional enteritis, 1565
"Lymphosarcoma-cell leukemia," 1824
Lyon hypothesis, 36, 37

Lysergic acid diethylamide, 703–705
  poisoning by, 712
Lysine hydrochloride, ingestion of, metabolic acidosis from, 1962
Lysis, bacterial, complement-mediated, 137
Lysosomal acid phosphatase deficiency, 43
Lysosomes, in shock, 1114, 1115
Lyssa, 833–836, *833, 835.* See also *Rabies.*

M protein, in streptococcal infections, 368
Machupo virus, 298, 299
Macleod's syndrome, 1004
Macrocytes, 1716
Macroglobulinemia, 1862–1863
  primary, 1862–1863
    vascular purpura in, 1880
  Waldenström's, 1862–1863
    electrophoretic patterns in, 1855, 1856, *1856*
    renal changes in, 1406
Macronodular cirrhosis, 1663
Macrophage(s), 129
  alveolar, bacterial ingestion by, 339, 340
    in immunocompromised patient, nosocomial pneumonia and, 363
  in host defense, 146
  in malnutrition, 1680
  in recovery from pneumococcal pneumonia, 351
Macular disciform lesions, in ocular histoplasmosis, 2324
Macule, 2273
Madura foot, 542
Madurella mycetomi, 542
Maduromycosis, 542
Maggots, infestation by, 111–112
"Magic mushrooms," 704
Magnesium
  excretion of, in chronic renal failure, 1356, *1357*
  nutrient value of, 1674
  recommended allowances of, *1671*
Magnesium citrate, in hepatic coma complicating cirrhosis, 1666
Magnesium hydroxide, in peptic ulcer, 1513
Magnesium sulfate, in malabsorption syndrome, *1536*
Magnetite miners, pneumoconiosis in, 987
"Magnification phenomenon," in chronic renal disease, 1349
Mal del pinto, *520,* **524–525**
Malabsorption syndrome, 1523–1550
  causes of, 1526
  classification of, *1526*
  clinical manifestations of, 1526–1528, *1527*
    pathophysiologic basis for, 1528–1530
  diagnosis of, 1530–1535
    laboratory, 1530, *1531*
  differential features and treatment of, 1535–1548
  disorders associated with, cutaneous signs of, *2298–2299*
  enteric loss of protein and, 1548–1549, *1548, 1549*

Malabsorption syndrome (*Continued*)
  hypocalcemia in, 1528, 2241
  in cancer patient, 1906
  in diabetes mellitus, 1547, 1548
  in regional enteritis, 1564
  management of, agents used in, *1536*
  osteomalacia in, 2249, 2250
  prognosis in, 1549–1550
Maladie des tics, 759
Malakoplakia, 1613
Malaria, 566–575
  algid, 572
  antimicrobial agents for, *558*
  antimicrobial prophylaxis in, *564*
  cerebral, 574
  chloroquine-resistant, 573, 574, 575
  chronic, syndromes associated with, 572
  clinical manifestations of, 571
  complications of, 571
  diagnosis of, 572
  differential diagnosis of, 573
  epidemiology of, 567
  falciparum, 567, 569
    clinical manifestations of, 571
    complications of, 571
    drug-resistant, 573
    erythrocyte forms of, *570*
    recrudescent, prevention of, 574
    supportive therapy in, 574
    vs. louse-borne typhus, 312
  hemolysis in, 1770
  host resistance in, 569
  immunity in, 569
  immunodiagnostic tests for, *565*
  malariae, 567
    clinical manifestations of, 571
  mixed infection in, 572
  ovale, 567
    clinical manifestations of, 571
    relapse of, 574
  parasitemia in, elimination of, 573
  pathogenesis of, 569
  prevention of, 574
    in community, 575
  quartan, 569, 571
  relapse of, due to persistent hepatic schizonts, 574
  tertian, 569, 571
  therapy of, 573
    supportive, 574
  vivax, 567
    clinical manifestations of, 571
    erythrocyte forms of, *570*
    relapse of, 574
  vs. hemorrhagic diseases caused by arenaviruses, 299
  vs. louse-borne relapsing fever, 527, 528
  vs. melioidosis, 470
  vs. typhoid fever, 448
  vs. visceral leishmaniasis, 586
Malariae malaria, 567
  clinical manifestations of, 571
Malayan filariasis, 634
"Male climacteric," 2174
Male genital tuberculosis, 496
Male hypogonadism, 2167–2172
Male infertility, 2170–2171, 2193, 2194
Male mid-life crises, 24
Male orgasm, 687
  dysfunction of, 688, 2198
Male pseudohermaphroditism, 2172–2173

Male reproductive maturation, *18,* 19, **2166**
Male sexual precocity, 2166–2167
Malformations, congenital, 48–49. See also names of specific congenital disorders.
Malignancy, internal, cutaneous manifestations of, 2295–2297, 2300, *2296–2297*
Malignant carcinoid syndrome, metastatic, malabsorption in, 1547
Malignant hypertension, 1204, 1205
  vs. primary aldosteronism, 2158
Malignant hyperthermia
  anesthetic agents causing, genetic basis of, 46
  myoglobinuria in, 924, 925
Malignant lymphoma
  idiopathic thrombocytopenic purpura in, 1876
  with high content of epithelioid histiocytes, 1832
Malignant melanomas, anal, 1618
Malignant pustule, 470
Malignant ulcer, 1508
Malingering, vs. hysteria, 678
Malleomyces, **diseases caused by, 468–470**
Malleomyces mallei, 468
Malleomyces pseudomallei, 469
Mallory-Weiss syndrome, 1478
Malnutrition
  effect of, on infection, 1679–1680
    protein, fatty liver in, 1660
  protein-calorie, 1680–1683
    clinical signs of, 1677
    effect of, on plasma amino acids, *2018*
    pubertal process and, 20
Malrotation, renal, 1457
Malum coxae senilis, 203
Mandrax. See *Methaqualone.*
Manganese
  nutrient value of, 1674
  poisoning by, 76
Mania
  in manic-depressive psychosis, 669, 670
    treatment of, 671
  vs. schizophrenia, 666, 667
Manic-depressive psychosis, 665, 669–672
  vs. depression, 677
Mannitol
  accumulation of, in extracellular fluid, 1955
  in bacterial meningitis, 416
  in cerebral edema complicating cerebral infarction, 791
  in cerebral edema complicating relapsing fever, 528
  in cramps complicating maintenance hemodialysis, 1381
  in differential diagnosis of acute renal failure, 1374
  in electric shock, 94
  in head injury, 882
  in prevention of acute tubular necrosis, 1374
  in renal complications of transfusion, 1788
  in thallium poisoning, 82
Mannosidosis, *41*
Mansonella ozzardi, 605, *632,* **635**

Mantoux test, in tuberculosis, 946
MAO inhibitors
  in depression of manic-depressive psychosis, 671
  poisoning by, *712*
  tyramine and, interaction of, hypertension from, 1209
Maple bark stripper's lung, *971*
Maple syrup urine disease, *41,* *2016–2017,* 2021
Marantic endocarditis, 387
Marasmus, 1680, **1681,** 1682
Marble bone disease, 2263
Marburg disease, 300–301
Marburg virus, 300
March hemoglobinuria, 924, **1767–1768,** 1783
Marchiafava-Bignami disease, 776
Marezine. See *Cyclizine.*
Marfan's syndrome, 2053–2054
  aortic lesion of, 1291
  aortic regurgitation in, 1194
  osteoporosis in, 2245
  vs. Ehlers-Danlos syndrome, 2055
Marie-Strümpell spondylitis, 194–195. See also *Ankylosing spondylitis.*
Marijuana, 702–703
Marine animals, venomous, 123–125
Maroteaux-Lamy syndrome, *41,* **2052, 2053**
Marrara syndrome, 120
Mass spectrometry, in critical care medicine, 1032
Massive spasms, infantile, 854
Mast cell disease, 2307–2308
Mastocytoma, 2307
Mastocytosis
  diffuse, 2307
  malabsorption in, 1548
  systemic, 161, *2296, 2298, 2302,* 2308
Mastoid bone, tuberculosis of, 492
Mastoiditis
  brain abscess from, 805
  in streptococcal pharyngitis, 373
Mastomys natalensis, 299
Masturbation, 690
Maternal deprivation syndrome, 2080
Matulane. See *Procarbazine.*
Maximal expiratory flow rate, 934, *934*
Maximal expiratory flow–volume curve, 934
Maximal mid-expiratory flow rate, 934, *934*
Mayaro fever, 279–280, *279*
Mayaro virus, 279
Mayer-Rokitansky-Küster-Hauser syndrome, amenorrhea from, 2185
Mayflies, allergic response to, 112
Mazzotti's test, in onchocerciasis, 636
McArdle's syndrome, vs. arteriosclerosis obliterans, 1301
McCune-Albright syndrome, 2167
Measles, 246–250, *248, 249*
  acute disseminated encephalomyelitis after, 836, 837
  German, **250–252.** See also *Rubella.*
  unfavorably modified, 249
  vs. Rocky Mountain spotted fever, 312, 323
  vs. rubella, 252
Measles vaccination, 250
Measles virus, 246
Measles-like virus, in subacute sclerosing panencephalitis, 841

Mebendazole
in ascariasis, 627
in capillariasis, 623
in enterobiasis, 629
in hookworm disease, 625
in intestinal nematodes, *559*
in trichuriasis, 629
Mechanical ventilation
in acute respiratory failure, 1040, 1041
indications for, 1039, *1039*
in critical care medicine, 1032, 1033
Mechlorethamine, in oncologic
treatment, 1931
Mecholyl test, in achalasia, 1486, 1487
Meckel's diverticulitis, 1500, 1501
Meckel's diverticulum, 1500–1501
radionuclide imaging in, 1470
Meclizine
in hyperactive labyrinths, 740
in motion sickness, 95
in vertigo, 739
Mediastinal collagenosis, pulmonary
venous hypertension from, 1145
Mediastinal emphysema, 1018
Mediastinal fibrosis, 224
Mediastinitis, 1018
hemorrhagic, in anthrax, 470, 471
Mediastinoscopy, in pulmonary disease,
950
Mediastinum
diseases of, 1018–1019
infections of, 1018
tumors of, 1018, 1019
Medical intensive care unit, 1031
instrumentation for, 1032–1033
Medical oncology, 1898–1948
Medicinal leeches, as agents of disease,
120
Medicine
clinical, biological science and, 6–8
laboratory investigation and, 4, 6, 7
psychologic testing in, 681–683
science, spectrum of disease and,
3–6
study of, 1–3
critical care, 1031–1058. See also
Critical care medicine.
geriatric, aging and, 25–30
in modern society, 8–10
internal, cancer and, 1898–1907
life-cycle perspective in, 16–17
nature of, 1–10
Mediterranean anemia, 1778
Mediterranean fever, familial,
2055–2057
arthritis in, 199
cutaneous signs of, *2299, 2300*
pericardial involvement by, 1276
Medium-chain triglycerides
after extensive small intestinal
resection 1544
in fat absorption, 1524
in malabsorption syndrome, 1538,
1539
Medroxyprogesterone acetate, in
evaluation of amenorrhea, 2183
Medulla
adrenal, 2199–2207
hormones of, 2199–2201
renal, cystic, nephronophthisis and,
1454–1455
Medullary carcinoma of thyroid, 2143,
2223–2224
carcinoid features of, 2212

Medullary cystic disease
adult-onset, 1454
volume depletion in, 1951
Medullary infarction, 788
Medullary necrosis, renal, 1412–1413
Medullary sponge kidney, 1455–1456
vs. adult polycystic kidney disease,
1454
Medullary thyroid carcinoma–
pheochromocytoma syndromes, detection of, in relatives, *58*
Medulloblastoma, 863
Megacolon, 1494–1496
acquired, 1496
vs. aganglionic megacolon, 1495
aganglionic, 1495–1496, *1495*
congenital, 1495–1496, *1495*
idiopathic, 1496
in Chagas' disease, 582, 583, 1496
psychogenic, 1496
secondary, 1496
toxic, in ulcerative colitis, 1569, 1570,
1570, 1574–1575
Megaesophagus, 1486–1488, *1487*
in Chagas' disease, 581, 582, 583
Megaloblastic anemias, 1719–1729
clinical manifestations of, 1724
differential diagnosis of, 1725, *1725*
etiologic classification of, 1719,
1720–1721
incidence and prevalence of, 1722
laboratory findings in, 1725
pathogenesis of, 1719
pathology of, 1723
therapeutic principles in, 1719
therapy of, 1726
"Megaloblastic madness," 1724,
1725
Megalopyge opercularis, 119
Megalourethra, 1458
Meglumine antimoniate, in visceral
leishmaniasis, 586
Meigs' syndrome, 1017, 1018
ascites in, 1593
Meiosis, 51, 52, *52*
Meiotic nondisjunction, 51–52, *52*
Mel B. See *Melarsoprol.*
Melanocytes, 2267
Melanocyte-stimulating hormone, 2090
function of, measurement of, 2094
Melanoma, 2310–2312
cutaneous, primary, 2310
juvenile, benign, 2312
lentiginous, acral, 2311
malignant, anal, 1618
nodular, 2311, *2311*
superficial spreading, 2311, *2311*
Melanoptysis, in complicated
pneumoconiosis, 993
Melanosis
diffuse, 2291
vs. pinta, 525
Melanosis coli, 1494, **1613–1614**
Melanotic freckle of Hutchinson, 2310,
2311
Melarsoprol
in African trypanosomiasis, 578,
579
in trypanosomiasis, *558*
Melasma, 2291, *2292*
Melatonin, 2112
biosynthesis of, *2113*
Melena, 1520
Meleney's synergistic gangrene, 367

Meleney's ulcers, hyperbaric oxygen
therapy in, 105
Melioidosis, 469–470
vs. glanders, 469
Melorheostosis, 2264
Melphalan, 1932
in multiple myeloma, 1861
Membranoproliferative
glomerulonephritis, 1327, **1398**
Membranous glomerular disease,
idiopathic, 1393
Memory, 658–659
anatomy of, 658
clinical disorders of, 659
disturbance of, in Alzheimer's
disease, 662
failure of, in dementia, 660
in hepatic encephalopathy, 1641
in hypothalamic dysfunction, 716
Menadione
in malabsorption syndrome, *1536*
in vitamin K deficiency, 1890
Menarche, *18, 19,* 2181
Mendelian disorders, common, *36*
Ménière's disorder, 739
hearing loss from, 736
vs. cerebral transient ischemic
attacks, 785
Meninges
anomalies of, 874–876
biopsy of, in intracranial
inflammatory disease, 804
metastatic disease of, vs. dementia in
cancer, 877
neoplasia of, diffuse, 867
suppurative diseases of, cerebrospinal
fluid findings in, *803*
tumors of, 863
Meningioma(s), 863
spinal cord, 896
Meningismus, vs. meningococcal
meningitis, 420, 421
Meningitis
"acute," brain abscess presenting as,
806
aseptic, 817, 818, 820
in Colorado tick fever, 280
in epidemic pleurodynia, 272
in leptospirosis, 533
in mumps, 262
vs. infectious mononucleosis, 267
"atypical" mycobacteria causing, 500
bacterial, 411–416
cerebrospinal fluid findings in, 413,
414, *803*
recurrent, 415
vs. arboviral encephalitis, 284
vs. poliomyelitis, 831
vs. viral meningitis, 820
Candida, 548
carcinomatous, 867
cerebrospinal, epidemic, 417
"chemical," vs. bacterial meningitis,
414
cryptococcal, 543, 544
cerebrospinal fluid findings in, *803*
enteric bacteria causing, 454
enterococcal, 416
epilepsy associated with, 852
fungal, vs. arboviral encephalitis, 284
vs. poliomyelitis, 831
vs. viral meningitis, 820
gonococcal, 410
gram-negative bacilli causing, 411

Meningitis (*Continued*)
  headache of, 729, 730
  Hemophilus influenzae, 411
    treatment of, 415
    type b, 424, 425
  hemorrhagic, in anthrax, 470, 471
  in cancer patient, 1901, 1903
  in coccidioidomycosis, 538, 539
  in listeriosis, 472, 473
  in miliary tuberculosis, 492, 493
  meningococcal, 411, 417
    clinical manifestations of, 420
    diagnosis of, 420, 421
    treatment of, 421
  Mollaret's, 842
    vs. bacterial meningitis, 415
  neoplastic, cerebrospinal fluid
    findings in, *803*
  nonsuppurative, cerebrospinal fluid
    findings in, *803*
  plague, 464, 465
  pneumococcal, 353, 411
    development of, factors associated
      with, 411
    treatment of, 415
  purulent, acute, 418
    in nocardiosis, 475
  pyogenic, 411
    vs. herpes simplex encephalitis, 824
  sarcoid, cerebrospinal fluid findings
    in, *803*
  serous, 817
  staphylococcal, 404, 411
    treatment of, 415, 416
  syphilitic, 813
    cerebrospinal fluid examination in,
      803, 813
  tuberculous, 481, **493–494**
    cerebrospinal fluid findings in, *803*
    vs. herpes simplex encephalitis,
      824
    vs. viral meningitis, 820
  tularemic, 467
  viral, 817–821
    cerebrospinal fluid findings, in,
      803, 820
    viruses associated with, 817, *817*, 818,
      818
Meningocele, 875–876
Meningococcal arthritis, 417
Meningococcal disease, 417–423
  antimicrobial prophylaxis for, *564*
Meningococcal endocarditis, 394
Meningococcal meningitis, 411, 417
  clinical manifestations of, 420
  diagnosis of, 420, 421
  treatment of, 421
Meningococcal vaccines, 423
Meningococcemia, 417
  adrenal apoplexy in, 2150
  clinical manifestations of, 418, 419,
    419
  fulminating, 419, *419*
    treatment of, 421
  pathogenesis and pathology of, 418
  treatment of, 421
  vs. dengue hemorrhagic fever, 297
  vs. rat-bite fever, 531
  vs. Rocky Mountain spotted fever,
    323
  vs. rubelliform exanthems, 274
  vs. smallpox, 257
  vs. tularemia, 467
Meningoencephalitis
  amebic, primary, 603–604

Meningoencephalitis (*Continued*)
  eosinophilic, *Angiostrongylus*
    cantonensis causing, 631
  in Chagas' disease, 581
  in cryptococcosis, 543, 544
  in rubella, 251
  viral, 817
    vs. meningococcal meningitis, 420,
      421
    vs. psittacosis, 338
Meningomyelitis, syphilitic, vs. vitamin
  B$_{12}$ deficiency, 776, 777
Meningomyelocele, 875
Meningonema peruzzii, 637
Meningonemiasis, 637
Meningovascular syphilis, 511, **813–814**
  treatment of, 516
  vs. transverse myelitis, 812
Menkes' kinky hair syndrome, *43*
  osteoporosis in, 2245
Menopausal urinary gonadotropin,
  human, in amenorrhea, 2192
Menopause, 2190, 2191
  mid-life crisis and, 24
Menstruation
  disorders of. See also *Amenorrhea.*
    in opiate addiction, 697
  gonadotropin secretion during, 2088,
    2088
  in systemic lupus erythematosus, 177
Mental changes
  in intracranial tumor, 865
  in metabolic brain disease, 647, 648
Mepacrine
  in cutaneous leishmaniasis of old
    world, 588
  in tapeworm infections, 608
Meperidine, 694
  in acute intermittent porphyria, 2047
  in acute pulmonary edema of heart
    failure, 1094
  in orchitis complicating mumps, 263
  in pain, *724*
  in shock, 1117
  poisoning by, *712*
Meprobamate
  in pain, *724*
  poisoning by, *712*, 713
MER, in oncologic treatment, 1940
Meralgia paresthetica, 902
Mercaptopurine, 1935
Mercury
  as nephrotoxin, 80, *1428*, 1430
  methyl, neuropathy from, 911
    poisoning by, 80
  organic intoxication from, 81
  poisoning by, 80–81
Mersalyl, in heart failure, *1104*
Mesangiocapillary glomerulonephritis,
  1398
Mescaline, 704
  poisoning by, *712*
Mesenchymal disease, neuropathy
  associated with, 908
Mesenteric adenitis, acute, vs. acute
  appendicitis, 1581
Mesenteric artery(ies)
  embolism of, 1589
  inferior, 1587, *1587*
  occlusion of, 1588, 1589
  superior, 1586, *1587*
  syndrome of, 1590
Mesenteric circulation, anatomy,
  physiology and pathophysiology of,
  1586–1587, *1586, 1587*

Mesenteric inflammatory disease, 1595,
  1596
Mesenteric lipodystrophy, 222
Mesenteric panniculitis, 222, 1596
Mesenteric venous thrombosis, 1589,
  1590
Mesenteritis, retractile, 1596
Mesentery
  cysts of, 1596
  diseases of, 1595–1596
  tumors of, 1596
Mesoblastic nephroma, congenital, 1460
Mesothelioma
  pleural, 1016
  primary, 1595
"Mess trick," 746
Messenger RNA, 31
  in protein synthesis, *32, 33*
Metabolic acidosis, 1322, **1961–1965**
  causes of, *1961*
  complicating chronic respiratory
    acidosis, 1968, *1968*
  in acute renal failure, 1372
  in cancer patient, 1904
  in hyperparathyroidism, 2216
  in shock, 1046
Metabolic alkalosis, 1322, 1961,
  1965–1967
  causes of, *1965*
  complicating chronic respiratory
    acidosis, 1967, 1968, *1968*
  in cancer patient, 1904
  potassium deficiency and, 1958
  tetany from, 2223
Metabolic brain disease, 644–651
  autonomic activity in, 648
  causes of, *644*
  causing coma, 642
  clinical features of, 647–649
  diagnosis of, 649–651
  electroencephalography in, 649
  laboratory evaluation of, 649, *649*
  mental changes in, 647, 648
  motor activity in, 648
  pathophysiologic aspects of, 645–647
  prognosis and treatment of, 651, *651*
  suspected, physical examination in,
    647
  ventilation in, 649
Metabolic complications of vomiting,
  1478
Metabolic encephalopathy, 645. See also
  Metabolic brain disease.
  causes of, *644*
  coma caused by, 642
  diagnosis of, 649–651
  endogenous, 645
  exogenous, 645
  in chronic liver disease, 1640, 1641
  vs. dementia in cancer, 877
Metabolic myopathies, vs. polymyositis,
  174
Metabolism. See also under
  Carbohydrate(s), Lipid(s), Protein(s),
  etc.
  abnormalities of, in liver disease,
    1642–1643
  basal, 1949
  diseases of, 1949–2059
    benign intracranial hypertension
      with, 871
    congenitai, in thyroid hormone
      formation, 2138–2140
    cutaneous manifestations of, *2300*
    epilepsy associated with, 853

Metabolism (*Continued*)
  diseases of, in cancer patient, 1903,
    1904
    in intracranial tumors, 866
    liver disease caused by, 1648–1650
    pericarditis in, 1272
    renal injury from, 1329–1330
    inborn errors of, 40–44, *41–44,* 1949
      amino acid, 2015–2029
      lipoprotein, 2004–2009
      screening for, 44
    intermediary, 1949
Metacentric chromosomes, 50, *50*
Metachromatic leukodystrophy, *42*
Metachromatic leukoencephalopathy,
850
Metagonimus yokogawai, 621
Metal nephropathies, 1428–1431, *1428*
Metals, heavy, poisoning by, 76–82
  vs. acute abdomen, 1581
Metaplasia, myeloid
  agnogenic, 1827–1829
    portal hypertension in, 1639
    vs. myelophthisic anemia, 1742
    myelofibrosis with, 1827
    vs. chronic granulocytic
      leukemia, 1822
Metaraminol bitartrate, in shock
  complicating relapsing fever, 528
Metastatic calcinosis, *2300*
Methacycline, *557, 562*
Methadone, 694
  illicit, use of, 695
  in narcotic withdrawal, 697
  in pain, *723, 724,* 725
  maintenance therapy with, 697–698
  poisoning by, *712*
Methamphetamine, abuse of, 701
Methaqualone
  abuse of, 698
  poisoning by, *712*
Methemoglobin, 1780
Methemoglobinemia, *42,* **1780–1782,**
  2302
  acquired, secondary polycythemia in,
    1799
  cyanosis caused by, 1777
  hereditary, 1780, 1781
  toxic, 1780, 1781
Methenamine mandelate and hippurate,
  556, 563
Methicillin, *557,* 559
  adverse reactions to, 560
  as nephrotoxin, 1426
  in infective endocarditis, 393
  in infective endocarditis prophylaxis,
    396
  in osteomyelitis, 2261
  in staphylococcal meningitis, 404
  in staphylococcal pneumonia, 402
Methimazole, in hyperthyroidism, 2123,
  2124
Methisazone, *556*
Methotrexate, 1933, 1934
  in eosinophilic granuloma, 1851
  in non-Hodgkin's lymphomas, *1836*
  in psoriatic arthritis, 197
  pulmonary hypersensitivity reactions
    from, 975
Methotrimeprazine, in pain, *724,* 725
Methoxyflurane
  anesthesia with, hepatitis after,
    1659–1660
  as nephrotoxin, 1433

Methyl alcohol, poisoning by, 75
  metabolic acidosis from, 1962
Methyl mercury
  neuropathy from, 911
  poisoning by, 80
Methylated nucleosides, as tumor
  markers, 1913
Methyl-CCNU, in oncologic treatment,
  1933
Methylcellulose, in Sjögren's syndrome,
  194
Methyldopa
  in arterial hypertension, *1212,* 1214
  in emergency reduction of blood
    pressure, 1216
  in hypertension of chronic renal
    failure, 1363
  in toxemia of pregnancy, 1415
α-Methyldopa
  "autoimmune" hemolysis due to,
    1766
  in Raynaud's disease, 1307
Methyldopa hepatitis, 1660
Methylene blue, in
  methemoglobinemia, 1782
Methylene THF reductase deficiency,
  2017
α-Methyl-β-hydroxybutyric acidemia,
  41
Methylmalonic aciduria
  homocystinuria with, *2017*
  prevention and management of, 55
  vitamin B$_{12}$ responsive, *41*
  vitamin B$_{12}$ unresponsive, *41*
Methylphenidate
  abuse of, 701
  in narcolepsy, 654
  poisoning by, *712*
Methylphenylethylhydantoin, in
  epilepsy, *859*
Methylprednisolone
  in chronic respiratory failure, 1029
  in rheumatoid arthritis, 192
  in septic shock, 1119
Methylprednisolone sodium succinate
  in acute respiratory failure, 1043
  in near-drowning, 107
Methyltestosterone
  in androgen deficiency, 2168
  in hypopituitarism, 2102
  intrahepatic cholestasis caused by,
    1658
Methyprylon, abuse of, 698
Methysergide
  in diarrhea of carcinoid syndrome,
    2213
  in erythromelalgia, 1309
  in malabsorption of metastatic
    malignant carcinoid syndrome, 1547
  in migraine, retroperitoneal fibrosis
    in, 223
  in migraine prophylaxis, 732
  pulmonary hypersensitivity reactions
    from, 975
  toxicity of, 1308
Metoclopramide
  in gastrointestinal symptoms of
    chronic renal failure, 1365
  in staphylococcal food poisoning, 65
Metoprolol, in arterial hypertension,
  1212
Metorchis conjunctus, 621
Metronidazole
  anaerobic susceptibility to, *445*

Metronidazole (*Continued*)
  in amebiasis, *558,* 592, 593
  in dracontiasis, 633
  in giardiasis, *558,* 602
  in malabsorption syndrome, *1536*
  in trichomoniasis, *558,* 603
  in tropical phagedenic ulcer, 530
  warfarin and, simultaneous use of,
    effects of, 2339
Metropathia hemorrhagica, 2193
Metyrapone
  in Cushing's syndrome with adrenal
    tumor, 2156
  in ectopic ACTH syndrome, 2156
MHA-TP test, in syphilis, 514
Mica workers, pneumoconiosis in, 987
Micelles, formation of, 1524
Michaelis-Gutmann bodies, in
  malakoplakia, 1613
Microangiopathic hemolytic anemia,
  1766–1767, *1767*
Microbes, drugs and, 549–553
Microbial diseases, 227–564
  bacterial, 307–535
  chemotherapy of, 549–564
  introduction to, 227–229
  mycotic, 535–549
  nature of, 227
  viral, 229–307
Microbial persistence, 550, 551
Microcirculation
  abnormalities of, hemolysis due to,
    1766–1767, *1767*
  in shock, 1112, 1113
Microhemagglutination assay for
  Treponema pallidum, 514
Microvacuoles, in metabolic brain
  disease, 645
Micturition syncope, 740, 744
Midbrain infarctions, 787–788
Midcervical spine, injuries of, 885
Middle ear
  infection of, brain abscess from, 805
  inflammation of. See *Otitis media.*
  tuberculosis of, 492
"Middle-age spread," 1693
Mid-esophageal diverticulum, 1499
Mid-expiratory flow rate, maximal, 934,
  934
Mid-life crisis, 23, 24
Midline granuloma, 220–221
  vs. Wegener's granulomatosis, 219
Mid-systolic click–late systolic murmur
  syndrome, 1188–1190
Migraine syndrome, 729, **731–732**
  vertiginous, 740
  vs. cerebral transient ischemic
    attacks, 785
Migration inhibition factor, 129
Migratory erythema, necrolytic, *2296,*
  2299
Miliaria crystallina, 2268
Miliaria profunda, 2268
Miliaria rubra, 2268
Miliary tuberculosis, 481, **492–493**
  hematologic disease and, 493
  vs. listeriosis, 473
  vs. psittacosis, 338
  vs. visceral leishmaniasis, 586
Milk, cow's, allergy to, 1499
Milk leg, in thrombophlebitis, 1126
Milk-alkali syndrome, 2237
Millard-Gubler syndrome, 788
Millipedes, dermatitis caused by, 117

Milroy's disease, 1314
Miltown. See *Meprobamate.*
Milzbrand, 470
Mineral(s). See also names of specific minerals.
    blood levels of, in acute infections, 1679
    nutrient value of, 1673–1674
    recommended allowances of, *1671*
Mineral oil
    in constipation, 1482
    vaporized, inhalation of, interstitial pneumonia from, 998, 999
Mineralocorticoids, in Addison's disease, 2150
Miner's anemia, 624–625
Minnesota Multiphasic Personality Inventory, 683
Minocycline, *557,* 562
Minoxidil, in arterial hypertension, *1212,* 1215
Miosis, in idiopathic autonomic insufficiency, 763
Mirizzi's syndrome, 1625
Mite-borne typhus, 327–328
Mites
    housedust, allergy to, 118
    trombiculid, dermatitis caused by, 113
Mithracin. See *Mithramycin.*
Mithramycin, 1937
    in hypercalcemia, 2239
    in hypercalcemia complicating hormonal treatment of breast cancer, 1920
    in Paget's disease, 2259
Mitochondrial function in shock, 1113
Mitogens, in T cell competence assay, 130
Mitomycin-C, 1937
Mitosis, 52, *52,* 53
Mitotane, in oncologic treatment, 1938
Mitotic nondisjunction, 52–53
Mitral regurgitation, 1185–1188
    general physiologic effects of, 1175, *1175*
    vs. aortic stenosis, 1193
    vs. atrial septal defect, 1162
Mitral stenosis, 1179–1185
    general physiologic effects of, *1175,* 1176
    mesenteric artery embolism in, 1589
    pulmonary circulation in, 1145–1146
    pulmonary hypertension and, vs. atrial septal defect, 1162
    silent, pulmonary hypertension and, 1140
    vs. idiopathic pulmonary hemosiderosis, 976
    vs. tricuspid stenosis, 1198
Mitral valve
    disorders of, left atrial hypertension from, 1144, 1145
    replacement of, in aortic stenosis, 1193
    in mitral stenosis, 1185
Mitral valve prolapse syndrome, 1187, 1188–1190
Mixed connective tissue disease, 171, 179
Mixed cryoglobulinemia, vs. periarteritis nodosa, 183
Mixed lymphocyte culture reaction, in T cell function assay, 130

MMPI, 683
Mobile spasms, 760
Molars, in congenital syphilis, 513
Mold(s)
    food contamination by, 69, 70
    spores of, allergic rhinitis from, 157
Mole(s), 2290–2291, *2290*
    hydatidiform, human chorionic gonadotropin levels in, 2181
Molecular biology, clinical medicine and, 7
Molecular disease, 40–44, 1949
Mollaret's meningitis, 842
    vs. bacterial meningitis, 415
Molluscs, stinging, 123, 124
Molluscum contagiosum, 2284
Moloney test, in diphtheria prevention, 433
Molybdenum, nutrient value of, 1674
Monge's disease, 101, 1799
Mongolism. See *Down's syndrome.*
Moniliasis, 547–549
Monkeys, green, in African hemorrhagic fever, 300
Monoamine oxidase inhibitors
    in depression of manic-depressive psychosis, 671
    poisoning by, *712*
    tyramine and, interaction of, hypertension from, 1209
Monoclonal gammopathy, benign, renal changes in, 1406
Monocytes, peripheral blood, increase in number of, 1813
Monocytic and plasmacytic dyscrasias, association between, 1867
Monocytic leukemia
    acute, 1814
    in multiple myeloma, 1867
Monocytopenia, 1812
Mononeuropathy, 900–902
    multiple, 902
Mononucleosis
    cytomegalovirus, 828
        vs. infectious mononucleosis, 267
    infectious, 264–268, *267*
        acute disseminated encephalomyelitis after, 836, 837
        cold agglutinin syndrome following, 1765
        liver disease and, 265, 1656
        vs. acute viral hepatitis, 1653, 1656
        vs. Chagas' disease, 582
        vs. cytomegalovirus mononucleosis, 828
        vs. diphtheria, 431
        vs. listeriosis, 472, 473
        vs. measles, *249*
        vs. psittacosis, 338
        vs. rubella, 252
        vs. secondary syphilis, 510
        vs. streptococcal pharyngitis, 372
        vs. toxoplasmosis, 597
        vs. tularemia, 467
Monosaccharides, malabsorption of, 1539
Montenegro test, in leishmaniasis, 584
"Moonshine" whiskey, lead poisoning caused by, 77
Morbilli, 246–250, *248, 249.* See also *Measles.*
Morerastrongylus costaricensis, 632
Morgagni, foramen of, herniation through, 1019

Morphine, 694–698
    in acute pulmonary edema of heart failure, 1094
    in orchitis complicating mumps, 263
    in pain, 723, 724, *724,* 725
    poisoning by, 75, *712*
Morphine sulfate
    in pain of myocardial infarction, 1233
    in pain of shock, 1117
Morquio's syndrome, *41,* **2052–2053,** *2052*
Mosaicism, 53, 2186
Moschcowitz's syndrome, 1401
Mosquitoes
    Aedes, in California encephalitis, 288
        in dengue, 277
        in dengue hemorrhagic fever, 297
        in eastern equine encephalitis, 286
        in yellow fever, 293, 294
    Anopheles, in malaria, 566, 567, 568
    Culex, in eastern equine encephalitis, 285
        in Japanese B encephalitis, 289, 290
        in Murray Valley encephalitis, 290
        in St. Louis encephalitis, 289
        in Venezuelan equine encephalitis, 286
        in West Nile fever, 278
        in western equine encephalitis, 284
    Haemagogus, in yellow fever, 294
Mossman fever, 327–328
Moths, dermatitis caused by, 118–119
Motilin
    in control of gastrointestinal motility, 1476
    in gastroduodenal motility, 1489
Motility
    colonic, disorders of, 1492–1498
        in ulcerative colitis, 1571
        normal, 1492, *1492,* 1493
    duodenal, disorders of, 1488–1490
        normal, 1488, 1489
    esophageal, disorders of, 1483–1488
        tests of, in achalasia, 1487
    gastric, disorders of, 1488–1490
        normal, 1488, 1489
    gastrointestinal, disorders of, 1475–1502
        pathophysiology and cardinal symptoms of, 1476–1483
        relation of symptoms to, 1476
        hormonal control of, 1476
        normal, 1475–1476
    intestinal, electrical control mechanisms for, 1475
    neural regulatory mechanisms for, 1475, 1476
Motility tests, in constipation, 1481
Motion sickness, 94–95
Motor activity, gastrointestinal. See *Motility.*
Motor and sensory neuropathies, hereditary, 912–913
Motor neuron diseases, 765–766
    after poliomyelitis, 832
    vs. leprosy, 503
    vs. multiple sclerosis, 847
    vs. polymyositis, 174
Motor polyradiculoneuropathy, inflammatory, acute, 906–907. See also *Guillain-Barré syndrome.*
Motor seizure, jacksonian, 855
Mountain sickness
    acute, 101

Mountain sickness (*Continued*)
  chronic, 101, 1799
  subacute, 101
Mouth
  in nutritional deficiency, 1676
  in scleroderma, 169
  procedures in, infective endocarditis
    prophylaxis in, 396
  tuberculosis of, 492
Mouth-to-mouth ventilation, in
  cardiopulmonary arrest, 1054, 1055
6-MP, 1935
mRNA, 31
  in protein synthesis, *32, 33*
MSH, 2090. See also
  Melanocyte-stimulating hormone.
Mucinosis, papular, 1865, *1865*
Mucocutaneous candidiasis, 548
Mucocutaneous leishmaniasis,
  American, *588,* **589**
Mucocutaneous lymph node syndrome,
  534, **2306**
Mucoepidermoid tumors, pulmonary,
  1012
Mucopolysaccharidoses, 2051–2053, *2052*
  aorta in, 1292
Mucopurulent bronchitis, 954
Mucor species, 545
Mucormycosis, 545–546
  in neutropenic patients on
    corticosteroid therapy, 149
  orbital, in diabetes mellitus, 2320
Mucosal cell abnormality,
  malabsorption syndrome from,
  1539–1544
Mucosal pemphigoid, benign, 2304
Mucous colitis, 1493
Mucous membranes
  in host defense, 145
  in host defense compromise, 146
  in syphilis, 509, *509*
Mucoviscidosis, 1559–1560
Mucus, cervical, examination of, 2180
  in infertility, 2194
Müller maneuver, in tricuspid stenosis,
  1198
Müllerian anomalies, amenorrhea from,
  2184, 2185
Multicentric reticulohistiocytosis, 201
Multiceps multiceps, 611
Multicystic kidney, congenital, 1450,
  1451, **1452**
    vs. childhood polycystic kidney
      disease, 1453
Multicystic renal dysplasia, 1452
Multifactorial inheritance, 44–45, *45*
Multifocal fibrosclerosis, 222–224
Multifocal leukoencephalopathy
  progressive, 841–842
    vs. brain tumor, 868
    vs. dementia in cancer, 877
Multifocal myoclonus, in metabolic
  brain disease, 648
Multi-infarct dementia, 661
Multinodular goiter, 2135–2137
  complications of, 2136–2137
Multiple enchondromatosis, 2264
Multiple endocrine adenomatosis, 2098
  detection of, in relatives, *58*
  hypercalcemia in, 2238
  in acromegaly, 2106
Multiple endocrine neoplasia, inherited,
  neuropathy with, 909
Multiple exostosis, hereditary, *1910,*
  2264, 2265

Multiple lipomatosis, 1697
Multiple lipoprotein–type
  hyperlipidemia, familial, 2007–2008
Multiple mononeuropathy, 902
Multiple myeloma, 1858–1862
  acute renal failure in, 1369
  cutaneous manifestations of, *2300,*
    2302
  electrophoretic patterns in, 1855, *1856*
  monocytic leukemia in, 1867
  neuropathy with, 910, 1860
    vs. acute inflammatory
      polyneuropathy, 907
  renal changes in, 1404–1405
  vascular purpura in, 1880
  vs. hyperparathyroidism, 2217
Multiple sclerosis, 845–848
  hearing loss in, 736
  HLA system and, 39
  pathogenesis of, 844
  possible variants of, 848–850
  possible viral cause of, 842
  symptoms and signs of, *846, 847*
  vertigo from, 739, 740
  vs. acute disseminated
    encephalomyelitis, 838
  vs. amyotrophic lateral sclerosis, 766
  vs. Friedreich's ataxia, 768
  vs. hysteria, 679
  vs. vitamin B_{12} deficiency, 776, 777
Multisensory dizziness, 741, 742
Mumps, 261–264
  acute disseminated encephalomyelitis
    after, 836, 837
Mumps meningitis, 262
Mumps virus, 261
  meningitis and encephalitis from,
    262, 818, *818, 819*
Mumps virus vaccine, 263
Munchausen syndrome, 678
Muramidase, secretion of, in acute
  myelocytic leukemia, 1816
Murchison type fever, in Hodgkin's
  disease, 1841
Murine typhus fever, 320–321
  clinical features of, *313*
  epidemiologic features of, *310*
Murmur(s)
  Austin Flint, in aortic regurgitation,
    1196
    vs. mitral stenosis, 1183
  in angina pectoris, 1225
  in aortic regurgitation, 1195, 1196
  in aortic stenosis, 1192
    congenital valvular, 1156
    discrete subvalvular, 1167
  in asymmetric septal hypertrophy,
    1278
  in atrial septal defect, 1161
  in carditis of rheumatic fever, 380
  in coarctation of aorta, 1158, 1290
  in congenital aneurysms of sinuses of
    Valsalva, 1170
  in congenital pulmonary
    arteriovenous fistula, 1168, 1169
  in Ebstein's anomaly, 1168
  in Fallot's tetralogy, 1165
  in hyperthyroidism, 2122
  in infective endocarditis, 389
  in mitral regurgitation, 1186
  in mitral stenosis, 1181, 1182
  in mitral valve prolapse syndrome,
    1188, 1189
  in myocardial infarction, 1230
  in patent ductus arteriosus, 1163

Murmur(s) (*Continued*)
  in pulmonic regurgitation, 1199
  in pulmonic stenosis, 1159
    supravalvular, 1168
  in tricuspid regurgitation, 1198
  in tricuspid stenosis, 1197, 1198
  vs. pericardial friction rub, 1272
Murray Valley encephalitis, 290
Muscle(s)
  anaerobic infection of, 443
  biopsy of, in differentiation of
    neurogenic and myopathic
    disease, 915
    in polymyositis and
      dermatomyositis, 172
    in trichinosis, 630, 631
  cramps in, 930
    in chronic renal failure, 1365
    in maintenance hemodialysis, 1381
  diseases of, 914–930
    inherited, 915–922
    primary, vs. amyotrophic lateral
      sclerosis, 766
    respiratory failure in, 1024
    sporadic, 923–930
  heart as, 1087
  in dystrophies, 916
  in radicular syndromes, 889
  in rheumatoid arthritis, 187, 188
  in scleroderma, 168, 169
  nonmetastatic effects of cancer on,
    879
  overactivity of, syndromes of, 930
  pain in, in nonparalytic poliomyelitis,
    830
  papillary, malfunction of, in
    myocardial infarction, 1231
  rigidity of, 751
    in paralysis agitans, 752
    in tetanus, 438
  weakness of, in cancer, 879
    in myasthenia gravis, 926
    in peripheral neuropathy, 903, 904
    in polymyositis and
      dermatomyositis, 172
Muscle fiber activity, continuous, 930
Muscle spasm(s)
  in paraplegia, 888
  in tetanus, 439, 440
Muscle tone, alterations in, 751
    in arteriosclerotic pseudo-
      parkinsonism, 754
Muscle-contraction headaches, 732
Muscular atrophy
  peroneal, vs. muscular dystrophies,
    918
  progressive, 765
Muscular dystrophy(ies), 915–918
  Becker, 917
  Duchenne, 915, 916, *916,* 917, 918
    cardiomyopathy in, 1280, 1281
    heterozygote detection in, 57, 58, *58*
  fascioscapulohumeral, 915, *916,* 917
  limb-girdle, 915, *916,* 917
  myotonic, 915, *916,* 917, 918
    cardiomyopathy in, 1281
    testicular atrophy in, 2170
  ocular, 918
  respiratory failure in, 1024
  vs. polymyositis, 173, 923
Muscular subaortic stenosis, 1278
Musculature, pubertal increase of, 18
Musculoskeletal system
  changes in, with aging, 27
  in Cushing's syndrome, 2154

Musculoskeletal system (*Continued*)
in maintenance hemodialysis, 1381
in paraplegia, 887
in scleroderma, 169
in systemic lupus erythematosus, 176
Mushroom worker's lung, *971*
Mushrooms
"magic," 704
poisoning by, 69
Mutation, genetic, selection and, 47
Mutism
akinetic, in midbrain infarctions, 787
vs. aphasia, 656
Myalgia
epidemic, 271–272
in influenza, 243
in periarteritis nodosa, 182
Myalgic encephalomyelitis, benign, 307
vs. poliomyelitis, 831
Myasthenia gravis, 925–929
bulbar, vs. hysteria, 679
crisis in, management of, 928, 929
immune mechanisms in, 133
respiratory failure in, 1024
vs. Eaton-Lambert syndrome, 929
vs. familial periodic paralysis, 921
Myasthenic syndrome, 929
cancer and, 879
Mycetoma, 542
Mycobacteria
"atypical," 498
clinically important, differentiation of, 480
diseases due to, 479–505
hypercalcemia in, 2238
other than *M. tuberculosis* and *M.
***leprae*, 498–500**
scotochromogenic, 480
Mycobacterium aquae, pulmonary disease caused by, 499
Mycobacterium avium, 480, 498
disseminated infection caused by, 500
lymphadenitis caused by, 500
pulmonary disease caused by, 499
Mycobacterium bovis, 479, 480
Mycobacterium chelonei
injection abscesses caused by, 500
pulmonary disease caused by, 499
Mycobacterium fortuitum, 498
disseminated infection caused by, 500
injection abscesses caused by, 500
pulmonary disease caused by, 499
Mycobacterium intracellulare, 480, 498
disseminated infection caused by, 500
lymphadenitis caused by, 500
pulmonary disease caused by, 499
Mycobacterium kansasii, 480, 498
disseminated infection caused by, 500
lymphadenitis caused by, 500
pulmonary disease caused by, 499
Mycobacterium leprae, 501
Mycobacterium marinum, 480, 498
skin infections caused by, 500
Mycobacterium scrofulaceum, 498
disseminated infection caused by, 500
lymphadenitis caused by, 500
pulmonary disease caused by, 499
Mycobacterium simiae, pulmonary disease caused by, 499
Mycobacterium szulgai, pulmonary disease caused by, 499
Mycobacterium tuberculosis, 479, 480
Mycobacterium ulcerans, skin infections caused by, 500

Mycobacterium xenopi, 498
pulmonary disease caused by, 499
Mycoplasma hominis, 346, 347
***Mycoplasma pneumoniae*, 343, 344**
respiratory diseases caused by, 343–346. See also *Mycoplasmal pneumonia.*
Mycoplasmal diseases, 343–347
genitourinary, 346–347
Mycoplasmal pneumonia, 343–346
cold agglutinin syndrome following, 1765
vs. coccidioidomycosis, 539
vs. pneumococcal pneumonia, 354
vs. psittacosis, 338
vs. tularemia, 467
Mycoplasmas
human, *343*
properties of, 343
T-, 346, 347
Mycoses, 535–549
antimicrobial agents for, *556–557*
superficial, vs. onchocerciasis, 636
vs. leprosy, 503
vs. listeriosis, 473
vs. melioidosis, 470
vs. pulmonary tuberculosis, 486
Mycosis fungoides, 2309–2310
Mycotic aneurysms
in infective endocarditis, 389, 390
intracranial hemorrhage from, 795
Mycotic arthritis, 186
Mycotoxicoses, 535
Mycotoxins, 69, 70
Mydriasis, in idiopathic autonomic insufficiency, 763
Myelin
biology of, 843
disorders of, 843, *843*
Myelin basic protein, 844
Myelinoclasis, perivascular, acute, 836
Myelinolysis, central pontine, 775–776
Myelitis
acute, vs. spinal epidural abscess, 811
transverse, 811–812, *811*
acute, 849
during nonpolio enteroviral infections, 270
vs. tick paralysis, 118
Myeloblastic leukemia, 1814
Myeloblasts, in acute leukemia, 1815
Myelocathexis, 1810
Myelocytic leukemia
acute, 1814
epidemiology of, 1816
pathogenesis of, 1816
treatment of, 1819, 1820
chronic, 1821–1824
subacute, vs. aplastic anemia, 1738
Myeloencephalitis, vs. meningococcal meningitis, 420, 421
Myelofibrosis with myeloid metaplasia, 1827
vs. chronic granulocytic leukemia, 1822
Myelogenous leukemia, chronic, 1821–1824
Myelography, 749
in intervertebral disc protrusion, 894
in intraspinal compression, 892
in transverse myelitis, 812
Myeloid leukemia, chronic, 1821–1824
Myeloid metaplasia
agnogenic, 1827–1829
portal hypertension in, 1639

Myeloid metaplasia (*Continued*)
agnogenic, vs. myelophthisic anemia, 1742
myelofibrosis with, 1827
vs. chronic granulocytic leukemia, 1822
Myeloma
multiple, 1858–1862
acute renal failure in, 1369
cutaneous manifestations of, *2300, 2302*
electrophoretic patterns in, 1855, *1856*
monocytic leukemia in, 1867
neuropathy with, 910, 1860
vs. acute inflammatory polyneuropathy, 907
renal changes in, 1404–1405
vascular purpura in, 1880
vs. hyperparathyroidism, 2217
plasma cell, 1858–1862
Myelomatosis, 1858–1862
Myelomeningocele, frequency and sex ratio of, *48*
Myelomonocytic leukemia, 1814
acute, in Hodgkin's disease, 1842, 1843
Myelopathy
cervical, 895
in cancer, 878
necrotizing, subacute, 849
radiation, 870
spondylosis causing, 894–895
transverse, **811–812,** *811*
Myeloperoxidase, 1802
deficiency of, *43,* **1806**
Myelophthisic anemia, 1742
in cancer patient, 1906
therapeutic principles in, 1719
vs. aplastic anemia, 1738
Myeloproliferative disorders, 1826–1829
Myeloptical neuropathy, subacute, 910
Myelosclerosis, vs. myelophthisic anemia, 1742
Myelosis, pseudoleukemic-pseudoerythremic, 1827
Myerson's sign, in paralysis agitans, 752
Myiasis, 111–112
Myleran. See *Busulfan.*
Myoadenylate deaminase deficiency, 2043
Myoblastomas, granular cell, of lung, 1013
Myocardial contractility, decreased, in shock, 1109, 1110
Myocardial depressant factors, in shock, 1110, 1114
Myocardial dysfunction, left ventricular, in aortic stenosis, 1191
Myocardial failure, 1080. See also *Heart failure.*
in louse-borne relapsing fever, 528
Myocardial infarction, 1223, 1229–1237
air travel after, 96
after myocardial revascularization procedures, 1240, 1241
clinical course of, 1230
clinical features of, 1229
complicating maintenance hemodialysis, 1381, 1382
complications of, early, 1230
late, 1237
surgical intervention in, 1239, 1240
diabetes mellitus and, 1981

Myocardial infarction (*Continued*)
diagnosis of, 1231
differential diagnosis of, 1232
digitalis in, 1099, 1100
Dressler's syndrome after, 1237, 1271
etiology and pathology of, 1229
oral contraceptive use and, 2195
pathophysiology of, 1229
pericarditis associated with, 1231, 1270, 1271
physical examination in, 1230
prognosis in, 1233
recurrent, prevention of, 1236
treatment of, 1233
unstable angina preceding, 1228
vs. acute appendicitis, 1581
vs. acute pericarditis, 1273
vs. angina pectoris, 1227
vs. dissecting aortic aneurysm, 1296
vs. peptic ulcer, 1507
vs. pulmonary embolism, 1133
Myocardial ischemia, in shock, 1110
Myocardial revascularization, surgical, 1238–1241
Myocardial sarcoidosis, 213
Myocarditis, 1281–1283
bacterial, 1282
diphtheritic, 431, 432, 1282
drug-induced, 1287
enteroviruses causing, 272–273
giant cell, 1283
in Chagas' disease, 581, 582, 583, 1283
in infective endocarditis, 389
in influenza, 243
in leptospirosis, 534
in mumps, 263
in potassium deficiency, 1284
in systemic lupus erythematosus, 177, 180
puerperal, 1287
radiation, 1287
Toxoplasma, 1282, 1283
viral, 1281, 1282
Myocardium
diseases of, 1276–1288
in infarction, 1229, 1231
Myochrysine. See *Sodium aurothiomalate.*
Myoclonic seizures, 854
Myoclonus, multifocal, in metabolic brain disease, 648
Myoclonus epilepsy, 854
Myofascial pain syndromes, 728
Myoglobin, 1743
Myoglobinuria
familial, 920–921
in alcoholic persons, 924
sporadic, 924–925
Myokymia, 930
facial, 900
Myonecrosis
clostridial, 433–435
differential diagnosis of, *435*
hyperbaric oxygen therapy in, 104
streptococcal, anaerobic, 434
treatment of, 435
vs. clostridial myonecrosis, *435*
Myopathy(ies), 914–930
acquired, 923–924
alcoholic, 924
carcinomatous, 923
centronuclear, 919
congenital, 919–920
distal, 918

Myopathy(ies) (*Continued*)
in bronchogenic carcinoma, 1007
in chronic renal failure, 1365
in multiple myeloma, 1860
inherited, 915–922
metabolic, vs. polymyositis, 174
myotubular, 919
nemaline, 919
rod, 919
thyrotoxic, 923
Myositis ossificans, 922
Myotonia congenita, 920
Myotonic muscular dystrophy, 915, *916, 917, 918*
cardiomyopathy in, 1281
testicular atrophy in, 2170
Myotonic pupil, Adie's, 900
Myotubular myopathy, 919
Myringitis, in mycoplasmal pneumonia, 344, 345, 346
Myxedema, 2132–2135
ascites in, 1593
hereditary factor in, 2121
pretibial, in Graves' disease, 2127, *2128*
primary, vs. hypopituitarism, 2102
Myxedema coma, 2134
Myxedema heart, 2134, 2135
Myxedema madness, 2133
Myxoma
atrial, left, vs. mitral stenosis, 1183
vs. infective endocarditis, 392
cardiac, 1288
Myxoviruses
associated with common cold, *230*
influenza from, 241

NADH–methemoglobin reductase deficiency, methemoglobinemia due to, 1780, 1781, 1782
Naegleria gruberi, 603, 604
Nafcillin, *557, 559*
in bacterial meningitis, 415
in infective endocarditis, 393
in infective endocarditis prophylaxis, 396
in osteomyelitis, 2261
in staphylococcal meningitis, 404
in staphylococcal pneumonia, 402
Nail(s)
in hyperthyroidism, 2122
in hypoparathyroidism, 2221
in iron deficiency anemia, 1748
Nail-patella syndrome, *2301*
Nalidixic acid, *556, 563*
Naloxone, in opiate poisoning, *712*
Naloxone HCl, in morphine poisoning, 75
Naltrexone, 698
Nandrolone decanoate, in anemia of chronic renal failure, 1364
Naproxen, in rheumatoid arthritis, 191
Narcolepsy, 653, 654
Narcotic analgesics, 694–698, 723, 724, *724*
Narcotic antagonists, 698
Nardil. See *Phenelzine.*
Nasal cannulas or prongs, for oxygenation in acute respiratory failure, 1027
Nasal diphtheria, anterior, 431
Nasal leeches, as agents of disease, 120

Nasal procedures, infective endocarditis prophylaxis in, 396
Nasal septum, in relapsing polychondritis, 218
Nasal structures, as sources of headache, 733
Nasogastric aspiration, in hemorrhage of peptic ulcer, 1516
Nasopharyngeal diphtheria, 431
Nasopharynx, in common cold, 232
Nausea, 1477
in chronic renal failure, 1364, 1365
in intracranial tumors, 865
in motion sickness, 94
Near-drowning, 105–108
Necator americanus, 559, 624
life cycle of, *621*
Neck
dermatologic diseases of, 2278–2279
in nutritional deficiency, 1676
stiff, in intracranial hemorrhage, treatment of, 800
in intracranial tumors, 865
in stupor or coma, 643
in subarachnoid hemorrhage, 797
veins of, examination of, in cardiovascular disease, 1073, *1073*
Necrobiosis lipoidica diabeticorum, 1980
Necrolysis, toxic epidermal, 2306
staphylococcal, 400
Necrolytic migratory erythema, *2296, 2299*
Necrosis
aseptic, of bone, after renal transplantation, 1385
fat, nodular, *2299*
papillary, in sickle cell hemoglobinopathy, 1404
renal cortical, acute renal failure from, 1368
renal medullary, 1412–1413
renal papillary, 1412–1413
acute renal failure from, 1369
in sickle cell hemoglobinopathy, 1404
vs. medullary sponge kidney, 1456
tubular, acute, 1367–1375
differential diagnosis of, 1373
pathogenesis of, 1369
pathologic physiology of, 1370
pathology of, 1370
prevention of, 1374
prognosis in, 1374
volume depletion in, 1951
Necrotizing angiitis, 165
classification of, 166–167, *166*
generalized, vs. classic periarteritis nodosa, 183
hepatitis B antigenemia and, 181
incidence of, at necropsy, *181*
Necrotizing angiopathy, 902
neuropathy associated with, 908
Necrotizing arteritis, in rheumatoid arthritis, 187
Necrotizing hemorrhagic encephalomyelitis, acute, 849
Necrotizing myelopathy, subacute, 849
Necrotizing nodular scleritis, 2315
Necrotizing papillitis, 1412–1413
Necrotizing pseudomembranous enterocolitis, acute, 405
Necrotizing sclerokeratitis, in periarteritis nodosa, 2317

Needle biopsy
of liver, 1647–1648
thyroid, 2119
Neisseria, **diseases caused by, 404–410**
Neisseria gonorrhoeae, 405, 406
in infective endocarditis, 387
Neisseria meningitidis
in bacterial meningitis, 411
in meningococcal disease, 417
Nelson's syndrome, 2098
Nemaline myopathy, 919
Nematodes, 621–637
intestinal, 622–630
antimicrobial agents for, *559*
life cycle of, *621*
prevalence of, *605*
prevalence of, *605*
tissue, 630–637
antimicrobial agents for, *559*
prevalence of, *605*
Nembutal. See *Pentobarbital.*
Neomycin, *556*, 561
adverse reactions to, 562
as nephrotoxin, 1425
in hepatic coma complicating
cirrhosis, 1666
malabsorption caused by, 1548
neuromuscular block caused by, 929
Neoplasia
associated with dust exposure,
994–995
meningeal, diffuse, 867
multiple endocrine, inherited,
neuropathy with, 909
Neoplasms. See also names of specific
neoplasms and of areas or
structures involved.
lymphoreticular, 1829–1848
classification of, *1830*
renal injury from, 1330
Neoplastic meningitis, cerebrospinal
fluid findings in, *803*
Neostigmine
in diagnosis of myasthenia gravis,
927
in diagnosis of neonatal myasthenia,
927
in myasthenia gravis, 928
Neovascular glaucoma, in diabetes
mellitus, 2321
Nephritic syndrome, acute, 1333–1334
Nephritis
anti-tubular basement membrane
antibody–mediated, *1324*, 1325
epimembranous, 1393
hereditary, 1402
in systemic lupus erythematosus, 177
interstitial, 1416–1422
chronic, etiologic types of,
1418–1422
idiopathic, 1422
penicillin-induced, 1426, 1427
poststreptococcal, acute, 1394
potassium-losing, vs. familial
periodic paralysis, 922
radiation, 1435
Nephroblastoma, 1460
Nephrocalcinosis, 1443
Nephrocarcinoma, 1458–1460
Nephrogenic diabetes insipidus,
1435–1437, 2064, 2110, 2111
Nephrolithiasis, 1443–1446
uric acid, 2030, 2037
treatment of, 2041
vs. hyperparathyroidism, 2217

Nephroma, mesoblastic, congenital,
1460
Nephron, distal, function of, 1319, 1320,
1320
Nephronophthisis, juvenile, familial,
1454
Nephronophthisis–cystic renal medulla
complex, 1454–1455
Nephropathy(ies)
analgesic, 1409, 1412, **1419–1420**
chronic renal failure and, 1352
Balkan, 1421–1422
diabetic, 1403, 1977, 1979
acute renal failure in, 1369
gouty, **1420–1421,** 2037, 2038
treatment of, 1421, 2040, 2041
hypercalcemic, 1438–1440
hypokalemic, 1437–1438
interstitial, 1416–1422
etiologic classification of, *1416*
metal, **1428–1431,** *1428*
obstructive, **1418–1419, 1447–1450**
causes of, *1448*
postobstructive, volume depletion in,
1951
reflux, 1409
toxic, **1328–1329,** *1328,* **1422–1435**
clinical syndromes associated with,
1424–1425
incidence of, 1423
pathogenic mechanisms in,
1423–1424, *1424*
urate, 1420–1421
uric acid, 1440
complicating treatment of
non-Hodgkin's lymphomas, 1837
Nephroptosis, 1457
Nephrosis, 1387
lipoid, 1327, **1391–1393**
quartan, 572
Nephrosonephritis, hemorrhagic, *293,*
301–302
Nephrotic syndrome, 1335, 1387–1390
causes of, 1387, *1387,* 1388
hypercholesterolemia in, 2009
in malaria, 572
in mercury poisoning, 80
in pregnancy, 1389, 1390, 1414
in systemic lupus erythematosus, 177
renal biopsy in, 1346
renal vein thrombosis in, 1408
toxic nephropathy with, 1425
vs. idiopathic membranous
glomerular disease, 1393
Nephrotoxins, 1425–1435
Nerve(s)
abducens, disorders of, 899
biopsy of, in peripheral neuropathy,
905
cranial, disorders of, 899–900
in bacterial meningitis, 412
in head injury, 883
nonmetastatic effects of cancer on,
876–878
facial, disorders of, 900
hypoglossal, disorders of, 900
in leprosy, 502, *502,* 503
oculomotor, disorders of, 899
olfactory, disorders of, 899
optic, disorders of, 899, **2327–2329**
glioma of, 868
in sarcoidosis, 2329
in sickle cell diseases, 2331
peripheral
in rheumatoid arthritis, 187, 189

Nerve(s) (*Continued*)
peripheral, nonmetastatic effects of
cancer on, 878
peroneal, acute and tardy palsy of,
902
radial, acute palsy of, 901, 902
trigeminal, disorders of, 900
trochlear, disorders of, 899
ulnar, palsy of, tardy, 901
Nerve blocks, in pain relief, 726
Nerve conduction, measurement of
in carpal tunnel syndrome, 901
in differential diagnosis of
neuropathy, 904
in differentiation of neurogenic and
myopathic disease, 915
Nerve growth factor, in
neurofibromatosis, 770
Nerve roots
compression of
disorders causing, 893
laboratory aids in, 892–893
management of, 893
spondylosis causing, 894
symptoms of, 889–892, *889, 890*
mechanical lesions of, 889–898
Nervous colon, 1493
Nervous system
autonomic, in diabetes mellitus, 1980
in heart failure, 1088
in tetanus, 439
behavior and, disorders of, 639–930
central
acute leukemia in, treatment of,
1818
depressants of, abuse of, 698–701
poisoning by, *712*
disorders of, amenorrhea due to,
2187–2188
in acute radiation syndrome, 88, 90
in acute renal failure, 1371, 1372
in alcohol abuse, 709
in arboviral encephalitis, 283
in cat scratch disease, 303, 304
in Colorado tick fever, 280
in meningococcal infections, 420
in periarteritis nodosa, 182
in Rocky Mountain spotted fever,
323
in schistosomiasis, 615
in systemic lupus erythematosus,
180
in western equine encephalitis, 285
infections and inflammatory
diseases of, 802–816
in cancer patient, 1901, 1903
lipidoses of, 850–851
stimulants of, abuse of, 701–702
poisoning by, *712*
suppurative diseases of,
cerebrospinal fluid findings in,
803
surgery of, in pain relief, 726, 727
syphilis of, 812–816. See also
Neurosyphilis.
vascular accident to, in diabetes
mellitus, 1980
changes in, with aging, 27
degenerative diseases of, inherited,
764–772
granulomas affecting, 864
higher functions of, focal
disturbances of, 656–659
in diabetes mellitus, 1979, 1980
in diphtheria, 432

Nervous system (*Continued*)
in scleroderma, 170
mycoplasmal infection of, 345
nonmetastatic effects of cancer on, 876–879, *877*
nutritional disorders of, 772–777
peripheral, diseases of, 899–913
in periarteritis nodosa, 182
radiation injury of, 869–870
slow infections of, 839–843
sympathetic, 2199–2207
hormones of, 2199–2201
viral diseases of, 816–843
Neural regulatory mechanisms for intestinal motility, 1475, 1476
Neuralgia
facial, atypical, 731
glossopharyngeal, 727
postherpetic, 728, 826
rectal, vs. proctalgia fugax, 1497
spreading, post-traumatic, 727
trigeminal, 727
Neurilemmoma, hearing loss from, 736
Neuritis
in malabsorption syndrome, 1530
intraocular, 848
optic, 848–849
acute, in cancer, 878
complicating ethambutol therapy of pulmonary tuberculosis, 488
peripheral, drugs causing, 156
in diphtheria, 432
vs. polymyositis, 173
retrobulbar, 848–849
Neuroblastoma(s), 2206, 2207
vs. nephroblastoma, 1460
Neurocirculatory asthenia, vs. angina pectoris, 1227
Neurocutaneous syndromes, 769–771
Neurodermatitis, vs. pinta, 525
Neuroendocrine control of puberty, 19, 20
Neuroendocrine diseases of pituitary gland, 2078–2081
Neuroendocrine transducers, 2074, *2075*
Neurofibromas
in neurofibromatosis, 769, 770
spinal cord, 896, 897
Neurofibromatosis, 769–770, *1910*
Crowe's sign of, 2290
skin in, 770, **2293–2294,** *2293, 2297, 2300*
vs. leprosy, 504
Neurologic diagnostic procedures, 746–750
Neurologic disorders
dysphagia in, 1483
hypothalamus and, 715–719
in acute intermittent porphyria, 2045
in adult celiac disease, 1541
in bronchogenic carcinoma, 1007
in heroin abuse, 697
in infective endocarditis, 390, 809
in multiple myeloma, 1860
in non-Hodgkin's lymphomas, 1834
in nonpolio enteroviral infections, 270
in regional enteritis, 1564
in systemic lupus erythematosus, 177
in tick-borne relapsing fever, 529
Neurologic examination, in epilepsy, 857
Neurologic symptoms, management of, 720–746

Neuroma, acoustic, 868
hearing loss from, 736
Neuromuscular block, unusual causes of, 929
Neuromuscular disorders, respiratory failure in, *1023,* 1024
Neuromuscular excitability, increased, after poliomyelitis, 832
Neuromuscular form of lead poisoning, 78
Neuromuscular junction
diseases of, 914–930
nonmetastatic effects of cancer on, 879
Neuromyasthenia
epidemic, 307
vs. poliomyelitis, 831
Neuromyelitis optica, 849
"Neuromyositis," 173
Neuromyotonia, 930
Neuron(s)
hypophysiotropic, 2074–2076
biogenic amine control of, 2076–2077
peripheral, inherited disorders of, 911
peripheral sensory, disorders of, 911–912
Neuronitis, vestibular, 738
Neuroparalytic accidents following antirabies vaccination, 838–839
Neuropathic joint disease, 200
Neuropathy(ies)
alcoholic, 772–773
esophagus in, 1488
ataxic, in diabetes mellitus, 908
autonomic, 909
inflammatory, acute, 907
diabetic, **908–909,** 1979, 1980
Charcot joints in, 200
esophagus in, 1488
vs. acute abdomen, 1581
femoral, 902, 909
hyperalgesic, 908, 909
hypertrophic, dominantly inherited, 912
recessively inherited, 913
lepromatous, vs. syringomyelia, 769
myeloptical, subacute, 910
optic, ischemic, in giant cell arteritis, 2319
peripheral, 899–913
alcohol-related, 709
diabetes mellitus and, 908–909, 1979, 1980. See also *Neuropathy(ies), diabetic.*
differential diagnosis of, 903–905
glossitis and, in malabsorption syndrome, 1529
in bronchogenic carcinoma, 1007
in chronic renal failure, 1365
in multiple myeloma, 910, 1860
respiratory failure in, *1023,* 1024
symptoms of, 903, 904
vs. amyotrophic lateral sclerosis, 766
vs. idiopathic autonomic insufficiency, 763
vs. myasthenia gravis, 927
vs. radiculopathy, 889, *890, 891*
with carcinoma, 910
with drug use, 910
with endocrine diseases, 909
with hepatic disease, 909

Neuropathy(ies) (*Continued*)
peripheral, with household and industrial poisons, 910
with infection, 905–906
with inflammation and presumed altered immunity, 906
with mesenchymal disease and necrotizing angiopathy, 908
with uremia, 909
plexus, 902–903
retrobulbar, nutritional, 774–775
sacral plexus, 902, 903
diabetic, 909
sarcoid, 908
sensory, hereditary, 911–912
vs. leprosy, 504
in cancer, 878
serum sickness, 906
vs. myopathies, 914–915
Neuropsychiatric abnormalities associated with liver disease, 1640–1641
Neurosarcoidosis, 213
Neurosecretion, hypothalamic, 2074–2076
Neurosis, anxiety, vs. angina pectoris, 1227
Neurosyphilis, 511, 512, **812–816**
Argyll Robertson pupil in, 512, 814, 815
asymptomatic, 511, 812, 813
congenital, 815–816
follow-up examinations in, 517
treatment of, 516, 816
Neurotensin, 2077, *2078*
Neurotic symptoms, 665, **672–680**
Neurovascular accidents, oral contraceptives and, 2195
Neurovascular dystrophy, reflex, 206
Neutropenia, 1807–1812
chronic benign, 1810
congenital, 1809, 1810
cyclic, 1810
in cancer patient with infection, 1901
infections in, *148,* 149
"pseudo," 1808
Neutrophil(s)
dysfunction of, syndromes of, 1803–1807, *1803*
function of, 1800–1802, *1801*
kinetics of, 1807, 1808
metabolism of, 1802, *1802*
response of, to microbial invasion, 1801, *1801*
transfusion of, in neutropenia, 1811
Neutrophil function tests, in chronic granulomatous disease, 1805
Neutrophilic dermatosis, febrile, acute, 2295
Neutrophilic leukemoid reactions, 1813
Nevoid basal cell syndrome, *1910*
Nevoid lentigines, 2290
Nevus(i)
congenital, 2312
internal malignancy and, *2297*
facial, in tuberous sclerosis, 770, 771
halo, 2291
intradermal, *2290,* 2291
melanoma arising in, 2312
pigmented, 2290–2291, *2290*
Spitz, 2312
Nevus spilus, 2290, *2290*

Newborn(s)
  hemolytic disease of, 131, **1763**
    kernicterus in, 1754
  hemorrhagic disease of, 1889
  hypocalcemia in, 2241
  impaired bilirubin conjugation in, 1649
  inclusion conjunctivitis of, 333
  jaundice in, 1638
  maternal diabetes and, 1988, 1989
  maternal varicella and, 254
  myasthenia gravis in, 927
  myocarditis of, enteroviral, 272, 273
  polycystic kidney disease in, 1453
  pulmonary arteries in, 1135
  purpura in, 1876
Newborn nursery epidemics, antimicrobial prophylaxis in, *564*
Nezelof's syndrome, 141
Niacin
  deficiency of. See also *Pellagra.*
    clinical signs of, *1677*
  nutrient value of, 1672
  recommended allowances of, *1671*
Niacinamide, in pellagra, 1688
Niclosamide, in tapeworm infections, *559*, 608, 609
Nicotinic acid
  in familial hypercholesterolemia, 2005
  in mixed hypertriglyceridemia, 2007
Niemann-Pick disease, *42, 2013,* **2014–2015**
Nifurtimox
  in Chagas' disease, 583
  in trypanosomiasis, *558*
Night terrors, 655
Nightshade, poisoning by, 70
Nigrospinodentatal degeneration, 765
Nikolsky's sign, 2303
  in pemphigus vulgaris, 2303
  in scalded skin syndrome, 400
  in toxic epidermal necrolysis, 2306
Niridazole, in schistosomiasis, *559,* 616
Nissl granules, dissolution of, in metabolic brain disease, 645
Nitrofurantoin, *556,* 563
  neuropathy from, 910
  pulmonary hypersensitivity reactions from, 975
Nitrofurazone, in African trypanosomiasis, 579
Nitrogen, oxides of, exposure to, pulmonary edema from, 1001
Nitrogen mustards, in oncologic treatment, 1931, 1932
Nitrogen narcosis, 103
Nitroglycerine
  in angina pectoris, 1228
  in heart failure, 1101, *1101*
Nitroprusside, in shock, 1121
Nitrosoureas, 1932, 1933
  in Hodgkin's disease, 1846
Nitrous oxide, recreational inhalation of, 705
Njovera, 522–523
Nocardia asteroides, 475
Nocardia brasiliensis
  in maduromycosis, 542
  in nocardiosis, 475
Nocardia caviae, 475
Nocardiosis, 474–475
Nocturnal dyspnea, paroxysmal, in left ventricular failure, 1090

Nocturnal hemoglobinuria, paroxysmal, **1768–1769**
  acute leukemia in, 1814
  aplastic anemia and, 1734, 1737
Nodose lesions of leg, 2295
Nodular collagenous pneumoconioses, **988–990**
Nodular fat necrosis, *2299*
Nodular goiter, toxic, 2136
Nodular liquefying panniculitis, 2295, *2297*
Nodular melanoma, 2311, *2311*
Nodular nonsuppurative panniculitis, **relapsing febrile, 221–222**
Nodular scleritis, necrotizing, 2315
Nodules
  episcleral rheumatoid, 2314, 2315
  subcutaneous, in rheumatic fever, 381
  subcutaneous or periosteal, in rheumatoid arthritis, 187, 188
Noise, hearing loss from, 736
Nonallelic genes, 40, *44*
Nonarticular rheumatism, 207–208
Nonbacterial endocarditis, verrucous, in systemic lupus erythematosus, 176, 177
Nonbacterial gastroenteritis, infectious, **acute, 305–306**
Nonbacterial regional lymphadenitis, **benign, 302–305,** *303, 304*
Nonbacterial thrombotic endocarditis, 387
  in cancer patient, 1905
  vs. infective endocarditis, 392
''Noncarcinoid'' tumor, carcinoid features of, 2212
Nonchromaffin paraganglioma, 867
Nonclostridial crepitant cellulitis, 434
Noncollagenous pneumoconioses, 984, **987–988,** *987*
Noncommunicating hydrocephalus, 873
Nondisjunction
  meiotic, 51–52, *52*
  mitotic, 52–53
Nonfluent aphasia, 656
Nongranulomatous ileojejunitis, 1542
  vs. eosinophilic gastroenteritis, 1543
Non-Hodgkin's lymphomas, 1830–1838
  clinical manifestations of, 1832
  epidemiology of, 1831
  etiology of, 1830
  lungs as primary site of, 1011, 1012
  pathology of, 1831
  prognosis in, 1837
  staging in, 1834, *1834*
  treatment of, 1835
Nonketotic hyperglycinemia, *41, 2017*
Nonketotic hyperosmolar coma, volume depletion in, 1951
Nonparalytic poliomyelitis, 829, 830
Nonpolio enteroviruses
  distinctive features of, 268–269
  infections with
    general aspects of, 269–270, *269*
    paralysis and other neurologic **complications of, 270**
Nonpuerperal galactorrhea, 2108
Nonreactive tuberculosis, 492, 493
Nonreticular neoplasms, plasma cell dyscrasia associated with, 1866–1867
Nonsporeforming anaerobic bacteria, **disease due to, 441–445**
Nonstreptococcal exudative pharyngitis, 237

Nonsuppurative meningitis, cerebrospinal fluid findings in, *803*
Nonsuppurative panniculitis, febrile **nodular, relapsing, 221–222**
Nonsyphilitic treponematoses, 518–525, *520*
Nonthrombocytopenic drug purpura, 1880
Nontropical sprue, 1539
  osteomalacia in, 2249
Nonvenereal childhood syphilis, **522–523**
Norepinephrine, 2199, 2200, *2200*
  in shock, 1115, 1119, 1120
  metabolic effects of, 2201
  pharmacology of, 2200, 2201
  secretion of, 2201
Norepinephrine-depleting agents, in arterial hypertension, *1212,* 1214
Norethandrolone, intrahepatic cholestasis caused by, 1658
Normochromic normocytic anemias, **1729–1742**
Normogammaglobulinemia, immunodeficiency with, *139*
Normogonadotropic normoestrogenic anovulation, 2193
North American blastomycosis, 540–541
North Asian tick-borne rickettsiosis, **324–325**
Norum disease, *42*
Norwalk-like agents, viral **gastroenteritis caused by, 305–306**
Norwegian scabies, 111
Nose. See *Nasal.*
Nosocomial pneumonia(s), 341, 361–364
  factors predisposing to, 362
  mechanisms and prevalence of, 361
  possible future management of, 363
Nosocomial staphylococcal infections, 398
Nothnagel's syndrome, in midbrain infarctions, 787
Novobiocin, *556,* 561
Nuclear imaging
  in angina pectoris, 1226, 1227
  in myocardial infarction, 1232
Nucleic acid, metabolism of, inborn errors of, *42*
Nucleosides, methylated, as tumor markers, 1913
5'-Nucleotidase, measurement of, in osteomalacia, 2248
Nutrient requirements, 1670–1674
Nutrients, individual, deficiencies of, **1684–1692**
Nutrition. See also *Diet(s).*
  abnormalities of, in liver disease, **1642–1643**
  after peptic ulcer surgery, 1520
  diseases of, 1670–1702
  in cancer patient, 1906
  in carcinoid syndrome, 2208, 2209
  in chronic renal failure, 1365
  in paraplegia, 887
  in regional enteritis, 1566
  in tetanus, 440
  infection and, 1678–1680
  intravenous, long-term, 1706, 1707, 1708
    short-term, 1706
  parenteral, 1705–1708
    total, 1706, 1707, 1708
Nutritional amblyopia, 774–775

Nutritional cardiomyopathy, 1283–1285
Nutritional disorders of nervous system, 772–777
Nutritional maintenance, in acute and chronic disease, 1703–1712
Nutritional polyneuropathy, 772–773
Nutritional retrobulbar neuropathy, 774–775
Nutritional status
  assessment of, 1675–1678
  biochemical tests of, 1677, 1678
  clinical examination of, 1675, 1676
  effect of infection on, 1678–1679
  evaluation of signs of, 1676, 1677
Nyctalopia, 1684
Nylen-Bárány maneuver, in evaluation of dizziness, 738
Nystagmus, positional vertigo and, 738, 738
Nystatin, 557
  in candidiasis, 548, 549

Obesity, 1692–1699
  adult-onset, 1693
  as cardiovascular risk factor, 1062
  atherosclerosis and, 1221
  clinical manifestations of, 1677, 1695, 1695
  clinical types of, 1693, 1694
  diabetes mellitus and, 1696, 1975, 1976
  diet in, 1697, 1710
  differential diagnosis of, 1696, 1696
  effect of, on plasma amino acids, 2018
  etiology of, 1694, 1694
  experimental, 1693
  fatty liver in, 1660
  hypothalamic, 718, 1697
  insulin resistance in, in diabetes mellitus, 1987
  lifelong, 1693
  measurement of, 1692
  metabolic abnormalities in, 1694, 1695
  pathogenesis of, 1693, 1694
  pathophysiology of, 1693
  prevalence and epidemiology of, 1692
  prevention of, 1698
  prognosis in, 1698
  treatment of, 1697
Obesity-hypoventilation syndrome, 1696
Obstruction
  airways, diseases associated with, 951–964
    respiratory failure in, 1022–1023, 1023
    due to organic particles, 997–998, 997
    in bullous disease, 1003
    localized, 964
    pathophysiology of, 952–953, 952
  arterial, organic, peripheral vascular diseases due to, 1299–1305
  bile duct
    extrahepatic, vs. biliary cirrhosis, 1666
    uncommon causes of, 1632–1633
  biliary, dyslipoproteinemia in, 2010
  esophageal, in esophageal carcinoma, 1597, 1598
  gastric outlet, 1490
    in peptic ulcer, 1507, 1517, 1518
    vs. acute appendicitis, 1580

Obstruction (Continued)
  intestinal, 1490–1492
    Ascaris causing, 627
    in congenital megacolon, 1495
  lymphatic, malabsorption in, 1544, 1545
  portal venous, portal hypertension in, 1639
  pseudo-, colonic, 1497–1498
    intestinal, 1497
      malabsorption in, 1538
  small intestinal, vs. acute appendicitis, 1580
  splenic vein, portal hypertension in, 1639
  superior vena cava, in bronchogenic carcinoma, 1006
  ureteral, vs. acute appendicitis, 1580
  urinary tract, 1335–1336, 1447–1450
    acute renal failure in, 1369
    chronic renal failure and, 1352, 1353
    common sites of, 1447
    renal injury from, 1330
Obstructive atelectasis, 964, 965
Obstructive bronchitis, chronic, 951, 960
Obstructive cardiomyopathy, hypertrophic, 1278
Obstructive cholangitis, 1631
Obstructive jaundice, 1638
  computerized tomography in, 1467
  cutaneous manifestations of, 1645
  ultrasonography in, 1465
Obstructive nephropathy, 1418–1419, 1447–1450
  causes of, 1448
Obstructive pulmonary disease, chronic, 951, 952, 960–964, 961
  pulmonary hypertension in, 1146, 1147
  secondary polycythemia in, 1799
  vs. asthma, 957
Obstructive ventilatory disorders, 935, 936, 936
Occlusion
  anterior cerebral artery, 787
  aortic, syndromes of, 1298–1299
  basilar artery, 788
  cavernous sinus, 789
  central retinal artery, 2317, 2318
  hepatic vein, 1661
  internal carotid artery, 786–787
  mesenteric arterial, 1588, 1589
  middle cerebral artery, 787
  posterior cerebral artery, 787
  posterior inferior cerebellar artery, 788
  renal artery or vein, acute renal failure in, 1369
  superior longitudinal sinus, in head injury, 884, 885
  superior sagittal sinus, 788
Occlusive disease, renal arterial, acute, 1407
Occult "normal pressure" hydrocephalus, 874
Occupational bronchitis, 995–996
Ocular. See also Eye(s) and names of specific ocular disorders.
Ocular albinism, 2029
Ocular dystrophy, 918
Ocular histoplasmosis, 2318, 2323–2325
Ocular sarcoidosis, 213, 2329–2330
Ocular toxoplasmosis, 596, 597, 598, 2318, 2334–2335

Ocular tuberculosis, 498
Oculocerebrorenal syndrome, Lowe's, 2021
Oculocutaneous albinism, 2029, 2293
Oculoglandular syndrome of Parinaud, in cat scratch disease, 303
Oculoglandular tularemia, 467
Oculomotor nerve, disorders of, 899
Oddi, sphincter of, stenosis of, 1636
Odynophagia, 1479
  in esophageal carcinoma, 1597, 1598
Oesophagostomiasis, 626
Oestrus ovis, 112
OHF virus, 290, 291
Olfactory nerve, disorders of, 899
Oligodendroglioma, 863
Oligomenorrhea, 2179
  functional, 2080
Oligospermia, 2171
Oliguria
  in acute renal failure, 1371
  in critically ill patient, 1050
  in epidemic hemorrhagic fever, 301
  in malaria, 574
Olivopontocerebellar degenerations, 768
Ollier's dyschondroplasia, 2264
Omentum
  diseases of, 1595–1596
  tumors of, 1596
Omsk hemorrhagic fever, 290–291, 293
Omsk hemorrhagic fever virus, 290, 291
Onchocerca volvulus, 559, 605, 632, 635
Onchocerciasis, 635–636
Oncofetal antigens, as tumor markers, 1911–1912
Oncologic treatment, principles of, 1922–1941
Oncology, medical, 1898–1948
Oncovin. See Vincristine.
Ondine's curse, 654, 726, 1147
"Onion skin lesions," splenic, in systemic lupus erythematosus, 176
Onycholysis, in hyperthyroidism, 2122
O'nyong-nyong fever, 279–280, 279
O'nyong-nyong virus, 279
Oophoritis, in mumps, 263
o,p'DDD, 1938
  in Cushing's syndrome with adrenal carcinoma, 2156
Ophthalmia neonatorum
  antimicrobial prophylaxis in, 564
  gonococcal, 410
Ophthalmopathy
  in Graves' disease, 2126, 2127
  thyroid, 2332–2333
Ophthalmoplegia
  bilateral external, 900
  in muscular dystrophy, 918
Opiates
  abuse of, 694–698
  action of, mechanism of, 696
  pharmacology of, 695
  poisoning by, 712
Opisthorchiasis, 618
Opisthorchis felineus, 605, 618
Opisthorchis viverrini, 618
Opisthotonos, 438
Opium, 694–698
  derivatives of, poisoning by, 75
  tincture of, in diarrhea, 1480
    in diarrhea after extensive small intestinal resection, 1544
    in malabsorption syndrome, 1536
Opsoclonus, 878

Opsonins, in pneumococcal pneumonia, 349
Optic atrophy, 813, **815**
hereditary motor and sensory neuropathy with, 913
Optic nerve
disorders of, 899, **2327–2329**
glioma of, 868
in sarcoidosis, 2329
in sickle cell diseases, 2331
Optic neuritis, 848–849
acute, in cancer, 878
complicating ethambutol therapy of pulmonary tuberculosis, 488
Optic neuropathy, ischemic, in giant cell arteritis, 2319
Oral cholecystography, 1622, *1623*
in chronic cholecystitis, 1625
Oral contraceptives, 2195–2197
cerebral infarction and, 781
contraindications to, 2197
hypertension and, 1211
side effects of, 2195, 2196
Oral hypoglycemic agents, in diabetes mellitus, 1986, *1986*
Oral-facial-digital-syndrome, *2300*
Orbit, pseudotumor of, 224
Orbital cellulitis
vs. cavernous sinus thrombosis, 808
vs. Romaña's sign in Chagas' disease, 582
Orbital mucormycosis, in diabetes mellitus, 2320
Orchitis, 2174
in epidemic pleurodynia, 272
in mumps, 262
Organic particles
acute airway reactions to, 996–997
airways obstruction due to, 997–998, *997*
pulmonary effects of, *984*
Organic solvents
as nephrotoxins, 1434
inhalation of, 705
Organomercurial diuretics, in heart failure, *1103, 1104,* 1105
Organophosphorus compounds, neuropathy from, 911
Orgasm, 687
female, dysfunction of, 688, 2198, 2199
male, dysfunction of, 688, 2198
Oriental cholangiohepatitis, 1633
Oriental sore, 587–589, *588*
Oriental tussock moth, dermatitis caused by, 119
Ornithine transcarbamylase deficiency, *2018,* 2022, 2044
Ornithinemia, 2022
Ornithodoros erraticus, 529
Ornithodoros hermsi, 529
Ornithodoros moubata, 526, 529
Ornithodoros tholozani, 529
Ornithodoros turicata, 529
Ornithosis, 336–338
Oropharyngeal tube, in acute respiratory failure, 1025, 1026
Orotic aciduria, *42,* 2044
prevention and management of, 55
Oroya fever, 331–332
Orthopedic surgery
in degenerative joint disease, 205
in rheumatoid arthritis, 193
Orthopnea, in left ventricular failure, 1089

Orthostatic hypotension, 742, 743
faintness in, 740
idiopathic, 762–763
in diabetes mellitus, 1980
Oscillopsia, in vertigo, 737
Osler's nodes, in infective endocarditis, 389
Osler-Weber-Rendu syndrome, 1880, *2298, 2301*
Osmium tetroxide, exposure to, respiratory effects of, 1000
Osmotic agents, in constipation, 1482
Osmotic diarrhea, 1479
Osmotic diuretics
in accidental poisoning, 74
in head injury, 882
Osseous hydatid, 609, 610
Osteitis deformans, 2257–2259
Osteitis fibrosa, in chronic renal failure, 1359, 1360
Osteitis fibrosa cystica, in hyperparathyroidism, 2215, *2216,* 2217
Osteoarthritis, 202–205, *203*
erosive, 204
hypertrophic, primary generalized, 204
vs. rheumatoid arthritis, 190
Osteoarthropathy, hypertrophic, 201, 2263
in bronchogenic carcinoma, 1007
Osteochondritis dissecans, 2260
Osteodystrophy, renal, 1360, **2254–2257**
Osteogenesis imperfecta, 2245
aorta in, 1292
vs. Ehlers-Danlos syndrome, 2055
vs. juvenile osteoporosis, 2246
Osteoid seams, 2247
Osteolysis, in Paget's disease, 2258
Osteomalacia, 2247–2254
anticonvulsant, 2253
axial, 2254
in cadmium poisoning, 82
in chronic renal failure, 1360, 2254
in malabsorption syndrome, 1528
vs. hyperparathyroidism, 2217
Osteomyelitis, 2260–2261
due to contiguous infection, 2261
in blastomycosis, 540
in subdural empyema, 807
pyogenic, subacute, 2260
refractory, hyperbaric oxygen therapy in, 105
Salmonella causing, 2260
in sickle cell anemia, 451
staphylococcal, 402–403, 2260
vs. sporotrichosis, 545
vs. actinomycosis, 474
Osteonecrosis, 2259–2260
dysbaric, of divers and caisson workers, 102
Osteopenia, disuse, 2236, 2237
Osteopetrosis, 2263
Osteopoikilosis, 2264
Osteoporosis, 2242–2246
endocrine, 2244
in adrenocorticosteroid therapy of rheumatoid arthritis, 192
in homocystinuria, 2028
in malabsorption syndrome, 1528
in multiple myeloma, 1858, *1859*
in rheumatoid arthritis, 189
juvenile, 2246
vs. osteogenesis imperfecta, 2245
painful, post-traumatic, 727

Osteoporosis (*Continued*)
postmenopausal, 2190, 2191, 2243, 2244
primary, 2243–2244
senile, 2243, 2244
treatment of, 2246
vs. hyperparathyroidism, 2217
Osteoporosis circumscripta, in Paget's disease, 2258
Osteoradionecrosis, hyperbaric oxygen therapy in, 104, 105
Osteosclerosis
in agnogenic myeloid metaplasia, 1828
in chronic renal failure, 1360
Ostium primum atrial septal defect, 1171
Ostium secundum atrial septal defect, 1160, 1161, 1162
Otitic hydrocephalus, 871
Otitis media
air travel and, 96
hearing loss from, 735
Hemophilus influenzae in, 425
in measles, 248
in streptococcal pharyngitis, 373
Otomycosis, 547
Otosclerosis, hearing loss from, 735
Ototoxic drugs
hearing loss from, 736
vertigo from, 739
Ouabain, in heart failure, *1096,* 1097
"Ouch-ouch" disease, 82, 1429
Ovale malaria, 567
clinical manifestations of, 571
relapse of, 574
Ovarian steroid biosynthesis, pathways of, 2178, *2178*
Ovary(ies), 2175–2199
cyst of, twisted, vs. acute appendicitis, 1581
disorders of, 2179–2199
amenorrhea due to, 2185–2186
ascites in, 1593
function of, 2175–2179
status of, breast cancer and, 1918
tests of, 2179, 2180, *2180,* 2181, *2181*
hormones of, function of, 2176, *2177,* 2177–2178
hyperfunction of, organic precocious pseudopuberty due to, 2182, 2183
polycystic, 2188–2190
resistant, syndrome of, 2186
sclerocystic, 2189
structure of, 2175–2179
tuberculosis of, 496
tumors of, carcinoid features of, 2212
Oversuppression syndrome, prolactin levels in, 2092
Oxacillin, *557,* 559
in bacterial meningitis, 415
in infective endocarditis, 393
in infective endocarditis prophylaxis, 396
in osteomyelitis, 2261
in staphylococcal meningitis, 404
in staphylococcal pneumonia, 402
Oxamniquine, in schistosomiasis, 616
Oxazolidinediones, as nephrotoxins, 1432
Oxprenolol
in arterial hypertension, *1212*
in hypertension of chronic renal failure, 1362
Oxycodone, in pain, *724*

Oxygen
  diffusion of, 936
  in cerebral metabolism, 646
Oxygen affinity
  abnormal, hemoglobins with,
    disorders caused by, 1777–1778,
    1778
  of red cells, 1771
Oxygen therapy
  hyperbaric, 103–105
    in clostridial myonecrosis, 435
    in acute respiratory failure, 1026–1027
    in chronic obstructive pulmonary
      disease, 963
    in chronic respiratory failure, 1028
    in decompression sickness, 103, 104
    in heart failure, 1094
    in myocardial infarction, 1234
    in shock, 1118
    in status asthmaticus, 959
Oxygen toxicity
    in acute respiratory failure treatment,
      1041
  in diving, 103
Oxygen-hemoglobin affinity, in shock,
  1113
Oxymetholone
  in agnogenic myeloid metaplasia,
    1828
  in aplastic anemia, 1740
  in paroxysmal nocturnal
    hemoglobinuria, 1769
Oxyphenbutazone, in acute gouty
  arthritis, 2039
Oxytetracycline, *557,* 562
  in balantidiasis, 603
  in malabsorption syndrome, *1536*
Oxyuriasis, 629–630

P wave, 1243, *1243*
Pacemakers, cardiac, 1267–1268, *1267,*
  1268
    in cardiopulmonary resuscitation,
      1057
Pachydermoperiostosis, 201, 2263
  acquired, *2296*
  vs. acromegaly, 2106
Pachymeningitis, hypertrophic, 813
Paddy-field foot, 1309
Paederus species, dermatitis caused by,
  114
Pagetic steal syndrome, 2258
Paget's disease
  of bone, 2257–2259
    vs. hyperparathyroidism, 2217
  of breast, 2287
    anal involvement in, 1618
    breast carcinoma and, *2296,* 2297
Pain, 720–728
  abdominal, 1476–1477
    referred, 1477
  anorectal, 1618
  chronic, management of, 722–727
  disorders causing, diagnosis of,
    721–722
  "gate control" theory of, 721, 725, 726
  hot, 727
  hysterical, 678
  in acute appendicitis, 1579, 1580
  in acute cholecystitis, 1626
  in acute intermittent porphyria, 2045
  in acute pancreatitis, 1552
  in acute pericarditis, 1272

Pain *(Continued)*
  in angina pectoris, 1223, 1224
    surgical relief of, 1238, 1239, 1241
  in ankylosing spondylitis, 194
  in anterior tibial compartment
    syndromes, 1305
  in arterial embolism, 1303
  in arteriosclerosis obliterans, 1300
  in bronchogenic carcinoma, 1006
  in chronic cholecystitis, 1624, 1625
  in chronic pancreatitis, 1555, *1555,*
    1557
  in colonic diverticulosis, 1501
  in cranial arteritis, 217
  in diffuse collagenous
    pneumoconioses, 991
  in diffuse esophageal spasm, 1486
  in dissecting aortic aneurysm, 1296
  in diverticulitis, 1582
  in epidemic pleurodynia, 271
  in erythromelalgia, 1308
  in Fabry's disease, 2011
  in familial Mediterranean fever 2056
  in gastric carcinoma, 1601
  in glossopharyngeal neuralgia, 727
  in herpes zoster, 825
  in intermittent cholangitis, 1629, 1630
  in intervertebral disc protrusion, 894
  in intraspinal compression, 893
  in irritable bowel syndrome, 1493
  in liver disease, 1645
  in malabsorption, 1527
  in multiple myeloma, 1858
  in myocardial infarction, 1229, 1230
    relief of, 1233, 1234
  in nonparalytic poliomyelitis, 830
  in obstructive nephropathy, 1448
  in Paget's disease, 2258
  in pancreatic carcinoma, 1558
  in paroxysmal nocturnal
    hemoglobinuria, 1768
  in peptic ulcer, 1507
  in pneumococcal pneumonia, 351
  in postherpetic neuralgia, 728
  in proctalgia fugax, 1497
  in pulmonary tuberculosis, 486
  in radicular syndromes, 889
  in reflex sympathetic dystrophies, 727
  in regional enteritis, 1563
  in rheumatoid arthritis, 188
  in shin splints, 1305
  in shock, 1117
  in shoulder, 205–207
  in sickle cell crises, 1774
  in spinal cord tumors, 896
  in spinal epidural infections, 810
  in strongyloidiasis, 623
  in syphilitic aortic aneurysm, 1294
  in tabes dorsalis, 727, 814
  in trigeminal neuralgia, 727
  in Zollinger-Ellison syndrome, 1508
  myofascial, syndromes of, 728
  on swallowing, 1479
  pathways of, 720–721, *720*
  phantom limb, 728
  pleural, 1013
  psychogenic, 723
  referred, 722
    abdominal, 1477
  relief of, analgesic agents in, 723–725,
    724
    physical methods for, 725–727
  specific syndromes of, 727–728
Painless diarrhea, 1493
Paint, lead, poisoning by, 77

Painter's colic, 78
Palate
  cleft, frequency and sex ratio of, *48*
  soft, paralysis of, in diphtheria, 432
Palindromic rheumatism, 198
Pallor, circumoral, in scarlet fever, 371
Palmar erythema, in liver disease, 1645
Palsy
  Bell's, 900
  bridegroom's, 902
  bulbar, progressive, 765
  cerebral, 760
  extraocular, pupillary disturbances
    and, 899, 900
  lateral rectus, in intracranial tumors,
    866
  peroneal nerve, acute and tardy, 902
  radial nerve, acute, 901, 902
  Saturday night, 901
  shaking, 752–756
  ulnar nerve, tardy, 901
Panacinar emphysema, 960
"Pancake kidney," 1457
Pancoast's syndrome, in bronchogenic
  carcinoma, 1006
Pancreas
  beta cells of, in diabetes mellitus,
    1972, 1973
  calcification of, in chronic
    pancreatitis, 1555, 1556
  carcinoma of, 1557–1559
    acinar cell, vs. Weber-Christian
      disease, 222
    acute pancreatitis and, 1551
    angiography in, *1470,* 1471
    percutaneous transhepatic
      cholangiography in, *1473*
  cystic fibrosis of, *43,* **1559–1560**
  cysts of, in chronic pancreatitis, 1556,
    1556
  diseases of, 1550–1560
    cutaneous signs of, 2299
    endoscopic retrograde
      cholangiopancreatography in,
      1472, *1472, 1473*
    eosinophilia in, 226
  function of, tests of, 2354
    in malabsorption syndrome, 1531
  insufficiency of, adult celiac disease
    and, 1541
    in chronic pancreatitis, 1554, 1555
    primary, 1535, 1536
      treatment of, 1538
    secondary, 1536
      treatment of, 1538
  islet cell tumors of
    carcinoid features of, 2212
    fasting hypoglycemia caused by,
      1993–1995
  pseudocyst of, ascites in, 1593
    in chronic pancreatitis, 1556, *1556*
    percutaneous transhepatic
      cholangiography in, *1473*
    ultrasonography in, *1465*
  radionuclide imaging of, 1470
  tuberculosis of, 498
Pancreatic extracts
  in chronic pancreatitis, 1557
  in postgastrectomy malabsorption,
    1546
Pancreatic juice, loss of, metabolic
  acidosis from, 1962
Pancreatic lipase, in fat absorption, 1524
Pancreatic oncofetal antigen, as tumor
  marker, 1912

Pancreatic supplements, oral, in malabsorption syndrome, *1536*
Pancreaticoduodenal arcades, 1586, *1586*
Pancreatitis, 1550–1557
  acute, 1550–1554
    etiologic factors in, 1551, *1551*
    hypocalcemia in, 1553, 2241
    mechanism of, 1552, *1552*
    vs. acute appendicitis, 1580, 1581
    vs. acute cholecystitis, 1627
    vs. choledocholithiasis, 1630
    vs. peptic ulcer, 1508
    bile duct obstruction by, 1632
  chronic, 1550, 1554–1557
    ascites in, 1593
    endoscopic retrograde cholangiopancreatography in, 1472, *1473*
    vs. pancreatic carcinoma, 1559
  clinical course of, 1550, *1550*
  diabetes mellitus in, 1982
  in chronic renal failure, 1366
  in familial lipoprotein lipase deficiency, 2006
  in hyperparathyroidism, 2214, 2215
  in mumps, 263
  pleural effusions in, 1017
  traumatic, 1551
  vs. acute pericarditis, 1273
  vs. chronic cholecystitis, 1625
  vs. myocardial infarction, 1233
  vs. Weber-Christian disease, 222
Pancytopenia, in aplastic anemia, 1733, 1737, 1739
Pandysautonomia, 907
Panencephalitis, sclerosing, subacute, 841
Panendoscopy, in gastrointestinal bleeding, 1522
Panhypopituitarism, 2100
Panic reaction, acute, in LSD use, 704, 705
Panniculitis, 221–222
  liquefying, nodular, 2295, *2297*
  mesenteric, 222, 1596
Panniculus adiposus, 2267
Pannus, in rheumatoid arthritis, 186, 187
Panstrongylus megistus, 580
Pantothenic acid
  deficiency of, 773
  nutrient value of, 1672, 1673
Papillary muscle, malfunction of, in myocardial infarction, 1231
Papillary necrosis, renal, 1412–1413
  acute renal failure from, 1369
  in sickle cell hemoglobinopathy, 1404
  vs. medullary sponge kidney, 1456
Papilledema, *2318,* **2327**
  in arterial hypertension, 1205
  in benign intracranial hypertension, 870, 872
  in intracranial tumors, 865
  in toxoplasmosis, 2334
  vs. optic neuritis, 849
  vs. pseudopapilledema, 2328
Papillitis, 848, 2328–2329
  in toxoplasmosis, 2334
  necrotizing, 1412–1413
Papilloma(s)
  bile duct, 1635
  choroid, 864
  of lung, 1013

Pappenheimer bodies, 1718
Paprika splitter's lung, *971*
Papular dermatitis of Spangler, 2305
Papular mucinosis, 1865, *1865*
Papule, 2273
Para-aminohippurate, in estimation of renal blood flow, 1340, 1341
Paracetamol, in louse-borne relapsing fever, 528
Paracentesis
  in ascites complicating cirrhosis, 1666
  volume depletion after, 1951
Parachlorophenylalanine, in carcinoid syndrome, 2213
Paracoccidioides brasiliensis, 541
Paracoccidioidomycosis, 541–542
Paradione. See *Paramethadione*.
Paraganglioma, nonchromaffin, 867
Paragonimiasis, 619–620
  antimicrobial agents for, *559*
  cerebral, vs. angiostrongyliasis, 631
Paragonimus africanus, 619
Paragonimus heterotremus, 619
Paragonimus skrjabini, 619
Paragonimus westermani, 559, 605, 619
Parahemophilia, *43, 1884,* 1888
Parainfluenza viral diseases, 239–240
Parainfluenza viruses, 239
Paraldehyde, poisoning by, metabolic acidosis from, 1962
Paralysis
  bulbar, in botulism, 67, 68
  diaphragmatic, 1019
  flaccid, in hyperkalemia, 1959
  general, of insane, 814
  in nonpolio enteroviral infections, 270
  in poliomyelitis, 829, 831
  in spinal epidural infections, 810
  in tuberculous spondylitis, 497
  of soft palate, in diphtheria, 432
  periodic, familial, 921–922
    hyperkalemic, 1959
    vs. hysteria, 679
  postical, 854
  sleep, 654
  swallowing, in poliomyelitis, 832
  tick, 117–118
    neuromuscular block caused by, 929
  Todd's, 854
Paralysis agitans, 752–756
Paralytic ileus
  in pneumococcal pneumonia, 354
  in spinal cord dysfunction, 887
  potassium deficiency inducing, 1958
Paralytic poliomyelitis, 829, 831
Paralytic shellfish poisoning, 68
Parameningeal infections, 804–809
  vs. bacterial meningitis, 414
  vs. viral meningitis, 820
Paramethadione
  as nephrotoxin, 1432
  in epilepsy, *859*
Paramethasone, in rheumatoid arthritis, 192
Paramyxoviruses associated with common cold, *230*
Paranasal sinuses, infection of
  brain abscess from, 805
  subdural empyema from, 807
Paranasal sinusitis, in streptococcal pharyngitis, 373
Paranasal structures, as sources of headache, 733

Parangi, 518–522, *520.* See also *Yaws.*
Paraphasias, 656
Paraplegia, 886–888
  air travel and, 96
  in diabetes mellitus, 1979
  spastic, hereditary, 768
    vs. vitamin B_{12} deficiency, 777
Paraprosthetic-enteric fistula, 1590
Paraproteinemias, 2010
Paraquat
  as nephrotoxin, 1435
  ingestion of, pulmonary edema from, 1001
Parasitemia, in malaria, elimination of, 573
Parasitic infections, 565–638. See also names of specific parasitic diseases.
  immunodiagnostic tests for, *565*
  of brain, vs. dementia in cancer, 877
Parathion, poisoning by, 75
Parathyroid, 2213–2224
  adenomas of, 2214
    preoperative localization of, 2218, *2219*
  in acromegaly, 2106
Parathyroid hormone, 2213–2214
  immunoreactive, circulating levels of, in vitamin D resistant rickets, 2250, 2251
  radioimmunoassay for, in hyperparathyroidism, 2218
  secretion of, in chronic renal failure, 1355, 1358
Paratyphoid fever, 449
  clinical manifestations of, 451
  diagnosis of, 452
  treatment of, 452
  vs. hemorrhagic diseases caused by arenaviruses, 299
Paregoric, in diarrhea, 1480
Parenchymatous cerebellar degeneration, 775
Parenteral nutrition, 1705–1708
  total, 1706, 1707, 1708
Paresis, general, 512, 813, 814
  treatment of, 516
Paresthesia, in radicular syndromes, 889
Pargyline, poisoning by, *712*
Parietal lobe abscess, 806
Parietal peritoneum, pain originating in, 1476
Parinaud's syndrome, 2113
  oculoglandular, in cat scratch disease, 303
Paris green, poisoning by, 76
Parkinsonism, 752–756
  course of, 756
  drug-induced, 753
  dysequilibrium in, 741
  management of, 754–756
  possible viral cause of, 842
  postencephalitic, 753
    vs. hysteria, 679
  seborrheic dermatitis in, 2278
  secondary, 753–754
  symptomatic, 753–754
    vs. senile tremor, 757
Parkinson's disease, 752–753
Paromomycin
  in intestinal amebiasis, 593
  in tapeworm infections, 608
Parotitis
  in mumps, 262, 263
  staphylococcal, 404

Parotitis (*Continued*)
  suppurative, vs. mumps, 263
Paroxysmal atrial tachycardia,
  1249–1251, *1249, 1251*
Paroxysmal cold hemoglobinuria,
  1765–1766, *2302*
  immune mechanisms in, 132
  in syphilis, 507
Paroxysmal hypothermia, 716
Paroxysmal nocturnal dyspnea, in left
  ventricular failure, 1090
Paroxysmal nocturnal hemoglobinuria,
  1768–1769
    acute leukemia in, 1814
    aplastic anemia and, 1734, 1737
Paroxysmal polyserositis, 2055–2057
Parrot fever, 336–338
Partial thromboplastin time, in
  hereditary coagulation disorders, *1884*
Particle agglutination tests, in
  protozoan and helminthic diseases,
  565
Passive transport, in normal absorption,
  1524
Passivity experiences, in schizophrenia,
  666
Patau's syndrome, clinical and
  cytogenetic characteristics of, *52*
Patchy atelectasis, 965
Patek, 518–522, *520.* See also *Yaws.*
Patent ductus arteriosus, 1162–1164
  pulmonary hypertension in, 1141,
  1142
Paterson–Brown Kelly syndrome, 1483
  in iron deficiency anemia, 1748
Pathologic left handers, 656
Pavor nocturnus, 655
"PCP," 704
Pectus carinatum, 1020, 1021
Pectus excavatum, 1020
Pediculosis, 108–110
Pediculus humanus, in relapsing fever,
  526
Pediculus humanus capitis, 108
  in epidemic typhus, 318
Pediculus humanus humanus, 108
  in epidemic typhus, 318
Pedigree analysis in inherited disease,
  34–40
Pel-Ebstein fever, in Hodgkin's disease,
  1841
Peliosis hepatis, 1658
Pelizaeus-Merzbacher disease, 850
Pellagra, 1687–1688, *1687*
  cutaneous lesions of, 1675, 1676,
  2299
  vs. transverse myelitis, 812
Pelvic abscesses, tuberculous, 492
Pelvic appendicitis, 1579
Pelvic endometriosis, vs. colorectal
  carcinoma, 1610
Pelvic infection, intrauterine device use
  and, 2197
Pelvic inflammatory disease,
  mycoplasmal, 346, 347
Pelvirectal abscess, 1617
Pemphigoid, *2303,* **2304**
Pemphigus, 2303–2304, *2303*
  familial chronic, benign, 2304
Pemphigus foliaceus, 2304
Pemphigus neonatorum, 400
Pemphigus vegetans, 2304
Pemphigus vulgaris, 2303
Pendred's syndrome, iodide
  organification defect in, 2139

Penetrance, genetic, 37
Penetration of peptic ulcer, 1518
D-Penicillamine
  as nephrotoxin, 1432
  in cystinuria, 2027
  in lead poisoning, 79
  in scleroderma, 171
  in Wilson's disease, 2050
Penicillin(s), 557, *557,* 558, 559, 560
  adverse reactions to, 559, 560
  benzathine. See *Benzathine penicillin.*
  derivatives of, as nephrotoxins, 1426
  hypersensitivity to, in treatment of
    infective endocarditis, 394
  in actinomycosis, 474
  in anaerobic infections, 444
  in bacterial meningitis, 415, 416
  in bejel, 523
  in brain abscess, 807
  in clostridial myonecrosis, 434
  in gonorrhea, 408, 409
  in hereditary spherocytosis, 1757
  in infective endocarditis, 392
  in louse-borne relapsing fever, 528
  in pneumococcal pneumonia, 355
  in psittacosis, 338
  in rheumatic fever, 383
  in subdural empyema, 808
  in syphilis, 515, *515,* 516
  in tetanus, 439
  in tropical phagedenic ulcer, 530
  penicillinase-resistant, *557,* 559
  penicillinase-sensitive, 557, *557,* 558,
    559
  phenoxymethyl, *557,* 558
    in acute poststreptococcal
      glomerulonephritis, 1396
  procaine. See *Procaine penicillin.*
  with gram-negative bacillary activity,
    557, 558
Penicillin G, 557, *557*
  adverse reactions to, 560
  aqueous, in congenital syphilis, 517
    in gonococcal disease, 409, 410
    in neurosyphilis, 516
  aqueous crystalline, 557, *557*
  in anaerobic infections, 444, *445*
  in anthrax, 471
  in diphtheria, 432
  in erysipeloid of Rosenbach, 473
  in group A streptococcal infections,
    376
  in infective endocarditis, 392, 393, 394
  in infective endocarditis prophylaxis,
    396
  in listeriosis, 473
  in lung abscess, 981, 982
  in meningococcal disease, 421
  in neurosyphilis, 516
  in osteomyelitis, 2261
  in pneumococcal pneumonia, 355
  in prophylaxis of streptococcal
    infection, 377
  in staphylococcal meningitis, 404
  in staphylococcal pneumonia, 402
  in Whipple's disease, 1542
Penicillin V
  in acute poststreptococcal
    glomerulonephritis, 1396
  in infective endocarditis prophylaxis,
    396
  in pneumococcal pneumonia, 355
  in streptobacillary rat-bite fever, 531
Penicillinase-resistant penicillins, *557,*
  559

Penicillinase-sensitive penicillins, 557,
  557, 558, 559
Pentagastrin, in gastric analysis, 1601
Pentamidine
  in African trypanosomiasis
    prevention, 579
  in babesiosis, 601
  in pneumocystosis, *558*
Pentamidine isethionate
  in pneumocystosis, 600
  in visceral leishmaniasis, 586
Pentastomiasis, 119–120
Pentavalent antimony
  in cutaneous leishmaniasis of new
    world, 589
  in cutaneous leishmaniasis of old
    world, 588
  in visceral leishmaniasis, 586
Pentazocine, 694, 696
  in pain, *724, 725*
  in pain of myocardial infarction, 1234
Pentobarbital
  abuse of, 698
  in insomnia, 653
Pentosuria, *41,* **2000**
Pepsins, secretion of, 1506
Peptic esophagitis
  vs. peptic ulcer, 1507
  with stricture, vs. esophageal
    carcinoma, 1598
Peptic ulcer, 1502–1520
  antacids in, 1513, 1514
  anticholinergic drugs in, 1515
  association of, with other diseases,
    1504
  back-diffusion of acid and, 1505
  chronic, 1502
  clinical manifestations of, 1507–1508
  complications of, 1516–1518
  diagnosis of, 1509–1513
  diet in, 1515
  differential diagnosis of, 1507, 1508
  drugs causing, 1504
  duodenogastric reflux and, 1507
  endocrine hyperfunction and,
    1508–1509
  endoscopy in, 1511, 1512
  environmental factors in, 1503
  epidemiology of, 1503
  gastric acid secretion in, 1506
  gastric carcinoma and, 1600
  gastric secretory tests in, 1512
  gastritis in, 1502, 1503
  genetic factors in, 1503
  hemorrhage in, 1516, 1517
  histamine H_2-receptor antagonists in,
    1514, *1514,* 1515
  hospital care in, 1515
  impaired gastric emptying in, 1507,
    1517, 1518
  in adrenocorticosteroid therapy of
    rheumatoid arthritis, 192
  in hyperparathyroidism, 2215
  medical therapy of, 1513–1516
  outlet obstruction in, 1517, 1518
  pathogenesis and pathophysiology of,
    1502–1507
  penetrating, 1518
  perforation in, 1518
    vs. acute cholecystitis, 1627
    vs. myocardial infarction, 1233
  physical examination in, 1507
  psychosomatic factors in, 1504
  recurrent, after surgical treatment,
    1520

Peptic ulcer (*Continued*)
roentgenography in, 1509, 1510, *1510,* 1511, *1511,* 1512, *1512*
stress causing, 1504
surgical treatment of, 1518–1520, *1519*
chronic postoperative morbidity in, 1520
symptoms of, 1507
vs. acute appendicitis, 1580
vs. angina pectoris, 1227
vs. chronic cholecystitis, 1625
Peptidergic neuron systems, central, 2077, *2078*
Peptococcus asaccharolyticus, 441
Peptococcus magnus, 441
Peptococcus prevotii, 441
Peptostreptococcus anaerobius, 441
Peptostreptococcus intermedius, 441
Peptostreptococcus micros, 441
Peptostreptococcus species, 367
Perchlorate discharge test, 2118, *2119*
Percutaneous antegrade pyelography, in obstructive nephropathy, 1449
Percutaneous transhepatic cholangiography, 1473–1474, *1473, 1474*
Percutaneous transtracheal aspiration, microbiologic diagnosis by, 342
Perennial allergic rhinitis, 157
Perforation
colonic, in amebiasis, 591
in ulcerative colitis, 1575
gallbladder, in acute cholecystitis, 1626, 1628
gastrointestinal, in cancer patient, 1906
ileal, in regional enteritis, 1564
intestinal, in typhoid fever, 447, 448
of peptic ulcer, 1518
vs. acute cholecystitis, 1627
vs. myocardial infarction, 1233
Perfusion, 932, **938**
impaired, radionuclide imaging in, 944, 945
in airways obstruction, 953
Perhexilene, in angina pectoris, 1228
Periactin. See *Cyproheptadine.*
Periampullary neoplasms, vs. choledocholithiasis, 1630
Perianal abscess, 1617
Periarteritis nodosa, 165, **180–183,** *2298*
cutaneous signs in, *2301*
drugs causing, 156
eyes in, 2317
malabsorption in, 1543
neuropathy in, 908
renal involvement in, 181, 1400
vs. toxocariasis, 628
vs. trichinosis, 631
Pericardial constriction, 1274–1275
Pericardial effusion, 1273–1274
chylous, 1276
in right ventricular failure, 1093
Pericardial friction rub, in acute pericarditis, 1272
Pericardiectomy, in constrictive pericarditis, 1275
Pericardiocentesis
in pericardial effusion, 1274
in tuberculous pericarditis, 494
Pericarditis
acute, 1269–1273
vs. myocardial infarction, 1233

Pericarditis (*Continued*)
allergic disorders associated with, 1272
amebic, 592
cholesterol, 1276
complicating maintenance hemodialysis, 1382
connective tissue disorders causing, 1271, 1272
constrictive, 1274–1275
protein-losing enteropathy and, 1549
enteroviruses causing, 272–273
idiopathic, 1269
benign, vs. rheumatic fever, 383
in bacterial meningitis, 414
in chronic renal failure, 1365
in pneumococcal pneumonia, 353, 354
treatment of, 356
in systemic lupus erythematosus, 180
in tularemia, 467
infectious, 1269–1270
metabolic disorders causing, 1272
nonspecific, 1269
physical or chemical agents causing, 1272
postmyocardial infarction, 1231, 1270, 1271
postsurgical, 1271
post-traumatic, 1271
staphylococcal, 404
tuberculous, 494–495, 1270
vs. acute appendicitis, 1581
vs. angina pectoris, 1227
vs. peptic ulcer, 1507
vs. pulmonary embolism, 1133
Pericardium
bacterial infections of, 1270
congenital absence of, 1276
congenital lesions of, 1276
disorders of, 1268–1276
etiology of, *1269*
diverticula of, 1276
in pneumococcal pneumonia, 349
tumors of, 1276
viral infections of, 1269
Perifolliculitis of ascorbic acid deficiency, 1675
Perihepatitis, gonococcal, 408, 409
vs. acute cholecystitis, 1627
Perinatal polycystic kidney disease, 1453
Perinephric abscess, 1410
Periodic catatonia, 668
Periodic fever, 2055–2057
Periodic paralysis
familial, 921–922
hyperkalemic, 921, 1959
vs. hysteria, 679
Periosteal nodules, in rheumatoid arthritis, 187, 188
Periostitis
in blastomycosis, 540
in syphilis, 510
in yaws, *520,* 521
Peripartum cardiomyopathy, 1287
Peripheral arteries, in diabetes mellitus, 1981
Peripheral arteritis, in systemic infections, 1305
Peripheral circulation, 1066–1067
Peripheral lymphatic vessels, diseases of, 1314–1315

Peripheral nerves
in rheumatoid arthritis, 187, 189
nonmetastatic effects of cancer on, 878
Peripheral nervous system
diseases of, 899–913
in periarteritis nodosa, 182
Peripheral neuritis
drugs causing, 156
in diphtheria, 432
vs. polymyositis, 173
Peripheral neurons, inherited disorders of, 911
Peripheral neuropathy(ies), 899–913
alcohol-related, 709
diabetes mellitus and, 908–909, 1979, 1980. See also *Neuropathy(ies), diabetic.*
differential diagnosis of, 903–905
glossitis and, in malabsorption syndrome, 1529
in bronchogenic carcinoma, 1007
in chronic renal failure, 1365
in multiple myeloma, 910, 1860
respiratory failure in, *1023,* 1024
symptoms of, 903, 904
vs. amyotrophic lateral sclerosis, 766
vs. idiopathic autonomic insufficiency, 763
vs. myasthenia gravis, 927
vs. radiculopathy, 889, *890, 891*
with carcinoma, 910
with drug use, 910
with endocrine diseases, 909
with hepatic disease, 909
with household and industrial poisons, 910
with infection, 905–906
with inflammation and presumed altered immunity, 906
with mesenchymal disease and necrotizing angiopathy, 908
with uremia, 909
Peripheral sensory neurons, disorders of, 911–912
Peripheral vascular diseases, 1299–1315
diabetes mellitus and, neuropathy in, 908
due to abnormal communications between arteries and veins, 1312–1313
due to abnormal vasoconstriction or vasodilatation, 1305–1309
due to exposure to cold, 1309–1312
due to organic arterial obstruction, 1299–1305
Peripheral vasoconstriction, in heart failure, 1088
Peripheral veins, diseases of, 1313–1314
Peripheral vestibulopathy
acute, 738
acute and recurrent, 738, 739
Periphlebitis, retinal, in sarcoidosis, 2329
Perirectal abscess(es)
enteric bacteria causing, 455
tuberculous, 492
Perirectal fistula, in regional enteritis, 1562
Peristalsis, esophageal, 1478
Peritoneal dialysis, 1377–1378
in accidental poisoning, 74
Peritoneoscopy, 1592

Peritoneum
  anatomy and physiology of, **1591**
  diseases of, 1591–1595
    diagnosis of, 1591, 1592
  infections of, 1593–1595
    parietal, pain originating in, 1476
  tumors of, 1595
Peritonitis
  acute, 1593–1594
    amebic, 590, 591, 592
    bile, in needle biopsy of liver, 1648
    in acute appendicitis, 1580
    in perforated peptic ulcer, 1518
    pain in, 1476
  practolol, 224
  spontaneous, 1594
  tuberculous, 495, 1594
Peritonsillar abscess, in streptococcal
  tonsillitis, 373
Periureteral fibrosis, 223–224
Perivascular myelinoclasis, acute, 836
Pernicious anemia, 1719
  adult, gastric carcinoma and, 1600
  clinical manifestations of, 1725
  cutaneous lesions in, *2302*
  eosinophilia in, 226
  immunologic aspects of, 133
  incidence and prevalence of, 1723
Pernio, 1310–1311
Peroneal muscular atrophy
  dominantly inherited hypertrophic
    neuropathy type of, 912
  neuronal type of, 913
  vs. muscular dystrophies, 918
Peroneal nerve, palsy of, acute and
  tardy, 902
Personality, 672, 682–683
  atherosclerosis and, 1221
  disorders of, 665, 672–680
    "hysterical," 678, 679
    hepatic encephalopathy and, 1641
    irritable bowel syndrome and, 1493,
      1494
    schizoid, 666
    sexual system and, 686
Perthes' disease, 2259, 2260
Pertussis, 426–428
Pertussis vaccine, 428
Pesticides, human health and, 61, 62
Pestis minor, 464
Petechiae
  in infective endocarditis, 389
  in scurvy, 1690, *1690*
Petit mal, 854
  vs. syncope, 745
Petit mal status, 856
Peutz-Jeghers syndrome, *1910, 2297,
  2298*
  colorectal carcinoma and, 1606
  lentigines in, 2290
Peyronie's disease, 224
Pfeiferella mallei, 468
Pfeiferella whitmori, 469
Phagedenic ulcer, tropical, 530–531
Phagocytes, circulating, in host defense,
  145, 146
Phagocytic activity, in malnutrition,
  1679
Phagocytosis, 1801, *1801*
  alveolar, 340, 341
  complement in, 136, 137
  defects of, 1804
    infections in, *148*

Phagocytosis (*Continued*)
  surface, in pneumococcal pneumonia,
    349
Phakomatoses, 769–771
Phalen's sign, in carpal tunnel
  syndrome, 901
Phallotoxins, 69
Phantom limb pain, 728
Pharmacogenetics, 45–46
Pharmacology, clinical, aging patient
  and, 29, 30
Pharyngitis
  adenoviral, vs. diphtheria, 431
    vs. streptococcal pharyngitis, 372
  exudative, nonstreptococcal, 237
    vs. streptococcal pharyngitis, 372
  febrile, acute, 237
    in listeriosis, 472
  gonococcal, 406, 407
  lymphonodular, acute, 271
  mycoplasmal, 343, 345
  staphylococcal, 404
  streptococcal, 371–374
    complications of, 373
    course of, 372
    diagnosis of, 372
    epidemiology of, 369, 370
    immunologic diagnosis of, 372
    pathogenesis of, 368
    rheumatic fever and, 378, 379, 382
    vs. diphtheria, 431
    vs. infectious mononucleosis, 266
    vs. influenza, 245
  viral, 235–236, *235*
    vs. infectious mononucleosis, 266
Pharyngoconjunctival fever, 237
Pharyngotonsillitis, toxic, infectious
  mononucleosis with, 267
Pharynx
  in swallowing act, 1478, *1478*
  lymphatic tissue of, tuberculosis of,
    492
Phenacemide, in epilepsy, *859*
Phenacetin
  in pain, *724*
  nephropathy from, 1419
Phencyclidine, 704
Phenelzine
  in depression, 678
  in pain, *724*
  poisoning by, *712*
Phenergan. See *Promethazine.*
Phenformin
  in diabetes mellitus, 1986, *1986*
  lactic acidosis from, 1962
Phenindione, as nephrotoxin, 1431, 1432
Phenmetrazine, abuse of, 701
Phenobarbital
  dexamethasone and, simultaneous
    use of, effects of, 2339
  hypocalcemia induced by, 2241
  in convulsions of chronic renal
    failure, 1366
  in epilepsy, *859,* 860
  in essential tremor, 757
  in heart failure, 1094
  in intracranial tumors, 869
  in muscle-contraction headaches, 732
  in thyroid storm, 2128
  in treatment of central nervous
    system depressant abuse, 700
  rickets or osteomalacia induced by,
    2253

Phenothiazines. See also names of
  specific agents.
  in pain, *724*
  in schizophrenia, 669
    tardive dyskinesia in, 669
  overdose of or sensitivity to, vs.
    tetanus, 439
  poisoning by, *712*
Phenoxybenzamine
  in carcinoid flush, 2212
  in pheochromocytoma, 2205
  in Raynaud's phenomenon of
    scleroderma, 171
Phenoxymethyl penicillin, *557,* 558
  in acute poststreptococcal
    glomerulonephritis, 1396
Phentolamine
  in heart failure, 1101, *1101*
  in pheochromocytoma, 2206
  in shock, 1121
Phenylalanine, metabolism of, 2024
Phenylbutazone
  aplastic anemia and, 1735
  as nephrotoxin, 1432
  in acute gouty arthritis, 2039
  in ankylosing spondylitis, 195
  in degenerative joint disease, 205
  in Reiter's syndrome, 198
  in rheumatoid arthritis, 191
Phenylketonuria, *41, 2016*
  atypical, *2016,* 2025
  classic, *2016,* 2024–2025
  dietary restriction in, 55
  "lethal," 2025–2026
  screening for, 44
  transient, *2016,* 2025
Phenylpropanolamine, monoamine
  oxidase inhibitors and, interaction of,
  hypertension from, 1209
Phenylpropanolamine hydrochloride, in
  common cold, 233
Phenytoin, 1265–1266. See also
    Diphenylhydantoin.
  in convulsions of chronic renal
    failure, 1366
  in trigeminal neuralgia, 727
Pheochromocytoma, 2201–2206
  diabetes mellitus in, 1982
  hypercalcemia in, 2237, 2238
  investigation for, in arterial
    hypertension, 1204, 1209
  neurofibromatosis in, 2294
  tumor localization in, 2204, 2205
Phialophora compactum, 542
Phialophora pedrosoi, 542
Phialophora verrucosa, 542
Philadelphia chromosome, in chronic
  granulocytic leukemia, 1822
Phlebectasias, *2298*
Phlebothrombosis, 1124–1129. See also
    Thrombophlebitis.
  in pneumococcal pneumonia, 354
Phlebotomus argentipes, 584
Phlebotomus ariasi, 584
Phlebotomus chinensis, 584
Phlebotomus longipes, 587
Phlebotomus major, 584
Phlebotomus martini, 584
Phlebotomus papatasii
  in cutaneous leishmaniasis of old
    world, 587
  in sandfly fever, 282
  in visceral leishmaniasis, 584

Phlebotomus perniciosus, 584
Phlebotomus sergenti, 587
Phlebotomus species, in bartonellosis, 331
Phlebotomus verrugarum, 331
Phlebotomy(ies)
  in hemochromatosis, 1791
  in polycythemia vera, 1797
Phlegmasia alba dolens, 1126
Phlegmasia cerulea dolens, 1126
  surgical management of, 1128, 1129
Phlyctenular keratoconjunctivitis, 498
  in pulmonary tuberculosis, 484
Phobic anxiety syndrome, 674
Phocomelia, 49
Phonemic paraphasias, 656
Phoneutria species, bites of, 115
Phonocardiography
  in acquired valvular heart disease, *1175*, 1178
  in aortic stenosis, 1192
  in mitral stenosis, *1175*, 1182
Phosgene, exposure to
  pulmonary edema from, 1001
  respiratory effects of, 1000
Phosphate
  absorption of, 2229
  depletion of, 2229
  excretion of, 2229
    in chronic renal failure, 1358, *1358*
    in hypercalcemia, 2240
    in vitamin D resistant rickets, 2251
  plasma, 2228–2229
Phosphate ester insecticides, poisoning by, 75
Phosphate salts, in renal calculi, 1446
6-Phosphogluconate dehydrogenase, deficiency of, 1761
Phosphorus, 2228–2230
  in Fanconi's syndrome, 2024
  in hyperparathyroidism, 2219
  plasma concentrations of, in osteomalacia, 2248
  recommended allowances of, *1671*
  requirements of, 2229–2230
Photoallergic contact dermatitis, 2289
Photoallergy, 2289
Photocoagulation, in diabetic retinopathy, 2321
Photodermatitis, polymorphous, 2288
Photoscanning, pulmonary isotopic, in pulmonary embolism, 1132, 1133
Photosensitive porphyria, congenital, 2045
Photosensitivity, 2288–2289
Phototoxicity, 2289
Phrynoderma, 1685
Phthalylsulfathiazole, 563
Phthirus pubis, 108
Phthisis florida, 485
Phycomycosis, 545
Physalia species, envenomation by, 123
Physical agents
  pericarditis caused by, 1272
  pulmonary infiltrative disease caused by, 979
Physical and chemical irritants to lungs, 983–1002, *984*
Physical factors, role of, in disease, 13
Physical injury, mononeuropathy from, 900, 901
Physical measures
  in degenerative joint disease, 205

Physical measures (*Continued*)
  in rheumatoid arthritis, 191
Physical therapy, in parkinsonism, 754
Physostigmine, in atropine poisoning, 75
Phytanic acid, excess of, recessively inherited hypertrophic neuropathy with, 913
Phytohemagglutinin
  in assessment of immune competence in cancer, 1925
  in chromosomal analysis, 49
  in T cell competence assay, 130
Phytonadione, in vitamin K deficiency, 1890
Pial arteries, small, involvement of, in bacterial meningitis, 412
Pian, 518–522, *520*. See also *Yaws*.
Pian bois, *588*
Pian dartre, 521
Pica, 77
  in iron deficiency anemia, 1748
"Pick cell," 661
Pick's disease, 662–663
  vs. hereditary chorea, 759
Pickwickian syndrome, 654, 655, 1696
Picornaviruses, 268, *268*
  associated with common cold, *230*
PIE syndrome, 225, 968–970, *969*
  drugs causing, 156
Piebald trait, 2029
Piebaldism, 2292
Pig-bel, 66, 436
Pigeon breast, 1020, 1021
Pigment gallstones, 1619, 1620
Pigmentation
  blotchy, 2291
  disturbances of, 2289–2293
  in chronic renal failure, 1366
  in liver disease, 1645
  patterned, 2291
Pigmented nevi, 2290–2291, *2290*
Pigmented villonodular synovitis, 202
Piles, 1617
Pilocarpine, in glaucoma, 2322
Pilosebaceous-apocrine apparatus, 2269–2271
Pineal, 2061, 2111–2113, *2112*, *2113*
  calcification of, 2112
  tumors of, 864, 2113
Pinealomas, 864, 2113
Ping-Pong vaginitis, 603
Pinguéculae, in chronic renal failure, 1366
"Pink disease," 80
"Pink puffers," in chronic obstructive pulmonary disease, 961
Pins' sign, in pericardial effusion, 1274
Pinta, *520*, **524–525**
Pinworm infection, 629–630
  antimicrobial agents for, *559*
Pipecolic acidemia, *2018*
Piperazine, in fasciolopsiasis, 620
Piperazine citrate, in ascariasis, 627
Piroplasma hominis, 600
Piroplasmosis, 600–602
Pit viper, bite of, 122
Pitressin. See *Vasopressin*.
Pituitary
  ablation of, in diabetic retinopathy, 2321
  adenomas of, excessive hormone secretion in, 2108

Pituitary (*Continued*)
  anterior, 2083–2108
    anatomy of, 2083
    disorders of, amenorrhea due to, 2186–2187
      diagnosis of, hypothalamic hormones in, 2081–2082, *2081*, *2082*
      diagnostic principles in, 2065
      vs. functional amenorrhea, 2080
    function of, 2084–2085, *2085*
      assessment of, 2091–2094
    hormones of, 2085–2091
      deficiency of, 2102, 2103
    secretion of, control of, 2074–2083
    hypothalamus and, 2074, *2075*
    insufficiency of, 2100–2105. See also *Hypopituitarism*.
    neuroendocrine diseases of, 2078–2081
  posterior, 2109–2111
  tumors of, 863, 868
    amenorrhea due to, 2187
    diagnosis and treatment of, 2094–2100
      guidelines for, 2099, 2100
      during pregnancy, 2098, 2099
      galactorrhea in, 2192
      radioimmunoassay in, 2092
Pituitary apoplexy, 2098
Pituitary dwarfism, 2103, 2104, 2105
  classification of, *2104*
  management of, 55
Pituitary gonadotropins, measurement of, 2180
Pituitary snuff lung, *971*
Pityriasis alba, vs. pinta, 525
Pityriasis rosea, 2279–2280, *2280*
  vs. secondary syphilis, 510
PK reaction, in urticaria, 161
Placebo effects, in chronic pain management, 723
Placental alkaline phosphatase, as tumor marker, 1913
"Placental bacteremia," 455
Placental lactogen, human, as tumor marker, 1912, 1913
Placental proteins, as tumor markers, 1912–1913
Plague, 463–465
  vs. lymphogranuloma venereum, 335
  yellow, 526–529
Plague meningitis, 464, 465
Plague vaccine, 465
Plants
  antithyroid compounds in, goiter caused by, 69
  poisonous, 69–70
Plaque
  atherosclerotic, 1218, 1219
  cutaneous, 2273
Plasma
  calcium in, 2225–2227
  composition of, in metabolic acidosis, 1962, *1962*
  donor, sensitivity to, transfusion reaction from, *1785*, 1788
Plasma cell dyscrasias, 1852–1867, *1852*
  clinical patterns of, 1858–1867
  of unknown significance, 1852, 1866–1867
    electrophoretic patterns in, 1857, *1857*

Plasma cell dyscrasias (*Continued*)
paraproteins of, 1853, *1853*
pathogenesis of, 1852
serum and urinary proteins in, electrophoretic patterns of, 1854, *1855, 1856, 1857*
Plasma cell leukemia, in multiple myeloma, 1859, 1860
Plasma cell myeloma, 1858–1862
Plasma chemical values, 2348
Plasma expanders, in gastrointestinal bleeding, 1522
Plasma lipoproteins
concentration of, normal regulation of, 2003–2004
properties of, 2002, *2002*
Plasma phosphate, 2228–2229
Plasma prekallikrein deficiency, *1884*
Plasma protein(s)
abnormalities of, *43*
drug binding to, 2337
in systemic lupus erythematosus, 178
purified, in shock, 1118
Plasma thromboplastin antecedent, 1881
deficiency of, *43, 1884, 1887*
Plasma volume, regulation of, in hypertension, 1208
Plasmacytic and monocytic dyscrasias, association between, 1867
Plasmid transfer, drug resistance characterized by, 551
Plasmin, fibrinogen digestion by, 1891, 1892
Plasmodium falciparum, 558, 566, 568, *570*
differentiation of, from *Plasmodium vivax, 570,* 572
resistance of, to chloroquine, 573
Plasmodium malariae, 558, 566, 568
Plasmodium ovale, 558, 566, 568
Plasmodium species, life cycle of, 568, *568*
Plasmodium vivax, 558, 566, 568, *570*
differentiation of, from *Plasmodium falciparum, 570,* 572
Platelets
abnormalities of
drug-induced, 1879
functional, acquired, 1879
qualitative, 1878–1879
quantitative, 1872–1878
decreased production of, 1872–1873
donor, sensitivity to, transfusion reaction from, *1785,* 1788
giant, syndrome of, 1878–1879
increased destruction of, 1873–1876
release reaction defects of, 1879
Plate-like atelectasis, 965
Platinosis, 999
Platinum coordination complexes, in oncologic treatment, 1938
Platybasia, 875
Pleiotropism, 38
Pleomorphic lymphomas, 1830, *1830,* 1832, *1833*
Plethysmography, body, 933
Pleura
biopsy of, 950, 1014
diseases of, 1013–1018
history and physical examination in, 1013, 1014
methods of examination in, 1013–1014

Pleura (*Continued*)
diseases of, radiologic examination in, 1014
respiratory failure in, *1023,* 1024
in asbestosis, 990, 991, 1017
in pneumococcal pneumonia, 349
mesothelioma of, 1016
metastatic carcinoma to, 1016
neoplasms of, 1016
pain in, 1013
in pulmonary tuberculosis, 486
tuberculosis of, 491, 1015–1016
Pleural effusion(s)
in cancer patient, 1904
in pneumococcal pneumonia, 353
in pulmonary infarction, 1130
in systemic diseases, 1017, 1018
with pneumonia, 1015
Pleural fibrosis, in asbestosis, 1017
Pleural fluid, examination of, 948–949, 1014
formation and removal of, 1013
in simple hydrothorax, 1014, 1015
roentgenographic appearance of, 942
Pleurisy
dry, 491
in pulmonary tuberculosis, 486
in chronic renal failure, 1366
in pneumococcal pneumonia, 353
vs. acute appendicitis or cholecystitis, 354
in systemic lupus erythematosus, 177, 180
serofibrinous, with effusion, 482, 491
tuberculous, effusion and, 485
vs. angina pectoris, 1227
vs. pulmonary infarction, 1133
Pleuritis
in familial Mediterranean fever, 2056
vs. peptic ulcer, 1507
Pleurodynia, epidemic, 271–272
Pleuropulmonary infection, anaerobic, 443
Plexus neuropathies, 902–903
Plummer's nails, in hyperthyroidism, 2122
Plummer-Vinson syndrome, 1483, *2298, 2302*
in iron deficiency anemia, 1748
Pneumatosis cystoides intestinalis, 1611–1612
in scleroderma, 169
Pneumaturia, 1443
in diverticulitis, 1583
Pneumococcal endocarditis, 353, 386
treatment of, 394
Pneumococcal lesions, suppurative, extrapulmonary, 351
Pneumococcal meningitis, 353, 411
development of, factors associated with, 411
treatment of, 415
Pneumococcal pneumonia, 347–357, *350*
acute glomerulonephritis from, 1397
bacteremia in, 349
bacteriology of, 347
clinical course of, 353
clinical manifestations of, 351
complications of, 353
treatment of, 356
differential diagnosis of, 354
early lesion of, 349
epidemiology of, 348

Pneumococcal pneumonia (*Continued*)
immunology in, 347, 348
interlobar spread in, 349
invasion of pleura and pericardium in, 349
laboratory findings in, 352
mechanism of recovery in, 349
pathogenesis and pathology of, 348
physical signs in, 351
prevention of, 357
prognosis in, 356
relapse of, 353
spreading lesion of, 349
symptoms of, 351
treatment of, 355
Pneumococcus, pneumonia caused by, 347–357, *350.* See also *Pneumococcal pneumonia.*
Pneumoconioses, 984
"benign," 987
coal workers', 987
pulmonary hypertension in, 1147
collagenous, 984
diffuse, 990–992
nodular, 988–990
complicated, 992–993
management of, 993
inorganic dust, diagnosis of, 986
treatment and prevention of, 993–994
noncollagenous, 984, 987–988, *987*
Pneumocystis carinii, 558
infection with, in cancer patient, 1901
Pneumocystis species, 598, 599
Pneumocystosis, *570,* 598–600
antimicrobial agents for, *558*
Pneumoencephalography, 749
in brain tumor, 867
in "empty" sella syndrome, 2099, *2099*
Pneumonia(s), 338–365
adenoviral, 237
vs. mycoplasmal pneumonia, 345
aerobic gram-negative bacilli causing, 361–365
bacterial. See also names of specific pneumonias.
in influenza, 245
recurrent, 340
vs. coccidioidomycosis, 539
vs. Goodpasture's syndrome, 976
vs. malaria, 573
vs. psittacosis, 338
vs. pulmonary tuberculosis, 487
Broad Street, 359
drug therapy in, choice of, 341
Escherichia coli causing, 361, 365
Friedländer's bacillus causing, 357–358
vs. pneumococcal pneumonia, 354
Hemophilus influenzae, vs. pneumococcal pneumonia, 354
hydrocarbon ingestion causing, 75
in aspergillosis, 547
in blastomycosis, 540
in legionnaires' disease, 359, 360
in measles, 248, 249
in psittacosis, 337
in typhoid fever, 447
influenza virus, bacterial pneumonia and, combined, 245
primary, 243, 244, *244*
vs. mycoplasmal pneumonia, 345

Pneumonia(s) (*Continued*)
  interstitial, 998–999
  Klebsiella pneumoniae **causing,**
    357–358
    vs. pneumococcal pneumonia, 354
  lipoid, 998–999
  mycoplasmal, 343–346
    cold agglutinin syndrome
      following, 1765
    vs. coccidioidomycosis, 539
    vs. pneumococcal pneumonia, 354
    vs. psittacosis, 338
    vs. tularemia, 467
  nonprimary, 341
  nosocomial, 341, 361–364
    factors predisposing to, 362
    mechanisms and prevalence of, 361
    possible future management of, 363
  patient management in, principles of,
    341
  pleural effusions with, 1015
  pneumococcal, 347–357, *350*
    acute glomerulonephritis from, 1397
    bacteremia in, 349
    bacteriology of, 347
    clinical course of, 353
    clinical manifestations of, 351
    complications of, 353
      treatment of, 356
    differential diagnosis of, 354
    early lesion of, 349
    epidemiology of, 348
    immunology in, 347, 348
    interlobar spread in, 349
    invasion of pleura and pericardium
      in, 349
    laboratory findings in, 352
    mechanism of recovery in, 349
    pathogenesis and pathology of, 348
    physical signs in, 351
    prevention of, 357
    prognosis in, 356
    relapse of, 353
    spreading lesion of, 349
    symptoms of, 351
    treatment of, 355
  primary atypical, vs. influenza, 245
  Proteus species causing, 365
  ***Pseudomonas*, 361, 364–365**
  rheumatic, 381
  routes of invasion in, 339
  staphylococcal, 401–402
    vs. melioidosis, 470
    vs. pneumococcal pneumonia, 354
  streptococcal, hemolytic, 375
    vs. pneumococcal pneumonia, 354
  tuberculous, 481, 482, 485
    vs. pneumococcal pneumonia, 354
  tularemic, 466, 467
    vs. pneumococcal pneumonia, 354
  viral, vs. Goodpasture's syndrome,
    976
    vs. psittacosis, 338
  vs. epidemic pleurodynia, 272
  vs. pulmonary infarction, 1133
Pneumonic plague, 463, 464, 465
Pneumonitis
  aspiration, 1478
  chemical, acute, 1000
  hypersensitivity, 970–972, *971*
  in coccidioidomycosis, 538
  in varicella, 254
  interstitial, desquamative, 978
    lymphocytic, 1011, 1012

Pneumonitis (*Continued*)
  interstitial, lymphoid, 979
    usual, 978–979
  radiation, 1002
  rheumatic, 381
Pneumothorax
  air travel and, 96
  roentgenographic appearance of, 942
  spontaneous, 1016–1017
    vs. myocardial infarction, 1233
    vs. pulmonary embolism, 1133
  tension, 1017
    vs. acute pericarditis, 1273
PNP deficiency, 2043
Poicilobdella species, as agents of
  disease, 120
Poikilocytosis, 1718
Poikilothermia, relative, 716
Poison(s)
  elimination of, from body, 74
  hemolysis induced by, 1769–1770
  household and industrial, neuropathy
    associated with, 910–911
  inactivation of, 74
  specific antidotes for, 75
Poisoning. See also names of specific
  poisoning agents, e.g., *Arsenic,*
  Mushrooms.
  accidental, common, 71–76
  carbon monoxide, 82–84
  drug, acute, 711–714, *712*
  food, 64–70
  heavy metal, 77–82
Poisonous plants and animals, 68–70
Pokeweed, roots and stems of,
  poisoning by, 70
Poliomyelitis, 829–833
  bulbar, 831
  myocarditis in, 1282
  nonparalytic, 829, 830
  paralytic, 829, 831
Poliomyelitis-like syndrome, in acute
  hemorrhagic conjunctivitis, 270, 275
Poliovirus(es), 829
Poliovirus vaccines, 832
Pollen(s)
  grass, allergic rhinitis from, 157
  identification of, 158
  ragweed, allergen of, 131
  timothy hay, allergen of, 131
  tree, allergic rhinitis from, 157
Polyamines, as tumor markers, 1913
Polyarteritis
  renal, 181
  with pulmonary involvement, 166,
    182
Polyarteritis nodosa, 180–183, *2298*. See
  also *Periarteritis nodosa.*
Polychondritis, relapsing, 218
  aortic regurgitation in, 1194
  arthritis in, 199
  eyes in, 2316
Polycystic kidney disease, 1450, 1451,
  1452–1454
  in adults, 1453–1454
  in children, 1452–1453
    vs. medullary sponge kidney, 1456
Polycystic liver disease, 1667
Polycystic ovary, 2188–2190
Polycythemia(s), 1792–1800
  abnormal hemoglobins causing, 1778,
    1779
  absolute, 1793–1800
  classification of, *1793*

Polycythemia(s) (*Continued*)
  cutaneous lesions in, *2302*
  in primary pulmonary hypertension,
    1140
  primary, 1794–1797. See also
    Polycythemia vera.
  relative, 1792–1793
  secondary, 1798–1800
    appropriate, 1798–1799
    inappropriate, 1799–1800
    vs. polycythemia vera, 1796, *1796*
  "stress," 1792, 1793
Polycythemia vera, 1794–1797
  diagnostic criteria for, *1796*
  hepatic vein occlusion in, 1661
  portal hypertension in, 1639
Polydipsia
  in diabetes insipidus, 2110
    nephrogenic, 1435, 1436
  in diabetes mellitus, 1976
  psychogenic, 1955
    vs. diabetes insipidus, 2111
Polygenic inheritance, 44–45, *45*
Polymenorrhea, 2179
Polymorphic variations in human
  karyotype, 51
Polymorphism(s)
  balanced, 47
  inherited, *44*
Polymorphonuclear leukocytes,
  neutrophilic
  antibacterial activity of, 340
  dysfunction of, syndromes of,
    1803–1807, *1803*
  function of, 1800–1802, *1801*
Polymorphous photodermatitis, 2288
Polymyalgia arteritica, 216–218
Polymyalgia rheumatica, 216–218
  vs. polymyositis, 174
Polymyopathy, 172
Polymyositis, 171–174, 923
  eyes in, 2319
  in cancer, 879
  pulmonary hypertension in, 1147
  pulmonary involvement in, 974
  vs. Eaton-Lambert syndrome, 929
  vs. familial periodic paralysis, 921
  vs. myasthenia gravis, 927
  vs. trichinosis, 631
  vs. Wohlfart-Kugelberg Welander
    disease, 766
Polymyxin(s), 557, 562
  malabsorption from, 1548
  neuromuscular block caused by, 929
Polymyxin B, *557, 562*
Polymyxin E, *557, 562*
  as nephrotoxin, 1426
Polyneuritis
  in cancer, 878
  vs. congenital myopathies, 920
  vs. Eaton-Lambert syndrome, 929
  vs. muscular dystrophies, 918
  vs. poliomyelitis, 831
  vs. tick paralysis, 118
Polyneuropathy(ies), 903–913
  in multiple myeloma, 910, 1860
  nutritional, 772–773
  sensorimotor, in cancer, 878
Polyps
  cholesterol, 1634
  gastric, gastric carcinoma and,
    1600
Polypeptide chains, in immunoglobulin
  structure, 126, *127*

Polypeptides
  ectopic, as tumor markers, 1913
  mode of action of, 2070, 2071, *2071*
Polypoid adenomas, colorectal
  carcinoma risk and, 1607, *1607*
Polyposis, familial
    colorectal carcinoma and, 1606
    detection of, in relatives, *58, 59*
Polyradiculoneuropathy(ies)
  inflammatory, acute, 906–907
    chronic, 908
    recurrent, 908
Polyserositis
  paroxysmal, 2055–2057
  recurrent, familial, 2055–2057
  tuberculous, 494
Polythiazide, in arterial hypertension,
  1212
Polytomography, in diagnostic
  evaluation of amenorrhea, 2184
Polyuria
  in chronic renal failure, 1355
  in diabetes insipidus, 2110
    nephrogenic, 1435, 1436
  in diabetes mellitus, 1976
Pompe's disease, 919, 1280, 1999
Ponos, 584–587
Pontine infarction, 788
Pontine myelinolysis, central, 775–776
Popliteal cysts, rupture of, in
  rheumatoid arthritis, 188
Population control, 2194–2197
Population genetics, 46–48
Pork tapeworm, 608
  antimicrobial agents for, *559*
  treatment of, 608–609
Porocephaliasis, 119–120
Porphobilinogen, in porphyria, 2044
Porphyria(s), 2044–2049
  acute, 2045
    vs. poliomyelitis, 832
  barbiturate sensitivity in, 46
  classification of, 2045
  constitutional, 2048
  **erythropoietic, congenital, *42*, 2045,
    *2302***
      hemolytic anemia in, 1761
  hepatic, 2045–2049
    mixed, 2047
    idiosyncratic, 2048
  intermittent, acute, *42*, 2045–2047
    vs. acute abdomen, 1581
    vs. acute inflammatory
      polyneuropathy, 907
    vs. hysteria, 679
    vs. lead poisoning, 78
    vs. variegate porphyria, 2048
  photosensitive, congenital, 2045
    South African genetic, 2047
    symptomatic, 2048
      cutaneous signs of, *2299*
  variegate, *42*, 2047–2048
**Porphyria cutanea tarda, *42*, 2047,
  2048–2049**
  photosensitivity in, 2288, *2288*
  vs. scleroderma, 170
Porphyria cutanea tarda symptomatica,
  2048
Porphyria hepatica, 2045
Porphyrin, metabolism of, inborn errors
  of, *42*
Portal hypertension, 1639–1640
  ascites in, 1593
  cirrhosis and, 1144, 1665

Portal hypertension (*Continued*)
  diagnostic procedures in, 1648
  gastrointestinal bleeding and, 1523
    in cirrhosis, 1665
  manifestations of, 1639, 1640
Portal venous obstruction, portal
  hypertension in, 1639
Portal-systemic collateral vessels, in
  portal hypertension, 1640
**Portal-systemic encephalopathy,
  1640–1641**
**Portopulmonary hypertension
  syndrome, 1144**
Portuguese man-of-war, 123
Portuguese type of inherited
  amyloidosis, 910
Positional vertigo, 738, *738*
  benign, 738
Positive end-expiratory pressure, in
  acute respiratory failure, 1041, 1042
Postcapillary vessels, in shock, 1112
**Postcholecystectomy syndrome,
  1635–1636**
Postconcussional syndrome, anxiety in,
  674
Postdysenteric colitis, 591
Postencephalitic parkinsonism, 753
  vs. hysteria, 679
Posterior pituitary, 2109–2111
Posterior uveitis, in sarcoidosis, 2329
Postgastrectomy malabsorption, 1538
Postgonococcal urethritis, 409
Posthepatitic cirrhosis, 1663
Postherpetic neuralgia, 728, 826
Postictal state, 853, 854
Postinfectious cold agglutinin
  syndrome, 1765
Postinfectious encephalitis, vs. arboviral
  encephalitis, 284
Postinfectious encephalomyelitis, 836
Postinfusion hypoglycemia, in total
  parenteral nutrition, 1707
Postmenopausal atherosclerosis, 2190
Postmenopausal osteoporosis, 2190,
  2191, 2243, 2244
Postmyocardial infarction syndrome,
  1237, 1271
Postnecrotic cirrhosis, 1663
Postobstructive nephropathy, volume
  depletion in, 1951
Postoperative gas gangrene, 435
Postpartum fever, mycoplasmal, 347
Postpartum renal failure, 1414
Postperfusion syndrome, 1785
Postpericardiotomy syndrome, 1271
**Postphlebitic syndrome, 1126,
  1313–1314**
  vs. arteriovenous fistula, 1312
"Post-pill amenorrhea, 2080, 2188
**Poststreptococcal glomerulonephritis,
  acute, 1394–1397**
Post-transfusion purpura, 1875–1876
Post-traumatic headache, recurrent, 732
Post-traumatic painful osteoporosis, 727
Post-traumatic pericarditis, 1271
**Post-traumatic pulmonary insufficiency,
  1033–1045**
Post-traumatic spreading neuralgia, 727
Postural proteinuria, 1332
Posture, disturbances in, 752
  in paralysis agitans, 753
Postvaccinal encephalitis, vs. arboviral
  encephalitis, 284
Postvaccinal encephalomyelitis, 836, 837

Postvaccinial encephalitis, 260
Postvaccination encephalomyelitis, 836
Postvagotomy diarrhea, 1520
Potassium
  deficiency of, 1957–1959
    causes of, *1957*
    myocarditis of, 1284
    depletion of, vs. diabetes insipidus,
      2110
    vs. familial periodic paralysis, 922
  **equilibrium of, disturbances of,
    1956–1960**
    excretion of, in chronic renal failure,
      1356, *1357*
      in interstitial nephritis, 1418
  homeostasis of, kidney in, 1323
    in diabetic ketoacidosis, 1984
    in hypokalemia, 1958
  intoxication with, 1959–1960
Potassium bromate, as nephrotoxin,
  1435
Potassium chloride
  in familial periodic paralysis, 922
  in gastric outlet obstruction
    complicating peptic ulcer, 1517
  in potassium deficiency, 1958, 1959
Potassium iodide
  in preparation for thyroidectomy,
    2125
  in simple chronic bronchitis, 955
  in sporotrichosis, 545
Potassium salts
  in digitalis toxicity, 1099
  in salicylate poisoning, 76
Potassium tartrate, poisoning by, 81
Potassium-losing nephritis, vs. familial
  periodic paralysis, 922
Potato plant, poisoning by, 70
Pott's disease, 185, 497
Pott's puffy tumor, 2261
  epidural abscess with, 808
Powassan virus, 290
Poxvirus bovis, 255
Poxvirus officinale, 255
Poxvirus variolae, 255
PPD of Seibert, in tuberculin test, 482
P-R interval, 1242, *1243*
  **short, with normal QRS complexes
    and supraventricular tachycardias,
    1256–1257**
Practolol peritonitis, 224
Prader-Willi syndrome, 920
Prausnitz-Küstner reaction, in urticaria,
  161
Prazosin
  in arterial hypertension, *1212*, 1215
  in hypertension of chronic renal
    failure, 1362
Precapillary sphincters, in shock, 1112
Precipitin test, in protozoan and
  helminthic diseases, *565*
Precocious pseudopuberty, 2080, 2167
  organic, due to adrenal and ovarian
    hyperfunction, 2182, 2183
Precocious puberty, 2080
  as manifestation of cancer, 1916
Precocity, sexual
  female, 2179, 2182–2183
  male, 2166–2167
Precoma, hepatic, 1640–1641
Precordial movements, evaluation of,
  1074, *1074*
Prednisolone
  in adult celiac disease, 1540

Prednisolone (*Continued*)
  in aplastic anemia, 1739
  in hypercalcemia complicating
    hormonal treatment of breast
    cancer, 1920
  in malabsorption syndrome, *1536*
  in minimal change glomerular
    disease, 1392
  in nongranulomatous ileojejunitis,
    1542
  in shock of pseudomembranous
    enterocolitis, 1585
  in ulcerative colitis, 1573
Prednisone
  in adult celiac disease, 1540
  in allergic rhinitis, 160
  in angioedema, 163
  in aplastic anemia, 1739
  in asthma, 958
  in autoimmune hemolytic anemia,
    1764
  in carcinoid flush, 2213
  in central nervous system in-
    volvement of systemic lupus
    erythematosus, 180
  in chronic active hepatitis, 1662
  in chronic lymphocytic leukemia,
    1825
  in chronic obstructive pulmonary
    disease, 963
  in dermatologic therapy, 2277
  in diphtheria, 432
  in drug allergy, 157
  in eosinophilic gastroenteritis, 1543
  in esoinophilic granuloma, 1851
  in exophthalmos complicating Graves'
    disease, 2127
  in glomerulitis and glomerulo-
    nephritis of systemic lupus
    erythematosus, 180
  in gold-induced dermatitis
    complicating rheumatoid arthritis
    therapy, 192
  in hypercalcemia, 2240
  in hyperthyroidism, 2125
  in idiopathic thrombocytopenic
    purpura, 1874
  in infectious mononucleosis with
    severe toxic pharyngotonsillitis,
    267
  in malabsorption syndrome, *1536*
  in multiple sclerosis, 847
  in myasthenia gravis, 928
  in nongranulomatous ileojejunitis,
    1542
  in non-Hodgkin's lymphomas, *1836*
  in ocular histoplasmosis, 2324
  in ocular toxoplasmosis, 2335
  in paroxysmal nocturnal
    hemoglobinuria, 1769
  in pemphigus, 2304
  in periarteritis nodosa, 183
  in polymyalgia rheumatica, 217
  in polymyositis and dermatomyositis,
    174
  in pulmonary tuberculosis, 489,
    490
  in regional enteritis, 1567
  in rheumatic fever, 384
  in rheumatoid arthritis, 192
  in sarcoidosis, 977
  in serum sickness, 154
  in shoulder-hand syndrome, 206
  in subacute thyroiditis, 2132
  in Sudeck's atrophy, 2246

Prednisone (*Continued*)
  in thrombotic thrombocytopenic
    purpura, 1877
  in thyroid eye disease, 2333
  in tuberculous meningitis, 494
  in typhoid fever, 448
  in ulcerative colitis, 1573
  in Wegener's granulomatosis, 220
Prednisone suppression test, in
  hyperparathyroidism, 2217
Preeclampsia, 1414
Preganglionic lumbar sympathectomy,
  in arteriosclerosis obliterans, 1301
Pregnancy
  air travel and, 96
  diabetes mellitus and, 1988, 1989
  Ehlers-Danlos syndrome and, 2055
  fasting hypoglycemia in, 1993
  fatty liver of, 1660
  glomerulonephritis in, 1414
  gonococcal disease in, treatment of,
    409, 410
  hypertension in, 1205, 1206, 1414,
    1415, 1416
  hyperthyroidism in, 2125, 2126
  influenza complications in, 244
  iron needs in, 1747, 1750
  jaundice of, recurrent, 1658
  listeriosis in, 472
  megaloblastic anemia of, 1723, 1726
  multiple sclerosis and, 845, 848
  mycoplasmal disease in, 347
  nephrotic syndrome and, 1389, 1390,
    1414
  obesity and, 1696
  opiate addiction and, 697
  pituitary tumors during, 2098, 2099
  "problem," counseling in, 690
  pyelonephritis in, 1414
  recommended dietary allowances in,
    1671
  renal disease in, 1414–1416
  sarcoidosis and, 214
  smallpox and, 256, 257
  syphilis in, treatment of, 516
  systemic lupus erythematosus and,
    177, 1414
  toxemia of, 1205, 1414–1416
  tubal, vs. gonococcal salpingitis, 408
  tuberculosis and, 483
Pregnanediol, urinary excretion of,
  values for, 2180, *2181*
Pregnanetriol, urinary excretion of,
  values for, 2180, *2181*
Preinfarction angina, 1228
Preleukemia, 1817
  vs. aplastic anemia, 1738
Preload, cardiac, 1064, 1065, 1083, 1084,
  1084
  reduction of, in shock, 1120
Premarital coitus, 690
Premature atrial beats, 1246
Premature ejaculation, 688, 2198
Premature ventricular beats, 1251
Prematurity, congenital heart disease
  and, 1150
Prenylamine, in angina pectoris,
  1228
Prerenal azotemia, 1369
  vs. acute tubular necrosis, 1373
Presbycusis, 736
"Presenile dementia," 662
  vs. brain tumor, 868
**Pressure, atmospheric, alterations in,
  97–103**

Pressure (*Continued*)
  **atmospheric, alterations in, direct
    effects of, 98–99**
    indirect effects of, 99–103
Pressure-volume relationships, in acute
  respiratory failure, 1035, *1035*
Pretibial fever, 534
Pretibial myxedema, in Graves' disease,
  2127, *2128*
Prickly heat, 2268
Primaquine
  in malaria, *558*
  in malaria prevention, 575
  in prevention of malaria relapse, 574
Primidone, in epilepsy, *859*, 860
Prinzmetal's angina, 1228, 1229
Proaccelerin, 1881
  deficiency of, 1888
    coexistent antihemophilic factor
     and, 1889
Probenecid
  in gonococcal disease, 409, 410
  in pregnancy, 409
  in tophaceous gout, 2040
Procainamide, 1264–1265
  in myotonia congenita, 920
  in myotonic dystrophy, 918
  in ventricular tachycardia, 1254
Procaine penicillin
  aqueous, in gonococcal disease, 409
    in group A streptococcal infection,
     376
    in syphilis, 516
     cardiovascular, 1295
  in infective endocarditis, 392
  in infective endocarditis prophylaxis,
    396
  in louse-borne relapsing fever, 528
  in streptobacillary rat-bite fever, 531
  in tropical phagedenic ulcer, 530
Procaine penicillin G, 557, *557*
  in congenital syphilis, 517
  in lung abscess, 981
  in neurosyphilis, 816
  in pinta, 525
  in rheumatic fever, 383
  in rheumatic fever prevention, 376
  in syphilis, *515*
  in yaws, 521
Procarbazine
  in Hodgkin's disease, 1846
  in non-Hodgkin's lymphomas, *1836*
  in oncologic treatment, 1938
Prochlorperazine
  in carcinoid flush, 2212
  in gastrointestinal symptoms of
    chronic renal failure, 1365
  in migraine syndrome, 732
  in staphylococcal food poisoning, 65
Proctalgia, 1618
Proctalgia fugax, 1497, 1618
Proctitis
  gonococcal, 407
  ulcerative, 1559, 1570, 1616
    vs. lymphogranuloma venereum,
     1572
Proctoscopy
  in colorectal carcinoma, 1608
  in diagnosis of constipation, 1481
Procyclidine, in parkinsonism, 755
Progeria
  vs. pituitary dwarfism, 2104
  vs. scleroderma, 170
Progesterone, plasma, values for, 2180,
  2180

Progesterone in oil, in evaluation of
amenorrhea, 2183
Progesterone withdrawal bleeding, in
evaluation of ovarian function, 2180
Proglutamic aciduria, *2019*
Progressive bulbar palsy, 765
Progressive chorea, chronic, 758–759
**Progressive multifocal
leukoencephalopathy, 841–842**
Progressive muscular atrophy, 765
Progressive stroke, 785
anticoagulant drugs or surgery in, 793
Progressive subcortical encephalopathy,
794
Progressive vaccinia, 260
Proinsulin, human, probable sequence
of, *1973*
Prolactin, 2087
ectopic production of, galactorrhea
from, 2192
function of, assessment of, 2092
secretion of, excessive, 2092, 2108,
2191
regulation of, 2077
Prolactin inhibitory factor, 2075
regulation of, disorders of, 2081
Prolactin-releasing factor, 2075
**Proliferative glomerulonephritis,
1394–1400**
in staphylococcal bacteremia and
endocarditis, 403
Proline-hydroxyproline-glycinuria, 2023
Prolixin. See *Fluphenazine.*
Promazine, in pain, *724*
Promethazine
in motion sickness, 95
in pain, *724*
Promyelocytic leukemia, 1814
hemorrhage in, 1817
Propantheline
in chronic pancreatitis, 1557
in colonic diverticulosis, 1501
in diarrhea after extensive small
intestinal resection, 1544
in malabsorption syndrome, *1536*
Properdin pathway of complement
activation, 135, *135*, 136
Propionibacterium acnes, 442
Propranolol, 1265
in angina pectoris, 1228
in arterial hypertension, *1212, 1213,
1214*
in dissecting aortic aneurysm, 1297
in essential tremor, 757
in hypertension of chronic renal
failure, 1362
in hyperthyroidism, 2125
in mitral valve prolapse syndrome,
1189
in multiple sclerosis, 848
in pheochromocytoma, 2205, 2206
in preparation for thyroidectomy,
2125
in tachycardia complicating tetanus,
440
in thyroid storm, 2128
Propranolol hydrochloride, in
lightheadedness from psychiatric
disorders, 742
Proptosis, in hyperthyroidism, 2122
Propylthiouracil, in hyperthyroidism,
2123, 2124
Prosector's wart, 479, 498
Prostacyclin, circulatory effects of, 1111

Prostaglandins, 2064
circulatory effects of, 1111
in peptic ulcer, 1515
Prostate
carcinoma of
hypofibrinogenemia in, 1894
medical treatment of, 1921–1922
tuberculosis of, 496
Prostatectomy, local fibrinolysis after,
1896
Prostatic acid phosphatase, as tumor
marker, 1913
Prostatitis, gonococcal, 407, 409
Prosthetic valve endocarditis, 391
Protamine sulfate, in bleeding
complicating heparin therapy of
thrombophlebitis, 1127
Protein(s)
absorption of, 1525
Bence Jones, in cardiac amyloidosis,
1286
C-reactive, complement activation by,
136
deficiency of, cutaneous lesions of,
1676
depletion of, in chronic renal failure,
1361
diets high in, in nephrotic syndrome,
1389
enteric loss of, malabsorption
syndrome and, 1548–1549, *1548,
1549*
in acute infections, 1678, 1679
in cerebrospinal fluid, in bacterial
meningitis, 413
M, in streptococcal infections, 368
metabolism of, impaired, in
malabsorption, 1528
in liver disease, 1643
mutant, modification of, in
management of genetic disease, 55
myelin basic, 844
nutrient value of, 1670
**placental, as tumor markers,
1912–1913**
plasma, abnormalities of, *43*
drug binding to, 2337
in systemic lupus erythematosus,
178
purified, in shock, 1118
serum, electrophoretic patterns of, in
plasma cell dyscrasias, 1854, *1855,
1856, 1857*
in kwashiorkor, 1681, 1682
synthesis of, derangements of, plasma
cell dyscrasias and, 1853, *1853*
gene and, 31
genetic control of, 32, *32*, 33
regulatory mechanisms of, 34
T, in group A streptococcal infections,
369
Tamm-Horsfall, 1337
urinary, electrophoretic patterns of, in
plasma cell dyscrasias, 1854, *1855,
1856, 1857*
Protein clearances, differential, in
nephrotic syndrome, 1389
Protein derivative, purified, in
tuberculin test, 482
Protein hormones, mode of action of,
2070, 2071, *2071*
Protein hydrolysate solutions, after
extensive small intestinal resection,
1544, *1544*

Protein malnutrition, fatty liver in, 1660
Protein-bound iodine, determination of,
2117
Protein-calorie deficiency, 1680–1683
clinical signs of, *1677*
effect of, on plasma amino acids, *2018*
**Protein-losing enteropathy, 1528,
1548–1549, *1548, 1549***
Proteinosis
lipoid, 2058
pulmonary alveolar, 978
Protein-restricted diets, 1711
Proteinuria, 1337–1338, *1338*
Bence Jones, in multiple myeloma,
1858, 1860
glomerular, 1337
in asymptomatic patient, 1331, 1332
in chronic renal failure, 1353
in diabetes mellitus, 1977
in glomerular disease, 1386
in γ heavy chain disease, 1865
in toxemia of pregnancy, 1414, 1415
persistent, 1331, 1337
postural, 1332
screening tests for, 1337
tubular, 1337
in chronic cadmium poisoning,
1429
Proteoglycans, 164, 165
Proteus morganii, 69
Proteus species, pneumonia caused by,
365
Prothrombin, deficiency of, 1888
Prothrombin time, in hereditary
coagulation disorders, *1884*
Protocoproporphyria hereditaria, 2047
Protoporphyria, 42, 2049
erythropoietic, 2049, *2302*
vs. variegate porphyria, 2048
Protozoan diseases, 565–604
antimicrobial agents for, *558*
hepatic, 1657
immunodiagnostic tests for, *565*
malabsorption in, 1546
Proximal gastric vagotomy, in duodenal
ulcer, 1519, *1519*
Prurigo gestationis, 2305
Pruritus
in biliary cirrhosis, 1666, 1667
in chronic renal failure, 1366
in Hodgkin's disease, 1841
in liver disease, 1645
intense, as sign of internal
malignancy, 2296
Pruritus ani, 1617–1618
Prussian blue, in thallium poisoning, 82
"Pseudochylous" ascites, 1593
Pseudocoarctation of aorta, 1290
Pseudocyst(s), pancreatic
ascites in, 1593
in chronic pancreatitis, 1556, *1556*
percutaneous transhepatic
cholangiography in, *1473*
ultrasonography in, *1465*
Pseudodeficiency rickets, 2252
Pseudodiabetes, uremic, 1361
Pseudofractures, in osteomalacia, 2248
Pseudogout, 201–202
**Pseudohermaphroditism, male,
2172–2173**
Pseudohyperkalemia, 1959
in essential thrombocythemia, 1878
"Pseudohyperparathyroid" syndrome,
2217

Pseudohyponatremia, 1955
Pseudohypoparathyroidism, 2064, **2221–2223**
    malabsorption in, 1547
Pseudohypophosphatasia, *2019*
Pseudoidiopathic hypoparathyroidism, 2064
Pseudoleukemic-pseudoerythremic myelosis, 1827
Pseudolymphoma of lung, 1011, 1012
Pseudomembranous enterocolitis, 1585
    necrotizing, acute, 405
Pseudomonas infections, unique features of, 456
Pseudomonas **pneumonia,** 361, **364–365**
Pseudomonas species, food poisoning by, 66
"Pseudomyotonia," 923
Pseudomyxoma peritonei, 1595
Pseudo-obstruction
    colonic, 1497–1498
    intestinal, 1497
        malabsorption in, 1538
Pseudopapilledema, 2327–2328
    vs. benign intracranial hypertension, 872
    vs. papilledema, 865
Pseudoparkinsonism, arteriosclerotic, 753–754
Pseudopolyps, in ulcerative colitis, 1569, 1571, *1571*
Pseudopseudohypoparathyroidism, 2221–2223
Pseudopuberty, precocious, 2080, 2167
    organic, due to adrenal and ovarian hyperfunction, 2182, 2183
Pseudotabes diabetica, 908
Pseudotumor(s)
    gallbladder, 1634, *1634*
    orbital, 224
Pseudotumor cerebri, 870–872, *871*
Pseudouridine, as tumor marker, 1913
Pseudo–vitamin D resistant rickets, 2252
Pseudoxanthoma elasticum, 2294–2295, *2298, 2301*
    aorta in, 1292
Psilocin, 704
Psilocybin, 704
    poisoning by, *712*
Psittacosis, 336–338
    vs. mycoplasmal pneumonia, 345
    vs. pneumococcal pneumonia, 354
    vs. tularemia, 467
Psoriasis, 2280–2281, *2281*
    in adult celiac disease, 1541
    vs. leprosy, 503
    vs. pinta, 525
    vs. secondary syphilis, 510
Psoriatic arthritis, 196–197, *197*
    vs. rheumatoid arthritis, 190
Psychedelics, 703–705
    poisoning by, *712*
Psychiatric disorders
    dizziness from, 742
    vs. metabolic encephalopathy, 649
Psychiatry, concept of disease in, 664–665
Psychogenic aerophagia, 1489
Psychogenic megacolon, 1496
Psychogenic pain, 723
Psychogenic polydipsia, 1955
    vs. diabetes insipidus, 2111

Psychogenic vomiting, 1477
    hypokalemia in, 1958
Psychologic factors in irritable bowel syndrome, 1493, 1494
Psychologic illness in medical practice, 664–680
Psychologic testing
    in clinical medicine, 681–683
    in epilepsy, 857
Psychomotor activity, in metabolic brain disease, 648
Psychomotor epilepsy, 855
    schizophrenia-like syndrome in, 668
    vs. syncope, 745
Psychomotor status, 856
Psychosis(es), 665
    alcohol abuse and, 709, 710
    amphetamine, 702
    cocaine, 702
    functional, 665–672
    in epilepsy, 856
    in myxedema, 2133
    Korsakoff's, 659, 774
        vs. dementia, 660, 661
        Wernicke's syndrome and, 773–774
    manic-depressive, 665, **669–672**
        vs. depression, 677
    psychedelic use and, 704, 705
    toxic, 645
        in chronic renal failure, 1366
Psychosocial development, adolescent, 20–22
Psychosocial problems of aging, 29
Psychosomatic factors in peptic ulcer, 1504
Psychotherapy
    in anorexia nervosa, 1702, 1703
    in anxiety, 675
    in epilepsy, 861
    in parkinsonism, 754
    in schizophrenia, 669
    in ulcerative colitis, 1574
PTA, 1881
    deficiency of, 43, *1884,* 1887
Pterois species, envenomation by, 124
Pteroylglutamic acid, in megaloblastic anemia, 1727, 1728
Ptosis, in myasthenia gravis, 926
Puberty
    biologic processes in, 17–20, *18*
    factors affecting, 20
    gonadotropin secretion in, 2176
    in female, *18,* 19, **2181–2182**
    in male, *18,* 19, **2166**
    neuroendocrine control of, 19, 20
    precocious, 2080
        as manifestation of cancer, 1916
    somatic changes in, 17, 18, 19
Pubic hair, development of, *18,* 19
Pubic louse, 108, 109
Puborectalis syndrome, 1618
Puerperal myocarditis, 1287
Puerperium, tuberculosis and, 483
Puffer fish, poisoning by, 69
Puffy tumor, Pott's, 2261
    epidural abscess with, 808
Pulmonary. See also *Lung(s).*
Pulmonary alveolar proteinosis, 978
Pulmonary angiography, 943
    in pulmonary embolism, 1132
Pulmonary arterial pressure
    at high altitude, 1137
    normal, 1135

Pulmonary arteriovenous fistula, congenital, 1168–1169
Pulmonary artery(ies), 1135
    in fetus and newborn, 1135
    stenosis of, 1143, **1167–1168**
    thrombosis of, vs. pulmonary embolism, 1133
Pulmonary aspergillosis, 547
Pulmonary atresia, Fallot's tetralogy with, 1164, 1165
Pulmonary blastoma, 1012
Pulmonary blastomycosis, primary, 540
Pulmonary blood flow, 1136
    distribution of, 938
Pulmonary blood volume, 1136
Pulmonary candidiasis, 548
Pulmonary capillaries, 1135
Pulmonary capillary blood volume, in diffusion, 937, 938
Pulmonary capillary wedge pressure, in acute respiratory failure, 1038, *1039*
Pulmonary circulation
    functions of, 938
    in mitral stenosis, 1145–1146
    normal, 1135–1137
Pulmonary complications
    in carcinoid syndrome, 2208
    in opiate addiction, 697
    in polyarteritis, 166, 182
    in rheumatoid arthritis, 187, 188
    in systemic lupus erythematosus, 177
Pulmonary cryptococcosis, 544
Pulmonary disease
    eosinophilia and, 225
    obstructive, chronic, 951, 952, **960–964,** *961*
        pulmonary hypertension in, 1146, 1147
        secondary polycythemia in, 1799
        vs. asthma, 957
    special diagnostic procedures in, 941–951
Pulmonary edema
    acute, in left ventricular failure, 1090
        management of, 1094
    chemical, 1001
        in acute chemical bronchitis or pneumonitis, 1000
        diseases causing, respiratory failure in, 1023–1024, *1023*
    high altitude, 101
    in chronic renal failure, 1363
    in malaria, 571, 572, 574
    "neurogenic," 717
    vs. Goodpasture's syndrome, 976
    vs. pulmonary embolism, 1133
Pulmonary emboli, pulmonary vascular disease in, 1143
Pulmonary embolism, 1015, **1129–1134**
    in myocardial infarction, 1231
    vs. myocardial infarction, 1232, 1233
Pulmonary embolization, vs. acute pericarditis, 1273
Pulmonary encephalopathy, benign intracranial hypertension in, 872
Pulmonary eosinophilia
    prolonged, 969–970, *969*
    simple, 969, *969*
    tropical, 225, **637,** *969,* **970**
    with asthma, *969,* **970**
    with periarteritis nodosa, *969,* **970**
Pulmonary fibrosis
    complicating cancer therapy, 1904

Pulmonary fibrosis (*Continued*)
in collagenous pneumoconioses, 990, 991
in paraquat ingestion, 1001
Pulmonary function tests
in left ventricular failure, 1091
in mitral stenosis, 1183
in sarcoidosis, 214
Pulmonary hemosiderosis, idiopathic, 976
pulmonary hypertension in, 1147
Pulmonary hypersensitivity reactions, drug-induced, 974–976
Pulmonary hypertension, 1135–1149
disorders of respiration and, 1146–1149
in atrial septal defect, 1161
in cirrhosis with portal hypertension, 1144
in coarctation of aorta, 1289
in congenital heart disease, 1141–1143
in mitral stenosis, 1180, 1181
vs. atrial septal defect, 1162
primary, 1137–1141
vs. mitral stenosis, 1183
Pulmonary infarction, 1015, 1129–1134
vs. acute appendicitis, 1581
vs. pnemococcal pneumonia, 354
Pulmonary infection, in cancer, 1901
Pulmonary infiltration
diseases of, 966–979
respiratory failure in, 1023, *1023*
with eosinophilia, 225, 968–970, *969*
drugs causing, 156
Pulmonary insufficiency, post-traumatic, 1033–1045
Pulmonary isotopic photoscanning, in pulmonary embolism, 1132, 1133
Pulmonary mucormycosis, 546
Pulmonary osteoarthropathy, hypertrophic, in bronchogenic carcinoma, 1007
Pulmonary overpressure accidents, 99
Pulmonary paragonimiasis, 619, 620
Pulmonary schistosomiasis, 614
Pulmonary surfactant, antibacterial activity of, 339
Pulmonary tropical eosinophilia, 637
Pulmonary trunk
anomalous origin of left coronary artery from, 1172
idiopathic dilatation of, 1167
congenital pulmonary regurgitation and, 1168
Pulmonary tuberculosis, 484–490
cavity formation in, 482
chronic, 482, 485–487
endobronchial spread of, 482
classification of, 487
lower and middle lobe, in aged, 487
progressive primary, 485
retreatment of, 490
symptomatic primary infection in, 484–485
treatment of, 487–490
bed rest in, 490
drug, 487
combined, 488
in noncompliant patient, 490
surgery in, 490
vs. pulmonary paragonimiasis, 620
Pulmonary tularemia, 467

Pulmonary valve
congenital regurgitation of, 1168
structural abnormalities of, regurgitation caused by, 1168
Pulmonary vascular disease
in congenital heart disease, 1141–1143
respiratory failure in, *1023*, 1024
Pulmonary vasculitis, 972–973
Pulmonary veno-occlusive disease, pulmonary venous hypertension from, 1145
Pulmonary venous connection, total anomalous, 1172, 1173
Pulmonary venous hypertension, 1144–1146
Pulmonary venules, 1135
Pulmonic regurgitation, 1199
vs. aortic regurgitation, 1197
Pulmonic stenosis, 1199
single ventricle with, 1174
subvalvular, 1167
supravalvular, 1167–1168
valvular, 1158–1160
ventricular septal defect with, 1164–1166
Pulmonic valve disease, 1199
Pulse(s)
arterial, examination of, 1074
in congenital heart disease, 1155
venous, examination of, 1073, *1073*
in congenital heart disease, 1155
water-hammer, in aortic regurgitation, 1195
Pulseless disease, 789, 1297. See also *Takayasu's syndrome.*
Pulsus alternans, in left ventricular failure, 1090
Punch biopsy of skin, 2273, 2274, *2274*
Punctate basophilia, 1718
Punctate keratitis
in onchocerciasis, 636
in Reiter's syndrome, 2316
Puncture, lumbar, 747–748. See also *Lumbar puncture.*
Pupil(s)
Adie's myotonic, 900
Argyll Robertson, 900
in neurosyphilis, 512, 814, 815
disturbances of, extraocular palsy and, 899, 900
Pupillary light reactions, in metabolic brain disease, 648
Purified protein derivative, in tuberculin test, 482
Purine, metabolism of, disorders of, 2029–2043
Purine analogues, in oncologic treatment, 1935
Purine nucleoside phosphorylase deficiency, 2043
Purine nucleotide synthesis, in gout, 2031, 2032, *2032*
Purine ring synthesis, interference with, *1721*
Purinethol. See *Mercaptopurine.*
Purpura(s)
anaphylactoid, renal involvement in, 1400, 1401
drug, 1873–1874, *1873*
nonthrombocytopenic, 1880
Henoch-Schönlein, 1880, *2298, 2301*
arthritis in, 201

Purpura(s) (*Continued*)
Henoch-Schönlein, renal involvement in, 1400, 1401
vs. periarteritis nodosa, 183
hyperglobulinemic, benign, 1880
immunologic, secondary, 1876
lung, nephritis and, 1401
neonatal, 1876
post-transfusion, 1875–1876
senile, 1879
thrombocytopenic
autoimmune, 1874
complicating rifampin treatment of pulmonary tuberculosis, 488
drugs associated with, 156, 1873–1874, *1873*
idiopathic, 1874–1875
immune mechanisms in, 132
thrombotic, 1876–1877
hypofibrinogenemia in, 1893
renal involvement in, 1401
vs. periarteritis nodosa, 183
vs. dengue hemorrhagic fever, 297
vascular, 1879–1880
causes of, *1879*
vs. coagulation disorders, 1871, *1872*
Purpura fulminans, 1893
Purpura hemorrhagica, in Crimean hemorrhagic fever, 298
Purpura simplex, 1879
Purulent arthritis, anaerobic, 444
Purulent meningitis
acute, 418
in nocardiosis, 475
Puss-caterpillar, dermatitis caused by, 119
Pustular acne vulgaris, 400
Pustule(s), 2273
malignant, 470
Putamen hemorrhage, clinical manifestations of, 797, 798
Putrescine, as tumor marker, 1913
Pyarthrosis, staphylococcal, 404
Pyelography
antegrade, 1343
intravenous, in nephrocarcinoma, 1459
percutaneous, in obstructive nephropathy, 1449
retrograde, 1343
Pyelonephritis, 1409–1413
chronic, 1422
in paraplegia, 888
in pregnancy, 1414
vs. acute appendicitis, 1581
vs. adult polycystic kidney disease, 1454
Pyloric stenosis, 1490
frequency and sex ratio of, *48*
Pyloromyotomy, in pyloric stenosis, 1490
Pyoderma, streptococcal, 374
epidemiology of, 370
pathogenesis of, 368
treatment of, 376
Pyogenic arthritis
gonococcal, 407
in bacterial meningitis, 414
Pyogenic liver abscesses, vs. hepatic amebiasis, 592
Pyogenic meningitis, 411
vs. herpes simplex encephalitis, 824

Pyogenic osteomyelitis, subacute, 2260
Pyomyositis
staphylococcal, 404
tropical, 404, **638**
Pyrantel embonate
in ascariasis, 627
in hookworm disease, 625
Pyrantel pamoate
in enterobiasis, 629
in hookworm disease, 625
in intestinal nematodes, *559*
Pyrazinamide, *557*
in pulmonary tuberculosis, 488, 490
Pyribenzamine. See *Tripelennamine.*
2-Pyridine aldoxime methiodide, in
poisoning by phosphate ester
insecticides, 75
Pyridostigmine, in myasthenia gravis,
928
Pyridoxal phosphate, 1673
deficiency of, 773
Pyridoxamine phosphate, 1673
Pyridoxine
deficiency of, in nutritional
polyneuropathy, 773
in homocystinuria, 2029
in primary hyperoxaluria, 2001
in pulmonary tuberculosis, 487
in sideroblastic anemia, 1741
in tuberculous meningitis, 494
in Wilson's disease, 2050
Pyridoxine-responsive sideroblastic
anemia, 1741
Pyrimethamine
in malaria, *558*
in malaria prophylaxis, 574, 575
in toxoplasmosis, *558*, 597
ocular, 2335
Pyrimidine
metabolism of, disorders of,
2043–2044
synthesis of, interference with, *1721*
Pyrimidine analogues, in oncologic
treatment, 1934
Pyrimidine 5'-nucleotidase deficiency,
2044
Pyrogenic transfusion reactions, *1785*,
1786
Pyropoikilocytosis, hereditary, 1758
Pyrosis, 1479
Pyrroloporphyria, Swedish type, 2045
Pyruvate carboxylase deficiency, *41*
Pyruvate decarboxylase deficiency, *41*
Pyruvate kinase deficiency, 1758–1759
Pyrvinium pamoate, in enterobiasis,
629, 630
Pyuria, in diverticulitis, 1583

Q fever, 309, **329–331**
clinical features of, *313*
epidemiologic features of, *310*
serologic responses in, *314*
vs. mycoplasmal pneumonia, 345
vs. pneumococcal pneumonia, 354
vs. psittacosis, 338
vs. tularemia, 467
Q fever endocarditis, 330
QRS complex(es), 1243, *1243*
normal, with short P-R interval and
supraventricular tachycardias,
1256–1257

Quäalude. See *Methaqualone.*
Qualitative screening test, in carcinoid
syndrome, 2209, *2211*
Quantal squander, 930
Quartan malaria, 569, 571
Quartan nephrosis, 572
Queensland tick typhus, 324–325
Quervain's syndrome, 207
Quervain's thyroiditis, 2131
Questionnaires, in personality
measurement, 683
Questran. See *Cholestyramine.*
Quinacrine
in giardiasis, *558*
in malabsorption from giardiasis,
1546
Quinacrine hydrochloride
in assessment of sex chromatin
pattern, 2165
in giardiasis, 602
in tapeworm infections, 608
Quincke's sign, in aortic regurgitation,
1195
Quinidine, 1265
sensitization caused by, 131
Quinine
in malaria, *558*
chloroquine-resistant, 573, 574
in myotonia congenita, 920
in myotonic dystrophy, 918
Quinine sulfate, in cramps, 930
nocturnal, of chronic renal failure,
1365
Quinsy sore throat, in streptococcal
tonsillitis, 373
Quintana fever, 329

Rabies, **833–836,** *833, 835*
vaccination against, neuroparalytic
accidents following, 838–839
vs. arboviral encephalitis, 284
Rabies vaccine, 835, *835*, 836
Rabies virus, 833, *833*
Raccoon eyes, in stupor or coma, 643
Race, blood pressure and, 1220, 1201
Rachischisis, complete, 875
Radial nerve palsy, acute, 901, 902
Radiation colitis, 1584–1585
vs. ulcerative colitis, 1572
Radiation enteritis, 1584–1585
malabsorption syndrome in, 1547
Radiation fibrosis, 1002
pulmonary hypertension in, 1147
Radiation injury, 86–92
acute, 88. See also *Radiation syndrome,*
acute.
aplastic anemia induced by, 1736,
1737
delayed effects of, 89
diagnosis of, 89
prognosis in, 91, 92
treatment of, 90, 91
local, 89
diagnosis of, 89
prognosis in, 91
treatment of, 90
of lungs, *984,* **1001–1002**
of nervous system, 869–870
prevention of, 92
Radiation leukemogenesis, 1814
Radiation myelopathy, 870

Radiation myocarditis, 1287
Radiation nephritis, 1435
Radiation pneumonitis, 1002
Radiation syndrome, acute, 88
diagnosis of, 89
prognosis in, 91
treatment of, 90
Radiation therapy, 1927–1930. See also
Radiotherapy.
Radiation-related eosinophilia, 226
Radicular syndromes, 889–890, *889, 890*
Radiculopathy
cervical, 895
vs. peripheral neuropathy, 889, *890,*
891
Radioactive iodine uptake
determination of, 2118
in hyperthyroidism, 2123, 2124, *2125*
Radioactive particles, airborne,
exposure to, neoplasia associated
with, 995
Radioallergosorbent test
in allergic rhinitis, 159
in Hymenoptera stings, 114
Radioimmunoassay
for parathyroid hormone, in
hyperparathyroidism, 2218
in endocrine disease, 2065, 2066,
2066, 2067
of lipotropins, 2094
of melanocyte-stimulating hormone,
2094
of plasma adrenocorticotropin, 2094
of plasma follicle-stimulating
hormone and luteinizing hormone,
2093, *2093*
of plasma growth hormone, 2091,
2092
in acromegaly, 2107
of plasma prolactin, 2092
of serum thyrotropin, 2093
Radioisotope cisternography, 749
Radionuclide bone toxicity, 2261
Radionuclide contamination
diagnosis of, 90
treatment of, 91
Radionuclide scanning. See also
Scanning.
in gastrointestinal disease, 1468–1470,
1468, 1469
in pulmonary disease, 944–945
of brain, 748–749
Radionuclide studies, in cardiovascular
disease, 1076, 1077, *1078*
Radiotherapy
biologic effects of, 1928–1929, *1928*
clinical applications of, 1929
in acidophilic adenoma with
acromegaly, 2097
in acromegaly, 2108
in basophilic adenoma with
Cushing's syndrome, 2098
in bronchogenic carcinoma, 1010
in Cushing's disease, 2155, 2156
in eosinophilic granuloma, 1850, 1951
in esophageal carcinoma, 1599
in exophthalmos complicating Graves'
disease, 2127
in gastric carcinoma, 1603
in Hodgkin's disease, 1845
chemotherapy and, 1846, 1847
in intracranial tumors, 869
in midline granuloma, 221

Radiotherapy (*Continued*)
in multiple myeloma, 1861
in non-Hodgkin's lymphomas, 1835
chemotherapy and, combined, 1836, 1837
in peptic ulcer, 1516
oncologic, 1927–1930
thyroid carcinoma following, 2141
toxic effects of, 1929–1930
Ragweed, allergic rhinitis from, 157
Ragweed pollen, allergen of, 131
Rales, post-tussic, in pulmonary tuberculosis, 486
Ramsay Hunt's syndrome, 768, 826, 900
Rapid eye movement sleep, 652, 653
Rapid plasma reagin test, in syphilis, *513, 514*
Rappaport classification of non-Hodgkin's lymphomas, *1830, 1831*
Rash
butterfly, in systemic lupus erythematosus, 174, 175, 176
drug, vs. measles, *249*
in bacterial meningitis, 412
in Chagas' disease, 581
in coccidioidomycosis, 538
in Colorado tick fever, 280
in dengue, 277
in drug allergy, 156
in epidemic louse-borne typhus, 319
in fevers caused by group A arboviruses, 279
in herpes zoster, 825
in infectious mononucleosis, 265
in juvenile rheumatoid arthritis, 196
in louse-borne relapsing fever, 527
in measles, 247, 248, *248*
in meningococcemia, 419, *419*
in onchocerciasis, 636
in polymyositis and dermatomyositis, 172, 173
in rat-bite fever, 531
in rickettsial diseases, *313*
in rickettsialpox, 326
in Rocky Mountain spotted fever, 322
in roseola-like exanthems, 274
in rubella, 251
in rubelliform exanthems, 274
in scarlet fever, 371
in syphilis, 509, *509*
in tick-borne rickettsioses of Eastern Hemisphere, 325
in tularemia, 467
in typhoid fever, 447
in varicella, 253, 254
in variola, 256
in West Nile fever, 278
Rasmussen's aneurysm, in pulmonary tuberculosis, 486
RAST procedure
in allergic rhinitis, 159
in Hymenoptera stings, 114
Rat tapeworm, 611
Rat-bite fever, 531–532
vs. louse-borne relapsing fever, 528
Rathke's pouch tumor, 2098
Rattus norvegicus, in typhus fever, 321
Rattus rattus, in typhus fever, 321
Raynaud's disease, 1305–1307
in primary pulmonary hypertension, 1138
vs. acrocyanosis, 1307
vs. ergotism and methysergide toxicity, 1308

Raynaud's disease (*Continued*)
vs. Raynaud's phenomenon in thromboangiitis obliterans, 1303
Raynaud's phenomenon, 1305–1307
in scleroderma, 168, 169, 171
in thromboangiitis obliterans, 1303
vs. cold agglutinin syndrome, 1765
Reactive hyperemia, in Raynaud's phenomenon, 1306
Reactive hypoglycemia, 1990
hypoglycemic coma in, 1991
Reagin(s), 128
Receptor sites, drug interactions at, 2337, 2338
Reciprocal translocation(s), 53, *53*
transmission of, 53, 54
Recklinghausen's disease, 769–770
pheochromocytomas in, 2201, 2203
skin in, 2293–2294, *2293, 2297*
Recruitment, in sensorineural hearing loss, 734, 735
Recruits, military, acute respiratory disease of, 236, 237
Rectal neuralgia, vs. proctalgia fugax, 1497
Rectovaginal fistulas, in ulcerative colitis, 1574
Rectum
biopsy of, in congenital megacolon, 1495
in schistosomiasis, 615
in ulcerative colitis, 1569
carcinoma of, 1606–1610
chancres near, in syphilis, 508
inflammatory or neoplastic lesions of, vs. lymphogranuloma venereum, 335
ulcer of, solitary, 1616
villous adenomas of, hypokalemia in, 1958
Recurrent fever, 526–529
Recurrent polyserositis, familial, 2055–2057
Red blood cells. See *Erythrocyte(s).*
Red bugs, dermatitis caused by, 113
Red cell aplasia, pure, 1735
Red eye, acute, differential diagnoses of, 2313–2314, *2313*
Red thrombus, 1122
Red whelk, paralytic poisoning by, 68
5α-Reductase deficiency, 2173
Reed-Sternberg cell, in Hodgkin's disease, 1839, 1840
Referred pain, 722
abdominal, 1477
Reflex cardiac standstill, syncope in, 743
"Reflex" epilepsy, 852
Reflex neurovascular dystrophy, 206
"Reflex spasms," in tetanus, 438
"Reflex sympathetic dystrophies," 727
Reflexes, stretch, hyperactive, in metabolic brain disease, 648
Reflux
duodenogastric, peptic ulcer and, 1507
eosphageal, vs. angina pectoris, 1227
vesicoureteral, after renal transplantation, 1385
Reflux esophagitis, 1484
hiatal hernia and, 1485
Reflux nephropathy, 1409
Refraction, errors of, headache from, 733
Refsum's disease, *42,* 913
vs. Friedreich's ataxia, 768

Regional enteritis, 1560–1567
ankylosing spondylitis in, 198, 1561
arthritis in, 198
clinical complications of, 1564
clinical manifestations of, 1562, 1563
diagnosis of, 1564
differential diagnosis of, 1565
epidemiology of, 1561
etiology of, 1561
eyes in, 2316
genetics in, 1561
laboratory studies in, 1563
malabsorption in, 1453, 1564
pathogenesis of, 1562
pathology of, 1562, *1562*
physical examination in, 1563
prognosis in, 1567
sclerosing cholangitis and, 1633
treatment of, 1566
Regional lymphadenitis, nonbacterial, benign, 302–305, *303, 304*
Regulatory genes, 34
Regurgitation, 1479
aortic, 1194–1197
Austin Flint murmur in, 1196
vs. mitral stenosis, 1183
general physiologic effects of, 1174, 1175, *1175*
ventricular septal defect with, 1171
mitral, 1185–1188
general physiologic effects of, 1175, *1175*
vs. aortic stenosis, 1193
vs. atrial septal defect, 1162
pulmonary valve, congenital, 1168
pulmonic, 1199
vs. aortic regurgitation, 1197
tricuspid, 1198–1199
vs. mitral regurgitation, 1187
Rehabilitation, after cerebral infarction, 792
Reichstein's substance S, 2146
Reiter's syndrome, 197–198, *2299, 2303*
eyes in, 2316
HLA system and, 39
vs. gonococcal arthritis, 408
Relapsing febrile nodular nonsuppurative panniculitis, 221–222
Relapsing fever, 526–530
louse-borne, 526–529
tick-borne, 526, 529–530
vs. malaria, 573
Relapsing polychondritis, 218
aortic regurgitation in, 1194
arthritis in, 199
eyes in, 2316
Relative polycythemia, 1792–1793
Relaxation atelectasis, 965
REM sleep, 652, 653
Renal. See also *Kidney(s).*
Renal acidosis, 1962, 1964, 1965
in interstitial nephritis, 1417, 1418
Renal arteriography, 1343, *1343*
Renal artery(ies)
aneurysm of, 1457
occlusion of, acute renal failure in, 1369
stenosis of, hypertension from, 1201, 1211
Renal blood flow, 1316
Renal calculi, 1443–1446
2,8-dihydroxyadenine, 2043
in gout, 2037
treatment of, 2041
in paraplegia, 888

Renal calculi (*Continued*)
  in regional enteritis, 1564
Renal candidiasis, 548
Renal colic, in renal calculi, 1444
Renal cortical necrosis, bilateral, acute
    renal failure from, 1368
Renal diabetes insipidus, *43*
Renal diseases, 1316–1462. See also
    names of specific diseases.
Renal failure
  acute, 1334, **1367–1375**
    causes of, 1368
    clinical manifestations of, 1371
    extracorporeal hemodialysis in,
      1380
    hypercalcemia in, 1369, 2237
    hyponatremia in, 1955
    in critically ill patient, 1050
    in malaria, 571, 572, 574
    in renal infarction, 1407
    renal biopsy in, 1346
    toxic nephropathy with, 1425
    treatment of, 1372
  as transfusion reaction, 1788–1789
  chronic, 1334–1335, **1351–1367**
    anemia in, 1363, *1363*, 1364, 1731
    causes of, 1351, *1352*
      classification of, *1351*
    clinical features of, management of,
      1362–1366
    degree of, assessment of, 1354
    diet in, 1711
    drug therapy in, 1367, *1367*
    extracorporeal hemodialysis in,
      1378, 1380
    general management of, 1366–1367,
      1367
    hyperkalemia in, 1959
    hyponatremia in, 1955
    incidence and prevalence of, 1351
    investigation of, 1352–1354, *1353*
    metabolic acidosis in, 1962
    osteodystrophy in, **2254–2257**
    osteomalacia in, 1360, 2254
    pathophysiology of, 1355–1362
    primary disease in, recognition of,
      1352
    rickets in, 1360, 2254
    secondary hyperparathyroidism in,
      2217, 2255
    toxic nephropathy with, 1425
    volume depletion in, 1951
    vs. acute renal failure, 1334
  hemoglobinuria and, 1783
  hemolysis in, 1770
  hemorrhagic phenomena in, 1891
  in acute poststreptococcal
    glomerulonephritis, 1395
  in cirrhosis and ascites, 1644
  in gout, 2030, 2037, 2038
  irreversible
    prevention of, 1376
    **treatment of, by transplantation
      and dialysis, 1375–1386**
  postpartum, 1414
  vs. diabetes insipidus, 2110
Renal glycosuria, *41*
Renal hyperaminoacidurias, **2023**
Renal hypertension, **1210–1211**
Renal infarction, from arterial thrombi
    and emboli, 1407
Renal medullary necrosis, 1412–1413
Renal osteodystrophy, **2254–2257**

Renal papillary necrosis, 1412–1413
  acute renal failure from, 1369
  in sickle cell hemoglobinopathy, 1404
  vs. medullary sponge kidney, 1456
Renal parenchymal injury
  coagulation-induced, 1327–1328
  immune-mediated, 1324–1327, *1324,
    1325*
  infection-mediated, 1329
  mechanisms of, 1323–1331
  toxin-mediated, 1328–1329, *1328*
Renal pelvis, candidiasis in, 548
Renal scintigraphy, 1344, *1344*
Renal syndromes, major, **1331–1336**
Renal transplantation, 1375, *1375, 1376,
    1376,* **1382–1386**
  biopsy after, 1346
  hypercalcemia after, 2237
  in cystinosis, 55
  in Fabry's disease, 55
  in scleroderma, 171
  rejected, acute renal failure in, 1369
    pathologic features of, 1384
  rejection crisis in, 1384
Renal tuberculosis, 496
Renal tubular acidosis, *43,* **1441–1442**
  rickets and osteomalacia in, 2252
Renal tubule(s)
  distal, function of, 1319, 1320, *1320*
  function of, defects of, 1336
    toxic nephropathy with, 1425
  elements of, 1316–1317
  **processing of glomerular filtrate by,
    1317–1320,** *1320*
  proximal, fluid reabsorption by, 1318,
    1320
Renal vascular disorders, 1407–1409
Renal vein thrombosis, 1408–1409
  vs. Goodpasture's syndrome, 976
Renal venography, 1344
Renal-retinal dysplasia, 1454
Renin
  angiotensin and, in blood pressure
    regulation, 1207, 1208
  circulatory effects of, 1111
  in chronic renal failure, 1361
Renin-dependent hypertension, 1210
Renography, 1345
Renoprival hypertension, 1207
Reoviruses associated with common
    cold, *230*
Reserpine
  in acrocyanosis, 1307
  in arterial hypertension, *1212,* 1214
  in chilblain and pernio, 1311
  in hypertension of dissecting aortic
    aneurysm, 1297
  in hypertensive encephalopathy,
    794
  in Raynaud's disease, 1307
  in Raynaud's phenomenon of
    scleroderma, 171
  in thyroid storm, 2128
Reservoir masks, for oxygenation in
    acute respiratory failure, 1027
Residual volume, 932, *932,* 933
Resistant ovary syndrome, 2186
Respiration, 931. See also *Breathing.*
  Cheyne-Stokes, in left ventricular
    failure, 1090
  **disorders of, pulmonary hypertension
    and, 1146–1149**
  in head injury, 882

Respiratory acidosis, 1961, **1967–1969**
  chronic, acid-base disturbances
    complicating, 1967, *1968*
  plasma composition in, *1967*
Respiratory alkalosis, 1961, **1969**
  plasma composition in, *1967*
Respiratory disease, **931–1030**
  acute, of military recruits, 236,
    237
  due to enteroviruses, 275
  nosocomial, 361–364
  rhinoviral, 234
  **special diagnostic procedures in,
    941–951**
Respiratory distress syndrome
  adult, 1024, **1033–1045**
    conditions associated with, *1024*
  after renal transplantation, 1385
Respiratory failure, **1021–1030**
  acute
    airway control in, 1039
    alveolar ventilation in, maintenance
      of, 1027
    clinical features of, 1033, 1034
    complicating massive blood
      transfusions, 1051
    condition underlying, identification
      and treatment of, 1027–1028
    critical care of, 1033–1045
    establishment of airway in,
      1025–1026
    etiologic factors in, 1033, *1033*
    fluid balance in, 1044
    hemodynamic responses in, 1038,
      1039
    hemodynamic support in, 1044
    infection in, 1044
    intermittent mandatory ventilation
      in, 1045, *1045*
    mechanical ventilation in, 1040,
      1041
      need for, evaluation of, 1039
    oxygen therapy in, 1026–1027
    pathologic changes in, 1034, 1035
    patient monitoring in, 1028
    physiology of, 1035, *1035,* 1036
    positive end-expiratory pressure in,
      1041, 1042
    Swan-Ganz catheter in, 1043
    treatment of, 1025–1028, 1039–1045
  causes of, 1022–1024, *1023*
  central, in intracranial tumors, 864
  chronic, treatment of, 1028–1030
  clinical manifestations of, 1024–1025
  in botulism, 67, 68
  in cancer patient, 1904, 1905
  in poliomyelitis, 832
  pathophysiology of, 1021–1022
  right heart failure from, 1022
Respiratory syncytial viral disease,
    238–239
Respiratory syncytial virus, 238
Respiratory tract
  changes in, with age, 26
  cultures of, in bacterial meningitis,
    413
  diffusion in, 936–938
  diseases of, 931–1030. See also
    Respiratory disease and names of
    specific diseases.
  gas exchange in, 939–**941**
  in cancer patient, 1904, 1905
  in control of breathing, 938–939

Respiratory tract (*Continued*)
in electric injury, 93
in measles, 247
in obesity, 1695, 1696
in paraplegia, 887
in Wegener's granulomatosis, 219
perfusion in, 938
structure and function of, 931–941
upper, in meningococcal infection,
418
sarcoidosis of, 212
ventilation in, 932–936
viral injections of, 230–246
prevalence of, factors related to,
236, *236*
vs. allergic rhinitis, 158
Restrictive cardiomyopathies, 1277
Restrictive ventilatory disorders, 935,
936, *936*
Resuscitation, cardiopulmonary,
1053–1058, *1054*
Retching, 1477
esophagogastric trauma from, 1478
Reticular dermis, in scleroderma, 168
Reticulocyte count, in hemolytic
disorders, 1752
Reticuloendothelial hyperplasia,
splenomegaly due to, 1869, 1870
Reticuloendothelial system
in host defense, 146
in typhoid fever, 446
neoplasms of, 1829–1848
overactivity of, hemolysis due to,
1770
Reticulohistiocytoma, *2297*
Reticulohistiocytosis, multicentric, 201
Retina
detachment of, in chronic renal
failure, 1366
in Rift Valley fever, 281
in arterial hypertension, 1203, 1205,
1206
in diabetes mellitus, 2320, 2321
in nephronophthisis–cystic renal
medulla complex, 1454
in scleroderma, 2317
in toxemia of pregnancy, 1415
stippling of, in lead poisoning, 78
Retinal artery, central, occlusion of,
2317, *2318*
Retinal periphlebitis, in sarcoidosis,
2329
Retinitis, toxoplasmic, recurrent, 2334,
2335
Retinitis pigmentosa, hereditary motor
and sensory neuropathy with, 913
Retinoblastoma, *1910*
Retinochoroiditis, toxoplasmic, 596, 597,
598
Retinol, 1670
in hypovitaminosis A, 1685
Retinopathy
central serous, in Rift Valley fever,
281
diabetic, 1976, 1977, *1978*, 2320, 2321
hypophysectomy and, 2103
in hypertension, 1206, *2318*, 2325,
2326, *2326*
accelerated, 1205
in chronic renal failure, 1366
Retinopathy, sickle, 2330, 2331, *2331*,
2332
Retractile mesenteritis, 1596

Retractile testes, vs. undescended
testes, 2173
Retrobulbar neuritis, 848–849
Retrobulbar neuropathy, nutritional,
774–775
Retrocecal appendicitis, 1579
Retrocollis, 761
Retrograde amnesia, 658
Retrograde cholangiopancreatography,
endoscopic, 1472–1473, *1472, 1473*
in biliary disease, 1622, 1623, *1623*
in chronic pancreatitis, 1556
Retrograde pyelography, 1343
Retroperitoneal fibrosis, 223–224
sclerosing cholangitis and, 1633
Retroperitoneal lymphangiography, in
non-Hodgkin's lymphomas, 1834,
1835
Rewarming, in hypothermia, 86
Reye's syndrome, 839
after influenza epidemics, 244
after varicella, 254
fatty liver in, 1660
Rhabdomyolysis, 924
Rheumatic disease, classification of, *184*
Rheumatic fever, 377–385
acute, epidemiology of, 370, *370*
vs. juvenile rheumatoid arthritis,
196
antimicrobial prophylaxis for, *564*
aortic regurgitation after, 1194, 1195
arteritis of, 166
clinical manifestations of, 379, *380*
death rates for, *1060*
diagnosis and differential diagnosis
of, 382
epidemiology of, 379, 1059
etiology of, 377
laboratory findings in, 381
mitral stenosis following, 1179, 1180
pathogenesis of, 377
pericarditis caused by, 1271
prevalence of, 1059
prevention of, 376, 384
prognosis in, 385
therapy of, 383
vs. gonococcal arthritis, 408
vs. infective endocarditis, 392
vs. rheumatoid arthritis, 190
Rheumatic heart disease
death rates for, *1060*
prevalence and epidemiology of, 1059
underlying infective endocarditis, 387
Rheumatic nodules, subcutaneous, in
rheumatic fever, 381
Rheumatic pneumonia, 381
Rheumatic pneumonitis, 381
Rheumatism, 184
nonarticular, 207–208
palindromic, 198
Rheumatoid arthritis, 186–193
adrenocorticosteroid therapy in, 192
anemia in, 189, 1732
aortic regurgitation in, 1194
Caplan's syndrome in, 187, 992, 993
clinical course of, 189
clinical manifestations of, 188
differential diagnosis of, 190
eosinophilia in, 226
epidemiology of, 186
extra-articular manifestations of, 187,
188, 189
eyes in, 2314, 2315

Rheumatoid arthritis (*Continued*)
gastric ulcer and, 1504
HLA system and, 39
immune mechanisms in, 133, 134
immunosuppressive therapy in, 193
incidence of, 186
juvenile, 195–196
eyes in, 2315
laboratory findings in, 189
management of, 190
mode of onset of, 188
neuropathy in, 908
neutropenia in, 1809
orthopedic surgery in, 193
pathogenesis of, 187
pathology of, 187
pericarditis caused by, 1271
physical measures in, 191
physical signs of, 188
pleura in, 1017
prognosis in, 189
pulmonary involvement in, 974
rest in, 191
roentgenographic findings in, 189
salicylates in, 191
skeletal manifestations of, 188, *188*,
189
splenomegaly in, 193
symptoms of, 188
variants of, 193–194
vs. degenerative joint disease, *203*,
204
vs. gonococcal arthritis, 408
vs. gout, 2039
vs. periarteritis nodosa, 183
vs. polymyalgia rheumatica, 217
vs. rheumatic fever, 383
vs. tuberculous arthritis, 186
Rheumatoid arthritis–lupus, 176
Rheumatoid factors, in rheumatoid
arthritis, 187, 189, 190
Rheumatoid nodules, episcleral, 2314,
2315
Rheumatoid spondylitis, 194–195. See
also *Spondylitis, ankylosing.*
Rhinitis
allergic, 157–160
perennial, 157
sensitization to external antigens
in, 131
vasomotor, 157, 160
Rhinopharyngitis mutilans, in yaws,
521
Rhinophyma, 2279, *2279*
Rhinorrhea
in bacterial meningitis, 415
in streptococcal pharyngitis in infants
and children, 371, 372
Rhinoviral respiratory disease, 234
Rhinoviruses, 234, 268
Rhipicephalus sanguineus
in boutonneuse fever, 325
in Rocky Mountain spotted fever, 322
Rhizopus species, in mucormycosis, 545
Rhodesian sleeping sickness, 576
clinical features of, 578
diagnosis of, 578
epidemiology of, 576
treatment of, 578, 579
vs. Gambian sleeping sickness, *577*
Rhodnius prolixus, 580
Rib, fracture of, vs. angina pectoris,
1227

Riboflavin
  deficiency of, 1686–1687
    clinical signs of, *1677*
    eyes in, 1675
    mouth in, 1676
  in ariboflavinosis, 1687
  nutrient value of, 1673
  recommended allowances of, *1671*
Ribonucleic acid, 31
  messenger, 31
    in protein synthesis, *32, 33*
  ribosomal, 32
  transfer, 31, 32
Ribonucleotide reductase, inhibition of,
  1721
Ribosomal RNA, 32
Rickets, 2247–2254
  anticonvulsant-induced, 2253
  clinical signs of, *1677*
  hypophosphatemic, X-linked, dietary
    treatment of, 55
  in chronic renal failure, 1360, 2254
  pseudodeficiency, 2252
  pseudo–vitamin D resistant, 2252
  vitamin D deficiency, 2248–2249
  vitamin D dependent, *43, 2021,* 2252
  vitamin D resistant, 2250–2252
  vs. pituitary dwarfism, 2104
Rickettsemia, patent, in rickettsial
  diseases, 310, 311
Rickettsia akari, 310, 326
Rickettsia australis, 324, 325
Rickettsia canada, 309
Rickettsia conorii, 310, 324, 325
Rickettsia mooseri, 309, *309,* 310, 321
Rickettsia prowazekii, 309, *309,* 310
  in Brill-Zinsser disease, 320
  in epidemic typhus, 318
Rickettsia rickettsii, 310, 322
Rickettsia sibirica, 324
Rickettsia tsutsugamushi, 310, 327
Rickettsiae
  biologic properties of, *309*
  direct demonstration of, in tissues,
    312
  isolation of, 312
Rickettsial antigens, demonstration of,
  in acute phase urine, 312
Rickettsial diseases, 309–332. See also
  names of specific diseases.
  clinical considerations in, 311, 312,
    313
  immunity in, 311
  laboratory diagnosis in, 312
  pathogenesis of, 310
  pathology of, 310
  serologic diagnosis of, 312, 313
  treatment of, 315
Rickettsialpox, 326
  clinical features of, *313*
  epidemiologic features of, *310*
  serologic responses in, *314*
Rickettsiosis(es)
  chigger-borne, 327–328
  tick-borne, North Asian, 324–325
    of Eastern Hemisphere, 324–325
Riedel's thyroiditis, 224, 2130–2131
  sclerosing cholangitis and, 1633
Rifampin, *557*
  as nephrotoxin, 1427
  effect of, on oral contraceptives, 2339
  in leprosy, 504
  in miliary tuberculosis, 493

Rifampin (*Continued*)
  in prophylaxis of meningococcal
    disease, 422
  in pulmonary disease caused by *M.
    kansasii,* 499
  in pulmonary tuberculosis, 487, 488,
    489, 490
  in tuberculous meningitis, 494
  in tuberculous pericarditis, 494
Rift Valley fever, *279, 281–282*
Rift Valley virus, 281
Right subclavian artery, aberrant, 1291
Right ventricle, double outlet, 1173
Right ventricular failure, 1081,
  1091–1093
  in acute respiratory failure, 1022
  in chronic respiratory failure,
    treatment of, 1029–1030
  in primary pulmonary hypertension,
    1140
  pulmonary hypertension and, in
    pulmonary disease, 1147, 1148
Right ventricular origin of both great
  arteries, 1173
Right hemisphere syndromes, 658
Right middle lobe syndrome, 965
Right-left disorientation, 658
Right-to-left shunting, 940, 1022
Rigidity, 751
  in paralysis agitans, 752
  in tetanus, 438
Riley-Day syndrome, 912, 2057–2058
  osteoporosis in, 2245, 2246
Ring, esophageal, lower, 1488, *1488*
Ringer's lactate, in shock, 1117, 1118
Rinne test, in hearing loss, 734
Riolan, arc of, 1587, *1587*
"Risk genes," 45
"Risus sardonicus," in tetanus, 438
Ritalin. See *Methylphenidate.*
Ritter's disease, 400
River blindness, 635–636
  antimicrobial agents for, *559*
RNA, 31
  messenger, 31
    in protein synthesis, *32, 33*
  ribosomal, 32
  transfer, 31, 32
Rochalimaea quintana, 309, *309,* 310, 329
Rocky Mountain spotted fever, 322–324
  clinical features of, *313*
  epidemiologic features of, *310*
  peripheral arteritis in, 1305
  vs. Colorado tick fever, 280
  vs. rat-bite fever, 531
  vs. tularemia, 467
Rod myopathy, 919
Roentgenography
  contrast media for, as nephrotoxins,
    1433–1434
  in abdominal aortic aneurysms, 1293
  in achalasia, 1487, *1487*
  in acquired valvular heart disease,
    1177
  in acromegaly, 2096, *2096, 2097*
  in acute abdomen, 1580, 1581
  in acute cholecystitis, 1626
  in acute pericarditis, 1272
  in adult celiac disease, 1532, *1533,*
    1540
  in alcaptonuria, 2026
  in angina pectoris, 1226
  in ankylosing spondylitis, 195

Roentgenography (*Continued*)
  in aortic regurgitation, 1196
  in aortic stenosis, 1192
  in asymmetric septal hypertrophy,
    1279
  in atrial septal defect, 1161
  in bacterial meningitis, 414
  in biliary disease, 1622–1623, *1623,*
    1648
  in bronchogenic carcinoma, 1007,
    1008
  in cardiovascular disease, 1075, 1076
  in cerebral infarction, 789
  in chronic pancreatitis, 1556
  in coarctation of aorta, 1158, 1290
  in colorectal carcinoma, 1608, *1608*
  in congenital aneurysms of sinuses of
    Valsalva, 1170
  in congenital coronary arteriovenous
    fistula, 1169
  in craniopharyngioma, *2084*
  in Crohn's disease of colon, 1577,
    1578
  in degenerative joint disease, 204
  in diffuse collagenous
    pneumoconioses, 991
  in diffuse esophageal spasm, 1486,
    1486
  in dissecting aortic aneurysm, 1296,
    1296
  in diverticulitis, 1583
  in Ebstein's anomaly, 1168
  in epilepsy, 857
  in esophageal carcinoma, 1598, *1598*
  in esophagitis, 1484
  in Fallot's tetralogy, 1165
  in gallstone ileus, 1629
  in gastric carcinoma, 1601, *1602*
  in head injury, 881
  in Hodgkin's disease, *1841,* 1844
  in hyperparathyroidism, 2215, *2216*
  in intestinal obstruction, 1491
  in intracranial inflammatory disease,
    804
  in intracranial tumors, 866, 867
  in intraspinal compression, 892
  **in investigation of renal structure and
    regional function, 1341–1344,** *1342,
    1343*
  in *Klebsiella* pneumonia, 358
  in left ventricular failure, 1091
  in legionnaires' disease, 360
  in Lutembacher's syndrome, 1169
  in malabsorption syndrome, 1532,
    1532, 1533
  in mast cell disease, 2308
  in mitral regurgitation, 1187
  in mitral stenosis, 1182
  in multiple myeloma, 1858, *1859*
  in mycoplasmal pneumonia, 345
  in neurologic diagnosis, 748
  in obstructive nephropathy, 1448
  in osteomalacia, 2247, 2248
  in Paget's disease of bone, 2258
  in patent ductus arteriosus, 1163
  in peptic ulcer, 1509, 1510, *1510,* 1511,
    1511, 1512, *1512*
  in pericardial constriction, 1275
  in pericardial effusion, 1274
  in peritoneal disease, 1591
  in PIE syndrome, *969*
  in pituitary tumors, 2095, *2095, 2096,
    2097*

Roentgenography (*Continued*)
  in pleural disease, 1014
  in primary pulmonary hypertension, 1140
  in pseudogout, 201
  in *Pseudomonas* pneumonia, 364
  in pulmonary disease, 941–944
  in pulmonary tuberculosis, 486
  in pulmonic stenosis, 1159
  in pyloric stenosis, 1490
  in regional enteritis, 1564, *1565*
  in renal colic, 1445
  in rheumatoid arthritis, 189
    juvenile, 196
  in scleroderma, 170
  in small intestinal malignancies, 1605, *1605*
  in syphilitic aortic aneurysm, 1294
  in total anomalous pulmonary venous connection, 1173
  in tricuspid regurgitation, 1198
  in tricuspid stenosis, 1198
  in ulcerative colitis, 1571, *1571*, *1572*
  in ventricular septal defect, 1170, 1171
Romaña's sign, in Chagas' disease, 581, 582
Romberg's sign
  in syringomyelia, 769
  in tabes dorsalis, 815
Rorschach test, 682
"Rose fever," 157
"Rose spots," in typhoid fever, 447
Rosenbach, erysipeloid of, 473
Roseola-like exanthems, 274
Rosetting procedure, in T cell detection, 129, 130
Ross River fever, 279–280, *279*
Ross River virus, 279
Rotator cuff, tears of, 206
Rotaviruses, viral gastroenteritis caused by, 305–306
Roth's spots, in infective endocarditis, 389
Rotor syndrome, 1638, 1650
Round window rupture, in divers, 99
Roundworms, 621–637
  antimicrobial agents for, *559*
  prevalence of, *605*
Roussy-Lévy syndrome, vs. Friedreich's ataxia, 768
Rowley-Rosenberg syndrome, *2021*
RS virus, 238
RSSE virus, 290, 291
Rubella, 250–252
  acute disseminated encephalomyelitis after, 836, 837
  congenital, 251, 252
    hearing loss from, 735
    vs. congenital cytomegalovirus infection, 828
  polyarthritis associated with, 186
  vs. infectious mononucleosis, 266, 267
  vs. measles, *249*
  vs. rat-bite fever, 531
  vs. rubelliform exanthems, 274
Rubella vaccine, 252
Rubella virus, 250
Rubelliform exanthems, 274
Rubeola, 246–250, *248*, *249*. See also *Measles*.
Rubeosis iridis, in diabetes mellitus, 1977, 2320
Rubin test, in infertility, 2194
Rumination, 1479

Rumpel-Leede sign, in scarlet fever, 371
Rumpel-Leede vascular fragility test, 1871
Runyon classification of mycobacteria, 480
Rupture
  cardiac, in myocardial infarction, 1231
  esophageal, vs. myocardial infarction, 1233
  hepatic, angiography in, 1471
  of arteriovenous anomaly, intracranial hemorrhage from, 795
    clinical manifestations of, 797
    prognosis in, 799
    treatment of, 801
  of graafian follicles, vs. acute appendicitis, 1581
  of synovial bursae, in rheumatoid arthritis, 188
  round window, in divers, 99
  splenic, angiography in, *1471*
    in infectious mononucleosis, 267
"Rural" leishmaniasis, 587
Rural typhus, 327–328
Russian spring-summer encephalitis, 290–291
Russian spring-summer encephalitis virus, 290, 291

"Saber shins," in congenital syphilis, 513
Sabethes mosquitoes, in yellow fever, 294
Sabin-Feldman dye test, in toxoplasmosis, 596, 597
Saccharopinuria, *41*, *2017*
Sacral plexus neuropathy, 902, 903
  diabetic, 909
Saddle emboli, in arterial embolism, 1303
Saddle-back caterpillar, dermatitis caused by, 119
Sagittal sinus, superior
  occlusion of, 788
  thrombosis of, 809
St. Louis encephalitis, 288–289
St. Louis encephalitis virus, 288
St. Vitus' dance, 757–758
Salicylates. See also names of specific agents.
  hypoglycemia induced by, 1996
  in ankylosing spondylitis, 195
  in Reiter's syndrome, 197, 198
  in rheumatoid arthritis, 191
  poisoning by, 75, 76
    metabolic acidosis from, 1962
Salicylazosulfapyridine, *557*, 563
  in regional enteritis, 1566
  in ulcerative colitis, 1573
Saline load test, for gastric emptying in peptic ulcer, 1518
Saline solution, in shock, 1117, 1118
Salivary electrolyte test, in digitalis toxicity, 1098
Salivary gland virus disease, generalized, 827–829
Salmonella agona, 449
Salmonella anatum, 450
Salmonella bacteremia, 449, 450
  clinical manifestations of, 451
  diagnosis of, 452
  treatment of, 452

Salmonella choleraesuis, 450, 451
Salmonella enteritidis, 449
Salmonella gastroenteritis, 449
  clinical manifestations of, 451
  diagnosis of, 452
  pathogenesis of, 450
  treatment of, 452
Salmonella heidelberg, 449
Salmonella infantis, 449
Salmonella javiana, 449
Salmonella newport, 449
Salmonella oranienburg, 449
Salmonella osteomyelitis, 2260
  in sickle cell anemia, 451
Salmonella paratyphi A, 451
Salmonella paratyphi B, 451
Salmonella saint-paul, 449
Salmonella typhi, 446, 449
Salmonella typhimurium, 449
Salmonellosis, 449–452
  chronic, in schistosomiasis, 615
  vs. amebic dysentery, 592
  vs. viral gastroenteritis caused by Norwalk-like agents and rotaviruses, 306
Salpingitis, gonococcal, 406, 407, 408, 410
  vs. acute appendicitis, 1581
Salt
  intake of, blood pressure and, 1201
  overload of, water overload and, hypertension from, 1210
  renal excretion of, factors controlling, 1321–1322
    in acute tubular necrosis, 1370, 1371
  restriction of, in heart failure, 1102
  retention of, in heart failure, 1089
Sandfly fever, 279, *282*
Sandfly viruses, 282
Sanfilippo's syndrome, 41, 2052, *2052*
Sansert. See *Methysergide*.
São Paulo typhus, 322–324
Sarasinula plebius, 632
Sarcocystis hominis, 604
Sarcocystis lindemanni, 604
Sarcoid meningitis, cerebrospinal fluid findings in, *803*
Sarcoid neuropathy, 908
Sarcoidosis, 209–216
  acute vs. chronic, 215, *216*
  arthritis in, 199
  biochemical findings in, 215
  bone in, 213, 214, 2235
  calcium metabolism in, 215
    disordered, renal disease secondary to, 1402
  cardiac involvement in, 1286
  clinical manifestations of, 211, 212, *213*
  complications of, 216
  course in, 215
  diagnosis of, 214
  differential diagnosis of, 215
  eosinophilia and, 226
  epidemiology of, 211
  etiology of, 209
  glomerulonephritis in, 1403
  granulomas of, 211, *211*, 864
    hepatic, 1667
  hypercalcemia in, 215, 2235–2236
  immunology in, 210
  in childhood, 214
  intrathoracic, 212, 213, *213*
  Kveim test for, 214, 946, 977

Sarcoidosis (*Continued*)
myocardial, 213
myopathy in, 924
neuro-, 213
ocular, 213, **2329–2330**
of upper respiratory tract, 212
pathogenesis of, 210
pathology of, 211
pericardial involvement by, 1276
physical examination in, 212, *212*
pregnancy and, 214
prognosis in, 215
pulmonary aspects of, 977
pulmonary hypertension in, 1141, 1143, 1147
renal changes in, 1402–1403
skin lesions in, 213, *2300*
treatment of, 216
vs. toxocariasis, 628
Sarcoma(s)
eosinophilia in, 226
granulocytic, 1822
hepatic, 1667–1668
Kaposi's, *2298*
Sarcoptes scabiei, 110, 111
Sarcoptic acariasis, 110–111
Sarcosinemia, *2017*
Sarcosporidiosis, 604
Saturday night palsy, 901
Saturnine gout, in lead poisoning, 78
"Sausage digits," in psoriatic arthritis, 196, *197*
Saxitoxin, 68
Scabies, 110–111
Norwegian, 111
vs. onchocerciasis, 636
vs. secondary syphilis, 510
Scalded skin syndrome, 400, 2306
Scale, cutaneous, 2273
Scalp, laceration of, 881, 882
Scanning
bone, in intraspinal compression, 892
brain, 748–749
in brain abscess, 806
in cerebral infarction, 790
in herpes simplex encephalitis, 823
in gastrointestinal disease, 1468–1470, *1468, 1469*
in pulmonary disease, 944–945
liver, 1468, *1468, 1469,* 1470, 1648
renal, 1344, *1344*
gamma camera, 1345, *1345*
thyroid, 2119, *2120*
in multinodular goiter, 2136
Scapuloperoneal syndrome, 918
Scarlet fever, 371–372
epidemiology of, 369, 370
staphylococcal, 400
vs. measles, *249*
vs. rubella, 252
Schatzki ring, 1488, *1488*
Scheie's syndrome, *41,* **2052,** *2052*
Schick test, in diphtheria, 430
Schilder's disease, 849
Schilling test, in vitamin B$_{12}$ deficiency, 777
Schirmer tear test, for kerato-conjunctivitis sicca, 2316
Schistosoma haematobium, 559, 605, 611, 612, 613, 614, 615
Schistosoma japonicum, 559, 605, 611, 612, 613, 614, 615

Schistosoma mansoni, 559, 605, 611, 612, 613, 614, 615
Schistosome dermatitis, 613
Schistosomiasis, 611–617
antimicrobial agents for, *559*
central nervous system, 615
chronic, 613, 614
clinical manifestations of, 613
diagnosis of, 615
epidemiology of, 612
etiology of, 611
hepatic, 614, 1657
hepatosplenic, 614
immunodiagnostic tests for, *565*
pathogenesis of, 613
prevention of, 616
prognosis in, 616
pulmonary, 614
treatment of, 615, 616
urinary tract, 615
vs. amebic dysentery, 592
vs. angiostrongyliasis, 631
vs. bancroftian filariasis, 634
vs. malaria, 573
vs. toxocariasis, 628
vs. visceral leishmaniasis, 586
Schizoid personality, 666
Schizophrenia, 665–669
Schizophrenia-like syndrome
in amphetamine intoxication, 668
in psychomotor epilepsy, 668
in withdrawal from excessive alcohol ingestion, 668
Schizophrenic word salad, vs. fluent aphasia, 657
Schüffner's dots, in malaria, *570, 572*
Schultz-Charlton reaction, in scarlet fever, 371
Schwannoma, vestibular, hearing loss from, 736
SCID, *139,* **141**
with adenosine deaminase deficiency, *139,* **141–142**
Science
biological, medical practice and, 6–8
clinical medicine, spectrum of disease and, 3–6
Scintigraphy, renal, 1344, *1344*
Sclera, in sarcoidosis, 2330
Scleredema, vs. scleroderma, 170
Scleritis
brawny, 2315
nodular, necrotizing, 2315
Sclerocystic ovaries, 2189
Scleroderma, 168–171
cutaneous signs in, 168, 169, *2298, 2301*
esophagus in, 169, 1488
eyes in, 2317
malabsorption in, 169, 171, 1538
pericarditis caused by, 1272
pulmonary hypertension in, 1143, 1144, 1147
pulmonary involvement in, 974
renal involvement in, 169, 170, 171, 1401
vs. rheumatoid arthritis, 190
Scleroderma heart disease, 170
"Sclerodermatomyositis," 923
Sclerokeratitis, necrotizing, in periarteritis nodosa, 2317
Scleromalacia perforans, 2315

Sclerosing cholangitis, 224, 1633
Sclerosing panencephalitis, subacute, 841
Sclerosis
amyotrophic lateral, 765–766
vs. multiple sclerosis, 847
vs. muscular dystrophies, 918
vs. myasthenia gravis, 927
diffuse, 849–850
multiple, 845–848
hearing loss in, 736
HLA system and, 39
pathogenesis of, 844
possible variants of, 848–850
possible viral cause of, 842
symptoms and signs of, *846, 847*
vertigo from, 739, 740
vs. acute disseminated encephalomyelitis, 838
vs. amyotrophic lateral sclerosis, 766
vs. Friedreich's ataxia, 768
vs. hysteria, 679
vs. vitamin B$_{12}$ deficiency, 776, 777
systemic, 168–171. See also *Scleroderma.*
transitional, 849
tuberous, 770–771, *1910*
adenoma sebaceum in, 770, 2292, *2292*
cutaneous manifestations of, *2300*
hypopigmentation in, 2292, *2292*
internal malignancy and, *2297*
Scoliosis, 1020
Scolopendra species, bites of, 117
Scombroid poisoning, 69
Scopolamine
in motion sickness, 95
ingestion of, 705
poisoning by, *712*
Scorbutic rosary, 1691
Scorpaena species, envenomation by, 124
Scorpaenopsis species, envenomation by, 124
Scorpion fishes, envenomation by, 124
Scorpion sting, 116–117
Scotoma, central, in Rift Valley fever, 281
Scrapie, 839, 840
Screening, genetic, 59
in inborn errors of metabolism, 44
Screening test, qualitative, in carcinoid syndrome, 2209, *2211*
Screw-worm, larvae of, infestation by, 112
Scrofula, 492, 495
Scrofuloderma, 498
Scrub typhus, 327–328
biologic properties of, 309, *309*
clinical features of, *313*
epidemiologic features of, *310*
serologic responses in, *314*
Scuba diving
air travel after, 96
hazards of, 98, 99, 102
Scurvy, 1689–1691, *1690*
vascular purpura in, 1880
Sea anemones, envenomation by, 123
Sea cucumbers, envenomation by, 124
Sea lilies, envenomation by, 124
Sea snake, bite by, 122

Sea urchins, envenomation by, 124
Sea wasps, envenomation by, 123
Seatworm infection, 629–630
Sebaceous glands, 2270
Seborrheic dermatitis, 2278
Seborrheic keratoses, 2291
Secobarbital
 abuse of, 698
 in insomnia, 653
Seconal. See *Secobarbital*.
Secretin
 in colonic motility, 1493
 in gastroduodenal motility, 1489
Secretin test, in chronic pancreatitis,
 1556
Sedatives, overdose of, 711–714
Segmental hyalinosis, 1393
Seibert, PPD of, in tuberculin test, 482
Seizure(s). See also *Epilepsy(ies)*.
 adversive, 855
 akinetic, 854
 autonomic, 855
 behavioral state between, 856
 classification of, *853*
 faintness in, 741
 focal, 851, 854, 855
 focal sensory, 855
 fragmentary, 854
 generalized, 851, 853, 854
 hysterical, vs. epilepsy, 679, 858
 in alcohol addiction, 709
 in bacterial meningitis, 412
 in brain tumor, 865
 in cancer, 876
 in cerebral infarction, 786
 in hypoparathyroidism, 2221
 in metabolic brain disease, 648
 jackknife, 854
 motor, jacksonian, 855
 myoclonic, 854
 partial, 854, 855
 psychomotor-temporal-limbic, 855
Selection, genetic, mutation and, 47
Selective hyperaldosteronism,
 hyperkalemia in, 1959
Selenium, nutrient value of, 1674
Sella, empty, 870, 2099, *2099*
 amenorrhea due to, 2187
Sella turcica, evaluation of, in
 amenorrhea, 2184
Semen
 examination of, in evaluation of
  testicular function, 2165
 normal values for, 2355
Seminal vesicles, tuberculosis of, 496
Seminal vesiculitis, gonococcal, 407, 409
Seminiferous tubule dysgenesis,
 2168–2170, *2169*
Seminoma, 2175
Semustine, in oncologic treatment, 1933
Sendai virus, 239
Senile chorea, 759
 vs. hereditary chorea, 759
Senile dementia, 30
Senile lentigo, 2289
Senile osteoporosis, 2243, 2244
Senile purpura, 1879
Senile tremor, 757
Sensorimotor polyneuropathy, in
 cancer, 878
Sensorineural hearing loss, 734, 735, 736
Sensory disturbances, in intracranial
 tumors, 865

Sensory neurons, peripheral, disorders
 of, 911–912
Sensory neuropathy(ies)
 hereditary, 911–912
  vs. leprosy, 504
 in cancer, 878
Sensory polyradiculoneuropathy,
 inflammatory acute, 907
Sensory-induced epilepsy, 852
Sepsis
 bacterial, vs. congenital
  cytomegalovirus infection, 828
 energy requirements in, 1704, 1705
 in total parenteral nutrition, 1707
 severe, hypofibrinogenemia in, 1894
Septal defect
 atrial, 1160–1162
  ostium primum, 1171
  ostium secundum, 1160, 1161, 1162
  pulmonary vascular disease in,
   1142, 1143
  vs. mitral stenosis, 1183
 ventricular, 1170–1171
  in myocardial infarction, surgical
   intervention in, 1240
  pulmonary hypertension in, 1141,
   1142
  vs. mitral regurgitation, 1187
  with aortic regurgitation, 1171
  with pulmonic stenosis, 1164–1166
Septal hypertrophy, asymmetric,
 1278–1279, *1280*
Septic abortion, hypofibrinogenemia in,
 1894
Septic granulomatous disease of
 childhood, chronic, 144
Septic shock, 1048, 1049, *1049*
 treatment of, 1119
Septicemia
 clostridial, 436
 gram-negative, liver disease in, 1656
 staphylococcal, vs. melioidosis, 470
Septicemic plague, primary, 464
Sequestran. See *Cholestyramine*.
Sequestration thrombocytopenia, 1877
Sequoiosis, *971*
Serofibrinous pleurisy with effusion,
 482, 491
Serologic procedures, normal values for,
 2352–2353
Serologic tests
 in amebiasis, 592
 in aspergillosis, 947
 in Chagas' disease, 582
 in coccidioidomycosis, 946
 in cryptococcosis, 947
 in pulmonary disease, 945, 946–947
 in syphilis, 513, *513*, 514
  false-positive, 514
 in trichinosis, 631
Serotonin
 circulatory effects of, 1111
 in control of gastrointestinal motility,
  1476
 synthesis and metabolism of, *2209*
Serous meningitis, 817
Serratia marcescens, pneumonia caused
 by, 361, 365
Serum chemical values, 2348
Serum enzymes
 concentrations of, in myocardial
  infarction, 1232
 in acute pericarditis, 1272

Serum enzymes (*Continued*)
 in differentiation of neurogenic and
  myopathic disease, 915
 in liver disease, 1647
Serum inhibitors, in sarcoidosis, 210
Serum iodoprotein defect, 2139
Serum sickness, 153–154
 Arthus reaction in, 131
 complicating rifampin treatment of
  pulmonary tuberculosis, 488
 vs. rheumatic fever, 383
Serum sickness neuropathy, 906
"Seven-year itch," 110
Sex
 as risk factor for atherosclerosis, 1219
 blood pressure and, 1200
Sex chromatin pattern, in evaluation of
 testicular function, 2165
Sex hormones, liver and, 1658
Sex play, childhood, 690
Sexual anhedonia, 689
Sexual desire, inhibited, 687
Sexual dysfunction
 classification of, 687–689, *687*
 "immediate" causes of, 688–689
 in chronic renal failure, 1362
Sexual excitement, inhibited, 687
Sexual function
 alcohol and, 708
 in middle life, 24
Sexual precocity
 female, *2179,* **2182–2183**
 male, 2166–2167
Sexuality, 686–687
 counseling in, 2197–2199
 medical aspects of, 684–692
 physician's role in, 684–686
Sézary's syndrome, 1834, *2302*, 2310
Shaking palsy, 752–756
Shaver's disease, 990
Sheehan's syndrome, 2098, 2100
Sheep cell agglutinins, in infectious
 mononucleosis, 266
Sheep red blood cells, in T cell
 detection, 129, 130
Shellfish, paralytic poisoning by, 68
Shiga bacillus, 457, 458
Shigella boydii, 457
Shigella dysenteriae, 457, 458
Shigella flexneri, 457, 458
Shigella sonnei, 457, 458
Shigellosis, 457–460
 vs. *Salmonella* gastroenteritis, 452
 vs. ulcerative colitis, 1572
 vs. viral gastroenteritis caused by
  Norwalk-like agents and
  rotaviruses, 306
Shin bone fever, 329
Shin splints, 1305
Shingles, 253, **824–827.** See also *Herpes
zoster.*
Ship fever, 318–320
Shock, 1107–1122
 acid-base disturbances in, 1046
 acidosis in, 1110
  correction of, 1118
 arrhythmias in, treatment of, 1118
 cardiogenic, surgical treatment in,
  1121, 1122
 causes and initiating mechanisms of,
  1108
 cellular and biochemical factors in,
  1113–1115

Shock (*Continued*)
cellular structure and function in, 1114
circulatory, hypotension and, in cancer patient, 1905
circulatory control in, 1108–1113, *1109*
complement activation in, 1115
critical care of, 1045–1050
diagnosis of, 1045, 1046
electric, 92–94, *93*
heart in, 1109, 1110
hypovolemia in, correction of, 1117, 1118
hypoxia in, 1109, 1110
correction of, 1118
in bacterial meningitis, 414
in clostridial myonecrosis, 434
in Crimean hemorrhagic fever, 298
in decompression sickness, *103*
in dengue hemorrhagic fever, 296, 297
in epidemic hemorrhagic fever, 301
in gastrointestinal bleeding, 1521, 1522
in gram-negative bacteremia, 455
in head injury, 882
in heat stroke, 85
in louse-borne relapsing fever, 528
in myocardial infarction, 1230, 1231
treatment of, 1236
surgical, 1239, 1240
in pneumococcal pneumonia, 354
treatment of, 356
in pseudomembranous enterocolitis, 1585
liver in, 1661
lysosomes in, 1114, 1115
microcirculation in, 1112, 1113
mitochondrial function in, 1113
oxygen-hemoglobin affinity in, 1113
patient assessment in, 1046, 1047, *1047*
"red," in transfusion reaction, 1786
refractory, 1050
septic, 1048, 1049, *1049*
treatment of, 1119
stages of, 1107, *1108*
transcapillary exchange in, 1112, 1113
treatment of, 1115–1122
general measures in, 1117, 1118
myths in, 1115, 1116
patient monitoring in, 1116
vascular factors in, 1110, 1111
vasoactive drugs in, 1048
Shock lung, 1113
Shohl's solution, in Fanconi's syndrome, 2024
Shoshin, 1689
Shoulder
frozen, 206–207
painful, 205–207
Shoulder-hand syndrome, 206, 727
after myocardial infarction, 1237
Shunt(s)
intrapulmonary, in acute respiratory failure, 1037
right-to-left, 940, 1022
Shunt hyperbilirubinemia, 1649
Shwartzman-Sanarelli phenomenon, 1328
Shy-Drager syndrome, 762–763
dizziness in, 740
Sibine stimulea, 119
Sick sinus syndrome, 1244
in myocardial infarction, 1235

Sickle cell anemia, 1773–1775
air travel and, 97
cutaneous lesions in, *2302*
heterozygote detection in, *58*
pneumococcal infections in, 348, 349
Salmonella infections in, 451
vs. rheumatic fever, 383
Sickle cell crises, 1773, 1774
Sickle cell disease
arthritis in, 200
cutaneous signs in, *2301*
eyes in, 2330–2332, *2331*
phagocytosis defects in, 1804
renal changes in, 1404
vs. acute abdomen, 1581
vs. infective endocarditis, 392
Sickle cell hemoglobin, screening for, 44
Sickle cell trait, 1775
genetic screening for, 59
vs. sickle cell anemia, 1774
Sickle cell–hemoglobin C disease, 1776
vs. sickle cell anemia, 1775
Sickle cell–hemoglobin D Punjab disease, 1776
Sickle cell–hemoglobin O Arab disease, 1776
Sickle cell–thalassemia, 1776
Sickle retinopathy, 2330, 2331, *2331*, 2332
Sickling disorders, 1773–1776
Sideroblastic anemia, 1740–1741, *1741*, 1751
therapeutic principles in, 1719
Sideropenic dysphagia, 1483
esophageal carcinoma and, 1597
Siderosis, 987, 1790
focal, 1790
Sigmoid colon
diverticulitis of, vs. Crohn's disease of colon, 1578
vs. ulcerative colitis, 1572
tuberculosis of, 492
Sigmoidoscopy
in Crohn's disease of colon, 1577
in diverticulitis, 1583
in radiation enterocolitis, 1584
in ulcerative colitis, 1571
Silicoproteinosis, acute, 990
Silicosis, *987*, **988–990**
host response to tuberculosis in, 483
management of, 993
pulmonary hypertension in, 1147
Silo-filler's disease, 1001
Simmonds' disease, 2100
Sinoatrial block, 1244–1245, *1245*
Sinoatrial node, 1242
Sinus(es)
carotid, hypersensitivity of, dizziness in, 740
stimulation of, in evaluation of dizziness, 737
cavernous, occlusion of, 789
thrombosis of, 780, 808
vs. Romaña's sign in Chagas' disease, 582
dural, major, thrombosis of, 808–809
lateral, thrombosis of, 789, 808, 809
of Valsalva, congenital aneurysms of, 1169–1170
paranasal, infections of, brain abscess from, 805
subdural empyema from, 807
superior longitudinal, occlusion of, in head injury, 884, 885

Sinus(es) (*Continued*)
superior sagittal, occlusion of, 788
thrombosis of, 809
transverse, thrombosis of, 789
venous, major, thrombophlebitis and thrombosis of, 808
Sinus arrhythmia, 1243
Sinus bradycardia, 1243
in myocardial infarction, 1230, 1235
in shock, 1118
in sick sinus syndrome, 1244
Sinus headache, 733
Sinus tachycardia, 1243–1244
in myocardial infarction, 1230
Sinus thrombosis, venous, intracranial, benign intracranial hypertension with, 871
Sinusitis
air travel and, 96
paranasal, in streptococcal pharyngitis, 373
Sipple's syndrome, *1910*, 2098, 2201, 2202, *2202*, 2203
internal malignancy and, *2296*
Sister, little, 587
Sister chromatids, 50, *50*
Situs inversus, 1166
Sjögren-like syndrome, in sarcoidosis, 213
Sjögren's syndrome, 193–194
eyes in, 2315, 2316
HLA system and, 39
immune mechanisms in, 133
in scleroderma, 169
neuropathy in, 908
Skeletal disease, hypocalcemia and, in malabsorption syndrome, 1528
Skeletal lesions, in multiple myeloma, 1858, *1859*
Skeleton, in Marfan's syndrome, 2053
Skerljevo, 522–523
Skin. See also *Cutaneous* and names of specific disorders affecting skin.
abscesses of, in heroin addiction, 696
anaerobic infection of, 443
biopsy of, 2273, 2274, *2274*
in systemic lupus erythematosus, 176
blood flow through, 2268
carcinoma of, squamous cell, 2309
changes in, with aging, 27, 2272
disease signs in, 2284–2301
diseases of, 2266–2312. See also names of specific diseases.
differential diagnosis of, 2277–2284
pathophysiology of, 2267–2272
prevalence of, *2266*
principles of therapy in, 2275–2277
superficial, "atypical" mycobacteria causing, 500
examination of, 2272–2275
supporting tests in, 2273, 2274
fungus infections of, 2281–2282, *2282*
heat loss through, 2269
hyperpigmentation of, associated with cancer, 1916, 2297
in adult celiac disease, 1541
in albinism, 2029
in anthrax, 470, 471
in arteriosclerosis obliterans, 1300
in bartonellosis, 331
in bejel, 523
in blastomycosis, 540
in chromomycosis, 543

Skin (*Continued*)
in chronic lymphocytic leukemia, 1824
in chronic renal failure, 1366
in coma, 643
in cryptococcosis, 544
in Cushing's syndrome, 2153, *2297*
in decompression sickness, *103*
in diabetes mellitus, 1980, 1981, *2300*
in diphtheria, 431
in drug allergy, 156
in Ehlers-Danlos syndrome, 2054, *2298*
in erysipelas, 375
in erysipeloid of Rosenbach, 473
in familial Mediterranean fever, 2056, *2299, 2300*
in fulminating meningococcemia, 419, *419*
in gastrointestinal disease, *2298–2299*
in gonococcal arthritis, 408, 409
in hematologic diseases, *2302*
in hemochromatosis, 1791, *2299*
in hereditary hemorrhagic telangiectasia, 1880
in herpes zoster, 825
in host defense, 145
in hyperthyroidism, 2122
in immersion foot, 1310
in iron deficiency anemia, 1748
in kwashiorkor, 1681, *1682*
in leprosy, 502, *502*, 503
in listeriosis, 472
in liver disease, 1645, *2299*
in non-Hodgkin's lymphomas, 1834
in nutritional deficiency, 1675, 1676
in obesity, 1696
in onchocerciasis, 636
in paracoccidioidomycosis, 541
in paraplegia, 887
in pellagra, 1675, 1676, *2299*
in periarteritis nodosa, 182
in pinta, *520*, 524, 525
in pneumococcal pneumonia, 352
in polymyositis and dermatomyositis, 172, 173, *2296*
in porphyria cutanea tarda, 2048, *2288, 2288*
in protoporphyria, 2049
in radiation injury, 89
in renal disease, *2300–2301*
in rheumatic disorders, *2303*
in rheumatic fever, 381
in sarcoidosis, 213, *2300*
in scarlet fever, 371
in scleroderma, 168, 169, *2298, 2301*
in specific system disorders, *2298–2303*, **2300–2301**
in sporotrichosis, 545
in streptococcal pyoderma, 374
in stupor, 643
in syphilis, 509, *509*
in thromboangiitis obliterans, 1303
in variegate porphyria, 2047, 2048
in visceral leishmaniasis, 585
in yaws, 519, *520, 521*
lesions of, viral diseases characterized by, 246–264
malignant change of, 2308–2312
mechanical properties of, 2268
mycoplasmal disease of, 345
neurofibromatosis of, 2293–2294, *2293, 2297, 2300*

Skin (*Continued*)
noncutaneous malignancy and, 2295–2297, 2300, *2296–2297*
pigmentary disturbances of, 2289–2293
scalded, syndrome of, 400, 2306
staphylococcal infections of, 399–401
in diabetes mellitus, 398
prevention of, 401
treatment of, 400–401
stimulation of, in pain relief, 725
streptococcal infections of, 368, **374–375**
structure of, 2267–2268, *2267, 2268*
sun damage to, 2272, 2288
sweat glands of, 2268–2272
tuberculosis of, 498
ulcers of, chronic, in rheumatoid arthritis, 187
water and electrolyte losses from, excessive, 1951
yeast infections of, 2282–2283
Skin grafts, impaired, hyperbaric oxygen therapy in, 105
Skin test(s)
for immune competence in cancer, 1925
in allergic rhinitis, 159
in brucellosis, 477, 478
in cat scratch disease, 303, 304
in coccidioidomycosis, 539, 946
in echinococcosis, 610
in histoplasmosis, 537, 946
in lymphogranuloma venereum, 336
in pulmonary disease, 945–946
in tuberculosis, 946
in tularemia, 466
Kveim-Siltzbach, in sarcoidosis, 214
Skin-sensitizing antibodies, 128
Skull
fracture of, basilar, 883
in Paget's disease, 2258
infections of, brain abscess from, 805
inspection of, in stupor or coma, 643
tumors of, 867
x-rays of, 748
in intracranial tumors, 866
SLE, 174–180. See also *Systemic lupus erythematosus.*
Sleep, 651–655
arousal and, hypothalamus in, 715
disorders of, 652–655
in dementia, 663
disturbed, 655
in manic-depressive psychosis, 670
physiology and pharmacology of, 652
rapid eye movement, 652, 653
slow wave, 652
"yen," in opiate addiction, 696
Sleep apnea, 654, 655
Sleep paralysis, 654
Sleeping sickness, 575, 576–579
Sleepwalking, 655
"Small airways disease," 951
Small intestine. See *Intestine(s), small,* and names of specific intestinal components.
Small left colon syndrome, 1498
Smallpox, 255–259
acute disseminated encephalomyelitis after, 836, 837
vaccination in, 259–260
Smallpox virus, 255

Smog, human health and, 62, 63
Smoke inhalation, hyperbaric oxygen therapy in, 104
Smoking
after myocardial infarction, 1234
as cardiovascular risk factor, 1062, 1220
dust exposure and, neoplasia associated with, 994, 995
in bronchogenic carcinoma, 1005
in chronic obstructive pulmonary disease, 960
in peptic ulcer, 1503, 1516
in simple chronic bronchitis, 953, 954
in "stress" polycythemia, 1793
in thromboangiitis obliterans, 1302
occupational bronchitis and, 995, 996
Snails, in schistosomiasis, 611, 612
Snakebite, 121–123
"Snowflake" cataract, in diabetes mellitus, 1976, 2320
Soaks, in dermatologic therapy, 2276
Soap colitis, 1614
Social factors, role of, in disease, 14
Sodium
depletion of, extracellular volume depletion and, defective water excretion from, 1953
excretion of, in chronic renal failure, 1355, 1356
loss of, water loss and, volume depletion from, 1950, 1951
reabsorption of, by renal tubules, 1317, 1318
renal conservation of, in interstitial nephritis, 1417
retention of, in chronic renal failure, 1355
serum, reduced concentration of, 1952. See also *Hyponatremia.*
transport of, 1525
Sodium amytal, in status epilepticus, *859*
Sodium aurothiomalate, in rheumatoid arthritis, 192
Sodium bicarbonate
in acidosis of shock, 1118
in chronic pancreatitis, 1557
in hyperkalemia, 1960
in metabolic acidosis, 1965
in near-drowning, 107
in peptic ulcer, 1513
in salicylate poisoning, 76
in ventricular fibrillation, 1056, 1057
Sodium chloride
hypertonic, in hyponatremia, 1953
in addisonian crisis, 2149
in Addison's disease, 2150
in gastric outlet obstruction complicating peptic ulcer, 1517
in heat exhaustion, 85
Sodium cyanate, neuropathy from, 910
Sodium fluoride, in osteoporosis, 2246
Sodium iodide, in thyroid storm, 2128
Sodium lactate, in metabolic acidosis, 1965
Sodium nitrite, in cyanide poisoning, 75
Sodium nitroprusside
in ergotism and methysergide toxicity, 1308
in heart failure, 1101, *1101*
Sodium phosphate, in hypercalcemia, 2239

Sodium phytate, in hypercalcemia, 2239
Sodium stibogluconate, in visceral leishmaniasis, 586
Sodium sulfate, isotonic, in hypercalcemia, 2240
Sodium thiosulfate, in cyanide poisoning, 75
Sodium-restricted diet, 1711, 1712
Sodoku, 531–532
Soft palate, paralysis of, in diphtheria, 432
Soft tissue(s), infection of
anaerobic, 443
gas-forming, differential diagnosis of, 435
Solanaceous plants, poisoning by, 70
Solanum species, poisoning by, 70
Solar urticaria, 161, 162
Soldier's heart, vs. angina pectoris, 1227
Soles, hyperkeratosis of, in yaws, 521
Solvents, organic
as nephrotoxins, 1434
inhalation of, 705
Somatic changes, pubertal, 17, 18, 19
Somatomedins, effect of, on growth hormone action, 2071
Somatostatin, 2075
Somatotropin, 2086–2087
Somatotropin release–inhibiting factor, 2075
Somnambulism, 655
Somogyi effect, in diabetes mellitus, 1987
Sopor. See Methaqualone.
Sorbitol, in hyperkalemia, 1960
Sore
bay, 588
Oriental, 587–589, 588
Sore throat
in infectious mononucleosis, 265
quinsy, in streptococcal tonsillitis, 373
streptococcal, 371–374. See also Streptococcal pharyngitis.
South African genetic porphyria, 2047
South American blastomycosis, 541–542
Spangler, papular dermatitis of, 2305
Spanish fly, 114
Sparganosis, 607
Sparganum proliferum, 607
Sparine. See Promazine.
Spasm(s)
esophageal, diffuse, 1485–1486, 1486
habit, 759–760
vs. acute chorea, 758
massive, infantile, 854
mobile, 760
muscle, in paraplegia, 888
in tetanus, 439, 440
"reflex," in tetanus, 438
Spasmodic torticollis, 761–762
Spastic colon, 1493
Spastic constipation, 1480
Spastic paraplegia, hereditary, 768
vs. vitamin B_{12} deficiency, 777
Spectinomycin, 557, 562
in gonococcal disease, 409, 410
in pregnancy, 409
Spectrometry, mass, in critical care medicine, 1032
Speech
disturbances of, in intracranial tumor, 865
in metabolic brain disease, 648
Speech area, isolation of, 657

Speech tests, in hearing loss, 735
Spermidine, as tumor marker, 1913
Spermine, as tumor marker, 1913
Spherocytosis, hereditary, 1756–1757
detection of, in relatives, 58
vs. pyruvate kinase deficiency, 1758, 1759
Sphincter(s)
anal, 1482
esophageal
in swallowing, 1478, 1478, 1479
lower, hypertensive, 1488
gastrointestinal, normal physiology of, 1475
ileocecal, 1492
of Oddi, stenosis of, 1636
precapillary, in shock, 1112
Sphincterotomy, transendoscopic, in choledocholithiasis, 1630
Sphingolipodystrophy, hematoside, 42
Sphingomyelin lipidosis, 2013, 2014–2015
Sphygmomanometer cuff pain test of Lowenberg, in thrombophlebitis, 1125
Sphygmomanometry, 1200
Spider angiomas, in liver disease, 1645
Spider bite, 114–115
Spina bifida, 875–876
syringomyelia and, 768, 769
Spina bifida occulta, 875
Spinal arachnoiditis, 897
vs. spinal epidural infections, 811
Spinal canal, disease of, vs. arteriosclerosis obliterans, 1301
Spinal cord
arteriovenous malformations of, 897–898
cavernous angiomas of, 898
compression of, disorders causing, 893–898
laboratory aids in, 892–893
levels of, 891–892
management of, 893
symptoms of, 890
vs. amyotrophic lateral sclerosis, 766
disorders of, respiratory failure in, 1024
vs. polymyositis, 173
dysfunction of, severe, 886–888
epidural granulomas of, 494
in decompression sickness, 103
in electric injury, 93
in vitamin B_{12} deficiency, 776, 777
lower, compressive lesions of, 891
mechanical lesions of, 889–898
nonmetastatic effects of cancer on, 878
tumors of, 896–897
vs. multiple sclerosis, 847
vs. tick paralysis, 118
vascular lesions of, 897–898
Spinal epidural abscess, 810, 811
cerebrospinal fluid findings in, 803
primary, 404
vs. transverse myelitis, 812
Spinal epidural hematoma, 898
Spinal epidural infections, 810–811
Spinal stenosis, lumbar, 895
Spine
anomalies of, 874–876
bamboo, in ankylosing spondylitis, 195

Spine (Continued)
cervical, compressive lesions of, 891
degenerative disease of, 204
hypertrophic spurs of, dysphagia from, 1483
injuries of, 885, 886
degenerative disease of, 204
fractures of, 885, 886
in epidural infections, 810, 811
injuries of, 885–886
lumbar, degenerative disease of, 204
stenosis of, 895
lumbosacral, compressive lesions of, 892
midcervical, injuries of, 885
thoracic, compression at, 891
thoracolumbar, injuries of, 886
x-rays of, 748
Spinocerebellar degenerations, 766–768
in bronchogenic carcinoma, 1007
vs. multiple sclerosis, 847
Spirillary and leptospiral diseases, 526–535
Spirillary rat-bite fever, 531–532
Spirillum minus, 531
Spirometra mansonoides, 607
Spironolactone(s)
hyperkalemia and, 1959
in ascites complicating cirrhosis, 1665
in heart failure, 1105
in primary aldosteronism, 2158
Spitz nevus, 2312
Spleen
diseases of, 1867–1871
enlargement of. See Splenomegaly.
function of, 1754, 1755, 1867, 1868
absent or reduced, 1869
in chronic granulocytic leukemia, 1821, 1822
in chronic lymphocytic leukemia, 1824
in hemolysis effected by immune reactions, 1762
in hemolytic anemia, 1754, 1755
in louse-borne relapsing fever, 527
in malaria, 571
in polycythemia vera, 1795
in schistosomiasis, 614
in sickle cell anemia, 1774
in systemic lupus erythematosus, 176, 177
in visceral leishmaniasis, 585
infarction of, vs. acute pericarditis, 1273
normal anatomy of, 1868, 1868
radionuclide imaging of, 1470
rupture of, angiography in, 1471
in infectious mononucleosis, 267
tuberculosis of, primary, 493
Splenectomy
consequences of, 1869
in agnogenic myeloid metaplasia, 1828, 1829
in hemolytic anemia, 1754, 1755
autoimmune, 1764
in hereditary spherocytosis, 1757
in Hodgkin's disease, 1842, 1844
in idiopathic thrombocytopenic purpura, 1874
indications for, 1871
pneumococcal pneumonia after, 348
Splenic fever, 470
Splenic venous obstruction, portal hypertension in, 1639

Splenomegaly, 1869–1871
causes of, 1869, 1870, *1870*
congestive, 1870
neutropenia in, 1809
in infectious mononucleosis, 265
in infective endocarditis, 389
in malaria, 571
in portal hypertension, 1639, 1640
in rheumatoid arthritis, 193
infiltrative, 1870
tropical, in malaria, 569, 572
portal hypertension and, 1639
vs. visceral leishmaniasis, 586
Splinter hemorrhages, in infective
endocarditis, 389
Splints, shin, 1305
Spondylitis
ankylosing, 194–195
aortic regurgitation in, 1194
eyes in, 2316
genetic factors in, 39, 194
pulmonary disability with, 1020
regional enteritis and, 198, 1561
ulcerative colitis and, 198, 1568
vs. degenerative joint disease, 205
vs. psoriatic arthritis, 196
Marie-Strümpell, 194–195. See also
Spondylitis, ankylosing.
rheumatoid, 194–195. See also
Spondylitis, ankylosing.
tuberculous, 185, 497
vs. staphylococcal infections of
vertebrae and intervertebral
discs, 403
Spondylosis, 894–895
cervical, 895
pain of, vs. angina pectoris, 1227
vs. multiple sclerosis, 847
vs. vitamin B_{12} deficiency, 776, 777
lumbar, 895
Sponge kidney, medullary, 1455–1456
vs. adult polycystic kidney disease,
1454
**Spongy degeneration of white matter,
850**
Spontaneous pneumothorax, 1016–1017
vs. myocardial infarction, 1233
vs. pulmonary embolism, 1133
Spoon nail, in iron deficiency anemia,
1748
**Sporadic goitrous hypothyroidism,
2138–2140**
Sporadic myoglobinuria, 924–925
Sporothrix schenckii, 544
Sporotrichosis, 544–545
vs. glanders, 469
vs. tularemia, 467
Spotted fever
meningococcal, 417
Rocky Mountain, 322–324
clinical features of, *313*
epidemiologic features of, *310*
peripheral arteritis in, 1305
vs. Colorado tick fever, 280
vs. rat-bite fever, 531
vs. tularemia, 467
Spotted fever group
biologic properties of, 309, *309*
clinical features of, *313*
epidemiologic features of, *310*
serologic responses in, *314*

**Spring-summer encephalitis, Russian,
290–291**
Sprue
celiac, 1539. See also *Celiac disease,
adult.*
collagenous, 1541
nontropical, 1539
osteomalacia in, 2249
tropical, 1545–1546
jejunal histology in, 1533
megaloblastosis in, 1723
Spurge laurel berries, poisoning by, 70
Sputum
examination of, in pulmonary
disease, 947–948
in bronchiectasis, 983
in bronchogenic carcinoma, 1006,
1008
in chronic respiratory failure, 1029
in *Klebsiella* pneumonia, 358
in pneumococcal pneumonia, 352, 353
in pulmonary tuberculosis, 486, 489
in simple chronic bronchitis, 954
Squamous cell carcinoma of skin, 2309
Squander, quantal, 930
"Squat-jump syndrome," 924
St. Louis encephalitis, 288–289
St. Louis encephalitis virus, 288
St. Vitus' dance, 757–758
Staggers, blind, 745
Stannosis, 987
Stapedius reflex measurement, in
hearing loss, 735
Staphylococcal bacteremia, 403–404
**Staphylococcal endocarditis, 386,
403–404**
treatment of, 393, 404
Staphylococcal enterocolitis, 404–405
Staphylococcal food poisoning, 64–65,
404
vs. *Salmonella* gastroenteritis, 452
Staphylococcal gastroenteritis, 404–405
bacteriology of, 396
cutaneous, 399–401
in diabetes mellitus, 398
prevention of, 401
treatment of, 400–401
epidemiology of, 397
hospital-acquired, 398
pathogenesis of, 397
treatment of, 398
Staphylococcal meningitis, 404, 411
treatment of, 415, 416
**Staphylococcal osteomyelitis, 402–403,
2260**
vs. sporotrichosis, 545
Staphylococcal parotitis, 404
Staphylococcal pericarditis, 404
Staphylococcal pharyngitis, 404
Staphylococcal pneumonia, 401–402
vs. melioidosis, 470
vs. pneumococcal pneumonia, 354
Staphylococcal pyarthrosis, 404
Staphylococcal pyomyositis, 404
**Staphylococcal scalded skin syndrome,
400,** 2306
Staphylococcal scarlet fever, 400
Staphylococcal septicemia, vs.
melioidosis, 470
Staphylococcal tonsillitis, 404

Staphylococcal toxic epidermal
necrolysis, 400
Staphylococcus albus. See *Staphylococcus
epidermidis.*
Staphylococcus aureus, 397
in bacterial meningitis, 411
in endocarditis in drug abusers, 390
in infective endocarditis, 386
in staphylococcal osteomyelitis, 402
in tropical pyomyositis, 638
Staphylococcus epidermidis, 397
in infective endocarditis, 386
Staphylococcus saprophyticus, 397
Starfishes, envenomation by, 124
Stargazers, envenomation by, 124
Starling forces, in control of renal salt
and water excretion, 1321
Starvation, 1684
accelerated, 1705
fatty liver in, 1660
fuel homeostasis in, 1704
Status asthmaticus, 957
treatment of, 959
Status demyelination, 760
Status epilepticus, 855, 856
treatment of, *859,* 860, 861
Status marmoratus, 760
Steatorrhea, clinical effects of, 1528
Stein-Leventhal syndrome, 2189
Stem cells, dysfunction of, in
polycythemia vera, 1794, 1795
Stenosing cholangitis, vs. biliary
cirrhosis, 1666
Stenosing tenovaginitis, 207
Stenosis
ampullary, 1636
aortic, 1190–1194
calcific, underlying infective
endocarditis, 387
differential diagnosis of, *1192, 1193*
general physiologic effects of, 1174,
1175, *1175*
subvalvular, discrete, 1167
supravalvular, 1167, 1289
valvular, congenital, 1156–1157
vs. mitral regurgitation, 1187
coronary artery, left main, surgical
treatment of, 1239, *1239*
internal carotid artery, ischemia from,
784, 785
lumbar spinal, 895
mitral, 1179–1185
general physiologic effects of, *1175,*
1176
mesenteric artery embolism in, 1589
pulmonary circulation in, 1145–1146
pulmonary hypertension and, vs.
atrial septal defect, 1162
silent, pulmonary hypertension
and, 1140
vs. idiopathic pulmonary
hemosiderosis, 976
vs. tricuspid stenosis, 1198
pulmonary artery, 1143, 1167–1168
pulmonic, 1199
single ventricle with, 1174
subvalvular, 1167
supravalvular, 1167–1168
valvular, 1158–1160
ventricular septal defect with,
1164–1166

Stenosis (*Continued*)
  pyloric, 1490
    frequency and sex ratio of, *48*
    renal artery, hypertension from, 1210, 1211
    subaortic, idiopathic hypertrophic, 1278, *1278*, 1279
      vs. aortic stenosis, *1192*, 1193
      vs. mitral regurgitation, 1187
      vs. mitral valve prolapse syndrome, 1189
    muscular, 1278
  tricuspid, 1197–1198
Stercobilin, 1637
Stercoral ulcer, 1615
Steroid contraception, 2195–2197. See also *Contraceptives, oral.*
Steroid hormones, mode of action of, 2070, *2071*
Stevens-Johnson syndrome, *2303*
  mycoplasmal infection and, 345
Stewart-Treves syndrome, *2296*, 2297
Stibine, poisoning by, 81
Stibocaptate, in schistosomiasis, 616
Stibophen, in erythema nodosum leprosum, 504
Stiff man syndrome, 930
Stiffness
  in ankylosing spondylitis, 194
  in neck, in intracranial hemorrhage, treatment of, 800
    in intracranial tumors, 865
    in stupor or coma, 643
    in subarachnoid hemorrhage, 797
  in polymyalgia rheumatica, 217
  in rheumatoid arthritis, 188
Still's disease, 196
  vs. rheumatic fever, 383
Stimulants, central nervous system
  abuse of, 701–702
  poisoning by, *712*
Sting(s)
  Hymenoptera, 113–114, 163
  mollusc, 123, 124
  scorpion, 116–117
Stingrays, envenomation by, 124
Stomach. See also *Gastric* and *Gastro-*
  adenoma of, 1604
  arterial supply to, 1586, *1586*
  carcinoid tumor of, 2210, *2211*, 2212
  carcinoma of, 1599–1603
  dilatation of, acute, 1489
    in pneumococcal pneumonia, 354
  diverticula of, 1500
  irradiation of, in peptic ulcer, 1516
  leiomyoma of, 1604
  leiomyosarcoma of, 1603
  lymphoma of, 1603
  motility in, disorders of, 1488–1490
    normal, 1488, 1489
  mucosa of, peptic ulcer and, 1504, 1505
  neoplasms of, benign, 1604
    malignant, 1599–1604
  outlet of, obstruction at, 1490
    in peptic ulcer, 1517, 1518
    vs. acute appendicitis, 1580
  pain originating in, 1476
  polyps of, gastric carcinoma and, 1600
  tuberculosis of, 492
  volvulus of, 1489–1490
Stomatitis
  denture, *Candida*, 548
  in mercury poisoning, 80
  vesicular, with exanthem, 274

Stomatocytosis, hereditary, 1757
Stonefishes, envenomation by, 124
  antivenin for, 125
Stool
  examination of, in amebiasis, *570*, 592
  fat in, measurement of, in malabsorption syndrome, 1530
Stoxil. See *Idoxuridine.*
STP, 704
  poisoning by, *712*
Strachan's syndrome, 775
Strawberry gallbladder, 1624
Strawberry hemangioma, *2302*
Streptobacillary rat-bite fever, 531
Streptobacillus moniliformis, 531
Streptocerciasis, 637
Streptococcal cellulitis
  vs. erysipeloid of Rosenbach, 473
  vs. glanders, 469
Streptococcal endocarditis, 386
  treatment of, 392, 393
Streptococcal infections, 366–385
  acute glomerulonephritis after, 1394–1397
  classification of, 366–367
  group A, 366, 367–371
    clinical syndromes of, 371–375
      rheumatic fever from, 377, 378, 379, 382
    treatment of, 375–376
  group B, 366
  group C, 367
  group D, 366, 367
  group G, 367
  of skin, 368, 374–375
  prophylaxis of, 376–377
Streptococcal myonecrosis
  anaerobic, 434
  treatment of, 435
  vs. clostridial myonecrosis, *435*
Streptococcal pharyngitis, 371–374
  complications of, 373
  course of, 372
  diagnosis of, 372
  epidemiology of, 369, 370
  immunologic diagnosis of, 372
  pathogenesis of, 368
  rheumatic fever and, 378, 379, 382
  vs. diphtheria, 431
  vs. infectious mononucleosis, 266
  vs. influenza, 245
Streptococcal pneumonia
  hemolytic, 375
  vs. pneumococcal pneumonia, 354
Streptococcal pyoderma, 374
  epidemiology of, 370
  pathogenesis of, 368
  treatment of, 376
Streptococcal sore throat, 371–374. See also *Streptococcal pharyngitis.*
Streptococcal tonsillitis
  complications of, 373
  epidemiology of, 369
Streptococci
  alpha-hemolytic, 366
  anaerobic, 367
  beta-hemolytic, 366
  "green," 367
  nonhemolytic, 367
  viridans group of, 367
    in infective endocarditis, 386
Streptococcus agalactiae, 366
Streptococcus bovis, 390
Streptococcus durans, 390
Streptococcus equinus, 390

Streptococcus faecalis, 366, 367
  in infective endocarditis, 390
Streptococcus faecium, 390
Streptococcus mitis, 367
  in infective endocarditis, 386
Streptococcus mutans, 367
Streptococcus pneumoniae
  in bacterial meningitis, 411
  in infective endocarditis, 386
  pneumonia caused by, 347–357, *350*
Streptococcus pyogenes, 366, 367
Streptococcus salivarius, 367
Streptococcus sanguis, 367
  in infective endocarditis, 386
Streptokinase, in thrombophlebitis, 1129
Streptomycin, 557, 561
  adverse reactions to, 562
  as nephrotoxin, 1425
  in brucellosis, 478
  in glanders, 469
  in infective endocarditis, 392, 393
  in infective endocarditis prophylaxis, 396
  in plague, 465
  in pulmonary disease caused by *M. kansasii*, 499
  in pulmonary tuberculosis, 488, 489, 490
  in tuberculous meningitis, 494
  in tularemia, 467
  neuromuscular block caused by, 929
Streptozotocin, 1933
  as nephrotoxin, 1432
Stress(es)
  atherosclerosis and, 1221
  cardiovascular response to, 1070, *1070*
  complicating maintenance hemodialysis, 1381
  galactorrhea due to, 2191
  Graves' disease and, 2120
  in addisonian patients, treatment during, 2149
  peptic lesions caused by, 1504
Stress diabetes, 1982
Stress hyperlipemia, 2009
"Stress polycythemia," 1792, 1793
Stress response, in acute infections, 1678
Stretch reflexes, hyperactive, in metabolic brain disease, 648
"Stretch syncope," 746
Striatonigral degeneration, 764–765
Stricture(s)
  biliary, 1631–1632
    vs. choledocholithiasis, 1630
    vs. malignant bile duct tumors, 1635
  colonic, in ulcerative colitis, 1574
  fibrous, in amebiasis, 591
  lye, esophageal, vs. carcinoma, 1598
Stroke, 784–789
  completed, 785–786
    anticoagulant drugs or surgery in, 793
  heat, 84–85
    vs. malaria, 573
  pituitary, 2098
  progressive, 785
    anticoagulant drugs or surgery in, 793
Stroke volume, cardiac, 1083, *1083*
  in shock, 1109, 1110
Stroke-in-evolution, 785
  anticoagulant drugs or surgery in, 793

Strongyloides fulleburni, 623
Strongyloides stercoralis, 559, 605, 621, 622
  life cycle of, *621*
Strongyloidiasis, 622–623
  vs. angiostrongyliasis, 631
Structural genes, 34
Stuart factor, 1881
  deficiency of, *1884,* 1888
    acquired, 1891
Stupor
  common causes of, *640*
  in acute drug poisoning, 713
  pathogenesis of, 640–643
  patient in, approach to, 642–643
Sturge-Weber disease, 771
Subaortic stenosis
  hypertrophic, idiopathic, 1278, *1278,* 1279
    vs. aortic stenosis, *1192,* 1193
    vs. mitral regurgitation, 1187
    vs. mitral valve prolapse syndrome, 1189
  muscular, 1278
Subarachnoid hemorrhage, 794
  clinical manifestations of, 796, 797
  pathology and pathogenesis of, 796
  with intracerebral extension, 794
Subclavian artery, right, aberrant, 1291
Subclavian steal syndrome, 785, 789
Subcortical encephalopathy, progressive, 794
Subcutaneous edema, in right ventricular failure, 1092
Subcutaneous nodules
  in rheumatic fever, 381
  in rheumatoid arthritis, 187, 188
Subdiaphragmatic abscess
  pleural effusion in, 1018
  vs. pneumococcal pneumonia, 354
Subdural effusions, in bacterial meningitis, 412
Subdural empyema, 807–808
  cerebrospinal fluid examination in, *803,* 807
Subdural hematoma
  complicating maintenance hemodialysis, 1381
  in head injury, 884
  vs. benign intracranial hypertension, 872
  vs. brain tumor, 868
  vs. California encephalitis, 288
  vs. cerebral infarction, 790
Suberosis, *971*
Subhyaloid hemorrhages, 797
Submetacentric chromosomes, 50, *50*
Submucous abscess, 1617
Subperiosteal hemorrhages, in scurvy, 1690
Subphrenic abscess, 1594
  radionuclide imaging in, *1469*
  vs. hepatic amebiasis, 592
Substance P, 2077, *2078*
Substance S, Reichstein's, 2146
Subtentorial mass lesions
  causing stupor or coma, *640,* 641–642
  vs. metabolic brain disease, 650
Subvalvular aortic stenosis, discrete, 1167
Subvalvular pulmonic stenosis, 1167
Succinylcholine sensitivity, 46
Succinylsulfathiazole, 563

Sucrase, deficiency of, 1539
Sucrase-isomaltase deficiency, *41*
Sucrose lysis test, in paroxysmal nocturnal hemoglobinuria, 1768, 1769
Sudanophilic leukodystrophy, 850
Sudden death, 1237–1238
  in aortic stenosis, 1191
Sudeck's atrophy, 206, 727, 2246
Suicide
  alcohol abuse and, 710
  drug overdosage in, 711
  inclination to, in depression, 677
    in manic-depressive psychosis, 670
Sulfadiazine, 563
  in glanders, 469
  in malaria, *558*
  in nocardiosis, 475
  in prophylaxis of streptococcal infection, 377
  in recrudescent falciparum malaria prevention, 574
  in toxoplasmosis, *558,* 597
  ocular, 2335
Sulfadimethoxine, 563
Sulfadoxine, in malaria prophylaxis, 575
Sulfamethoxazole, 563
  trimethoprim and, *556,* 563
    in gonococcal disease, 410
    in pneumocystosis, *558,* 600
Sulfamethoxypyridazine, 563
Sulfate, in chronic renal failure, 1360
Sulfatide lipidoses, 850
Sulfhemoglobin, 1782
Sulfhemoglobinemia, 1782
Sulfinpyrazone
  as nephrotoxin, 1432
  in tophaceous gout, 2040
Sulfisoxazole, *557,* 563
  in malabsorption syndrome, *1536*
Sulfite oxidase deficiency, *43*
Sulfobromophthalein sodium clearance, 1646
Sulfonamide(s), *557,* 562. See also names of specific agents.
  as nephrotoxins, 1427
  contraindications to, 553
  in prophylaxis of streptococcal infection, 377
Sulfonamide-streptomycin form of drug resistance, 551
Sulfonylureas
  hypoglycemic coma induced by, 1996
  in diabetes mellitus, 1986, *1986*
Sulfur aminoacidemias, *2017*
Sulfur dioxide, exposure to, respiratory effects of, 1000
"Summer grippe," 275
Superior longitudinal sinus, occlusion of, in head injury, 884, 885
Superior mesenteric artery, 1586, *1587*
Superior mesenteric artery syndrome, 1590
Superior sagittal sinus occlusion, 788
Superior sagittal sinus thrombosis, 809
Superior vena cava
  angiography of, 944
  compression or obstruction of, in bronchogenic carcinoma, 1006
Superior vena caval syndrome, 1018
Suppurative cholangitis, 1631
  liver abscess in, 1657
Suppurative complications of streptococcal pharyngitis, 373

Suppurative parotitis, vs. mumps, 263
Suppurative thyroiditis, 2131
Supratentorial mass lesions
  causing stupor or coma, *640,* 641
  vs. metabolic brain disease, 650
Supravalvular aortic stenosis, 1167, 1289
Supravalvular pulmonic stenosis, 1167–1168
Supraventricular tachycardias
  in Wolff-Parkinson-White syndrome, *1258,* **1259–1260,** *1259*
  with short P-R interval and normal QRS complexes, 1256–1257
Suramin
  in African trypanosomiasis, *558,* 578
  in onchocerciasis, 636
  in river blindness, *559*
Surfactant
  alveolar, 932
  pulmonary, antibacterial activity of, 339
Surgical decompression, in spinal injuries, 886
Surgical treatment of coronary artery disease, 1238–1241
Sustanon, in anemia of chronic renal failure, 1364
Suxamethonium sensitivity, *43,* 46
SW sleep, 652
Swallowing
  air, 1479, 1489
  difficulty in, 1479. See also *Dysphagia.*
  disorders of, 1478–1479
  normal, 1478, *1478, 1479*
  pain with, 1479
    in esophageal carcinoma, 1597, 1598
Swallowing paralysis, in poliomyelitis, 832
Swan-Ganz catheterization
  in acute respiratory failure, 1043
  in shock, 1116
Sweat, formation of, 2269
Sweat glands, 2268–2272
Sweating, excessive, volume depletion in, 1951
Swimmer's itch, 613
Swine influenza, 241, 242, 246
Swiss type immunodeficiency, 141
Swyer-James syndrome, 1004
Sycosis barbae, 400
Sydenham's chorea, 757–758
  in rheumatic fever, 381
  vs. African trypanosomiasis, 578
Sylvan yellow fever, 293, *293,* 294
Sylvest's disease, 271–272
Sympathectomy, lumbar, preganglionic, in arteriosclerosis obliterans, 1301
Sympathetic nervous system, 2199–2207
  hormones of, 2199–2201
Sympathomimetic amines. See also names of specific agents.
  in heart failure, 1100
  in shock, 1119, 1120
Synanceja species, envenomation by, 124, 125
Syncope, 742–745
  carotid sinus, 743, 744
  cough, 740, 744
  effort, 744
  heat, 85
    vs. heat stroke, 84
  in aortic stenosis, 1191
  in asymmetric septal hypertrophy, 1278

Syncope (*Continued*)
in myocardial disease, 744
in primary pulmonary hypertension, 1139
micturition, 740, 744
"stretch," 746
vasodepressor, 743
vs. hysterical fainting, 744
vs. idiopathic autonomic insufficiency, 763
vasovagal, 740
vs. epilepsy, 858
Syndrome. See names of specific syndromes.
Synergistic gangrene, Meleney's, 367
Synovial bursae, extension or rupture of, in rheumatoid arthritis, 188
Synovial chondromatosis, 202
Synovial chondrosarcoma, 202
Synovial fluid
in rheumatoid arthritis, 189
normal values for, 2355
Synovioma, 202
Synovitis, pigmented villonodular, 202
Synovium
in scleroderma, 168
tumors of, 202
Syphilis, 505–518
aortic aneurysm in, 511, 1294, 1295
aortic regurgitation in, 1194
cardiovascular, 511, 1294–1295, *1295*
treatment of, 516, 1295
cerebral infarction from, 779
chancre in, 508, *509*
clinical manifestations of, 508
congenital, 512, 513
follow-up examinations in, 517
IgM FTA-ABS test for, 515
treatment of, *515,* 516, 517
darkfield examination in, 513
diagnosis of, 513, 514, 515
early, treatment of, 516
endemic, 522–523
epidemiologic investigation and treatment in, 517
epidemiology of, 507
etiology of, 505
gummas in, 510, 511, 813, 815, 864
host response in, 506
in pregnancy, treatment of, 516
Jarisch-Herxheimer reaction in, 517
late, 510
benign, 510
treatment of, 516
vs. lupoid leishmaniasis, 588
latent, 510
treatment of, *515,* 516
meningovascular, 511, 813–814
treatment of, 516
vs. transverse myelitis, 812
neuro-, 511, 512, 812–816. See also *Neurosyphilis.*
nonvenereal childhood, 522–523
orchitis in, 2174
pathogenesis of, 506
peripheral vascular complications of, 1305
prevention of, prospects for, 518
primary, 508, *509*
relapsing, 510
secondary, 508, 509, *509,* 510
liver disease in, 1656
vs. leprosy, 504
vs. yaws, 521

Syphilis (*Continued*)
serologic tests in, 513, *513,* 514
false-positive, 514
in gonorrhea, 410
tertiary, 510
treatment of, 515–518, *515*
follow-up examinations in, 517
persistence of treponemes after, 517
untreated, natural course of, 507
vs. bejel, 523
vs. Chagas' disease, 582
vs. chromomycosis, 543
vs. lymphogranuloma venereum, 335
vs. paracoccidioidomycosis, 541
vs. pinta, 525
Syphilitic aortic aneurysm, 511, 1294, 1295
Syphilitic aortitis, 511, 1294–1295, *1295*
Syphilitic arthritis, 186
Syphilitic heart disease, 1294–1295
Syphilitic infections of central nervous system, 812–816. See also *Neurosyphilis.*
Syphilitic meningitis, 813
cerebrospinal fluid examination in, *803,* 813
Syphilitic meningomyelitis, vs. vitamin B_{12} deficiency, 776, 777
Syringobulbia, 768, 769
Syringomyelia, 768–769
vs. idiopathic autonomic insufficiency, 763
vs. leprosy, 503
vs. tick paralysis, 118
Syringomyelia-like syndrome, 890
Syrup of ipecac, in accidental poisoning, 74
Systemic candidiasis, in neutropenia, 149
Systemic diseases, chronic, anemia associated with, 1731–1733
Systemic hypertension
eyes in, 2325–2326, *2326*
in intracranial tumors, 864
severe, aortic regurgitation in, 1194
Systemic lupus erythematosus, 174–180
autoantibodies in, 178, *179*
autoimmune thrombocytopenia in, 1876
clinical symptoms in, frequency of, *176*
cutaneous signs in, *2301, 2302*
drug-induced, 156, 179, 975, *975*
eyes in, 177, 2317, *2318*
immune complexes in, 134
immune mechanisms in, 132
laboratory abnormalities in, 178, *178*
malabsorption in, 1543
pericarditis caused by, 1271
photosensitivity in, 2289
pleura in, 1017
pregnancy and, 177, 1414
pulmonary hypertension in, 1141, 1143
pulmonary involvement in, 974
renal involvement in, 175, 176, 177, 178, 1400
vs. infective endocarditis, 392
vs. leprosy, 503
vs. periarteritis nodosa, 183
vs. rheumatic fever, 383
vs. rheumatoid arthritis, 190
Systemic lupus erythematosus–related syndrome, 137

Systemic mastocytosis, 161, *2296, 2298, 2302,* 2308
Systemic sclerosis, 168–171. See also *Scleroderma.*
Systemic venous congestion, in right ventricular failure, 1092
Systemic Weber-Christian disease, 222
Systoles, premature
atrial, 1246
ventricular, 1251
Systolic hypertension, 1209

T cells, 126, 128
alterations of, in disease states, 130
characteristics and estimation of, 129–130, *129*
deficiency of, treatment of, 152
deficiency or dysfunction of, infections in, *148,* 150
development of, *128*
in host defense, 146
diagnostic evaluation of, 150, 151, *151*
in sarcoidosis, 210, *210,* 211
primary immunodeficiency diseases and, 138–143
T proteins, in group A streptococcal infections, 369
T_3, 2114, 2115, 2116
T_3 resin uptake, determination of, 2118
T_3 suppression test, 2119
T_3 toxicosis, 2064, 2123
T_4, 2114, 2115, 2116
Tabardillo, 318–320
Tabes dorsalis, 512, 813, 814–815
lightning pains of, 727, 814
neuropathic joint disease in, 200
treatment of, 516
vs. acute abdomen, 1581
vs. idiopathic autonomic insufficiency, 763
Taboparesis, 814, 815
Tache noire, in tick-borne rickettsioses of Eastern Hemisphere, 325
Tachycardia(s)
atrial
in myocardial infarction, 1235
paroxysmal, 1249–1251, *1249, 1251*
bidirectional, 1254, *1255*
chronic, in heart failure, 1086
in shock, 1009
in tetanus, 440
sinus, 1243–1244
in myocardial infarction, 1230
supraventricular, in Wolff-Parkinson-White syndrome, *1258,* **1259–1260,** *1259*
with short P-R interval and normal QRS complexes, 1256–1257
ventricular, 1252–1254, *1253*
DC electroshock in, 1267
in myocardial infarction, 1230, 1235
in shock, 1118
Taenia brauni, 611
Taenia saginata, 559, *605, 606,* **607–608**
Taenia solium, 559, *605,* 606, *606,* **608**
Takahara's disease, 2057
Takayasu's syndrome, 789, 1297, 1298, *1298*
cerebral infarction from, 779
Talcosis, 990
Talipes equinovarus, frequency and sex ratio of, *48*

Talwin. See *Pentazocine*.
Tamm-Horsfall protein, 1337
Tamponade
cardiac, 1273
esophageal, in portal hypertension
with gastrointestinal bleeding, 1523
Tangier disease, *42*, **2008**
Tapeworm(s), 606–611, *606*
antimicrobial agents for, *559*
beef, 607–608
dog, 611
dwarf, 609
fish, 607
pork, 608
prevalence of, *605*
rat, 611
treatment of, 608–609
Tarantulas, 114
Tardive dyskinesia, 669, 753
Target cell anemia, 1778
Target cells, significance of, 1718
Tarsal tunnel syndrome, 902
Tartar emetic, poisoning by, 81
Tatara vicina, in visceral leishmaniasis,
584
Taussig-Bing complex, 1173
Tay-Sachs disease, 850, 851
heterozygote detection in, 58, *58*
screening for, 44, 59
TDI sensitivity, 999
Teeth
caries of, pathogenesis of, 367
disease of, headache from, 733
Hutchinson's, in congenital syphilis,
513
in hypoparathyroidism, 2221
in nutritional deficiency, 1676
procedures on, infective endocarditis
prophylaxis in, 396
Tegretol. See *Carbamazepine*.
Teichoic acid, serum antibodies to, in
infective endocarditis, 391
Telangiectasia
fine, 2273
hemorrhagic, hereditary, 1880
in congenital pulmonary
arteriovenous fistula, 1168, 1169
Telangiectases, in Fabry's disease, 2011
Telogen, 2270
Telogen effluvium, 2271
Temperature, body, basal, in evaluation
of ovarian function, 2180
Temporal arteritis, 216–218
Temporal artery biopsy, in polymyalgia
rheumatica, 217
Temporal lobe abscess, 806
Temporal lobe status, 856
Tempra. See *Acetaminophen*.
Tendinitis
bicipital, 206
calcific, bursitis and, 206
Tendon sheaths, tuberculosis of, 497
Tendons, in scleroderma, 168
Tenesmus, in carcinoid syndrome, 2213
Tennis elbow, 207
Tenosynovitis, 207
in gonococcal arthritis, 407
Tenovaginitis, stenosing, 207
Tension pneumothorax, 1017
Teratomas, 864
Terbutaline, in asthma, 958
**Terminal illness, patient with, care of,
1941–1948**
Terminator codons, 33, *33*

Ternidens deminutus, vs. hookworm ova,
625
Terpin hydrate with codeine, in
common cold, 233
Terrors, night, 655
Tertian malaria, 569, 571
Test(s). See names of specific tests.
Testicular feminization, 2064, 2172–2173
amenorrhea in, 2185
incomplete, 2173
Testicular hormones, chemistry and
physiology of, 2163–2164
Testis(es), 2162–2175
absence of, 2170
biopsy of, in evaluation of testicular
function, 2165
fetal development of, 2162, *2163*
function of, evaluation of, 2164–2165
primary failure of, 2168–2171
pubertal development of, 2166
retractile, vs. undescended testes,
2173
tuberculosis of, 496
tumors of, 2174–2175, *2175*
interstitial cell, 2175
sexual precocity caused by, 2167
undescended, 2173–2174
Testosterone, 2163
biosynthesis of, 2164
plasma and urinary, in evaluation of
testicular function, 2164, 2165
secondary polycythemia caused by,
1799
Testosterone cyclopentylpropionate, in
androgen deficiency, 2168
Testosterone cypionate, in anemia of
chronic renal failure, 1364
Testosterone enanthate
in agnogenic myeloid metaplasia,
1828
in androgen deficiency, 2168
in aplastic anemia, 1740
in hypopituitarism, 2102
Testosterone propionate
in androgen deficiency, 2168
in hypopituitarism, 2102
Tetanolysin, 437
Tetanospasm, 437
Tetanus, 436–441
Tetanus antitoxin, 437, 438
Tetanus immune globulin, in snakebite,
122
Tetanus toxoid, 437
Tetany, 930, 2223
differential diagnosis of, *2223*
in hypocalcemia, 2241, 2242
in hypoparathyroidism, 2220, 2221
postoperative, in
hyperparathyroidism, 2220
Tetrachloroethylene, in fasciolopsiasis,
620
Tetracycline(s), *557*, 562
adverse reactions to, 563
as nephrotoxin, 1427
contraindications to, 553
deposition of, in bone tissue, 2247
fatty liver from, 1660
in acne, 2279
in amebiasis, 593
in anthrax, 471
in bartonellosis, 332
in brucellosis, 478
in cholera, 462
in chronic respiratory failure, 1029

Tetracycline(s) (*Continued*)
in gonococcal disease, 409, 410
in louse-borne relapsing fever, 528
in louse-borne relapsing fever
prevention, 529
in lymphogranuloma venereum, 336
in malabsorption of scleroderma, 171
in malabsorption syndrome, *1536*
in melioidosis, 470
in mycoplasmal pneumonia, 346
in mycoplasmal urethritis, 347
in plague, 465
in postgastrectomy malabsorption,
1546
in postgonococcal urethritis, 409
in psittacosis, 338
in regional enteritis, 1566
in rickettsial diseases, 315
in simple chronic bronchitis, 954, 955
in syphilis, 516
in tetanus, 439
in tick-borne relapsing fever, 529
in trachoma and inclusion
conjunctivitis, 334
in tropical sprue, 1546
in tularemia, 468
in Whipple's disease, 1542
malabsorption caused by, 1548
Tetralogy, Fallot's, 1164–1166
cyanotic, classic, 1164, 1165
vs. right ventricular origin of
both great arteries, 1173
Tetraodon poisoning, 69
Tetrodotoxin, 69
Thalamic hemorrhage, clinical
manifestations of, 798
Thalassemia(s), 1751, 1772, 1778–1780
alpha, 1779
beta, heterozygous, 1778–1779
homozygous, 1778
molecular basis of, 34
Thalassemia major, 1778
heterozygote detection in, *58*
Thalassemia minor, 1778, 1779
Thalidomide
congenital malformation from, 49
in leprosy reactions, 504
in Weber-Christian disease, 222
Thallium
nephrotoxicity from, *1428*, 1431
poisoning by, 82
neuropathy from, 911
Theophylline, in heart failure, *1104*
Therapeutic hyperbaric oxygen, 103–105
Thermal burns, hyperbaric oxygen
therapy in, 105
Thermodilution technique, cardiac
output determination by, 1032
**Thermoregulation, hypothalamic
dysfunction and, 716–717**
Thiabendazole
in cutaneous larva migrans, 625
in intestinal nematodes, *559*
in malabsorption syndrome, *1536*
in protein-losing enteropathy of
capillariasis, 1549
in strongyloidiasis, 623
in toxocariasis, 628
in trichinosis, *559*, 631
in trichuriasis, 629
Thiamin
deficiency of, 1688–1689. See also
Beriberi.
clinical signs of, *1677*

Thiamin (*Continued*)
in nutritional polyneuropathy, 773
in Wernicke-Korsakoff syndrome, 774
nutrient value of, 1673
recommended allowances of, *1671*
Thiazides
in arterial hypertension, 1212, *1212*, 1213
in heart failure, *1103*, 1104, *1104*
Thibierge-Weissenbach syndrome, 169
Thiethylperazine, in gastrointestinal symptoms of chronic renal failure, 1365
Thioguanine, in oncologic treatment, 1935
Thioridazine, in dementia, 663
Thirst, in chronic renal failure, 1355
Thirst center, 2109
Thomsen's disease, 920
Thoracic actinomycosis, 474
Thoracic outlet syndrome, 902
Thoracic spine, compression at, 891
Thoracolumbar spine, injuries of, 886
Thoracotomy, open, in microbiologic diagnosis, 342
Thorax, dermatologic diseases affecting, 2279–2283
Thorazine. See *Chlorpromazine.*
Thorn apple, poisoning by, 70
"Threshold effect," in polygenic inheritance, 45, *45*
Throat
procedures in, infective endocarditis prophylaxis in, 396
sore
in infectious mononucleosis, 265
quinsy, in streptococcal tonsillitis, 373
streptococcal, 371–374. See also *Streptococcal pharyngitis.*
Thrombasthenia, 1878
Thrombectomy, in phlegmasia cerulea dolens, 1128, 1129
Thrombin
formation of, 1881, *1882*
disorders of, *1884*
generation of, inhibition of, 1897
Thrombin time, in hereditary coagulation disorders, *1884*
Thromboangiitis obliterans, 1302–1303
Thrombocythemia, essential, 1878
Thrombocytopenia, 1872–1877
classification of, *1873*
dilutional, 1877
hypersplenic, 1877
in acute infection, 1877
in aplastic anemia, 1737
in critically ill patient, 1052
in liver disease, 1643
in multiple myeloma, 1859
intracranial hemorrhage from, 795
sequestration, 1877
Thrombocytopenic purpura
autoimmune, 1874
complicating rifampin treatment of pulmonary tuberculosis, 488
drugs associated with, 156, 1873–1874, *1873*
idiopathic, 1874–1875
immune mechanisms in, 132
thrombotic, 1876–1877
hypofibrinogenemia in, 1893
renal involvement in, 1401
vs. periarteritis nodosa, 183
vs. dengue hemorrhagic fever, 297

Thrombocytosis, 1877–1878
postsplenectomy, 1869
Thromboembolic diseases, 1122–1134
Thromboembolism, 1122, 1123
in homocystinuria, 2028
in myocardial infarction, 1231
Thrombolytic agents. See also names of specific agents.
in pulmonary embolism, 1133
in thrombophlebitis, 1129
Thrombophlebitis, 1124–1129
acute, vs. lymphangitis, 1315
cerebrospinal fluid findings in, *803*
cortical, 808
in bacterial meningitis, 412
iliofemoral, acute, vs. arterial embolism, 1304
in bronchogenic carcinoma, 1007
in cancer patient, 1906
in heroin addiction, 696
of major venous sinuses, 808
vs. arteriovenous fistula, 1312
Thrombophlebitis migrans, *2297*
Thromboplastin time, partial, in hereditary coagulation disorders, *1884*
Thrombosis, 1122–1124
carotid artery, internal, in head injury, 884
cavernous sinus, 780, 808
vs. Romaña's sign in Chagas' disease, 582
cerebral artery, middle, in head injury, 884
cerebral venous, cerebral infarction from, 780
deep, of leg, oral contraceptives and, 2195
in myocardial infarction, 1229
in paroxysmal nocturnal hemoglobinuria, 1768
lateral sinus, 789, 808, 809
localized, hypofibrinogenemic syndromes associated with, 1893
of major dural sinuses, 808–809
of major venous sinuses, 808
pulmonary artery, vs. pulmonary embolism, 1133
renal vein, 1408–1409
vs. Goodpasture's syndrome, 976
superior sagittal sinus, 809
transverse sinus, 789
venous, 1124, 1125, 1126
cerebral, 788–789
mesenteric, 1589, 1590
venous sinus, intracranial, benign intracranial hypertension with, 871
Thrombotic endocarditis, nonbacterial, 387
in cancer patient, 1905
vs. infective endocarditis, 392
Thrombotic thrombocytopenic purpura, 1876–1877
hypofibrinogenemia in, 1893
renal involvement in, 1401
vs. periarteritis nodosa, 183
Thromboxane A$_2$, circulatory effects of, 1111
Thrombus(i), 1122
arterial, renal infarction from, 1407
formation of, cerebral infarction from, 781
leg vein, 1124, 1125
red, 1122
white, 1122

Thrush, 547–549
vs. secondary syphilis, 510
Thuja plicata, asthma-like reactions to, 996
Thymic hypoplasia, *139*, 140
Thymoma
immunodeficiency with, *139*, 142
in myasthenia gravis, 926
Thymoma-agammaglobulinemia syndrome, 142
Thymus, endocrine functions of, 2061
Thyroglobulin, 2114, 2115
Thyroid, 2114–2144
adenomas of, 2141, 2142
carcinoma of, 2141, 2143–2144, *2144*
medical treatment of, 1922
medullary, 2143, 2223–2224
carcinoid features of, 2212
desiccated, in hypothyroidism, 2133
development and anatomy of, 2114
disease of, eyes in, 2332–2333
function of, 2114–2117
controls of, 2116, 2117
tests of, 2117–2120, 2355
selection of, 2119, 2120
in acromegaly, 2106
in hyperthyroidism, 2122
needle biopsy of, 2119
neoplasms of, 2141–2144
scans of, 2119, *2120*
in multinodular goiter, 2136
solitary nodule of, 2142
tuberculosis of, 498
Thyroid hormone
action of, hereditary resistance to, 2140–2141
formation of, congenital metabolic defects in, 2138–2140
free, determination of, 2118
metabolic action of, 2116
metabolism of, 2114, *2114*, 2116
mode of action of, 2070, *2071*
secretion of, 2115
synthesis of, defects of, 2138, 2139
transport of, 2115, *2115*
defects in, 2140
Thyroid myopathy, chronic, vs. polymyositis, 174
Thyroid storm, in Graves' disease, 2127, 2128
Thyroidectomy
in hyperthyroidism, 2125
in thyroid cancer, 2143
Thyroiditis, 2128–2132
acute, 2131
vs. subacute thyroiditis, 2131, 2132
autosensitization in, 132
de Quervain's, 2131
granulomatous, 2131
Hashimoto's, 2128–2130, *2130*
autosensitization in, 132
hereditary factor in, 2121
hypothyroidism developing from, 2132
vs. multinodular goiter, 2135, 2136
Riedel's, 224, 2130–2131
sclerosing cholangitis and, 1633
subacute, 2131–2132
suppurative, 2131
Thyroid-stimulating hormone, 2089
action of, on thyroid, 2117
function of, assessment of, 2093
serum, assay of, 2118
Thyroid-stimulating hormone stimulation test, 2119

Thyrotoxic myopathy, 923
Thyrotoxicosis, 2120
  diabetes mellitus in, 1982
  differentiation of, from other
    mitochondrial diseases, 2123
  in children, 2126
  in endemic goiter, 2138
  myasthenia gravis and, 927
  T₃, 2064, 2123
  vs. familial periodic paralysis, 922
Thyrotropic hormone, 2089
Thyrotropin, 2089
  function of, assessment of, 2093
Thyrotropin-releasing hormone, 2075,
  2117
  synthetic, in diagnosis of anterior
    pituitary disease, 2081, *2081*
Thyrotropin-releasing hormone test,
  2081, *2081*, 2119, *2119*
Thyroxine, 2114, 2115, 2116
  in myxedema coma, 2134
  serum, determination of, 2117, 2118
L-Thyroxine
  in hypophysectomy-induced
    hypopituitarism, 2103
  in hypopituitarism, 2102
  in hypothyroidism, 2133
Thyroxine-binding globulin, abnormal
  quantities of, thyroid hormone
  transport defect from, 2140
Tibial compartment syndromes,
  anterior, 1305
Tic(s), 759–760
  vs. acute chorea, 758
Tic douloureux, 727
Ticarcillin, *557*, 559
Tick fever, 526, 529–530
  Colorado, *279*, 280–281
Tick paralysis, 117–118
  neuromuscular block caused by, 929
Tick typhus, 322–324
  African, 324–325
  Indian, 324
  Queensland, 324–325
Tick-borne group B arbovirus diseases,
  290–291
Tick-borne relapsing fever, 526, 529–530
Tick-borne rickettsioses of Eastern
  Hemisphere, 324–325
Tidal volume, 932
Tietze's syndrome, 207–208
  vs. angina pectoris, 1227
Tifus exantemático, 318–320
Time zones, changes of, effects of, 96
Timothy hay pollen, allergen of, 131
Tinea capitis, 2282
Tinea versicolor, 2281, *2282*
  vs. pinta, 525
Tinel's sign, in carpal tunnel syndrome,
  901
Tissue integrity, in malnutrition, 1680
Tissue nematodes, 630–637
  antimicrobial agents for, *559*
  prevalence of, *605*
Tissues, in aging process, 26
Tityus serrulatus, 116
T-mycoplasmas, 346, 347
Toadfishes, envenomation by, 124
Tobacco-alcohol amblyopia, 774–775
Tobramycin, *557*, 561
  adverse reactions to, 562
  as nephrotoxin, 1426

Todd's paralysis, 854
Toes
  clubbing of, in hypertrophic
    osteoarthropathy, 201
  curled up, 903
Tofranil. See *Imipramine.*
Tolazamide, in diabetes mellitus, *1986*
Tolazoline, in acrocyanosis, 1307
Tolbutamide, in diabetes mellitus, 1986,
  1986
Tolmetin, in rheumatoid arthritis, 191
Toluene, inhalation of, 705
Toluene di-isocyanate, asthma-like
  reactions to, 999
Tomography, computerized
  in brain abscess, 806
  in brain tumor, 867
  in cerebral infarction, 789, 790
  in chronic pancreatitis, 1556
  in epilepsy, 857
  in evaluation of jaundice, 1622
  in fatty infiltration of liver, *1467*
  in gastrointestinal diseases,
    1466–1468, *1467*
  in head injury, 881
  in hepatic abscess, *1467*
  in herpes simplex encephalitis,
    823
  in intracranial hemorrhage, 798
  in intracranial inflammatory
    disease, 804
  in intraspinal compression, 892
  in nephrocarcinoma, 1459
  in neurologic diagnosis, 747
  in obstructive jaundice, *1467*
  in peritoneal disease, 1592
  in pulmonary disease, 944
  in renal investigation, 1344
Tone decay, in sensorineural hearing
  loss, 734, 735
Tongue
  in ariboflavinosis, 1686
  in nutritional deficiency, 1676
  in scarlet fever, 371
  tuberculosis of, 492
Tonsil, tuberculosis of, 492
Tonsillar diphtheria, 431
Tonsillitis
  exudative, 443
  staphylococcal, 404
  streptococcal, complications of, 373
    epidemiology of, 369
Tooth. See *Teeth.*
Tophaceous gout, 2030, *2036*, 2037
  treatment of, 2039, 2040
Topical dermatologic therapy, 2276,
  2277, *2277*
Topical steroids, in dermatologic
  therapy, 2277
Torres bodies, in yellow fever, 294
Torsion dystonia, 760–761
Torticollis, spasmodic, 761–762
Toruloma, 864
Torulosis, 543–544
Total lung capacity, 932, *932*
Tourette's disease, 759
Toxemia
  in clostridial myonecrosis, 434
  in pneumococcal pneumonia, 351
  of pregnancy, 1205, 1414–1416
Toxic disorders, epilepsy associated
  with, 853

Toxic encephalopathies, vs. arboviral
  encephalitis, 284
Toxic epidermal necrolysis, 2306
  staphylococcal, 400
Toxic hepatitis, 1657–1659
  cirrhosis in, 1663
  vs. acute viral hepatitis, 1653
Toxic megacolon, in ulcerative colitis,
  1569, 1570, *1570*, 1574–1575
Toxic methemoglobinemia, 1780, 1781
Toxic nephropathy, 1328–1329, *1328,*
  1422–1435
  clinical syndromes associated with,
    1424–1425
  incidence of, 1423
  pathogenetic mechanisms in,
    1423–1424, *1424*
Toxic nodular goiter, 2136
Toxic pharyngotonsillitis, infectious
  mononucleosis with, 267
Toxic psychosis, 645
  in chronic renal failure, 1366
Toxicosis, T₃, 2064, 2123
Toxins, bacterial, destruction of, in
  malnutrition, 1680
Toxocara canis, 627
Toxocara cati, 627
Toxocariasis, 627–628
  immunodiagnostic tests for, *565*
Toxoplasma gondii, 558, 594, 595
Toxoplasma myocarditis, 1282, 1283
Toxoplasmic retinitis, recurrent, 2334,
  2335
Toxoplasmic retinochoroiditis, 596, 597,
  598
Toxoplasmosis, 594–598
  antimicrobial agents for, *558*
  congenital, 595, 596, 597, 598
  immunodiagnostic tests for, *565*
  ocular, 596, 597, 598, *2318*, **2334–2335**
  vs. Chagas' disease, 582
  vs. congenital cytomegalovirus
    infection, 828
  vs. infectious mononucleosis, 267
  vs. pneumocystosis, 599
  vs. polymyositis, 174
Trace elements, accumulation of, in
  chronic renal failure, 1360
Tracheobronchitis, mycoplasmal, 345
Tracheostomy
  in acute respiratory failure, 1026, 1040
  nosocomial pneumonia and, 362
Trachoma and inclusion conjunctivitis,
  332–335
Tranquilizers. See also names of specific
  agents.
  abuse of, 698
Transcapillary exchange, in shock, 1112,
  1113
Transducers, in critical care medicine,
  1032
Transendoscopic sphincterotomy, in
  choledocholithiasis, 1630
"Transfer factor," 129
  in delayed-type hypersensitivity, 130
  in therapy of immune response
    disorders, 152
Transfer RNA, 31, 32
Transferrin, 1743
  in iron absorption, 1526
Transfusion(s)
  disease transmission in, 1785

Transfusion(s) (*Continued*)
exchange, in accidental poisoning, 74
in anemia, 1719
  acute hemorrhagic, 1730
  hemolytic, 1754
    autoimmune, 1764
  of chronic renal failure, 1364
  sickle cell, 1775
  sideroblastic, 1741
in chronic granulomatous disease, 1806
in reaction-prone patient, 1789
iron overload from, 1790
massive, 1051–1052
  complications of, 1051, 1785, 1786
  metabolic alkalosis in, 1966
neutrophil, in neutropenia, 1811
purpura following, 1875–1876
Transfusion hemosiderosis, 1785
Transfusion reactions, 1785–1789
categories of, *1785*
Transhepatic cholangiography, 1622, 1623
percutaneous, 1473–1474, *1473, 1474*
Transitional sclerosis, 849
Transketolase, genetic abnormality of, in Wernicke-Korsakoff syndrome, 774
Translocation(s)
centric fusion, 53, *53*
reciprocal, 53, *53*
  transmission of, 53, 54
"Transplant lung" syndrome, 1385
Transplantation
bone marrow, in aplastic anemia, 1738, 1739
  in hematologic form of acute radiation syndrome, 90
  in neutropenia of aplastic anemia, 1810
renal, 1375, *1375,* 1376, *1376,* **1382–1386**
  biopsy after, 1346
  hypercalcemia after, 2237
  in cystinosis, 55
  in Fabry's disease, 55
  in scleroderma, 171
  rejected, acute renal failure in, 1369
    pathologic features of, 1384
  rejection crisis in, 1384
Transport, active and passive, in normal absorption, 1524
Transposition of great arteries
complete, 1172
congenitally corrected, 1166–1167
Transsexuality, 686
Transtracheal aspiration, percutaneous, microbiologic diagnosis by, 342
Transverse colon, tuberculosis of, 492
Transverse myelitis, 811–812, *811*
acute, 849
  during nonpolio enteroviral infections, 270
Transverse myelopathy, 811–812, *811*
Tranylcypromine, poisoning by, *712*
Traumatic cardiac hemolytic anemia, 1767
Tree pollen, allergic rhinitis from, 157
Trematodes
antimicrobial agents for, *559*
diseases caused by, 611–621
prevalence of, *605*
Tremor(s), 751
essential, 756–757

Tremor(s) (*Continued*)
familial, 756–757
in alcohol withdrawal state, 709
in chronic renal failure, 1365
in mercury poisoning, 80
in metabolic brain disease, 648
in paralysis agitans, 752
in Wilson's disease, 2049
senile, 757
Trench fever, 309, **329**
epidemiologic features of, *310*
Trench foot, 1309–1310
Treponema carateum, 524
Treponema pallidum, 505, 506
Treponema pertenue, 518, 519
Treponemal antibody tests, in syphilis, 514
Treponemal diseases, 505–525
nonsyphilitic, 518–525, *520*
Triacetyl-6-azauridine, in oncologic treatment, 1934, 1935
Triacetyloleandomycin, 560
Triamcinolone, in rheumatoid arthritis, 192
Triamterene
hyperkalemia and, 1959
in heart failure, *1104,* 1105
Triatoma infestans, 580
Triazenes, in oncologic treatment, 1933
Trichinella spiralis, 559, 605, 621, 630
life cycle of, *621*
Trichinellosis, 630–631
Trichiniasis, 630–631
Trichinosis, 630–631
antimicrobial agents for, *559*
immunodiagnostic tests for, *565*
myocardial involvement in, 1283
vs. angiostrongyliasis, 631
vs. polymyositis, 174
Trichlormethiazide, in hypoglycemia caused by functioning islet cell tumors, 1995
Trichocephaliasis, 628–629
Trichomonas hominis, 602
Trichomonas tenax, 602
Trichomonas vaginalis, 558, 602, 603
Trichomoniasis, 602–603
antimicrobial agents for, *558*
Trichophytosis of glabrous skin, vs. pinta, 525
Trichostrongyliasis, 626
vs. hookworm disease, 625
Trichothecenes, alimentary toxic aleukia caused by, 70
Trichuriasis, 628–629
Trichuris trichiura, 559, 605, 629
life cycle of, *621*
Tricuspid atresia, 1171–1172
Tricuspid regurgitation, 1198–1199
vs. mitral regurgitation, 1187
Tricuspid stenosis, 1197–1198
Tricuspid valve
disease of, 1197–1199
Ebstein's anomaly of, 1168
Tricyclic antidepressants, in depression of manic-depressive psychosis, 671
Tridione. See *Trimethadione.*
Triethylene tetramine dihydrochloride, in Wilson's disease, 2050
Trifluorothymidine, in oncologic treatment, 1934
Trigeminal nerve, disorders of, 900
Trigeminal neuralgia, 727

Triglyceride(s)
elevated, as risk factor for atherosclerosis, 1220
medium-chain, after extensive small intestinal resection, 1544
  in fat absorption, 1524
  in malabsorption syndrome, 1538, 1539
metabolism of, in liver disease, 1642
transport of, 2002
Trihexyphenidyl, in parkinsonism, 755
Triiodothyronine, 2114, 2115, 2116
determination of, 2117, 2118
L-Triiodothyronine, in hypothyroidism, 2133
Trimellitic anhydride, exposure to, respiratory effects of, 1000
Trimethadione
as nephrotoxin, 1432
in epilepsy, *859*
Trimethaphan
in heart failure, *1101*
in hypertension of dissecting aortic aneurysm, 1297
Trimethobenzamide hydrochloride, in vertigo, 739
Trimethoprim-sulfamethoxazole, *556,* 563
in gonococcal disease, 410
in pneumocystosis, *558,* 600
Tri-ortho-cresyl phosphate, neuropathy from, 911
Tripelennamine
in angioedema, 163
in urticaria, 162
Triple X syndrome, clinical and cytogenetic characteristics of, *52*
Trismus, in tetanus, 438, 439
Trisomy, 53
Trisomy 13, clinical and cytogenetic characteristics of, *52*
Trisomy 18, clinical and cytogenetic characteristics of, *52*
Trisomy 21, clinical and cytogenetic characteristics of, *52*
Trisulfapyrimidines
in lymphogranuloma venereum, 336
in trachoma and inclusion conjunctivitis, 334
Trivalent antitoxin, in botulism, 68
Trochlear nerve, disorders of, 899
Trombiculid mites, dermatitis caused by, 113
Tropical eosinophilia, 225, **637,** *969,* **970**
Tropical immersion foot, 1309
Tropical phagedenic ulcer, 530–531
Tropical pyomyositis, 404, **638**
Tropical splenomegaly syndrome
in malaria, 569, 572
portal hypertension and, 1639
vs. visceral leishmaniasis, 586
Tropical sprue, 1545–1546
jejunal histology in, 1533
megaloblastosis in, 1723
Tropical typhus, 327–328
Tropical ulcer, vs. yaws, 521
Truncal vagotomy and antrectomy, in duodenal ulcer, 1519, *1519*
Truncal vagotomy and "drainage," in duodenal ulcer, 1519, *1519*
Truncus arteriosus, 1173
Trypanosoma brucei, 566, 576
Trypanosoma cruzi, 558, 566, 575, *576,* 579, 580

Trypanosoma gambiense, 558, 576, 576
Trypanosoma rangeli, 575, 576
Trypanosoma rhodesiense, 558, 570, 576, 576
Trypanosomiasis(es), 566, 575–583
  African, 575, 576–579
  American, 579–583. See also *Chagas' disease.*
  antimicrobial agents for, *558*
  differences between, 575, *576*
  myocarditis in, 1283
Trypsin, in protein absorption, 1525
Trypsinogen, in protein absorption, 1525
Tryptophan metabolites, measurement of, in malabsorption syndrome, 1531
Tsetse flies, 576
TSH, 2089. See also *Thryoid-stimulating hormone.*
Tsutsugamushi disease, 327–328
  clinical features of, *313*
  epidemiologic features of, *310*
Tubal pregnancy, vs. gonococcal salpingitis, 408
Tubercle baccillus(i), 481
  disappearance rate of, after drug therapy, 489
Tubercles, choroidal, in disseminated tuberculosis, 498
Tuberculids, 498
Tuberculin hypersensitivity, 481
Tuberculin reaction, in sarcoidosis, 214
Tuberculin test, in tuberculosis, 482
Tuberculoid leprosy, 502, *502*
Tuberculoma(s), 494, 864
Tuberculosa multiplex cystica, 497
Tuberculosis, 479–484
  amenorrhea in, 2184
  bacteriology of, 479, 480
  chemoprophylaxis of, 483, 484
  complicated pneumoconiosis and, 992
  control of, in working populations, 994
  course of, factors modifying, 483
  cutaneous, 498
    vs. lupoid leishmaniasis, 588
  delayed-type hypersensitivity in, 130
  disseminated, vs. glanders, 469
  endobronchial, 491
  endosalpingeal, 496
  epidemiology of, 480
  extrapulmonary, 491–498
    drug therapy in, 491
  female genital, 496
  gastrointestinal, 492
  genitourinary, 496
  hematogenous, chronic, 492
    generalized acute, 481
  hepatic, primary, 493
  hepatic granulomas in, 1667
  Hodgkin's disease and, 483, 1844
  hypercalcemia in, 2238
  ileocecal, 492
    vs. regional enteritis, 1565
  immunologic response in, 480, 481
  incidence of, 480
  intestinal, malabsorption in, 1545
  male genital, 496
  Mantoux test in, 946
  miliary, 481, **492–493**
    hematologic disease and, 493
    vs. listeriosis, 473
    vs. psittacosis, 338
    vs. visceral leishmaniasis, 586

Tuberculosis (*Continued*)
  nonreactive, 492, 493
  ocular, 498
  of adrenals, 498
  of bones, 496–497
    cystic, 497
  of breast, 498
  of bursae, 497
  of cervix, 496
  of colon, 492
  of costochondral junction, 497
  of duodenum, 492
  of endometrium, 496
  of epididymides, 496
  of esophagus, 492
  of joints, 496–497
  of larynx, 491
  of mastoid bone, 492
  of middle ear, 492
  of mouth, 492
  of ovary, 496
  of pancreas, 498
  of peripheral arteries, 1305
  of pharyngeal lymphatic tissue, 492
  of pleura, 491, 1015–1016
  of prostate, 496
  of seminal vesicles, 496
  of small intestine, 492
  of spleen, primary, 493
  of stomach, 492
  of tendon sheaths, 497
  of testes, 496
  of thyroid, 498
  of tongue, 492
  of tonsil, 492
  pathogenesis of, 481, 482
  pathologic features of, 480, 481
  prevalence of, 480
  prevention of, 483–484
  primary infection in, fate of, 481
  pulmonary, 484–490
    cavity formation in, 482
    chronic, 482, 485–487
      endobronchial spread of, 482
    classification of, 487
    lower and middle lobe, in aged, 487
    progressive primary, 485
    retreatment of, 490
    symptomatic primary infection in, 484–485
    treatment of, 487–490
      bed rest in, 490
      drug, 487
        combined, 488
        in noncompliant patient, 490
      surgery in, 490
    vs. pulmonary paragonimiasis, 620
  pulmonary hypertension in, 1147
  rare forms of, 498
  renal, 496
  skin tests in, 946
  splenic, primary, 493
  tuberculin test in, 482
  vs. actinomycosis, 474
  vs. bancroftian filariasis, 634
  vs. chromomycosis, 543
  vs. coccidioidomycosis, 539
  vs. eosinophilic gastroenteritis, 1543
  vs. histoplasmosis, 537
  vs. lung abscess, 981
  vs. maduromycosis, 542
  vs. melioidosis, 470
  vs. psittacosis, 338
  vs. sporotrichosis, 545

Tuberculosis (*Continued*)
  vs. toxoplasmosis, 597
  vs. Whipple's disease, 1541
  vs. yaws, 521
Tuberculosis cutis miliaris acuta disseminata, 498
Tuberculosis orificialis, 498
Tuberculosis vaccination, 483
Tuberculosis verrucosa cutis, 498
Tuberculous adenitis, vs. paracoccidioidomycosis, 541
Tuberculous anorectal abscess, 1617
Tuberculous arthritis, 185–186, **497**
Tuberculous caries, 497
Tuberculous fistula in ano, 492
Tuberculous lymphadenitis, 495
  malabsorption in, 1545
  vs. bancroftian filariasis, 634
Tuberculous meningitis, 481, **493–494**
  cerebrospinal fluid findings in, *803*
  vs. herpes simplex encephalitis, 824
  vs. viral meningitis, 820
Tuberculous pericarditis, 494–495, 1270
Tuberculous perirectal and pelvic abscesses, 492
Tuberculous peritonitis, 495, 1594
Tuberculous pleurisy and effusion, 485
Tuberculous pneumonia, 481, 482, 485
  vs. pneumococcal pneumonia, 354
Tuberculous polyserositis, 494
Tuberculous spondylitis, 185, **497**
  vs. staphylococcal infections of vertebrae and intervertebral discs, 403
Tuberous sclerosis, 770–771, *1910*
  adenoma sebaceum in, 770, 2292, *2292*
  cutaneous manifestations of, *2300*
  hypopigmentation in, 2292, *2292*
  internal malignancy and, *2297*
Tubular defects, in glomerular disease, 1387
Tubular necrosis, acute, 1367–1375
  differential diagnosis of, 1373
  pathogenesis of, 1369
  pathologic physiology of, 1370
  pathology of, 1370
  prevention of, 1374
  prognosis in, 1374
  volume depletion in, 1951
Tubular proteinuria, 1337
  in chronic cadmium poisoning, 1429
Tubules, renal
  distal, function of, 1319, 1320, *1320*
  function of, defects of, 1336
    toxic nephropathy with, 1425
  elements of, 1316–1317
  processing of glomerular filtrate by, 1317–1320, *1320*
  proximal, fluid reabsorption by, 1317, 1318, *1320*
Tubulointerstitial disease, immune complex–mediated, *1324, 1326*
Tularemia, 465–468
  vs. lymphogranuloma venereum, 335
  vs. plague, 464
  vs. psittacosis, 338
  vs. sporotrichosis, 545
  vs. toxoplasmosis, 597
Tularemia vaccines, 468
Tularemic pneumonia, 466, 467
  vs. pneumococcal pneumonia, 354
Tumor(s). See also names and locations of specific tumors.

Tumor(s) (*Continued*)
adnexal, 864
adrenal
Cushing's syndrome resulting from, 2152
treatment of, 2156
feminizing, 2162
virilizing, 2161–2162
anal, malignant, 1618
bile duct, benign, 1635
common, carcinoid features of, 2212
malignant, 1634–1635
brain, 863–869
epilepsy associated with, 853
headache in, 730, 864, 865
intracranial hemorrhage in, 795
arteriography in, 799
metastatic, 864, 868
primary, 863
vs. benign intracranial hypertension, 872
vs. cerebral infarction, 790
brainstem, 868
carcinoid, 2207
bronchial, 1011, 2210, *2211*
gastric, 2210, *2211,* 2212
ileal, 2210, *2211*
vs. regional enteritis, 1565
cardiac, 1288
cauda equina, anal pain from, 1618
vs. hysteria, 679
cerebellar, 867
cerebellopontine angle, 868
vertigo caused by, 740
cutaneous signs of, 2296
epidural, in Hodgkin's disease, 1844
gallbladder, 1633–1634, *1634*
gastrin-secreting, in Zollinger-Ellison syndrome, 1508, 1509
gastrointestinal, 1596–1610
glomus, 1313
glomus jugulare, 867
hepatic
angiography in, *1470,* 1471
benign, 1667
malignant, 1667–1668
intracranial, 863–869
islet cell
carcinoid features of, 2212
functioning, fasting hypoglycemia caused by, 1993–1995
juxtaglomerular cell, hypokalemia in, 1957
Klatskin, 1634, 1635
lung, hormonal secretion by, 2061, *2062*
mediastinal, 1018, 1019
meningeal, 863
mesenteric, 1596
mucoepidermoid, pulmonary, 1012
"noncarcinoid," carcinoid features of, 2212
of cerebral hemispheres, 867
omental, 1596
ovarian, carcinoid features of, 2212
pericardial, 1276
peritoneal, 1595
pineal, 864, 2113
pituitary, 863, 868
amenorrhea due to, 2187
diagnosis and treatment of, 2094–2100
guidelines for, 2099, 2100
during pregnancy, 2098, 2099

Tumor(s) (*Continued*)
pituitary, galactorrhea in, 2192
radioimmunoassay in, 2092
Pott's puffy, 2261
epidural abscess with, 808
Rathke's pouch, 2098
recurrent, vs. radiation injury of nervous system, 870
renal, 1458–1462
benign, 1461, 1462
classification of, 1458, *1458*
single, multiple hormones produced by, 1918
spinal cord, 896–897
vs. multiple sclerosis, 847
vs. tick paralysis, 118
synovial, 202
testicular, 2174–2175, *2175*
interstitial cell, 2175
sexual precocity caused by, 2167
urothelial, 1461
vascular, 863
Wilms', 1460
Tumor lysis syndrome, 1904
Tumor markers, 1911–1914, 1926, 1927

Tunga penetrans, 110
Turbinaire. See *Dexamethasone spray.*
Turcot syndrome, colorectal carcinoma and, 1606
Turner's syndrome, 2185, 2186, *2186*
clinical and cytogenetic characteristics of, *52*
coarctation of aorta with, 1157
vs. pituitary dwarfism, 2104
Tylenol. See *Acetaminophen.*
Tylosis, *2297*
Tylosis palmaris et plantaris, *1910*
Tympanometry, in hearing loss, 735
Typhoid, bilious, 526–529
Typhoid carriers, 447
treatment of, 448
Typhoid fever, 446–449
liver disease in, 446, 447, 1656
vs. Chagas' disease, 582
vs. hemorrhagic diseases caused by arenaviruses, 299
vs. listeriosis, 473
vs. louse-borne typhus, 312
vs. malaria, 573
vs. melioidosis, 470
vs. psittacosis, 338
vs. visceral leishmaniasis, 586
Typhoid vaccine, 449
Typhoidal tularemia, 466
Typhus
classic, 318–320
European, 318–320
flea-borne, 320–321
historic, 318–320
louse-borne, epidemic, 318–320
clinical features of, *313*
epidemiologic features of, *310*
mite-borne, 327–328
murine, 320–321
clinical features of, *313*
epidemiologic features of, *310*
peripheral arteritis in, 1305
recrudescent, 320
rural, 327–328
São Paulo, 322–324
scrub, 327–328
biologic properties of, 309, *309*
clinical features of, *313*

Typhus (*Continued*)
scrub, epidemiologic features of, *310*
serologic responses in, *314*
tick, 322–324
African, 324–325
Indian, 324
Queensland, 324–325
tropical, 327–328
vs. hemorrhagic diseases caused by arenaviruses, 299
vs. malaria, 573
vs. smallpox, 257
Typhus abdominalis, 318
Typhus exanthématique, 318–320
Typhus group, 318–321
biologic properties of, 309, *309*
clinical features of, *313*
epidemiologic features of, *310*
serologic responses in, *314*
Typhus vaccines, 320
Tyramine, monoamine oxidase inhibitors and, interaction of, hypertension from, 1209
Tyrosinase-negative albinism, 2029
Tyrosinase-positive albinism, 2029
Tyrosinemia, *41*
hereditary, *2016, 2020*
neonatal, *2016*
Tyrosinosis, *41, 2016*
Tzanck smear, 2273
in toxic epidermal necrolysis, 2306

Ulcer(s)
aphthous, 149
Barrett's, 1484
Buruli, 500
vs. tropical phagedenic ulcer, 530
chicle, *588*
colonic, nonspecific or solitary, 1615–1616
Cushing's, in intracranial tumors, 866
decubitus, enteric bacteria in, 455
in aging patient, 30
in paraplegia, 887
duodenal. See also *Ulcer(s), peptic.*
duodenitis and, 1508
hyperparathyroidism and, 1504
pain in, radiation of, 1477
pathogenesis of, 1503, 1504
pathophysiology of, 1504, 1505, 1506, 1507
radiographic appearance of, 1511, *1511, 1512*
surgical treatment of, indications for, 1519
types of, 1519, *1519*
esophageal, radiographic appearance of, 1509, *1510*
gastric. See also *Ulcer(s), peptic.*
malignant, 1508
pathogenesis of, 1503, 1504
pathophysiology of, 1504, 1505, 1506, 1507
radiographic appearance of, 1510, *1510*
rheumatoid arthritis and, 1504
surgical treatment of, indications for, 1519
types of, 1520
gastrointestinal, neurogenic, 717
herpetic, vs. syphilitic chancre, 508

Ulcer(s) (*Continued*)
Hines', vs. ischemic ulcers of
  arteriosclerosis obliterans, 1301
Meleney's, hyperbaric oxygen therapy
  in, 105
peptic, 1502–1520
  antacids in, 1513, 1514
  anticholinergic drugs in, 1515
  association of, with other diseases,
    1504
  back-diffusion of acid and, 1505
  chronic, 1502
  **clinical manifestations of,
    1507–1508**
  complications of, 1516–1518
  diagnosis of, 1509–1513
  diet in, 1515
  differential diagnosis of, 1507, 1508
  drugs causing, 1504
  duodenogastric reflux and, 1507
  **endocrine hyperfunction and,
    1508–1509**
  endoscopy in, 1511, 1512
  environmental factors in, 1503
  epidemiology of, 1503
  gastric acid secretion in, 1506
  gastric carcinoma and, 1600
  gastric secretory tests in, 1512
  gastritis in, 1502, 1503
  genetic factors in, 1503
  hemorrhage in, 1516, 1517
  histamine H_2-receptor antagonists
    in, 1514, *1514*, 1515
  hospital care in, 1515
  impaired gastric emptying in, 1507,
    1517, 1518
  in adrenocorticosteroid therapy of
    rheumatoid arthritis, 192
  in hyperparathyroidism, 2215
  medical therapy of, 1513–1516
  outlet obstruction in, 1517, 1518
  **pathogenesis and pathophysiology
    of, 1502–1507**
  penetrating, 1518
  perforation in, 1518
    vs. acute cholecystitis, 1627
    vs. myocardial infarction, 1233
  physical examination in, 1507
  psychosomatic factors in, 1504
  recurrent, after surgical treatment,
    1520
  roentgenography in, 1509, 1510,
    1510, 1511, *1511*, 1512, *1512*
  stress causing, 1504
  **surgical treatment of, 1518–1520,
    *1519***
    chronic postoperative morbidity
      in, 1520
  symptoms of, 1507
  vs. acute appendicitis, 1580
  vs. angina pectoris, 1227
  vs. chronic cholecystitis, 1625
phagedenic, tropical, 530–531
rectal, solitary, 1616
skin, chronic, in rheumatoid arthritis,
  187
stercoral, 1615
tropical, vs. yaws, 521
varicose, enteric bacteria in, 455
  vs. tropical phagedenic ulcer, 530
Ulceration. See also *Ulcer(s)*.
amebic, 590, 591

Ulceration (*Continued*)
  small intestinal
    in adult celiac disease, 1541
    primary nonspecific, 1585–1586
Ulcerative colitis, 1568–1576
  ankylosing spondylitis in, 198, 1568
  arthritis in, 198, 1575
  clinical manifestations of, 1570
  colorectal carcinoma and, 1607
  complications of, 1574
  cutaneous signs of, *2298*
  diagnosis of, 1571
  differential diagnosis of, 1572
  disease manifestations of,
    mechanisms of, 1571
  eosinophilia in, 226
  epidemiology of, 1568
  etiology of, 1568
  eyes in, 2316
  genetics in, 1568
  incidence and prevalence of, 1568
  laboratory studies in, 1571
  pathology and pathogenesis of, 1569
  physical examination in, 1570
  regional enteritis and, 1561, 1562
  sclerosing cholangitis and, 1633
  toxic megacolon in, 1569, 1570, *1570*,
    1574–1575
  treatment of, 1572
    surgical, 1575
  vs. amebic dysentery, 592
  vs. balantidiasis, 603
  vs. Crohn's disease of colon, 1576
  vs. shigellosis, 459
Ulcerative proctitis, 1569, 1570, 1616
  vs. lymphogranuloma venereum, 1572
Ulceroglandular tularemia, 466
Ulnar nerve palsy, tardy, 901
Ultrasonography
  abdominal, 1465–1466, *1465*, *1466*
    in abdominal aortic aneurysm, *1466*
    in biliary disease, 1623
    in chronic pancreatitis, 1556
    in evaluation of jaundice, 1622
    in gallstones, *1466*
    in nephrocarcinoma, 1459
    in obstructive jaundice, *1465*
    in pancreatic pseudocyst, *1465*
    in pulmonary disease, 945
Uncal herniation, in intracranial
  tumors, 864
Uncinaria stenocephala, 625
Unconjugated hyperbilirubinemia, 1638,
  1648, 1649
  idiopathic, 1649
Undernutrition, 1684
  clinical signs of, *1677*
Undescended testes, 2173–2174
"Universal antidote," 74
Universal donor, dangerous, transfusion
  reaction from, 1787, 1788
Unstable angina, 1228, 1229
  vs. myocardial infarction, 1232
Unstable colon, 1493
Unverricht, myoclonus epilepsy of, 854
Uracil mustard, in oncologic treatment,
  1932
Uranium, nephrotoxicity from, *1428*,
  1430
Urate
  precipitation of, 2033
  serum, levels of, in gout, 2031, *2031*

Urate nephropathies, 1420–1421
"Urban" leishmaniasis, 587
Urban yellow fever, 293, *293*, 294
Urea
  clearance rates for, with peritoneal
    dialysis, 1378
  in cerebral edema complicating
    cerebral infarction, 791
  in chronic renal failure, 1360
  in head injury, 882
Urea cycle, diseases of, 2022, *2022*
Urea solution, in lead encephalopathy,
  79
Urea stibamine, in visceral
  leishmaniasis, 586
Ureaplasma urealyticum, 346, 347
Urecholine, in esophagitis, 1484
Uremia
  in acute poststreptococcal
    glomerulonephritis, 1396
  in acute renal failure, 1371
  in chronic renal failure, 1362
    bleeding in, 1364
  neuropathy associated with, 909
  osteodystrophy in, 2254–2257
  pericarditis in, 1272
  platelet abnormalities in, 1879
Uremic pseudodiabetes, 1361
Ureter
  anomalies of, 1457–1458
  in retroperitoneal fibrosis, 223
  obstruction of, vs. acute appendicitis,
    1580
Ureteral colic, in analgesic nephropathy,
  1420
Urethra, anomalies of, 1458
Urethritis
  gonococcal, 406, 407
  mycoplasmal, 346
  nongonococcal vs. gonococcal, 408
  postgonococcal, 409
  trachomatous, 333, 334
Uric acid
  in chronic renal failure, 1361
  in sarcoidosis, 215
  synthesis of, 2031, *2031*
    in gout, 2032
Uric acid nephrolithiasis, 2030, 2037
  treatment of, 2041
Uric acid nephropathy, 1440
  complicating treatment of
    non-Hodgkin's lymphomas, 1837
Urinalysis
  **abnormal, in asymptomatic
    individuals, 1331–1333**
  in acute abdomen, 1580
  in interstitial nephritis and interstitial
    nephropathy, 1417
Urinary bladder
  anomalies of, 1458
  function of, after myocardial
    infarction, 1234
  in diabetes mellitus, 1980
  inflammation of, 1409, 1410
  lining of, candidiasis in, 548
Urinary casts, in chronic renal failure,
  1353, 1354
Urinary catheterization
  in paraplegia, 888
  in shock, 1116
Urinary concentrating power,
  estimation of, 1341

Urinary excretion of bile pigments, 1638–1639
  measurement of, 1646
Urinary tract
  anomalies of, 1456–1458
  hemoglobinuria originating in, 1783
  in paraplegia, 888
  in schistosomiasis, 615
  infection of, 1335, 1409–1413
    after renal transplantation, 1385
    in chronic renal failure, 1354
  obstruction of, 1335–1336, 1447–1450
    acute renal failure in, 1369
    chronic renal failure and, 1352, 1353
    common sites of, 1447
    renal injury from, 1330
Urinary vanillylmandelic acid, measurement of, in arterial hypertension, 1204, 1209
Urine
  alkalinization of, in acute drug poisoning, 714
  bilirubin in, tests for, 1645
  casts in, 1338, 1339
  concentrated, production of, mechanisms of, 1317–1320, 1320
  crystalloids in, 1443, 1444
  in acute poststreptococcal glomerulonephritis, 1395
  microscopy of, 1338–1339
  normal values for, 2349–2350
  osmolality of, in differential diagnosis of acute renal failure, 1374
  protein in, 1337–1338, 1338. See also Proteinuria.
  volume of, in differential diagnosis of acute renal failure, 1374
Urine ascites, 1593
Urobilin, 1637
Urobilinogen, urinary and fecal, 1639
  measurement of, 1646
Urogenital. See Genitourinary.
Urography
  in interstitial nephritis, 1418
  intravenous, 1342, 1342, 1343
    in analgesic nephropathy, 1420
Urokinase, in thrombophlebitis, 1129
Uropathy, obstructive, 1447–1450
Urothelial tumors, 1461
Urticaria, 160–162, 2273
  caterpillars and moths causing, 119
  cholinergic, 161
  cold, 161, 162
  solar, 161, 162
Urticaria pigmentosa, 161, 2307, 2308
Uta, 588
Uterus, clostridial infections of, postabortion and postpartum, 435
Uveitis
  anterior, acute, 2313, 2314
    in ankylosing spondylitis, 2316
    in Behçet's disease, 2316
    in juvenile rheumatoid arthritis, 2315
    in enteritis with arthritis, 198
    in sarcoidosis, 213, 2329
Uveoencephalitic syndrome, 842
Uveoparotid fever, 2329

Vaccination, antirabies, neuroparalytic accidents following, 838–839

Vaccine(s), 230
  adenovirus, 237
  cholera, 462
  common cold, 233
  encephalitic complications of, 836–839
  influenza, 245, 246
  measles, 250
  measles modified by, 249
  meningococcal, 423
  mumps virus, 263
  pertussis, 428
  plague, 465
  pneumococcal pneumonia, 357
  poliovirus, 832
  rabies, 835, 835, 836
  rubella, 252
  tetanus, 437
  tuberculosis, 483
  tularemia, 468
  typhoid, 449
  typhus, 320
  variola, 258, 259, 260
  yellow fever, 296
Vaccinia, 255, 259–260
  progressive, 260
Vaccinia gangrenosa, 260
Vaccinia virus, 255
Vaccinia-immune globulin
  in complications of smallpox vaccination, 260
  in smallpox exposure, 258
Vagabond fever, 526–529
Vagina, epithelial cornification of, as test of ovarian function, 2180
Vaginismus, 689, 2199
Vaginitis
  Candida, 548
  mycoplasmal, 347
  Trichomonas, 603
Vaginulus plebius, 632
Vagotomy
  diarrhea after, 1520
  proximal gastric, in duodenal ulcer, 1519, 1519
  truncal, antrectomy and, in duodenal ulcer, 1519, 1519
  "drainage" and, in duodenal ulcer, 1519, 1519
Valium. See Diazepam.
Valley fever, 537–540
Valproic acid, in epilepsy, 859
Valsalva, sinuses of, congenital aneurysms of, 1169–1170
Valsalva maneuver
  abnormal response to, in heart failure, 1088
  hyperventilation combined with, 746
Valvular aortic stenosis, congenital, 1156–1157
Valvular heart disease, acquired, 1174–1199
  cardiac catheterization and operation in, 1178–1179
  evaluation of, 1176–1178
  physiologic effects of, 1174–1176, 1175
Valvular pulmonic stenosis, 1158–1160
Valvuloplasty, in mitral stenosis, 1185
Vanadium pentoxide, exposure to, respiratory effects of, 1000
Vancomycin, 557, 560
  adverse reactions to, 560

Vancomycin (Continued)
  in bacterial meningitis, 416
  in infective endocarditis, 392, 393
  in infective endocarditis prophylaxis, 396
  in pseudomembranous enterocolitis, 1585
  in staphylococcal gastroenteritis and enterocolitis, 405
  in staphylococcal infections, 399
  in staphylococcal pneumonia, 402
Vanillylmandelic acid, urinary, measurement of, in arterial hypertension, 1204, 1209
Variable immunodeficiency, common, 142–143
Variant angina, 1229
Varicella, 253–255, 824, 825
  acute disseminated encephalomyelitis after, 836, 837
  vs. mild smallpox, 257
  vs. rickettsialpox, 326
Varicella-zoster virus, 253, 824, 825
Varices
  esophageal, bleeding, 1523
    in cancer patient, 1905
    in schistosomiasis, 614
    in portal hypertension, 1640
  gastric, in portal hypertension, 1640
Varicocele, infertility and, 2171
Varicose ulcers
  enteric bacteria in, 455
  vs. tropical phagedenic ulcer, 530
Varicose veins, 1313–1314
Variegate porphyria, 42, 2047–2048
Variola, 255–259
  acute disseminated encephalomyelitis after, 836, 837
  vaccination in, 259–260
Variola minor, 257
Variola sine eruptione, 256
Variola vaccine, 258, 259, 260
Vascular autoregulation of blood pressure, 1208
Vascular disease(s)
  atherosclerotic, hyperlipoproteinemia in, 2010–2011
  intestinal, 1586–1591
  of kidney, 1407–1409
  peripheral, 1299–1315
    diabetes mellitus and, neuropathy in, 908
    due to abnormal communications between arteries and veins, 1312–1313
    due to abnormal vasoconstriction or vasodilatation, 1305–1309
    due to exposure to cold, 1309–1312
    due to organic arterial obstruction, 1299–1305
  prediction of, risk factors for, 1201, 1202, 1202
  pulmonary, in congenital heart disease, 1141–1143
  vs. brain tumor, 868
Vascular ectasias, colonic, 1590
Vascular headaches, 730–731
Vascular lesions
  disseminated, in rickettsial diseases, 311
  of spinal cord, 897–898

Vascular occlusive disease, hearing loss from, 736
Vascular purpura, 1879–1880
  causes of, *1879*
Vascular spiders, in liver disease, 1645
Vascular tumors, 863
Vasculitis, 165
  granulomatous, 972–973
  pulmonary, 972–973
Vasoactive drugs, in shock, 1048
Vasoconstriction
  abnormal, peripheral vascular disease due to, 1305–1309
  peripheral, in heart failure, 1088
Vasodepressor syncope, 743
  vs. hysterical fainting, 744
  vs. idiopathic autonomic insufficiency, 763
Vasodilatation, abnormal, peripheral vascular disease due to, 1305–1309
Vasodilators. See also names of specific agents.
  in arterial hypertension, *1212,* 1214, 1215
  in heart failure, 1100–1102, *1100, 1101*
  in shock, 1120, 1121
Vasogenic brain edema, 864
Vasomotor rhinitis, 157, **160**
Vasopressin, 2109
  circulatory effects of, 1111
  in diabetes insipidus, 2111
  in gastrointestinal bleeding, 1522
  in portal hypertension with gastrointestinal bleeding, 1523
Vasovagal syncope, 740
Vasquez-Osler disease, 1794
VDRL test, in syphilis, 513, *513,* 514
Vegetative state, after head injury, 885
Veins
  arteries and, abnormal communications between, peripheral vascular diseases due to, 1312–1313
  autologous, for coronary bypass graft, 1240
  peripheral, diseases of, 1313–1314
  varicose, 1313–1314
Velban. See *Vinblastine.*
Vena cava, superior
  angiography of, 944
  compression or obstruction of, in bronchogenic carcinoma, 1006
Vena cava syndrome, superior, 1018
Vena caval to left atrial connection, 1170
Venereal Disease Research Laboratories Test, in syphilis, 513, *513,* 514
Venezuelan equine encephalitis, 286–288
Venezuelan equine encephalitis virus, 286
Venography
  in thrombophlebitis, 1126
  renal, 1344
Venomous marine animals, 123–125
Veno-occlusive disease, pulmonary, pulmonary venous hypertension from, 1145
Venous congestion, systemic, in right ventricular failure, 1092
Venous hypertension, in heart failure, 1087, 1088
Venous pressure, in cardiovascular physical examination, 1073
Venous pulse, examination of, 1073, *1073*
  in congenital heart disease, 1155

Venous return, factors determining, 1068, 1069
Venous sinus thrombosis, intracranial, benign intracranial hypertension with, 871
Venous sinuses, major, thrombophlebitis and thrombosis of, 808
Venous system, 1067
Venous thrombosis, 1124, 1125, 1126
  cerebral, 788–789
  mesenteric, 1589, 1590
Ventilation, 932–936
  abnormalities of, 935–936, *936*
  alveolar, maintenance of, in acute respiratory failure, 1027
  artificial, in cardiopulmonary arrest, 1054, 1055
  continuous positive pressure, in acute respiratory failure, 1027
  distribution of, 935
  evaluation of, radionuclide imaging in, 945
  in acute respiratory failure, 1036, 1045, *1045*
  in airways obstruction, 953
  in metabolic brain disease, 649
  in sedative overdose, 713
  intermittent positive pressure, in acute respiratory failure, 1027
  intubation-assisted, in chronic respiratory failure, 1028–1029
  mechanical, in acute respiratory failure, 1027, 1040, 1041
    indications for, 1039, *1039*
Ventilation-perfusion mismatching, 940, 1022
Ventilators, mechanical, in critical care medicine, 1032, 1033
Ventricle(s)
  functional anatomy of, 1064
  right, "atrialized," 1168
    double outlet, 1173
    single, 1174
Ventricular aberration, 1246
Ventricular aneurysm, after myocardial infarction, 1237
Ventricular beats, premature, 1251
Ventricular bigeminy, 1252, *1252*
Ventricular contractions, premature, 1246
Ventricular ectopic beats, in myocardial infarction, 1230, 1235
Ventricular empyema, cerebrospinal fluid findings in, *803*
Ventricular end-diastolic pressure, 1084
Ventricular extrasystoles, 1251–1252, *1252*
Ventricular failure. See also *Heart failure.*
  left, 1081, 1089–1091
    acute pulmonary edema in, 1090
      management of, 1094
    hypertensive, 1206
    in myocardial infarction, 1231
  right, 1081, 1091–1093
    in acute respiratory failure, 1022
    in chronic respiratory failure, treatment of, 1029–1030
    in primary pulmonary hypertension, 1140
    pulmonary hypertension and, in pulmonary disease, 1147, 1148
Ventricular fibrillation, 1255, *1255*
  cardiac arrest from, 1056, 1057
  DC electroshock in, 1267

Ventricular fibrillation (*Continued*)
  in digitalis toxicity, 1098, 1099
  in myocardial infarction, 1230, 1235
  sudden death due to, 1237, 1238
Ventricular function curves, 1065, *1065*
  1066, *1066*
Ventricular hypertrophy, in heart failure, 1086, 1087
Ventricular septal defect, 1170–1171
  in myocardial infarction, surgical intervention in, 1240
  pulmonary hypertension in, 1141, 1142
  vs. mitral regurgitation, 1187
  with aortic regurgitation, 1171
  with pulmonic stenosis, 1164–1166
Ventricular tachycardia, 1252–1254, *1253*
  DC electroshock in, 1267
  in myocardial infarction, 1230, 1235
  in shock, 1118
Ventricular wall, thickness of, 1064
Ventriculitis, in bacterial meningitis, 412
Ventriculography, in brain tumor, 867
Venturi masks, for oxygenation in acute respiratory failure, 1027
Venular resistance, in shock, 1112
Venules, pulmonary, 1135
Verapamil, in angina pectoris, 1228
Verbal paraphasias, 656
Verruca vulgaris, 2284
Verrucous nonbacterial endocarditis, in systemic lupus erythematosus, 176, 177
Verruga peruana, 331–332
Vertebrae
  cervical, congenital fusion of, 875
    syringomyelia and, 769
    staphylococcal infections of, 402
Vertebral arteries, 782–783, *783*
  ischemia of, 784, 785
Vertebral degenerative joint disease, 204
Vertiginous migraine, 740
Vertigo, 737–742
  central causes of, 739, 740
  cervicogenic, 739
  peripheral causes of, 738, 739
  positional, 738, *738*
    benign, 738
Vesicle, 2273
Vesicoureteral reflux, after renal transplantation, 1385
Vesicular stomatitis with exanthem, 274
Vestibular neuronitis, 738
Vestibular schwannoma, hearing loss from, 736
Vestibulogenic epilepsy, 741
Vestibulopathy, peripheral
  acute, 738
  acute and recurrent, 738, 739
Vibrio cholerae, 460
Vibrio parahaemolyticus food poisoning, 66
Villonodular synovitis, pigmented, 202
Villous adenomas, 1610
  rectal, hypokalemia in, 1958
Vinblastine, 1935, 1936
  in eosinophilic granuloma, 1851
  in Hodgkin's disease, 1846
  neuropathy from, 910
Vinca alkaloids, in oncologic treatment, 1935, 1936
Vincent's angina, 443
  vs. diphtheria, 431
  vs. infectious mononucleosis, 266

Vincristine, 1936
hyponatremia induced by, 1954
in Hodgkin's disease, 1846
in non-Hodgkin's lymphomas, 1836
neuropathy from, 910
Viomycin, 557
in pulmonary tuberculosis, 488, 490
Viper, bite of, 122
Viral arthritis, 186
Viral diseases, 299–307. See also names
of specific viral diseases.
acute pancreatitis and, 1551
antimicrobial agents for, 556–557
characterized by cutaneous lesions,
246–264
encephalitic complications of, 836–839
of nervous system, 816–843
parainfluenza, 239–240
presumptive, 302–307
respiratory, 230–246
prevalence of, factors related to,
236, 236
vs. allergic rhinitis, 158
respiratory syncytial, 238–239
vertigo caused by, 740
Viral encephalitis, 817–821
arthropod-borne, 283–291
vs. malaria, 573
vs. poliomyelitis, 831
Viral fevers, arthropod-borne,
undifferentiated, 277–282, 279
Viral gastroenteritis, Norwalk-like
agents and rotaviruses causing,
305–306
Viral hemorrhagic fevers, 292–302, 293
Viral hepatitis
acute, 1650–1655
cirrhosis in, 1663
vs. acute cholecystitis, 1627
complicating maintenance
hemodialysis, 1382
in opiate addiction, 697
non-A, non-B, 1656
polyarthritis associated with, 186
type A, 1650, 1651
prophylaxis of, 1654, 1655
vs. cytomegalovirus mononucleosis,
828
type B, 1650, 1651
in chronic renal failure, 1366
prophylaxis of, 1655
vs. cytomegalovirus mononucleosis,
828, 829
types A and B, differentiation of, 1654
vs. hepatic amebiasis, 592
vs. jaundice of malaria, 573
vs. leptospirosis, 534
vs. louse-borne relapsing fever, 528
vs. rat-bite fever, 531
Viral labyrinthitis, hearing loss from,
736
Viral laryngitis, 235–236
Viral meningitis, 817–821
cerebrospinal fluid findings in, 803,
820
Viral meningoencephalitis, 817
vs. meningococcal meningitis, 420,
421
vs. psittacosis, 338
Viral myocarditis, 1281, 1282
Viral pharyngitis, 235–236, 235
vs. infectious mononucleosis, 266
Viral pneumonia(s)
vs. Goodpasture's syndrome, 976
vs. psittacosis, 338

Viridans streptococci, 367
in infective endocarditis, 386
Virilism, in Cushing's syndrome, 2157
Virilizing adrenal tumors, 2161–2162
Virus(es). See also names of groups of
viruses, e.g., Arboviruses,
Enteroviruses.
arthropod-borne, 276–302. See also
Arboviruses.
associated with meningitis and
encephalitis, 817, 817, 818, 818
California arbovirus complex, 288
cancer and, 1910
CHF-Congo, 298
chikungunya, 279
Colorado tick fever, 280
common cold, 230, 230, 231
cowpox, 255
dengue, 277
hemorrhagic fever caused by, 296
eastern equine encephalitis, 285
Ebola, 300
Epstein-Barr, in Burkitt's lymphoma,
1838
in infectious mononucleosis, 264
hepatitis A, 1650, 1651
hepatitis B, 1650, 1651
herpes simplex, encephalitis from,
818, 818, 821 822
meningitis from, 818, 818
in etiology of acute leukemia, 1814,
1815
influenza, 241, 241, 242
Japanese B, 289
JC, 842
Junin, 298, 299
KFD, 290, 291
La Crosse, 288
Lassa, 298, 299
louping ill, 291
Machupo, 298, 299
Marburg, 300
Mayaro, 279
measles, 246
measles-like, in subacute sclerosing
panencephalitis, 841
mumps, 261
meningitis and encephalitis from,
262, 818, 818, 819
OHF, 290, 291
O'nyong-nyong, 279
parainfluenza, 239
Powassan, 290
properties of, 229
rabies, 833, 833
respiratory syncytial, 238
Rift Valley, 281
Ross River, 279
RS, 238
RSSE, 290, 291
rubella, 250
St. Louis encephalitis, 288
sandfly, 282
Sendai, 239
smallpox, 255
systemic lupus erythematosus and,
175
vaccinia, 255
varicella-zoster, 253, 824, 825
Venezuelan equine encephalitis, 286
West Nile, 278
western equine encephalitis, 284
yellow fever, 292, 293
Visceral angiography, 1470–1471, 1470,
1471

Visceral crises, in tabes dorsalis, 814
Visceral larva migrans, 627–628
vs. clonorchiasis, 618
Visceral leishmaniasis, 583, 584–587
vs. malaria, 573
Visna, 839, 840
Vital capacity, 932, 932
determination of, 933
forced, 934, 934
Vitamin(s)
blood levels of, in acute infections,
1679
in kwashiorkor, 1682, 1683
fat-soluble, nutrient value of, 1670,
1672
recommended allowances of, 1671
metabolism of, inborn errors of, 43
water-soluble, nutrient value of,
1672–1673
recommended allowances of, 1671
Vitamin A
benign intracranial hypertension
from, 871
deficiency of, 1684–1686
clinical signs of, 1677
eyes in, 1675
in malabsorption syndrome, 1529
in biliary cirrhosis, 1666
in kwashiorkor, 1682
in malabsorption syndrome, 1536
intoxication with, 1691–1692
hypercalcemia in, 2235
nutrient value of, 1670, 1672
recommended allowances of, 1671
Vitamin B complex
deficiency of, in malabsorption
syndrome, 1530
in malabsorption syndrome, 1536
Vitamin B₁. See Thiamin.
Vitamin B₆
nutrient value of, 1673
recommended allowances of, 1671
Vitamin B₁₂
absorption of, 1525
tests of, in malabsorption
syndrome, 1532
deficiency of, 776–777
causes of, 1720
in malabsorption syndrome, 1529,
1529
neurologic disorders associated
with, 1724, 1725
neutropenia in, 1809
vs. folate deficiency, 1725, 1725
vs. transverse myelitis, 812
in malabsorption syndrome, 1536
in megaloblastic anemia, 1726, 1727,
1727, 1728
in postgastrectomy malabsorption,
1546
malabsorption of, 1539
tests of, 1726
metabolism of, 1719, 1722
nutrient value of, 1673
recommended allowances of, 1671
Vitamin C. See also Ascorbic acid.
nutrient value of, 1672
recommended allowances of, 1671
Vitamin D, 2232–2233
calcium absorption by, 1526
deficiency of, clinical signs of, 1677
in malabsorption syndrome, 1528
in anticonvulsant-induced rickets or
osteomalacia, 2253
in biliary cirrhosis, 1666

Vitamin D (*Continued*)
  in malabsorption syndrome, *1536*
  in osteomalacia of nontropical sprue,
    2249
  in osteoporosis, 2246
  in postoperative tetany complicating
    hyperparathyroidism, 2220
  in renal osteodystrophy, 2256
  in vitamin D deficiency rickets, 2249
  in vitamin D resistant rickets, 2251
  metabolism of, in vitamin D resistant
    rickets, 2250
  nutrient value of, 1672
  overdosage of, 1691, 1692
    hypercalcemia in, 2234–2235
  recommended allowances of, *1671*
Vitamin D$_2$, 2232
  in hypoparathyroidism, 2221
Vitamin D$_3$, 2232
Vitamin D deficiency rickets, 2248–2249
Vitamin D dependent rickets, *43, 2021,*
  2252
Vitamin D resistance, in uremia, 2255
Vitamin D resistant rickets, 2250–2252
  pseudo-, 2252
Vitamin diseases, 1684–1692
Vitamin E
  deficiency of, in malabsorption
    syndrome, 1529
  nutrient value of, 1672
  recommended allowances of, *1671*
Vitamin K
  deficiency of, 1889–1890
    in malabsorption syndrome, 1529
  depletion of, in critically ill patient,
    1053
  in louse-borne relapsing fever, 528
  in malabsorption syndrome, *1536*
  nutrient value of, 1672
Vitamin K$_1$
  in biliary cirrhosis, 1666
  in bleeding complicating
    anticoagulant therapy of
    thrombophlebitis, 1128
  in vitamin K deficiency, 1890
Vitiligo, 2292–2293
  vs. albinism, 2029
  vs. leprosy, 503
  vs. pinta, 525
Vitreous body, in sarcoidosis, 2329
Vitreous hemorrhage, in sickle cell
  diseases, 2332
Vivax malaria, 567
  clinical manifestations of, 571
  erythrocyte forms of, *570*
  relapse of, 574
Vogt-Koyanagi-Harada syndrome, 842
Volhynian fever, 329
Volume depletion, 1950–1952
  causes of, *1950*
  sodium depletion and, defective
    water excretion from, 1953
Volume-pressure relationships of chest
  wall and lungs, 932, *932*
Volvulus, gastric, 1489–1490
Vomiting, 1477–1478
  bilious, after peptic ulcer surgery,
    1520
  clinical types of, 1477, 1478
  in anorexia nervosa, 1477, 1700, 1701
  in chronic renal failure, 1364, 1365
  in impaired gastric emptying
    complicating peptic ulcer, 1517,
    1518

Vomiting (*Continued*)
  in intracranial tumors, 865
  in staphylococcal food poisoning, 65
  in yellow fever, 295
  metabolic alkalosis caused by, 1965,
    1966
  metabolic complications of, 1478
  psychogenic, 1477
    hypokalemia in, 1958
  treatment of, 1478
Vomiting disease, winter, 305–306
von Bechterew's syndrome, 194–195.
  See also *Spondylitis, ankylosing.*
von Economo's disease, parkinsonism
  secondary to, 753
von Hippel–Lindau disease, 771, *1910*
  cutaneous manifestations of, *2300*
  internal malignancy and, *2296*
von Recklinghausen's disease, 769–770
  pheochromocytomas in, 2201, 2203
  skin in, 2293–2294, *2293, 2297*
von Willebrand's disease, *43, 1884,*
  1886–1887, 2302
  vs. classic hemophilia, 1885
Vulvovaginitis, gonococcal, 406
V-Z virus, 253

Wada test, 656
WAIS, 681, 682
  in diagnosis of dementia, 661
Waldenström's macroglobulinemia,
  1862–1863
  electrophoretic patterns in, 1855,
    1856, *1856*
  renal changes in, 1406
Waldenström's syndrome, 213
Wallenberg's syndrome, 788
War fever, 318–320
Warfarin
  in thrombophlebitis, 1128
  metronidazole and, simultaneous use
    of, effects of, 2339
Warm water immersion foot, 1309, 1310
Warming, in hypothermia, 86
Warm-reacting antibodies, hemolysis
  due to, 1763–1764
Wart, prosector's 479, 498
Wasp stings, 113–114, 163
Wassermann test, in syphilis, 513
Water
  absorption of, 1525
    diminished, in malabsorption
      syndrome, 1529
  chemical contamination of, 60–64
  compulsive drinking of, vs. diabetes
    insipidus, 2111
  excessive intake of, with normal renal
    function, 1955
  excretion of, defective, functional
    disorders leading to, 1953, 1954
    in acute tubular necrosis, 1370, 1371
  exposure of extremities to, prolonged,
    1309, 1310
  loss of, volume depletion from, 1950,
    1951
  overload of, salt overload and,
    hypertension from, 1210
  restriction of, in heart failure, 1102
  retention of, in heart failure, 1089
Water balance
  hypothalamic dysfunction and,
  718–719
  physiology of, 718

Water deprivation test, in diabetes
  insipidus, 2110, 2111
Water hemlocks, poisoning by, 70
Water intoxication, 719
Water-hammer pulse, in aortic
  regurgitation, 1195
Waterhouse-Friderichsen syndrome
  adrenal apoplexy in, 2150
  hypofibrinogenemia in, 1894
  in meningococcemia, 418, 419
  vs. dengue hemorrhagic fever, 297
Water-soluble vitamins
  nutrient value of, 1672–1673
  recommended allowances of, *1671*
Watson-Crick model for DNA, 31
Watson-Schwartz test, in acute
  intermittent porphyria, 2046
Weakness
  hysterical, vs. myasthenia gravis, 927
  in hyperkalemia, 1959
  in malabsorption syndrome, 1529
  in metabolic brain disease, 648
  in multiple sclerosis, 846
  in myasthenia gravis, 926
  in peripheral neuropathy, 903, 904
  in polymyositis and dermatomyositis,
    172
  in right ventricular failure, 1093
  in spinal epidural infections, 810
  in transverse myelitis, 812
  muscular, in cancer, 879
Weber test, in hearing loss, 734
Weber-Christian disease, 221–222
Weber's syndrome, in midbrain
  infarctions, 787
Wechsler Adult Intelligence Scale, 681,
  682
  in diagnosis of dementia, 661
Weeverfishes, envenomation by, 124
Wegener's granulomatosis, 166,
  218–220, 972–973
  cutaneous signs in, *2301*
  eyes in, 219, 2317
  neuropathy in, 908
  renal involvement in, 219, 1400
  vs. allergic angiitis and
    granulomatosis, 183
  vs. Goodpasture's syndrome, 976
  vs. midline granuloma, 221
Weight
  as factor in antimicrobial agent
    selection, 553
  blood pressure and, 1201
  desirable, according to height and
    frame, *1692*
  gain of, with oral contraceptive use,
    2196
  loss of, in anorexia nervosa, 1700
    in bronchogenic carcinoma, 1006
    in gastric carcinoma, 1601
    in liver disease, 1642
    in malabsorption, 1528, *1528*
  pubertal spurt of, 17, 18
"Weightlifter's blackout," 746
Weil-Felix reaction, in rickettsial
  diseases, 313, *314*
Weil's syndrome, 532, 533
Weingarten's syndrome, 637
"Welch abscess," 434
Wenckebach phenomenon, in second
  degree atrioventricular block, 1261,
  1261
Werdnig-Hoffmann disease, 765, 766,
  920

Wermer's syndrome, 2098
Werner's syndrome, *1910*, **2058–2059**
  vs. scleroderma, 170
Wernicke-Korsakoff syndrome, 773–774
Wernicke's aphasia, 657
Wernicke's disease, 773
  in beriberi, 1688, 1689
West African sleeping sickness, 576
West Nile fever, 278, *279*
West Nile virus, 278
Western equine encephalitis, 284–285
Western equine encephalitis virus, 284
Wet dressings, in dermatologic therapy,
  2275, *2275*, 2276
Wheal-and-flare reaction
  in allergic rhinitis, 157
  in drug allergy, 155
Wheat weevil disease, *971*
Wheezing
  as reaction to organic particles, 997
  in asthma, 956, 957
  in bronchogenic carcinoma, 1006
  in simple chronic bronchitis, 953, 954
Whelk, red, paralytic poisoning by, 68
"Whip-lash dermatitis," 114
Whipple's disease, 1541–1542
  arthritis in, 199
  jejunal histology in, 1535, *1535*
Whipworm infection, 628–629
  antimicrobial agents for, *559*
White arsenic, poisoning by, 76
White blood cells, diseases of,
  1800–1829
White matter, spongy degeneration of,
  850
White thrombus, 1122
Whooping cough, 426–428
Widal test, in typhoid fever, 448
Willebrand's disease, *43*, *1884*,
  1886–1887, *2302*
  vs. classic hemophilia, 1885
Williams trait, 1888
Willis, circle of, anomalies of, cerebral
  infarction and, 779
Wilms' tumor, 1460
Wilson's disease, *43*, *2020*, **2049–2051**
  acute liver disease in, vs. chronic
    active hepatitis, 1662
  prevention and management of, 55
Winter vomiting disease, 305–306
Wiskott-Aldrich syndrome, *1910*
  immunodeficiency with, *139*, **143–144**
    internal malignancy and, *2296*
Withdrawal syndrome
  in alcohol abuse, 668, 709, 710
  in central nervous system depressant
    abuse, 699, 700
  in opiate abuse, 695, 696
Wohlfart-Kugelberg-Welander disease,
  765, 766
  vs. congenital myopathies, 920
  vs. muscular dystrophies, 918
Wolf spiders, bites of, 115

Wolff-Parkinson-White syndrome,
  1257–1260, *1257*, *1258*, *1259*
Wolman's disease, *42*
Wood's light, in skin examination, 2273
Woody nightshade, poisoning by, 70
Woolsorters' disease, 470
Word salad, schizophrenic, vs. fluent
  aphasia, 657
Word-deafness, pure, 657
Wound(s)
  care of, in electric injury, 94
  clostridial contamination of, 434
  healing of, in chronic renal failure,
    1366
    in malnutrition, 1680
    in scurvy, 1691
  infected, vs. malaria, 573
Wrist drop, in lead poisoning, 78
Wrists, in rheumatoid arthritis, 188
Wuchereria bancrofti, *559*, *605*, *632*, *633*

Xanthelasma(s)
  in familial hypercholesterolemia, 2005
  in liver disease, 1645
Xanthine oxidase
  in uric acid synthesis, 2031, *2031*
  inhibition of, by allopurinol, 2340
Xanthinuria, *42*, **2041–2042**
Xanthoma(s)
  in familial dysbetalipoproteinemia,
    2005, 2006
  in familial hypercholesterolemia, 2005
  in familial lipoprotein lipase
    deficiency, 2006
  in liver disease, 1645
Xanthoma diabeticorum, 1981
Xanthomatosis
  cerebrotendinous, *42*
  eruptive, in diabetes mellitus, 1981
Xanthurenic aciduria, *42*
Xenodiagnostic test, in Chagas' disease,
  582
Xenopsylla cheopis
  in murine typhus fever, 320, 321
  in plague, 463
Xeroderma pigmentosum, *42*, *1909*,
  1910, 2288
Xerophthalmia, 1675, **1684–1686**, *1685*
Xerosis, 1675
Xerosis conjunctivae, *1685*
X-linked diabetes insipidus, prevention
  and management of, 55
X-linked hypophosphatemic rickets,
  dietary treatment of, 55
X-linked ichthyosis, *2286*
X-linked immunodeficiency with
  increased IgM, *43*, *139*
X-linked infantile agamma-
  globulinemia, *43*, **139–140**,
  139, *140*
  Bruton type of, 139, 150, *1910*

X-linked inheritance, 36, *36*
X-linked traits
  dominant, 36, *36*
  recessive, 36, *36*
d-Xylose absorption, measurement of,
  in malabsorption syndrome, 1530
XYY syndrome, 2170
  clinical and cytogenetic characteristics
    of, *52*

Yaws, **518–522**, *520*
  "forest," *588*
  vs. bejel, 523
  vs. chromomycosis, 543
  vs. leprosy, 504
  vs. maduromycosis, 542
  vs. paracoccidioidomycosis, 541
  vs. pinta, 525
  vs. tropical phagedenic ulcer, 530
Yeast infections of skin, 2282–2283
Yellow atrophy, acute
  in fulminant hepatitis, 1655
  in viral hepatitis, 1652
Yellow famine fever, 526–529
Yellow fever, **292–296**, *293*
  sylvan, 293, *293*, 294
  urban, 293, *293*, 294
  vs. hemorrhagic diseases caused by
    arenaviruses, 299
  vs. louse-borne relapsing fever, 528
Yellow fever vaccine, 296
Yellow fever virus, 292, 293
Yellow plague, 526–529
"Yen sleep," in opiate addiction, 696
Yersinia pestis, 463
Y-linked inheritance, 37

Zebra fishes, envenomation by, 124
Zenker's diverticulum, 1499
Ziehl-Neelsen method, in sputum
  examination, 948
Zieve's syndrome, 1643, 1664
Zinc
  nutrient value of, 1674
  recommended allowances of, *1671*
Zinc chloride, exposure to, respiratory
  effects of, 1000
Zirconium, sarcoidosis and, 210
Zollinger-Ellison syndrome, **1508–1509**
  hyperparathyroidism and, 1509, 2215,
    2216
Zona, **824–827**. See also *Herpes zoster*.
Zoster immune globulin, in prevention
  of varicella, 254, 255
Zoster sine herpete, 826
Zyloprim. See *Allopurinol*.